1989-1990 ASHA

MEMBERSHIP

DIRECTORY

January, 1989

Editor
Frederick T. Spahr, Ph.D.

American Speech–Language–Hearing Association
10801 Rockville Pike
Rockville, Maryland 20852

Published by the American Speech-Language-Hearing Association
10801 Rockville Pike
Rockville, Maryland 20852

ISBN 0-910329-45-1 (Hardbound)
ISBN 0-910329-44-3 (Softbound)

Printed in the United States of America
Library of Congress Catalog Card No. 86-657543

Copies of the 1989-1990 *ASHA Membership Directory* may be ordered from:

Publications Sales Office
American Speech-Language-Hearing Association
10801 Rockville Pike
Rockville, Maryland 20852
(301) 897-5700

CONTENTS

PREFACE

Let me begin by thanking the overwhelming majority of the membership who responded on a timely basis to the *1989-1990 ASHA Membership Directory* update form. It was mailed in September, 1988 to all members of record as of August 5, 1988. Your response has enabled us to achieve our goal of getting this Directory to you at the beginning of 1989.

In compliance with the "Issues In Ethics Statement" published in *Asha* (June, 1987, p. 42), the *1989-1990 ASHA Membership Directory* contains for the first time the doctoral field of study for all members listed with doctoral degrees. For members who did not return the update form, or did not indicate the doctoral field of study as requested, the designation "NS" (Not Specified) appears indicating that non-response.

Otherwise, in a content sense, the *1989-1990 ASHA Membership Directory* follows closely the format of earlier editions: front-matter covering a wide variety of reference material which we hope will be of interest both to the membership and the public; an alphabetical listing of members; and, finally, a geographical listing of members. The Geographical Section in this edition concentrates on the state and city each member specified for his/her directory address, and does not list groups of members by employer within a city. The Table of Contents provides specific details and page references for each section.

The *1989-1990 ASHA Membership Directory,* not suprisingly, is just what it purports to be–a list of members. Further, like all similar lists, it is a list as of a particular date. In this instance, that date is August 5, 1988. For all members who responded with updated information by the stated deadline near the end of September, we updated any new information sent us to the best of our ability to do so within the parameters established for this publication. For those who did not respond as requested, the *1989-1990 ASHA Membership Directory* merely reflects the information already existing in the membership files in the National Office. Those who joined ASHA after the closing date for processing information for this Directory; or those who may subsequently have become certified or improved their certification status may look forward to appropriate inclusion in the next full biographical/geographical listing which is scheduled to be published in 1992.

Instructions for understanding the listings in this Directory will be found in the section specified as "Directory Instructions". The user is urged to examine that section carefully in order to make maximum use of this Directory.

It should be noted that *Directory* listings are intended to include only **earned** degrees, and ASHA relies on each member to indicate only such degrees for that purpose.

The Editor wishes to express his gratitude to the staff of the National Office for its essential help in the preparation of the *1989-1990 ASHA Membership Directory.* With any listing of this nature, however, we know there certainly will be some errors. Let us say now that we regret their occurrence. If one of those errors is in a personal listing, please *write* us providing the correct information so that we may update our membership base and, hopefully, avoid duplicating the error in future editions.

Rockville, Maryland
December 2, 1988

FREDERICK T. SPAHR, Ph.D.
Executive Director

AMERICAN SPEECH-LANGUAGE-HEARING ASSOCIATION

The American Speech-Language-Hearing Association is a scientific and professional association with a current membership of over 51,000. Activated in 1925 as the American Academy of Speech Correction, the organization became the American Society for the Study of Disorders of Speech in 1927, the American Speech Correction Association in 1934, the American Speech and Hearing Association in 1947, and assumed its present name in 1978. Formal annual conventions have been held since 1925, and membership records have been kept since 1926.

PURPOSES

The purposes of this Association shall be: (1) To encourage basic scientific study of the processes of individual human communication with special reference to speech, language and hearing; (2) To promote appropriate academic and clinical preparation of individuals entering the discipline of human communication sciences and disorders and promote the maintenance of current knowledge and skills of those within the discipline; (3) To promote investigation and prevention of disorders of human communication; (4) To foster improvement of clinical services and procedures concerning such disorders; (5) To stimulate exchange of information among persons and organizations thus engaged and to disseminate such information; (6) To advocate the rights and interests of persons with communication disorders; and (7) To promote the individual and collective professional interests of the members of the Association.

MEMBERSHIP, FELLOWS, LIFE MEMBERS AND INTERNATIONAL AFFILIATES

Members must hold: (1) a Master's degree or equivalent with major emphasis in speech-language pathology, audiology, language, or speech and hearing science; or (2) a Master's degree or equivalent, and present evidence of active research, interest, and performance in the field of human communication. Persons applying for membership under (2) above must provide names of two members attesting to their interest in the field of human communication. Members assume the ethical responsibilities designated in the Code of Ethics of the American Speech-Language-Hearing Association.

Members who have demonstrated unusual professional or scientific achievement may be elected to Fellowship by the Committee on Honors. Members who have held membership for the ten consecutive years immediately prior to attaining the age of 65 may apply for and automatically receive Life Membership with full membership privileges and exemption from dues payments for any years subsequent to the year in which age 65 is attained. Persons who are citizens of foreign countries, reside abroad, and meet specified educational requirements may affiliate with the Association as an International Affiliate. International Affiliates, while not members of ASHA, are afforded all benefits of membership except voting and holding office.

CLINICAL CERTIFICATION

The Association provides a Certificate of Clinical Competence (CCC) to qualified Speech-Language Pathologists and Audiologists. Requirements for the Certificate of Clinical Competence include a graduate degree, supervised clinical experience, and a passing score on the National Examination. Certification permits the holder to provide independent clinical services, and to supervise the clinical practice of students and uncertified clinicians. Individuals who meet requirements in Speech-Language Pathology and Audiology may be issued both certificates.

CONTINUING EDUCATION

The Association provides a voluntary Continuing Education Program. An Award for Continuing Education (ACE) is offered to ASHA members and nonmember Certificate holders who complete the requirements established by the Continuing Education Board (CEB). The ACE is valid for a three year period during which time the requirements may be completed for a subsequent ACE. The CEB offers Sponsor Approval to providers of continuing education activities for speech-language pathologists and audiologists. ASHA, as an Approved Sponsor, conducts a wide range of continuing education activities such as workshops, seminars, conferences, convention, etc. The Association maintains the Continuing Education Registry, a computerized record-keeping system for activities offered by Approved Sponsors.

EMPLOYMENT SERVICE

Employment Opportunities (classified advertisements) are published each month in *Asha.* Members seeking employment and persons and agencies desiring to secure the services of ASHA members should request information on classified advertising rates and schedules. Employment opportunities are available also through ASHA's computerized Employment Referral Service.

PUBLICATIONS

The Association publishes four journals: the *Journal of Speech and Hearing Disorders;* the *Journal of Speech and Hearing Research; Language, Speech, and Hearing Services in Schools;* and *Asha.* The *Journal of Speech and Hearing Disorders,* a quarterly journal, was first issued in 1936 as the *Journal of Speech Disorders* and appeared under that title through Volume 12, 1947. The *Journal of Speech and Hearing Research,* also a quarterly journal, was first issued in 1958. *Language, Speech, and Hearing Services in Schools* was formerly called *Speech and Hearing Services in Schools,* Volume 1, Numbers 1-3, and *Language, Speech, and Hearing Services in Schools,* Volume 2, Numbers 4 and 5. Volumes 1 and 2 were published irregularly during 1970 and 1971. Regular publication of *LSHSS* began in January, 1972. *Asha* is a monthly journal and was first issued in 1959. The *ASHA Membership Directory,* the *Guide to Professional Services in Speech-Language Pathology and Audiology,* and the *Guide to Graduate Education in Speech-Language Pathology and Audiology* are published biennially. *ASHA Monographs* and *ASHA Reports* are published irregularly. *JSHD, JSHR, LSHSS,* and *Asha* are distributed to Members as part of their dues.

THE AMERICAN SPEECH-LANGUAGE-HEARING FOUNDATION

The American Speech-Language-Hearing Foundation is a nonprofit charitable trust established in 1956 by the American Speech-Language-Hearing Association.

The Mission of the American Speech-Language-Hearing Foundation is to generate and allocate funds in support of the advancement of knowledge and improvement of practice in serving children and adults who have speech, language or hearing disorders and to support the role of the Association.

The allocation of funds has three goals:

(1) To further education in speech-language and hearing through the provision of financial assistance;

(2) To recognize and support research and similar endeavors which contribute to the advancement of knowledge and improvement of practice in serving children and adults who have speech-language-hearing disorders; and

(3) To facilitate new directions in the field of communication sciences and disorders through support of such vehicles as conferences, publications and other media.

THE COUNCIL ON PROFESSIONAL STANDARDS IN SPEECH-LANGUAGE PATHOLOGY AND AUDIOLOGY

The American Speech-Language-Hearing Association established the American Boards of Examiners in Speech Pathology and Audiology (ABESPA) in 1959 to ensure the provision of quality services to the communicatively handicapped. The Association's Bylaws (Article IX) were amended to replace ABESPA with the Council on Professional Standards in Speech-Language Pathology and Audiology (Standards Council) effective January 1, 1980. The Standards Council is responsible for establishing standards, monitoring the implementation of the standards, and arbitrating appeals of decisions rendered by the Clinical Certification Board, the Educational Standards Board, and the Professional Services Board.

The operating boards of examiners in speech-language pathology and audiology (Clincial Certification Board, Professional Services Board, Educational Standards Board) administer the Association's certification and accreditation programs, and interpret and apply standards by the Standards Council.

ASHA POLITICAL ACTION COMMITTEE

The American Speech-Language-Hearing Association Political Action Committee (ASHA-PAC) is a nonprofit, unincorporated, and nonpartisan committee of speech-language pathologists and audiologists. Established by the Legislative Council in 1985, the Committee was organized and began fundraising the following year. The main purpose of ASHA-PAC is to support candidates for federal elective office who indicate an awareness and interest in addressing issues of importance to persons with communicative disorders. Further, ASHA-PAC encourages and facilitates participation by members of the profession in the policymaking process.

ASHA-PAC is registered with the Federal Election Commission (FEC) and complies with laws and regulations governing the activities of federal political action committees.

BYLAWS OF THE AMERICAN SPEECH-LANGUAGE-HEARING ASSOCIATION
(As Approved by Legislative Council - 11/88)
TABLE OF CONTENTS

ARTICLE I

NAME AND SEAL

1.1. The name of this corporation shall be American Speech-Language-Hearing Association (hereinafter called "the Association") and the Seal of the Association shall be:

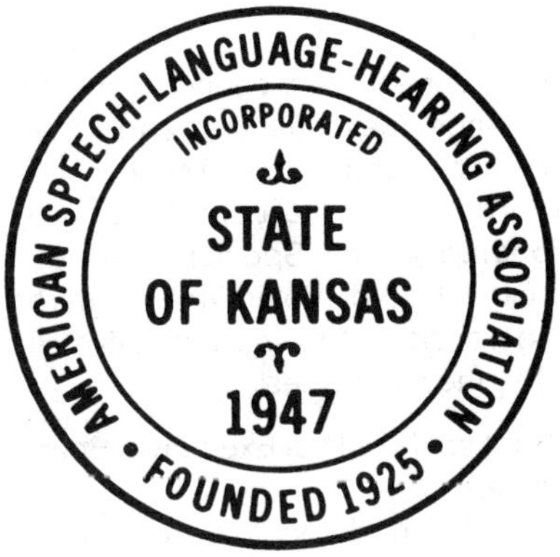

ARTICLE II

PURPOSES

2.1. The purposes of this Association shall be:
- (1) To encourage basic scientific study of the processes of individual human communication with special reference to speech, language and hearing;
- (2) To promote appropriate academic and clinical preparation of individuals entering the discipline of human communication sciences and disorders and promote the maintenance of current knowledge and skills of those within the discipline;
- (3) To promote investigation and prevention of disorders of human communication;
- (4) To foster improvement of clinical services and procedures concerning such disorders;
- (5) To stimulate exchange of information among persons and organizations thus engaged and to disseminate such information;
- (6) To advocate the rights and interests of persons with communication disorders; and
- (7) To promote the individual and collective professional interests of the members of the Association.

ARTICLE III

MEMBERSHIP

3.1. Eligibility

3.1.a. Members must hold: (1) a master's degree or its equivalent with major emphasis in speech-language pathology, audiology, or speech, language, or hearing science; or (2) a master's degree or its equivalent and present evidence of active research, interest, and performance in the field of human communication.

3.1.b. The requirements for membership may be waived in special instances by recommendation of the Executive Board and a majority vote of the Legislative Council.

3.1.c. Members must agree to abide by the Code of Ethics of the Association.

3.2. Dues

3.2.a. The annual dues for members of the Association shall be determined by the Legislative Council following recommendation by the Executive Board.

3.2.b. In accordance with the policies of the Association adopted from time to time, dues may be waived for members who (1) are eligible for Life Membership or (2) become totally disabled.

3.3. Rights Reserved to Members

The following rights are reserved to the members of the Association:

3.3.a. Election of voting members of the Executive Board.

3.3.b. Nomination and election of Councilors to the Legislative Council.

3.3.c. Privilege of removal of voting members of the Executive Board, pursuant to Section 4.2.g. and of Legislative Councilors pursuant to Section 4.1.g.

3.3.d. Initiation of amendments to these Bylaws pursuant to Section 11.2.

ARTICLE IV

GOVERNMENT

Section 1. Legislative Council

4.1.a. Powers
The Legislative Council is the governing body of the Association. It establishes the policies of the Association and exercises all powers except those reserved to the membership or assigned to the Executive Board by these Bylaws. The Legislative Council may delegate such powers as it may determine from time to time.

4.1.a.1. Delegation of Powers
If there is no quorum (see Section 4.1.h.) of the Legislative Council at a meeting, or if the meeting is not held for reasons of war, riot, or other reason, or if an emergency is declared to exist by a two-thirds vote of both the Executive Board and the Association Advisory Committee, the powers of the Legislative Council are hereby assigned to and shall be exercised by the Executive Board until the next meeting of the Legislative Council. The Executive Board shall make a report of any such emergency transactions to the Legislative Council as soon as possible.

4.1.b. Composition
The Legislative Council shall consist of not more than 150 voting members of the Association representing the following fifty-three Constituencies:

(1) members residing in each of the fifty states of the United States and the District of Columbia:

(2) members residing outside the United States; and

(3) other representatives as specified in Section 9.2.

The Legislative Council shall also include (1) the President who shall serve as Chair, and (2) the other members of the Executive Board who will serve ex officio and without vote. The Legislative Council shall from time to time establish a schedule denoting the number of representatives for each constituency.

4.1.c. Nominations
A member of the Association may submit nominations and be a candidate for election to the Legislative Council only from the Constituency in which the member resides. Each member is entitled to nominate as many individuals from that member's Constituency as that Constituency is authorized to elect to the Legislative Council in the next election.

4.1.d. Elections
Each member shall receive an election ballot and may vote for as many nominees on that ballot from that member's Constituency as that Constituency is authorized to elect.

4.1.e. Terms of Office
Councilors shall be elected to three-year terms with approximately one-third of the Councilors from each Constituency and insofar as possible, the Councilors within each state of the United States, elected per year and approximately one-third of the total number of Councilors being elected each year, all terms of office being on a calendar year basis.

4.1.f. Vacancies
If a Councilor (1) changes residence to another Constituency or (2) for any reason no longer fulfills the requirement for election to his or her seat or (3) advises the Chair of the Legislative Council that he or she is no longer willing to serve, the member shall no longer serve as a Councilor, and a committee so charged by the Legislative Council shall designate as a replacement for the unexpired term of that Councilor, the highest ranking alternate in the most recent election, and if there is no alternate, the committee shall designate a replacement and an alternate for the replacement from among the members of the Association within that Councilor's Constituency.

4.1.g. Removal from Office
Any elected Councilor, except those elected pursuant to Section 9.2, may be removed from office by (1) a written petition for removal signed by 10 percent of the total number of members residing in the Councilor's Constituency submitted to the Chair of the Legislative Council and (2) approval of the petition by 75 percent of the members of the Association residing in that Councilor's Constituency who vote in response to the mail submission of the petition.

4.1.h. Meetings
The Legislative Council shall meet at least once a year. Additional meetings may be held. A quorum shall consist of 51 percent of the members of the Legislative Council. Once a quorum has been established, the Legislative Council shall have the power to conduct all business throughout subsequent session of the meeting, regardless of the number of Councilors in attendance at the meeting.

4.1.i. Committees
The Legislative Council shall create and dissolve standing committees, councils, and boards, designate and change their charges, and determine their size, composition, and terms. Those committees charged with functions of the Legislative Council shall be so designated in the Special Rules of the Legislative Council. All other committees, boards, and councils shall be assigned to the Executive Board which shall monitor their activities.

Section 2. The Executive Board

4.2.a. Powers

4.2.a.1. The Executive Board is the management body and shall supervise, control, and direct the affairs of the Association, and shall actively prosecute the objectives of the Association, operating in accordance with and administering and implementing the programs and policies established by these Bylaws and by the Legislative Council. The Executive Board shall manage and operate the American Speech-Language-Hearing Foundation through the power to appoint and remove the Board of Trustees of the Foundation.

4.2.a.2. The Executive Board shall have discretion in the disbursement of funds under the policies established by the Legislative Council. The actions of the Executive Board shall be reported to the Legislative Council at its next meeting.

4.2.b. Composition
The Executive Board shall consist of ten officers, as follows:

(1) The President, who shall serve as Chair of the Legislative Council and Chair of the Executive Board, and who shall coordinate the functions of both bodies, and who shall automatically become Past President at the end of the term as President;

(2) The President-Elect, who shall serve as Chair of the Legislative Council and Chair of the Executive Board in the absence of the President, and who shall automatically become President at the end of the term of President-Elect;

(3) The Past President;

(4) The Vice-President for Administration and Planning, who shall serve as treasurer;

(5) The Vice-President for Research and Technology;

(6) The Vice-President for Quality of Service;

(7) The Vice-President for Professional Practice;

(8) The Vice-President for Academic Affairs;

(9) The Vice President for Governmental and Social Policies;

(10) The Executive Director of the Association who shall serve as nonvoting member.

4.2.c. Nominations

A committee consisting of six members elected annually by the Legislative Council and the Past President serving as Chair shall present in writing prior to the annual meeting of the Legislative Council a slate of three nominees for each office to be filled.

The Legislative Council may, by two-thirds vote, make no more than two additional nominations for each office. A nominee may be any member of the Association including a Councilor who must express willingness to serve if elected.

4.2.d. Elections

Election to each office shall be by mail ballot of the entire membership of the Association conducted by the National Office and supervised by a committee appointed by the Executive Board at such time and in such manner as to permit and require completion and counting of the balloting prior to the next meeting of the Legislative Council. The nominee for each office receiving the most votes shall be elected. In each case where a nominee withdraws from a national election after the ballots have been mailed to the membership, the candidates remaining will constitute the slate of nominees, and the person with the largest number of votes shall be declared the winner. In the event of a tie, a separate tie-breaking mail ballot shall be prepared by a committee so charged and submitted to the voting members of the Legislative Council. The nominee receiving the most votes in this tie-breaking election shall be elected. A member of the Executive Board may not serve simultaneously as an elected Legislative Councilor.

4.2.e. Terms of Office

(1) The President-Elect shall serve three consecutive one-year terms, as President-Elect, President, and Past President, respectively.

(2) Each Vice-President shall be elected for a term of three years.

(3) No elected officer shall serve two full terms in the same office successively.

(4) All terms of office shall be on a calendar year basis.

4.2.f. Vacancies

Should a vacancy in the Executive Board be created by the resignation, death, removal from office, or inability to serve of any member of the Executive Board arising at any time subsequent to the member's election, the resultant vacancy shall be filled in accordance with the following procedure:

(1) If the vacancy is in the presidency, the President-Elect shall automatically become and serve as President for the remainder of the year in addition to the term to which the officer was previously elected. The resultant vacancy in the office of the President-Elect shall not be filled until the next election.

In the event there is a vacancy in the office of the President-Elect, another Executive Board member shall become President in accord with an order of succession to be established by the Legislative Council and shall serve for the remainder of the year.

(2) If the vacancy is in the office of President-Elect, including a vacancy which occurs in this office pursuant to the previous paragraph, the Vice-President for Administration and Planning shall assume the duties of the President-Elect for the remainder of the year.

(3) If the vacancy is in the office of a Vice-President, the Executive Board shall elect a member of the Association to serve for the unexpired portion of the term of that Vice President.

(4) If the vacancy occurs in the office of Past President, the most immediate Past President willing to serve shall complete the unexpired portion of the term.

4.2.g. Removal from Office

Any elected member of the Executive Board may be removed from office by (1) a written petition signed by 250 members of the Association or by one-third of the members of the Legislative Council submitted to the Chair of the Legislative Council, or, in the instance where the President is the object of the removal petition, to the President-Elect, (2) approval of the petition by 75 percent of the members of the Legislative Council voting, and (3) approval of the petition by 75 percent of the members of the Association voting. All ballots to be by mail and all procedures to be established by the Legislative Council.

4.2.h. Meetings

The Executive Board shall meet at least three times each year at such times and places as the President may determine. A quorum shall consist of six members of the Executive Board. At the discretion of the Executive Board, its business may be conducted by mail or telephone or other appropriate means.

4.2.i. Committees

4.2.i.1. The Executive Board may establish interim standing committees, designating their charges, size, composition and terms. Any such committee shall function until approved by the Legislative Council at its next meeting.

4.2.i.2. The Executive Board may establish task forces, ad hoc committees, networks, and working groups designating their charges, size, composition, terms, and budgets.

4.2.i.3. Vice-Presidents may establish subcommittees of existing committees assigned to them by the Executive Board, specify their charges, and appoint members to them, including persons not originally members of the existing committees, such action being taken only after securing the advice of the Chair of the committee.

4.2.i.4. The six Vice-Presidents and the President-Elect shall constitute a Committee on Committees, the President-Elect serving as Chair, which shall appoint members to all committees, boards, working groups, councils, and task forces (except the Executive Board, the Association Advisory Committee, Committees of the Legislative Council, and those Legislative Council positions on the Committee on Financial Planning and the Committee on Long Range Planning). The Committee on Committees shall complete periodic reviews of all committees and boards and shall make recommendations on such committees to the Legislative Council when issues of policy are concerned.

Section 3. National Office

4.3.a. Responsibilities
The Association shall maintain a National Office which shall constitute a permanent repository for Association records and shall carry out the procedures and policies of the Association under the guidance of the Executive Board. An annual audit of all accounts administered by the National Office shall be conducted by an independent firm of certified public accountants selected by the Executive Board, and the report thereof shall be available to all members and others as appropriate.

4.3.b. Executive Director
The Executive Director shall be appointed by the Executive Board and shall serve as the chief administrative officer of the Association. The Executive Director (or designee) shall serve as an ex-officio nonvoting member, unless otherwise stipulated, of all committees, boards, and councils of the Executive Board.

ARTICLE V

PROFESSIONAL STANDARDS

5.1. Certification and Accreditation
The Association, by action of the Legislative Council, shall establish and maintain programs of certification and accreditation according to standards specified by the Council on Professional Standards in Speech-Language Pathology and Audiology (hereafter the "Council") and shall maintain a registry of holders of certification and accreditation.

5.2. Council on Professional Standards in Speech-Language Pathology and Audiology
The Association shall establish the Council which shall define the standards for certification and for the accreditation of graduate educational programs and of professional service programs, and shall monitor the interpretation and application of these standards. The Council shall decide appeals from decisions rendered by such operating boards as the Legislative Council may establish. The decisions of the Council, insofar as they involve the award or denial of certification or accreditation, shall be final.

5.3. Code of Ethics
The Association shall establish a Council on Professional Ethics in Speech-Language Pathology and Audiology (hereinafter referred to as the "Ethics Council") which shall formulate, and publish, and, from time to time, amend (a) a Code of Ethics (hereinafter the "Code") containing the professional responsibilities by which members and certificate holders shall be bound and (b) educational programs in ethics for distribution to members and certificate holders and to educational programs. The Code and all amendments shall be subject to approval by the Legislative Council. The Association shall establish an Ethical Practice Board which shall formulate and publish procedures which shall be used for the processing of alleged violations of the Code including a reasonable opportunity to be heard through counsel of one's own choosing. The Ethical Practice Board shall determine sanctions for violations in its discretion as it deems appropriate including revoking and/or suspending membership and/or certification. All appeals of Ethical Practice Board actions shall be decided by the Executive Board or a panel thereof, whose decisions shall be final.

ARTICLE VI

PUBLICATIONS

6.1. Official Publications

6.1.a. The Association shall: (1) publish periodicals entitled *Journal of Speech and Hearing Disorders, Journal of Speech and Hearing Research, Asha* and *Language, Speech, and Hearing Services in Schools;* (2) issue irregularly *ASHA Reports* and *ASHA Monographs* at the discretion of the Publictions Board; (3) publish a Directory and other publications recommended by the Executive Board and approved by the Legislative Council

6.1.b. Members shall receive the *Journal of Speech and Hearing Disorders;* the *Journal of Speech and Hearing Research; Language, Speech, and Hearing Services in the Schools; Asha,* and such other publications as the Legislative Council may designate. Members who have received life membership may elect not to receive selected publications of the Association.

ARTICLE VII

DISCRIMINATION

7.1. The Association shall not discriminate on the basis of race, national origin, religion, age, sex, sexual orientation, or handicapping condition. All programs and activities of the Association shall be conducted in furtherance of this policy.

ARTICLE VIII

HONORS

8.1. The Honors of the Association
The Honors of the Association recognize distinguished contribution to the field of speech, language and hearing

and is the highest honor the Association can give. It may be presented to an individual upon recommendation by the Committee on Honors and approval by 75 percent vote of the Legislative Council voting on the recommendation.

8.2. Fellowship
Fellowship is an award recognizing professional or scientific achievement and may be given to a member on approval by two-thirds vote of the Committee on Honors. The status of Fellow shall be retained by the individual to whom it is awarded as long as the person remains a member in good standing of the Association.

ARTICLE IX

RECOGNITION OF OTHER ORGANIZATIONS

9.1. State Speech-Language Hearing Associations

9.1.a. Purpose
Recognition offers official identification of state speech-language-hearing associations.

9.1.b. Method of Recognition
A state association which desires recognition shall petition in writing to the Executive Board. Recognition shall be granted and maintained at the discretion of the Executive Board to only one association in each state and shall be available only to those state associations with purposes and membership requirements which are both consistent with those of the Association and which are independent and not controlled, directly or indirectly, by any other organization.

9.2. National Student Speech Language Hearing Association
The Association recognizes the National Student Speech Language Hearing Association as the sole national student association in the field of speech, language and hearing. The Legislative Council shall include two (2) elected representatives of the National Student Speech Language Hearing Association with full voting privileges.

ARTICLE X

PARLIAMENTARY AUTHORITY

10.1. The rules contained in the current edition of Robert's Rules of Order Newly Revised, as it may be amended from time to time, shall govern the Association in all cases to which they are applicable and in which they are not inconsistent with these Bylaws, or with the Articles of Incorporation or with any special rules of order the Association may adopt.

ARTICLE XI

AMENDMENTS

These Bylaws may be amended by either of the following procedures:

11.1. By the Legislative Council, pursuant to notice in the call of a meeting or at a session of a meeting pursuant to notice not later than the prior session of that meeting, by two-thirds vote of its members voting, except that any amendment involving a matter reserved to members under Section 3.3 shall, after the required Council approval, be submitted to members for vote by mail ballot and shall require for adoption a two-thirds vote of those members of the Association voting within 21 days from the mailing of the ballot.

11.2. By written petition by 175 members of the Association submitted to the Legislative Council and adopted by a two-thirds vote of its members voting at that meeting, except that if any amendment involving a matter reserved to the members under Section 3.3 shall, after the required approval of the Legislative Council, be submitted to the members as prescribed in Section 11.1.

"1988 DELETIONS FROM BYLAWS"

The following policies of the American Speech-Language-Hearing Association (ASHA) were contained in the Association's Bylaws. In 1988, by action of the Legislative Council, the policies were removed from the Bylaws and continue in effect.

Life Membership: Any member who has attained the age of 65 and who has held membership for twenty-five consecutive years immediately prior to attaining age 65 may apply for and automatically receive life membership with all privileges of a member without payment of annual dues for any years subsequent to the year in which age 65 is attained, effective January 1, 1991. Until December 31, 1990, a member must have held membership for 10 years immediately prior to attaining age 65.

Disability: Any member who becomes totally disabled and who has held membership for five consecutive years immediately prior to disability may make application for disability life membership with all privileges of a member without payment of annual dues for any years subsequent to the year in which disability life membership is granted and periodically verified.

Dues/Fees: All applications for membership received at ASHA with required dues/fees: (1) on March 1 through August 31 shall be assigned to the July membership year which shall run from July 1 through June 30 of each year; or (2) on September 1 through February 28 (or 29) shall be assigned to the January membership year which shall run from January 1 through December 31 of each year. Annual renewal dues/fees shall be payable in full in advance of each membership year/billing cycle, either on January 1 or on July 1, depending upon the membership year/billing cycle to which the applicant has been assigned.

Termination of Membership and Privileges: a. Any member who violates the Code of Ethics of the Association may be dropped from membership by a two-thirds vote of the Ethical Practice Board. Persons who have thus been dropped may be reinstated after one year by a two thirds vote of the Ethical Practice Board.

b. A member whose dues are not paid shall not receive the publications of the Association until dues have been paid for the current membership year to which assigned.

c. A member whose dues are in arrears on April 1 if assigned to the January membership year; or on October 1, if assigned to the July membership year, automatically shall be dropped from the rolls of the Association.

Residence For all purposes regarding member participation in the governance of the Association, a member's residence shall be the mailing address designated by the member in writing to the National Office.

Those members whose mailing address is an APO or FPO shall designate their residence in writing.

Nominations for Legislative Council: The size of the Legislative Council per state shall remain the same as in effect for the year 1978, by the election of appropriate replacements, without increasing the size of any state delegation.

Members of the Association whose mailing addresses are outside of the United States shall choose Councilors from among themselves according to the schedule of representation.

The National Office shall conduct the procedures for nominating and electing Councilors. The National Office shall send nomination ballots to individual members.

Nomination ballots shall be returned for tabulation to the National Elections Committee. The committee shall secure agreement from nominees to serve if elected.

Nominees will be ranked according to the number of nominations received. A slate will be prepared of the highest ranked nominees comprising twice the number of candidates required to fill the available seats. When ties preclude immediate identification of the specified number of candidates, the slate shall be increased to include all nominees tied for the final position on the slate. In the event that fewer than the specified number of candidates are nominated, all qualified nominees shall be placed on the ballot and the additional number, if any, required to equal the number of nominees authorized by the state shall be designated by the National Elections Committee. Candidates for election to the Council shall be listed alphabetically on the state election ballot prepared by the National Elections Committee. The nominees receiving the largest number of votes up to the number of Councilors authorized shall be designated as duly elected Councilors by the National Elections Committee. When ties prevent the immediate identification of the Councilor(s) to fill the available seats, a separate tie-breaking mail ballot shall be prepared by the National Elections Committee and submitted to the voting members residing in that state. The nominee(s) receiving the largest number of votes from this tie-breaking election shall be designated as duly elected Councilor(s). The remaining nominees shall be designated as Alternate I, Alternate II, et cetera, in descending rank order, beginning with the nominee receiving the next highest number of votes.

For the purposes of Section 4.1.f. of the Bylaws, the committee charged with filling vacancies on the Legislative Council shall be the National Elections Committee.

Executive Board: Election to each office shall be by mail ballot of the entire membership of the Association, conducted for the National Elections Committee by the National Office at such time and in such manner as to permit and require completion and counting of the balloting prior to the annual convention of the Association. The nominee for each office receiving the most votes shall be elected. In the event of a tie, a separate tie-breaking mail ballot shall be prepared by the National Elections Committee and submitted to the voting members of the Legislative Council. The nominee receiving the most votes in this tie-breaking election shall be elected. In each case where a nominee withdraws from a national election after the ballots have been mailed to the Membership, the candidates remaining will constitute the slate of nominees and the person with the highest number of votes shall be declared the victor.

The Executive Board shall perform its functions through the officers of the Association and through the committees and boards that report to the Executive Board.

The Executive Board shall assign each ad hoc committee to a Vice-President who shall monitor its activities and to the Executive Director (or the Executive Director's designee) who shall provide liaison with the National Office. The Executive Board shall assign each task force to the Executive Director (or the Executive Director's designee) who shall serve as coordinator and to an officer who shall provide liaison with the Executive Board. The establishment of a subcommittee, its size, and the determination of its charge shall be subject to the approval of the Executive Board at its next meeting.

Each Vice-President shall recommend to the Committee on Committees candidates to fill vacancies on committees, boards and task forces assigned to that officer.

Each committee, board and council shall submit an annual written report of its activities and recommendations to the individual or body to whom it is assigned, who in turn shall report to the Executive Board in a manner and form and at such time as the Executive Board shall require. The Executive Board shall report to the Legislative Council all significant committee activities during the year.

In regard to removal of a member of the Executive Board, the Legislative Council shall establish appropriate procedures to include the conduct of fair hearings.

Association Conventions: Conventions of the Association shall be held annually at a time and place determined by the Executive Board. Conventions shall be held only in establishments in which meetings can be held without discrimination on the bases of race, national origin, religion, sex, age, or handicapping condition. The responsibility for arranging the Conventions shall be shared by the Scientific and Professional Programs Board and the Executive Board.

Council on Professional Standards: The Executive Board shall appoint the Council which shall consist of at least 11 members who shall serve three-year, staggered terms. At least five Council members shall represent clinical services settings, three of those representing non-university settings, at least four shall represent graduate education programs, and at least one shall be a person who is a representative of the public. Further, at least three Council members shall hold the Certificate of Clinical Competence in Speech-Language Pathology and at least three shall hold the Certificate of Clinical Competence in Audiology, at least one shall be recognized as a speech and hearing scientist. Association accredited educational and professional services programs shall be represented. These members need not be members of the Association. The Council shall elect from among its members a chair, a vice chair and a secretary. The Council shall publish an Annual Report.

The operating boards of examiners in speech-language pathology and audiology (Clinical Certification Board, Professional Services Board, Educational Standards Board) shall administer the Association's certification and accreditation programs; shall interpret and apply standards established by the Council to individuals, institutions and organizations; and shall formulate procedures, including the conduct of examinations, for the determination of qualifications of individuals applying for Certificates of Clinical Competence, and institutions and organizations applying for accreditation.

Publications: The Publications Board shall be responsible to the Executive Board. The Executive Director (or designee) of the American Speech-Language-Hearing Association shall be Editor of *Asha* and shall be responsible to the Executive Board for these editorial duties. The Editors of all other publications shall be appointed by the Executive Board, on recommendation of the Publications Board for terms of four years. These Editors shall have immediate editorial responsibility for their respective publications. They shall be responsible to the Publications Board. The staff of each Editor shall consist of such Associate Editors, Department Editors, Assistant Editors, and other personnel as are considered necessary by the Editor, these to be appointed by the Editor, subject to approval by the Publications Board. Each Editor shall make an annual report to the Publictions Board for inclusion in that Board's annual report.

Recognition of Other Associations, Procedures for Denial, Withdrawal, Appeal: Basis and Procedure for Denial or Withdrawal of Recognition and Appeal: A state association seeking recognition may have student representation on the governing body of the state association with full rights and privileges, including voting privileges. At the discretion of the Executive Board, recognition shall be denied or withdrawn from a state association which does not meet the criteria for recognition.

The Executive Board shall address in writing the state association which has had its recognition denied or withdrawn.

The statement shall include reasons for denial or withdrawal of recognition and shall outline the following procedures for appealing the decision.

(1) A state association may register formal request for reconsideration to the Executive Board. The Executive Board or its appointed representatives must review all such requests.

(2) If the Executive Board upholds its original decision, the state association may request the Board to appoint an ad hoc committee to review the appeal. Such committee shall consist of five voting members all of whom are Association members and three of whom are members of the Legislative Council. This ad hoc committee shall be formed in the following manner. The Executive Board will submit to the state association the names of ten qualified and available persons recommended for appointment and the state association may select the five committee members from the list or may recommend that the Executive Board appoint five committee members from the list.

(3) The ad hoc committee, under such procedures as it may adopt, will consider the appeal of the state association and will act by majority vote. The decision of the committee will be based on information submitted by the state association and the Executive Board.

(4) The majority vote of the ad hoc committee will be binding on the Executive Board.

Executive Director The Executive Director is appointed by the Executive Board for a contract period of up to four years which may be renewed as deemed appropriate by the Board. The Executive Director functions as the director of the National Office staff and operations, chief liaison and public information agent of the Association, contracting and financial officer of the Association with authority to collect and disburse all funds of the Association, and the business manager of the Association and its publications. The Executive Director records the minutes of all meetings of the Legislative Council and of the Executive Board. The Executive Director and any additional persons disbursing Association funds shall also be bonded.

Council on Professional Ethics: The Executive Board shall appoint the Council on Professional Ethics which shall consist of no more than 10 members who shall serve three-year staggered terms. The Council members shall represent a variety of clinical practice settings and research and academic settings and at least one shall be a person who is representative of the public. At least five Council members shall have had previous experience as members of the Ethical Practice Board. Further, at least three Council members shall hold the Certificate of Clinical Competence in Speech-Language Pathology and at least three shall hold the Certificate of Clinical Competence in Audiology.

CODE OF ETHICS of the AMERICAN SPEECH-LANGUAGE-HEARING ASSOCIATION 1986

(Revised January 1, 1986)

Preamble

The preservation of the highest standards of integrity and ethical principles is vital to the successful discharge of the professional responsibilities of all speech-language pathologists and audiologists. This Code of Ethics has been promulgated by the Association in an effort to stress the fundamental rules considered essential to this basic purpose. Any action that is in violation of the spirit and purpose of this Code shall be considered unethical. Failure to specify any particular responsibility or practice in this Code of Ethics should not be construed as denial of the existence of other responsibilities or practices.

The fundamental rules of ethical conduct are described in three categories: Principles of Ethics, Ethical Proscriptions, Matters of Professional Propriety.

1. *Principles of Ethics.* Six Principles serve as a basis for the ethical evaluation of professional conduct and form the underlying moral basis for the Code of Ethics. Individuals[1] subscribing to this Code shall observe these principles as affirmative obligations under all conditions of professional activity.

2. *Ethical Proscriptions.* Ethical Proscriptions are formal statements of prohibitions that are derived from the Principles of Ethics.

3. *Matters of Professional Propriety.* Matters of Professional Propriety represent guidelines of conduct designed to promote the public interest and thereby better inform the public and particularly the persons in need of speech-language pathology and audiology services as to the availability and the rules regarding the delivery of those services.

PRINCIPLE OF ETHICS I

Individuals shall hold paramount the welfare of persons served professionally.

A. Individuals shall use every resource available, including referral to other specialists as needed, to provide the best service possible.

B. Individuals shall fully inform persons served of the nature and possible effects of the services.

C. Individuals shall fully inform subjects participating in research or teaching activities of the nature and possible effects of these activities.

D. Individuals' fees shall be commensurate with services rendered.

E. Individuals shall provide appropriate access to records of persons served professionally.

F. Individuals shall take all reasonable precautions to avoid injuring persons in the delivery of professional services.

G. Individuals shall evaluate services rendered to determine effectiveness.

Ethical Proscriptions

1. Individuals must not exploit persons in the delivery of professional services, including accepting persons for treatment when benefit cannot reasonably be expected or continuing treatment unnecessarily.

2. Individuals must not guarantee the results of any therapeutic procedures, directly or by implication. A reasonable statement of prognosis may be made, but caution must be exercised not to mislead persons served professionally to expect results that cannot be predicted from sound evidence.

3. Individuals must not use persons for teaching or research in a manner that constitutes invasion of privacy or fails to afford informed free choice to participate.

4. Individuals must not evaluate or treat speech, language or hearing disorders except in a professional relationship. They must not evaluate or treat solely by correspondence. This does not preclude follow-up correspondence with persons previously seen, nor providing them with general information of an educational nature.

5. Individuals must not reveal to unauthorized persons any professional or personal information obtained from the person served professionally, unless required by law or unless necessary to protect the welfare of the person or the community.

6. Individuals must not discriminate in the delivery of professional services on any basis that is unjustifiable or irrelevant to the need for and potential benefit from such services, such as race, sex, age, or religion.

7. Individuals must not charge for services not rendered.

PRINCIPLE OF ETHICS II

Individuals shall maintain high standards of professional competence.

[1] "Individuals" refers to all Members of the American Speech-Language-Hearing Association and non-members who hold Certificate of Clinical Competence from this Association.

A. Individuals engaging in clinical practice shall or supervision thereof shall hold the appropriate Certificate(s) of Clinical Competence for the area(s) in which they are providing or supervising professional services.

B. Individuals shall continue their professional development throughout their careers.

C. Individuals shall identify competent, dependable referral sources for persons served professionally.

D. Individuals shall maintain adequate records of professional services rendered.

Ethical Proscriptions

1. Individuals must neither provide services nor supervision of services for which they have not been properly prepared, nor permit services to be provided by any of their staff who are not properly prepared.

2. Individuals must not provide clinical services by prescription of anyone who does not hold the Certificate of Clinical Competence.

3. Individuals must not delegate any service requiring the professional competence of a certified clinician to anyone unqualified.

4. Individuals must not offer clinical services by supportive personnel for whom they do not provide appropriate supervision and assume full responsibility.

5. Individuals must not require anyone under their supervision to engage in any practice that is a violation of the Code of Ethics.

PRINCIPLE OF ETHICS III

Individuals' statements to persons served professionally and to the public shall provide accurate information about the nature and management of communicative disorders, and about the profession and services rendered by its practitioners.

Ethical Proscriptions

1. Individuals must not misrepresent their training or competence.

2. Individuals' public statements providing information about professional services and products must not contain representations or claims that are false, deceptive or misleading.

3. Individuals must not use professional or commercial affiliations in any way that would mislead or limit services to persons served professionally.

Matters of Professional Propriety

1. Individuals should announce services in a manner consonant with highest professional standards in the community.

PRINCIPLE OF ETHICS IV

Individuals shall maintain objectivity in all matters concerning the welfare of persons served professionally.

A. Individuals who dispense products to persons served professionally shall observe the following standards:

(1) Products associated with professional practice must be dispensed to the person served as a part of a program of comprehensive habilitative care.

(2) Fees established for professional services must be independent of whether a product is dispensed.

(3) Persons served must be provided freedom of choice for the source of services and products.

(4) Price information about professional services rendered and products dispensed must be disclosed by providing to or posting for persons served a complete schedule of fees and charges in advance of rendering services, which schedule differentiates between fees for professional services and charges for products dispensed.

(5) Products dispensed to the person served must be evaluated to determine effectiveness.

Ethical Proscriptions

1. Individuals must not participate in activities that constitute a conflict of professional interest.

Matters of Professional Propriety

1. Individuals should not accept compensation for supervision or sponsorship from the clinical fellow being supervised or sponsored beyond reasonable reimbursement for direct expenses.

2. Individuals should present products they have developed to their colleagues in a manner consonant with highest professional standards.

PRINCIPLE OF ETHICS V

Individuals shall honor their responsibilities to the public, their profession, and their relationships with colleagues and members of allied professions.

Matters of Professional Propriety

1. Individuals should seek to provide and expand services to persons with speech, language and hearing handicaps as well as to assist in establishing high professional standards for such programs.

2. Individuals should educate the public about speech, language and hearing processes, speech, language and hearing problems, and matters related to professional competence.

3. Individuals should strive to increase knowledge within the profession and share research with colleagues.

4. Individuals should establish harmonious relations with colleagues and members of other professions, and endeavor to inform members of related professions of services provided by speech-language pathologists and audiologists, as well as seek information from them.

5. Individuals should assign credit to those who have contributed to a publication in proportion to their contribution.

PRINCIPLE OF ETHICS VI

Individuals shall uphold the dignity of the profession and freely accept the profession's self-imposed standards.

A. Individuals shall inform the Ethical Practice Board when they have reason to believe that a member or certificate holder may have violated the Code of Ethics.

B. Individuals shall cooperate fully with the Ethical Practice Board concerning matters of professional conduct related to this Code of Ethics.

Ethical Proscriptions

1. Individuals shall not engage in violations of the Principles of Ethics or in any attempt to circumvent any of them.

2. Individuals shall not engage in dishonesty, fraud, deceit, misrepresentation, or other forms of illegal conduct that adversely reflect on the profession or the individuals' fitness for membership in the profession.

AMERICAN SPEECH-LANGUAGE-HEARING ASSOCIATION ETHICAL PRACTICE BOARD STATEMENT OF PRACTICES AND PROCEDURES

(Effective February 15, 1986)

The Ethical Practice Board (EPB) is charged by the Bylaws of the American Speech-Language-Hearing Association with the responsibility to interpret, administer, and enforce the Code of Ethics of the Association. Accordingly, the EPB hereby adopts the following practices and procedures to be followed in administering and enforcing that Code.

A fundamental precept that guides the EPB in the discharge of its responsibility is that an effective Code of Ethics requires an orderly and fair administration and enforcement of its terms and requires full compliance by all members of the Association and all holders of Certificates of Clinical Competence. The EPB recognizes that each case must be judged on an individual basis, and that no two cases are likely to be identical. Thus, the EPB has the responsibility to exercise its judgment on the merits of each case and on its interpretation of the Code.

A. Definition of Terms

1.	EPB:	Ethical Practice Board
2.	Association:	American Speech-Language-Hearing Association
3.	Code:	Code of Ethics of the Association
4.	Certificate(s):	Certificate(s) of Clinical Competence
5.	Respondent:	The alleged offender
6.	Complainant(s):	The person(s) alleging that a violation occurred
7.	Initial Determination:	Initial Determination by the EPB, subject to Further Consideration and appeal, of the (a) finding, (b) proposed sanction, and (c) extent of disclosure
8.	Sanction(s):	Penalties imposed by the EPB
9.	Disclosure:	Announcement of the final EPB Decision to other than Respondent
10.	Further Consideration:	Further Consideration by the EPB of its Initial Determination
11.	EPB Decision:	Final decision of the EPB after: 1) Further Consideration; or 2) 30 days from the date of notice of the Initial Determination by the EPB if no request for Further Consideration is received
12.	Appeal:	Written request from Respondent to EPB alleging error in the EPB Decision and asking that it be reversed in whole or in part by the Executive Board

B. Investigative Procedures

1. Alleged violations shall be reviewed by the EPB in such manner as the EPB may, in its discretion, deem necessary and proper. If, after review, the EPB elects to investigate the allegation, the EPB shall notify Respondent of the alleged offense in writing and shall advise Respondent that Respondent's answer to the allegation shall be in writing and must be *received* by the EPB no later than 45 days after the date of the EPB notice to Respondent. Voluntary resignation of membership and or voluntary surrender of the Certificate(s) shall not preclude the EPB from continuing the process the alleged violation to conclusion, and the notice from the EPB to Respondent requesting an answer shall so advise Respondent.

2. At the discretion of the EPB, the Director of the Professional Affairs Department of the Association's National Office may be informed that respondent is under investigation by the EPB for alleged violation of the Code and may be instructed that no change in membership and/or certification status shall be permitted without approval of the EPB.

3. The EPB shall consider all information secured from its investigation, including Respondent's answer to the allegation, and shall base its initial Determination on that information.

4. If the EPB finds that there is not sufficient evidence to warrant further proceedings, Respondent and Complainant(s) shall be so advised and the investigation shall be terminated.

5. If the EPB finds that there is sufficient evidence to warrant further proceedings, the EPB shall make an Initial Determination, which includes (a) the finding of violation, (b) the proposed sanction, and (c) the proposed extent of disclosure. In this regard, the final decision of any State, Federal, regulatory, or judicial body may be considered sufficient evidence that the Code was violated.

6. The EPB may, as part of its Initial Determination, order that the Respondent cease and desist from any practice found to be a violation of the Code. Failure to comply with such a Cease and Desist Order is, itself, a violation of the Code, and shall normally result in Revocation of Membership and or Revocation of the Certificate(s).

7. The EPB shall give Respondent notice of its Initial Determination, with copy to Complainant(s). The notice shall also advise Respondent of the right to request Further Consideration by the EPB and of the right, *after Further Consideration,* to an appeal to the Executive Board. The procedures to be followed in exercising those rights are described in Sections F and G of this statement.

C. Notices and Answers

All notices and answers shall be in writing and considered to be given or furnished (1) to Respondent when *sent*—Certified Mail, Addressee Only. Return Receipt Requested—to the address then listed in the ASHA membership records, and (2) to EPB when *received* by the EPB.

D. Sanctions

Sanctions shall consist of one or more of the following: Reprimand; Censure; Withhold, Suspend, or Revoke Membership;

Withhold, Suspend, or Revoke the Certificate(s); or other measures determined by the EPB at its discretion.

E. Disclosure

1. The EPB Decision, upon becoming final, shall be published in the Journal *Asha* unless the sanction is Reprimand. In the case of Reprimand, the EPB Decision normally shall be disclosed only to Respondent, Respondent's counsel, Complainant(s), witnesses at the EPB Further Consideration Hearing and/or at the Executive Board Hearing, staff, Association counsel, and the Coordinator of the Professional Ethics Section of the Association's National Office, each of whom shall be advised that the decision is strictly confidential and that any breach of that confidentiality by any party who is a member and/or certificate holder of the Association is, itself, a violation of the Code.

2. In appropriate cases, including when the sanction is Reprimand, the EPB may also determine that its Decision shall be disclosed to aggrieved parties and/or other appropriate individuals, bodies, or agencies.

F. Further Consideration by the EPB of the Initial Determination

1. When the notice of Initial Determination from the EPB states that Respondent has violated the Code and announces a proposed sanction and extent of disclosure, Respondent may request that the EPB give Further Consideration to the Initial Determination.

2. Respondent's request for further Consideration shall be in writing and must be *received* by the EPB Chair no later than 30 days after the date of notice of Initial Determination. *The request for Further Consideration must specify in what respects the Initial Determination was allegedly wrong and why.* In the absence of a timely request for Further Consideration, the Initial Determination shall be the EPB Decision, which decision shall be final, there shall be no further right of appeal to the Executive Board.

3. If Respondent submits a timely request for Further Consideration by the EPB, the EPB shall schedule a hearing and notify Respondent. At the hearing, Respondent shall be entitled to submit a written brief or to appear personally to present evidence and to be accompanied by counsel. The proceeding shall be informal; strict adherence to the rules of evidence shall not be observed, but all evidence shall be accorded such weight as it deserves. As an alternative to personal appearance at the hearing, the EPB shall afford Respondent the opportunity to make a presentation to the EPB and to respond to questions from the EPB via a conference telephone call placed to Respondent by the EPB. All personal costs in connection with the Further Consideration hearing, including travel and lodging costs incurred by Respondent, Resondent's counsel and witnesses, and counsel and other fees, shall be Respondent's sole responsibility. The hearing shall be transcribed in full and, upon request, a copy of the transcript shall be made available to Respondent at Respondent's sole expense.

4. After the Further Consideration Hearing, the EPB shall render its decision and notify Respondent. If evidence presented at the hearing warrants, the EPB may modify the finding, increase or decrease the severity of the sanction, and/or modify the extent of disclosure that was announced to Respondent in the notice of Initial Determination. This decision shall be the EPB Decision, and in the absence of a timely appeal to the Executive Board, the EPB Decision shall be final.

G. Appeal of EPB Decision to Executive Board

1. Respondent may appeal the EPB Decision to the Executive Board. The request for appeal shall be in writing and must be *received* by the EPB Chair no later than 30 days after the date of notice of the EPB Decision. *The request for appeal shall specify in what respects the EPB Decision was allegedly wrong and why.*

2. The procedures for a hearing before the Executive Board are described in the Executive Board Statement of Practices and Procedures for Appeals of Decisions of the Ethical Practice Board.

H. Reinstatement

Persons whose membership or certification has been revoked may, upon application therefore, be reinstated after one year upon a two-thirds vote of the EPB. The applicant bears the burden of demonstrating that the reason(s) for revocation no longer exist and that, upon reinstatement, applicant will abide by the Code.

I. Amendment

This *Statement of Practices and Procedures* may be amended upon recommendation of the EPB and a vote of the Executive Board. All such changes will be given appropriate publicity.

EXECUTIVE BOARD STATEMENT OF PRACTICES AND PROCEDURES FOR APPEALS OF DECISIONS OF THE ETHICAL PRACTICE BOARD

(Effective May 1, 1987)

Pursuant to Article V of the Bylaws, the Executive Board (EB) hereby adopts this procedure governing an appeal from a Decision of the Ethical Practice Board (EPB).

Appeals to the Executive Board are only permitted from EPB Decisions following an EPB Further Consideration Hearing.

Such appeal shall be heard by an EB Appeals Panel consisting of three EB members appointed by the EB chair.

The EB Appeals Panel shall given written notice to the appellant and to the EPB of the time and place of the hearing. Said notice shall be given at least 30 days in advance of the hearing, by certified mail, return receipt requested, and shall advise of the right to counsel, of the right to submit in advance a written brief, of the right to oral argument at the hearing either in person or by conference call. The notice shall also advise that the Executive Board Appeals Panel will not consider any evidence except that which was presented at the Further Consideration Hearing before the EPB. The Executive Board Appeals Panel shall render its decision promptly after the hearing and shall state it in writing.

All costs in connection with the appeal, including travel and lodging costs incurred by appellant and appellant's counsel (and witnesses), and appellant's counsel and other fees shall be appellant's sole responsibility.

Said decision shall be final and shall be subject to normal or Special Publication as determined by the Executive Board Appeals Panel.

This procedure may be amended by a two-thirds vote of the Executive Board.

REQUIREMENTS for the CERTIFICATES OF CLINICAL COMPETENCE

(Revised January 1, 1988)

The American Speech-Language-Hearing Association issues Certificates of Clinical Competence to individuals who present satisfactory evidence of their ability to provide independent clinical services to persons who have disorders of communication (speech, language, and/or hearing). An individual who meets these requirements may be awarded a Certificate in Speech-Language Pathology or in Audiology, depending upon the emphasis of preparation; a person who meets the requirements in both professional areas may be awarded both Certificates.

I. STANDARDS

The individual who is awarded either, or both of the Certificates of Clinical Competence must hold a master's degree or equivalent[1] with major emphasis in speech-language pathology, audiology, or speech language and hearing science. The individual must also meet the following qualifications:

I,A. General Background Education

As stipulated below, applicants for a certificate should have completed specialized academic training and preparatory professional experience that provides an in-depth knowledge of normal communication processes, development and disorders thereof, evaluation procedures to assess the bases of such disorders, and clinical techniques that have been shown to improve or eradicate them. It is expected that the applicant will have obtained a broad general education to serve as a background prior to such study and experience and demonstrates adequate oral and written communication skills. The specific content of this general background education is left to the discretion of the applicant and to the training program attended. However, it is highly desirable that it include study in the areas of human psychology, sociology, psychological and physical development, the physical sciences (especially those that pertain to acoustic and biological phenomena) and human anatomy and physiology, including neuroanatomy and neurophysiology.

I,B. Required Education

A total of 60 semester hours[2] of academic credit must have been accumulated from accredited colleges or universities that demonstrate that the applicant has obtained a well-integrated program of course study dealing with the normal aspects of human communication, development thereof, disorders thereof, and clinical techniques for evaluation and management of such disorders.

[1]Equivalent is defined as holding a bachelor's degree from an accredited college or university, and at least 42 post baccalaureate semester hours acceptable toward a master's degree, of which at least 30 semester hours must be in the areas of speech-language pathology, audiology, or speech-language and hearing science. At least 21 of these 42 semester hours must be obtained from a single college or university, none may have been completed more than 10 years prior to the date of application and no more than six semester hours may be credit offered for clinical practicum.

[2]In evaluation of credits, one quarter hour will be considered the equivalent of two-thirds of a semester hour. Transcripts that do not report credit in terms of semester or quarter hours should be submitted for special evaluation.

Twelve (12) of these 60 semester hours must be obtained in courses that provide information that pertains to normal development and use of speech, language and hearing.

Thirty (30) of these 60 semester hours must be in courses that provide (1) information relative to communication disorders, and (2) information about and training in evaluation and management of speech, language and hearing disorders. At least 24 of these 30 semester hours must be in courses in the professional area (speech-language pathology or audiology) for which the certificate is requested, and at least six (6) must be in audiology for the certificate in speech-language pathology or in speech-language pathology for the certificate in audiology. Moreover, no more than six (6) semester hours may be in courses that provide credit for clinical practicum obtained during academic training.

Credit for study of information pertaining to related fields that augment the work of the clinical practitioner of speech-language pathology and/or audiology may also apply toward the total 60 semester hours.

Thirty (30) of the total 60 semester hours that are required for a certificate must be in courses that are acceptable toward a graduate degree by the college or university in which they are taken.[3] Moreover, 21 of those 30 semester hours must be within the 24 semester hours required in the professional area (speech-language pathology or audiology) for which the certificate is requested or within the six (6) semester hours required in the other area.

I,C. Academic Clinical Practicum

The applicant must have completed a minimum of 300 clock hours of supervised clinical experience with individuals who present a variety of communication disorders, and this experience must have been obtained within the training institution or in one of its cooperating programs.

I,D. The Clinical Fellowship Year

The applicant must have obtained the equivalent of nine (9) months of full-time professional experience (the Clinical Fellowship Year) in which bona fide clinical work has been accomplished in the major professional area (speech-language pathology or audiology) in which the certificate is being sought. The Clinical Fellowship Year must have begun after completion of the academic and clinical practicum experiences specified in Standards I,A., I,B., and I,C. above.

[3]This requirement may be met by courses completed as an undergraduate providing the college or university in which they are taken specifies that these courses would be acceptable toward a graduate degree if they were taken at the graduate level.

I,E. The National Examinations in Speech-Language Pathology and Audiology

The applicant must have passed one of the National Examinations in Speech-Language Pathology and Audiology, either the National Examination in Speech-Language Pathology or the National Examination in Audiology.

II. EXPLANATORY NOTES

II,A. General Background Education

While the broadest possible general educational background for the future clinical practitioner of speech-language pathology and/or audiology is encouraged, the nature of the clinician's professional endeavors suggests the necessity for some emphasis in general education. For example, elementary courses in general psychology and sociology are desirable as are studies in mathematics, general physics, zoology, as well as human anatomy and physiology. Those areas of introductory study that do not deal specifically with communication processes are not to be credited to the minimum 60 semester hours of education specified in Standard I,B.

II,B. Required Education

II,B,1. Basic Communication Processes Area. The 12 semester hours in courses that provide information applicable to the normal development and use of speech, language, and hearing should be selected with emphasis on the normal aspects of human communication in order that the applicant has a wide exposure to the diverse kinds of information suggested by the content areas given under the three broad categories that follow: (1) anatomic and physiological bases for the normal development and use of speech, language, and hearing such as anatomy, neurology, and physiology of speech, language, and hearing mechanisms; (2) physical bases and processes of the production and perception of speech, language and hearing, such as (a) acoustics or physics of sound, (b) phonology, (c) physiologic and acoustic phonetics, (d) perceptual processes, and (e) psychoacoustics; and (3) linguistic and psycholinguistic variables related to normal development and use of speech, language, and hearing, such as (a) linguistics (historical, descriptive, sociolinguistics, urban language), (b) psychology of language, (c) psycholinguistics, (d) language and speech acquisition, and (e) verbal learning or verbal behavior.

It is emphasized that the three broad categories of required education given above, and the examples of areas of study within these classifications, are not meant to be analogous to, or imply, specific course titles. Neither are the examples of areas of study within these categories meant to be exhaustive.

At least two (2) semester hours of credit must be earned in each of the three categories.

Obviously, some of these 12 semester hours may be obtained in courses that are taught in departments other than those offering speech-language pathology and audiology programs. Courses designed to improve the speaking and writing ability of the student will not be credited.

II,B,2. Major Professional Area, Certificate in Speech-Language Pathology. The 24 semester hours of professional education required for the Certificate of Clinical Competence in Speech-Language Pathology should include information pertaining to speech and language disorders as follows: (1) understanding of speech and language disorders, such as (a) various types of disorders of communication, (b) their manifestations, and (c) their classifications and causes; (2) evaluation skills such as procedures, techniques, and instrumentation used to assess (a) the speech and language status of children and adults, and (b) the bases of disorders of speech and language, and (3) management procedures, such as principles in remedial methods used in habilitation and rehabilitation for children and adults with various disorders of communication.

Within these categories at least six (6) semester hours must deal with speech disorders and at least six (6) semester hours must deal with language disorders.

II,B,3. Minor Professional Area, Certificate in Speech-Language Pathology. For the individual to obtain the Certificate in Speech-Language Pathology, at least six (6) semester hours of academic credit in audiology are required. Where only the minimum requirement of six (6) semester hours is met, three (3) semester hours must be in habilitative/rehabilitative procedures with speech and language problems associated with hearing impairment, and three (3) semester hours must be in study of the pathologies of the auditory system and assessment of auditory disorders. However, when more than the minimum six (6) semester hours is met, study of habilitative/rehabilitative procedures may be counted in the Major Professional Area for the Certificate in Speech-Language Pathology (see *Section II,B,8).*

II,B,4. Major Professional Area, Certificate in Audiology. The 24 semester hours of professional education required for the Certificate of Clinical Competence in Audiology should be in the broad, but not necessarily exclusive, categories of study as follows: (1) auditory disorders, such as (a) pathologies of the auditory system, and (b) assessment of auditory disorders and their effect on communication; (2) habilitative/rehabilitative procedures, such as (a) selection and use of appropriate amplification instrumentation for the hearing impaired, both wearable and group, (b) evaluation of speech and language problems of the hearing impaired, and (c) management procedures for speech and language habilitation and/or rehabilitation of the hearing impaired (that may include manual communication); (3) conservation of hearing, such as (a) environmental noise control, and (b) identification audiometry (school, military, industry); and (4) instrumentation, such as (a) electronics, (b) calibration techniques, and (c) characteristics of amplifying systems.

Not less than six (6) semester hours must be in the auditory pathology category, and no less than six (6) semester hours must be in the habilitation/rehabilitation category.

II,B,5. Minor Professional Area, Certificate in Audiology. For the individual to obtain the Certificate in Audiology, at least six (6) semester hours must be in the area of speech-language pathology. Of these, three (3) hours must be in the area of speech pathology and three (3) hours in the area of language pathology. It is suggested that where only this minimum requirement of six (6) semester hours is met, such study be in the areas of evaluation procedures and management of speech and language problems that are not associated with hearing impairment.

II,B,6. Related Areas. In addition to the 12 semester hours of course study in the Basic Communication Processes Area, the 24 semester hours in the Major Professional Area and the six (6) semester hours in the Minor Professional Area, the applicant may receive credit toward the minimum requirement of 60 semester hours of required education through advanced study in a variety of related areas. Such study should pertain to the understanding of human behavior, both normal and abnormal, as well as services available from related professions, and, in general should augment the background for a professional career. Examples of such areas of study are as follows: (a) theories of learning and behavior, (b) services available from related professions that also deal with persons who have disorders of communication, and (c) information from these professions about the sensory, physical, emotional, social, and/or intellectual status of a child or an adult.

Academic credit that is obtained from practice teaching or practicum work in other professions will not be counted toward the minimum requirements.

In order that the future applicant for one of the certificates will be capable of critically reviewing scientific matters dealing with clinical issues relative to speech-language pathology and audiology, credit for study in the area of statistics, beyond an introductory course, will be allowed to a maximum of three (3) semester hours. Academic study of the administrative organization of speech-language pathology and audiology programs also may be applied to a maximum of three (3) semester hours.

II,B,7. Education Applicable to All Areas. Certain types of course work may be acceptable among more than one of the areas of study specified above, depending upon the emphasis. For example, courses that provide an overview of research, e.g., introduction to graduate study or introduction to research, that consist primarily of a critical review of research in communication sciences, disorders, or management thereof, and/or a more general presentation of research procedures and techniques that will permit the clinician to read and evaluate literature critically will be acceptable to a maximum of three (3) semester hours. Such courses may be credited to the Basic Communication Processes Area, or one of the Professional Areas or the Related Area, if substantive content of the course(s) covers material in those areas. Academic credit for a thesis or dissertation may be acceptable to a maximum of three (3) semester hours in the appropriate area. An abstract of the study must be submitted with the application if such credit is requested. In order to be acceptable, the thesis or dissertation must have been an experiment or descriptive investigation in the areas of speech, language and hearing science, speech-language pathology or audiology; that is, credit will not be allowed if the project was a survey of opinions, a study of professional issues, an annotated bibliography, biography, or a study of curricular design.

As implied by the above, the academic credit hours obtained from one course or one enrollment may, and should, be in some instances divided among the Basic Communication Processes Area, one of the Professional Areas, and/or the Related Area. In such cases, a description of the content of that course should accompany the application. This description should be extensive enough to provide the Clinical Certification Board with information necessary to evaluate the validity of the request to apply the content to more than one of the areas.

II,B,8. Major Professional Education Applicable to Both Certificates. Study in the area of understanding, evaluation, and management of speech and language disorders associated with hearing impairment may apply to the 24 semester hours of Major Professional Area required for either certificate (speech-language pathology or audiology). However, no more than six (6) semester hours of that study will be allowed in that manner for the certificate in speech-language pathology.

II,C. Academic Clinical Practicum

It is highly desirable that students who anticipate applying for one of the Certificates of Clinical Competence have the opportunity, relatively early in their training program, to observe the various procedures involved in a clinical program in speech-language pathology and audiology, but this passive participation is not to be construed as direct clinical practicum during academic training. The student should participate in supervised, direct clinical experience during that training only after the student has had sufficient course work to qualify for work as a student clinician and only after the student has sufficient background to undertake clinical practice under direct supervision. A minimum of 150 clock hours of the supervised clinical experience must be obtained during graduate study. Once this experience is undertaken, a substantial period of time may be spent in writing reports, in preparation for clinical sessions, in conferences with supervisors, and in class attendance to discuss clinical procedures and experiences; such time may not be credited toward the 300 minimum clock hours of supervised clinical experience required.

All student clinicians are expected to obtain direct clinical experience with both children and adults, and it is recommended that some of their direct clinical experience be conducted with groups. Although the student clinician should have experience with both speech-language and hearing disorders, at least 200 clock hours of this supervised experience must be obtained in the major professional area (speech-language pathology or audiology) in which certification is sought, and not less than 35 clock hours must be obtained in the minor area. At least 50 supervised clock hours of the required 300 hours of clinical experience must be obtained in each of two distinctly different clinical settings. (The two separate clinical settings may be within the organizational structure of the same institution and may include the academic program's clinic and affiliated medical facilities, community clinics, public schools, etc.)

For certification in speech-language pathology, the student clinician is expected to have experience in both the evaluation and management of a variety of speech and language problems. The student must have at least 50 clock hours of experience in evaluation of speech and language problems. The applicant must also have at least 75 clock hours of experience in management of language disorders of children and adults, and at least 25 clock hours each of experience in management of children and adults with whom disorders of (1) voice, (2) articulation, and (3) fluency are significant aspects of the communication handicap.[4]

Where only the minimum 35 clock hours of clinical practicum in audiology is met that is required for the persons seeking certification in speech-language pathology, that practicum must include 15 clock hours in assessment and/or management of speech and language problems associated with hearing impairment, and 15 clock hours must be in the assessment of

[4]Work with multiple problems may be credited among these types of disorders. For example, a child with an articulation problem may also have a voice disorder. The clock hours of work with that child may be credited to experience with either articulation or voice disorders, whichever is most appropriate.

auditory disorders. However, where more than this minimum requirement is met, clinical practicum in assessment and/or management of speech and language problems associated with hearing impairment may be counted toward the minimum clock hours obtained with language and/or speech disorders.

For the student clinician who is preparing for certification in audiology, 50 clock hours of direct supervised experience must be obtained in identification and evaluation of hearing impairment, and 50 clock hours must be obtained in habilitation or rehabilitation of the communication handicaps of the hearing impaired. It is suggested that the 35 clock hours of clinical practicum in speech-language pathology required for certification in audiology be in the evaluation and management of speech and language problems that are not related to hearing impairment.

Supervisors of clinical practicum must be competent professional workers who hold a Certificate of Clinical Competence in the professional area (speech-language pathology or audiology) in which supervision is provided. This supervision must entail the personal and direct involvement of the supervisor in any and all ways that will permit the supervisor to attest to the adequacy of the student's performance in the clinical training experience. At least 25% of the therapy sessions conducted by a student clinician must be directly supervised, with such supervision being appropriately scheduled throughout the training period. (Direct supervision is defined as on-site observation or closed-circuit TV monitoring of the student clinician.) At least one-half of each diagnostic evaluation conducted by a student clinician must be directly supervised. (The amount of direct supervision beyond these minima should be adjusted upward depending on the student's level of competence.) The first 25 hours of a student's clinical practicum must be supervised by a qualified clinical supervisor who is a member of the program's professional staff (i.e., a primary employee of the training program). In addition to the required direct supervision, supervisors may use a variety of other ways to obtain knowledge of the student's clinical work such as conferences, audio- and videotape recordings, written reports, staffings, and discussions with other persons who have participated in the student's clinical training.

II,D. The Clinical Fellowship Year

Upon completion of professional and clinical practicum education, the applicant must complete a Clinical Fellowship Year under the supervision of one who holds the Certificate of Clinical Competence in the professional area (speech-language pathology or audiology) in which that applicant is working (and seeking certification).

Professional experience is construed to mean direct clinical work with patients, consultations, record keeping, or any other duties relevant to a bona fide program of clinical work. It is expected, however, that a significant amount[5] of clinical experience will be in direct clinical contact with persons who have communication handicaps. Time spent in supervision of students, academic teaching, and research, as well as administrative activity that does not deal directly with management programs of specific patients or clients will not be counted as professional experience in this context.

The Clinical Fellowship Year is defined as no less than nine months of full-time professional employment with full-time employment defined as a minimum of 30 clock hours of work a week. This requirement also may be fulfilled by part-time employment as follows: (1) work of 15-19 hours per week over 18 months; (2) work of 20-24 hours per week over 15 months; or, (3) work of 25-29 hours per week over 12 months. In the event that part-time employment is used to fulfill a part of the Clinical Fellowship Year, 100% of the minimum hours of the part-time work per week requirement must be spent in direct professional experience as defined above. The Clinical Fellowship Year must be completed within a maximum period of 36 consecutive months. Professional employment of less than 15 hours per week will not fulfill any part of this requirement. If the CFY is not initiated within two years of the date the academic and practicum education is completed, the applicant must meet the academic and practicum requirements current when the CFY is begun. Whether or not the Clinical Fellow (CF) is a Member of ASHA, the CF must understand and abide by the ASHA Code of Ethics.

CFY supervision must entail the personal and direct involvement of the supervisor in any and all ways that will permit the CFY supervisor to monitor, improve, and evaluate the CF's performance in professional employment. The CFY supervisor must base the total evaluation on no less 36 supervisory activities during the CFY. The supervisor must include 18 on-site observations of the CF (1 hour=one on-site observation; up to 6 hours may be accrued in one day; at least 6 on-site observations must be accrued during each third of the experience). The CFY supervisor must complete 18 other monitoring activities (at least one per month). These other monitoring activities may be executed by correspondence and include conferences with the CF, evaluation of written reports, evaluations by professional colleagues, etc. If multiple sites are utilized in the CFY experience, at least one on-site observation must be conducted at each site of the same provider type[6] during two of the three (1/3) segments. (NOTE: Requests for utilizing alternative mechanisms for meeting the CFY requirements stated in this paragraph must be submitted in writing to the Clinical Certification Board for prior approval.)

Should any supervisor suspect at any time during the Clinical Fellowship Year that the CF under supervision will not meet requirements, the CFY supervisor must counsel the CF both orally and in writing and maintain careful written records of all contacts and conferences in the ensuing months.[7]

II,E. The National Examinations in Speech-Language Pathology and Audiology

The National Examinations in Speech-Language Pathology and Audiology are designed to assess, in a comprehensive fashion, the applicant's mastery of professional concepts as outlined above to which the applicant has been exposed throughout professional education and clinical practicum. The applicant must pass the National Examination, in either Speech-Language Pathology or Audiology that is appropriate to the certificate being sought. An applicant will be declared eligible for the National Examination on notification of the acceptable completion of the educational and clinical practicum requirements. The Examination must be passed within three years after the first administration for which an applicant is notified of eligibility.

---

[5] The Clinical Certification Board Interpretation is that a "significant amount" is 80% of the CFY work week.

[6] Provider type: defined as one or more physical settings in which the client populations are similar (e.g., nursing homes, hospitals, schools, industrial locations, hearing aid provider offices, etc.)

[7] Further requirements for the Clinical Fellowship Year are included in the ASHA Membership and Certification Handbook.

In the event the applicant fails the examination, it may be retaken. If the examination is not successfully completed within the above mentioned three years, the person's application for certification will lapse. If the examination is passed at a later date, the person may reapply for clinical certification.[8]

II,F. Applicants Educated in Other Countries.

In the case of an applicant who has received all or most of his/her professional education in another country, and who has qualified under the standards of another country as an independent practitioner in speech-language pathology and/or audiology, the Clinical Certification Board has the discretion to waive all or part of Standards I,A through I,D provided that the Board is satisfied that the applicant has received fairly equivalent professional preparation. In all such cases however, Standard I,E shall not be waived.

(Note:
Standard I,A—General Background Education
Standard I,B—Required Education
Standard I,C—Academic Clinical Practicum
Standard I,D—The Clinical Fellowship Year
Standard I,E—The National Examinations in Speech-Language Pathology and Audiology.)

III. PROCEDURES FOR OBTAINING THE CERTIFICATES

III,A. The applicant must submit to the Clinical Certification Board, a description of professional education and academic clinical practicum on the form provided for that purpose. The applicant should recognize that it is highly desirable to list upon this application form the entire professional education and academic clinical practicum training.

No credit may be allowed for courses listed on the application unless satisfactory completion is verified by an official transcript. *Satisfactory completion* is defined as the applicant's having received academic credit (i.e., semester hours, quarter hours, or other unit of credit) with a passing grade as defined by the training institution. If the majority of an applicant's professional training is received at a program accredited by the Educational Standards Board (ESB) of the American Speech-Language-Hearing Association (ASHA), approval of education and academic clinical practicum requirements will be automatic.

The applicant must request that the director of the training program where the majority of graduate training was obtained sign the application. In the case where the training program is not accredited by ESB of ASHA that director (1) certifies that the applicant has met the educational and clinical practicum requirements, and (2) recommends that the applicant receive the certificate upon completion of all the requirements.

In the event that the applicant cannot obtain the signature of the director of the training program, the applicant should send with the application a letter giving in detail the reasons for the inability to do so. In such an instance, letters of recommendation from other faculty members may be submitted.

Application for approval of educational requirements and academic clinical practicum experiences should be made (1) as soon as possible after completion of these experiences, and (2) either before or shortly after the Clinical Fellowship Year is begun.

III,B. Upon completion of education and academic clinical practicum training, the applicant should proceed to obtain professional employment and a supervisor for the Clinical Fellowship Year. Although the filing of a CFY Plan is not required, applicants may submit such a plan to the Clinical Certification Board (CCB) if they wish prior approval of the planned professional experience.

Within one month following completion of the Clinical Fellowship Year, the CF and the CFY supervisor must submit a CFY Report to the Clinical Certification Board. If the CFY was completed in a program accredited by the Professional Services Board (PSB) of ASHA, approval of the CFY will be automatic. In such instance, the director of the PSB program must sign the CFY Report verifying compliance with requirements.

III,C. Upon notification by the Clinical Certification Board of approval of the academic course work and clinical practicum requirements the applicant will be sent registration material for the National Examinations in Speech-Language Pathology and Audiology. Upon approval of the Clinical Fellowship Year, achieving a passing score on the National Examination, and payment of all fees the applicant will become certified.

III,D. As mentioned in Footnote 9, a schedule of fees for certification may be obtained, and payment of these fees is requisite for the various steps involved in obtaining a certificate. Checks should be made payable to the American Speech-Language-Hearing Association.

III,E. After certification has been awarded, an Annual Certification Fee (ACF) is payable in advance each year. A certificate holder whose ACF is in arrears will be dropped from the registry of certificate holders.

IV. APPEALS

In the event that at any stage the Clinical Certification Board informs the applicant that the application has been rejected, the applicant has the right of formal appeal. In order to initiate such an appeal, the applicant must write to the Chair of the Clinical Certification Board and specifically request a formal review of the application. If that review results, again, in rejection, the applicant has the right to appeal the case to the Council on Professional Standards in Speech-Language Pathology and Audiology (the Standards Council) by writing to the Chair of the Standards Council at the National Office of the American Speech-Language-Hearing Association. The applicant must submit a letter of intent to appeal within 30 days and a memorandum specifying the grounds of the appeal within 60 days from the date of the rejection letter. The decision of the Standards Council will be final.

---

[8] Upon such reapplication, the individual's application will be reviewed and current requirements will be applied. Appropriate fees will be charged for this review.

[9] Application material for certification, including a schedule of fees, may be obtained by writing to the American Speech-language-Hearing Association, 10801 Rockville Pike, Rockville, Maryland 20852.

REQUIREMENTS for the AWARD FOR CONTINUING EDUCATION

The American Speech-Language-Hearing Association offers an Award for Continuing Education (ACE) to ASHA members and nonmember holders of the Certificate of Clinical Competence. Requirements for the ACE are established by the Continuing Education Board (CEB) and must be met within the current three year period. The ACE is valid for three years, during which time the requirements may be completed for renewal of the Award.

Requirements

(1) Earn seven Continuing Education Units (CEUs) within the three year period immediately preceding application for the ACE. CEUs must be earned in the specified content areas from Sponsors of continuing education activities who have been approved by the CEB.

(2) Complete six semester hours (9 quarter hours) of academic coursework in the specified content areas from an ASHA Approved Sponsor or an ASHA Educational Standards Board (ESB) accredited training program within the three year period immediately preceding application for the ACE. No more than three semester hours may be applied from the related areas. Coursework other than graduate level must be justified in a statement of relevance for the ACE.

(3) Earn a combination of CEUs and academic credits in one of the following ratios within the three year period immediately preceding application for the ACE: 7 CEUs/0 credits; 6 CEUs/1 credit; 5 CEUs/2 credits; 4 CEUs/3 credits; 3 CEUs/4 credits; 2 CEUs/5 credits; 0 CEUs/6 credits. All CEUs and academic credit must be earned from Approved Sponsors or ESB accredited programs. Participants may not apply both academic credit and CEUs earned for the same activity towards the ACE. If both types of credits are earned, participants must decide whether to apply CEUs or academic credit to the ACE. There is no conversion of academic credit into CEUs.

(4) Successfully retake the National Examination in Speech-Language Pathology and/or Audiology (NESPA) within a year of application for the ACE and not sooner than three years after the previous examination was passed. This option is available only to holders of ASHA's Certificate of Clinical Competence. The passing score is the same as for ASHA certification.

Content Areas

CEUs for the ACE must be obtained for participation in education activities that incorporate knowledge from specific content areas: Basic Communication Processes Area, Professional Area and Related Areas. At least four of the total seven CEUs must be obtained in the Basic Communication Processes and/or Professional Areas. The remaining three CEUs may be obtained from any of the three areas. The three content areas are described below.

Basic Communication Processes Area: Information (beyond the basic certification requirements) applicable to the normal development and use of speech, language, and hearing, i.e., (1) anatomic and physiological bases for the normal development and use of speech, language, and hearing; (2) physical bases and processes of the production and perception of speech, language, and hearing; (3) linguistic and psycholinguistic variables related to normal development and use of speech, language and hearing; and (4) technological, biomedical, engineering, and instrumentation information (such as computer programming and microprocessor adaptations) which enable expansion of knowledge in the basic communication processes.

Professional Area: Information pertaining to disorders of speech, language, and hearing, e.g., (1) various types of disorders of communication, their manifestations, classifications, and causes; (2) evaluation skills, including procedures, techniques and instrumentation for assessment; and (3) management procedures and principles in habilitation and rehabilitation of communication disorders.

Related Areas: Study pertaining to the understanding of human behavior, both normal and abnormal, as well as services available from related professions which apply to the contemporary practice of speech-language pathology/audiology, e.g., (1) theories of learning and behavior; (2) services available from related professions that also deal with persons who have disorders of communication; and (3) information from these professions about the sensory, physical, emotional, social and/or intellectual states of child or adult; and (4) other areas such as program management, economics of professional practice, professional ethics, clinical supervision, counseling and interviewing, application of computers, and modern technology and statistics.

MEMBERSHIP IN THE AMERICAN SPEECH-LANGUAGE-HEARING ASSOCIATION 1926-1988 (Est.)

Year	*Associate*	*Clinical*	*Professional*	*Fellow*	*Total*
1926	3			19	22
1927	3			19	22
1928	3			19	22
1929	2			23	25
1930	2			23	25
1931	2			27	29
1932	9			28	37
1933	25			27	52
1934	20			37	57
1935	53			34	87
1936	72			43	115
1937	125			60	185
1938	176			72	248
1939	190			61	251
1940	261			69	330
1941	302			72	374
1942	409			72	481
1943	496	5	13	73	587
1944	451	31	24	78	584
1945	498	65	47	74	684
1946	488	120	67	83	758
1947	606	213	84	91	994
1948	603	340	99	102	1,144
1949	816	389	126	101	1,432
1950	812	566	147	98	1,623

Year	*Associate*	*Members*	*Total*
1951	789	1,070	1,859
1952	631	1,602	2,233
1953	748	2,068	2,816
1954	788	2,373	3,161
1955	713	2,947	3,660
1956	601	3,373	3,974
1957	635	4,070	4,705
1958	504	4,263	4,767
1959	635	4,805	5,440
1960	416	5,833	6,249
1961	817	6,770	7,587
1962	1,064	8,154	9,218
1963	1,553	9,185	10,738
1964	1,451	10,252	11,703
1965[1]		13,617	13,617
1966		12,781	12,781
1967		11,858	11,858
1968		11,975	11,975
1969		12,193	12,193
1970		12,873	12,873
1971		13,741	13,741
1972		14,650	14,650

[1] Associate category eliminated in 1965

Membership

Year	Associate	Members	Total
1973		16,306	16,306
1974		18,621	18,621
1975		21,435	21,435
1976		24,466	24,466
1977		27,642	27,642
1978		30,397	30,397
1979		33,143	33,143
1980		34,840	34,840
1981		34,772	34,772
1982		36,686	36,686
1983		37,806	37,806
1984		41,474	41,474
1985		44,067	44,067
1986		46,623	46,623
1987		49,501	49,501
1988 (Est.)		52,600	52,600

Note: Counts through 1985 are as of July 1 of the year indicated. Beginning in 1986, counts (or estimate for the final year shown) are as of December 31.

LEGISLATIVE COUNCIL
1989

Alabama (2)
Clark-Lewis, Sandra
Cooper, Eugene B.

Alaska (1)
Olmstead, Patricia J.

Arizona (2)
Meyer, Judith P.
Whaley, Patricia

Arkansas (2)
McGrail, Louis, J.
Roberts, Kathleen B.

California (9)
Arnst, Dennis J.
Breakey, Lisa K.
Darby, John L.
Dickerson, Mary V.
Flower, Wilda M.
Heffernan, H. Patricia
Montgomery, Judith K.
Thies, Terry L.
Wolf, Kenneth E.

Colorado (3)
Casey, Pauline E.
Moore, Susan M.
Pike, Patricia

Connecticut (3)
Aronin, Meryl W.
Gist, Kenneth T.
Ulrich, Sandra R.

Delaware (1)
Westerhouse, Janice J.

District of Columbia (2)
Baquet, Glenn M.
Pietranton, Arlene A.

Florida (4)
Ehren, Barbara J.
Kennedy, June F.
Ratcliff, L. Gay
Work, Rhonda S.

Georgia (3)
Reeves, Rebecca K.
Smith, Susan P.
Steward, Noreen

Hawaii (1)
Craven, Dorothy D.

Idaho (1)
Anderson, Kathleen C.

Illinois (6)
Block, Frances K.
Cassidy, Robert D.
Dunn-Engel, Elaine S.
LeDuc, Judith A.
Lee, Corinne C.
Phillips, Nevis C.

Indiana (3)
Binnie, Carl A.
Sapp, Helen D.
Solomon, Barbara S.W.

Iowa (3)
Barker, Kenneth D.
Bennett-Porter, Sandra M.
Jordan, Herbert N.

Kansas (3)
Britten, Frederick
Gatlin, Kaye L.
Scudder, Rosalind

Kentucky (2)
Steckol, Karen F.
Swigert, Nancy B.

Louisiana (3)
Baxter, Kelmer D.
Miller, Paul S.
Pannbacker, Mary D.

Maine (1)
Olsen, Bruce D.

Maryland (4)
Gladstone, Vic S.
Greyerbiehl, Dianne H.
Laufer, M. Barbara
Sloan, John M.

Massachusetts (4)
Arnold, Barbara J.
Cumpata, Joellen F.
Quin, Paul E.
Sanderson, Robert G.

Michigan (5)
Dreyer, Dorothy E.
Eldis, Frances E.
Laeder, Ronald L.
Nelson, Nickola
Smith, Linda Lou

Minnesota (3)
Goulett, Diane M.
Kozan, Anita L.
Mueller, Rita J.

Mississippi (2)
Kellum, Gloria D.
Wylde, Margaret

Missouri (3)
Brennan, Donald G.
Carver, William F.
Hamlin, Jeanne F.

Montana (2)
Boehmler, Richard M.
DeVoe, Shirley J.

Nebraska (2)
Konz, Ruth A.
McCulloch, Barbara J.

Nevada (1)
Cremen, Lynn

New Hampshire (1)
Lister, Paul B.

New Jersey (4)
Aitchison, Carole J.
Binney, Jan
Kandel, Ellen B.
Pietro, Maryjo Santo

New Mexico (2)
Bolton-Koppenhaver, Mary L.
Westby, Carol E.

New York (9)
Battle, Dolores
Bernstein, Deena K.
Butler, Katharine G.
Casper, Janina K.
Huffman, Nancy P.
Kerman-Lerner, Patricia
Metz, Dale E.
O'Brien, Mary Ann
Stark, Joel

North Carolina (3)
Bartels, David D.
Muzzarelli, Robert A.
Pearson, Patricia A.

North Dakota (1)
Schill, Mary Jo

Ohio (5)
Leslie, Carol P.
Nodar, Richard H.
Plummer, Sally Ann
Roberts, Margaret M.
Wegener, John G.

Oklahoma (2)
LaCroix, Zane E.
Mencke, Eugene O.

Oregon (3)
Casteel, Robert L.
Horner, Nancy S.
Levinson, Philip J.

Pennsylvania (6)
Dellegrotto, John T.
Eger, Diane Levy
Krieger, Richard C.
Lovrinic, Jean
Towne, Carol C.
Von Drach, Robert B.

Rhode Island (1)
Stoskopf, Colette M.

South Carolina (2)
Carney, R. John
Powell, Harold

South Dakota (1)
Samuelsen, Ruth A.

Tennessee (3)
Coscarelli-Buchanan, Janet E.
King, Deborah A.
Wark, David J.

Texas (6)
Formby, Ellen S.F.
Friel-Patti, Sandy
Hanke, Gilbert C.
Higdon, Lawrence W.
Larson, D. Jayne
Wood, Mary Lovey

Utah (1)
Nielson, Harriet R.

Vermont (1)
Cohen, Brenda P.

Virginia (3)
Bountress, Nicholas G.
Cluver, Elizabeth
O'Hare, Nancy K.

Washington (3)
Kelley, Roberta Ann
McRandle, Carol C.
Rosendahl, Pamela D.

West Virginia (2)
Cartwright, Lynn R.
Olson, Robert D.

Wisconsin (4)
Ewanowski, Stanley J.
Marks, Susan M.
Mueller, Lois G.
Weismer, Susan Ellis

Wyoming (1)
Jelinek, Janis A.

International (3)
Martin, Virginia E.
Mencher, George T.
Ward, Betty Jane

National Student Speech Language Hearing Association (2)
Reinhart, Victoria L.
Vogt-Fisher, Kimberly C.

EXECUTIVE BOARD
AMERICAN SPEECH-LANGUAGE-HEARING ASSOCIATION
1989

President
Gilbert R. Herer, Ph.D.
Children's Hospital National Medical Center
Children's Hearing and Speech Center
Washington, D.C.

President-Elect
Roy A. Koenigsknecht, Ph.D.
The Ohio State University - Columbus

Past President
Sandra C. Holley, Ph.D.
Southern Connecticut State University - New Haven

Vice President for Administration
Thomas J. O'Toole, Ed.D.
Montgomery County Public Schools
Rockville, Maryland

Vice President for Clinical Affairs
Teris K. Schery, Ph.D.
California State University at Los Angeles

Vice President for Education and Scientific Affairs
Theodore J. Glattke, Ph.D.
University of Arizona - Tucson

Vice President for Planning
Robert L. Douglass, Ph.D.
Los Angeles, California

Vice President for Professional and Governmental Affairs
Ann L. Carey, Ph.D.
Southern Illinois University - Edwardsville

Vice President for Standards and Ethics
Patrick J. Carney, Ph.D.
University of Tennessee - Knoxville

Executive Director
Frederick T. Spahr, Ph.D.

LIST OF PRESIDENTS, SECRETARIES, VICE PRESIDENTS, AND EDITORS

PRESIDENTS

Robert W. West	1925-28
Elmer L. Kenyon	1929-32
Smiley Blanton	1933-34
Lee E. Travis	1935-36
Max A. Goldstein	1937-38
Sara Stinchfield Hawk	1939-40
Samuel D. Robbins	1941-42
Bryng Bryngelson	1943-44
Harry Heltman	1945
Clarence T. Simon	1946
Herbert Koepp-Baker	1947
Martin F. Palmer	1948
D. W. Morris	1949
Wendell Johnson	1950
M. D. Steer	1951
Harold Westlake	1952
S. Richard Silverman	1953
Margaret Hall Powers	1954
Harlan Bloomer	1955
James A. Carrell	1956
Raymond Carhart	1957
Jon Eisenson	1958
George A. Kopp	1959
Stanley Ainsworth	1960
Paul Moore	1961
James F. Curtis	1962
Jack Matthews	1963
Hayes A. Newby	1964
Duane C. Spriestersbach	1965
William G. Hardy	1966
Leo G. Doerfler	1967
John V. Irwin	1968
John J. O'Neill	1969
Frank R. Kleffner	1970
Jack L. Bangs	1971
Robert Goldstein	1971-72
Sylvia O. Richardson	1973
Kenneth L. Moll	1974
Phillip A. Yantis	1975
Daniel R. Boone	1976
Rolland J. Van Hattum	1977
Katharine G. Butler	1978
Norma S. Rees	1979
Margaret C. Byrne	1980
Alan S. Feldman	1981
Laura Ann Wilber	1982
Fred D. Minifie	1983
David E. Yoder	1984
Richard M. Flower	1985
Betty Jane Philips	1986
Patricia R. Cole	1987
Sandra C. Holley	1988
Gilbert R. Herer	1989

SECRETARIES

Sara Stinchfield Hawk	1925-30
Samuel D. Robbins	1931-40
D. W. Morris	1941-42

TREASURERS

Richard Borden	1925-28
Alvin T. Busse	1929-32
Bryng Bryngelson	1933-42

SECRETARY-TREASURERS

D. W. Morris	1943-47
George A. Kopp	1948-57

EXECUTIVE VICE PRESIDENTS

Ernest H. Henrikson	1951-54
Stanley Ainsworth	1955-58
Jack Matthews	1959-62
John V. Irwin	1963-66
Jack L. Bangs	1967-68

EXECUTIVE SECRETARY

Kenneth O. Johnson	1957-79
Frederick T. Spahr	1980

EXECUTIVE DIRECTOR

Frederick T. Spahr	1980-

VICE PRESIDENT FOR ADMINISTRATION

Theodore D. Hanley	1969-70
Harold L. Luper	1971-73
Sara E. Conlon	1974
Donald T. Counihan	1975-76
Jerome G. Alpiner	1977-79
Richard W. Stream	1980-82
Sandra C. Holley	1983-85
Roy Koenigsknecht	1986-88
Thomas J. O'Toole	1989-

VICE PRESIDENT FOR CLINICAL AFFAIRS

Daniel R. Boone	1969
Gerald G. Freeman	1970-72
Doris P. Bradley	1973-75
Alan S. Feldman	1976-78
David E. Yoder	1979-81
Hughlett L. Morris	1982-84
Gilbert R. Herer	1985-87
Teris K. Schery	1988-

VICE PRESIDENT FOR EDUCATION AND SCIENTIFIC AFFAIRS

William R. Tiffany	1969-70
Rolland J. Van Hattum	1971-73
Fred D. Minifie	1974-76
Jerry V. Tobias	1977-79
Richard L. Schiefelbusch	1980-82
Steffi B. Resnick	1983-85
Charles I. Berlin	1986-88
Theodore J. Glattke	1989-

VICE PRESIDENT FOR PLANNING

Phillip A. Yantis	1969-71
Thelma P. Albritton	1972-74
Norma S. Rees	1975-77
Ronald Goldman	1978-80
Patricia R. Cole	1981-83
Carol P. Leslie	1984-86
Robert L. Douglass	1987-

VICE PRESIDENT FOR PROFESSIONAL AND GOVERNMENTAL AFFAIRS

Marie Love Johnson	1977-78
Rhonda S. Work	1979-81
Mariana Newton	1982-84
Nancy G. Becker	1985-87
Ann L. Carey	1988-

VICE PRESIDENT FOR STANDARDS AND ETHICS

Katherine F. Thorn	1969
Kenneth L. Moll	1970-71
Frederick E. Garbee	1972-74
Richard M. Flower	1975-77
Laura Ann Wilber	1978-80
Betty Jane Philips	1981-83
Jane R. Madell	1984-86
Patrick J. Carney	1987-

EDITOR OF THE ASSOCIATION

Robert W. West	1955-58

CHAIRS, PUBLICATIONS BOARD

Wendell Johnson	1959-62
Paul Moore	1963-66
Ira Hirsh	1967-69
Frederic L. Darley	1970-75
James F. Curtis	1975-79
Jerry V. Tobias	1980-83
Robert C. Bilger	1983-87
Tanya M. Gallagher	1988-

EDITORS

Journal of Speech Disorders

G. Oscar Russell	1936-42
Wendell Johnson	1943-47

Journal of Speech and Hearing Disorders

Wendell Johnson	1947-48
Grant Fairbanks	1949-54
Gordon Peterson	1955-57
Mary Huber	1958-61
William R. Tiffany	1962-65
Margaret C. Byrne	1965-68
Elizabeth Carrow	1969-74
Ralph L. Shelton	1974-78
William H. Perkins	1978-81
Janis M. Costello Ingham	1982-85
Laurence B. Leonard	1986-

Journal of Speech and Hearing Research

Dorothy Sherman	1958-62
James Jerger	1963-70
Robert Bilger	1970-74
Thomas J. Hixon	1974-78
Raymond D. Kent	1978-80
Tanya Gallagher	1981-83
Theodore J. Glattke	1984-87
Dianne J. Van Tasell	1988-

Asha

Kenneth O. Johnson	1959-79
Frederick T. Spahr	1980-

ASHA Monographs

Frederic L. Darley	1952-62
Maryjane Rees	1964-66
Gerald M. Siegel	1968-73
James C. Hardy	1974-79
Charles Speaks	1980-83
Robin S. Chapman	1984-88
Lawrence J. Feth	1989-

ASHA Reports

Frederic L. Darley	1968-69
Robert T. Wertz	1970-78
Theodore J. Glattke	1979-83
Arnold M. Small	1984-

Language, Speech, and Hearing Services in Schools (formerly *Speech and Hearing Services in Schools)*

Thelma P. Albritton	1970
William C. Healey	1971-73
Elinor Zaslow	1973-75
Gerald G. Freeman	1975-78
Patricia A. Broen	1978-86
Alan G. Kamhi	1987-

HONORS OF THE ASSOCIATION
1944-1988

The Honors of the Association may be awarded upon the recommendation of the Committee on Honors with the approval of the Council in recognition of distinguished service to the profession.

1944
Carl Emil Seashore

1946
Wendell Johnson

1947
Robert West
Lee E. Travis
Walter Hughson

1949
Harvey Fletcher
Delyte W. Morris

1950
Clarence T. Simon

1951
Hallowell Davis

1953
Sara Stinchfield Hawk
R. H. Stetson

1954
S. Richard Silverman

1955
Grant Fairbanks

1956
Margaret Hall Powers
Charles Van Riper

1957
George A. Kopp

1958
Mack D. Steer

1959
Martin F. Palmer

1960
Charles S. Bluemel
Raymond Carhart

1961
Gordon E. Peterson

1962
Stanley H. Ainsworth

1963
Bryng Bryngelson

1965
Herbert Koepp-Baker
Paul Moore

1966
Georg von Bekesy
Franklin S. Cooper
Harold Westlake

1967
Jon Eisenson
Kenneth O. Johnson
Richard Masland
E. Glen Wever

1968
John Wilson Black
William G. Hardy
Ira J. Hirsh
Lou Kennedy

1969
James F. Curtis
Frederic L. Darley
Scott N. Reger
D. C. Spriestersbach

1970
John V. Irwin
Jack Matthews
Robert L. Milisen
Hildred Schuell

1971
Jack L. Bangs
Mildred F. Berry

1972
Dorothy Helen Sherman

1973
H. Harlan Bloomer

1974
James A. Carrell

1975
Leo G. Doerfler
Helen Sullivan Knight
Paul D. Knight

1976
Eugene T. McDonald
Richard L. Schiefelbusch

1977
Freeman E. McConnell
Joseph M. Wepman

1978
Hayes A. Newby

1979
Marion P. Downs
James F. Jerger
Laura L. Lee
John J. O'Neill

1980
Louis M. DiCarlo
Ruth Beckey Irwin
Herbert J. Oyer
Charlotte G. Wells

1981
Friedrich S. Brodnitz
Cornelius P. Goetzinger
Herold S. Lillywhite
Mildred C. Templin

1982
Godfrey E. Arnold
Moe Bergman
Elise Hahn

1983
William H. Perkins
Ira M. Ventry

1984
Daniel R. Boone
Margaret C. Byrne
Kenneth L. Moll
Rolland J. Van Hattum

1985
Frank R. Kleffner

1986
Robert Goldstein
Norma S. Rees

1987
Katharine G. Butler
Richard Merrill Flower
Phillip A. Yantis

1988
Katherine Safford Harris
Sylvia Onesti Richardson

DISTINGUISHED SERVICE AWARDS 1969-1988

The Distinguished Service Award recognizes significant contributions to the field of speech-language pathology and audiology by persons who are not Members of the American Speech-Language-Hearing Association.

1969
Powrie V. Doctor
Mary E. Switzer

1973
Thomas E. Poag

1974
Gunnar Fant
Cecile Hillyer
Children's Television Workshop

1975
John Brademas
Karl D. Kryter
Margaret Kuhn
Charles H. Percy

1976
Samuel A. Kirk
George A. Miller

1977
James L. Flanagan
Lipman Redman
Louise T. Tracy
Bureau of Education for the Handicapped, U.S. Office of Education

1978
Edith L. R. Corliss
Samuel F. Lybarger
Speech Foundation of America

1979
William C. Geer
Lloyd A. Jeffress

1980
John E. D. Ball
Patria G. Forsythe
Richard S. Schweicker

1981
Lowell P. Weicker
Psi Iota Xi Sorority

1982
Army Surgeon General and the Army Audiology Program
Harold Goodglass
Haskins Laboratory
Claude Pepper
Scottish Rite Aphasia Program

1983
American Cleft Palate Association
Veterans Administration Audiology and Speech Pathology Program
The Voice Foundation

1984
Roger Brown
Silvio O. Conte

1985
Norman Lear, ABC Television
Sertoma Foundation
Volunteer boards of directors of clinics certified by ASHA's Professional Services Board

1986
International Association of Lions Clubs, Inc.
National Theatre of the Deaf

1987
American Business Clubs
Purple Cross Deaf Detection and Development Fund
Howard "Rocky " Stone and Self-Help for Hard of Hearing People, Inc.
Representative Pat Williams (Montana)

1988
Hampton Inns
Robert Wood Johnson Foundation
Las Floristas Womens Guild
Rona Mirmelstein
Quota International and Kathleen Thomas

FELLOWS OF THE ASSOCIATION

Fellowship is an honor which may be awarded to a Member in recognition of achievement in the directions indicated by the statement of the purposes of the Association as recorded in the Bylaws. It has no fixed requirements, and it may not be applied for or proposed by a Member for himself. It is not a class of membership, is not awarded to any arbitrary percentage of the membership, and is not applicable to non-Members.

A Fellow shall have been active in the Association, as evidenced by publications, appearance on the convention programs or service on committees, and shall have a record of achievement, unquestionable and sustained, of one or more of the following types: (1) original contributions to the advancement of knowledge; (2) distinguished educational, professional, or administrative activity; (3) outstanding service to the Association. — *Extract from the Report of the Committee on Honors, 1951.*

A

Abbott, Thomas B.
Adams, Larry E.
Adams, Martin R.
Adler, Sol
Agnello, Joseph G.
Agranowitz, Aleen C.
Ainsworth, Stanley H.
Albritton, Thelma
Allen, Evelyn Y.
Allen, Madge B.
Allen, Nell R.
Alpiner, Jerome G.
Ambroe, Mary H.
Amster, Walter W.
Anderman, Bernard
Anderson, Bernard A.
Anderson, Charles V.
Anderson, Jean L.
Anderson, Ruth M.
Anderson, Virgil
Andrews, James R.
Ansberry, Merle
Arnold, Godfrey E.
Aronson, Arnold E.
Ashmore, Lear Lee
Asp, Carl W.
Aten, James L.
Attanasio, Frederick G.
Austin, Carolyn S.
Avery, Charlotte B.

B

Backus, Ollie L.
Baken, Ronald J.
Bangs, Tina E.
Bankson, Nicholas W.
Barker, Kenneth D.
Barrett, Lyman S.
Barry, S. Joseph
Battin, R. Ray
Battle, Dolores
Bayles, Kathryn A.
Beasley, Daniel S.
Becker, Nancy G.
Bell-Berti, Fredericka
Berg, Frederick S.
Berger, Kenneth W.
Bergman, Moe
Berlin, Charles I.
Bernthal, John E.
Berry, Mildred F.
Bersinger, Don D.
Bess, Fred H.
Betts, Carl E.
Beukelman, David R.
Bilger, Robert C.
Bingham, Dale S.
Binnie, Carl A.
Blakeley, Robert W.
Block, Frances K.
Bloodstein, Oliver
Bloom, Lois
Bloomer, H. Harlan
Boehmler, Richard M.
Boland, John L., Jr.
Bollinger, Rick L.
Boomsliter, Paul C.
Boone, Daniel R.
Boothroyd, Arthur
Bowling, Lloyd S.
Brackett, Isaac P.
Bradford, Larry J.
Bradley, Doris P.
Bralley, Ralph C.
Brandt, John F.
Brennan, Donald G.
Brett, Richard J.
Brewer, Diane M.
Bridgeford, Ethel
Brittin, Marie E.
Brodnitz, Friedrich S.
Broen, Patricia A.
Bronstein, Arthur J.
Brookshire, Robert H.
Brown, Jerome D.
Brown, Loretta G.
Brown, William S., Jr.
Brown-Grant, Elaine L.
Brutten, Gene J.
Burgess, Eleanor H.
Burgi, Ernest J.
Burk, Kenneth W.
Burkland, Marjorie B.
Burr, Helen G.
Butler, Katharine G.
Byers, Vincent W.
Bynum, Donald F.
Bzoch, Kenneth R.

C

Calvert, Donald R.
Cancel, Cruz A.
Canfield, Norton
Canfield, William H.
Canter, Gerald J.
Canterbury, David R.
Capano, Richard F.
Carey, Ann Lee
Carnell, Claude M., Jr.
Carney, Patrick J.
Carroll, Anne W.
Carver, William F.
Case, James L.
Casteel, Robert L.
Castle, Diane Sklar
Castle, William E.
Catlin, Francis Irving
Causey, G. Donald
Chaiklin, Joseph B.
Chial, Michael R.
Christensen, Ned J.
Clifford, Sylvester
Coates, Nadine H.
Cofey, Carol J.
Cohen, Carol G.
Cole, Lorraine T.
Cole, Patricia R.
Coleman, Ralph O.
Coleman, Robert F.
Collins, Michael J.
Collins, M. Jane
Colton, Raymond H.
Conlon, Sara
Cooper, Crystal S.
Cooper, Eugene B.
Cooper, William A., Jr.
Costello, Mary R.
Coston, Gale Norman
Counihan, Donald T.
Covington, Ann J.
Craven, Dorothy D.
Creaghead, Nancy A.
Crotty, Carol M.
Culatta, Richard A.
Cullinan, Walter L.
Curlee, Richard F.
Curry, E. Thayer
Curtis, James F.

D

Dahle, Arthur J.
Dalston, Rodger M.
Daly, David A.
Daniloff, Raymond
Danwitz, Mary Winifred
Darby, John L.
Darley, Frederic L.
D'Asaro, Michael J.
Davis, Donald C.
Davis, Julia M.
Davison, Louise M.
De Hirsch, Katrina
Deal, Leo V.
Dennis, J. Michael
DiCarlo, Louis M.
Dickerson, Mary V.
Dickson, David R.
Dickson, Stanley
Diedrich, William M.
Dirks, Donald D.
Dixon, Richard F.
Doerfler, Leo G.
Donnelly, Kenneth G.
Dopheide, William R.
Douglass, Robert L.
Downs, Marion P.
Dreyer, Dorothy E.
Dublinske, Stan
Duchan, Judith F.
Duffy, Marjorie R.
Duguay, Marshall J.

E

Earnest, Sue W.
Eblen, Roy E.
Eckelmann, Dorathy
Edwards, Elsie M.
Egan, James P.
Egan, Katherine P.
Eger, Diane Levy
Ehrlich, Carol H.
Eisenson, Jon
Eisenstadt, Arthur A.

Elbert, Mary F.
Eldis, Frances E.
Emanuel, Floyd W.
Engel, Dean C.
English, Robert H.
Engnoth, Gloria
Epstein, Aubrey
Erickson, Robert L.
Eshelman, Mary P.
Ewanowski, Stanley J.

F

Falconer, George A.
Falk, Mervyn L.
Farquhar, Mary S.
Favors, Aaron
Fay, Thomas H.
Feldman, Alan S.
Fisher, Cletus G. (Raydon)
Fisher, Hilda B.
Fisher, Lee I.
Fitch, James L.
Fitzgerald, Rita A.
Fitzsimons, Ruth N.
Fletcher, John Lynn
Fletcher, Samuel G.
Florance, Cheri L.
Flower, Richard M.
Flower, Wilda M.
Formaad, William
Fox, Donna R.
Frank, Thomas A.
Freeman, Gerald G.
Freilinger, J. Joseph
Frick, James V.
Fristoe, Macalyne
Fritzell, Bjorn
Fucci, Donald J.
Fudala, Janet B.
Fuller, Carl W.

G

Gallagher, Tanya M.
Garrett, Edgar R.
Garstecki, Dean C.
Garwood, Victor P.
Geffner, Donna S.
Gelfand, Stanley A.
Gens, George W.
Gerber, Adele
Gerber, Sanford E.
Gerstman, Hubert L
Gholson, Sibyl G.
Gilbert, Harvey R.
Gilmore, Stuart I.
Giolas, Thomas G.
Givens, Gregg D.
Gladstone, Vic S.
Glasner, Philip J.
Glattke, Jean B.
Glattke, Theodore J.
Glorig, Aram
Goates, Wallace A.
Goda, Sidney
Goetzinger, Cornelius Peter
Goldman, Ronald
Goldstein, David P.
Goldstein, Robert
Golper, Lee Ann C.
Goodding, Patricia J.
Goodhill, Victor
Goodman, Allan C.
Graham, A. Bruce
Graham, J. Keith
Graham, James T.
Graunke, W. Lloyd
Gray, Burl B.
Green, William W.
Greenberg, Frederick R.
Gregory, Hugo H.
Griffin, Kathleen F.
Griffith, Francis A.
Grimm, William A., III
Guilford, Arthur M.
Guilar, Barry
Guttman, Newman

H

Hadjian, Sophia
Hagen, Chris
Hahn, Elise S.
Hale, Lester L.
Halfond, Murray M.
Halper, Anita S.
Halpern, Harvey
Ham, Richard E.
Hammer, Lowell C.
Hamre, Curtis E.
Haney, Russell
Hanley, Theodore D.
Hanson, Marvin L.
Hanson, Wayne R.
Hardy, James C.
Hardy, Miriam P.
Harford, Earl R.
Harrington, Don A.
Harris, Dean A.
Harris, Gail A. S.
Harris, Katherine
Harrison, Peggy R.
Harrison, R. J.
Haspiel, George S.
Hayes, Claude S.
Healey, William C.
Heaton, Elaine M.
Hedgecock, Leroy D.
Hedrick, Dona Lea
Heffernan, H. Patricia
Heller, Joyce C.
Helmick, Joseph W.
Henrikson, Ernest H.
Herbert, Esther L.
Herer, Gilbert R.
Hess, Carla W.
Hess, Donald A.
Higdon, Lawrence W.
Higgins, Mary K.
Hillis, James W.
Hirsh, Ira J.
Hixon, Thomas J.
Hochberg, Irving
Hodgson, William R.
Hodson, Barbara W.
Hoffman, Jeanette A.
Holley, Sandra C.
Hood, Stephen B.
Hoops, H. Ray
Hopkinson, Norma T.
Horowitz, Leola S.
House, Arthur S.
Hoversten, Gloria H.
Huber, Mary W.
Huffman, Nancy P.
Hull, Raymond H.
Hurst, Charles G., Jr.
Hutchinson, Edward C.
Hyman, Melvin

I

Ickes, William K.
Iglesias, Aquiles
Ingham, Janis Costello
Ingham, Roger J.
Irwin, John V.
Irwin, Ruth B.

J

Jelinek, Janis A.
Jensen, Jay R.
Jensen, Paul J.
Jerger, James F.
Johns, Donnell F.
Johns, Elizabeth
Johnson, Donald D.
Johnson, Doris J.
Johnson, Kenneth O.
Johnson, Marie Love
Johnson, Robert M.
Johnson, T. Earle
Johnson, Warren E.
Johnston, Judith Rae
Jones, Mamie J.
Jones, Shirley A.

K

Kasten, Roger N.
Katz, Jack
Kavanagh, James F.
Keaster, Jacqueline
Keith, Robert L.
Keith, Robert W.
Kellum, Gloria D.
Kemker, Francis J.
Kemp, James C.
Kent, Raymond D.
Kerman-Lerner, Patricia
Kleffner, Frank R.
Klim, Charles J.
Klinger, Herbert
Knepflar, Kenneth J.
Knight, Elmo L.
Knight, Helen Sullivan
Knight, Paul D.
Knobeloch, F. X. Calvin
Knox, Albert W.
Koenigsknecht, Roy A.
Koepp-Baker, Herbert
Kopp, Harriet G.
Kopra, Lennart L.
Kramer, Marc B.
Krebs, Donald F.
Kruger, Barbara
Kuchon, Patricia P.
Kuehn, David P.
Kunze, Luvern H.

L

Labudde, Dorothy E.
Ladefoged, Peter N.
Laeder, Ronald L.
Laguaite, Jeannette
Lahey, Margaret M.
Landes, Bernard A.
Lane, Helen S.
LaPointe, Leonard L.
Larson, Vernon D.
Lass, Norman J.
Lassman, Frank M.
Lau, Aileen C.
Leach, Edwin A.
Lee, Corinne C.
Leeper, Herbert A., Jr.
Lefevre, Margaret C.
Leith, William R.
Lemme, Margaret L.
Leonard, Laurence
Lerea, Louis
Lerman, Jay W.
Leslie, Carol P.
Levitt, Harry
Lilly, David J.
Lillywhite, Herold
Ling, Daniel
Lingwall, James B.
Linke, Charles E.
Lipscomb, David M.
Lloyd, Lyle L.
Loavenbruck, Angela M.
Locke, John L.
Lockwood, Dean D.
Logemann, Jerilyn A.
Longerich, Mary C.
Love, Russell J.
Lovrinic, Jean Hahn
Lowell, Edgar L.
Lubinske, Rosemary B.
Lubker, James F.
Ludlow, Christy L.
Luper, Harold L.
Luse, Eleanor M.

Luterman, David M.
Lynch, Joan I.

M

MacLearie, Elizabeth
Madell, Jane R.
Maisel, Clare G.
Malone, Russell L.
Mandell, Theodore
Mann, Mary B.
Marge, Michael
Marshall, Robert C.
Martin, Edwin W.
Martin, Frederick N.
Martin, Richard R.
Mase, Darrel J.
Mason, Robert M.
Massengill, Raymond, Jr.
Matkin, Noel D.
Matsko, Thomas A.
Matthews, Jack
Maurer, James F.
McCall, Gerald N.
McConnell, Freeman E.
McCroskey, Robert L.
McDermott, Richard P.
McDonald, Eugene T.
McDonald, F. Douglas
McDowell, Elizabeth
McElroy, Margaret D.
McFarlane, Stephen C.
McLauchlin, Robert M.
McLean, James E.
McReynolds, Leija V.
McWilliams, Betty J.
Mecham, Merlin J.
Meek, Merry M.
Melnick, William
Melrose, Jay
Mencher, George T.
Mencke, Eugene O.
Mendel, Maurice I.
Menyuk, Paula
Merten, Karol K.
Michael, Paul L.
Milisen, Robert
Miller, June B.
Miller, Maurice H.
Miller, Paul S.
Millin, Joseph P.
Miner, Adah L.
Minifie, Fred D.
Moeller, Mary P.
Moll, Kenneth L.
Moller, Karlind T.
Moncur, John P.
Montague, James C., Jr.
Montgomery, Judith K.
Moore, G. Paul
Moore, Mary Virginia M.
Morley, Alonzo J.
Morley, D. E.
Morley, Russell D.
Morris, Hughlett L.
Mowrer, Donald
Mueller, H. Gustav
Mullendore, James M.
Muma, John R.
Murray, Elwood
Murray, Frederick
Murry, Thomas
Musiek, Frank E.
Mysak, Edward D.

N

Naremore, Rita
Nathanson, Yale S.
Nation, James E.
Naunton, Ralph F.
Neal, W. Ray, Jr.
Nelson, C. Donald
Nelson, Lois A.
Nelson, Max
Nelson, Nickola W.
Nerbonne, Michael A.
Newby, Hayes A.
Newman, Parley W.
Newton, Mariana
Nober, E. Harris
Nodar, Richard H.
Noll, J. Douglas
Northern, Jerry L.
Nuru, Njeri J.

O

O'Hare, Nancy K.
O'Neill, John J.
O'Toole, Thomas J.
Ochsner, Glenda F.
Oliver, Jean G.
Olsen, Wayne O.
Olson, Don A.
Olson, Robert D.
Osborn, Courtney D.
Owens, Elmer
Oyer, Herbert J.

P

Paden, Elaine P.
Paesani, Andrew, Jr.
Palmer, John M.
Panagos, John M.
Pannbacker, Mary D.
Parish, Robbin
Parker, Charles D.
Paruzynski, Thad F.
Patterson, Ramelle F.
Payne, Peter D.
Paynter, Earlene T.
Peacher, William G.
Pearson, Margaret D.
Peets, Ruth Du Puis
Peins, Maryann
Pendergast, Kathleen K.
Perkins, William H.
Perrin, Kenneth L.
Peters, Robert W.
Peterson, Harold A.
Peterson-Falzone, Sally J.
Philips, Betty Jane
Pierce, Bruce R.
Pierce, Robert
Pike, Harriet H.
Pinheiro, Marilyn L.
Plotkin, William H.
Popelka, Gerald R.
Porch, Bruce E.
Potter, Robert E.
Powell, Harold
Powers, Gene R.
Prather, Elizabeth M.
Prather, William F.
Pressel, Gene
Pronovost, Wilbert
Prutting, Carol Ann

Q

Querry, Patricia H.
Quintana, Marilyn M.
Quigley, Stephen P.

R

Radus, Libby
Rampp, Donald L.
Ranney, J. B.
Rassi, Judith A.
Raubicheck, Letitia E.
Reed, L. Deno
Rees, Maryjane
Rees, Norma S.
Reid, Philip
Resnick, David M.
Resnick, Steffi B.
Rice, Mabel L.
Richardson, Sylvia O.
Rigrodsky, Seymour
Riley, Glyndon D.
Ringel, Robert L.
Rintelmann, William F.
Ritter, E. Gene
Rittmanic, Paul A.
Roach, Robert E.
Robertson, Mary Lu
Robinson, Frank B.
Roeser, Ross J.
Rose, Darrell E.
Rosen, Jack
Rosenbaum, S. Steve
Rosenbek, John C.
Ross, Mark
Rousey, Clyde L.
Rubin, Herbert
Rubin, Martha T.
Ruhm, Howard B.
Runyan, Charles M.
Rupp, Ralph R.
Ruscello, Dennis M.
Russell, Lorraine H.
Rutherford, Berneice R.
Rutherford, David R.
Ryan, Bruce P.

S

Salmon, Shirley J.
Sanders, Derek A.
Sanders, Jay W.
Sands, Elaine S.
Saricks, Margaret Byrne
Sarno, Martha Taylor
Schendel, Laurel L.
Schery, Teris Kim
Schiefelbusch, Richard L.
Schlanger, Bernard B.
Schlanger, Phoebe H.
Schlitt, Robert
Scholl, Harold M.
Schubert, George W.
Schuckers, Gordon H.
Schwartz, Arthur H.
Schwartz, Daniel M.
Scott, Cheryl M.
Screen, Robert M.
Sedge, Roy K.
Seidemann, Michael F.
Seitz, Michael R.
Seltz, Anne Eleanor
Sergeant, Russell L.
Seymour, Charlena M.
Seymour, Harry N.
Shaffer, George
Shallop, Jon K.
Shames, George H.
Shank, Kennon H.
Shanks, James C., Jr.
Sheehan, Vivian
Sheldon, Neil
Shelton, Ralph L., Jr.
Shepherd, David C.
Sherman, Dorothy
Shervanian, Chris C.
Shewan, Cynthia M.
Shimizu, Hiroshi
Shipp, Thomas
Showalter, Robert G.
Shriberg, Lawrence D.
Siegel, Gerald M.
Siegenthaler, Bruce M.
Silliman, Elaine R.
Silman, Shlomo
Silverman, Ellen M.
Silverman, Franklin H.
Silverman, S. Richard
Simmons-Martin, Audrey
Simonson, Josephine
Singh, Sadanand

Skelly-Hakanson, Madge
Small, Arnold M.
Smead, Lucille J.
Smith, Frances S.
Smith, Jeanne K.
Smith, Linda L.
Sokolnicki, Alfred J.
Soliman, Salah
Sommers, Ronald K.
Sonday, Francis L.
Sonies, Barbara C.
Spahr, Frederick T.
Speaks, Charles E.
Spriestersbach, Bette
Spriestersbach, D. C.
Spuehler, H. E.
Stark, Earl W.
Stark, Joel
Stark, Rachel E.
Starkweather, C. Woodruff
Starr, Clark D.
Steer, Mack D.
Stein, Laszlo K.
Stephenson, William T.
Stoia, Louis
Stone, Robert E., Jr.
Stream, Kathryn S.
Stream, Richard W.
Stromsta, Courtney
Studebaker, Gerald A.
Subtelny, Joanne D.
Sullivan, Roy F.
Swisher, Linda P.

T

Talbott, Richard E.
Taylor, Orlando L.
Tekieli, Mary Ellen
Templin, Mildred C.
Terango, Larry
Thomas, William G.
Thompson, Jesse J.
Thurman, Wayne L.
Tikofsky, Ronald S.
Tillman, Tom W.
Tobey, Emily A.
Tobias, Jerry V.
Tomblin, J. Bruce
Toubbeh, Jamil I.
Trombly, Thelma
Trost-Cardamone, Judith E.

U

Ulrich, Sandra R.

V

Vallon, Jerome M.
Van Demark, D. R.
Van Dusen, C. Raymond
Van Riper, Charles
Van Tasell, Dianne J.
Vaughn, Gwenyth R.
Von Drach, Robert B.
Von Leden, Hans V.

W

Walden, Brian E.
Wallace, Elizabeth M.
Ward, Louise M.
Ward, W. Dixon
Warren, Donald W.
Waryas, Carol L.
Waryas, Paul A.
Weber, Bruce A.
Webster, Elizabeth
Webster, John C.
Webster, Michael
Weidner, William E.
Weinberg, Bernd
Weiss, Arthur I.
Welch, Lin
Wells, Charlotte
Wertz, Robert T.
Westby, Carol E.
Westlake, Harold
Weston, Alan Jay
Whaley, Patricia
Wheelden, Julie A.
Whitehead, Robert L.
Whitlock, Beverly H.
Wiig, Eilsabeth H.
Wilber, Laura Ann
Wiley, Terry L.
Willeford, Jack A.
Williams, Dean E.
Wilson, D. Kenneth
Wilson, Frank B.
Wilson, Mary S.
Wilson, Wesley R.
Winitz, Harris
Wischner, George J.
Wolfe, Virginia S.
Wood, Kenneth Scott
Wood, Mary Lovey
Woolfolk, Elizabeth Carrow
Work, Rhonda S.
Worthington, Don W.
Wright, H. N.
Wright, Laura F.

Y

Yairi, Ehud
Yantis, Phillip A.
Yates, James T.
Yates, Jo Ann R.
Yoder, David E.
Yoss, Kathe A.
Young, Elizabeth Bell
Young, Martin A.
Young, Norton B.

Z

Zaner, Annette R.
Zedler, Empress
Zemlin, Willard R.
Zimmer, Catherine H.
Zwislocki, Jozef J.

LIFE MEMBERS OF THE ASSOCIATION

A Member who has held membership for the 10 consecutive years* immediately prior to attaining the age of 65 may apply for and automatically receive Life Membership with all the privileges of a member. Annual dues/fees are waived.

* Effective 1/1/91, this changes to 25 consecutive years.

A

Abraham, Annabel S.
Adams, Esther Y.
Aden, Frances A.
Adler, Raphael
Agnello, Virginia
Ahrendts, Harold L.
Ainsworth, Stanley H.
Alberts, Cecil D.
Albright, Joy S.
Allen, Catherine
Allen, Emma M.
Allen, Evelyn Y.
Allen, Madge B.
Allen, Mildred
Allman, Jeanette
Anderman, Bernard
Anderson, Bernard A.
Anderson, Jean L.
Anderson, John O.
Anderson, Robert H. N.
Anderson, Ruth M.
Anderson, Virgil
Ansberry, Merle
Argetsinger, Elaine
Arlt, Phyllis B.
Arnold, Genevieve
Arnold, Godfrey E.
Arnold, Julia L.
Aronoff, Rebecca C.
Aronson, Hannah U.
Ashmead, Allez M.

B

Backus, Ollie L.
Badick, Martha
Baer, Mildred
Baisinger, Wilbur H.
Baisler, Perry E.
Baker, Ida C.
Baker, Marjorie L.
Bangs, Dorothy Z.
Bangs, Tina E.
Banikiotes, Florence G.
Bardanouve, Venus T.
Bargemeyer, Kurt E.
Barrett, Sarah D.
Barritt, Virgil C.
Barton, Amy V.
Bartram, Margaret
Bass, Robbie A.
Bassin, Beatrice K.
Batza, Eugene M.
Bauquier, Oliver W.
Bealmear, Mary K.
Beamer, Mary W.
Beckelheimer, Alice F.
Beckett, Lyda B.
Beckett, Ralph L.
Beebe, Helen H.
Beitsch, Estelle L.
Belak-Plenger, Barbara J.
Bell, Dorothy M.
Bell, Jeannette
Bell Joan L.
Bender, Ruth E.
Benjamin Ruth
Bennett, Audrey
Bennett, Clayton L.
Bettett Daphne N.
Bennett, Floy L.
Bennetts, Genevieve G.
Benson, Mary E.
Berg, Viola G.
Berger, Mildred B.
Bergl, Burkett K.
Bergman, Moe
Berlin, Asa J.
Berntsen, Harold R.
Berry, Mildred F.
Bielski, Lee S.
Bingham, Carol C.
Bingham, Dale S.
Blair, Greta B.
Bledsole, Irma M.
Bleiberg, Aaron H.
Blizard, Dorothy E.
Bloodstein, Oliver
Bloomer, H. Harlan
Bock, Margaret B.
Bognar, Phyllis, M.
Bohannon, Dorothy E.
Bokelmann, Dorothy T.
Boland, M.
Boland, Jr., John L.
Bolson, Virginia A.
Bond, Jean M.
Boomsliter, Paul C.
Bordman, Martin
Bosley, Elizabeth
Bost, Katherine
Bowe, Angela J.
Bowlen, James H.
Bowler, Ned W.
Brackett, Isaac P.
Brady, Margaret S.
Bragg, Vernon C.
Brand, Madeline
Branson, Virginia M.
Breakey, Margaret R.
Bridgeford, Ethel B.
Brigham, DO, Fleda M.
Brisbane, Arlene
Brittin, Marie E.
Britton, Jean M.
Brodnitz, Friedrich S.
Broida, Helen
Bronstein, Arthur J.
Brooks, Francis D.
Brown, C. Rebecca
Brown, Helen E. D.
Brown, Melba V.
Brown, Phyllis F.
Bruce, Helen B.
Bruner, Thelma J.
Brungard, Maude O.
Buchanan, Dorothea
Buhr, Barbara
Burdick, Eve C.
Burgess, Carla D.
Bukland, Marjorie B.
Burnstad, Evelyn G.
Burr, Helen G.
Buzash, Lola H.
Bycraft, Helen B.
Byrnes, Nona J.
Bywaters, Eleanor B.

C

Calamaras, Peter
Camardo, Joan L.
Campbell, Alice L.
Campbell, Marcia
Campbell, Marian F.
Canales, Betty H.
Canfield, Dana W.
Canfield, Norton
Canfield, William H.
Carney, R. John
Carson, Loretta S.
Carstensen, Gustav V.
Carter, Cleo I.
Carter, Eunice T.
Carver, Phyllis W.
Casebier, Gabrielle
Castner, Marguerite L.
Caughey, Mary B.
Cavanagh, George, J.
Chamberlain, Ruth I.
Chambers, Dorothy L.
Chambers, Helen G.
Champion, William N.
Chaplin, Ruth T.
Chapman, Verna J.
Cheskin, Adele
Christensen, Arden H.
Christman, Josephine E.
Church, Rose M.
Claeys, Wanda M.
Clark, Dorothy W.
Clark, Ione A.
Clark, Jeanne
Clark, Pearl M.
Clements, Elizabeth
Clemons, M. Elaine
Clift, Mildred A.
Cloud, Zletta K.
Coates, Madine H.
Cochran, Evelyn C.
Cochran, Ione M.
Cochran, Jane D.
Cochran, John R.
Cofey, Carol J.
Coffield, Eleanor
Cohen, Garland J.
Cohen, Lillian K.
Cole, Madeline B.
Cole, Ross G.
Collins, Lula M.
Colton, Sophia S.
Colville, Mary B.
Connell, Jane S.
Connelly, Helen L.
Cook, Mildred B.
Cooper, Georgia T.
Cooper, Reuben
Copeland, Marie E.
Copeland, Pauline B.
Corcoran, John A.
Coreys, Esther
Cosart, Anne R.
Costello, Mary R.
Cowart, Rosa C.
Crabtree, Margaret
Craig, Rebecca S.
Craig, Sam B.
Crary, Margaret A.
Crawford, Gladys H.
Crickmay, Marie C.
Crotty, Carol M.
Crutchfield, Verna M.
Cubert, Catherine L.
Cummings, Marjorie D.
Curry, E. Thayer
Curtis, James F.
Curtis, Ruth
Cutler, S. James

D

Daggett, Helen C.
Daly, Cynthia
Danko, Angela N.
Dardas, RN, Kathryn D.
Dardick, Leila R.
Darley, Frederic L.
Dasaro, Michael J.
Davidson, Dora L.
Davidson, Keith, C.
Davis, Donald C.
Davis, Margaret W.
Davison, Louise D.
Dawson, Warren, R.
de Hirsch, Katrina
De Laubenfels, Richard J.
De Voe, Anne S.
DeLacy, Hester S.
De Luca, Joseph A.
Denny, Martha Q.
Deupree, Robert M.
Di Russo, Irma B.
Diamond, Matthew
DiCarlo, Louis M.
Dickinson, Barbara
Diel, Dorothy L.
Digby, Matthew J.
Dixon, Carmen C.
Dobson, Patricia T.
Doerfler, Leo G.
Dolan, Leo F.
Donewald, Marian
Donohue, Helen S.
Doob, Dorothy
Dorn, Israel J.
Dorval, Bertha M.
Doudna, Mark E.
Dougherty, Leona Mae
Douglass, Lois W.
Douglass, Robert L.
Downs, Marion P.
Drake, Jack
Drake, Marion E.
Drexler, Hazel G.
Drogin, Brodea M.
Dubard, Etoile
Duffy, John K.
Duncan, Melba H.
Dvosin, Edna
Dyer, Helen A.
Dyer, Ruth S.
Dzuba, Selma S.

E

Earnest, Sue W.
Eblen, Roy E.
Eckelmann, Dorothy
Economou, Helen M.
Edmund, Elizabeth G.
Edwards, Ellen C.
Edwards, Elsie, M.
Edwards Rosemary C.
Egan, James P.
Egan, Katherine S.
Egbert, James H.
Ehrenfreund, Joseph
Ehrlich, Pauline
Eisenson, Jon
Eisenstadt, Arthur A.
Elliott, Charles R.
Elliott, Margaret L.
Elliott, Marian
Ellis, Mary M.
Emanuel, Permelia R.
Engelson, Henriette
English, Robert H.
Epstein, Aubrey
Erickson, Ellen A.
Ervin, Jean C.
Esber, Elizabeth C.
Esch-Johnson, Geraldine G.
Eshelman, Mary P.
Eskew, Lorraine W.
Evans, Virginia F.
Even, Helen H.

F

Fabian, Eulalia W.
Falconer, George A.
Farley, Dollie O.
Farley, Joyce J.
Farquhar, Mary S.
Farrant, R. H.
Farrington, Mitzi G.
Farris, Ruth B.
Faust, Ruth S.
Feinsod, Miriam G.
Feldman, Irene R.
Ferguson, Marie N.
Fischer, Clare O.
Fishbein, Gloria B.
Fisher, Cletus G.
Fisher, Hilda B.
Fishman, Sally W.
Fitch, Waring J.
Fitzsimons, Ruth N.
Fletcher, Rose
Fletchinger, M. Therese
Flory, William C.
Flowers, Elsie A.
Fogelstrom, Suzanne S.
Foreman, Lydia Marie
Forster, Charlotte F.
Fossum, Ernest C.
Fouts, Ann P.
Fowler, Mary M.
Fox, Vernie R.
Fraser, Malcolm H.
Frazier, Barbara
Frazier, Mary E.
Frederick, Lois K.
Freeman, Beatrice D.
Freeman, Ben
Freeman, Gertrude A.
Freeman, Patty L.
Frevert, Corine T.
Frick, James V.
Fried, Leonard
Fried, Marla G.
Friedman, Pacy
Friedman, Ruth F.
Froslie, Lucille L.
Fuller, Carl W.
Fulton, Helen L.
Furuheim, Frances W.

G

Gage, LaVada W.
Gallagher, Betty
Garbutt, Cameron W.
Gardner, Lela
Garrett, Edgar R.
Garrigan, Verita M.
Garrison, Lola M.
Garwood, Victor P.
Gasaway, Jane
Gay, Helen S.
Geddes, Elsie M.
Geldin, Irving H.
Gendelman, Evelyn G.
Gens, George W.
Gerber, Adele
Getlin, Jules P.
Gholson, Sibyl G.
Gibbs, Inez G.
Gilchrist, Florence S.
Giles, Gerald, L.
Gilmartin, Eva Marie
Gilmore, Marian L.
Glasner, Philip J.
Glenn, Almetta M.
Glorig, Aram
Goebel, Elizabeth
Goetzinger, Cornelius P.
Goldberger, Rhoda S.
Goldstein, Marion B.
Gomer, Betty J.
Gooch, Gilbert E.
Goodhill, Victor
Goodman, Allan C.
Gordon, Henrietta
Gordon, Miriam M.
Goulding, Virginia R.
Gousha, Catherine
Graham, A. Bruce
Graham, Harriet J.
Graham, Margaret S.
Grant, Naomi M.
Granum, Arline S.
Graunke, W. Lloyd
Gray, Marnetta J.
Green, Evelyn M.
Green, Martha H.
Greenberg, Sylvia
Greenwell, Alice R.
Grieg, Diana H.
Grier, Tose F.
Grilley, Beryl H.
Groginski, Beatrice B.
Guerra, Maria Z.
Gunderson, Herbert E.
Gunn Kathleen

H

Hageman, Ruth A.
Hahn, Elsie S.
Haines, Harold H.
Hale, Lester L.
Hall, Cora B.
Hall, Rubye M.
Hall, William F.
Hallock, Viola K.
Halpert, Helen V.
Hamberg, Mildred S.
Hamilton, Ruth G.
Hankammer, S. Bonnie
Hanley, Theodore D.
Hanning, Luella M.
Hanses, Mary C.
Hanson, Grace H.
Hanson, Lyle D.
Harada, Clark
Hardy, Miriam P.
Harper, Edith
Harrigan, Christine
Harris, Beatrice G.
Harris, Charles N.
Harris, Elizabeth
Harris, Kathleen P.
Harris, Lester L.
Harris, Maude M.
Harris, Willie V.
Harrison, Anne
Harrison, John P.
Harrison, Peggy R.
Hartsough, Kathleen F.
Hatcher, Caro C.
Haug, C. Olaf
Hawk, Dorothy M.
Hawk, Elizabeth
Hawk, Eloise B.
Hawkins, Margaret C.
Haworth, Freda
Hayes, Claude
Hayes, Harriet M.
Healey, Grace D.
Healey, Patricia
Heath, Marguerite
Hedgecock, Leroy D.
Hembree, Margaret E.
Hendrickson, Jr. Joseph G.
Henretig, Max D.
Henrikson, Ernest H.
Henry, Andrell W.
Henry, Betsy W.
Henry, Frances V.
Henson, Evelyn B.
Herbert, Esther L.
Herndon, Geneva
Herrick, Margaret H.
Herzog, Winifred P.

Hess, Donald A.
Heyer, Mary H.
Higley, Beulah S.
Hildebrandt, Emery V.
Hill, Wathina S.
Hill, Jr., George E.
Hinman, Mary P.
Hinnant, Elizabeth
Hinson, Mary C.
Hirsh, Ira J.
Hiser, Velma B.
Hitschman, Hedwig
Hoberman, Shirley E.
Hodges, Monetta G.
Hofflund, Violet
Hoffman, Harleene S.
Hoffman, Jeanette A.
Hoffmann, Dale E.
Holmes, Imogene L.
Hornaday, Nila
Horowitz, Leola S.
Hoshiko, Michael
House, Arthur S.
House, Mary R.
Houston, Mary A.
Hoversten, Gloria H.
Huber, Mary W.
Hubschman, Eva W.
Hudson, Atwood
Huffman, Elna S.
Hull Mary E.
Hunt, Mary I.
Hunte, Frances
Huot, Germaine
Hurd, Mary E.

I

Iandoli, Edward W.
Indursky, Beatrice
Ingram, Maria M.
Irwin, John V.
Irwin, Ruth B.
Ivey, Lillian P.
Ivey, Sara M.

J

Jackson, Bernard R.
Jackson, Charline B.
Jackson, Janancy S.
Jackson, Ruth M.
Jacobs, Mary T.
Jacoby, Beatrice F.
Jefers, Florence K.
Jemelka, Victor J.
Jenkins, Edna M.
Jensen, Senta H.
Jerome, Eldon K.
Johnson, Alice L.
Johnson, Constance C.
Johnson, Dorothy C.
Johnson, E. W.
Johnson, Georgiana
Johnson, Kenneth O.
Johnson, Louise C.
Johnson, Mary E.
Johnson, T. Earle
Johnston, Elizabeth
Johnston, Virginia J.
Jolly, Faith
Jones, Lucille W.
Jones, Mamie J.
Jones, Martha E.
Jones, Morris V.
Jones, Ruth E.
Jordan, Ethel S.

K

Kaltenborn, Jr., Arthur L.
Kaplan, Donald E.
Katz, Erica J.
Kauffman, Ellen K.
Kavanaugh, Heddy L.
Keaster, Jacqueline
Keeler, Darlene D.
Kelleher, Loleati, A.
Kelly, Delores, L.
Kelmenson, Florence
Kemble, Carita
Kemster, Marjory I.
Kennedy, Alicia Q.
Kennedy, Grace M.
Kennedy, Kathleen D.
Kennedy, Margaret F.
Kennedy, William W.
Kent, Margaret S.
Kierstead, James M.
Killam, Alma E.
Kilpatrick, Janet I.
King, Fannie E.
Kinney-White, Barbara A.
Kinstler, Donald B.
Kirby, Kathleen F.
Kishter, Helen H.
Klinger, Herbert
Knauf, Loren W.
Knauf, Vincent H.
Knight, Elmo L.
Knight, Helen S.
Knight, Marion H.
Knight, Paul D.
Knox, Albert W.
Knox, Barbara D.
Knox, Thomas E.
Kodama, Mildred R.
Koepp-Baker, Herbert
Kohl, Evelyn P.
Kohrs, Charlotte
Kopp, Harriet G.
Kosh, Zelda H.
Krantz, Henrietta C.
Krantz, Miriam L.
Krieger, Miriam R.
Krug, Richard F.
Kunken, Naomi S.
Kuper, Eolin C.

L

Laguaite, Jeannette
Lahaie, Ralph V.
Laky, Mildred H.
Lamb, Mary L.
Lambert, Alice M.
Lampe, Henrica C.
Lande, Anita
Landers, Madie L.
Landers, Millard T.
Lane, Helen S.
Lang, Elizabeth
Larson, Mark H.
Larson, Thalia W.
Laub, Clarice C.
Lauder, Edmund
Lawrence, Telete Z.
Lefevre, Margaret C.
Leidecker, Catherine B.
Leiper, Norah M.
Lennon, E. James
Lessac, Arthur
Levine, Nioma K.
Lewis, Mary C.
Lewis, Mary G.
Lieberman, Elaine F.
Liljeblad, Astrid
Lillywhite, Herold
Linander, Esther S.
Linke, Charles E.
Linn, George B.
Linter, Mary E.
Lisemby, Doris M.
Livesay, Laurel Y.
Longerich, Mary C.
Lore, James I.
Loughery, James H.
Loughery, Jean M.
Lovestedt, Lucille K.
Low, Gordon M.
Lowe, Raymond L.
Lowell, Edgar L.
Luckern, Marie P.
Ludden, Mary A.
Lundeen, Dale J.
Luse, Eleanor, M.
Lux, Elizabeth P.
Lyndes, Kellogg O.
Lytton, Beverly J.

M

MacIntosh, Rita G.
MacIver, Margaret L.
MacLearie, Elizabeth
MacPherson, Helen M.
Magers, Mary A.
Mahon, Florence L.
Mahoney, Melanie
Maloney, Nina B.
Mamolen, Eleanor G.
Mandell, Theodore
Mann, Mary B.
Manucia, Charles F.
March, Harold H.
Marquardt, Lillian A.
Marsh, Lucille T.
Martin, Katherine
Marx, Francis N.
Mase, Darrel J.
Masland, Mary W.
Mathews, Bertha B.
Matis, Edward E.
Matis, Mary J.
Matthews, Hannah
Matthews, Jack
Mattox, Helen M.
Mawhinney, Clara K.
McAllister, Mary E.
McAlphine, Catherine A.
McConnell, Freeman E.
McDearmon, James R.
McDonald, Eugene T.
McDonald, Gertrude R.
McDonald, Margaret M.
McDonald, Ryta E.
McDowell, Elizabeth
McDowell, Mary L.
McGuire, Marion
McIntyre, Christine
McKeown, Milfred R.
McKnight, Laura W.
McLaughlin, Florence E.
McMillan, Olga C.
McMillen, Anne P.
McPhillips, M. Regina
McReynolds, Leija V.
Mecham, Merlin J.
Meisler, Beatrice R.
Meissner, James H.
Mellencamp, Virginia L.
Menzel, Otto J.
Messick, Anna M.
Metcalf, Jean V.
Metraux, Ruth W.
Metz, Mary A.
Miksak, Joseph A.
Milisen, Robert
Millard, Robert T.
Miller, A. Elizabeth
Miller, Charles J.
Miller, Earl L.
Miller, John R.
Miller, June B.
Miller, Louise H.
Miller, Madge B.
Millin, Joseph P.
Mills, Charlotte
Millward, Dorothy D.
Miner, Adah L.
Mines, Ethel S.
Minifie, Ferne
Mitchell, Oscar, Jr.
Molloy, Julia S.
Molloy, R.
Moncur, John P.

Monroe, Alice D.
Monteith, Martha
Moody, Pauline F.
Moore, Edith Y.
Moore, Ellen H.
Moore, G. Paul
Moore, Marguerite
Moran, Marion C.
Morley, Alonzo J.
Morley, D. E.
Morren, Jeanette A.
Morriconi, Alfonso
Morris, Marion G.
Moseley, Faye
Moser, Henry M.
Moser, Miriam T.
Moses, Jr., Elbert R.
Moss, Margaret L.
Mueh, Ferne H.
Mulholland, Ann M.
Mullendore, James M.
Multer, Patricia C.
Munneke, Margaret F.
Murdock, Betty J.
Murphy, Blanche M.
Murray, Barbara E.
Murray, Elwood
Mussen, Ethel F.
Myers, Dorothy E.
Myers, Gladys I.

N

Nagel, Robert F.
Nailor, Audrey
Nathanson, Yale S.
Nation, Alta G.
Naylor, Rex V.
Needham, Thyria H.
Neidecker, Elizabeth
Nelson, Max
Neugebauer, Freda W.
Newby, Hayes A.
Newkirk, Alice B.W.
Newton, Kathryn K.
Nicholas, Rosalind H.
Norbury, Aaron, W.
Nordheim, Lee T.
Norrix, James M.
Norton, Max C.
Novack, Harry S.
Nowinski, Hazel, Y.
Nystrom, Clarence L.

O

O'Brien, Audrey
O'Brien, Mary R.
O'Connor, Pearl M.
Obermann, C. Esco
Offill, Elinor B.
Ohlweiler, Zita
Oleary, Roberta M.
Olsen, Betty
Omer, Jane L.
Oppenheim-Errera, Gabrielle
Orion, Gertrude
Osborn, Courtney D.
Osborn, Emma L.
Ottaway, Ruth
Owens, Katharine
Oxman, Emily K.
Oyer, Herbert J.

P

Paden, Elaine P.
Palen, Sharon B.
Palmer, John M.
Pals, Marjorie E.
Pappafava, Kathryn B.
Parker, Jayne H.
Parks, Mary D.
Parry Iola M.J.
Parsons, Charlotte
Parsons, Helene
Partridge, Lyman M.
Paruzynski, Thad F.
Patterson, Robert E.
Patton, Eleanor M.
Paul, John E.
Pawling, Helen M.
Payne, Virginia M.
Peacher, Georgiana M.
Peake, Mary L.
Pearce, Margaret C.
Pearlstine, Edelu G.
Pearman, Sophia L.
Pearson, Margaret D.
Peets, Ruth D.
Pendergast, Kathleen K.
Penn, Erta V.
Penn, Jacques P.
Pennington, Gwendolyn
Pennington, R. Corbin
Perkins, Charlotte
Perkins, William H.
Perry, Alberta H.
Peters, Dorothy M.
Peters, Robert M.
Peters, Robert W.
Peterson, Ila C.
Peterson, Mary B.
Phillips, Erva J.
Phillips, Sylvia D.
Phoebus, Maudie P.
Pierce, Robert
Pierini, M. Paul
Pike, Harriet H.
Pinheiro, Marilyn L.
Pitman, Rosamond M.
Pittman, Laura M.
Pitts, WIlliam M.
Pitts, Jr., Willis N.
Platt, James H.
Platt, Mary
Plumb, Norma H.
Pollack, Doreen M.
Pomerantz, Bonnie K.
Porter, Wyne W.
Postove, Mary A.
Poulos, Thomas H.
Powell, Orpha L.
Prall, Josephine
Primley, Alice A.
Proctor, Minnie B.
Pronovost, Wilbert
Pruett, Ruby T.
Puglisi, Elizabeth A.
Pulliam, Louis L.

Q

Quine, Doris M.

R

Rabinowitz, Marcia G.
Radus, Libby
Rafkind, Shirley M.
Ramedia, Mary A.
Ransaw, Anna K.
Rasmus, Ward
Raubicheck, Letitia E.
Redding, Marguerite S.
Redwine, Ruth W.
Reed, Dora R.
Reed, Martha K.
Rees, Muriel
Regan, M. Clare
Reiz, Zelda L.
Retzlaff, Wesley
Revis, Margaret F.
Rhoades, Inez B
Richard, Isabel
Richards, Doris M.
Richardson, Sylvia O.
Richmond, Jr., Thomas E.
Richter, Katherine
Rickler, Irwin
Rintoul, Dorothy B.
Roach, Robert A.
Roach, Robert E.
Roberts Kathylene
Roberts, William H.
Robertson, Helen
Robinson, Frank B.
Robinson, John E.
Roblee, Lorraine A.
Ronnei, Eleanor C.
Rose, Opal L.
Rosen, Arlene S.
Rosen, Jack
Rosenfeld, Laura S.
Rosenstein, Beverly B.
Ross, Dorothy E.
Ross, Francie
Ross, Jean C.
Rosson, Grace L.
Roth, Hazel F.
Rothman, Frederick
Rothman, Ruth A.
Rotter, Paul
Rouse, Lucy W.
Rowe, Margaret L.
Rudisill, Harlene C.
Rue, Hazel M.
Runion, Howard L.
Rutherford, Berneice R.
Rutherford, Gorin
Rutstein, Irving T.

S

Sack, Leo P.
Sadler, Dorothy O.
Sanderson, Virginia S.
Saricks, Margaret C.
Savell, Mildred S.
Scantlin, Dorothy L.
Schaffer, Elliott J.
Schapiro, Dorris B.
Schendel, Laurel L.
Schinske, Erhart A.
Schlanger, Bernard B.
Schlanger, Phoebe H.
Schlosser, Frances D.
Schmidt, John H.
Schneider, Lianne P.
Schneider, Marie J.
Schrader, Clarence H.
Schrock, Adeleen S.
Schroeder, Tamara P.
Schumacher, Walter C.
Schwab, Constance
Schwartz, Edith M.
Schwartz, Ralph J.
Scott, Duncan R.
Scott, Elizabeth
Seitz, Gail M.
Semple, Jean E.
Sevigny, Barbara H.
Shaffer, Chester M.
Shaffer, George
Shank, Kennon H.
Shanks, Jr., James C.
Shapiro, Gertrude
Shapley, James
Sharp, Florence A.
Shea, William L
Sherman, Dorothy
Shields, Dorothy D.
Shippee, Frank H.
Shopwin, Charles D.
Shotwell, Jeannette
Shulman, Edward
Siegenthaler, Bruce M.
Silverman, Eleanor T.
Silverman, Irving
Silverman, S. Richard
Silverman, Sidney I.
Simmons, Harriet A.
Simmons, Ruby K.
Simmons-Martin, Audrey
Simonson, Josephine
Simpson, Bessie C.

Singer, Louis
Skelly-Hakanson, Madge
Sklar, Maurice
Slate, Suzanne I.
Slind, Margaret A.
Slipakoff, Ethel L.
Smayling, Lyda M.
Smead, Lucille J.
Smith, Barbara M.
Smith, Clarissa R.
Smith, D. Wayne
Smith, Evelyn H.
Smith, Frances G.
Smith, Glenn L.
Smith, Jeanne K.
Smith, Loretta W.
Snedeker, Jr., Leo W.
Snell, Helen P.
Snodgrass, R. E.
Soisson, Margaret
Sokolnicki, Alfred J.
Sokoloff, Martin A.
Solomon, Arthur L.
Sonday, Francis L.
Sorensen, Eugenia R.
Spates, Eleanor F.
Spear, Barbara H.
Spriestersbach, Bette
St. Onge, Keith R.
Stansell, Barbara J.
Stanton, Fred E.
Steer, Mack D.
Steer, Ruth P.
Stein, Shirley P.
Steinau, Stanley J.
Stennett, Nadine E.
Stiebel, Hart H.
Stiles, Louise C.
Stitt, Clyde L.
Stocker, Beatrice
Stocker, Harold S.
Stoia, Louis
Stolp, Lauren E.
Stone, Welton S.
Storey, Mary F.
Storm, Florence R.
Stovall, Janice J.
Strait, Rose
Streng, Alice H.
Stromsta, Courtney
Sudaka, Martha F.
Sullivan, E. Barbara
Sullivan, Helen A.
Summers, Janet
Sumner, Florence G.
Suppan, Josephine
Suppan, Vincent V.
Sutherland, Laverne
Swallom, Alice
Sweeney, Marian K.
Sweeney, Mary G.
Szymoniak, Eliaine F.

T

Taylor, Irma S.
Taylor, Margaret F.
Taylor, Myra J.
Templin, Mildred C.
Tew, Roy E.
Thaxton, Loree D.
Thompson, Jesse J.
Thompson, Traudl
Thompson, Virginia L.
Thurman, Wayne L.
Tieszen, Marion V.
Tjomsland, Lily C.
Tockert, M.
Todd, Eleanor F.
Tonn, Martin
Trail, Wayne D.
Trattner, Naoma H.
Trombly, Thelma
Trotter, William D.
Trumbo, Charles R.
Tuch, Claire H.
Turner, Jayne S.
Turner, Martha P.
Twichell, Doris Y.

U

Ulrich, Miriam N.
Umble, Ray H.
Unger, Dorothy M.

V

Valentine, Courtney H.
Van Dusen, C. Raymond
Van Luven, Elizabeth
Van Riper, Charles
Van Tine, Ruth H.
Varner, Harriet K.
Vaughn, Gwenyth R.
Vaurio, Kathryn P.
Vernon, Jean C.
Vickers, William E.
Vickroy, Mildred R.
Villarreal, Jesse J.
Voelker, Evelyn G.
Volkland, Effie E.
Von Leden, Hans V.
Vonherman, Jean O.
Vorce, Eleanor R.

W

Wagner, Charlotte
Wainer, Marilyn F.
Walcher, Helen R.
Waldron, Daryle, L.
Walker, Clara E.
Walker, Maude J.
Wallace, Doris D.
Wallenius, Wesley A.
Walpole, Elizabeth
Walsh, Dorothy W.
Ward, Dolores M.
Ward, Louise M.
Warren, Berniece B.
Washa, Laura K.
Washington, Dorothy M.
Watts, Vivian G.
Weaver, Ella H.
Webber, Ava L.
Weber, Mary A.
Webster, John C.
Weers, Werdna E.
Weiner, Adeline E.
Weiner, Ruth H.
Weir, Clara B.
Wells, Charlotte
Werner, Lorna S.
Wertz, Florence C.
Wertz, Mildred B.
West, Hazel H.
Westlake, Harold
Whalen, M. Clare E.
Wheeler, Grete M.
White, Ethel B.
White, David L.
White Ethel B.
White, Margaret J.
Whitten, Ida E.
Wick, Laura M.
Wickens, Alice R.
Wight, Marallyn
Wilcox, Edna B.
Wilkinson, Esther R.
Willeford, Jack A.
Williams, Caroline M.
Williams, Frances G.
Williams J. David
Williams, Mary H.
Williams, William N.
Wilson, Beverley L.
Wilson, D. Kenneth
Wilson, Donald M.
Wilson, Elizabeth
Wilson, Frances P.
Wilson, Mary L.
Winchester, Madonna R.
Winder, Surline A.
Winters, Ellura H.
Wischner, George J.
Witkin, Belle R.
Woerl, Mary L.
Wood, Kenneth S.
Wood, Mary H.
Wood, Mildred H.
Woods, Catherine
Woods, M. Lucy
Woods, Roland E.
Wortley, John S.
Wray, Elinor C.
Wright, Ferne E.
Wright, Laura F.
Wyatt, Eldean L.
Wyatt, Gertrud L.

Y

Yacks, Colin
Yanchus, Elizabeth
Ylvisaker, Velma S.
Young, Jacqueline S.
Youse, Lillian D.

Z

Zachar, Rosalie T.
Zarwell, Lillian H.
Zedler, Empress
Zeitlin, Rosalyn R.
Zelman, Betty M.
Zimmer, Catherine H.
Zimmerman, Susan

AMERICAN SPEECH-LANGUAGE-HEARING FOUNDATION 1988 FOUNDATION FOUNDERS

Foundation Founders have contributed at least $100 annually to the American Speech-Language-Hearing Foundation. Founder support underwrites the mission of the Foundation: to improve the knowledge base in communication sciences and disorders.

A

Adams, Larry E.
**Adler, Leslie
Adler, Sol
Albritton, Thelma
Allen, Madge B.
Allen, Nell
Anderman, Bernard
Anderson, Charles V.
Anderson, Ruth M.
Angelelli, Roger M.
Armbruster, Joan M.
Ashmore, Lear
Aten, James L.

B

Bain, Barbara A.
Baker, Robert H.
Balko, John
Bangs, Tina E.
Bashir, Anthony S.
Battle, Dolores E.
Baxter, Jane H.
Beadle, Kathryn R.
Beasley, Daniel S.
Beauchamp, James A.
Bernthal, John E.
Berryman, Joan D.
Bess, Fred H.
Betts, Carl E.
Bevan, Marlene
Blackstone, Sarah
Blakeley, Robert W.
Blau, Andrea
Bless, Diane McQueen
Bloomer, H. Harlan
Boehmler, Richard M.
Bolton-Koppenhaver, Mary
Boone, Daniel R.
Boothroyd, Arthur
Borden, Gloria
Borton III, Thomas E.
Boysen, Allen
Brazier, Susan H.
Bregstone, Andrea P.
Brittin, Marie E.
Brown, Loretta G.
Bull, Glen L.
Burgess, Eleanor H.
Burkland, Marjorie
Burkowsky, Mitchell R.
Burtis, Mary Irene
Butler, Katherine G.

C

Canter, Gerald J.
Carey, Ann
Carney, Patrick J.
Casteel, Robert L.
Castle, Diane Sklar
Castle, William E.
Catlett, Camille
Cayne, Patricia Donner
Cherow, Evelyn
Chisholm, Mary C.
Citron III, David
Clark, Michael J.
Cohen, Carol
Cole, Lorraine
Cole, Patricia
Cole, Sarah
Conlon, Sara
Cook, Sally J.
Cooper, Crystal S.
Cooper, Eugene B.
Cooper, Jr., J.C.
Counihan, Donald T.
Cremen, Lynn K.
Culatta, Richard A.
Curran, Michael F.
Curtis, James F.
Czvik, Patsy S.

D

Dahle, Arthur
Dalzell, Larry E.
Dalzell, Sheila M.
Danhauer, Jeffery L.
Darby, John L.
Darley, Frederic L.
D'Asaro, Michael J.
Davis, F. Teresa Runzo
Davis, Julia M.
Dawgert, Grace F.
Deal, Leo V.
DeBole, S. Mario
Demetras, Martha J.
Demorest, Marilyn Elizabeth
Deutsch, Lawrence
Dickerson, Mary V.
Dickman, Harriet B.
Dickson, Stanley
Diedrich, William M.
Dinner, M. Bernice
Dixon, Richard F.
Doerfler, Leo G.
Dopheide, William R.
Douglass, Lois W.
Douglass, Robert L.
Downs, Marion P.
Dreyer, Dorothy E.
Dublinske, Stan
Duffy, Marjorie R.
Dunn, Marianne
Dunn-Engel, Elaine

E

Eblen, Roy E.
Eger, Diane Levy
Ehrlich, Carol H.
Ehrlich, Pauline
English, Joy
Engman, Margaret Wyatt

F

Falconer, George A.
Falk, Merwyn
Feldman, Alan S.
Ferullo, Robert J.
Feuerberg, Lydia E.
Finch, Amy
Finitzo, Terese
Firestone, Barbara
Fitch, James L.
Fitz-Armstrong, Linda C.
Fitzgerald, Mary Trabue
Florentine, Mary
Fowler, Carol
Fox, Donna R.
Fox, Joseph P.
Fox, Robert L.
Fraser, Malcolm
Freilinger, J. Joseph
Friedrich, Lorraine P.
Fujikawa, Sharon
Fuller, Carl W.

G

Garrett, Edgar R.
Garstecki, Dean C.
Gelatt, James P.
Gist, Kenneth T.
Glattke, Jean B.
*Glattke, Theodore J.
Glickenhaus, Sarah Brody
Golanka, Janet M.
Goldman, Ronald
Goldring, Sondra K.
Goldstein, David P.
Goldstein, Howard
Goldwasser, Marilyn
Golper, Lee Ann
Goodhill, Victor
Goodman, Sharlene
Goodstein, R. Sarah
Gordon, Mary E.
Graham, A. Bruce
Grant, Dorothy E.
Grason, Rufus
Gray, Burl B.
Green, William W.
Grey, Howard A.
Griffin, Kathleen M.
Griffith, Francis A.
Griffith, Twila E.
Grimes, Charles T.
Gudmundsen, Gail I.
Guilford, Arthur M.

H

Halper, Anita S.
Halpert, Helen V.
Ham, Richard E.
Hammer, Lowell C.
Hampton, Dennis C.
Hansard, Victoria
Hanson, Wayne R.
Harada, Clark
Hardy, Miriam P.
Harris, J. Donald
Harris, Katherine S.
Harris Ruth L.
Harrison, Peggy
Haslett, Elizabeth J.
Heffernan, Patricia
Heller, Joyce
Herer, Gilbert R.
Hess, Carla W.
Hoadley, Barbara R.
Hodson, Barbara W.
Hoffa, Jr., Daniel C.
Holland, Audrey L.

Holley, Sandra C.
Hood, Richard B.
Hood, Stephen B.
Hutchinson, Edward C.

I

Irwin, Ruth B.

J

Jerger, James F.
Johns, Donnell F.
Johnson, Kenneth O.
Johnson, Kenneth R.
Johnson, T. Earle
Jones, Bobby D.
Julis, Melvin

K

Kahl, W. Bailey
Kalas, Beth
Kasden, Stephen D.
Kau, Darlene M.
Keith, Robert W.
Keller, Geraldine B.
Kleffner, Frank R.
Klim, Charles J.
Knight, Paul D.
Koenigsknecht, Roy A.
Kretschmer, Laura W.
Kruger, Barbara
Kuba, Janis M.
Kunze, Luvern H.

L

Laguaite, Jeannette K.
Landes, Bernard
Larkin, Marilyn K.
Larson, Lillian
Lassman, Frank
Lathrop, Jennifer Fargo
Laufer, Marsha Z.
Law, Deborah
Lee, Corinne C.
Lehner, Leslie H.
Lehrhoff, Irwin
Leith, William R.
Leonard, Laurence
Leonard, Rebecca
Lingwall, James B.
Loavenbruck, Angela
Logemann, Jerilyn A.
Lorell, Daryl M.
**Louis, Timothy
Lovrinic, Jean Hahn
Lovrinic, William S.
Ludlow, Christy L.
Lustig, Vincent
Lynch, Joan I.

M

Madell, Jane Reger
Mahaffey, Robert B.
Malone, Russell
Marillo, Marie
Markwitz, Adele
Marshall, Mary H.
Marzell, Miriam
Massey, Holly J.
Matkin, Noel D.
May, Annette Anisman
McAlpine, Catherine A.
McClatchie, Adeline
McClelland, William
McConnell, Freeman
McFarlane, Stephen C.
McLauchlin, Robert M.
Melcher, Joe A.
Mencke, Eugene O.
Mendel, Maurice I.
Menyuk, Paula
Miller, Jon F.
Miller, June
Miller, Maurice H.
Mills, Jack R.
Minghetti, Nancy J.
Minifie, Fred D.
Moll, Kenneth L.
Monteleone, Ila K.
Montgomery, Allen A.
Moore, G. Paul
Murphy, C.W.
Mussen, Ethel F.
Myers, Margaret A.
Mysak, Edward D.

N

Naliboff, Ellen C.
Nathanson, Susan
Nelson, Lois A.
Nelson, Nickola W.
Newby, Hayes A.
Newton, Mariana
Noeth, Carolyn F.
Noffsinger, P. Douglas
Noll, J. Douglas
Northern, Jerry L.
Nuru, Njeri

O

O'Neill, John J.
O'Toole, Thomas J.
Olsen, Wayne
Olson, Don A.
Olson, Robert
Olswang, Lesley Barrett
Oyer, Herbert

P

Paesani, Jr., Andrew
Parish, Marion Robbins
Pendergast, Kathleen K.
Perkins, William
Peters, Theodore J.
Peterson, John L.
Pettas, Mary
Petty, Sr. Alice
Pickering, Marisue
Pike, Patricia
Plum, Marion K.
Podwall, Arthur
Popejoy, Maurice E.
Powell, Harold
Powers, Gene R.
Pressman, D. Elaine
Prins, David

R

Ratusnik, David L.
Reed, Andrea Brown
Rees, Norma S.
Reid, Philip
Revoile, Sally G.
Richardson, Sylvia O.
Riedman, Richard M.
Riley, Glyndon
Ringel, Robert L.
Rintelmann, William F.
Ripich, Danielle
Robinette, Martin S.
Rosen, Jack
Rosenstein, Joseph
Ross, Mark
Rosson, Grace L.
Rubin, Herbert

S

Salkowitz, Bobbe Bank
Sarno, Martha Taylor
Schiller, Newton M.
Schmidt, Robert K.
Schmitt, John F.
Schoen, Rosanne Z.
Scholl, Harold
Schultz, Adeline R.
Schwartz, Arthur H.
Schwartz, Ralph J.
Schwartz, Roberta
Scudder, Rosalind R.
Secord, Wayne A.
Seymour, Charlena
Shanks, Jr., James C.
Shapiro, Irving
Sheehan, Vivian M.
Shewan, Cynthia M.
Shifman, Suzanne
Shimizu, Hiroshi
Short, Mary G.
Shriberg, Lawrence D.
Shulman, Audrey O.
Shulman, Brian B.
Singer, Louis
Singh, Sadanand
Smith, Linda Lou
Smitheimer, Luella Sude
Snavely, Jan Allyson
Spahr, Frederick T.
Spriestersbach, Bette
Spriestersbach, D.C.
Stark, Rachel
Steer, Mack D.
Stein, Laszlo
Stephens, Myrna Mannila
Stockman, Ida S.
Stream, Kathryn S.
Sue-O'Brien, Debra
Sullivan, Jean A.

T

Telega, Mildred C.
Teter, Darrel Lee
Tompkins, Connie A.
Traynor, Robert M.
Trombly, Thelma
Tye-Murray, Nancy

U

Ulrich, Sandra R.
Uyehara-Isono, June M.

V

Van Vliet, Louise
Vaughn, Gwenyth R.
Ventry, Nona B.
Victor, Shelley

W

Wallace, Elizabeth
Walsh, Patricia S.
Wells, Charlotte
Westby, Carol
Whatley, Inez W.
White, Steven C.
Wiig, Elisabeth
Wilber, Laura Ann
Williams, Peggy S.
Wilson, Mary S.
Wisnia, Judith F.
Wolf, Kenneth E.
Wolf, Patricia L.
Wood, Mary Lovey
*Work, Rhonda Sue

Y

Yantis, Elna M.
Yantis, Phillip A.
Yoder, David E.

Z

Zaner, Annette R.
Zaslow, Elinor L.
Zinberg, Mildred
Zwislocki, Jozef

* Silver Founder
** Gold Founder

PRESIDENT'S CIRCLE

President's Circle members have contributed an aggregate of $1000.

A

Adler, Leslie

B

Barr, Nona Lee
Bon, Isidor
Boone, Daniel R.
Burkland, Marjorie B.

C

Castle, Diane S.
Castle, William E.

D

Dalzell, Larry E.
Dalzell, Sheila M.
Davison, Louise D.
DiCarlo, Louis M.

E

Ehrlich, Carol H.

F

Feldman, Alan S.
Fraser, Malcolm H.

G

Gelatt, James P.
Glattke, Theodore
Goldman, Ronald
Grason, Rufus L.
Griffin, Kathleen M.

H

Harden, Sheila H.

K

Kleffner, Frank R.

L

Laguaite, Jeannette K.
Lockwood, Herbert

M

Mason, LaRita
Matkin, Noel D.
Mussen, Ethel F.

O

Olson, Robert D.

S

Schwartz, Arthur H.
Shifman, Suzanne
Singh, Sadanand

V

Ventry, Nona B.

W

Work, Rhonda S.

Y

Yackel, John P.

1988 FOUNDATION ASSOCIATES

Foundation Associates have contributed at least $50 within the year.

A

Anderson, Bernard
Aram, Dorothy W.
Arzt, Aliza C.P.

B

Beere, Adele
Black, Helen
Burton, Wendy

C

Caplan, Francis A.
Cohen, Marla S.
Colodzin, Louise M.

D

Davis, Lynne
DeShaw, Donna
DeSola, Deborah

F

Favors, Aaron
Feldman, Irene R.
Florence, Mary L.

G

Gladwin, Helen J.
Gottfred, Catherine H.

H

Haas, William H.
Hagerman, Evie
Hayes, Deborah
Hewitt, Joan T.
Hoy, Sharon Ann

J

Jackson-Colando, Pat
Jerger, Susan W.

K

Kagel, Marion C.
Kamhi, Alan G.

L

Landsman, Carol
LaPointe, Leonard L.
Lesner, Sharon
Lipscomb, David M.

M

Malsbary, Anne G.
Morley, Russell D.
Munneke Margaret F.

N

Norton, Barbara

O

Orme, Cheryl L.

P

Peizer, Elaine

R

Rassi, Judith A.
Ritter, E. Gene
Royal, Carolyn A.

S

Sanderson, M.E.
Shelton, Jr., Ralph
Soll, Edward L.
Suematsu, Kikuyo

W

Watnick, Myra
Weiner, Fredrick F.
Wertz, Robert T.
Wolfe, Virginia

Y

Young, Edna C.

1988 FOUNDATION CORPORATE SPONSORS

Adaptive Communication Systems, Inc.
AGS/American Guidance Service, Inc.
Apple Computer, Inc.
Aspen Publishers, Inc.
Cochlear Corporation
Communi-Care, Inc.
Communication Skill Builders, Inc.
DLM Teaching Resources
Electone, Inc.
Etymotic Research, Inc.
Grason-Stadler, Inc.
Hear$_x$ Ltd.
InSpeech, Inc.
International Business Machines Corporation
Laureate Learning Systems, Inc.
LinguiSystems, Inc.
Mindscape, Inc.
Phonic Ear, Inc.
Prentke Romich Company
Psychological Corporation
United Educational Services, Inc.
Words+, Inc.
Xomed, Inc.

1988 STATE ASSOCIATION FOUNDERS

Arizona Speech-Language-Hearing Association
Arkansas Speech-Language-Hearing Association
California Speech-Language-Hearing Association
Connecticut Speech-Language-Hearing Association
District of Columbia Speech-Language-Hearing Association
Florida Language, Speech, and Hearing Association
Illinois Speech-Language-Hearing Association
Kentucky Speech-Language-Hearing Association
Louisiana Speech-Language-Hearing Association
Maine Speech-Language-Hearing Association
Massachusetts Speech-Language-Hearing Association
Mississippi Speech-Language-Hearing Association
Missouri Speech-Language-Hearing Association
Nebraska Speech-Language-Hearing Association
New Hampshire Speech-Language-Hearing Association
New Jersey Speech-Language-Hearing Association
New York State Speech-Language-Hearing Association
Ohio Speech and Hearing Association
Oregon Speech and Hearing Association
Pennsylvania Speech-Language-Hearing Association
Texas Speech-Language-Hearing Association
Utah Speech-Language-Hearing Association
Wisconsin Speech-Language-Hearing Association

1988 ORGANIZATIONAL SUPPORT

Academy of Rehabilitative Audiology
AGS/American Guidance Service, Inc.
Apple Computer, Inc.
Communi-Care, Inc.
Communication Skill Builders, Inc.
DLM Teaching Resources
InSpeech, Inc.
LinguiSystems, Inc.
Little, Brown & Company
Phonic Ear, Inc.
Prentke Romich Company
Psi Iota Xi
Todd Allan Printing, Inc.

ACCREDITED PROGRAMS EDUCATIONAL STANDARDS BOARD

September, 1988

The following list specifies those institutions of higher learning in which the master's degree program in speech-language pathology and/or audiology has been accredited by the Educational Standards Board (ESB) of the American Speech-Language-Hearing Association. ESB accreditation is sought voluntarily by educational programs that offer master's degrees in speech-language pathology, audiology, or both. The ESB accreditation program is recognized by the Council on Post-secondary Accreditation (COPA) and the U.S. Office of Education.

The area in which a program has been accredited by ESB is indicated by the letters SLP (speech-language pathology), A (audiology), or SLP/A (both) that appear to the right of each entry.

ESB accreditation offers a graduate the assurance that the academic and clinical practicum experience obtained in an accredited program meets nationally established standards. ESB accreditation means that a program has:

- engaged in extensive self-study often over a period of years;
- prepared and submitted a complex application often as much as a hundred pages long;
- undergone an on-site visit by a team of specially trained peers;
- received, and responded to, a digest of the report submitted by the site visitors;
- had their application, the site visit report, and their response thereto studied by ESB;
- undergone final evaluation and approval by ESB; and
- submitted annual reports during the period of their accreditation.

For information relative to a specific educational program, write to the director of the speech-language pathology and audiology program in care of the institution listed. Additional information about the profession can be obtained by writing to the American Speech-Language-Hearing Association, 10801 Rockville Pike, Rockville, Maryland 20852.

Alabama

Auburn University — SLP/A
Department of Communication Disorders
1199 Haley Center
Auburn 36849

University of Alabama — SLP/A
Department of Communicative Disorders
P.O. Box 870242
Tuscaloosa 35487

University of Montevallo — SLP/A
Department of Communication Science and Disorders
Montevallo 35115

University of South Alabama — SLP/A
Department of Speech Pathology and Audiology
Mobile 36688

Arizona

Arizona State University — SLP/A
Department of Speech and Hearing Science
Tempe 85281

University of Arizona — SLP/A
Speech and Hearing Sciences Department
104 Speech Bldg., #25
Tucson 85721

Arkansas

University of Central Arkansas — SLP
Speech Pathology/Communication Disorders
Box U 1745
Conway 72032

University of Arkansas at Fayetteville — SLP
Speech Pathology-Audiology Program
410 Arkansas Avenue
Fayetteville 72701

University of Arkansas at Little Rock — SLP/A
Department of Communicative Disorders
2601 S. University
Little Rock 72204

California

California State University, Chico — SLP
Speech Pathology and Audiology
Chico 95929-0222

California State University, Fresno — SLP/A
Department of Communicative Disorders
Fresno 93740

California State University, Fullerton — SLP
Department of Speech Communication
800 North State College Boulevard
Fullerton 92634

California State University, Los Angeles — SLP
Dept. of Communication Disorders
5151 State University Drive
Los Angeles 90032

California State University, Northridge — SLP/A
Department of Communicative Disorders
18111 Nordhoff Street
Northridge 91330

San Diego State University SLP/A
Department of Communicative Disorders
San Diego 92182

San Francisco State University SLP/A
Communicative Disorders Program
1600 Holloway Avenue
San Francisco 94132

San Jose State University SLP/A
Speech and Hearing Center
Washington Square
San Jose 95192

University of California, Santa Barbara SLP/A
Department of Speech and Hearing Sciences
Speech and Hearing Center
Santa Barbara 93106

University of the Pacific SLP
Department of Communicative Disorders
3601 Pacific Avenue
Stockton 95211

California State University, Long Beach SLP/A
Communicative Disorders
1250 Bellflower Boulevard
Long Beach 90840

California State University, Sacramento SLP/A
Department of Speech Pathology and Audiology
6000 J Street
Sacramento 95819

Colorado

University of Colorado SLP/A
Department of Communication Disorders and Speech Science
Campus Box 409
Boulder 80309

Colorado State University SLP/A
Department of Communication Disorders
Fort Collins 80523

University of Northern Colorado SLP/A
Department of Communication Disorders
Greeley 80639

Connecticut

Southern Connecticut State University SLP
Department of Communication Disorders
501 Crescent Street
New Haven 06515

University of Connecticut SLP/A
Department of Communication Sciences U-85
Storrs 06268

District of Columbia

University of the District of Columbia SLP
Department of Communication Sciences
916 G Street, N.W.
Washington 20001

Gallaudet University A
Department of Audiology and Speech-Language Pathology
800 Florida Avenue, N.E.
Washington, DC 20002

George Washington University SLP/A
Department of Speech and Hearing
2201 G Street, N.W.
Washington 20052

Howard University SLP
Department of Communication Arts and Sciences
Washington 20059

Florida

University of Florida SLP/A
Speech-Language Pathology and Audiology Program
Department of Speech
335 ASB (Speech)
Gainesville 32611

University of Central Florida SLP/A
Dept. of Communicative Disorders
4000 Central Florida Boulevard
Orlando 32816

Florida State University SLP/A
Department of Communication Disorders
304 Regional Rehabilitation Center
Tallahassee 32306

University of South Florida SLP/A
Department of Communicology
4202 E. Fowler Avenue
Tampa 33620

Georgia

University of Georgia SLP/A
Communication Sciences and Disorders
Aderhold Hall
Athens 30602

Hawaii

University of Hawaii at Manoa SLP/A
Division of Speech Pathology and Audiology
John A. Burns School of Medicine
1410 Lower Campus Drive
Honolulu 96822

Idaho

Idaho State University SLP/A
Department of Speech Pathology and Audiology
Box 8116
Pocatello 83209

Illinois

Southern Illinois University, Carbondale SLP
Communication Disorders and Sciences
Carbondale 62901

University of Illinois SLP/A
Speech and Hearing Science
220 Speech and Hearing Science Building
901 South 6th Street
Champaign 61820

Eastern Illinois University SLP
Department of Communication Disorders and Sciences
Charleston 61920

Northern Illinois University SLP/A
Department of Communicative Disorders
DeKalb 60115

Southern Illinois University at Edwardsville SLP
Department of Speech Pathology and Audiology
Box 1776
Edwardsville 62026

Northwestern University SLP/A
Department of Communicative Disorders
Francis Searle Building
2299 Sheridan Road
Evanston 60201

Western Illinois University SLP/A
Communication Arts and Sciences
Memorial Hall 121
Macomb 61455

Illinois State University SLP/A
Department of Speech Pathology and Audiology
Fairchild Hall, #204
Normal 61761

Governors State University SLP
Division of Communication Disorders
University Park 60466

Indiana

Indiana University SLP/A
Department of Speech and Hearing Sciences
Bloomington 47405

Ball State University SLP/A
Department of Speech Pathology and Audiology
200 University Avenue
Muncie 47306

Indiana State University SLP
Department of Communication Disorders
8th and Sycamore
Terre Haute 47809

Purdue University SLP/A
Department of Audiology and Speech Sciences
Heavilon Hall
West Lafayette 47907

Iowa

University of Northern Iowa SLP/A
Department of Communicative Disorders
Cedar Falls 50614

University of Iowa SLP/A
Department of Speech Pathology and Audiology
Wendell Johnson Speech and Hearing Center
Iowa City 52242

Kansas

Fort Hays State University SLP
Area of Communication Disorders
600 Park Street
Hays 67601

University of Kansas SLP/A
Intercampus Program in Speech-Language Pathology
Audiology and Speech and Hearing Science
290 Haworth Hall
Lawrence 66045

Kansas State University SLP
Leasure Hall
Department of Speech
Manhattan 66506

Wichita State University SLP/A
Department of Communicative Disorders
and Sciences
Box 75
Wichita 67208

Kentucky

Eastern Kentucky University SLP
Communication Disorders Program
Department of Special Education
Richmond 40475

University of Louisville SLP/A
Division of Communicative Disorders
Meyers Hall
129 E. Broadway
Louisville 40292

University of Kentucky SLP
Program in Speech and Communication Disorders
229 Taylor Education Building
Lexington 40506

Murray State University SLP
Division of Communication Disorders
16th and Main Streets
Murray 42071

Louisiana

Louisiana State University and Agricultural
and Mechanical College SLP
Division of Communication Disorders
Music and Dramatic Arts Bldg.
Baton Rouge 70803-2606

University of Southwestern Louisiana SLP
Department of Communicative Disorders
P.O. Box 43170
Lafayette 70504

Louisiana State University Medical Center SLP/A
Department of Communication Disorders
1900 Gravier Street
New Orleans 70112

Louisiana Tech University SLP
Department of Speech
Ruston 71272

Maine

University of Maine — SLP
Conley Speech and Hearing Center
North Stevens Hall
Orono 04469

Maryland

University of Maryland at College Park — SLP/A
Hearing and Speech Sciences
College Park 20742

Massachusetts

University of Massachusetts — SLP/A
Department of Communication Disorders
Arnold House, Room 6
Amherst 01003

Emerson College — SLP
Department of Communication Disorders
168 Beacon Street
Boston 02116

Northeastern University — SLP/A
Department of Speech-Language Pathology and Audiology
360 Huntington Avenue
Boston 02115

Boston University — SLP
Department of Communication Disorders
36 Cummington Street
Boston 02215

Worcester State College — SLP
Communication Disorders Department
486 Chandler Street
Worcester 01602-2597

Michigan

Wayne State University School of Medicine — A
Department of Audiology
5E University Health Center
540 East Canfield
Detroit 48201

Wayne State University — SLP
Communication Disorders and Sciences
555 Manoogian Hall
Detroit 48202

Michigan State University — SLP/A
Department of Audiology and Speech Sciences
378 Communication Arts and Science Bldg.
East Lansing 48824-1212

Western Michigan University — SLP/A
Department of Speech Pathology and Audiology
Kalamazoo 49008

Northern Michigan University — SLP
Department of Communication Disorders
Marquette 49855

Central Michigan University — SLP/A
Communication Disorders
Moore Hall 442
Mt. Pleasant 48859

Eastern Michigan University — SLP
Speech Pathology Program
Ypsilanti 48197

Minnesota

University of Minnesota, Duluth — SLP
Department of Communicative Disorders
2400 Oakland Avenue
Duluth 55812

University of Minnesota — SLP/A
Department of Communication Disorders
115 Shevlin Hall
164 Pillsbury Drive, S.E.
Minneapolis 55455

St. Cloud State University — SLP
Dept. of Communication Disorders
St. Cloud 56301

Mississippi

University of Southern Mississippi — SLP/A
Department of Speech and Hearing Sciences
P.O. Box 5092, Southern Station
Hattiesburg 39406

University of Mississippi — SLP/A
Department of Communicative Disorders
University 38677

Missouri

Southeast Missouri State University — SLP
Department of Speech Communication and Theatre
Cape Girardeau 63701

University of Missouri – Columbia — SLP
Program in Communicative Disorders
125 Parker Hall
Columbia 65211

Northeast Missouri State University — SLP
Department of Communication Disorders
Kirksville 63501

St. Louis University — SLP
Department of Communicative Disorders
3733 West Pine Boulevard
St. Louis 63108

Central Institute For the Deaf-Washington University — A
818 South Euclid Avenue
St. Louis 63110

Central Missouri State University — SLP/A
Speech Pathology and Audiology Department
Warrensburg 64093

Montana

University of Montana — SLP/A
Department of Communication Sciences and Disorders
Missoula 59812

Nebraska

Kearney State College — SLP
Communication Disorders Program
Kearney 68849-0507

University of Nebraska – Lincoln — SLP/A
Department of Special Education and Communication Disorders
202 Barkley Memorial Center
Lincoln 68583-0731

University of Nebraska at Omaha — SLP
Speech and Language Pathology
Department of Counseling and Special Education
Omaha 68182

Nevada

University of Nevada-Reno — SLP
Dept. of Speech Pathology and Audiology
Mackey Science Building
Reno 89557

New Jersey

Trenton State College — SLP
Graduate Programs in Speech Pathology and Audiology
Hillwood Lakes, CN 4700
Trenton 08650-4700

Montclair State College — SLP
Communication Sciences and Disorders
Upper Montclair 07043

William Paterson College — SLP
Department of Communication Disorders
300 Pompton Road
Wayne 07470

New Mexico

University of New Mexico — SLP/A
Department of Communicative Disorders
901 Vassar, N.E.
Albuquerque 87131

New Mexico State University — SLP
Communication Disorders
Las Cruces 88003

New York

Lehman College of the City University of New York — SLP
Department of Speech and Theatre
Speech and Hearing Center
Bedford Park Boulevard, West
Bronx 10468

Brooklyn College, City University of New York — SLP/A
Speech and Hearing Center
Bedford Avenue and Avenue H
Brooklyn 11210

State University College at Buffalo — SLP
Communication Disorders Program
1300 Elmwood Avenue
Buffalo 14222

State University of New York at Buffalo — SLP/A
Department of Communicative Disorders and Sciences
109 Park Hall
Buffalo 14260

Queens College of the City University of New York — SLP/A
Communication Sciences and Disorders
65-30 Kissena Blvd.
Flushing 11367

Adelphi University — SLP
Department of Speech Arts and Communicative Disorders
South Avenue
Garden City 11530

State University of New York College of Arts and Sciences — SLP/A
Department of Speech Pathology and Audiology
218 Sturges Hall
Geneseo 14454

Hofstra University — SLP/A
Department of Speech Arts and Sciences
Room 108 Roosevelt Hall
Hempstead 11550

Ithaca College — SLP/A
Department of Speech Pathology and Audiology
Ithaca 14850

Hunter College of City University of New York — SLP/A
Communication Sciences Program
School of Health Sciences
425 E. 25th Street
New York 10010

New York University — SLP
Speech Pathology and Audiology
Department of Communication Arts and Sciences
50 West 4th Street
New York 10003

Teachers College, Columbia University — SLP/A
Department of Speech and Language Pathology and Audiology
525 West 120th Street
New York 10027

Syracuse University — SLP/A
Communication Sciences and Disorders Programs
805 South Crouse Avenue
Syracuse 13210

North Carolina

East Carolina University — SLP/A
Dept. of Speech-Language and Auditory Pathology
Greenville 27834

University of North Carolina at Greensboro SLP
Division of Communication Disorders
FERG 300, UNCG
Greensboro 27412

North Dakota

University of North Dakota SLP
Department of Communication Disorders
P.O. Box 8040
Grand Forks 58202-8040

Minot State University SLP
Dept. of Communication Disorders
500 Nineth Avenue, N.W.
Minot 58701

Ohio

University of Akron SLP/A
Department of Communicative Disorders
302 E. Buchtel Avenue
Akron 44325

Ohio University SLP/A
School of Hearing and Speech Sciences
207 Lindley Hall
Athens 45701

Bowling Green State University SLP/A
Programs in Communication Disorders
Bowling Green 43403

University of Cincinnati SLP/A
Communication Disorders
Mail Station 379
Cincinnati 45221

Case Western Reserve University SLP
Department of Communication Sciences
11206 Euclid Avenue
Cleveland 44106

Cleveland State University SLP/A
Department of Speech and Hearing
Main Classroom 430
Euclid Avenue and E. 22nd Street
Cleveland 44115

Ohio State University SLP/A
Speech and Hearing Science
154 North Oval Mall
Columbus 43210

Kent State University SLP/A
School of Speech Pathology and Audiology
A104 Music and Speech Center
Kent 44242

Miami University SLP
Speech Pathology and Audiology
Bachelor Hall
Oxford 45056

Oklahoma

University of Oklahoma Health Sciences Center SLP/A
Department of Communication Disorders
825 N.E. 14th
Oklahoma City 73190

Oklahoma State University SLP
Speech and Language Pathology and Audiology
120 Hanner Hall
Stillwater 74078

University of Tulsa SLP
Dept. of Communicative Disorders and Sciences
600 South College Avenue
Tulsa 74104

Oregon

Portland State University SLP/A
Speech and Hearing Sciences Program
P.O. Box 751
Portland 97207

Pennsylvania

Temple University SLP/A
Division of Speech-Language and Hearing Sciences
Department of Speech
Philadelphia 19122

University of Pittsburgh SLP/A
Division of Speech Pathology – Audiology
5th Avenue and Bigelow Boulevard
1116 Cathedral of Learning
Pittsburgh 15260

Pennsylvania State University SLP/A
Communication Disorders Programs
110 Moore Building
University Park 16802

Puerto Rico

University of Puerto Rico SLP
Department of Communicology
Medical Sciences Campus
GPO 5067
San Juan 00936

Rhode Island

University of Rhode Island SLP/A
Dept. of Communicative Disorders
Kingston 02881

South Carolina

University of South Carolina SLP/A
Department of Communicative Disorders
Columbia 29208

South Dakota

University of South Dakota SLP
Communication Disorders Program
Department of Communication
Vermillion 57069

Tennessee

University of Tennessee SLP/A
Department of Audiology and Speech Pathology
457 South Stadium Hall
Knoxville 37996-0740

Memphis State University — SLP/A
Department of Audiology and Speech Pathology
807 Jefferson Avenue
Memphis 38105

Vanderbilt University — SLP/A
Division of Hearing and Speech Sciences
1114 19th Avenue, South
Nashville 37232

Tennessee State University — SLP
Department of Speech Pathology and Audiology
3500 John Merritt Boulevard
Nashville 37203

Texas

University of Texas at Austin — SLP/A
Program in Communication Disorders
Austin 78712

Lamar University — SLP
Department of Communication
Box 10076 – Lamar Station
Beaumont 77710

University of Texas at Dallas — SLP/A
Program in Communication Disorders
Callier Center for Communicative Disorders
1966 Inwood
Dallas 75235

University of North Texas — SLP/A
Division of Communication Disorders
Denton 76203

Texas Christian University — SLP
Dept. of Speech Communication
2800 S. University Drive
Ft. Worth 76129

University of Houston — SLP
Communication Disorders
Houston 77004

Texas Tech University — SLP/A
Speech and Hearing Sciences
Lubbock 79409

Our Lady of the Lake University — SLP
Communication and Learning Disorders
411 Southwest 24th Street
San Antonio 78285

Southwest Texas State University — SLP
Communication Disorders Program
San Marcos 78666

Utah

Utah State University — SLP/A
Department of Communicative Disorders
UMC 10
Logan 84322

Brigham Young University — SLP/A
Communication Sciences and Disorders
136 John Taylor Building
Provo 84602

University of Utah — SLP/A
Department of Communication Disorders
1201 Behavioral Science Building
Salt Lake City 84112

Vermont

University of Vermont — SLP
Department of Communication Sciences and Disorders
Allen House
Burlington 04505

Virginia

University of Virginia — SLP/A
Speech Pathology and Audiology
132 Emmet Street
Charlottesville 22906

James Madison University — SLP/A
Department of Speech Pathology and Audiology
Harrisonburg 22807

Hampton University — SLP
Dept. of Communication Disorders
Hampton 23668

Radford University — SLP/A
Dept. of Communication Sciences and Disorders
Radford 24142

Washington

Washington State University — SLP
Communications Disorders Program
Department of Speech, 218 Daggy Hall
Pullman 99164

Western Washington University — SLP/A
Department of Speech Pathology and Audiology
Bellingham 98225

University of Washington — SLP/A
Department of Speech and Hearing Sciences
4101 N.E. 15th
Seattle 98195

West Virginia

West Virginia University — SLP/A
Department of Speech Pathology and Audiology
P.O. Box 6122
Morgantown 26506-6122

Wisconsin

University of Wisconsin – Eau Claire — SLP
Department of Communication Disorders
Eau Claire 54702

University of Wisconsin – Madison — SLP/A
Department of Communicative Disorders
1975 Willow Drive
Madison 53706

Marquette University — SLP
Speech Pathology and Audiology
619 North 16th Street
Milwaukee 53233

University of Wisconsin – Milwaukee SLP
Department of Speech Pathology and Audiology
P.O. Box 413
Milwaukee 53201

University of Wisconsin – River Falls SLP
Dept. of Communicative Disorders
Kleinpell Fine Arts Building
River Falls 54022

University of Wisconsin – Stevens Point SLP/A
School of Communicative Disorders
2100 Main Street
Stevens Point 54481

University of Wisconsin – Whitewater SLP
Program in Communicative Disorders
Whitewater 53190

Wyoming

University of Wyoming SLP/A
Department of Speech-Language Pathology and Audiology
P.O. Box 3311 – University Station
Laramie 82071

ACCREDITED PROGRAMS PROFESSIONAL SERVICES BOARD

January, 1989

The following programs offering clinical services in speech-language pathology and/or audiology have been approved for accreditation by the Professional Services Board (PSB) of the American Speech-Language-Hearing Association. Accreditation in speech-language pathology, or audiology, or both is shown by the letters, SLP, A, or SLP/A to the right of each entry.

Accreditation by PSB signifies to the consumer, to referring agencies, and professionals, to third party payors and to the public and profession-at-large that the program meets exacting standards of professional service relating to governance, administration, staffing, clinical practices, and procedures, record-keeping, equipment and facilities. In order to attain accreditation the program must engage in a self-study and file an application; undergo a visit by peer reviewers drawn from other ASHA PSB-accredited programs; receive the approval of ASHA PSB following review of the application, site visit report and response of the program; file an annual report.

ASHA PSB accreditation is voluntarily initiated by making application to: Chair, Professional Services Board, American Speech-Language-Hearing Association, 10801 Rockville Pike, Rockville, Maryland 20852.

Alabama

University of Alabama-Birmingham — SLP/A
UAB Speech and Hearing Clinic
University Station
Box 187
Birmingham 35294

Lakeshore-Huntsville Rehabilitation Center — SLP/A
Speech Department
316 Longwood Drive, S.W.
Huntsville 35801

University of South Alabama-Mobile — SLP/A
Speech and Hearing Center
Humanities Building
Mobile 36688

Alaska

Alaska Department of Health and Social Services — SLP/A
Communicative Disorders Program
1231 Gambel
Anchorage 99501

Arizona

Good Samaritan Medical Center — A
Audiology Department
1111 East McDowell Road
Phoenix 85006

Good Samaritan Medical Center — SLP
Speech-Language Pathology Department
1111 East McDowell Road
Phoenix 85006

St. Joseph's Hospital and Medical Center — SLP/A
Speech-Language-Hearing Department
350 West Thomas Road
Phoenix 85013

Carondelet Health Services, Inc. — SLP
Speech-Language-Hearing Clinic
1601 West St. Mary's Road
Tucson 85703

California

Rancho Los Amigos Medical Center — SLP/A
Communication Disorders Service
7601 East Imperial Highway
Downey 90242

Community Speech and Hearing Center — SLP/A
7140 Balboa Boulevard
Van Nuys 91406

California State University, Fresno — SLP/A
Language, Hearing & Speech Clinic
Department of Communicative Disorders
Maple and Shaw Avenues
Fresno 93740

Valley Children's Hospital — SLP/A
Department of Speech-Language Pathology and Audiology
3151 North Millbrook
Fresno 93703

Veteran's Administration Hospital — SLP/A
Audiology and Speech Pathology Service
5901 East 7th Street
Long Beach 90822

VA Medical Center, West Los Angeles — SLP/A
Audiology and Speech Pathology Service (W126)
Wilshire and Sawtelle Boulevards
Los Angeles 90073

UCLA Medical School — SLP/A
Audiology and Speech Clinic
62-202 CHS
10833 LeConte Avenue
West Los Angeles 90024

Providence Speech and Hearing Center — SLP/A
Speech Pathology and Audiology Service
1308 Providence Avenue
Orange 92668

Letterman Army Medical Center — SLP/A
Speech Pathology and Auditory Evaluation and Treatment Clinic
Presidio of San Francisco 94129-6700

San Diego State University — SLP/A
Communications Clinic
Department of Communicative Disorders
5300 Campanile Drive
San Diego 92182

Speech, Hearing, Neurosensory Center — SLP/A
8001 Frost Street
San Diego 92123

Stanford University School of Medicine — A
Audiology Clinic
Division of Otolaryngology
R-135, 300 Pasteur Drive
Stanford 94305

Colorado

Memorial Hospital, Boulder — SLP
Department of Speech Pathology and Audiology
311 Mapleton Avenue
Boulder 80302

Porter Memorial Hospital — SLP/A
Speech and Hearing Department
2525 South Downing Street
Denver 80210

Children's Hospital — SLP/A
Audiology and Speech Pathology Department
1056 East 19th Avenue
Denver 80218

The University of Northern Colorado — SLP/A
Speech-Language Pathology and Audiology Clinics
Department of Communication Disorders
Greeley 80639

Connecticut

East Hartford Board of Education — SLP
Language, Speech and Hearing Services
110 Long Hill Road
East Hartford 06168

Southern Connecticut State University — SLP
Center for Communication Disorders
501 Crescent Street
New Haven 06515

Stamford Public Schools — SLP
Speech, Language, Hearing Program
195 Hillandale Avenue
Stamford 06902

Stamford Private School Health Program — SLP
Language, Speech and Hearing Services
888 Washington Boulevard
Stamford 06904-2152

The University of Connecticut-Storrs — SLP/A
Speech and Hearing Clinic
Department of Communication Sciences
Box U-85, Communication Sciences Building
Storrs 06268

Gaylord Hospital — SLP/A
Communication Disorders Department
P.O. Box 400
Wallingford 06492

Wethersfield Public Schools — SLP
Department of Communication Development
51 Willow Street, Webb Building
Wethersfield 06109

Delaware

Delaware Curative Workshop — SLP
Speech Department
1600 Washington Street
Wilmington 19802

The Medical Center of Delaware — SLP/A
Speech and Hearing Center
501 West 14th Street
Wilmington 19899

Riverside Hospital — A
Hearing Center
700 Lea Boulevard
Wilmington 19899

District of Columbia

Walter Reed Army Medical Center — SLP/A
Army Audiology and Speech Center
The Department of the Army
Washington, D.C. 20307-5001

Washington Hospital Center — SLP/A
Hearing and Speech Center
110 Irving Street, N.W.
Washington, D.C. 20010

Florida

Morton F. Plant Hospital — SLP/A
Dept. of Speech, Hearing and Learning Services
430 Pirellas Street
Clearwater 33516

Speech and Hearing Center, Inc. — SLP/A
1128 Laura Street
Jacksonville 33206

Central Florida Speech and Hearing Center, Inc. — SLP/A
710 East Bella Vista Street
Lakeland 33805

Munroe Regional Medical Center — SLP
Speech Pathology Services
Department of Rehabilitation
131 S.W. 15th Street
P.O. Box 6000
Ocala 32678

Baptist Hospital — SLP/A
Speech and Hearing Clinic
1000 West Moreno Street
Pensacola 32501

All Children's Hospital — SLP/A
Speech-Language-Hearing Centers
P.O. Box 31020
St. Petersburg 33731-8920

Florida State University — SLP
The Speech and Hearing Clinic
Department of Communication Disorders
Room 113
Regional Rehabilitation Center
Tallahassee 32306

Georgia

Atlanta Speech School, Inc. — SLP/A
3160 Northside Parkway, N.W.
Atlanta 30327

The Davison School, Inc. — SLP
1500 North Decatur Road, N.E.
Atlanta 30306

Easter Seal Speech and Hearing Center — SLP
Georgia Easter Seal Society
2228 Starling Street
Brunswick 31520

Northeast Georgia Speech Center — SLP
621 East Spring Street
P.O. Box 1482
Gainesville 30503

Gracewood State School and Hospital — SLP/A
Speech and Hearing Clinic
Gracewood 30812-1299

Hawaii

Tripler Army Medical Center — SLP/A
Audiology and Speech Pathology Clinic
Honolulu 96859-5000

Illinois

University of Illinois at Urbana-Champaign — SLP/A
Speech and Hearing Clinic
901 South Sixth Street
Champaign 61820

Henry Horner Children's Center — SLP/A
Speech-Language-Hearing Service
Institute for Juvenile Research
4201 North Oak Park Avenue
Chicago 60634

David T. Siegel Institute for Communicative Disorder — SLP/A
Michael Reese Medical Center
3033 South Cottage Grove
Chicago 60616

Rush Presbyterian-St. Luke's Medical Center — SLP/A
Section of Communication Disorders
1753 West Congress Parkway
Chicago 60612

Rehabilitation Institute of Chicago — SLP/A
Speech Pathology and Audiology
Department of Communicative Disorders
345 East Superior Street
Chicago 60611

Schwab Rehabilitation Center — SLP/A
Department of Communicative Disorders
1401 South California Boulevard
Chicago 60608

Northern Illinois University — SLP/A
Speech and Hearing Clinic
DeKalb 60115

Jayne Shover Easter Seal Rehabilitation Center, Inc. — SLP/A
Communication Disorders Department
799 South McLean Boulevard
Elgin 60120

Elaine S. Dunn, Ph.D., Ltd. — SLP
Disorders of Speech and Language
636 Church Street
Evanston 60201

Northwestern University — SLP/A
Speech Language Pathology and Audiology
Department of Communicative Disorders
Frances Searle Building
2299 Sheridan Road
Evanston 60201

Foster G. McGaw Hospital — SLP/A
Loyola University Medical Center
Communicative Disorders
Speech Pathology and Audiology
2160 South First Avenue
Maywood 60153

Marianjoy Rehabilitation Hospital — SLP
Speech Pathology Department
26 West 171 Roosevelt Road
Wheaton 60187

Iowa

Mississippi Bend Area Education Agency — SLP/A
Department of Hearing Conservation-Educational Services
Department of Clinical Speech and Language Services
729 21st Street
Bettendorf 52722

St. Luke's Methodist Hospital — SLP/A
Department of Speech Pathology and Audiology
1026 A Avenue, N.E.
Cedar Rapids 52402

Des Moines Hearing and Speech Center — SLP/A
3004 30th Street
Des Moines 50310

VA Medical Center — SLP/A
Audiology-Speech Pathology Service
1515 West Pleasant Street
Knoxville 50138

Kansas

The Capper Foundation for Crippled Children — SLP
Speech Pathology Department
3500 West 10th Street
Topeka 66604

Institute of Logopedics — SLP/A
Client Services
2400 Jardine Drive
Wichita 67219

Kentucky

Geiger Easter Seal Speech and Hearing Center — SLP/A
2201 Lexington Avenue
P.O. Box 151
Ashland 41105-0151

Northern Kentucky Easter Seal Center — SLP
Speech and Hearing Center
212 Levassor Avenue
Covington 41014

Cardinal Hill Hospital — SLP
Department of Speech/Language Pathology
2050 Versailles Road
Lexington 40504

Kentucky Easter Seal Society — SLP/A
Hearing and Speech Center
233 East Broadway
Louisville 40202

Murray State University — SLP/A
Speech and Hearing Clinic
Murray 42071

Eastern Kentucky University — SLP
Communication Disorders Program
Speech, Language, Hearing Clinic
Wallace 245
Richmond 40475

Louisiana

Children's Hospital — SLP/A
Speech, Language and Audiology Department
200 Henry Clay Avenue
New Orleans 70118

Louisiana State University Medical Center — SLP/A
Department of Communication Disorders
School of Allied Health Professions
1900 Gravier Street
New Orleans 70119

New Orleans Speech and Hearing Center — SLP/A
1636 Toledano Street
New Orleans 70115

Maine

Pine Tree Society for Crippled Children and Adults, Inc. — SLP/A
Speech and Hearing Services
P.O. Box 518
Bath 04530

Northeast Hearing and Speech Center, Inc. — SLP/A
43 Baxter Boulevard
Portland 04101

York County Counseling Services, Inc. — SLP/A
Speech and Hearing Program
P.O. Box 1010
Saco 04072

F. T. Hill Center for Communication Disorders — SLP/A
Mid-Maine Medical Center
Waterville 04901

Maryland

Easter Seal Society of Central Maryland — SLP
Communication Disorders Program
3700 Fourth Street
Baltimore 21225

University of Maryland at Baltimore — SLP
Shock Trauma Center and Montebello Rehabilitation Hospital
Maryland Institute for Emergency Medical Services System (MIEMSS)
Speech-Communication Disorders Program
22 S. Greene Street
Baltimore 21201

John F. Kennedy Institute — SLP/A
Communication Sciences and Disorders
707 North Broadway
Baltimore 21205

St. Agnes Hospital — SLP/A
Audiology Speech/Language Section
900 Caton Avenue
Baltimore 21229

Kilby Easter Seal Center — SLP
Easter Seal Society for Disabled Children and Adults, Inc.
Speech and Language Program
6400 Laurel-Bowie Road
Bowie 20715

Prince George's County Health Department — SLP/A
Division of Speech and Audiology
Cheverly 20785

Baltimore County Department of Health — SLP/A
Division of Speech, Language and Hearing
Eastern Regional Health Center
9100 Franklin Square Drive
Baltimore 21237

Leo Kanner Speech and Hearing Center — SLP/A
Rosewood Center
Owings Mills 21117

Montgomery County Public Schools — SLP
Division of Speech and Language Programs
850 Hungerford Drive
Rockville 20850

The Treatment and Learning Centers — SLP/A
9975 Medical Center Drive
Rockville 20850

Baltimore County Public Schools — SLP/A
Speech, Hearing and Language Therapy Program
6901 North Charles Street
Towson 20204

Massachusetts

Acton Boxborough Regional Schools — SLP
Speech and Language Department
96 Haywood Road
Acton 01720

Amherst Regional Schools and
Amherst-Pelham Schools — SLP
Language and Speech Services
Chestnut Street
Amherst 01002

University of Massachusetts — SLP/A
Communication Disorders Clinic
Arnold House, Room 6
Amherst 01003

Beverly Hospital — SLP/A
Center for Communication Disorders
Herrick Street
Beverly 01915

Beth Israel Hospital — A
Department of Audiology
330 Brookline Avenue
Boston 02215

Boston Guild for the Hard of Hearing — A
Audiology Services
283 Commonwealth Avenue
Boston 02115

Daniels Speech and Language Clinic — SLP
University Hospital
Boston University Medical Center
75 East Newton Street
Boston 02118

The Children's Hospital Medical Center — SLP/A
Hearing and Speech Division
300 Longwood Avenue
Boston 02115

Massachusetts Eye and Ear Infirmary — A
243 Charles Street
Boston 02114

Massachusetts General Hospital — SLP
Speech-Language Pathology Department
Boston 02114

Spaulding Rehabilitation Hospital — SLP
Speech-Language Pathology Department
125 Nashua Street
Boston 02114

New England Medical Center Hospitals — SLP/A
Speech, Hearing, and Language Center
185 Harrison Avenue
Boston 02111

Northeastern University — SLP/A
Department of Speech-Language Pathology
and Audiology
360 Huntington Avenue
Boston 02115

Brigham and Women's Hospital — SLP/A
Speech and Hearing Division
75 Francis Street
Boston 02115

Braintree Hospital — SLP/A
Center for Communication Disorders
250 Pond Street
Braintree 02184

Kennedy Memorial Hospital for Children — SLP/A
Speech-Language Pathology
and Audiology Departments
30 Warren Street
Brighton 02135

Clinton Hospital — SLP/A
Speech, Language and Hearing Department
201 Highland Street
Clinton 01510

Dracut Public Schools — SLP/A
Speech-Language Pathology Program
2063 Lakeview Avenue
Dracut 01826

Burbank Hospital — SLP/A
Speech Language and Hearing Center
Nichols Road
Fitchburg 01420

The Learning Center for Deaf Children — A
Audiological Evaluation Unit
848 Central Street
Framingham 01701

Franklin Medical Center — SLP/A
Communication Disorders Department
164 High Street
Greenfield 01301

The Faulkner Hospital — A
Audiology Department
1153 Centre Street
Jamaica Plain 02130

North Shore Children's Hopsital — SLP/A
Department of Language, Speech, and Hearing
57 Highland Avenue
Salem 01970

Mercy Hospital — SLP/A
Speech, Hearing, and Language Center
P.O. Box 90126 - 271 Carew Street
Springfield 01102-9012

New England Memorial Hospital — SLP/A
Department of Speech-Language
Pathology & Audiology
Five Wodland Road
Stoneham 02180

New England Sinai Hospital — SLP/A
Speech, Language and Hearing Clinic
150 York Street
P.O. Box 647
Stoughton 02072

Morton Hospital — SLP/A
Speech, Hearing, and Language Center
88 Washington Street
Taunton 02780

The Waltham-Weston Hospital and Medical Center — SLP/A
Center for Speech, Language and Hearing
9 Hope Avenue
Waltham 02254-9116

University of Massachusetts Medical Center — SLP/A
Audiology and Speech-Language Pathology Departments
55 Lake Avenue
Worcester 01605

Hahnemann Rehabilitation Center — SLP/A
Audiology/Speech Pathology Department
Worcester Hahnemann Hospital
Lincoln Plaza – 535 Lincoln Street
Worcester 01605

Worcester State College — SLP
Communications Disorders Clinic
486 Chandler Street
Worcester 01602-2597

Michigan

University of Michigan Hospitals — SLP
Division of Speech/Language Pathology
Department of Physical Medicine and Rehabilitation
1500 East Medical Center Drive
Ann Arbor 48109

Marie Carls Communication Disorders Center — SLP/A
Children's Hospital of Michigan
3901 Beaubien
Detroit 48201

Sinai Hospital of Detroit — SLP/A
Department of Rehabilitation Medicine
Section of Speech-Language Pathology and Audiology
6767 West Outer Drive
Detroit 48235-2899

McLaren General Hospital — SLP/A
Speech and Hearing Department
401 Ballenger Highway
Flint 48502

Mott Children's Health Center — SLP/A
Speech and Hearing Service
806 West Sixth Avenue
Flint 48503

Hurley Medical Center — SLP
Speech Pathology
One Hurley Place
Flint 48502

Comprehensive Audiologic Services — A
2566 Woodmeadow Drive, SE
Grand Rapids 49506

Psychiatric Consultation Services — SLP
Speech and Language Services
825 Parchment Drive, S.E.
Grand Rapids 49506

West Michigan Hearing Ctr. — A
111 West 24th Street
Holland 49423

Contance Brown Hearing and Speech Center — SLP/A
Borgess Medical Center
1521 Gull Road
Kalamazoo 49001

VanBuren Intermediate School District — SLP/A
Special Education Services
701 So. Paw Paw Street
Lawrence 49064

Central Michigan University — SLP/A
Speech-Language-Hearing Clinic
Mt. Pleasant 48859

Cognitive Restructuring Center — SLP
Total Therapy Management
28511 Orchard Lake Road – Suite A
Farmington Hills 48018

Oakland Schools Intermediate District — SLP/A
Speech and Hearing Clinic
2100 Pontiac Lake Road
Pontiac 48054

William Beaumont Hospital — SLP
Speech/Language Pathology Department
3601 West Thirteen Mile Road
Royal Oak 48072

Providence Hospital — A
Department of Audiology and Neurological Evoked Potentials
16001 West Nine Mile Road
P.O. Box 2043
Southfield 48037

Providence Hospital — SLP
Department of Speech-Language Pathology
16001 West Nine Mile Road
P.O. Box 2043
Southfield 48037

Eastern Michigan University — SLP/A
Speech and Hearing Program
Rackham Building
Ypsilanti 48197

Mississippi

Mississippi University for Women — SLP/A
Speech and Hearing Clinic
P.O. Box W-1340
Columbus 39701

University of Southern Mississippi — SLP/A
Speech and Hearing Clinic
Box 5092, Southern Station
Hattiesburg 39401

Easter Seal Speech and Language Clinic — SLP
Mississippi Easter Seal Society
P.O. Box 4221
3226 North State Street
Jackson 39216

The University of Mississippi — SLP/A
Speech and Hearing Center
University 38677

Missouri

University of Missouri-Columbia Hospital and Clinics — SLP
Communication Disorders Unit
One Hospital Drive
Columbia 65212

Children's Mercy Hospital — SLP/A
Hearing and Speech Department
24th and Gillham Road
Kansas City 64108

Central Institute for the Deaf — SLP/A
Hearing, Language and Speech Clinic
818 South Euclid
St. Louis 63112

The Special School District of St. Louis County — SLP/A
Speech, Language, Hearing Programs
12110 Clayton Road
Town and Country 63131

Montana

University of Montana — SLP/A
Speech, Hearing and Language Clinic
Missoula 59812

Nebraska

Educational Service Unit #9 — SLP
Speech and Language Services Program
1117 East South Street
P.O. Box 2047
Hastings 68901

University of Nebraska-Lincoln — SLP/A
Special Education and Communication Disorders
301A Barkley Memorial Center
Lincoln 68583-0731

Boys Town National Institute for Communication Disorders in Children — SLP/A
555 North 30th Street
Omaha 68131

New Jersey

The Robert Wood Johnson, Jr. Rehabilitation Institute — SLP/A
Speech and Hearing Department
John F. Kennedy Medical Center
James Street
Edison 08817

Hunterdon Medical Center — SLP/A
Speech and Hearing Department
Route 31
Flemington 08822

Hackensack Medical Center — SLP/A
Institute for Child Development
30 Prospect Avenue – Johnson Hall
Hackensack 07601

Saint Barnabas Medical Center — SLP/A
Rehabilitation Center for Speech and Hearing
Old Short Hills Road
Livingston 07039

Roosevelt Hospital — SLP
Speech Pathology and Audiology Department
P.O. Box 151
Metuchen 08840

The Matheny School/Hospital — SLP
Speech and Language Department
Main Street
Peapack 07977

North Jersey Developmental Center — SLP/A
Department of Speech Pathology/Audiology
P.O. Box 169
Totowa 07511

William Paterson College — SLP
Speech Pathology Clinic
300 Pompton Road
Wayne 07470

Kessler Institute — SLP
Speech and Audiology Department
Pleasant Valley Way
West Orange 07052

Children's Specialized Hospital — SLP/A
Speech and Hearing Department
New Providence Road
Westfield-Mountainside 07091

New Mexico

Lovelace Medical Center — A
Audiology Section
5200 Gibson Avenue, S.E.
Albuquerque 87108

New York

Easter Seal Speech and Hearing Center — SLP
107 Washington Avenue
Albany 12210

Mount Saint Ursula Speech Center — SLP
200th Street and Marion Avenue
Bronx 10458

Montefiore Hospital and Medical Center — SLP/A
Speech and Hearing Center
111 East 210th Street
Bronx 10467

North Central Bronx Hospital — SLP
Speech-Language Pathology
Rehabilitation Medicine (4F)
3424 Kossuth Avenue
Bronx 10467

Hospital of the Albert Einstein College of Medicine and Montefiore Medical Center — A
Audiology Clinic 2S51-RDC
1825 Eastchester Rd.
Bronx 10461

The Brooklyn Hospital — SLP/A
Speech and Hearing Center
121 DeKalb Avenue
Brooklyn 11201

SUNY, Buffalo — SLP/A
Speech Pathology & Audiology Clinic
Department of Communication Disorders & Sciences
130 Park Hall
Buffalo 14260

Queens College - CUNY — SLP/A
Speech and Hearing Center
65-30 Kissena Boulevard
Flushing 11367

Hy Weinberg Center for Communication Disorders — SLP/A
Adelphi University
P.O. Box 701
158 Cambridge Ave.
Garden City 11530

Hofstra University — SLP
Speech and Hearing Center
Hempstead 11550

Lexington Hearing and Speech Center — SLP/A
74-20 25th Avenue
Jackson Heights 11370

North Shore University Hospital — SLP/A
Speech Pathology and Audiology Services
300 Community Drive
Manhasset 11030

Long Island Jewish Medical Center — SLP/A
Audiology and Speech Pathology
New Hyde Park 11042

City School District of New Rochelle — SLP
Speech and Hearing Department
515 North Avenue
New Rochelle 10801

Beth Israel Medical Center — SLP/A
Speech & Hearing Division
Department of Surgery
Nathan D. Perlman Place
New York 10003

Hunter College - CUNY — SLP/A
Communication Disorders
School of Health Sciences
425 East 25th Street
New York 10010

ICD-International Center for the Disabled — SLP
Speech and Hearing Department
340 East 24th Street
New York 10010

Lenox Hill Hospital — SLP/A
Center for Communication Disorders
100 East 77th Street
New York 10021

Marymount Manhattan College — SLP
Communication and Learning Center
221 East 71st Street
New York 10021

Mount Sinai Medical Center — SLP/A
Communication Disorders Center
One Gustave L. Levy Place
New York 10029

New York Eye and Ear Infirmary — A
310 East 14th Street
New York 10003

New York League for the Hard of Hearing — SLP/A
71 West 23rd Street
New York 10010

Institute of Rehabilitation Medicine — SLP
New York University Medical Center
Speech/Language Pathology Service
400 East 34th Street
New York 10016

Teachers College, Columbia University — SLP/A
Speech and Hearing Center
525 West 120 Street
New York 10027

Hearing and Speech Center of Rochester — SLP/A
1000 Elmwood Avenue
Rochester 14620

Strong Memorial Hospital — SLP/A
Department of Audiology and Speech Pathology
601 Elmwood Avenue
Rochester 14642

Goldwater Memorial Hospital — SLP/A
Speech Pathology and Audiology Services
New York University Medical Center
Roosevelt Island 10044

Arthur Podwall, M.S. & Associates — SLP/A
222 East Main Street
Smithtown 11787

Syosset Speech and Hearing Center — SLP/A
Syosset Medical Building
175 Jericho Turnpike
Syosset 11791

SUNY - Upstate Medical Center — SLP/A
State University Hospital
Communication Disorder Unit
766 Irving Avenue
Syracuse 13210

VA Medical Center — SLP/A
Audiology and Speech Pathology Service
800 Irving Avenue
Syracuse 13210

Blythedale Children's Hospital — SLP/A
Department of Speech Pathology and Audiology
Bradhurst Avenue
Valhalla 10595

Wassaic Developmental Center — SLP/A
Communication Disabilities Department
Station A
Wassaic 12592

The Burke Rehabilitation Center — SLP/A
Speech/Language and Audiology Department
785 Mamaroneck Avenue
White Plains 10605

St. Agnes Hospital — SLP
Children's Rehabilitation Center
Speech Pathology Department
305 North Street
White Plains 10600

North Carolina

Partin Speech and Hearing Center — SLP
Thoms Rehabilitation Hospital, Inc.
of Western North Carolina
One Rotary Drive
Asheville 28803

Charlotte Speech and Hearing Center — SLP/A
300 South Caldwell Street
Charlotte 28202

Southeastern Speech and Hearing — SLP/A
Services of North Carolina, Inc.
226 Bradford Avenue, P.O. Box 53415
Fayetteville 28315

North Dakota

University of North Dakota — SLP/A
Medical Center Rehabilitation Hospital
Department of Communication Disorders
1300 South Columbia Road
Grand Forks 58201

Ohio

University of Akron — SLP/A
Speech and Hearing Center
West Hall
Akron 44325

Ohio University — SLP/A
Speech and Hearing Clinic
Lindley Hall
Athens 45701

Bes-Mont Speech, Hearing and Language Center — SLP
Wells Professional Building
515 Third Street, N.W.
Canton 44703

South Central Ohio Speech & Hearing Center — SLP/A
30 North Walnut Street
Chillicothe 45601

Cincinnati Speech and Hearing Center — SLP/A
3021 Vernon Place
Cincinnati 45219

University of Cincinnati Medical Center — SLP/A
Division of Audiology and Speech Pathology
234 Goodman Street
Cincinnati 45267

Cleveland Clinic Foundation — SLP/A
Dept. of Otolarynology & Comm. Disorders
Section of Communicative Disorders
9500 Euclid Avenue
Cleveland 44106

Cleveland Hearing and Speech Center — SLP/A
11206 Euclid Avenue
Cleveland 44106

Cleveland Metropolitan General/Highland — SLP/A
View Hospital
Communication Disorders
3395 Scranton Road
Cleveland 44109

Cleveland State University — SLP/A
Speech and Hearing Clinic
Main Classroom Building, Room 418
Euclid and East 22nd Street
Cleveland 44115

Fairview General Hospital — SLP/A
Speech Pathology and Audiology Department
18101 Lorain Avenue
Cleveland 44111

The Ohio State University — SLP/A
Speech and Hearing Clinic
154 North Ovall Mall
318 Derby Hall
Columbus 43210

Columbus Speech & Hearing Center — SLP/A
4410 North High Street
Columbus 43214

Hearing and Speech Center for Children — SLP/A
and Adults of Metropolitan Dayton
730 Valley Street
Dayton 45404

Delaware Speech and Hearing Center — SLP/A
27 West Central Avenue
Delaware 43015

Lima Memorial Hospital — SLP/A
Speech and Hearing Clinic
1001 Bellefontaine Avenue
Lima 45804

The Marion Therapy Center — SLP/A
Speech and Hearing Clinic
269 Rose Avenue
Marion 43302

West Central Ohio Hearing and Speech Center — SLP/A
2612 Elmore Drive
Springfield 45505

Medical College of Ohio Hospital SLP/A
Speech Language Pathology and Audiology Services
3000 Arlington Avenue
C.S. #10008
Toledo 43699

Toledo Hearing and Speech Center SLP/A
Community Services Building
One Stranahan Square
Toledo 43604

Toledo Hospital SLP/A
Communication Disorders Program
2142 North Cove Boulevard
Toledo 43606

Oklahoma

University of Oklahoma Health Sciences Center SLP/A
Speech and Hearing Clinic
825 Northeast 14th Street
Oklahoma City 73100

Oregon

Clatsop City Education Service District SLP
Speech, Language, and Hearing Program
3194 Marine Drive
Astoria 97103

Eugene Hearing and Speech Center SLP/A
1202 Almaden Street
P.O. Box 2087
Eugene 97402

Umatilla Education Service District SLP/A
Speech-Language & Hearing Services
P.O. Box 38
412 Southeast Dorion
Pendleton 97801

Portland Center for Hearing & Speech SLP/A
3515 S.W. Veterans Hospital Road
Portland 97201

The Oregon Health Sciences University SLP/A
Speech Pathology/Audiology Section
Crippled Children's Division
P.O. Box 574
Portland 97207

Pennsylvania

Sacred Heart Hospital SLP/A
Speech and Hearing Center
421 Chew Street
Allentown 18102

Bloomsburg University SLP/A
Speech, Hearing and Language Clinic
Bloomsburg 17815

Capital Area Intermediate Unit SLP/A
Department of Communication Disorders
2929 Old Gettysburg Road
Camp Hill 17011

Geisinger Medical Center SLP/A
Audiology and Speech Pathology
Danville 17822

Polyclinic Medical Center SLP/A
Speech and Hearing Center
2601 North Third Street
Harrisburg 17105

Hearing Conservation/Deaf Services Center, Inc. A
630 Janet Avenue
Lancaster 17601

Robinson Developmental Center SLP
Speech Pathology and Audiology Services
Clever Road
McKees Rocks 15136

Moss Rehabilitation Hospital SLP/A
Center for Comm. Disorders
12th and Taber Road
Philadelphia 19141

Philadelphia College of Osteopathic Medicine SLP/A
Division of Speech and Hearing
4150 City Avenue
Philadelphia 19131

University of Pittsburgh SLP
Speech & Hearing Clinic
1109 Cathedral of Learning
Pittsburgh 15269

Children's Hospital of Pittsburgh SLP
Department of Communication Disorders
125 DeSoto Street
Pittsburgh 15213

The Pennsylvania State University SLP/A
Speech and Hearing Clinic
111 Moore Building
University Park 16802

Rhode Island

Rhode Island Hospital SLP/A
Hearing and Speech Center
593 Eddy Street
Providence 02902

South Carolina

University of South Carolina
Speech and Hearing SLP/A
1601 St. Julian Place
Middleburg Office Park
Columbia 29204

Pee Dee Speech and Hearing Center SLP/A
153 North Baroody Street
P.O. Box 804
Florence 29503

Tennessee

University of Tennessee SLP/A
Hearing and Speech Center
Stadium Drive at Yale Avenue
Knoxville 37996

Memphis State University — SLP/A
Speech and Hearing Center
807 Jefferson Avenue
Memphis 38105

Bill Wilkerson Hearing and Speech Center — SLP/A
1114 19th Avenue, South
Nashville 37212

Texas

South Texas Speech, Hearing, and Language Center — SLP/A
P.O. Box 331246
1415 Third Street, Suite 307
Corpus Christi 78404

The Callier Center for Communication Disorders — SLP/A
The University of Texas at Dallas
1966 Inwood Road
Dallas 75235

North Texas State University — SLP/A
Speech and Hearing Center
Division of Communication Disorders
P.O. Box 5008, NTSU Station
Denton 76203

The University of Texas Medical Branch — SLP/A
Center for Audiology and Speech Pathology
Department of Otolaryngology
Galveston 77550

The Battin Clinic — SLP/A
3931 Essex Lane, Suite G
Houston 77027

Baylor College of Medicine - Methodist Hospital — SLP/A
Audiology & Speech Pathology Programs
6501 Fannin Street, NA 200
Houston 77030

University of Texas Health Science Center at Houston — SLP/A
Speech and Hearing Institute
1343 Moursund Avenue
Houston 77030

Richardson Independent School District — SLP
Speech-Language Services
400 South Greenville Avenue
Richardson 75080

Brooke Army Medical Center — A
Audiology Evaluation and Treatment Clinic
Otolaryngology Service, Beach Pavillon
Fort Sam Houston
San Antonio 78234

Harry Jersig Center for Language, Speech, Hearing, Learning Disorders — SLP/A
Our Lady of the Lake University
411 S.W. 24th Street
San Antonio 78285

Southwest Texas State University — SLP
Speech-Hearing-Language Clinic
NED 2040 - SWTSU
San Marcos 78666

Vaughn Memorial Speech and Hearing Center — SLP/A
P.O. Drawer 6400
Tyler 75711

Texas Tech University — SLP/A
Speech Pathology and Audiology
Box 4266
Lubbock 79409

Utah

Utah State Department of Health — SLP/A
Bureau of Communicative Disorders
44 Medical Drive
Salt Lake City 84113

Vermont

Eleanor M. Luse Center for Communication Disorders — SLP/A
University of Vermont
Burlington 05405

Virginia

The Mount Vernon Hospital — SLP
Speech-Language Pathology Service
Physical Medicine and Rehabilitation Department
2501 Parker's Lane
Alexandria 22306

University of Virginia — SLP/A
Speech and Hearing Center
109 Cabell Hall
Charlottesville 29903

Woodrow Wilson Rehabilitation Center — SLP/A
Department of Communication Services
Fisherville 22939

James Madison University — SLP/A
Speech and Hearing Center
Harrisonburg 22807

Central Virginia Speech and Hearing Center, Inc. — SLP/A
Virginia Baptist Hospital
Lynchburg 24503

Roanoke Valley Speech and Hearing Center, Inc. — SLP/A
2030 Colonial Avenue, S.W.
Roanoke 24015

Danville Speech and Hearing Center — SLP
610 Upper Street
Danville 24541

Washington

Hearing, Speech and Deafness Center — SLP/A
Speech/Language and Audiology Services
1620 18th Avenue
Seattle 98122

Speech and Hearing Clinic — SLP/A
University of Washington
4131 15th NE, JH-40
Seattle 98195

Wisconsin

St. Elizabeth Hospital — SLP
Department of Speech Pathology
1506 South Oneida Street
Appleton 54911

St. Francis Medical Health Corporation — SLP
Department of Speech Pathology
700 West Avenue South
LaCrosse 54601

Marshfield Clinic — SLP/A
Department of Speech Pathology/Audiology
1000 North Oak
Marshfield 54449

LaCrosse Lutheran Hospital/Gundersen Clinic, Inc. — SLP
Speech Pathology Services
1910 South Avenue
La Crosse 54601

Canada

Glenrose Rehabilitation Hospital — A
Department of Audiology
Dept. of Communication Disorders
10230 111th Avenue
Edmonton, Alberta T5G 0B7

Glenrose Rehabilitation Hospital — SLP
Department of Speech Pathology
Dept. of Communication Disorders
10230 111th Avenue
Edmonton, Alberta T5G 0B7

University Hospital — SLP
Speech Pathology Services
339 Windermere Road
London, Ontario N6A 5A5

APPROVED SPONSORS CONTINUING EDUCATION BOARD

October, 1988

The following sponsors have been approved by the Continuing Education Board (CEB) of the American Speech-Language-Hearing Association to offer continuing education activities to speech-language-pathologists and audiologists. These ASHA Approved Sponsors offer activities which provide participants with the opportunity to earn Continuing Education Units (CEUs) applicable toward the Award for Continuing Education. Approved Sponsors who are also Independent Study Sponsors are designated with an asterisk (*).

Quality continuing education is assured by initial sponsor application review and ongoing monitoring by the CEB. ASHA approval for continuing education sponsorship does not imply endorsement of a specific product or clinical practice.

ASHA CE Sponsor Approval is voluntarily initiated. Applications and additional information may be obtained by contacting: Continuing Education Branch, American Speech-Language-Hearing Association, 10801 Rockville Pike, Rockville, MD 20852.

Alabama

*Communication Concepts & Consulting
P.O. Box 131058
Birmingham 35213

*Med Therapy, Inc.
2 Metroplex Drive
Suite 214
Birmingham 35209

*Speech and Hearing Association of Alabama
c/o Program for Exceptional Children and Youth
1020 Monticello Court
Montgomery 36117

Alaska

*Alaska Speech and Hearing Association
HC79, Box 6438
Chugiak 99567

Arizona

*Arizona Speech and Hearing Association
6134 West Corrine Drive
Glendale 85304

Good Samaritan Medical Center
Speech-Language Pathology Department
1111 East McDowell Road, P.O. Box 2989
Phoenix 85062

Tucson Audiology Institute
1980 W. Hospital Drive, Suite 109
Northwest Hospital
Medical Plaza Building
Tucson 85704

University of Arizona
Department of Speech and Hearing Sciences
Tucson 85721

Arkansas

Arkansas Speech-Language-Hearing Association
510 North Bryan
Little Rock 72205

NSSLHA-University of Central Arkansas Chapter
Post Office Box U 1745
Conway 72032

*UALR-UAMS Consortium Program
c/o Speech-Language-Hearing Clinic
2801 South University
Little Rock 72204

California

Access Speech and Language
362 Capp Street
San Francisco 94110

California-Hawaii Elks Major Project, Inc.
P.O. Box 7823
Ventura 93003-7823

California Speech-Language-Hearing Association
2631 Capitol Avenue
Sacramento 95816

California State University – Los Angeles
Department of Communication Disorders
51251 State University Drive
Los Angeles 90032

*California State University – Northridge
Department of Communicative Disorders
18111 Nordhoff Street
Northridge 91330

*Crippled Children's Society of Santa Clara County, Inc.
2851 Park Avenue
Santa Clara 95050

House Ear Institute
256 South Lake Street
Los Angeles 90057

*Independent Study Sponsors

Institute for Cortext Research and Development
3903 D Middlefield Road
Palo Alto 94303

Institute of Child Language and Phonology
2140 Pierce Street
San Francisco 44115

*Los Angeles Center for Therapy and Education
13130 Burbank Boulevard
Van Nuys 91401

MSP Communications, Inc.
140 University Avenue, Suite 127
Palo Alto 94301

National Black Association for Speech, Language and Hearing
P.O. Box 7856
San Jose 95101-9612

Newport Language, Speech and Audiology Center, Inc.
24953 Paseo de Valencia #14C
Languna Hills 92653

NSSLHA – San Francisco State University Chapter
Communicative Disorders Clinic
Department of Special Education, SFSU
1600 Holloway Avenue
San Francisco 94132

Paradise Valley Hospital
2400 East Fourth Street
National City 92050

Professional Seminars International (PSI)
P.O. Box 545
La Mesa 92041

Project Hear
1801 Page Mill Road
Palo Alto 94304

*Rancho Los Amigos Med Center
Communication Disorders Department
7601 East Imperial Highway
Downey 90242

Robert H. Ballard Center for Rehabilitation
Department of Speech-Language Pathology
San Bernardino Community Hospital
1500 West 17th Street
San Bernardino 92411

*Saint John's Hospital and Health Center
Speech and Hearing Services
1328 22nd Street
Santa Monica 90404

San Diego State University
Department of Communicative Disorders
5300 Companile Drive
San Diego 92182

San Francisco Bay Area Audiology Group
3550 California Street, #3
San Francisco 94118

San Jose State University
Speech and Hearing Center
Washington Square
San Jose 95192

Stanford University Medical Center
Audiology Clinic
Edwards Building, R135
Stanford 94305

The Orton Dyslexia Society
131 Hillbrook Drive
Los Gatos 95030

*The Professional Continuum
P.O. Box 5667
Concord 94522-0567

The Voice and Speech Company of America
10921 Wilshire Boulevard, Suite 400
Los Angeles 90024

Whittier College
Department of Communicative Disorders
13724 Earlham Drive
Whittier 90608

Colorado

The Children's Hospital
Audiology and Speech Pathology
1056 East 19th Avenue
Denver 80218

Colorado Hearing Foundation
4200 E. Ninth Avenue, Box B210
Denver 80262

*Colorado Speech-Language-Hearing Association
1325 South Colorado Blvd., B-401
Denver 80222

Seminars in Speech and Language;
Seminars in Hearing
4200 East Ninth Avenue, Box B-210
Denver 80262
(Journal Study)

University of Colorado
Department of Communication Disorders and Speech Science
Campus Box 409
Boulder 80309

Connecticut

*Connecticut Speech-Language-Hearing Association
46 Peddlers Drive
Branford 06405

**Independent Study Sponsors*

Southern Connecticut State University
Department of Communication Disorders
501 Crescent Street
New Haven 06515

Delaware

*Delaware Speech and Hearing Association
c/o Alfred I. DuPont Institute
Rockland Road
Wilmington 19899

District of Columbia

*Alexander Graham Bell Association for the Deaf, Inc.
3417 Volta Place, N.W.
Washington 20007

*Army Audiology and Speech Center
Walter Reed Army Medical Center
Washington 20307-5001

Children's Hospital National Medical Center
Children's Hearing and Speech Center
111 Michigan Avenue, N.W.
Washington 20010

District of Columbia Speech-Language-Hearing Association
835 Crittenden Street, NE
Washington 20017

Gallaudet College
Department of Audiology
7th and Florida Avenue, NE
Washington 20002

*George Washington University
Speech and Hearing Clinic
2201 G Street, N.W., Room 407
Washington 20052

*Georgetown University Child Development Center
3800 Reservoir Road, N.W.
Washington 20007

Howard University
Department of Communication Arts and Sciences
P.O. Box 65
Washington 20059

*National Rehabilitation Hospital
Speech-Language Pathology Services
102 Irving Street, NW
Washington, DC 20010-2949

University of the District of Columbia
Dept. of Communication Sciences
4200 Connecticut Ave., NW
Washington 20008

Florida

Academy/Dispensing Audiologists
c/o Med Gardens Hearing Center
215 Palermo
Venice 34285

Cedars Medical Center
J. Freeman Hearing and Speech Center
1400 NW 12th Avenue
Miami 33136

Easter Seal Society of Broward County
6951 West Sunrise Boulevard
Plantation 33317

Florida Diagnostic Learning Resources System-South
9220 SW 52nd Terrace
Miami 33165

*Florida Language Speech and Hearing Association
c/o H. Lee Moffitt Cancer Center
12902 Magnolia Drive
Tampa 33624

Florida State University
Center for Professional Development
Florida State Conference Center
Tallahassee 32306-2007

Hearing Education and Research Foundation
408 Mercy Professional Building
3661 South Miami Avenue
Miami 33133

*Institute for Myofunctional Therapy
1450 Madruga Avenue, Suite 404
Coral Gables 33146

*Miami Association of Communication Specialists
1925 NE 117th Road
North Miami 33181

*Morton F. Plant Hospital
323 Jeffords
Clearwater 33517

Munroe Regional Medical Center
131 SW 15th Street
P.O. Box 6000
Ocala 32671

Nova University
Speech-Language Pathology Masters Program
3375 SW 75th Avenue
Fort Lauderdale 33314

S. Allen Smith Clinic
230 Arlington Road, North
Jacksonville 32211

*Speech and Hearing Center, Inc.
1128 Laura Street
Jacksonville, Florida 32206

University of Florida, Department of Speech
355 Dauer Hall
Gainesville 32611

Independent Study Sponsors

*University of Central Florida
Department of Communicative Disorders
Alfaya Trail
Orlando 32816

*The University of South Florida
Department of Communicology
College of Social and Behavioral Sciences, CAB 255
Tampa 33620

Georgia

Audiological Consultants of Atlanta, Inc.
2550 Windy Hill Road, Suite 305-A
Marietta 30067

Georgia Speech and Hearing Association
West Georgia Medical Center Audiology Department
1514 Vernon Road
La Grange 30240

Hawaii

Hawaii Speech-Language-Hearing Association
4921 Waa Street
Honolulu 96813

Idaho

International Association for Orofacial Myology
6700 Emerald Street
Boise 83704

Illinois

Cadwell Laboratories, Inc.
c/o Neurological Associates, SC
214 NE Glen Oak Avenue, Suite 502
Peoria 61603

Carle Clinic Association
602 West University Avenue
Urbana 61801

*Center for Speech and Language Disorders
479 Spring Road
Elmhurst 60126

Continuing Education Programs of America
Division of Innovation and Development
16 Cherry Lane, Suite #1
Morton 61550

Continuing Education Resource, Inc.
P.O. Box 210
Glen Ellyn 60138

*David T. Siegel Institute for Communicative Disorders
Michael Reese Hospital and Medical Center
Lake Shore Drive and 31st Street
Chicago 60616

*Governors State University
College of Health Professions
Division of Communication Disorders
University 60466-0975

*Illinois Speech Language Hearing Association
Department of Speech Pathology & Audiology
Southern Illinois University
P.O. Box 1776
Edwardsville 62026

Lake-McHenry Regional Program
394 Peterson Road
Libertyville 60048

Linguisystems, Inc.
716 17th Street
Moline 61265

Marianjoy Rehabilitation Hospital
26W171 Roosevelt Road
P.O. Box 795
Wheaton 60189-0795

Midwest Orofacial Myology
4313 DuBois Boulevard
Brookfield 60513

Neuro-Developmental Treatment Association
P.O. Box 70
Oak Park 60300

*Northwestern University
Communication Sciences and Disorders
2299 Sheridan Road
Evanston 60201

*Rehabilitation Institute of Chicago
345 East Superior Street
Chicago 60611

*Rush-Presbyterian-St. Luke's Medical Center
Rush University
1753 West Congress Parkway
Chicago 60612

*Schwab Rehabilitation Hospital
Communication Disorders Department
1401 South California Boulevard
Chicago 60608

Sertoma Center for Communicative Disorders
7330 College Drive
Palos Heights 60463

Southern Illinois University at Carbondale
Department of Communication Disorders and Sciences
Room 1003, Communications Building
Carbondale 62901-6616

*Southern Illinois University at Edwardsville
Department of Speech Pathology and Audiology
P.O. Box 1776
Edwardsville 62026

**Independent Study Sponsors*

University of Illinois at Urbana/Champaign
Department of Speech and Hearing Sciences
901 S. Sixth Street
Champaign 61820

Veterans Administration Medical Center
Audiology/Speech Pathology
Service (126)
3001 Green Bay Road
North Chicago 60064

Indiana

*CNR Research Institute
CTR/Neuropsychological Rehabilitation
8925 N. Meridian Street, Suite 210
Indanapolis 46260

Indiana Speech-Language-Hearing Association
c/o Department of Audiology and Speech Sciences
Purdue University
West Lafayette 47907

Purdue University
Department of Audiology and Speech Sciences
West Lafayette 47907

Iowa

*Audiology Consultants, Inc.
3319 Spring Street
Suite 104
Davenport 52807

Kansas

*Bethany Medical Center
Allied Health CE Programs
51 North 12 Street
Kansas City 66102

Intercampus Program in Communication Disorders
Department of Hearing and Speech
Kansas University Medical Center
39th and Rainbow Boulevard
Kansas City 66103

Kansas Speech-Language-Hearing Association
310 North Delrose
Wichita 67208

*Wichita State University
Department of Communicative Disorders and Sciences
1845 North Fairmount
Wichita 67208

Kentucky

Cardinal Hill Hospital
Department of Speech/Language Pathology
2050 Versailles Road
Lexington 40504

*Kentucky Speech-Language Hearing Association
3382 Buckhorn Drive
Lexington 40515

Murray State University
Division of Communicative Disorders
Department of Special Education
Murray 42071

University of Kentucky Medical Center
Neurosensory and Communicative Disorders
800 Rose Street
Lexington 40536-0084

*University of Louisville
Graduate Program in Communicative Disorders
Department of Surgery
Myers Hall
129 East Broadway
Louisville 40292

Louisiana

Louisiana Board of Examiners for Speech Pathology and Audiology
P.O. Box 355
Prairieville 70767

Maine

*F. T. Hill Center for Communication Disorders
Mid-Maine Medical Center
Chase Avenue
Waterville 04901

York County Counseling Services
Speech and Hearing Program
23 Water Street
Saco 04072

Maryland

American Speech-Language-Hearing Association
10801 Rockville Pike
Rockville 20852

American Speech-Language-Hearing Foundation
10801 Rockville Pike
Rockville 20853

*Bilingual Language-Speech-Hearing Association, Inc.
13902 Shippers Lane
Rockville 20853

*Clarion Foundation for Continuing Education
8715 Garfield Street
Bethesda 20817

Hearing and Speech Agency of Metropolitan Baltimore, Inc.
2220 St. Paul Street
Baltimore 21218

**Independent Study Sponsors*

*The John F. Kennedy Institute
Department of Communication Sciences and Disorders
707 North Broadway
Baltimore 21205

Loyola College
Department of Speech-Language Pathology/Audiology
4501 North Charles Street
Baltimore 21210

Maryland Institute for Emergency Medical Services Systems
University of Maryland Medical Systems
Speech-Communication Disorders
22 South Greene Street
Baltimore 21201

Maryland Speech-Language-Hearing Association
404 Waveland Road
Baltimore 21228

*M. J. Dance Cancer Rehabilitation Center
6701 North Charles Street
Baltimore 21204

*Prince George's County Health Department
Division of Speech and Audiology
6490 Landover Road, Suite E
Landover 20785

Self Help for Hard of Hearing
7800 Wisconsin Avenue
Bethesda 20814

Topics in Language Disorders
Aspen Publishers, Inc.
1600 Research Boulevard
Rockville 20850
(Journal Study)

*Towson State University
Department of Communication Sciences and Disorder
York Road
Towson 21204

Treatment Centers
Outpatient Speech and Language Service
1000 Twinbrook Parkway
Rockville 20851

University of Maryland
Department of Hearing and Speech Sciences
Lefrak Hall, Room 0100
College Park 20742

Massachusetts

Beth Israel Hospital
Neurological Unit
330 Brookline Avenue
Boston 02215

Boston Area Clinical Aphasilogy Group (BCAG)
c/o G. Gramigna
ENRM Veterans' Hospital
Audiology/Speech Pathology Section
Bedford 01730

*Boston University
Department of Communication Disorders
48 Cummington Street
Boston 02215

Braintree Hospital
Center for Communication Disorders
250 Pond Street
Braintree 02184

Emerson College
Division of Communication Disorders
168 Beacon Street
Boston 02116

Framingham Rehabilitation Center
P.O. Box 2007
Framingham 01701

*Franciscan Childrens' Hospital Rehabilitation Center
Speech Language Pathology Department
30 Warren Street
Brighton 02135

Hahnemann Rehabilitation Center
535 Lincoln Street
Worcester 01605

Massachusetts Eye and Ear Infirmary
243 Charles Street
Boston 02114

*Massachusetts General Hospital
Speech-Language Pathology Dept.
Boston 02114

Massachusetts Speech Language Hearing Association
Hahnemann Rehabilitation Center
535 Lincoln Street
Worcester 01605

Morton Hospital and Medical Center
Speech, Hearing and Language Center
88 Washington Street
Taunton 02780

*New England Medical Center Hospital
Speech, Hearing and Language Center
750 Washington Street
Box 823
Boston 02111

New England Rehabilitation Hospital
Department of Communication Disorders
Rehabilitation Way
Woburn 01801

Northeastern University
Department of Speech-Language Pathology and Audiology
360 Huntington Avenue
Boston 02115

Spaulding Rehabilitation Hospital
Speech-Language Pathology Department
125 Nashua Street
Boston 02114

**Independent Study Sponsors*

*University of Massachusetts
Division of Continuing Education
Goodell, Room 608
Amherst 01003

*Worcester State College
486 Chandler Street
Worcester 01602

Michigan

*Central Michigan University
Department of Communication Disorders
Moore Hall 4411
Mt. Pleasant 48859

*Head Injury Therapy Services, Inc.
613 Ashman Street
Midland 48640

Hearing Aid Center of Kalamazoo
3130 Protage Street
P.O. Box 3055
Kalamazoo 49003

McLaren General Hospital
Speech and Hearing Department
401 South Ballenger Highway
Flint 48523

*Michigan Speech Language and Hearing Association
44001 Garfield Road
Mt. Clemens 48044

Michigan Speech Pathologists in Clinical Practice
7249 Oak Forest
Clarkston 48016

Michigan State University
Department of Audiology and Speech Sciences
378 Communication Arts and Sciences Building
East Lansing 48824-1212

Northern Speech Services, Inc.
117 North Elm Street
P.O. Box 1036
Gaylord 49735

Rehabilitation Network, Inc.
29275 Northwestern Highway
Suite 208
Southfield 48034

Unitron Industries, Inc.
3555 Walnut Street
P.O. Box 6010
Port Huron 48060

*Western Michigan University
Department of Speech Pathology and Audiology
Kalamazoo 49008

*William Beaumont Hospital
Speech and Language Pathology
3601 West Thirteen Mile Road
Royal Oak 48072

Minnesota

*3M Hearing Health
3M Center, Building 552-2W-02
St. Paul 55144

Mayo Clinic
200 First Avenue, S.W.
Rochester 55901

Minnesota Speech-Language and Hearing Association
P.O. Box 26115
St. Louis Park 55426

*Professional Development Programs
12015 July Avenue North
Hugo 55038

*Telex Communications, Inc.
Hearing Instruments Group
9600 Aldrich Avenue South
Minneapolis 55420

*University of Minnesota, Duluth
Department of Allied Clinical Health
19 School/Business, 10 University Drive
Duluth 55812

Mississippi

Language/Speech Services, Inc.
312 Marion Avenue
McComb 39648

Mississippi Speech and Hearing Association
P.O. Box 5361, Fondren Station
Jackson 39216

*Mississippi University for Women
Speech and Hearing Center
P.O. Box W-1340
Columbus 39701

The University of Mississippi
Department of Communicative Disorders
George Hall
University 38677

*University of Southern Mississippi
Department of Speech and Hearing Sciences
Box 5092 Southern Station
Hattiesburg 39401

Missouri

*Central Institute for the Deaf
818 South Euclid Avenue
St. Louis 63110

Missouri Speech-Language-Hearing Association
c/o MSHA Central Office
Route 1, Box 346
Rocheport 65279

**Independent Study Sponsors*

Northeast Missouri State University
East Normal Street
Kirksville 63501

Research Medical Center
2316 East Meyer Boulevard
Kansas City 64132

Saint Louis University
Department of Communication Disorders
3733 West Pine
St. Louis 63108

St. Luke's Hospital
Speech Pathology & Audiology
44th and Wornall
Kansas City 64111

Montana

Missoula Community Medical Center
Cognitive Remediation Department
2827 Forth Missoula Road
Missoula 59801

Montana Speech, Hearing and Language Association
Post Office Box 515
Broadus 59317

*University of Montana
Communication Sciences and Disorders
634 Eddy Avenue
Missoula 59812

Nebraska

Boys Town National Institute for Communication Disorders
555 North 30th Street
Omaha 68131

*The University of Nebraska Medical Center
Center for Continuing Education
42nd and Dewey
Omaha 68105

New Hampshire

*New Hampshire Speech-Language-Hearing Association
Dartmouth Hitchcock Medical Center
2 Maynard Street
Hanover 03756

New Jersey

Children's Specialized Hospital
150 New Providence Road
Mountainside 07091

Institute of Child Development
Hackensack Medical Centers
30 Prospect Avenue
Hackensack 07601

*Johnson Rehabilitation Institute
John F. Kennedy Medical Center
James Street
Edison 08817

*Kean College of New Jersey
Speech Pathology-SCI Building
Morris Avenue
Union 07083

Kessler Institute for Rehabiliation, Inc.
1199 Pleasant Valley Way
West Orange 07052

Montclair State College
Department of Communication Sciences and Disorders
Upper Montclair 07043

New Jersey Speech-Language-Hearing Association
515 Avon Lane
Saddle Brook 07662

Overlook Hospital
Speech-Language Pathology
99 Beauvoiir Avenue
Summit 07901

Siemens Hearing Instruments, Inc.
10 Corporate Place South
Piscataway 08854

Speech and Hearing Associates
315 Lenox Avenue
Westfield 07090

*St. Lawrence Rehabilitation Center
2381 Lawrenceville Road
Lawrenceville 08648

Trenton State College
Department of Speech Pathology, Audiology, Education for the Hearing Impaired
Hillwood Lakes CN4700
Trenton 08650-4700

*William Paterson College
Department of Speech Pathology and Audiology
300 Pompton Road
Wayne 07470

New Mexico

*New Mexico Speech-Language-Hearing Association
2745 Tramway Circle
Albuquerque 87123

Pica Programs
713 Parkland Circle, S.E.
Albuquerque 87108

**Independent Study Sponsors*

Professional Seminar Consultants, Inc.
Office of Continuing Professional Education
Heritor Square
4171 Montgomery, NE
Albuquerque 87109

University of New Mexico
Department of Communicative Disorders
901 Vassar NE
Albuquerque 87131

New York

Adelphi University
Department of Speech Arts and Communicative Disorders
Box 701
Garden City 11530

Beth Israel Medical Center
Department of Rehabilitation Medicine
10 Nathan D. Perlman Place
New York 10003

Brooklyn College of CUNY
Program in Speech Pathology-Audiology
Speech and Hearing Sciences
Bedford Avenue and Avenue H
Brooklyn 11210

*CUNY Graduate School
Ph.D. Program in Speech and Hearing Sciences
33 West 42nd St.
New York 10036

Donald R. Reed Speech Center, Inc.
Phelps Memorial Hospital
North Tarrytown 10591

*Hofstra University
Department of Speech Arts and Sciences
Hempstead 11550

Hunter College of the City University of New York
Communication Sciences Program
425 East 25th Street
New York 10010

Ithaca College
Office of Continuing Education
Ithaca 14850

Kingsbrook Jewish Medical Center
Department of Rehabilitation Medicine
585 Schenectady Avenue
Brooklyn 11203

Lexington Hearing and Speech Center
74-20 25th Avenue, Jackson Heights
Queens 11370

*Long Island Speech-Language-Hearing Association
54 Hollyhock Road
Levittown 11756

Marymount Manhattan College
Communication & Learning Center
221 East 71st Street
New York 10021

Mill Neck Manor Lutheran School for the Deaf
Box 12, Frost Mill Road
Mill Neck 11765

Mount Sinai Medical Center
Communication Disorders Center
One Gustave Levy Place
New York 10029

*New York City Speech, Hearing and Language Association
36 Sutton Place South
New York 10022

*New York League for the Hard of Hearing
71 West 23rd Street
New York 10010

New York State Speech-Language-Hearing Association
111 Washington Ave., Suite 600
Albany 12210

*New York University
Department of Communication Arts & Sciences
829 Shimkin Hall
50 West 4th Street
New York 10003

New York Univeristy Medical Center
Speech Pathology Services
Howard A. Rusk Institute of Rehabilitation
400 East 34th Street
New York 10016

*Queens College of the City University of New York
Speech and Hearing Sciences
65-30 Kissena Boulevard
Flushing 11367

*South Tier Area Speech-Language-Hearing Association
Box 137, RD #5
Upper Stella Ireland Road
Binghamton 13905

Speech and Hearing Association of Western New York
S 3464 Timothy Lane
East Aurora 14052

*SUNY College at Fredonia
Department of Speech Pathology/Audiology
Thompson Hall
Fredonia 14063

*SUNY College of Arts and Science
Department of Speech Pathology & Audiology
218 Sturges Hall
Geneseo 14454

State University of New York
Department of Communication Disorders and Sciences
106 Park Hall
Buffalo 14260

Independent Study Sponsors

*Teachers College, Columbia University
Department of Speech Pathology and Audiology
Box 3, 525 West 120th Street
New York 10027

V.A. Medical Center – Syracuse
Audiology and Speech Pathology Serives (126)
800 Irving Avenue
Syracuse 13210

North Carolina

*East Carolina University
Department of Speech-Language & Auditory Pathology
School of Allied Health Sciences
Greenville 27858-4353

North Carolina Speech, Hearing and Language Association
Department of Speech-Language and Auditory Pathology
East Carolina University
School of Allied Health Sciences
Greenville 27858-4353

*University of North Carolina
Division of Speech and Hearing Sciences
Dept./Med. Allied Health Professions
78 Wing D Medical School, 208H
Chapel Hill 27514

*University of North Carolina at Greensboro
Office of Continuing Education
1000 Spring Garden Street
Greensboro 27412

North Dakota

*State University of North Dakota at Minot
Department of COmmunication Disorders
Box 86
Minot 58701

Ohio

Case Western Reserve University
Department of Communication Sciences
The Cleveland Hearing and Speech Center
11206 Euclid Avenue
Cleveland 44106

Cleveland Clinic Educational Foundation
Section of Communicative Disorders
9500 Euclid Avenue
Cleveland 44106

Cleveland State University
Department of Speech and Hearing
Euclid and East 22nd Street
Main Classroom, Building #430
Cleveland 44115

Kent State University
Division of Speech Pathology and Audiology
Speech and Hearing Clinic
A-104 Music and Speech Building
Kent 44242

Ohio Speech and Hearing Association
3683 Riedham Road
Shaker Heights 44120

*Ohio State University
324 Derby Hall
154 North Oval Mall
Columbus 43210

Prentke Romich Company
1022 Heyl Road
Wooster 44691

*St. Elizabeth Medical Center
Education and Training Department
601 Edwin C. Moses Boulevard
Dayton 45408

Toledo Hearing and Speech Center
One Stranahan Square
Suite 342
Toledo 43604

Toledo Hospital
Division of Communication Disorders
2142 North Cove Boulevard
Toledo 43606

*University of Akron
West Hall
Akron 44325

*University of Cincinnati Medical Center
Division of Audiology and Speech Pathology
University Hospital
Mail Location #780
Cincinnati 45267-0780

Oklahoma

Oklahoma Speech-Language-Hearing Association
Muskogee Guidance Center
530 South 34th Street
Muskogee 74401

Oklahoma State University
Department of Speech-Language Pathology/Audiology
120 Hanner Hall
Stillwater 74078

*University of Oklahoma Health Sciences Center
Department of Communication Disorders
825 NE 14th
P.O. Box 26901
Oklahoma City 73190

Oregon

APRICOT, Inc.
P.O. Box 18191
Portland 97218

*Oregon Speech and Hearing Association
10715 S.W. 63rd Place
Portland 97219

Independent Study Sponsors

*Portland State University
Program in Speech and Hearing Sciences
P.O. Box 751
Portland 97207

Starkey Laboratories
Starkey Northwest
2255 NE 194th Avenue
Portland 97230

Pennsylvania

American Academy/Private Practice
Speech Pathology and Audiology
1602 Overbrook Drive, Box 474
Gwynedd Valley 19437

American Cleft Palate Association Educational Foundation
The University of Pittsburgh
1218 Grandview
Pittsburgh 15211

*Capital Area Intermediate Unit
Department of Communication Disorders
2929 Gettysburg Road
Camp Hill 17011

*Children's Seashore House/Children's Hospital of Philadelphia
Division of Child Development and Rehabilitaion
34th Street and Civic Center Boulevard
Philadelphia 19104

*Communication Skills, Inc.
1241 Cox Road
Rydal 19046

*Edinboro University of Pennsylvania
Department of Speech Communication
Speech-Language Pathology Program
Taylor House
Edinboro 16444

The Good Shepherd Rehabilitation Hospital
Department of Speech and Communication
5th and St. John Streets
Allentown 18103

Hahnemann University
Division of Graudate Studies in Speech Pathology and Audiology
Department of Otorhinolaryngology
Mail Station 419, Broad and Vine
Philadelphia 19102

InSpeech, Inc.
P.O. Box 928
Valley Forge 19482-0928

*Moss Rehabilitation Hospital
12th Street and Tabor Road
Philadelphia 19141

The Pennsylvania Speech and Hearing Association
Barclay Street
RD 2, Box 298B
Hertztown 19539

The Pennsylvania State University
Division of Continuing Education
209 J. Orvis Keller Building
University Park 16802

The Reading Hospital and Medical Center
Speech and Hearing Center
6th Avenue and Spruce Street
Reading 19603

*Technical Assistance for Sensory Impaired Programs
150 South Progress Avenue
Harrisburg 17109

*Temple University
Department of Speech
Speech and Hearing Science Division
Philadelphia 19122

University of Pittsburgh
244 Blvd. of Allies at Wood Street
Pittsburgh 15222

Rhode Island

*Bradley Hospital
1011 Veterans Memorial Pkwy.
East Providence 02915

*Rhode Island Speech and Hearing Association, Inc.
P.O. Box 9241
Providence 02940

South Carolina

South Carolina Speech and Hearing Association
University of South Carolina
112 Tyborne Circle
Columbia 29210

*University of South Carolina
Department of Communicative Disorders
1601 St. Julian Place
Columbia 29204

South Dakota

South Dakota Speech-Language-Hearing Association
1410 South Center Avenue
Sioux Falls 57105

Tennessee

Bill Wilkerson Hearing and Speech Center
Division of Hearing and Speech Sciences
Vanderbilt University School of Medicine
1114 19th Avenue South
Nashville 37212

*Fort Sanders Regional Medical Center
1901 Clinch Avenue, S.W.
Knoxville 37916

**Independent Study Sponsors*

NSSLHA Memphis State University Chapter
807 Jefferson Avenue
Memphis 38105

Tennessee Speech, Language and Hearing Association
1929 Lapaloma Street
Memphis 38105

*The University of Tennessee
Department of Audiology and Speech Pathology
457 South Stadium Hall
Knoxville 37996-0740

Texas

Bruel and Kjaer Instruments, Inc.
2411 Gateway Drive, Suite 100
Irving 75063

*Callier Center for Communication Disorders
1966 Inwood Road
Dallas 75235

Language and Learning Institute
4304 Shoalwood Avenue
Austin 78756

Methodist Hospital
Division of Audiology and Speech-Language Pathology
6501 Fannin, NA 200
Houston 77030

Our Lady of the Lake University
Communication and Learning Disorders
411 S.W. 24th Street
San Antonio 78285

*Southwest Texas State University
Communication Disorders Program
2040 New Education
San Marcos 78666

Speech and Hearing Institute
University of Texas Health Science Center at Houston
1343 Moursund
Houston 77030

*Texas Speech, Language and Hearing Association
c/o Bonks Miller & Associates
P.O. Box 610250
Austin 78761

*Texas Tech University
Speech and Hearing Clinic
P.O. Box 4266
Lubbock 79409

The Psychological Corporation
555 Academic Court
San Antonio 78204

*University of North Texas
Division of Communication Disorders
Denton 76203

*University of Texas at Austin
Program in Communication Disorders
Austin 78712

Utah

Jordan School District
9361 South 400 East
Sandy 84070

*Utah State University
Department of Communicative Disorders
Logan 84322-1000

Vermont

University of Vermont
Department of Communication Science & Disorders
461 Main Street
Allen House
Burlington 05405

Virginia

*James Madison University
Speech Pathology and Audiology
Harrisonburg 22807

Medical College of Virginia, VCU
Audiology/Speech Pathology
Department of Otolaryngology
Box 545 MCV Station
Richmond 23298-0545

Mount Vernon Hospital
Physical Medicine and Rehabilitation
2501 Parker's Lane
Alexandria 22306

*New Visions
Route 1, Box 175-S
Faber 22938

Speech and Hearing Association of Virginia, Inc.
c/o University of Virginia
Communication Disorders Program
132 Emmet Street
P.O. Box 9022
Charlottesville 22906-9022

University of Virginia
Communication Disorders Program
132 Emmet Street
P.O. Box 9022
Charlottesville 22906-9022

Washington

*Eastern Washington University
Department of Communication Disorders
MS-106
Cheney 99004

**Independent Study Sponsors*

*Hearing, Speech and Deafness Center
1620 18th Street
Seattle 98122

University of Washington
Department of Speech and Hearing Sciences
1417 N.E. 42nd Street, JG-15
Seattle 98195

Virginia Mason Clinic
1100 9th Avenue
Seattle 98111

*Washington Speech and Hearing Association
c/o Lynwood Medical Center
2200 54th Avenue West
Lynwood 98036

*Washington State University
Communication Disorders Program
Pullman 99164

Western Washington University
Speech Pathology and Audiology
017 Parks Hall
Bellingham 98225

Wisconsin

*Gundersen Clinic, Ltd./LaCrosse Lutheran Hospital
1836 South Avenue
LaCrosse 54601

Marshfield Clinic
Section of Speech-Language Pathology and Audiology
1000 North Oak Avenue
Marshfield 54449

*University of Wisconsin, Madison
University Outreach
217 Lowell Hall
610 Langdon Street
Madison 53706

*Wisconsin Speech-Language-Hearing Association, Inc.
1126 G Division
River Falls, 54022

Wyoming

Wyoming Speech-Language-Hearing Association
Rural Route 1, Box 203G
14 Sage Drive
Riverton 82501

Canada

*Chedoke-McMaster Hospitals
Box 2000, Station "A"
Hamilton, Ontario L8N 3Z5

*Easter Seals Communication Institute
Blissymbolics Communication Institute
24 Ferrand Drive
Don Mills, Ontario
Canada M3C 3N2

Glenrose Rehabilitation Hospital
Audiology Department
10230 – 111th Avenue
Hamilton, Ontario
Canada L8N 3Z5

*Ontario Association for Speech-Language Pathology and Audiology
126 Catalina Court
Sudbury, Ontario
Canada P3E 5T8

**Independent Study Sponsors*

STATE ORGANIZATIONS RECOGNIZED BY THE AMERICAN SPEECH-LANGUAGE-HEARING ASSOCIATION

January 1, 1989

Speech and Hearing Association of Alabama

President:
Betty Faircloth
3555 Lancaster Lane
Montgomery, Alabama 36106
Office: (205) 264-7786
Association Address:
(Same as current President)

Alaska Speech-Language-Hearing Association

President:
Linette Finstad
1606 Marika, #4
Fairbanks, Alaska 99709
Office: (907) 456-5775
Association Address:
(Same as current President)

Arizona Speech-Language-Hearing Association

President:
Kathleen Evans Peterson
2034 E. Southern, Ste. 9
Tempe, Arizona 85282
Office: (602) 820-3910
Association Address:
7622 North 48th Drive
Glendale, Arizona 85301
(602) 435-0373

Arkansas Speech-Language-Hearing Association

President:
Carolane Jones
So. Arkansas Professional Plaza
403 West Oak, Ste. 303
El Dorado, Arkansas 71730
Office: (501) 863-2666
Association Address:
P.O. Box 22635
Little Rock, Arkansas 72221-2635

California Speech-Language-Hearing Association

President:
Judy K. Montgomery
Fountain Valley School District
17210 Oak Street
Fountain Valley, California 92708
Office: (714) 843-3280
Association Address:
825 University Avenue
Sacramento, California 95825
(916) 921-1568

Colorado Speech-Language-Hearing Association

President:
Fran Lowry-Romero
1325 S. Colorado Blvd.
Suite B401
Denver, Colorado 80222
Office: (303) 361-8120
Association Address:
1325 S. Colorado Blvd., Suite B401
Denver, Colorado 80222
(303) 753-1221

Connecticut Speech-Language-Hearing Association, Inc.

President:
Antonia Maxon
131 Chaffeeville Road
Mansfield Center, Connecticut 06250
Office: (203) 486-3687/486-2629
Association Address:
P.O. Box 7-23
West Hartford, Connecticut 06107
(203) 522-4520

Delaware Speech and Hearing Association

President:
Jane Eareckson
102 West 37th Street
Wilmington, Delaware 19802
Office: (302) 428-2921
Association Address:
P.O. Box #662
Dover, Delaware 19903

District of Columbia Speech-Language-Hearing Association

President:
Glen Baquet
8830 Dollyhyde Road
Union Bridge, Maryland 21791
Office: (202) 636-6990
Association Address:
P.O. Box 53159
Washington, D.C. 20009
(202) 651-5328

Florida Language, Speech, and Hearing Association

President:
Frederick Rahe
201 NW 82nd Avenue, #103
Plantation, Florida 33324
Office: (305) 472-1212

Association Address:
P.O. Box 10523
Tallahassee, Florida 32302
(904) 222-1907

Georgia Speech and Hearing Association
President:
Noreen K. Steward
1824 Druid Oaks
Atlanta, Georgia 30329
Office: (404) 658-2310
Association Address:
2786 N. Decatur Road, Ste. 200
Decatur, Georgia 30033
(404) 292-3074

Hawaii Speech-Language-Hearing Association
President:
Jean Stewart
1731 Halekoa Drive
Honolulu, Hawaii 96821
Office: (808) 735-0434
Association Address:
P.O. Box 1303
Kailua, Hawaii 96734
(808) 732-0672

Illinois Speech, Language and Hearing Association
President:
Robert Augustine
Eastern Illinois University
7th & Hayes
Charleston, Illinois 61920
Office: (217) 581-2712
Association Address:
United Way Building, Room 111
730 E. Vine Street
Springfield, Illinois 62703
(217) 789-1876

Indiana Speech and Hearing Association
President:
Richard Hoops
Speech Pathology and Audiology
Ball State University
Muncie, Indiana 47306
Office: (317) 285-8162
Association Address:
P.O. Box 731
Greenwood, Indiana 46142
(317) 881-6070

Iowa Speech-Language and Hearing Association
President:
Linda Jordan
Department of Neurology
University of Iowa Hospitals
Iowa City, Iowa 52242
Office: (319) 356-2031
Association Address:
520 35th Street
Des Moines, Iowa 50312
(515) 274-5918

Kansas Speech-Language-Hearing Association
President:
Teresa Kennalley
427 N. Hillside
Wichita, Kansas 67214
Office: (316) 686-6608
Association Address:
3117 28th
Great Bend, Kansas 67530
(316) 793-6550

Kentucky Speech-Language-Hearing Association
President:
Mary Gray
3776 Belleauwood Drive
Lexington, Kentucky 40503
Office: (606) 233-4511, ext. 3130
Association Address:
P.O. Box 4098
Lexington, Kentucky 40544

Louisiana Speech-Language-Hearing Association
President:
Rosalie Lott
7735 Millicant Circle
Shreveport, Louisiana 71105
Office: (318) 631-5842
Association Address:
P.O. Box 2085
Lafayette, Louisiana 70502-1344

Maine Speech-Language-Hearing Association
President:
Rosemarie De Angelis
16 Franklin Street
Saco, Maine 04072
Office: (207) 284-8344
Association Address:
(Same as current President)

Maryland Speech-Language-Hearing Association
President:
Paul Rao
12 Elkwood Court
Catonsville, Maryland 21228
Office: (202) 877-1440
Association Address:
P.O. Box 234
Columbia, Maryland 21044
(301) 997-7775

Massachusetts Speech-Language-Hearing Association
President:
Barbara Arnold
10 Wentworth Drive
Amherst, Massachusetts 01002
Office: (413) 772-0211 ext. 2360
Association Address:
518 N. Main Street
Randolph, Massachusetts 02368
(617) 986-8177

Michigan Speech-Language-Hearing Association

President:
Robert McLauchlin
Communication Disorders
Central Michigan University
Mt. Pleasant, Michigan 48859
Office: (517) 332-5691
Association Address:
855 Grove Street
E. Lansing, Michigan 48823
(517) 332-5691

Minnesota Speech-Language-Hearing Association

President:
Janet Jacobs
3064 Mildred Drive
Roseville, Minnesota 55113
Office: (612) 298-8288
Association Address:
P.O. Box 26115
St. Louis Park, Minnesota 55426
(612) 935-5057

Mississippi Speech-Language-Hearing Association

President:
Lynn Bishop
5155 Keele, #12A
Jackson, Mississippi 39206
Office: (601) 353-4331
Association Address:
P.O. Box 5361
Foundren Station
Jackson, Mississippi 39216

Missouri Speech-Language-Hearing Association

President:
James Wilson
113 Fairview Dirve
Warrensburg, Missouri 64093
Office: (816) 429-4993
Association Address:
Route 1, Box 346
Rocheport, Missouri 65279
(314) 445-8805

Montana Speech, Language, and Hearing Association

President:
Rosemary Harrison
217 Woodworth Avenue
Missoula, Montana 59801
Office: (406) 721-6096
Association Address:
(Same as current President)

Nebraska Speech-Language-Hearing Association

President:
Peter Hixson
3820 Burt Street
Omaha, Nebraska 68131
Office: (402) 558-5768
Association Address:
1033 K Street
Lincoln, Nebraska 68508
(402) 476-9573

Nevada Speech-Language-Hearing Association

President:
Lindy Spuhler
P.O. Box 3434
Sparks, Nevada 89432-3434
Office: (702) 789-3268
Association Address:
(Same as current President)

New Hampshire Speech-Language-Hearing Association

President:
Trudi Ocenasek
24 Nottingham Road
Deerfield, New Hampshire 03037
Office: (603) 463-7422
Association Address:
Box 7202
Concord Heights Station, New Hampshire 03301

New Jersey Speech-Language-Hearing Association

President:
Laura Hartner
656 Elliot Court
Somerville, New Jersey 08876
Office: (201) 218-4117
Association Address:
120 Finderne Avenue
Bridgewater, New Jersey 08807
(201) 725-0660

New Mexico Speech, Language and Hearing Association

President:
Carol Westby
328 Solano, NE
Albuquerque, New Mexico 87108
Office: (505) 843-2192
Association Address:
Box 4720
Albuquerque, New Mexico 87196-4720

New York State Speech-Language-Hearing Association

President:
Mary Ann O'Brien
497 Whiting Road
Webster, New York 14580
Office: (716) 377-4660
Association Address:
111 Washington Avenue
Albany, New York 12210
(518) 463-5272

North Carolina Speech, Hearing and Language Association

President:
P. David Blalock
North Carolina Baptist Hospital
300 Hawthorne Road
Winston-Salem, North Carolina 27103
Office: (919) 748-3103
Association Address:
White/Holman House
206 New Bern Avenue
P.O. Box 28446
Raleigh, North Carolina 27611-8446
(919) 833-3984

North Dakota Speech-Language-Hearing Association
President:
Diane Carriere
Medical Center Rehabilitation Hospital
1300 S. Columbia Road
Grand Forks, North Dakota 58202
Office: (701) 780-2447
Association Address:
P.O. Box 5175
Grand Forks, North Dakota 58206-5175
(701) 780-2447

Ohio Speech and Hearing Association
President:
Kathy Kelley-Ohlrich
75 Easton Lane
Moreland Hills, Ohio 44022
Office: (216) 421-1585
Association Address:
9331 South Union Road
Miamisburg, Ohio 45342
(513) 866-4972

Oklahoma Speech-Language-Hearing Association
President:
Kelli Vestal
7214 E. 73rd Street
Tulsa, Oklahoma 74133
Office: (918) 494-1474
Association Address:
Box 53217, State Capital Station
Oklahoma City, Oklahoma 73105

Oregon Speech and Hearing Association
President:
Marie T. Rau
3610 SW Alice Street
Portland, Oregon 97219
Office: (503) 222-9221, ext. 5717
Association Address:
P.O. Box 523
255 13th Street, N.E.
Salem, Oregon 97308

Pennsylvania Speech-Language-Hearing Association
President:
Thomas Matsko
Center for Communication Disorders
Moss Rehabilitation Hospital
12th & Tabor Road
Philadelphia, Pennsylvania 19141
Office: (215) 329-5715
Association Address:
P.O. Box 1385
North Wales, Pennsylvania 19454-1385
(215) 375-8586

Rhode Island Speech and Hearing Association, Inc.
President:
Toni Salisbury
67 Prospect Avenue #6
Wickford, Rhode Island 02852
Office: (401) 294-4561, ext. 396
Association Address:
P.O. Box 9241
Providence, Rhode Island 02940
(401) 724-0550

South Carolina Speech and Hearing Association
President:
Emily Johnson
199 Kent Court
Summerville, South Carolina 29483
Office: (803) 761-8631
Association Address:
3008 Millwood Avenue
Columbia, South Carolina 29205
(803) 252-5646

South Dakota Speech-Language-Hearing Association
President:
Sylvester Clifford
424 E. Main
Vermillion, South Dakota 57069
Office: (605) 677-5474
Association Address:
(Same as current President)

Tennessee Speech-Language-Hearing Association
President:
Gene Bratt
Audiology & Speech Pathology (126)
1310 24th Avenue, South
Nashville, Tennessee 37203
Office: (615) 327-5325
Association Address:
P.O. Box 121255
Nashville, Tennessee 37212
(615) 254-3687

Texas Speech-Language-Hearing Association
President:
Martha McGlothlin
8414 Stillwood Lane
Austin, Texas 78758
Office: (512) 450-1177
Association Address:
P.O. Box 610250
Austin, Texas 78761
(512) 452-4571

Vermont Speech, Language and Hearing Association
President:
Mitchell Kramer
69 Allen Street, Ste. 4
Rutland, Vermont 05701
Office: (802) 775-3314
Association Address:
P.O. Box 242
Montpelier, Vermont 05602

Speech and Hearing Association of Virginia
President:
James Nicely
191 Dogwood Lane
Redford, Virginia 24142
Office: (703) 831-5453
Association Address:
Professional Edge
7206 Hull Street Road, Suite 101A
Richmond, Virginia 23235
(804) 745-8420

Washington Speech and Hearing Association

President:
Jack M. Snyder
Department of Otolaryngology, RL-30
Seattle, Washington 98195
Office: (206) 543-5230

Association Address:
P.O. Box 15151
Seattle, Washington 98115

West Virginia Speech-Language-Hearing Association, Inc.

President:
Cheryl Pritchard
Rt. #6, Box 231-C
Cherry Hill Road
Morgantown, West Virginia 26505
Office: (304) 293-4242

Association Address:
(Same as current President)

Wisconsin Speech-Language-Hearing Association, Inc.

President:
Alma Peters
Therapy Associates
1516 W. Mequon Road
Mequon, Wisconsin 53092
Office: (414) 241-4240

Association Address:
Box 199
Medical College of Wisconsin
8700 West Wisconsin Avenue
Milwaukee, Wisconsin 53226
(414) 257-5870

Wyoming Speech-Language-Hearing Association

President:
Ken Logan
510 Fremont Street
Laramie, Wyoming 82070
Office: (307) 766-5707

Association Address:
(Same as current President)

DIRECTORY INSTRUCTIONS

The following information is provided to assist the user of this *Membership Directory*. The user should keep in mind that in most cases, the biographical and geographical information was obtained from the directory questionnaires mailed to the membership in September, 1988. Members who did not return their questionnaires are listed according to information contained in the National Office membership records as of August 5, 1988.

Name, address, educational history, present employment, certification and awards are printed for all included members. Other information is printed at the option of the member.

Sample Alphabetical Listing

Jones, Betty F.[1] 7645 North Elm St. Athens, OH 45056[2]. (305) 562-2871[3] BA 49 IN Univ; MA 53 Univ MN; PhD 60 (Speech Pathology and Audiology) OH State Univ[4] 85-Dir, SP and Hrng Dept, OH Med Ctr, [5] **SLP A**[6] **F**[7] **H**[8] **LM**[9] **ACE**[10]

NAME: [1]Member's full name and middle initial.

ADDRESS: [2]Member's preferred directory address.

TELEPHONE LISTING: [3]Member's preferred telephone listing. It may be either residence or place of employment.

EDUCATIONAL HISTORY: [4]The three highest earned degrees are listed. Certificates of advanced study are not listed. Immediately following the earned degree is the year the degree was conferred and the name of the university or college granting the degree. For members listing a doctoral degree, the field of study is indicated. "NS" (not specified) appears when members did not provide that requested information. Standard codes of PH, ED, MD and DD are used at the doctoral level; MA, MS, ME and ES at the master's level; and BA or BS at the bachelor's level. The letters "OB", "OM", and "OD" indicate those bachelor, master, and doctorate degrees that are not one of the standard codes. Names of the universities and colleges are listed in two-letter state abbreviations.

PRESENT EMPLOYMENT: [5]Member's current place of employment and job title. The number preceding the position indicates the year of the employment.

CLINICAL CERTIFICATION: [6]The area in which the member holds the Certificate of Clinical Competence: **SLP** - Speech-Language Pathology; **A** - Audiology. The Certificate of Clinical Competence permits the holder to provide independent clinical services, and to supervise the clinical practice of students and non-certified clinicians.

FELLOWSHIP: [7]The letter **"F"** indicates those members who are Fellows of the Association. Fellowship is an award recognizing professional or scientific achievement and is given to a member on approval by the Committee on Honors.

HONORS OF THE ASSOCIATION: [8]The letter **"H"** indicates those members awarded the Honors of the Association. The Honors of the Association may be awarded upon the recommendation of the Committee on Honors with the approval of the Legislative Council in recognition of distinguished service to the profession. Honors of the Association is the highest award a member can receive.

LIFE MEMBERS: [9]The letters **"LM"** designates those individuals who are Life Members of the Association. Any member who has held membership for the ten consecutive years* immediately prior to attaining the age of 65, may apply for and automatically receive Life Membership with all privileges of a member. Annual dues/fees are waived. *Effective 1/1/91, this changes to 25 consecutive years.

AWARD FOR CONTINUING EDUCATION: [10]The letters **"ACE"** indicate that the individual participated in continuing professional education approved by the Continuing Education Board and has met all requirements necessary to receive an Award for Continuing Education. The award is valid for a three-year period from the date of issue. Individuals having this designation in this *Membership Directory* have been awarded an ACE 1/1/86 or later.

GEOGRAPHICAL DIRECTORY OF MEMBERS

Members are listed by state and city. The Geographical Section in this edition concentrates on the state and city each member specified for his/her directory address, and does not list groups of members by employer within a city. The clinical certification codes and awards are repeated in the geographical section.

DIRECTORY ABBREVIATIONS

State Abbreviations

AL	Alabama
AK	Alaska
AZ	Arizona
AR	Arkansas
CA	California
CO	Colorado
CT	Connecticut
DE	Delaware
DC	District of Columbia
FL	Florida
GA	Georgia
HI	Hawaii
ID	Idaho
IL	Illinois
IN	Indiana
IA	Iowa
KS	Kansas
KY	Kentucky
LA	Louisiana
ME	Maine
MD	Maryland
MA	Massachusetts
MI	Michigan
MN	Minnesota
MS	Mississippi
MO	Missouri
MT	Montana
NE	Nebraska
NV	Nevada
NH	New Hampshire
NJ	New Jersey
NM	New Mexico
NY	New York
NC	North Carolina
ND	North Dakota
OH	Ohio
OK	Oklahoma
OR	Oregon
PA	Pennsylvania
RI	Rhode Island
SC	South Carolina
SD	South Dakota
TN	Tennessee
TX	Texas
UT	Utah
VT	Vermont
VA	Virginia
WA	Washington
WV	West Virginia
WI	Wisconsin
WY	Wyoming

Territorial

AS	American Samoa
GU	Guam
MR	Mariana Islands
PR	Puerto Rico
VI	Virgin Islands

Canada

AB	Alberta
BC	British Columbia
MB	Manitoba
NB	New Brunswick
NF	Newfoundland
NT	Northwest Territories
NS	Nova Scotia
ON	Ontario
PE	Prince Edward island
PQ	Quebec
SK	Saskatchewan
YT	Yukon Territory

ASHA Certification/Membership Awards

A	Certificate of Clinical Competence in Audiology
ACE	Award for Continuing Education
F	Fellow of the Association
H	Honors of the Association
LM	Life Member of the Association
SLP	Certificate of Clinical Competence in Speech-Language Pathology

Acronyms

AEA	Area Educational Agency
AMC	Army Medical Center
ASHA	American Speech-Language-Hearing Association
BOCES	Board of Cooperative Education Services
CEC	Council for Exceptional Children
CID	Central Institute for the Deaf
CUNY	City University of New York
ENT	Ear, Nose & Throat
ISD	Independent School District Intermediate School District
IU	Intermediate Unit
MIT	Massachusetts Institute of Technology
NICHD	National Institute of Child Health and Human Development
NIDR	National Institute of Dental Research
NIH	National Institutes of Health
NIMH	National Institute of Mental Health
NINCDS	National Institute of Neurological and Communicative Disorders and Stroke
NSDSP	Neurological and Sensory Diseases Service Program
PA	Professional Associate(ion)
SMU	Southern Methodist University
UCLA	University of California at Los Angeles
UCP	United Cerebral Palsy
USAF	United States Air Force
USC	University of Southern California
USD	Unified School District; United School Dirstrict
USPHS	United States Public Health Service
UW	United Way
VA	Veterans Administration
VNA	Visiting Nurses Association
VRA	Vocational Rehabilitation Administration
WRAMC	Walter Reed Army Medical Center

General Abbreviations

A

adj	adjunct
admin	administration
agcy	agency
Amer	American
Asst	Assistant
Assoc	Associate
Assn	Association
aud	audiology, audiologist

B

bd	board
blvd	boulevard

C

cen	central
ch	chief
chldn	children
cnty	county
coll	college
comm	commission, community
commun	communication
consult	consultant
coop	cooperative
coord	coordinator
corp	corporation
counsl	counseling, counselor
ctr	center

D

dep	dependent
dept	department
dev	development, developmental
dir	director
dis	disorders
dist	district
div	division

E

educ	educator, education
elem	elementary
emer	emeritus
excep	exceptional
exec	executive

General Abbreviations (cont.)

F

found	foundation

G

gen	general
grad	graduate
guid	guidance

H

hlth	health
hndcpd	handicapped
hosp	hospital, hospitals
hrng	hearing
hts	heights

I

impr	impaired
imprv	improvement
inc	incorporated
inst	institute
instr	instructor
intermed	intermediate
intl	international

L

lab	laboratory
lang	language
lrng	learning

M

med	medical, medicine
mem	memorial
mentl	mental, mentally
mgmt	management

N

natl	national
neur	neurological, neurology

O

occup	occupational
ofc	office
org	organization
ortho	orthopedic
otol	otolaryngology
otor	otorhinolaryngology

P

path	pathology, pathologist
ped	pediatrics
pers	personnel
phys	physician
prac	practice
presch	preschool
priv	private
prof	professor, professional
prog	program
proj	project
prov	province
pub	public

R

rdng	reading
reg	region, regional
rehab	rehabilitation
rem	remedial
resch	research
ret	retardation, retarded

S

sch	school
sect	section
soc	society
sp	speech
spec	special, specialist
Sr	senior, Sister
st	saint, state, street
supt	superintendent
supvr	supervisor
svc	service
syst	system

T

tchr	teacher
tchng	teaching
tech	technology
ther	therapy
treat	treatment

U

unif	unified
univ	university

V

voc	vocational

1989-1990 ASHA

MEMBERSHIP

DIRECTORY

ALPHABETICAL LIST OF MEMBERS

A

Aach, Mrs Lori Fishman 1188 Royal Glen Drive, #110A, Glen Ellyn, IL 60137, (312) 495-2287, BS 86 Fontbonne Coll; MA 87 Saint Louis Univ; Sp-Lang Path, Private Practice

Aarni, John D 1030 Dry Creek Lane, Marion, IA 52302

Aaron, Lee R 950 Yeadon Avenue, Yeadon, PA 19050, (215) 351-7036, BA 76 Hofstra Univ; MA 81 West Chester Univ of PA; Sp-Lang Path, Sch Dist of Philadelphia, **SLP**

Aaron, Mrs Marilyn B 4123 Fawn Hollow Drive, Dallas, TX 75244, (214) 350-8207, BA 59 Univ of MI - Ann Arbor; MS 78 Univ of TX - Dallas; Dir, Shelton Speech Language & Hearing Clinic, **SLP**

Aaron, Roxanne Jennemann 9528 Koerber Lane, St Louis, MO 63123, (314) 631-1639, BA 81 Southern IL Univ-Edwardsvill; MA 83 Memphis St Univ; Aud, **A**

Aaron, Sheryl A 28675 Franklin Road #213, Southfield, MI 48034, (312) 878-4300, BS 79 Eastern MI Univ; MA 80 Eastern MI Univ; Sp-Lang Path, Medi-Speech Serv Inc, **SLP**

Aarons, Marlene 2920 Chapel Hill Road, Apartment 49B, Durham, NC 27707, (919) 490-1054, BA 79 Univ of FL; MS 82 Univ of NC - Chapel Hill; SLP, Hearing and Speech Agency, **SLP ACE**

Aarts, Nancy Lee 530 Washington Boulevard #2E, Oak Park, IL 60302, (312) 386-1293, BS 82 FL St Univ; MA 84 Univ of FL; 87–Aud, IL Eye & Ear Infirmary, **A**

Aasby, Mrs Susan McGuinn 2165 East Swallow, Springfield, MO 65804, (417) 725-2637, BS 81 Southwest MO St Univ; MS 82 Univ of MO - Columbia; Sp/Lang Path, Nixa Pub Sch, **SLP**

Abahazi, Dr Dennis A 5715 Forest Ridge Drive, North Olmsted, OH 44070, (216) 476-7104, BS 67 Bowling Green St Univ; MA 69 Bowling Green St Univ; PH 75 (NS) Bowling Green St Univ; Dir SLP & Aud, Fairview General Hosp, **SLP A**

Abate, Mrs Mary A 4627 172nd Avenue S E, Issaquah, WA 98027, (206) 644-2487, BS 75 Univ of OR; MA 77 Univ of CA - Santa Barbara; 88–Sp-Lang Path, Sp-Lang & Hrng Svcs, **SLP**

Abba, Mrs Deborah Graham 1124 Lexington Avenue, Schenectady, NY 12309, (518) 370-4619, BS 80 SUNY - Coll at Geneseo; MA 81 SUNY - Coll at Geneseo; 88–Prog Coord, Saratoga Preschool Prog, **SLP**

Abbanat, Mrs Ginette Rand 442 High Street, Salem, VA 24153, (203) 487-1204, BS 81 Univ of NH; MA 87 Univ of CT; 87–Sp-Lang Path, Rehab Svc of Roanoke, **SLP**

Abbott, Mrs Christine Malone 3027 Sleepy Hollow Drive, Stockton, CA 95209, (209) 944-4294, BA 78 CA St Univ - Sacramento; MA 79 Univ of the Pacific; Sp-Lang Path, Stockton USD, **SLP**

Abbott, Cynthia D Lahey Clinic Medical Center, Box 541, 41 Mall Road, Burlington, MA 01805, (617) 273-8450, BA 72 Univ of NH; ME 75 Northeastern Univ; Chief of Aud, Lahey Clinic Med Cen, **A**

Abbott, Harry D 1200 Edward Street, State College, PA 16801, (215) 327-7088, BA 74 Heidelberg Coll; MA 83 West Chester Univ of PA; Chief Communicative Disorders, Lewistown Hospital, **SLP ACE**

Abbott, Mrs Laura Jean 1943 North Lexington Avenue, Apartment 8, Roseville, MN 55113, (612) 489-8300, BS 83 Univ of IA; MA 85 Univ of MN - Minneap-St Paul; Sp-Lang Path, Achievement Rehab Corp, **SLP**

Abbott, Mrs Marcia Staggs 3853 Butterfield, San Angelo, TX 76904, (915) 944-7398, MS 80 Univ of North TX; 87–Sp-Lang Path, Private Practice, **SLP**

Abbott, Nancy Jean 218 Beverly Road, Pittsburgh, PA 15216, (412) 745-8000, BA 82 Univ of Pittsburgh - Pittsburgh; MA 84 Univ of Pittsburgh - Pittsburgh; Sp-Lang Path, Meadowlands Health Care Ctr, **SLP**

Abbott, Mrs Pamela P 1605 Avondale, Jacksonville, FL 32205, (215) 565-1425, BS 70 Western MI Univ; MA 73 Univ of IL - Urbana

Abbott, Mrs Phyllis Annette 1061 Hill Place, Macon, GA 31210, (912) 474-4115, **A**

Abbott, Mrs Robin K 41 Fairlee Road, West Hartford, CT 06107, (203) 628-0364, BS 75 Boston Univ; MA 80 Montclair St Coll; 87–Sp-Lang Path, Woodmere Health Care Fac, **SLP**

Abbott, Susan Elayne 2538 Yorktown Road #282, Houston, TX 77056, (713) 461-3822, BS 84 East TX St Univ - Commerce; MA 86 Northwestern Univ; Aud, Ctr for Sp-Hrng & L, **A**

Abbott, Mrs Susan Harvey 12 Sudbury Lane, Williamsville, NY 14221, (716) 941-5991, BS 75 Indiana Univ of PA; MS 78 WV Univ; Sp-Lang Path, **SLP**

Abbott, Dr Thomas B Department Of Speech, University Of Florida, 356 Dauer Hall/ASB, Gainesville, FL 32611, (904) 392-2113, BA 43 Muskingum Coll; MA 48 Case Western Reserve Univ; PH 57 (NS) Univ of FL; Prof, U of FL, **SLP F ACE**

Abbott, Thomas M 815 North 2nd Street, Ozark, AR 72949, (501) 667-4745, OM 82 AR St Univ; Sp-Lang Path, Ozark Pub Sch, **SLP**

Abbott, Virginia Miller 498 Valley Road, Mason, NH 03048, (603) 878-2000, BA 64 George Washington Univ; ME 72 Fitchburg St Coll; 87–Sp-Lang Path, Private Practice, **SLP**

Abbott-Cason, Susan Box 52 Larmc, APO New York, NY 09180, OB 72 Univ of FL; ME 75 Univ of Miami; Chf Sp-Lang Path, Lanstuhl Army-Reg Med Cen, **SLP**

Abbs, James Howard 1508 Capital Avenue, Madison, WI 53705, (608) 238-9399

Abdala, Caroline 5233 15th Avenue N E #205, Seattle, WA 98105, (206) 523-5044, BA 84 CA St Univ - Fullerton; MA 86 Univ of CA - Santa Barbara; Grad, **A**

Abdale, Mrs Edna K V 56 Ward Street, Westbury, NY 11590, (516) 997-6907, BA 71 Fordham Univ; MA 73 CUNY - Queens Coll; **SLP**

Abdelahad, Linda L 2 Francis Drive #210, Randolph, MA 02368, (617) 986-1519, BS 78 Northeastern Univ; ME 80 Northeastern Univ; Sp-Lang Path, Braintree Hospital, **SLP ACE**

Abdelhak, Catherine Ann 816 East Fishers Creek, Smithville, NJ 08201, (609) 652-0740, BA 83 SUNY - Coll at New Paltz; ME 85 Univ of VA - Charlottesville; Sp-Lang Path, Betty Bacharach Rehabilitation, **SLP**

Abdel-Wahab, Dr Aly Ezzat 32 Pinehurst Road, Holyoke, MA 01040, PH (NS); **SLP**

Abderrahman, Mrs Carole Jean Route 1 Box 73, Clermont, FL 32711, (904) 372-3316, **SLP**

Abdullah, Shireen B No 12 Jalan 12/16B, Petaling Jaya 46200, Selangor, Malaysia, BA 79 WA St Univ; MA 83 WA St Univ; **SLP**

Abe, Mrs Agnes O P O Box 365, Kahului Maui, HI 96732, BA 59 Univ of HI - Manoa; Sp-Lang Path, Hi Dept of Ed, **SLP**

Abecassis, Nancy F 2430 N E 197th Street, North Miami, FL 33180, (305) 937-0961, BS 75 Salem St Coll; ME 77 Northeastern Univ; **SLP**

Abegg, Mrs Michelle Lynn 1940 Heatherwood Drive, Apartment 306, Lawrence, KS 66044, (913) 594-2737, BS 83 PA St Univ - Univ Park; MA 84 Edinboro Univ of PA; Sp-Lang Path, East Central Kansas Coop in Educ, **SLP**

Abel, Cullen D 564 Staples Street, East Taunton, MA 02718, (617) 238-1441, SUNY - Coll at Geneseo; Consult Sp-Lang Path, **SLP**

Abel, Debra B 8865 Lynnett Street N E, Alliance, OH 44601, (216) 823-1680, BS 75 Kent St Univ; MA 77 Kent St Univ; Aud, Alliance Eye & Ear Cl, **A ACE**

Abel, Joseph H, Jr 8521 Visby Place, Sun Valley, CA 91352, (213) 732-1976, BS 54 George Washington Univ; Sp-Lang Path, Los Angeles City Schools, **SLP**

Abel, Judith S P O Box 904, Cottage Grove, OR 97424, (503) 942-8602, BA 63 CUNY - Queens Coll; MS 66 CUNY - Queens Coll; Dir, Abel Ctr for Rehab Therapies, **SLP**

Abele, Mary E P 53 Elm Street, Woburn, MA 01801, (617) 273-1870, BA 60 Elmhurst Coll; MS 80 Boston Univ; SLP, Burlington Public Sch, **SLP**

Abell, Mrs Jacqueline 1405 East Revere Road, Fresno, CA 93710, (209) 449-3603, BA 49 Univ of CA - Berkeley; MA 63 CA St Univ - Fresno; Dir, Abell Speech-Language Center, **SLP**

Abell, Mrs Jean C 2304 Keri Lane, Chico, CA 95926, (916) 891-2724, BS 68 OR St Univ; MA 79 CA St Univ - Chico; SLP, Butte Co Supt of Sch, **SLP**

Abeloff, Suzanne P 382 Central Park West, New York, NY 10025, (212) 852-3220, BA 63; MA 66 Columbia Univ Teachers Coll; Sp-Lang Path, League Center, **SLP**

Abels, Mrs Jeanne Route 1 Box 488, Colrain, MA 01340, (413) 584-8271, BA 73 Glassboro St Coll; MA 75 Western MI Univ; 88–Prog Case Mgr, Pioneer Valley Head Injury Cen, **SLP ACE**

Abelson, Mrs Lori Haskins 108 Garnet Street, Waterford, NY 12188, (518) 272-0767, BA 80 SUNY - Coll at Plattsburgh; MA 84 Univ of ME - Orono; **SLP**

Abenis-Cintron, Anna M 17 Wafer Lane, Wantagh, NY 11793, (212) 579-5440, BA 75 CUNY - Hunter Coll; MS 77 Columbia Univ Teachers Coll; SLP, Chldn's Eval & Rehab Cl, **SLP**

Aber, William 18 Morningside Drive, Livingston, NJ 07039, (201) 992-0820, BA 53 CUNY - Brooklyn Coll; MA 57 Columbia Univ Sch of Gen St; Aud, Private Practice, **SLP A**

Abernathy, Mrs Barbara M 5445 Eastwind Road, Wilmington, NC 28403, (919) 799-1048, BS 72 Univ Southern MS-Hattiesburg; MS 76 Univ Southern MS-Hattiesburg; Sp-Lang Path, UCP Center, **SLP**

Abernathy, Donna Carol 4305 North Hill Parkway, Atlanta, GA 30341-1241, Aud, Atlanta Hearing Aid Service

Abernathy, Mrs Dorothy E 306 Glenn Avenue, Rockwall, TX 75087, (214) 771-0765, OB 72 Southern Methodist Univ; MS 74 Southern Methodist Univ; **SLP**

Abernathy, Mrs Robin C 3324 Stoneybrook, Oklahoma City, OK 73120, (405) 949-3280, BA 77 Univ of OK - Norman; MS 79 Univ of OK Medical Center; Sp-Lang Path, Baptist Med Cen, **SLP**

Abernathy, Susan Gower 1832 Forest Road, Durham, NC 27705, (919) 286-2446, MS 86 Univ of NC - Chapel Hill; **SLP**

Abernethy, Pearl Mary 744 20th Avenue, Honolulu, HI 96816, (808) 262-5115, BA 73 Seattle Pacific Univ; MS 77 Western OR St Coll; SLP, Hi Dept Ed/Windward Dist, **SLP**

Aberwald, Leslie Allison 2925 Riverside Avenue #1, Jacksonville, FL 32205, (904) 387-1460, MA 84 Univ of FL; Audiologist, University Hospital, **A**

Abes, Karen Susan 2527 Malibu Road, Bellmore, NY 11710, (718) 471-0200, BS 84 SUNY - Coll at Oneonta; MS 85 Adelphi Univ; 86–Sp-Lang Path, Valley Stream Union Free Sch, **SLP**

Abeyounis, Elizabeth Cardwell 1065 Willow Green Drive, Newport News, VA 23602, (804) 595-5905, BS 80 FL St Univ; MS 81 FL St Univ; Sp/Lang Path, Riverside Hosp, **SLP**

Abikoff, Laurence 266 Union Avenue, Laconia, NH 03246, (603) 524-7080, BA 72 CUNY - Grad Sch & Univ Cntr; MA 83 Univ of TN - Knoxville; Aud, Community Hearing Services, **A**

Abila, Amparo 5005 S E 109th Street, Portland, OR 97266, (503) 280-6181, BS 73 Portland St Univ; MS 76 Portland St Univ; Sp-Lang Path, Portland PS, **SLP**

Abjanich, Patricia B 2858 Cathy Lane, Clearwater, FL 33520, **SLP**

Abkarian, G G Dept Of Communicative Disorder, Colorado State University, Fort Collins, CO 80523, (303) 491-6981, BS 63 SUNY - Coll at Buffalo; MS 64 Univ of WI - Madison; PH 75 (Commun/Sci/Dis) SUNY - Center at Buffalo; Assoc Prof, Co St Univ, **SLP**

Ablonczy-Popeson, Joanne 217 West Forest Drive, Linwood, NJ 08221, (609) 926-1369, BA 75 Montclair St Coll; MA 80 Trenton St Coll; Cl Instr, Stockton St Coll, **SLP**

Abood, Valerie L 3091 West Dean Road, Lambertville, MI 48144, **SLP**

Abott, Ellen Fran 2224 East 65th Street, Brooklyn, NY 11234, (718) 763-1445, BA 85 CUNY - Brooklyn Coll; MS 87 CUNY - Brooklyn Coll; **A**

Abraham, Annabel S 1131 North Oak Park Avenue, Oak Park, IL 60302, (312) 656-2300, BA 40 Northwestern Univ; MA 42 Northwestern Univ; Sp-Lang Path, J Sterling Morton HS, **SLP LM**

Abraham, Mrs Melinda Sue P O Box 371, Waterloo, NY 13165, (315) 539-3240, MA 85 CUNY - Hunter Coll; Sp-Lang Path, Wayne-Finger Lakes BOCES, **SLP**

Abraham, Mrs Sheradine 2934 Villa Sur Trail, Dallas, TX 75228, (214) 324-4626, BA 74 SC St Coll; MA 78 SC St Coll; SLP, Dallas ISD, **SLP**

Abraham, Dr Suzanne Stephanie Teachers College, Columbia University, Dept Of Spec Ed Box 223, New York, NY 10027, (212) 678-3864, BS 68 PA St Univ - Univ Park; MS 74 PA St Univ - Univ Park; PH 84 (Communication Disorders) PA St Univ - Univ Park; Coord/Supvr of Masters Prog, Teachers College

Abrahams, Arlene G Sp-Lang & Hrng Ctr Of Li Inc, 444 Lakeville Road, Lake Success, NY 11040, (516) 354-5412, BS 55 Northwestern Univ; MA 72 Hofstra Univ; Co-Dir, Sp Lang & Hrng Cent of Li, **SLP**

Abrahams, Mrs Karen Joy 56 Maegan Place #9, Thousand Oaks, CA 91362, (805) 497-9511, MA 86 CA St Univ - Northridge; 86–Sp-Lang Path, Conejo Valley USD, **SLP**

Abrahamsen, Dr Eileen P 732 Maryland Avenue, Norfolk, VA 23508, (804) 683-4117, BS 68 Elmira Coll; MA 72 SUNY - Center at Albany; ED 80 (Sp Path) Columbia Univ Teachers Coll; Associate Professor, Old Dominion U, **SLP**

Abrahamsohn, Mrs Freida 13 Heytor Road, Victory Park, Johannesburg, South Africa 2195, BA 60; 81–Aud, Soc for the Hard of Hrng Child, **SLP**

Abrahamson, Debbie Lynn 1595 Highway A1A #102, Satellite Beach, FL 32937, (407) 676-1431, BS 83 Southwest MO St Univ; MA 85 Southwest MO St Univ; Sp-Lang Path, Brevard Speech & Lang Ctr, **SLP**

Abrahamson, Judy E 1200 Madison Avenue, Austin, TX 78757-1928, MS 73 Univ of TX - Austin; Aud, Assoc in Otolaryngology, **A**

Abrahamson, Marilyn Samberg 144-55 Melbourne Avenue, #4F, Kew Gardens, NY 11367, (718) 990-8883, BA 86 Kean Coll of NJ; MA 87 Kean Coll of NJ

Abramovitz, Dr Rachelle S 75-19 190th Street, Fresh Meadows, NY 11366, (212) 464-5422, BA 71 CUNY - Queens Coll; MA 73 CUNY - Queens Coll; PH 79 (Aud & Hrng Science); 88–Aud, Bernard Finenson Dev Ctr, **A**

Abramowitz, Judith Sarah 82-31 Little Neck Parkway, Floral Park, NY 11004, (212) 360-5600, **SLP**

Abramowitz, Marvin R 12082 Long Lake Drive, Owings Mills, MD 21117, (301) 225-8380, BS 72 Towson St Univ; MS 74 Towson St Univ; Director of Rehabilitation, Maryland Gen Hosp, **SLP**

Abrams, Annette 2927 32nd St, San Diego, CA 92104, (619) 280-8667, MA 87 San Diego St Univ

Abrams, Beth L 333 East 56th Street #11C, New York, NY 10022, (212) 223-3775, BS 77 Northwestern Univ; MS 79 Univ of WI - Madison; 87–Sp-Lang Path, Herbert G Birch Sch for Exceptional Children Inc, **SLP**

Abrams, Deborah Shanok 5288 South Kenton Way, Englewood, CO 80111, (303) 798-2438, BS 72 OH St Univ; MA 79 Univ of CO - Boulder; Sp-Lang Path, Littleton Sch Dist/Arapahoe #6, **SLP**

Abrams, Mrs Ellen J 118 Three Mile Road, Glastonbury, CT 06033, (203) 632-2158, BA 61 Univ of CT; MA 63 CUNY - Brooklyn Coll; Sp-Lang Path, Middletown Bd of Educ, **SLP**

Abrams, Dr Harvey B Audiology/Speech Pathology Service, VA Medical Center, Bay Pines, FL 33504, (813) 398-9395, BA 70 George Washington Univ; MA 71 Univ of FL; PH 80 (Aud) Univ of FL; Chief, VA Med Cen Bay Pines FL, **A**

Abrams, Mrs Jane F 9905 Barstow Court, Potomac, MD 20854, (301) 762-2668, BS 66 Boston Univ; MA 68 Univ of MD - College Park; 88–Sp-Lang Path, Private Practice, **SLP**

Abrams, Mrs Kathleen M 54 Eldrid Drive, Silver Spring, MD 20904, (301) 680-9433, BS 66 Georgetown Univ; MA 70 Catholic Univ of America; Sp-Lang Path, Mont Co Pub Sch-Div/Sp-Lang, **SLP**

Abrams, Marjorie C 1307 Providence Road, Baltimore, MD 21204, **SLP**

Abrams, Michele R 38 Cadwallader Court, Yardley, PA 19067, (215) 860-2803, Newton Audiology, **A**

Abrams, Nellie 10304 Alicia Drive, Midwest City, OK 73130, (405) 732-9873, BA 80 Univ of OK - Norman; MS 82 Univ of OK - OK City; Sp-Lang Path, Oklahoma City Public Schools, **SLP**

Abrams, Peter C 25 Zenas Drive, Glens Falls, NY 12801, (518) 792-3336, MS 72 SUNY - Center at Albany; 70–Sp-Lang Path, WA-Warren Hamilton/BOCES, **SLP**

Abrams, Mrs Rosalie Gelfand 266 Newman Street, Metuchen, NJ 08840, (201) 494-0359, BA 73 CUNY - Lehman Coll; MA 75 CUNY - Lehman Coll; 88–Sp-Lang Path, Union Co Day Training Ctr

Abrams, Scott David 73-63 Bell Boulevard, Bayside, NY 11364, (718) 464-3265, MA 87 CUNY - Lehman Coll; 88–Sp-Lang Path, NY City Bd of Educ

Abrams, Mrs Susan L S 12327 Overcup Drive, Houston, TX 77024, (713) 932-6719, BS 75 Univ of TX - Austin; MS 77 Baylor Coll of Medicine; **A**

Abrams, Susan M 713 Hurley Avenue, Rockville, MD 20850, (301) 294-0146, BA 74 Hofstra Univ; MA 75 Hofstra Univ; MA 77 George Washington Univ; Sp-Lang Path, Private Practice, **SLP**

Abrams, Suzanne Lori 532 East 83rd Street #2F, New York, NY 10028, (212) 838-4333, MS 83 Columbia Univ Teachers Coll; 86–Sp-Lang Path, Karen Horney Cl-Ther Nursery, **SLP**

Abrams, Mrs Wendy Chukerman 515 West Belden, Chicago, IL 60614, (312) 943-5511, **SLP**

Abramson, Mrs Arlene F 18 Cross Street, South Easton, MA 02375, (508) 676-3411, BA 74 Univ of MA - Amherst; ME 75 Northeastern Univ; 75–Aud, R H Fitton Jr MD Inc, **A**

Abramson, Dr Arthur S University Of Connecticut, Linguistics U-145 Room 230, 341 Mansfield Road, Storrs, CT 06268, (203) 486-4229, BA 49 Yeshiva Univ; MA 50 Columbia Univ Teachers Coll; PH 60 (Linguistics) Columbia Univ Teachers Coll; Prof of Linguistics, U of CT

Abramson, Lois Michele 341 Clearmeadow Drive, East Meadow, NY 11554, (516) 796-2003, MS 87 Adelphi Univ; **SLP**

Abramson, Maria L K 33292 Astoria, Dana Point, CA 92629, (714) 640-5702, BS 77 Northwestern Univ; MS 79 Univ of WA; Director of Audiology, Hearing Professionals/Irvine, **A**

Abramson, Mrs Myrna G 14 North Crest Road, Chattanooga, TN 37404, (615) 698-4201, BS 60 PA St Univ - Univ Park; MS 64 Tulane Univ; **SLP**

Abrassart, Mrs Joanne Y 2502 Rainbow Lane, Brea, CA 92621, (714) 529-3916, BA 72 Univ of Redlands; MS 73 Univ of Redlands; **SLP**

Abrassart, Richard A 2502 Rainbow Lane, Brea, CA 92621, (714) 891-8290, BA 70 Univ of Redlands; MS 71 Univ of Redlands; SLP, California State U Fullerton, **SLP**

Abreu, Katherine Oconnor 3170 Spawn Road, Schenectady, NY 12303, (518) 374-4551, BA 71 SUNY - Center at Binghamton; MS 82 Coll of Saint Rose; SLP, Center for Human Capabilities, **SLP**

Abreu, Rosa A 150 Paulison Avenue, Unit 4, Passaic, NJ 07055, (201) 473-7519, BA 81 Fairleigh Dickinson U-Ruther; MA 84 CUNY - Grad Sch & Univ Cntr; 86–Sp-Lang Path, St Francis Hosp, **A**

Abromaitis, Mrs Kay Marie 4605 Leesburg Court, Louisville, KY 40241, (502) 425-7727, BS 72 Western MI Univ; MS 85 Univ of Louisville; 85–Sp-Lang Path, Private Practice, **SLP**

Abruzzese, Rosalie Mary 114 Huemmer Terrace, Clifton, NJ 07013, (201) 773-1786, BA 79 Montclair St Coll; MA 84 Montclair St Coll; **SLP**

Abruzzo, Lynette 148-54 Huxley Street, Rosedale, NY 11422, BA 81 Saint John's Univ - Jamaica; MA 83 CUNY - Queens Coll; Sp-Lang Path, Long Island Jewish Preschool, **SLP**

Absher, Mrs Fern S 704 9th Street, North Wilkesboro, NC 28659, BS 73 Appalachian St Univ; MA 74 Appalachian St Univ; 76–Sp-Lang Path, Alexander Co Sch, **SLP**

Abshez, Mrs Wendy Ann 827 South Stanley Avenue, Los Angeles, CA 90036, (213) 857-1372, **SLP**

Abshier, Victoria Plunkett 937 Edgefield Trail, Lewisville, TX 75028, (817) 370-3407, MS 84 Univ of North TX; Sp-Lang Path, Lewisville ISD, **SLP**

Abshire-Jumonville, Mrs Wendy Marie 1425 South Alameda, Baton Rouge, LA 70815, (504) 388-2991, BS 81 Saint Mary's Dominicon Coll; MS 83 Purdue Univ - West Lafayette; 88–Instr, Louisiana State Univ, **A**

Abu-Rayyan, Mrs Rebecca G 4103 Walhill Lane, Austin, TX 78759, (512) 892-0886, BS 67 Univ of IL - Urbana; MA 68 Univ of IL - Urbana; 88–Sp-Lang Path, Central TX Aud & Sp Path Svcs, **SLP**

Accardi, Clare Mercier 45 Beth Avenue, Warren, RI 02885, (617) 992-4756, **SLP**

Acevedo, Mrs Ann M 96 East Cherbourg, Cheektowaga, NY 14227, (716) 674-6300, BS 75 SUNY - Coll at Buffalo; MS 77 SUNY - Coll at Buffalo; Team Leader, West Seneca Develop Cen, **SLP**

Acevedo, Mary Ann 1903 Pompton, Austin, TX 78758, (512) 245-2330, BA 65 Univ of TX - Austin; MA 67 Univ of TX - Austin; PH 79 (Communication Disorders) Univ of TX - Austin; 86–Asst Prof, Southwest Texas State Univ, **SLP ACE**

Achilles, Mrs Judith 424 West Scotland Drive, Irving, TX 75062, (214) 368-5823, BA 75 Univ of CA - Riverside; MA 79 Univ of North TX; SLP, Dallas ISD, **SLP**

Achilles, Dr Robert F Speech And Hearing Center, Lamar University, Box 10076, Beaumont, TX 77710, (409) 838-8173, BS 49 McPherson Coll; MA 55 Wichita St Univ; PH 68 (NS) Wichita St Univ; Prof, Lamar U, **SLP**

Achiron, Mrs Michele R 18 Holbrooke Road, White Plains, NY 10605, (914) 965-6700, BS 74 SUNY - Center at Albany; MA 76 NY Univ; Supervisor Speech & Audiology, St Josephs Med Cen, **SLP**

Achord, Mrs Sara H 1216 Cherry Lane, Calimesa, CA 92320, (714) 795-5130, BA 65 Union Coll; MS 80 Univ of Redlands; SLP, Beaumont USD, **SLP**

Acimovic, Mary Lou 1309 Centaur Circle, Lafayette, CO 80026, (303) 665-7840, BA 71 Univ of CO - Boulder; MA 75 Univ of CO - Boulder; Sp/Lang Path, Louisville Therapy Clinic, **SLP**

Acinger, Mrs Rhonda R R 1 Box 86, Spring Hill, KS 66083, (913) 884-7101, BS 76 KS St Univ; MA 78 KS St Univ; Sp-Lang Path, USD 231, **SLP**

Acker, Mrs Jane M 2420 Chip Road, Kawkawlin, MI 48631, MS 71 MI St Univ; Sp-Lang Path, Tuscola Intermed School Dist, **SLP**

Acker-Bailey, Patricia G 5243 Terrace Road, Mechanicsburg, PA 17055, (717) 737-7589, BS 79 Univ of WI - Madison; MS 83 Emerson Coll; 88–Clin Supvr, InSpeech Inc, **SLP**

Ackeret, Mrs Rosalind Marie 9401 W Calumet Road #201, Milwaukee, WI 53224, (414) 263-6732, BS 82 Univ of WI - Eau Claire; MS 86 Marquette Univ; 87–Sp-Lang Path, Curative Rehab Ctr, **SLP**

Ackeret, Ruth E 1377 Eminence Street, Green Bay, WI 54313, (414) 469-4811, BS 72 Univ of WI - River Falls; MS 77 Univ of WI - Eau Claire; Sp-Lang Path, Green Bay Bd of Ed, **SLP**

Ackerman, Carol A 9911 West Pico Boulevard #1040, Los Angeles, CA 90035, (213) 201-6562, BS 69 Bowling Green St Univ; MA 75 CA St Univ - Los Angeles; Sp-Lang Path, Private Practice, **SLP**

Ackerman, Marjorie Cimmet 2075 Salisbury Park Drive, Westbury, NY 11590, (516) 667-5353, BA 50 Univ of MD - College Park; SLP, Suffolk Co BOCES #3, **SLP**

Ackerman, Martha G 1356 East Hyde Park Blvd, Chicago, IL 60615, (312) 268-1356, BA 63 Univ of CA - Los Angeles; MA 70 Columbia Univ Teachers Coll; 88–Acct Exec, CEBCOR Employee Leasing Co, **SLP**

Ackerman, Mindy W 97 Wilson Drive, New Rochelle, NY 10801, (914) 632-1412, BA 73 SUNY - Center at Buffalo; MS 74 Univ of MI - Ann Arbor; **SLP**

Ackerman, Mrs Randa R 1035 South Dove Place, Anaheim, CA 92805, (213) 336-5061, BS 71 Bowling Green St Univ; MA 72 Bowling Green St Univ; 75–Sp-Lang Path, Los Angeles County Office of Educ, **SLP**

Ackerman, Dr Robert J Dept Speech Path & Audiology, East Stroudsburg Univ, East Stroudsburg, PA 18301, (717) 424-3681, BA 72 SUNY - Center at Albany; MS 76 Towson St Univ; PH 82 (NS) Wichita St Univ; Assistant Professor, East Stroudsburg University, **SLP**

Ackerman, Mrs Sonia Sperry 4317 W Poinsettia, Glendale, AZ 85304, (602) 967-6473, **SLP**

Ackermann, Diane Lillian 6826 Chesapeake Drive, Apt E, Florissant, MO 63033, MA 86 Saint Louis Univ; **SLP**

Ackermann, Lynne Marie 3848 Windemer Drive, Florissant, MO 63033, (314) 831-3898, BS 85 Southwest MO St Univ; MA 87 Saint Louis Univ

Ackles, Mrs Mary Egan 15999 Highway 66, Ashland, OR 97520, (503) 482-0920, BA 78 CA St Univ - Long Beach; MA 81 CA St Univ - Long Beach; Sp-Lang Path, Jackson Co Ed Serv Dist, **SLP**

Ackley, Diane D 1723 Kingston Circle, Redlands, CA 92374, (714) 788-7374, BA 72 Loma Linda Univ - Riverside; MA 73 Univ of Denver; SLP, Riverside USD, **SLP**

Ackley, Mrs Dolores Shuler 5601 New Haven, Greenville, TX 75401, (214) 455-5373, BS 79 East TX St Univ - Commerce; MS 82 Univ of TX - Dallas; **SLP**

Ackley, Robert S 1129 West Mulberry, Fort Collins, CO 80521-3518, **A**

Acord, Mrs Tera S 3005 Glenhollow Circle, Carrollton, TX 75007, (214) 245-8685, BA 64 Baylor Univ; MS 76 Baylor Univ; Sp-Lang Path, Carrollton-Farmers-Branch ISD, **SLP**

Acosta, Lorena HC-01 Box 4871, Lajas, PR 00667, BS 84 Univ of RI; MS 86 TX Christian Univ; 88–Sp-Lang Path, Centro de Educ Esp del Oeste, **SLP**

Acosta, Sharon Trimble 6383 Northampton, Memphis, TN 38134-3749, (901) 373-5359, BA 74 MS St Univ - MS State; MA 76 Memphis St Univ; Sp/Lang Path, Baptist Memorial Hospital, **SLP**

Acree, Jo Nell Route 4 Box 301, Lynchburg, VA 24503, (804) 522-4520, BS 84 Radford Univ; MS 85 Radford Univ; 85–Aud, Central VA Sp & Hrng Cntr, **A**

Acree, Laura 5633 Rock Road, Union City, GA 30291, (404) 969-1595, BA 70 Hampton Univ; MS 71 PA St Univ - Univ Park; Sp-Lang Path, Atlanta Bd of Ed, **SLP**

Acri, Jane B 8816 Maywood Avenue, Silver Spring, MD 20910, (202) 576-1649, BA 73 Washington Univ; MA 77 Catholic Univ of America; Aud, Wramc, **A**

Acton, Lynn M 42 Edgewood Road, Robbinsville, NJ 08691, (609) 259-9168, MS 88 PA St Univ - Univ Park

Acton, Shari Kay 1112 West McGee Street, Springfield, MO 65807, (417) 887-5750, BS 82 Univ of NE - Lincoln; MS 83 Univ of NE - Lincoln; Aud, Reg Ear Nose & Throat Ctr, **A**

Acutt, Mrs Margaret S Cliff House Flat #6, Bonchurch Shute, Ventnor PO 38 Inu, Isle of Wight, England, BA 69 Case Western Reserve Univ; MA 73 Univ of TX - Austin; SLP, Isle of Wight Hlth Auth, **SLP**

Adair, Dr Joe B R R 3 Box 805, Gatlinburg, TN 37738, (615) 436-6561, BA 69 OK St Univ; MS 71 Phillips Univ; PH 81 (NS) Univ of IA; VP, Mountainbrook Resch & Training, **A**

Adair, Melanie N R R 3 Box 805, Gatlinburg, TN 37738-9803, (615) 822-9010, BS 68 OK St Univ; MA 69 OK St Univ; 86–Ex VP/Rehab Svcs, Rebound Inc, **SLP**

Adair, Sharon 149 Rowayton Woods, Norwalk, CT 06854-3941, (203) 852-9613, BS 62 Univ of KS; MA 69 Univ of KS; Sp-Lang Path, Norwalk Pub Sch, **SLP**

Adair, Mrs Victoria Lynne HCR 72, P O Box 350, Wasola, MO 65773, (417) 265-3439, MS 87 Central MO St Univ

Adam, Arlie J 4612 S E 44th Street, Portland, OR 97206, (503) 235-6551, BA 74 Portland St Univ; MS 78 Portland St Univ; Aud, Audiology Cl, **A**

Adam, Mrs Colleen 1101 North Lincoln, Hastings, NE 68901, (402) 463-4358, BS 70 Univ of NE - Lincoln; MA 72 Univ of NE - Lincoln; **A**

Adam, Mrs Kathryn L 6835 West Evergreen, Palos Heights, IL 60463, (312) 361-6065, BA 73 Elmhurst Coll; MA 74 Southern IL Univ -Carbondale; Dir Sp-Lang Path Dept, Mercy Hosp and Med Ctr, **SLP ACE**

Adam, Linda Peebles 630 N W 214th Street #105, Miami, FL 33169, (305) 324-3148, BS 74 East Carolina Univ; MA 80 Appalachian St Univ; 88–Mgmt Asst/Sp-Lang Path, Veterans Administration Med Ct, **SLP**

Adamczak, Jeffrey E 4980 North Marine Drive, Apt #1231, Chicago, IL 60640, BS 75 Western MI Univ; MA 79 Wayne St Univ; SLP, Chicago Public Schools, **SLP**

Adamczyk, Deborah Fischer 149 Briarwood Lane, Mars, PA 16046, (412) 961-0295, BS 73 Edinboro Univ of PA; MA 78 Univ of Pittsburgh - Pittsburgh; SLP, Allegheny Intermed Unit, **SLP**

Adamo, Brian 5664 Montezuma Road, San Diego, CA 92115, (619) 589-4108, BA 79 San Diego St Univ; MA 87 San Diego St Univ; 88–Sp-Lang Path, Grossmont Dist Hosp

Adamousky, Dawn Julie 540 Ocean Parkway, Brooklyn, NY 11218, (718) 436-9869, BA 83 CUNY - Brooklyn Coll; MS 86 CUNY - Brooklyn Coll

Adamovich, Dr Brenda L B 9 Butternut Road, Westfield, MA 01085, (413) 781-9100, BS 72 OH St Univ; MS 73 OH St Univ; PH 76 (NS) OH St Univ; Dir Ambulatory Ser Div, New Medico Assoc Inc, **SLP**

Adamowicz, Michael F 3820 N W 83rd Terrace, Coral Springs, FL 33065, (305) 497-1850, BS 75 Bloomsburg Univ of PA; ME 76 Bloomsburg Univ of PA; Aud, Sch Bd of Broward Cty, **A**

Adams, A Barbara Box 811, Kinston, NC 28501, (919) 527-9561, BS 82 Trenton St Coll; MA 84 Trenton St Coll; 86–Sp-Lang Path, Home Health & Hospice Care, **SLP ACE**

Adams, Amanda Wallin 720 North K Street #B, Tacoma, WA 98403, (206) 572-5252, BA 84 Univ of WA; MS 86 Univ of WA; Sp-Lang Path, Multicare Med Ctr, **SLP**

Adams, Amy Kathryn 2000 North Meridian Road, Apartment 144, Tallahassee, FL 32303, (904) 627-9651, BS 84 FL St Univ; MS 85 FL St Univ; SLP, Gadsden Co P S, **SLP**

Adams, Amy L 12997 West Cedar #307, Lakewood, CO 80228, (303) 988-3297, BS 85 Western IL Univ; MA 86 Western IL Univ; **SLP**

Adams, Mrs Barbara M Rd #1 Box 234B, Woodbine, NJ 08270, (609) 861-2164, BS 84 Bloomsburg Univ of PA; MS 85 Bloomsburg Univ of PA; 88–Sp-Lang Path, Woodbine Developmental Center, **SLP**

Adams, Bonnie Stalians 2305 Coffee Road, Modesto, CA 95355, (209) 578-0888, BA 75 CA St Univ - Stanislaus; MA 77 CA St Univ - Stanislaus; Director, Speech Therapy Services, **SLP**

Adams, Carol M 2715 S W Stanley Court, Portland, OR 97219, (503) 245-3204, BS 76 Portland St Univ; MA 77 San Diego St Univ; Sp-Lang Path, Good Samaritan Hosp & Med Cen, **SLP**

Adams, Carolyn A 12711 Nettles Drive #16, Newport News, VA 23606, **SLP**

Adams, Carroll M 3904 Willow Ridge Drive, Helena, AL 35080, (205) 669-4158, BS 76 Univ Southern MS-Hattiesburg; MS 77 Univ Southern MS-Hattiesburg; Sp-Lang Path, Shelby Co Bd of Ed, **SLP**

Adams, Clarinda T 12912 Archdale, Detroit, MI 48227, (313) 433-1844, BA 77 Univ of MI - Ann Arbor; MA 79 Wayne St Univ; Sp-Lang Path, Harriet Cooper Neurohab Ctr, **SLP**

Adams, Debbie M 31 East Firestone Blvd, Apartment 7A, Akron, OH 44301, (216) 489-1135, BA 79 Univ of Akron; MA 81 Univ of Akron; 86–Sp-Lang Path, Timken Mercy Med Ctr, **SLP**

Adams, Mrs Deborah A 1714 Carolina, Marysville, MI 48040, (313) 364-8990, BS 73 Eastern MI Univ; MA 74 Eastern MI Univ; Sp-Lang Path, **SLP**

Adams, Deborah Lynn M-205 Rogers Road, Athens, GA 30605, (404) 543-4839, BS 82 Univ of GA; ME 84 Univ of GA; 88–Parent Advisor, Georgia Pines, **A**

Adams, Denise S P O Box 936, Starke, FL 32091, (904) 964-6800, BS 75 FL St Univ; MS 76 FL St Univ; 87–Exceptional Stu Educ Dir, Bradford Co Sch Bd, **SLP**

Adams, Eleanor 530 West Routt, Pueblo, CO 81004, (719) 542-2419, BA 74 Hollins Coll; MA 76 Univ of TN - Knoxville; Dept Head Sp-Lang Path, H & W Therapy PC, **SLP**

Adams, Elizabeth Mantione 196-50 67th Avenue, Fresh Meadows, NY 11365, (212) 750-4942, BA 84 CUNY - Queens Coll; MA 86 CUNY - Queens Coll; **SLP**

Adams, Mrs Esther Young 100 West 12th Street, Hutchinson, KS 67501, (316) 662-6116, BS 53 Univ of KS; MS 57 Univ of KS; Sp-Lang Path, Private Practice, **LM**

Adams, H Gregory 412 East Street, Athens, AL 35611, (205) 534-6421, BA 70 Auburn Univ - Auburn; MA 73 Auburn Univ - Auburn; 87–Dir of Audiology, Lakeshore Huntsville Rehab Ctr, **A**

Adams, Heidi Marie 910 Longmeadow Drive, Geneva, IL 60134, (312) 232-8218, BS 63 Northwestern Univ; MA 64 Northwestern Univ; Sp-Lang Path, East Aurora Pub Sch Dist 131, **SLP**

Adams, Mrs Janet Olive 13801 East Ashlan, Sanger, CA 93657, (209) 875-5013, MA 86 Montclair St Coll; **SLP**

Adams, Janet Rose 508 West 57th Street, Erie, PA 16509, (814) 864-3725, BS 74 Edinboro Univ of PA; MA 79 Edinboro Univ of PA; Sp-Lang Path, St Vincent's Hlth Cen, **SLP**

Adams, John (Jack) H Audiology Consultants, 625 Del Prado Boulevard, Cape Coral, FL 33990, (813) 772-0940, MS 76 Tulane Univ; Aud, Aud Consultants, **A**

Adams, Judy K 1368 Laurel Avenue, St Paul, MN 55104, (612) 644-6168, BS 72 Univ of TX - Austin; MA 74 Univ of TX - Austin; 78–Sp/Lang Path, St Paul Pub Sch, **SLP**

Adams, Mrs Julia G 2845 Denver, San Diego, CA 92117, (619) 274-9871, BS 63 Univ of ID; MA 65 Univ of IA; Sp-Lang Path, San Diego USD, **SLP**

Adams, June B 4109 Shiloh Drive, Birmingham, AL 35213, (205) 252-6041, BA 73 Univ of AL- Tuscaloosa; MA 74 Univ of AL- Tuscaloosa; Sp/Lang Path, Birmingham Cty Sch, **SLP**

Adams, Karen Mary 6022 Rock Glen Drive, Baltimore, MD 21227, (301) 796-7572, BA 71 PA St Univ - Univ Park; MS 78 Loyola Coll; **SLP**

Adams, Kathryn L 11957 Brook Road, Golden, CO 80403, (303) 426-2151, SLP, St Anthonys Hosp, **SLP**

Adams, Dr Larry 3904 Willow Ridge Drive, Helena, AL 35080, (205) 934-4467, BS 72 Henderson St Univ; PH 76 (NS) Northwestern Univ; V-Chair Dept of Communication, University of Alabama, **SLP**

Adams, Lennon C, Jr Southeastern Hearing Conservation Inc, 19920 SW 87th Place, Miami, FL 33157, (305) 253-3832, MS 73 Univ of South FL; **A**

Adams, Leslie Anderson 13326 Point Rider Lane, Herndon, VA 22071, (703) 435-0896, BA 72 Univ of Redlands; MS 74 Univ of Redlands; Sp-Lang Path, Fairfax County Schools, **SLP**

Adams, Leslie J Basic Educational Tutors, 2623 East Madison, Seattle, WA 98112, (206) 322-2113, BA 75 Univ of WA; MS 77 Univ of WA; Sp-Lang Path, Basic Educational Tutors, **SLP**

Adams, Linda 55 King Street, Watertown, MA 02172, (617) 531-1600, BS 81 Northeastern Univ; ME 83 Northeastern Univ; Sp-Lang Path, Peabody School Dept, **SLP**

Adams, Mrs Linda G 513 Highway 9, #163, Lake Stevens, WA 98258, (206) 334-3702, BA 74 Univ of the Pacific; MA 76 Univ of the Pacific; SLP, Lake Stevens School District 4, **SLP**

Adams, Lisa Ann 9410 North 31st Avenue, Apartment 1001, Phoenix, AZ 85051, (602) 870-4055, BS 84 Univ of Montevallo; MA 86 Memphis St Univ; **SLP**

Adams, Mrs Marla R 9 Christine Avenue, Franklin, MA 02038, (617) 528-2457, BA 72 Univ of WI - Eau Claire; MS 78 Univ of WI - Eau Claire; Sp-Lang Path, Spoke Collaborative, **SLP**

Adams, Marsha Lee 720 North 92nd, Seattle, WA 98103, (206) 782-8734, BS 84 Univ of WA; MS 87 Univ of WA; **SLP**

Adams, Dr Martin R 12910 Figaro, Houston, TX 77024, (713) 749-4553, BA 57 Univ of Redlands; MA 58 Univ of Redlands; PH 67 (NS) Southern IL Univ -Carbondale; Prof, U of Houston, **SLP F**

Adams, Mrs Mary Beth Kane 1122 Sara Court, Erie, PA 16504, (814) 825-3295, BS 80 Indiana Univ of PA; MA 83 Univ of Pittsburgh - Pittsburgh; Sp/Lang Path, Associates In Communication, **SLP**

Adams, Mary M 4428 East Justice Circle, Orange, CA 92669, (714) 737-4200, BS 75 Towson St Univ; MA 78 Univ of CT; 86–Aud, Communication Health Services, **A**

Adams, Maryln Allen 4015 Clifton Avenue, Cincinnati, OH 45220, (513) 729-0130, OB 68 Univ of WI - Whitewater; MA 75 Univ of Cincinnati; Sp-Lang Path, Mt Healthy Pub Sch, **SLP**

Adams, McKinnie D P O Box 17241, Winston-Salem, NC 27116, (919) 761-0786, BS 86 Univ of NC - Greensboro; MA 87 Univ of NC - Greensboro

Adams, Mrs Nancy Engel 4226 Fort Donelson, Stockton, CA 95209, (209) 467-6345, BA 80 Univ of the Pacific; MA 81 Univ of the Pacific; Sp-Lang Path, St Joseph's Hosp, **SLP**

Adams, Mrs Pamela Martin Rd 1 Box 231-B, Grantsville, MD 21536, (301) 895-3251, BS 77 CA Univ of PA; MS 80 PA St Univ - Univ Park; 88–Aud, Private Practice, **A**

Adams, Patricia Agnes 594 Cambridge Street #2, Allston, MA 02134, (617) 787-2471, BA 85 Univ of WA; MS 87 Univ of WA; **SLP**

Adams, Mrs Patricia S 1901 Cathy Avenue, Fairmont, WV 26554, (304) 366-2070, BS 76 WV Univ; MS 78 WV Univ; Aud/SLP, Marion County Schools, **A**

Adams, Mrs Phyllis S 1615 Paseo, DE La Conquistadora, Santa Fe, NM 87501, (505) 982-2345, BA 73 NM St Univ; MA 75 NM St Univ; **SLP**

Adams, R Kathleen 322 East Antietam Street, Suite 101, Hagerstown, MD 21740, (301) 733-1190, BA 81 Univ of Northern CO; MA 82 Univ of Northern CO; Aud, The Hearing Care Center, **A**

Adams, Mrs Renee P S 5723 Eugenia Lane, Peoria Heights, IL 61614, (309) 274-4841, BS 74 Western IL Univ; MS 75 IL St Univ - Normal; Sp-Lang Path, IL Valley Cen Sch Dist #321, **SLP**

Adams, Richard T 15 Millstone Road, Randallstown, MD 21133, **SLP**

Adams, Rita Lynn 108 9th Court South, Bessemer, AL 35020, (205) 426-0349, BS 84 Central MO St Univ; MS 86 Univ of Montevallo; **SLP**

Adams, Robert J 994 Summer N E, Salem, OR 97301, (303) 399-3145, BA 55 Univ of Northern CO; MA 58 Univ of Northern CO; **SLP**

Adams, Mrs Ruth W 3905 South Washburn Avenue, Minneapolis, MN 55410, (612) 920-5397, BA 57 Hamline Univ; **SLP**

Adams, Sally Lynne 479 Grand Street, Allegan, MI 49010, (616) 673-4805, BS 77 Western MI Univ; MA 85 Western MI Univ; **SLP**

Adams, Susan E 37 Green Street - Rear, Augusta, ME 04330, (207) 872-4383, MS 78 Ithaca Coll; Aud, Mid ME Med Cen, **A**

Adams, Susan L 60-C North Mountain Road, New Britain, CT 06053, (203) 233-1455, BA 80 Univ of CT; MA 82 IN Univ - Bloomington; 88–Sp/Lang Path, West Hartford PS, **SLP**

Adams, Terri Ruth P O Box 7, Chinle, AZ 86503, (602) 674-3481, MS 81 Univ of South FL; Sp-Lang Path, Chinle Shcl Dist, **SLP**

Adams, Mrs Vickie L 730 Valley Street, Dayton, OH 45404, (513) 222-5597, BS 80 Univ of Cincinnati; MA 83 Univ of Cincinnati; 88–Aud, Hearing & Speech Ctr, **A**

Adams, Virginia S 504 South Oak Street, Fergus Falls, MN 56537, (218) 736-4842, BA 48 Carleton Coll; MS 73 Moorhead St Univ; Sp-Lang Path, Pvt Voice Therapy, **SLP**

Adams-Davis, Mrs Pamela M 2334 Ridgewood Avenue, Omaha, NE 68124, (402) 691-1335, BS 75 Univ of NE - Lincoln; MS 76 Univ of AZ; Sp-Lang Path, Millard PS, **SLP**

Adams-Ethridge, Donna E 5603 Glen Mist Lane, Houston, TX 77069, (713) 462-2686, BS 75 Univ of TX - Austin; MA 77 Univ of Houston - Univ Park; 88–Coord of Spec Educ Prog, Cypress-Fairbanks ISD, **SLP**

Adamski, Mrs Jeanette Johnson 614 109th Avenue N W, Coon Rapids, MN 55433, (215) 631-9300, BA 85 Mayville St Coll; MS 87 Mayville St Coll; **SLP**

Adamson, Benita McCarthy 226 S E 1st Circle, Boynton Beach, FL 33435, (305) 655-7268, BA 76 Univ of FL; MS 80 FL St Univ; Sp-Lang Path, Bethesda Mem Hosp, **SLP ACE**

Adamson, Cathy 17 Woodland Village, Leeds, AL 35094, (205) 939-5917, BS 75 Auburn Univ - Auburn; OM 77 Auburn Univ - Auburn; Aud, Crippled Chldn Serv, **A**

Adamson, Clark R Box 382, Silverton, ID 83867, (208) 556-1531, BS 72 Central St Univ; BA 66 Eastern WA Univ; OM 83 Univ of ID; Dir of Spec Serv, Sch Dist 391-2&3, **SLP**

Adasko, Mrs Mary Hardy 1797 East 22nd Street, Brooklyn, NY 11229, (212) 376-0947, BA 69 CUNY - Brooklyn Coll; MS 76 CUNY - Brooklyn Coll; SLP, NYC Bd of Ed, **SLP ACE**

Adcock, Aleta Millet 407 West Woodgate Court, Baton Rouge, LA 70808, (504) 381-6525, BA 76 LA St Univ - Baton Rouge; MA 78 Memphis St Univ; Sp-Lang Path, Baton Rouge General Med Ctr, **SLP**

Adcock, Ava L 618 Laurel Avenue, South Pittsburg, TN 37380, **SLP**

Addicks, Connie S 406 South 3rd Avenue, Arcadia, CA 91006, (818) 445-2987, BA 69 Univ of LA Verne; MA 70 Univ of Redlands; 88–Human Resource Rep, InSpeech Inc, **SLP**

Addicott, John P 3858 Las Pasas Way, Sacramento, CA 95864, (916) 454-6601, BA 65 Moorhead St Univ; MA 67 Univ of WA, PH 73 (NS) Univ of WA; 74–Prof, California St Univ Sacramento, **SLP**

Addicott, Mrs Margaret A 3858 Las Pasas Way, Sacramento, CA 95864, (916) 363-9650, BA 67 Univ of WA; MA 69 Univ of WA; Sp-Lang Path, San Juan USD, **SLP**

Addis, Ann Buckler 330 Bryn Mawr Avenue, Bala-Cynwyd, PA 19004, (215) 587-3143, BA 74 Cornell Univ; MA 76 Northwestern Univ; 87–Sp-Lang Path, Magee Rehab Hosp, **SLP**

Addis, Dr Judith T PO Box #96, Hewlett Plaza, Hewlett, NY 11557, (516) 997-8700, BA 69; MA 83; PH 86 (Psychotherapy); 88–SLP, Tropic Doc Inc

Addison, C Lewis Tenn Valley Authority, Edney Bldg Third Floor, Chattanooga, TN 37402-2801, (615) 751-7655, BS 72 Univ of GA; 82–Aud, TN Valley Authority, **A**

Addison, Tina Marie 415-H Tradewinds Drive, Fayetteville, NC 28304, (919) 323-6093, BS 84 Univ of NC - Greensboro; ME 86 Univ of NC - Greensboro; **SLP**

Adducci, Helen Josephine 7708 Vine Street, River Forest, IL 60305, (312) 366-2155, BS 81 Minot St Univ; MS 82 Minot St Univ; **A**

Addy-Cantieri, Carol 1533 Highland Avenue, Wilmette, IL 60091, (312) 880-3430, BA 75 George Washington Univ; MA 77 George Washington Univ; Sp-Lang Path, Chldrns Mem Hosp, **SLP**

Aden, Mrs Frances A 8106 70th Court S W, Tacoma, WA 98499, (206) 588-3489, BA 29 OR St Univ; MA 36 Univ of WA; **SLP A LM**

Adermann, Annette 705 1/2 Diagonal Street, Apt #1, Algona, IA 50511, (515) 295-7887, BA 85 Univ of ND; MA 87 Univ of SD - Vermillion; Sp-Lang Path, Lakeland AEA, **SLP**

Adham, Mrs Mary Lenschow P O Box 542, 260 East Jackson, Hampshire, IL 60140, (312) 859-6105, BS 81 Northern IL Univ - De Kalb; MA 84 Western MI Univ; **A**

Adicks, Jennifer E 2500 West Lee Road, Apt 133, Winter Park, FL 32789, (305) 365-5269, BA 86 Univ of Central FL; MS 87 FL St Univ; 88–Sp-Lang Path, Ctr for Sp & Lang

Adkins, Bonnie Riepe Tom Sawyer Road, Mark Twain Meadows, Muscatine, IA 52761, (319) 263-8476, BA 76 Univ of Northern IA; MA 77 Univ of Northern IA; Sp-Lang Path, Mbaea #9, **SLP**

Adkins, Mrs Dawna Dutton 2015 Martingale Drive, Norman, OK 73072, (405) 340-7034, BA 77 Univ of OK - Norman; MS 87 Univ of OK Medical Center; 87–Sp-Lang Path Assoc, Sp & Hrng Assoc, **SLP**

Adkins, Gail M 5827 South 76th East Avenue, Tulsa, OK 74145, (918) 341-3653, BS 78 OK St Univ; MA 80 Univ of Tulsa; Aud, Gail M Adkins, **A**

Adkins, Mrs J Pamela 29 Riverdale, Winfield, WV 25213, (304) 344-3974, BA 75 Marshall Univ; MA 76 Marshall Univ; 86–Sp-Lang Path, Putnam Co Sch, **SLP A**

Adkins, Laura Westerberg Rd 1 Box 665CK Road, Hill Street, Felton, PA 17322, (717) 757-1035, MA 84 Univ of MD - College Park; Sp-Lang Path, Trans-York & Comm Inter & Rehab Inc, **SLP**

Adkins, Laurie Murray 9501 Chadwick Drive, Boise, ID 83704, (208) 338-3655, BS 74 ID St Univ; MS 78 ID St Univ; SLP, Boise Pub Sch, **SLP**

Adkins, Lynda Compton 421 Homestead Trail, Collinsville, VA 24078, (703) 647-3315, BS 77 James Madison Univ; MS 81 James Madison Univ; Sp-Lang Path, Private Practice, **SLP**

Adkins-Smith, Julie S 4302B 52nd, Lubbock, TX 79413-3822, (806) 796-0791, BA 75 Univ of TX - El Paso; MA 77 Univ of TX - El Paso; Sp-Lang Path, Lubbock ISD, **SLP**

Adkisson, Carol D 1448 Waterside Drive, North Little Rock, AR 72116, (501) 663-8331, BS 74 Evangel Coll; MS 82 Univ of AR - Little Rock; Sp-Lang Path, Easter Seals Rehab Center, **SLP**

Adler, Anne Joyce 696 Mowbray Arch #420, Norfolk, VA 23507, (804) 623-5857, BS 78 Boston Univ; ME 80 Univ of VA - Charlottesville; Aud, VA Sch for Deaf & Blind, **A**

Adler, Beryl T 2425 Kings Highway, Brooklyn, NY 11229, (718) 338-1729, BS 67 CUNY - Brooklyn Coll; MS 69 CUNY - Brooklyn Coll; Dir, Private Practice, **SLP**

Adler, Carol R 25 Green Street #3, Brookline, MA 02146, (617) 566-7754, BS 66 Columbia Univ Sch of Gen St; ME 80 Northeastern Univ; 84–Sp-Lang Path, Cambridge PS, **SLP**

Adler, Mrs Dianne L 2 Pine Hill Trail West, Tequesta, FL 33469, (305) 575-4944

Adler, Mrs Elaine T 835 N E 171 Street, North Miami Beach, FL 33162, (305) 654-9928, BA 73 SUNY - Center at Buffalo; MS 74 Univ of WI - Madison; 80–Sp-Lang Path, Private Practice, **SLP**

Adler, Ellen T 9837 N W 3rd Court, Plantation, FL 33324, (305) 761-8110, BA 68 NY Univ; MA 72 NY Univ; 75–Sp-Lang Path, ARC of Broward Inc, **SLP**

Adler, Eve 49 Newbrook Circle, Chestnut Hill, MA 02167, BA 75 Univ of MA - Amherst; MS 78 Boston Univ; Aud, Newton Pub Hlth Dept, **A**

Adler, Jacqueline 12698 Monterey Cypress Way, San Diego, CA 92130, **A**

Adler, Mrs Janet Louis 11119 Valley Heights Drive, Owings Mills, MD 21117, BS 67 Boston Univ; ME 68 Univ of VA - Charlottesville; Sp-Lang Path, Private Practice, **SLP**

Adler, Mrs Jean L 3 Sam Law Drive, Monsey, NY 10952, (914) 352-7933, OB 71 Yeshiva Univ; BA 71 CUNY - Brooklyn Coll; MS 74 CUNY - Brooklyn Coll; Sp-Lang Path, Private Practice, **SLP ACE**

Adler, Julie A 20 Dorothy Drive, Spring Valley, NY 10977, (914) 285-7294, BA 84 CUNY - Queens Coll; MA 88 CUNY - Queens Coll; 88–Sp-Lang Path, Westchester County Med Ctr

Adler, Mrs Kathleen 37 Wilmore Road, Little Falls, NJ 07424, (201) 785-1486, BA 67 Montclair St Coll; MA 69 William Paterson Coll; 69–Sp-Lang Path, Montclair Bd Ed, **SLP**

Adler, Nancy Ford 6333 Fairfield Drive, Flourtown, PA 19031, (215) 233-3618, BS 78 SUNY - Coll at Buffalo; MS 80 Hahneman Medical Coll; 88–Sp-Lang Path/Aud, Nancy Ford Assoc, **SLP A**

Adler, Mrs Nancy H 190 West 21st Street, Huntington Station, NY 11746, (516) 921-7650, BA 75 SUNY - Coll at Cortland; MS 77 Adelphi Univ; Asst Director Sp-Lang Path, Nassau Cen for Dev Disabl, **SLP**

Adler, Dr Raphael 21819 Virginia Drive, Southfield, MI 48076, (313) 360-3054, BA 53 Wayne St Univ; ME 62 Wayne St Univ; PH 80 (NS) Walden Univ; Prof, Oakland Commun Coll, **SLP LM**

Adler, Dr Richard K 2520 Windy Hill Road, Suite 101, Marietta, GA 30067, (404) 953-6808, MA 70 NY Univ; MA 76 Univ of Akron; PH 80 (Psycholinguistics) OH Univ - Athens; 86–Sp-Lang Path, Communication Improvements Inc, **SLP ACE**

Adler, Robin Birnbaum 178 East 80th Street #14-A, New York, NY 10021, (914) 472-2852, **SLP**

Adler, Dr Sol Dept Audiology & Speech Path, University Of Tennessee, Knoxville, TN 37996, (615) 974-5019, BA 52 CUNY - Brooklyn Coll; MA 53 CUNY - Brooklyn Coll; PH 56 (NS) OH St Univ; Prof, Dept Aud & Sp-Lang Path, **SLP F**

Adler, Vivian Kahn 70-25 Yellowstone Blvd, Apartment 3-C, Forest Hills, NY 11375, BS 80 NY Univ; MA 82 NY Univ; **SLP**

Adley, Mrs Luz Marina 160 Alexander Street, North Providence, RI 02904, (401) 277-3525, MA 85 Univ of Akron; 88–Aud, Rhode Island Sch for the Deaf, **A**

Adolf, Kathryn A 22757 E Lakeway Drive #424, Diamond Bar, CA 91765-4444, (714) 860-4402, BS 79 Western IL Univ; MA 80 Western IL Univ; Sp-Lang Path, Rowland USD, **SLP**

Adolph, Mrs Melinda Rae 680 West Tenaya, Clovis, CA 93612, (209) 439-0520, BA 77 CA St Univ - Fresno; MA 80 CA St Univ - Fresno; 80–Sp-Lang Path, Clovis USD, **SLP**

Adomaitis, Christine Marie 143 Hartshorn Drive, Painesville, OH 44077, (216) 632-0261, BS 83 John Carroll Univ; MA 86 Cleveland St Univ; 88–Sp-Lang Path, Cardinal Sch Dist, **SLP**

Adornato, Denise Marie 42C Pennwood Drive, Rochester, NY 14625, (716) 377-4660, BS 79 SUNY - Coll at Buffalo; MA 81 SUNY - Center at Buffalo; **SLP**

Adornato, Viki Ann 247 Copper Creek Circle, Louisville, KY 40222-6806, (502) 582-7483, BS 84 Northwestern Univ; MA 85 Northwestern Univ; 85–SLP, Frazier Rehab Cen, **SLP**

Adrian, Marjorie R 17163 Beaver Springs Drive, Houston, TX 77090, (713) 537-1008, BS 72 SUNY - Center at Buffalo; MS 82 LA St Univ - Shreveport; 85–Sp-Lang Path, Spring ISD, **SLP**

Adriance, Carolyn Ruth 6917 Robin Willow, Dallas, TX 75248, (214) 348-1210, BS 76 Univ of North TX; MS 79 Univ of North TX; Sp-Lang Path, Richardson ISD, **SLP**

Adriansen, Therese J 2678 Knightsbridge Avenue, Thousand Oaks, CA 91362-5316, BS 77 Northern IL Univ - De Kalb; MA 79 Northern IL Univ - De Kalb; SLP, Corejo Valley USD, **SLP**

Adriatico, Terry 35 East Augusta Avenue, Staten Island, NY 10308, (718) 317-0649, BA 73 CUNY - Hunter Coll; MS 75 Columbia Univ Teachers Coll; 87–Aud, NYC Dept of Health, **A**

Adshead, Mrs Jeanne Weiss 1828 Allen Lane, Abington, PA 19001-1202, (215) 247-4404, BS 79 PA St Univ - Univ Park; MA 82 2919; Aud, Hrng Hlth Care Inc, **A**

Adsit, Paula S 5929 North Arlington, Richmond, CA 94806, (419) 236-1635, BA 65 Bowling Green St Univ; MA 70 San Francisco St Univ; Sp-Lang Path, Rich USD, **SLP**

Adubato, Felicia A 935 Broad Street #64-A, Bloomfield, NJ 07003, (201) 633-3149, BA 73 Seton Hall Univ; MS 74 Seton Hall Univ; Sp-Lang Path, Private Practice, **SLP**

Adzovich, Mrs Nancy Lea 370 Via Vaquero, San Dimas, CA 91773, (714) 592-7155, MA 85 CA St Univ - Los Angeles; Aud, El Monte Compreh Health Ctr, **A**

Aeder, Mrs Nancy G 5277 Ruthton, Columbus, OH 43220, (614) 459-9291, SLP, **SLP**

Affholder, Thomas G 427 East Second Street, Ottawa, OH 45875, **SLP**

Affleck, Christine Anne 180 West Ackerman #39, Monmouth, OR 97361, (503) 838-4816, ME 88 Western OR St Coll

Afflerbaugh, Carol P 22800 Lisa Court, Farmington Hills, MI 48024, (313) 478-4068, BS 68 Univ of CA - Santa Barbara; MA 71 Univ of CA - Santa Barbara; **SLP**

Afroilan, Mrs Rebecca F 101 Juniper Road, Havertown, PA 19083, (215) 446-6900, BS 73 SUNY - Coll at Geneseo; MS 75 Gallaudet Coll; 86–Aud, Head & Neck Assoc of S/E Penn, **A**

Agee, Mrs Lisbeth Ann 1527 Kathwood Drive, Columbia, SC 29206, (803) 787-1910, BS 70 Univ of GA; OM 84 Univ of SC - Columbia; 84–Sp-Lang Path, Richland Sch Dist Two, **SLP**

Agee, Mrs Teresa McGowan 1524 Coffee, Pampa, TX 79065, (802) 665-6228, BS 80 Stephen F Austin St Univ; ME 81 Stephen F Austin St Univ; 87–Sp-Lang Path, Pampa ISD, **SLP**

Agee-Burton, Debra Lynn 4828 Marshall Drive, Santa Rosa, CA 95409, (707) 538-3092, BA 78 Towson St Univ; MA 87 San Jose St Univ; 88–Sp-Lang Path, Northcoast Rehab Ctr, **SLP**

Agemy, Evangeline 6312 Campus, Dearborn Heights, MI 48127, (313) 277-0663, BS 76; MA 77 Eastern MI Univ; Sp-Lang Path, Detroit PS, **SLP**

Aggen, Carol J 6621 Plymouth Avenue North, Golden Valley, MN 55427, **SLP**

Aggen, Mrs Janet S 216 Webster Court, Algonquin, IL 60102, (312) 658-6968, BS 72 Elmhurst Coll; MA 73 Western MI Univ; Sp-Lang Path, School District U46, **SLP**

Agi, Mrs Esta-Dara 1730 Crescent Drive, Anchorage, AK 99508, (907) 562-0079, BA 71 CUNY - Brooklyn Coll; MS 73 Columbia Univ Teachers Coll; Sp-Lang Path, **SLP**

Agin, Dr Rhoda Leah 2552 Le Conte Avenue, Berkeley, CA 94709, (415) 549-1359, BA 68 CUNY - Brooklyn Coll; MA 71 Univ of IL - Urbana; PH 76 (NS) Univ of IL - Urbana; Professor, California State Univ-Hayward, **SLP ACE**

Agins-Bochetto, Paula The Academy House, 1420 Locust Street #6A, Philadelphia, PA 19102, (215) 545-2540, BS 74 Boston Univ; MS 76 Emory Univ; Sp-Lang Path, Private Practice, **SLP**

Agliata, Dana Ann 429 Forest Avenue, Oak Park, IL 60302, (312) 824-1136, BA 82 Augustana Coll; MA 83 Western MI Univ; Sp/Lang Path, Comm Consol Sch Dist #62, **SLP**

Aglieco-McDonald, Mrs Susan M 52 Villa Roma Drive, Tewksbury, MA 01876, (617) 267-4730, BS 81 Univ of MA - Amherst; MA 82 OH Univ - Athens; 84–Aud, Boston Guild for the HOH, **A**

Agnello, Dr Joseph G 364 Plum Street, Cincinnati, OH 45246, PH 63 (NS) OH St Univ; **SLP F**

Agnello, Virginia L 466 Winding Wood Way, Sebastopol, CA 95472, (707) 829-1736, BA 66 CA St Univ - Northridge; MA 68 CA St Univ - Northridge; Sp-Lang Path, Private Practice, **SLP LM**

Agnes, Stephanie 6383 Brooks Drive, Arvada, CO 80004, **SLP**

Agnew, Sue Ann P O Box 72, Vestal, NY 13851, (607) 773-3111, BA 80 SUNY - Coll at Potsdam; MA 82 SUNY - Coll at Geneseo; Sp-Lang Path, Broome Development Center, **SLP**

Agone, Mary Sue P O Box 41, Lake Elmore, VT 05657, (802) 888-3198, BA 73 SUNY - Coll at Oswego; MS 81 Univ of VT; Sp/Lang Path, Lamoille So Supervisory Union, **SLP**

Agranowitz, Aleen C 4623 Harvey Way, Long Beach, CA 90808, (714) 821-3620, MA 74 Univ of Southern CA; Dir, Sp and Lang Develop Cen, **SLP F**

Agranowitz, Sara 4700 Harvey Way, Long Beach, CA 90808, (714) 821-3620, BA 76 Chapman Coll; MS 78 Chapman Coll; Sp-Lang Path, Spch-Language Development Cen, **SLP**

Agresta, Mrs Lillian P 904 4th Street, East Northport, NY 11731, (516) 757-9669, BA 72 Long Island U - CW Post Ctr; MS 77 Adelphi Univ; Sp-Lang Path, Private Practice, **SLP**

Agricola, Mrs Susan Merrill 5194 East Pinehurst, Eden, UT 84310, (801) 350-4682, MS 77 UT St Univ; 88–Aud, Holy Cross Hosp, **A**

Aguilera-Posen, Judith Diana 1925 Pritchard Way, Hacienda Heights, CA 91745, (213) 940-8297, BA 81 Univ of the Pacific; MA 83 Univ of IA; Sp-Lang Path, Rancho Los Amigos Medical Cen, **SLP**

Aguillard, Mary Christie 3964 Emily Drive, Port Allen, LA 70767, (504) 346-8598, MA 80 LA St Univ - Baton Rouge; BS 78 LA St Univ - Baton Rouge; Sp-Lang Path, E Baton Rouge Parish Sch Bd, **SLP**

Aguirre, Guadalupe Maria 731-B Durham Lane, Ventura, CA 93004, (805) 648-5391, BA 76 San Diego St Univ; MS 85 Univ of Redlands; 79–Sp-Lang Path, Ventura USD, **SLP**

Aguirre, Marguerite 728 Taylor, Las Cruces, NM 88005, (505) 524-8656, BA 81 NM St Univ; MA 83 NM St Univ; 86–Sp-Lang Path, Las Cruces PS, **SLP**

Ahart, Mrs Alice G 903 East Harmon Street, Urbana, IL 61801, (217) 877-3410, BA 54 Marietta Coll; MA 66 Univ of MN - Minneap-St Paul; Supervisor Sp-Lang-Hrng Prog, Adolf Meyer Mental Health Cen, **SLP**

Ahaus, Dr William Hoffman VA Medical Center (126), 921 N E 13th Street, Oklahoma City, OK 73104, (405) 270-5164, BS 64 IN Univ - Bloomington; MA 67 IN Univ - Bloomington; PH 73 (NS) Univ of MN - Minneap-St Paul; Ch, Aud & SLP Serv, VA Med Cen, **A**

Ahearn, Barbara Lynne 56 Houston Drive, Groton, CT 06340, (203) 449-1632, BA 74 Univ of Northern IA; MA 75 Univ of Northern IA; **SLP**

Ahearn, Mary E Speech Pathology Department, St Josephs Hospital, 555 East Market Street, Elmira, NY 14902, (607) 733-6541, BS 78 Marywood Coll; MA 81 OH Univ - Athens; Sp-Lang Path, St Joseph's Hosp, **SLP**

Ahearn, Natalie D 6 Bronson Avenue, Scarsdale, NY 10583, (914) 723-5137, BA 66 CUNY - Hunter Coll; ME 86 Columbia Univ Teachers Coll; ED 88 (Educational Adminis) Columbia Univ Teachers Coll; 79–Sp-Lang Path, Eastchester PS, **SLP**

Ahern, Ellen Louise P O Box 7084, San Carlos, CA 94070-3029, (415) 592-6637, MA; SLP, Private Practice, **SLP**

Ahern, Janis C 120 San Luis Way, Novato, CA 94947, **SLP**

Aherne-Lang, M Theresa 105 Pratt Street, West Babylon, NY 11704-7908, (516) 562-4600, BA 83 Molloy Coll; MA 85 CUNY - Queens Coll; **SLP**

Ahlbrand, Mrs Karen P 107 Olde Newburgh Place, Newburgh, IN 47630, (812) 479-1411, MA 87 Ball St Univ; SLP, The Rehab Ctr, **SLP**

Ahlgren, Mrs Marianne Collins Box C, APO San Francisco, CA 96346-4040, BA 62 Saint Xavier Coll; MA 64 Univ of IL - Urbana; **A**

Ahlijanian, Mrs Zarie K 93 Apple Tree Lane, Warwick, RI 02888, (401) 737-3300, BA 76 Univ of RI; MS 79 Univ of RI; Sp/Lang Path, Warwick Public Schools, **SLP**

Ahlman, Mrs Pamela S 701 East Vaughn Avenue, Gilbert, AZ 85234, (602) 497-2542, BA 73 Elmira Coll; MA 74 Univ of Northern CO; Sp/Lang Path, Gilbert PS, **SLP**

Ahlschlager, Elizabeth Dawn 13 Mount Sheraton, Star Route B, Lawton, OK 73501, (405) 529-2805, MS 88 Baylor Univ

Ahlstedt, Gayla Blythe 332 Navarre Drive, Stone Mountain, GA 30087, (904) 784-4878, BS 85 Univ of GA; ME 86 Univ of GA; **SLP**

Ahlstrom, Jayne B 3906 Creekwood Lane, Martinez, GA 30907, (404) 721-6009, BS 79 Bradley Univ; MS 81 Vanderbilt Univ; 86–Aud, Medical Coll of GA, **A**

Ahnert, Mrs Alice C 620 North Alleghaney, Odessa, TX 79761, (915) 368-5689, BS 85 Univ of North TX; MS 87 Univ of North TX; Sp-Lang Path, Permian Basin Rehab Ctr, **SLP**

Ahonen, Judi Elizabeth 17 Peralta Avenue, San Francisco, CA 94110, (415) 824-9024, BA 76 Univ of WA; OM 77 Univ of WA; MA 83 Univ of MN - Minneap-St Paul; 86–Sp-Lang Path, San Mateo Co Ofc of Educ, **SLP A**

Ahonen, Michele A 1843 Polk Street, Concord, CA 94521, (415) 458-3216, BS 74 Central MI Univ; MA 76 Northwestern Univ; Spec Day Class Tchr, Mt Diablo USD, **SLP**

Ahrendts, Dr Harold L Dept Of Speech Communication, Kearney State College, Kearney, NE 68847, (308) 236-4078, BA 38 NE Wesleyan Univ; MA 42 Univ of MI - Ann Arbor; PH 62 (NS) Univ of Denver; **SLP LM**

Ahrens, Jill Ann 7983 Woodridge Drive #212, Woodridge, IL 60517, (312) 968-9421, BS 83 Univ of IL - Urbana; MS 84 Univ of IL - Urbana; Sp-Lang Path, Sased, **SLP**

Ahrens, Mrs Joan Ellen 6216 Seminole Place, Berwyn Heights, MD 20740, (301) 894-2600, MA 83 Univ of MD - College Park; 88–Sp-Lang Path, Prince George's Co PS, **SLP**

Ahrens, Mrs L Ann D 3416 Fairmeadows Lane, Fort Worth, TX 76123-1213, PH (NS); **SLP**

Ahrens, Sandra F 24 Home Road, Hatboro, PA 19040-2026, BS 66 Ithaca Coll; MA 70 Temple Univ-Tyler Sch of Art; SLP, Sch Dist of Phila, **SLP**

Ahrndt, Gretchen Mary 500 110th Avenue North #611, St Petersburg, FL 33716, (813) 579-4693, BA 84 Univ of WI - Eau Claire; MS 86 Marquette Univ; **SLP**

Aiello, Arlene R 35 Appleton Street, Salem, MA 01970, (508) 745-6146, BS 77 Salem St Coll; ME 79 Northeastern Univ; 78–Sp-Lang Path, Beverly PS, **SLP**

Aiello, Dr Francis A Columbia Basin Sp Lang Hrng, Medical Arts Bldg Suite 4, 750 Swift, Richland, WA 99352, (509) 943-2682, BS 63 Mansfield Univ of PA; MS 70 Southern IL Univ -Carbondale; PH 74 (NS) Univ of WA; Aud, Columbia Basin Sp-Lang-Hrng, **A**

Aiello, Margaret Guinan 5204 S W 153rd Place North, Miami, FL 33185, (305) 553-2693, BA 79 Adelphi Univ; MS 80 Adelphi Univ; 83–Sp/Lang Path, Sch Bd of Dade Co FL, **SLP**

Aiello, Maribeth Ann 1912-35th Street, Kenosha, WI 53140, (414) 654-8283, BS 86 Univ of WI - Milwaukee; MS 88 Marquette Univ; 88–Sp-Lang Path, NM Rehab Ctr WI

Aiken, Cynthia Lou 430 School Street, Webster, MA 01570, (508) 943-4889, BS 82 TX Christian Univ; MA 85 Univ of MA - Amherst; 88–Sp-Lang Path, MA Easter Seal Society, **SLP**

Aiman, Eliece B Charlevoix-Emmet Int Sch Dist, Mercer Boulevard, Charlevoix, MI 49720, (616) 547-9947, BA 73 Western MI Univ; MA 78 Western MI Univ; SLP, Charlevoix-Emmet ISD, **SLP**

Aine, Mrs Lavera F 13462 Montserrat Court, Chino Hills, CA 91709, (714) 590-7227, BA 76 CA St Univ - Los Angeles; MA 79 CA St Univ - Los Angeles; Dir, Ainesworth Sp - Lang Serv, **SLP**

Ainslie, Mrs Ann Ironside 19 Ironside Drive, Hastings, MI 49058, (616) 948-2997, BA 74 Univ of MI - Ann Arbor; MS 75 Univ of MI - Ann Arbor; Sp-Lang Path, Barry Intermediate Sch Dist, **SLP**

Ainsworth, Dr Stanley H Route HC 61 Box 199, Tahlequah, OK 74464, (918) 458-9450, BA 33 Eastern MI Univ; MA 37 Univ of IA; PH 49 (Sp Path Aud and Cl Psychology) Northwestern Univ; **SLP A F H LM**

Air, Dr Dorothy H 39 Linden Hill Drive, Crescent Springs, KY 41017, (513) 872-5353, BS 66 Marquette Univ; MS 68 Marquette Univ; PH 79 (NS) Univ of Cincinnati; Assoc Dir of Aud/SLP, U of Cinn Med Cen, **SLP**

Airola, Catherine E 721 Esplanade #303, Redondo Beach, CA 90277, (213) 540-6363, SLP, LA County Superint/Schools, **SLP**

Aisenberg, Sondra Lee 4935 Columbia Road #F, Columbia, MD 21044, (301) 596-0437, BA 81 Univ of MI - Ann Arbor; MS 83 Univ of MI - Ann Arbor; 88–Sp-Lang Path, Mont Co PS, **SLP**

Aisner, Claudia Gail 3060 Edwin Avenue #4D, Fort Lee, NJ 07024, (201) 585-7487, BS 81 Ithaca Coll; MA 82 Hofstra Univ; Aud, The Hrng Lab, **A**

Aistrup, Suzann 3610 Gabriel #337, Parsons, KS 67357, (316) 421-1178, MA 87 Fort Hays St Univ; **SLP**

Aitchison, Dr Carole J 82 Pine Street, Chatham, NJ 07928, (201) 277-6350, BA 73 Univ of ND; MA 74 Univ of ND; PH 81 (Spec Educ) Univ of ND; Prin, The Winston Sch, **SLP**

Aitken, Mrs Karen B 3556 E Nugget Canyon Place, Tucson, AZ 85718, (602) 299-0761, BA 72 Univ of CA - Santa Barbara; MS 74 Univ of AZ; 74–Sp-Lang Path, Tucson USD, **SLP**

Aitken, Mrs Paula Robertson 124 East Lake Drive, Monroe, LA 71203-6402, (318) 325-0601, **SLP**

Aitken, Mrs Sheryl Hooper 3426 Rio Hato Court, Camarillo, CA 93010, (805) 482-6544, BS 83 Southwest MO St Univ; MA 87 CA St Univ - Northridge

Aitken, Susan E 1000 River Reach Drive, Apartment 215, Fort Lauderdale, FL 33315, (305) 581-3740, BS Northwestern Univ; MA Northwestern Univ; Sp-Lang Path, Sch Bd of Broward Co FL, **SLP ACE**

Aitro, Moira O'Neill 1423 Quinnipiac Avenue, Apartment 113, New Haven, CT 06513, (203) 272-3577, MS 83 Southern CT St Univ; Sp-Lang Path, Cheshire Early Interven Ctr, **SLP**

Ajdinovich, Mrs Suzanne P 8701 Monroe, Munster, IN 46321, (219) 933-2004, BS 76 Purdue Univ - West Lafayette; MA 77 Ball St Univ; Ch Sp-Lang Path, St Margaret Hospital, **SLP**

Akama-Lapinta, Jean E 2696 Ainaola Road, Hilo, HI 96720, (808) 961-7537, BA 76 Univ of HI - Hilo; MS 78 Univ of HI - Manoa; Sp/Lang Path, Dept of Ed Spec Ed St of Hi, **SLP**

Akar, Mrs Christine Hintz 1087 N W 96th Avenue, Plantation, FL 33324, (305) 474-9768, **SLP**

Aker, Mrs Adelyn Ramoni P O Box 231, APO New York, NY 09210-5360, (415) 222-2161, BA 66 Montclair St Coll; MA 70 Northwestern Univ; Teacher, Full Potential Richmond USD, **SLP**

Aker, Dr Charles Randall 1498 Beche Street S E, Palm Bay, FL 32909, (305) 676-2160, BS 75 Memphis St Univ; MS 78 FL St Univ; PH 81 (NS) FL St Univ; Sp-Lang Path, Multi Services Inc, **SLP**

Akerlund, Paula M 408 3rd Avenue, Aberdeen, WA 98520, (206) 872-4458, BA 75 9298; MA 77 Univ of OR; SLP, Grays Harbor Pupil Services, **SLP**

Akerman, Mrs Cynthia I Route 7 Box 816, Columbus, MS 39701-9222, **SLP**

Akerman, Judith L 1170 Woodstream Drive, Lawrenceville, GA 30244, BA 75 Augustana Coll; ME 76 Univ of GA; Sp-Lang Path, Gwinnett Co Schs, **SLP**

Akers, Edwin L 1010 East Oak, Taylorville, IL 62568, (217) 824-8121, BS 64 Southern IL Univ -Carbondale; MS 74 Southern IL Univ-Edwardsvill; Sp-Lang Path, Taylorville Commun Ut Sch, **SLP**

Akers, Susan Gail Rt 1 Box 845, Bassett, VA 24055, (703) 629-7106, BS Radford Univ; MS 86 Radford Univ; **SLP**

Akeson, Marcia L 18 Olive Street, Danbury, CT 06810, (203) 355-2611, BA 78 Southern CT St Univ; MA 81 Kent St Univ; Sp-Lang Path, New Milford Hosp, **SLP**

Akey, Phyllis Irene 100 South Parkway Blvd, Unit D, Liberal, KS 67901, (319) 273-8250, MA 85 Univ of Northern CO; **A**

Akin, Wendla R W 11942 Barkman Drive, St Louis, MO 63146-5476, BA 74 Hendrix Coll; MA 77 Univ of AR - Fayetteville; **SLP**

Akins, Joan M 1507 Salem Road, Point Pleasant, NJ 08742, (201) 295-4287, BA 74 Kean Coll of NJ; MA 75 Kean Coll of NJ; Sp-Lang Path, Private Practice, **SLP ACE**

Akins, Mrs Myra Jean C 4144 Louisiana Street, Gary, IN 46409, (219) 884-2659, BA 70 IN Univ - Bloomington; OM 80 Governors St Univ; Sp/Lang Path, Gary Comm Sch Corp, **SLP ACE**

Akins, Mrs Tanya M P 5700 St Anthony #109, New Orleans, LA 70122, (504) 288-0952, BS 78 Univ of TN - Chattanooga; ME 80 GA St Univ; Sp/Lang Path, St Bernard Parish Schs, **SLP**

Akre, Mrs Marie Patricia 320 Oakwood Drive, Delafield, WI 53018, (414) 646-3866, BS 82 Marquette Univ; MS 84 Marquette Univ; SLP, M J Therapy Services, **SLP**

Akridge, Jeanie Dupuy P O Box 12353, Alexandria, LA 71315, (318) 442-1645, BS 84 LA St Univ - Baton Rouge; MS 85 Univ of Southwestern LA; Sp-Lang Path, People Plus Inc, **SLP**

Akridge, Mrs Jill J 4688 Shawn Terrace, Norcross, GA 30092, (404) 642-9630, BS 85 Murray St Univ; MS 87 Murray St Univ; **SLP**

Akrin, Donna C 32 Liberty Street, Dansville, NY 14437, **SLP**

Alabovitz, Sanford R 111 Chestnut Street, Shillington, PA 19607, (215) 777-8084, BS 69 PA St Univ - Univ Park; ME 72 Bloomsburg Univ of PA; Aud, Private Practice, **A**

Alagna, Mrs Pauline R 418 North Village Avenue, Rockville Centre, NY 11570, (212) 988-9500, BA 53 OH St Univ; MA 56 CUNY - Brooklyn Coll; Dir Sp-Lang Dept, Kennedy Child Study Cen, **SLP A**

Aland, Mrs Caroline Holland 607-B Harbor Drive, Route 2, Chester, MD 21619, (301) 643-5847, BS 84 East TN St Univ; MS 85 Univ of NC - Chapel Hill; 86–Aud, Chesapeake Hearing Ctrs Inc, **A**

Albala, Brent M 29 Vera Avenue, Plainview, NY 11803, (516) 385-2118, BA 77 SUNY - Coll at Oswego; MA 81 Long Island U - CW Post Ctr; 80–Sp-Lang Path, Long Island Dev Cen, **SLP**

Albamonte, Stefanie J 7 Campbell Lane, Berkeley Heights, NJ 07922, MS 84 Indiana Univ of PA; SLP, Childrens Specialized Hospital, **SLP**

Albanese, Santina D 2863 Marshall, Cincinnati, OH 45225, (513) 742-2200, BS 77 Bowling Green St Univ; MA 79 Bowling Green St Univ; 80–Sp-Lang Path, Hamilton Co Offi of Ed, **SLP ACE**

Albanese, Susan Gillis Woodfield Drive, Middlebury, CT 06762, (203) 574-8004, BA 82 Southern CT St Univ; MS 85 Southern CT St Univ; **SLP**

Albaugh, Julie A 49 Charleston Street, Wellsboro, PA 16901, (717) 724-3913, BA 82 Univ of Pittsburgh - Pittsburgh; MS 84 Univ of WI - Stevens Point; SLP, InSpeech Inc, **SLP**

Albee, David C 6130 Sherwood Glen Way, Apartment 7, West Palm Beach, FL 33415, (305) 935-6261, BA 74 FL Atlantic Univ; MS 80 Washington Univ; 88–Aud, Pro Hrng Aid Ctr, **A**

Alber, Denise Marie Little Co Of Mary, Evergreen Park, IL 60642, (312) 343-7200, BS 84 Bradley Univ; MS 86 Rush Univ; 86–Dir of Aud, Little Co of Mary, **A**

Albernaz, Dr Pedro L M Avenue Faria Lima 830, Sao Paulo Sp, Brazil 01452, MA 60 Washington Univ; MA 60 Washington Univ; MD 55 (NS); Prof & Hd/Otol, Escola Paulista De Medicina

Albers, Mrs Carol Somerset Medical Center, Speech And Hearing Dept, 110 Rehill Avenue, Somerville, NJ 08876, (201) 685-2946, BA 75 George Washington Univ; MA 76 George Washington Univ; Aud, Hrng & Sp Consult of Westfield, **A**

Albersworth, Linda J M 2745 Memory Lane, Brookfield, WI 53005, (414) 797-8574, BA 76 Elmhurst Coll; MS 78 Univ of WI - Milwaukee; Sp-Lang Path, Racine Co Sch, **SLP**

Albert, Mrs Judith I 164 Great Hollow Road, Woodbury, CT 06798, (203) 263-0612, BS 79 Boston Coll; MS 81 Southern CT St Univ; Sp-Lang Path, Regional School District 15, **SLP**

Albert, Mrs Lu-Anne M 3750 Bays Ferry Way, Marietta, GA 30062, (404) 971-5758, BS 76 Ithaca Coll; MA 78 Univ of MD - College Park; 87–Aud, VA Med Ctr, **A**

Albert, Susan 14 James Street, Shoreham, NY 11786, (516) 499-5655, BS 68 Ithaca Coll; MA 70 NY Univ; Dir Sp-Lang Path, Ctr for Rehab, **SLP**

Albertelli, Mrs Aprile Antosh 299 Village Street, Medway, MA 02053, (617) 533-2251, BS 83 Worcester St Coll; MS 87 Northeastern Univ; 83–Sp-Lang Path, Franklin PS, **SLP**

Alberti, Deborah Ann 154 Seaside Avenue, Stamford, CT 06902, BA 79 Pace U -NY City; MA 83 NY Univ; Sp-Lang Path, Westchester County Medical Cen, **SLP**

Alberti, Mrs Gail G G 228 Tinton Place, East Northport, NY 11731, (516) 266-2261, BA 76 Adelphi Univ; MS 80 Adelphi Univ; Sp-Lang Path, BOCES III Suffolk Co, **SLP**

Alberts, Mrs Alice S 2S 268 Valley Road, Lombard, IL 60148, MS 67 Western MI Univ; Public School Clinician, School District 48, **SLP**

Alberts, Carol Ann Great Plains ENT/HNS Institute PC, 630 North Cotner Boulevard, Lincoln, NE 68505, (402) 464-8385, BS 69 Univ of NE - Lincoln; MA 73 Univ of NE - Lincoln; 82–Aud/Sp-Lang Path, Great Plains ENT/HNS Inst PC, **SLP A**

Alberts, Cecil D 3177 Hogarth, Sacramento, CA 95827, (916) 369-2032, BS 50 Univ of Southern CA; MS 63 Univ of Southern CA; Manager, Spin-A-Test Pub Co, **SLP A LM**

Alberts, Mrs Novela Pinckney 808 Cleveland Avenue, Scotch Plains, NJ 07076, (201) 558-3466, BA 69 Savannah St Coll; MA 83 Kean Coll of NJ; SLP, Elizabeth Bd of Ed

Alberts, Dr Ruby W 22 West Parkway, Wichita, KS 67206, (316) 682-1722, BS 46 KS St Univ; MA 51 Wichita St Univ; PH 84 (Sp-Lang Path) Walden Univ - Minneapolis; 84–Sp-Lang Path, St Joseph Med Ctr

Albertson, Nancy 25 Ashmont Road, Wellesley, MA 02181, (617) 965-0987, BA 73 Ithaca Coll; ME 80 Northeastern Univ; Sp-Lang Path, Wellesley Pub Sch, **SLP**

Albino, Susan G P O Box 292, East Hampton, MA 01027, (413) 247-5010, BA 70 Univ of MA - Amherst; MA 71 Univ of MA - Amherst; Sp-Lang Path, Smith Academy, **SLP**

Albinson, Mrs Sharon J 4222 38th Street N W, Washington, DC 20016, (202) 966-2494, BA 66 Rutger's St Univ - Douglas Coll; MA 77 Catholic Univ of America; 86–Sp-Lang Path, Private Practice, **SLP A**

Albonico, Sharon Lee 10209 San Luis Rey Pl N E, Albuquerque, NM 87111, (505) 298-8299, BS 76 IL St Univ - Normal; MS 78 Southern IL Univ -Carbondale; 87–Sp-Lang Path, Pediatric Sp-Lang Therapy, **SLP**

Albosta, Karen 5104 Hayter Avenue #4, Lakewood, CA 90712, (517) 323-3482, BA 84 MI St Univ; OM 85 MI St Univ; **SLP**

Albrecht, Dana Sue 3501 Apollo Drive #E-338, Metairie, LA 70003, (504) 826-2400, BS 85 Purdue Univ - West Lafayette; MS 87 Purdue Univ - West Lafayette; 87–Aud, LA St Dept of Health & Hosp

Albrecht, Mrs Elizabeth 161 Acorn Lane, Libertyville, IL 60048, (312) 432-7936, BS 60 Univ of WI - Madison; MS 69 Univ of WI - Milwaukee; Sp-Lang Path, School District 108, **SLP**

Albrecht, Judith L Lewiston Hospital, Highland Avenue, Lewistown, PA 17044, (717) 248-5411, BS 70 Univ of IA; MS 71 FL St Univ; PH 83 (NS) FL St Univ; Audiologist, Lewiston Hospital, **SLP A**

Albrecht, Judy R 1125 Oakton, Evanston, IL 60202, (312) 492-5866, BA 68 Univ of MI - Ann Arbor; MA 70 Northwestern Univ; Sp-Lang Path Supvr, Evanston PS Dist 65, **SLP**

Albrecht, Phyllis H 217 East Sheridan Place, Lake Bluff, IL 60044, MA 71 Northwestern Univ; Lect Sp-Lang Path, Northwestern U, **SLP**

Albright, Doris Ann 8055 East 50th Street, Indianapolis, IN 46226, (317) 545-2128, **SLP**

Albright, Janet Juracich 7699 Fletcher Bay Road, Bainbridge Island, WA 98110, (206) 340-8255, **A**

Albright, Mrs Joy S 702 Roosevelt Street, Tempe, AZ 85281, (602) 968-6461, BA 40 Univ of WA; Sp-Lang Path, AZ Chldns Serv Dep Fam Hlth, **SLP LM**

Albright, Kathryn Bills 4510 Briarbend, Houston, TX 77035, (713) 797-3277, BS 82 Univ of TX - Austin; MA 87 Univ of TX - Austin; 88–Aud, Hermann Hosp, **A**

Albright, Mrs Linda M 1509 Woodridge Lane, Sykesville, MD 21784, (301) 795-4060, BS 76 Towson St Univ; MS 79 Towson St Univ; Sp-Lang Path, Baltimore Co Bd of Ed, **SLP**

Albright, Melissa De Shong 229 South Cortez, New Orleans, LA 70119, (504) 486-0872, BS 80 LA St Univ - Baton Rouge; MA 82 LA St Univ - Baton Rouge; Aud, Dr Daniel Mouney, **A**

Albright, Mrs Paulette A 4617 Stuart Avenue, Richmond, VA 23226, (804) 786-0431, BA 67 Univ of San Diego; MA 71 IN Univ - Bloomington; Aud, Virginia Commonwealth Univ, **SLP A**

Albright, Shirley Mona 2604 Northwestern, Ames, IA 50010, (515) 233-1367, BA 72 Univ of CA - Santa Barbara; MA 74 CA St Univ - Fresno; 88–Aud, Ames Hearing Aid Ctr, **A**

Albright, Mrs Susan Colson 9027 Arrowwood Court, Terre Haute, IN 47802, (812) 299-8225, BS 86 IN St Univ - Terre Haute; **SLP**

Albright, Mrs Susan M 48 Lerner Court, Baltimore, MD 21236, (301) 668-0893, BS 76 Towson St Univ; MS 78 Towson St Univ; Sp-Lang Path, **SLP**

Albrigo, Angela Marie 608 Maple Brook Road, Bellingham, MA 02901, (617) 872-2877, BS 83 SUNY - Center at Buffalo; MS 84 Syracuse Univ; 88–Sp-Lang Path, Cumberland Sch Sys, **SLP**

Albritton, Mrs Elizabeth Marshall 2315 Cherry Bend, Houston, TX 77077, (713) 556-8478, BS 81 Univ of TX - Austin; MA 88 Univ of TX - Austin; 85–Mainstream Specialist, Houston School for Deaf Children, **SLP**

Albritton, Dr Evelyn G 4101 Crescent Drive, Sioux Falls, SD 57106, (605) 361-7733, PH (NS); Prof, U of AR Med Sciences, **SLP A ACE**

Albritton, Thelma Nova Univ, 3375 S W 75th Avenue, Fort Lauderdale, FL 33314, (305) 475-7075, BA 56 Greensboro Coll; ME 61 Univ of OR; Sp-Lang Path, Nova Univ, **SLP F**

Albus, Marianne L 1863-113th Lane N W, Coon Rapids, MN 55433, (612) 753-2740, BS 78 Univ of WI - Madison; MS 80 Univ of WI - Madison; Sp-Lang Path, ISD #15, **SLP**

Alcala, Mrs Sheri Kae 115 W Brunswick Avenue, Indianapolis, IN 46217, (317) 784-9626, BA 86 Univ of TN - Knoxville; MA 87 Univ of TN - Knoxville; 87–Sp-Lang Path, Hendricks Comm Hosp, **SLP**

Alcan, Christine Lynn 310 North Beachwood Drive, Los Angeles, CA 90004, (213) 856-8020, BA 78 CA Lutheran Coll; MA 86 CA St Univ - Los Angeles; **SLP**

Alcorn, Stephen R 3666 Chatham Drive, Palm Harbor, FL 34684, (813) 381-1292, OB 68 Eastern IL Univ; MS 71 Eastern IL Univ; MS 81 Vanderbilt Univ; 88–Aud/Sp-Lang Path, Pinellas Hrng & Sp Inc, **SLP A ACE**

Alden, Carol L 80 Mears Avenue, Quincy, MA 02169, (617) 848-5353, BA 71 Montclair St Coll; MA 72 Montclair St Coll; Assist Cl Superv, Braintree Hosp, **SLP**

Alden, Judith Ann RR 1 Box 215, Hamilton, MO 64644, (816) 583-2520, MS 86 Northwest MO St Univ; 88–Sp-Lang Path, Hamilton PS, **SLP**

Alderfer, Maureen C Summer Hill Estates, Rd 5 #5 Box 525, Bloomsburg, PA 17815, (717) 759-1237, BS 76 OH Univ - Athens; MS 77 Bloomsburg Univ of PA; SLP, Columbia/Sullivan Co Hd, **SLP**

Alderson, Mrs Carol Vagge 7537 E Mineral Place, Englewood, CO 80112, (303) 688-4102, BS 81 CO St Univ; MS 83 CO St Univ; Sp/Lang Path, Douglas Coy Pub Sch, **SLP**

Alderson, Tracy Breitbach 821 Ridgeway Avenue, Morgantown, WV 26505, (304) 329-0580, BA 80 Frostburg St Coll; MS 82 WV Univ; Sp-Lang Path, Preston Co Bd of Ed, **SLP**

Aldes, Maureen E 6033 Cedar Knot Court, Mobile, AL 36609, (205) 342-7125, BS 73 Univ of MN - Minneap-St Paul; MS 77 CO St Univ; Dir, Sp and Lang Specialists, **SLP**

Aldrich, Donna Reed 507 Vanden Bosch Parkway, Gallup, NM 87301, (505) 863-4808, BS 77 AZ St Univ; MS 80 CO St Univ; Sp-Lang Path, **SLP**

Aldrich, Mrs Mary K St Francis Medical Center, Rehabilitation Department, 530 Northeast Glen Oak Avenue, Peoria, IL 61637, (309) 655-3777, BA 77 Northern IL Univ - De Kalb; MA 78 Northern IL Univ - De Kalb; 84–Sp/Lang Path & Dir SLP, St Francis Medical Center, **SLP**

Aldrich, Richard S 2547 Salee Lane, Visalia, CA 93277-6168, **SLP**

Aldrich, Dr William M 4704 N Laurel Drive, Peoria, IL 61614, (309) 672-2616, MS 70 Univ of AR - Little Rock; MS 73 Univ of OK Medical Center; PH 75 (NS) Univ of OK Medical Center; Clin Neurophysiologist, Neurological Associates, **A**

Aldridge, Mrs Augusta S 1724 N Scenic Heights Road, Oak Harbor, WA 98277, (206) 675-7560, BA 62 San Jose St Univ; MA 69 San Jose St Univ; 88–Lrng Prob Consult, Private Practice, **SLP**

Aleksa-Parr, Mrs Barbara 1284 Williver Drive, Decatur, GA 30033, (404) 257-2076, BA 76 Kenyon Coll; MA 80 Case Western Reserve Univ; Sp-Lang Path, Scotish Rite Chldn's Hosp, **SLP**

Aleman, Mrs Malisa D 96 Murdock Street, Richmond, CA 94804, (415) 236-1019, MS 88 CA St Univ - Hayward

Aleman, Martha M Centro Pediatrico Isla Verde, Marginal AO-21 Ext Villamar, Isla Verde, PR 00913, (809) 727-7190, BA 80 Univ of PR - Rio Piedras; MS 82 Tulane Univ; Sp-Lang Path, Centro Pediatrico Isla Verde, **SLP**

Aleo, Dr Edward L 206 Henry Street, Kingston, NY 12401, (914) 338-8686, BA 66 ID St Univ; MA 68 OH St Univ; PH 70 (NS) OH St Univ; Aud/Sp-Lang Path, Edward L Aleo Phd & Assoc, **SLP A**

Alesnik, Christina 5929 South Park Boulevard, Parma, OH 44134, (216) 362-6450, BA 76 Cleveland St Univ; MA 78 Cleveland St Univ; Sp-Lang Path, Cuyahoga Co Bd of Ment Ret, **SLP**

Alessandroni, Mrs Gale M 17 Linden Place, New Rochelle, NY 10805, BS 68 Saint Louis Univ; MA 70 Saint Louis Univ; **SLP**

Alessio, Charles Rd 5 Box 343, Belle Vernon, PA 15012, (412) 929-3451, BS 61 CA Univ of PA; MA 63 WV Univ; Sp-Lang Path, Westmoreland I V #7, **SLP**

Alex, Cathleen A Neil Lindenman Md DMD Pc, Pomperaug Office Park, Suites 203 & 204, Southbury, CT 06488, (203) 264-2909, BS 77 PA St Univ - Univ Park; MS 78 PA St Univ - Univ Park; Aud, Neil Lindenman, **A**

Alexander, Anna S 1436 Central, Superior, NE 68978, MS 77; Sp-Lang Path, Esu #9, **SLP**

Alexander, C Joy 505 Fairlane Drive, Shelbyville, TN 37160, (615) 684-7970, BS 75 Southwest TX St Univ; ME 76 Southwest TX St Univ; 88–Sp-Lang Path, Bedford County Sch Sys, **SLP**

Alexander, Mrs Eldonna Marie 1511 Belmont Drive, Murray, KY 42071, (502) 753-7629, BS 80 Murray St Univ; MS 82 Murray St Univ; 86–Sp-Lang Path, Murray ISD, **SLP**

Alexander, Elizabeth Ann 4850 N W 53rd Court, Des Moines, IA 50310, (515) 276-2607, BS 76 MacMurray Coll; MA 85 Western IL Univ; Aud, Heartland AEA #11, **A**

Alexander, Elizabeth W 191 Old Post Road, P O Box 185, Centerville, MA 02632-0920, (617) 771-2854, BS 73 Univ of Central AR; ME 80 GA St Univ; Sp-Lang Path, Cape Cod Collaborative, **SLP**

Alexander, Genevieve C 807 Jefferson Avenue, Memphis, TN 38105, (901) 525-2682, **A**

Alexander, James H 1426 East Oklahoma, Enid, OK 73701, (405) 233-2200, BS 70 OK St Univ; MA 80 OH Univ - Athens; 85–Aud, J M Dilling Jr MD Inc, **A**

Alexander, Jan Wrather Post Office Box 1366, Kayenta, AZ 86033, (602) 697-8187, BS 73 Murray St Univ; MS 87 Northern AZ Univ

Alexander, Jane E P O Box 1275, Chiefland, FL 32626, **SLP**

Alexander, Mrs Jeran D 711 Scottsdale, Richardson, TX 75080, (214) 231-5058, BA 68 Stephen F Austin St Univ; MS 73 Southern Methodist Univ; **SLP**

Alexander, Joan W H 548 Leeanne, Yuba City, CA 95991, MS 66

Alexander, Kathleen 2833 Central Park Way NE #103, Grand Rapids, MI 49505, (616) 361-6102, BS 86 Central MI Univ; MA 87 Central MI Univ; 88–Sp-Lang Path, Rockford PS, **SLP**

Alexander, Kenmar Campbell 725 Selma Boulevard, Staunton, VA 24401, (703) 885-8153, BS 84 James Madison Univ; ME 86 James Madison Univ; Aud, Augusta Co Ps, **A**

Alexander, Linda Lamison 2019 Lac Du Mont, Haslett, MI 48840-9533, (517) 676-3401, BS 61 Oakland Univ; MA 80 MI St Univ; **SLP**

Alexander, Lynn Gunn 4810 Polk Street, Omaha, NE 68117, (402) 733-3237, BS 77 SUNY - Coll at Buffalo; MS 81 SUNY - Coll at Buffalo; 88–Sp-Lang Path, Educational Service Unit #4, **SLP**

Alexander, Marcia L 2806 Lenoir Drive, Greensboro, NC 27408, **SLP**

Alexander, Mrs Marilyn K P O Box 888082, Atlanta, GA 30338, (404) 394-6673, BA 63 CUNY - Brooklyn Coll; ME 78 Univ of GA; Sp-Lang Path, Dekalb Cty Sch, **SLP**

Alexander, Martha E 91 Rumson Road #A12, Atlanta, GA 30305, (404) 321-4104, Com Coor Hra Project, Emory Univ, **SLP**

Alexander, Nancy J P O Box 3741, Estes Park, CO 80517, (303) 586-6812, BA 79 Univ of Northern CO; MA 82 Univ of Denver; **A**

Alexander, Mrs Patricia 1621 South Chestnut, Broken Arrow, OK 74012, (918) 258-6158, BS 73 OK St Univ; MA 76 Univ of KS; Sp-Lang Path, Private Practice, **SLP**

Alexander, Dr Patrick T 21 Carlyle Bay, Winnipeg, MB, Canada R3K OH2, (604) 479-3711, BS 67 Minot St Univ; MS 68 Minot St Univ; PH 74 (NS) Univ of UT; 84–Dir-Dept of Commun Dis, Health Sciences Ctr, **SLP**

Alexander, Mrs Rebecca Lynn R R 1 Box 99-Ab, Neoga, IL 62447-9720, (217) 895-3526, BS 82 Radford Univ; MS 83 Radford Univ; Aud, Link Clinic

Alexander, Mrs Rise Barnett 1815 Nemoke Trails #6, Haslett, MI 48840, (513) 222-5597, BS 79 Univ of MN - Minneap-St Paul; MA 81 Ball St Univ; Sp-Lang Path, E W Sparrow Hospital 8, **SLP**

Alexander, Dr Rona P P O Box 26734, Wauwatosa, WI 53226, (414) 771-8117, BA 71 IN Univ - Bloomington; MA 72 NY Univ; PH 76 (Sp-Lang Path) Univ of IL - Urbana; 85–Sp-Lang Path, Private Practice, **SLP**

Alexander, Rosanne Lessin 5 Blueburry Ridge Court, Potomac, MD 20854, (301) 251-9833, BA 70 Kean Coll of NJ; ME 71 Boston Univ; **SLP**

Alexander, Sharon Z 10104 West 80th #84, Overland Park, KS 66204-4703, (913) 383-1549, BA 85 OK St Univ; MA 86 OK St Univ; **SLP**

Alexander, Shirley J 1038 East Idahome Street, West Covina, CA 91790, (818) 966-9393, BA 84 CA St Univ - Los Angeles; MA 85 CA St Univ - Los Angeles; **A**

Alexander, Mrs Susan Killen 1265 Union Avenue, Memphis, TN 38104, (901) 726-8472, BA 85 Univ of MS; MA 87 Memphis St Univ; Sp-Lang Path, Mthodist Rehab Ctr, **SLP**

Alexander, Mrs Susan S 1113 Sirroco, Pampa, TX 79065, (806) 669-2792, BS 82 Baylor Univ; MS 83 Univ of North TX; Sp-Lang Path, Pampa ISD, **SLP**

Alexander, Suzanne 10 Butternut Road, Allendale, NJ 07401-1818, **SLP**

Alexander, Mrs Twylla B P O Box 23, Barrow, AK 99723-0023, (501) 967-2322, BA 74 Henderson St Univ; MA 76 Memphis St Univ; Sp-Lang Path, Friendship Servs Cen, **SLP**

Alexander, Valerie M 3303 Foster Avenue #4-E, Brooklyn, NY 11203, (718) 284-1296, MS 88 CUNY - Brooklyn Coll

Alexander-Feasley, Mrs Margaret A 904 Prospect Street, Takoma Park, MD 20912, (202) 541-6717, BS 78 Middle TN St Univ; MS 80 Purdue Univ - West Lafayette; Sp-Lang Path, Wash Hospital Ctr Hrng-Sp Ctr, **SLP**

Alexander-Stone, Elise 3097 North Lake Avenue, Altadena, CA 91001, (818) 397-5458, BA 83 CA St Univ - Northridge; MS 85 CA St Univ - Northridge; 85–Sp-Lang Path, Huntington Mem Hosp, **SLP**

Alexander-Whiting, Mrs Harriett 4010 Rocky Mount Drive, Temple Hills, MD 20748, (202) 651-5326, BS 68 Northern IL Univ - De Kalb; MA 70 Kent St Univ; Coord Commun Unit/Sp-Lang Path, Gallaudet Univ, **SLP**

Alexopulos, Janet Vitelozzi 1811 Viewtop Court, Annapolis, MD 21401, **SLP**

Alfera, Mrs Valerie A 767 S E Albatross Avenue, Port St Lucie, FL 34983, (407) 879-1357, BA 76 SUNY - Coll at Cortland; OM 83 LA St Univ - N O Medical Ctr; **SLP**

Alfieri, Linda M 256 West Spruce Street, East Rochester, NY 14445, (716) 586-6288, MS 88 Nazareth Coll of Rochester; 87–Sp-Lang Path, BOCES #1 Monroe Co

Alfiero-Bavasso, Mrs Susan Jane 38 Clark Street, Westerly, RI 02891, (401) 596-9265, BA 76 Emmanuel Coll; MA 79 Univ of RI; MS 83 Univ of RI; Sp-Lang Path, Chariho Regional Sch Dist, **SLP**

Alfin, Marlene V 143 King Philip Drive, West Hartford, CT 06117, **SLP**

Alfirevic, Janine R 9221 South 52nd Avenue, Oak Lawn, IL 60453, (312) 687-7200, BA 79 Mundelein Coll; MS 81 Univ of WI - Madison; Sp-Lang Path, Ingalls Memorial Hosp, **SLP**

Alfke-Norman, Dorothy C 36 Westfield Road, West Hartford, CT 06119, (203) 561-2200, BS 73 SUNY - Coll at New Paltz; MA 74 Bowling Green St Univ; SLP, West Hartford Pub Sch, **SLP**

Alfonso, Mrs Jilana B 5803 N W 66th Avenue, Parkland, FL 33067, (305) 765-6747, BS 78 Indiana Univ of PA; MS 79 PA St Univ - Univ Park; 80–Sp-Lang Path, Private Practice, **SLP**

Alfonso, Dr Peter J Haskins Laboratories, 270 Crown Street, New Haven, CT 06510, (203) 486-2628, BA 72 Univ of CT; MA 73 Western MI Univ; PH 77 (NS) Purdue Univ - West Lafayette; 83–Assoc Prof, Univ of Connecticut, **SLP**

Alfonso, Rosa Maria 2255 West Orange Grove Rd, #12203, Tucson, AZ 85741-3116, (602) 622-5833, BA 80 Univ of OK - Norman; MA 85 Univ of IA; **SLP**

Alford, Denise A 481 Ruttedge Road, Tallahassee, FL 32301, **SLP**

Alford, Emily Cheryl 3544 Creekwood Drive, Apartment 9, Lexington, KY 40502, BA 81 Univ of MS; MS 85 Univ of MS; **SLP**

Alford, Mrs P Wynn Ear Nose & Throat Assoc Pa, 101 Courtenay Circle, Hattiesburg, MS 39401, (601) 264-5684, BS 82 Univ Southern MS-Hattiesburg; MS 84 Univ Southern MS-Hattiesburg; 84–Aud, Ear Nose & Throat Assoc Pa, **A**

Alfson, Karen K 1813 Duke Drive, Richardson, TX 75081, (316) 686-0090, BA 74 Wichita St Univ; MA 75 Wichita St Univ; Sp-Lang Path, Private Practice, **SLP**

Algeo, Mark A 1506 Eden Drive, Inverness, FL 32650, (904) 344-1822, MS 74 Univ of South FL; Sp-Lang Path, Citrus Co Sch Bd, **SLP**

Algiere, Elaine Catherine 36 Village Road, Milford, CT 06460, (203) 874-8830, BA 83 Univ of RI; MS 85 Southern CT St Univ; SLP, Shelton Ps, **SLP**

Ali, Mrs Angela Catherine 1118 Superior Avenue, Dayton, OH 45407, (513) 278-1974, BA 83 IN Univ - Bloomington; **SLP**

Alicea, Eileen E 2959 North Damen #3D, Chicago, IL 60618, (312) 327-2546, BS 77 FL St Univ; MA 78 Univ of IL - Urbana; SLP, Private Practice, **SLP**

Alimaras, Constance Siomkos 56-12 206th Street, Bayside, NY 11364, BA 79 CUNY - Queens Coll; MA 81 CUNY - Queens Coll; Sp/Lang Path, Shield I/Ment Ret & Dev Disabl, **SLP**

Aliminosa, Donna 5210 Eliots Oak, Columbia, MD 21044, (301) 730-4075, BA 73 Goucher Coll; MA 75 Catholic Univ of America; 85–Patient Tester, The Johns Hopkins Univ, **SLP**

Aliza, Barbara E Needham Road, R R 1 Box 296-D, Norwich, VT 05055, (603) 646-8302, BA 67 Univ of CA - Los Angeles; MA 75 Catholic Univ of America; 86–Assoc Dir Maternal & Child Health, Dartmouth Med Sch, **SLP**

Alkistis, Charalambo W322 Owen Hall, East Lansing, MI 48823, (517) 353-3583

Allaire, Mrs Janet H 805 Emerson Drive, Charlottesville, VA 22901, (804) 924-8239, BS 69 1023; MA 70 Univ of IL - Urbana; Asst Prof & Dir, Univ of VA, **SLP**

Allamanno, Mrs Judith Carole 1977 Cardigan Avenue, Columbus, OH 43212, (614) 488-3897, BA 80 OH St Univ; MA 82 OH St Univ; SLP, Franklin Co Bd of Mr/Dd, **SLP**

Allan, Joan 7802 Big Sky Drive #209, Madison, WI 53719, (608) 271-3333, BS 78 Univ of WI - Madison; MS 80 Univ of South FL; Aud, Nicolet Instrument Corp, **A**

Allan, Mrs Maryanne Miller 28 William Drive, Middletown, RI 02840, (401) 849-2124, BA 78 Univ of RI; ME 80 Northeastern Univ; Sp-Lang Path, Middletown Sch Syst, **SLP**

Allard, Mrs Elinor T 2443 South Neel, Rural Route 5, Rapid City, SD 57701, (605) 394-4036, BS 64 Minot St Univ; MS 69 Minot St Univ; Sp-Lang Path, Rapid Cty Area Sch Dist 51/4, **SLP**

Allard, Elizabeth 75 Giles Drive, Bedford, NS, Canada B4B 1B9, BA 70 Univ of CT; MA 71 Western MI Univ; **SLP**

Allard, Dr Juan Bradley R R 1 Box 346, Rocheport, MO 65279, (314) 445-2365, **A**

Allard, Laura Ann 315 North Associated Road, Apartment 1102, Brea, CA 92621, (714) 826-0824, BS 82 Purdue Univ - West Lafayette; MA 83 Univ of Northern CO; California Reg Rep, Starkey California, **A**

Allega, Nancy Louise 8062 Greenwood Court #F, Terre Haute, IN 47802, (317) 832-3179, BA 82 IN Univ - Bloomington; MS 84 IN St Univ - Terre Haute; SLP, Covered Bridge Special Ed Dist, **SLP**

Allen, Mrs Ana Elena 901 Robinson, El Paso, TX 79902, BA 76 Univ of TX - El Paso; MA 80 Univ of TX - El Paso; Sp-Lang Path, El Paso School District, **SLP**

Allen, Angela Raphael 17967 Wood, Melvindale, MI 48122, (313) 557-5440, **SLP**

Allen, Annalee A 2616 Beartooth Drive, Billings, MT 59102, (406) 657-2054, BA 70 Rocky Mountain Coll; MA 75 KS St Univ; Sp-Lang Path, Mt Cen for Hndcpd Chldn, **SLP**

Allen, Barbara 815 Prescott Lane, Springfield, OR 97477, (503) 726-3387, BS 76 Univ of OR; MS 77 Univ of OR; Sp-Lang Path, Communication Innovations, **SLP**

Allen, Mrs Barbara Anne 805 South 27th Street, Mount Vernon, IL 62864, (618) 244-3404, BS 84 Fontbonne Coll; MS 85 Fontbonne Coll; 88–Sp-Lang Path, Good Samaritan Reg Hlth Ctr, **SLP**

Allen, Barbara E 803 Coddington Road, Ithaca, NY 14850, (607) 277-5474, MS 85 Ithaca Coll; Sp-Lang Path, Empire Rehab Associates, **SLP**

Allen, Brenda May 11968 Avenida Marcella, San Diego, CA 92019, (619) 464-5308, BA 77 CA St Univ - Long Beach; MA 82 San Diego St Univ; SLP, San Diego USD, **SLP**

Allen, Mrs Carletta M Star Route 3 Box 113-A, Cottonwood, ID 83522, (208) 962-7173, BA 75 Northwest Nazarene Coll; MS 78 ID St Univ; Sp-Lang Path, Adult Chld Dev Cen, **SLP**

Allen, Carol S 1702 North 7th, Boise, ID 83702, (208) 386-9385, BS 74 ID St Univ; MS 76 ID St Univ; SLP, Canyon-Owyhee Sch Serv Agency, **SLP**

Allen, Mrs Catherine 2670 West Pueblo Avenue, Napa, CA 94558, (707) 226-2731, OB 62 San Francisco St Univ; MA 67 San Francisco St Univ; **SLP LM**

Allen, Charlotte Anne Route 2 Box 09, Ronda, NC 28670, (919) 984-2606, BS 83 Appalachian St Univ; MA 86 Univ of TN - Knoxville; **SLP**

Allen, Christy Denise 13214 Laurel Oaks, Little Rock, AR 72211, (501) 661-2320, BS 84 Univ of AR - Fayetteville; MS 86 Univ of AR - Little Rock; 87–Sp-Lang Path, AR Dept of Health, **SLP**

Allen, Mrs Claudia Koller 230 Cheyenne Drive, Vacaville, CA 95688, (707) 429-5075, BA 83 CA St Univ - Sacramento; MA 84 Univ of the Pacific; **SLP**

Allen, Constance 17634 Ridge Creek Road, Strongsville, OH 44136, MS 72 Univ of Akron; Prof/Speech Cpommunication, Baldwin-Wallace College, **SLP**

Allen, Mrs Cynthia Marie 6018 Burlingame Avenue, Richmond, CA 94804, (415) 222-2161, BS 79 CA St Univ - Hayward; MA 84 Univ of San Francisco; **SLP**

Allen, Mrs Darla Rae Marie 4901 South Marion Road, Apt 1, Sioux Falls, SD 57106, (605) 361-7999, MS 87 Univ of ND; SLP, Sioux Falls Ps

Allen, Deborah W P O Box 329, Meriden, NH 03770-0329, (603) 646-5978, BA 77 Wellesley Coll; MA 79 Univ of Denver; Chief Sp-Lang Path, Dartmouth-Hitchcock Med Center, **SLP**

Allen, Debra Betschart 594 Farm To Market Road, Bow, WA 98232, (206) 384-3591, BA 74 Western WA Univ; MA 76 Western WA Univ; SLP, Ferndale School District, **SLP**

Allen, Deidre J 405 Red Oak Drive, Palisades, NY 10964, (914) 365-2192, BA 74 CUNY - Queens Coll; MA 75 CUNY - Queens Coll; Sp/Lang Path, Private Practice, **SLP**

Allen, Doris Virginia P O Box 8278, Royal Oak, MI 48068, (313) 577-1393, BS 50 Univ of MI - Ann Arbor; MA 63 Wayne St Univ; PH 65 (Psychology (Exp)) Wayne St Univ; 78–Prof, Wayne St U

Allen, Dr Elizabeth Speech Pathology & Audiology, New York University, 733 Shimkin Hall Wash Sq, New York, NY 10003, (212) 598-3233, BA 58 Linfield Coll; MA 60 Univ of IA; PH 72 (NS) Univ of FL; Assoc Prof, NYU, **SLP**

Allen, Elizabeth Dept Communicative Disorders, San Diego State University, San Diego, CA 92182, (619) 265-6775, BA 60 Seattle Pacific Univ; MA 62 LA St Univ - Baton Rouge; PH 72 (NS) LA St Univ - Baton Rouge; Assoc, San Diego St U, **SLP ACE**

Allen, Mrs Elizabeth 3816 East Donner Avenue, Fresno, CA 93726, (209) 488-3306, BA 73 CA St Univ - Fresno; MA 76 CA St Univ - Fresno; 76–Sp-Lang Path, Fresno County Dept Education, **SLP**

Allen, Mrs Elizabeth Alice 2970 Whitegate Drive, Merced, CA 95340, (209) 722-4581, BA 79 CA St Univ - Stanislaus; MA 82 CA St Univ - Stanislaus; SLP, Merced River School District

Allen, Mrs Elizabeth Bishop 13337 Tiverton Road, San Diego, CA 92130, (619) 755-0961, BS 84 ID St Univ; MA 86 CA St Univ - Chico; Sp-Lang Path, Solana Beach/Oceanside Sch Dist, **SLP**

Allen, Mrs Elizabeth Carter 1612 Long Wood Road, Mobile, AL 36609, (205) 639-0201, BA 70 MS Coll; MS 71 MS Univ for Women; 85–Sp-Lang Path, Neurology Ctr PC, **SLP ACE**

Allen, Dr Emma M 3889 Oxford Place, Oceanside, CA 92056, (619) 726-8789, BA 40 CUNY - Hunter Coll; MA 46 Univ of WI - Madison; PH 57 (NS) Univ of WI - Madison; 82–Retired, **SLP LM**

Allen, Mrs Evelyn Y Kingswood Manor #4415, 10000 Wornall Road, Kansas City, MO 64114, (816) 942-1366, BS 34 Northwestern Univ; MA 46 Univ of IA; **SLP F LM**

Allen, George D Purdue University, Dept Audiology/Speech Sci, Lafayette, IN 47907, BA 59 Yale Univ; MA 60 Yale Univ; PH 66 (NS) Univ of MI - Ann Arbor; Associate Professor, Purdue University

Allen, Mrs Ima Jean Star Route Box 2096, Gainesville, TX 76240, (817) 665-6414, BS 62 TX Woman's Univ; ME 72 TX Woman's Univ; Sp-Lang Path, Gainesville ISD, **SLP**

Allen, Jacqueline F 10464 Andora Avenue, Chatsworth, CA 91311, (818) 363-9558, MS; SLP, Los Angeles USD, **SLP**

Allen, Mrs Jane Law 68 North Muscogee Avenue N W, Atlanta, GA 30305, (404) 237-4119, BA 60 Agnes Scott Coll; ME 61 Emory Univ; Sp-Lang Path, Private Practice, **SLP**

Allen, Jo Ann 111 Wilkshire Drive, Greenville, NC 27834, (919) 756-3707, MS 73 East Carolina Univ; Sp-Lang Path, Pitt Co Sch, **SLP**

Allen, Mrs Joan L 610 Erin Drive, Jeffersonville, IN 47130, (502) 625-6673, BA 79 IN Univ - Bloomington; MA 82 IN Univ - Bloomington; Aud, Jefferson Co Bd of Hlth, **A**

Allen, Maj John R Psc 2 Box 181, APO New York, NY 09220, (301) 981-4928, BA 75 Univ of MD - College Park; MA 77 Catholic Univ of America; Chief of Audiology, Malcolm Grow Usaf Med Cen, **SLP A ACE**

Allen, Mrs Karen L 8601 Dorotha Court, Austin, TX 78759, (512) 346-1336, BS 80 6852; MA 82 Univ of KS; Sp-Lang Path, St Davids Community Hospital, **SLP**

Allen, Kelly A 1430 W George Street, Chicago, IL 60657, (312) 398-3210, BS 80 Univ of WI - Madison; MA 82 Univ of IL - Urbana; 84–Sp-Lang Path, NW Suburban Special Ed Org, **SLP**

Allen, Kerry L 53 Cunningham Avenue, Cadiz, KY 42211-9143, (502) 522-6071, BS 81 Western KY Univ; MS 82 Western KY Univ; 84–Sp-Lang Path, Trigg Co Sch Syst, **SLP**

Allen, Kimberlee M P O Box 9187, 15 Looking Glass Lane, Asheville, NC 28815, (704) 298-3358, BS 86 Western Carolina Univ; MA 87 Western Carolina Univ

Allen, Mrs Korie L 212 Hunt Drive, Fayetteville, NY 13066-1226, (315) 476-7441, BA 77 SUNY - Coll at Cortland; MS 80 Ithaca Coll; Sp-Lang Path, Cicero N Syracuse School Sys, **SLP**

Allen, Mrs Lauri Marie P O Box 2405, Culver City, CA 90230, (213) 936-2153, BS 84 Univ of TX - Austin; MA 86 Univ of TX - Austin; Sp-Lang Path, L A Scottish Rite Pro Chld Dis, **SLP**

Allen, Laurie A Keystone Area Education Agency, 1473 Central Avenue, Dubuque, IA 52001, (319) 588-0538, BA 76 Univ of IA; MA 78 Univ of IA; Aud, Keystone AEA, **A**

Allen, Laurie E R R 1 Box 2351A, Lisbon Falls, ME 04252, (207) 783-3390, BA 77 Univ of ME - Orono; MA 79 OH Univ - Athens; SLP, Lewiston Sch Dept, **SLP**

Allen, Mrs Linda Bronerwine 9 North Sunset Blvd, Gulf Breeze, FL 32561, (904) 934-1280, BA 76 George Washington Univ; MS 78 Tulane Univ; 81–Aud Cl Dir, Sch Dist/Escambia Co, **A ACE**

Allen, Mrs Lois N 3970 Teale Avenue, San Jose, CA 95117, BA 75 San Jose St Univ; MA 77 San Jose St Univ; Tchr, San Jose USD, **SLP**

Allen, Dr Madge B P O Box 2193, Petersburg, VA 23804, (804) 861-6032, BA 37 Langston Univ; MA 46 Univ of Southern CA; PH 60 (Sp Path) Univ of Southern CA; **SLP F LM**

Allen, Mrs Margaret F 59 Passaic Lane, Richmond Hill, GA 31324, (912) 727-2257, BA 73 Creighton Univ; MA 74 Northern IL Univ - De Kalb; 84–Clin Supvr, InSpeech Inc, **SLP**

Allen, Mark Eugene 12723 Barlin Avenue, Downey, CA 90242, (213) 862-2628, BA 83 Univ of the Pacific; MA 84 Univ of the Pacific; **SLP**

Allen, Mary Kay 118 Candlewyck #1009, Kalamazoo, MI 49001, (616) 342-8099, MA 88 Western MI Univ

Allen, Mrs Mary Kay DeBoer 1102 Village Circle Drive-N, Phoenix, AZ 85022, (602) 993-2124, BA 73 Univ of WI - Stevens Point; MS 74 Creighton Univ; **SLP**

Allen, Mary W P O Box 661, Jonesville, VA 24263, (703) 346-3217, BA 75 Univ of TN - Knoxville; MA 77 Univ of TN - Knoxville; Sp/Lang Path, Lee Co Pub Sch, **SLP**

Allen, Mildred P O Box 5021, Modesto, CA 95352, (209) 523-6750, BA 42 LA St Univ - Baton Rouge; MA 47 LA St Univ - Baton Rouge; Private Practice, **SLP LM**

Allen, Nancy R Atlanta Area School For Deaf, 890 North Indian Creek Dr, Clarkston, GA 30021, BA 71 Univ of NC - Greensboro; ME 79 Univ of GA; Aud, Atlanta Area Sch for Deaf, **A**

Allen, Nell R 6755 River Road, New Orleans, LA 70123, (504) 737-0260, BA 50 Northwestern St Univ; ME 57 Wayne St Univ; Sp-Lang Path, **SLP A F**

Allen, Patricia Lee 5212 N Lovers Lane #4, Milwaukee, WI 53225, (414) 241-4240, BA 72 Univ of WI - Madison; MA 76 Univ of West FL; MS 86 Univ of WI - Milwaukee; **SLP**

Allen, Paula H Carpenter 510 Oak Hill Circle S E, Marietta, GA 30067, (404) 953-3316, BS 62 Auburn Univ - Auburn; MS 66 Auburn Univ - Auburn; Sp-Lang Path, Comprehensive Physical Ther Svcs, **SLP**

Allen, Prudence Waisman Center Mental Retardation & Human Development, 1500 Highland Avenue Room 319, Madison, WI 53706, (608) 263-3301, BS 76 SUNY - Coll at Buffalo; MA 79 SUNY - Center at Buffalo; Aud, Hearing Dev Research Lab, **A**

Allen, Ralph Charles Route 1 Box 760, Goshen Mt Road, Clarkesville, GA 30523, (404) 754-2913, BS 74 Central MI Univ; MA 77 Central MI Univ; **SLP**

Allen, Rhonda Yvonne Star Route, Brenton, WV 24818, (304) 436-3161, BA 79 Marshall Univ; MA 80 Marshall Univ; Sp-Lang Path, Stevens Cl Hosp Inc, **SLP**

Allen, Robin Janine 777 Riverside Drive, Apartment 1535, Coral Springs, FL 33071, (305) 341-7382, MS 83 FL St Univ; Sp-Lang Path, Communicare, **SLP**

Allen, Rose L #7 Greenfield, R R 2 Box 724-B1, Mulvane, KS 67110, (316) 682-9578, BA 74 Wichita St Univ; MA 75 Wichita St Univ; MA 79 Wichita St Univ; 87–Aud, Radionic Hearing Aid Svc, **SLP A**

Allen, Mrs Sharon A Terrebonne Association For, Retarded Citizens, 1 McCord Road, Houma, LA 70363, (504) 868-2455, BS 65 Northwestern St Univ; MA 68 Northwestern St Univ; Exec Dir, Special School, **SLP**

Allen, Sonia Rodriguez 740 9th Avenue South, Hopkins, MN 55343, (612) 938-2337, BA 81 Univ of ND; MA 82 Univ of Northern CO; 88–Aud, Courage Ctr, **A**

Allen, Mrs Sue Sharp c/o David Allen, A Company 2-4 Avenue Reg, APO New York, NY 09815-2370, 11-49 -6132, BS 70 KS St Univ; MA 71 KS St Univ; Sp-Lang Path, **SLP**

Allen, Mrs Susan E 3505 Ashford, Fort Worth, TX 76133, (817) 465-9581, BS 75 TX Tech Univ; MS 80 TX Tech Univ; 80–Sp-Lang Path, Arlington ISD, **SLP**

Allen, Mrs Susan G 2887 Evercharm Place, Jacksonville, FL 32217, (904) 824-1654, OB 64 Univ of MI - Ann Arbor; ME 65 Smith Coll; ME 87 Univ of North FL; **SLP**

Allen, Mrs Suzanne S 134 Prospect Hill, Nashville, TN 37205, (615) 297-2192, BA 69 Vanderbilt Univ; MA 70 Vanderbilt Univ; 88–Sp-Lang Path, Vanderbilt Univ Med Ctr, **SLP**

Allen, Dr Sylvia K 1309 Carrollton Avenue #105, Metairie, LA 70005, (504) 568-4785, BA 71 Univ of Pittsburgh - Pittsburgh; MS 73 Univ of Pittsburgh - Pittsburgh; PH 81 (NS) Vanderbilt Univ; Asst Prof, Marshall U, **A**

Allen, Tedi 10419 Annapolis, San Antonio, TX 78230-2301, (512) 655-3401, BS 70 Southwest TX St Univ; ME 73 Southwest TX St Univ; Sp-Lang Path, **SLP**

Allen, Mrs Teresa Grant P O Box 1752, St Francisville, LA 70775, (504) 635-3373, BS 70 Univ Southern MS-Hattiesburg; MS 72 MS Univ for Women; Sp-Lang Path, Private Practice, **SLP**

Allen, Wendy Leyfert 702 Del Ray Drive, Kissimmee, FL 32758, (407) 423-9293, BS 82 PA St Univ - Univ Park; MS 83 Bloomsburg Univ of PA; Sp-Lang Path, Orange County PS, **SLP**

Allen-Peoples, Mrs Yvonne 11309 Winthrop, Detroit, MI 48227, (313) 838-8542, BA 74 MI St Univ; MA 77 MI St Univ; SLP, Detroit Bd of Ed, **SLP**

Allen-Smith, Mrs Charlotte J 22 Upton Road, Westborough, MA 01581, (617) 829-6631, MS 87 Worcester St Coll

Allen-Talley, Antoinette 12280 Green Meadow Drive, Apartment H, Columbia, MD 21044, (301) 730-8579, BA 79 Univ of MD - College Park; MA 83 Univ of MD - College Park; Sp-Lang Path, Balt Cty Pub Sch, **SLP**

Aller, Kathleen L 245 23rd Street Drive S E, Cedar Rapids, IA 52403, (319) 399-6829, BA 71 Creighton Univ; MA 72 Univ of IA; 75–Sp-Lang Path, Grant Wood AEA, **SLP**

Aller, Dr Sonia Konialian 17745 Stagg Street, Reseda, CA 91335, (213) 669-4593, BA 66; PH 78 (NS) IN Univ - Bloomington; 87–Sp-Lang Path, Childrens Hosp of Los Angeles, **SLP**

Aller, Mrs Virginia K RD #2 Hillcrest Box 485A, Wallkill, NY 12589, (914) 564-1590, BA 57 Coll of New Rochelle; MA 63 NY Univ; Sp-Lang Path, Newburgh Cty Pub Sch, **SLP**

Allerton, Leslie Ruth 201 Van Ostrand Road, Rd #1, Groton, NY 13073, (607) 533-4243, BS 83 SUNY - Coll at Geneseo; MS 85 Ithaca Coll

Alles, Catherine Dykstra 2187 Timothy Drive, Westminster, MD 21157, (301) 635-6348, BS 76 NY Univ; MA 78 Univ of MD - College Park; **A**

Alley, Deborah Justice 3890 Tremont Place, Ann Arbor, MI 48105, (313) 553-4135, BS 78 Purdue Univ - West Lafayette; MS 80 Univ of WA; Sp-Lang Path, Commun Hlth Care Assoc, **SLP**

Alley, James R 1067 Chula Vista Court, Greenwood, IN 46143, BS 58; MA 61 IN Univ - Bloomington; 88–Case Mgr, Ind Advocacy Svcs, **SLP**

Alley, Lynda Laura 14603 McKnew Road, Burtonsville, MD 20866, (301) 498-3532, BA 85 San Francisco St Univ; MS 86 San Francisco St Univ; 86–Dist Supvr, The Hrng Lab at Pearle Vision Center, **A**

Allie, Kathleen Marie 2610 Jefferson Street, Duluth, MN 55812, (715) 634-8924, BA 84 Univ of MN - Duluth; MA 85 Univ of MN - Duluth; **SLP**

Alliker, Mrs Esta R 2218 Shaded Brook Drive, Owings Mills, MD 21117, (301) 687-6500, BA 70 Towson St Univ; MS 73 Univ of MI - Ann Arbor; Sp-Lang Path, Baltimore Cty Hlth Dept, **SLP**

Allison, Mrs Carolyn Barth 5155 Mayweed Court, Colorado Springs, CO 80917, (303) 598-2575, BS 76 Univ of Southern CO; MA 77 Adams St Coll; Sp-Lang Path, Academy Dist #20

Allison, Mrs Cathi Pierce 12635 Sand Ridge Drive, Jacksonville, FL 32223, (904) 731-2653, BS 79 Univ of GA; ME 80 Univ of GA; Sp/Lang Path, Duval Co Pub Sch, **SLP**

Allison, Mrs Frances T 8604 West Progress Place, Littleton, CO 80123, (303) 978-9319, BS 73 CO St Univ; MA 74 Univ of Denver; Sp-Lang Path, Jefferson County Schools, **SLP**

Allison, Geraldine 9964 Meadowcrest Court, Elk Grove, CA 95624, (916) 685-5799, BA 62 CA St Univ - Chico; MS 72 Central WA Univ; 76–SLP, Sacramento Cty Unif Sch Dist, **SLP**

Allison, Jane Mathys 9734 Woodleaf Drive, Rancho Cucamonga, CA 91730, (714) 829-5950, BA 80 CA St Univ - Long Beach; MA 84 CA St Univ - Long Beach; 84–Aud, Kaiser Permanente, **A**

Allison, Lynn M 4417 North Emerald Drive, Cohutta, GA 30710, (404) 694-8553, BS 78 Univ of GA; ME 79 Univ of GA; Sp-Lang Path, Looper Sp & Hrng Cen, **SLP**

Allison, Paula 902 Frostwood Suite 303, Houston, TX 77024, (713) 932-3619, BA 77 SUNY - Coll at Plattsburgh; MS 83 Lamar Univ; 83–Dir,Aud, Memorial City Med Cen, **A**

Allison, Regina M 755 Via Otogic, San Clemente, CA 92672, (714) 586-1234, MA 83 CA St Univ - Fullerton; BA 81 CA St Univ - Fullerton; Sp-Lang Path, Saddleback Valley USD, **SLP**

Allison, Richard E 2215 Pleasant Avenue, Lake View, NY 14085, (716) 627-9817, BS 52 Eastern IL Univ; MA 58 IN Univ - Bloomington; Aud/Sp-Lang Path, Language Development Sch, **SLP A**

Allison, Mrs Scarlett M Box 324, Pinehurst, NC 28374, Consultant, Moore County Schools, **SLP**

Allman, Mrs Jean Wheeler 3428 Sea Eagle Court, Wilmington, NC 28403, (919) 762-0234, BS 78 Campbell Univ; MS 84 Univ of NC - Chapel Hill; Aud, Drs Botros & Pollock, **A**

Allman, Mrs Jeannette 836 34th Street N W #208, Canton, OH 44709, BS 47 Kent St Univ; MA 53 Kent St Univ; **SLP LM**

Allmaras, Geri Anne 1052 Sunflower Lane, Sidney, MT 59270, (406) 482-2530, BS 82 Univ of ND; MS 83 Minot St Univ; Super Sp-Lang Path, Sidney Pub Sch Sys, **SLP**

Allmayer-Beck, Rosemary 6540 Kirkville Road #156, East Syracuse, NY 13057, (315) 656-7236, BA 62 Syracuse Univ; OM 64 Middlebury Coll; MA 72 Coll of Saint Rose; Sp-Lang Path, E Syracuse-Minoa Sch Dist, **SLP**

Alloy, Linda K 10 Hawthorne Court, Fishkill, NY 12524, (914) 832-6611, BS 75 Towson St Univ; MA 76 Bowling Green St Univ; OM 80 Johns Hopkins Univ; Coord SLP & Audiology, Weschester Development Center, **SLP**

Allred, Elizabeth 14010 Ella Lee Lane, Houston, TX 77077, (713) 493-5838, BS 72 Southwest TX St Univ; MA 78 Univ of Houston - Univ Park; **SLP**

Allred, Julia D 101 Westbury Drive, Chapel Hill, NC 27514, **SLP**

Allred, Mrs Patricia Choate Rt 5 Box 1346, Hickory, NC 28601, (704) 324-3378, BS 77 Western Carolina Univ; ME 83 Univ of NC - Greensboro; Prog Manager Sp & Hrng, Frye Reg Med Ctr, **SLP**

Allred, Mrs Penelope Graves 73 Mar-Ree Drive, Laurel, MS 39440, (601) 649-6391, BS 75 Univ Southern MS-Hattiesburg; MS 87 Univ Southern MS-Hattiesburg

Allred, Dr Phillip L A S Hearing & Vision Center, 1320 10th Street, P O Box 6073, Huntsville, TX 77340, (409) 291-2414, BS 69 Brigham Young Univ; MS 74 Brigham Young Univ; PH 80 (NS) Univ of UT; Owner, A S Hrng & Vision Ctr, **A**

Allsman, Catherine 256 South Lake, Los Angeles, CA 90057, (213) 483-4431, BA 84 CA St Univ - Fresno; MA 86 Wichita St Univ; 87–Aud, House Ear Inst, **A**

Allsop, Terilee 6235 Swayne Drive N E, Olympia, WA 98506, (206) 753-8962, OM 77 Univ of WA; SLP, Olympia Public Schools, **SLP**

Allsup, Debra L 206 Hickory Street, Rossville, GA 30741, (615) 267-5641, OM 86 Auburn Univ - Auburn; Aud, Hamilton Co Sp & Hrng Cntr, **A**

Allsup-Armstrong, Peggy 22881 WCR 70, Eaton, CO 80615, (303) 339-5360, BA 80 Univ of Northern CO; MA 81 Univ of Northern CO; Sp-Lang Path, Weld County School District 6, **SLP ACE**

Allway, Linda J L Rural Delivery 3, Cazenovia, NY 13035, (315) 682-9192, BS 64 SUNY - Coll at Buffalo; MS 78 Syracuse Univ; Sp/Lang Path, Fayetteville-Manlius Schs, **SLP**

Alm, Mrs Janice M R R 3 Box 185, Moorhead, MN 56560, (218) 233-8385, BS 60 ND St Univ; MS 72 Moorhead St Univ; **SLP**

Alman, Martha Hirsch 41 Sherrill Heights, Little Rock, AR 72202, (501) 661-0558, BA 74 Univ of AR - Little Rock; MS 75 Southern Methodist Univ; Sp/Lang Path, AR Ped Cl, **SLP**

Almerico, Rebecca Garda 10154 S Bannor Hill Road, Sandy, UT 84092, (801) 566-1521, BA 77 Univ of KY; MA 78 OH St Univ; **SLP**

Almerico, Thomas P 10154 South Banner Hill Rd, Sandy, UT 84092-3950, (801) 566-1142, BS 77 Univ of UT; MA 79 OH St Univ; **SLP**

Almog, Donna Raspa 12 Marlee Drive, Spotswood, NJ 08884, (201) 668-2454, BA 78 Kean Coll of NJ; MA 80 Univ of CT; Sp-Lang Path, Muhlenberg Hosp, **SLP ACE**

Almon, Mrs Grace M 730 Ashbury Street, San Francisco, CA 94117, (415) 565-6150, BA 53 Vanderbilt Univ; Dept Hd/Sp-Lang, Ralph K Davies Med Cen, **SLP**

Almon, Mrs Ledonna H 412 Hermitage Drive, Altamonte Springs, FL 32701, (305) 834-5585, BS 76 Auburn Univ - Auburn; MA 77 Memphis St Univ; **SLP**

Almon-Matangos, Mrs Susan Elizabeth 40 Bayberry Drive, Mechanicsburg, PA 17055, (215) 631-9300, BA 79 Jacksonville St Univ; MS 82 Univ of AL- Tuscaloosa; Sp/Lang Path, InSpeech Inc, **SLP ACE**

Almost, Deborah Gilchrist Rural Route 7, Woodstock, ON, Canada N4S 7W2, (519) 537-6970, OB 80 Univ of Western Ontario; OM 82 Univ of Western Ontario; Sp/Lang Path, Woodstock General Hosp, **SLP**

Almquist, Mrs Bonnie Bricker 435 Fleming Road, Sarver, PA 16055, (412) 394-5815, BS 77 PA St Univ - Univ Park; MA 83 Univ of Pittsburgh - Pittsburgh; **SLP**

Almy, Judith K 216 North Hillside Drive, Exton, PA 19341, (215) 524-1058, MS 73 Ithaca Coll; BS 68 SUNY - Coll at Geneseo; 83–Sp-Lang Path, Exton Sp Path, **SLP**

Alper, Beth Sheckman 905 Melrose Avenue, Melrose Park, PA 19126, (215) 928-7445, BA 75 Temple Univ; MA 77 Temple Univ; 79–Sp-Lang Path, Thomas Jefferson U Hosp, **SLP**

Alper, Dina Pachino 50 Overlook Terrace #6H, New York, NY 10033, (212) 923-1223, BA 81 Yeshiva Univ; MS 83 Columbia Univ Teachers Coll; **SLP**

Alper, Mrs Elaine G 226 North Austin Blvd, Oak Park, IL 60302, (312) 383-7448, BS 59 PA St Univ - Univ Park; ME 64 PA St Univ - Univ Park; Sp-Lang Path, Chicago Board of Education, **SLP**

Alper, Randi R 191 Griggs Avenue, Teaneck, NJ 07666, (212) 523-6817, BA 78 CUNY - Queens Coll; MS 80 Univ of UT; Aud, St Luke's/Roosevelt Hosp Ctr, **A**

Alpern, Dr Carol Sober 571 Laurelton Boulevard, Long Beach, NY 11561, (212) 488-1441, BA 67 Adelphi Univ; MA 68 Columbia Univ Teachers Coll; PH 84 (Sp-Lang Path) CUNY - Grad Sch & Univ Cntr; 87–Asst Prof, Pace Univ, **SLP**

Alpern, Jane A 742 West Bittersweet #2W, Chicago, IL 60613, (312) 929-3808, BA 85 IN Univ - Bloomington; OM 87 IN Univ - Bloomington

Alpern, Mrs Ramona L Box R 14, 220 Gulph Hills Road, Radnor, PA 19087, (215) 525-2460, BS 48 NY Univ; MA 49 Northwestern Univ; Pres, Alpern and Associates, **SLP**

Alpert, Cynthia M 190 S Avenue, Glencoe, IL 60022, **SLP**

Alpert, Fay Ellen 18414 Collins Street #204, Tarzana, CA 91356, (213) 939-7322, MA 83 CA St Univ - Northridge; BA 76 CA St Univ - Northridge; Los Angeles City Schools, **SLP**

Alpiner, Dr Jerome G 1217 Edinborough Lane, Birmingham, AL 35226-3001, (205) 933-8101, BA 54 OH Univ - Athens; MA 59 Case Western Reserve Univ; PH 61 (NS) OH Univ - Athens; 87–Chief-Audiology Sec, VA Med Ctr, **A F**

Alprin, Mrs Linda Ann 6604 31st Street N W, Washington, DC 20015, (301) 652-3922, **SLP**

Alric, Mrs Ellen M Rd 2 Box 711, Gloversville, NY 12078, (518) 725-5062, BS 76 Bloomsburg Univ of PA; MA 77 Bowling Green St Univ; 86–Supvg Sp-Lang Path, Private Practice, **SLP**

Al-Saadi, Karen S 1302 Olivia Street, Ann Arbor, MI 48104, (313) 996-1734, BA 64 Univ of MI - Ann Arbor; MS 70 Univ of MI - Ann Arbor; Sp/Lang Path, Private Practice, **SLP**

Alsaker, Nora V 2620 Shannon Road, Northbrook, IL 60062, (312) 520-2745, BA 70 Elmhurst Coll; MA 72 Northern IL Univ - De Kalb; Sp-Lang Path, Wheeling Comm Consol Sc DIST21, **SLP**

Alsbrooks, Sharon W Route #2 Box 264, Orange Grove, TX 78372, (512) 384-9221, BS 74 Southwest TX St Univ; ME 75 Southwest TX St Univ; Sp-Lang Path, Brush Co Co Op, **SLP**

Alson, Leila B 210 Locust Street, Philadelphia, PA 19106, (215) 436-3404, BA 50 CUNY - Hunter Coll; MA 51 OH Univ - Athens; Sp-Lang Path, West Chester Univ, **SLP ACE**

Alspector, Mrs Helen W 716 Belvedere Avenue, Westfield, NJ 07090, (201) 233-6048, BS 70 Russell Sage Coll; MS 73 Rutgers St Univ -N Brunswick; Sp-Lang Path, Shapiro Cen for Infant Dev, **SLP**

Alsum, Mrs Terese Diane 1744 Sherwood S E, Grand Rapids, MI 49506, (616) 942-1660, BA 84 MI St Univ; MA 85 MI St Univ; **A**

Alt, Mrs Lisa Wojcik 2510 Kimberly Drive, Garland, TX 75040, (214) 270-8807, BA 80 TX Tech Univ; MS 88 Univ of TX - Dallas; 88–Aud, Mesquite Reg Day Sch for Deaf

Alt, Patricia E P O Box 1752, Cullowhee, NC 28723, (704) 227-7251, BS 72 Old Dominion Univ; MA 76 Univ of AL- Tuscaloosa; 77–Sp-Lang Path, Wn Carolina U, **SLP**

Alt, Phillip J 2202 Goff Street, Tifton, GA 31794, (912) 382-5114, BS 74 WV Univ; MS 77 WV Univ; 86–Audiologist, Tifton ENT Clinic & Hd Nck Sur, **A**

Alt, Mrs Susan P 981 Longstreet Drive, Bartlett, IL 60103, (312) 289-5210, BS 74 Northern IL Univ - De Kalb; MA 76 Northern IL Univ - De Kalb; **SLP**

Altepeter, Mrs Audrey E 471 Brightspur Lane, Ballwin, MO 63011, (314) 394-9624, BA 75 Loyola Coll; MS 77 Loyola Coll; **SLP**

Alter, Mrs Kathryn Satterfield 2207 Rural Point Drive, Mechanicsville, VA 23111, (804) 329-1765, BS 78 James Madison Univ; MS 83 James Madison Univ; Sp-Lang Path, Henrico Co Pub Schs, **SLP**

Alter, Mrs Susan White 79 Briarwood Court, Howell, NJ 07731, (201) 431-2240, BA 84 Montclair St Coll; MA 87 Trenton St Coll; **SLP**

Alterbaum, Irene P 101 Clark Street, Brooklyn, NY 11201, **SLP**

Alterman, Mrs Lorraine 10 Rockwell Circle, Marlboro, NJ 07746, (201) 972-1576, BA 74 CUNY - Queens Coll; MS 76 CUNY - Brooklyn Coll; **SLP**

Alterman, Mrs Maureen M 11554 West Highland Road, Hartland, MI 48029, (313) 632-6588, BA 72 Central MI Univ; MS 76 Univ of MI - Ann Arbor; Director, Sp-Lang & Reading Services Inc, **SLP**

Alterman, Merrill J 1864 Autumn Frost Lane, Baltimore, MD 21209, (301) 653-0134, BS 68 Ithaca Coll; MA 71 NY Univ; Aud, Baltimore City Schs, **A**

Alters, Mrs Laura Lynn 12702 Barbara Avenue, Garden Grove, CA 92640, (714) 530-3401, BA 83 CA St Univ - Fullerton; MA 86 CA St Univ - Fullerton; **SLP**

Altersohn, Mrs Kathleen Ann 2310F Century Pointe Lane, Glendale Heights, IL 60139, (312) 529-2187, BS 78 Marquette Univ; MS 80 Southern IL Univ -Carbondale; Sp-Lang Path, DuPage West Cook Spec Educ Org, **SLP**

Althouse, Susan R Good Samaritan Hospital, Speech & Language Path, 4th & Walnut Streets, Lebanon, PA 17042, (717) 272-7611, BS 78 Bloomsburg Univ of PA; MS 79 Bloomsburg Univ of PA; Sp-Lang Path, Good Samaritan Hosp, **SLP**

Altman, Betsy Jean The Watson Clinic, 1600 Lakeland Blvd, Lakeland, FL 33805, (813) 680-7195, BS 82 Western Carolina Univ; MA 84 Univ of SC - Columbia; Aud, Watson Clinic, **A**

Altman, Elaine K 100 Bleecker Street #19A, New York, NY 10012, (212) 228-2749, BA 66 Univ of CA - Los Angeles; MA 79 NY Univ; Sp-Lang Path, Private Practice, **SLP**

Altman, Holly M 947 Burts Pit Road, Northampton, MA 01060, (413) 584-3450, MA 83 Univ of MA - Amherst; Audiologist, Clarke School for the Deaf, **A**

Altman, Mrs Jill Cook 728 North Foote Avenue, Colorado Springs, CO 80909, (303) 576-0274, BA 76 Univ of FL; MS 78 Miami Univ - Oxford; Sp-Lang Path, Harrison Sch Dist #2, **SLP**

Altman, Mary Ellen 538 East 8th Street, Tucson, AZ 85705, (602) 623-1191, MS 87 Univ of AZ; 87–Sp-Lang Path, AZ Sch for Deaf & Blind, **SLP**

Altman, Dr Mickey D Wasilla High School, 701 Bogard, Wasilla, AK 99687-8555, (907) 376-5341, ED 85 WA St Univ; BA 64 WA St Univ; MA 68 (Educational Administration) WA St Univ; Asst Prin, Wasilla High School, **SLP**

Altman, Mrs Pamela Ruth 4061 Stilmore Road, South Euclid, OH 44121, (216) 231-8787, BS 84 Kent St Univ; MA 84 Kent St Univ; Sp-Lang Path, Cleveland Hrng & Sp Ctr, **SLP**

Altman, Mrs Sharon Demme 5 Wynngate Court, Fredericksburg, VA 22405, (804) 225-2068, BS 80 Clarion Univ of PA; MS 84 Clarion Univ of PA; 88–Supvr-Sp-Lang Hrng, VA Dept of Educ, **SLP**

Altman, Mrs Stephanie R 19501 N E 18th Court, North Miami Beach, FL 33179, (305) 935-5095, BS 62 Temple Univ-Tyler Sch of Art; MS 71 Loyola Coll; Sp-Lang Path, Dade Co Bd of Ed, **SLP**

Alto, Mrs Carolyn L 4389 Cypress Cove, Rock Hill, SC 29730, (803) 366-2994, BA 79 Rutger's St Univ - Douglas Coll; MA 81 Montclair St Coll; Aud, **A**

Altomare, Diane T 240 West Olive Street, Mount Carmel, PA 17851, (717) 644-0847, BS 81 Kutztown Univ of PA; MS 86 Bloomsburg Univ of PA; 84–Sp-Lang Path, Cen Susquehanna Interm Unit

Altomare, Lynn Woods 5116 Park West Avenue, San Diego, CA 92117, (619) 278-7470, **SLP**

Altringer, Kerry Mack 1405 Lochedem, Storm Lake, IA 50588, MS 72 Minot St Univ; SLP, Arrowhead AEA 5, **SLP**

Altschuler, Dr Sherry Levin 931 Waverly Road, Bryn Mawr, PA 19010, (215) 823-5853, BA 64 Temple Univ-Tyler Sch of Art; MA 65 OH St Univ; PH 73 (NS) Temple Univ-Tyler Sch of Art; 67–Chief Audiology-SLP, Phila VA Med Ctr Hosp Sect, **SLP**

Altshuler, Dr Morton W VA Hospital (126), 1421 Cherry Street, Philadelphia, PA 19102, (215) 597-7167, BS 57 PA St Univ - Univ Park; MS 58 PA St Univ - Univ Park; ED 63 (NS) Boston Univ; Ch-Aud & SLP Serv, VA, **SLP A**

Alvarenga, Joyce E 58 North Columbus Avenue, Mount Vernon, NY 10553, (212) 822-5345, BA 70 Pace U -NY City; MA 71 CUNY - Lehman Coll; Sp-Lang Path, Bd of Ed NYC Sp Serv Ut, **SLP**

Alverson, Robin P M Edwin Davis Md, 29 S W Upper Riverdale Road, Suite 130, Riverdale, GA 30274, (404) 991-1170, BS 80 Univ of GA; OM 82 Emory Univ; Aud, M Edwin Davis MD, **A**

Alvey, Mrs Charlene R 412 Perkins Drive, Franklin, TN 37064, BS 77 James Madison Univ; ME 79 James Madison Univ; Aud, Franklin Spec Sch Dist, **A**

Alvig, Kathleen 10390 Lancaster Lane, Maple Grove, MN 55369, (612) 535-2015, BS 71 Univ of MN - Minneap-St Paul; MS 72 Saint Cloud St Univ; Sp-Lang Path, Hennepine T Cen 287, **SLP**

Alvord, Dr Lynn S 2435 Falcon Way, Sandy, UT 84093, (801) 756-5291, BA 75 Weber St Coll; PH 80 (NS) Univ of UT; Owner, Alpine Aud Consul, **A**

Alworth, Mrs Lois Anne 4524 South Galvez, New Orleans, LA 70125, (504) 363-2224, BA 64 Univ of CA - Berkeley; MA 80 Tulane Univ; 85–Sp-Lang Path, F Edward Hebert Rehab Inst, **SLP**

Alzos-Howe, Elaine I May Whitney Elementary School, 120 Church Street, Lake Zurich, IL 60047, (312) 438-2351, BS 72 Purdue Univ - West Lafayette; MA 74 Northern IL Univ - De Kalb; Sp-Lang Path, Comm Ut Sch Dist 95, **SLP**

Amabile, Mrs Lisa Boardman 74 Baldwin Avenue, Jersey City, NJ 07306, (201) 333-8698, BS 85 Trenton St Coll; MA 87 Hahnemann Univ Grad Sch; SLP, Garden State Rehab Hosp, **SLP**

Amabile, Mrs Michelle Rico 1521 6th Street, Los Banos, CA 93635, (209) 357-6100, BA 80 CA St Univ - Stanislaus; MA 82 CA St Univ - Stanislaus; Sp-Lang Path, Office of Merced Co Sch Supt, **SLP**

Amadio, Phillip H 1800 Middlesbrough Court, Apartment G-1, Maumee, OH 43537, (419) 698-7230, MA 78 OH Univ - Athens; 88–Mktg Rep, St Charles Hosp, **SLP**

Amano, Mrs Sandra E 98-625 Kilinoe Street, Apartment 3B1, Aiea, HI 96701, (808) 488-8075, **SLP**

Amato, John J 17 Little Harbor Road, Mount Sinai, NY 11766, (516) 724-3626, BA 70 Hofstra Univ; MS 71 Ithaca Coll; Dir/Dept of Commun Dis, Suffolk Child Dev Cen, **SLP**

Amato, Mrs Sylvia R 172 Vose Avenue, South Orange, NJ 07079, (201) 762-5891, BA 55 CUNY - Brooklyn Coll; MA 73 Kean Coll of NJ; 70–Sp-Lang Path, East Orange Board of Education, **SLP**

Ambalong, Mrs Gaudencia 7423 Golden Oak Way, Sacramento, CA 95831, BA 53 Pacific Univ; MS 56 Univ of OR; SLP, Yolo County Supt of Schools, **SLP**

Amberg, Cheryl D 7783 Wayfaring Court, Reynoldsburg, OH 43068, (614) 687-6666, BA 76 OH St Univ; MA 78 OH St Univ; Sp-Lang Path, Septa Inc, **SLP**

Amberg, Susan Michele 1412 Edmonson Circle, Nashville, TN 37211, (615) 331-3907, BA 83 Univ of MI - Ann Arbor; MA 84 MI St Univ; Clinical Director/Aud, N Rocky Mountain Easter Seal, **A**

Ambro, Mrs Lilli Moore 5421 Guida Drive, Greensboro, NC 27401, (919) 373-3157, OB 79 Salem Coll; MA 83 Univ of NC - Greensboro; SLP, Guilford Co Hlth Dept, **SLP**

Ambroe, Mary H 8446 Humboldt Avenue South, Bloomington, MN 55431, (612) 936-4025, BA 62 Univ of MN - Minneap-St Paul; MA 67 Univ of MN - Minneap-St Paul; Pres, Exec Admin Svcs Inc, **SLP F**

Ambrose, Mrs Bobbie Robertson 2536 Bittle Road, Owensboro, KY 42301, (502) 685-1277, BA 52 Georgetown Coll; Dir SLP Serv, **SLP**

Ambrose, Mrs Carolyn E 3815 Bennett Avenue, Bellingham, WA 98226, (206) 676-6514, BA 68 Western WA Univ; OM 69 Univ of WA; Sp-Lang Path, Bellingham Pub Sch, **SLP**

Ambrose, Cheryl Lee 26255 Rainbow Glen Drive, Newhall, CA 91321, (818) 795-6981, MA 82 CA St Univ - Northridge; SLP, Pasadena USD, **SLP**

Ambrose, David L 434 East Norwegain Street, Pottsville, PA 17901, (717) 622-1435, BS 72 PA St Univ - Univ Park; ME 74 Bloomsburg Univ of PA; Aud/Owner, Ambrose Hearing Center, **A**

Ambrose, Dr William Rufus 6064 Millstone Run, Stone Mountain, GA 30087, (404) 325-5978, BS 60 Centenary Coll of LA; ME 64 Univ of VA - Charlottesville; PH 68 (Aud) Syracuse Univ; Aud, Dekalb Co Bd of Ed, **A**

Ambrosi, Denise Maria 10 Bradbury Avenue, Medford, MA 02155, (617) 720-6727, MS 85 Univ of TX - Dallas; **SLP**

Ambrosino, Mrs Barbara Marie 4 Karista Spring Drive, Saratoga Springs, NY 12866, (518) 583-1488, BS 80 SUNY - Coll at Fredonia; MS 82 Coll of Saint Rose; SLP, Glens Falls City Schools, **SLP**

Ambrosio, Mrs Susan Ellenis 9 Roosevelt Avenue, East Northport, NY 11731, (516) 549-4900, BA 82 SUNY - Coll at Oswego; MS 84 Adelphi Univ; SLP, BOCES III, **SLP**

Ambrozy, Dr Carol A 211 Riverview Avenue, Athol, MA 01331, (617) 249-3806, BA 73 Univ of MA - Amherst; MA 74 Univ of MA - Amherst; ED 83 (NS) Nova Univ; Spec Ed Admin, Athol-Royal Reg Sch Dist, **SLP**

Amdur, Mrs Judith Ann 12209 Quorn Lane, Reston, VA 22091, (703) 698-7500, BA 59 CUNY - Brooklyn Coll; Sp-Lang Path, Fairfax Co Pub Sch, **SLP**

Amen, Linde Ann 727 Rio Grande, Raton, NM 87740-9801, (505) 445-5184, MS 87 CO St Univ

Amend, Mrs Gaylee M 702 East Home Avenue, Fresno, CA 93728, (209) 442-3967, BA 70 CA St Univ - Fresno; MA 71 CA St Univ - Fresno; 71–Sp-Lang Path, Fresno Comm Hosp & Med Cen, **SLP**

Amend, Mrs Mary J 33024 N E 142nd Street, Rural Route 2, Duvall, WA 98019, (715) 832-9980, **SLP**

Amenson, Mrs Gail Arlene 6110 East Janice Way, Scottsdale, AZ 85254, (602) 483-8254, OM 85 AZ St Univ; 87–SLP, Deer Valley USD, **SLP**

Ament, Annemarie 309 Maleza Way, Santa Barbara, CA 93111, (805) 683-1928, MA 88 Univ of CA - Santa Barbara

Ament, George D, Jr 1450 Conway Drive, Swarthmore, PA 19081, (215) 544-4860, BS 82 Kutztown Univ of PA; MA 86 Temple Univ-Tyler Sch of Art; Sp-Lang Path, Delaware Curative Workshop, **SLP**

Americo, Peter K 1507 Byng Drive, South Charleston, WV 25303, (304) 348-7626, BS 66 CA Univ of PA; MS 67 WV Univ; Sp-Lang Path, Charleston Area Medical Center, **SLP**

Ameris, Mrs Kimberly Kay 863 Ardmore Avenue, Akron, OH 44302, (216) 434-1703, BA 84 Univ of Akron; MA 87 Univ of Akron; **SLP**

Amerman, Dr James D University Of Missouri, Commun Disorders Program, 106 Parker Hall, Columbia, MO 65211, BA 66 Univ of NE - Lincoln; MS 69 Univ of IL - Urbana; PH 70 (NS) Univ of IL - Urbana; Dir, U of MO - Columbia

Ames, Janis G 33 Heather Road, Bangor, ME 04401, (207) 942-2474, BA 67 Univ of ME - Orono; MA 80 Univ of ME - Orono; Sp-Lang Path, Private Practice, **SLP**

Amesquita, Mrs Rikki K 5839 Lincoln #B, Morton Grove, IL 60053-3346, BS 80 Univ of IL - Urbana; MS 81 Univ of IL - Urbana; 88–Sp-Lang Path, Northwest Suburban Spec Educ Org, **SLP**

Amick, David K 10623 Wadsworth Court, Fort Wayne, IN 46825, (219) 425-7463, BA 69 Ball St Univ; MA 72 Ball St Univ; **SLP**

Amick, Jeana M 172 West Zaun, Blue Springs, MO 64015, (816) 833-2088, BS 84 Central MO St Univ; MS 88 Central MO St Univ; 87–Sp-Lang Path, Sunshine Ctr Inc

Amick, Katherine Ann 401 East Lincoln Way, Libson, OH 44432, (216) 424-9591, BS 81 Purdue Univ - West Lafayette; MA 83 IN Univ - Bloomington; 83–Sp-Lang Path, Columbiana Co Board of Educ, **SLP ACE**

Amidon, Mrs Joy W 47 Andersen Drive, Boxford, MA 01921, (508) 468-2626, BS 59 SD St Univ; MS 77 Univ of VT; 86–Sp-Lang Path, Hamilton-Wenham Sch Dist, **SLP**

Amira, Carol J 152 Greenmeadow Drive, Deer Park, NY 11729, (516) 434-5200, BA 75 SUNY - Center at Buffalo; MA 77 OH St Univ; Sp-Lang Path, Pilgrim Psychi Cen, **A**

Amis, Mrs Jane Wiggins Surgical Associates ENT, 1 South Prospect Street, Burlington, VT 05401, (802) 656-4535, BS 82 Univ of VT; Aud, Surgical Assoc Foundation, **A**

Amis, Judith L North Fulton Regional Hospital, 11585 Alpharetta Highway, Roswell, GA 30076, BS 73 Univ of GA; ME 74 Univ of GA; 88–Dir of Rehab, North Fulton Reg Hosp, **SLP**

Amish, Mrs Frances J 3087 Lazy Creek Drive, Medford, OR 97504, (503) 779-0530, BA 70 CA St Univ - Long Beach; MA 74 CA St Univ - Long Beach; Sp-Lang Path, Josephine Co Mental Health Div, **SLP**

Amling, Mrs Frances Williamson 207 Kitchell Avenue, Pana, IL 62557, (618) 283-3659, BS 81 Eastern IL Univ; MS 82 Eastern IL Univ; Sp-Lang Path, Mid State Special Education, **SLP**

Amman, Debra A 2901 Lake Joanna Drive, Eustis, FL 32726, (904) 589-1856, BS 71 FL St Univ; MS 73 FL St Univ; Sp-Path Commun Dis Classrm, Lake Co Bd of Pub Inst, **SLP**

Ammann, Mrs Susan Indian Lake Road, Putnam Valley, NY 10579, (914) 628-3415, BA 76 SUNY - Coll at New Paltz; MA 82 CUNY - Hunter Coll; Sp-Lang Path, Mahopac Ctrl Sch Dist, **SLP**

Ammons, Dr Robert B Box 9229, Missoula, MT 59807, BA 39 San Diego St Univ; MA 41 Univ of IA; PH 46 (NS) Univ of IA; 57–Prof, Univ of Montana

Amo, Kathleen Marie P O Box 1236, Rhinelander, WI 54501, (715) 362-7654, **SLP**

Amorillo, Thomas P 12-A Christine Lane, East Northport, NY 11731, (516) 385-2867, BA 72 Iona Coll; MA 78 Long Island U - CW Post Ctr; Chief of Sp & Hrng, Long Is Dev Cen, **SLP A**

Amoroso, Patricia 17 Charles Drive, Franklin, MA 02038, (617) 528-1677, BS 70 Northeastern Univ; ME 74 Northeastern Univ; SLP, Foxborough Public Schools, **SLP**

Amos, Mrs Bonnie W 3709 Wynnewood Drive, Greensboro, NC 27408, (919) 288-4164, BA 66 Greensboro Coll; MA 72 Univ of NC - Greensboro; Sp-Lang Path, Greensboro Pub Sch, **SLP**

Amos, Mrs Opal Chavis 312 Branchwood Court, Jacksonville, NC 28540, (919) 455-2057, BS 80 East Carolina Univ; MS 82 East Carolina Univ; 86–Sp-Lang Path, Onslow County School System, **SLP**

Amos-King, Phyllis W 531 Maude Avenue, Baltimore, MD 21225-1027, (301) 396-7107, BA 71 Univ of CO - Boulder; MS 72 FL St Univ; Sp-Lang Path, Cty of Balto Pub Sch, **SLP**

Amprimo-Beer, Mrs Arlene Mary Cornfield Road, Spencer, MA 01562, (508) 885-9449, BA 80 Elms Coll; MA 82 Univ of MA - Amherst; Sp-Lang Path, Spencer Sch Sys, **SLP**

Amsel, Mrs Lynn J 11 Cameo Lane, Westbury, NY 11590, (212) 526-1000, BA 77 Hofstra Univ; MA 78 NY Univ; **A**

Amspaugh, Gilbert D 2311 Dora Drive, Clearwater, FL 34625, (813) 799-3241, BS 69 Ball St Univ; MA 76 Ball St Univ; SLP, Private Practice, **SLP**

Amster, Dr Barbara J 26 Eldon Road, Lansdowne, PA 19050, BA 69 CUNY - Brooklyn Coll; MS 71 Univ of Pittsburgh - Pittsburgh; PH 84 (NS) Temple Univ; 75–Asst Prof, Med Coll of PA, **SLP**

Amster, Dr Walter W Chief Aud & Speech Path Serv, VA Medical Center, 800 Irving Avenue, Syracuse, NY 13210, (305) 321-3148, BS 48 IN Univ - Bloomington; MA 50 Univ of IA; PH 54 (NS) Syracuse Univ; Chf Aud & SLP, VA, **SLP F**

Amundsen, Joanne E 10364 Princess JoAnn Road, Santee, CA 92071, (619) 448-1630, BA 75 Univ of MI - Ann Arbor; MA 76 Central MI Univ; MA 81 4689; Sp-Lang Path, San Diego City Sch, **SLP**

Amundsen, Mrs Judith A 2030 Webster Street, Racine, WI 53403, (414) 632-6478, BS 65 Univ of WI - Madison; MS 74 Univ of WI - Milwaukee; Sp-Lang Path, Racine USD, **SLP**

Amundson, Jill Katherine 784 Springwood Street, Apartment N, Corona, CA 91720, (714) 371-6804, BS 84 Univ of ND; MS 86 Univ of WI - Madison; **SLP**

Amundson, Martha Z 502 Fremont Street East, Northfield, MN 55057, (507) 332-3387, BS 73 Moorhead St Univ; MS 76 Moorhead St Univ; Sp-Lang Path, Faribault St Hosp, **SLP**

Amundson, Martin A Park Avenue Suites, 400 Park Avenue, Bldg D, Paducah, KY 42001, (502) 443-3651, BA 76 Eastern IL Univ; BS 76 Eastern IL Univ; MS 76 Eastern IL Univ; Aud, Comm for Handicapped Children, **A**

Amy, Mrs Sandra L Rd 2 Box 253, Monongahela, PA 15063, (412) 258-8456, BS 66 CA Univ of PA; MA 75 Cleveland St Univ; Sp-Lang Path, CA Univ of PA, **SLP**

Anae, Mrs Annabel Porter 55-470 Joseph Street, Laie, HI 96762, (808) 732-1853, **A**

Anastario, Patricia Kelley 12 Heritage Cove, Casselberry, FL 32707, (407) 831-8989, BS 76 Kent St Univ; MA 84 Univ of Central FL; Sp-Lang Path, **SLP ACE**

Anastasia, Antoinette Marie 759 Jersey Avenue, Elizabeth, NJ 07202, (201) 355-0359, MA 85 Kean Coll of NJ; **SLP**

Anastasia, Mrs Stefanie Carol 5180 Winona Lane, Gurnee, IL 60031, (312) 336-4311, BS 82 IL St Univ - Normal; OM 84 Governors St Univ; Sp-Lang Path, Waukegan PS, **SLP**

Anastasio, Joan 245 Forsgate Drive, Jamesburg, NJ 08831, (201) 521-1096, BS 84 Trenton St Coll; MA 87 Trenton St Coll

Ancell, Mrs Gale Skalsky 205 Goldbrier Drive, Sikeston, MO 63801, (314) 471-8854, BS 69 Southeast MO St Univ; MA 79 Southeast MO St Univ; 86–Sp-Lang Path, Sikeston PS, **SLP**

Ancheta, Maria Celeste 4274 Mahogany Run S E, Winter Haven, FL 33884, (813) 324-7061, MS 87 Univ Southern MS-Hattiesburg; 88–Sp-Lang Path, The Vanguard Sch

Anchin, Mrs Ellen 616 Seney Avenue, Mamaroneck, NY 10543, (914) 285-7294, BS 56 Kent St Univ; MS 76 Columbia Univ Teachers Coll; Chief of Sp-Lang Path, Westchester Co Med Cen, **SLP ACE**

Ancona, Beverly Wolfe P O Box 31847, Palm Beach Gardens, FL 33410-7847, (713) 789-1891, MA 75 Marshall Univ; Sp/Lang Path, Palm Beach Co Schs, **SLP**

Andary, Diane Kelly 3284 Roosevelt Road #J-11, Muskegon, MI 49441-3958, (616) 744-1493, MA 86 Central MI Univ; BA 84 MI St Univ; **SLP**

Andela, Mrs Christine Rita 11 Newark Street, Sodus, NY 14551, (315) 597-3469, BA 81 SUNY - Coll at Cortland; MS 85 Ithaca Coll; Sp-Lang Path, Palmyra-Macedon Central Schs, **SLP**

Andelman, Mrs Fani 6 Elyahu Hakim Str, Apartment 32 B, Tel Aviv, Israel 69120, 3-541-1127, BA 76; MA 79; MS 82 Boston Univ; **SLP**

Andereck, Amy 12408 South Hobart Avenue, Palos Park, IL 60464, (312) 448-3637, BA 73 TX Christian Univ; MA 75 TX Christian Univ; **SLP**

Anderegg, Mrs Pamela P Route 1 Box 196, Rincon, GA 31326, (912) 754-6137, BA 77 Univ of Southwestern LA; MS 79 Univ of Southwestern LA; 85–Sp-Lang Path, Effingham Co Bd of Educ, **SLP**

Anderle, Mrs Dawn Dershem P O Box 4923, Carmel, CA 93921, (408) 625-5281, BA 80 San Diego St Univ; MA 82 Memphis St Univ; 87–Sp-Lang Path/Dir, **SLP**

Anderman, Barbara B 158 Danefield Place, Moraga, CA 94556, (415) 947-5300, BA 72 Long Island U - CW Post Ctr; MA 76 Univ of CO - Boulder; Dir/Sp-Lang Path, John Muir Med Ctr, **SLP**

Anderman, Dr Bernard 4601 North Park Avenue, Apartment 107, Chevy Chase, MD 20015, (301) 654-3549, BA 37 CUNY - Brooklyn Coll; MA 39 Columbia Univ Teachers Coll; ED 56 (NS) Columbia Univ Teachers Coll; **SLP A F LM**

Anders, Linda Dovalina 308 South McKinney, Mexia, TX 76667, (817) 562-2267, **SLP**

Anders, Victoria Meighan 158 Wolseley North, Montreal, PQ, Canada H4X 1V9, (514) 487-7643, BS 76 West Chester Univ of PA; MA 85 SUNY - Coll at Plattsburgh; 80–Sp-Lang Path, Canadian Inst for Neuro-Integrative Dev

Andersen, Allan L Alta View Hearing Services, 9690 South 1300 East, Suite 200, Sandy, UT 84092, (801) 572-0041, BS 77 Univ of UT; MS 78 Univ of UT; Aud, Alta View ENT Assoc, **A**

Andersen, Beverly H 6250 East Pershing, Scottsdale, AZ 85254, (602) 255-3448, BS 70 CO St Univ; MS 72 CO St Univ; Aud, Phoenix Day Sch for the Deaf, **SLP A**

Andersen, Carol L 105 Edgemoor Avenue, Wellesley, MA 02181, (619) 459-7307, BA 69 Univ of CA - Berkeley; MS 79 San Francisco St Univ; Aud, **A**

Andersen, Dr Catherine Finneran 4305 Sir Walter Lane, Olney, MD 20832, (202) 722-5823, BS 73 OH Univ - Athens; MA 75 Hofstra Univ; PH 81 (NS) IN Univ - Bloomington; Sp-Lang Path, Gallaudet College, **SLP A**

Andersen, Debra S P O Box 698, Clinton, OK 73601, (405) 323-2100, BA 77 KS St Univ; MA 80 KS St Univ; Sp/Lang Path, OK St Dept of Hlth, **SLP**

Andersen, Douglas E 1409 Longway Lane, Bakersfield, CA 93309, (805) 832-3586, MA 79 CA St Univ - Los Angeles; Aud, Mercy Hosp, **A**

Andersen, Dr Helen G 6427 S W 37th Way, Gainesville, FL 32608, (904) 376-2800, BS 64 Univ of FL; ME 69 Univ of FL; PH 81 (NS) Univ of FL; Sp-Lang Path, Private Practice, **SLP**

Andersen, Jacqueline Barsoom 1514 Newlands Avenue, Burlingame, CA 94010, (415) 573-2234, BA 73 Univ of the Pacific; MA 74 Univ of the Pacific; SLP, San Mako Co Supt/Sch, **SLP**

Andersen, Mrs Julia 3000 South Carpenter, Appleton, WI 54915, (414) 779-4043, BA 75 Univ of WI - Eau Claire; MS 82 Univ of WI - Oshkosh; Sp-Lang Path, Hortonville Comm Sch, **SLP**

Andersen, Mrs Katherine Kiehn 1603 East Chestnut Avenue, Orange, CA 92667, (714) 637-4308, BA 55 Univ of the Pacific; BA 80 CA St Univ - Fullerton; MA 82 CA St Univ - Fullerton; Spec Day Class/Commun Hndcpd, Santa Ana USD, **SLP**

Andersen, Lucie C P O Box 13843, Reno, NV 89507, (702) 265-3812, MS 87 Univ of NV - Reno

Andersen, Monica K Houston ENT Clinic, One Memorial Southwest Suite 820, 7777 Southwest Freeway, Houston, TX 77074-1864, (713) 776-2211, BA 71 Univ of IA; OM 81 Houston Baptist Univ; MA 75 Univ of Northern CO; 76–Dir of Aud, Houston ENT Clinic, **A**

Andersen, Mrs Pamela Mary S 5221 Pony Creek Circle, Colorado Springs, CO 80919, (303) 590-7290, BA 77 Univ of Northern CO; MA 78 Univ of Denver; Dir/Augmentative Communication, Penrose Hospital, **SLP**

Anderson, Amy Beth 9550 Ella Lee Lane #2033, Houston, TX 77063, (713) 467-4696, BS 84 TX Woman's Univ; MS 86 Univ of TX - Houston; **SLP**

Anderson, Andrea Stockard 436 Marengo #202, Pasadena, CA 91101, (818) 885-5330, BA 83 Univ of the Pacific; MA 84 Univ of the Pacific; Sp-Lang Path, Northridge Hosp Med Ctr, **SLP**

Anderson, Angela 8 Rochambeau, Pompton Plains, NJ 07444, (904) 678-3224, BA 67 Univ of KY; MS 69 Vanderbilt Univ; **SLP**

Anderson, Anita J 6811 DE Paul Cove, Austin, TX 78723, (512) 450-3195, BA 66 Southern Methodist Univ; MA 68 Southern Methodist Univ; Coord/Sers for Disabld, TX Dept of Human Svcs, **A**

Anderson, Mrs Ann Brown 2421 60th Street N W, Rochester, MN 55901, (507) 284-2577, BS 82 Univ of MN - Minneap-St Paul; MS 84 Univ of AZ; 84–Aud, Mayo Clinic, **A**

Anderson, Mrs Ann Catlett 819 Summerdale Drive, Knoxville, TN 37922-5055, (615) 435-2519, BS 80 Univ of TN - Knoxville; MA 81 Univ of TN - Knoxville; 86–Sp-Lang Path, Anderson Co Schs, **SLP**

Anderson, Ann L 1885 113th Avenue N W, Coon Rapids, MN 55433, (612) 295-2934, BA 72 Univ of MN - Minneap-St Paul; MA 75 Univ of MN - Duluth; SLP, Monticello School District 882, **SLP**

Anderson, Mrs Ann N 2917 Meadow Park Drive, Dayton, OH 45440, (513) 254-8425, BS 57 OH Univ - Athens; MA 74 Univ of Cincinnati; Resource Person Multi-Hndcpd, Dayton Bd Ed, **SLP**

Anderson, Anne F Martinsville City Schools, Martinsville, VA 24112, **SLP**

Anderson, Annette McKenzie 4850 Connecticut Avenue N W, Washington, DC 20008, (202) 576-6090, BS 63 Hampton Univ; MS 74 Univ of the DC; Sp/Lang Path, Dc Pub Sch, **SLP**

Anderson, Mrs Arlene K 4935 Iron House Trail, Colorado Springs, CO 80917, (719) 591-2152, BS 73 WV Univ; MA 74 Univ of FL; Sp-Lang Path, Sch Dist 11 Colorado Springs, **SLP**

Anderson, Mrs Barbara B 840 Kings Point Drive West, Addison, IL 60101, (312) 653-7000, BS 53 Univ of WI - Madison; MA 72 OH St Univ; MA 85 Roosevelt Univ; Sp-Lang Path, Glenbard Township Hs Dist 87, **SLP**

Anderson, Barbara H 2833 Iris Avenue N W, Cedar Rapids, IA 52405, **SLP**

Anderson, Dr Bernadette The Speech Excel Center, 30 West Washington, Suite 1132, Chicago, IL 60602, (312) 236-0911, BS 70 Univ of IL - Urbana; MA 71 Univ of IL - Urbana; PH 81 (NS) Northwestern Univ; Director, The Speech Excel Ctr, **SLP**

Anderson, Dr Bernard A 220 Brownstone Drive, Reno, NV 89512, (702) 323-3767, BA 33 Univ of WA; MA 37 Univ of WA; PH 50 (NS) Univ of WI - Madison; Professor Emeritus, University of Nevada, **SLP F LM**

Anderson, Beth Louise 20037 Avenue Of The Oaks, Newhall, CA 91321, BA 72 Univ of CA - Santa Cruz; MA 83 CA St Univ - Northridge; Sp-Lang Path, LA USD, **SLP**

Anderson, Betty D Sacramento Biofeedback Center, 6600 Mercy Court, Suite 250, Fair Oaks, CA 95628-3133, (916) 967-1115, BA 71 CA St Univ - Sacramento; MA 73 CA St Univ - Sacramento; Co-Dir, Sacramento Biofdbck&Behav Mod, **SLP**

Anderson, Bettye E 18949 Springfield Avenue, Flossmoor, IL 60422, (312) 799-6552, BS 74 Univ of VA - Charlottesville; ME 75 Univ of VA - Charlottesville; **SLP**

Anderson, Cara Wright 1401-A University N E, Albuquerque, NM 87102, (505) 242-4995, BA 66 AZ St Univ; MA 70 Univ of NM; Director/Owner, Albuquerque Aphasia&Sp Consult, **SLP**

Anderson, Carey Lynn 916 Dartmouth Road, Baltimore, MD 21212, (301) 687-8853, BS 83 Towson St Univ; MS 85 Towson St Univ; 88–Sp-Lang Path, Ft Howard VA Med Ctr, **SLP**

Anderson, Carol A 1334 Greenhills Road, Greenfield, IN 46140, (317) 462-0503, BS 69 CO St Univ; MS 70 Univ of WI - Madison; Sp-Lang Path, Hancock Mem Hosp, **SLP**

Anderson, Carol B 512 East Foster Avenue, State College, PA 16801, (717) 242-7343, BA 64 Oberlin Coll; MA 66 Case Western Reserve Univ; PH 86 (Linguistics); 88–Dir-SLP Dept, Lewistown Hosp, **SLP**

Anderson, Carol Jane 521 Mildred Place, Oradell, NJ 07649, (201) 441-2161, BS 81 Stockton St Coll; MA 84 Montclair St Coll; **A**

Anderson, Mrs Caroline A County Road 460, Box 825, Newberry, MI 49868, (906) 293-5421, BS 64 Central MI Univ; MA Central MI Univ; Sp/Lang Path, Tahquamenon Area Sch, **SLP**

Anderson, Catherine Howley 11 Buckingham Street #3, Rochester, NY 14607, (716) 244-9678, BA 83 Univ of Western Ontario; MA 85 SUNY - Coll at Geneseo; 86–Sp-Lang Path, Rochester City Sch Dist, **SLP**

Anderson, Charles A 1406 East Church, Pierre, SD 57501, (605) 677-5311, BA 64 Univ of SD - Vermillion; MA 66 Univ of SD - Vermillion; ED 83 (NS) Univ of SD - Vermillion; Dir, U of SD Sch of Med, **SLP**

Anderson, Charles V Wendell Johnson Sp & Hrng Ctr, Dept Of Speech Path & Aud, University Of Iowa, Iowa City, IA 52242, (319) 335-8700, BS 55 Univ of NE - Lincoln; MA 57 Univ of NE - Lincoln; PH 62 (NS) Univ of Pittsburgh - Pittsburgh; Assoc Prof, U of Iowa, **A F**

Anderson, Charone B 8580 Hague Road, Indianapolis, IN 46256, (317) 849-6262, BA 79 Ball St Univ; MA 80 Ball St Univ; Sp-Lang Path, Community Hospital North, **SLP**

Anderson, Cheryl C 30031 Troutdale Ridge Road, Evergreen, CO 80439, (303) 670-3268, MS 73 Vanderbilt Univ; Sp-Lang Path, Private Practice, **SLP**

Anderson, Cheryl L Mississippi Valley Rehab Serv, 2 St Anthony's Way, Suite 111, Alton, IL 62002, (618) 465-0105, BA 73 Univ of IL - Urbana; MA 74 Univ of IL - Urbana; Coord of Field Services, Mississippi Valley Rehab Serv, **SLP**

Anderson, Mrs Christina Susanne 215 West Kathleen, Phoenix, AZ 85023, (602) 993-1584, BS 72 AZ St Univ; MS 76 AZ St Univ; Sp-Lang Path, Washington Elem Sch Dist, **SLP ACE**

Anderson, Christine P O Box 1044, Damariscotta, ME 04543, BS 77 Portland St Univ; ME 80 Trenton St Coll; Sp-Lang Path, Sad #61, **SLP**

Anderson, Coleen P 11875 91st Avenue North, Maple Grove, MN 55369, (612) 781-6571, BA 80 Univ of MN - Minneap-St Paul; MS 83 Saint Cloud St Univ; Sp-Lang Path, Sister Kenny Institute, **SLP**

Anderson, Colleen 127 Hollywood Lane, Kirkwood, MO 63122, (314) 966-8872, **SLP**

Anderson, Cynthia A Box 1805, 3321 Avenue A, Kearney, NE 68847, (305) 234-4586, BA 74 Univ of NE - Lincoln; MA 76 Univ of NE - Lincoln; Aud, Mid-NE ENT Assoc, **A**

Anderson, Mrs Cynthia R 9702 Palantine North, Seattle, WA 98103, (206) 771-0667, BA 76 Univ of WA; OM 78 Univ of WA; SLP, Edmonds Sch Dist #15, **SLP**

Anderson, Daniel G 116 Myrtle Road #4, Burlingame, CA 94010, (415) 375-1039, BA 73 San Jose St Univ; MA 82 San Jose St Univ; Sp-Lang Path, Mills Hosp, **SLP**

Anderson, Dr Daryl E 3761 S E Kelly, Portland, OR 97202, (503) 279-8356, BS 65 Portland St Univ; MS 69 Portland St Univ; PH 73 (NS) Univ of WA; Assoc Prof/Sp-Lang Path, Child Development & Rehab Ctr, **SLP**

Anderson, Daryrene 1152 E 7th Place, Mesa, AZ 85203, (602) 986-1977, BS 83 Brigham Young Univ; OM 85 Brigham Young Univ

Anderson, David E 3006 Maryland Parkway, Suite 215-A, Las Vegas, NV 89109, (702) 732-4317, BS 74 UT St Univ; MS 75 UT St Univ; Aud, Private Practice, **A**

Anderson, Deborah Gertrude Chedoke-McMaster Hospital, Box 2000 Station A, Hamilton, ON, Canada L8N 3Z5, (416) 521-7951, BA 85 Univ of Western Ontario; MA 87 Central MI Univ; 87–Sp-Lang Path, Chedoke-McMaster Hosp

Anderson, Mrs Deborah Phillips 10 Bannister Court, Poquoson, VA 23662, (804) 868-0097, MA 75 Univ of TN - Knoxville; 86–Sp-Lang Path, InSpeech Inc, **SLP ACE**

Anderson, Mrs Debra P 77 Hermitage, Conroe, TX 77302, (409) 273-3478, BA 73 Univ of Houston - Univ Park; MA 79 Univ of Houston - Univ Park; 88–Sp-Lang Path, Spring Branch ISD, **SLP**

Anderson, Debra Sue 5715 East 22nd Street, Tulsa, OK 74114, (918) 245-3429, BS 78 OK St Univ; MA 79 Univ of AR - Fayetteville; Sp-Lang Path, Sand Springs Ok Public Schools, **SLP**

Anderson, Delmarine 9290 Woodfair #410, Houston, TX 77036, (713) 777-1258, BA 80 Wichita St Univ; MS 85 Fort Hays St Univ; 88–Sp-Lang Path, PsyCog Associates Inc, **SLP**

Anderson, Diana Best 1270 Le Conte Drive, Riverside, CA 92507, **SLP A**

Anderson, Mrs Diane Carolan 2268 Felspar, San Diego, CA 92109, (619) 541-3088, BA 79 Tulane Univ; MA 85 San Diego St Univ; 86–Sp-Lang Path, Children's Hosp & Health Ctr, **SLP**

Anderson, Dierdre M 15 Beck Street, Newburyport, MA 01950, (508) 465-5321, BA 85 Univ of CA - Santa Barbara; MA 87 Univ of MA - Amherst; 88–Aud, NorthShore Hearing, **A**

Anderson, Mrs Dona C 83 Bouse Lane, Edwardsville, IL 62025, (618) 656-8480, BS 68 Univ of MO - Columbia; MA 69 Univ of MO - Columbia; Early Childhood Teacher, Edwardsville District 7, **SLP**

Anderson, Mrs Donna L 3206 Grischy Lane, Cincinnati, OH 45208, (513) 321-4297, BS 76 Univ of Cincinnati; MA 78 Univ of Cincinnati; Sp-Lang Path, Cincinnati Bd of Ed, **SLP**

Anderson, Dr Duane I 2018 N E Alameda Drive, Portland, OR 97212, (503) 282-4108, BA 52 Western WA Univ; MS 54 Univ of OR; ED 67 (NS) Univ of OR; 87–Aud, Hearing Conservation Svcs Inc, **SLP A**

Anderson, Dr Elaine R 10460 Longwood Drive, Largo, FL 34647, (813) 393-1411, BS 53 Cedar Crest Coll; MS 57 Syracuse Univ; PH 70 (NS) Syracuse Univ; Sp-Lang Path, **SLP**

Anderson, Elaine Rohde 25 Birch Hill Road, Belmont, MA 02178, (617) 484-5929, BS 72 UT St Univ; MS 74 UT St Univ; **SLP**

Anderson, Eleanor I Rural Route 1, St Patricks Road, Hunter River, PE, Canada C0A 1N0, (902) 368-4954, BS 75; MS 77 Purdue Univ - West Lafayette; Coord of Sp-Lang Path, Dept/Hlth & Soc Serv, **SLP**

Anderson, Elizabeth 824 Hilma Circle, Tarboro, NC 27886, **SLP**

Anderson, Mrs Elizabeth J 7102 Guilford Road, Clarksville, MD 21029, (301) 531-5074, BA 71 Univ of MD - College Park; MA 73 Univ of MD - College Park; Sp-Lang Path, Prince George Co Pub Sch, **SLP**

Anderson, Mrs Elizabeth S 511 Woodcrest Boulevard, O'Fallon, MO 63366, (314) 324-2174, BS 77 Southeast MO St Univ; ME 82 Southeast MO St Univ; Sp-Lang Path, Lincoln County R-IV Sch Dist, **SLP**

Anderson, Ellen Biddle 1205 North Etta Court, Liberty Lake, WA 99019, (509) 926-0214, BS 72 Purdue Univ - West Lafayette; MA 74 Western MI Univ; **SLP**

Anderson, Ellen K 2275 Feather Hill Road, Santa Barbara, CA 93108, (805) 963-8841, BS 75 Wayne St Univ; MA 76 Wayne St Univ; Playwriter, Self Employed, **SLP**

Anderson, Ellen L 2537-1/2 Prairie #208, Evanston, IL 60201, (312) 328-1009, BS 86 Northwestern Univ; MA 87 Northwestern Univ; 87–Sp-Lang Path, Schaumburg Sch Dist #54, **SLP**

Anderson, Dr Elwood G 552 Robin Avenue, Alpena, MI 49707, (517) 354-8967, BA 52 Albion Coll; ME 53 Wayne St Univ; ED 68 (NS) Wayne St Univ; Sp-Lang Path, Alpena Pub Sch, **SLP ACE**

Anderson, Mrs Emily T 703 Flamingo Way, Duncanville, TX 75116, (214) 298-6634, BA 68 Southern Methodist Univ; OM 70 Southern Methodist Univ; **SLP**

Anderson, Erin Gaye 1000 Pine Gate Drive, Apartment J-199, Spartanburg, SC 29303, (803) 269-9239, BS 82 Univ of TN - Knoxville; MA 84 Univ of TN - Knoxville; Sp-Lang Path, Pro Rehab Agency, **SLP**

Anderson, Eunice 933 North Euclid Avenue, Oak Park, IL 60302, (312) 386-0933, BA 45 Augustana Coll; **SLP**

Anderson, Frances S 27 W 205 Providence Lane, Winfield, IL 60190, (312) 682-2095, BS 56 Univ of IL - Urbana; MA 80 MI St Univ; Sp-Lang Path, Sased, **SLP**

Anderson, Francis Martin 6013 Benalder Drive, Bethesda, MD 20816, (301) 762-0632, BS 62 Georgetown Univ; MA 72 Catholic Univ of America; Sp/Lang Path, Montgomery Co Pub Sch, **SLP**

Anderson, Galen B 318 West 12th, Newton, KS 67114, (316) 283-5011, BA 76 Fort Hays St Univ; MS 79 Fort Hays St Univ; Sp-Lang Path, Harvey County Spec Ed Coop, **SLP**

Anderson, Georgiana 183 Masters Avenue, Riverside, CA 92507, (714) 787-0204, BA 82 CA St Univ - Fullerton; MA 85 CA St Univ - Fullerton; Sp-Lang Path, Communication Health Services, **SLP**

Anderson, Gloria M 2010 Tomahawk, Okemos, MI 48864, (517) 676-1051, BA 72 Nazareth Coll of Rochester; MA 77 MI St Univ; 87–Supvr, Ingham ISD, **SLP**

Anderson, James Russell 415 East Citrus, Redlands, CA 92373, (714) 793-5646, BA 83 CA St Univ - Fresno; MA 85 CA St Univ - Fresno; 88–Aud, Jacobs & Saline Cl Aud Inc, **A**

Anderson, Jan P 1516 Santiago Court, Bakersfield, CA 93307, (805) 835-1017, BS 62 Ball St Univ; Sp-Lang Path, Bakers Field Cty Sch Dist, **SLP**

Anderson, Jane 404 North Elder, Broken Arrow, OK 74012, (918) 252-5750, BS 78 Univ of Tulsa; MA 80 Univ of Tulsa; SLP, Union Pu Sch Dist, **SLP**

Anderson, Janet E 2209 Lincoln Drive #605, Arlington, TX 76011, (817) 460-4691, BS 73 Univ of North TX; MS 74 Univ of North TX; Sp-Lang Path, Arlington ISD JL Hill Elem, **SLP**

Anderson, Mrs Janice Ann 9011 31st W, Tacoma, WA 98466, (206) 565-3411, BA 84 WA St Univ; MA 84 WA St Univ; Sp-Lang Path, Clover Park Sch Dist, **SLP**

Anderson, Mrs Janice S 4442 Gilbert, Western Springs, IL 60558, (312) 996-4722, BS 72 IL St Univ - Normal; MA 73 Univ of IL - Urbana; SLP/Aud, U of IL, **A**

Anderson, Jean L 4218 Saratoga Drive, Bloomington, IN 47401, (812) 336-3334, BS 43 Western MI Univ; MS 51 IN Univ - Bloomington; ED 69 (NS) IN Univ - Bloomington; Emeritus Prof, IN V, **SLP F LM**

Anderson, Jenifer Lyn 208 Woodside Road, Riverside, IL 60546, (312) 447-9539, BS 86 Northeast MO St Univ; MA 87 Northeast MO St Univ; 88–Sp-Lang Path, Therapeutic Sys/Hawthorn Svcs

Anderson, Jill Marie 3400 Chateau Boulevard, #217, Kenner, LA 70065, (504) 595-6152, BS 85 Univ of South AL; MS 87 Univ of South AL; **A**

Anderson, Mrs Joann Wanda 425 Columbia Center Boulevard #H206, Kennewick, WA 99336, (701) 282-5276, BS 84 Moorhead St Univ; MS 86 Moorhead St Univ; 88–Sp-Lang Path, Benton Franklin Dev Ctr, **SLP**

Anderson, Joanne C 147 Highland Street, Marshfield, MA 02050, (617) 569-5800, BS 77 Boston Univ; MS 80 Boston Univ; 81–Aud, E Boston Neigh Health Ctr, **A**

Anderson, John O Dept Communication Dis & Sci, Southern Illinois Univ, Carbondale, IL 62901, (618) 453-4301, BA 44 CO Coll; MS 48 UT St Univ; PH 50 (Sp Path) OH St Univ; 86–Prof Emeritus, Sn IL U at Carbondale, **SLP LM**

Anderson, Joy E 1600 South Eads Street, Apartment 910-N, Arlington, VA 22202, (703) 685-4193, MA 88 George Washington Univ

Anderson, Mrs Judy Annbrenner 1045 Schafer Drive, Onalaska, WI 54650, (608) 783-6659, BS 73 Univ of WI - Eau Claire; MS 77 Univ of WI - Eau Claire; SLP, Onalaska Pub Schs, **SLP**

Anderson, Juel H WM Beaumont Army Medical Ctr, Audiology Clinic, El Paso, TX 79920, (915) 569-2065, BS 65 ND St Univ; MS 69 ND St Univ; Audiologist, William Beaumont Army Med Cen, **A**

Anderson, Mrs June Elizabeth 598 Tilden Avenue, Teaneck, NJ 07666, (914) 634-4941, MS 83 Columbia Univ Teachers Coll; Sp-Lang Path, Clarkstown Central School Dist, **SLP**

Anderson, Karen Alanna 1130 Fourth Street #207, Santa Rosa, CA 95404, (707) 579-3498, BS 80 Univ of TX - Austin; ME 82 Southwest TX St Univ; SLP, Belle Chasse State Sch, **SLP**

Anderson, Karen C 6809 Bellaire Court South, Fort Worth, TX 76132, (817) 737-8783, BA 73 TX Christian Univ; MS 76 TX Christian Univ; **SLP**

Anderson, Karen Gail 1612 Franklin Street, Bellevue, NE 68005, (402) 397-3150, BS 81 Univ of NE - Omaha; MS 82 Univ of NE - Omaha; Meth Midtown Post-Acute Servs, **SLP**

Anderson, Karen L Rt 2 Box 2254, Hager City, WI 54014, (715) 386-4242, BS 86 Univ of WI - River Falls; OM 87 Univ of WI - River Falls; Sp-Lang Path, Hudson Sch Dist

Anderson, Karen Lynn 3108 161st Street East, Spanaway, WA 98387, (218) 724-2804, OB 79 Univ of MN - Duluth; ME 81 Univ of MN - Duluth; Aud Consult, NE MN Ed Coop Serv Ut, **A**

Anderson, Karen M 3120 Westside, Grand Island, NE 68803, (402) 463-1518, BS 76 Kearney St Coll; MS 78 Kearney St Coll; Sp-Lang Path, U NE-Lincoln, **SLP**

Anderson, Mrs Karen Maxton 1835 Greenhaven Lane, Owatonna, MN 55060, (507) 332-3397, BS 78 Moorhead St Univ; MS 80 Moorhead St Univ; Sp-Lang Path, Faribault Reg Cen, **SLP**

Anderson, Katherine Mary 942 Viking Drive, Valley City, ND 58072, (701) 845-3261, BA 84 Univ of ND; MS 85 Moorhead St Univ; **SLP**

Anderson, Mrs Kathleen 1580 Oakwood, Roswell, GA 30075, (404) 992-2030, BS 67 IN Univ - Bloomington; MA 74 Saint Louis Univ; **SLP**

Anderson, Mrs Kathleen Ann 121 Brookwood Drive, La Grange, GA 30240, (404) 884-1974, BA 81 Univ of FL; ME 86 Columbus Coll

Anderson, Kathleen C 1207 Glenn Avenue, Augusta, GA 30904-4615, (404) 738-7055, **SLP**

Anderson, Kathleen Caliendo 1124 Vineyard Drive, Lewiston, ID 83501, (208) 799-3460, BA 66 OH St Univ; MA 71 Case Western Reserve Univ; Region II Adult/Chld Dev Super, ID Dept of Hlt & Wlfr, **SLP**

Anderson, Mrs Kathleen M 10107 South Harding, Chicago, IL 60642, BA 75 Saint Xavier Coll; MS 76 Southern IL Univ-Edwardsvill; **SLP**

Anderson, Mrs Kathryn Larson 1812 Mountain View Place, Los Alamos, NM 87544, (505) 662-2788, BS 80 TX Christian Univ; MA 85 Univ of TX - Austin; Sp-Lang Path, Private Practice, **SLP**

Anderson, Kenneth E 6453 Portage Avenue, Portage, IN 46368, BS 64 IN St Univ - Terre Haute; MS 68 IN St Univ - Terre Haute; Pres, N Ctrl Sp Path Serv Inc, **SLP**

Anderson, Laura Jean 2435 Oxford Road, Montgomery, AL 36111, (205) 567-8471, MA 71 Univ of AL- Tuscaloosa; Aud, Central Ala ENT Assoc, **A**

Anderson, Laura O 35 Lincoln Street, Greenfield, MA 01301, **SLP**

Anderson, Mrs LaVae M Hoffman 107 East Paradise Lane, Phoenix, AZ 85022, (602) 866-2215, BA 82 Univ of MN - Duluth; MA 83 Univ of MN - Duluth; 87–Sp-Lang Path, Peoria USD, **SLP**

Anderson, Mrs Leslie Giles 4347 Yosemite Street, Carlsbad, CA 92008, BA 77 Univ of Redlands; MS 79 Univ of Redlands; Sp-Lang Path, Oceanside USD, **SLP**

Anderson, Linda Christine 421-H Tradewinds Drive, Fayetteville, NC 28304, (919) 864-9729, BA 83 North Park Coll; BS 86 SUNY - Coll at Fredonia; MS 86 SUNY - Coll at Fredonia; 88–Sp-Lang Path, Cumberland Co Sch Sys, **SLP**

Anderson, Mrs Linda D 78 Main Street, Fair Oaks, PA 15003, (412) 262-2700, BS 70 CA Univ of PA; ME 74 CA Univ of PA; Sp-Lang Path, Alleg Inter Ut, **SLP**

Anderson, Lisa Kay 2929 Lambert, Mesquite, TX 75150, (214) 270-9791, MS 88 Baylor Univ

Anderson, Lloyd C 1033 Springfield Drive, Millbrae, CA 94030, (415) 697-3884, BA 65 San Francisco St Univ; MA 69 San Francisco St Univ; Sp-Lang Path, Millbrae Elem Sch Dist, **SLP**

Anderson, Mrs Lois L 2323 Cherry Street, Bellingham, WA 98225, (206) 676-6514, BA 72 Western WA Univ; MA 74 Western WA Univ; SLP, Bellingham Sch Dist, **SLP**

Anderson, Lynn Froehling 2004 North Northcrest, Peoria, IL 61604, (309) 682-0618, BS 83 Bradley Univ; MS 85 Bradley Univ; **SLP**

Anderson, Mrs Lynn Lowe 811 East Laurel Avenue, Hattiesburg, MS 39401, (601) 582-3732, BS 79 Univ Southern MS-Hattiesburg; MS 81 Univ Southern MS-Hattiesburg; **A**

Anderson, M Lynn 1608 Peters Colony Road, Carrollton, TX 75007, (214) 492-7868, BS 78 Southern Methodist Univ; MS 79 Southern Methodist Univ; Sp-Lang Path, Private Practice, **SLP**

Anderson, Mrs Marcia Alexander 8609 Julian Road, Richmond, VA 23229, (804) 323-2615, BA 74 Mary Washington Coll; ME 75 Univ of VA - Charlottesville; Sp-Lang Path, Dept Correctional Education, **SLP**

Anderson, Marcia L 29 Elliot Road, Great Neck, NY 11021, (516) 482-8778, BA 73 Hofstra Univ; MA 74 Hofstra Univ; Aud, Private Practice, **A**

Anderson, Mrs Margaret Keating 192 Hancock Street, Apartment C, Everett, MA 02149, (617) 387-1769, BA 81 MI St Univ; OM 84 LA St Univ - N O Medical Ctr; Sp-Lang Path, **SLP**

Anderson, Mrs Marilynne Anne 19 Lake Drive, Darien, CT 06820, (203) 324-9816, BS 83 WV Univ; MS 84 WV Univ; **SLP**

Anderson, Mrs Marlis E 11505 37th Avenue North, Plymouth, MN 55441, BS 61 Saint Cloud St Univ; Sp-Lang Path, School District 281, **SLP**

Anderson, Dr Martha W 116 Evonshire, Arkadelphia, AR 71923, (501) 246-5511, BS 59 East TX St Univ - Commerce; MS 66 Univ of Houston - Univ Park; PH 74 (Sp Path) Univ of FL; Prof, Henderson State U, **SLP A**

Anderson, Mary Kathryn 2119 Lumpkin #C-4, Augusta, GA 30906-3439, (404) 793-1462, BS 81 Southwest MO St Univ; MA 87 Southwest MO St Univ; 87–Sp-Lang Path, InSpeech Inc, **SLP**

Anderson, Mrs Mary Lou Route 1 Box 142-C, Munfordville, KY 42765, (502) 524-1340, BS 81 Western KY Univ; MS 84 Western KY Univ; **SLP**

Anderson, Mary S 10530 Idlebrook, Houston, TX 77070, **SLP**

Anderson, Marzene Elizabeth 2245 College Drive #147, Baton Rouge, LA 70808, (504) 769-8160, BS 52 Hampton Univ; MS 58 Univ of TN - Knoxville; Principal, LA Sch for Deaf

Anderson, Mrs Maureen 2684 A Buckner Avenue, Fort Meade, MD 20755, (301) 672-1566, BS 78 Miami Univ - Oxford; MA 79 Univ of Houston - Univ Park; Sp/Lang Path, Chldrn Cent, **SLP**

Anderson, Mrs Maureen J 912 Glencove Road, Syracuse, NY 13206, (315) 463-0415, BA 70 MI St Univ; MS 76 Columbia Univ Teachers Coll; 88–Sp-Lang Path, Syracuse City Sch Dist, **SLP**

Anderson, Mrs Maxine Ulyate 16119 County Road 28 2, Dolores, CO 81323, (303) 882-7051, BA 74 Univ of CA - Riverside; MS 79 Loma Linda Univ - Riverside; Sp-Lang Path, Montezuma Cortez School Dist, **SLP**

Anderson, Melanie Gayle 106 Lincreek Drive, Columbia, SC 29210, (803) 732-1391, BS 75 Columbia Coll; OM 76 Univ of SC - Columbia; **SLP**

Anderson, Mrs Nancy A D 15 Wilmette Drive, Normal, IL 61761, (309) 827-4321, BS 75 IL St Univ - Normal; MS 76 IL St Univ - Normal; 78–Sp-Lang Path, BroMenn Healthcare, **SLP**

Anderson, Mrs Nancy Bales 1215 Orchard Drive, Ames, IA 50010, (515) 233-5707, BS 78 Univ of WI - Madison; MS 80 Univ of WI - Madison; SLP, SLP, **SLP**

Anderson, Dr Noma B 13920 Castle Boulevard #L1, Silver Spring, MD 20904, (202) 636-6990, BA 71 Hampton Univ; MS 72 Emerson Coll; PH 79 (Lang Development & Disorders) Univ of Pittsburgh - Pittsburgh; 85–Asst Prof Comm Disorders, Howard University, **SLP**

Anderson, Pamala 7778 Grindstone Hill Road, Chambersburg, PA 17201, (717) 267-7720, BS 77 IL St Univ - Normal; MS 79 IL St Univ - Normal; 86–Dir Sp-Lang Path, The Chambersburg Hosp, **SLP ACE**

Anderson, Pamela J 6918 Raven Court, Eden Prairie, MN 55344, BA 76 Univ of ND; MA 77 Univ of ND; Sp-Lang Path, Indepen Sch Dist #112-Chaska, **SLP**

Anderson, Patricia A 3446 Buford Highway #I-8, Atlanta, GA 30329, (404) 589-4679, BA 78 Univ of FL; ME 79 Univ of FL; Sp-Lang Path, Grady Mem Hosp, **SLP**

Anderson, Patricia Anne 8349 East D Avenue, Richland, MI 49083, (616) 629-4332, BS 84 Western MI Univ; MA 85 Western MI Univ; 86–Sp-Lang Path, Comstock Public Schools, **SLP**

Anderson, Patricia Lynn 6230 Turpin Street, Murray, UT 84107, (801) 533-3830, BS 85 Brigham Young Univ; MA 87 Univ of FL; 88–Sp-Lang Path, Ther Management

Anderson, Mrs Patricia M P O Box 2246, Fallon, NV 89406, (702) 423-4073, BS 74 CO St Univ; 86–Sp-Lang Path, Churchill Co Sch Dist, **SLP**

Anderson, Patti W 316 North Parkside, Normal, IL 61761, (309) 454-3973, BS 73 Univ of IL - Urbana; MS 75 Bradley Univ; Sp/Lang Path, Normal Comm Unit #5, **SLP**

Anderson, Paula Lynette 4420 Willowpoint, Norman, OK 73070, (405) 360-2610, BS 81 OK St Univ; MS 84 Univ of OK Medical Center; Sp-Lang Path, Pauls Valley State School, **SLP**

Anderson, Randy L 4347 Yosemite Street, Carlsbad, CA 92008, (619) 758-1620, BS 74 Univ of UT; MS 75 Univ of UT; Clinical Super, Chldn Hosp & Hlth Cen, **SLP**

Anderson, Dr Raquel Teresa Las Caobas #182, Hyde Park, Rio Piedras, PR 00927, (809) 764-4936, BA 80 Oberlin Coll; MS 82 Univ of PR - Rio Piedras; PH 87 (Sp-Lang Path) Northwestern Univ; 87–Asst Prof, Univ of Puerto-Med Sci Campus, **SLP**

Anderson, Mrs Rebecca D 38 Cambell Lane, Los [illegible] NM 87031, (505) 865-7076, BA 75 Univ of NM; MS [illegible] of NM; Sp-Lang Path, Albuquerque Public Schools

Anderson, Mrs Rebecca S 8485 Boca Rio Drive, Boca Raton, FL 33433-7960, (407) 737-7733, BA 79 MI St Univ; MA 80 MI St Univ; Aud, Bethesda Memorial Hosp, **A**

Anderson, Regina W 440 South Gulfview Blvd, Apartment 1702, Clearwater, FL 33515, **SLP**

Anderson, Mrs Renata Appel 1601 Center Street, Walla Walla, WA 99362, (509) 529-5010, BS 82 WA St Univ; MA 83 WA St Univ; Aud, Joanne Price Ma Ccc-A, **A**

Anderson, Robert H N 33946 Harroun, Wayne, MI 48184, (313) 326-2541, BS 50 Univ of OK - Norman; ME 51 Univ of OK - Norman; **SLP LM**

Anderson, Robert M 2145 Brierbrook, Germantown, TN 38138, **SLP**

Anderson, Mrs Robyn Lynette 8535 Eby, Overland Park, KS 66212, (913) 621-5155, **SLP**

Anderson, Roger P 560 Newberry Drive, Elk Grove, IL 60007, (312) 543-4494, BS 77 IA St Univ; MA 78 Univ of Northern IA; Sp-Lang Path, Graham Assoc for Hndcpd, **SLP**

Anderson, Roy Bruce Star Route Box 1699, Eagle River, AK 99577, (907) 561-1133, BA 70 OR St Univ; MA 71 OR St Univ; Prog Dir, Employnt & Trng Cen of Ak, **A**

Anderson, Roy K 31708 Sunrise Avenue, Dowagiac, MI 49047-9233, (616) 926-8028, BS 63 Western MI Univ; MA 65 Western MI Univ; Sp-Lang Path, Anderson Sp/Hrng Serv Inc, **SLP**

Anderson, Ruth M 2609 Croyden, Tucson, AZ 85716, (602) 327-7855, OB 37; MA 47 Wichita St Univ; **SLP F LM**

Anderson, Mrs Sally B 604 30th Street N W, Winter Haven, FL 33880, (813) 293-3206, BA 64 Univ of Northern IA; MA 69 Univ of South FL; SLP, Polk Co Schs, **SLP**

Anderson, Samantha G Route 2 Box 67-A, Mc Gregor, TX 76657, **SLP**

Anderson, Samira B 35 S W 2nd Street, Faribault, MN 55021, (507) 332-3593, BA 79 IN Univ - Bloomington; MA 81 IN Univ - Bloomington; Aud, Faribault Reg Ctr, **A**

Anderson, Shirley Mae Route 1 Box 17, Milan, MN 56262, (612) 598-7556, BA 76 Saint Cloud St Univ; MA 85 Univ of MN - Minneap-St Paul; Audiologist, Madison Hospital, **A**

Anderson, Sue Ellen 533 East Lawndale, Peoria, IL 61603, (309) 672-6665, BS 84 Bradley Univ; MS 85 Bradley Univ; 86–Sp-Lang Path, Peoria PS, **SLP**

Anderson, Susan Alice 6842 Louisiana N E, Albuquerque, NM 87109, (505) 822-8952, BA 78 Univ of NE - Lincoln; MS 83 Univ of OK - OK City; Sp/Lang Path, Albuquerque Public Schools, **SLP**

Anderson, Susan B 130 Yarnell Street, Kane, PA 16735, (814) 837-8590, BS 73 Indiana Univ of PA; MS 80 PA St Univ - Univ Park; Sp-Lang Path, Seneca Highlands Interm Unit 9, **SLP**

Anderson, Mrs Susan Elizabeth Covenant Medical Center, 2101 Kimball Avenue, Waterloo, IA 50702, (319) 291-3336, BA 83 Univ of Northern IA; MA 85 Univ of Northern IA; 86–Sp-Lang Path, Covenant Med Ctr, **SLP**

Anderson, Susan H 82 East Farmland Drive, Valparaiso, IN 46383, (219) 464-7098, BS 77 Bucknell Univ; MS 79 Syracuse Univ; Sp/Lang Path, CARES Head Injury Rehab, **SLP**

Anderson, Susan Marie 26511 New Road, North Liberty, IN 46554-9452, (219) 656-3256, MA 88 IN Univ - Bloomington; 88–Sp-Lang Path, Arrabright Comm

Anderson, Susan Ruth 1507 West Atlantic Avenue Apartment 73, Manasquan, NJ 08736, BA 84 Univ of Pittsburgh - Pittsburgh; MS 86 PA St Univ - Univ Park; 87–Sp-Lang Path, Garden State Rehab Hosp, **SLP**

Anderson, Susan S 28 Kingery, El Paso, TX 79902, BS 73 Univ of Houston - Univ Park; MA 75 Univ of TX - El Paso; **SLP**

Anderson, Mrs Susanne R P O Box 894, Malibu, CA 90265, (818) 991-4709, BA 68 Occidental Coll; MA 69 CA St Univ - Los Angeles; Private Practice, **SLP**

Anderson, Mrs Therese Ann 675 Wells Landing Drive, Orange Park, FL 32073, (904) 725-8972, BA 80 Univ of FL; ME 83 Univ of FL; Sp-Lang Path, S Allen Smith Cl, **SLP**

Anderson, Mrs Vera L 1075 Maple Lane, Manhasset, NY 11040, (516) 741-1145, BA 71 CUNY - Queens Coll; MA 72 Hofstra Univ; Aud, **A**

Anderson, Mrs Vicki Driver 4723 Chablis Way, Birmingham, AL 35244, (205) 934-4467, BA 81 Univ of AL- Tuscaloosa; MS 82 Univ of AL- Tuscaloosa; Sp-Lang Path, UAB Sp and Hrng Cl, **SLP**

Anderson, Vicki M 12824 88th Avenue North, Maple Grove, MN 55369, (612) 420-8622, BA 75 Univ of MN - Minneap-St Paul; MA 80 Univ of MN - Minneap-St Paul; Aud, Hennepin County Med Ctr, **SLP A**

Anderson, Dr Virgil 01152 Winchuck Road, Brookings, OR 97415, (415) 857-1017, BA 23; MA 32 Stanford Univ; PH 37 (NS) Saint Norbert Coll; **SLP F LM**

Anderson, Vivian Denise Route 2 Box 238, Mineral, VA 23117, (703) 894-4193, BS 83 Longwood Coll; ME 85 Univ of VA - Charlottesville; **SLP**

Anderson, William O 5700 Ming Avenue #65, Bakersfield, CA 93309, (805) 397-9209, SLP, Office of Kern Co Supt of Schl, **SLP**

Anderson-Balch, Rhonda 518 58th Street, Des Moines, IA 50312, MS 76 Univ of NE - Lincoln; SLP, AEA 11, **SLP**

Anderson-Pelec, Karen Marie 2160 South First Avenue, Maywood, IL 60153, (312) 531-3771, BA 83 Saint Xavier Coll; MS 86 Governors St Univ; 86–Sp-Lang Path, Loyola Univ Med Ctr, **SLP**

Anderson-Smith, Mrs Cheryl Joy 5700 North Beach #303, Fort Worth, TX 76137, (214) 790-4778, MS 88 Univ of TX - Dallas; 88–Sp-Lang Path, Irving ISD

Andes-Viski, Suzanne Evelyn Rt 9 Box 1196, Morgantown, WV 26505, (304) 329-0850, BS 82 WV Univ; MS 83 WV Univ; Sp/Lang Path, Preston Co Bd of Ed, **SLP**

Andis, Jennifer Jean 5041 East Sherwood, Newburgh, IN 47630-3023, (812) 426-3353, BS 78 IN St Univ - Terre Haute; MS 84 Western KY Univ; Sp-Lang Path, Deaconess Hospital, **SLP**

Andraska, Ann K Chelsea School District, South Elementary, Pierce Street, Chelsea, MI 48118, (313) 475-3715, BS 77 CA Univ of PA; MA 82 Eastern MI Univ; 83–Sp-Lang Path, Chelsea Sch Dis, **SLP**

Andrasko, Gay B 5753 East 25th Street, Tulsa, OK 74114, (918) 744-0859, BS 71 Univ of Tulsa; MA 82 OK St Univ; Sp-Lang Path, Public Schools, **SLP**

Andre, Janice J 536 Glenmont Drive, Solana Beach, CA 92075, (619) 589-4108, BA 73 San Diego St Univ; MA 81 San Diego St Univ; Sp-Lang Path, Grossmont Hosp, **SLP**

Andre, Susan L 6886 South Cook Way, Littleton, CO 80122, (303) 721-1143, BS 75 West Chester Univ of PA; MS 78 Univ of VT; 87–Sp/Lang Path, Littleton PS, **SLP ACE**

Andre, Vicki Linn 49 Harvard Street, Waltham, MA 02154, (406) 243-5467, MA 84 Univ of MT; Sp-Lang Path, Concord Area Early Inter Prog, **SLP**

Andreani, Bonita K Kent State University, Speech & Hearing Clinic #A147, Kent, OH 44240, (216) 672-2672, BS 66 CA Univ of PA; MS 67 WV Univ; Instr/Cl Superv, Kent St U, **SLP**

Andregg, Mrs Karen Jan 2933 Wickersham Lane, Austin, TX 78741-7354, (512) 474-2401, OB 84 Univ of KS; MA 86 Univ of KS; **A**

Andrejasich, Mrs Deirdre Kogan 2802 West Gilbert, Peoria, IL 61604, (309) 671-2933, BS 83 Bradley Univ; MS 84 Bradley Univ; Sp-Lang Path, Institute Phys Med & Rehabiltn, **SLP**

Andres, Mrs Cecilia Basilio 95-658 Makaunulau Street, Mililani Town, HI 96789, (808) 625-1911, BS 82 Univ of HI - Manoa; MS 84 Univ of HI - Manoa; Sp-Lang Path, Dept of Ed Ctrl Oahu Dist, **SLP**

Andres, Mrs Sandra A 24 Woodland Glen, Park Forest, IL 60466, (312) 895-2450, BS 71 Ball St Univ; MS 76 IN St Univ - Terre Haute; 87–Coord of Spec Educ, Sandridge Sch Dist #172, **SLP**

Andreski, Mrs Mary K N-793 Center Road, Merrill, WI 54452, (715) 536-9600, BS 79 Univ of WI - Madison; MS 81 Univ of WI - Whitewater; SLP, Merrill Area Pub Schs, **SLP**

Andress, Diane 1514 Fernwood-Glendale Rd, Seville Apartment #1109, Spartanburg, SC 29302, (803) 591-6480, BS 77 Clemson Univ; MS 83 Univ of SC - Columbia; 85–Sp/Lang Path, Spartanburg Reg Med Ctr, **SLP**

Andress, Mrs Marilyn Miller 721 Bushkill Center Road, Nazareth, PA 18064, (215) 759-7600, BS 77 East Stroudsburg Univ of PA; MS 84 Bloomsburg Univ of PA; Sp-Lang Path, Colonial Northampton In Unt 20, **SLP**

Andrew, Diane Valdosta State College, 107 Ed Bldg, Valdosta, GA 31698, (912) 333-5931, BS 73 Univ of WI - Whitewater; MS 77 Univ of WI - Whitewater; Instr/Supv, Valdosta St Coll, **SLP**

Andrew, Lisa M 247 East Chestnut Unit 404, Chicago, IL 60611, (312) 664-9173, BS 85 Fontbonne Coll; MS 86 Fontbonne Coll; 86–Sp-Lang Path, Therapeutic Sys, **SLP**

Andrew, Mrs Margarette White Box 230, Weston, VT 05161, (802) 824-6811, Sp-Lang Path, Windham Southwest School Dist, **SLP**

Andrews, Alice E 1904 Houston Avenue, Valdosta, GA 31601, (912) 244-1754, BS 73 Northeast MO St Univ; MA 74 Northeast MO St Univ; Sp-Lang Path, Tift Co Bd of Ed, **SLP**

Andrews, Mrs Amy Correan 227 Roosevelt Drive, Beloit, KS 67420, (913) 738-6540, BA 85 Fort Hays St Univ; MS 87 Fort Hays St Univ; 87–Sp-Lang Path, Beloit Spec Educ Coop, **SLP**

Andrews, Betsy Jean 1324 South Fremont, Springfield, MO 65804, (417) 831-0814, BS 74 Univ of MO - Columbia; MS 87 Northwest MO St Univ; 88–Sp-Lang Path, Springfield R-XII Sch Dist, **SLP**

Andrews, Carol L 10336 Coppedge Lane, Dallas, TX 75229, **SLP**

Andrews, Cheryl H 6706 Haycock Road, Falls Church, VA 22043, (703) 941-7705, BS 75 Southern Methodist Univ; MA 81 George Washington Univ; SLP, Sch for Contemporary Ed, **SLP**

Andrews, Christine Marie 4157 South Harvard, Suite 109, Tulsa, OK 74135, (918) 747-9387, BS 82 TX Christian Univ; MS 84 Univ of OK - OK City; SLP, The Tulsa Child Guidance Ctr, **SLP**

Andrews, Claudia B 21105 21st Avenue West, Lynnwood, WA 98036, (206) 776-3564, BA 79 Univ of WA; OM 81 Univ of WA; Sp-Lang Path, Providence Hospital Pdtc, **SLP**

Andrews, D Karen 22927 Hollander, Dearborn, MI 48128, BS 63 Western MI Univ; MS 67 Univ of MI - Ann Arbor; SLP, Wayne Westland Comm Sch, **SLP**

Andrews, Mrs Dale Joan 105 Clamar Avenue, Havertown, PA 19083, (215) 891-2211, BS 75 Univ of Montevallo; ME 76 Bloomsburg Univ of PA; Sp-Lang Path, Elwyn I, **SLP**

Andrews, Diana L 7 Pegs Lane, Huntington, NY 11743, (516) 271-7971, BA 71 Georgetown Univ; MS 74 Boston Univ; MD 85 (Medicine) NY Univ; 80–Pediatrician, Private Practice, **SLP**

Andrews, Dianne G 15522 Bennington Place, Granger, IN 46530, (219) 234-3136, BS 72 Bowling Green St Univ; MA 73 Bowling Green St Univ; Sp-Lang Path, United Health Services, **SLP**

Andrews, Mrs Evalin W P O Box 46, 1620 5th Avenue, Nebraska City, NE 68410, (402) 873-3531, BS 60 Peru St Coll; MA 71 Univ of NE - Lincoln; Sp-Lang Path, St Mary Hosp Home Hlth Care, **SLP**

Andrews, Frank D 5319 Morning Dove Lane, Cross Lanes, WV 25313, MS 68 Univ of WI - Madison; Assistant Director Spec Educ, West Virginia Dept Education, **SLP**

Andrews, Dr James R Dept Communicative Disorders, Northern Illinois Univ, De Kalb, IL 60115, (815) 753-1486, BS 62 Univ of MN - Minneap-St Paul; MA 63 Northwestern Univ; PH 67 (NS) Northwestern Univ; Prof/Dept Chmn, Nn IL U, **SLP F**

Andrews, Mrs Jane W 10839 Granada Road, Richmond, VA 23235, BS 71 Univ of GA; ME 72 Univ of GA; Sp-Lang Path, Richmond Public Schools, **SLP**

Andrews, Janet Patricia Route 4 Box 166 Dumas Rd, Forsyth, GA 31029, (912) 745-5497, MS 82 FL St Univ; Aud, Central GA Speech & Hring Ctr, **A**

Andrews, Jo Lynn 1337 Cedar Avenue, Sheridan, WY 82801, (307) 672-9592, BA 70 OH Wesleyan Univ; MA 74 OH St Univ; 74–Sp-Lang Path, The Children's Ctr Region #2, **SLP ACE**

Andrews, Jonni Anne Rt 3 Box 5B, Deming, NM 88030, (505) 522-7977, MS 86 Grand Canyon Coll; 88–Aud, Private Practice, **A**

Andrews, Mrs Martha G R R 2 Box 256-A1, Bunganut Lake, Alfred, ME 04002, (207) 324-8483, BA 68 Univ of CT; MA 69 Univ of CT; Aud, York Co Couns Serv Inc, **A**

Andrews, Mrs Mary J 2216 Clermont Circle, Plano, TX 75023, BS 68 Univ of IL - Urbana; MS 69 Univ of WI - Madison; Sp-Lang Path, Richardson ISD, **SLP**

Andrews, Dr Moya L Speech And Hearing Center, Indiana University, Bloomington, IN 47405, (812) 335-3375, BA 64 Univ of Queensland - Australi; MA 67 Univ of CA - Santa Barbara; ED 71 (NS) Columbia Univ Teachers Coll; 72–Prof/Sp & Hrng Sci, IN U, **SLP**

Andrews, Mrs Nancy A Lunde 621 North Colorado Street, Chandler, AZ 85225, BA 75 Univ of Northern CO; MS 79 Univ of Redlands; Sp-Lang Path, **SLP**

Andrews, Mrs Pamela K R R 5 Box 162, Newton, IA 50208, (515) 792-4870, BS 73 Northeast MO St Univ; MA 73 Northeast MO St Univ; Sp-Lang Path, Heartland AEA, **SLP**

Andrews, Mrs Rachel E 340 South Kenilworth #3, Oak Park, IL 60302, (312) 524-9287, BA 79 Elmhurst Coll; MA 80 Univ of IL - Urbana; Sp-Lang Path, Cooperative Assn for Spec Educ, **SLP**

Andrews, Robin S 5880 Huddersfield Road, Macon, GA 31210, (912) 743-8953, BS 73 Western MI Univ; MS 80 Univ of AL- Tuscaloosa; Aud, Audiologic Health Services, **A**

Andrews, Mrs Susan Beth 145 Canady Drive, Athens, GA 30607, (404) 769-7764, **SLP**

Andrews, Valerie Elizabeth 4307 Elmwood Road, Beltsville, MD 20705, (301) 937-1531, BA 85 Univ of MD - College Park; MA 87 Univ of MD - College Park; **SLP**

Andrews-O'Hearn, Mrs Joanne 2556 Arleigh Road, East Meadow, NY 11554, (516) 579-6557, BA 81 Hofstra Univ; MA 83 Hofstra Univ; Sp-Lang Path, NY Cty Bd of Ed Sp Serv Ut, **SLP**

Andriacchi, Catherine 821 E Cochise Drive A, Phoenix, AZ 85020, (602) 943-8517, **SLP**

Andrich, Margo Louise 534 Goldwood, Ballwin, MO 63011, (314) 441-6465, BS 82 Fontbonne Coll; MS 85 Fontbonne Coll; **SLP**

Andries, Julie Gement P O Box 606, Abita Springs, LA 70420, (504) 898-3311, BA 83 Southeastern LA Univ; ME Southeastern LA Univ; 84–Sp-Lang Path, St Tammany Parish Schl Bd, **SLP**

Andriopoulos, Cheryl Lynn 744 Schooner Lane, Elk Grove Village, IL 60007-6909, (312) 529-2223, BS 83 Univ of IL - Urbana; MS 84 Univ of IL - Urbana; 84–Sp-Lang Path, Bloomingdale Elem Sch Dist #13, **SLP**

Andriot, Celeste F 97 Marshall Avenue, Trenton, NJ 08610, (609) 292-5676, BS 75 Trenton St Coll; MA 77 Trenton St Coll; SLP/Aud Consult, NJ Dept of Hlth, **SLP**

Andrues, James W Multicare Spch & Hrng Cen, 1220 Division, Tacoma, WA 98403, BA 64 San Jose St Univ; MA 65 San Jose St Univ; PH 70 (NS) Univ of WA; Aud, Mary Bridge Sp & Hrng Cen, **A**

Andrus, Gary Wyatt Ukiah Hearing Care, 1165 South Dora, Suite B2, Ukiah, CA 95482, (707) 468-0400, BS 82 Brigham Young Univ; OM 83 Brigham Young Univ; Aud, Ukiah Hearing Care, **A**

Andrus, Mrs Pamela Bergkamp 7600 Devonshire Avenue, St Louis, MO 63119-2805, (314) 781-6354, BS 81 Northwestern Univ; MA 83 Saint Louis Univ; Sp/Lang Path, Good Shepard School for Child, **SLP**

Andrzejewski, Sally Ann 1608 31st Street, Bay City, MI 48706, (219) 234-3136, BS 80 Central MI Univ; MA 83 Central MI Univ; Sp/Lang Path, Utd Hlth Serv, **SLP**

Anello, Denise Marie 116 Wilmington Avenue, Tonawanda, NY 14150, BA 84 0684; MA 86 0686; **SLP**

Anello, Mrs Elizabeth Lois 23 Valarian Ct, Rockville, MD 20852, (301) 279-0441, BS 74 Univ of MD - College Park; MA 77 Univ of MD - College Park; Sp-Lang Path, Montgomery Co Public Schools, **SLP**

Aneshansley, Mrs Melaine Kim 145 Sandra Road, Clinton, OK 73601, (405) 323-5495, BS 78 OK St Univ; ME 81 Southwestern OK St Univ; ME 84 Central St Univ

Angel, Mrs Amelia Ayala 10427 Valtierra S W, Albuquerque, NM 87105, (505) 345-8531, BS 77 TX Woman's Univ; MS 84 Univ of NM; **SLP**

Angelelli, Dr Roger M Southwestern Hrng Health Serv, 500 Lewis Run Road, P O Box 18066, Pittsburgh, PA 15236, (412) 466-5550, BS 64 CA Univ of PA; MS 66 WV Univ; PH 75 (NS) Univ of Pittsburgh - Pittsburgh; Owner, Southwestern Hrng Hlth Servs, **A**

Angell, Robin L 4467 Cox Drive, Stow, OH 44224, (216) 349-1803, BS 86 Clarion Univ of PA; MS 87 Bowling Green St Univ; **SLP**

Angell, Steven N 3231 S National, Springfield, MO 65807, (417) 883-7422, BA 55 Park Coll; MA 64 Univ of KS; Aud, **A**

Angello, Martha J 7120 Contreras Road, Oxford, OH 45056, BS 73 OH Univ - Athens; MA 74 Cleveland St Univ; **SLP**

Angelo, Dr Dianne H Dept Of Comm Dis And Spec Educ, Room 4 Navy Hall, Bloomsburg University, Bloomsburg, PA 17815, (717) 389-4448, BS 73 Clarion Univ of PA; ME 76 Clarion Univ of PA; PH 88 (Communications) Univ of Pittsburgh - Pittsburgh; 85–Assistant Professor, Bloomsburg University, **SLP**

Angelo, Mary Ann 8165 South Newport Way, Englewood, CO 80112, **A**

Angelo, Dr Richard Dept Communication Disorders, Bloomsburg University, Bloomsburg, PA 17815, BS 70 Mansfield Univ of PA; ME 72 Bloomsburg Univ of PA; ED 80 (NS) Lehigh Univ; Assistant Professor Audiology, Bloomsburg University, **A**

Angelo, Robert J 303 Elm Street, Hamburg, PA 19526, (215) 562-6109, BS 74 Bloomsburg Univ of PA; MS 77 Bloomsburg Univ of PA; Coord Sp-Lang Path & Aud, Hamburg Cen, **SLP**

Angelo, Mrs Valerie T 79 Elmira Street, South Waverly, PA 18840, (717) 888-7326, BA 71 Temple Univ-Tyler Sch of Art; MA 73 Temple Univ-Tyler Sch of Art; **SLP**

Angelo, Veronica Rose 2716 Sipp Avenue, Medford, NY 11763, (516) 289-4459, BA 80 Long Island U - CW Post Ctr; MS 86 Northeastern Univ; 87–SLP, UCP of Greater Suffolk, **SLP**

Angelo, Victor M Route 12 Box 72-Aa, Goldsboro, NC 27530, (919) 731-3599, BA 76 Univ of MS; OM 77 Univ of MS; Sp & Hrng Prog Dir, Oberry Center, **SLP**

Angelocci, Dr Angelo A 9883 Leach Lane, Dexter, MI 48130, (313) 426-2506, BS 50 Eastern MI Univ; MA 51 Univ of MI - Ann Arbor; PH 62 (Sp-Lang Path/Aud) Wayne St Univ - Sch of Med; Prof, En MI U, **SLP**

Anger, Carol Ann 2614 Bauer Street, Eau Claire, WI 54701, (715) 839-4365, BA 83 Univ of WI - Eau Claire; MS 84 Univ of WI - Eau Claire; **SLP**

Anger, Pamela J Mertz 463 Irvington Road, Drexel Hill, PA 19026, (215) 284-3063, BS 77 WV Univ; MS 79 Purdue Univ - West Lafayette; 87–Dir of Aud, Team Rehabilitation Inc, **SLP A**

Angermeier, Dr Cynthia B 306 Dawn Court #C, Bloomingdale, IL 60108, (312) 980-7250, BS 70 Purdue Univ - West Lafayette; MA 72 Univ of CT; PH 79 (NS) Purdue Univ - West Lafayette; **SLP**

Anghelone, Mrs Joyce G Rd 2 Box 328, Columbus, NJ 08022, (609) 298-0308, BA 72 Montclair St Coll; MS 73 Rutgers St Univ -N Brunswick; Sp/Lang Path, Columbus Elem School, **SLP**

Angiulo-Pugnali, Jayne Ann Traver Road, Pleasant Valley, NY 12569, (914) 471-8800, BS 82 SUNY - Coll at New Paltz; MA 84 CUNY - Queens Coll; **SLP**

Angle, Mrs Ann M 8211 Burnley Road, Towson, MD 21204, (301) 828-2433, BS 69 Towson St Univ; MS 70 Loyola Coll; MS 72 Johns Hopkins Univ; Sp/Lang Path, Gtr Balt Med Cen, **SLP**

Angle, Pamela Marie 5538 Southfield Drive Apartment E, St Louis, MO 63129, (314) 865-3333, BS 81 Central MO St Univ; MS 83 Central MO St Univ; 83–Aud, Alexian Brothers Hosp, **A**

Anglero, Olga M Calle Enseneda 561, Cond San Rafael 5C, Miramar, PR 00907, (809) 722-1605, BA 70 Univ of PR - Rio Piedras; MS 76 Univ of PR - Rio Piedras; Spec Educ Prof, Metropolitan Univ

Anglin, Colleen Sue 300 West Carter Drive, Glendora, CA 91740, (818) 335-3080, BA 78 CA St Univ - Los Angeles; Sp-Lang Path, Glendale USD, **SLP**

Anglin, Joyce Ann 3554 Lynnfield Road, Shaker Heights, OH 44122, (216) 946-5000, BS 69 Ball St Univ; MS 75 IN Univ - Bloomington; MA 83 Kent St Univ; Aud, Willoughby-Eastlake Schools, **A**

Anglin, Mrs Michele Susan 1903 Gainsboro Road, Rockville, MD 20851, (301) 261-3174, BA 84 Univ of MD - College Park; MS 86 Loyola Coll; **SLP**

Angstman, Mrs Jean Ward 2945 South Clayton Street, Denver, CO 80210-6701, (303) 399-0603, BA 80 Grinnell Coll; MA 84 Univ of Denver; Sp-Lang Path, Aurora Pub Sch, **SLP**

Anik, Mrs Margie Abrahamson 91 Stratford Avenue, White Plains, NY 10605, (914) 948-0050, BS 78 SUNY - Coll at Buffalo; MS 79 PA St Univ - Univ Park; Sp-Lang Path, Private Practice, **SLP**

Anis, Helen 1315 Commonwealth Avenue, Allston, MA 02134, (617) 437-2492, BA 69 CUNY - City College; MA 71 Univ of CT; Cl Asst Prof, Nen U, **SLP**

Ankenbruck, Paula Jean 11107 South Hoyne Apartment 3-W, Chicago, IL 60643, (312) 445-3627, BS 83 Ball St Univ; MS 84 Ball St Univ; 88–Sp-Lang Path, SW Cook Co Coop Assoc Spec Educ, **SLP**

Anketell, Mary T 865 Northwest Blvd, Columbus, OH 43212, (614) 447-8444, BA 82 Elms Coll; MA 84 Univ of CT; Sp-Lang Path, Great Lakes Reg Ctr Df/Bl Ed, **SLP**

Ankney, Enid Elaine Sherry Like Apartment, 150 Greenwich House, Conshohocken, PA 19428, (215) 941-0654, BS 82 WV Univ; MS 84 Kent St Univ; Sp-Lang Path, Montgomery County Intermed, **SLP**

Ankney, Teresa M 5711 Melvin Street, Pittsburgh, PA 15217, (412) 941-9500, BS 76 PA St Univ - Univ Park; MA 80 Univ of Pittsburgh - Pittsburgh; **SLP**

Ankrom, Judith M 3401 East Prairie, Decatur, IL 62521, BS 72 Eastern IL Univ; MS 73 Eastern IL Univ; Sp-Lang Path, Decatur PS Dist #61, **SLP**

Annen, Mrs Lonette Marie 2952 South State Road 2, Valparaiso, IN 46383, (218) 987-2789, BA 83 Valparaiso Univ; MS 85 Purdue Univ - West Lafayette; 85–Sp-Lang Path, Demotte Elementary School, **SLP**

Annison, Mrs Marguerite Route 1 Box 170, Ethel, LA 70730, (504) 683-3318, BS 51 LA St Univ - Baton Rouge; MA 59 LA St Univ - Baton Rouge; Superv of Spec Ed, E Feliciana Parish Sch Bd, **SLP**

Annunziata, Christine Russo 1527 East 33rd Street, Brooklyn, NY 11234, (201) 676-1000, MS 87 CUNY - Brooklyn Coll; **A**

Ansai, Patricia Susan c/o Eddow Ansai, 312 Douglas Street, Park Forest, IL 60466, (312) 733-2827, BA 80 Coll of Saint Francis; MS 85 Rush Univ; SLP, Bd of Ed, **SLP**

Ansbacher, Mrs Riva Hankel 1586 East 26th Street, Brooklyn, NY 11229, (212) 253-3612, BS 76 CUNY - City College; MS 84 CUNY - Brooklyn Coll; 86–Sp-Lang Path, P'Tach, **SLP**

Ansberry, Dr Merle 5530 Haleola Street, Honolulu, HI 96821, (808) 373-1760, BA 29 Univ of CA - Berkeley; MA 31 Univ of CA - Berkeley; PH 37 (NS) Univ of WI - Madison; **A F LM**

Ansel, Dr Beth Mindy 1200 Happy Hollow Road, #508, West Lafayette, IN 47906, (317) 494-3800, BS 77 SUNY - Center at Stony Brook; MS 81 Univ of WI - Madison; PH 85 (Sp Path-Neurogenics) Univ of WI - Madison; Sp-Lang Path, Purdue University, **SLP**

Ansell, Dr Barbara J Communicative Disorders Prog, Univ Of Wisconsin-Oshkosh, Oshkosh, WI 54901, BA 63 Temple Univ; MS 64 Univ of MI - Ann Arbor; PH 80 (Sp & Hrng Sciences) Univ of WA; 88–Asst Prof, Univ of WI, **SLP**

Anserello, Mrs Kathi Vogt 104 Graceland Drive, La Porte, IN 46350, (219) 362-2052, BA 83 Ball St Univ; MA 88 Ball St Univ; 88–Sp-Lang Path, South LaPorte Spec Educ Coop, **SLP**

Ansfield, Mrs Sandra 1135 Maricopa Drive, Oshkosh, WI 54904, BS 60 Univ of WI - Milwaukee; MS 61 Purdue Univ - West Lafayette; MS 86 Univ of WI - Oshkosh; Sp-Lang Path, Neenah Joint Sch Dist, **SLP**

Anshell, Susan Ellen 6802 Bonnie Ridge Drive, Apartment 102, Baltimore, MD 21209, (301) 486-2917, BA 81 Univ of MD - College Park; MS 85 Towson St Univ; **A**

Ansley, Mrs Ellen R 5 Jonathan Lane, Poughkeepsie, NY 12603, (914) 452-0910, BS 72 Cornell Univ; MS 74 Ithaca Coll; Sp/Lang Path, Arlington Ctrl Sch Dist, **SLP**

Anslow, Barbara Ellen 330 New Scotland Avenue, Albany, NY 12208, (518) 438-6294, BS 85 SUNY - Coll at Geneseo; MS 86 Coll of Saint Rose; 88–Sp-Lang Path, The Village Preschool, **SLP**

Anson, Holly PO Box 632662, Nacogdoches, TX 75963, (409) 564-9673, BS 74 Stephen F Austin St Univ; ME 79 Stephen F Austin St Univ; Deaf Education Teacher, Nacogdoches Reg Day Sch/Deaf, **SLP**

Anson, Lynn T 97-02 125th Street, Richmond Hill, NY 11419, (718) 377-5090, BA 85 SUNY - Coll at Oneonta; MA 88 Long Island U - CW Post Ctr

Antanaitis, Robert J 14 High Street, Bethel, CT 06801, (203) 255-8300, BS 53 Indiana Univ of PA; ME 58 PA St Univ - Univ Park; SLP/Aud, Fairfield Pub Schs, **SLP**

Anthenelli, Mrs Monica H 21 Devonshire Drive, Salisbury, MD 21801, (301) 749-9077, BA 72 Univ of MD - College Park; MS 74 Loyola Coll; Sp-Lang Path, **SLP**

Anthony, Gene M 1303 13th Street, Auburn, NE 68305, (402) 274-4284, BA 65 SD St Univ; MA 68 SD St Univ; SLP/Coord, Ed Serv Ut #4, **SLP**

Anthony, Jackie Gail Box 279, Oran, MO 63771, (618) 734-1027, BS 84 Southeast MO St Univ; MA 86 Southeast MO St Univ

Anthony, Mrs Julie Virginia 18788 Rivers Edge West, Chagrin Falls, OH 44022, (216) 543-9380, BA 66 Bowling Green St Univ; MA 67 Case Western Reserve Univ; 81–Sp-Lang Path, Kenston Bd of Educ, **SLP**

Anthony, Karen Jane 122 Cypress Road, Newington, CT 06111, BA 82 Univ of CT; MA 84 Univ of CT; Sp-Lang Path, Newington Children's Hosp, **SLP**

Anthony, Mrs Lea Love 21410 Talisman Street, Torrance, CA 90503, BA 74 CA St Univ - Northridge; MA 76 CA St Univ - Northridge; Sp-Lang Path, Off of Los Ang Co Supt of Sch, **SLP**

Anthony, Mrs Margaret Fuller 411 Ridgewood Road, Shippenville, PA 16254, (814) 226-4736, BS 83; MS 84 Indiana Univ of PA; 88–Sp-Lang Path, Crossroads Speech & Hrng Inc, **SLP**

Anthony, Mrs Marilyn H 34 Patten Terrace, Cedar Grove, NJ 07009, (201) 838-5500, MA 82 Montclair St Coll; SLP, Kinnelon Schs Spec Servs, **SLP**

Antignano, Mrs Karin 61 Greatwater Avenue, Massapequa, NY 11758, (516) 799-2950, BA 71 CUNY - Queens Coll; MA 76 Hofstra Univ; OM 86 Hofstra Univ; SLP, Massapequa Pub Sch, **SLP**

Antinore, Deborah Ann 501 French Road #5, Rochester, NY 14618-5320, **SLP**

Antolick, Sharron Andeara 6504 Ducketts Lane, Elkridge, MD 21227, (301) 796-1963, BS 84 PA St Univ - Univ Park; MS 86 PA St Univ - Univ Park; **SLP**

Anton, Larry J 13529 Josephine Street, Omaha, NE 68138, (402) 895-4927, BA 72 Northwestern OK St Univ; MS 75 Central MO St Univ; Aud, Immanuel Med Cen, **A**

Anton, Mrs Linda 2420 North 94th Street, Milwaukee, WI 53226, (414) 475-6702, BS 78 Marquette Univ; MS 79 Marquette Univ; Sp/Lang Path, Shared Therp Serv of Wisc, **SLP**

Antonak, Carol Christine RR 1 Box 857, Wolfeboro, NH 03894, (603) 569-6410, BS 79 Univ of NH; MS 83 Univ of NH; 87–Asst Clin Dir, Highwatch Rehabilitation Ctr, **SLP**

Antone, Deborah C 148 South Detroit Street, Los Angeles, CA 90036, (213) 477-8069, BA 74 Fordham Univ; MA 78 CA St Univ - Los Angeles; Sp-Lang Path, Julia Hobbs, **SLP**

Antonellis, Mrs Susan A 1067 Esther Street, Franklin Square, NY 11010, (516) 352-0974, BA 81 Saint John's Univ - Jamaica; MS 83 Adelphi Univ; 88–Asst Dir, Hy Weinberg Ctr/Adelphi Univ, **A**

Antoniadis, Anastasia 101 East Bells Mill Road, Philadelphia, PA 19118, (215) 427-5590, BS 75 Mercy Coll; MA 77 CUNY - City College; 87–Mgr Sp-Lang Svcs, Phila Early Childhood Eval Ctr, **SLP ACE**

Antonik, Susan P 339 Hazelwood Terrace, Rochester, NY 14609, (716) 377-0488, BS 83 SUNY - Coll at Geneseo; MA 86 SUNY - Center at Buffalo; **SLP**

Antonucci, Mrs Lorraine D 340 Auburn Way #15, San Jose, CA 95129, (408) 243-6769, BA 75 Vassar Coll; MS 79 San Francisco St Univ; **SLP**

Antony, Mrs Christine Holly 20 Romar Drive, Brownsburg, IN 46112, (317) 852-6787, BA 83 Butler Univ; MA 84 Western MI Univ; **SLP**

Antrobus-Kendall, Sarah A 211 South Itasca, Plainview, TX 79072-6663, (806) 296-6688, BA 64 West TX St Univ; MA 67 TX Tech Univ; Sp-Lang Path, Plainview ISD, **SLP**

Antunes-Smith, Katherine 9923 Forestglen Drive, Cincinnati, OH 45242-5115, **SLP**

Antwine, Brenda M 807 Jefferson Avenue, Memphis, TN 38105, (901) 525-2682, BA 71 Univ of AR - Little Rock; MA 75 Memphis St Univ; 87–Asst Prof, Memphis State U, **SLP**

Anuber, Susan Elizabeth 7851 Wildridge Drive, Fair Oaks, CA 95628, (916) 486-2145, BS 85 CA St Univ - Sacramento; MA 86 Univ of the Pacific; Slp, American River Hosp, **SLP**

Anzelmo, Mrs Mary E 3301 Hewitt Avenue #105, Silver Spring, MD 20906, (301) 871-3944, BA 70 George Washington Univ; MA 75 Catholic Univ of America; Sp-Lang Path, Fancis Fuchs Spec Ctr, **SLP**

Anzelone, Deborah Kristen 4610 Quimby Avenue, Beltsville, MD 20705, (202) 722-5860, MS 87 Gallaudet Coll; 87–Aud, Gallaudet Univ-Sch of Prep Stu, **A**

Anzovino, Mrs Sharon Weber R R 1 Box 317, Overhill Road, Stormville, NY 12582, BA 79 SUNY - Coll at Cortland; MA 80 Bowling Green St Univ; Sp-Lang Path, Putnam Valley Central Schools, **SLP**

Apa, Mrs Marty Ann 71 Charles, Deadwood, SD 57732, (605) 578-2364, BA 70 SD St Univ; MA 75 Univ of Northern CO; Aud, Black Hills Medical Center, **A**

Apel, Mrs Carolann D 345 West Dickens Avenue, Chicago, IL 60614, (312) 975-5000, BA 59 MacMurray Coll; MA 68 MI St Univ; Sp-Lang Path, Augustana Hosp, **SLP**

Apel, Dr Kenn Whittier College, Department Of Communication Disorders, PO Box 634, Whittier, CA 90608, (213) 693-0771, BA 81 4482; MA 83 San Diego St Univ; PH 86 (Sp-Lang Path) Memphis St Univ; Asst Prof, Whittier College, **SLP**

Apfelbeck, Mrs Jean Glover 321-B Santiago Road, Virginia Beach, VA 23459, (804) 628-7182, BS 85 Miami Univ - Oxford; MS 87 Old Dominion Univ; 87–Sp-Lang Path, Childrens Hosp Kings Daughters, **SLP**

Apicella, Mrs Susan Ellen 5 Ballou Road, Hopedale, MA 01747, (617) 234-6346, BA 82 Bridgewater St Coll; MS 85 Worcester St Coll; Sp-Lang Path, Northbridge Public Schools, **SLP**

Apilado, Benjamin C 440 East Mill Avenue, Porterville, CA 93257, (209) 784-2000, BA 75 San Francisco St Univ; MA 76 San Francisco St Univ; **A**

Apkon, Susan Debra 12 Merriam Road, Framingham, MA 01701, (617) 787-3390, MA 87 Northwestern Univ; SLP, Greenery Rehab & Skilled N Ctr, **SLP**

Apodaca, Anna Rose 991 East Jasper Road, Heber, CA 92249, (619) 357-0122, BS 77 Loma Linda Univ - Riverside; MS 82 Loma Linda Univ - Riverside; Sp-Lang Path, Calexico USD

Apodaca, Mrs Jane F 701 West Roselawn, Danville, IL 61832, (217) 443-2900, BS 78 Saint Louis Univ; MA 80 Saint Louis Univ; SLP, Danville Sch Dist 118, **SLP**

Appaya, Monjula N 1409 Wilson Avenue, Lima, OH 45805, (419) 228-3335, BA 82 OH St Univ; MA 85 OH St Univ; **SLP**

Appelbaum, Mrs Beth Rosenau 3844 Byron Road, Huntingdon Valley, PA 19006, (215) 947-7472, BS 78 PA St Univ - Univ Park; BS 78 PA St Univ - Univ Park; MA 80 Temple Univ; Sp-Lang Path, Private Practice, **SLP**

Appelbaum, Maris Joan 1A East 69th Street, New York, NY 10021, (212) 535-5392, BS 79 Georgetown Univ; MS 82 Columbia Univ Teachers Coll; Aud, Private Practice, **A**

Apper, Cheryl Wenkart 1128 South Holt #6, Los Angeles, CA 90035, (213) 854-5442, BA 78; MA 86 CA St Univ - Northridge; 88–Sp-Lang Path, San Fernando Child Guid Cl, **SLP**

Appert, Mrs Alice M 6 Woodmont Court, Medford, NJ 08055, **SLP**

Applbaum, Robyn Sue 954 Palo Verde Avenue, Long Beach, CA 90815, (714) 964-2057, BA 77 Univ of the Pacific; MA 78 Univ of the Pacific; SLP, Orange Co Dept of Ed, **SLP**

Applbaum, Dr Ronald Lee 1320 Tulip Circle, Mc Allen, TX 78504, (512) 631-4406, BA 65 CA St Univ - Long Beach; MA 66 CA St Univ - Long Beach; PH 69 (NS) PA St Univ - Univ Park

Apple, Mrs Janice Kanter 2 Windsor Drive, Voorhees, NJ 08043, (609) 772-1507, BA 80 Tulane Univ; MA 81 Tulane Univ; Sp-Lang Path, Private Practice, **SLP**

Apple, Mrs Jill Elizabeth 3847 Timberglen #2624, Dallas, TX 75252, (214) 306-7754, MS 88 Univ of North TX; 88–Sp-Lang Path, Richardson ISD

Apple, Linda G 2912 Claremont Avenue #33, Berkeley, CA 94705, (415) 845-3509, BA 84 Barnard Coll; MS 87 Columbia Univ Teachers Coll; 88–Sp-Lang Path, Scottish Rite Clinic

Applebaum, Fredrica 11841 S W 57 Court, Miami, FL 33156, (305) 666-5013, ME 75 Univ of Miami; **SLP**

Applebaum, Merle S 5604 Greenly NE, Albuquerque, NM 87111, (505) 293-4270, BS 71 IN Univ - Bloomington; MS 73 Univ of NM; Sp-Lang Path, Albuquerque PS, **SLP**

Applebaum, Mrs Nikki A R 2210 El Baile Place, Hacienda Heights, CA 91745, (818) 336-6939, BA 72 CA St Univ - Los Angeles; MA 74 CA St Univ - Los Angeles; 86–Tchr, Hacienda La Puente Adult Sch, **SLP**

Applebaum, Mrs Valerie K 2708 Mill Avenue, Brooklyn, NY 11234, (212) 241-9748, BA 67 CUNY - Hunter Coll; MS 68 Univ of MI - Ann Arbor; 75–Sp-Lang Path, Private Practice, **SLP**

Appleby, Annette 2417 Hayden Street, Amarillo, TX 79109, (806) 373-4880, BA 46 Grinnell Coll; MS 60 Univ of MI - Ann Arbor; Retired, Chldns Rehab Cen, **SLP**

Appleby, Mrs Maribelle F 11225 Lewis Court, Burnsville, MN 55337, (612) 895-7292, BS 63 Univ of NE - Lincoln; Sp-Lang Path, ISD #191, **SLP**

Appleby, Mary Patricia 877 Homedale, New Orleans, LA 70124-2737, (504) 737-8982, BS 79 SUNY - Coll at Buffalo; OM 83 LA St Univ - N O Medical Ctr; 87–Sp-Lang Path, Health South Rehab Ctr, **SLP**

Appleby, Rena Beth 0, 5450 Astor Lane, Rolling Meadows, IL 60008, (312) 532-7000, BS 84 Northern IL Univ - De Kalb; MA 87 Northern IL Univ - De Kalb

Applegate, Mrs Debra Ann K-5 Garden Lane, Flemington, NJ 08822, (201) 735-4031, BS 80 Elmira Coll; MA 84 Montclair St Coll; SLP, Hunterdon Development Center, **SLP**

Applegate, Dr John A 147 Violette Hall-NMSU, Kirksville, MO 63501, (816) 785-4675, BA 66 Muskingum Coll; MA 68 OH Univ - Athens; PH 84 (Sp Path) Kent St Univ; Asst Prof of Sp-Lang Path, NE MO State U, **SLP**

Applegate, Mrs Mary P 25315 Pepper Ridge, Spring, TX 77373, (713) 353-8873, BA 72 Univ of Houston - Univ Park; MA 73 Univ of Houston - Univ Park; Sp-Lang Path, Spring ISD, **SLP**

Applestein, Mrs Shiela A 605 Farmhurst Road, Baltimore, MD 21208, (301) 486-8644, BA 52 Univ of MD - College Park; MS 74 Loyola Coll; Baltimore City Pub Schs, **SLP**

Appletoft, Mrs Nancy C 2507 West 19th, Sioux City, IA 51103, (712) 252-2371, BS 80; MA 82; Aud & Sp-Path, Siouxland Easter Seal Soc, **SLP A**

Appleton, Rita Anne 94-2915 Norman Avenue, Point Coquitlam, BC, Canada V3C 4H8, (604) 596-7733, MA 84 Western WA Univ; 79–Sp-Lang Path, Sch Dist 36 Surrey, **SLP**

Appleton, Rozanne S P O Box 305, Amenia, NY 12501, (914) 877-6821, BA 71 Paterson St Coll; MA 74 CUNY - City College; SLP, Wassaic Dev Cen, **SLP**

Apt, Mrs Norma Abramson 5638 Del Roy Drive, Dallas, TX 75230, (214) 987-0064, BA 51; MA 53; Sp-Lang Path, Private Practice, **SLP**

Aptaker, Ruth 515 North Avenue, New Rochelle, NY 10801, (914) 632-9000, BA 55 Adelphi Univ; Sp-Lnag Path, Cty Sch Dist-New Rochelle, **SLP**

Aptakin, Sammye Jean 21620 Burbank Boulevard #4, Woodland Hills, CA 91367, (818) 348-3967, BA 69 Univ of CA - Los Angeles; MA 82 CA St Univ - Northridge; Sp-Lang Path, Los Angeles USD, **SLP**

Arab, Margaret Mary PO Box 265, Munster Hamlet, ON, Canada K0A 3P0, (613) 838-4454, MS 87 Dalhousie Univ - Nova Scotia; 88–Sp-Lang Path, Lanark Co Lang & Dev Prog

Arabia, Janet C 1202 Shore Road, Linwood, NJ 08221, (609) 927-9116, BS Syracuse Univ; MA Trenton St Coll; Sp-Lang Path, Somers Pt Bd Educ, **SLP**

Aradine, Rebecca A 526 East Union Street, Newark, NY 14513, (315) 331-1700, BS 86 SUNY - Coll at Fredonia; MS 87 SUNY - Coll at Fredonia; Asst SLP, Newark Dev Ctr

Arakaki, Gaye Keiko 94-917 Kaaholo Street, Waipahu, HI 96797-4523, (808) 455-2885, BS 80 Univ of HI - Manoa; MS 82 Univ of HI - Manoa; 82–Sp-Lang Path, State of Hawaii-Dept of Educ, **SLP**

Aram, Dr Dorothy W Rainbow Babies & Children's Hosp, Department Of Pediatrics, 2101 Adelbert Road, Cleveland, OH 44106, (216) 844-3669, BS 64 Northwestern Univ; MA 65 Northwestern Univ; PH 72 (Sp-Lang Path) Case Western Reserve Univ; Assoc Prof, Case Western Reserve Univ Sch of Med, **SLP**

Arambula, Gustavo Guerrero 963 Franquette Avenue, San Jose, CA 95125, (408) 998-3212, BA 81 San Jose St Univ; MA 83 San Jose St Univ; Sp-Lang Path, San Jose Hosp, **SLP**

Arana, Margot A 303 Caselli Street, San Francisco, CA 94114, (415) 326-5530, BA 78 Univ of ME - Orono; MA 80 Univ of FL; Sp/Lang Path, Chldrns Hlth Council, **SLP**

Arbanas, Marybeth 215 Washington Street, Glenview, IL 60025, (312) 965-6200, BS 73 Saint Louis Univ; MA 74 Univ of IL - Urbana; Sp-Lang Path, Morton Grove Pub Sch, **SLP**

Arbeit, Holley S 617 Quail Park Court, Bakersfield, CA 93309, (805) 832-4332, BS 76 SUNY - Coll at Fredonia; MA 80 OH Univ - Athens; 75–Sp-Lang Path, Kern HS Dist, **SLP**

Arbib, Brenda Sullivan Box 54, Main Street, Cummington, MA 01026, (413) 586-8353, BA 74 SUNY - Coll at Plattsburgh; MA 81 Univ of MA - Amherst; Sp/Lang Path, Hampshire Educ Collaborative, **SLP**

Arbter, Mrs Jody Ann 822 North 5th Avenue, Sturgeon Bay, WI 54235-2006, (414) 743-8176, BA 81 Univ of WI - Eau Claire; MS 85 Univ of WI - Oshkosh; SLP, Southern Door Schools, **SLP**

Arbuckle, Priscilla 82 Fairlawn Street, Whitinsville, MA 01588, (617) 478-2240, BA 62 Univ of NM; MS 74 Univ of RI; Sp-Lang Path, Mendon Upton Reg Sch, **SLP ACE**

Arcell, Paul C 17 Miller Street, Caldwell, NJ 07006, (201) 227-2000, BA 79 Univ of Charleston; MS 83 Southern CT St Univ; Product Specialist, Kay Elematrics Corp, **SLP**

Arceneaux, Judith D 2011 Spenwick Drive #726, Houston, TX 77055, (713) 428-7039, BS 75 Xavier Univ of LA; MA 77 Univ of Houston - Univ Park; 82–Sp/Lang Path, Pj Johnson Phd & Assoc Pc, **SLP ACE**

Arch, Robyn Joan 306 Wyandotte Street, Apt E, Bethlehem, PA 18015, (215) 865-6077, BS 85 Bloomsburg Univ of PA; MS 86 Bloomsburg Univ of PA; 87–Sp-Lang Path, InSpeech Inc, **SLP**

Archambault, Gayle M 40 Charles River Road, Waltham, MA 02154, (617) 893-9938, **SLP**

Archer, Mrs Cassandra Apostolou 4 Militia Hill Drive, Wayne, PA 19087, (215) 889-1764, BA 72 Univ of RI; MS 75 Univ of VT; **SLP**

Archer, Mrs Jane B 12331 Oakwood, Garden Grove, CA 92640, (714) 663-6384, BS 55 Univ of IL - Urbana; MS 58 Univ of IL - Urbana; Sp-Lang Path, Garden Grove USD, **SLP**

Archer, Judith Ann 5370 S W 97th Coure, Miami, FL 33165, (305) 595-7275, BA 84 Univ of FL; MS 87 Nova Univ

Archer, Susan E 5 Woodside Park Blvd, Pleasant Ridge, MI 48069-1042, (800) 638-2680, BA 71 Marymount Coll; MA 73 Eastern MI Univ; Aud, Phonic Ear Inc, **A**

Archer-Chmela, Mrs Kristin Marie 592 Chesterfield Lane, Barrington, IL 60010, (312) 272-6303, BA 85 AZ St Univ; MA 87 Northwestern Univ; 87–Sp-Lang Path, Comm Consolidated Dist 15

Archibald, Judith A 10 Clinton Avenue, Ridgewood, NJ 07450, (201) 444-6305, BA 60 Denison Univ; MS 75 William Paterson Coll; Dir, Ridgewood Sp/Lang Cen, **SLP ACE**

Archie, Mrs Lori Longfellow 1078 Horseshoe Creek Road, Glendo, WY 82213, (307) 322-4327, BS 77 AZ St Univ; MS 78 Fort Hays St Univ; 88–Sp-Lang Path, Northfork Sp/Hrng Svc, **SLP**

Arcidiacono, Nancy Century Village, 98 Winterwood Drive, Londonderry, NH 03053, (603) 893-2900, BA 74 Univ of MA - Amherst; MA 76 Case Western Reserve Univ; Dir Commun Disorders Dept, Northeast Rehab Hosp, **SLP ACE**

Arcidiacono, Nina A P O Box 7491, Hemet, CA 92343, BA 76 Univ of HI - Hilo; MA 79 Univ of Redlands; MS 79 Univ of Redlands; Sp-Lang Path, Hemet USD, **SLP**

Arcus, Doreen M Harvard University, William Sames Hall, 33 Kirkland Street, Cambridge, MA 02138, (312) 996-3186, BA 76 Saint Xavier Coll; MA 77 Western MI Univ; Sp-Lang Path, Private Practice, **SLP**

Ardito, Vito 47 Sparrow Lane, Levittown, NY 11756, (212) 741-3164, BA 74 CUNY - Queens Coll; MA 76 CUNY - City College; Mobile Unit Aud, NY League for Hard of Hrng, **A**

Ard-Manka, Mrs Sarah Margaret 6204 N W Cheyenne Avenue, Lawton, OK 73505, (405) 536-5618, BA 76 Trinity Univ; MS 83 Univ of OK - OK City; 88–Aud, Comanche Co Health Dept, **A**

Ardys, Inore A 19051 Meredith Avenue, Euclid, OH 44119, (216) 481-1376, MA 88 Case Western Reserve Univ

Arechavaleta, Maria Teresa 6024 S W 26th Street #206, Miramar, FL 33023, (305) 666-6511, BA 82 Univ of Northern CO; MA 84 Univ of Northern CO; 84–Sp-Lang Path, Miami Childrens Hospital, **SLP ACE**

Arectos, Linda A 14 North Hill Drive, North Falmouth, MA 02556, (508) 540-2686, BS 68 Saint John's Univ - Jamaica; OM 73 NY Univ; MS 79 Columbia Univ Teachers Coll; Aud, Cape Cod ENT Assoc Inc, **A**

Areeda, Laura A Carlisle Hospital, Speech & Hearing Dept, 246 Parker Street, Carlisle, PA 17013, (717) 245-5332, BS 74 Bloomsburg Univ of PA; MS 76 Indiana Univ of PA; Sp-Lang Path, Carlisle Hosp, **SLP**

Arehole, Dr Shalini Dept Of Communicative Dis, P O Box 43170 Usl, Lafayette, LA 70504-3170, (318) 231-5241, BS 77; MS 79; PH 86 (Commun Dis) Univ of TX - Dallas; 87–Asst Prof-Aud, Univ of SW Louisiana, **A**

Arellano, Mrs Joan Sheridan 344 Glorietta Boulevard, Orinda, CA 94563, (415) 685-1960, BA 66 San Francisco St Univ; MA 68 San Francisco St Univ; SLP, Mt Diablo Sch Dist, **SLP**

Arena, Ann Marie 1131 Summerwood Drive, Harrisburg, PA 17111-4702, (717) 545-7228, BA 84 Loyola Coll; MS 86 James Madison Univ; **SLP**

Arena, Maria Lynn 1621 North 35th Street, Apartment D, Sheboygan, WI 53081, (414) 459-3534, BS 85 Univ of WI - Milwaukee; MS 86 Marquette Univ; 86–Sp-Lang Path, Sheboygan Area Sch Dist, **SLP**

Arends, Mrs Jill Gallup 308 Whytegate Court, Lake Forest, IL 60045, (312) 234-5760, BA 75 Univ of MD - College Park; MA 77 Univ of IL - Urbana; Sp-Lang Path, Private Practice, **SLP**

Arensberg, Karen Elizabeth 60 Second Avenue #507, Orangeville, ON, Canada L9W 3R2, (519) 942-0170, BA 84 Univ of TN - Knoxville; MA 86 Univ of North TX; 87–Sp-Lang Path, Wellington-Dufferin-Guelph Health Unit, **SLP**

Arenson, Mrs Diane K 5216 Duggan Plaza, Edina, MN 55435, (612) 829-0810, BA 75 Univ of MN - Minneap-St Paul; MA 77 Univ of IA; **SLP**

Arey, H Regina Smith 24 Le June Road, Cinnaminson, NJ 08077, (609) 871-7790, BS 75 Carlow Coll; MS 78 UT St Univ; Sp-Lang Path, Prep Prog-Preschool, **SLP**

Argabright, Margaret L 631 Franklin Square Suite 104, Michigan City, IN 46360, (219) 879-6221, BS 75 Purdue Univ - West Lafayette; MS 79 Governors St Univ; Sp/Lang Path, Argabright Communications, **SLP**

Argentiere, Mrs Barbara Elaine 149 Villa Place, Rahway, NJ 07065, (201) 745-5405, BA 82 Kean Coll of NJ; MA 85 Kean Coll of NJ; 88–Sp-Lang Path, New Brunswick Bd of Educ

Arger, Mrs Janice L 800 19th Street #6, Menominee, MI 49858, (906) 863-5665, MS 80 Univ of WI - River Falls; Sp-Lang Path, Menominee Co ISD, **SLP**

Argetsinger, Elaine 4124 Raleigh Avenue, Minneapolis, MN 55416, (612) 926-7287, MA 65 Univ of MN - Minneap-St Paul; **SLP LM**

Argon, Janet Lynn 1130 West Olive, Redlands, CA 92373, (714) 653-2141, BA 81 Chapman Coll; MS 83 Chapman Coll; Sp-Lang Path, Moreno Valley USD, **SLP**

Arguello, Nancy Kathryn 940 Carob Street, Redlands, CA 92373, (714) 798-0599, BA 69 Univ of Redlands; MA 70 Univ of Redlands; Sp-Lang Path, Private Practice, **SLP**

Arguijo, Edward Valley View Speech Path Serv, 5300 Orange Avenue, Suite 115, Cypress, CA 90630, (714) 826-1025, BA 67 CA St Univ - Los Angeles; MA 69 CA St Univ - Los Angeles; Dir, Valley View Sp Path Ser Inc, **SLP**

Arguijo, Mrs Rebecca Lou 5300 Orange Avenue #115, Cypress, CA 90630, (714) 826-1025, BA 74 CA St Univ - Long Beach; MA 81 CA St Univ - Long Beach; **SLP**

Ariail, Alison Millet 4041 Idaho #B, Kenner, LA 70065, (504) 443-6442, BS 83 LA St Univ - Baton Rouge; MS 86 LA St Univ - N O Medical Ctr; 84–Sp-Lang Path, Jefferson Parish PS Sys, **SLP**

Arias, Carmen M 4757-F Walden Circle, Orlando, FL 32805, (407) 351-8500, BA 83 Tufts Univ; MA 88 Univ of FL; **SLP**

Arichibald, Cynthia Austin 987 Castlebury, Yukon, OK 73099, (405) 354-8302, MS 88 Univ of OK Medical Center

Arick, Judith T Brookline Hearing Services Inc, 115 Marion Street, Brookline, MA 02146, (617) 232-1299, BA 63 Univ of CT; MA 65 Univ of IA; Owner, Brookline Hearing Services Inc, **A**

Arieux, Mrs Donna P 1146 Appian Way, Dothan, AL 36303, (205) 794-7723, BS 74 Auburn Univ - Auburn; MS 76 Auburn Univ - Auburn; Sp-Lang Path, Dothan Cty Sch, **SLP**

Ariff-Karrberg, Judy A 1111 Laurel Avenue, Sea Girt, NJ 08750, (201) 899-3737, BA 76 Rutger's St Univ - Douglas Coll; MA 77 Univ of MD - College Park; 79–Sp-Lang Path, Pt Pleasant Bch Sch, **A**

Arin, Merle Allan Box 131, Nome, AK 99762, (907) 443-5299, BA 79 Saint John's Univ; MA 85 Coll of St Thomas; MS 85 Univ of ND; Sp-Lang Path, Nome Pub Sch, **SLP**

Aring, Mrs Mary Root 2953 Gracewood, Toledo, OH 43613, (313) 856-1950, OB 75 Univ of Toledo; BA 75 Univ of Toledo; MA 76 Kent St Univ; Sp-Lang Path, Bedford Pub Sch, **SLP**

Arismendi, Mrs Cheryl A 20815 South Norwalk Blvd, Suite 5, Lakewood, CA 90715-1569, (213) 865-7314, BA 83 CA St Univ - Fullerton; MA 87 CA St Univ - Fullerton; **SLP**

Arista, Yolanda 9365 Pinyon Tree Lane #149, Dallas, TX 75243, **SLP**

Ark, Mary P 2053 Lake Road P O Box 393, Silver Creek, NY 14136, (716) 934-2648, BS 67 SUNY - Coll at Buffalo; MS 71 SUNY - Coll at Buffalo; **SLP**

Arkebauer, Dr Herbert J 945 East Evans, Springfield, MO 65810, (417) 836-5275, BS 51 Concordia Coll; MA 53 Columbia Univ Teachers Coll; PH 64 (Sp Path) Univ of IA; 78–Chmn Comm Dis, SW Mo St U, **SLP**

Arker, Dina 804 Porter Place, Woodsburgh, NY 11598, (516) 569-7830, **SLP**

Arkis, Peter N 14004 Watt Road, Novelty, OH 44072, (216) 856-4000, BS 74 Kent St Univ; MA 76 Kent St Univ; Aud, Warren Otologic Group, **A**

Arkwright, Mrs Judy C 6471 Larme, Allen Park, MI 48101, (313) 381-8087, BA 77 MI St Univ; MA 78 MI St Univ; Sp-Lang Path, Wayne County Inter Sch Dist, **SLP**

Arlt, Mrs Phyllis B 947 Narcissus, Clearwater Beach, FL 34630, (813) 447-4642, BA 37 Cornell Univ; MA 39 Cornell Univ; **SLP LM**

Arm, Janine I 1632 Mill Pond Drive, Salem, VA 24153, (703) 382-5137, BS 78 James Madison Univ; MS 81 Radford Univ; Sp-Lang Path, Montgomery Co Sch Syst, **SLP**

Armbruster, Joan M 159 East 69th Street, New York, NY 10021, (212) 734-8900, BS 72 Marquette Univ; MS 73 Columbia Univ Teachers Coll; 80, Private Practice, **A**

Armel, Joyce P Moshav Shorashim, DN Misgar, Israel 20164, BA 75 CUNY - Lehman Coll; MS 79 Univ of TX - Houston; Sp-Lang Path, Misgav Health Center, **SLP**

Armel, Sarah Douek 11 Hawthorn Drive, North Edison, NJ 08820, (201) 756-4946, BA 74 CUNY - Brooklyn Coll; MS 76 CUNY - Brooklyn Coll; Sp-Lang Path, NYC Bd of Ed- Sp Serv Ut, **SLP**

Armentrout, Carolyn Clement 11879 St Trinians Court, Reston, VA 22091, (703) 777-2290, BS 84 James Madison Univ; MS 85 James Madison Univ; 88–Spec Educ Coord, Loudoun County Pub School Syst, **SLP**

Armgardt, Mrs Colleen K 2921 94th Street, Sturtevant, WI 53177, (312) 662-1877, BA 77 Marquette Univ; MA 79 Univ of IL - Urbana; Aud, Lk McHenry Reg Prog, **A**

Armin, Mary Jo 9034 Woodmoss Lane #2A, Indianapolis, IN 46250-1038, (317) 353-5429, BS 79 Ball St Univ; MA 80 Ball St Univ; 80–Sp-Lang Path, Comm Hosp of Indpls Inc, **SLP**

Armor, Robin A Route 4 Box 242, Lexington, VA 24450, (804) 745-3583, BS 78 WV Univ; MS 79 WV Univ; Aud, John A Wade MD Inc, **A**

Armour, Mrs Betsy Crane 1800 Montgomery Avenue, Villanova, PA 19085, (215) 525-6449, BA 49 Wellesley Coll; MA 84 West Chester Univ of PA; Sp-Lang Path, Sp Path Assoc, **SLP**

Armour, Jill Ann 2981 Plateau Drive, Salt Lake City, UT 84109-2318, (801) 485-4554, BS 80 Phillips Univ; MA 81 Univ of Denver; PH 88 (Aud) Univ of UT; 88–Aud, Private Practice, **SLP A ACE**

Armour, Lucinda G 7543 West Beryl Avenue, Peoria, AZ 85345, (602) 878-8508, BA 79 MI St Univ; MS 83 AZ St Univ; Sp-Lang Path, Peoria Sch Dist, **SLP**

Armson, Joy M School Of Human Communication Disorders, Dalhousie University, 5599 Fenwick Street, Halifax, NS, Canada B3H 1R2, BA 72 Dalhousie Univ - Nova Scotia; MS 74 Univ of WI - Madison; 88–Asst Prof, Dalhousie Univ, **SLP**

Armstead, Dr Kay A G 675 Jarvis Drive, Suite B, Morgan Hill, CA 95037, (408) 779-6769, BA 55 San Jose St Univ; MA 65 San Jose St Univ; ED 81 (NS) Univ of San Francisco; Assoc Prof, San Jose St U, **SLP**

Armstrong, Andrea F 150 Paulison Avenue, Unit 4, Passaic, NJ 07055, (201) 863-0646, BS 78 SUNY - Coll at Geneseo; MS 79 IN St Univ - Terre Haute; Milestones Child Dev Ctr, **SLP**

Armstrong, Mrs Ann H 1113 North Elmwood Avenue, Oak Park, IL 60302, (312) 922-5616, BA 64 Univ of WI - Madison; MA 66 Stanford Univ; **SLP**

Armstrong, Barbara L 1247 Llewellyn Road, Mount Pleasant, SC 29464, (803) 792-3190, BS 78 OH Univ - Athens; MA 80 OH Univ - Athens; Instr of Ped, Medical Univ of SC, **SLP**

Armstrong, Catherine Ann 552 West Deming Place Apartment #3, Chicago, IL 60614, (312) 248-2835, BS 85 Marquette Univ; MS 87 Marquette Univ; 88–Sp-Lang Path, Rehab Inst of Chicago, **SLP**

Armstrong, Mrs Chandler Loomis 1365 Virginia Road, Santa Barbara, CA 93108, (805) 963-4331, BA 72 Univ of CA - Los Angeles; MA 76 Univ of CA - Santa Barbara; Sp-Lang Path, Santa Barbara Cty Schs, **SLP**

Armstrong, Charlotte Butterfield 208 Old Kings Highway No, Darien, CT 06820, (203) 655-5105, BS 64 Bowling Green St Univ; MA 66 OH St Univ; 81–Sp-Lang Path, Private Practice, **SLP**

Armstrong, Daryl Vesper 1164 Bishop Street, Suite 124, Honolulu, HI 96813, (808) 547-4578, BS 81 Baylor Univ; MS 83 Univ of WI - Madison; Sp-Lang Path, The Queen's Med Ctr, **SLP**

Armstrong, Debra J 407F Tradewinds Drive, Fayetteville, NC 28304, (919) 323-6079, BA 80 Univ of NC - Chapel Hill; MS 82 Univ of NC - Chapel Hill; 88–Sp-Lang Path, Southeastern Reg Rehab Cntr, **SLP**

Armstrong, Mrs Donna C Star Route 1, Ozark, AR 72949, BA 74 Univ of AR - Fayetteville; MA 79 Univ of AR - Fayetteville; **SLP**

Armstrong, Elizabeth Gale 441 South Ham Lane, Suite B, Lodi, CA 95240, (209) 368-9222, MA 83 CA St Univ - Sacramento; Aud, Hearing Services Center, **A**

Armstrong, Jane E Speech Path & Audiology Serv, Medical College Of Georgia, Augusta, GA 30912, (404) 828-3505, BS 57 Univ of GA; Sp-Lang Path/Instr, Med Coll of GA, **SLP**

Armstrong, Joyce A 4516 46th Avenue N E, Salem, OR 97305, (503) 378-5286, **SLP**

Armstrong, Mrs Karen Marie 1042 Ada, Muskegon, MI 49442, (616) 744-4736, BS 84 Northern MI Univ; MA 86 MI St Univ; 88–Sp-Lang Path, Reeths Puffer Schs, **SLP**

Armstrong, Mrs Marcia J Rd 2 Box 67, Richfield Spring, NY 13439, (315) 823-0808, BA 65 SUNY - Coll at Geneseo; MS 69 Syracuse Univ; Sp-Lang Path, Leatherstocking Learn Ladder, **SLP**

Armstrong, Mrs Marjorie K 313 Midland Drive, Council Bluffs, IA 51501, (515) 322-7354, BA 80 Univ of Northern IA; MA 81 Univ of Northern IA; Sp-Lang Path, Loess Hills AEA 13, **SLP**

Armstrong, Mary B 106 Garden Circle, Thibodaux, LA 70301, (504) 446-8111, BS 74 Tulane Univ; OM 76 LA St Univ - N O Medical Ctr; Asst Prof, Nicholls St U, **SLP**

Armstrong, Mrs Nancy Monack 370 Lake Luanna Estates, Dyersburg, TN 38024, (901) 286-1723, BS 77 Murray St Univ; MA 82 Kent St Univ; 80–Aud, Dyer County Board of Education, **A**

Armstrong, Mrs Paula Johnston 8111 Barrett Road, West Chester, OH 45069, (513) 398-0474, BS 76 Miami Univ - Oxford; MS 82 Miami Univ - Oxford; Sp-Lang Path, Mason Local Sch, **SLP**

Armstrong, Sharon Kay 7610-14 Antlers Lane, Charlotte, NC 28210, (704) 552-5320, BS 85 East Carolina Univ; MS 86 East Carolina Univ; **SLP**

Armstrong, Sheri A 6540 Ralston Road, Indianapolis, IN 46241, (317) 637-1303, BA 78 IN Univ - Bloomington; MA 80 IN Univ - Bloomington; **A**

Armstrong, Susan 401 Jackman Street, San Marcos, TX 78666, (512) 396-2058, BS 81 Univ of North TX; MS 85 Univ of IL - Urbana; 87–Sp-Lang Path, Homespun Early Child Inter Prog, **SLP**

Armstrong, Mrs Susan J P O Box 122, Williamstown, WV 26187, (304) 375-7675, BS 74 OH Univ - Athens; MS 80 OH Univ - Athens; Sp-Lang Path, Wood County Schools, **SLP**

Armstrong, Suzanne Elaine 3201 Golden Avenue, Apartment #5, Cincinnati, OH 45226, (513) 559-4601, BS 84 Miami Univ - Oxford; MA 86 Univ of Cincinnati; **SLP**

Armstrong, Timothy Patrick 2663 Rio Bravo Circle, Sacramento, CA 95826-2248, (916) 929-2277, BA 80 CA St Univ - Sacramento; MA 83 CA St Univ - Sacramento; Aud, Sutter Hearing & Speech Center, **A**

Armstrong, W Jean 56 Rackleff Street #1, Portland, ME 04103-3033, (207) 879-1886, BA 76 Univ of ME - Orono; MS 81 Emerson Coll; Sp-Lang Path, Northeast Hrng & Sp Cen, **SLP**

Armus, Sharon Roberta 1160 Grand #9, St Paul, MN 55105, (612) 291-0194, BA 80 Univ of MI - Ann Arbor; MA 86 Univ of MN - Minneap-St Paul; **SLP**

Arnaboldi, Loren Joseph 81/2 Chestnut Street, Binghamton, NY 13905, (607) 724-4918, BS 80 SUNY - Coll at Oneonta; MA 82 Western MI Univ; Sp-Lang Path, Hca of Southern NY, **SLP**

Arnao, Susan Geri St Vincent's Medical Center Of Richmond, Speech & Hearing Center, 355 Bard Avenue, Staten Island, NY 10310, (718) 390-1480, MS 84 Ithaca Coll; 87–Aud, St Vincent's Med Ctr, **A**

Arndt, Donna K Morehead 4820 Howell Street, Golden, CO 80403, (303) 422-2334, BA 76 Univ of Northern CO; MA 77 Univ of Northern CO; Sp-Lang Path, Jefferson Co Pub Sch, **SLP**

Arndt, Mrs Kristine K 405 Moreland Avenue, Mankato, MN 56001, (507) 345-3015, BA 84 Mankato St Univ; MS 86 Mankato St Univ; 88–Sp-Lang Path, ISD #77, **SLP**

Arndt, Patti L 803 West 101st Terrace, Kansas City, MO 64114, (816) 942-9738, Aud, St Luke's Hosp of KC, **A**

Arnesen, Carol B Orange Cnty Dept Of Education, 200 Kalmus Drive, P O Box 9050, Costa Mesa, CA 92628, (714) 966-4120, BA 63 OH St Univ; MA 77 CA St Univ - Fullerton; 86–Dir-Spec Educ, Orange Co Dept of Ed, **SLP**

Arneson, Debra J 1101 Westwood #212, Bismarck, ND 58504, (701) 224-6051, BS 83 Moorhead St Univ; OM 85 Univ of MT; 85–Aud, Medcenter One, **A**

Arneson, James 1045 Jasmine, Lompoc, CA 93436, (805) 736-2371, BA 54 Univ of WA; Dept Head/Sp Therapy, Lompoc USD, **SLP A**

Arnett, Patricia 1070 Boonville Road, Ukiah, CA 95482, (707) 463-0208, BA 70 Univ of CA - Santa Barbara; MA 73 Humboldt St Univ; Resource Spec, Mendecere USD, **SLP**

Arnett, Tammy Ann Box 271, Hager, KY 41439, (606) 349-6117, MS 83 Univ of KY; Sp-Lang Path, Magoffin County Board of Educ, **SLP**

Arney, Mary Shepard 5306 Brookstone Lane, Virginia Beach, VA 23455, (804) 431-4015, BS 68 Longwood Coll; MS 75 Old Dominion Univ; Sp-Lang Path, VA Beach Pub Sch, **SLP**

Arnhold, Mrs Linda M 19357 Dairen Street, Rowland Heights, CA 91748, (714) 983-9501, BA 74 CA St Univ - Los Angeles; MA 80 CA St Univ - Los Angeles; 87–Sp-Lang Path, Ontario-Montclair Sch Dist, **SLP**

Arnn, Cheryl McDougall 8058 Camino Tranquilo, San Diego, CA 92122, (619) 747-1245, BA 75 Univ of WA; MA 77 Univ of WA; SLP, Escondido Elem Sch Dist, **SLP**

Arnoff, Mrs Judith B 9006 Horton Road, Laurel, MD 20708, (301) 772-0990, BA 59 Univ of MD - College Park; MA 61 Case Western Reserve Univ; 75–Aud, Pr George's Co Hlth Dept, **A**

Arnold, Barbara J 10 Wentworth Drive, Amherst, MA 01002, (413) 253-2010, BS 77 Univ of MA - Amherst; MA 81 Univ of MA - Amherst; Aud, Franklin Med Cen, **A**

Arnold, Carol Brown 1708 North Barton Street, Arlington, VA 22201

Arnold, Mrs Claire L 11 Club Lane, Littleton, CO 80123, (303) 233-1666, BA 71 Elmira Coll; MA 72 Univ of Denver; VP-Prog, Co Er Sl So, **SLP**

Arnold, David Middle Tennessee State Univ, Box 364, Murfreesboro, TN 37132, (615) 898-2661, BA 52 David Lipscomb Coll; MA 62 LA St Univ - Baton Rouge; Assoc Prof, Mid TN St U, **SLP**

Arnold, Deborah A 130 Echol Lane, Travelers Rest, SC 29690, (803) 834-9735, MS 78 East TN St Univ; Sp-Lang Path, Greenville Co Sch, **SLP**

Arnold, Genevieve 4926 Culmore Drive, Houston, TX 77021, (713) 747-9159, BA 34 Univ of MN - Minneap-St Paul; MA 36 Univ of MN - Minneap-St Paul; PH 55 (NS) Univ of Houston - Univ Park; **SLP LM**

Arnold, Dr Godfrey E P O Box 906, Clinton, MS 39056, (601) 924-5400, MA 36 0109; MD 37 (NS) 0108; **F H LM**

Arnold, Mrs Janice M 3588 Betty Ford Road, Murfreesboro, TN 37130, (615) 893-7604, BS 63 Middle TN St Univ; ME 76 Middle TN St Univ; 63–Sp-Lang Path, Rutherford Co Sch, **SLP**

Arnold, Mrs Julia L 2267 Cedardale Avenue, Baton Rouge, LA 70808, (504) 387-1259, BS 44 GA Southern Coll; ME 54 LA St Univ - Baton Rouge; **SLP LM**

Arnold, Kathy L 1155 Rickey Drive, Yuba City, CA 95991, (916) 674-9911, **SLP**

Arnold, Kay L 7603 Nantucket, Wichita, KS 67212, (316) 721-2030, BA 85 Wichita St Univ; 86–Sp-Lang Path, Wichita Child Care Assoc, **SLP**

Arnold, Kelly Ann 1016 Connecticut Apartment 2, Joplin, MO 64801, (417) 649-7011, OB 85 Univ of MO - Columbia; OM 87 Univ of MO - Columbia; 87–Sp-Lang Path, Carl Junction R-1 Sch Dist, **SLP**

Arnold, Laura Jean Trover Clinic, Clinic Drive, Madisonville, KY 42431, (502) 825-7279, BA 85 Univ of Northern CO; MA 86 Univ of Northern CO; 87–Aud, Trover Clinic, **A**

Arnold, Linda Jean 430 Northwest 46th Avenue, Plantation, FL 33317-2038, (305) 325-0470, BS 84 FL St Univ; MS 87 FL St Univ; **SLP**

Arnold, Mrs Lynn C Audiology Speech Pathology 126, Vamc, 700 South 19th Street, Birmingham, AL 35233, (205) 933-1857, BA 69 Univ of AL- Tuscaloosa; MA 71 Univ of AL- Tuscaloosa; Audiologist, VA Hospital, **SLP A**

Arnold, Marcia L 11918 Cameo Place, Granada Hills, CA 91344, (818) 360-8911, BA 69 Univ of CA - Berkeley; MA 81 CA St Univ - Los Angeles; Sp-Lang Path, Los Angeles USD, **SLP**

Arnold, Marcia M Route 3 Box 158, Leesburg, GA 31763, (912) 759-6278, BS 69 Univ of GA; ME 73 Univ of GA; 85–Sp-Lang Path /Spec Ed Coord, Lee Co Schs, **SLP**

Arnold, Maretta J 44 Forest Boulevard, Park Forest, IL 60466, MS; **SLP**

Arnold, Mary Beth Shick 4525 Mockingbird Lane, Dallas, TX 75205, (713) 462-6192, BS 78 SUNY - Coll at Geneseo; MA 80 Univ of Houston - Univ Park; Dir, Assoc In Sp-Lang & Lrng, **SLP**

Arnold, Mary Duncan 1613 Skyline Drive, Gautier, MS 39553, (601) 388-1376, BA 84 Univ of MS; MS 85 Univ of MS; Aud, Aud Sp & L Clinic, **A**

Arnold, Peggy Lee 1020 Bay Street #A, Santa Monica, CA 90405, (213) 452-2457, MA 83 CA St Univ - Northridge; BA 81 CA St Univ - Northridge; SLP, Los Angeles USD, **SLP**

Arnold, Ruth H 10018 Wayne Road, Cheyenne, WY 82009, BA 68; MS 69; 80–Sp-Lang Path, Laramie Co Sch Dist #1, **SLP**

Arnold, Ruth Levine 42 Annawan Road, Waban, MA 02168, (617) 965-3171, BS 70 Boston Univ; MS 72 Univ of Pittsburgh - Pittsburgh; Sp/Lang Path, Private Practice, **SLP**

Arnold, Dr Sally A Children's Sph & Hearing Clinic, 936 Delaware Avenue, Buffalo, NY 14209, (716) 878-7371, BS 74 SUNY - Coll at Buffalo; MS 75 Syracuse Univ; PH 84 (Aud & Hrng Impairment) Northwestern Univ; 87–Aud, Children's Hosp of Buffalo, **A**

Arnold, Mrs Shirley Ann 532 Northlawn Drive, Youngstown, OH 44505, (216) 743-1151, BS 58 OH St Univ; SLP, Youngstown Sch, **SLP**

Arnold-Cockburn, Mrs Shelley 6930 Southeast Norbert Dr, Milwaukie, OR 97222, (503) 654-5183, BS 83 Univ of OR; MS 87 Portland St Univ; 88–Sp-Lang Path, Portland PS, **SLP**

Arnott, Mrs Lora Lynn 3313 O' Henry Road, Brooklyn Center, MN 55429, (612) 566-7015, BA 79 Univ of MO - KS City; MA 82 Univ of MN - Minneap-St Paul; Sp-Lang Path, **SLP**

Arnott, Mary Ann 318 Canary Lane, Iola, KS 66749, (316) 365-6605, BS 69 Univ of Houston - Univ Park; MA 71 Univ of KS; Sp-Lang Path, Anw Special Education Coop, **SLP**

Arnovitz, Mrs Elaine S 5331 Highmeadow Lane, Dayton, OH 45415, (513) 277-0400, BS 81 Univ of Cincinnati; MA 82 Northwestern Univ; Sp-Lang Path, Doty House Inc, **SLP**

Arnovitz, Mrs Laura Mazo 2205 Deodara Cove, Memphis, TN 38138, (901) 767-5571, BS 76 SUNY - Center at Buffalo; MA 78 SUNY - Center at Buffalo; V P for Advertising & Sales, Workbench, **A**

Arnson, Cheryl Byer 18 Springdale Road, Kendall Park, NJ 08824, (201) 321-7063, BA 80 MI St Univ; MA 81 MI St Univ; Aud, JFK Medical Ctr, **A**

Arnst, Dr Dennis James Hearing Services & Consultants, 1040 East Herndon, Fresno, CA 93710, (209) 435-4678, BA 68 Univ of WI - Madison; MA 70 OH Univ - Athens; PH 73 (NS) OH Univ - Athens; Dir, Hrng Serv & Consult, **A ACE**

Arntson, Mrs Rachel M 19203 81st Place North, Corcoran, MN 55369, (612) 420-3050, BS 78 Northern St Coll; MS 80 Phillips Univ; 88–Sp-Lang Path, Park Nicollet Med Ctr, **SLP**

Aroesty, Mrs Fern 17228 Bullock Street, Encino, CA 91316, (818) 997-2357, BA 61 Univ of CA - Los Angeles; SLP, LA USD, **SLP**

Aron, Mrs Arlis 36 Woodside Avenue, Westport, CT 06880-3028, (203) 454-3986, BA 68 Univ of Pittsburgh - Pittsburgh; ME 70 Boston Univ; Sp/Lang Path, Westport Sch Sys, **SLP**

Aron, Mrs Elizabeth Foreman 4128 North Monitor, Chicago, IL 60634, (312) 283-7219, BS 83 Bradley Univ; MS 84 Bradley Univ; 88–Sp-Lang Path, Our Lady Resurrection Med Ctr, **SLP**

Aron, Prof Myrtle L Dept Speech Path & Audiology, Univ Of The Witwatersrand, Milner Park, Johannesburg, South Africa, BA 52 Witwatersrand Univ S Africa; MA 59 Witwatersrand Univ S Africa; PH 64 (Sp Path (Stuttering)) Witwatersrand Univ S Africa; 72–Sp-Lang Path, U of the Witwatersrand, **SLP**

Aronin, Meryl W 172 Dannell Drive, Stamford, CT 06905, (203) 977-4848, BA 67 Univ of WI - Whitewater; MA 71 Univ of KS; OM 80 Univ of Bridgeport; Supvr Lang Sp & Hrng Svcs, Stamford Hlth Dept, **SLP**

Aronoff, Mrs Rebecca C 4538 Narraganset Trail, Sarasota, FL 34233, (813) 924-7040, BA 60 Miami Univ - Oxford; ME 65 Miami Univ - Oxford; **SLP LM**

Arons, Mrs Lauri Jill 6304 Kerryhill Court, Agoura Hills, CA 91301, (818) 889-4004, BA 74 Univ of CA - Los Angeles; MA 83 CA St Univ - Northridge; **SLP**

Aronson, Anne Jody 18 Pleasant Gardens Road, Canton, MA 02021, BS 76 Univ of MA - Amherst; MS 78 Boston Univ; Sp-Lang Path, City of Boston, **SLP**

Aronson, Dr Arnold E Mayo Clinic, 200 1st Street S W, Rochester, MN 55901, (507) 284-3112, BS 51 Univ of WI - Madison; MS 52 Univ of WI - Madison; PH 57 (Speech Pathology) Univ of WI - Madison; Head, Sect of Sp-Path, Mayo Clinic, **SLP F**

Aronson, Hannah U 9 Riverview Drive West, Upper Montclair, NJ 07043, (201) 744-6112, BA 30 CUNY - Hunter Coll; MA 32 Columbia Univ Teachers Coll; Sp-Lang Path, Private Practice, **SLP LM**

Aronson, Joan Leach 655 Exchange Place Ste C-1, Lilburn, GA 30247, (404) 381-1772, BA 73 Univ of Miami; ME 74 Univ of Miami; Dir, Gr Atlanta Sp/Lang Clinics, **SLP**

Aronson, Mrs Nola Clark 26153 Las Lanas Court, Valencia, CA 91355, (805) 259-1687, BS 75 Univ of Hartford; MA 82 CA St Univ - Long Beach; Aud, **A**

Arps, Ritalyn K 708 Merlin Drive, Green Bay, WI 54301, (414) 336-0225, BA 71 Univ of WI - Oshkosh; MA 73 Univ of IA; 87–Sp-Lang Path, Green Bay Area PS, **SLP A**

Arras, Mrs Patricia Gail 135 Mesquitewood, Coppell, TX 75019, (214) 270-8807, BS 82 Southern Methodist Univ; MS 84 Univ of TX - Dallas; Aud, Mesquite ISD, **A**

Arrington, Mrs Roberta Barker 8137 Meadowdale Lane, Charlotte, NC 28212, (803) 328-1864, BS 82 James Madison Univ; ME 84 James Madison Univ; 86–Aud, ENT Clinic PA, **A**

Arrow, Mrs Donna K 2 Edna Place, New Rochelle, NY 10804, (914) 793-6130, BA 70 Temple Univ; MA 72 Northwestern Univ; Sp-Lang Path, Eastchester Un-Free Sch Dist, **SLP**

Arrowsnith, Amy L 845 North 29th, Lincoln, NE 68503, (402) 477-6491, MS 88 Univ of NE - Lincoln

Arroyo, Mrs Marian L 1301 S W 74th Terrace, Plantation, FL 33317, (305) 581-4630, BS 68 Univ of IL - Urbana; MA 73 Univ of Tulsa; Sp-Lang Path, Sch Bd of Broward County, **SLP**

Arruda, Patricia A P O Box 740, West Hyannisport, MA 02672, (508) 778-7979, BS 76 Bridgewater St Coll; MA 81 Southeastern MA Univ; MS 82 Univ of RI; 88–Sp-Lang Path, Dennis/Yarmouth PS, **SLP**

Arsanis, David J 1416 West Lincoln Road, Stockton, CA 95207, (209) 474-1499, BA 70 CA St Univ - Fresno; MA 72 Univ of the Pacific; SLP, Stockton USD, **SLP**

Arsenault, Joan Kelly Massachusetts General Hospital, Language Disorders, Ambulatory Care Center 637, Boston, MA 02114, (617) 726-2763, BA 79 Stockton St Coll; MA 81 Memphis St Univ; Supvr/Coord of In-Patients, Mass General Hosp, **SLP**

Arsenault, Michael Dennis #305 Professional Bldg, 2171 Jefferson, Trenton, MI 48183, (313) 577-1393, BS 83 Wayne St Univ; MA 85 Wayne St Univ - Sch of Med; Audiologist, Custom Hearing Aid Center, **A**

Arsenault, Patricia Ann 2171 West Jefferson, Suite 305, Trenton, MI 48183, (313) 676-7442, BS 82 Oakland Univ; MA 87 Wayne St Univ; **A**

Arshen, Beverly S 501 East 87th Street #3-J, New York, NY 10128, (212) 794-1704, BA 68 CUNY - City College; MA 69 Univ of FL; Sp-Lang Path, NYC Bd of Educ Dist 2-Manhattan, **SLP**

Arshen, Mrs Joan R 11 Huyler Road, Somerville, NJ 08876, (201) 685-1055, BA 75 Rutger's St Univ - Douglas Coll; MS 76 Columbia Univ Teachers Coll; Sp-Lang Path, Private Practice, **SLP**

Arst, Linda B P O Box 1382, Marblehead, MA 01945-5382, **SLP**

Artemenko, Sherry Younger 105 Sturbridge, Southport, CT 06490, (203) 259-6161, BS 73 Northwestern Univ; MA 74 Northwestern Univ; 88–Sp-Lang Path, Fairfield PS, **SLP**

Arterbury, Mrs Tammy S 5185 Pony Creek Circle, Colorado Springs, CO 80919, (719) 598-9563, BA 80 Wichita St Univ; MA 81 Wichita St Univ; 85–Sp-Lang Path, Widefield School District 3, **SLP**

Artes, Dr Richard 401 North Taft Road, Muncie, IN 47304, (317) 285-6571, BA 49 AZ St Univ; MA 51 Univ of IA; PH 67 (NS) Univ of IA; Prof & Cl Coor, Ball St U, **SLP**

Arthur, Deborah W University Of Tennessee, Dept Of Audiology, Knoxville, TN 37996-0740, (615) 974-5453, BS 71 East TN St Univ; MA 73 Univ of TN - Knoxville; Asst Prof, U of TN, **A**

Arthur, Gail Wimp 23 Cherry Lane Drive, Englewood, CO 80110, **SLP**

Arthur, Priscilla S 307 17th Street S E, Washington, DC 20003, (202) 675-7324, **A**

Arthur, Susan Ann 2559 North Tucson Blvd, Apartment 2202, Tucson, AZ 85716-2461, (602) 326-7569, BS 83 CA St Univ - Hayward; MS 85 Univ of AZ; **SLP**

Artigliere, Julia Marie 5607 Mt Audubon Place, Longmont, CO 80501, (303) 530-9212, BS 76 West Chester Univ of PA; MA 79 West Chester Univ of PA; PhD Cand/Rsrch Asst, U of CO, **SLP**

Artis, Mrs Carmen W Bb-147 Stedwick Drive, Budd Lake, NJ 07828, (201) 361-0800, BA 70 Univ of MD - College Park; MA 71 George Washington Univ; Sp-Lang Path, Randolph Twsp Pub Sch, **SLP**

Aruta, Donna Marian 29-11 169th Street, Flushing, NY 11358, (718) 359-7138, BS 83; MS 84; 88–Sp-Lang Path, Sch for Lang and Commun Devel, **SLP**

Arvedson, Dr Joan Carol Department Of Speech Language And Hearing, Children's Hospital, 219 Bryant Street, Buffalo, NY 14209, (716) 878-7371, BS 63 Univ of WI - Madison; MS 64 Univ of WI - Madison; PH 86 (Sp-Lang Path) Univ of WI - Madison; 88–Dir, Children's Hosp of Buffalo, **SLP**

Arvin, Regina S B 7745 East 95th Terrace Dr, Kansas City, MO 64134, **SLP**

Arvold, Joan P 5009 Proctor Avenue, Oakland, CA 94618, (415) 547-0951, BA 63 William Paterson Coll; **SLP**

Arwood, Dr Ellyn Lucas P O Box 18191, Portland, OR 97218-0191, (503) 283-7135, BA 71 Univ of OR; MA 73 WA St Univ; ED 77 (NS) Univ of GA; Assoc Prof/Dir Human Svcs, Univ of Portland, **SLP**

Arwood, Thomas Wheeler P O Box 18191, Portland, OR 97218, (503) 235-4119, BA 72 Univ of TX - Austin; MA 77 TX Tech Univ; OD 82 (Law) TX Tech Univ; 88–Pres, Arwood Pragmat Inst for Comm Therapy Inc

Arzt, Aliza C P 104 Josephine Avenue, Somerville, MA 02144, (617) 566-1408, BA 77 Univ of PA; MS 81 Boston Univ; Sp/Lang Path, University Hospital, **SLP**

Asamen, Julie Kimiko 185 West D Street #5, Brawley, CA 92227, (619) 344-8113, BA 81 CA St Univ - Northridge; MA 83 CA St Univ - Northridge; 83–Sp-Lang Path, Brawley Sch Dist, **SLP**

Asaro, Danna Valdin 5108 Pike Drive, Metairie, LA 70003, (504) 367-3120, BA 76 Univ of Southwestern LA; OM 78 LA St Univ - N O Medical Ctr; Sp/Lang Path, Jefferson Parish Sch Bd, **SLP**

Asato, Joanne Chiemi 98 Airako Avenue, Hilo, HI 96720, (808) 732-1725, BA 81 Univ of CO - Denver; MA 83 Univ of CO - Denver; Audiologist, Hawaii State Dept of Health, **A**

Asby, Robert S Suite 320 Medical Arts Bldg, 35 West Linden Street, Wilkes-Barre, PA 18702, (717) 826-6892, BS 59 Bloomsburg Univ of PA; MS 66 WV Univ; 68–Sp-Lang Path/Aud, Private Practice, **SLP A**

Aschbacher, Mrs Julie Agnes 6520 Marble 23-25 Lane, Gladstone, MI 49837, (906) 428-1608, BS 82 Univ of WI - Stevens Point; MS 84 Univ of WI - Stevens Point; 84–Sp-Lang Path, Gladstone Area Schs, **SLP**

Ascher, Christine Ann 1010 West Springfield #206, Urbana, IL 61801, MA 88 Univ of IL - Urbana

Aschliman, Mrs Teri L 3486 Thornhill Drive, Jacksonville, FL 32211, (904) 721-2144, MA 70 Univ of South FL; Principal, Diocese of St Augustine

Asciutto, Mrs Marium Al-Oboudi 2257 South 11th Street, Kalamazoo, MI 49009, (616) 375-1861, MA 88 Western MI Univ

Ash, Carol Diane 8655 Belford Avenue, #162, Los Angeles, CA 90045, (213) 216-1613, BA 81 Univ of CA - Santa Barbara; MA 83 CA St Univ - Los Angeles; Aud, Private Practice, **A**

Ash, Harry B 1425 Ellis Hollow Road, Ithaca, NY 14850-9601, (607) 733-6541, MS 75 Univ of South FL; 86–Admin, Health Resources Inc, **SLP**

Ash, Kathryn Lynn Route 1 Box 100, Sistersville, WV 26175, (304) 652-2267, MA 87 WV Univ

Ash, Mrs Mary S 6561 Clays Mill Road, Lexington, KY 40514-1242, (606) 223-7554, BA 64 Univ of IA; MA 75 Univ of IA; Early Childhood Consult, Mid-South Reg Resource Ctr, **SLP**

Ash, Pamela Helen 1234 South 89th Street, West Allis, WI 53214, (414) 327-3939, BS 80 Saint Louis Univ; MS 82 Univ of WI - Milwaukee; Director Sp-Lang Path, Shared Theraputic Serv, **SLP**

Ash, Wendy Lynn 1525 Amherst Manor Drive, Apartment 810, Buffalo, NY 14221, (716) 632-5479, BA 86 SUNY - Center at Buffalo; MA 81 SUNY - Center at Buffalo; 87–Sp-Lang Path, Millard Fillmore Hosp, **SLP**

Ashbaugh, Mrs Judith A 1535 South Gillette, Tulsa, OK 74104, (918) 631-2898, BA 60 Univ of OK - Norman; OM 65; Asst Prof, University of Tulsa, **SLP**

Ash-Bernstein, Melissa Hillary 6740 Yellowstone Boulevard, Apartment 30, Forest Hills, NY 11375-2623, (516) 338-4204, MA 83 George Washington Univ; SLP, North Shore Hospital, **SLP**

Ashby, Dr Jon K Abilene Christian University, Station Box 8058, Abilene, TX 79699, (915) 677-1911, BS 64 Abilene Christian Univ; MA 66 LA St Univ - Baton Rouge; PH 72 (NS) LA St Univ - Baton Rouge; Prof/Dir Commun Dis Prog, Abilene Christian U, **SLP A**

Ashcom, Mrs Pamela H 4748 153rd Avenue Southeast, Bellevue, WA 98006, (206) 641-4965, BA 71 Valparaiso Univ; MS 75 Loma Linda Univ - Riverside; Sp-Lang Path, Private Practice, **SLP**

Ashcraft, Paula S 3379 Rexford Place, Salt Lake City, UT 84121, (801) 943-0862, BS 72 Univ of UT; MS 74 Univ of UT; Resource Teacher, Salt Lake City Sch Dist, **SLP**

Ashe, Betty C Route 10, 86 Simpson Road, Gulfport, MS 39503, (601) 467-1021, BA 57 Northwestern St Univ; MA 60 Northwestern St Univ; MA 70 Univ of KY; Superv of Sp Ed, Bay St Louis Sep Sch Dist, **SLP**

Ashe, Mrs Frances Marie 46 Tracy Lyn Road, Holliston, MA 01746, MS 85 Worcester St Coll; Sp-Lang Path, Walpole Area Visiting Nurses, **SLP**

Ashelin, Cynthia A 539 5th Street N W, Sioux Center, IA 51250, (712) 722-4374, BA 79 Coll of Saint Teresa; MS 80 Univ of WI - Eau Claire; 82–Sp-Lang Path, AEA 4, **SLP**

Asher, Margaret 1369 West 23rd Avenue, Golden, CO 80401, (303) 424-8439, BS 69 Univ of CO - Boulder; MA 74 Univ of CO - Boulder; Sp-Lang Path, Jefferson Co Sch, **SLP**

Ashford, John R 304 Country Court, Antioch, TN 37013, BS 67 Univ Southern MS-Hattiesburg; MS 68 Univ Southern MS-Hattiesburg; Sp-Lang Path, VA Medical Center, **SLP**

Ashford, Mrs Pamela C 9260 Alcosta Boulevard Suite 14B, San Ramon, CA 94550, (415) 830-9333, BS 78 CA St Univ - Hayward; MS 81 San Francisco St Univ; Sp-Lang Path, Bay Area Sp/Lang/Hrng Clinic, **SLP**

Ashinoff, Mrs Ellen Herbst 3452 Steven Road, Baldwin Harbor, NY 11510, (718) 851-3700, BS 77 SUNY - Center at Albany; MS 78 Adelphi Univ; Sp-Lang Path, Metro Jewish Geriatric Center, **SLP ACE**

Ashkinaze, Barbara 500 East 77th Street #327, New York, NY 10162, (212) 439-9127, BA 80 George Washington Univ; MS 82 Boston Univ; Audiologist, **A**

Ashland, Jean E 484 Commercial St #2, Boston, MA 02109, (617) 726-2762, BS 81 Univ of WY; MA 83 San Diego St Univ; Sp-Lang Path, MA Gen Hosp, **SLP**

Ashley, Betty Ann Marie 134-07 101st Avenue, Richmond Hill, NY 11419, (212) 430-2441, BA 83 Barnard Coll; MS 86 Columbia Univ Teachers Coll; Sp-Lang Path, J F Kennedy Ctr, **SLP**

Ashley, Betty Thomas 511 Hodges Drive N W, Orangeburg, SC 29115, (803) 536-4566, BA 78 Columbia Coll; MA 81 SC St Coll; SLP, Orangeburg City Schools, **SLP**

Ashley, Debra Lynn West 113 Florence, Spokane, WA 99218, (509) 467-6858, BA 86 Eastern WA Univ; MA 87 WA St Univ; 88–Aud, Spokane ENT Clinic PS

Ashley, Donna Debolt 274 Bay West Neighbors Ct, Orlando, FL 32811, (305) 298-4622, BA 76 Univ of FL; MA 87 Univ of Central FL; **SLP**

Ashley, Mark J Centre For Neuro Skills, 2658 Mt Vernon, Bakersfield, CA 93306, (805) 872-3408, BS 77 SUNY - Coll at Geneseo; MS 79 Southern IL Univ -Carbondale; Exec Dir, Centre for Neuro Skills, **SLP**

Ashley, Mrs Melinda Varda 17 Chippendale Court, Horse Shoe, NC 28742, (704) 891-4581, BS 81 WV Univ; MS 82 WV Univ; 86–Sp-Lang Path, Private Practice, **SLP**

Ashley, Stephen J 3503 Dauphine Street, Sebring, FL 33870, (813) 385-4980, BA 72 King's Coll; MS 76 SUNY - Coll at Fredonia; SLP, Highlands Co Sch Sys, **SLP**

Ashley, Susan M 1901 Haggin Oaks Drive, Bakersfield, CA 93311-1529, (805) 872-3408, BS 77 SUNY - Coll at Geneseo; MS 79 Southern IL Univ -Carbondale; SLP Dept Head, Cen for Neuro Skills, **SLP**

Ashley-Smutko, Mrs Nan N Capron Rehab Center, P O Box 7021, Colorado Springs, CO 80933, (303) 630-5200, BS 70 Bowling Green St Univ; MA 72 Bowling Green St Univ; 86–Mgr Sp-Lang Path, Penrose Hosp, **SLP**

Ashmar, Sharon Miller 1069 Spruce Road #3C, Wescosville, PA 18106, (215) 995-3727, BS 84 Bloomsburg Univ of PA; MS 85 Bloomsburg Univ of PA; Sp-Lang Path, Cedarbrook County Home, **SLP**

Ashmead, Dr Allez M 719 East Center Street, Kaysville, UT 84037, (801) 544-3066, BS 38 UT St Univ; MS 50 Univ of UT; PH 70 (Secondary Stuttering) Univ of UT; Sp-Lang Path, Harrison Prof Cen, **SLP LM ACE**

Ashmont, Janice Gomez 5 Chestnut Lane, Unionville, CT 06085, (203) 563-8181, BA 75 Univ of MA - Amherst; MA 76 Univ of MA - Amherst; Sp-Lang Path, Wethersfield Pub Sch, **SLP**

Ashmore, Lear Lee Speech Department, University Of Texas, Austin, TX 78712, (512) 450-1177, BA 49 Univ of TX - Austin; ME 53 Univ of TX - Austin; PH 58 (Sp Path) Univ of WI - Madison; Prof Emeritus, U TX Austin, **SLP F**

Ashmore, Mrs Susan H 375 West Broad Street, Souderton, PA 18964, (215) 539-8550, BS 70 Bloomsburg Univ of PA; MA 73 Kent St Univ; SLP, Montgy Co Inter Ut #23, **SLP**

Ashton, Carol G 2225 Ashley River Road, Apartment 268, Charleston, SC 29414-9754, (803) 766-7358, BS 63 Univ of CA - Davis; MS 79 William Paterson Coll; Dir of Sp-Lang Serv, **SLP**

Ashton, Lori Jean c/o Patricia Ashton, 125 Oak Hill Drive, Willimantic, CT 06226-1224, (215) 242-4320, BA 83 Univ of VT; MA 85 Temple Univ-Tyler Sch of Art; **SLP**

Ashworth, Kathleen F P O Box 62, Totowa Boro, NJ 07512, (201) 785-3060, MA 68 William Paterson Coll; MS 78 William Paterson Coll; 88–Sp-Lang Path, Private Practice

Ashworth, Mrs Michelle A 528 E Madison Street, Villa Park, IL 60181, (312) 941-1305, BS 82 Elmhurst Coll; ME 87 Univ of VA - Charlottesville; 87–Aud, Mercy Hosp & Med Ctr, **A**

Ashworth, Myra Y Pacific Asia Christian Univ, P O Box Ywam, Kailua Kona, HI 96745, (808) 329-7784, BS 75 Southern IL Univ -Carbondale; MS 79 Southeast MO St Univ; Early Childhood, Pacific Asia Christ U, **SLP**

Askeland, Mrs Susan R 4408 Applewood Avenue, Sioux City, IA 51106, (712) 274-6040, BS 73 Univ of NE - Lincoln; MA 74 Univ of NE - Lincoln; Sp-Lang Path, Wn Hills AEA 12, **SLP**

Askew, Benna L 7148 Rothland Street, Dallas, TX 75227-1832, (214) 372-7013, BS 65 Univ of TX - Austin; MS 71 Univ of North TX; 75–Sp-Lang Path, VA Med Center, **SLP**

Askew, Wanda 2065 Canakin Court #24, St Louis, MO 63146, (314) 652-3600, BS 78 Memphis St Univ; MA 80 Memphis St Univ; Sp-Lang Path, Cardinal Ritter I, **SLP**

Askins, Mrs Judith C 5687 Running Brook Road, Farmington, NY 14425, (716) 398-3012, BS 73 Indiana Univ of PA; MS 75 Indiana Univ of PA; **SLP**

Aslin, Larry W 2884 Sunny Lane, Fayetteville, AR 72703, (501) 575-4918, BA 70 Univ of MO - Columbia; MA 73 Univ of MO - Columbia; Res Asst - Cl Coord, U of Arkansas, Fayetteville, **SLP**

Aslin, Mary E 2884 Sunny Lane, Fayetteville, AR 72703, BS 72 Southwest MO St Univ; MA 73 Univ of MO - Columbia; Sp-Lang Path, Fayetteville Pub Schs, **SLP**

Asmussen, Anita Ruth 1534 Northeast 26th #8, Portland, OR 97232, (206) 533-0450, BA 81 Eastern WA Univ; MA 84 Western WA Univ; Sp-Lang Path, Visiting Nurse Association, **SLP**

Asp, Dr Carl W Dept Audiology & Speech Path, University Of Tennessee, 457 South Stadium, Knoxville, TN 37996-0740, (615) 523-0969, BS 63 OH St Univ; MA 64 OH St Univ; PH 67 (NS) OH St Univ; Professor, University of Tennessee, **SLP A F**

Aspan, Mary Ann W302 N970 Maple Avenue, Waukesha, WI 53188, (414) 778-6588, BS 82 SUNY - Coll at Buffalo; MS 84 SUNY - Coll at Buffalo; 86–Sp-Lang Path, Wauwatosa Sch Dist, **SLP**

Aspelund, Mrs Leanna C 20626 Castle Bend Drive, Katy, TX 77450, (713) 578-7110, BS 74 Saint Mary's Dominican Coll; OM 75 LA St Univ - N O Medical Ctr; **SLP**

Asper, Nancy Jo NC Hospital, 1100 West 38th Street, Bemidji, MN 56601, (218) 751-5430, MS 83 Moorhead St Univ; Sp-Path, North Country Health Services, **SLP**

Asperheim, Kelly Lynn 1410 A Avenue East, Oskaloosa, IA 52577, (515) 682-8591, BA 84 Augustana Coll; MA 85 Northeast MO St Univ; 85–Sp-Lang Path, Southern Prairie AEA 15, **SLP**

Aspinall, Dr Kenneth B Usareur-Audiology Center, Landstuhl Army Medical Ctr, Box 52, APO New York, NY 09180-5300, BS 65 Univ of NE - Lincoln; MA 66 Univ of KS; PH 73 (NS) Univ of CO - Boulder; Ch/Aud Cl, Usareur-Audiology Ctr, **A ACE**

Aspiras, Rose Angela 2219 Port Trinity Circle, Stockton, CA 95206-4803, (209) 943-5628, BA 83 CA St Univ - Fresno; MA 88 CA St Univ - Fresno

Asplund, Mrs Janet Pochailo Rural Route 1, Fort Frances, ON, Canada P9A 1M1, 77–Sp-Lang Path, Ft Francis Rainy River Boe, **SLP**

Aster, Christine Pampush 25261 Margot Court, Beachwood, OH 44122, (216) 942-0260, BS 75 Miami Univ - Oxford; MA 76 Kent St Univ; Sp-Lang Path, Lake Co Bd of Men Ret, **SLP**

Asthana, Mrs Pamela Sulochini 117 West Glencrest Drive, Mankato, MN 56001, (507) 388-2994, BS 70 PA St Univ - Univ Park; MS 77

Astorino, Marylou 160 Engbert Road, Johnstown, PA 15902, (814) 536-0401, BS 79 Indiana Univ of PA; MS 80 PA St Univ - Univ Park; Aud, David R Rogerson MD, **A**

Astrue, Carol Marie 1627 Laramie Street #1, Manhattan, KS 66502-4045, BS 80 SD St Univ; MA 82 Univ of SD - Vermillion; **SLP**

Atack, Dr Rodney M 13208 Osterport Drive, Silver Spring, MD 20906, (202) 576-2413, BS 63 Brigham Young Univ; MS 72 Brigham Young Univ; PH 83 (Aud) Univ of UT; 86–Dir Army Aud and Sp Ctr, Walter Reed Army Med Ctr, **A ACE**

Atanowsky, Orysia I 1024 South Peale Avenue, Park Ridge, IL 60068, (312) 398-4288, BA 70 Univ of IL - Chicago; MA 74 Northern IL Univ - De Kalb; SLP, Arlington Hts Pub Schs, **SLP**

Atcheson, Dr Barbara A 19536 S E 51st Street, Issaquah, WA 98027, (206) 326-4075, BS 62 Univ of WI - Madison; MS 63 Univ of WI - Madison; PH 76 (NS) Univ of WA; Aud, Pacific Hlth Assoc of Seattle, **SLP A**

Atchison, Mrs Shirley A 525 Highland Woods Drive E, Mobile, AL 36608, (205) 478-5266, BA 66 Univ of AL-Tuscaloosa; MS 79 Univ of South AL; SLP, Mobile Co Public Schools, **SLP**

Atchison, Susan L 3017 Gilmer, Abilene, TX 79606, (915) 670-2134, BA 75 Northeast LA Univ; MA 77 Univ of SD - Vermillion; Aud, Hendrick Medical Center, **A**

Atchley, Pamela Sue R R 2 Box 179, Tipton, IN 46072, (317) 675-8050, **SLP**

Atchue, Catherine Mary 18 Hooper Street, Westwood, MA 02090, (617) 326-6336, BS 84 Univ of NH; MA 86 Univ of MA - Amherst; **SLP**

Aten, Dr James L Audiology/Sp Path Serv (126), Long Beach VA Medical Ctr, 5901 East 7th Street, Long Beach, CA 90822, (213) 494-5415, BA 53 Univ of Redlands; MA 56 Univ of Redlands; PH 60 (Sp Path) Univ of WA; Chief Sp-Path/Aud Svc, Long Beach VA Med Cen, **SLP F**

Atencio, Rebecca Leora P O Box 1223, Aztec, NM 87410, (505) 334-2621, BS 82 Eastern NM Univ; MS 83 Eastern NM Univ; 84–Sp-Lang Path, Aztec Municipal Schs, **SLP**

Ater, Mrs Jacquelyn 181 Beaconview Court, Rochester, NY 14617, (716) 342-7867, BS 74 SUNY - Coll at Brockport; MA 75 SUNY - Coll at Geneseo; 78–Sp-Lang Path, Genesee Hospital, **SLP**

Ater, Judy A 1400 Moonstone Way #2, Louisville, KY 40222, (502) 588-5331, BS 76 Univ of GA; MS 78 Univ of Louisville; Coord Early Diag & Interv Prgm, Chld Eval Cen, **SLP**

Atha, Mrs Karen J B 2555 Ranfield Road, Mogadore, OH 44260, (216) 724-1227, BS 74 Univ of Akron; MA 78 Univ of Akron; Sp-Lang Path, Akron Pub Sch, **SLP**

Athans, Olga 5854 Marble Drive, Troy, MI 48098, (313) 879-2786, MA 84 MI St Univ; **SLP**

Atherton, Deanna J 7520 Clear Sky Road, San Diego, CA 92120, (619) 583-5514, BS 65 Univ of MN - Duluth; MA 66 Western MI Univ; **SLP**

Atherton, Nancy J 44 Lettington Drive, Rochester, NY 14624, (716) 475-6267, BS 67 OH St Univ; MA 79 SUNY - Coll at Geneseo; SLP/Instr, NTID, **SLP**

Athey, Joseph T PO Box 7215, Napa, CA 94558, (707) 253-5845, MA 76 Univ of IA; Aud, Napa State Hospital, **A**

Athman, Teresa M 601 S E Foley Lane, Hamilton, MT 59840, (406) 363-6681, BA 71 Saint Cloud St Univ; MS 73 Saint Cloud St Univ; **SLP**

Atkin, Leanne Lynn 360 Timber Way East, Marietta, GA 30066, (404) 971-6060, BS 75 Univ of WI - Oshkosh; MS 83 Marquette Univ; Sp-Lang Path, Cobb County Public Schools, **SLP**

Atkins, Alice E 8 Malverna Road, Roslindale, MA 02131, (617) 325-0269, ME 83 Northeastern Univ; Speech Language Pathologist, New England Rehab Hospital, **SLP**

Atkins, Mrs Carol J 23442 Via Cordorniz, Trabuco Canyon, CA 92679, (619) 758-1620, BA 65 San Diego St Univ; MA 67 San Francisco St Univ; 86–Aud, Sp Hrng Neurosensory Ctr, **A**

Atkins, Dr Carolyn P 868 Vandalia Road, Morgantown, WV 26505, (304) 293-4241, BA 69 WV Univ; MA 70 WV Univ; ED 77 (NS) WV Univ; Assoc Prof/SLP, West Virginia University, **SLP**

Atkins, Mrs Elizabeth C 9000 West Wilderness Way, Apartment 72, Shreveport, LA 71106, (318) 865-5675, BA 81 LA St Univ - Shreveport; OM 82 LA St Univ - N O Medical Ctr; SLP, Caddo Parish Sch Bd, **SLP**

Atkins, Mrs Janet L 410 Margate, Atlanta, GA 30328, (404) 351-0351, BA 70 SUNY - Coll at Cortland; MA 76 CA St Univ - Los Angeles; Sp-Lang Path, W Paces Ferry Hosp, **SLP**

Atkins, Mary D 111 Eastern Avenue, Somerville, NJ 08876, (201) 526-0538, BS 80 PA St Univ - Univ Park; MS 82 Boston Univ; Sp-Lang Path, The Midland Sch, **SLP**

Atkins, Mrs Naomi R 1050 Wellington Road, Jenkintown, PA 19046, BA 77 CUNY - Brooklyn Coll; MS 79 Columbia Univ Teachers Coll; **SLP**

Atkins, Mrs Patricia Lynn 3608 Kirkfield Street, Fort Wayne, IN 46815, (219) 484-6636, BS 83 Purdue Univ - West Lafayette; MA 84 Ball St Univ; Sp-Lang Path, Parkview Reginal Outreach, **SLP**

Atkins, Mrs Pennie L 917 Frontier Park Avenue, Cheyenne, WY 82001, (307) 634-0556, MS 75 Univ of WY; **SLP**

Atkins, Wendy F 4750 Bedford Avenue #1K, Brooklyn, NY 11235, **SLP**

Atkinson, Connie G 3324 South Lamar Boulevard, Oxford, MS 38655, (601) 232-3766, BA 72 Univ of MS; OM 73 Univ of MS; 87–Instr/Clin Supvr, Univ of MS Sp and Hrng Ctr, **SLP**

Atkinson, Mrs Eleanor R Box 96, Penns Park, PA 18943, (215) 598-7717, BS 65 Temple Univ; MA 67 Temple Univ; SLP, Bucks Co Sch I U 22, **SLP**

Atkinson, Dr James Edward Metavox Inc, 8375 Leesburg Pike, Suite 421, Vienna, VA 22180, (703) 759-2995

Atkinson, Mrs Karen Staicer 15935 Bent Tree Forest Circle, #2065, Dallas, TX 75248, (214) 590-8139, BS 84 Univ of North TX; MS 87 Univ of North TX; 87–Sp-Lang Path, Parkland Mem Hosp, **SLP**

Atkinson, Mrs Kimberly Harder 29 Spotted Deer Drive, Tallahassee, FL 32304, (904) 482-9381, BS 82 FL St Univ; MS 84 FL St Univ; Sp-Lang Path, Florida A & M University, **SLP**

Atkinson, Mrs Lanoma 12900 Charing Cross Road, Lenexa, KS 66215, (913) 894-4248, BS 71 Univ of NE - Lincoln; MA 73 Univ of NE - Lincoln; Aud, **A**

Atkinson, Mrs Lavonne Lynne 41 Linda Lane, Bethel, CT 06801, (203) 938-2519, BS 73 Univ of SD - Vermillion; MA 77 Northern St Coll; Sp-Lang Path, Redding Sch, **SLP**

Atkinson, Mary Wray 1702 Guilford Lane, Oklahoma City, OK 73120, (405) 755-6174, BA 58 Univ of AR - Fayetteville; MS 60 Tulane Univ; Sp-Lang Path, Private Practice, **SLP ACE**

Atkinson, Mrs Pamela M 1099 6th Avenue N E, Largo, FL 34640, (813) 584-8063, BA 66 FL St Univ; MS 67 FL St Univ; Sp-Lang Path, Private Practice, **SLP**

Atkinson, Mrs Susan Ingram P O Box 294 Station A, Goose Bay, Labrador, NF, Canada A0P 1S0, (709) 896-3841, BA 77 Saint Francis Xavier Univ-Ns; MS 79 Dalhousie Univ - Nova Scotia; 87–Sp-Lang Path, Labrador E Integrated Sch Bd, **SLP**

Atkinson-Goward, Mrs Kathryn B 110 Crane Street, Alma, MI 48801, (517) 773-1209, BA 84 Valparaiso Univ; MA 85 Central MI Univ; 87–Sp-Lang Path, Allied Health Services Inc, **SLP**

Atkisson, Beth St Joseph Medical Center, Department Of Speech Pathology, Buena Vista & Alameda, Burbank, CA 91505, (818) 840-7900, BA 76 CA St Univ - Los Angeles; MA 79 CA St Univ - Los Angeles; Director Speech Pathology, St Joseph Medical Center, **SLP**

Atkisson, Nancy L 1359 Stephora Lane, Glendora, CA 91740, (213) 861-4357, BA 80 CA St Univ - Los Angeles; MA 82 CA St Univ - Los Angeles; Sp-Lang Path, Los Angeles Co Supt of Sch, **SLP**

Atlas, Deborah 3364 Quail Lake Road #128, Colorado Springs, CO 80906, (719) 560-5005, BS 74 Syracuse Univ; MA 76 Case Western Reserve Univ; Sp-Lang Path, St Mary Corwin Hospital, **SLP**

Attanasio, Dr Frederick G 78 Roosevelt Road, Hyde Park, NY 12538, (914) 431-8299, BS 56 OH Univ - Athens; MA 57 OH Univ - Athens; PH 61 (NS) OH Univ - Athens; Director/Dept of Communication, St Francis Hospital, **SLP F**

Attanasio, Joseph S 32 Normal Avenue, Upper Montclair, NJ 07043, (201) 893-4232, BA 62 Montclair St Coll; MA 65 Montclair St Coll; PH 77 (Sp Path) NY Univ; 88–Prof, Montclair State Coll, **SLP**

Attar, Vickie Lynne C-45 Canterbury Court, New Albany, IN 47150-5478, (219) 484-9846, BA 83 Ball St Univ; MA 84 Ball St Univ; **SLP**

Attaway, Mrs Judith Marie 2541 Sidon Avenue, La Habra, CA 90631, (714) 522-0150, BS 80 Univ of CA - Riverside; MA 82 CA St Univ - Los Angeles; Aud, La Palma Intercom Hosp, **A**

Attermeier, Julie A 5426 Somerset Lane South, Greenfield, WI 53221, **SLP**

Attisani, Donna M 57 September Lane, Weston, CT 06883, (203) 454-1325, BS 76 Emerson Coll; MS 77 Univ of MI - Ann Arbor; 85–Dir Communication Sciences, New Rochelle Hosp Med Cen, **SLP**

Attorri, Judith Treadwell 907 Sixth Street S W, Apartment #911-C, Washington, DC 20024, (202) 554-2951, MS 85 Univ of VT; 87–SLP, Mt Vernon Hosp, **SLP**

Atwater, Tonja Fayette 1 Pheasant Lane, Willingboro, NJ 08046, (215) 222-1300, BA 83 NC St Univ at Raleigh; MS 84 East Carolina Univ; Sp-Lang Path, Home Merciful Savior Crip Chdn, **SLP**

Atwood, Elizabeth May 5 Alamo Court, Lake City, FL 32055, (904) 599-9190, MS 86 FL St Univ; **SLP**

Atwood, Iris Brastow 41 Pembroke Avenue, Attleboro, MA 02703, (508) 222-1193, BS 86 Eastern KY Univ; ME 87 Eastern KY Univ; 88–Sp-Lang Path, Attleboro PS Sys

Atwood, Karen Hoffman 406 Kent Drive, Mechanicsburg, PA 17055, (717) 232-0101, BA 78 Wellesley Coll; ME 83 Univ of VA - Charlottesville; 87–Sp-Lang Path, Private Practice, **SLP**

Atwood, Mrs Kathryn P 812 Saturn Circle, Temple, TX 76502, (817) 939-5731, BA 66 TX Tech Univ; MA 67 TX Tech Univ; Sp-Lang Path, Belton ISD, **SLP**

Auber, Patricia Anne 21 West Maxwell Drive, West Hartford, CT, BA 80 Univ of CT; MS 83 Southern CT St Univ; Sp-Lang Path, West Hartford PS, **SLP**

Aubertine, Mrs Jane Sullivan Rd 1 Box 6, Holland Patent, NY 13354-9702, (315) 896-2654, BS 81 SUNY - Coll at Geneseo; MA 82 SUNY - Coll at Geneseo; Sp-Lang Path, UCP Center, **SLP**

Aubin, Mrs Myra L 112 Douglas Drive, Maurice, LA 70555, (318) 898-1151, MS 87 Univ of Southwestern LA; SLP, Vermilion Parish Schl Bd

Aubrey, Mrs Joan A V 33 Wild Duck Road, Wilton, CT 06897, (203) 797-4861, BA 74 Univ of Houston - Univ Park; MA 77 LA St Univ - Baton Rouge; Sp-Lang Path, Danbury Public Schools, **SLP**

Aubuchon, Mrs Pamela R 11 Algonquin Forest, Millstadt, IL 62260-1713, (618) 476-7880, BS 83 Southern IL Univ-Edwardsvill; MS 84 Southern IL Univ-Edwardsvill; Sp-Lang Path, Special School District, **SLP**

Auburn, Dr Sandra K 2510 East Drive, Fort Wayne, IN 46805, (219) 484-9746, BA 67 Univ of Akron; MA 68 Univ of Akron; PH 78 (NS) OH St Univ; Consult-Aging, Private Practice, **SLP**

Aucoin, Cheryl Lynne Hearing And Sp Center Of Roch, 1000 Elmwood Avenue, Rochester, NY 14620, (716) 271-0680, BS 83 SUNY - Coll at Geneseo; MA 84 SUNY - Coll at Geneseo; 85–Aud, Hrng & Sp Ctr of Rochester, **A**

Audet, Lisa R 200 Vine Street, Pawtucket, RI 02861, BS 81 RI Coll; MS 86 Univ of RI; Sp-Lang Path, Bradley Hosp, **SLP**

Audiffred, Martin J 300 Steeple Chase, Lafayette, LA 70506, (318) 265-5311, BA 75 Univ of Southwestern LA; MS 78 Univ of Southwestern LA; Aud, LA St Dept of Hlth, **A**

Auer, Karla M 2179 La Granada, Thousand Oaks, CA 91360, (818) 341-0931, BA 65 CA St Univ - Northridge; MA 75 CA St Univ - Northridge; Sp-Lang-Hrng Spec, LA USD, **SLP**

Auerbach, Dr Lawrence 108 Clinton Park Drive, Bergenfield, NJ 07621, (201) 384-0212, MA 54 Columbia Univ Teachers Coll; MA 73 Montclair St Coll; PH 60 (Speech) Univ of WI - Madison; 88–Prof, Fairleigh Dickinson Univ, **SLP**

Auerbach, Robin E Audiology & Hearing Clinic, 404 Walnut Street, Gadsden, AL 35901, (205) 543-3221, BA 80 Auburn Univ - Montgomery; OM 82 Auburn Univ - Auburn; Owner, Audiology & Hearing Clinic, **A**

Auerbach, Sylvia S 3733 West 173rd Street, Torrance, CA 90504, (213) 515-3084, BA 75 CA St Univ - Northridge; MA 77 CA St Univ - Northridge; SLP, Los Angeles USD, **SLP**

Auffenberg, Mrs Nancy Ann Whatley 229 River Lane, Dearborn, MI 48124, BS 76 Western MI Univ; MA 81 Eastern MI Univ; SLP, Wayne County Inter School Dist, **SLP**

Aufiero-Sanchez, Joanne 222 Brook Road, Mahopac, NY 10541, (212) 379-5020, BA 74 CUNY - Lehman Coll; MS 76 Columbia Univ Teachers Coll; Dir-SLP/Aud, Hebrew Hosp for Chronic Ill, **SLP**

Aufrecht, Joan B 2127 East 37th Avenue, Anchorage, AK 99508, BA 69 Univ of CA - Los Angeles; OM 76 CA St Univ - Los Angeles; Ed Consult, Totline

Aufricht, Dr Hedda 5451 North East River Road, Apartment 1011, Chicago, IL 60656, (312) 633-2169, BA 50 CUNY - Queens Coll; MA 51 Northwestern Univ; PH 59 (Sp Path) Northwestern Univ; Chief/Aud-SLP Ser, VA Med Cen, **SLP A**

Aufrichtig, Sandra Joseph 53 Amber Drive, Croton on Hudson, NY 10520, (914) 681-4678, BA 80 Hofstra Univ; MA 81 Hofstra Univ; Sp-Lang Path, St Agnes Childrens Rehab Cen, **SLP**

Augsburger, Julie B 1114 Priscilla Lane, Cincinnati, OH 45208, (513) 871-9084, BS 80 Miami Univ - Oxford; MS 81 Miami Univ - Oxford; Sp-Lang Path/Consultant, Cincinnati Ctr for Devel Dis, **SLP**

Augspurger, Mrs Jane Schmida 9500 Winston Avenue, Des Moines, IA 50322, (515) 224-0979, BS 83 Univ of IA; MA 85 Univ of Northern IA; Sp-Lang Path, Central Sp & Lang Services, **SLP**

August, Chandler I PO Box 701953, Tulsa, OK 74170, (918) 744-1184, BA 69 Univ of NM; MA 70 Univ of NM; Sp-Lang Path, Private Practice, **SLP**

Augustine, Joanne 1035 West Independence St, Shamokin, PA 17872, (717) 648-2904, BS 85 Bloomsburg Univ of PA; MS 86 Bloomsburg Univ of PA; **SLP**

Augustine, Dr Lloyd E 100 Norman, Lafayette, LA 70508, (318) 231-6721, BS 63 Brigham Young Univ; MS 64 Brigham Young Univ; PH 72 (NS) Univ of WA; Assoc Prof, U of LA, **SLP**

Augustine, Dr Robert M 2102 University Drive, Charleston, IL 61920, (217) 581-2712, BS 75 IL St Univ - Normal; MS 76 IL St Univ - Normal; PH 85 (NS) Southern IL Univ -Carbondale; 78–Assoc Prof, Eastern IL Univ, **SLP**

Augustine, Russell Albert 50 Robert Drive, East Haven, CT 06512, (203) 467-3668, MA 84 Univ of Akron; BA 75 Southern CT St Univ; **SLP**

Augustine, Mrs Suzanne Renee 10345 Centinella, La Mesa, CA 92041, (919) 633-0775, BA 82 Miami Univ - Oxford; MS 83 East Carolina Univ; Sp-Lang Path, Dev Eval Cen, **SLP**

Augustyniak, Carol Ann 64 Gaslight Lane, Easton, MA 02334-9999, (617) 762-1319, **SLP**

Aulbach, Melanie B 621 Dunberry Drive, Arnold, MD 21012, (301) 757-2600, BS 73 Indiana Univ of PA; ME 74 Univ of VA - Charlottesville; Sp-Lang Path, Anne Arundel Co Bd of Ed, **SLP**

Auld-Whalen, Mrs Linda A 75 Meadowview Road, Millington, NJ 07946, (201) 647-6518, BS 79 Mercy Coll; MA 81 CUNY - Hunter Coll; Sp-Lang Path, Assn for Mentally Ill Children, **SLP**

Aulis, Patricia S HC 61 Box 195DDD, Laurel Street, Etna, NH 03750, (603) 643-5208, OM 73 Univ of VT; MS 80 Univ of VT; 88–Sp-Lang Path, Dresden Sch Dist, **SLP**

Ault-Teeters, Ronna L Box 1453, Dickinson, ND 58602, (701) 225-3172, BA 70 Univ of MI - Ann Arbor; OM 74 Univ of WA; Sp-Lang Path, Dickinson Pub Sch/Roosevelt El, **SLP**

Aungst, Dr Lester F, Jr 127 Elmwood Avenue, Narberth, PA 19072, (215) 436-3388, BA 60 Augustana Coll; MS 61 PA St Univ - Univ Park; PH 65 (Sp Path & Aud) PA St Univ - Univ Park; Assoc Prof/Coord Clin Svcs, W Chester U, **SLP**

Aungst, Mrs Roberta B 127 Elmwood Avenue, Narberth, PA 19072, (215) 275-4151, BS 61 Emerson Coll; MS 66 PA St Univ - Univ Park; Dir of Aud, Aud Diag & Rehab Ctr, **A**

Aurand, Barbara S 422 Burleigh Avenue, Norfolk, VA 23505, (804) 481-4004, BS 79 Univ of VA - Charlottesville; ME 81 Univ of VA - Charlottesville; Sp-Lang Path, Virginia Speech & Lang Assocts, **SLP**

Aurelia, Joseph C 65 Garfield Road, Melrose, MA 02176, Director, Diagnostic Hrng & Lang Assoc, **SLP**

Aurelio, Katherine Spiers 16 Warner Road, Ipswich, MA 01938, (617) 745-9000, BA 74 Univ of MA - Amherst; MS 75 Purdue Univ - West Lafayette; Dir Sp/Lang Dept, Shaughnessy Rehab Hosp, **SLP**

Aurich, Carol Diane 8523 23rd Avenue N E, Apartment 1, Seattle, WA 98115, (206) 622-9916, BS 82 Univ of WA; MS 84 Univ of WA; **A**

Auriemma, Mrs Donna M S 11 Overlook Road, Chatham Township, NJ 07928, (201) 593-3153, BS 73 Seton Hall Univ; MA 78 Seton Hall Univ; 75–Sp-Lang Path, Madison Boro Pub Sch, **SLP**

Auriemma, Joseph R 196 Birch Lane, Scotia, NY 12302, (518) 399-8100, BS 66 SUNY - Coll at Geneseo; MS 67 SUNY - Coll at Geneseo; **SLP**

Auriemmo, Jane 89-33 201st Street, Hollis, NY 11423, (212) 689-7503, BA 84 CUNY - Queens Coll; MA 86 CUNY - Hunter Coll; **A**

Auslander, Martha Clifford 555 North 30th Street, Omaha, NE 68131, (402) 449-6529, BA 67 Sarah Lawrence Coll; ME 69 Univ of AZ; MS 82 Univ of AZ; Aud, Boystwn Natl I for Commundis, **A**

Auslander, Susanne 67-12 Yellowstone Blvd, Apartment D-5, Forest Hills, NY 11375, (718) 240-5819, BA 84 CUNY - Queens Coll; MS 86 Columbia Univ Teachers Coll; SLP, Brookdale Hosp, **SLP**

Auslander-Chroman, Mrs Barbara 20 Cherry Hill Road, Livingston, NJ 07039, (201) 535-3547, MS 79 PA St Univ - Univ Park; Sp-Lang Path, Private Practice, **SLP**

Aussenberg, Mrs Elizabeth G Associates In Comm Disorders, 5239 Lymbar, Houston, TX 77096, (713) 721-8292, BS 80 Univ of TX - Austin; MA 81 George Washington Univ; Sp-Lang Path Dir, Assoc In Commun Dis, **SLP**

Austen, Stacey L 16 Roderick Court, East Northport, NY 11731, (516) 260-4400, BA 85 SUNY - Coll at New Paltz; MS 86 FL St Univ; 87–Sp-Lang Path, The Opportunity Pre-School, **SLP**

Austerlitz, Mrs Francine S 10046 Fuerte Drive, La Mesa, CA 92041, (619) 532-9644, BS 70 Syracuse Univ; ME 71 Boston Univ; 76–Head-SLP Dept, Naval Hosp-San Diego, **SLP**

Austin, Allen A 25 East Park Road, Pittsford, NY 14534, (716) 475-6259, MA 71 Univ of IL - Urbana; BA 69 IN Univ - Bloomington; 72–Asst Prof, NTID, **SLP ACE**

Austin, Mrs Barbara A 34475 Ada Drive, Solon, OH 44139, BA 76 Cleveland St Univ; MA 78 Cleveland St Univ; Sp-Lang Path, Cleveland Bd of Ed, **SLP**

Austin, Mrs Carolyn S 401 East 32nd Street #1214, Chicago, IL 60616, (312) 842-7973, BS 53 Northwestern Univ; MS 57 Univ of WI - Madison; Retired, Evanston Pub Sch Dist, **SLP F**

Austin, Elizabeth 563 Lees Trace, Marietta, GA 30064, (404) 424-1938, BS 75 OH St Univ; MS 78 GA St Univ; **SLP**

Austin, Mrs Ellen L 5187 Mt Vernon Way, Dunwoody, GA 30338, (404) 394-7797, ME 68 Temple Univ-Tyler Sch of Art; MA 73 Temple Univ-Tyler Sch of Art; **SLP**

Austin, Mrs Jane E P O Box 325, New Boston, NH 03070, (603) 487-2744, BS 76 James Madison Univ; ME 81 Northeastern Univ; Sp/Lang Path, Merrimack/Bedford Pub Sch, **SLP**

Austin, Janet H The Marvelwood School, Cornwall, CT 06753, (215) 842-6596, BA 73 SUNY - Center at Binghamton; MA 81 George Washington Univ; SLP Section Head, Hosp of the Med Coll of Pa, **SLP**

Austin, Jeannine P O Box 334, Locust, NC 28097, (704) 888-2225, BS 69 Appalachian St Univ; MA 72 Univ of NC - Greensboro; **SLP**

Austin, Jill M 711 Lake Mead Place, San Ramon, CA 94583, (415) 866-9486, BA 78 San Jose St Univ; MA 81 San Jose St Univ; Sp-Lang Path, **SLP**

Austin, Mrs Jolynn Sanborn 61 Cragmont Court, Walnut Creek, CA 94598, (415) 934-6598, BA 76 Chapman Coll; MS 83 Chapman Coll; **SLP**

Austin, Juanita T 19 Arms Boulevard #7, Niles, OH 44446, (216) 856-2107, BS 81 Trenton St Coll; MS 82 Indiana Univ of PA; Sp-Lang Path, Chldn Rehab Cen, **SLP**

Austin, Mrs Judith K 8600 Starboard Drive, Apartment 2056, Las Vegas, NV 89117, (702) 486-5223, BA 65 Western MI Univ; MA 70 Western MI Univ; SLP, Special Childrens Clinic, **SLP**

Austin, Mrs Katharine Thorne 304 Mansfield Parkway, Morehead City, NC 28557-2724, (919) 638-2666, BA 80 Univ of SC - Columbia; OM 84 Univ of SC - Columbia; Aud, Coastal ENT, **A**

Austin, Lisa L 61 Bienville Avenue, Mobile, AL 36606, (205) 476-4895, BS 76 Auburn Univ - Auburn; MS 77 Auburn Univ - Auburn; **SLP**

Austin, Mrs Lynette Blackburn 500 North Judge Ely, Apartment 3-206, Abilene, TX 79601, (915) 691-7300, BS 85 Abilene Christian Univ; MA 87 Abilene Christian Univ; 88–Sp-Lang Path, West Texas Rehab Ctr, **SLP**

Austin, Mrs Lynn Hogsed 2573 Old Hendersonville Hwy, Pisgah Forest, NC 28768, (704) 877-4235, MA 87 Appalachian St Univ

Austin, Mrs Meredith Hall 3920 Cortlandt, Houston, TX 77018, (713) 694-8379, BS 77 TX Woman's Univ; MS 78 Univ of North TX; **SLP**

Austin, Mrs Patricia H 313 Westview Street, Kannapolis, NC 28081, (704) 938-3151, BS 79 Western Carolina Univ; ME 80 Univ of NC - Greensboro; Sp-Lang Path, Kannapolis City Schools, **SLP**

Austin, Paul W 74 Colburn Street, North Attleboro, MA 02760, (401) 277-5485, ME 72 Boston Univ; OM 82 Northeastern Univ; SLP, Ri Hosp, **SLP A ACE**

Austin, Mrs Sue Ann Southeast Missouri Hospital, 1701 Lacey, Cape Girardeau, MO 63701, (314) 651-5523, BS 77 Southeast MO St Univ; ME 78 Southeast MO St Univ; Sp/Lang Path, Southeast Mo Hosp, **SLP**

Austin, Mrs Sue M 1401 Terral Island Road, Farmerville, LA 71241, (318) 824-6741, BA 69 Univ of North TX; MA 73 Univ of North TX; **SLP**

Austin, Teresa Dawn 10929 Buggy Whip Drive, Jacksonville, FL 32223, (904) 262-9251, BS 83 Univ of GA; ME 85 GA St Univ; **SLP**

Austing, Elisa M Patterson Kennedy School, 258 Wyoming Street, Dayton, OH 45409, (513) 228-8484, BA 78 Coll of Mount Saint Joseph; MA 86 Univ of Cincinnati; Aud, Dayton Bd of Ed, **A**

Auten, Mrs Laura H 2811 South 137th East Avenue, Tulsa, OK 74134, (918) 437-4264, BA 75 Univ of OK - Norman; MS 77 Univ of OK Medical Center; Sp-Lang Path, ISD #1, **SLP**

Auton, Mrs Vicky A 402 Auber Drive, Manchester, MO 63011, (314) 394-8420, BA 61 Univ of Science & Arts of OK; MS 78 Fontbonne Coll; SLP, Spec Sch Dist/St Louis Co, **SLP**

Autrey, Theresa Lynn 7110 Fordshire Lane, Hazelwood, MO 63042, (314) 895-1976, BS 82 Southeast MO St Univ; MA 84 Saint Louis Univ; **SLP**

Autry, Mrs Alice M 2205 Shorefield Road #831, Wheaton, MD 20902, (301) 424-5200, BA 72 Univ of WI - Whitewater; MS 77 Univ of WI - Milwaukee; 87–Sp-Lang Path, Treatment & Learning Centers, **SLP**

Autry, Mrs Sarah B 5704 Northwood Drive, Edmond, OK 73034, (405) 341-0405, BA 69 Univ of MO - Columbia; MS 74 Central MO St Univ; 84–Sp-Lang Path, Edmond Public Schools, **SLP**

Avallone, Mrs Margaret T 5 Maplevale Court, East Haven, CT 06512, (203) 787-8646, BS 69 Univ of KS; ME 70 PA St Univ - Univ Park; Sp/Lang Path, New Haven Bd of Ed, **SLP**

Avallone, Paula 27 Pleasant Hill Road, Falmouth, ME 04105, BS 75 Boston Univ; OM 83 Univ of MT; Sp-Lang Path, South Portland Sch Sys, **SLP**

Avallone, Sharon Rose 2100 West Barnett Springs, Apartment 130, Ruston, LA 71270, (318) 362-4049, BA 84 LA Tech Univ; MA 86 LA Tech Univ; Sp-Lang Path, St Francis Med Ctr, **SLP**

Avant, Mrs Susan L 1218 Centoni, Lake Zurich, IL 60047, (312) 438-3428, BS 72 OK St Univ; MA 73 Memphis St Univ; **SLP**

Avari, Dinci N 7 4th Street, Norwood, NJ 07648, **SLP**

Avella, Richard D 42 Essex Street, Buffalo, NY 14213, BS 72 SUNY - Coll at Fredonia; MS 73 SUNY - Coll at Fredonia; OM 83 SUNY - Coll at Buffalo; Sp-Lang Path, Niagara Falls Board of Educatn, **SLP**

Avent, Fayma L H 102 Peach Orchard Drive, Greensboro, NC 27405, (919) 370-8270, BA 72 Univ of NC - Greensboro; ME 74 Univ of NC - Greensboro; 76–Sp-Lang Path, Greensboro Pub Sch, **SLP**

Averell, Lois H 815 Washington Street, Whitman, MA 02382, (617) 447-3224, BS 42 Boston Univ; ME 53 Boston Univ; Sp/Lang Path/Aud, Mayflower House Chld Care Cen, **SLP A**

Avers, Kenneth William 1725 Chittenden Circle N E, Massillon, OH 44646, (216) 837-4346, BA 63 Elmhurst Coll; MA 67 De Paul Univ; 86–Sp-Lang Path, Apple Creek Dev Ctr, **SLP**

Aversano, Anthony Michael 114th Avenue #T, Brooklyn, NY 11223, (718) 266-0036, BA 84 CUNY - Brooklyn Coll; MS 86 CUNY - Brooklyn Coll; **SLP**

Averto, Mrs Christine Rd 4 Box 80, Belle Aire Acres, Lake Ariel, PA 18436, (717) 348-3455, BA 73 Marywood Coll; ME 75 Bloomsburg Univ of PA; 73–SLP, Scranton Sch Dist, **SLP**

Avery, Charlotte B 220 North Dithridge Street, Apartment 601, Pittsburgh, PA 15213, (412) 647-5580, BA 43 Univ of WI - Milwaukee; MA 47 Northwestern Univ; 77–Coor-Post Assess Act, Chldn Hosp of Pgh, **A F**

Avezzano, Karen Hillman 2510-B South Walter Reed, Arlington, VA 22206, (703) 660-7100, BA 82 SUNY - Coll at Plattsburgh; MS 84 Columbia Univ Teachers Coll; SLP, Fairfax Co Hlth Dept, **SLP**

Avignone, John L 16420 Highland Avenue #4, Jamaica, NY 11432-3561, (212) 380-3000, BA 76 CUNY - Queens Coll; MA 77 Hofstra Univ; Sp-Lang Path, UCP-Queens, **SLP**

Avignone, Olympia 43-36 Robinson Street #5H, Flushing, NY 11355, (516) 997-7004, BA 76 CUNY - Queens Coll; MA 77 Hofstra Univ; 84–Sp-Lang Path, Northshore Univ Hosp Dev Prog, **SLP**

Avino, Mrs Gail J 33 Lorraine Drive, Tolland, CT 06084, (203) 872-4375, BS 70 Univ of CT; MS 73 Univ of CT; **SLP**

Avishar, Mrs Nancy J 473 Le Parc Circle, Buffalo Grove, IL 60089, (312) 966-8600, BA 69 MI St Univ; MA 70 MI St Univ; ME 82 Univ of IL - Chicago; Teacher of Hearing Impaired, Julia S Molloy Ed Ctr, **A**

Avne, Mrs Laura 22232 Crane Street, El Toro, CA 92630, (714) 855-1217, BA 79 CA St Univ - Fullerton; MA 83 CA St Univ - Fullerton; Director of SLP, Healthtech Rehab Inc, **SLP**

Avner, Ellen Rosenblatt 3274 Prestwick Lane, Northbrook, IL 60062, (312) 205-0313, BA 77 Univ of IL - Chicago; MA 81 CUNY - Hunter Coll; Sp/Lang Path, **SLP**

Avni, Nitza Movshovitch 14 Warwick Road, Brookline, MA 02146, (617) 738-6915, BA 71; OM 83 Harvard Univ; **A**

Avolio, Mrs Wendy F 3532 N Fiesta Del Sol East, Tucson, AZ 85715, (602) 622-5734, BS 73 Bradley Univ; MA 75 Northern IL Univ - De Kalb; Sp-Lang Path, S AZ Spec Educ Coop, **SLP**

Avriett, Mrs Paula Hayes 1338 Stonewood Court, San Pedro, CA 90732-1550, BA 84 Univ of the Pacific; MA 85 Univ of the Pacific

Avrin, Mrs Lois Silver 23 Kearney Drive, Middletown, NJ 07748, (201) 671-3850, BA 65 CUNY - Hunter Coll; MA 84 Kean Coll of NJ; 83–Sp-Lang Path, Middletown Township PS, **SLP**

Awan, Karen Judith 507 Old Forge Road, Kent, OH 44240, (215) 631-9300, BA 85 Clarion Univ of PA; MA 86 Clarion Univ of PA; Sp-Lang Path, Robinson Memorial Hosp, **SLP**

Awan, Shaheen Nazir 507 Old Forge Road, Kent, OH 44240, (216) 672-2672, BA 84 Univ of Western Ontario; MS 86 Clarion Univ of PA; **SLP**

Awerbuch-Schwartz, Felicity Broadpark Lodge, 2 Westchester Avenue #5P, White Plains, NY 10601, (914) 698-7805, **SLP**

Axelrod, Jennifer K 1047 West Belden Avenue, Chicago, IL 60614, BA 68 Univ of MI - Ann Arbor; MA 70 Northwestern Univ; Sp-Lang Path, Holy Cross Hosp, **SLP**

Axelrod, Mrs Lauren Sherri 15 First Street #3B, Hackensack, NJ 07601, (201) 533-5000, BA 83 Kean Coll of NJ; MA 84 Kean Coll of NJ

Axelrod, Natalie 72 Jackman Avenue, Toronto, ON, Canada M4K 2Y9, **SLP**

Axelrod, Susan Breazzano 1006 Serpentine Lane, Wyncote, PA 19095, **SLP**

Axelson, Mrs Audrey M 249-20 57 Avenue, Little Neck, NY 11362, (718) 380-3000, BA 71 Long Island U - Brooklyn Ctr; MA 73 Hofstra Univ; Sp-Lang Path, UCP of Queens, **SLP**

Axtell, Sherri Lee 904 Norwood Street, Apartment 1, Fayetteville, NC 28305, (919) 738-6071, BS 84 CA Univ of PA; MS 86 CA Univ of PA; 87–Sp-Lang Path, Sp Path Svcs, **SLP**

Ayala, Aurea Margarita 911 Maybelle N E, Grand Rapids, MI 49503, (616) 458-8688, BS 82 Univ of PR - San Juan; MA 84 MI St Univ; Sp-Lang Path, Grand Rapids Public Schools, **SLP**

Ayer, Edith Annette 3000 Cowell Blvd #273, Davis, CA 95616-4836, (707) 425-8451, BA 82 CA St Univ - Sacramento; MA 84 CA St Univ - Sacramento; Sp-Lang Path, Fairfield-Susan USD, **SLP**

Ayers, Cathi Anne 1146 17th Avenue North, St Petersburg, FL 33704, BS 72 FL St Univ; MS 73 5216; Coord Sp/Lang Path Serv, All Chldn's Hosp, **SLP**

Ayers, Shelley B P O Box 4277, Federal Way, WA 98063, (206) 874-1604, BA 71 WA St Univ; MA 72 WA St Univ; Private Practice, **SLP**

Ayers, Mrs Susan Kay 1607 Calhoun Road, Rome, GA 30161, (404) 235-3892, BA 81 Univ of AL- Tuscaloosa; MS 82 Univ of AL- Tuscaloosa; Sp/Lang Path, Floyd Co Bd of Ed, **SLP**

Aylesworth, Dr Donald L Sch Of Communicative Disorders, University Of Wisconsin, Stevens Point, WI 54481, PH 71 (NS) MI St Univ; **SLP**

Aylesworth, Mrs Margaret R 3230 Harrison, Evanston, IL 60201, (312) 492-5012, BS 60 Northwestern Univ; MA 65 Northwestern Univ; Asst Prof, Northwestern University, **SLP ACE**

Ayres, Mrs Deborah Ann 78 Miami Trail, Rockaway, NJ 07866-1036, **SLP**

Ayres, Mrs Ruth Young 2809 Marquette Avenue, Natchez, MS 39120, (601) 445-8678, BS 81 Univ Southern MS-Hattiesburg; MS 82 Univ Southern MS-Hattiesburg; Sp-Lang Path, Natchez Public Schools, **SLP**

Azimi-Bolourian, Carol Lacava P O Box 1420, Norman, OK 73070, (405) 271-6816, BS 74; MS 79 Univ of OK Medical Center; Sp-Lang Path, Child Study Ctr Ok Teach Hosp, **SLP**

Aziza, Mrs Elana Flori 249-A South Eighth Avenue, Highland Park, NJ 08904, (716) 638-0189, BS 83 Univ of Toronto - Ontario; OM 84 Univ of Toronto - Ontario; **SLP**

Aznavoorian, Karen Lea 322-C Marguerite Place, Corona Del Mar, CA 92625, (714) 675-8926, BA 77 CA St Univ - Fullerton; MA 86 CA St Univ - Fullerton; **SLP**

Azure, Mrs Linda S 14401 NE 30th Place #B, Bellevue, WA 98007, (206) 881-5285, BS 84 Minot St Univ; MS 88 Univ of WA; 88–Sp-Lang Path, Children's Hosp & Med Ctr

Azzara, Alice C G 69 Clover Avenue, Floral Park, NY 11001, BA 74 CUNY - Queens Coll; MA 75 CUNY - Queens Coll; OD 88 (Educ Admin) Saint John's Univ; 82–Sp-Lang Path, NYC Bd of Ed, **SLP**

Azzara, John P 238 Tinsley Court, Salem Woods, Newark, DE 19702, (302) 999-0301, BA 77 SUNY - Center at Binghamton; ME 80 Univ of VA - Charlottesville; Super Sp Therapy Serv, Delaware Speech Hrng Ctr, **SLP**

Azzara, Mrs Marie Randolph 238 Tinsley Court, Salem Woods, Newark, DE 19702, (302) 429-4062, **SLP**

Azzaretti, Anne 14 Sejon Drive, Sayville, NY 11782, (516) 727-8080, BA 71 Long Island U - CW Post Ctr; MA 75 Hofstra Univ; Sp-Lang Path, Riverhead Ctrl Sch Dist, **SLP**

B

Baack, Kris L 2902 Raleigh, Lincoln, NE 68512, (402) 472-2075, BS 75 Univ of NE - Lincoln; MA 76 Univ of NE - Lincoln; Instructor/Superv, Univ of Neb-Lincoln, **SLP**

Baalke, Mrs Nancy Wiedmeyer 2003 South 16th Street, Sheboygan, WI 53081, (414) 459-9058, BS 76 Univ of WI - Madison; MS 77 Univ of WI - Milwaukee; Sp-Lang Path, **SLP**

Baalman, Lee 824 West, Emporia, KS 66801, (316) 343-2302, BS 78 Fort Hays St Univ; MS 80 Fort Hays St Univ; Sp-Lang Path, Flint Hills Special Ed Coop, **SLP**

Baarslag-Benson, Ross Edward 3534 N E 123rd, Seattle, WA 98125, (206) 326-7330, BA 82 Univ of WA; MS 85 Univ of WA; **SLP**

Baba, Ann Harumi 212 N Valley Street, Unit 15, Burbank, CA 91505-3938, (213) 625-4183

Babas, Linda 269 Clearwater Drive, East Meadow, NY 11554, BA 63 Adelphi Univ; MS 66 Adelphi Univ; SLP, BOCES III, **SLP**

Babb, Agatha B Route 2 Box 764, Belton, SC 29627, (803) 224-2173, BA 67 Erskine Coll; ME 81 Univ of GA; ME 73 Clemson Univ; Sp-Lang Path, Anderson Sch Dist #5, **SLP**

Babb, Carol 32 Gramercy Park South, Apartment 18E, New York, NY 10003, (212) 777-5977, BA 81 San Francisco St Univ; MS 83 San Francisco St Univ; 88–Sp-Lang Path, Port Washington PS, **SLP**

Babb, Mrs Elizabeth 5 Robinwood Lane, Anniston, AL 36201, (205) 236-5560, BS 65 G Peabody Coll-Vanderbilt U; MS 66 Vanderbilt Univ; **SLP**

Babb, Maxine Althea 550 Crown Street, Brooklyn, NY 11213, (718) 756-0035, **SLP**

Babb, Mrs Pamela Bobich First Tennessee Reg Health Off, 1233 Southwest Avenue Ext, Johnson City, TN 37601, (615) 929-5939, BS 77 Indiana Univ of PA; MA 79 Univ of TN - Knoxville; Reg Coord/Sp & Hrng Ser, TN-Dept Hlth & Envrn, **A**

Babbitt, Douglas A 59 Holten Street, Danvers, MA 01923, (508) 777-5441, BS 81 Univ of ME - Farmington; MS 86 PA St Univ - Univ Park; Sp-Lang Path, Private Practice, **SLP**

Babbitt, Susan 225 Davisville Avenue #2515, Toronto, ON, Canada M4S 1G9, (416) 229-5800, BA 63 Queens Univ - Ontario; MA 65 Univ of Toronto - Ontario; 81–Supervisor / Sp-Lang Path, Home Care Prog Met Toronto, **SLP**

Babbs, Barbara S 2712 Wisconsin Avenue N W, Apartment 712, Washington, DC 20007, (202) 727-3866, BA 65 Univ of HI - Manoa; MA 80 George Washington Univ; **SLP**

Babcock, Shirley Joan 2929 Landrum Drive S W, Apartment H-50, Atlanta, GA 30311, (404) 349-4198, BS 71 Univ of WI - Stevens Point; MS 77 Univ of WI - Stevens Point; Rehab Servs Coord, Botswana Natl Council/Disable, **SLP**

Babcock, Susan L 6876 Country Woods Circle, Midvale, UT 84047, (801) 571-1223, MS 79 CO St Univ; BS 77 CO St Univ; Sp/Lang Path, Primary Chldn's Med Cen, **SLP**

Babey, Lois J 46 Peddlers Drive, Branford, CT 06405, (203) 272-3577, OM 85 Southern CT St Univ; BA 75 Univ of CT; MS 78 Southern CT St Univ; Sp-Lang Path, Cheshire Early Interven Cen, **SLP**

Babiak, Mrs Joann U 9250 Oak Leaf Way, Roseville, CA 95661, (916) 791-2172, BS 77 Boston Univ; MA 80 Univ of the Pacific; Sp-Lang Path, Private Practice, **SLP**

Babik, Mrs Rebecca A 3107 South Park Road, Bethel Park, PA 15102, BS 74 CA Univ of PA; MS 77 Indiana Univ of PA; Sp-Lang Path, Crossroads Sp & Hrng Ctr, **SLP**

Babin, Mrs Sharon B 760 Rue Crozat, Baton Rouge, LA 70810, (504) 342-4756, BA 68 LA St Univ - Baton Rouge; MA 72 LA St Univ - Baton Rouge; Sp/Lang Path, Louisiana Sch-Visually Imp, **SLP**

Babineau, Mary Kathleen Windsor 206, 1465 Hooksett Road, Hooksett, NH 03106, (603) 883-5521, BS 84 Ithaca Coll; MS 86 Boston Univ; **SLP**

Babington, Vicki L 614 Shenandoah Drive, Spring, TX 77381-1042, (713) 292-6387, BS 71 McMurry Coll; MS 76 Univ of North TX; Sp-Lang Path Owner, Sp-Lang Cl, **SLP**

Babl, Linda C 574 Hillcrest Drive, Verona, WI 53593, **SLP**

Babon, Mrs Wendy Diane 100 Granitevilla Road, Chelmsford, MA 01824, (617) 251-8384, BS 75 Framingham St Coll; ME 83 Northeastern Univ; Sp/Lang Path, Chelmsford Sch Syst/Spec Ed, **SLP**

Baca, Ann H 4829 Alicia Drive, Fort Worth, TX 76133-6707, (817) 292-2370, BA 73 Loretto Heights Coll; MS 77 TX Christian Univ; Sp-Lang Path, Fort Worth ISD, **SLP**

Baca, Capt Margaret Louise P O Box 5, Fort Polk, LA 71459-5000, (303) 456-0598, MS 82 Eastern NM Univ; Commander Spec Security Detach, US Army Special Security Group

Baca, Maria Langereis 465 Milton Avenue, Las Cruces, NM 88005, (505) 524-2247, OM 85 NM St Univ; MA 85 NM St Univ; Sp-Lang Path, Hatch Valley Mun Schs, **SLP ACE**

Bacca, Glenda G 318 Locust Street, Turlock, CA 95380, (209) 538-0164, BA 78 CA St Univ - Stanislaus; MA 80 Univ of IL - Urbana; Sp-Lang Path, Stanislaus Co Dept Ed, **SLP**

Baccaro, Paul Michel 5810 Willow Bend, Houston, TX 77096, (713) 795-0111, BA 53 Univ of MS; MA 55 Univ of MS; Aud-SLP, Med Cen ENT Assoc, **SLP A**

Bacchus, Mrs Cathy P O Box 343, 117 Jeweled Mesa, Santa Teresa, NM 88008, BS 78 Baylor Univ; MA 80 Univ of TX - El Paso; Sp-Lang Path, El Paso Public Schools, **SLP**

Bach, Mrs Barbara 22 Rolling Way, New Rochelle, NY 10804, (212) 939-8700, BA 72 Univ of Pittsburgh - Pittsburgh; MS 73 Columbia Univ Teachers Coll; Sp-Lang Path, Bd Comb Ed Serv S Westchester, **SLP**

Bach, Nancy H 3407 Commander Court, Arlington, TX 76017, (817) 334-0200, BA 78 TX Tech Univ; MA 79 Univ of North TX; Aud, Howard Shaffer MD Pa, **A**

Bachand, Mrs Patricia S P O Box 546, St Anne, IL 60964, (815) 932-0061, BS 77 IL St Univ - Normal; MA 78 Univ of IL - Urbana; Sp-Lang Path, Kankakee Area Spec Ed Coop, **SLP**

Bachelder, Mrs Katherine P O Box 924, Portland, ME 04104, (207) 773-3415, BS 78 Univ of ME - Farmington; MS 79 Ithaca Coll; Sp-Lang Path, S Portland Sch Syst, **SLP**

Bache-Wiig, Mrs Barbara J 1100 Grant Street, Waukesha, WI 53186, (414) 547-9014, BS 47 Univ of MN - Minneap-St Paul; OM 56; MS 52 Univ of MN - Minneap-St Paul; Instr, Waukesha Co Tech Coll, **SLP**

Bachi, Dr Ilana Misgav Ladach Ii, Jewish Quarters Old City, Jerusalem, Israel, BA CUNY - Hunter Coll; Sp-Lang Path/Aud, Private Practice, **SLP A**

Bachman, David M 1409 Morning Glory Drive, Petaluma, CA 94952, (707) 765-2714, BA 74 Univ of CA - Irvine; MA 81 CA St Univ - Sacramento; Sp-Lang Path, North Coast Rehab Center, **SLP**

Bachman, Mary Elizabeth 3177 East 17th Street, Highland, CA 92346, (213) 273-8480, BA 80 Univ of CA - Riverside; MS 83 Univ of Redlands; Sp-Lang Path, I Lehrhoff PhD & Associates, **SLP**

Bachman, Mary L 1905 Wahalaw Court, Tallahassee, FL 32301, (904) 488-4150, BS 58 FL St Univ; MS 73 FL St Univ; Sp-Lang Path, FL Diag Lrng Res Sys, **SLP ACE**

Bachmann, Glenda J 5733 Elm, Raytown, MO 64133, (913) 651-6466, BA 77 Univ of MO - Columbia; MA 78 Univ of MO - Columbia; Sp-Lang Path, Leavenworth Co Spec Ed Coop, **SLP**

Bachmann, Mrs Grace 5 Fleetwood Avenue, Fairfield, NJ 07006, (201) 272-9100, BA 62 Montclair St Coll; MA 65 Montclair St Coll; Sp-Lang Path, Cranford Bd of Ed, **SLP**

Bachner, Mrs Lisa Dawn 3616 Sutherland Road, Shaker Heights, OH 44122, (216) 295-0870, BS 83 Ithaca Coll; MA 85 Hofstra Univ; 87–Sp-Lang Path, Cleveland Hrng & Sp Ctr, **SLP**

Bachnivsky, Mrs Valentina H ENT And Facial Surgery Inc, 711 River Drive, Marion, IN 46952, (317) 662-3995, BA 74 IN Univ - Bloomington; MA 75 IN Univ - Bloomington; Aud, ENT & Facial Surgery Inc, **A**

Bachrach, Annette M 6700 East Mississippi Avenue, Unit E, Denver, CO 80224, (303) 837-1000, BA 68 Univ of CO - Boulder; MA 71 Univ of Northern CO; SLP, Denver Pub Sch, **SLP**

Bachtell, Cheryl Lee 4330 South Lenox Street, Milwaukee, WI 53207-5240, (414) 481-6478, BS 81 Univ of WI - Milwaukee; MS 83 Univ of WI - Milwaukee; 83–Sp-Lang Path, Milwaukee Public Schools, **SLP**

Bachyrycz, Mrs Jayne J 88 Captain Wooster Road, Oxford, CT 06483, (203) 789-3362, BA 77 Univ of NC - Greensboro; MS 80 Southern CT St Univ; Sp-Lang Path, Hospital of St Raphael, **SLP**

Backer-Conklin, Sue 3006 Silver Bow Court, St Louis, MO 63129, (314) 846-5307, BS 80 Univ of MO - Columbia; MS 81 Central MO St Univ; Sp-Lang Path, Natl Hlth Corp, **SLP**

Backes, Jeanne M 1754 Hunter Avenue, Mobile, AL 36604, (205) 478-0710, BA 77 MI St Univ; MA 78 Wayne St Univ; 85–Sp/Lang Path, Speech and Language Specialists, **SLP**

Backiel, Thomas C Box 1245, Bangor, ME 04401, (207) 941-4360, BA 77 Temple Univ-Tyler Sch of Art; MS 79 Phillips Univ; 79–Sp-Lang Path, Bur of Ment Ret, **SLP**

Backlar, Annette Warren Psc, Box 2319, APO San Francisco, CA 96293, BS 78 OK St Univ; MS 80 Univ of OK Medical Center; Sp-Lang Path, Yokota West Elementary School, **SLP**

Backman, Nancy S 235 South Avenue, Webster, NY 14580, (716) 872-1903, BS 67 Ithaca Coll; MA 69 Univ of TN - Knoxville; Sp/Lang Path, Monroe BOCES #1, **SLP**

Backner, Kathleen A 37 Crescent Drive, Washington, PA 15301, (412) 223-3290, BS 75 Carlow Coll; ME 78 CA Univ of PA; Sp-Lang Path, Washington Hospital, **SLP ACE**

Backoff, Lori S 2749 West 61st Place, Apt 1-B, Merrillville, IN 46410, (219) 884-3730, BS 86 IL St Univ - Normal; MS 88 IL St Univ - Normal; 88–Sp-Lang Path, Southlake Speech & Hearing Ctr

Backoff, Patricia M 320 Larkspur, Ann Arbor, MI 48105, (313) 769-6471, BA 76 MI St Univ; MS 78 Univ of AZ; 85–Aud, McAuley Audiology Svcs, **A**

Backstrom, Melissa Katherine 333 N University #12, Redlands, CA 92374, (714) 887-6333, BA 85 Chapman Coll; MS 87 Univ of Redlands; 87–Sp-Lang Path, San Bernardino Comm Hosp, **SLP**

Backus, Mrs Marcia L 1513 North Hague Avenue, Columbus, OH 43204, (614) 476-0530, BS 80 Bowling Green St Univ; MA 81 Bowling Green St Univ; SLP, Franklin Co Board of Mental Re, **SLP**

Backus, Dr Ollie L 650 West Harrison Avenue, Claremont, CA 91711, (714) 625-2378, BA 29 Univ of MI - Ann Arbor; MA 30 Univ of MI - Ann Arbor; PH 33 (Sp Disorders-major Neuroanatomy & Physiology-minors) Univ of WI - Madison; Psychotherapy, Private Practice, **SLP F LM**

Baclawski, Mrs Darlene C 1530 Whitman Street, Williamsport, PA 17701, (717) 323-4555, **SLP**

Bacolini, Paula 11 Garland Drive, Glastonbury, CT 06033, (203) 284-2880, BA 70 Adelphi Univ; MS 76 CUNY - Queens Coll; Sp-Lang Path, Gaylord Hosp, **SLP**

Bacon, Hope H 1302 Valencia Way, Dalton, GA 30720, (404) 278-8143, BA 70 Baylor Univ; MA 71 Vanderbilt Univ; Prog Superv, Cheerhaven Inc, **SLP**

Bacon, Mrs Karen Elizabeth Route 1 Box 188-A, Fair Grove, MO 65648, (417) 864-3657, **SLP**

Bacon, Linda A M 6 Reynard Court, Little Rock, AR 72207, (501) 758-6560, BA 77 Univ of AR - Fayetteville; MA 79 Univ of KS; **A**

Bacon, Mrs Mariana Goytisolo 22 Gray Squirrel Court, Timonium, MD 21093, (301) 252-7792, BA 83 Loyola Coll; MS 84 Loyola Coll; 84–Sp-Lang Path, Baltimore City Schs, **SLP**

Bacon, Marilee J 15 Maywood Place, Buffalo, NY 14210, (716) 822-7208, BA 80 SUNY - Coll at Cortland; MA 85 SUNY - Center at Buffalo; 88–Sp-Lang Path, Lang Dev Prog, **SLP**

Bacon, Mary J 4030 Lawn Avenue, Western Springs, IL 60558, (312) 942-5332, BS 71 Miami Univ - Oxford; MA 72 Northern IL Univ - De Kalb; Sp-Lang Path Asst Prof, Rush-Presby St Lukes Med Cen, **SLP**

Bacon, Dr Sid P Department Of Speech & Hearing Science, Arizona State University, Tempe, AZ 85287-0102, (602) 965-3345, OB 77 Univ of KS; MA 79 Univ of KS; PH 85 (NS) Univ of MN - Minneap-St Paul; 88–Assoc Prof, AZ State Univ

Bacon, Susanellen 364 Wilson Avenue, Kent, OH 44240, (216) 672-2672, BA 67 Western WA Univ; MS 80 Marquette Univ; Asst to Director/SLP, Kent State University, **SLP**

Badam, Kimberly K 10770 Black Mountain Road, Apartment 231, San Diego, CA 92126-2919, (801) 375-3636, **SLP**

Badanes, Mrs Amy L 8089 Hetz Drive, Cincinnati, OH 45242, (513) 867-5960, BS 79 Miami Univ - Oxford; MS 80 Miami Univ - Oxford; SLP, Butler Co Bd of Ment Ret, **SLP**

Badders, Mrs Bonnie Barrett R R #1 Box 36B, Portland, IN 47371, (219) 726-8890, BS 74 Purdue Univ - West Lafayette; MA 78 Ball St Univ; SLP, Jay Sch Corp, **SLP**

Badders, Mrs Debra M R R 2 Box 213P, Effingham, IL 62401, (217) 258-2568, BS 80 Purdue Univ - West Lafayette; MA 81 Northern IL Univ - De Kalb; Sp-Lang Path, Sarah Bush Lincoln Health Cen, **SLP**

Bade, Mrs Joan Elaine 208 Capital Lane, Findlay, OH 45840, (419) 226-5070, BA 85 Bowling Green St Univ; MA 87 Ball St Univ; 88–Sp-Lang Path, Lima Mem Hosp, **SLP**

Bade, Marlane T 44 Hance Road, Fair Haven, NJ 07701, **SLP**

Baden, Nancy A 6122 Wagon Bend, Austin, TX 78744, (512) 453-0037, BS 75 Univ of TX - Austin; MA 78 Univ of TX - Austin; Sp-Lang Path, Pediatric Therapy Svcs, **SLP**

Baden, Phyllis M 185 East 85th Street, New York, NY 10028, (212) 722-3104, BS 70 CUNY - Queens Coll; MS 74 Columbia Univ Teachers Coll; 70–Sp-Lang Path, St Joseph's Sch for the Deaf, **SLP**

Bader, C Sarah 15 Jesswig Drive, Hamden, CT 06517, (203) 488-5000, BA 58 0500; ME 60 0500; MS 86 Southern CT St Univ; **SLP**

Bader, Ellen K 60 Greenway South, Forest Hills, NY 11375, BA 75 CUNY - Queens Coll; MA 77 CUNY - Queens Coll; SLP, New York City Board of Educ, **SLP**

Bader, Paula D 2351 Heather Way, Lexington, KY 40503, (606) 278-7150, BA 73 Univ of KY; MA 78 Univ of KY; SLP, Fayette Co Sch, **SLP**

Bader, Mrs Shellie Sue LA West Speech Communication, 6380 Wilshire Boulevard Suite 911, Los Angeles, CA 90048, (213) 653-3020, BA 79 Univ of CA - Los Angeles; MA 82 CA St Univ - Northridge; 88–Dir, LA West Speech Communication, **SLP**

Bader, Sheryl 1800 East 12th Street, Brooklyn, NY 11229, (718) 375-8417, BA 78 CUNY - Brooklyn Coll; MS 82 CUNY - Brooklyn Coll; Sp/Lang Path, Milestone Sch for Chld Dev, **SLP**

Bader, Virginia T 2111 Key West Cove, Austin, TX 78746, (512) 329-4807, BA 70; MA 80; **SLP**

Badger, Mrs Shelli M 162 East Greer Drive, Newark, OH 43055, (614) 393-9860, SLP, Colin Anderson Center, **SLP**

Badgett, Carol Elizabeth Rt 4 Box 57-C, Madisonville, KY 42431, (502) 821-5446, BS 78 Brescia Coll; MA 81 Memphis St Univ; Admin, **SLP**

Badgley, Mrs Janelyn Voigt 7190 Chadwood Lane #2D, Columbus, OH 43235, (614) 761-9055, BA 82 Univ of Toledo; MA 83 Bowling Green St Univ; Aud, InSpeech Inc, **SLP A**

Badick, Martha 2430 Owen Drive, Wilmington, DE 19808, (302) 994-6171, BS 46 Lock Haven St Coll; ME 53 PA St Univ - Univ Park; SLP, Chldn Beach House Inc, **SLP LM**

Badman, Arlene Luberoff 10117-A Oakbrook Drive, Charlotte, NC 28210, (704) 332-4834, BA 83 Columbia Coll; MA 85 Univ of MD - College Park; 88–Sp-Lang Path, Child & Family Dev Assoc Inc, **SLP**

Badofsky, Mrs Ellen Potischman 5044 N Marine Drive #A-2, Chicago, IL 60640, (312) 989-0778, BS 85 Ithaca Coll; MA 87 Northwestern Univ; **SLP**

Badolato, Sheryl Ann 907 McKinley Avenue, Rome, NY 13440, (315) 337-8400, BS 84 SUNY - Coll at Geneseo; MS 85 Coll of Saint Rose; **SLP**

Badon, Linda Cain 215 Choctaw Road, Lafayette, LA 70501, (318) 235-0768, BA 73 Univ of Southwestern LA; MS 80 Univ of Southwestern LA; Sp-Lang Path, Vermilion Par Sch Bd

Bady, Harold L 2500 West 80th Street, Chicago, IL 60652, (312) 567-5557, **SLP**

Bady, Janet A 7192 West Mission Hills Dr, Las Vegas, NV 89113, (702) 873-8777, BS 77 Univ of WI - Madison; MS 78 Marquette Univ; Sp-Lang Path, Clark Co Sch Dist, **SLP**

Baecker, Frederick W 731 Hunt Way, Davis, CA 95616-2322, (916) 454-8183, BA 71 Univ of WI - Madison; MS 81 Univ of WI - Madison; Sp-Lang Path, Sacramento City USD, **SLP**

Baecker, Phyllis J 731 Hunt Way, Davis, CA 95616, (916) 678-5573, BS 77 Univ of MN - Minneap-St Paul; MS 79 Univ of WI - Madison; SLP, Solano Co Offi of Ed Ca, **SLP**

Baehr, Bonnie 17308 Avenue DE La Herradvra, Pacific Palisades, CA 90272, (213) 276-8585, BA 72 CA St Univ - Northridge; MA 74 CA St Univ - Los Angeles; Aud, Beverly Hills Hrng Aid Cen, **A**

Baer, Elizabeth Cardwell Route 2 Box 291, White Pines Farm, Centerville, MD 21617, Sp-Lang Path, Queen Annes County Board of Ed, **SLP**

Baer, Juli Ann Department Speech Pathology A-208, Loma Linda University Medical Center, Barton & Anderson Roads, Loma Linda, CA 92354, (714) 824-4401, BA 74 Univ of Redlands; MS 76 Univ of Redlands, 76–Sp-Lang Path, Loma Linda University Med Ctr, **SLP**

Baer, Karen Marie Route 2 Box 540-Aa, Berlin, MD 21811, (301) 289-4112, BS 80 Bloomsburg Univ of PA; MA 82 Univ of TN - Knoxville; Sp-Lang Path, Worcester County Sch, **SLP**

Baer, Mildred I 4712 West 6th, Topeka, KS 66606, (913) 272-6756, OB 51 Washburn Univ; MS 59 Univ of KS; **SLP LM**

Baer, Dr Sherwin H Dept Communication Disorders, Indiana State University, School Of Educ Bldg #420, Terre Haute, IN 47809, (812) 237-2807, BS 54 Univ of UT; MS 55 Brigham Young Univ; PH 58 (NS) OH St Univ; Prof-Commun Dis, IN St U, **SLP A**

Baer, Dr William P 128 Chisholm Trail, Redlands, CA 92373, BS Univ of MN - Minneap-St Paul; MA Univ of MN - Minneap-St Paul; PH (NS) Case Western Reserve Univ; Chief Aud/SLP Svc, VA Hosp/Loma Linda Ca, **SLP**

Baer-Forman, Mrs Mary Ann 13901 Olive View Lane #57, Sylmar, CA 91342, (818) 362-5222, MA 79 CA St Univ - Los Angeles; SLP, LA Co Schs, **SLP**

Baernstein, Mrs Denise Marie C 12304 3rd Street, Yucaipa, CA 92399, (714) 793-6841, BA 76 Univ of Redlands; MS 81 Univ of Redlands; Sp-Lang Path, Redlands USD, **SLP**

Baessler, Jane K 416 East Wayne Street, Maumee, OH 43537, (419) 893-1483, BA 69 Coll of Wooster; MA 71 MI St Univ; Sp-Lang Path, Sunshine Chldns Home, **SLP**

Baete, Mrs Phyllis Pharis 2580 Charlestown Road, New Albany, IN 47150, (812) 948-1336, BS 68 Murray St Univ; MS 71 Murray St Univ; Aud, Southeast IN Rehab Ctr, **A**

Bagan, Mary Ann Box 211, Gage Hill, Luzerne, NY 12846, (518) 584-3110, BA 69 SUNY - Center at Albany; MS 76 SUNY - Center at Albany; 82–Discipline Coord/Sp-Lang Path-Aud, Wilton Developmental Center, **SLP**

Bagarella, Diane R 62 Glen Street, Melrose, MA 02176, **SLP**

Bagby, Mrs Jill Rebecca G PO Box 2247, Shelby, NC 28150, (704) 487-5225, BS 76 Univ of WI - Stevens Point; MS 78 Univ of WI - Eau Claire; Sp-Lang Path, Cleveland Home Health Agency, **SLP**

Baggett, Donna D Lake Arrowhead Station 3024, Waleska, GA 30183, (404) 226-4623, ME 86 Univ of GA; 88–Clinical Svcs Coord, Looper's Speech & Hearing Clinic, **SLP**

Baggett, Jewell M 2415 Xenium Lane, Plymouth, MN 55441, (612) 553-0787, BA 81 Univ of Southwestern LA; OM 82 LA St Univ - N O Medical Ctr; Aud, Rexton, **A**

Baggett, Julie Evan 323 SE Baublits Road, Pensacola, FL 32507, (904) 455-6240, BS 83 Univ of South AL; OM 85 Auburn Univ - Auburn; 87–Sp-Lang Path, Escambia Co PS, **SLP**

Baggs, Terry W 4540 Flamingo Road, Memphis, TN 38117-1148, (901) 525-2682, BA 77 Freed-Hardeman Coll; MS 81 Univ of AR - Fayetteville; Phd Stud, Memphis St U, **SLP**

Baghdassarian, Mrs Kathleen 1960 Starvale Road, Glendale, CA 91207, (818) 500-8911, BS 73 Univ of IL - Urbana; MA 74 Univ of IL - Urbana; **A**

Bagley, Christine Maria 1033 Golf Course Drive, Rohnert Park, CA 94928, (707) 762-6601, BA 74 CA St Univ - Sacramento; MA 76 Humboldt St Univ; **SLP**

Bagli, Dr Zenobia R 727 Woodmere Drive, Nashville, TN 37217, (615) 320-3049, BS 70 Bombay Univ - India; MA 72 Univ of Cincinnati; PH 77 (Aud) Univ of Cincinnati; 77–Associate Professor/Coord Aud, Tennessee State University, **SLP A ACE**

Bagnall, Mrs Tracy Ann 7323 South Teller Court, Littleton, CO 80123, (303) 270-7856, BA 86 Univ of Northern CO; MA 87 Univ of Northern CO; 88–Aud, U of CO Hlth Sci Ctr, **A**

Bagni, Martha J 5 Pine Street, Newburyport, MA 01950, (617) 462-0687, MS 86 Univ of NH; 87–Sp-Lang Path, Pvt Cont Practice, **SLP**

Bagniefski, Susan Mary 915 Park, Kemmerer, WY 83101, BS 77 Univ of WI - Eau Claire; MS 80 Univ of WI - Eau Claire; SLP, Sandstone Pub Schs, **SLP**

Bagwell, Cynthia L 214 Chandler Avenue, Oxford, MS 38655, (601) 234-1476, BA 77 Univ of MS; MA 80 Univ of MS; Dir Diag Svc, N MS Retard Cen, **A**

Bahas-Horattas, Mrs Karen Marie 414 St Leger Avenue, Akron, OH 44305, (216) 379-8264, BA 84 Univ of Akron; MA 86 Univ of Akron; **SLP**

Bahmani, Amy Frances 380 West Glen Drive, Glen Carbon, IL 62034, BS 80 Southern IL Univ-Edwardsvill; MS 82 Southern IL Univ-Edwardsvill

Bahra, Mrs Joan A 36221 Grand River Avenue, Apartment 103, Farmington Hills, MI 48024-1438, (313) 421-1585, BA 80 MI St Univ; MA 81 Western MI Univ; 87–Clin Dir, Lake Forest Health Svcs, **SLP**

Bahrainwala, Lubaina E Kumc Student Union #268, Kansas City, KS 66103, (312) 303-5362, MA 88 Univ of KS

Bahruth-Poskey, Mary E 117 Patton Drive, Ponca City, OK 74601, (405) 765-8073, BS 78 Fort Hays St Univ; MS 80 Fort Hays St Univ; Sp/Lang Path, Sp Path Assoc of N Central Oklahoma, **SLP**

Baidowsky, Pamela Michele 2 Medallion Road, Kiamesha Lake, NY 12751, (914) 338-8686, BA 84 SUNY - Center at Buffalo; MA 86 Univ of CT; 86–Dir of Aud, Aud & Hearing Aid Svcs, **A**

Baier, Mrs Mary S Rural Route 1, Hager City, WI 54014, (612) 388-8875, BS 74 Univ of WI - River Falls; MS 76 Univ of WI - River Falls; 80–Sp-Lang Path, Red Wing District 256, **SLP**

Baier, Pamela Louise 104 NW 8th Street, Pocahontas, IA 50574, (712) 335-3588, BA 81 Univ of Northern IA; MA 82 Univ of SD - Vermillion; Sp-Lang Path, Arrowhead AEA, **SLP**

Bailets, Mrs Ann Britt 208 West Courtland Avenue, Shiremanstown, PA 17011, (717) 737-6960, BS 79 Bloomsburg Univ of PA; MS 80 Bloomsburg Univ of PA; 80–Sp-Lang Path, Capital Area Intermed Unit 15, **SLP ACE**

Bailey, Mrs Alice G 2007 Bob White Lane, West Columbia, SC 29169, (803) 252-2538, BS 64 Univ of GA; ME 65 Univ of GA; Dir, Palmetto Sp Path Assoc Consult, **SLP**

Bailey, Mrs Anita S 2436 Aloma, Wichita, KS 67211, (316) 262-4021, BA 67 Wichita St Univ; MS 71 CO St Univ; Sp-Lang Path, Black Hills Rehab Hosp, **SLP**

Bailey, Mrs Annmarie Doyle 3317 Larchmore Avenue, Wayzata, MN 55391, (612) 546-5411, BA 81 Saint Cloud St Univ; MA 82 Univ of WI - River Falls; SLP, Ebenezer Caroline Center, **SLP**

Bailey, Beryl Irene 80 Thompson Street, First Floor, New Haven, CT 06511, (203) 576-7426, BA 81 Simmons Coll; MS 87 Southern CT St Univ; 88–Sp-Lang Path, Hartford PS

Bailey, Mrs Beth Ann 4308 Donnelly Road, Anderson, IN 46017, (317) 529-0900, BS 81 Ball St Univ; MA 83 Ball St Univ; Sp-Lang Path, New Castle State Devel Center, **SLP**

Bailey, Beverly S Concourse Centre Suite B, 401 West Pike Street, Lawrenceville, GA 30245, (404) 995-5327, BS 67 Clarion Univ of PA; MS 72 Univ of Pittsburgh - Pittsburgh; 83–Dir, Bailey Sp & Lang Svcs, **SLP**

Bailey, Mrs Cherie Campagna 2800 Hirschfield #77, Spring, TX 77373, (913) 350-8341, BS 85 LA St Univ - Baton Rouge; MA 87 Univ of Houston - Univ Park; Sp-Lang Path, Northwest Memorial Hosp, **SLP**

Bailey, Deborah Hinton 185 Pulpit Road, Bedford, NH 03102, (603) 624-6422, BS 78 Univ of NH; MA 80 OH Univ - Athens; Sp-Lang Path, Manchester Prog for Hrng Imp, **SLP**

Bailey, Mrs Demetriel Poche 2620 Kismet Street, Marrero, LA 70072, (504) 362-3644, BA 81 Univ of Southwestern LA; ME 86 Southeastern LA Univ; 82–Sp-Lang Path, New Orleans PS, **SLP**

Bailey, Dena A 31 Northfield Road, Longmeadow, MA 01106, (413) 567-7431, BA 67 Univ of VT; MS 68 Univ of VT; SLP, Early Childhood Serv Team, **SLP**

Bailey, Dr Donn Fritz 5626 Dorchester, Chicago, IL 60637, (312) 268-7500, BS 54 IN Univ - Bloomington; MA 62 IN Univ - Bloomington; PH 74 (Sp Comm Soc Linguistics) PA St Univ - Univ Park; 74–Dir/Prof, Northwestern IL Univ, **SLP**

Bailey, Elizabeth 418 Belvue Lane, Balboa, CA 92661, BA 70 Univ of CA - Irvine; MA 86 CA St Univ - Fullerton

Bailey, Mrs Elizabeth P P O Box 88037, Dunwoody, GA 30356, **SLP**

Bailey, Jean F 2320 Eastgate Way, Tallahassee, FL 32308, (904) 385-5575, BS 73 FL St Univ; MS 72 FL St Univ; Prog Spec for Sp-Lang Prog, Leon Co Sch, **SLP**

Bailey, Mrs Jill Anne 8971 Yukon Street, Westminster, CO 80020, (303) 423-3985, BS 83 CO St Univ; MS 86 CO St Univ; 86–Sp-Lang Path, Aurora PS, **SLP**

Bailey, Jill M 216 Van Buren Drive, Mason, OH 45040, (606) 292-4020, BS 80 WV Univ; MA 83 Univ of Cincinnati; 84–Sp-Lang Path, St Elizabeth Med Cen, **SLP**

Bailey, Mrs Jolan Nagy Rd 2 Box 62-Ab, Ligonier, PA 15658, (412) 459-8000, BS 71 Indiana Univ of PA; ME 72 Indiana Univ of PA; **SLP**

Bailey, Mrs Kathryn C 3620 Double Rock Lane, Baltimore, MD 21234, (301) 939-2410, BA 80 Loyola Coll; MS 81 Loyola Coll; Sp-Lang Path, Harford County Schools, **SLP**

Bailey, Kristi Anne 15 Holbrook Avenue, North Attleboro, MA 02760, (617) 695-4857, MA 83 Central MI Univ; Sp-Lang Path, Mansfield Public School, **SLP**

Bailey, Larry Jerome 851 1/2 Golden Street, Tallahassee, FL 32304-2473, (904) 224-6246, SLP, **SLP**

Bailey, Laura Miller 711 Kottke, Madison, WI 53719, (608) 271-4631, MA 85 MI St Univ; **SLP**

Bailey, Leslie Ann 668 Yoeman Hall Road, Kalispell, MT 59901, (406) 752-3346, MA 83 Humboldt St Univ; 85–Sp-Lang Path, Private Practice, **SLP**

Bailey, Mrs Linda K 976 West Foothill, Suite 507, Claremont, CA 91711, (714) 626-5766, BA 74 CA St Univ - Fullerton; MS 78 Univ of LA Verne; Tchr, San Bernardino Co Sch, **SLP**

Bailey, Lorena 10601 South Drive #102, Houston, TX 77099, BS 72 Univ Southern MS-Hattiesburg; MA 74 Wichita St Univ; Sp-Lang Path, Lamar Cons ISD, **SLP**

Bailey, Mrs Madeleine Marie L 102 Euclid Avenue, Somerset, MA 02726, (617) 679-5840, BS 75 Boston Univ; MS 80 Univ of RI; Sp-Lang Path, Somerset Sch Dept, **SLP**

Bailey, Mrs Marie A 1850 Kehrswood Drive, Chesterfield, MO 63005, (314) 537-9447, BS 62 Purdue Univ - West Lafayette; MS 66 Purdue Univ - West Lafayette; Sp-Lang Path, **SLP**

Bailey, Mrs Martha Yvette 305 Royal Street, Gulfport, MS 39503, (601) 832-2165, BS 82 Univ Southern MS-Hattiesburg; MS 84 Univ Southern MS-Hattiesburg; SLP, Keesler Air Force Base, **SLP**

Bailey, Mary Ellen 7351 East Speedway #34E, Tucson, AZ 85710, (602) 621-7069, OB 68 Emporia St Univ; MA 70 Wichita St Univ; Cl Instr, U of AZ, **SLP**

Bailey, Melinda Robin 4593 Lavista Road, Tucker, GA 30084, (404) 279-5140, BS 85 Univ of GA; ME 86 GA St Univ; **SLP**

Bailey, Pauline G 79 Gary Road, Stamford, CT 06903, (203) 322-2942, BA 70 MI St Univ; MA 71 MI St Univ; Aud, Private Practice, **A**

Bailey, Peggy L 2249 West Whittier Blvd, La Habra, CA 90631, (213) 691-0827, BA 72 CA St Univ - Long Beach; MA 75 Whittier Coll; 77–Sp-Lang Path, La Habra Rehab Assoc, **SLP**

Bailey, Mrs Suzanne B 55 Pharr Road N W #A-112, Atlanta, GA 30305, (404) 378-5433, BA 80 FL St Univ; OM 82 Emory Univ; Sp-Lang Path, Visiting Nurse Ass of Atlanta, **SLP**

Bailey, Mrs Tyyna M 28 1/2 North 100 East, Apartment 7, Logan, UT 84321, (801) 753-0352, BA 86 Henderson St Univ; MS 88 UT St Univ

Bailey-Jones, Karen E 73 Carriage Road, Clifton Park, NY 12065, (518) 383-0962, BA 73 SUNY - Coll at Buffalo; MA 76 SUNY - Center at Buffalo; 86–Sp-Lang Path, Albany County Nursing Home, **SLP**

Bailin, Janet H G 1410 South Center Avenue, Sioux Falls, SD 57105, (605) 331-7956, BA 51 Vassar Coll; MA 72 Augustana Coll; SLP, Sioux Falls Pub School System, **SLP**

Bailis, Barbara L 239 Marilynn Street, East Islip, NY 11730, (516) 541-7400, BA 52 CUNY - Brooklyn Coll; Sp-Path, BOCES-Nassau, **SLP**

Baillargeon, Jocelyne G 234 Wareham Street, Middleboro, MA 02346, (617) 947-3634, BS 76 Univ of ME - Farmington; ME 81 Northeastern Univ

Baily, Mrs Linda B 4445 Roxborough Place, Pensacola, FL 32514, (904) 474-5358, BA 75 Univ of MI - Ann Arbor; MA 77 Univ of Houston - Univ Park; Sp-Lang Path, Rehab I of West FL, **SLP**

Bailys, Wendy Susan 6811 Mayfield Road #695, Mayfield Heights, OH 44124, (216) 526-5000, BA 79 OH St Univ; MA 84 Cleveland St Univ; SLP, Warrensville Developmental Cen, **SLP**

Bain, Dr Barbara A Communication Sci & Disorders, University Of Montana, Missoula, MT 59812, (406) 243-4131, BS 63 KS St Univ; MA 65 Univ of IA; PH 81 (NS) Univ of WA; Assoc Prof & Chair, U of MO, **SLP A ACE**

Bain, Donna McDade 3/5 Swanbourne Street, Fremantle, West Australia, Australia 6160, (616) 343-2601, BA 83 Univ of VT; MA 85 Univ of ME - Orono; **SLP**

Bain, Sue McDevett 1910 York Street, Kinston, NC 28501, (919) 523-0687, BS 81 East Carolina Univ; MS 85 East Carolina Univ; 85–Aud, Kinston Head & Neck Phys, **A**

Bainbridge, Mrs Patricia P 50 Audubon Drive, Synder, NY 14226, (716) 839-5050, BA 66 MI St Univ; MA 67 MI St Univ; 86–Coord, UCP Assoc, **SLP**

Baines, Kathleen Anderson 3940 Holden Drive, Ann Arbor, MI 48103, (313) 475-1311, BS 69 OH Univ - Athens; MS 70 Univ of MI - Ann Arbor; Dir SLP Dept, Chelsea Comm Hosp, **SLP**

Bair, Deborah L 93 Chase Street, Burlington, VT 05401-1519, (802) 863-4521, MS 81 Univ of VT; 83–Sp-Lang Path, Burlington PS, **SLP**

Bair, Mrs Janice J Route 3 Box 442-A, Trinity, NC 27370, (704) 731-3361, BA 80 Univ of TN - Knoxville; MA 81 Marshall Univ; Sp-Lang Path, Davidson Co Pub Sch, **SLP**

Bair, Sharon Mutchler 501 Tara Court, De Forest, WI 53532, (608) 742-4131, BS 79 Univ of WI - Madison; MA 81 Univ of IA; Sp-Lang Path, Divine Savior Hosp & Nurs Home, **SLP**

Baird, Allison J 1-38 Home Street, Winnipeg, MB, Canada R3G 1W6, (416) 256-4301, MA 79 Univ of ND; Sp-Lang Path, St Amant Center Inc, **SLP**

Baird, Ann Elizabeth 1757 S E Laconia Avenue, Des Moines, IA 50320-1166, (515) 243-1297, BS 82 IA St Univ; MA 84 Northeast MO St Univ; SLP, Des Moines ISD, **SLP**

Baird, Mrs Barbara H 14 Starr Lane, Bethel, CT 06801, (203) 792-1936, BS 71 Lamar Univ; MS 76 Lamar Univ

Baird, Mrs Beverly 321 Flurnoy Avenue, Florence, AL 35630, (205) 766-1618, BS 70 MS Coll; MA 72 Univ of TN - Knoxville; Instructor, MS Coll, **SLP**

Baird, Mrs Bonnie Stuart 4 Haines Court, Franklin, NJ 07416, (717) 296-9261, MA 84 Montclair St Coll; Sp-Lang Path, Head Injury Recov Ctr Hillcrst, **SLP ACE**

Baird, Deborah Gustafson Physical Medicine & Rehab, St Paul-Ramsey Medical Ctr, 640 Jackson Street, St Paul, MN 55101, (612) 221-2053, BA 76 Bethel Coll; MA 82 Univ of MN - Minneap-St Paul; Sp/Lang Path, St Paul-Ramsey Med Cen, **SLP**

Baird, Diane J 91 Fallon Avenue, Providence, RI 02908, **SLP**

Baird, Mrs Judy File R R 1 Box 86-E, Edgerton, KS 66021, (913) 782-8950, BA 74 KS St Univ; MS 75 KS St Univ; Sp-Lang Path, Olathe Dist Sch, **SLP**

Baird, Mary P 2151 Wildwood, Jackson, MI 49202, (517) 787-1468, BA 71 Mercy Coll of Detroit; MA 73 Central MI Univ; Exec Dir, Jackson Sp Hrng Cl, **A**

Baird, Patricia M 4939 Garfield Street, La Mesa, CA 92041, MA 70 Univ of CA - San Diego; Chief/Audiological Services, Univ Calif-San Diego Med Ctr, **A**

Baird, Dr Samera M Auburn University, Dept Rehab & Special Educ, 1234 Haley Center, Auburn, AL 36849, (205) 826-5943, BS 72 Univ of TN - Knoxville; MA 73 Univ of TN - Knoxville; PH 87 (Speical Education Early Childhood); Asst Prof, Auburn University, **SLP**

Baird, Mrs Virginia G 58 Barbara Lane N W, Atlanta, GA 30327, (404) 351-1530, BA Wesleyan Coll; BA Wesleyan Coll; ME Emory Univ; Liaison Specialist Prog Ex Chi, Atlanta Pub Sch, **SLP**

Baisden, Terese Horning 903 Richards Avenue, Watertown, WI 53094, (414) 262-0063, BS 79 Marquette Univ; MS 80 Marquette Univ; 87–Sp-Lang Path, Oconomowoc Area Sch Dist, **SLP**

Baisinger, Dr Wilbur H 1014 North Union Avenue, Tacoma, WA 98406, PH 58 (NS) Northwestern Univ; Professor Emeritus, University of Puget Sound, **SLP LM**

Baisler, Perry E 23033 Westchester Boulevard, Apartment D-401, Port Charlotte, FL 33980, (813) 743-6428, BA 32 Univ of WA; MA 38 Univ of WA; PH 50 (NS) Northwestern Univ; Retired, **SLP LM**

Bajusz, Mrs Goldie A 1125 Huntleigh Drive, Naperville, IL 60540, (312) 961-3060, BA 54 Coll of Saint Francis; MA 55 Marquette Univ; Sp/Lang Path, Bromberek Sch-Dist 65, **SLP**

Bakaysza, Mrs Donna 8358 Elaine Drive, Pittsburgh, PA 15237, BS 76 Edinboro Univ of PA; MA 77 Edinboro Univ of PA; **SLP**

Baken, Dr Ronald J Columbia University, Teachers College Box 3, 525 West 120th Street, New York, NY 10027, (212) 678-3894, BA 63 Columbia Univ Teachers Coll; MS 65 Univ of NE - Omaha; PH 69 (NS) Columbia Univ Teachers Coll; Prof, Tchr Coll Columbia U

Baker, Mrs Alyse Otvos 10145 Grubbs Road, Wexford, PA 15090, (412) 935-2044, BA 72 Yale Univ; ME 73 Univ of MI - Ann Arbor; MS 74 Univ of MI - Ann Arbor; 88–Sp-Lang Path, InSpeech Inc, **SLP ACE**

Baker, Mrs Arlene M 30 Richland Street, South Portland, ME 04106, (207) 871-1205, MS 74 Univ of AZ; Sp-Lang Path, Spurwink School, **SLP**

Baker, Mrs Arlene P 2315 Bondy Street, Windsor, ON, Canada N9H 1J4, (519) 966-5668, BA 66 Wayne St Univ; MA 87 Wayne St Univ

Baker, Ashley H 10 Tregunter Path, Apartment 1201, Tavistock, Hong Kong, MA 72 Univ of Denver; **A**

Baker, Audrey Vendeland 617 Surfside Drive, Akron, OH 44319, (216) 644-0699, BS 82 Kent St Univ; MA 82 Kent St Univ; Sp-Lang Path, Coventry Local Sch, **SLP**

Baker, Mrs Beth 814 Tanager #25, Fort Walton Beach, FL 32548, (904) 474-0666, BA 74 FL St Univ; MS 77 FL St Univ; Sp-Lang Path Consul, **SLP**

Baker, Mrs Beverly H 1505 Stagecoach Drive, Arlington, TX 76013, (504) 291-6370, BA 73 Eastern WA Univ; BA 74 Eastern WA Univ; MS 75 Eastern WA Univ; **SLP**

Baker, Billie Ruth P O Box 79, San Marcos, TX 78667-0079, BA 79 Univ of MS; MA 81 Univ of MS; Audiologist, J P Bordelon MD & Assoc, **A**

Baker, Carla Jean 232 Randall Drive, Folsom, CA 95630, (916) 644-2096, BA 79 CA St Univ - Sacramento; MA 81 CA St Univ - Sacramento; Sp-Lang Path, Pollock Pines Elemen Sch Dist, **SLP**

Baker, Carol Putman Rt 4 Box 4445, Joelton, TN 37080, (615) 327-3040, BS 84 Univ of TN - Knoxville; MA 86 Memphis St Univ; 88–Aud, The Otology Group, **A**

Baker, Catherine S 926 The Alameda, Berkeley, CA 94707, (415) 527-7045, BA 74 Washington Univ; MS 81 San Francisco St Univ; Sp-Lang Path, Private Practice, **SLP**

Baker, Charlotte Pierce 630 Belfry Drive, Centre Square, PA 19422, (215) 438-5714, BA 65 Howard Univ; MA 66 OH St Univ; PH 85 (Sp/Linguistics) Temple Univ; 84–Tchr, Germantown Friends Sch, **SLP**

Baker, Christopher 207 W Audubon, Fresno, CA 93711, (209) 229-9206, BS 78 Wheeling Coll; MS 81 WV Univ; 81–Sp-Lang Path, InSpeech Inc, **SLP ACE**

Baker, Mrs Connie K 3707 Sweetwater Drive, Rocklin, CA 95677, (916) 624-2907, BA 71 San Diego St Univ; MA 73 San Diego St Univ; **A**

Baker, Correan M 6311 Linus Drive, Baltimore, MD 21207, (301) 788-8007, BA 72 Univ of MD - College Park; MA 73 Univ of MD - College Park; SLP, Balt Cty Pub Schs, **SLP**

Baker, Mrs Cynthia S 2204 Wilkinson Place, Alexandria, VA 22306, (703) 360-0929, BS 74 Univ of MD - College Park; MS 76 Towson St Univ; SLP, Fairfax County Pub Sch, **SLP**

Baker, Deborah E 643 Naugher Road, Huntsville, AL 35811, (205) 532-4718, BS 75 Univ of AL- Tuscaloosa; MS 79 Univ of AL- Tuscaloosa; Coord Hrng Impaired Program, Huntsville City Schs, **A**

Baker, Deborah Prince 312 East 7th Street, Mountain Home, AR 72653, (501) 424-4327, BA 76 Univ Southern MS-Hattiesburg; MS 77 Univ Southern MS-Hattiesburg; 88–Aud, Private Practice, **A**

Baker, Dian Gail 3626 Elmridge, Houston, TX 77025, (713) 661-2369, BA 78 Univ of Houston - Univ Park; MA 87 Univ of Houston - Univ Park; 88–Sp-Lang Path, Alief ISD, **SLP**

Baker, Dr Donald J 9913 Edgehill Lane, Silver Spring, MD 20901, (301) 454-5831, BS 54 OH St Univ; MA 56 OH St Univ; PH 62 (Hrng & Sp Science) OH St Univ; Aud, Univ of MD-College Pk, **A**

Baker, Mrs Dorothy A C 222 North Clay Street, Zelienople, PA 16063, (412) 452-0650, BA 79 Univ of Pittsburgh - Pittsburgh; MA 81 Memphis St Univ; Sp-Lang Path, **SLP**

Baker, Dorothy E 1628 19th Street, Lubbock, TX 79401, (806) 766-1214, BS 77 Abilene Christian Univ; MS 78 TX Tech Univ; Coord Diagnostic, Lubbock ISD, **SLP**

Baker, Elizabeth 414 Langhorlm Drive, Winter Park, FL 32789, (305) 322-8823, BS 73 SUNY - Coll at Geneseo; MA 81 Univ of Central FL; SLP, Seminole Co Sch Bd, **SLP**

Baker, Ellen P B 1503 East 22nd Street, Brooklyn, NY 11210, (212) 338-1736, BA 73 CUNY - Brooklyn Coll; MS 76 CUNY - Brooklyn Coll; Sp/Lang Path, Ellen Baker, **SLP**

Baker, Dr Elmer E, Jr 330 East 63rd Street #4E, New York, NY 10021, (212) 598-2938, MA 49 NY Univ; PH 54 NY Univ; OD 69 (NS) Emerson Coll; Prof, New York U, **SLP**

Baker, Helen L P O Box 48, Otterbein, IN 47970, (317) 583-4504, MA 62 IN Univ - Bloomington; **SLP**

Baker, Mrs Ida Carter 12927 South Lowe Avenue, Chicago, IL 60628, BS; **SLP LM**

Baker, Jane Meier 3172 Quentin Street, Aurora, CO 80011, (303) 778-5817, BS 84 CO St Univ; MS 86 CO St Univ; **A**

Baker, Mrs Janet Ann 11 Devon Court, Wilmington, DE 19810, (215) 447-2428, BS 77 Northwestern Univ; MA 78 Northwestern Univ; Sp-Lang Path, Crozer-Chester Med Cen, **SLP**

Baker, Janet L 9 Breckinridge Square, Louisville, KY 40220, (502) 588-5331, BA 83 Univ of KY; MS 84 Univ of KY; 88–Sp/Lang Path, Univ of Louisville, **SLP**

Baker, Jennifer Cox 3408 Redbud Lane, Lima, OH 45806, (419) 228-4271, BS 77 Miami Univ - Oxford; MA 82 OH St Univ; Sp-Lang Path, Allen County Public Schools, **SLP**

Baker, Jill Andrea 5064 Imperial, Richton Park, IL 60471, (312) 747-1879, MS 88 Eastern IL Univ; 88–Sp-Lang Path, Ctr for Comm Dis Ltd

Baker, Judith Ann 7845 South Nagle Avenue, Burbank, IL 60459, (312) 629-8900, BS 86 Bradley Univ; MA 88 OH Univ - Athens; 88–Aud, MTS Associates Inc

Baker, Judith Diane 905 East Michigan Street, Mount Pleasant, MI 48858, (517) 773-1209, BS 83 Central MI Univ; MA 86 Central MI Univ; 86–Aud/Prog Dir, Allied Hlth Svcs Inc, **A**

Baker, Karen Ann 221 North Downtown Mall, Las Cruces, NM 88001, (505) 523-0661, MA 86 NM St Univ; 87–Sp-Lang Path, Baker & Stern, **SLP**

Baker, Karen Lee 738 North Palo Verde Avenue, Tucson, AZ 85716, (602) 326-5725, BS 85 Baylor Univ; MS 86 Univ of TX - Dallas; 87–Sp-Lang Path, Carondelet St Mary's Hosp, **SLP**

Baker, Mrs Karen M 34 Kennedy Drive, North Chelmsford, MA 01863, (508) 251-0381, BA 80 SUNY - Coll at Cortland; MS 82 Adelphi Univ; 88–Sp-Lang Path, Mass Easter Seal Society, **SLP**

Baker, Karen P 619 Aster Boulevard, Rockville, MD 20850, (301) 340-3025, BS 63 Syracuse Univ; MA 65 IN Univ - Bloomington; **SLP**

Baker, Mrs Karin S 2285 S W Cedar Hills Blvd, Portland, OR 97225, (503) 643-4371

Baker, Mrs Katherine Perez 5535 Virginia Beach Blvd, Norfolk, VA 23502, (804) 466-7566, BS 77 Univ of South AL; MS 79 Univ of AL- Tuscaloosa; Sp-Lang Path, Rotary Rehab Hosp, **SLP**

Baker, Kathy L 63 John Street, Winsted, CT 06098, (203) 482-0196, BA 83 Central CT St Univ; MA 87 SUNY - Coll at Plattsburgh; 88–Sp-Lang Path, Northwest Ctr, **SLP**

Baker, Kathy Sue The Children's Hospital, 1056 East 19th Avenue, Denver, CO 80218-1088, (303) 861-6800, BA 77 Univ of Northern CO; MA 81 Univ of Northern CO; 87–Aud, The Children's Hosp, **A**

Baker, Kelley D 2419 Hickory Hollow Lane, Spring, TX 77386, (713) 353-2345, BS 83 Baylor Univ; MS 84 Baylor Univ; 88–Kindergarten Tchr, Spring ISD, **SLP**

Baker, Kelly Taylor Oakwood Village, Bldg 75 Apartment 6, Flanders, NJ 07836, (215) 631-9300, BA 85 Univ of Pittsburgh - Pittsburgh; MA 87 Univ of Pittsburgh - Pittsburgh; **SLP**

Baker, Dr La Verne L Univ Southwest Louisiana, Dept Comm Disorders, Lafayette, LA 70504, (318) 231-6721, BA 56 Wichita St Univ; MS 60 6131; PH 81 (Communicative Disorders & Sciences) Wichita St Univ; Asst Prof Commun Dis Sciences, Univ of Southwestern Louisiana, **SLP**

Baker, Mrs Laura L 9162 Emerson's Reach, Columbia, MD 21045, (301) 687-8151, BA 76 Loyola Coll; MS 77 Loyola Coll; Sp Ed Dept Chairmn/Sp-Lng Path, Baltimore County Board of Educ, **SLP**

Baker, Linda T R643 Hale Street, Beverly Farms, MA 01915, **SLP**

Baker, Linda Veronica 12345 N I-10 Service Road, Apartment 902, New Orleans, LA 70128, (504) 944-5877, BS 74 Univ Southern MS-Hattiesburg; ME 85 Southeastern LA Univ; **SLP**

Baker, Lisa Ann 2457 East 19th Street, Brooklyn, NY 12354, (718) 769-2907, BA 84 CUNY - Brooklyn Coll; MS 86 CUNY - Brooklyn Coll; **SLP**

Baker, Lorie H 1201 Adell, Little Rock, AR 72212, (501) 224-4457, **SLP**

Baker, Lynn S 131 Evelyn Place, Asheville, NC 28801, (704) 274-9136, BS 72 Western Carolina Univ; ME 87 Western Carolina Univ; 87–Sp-Lang Path, Buncombe County PS, **SLP**

Baker, Mrs Marcia T P O Box 698, Cashiers, NC 28717, (704) 743-3940, BA 79 Lenoir-Rhyne Coll; ME 81 Univ of Cincinnati; **SLP**

Baker, Margaret L 204 Idlewild Lane, Media, PA 19063, (215) 237-4388, BA 69 Hobart-William Smith Coll; MA 82 Temple Univ; 83–Sp-Lang Path, Mercy Catholic Med Ctr, **SLP**

Baker, Marilyn Ruth 3525 Middleton Avenue #3, Cincinnati, OH 45220, (606) 341-2044, BS 78 Northwestern Univ; ME 79 Boston Univ; Sp-Lang Path, American Hosp for Rehab-Edgewood, **SLP**

Baker, Mrs Marjorie L Route 2 Box 38, Venture Out on Cudjoe Cay, Summerland Key, FL 33042, (305) 745-1779, BS 54 Johns Hopkins Univ; MA 61 Univ of MD - College Park; **SLP LM**

Baker, Mrs Marletta A 902 Warner, Lemont, IL 60439, (312) 687-0900, BS 71 Pacific Union Coll; MA 72 Pacific Union Coll; Sp-Lang Path, SW Cook Co Coop Assoc Spec Ed, **SLP**

Baker, Mrs Martha E 2120 Hidden Springs Court, West Linn, OR 97068, (503) 655-3833, BA 48 Bob Jones Univ; MA 72 CA St Univ - Fresno; Sp-Lang Path, Private Practice, **SLP**

Baker, Martha Sue 149 Portland Avenue #92, Dover, NH 03820, (603) 742-2146, BA 85 Northern MI Univ; MA 86 MI St Univ; 88–Sp-Lang Path, SAU #33 Raymond NH Sch Dist, **SLP**

Baker, Mary Blank 129 Adams Lane, Richmond, KY 40475, (606) 792-3047, BS 75 Eastern KY Univ; ME 80 Eastern KY Univ; SLP, Garrard Co Schs, **SLP**

Baker, Mrs Mary G 416 Duff Road, Sewickley, PA 15143, (412) 741-0803, BS 78 CA Univ of PA; ME 81 CA Univ of PA; Sp-Lang Path, Albert Gallatin Human Serv Agc, **SLP**

Baker, Dr Nancy E Dept Communication Sci & Dis, University Of Vermont, Allen House, Burlington, VT 05405, (802) 656-3861, BS 66 Tufts Univ; MS 69 Univ of Pittsburgh - Pittsburgh; PH 81 (NS) Univ of Pittsburgh - Pittsburgh; U of VT, **SLP**

Baker, Nancy Mae American Hearing Center, 1809 SW H K Dodgen Loop, Temple, TX 76502, (817) 774-7727, BA 83 TX Tech Univ; MS 86 Univ of TX - Dallas; 87–Dir of Aud, American Hearing Center/ENT, **A**

Baker, Nora Mandell 1112 Quaker Ridge Drive, Austin, TX 78746, (512) 327-6532, BA 76 MI St Univ; MA 77 Eastern MI Univ; MA 78 MI St Univ; Audiologist, J P Bordelon MD, **SLP A**

Baker, Mrs Norma Jean 1117 South Ferguson, Springfield, MO 65807, (417) 589-2171, MA 83 Southeast MO St Univ; SLP, Laclede County R-1, **SLP**

Baker, Palma C 4542 Mountain View Trail, Clarkston, MI 48016, (313) 628-4417, BA 75 MI St Univ; MA 77 LA St Univ - Baton Rouge; Prog Dir, Total Therapy Management, **SLP**

Baker, Mrs Pattie W 1721 Montgomery Road, Thousand Oaks, CA 91360, (805) 497-9606, BA 78; MA 81 CA St Univ - Long Beach; Dir Sp-Lang Path, Burnwall Clinic, **SLP**

Baker, Rachelle D S 2621 Palisade Avenue, Riverdale, NY 10463, (212) 548-3624, BA 74 CUNY - City College; MS 75 Columbia Univ Teachers Coll; Sp-Lang Path, Fairfld Div/Heb Home for Aged, **SLP**

Baker, Richard D 1261 S E Skyline Drive, Santa Ana, CA 92705, (714) 731-0044, BS 64 UT St Univ; MS 66 UT St Univ; **SLP**

Baker, Mrs Rita Arlene 3615-C Camp Bowie, Fort Worth, TX 76107, (817) 735-8505, MS 75 Univ of North TX; SLP, Private Practice, **SLP**

Baker, Rita J 510 North Beverly, Arlington Heights, IL 60004, MS; **SLP**

Baker, Mrs Rita T P O Box 99, Bellwood, AL 36313, (205) 588-3793, BA 71 Auburn Univ - Auburn; MA 72 Univ of AL- Tuscaloosa; Sp-Lang Path, Daleville City Schools, **SLP**

Baker, Robert 4516 Boastfield Lane, Olney, MD 20832, (301) 774-1076, BS 78 Towson St Univ; MS 80 Towson St Univ; Aud, **A**

Baker, Dr Rochelle A 412 Beach Avenue, Half Moon Bay, CA 94019, (415) 726-3363, BA Emmanuel Coll; MS 72 MI St Univ; PH 86 (Commun Disorders) Univ of TX - Dallas; Sp-Lang Path, Private Practice, **SLP**

Baker, Sara Ann 6122 Foster #223, Overland Park, KS 66202, (816) 756-2250, BA 82 Univ of Northern IA; MA 85 Univ of KS; SLP, Rehab Institute, **SLP**

Baker, Mrs Susan K 1707 Chaise Court, Carson City, NV 89701-2335, BS 79 Univ of NV - Reno; MS 82 Univ of NV - Reno; Sp-Lang Path, Carson City Sch Dist, **SLP**

Baker, Susan Kay 608 Conneaut Avenue #14, Bowling Green, OH 43402, (419) 875-6965, BS 82 Western MI Univ; MA 83 Western MI Univ; Sp-Lang Path, Maumee Youth Cen, **SLP**

Baker, Tarrah M 5004 228th S E, Issaquah, WA 98027, (206) 392-1030, BS 79 Univ of WA; MS 81 Univ of WA; Sp-Lang Path, Issaquah Sch Dist, **SLP**

Baker, Terry L 1015 Barberry Lane, Kirkwood, MO 63122-5137, (314) 821-4220, BS 72 IL St Univ - Normal; MS 74 Southern IL Univ-Edwardsvill; Sp-Lang Path, Child Enrichment Center, **SLP**

Baker, Mrs Trudy Annette 1128 South John, Springfield, MO 65804, (417) 886-0011, BS 82 Southwest MO St Univ; MA 84 Memphis St Univ; 87–Aud, Reg Ear Nose and Throat Ctr, **A**

Baker-Buchalter, Mrs Darlene 806 North Stone Avenue, La Grange Park, IL 60525, (312) 863-4856, OB 57 Northern IL Univ - De Kalb; ME 77 De Paul Univ; Early Chldhood Sp & Lang Path, Bd of Ed-Cicero Sch Dist 99, **SLP**

Bakhit, Lily Mary 4309 Aliso Circle, La Verne, CA 91750, MA 86 CA St Univ - Fullerton; **SLP**

Bakhshi, Christine Lowe 2115 Honeytree Court, Columbus, OH 43229, (614) 365-5230, BS 72 OH St Univ; MA 81 OH St Univ; Sp-Lang Path, Columbus Pub Schs, **SLP**

Bakie, Bruce E 4105 Ballard Avenue, Cincinnati, OH 45209, BS 73 Univ of Cincinnati; MA 75 Univ of Cincinnati; Sp-Lang Path, Private Practice, **SLP**

Bakke, Matthew H 3114 Avenue P, Brooklyn, NY 11234, (212) 998-7714, MA 74 Columbia Univ Teachers Coll; MS 86 CUNY - Brooklyn Coll

Bakke-Horton, Mary G 221 Taylor Street, Rock Springs, WY 82901, (307) 362-2474, BS 73 CO St Univ; MA 74 Memphis St Univ; SLP, Sweetwater Co Sch Dist 1, **SLP**

Bakker, Connie Reddick Box 3114, Spruce Grove, AB, Canada T7X 3A4, (403) 482-8161, BS 79 Univ of Alberta - Alberta; MA 86 Univ of TX - Austin; 88–Sp-Lang Path, Edmonton Gen Hosp, **SLP**

Bakker, Dr Klaas 9042 North Park Plaza Court, Milwaukee, WI 53223, (414) 229-4810, PH 87 (NS) Southern IL Univ -Carbondale; 88–Asst Prof, Univ of WI at Milwaukee

Bakonyi, Susan Marie 4035 Three Oaks Blvd #4-B, Troy, MI 48098, (313) 632-0863, BA 84 MI St Univ; MA 86 Univ of CO - Boulder; **SLP**

Bakst, Julie S 459 Sierra Vista Lane, Bldg 11, Valley Cottage, NY 10989, (914) 358-0387, BA 75 SUNY - Coll at New Paltz; MA 79 Montclair St Coll; OM 84 SUNY - Coll at New Paltz; Chairpsn Speech Lang & Hearing, E Ramapo Central School Dist, **SLP**

Bala, Mrs Sandra M 104 Saratoga Road, Amherst, NY 14226, (716) 876-5918, BA 72 SUNY - Coll at Buffalo; MA 73 SUNY - Coll at Buffalo; SLP, Buffalo Bd of Ed, **SLP**

Balaban, Dr Mae J 100 State Street, Teaneck, NJ 07666, (201) 833-0655, ED 75 (Learning Disabilities) Columbia Univ Teachers Coll; 83–Director, Bergen Independent Child Study, **SLP A**

Balakrishnan, Uma Box 235 RFD 2, Putney, VT 05346, (413) 967-6211, MA 84 Univ of MA - Amherst; **SLP A**

Balanay, Mrs Cheryl A 8033 Bonnie Circle, Abilene, TX 79605, (915) 692-4053, BS 73 Loma Linda Univ - Riverside; MA 80 San Diego St Univ; 83–Supvr-Commun Ther, Abilene State School 676, **SLP**

Balas, Dr Robert F Sch Of Communicative Disorders, University Of Wisconsin, Stevens Point, WI 54481, (715) 346-2739, BA 61 Valparaiso Univ; MA 63 Northern IL Univ - De Kalb; PH 66 (NS) Univ of Denver; Prof, U of Wisconsin, **A**

Balash, Joan M 513 Pecan Grove Road #209, Austin, TX 78704, (512) 442-9379, BA 84 IN Univ - Bloomington; MA 87 Univ of TX - Austin; **A**

Balasubramanian, Dr Venugopal 58 North East St B-2 A4, Amherst, MA 01002, (413) 253-2176, PH 86 (Sp-Lang Path) SUNY - Center at Buffalo; 87–Sp-Lang Path, Valley Rehab Inc, **SLP**

Balay, Catherine Nolan 1123 N Clinton, Dallas, TX 75208, (214) 943-5241, MS 86 Univ of TX - Dallas; 87–Sp-Lang Path, Callier Ctr Univ of TX-Dallas, **SLP**

Balay, Georgean 2044 Devonshire Road, Bloomfield Hills, MI 48013-1590, (313) 478-8616, MS 68 Univ of Pittsburgh - Pittsburgh; **A**

Balbach, Mrs Julia Jochum 3811 Charles Drive, Evansville, IN 47711-9346, (812) 425-9404, BA 80 IN Univ - Bloomington; MA 81 IN Univ - Bloomington; Aud, Rehab Ctr, **A**

Balber, Bethel 6000 Canterbury #D314, Culver City, CA 90230, (213) 641-1721, BA 74 Univ of CA - Los Angeles; MA 80 CA St Univ - Los Angeles; SLP, LA USD, **SLP**

Balbierer, Mrs Karen Kingsley 4 Rockland Way, Glenmoore, PA 19343, (215) 942-3572, BS 86 Bloomsburg Univ of PA; MS 87 Bloomsburg Univ of PA; 88–Sp-Lang Path, Delaware Co Interm Unit, **SLP**

Balbo, John M VA Medical Center, Memorial Drive #117-H, Waco, TX 76703, (817) 752-6581, BS 76 Northern IL Univ - De Kalb; MS 78 IL St Univ - Normal; Aud, VA Med Cen, **A**

Balcena, Alice M 634 Canyon Road, Logan, UT 84321, (801) 752-6546, MS 88 UT St Univ; Sp-Lang Path, Cache Co Sch Dist

Baldes, Robert A Miss Bend Area Education Agency #9, 729 21st Street, Bettendorf, IA 52722, OB 66 Northeast MO St Univ; MA 66 Northeast MO St Univ; Supvr of Sp-Lang Path, Miss Bend AEA, **SLP**

Baldinger, Wendy R 479 Darla Court, West St Paul, MN 55118, (612) 455-2857, BS 78 Univ of MN - Minneap-St Paul; MA 80 Northwestern Univ; **SLP**

Baldovin, Mrs Jill RD 4 Box 219 Ridge Road, Vestal, NY 13850, (607) 785-2400, BS 78 SUNY - Coll at Geneseo; MA 79 IN Univ - Bloomington; Sp-Lang Path, Speech & Hearing Assoc, **SLP**

Baldwin, Ann M 12361 Oak Park Boulevard #305, Blaine, MN 55434, (612) 786-5570, OB 86 Univ of MN - Duluth; MA 87 Univ of MN - Duluth; 88–Sp-Lang Path, Spring Lake Park PS, **SLP**

Baldwin, Mrs Anne C 22593 Brookdale, Farmington Hills, MI 48024, (313) 851-2000, BS 77 Eastern MI Univ; MA 78 Eastern MI Univ; SLP, Bloomfield Hills Schs, **SLP**

Baldwin, Anne L Rangeway East, 2 Carle Apartment 5, Waterville, ME 04901, (207) 873-7186, BS 85 Coll of Saint Rose; MS 87 Indiana Univ of PA; 87–Sp-Lang Path, Elaine R Stevens Assoc, **SLP**

Baldwin, Barbara A Van Hogendorplaan 20, 3771 CP, Barneveld, Netherlands, BS 76 Fontbonne Coll; MS 77 Southern IL Univ -Carbondale; 88–Dir, American Red Cross, **SLP**

Baldwin, Mrs Barbara S P O Box 352, Unionville, CT 06085, (203) 673-2511, BA 66 FL St Univ; MS 67 FL St Univ; Sp-Lang Path, Reg Sch Dist #10 Harw/Burl Ct, **SLP**

Baldwin, Janice Louise Box 174B, North Creek Road, Greenfield Center, NY 12833, **SLP**

Baldwin, Kathleen A 1811 East Kenwood Blvd, Milwaukee, WI 53211, **SLP**

Baldwin, Laurel R 405 Harris Street, Spruce Pine, NC 28777, (704) 765-6999, BA Appalachian St Univ; MS Bowling Green St Univ; Sp-Lang Path, Avery County PS, **SLP**

Baldwin, Linda Mae Apt 9, 7601 32nd Avenue, Crystal, MN 55427, (612) 541-4747, BS 81 WV Univ; MA 82 Western MI Univ; 87–Sp-Lang Path, Achievement Rehab Corp, **SLP**

Baldwin, Martha Lynne 1017 Woodmont Blvd, Nashville, TN 37204, (615) 269-9294, BS 82 Abilene Christian Univ; MA 85 Memphis St Univ; SLP, Vanderbuilt Hosp, **SLP**

Baldwin, Dr Nona B 237 Balsam Road, Wakefield, RI 02879, (401) 294-4561, BS 61 Bloomsburg Univ of PA; MS 65 Bucknell Univ; PH 74 (Spec Ed and Rehab) Univ of Pittsburgh - Pittsburgh; Superv Spec Ed, Ladd Cen, **SLP**

Baldwin, Mrs Rachel Anne 2210 Wintergreen Place, Durham, NC 27707, (919) 596-8077, BA 75 NC Central Univ; MA 76 NC Central Univ; 83–Sp-Lang Path, Orange County Schs, **SLP**

Baldwin, Steven J 405 Harris Street, Spruce Pine, NC 28777, (704) 765-6999, 88–VP-Oper, Pro-Rehab Communi-care Inc, **SLP**

Baldwin, Susan 1108 Indian Prairie, Victor, MT 59875, BA 72 Univ of MT; MA 75 Univ of MT; Sp-Lang Path, **SLP**

Baldwin, Virginia H 68 Maple Avenue, PO Box 701, Norfork, CT 06058, (203) 727-1320, BA 50 Univ of NC - Chapel Hill; MS 78 Southern CT St Univ; **SLP**

Balent, Jerilyn W 1 Sycamore Street #3B, Newtown, PA 18940, (215) 757-7300, BS 79 Trenton St Coll; MS 83 Bloomsburg Univ of PA; Aud, ENT & Facial Plastic Surg Assoc Ltd, **A**

Bales, Mrs Debra Nicosia 1165 Saltaire Way, Mattituck, NY 11952, (516) 298-4304, BA 76 WV Univ; MA 81 Hofstra Univ; MA 84 Hofstra Univ; Sp-Lang Path, Mattituck-Cutchogue School, **SLP**

Bales, Joel D Army Aud & Speech Center, Walter Reed Army Med Ctr, Washington, DC 20307, BA 78 Univ of TN - Knoxville; MA 79 Univ of TN - Knoxville; 79–Aud, US Army, **A**

Bales, Mrs Julia Ann 2407 South Troost, Tulsa, OK 74114, (918) 749-1326, BS 77 Southwest MO St Univ; MA 85 Univ of Tulsa; Sp-Lang Path, Town and Country School, **SLP**

Bales, Tammy Lynn 380-A Peachtree Road, Spartanburg, SC 29302, (803) 573-6480, BS 80 Baylor Univ; MA 81 Univ of TN - Knoxville; SLP, Spartanburg Gen Hosp, **SLP**

Balfour, Patricia University Of South Carolina, Green & Pickens, Dept Of Commun Disorders, Columbia, SC 29208, (803) 777-4813, BA 78 Univ of MD - College Park; MS 80 Gallaudet Coll; 87–Aud, Univ of South Carolina, **A**

Balick, Dr Sylvia G 28 East 10th Street, New York, NY 10003, (212) 420-2760, BA 46 CUNY - Hunter Coll; MA 64 NY Univ; PH 77 (NS) NY Univ; Chief Speech-Lang Pathology, Beth Israel Medial Center, **SLP**

Baliga, Mrs Gayathri Bantwal 501 North Gardner Avenue, Lubbock, TX 79416, (806) 766-1198, MA 77 Kent St Univ; 88–Sp-Lang Path, Lubbock ISD, **SLP**

Balin, Mrs Betty W 2207 Touchstone Court, Silver Spring, MD 20904-5239, (301) 622-4354, **SLP**

Balinskas, Carolyn 10 Conwell Street, Somerville, MA 02143, (617) 628-2592, MS 88 Northeastern Univ

Balisy, Mrs Diane Elizabeth 4944 Angeles Crest, La Canada, CA 91011, (213) 625-4183, BA 83 CA St Univ - Northridge; MA 85 CA St Univ - Northridge; 88–Sp-Lang Path, Los Angeles USD, **SLP**

Balius, Mrs Andrea S VA Medical Center, Routing Symbol 126, Biloxi, MS 39531, (601) 388-5541, BA 69 Catawba Coll; ME 71 Univ of VA - Charlottesville; Sp-Lang Path, VA Hosp, **SLP**

Balkin, Barbara Hollis 630 West 246th Street, Apartment 530, Riverdale, NY 10471, (212) 601-2436, BS 73 SUNY - Center at Albany; MS 74 Columbia Univ Teachers Coll; **SLP**

Balko, John P 3621 Cardinal Drive, Sharpsville, PA 16150, (412) 981-2535, BS 70 Clarion Univ of PA; MA 73 Kent St Univ; Aud, Hearing Healthcare Associates, **A ACE**

Balko, Karla Ann 1725 W Glendale Avenue, Apartment 3090, Phoenix, AZ 85021, (602) 239-4577, BS 83 Northern AZ Univ; MS 85 Purdue Univ - West Lafayette; **A**

Ball, Arnetha 592 Chardonnay Drive, Fremont, CA 94539, (415) 232-4064, MS; Sub, Richmond USD, **SLP**

Ball, Barbara Anne 5101 N Casa Blanca Road, Apartment 229, Scottsdale, AZ 85253, (602) 285-3284, BA 73 Univ of AZ; OM 85 AZ St Univ; **SLP**

Ball, Grace Ann Calle A, 99 Ext Mariani, Ponce, PR 00731, (809) 844-9017, MS 88 Univ of PR - San Juan

Ball, Jennifer Leigh 810 North Fourth, P O Box 61, St Joseph, IL 61873, (217) 469-2291, BS 85 Eastern IL Univ; MS 86 Eastern IL Univ; 88–Sp-Lang Path, St Joseph Comm Sch Dist 169, **SLP**

Ball, Mrs Joyce S 3305 Turfwood Drive, Greensboro, NC 27410, (919) 761-2390, BA 55 Grove City Coll; MA 71 Univ of NC - Greensboro; Maternal & Chld Care Superv, St of NC-Div of Hlth Serv, **SLP**

Ball, Judith K 328 Argyle Street, Thunder Bay, ON, Canada P7A 3P6, **SLP**

Ball, Karen A 6 Fulmer Street, Mohawk, NY 13407, (603) 883-5521, BS 80 SUNY - Coll at Geneseo; MS 82 Boston Univ; SLP, Nashua Mem Hosp, **SLP**

Ball, Laura J 34th General Hospital, Box 304 EFMS, APO New York, NY 09178, BA 80 WV Univ; BS 80 WV Univ; MA 81 Univ of TN - Knoxville; Sp-Lang Path, US Army Hosp, **SLP**

Ball, Mary M 558 Madison Street, Denver, CO 80206, (303) 770-4327, BA 74 Univ of Northern CO; MA 75 Univ of Northern CO; Owner, Arapahoe Hrng Assoc, **A**

Ball, Nadine Ann 261 West Walnut Lane, Philadelphia, PA 19144, (609) 921-7700, BS 85 PA St Univ - Univ Park; MS 87 Rutgers St Univ -N Brunswick; 87–Sp-Lang Path, The Med Ctr of Princeton, **SLP**

Ball, Mrs Nancy J 2025 Kynwyd Road, North Graylyn Crest, Wilmington, DE 19810, (302) 475-1912, BA 75 CUNY - Queens Coll; MA 77 SUNY - Center at Buffalo; Sp-Lang Path, **SLP**

Ball, Susan R 53 Old Main Road, North Falmouth, MA 02556, (508) 548-0151, BA 74 Univ of ME - Orono; OM 78 Univ of WA; Sp-Lang Path, Falmouth Pub Sch, **SLP**

Ball, Mrs Theresa L 5403 Fantail Drive, Sykesville, MD 21784, (301) 848-3900, BA 75 Loyola Coll; MS 76 Loyola Coll; Sp-Lang Path, Carroll County Public Schools, **SLP**

Ballagh, Brenda Johnson 5541 Pentail Circle, Tampa, FL 33624, (813) 870-1300, BS 71 FL St Univ; MS 72 FL St Univ; Dir/Sp-Lang Path, J Clifford MacDonald Cen, **SLP**

Ballantine, George Herbert 4601 Mantano N W #175, Albuquerque, NM 87120, (505) 897-1837, BA 80 Univ of NM; MS 82 Univ of NM; Consultant, CES, **SLP**

Ballantyne, Margaret Morgan 2416 North Greenwood, Pueblo, CO 81003, (303) 543-1170, BS 79 SUNY - Coll at Fredonia; MA 80 Bowling Green St Univ; Sp-Lang Path, Sch District #60, **SLP**

Ballard, Mrs Dail Daly P O Box 672, Hillsborough, NC 27278, (919) 966-1006, MS 83 Univ of NC - Chapel Hill; Cl Instrctr, U Chapel Hill, **SLP**

Ballard, Deborah Denise 1409 Claxton Road, Richmond, VA 23233, (804) 266-1642, BS 84 Hampton Univ; MS 86 Univ of MI - Ann Arbor; **SLP**

Ballard, Katheryn Lynn 1610 East McKinney #1707, Denton, TX 76201, (817) 387-3031, BS 84 Univ of TX - Dallas; MA 87 TX Woman's Univ; 88–Sp-Lang Path, Denton St Sch, **SLP**

Ballard, Mrs Kathleen Schwarz 8836 Carriage, Lenexa, KS 66215, (913) 782-3299, BS 73 Northwest MO St Univ; MS 76 TX Christian Univ; Sp-Lang Path, Olathe Dist Sch, **SLP**

Ballard, Mara L 217 Anderson Avenue, Fort Valley, GA 31030, (912) 825-2479, BA 73 Ball St Univ; MS 75 Purdue Univ - West Lafayette; Aud, Macon Hrng & Sp Cen, **A**

Ballard, Melissa J 2661 Ashton Road, Cleveland Heights, OH 44118, (216) 932-8143, BA 77 Cleveland St Univ; MA 79 Cleveland St Univ; Sp-Lang Path, Private Practice, **SLP**

Ballard, Paige Marten 390 Woodside Drive #104, Altamonte Springs, FL 32701, (305) 422-3709, BS 82 FL St Univ; MS 84 FL St Univ; **SLP**

Ballato, Mrs Pamela R 2525 Brofferton Court, Herndon, VA 22071, (703) 378-4800, BA 68 SUNY - Center at Albany; MA 72 SUNY - Center at Albany; Sp-Lang Path, Fairfax Co PS, **SLP**

Ballein, Kathleen C Box 35, River Hill, Monongahela, PA 15063, (412) 653-5600, BS 75 Carlow Coll; ME 80 CA Univ of PA; Sp-Lang Path, Jefferson Home Care-South Hills Health Sys, **SLP**

Ballew, Dr Laurie Kay 540 Oakland Circle, Paducah, KY 42001, (502) 442-4396, BS 71 Murray St Univ; MS 72 Murray St Univ; ED 83 (NS) Vanderbilt Univ; Sp-Lang Path, Rehab Assoc, **SLP**

Ballinger, Mrs Susan E 5776 Lentzier Trace, Jeffersonville, IN 47130, (812) 284-5317, BA 78 CA St Univ - Sacramento; MA 80 Univ of the Pacific; 86–Sp-Lang Path, Private Practice, **SLP**

Ball-Kimball, Pamela L Golden State Audiology Assoc, 877 West Fremont Avenue, Suite I-4, Sunnyvale, CA 94087, (408) 773-0204, BA 74 San Jose St Univ; MA 76 San Jose St Univ; President, Golden State Audiology Assoc, **A**

Ballmer, Mrs Irene Mary 850 Marjan Street, Anaheim, CA 92806, (714) 630-2588, BA 81 CA St Univ - Fullerton; MA 83 CA St Univ - Fullerton; **SLP**

Balloun, Lois Ann 2102 Greenbriar Drive, Ruston, LA 71270, (318) 251-3126, BS 72 Miami Univ - Oxford; MS 73 Univ of WI - Milwaukee; 88–Supvr of Sp-Lang Path, No LA Rehab Hosp, **SLP**

Ballow, Mrs Judith G 6950 Radcliffe Street, Bristol, PA 19007, (215) 946-2572, BS 62 Syracuse Univ; MA 64 Northwestern Univ; 84–Aud, ENT/Facial Plastic Surg Assoc, **A**

Bally, Scott J Gallaudet Univ Kendall Green, Department Of Audiology, 7th & Florida Avenue N E, Washington, DC 20002, (202) 651-5328, BS 67 Northeast MO St Univ; MS 69 CO St Univ; Cl Superv, Gallaudet Univ, **SLP**

Balmer, Irene W 195 Barton Drive, Ann Arbor, MI 48105, (313) 572-2400, BS 75 Eastern MI Univ; MA 76 Eastern MI Univ; 80–Sp-Lang Path, St Josephs Mercy Hosp, **SLP**

Balmert, Donna M 8105 Pocket Hollow Court, Indianapolis, IN 46256, (317) 353-5429, BS 77 Indiana Univ of PA; MA 79 Univ of Pittsburgh - Pittsburgh; Sp-Lang Path, Community Hospital of Indpls, **SLP**

Balmforth, Mrs Marlene L 1718 N E 64th, Portland, OR 97213, (503) 282-8368, BA 78 Univ of CA - Santa Barbara; MS 80 Univ of OR; Sp-Lang Path, Parkrose Sch Dist, **SLP**

Balmuth, Stacy Brucker 48 La Frentz Road, Greenwich, CT 06830-2610, MA 79 Kean Coll of NJ; Aud, Manhattan Med Group, **A**

Balog, Katherine Marie 1117 Marquette Avenue, Apartment 2409, Minneapolis, MN 55403, (612) 333-4155, MA 87 MI St Univ

Balogh, Mrs Lucille M 11231 White Oak Lane, Port Richey, FL 34668, (813) 848-3402, BS 77 SUNY - Coll at Buffalo; MS 79 SUNY - Coll at Buffalo; Sp/Lang Path, Cypress Elem Sch, **SLP**

Balogh, Mrs Trudy C 370 Southbury Court, Schaumburg, IL 60193, (312) 893-4729, BS 79 Eastern MI Univ; MA 80 Eastern MI Univ; 81–Sp-Lang Path, Bensenville Dist #2 Pub Sch, **SLP**

Balsavage-Fritzinger, Lynn 201 Calvert Boulevard, Tonawanda, NY 14150, (716) 692-8330, BA 80 SUNY - Center at Buffalo; MA 81 SUNY - Center at Buffalo; Sp-Lang Path, Williamsville Central Schools, **SLP**

Balsavich, Mrs Donna Marie 13817 Lincolnshire Drive, Orland Park, IL 60462, (312) 460-1805, BS 75 Southern IL Univ -Carbondale; MS 76 Southern IL Univ -Carbondale; **SLP**

Balser, Elnora M 305 South McKemy, Apartment #H, Tempe, AZ 85281, (602) 829-9003, BA 74 Cleveland St Univ; MA 77 Cleveland St Univ; President, Sound Audiologics Inc, **SLP A**

Baltazar, Shirley Amaral 15422 Skyline Drive, Dumfries, VA 22026, (703) 791-7775, BA 69 CA St Univ - Fresno; MA 71 CA St Univ - Sacramento; **SLP**

Balthazor, Mrs Patricia N P O Box 6977, San Bernardino, CA 92412, (714) 793-5914, BS 75 Purdue Univ - West Lafayette; MS 77 Purdue Univ - West Lafayette; Sp-Lang Path, Lang Ser for Preschoolers, **SLP**

Balthazor, Dr Ronald J 1421 Frances, Redlands, CA 92374, (714) 825-7084, BA 68; MA 72 Coll of Saint Rose; PH 75 (NS) Purdue Univ - West Lafayette; 88–Aud, VA Hosp, **A**

Baltowski, Marianne 607 Sutton Court, Wheeling, IL 60090, (312) 696-6274, BS 82 Univ of IL - Urbana; MA 84 Northern IL Univ - De Kalb; Aud, Lutheran General Hospital, **A**

Baltzell, David R 472 Ridgecrest Road, Atlanta, GA 30307, **A**

Balutis, Karen A 806 Newell Street, Utica, NY 13502, (305) 268-0468, BS 78 SUNY - Coll at Fredonia; MS 80 Univ of ND; Sp-Lang Path, Valleyspeech Enterprises, **SLP**

Balzer, Lorie A 1649 Carbon Canyon Road, Chino Hills, CA 91709, (714) 524-3223, MS 76 Rutgers St Univ - Newark; Admin, Chino HealthCare Ctr, **SLP**

Bamberg, Mrs Gail A 1360 Dalarna Way, Turlock, CA 95380, MS 76 Northern IL Univ - De Kalb; Sp-Lang Path, Merced County Office Supt Sch, **SLP**

Ban, Dr Paul K 1110A Akipohe Street, Kailua, HI 96734, (808) 423-1720, BS 73 Univ of HI - Manoa; MA 75 Univ of HI - Manoa; PH 79 (NS) Univ of HI - Manoa; Sch Psychologist Sp-Lang Path, Dept Education Windward Dist, **SLP**

Banajee, Mrs Meher Hormazd 4625 Yale Street #B, Metairie, LA 70006, (504) 899-9511, BS 75 Topiwala Nat'l Med Coll Bombay Univ - India; MS 77 All India Inst of Sp & Hrng; Sp-Lang Path, Childrens Hosp, **SLP ACE**

Banas, Mrs Adele S P O Box 47, Colebrook, CT 06021, (203) 379-2140, BA 70 Univ of CT; MA 72 Univ of CT; SLP, Shared Services, **SLP**

Banas, Mrs Debbie 11660 115th Street No, Stillwater, MN 55082, (612) 457-7245, MA 77 Univ of TN - Knoxville; SLP, Inver Grove Hghts Sch Dist 199

Banas, Patricia A 2245 Valencia Street #3, Bellingham, WA 98225, (206) 647-3834, BA 78 Western WA Univ; MA 85 Western WA Univ; Sp-Lang Path, Visiting Nurse Home Health, **SLP**

Bance-Davis, Mrs Angela Velma 2218 Pansy Avenue, Upland, CA 91786, (714) 735-7466, MS 83 Chapman Coll; Special Education Teacher, Norwalk USD, **SLP**

Banchefsky, Mrs Debra Kirshner 154 South Dawson, Columbus, OH 43209, (614) 235-8155, BS 79 Boston Univ; MA 81 OH St Univ; Sp-Lang Path, Doctor's Hosp, **SLP**

Banchi, Charlotte A 11383 Tortuga Street, Cypress, CA 90630, (714) 898-8471, MA 88 CA St Univ - Long Beach; 88–Aud, CSULB Foundation/Hearing Clinic

Bancroft, Kathleen Stanton 1665 Hood Court, Kennesaw, GA 30144, (404) 427-4705, BS 64 IL St Univ - Normal; ME 86 GA St Univ; 78–Sp-Lang Path, Bartow Co Bd of Educ, **SLP**

Bancroft, Robert L 3697 Brentwood, Muskegon, MI 49441, (616) 777-2581, BA 66 Western MI Univ; MA 69 Western MI Univ; Aud, Muskegon Hrng & Sp Cen, **SLP A**

Banda, Cynthia Ann 608 Pine Street, Johnstown, PA 15902, (814) 536-9031, BS 74 CA Univ of PA; MS 84 Indiana Univ of PA; 79–Sp-Lang Path, Cambria Co Head Start, **SLP**

Bandera, Elizabeth Ann 15704 Orlan Brook Drive, Apartment 164, Orland Park, IL 60462, (312) 460-7749, BS 82 Northwestern Univ; MA 83 Northwestern Univ; **SLP**

Bandur, Donna 54 Nanette Crescent, London, ON, Canada N5X 3L1, (519) 663-3517, BS 74 Univ of Western Ontario; OM 75 Univ of Western Ontario; Manager, University Hosp, **SLP**

Bandy-Palmer, Elizabeth Neoserrc, 409 Harmon Street N W, Warren, OH 44483, (216) 394-0310, BS 74 Kent St Univ; MA 75 Kent St Univ; Ed Assessment Proj Coord, Neo/Serrc, **SLP**

Bane, Mary J 5390 South Garland Way, Littleton, CO 80123, (303) 978-9511, BS 76 Univ of WI - Whitewater; MA 79 Univ of CO - Boulder; SLP, SW Pediatric Habilitation Ctr, **SLP**

Banford, Rhonda J 16555 Birch Forest Drive, Ballwin, MO 63011, (314) 458-3438, BA 80 Newcomb Coll Tulane Univ; OM 81 Tulane Univ; Sp-Lang Path, Private Practice, **SLP**

Bangar, Diane M 955 East 3rd Street #318, Long Beach, CA 90802, (213) 940-7682, BA 76 Univ of Southern CA; MA 78 Whittier Coll; Training Educ Coordinator, Rancho Los Amigos Medical Cen, **SLP**

Banghart-Bragg, Mrs Denise Helen 2200 Arnhem Place, Modesto, CA 95356, (209) 525-5143, BA 78 CA St Univ - Stanislaus; MA 80 CA St Univ - Stanislaus; SLP, Stanislaus Co Dept of Ed, **SLP**

Bangs, Mrs Dorothy Z 104 Highland Circle, Chambersburg, PA 17201, (717) 263-8203, ME 63 Western MD Coll; BS 60 Bloomsburg Univ of PA; Retired, Chambersburg Area Sch Dist, **SLP LM**

Bangs, Dr Tina E 7532 Chevy Chase, Houston, TX 77063, (713) 782-1840, BA 37 Univ of WA; MA 41 Univ of WA; PH 58 (NS) Stanford Univ; Retired, **SLP A F LM**

Banick, Patricia L 8 Shamrock Road, Bel Air, MD 21014, (301) 838-7690, BS 76 James Madison Univ; MA 87 Southwest MO St Univ; 88–Sp-Lang Path, Harford County Bd of Educ, **SLP**

Banigan, Dr Rae Loraine Talking With Children Inc, PO Box 839, Palmer, MA 01069, (413) 283-9240, BA 71 SUNY - Center at Albany; MA 75 Coll of Saint Rose; PH 87 (Comm Disord-Ear Child Lang Develop) Univ of MA - Amherst; 87–Sp-Lang Path/Pres, Talking with Children Inc, **SLP ACE**

Banik, Mrs Jan M 15 Le Man Lane, Hopkinton, MA 01748, BA 75 Saint Xavier Coll; MS 76 Marquette Univ; **SLP**

Banikiotes, Florence G 4030 Starwreath Way, Ellicott City, MD 21043, (301) 461-5049, BS 68 CUNY - City College; MS 70 Purdue Univ - West Lafayette; OM 82 Univ of Notre Dame; **SLP LM**

Banis, Mrs Carolyn J 2919 Reiger Court, Las Vegas, NV 89117, BA 67 Univ of NV - Reno; MS 78 Univ of NV - Reno; **SLP**

Bank, Mrs Nancy 3305 Woodview Lake Road, West Bloomfield, MI 48033, (313) 851-7605, BA 63 Univ of MI - Ann Arbor; MS 66 CUNY - Queens Coll; Sp-Lang Path, W Bloomfield Pub Sch, **SLP**

Bank, Mrs Robin M 1575 Alex Lane, Bayside, CA 95524, (707) 822-3849, BA 74 Univ of CA - Irvine; MA 83 Humboldt St Univ; SLP, Ferndale Elem Sch Dist, **SLP**

Banker, Mrs Melinda Sanders 7903-B Hunnicut, Dallas, TX 75228, (214) 320-9691, BS 83 Stephen F Austin St Univ; MS 87 Univ of TX - Dallas; 87–Sp-Lang Path, Oak Hill Academy, **SLP**

Banker, Dr Michele S 79 Scott Road, Belmont, MA 02178, (617) 484-0707, BS 66 Boston Univ; ME 73 Boston Univ; ED 85 (NS) Boston Univ; **SLP**

Banker-Trotter, Anne 1056 Manzana Place, Lafayette, CA 94549, **SLP**

Bankhead, Lorna Marian Rt 2 1230 1st South, Okanogan, WA 98840, (509) 826-0320, BA 72 Eastern WA Univ; MS 82 Eastern WA Univ; 87–Sp-Lang Path, Omak Sch Dist, **SLP**

Bankoski, Susan Marie Hampden Hearing Center E, 219 North Main Street, East Longmeadow, MA 01028, (413) 525-7979, BA 81 Univ of CT; MA 83 Univ of CT; 84–Aud, Hampden Hearing Center East, **A**

Banks, Mrs Carolyn G 20296 South Mountain Road, Santa Paula, CA 93060, (805) 487-0055, BA 72 Univ of CA - Santa Barbara; MA 84 CA Lutheran Coll; MA 78 CA St Univ - Northridge; 88–Learning Dir, Oxnard Sch Dist, **SLP**

Banks, Mrs Cheryl P O Box 14441, Omaha, NE 68124, Sp-Lang Path, Iowa School for the Deaf, **SLP**

Banks, Diane Moody 4410 Township Line #K-1C, Drexel Hill, PA 19026, (215) 622-0091, BS 74 PA St Univ - Univ Park; MS 75 Univ of the DC; 84–Sp-Lang Path, Elwyn Institutes, **SLP**

Banks, Mrs Frances M 243 Evergreen Drive, Poland, OH 44514, (216) 757-1848, BA 74 Cleveland St Univ; MA 76 Cleveland St Univ; Sp/Lang Path, Boardman City Schs, **SLP**

Banks, Nora Jacqueline 1063 Crisfield Drive, Cincinnati, OH 45245, (513) 232-7216, BS 81 Univ of Cincinnati; MA 83 Univ of Cincinnati; SLP, Bethesda Hospital, **SLP**

Banks, Pamela Fallon P O Box 742, 61 Ridge Road, Hollis, NH 03049, (603) 465-3319, BS 81 Boston Univ; MA 83 Univ of CT; Sp-Lang Path, St Joseph Hosp, **SLP**

Banks, Mrs Rhonda E 40 Heritage Park Circle, North Little Rock, AR 72116, (501) 758-8467, BA 74 Baylor Univ; MS 75 Baylor Univ; **SLP**

Banks, Mrs Sandra Garrity 3961 Grilletta, Marrero, LA 70072, (504) 340-3936, BA 81 Southeastern LA Univ; OM 87 LA St Univ - N O Medical Ctr; **SLP**

Banks, Mrs Tabitha Owens 3116 Laurel Ridge Circle, Bridgeville, PA 15017, (412) 257-4661, **SLP**

Banks, Mrs Teresa M 544 Ranch Drive, Eagle, ID 83616, (208) 939-8833, BS 71 Brigham Young Univ; MA 74 Our Lady Lake Univ-San Anton; **SLP**

Banks, Walter G 1152 North 6th Street, Coos Bay, OR 97420, (503) 267-3104, BA 50 Univ of OR; MA 55 Univ of OR; Sp-Lang Path, Private Practice, **SLP**

Bankson, Dr Nicholas Webb 36 Cummington St, Boston, MA 02215, (617) 353-3252, BS 60 Univ of KS; MA 61 Univ of KS; PH 70 (Sp-Lang Path) Univ of KS; Prof & Chmn, Boston Univ, **SLP F**

Bankston, Debra W P O Box 632161, Nacogdoches, TX 75963, (409) 569-6182, BA 74 LA Tech Univ; MA 75 Memphis St Univ; Instr/Cl Supvr, Stephen F Austin State Univ, **SLP**

Bankus, Mrs Carol A Rd 2 Box 299-A, Millville, PA 17846, BS 74 Bloomsburg Univ of PA; MS 80 Bloomsburg Univ of PA; Sp-Lang Path, Berwick Hosp Corp, **SLP**

Banner, Barbara C 225 Bentwood Court West, Albany, NY 12203, (518) 783-1644, BS 74 SUNY - Center at Albany; MS 76 Columbia Univ Teachers Coll; 84–Sp-Lang Path Dept Chairperson, Wildwood School, **SLP**

Bannister, Kay A 9016 N E 186th, Bothell, WA 98011, MS 86 Univ of WA; 87–Sp-Lang Path, Private Practice, **SLP**

Bannister, Dr Marcia L Fort Hays State University, 600 Park, Hays, KS 67601, BS 61 Fort Hays St Univ; MS 62 Fort Hays St Univ; PH 73 (Sp-Lang Path) Univ of KS; Prof of Commun Dis, Ft Hays St U, **SLP**

Bannister, Stacy G 1038 North Ohio Avenue, Atlantic City, NJ 08401, (609) 345-9027, MA 87 Univ of MA - Amherst

Bannister, Susan Marie 11502 Holmes #2, Kansas City, MO 64131, (816) 932-3262, BS 85 Univ of MO - Columbia; MS 86 Univ of MO - Columbia; Sp-Lang Path, St Lukes Hosp, **SLP**

Bannon, Kelley Ann 458 East Wilbur Road #204, Thousand Oaks, CA 91360, (818) 719-3710, BS 84 CO St Univ; MA 86 CA St Univ - Northridge; Aud, Kaiser Permanente, **A**

Bante, Alice J 31 Wilshire Terrace, St Louis, MO 63119, (314) 966-7537, BS 50 Saint Louis Univ; MA 71 Saint Louis Univ; Associate Professor, St Louis Community College, **SLP**

Banton, Mrs Ann E 3905 Weber Way, Lexington, KY 40514, (606) 223-4302, BA 80 Univ of KY; MS 81 Univ of KY; 87–Sp-Lang Path, Surgert & Associates Inc, **SLP**

Baquet, Glenn M Howard University Director, Speech & Hearing Clinic, 4th & Bryan Street N W, Washington, DC 20059, (202) 636-6990, BS 70 Xavier Univ of LA; MS 72 WV Univ; Cl Dir, Howard U Sp & Hrng Cl, **A**

Barabell, Mrs Fran H 15 Concord Drive, New City, NY 10956, BA 72 CUNY - Queens Coll; MA 74 CUNY - Queens Coll; Sp-Lang Path, Clarkstown Sch Dist, **SLP**

Barach, Mrs Carol M 541 Hickory Trail Drive, Nashville, TN 37209, (615) 353-0149, BA 57 Vassar Coll; MA 71 Vanderbilt Univ; Sp-Lang Path, Private Practice, **SLP**

Barad, Mrs Dianne D 2 Brandywine Road, South Barrington, IL 60010, (312) 377-4857, BS 54 NY Univ; MA 70 CA St Univ - Northridge; 87–Sp-Lang Path, Mid-Valley Spec Educ Coop, **SLP**

Barada, Mrs Patricia Beam 380 West Main Street, Chillicothe, OH 45601, (614) 774-2717, BA 51 Univ of MI - Ann Arbor; Sp-Lang Path, **SLP**

Barajas, Mrs Dorinda Ann E 1838 Spruce Knob, Kingwood, TX 77339, BA 75 CA St Univ - Los Angeles; MA 80 CA St Univ - Los Angeles; Sp-Lang Path, Aldine ISD, **SLP**

Barakat, Zeina Christine 12050 Eaglewood Court, Silver Spring, MD 20902, (202) 877-1440, BA 83 Am Univ of Beirut - Lebanon; MS 86 Columbia Univ Teachers Coll; **SLP**

Baral, Mrs Sydell 3140 Butler Avenue, Los Angeles, CA 90066, (213) 398-0053, BA 48 CUNY - Brooklyn Coll; MA 65 Univ of CA - Los Angeles; Prof Sp Dept, La Harbor Coll, **SLP**

Baran, Dr Jane A Dept Communication Disorders, Univ Of Massachusetts, 18 Arnold House, Amherst, MA 01003, (413) 545-0565, BA 72 Univ of MA - Amherst; MA 74 Univ of MA - Amherst; PH 79 (NS) Purdue Univ - West Lafayette; 79–Assoc Prof, Univ of MA Dept of Comm Disorders, **SLP A**

Baran, Judith M 57197 Beaconsfield, Washington, MI 48094, (313) 781-6503, BA 75 MI St Univ; MA 76 Wayne St Univ - Sch of Med; Sp/Lang Path, Romeo Community Sch, **SLP**

Baran, Lorelei Jeane 2326-3 Treescape Drive, Charleston, SC 29414, (803) 724-7798, BS 75 Purdue Univ - West Lafayette; MA 84 IN Univ - Bloomington; **SLP**

Baranchik, Debra H K 8704 North Trumbull Avenue, Skokie, IL 60076, **SLP**

Baranek, Thomas Paul 6606 York Road, Parma Heights, OH 44130, (216) 888-9445, Self Employed, **A**

Baranowski, Maryanne V 728 Campbell Street, P O Box 21, South Amboy, NJ 08879, (201) 727-1568, BA 74 Rutger's St Univ - Douglas Coll; MA 79 Kean Coll of NJ; 74–Sp-Lang Path, Old Bridge Township Pub Sch, **SLP**

Baraz, Julie E 8700 25th Avenue, Brooklyn, NY 11214, (718) 996-1792, BA 63 Goucher Coll; MA 65 Columbia Univ Teachers Coll; Sp-Lang Path, Julie Baraz, **SLP ACE**

Barba, Caressa Maria 1206 Ingleside Avenue, Baltimore, MD 21207, (301) 744-6512, MS 88 Loyola Coll

Barbare, Diane E 1309 North Alabama, De Land, FL 32724, (904) 738-1112, BA 77 Univ of FL; MS 78 Univ of AL- Tuscaloosa; Tchr, Blue Lake Elem Sch -Volusia Co, **SLP**

Barbaria, Lynn 3667 Cutter Way, Sacramento, CA 95818, (916) 663-2096, BA 76 CA St Univ - Sacramento; MA 79 CA St Univ - Sacramento; SLP, Placer Co Offied, **SLP**

Barbaro, Anne L 7 Crestline Circle, Danvers, MA 01923, (617) 774-3664, BS 85 Univ of MA - Amherst; MS 87 Northeastern Univ; 87–Aud, VA Outpatient Clinic, **A**

Barbatsis, D Lynne 1620 River Terrace East, Minneapolis, MN 55414-3648, (612) 786-7100, BA 70 Univ of WI - Madison; MS 72 Univ of WI - Madison; Aud, ENT Prof Assoc Ltd, **A**

Barbay, Judy Hammonds 420 Corby Dr, Baton Rouge, LA 70810-4505, (504) 343-6087, BS 77 LA St Univ - Baton Rouge; OM 86 LA St Univ - Baton Rouge; 88–Sp-Lang Path, E Baton Rouge Parish Sch Bd, **SLP**

Barbe, Joann 7007 Gulf Drive, Holmes Beach, FL 34217, (813) 778-1629, BS 84 FL St Univ; MS 86 FL St Univ; SLP, **SLP**

Barbee, Jeanette Patterson 4100 Morris Road #1113, Flower Mound, TX 75028, (214) 539-0803, BA 39 Hardin-Simmons Univ; MA 79 TX Woman's Univ; 88, Private Practice, **SLP**

Barbee, Mrs Lynda Jean 2712 Westridge Drive, Plano, TX 75075, (214) 867-0010, MS 84 Univ of TX - Dallas; Sp-Lang Path, Plano ISD, **SLP**

Barbee, Mrs Mary Ann F 17 Central Close, Auburndale, MA 02166, (617) 757-2756, BA 62 Greensboro Coll; ME 69 Northeastern Univ; **SLP**

Barber, Mrs Aagje V Swaay 1839 Putnam, Bartlesville, OK 74006, (918) 333-4210, BA 76 Univ of Houston - Univ Park; MA 78 Univ of Houston - Univ Park; **SLP**

Barber, Mrs Aleisa Dolloph 8300 Summer Place Drive, Austin, TX 78759, (512) 343-2065, BA 84 Marshall Univ; MA 85 Marshall Univ; 88–Sp-Lang Path, Austin ISD, **SLP**

Barber, Carol Maynard Children's Health Care, 3580 Peach Street, Erie, PA 16508, (814) 868-9633, ME 79 Univ of VA - Charlottesville; 88–Aud, Children's Health Care, **A**

Barber, Diana Linda 4413 East Shelby Road, Medina, NY 14103, (716) 798-1243, BS 82 SUNY - Coll at Brockport; MA 85 SUNY - Coll at Geneseo; 86–Sp-Lang Path, Orleans-Niagara BOCES, **SLP**

Barber, Mrs Ellen J 860 Stratford Drive East, Apartment 2, Bourbonnais, IL 60914, (815) 932-0623, BS 79 Univ of WI - Stevens Point; MA 81 Western MI Univ; Sp/Lang Path, New Lenox District 122, **SLP**

Barber, Dr J Manford, III 11530 S W 13th, Topeka, KS 66615, (913) 233-5033, MA 72 Univ of FL; ME 73 Harvard Univ; OD 77 (NS) Johns Hopkins Univ; Sp-Lang Path/Aud, Menninger Found, **SLP A**

Barber, James L 816 4th Avenue, Dixon, IL 61021, **SLP**

Barber, Judith Louise 1138 Elm Street, Grinnell, IA 50112, (515) 236-5560, **SLP**

Barber, Kathy L 519 Cleveland Boulevard, Fayetteville, NY 13066, (315) 488-2951, BS 78 SUNY - Coll at Buffalo; MS 80 PA St Univ - Univ Park; 81–Sp-Lang Path, St Camillus Hlth & Rehab Cen, **SLP**

Barber, Linda L 1400 Meridian Avenue #3, Colonial Heights, VA 23834, (804) 520-7557, BS 74 Longwood Coll; ME 76 Univ of VA - Charlottesville; Sp-Lang Path, Communi-Care Inc, **SLP**

Barber, Marian E 1126 Highland Avenue, Oak Park, IL 60304-2210, BS 84 Eastern MI Univ; MA 86 Eastern MI Univ; Sp-Lang Path, Chicago Bd of Educ, **SLP**

Barber, Sr Mary Nora 13105 Watertown Plank Road, Elm Grove, WI 53122, (414) 782-1450, ME 82 Univ of FL; MA 57 Univ of Detroit; PH 64 (NS) Catholic Univ of America; Sp-Lang Path, Notre Dame Health Care Center

Barber, Mrs Prudence S 816 4th Avenue, Dixon, IL 61021, (815) 284-7722, BA 61 MI St Univ; MS 67 Northern IL Univ - De Kalb; Sp-Lang Path, Dixon Pub Sch, **SLP A**

Barber, Mrs Ronda Joyce 8321 South Upham Way #210, Littleton, CO 80123, (303) 972-4911, BA 82 Univ of Denver; MS 85 Boston Univ; SLP, St Anthonys Hosp, **SLP**

Barber, Russell James Speech & Hearing Department, Whitten Center, Clinton, SC 29325, (803) 833-2733, MS 81 Univ of SC - Columbia; Audiologist, S Carolina Dept Mental Retardn

Barber, Mrs Sheila J W 459 Sybille Creek Road, Wheatland, WY 82201, (307) 322-3836, BS 77 Fort Hays St Univ; MS 78 Fort Hays St Univ; Sp-Lang Path, Platte County Sch Dist 1, **SLP**

Barber, Sylvia E V 334 Hawthorn Street, New Bedford, MA 02740, **SLP**

Barber, Winde Jeanne 4634 Twin Oak, Macon, GA 31210, (912) 743-1133, ME 85 Univ of GA; Sp-Lang Path, Bibb Co Bd of Educ/Healthmaster, **SLP**

Barbera-Hanson, Cheriann 56 Voyagers Lane, Ashland, MA 01721, (617) 881-3520, BS 78 WV Univ; MS 79 FL St Univ; SLP, Summit Ctr Human Development, **SLP**

Barberino, Mrs Lorraine E P O Box 419, Granby, CT 06035, (203) 653-2167, MS 76 Southern CT St Univ; **SLP**

Barber Kwolek, Mrs Cathleen M 412 Bostwick Lane, Gaithersburg, MD 20878, (301) 493-4884

Barbetta, Christine RR 2 Box 520, Lincolnville, ME 04849, (207) 236-3144, BA 77 CA St Univ - Stanislaus; MA 79 CA St Univ - Stanislaus; 87–Sp-Lang Path, MSAD #28, **SLP**

Barbieri-Welge, Rene L 10011 Paseo Montril, San Diego, CA 92129, (619) 477-1129, BA 80 CA St Univ - Sacramento; MA 83 CA St Univ - Sacramento; SLP, Natl Sch Dist, **SLP**

Barbiero, Denise Celeste 222 Elm Street #504, Toronto, ON, Canada M5T 1K5, (416) 979-3752, BS 84 Univ of MS; MS 85 Univ of MS; **A**

Barbosa, Maureen McLean 879 South Lincoln Avenue, Monterey Park, CA 91754-4047, (213) 223-1336, BA 78 CA St Univ - Los Angeles; MA 81 CA St Univ - Los Angeles; Sp-Lang Path, Los Angeles USD, **SLP**

Barbour, Mrs Elaine J 325 Auckland Lane, Matthews, NC 28105, (704) 821-7953, MA 64 Univ of NC - Greensboro; Sp-Lang Path, **SLP**

Barbour, Mrs Lloydene J 3874 N E Rene, Gresham, OR 97030, BA 57 Univ of OR; MS 76 AZ St Univ; Sp-Lang Path, Centennial School District, **SLP**

Barbour, Myra Maxwell 3056 Fairland Road, Silver Spring, MD 20904, (301) 595-5000, BS 72 Univ of the DC; MS 73 Univ of the DC; Dir of Sp & Hrng Dept, Dept Hlth & Ment Hyg-Gr Oaks C, **SLP**

Barbour, Mrs Ruth A 1307 Cantebury Circle, Brookfield, WI 53005, (414) 545-7910, BA 67 Univ of Science & Arts of OK; MA 68 Univ of WI - Milwaukee; Sp-Lang Path, West Allis Pub Sch, **SLP**

Barclay, Mrs Pamela Harford 635 Sea Lane, La Jolla, CA 92037, (619) 456-9941, BA 82 CA St Univ - Fullerton; MA 87 San Diego St Univ; **SLP**

Barco, Diana C 3839 Briarcliff Road, Kansas City, MO 64116, BS 69 Univ of MO - KS City; MA 72 Univ of KS; Sp-Lang Path, Liberty Pub Sch, **SLP**

Barcus, Janet Sue 2329 South Ozark, Joplin, MO 64804, (417) 624-9261, BS 79 Central MO St Univ; MS 81 Central MO St Univ; Sp-Lang Path, Joplin Regional Center, **SLP**

Bard, Dr Barbara 400 North Quaker Lane, West Hartford, CT 06117, (203) 827-7558, BA 54 CUNY - Brooklyn Coll; MA 55 Univ of MI - Ann Arbor; PH 65 (NS) NY Univ; Professor, Central Connecticut State Univ, **SLP**

Bard, Madeline 1 Huckleberry Lane, Oyster Bay, NY 11771, (516) 922-3934, BA 77 SUNY - Coll at Plattsburgh; MS 79 Adelphi Univ; SLP, Huntington Pub Sch Dist 3, **SLP**

Bardanouve, Mrs Venus T Box 367, Harlem, MT 59526, (406) 353-2397, BA 47 Univ of NE - Lincoln; MA 55 Saint Louis Univ; **SLP A LM**

Bar-David, Mrs Dahlia 30 Frank Peleg Street, Haifa, Israel 34987, **SLP A**

Barden, Dr Elaine 11 Carlisle Road, Upper Montclair, NJ 07043, (201) 893-4227, BA 55 Rutger's St Univ - Douglas Coll; MA 64 Seton Hall Univ; PH 72 (NS) Columbia Univ Teachers Coll; Assoc Prof, Montclair St Coll, **SLP**

Barden, Randall Glen 1535 Parent Avenue, Windsor, ON, Canada N8X 4J8, (313) 838-7150, **A**

Bardon, Constance Lynn 2021 Milan Street, New Orleans, LA 70115, (504) 899-1993, **SLP**

Bardorf, Mary Catherine 26 South Drive, Middletown, RI 02840, (401) 849-2122, BA 61 Univ of Toronto - Ontario; OB 62 Univ of Montreal - Quebec; MS 84 Univ of RI; 86–Sp-Lang Path, Newport Co Reg Spec Educ, **SLP**

Bardsley, Ellen M 14 Magnus Avenue, Somerville, MA 02143, (617) 642-0217, MS 87 Emerson Coll; 87–Sp-Lang Path, Eunice Kennedy Shriver Ctr, **SLP**

Bardsley, Mrs Karen L 5110 Crestmont, Troy, MI 48098, (313) 641-7809, BS 65 IL St Univ - Normal; MA 80 Eastern MI Univ; Sp-Lang Path, Atherton Comm Sch, **SLP**

Bardwell, Mrs Marianne K 2 Governors Drive S W, Leesburg, VA 22075, (703) 771-1960, BS 67 Northwestern Univ; MS 69 Purdue Univ - West Lafayette; 88–Sp-Lang Path, ACRE Ctr, **SLP**

Barefoot, Mrs Myrna C 54 Hillside Drive, Carlisle, PA 17013, (717) 243-3083, BS 55 CA Univ of PA; MS 76 PA St Univ - Univ Park; SLP, Capital Area Interm Unit #15, **SLP**

Barefoot, Sidney M 9306 Warsaw Road, Leroy, NY 14482, (716) 475-6263, BS 72 SUNY - Coll at Geneseo; MS 73 PA St Univ - Univ Park; SLP, NTID, **SLP**

Bareither, Mrs Joan McCarthy 106 Falling Leaves Drive, Warner Robins, GA 31088, (912) 929-7800, BS 72 Purdue Univ - West Lafayette; MS 81 MS Univ for Women; 88–Sp-Lang Path, Houston Co Sch Sys, **SLP**

Bareither, Mrs Theresa M 7046 Bexley Drive East, Indianapolis, IN 46256, BS 70 Purdue Univ - West Lafayette; MS 73 Southern IL Univ-Edwardsvill; Mgr Sp-Lang Path & Aud, St Francis Hosp, **SLP**

Baren, Mrs Robin Prince 200 Atlantic Avenue #404, Lynbrook, NY 11563, (516) 643-1161, BS 84 Boston Univ; MS 85 Adelphi Univ; Sp-Lang Path, BOCES 3, **SLP**

Barfield, Judy T 103 Nottingham Way, Prescott, AR 71857, (501) 246-5511, BS 76 Henderson St Univ; MS 78 Southern Methodist Univ; 86–Sp-Lang Path, Henderson State Univ, **SLP**

Barforoush, Kathleen Bauman 12802 West 57th Terrace, Shawnee, KS 66216, (816) 228-5929, MA 84 Univ of KS; Aud, Multi-Dist Hrng Imp Prog, **A**

Bargas, Lori R 17735 Fieldbrook Circle N, Boca Raton, FL 33496, (305) 997-6323, MA 84 Univ of CO - Boulder; Sp-Lang Path, Private Practice, **SLP**

Bargelt, Hal James 2451 Laurel Pass, Los Angeles, CA 90046, (213) 654-9694, BA 42 Univ of Southern CA; MA 50 Univ of Southern CA; PH 59 (NS) Univ of Southern CA; Dir, CA Sp-Lang Lab, **SLP**

Bargelt, Dr James Hager 5441 Fulton Avenue, Van Nuys, CA 91401, (818) 994-7129, BA 80 Univ of CA - Santa Barbara; MA 82 Univ of TN - Knoxville; PH 85 (NS) Univ of TN - Knoxville; Sp-Lang Path, California Sp-Lang Laboratory, **SLP**

Barger, Mary Jane 406 Pineridge Street, Brea, CA 92621, (213) 943-0211, BA 72 CA St Univ - Fullerton; MA 76 CA St Univ - Fullerton; 76–Sp-Lang Path, Lowell Joint Sch Dist, **SLP**

Bargman, Kathleen 1496 14th Avenue, San Francisco, CA 94122, **SLP**

Bargmeyer, Kurt Erwin 2325 126th Avenue Court E, Puyallup, WA 98372, BA 40 Univ of WA; **LM**

Bargones, Jill Yvette University Of Washington, Speech & Hearing Sci Jg-15, Seattle, WA 98195, (805) 543-6934, BA 83 Univ of CA - Santa Barbara; MS 86 Univ of WA; 88–Research Assoc, Univ of Washington, **A**

Bargstadt, Mrs Grace H 811 Taylor Street, Papillion, NE 68046, (402) 330-2770, BA 73 Augusta Coll; MS 76 ID St Univ; Special Ed Coordinator, Ed Service Unit #3, **SLP**

Barham, Mrs Renay Painter 201 Valencia Court, Jacksonville, NC 28540, (919) 577-4270, BS 81 East Carolina Univ; MS 83 East Carolina Univ; Sp-Lang Path, **SLP**

Barhorst, Annette Marie 8303 Partlow Lane, Houston, TX 77040, BS 85 Stephen F Austin St Univ; MS 87 Univ of North TX; 87–Sp-Lang Path, Speech & Lang Svcs, **SLP**

Bari-Bayci, Mrs Anna M 406 East Bevan Drive, Joliet, IL 60435, (815) 744-3500, BS 78 Univ of IL - Urbana; MS 79 Univ of IL - Urbana; Sp-Lang Path, UCP, **SLP**

Baribeau, Larry J Route 3, Tomah, WI 54660, (608) 372-3971, BS 67 Univ of WI - Eau Claire; ME 71 Univ of WI - Eau Claire; **SLP**

Barickman, Barbara L 3 Cornflower, Pueblo, CO 81001, (303) 544-2269, BA 75 Univ of Northern CO; MA 76 Univ of Northern CO; Sp-Lang Path, Pueblo Sch Dist #60, **SLP**

Barickman, Julia A P O Box 1871, Bonita Springs, FL 33959-1871, (813) 992-0657, BS 78 Eastern IL Univ; MS 79 Eastern IL Univ; 86–Sp-Lang Path, Naples Comm Hosp, **SLP ACE**

Barile, Veronica Maria 51-36 30th Avenue, Woodside, NY 11377, (212) 726-6754, BA 82 CUNY - City College; MA 84 CUNY - City College; 85–Sp-Lang Path, Jewish Guild for the Blind, **SLP**

Barilko, Margaret R 1041 Steele Street, Denver, CO 80206, (303) 320-2140, BS 80 Univ of Alberta - Alberta; MA 83 Univ of Denver; Sp-Lang Path, Rose Medical Center, **SLP**

Barillaro, Mrs Judith Ann 619 Finch Avenue, Meriden, CT 06450, (203) 777-2000, BS 66 Central CT St Univ; MS 84 Southern CT St Univ; **SLP**

Barimo, Joseph Patrick 14550 Bruce B Downs Blvd, Bldg #31 Unit 69, Tampa, FL 33613, (813) 680-7719, MS 85 Univ of South FL; SLP, Polk County School Bd, **SLP**

Barina, Jean Louise 1313 East Harriet Street, Apartment 7, Appleton, WI 54915, (414) 731-6905, BS 83 Univ of WI - Stevens Point; MS 85 Univ of WI - Stevens Point; **SLP**

Barinotti, Mrs Margaret 1601 Hemingway, St Charles, MO 63303, (314) 447-4232, BA 69 Fontbonne Coll; MS 77 Fontbonne Coll; SLP, Francis Howell School District, **SLP**

Barkan, Merle Beth 123 South Figueroa Street, Apartment 510, Los Angeles, CA 90012-2465, (714) 581-2800, BA 79 Univ of CA - Santa Barbara; BA 82 CA St Univ - Long Beach; MA 84 CA St Univ - Long Beach; Sp-Lang Path, Newport Lang Sp Aud Ctr, **SLP**

Barkan, Vicki Lee 4900 Sunset Boulevard, Speech/ENT Department, Los Angeles, CA 90027, (213) 667-8193, BA 81 CA St Univ - Northridge; MA 83 Univ of CO - Boulder; Sp-Lang Path, Kaiser Permanente Med Group 8, **SLP**

Barkand, Dixie 109 Ramblewood Parkway, Mount Laurel, NJ 08054, (609) 983-4165, BS 73 Clarion Univ of PA; MA 86 Trenton St Coll; **SLP**

Barkell, Nancy Leigh 1040 Bennett Avenue #2, Long Beach, CA 90804, (213) 691-0827, BA 80 San Diego St Univ; MA 83 CA St Univ - Long Beach; **SLP**

Barkemeyer, Maudene Wheeler 44-833 Oro Grande Circle, Indian Wells, CA 92210, (619) 346-3919, BS 56 Southeast MO St Univ; MA 62 Univ of MO - Columbia; **SLP**

Barker, Mrs Ann C 615 South Jackson, Pratt, KS 67124, (316) 672-5816, MA 87 Wichita St Univ

Barker, Mrs Ann M Audiology Consultants, 3319 Spring Street, Suite 104, Davenport, IA 52807, (319) 355-7712, BA 68 Univ of IA; MA 70 Univ of IA; Aud, Aud Consult, **A**

Barker, Constance J 3301 S W Archer Road #9B, Gainesville, FL 32608, (904) 392-2041, BA 73 Western WA Univ; MA 78 Western WA Univ; Aud, Univ of Florida, **A**

Barker, Daniel Edward 3280 56th Way North, St Petersburg, FL 33710, (813) 391-9771, Aud, Suncoast ENT Associates, **A**

Barker, David James 1333 Gorman Bridge Road, Asheville, NC 28806, (704) 258-1651, MA 87 Western Carolina Univ; Sp-Lang Path, Asheville City Schs, **SLP**

Barker, Mrs Deborah Anne 9641 Village Drive, Oklahoma City, OK 73120, (405) 752-0026, BA 72 OK Christian Coll; ME 87 Central St Univ; **SLP**

Barker, Diane Shelton 901 Maupin Drive, Columbia, MO 65203, (314) 443-1085, 87–Sp-Lang Path, Columbia PS, **SLP ACE**

Barker, Dianne Lynne 496 Hammond Street, Corning, NY 14830, (607) 324-5893, BS 80 Elmira Coll; MA 83 SUNY - Coll at Geneseo; Sp-Lang Path, Steuben-Alleghany BOCES, **SLP**

Barker, Elisabeth 79 Courtland Lane, Boxborough, MA 01719, BA 63 CT Coll; MS 81 Towson St Univ; Sp-Lang Path Parent-Infnt Prog, Hearing/Sp Agcy Met Baltimore, **SLP**

Barker, Mrs Francine P 1333 Gorman Bridge Road, Asheville, NC 28806, (704) 255-5367, BS 81 Western Carolina Univ; ME 82 Western Carolina Univ; Sp-Lang Path, Asheville City Schs, **SLP**

Barker, Kenneth D R R 3 Box 118-A, Mount Pleasant, IA 52641, Northeast MO St Univ; Superv/Speech-Lang Services, AEA 16, **SLP F**

Barker, Lynette Mae 1649 Lee Highway, Bristol, VA 24201, (703) 628-1842, BS 81 East TN St Univ; OM 85 Univ of SC - Columbia; Sp-Lang Path, Washington Co Public Schools, **SLP**

Barker, Lynn D 30 Heritage Drive, Terre Haute, IN 47803-2374, **SLP**

Barker, Mary Elizabeth 610 Linden Street #2, Waukesha, WI 53186, (414) 548-0090, BS 84 Univ of WI - Madison; MS 86 Univ of WI - Madison; 86–Sp-Lang Path, Sch Dist of Waukesha, **SLP**

Barker, Mrs Mary Jean P O Box 255, Parker, CO 80134, MS 84 Univ of NM; Aud, Cochlear Corporation, **A ACE**

Barker, Nancy Tripp 6605 Orford Court, Raleigh, NC 27615, (919) 832-8301, BA 80 Elon Coll; MS 84 Univ of NC - Chapel Hill; Sp-Lang Path, Rehab Services of Wake Co Inc, **SLP**

Barker, Dr Rebecca Providence Medical Center, Rehabilitation Department, 500 17th Avenue, Seattle, WA 98124, (206) 326-5100, BA 73 CA St Univ - Sacramento; MA 74 CA St Univ - Sacramento; PH 84 (Sp Lang Path) Univ of WA; 76–Dir-Sp-Lang Path Dept, Providence Med Cen, **SLP**

Barker, Mrs Ruth A 3635 Partition Road, Woodside, CA 94062, (415) 851-0992, BA 65 San Jose St Univ; MA 69 San Jose St Univ; **SLP**

Barker, Mrs Susan Leigh 11540 Hardtner, Wichita, KS 67212, (316) 886-3425, BA 74 Wichita St Univ; MA 75 Wichita St Univ; **SLP**

Barker, Verla Lee R R #3 Box 118A, Mount Pleasant, IA 52641, (319) 753-6561, **SLP**

Barkey-Kasminsky, Mrs Deborah Ann P O Box 1526, West Point, VA 23181, (804) 843-2030, BA 84 Baldwin-Wallace Coll; MA 86 Kent St Univ; 86–Sp-Lang Path, West Point PS, **SLP**

Barkmeier, Julie 2730 Wayne Avenue #1, Iowa City, IA 52240, (319) 354-1175, MA 88 Univ of IA

Barksdale, Mrs Ethelyn Burton 4225 Williamsburg Drive, College Park, GA 30337-4527, (404) 762-1557, OM 84 Emory Univ; Sp-Lang Path, Atlanta Board of Education, **SLP**

Barksdale, Mrs Linda M 12022 S W 105th Lane, Miami, FL 33186, (305) 552-1320, BS 69 FL St Univ; MS 70 FL St Univ; Sp-Lang Path, Dade Co Pub Sch, **SLP**

Barlow, Elizabeth K 1071 Fielding Way, Marietta, GA 30068, BS 82 Bradley Univ; MS 83 Bradley Univ; Aud, **A**

Barlow, Karen S 1120 Brookside, Plainfield, IN 46168, (817) 932-6586, BS 73 IN Univ - Bloomington; MA 74 IN Univ - Bloomington; Sp-Lang Path, Oral Funtion & Speech Therapy, **SLP**

Barlow, Kathleen G 1020 Washington Street, Brighton, MI 48116, (313) 229-5714, BS 78 Univ of WI - Madison; MA 81 Univ of KS; Sp-Lang Path, Private Practice, **SLP**

Barlow, Kevin Thomas 539 Central Avenue East, Winter Haven, FL 33880, (813) 293-8998, **A**

Barlow, Dr Steven Michael Boys Town Natl Institute, 555 North 30th Street, Omaha, NE 68131, (402) 498-6701, BS 76 Univ of WI - Madison; MS 80 Univ of WI - Madison; PH (Sp Physiology) Univ of WI - Madison; 83–Sci, Boystown National Institute

Barlow, Virginia L 7423 Century Avenue #7, Middleton, WI 53562, (608) 798-3191, BS 76 Univ of WI - Madison; MS 77 Univ of WI - Whitewater; SLP, Middleton School District, **SLP**

Barlund, Mrs Sarah L 4 Heritage Court, Little Rock, AR 72211, (501) 227-5550, BS 62 Univ of MO - College Park; MS 87 Univ of AR - Medical Sci; 88–Sp-Lang Path, Little Rock Sch Dist, **SLP**

Barmeier, Janet M 309 Royal Village Drive, Manchester, MO 63011, **SLP**

Barna, Mrs Theresa Elizabeth 201 Ridgeview-Eastlawn, Danville, PA 17821, (717) 275-0709, BS 81 Marywood Coll; MS 83 Hahneman Medical Coll; Aud, **A**

Barnard, Gail Engels 2804 N E 31st Street, Portland, OR 97212, (503) 282-2638, MA 76 Univ of MN - Minneap-St Paul; Sp-Lang Path, Private Practice, **SLP**

Barnard, Laurie W P O Box 183, East Glacier Park, MT 59434, (406) 338-2715, BA 78 MI St Univ; MA 79 MI St Univ; 88–Aud/Sp-Lang Path, Browning Pub Sch Dist #9, **A ACE**

Barnard, Dr Logan W Orthodontic Department, School Of Dentistry, Loma Linda, CA 92354, (714) 797-4592, BA 57 Brigham Young Univ; MA 59 Brigham Young Univ; PH 71 (Sp-Dental Research) Univ of UT; 73–Sp-Lang Path, Loma Linda U Sch of Dentistry, **SLP**

Barnard, Mrs Norma J 9836 S Campbell Avenue, Evergreen Park, IL 60642, (312) 423-5639, BA 77 Elmhurst Coll; MA 79 Northwestern Univ; Sp-Lang Path, **SLP**

Barnartt, Elaine R BA 73 Brandeis Univ; ME 77 Northeastern Univ; **SLP ACE**

Barnes, Ann Marie 106 East Roumfort Road, Philadelphia, PA 19119, (215) 242-3266, BS 84 Coll of Saint Rose; MA 86 Temple Univ-Tyler Sch of Art; 87–Sp-Lang Path, Montgomery Cty Interm Unit, **SLP**

Barnes, Beth L 7616 18th Avenue N W, Bradenton, FL 34209, (813) 792-5552, BS 59 Miami Univ - Oxford; MA 62 Northwestern Univ; Sp/Lang Path, Sch Bd of Manatee Co, **SLP**

Barnes, Beverly Gaither P O Box 201, Sanatorium, MS 39112, (601) 849-3321, OB 75 Millsaps Coll; OM 84 Univ Southern MS-Hattiesburg; **SLP**

Barnes, Mrs Charla Kaye Route 5 Box 5624, Farmington, MO 63640, (314) 358-2281, BS 82 Southeast MO St Univ; MS 87 Central MO St Univ; Sp-Lang Path, North County School District, **SLP**

Barnes, Cherise Crozier 3146 West Calhoun Blvd, Apartment 509, Minneapolis, MN 55416, (612) 920-6377, BA 86 Univ of WI - Eau Claire; MS 87 Univ of WI - Eau Claire; 88–Sp-Lang Path, Groves Learning Ctr, **SLP**

Barnes, Christine Cheryl 2323 West Tremont Court, Richmond, VA 23225, (804) 321-7474, BS 84 James Madison Univ; MA 86 Univ of CT; 88–Sp-Lang Path, Children's Hosp of Richmond, **SLP**

Barnes, Mrs Cynthia Lillian 3165 Russell Street #504, Windsor, ON, Canada N9C 1E3, (519) 354-5170, BS 83 Northern MI Univ; MA 86 Northern MI Univ; 86–Sp-Lang Path, Kent Co Catholic Sch Bd, **SLP**

Barnes, Dr Gary J Vamc Ausp(126), 3350 La Jolla Village Dr, San Diego, CA 92161, (619) 453-7500, BA 78 San Diego St Univ; MA 79 San Diego St Univ; PH 83 (Speech Pathology) Memphis St Univ; 82–Sp-Lang Path/Prog Mgr, VA Med Ctr, **SLP**

Barnes, Gertha Roberts 3310 Stonebrook Circle, Huntsville, AL 35810, (205) 852-5996, BS 76 AL A & M Univ; MA 79 Saint Louis Univ; 85–Sp-Lang Path, Huntsville City Sch Sys, **SLP**

Barnes, Glynda PO Box 356, Monroe, VA 24574, (804) 237-4658, BA 69 Univ of Richmond; MA 71 LA St Univ - Baton Rouge; 88–Sp-Lang Path, Central Virginia Training Ctr, **SLP**

Barnes, Gwendolyn 9347 South Forest Avenue, Chicago, IL 60619, (312) 734-7915, BS 67 IL St Univ - Normal; MA 76 Governors St Univ; Sp-Lang Path, Chicago Bd of Ed, **SLP ACE**

Barnes, Mrs Helen H 102 Maid Marion Court, Warner Robins, GA 31088, (912) 926-3671, BS 70 Univ of Montevallo; MS 73 Univ of Montevallo; Sp-Lang Path, Robins AFB Sch Syst, **SLP**

Barnes, Janet C James 751 Sandpiper Circle, Longwood, FL 32750, (407) 774-5148, BS 64 Bowling Green St Univ; MA 87 Univ of Central FL; 88–Aud, Orange Co PS, **A**

Barnes, Dr Janice B 791 Macon Alley, Columbus, OH 43206, (614) 261-5364, BS 59 Bowling Green St Univ; MA 69 OH St Univ; PH 75 (NS) OH St Univ; Dir-SLP Dept, Riverside Methodist Hosp, **SLP**

Barnes, Mrs Jill Harwood 1500 Seminole Drive, Pecan Court #12, Johnson City, TN 37604, (615) 928-5771, BS 84 East TN St Univ; MA 85 Univ of TN - Knoxville; 88–Aud, Daniel R Schumaier & Assoc, **A**

Barnes, Judith E M 9105 Snowheights N E, Albuquerque, NM 87112, (505) 883-0131, 84–Sp-Lang Path, Barnes & Elledge, **SLP**

Barnes, Mrs Kandace Leigh 5480 Oak Hollow #1, Memphis, TN 38116, (901) 332-2075, BA 84 Harding Univ; MS 87 Univ of MS

Barnes, Mrs Kimberly M 1970 East Princeton, Salt Lake City, UT 84108, (801) 565-6545, BS 77 Univ of UT; MA 79 CA St Univ - Long Beach; 88–Dir Speech Pathology & Aud, Western Rehab Institute, **SLP**

Barnes, Laura Ann 6318 Joel Court, Rowlett, TX 75088-3474, (214) 285-1231, BS 82 East TX St Univ - Commerce; MA 85 TX Woman's Univ; **SLP**

Barnes, Mrs Leigh C Route 3 Box 75, Harbor Heights, Ninety Six, SC 29666, (803) 223-4862, BA 70 Univ of TN - Knoxville; MA 73 Univ of TN - Knoxville; Exec Dir, St Nicholas Sp & Hrng Cen, **SLP**

Barnes, Mrs Lisa C 4002 Garden Court, Cheyenne, WY 82001-2352, (307) 632-6411, BS 85 CO St Univ; MS 87 CO St Univ; 88–Sp-Lang Path, DePaul Hosp, **SLP**

Barnes, Margaret L 141-A Cornerbrook Crescent, Waterloo, ON, Canada N2V 1L3, (519) 893-6800, **A**

Barnes, Martha D Toute 3 Box 525, Clinton, IN 47842, (317) 832-3516, **SLP**

Barnes, Mrs Mary Jane 953 B Street, Virginia Beach, VA 23451, (804) 428-4643, BS 63 Old Dominion Univ; Sp-Lang Path, Private Practice, **SLP**

Barnes, Mary Z 23271 Stoneybrook Drive, North Olmsted, OH 44070, (216) 331-5500, BS 78 Bowling Green St Univ; MA 79 Bowling Green St Univ; 86–Sp-Lang Path, Fairview Park City Schs, **SLP**

Barnes, Nancy Jean G 12651 Scandia, Garden Grove, CA 92645, (714) 962-8828, BS 74 Univ of Southern CA; MA 77 CA St Univ - Long Beach; SLP, Fountain Valley Sch Dist, **SLP**

Barnes, Dr Norman S 50 Irving Street N W, Washington, DC 20422, (202) 745-8270, BS 54 Western MI Univ; MS 57 Purdue Univ - West Lafayette; PH 66 (NS) Purdue Univ - West Lafayette; Super/SLP, VA Med Cen, **SLP**

Barnes, Phyllis Julie P O Box 851, Corona, CA 91718, (714) 369-5945, BA 75 Southern IL Univ-Edwardsvill; MA 77 Northern IL Univ - De Kalb; 79–Sp-Lang Path, Corona Norco USD, **SLP**

Barnes, Ruth A 6401 Rural Point Court, Mechanicsville, VA 23111, (804) 730-8006, BS 75 James Madison Univ; MS 79 James Madison Univ; Reg Mgr, Communicare, **SLP**

Barnes, Mrs Suzanne M 557 Gloria Road, Arcadia, CA 91006, (818) 355-3882, BA 66 Univ of OK - Norman; MA 67 Columbia Univ Teachers Coll; Sp-Lang Path, Private Practice, **SLP**

Barnes-Shankel, Loretta Ann P O Box 5010, Kahului, Maui, HI 96732, (808) 877-7288, BA 81 CA St Univ - Sacramento; MA 82 Univ of the Pacific; Sp/Lang Path, Dept of Ed, **SLP**

Barnett, Carol Jane 11607 Rowan, Houston, TX 77072, (713) 797-1551, BS 84 Brigham Young Univ; OM 85 Brigham Young Univ; **A**

Barnett, Carol L 1215 Anchors Way Drive #54, Ventura, CA 93001, (805) 644-1586, BS 67 Fort Hays St Univ; MA 77 Phillips Univ; Sp-Lang Path, Easter Seal Infant Program, **SLP**

Barnett, Claudette S 6514 Spanish Earth, San Antonio, TX 78233, (512) 224-2181, BS 73 Univ Southern MS-Hattiesburg; MS 74 Univ Southern MS-Hattiesburg; Sp/Lang Path, Fort Sam Houston ISD, **SLP**

Barnett, Constance 2990 Weatherly, Howell, MI 48843, (517) 548-1447, BA 75 MI St Univ; MA 76 Central MI Univ; Sp-Lang Path, Private Practice, **SLP**

Barnett, Deborah S 1015 North Willow, Pierre, SD 57501, **SLP**

Barnett, Mrs Debra L 10625 Vista Lago Place, San Diego, CA 92131, (619) 466-3398, BA 76 San Diego St Univ; MA 80 San Diego St Univ; Sp-Lang Path, Private Practice, **SLP**

Barnett, Mrs Denise Derrick 903 Northwest 11th, Andrews, TX 79714, (915) 524-3485, BS 81 Abilene Christian Univ; MA 82 Abilene Christian Univ; Sp-Lang Path, Private Practice, **SLP**

Barnett, Janie P 647 East 14th Street #M-B, New York, NY 10009, (212) 460-8929, BA 72 Hofstra Univ; MS 74 Columbia Univ Teachers Coll; Aud, J P B Audiology, **A**

Barnett, Kathleen Ann 3014 Dale Ann Drive, Louisville, KY 40220, (502) 456-3444, BA 83 Univ of KY; MS 87 Univ of Louisville

Barnett, Mrs Lorrie Colleen 2708 Portsmouth Lane, Modesto, CA 95355, (209) 526-4500, 82–Sp-Lang Path, Strand-Kelly Sp Path, **SLP**

Barnett, Marsha S 2 Polaris Drive, Newark, DE 19711, (302) 239-2513, BS 66 Univ of IL - Urbana; MA 68 Northwestern Univ; Sp/Lang Path, Hockessin U Meth Ch, **SLP**

Barnett, Mary Barbara 11530 Vance Jackson, Apartment 705, San Antonio, TX 78230, (512) 691-0737, BS 82 Univ of TX - Austin; MS 84 Univ of TX - Dallas; 88–Sp-Lang Path, Rehab Inst of San Antonio, **SLP**

Barnett, Rebecca Sue 314 Runaway Bay Circle, Apartment 1-A, Mishawaka, IN 46545-8056, (219) 237-7246, SLP, St Joseph Med Cntr, **SLP**

Barnett, Rebekah Lyn 7717 East 57 Street, Tulsa, OK 74145, (205) 492-0760, BS 85 Univ of AR - Fayetteville; OM 86 Auburn Univ - Auburn; **A**

Barnett-Frazier, Amy Frances 10831 113th Court N E, Apartment G-207, Kirkland, WA 98033, (206) 828-3586, BA 81 SUNY - Coll at Oneonta; MS 85 Northeastern Univ; **SLP**

Barnewold, Mrs Melinda Magruder 351 Duperier Avenue, New Iberia, LA 70560, (318) 365-2341, BA 75; OM 75; Sp-Lang Path, Iberia Parish Sch Bd, **SLP**

Barney, L Gayle 225 Hilltop View Way, Elizabethtown, PA 17022, (717) 767-6941, BS 75 Wheeling Coll; MA 78 OH St Univ; Dir Outpatient Svcs, Rehab Hosp of York, **SLP**

Barney, Riley J 11101 East Rusty Spur, Tucson, AZ 85749, (602) 294-4471, **A**

Barnhart, Kimberly Marie 2271 Clover Drive, Tustin, CA 92680-6803, (817) 283-1583, **SLP**

Barnhart, Laura Drewyer 4112 Efkew Drive, Austin, TX 78749, (512) 280-3182, ME 83 Univ of FL; Sp-Lang Path, Health Care Rehab Ctr, **SLP**

Barnhart, Susan E 6810 Juniata Place, Pittsburgh, PA 15208, (412) 622-4484, BS 81 PA St Univ - Univ Park; MA 83 Memphis St Univ; 88–Sp-Lang Path, Saint Francis Med Ctr, **SLP**

Barnhill, Mrs Kathy Harrison 3819 Linklea, Houston, TX 77025, (713) 667-4922, BS 83 Univ of Houston - Univ Park; MA 85 Univ of Houston - Univ Park; 88–Sp-Lang Path, HCA Med Ctr Hosp, **SLP**

Barnkow, David Scott 5033 Chippewa Street, St Louis, MO 63109, (314) 353-5873, BS 82 CO St Univ; MA 86 Univ of Northern CO; Aud, Washington University/Div Orth, **A**

Barno, Jeanne Ellen 33 Lake Vista Trail #207, Port St Lucie, FL 34952, (407) 879-3506, BA 79 OH St Univ; MA 82 Cleveland St Univ; Aud, R Allen, **A**

Barnowsky, Mrs Joyce C P O Box 9, Fly Creek, NY 13337, (607) 547-5415, BA 76 SUNY - Coll at Oneonta; MS 78 SUNY - Center at Albany; Sp/Lang Path, Otsego Co/N Catskills BOCES, **SLP**

Barnum, Lawrence Dean 2621 North 1600 East, Layton, UT 84041, (801) 777-5210, BS 76 Brigham Young Univ; OM 78 Brigham Young Univ; Hrng Conserv/Aud, US Air Force Hospital, **A**

Barnum, Rebecca A 9696 Walnut #1512, Dallas, TX 75243, (214) 231-7260, BS 70 OK St Univ; MA 72 OK St Univ; Appraisal Spec, Richardson ISD, **SLP**

Barnwell, Mrs Elizabeth Ogier 119 Live Oak Drive, Mount Pleasant, SC 29464, (803) 884-3138, BA 77 Univ of SC - Columbia; OM 81 Univ of SC - Columbia; Sp-Lang Path, Private Practice, **SLP**

Barnwell, Veronica Bernadette 2707 Fox Road, Baldwin, NY 11510, (516) 239-6400, BS 82 SUNY - Coll at Geneseo; MA 84 CUNY - Queens Coll; Aud, Wilks Hrng Cen Inc, **A**

Barnwell, Dr Ysaye Maria 1833 Summit Place N W #201, Washington, DC 20009, (202) 387-5990, ME 68 SUNY - Coll at Geneseo; OM 81 Howard Univ; PH 75 (NS) Univ of Pittsburgh - Pittsburgh; 88–Proj Mgr, Gallaudet Univ, **SLP**

Baron, Barbara Schwartz 100-17 Debs Place, Bronx, NY 10475, (212) 671-8119, BA 83 CUNY - Lehman Coll; MA 85 CUNY - Lehman Coll; 84–Tchr, New York City Board of Educ, **SLP**

Baron, Billie Lynn 36 E Mills Avenue, Cincinnati, OH 45215, (513) 331-0880, MA 87 Vanderbilt Univ; 87–Sp-Lang Path, Redwood Sch & Rehab Ctr, **SLP**

Baron, Christine Rochelle National Rehab Hospital, Speech-Lang Pathology SVC, 102 Irving Street N W, Washington, DC 20010-2949, (202) 877-1440, BS 82 Univ of MN - Minneap-St Paul; MA 85 Univ of MN - Minneap-St Paul; 87–Sp-Lang Path, Natl Rehabilitation Hosp, **SLP**

Baron, Fern A 2843 South Home Avenue, Berwyn, IL 60402, (312) 795-2332, BS 75 Univ of IL - Urbana; MS 76 Univ of IL - Urbana; Sp-Lang Path, Sch Dist 100, **SLP**

Baron, Helen 161 Pearsall Drive Apt 6C, Mount Vernon, NY 10552, (914) 949-7219, BS 78 Mercy Coll; MA 85 Hofstra Univ; **A**

Baron, Marla Balak 762 Brandlwood Way, Lilburn, GA 30247, (404) 963-6713, BA 76 Univ of MD - College Park; OM 78 Emory Univ; Aud, Gwinnett Co Sch Syst, **A**

Baron, Mrs Marleen Ann 801-H South Street, Philadelphia, PA 19147, (215) 596-9125, BA 67 Temple Univ; MA 69 Temple Univ; Sp/Lang Path, Childrens Seashore House, **SLP**

Baron, Mrs Phyllis G 15 Van Winkle Road, Monsey, NY 10952, (914) 354-1398, BA 73 CUNY - Brooklyn Coll; MS 76 CUNY - Brooklyn Coll; Sp/Lang Path, Greenburgh Cen Sch Dist #7, **SLP**

Baron, Rori Faith 13221 Coralberry Drive, Fairfax, VA 22033, (703) 538-4480, BA 80 Univ of PA; MA 85 Univ of MD - College Park; 87–Sp-Lang Prog Coord, Easter Seal Soc of N VA, **SLP**

Barone, Mrs Deborah Sue 877 Corcoran Court, Benicia, CA 94510, (707) 746-6700, BA 71 CA St Univ - Sacramento; MA 82 Univ of San Francisco; 79–Spec Educ Tchr, Richmond USD, **SLP**

Barousse, Mrs Melanie S Route 1 Box 334, Carencro, LA 70520, (318) 896-3263, BA 74 Univ of Southwestern LA; MS 80 Univ of Southwestern LA; SLP, Lafayette Parish School Board, **SLP**

Barr, Mrs Audrey L C 116 Fig Avenue, Fairhope, AL 36532, (205) 928-8809, BA 71 LA Tech Univ; BA 76 LA St Univ - Shreveport; OM 77 LA St Univ - N O Medical Ctr; Sp-Lang Path, Baldwin County Bd of Educ, **SLP**

Barr, Beth Kalman 340 Ocean Avenue, Lawrence, NY 11559, (212) 647-2100, BA 69 CUNY - Brooklyn Coll; MS 72 CUNY - Brooklyn Coll; SLP, Bd of Ed Sp Serv U, **SLP**

Barr, Dr David F 1099 Florida Avenue, Rockledge, FL 32955, (407) 632-6900, BS 64 Univ of TN - Knoxville; MA 67 Univ of TN - Knoxville; PH 74 (Neurolinguistics) Patna Univ - India; Aud, Private Practice, **A**

Barr, David Joseph 751 King St West, Suite 311, Kitchener, ON, Canada N2G 1E5, (519) 742-3220, BA 79 Univ of Western Ontario; MA 81 Wayne St Univ; **A**

Barr, Mrs Delores 148-30 58th Road, Flushing, NY 11355, (212) 461-7248, BA 52 CUNY - Brooklyn Coll; MA 53 Columbia Univ Teachers Coll; Tchr, Bd of Ed NYC, **SLP**

Barr, Mrs Jennifer Kay 2432 15th Street, Cuyahoga Falls, OH 44223, (216) 297-2780, BA 84 Valparaiso Univ; MA 86 Kent St Univ; Sp-Lang Path, Robinson Mem Hosp, **SLP**

Barr, Lynn H 1010 Pearl, Ypsilanti, MI 48197, (313) 482-2870, BA 75 Emory Univ; MA 82 Eastern MI Univ; Sp/Lang Path, Willow Run Sch Dist, **SLP**

Barr, Mark Edward 764 East 7th Street, Chico, CA 95928-5649, (916) 896-5381, BA 83 CA St Univ - Chico; MA 85 CA St Univ - Chico; **SLP**

Barr, Dr Nona Lee 2509 Ingrid Lane, Metairie, LA 70003, (504) 455-6690, BS 65 Univ of Houston - Univ Park; MA 68 Univ of Houston - Univ Park; PH 78 (NS); Sp-Lang Path, Jefferson Par Pub Sch Syst, **SLP**

Barr, Mrs Rebecca Welch 9924 Cedar, Overland Park, KS 66207, (913) 642-2812, BS 78 Univ of KS; MA 80 Univ of KS; Sp-Lang Path, St Michael's Day Sch, **SLP**

Barragan, Mrs Connie L 2801 Walnutbend Lane, Apartment 253 C, Houston, TX 77042, (713) 781-0983, MS 80 Univ of South AL; Aud, Houston ISD, **A**

Barrager, Dr Diane Copeland 13220 Robleda Road, Los Altos Hills, CA 94022, (415) 338-1001, BS 64 Northwestern Univ; MA 65 Northwestern Univ; PH 74 (NS) Stanford Univ; Prof, San Francisco St Univ, **A**

Barranco, Jody 114 Hyacinth Street, Metairie, LA 70005, (504) 832-1527, BS 78 LA St Univ - Baton Rouge; MA 80 LA St Univ - Baton Rouge; Sp-Lang Path, Jefferson Parish School System, **SLP**

Barranti, Mary F 2148 Hillside Circle, San Leandro, CA 94577, **SLP**

Barras, June M 15 Thomas Road, Lynnfield, MA 01940, (617) 334-6744, BA 72 Vanderbilt Univ; MA 68 Vanderbilt Univ; Aud, **A**

Barrera, Deborah E 3700 McKamy Oaks Trail, Arlington, TX 76017, **SLP**

Barrere, Mrs Eleni 2701 Park Avenue, Baldwin, NY 11510, (516) 868-7726, BA 86 Adelphi Univ; MS 87 Adelphi Univ; **SLP**

Barresi, Barbara A P O Box 702, Needham, MA 02192, (617) 455-6875, BA 64 Bowling Green St Univ; MS 67 Emerson Coll; Sp-Lang Path, Private Practice, **SLP**

Barrett, Betty A 3436 Jasmine #4, Los Angeles, CA 90034, (213) 559-2200, **SLP**

Barrett, Jean Lorene 6518-4 East Camino Vista, Anaheim Hills, CA 92807, (714) 974-4580, MA 80 CA St Univ - Fullerton; BA 75 CA St Univ - Fullerton; SLP, Orange USD, **SLP**

Barrett, Julia Jeanne 2813 Occidental Street, Bakersfield, CA 93305, (805) 398-8350, MA 83 Univ of the Pacific; SLP, Kern County Supt/Schools, **SLP**

Barrett, Kathleen Krock 428 Vista Roma, Newport Beach, CA 92660, (714) 997-6229, **SLP**

Barrett, Kathryn A 2915 Stevens Street, Madison, WI 53705, (608) 238-2677, BS 75 East Carolina Univ; MS 79 East Carolina Univ; **A**

Barrett, Dr Lyman Stewart VA Medical Center (126), 4150 Clement Street, San Francisco, CA 94121, (415) 750-2124, BA 43 Univ of CA - Berkeley; PH 59 (Sp Path Aud) Stanford Univ; 55–Chief, Aud & Speech Pathology, Veterans Administration, **SLP A F**

Barrett, Mark D LinguiSystems Inc, 716 17th Street, Moline, IL 61265, (309) 762-5112, BS 71 IA St Univ; MA 72 Northeast MO St Univ; Editor In Chief, LinguiSystems Inc, **SLP**

Barrett, Ross S Eastern Virginia Medical Sch, Ctr For Comm Disorders, 855 West Brambleton Avenue, Norfolk, VA 23510, (804) 446-5938, BA 70 Univ of Cincinnati; MA 76 Univ of Cincinnati; Consult/Dir of Fluency Prog, En VA Med Sch, **SLP**

Barrett, Mrs Sarah Davison 120 Colonial Drive, St Simons Island, GA 31522, (912) 638-3181, BS 39 Washington Univ; Sp/Lang Path, Private Practice, **SLP LM**

Barrett, Mrs Vivian Thompson 1265 Brennan Drive, Warminster, PA 18974, (215) 351-7213, BS 56 West Chester Univ of PA; ME 61 Temple Univ; Dir-Tech Support/Spec Educ, Sch Dis of Phila, **SLP**

Barrett-Ensby, Cherilyn 328 Umstead Drive, Chapel Hill, NC 27514, **SLP**

Barrick, Mrs Marcia Lee 7810 Cervin Drive, Amarillo, TX 79121, (806) 354-4200, BS 73 TX Tech Univ; MA 85 West TX St Univ; Sp-Lang Path, Amarillo ISD, **SLP**

Barrick, Mrs Wendy Laura 460 Bohemia Parkway, Sayville, NY 11782, (516) 563-4156, BA 81 SUNY - Coll at Cortland; MS 83 Adelphi Univ; Sp-Lang Path, Sayville PS, **SLP ACE**

Barricklow, Susan R Hilltop School, 24524 Hilltop Drive, Beachwood, OH 44122, (216) 831-2080, BS 83 Kent St Univ; MA 84 Kent St Univ; Sp-Lang Path, Beachwood Bd of Educ, **SLP**

Barrie-Blackley, Sandie Tri-County Speech & Language, Box 782, Elkin, NC 28621, (919) 835-3722, BA 68 Univ of MO - Columbia; MA 69 Univ of MO - Columbia; Dir, Trico Sp-Lang Ser, **SLP**

Barrios, Cynthia Flesher 431 Austin, Mount Lebanon, PA 15243, BA 84 Univ of Northern IA; MA 85 Univ of Northern IA; **SLP**

Barrios, Martha E 5212 Forest Brook, Marietta, GA 30068, (404) 992-7355, BA 74 San Diego St Univ; MA 76 CA St Univ - Los Angeles; Sp-Lang Path, Private Practice, **SLP**

Barritt, Virgil C 562 River Shore Drive, Roseburg, OR 97470, (503) 496-0531, BA 37 Univ of KS; 82–Sp-Lang Path, Private Practice, **SLP LM**

Barron, Cynthia Patricia 37 Brook Road, Milton, MA 02186, (617) 926-8064, BS 84 Northeastern Univ; MS 86 Northeastern Univ; **SLP**

Barron, David Pitt 334 Brook Street, Noank, CT 06340, (203) 536-2887, BA 54 Emerson Coll; MA 55 Emerson Coll; Dir, Prof Sp & Hrng Serv, **SLP A**

Barron, Diana R 9100 Wornall Road, Kansas City, MO 64114, (816) 361-3583, BS 71 Central MO St Univ; MS 76 Central MO St Univ; Sp-Lang Path, Private Practice, **SLP**

Barron, Joan S 1701 North Sibley Street, Metairie, LA 70003, (504) 467-4726, BS 74 Saint Mary's Dominican Coll; OM 76 LA St Univ - N O Medical Ctr; SLP, Jefferson Parish Sch Bd, **SLP**

Barron, Mrs Nancy J 517 East 50th, Loveland, CO 80538, (303) 490-4190, BS 74 CO St Univ; MS 77 CO St Univ; 85–Sp-Lang Path, Poudre Valley Mem Hosp, **SLP**

Barron, Peter Bedford 4538 Obsidian Place N E, Rio Rancho, NM 87124, (505) 892-8914, MA 83 OK St Univ; Sp-Lang Path, Coop Educational Services, **SLP**

Barron, Mrs Sara 106 West Montgomery Avenue, Unit 9, Ardmore, PA 19003, (215) 895-5710, BS 82 NY Univ; MS 84 Columbia Univ Teachers Coll; 85–Aud, Elwyn Inst Natl Rehab Ctr, **A**

Barron, Mrs Sara Elizabeth 6668 Patricia Street, Point 07, Wells, MI 49894, (906) 786-3192, BS 82 Western MI Univ; MA 83 Western MI Univ; **SLP**

Barron, Sharon C 3220 Fortunes Ridge Road, Midlothian, VA 23113, (804) 744-1228, BA 68 Albion Coll; MS 70 Univ of IL - Urbana; **SLP**

Barron, Mrs Toni Ross 7214 S W Oxford Avenue, Lawton, OK 73505, (405) 357-6900, BS 79 TX Christian Univ; MA 83 Univ of TX - Austin; **SLP**

Barron, Mrs Verna S 28 Eldon Avenue, Lansdowne, PA 19050, (215) 626-4990, BA 54 Univ of PA; MA 58 Temple Univ; 78–Sp-Lang Path, Private Practice, **SLP**

Barrouk, Marie Martin 113 Brown Street, Wilkes-Barre, PA 18702, (717) 825-9152, BS 83 Covenant Coll; MS 86 Columbia Coll; **SLP**

Barrow, Mrs Irene Marie 504 Kings Neck Cove, Virginia Beach, VA 23452-5841, (804) 468-3140, Program Coordinator, Easter Seal Soc of VA, **SLP**

Barrow, Jeannette Carr 6399 South Oneida Court, Englewood, CO 80111, **SLP**

Barrow, Mrs Kathy Glass 3847 Timberglen #3814, Dallas, TX 75252, (214) 306-4208, BS 80 Baylor Univ; MS 82 Univ of North TX; Sp-Lang Path, Private Practice, **SLP**

Barrow, Mrs Mary Hunter 1874 Greenwood Road S W, Roanoke, VA 24015-2820, (703) 343-3479, BS 74 Univ of VA - Charlottesville; MS 82 Syracuse Univ; **SLP**

Barrow, Mrs Meryl B 951 Jerome Street, Baldwin Harbor, NY 11510, (516) 228-7997, BS 77 SUNY - Center at Albany; MS 78 Adelphi Univ; MS 78 Adelphi Univ; Cl Supvr, Adelphi, **SLP ACE**

Barrows, Jane Deringer 1415 Grevelia, South Pasadena, CA 91030, (714) 624-1631, OM 85 Brigham Young Univ

Barrows, Susan Miller 3071 South Birch, Denver, CO 80222, (303) 861-0504, BA 77 IL St Univ - Normal; MS 79 Univ of WI - Stevens Point; Sp-Lang Path, Spaulding Rehabilitation Hosp, **SLP**

Barrows-Butler, Mrs Dorothy 1008 Bear, Mountain Home, AR 72653-4909, (316) 682-3363, MS 88 Wichita St Univ

Barr-Silk, Mary Jane Box 183, Pipersville, PA 18947, (215) 691-4204, MS 77 PA St Univ - Univ Park; 78–Sp-Lang Path, St Luke's Hosp, **SLP**

Barry, Ann Marie 445 Cross Creek Road, Racine, WI 53402, (414) 637-4623, BS 77 Marquette Univ; MS 78 Marquette Univ; Sp/Lang Path, Racine USD, **SLP**

Barry, Barbara Emilie 4845 N W Crescent Valley Dr, Corvallis, OR 97330, (503) 367-6111, BA 83 Univ of CA - Santa Barbara; MS 86 Univ of WA; **SLP**

Barry, Mrs Carol B 1236 Carlisle Road, North Brunswick, NJ 08902, (201) 247-6575, BS 71 Southern IL Univ -Carbondale; MS 73 Southern IL Univ -Carbondale; Sp-Lang Path, Private Practice, **SLP**

Barry, Cheryl A 240 East Washington Avenue, Lake Bluff, IL 60044-2157, (312) 295-6232, BS 72 CUNY - Queens Coll; MS 70 CUNY - Queens Coll; **SLP**

Barry, Dorothy A 155 Noanett Road, Needham, MA 02194, (617) 745-2100, BA 84 Bridgewater St Coll; MS 86 Southern CT St Univ; **SLP**

Barry, Mrs Jane D 2006 South Race Street, Urbana, IL 61801, (217) 384-3602, BS 66 Western IL Univ; MS 69 Univ of IL - Urbana; Sp-Lang Path, Urbana School District #116, **SLP ACE**

Barry, Mrs Jean Kaer 4402 Central Avenue, Kearney, NE 68847, (308) 237-5927, BA 72 Kearney St Coll; MS 87 Kearney St Coll; 78–Sp-Lang Path, Educ Svc Unit #10, **SLP**

Barry, June D 709 W Lower Springboro Rd, Lebanon, OH 45036, (513) 748-1161, BS 69 Univ of MO - Columbia; MA 70 Univ of MO - Columbia; Sp/Lang Path, Family Hlth Center, **SLP**

Barry, Mrs Karen McNaught P O Box 793, 12 Parker River Drive, Byfield, MA 01922, (617) 465-1558, BS 81 Northeastern Univ; ME 78 Northeastern Univ; Sp-Lang Path, Communicative Health Care Assc, **SLP**

Barry, Mrs Linda H 5 Century Parkway, Neodesha, KS 66757, (316) 331-6303, BA 67 Univ of MI - Ann Arbor; MA 72 CA St Univ - Sacramento; Sp-Lang Path, Tri Co Spec Ed Coop, **SLP**

Barry, Marianne B 239 High Street, Northville, MI 48167, (313) 967-4120, BS 75 Eastern MI Univ; MA 76 Eastern MI Univ; Sp-Lang Path, Oak Park Sch Dist, **SLP**

Barry, Mrs Martha L 613 Lakemont Court, Fort Wayne, IN 46845, (219) 436-6000, BA 70 Marygove Coll; MS 71 Purdue Univ - West Lafayette; Sp-Lang Path Coord, Smith-Green W Allen Spec Ed Co, **SLP**

Barry, Mrs Mary Chiodo 7801 Brompton Drive, Darien, IL 60559-4359, (312) 971-3344, BS 79 Northern IL Univ - De Kalb; MA 80 Northern IL Univ - De Kalb; Sp-Lang Path, Cen Cass Sch Dist 66, **SLP**

Barry, Mary M Department Of Audiology, Gallaudet College, Florida Avenue & 7th St N E, Washington, DC 20002, (202) 651-5328, MA 78 CA St Univ - Long Beach; Aud, Dept Aud/Gallaudet Coll, **A**

Barry, Nancy W 4354 Dalerosa Court, Fort Worth, TX 76126, **SLP**

Barry, Pamela 586 Defense Highway, Crownsville, MD 21032, (301) 266-6136, BS 77 WV Univ; MS 79 WV Univ; Sp-Lang Path, Baltimore City PS, **SLP**

Barry, Pamela Jeanne 5585 First Statesman Lane, Alexandria, VA 22312, (202) 651-5018, BA 82 George Washington Univ; MS 86 Univ of the DC; **SLP**

Barry, Dr S Joseph Keys Speech & Hearing Center, Health Sci Ctr Univ Of Ok, P O Box 26901, Oklahoma City, OK 73190, (405) 271-3378, BA 55 Saint John's Univ - Jamaica; MA 60 NY Univ; PH 66 (NS) Northwestern Univ; Prof of Aud, Univ of Ok Hlth Sci Cen, **A**

Barsch, Ann E 510 South Adams Street, Fredericksburg, TX 78624, (512) 997-9825, BA 77 Univ of IA; MS 79 Purdue Univ - West Lafayette; 84–Aud, Private Practice, **A**

Barse, Mrs Elinor A S 47 Magnolia Lane, Roslyn Heights, NY 11577, (212) 470-2556, BA 57 CUNY - Brooklyn Coll; MA 72 Hofstra Univ; Aud, Li Jewish Hillside Med Cen, **A**

Barshop-Molberger, Jill E 10 Surrey Drive, Riverside, CT 06878, BA 76 SUNY - Center at Buffalo; MS 78 Columbia Univ Teachers Coll; Sp-Lang Path, **SLP**

Barsky, Dr Lisa 822 Westminster Avenue, Hillside, NJ 07205, (201) 574-3550, BA 77; MA 78; PH 87 (Deafness Rehabilitation) NY Univ; 86–Dir, Speech & Hearing Inst

Barsky, Mrs Shari Lisa 250 N Arcadia Avenue #1516, Tucson, AZ 85711, (602) 571-0451, BA 84 Rutgers St Univ -N Brunswick; MS 86 Rutgers St Univ -N Brunswick; 88–Sp-Lang Path, Sunnyside USD, **SLP**

Barsky, Steven S 259 Juniper Court, Middle Island, NY 11953, (516) 924-1911, BA 77 SUNY - Coll at Brockport; MS 78 Adelphi Univ; SLP, Suffolk BOCES 1, **SLP**

Barson, Mrs Gay Lynn Flanders P O Box 549, Fort Rucker, AL 36362, OB 76 Univ of MI - Ann Arbor; MA 79 Univ of Tulsa; Sp-Lang Path, Scott & White Clinic, **SLP**

Barsook-Schwartz, Barbara 10434 Whipple Street, Toluca Lake, CA 91602, (213) 894-3850, BA 78 CA St Univ - Northridge; MA 82 CA St Univ - Northridge; Aud, Private Practice, **A**

Barsoumian, Vergine 5904 Mt Eagle Drive #602, Alexandria, VA 22303, (703) 323-4000, MA 69; MS 73 Columbia Univ Teachers Coll; Chief/SLP & Aud Services, North Virginia Training Center, **A**

Bartell, Carol W 1202 Beaver Creek Road, Chesterfield, MO 63017, (314) 569-8103, BA 66 CUNY - Hunter Coll; MA 71 CUNY - Hunter Coll; Aud, Spec Sch Dist of St Louis Co, **A**

Bartels, Charles E Speech And Hearing Clinic, 6900 Paradise Lane North, Brainerd, MN 56401, (218) 828-2367, BS 64 ND St Univ; MS 71 Bradley Univ; Dir Sp & Hrng Cl, Brainerd St Hosp/St Joseph Med, **SLP**

Bartels, David D Audiologist Services Incorporated, PO Box 35336, Charlotte, NC 28235, (704) 332-1574, BS 68 Univ of WI - River Falls; MS 69 Univ of MI - Ann Arbor; Aud, Aud Serv Inc, **A**

Bartels, Mrs Jane Lennon 2826 22nd Street Road, Greeley, CO 80631, (303) 339-5360, BA 81 Univ of Northern CO; MA 82 Univ of Northern CO; Sp-Lang Path, Centennial Dev Svcs Inc, **SLP**

Bartels, Kathleen Southeastern La University, P O Box 879, University Station, Hammond, LA 70402, (504) 549-2215, BA 75 LA St Univ - Baton Rouge; OM 76 LA St Univ - N O Medical Ctr; PH 86 (Special Educ) Univ of New Orleans; Assist Prof, Southeastern LA Univ, **SLP A**

Bartels, Mary Jo 7144 N W Thompson Road, Portland, OR 97229, (503) 280-5757, BA 71 Saint Louis Univ; MS 78 Portland St Univ; **SLP**

Bartelt, Rosalyn M 10038 Co Tkv, Marshfield, WI 54449, (715) 387-5128, BS 75 Univ of WI - Oshkosh; MS 80 Univ of WI - Stevens Point; Sp-Lang Path, Marshfield Clinic, **SLP**

Bartelt, Susan M 453 Queen Street East, Toronto, ON, Canada M5A 1T6, (416) 820-7111, BS 78 SUNY - Coll at Geneseo; MA 79 MI St Univ; Dir, Erinoak, **SLP**

Bartfeld, Leslie M 150 East 69th Street #15T, New York, NY 10021, (212) 981-6020, BA 73; MA 75 CUNY - Queens Coll; Aud, Staten Island Audiological Ser, **A**

Barth, Craig T 19 Galway Drive, Mendham, NJ 07945, (201) 543-4205, BA 76 CT Coll; MA 81 CUNY - Grad Sch & Univ Cntr; 86–Aud, Private Practice, **A ACE**

Barth, Mrs Jeanne M 15707 Gardenside, Tampa, FL 33624, (813) 875-7884, BA 73 Univ of IL - Chicago; MA 75 Northwestern Univ; Sp-Lang Path, Private Practice, **SLP ACE**

Barth, Sherry L HCR 75 Box 17, Lock Haven, PA 17745, (717) 748-4660, BS 76 Bloomsburg Univ of PA; MS 77 Bloomsburg Univ of PA; 77–Sp-Lang Path, Cen Intermediate Ut #10, **SLP**

Barth, Susan L 2206 Lincoln Green #1215, Arlington, TX 76011, (817) 283-4611, BA 77 Trinity Univ; MA 78 Univ of North TX; 87–Aud, Arlington ISD, **A**

Barth, Tami Feland 3415 Federal Drive, #213, Eagan, MN 55122, (612) 452-0428, BS 85 Moorhead St Univ; MS 86 Moorhead St Univ; **SLP**

Bartholme, Susan Elaine 137 East Third Street, Waterford, PA 16441, (709) 651-2500, BS 77 Indiana Univ of PA; MA 83 Edinboro Univ of PA; Sp-Lang Path, Home Health Services Erie Cnty, **SLP**

Bartholome, Kim Marie 2261 North Oxford Avenue, Claremont, CA 91711, (213) 940-8258, BA 84 Univ of CA - Santa Barbara; MA 85 Univ of Northern CO; Audiologist, Rancho Los Amigos Med Ctr, **A**

Bartholomew, Carol I 2711 Bushkill Drive, Easton, PA 18042, (215) 253-2488, BS 79 Bloomsburg Univ of PA; MS 83 PA St Univ - Univ Park; Sp-Lang Path, InSpeech Inc, **SLP**

Bartholomew, Mrs Karen Case 1100 South 228 East, Orem, UT 84058, (801) 378-7747, BS 83 Univ of UT; OM 85 Brigham Young Univ; 85–Supvr, Brigham Young Univ, **A**

Bartholomew, Karen Jane 922 Cypress Pointe Drive, Apartment C-91, Crown Point, IN 46307, (219) 769-4000, BA 85 MI St Univ; MA 86 MI St Univ; 86–Sp-Lang Path, Northwest Ind Spec Educ Coop, **SLP**

Bartholomew, Patrick Cary 111 Old Shelby Road, Morganton, NC 28655, (704) 734-1122, BS 84 Western Carolina Univ; MA 86 Western Carolina Univ; 86–Sp-Lang Path, Family Infant Pre Schl Prgrm, **SLP**

Bartholomy, Dr John M President, William Woods College, Fulton, MO 65251, (314) 642-2251, BS 62 Western MI Univ; MA 63 Western MI Univ; PH 69 (NS) OH Univ - Athens; Pres, William Woods College, **SLP**

Bartishevich, Karen Y 1216 Trumansburg Road, Ithaca, NY 14850, BS 83 SUNY - Coll at Geneseo; ME 85 Univ of VA - Charlottesville; 87–Sp-Lang Path, Special Children's Ctr, **SLP**

Bartkowiak, Mrs Elaine P 175 Messer Avenue, Depew, NY 14043, (716) 891-6433, BA 65 SUNY - Center at Buffalo; MA 75 SUNY - Coll at Buffalo; OM 83 SUNY - Coll at Buffalo; Sp/Lang Path Presch Dir, Cheektowaga Un Free Sch Dist 9, **SLP**

Bartlebaugh, Susan C 191 Elmdale Avenue, Akron, OH 44313, (216) 836-3470, BS 83 James Madison Univ; MA 85 Kent St Univ; 86–Sp-Lang Path, Bedford Bd of Educ, **SLP**

Bartlett, Mrs Cynthia Denise L 9231 N W 12th Place, Gainesville, FL 32606, (904) 495-2111, BA 68 Univ of MI - Ann Arbor; MA 71 Eastern MI Univ; 82–Sp-Lang Path, Alachua Co Schs, **SLP**

Bartlett, Cynthia L 18 Webster Street, Medford, MA 02155, (617) 578-8732, BA 67 IN Univ - Bloomington; MA 69 IN Univ - Bloomington; PH 82 (Sp-Lang Path) Univ of Pittsburgh - Pittsburgh; Asst Prof, Emerson College, **SLP ACE**

Bartlett, Jennifer L 510 Bedford Lane, New Castle, DE 19720, (302) 323-9688, BS 85 Western MI Univ; MA 86 Western MI Univ; 87–Aud, Aud Svcs of DE, **A**

Bartlett, Susan E 85 Ladyslipper Lane, Glastonbury, CT 06033-1739, (203) 486-2629, BA 72 Elmira Coll; MA 74 Univ of CT; Sp-Lang Path, U of CT, **SLP ACE**

Bartley, Cynthia Ann 4750 Southern Southeast, Albuquerque, NM 87108, (505) 255-6983, BA 71 NM St Univ; MS 83 Univ of NM; Sp-Lang Path, Albuquerque Public Schools, **SLP**

Bartlinski, Jonette Ann 5290-G Gatehouse Drive, Columbus, OH 43213, (614) 222-3466, BA 83 Loyola Coll; MS 86 Towson St Univ; Aud, Central Oh Med Group, **A**

Bartok, Mrs Susan V 956 Wyandotte Trail, Westfield, NJ 07090, (201) 469-4497, BA 57 McGill Univ - Quebec; MA 72 Kean Coll of NJ; **SLP**

Bartol, Pamela K 31 Greenwood Avenue, Rumford, RI 02916, (401) 438-6590, BA 72 Univ of MA - Amherst; MA 78 Univ of CT; Aud, J Barry Regan-Dir Hrng&Sp Dept, **A ACE**

Bartoletto, Nancy E HCR Box 17, East Thetford, VT 05043, (603) 646-5976, BS 81 Northern MI Univ; MS 87 Boston Univ; 87–Sp-Lang Path, Mary Hitchcock Mem Hosp, **SLP**

Bartoli-Izquierdo, Mrs Paula 1208 Country Court, Cary, NC 27511, (919) 790-2502, BA 80 Univ of FL; ME 82 Univ of FL; 88–Sp-Lang Path, Wake Co Sch Bd, **SLP**

Bartolotta, Mrs Theresa E 16 Poplar Avenue, Bronx, NY 10465, (212) 931-3072, BS 80 Mercy Coll; MA 82 CUNY - Queens Coll; 86–Sp-Lang Path, Private Practice, **SLP ACE**

Barton, Amy Veerhoff 2 Pine Lane, Rye, NY 10580, (914) 967-0539, BS 35 Northwestern Univ; MA 67 Columbia Univ Teachers Coll; 75–Sp-Lang Path, Private Practice, **SLP LM**

Barton, Debbie Elaine 11 Balcome Drive #5, Halifax, NS, Canada B3N 1H9, (506) 855-1600, BA 76 Univ of New Brunswick - Nb; MA 81 MI St Univ; 85–Sp-Lang Path, Private Practice, **SLP**

Barton, Deborah S 1405 Fairbanks Drive, Hanover, MD 21076, (301) 483-4355, BA 73 Skidmore Coll; MA 78 Catholic Univ of America; Sp-Lang Path, Baltimore Cty Pub Sch, **SLP**

Barton, Dr James P 3411 San Felipe Drive, Baton Rouge, LA 70809, (504) 769-5664, BS 69 Coll of Great Falls; MA 71 Northern St Univ; PH 77 (NS) Univ of UT; Sp-Lang Path, Clinical Affiliates, Inc, **SLP**

Barton, Jesse M, Jr 4104 Staunton Avenue S E, Charleston, WV 25304, (304) 766-3997, BA 47 Bethany Coll; MA 53 Northwestern Univ; Consultant, Private Practice, **SLP ACE**

Barton, Mrs Jill H 1169 North 1100 West, Farmington, UT 84025, (801) 451-6646, MS 88 Univ of UT

Barton, Johnny L Northwestern State College, 700 Oklahoma Boulevard, Alva, OK 73717, (405) 327-1700, BA 64 Northwestern OK St Univ; MS 66 Univ of OK - Norman; Assoc Professor/Divn Director, Northwestern State University, **SLP**

Barton, Kathleen Ann 2627 North 69th Street, Omaha, NE 68104, (402) 895-8350, BS 81 Univ of NE - Omaha; MS 82 Univ of NE - Omaha; Sp/Lang Path, Millard Pub Schs, **SLP**

Barton, Kay Humphreys Route 64 North Box 27, Fox, AR 72051, BA 72 MS St Univ - MS State; OM 82 Univ of MS; Sp-Lang Path, West Side Public School, **SLP**

Barton, Lori Jean 47 Harbor Oaks Circle, Safety Harbor, FL 33572, (614) 753-1973, BS 81 OH Univ - Athens; MA 82 Kent St Univ; Sp-Lang Path, Commonwealth Rehabilitaion, **SLP**

Barton, Marion Elizabeth Route 4 Box 387, Hamilton, AL 35570, (205) 921-7240

Barton, Mrs Vicki Parrish 1394 Belmont Lane, Helena, AL 35080, (205) 491-1752, BS 76 Auburn Univ - Auburn; MS 83 Univ of South AL; SLP, Jefferson Co Sch Syst, **SLP**

Bartosiewicz, Mrs Sharon Rosa Rd 2 Glendale, Box 176-H, Avoca, PA 18641, (717) 443-9564, BS 76 Bloomsburg Univ of PA; MS 77 Bloomsburg Univ of PA; Sp-Lang Path, White Haven Cen, **A**

Bartoul, Millet J Advanced Hearing Systems Inc, 5579 Pearl Road, Suite 105, Parma, OH 44129, (216) 888-8050, BA 71 Cleveland St Univ; MA 73 Cleveland St Univ; Pres/Aud, Adv Hrng Sys Inc, **A**

Bartram, Margaret Lynne 500 Oxcart Road #103, Ashland, KY 41101, (606) 324-1656, BA 63 Marshall Univ; Sp-Lang Path, Warren Consolidated Schs, **SLP LM**

Bartrug, Donna Briddell 332 Tourmaline Drive, Hebron, MD 21830, (301) 742-4977, BS 77 James Madison Univ; MS 79 James Madison Univ; Sp-Lang Path, Chesapeake Speech Hearing Clin, **SLP**

Bartsch, Mrs Nancy R A 1804 South Mariposa Lane, Billings, MT 59102, (406) 252-3927, BA 73 Univ of MN - Duluth; MA 75 Univ of MN - Duluth; SLP, Sch Dist #2, **SLP**

Bartsh, Lorrie Lynette 10650 Brunswick Road #205, Bloomington, MN 55438, (612) 881-4804, BA 85 Univ of WI - Eau Claire; MS 86 Univ of WI - Eau Claire; **SLP**

Bartshe, Judy Diann 2204 Aqueduct Place, Independence, MO 64057-1009, (417) 781-2311, BS 81 Central MO St Univ; MS 84 Central MO St Univ; Sp-Lang Path, Area Hearing and Speech Clinic, **SLP**

Bartusch, Mrs Mary Ann R 8750 West Taos Drive, Palos Hills, IL 60465, (312) 284-1102, BS 62 Bradley Univ; Sp-Lang Path, Chicago Bd of Ed, **SLP**

Bartz, Mrs Lynn O'Brien 349 Joslyn Drive, Elgin, IL 60120, (312) 741-5440, BS 84 Univ of IL - Urbana; MS 85 Univ of IL - Urbana; Sp-Lang Path, McHenry Co Spec Ed Dist, **SLP**

Bartz, Mrs Patricia R 2522 Southridge, Helena, MT 59601, (406) 443-0467, BA 75 Univ of WY; BA 75 Univ of WY; MS 80 Univ of HI - Manoa; Sp-Lang Path, Private Practice, **SLP**

Barwell, David R 9424 Horizon Run Road, Gaithersburg, MD 20879, (301) 530-8606, MA 72 Univ of MD - College Park; Aud, Private Practice, **A**

Barwick, Steven A 18423 Santa Carlotta, Fountain Valley, CA 92708, (714) 963-4358, BA 73 CA St Univ - Fullerton; MS 77 Univ of AZ; Pres, Vector Hrng Mangement Inc, **A**

Barwise, Kathryn T 8218 Wisconsin Avenue N W, Bethesda, MD 20814, **SLP**

Baryla, Joanne 2406 Milltown Road #3-A, Wilmington, DE 19808, (302) 323-2935, BS 81 Bloomsburg Univ of PA; MS 82 Bloomsburg Univ of PA; 85–Sp-Lang Path, Colonial School District, **SLP**

Barzey, Mrs Beverly F 300 First Avenue #9F, New York, NY 10009, BS 59 CUNY - Brooklyn Coll; SLP, Visiting Nurse Service of NY, **SLP**

Bas, Helen S 4014 Park Forest Drive, Flint, MI 48507, (313) 767-1291, BS 79 Univ of MI - Flint; MA 84 MI St Univ; Sp-Lang Path, **SLP**

Basalyga, Mrs Michele Dunne 516 Highland Avenue, Clarks Summit, PA 18411-2528, (717) 586-4285, BS 82 Marywood Coll; MA 86 Montclair St Coll; **SLP**

Basham, Jean Carla 240 Central Avenue, South Charleston, WV 25303, (304) 766-4870, BA 83 Marshall Univ; MA 84 Univ of TN - Knoxville; 88–Sp-Lang Path, West VA Rehab Ctr, **SLP**

Bashir, Anthony 300 Longwood Avenue, Boston, MA 02115, MS 63 Northwestern Univ; PH 68 (NS) Northwestern Univ; Sp-Lang Path, The Childrens Hospital, **SLP**

Bashista, Mrs Kathleen F 2574 Mount Gretna Road, Elizabethtown, PA 17022, (717) 367-4863, BS 68 PA St Univ - Univ Park; ME 70 PA St Univ - Univ Park; SLP, Milton S Hershey Med Cen, **SLP**

Bashor, Pamela H Speech Pathologist, Doctors Bldg Suite 221, 1012 South Kings Drive, Charlotte, NC 28283, (704) 375-5231, BA 69 FL St Univ; MS 70 FL St Univ; Sp-Lang Path, Private Practice, **SLP**

Bashore, Samuel R 5703 Cricket Lane, Harrisburg, PA 17112, (717) 783-6913, ME 68 PA St Univ - Univ Park; Chief, Div of Regional Review, Pennsylvania Dept of Education, **A**

Basik, Carleen P 117 A Morningside Drive, Manhattan Beach, CA 90266, **A**

Basil, Sherwin A Riverview Hrng Sp & Lang Ctr, 1165 East San Antonio, Suite A, Long Beach, CA 90807, (213) 422-3388, BS 65 Northern IL Univ - De Kalb; MA 74 CA St Univ - Long Beach; Dir, Riverview Hrng Sp & Lang Cen, **SLP A**

Basili, Dr Annanmaria 400 Grist Mill Crossing, Severna Park, MD 21146, (301) 477-1800, BA 65; MA 67 Columbia Univ Teachers Coll; PH 71 (NS) Purdue Univ - West Lafayette; Ch/Aud & SLP, VA Med Cen, **SLP**

Basilone, Frank J 194 Elm Crest Drive, Wheeling, WV 26003, (304) 243-0363, BS 74 Edinboro Univ of PA; MA 78 Edinboro Univ of PA; 86–Coord Comm, Ohio County Schs, **SLP**

Basinger, Sherry Marie 5844-D Westower Drive, Richmond, VA 23225, (804) 524-7354, MS 87 Radford Univ; 87–Sp-Lang Path, Southside Vir Training Ctr, **SLP**

Baskervill, Mrs Maxine A 167 Berkshire Avenue, Buffalo, NY 14215, (716) 631-5586, BS 64 SUNY - Coll at Geneseo; MA 68 OH Univ - Athens; SLP, Baskervill Assoc for Comm Dis, **SLP**

Baskervill, Dr Robert David 167 Berkshire Avenue, Buffalo, NY 14215, (714) 631-5586, BS 60 Hampton Univ; MA 68 Coll of Saint Rose; PH 79 (NS) SUNY - Center at Buffalo; Dir, Bacd, P C, **SLP**

Baskies, Susan Baer 1235 Sequoia Road, Cherry Hill, NJ 08003, ME 73 Northeastern Univ; Sp-Lang Path, Private Practice, **SLP**

Baskin, Barbara Jane 7116 Cresheim Road, Philadelphia, PA 19119, (215) 284-8570, BS 80 Univ of WA; OM 82 Hahneman Medical Coll; Chief/Sp-Lang Path, Deco Mem Hosp-Hrng Sp Cen, **SLP**

Baskin, Cynthia Mae Rt 4 Box 486, Clarksburg, WV 26301, (304) 622-1837, BS 82 WV Univ; MS 83 WV Univ; Audiologist, Audiology & Hrng Aid Services, **A**

Baskin, Roger B PO Box 2007, Framingham, MA 01701, (617) 620-1552, BS 74 Syracuse Univ; MS 76 SUNY - Coll at Buffalo; Director, Framingham Rehabilitation Ctr, **SLP**

Basner, Anne M 4509 Jasmine Avenue, Culver City, CA 90230, **A**

Basner, Barry 8105 Raintree Circle #105, Culver City, CA 90230, (213) 986-1977, BA 79 Univ of CA - Los Angeles; MA 82 CA St Univ - Los Angeles; Irwin Lehroff and Associates, **SLP**

Basom, Mrs Susan Marckese 4864 Heights Drive Drive, Stow, OH 44224, (216) 630-3042, BS 72 Kent St Univ; MA 74 Kent St Univ; 75–Sp-Lang Path, Co of Summit Bd of Ment Ret, **SLP**

Bass, Mrs Emily Anne 3772 Ingold, Houston, TX 77005, (713) 665-6112, MS 71 George Washington Univ; 88–Sp-Lang Path, Houston ISD, **SLP**

Bass, Mrs Iris Goldberh 3801 Louise Street, Skokie, IL 60076-3425, BA 81 Univ of WI - Madison; MA 84 Northwestern Univ; Sp-Lang Path, Infant Welfare Soc, **SLP**

Bass, Mrs Janice Heller 12408 Buckley Drive, Silver Spring, MD 20904, (301) 622-5844, BS 51 Syracuse Univ; MA 55 Columbia Univ Teachers Coll; **SLP A**

Bass, Mrs M Virginia 8503 Douglas Court, St Louis, MO 63144, (314) 968-3591, BA 68 Fontbonne Coll; MA 70 Saint Louis Univ; Sp/Lang Path, Private Practice, **SLP**

Bass, Mrs Nancy F 2866 Sedgewick Road, Shaker Heights, OH 44120, MA 77 Case Western Reserve Univ; Asst Coord Ocs, Clev Hrbg & Sp Ctr, **SLP**

Bass, Pamela M 3120 S W Freeway Ste 205, Houston, TX 77098, (713) 529-5111, BS 66 Univ of Houston - Univ Park; MA 68 Univ of Houston - Univ Park; Sp-Lang Path, Private Practice, **SLP**

Bass, Mrs Robbie A 3053 Stanton Circle, Carmichael, CA 95608, BA CA St Univ - Sacramento; MA CA St Univ - Sacramento; **SLP LM**

Bassen, Mrs Alice M P O Box 801, Lee, MA 01238, (413) 243-4551, BA 80 Empire St Coll; MA 85 Univ of MA - Amherst; **A**

Basser, Mrs Roberta Ilene 4335-100 Nobel Drive, San Diego, CA 92122, (619) 546-0168, BA 76 PA St Univ - Univ Park; ME 78 Trenton St Coll; 87–Sp-Lang Path, San Dieguito Jr HS Dist, **SLP**

Bassett, Mrs Jane T 32 Stiles Road, Suite 210, Salem, NH 03079, (603) 893-1519, BA 70 Denison Univ; MA 72 OH Univ - Athens; **SLP**

Bassett, Katherine Evans 2000 Crowfoot Drive, Lafayette, IN 47905, (317) 423-6336, BS 76 Purdue Univ - West Lafayette; MA 77 Ball St Univ; 78–Sp-Path, St Eliz Hosp Med Cen, **SLP**

Bassett, Michele 8378 East San Sabastian, Scottsdale, AZ 85258, (602) 998-7545, BS 78 Towson St Univ; MS 81 Vanderbilt Univ; 87–Aud, East Valley ENT, **A**

Bassett, Mrs Nancy L 14641 Woodridge, Grand Haven, MI 49417, (616) 842-3571, BS 71 Western MI Univ; MA 72 Western MI Univ; Sp-Lang Path, Grand Haven Pub Schools, **SLP**

Bassett, Sandra S 4920 South Pittsburgh, Spokane, WA 99223, (509) 455-3306, MS 73 Univ of AZ; Sp-Lang Path, Sacred Heart Med Cen, **SLP**

Bassett, Mrs Wendy Bendrick P O Box 872, Minequa, WI 54548, (715) 356-4413, BS 81 Univ of WI - Madison; MS 83 Univ of WI - Madison; Sp-Lang Path, School District of Rhinelander, **SLP**

Bassham, Mrs Geanifer Jo 2514 Hardwood, Bryan, TX 77803, (409) 778-0843, BS 82 Abilene Christian Univ; MA 83 Abilene Christian Univ; SLP, Brenham State Sch, **SLP**

Bassich, Celia J 25 Buchanan Road, Baltimore, MD 21212, (301) 496-5061, BA 75 Catholic Univ of America; MA 77 Catholic Univ of America; Sp-Lang Path, Nat Inst Neur/Commun Dis, **SLP**

Bassin, Mrs Beatrice Kellner 2891 Audubon Terrace N W, Washington, DC 20008, (202) 686-0325, BA 35 CUNY - Brooklyn Coll; ME 37 CUNY - City College; Retired, **SLP LM**

Bassin, Mrs Randee Levick 4398 Hickory Court, Orchard Lake, MI 48033, (313) 683-2022, BA 72 MI St Univ; MA 77 Eastern MI Univ; **SLP**

Basso, Mrs Barbara May 674 School Road, Nazareth, PA 18064, (215) 868-6900, MS 84 Bloomsburg Univ of PA; BS 83 East Stroudsburg Univ of PA; Audiologist, Priv Pract, **A**

Bassoul-Restivo, Regina 9 Ridge Way, Fanwood, NJ 07023, (201) 889-8478, BS 71 Boston Univ; ME 72 Boston Univ; 87–Sp-Lang Path, Private Practice, **SLP**

Basta, Susan Cohick 119 Wood Haven Road, Pawtucket, RI 02861, MS 84 Univ of WI - Madison; BS 80 Ithaca Coll; SLP, R E A D S, **SLP**

Bastardo, Mrs Susan Marie 7 Marsh Avenue, Worcester, MA 01605, (617) 853-6631, BA 81 Worcester St Coll; MS 85 Worcester St Coll; Sp-Lang Path, Shrewsbury PS, **SLP**

Bastean, Judith Ann P Route 5, Fulton, MO 65251, (314) 642-3301, BA 80 CA St Univ - Sacramento; MS 81 Univ of MO - Columbia; Head of Aud, Mo School for the Deaf, **A**

Bastian, Jalinda A 7420 Monte Vista Avenue, La Jolla, CA 92037, (619) 589-4108, BA 73 Univ of IA; MA 75 Univ of IA; 77–Dir Sp Lang Cognitive Serv, Grossmont Hosp, **SLP ACE**

Bastiani, Robert 245 North Columbia Blvd, Brookfield, WI 53005, BS 52; MS 54 Syracuse Univ; SLP, Milwaukee Public Schools, **SLP**

Bastidas, Deborah Ann 5415 Braesvalley #794, Houston, TX 77096, (713) 792-4500, BS 77 Univ of WI - Madison; MS 79 Univ of WI - Madison; Sp-Lang Path, Univ TX Sp&Hrg Institute, **SLP**

Bastin, Mrs Carol E 7548 Graystone Court, West Chester, OH 45069, (513) 777-4691, OB 82 Miami Univ - Oxford; OM 84 Miami Univ - Oxford; 84–Sp-Lang Path, Hamilton Co Bd of Educ, **SLP**

Bastin, Mrs Lana L 5350 Huffmans Mill Road, Hopkinsville, KY 42240, (502) 887-1280, BS 75 Murray St Univ; MS 77 Murray St Univ; OM 78 Murray St Univ; Sp-Lang Path, Christian Co Bd of Ed, **SLP**

Baszler, Stephanie Ann 1404 McHenry, Urbana, IL 61801, (701) 280-4493, BS 81 IA St Univ; MS 84 Moorhead St Univ; Coord of Sp-Lang Path, Christie Clinic Association, **SLP**

Batalia, Eugenia Rabias 502 Redondo Drive, Downers Grove, IL 60516, (312) 352-0145, BA 74 Elmhurst Coll; MS 78 Southern IL Univ -Carbondale; Sp-Lang Path, La Grange Park PS, **SLP**

Batchelor, Barbara M Route 3 Box 693, Ringgold, LA 71068, (318) 894-2911, BA 81 LA St Univ - Shreveport; OM 85 LA St Univ - N O Medical Ctr; 81–Sp-Lang Path, Bienville Parish Sch Bd, **SLP**

Batchelor, Mrs Maureen C 2452 Greensward North, Warrington, PA 18976, (215) 343-5189, BS 75 Marquette Univ; MS 76 Marquette Univ; **SLP**

Batchelor, Mrs Valerie W 3610 Powell, Memphis, TN 38122, (901) 525-2682, BS 79 Middle TN St Univ; MA 81 Memphis St Univ; Clinical Instructor, Memphis Speech-Hearing Center, **A**

Bate, Mrs Christine Porter 23344 Camino Hermoso, Los Altos Hills, CA 94022, (415) 326-5530, BA 51; MA 72 Univ of CO - Boulder; Sp-Lang Path, The Chldn Hlth Council, **SLP**

Bate, Dr Harold L Western Michigan University, Kalamazoo, MI 49008, (616) 383-0963, BA 59 Butler Univ; MA 61 Univ of FL; PH 64 (NS) Univ of WI - Madison; Prof, Wn MI U/Dept Sp Path & Aud, **A**

Bateman, Dr Hugh Elton University Of Mississippi, 105 Labauve, University, MS 38677, (601) 232-5970, BA 61 William Carey Coll; MS 66 Univ Southern MS-Hattiesburg; PH 69 (NS) Univ Southern MS-Hattiesburg; Prof of Commun Dis & Asst Dean, U of MS, **SLP**

Bateman, Mrs Julie 60 Rathbun Hill Road, Salem, CT 06415, (203) 859-0299, BA 64 Univ of Northern IA; ME 69 Bloomsburg Univ of PA; Sp-Lang Path, Montville Sch Dist, **SLP**

Bateman, Mrs Sally F Box 545, Sidney, IA 51652, (712) 527-5261, BA 69 Univ of NE - Lincoln; ME 71 Univ of NE - Lincoln; SLP, AEA 13, **SLP**

Bateman, Mrs Susan Blair 15237 Dufief Drive, Gaithersburg, MD 20878, (301) 972-9620, BA 80 Catholic Univ of America; MA 81 George Washington Univ; Sp/Lang Path, Montgomery Co Pub Sch, **SLP**

Bates, Mrs Ann Lloyd 139 Greenwood Circle, Harvest, AL 35749, (303) 366-2553, BA 80 Univ of CA - Davis; MA 83 Univ of Denver; **SLP**

Bates, Bette B 1425 Villa Drive, Los Altos, CA 94022, (415) 493-5000, BA 61 Stanford Univ; MA 62 Stanford Univ; Aud, VA, **A**

Bates, Beverly G Bates Learning Center, P O Box 102, Newfane, VT 05345, (802) 365-4294, BS 58 Boston Univ; ME 58 Boston Univ; Dir, Bates Lrng Cen, **SLP A**

Bates, Dana Marie 2707 S Emporia #1109, Wichita, KS 67216, (316) 264-3832, BA 85 Wichita St Univ; MA 86 Wichita St Univ; **SLP**

Bates, Dawn 546 West Spencer Road, Ithaca, NY 14850-5108, (518) 272-3991, BA 85 SUNY - Coll at Plattsburgh; MS 86 Ithaca Coll; **SLP**

Bates, Mrs Diane E 12 Moro Terrace, Wayne, NJ 07470, (201) 696-2885, BA 74 William Paterson Coll; MS 77 William Paterson Coll; Sp/Lang Path, Elmwood Park Board of Ed, **SLP**

Bates, Elsie C 11 Sunset Drive East, Nutley, NJ 07110, (201) 239-5146, BS 58 Jersey City St Coll; MA 62 Newark St Coll; 62–Sp-Lang Path, Cedar Grove Bd of Ed, **SLP**

Bates, Fredra D 21805 Rushford Drive, El Toro, CA 92630, (714) 458-5759, BS 77 Wichita St Univ; MA 78 Wichita St Univ; Coord Sp/Lang Serv, Peoria Sch Dist, **SLP**

Bates, Mrs Joyce W 312 Marion Avenue, McComb, MS 39648, (601) 249-3254, MS 80 Univ Southern MS-Hattiesburg; Dir/SLP, Speech and Hearing Center, **SLP**

Bates, Karen L 9313 S E Morrison Street, Portland, OR 97216-2117, (503) 256-5178, BA 78 Univ of WI - Eau Claire; MS 79 Univ of WI - Eau Claire; Sp-Lang Path, **SLP**

Bates, Dr Kathie Berles 8043 Via Palma, Scottsdale, AZ 85258, PH 76 (Speech) Univ of IL - Urbana; **SLP**

Bates, Mrs Kim M 1528 Sand Point Drive, Lansing, MI 48917, (517) 321-7265, BA 78 MI St Univ; MA 79 MI St Univ; 80–SLP, Waverly Comm Sch, **SLP**

Bates, Kimberly K 4900 Derussey Parkway, Chevy Chase, MD 20815, (301) 652-0796, BS 71 Western MI Univ; MA 77 Univ of MD - College Park; Sp-Lang Path, Mongomery Co Pub Sch, **SLP**

Bates, Susan M V 57 Peachtree Hills Avenue, Atlanta, GA 30305, (404) 763-0580, MS 74 Univ of South FL; Consultant-Presch, Fulton Co Bd of Ed, **SLP**

Bates, Tempie M Saint Joseph Medical Center, 333 North Madison Street, Joliet, IL 60435, (815) 722-3078, BA 75 Southern IL Univ-Edwardsvill; MS 76 Southern IL Univ-Edwardsvill; Dir/Dept Sp-Lang Path & Aud, St Josephs Med Ctr, **SLP ACE**

Bateson, Mrs Cynthia Lee 18 Albion Street, Lawrence, MA 01841, (508) 681-8722, BA 80 Bucknell Univ; MA 84 Northwestern Univ; 86–Sp-Lang Path, Laura Lee Sch, **SLP**

Bateson, Lynn Malene Com Health Services E I Wood Bldg, 350 Cheadle Street West, Swift Current, SK, Canada S9H 2S9, (306) 773-8301, OB 81 Univ of Regina -Saskatchewan; MS 87 Minot St Univ; 87–Sp-Lang Path, Saskatchewan Health

Bates-Stokes, Barbara A 1705 East Madison, Petaluma, CA 94952, (707) 996-6774, BA 75 CA St Univ - Sacramento; MS 78 Univ of NE - Omaha; SLP, Sonoma Valley USD, **SLP**

Batezel, Mrs Roxanne Kay 9303 Beowulf, San Antonio, TX 78250-2251, (512) 434-6711, BS 75 Phillips Univ; MS 77 CO St Univ; 85–Faculty Assoc, Harry Jersig Ctr, **SLP**

Bathey, Janet Rose 15700 Lexington Boulevard #305, Sugar Land, TX 77478, (713) 341-3366, BS 84 Univ of Houston - Univ Park; MA 87 Univ of Houston - Univ Park; **SLP**

Bathke, Robert E 5224 12th Avenue South, Minneapolis, MN 55417, (612) 457-1138, BA 77 Univ of WI - Eau Claire; MA 78 Univ of MN - Duluth; 87–Sp-Lang Path, Dakota Inc, **SLP**

Batie, Ramona L 509 North Cedar, Little Rock, AR 72204, (501) 843-3562, BS 81 Univ of AR - Little Rock; MS 82 AR St Univ; Sp/Lang Path, Cabot Publ Schs, **SLP**

Batill, Anthony Scott 17 Monroe Avenue, Oneonta, NY 13820, (607) 547-3264, BA 78 CA St Univ - Sacramento; MA 79 CA St Univ - Los Angeles; Chief of Aud & Sp-Lang Path, M I Bassett Hospital, **A**

Batista, Mrs Lourdes 12530 S W 22nd Terrace, Miami, FL 33175, (305) 226-9734, BA 78 Univ of Miami; MA 79 Univ of Miami; 88–Sp-Lang Path, Ctr for Pediatric Therapy, **SLP**

Batiste, Dierdra M 12345 North I-10 SVC Road, Apartment 617, New Orleans, LA 70128, (504) 242-5744, BA 82 Southern Univ - New Orleans; MS 84 Murray St Univ; **SLP**

Bator, Mrs Cecilia J 31235 West Rutland, Birmingham, MI 48009, (313) 283-8220, BS 77 Wayne St Univ; MA 78 Wayne St Univ; Sp-Lang Path, Wyandotte Public Schools, **SLP**

Batory, Mrs Nancy Anderson 227 Cricket Knoll, Wethersfield, CT 06109, (203) 659-2759, BS 75 Ithaca Coll; MA 77 MI St Univ; Aud, Private Practice, **A**

Batshaw, Marilyn Seidner 166 Westgate Drive, Edison, NJ 08820, (201) 549-5580, BA 68 Kean Coll of NJ; MA 72 Kean Coll of NJ; 86–Dir of Educ/Prin, Lakeview Sch-Cerebral Palsy Assn, **A**

Batson, Dr Delaina W Texas Womans University, Box 23775, Denton, TX 75230, (817) 387-6169, BA 60 Southern Methodist Univ; MS 68 Univ of UT; PH 80 (NS) Univ of TX - Austin; Asst Prof, TX Womans U, **SLP**

Batson, Laura Guthrie 1722 Skyview, Wichita, KS 67212, (316) 721-2527, BA 82 Wichita St Univ; MA 84 Wichita St Univ; **A**

Batson-Magnuson, Mrs Luann 127 Northhmpton Street, Bangor, PA 18013, (201) 475-5118, BS 82 East Stroudsburg Univ of PA; MS 87 Bloomsburg Univ of PA; 83–Sp-Lang Path, Knowlton Twp Bd of Educ, **SLP**

Batten, Claudia P 502 Whitney Avenue, Glassboro, NJ 08028, (609) 881-1661, BA 72 Marymount Coll; MS 75 Columbia Univ Teachers Coll; Sp-Lang Path, Private Practice, **SLP**

Batten, Mrs Jennifer Swartley 837 Poplar Street, Pottstown, PA 19464, (215) 970-5100, BA 81 Loyola Coll; MS 83 Towson St Univ; Sp-Lang Path, The Reading Hosp & Med Ctr, **SLP**

Batterman, Mrs Laurel Kay 12750 West National Avenue, Apartment 106, New Berlin, WI 53151-4073, (414) 542-8036, BS 84 Univ of WI - Stevens Point; MS 87 Univ of WI - Stevens Point; **SLP**

Battin, Dr R Ray The Battin Clinic, 3931 Essex Lane, Houston, TX 77027, (713) 621-3072, BA 48 Univ of Denver; MS 50 Univ of MI - Ann Arbor; PH 59 (NS) Univ of FL; 59–Dir, The Battin Cl, **SLP A F**

Battle, Dr Dolores 141 South Lane, Orchard Park, NY 14127, (716) 878-5719, BS 63 Univ of MA - Amherst; ME 71 SUNY - Coll at Buffalo; PH 78 (Commun Dis & Sciences) SUNY - Center at Buffalo; 70–Assoc Prof, SUNY Coll at Buffalo, **SLP F ACE**

Battle, Marie Josephine 2853 Corpus Christie, Simi Valley, CA 93063, (805) 527-0092, BA 75; MA 77 CA St Univ - Northridge; SLP, Los Angeles USD, **SLP**

Battles, James F 4401 North Ardmore Avenue, Shorewood, WI 53211, (414) 781-5280, BS 72 Univ of WI - Milwaukee; MS 74 Univ of WI - Milwaukee; Sp-Lang Path, Elmbrook Sch Dist, **SLP**

Battles, Kathy J 816 Old Strawberry Hill Road #3A, Centerville, MA 02632, (508) 771-0612, BS 79 Univ of MN - Minneap-St Paul; MA 83 Univ of KS; SLP, Head Injury Ctr at Lewis Bay, **SLP**

Batts, Kathryn P 1036 Sycamore Street, Rocky Mount, NC 27801, (919) 443-8048, BS 74 Western Carolina Univ; MS 77 East Carolina Univ; Sp-Lang Path, Nash General Hosp, **SLP**

Batza, Dr Eugene M 14975 Hill Drive, Novelty, OH 44072, (216) 338-6051, BA 37 Coll of Wooster; MA 51 Northwestern Univ; PH 56 (NS) Northwestern Univ; **SLP A LM**

Bauch, Chris D Section Of Audiology, Mayo Clinic, Rochester, MN 55905, (507) 284-2577, BA 72; MS 73; PH 77 (Aud); 78–Aud, Mayo Cl, **A**

Bauchiero, Rosemary 1035 West Third Street, Dubuque, IA 52001, (319) 588-0506, BS 83 Elmira Coll; MA 85 OH Univ - Athens; 85–Aud, Dubuque Otolaryngology Head & Neck Surgery PC, **A**

Baucum, Kay 2634 July Street, Baton Rouge, LA 70808, **SLP**

Baudoin-Chial, Dr Sonia T 24 Rue Durantin 75018, Paris, France, 42-55-87-87, BA 73 Tulane Univ; MS 75 2162; OD 82 (Neuropsychology) 8146; **SLP**

Bauer, Ann M 3104 Bob-O-Link Avenue, Wausau, WI 54401, (715) 845-3944, BS 80 Univ of WI - Stevens Point; MS 82 Univ of WI - Eau Claire; Sp-Lang Path, N Ctrl Hlth Care Facility, **SLP**

Bauer, Mrs Carmille A 16 Bondcroft Drive, Eggertsville, NY 14226, BS 60 SUNY - Coll at Buffalo; MS 66 SUNY - Coll at Buffalo; SLP, BOCES #1, **SLP**

Bauer, Mrs Cathy Lynn 112 Woodland, Rittman, OH 44270, (216) 925-7167, Multihandicapped-Lang Teacher, Brunswick City Schools, **SLP**

Bauer, Dr Cherie 7436 Nada, Downey, CA 90241, (714) 821-0800, BA 71 CA St Univ - Fullerton; MA 75 CA St Univ - Fullerton; ME 85 Univ of Southern CA; Prog Spec, Greater Anaheim Spec Ed Area, **SLP**

Bauer, David A 5002-B Foothills Road, Lake Oswego, OR 97034, (503) 252-0966, BA 65 Western OR St Coll; MS 69 Western OR St Coll; Sp-Lang Path, Assoc-Total Home Hlth Serv, **SLP**

Bauer, Mrs Debra B A 993 Dove Meadow, Keller, TX 76248, (817) 379-6883, BA 75 IN Univ - Bloomington; MA 76 IN Univ - Bloomington; 87–Aud, Child Study Ctr, **A**

Bauer, Doris S 15 Brookland Avenue #205, Aurora, ON, Canada L4G 2H7, (416) 895-4521, BA 78 York Univ - Ontario; OM 81 Univ of Western Ontario; Sp-Lang Path, York County Hospital, **SLP**

Bauer, Dr Harold R OH State Univ Sp & Hrng Sci, 324 Derby Hall, 154 North Oval Mall, Columbus, OH 43210, (614) 422-8207, BA 68 SUNY - Coll at Plattsburgh; MA 70; PH 77 (NS) Stanford Univ; Asst Prof, Sp & Hrng Science Sect

Bauer, Janetta M 3411 Buffalo Springs Trail, Georgetown, TX 78626, (512) 869-1235, MS; **SLP**

Bauer, Karen E 1213 Subella Drive, Columbia, MO 65203, (314) 882-1571, BS 79 Univ of MN - Minneap-St Paul; MA 83 Univ of MN - Minneap-St Paul; 87–Aud, Univ of MO Hosp & Clinics, **A**

Bauer, Mrs Laurie Marie 2838 Woodridge Lane, Stillwater, MN 55082, (715) 684-3393, BS 83 Univ of WI - River Falls; MS 84 Univ of WI - River Falls; 84–Sp-Lang Path, Midwest Rehab Specialists Inc, **SLP**

Bauer, Mrs Lynn G 47 Mountain View, Fairfax, CA 94930, (415) 897-4250, BA 68 Univ of CA - Santa Barbara; BA 68 Univ of CA - Santa Barbara; Sp-Lang Path, Novato USD, **SLP**

Bauer, Mrs Mary L 203 West Green Street, Winterset, IA 50273, (312) 355-3545, BS 59 Univ of IL - Urbana; **SLP**

Bauer, Meier H 4244 Cloverhill Terrace, Cincinnati, OH 45238, (513) 251-4444, BS 66 Univ of Cincinnati; MA 75 Univ of Cincinnati; Sp-Lang Path, Hamilton Co Offi of Ed, **SLP**

Bauer, Monica Lynn 3945 Utah, Apt A, St Louis, MO 63116, (314) 771-5031, BS 85 Fontbonne Coll; MA 86 Saint Louis Univ; 86–Sp-Lang Path, Cardinal Glennon Child Hosp, **SLP**

Bauer, Mrs Nancy S 437 Abbey Circle, Abingdon, MD 21009, (301) 396-6478, BS 74 Towson St Univ; MS 77 Towson St Univ; Sp-Lang Path, Baltimore Cty Pub Sch, **SLP**

Bauer, Pamela Rae 29 Rushmore, Glen Carbon, IL 62034, (618) 259-7150, BS 80 Southern IL Univ-Edwardsvill; MS 81 Southern IL Univ-Edwardsvill; Sp-Lang Path, Region III Spec Educ Co-op, **SLP**

Bauer, Renata 1235 Avenue Road #3, Toronto, ON, Canada M5N 2G5, (416) 890-1221, BA 79 Univ of Toronto - Ontario; MS 81 Emerson Coll; 81–Sp/Lang Path, Dufferin-Peel RCSS Bd, **SLP**

Bauer, Steven 2000 Quinn Court, Tallahassee, FL 32308, (904) 681-5482, BA 73 CUNY - Queens Coll; OM 83 NY Inst of Tech - NY City; MA 74 Hofstra Univ; Chief of Speech Pathology, Tallahassee Mem Reg Med Center, **SLP**

Bauersfeld, Mrs Margaret M 40 Dunkirk Road, Baltimore, MD 21212, (301) 377-4126, MS 88 Towson St Univ

Baughman, Amy 3802 North Hamilton #2, Chicago, IL 60618, (312) 848-9750, MA 86 Northwestern Univ; **SLP**

Baughman, Jane Kirsten 1525 Dara Drive, Lebanon, MO 65536, (417) 588-4448, BS 79 Northeast MO St Univ; MA 87 Southwest MO St Univ; 83–Sp-Lang Path, Waynesville R-VI Schs, **SLP**

Baughman, Sherry L 3150 Johnson Road #B-5, Steubenville, OH 43952, (614) 283-3674, BS 85 OH Univ - Athens; MA 87 OH Univ - Athens; 87–Sp-Lang Path, Eastern Ohio Sp Hrng Ctr Inc, **SLP**

Baughn, Cynthia E 97 Myrtle Avenue, Ansonia, CT 06401, (203) 389-4561, BA 76 Univ of CT; ME 78 Univ of VA - Charlottesville; Superv Sp-Lang Path Dept, Easter Seal Rehab Cen, **SLP**

Baughn, Helen Mankato Rehabilitation Center, P O Box 328, 15 Map Drive, Mankato, MN 56001, (507) 345-4507, BA 56 Coll of Saint Benedict; BS 72 Mankato St Univ; MA 73 Mankato St Univ; Superv Dept of Commun Dis, Mankato Rehab Cen Inc, **SLP**

Baum, Mrs Bonnie L 19 Rose Lane, Flourtown, PA 19031, (215) 233-4144, BS 73 IL St Univ - Normal; MA 75 Univ of FL; Ed Consult, Wm Penn Charter Sch, **SLP**

Baum, Mrs Ginette A 23261 Wendover Drive, Beachwood, OH 44122-1444, (216) 381-2077, BA 79 CUNY - Queens Coll; MA 81 CUNY - Queens Coll; Clinical Supervisor, Cleveland State Univ, **SLP**

Baum, Helen C P O Box 204, Manteo, NC 27954, **SLP**

Baum, Lori Jean 6529 Langley Court, Woodridge, IL 60517, (312) 968-0294, BS 82 Elmhurst Coll; MA 84 Northern IL Univ - De Kalb; Sp-Lang Path, Puffer-Hefty School Dist 69, **SLP**

Baum, Mrs Meryl 43 Drayton Lane, Plainsboro, NJ 08536, (201) 267-2642, BS 76 Ithaca Coll; MS 77 Adelphi Univ; Sp-Lang Path, Center School, **SLP**

Baum, Dr Shari R School Of Human Com Disorders, McGill University, 1266 Pine Avenue West, Montreal, PQ, Canada H3G 1A8, (514) 398-4137, BA 80 Cornell Univ; MS 82 Univ of VT; PH 86 (Linguistics) Brown Univ; 88–Asst Prof, McGill Univ, **SLP**

Baum, Mrs Sherry Ann 178 Monarch, Louisville, CO 80027, (303) 270-8315, BS 81 Old Dominion Univ; MA 85 Univ of CO - Boulder; 86–Sp-Lang Path, Univ of CO Health Sciences Ctr, **SLP**

Bauman, Gary M 181 Alexander Avenue, Nesconset, NY 11767, (516) 724-7854, BA 74 Pace U -NY City; MA 76 Hofstra Univ; 82–Sp-Lang Path, Private Practice, **SLP**

Bauman, Dr Natan 625 Redstone Drive, Cheshire, CT 06410, (203) 785-2467, MS 69; MS 75 Columbia Univ Teachers Coll; ED 84 (NS) Columbia Univ Teachers Coll; 88–Pres, Hearing Balance & Speech Ctr, **A**

Bauman, Sheila M 8708 West 90th Street, Overland Park, KS 66212, (913) 884-8711, BS 78 Univ of KS; MA 80 Univ of KS; 87–Sp-Lang Path, Meadowbrook Hosp, **SLP**

Baumann, Mrs Ann Arends 611 Sitka #5, Newberg, OR 97132, (503) 623-6691, BA 81 Univ of Northern IA; MS 83 Univ of WI - Stevens Point; Sp-Lang Path, Polk Educ Svc Dist, **SLP**

Baumann, Carolyn A Box 349, CFAS, FPO Seattle, WA 98766, BA 83 Univ of North TX; MA 87 Univ of CO - Boulder; 87–Tchr, DOD Dependents Schs

Baumann, Mary Ellen 3263 Cherrywood Drive, Wantagh, NY 11793, (516) 922-4100, BS 84 Long Island U - CW Post Ctr; MS 85 Adelphi Univ; 85–Sp-Lang Path, Mll Nck Manr Luther Sch for the Deaf, **SLP**

Baumann, Mrs Pamela Dunn 15 Cherry Lane, Pomona, NY 10970, (914) 362-1431, BS 78 Bradley Univ; MS 79 Bradley Univ; SLP, Ramapo Central Sch Dist, **SLP**

Baumann, Mrs Patricia B 112 Pine Avenue, Ossining, NY 10562, (914) 631-4144, BA 73 Univ of NC - Chapel Hill; MS 76 Univ of NC - Chapel Hill; Sp-Lang Path, Pu Sch of the Tarrytowns, **SLP**

Bauman-Waengler, Dr Jacqueline Ann 26301 State Line Road, Lucedale, MS 39452, (205) 460-6327, BS 72 CO St Univ; MA 75 Univ of CO - Boulder; PH 78 (NS) Univ of CO - Boulder; 88–Prof, Univ of South AL, **SLP**

Baumbich, Brenda 807 Country Lane, Des Plaines, IL 60016, (312) 825-7711, BA 61 Elmhurst Coll; MA 68 Northern IL Univ - De Kalb; Sp-Lang Path, Maine Twsp Hs Dist 207, **SLP**

Baumblatt, Mrs Gladys R 2108 Arms Drive, Girard, OH 44420, BS 54 Univ of WI - Madison; **SLP**

Baumeister, Marilyn E 23916 Malibu Knolls Road, Malibu, CA 90265, (213) 456-6872, BS 59 CA St Univ - Los Angeles; MA 65 IL St Univ - Normal; **SLP**

Baumel, Mrs Deborah W 2042 Redood Crest, Vista, CA 92083, BA 80 George Washington Univ; MS 82 James Madison Univ; Sp-Lang Path, Visiting Nurses Association, **SLP**

Baumer, Mrs Judith E 639 Huntwood Lane, Kirkwood, MO 63122, (314) 239-8000, BA 62 Denison Univ; MA 66 Case Western Reserve Univ; 86–Aud, St John's Mercy Hosp, **A**

Baumert, Kathleen A 362 Kenmore, Council Bluffs, IA 51501, (712) 322-7354, BS 76 Univ of NE - Lincoln; MS 77 Univ of NE - Omaha; Sp-Lang Path, Loess Hills AEA, **SLP**

Baumgardner, Ruth E 107 Linden Avenue, Hampton, VA 23669, BS 79 Univ of IL - Urbana; MS 80 Univ of IL - Urbana; **SLP**

Baumgart, Margaret S 3233 Mayer Drive, Murrysville, PA 15668, (412) 327-4926, MA 75 SUNY - Coll at Buffalo; **SLP**

Baumgarten, Deborah Susan 2819 Toledo Avenue South, St Louis Park, MN 55416, (612) 929-7899, BS 81 Univ of MN - Minneap-St Paul; BA 81 Univ of MN - Minneap-St Paul; MA 85 Univ of MN - Minneap-St Paul; Sp-Lang Path, Mercy Med Ctr, **SLP**

Baumgarten, Mrs Rachel Bazant 470 Summit Drive, Orange, CT 06477, (203) 795-0627, MS 86 Southern CT St Univ

Baumgartner, Carolyn 237 Kent Lane, Homewood, AL 35209, (205) 631-3277, BS 77 Auburn Univ - Auburn; MA 79 Univ of Montevallo; SLP, Jefferson Co Bd Ed, **SLP**

Baumgartner, Mrs Dawn M Route 1 Box 286, Ferndale, CA 95536-0286, (707) 786-4160, BS 72 Pacific Union Coll; MS 74 Univ of Redlands; Sp-Lang Path, Humboldt Bay Adventist Sch, **SLP**

Baumgartner, Mrs Holly Fisher 3519 Meadowbrook Road, Antioch, CA 94509, (415) 754-6704, BA 80 CA St Univ - Chico; MA 82 CA St Univ - Chico; Sp-Lang Path, Sp Path Serv, **SLP**

Baumgartner, Dr John M Dept Of Communicative Dis, Presbyterian St Lukes Hosp, 1753 W Congress Parkway, Chicago, IL 60612, (312) 942-5332, BS 72 Univ of WI - Stevens Point; MS 73 Univ of WI - Stevens Point; PH 78 (NS) Southern IL Univ -Carbondale; Sp-Lang Path, Pres St Lukes, **SLP**

Baumgartner, Linda Strear 259 Maple Avenue, Elmhurst, IL 60126, (312) 279-2420, BA 82 Univ of CO - Boulder; MA 85 Univ of Denver; **SLP**

Baumwohl, Dana 11633 Gorham Avenue #17, Los Angeles, CA 90049, (213) 207-9339, BA 81 San Diego St Univ; MA 83 CA St Univ - Northridge; Aud, **A**

Bauquier, Oliver W 2444 Raleigh Drive, San Jose, CA 95124, (408) 269-0841, BA 43 San Jose St Univ; MA 51 San Jose St Univ; **SLP LM**

Baurys, Karl J New Highway, Aristes, PA 17920, (717) 875-3273, BA 85 Bloomsburg Univ of PA; MS 86 Bloomsburg Univ of PA; **A**

Baustien, Mrs Julie B 9314 Walhampton Drive, Louisville, KY 40242, (502) 426-1249, BA 80 Univ of KY; MS 81 Univ of Louisville; SLP, Shelby Ct Pub Sch Syst, **SLP**

Bautch-Daniels, Doreen A 1062 Plymouth Drive, Sunnyvale, CA 94087, (408) 378-6131, BS 75 IL St Univ - Normal; MS 76 Purdue Univ - West Lafayette; Sp-Lang Path, Los Gatos Rehab Ctr, **SLP**

Bautista, Christina Diane 1941 S W 82nd Avenue, Davie, FL 33324, (813) 474-9043, MS 84 Univ of South FL; **SLP**

Baval, Bonnie D 1205 Estates Lane, Bayside, NY 11360-1141, (212) 246-4100, BA 75 CUNY - Brooklyn Coll; MA 78 Queens Coll; Agent, Phoenix Mutual Life Ins, **SLP**

Baxley, Mary Beth Box 358, Cullowhee, NC 28723, (704) 227-7251, MS 84 Western Carolina Univ; 87–Sp-Lang Path, Western Carolina Univ, **SLP**

Baxter, Jane H Pacific Hearing Service, 960 N San Antonio Road, Suite 101, Los Altos, CA 94022, (415) 497-6818, BA 76 Univ of CA - Santa Barbara; MS 81 San Francisco St Univ; 86–Aud, Pacific Hearing Svcs, **A**

Baxter, Mrs Katherine R 49 Orchard Park, Tiffin, OH 44883, (419) 447-5390, BA 65 Heidelberg Coll; MA 68 OH St Univ; Sp-Lang Path, Betty Jane Rehabilitation Ctr, **SLP**

Baxter, Dr Kelmer D Speech And Hearing Center, Univ Of Southwestern Louisiana, PO Box 43170, Lafayette, LA 70504, (318) 231-6721, BA 49 Univ of FL; MA 50 Univ of FL; PH 72 (NS) OH St Univ; Assoc Prof, Univ of Southwestern Louisiana, **SLP**

Baxter, Lisa R 189 Jefferson Avenue, Island Park, NY 11558, (516) 431-0962, BS 85 SUNY - Coll at Geneseo; MS 87 Emerson Coll; 87–Sp-Lang Path, St Charles Hosp & Rehab Ctr

Baxter, Martha Ann 1701 East Farrell #74, Shawnee, OK 74801, (405) 275-0587, **SLP**

Baxter, Mrs Sandra D 8717 Apple Tree Lane, Cherry Valley, CA 92223, (714) 358-4125, MA 75 CA St Univ - Fullerton; MS 85 Trinity Univ; OD 87 (NS) 4802; Deputy Cty Counsel, Riverside County, **SLP**

Baxter, Mrs Theresa G 9203 Beach Way Lane, Springfield, VA 22153, (703) 538-4480, BA 68 Adelphi Univ; MA 74 Catholic Univ of America; **SLP**

Baxter-Fiorella, Alison Elizabeth 703 Niagara Blvd, Fort Erie, ON, Canada L2A3J1, (416) 732-6111, BS 84 SUNY - Coll at Fredonia; OM 86 Univ of Western Ontario; 86–Chief Sp-Lang Path, Welland County Gen Hosp, **SLP**

Baxter-Saari, Deborah 3854 West Elgin, Chandler, AZ 85226, (602) 899-4415, BS 80 FL St Univ; MS 83 5210; Aud, E Valley Otol Consultants PC, **A**

Bay, Carolyn Amelia 1309 East Shore Drive, Alameda, CA 94501, (415) 922-9514, BA 83 Holy Names Coll; MA 84 Univ of the Pacific; **SLP**

Bay, Jean E 5927 Archwood, San Antonio, TX 78239, ME; Sp-Lang Path, NE ISD, **SLP**

Baye-Kaye, Lisa 914 High Street, Dedham, MA 02026, (617) 344-0600, BS 78 Univ of MA - Amherst; OM 82 Univ of MT; 88–Aud, New Eng Sinai Hosp & Rehab Ctr, **A**

Bayer, Mrs Gail V 452 Roundhill Road, East Hills, NY 11577, (516) 621-2786, BA 77 CUNY - Queens Coll; MA 76 Hofstra Univ; Sp-Lang Path, Self Employed, **SLP**

Bayer, Mrs Helen K 1054 Toreador Drive, Creve Coeur, MO 63141, (314) 569-8214, BS 69 Univ of IL - Urbana; MA 70 Univ of IL - Urbana; Area Coordinator, Spec School Dist/St Louis Co, **SLP**

Bayleran, Mrs Ann Sarkis 5620 Crabtree, Birmingham, MI 48010, (313) 626-2405, **SLP**

Bayles, Dr Kathryn A 5321 North Via Condesa, Tucson, AZ 85718, (602) 629-9747, BS 63 Univ of NE - Lincoln; MS 74 AZ St Univ; PH 79 (NS) Univ of AZ; Assoc Prof, University of Arizona, **SLP**

Bayless, Mrs Barbara 3565 Oakwood Court, Morgan Hill, CA 95037, (408) 842-8292, BS 67 Purdue Univ - West Lafayette; MS 69 Purdue Univ - West Lafayette; Sp-Lang Path, Gilroy USD, **SLP**

Bayless, Becky Lynn 407 Southland #5, Greenville, IL 62246, (618) 283-3659, BS 80 Eastern IL Univ; MS 81 Eastern IL Univ; Sp-Lang Path, Mid State Spec Ed Dstr, **SLP**

Bayless, Elizabeth Marie 2921 South Richmond, Wichita, KS 67217, (316) 943-9756, BA 84 Wichita St Univ; MA 86 Wichita St Univ; 86–Sp-Lang Path, USD #259, **SLP**

Bayley, Mrs Bonnie Z 1500 Sherwin, Chicago, IL 60626, (312) 522-2010, BS 79 Univ of WI - Stevens Point; MS 81 Univ of WI - Madison; 86–Dir of Comm Disorders, Schwab Rehabilitation Ctr, **SLP**

Bayley, Geraldine 269 Southaven Avenue, Medford, NY 11763, (516) 338-4204, BA 79 Saint John's Univ - Jamaica; MS 80 PA St Univ - Univ Park; Sp-Lang Path, Pre School Development Program, **SLP**

Bayliss, Mrs Kim I M 2953 Aquadale Lane, Cincinnati, OH 45211, (513) 922-3223, BS 77 Univ of Cincinnati; MS 78 Miami Univ - Oxford; Sp/Lang Path, Hamilton Co Offi of Ed, **SLP**

Baylor, Charles Morgan 607 Fourth Street, West Pittston, PA 18643, (717) 288-9386, BA 83 Wilkes Coll; BA 83 Wilkes Coll; MS 85 PA St Univ - Univ Park; **SLP**

Bayly, Mrs Debra Ann 101 Windsong Court, Lake Mary, FL 32746, (305) 323-1813, BA 77 MI St Univ; MA 78 Memphis St Univ; SLP Self-Contained Lang Cl, Orange County Pub Sch, **SLP**

Bayme, Mrs Anne B 174 New Street, Macon, GA 31201, (912) 746-2406, BS 74 Univ of GA; ME 75 Univ of GA; Sp/Lang Path, Private Practice, **SLP**

Baynard, Catherine Elizabeth 6945 South Lowe Avenue, Chicago, IL 60621, (312) 874-3286, BS 80 Northern IL Univ - De Kalb; MA 85 Univ of Northern IA

Bayone Cook, Ilene 67-57 211th Street, Bayside, NY 11364, (718) 229-6661, BA 73 SUNY - Coll at New Paltz; MA 76 CUNY - Queens Coll; 87–Sp-Lang Path, SteppingStone Day Sch Inc, **SLP**

Baysinger, Mrs Kathleen S 2711 Dexter Avenue, Terre Haute, IN 47805, (812) 238-7577, BA 74 IN St Univ - Terre Haute; MS 77 IN St Univ - Terre Haute; Dir Sp-Lang Path, Union Hosp, **SLP**

Bayton-Langford, Angela Joann 2735 Gillham #1 South, Kansas City, MO 64108, (816) 474-1128, BS 83 Central MO St Univ; MA 85 Univ of KS; **A**

Bazan, Mrs Theresa Caruso 1409 Calcutta Ln, Naperville, IL 60540, (312) 416-0754, BS 80 Univ of IL - Urbana; MS 82 Univ of IL - Urbana; SLP, Spec Ed Serv Aurora Ed Cen, **SLP**

Bazell, Cindy Lynn 13680 Wales, Oak Park, MI 48237, (313) 545-4642, MA 80 Wayne St Univ - Sch of Med; Aud, Chldrns Hosp, **A**

Bazil, Mrs Connie Audiology Assoc Inc, 221 North East Glen Oak Avenue, Peoria, IL 61636, (309) 672-5788, **A**

Beach, Carol D Roseburg Audiology Center, 1367 West Harvard, Roseburg, OR 97470, (503) 672-8868, BS 73 Univ of NE - Lincoln; MA 77 Univ of NE - Lincoln; Aud, Roseburg Aud Cen, **A**

Beach, Cynthia M P O Box 319, West Mystic, CT 06388, (203) 572-7123, BS 84 Bowling Green St Univ; MA 87 Kent St Univ; 87–Sp-Lang Path, Dept of Men Ret/State of CT, **SLP**

Beach, Danna Kay 111 East Arapahoe #1, Thermopolis, WY 82443, (307) 864-2147, MS 86 Univ of UT; 86–Sp-Lang Path, The Gottsche Rehab Ctr, **SLP**

Beach, Kimberlee K 12004 53rd SE, Everett, WA 98204, (206) 258-7512, BS 82 Univ of WA; MS 87 Univ of WA; 87–Sp-Lang Path, Providence Hosp of Everett, **SLP**

Beach, Mrs Mary Nisbet 6615 Tupelo Drive, Bedford Heights, OH 44146, (216) 439-1746, BS 49 Univ of WI - Madison; MS 54 Syracuse Univ; Sp/Lang Path, Psi Associates Inc, **SLP**

Beach, Rita Marie 2603 Finley Street, Silver Spring, MD 20902, **SLP**

Beach, Suzanne Lynn 552 Eastern Avenue, Bellefontaine, OH 43311, (513) 592-2164, BS 83 WV Univ; MS 85 WV Univ; 88–Sp-Lang Path, Private Practice, **SLP**

Beach, Woodford A 2506 Huguenot Springs Road, Midlothian, VA 23113, (804) 786-0207, BA 75 Cornell Univ; MS 82 WV Univ; Sp-Lang Path, The Medical College of VA, **SLP ACE**

Beachler, Cindy Robbins 6092-3 Woodfield Drive, Grand Rapids, MI 49508, (616) 455-3804, BS 78 Purdue Univ - West Lafayette; MS 81 Purdue Univ - West Lafayette; Audiologist, Constance Brown Ctr, **A**

Beachler, Jeanne C 1222 Highland Avenue, Langhorne, PA 19047, (215) 741-1252, BA 77 Univ of DE; MS 78 PA St Univ - Univ Park; Sp-Lang Path, Private Practice, **SLP**

Beachy, Mrs Jane Ellen 2434 Prendergast Place, Reynoldsburg, OH 43068, (614) 867-1950, BS 86 McMurry Coll; MS 87 Miami Univ - Oxford; **SLP**

Beachy, Mrs Teresa S 17 Godwin Lane, St Louis, MO 63124, (314) 993-9349, BA 70 MI St Univ; MA 71 MI St Univ; Sp-Lang Path, Special School District, **SLP**

Beadle, Dr Kathryn R 3935 Duncan Place, Palo Alto, CA 94306, (415) 493-8111, BS 59 Univ of WI - Madison; MA 62 Univ of HI - Manoa; PH 70 (NS) Stanford Univ; Exec Dir, Midpeninsula Sp & Lang Cl, **SLP**

Beagle, Mrs Linda D Boc 4789 D S, Portland, ME 04112, (207) 775-3314, BA 70 Univ of San Diego; MA 72 Univ of Southern CA; Sp/Lang Path, Private Practice, **SLP**

Beale, Catherine 3802-B Chestnut, New Orleans, LA 70115, (504) 436-2474, BA 70 Mary Washington Coll; ME 74 Univ of VA - Charlottesville; Sp-Lang Path, Jefferson Parish Sch Syst, **SLP**

Beale, Dr Cecilia R 25 University Avenue West, Minot, ND 58701, (701) 857-3030, BS 71 Southeast MO St Univ; MA 72 Univ of MO - Columbia; PH 76 (NS) Univ of MO - Columbia; 88–Assoc Prof, Minot State Univ, **SLP**

Beall, Mrs Carolyn R 1414 Country Club Drive, Midland, TX 79701, (915) 686-0100, BA 74 Univ of OK - Norman; MA 78 Univ of Denver; **A**

Beall, Mrs Robbin J 11 Belvedere Drive, Mechanicsburg, PA 17055, (717) 737-6728, BS 83 Bloomsburg Univ of PA; MS 84 Bloomsburg Univ of PA; Aud, Capital Area Intermed Unit, **A**

Beall, Scott Gregory 1501 Market Street, Camp Hill, PA 17011, (717) 761-7200, BS 83 Bloomsburg Univ of PA; MS 84 Bloomsburg Univ of PA; 84–Pres, Bell Hearing Aid Centers Inc, **A**

Beall, Mrs Shelley Campbell 2500 Spring Valley Drive, Bedford, TX 76021, BA 79 Univ of OK - Norman; MS 81 Univ of OK Medical Center; **SLP**

Bealmear, Dr Mary K 3541 Ranch House Road, Weatherford, TX 76086, (817) 441-8915, PH (NS); **SLP LM**

Beam, Mrs Mary P 821 Conestoga Drive, Charlotte, NC 28226, (704) 847-7632, BA 82 Univ of AL- Tuscaloosa; MS 83 Univ of AL- Tuscaloosa; 87–Sp-Lang Path, Charlotte-Mecklenburg Bd of Educ, **SLP**

Beam, Mrs Susan Dickey 1060 Terrace Court, Zanesville, OH 43701, (614) 454-5256, BS 80 Indiana Univ of PA; MA 82 Kent St Univ; Aud/Mgr, Good Samaritan Med Cen, **A**

Beaman, Kimberly Elaine 1907 Highview Street #I-6, Burlington, NC 27215, (919) 226-4373, BA 82 Univ of NC - Greensboro; ME 83 Univ of NC - Greensboro; Sp-Lang Path, Grove Park Sch, **SLP**

Beaman, Wynne B 8502 16th Street #402, Silver Spring, MD 20910, (301) 649-5555, OB 83 Univ of MD - College Park; MS 87 Univ of WA; **A**

Beamer, Mrs Mary W 2500 Hinkle Drive #327, Denton, TX 76201, (817) 382-5378, BA 29 William Jewell Coll; MA 54 TX Woman's Univ; **SLP LM**

Beamer, Sharon L HHC 6th Asg, Box 13, APO New York, NY 09154, BA 79 Univ of HI - Manoa; BS 79 Univ of HI - Manoa; MA 81 Univ of MD - College Park; Aud, Department of the Army, **A ACE**

Beamon, Lehua L 5904 Highgate, East Lansing, MI 48823, (517) 394-5100, BA 79 MI St Univ; MA 80 MI St Univ; Sp-Lang Path, Comm Ment Hlth, **SLP**

Beamsley, Virginia Bacon 1706 Kiva Drive, Gallup, NM 87301, (505) 722-2844, BS 76 Elmira Coll; MS 83 Univ of NM; 85–Sp-Lang Path, Private Practice, **SLP**

Bean, Carolyn 2027 9th Street #2, Coralville, IA 52241, (319) 351-5571, BS 81 Southwest TX St Univ; ME 82 Southwest TX St Univ; Sp-Lang Path, St Luke's Hosp, **SLP**

Bean, Donald R 19702 Encino Way, San Antonio, TX 78259, (512) 221-2878, BS 62 Minot St Univ; MS 69 CO St Univ; Dir SLP Cl, Brooke Army Med Cen, **SLP ACE**

Bean, Jerrilyn Akins 118 Vermont Court East, Matawan, NJ 07747, (201) 287-4400, BS 68 Univ of GA; MA 79 Trenton St Coll; Sp/Lang Path, Edison Township Pub Schs, **SLP**

Bean, Melinda Joyce Communicative Disorders Lab, University Of MS Medical Center, 2500 North State Street, Jackson, MS 39216, (601) 984-4550, BS 81 Univ Southern MS-Hattiesburg; MS 83 Univ Southern MS-Hattiesburg; 87–Aud, Univ MS Med Ctr, **A**

Bean, Mrs Patricia A Route 3 Box 288, Fort Worth, TX 76140, (817) 295-8191, BS 75 Univ of North TX; MS 79 Univ of North TX; Sp-Lang Path, Burleson Independent Sch Dist, **SLP**

Bean, Sandra L 553 Pennsylvania Avenue, York, PA 17404, (717) 757-1227, BS 80 Edinboro Univ of PA; MS 87 Towson St Univ; Sp-Lang Path, Luth Social Svcs South Reg, **SLP**

Bean, Susan M Audiology Department, Massachusetts Eye & Ear Infirmary, 243 Charles Street, Boston, MA 02114, (617) 573-3266, BA 74 Univ of MA - Amherst; MS 75 Univ of NM; 87–Aud, MA Eye & Eye Infirmary, **A**

Bear, Mrs Annette Marie 944 Manchester Street, Cary, IL 60013-1839, (312) 358-4193, MS 83 IL St Univ - Normal; Sp-Lang Path, Cary Sch Dist 26, **SLP**

Bear, Mary C Route 1 Box 231, Tippecanoe, OH 44699-9625, (614) 269-2141, BS 74 Kent St Univ; MA 75 Kent St Univ; Sp-Lang Path, Harrison Co Sch, **SLP**

Bear, Ronald D 2036 East 48th Street, Davenport, IA 52807, (319) 383-1499, BA 74 Augustana Coll; MA 75 Univ of IL - Urbana; Dir Dept of Sp & Hrng, Mercy Hosp, **SLP**

Beard, Dr Anne Evans 532 East Main Street, Rock Hill, SC 29730, (804) 323-2387, BA 50 Columbia Coll; MS 70 Univ of SC - Columbia; ED 74 (NS) Univ of GA; Assoc Prof, Winthrop Coll, **SLP**

Beard, Mrs Diane Y 501 Georgia Parkway, Washington, IL 61571, (309) 672-6308, BS 81 Bradley Univ; MS 82 Bradley Univ; 84–Sp-Lang Path, Peoria Assoc/Ret Citizens, **SLP**

Beard, Ellen Kay 725 Kingsland #210, St Louis, MO 63130, (314) 361-1212, BS 79 Murray St Univ; MA 81 Saint Louis Univ; Chief/Sp-Lang Pathology, Incarnate Word Hospital, **SLP**

Beard, Janice Holcomb 1412 Munal, Baton Rouge, LA 70816, MS 86 Univ of WI - Madison; **SLP**

Beard, Kim G Rd 5 Box 115, Dillsburg, PA 17019, (717) 432-8369, BS 77 Bloomsburg Univ of PA; MS 78 Bloomsburg Univ of PA; Sp-Lang Path, **SLP ACE**

Beard, Maria Cherie 16400 Henderson Pass #435, San Antonio, TX 78232, (512) 231-8633, OB 86 Southwest TX St Univ; MS 87 Southwest TX St Univ

Beard, Mrs Raquel Tomic P O Box 7424, Odessa, TX 79707, (915) 544-6868

Beardemphl, Jessica W 1004 Hermosa, Artesia, NM 88210, **SLP**

Bearden-Rettger, Theresa Faye 170 North Hazel, St Paul, MN 55119, (612) 731-2652, BA 77 MI St Univ; MA 78 MI St Univ; Sp-Lang Path, **SLP**

Beardslee, Mary Lou L 2215 S E 53rd, Topeka, KS 66605, (913) 272-3636, BS 73 Fort Hays St Univ; MS 74 Fort Hays St Univ; Sp-Lang Path, Auburn USD 437, **SLP**

Beardsley, Amy Neel 2309 Chelmsford Court, Alvin, TX 77511, (409) 761-2711, MS 84 Univ of OK - OK City; Sp-Lang Path, Univ of TX Med Branch, **SLP**

Beartrack, Susan K Route 2 Box 11, Fairfax, OK 74637, **SLP**

Bearup, Patricia H 322 Birchwood, Traverse City, MI 49684, (616) 922-6200, BA 75 Univ of MI - Ann Arbor; MA 77 Western MI Univ; Sp-Lang Path, Traverse Bay Area Sch Dist, **SLP**

Beary-Stolle, Jean 2414 N E 102nd Street, Vancouver, WA 98686, (206) 696-6248, BA 75 Univ of MT; MS 77 Univ of WA; Sp-Lang Path, WA St Sch Blind, **SLP**

Beasley, Cynthia Oslin 1095 Kennesaw Springs Ct, Kennesaw, GA 30144-5601, (404) 386-3417, BS 85 Univ of GA; ME 86 Univ of GA; 86–Sp-Lang Path, Cartersville City Schs, **SLP**

Beasley, Dr Daniel S 302 North Stonewall, Memphis, TN 38112, (901) 525-2682, BA 66 Univ of Akron; MA 68 Univ of IL - Urbana; PH 70 (Sp & Hrng Science) Univ of IL - Urbana; Prof/Chmn, Memphis St U, **SLP F**

Beasley, Mrs Jean L 3803 Langdon Drive, Greensboro, NC 27410, (919) 229-0870, BA 70 Univ of MS; MS 72 Univ of MS; SLP, Michelle Jensen PhD, **SLP A**

Beasley, Mrs Joyce Bramley 214 North Miles Street, Elizabethtown, KY 42701, (502) 769-1599, BS 76 Murray St Univ; MS 87 Western KY Univ; 78–Sp-Lang Path, ISD, **SLP**

Beasley, Lillian Elaine Roanoke Ear Nose & Throat Inc, P O Box 8306, Roanoke, VA 24014, (705) 982-6800, BS 75 James Madison Univ; ME 83 Univ of VA - Charlottesville; Aud, Roanoke ENT Cl, **A**

Beasley, Mrs Mary J 236 North Pershing, Wichita, KS 67208, (316) 685-1046, BA 78 Wichita St Univ; MA 79 Wichita St Univ; Sp-Lang Path, USD #259, **SLP ACE**

Beastrom, Mrs Diane Reynolds 1425 Wagar Avenue, Cleveland, OH 44107, (216) 582-1085, BA 77 Cleveland St Univ; MA 79 Cleveland St Univ; Asst Director, OH Reside Serv, **SLP**

Beastrom, Susan Lynn 1408 West Warner, Garden West, Chicago, IL 60613, (312) 791-4240, BS 83 Central MO St Univ; MA 85 Univ of KS; SLP, Michael Reese Hosp, **SLP**

Beatch-Tilden, Susan C 5 Crosby Circle, Framingham, MA 01701, (617) 875-7132, BA 76 Boston Coll; MA 78 MI St Univ; Aud, Joint Ctr for Otolarygology, **A**

Beaton, Janice M C 103 Karyl Street, Waterville, OH 43566, (419) 698-7616, BS 74 Marquette Univ; MS 76 Purdue Univ - West Lafayette; Aud, St Charles Hospital, **A**

Beaton, Mrs Lillian L 15725 S W 82th Court, Miami, FL 33157, (305) 238-5194, BS 52 Bowling Green St Univ; MA 56 OH St Univ; Sp-Lang Path, Dade Co Pub Sch, **SLP**

Beaton, Mrs Susan L 45547 Emerald Forest Drive, Novi, MI 48050, (313) 295-4200, BA 79 MI St Univ; MA 81 Wayne St Univ - Sch of Med; Aud, Assoc Physicians Med Cen, **A**

Beaton, Suzanne Kay 210 Viewmont, Vallejo, CA 94590, (303) 839-6760, OM 83 Univ of CO - Boulder; **SLP**

Beaton, Mrs Wendy Sue P O Box 546, East Setauket, NY 11733, (516) 698-8679, BA 80 CUNY - Queens Coll; MA 85 CUNY - Queens Coll; **SLP**

Beattie, Randall C Dept Of Communicative Disorder, Ca State Univ Long Beach, Long Beach, CA 90840, (213) 985-5281, PH (NS); Prof, CA State Univ, **A**

Beattie, Mrs Rosanne Thubauvill 202 8th Avenue South, Princeton, MN 55371, (612) 389-3316, BS 70 Univ of WI - Madison; MS 71 Univ of WI - Madison; Sp-Lang Path, Princeton Pub Sch, **SLP**

Beatty, Beth Marinne 803 Grove, Atwater, CA 95301, (209) 358-2766, BA 83 CA St Univ - Stanislaus; MA 85 CA St Univ - Stanislaus; **SLP**

Beatty, Mrs Gertrude D 710 West 28th, Kearney, NE 68847, (308) 237-5927, BS 53 Univ of NE - Lincoln; Sp-Lang Path, Educational Service Unit #10, **SLP**

Beatty, Janet G 3200 Longwood Avenue, Boulder, CO 80303, (303) 441-0437, BA 82 Univ of CA - Santa Barbara; MA 87 Univ of CO - Boulder

Beatty, Janice K 8840 Wellerstation Drive, Cincinnati, OH 45249, (513) 872-2481, BA 70 Western MI Univ; MA 72 MI St Univ; Sp-Lang Path, Good Samaritan Hosp, **SLP**

Beatty, Kathy V 401 Northampton Court, Huron, OH 44839, BS 74 Kent St Univ; MA 75 Kent St Univ; Sp-Lang Path, Erie Co Bd of Ed, **SLP**

Beatty, Lizabeth Mary 228 Weber Street, Stratford, CT 06497, (203) 336-5034, MS 85 Southern CT St Univ; **SLP**

Beatty, Raymond L, Jr 20 Hilson Drive, Rome, NY 13440, (315) 488-2951, BS 71 SUNY - Coll at Brockport; MS 72 SUNY - Coll at Geneseo; Sp-Lang Path, St Camillus Hlth Rehab Cen, **SLP**

Beatty, Sherry M 5121 Willow Oak Road, Bismarck, ND 58501, **SLP**

Beatty-Hanko, Maya P 1011 Elk Valley Road, Crescent City, CA 95531, (707) 464-5322, BA 72 San Francisco St Univ; MA 77 San Francisco St Univ; Sp-Lang Path, Harmony Speech & Lang Svcs, **SLP**

Beaty, Carol A 5021 Claire, Lincoln, NE 68516, (402) 786-2341, BS 72 Univ of NE - Lincoln; MA 73 Univ of NE - Lincoln; Sp/Lang Path, Sch Dist #145, **SLP**

Beaubien, Marilyn R 13047 Glenside Drive, Dallas, TX 75234, BA 57 Southern Methodist Univ; MA 70 Southern Methodist Univ; 71–Aud, Dallas Easter Seal Soc for Children, **A**

Beauchaine, Kathryn A Btni, 555 North 30th Street, Omaha, NE 68131, (402) 449-6520, BS 77 Univ of WI - Oshkosh; MA 79 Univ of Denver; Aud, Boystown Nat'l I, **A**

Beauchamp, Angel Dexter Calle Rio Corozal A11, Bayamon, PR 00619, (809) 751-5609, BA 65 Univ of PR - Rio Piedras; MA 71 NY Univ; MS 73 Univ of PR - Rio Piedras; **A**

Beauchamp, James A W D Clinite Cen For Hrng Imprd, 1073 West Sonora Avenue, Tulare, CA 93274, (209) 688-7424, BA 73 CA St Univ - Fresno; MA 74 CA St Univ - Fresno; Aud, Tulare Co Dept of Ed, **A ACE**

Beauchamp, Mrs Terese D 609 Worcester Road, Towson, MD 21204, (301) 321-6912, BA 72 George Washington Univ; ME 74 Northeastern Univ; **A**

Beauclair, Lynette M 151 Sunset Boulevard, Suite 11, New Port Richey, FL 34652, (813) 847-9237, BA 76 Univ of Northern CO; MA 78 Univ of Northern CO; Admin, Commun Dis Cl, **SLP**

Beaudet, Rudy R 12180 Shenandoah Road, Middletown, CA 95461, (707) 928-5687, BA 68 CA St Univ - Long Beach; MA 70 CA St Univ - Long Beach; Sp/Lang Path, Private Practice, **SLP**

Beaudette, Mrs Jane Irene 196 Pleasant Street, Hooksett, NH 03106, (603) 225-0844, BA 74 Univ of NH; MS 83 Univ of NH; Sp-Lang Path, **SLP**

Beaudette, Mrs Kristine M 719 White Willow Bay, Palatine, IL 60067, (312) 358-7232, BS 76 Univ of IL - Urbana; MS 77 Univ of IL - Urbana; Sp-Lang Path, Schaumburg Twsp Elem Schs, **SLP**

Beaudette, Paula A 324 Millpond Village Road, Hamden, CT 06514, (203) 384-8681, BS 67 Northern MI Univ; MA 68 Northern MI Univ; Coord/Cl Ser, Rehab Assoc Inc, **SLP**

Beaufait, Kathleen B 11679 Montana #10, Los Angeles, CA 90049, **SLP**

Beaulieu, Jacqueline Johnson 1920 West Tarrant Road, Apartment 61-E, Grand Prairie, TX 75050, (714) 787-1199, BS 82 Pacific Union Coll; **SLP**

Beaulieu-Chalke, Mrs Norma J 56 Chiswick Street, Longmeadow, MA 01106, (413) 567-6087, BS 82 PA St Univ - Univ Park; ME 84 Univ of VA - Charlottesville; 88–Sp-Lang Path, Gengras Ctr at St Joseph Coll, **SLP**

Beauparlant, Mrs Pamela Ann 6421 Concordia N E, Albuquerque, NM 87111, (505) 247-0301, BA 81 San Diego St Univ; MS 83 Univ of NM; Aud, Karl L Horn MD, **A**

Beaupre, Dr Walter J P O Box 8, Kingston, RI 02881, (401) 792-5969, BA 47 Bates Coll; MA 51 Lehigh Univ; PH 62 (Sp Path & Aud) Columbia Univ Teachers Coll; Prof/Commun Dis, Univ of Rhode Island, **SLP A**

Beauregard, Barbara Ann 1002 South Washington, Royal Oak, MI 48067, (313) 779-7610, BA 83 Northern MI Univ; MA 85 Wayne St Univ; 86–Coord, Lakeshore ENT Center PC, **SLP**

Beauregard, Cynthia 33 Ashton Lane, South Hadley, MA 01075-2179, (413) 534-0948, MA; **A**

Beauregard, Roxann 2496 South 550 East, Bountiful, UT 84010, (801) 295-8069, BS 82 Univ of UT; MS 86 Univ of UT; **SLP**

Beaver, Elizabeth P O Box 5632, Santa Barbara, CA 93108, **SLP**

Beaver, Harold G Scott And White Medical Clinic, 2801 South 31st, Temple, TX 76508, BA 56 Baylor Univ; MA 61 Univ of IA; Aud, Scott & White Med Cl & Hosp, **SLP A ACE**

Beaver, Mrs Jennifer Bennett 42 West Luzon Drive, Fort Bragg, NC 28307, (919) 497-4128, BS Univ of GA; ME 85 Univ of GA; **A**

Beaver, Lora L 113 South Douglas, Lyons, KS 67554, (316) 257-5196, BA 77 Wichita St Univ; MA 78 Wichita St Univ; SLP, USD 405 Rice Co Spec Serv Coop, **SLP**

Beavers, Mrs Renee Marie 3702 Williamsburg Court, Apartment 6E, Columbus, IN 47203, (317) 264-6991, BA 81 OH St Univ; MA 83 OH Univ - Athens; OM 85 IN Univ - Bloomington; 85–Sp/Lang Path, **SLP**

Beavers, Rosemarie Joyce 2102 1/2 West 39th Street, Apartment 3, Kearney, NE 68847, (308) 236-7678, BS 85 Kearney St Coll; MS 87 Kearney St Coll; 88–Sp-Lang Path, Grand Island Veteran's Hosp

Bebb, Gretchen E 5604 A Chaucer, Houston, TX 77005, (713) 621-1658, **SLP**

Bebensee, Julia Gaudineer 209 Holiday Road, Apt #332, Coralville, IA 52241, (319) 351-2510, BS 84 Univ of IA; MA 86 Northeast MO St Univ; 88–Sp-Lang Path, Grantwood AEA, **SLP**

Beber, Mrs Pamela Sue 6531 Espanita Street, Long Beach, CA 90815, (714) 972-8144, MA 83 CA St Univ - Long Beach; 83–Sp-Lang Path, Julia Hobbs Sp Path Inc, **SLP**

Bebout, Dr Linda Joyce English Department, University Of Windsor, Windsor, ON, Canada N9B 3P4, (519) 253-4232, BA 69 Central Univ of IA; MS 87 San Francisco St Univ; PH 74 (Linguistics) Cornell Univ; 77–Asst Prof, Univ of Windsor

Beccia-Blakeslee, Marisa Ann 233 South Main Street, Thomaston, CT 06705, (203) 574-8182, BA 82 Southern CT St Univ; MA 85 Southern CT St Univ; Sp-Lang Path, Waterbury Board of Education, **SLP**

Becerra, Mrs Candice 46 Sundial Lane, Bellport, NY 11713, (516) 286-3506, BA 78 Univ of FL; MS 80 Adelphi Univ; 88–Sp-Lang Path, Private Practice, **SLP**

Bechard, Mrs Maria Fotias 9204 Trentham Lane, Louisville, KY 40222, (319) 277-9654, **SLP**

Becher, Diane L 4570 Red Maple Road, Bradenton, FL 34210, (813) 795-2723, BS 72 Kent St Univ; MA 74 Kent St Univ; Aud, **A**

Becher, Donna K 824 St James Avenue, Park Hills, KY 41011, (606) 331-0880, BS 76 Ball St Univ; MS 79 Univ of Louisville; Sp-Lang Path, Pediatric Care Psc, **SLP**

Becher, Leitsa K 2080 Cheshire Road, Columbus, OH 43221, BS 58 OH St Univ; MS 61 Univ of MI - Ann Arbor; 87–Sp-Lang Path, Dublin City Sch Dist, **SLP**

Becher, Mrs Nancy A 1813 Meadow Lane, Edwardsville, IL 62025, (618) 692-0492, BS 82 Southern IL Univ-Edwardsvill; MS 83 Southern IL Univ-Edwardsvill; Sp-Lang Path, Collinsville Unit 10 Sd, **SLP**

Becht, Kelly Marie 305 Lindenhurst Drive, Apartment 2044, Lexington, KY 40509-1632, (606) 263-4920, BA 86 Univ of KY; MS 87 Univ of Louisville

Bechthold, Mary Lee 5525 Cedar Point Drive #C-66, Crown Point, IN 46307, (219) 769-3807, BA 85 Univ of IA; MA 88 KS St Univ; 88–Sp-Lang Path, InSpeech Inc

Bechtol, Linda S 5111 Centennial Road, Sylvania, OH 43560, (419) 866-6500, SLP, Decem Center, **SLP**

Bechtold, Janice M 5311-I Forest Creek Drive, Hazelwood, MO 63042, (314) 741-0698, BS 77 Southern IL Univ-Edwardsvill; MS 78 Southern IL Univ-Edwardsvill; SLP, Spec Sch Dist of St Louis Co, **SLP**

Bechtold, Mrs Judith Alexander 3531 Kimmer Rowe Road, Tallahassee, FL 32308, (904) 488-4673, BS 66 Purdue Univ - West Lafayette; BS 83 FL St Univ; MS 84 FL St Univ; 84–Sp-Lang Path, Leon Co Schs

Bechtold, Patricia A 3658 Queen Ann Way, Colorado Springs, CO 80917, (719) 550-1027, BS 85 Baylor Univ; MS 86 Baylor Univ; **SLP**

Beck, Allan L 3413 Crawford St S E, Salem, OR 97302, (503) 399-3193, BS 73 Western OR St Coll; MS 74 Western OR St Coll; 74–Sp-Lang Path, Salem Pub Schs, **SLP**

Beck, Dr Ann R 206 Denvale Drive, Danville, IL 61832, (217) 442-8000, BS 73 Southern IL Univ -Carbondale; MS 75 Southern IL Univ -Carbondale; PH 81 (Sp-Lang Path) Univ of IL - Urbana; Sp-Lang Path, Danville Dist 118 Sch, **SLP**

Beck, Mrs Beverly Atwood Route 7 Wedgewood Drive, Whiteville, NC 28472, (919) 642-5964, BS 74 Longwood Coll; ME 75 Univ of VA - Charlottesville; Sp-Lang Path, Comprehensive Homehealth Care, **SLP**

Beck, Mrs Blanche F 51 Cold Spring Circle, Shelton, CT 06484, (203) 929-7115, BA 68 SUNY - Center at Albany; MS 73 Southern CT St Univ; Sp-Lang Path, Shelton Bd of Ed, **SLP**

Beck, Mrs Bonnie R 9420 N W 33rd Manor, Sunrise, FL 33351, (305) 791-9569, BS 69 Syracuse Univ; MS 70 SUNY - Center at Albany; Sp/Lang Path, Private Practice, **SLP ACE**

Beck, Mrs Darlene Iverson 6875 N W Trail Ridge Drive, Johnston, IA 50131, (515) 274-3873, BA 62 Univ of IA; MA 66 Univ of IA; Sp-Lang Path, Des Moines Pub Schs, **SLP**

Beck, Mrs Diane Elizabeth 235 Hooks Road, Silsbee, TX 77656, (318) 463-4534, **SLP**

Beck, Edwin L P O Box 3079, Annapolis, MD 21403, MA 76 Univ of FL; **A**

Beck, Mrs Janet Anderson 1607 S 70th Avenue, Yakima, WA 98908, (509) 965-2080, BA 79 WA St Univ; MA 81 WA St Univ; SLP, West Valley School Dist #208, **SLP**

Beck, Janet Ann Rd 2 Box 810, Ruffs Dale, PA 15679, (412) 925-7015, ME 73 PA St Univ - Univ Park; BS 59 CA Univ of PA; Sp/Lang Path, Westmoreland Iu #7, **SLP**

Beck, Janice Nutt 1332 Menominee Drive, Oshkosh, WI 54901, MS 77 Western IL Univ; SLP, Oshkosh Public Schools, **SLP**

Beck, Joan Karen 600 Firestone #214, Muscle Shoals, AL 35661, (205) 381-2587, BA 63 Vanderbilt Univ; MA 68 Vanderbilt Univ; Sp-Lang Path, Muscle Shoals Bd of Ed, **SLP**

Beck, Mrs Judith A 27 Wade Trail, Texarkana, AR 75502, (214) 793-0691, OB 69; MS 78 AR St Univ; Sp-Lang Path, Sp Path Serv, **SLP**

Beck, Judith E 324 Winnebago, Menasha, WI 54952, (414) 738-2580, BS 75 Univ of WI - Stevens Point; MS 76 Univ of WI - Stevens Point; Director Sp-Lang Path, St Elizabeth Hospital, **SLP**

Beck, Mrs Karen S 4829 Mays Avenue, Reading, PA 19606, (215) 779-4897, BS 81; MS 82 Bloomsburg Univ of PA; Sp-Lang Path, Reading Rehab Hosp, **SLP**

Beck, Karla Luise 395 South Los Robles Avenue, Apartment 29, Pasadena, CA 91101-3224, (818) 796-9001, MA 86 CA St Univ - Los Angeles; 86–Sp-Lang Path, InSpeech Inc, **SLP**

Beck, Dr Lucille B 6000 Western Avenue, Chevy Chase, MD 20815, (202) 745-8270, BA 71 Adelphi Univ; MA 73 Univ of MD - College Park; PH 78 (NS) Univ of MD - College Park; Sp-Lang Path, VA Med Cen, **A**

Beck, Michael David 15263 Las Flores, La Mirada, CA 90638, (213) 943-1640, BA 80 Abilene Christian Univ; MS 82 Univ of OK Medical Center; **SLP**

Beck, Dr Robert Nels 420 D Winston Street, Farmville, VA 23901, (804) 392-9280, BA 65 Univ of FL; MA 76 Univ of FL; PH 70 (Sp Path & Aud) Univ of KS; 88–Assoc Prof, Longwood Coll, **SLP**

Beck, Mrs Sherri Madden 5601 N Heatherstone Drive, Shreveport, LA 71129, (318) 226-9441, BA 79 LA St Univ - Shreveport; MA 83 LA Tech Univ; **A**

Beck, Sydney Leighann 8541 Cap Of TX Hwy North, Apartment 2083, Austin, TX 78759, (512) 338-0467, BS 83 OK St Univ; MS 85 Univ of OK Medical Center; 87–Sp-Lang Path, The Oaks Treatment Center, **SLP**

Beck, William Gregory 2910 Scott Avenue North, Golden Valley, MN 55422-2742, (612) 624-3322, BS 74 Univ of TX - Austin; MA 76 Univ of TX - Austin; 76–Aud, US Army, **A**

Beckelheimer, Alice F 308 Plumtree Road, Bel Air, MD 21014, (301) 687-8311, BS 38 Converse Coll; MA 56 Univ of AL- Tuscaloosa; Sp-Lang Path/Chmn, Bd of Ed-Baltimore Co, **SLP LM**

Becker, Alan M 2201 South 10th Street #B, Fort Pierce, FL 34950, (407) 461-3266, OB 72 Univ of MS; MA 80 Univ of MS; 80–Aud, Hearing Aid Cen Ft Pierce In, **A**

Becker, Mrs Andrea 11108 Audubon Avenue, Philadelphia, PA 19116, (215) 969-3227, BA 84 Hofstra Univ; MS 86 PA St Univ - Univ Park; 87–Sp-Lang Path, CORA Services, **SLP**

Becker, Beverly Adelaide Box 83 USAMEDDAC, APO New York, NY 09801, 011 0931 286 241, BA 77 Univ of MS; MS 84 AR St Univ; Sp-Lang Path, Dept of the Army, **SLP**

Becker, Carolyn A 426 Setter Trail, Winter Park, FL 32789, (305) 628-3364, BA 73 Univ of Central FL; MA 87 Univ of Central FL; **SLP**

Becker, Mrs Carolyn F 620 Hobbs Road, Jefferson City, MO 65101, (314) 893-6033, BS 72 Lincoln Univ; MS 75 Central MO St Univ; Sp-Lang Path, Jefferson Cty Pub Sch, **SLP**

Becker, Catherine 33802 Zarzito Drive, Dana Point, CA 92629, (714) 661-2837, MS 72 Northwestern Univ; **SLP**

Becker, Mrs Chris Nunn 965 Briarcrest Way, Sacramento, CA 95831, BS 75 SUNY - Coll at Geneseo; MS 77 Univ of WY; 86–Sp-Lang Path, Mercy Hosp of Sacramento, **SLP**

Becker, Mrs Christine Anne Arundel Cnty Health Dept, 3 Harry Truman Parkway, Annapolis, MD 21401, (301) 224-7153, MA 74 George Washington Univ; Aud, A A Co Hlth Dept, **A**

Becker, Helen Kay 361 I Avant Drive, Hazelwood, MO 63042, (314) 839-0153, BS 75 Southwest MO St Univ; MS 86 Central MO St Univ; 88–Sp-Lang Path, Spec SD of St Louis Co, **SLP**

Becker, Mrs Irene A 2155 82nd Street #6-L, Brooklyn, NY 11214, (212) 259-4592, BA 74 Temple Univ-Tyler Sch of Art; MS 76 Adelphi Univ; SLP, NY Cty Bd of Ed, **SLP**

Becker, Irene M 1 Farmington Court, Madison, WI 53717, (414) 549-3467, BS 76 Univ of WI - Madison; MS 77 Univ of WI - Milwaukee; Sp-Lang Path, St Lukes Hosp, **SLP**

Becker, Mrs Irma Weiss 11 Chittenden Road, Fair Lawn, NJ 07410, (201) 261-5346, BA 56 CUNY - Queens Coll; MS 75 William Paterson Coll; 76–Sp-Lang Path, Bergen Co Bd of Voc Ed, **SLP**

Becker, Mrs Jill J 6386 N W 65th Terrace, Parkland, FL 33067, (305) 344-1646, **SLP**

Becker, Kathleen Marie 31 Graves Avenue, Northampton, MA 01060, (413) 586-8746, BA 73 SUNY - Center at Buffalo; MA 76 SUNY - Center at Buffalo; Co-Dir, Open Pathways, **SLP**

Becker, Katie Ann 10407 West 117th Terrace, #48, Overland Park, KS 66210, (913) 621-5155, OB 84 Univ of KS; MA 86 Wichita St Univ; 88–Sp-Lang Path, Kansas City Kansas PS, **SLP**

Becker, Laurence R 2652 Brown Street, Brooklyn, NY 11235, (718) 998-7084, BA 52 CUNY - Brooklyn Coll; MA 57 CUNY - Brooklyn Coll; SLP, Bd of Ed Cty of NY Dist 21, **SLP**

Becker, Leanne Marie 12 Spring Cove Road, Nashua, NH 03062, (303) 499-6238, BS 84 Marquette Univ; MA 86 Univ of CO - Boulder; **SLP**

Becker, Leonard V 1215 Sorolla Avenue, Coral Gables, FL 33134, **SLP A**

Becker, Leslie A 1906 Bainbridge Row Drive, Louisville, KY 40207, (812) 283-2210, BA 74 SUNY - Coll at Cortland; MA 75 Montclair St Coll; Sp-Lang Path, Rehab Care Clark Co Mem Hosp, **SLP**

Becker, Marianne P O Box 2069, Kingston, ON, Canada K7L 5J8, (613) 542-5040, OB 75 Edinboro Univ of PA; OM 84 Univ of Western Ontario; 87–Sp-Lang Path, Private Practice, **SLP**

Becker, Mrs Marilyn H 24 Preston Beach Road, Marblehead, MA 01945, (508) 937-7648, BA 46 Cornell Univ; ME 60 Boston Univ; 84–Sp-Lang Path, Lowell Public Schools, **SLP**

Becker, Mark M 16257 Tuba Street, Sepulveda, CA 91343, **A**

Becker, Mary R 191 Avenida Malaga, Anaheim Hills, CA 92808, (213) 922-7951, BA 79 CA St Univ - Fullerton; MA 81 CA St Univ - Fullerton; SLP, Rancho Los Amigos Hosp, **SLP**

Becker, Mrs Mary Sheldon 368 Northern Pines, Gansevoort, NY 12831, (518) 583-1315, BS 82 Univ of WI - River Falls; MS 83 Univ of WI - Milwaukee; Sp-Lang Path, Community Workshop Inc, **SLP**

Becker, Mary T 9833 Beard Avenue South, Bloomington, MN 55431, (612) 893-0566, BS 71 Univ of MN - Minneap-St Paul; MA 73 Univ of MN - Minneap-St Paul; 83–Admin Mgr, VanWagner & Associates Inc, **SLP**

Becker, Michelle Ann 2302 30th Avenue South, #506, Grand Forks, ND 58201, (701) 780-9983, BS 83 Moorhead St Univ; MS 85 Moorhead St Univ; Sp-Lang Path, **SLP**

Becker, Mrs Myra M 1771 Country Knolls Lane, Elgin, IL 60120, BS 46 Univ of IA; MA 47 Univ of IA; **SLP**

Becker, Dr Nancy G 5559 W Van Buren Street, Chicago, IL 60644, (312) 633-8867, BA 64 Juniata Coll; MA 68 Northwestern Univ; PH 73 (NS) Northwestern Univ; Director/ Sp-Lang-Hrng, Cook Co Hospital, **SLP F**

Becker, Mrs Rosalind 807 Seamas Avenue, Sacramento, CA 95822, (916) 442-1850, MA 88 Univ of the Pacific; 88–Sp-Lang Path, Sacramento City USD

Becker, Sandra K H 117 Carol, Tahlequah, OK 74464-6211, (918) 456-5511, BS 68 Central MO St Univ; OB 74 Northwest MO St Univ; MS 76 Central MO St Univ; Instr/Clinic Dir, Northeastern State Univ, **SLP**

Becker, Mrs Shari Brown 177 Browns Road, Nesconset, NY 11767, (516) 271-6263, MS 86 CUNY - Brooklyn Coll; 87–Aud, Huntington Hrng & Sp Ctr

Becker, Stephanie P O Box 10, Meridian, CA 95957, (916) 961-2266, BA 76 CA St Univ - Sacramento; MA 78 CA St Univ - Sacramento; 77–Aud, ENT Surgical & Med Gp/N Area, **A**

Becker, Susan Nancy 2285 South Langspur, Hacienda Heights, CA 91745, (714) 981-7616, BA 79 Univ of CA - Los Angeles; MA 83 CA St Univ - Northridge; Audiologist, Pacific Hrng Serv, **A**

Becker, Tim Richard 1635 Fox River Parkway, Waukesha, WI 53186-7196, (414) 544-0174, **A**

Becker Caplan, Laura 40 Littlefield Road, Newton Center, MA 02159, (617) 332-6233, BA 70 Univ of Northern CO; MA 71 Univ of Denver; Sp-Lang Path, Private Practice, **SLP**

Beckerleg, Mrs Wendy 24780 West Woodside, Farmington Hills, MI 48331, (313) 242-7214, BA 79 MI St Univ; MA 80 MI St Univ; Dir Sp /Lang Dept, Mercy Mem Hosp, **SLP ACE**

Beckerman, Lynn P 21850 Potomac, Southfield, MI 48076, (313) 353-9684, BA 72 Univ of MI - Ann Arbor; MS 73 Univ of MI - Ann Arbor; SLP, Livonia Pub Schs, **SLP**

Becker-Olans, Mrs Jacquie Michelle 23 Meadowood Drive, Stoughton, MA 02072, (617) 893-8050, BS 82 Boston Univ; MS 85 Emerson Coll; **SLP**

Beckett, Mrs Lyda B 1330 El Solyo, Campbell, CA 95008, BA 61 San Jose St Univ; MA 63 San Jose St Univ; **SLP LM**

Beckett, Dr Ralph L 1238 Venice Avenue, Placentia, CA 92670, (714) 773-3617, BA 50 Univ of Southern CA; MA 52 Univ of Southern CA; PH 68 (NS) Univ of Southern CA; Retired, CA State University, **SLP LM**

Beckett, Mrs Rebecca Justus 2644 Parkview Drive, Vinton, VA 24179, (703) 890-5505, BS 78 WV Univ; MS 83 James Madison Univ; 88–Sp-Lang Path, Pro Therapies of Roanoke Inc, **SLP**

Beckford, Andrea Marcelle 815 Thayer Avenue #504, Silver Spring, MD 20910, (301) 585-7106, MS 88 Univ of the DC

Beckham-Woodward, Mrs Paula L 7409 Olympia Drive #D, Bakersfield, CA 93309, (805) 835-0422, BA 82 Univ of CA - Santa Barbara; MA 85 CA St Univ - Chico; **SLP**

Beckler, Deanne Mary 827 Thomas Road, Columbus, OH 43212, (614) 272-0509, MA 83 OH St Univ; Sp-Lang Path, Affilited Aud & Sp Path, **SLP**

Beckler, Mrs Lynn L 2129 Bennigan Street, League City, TX 77573, (808) 521-3562, BS 83 Univ of HI - Manoa; MS 84 Univ of HI - Manoa; **SLP**

Beckley, Mrs Debby P 503 Jackson Avenue, Lexington, VA 24450, (703) 463-2041, BS 71 G Peabody Coll-Vanderbilt U; MS 72 Vanderbilt Univ; Sp-Lang Path, Lexington Cty Sch, **SLP**

Beckley, Mrs Karen W 2 Sunbury Lane, Savannah, GA 31406, (912) 355-4601, BS 69 Univ of NE - Lincoln; MA 70 Univ of NE - Lincoln; 84–Sp-Lang Path, Savannah Sp Hrng Cen, **SLP**

Beckley, Linda S 7009 Twelve Oaks Blvd, Tampa, FL 33634, (813) 893-6727, BS 80 FL St Univ; MS 81 FL St Univ; 87–Coord of Dysphagia Svcs, Bayfront Med Ctr, **SLP ACE**

Beckman, Debra S 1210 Ridge Road, Longwood, FL 32750, (407) 332-7409, BS 75 AR St Univ; MS 80 Univ of AR - Little Rock; Consultant, Private Practice, **SLP**

Beckman, Mrs Debra Sue 1201 College, Tarkio, MO 64491, (816) 736-4177, BS 77 Northwest MO St Univ; MS 84 Northwest MO St Univ; 79–Sp-Lang Path, Tarkio R-1 Sch Dist, **SLP ACE**

Beckman, John Thomas Don Duplan Md, 3400 Hwy 365 Ste 300, Port Arthur, TX 77642, (409) 722-5000, BS 82 Lamar Univ; MS 87 Lamar Univ; Aud, Don Duplan

Beckman, Sandra L 21 Gramercy Park S-6A, New York, NY 10003, (212) 340-6025, BA 57 Univ of Rochester; MA 74 San Francisco St Univ; Asst Research Sci, Rusk Institute, **SLP**

Beckmann, Dr Dorothy A 79-38 77th Avenue, Glendale, NY 11385, (718) 934-5000, BA 53 CUNY - Queens Coll; MA 54 CUNY - Queens Coll; PH 70 (NS) Columbia Univ Teachers Coll; Assoc Prof/Sp, CUNY-Kingsborough Com Coll, **SLP**

Beckmann, Frieda J 79-38 77th Avenue, Glendale, NY 11385, (516) 785-3637, BS 62 CUNY - Bernard M Baruch Coll; ME 65 CUNY - Queens Coll; Sp-Lang Path, N Bellmore Pub Sch, **SLP**

Beckoff, Esther Miller 110-50 71st Road #8-E, Forest Hills, NY 11375, (718) 575-8871, BA 78 CUNY - Brooklyn Coll; MA 80 SUNY - Center at Buffalo; Sp-Lang Path, NY League For the Hard of Hearing, **SLP**

Beckstead, Debra Ann 4817 South 7th, Tacoma, WA 98405, (206) 829-0600, **SLP**

Beckwith, Mrs Barbara Ann 18488 Beverly, Birmingham, MI 48009, (313) 546-4810, BA 80 Univ of MI - Ann Arbor; MA 82 Wayne St Univ; Systems Dir, Neurological Recovery Sys, **SLP**

Beckwith, Rosalind Lorraine 5262 Timuquana Road #711, Jacksonville, FL 32210, (904) 390-2079, MS 85 FL St Univ; **SLP**

Beckworth, Ralph M 2655 Hackwood Place, Birmingham, AL 35226, BS 74 Univ of AL- Tuscaloosa; MS 85 Univ of AL- Tuscaloosa; **A**

Bedard, Janet Linda 1298 Commonwealth Avenue, Newton, MA 02165, (617) 792-8500, BA 81 Univ of CT; ME 84 Northeastern Univ; Sp-Lang Path, Hahnemann Rehabilitation Cen, **SLP**

Bedard, Laurie Gay 191 North Second Street, Bethpage, NY 11714, (516) 433-6537, BA 83 Univ of MD - College Park; MA 85 Hofstra Univ; 87–Aud, Dr David A Abraham, **A**

Bedder-Manley, Carrie Elise 89 Brickstone Circle, Thornhill, ON, Canada L4J 6M5, (416) 738-8660, BA 82 York Univ - Ontario; MA 85 SUNY - Center at Buffalo; 88–Sp-Lang Path, Hosp for Sick Children, **SLP**

Bedell, Mrs Beverly Lynn 2876 10th Street, Cuyahoga Falls, OH 44221, (216) 724-1139, MA 84 Univ of Akron; BA 83 Univ of Akron; SLP, Lake County Soc Crpld Chn & Ad, **SLP**

Bedell, Joy Anne 410 East Chicago Avenue, Naperville, IL 60540, (312) 896-1961, MA 84 Butler Univ; **SLP**

Bedford, Mrs Leslie V 85 Jefferson Road, Farmingdale, NY 11735, (516) 752-6514, BA 71 CUNY - Queens Coll; MA 72 Univ of MA - Amherst; 88–Chairperson of Educ Prog, Ufsd #22 Farmingdale Pub Sch, **SLP**

Bedient, Laurie K White P O Box 123, Gerry Levant Rd, Gerry, NY 14740, (716) 487-0141, BA 79 SUNY - Coll at Plattsburgh; MA 81 SUNY - Coll at Plattsburgh; 82–Aud, WCA Hosp, **A**

Bednarik, Patricia Ann 673 Sloop Road, Pittsburgh, PA 15237, (412) 521-9000, BS 81 Bowling Green St Univ; MS 85 Miami Univ - Oxford; **SLP**

Bednarz, Maryann 4556 Kings Crossing Dr N E, Kennesaw, GA 30144, (404) 924-4996, BS 77 Elmhurst Coll; MA 79 Univ of WI - Madison; Aud, **A**

Bednarz, Therese F 6524 West 157th Street, Oak Forest, IL 60452, (312) 596-3200, BS 76 Univ of IL - Urbana; MS 77 Univ of IL - Urbana; 88–Sp-Lang Path, ECHO, **SLP**

Bedore, Joan McGarry 126 North Waiola, La Grange, IL 60525, (312) 354-5730, BA 82 Saint Xavier Coll; OM 85 Governors St Univ; **SLP**

Bedrosian, Dr Janice L 905 Kearney Street, Manhattan, KS 66502, (913) 532-6879, BA 74 Univ of CA - Santa Barbara; MA 76 Univ of CA - Santa Barbara; PH 81 (NS) Univ of WI - Madison; Asst Prof, Kansas St U, **SLP**

Bedwinek, Anne Plummer 1624 Cove Creek Lane, Knoxville, TN 37919, (615) 588-0906, BA 69 Univ of MI - Ann Arbor; MA 72 Northwestern Univ; Instructor, U TN, **SLP**

Bee, Norma M 52 Mountaineer Heights, Elkview, WV 25071, (304) 965-6244, BA 67 Coll of Mount Saint Vincent; MS 69 Rutgers St Univ -N Brunswick; Sp-Lang Path, Kanawha Cnty Dept Exceptnl Stu, **SLP**

Beebe, Mrs Helen Hulick 608 Porter Street, Easton, PA 18042, (215) 252-3461, Exec Dir, Helen Beebe Sp Hrng Cen, **SLP LM**

Beebe, Mrs Judith P 11492 Tomarsue Drive, Marilla, NY 14102, (716) 652-1845, BA 76 SUNY - Center at Buffalo; MS 87 SUNY - Coll at Buffalo; 88–Sp-Lang Path, BOCES of Erie 2-Chautauqua-Cattaraugus Counties, **SLP**

Beebe, Karen M 6312 Redbird Lane, Crystal Lake, IL 60014, (815) 459-6238, BS 85 Northern IL Univ - De Kalb; MA 86 Northern IL Univ - De Kalb; **SLP**

Beebe, Kary Lynn 7429 Vernon Square Drive, Apartment 102, Alexandria, VA 22306, (703) 664-7190, BA 83 Univ of CT; MS 85 Southern CT St Univ; Sp-Lang Path, Mount Vernon Hosp, **SLP**

Beebe, Margaret W 283 Regulus Avenue, Lompoc, CA 93436, (805) 733-1239, BA 73 San Jose St Univ; MA 75 Univ of CA - Santa Barbara; Sp-Lang Path, Lompoc USD, **SLP**

Beeby, Gary James Speech & Hearing Clinic, Oklahoma State University, Hanner Hall, Stillwater, OK 74078, (405) 744-6021, BS 63 Phillips Univ; MA 65 Univ of IL - Urbana; Assist Prof, OK St U, **SLP A**

Beeby, Marilyn G Department Speech-Language Services, PO Box 773, Shattuck, OK 73858, (405) 938-2830, BS 61 Phillips Univ; Sp-Lang Path, OK Public Schools, **SLP**

Beech, Mrs Marjorie M 5201 Berkeley Way, Vancouver, WA 98661, (206) 695-4627, BA 59 Univ of IA; Sp-Lang Path, Clackamas Co Educ Service Dist, **SLP**

Beecher, Robert Best Childrens Hospital Of WI, P O Box 1997, Milwaukee, WI 53201, (414) 931-4065, BA 66 Marietta Coll; MS 74 Emerson Coll; Sp-Lang Path, Childrens Hospital of Wisc, **SLP**

Beecher, Mrs Valerie P R R 1 Box 573, Farm Road, Windsor, VT 05089, (802) 295-8605, BA 74 SUNY - Coll at Oswego; MS 76 SUNY - Coll at Geneseo; 84–Sp/Lang Path, Hartford School District, **SLP**

Beechler, Margaret Lydia 211 N E 8th Avenue #109, Hallandale, FL 33009, (305) 765-6000, BA 79 Univ of FL; MS 85 Nova Univ; **SLP**

Beechley, Mrs Rena Bryant 35 Sejon Drive, Sayville, NY 11782, (516) 567-3033, BA 63 Univ of FL; ME 71 Univ of FL; Sp-Lang Path, Sayville Public Schools, **SLP**

Beedle-Johnson, Debra Leah 14308 Northville Road, Plymouth, MI 48170, (313) 453-1939, BS Eastern MI Univ; MA Eastern MI Univ; Sp-Lang Path, Wyandotte Schools, **SLP**

Beegle, Barbara B 3673 Randall Mill Road N W, Atlanta, GA 30327, BS 76 Univ of GA; ME 74 Univ of GA; Sp-Lang Path, **SLP**

Beekman, Mrs Jane Kyhl 2702 Euclid Avenue, Muncie, IN 47304, (317) 288-2479, BA 54 Univ of IA; **SLP**

Beeler, Mrs Charlene C 600 Polaris Drive, Upper Sandusky, OH 43351, (419) 294-5261, BA 72 Heidelberg Coll; MA 74 Univ of Cincinnati; Sp-Lang Path, Upper Sandusky Public Schools, **SLP**

Beeman, Marsha L 5950 Old Spanish Trail #29, Pensacola, FL 32504-8561, (904) 474-3732, BS 83 FL St Univ; MS 85 FL St Univ; Sp-Lang Path, Rehabilitation Inst West Fla, **SLP**

Beemsterboer, Priscilla 20428 Hellenic Drive, Olympia Fields, IL 60461, (312) 748-3932, BA 71 Knox Coll; MS 78 Governors St Univ; Sp/Lang Path, Speed Joint Agreement, **SLP**

Beermann, Martha L L 1411 McClaren Drive, Carmichael, CA 95608, BA 69 San Diego St Univ; MS 75 Univ of NV - Reno; Resource Specialist, Washington USD, **SLP**

Beers, Mrs Ann Mackey 18605 Mc Coy Avenue, Port Charlotte, FL 33948, (813) 743-3148, BS 60 Univ of OR; ME 65 Univ of OR; 88–Retired, **SLP ACE**

Beers, Mrs Kathleen B 108 Apache Drive, Indiana, PA 15701-8958, (412) 349-9493, BS 79 Indiana Univ of PA; MA 81 Memphis St Univ; SLP, Audiological & Speech Assoc, **SLP**

Beery, Dr Quinter C Center For Speech Language And Voice Pathology, Eye And Ear Hospital, 230 Lothrop Street, Pittsburgh, PA 15213, (412) 647-2030, BA 62 Univ of LA Verne; MA 64 Univ of Redlands; PH 72 (NS) Univ of Pittsburgh - Pittsburgh; Assoc Prof/Sp-Lang Path, Univ of Pittsburgh, **SLP**

Beeson, Mrs Cheryl A HC 1 Box 155-A, Soldotna, AK 99669, (907) 262-9026, BA 77 WA St Univ; MA 78 WA St Univ; SLP, Kenai Penninsula Boro Sch Dist, **SLP**

Beeson, Joann Regina 432 Edgewood Drive, Slidell, LA 70460, (504) 643-5629, ME 87 Southeastern LA Univ

Beeson, Pelagie M 1531 West Dutton Place, Tucson, AZ 85737, (602) 621-1644, BS 75 Univ of KS; MA 76 Univ of KS; **SLP**

Beeson-Holmes, Melissa 2931 Rockford Avenue, Stockton, CA 95207, (209) 951-5525, BA 75 San Diego St Univ; MA 78 San Diego St Univ; Sp-Lang Path, Delta College, **SLP**

Beetz, Ann L 4200 Westview Road, Baltimore, MD 21218, (301) 323-1010, BA 71 Loyola Coll; MS 75 Loyola Coll; 75–Sp-Lang Path, Balt Cty Pub Sch, **SLP**

Befus, Mrs Barbara H 4235 Edinburgh S E, Grand Rapids, MI 49506, BA 76 Augustana Coll; MA 77 Western MI Univ; Sp-Lang Path, Private Practice, **SLP**

Begeal, Mrs Anne T Rd 2 Box 36, Northville, NY 12134-9616, (518) 863-4807, MS 79 Coll of Saint Rose; BS 77 SUNY - Coll at Geneseo; Sp-Lang Path, Fonda-Fultonville Cen Sch, **SLP**

Begen-Peltz, Linda Gail 16 Dorothy Place, Berkeley, CA 94705, (415) 845-4826, BA 67 San Francisco St Univ; MA 68 San Francisco St Univ; 77–Owner/Aud, Berkeley Aud Serv, **A**

Beggs, Fred R 4815 West Markham Street, Little Rock, AR 72205, (501) 661-2328, BA 70 Univ Southern MS-Hattiesburg; MS 71 Univ Southern MS-Hattiesburg; Dir Hrng Sp & Vision Serv, AR Dept of Hlth, **A**

Beggs, Mary Ann 2988 Madison, Eugene, OR 97405, (503) 687-3375, BA 61 KS St Univ; MS 69 Univ of OR; SLP, Eugene Pub Schs, **SLP**

Begines, Mrs Terry Walker R R 21 Box 256, Terre Haute, IN 47802, (812) 234-3788, BA 80 IN Univ - Bloomington; MA 82 IN Univ - Bloomington; 84–Aud, Fred D Drake MD, **A**

Begley, Liz H 8 Asbury Drive, Ithaca, NY 14850, BA 77 CA St Univ - Long Beach; MA 80 CA St Univ - Long Beach; SLP, Charmss Collaborative, **SLP**

Begley, Mrs Michelle M 2161 Rush Road, Abington, PA 19001, (215) 884-7910, MA 79 Kent St Univ; SLP, Mont Co Inter Unit, **SLP**

Begner, Mrs Patricia 290 Chestnut Ridge Road, Rochester, NY 14624, (716) 325-4560, BA 67 SUNY - Center at Albany; OM 77 SUNY - Coll at Brockport; MS 71 SUNY - Coll at Geneseo; Dir/Pupil Per Ser, Rochester Cty Sch Dist, **SLP**

Beha, Deborah Mary Rd 2 Route 49, Box 50-A, Marcy, NY 13403, (315) 336-2300, BS 80 East Stroudsburg Univ of PA; MS 86 Coll of Saint Rose

Beh-Arendshorst, Monica 785 Concord, Holland, MI 49423, (616) 335-5590, BS 73 Wayne St Univ; MA 74 Wayne St Univ; Sp-Lang Path, Private Practice, **SLP**

Behm, Mrs Julia A 4821 34th Street, Columbus, NE 68601, (402) 563-3784, BA 76 Univ of WI - Eau Claire; MA 78 Univ of MN - Duluth; 88–Sp-Lang Path, Columbus City Schs, **SLP**

Behnke, Mrs Barbara Johnson 2105 Preston, Salt Lake City, UT 84106, (801) 521-1688, BA 80 Univ of WI - Eau Claire; MS 82 CO St Univ; Sp-Lang Path, Primary Chldns Med Cen, **SLP**

Behnke, Charles R 7510 Farmingdale Drive, Darien, IL 60559, (312) 633-2169, BA 67 Milton Coll; MA 73 Northern IL Univ - De Kalb; 72–Aud, VA Wside Med Cen, **A**

Behnke, Kim L 3534 Ridge Road, Lockport, NY 14094, (716) 434-8911, MA 88 SUNY - Center at Buffalo

Behnke, Sue E 3312 North 32nd, Waco, TX 76708, (214) 353-9921, BS 82 TX Woman's Univ; BS 73 Southwest TX St Univ; ME 75 Southwest TX St Univ; Registered Nurse, Parkland Mem Hosp, **SLP ACE**

Behnken, Susan A 685 Grove Drive #203, Buffalo Grove, IL 60089-4040, BA 79 Elmhurst Coll; MA 80 Univ of IL - Urbana; Sp-Lang Path, Behavioral Ed Cen, **SLP**

Behr, Tina 36 James Street, Shrewsbury, NJ 07702, (201) 577-1280, BS 71 Trenton St Coll; MA 74 Montclair St Coll; Coord Sp-Lang Prog Chr Ed Dept, CPC Mental Health Services, **SLP**

Behrends, Bernadette Cotta 26 Maryland Avenue, Woodland, CA 95695, (916) 662-8562, BA 74 CA St Univ - Fresno; MA 76 CA St Univ - Fresno

Behrends, William H, Jr 1050 West Carlton Road, Pensacola, FL 32514, (904) 474-8328, BA 72 Univ of South AL; MA 73 Univ Southern MS-Hattiesburg; 76–Dir of Aud, Med Ctr Clinic, **A**

Behrendsen, Mrs Lynn L Route 1 Box 571-A, N E Vista, Woodland, WA 98674, (206) 225-9265, MS 88 Portland St Univ

Behrendt, Karen Lynne 102 Woodview Drive, Laurens, SC 29360, (803) 833-2733, MA 83 Central MI Univ; BS 82 Central MI Univ; **SLP**

Behrendt, Mrs Linda Lane 5820 Hermitage Road, Richmond, VA 23228, BA 63 Univ of MA - Amherst; MA 66 Univ of MA - Amherst; **SLP**

Behrens, Denise P O Box 5869, Caracas, Venezuela 1010-A, MS 80 Syracuse Univ; 74–Sp-Lang Path, **SLP**

Behrens, George R PO Box #326, Chestertown, NY 12817, (518) 494-7439, MA 66 Syracuse Univ; BA 50 Emerson Coll; Retired, **SLP**

Behrens, Kathleen Ann 5368 Locksley Avenue, Oakland, CA 94618, (415) 682-9000, MS 84 San Francisco St Univ; BA 80 Univ of MI - Ann Arbor; 88–Sp-Lang Path, Neuro Care Inc, **SLP**

Behrens, Leilani 1929 Branding Iron Way, Roseville, CA 95661, (916) 447-5468, MA 82 CA St Univ - Sacramento; **SLP**

Behrens, Thomas R 3630 North Nelson Street, Arlington, VA 22207, (202) 732-1170, PH 63 (NS) Northwestern Univ; Dir Div of Innovation, US Dept of Ed, **A**

Behringer, Mrs Sandra M 838 Claridge Court, Indianapolis, IN 46260, (317) 251-9731, BA 59 Mundelein Coll; MA 60 Northwestern Univ; Clinical Supervisor, InSpeech Inc, **SLP**

Behrman, Eileen Ann 6100 NW 32 Terrace, Fort Lauderdale, FL 33309, (305) 390-0780, BA 72 CUNY - Brooklyn Coll; MS 76 CUNY - Brooklyn Coll; 77–Sp-Lang Path, Broward Co Schs

Behrmann, Georgette E 54 Fuller Road, Albany, NY 12203, (518) 489-4283, MS 86 Coll of Saint Rose; 86–Sp-Lang Path, Wilton Developmental Center, **SLP**

Behun, Elizabeth K 1202E County House Lane, Marietta, OH 45750, (412) 439-1444, BA 86 Thiel Coll; MA 88 OH Univ - Athens; 88–Sp-Lang Path, SG Rehab Agency Inc

Beich, Diane L 20001 Edmunton, St Clair Shores, MI 48080, (313) 664-2951, Self Employed, **SLP**

Beichel, Mrs Pamela Lory 8100-154 East Camelback Rd, Scottsdale, AZ 85251, (602) 239-4755, BS 72 Southern IL Univ-Edwardsvill; MS 71 Southern IL Univ-Edwardsvill; SLP, Good Samaritan Med Cen, **SLP**

Beier, Pamela Marie 1557 Oakland, St Clair, MI 48079, (313) 329-7534, **A**

Beighley, Melody F 14 Sandalwood Court, Racine, WI 53402, (414) 637-3179, BS 76 Miami Univ - Oxford; MS 77 Univ of IL - Urbana; Sp-Lang Path, Racine USD, **SLP**

Beighley, Nancy Ruttenberg South Valley Speech & Lang Ser, 6911 South Yosemite, Suite 104, Englewood, CO 80112, (303) 850-7717, BA 73 Univ of Denver; MA 74 Univ of Denver; Sp-Lang Path, South Valley Sp & Lang Serv, **SLP**

Beil, Janice Krempasky 400 Main Street, Mohnton, PA 19540, (215) 683-5422, BS 79 Bloomsburg Univ of PA; MS 82 PA St Univ - Univ Park; Sp-Lang Path, Berks Co Intermed Unit, **SLP**

Beilis, Mrs Rosalie 8 Dogwood Circle, Matawan, NJ 07747, (212) 266-9800, BA 72 CUNY - Brooklyn Coll; MS 74 Columbia Univ Teachers Coll; 74–Sp-Lang Path, Bd of Educ NYC, **SLP**

Beilke, Richard Marshall 150 Font Boulevard M K, San Francisco, CA 94132, (415) 333-1843, BA 79 Univ of CA - Santa Cruz; MS 86 San Francisco St Univ; 86–Sp-Lang Path, Oakland USD, **SLP**

Beiriger, Mrs Antonia A 555 Lorraine Avenue, Waukegan, IL 60085, (312) 623-9300, BS 80 Northwestern Univ; MA 82 Univ of IL - Urbana; Sp-Lang Path, Beach Park Sch Dist #3, **SLP**

Beisler, Jean Madsen Rural Route 6, 14 Valley View, Iowa City, IA 52240, (319) 356-0445, BA 72 Luther Coll; MA 74 Univ of IA; Sp-Lang Path, U of IA Hosp, **SLP**

Beiter, Anne L Cochlear Corp, 61 Inverness Dr E Ste 100, Englewood, CO 80112, (303) 790-9010, BA 70 Univ of IA; MS 75 Univ of WI - Madison; 86–Aud, Cochlear Corp, **SLP A**

Beiter, Dr Robert C 112 Pamela Drive, Bensenville, IL 60106, (312) 804-0550, BA 65 SUNY - Center at Buffalo; MA 67 Univ of WI - Madison; PH 74 (Aud/Hrng Science) Univ of MI - Ann Arbor; 81–Aud, Consult Aud Assoc, **A**

Beitsch, Mrs Estelle L 135 Riverside Road, Baltimore, MD 21221, (301) 686-7641, BA 36 CUNY - Brooklyn Coll; MA 62 Univ of MD - College Park; **SLP LM**

Beittel, Mrs Marylin P 16 North Bausman Drive, Lancaster, PA 17603, (717) 394-6014, BA 57 Oberlin Coll; MS 59 Purdue Univ - West Lafayette; Sp-Lang Path, Chld Dev Prog-Headstart, **SLP**

Bejoian, Linda C 544 Huron Avenue, Cambridge, MA 02138, (617) 354-4435, **SLP**

Bejtlich, Mrs Janet Lynne 116 Armour Street, New Bedford, MA 02740, (617) 992-4756, BS 83 Univ of NH; MS 85 Emerson Coll; **SLP**

Bekemeier, Linda Grace 914 12th Street, Eldora, IA 50627, (515) 539-8550, BA 63 Univ of IA; 87–Sp-Lang Path, AEA 6, **SLP**

Belak-Plenger, Barbara J 735 Beaverbrook Lane, Glendora, CA 91740, (818) 914-2398, MA 73 Univ of IL - Urbana; BS 72 Univ of IL - Urbana; **SLP LM**

Belanger, Steven A 189 Winter Street, Laconia, NH 03246, (603) 524-0729, BS 77 Boston Univ; MA 79 Univ of MN - Minneap-St Paul; **SLP ACE**

Belasco, Mrs Carol W 1004 Providence Lane, Buffalo Grove, IL 60089, (312) 381-7850, BS 76 Northwestern Univ; MA 78 Northwestern Univ; 78–Sp-Lang Path, Barrington Comm Ut Sch DIST220, **SLP**

Belcastro, Mary Elizabeth 8425-A Captons Lane #2-S, Darien, IL 60559, (312) 963-8760, BA 85 IN Univ - Bloomington; OM 87 Governors St Univ; 88–Sp-Lang Path, Oak Leyden Dev Svcs, **SLP**

Belcher, Jane Marie 445 East Broadway, Danville, IN 46122, (317) 929-3311, BS 81 Purdue Univ - West Lafayette; MS 83 Purdue Univ - West Lafayette; 84–Aud, Methodist Hosp, **A**

Belcher, Louise A 822 Mill Landing Road, Chesapeake, VA 23320, (804) 467-8283, BS 69 Western MI Univ; MA 70 Western MI Univ; Assistant-Resource Services, Southeastern VA Training Cen, **SLP**

Belcher, Marsha Davis Speech Path & Language Clinic, Gracewood State Sch & Hosp, Gracewood, GA 30812, (404) 790-2197, BS 78 Bloomsburg Univ of PA; MS 79 Bloomsburg Univ of PA; ED 84 (NS) Univ of GA; Sp/Lang Path, Gracewood St Sch/Hosp, **SLP**

Belcher, Mrs Patricia Y P O Box 1891, Dublin, GA 31040, (912) 272-8612, BA 48 FL St Univ; ME 60 Univ of GA; Sp-Lang Path, Laurens Co Sch, **SLP**

Belcher, Mrs Suzanne W 3255 Wilmington Road, Montgomery, AL 36105, (205) 265-8922, BS 79 Univ of Montevallo; MS 87 Univ of Montevallo; **SLP**

Belden, Christine Shanks 500 Scott Drive, Ormond Beach, FL 32074, (904) 767-0221, BS 74 FL St Univ; MA 75 FL St Univ; Sp-Lang Path, Volusia County School Board, **SLP**

Belden-Pope, Mrs Lori 7466 South Englehart, Reedley, CA 93654, (619) 243-1240, BA 79 Wichita St Univ; MA 81 CA St Univ - Chico; Sp-Lang Path/Coord, Kings Co USD, **SLP**

Beldin, Annette Teresa 92 Greatbrook Road, Milford, NH 03055, (617) 345-3204, BA 83 Univ of FL; ME 85 Univ of FL; 87–Sp-Lang Path, Fitchburg PS, **SLP**

Beldin, Mrs Nancy J C 1071 Mulbury Mansion, Yukon, OK 73099, (405) 354-6545, BS 80 Loma Linda Univ - Riverside; MA 82 Wichita St Univ; Sp-Lang Path, Putnam City Sch Dist, **SLP**

Belding, Donna Lynn 1707 2nd Street #3, New Orleans, LA 70113, (504) 891-7567, BS 82 Univ Southern MS-Hattiesburg; MS 84 Univ Southern MS-Hattiesburg

Belenchia-Huggins, Mrs Patricia Laura 108 McGuire Cove, Clarksdale, MS 38614, (601) 627-5247, BA 82 Univ of MS; MS 84 Univ of MS; SLP, Clarksdale Sp & Hrng Cntr, **SLP**

Belf, Lee A 35 East County Road C #308, Little Canada, MN 55117, (612) 490-0547, Audiologist, Special Int School Distr 916, **A**

Belfanti, Mrs Debra J 2836 Frink Street, Scranton, PA 18504, (717) 348-1321, BS 78 Marywood Coll; MS 80 Rutgers St Univ - Newark; Sp/Lang Path, Allied Serv for Hndcpd, **SLP**

Belford, Mrs Linda Morris 6441 West Cimarron Trail, Flint, MI 48532, (313) 762-6663, BA 74 Univ of MI - Ann Arbor; OM 84 Univ of MI - Flint; MA 75 MI St Univ; 88–Sys Analyst, Hurley Med Cen, **SLP**

Belgard, Karen Lyn 5433 West National Avenue, Apartment 210-A, West Milwaukee, WI 53214, (414) 241-8000, BS 85 Marquette Univ; MA 86 Northwestern Univ; 86–Aud, Milwaukee ENT Cl, **A**

Belin-Frost, Mrs Gayle 47 Hillcrest Road, Burlington, VT 05401, (802) 658-5017, BA 75 MI St Univ; MA 76 MI St Univ; Sp-Lang Path, **SLP**

Belinski, Theresa M 2506 Winfield Avenue, Scranton, PA 18505, (717) 282-9200, BS 78 Marywood Coll; MS 81 Bloomsburg Univ of PA; Sp-Lang Path, Nen Ed Inter U #19, **SLP**

Belitz, Mrs Leslie 8813 Freedom Way NE, Albuquerque, NM 87109, (505) 821-2671, BA 77 CUNY - Lehman Coll; MA 78 CUNY - Lehman Coll; Sp/Lang Path, Alta Mira, **SLP**

Belk, Dr Judith B 2204 East Fort Lowell Road, Tucson, AZ 85719, (602) 325-2300, MA 64 Syracuse Univ; MS 69 Univ of CA - Los Angeles; PH 74 (Special Education: Learning Disabilities) Univ of Southern CA; Sp-Lang Path, Judith B Belk Phd Inc, **SLP A ACE**

Belkin, Dr Amy S 205 West End Avenue #7-D, New York, NY 10023, (212) 369-2821, OB 65 Carnegie-Mellon Univ; MA 68 Columbia Univ Teachers Coll; ED 75 (NS) Columbia Univ Teachers Coll; Sp/Lang Path, The Dalton Sch, **SLP**

Belkin, Mrs Marlene R 810 Elmway Circle, Norristown, PA 19401, (215) 668-9012, BA 80 Temple Univ; MA 82 Hofstra Univ; 87–Sp-Lang Path, PASS Program, **SLP**

Belknap, Barbara A 2314 West Jefferson Street, Boise, ID 83702-4809, (208) 486-0078, **SLP**

Bell, Alicia A A Route 5 Box 58E, Nashville, AR 71852, (713) 621-3072, BA 75 Henderson St Univ; MA 78 Univ of AR - Fayetteville; 87–Sp-Lang Path, The Battin Clinic Memorial Hall Sch, **SLP**

Bell, Mrs Alison C 218 Maryland, Waterloo, IA 50701, (319) 232-4529, BA 74 Univ of IA; MA 75 Univ of Northern IA; SLP, AEA #7, **SLP**

Bell, Mrs Alison Louise 89 Peel Street, Barrie, ON, Canada L4M 3L5, (705) 728-9802, **SLP**

Bell, Ann Elizabeth 11909 Locust Road, Louisville, KY 40243-1412, (502) 484-3417, MS 83 Univ of Louisville; Sp-Lang Path, Eminence ISD, **SLP**

Bell, Barbara Ann 11 Byfield Street, Bristol, RI 02809, (617) 992-4756, BA 79 RI Coll; MA 82 Univ of ME - Orono; **SLP**

Bell, Barbara Anne 148 El Nido #B, Monrovia, CA 91016, BA 83 Univ of CA - Santa Barbara; MA 85 Univ of Northern CO; 87–Aud, Otologic Med Ctr, **A**

Bell, Bert H Saginaw Board Of Education, 550 Millard, Saginaw, MI 48607, (517) 776-0289, BA 68; MS 70 Western OR St Coll; PH 82 (NS); Program Director Sp & Hrng, Saginaw Board of Education, **SLP**

Bell, Brenda Lynn 600 North Dwyer Drive, Anaheim, CA 92801, (714) 956-3845, BA 85 Univ of CA - Santa Barbara; MS 88 UT St Univ

Bell, Carolyn Baumwart 311 West Georgia, Anadarko, OK 73005, (405) 247-6607, **SLP**

Bell, Mrs Cheryl J 213 N Willow Springs Road, Orange, CA 92669, (714) 771-6546, BA 77 CA St Univ - Long Beach; MA 79 CA St Univ - Los Angeles; **A**

Bell, Constance S 6307 Chimney Wood Court, Alexandria, VA 22306, (703) 768-0378, BS 75 WV Univ; MA 76 OH St Univ; 88–Sp-Lang Path, Birth-Four Eval & Treat Ctr, **SLP ACE**

Bell, David J 173 Sweet Acres Dr, Rochester, NY 14612, (716) 392-5765, MA; **SLP**

Bell, Deborah A 215 Columbia Street, Santa Cruz, CA 95060, (408) 425-8840, BA 76 CA St Univ - Northridge; MA 78 CA St Univ - Northridge; 88–Sp-Lang Path, Private Practice, **SLP**

Bell, Delores C 17860 Springfield, Country Club Hills, IL 60477, **SLP**

Bell, Mrs Doris C 5427 Bartlett Street, Pittsburgh, PA 15217, (412) 683-7100, BA 49 Monmouth Coll; MS 50 Univ of IL - Urbana; Sp-Lang Path, UCP Assoc, **SLP**

Bell, Dr Dorothy M 2314 Willing Street, Fort Worth, TX 76110, (817) 924-2822, **SLP A LM**

Bell, Ellen R 3164 Beach Boulevard, Cicero, IN 46034, (317) 773-9201, MS 70 IN Univ - Bloomington; 88–Tchr, Hamilton Heights Sch Corp, **SLP**

Bell, Fred E 4705 Palmetto Point Drive, Bay Colony, Palmetto, FL 33561, (813) 729-3758, BA 51 MI St Univ; MA 63 MI St Univ; Retired, Lw Blake Mem Hosp, **SLP**

Bell, Dr Hannah R 556 St Davids Avenue, St Davids, PA 19087, (512) 434-6711, BA 66 Northwest Nazarene Coll; MS 74 Limestone Coll; PH 80 (NS) Univ of TX - Dallas; Temple Univ, **SLP**

Bell, Mrs Jean L , New Castle, KY 40050, BA 52 Univ of KY; ME 57 Univ of KY; Retired, Ky Dep of Ed-Off of Ed Excp Ch

Bell, Jeannette P O Box 155, Zuni, NM 87327, (505) 782-5511, BA 60 TX Christian Univ; MA 62 TX Christian Univ; Sp/Lang Path, Zuni PS, **SLP LM**

Bell, Mrs Joan L 19408 Keswick Street, Reseda, CA 91335, (213) 885-8921, BA 43 Bowling Green St Univ; MA 69 CA St Univ - Northridge; SLP, LA Cty USD, **SLP LM**

Bell, Julie Ann 901 Gatepost Lane, Apartment 3A, Frederick, MD 21701, (301) 371-5700, BS 84 Indiana Univ of PA; MS 85 James Madison Univ; Sp-Lang Path, Frederick Co Board of Educ, **SLP**

Bell, Karen J 10445 Wilshire Boulevard, Apartment 605, Los Angeles, CA 90024, (213) 470-6756, **SLP A**

Bell, Kathryn J 423 South Scoville #3N, Oak Park, IL 60302, (312) 383-1203, BS 79 Eastern IL Univ; MS 80 Eastern IL Univ; Sp-Lang Path, Proviso Area for Execp Chldn, **SLP**

Bell, Linda C 2327 Peytonsville Road, Franklin, TN 37064, (615) 790-0154, MS 87 Vanderbilt Univ; Sp-Lang Path, Pro Health Svcs, **SLP**

Bell, Mrs Lisa Barnes 3416 Cavalier Court, Irving, TX 75062, (214) 255-1659, BS 83 Univ of North TX; MS 86 Univ of TX - Dallas; 86–Sp-Lang Path, Arlington ISD, **SLP**

Bell, Lisa Conover 56 Phillips Avenue, Ponte Vedra Beach, FL 32082, (904) 285-6022, OB 83 Univ of FL; MA 86 Univ of FL; 87–Sp-Lang Path, St Johns County Sch Bd, **SLP**

Bell, Mrs Lynda G 271 Hillcrest Drive, Mobile, AL 36609, (205) 666-0047, BS 81 Univ of AL- Tuscaloosa; MS 85 Univ of South AL; Sp-Lang Path, Mobile County Pub Sch, **SLP**

Bell, Mrs Margaret L 569 Julia Circle, Leeds, AL 35094, (205) 699-6871, BS 75 Univ of Montevallo; MS 76 Univ of Montevallo; **SLP**

Bell, Mrs Martha Groenendyk 1902 Deerpath Road, Dothan, AL 36303, (205) 983-3521, BA 60 Univ of AL-Tuscaloosa; ME 78 Univ of AL-Birmingham; 87–Coord Sp-Lang Path, Wallace Coll, **SLP**

Bell, Mary W 627 Pine Street, Vienna, VA 22180, (703) 378-6100, BA 74 George Washington Univ; MA 75; **SLP**

Bell, Niki Sue 1319 South 6th Avenue East, Newton, IA 50208, (515) 792-4870, BA 72 Univ of Northern IA; MA 73 Univ of Northern IA; SLP, AEA II, **SLP**

Bell, Pamela 1808 El Dorado Terrace, Escondido, CA 92025, BA 73 Univ of Denver; MA 76 San Jose St Univ; **SLP**

Bell, Mrs Patricia Gail 518 Lowewood Place, Chula Vista, CA 92010, (619) 589-5600, BA 77 San Diego St Univ; MA 84 San Diego St Univ; 81–Sp-Lang Path, Lemon Grove Sch Dist, **SLP**

Bell, Raylene 1426 Wayside Drive, Tyler, TX 75701, (214) 593-8313, BS 76 TX Tech Univ; MS 77 TX Tech Univ; Sp-Lang Path, Bell & Mitchell Inc, **SLP**

Bell, Mrs Sandra A 1509 Pine Meadow Court, Lexington, KY 40504, (606) 885-4179, BA 72 Univ of KY; MA 74 Univ of KY; MA 74 Univ of KY; Sp-Lang Path, Jessamine County Board of Educ, **SLP**

Bell, Mrs Sandra Sue Rt 2 Box 34, Pine Bluff, AR 71603, (501) 534-3715, BS 77 Lincoln Univ; OM 85 Univ of Central AR; 81–Sp-Lang Path, Pine Bluff Public Schools, **SLP**

Bell, Susan F 15506 Sungold Court, Houston, TX 77095, BA 71 Univ of CA - Santa Barbara; MA 73 Univ of CA - Santa Barbara; Sp-Lang Path, Klein ISD, **SLP**

Bell, Tina A Denver Ctr For Comm Dis Inc, 6000 East Evans Avenue, Bldg #1 Suite 250, Denver, CO 80222, (303) 757-2662, BA 70 Hollins Coll; MA 74 Univ of Denver; Dir, Denver Cen/Commun Dis Inc, **SLP**

Bell, Walter J 733 Derby Milford Road, Orange, CT 06477, **SLP**

Bellaire, Karen J 5489 Martina Way, Dunwoody, GA 30338, (404) 668-0923, BA 79 Univ of MT; MA 82 Univ of MT; 86–Sp-Lang Path, Atlanta VA Med Ctr, **SLP**

Bellairs-Salemi, Mrs Luanna Lee 6414 Baseline #84, Little Rock, AR 72209, (501) 562-9106, BS 82 Univ of Central AR; MS 83 Univ of Central AR; **SLP**

Bellanti, Carolyn A 433 West Hillcrest Avenue, State College, PA 16803, (814) 231-1076, BA 61 Hamline Univ; OM 62 Johns Hopkins Univ; MS 74 PA St Univ - Univ Park; 74–Sp-Lang Path, State Coll Area Sch Dist, **SLP**

Bellassai, Mrs Kimberly Ann 617 West 88th Terrace, Kansas City, MO 64114, (816) 363-2602, BS 84 Northeast MO St Univ; MS 87 Central MO St Univ; **SLP**

Bell-Berti, Dr Fredericka St Johns University, Grand Ctrl & Utopia Pkwy, Jamaica, NY 11439, (212) 990-6161, BS 67 CUNY - City College; PH 73 (Sp Science) CUNY - Grad Sch & Univ Cntr; Assoc Prof, St Johns Univ, **F**

Bellefleur, Dr Philip A VA School Hampton, 700 Shell Road, Hampton, VA 23661, (804) 247-2032, BS 58 Central MI Univ; MA 62 Wayne St Univ - Sch of Med; PH 64 (NS) Wayne St Univ - Sch of Med; Super, Virginia School/Deaf & Blind, **A**

Bellerose, Betty 5421 Wormall, Kansas City, MO 64112, (816) 531-1200, BS 56 Univ of KS; MS 63 Univ of KS; Sp-Lang Path, Truman Medical Center West, **SLP**

Bellevue, Beverly Walker Ctr For Communication Disorder, Beverly Hospital, Herrick & Heather Streets, Beverly, MA 01915, (617) 922-3000, BS 78 Southern IL Univ -Carbondale; MA 80 IN Univ - Bloomington; Dir Comm Disorders, Beverly Hospital, **SLP**

Bellevue, Mrs Dorothy I 5619 Calle DE Arboles, Torrance, CA 90505, (213) 533-4532, BA 62 CA St Univ - Long Beach; MA 69 CA St Univ - Long Beach; SLP, LA Co Supt of Schs, **SLP**

Bell-Hiett, Cynthia J 6171 Idlewyle, Birmingham, MI 48010, (313) 540-8085, BS 75 Central MI Univ; MA 78 Central MI Univ; SLP, Birmingham Public Schools, **SLP**

Belli, Mrs Sharon Catherine 1821 Compass Ct, Toms River, NJ 08753, (201) 499-5362, BA 82 Kean Coll of NJ; MA 83 Kean Coll of NJ; 83–Sp-Lang Path, Woodbridge Dev Ctr, **SLP**

Belling, Erlene D 2325 N W 121st, Oklahoma City, OK 73120, (405) 521-3351, BS 59 Northeastern OK St Univ; ME 63 Northeastern OK St Univ; Consult-Sp-Lang-Hrng, St Dept Ed, **A**

Bellinger, Joyce H 117 South Waterwheel Way, Orange, CA 92669, (714) 997-6315, BA 70 Univ of Southern CA; MA 74 Univ of Southern CA; Sp-Lang Path, Orange USD, **SLP**

Bellini, Patricia Iafrate 77 Hawthorne Place, North Providence, RI 02904, (401) 353-7893, BA 79 RI Coll; MS 81 Boston Univ; Sp-Lang Path, Central Falls School Dept, **SLP**

Bellis, Mrs Teri James 1816 Van Diest Road, Colorado Springs, CO 80915, (719) 630-5200, BA 83 Univ of Northern CO; MA 85 Univ of CA - Santa Barbara; 86–Aud, Capron Inst, **A**

Bellissima, Mary Ann L 922 North Chrysler Drive #8, Tucson, AZ 85716, (602) 298-4358, BS 75 Nazareth Coll of Rochester; MS 78 Univ of AZ; Aud, Tucson Ear Nose & Throat Assoc, **A**

Bellissimo, Mary A 340 Abbeyville Road #B, Pittsburgh, PA 15228, (412) 664-5020, BS 75 Indiana Univ of PA; MS 77 WV Univ; Sp-Lang Path, S Hills Hlth Syst, **SLP ACE**

Bell-McGhee, Mary Elizabeth 2608 North 17th Street, Milwaukee, WI 53206, (414) 383-4490, BS 79 Marquette Univ; MS 82 Marquette Univ; Sp-Lang Path, Sinai Samaritan Med Ctr, **SLP**

Bellows, Liz Nathan 648 Monterey Road, Palm Springs, CA 92262, (712) 623-3237, BA 81 Univ of CA - Santa Barbara; MA 85 Univ of IA; Aud, Audiological Services, **A**

Bellugi, Dr Ursula The Salk Institute, P O Box 85800, San Diego, CA 92138, (619) 453-4100

Bellville, Judith Gail 425 South Hubbards Lane, Apartment 135, Louisville, KY 40207, (502) 893-9563, BA 84 Augustana Coll; MS 85 Univ of Louisville; Sp-Lang Path, Univ Speech Pathology Assoc, **SLP**

Bell-Vollandt, Clarice Angela 2550 Independence Avenue, Apartment 7-K, Riverdale, NY 10463, (212) 590-5302, BA 80 SUNY - Center at Stony Brook; MA 84 CUNY - Lehman Coll; 82–Sp-Lang Path, NY City Bd of Educ Sp Svcs Unit

Belmont, Suzanne Snipes 343 East 30th Street #2-M, New York, NY 10016, (212) 722-7224, BA 80 Univ of MS; MA 82 Univ of MS; Aud, Manhattan ENT Hosp, **A**

Belobradic-Joyce, Lynn Christine 39100 Chagrin Boulevard, Chagrin Falls, OH 44022, (216) 247-8788, BS 76 Inter American Univ; MS 80 Univ of Philippines; **SLP**

Belozerco, Laura Gail 79-27 68th Avenue, Middle Village, NY 11379, (718) 326-2695, 88 CUNY - Queens Coll; MA; 88–Sp-Lang Path, St Joseph's Med Ctr

Belpedio, Katherine Elizabeth 1310 118th Avenue N W, Coon Rapids, MN 55433, (612) 755-8220, BS 79 Univ of WI - River Falls; MS 84 Univ of WI - River Falls; **SLP**

Belsante, Mrs Susan Zohn 542 Brian Dean Drive, Glen Gardner, NJ 08826, (201) 537-4933, BS 78 Ithaca Coll; MA 79 Bowling Green St Univ; Sp-Lang Path, W Essex Comm Hlth Svc, **SLP**

Belshe, Susan Graham 317 Jastram Street, Providence, RI 02908, (401) 272-3876, BA 78 MacAlster Coll; MS 82 Saint Cloud St Univ; Sp-Lang Path, Lincoln Sch Dept, **SLP**

Belsjoe, Frances W 9231 Oak Ledge Drive, San Antonio, TX 78217, (512) 734-5721, BA 58 Baylor Univ; Sp/Lang Path, San Antonio ISD, **SLP**

Belsky, Mrs Susan K 310 Kerrwood Drive, Wayne, PA 19087, (215) 296-5090, BA 71 Univ of MD - College Park; MA 72 Univ of MD - College Park; Sp-Lang Path, Mont Co Interm Unit-Preschool Div, **SLP**

Belson, Mrs Muriel F 7112 East Prairie Road, Lincolnwood, IL 60645, (312) 791-2900, BS 46 Northwestern Univ; MA 67 Northwestern Univ; 67–Coord, Adult Neur Sp-Lang Serv, David T Siegel I-Commun Dis, **SLP**

Belsterling, Ralph John 3525 Middleboro Road, Castle Shannon, PA 15234, (412) 466-5550, BS 78 CA Univ of PA; MS 86 Clarion Univ of PA; ME 80 CA Univ of PA; Aud, Southwestern Hrng Health Svcs, **SLP A**

Belt, Charles William 1202 Bancroft Court, Bel Air, MD 21014, (302) 429-4410, BS 76 West Chester Univ of PA; MS 81 Loyola Coll; Sp-Path, Charles W Bush Sch, **SLP**

Belt, Dr Donald A 920 Riverside Road, Hollister, CA 95023, (408) 730-4220, BA 61 Univ of Redlands; MA 62 Univ of Redlands; PH 67 (NS) Univ of WA; Owner, Private Practice, **SLP A**

Belus, Gail Seiler 1910 East Manhattan Drive, Tempe, AZ 85282, (602) 461-2781, BS 78 Eastern IL Univ; MS 78 Eastern IL Univ; MS 86 Rush Univ; 87–Sp-Lang Path/Manager, Mesa Lutheran Hosp, **SLP A**

Belveal, Mrs Sally Squires 7820 West Capitol #1006, Little Rock, AR 72205, (501) 847-3506, BS 83 Delta St Univ; MS 85 Univ of AR - Little Rock; Instr Supvr, Alexander Human Dev Ctr, **A**

Belvoir, Mary Elizabeth 3710 South Urbana, Tulsa, OK 74135, (918) 492-8200, BA 78 Univ of WI - River Falls; MS 81 Phillips Univ; Sp-Lang Path, Shadow Mountain Institute, **SLP**

Bem, Denise Chippo Rd 2 Box 453, Portage, PA 15946, (814) 736-3659, BS 77 Indiana Univ of PA; ME 82 Indiana Univ of PA; Sp/Lang Path, Applachia Inter Ut 08, **SLP**

Bement, Linda Bryant 29 Kramer St, Rochester, NY 14623, (716) 475-6554, BS 81 Nazareth Coll of Rochester; MS 83 Gallaudet Coll; Rehab Audiologist/Instructor, NTID, **A**

Bemski, Mrs Sandra L 1974 South Perry, Denver, CO 80219, (303) 936-0371, BA 83 Univ of CO - Boulder; MS 85 Univ of WA; **A**

Ben'Ary, Adele N 820 Mountain Avenue, Berkeley Heights, NJ 07922, (201) 464-2771, BA 68 Marywood Coll; MA 72 Newark St Coll; 84–Sp-Lang Path, Ben' Ary Assoc, **SLP ACE**

Benas, Jacquelyn P O Box 473, West Boxford, MA 01885, (617) 352-6354, BS 74 Salem St Coll; ME 81 Northeastern Univ; 88–Sp-Lang Path, Lynn PS Syst, **SLP**

Ben-Azay, Marcie Lyn 193 Upland Avenue, Newton, MA 02161, (617) 734-1111, MA 84 Hofstra Univ; SLP, Brookline Public Schools, **SLP**

Benbow, Mrs Pamela Jean 809 Shirley Drive, Myrtle Beach, SC 29577, (803) 448-2913, **A**

Benci, Mrs Dee Yvonne 529 South Highway 22A, Panama City, FL 32404, (904) 785-0822, BS 87 Univ Southern MS-Hattiesburg; MS 88 Univ Southern MS-Hattiesburg; 88–Sp-Lang Path, InSpeech Inc, **F**

Bencin, Maryann E 773 Cherokee Trail, Willoughby, OH 44094, (216) 255-0800, BS 80 Univ of Toledo; MA 85 Cleveland St Univ; 88–Aud, Mednet Clinics, **A**

Bencivenga, Anthony J 5455 Pepperwood Road, Santa Rosa, CA 95405, **A**

Benda, Mary G 7800 Lake Forest Drive, Richmond, VA 23235, (804) 276-9596, BS 72 Bowling Green St Univ; MA 74 Marshall Univ; SLP, Med Facilities of Amer, **SLP**

Benda, Mrs Teresa Ann 1800 Center #10, St Maries, ID 83861, (208) 245-2508, BA 83 Eastern WA Univ; MS 84 Eastern WA Univ; **SLP**

Bendana, Frances B 1406 Henry Clay Avenue, New Orleans, LA 70118, (504) 897-0328, BA 63 Univ of Southwestern LA; MS 77 Tulane Univ; **A**

Bender, Barbara Lynn 10155 Northwest 9th St, Circle #205, Miami, FL 33172, (305) 221-1947, BA 76 Univ of NC - Greensboro; ME 78 Univ of NC - Greensboro; Sp-Lang Path, Dade County Schools, **SLP**

Bender, Mrs Dianne C 302-A Overlook Drive, Wading River, NY 11792, (516) 924-0191, BA 76 SUNY - Coll at Plattsburgh; MA 80 Hofstra Univ; Sp-Lang Path, Mid Island Cen Sch, **SLP**

Bender, Dr Donald R Chief-Audiology Section, Brooke Army Medical Center, Ft Sam Houston, San Antonio, TX 78234, (512) 221-5054, BA 69 William Paterson Coll; MA 70 Seton Hall Univ; PH 77 (NS) Univ of MD - College Park; Aud, US Army, **A**

Bender, Mrs Jessica D 509 Warren Avenue, St Louis, MO 63130, (314) 726-2396, BA 64 Cornell Univ; OM 65 Harvard Univ; MA 81 Saint Louis Univ; Sp-Lang Path, Sp Sch Dist of St Louis Co Mo, **SLP**

Bender, Mrs Kathleen O 7000 Hillswick Drive, Charlotte, NC 28215, BA 70 SUNY - Coll at New Paltz; MA 72 PA St Univ - Univ Park; MS 74 Winthrop Coll; Sp/Lang Path, Charlotte Mecklenberg Sch, **SLP**

Bender, Lisa H 926 Buchholz, Wooster, OH 44691, (614) 397-4548, BS 78 Bowling Green St Univ; MS 82 IL St Univ - Normal; Sp-Lang Path/Aud, Deborah B Romas, **SLP A**

Bender, Lisa J P O Box 783, New Paltz, NY 12561, (914) 255-0772, BS 83 SUNY - Coll at New Paltz; ME 87 SUNY - Coll at New Paltz; 86–SLP, Wallkill Central Sch Dist, **SLP**

Bender, Martha A M 11923 Rocky Knoll, Houston, TX 77077, (713) 870-1618, BS 75 Southern Methodist Univ; MA 78 Univ of TX - Austin; **SLP**

Bender, Mrs Pamela A Z Head & Neck Surgical Assoc, 1622 11th Street, Wichita Falls, TX 76301, (817) 322-6953, BS 74 Univ of North TX; MS 75 Univ of North TX; Chief Aud, Head & Neck Surgical Assoc, **A**

Bender, Ron G 1620 11th Street, Wichita Falls, TX 76301, (817) 767-3215, MS 75 Baylor Univ; Owner, Private Practice, **SLP**

Bender, Ruth E 1425 Greencroft Drive, Apartment #237, Goshen, IN 46526, (212) 533-6594, PH 56 (Aud) Case Western Reserve Univ; **A LM**

Bender, Mrs Wendy E A 39 Woodbine Lane, Fairfield, CT 06432, (203) 372-3066, BA 68 CT Coll; MA 70 Columbia Univ Teachers Coll; **SLP**

Bendet, Dr Roslyn M 105 Morningside Center, 1802 Jancey Street, Pittsburgh, PA 15206, (412) 665-4953, BS 59 Vanderbilt Univ; MS 62 Univ of Pittsburgh - Pittsburgh; PH 77 (Special Educ/Supervis) Univ of Pittsburgh - Pittsburgh; Aud, Pittsburg Pub Sch, **A**

Bendikas, Sylvia C 1335 Sunburst Lane, Northbrook, IL 60062, (312) 696-6274, BS 76 Northwestern Univ; MS 78 Univ of WI - Madison; 78–Sp-Lang Path, Lutheran General Hospital, **SLP**

Bendroff, Mrs Ann Denise 3840 Blue Gum Drive, Yorba Linda, CA 92686, (714) 779-5589, BA 83 San Diego St Univ; MA 85 Memphis St Univ; 88–Sp-Lang Path, Assoc Sp & Lang Svcs, **SLP**

Bene, Mrs Julie Barber 407 14th Avenue SE, Puyallup, WA 98371, (206) 841-7414, BA 82 Univ of WA; MS 86 Univ of WA; Sp-Lang Path, Good Samaritan Hosp, **SLP**

Bene, Mrs Kay 28 Twin Springs, St Louis, MO 63124, (314) 851-0094, BS 73 Univ of MO - Saint Louis; MA 77 Saint Louis Univ; 77–SLP, Spec School Dist St Louis Cnty, **SLP**

Benedek, Diane K 5727 Woodland Drive, Western Springs, IL 60558-2138, (312) 531-3771, BS 68 Northern IL Univ - De Kalb; MA 71 Northwestern Univ; Dir of Dept of SLP/Aud, Loyola University/McGaw Hosp, **A**

Benedetti, Nancy L 368 Deer Trace #201, Pineville, LA 71360, (318) 640-0754, MA 85 Western MI Univ; 86–Sp-Lang Path, Pinecrest State School, **SLP**

Benedict, Ellen T 340 Hager Lane, Glenview, IL 60025, (312) 998-5668, BA 82 Univ of MT; OM 85 Univ of MT; **A**

Benedict, Kathleen Whalen 9412 Kennerly Street, Temple City, CA 91780, (202) 265-7335, BA 80 Univ of CA - Santa Barbara; MS 83 Boston Univ; **SLP**

Benedict, Lois Anne 24-E Colonial Parkway, Pittsford, NY 14534, (716) 271-0680, BS 64 Kent St Univ; MA 66 Case Western Reserve Univ; 70–Dir Sp-Lang Path, Hrng & Sp Cen of Rochester Inc, **SLP**

Benedict, Mary K Box 238, APO New York, NY 09238, **SLP**

Benedict, Pamela H Milwaukee Ear Nose & Throat Cl, 10520 North Prt Washington Rd, Mequon, WI 53092, (414) 241-8000, BS 76 Marquette Univ; MA 77 OH St Univ; Aud, Milwaukee ENT Cl, **A**

Benedict, Mrs Paula Maria 4231 Ridgemont Court, Oakland Hills, CA 94619, (415) 651-1190, BA 74 MI St Univ; MA 75 MI St Univ; Sp-Lang Path, Fremont USD, **SLP ACE**

Benedict, Dr William S R R 1 Box 1111, Maryland, NY 12116, (607) 431-2474, BS 59 SUNY - Coll at Geneseo; MS 65 Syracuse Univ; PH 79 (NS) SUNY - Center at Buffalo; Assoc Prof/Sp, St U of NY-Oneonta, **SLP**

Beneroski, Kimberly Jo 136 43rd Avenue, Vero Beach, FL 32962, (305) 778-2100, BS 83 Edinboro Univ of PA; MA 84 Edinboro Univ of PA; 86–Sp-Lang Path, Treasure Coast Rehab Hosp, **SLP**

Benfield, Kathy Jean Coastal ENT, 445 Western Blvd, Suite O, Jacksonville, NC 28540, (919) 455-9884, BS 82 Appalachian St Univ; MS 84 East Carolina Univ; Aud, Coastal Hrng Ser, **A**

Bengala, Mrs Deborah E Speech-Lang-Auditory-Path Dept, East Carolina University, Greenville, NC 27858, BA 71 OH Univ - Athens; MA 76 Western MI Univ; Cl Asst Prof, East Carolina Univ, **SLP**

Benge, Mrs Mary Riley 7401 West Bloomfield Road, Peoria, AZ 85345-5362, (602) 978-3860, BS 75 Northern AZ Univ; MS 79 Univ of AZ; Sp/Lang Path, Glendale USD, **SLP**

Bengel, Mrs Patricia Ellen 37495 Dale Drive #104, Westland, MI 48185, (313) 455-0943, BS 84 Purdue Univ - West Lafayette; MA 87 Wayne St Univ; **SLP**

Bengston, Susan D 737 Tuckahoe Road, Apartment #14, Yonkers, NY 10710-5201, BS 71 NY Univ; MA 78 NY Univ; Sp-Lang Path, NYC Bd of Ed, **SLP**

Benham, Deborah Marie 372 Mountain View Avenue, Mountain View, CA 94040-1114, (415) 329-2857, MA 83 San Jose St Univ; Sp-Lang Path, Ravenswood City Sch Dist, **SLP**

Benham, Jayne Ann 460 Catalpa Avenue, North Plainfield, NJ 07060, (201) 584-8145, BA 83 Rutger's St Univ - Douglas Coll; MA 85 Kean Coll of NJ; 85–SLP, Welkind Rehab Hosp, **SLP**

Benham, Mrs Laura L 1830 East 17th, Ada, OK 74820, (405) 332-6528, BA 79 Univ of OK - Norman; MS 81 Univ of OK Medical Center; Sp/Lang Path, Pontotoc Co Guidance Clin, **SLP**

Benishek, Mrs Lois Ann 2803 Wayne, Iowa City, IA 52240, (319) 356-1169, BS 73 CO St Univ; MS 75 CO St Univ; Sp-Lang Path, Univ of Iowa Hosp Sch, **SLP**

Benitez, Mercedes J 2213 Washington Avenue, Chevy Chase, MD 20910, (202) 865-6100, BS 76 George Washington Univ; MS 78 George Washington Univ; 82–Dir Sp-Lang Path, Howard U Med Cen, **SLP**

Benjamin, Dr Barbaranne J 5825 Tantallon Circle, Sylvania, OH 43560, (419) 537-2055, MA 73 PA St Univ - Univ Park; MS 74 PA St Univ - Univ Park; PH 80 (NS) PA St Univ - Univ Park; Dept Chmn, U of Toledo, **SLP ACE**

Benjamin, Carolyn D 7020 Kamilo Street, Honolulu, HI 96825, (808) 547-4277, BS 73 Miami Univ - Oxford; MA 78 TX Woman's Univ; Sp-Lang Path, Queens Medical Ctr, **SLP**

Benjamin, Francine H Brooklyn Audiology Association, 3003 Ocean Parkway, Brooklyn, NY 11235, (718) 449-9800, BA 82 CUNY - Brooklyn Coll; MS 84 CUNY - Brooklyn Coll; Aud, Montefiore Med Ctr, **A**

Benjamin, Helise I 14 Millrock Road, New Paltz, NY 12561, **SLP**

Benjamin, Kathleen M 2841 Kelling Street, Davenport, IA 52804, (319) 391-1292, BS 73 Boston Univ; MS 75 Univ of VT; **SLP**

Benjamin, Ruth 1214 Hookston Road, Concord, CA 94518, **SLP**

Benko, Judy Kadell 196 Southwest Raymond, West Linn, OR 97068, (503) 279-4206, BA 78 Muskingum Coll; MA 80 Bowling Green St Univ; 87–Sp-Lang Path, Infant Hrng Resource, **SLP**

Benko, Mrs Kay Lynn 12333 Sunnyglen Drive, Moorpark, CA 93021, (818) 894-4588, MS 84 San Francisco St Univ; Aud, Auditory-Vestibular Ctr, **A**

Ben-Moshe, Mrs Felice 445 North Formosa Avenue, Los Angeles, CA 90036, (213) 936-7004, BA 76 CUNY - Queens Coll; MS 79 Univ of WI - Madison; SLP, Private Practice, **SLP**

Bennardo, Lois Mary 126 East 19th Street, New York, NY 10003, (212) 529-5806, BA 77 Saint John's Univ - Jamaica; MS 83 Columbia Univ Teachers Coll; Aud, Private Practice, **A**

Bennefield, Mrs Susan Carol 23939 Winifred, Warren, MI 48091, (313) 689-9539, BS 80 Eastern MI Univ; MA 81 Eastern MI Univ; Sp-Lang Path, Advncd Prof Home Hlth Care Inc, **SLP**

Benner, Mrs Nancy L 2820 234th Place NE, Redmond, WA 98053, (206) 868-2119, BS 77 Eastern WA Univ; MS 78 Eastern WA Univ; Sp-Lang Path, Mead Sch Dist, **SLP**

Benners, Ann Ownby 4013-A Lewis Lane, Austin, TX 78756, (512) 459-6930, BA 80 Univ of the South; MA 85 Univ of TX - Austin; Sp-Lang Path, Austin ISD, **SLP**

Bennett, Ana Aurora 94-364 Hokuala Street #181, Mililani Town, HI 96789, (808) 668-7777, BA 75 Univ of HI - Manoa; MS 84 Univ of HI - Manoa; Sp-Lang Path, Hi Dept of Ed, **SLP**

Bennett, Mrs Angela Shaddock 1004 Crestwood, El Dorado, AR 71730, (501) 864-0650, BS 81 AR St Univ; MS 83 Univ of AR - Medical Sci; Sp-Lang Path, Union Co Ctr for Hndcpd, **SLP**

Bennett, Audrey 29 St Helens #506, Tacoma, WA 98402, (206) 627-8353, BS 61; **SLP LM**

Bennett, Barbara A 187 Irwin Street, Brooklyn, NY 11235, **SLP**

Bennett, Barbara E 1208 Kost, Alvin, TX 77511, **SLP**

Bennett, Becky Bounous 134 East 26th Street, Tulsa, OK 74114-2416, (918) 584-2921, BA 80 Wichita St Univ; MA 81 Wichita St Univ; Sp/Lang Path, USD 373 Newton Ks Pub Sch, **SLP**

Bennett, Carissa D 4116 Perlita Avenue, Los Angeles, CA 90039, (818) 244-7653, BA 79 Univ of CA - Santa Barbara; MS 81 Univ of WA; Aud, Private Practice, **A**

Bennett, Mrs Carol L M 3051 West 69th Place, Tulsa, OK 74132, (918) 663-2506, BS 77 Univ of Tulsa; MA 80 Univ of KS; Sp-Lang Path, Tulsa Co Supt of Sch, **SLP**

Bennett, Caroline T #3 Linrose Circle, Lonoke, AR 72086, (501) 676-6879, BS 78 Southern Methodist Univ; MS 79 Southern Methodist Univ; Sp-Lang Path, Private Practice, **SLP**

Bennett, Capt Carolyn Sydnee 92nd Stat Hospital Fairchild, Fairchild AFB, WA 99011, (509) 247-5698, BS 72 UT St Univ; MS 77 UT St Univ; 86–Chief Aud Svcs, 92nd Stat Hosp Fairchild AFB, **A**

Bennett, Cecile S 605 Dafney Drive, Lafayette, LA 70503, (318) 984-3653, BA 64 Univ of Southwestern LA; SLP, Lafayette Parish Sch Bd, **SLP**

Bennett, Dr Clayton L 4783 Aberdeen Street, San Diego, CA 92117, (714) 481-8304, OB 48 Univ of Southern CA; MA 49 Univ of Southern CA; PH 52 (NS) Univ of Southern CA; Private Practice, **SLP LM**

Bennett, Dr Clinton Dept Of Speech Pathology, James Madison University, Harrisonburg, VA 22801, (703) 568-3867, BS 69 CO St Univ; MS 70 Univ of KS; PH 73 (NS) McGill Univ - Quebec; Prof, James Madison U, **SLP ACE**

Bennett, Mrs Cynthia Wright 3108 Alachua Lane, Albany, GA 31707, (409) 693-3326, BS 81 Auburn Univ - Auburn; MS 83 Auburn Univ - Auburn; Sp-Lang Path, College Sta ISD, **SLP**

Bennett, Daphne N 306 East California Street, Arcadia, CA 91006, (213) 265-8943, BA 42 0125; MA 53 Univ of UT; PH 55 (NS) Univ of Southern CA; **SLP LM**

Bennett, Debra G 110 Cushing Street, Waltham, MA 02154, **SLP**

Bennett, Mrs Debra K 3204 T Street, Lincoln, NE 68503, (402) 435-8198, BS 77 Clarion Univ of PA; ME 78 Clarion Univ of PA; **SLP**

Bennett, Mrs Diane E H 2300 Burgan Avenue, Clovis, CA 93612, (209) 896-6500, BA 76 San Jose St Univ; Sp-Lang Path, Fresno Co Schs, **SLP**

Bennett, Mrs Donna Faye 4942 Silver Ranch Way, Carmichael, CA 95608, MA 80 CA St Univ - Sacramento; SLP, North Sacramento School Dist, **SLP**

Bennett, Dorothy J 7700 East 13th #14, Wichita, KS 67206-1254, (316) 683-2129, BA 56 Wichita St Univ; MS 75 Wichita St Univ; SLP, Wichita Pub Schs USD #259, **SLP**

Bennett, Mrs Dyann D 5020 East 68th Street, Tulsa, OK 74136, (918) 492-3636, BS 67 Univ of Tulsa; MS 69 UT St Univ; Aud, En OK ENT Cl, **A**

Bennett, Mrs Floy L 1600 West White Oak #211, Independence, MO 64050, (816) 254-3530, BA 36 Southern IL Univ -Carbondale; MA 39 Univ of IL - Urbana; Retired, **LM**

Bennett, Dr Gladys H 504 Hermits Trail, Altamonte Springs, FL 32701, (305) 671-9321, BS 49 Ithaca Coll; ME 62 Boston Univ; PH 72 (NS) Syracuse Univ; Private Practice, **SLP**

Bennett, Howard D P O Box 5325, APO New York, NY 09057, OB 62 OH Univ - Athens; Sp-Lang Path, Dod Depends Schs, **SLP**

Bennett, Ida L Toronto General Hospital, 200 Elizabeth Street, 7EN-209, Toronto, ON, Canada M5G 2C4, (416) 595-3666, BA 77 Univ of Northern CO; MA 78 Univ of Northern CO; Aud, Toronto Gen Mt Sinai Hosp, **A**

Bennett, Mrs Jana C 580 High Street, Medford, MA 02155, (617) 488-6241, BS 79 Brigham Young Univ; ME 83 Univ of VA - Charlottesville; **SLP**

Bennett, Mrs Janet M 50 Russell Avenue, Asheville, NC 28806, (704) 253-0191, BA 75 Univ of NC - Greensboro; ME 76 Univ of NC - Greensboro; Sp-Lang Path, Private Practice, **SLP**

Bennett, Jerry J 4 Little John Road, Dundas, ON, Canada L9H 4G6, **A**

Bennett, Joel 3 Kinckerbocker Road South, Plainview, NY 11803, **SLP**

Bennett, John M 313 Southeast English, Moore, OK 73160, (405) 793-1901, BS 74 East TX St Univ - Commerce; MS 76 East TX St Univ - Commerce; Sp-Lang Path, **SLP**

Bennett, Karen Isaacs P O Box 14, Eastwood, KY 40018, (502) 454-8327, BS 76 Eastern KY Univ; MS 80 Univ of Louisville; Sp-Lang Path, Jefferson Co Bd of Ed, **SLP**

Bennett, Kathy Lee 3507 Peachwood Road, Knoxville, TN 37921, (615) 525-0757, BS 82 Univ of TN - Knoxville; MA 86 Univ of TN - Knoxville; **SLP**

Bennett, Laurie Floren 901 South 6th Street, Champaign, IL 61820, (217) 244-2552, BA 76 IA St Univ; MS 82 Purdue Univ - West Lafayette; 87–Dir-Hearing Clin, University of Illnois, **A**

Bennett, Leann W 2719 Meadowcreek, Missouri City, TX 77459, (713) 437-1988, BA 71 Baylor Univ; MA 73 Univ of Houston - Univ Park; Sp-Lang Path, Ft Bend ISD, **SLP**

Bennett, Leigh Holtby 4610 Webber Street, Sarasota, FL 34232, (813) 355-7637, BS 80 Ithaca Coll; MA 82 SUNY - Coll at Buffalo; **SLP**

Bennett, Leslie A 4448 West 9th Avenue, Vancouver, BC, Canada V6R 2E1, (604) 222-1369, BA 80 Univ of Ottawa - Ontario; MS 82 Syracuse Univ; Aud, School District #43, Coquitlam, **A**

Bennett, Linda A 2617 White Oak Court, Arlington, TX 76012, (817) 294-8408, BS 79 TX Christian Univ; MS 81 Phillips Univ; Sp-Lang Path, Overton Sp & Lang Cen, **SLP**

Bennett, Mrs Linda Angst Route 2, Box 555, Broadway, VA 22815, (703) 667-7200, BS 84 Bloomsburg Univ of PA; ME 86 James Madison Univ; 86–Aud, ENT Consults of Winchester Inc, **A**

Bennett, Lisa J W 2314 Arcola Avenue, Wheaton, MD 20902, (301) 949-3764, BA 77 MI St Univ; MA 78 Univ of Houston - Univ Park; Sp-Lang Path, Montgomery Co Pub Sch, **SLP**

Bennett, Marilyn S 3720 Francis Avenue, Cincinnati, OH 45211-4613, (513) 574-0990, BS 75 G Peabody Coll-Vanderbilt U; MS 80 Univ of WI - Madison; SLP, Hamilton Co Bd of Ment Retard, **SLP**

Bennett, Mary S 214 Trafalgar Street, Rochester, NY 14619, (716) 647-2960, BS 78 Radford Univ; MA 80 Univ of TN - Knoxville; Sp-Lang Path, Rochester Cty Sch Dist, **SLP**

Bennett, Mary Slattery 142 Connecticut Street, Jamestown, NY 14701, (716) 487-0141, BS 80 SUNY - Coll at Geneseo; ME 81 SUNY - Coll at Fredonia; Sp-Lang Path, Wca Hosp, **SLP**

Bennett, Mrs Nellie Mae 17412 N E 10th Street, Bellevue, WA 98008, (206) 641-0268, BA 55 Seattle Pacific Univ; ME 68 Univ of OR; Sp-Lang Path, Private Practice, **SLP LM**

Bennett, Pama L 2111 Kennedy Drive, Sioux City, IA 51104, (712) 274-6040, BA 73 Univ of IA; MA 76 Univ of IA; Sp-Lang Path, Wn Hills AEA, **SLP**

Bennett, Mrs Patricia Petrich Broad & Frederick Streets, Sewickley, PA 15143, (412) 741-4087, BA 82 Univ of Pittsburgh - Pittsburgh; MS 84 Univ of Pittsburgh - Pittsburgh; 87–Dir of Sp-Lang Dept, Laughlin Child Ctr, **SLP**

Bennett, Steven R 1401 Ottawa Court, Fort Collins, CO 80526, (303) 778-5645, BS 77 CO St Univ; MS 79 CO St Univ; 87–Sp-Lang Path, Porter Memorial Hosp, **SLP**

Bennett, Susan G 2024 Damon Drive, Florence, SC 29501, **SLP**

Bennett, Mrs Susan N 21172 Whitebark, Mission Viejo, CA 92692-4055, (714) 768-2088, BA 68 CA St Univ - Long Beach; MA 74 CA St Univ - Long Beach; Chprs/Early Interventn Prog, ABC USD, **SLP**

Bennett, Dr Suzanne Div Of Communication Disorders, Emerson College, 168 Beacon Street, Boston, MA 02116, (617) 578-8734, BS 65 Southern IL Univ -Carbondale; MS 69 Western MI Univ; PH 77 (NS) Purdue Univ - West Lafayette; Assoc Prof, Emerson Coll/Div of Commun Dis, **SLP**

Bennett, Tammy Warren 20 Buttermilk Road, Little Rock, AR 72207, (501) 223-9401, BA 80 Univ of AR - Fayetteville; MS 82 Univ of AR - Fayetteville; 87–Sp-Lang Path, Little Rock Sch Dist, **SLP**

Bennett, Trudy B Trudy Bennett & Associates, 2674 East Main, Ventura, CA 93003, (805) 653-7334, BS 76 ID St Univ; MS 77 ID St Univ; Director, T Bennett Assoc, **SLP ACE**

Bennett, Mrs Virginia Gallup 6130 Oak Street, Kansas City, MO 64113, (816) 363-1047, BS 75 MI St Univ; MA 76 Wayne St Univ; Teacher/Special Day Class, USD, **SLP**

Bennett-Briscoe, Edna A 14159 Dickens Street #107, Sherman Oaks, CA 91423, (818) 892-4388, BA 74 CA St Univ - Los Angeles; MA 82 CA St Univ - Los Angeles; Sp-Lang Path, LA USD, **SLP**

Bennett-Kastor, Dr Tina L Wichita State University, Box 14, Wichita, KS 67208, (316) 689-3130, OB 73 CA Inst of the Arts; MA 76 Univ of Southern CA; PH 78 (Linguistics) Univ of Southern CA; 78–Prof Linguistics & Eng, Wichita St U

Bennett-Porter, Sandra M 406 New Salem Road, Marshalltown, IA 50158, (515) 752-6731, BA 69 Wichita St Univ; MA 70 Wichita St Univ; Sp-Lang Path, AEA 6, **SLP**

Bennetts, Mrs Genevieve Gillett 24 Telegraph Drive, Virginia, MN 55792, (218) 741-1878, BS 39 Univ of WI - Madison; MA 69 Univ of MN - Duluth; **SLP LM**

Benning, Caryl M 732 Borello Way, Mountain View, CA 94041, (408) 249-1919, BA 69 CA St Univ - Fullerton; MA 71 CA St Univ - Fullerton; Sp-Lang Path, Private Practice, **SLP**

Benning, Mrs Lori Joan 715 Balzar Circle, Reno, NV 89502, (702) 322-2469, BS 81 Northern IL Univ - De Kalb; MA 83 Northern IL Univ - De Kalb; Sp-Lang Path, Washoe County Schs, **SLP**

Bennion, Martell S 3291 Chaparral Drive, St George, UT 84770, (801) 673-6274, MA 85 UT St Univ; 88–Sp-Lang Path, Wash Co Sch Dist, **SLP**

Bennitt, Barbara A 5009 Hemlock Street, Sacramento, CA 95841, **A**

Benoit, Mrs Jeannine Brayer 4226 Lake Avenue, Lockport, NY 14094, (716) 433-7593, BS 73 SUNY - Coll at Brockport; MS 78 SUNY - Coll at Buffalo

Bensen, Court M 3465 Rauscher Drive, Reno, NV 89503, (702) 747-2042, BA 65 Univ of NV - Reno; MA 74 Western WA Univ; **SLP**

Benshoof, Mrs Geraldine 2387 Badger Road, North Pole, AK 99705, (907) 488-2889, BS 62 Saint Cloud St Univ; ME 72 Univ of AK - Fairbanks; SLP, Fairbanks N Star Borough Sch D, **SLP**

Benshoof, Patricia G 1224 Steel Road, Havertown, PA 19083-4201, MS 80 PA St Univ - Univ Park; 87–Dir of Pro Svc, Team Rehabilitation Inc, **SLP**

Bensman, Mrs Harriet L 8391 Westfair Circle North, Germantown, TN 38138, (901) 754-1879, BS 63 Boston Univ; MS 65 Univ of WI - Madison; Sp-Lang Path, St Joseph Hosp, **SLP**

Benson, Betty Dilley 2110-B Sims Place, La Crosse, WI 54601, (608) 784-1875, BS 84 Northern St Coll; MA 86 Univ of SD - Vermillion; 88–Sp-Lang Path, St Francis Health Svcs, **SLP**

Benson, Mrs Bonnie Kramer 526 N Wynnewood Avenue, Wynnewood, PA 19096-1312, BS 81 Boston Univ; MA 83 Temple Univ; SLP, **SLP**

Benson, Darcy E P O Box 2040, El Granada, CA 94018, (415) 494-1000, BA 77 Univ of CA - Santa Barbara; MS 80 CO St Univ; 80–Director of Audiology, California Ear Institute, **A**

Benson, Donna M 7202 Orchid Lane, Eldersburg, MD 21784, (301) 795-3275, BA 82 Loyola Coll; MS 86 Loyola Coll; **SLP**

Benson, Donna Patricia 4306 Cowan Place, Belcamp, MD 21017, (301) 398-0400, BS 83 Towson St Univ; MS 85 Towson St Univ; 85–Sp-Lang Path, Cecil Co PS, **SLP**

Benson, Mrs Janice T 4517 White Aspen, Madison, WI 53704, (608) 244-6575, BS 75 Northeast MO St Univ; MA 76 Northeast MO St Univ; **SLP**

Benson, Mrs Mary Elizabeth 4412 North 56th Street, Phoenix, AZ 85018, (602) 952-1718, BA 40 IL Wesleyan Univ; **SLP LM**

Benson, Mrs Nancy K 109 Warwick Road, De Witt, NY 13214, (315) 470-3277, BA 70 NY Univ; MS 72 Ithaca Coll; Sp-Lang Path, North Syracuse Sch, **SLP**

Benson, Mrs Nancy S 505 Los Palmas Drive, Orange Park, FL 32073, (904) 264-6732, BA 77 Univ of IA; MA 78 Univ of SD - Vermillion; **SLP**

Benson, Mrs Pamela 8 Red Maple Road, Shokan, NY 12481, (914) 657-2354, BS 79 Elmira Coll; ME 82 Coll of Saint Rose; SLP, Onteora Cen Sch, **SLP**

Benson, Mrs Sheri H N-8493 Norton Road, Mauston, WI 53948-9726, (608) 562-5112, BS 80 Univ of WI - Madison; MS 81 Univ of WI - Stevens Point; Sp-Lang Path, Sch Dist of Wisconsin Dells, **SLP**

Bensussen, Jane O 365 25th Street, Santa Monica, CA 90402, (213) 674-7050, BA 67 Univ of MO - Columbia; MA 69 Univ of Southern CA; Dir Commun Dis, Daniel Freeman Mem Hosp, **SLP**

Bentler, Ruth A Wendell Johnson Speech & Hearing Clinic, Iowa City, IA 52242, (319) 353-5081, BS 71 Univ of IA; MA 73 Univ of IA; PH 87 (Aud) Univ of IA; Asst Prof, Univ of Iowa, **A ACE**

Bentley, Bruce O, Jr 813 St Anne's Drive, Iowa City, IA 52245, (319) 338-0581, OB 71 Univ of IA; MA 74 Univ of IA; Aud, Veterans Administration, **A**

Bentley, Carolyn Sullivan 279 Emerson Place, Valley Stream, NY 11580, (212) 889-6705, BS 75 SUNY - Coll at Fredonia; MS 79 Adelphi Univ; Aud, District Council 37, **A**

Bentley, Julie A 1004 Hertige Court East, Vadnais Height, MN 55127, (612) 426-3340, BS 79 Moorhead St Univ; MS 80 Univ of WI - Eau Claire; Sp-Lang Path, Roseville Area Sch, **SLP**

Bentley, Mrs Patricia K 931 Twisted Oak, Buffalo Grove, IL 60089, (312) 541-8084, BS 64 Marquette Univ; ME 88 Nat'l Coll of Ed - Evanston; Sp-Lang Path, Comm Consolidated Dist 102, **SLP**

Bentley, Mrs Peggy Weakland 263 Mentor Drive, Naples, FL 33942, (813) 598-4094, BS 82 Eastern MI Univ; MA 82 Eastern MI Univ; Sp-Lang Path, Collier Co Schools, **SLP**

Bentley, Mrs Rebecca D Route 1 Box 237-M, Eldorado, IL 62930, (618) 273-9544, BS 85 Southern IL Univ -Carbondale; MS 87 Southern IL Univ -Carbondale; 87–Sp-Lang Path, Hamilton Co Sch Unit #10, **SLP**

Benton, Steven Lamar 634 Esplanade Avenue #5, New Orleans, LA 70116, (504) 589-5566, BA 83 LA Tech Univ; MS 84 Univ of AL- Tuscaloosa; Aud, VA Med Ctr, **A**

Bentrum, Sheila M 2724 Glenbridge Court, Ann Arbor, MI 48104, (517) 423-2141, BS 79 Eastern MI Univ; MA 80 Eastern MI Univ; Dept Hd-Herrick Mem Hosp, Bentrum Sp-Lang Ther Serv, **SLP**

Bentrup, Sarah Kickham 559 Matianuck Avenue, Windsor, CT 06095, (203) 722-8635, OB 83 Univ of MO - Columbia; MS 85 Southern IL Univ-Edwardsvill; SLP, Hartford Pub Schs, **SLP**

Bentur, Dr Esther Eden 121 Einstein Street, Haifa, Israel 34601, MA 77; MA 84; PH 78 (NS); **SLP**

Bentwood, Mrs Judy J 1-A Bunyula Road, Bellevue Hill, New South Wales, Australia 2023, BS 75; MS 79 Emerson Coll; Sp/Lang Path, Private Practice, **SLP**

Bentz, Jocelyn Gillen 20426 73rd Place Northeast, Bothell, WA 98011, (206) 771-4374, BS 72 OH Univ - Athens; MA 79 Univ of Cincinnati; Sp-Lang Path, Edmonds Sch Dist, **SLP ACE**

Bentzen, Ernestine 19975 Westphalia, Detroit, MI 48205, (313) 371-0070, BA 50 Capital Univ; MA 69 Eastern MI Univ; MA 82 MI St Univ; Retired, **SLP**

Benvenutti, Mrs Elizabeth 203 Leonhard Avenue, Bay St Louis, MS 39520, (601) 467-2962, BA 75 Univ of MS; MA 76 Univ of MS; Sp-Lang Path, Language & Sp Serv, **SLP**

Benya, Dr John, Jr R R 1 Box 239, Convoy, OH 45832, (419) 238-0538, BA 55 Miami Univ - Oxford; MS 64 Bowling Green St Univ; PH 70 (NS) Wayne St Univ; SLP, Private Practice, **SLP**

Benz, Mrs Patricia W Route 1, Baltimore Pike, Wallingford, PA 19063, (215) 459-4514, BS 74 West Chester Univ of PA; MA 79 West Chester Univ of PA; Sp-Lang Path, Haverford Twp Sch Dist, **SLP**

Benziger, Lise M 3100 Erindale Station Road, Apartment 605, Mississauga, ON, Canada L5C 1Y4, (902) 566-6132, BA 79 SUNY - Center at Buffalo; MA 81 SUNY - Center at Buffalo; Aud, Dept of Hlth & Social Serv, **A**

Bequest, Mrs Julie A 509 North Honey Lake Road, Burlington, WI 53105, (414) 534-3557, **SLP**

Beran, Janine Ann 2200 Pierce #1, Sioux City, IA 51104, (712) 255-7326, MA 83 Univ of SD - Vermillion; Sp-Lang Path, Marian Health Ctr, **SLP**

Berardino, John T VA Outpatient Clinic, West Columbia Street, Orlando, FL 32806, (813) 972-2000, MS 76 Univ of South FL; Aud, VA Hospital, **A**

Berardino, Mrs Mary Baldi 131 Roberta Drive #1, Pittsburgh, PA 15221, (412) 243-9394, BS 84 Indiana Univ of PA; MS 86 Indiana Univ of PA; 86–Sp-Lang Path, Allegheny Inter Unit-Proj DART

Berasi, Karen Marie 1106 Golden Rain Street, Upland, CA 91786-3717, (714) 627-9817, BA 72 OH Univ - Athens; MA 73 OH Univ - Athens; SLP, Chino USD, **SLP**

Berberet, Mrs Susan Buss 17460 Inland Circle, Lakeville, MN 55044, (612) 892-1006, BA 82 Univ of WI - Eau Claire; MS 83 Univ of WI - River Falls; Sp-Lang Path, **SLP**

Berberich, Mary E 1711 North 91st Street, Omaha, NE 68114, (402) 978-7316, BA 73 Briar Cliff Coll; MS 75 Univ of NE - Omaha; Sp-Lang Path, Omaha Pub Sch, **SLP**

Bercaw, Mrs Maggi Delaney Chattanooga-Hamilton Company, Speech/Hearing Center, 529 Oak Street, Chattanooga, TN 37403, (615) 267-5641, BS 71 Univ of TN - Knoxville; MA 75 Univ of TN - Knoxville; 86–Aud, Chattanooga-Hamilton Co Speech & Hearing Ctr, **A ACE**

Bercovitz, Karin R 22744 Wildwood Street, Hayward, CA 94541, (415) 784-2814, BA 70 Univ of Southern CA; MA 72 Univ of Southern CA; **SLP**

Beremana, Mrs Pamela J 6805 Mayfield Road, Apartment 1123, Mayfield Heights, OH 44124, (216) 944-9400, BA 84 OH St Univ; MA 86 OH St Univ; 86–Sp-Lang Path, InSpeech Inc, **SLP**

Berendsen, Mrs Madeline Geary 428 State Street, Ripon, WI 54971-1426, (414) 748-5509, BS 80 Marquette Univ; MS 81 Univ of WI - Eau Claire; 88–Sp-Lang Path, Private Practice, **SLP**

Berenhaus, Sandra R 2440-24 Hunter Avenue, Bronx, NY 10475, (212) 916-8348, **A**

Berenson, Mrs Ann Berlin 1420 Locust Street Unit 25, Philadelphia, PA 19102, (609) 854-6525, BA 59 Temple Univ; MA 82 Trenton St Coll; Sp-Lang Path, Haddon Twp Board of Education, **SLP**

Berezow, Mrs Adeana Tova 144-23 68 Road, Flushing, NY 11367, (718) 471-8519, BA 82 CUNY - Queens Coll; MS 84 Loyola Coll; **SLP**

Berg, Abbey L F 245 West 107th Street #2-F, New York, NY 10025, (212) 866-6533, BA 72 George Washington Univ; MS 74 Purdue Univ - West Lafayette; Cl Instr of Pediatrics, New York Medical College, **A**

Berg, Mrs Cecilia A 6602 Treadwell, Austin, TX 78731, (512) 385-3330, BA 70 Our Lady Lake Univ-San Anton; MA 71 Our Lady Lake Univ-San Anton; Sp-Lang Path, Austin ISD, **SLP**

Berg, Mrs Cherie Jo 4031 Bethel Drive Apartment 22, Arden Hills, MN 55112, (612) 866-3351, BA 85 Univ of WI - Eau Claire; MS 86 Marquette Univ; 88–Sp-Lang Path, Hennepin Technical Institute Dist #287, **SLP**

Berg, Dr Frederick S Dept Communicative Disorders, Utah State University, Umc 10, Logan, UT 84322, (801) 750-1378, BS 52 Washington Univ; MS 56 Southern IL Univ -Carbondale; PH 60 (NS) Southern IL Univ -Carbondale; Prof, UT St U, **A F**

Berg, Janet Beth 6327 Nicolet Avenue South, Minneapolis, MN 55423-1605, (612) 451-7981, BS 82 Univ of MN - Minneap-St Paul; MA 85 Univ of MN - Minneap-St Paul; **SLP**

Berg, Jeanette M 532 Pontiac Lane, Bolingbrook, IL 60439, (312) 887-1130, BS 79 Northern IL Univ - De Kalb; MS 81 IL St Univ - Normal; Aud, Shambaugh Ear & Allergy, **A**

Berg, Joanne Kaye 508 South 16th Street, Hot Springs, SD 57747, (605) 745-4149, MA 85 Univ of SD - Vermillion; 86–Sp-Lang Path, Hot Springs Sch Dist, **SLP**

Berg, Jody Lynn 630 Glen Echo Road, Philadelphia, PA 19119, (215) 627-3830, **SLP**

Berg, Joyce Kennedy 1568 Avenida La Posta, Encinitas, CA 92024, (619) 436-5354, MA 83 Eastern MI Univ; 88–Sp-Lang Path, Private Practice, **SLP**

Berg, Kristi 4520 Westwood Lane, Golden Valley, MN 55416, OM 77 Emory Univ; Sp-Lang Path, Sister Kenny I, **SLP**

Berg, Roberta J 4541 Alla Road #5, Marina Del Rey, CA 90292, (213) 670-1789, MA 75; Aud, Private Practice, **A**

Berg, Mrs Ruth R P O Box 1628, Los Fresnos, TX 78566, (512) 546-0411, BA 60 Temple Univ; Sp-Lang Path, Brownsville ISD, **SLP**

Berg, Mrs Sheryl Swofford 1900 Papeete, Plano, TX 75075, (512) 992-5265, BA 77 Univ of MN - Minneap-St Paul; MA 81 Univ of TX - Austin; Sp/Lang Path, Costal Bend Sp Lang Assoc, **SLP**

Berg, Viola G 6326 Island View Terrace, Gig Harbor, WA 98335, MS 65 CA St Univ - Long Beach; Sp-Lang Path, Private Practice, **SLP LM**

Berg, Virginia K 1280 Claas Avenue, Holbrook, NY 11741, BA 77 Long Island U - CW Post Ctr; MA 80 Long Island U - CW Post Ctr; Sp-Lang Path, Sachem Un Free Sch Dist, **SLP**

Bergamini, Mrs Marcia Higney 63 Lucien Drive, Hamden, CT 06518, (203) 288-8473, BS 59 Southern CT St Univ; MS 83 Southern CT St Univ; Sp-Lang Path, Hamden Bd of Educ, **SLP**

Bergart, Mrs Marlene H 26 Alcott Street, Acton, MA 01720, (617) 263-4112, BS 71 Emerson Coll; ME 76 Northeastern Univ; Sp-Lang Path, Stow Pub Sch, **SLP**

Bergauer, Judith H 2063 Midlothian Road, Roseville, MN 55113, (612) 633-8150, BA 70 Univ of WI - Eau Claire; MS 71 Univ of WI - Eau Claire; Sp Ed Prog Superv, Roseville Ar Sch, **SLP**

Bergen, Mrs Geraldine Gibbia 105 Sylvester Avenue, Hawthorne, NJ 07506, (201) 595-2207, BA 74 Marymount Coll; MA 76 CUNY - Queens Coll; OM 85 CUNY - Grad Sch & Univ Cntr; Dir of Sp & Hearing Clinic, William Paterson Coll, **SLP**

Bergen, Karen Koppel 2426 Benjamin Drive, Mountain View, CA 94043, (415) 961-3389, BA 71 Univ of CA - Berkeley; MA 74 San Francisco St Univ; 88–Tchr, Sunnyvale Elem Sch Dist, **SLP**

Berger, Mrs Barbara B 3736 Laguna Way, Sacramento, CA 95825, (916) 666-8710, BA 55 LA Tech Univ; MA 59 Univ of AR - Fayetteville; Sp-Lang Path, Yolo County Schools, **SLP**

Berger, Charlene B 3069 Rio Bonita Street, Indialantic, FL 32903, (407) 777-0686, BA 65 Univ of FL; MA 77 George Washington Univ; 88–Sp-Lang Path, Brevard County Sch Sys, **SLP**

Berger, Cynthia D 267 Maple Street, East Longmeadow, MA 01028, (413) 525-1570, BS 68 Boston Univ; ME 70 Northeastern Univ; SLP, Lower Pioneer Val Ed Collabtv, **SLP**

Berger, Elliott H 4707 Washington Boulevard, Indianapolis, IN 46205, (317) 872-1111, BS 74; MS 76 NC St Univ at Raleigh; Mgr, E-A-R Div

Berger, Mrs Jeri Skolkin 4301 Lizshire Lane #C-202, Orlando, FL 32822, (305) 281-8767, MS 85 Univ of South FL; 88–Sp-Lang Path, Orange Co Sch Sys, **SLP**

Berger, Jill Melodie 1455 Beacon Street #53, Brookline, MA 02146, (617) 246-3549, BA 83 SUNY - Center at Buffalo; MS 84 Boston Univ; **SLP**

Berger, Mrs Julie Ann Marshfield Clinic, 1000 North Oak Avenue, Marshfield, WI 54449, (715) 387-5371, BS 83 Univ of WI - Oshkosh; MS 85 Univ of WI - Oshkosh; 85–Aud, Marshfield Clinic, **A**

Berger, Kathy M 113 North 2nd Street, Milwaukee, WI 53226, (414) 774-3312, MS 88 Univ of WI - Milwaukee

Berger, Kenneth W 647 Longmere Drive, Kent, OH 44240, (216) 673-5654, BA 49 Univ of Evansville; MS 60 Southern IL Univ -Carbondale; PH 62 (Sp Path & Aud) Southern IL Univ -Carbondale; Prof Emeritus, Kent St U, **SLP A F**

Berger, Linda C 10 Esperanza Drive, Lexington Park, MD 20653, (301) 475-3084, BA 62 Bates Coll; MA 65 Univ of Rochester; MA 77 CUNY - Hunter Coll; 77–Sp-Lang Path, St Mary's Co PS, **SLP**

Berger, Linda S 7950 Henry Avenue #4-C, Philadelphia, PA 19128, (215) 539-8550, BA 82 Temple Univ-Tyler Sch of Art; MA 84 Temple Univ-Tyler Sch of Art; **SLP**

Berger, Mrs Mary B 37 Willowbrook Road, Asheville, NC 28805, (704) 253-5909, BS 77 Appalachian St Univ; OM 79 Auburn Univ - Auburn; Sp-Lang Path, Private Practice, **SLP**

Berger, Mrs Mary I 2222 North Orchard Street, Chicago, IL 60614, (312) 871-1080, BS 63 Northwestern Univ; MA 68 Northwestern Univ; **SLP**

Berger, Mary K Speech-Language Pathology Box 0050, Department Of Physical Medicine And Rehabilitation, University Of Michigan Hospital, Ann Arbor, MI 48109, (313) 936-7080, BA 79 Univ of MI - Ann Arbor; MS 81 Univ of MI - Ann Arbor; Sp-Lang Path, U of MI Med Ctr, **SLP**

Berger, Mildred B P O Box 49948, Sarasota, FL 33578, (813) 955-8321, BS 45 Case Western Reserve Univ; MA 50 Kent St Univ; **SLP LM**

Berger, Phyllis N 42 South Barneburg Road, Medford, OR 97504, (503) 826-3364, BA 62 CUNY - Queens Coll; MA 65 Northern IL Univ - De Kalb; Sp-Lang Path, Jackson Ed Serv Dist, **SLP**

Berger, Mrs Rochelle 5 Lyncrest Road, Peekskill, NY 10566, (914) 739-2152, BS 78 SUNY - Center at Albany; MA 80 CUNY - Hunter Coll; 79–Sp/Lang Path, Putnam/N Westchester BOCES, **SLP**

Berger, Shelley Carpman 85 Colleen Street, Thornhill, ON, Canada L4J 3K2, (416) 747-3093, MS 81 Univ of VT; 88–Sp-Lang Path, York Reg Bd of Educ, **SLP**

Berger, Shirley L 2706 Woodruff Heights, Avon Park, FL 33825, (813) 773-2857, BA 50 IN Univ - Bloomington; MA 54 Univ of IA; 87–Sp-Lang Path, New Medico Rehab Cntr, **SLP**

Berger, Mrs Sue C P O Box 1284, 501 S E 5th Street, Ava, MO 65608, (417) 683-5105, BS 78 Central MO St Univ; MS 83 Central MO St Univ; Sp-Lang Path, Ava R I Pub Sch, **SLP**

Berger, Vicki J Route 1 Box 1219, Hayward, WI 54843, **SLP**

Berger-Landau, Janice M 11810 S W 92nd Terrace, Miami, FL 33186, (305) 274-7198, BS 73 Emerson Coll; MS 74 Baylor Univ; Sp-Lang Path, Private Practice, **SLP**

Berger-Morra, Rita 304 Wellesley Road, Philadelphia, PA 19119, (215) 242-6705, BS 73 Univ of RI; MS 77 CA St Univ - Fresno; Sp-Lang Path, Pub Schs of Philadelphia, **SLP**

Bergeron, Laura 2573-4 Douglas Highway, Juneau, AK 99801, (907) 364-2873, BA 85 OR St Univ; MS 87 Emerson Coll; 88–Sp-Lang Path, Juneau Sch Dist, **SLP**

Bergeron, Linda P Hq Usareur And Seventh Arm, Psc Box 2407, APO New York, NY 09063, BS 73 Univ Southern MS-Hattiesburg; MA 82 Hampton Univ; Tchr, DODDS-Germany, **SLP**

Bergeron, Sena M 1360 Fraser Drive, Fayetteville, NC 28303, (919) 432-3233, BS 77 Univ of Montevallo; MA 80 Univ of TN - Knoxville; Aud, US Govt DOD, **A ACE**

Berger-Reynolds, Mrs Lisa C 4602 Hickory Run Court, Acworth, GA 30101-6407, (404) 971-5870, BA 83 Univ of South FL; BS 84 FL St Univ; MS 86 FL St Univ; 88–Sp-Lang Path, MedTherapy, **SLP**

Bergerson, Jane T S 1013 Steeplechase Drive, Brentwood, TN 37027, (503) 397-5780, BA 73 Univ of WA; OM 75 Univ of WA; **SLP**

Bergert, Mrs Sandra G V 4942 Casa Oro Drive, Yorba Linda, CA 92686-3609, BS 78 Augustana Coll; MS 79 Univ of Northern IA; Sp-Lang Path, Westminster Sch Dist, **SLP**

Bergeson, Mary H P 12720 S W 71st Terrace, Miami, FL 33183, **SLP**

Bergeson, Mrs Rebecca A 9752 Arrowsmith Avenue S, Seattle, WA 98118, (206) 722-7969, BS 65 Univ of OR; ME 71 Northeastern Univ; SLP, Tacoma Pub Schs, **SLP**

Bergey, Mrs Patricia S 2812 Shawn Leigh Drive, Vienna, VA 22180, (703) 938-5536, BA 81 San Francisco St Univ; MS 83 San Francisco St Univ; 87–Sp-Lang Path, Private Practice, **SLP**

Berghauer, Jaye R 2350 North 91 Street, Wauwatosa, WI 53226, (414) 459-8454, **SLP**

Bergin, Eileen Celeste 100 Dudley Street, Dudley Audiology Services, Providence, RI 02905, (401) 331-5511, BA 82 SUNY - Coll at Cortland; MA 84 Univ of Northern CO; 88–Aud, Dudley Aud, **A**

Bergin, Dr Kendall R 10406 Lovell Center Drive, Knoxville, TN 37922, (615) 690-5399, BS 77 Univ of Montevallo; MS 78 Univ of Montevallo; PH 88 (Sp & Hrng Sciences) Univ of TN - Knoxville; 85–Owner, Knoxville Ctr for Early Educ, **SLP**

Bergin, Leslie Ann 11209 Markwell Drive, Oklahoma City, OK 73162, (405) 720-7978, BA 81 Univ of KS; MA 86 Wichita St Univ; **SLP**

Bergin, Mary P 27 Braunston Drive, Fairport, NY 14450, (716) 586-4880, BS 70 Nazareth Coll of Rochester; MS 75 Nazareth Coll of Rochester; Sp-Lang Path, Monroe Cnty Bd Coop Ed Serv 1, **SLP**

Bergl, Mrs Burkett K 101 South Anderson Street, Apartment B, Morganton, NC 28655, (704) 437-5207, BA 49 Univ of CA - Santa Barbara; MA 66 Appalachian St Univ; **SLP A LM**

Bergman, Ingrid R 2581 Gazebo Court, Mississauga, ON, Canada L5L 3M8, (416) 848-7286, OB 73 York Univ - Ontario; OM 75 McGill Univ - Quebec; Dir Sp-Lang Path, Mississauga Hosp, **SLP**

Bergman, Judith L 49 Autumn Lane, Amherst, MA 01002, (413) 637-3280, BA 62 Barnard Coll; MA 65 CUNY - Hunter Coll; Sp-Lang Path, Children's Lang Inst, **SLP**

Bergman, Mrs Judy Merlin 127 Forest Ridge Drive, Sterling Park, VA 22170, (703) 471-4181, BA 71 Univ of Pittsburgh - Pittsburgh; MA 73 Univ of Pittsburgh - Pittsburgh; SLP, Fairfax Co Pub Schs, **SLP**

Bergman, Kathleen S 107 Verde Court, Los Gatos, CA 95030, MS 71 KS St Univ; Sp-Lang Path, **SLP**

Bergman, Mrs Lisa Marie 1911 4th Street #1, Altoona, PA 16601, (814) 942-3629, MS 88 Clarion Univ of PA

Bergman, Mrs Marla Darefsky 439 Pinebrook Boulevard, New Rochelle, NY 10804, (203) 977-4833, BA 77 Hofstra Univ; MA 78 NY Univ; Sp/Lang Path, Stamford Bd of Ed, **SLP**

Bergman, Dr Moe 10 Wissotzky Street, Tel Aviv, Israel, BA 37 Univ of IL - Urbana; MA 39 Columbia Univ Teachers Coll; ED 49 (NS) Columbia Univ Teachers Coll; Prof, Tel-Aviv Univ, **A F H LM**

Bergman, Nikki K 1004 East Ludington Avenue, PO Box 395, Ludington, MI 49431, (616) 843-8430, BS 85 Western MI Univ; MA 88 Western MI Univ; 88–Aud, Tinsley Sp-Lg-Hrg Cons

Bergman, Stephanie 1029 Ackerman Avenue, Syracuse, NY 13210, (315) 487-4653, BA 66 Newark St Coll; ME 67 PA St Univ - Univ Park; Sp-Lang Path, W Genesee Ctrl Sch Dist, **SLP**

Bergman, Wendy O 16926 Rinaldi Street, Granada Hills, CA 91344, (213) 368-5602, **SLP**

Berg-Mattos, Wendy Marie 2091 North Candlewood Lane, Hanford, CA 93230, (209) 584-9782, BA 83 CA St Univ - Fresno; MA 86 CA St Univ - Fresno; 87–Sp-Lang Path, Valley Chldn Hosp-Sp & Hrng Dept, **SLP**

Bergner, Mrs Carla Muntz 512 A Alexander Place, West Point, NY 10996, (914) 446-2406, BS 79 Baylor Univ; ME 80 Univ of GA; **SLP**

Bergounous, Paulette M 2216 New Castle Gap Drive, Gold River, CA 95670, BS 68 De Paul Univ; MS 76 Univ of WI - Stevens Point; Sp-Lang Path, San Juan USD, **SLP**

Bergren, Rebecca 5716 8th Avenue South, Birmingham, AL 35212, MA 80 Eastern MI Univ; SLP, Wayne County Intermed Sch Dist, **SLP**

Bergsagel, Mrs Judith Anna 1803 11th Avenue West, Seattle, WA 98119, (915) 544-2002, BS 74 East TN St Univ; MS 81 Univ of NC - Chapel Hill; SLP, Dept Defense Dependent Schools, **SLP ACE**

Bergstrand, Mrs Cynthia M 17855 Atlas Lane, Granger, IN 46530, (219) 277-6160, BS 74 Northwestern Univ; MA 75 Northwestern Univ; **SLP**

Bergstresser, Mrs Rene Marie 50 Putnam Street, West Newton, MA 02165, (617) 965-5820, BA 71 Rutgers St Univ - Newark; MS 87 Northeastern Univ; 88–Sp-Lang Path, Learning Prep Sch, **SLP**

Bergstrom, Mrs Larrabeth Fendler 102 East 6th Street, Box 245, Milledgeville, IL 61051, (815) 225-7141, BS 83 Northern IL Univ - De Kalb; MA 85 Northern IL Univ - De Kalb; **SLP**

Bergstrom, Sue A 6190 Pinewood Court #304, Willowbrook, IL 60514, Univ of IL - Urbana; Sp-Lang Path, Schaumburg Elememtary Schools, **SLP**

Beridon, Brenda T 4531 Essington, Baton Rouge, LA 70816, (504) 292-3574, BA 72 Southeastern LA Univ; MS 80 Univ of Southwestern LA; Sp-Lang Path, Ascension Parish School Board, **SLP**

Berinbaum, Mrs Penelope V 8300 Sunnycroft Road, Richmond, BC, Canada V6Y 1X6, (604) 277-8590, BS 66 Ithaca Coll; MA 68 Columbia Univ Teachers Coll; SLP, Private Practice, **SLP**

Bering, Charles W 2198 Carlyle Drive N E, Marietta, GA 30062, (404) 973-3003, BS 68 Miami Univ - Oxford; MS 69 Miami Univ - Oxford; Southern Reg Mgr, Siemens Hrng Instruments Inc, **SLP A**

Berins, Mrs Jane Z 4707 Hessmer Avenue, Metairie, LA 70002, (504) 455-4707, BA 64 Univ of FL; **SLP**

Berk, Mrs Barbara B Cornelia Drive, Greenwich, CT 06830, (203) 622-9364, BS 59 Boston Univ; MA 60 Columbia Univ Teachers Coll; Sp-Lang Path, Greenwich Bd of Ed, **SLP**

Berke, Mrs Lisa A 52 Blue Ridge Drive, Simsbury, CT 06089, (203) 658-1239, BS 79 SUNY - Center at Albany; MS 82 Southern CT St Univ; Sp-Lang Path, Hartford Pub Sch, **SLP**

Berkey, David A 11600 Wilshire Boulevard, Suite 114, Los Angeles, CA 90025, (213) 477-1519, BS 74 Boston Univ; MA 76 Univ of CT; Pres/Mgr, Hrng Cen of W Los Angeles Inc, **A**

Berkin, Alissa M 4901 East Sunrise Drive, Tucson, AZ 85718, (602) 577-9057, BA 84 Univ of CA - Santa Barbara; MS 86 Univ of AZ; **SLP**

Berkler, Carla S 408 Chestnut Avenue, Lytton, IA 50561, (712) 297-8913, BA 74 Moorhead St Univ; MS 77 Moorhead St Univ; Sp-Lang Path, Arrowhead AEA, **SLP**

Berkley, Rita K 6855 East Edgewater Drive, Coral Gables, FL 33133, (305) 667-6359, MS 63 Barry Univ; Sp-Lang Path, Dade Co Bd of Pub Instr, **SLP**

Berkman, Mrs Laurel H 620 Wyngate Drive West, North Valley Stream, NY 11580, (718) 670-8000, 51 CUNY - Hunter Coll; 52 OH St Univ; 70–Sp-Lang Path, Visiting Nurse Service of NY-Home Care, **SLP**

Berkman, Linda S 279 South Drexel Avenue, Columbus, OH 43209, BA 73 George Washington Univ; MS 74 SUNY - Center at Albany; **SLP**

Berkman, Sheryl A 66-01 Burns Street #61, Forest Hills, NY 11374, BA 77 SUNY - Center at Buffalo; MS 79 Boston Univ; Sp-Lang Path, BOCES III, **SLP**

Berko, Mrs Deborah R 895 Ridgewood Road, Millburn, NJ 07041, (201) 564-9539, BA 78 George Washington Univ; MS 81 Columbia Univ Teachers Coll; Aud, Neurotologic Assoc Pc, **A**

Berkowitz, Dr Alice O 39 Gramercy Park, New York, NY 10010, (212) 674-9182, BA New York Univ; MA New York Univ; PH 70 (NS) NY Univ; 88–Reg Mgr, Telex Comm Memorex-Telex Inc, **SLP A**

Berkowitz, Helene Rapp 155 West 68th Street, New York, NY 10023, BS 75 NY Univ; MA 77 NY Univ; Sp/Lang Path, Private Practice, **SLP**

Berkowitz, Joyce R 316 South Plum Street, Media, PA 19063, (609) 342-7600, BA 80 Univ of Pittsburgh - Pittsburgh; OM 84 Hahneman Medical Coll; Sp-Lang Path, Head Trauma Ctr Devereux Fndtn, **SLP**

Berkowitz, Mrs Laurie S 21 Maynard Farm Road, Sudbury, MA 01776, (617) 443-4576, BA 80 Univ of MI - Ann Arbor; MS 82 Boston Univ; **SLP**

Berkowitz, Marjorie B 5701 South Colorado Blvd, Littleton, CO 80121, (303) 694-1237, BA 58 CUNY - City College; SLP, Cherry Creek Sch Dist #5, **SLP**

Berkowitz, Michael A 8107 Furlong, Houston, TX 77071, (713) 776-9922, BS 74 Univ of WI - Madison; MS 76 Univ of AZ; Sp-Lang Path, Private Practice, **SLP**

Berkowitz, Mrs Mozelle 82 Wayne Road, Newton, MA 02159, (617) 552-7657, MS 80 Boston Univ; Sp-Lang Path, Newton Pub Sch, **SLP**

Berkowitz, Mrs Nancy E 19 Berkley Lane, Rye Brook, NY 10573, (914) 698-9000, BA 67 SUNY - Center at Buffalo; MS 68 SUNY - Coll at Buffalo; Sp-Lang Path, Sch Dist Spec Prog, **SLP**

Berkowitz, Sherry Lee 50-48 175th Place, Fresh Meadows, NY 11365-1626, BA 81 CUNY - Queens Coll; MA 83 Hofstra Univ; ME 85 CUNY - Queens Coll; 82–Sp-Lang Path, NYC Bd of Educ, **SLP**

Berkowitz, Susan 33 Turnpike Road, New England Center For Autism, Southborough, MA 01772, (617) 481-1015, BA 75 Clark Univ; ME 83 CA St Univ - Fullerton; MS 78 Tulane Univ; 87–Dir Sp-Lang Path Dept, New England Center/Autism, **SLP**

Berkun, Elaine Rose 587 Broadway #G-6, Menands, NY 12204, (518) 399-8100, BS 81 Syracuse Univ; MS 84 Coll of Saint Rose; 84–Sp-Lang Path, Sp & Reading Imprv Ctr Inc, **SLP**

Berlad, Tina Beth 14 Wallis Road, Chestnut Hill, MA 02167, (617) 469-0867, BS 68 Emerson Coll; MS 87 Northeastern Univ; 68–Sp-Lang Path, Westborough MA PS, **SLP**

Berlau, Mrs Marcia L 4205 West 94th Terrace, Prairie Village, KS 66207, (913) 649-4975, **SLP**

Berliant, Yola 6550 Wetherole Street #1-C, Rego Park, NY 11374, (212) 897-2716, BA 73 CUNY - Queens Coll; MA 75 CUNY - Queens Coll; Sp/Lang Path Tchr, NYC Bd Ed, **SLP**

Berlin, Dr Asa J 550 Glenn Road, State College, PA 16803, (814) 237-3487, BA 42 CUNY - Brooklyn Coll; MA 43 Univ of WI - Madison; PH 54 (NS) Northwestern Univ; Prof/Sp-Lang Path, PA St U/Private Practice, **SLP LM**

Berlin, Dr Charles I 2020 Gravier Street, Suite A, New Orleans, LA 70112, (504) 568-4785, BS 53 NY Univ; MS 54 Univ of WI - Madison; PH 58 (NS) Univ of Pittsburgh - Pittsburgh; Prof & Dir Kresge Hrng Labs, Lsu Med Cen, **SLP A F**

Berlin, Donna Susan 179 South Bailey, Romeo, MI 48065, (313) 752-5685, BA 82 MI St Univ; MA 85 MI St Univ; 88–Aud, Woodland Medical Group, **A**

Berlin, Faye M 1202 Robin Hill Apts, 4th Avenue, Voorhees Township, NJ 08043, (609) 541-1181, BA 66 Rutger's St Univ - Douglas Coll; MA 70 Temple Univ; Sp-Lang Path, Camden Cty Pub Sch, **SLP**

Berlin, Melanie Ann 5612-313 Weslo Willow Crc, Greensboro, NC 27409, (919) 768-0886, BS 84 Univ of NC - Greensboro; MA 86 Univ of NC - Greensboro; 86–Aud, Forsyth Head and Neck Assoc PA, **A**

Berlin, Nancy L 7307 Woodley Place, Falls Church, VA 22046, (703) 698-5403, BS 78 James Madison Univ; ME 81 James Madison Univ; 88–Consult/Speechreading Tchr, Private Practice, **A**

Berliner, Ronna 55 Blake Road, Brookline, MA 02146, (617) 731-9566, BA 67 SUNY - Coll at Buffalo; MA 71 Northeastern Univ; Sp-Lang Path, Private Practice, **SLP**

Berlinger, Susan M 3450 Palencia Drive #1407, Tampa, FL 33618-1853, (813) 996-3122, SLP, Pasco County School System, **SLP**

Berlinsky, Dr Stanley L 2829 Connecticut Avenue N W, Washington, DC 20008, PH; **SLP**

Berlin-Stern, Mrs Euna 2001 Granada Drive #0-1, Coconut Creek, FL 33066, (305) 973-1284, BA 51 Adelphi Univ; MA 56 NY Univ; Sp/Lang Path, **SLP**

Bermack, Dr Elaine 70 Knolls Drive North, Manhasset, NY 11040, (516) 627-7679, BA 51 NY Univ; MA 69 Columbia Univ Teachers Coll; PH 88 (NS) NY Univ; Adjunct Asst Prof, St John's Univ, **SLP**

Berman, Beth D 1419 Sylvan Lane, East Meadow, NY 11554, (516) 921-7171, MA 70 NY Univ; Sp-Lang Path, Variety Preschoolers Workshop, **SLP**

Berman, Bonnie 1422 San Vicente Boulevard, Santa Monica, CA 90402-2204, BS 73 Univ of IL - Urbana; MA 74 Northwestern Univ; Sp/Lang Path, St Johns Hosp/Private Practice, **SLP**

Berman, Carol Bauer 1302 Meridene Drive, Baltimore, MD 21239, (301) 435-0392, BS 67 Northwestern Univ; MA 68 Univ of IL - Urbana; Sp-Lang Path, Private Practice, **SLP**

Berman, Mrs Carol P 2801 New Mexico Avenue N W, Apartment 816, Washington, DC 20007, (202) 347-0308, BS 62 Syracuse Univ; MA 64 IN Univ - Bloomington; Dir of Develop, Nat Cen for Cl Infant Prog, **SLP A**

Berman, Deborah A Box 30, Bath, ME 04530, (207) 443-3341, BA 72 Allegheny Coll; MS 74 PA St Univ - Univ Park; Aud, Pine Tree Soc Hndcpd Chld & Ad, **A**

Berman, Mrs Dorothy M 1500 Tyler Avenue, East Meadow, NY 11554, (516) 549-4900, BA 62 Adelphi Univ; MS 65 Adelphi Univ; SLP, BOCES III, **SLP**

Berman, Ira Isaac 25588 Oak Street, Lomita, CA 90717, (213) 326-9328, BA 79 Univ of CA - Los Angeles; MA 84 CA St Univ - Long Beach; 85–Sp-Lang Path, LA USD, **SLP**

Berman, Mrs Jennifer Farmer 1003 Easton Road, Apartment 220C, Willow Grove, PA 19090, (215) 631-9300, BA 82 Univ of CT; ME 84 Univ of VA - Charlottesville; Sp-Lang Path, InSpeech Inc, **SLP**

Berman, Mrs Jeri K 11416 Hounds Way, Rockville, MD 20852, (301) 937-6600, BS 70 Univ of GA; MA 71 Univ of MD - College Park; Sp-Lang Path, Prince Georges Co Board of Ed, **SLP**

Berman, Judy B 3305 Garrison Farms Road, Baltimore, MD 21208, (301) 323-1010, BA 69 Towson St Univ; MS 78 Towson St Univ; Clin Supvr/Instr, Loyola Coll, **SLP**

Berman, Judy S c/o Normas S Berman, Md, 5555 Reservoir Drive #301, San Diego, CA 92120-5138, (619) 449-4301, BS 71 OH St Univ; OM 73 Emory Univ; **SLP A**

Berman, Julie Seibert 30 West 93rd Street Apartment 302 A, Bloomington, MN 55420, (612) 884-2677, BS 83 IL St Univ - Normal; MS 85 Vanderbilt Univ; 88–Sp-Lang Path, Courage Ctr, **SLP**

Berman, Laura B 94 Poplar Street, Nanuet, NY 10954, (212) 360-3720, BA 73 CUNY - City College; MA 77 CUNY - City College; Dir Cl Communicology, Cardinal Cooke Health Care Ctr, **SLP**

Berman, Mrs Laura N 1541 Chalet Drive, Cherry Hill, NJ 08003, (609) 778-0559, BA 73 CUNY - Lehman Coll; MS 74 Columbia Univ Teachers Coll; Aud, Regional ENT Assoc, **A**

Berman, Leslie W 11 Deerfield Road, Sharon, MA 02067, **SLP**

Berman, Mrs Lois M 9524 North Leclaire, Skokie, IL 60077, (312) 676-3995, BS 61 Univ of WI - Madison; MA 65 Northwestern Univ; SLP, Chicago Bd of Ed, **SLP**

Berman, Lynne Winter 95 Ford Avenue, Oneonta, NY 13820, (607) 432-8200, BA 65 Univ of MI - Ann Arbor; MA 67 Univ of WA; Sp-Lang Path, Oneonta City School District, **SLP ACE**

Berman, Dr Marilyn S Audiology Speech Path Service, VA Medical Center, 1670 Clairmont Road, Decatur, GA 30033, (404) 321-6111, BA 61 Univ of MI - Ann Arbor; MA 63 Univ of MI - Ann Arbor; PH 69 (NS) Univ of MI - Ann Arbor; Coord Sp-Lang Path, Vamc Atlanta, **SLP**

Berman, Rachel G 873 Davidson Road, Johnson Apartment, Piscataway, NJ 08854, (201) 932-1333, BA 81 Rutger's St Univ - Douglas Coll; MS 82 Rutgers St Univ -N Brunswick; Sp-Lang Path, Early Intervent Prog Inc, **SLP**

Berman, Mrs Rita W 1111 University Blvd West, Apartment 705, Silver Spring, MD 20902, BA 60 George Washington Univ; MA 66 Catholic Univ of America; Sp-Lang Path, D C Pub Sch, **SLP**

Berman, S Sue W220 S3750 Hidden Court, Waukesha, WI 53186, (414) 224-7349, BA 67 Univ of MI - Ann Arbor; MA 69 Northwestern Univ; 74–Cl Supvr, Marquette U-Sp Path & Aud, **SLP**

Berman, Sheree Ilene 212 Two Independence Place, 6th Street & Locust Walk, Philadelphia, PA 19106, (215) 925-2833, BS 80 Boston Univ; MA 82 NY Univ; Sp-Lang Path, Cooper Hospital/Univ Med Ctr, **SLP**

Berman, Sondra P Monmouth Rehabilitation Pa, Northern Ocean Prof Plaza, 525 Route 70, Lakewood, NJ 08701, (201) 370-8010, BS 71 Trenton St Coll; MA 75 Trenton St Coll; Sp-Lang Path, Monmouth Rehab Pa, **SLP**

Berman, Dr Steven E Medical College Of Pa, 3300 Henry, Philadelphia, PA 19129, (215) 842-6631, OB 70 Univ of Miami; MA 72 Kean Coll of NJ; PH 76 (NS) FL St Univ; Dir of Aud, Med Coll of PA, **SLP A**

Bermejo, Dr Juan J 9001 Duncanson Drive, Bakersfield, CA 93311, (805) 664-1989, PH 84 (Aud) OH Univ - Athens; 87–Aud, Private Practice, **A**

Bermejo, Mrs Kathy Fletcher 9001 Duncanson Drive, Bakersfield, CA 93311, (805) 872-3408, BS 80 OH Univ - Athens; MA 82 OH Univ - Athens; 87–Asst Clinical Supervisor-Slp, Ctr for Neuro Skills, **SLP**

Bermudez, Mrs Leona Brauns 12931 Bubbling Well Road, Santa Ana, CA 92705, (714) 529-2185, BS 66 Towson St Univ; MA 82 CA St Univ - Fullerton; Tchr, Brea-Olinda USD, **SLP**

Bern, Martha Graham 1040 Arlington Way, Martinez, CA 94553, (707) 643-0341, BA 64 Univ of IA; MA 72 CA St Univ - Long Beach; SLP, Vallejo Cty USD, **SLP**

Bernacchio, Mrs Carmela Granata 259 Mineola Boulevard, Mineola, NY 11501, (516) 741-5141, BA 75 CUNY - Queens Coll; MS 79 Adelphi Univ; **SLP**

Bernard, Annella K 3973 Windhaven, Fort Worth, TX 76133, (612) 252-0415, BS 77 Univ of MN - Minneap-St Paul; MS 78 Saint Cloud St Univ; SLP, Fort Worth ISD, **SLP**

Bernard, Carolyn Nicrosi 7230 East Broad Street, Blacklick, OH 43004, (304) 594-1008, **SLP**

Bernard, Dorothy Jean 712 Atalin Street, Mandeville, LA 70448, (504) 626-8546, ME 85 Southeastern LA Univ; 83–Coord, St Tammany Parish Sch Bd, **SLP**

Bernard, Kathryn Ann 809 N Wabash #2W, Chicago, IL 60611, (312) 908-6134, BA 82 Valparaiso Univ; MA 83 Univ of IL - Urbana; Sp-Lang Path, Rehab Inst of Chg, **SLP**

Bernard, Patricia Jane 1490 South Columbine Street, Denver, CO 80210, (303) 733-2361, MS 74 Southern IL Univ -Carbondale; Sp-Lang Path, Denver PS, **SLP**

Bernardin, Lisa R 81 Susie Wilson Road, Essex Junction, VT 05453, (802) 878-7807, BS 76 Miami Univ - Oxford; MS 77 Univ of VT; 88–Sp-Lang Path, Colchester EEE, **SLP**

Bernardini, Deborah M 137 11th Street, La Salle, IL 61301, (815) 434-0857, BS 74 Eastern IL Univ; MS 75 Eastern IL Univ; Sp-Lang Path, Reg Educ Svc Agency, **SLP**

Bernard-Morris, Mrs Laura M 37-27 86th Street, Apartment 2-O, Jackson Heights, NY 11372, (212) 986-6470, BS 79 Coll of Saint Rose; MS 80 Syracuse Univ; Aud-Consult, Precision Acoustic Indust Inc, **A**

Bernardo, Mrs Anita R 438 Commonwealth Avenue, Erlanger, KY 41018, (606) 586-7120, BS 83 Eastern KY Univ; MA 84 Eastern KY Univ; 85–Sp-Lang Path, Boone Co Bd of Educ, **SLP**

Berndt, Alice 424 East Main, Vermillion, SD 57069, (605) 624-2860, MA 83; Aud, Private Practice, **A**

Berndtson, Deborah L 141 Belmont Street, Reading, MA 01867, (617) 942-0050, BA 74 Univ of MA - Amherst; MS 77 Emerson Coll; Aud, Chestnut Hill ENT, **A**

Bernero, Dr Raymond J Crippled Children's Service, DC General Hospital, 19th & Mass Avenue S E, Washington, DC 20003, (202) 675-7324, BS 56 Northwestern Univ; MA 57 Northwestern Univ; PH 82 (Spec Ed Admin) Gallaudet Coll; Ch Aud & Sp-Lang Path, Dc Govt Dept of Human Serv, **A**

Bernhard, Beth A 3816 South Lamar Boulevard, Apartment 1810, Austin, TX 78704, (512) 443-1141, BS 79 Univ of TX - Austin; MA 82 Univ of TX - Austin; 82–Sp-Lang Path, Austin ISD, **SLP**

Bernhardt, Mrs Ann S 2070 Fixlini Street, San Luis Obispo, CA 93401, (805) 543-7694, BA 64 Univ of CA - San Diego; MA 65 Stanford Univ; 88–Sp-Lang Path, Comm Coll Foundation, **SLP**

Bernhardt, Linda Elsie 1220 North 44th Street, Seattle, WA 98103, (206) 547-1846, BS 77 SUNY - Coll at Geneseo; MS 84 Univ of OR; Sp-Lang Path, Valley Med Ctr, **SLP**

Bernholz-Balsam, Lisa H 2316 East 13th Street, Brooklyn, NY 11229, (718) 648-3511, BA 81 CUNY - Brooklyn Coll; MS 84 CUNY - Brooklyn Coll; Audiology, Brooklyn College Speech & Hrng, **SLP A**

Berniard, Terry Peterson 6519 Buene Aire Drive, Charlotte, NC 28212, (318) 828-1767, BA 79 Univ of Southwestern LA; MS 81 Univ of Southwestern LA; Supervisor of Speech Therapy, St Mary Parish School Board, **SLP**

Bernier, Carla Ann 109 Beacon Street, Greenfield, MA 01301, (413) 781-9100, BS 82 Univ of MA - Amherst; MA 84 Univ of MA - Amherst; 86–Sp-Lang Path, Mercy Hosp Sp Hrng Lang Ctr, **SLP**

Bernier, Mrs Cheryl E 36 Norman Street, New Bedford, MA 02744, (617) 997-4511, BA 78 Bridgewater St Coll; MS 80 PA St Univ - Univ Park; Sp-Lang Path, New Bedford Sch Dept, **SLP**

Bernier, Mrs Judith C 84 Railroad Avenue, Rowley, MA 01969, (508) 745-9000, BA 68 Univ of MA - Amherst; MS 69 Emerson Coll; 88–Sp-Lang Path, Shaughnessy-Kaplan Rehab Hosp, **SLP ACE**

Bernier, Karen Marie 244 Lathrop Street, South Hadley, MA 01075, (413) 527-0037, BS 64 Emerson Coll; MA 67 Univ of MA - Amherst; **SLP**

Bernier-Gawle, Carol A 26 Line Street, Easthampton, MA 01027, (413) 527-9295, BS 78 Univ of MA - Amherst; MA 80 Univ of MA - Amherst; Sp-Lang Path, Wn MA Sp/Lang Serv Assoc Inc, **SLP**

Berniger, Therese Marie New England Rehab Hospital, Communication Disorders, 2 Rehabilitation Way, Woburn, MA 01801, (617) 935-5050, BA 82 Our Lady Lake Univ-San Anton; MS 85 Univ of TX - Dallas; **SLP**

Berning, Mrs Alison Ruese 7335 Wells Road, Anna, OH 45302, (419) 628-4080, BS 84 Miami Univ - Oxford; MS 85 Miami Univ - Oxford; **SLP**

Berns, Donna B 1316 DE La Guerra Road, Santa Barbara, CA 93103, (805) 963-4331, BA 74 IN Univ - Bloomington; MA 76 IN Univ - Bloomington; Sp-Lang-Hrng Spec, Santa Barbara Hs Dist, **SLP**

Bernstein, Abby Lou 154 Murray Drive, Oceanside, NY 11572, (516) 536-3635, BA 85 SUNY - Coll at Cortland; MA 86 Hofstra Univ; 87–Aud, NY League for the Hard of Hrng, **A**

Bernstein, Bonnie Lynn 7347 Grant #12, Omaha, NE 68134, (402) 449-6617, BA 82 Univ of Denver; MS 85 Univ of WI - Madison; SLP, Boys Town, **SLP**

Bernstein, Dr Claire M Honey Tree Apartment, 1526-H Split Oak Lane, Richmond, VA 23229, (804) 288-3357, BA 76 CUNY - Queens Coll; MS 78 Columbia Univ Teachers Coll; PH 84 (Aud) Columbia Univ Teachers Coll; 88–Aud, Private Practice, **A**

Bernstein, Dr Deena K 69 Sutton Place, Lawrence, NY 11559, (212) 960-8138, BA 63 CUNY - Brooklyn Coll; MA 67 Temple Univ-Tyler Sch of Art; PH 78 (Sp & Hrng Sciences) CUNY - Grad Sch & Univ Cntr; Assoc Prof, Lehman College City University, **SLP ACE**

Bernstein, Mrs Diane Elizabeth 1749 So Stearns Drive, Los Angeles, CA 90035, (213) 290-1051, BA 81 CA St Univ - Los Angeles; MA 84 CA St Univ - Los Angeles; **SLP**

Bernstein, Mrs Jo Ellen 5628 Appomattox Road, Davenport, IA 52806, (319) 388-9916, BS 66 Purdue Univ - West Lafayette; OM 68 IN Univ - Bloomington; **SLP**

Bernstein, Dr Joyce Edens 3517 Carroll Circle, Huntsville, AL 35801-6102, (205) 536-9741, BS 59 Middle TN St Univ; MA 63 Univ of TN - Knoxville; ED 81 (NS) Vanderbilt Univ; Coord, Al A & M U, **SLP**

Bernstein, Lois M 5939 North 83rd Street, Scottsdale, AZ 85253, (602) 943-3484, BS 66 Univ of Bridgeport; ME 68 Univ of VA - Charlottesville; SLP, Gompers Rehab Cen, **SLP**

Bernstein, Mrs Patricia E 4277 Jackdaw Street, San Diego, CA 92103, (619) 274-9720, BA 54 San Diego St Univ; ME 57 Wayne St Univ; 76–Sp/Lang Path, Sd Unif Sch Dist, **SLP**

Bernstein, Mrs Phyllis Carol 34 Niles Place, Staten Island, NY 10314, (718) 698-3010, BA 74 Kean Coll of NJ; MS 76 CUNY - Brooklyn Coll; Coord of Sp & Hearing Serv, Child Study Center of New York, **SLP**

Bernstein, Mrs Phyllis F 6004 Warm Mist, Dallas, TX 75248, (214) 233-6913, BA 64 Tulane Univ; MA 67 Univ of TX - Austin; **A**

Bernstein, Mrs Rena S 1135 Carrigan Boulevard, Merritt Island, FL 32952, (407) 452-1126, BS 55 NY Univ; MA 74 Seton Hall Univ; Retired, Ridgewood Bd of Ed, **SLP**

Bernstein, Sharon P 110 Monroe Street, Dedham, MA 02026, BS 77 Boston Univ; MS 83 Worcester St Coll; Sp-Lang Path, Private Practice, **SLP**

Bernstein, Sheila H 145-30 22nd Avenue, Whitestone, NY 11357, (718) 359-3110, BA 76 SUNY - Coll at Brockport; MA 80 Long Island U - CW Post Ctr; Sp-Lang Path, Hunter College/Private Practice, **SLP ACE**

Bernstein, Mrs Susan R 2175 Batchelder Street, Brooklyn, NY 11229, (212) 998-3951, BA 72 CUNY - Brooklyn Coll; MS 75 CUNY - Brooklyn Coll; SLP, New York City Bd of Education, **SLP**

Bernstein-Ellis, Ellen Gay 4426 Canoe Birch Court, Concord, CA 94521, (415) 228-6800, BA 81 Univ of CA - Santa Barbara; MS 84 Univ of CA - Santa Barbara; 84–Sp-Lang Path, VA Med Ctr, **SLP**

Bernthal, Mrs Gail 5349 Orchard Street North, Fresno, CA 93710, (209) 225-5052, BS 77 Univ of WA; OM 78 Univ of WA; **A**

Bernthal, John E University Of Nebraska-Lincoln, Lincoln, NE 68583-0738, (402) 472-2145, BA 62 Wayne St Coll; MA 64 Univ of KS; PH 71 (Communciative Disorders) Univ of WI - Madison; Chair Dept Sp Ed Comm Disord, Univ of NB-Lincoln, **SLP A F**

Berntsen, Harold R 706 Heinel Drive, St Paul, MN 55113, (612) 484-9135, MS; **SLP LM**

Berntsen, Jilayne Susan 3706 Grand Avenue #4, Minneapolis, MN 55409, (612) 823-6361, BA 83 Univ of Northern CO; MS 85 IL St Univ - Normal; Sp-Lang Path, Courage Ctr, **SLP**

Bero, Judy A Oxford Towne Apartment E3, Gateshead Road, New Hartford, NY 13413, (315) 724-5101, BS 84 Ithaca Coll; MS 86 FL St Univ; **A**

Berquist, Rebecca Bonini 2143 Robin Road, Lewisville, TX 75067, (214) 436-0418, BA 76 Northern MI Univ; MA 82 Univ of North TX; Aud, Univ of North Texas, **A**

Berreth-Brazier, Lorraine Shelley 1730 Tembroke Street, Topeka, KS 66604, (913) 296-5451, BA 77 Simpson Coll; MA 81 KS St Univ; Qualified Mr Professional, Kansas Neurological Institute, **SLP**

Berrett, Dr M Victor 200 Medical Parkway, Suite 303, Chesapeake, VA 23320, (804) 547-8986, BS 68 UT St Univ; MS 69 UT St Univ; PH 73 (Aud) Univ of IA; Aud, Chesapeake ENT Assoc, **A**

Berrie, Mrs Elaine B 344 Cindy Drive, Fairbanks, AK 99701, (907) 356-2721, BA 64 Univ of CT; ME 74 Univ of GA; 85–Sp-Lang Path, Fairbnk/N Star Borough Sch Dist, **SLP**

Berris, Anastasia 248 Copper Road, San Ramon, CA 94583, (209) 831-5029, BA 80 San Jose St Univ; MA 87 San Jose St Univ

Berry, Mrs Anna Whitley 5001 Lakefront Drive, #C-3, Tallahassee, FL 32303, (904) 562-8141, MA 76 FL St Univ; Sp-Lang Path, Leon Co Pub Sch, **SLP**

Berry, Barbara Suzanne 8 Poplar Place, Fanwood, NJ 07023, (201) 233-3720, BS 78 Old Dominion Univ; MA 84 Kean Coll of NJ; Sp-Lang Path, Chldrns Specialized Hosp, **SLP**

Berry, Mrs Betsy L S 5646 Medeabrook, Agoura, CA 91301, (805) 496-4451, BA 56 PA St Univ - Univ Park; MA 61 San Francisco St Univ; Coord Spec Ed/Esl, Conejo Valley USD, **SLP**

Berry, Bette J Tn State Dept Of Education, 132 Cordell Hull Bldg, Nashville, TN 37219, (615) 741-2851, BA 49 G Peabody Coll-Vanderbilt U; MS 65 G Peabody Coll-Vanderbilt U; Dir/Sp Lang Prog, TN St Dept of Ed, **SLP A**

Berry, Dr Bill 6943 Fords Station, Germantown, TN 38138, (901) 523-8990, BA 66 Wabash Coll; MS 68 Univ of HI - Manoa; PH 71 (Sp Path) Purdue Univ - West Lafayette; Ch Aud/SLP Serv, VA Med Cen, **SLP**

Berry, Cheryl Denise 4238 8th Avenue #202, Los Angeles, CA 90008, (213) 294-5976, MA 87 CA St Univ - Los Angeles; **SLP**

Berry, Debra Marie 612 West Patterson #301, Chicago, IL 60613, (312) 472-6657, OB 83 Univ of MO - Columbia; MA 84 Saint Louis Univ; Sp-Lang Path, La Rabida Children Hospital, **SLP**

Berry, Dr Galen W Audiology Associates, 321 North 2nd Street, Box 207, River Falls, WI 54022, (715) 425-7905, BS 72 KS St Univ; MS 73 KS St Univ; PH 77 (NS) Univ of KS; Pres, Aud Assoc, **A**

Berry, Grant A Speech And Hearing Center, Hospital Of The University Of Pennsylvania, 3400 Spruce Street, Philadelphia, PA 19104, (215) 662-2784, BS 76 Central MI Univ; MA 78 Central MI Univ; Aud, Hosp of the Univ of Pa, **A**

Berry, Jana Marie HC-01 Box 46, Monument, KS 67747, (913) 462-8282, BA 81 Fort Hays St Univ; MS 83 Fort Hays St Univ; Sp-Lang Path, Nkesc, **SLP**

Berry, John S Blount Hearing & Speech Serv, 404 Church Avenue, Professional Bldg Suite 1, Maryville, TN 37801, (615) 982-8557, BA 68 Saint Edward's Univ; MS 72 Univ of TN - Knoxville; Aural Rehab, Blount Hrng & Sp Servs

Berry, Judy O 1392 East 26th Place, Tulsa, OK 74114, (918) 631-2834, BA 66 Univ of OK - Norman; MA 68 KS St Univ; ED 82 (Counseling Psychology) Univ of Tulsa; 87–Prof, The Univ of Tulsa, **SLP**

Berry, Mrs Kathleen M 10632 South Ridgeway, Chicago, IL 60655, (312) 233-6301, BS 69 Western IL Univ; MA 72 CA St Univ - Fullerton; Tchr, St Linus Sch, **SLP**

Berry, Mrs Maryann B 1500 St James Place, Kinston, NC 28501, (617) 726-2762, BA 76 Univ of NC - Chapel Hill; MA 77 George Washington Univ; **SLP**

Berry, Maureen M 57 Pratt Road, Scituate, MA 02066, **SLP**

Berry, Dr Mildred F 4332 Pine Crest Road, Rockford, IL 61107, (815) 399-1131, BA 22 Univ of IA; MA 25 Univ of IA; PH 37 (NS) Univ of WI - Madison; Self Employed, **SLP F H LM**

Berry, Nina J 2909 West 11th, Plainview, TX 79072, (806) 293-7071, BS 74 TX Tech Univ; MS 76 TX Tech Univ; Sp-Lang Path, Plainview ISD, **SLP**

Berry, Patricia 501 Dahlia Avenue, Corona Del Mar, CA 92625, (213) 860-2451, BA 74 CA St Univ - Fullerton; MA 78 CA St Univ - Fullerton; Asst Prof/Sp-Lang Path, Cerritos College, **SLP**

Berry, Mrs Patsy A 4924 Pershing, Fort Worth, TX 76107, (817) 732-1539, BA 50 6841; MA 79 6841; Sp-Lang Path, Ft Worth ISD, **SLP ACE**

Berry, Richard C P O Box 841, Pomona, NJ 08240, (609) 645-7400, BA 67 Univ of MA - Amherst; MA 68 Univ of MA - Amherst; PH 70 (NS) Univ of IL - Urbana; Prog Coord SLP/Aud, Stockton St Coll, **SLP A**

Berry, Robert A Exeter Hearing Clinic, 21 Hampton Road, Exeter, NH 03833, (603) 778-1780, BA 69 Univ of South FL; MS 70 Univ of South FL; Owner/Aud, Exeter Hearing Clinic, **SLP A**

Berry, Sarah E 1610 Saint Ann Street, Jackson, MS 39202, (601) 944-0711, BA 76 Univ of MS; OM 77 Univ of MS; **SLP**

Berry, Mrs Susan Lynn 606 Silver Hill Apartment, Milford, DE 19963, (302) 422-0809, BA 85 Marshall Univ; MA 86 Marshall Univ; 86–Sp-Lang Path, Cape Henlopen Sch Dist, **SLP**

Berry, Virginia S 11701 St Charles Boulevard, Little Rock, AR 72211, (501) 371-2554, BA 71 LA St Univ - Baton Rouge; MS 72 Vanderbilt Univ; 85–Aud, Arkansas Dept of Ed, **A ACE**

Berryman, Mrs Ann Jaleen Foster High School, Attn Ann Berryman, 4242 South 144th Street, Seattle, WA 98168, (206) 246-1277, SLP, South Central Public Schools, **SLP**

Berryman, Mrs Dolores S 510 West Dana Lane, Houston, TX 77024, **SLP**

Berryman, Erika Linette 242 East Hamilton Avenue, El Centro, CA 92243, (619) 353-1445, BS 84 Loma Linda Univ - Riverside; MA 85 Univ of the Pacific; Sp-Lang Path, Central Union HS Dist, **SLP**

Berryman, Janice Lynn 3151 Village Blvd Apt 307, West Palm Beach, FL 33409, (305) 641-1266, BA 82 MI St Univ; MA 84 Wayne St Univ; Sp-Lang Path, School Bd/Palm Beach County, **SLP**

Berryman, Joan D University Of Georgia, 570 Aderhold Hall, Athens, GA 30602, (404) 542-1685, BA 59 Centre Coll of KY; ME 63 Univ of GA; ED 66 (NS) Univ of GA; Assoc Prof, U of GA, **SLP**

Berryman, Joyce Lanham 265 Hoffman Avenue, Morgantown, WV 26505, (304) 293-4258, BS 77 WV Univ; MS 78 Univ of NC - Chapel Hill; Cl Asst Prof, West Virginia U Med Cen, **SLP**

Berry-Shawver, Sally Lu 4359 Garst Mill Road, Apartment D, Roanoke, VA 24018, BS 80 Radford Univ; MS 87 Radford Univ; **SLP**

Bersinger, Don D 1517 East Ridgeway Drive, Fayetteville, AR 72701, (501) 575-4919, BS 52 PA St Univ - Univ Park; MS 55 PA St Univ - Univ Park; PH 73 (NS) PA St Univ - Univ Park; Professor SLP/Aud, University of Arkansas, **SLP A F**

Berson, Ellen M 636 Bernardston Road, Greenfield, MA 01301, (413) 774-2607, BS 69 Boston Univ; ME 70 Boston Univ; Sp-Lang Path, Amherst-Pelham Pub Schs, **SLP**

Berson, Esther 748 Pine Street, Seekonk, MA 02771, (617) 761-7394, BS 84 Worcester St Coll; MS 85 Boston Univ; 88–Sp-Lang Path, Ocean State Rehab Svcs, **SLP**

Berson, Mrs Lauren Goldfarb 2313 Grove Street, Allentown, PA 18104, (215) 799-4111, BS 82 Northeastern Univ; MA 84 Temple Univ; Sp-Lang Path, Carbon Lehigh Inter Unit, **SLP**

Bersson, Robin S Dimensions Sp Lang & Lrng Serv, 20855 N W 1st Avenue, Miami, FL 33169, (305) 653-3764, BA 77 Univ of Miami; MA 80 Univ of Miami; Sp-Lang Path, Dimensions Sp-Lang & Lrng Ser, **SLP**

Berta, Mrs Susan Lea 414 Lantern Way, Windsor, CT 06095, BA 72 MI St Univ; MA 76 Coll of Saint Rose; 88–Sp-Lang Path, Windsor PS Sys, **SLP**

Bertaccini, Ruona M 536 West 111th Street #64, New York, NY 10025, (212) 340-6024, BA 69 Univ of TX - El Paso; MS 71 Univ of Pittsburgh - Pittsburgh; Sp-Lang Path, Private Practice, **SLP**

Bertelsen, Mrs Beth Billman 8006 Kurtland Court, Dexter, MI 48130, (517) 787-1468, BA 84 Univ of MI - Ann Arbor; MA 87 IN Univ - Bloomington; Sp-Lang Path, Jackson Sp & Hrng Clinic, **SLP**

Berthiaume, Mrs Mary Ann 3492 Agnes Street, Jackson, MI 49203, (517) 787-2800, BS 68 Eastern MI Univ; MA 83 Eastern MI Univ; Sp/Lang Path, Jackson Co ISD, **SLP**

Berti, Martha Carol 500 East 73rd Street #C-2, New York, NY 10021, (212) 734-5579, BS 84 SUNY - Coll at Geneseo; MS 85 Syracuse Univ; **SLP ACE**

Bertoldi, Janet Thayer 3420 Santa Maria Way #202, Santa Maria, CA 93455, (805) 937-2511, BA 81 CA St Univ - Fresno; MA 83 Univ of CA - Santa Barbara; Tchr, Orcutt School District, **SLP**

Bertoni, Mrs Martina B 7 Cornwall Circle, St Davids, PA 19087, (215) 688-0727, BS 67 Northwestern Univ; MS 68 Univ of MI - Ann Arbor; Sp/Lang Path, Private Practice, **SLP**

Bertram, Christie C 453 West 3rd Apartment D, Lexington, KY 40508, (606) 254-0265, BA 84 Univ of KY; MS 86 Univ of KY; 88–Sp-Lang Path, Horn Richardson & Assoc, **SLP**

Bertrand, Mrs Judy Davidson 1221 Algonquin Avenue, Suite 304, North Bay, ON, Canada P1B 4Y3, **A**

Bertsch-Hill, Paula 37 Toftree Lane, Dover, NH 03820, **SLP**

Bertucci-Maratea, Susan 4927 West Louise #3, Skokie, IL 60077, (312) 696-6274, BA 80 Saint Xavier Coll; MA 81 Northern IL Univ - De Kalb; 86–Sp/Lang Path, Lutheran Gen Hosp, **SLP**

Berube, Michele E 52 Second Street, South Glens Falls, NY 12803, (518) 761-5333, BS 82 SUNY - Coll at Geneseo; MS 86 Syracuse Univ, SLP, Glen Falls Hospital, **SLP**

Berumen, Sharon 9314 East 49th Street, Tulsa, OK 74145, (918) 663-6397, BS 74 Univ of Tulsa; MA 76 Univ of Tulsa; Sp-Lang Path, Sand Springs Sch, **SLP**

Berwald, Rosemary Rhines 16455 Ferris Avenue, Los Gatos, CA 95030, (408) 356-7224, BA 73 Univ of NH; MA 75 Univ of CT; Sp-Lang Path, Private Practice, **SLP**

Berwick, Mary Jo Route 2 Box 5D, Rociada, NM 87742, (505) 425-8561, BS 81 Eastern MI Univ; MA 82 Eastern MI Univ; Sp-Lang Path, Las Vegas City Schools, **SLP**

Berz, Mrs Sherry K 6832 Wilson Lane, Bethesda, MD 20817, (301) 229-6458, BA 71 George Washington Univ; MA 72 George Washington Univ; 84–Sp-Lang Path, Montgomery Co Public Schools, **SLP**

Berzin, Audrey E 3516 Witherspoon Green, Fremont, CA 94538-3512, (415) 657-2350, BA 60 San Jose St Univ; MA 74 San Jose St Univ; SLP, Fremont USD, **SLP**

Besetzny-Holub, Diane Marie 8938 High Haven, Houston, TX 77083-5812, (713) 467-3911, BS 79 Southwest TX St Univ; ME 80 Southwest TX St Univ; Sp-Lang Path, S/P Assoc, **SLP**

Beshear, Mrs Deborah Wood 151 Carlisle Drive, Madisonville, KY 42431, (502) 825-6038, BS 74 Murray St Univ; MS 83 Western KY Univ; Sp-Lang Path, Hopkins Co Bd of Ed, **SLP**

Beshir, Mary 18 12th S E, Mason City, IA 50401, (515) 423-4436, BS 74 Mankato St Univ; MS 75 Moorhead St Univ; Sp-Lang Path, Nn Trails AEA, **SLP**

Besing, Joan M MIT-RLE, Room 36-747, Cambridge, MA 02139, (617) 253-8134, BA 77 Univ of IA; MS 79 IL St Univ - Normal; PH 88 (Aud/Hrng Science) LA St Univ - Baton Rouge; 88–Post Doctoral Trainee, Mass Inst of Tehc, **A**

Besly, Mrs Nancy S 3311 Otsego, Amarillo, TX 79106, (806) 359-5341, BA 70 Univ of OK - Norman; MA 71 Univ of OK - Norman; Sp/Lang Path, Swisher-Briscoe Educatnl Coop, **SLP**

Besmark, Anna Marie 3671 Lincoln Street, Gary, IN 46408, (219) 886-6510, BS 68 Ball St Univ; MS 73 IN St Univ - Terre Haute; MS 78 Purdue Univ - West Lafayette; Central Office Coord Spec Educ, Gary Community Schools Corp, **SLP**

Besozzi, Ella June 3037 Conlin Drive, Akron, OH 44319, (216) 499-1805, MA 85 Univ of Akron; 71–Sp-Lang Path, Jackson Local Schs, **SLP**

Besozzi, Thomas E 1235 7th Street N E, North Canton, OH 44720-2005, (216) 455-0022, BS 62 Kent St Univ; MA 68 Kent St Univ; Executive Director, Bes-Mont Speech & Language Ctr, **SLP**

Bess, Mrs Christine 3421 Cross Creek Drive, Montgomery, AL 36116, (205) 288-2594, BS 76 Eastern IL Univ; MS 77 Eastern IL Univ; Sp-Lang Path, Auburn U/Montgy, **SLP**

Bess, Fred H Vanderbilt Univ School Of Med, Wilkerson Hrng & Sp Center, 1114 19th Avenue South, Nashville, TN 37212, (615) 322-4099, PH (NS); **A F**

Bess, Laura Ann 45 Litchfield Street #3, Brighton, MA 02135, (617) 862-1004, BA 85 Univ of Northern CO; MA 86 Univ of Northern CO; **SLP**

Bess, Mrs Nanette Monygomery Rural Route 1, Pearl, IL 62361, (217) 723-4093, BA 78 IL Coll; MA 80 Western IL Univ; SLP, Griggsville Comm Unit #4, **SLP**

Bess-Berg, Mrs Doris F 9026 N E 19th Street, Bellevue, WA 98004, (206) 281-6943, BA 69 Univ of WA; OM 70 Univ of WA; Sp-Lang Path, Seattle Pub Sch, **SLP**

Bessel, Harriet W 8601 Cottington Road, Baltimore, MD 21236, (301) 444-5000, BA 70 CUNY - Queens Coll; MA 72 CUNY - Queens Coll; Prog Dir, The MD Sch for the Blind, **SLP**

Bessell, Laura Anne 4294 Greensboro, Troy, MI 48098, (313) 627-4981, BS 85 Central MI Univ; MA 87 Central MI Univ; **SLP**

Besser, Joyce A T 14766 Oak Run Lane, Burnsville, MN 55337, (612) 423-9427, BS 59 Univ of MN - Duluth; MA 80 Univ of MN - Duluth; Dir of Spec Educ, Rosemount/Apple Valley Schls, **SLP**

Bessler, Mrs Ramona M 2330 West Sumner, Lincoln, NE 68522, (402) 473-0278, BA 76 Kearney St Coll; MS 79 Univ of NE - Omaha; Sp-Lang Path, Lincoln Public Schools, **SLP**

Bessom, Mrs Kathy K 1901 Elmhurst Drive, Athens, TN 37303, (615) 745-6313, BS 75 Univ of TN - Knoxville; MA 77 Univ of TN - Knoxville; Sp-Lang Path, Private Practice, **SLP**

Best, Karen P Lincoln Way Spec Ed Res Center, 1450 West Main Street, P O Box 166, Louisville, OH 44641, (216) 875-9996, BS 75 OH Univ - Athens; MA 79 Kent St Univ; Sp-Lang Path, Lincoln Way Spec Ed Res Center, **SLP**

Best, Lorraine D Route 2 Box 421, Tuscola, IL 61953, (217) 253-4505, MS 84 Eastern IL Univ; 85–Sp-Lang Path, Champaign Unit 4 Sch Dist, **SLP**

Best, Mrs Pamela O'Bryan 4951 Clairemont Square Suite 306, San Diego, CA 92117, (619) 273-3277, MA 86 Univ of CO - Boulder; 88–Aud, HearCare

Best, Robin 3 Annandale Road, Commack, NY 11725, (516) 938-5400, BA 79 Adelphi Univ; MA 81 Hofstra Univ; Sp/Lang Path, Plainview Old Bethpage Sch Dst, **SLP**

Best, Sharon Larson 1325 Whenona Drive, Madison, WI 53711, (608) 267-6174, BA 76 Univ of WI - Madison; MS 85 Univ of WI - Madison; Sp-Lang Path, Meriter Hosp, **SLP**

Beste, Ann Margaret Rt 1 Box 65, Civa, MT 59274, (406) 525-3377, MA 84 Univ of MN - Duluth; Sp-Lang Path, Roof Valley Spec Ed Coop, **SLP**

Beste, Patrick D Immanuel Rehab Center, 6901 North 72nd Street, Omaha, NE 68122, (402) 572-2197, BS 72 Univ of NE - Lincoln; MA 73 Univ of NE - Lincoln; 88–Admin Dir, Immanuel Rehab Ctr, **SLP**

Besten, Mrs Michelle Borror 1621 Lindy Lane, Lexington, KY 40502, (606) 234-1001, BA 81 Univ of KY; MS 85 Univ of KY; 85–Sp-Lang Path, Harrison Co Bd of Educ, **SLP**

Beswick, Jane D 23 Hale Street, Beverly, MA 01915, (508) 922-0128, BA 64 Elms Coll; MA 70 Emerson Coll; Sp-Lang Path, Ipswich Pub Sch, **SLP**

Betancourt, Lisette M Miami Children's Hosp, 6125 SW 31st, Miami, FL 33155, (305) 666-6511, MA 85 Northwestern Univ; 86–Sp-Lang Path, Miami Children's Hosp, **SLP**

Betancourt, Susan Wahl 6412 Malibu Drive, Raleigh, NC 27603, (919) 733-0762, BS 79 SUNY - Coll at Geneseo; MS 83 East Carolina Univ; 88–Sp-Lang Path, Dorothea Dix Hosp, **SLP**

Bethel, Mrs Patsy M 2377 Rullion Greenway, Henderson, KY 42420, (812) 479-1411, BS 77 Murray St Univ; MS 80 Vanderbilt Univ; Aud, The Rehabilitation Ctr, **A**

Bethke, Mrs Darla H 28421 Ronea, Mission Viejo, CA 92692, (213) 865-7474, BS 62 Univ of WI - Madison; Sp-Lang Path, Cypress ISD, **SLP**

Bethke, Mrs Dorothy P 1121 Fox Chase, Centerville, OH 45459, (513) 433-6355, BS 64 Univ of WI - Madison; Sp-Lang Path, Private Practice, **SLP**

Bethke, Nancy Lanell 3611 Keystone Avenue, Baltimore, MD 21211, (301) 396-8987, MS 86 Towson St Univ; 86–Sp-Lang Path, Balt City PS, **SLP**

Betines, Mary Alice 403 Cindy Street, Old Bridge, NJ 08857, (201) 679-4312, BA 85 Univ of DE; MA 86 Northwestern Univ; Aud, Children's Specialized Hosp, **A**

Betit, Suzanne L 4012 Ridgeway, Juneau, AK 99801, BS 74 Univ of VT; ME 77 Univ of VA - Charlottesville; Res Analyst, Dept of Transp/Pub Facilities, **A**

Betley, Nora 7341 Revere Street, Philadelphia, PA 19152, (215) 338-9766, BA 84 Temple Univ; MA 87 Temple Univ; **SLP**

Betros, Cecil G, Jr Communication Concepts & Consulting, PO Box 131058, 201 Morningside Circle, Birmingham, AL 35213, (205) 871-3626, BS 74 Univ of Montevallo; MS 75 Univ of Montevallo; Pres, Comm Concepts & Consulting, **SLP**

Betsworth, Mrs Anne Hogue Aud Clinic Ctr For Health Science, 10833 Le Conte Avenue, Room 62-202, Los Angeles, CA 90024, (213) 825-5721, BS 65 Univ Southern MS-Hattiesburg; MS 66 Univ Southern MS-Hattiesburg; Aud, UCLA Medical Center, **A**

Bettigole, Donna Klein 4421 45th Street N W, Washington, DC 20016, (202) 362-2403, BA 77 SUNY - Center at Stony Brook; MS 81 Columbia Univ Teachers Coll; Sp-Lang Path, Mount Vernon Hosp, **SLP**

Betts, Dr Carl E University Hospital School, University Of Iowa, Iowa City, IA 52241, (319) 353-3649, BA 51 Univ of IA; MA 55 Univ of IA; PH 63 (NS) Univ of IA; Dir SLP & Aud Serv, U of IA-Spec Chld Hlth Serv, **SLP F**

Betts, Jeri-Lynn 107-1/2 North Montgomery, Watertown, WI 53094, (414) 261-3050, BS 76 Univ of WI - Oshkosh; MS 77 Univ of WI - Stevens Point; 88–Tchr, Watertown Sch Dist, **SLP**

Betty, Charles Jones 1406 55th Street, Columbus, GA 31904, (404) 327-8630, BA 50 Univ of the South; MA 56 Univ of AL- Tuscaloosa; ME 84 Columbus Coll; Sp-Lang Path, Oak Manor Nursing Home, **SLP**

Betz, Susan E 1610 East 3rd Street, Duluth, MN 55812, (218) 728-4951, BA 74 Univ of MN - Duluth; MA 87 Univ of MN - Duluth; 87–Sp-Lang Path, InSpeech Inc, **SLP**

Betzig, Lynn Louise 3721 Mount Ashmun Place, San Diego, CA 92111, (619) 571-0453, BA 83 Univ of WI - Madison; MS 87 Univ of WI - Oshkosh; **A**

Beuckman, Sharon P Memorial Hospital, 4501 North Park Drive, Belleville, IL 62223, MS; **SLP**

Beukelman, Dr David R 7630 Cooper Avenue, Lincoln, NE 68506-0731, (402) 472-5463, BA 65 Western MI Univ; MS 68 Univ of WI - Madison; PH 71 (NS) Univ of WI - Madison; Prof, Univ of NE, **SLP F**

Beukema, Hermine 1467 West Catalpa Avenue, Apartment 3, Chicago, IL 60640, (312) 943-5511, OB 55 Northwestern Univ; MA 59 Univ of Chicago; MA 60 Northwestern Univ; **SLP**

Beutke, Kenneth Paul 1513 Manhattan Drive, Streator, IL 61364, (815) 672-4320, BS 84 IL St Univ - Normal; MS 85 IL St Univ - Normal; Sp-Lang Path, St Marys Hosp, **SLP**

Beuttler, Deborah B 511 Crest View #131, Belmont, CA 94002, (415) 282-2551, BA 80 Univ of Redlands; MS 82 San Francisco St Univ; Sp/Lang Path, St Lukes Hrng & Sp Cen, **SLP**

Bevacqua, Yvette Lynn 6809 Bonnie Ridge Drive, Apt T-2, Baltimore, MD 21209, (301) 578-5602, BA 83 Univ of RI; MA 84 George Washington Univ; Sp-Lang Path, Sinai Hosp of Baltimore, **SLP**

Bevan, Mrs Debora Lee 61 South 700 West, Blackfoot, ID 83221, (208) 684-3430, BA 81 Brigham Young Univ; OM 83 Brigham Young Univ; 88–Sp-Lang Path, Blackfoot Sch Dist, **SLP**

Bevan, Mrs Joann L 100 East Oak Avenue #A-9, Glenolden, PA 19036, (215) 985-4964, BS 86 Bloomsburg Univ of PA; MS 87 Bloomsburg Univ of PA; **A**

Bevan, Dr Marlene A Audicare Hearing Center, 802 A South Garfield Avenue, Traverse City, MI 49684, (616) 947-2324, BA 72 CA St Univ - Los Angeles; MS 73 Univ of Redlands; PH 80 (Aud) Univ of CT; Dir/Aud, Audicare Hrng Ctr, **A**

Bevan, Richard C Newtown Park Plaza Apt G-1, Newtown, PA 18940, MS

Bevan, Ronnie E 1075 Brown Road, Bridgewater, NJ 08807, (201) 725-3788, **SLP**

Bevans, Denise Dardaris 31 Brenner Road, Coram, NY 11727, (214) 522-8220, BS 78 Kutztown Univ of PA; MA 85 Trenton St Coll; **SLP**

Bever, Mrs Donna J 13 Beech Hill Drive, Londonderry, NH 03053, (603) 432-6929, BA 77 Bridgewater St Coll; MA 79 OH Univ - Athens; Sp-Lang Path, Londonderry Sch Dist, **SLP**

Beveridge, Lynn Ruth 47 Broadview Street, Newington, CT 06111, (203) 666-9529, BS 75 Univ of Hartford; MS 79 Southern CT St Univ; Sp-Lang Pathologist, CT Dept Mental Retardation, **SLP**

Beveridge, Susan Eileen 1847 Silvana Lane, Santa Cruz, CA 95062, (408) 462-9109, BA 76 CA St Univ - Fresno; MA 79 CA St Univ - Fresno; Sp-Lang Path, Scotts Valley Un Sch Dist, **SLP**

Beveridge-Wavering, Mrs Agnes 511 West Reynolds, Springfield, IL 62702, (217) 525-3176, BS 70 IL St Univ - Normal; MS 73 IL St Univ - Normal; SLP, Springfield Sch Dist #186, **SLP**

Beverly, Brenda Lee 106 Hillcrest Terrace, Florence, SC 29501, (803) 662-7602, BS 85 Bloomsburg Univ of PA; MS 86 Bloomsburg Univ of PA; 86–Sp-Lang Path, Pee Dee Speech & Hearing Ctr, **SLP**

Beverly, Robin C 29 Paseo, Lamar, CO 81052, (719) 336-2022, BA 75 Univ of Northern CO; MA 76 Univ of Northern CO; Sp-Lang Path, Southeast BOCES, **SLP**

Beverly-Ducker, Mrs Karen L 19821 Cochrane Way, Gaithersburg, MD 20879, (202) 387-3776, BA 76 Univ of MD - College Park; MA 77 Univ of MD - College Park; **A**

Beverly-Walker, Amy S 11205 Quietwood Court, Charlotte, NC 28226, (704) 372-7790, BS 77 WV Univ; MS 78 WV Univ; 85–Sp-Lang Path, Mecklenburg Co Cnt Human Dev, **SLP**

Beverung, John William 100 Glasgow Court, Greenville, SC 29607, (803) 292-5154, BS 82 Univ of WI - Madison; BS 82 Univ of WI - Madison; MA 83 Univ of FL; 86–Sp-Lang Path, Sp L P Services, **SLP**

Bevins, Carla McKenzie 2912 N W 104th Court #1, Gainesville, FL 32606, (813) 996-3600, MS 86 Univ of South FL; **SLP**

Bewley, Mrs Nancy A 1928 Wren Drive, Munster, IN 46321, (312) 333-7812, BA 76 IN Univ - Bloomington; MA 78 IN Univ - Bloomington; 80–Sp-Lang Path, S Metro Asson, **SLP**

Bex, Mrs Margaret Ann 35 Pearl Street, Camden, ME 04843, (207) 236-2101, BS 61 Univ of IL - Urbana; **SLP**

Bey, Krista M P O Box 1593, Camden, NJ 08101, **SLP**

Beyer, Mrs Elaine M Box 42, 93 Cattaraugus T, Springville, NY 14141, (716) 662-0135, BS 58 SUNY - Coll at Buffalo; MS 70 SUNY - Coll at Buffalo; Supervisor of Special Educ, Erie #2 Chautauqua-Cattaraugus BOCES, **SLP**

Beyer, Kerry Lee 2090 Wyndham Hill Drive NE #302, Grand Rapids, MI 49505, (616) 776-2034, BS 84 Marquette Univ; MS 86 Marquette Univ; Sp-Lang Path, Butterworth Hosp, **SLP**

Beyer, Norman L Hearing & Speech Care Incorporated, Rt 1 Box 98, Centertown, MO 65023, (314) 796-3279, BA 59 Univ of Northern CO; MA 71 Univ of MO - Columbia; Sp-Lang Path/Aud, Hrng & Sp Care, **SLP A**

Beyer, Willena A 8512 Golden Avenue, Lemon Grove, CA 92045, **A**

Beykirch, Dr Hugh L 2122 Bicentennial Drive, Cedar Falls, IA 50613, (319) 273-2496, BA 68 Wayne St Univ; MA 69 Wayne St Univ; PH 74 (NS) Wayne St Univ; 79–Assoc Prof of Aud, U of Northern Iowa, **A**

Bezdek, Kathleen Terese 2052 West Parkway, De Land, FL 32724, (904) 734-4327, BA 81 LA St Univ - Baton Rouge; MA 82 LA St Univ - Baton Rouge; 85–Aud/Owner, DeLand Hearing Clinic, **A**

Bezdeny, Barbara Drake 45 Needham Street, North Chelmsford, MA 01863, (617) 454-5431, BA 62 Univ of MA - Amherst; MA 61 Univ of MA - Amherst; Sp-Lang Path, Lowell Pub Sch Dept, **SLP**

Bezonsky, Deborah A 15453 Sutton Street, Sherman Oaks, CA 91403, (818) 501-6636, **SLP**

Bezozo, Sheila G 2072 Lawry Lane, Merrick, NY 11566, (516) 791-5490, BA 71 Hofstra Univ; MS 74 Hofstra Univ; MA 79 Hofstra Univ; Sp-Lang Path, Valley Strm Ufsd #24, **SLP**

Bhardwaj, Mrs Kathern A 366 Cannon Green, Goleta, CA 93117, (805) 968-6938, BA 70 Univ of CA - Santa Barbara; MA 76 Univ of CA - Santa Barbara; SLP, Goleta Union Sch Dist, **SLP**

Bhathal, Inderjit Kaur 5703 Seminole Street, College Park, MD 20740, (202) 529-7600, BA 83 Univ of MD - College Park; **SLP**

Bhatnagar, Dr Subhash C Speech Path & Audiology Dept, Marquette University, Milwaukee, WI 53233, (414) 224-7349, MA 74 Univ of Rochester; MA 76 SUNY - Center at Buffalo; PH 79 (NS) Univ of Rochester; Asst Prof, Marquette Univ, **SLP**

Biagini, Mrs Elizabeth Duffy 100 Bryn Mawr Court, West 416, Pittsburgh, PA 15221, (412) 241-2467, BA 81 Duquesne Univ; MA 83 Univ of Pittsburgh - Pittsburgh; Aud, Pittsburg ENT Assoc, **A**

Bialas, Susan Nallen 19 Barbara Avenue, Auburn, MA 01501, (508) 832-7431, BS 78 Univ of MA - Amherst; MS 80 Southern CT St Univ; 87–Sp-Lang Path, VNA of Southern Worcester Co, **SLP**

Biales, Mrs Cynthia Dipaola 40 Sylvan Park Court, Baltimore, MD 21236, (301) 396-9274, BS 79 SUNY - Coll at Buffalo; MS 83 Towson St Univ; 80–Sp/Lang Path, Baltimore Cty Pub Sch, **SLP**

Bialo, Nancy Kaye 37 Locust Avenue, Larchmont, NY 10538, **SLP**

Bialostozky, Franklin 10207 Lariston Lane, Silver Spring, MD 20903, (301) 434-4300, BS 72 CUNY - Brooklyn Coll; MA 76 Northwestern Univ; Aud, Auditory Services Inc, **A**

Bialzik, Barb J 357 Heritage Lane, Rosholt, WI 54473, (715) 446-2093, BS 79 Univ of WI - River Falls; MS 86 Univ of WI - Stevens Point; 87–Sp-Lang Path, DC Everest Sch Dist, **SLP**

Biamon, Carmen Teresa Zone M-243, Villa Caparra, Guaynabo, PR 00657, (809) 781-7077, BS 76; ME 78 Clarion Univ of PA; Sp-Lang Path, Inst De Orientacion & Terapia, **SLP**

Biancardi Krukowski, Mrs Dawn P O Box 317, Washington Depot, CT 06794, (203) 868-0156, **SLP**

Bianchi, Patricia 1128 Wavell Road, Schenectady, NY 12303, (518) 861-8528, BA 65 SUNY - Center at Albany; MS 66 PA St Univ - Univ Park; Aud, Guilderland Ctrl Sch, **A**

Bianco, Carol 1740 N W 97th Terrace, Plantation, FL 33322, (305) 370-7513, BA 72 Univ of Miami; ME 73 Univ of Miami; Except Stu Educ Spec, Sch Bd of Broward County FL, **SLP ACE**

Bianco, Ellenbeth One Bay Club Drive #1S, Bayside, NY 11360, (212) 225-8651, BA 77 Adelphi Univ; MS 78 Rutgers St Univ -N Brunswick; 78–Sp-Lang Path, Northshore Commun Consult, **SLP**

Bianco, Penny L 85 Packard Street, Rochester, NY 14609, (716) 328-0120, BA 80 SUNY - Coll at Cortland; MS 83 Nazareth Coll of Rochester; Sp-Lang Path, Rochester City Sch Dist, **SLP**

Bianco-Vasquez, Andrea Louise 11723 Jonny Lane, San Diego, CA 92126, (619) 449-2363, BS 78 CA St Univ - Hayward; MA 85 San Diego St Univ; **SLP**

Biancuzzo, Mrs Marjorie Beth 48 Whitney Circle, Swansea, MA 02777, (401) 253-4000, Sp-Lang Path, Bristol Pub Schs, **SLP**

Biasatti-Croak, Lynne 3208 Nogales Court, Lafayette, CA 94549, (415) 937-4595, BS 80 CA St Univ - Hayward; MA 83 San Jose St Univ; SLP, Fairfield USD, **SLP**

Bias-Scott, Mary Ellen 1918 West 112th Street, Los Angeles, CA 90047, (213) 757-4181, BA 71 Univ of MA - Amherst; MA 72 Univ of MA - Amherst; SLP, Los Angeles USD, **SLP ACE**

Biberdorf, Peggy Schorsch 1415 8th Avenue S #16, Grand Forks, ND 58201, (701) 775-2694, BA 80 Univ of ND; MS 82 Minot St Univ; Sp-Lang Path, Human Comm Assoc Ltd, **SLP**

Biberdorf, Vicki Lynn 152 Country Wood Circle, Nashville, TN 37214, (615) 885-9431, BA 84 Valparaiso Univ; MA 85 Saint Louis Univ; Sp-Lang Path, Rebound Inc, **SLP**

Bible, Judith Anne 2223 McClintock Road, Charlotte, NC 28205, (704) 372-3300, BS 82 Bowling Green St Univ; MA 85 Kent St Univ; Aud, Mecklenburg Ctr for Human Dev, **A**

Bichler, Amy C 10025 Queens Boulevard #3P, Flushing, NY 11375-2454, (516) 378-2000, BA 80 Hofstra Univ; MA 82 CUNY - Queens Coll; Sp/Lang Path, UCP-Nassau Co, **SLP**

Bickerstaff, Mrs Jane Hanneman 5057 Cooper Road, Stockbridge, MI 49285, (517) 483-2700, BA 85 MI St Univ; MA 86 MI St Univ

Bickett, Jeanne Lanovara 4021 Milo Avenue, Bakersfield, CA 93313, (805) 397-8814, BA 81 CA St Univ - Stanislaus; MA 85 CA St Univ - Stanislaus; **SLP**

Bickford, David L 96 Dunphy Drive, Northampton, MA 01060, (413) 323-6311, BA 70 Univ of MA - Amherst; MA 76 Univ of MA - Amherst; Clinical Specialist, Head Injury Ctr/Pioneer Valley, **SLP**

Bickford, Mrs Vernenna Donell 21 Setzer Drive, Barboursville, WV 25504, (614) 532-6451, BA 83 Marshall Univ; MA 84 Marshall Univ; 84–Sp-Lang Path, Dawson-Bryant Local Schs, **SLP**

Bickham, Carol M 905 Baldwin #D-8, Waukegan, IL 60085, (312) 360-5437, BA 76 Augustana Coll; MS 77 Eastern IL Univ; 78–Head Sp-Lang Path Dept, Waukegan Pub Sch Dist #60, **SLP**

Bickings, Mrs Jayme J 36 Kinkle Road, Bridgeton, NJ 08302, (609) 453-0076, BS 76 TX Woman's Univ; MA 77 TX Woman's Univ; Sp-Lang Path, Hopewell Crest Sch-R Gable, **SLP ACE**

Bickley, Mrs Minda S 338 East Allen Street, Lancaster, OH 43130, (614) 422-9920, BA 82 OH St Univ; MA 83 OH St Univ; **SLP**

Bicknell, Mrs Gertrude L P O Box 6604, Hamden, CT 06517, (203) 288-2464, BS 70 Western CT St Univ; MS 75 Southern CT St Univ; SLP, Trumbull Board of Education, **SLP**

Bicky, Linda 251 174th Street #1417, North Miami Beach, FL 33160, (305) 931-4616, BA 82 Univ of FL; MA 87 George Washington Univ; 87–Sp-Lang Path, Hearing & Speech Ctr of FL, **SLP**

Bidoli, Diane E 170 Promenade Street, Ridge Vue Manor #1, Crafton, PA 15205, (412) 621-0100, **SLP**

Bidwill, Bettye J 800 Happ Road, Northfield, IL 60093, BS 73 OK St Univ; MA 75 Univ of Denver; **SLP**

Bieber, Catherine R 1136 North Dunton Avenue, Arlington Heights, IL 60004, (312) 259-8500, BS 72 Northern IL Univ - De Kalb; MA 74 Northern IL Univ - De Kalb; MA 83 Univ of Reading - England; 76–SLP, Township Hs Dist #214, **SLP**

Bieber, Karen M 10253 Yorktown Lane, Maple Grove, MN 55369, (612) 425-0577, BS 69 Mankato St Univ; MS 79 Mankato St Univ; Sp-Lang Path, Osseo ISD #279, **SLP**

Biedscheid, Melia Collette c/o Medical Arts Hearing Services, 210 Sunnyview Lane, Suite 101, Kalispell, MT 59901, (406) 752-1014, BA 80; 86–Aud, Med Arts Hearing Svcs, **SLP A**

Biegert, Mrs Janice L 1767 Wood Lane, Mount Prospect, IL 60056, (312) 794-3965, BA 59 Carleton Coll; MA 61 Univ of IA; 74–Sp-Lang Path, Henry Horner Childrens Ctr, **SLP**

Biegner, Laura Marie 966 Vetch Circle, Lafayette, CO 80026, (303) 492-8551, MA 85 Univ of CO - Boulder; BA 82 Univ of CO - Boulder; **SLP**

Biegun, Deborah Lee 11730 Washington Blvd #2, Los Angeles, CA 90066, (213) 397-8990, BA 79 Univ of CA - Los Angeles; MA 84 CA St Univ - Northridge; 86–Sp-Lang Path, Los Angeles Co Ofc of Educ, **SLP**

Biehl, Larry V Area Education Agency 4, 102 South Main Avenue, Sioux Center, IA 51250, (712) 722-4374, BA 70 Kearney St Coll; MS 72 Univ of NE - Lincoln; 75–Superv/Speech-Lang Services, AEA 4, **SLP**

Biehn, Susan S 101 11th Avenue North, South St Paul, MN 55075, (612) 293-7635, BS 75 Mankato St Univ; MS 79 Univ of WI - River Falls; SLP, Bridgeview School, **SLP**

Bieker, Rebecca R 5440 Netherland Avenue, Bronx, NY 10471, (212) 904-2677, BA 75 Univ of MO - Columbia; MA 78 Northern IL Univ - De Kalb; Aud, A Einstein Coll of Med, **A**

Biel, Mrs Claire D 24151 Letchworth Road, Beachwood, OH 44122, (216) 371-7312, BS 55 Northwestern Univ; MA 75 Cleveland St Univ; Sp-Lang Path, Cleveland Hts - U Hts Bd of Ed, **SLP ACE**

Biel, Mrs Joanne Ring 4965 Forestview Lane, Plymouth, MN 55442, (612) 927-3838, BS 80 Univ of MN - Minneap-St Paul; MA 82 Northwestern Univ; Sp-Lang Path, Park Nicollet Medical Center, **SLP ACE**

Bielak, Mrs Elizabeth Ann 26237 Springland Drive, Farmington Hills, MI 48018, (313) 477-4196, BS 81 Wayne St Univ; MA 83 Wayne St Univ; Sp/Lang Path, Health Care Pro Ltd, **SLP**

Bielecki, Debra Shiro 1515 Nuuanu Avenue, Queen 73, Honolulu, HI 96817, (808) 947-8235, BS 73 Univ of HI - Manoa; OM 76 Univ of WA; Sp-Lang Path, Kapiolani Med Ctr, **SLP**

Bielefeldt, John M 2106 7th Avenue #4, Moline, IL 61265, (309) 793-2009, BS 75 IL St Univ - Normal; MS 76 IL St Univ - Normal; Chief/SLP, Franciscan Med Cen-Rehab Cen, **SLP**

Bielinski, Mrs Di Anne S 5613 West 99th Street, Oak Lawn, IL 60453, (312) 422-1325, BS 69 Marquette Univ; MA 75 Governors St Univ; Sp-Lang Path, Chicago Bd of Ed, **SLP**

Bielitz, Roberta Ann 1003 Justin Lane #1099, Austin, TX 78757, (512) 483-3115, BS 81 LA St Univ - Baton Rouge; MA 84 LA St Univ - Baton Rouge; 87–Sp-Lang Path, Austin ISD, **SLP**

Bielmaier, Catherine Ann PO Box 2369, Avon, CO 81620, (303) 949-6382, BS 83 SD St Univ; MA 86 Univ of Northern CO; 88–Sp-Lang Path, Eagle County Sch Dist

Bielski, Mrs Lee S 5035 Klingle Street N W, Washington, DC 20016, (202) 676-6352, BS 40 OH Univ - Athens; MA 44 Univ of MI - Ann Arbor; Prof of Sp, George Washington U, **SLP LM**

Biemer, Carole Ann 10870 North Stelling Road, Apartment 28E, Cupertino, CA 95014, (408) 998-7277, BS 65 PA St Univ - Univ Park; MS 69 Purdue Univ - West Lafayette; SLP, Santa Clara Co Ofc of Educ, **SLP**

Bienvenue, Dr Gordon R Dept Of Speech Communication, State Univ Of New York, College At New Paltz, New Paltz, NY 12561, (914) 257-2030, BA 68 Univ of MA - Amherst; MA 69 MI St Univ; PH 75 (NS) PA St Univ - Univ Park; Assoc Prof, SUNY-New Paltz, **A**

Bier, Barbara N 45 Nutmeg Ridge, Ridgefield, CT 06877, (201) 431-3614, BA 75 SUNY - Center at Buffalo; MA 77 CUNY - Queens Coll; 87–SLP, Ridgefield PS, **SLP**

Bier, Margaret C Route 3 Box 225-B, Crowley, LA 70526-9413, **SLP**

Bierbaum, Mrs Agnes M 2627 Sugar Bush Lane, Dryden, NY 13053, (607) 753-9301, BS 55 Southeast MO St Univ; MA 65 Univ of MO - Columbia; Sp-Lang Path, Onondaga-Cortland-Madison BOCES, **SLP**

Biere, Julia Ann 705 Vendome Lane, Manchester, MO 63011, (314) 391-8882, MS 87 Fontbonne Coll

Bierly, Mrs Debra Roth 208 Pembroke Drive, Reading, PA 19607, (717) 569-7331, BS 76 Kutztown Univ of PA; MA 84 Univ of MD - College Park; 76–SLP, Lancaster Leb Intermed Unit 13, **SLP**

Bierman, Mrs Marie S 189 Old Spofford Road, Winchester, NH 03470, (603) 239-6879, BS 50 Fordham Univ; MA 52 Columbia Univ Teachers Coll; Dir of Pupil Personnel Serv, Greenwich Ct Pub Schs, **SLP**

Biety, Karen Ann 909 North Oakwood Avenue, Lake Forest, IL 60045, (312) 690-8580, BS 64 Northwestern Univ; MA 80 Univ of Pittsburgh - Pittsburgh; Superv, Suburban Sp Lang Hrng Assoc, **SLP**

Biever, Dawn Marie 530 North Eau Claire Avenue, Apartment 205, Madison, WI 53705, (402) 449-6538, BS 81 Univ of WI - Madison; MS 85 Univ of WI - Madison; SLP, Boys Town National Institute, **SLP**

Biga, Judith M 4617 Chicory, Colorado Springs, CO 80917, (719) 574-2234, MS 87 IL St Univ - Normal

Bigelow, Mrs Joanne Leduc 58 Manton Street, Fall River, MA 02724, (617) 823-5327, BA 83 Bridgewater St Coll; MS 86 Boston Univ; **SLP**

Biggam, Mrs Lynn Lincoln 2225 Westfield Avenue, Winston-Salem, NC 27103-3640, BA 79 Univ of NC - Chapel Hill; MA 82 Univ of TN - Knoxville; **SLP**

Bigger, Mrs Ruth Ann W 808 Clay Street, Franklin, VA 23851, (804) 569-8400, BA 68 Old Dominion Univ; MA 70 Univ of TN - Knoxville; **A**

Biggerstaff, Karen Diane 14342 Hill Prince Street, San Antonio, TX 78248, (512) 824-2651, BS 75 Southwest TX St Univ; MA 78 Univ of TX - San Antonio; MA 85 Our Lady Lake Univ-San Anton; 79–Sp-Lang Path, North East ISD, **SLP**

Biggerstaff, Michele Ann 11588 Calle Albara, El Cajon, CA 92019, (619) 221-6000, BA 73 Univ of West FL; **SLP**

Biggins, Anne R 3536 Queen Anne Drive, Fairfax, VA 22030, **SLP**

Biggins, Mrs Nancy Antonino 320 Robertson Road, Hermitage, PA 16148, (412) 347-3153, BS 72 Clarion Univ of PA; ME 73 Clarion Univ of PA; Consultant, Area Nursing Homes, **SLP**

Biggio, Stacey Margaret 945 Watervliet Shaker Road, Albany, NY 12205, (518) 452-0428, BA 86 SUNY - Coll at New Paltz; MS 87 Coll of Saint Rose

Biggs, Gail R 101 North Spring Street, Suite 105, Searcy, AR 72143, (501) 268-3378, BA 72 Univ of AR - Fayetteville; MS 75 Univ of AR - Medical Sci; 86–Sp-Lang Path, Private Practice, **SLP**

Bigham, Artan 25341 Shawassee Circle #105, Southfield, MI 48034, BA 77 Univ of MI - Ann Arbor; MA 79 Wayne St Univ; **SLP**

Bigham, Caryl L 1311 Briarcliff Boulevard, Austin, TX 78723, (512) 454-4731, BA 77 TX Tech Univ; MA 79 Kent St Univ; Aud, Austin State Sch, **A**

Bigham, Mrs Dona E 5512 Dundee Road, Edina, MN 55436, (612) 925-0151, BS 72 SUNY - Coll at Buffalo; MS 73 Univ of WI - Madison; 77–Sp-Lang Path, Courage Center, **SLP**

Bigiarelli, Michele Ann 129 Wells Point Drive, Irmo, SC 29063, (803) 254-2495, BS 77 James Madison Univ; ME 82 James Madison Univ; Aud, Midland ENT PA, **A**

Bigler-Burke, Mrs Linda G 1215 Victor Road, Macedon, NY 14502, (716) 272-2111, BS 79 SUNY - Coll at Geneseo; MA 81 SUNY - Coll at Geneseo; Sp-Lang Path, Monroe Developmental Center, **SLP**

Bihldorff, Mary F 37 Normand Street, North Dartmouth, MA 02747, (508) 994-6239, BS 71 Boston Univ; MA 72 IN Univ - Bloomington; **A**

Bihr, Mrs Roxann P 13961 East Arkansas Drive, Aurora, CO 80012, (303) 690-1133, BS 72 CO St Univ; MS 74 CO St Univ; Sp-Lang Path, Aurora Pub Sch, **SLP**

Bihum, Virginia C 3830 Folsom, Boulder, CO 80302, (303) 441-0437, BS 73 Indiana Univ of PA; MA 75 Central MI Univ; Program Director Ped Rehab Ser, Boulder Mem Hosp, **SLP**

Bikulcs, Lucy P O Box 875643, Wasilla, AK 99687, (907) 376-5371, BA 81 Eastern IL Univ; BS 81 Eastern IL Univ; MS 82 Eastern IL Univ; Sp-Lang Path, Mat-Su Borough Sch Dist, **SLP**

Biladeau, Mrs Julie A 20 Phelps Street, Easthampton, MA 01027, (413) 527-6611, BA 75 Univ of MA - Amherst; MA 78 Univ of MA - Amherst; 82–Sp-Lang Path, Easthampton Pub Sch, **SLP**

Bilberry, Tina M 1901 Sycamore, Abilene, TX 79602, (915) 677-7644, BS 76 Univ of TX - Austin; ME 79 Southwest TX St Univ; 87–Sp-Lang Path, Abilene ISD, **SLP**

Bilderback, Mrs Linda Lyon 1545 North Magnolia Avenue, Rialto, CA 92376, (714) 874-8970, BS 64 Univ of IA; MS 70 PA St Univ - Univ Park; SLP, San Bernardino Co Sch, **SLP**

Bildner, Betty R 13876 Valley Vista, Sherman Oaks, CA 91423, (818) 905-1388, BA 77 Univ of CA - Los Angeles; MA 81 CA St Univ - Los Angeles; Sp-Lang Path, Tarzana Sp & Lang Ctr, **SLP**

Bilecki, Mary Ann Schiffer Herrick Hospital, 2001 Dwight Way, Berkeley, CA 94704, (415) 845-0130, BS 79 Stockton St Coll; MA 81 Univ of TN - Knoxville; Aud, Herrick Hospital, **A**

Biles, Patricia Ann 3412 Arnold Lane, Falls Church, VA 22042, (703) 641-0256, MS 73 Murray St Univ

Bilger, Robert C Dept Of Speech & Hearing Sci, University Of Illinois, 901 South 6th Street, Champaign, IL 61820, (217) 244-4140, BS 49 Purdue Univ - West Lafayette; MS 51 Purdue Univ - West Lafayette; PH 54 (Exptl Psychol) Purdue Univ - West Lafayette; Prof, Univ of Illinois, **F**

Bilina, Faith B 8960 Leslie Drive, Orland Hills, IL 60477, (312) 333-7812, BS 78 Southern IL Univ -Carbondale; MS 83 Governors St Univ; 85–Sp-Lang Path, South Metropolitan Assoc, **SLP**

Bilko, Mrs Sheila Monica 9 Walnut Street, Glenhead, NY 11545, BA 82 Saint John's Univ - Jamaica; MS 84 Adelphi Univ; Sp-Lang Path, Little Village School, **SLP**

Bilkovsky-Johnson, Margie Renee 5634 Deville, East Lansing, MI 48823, (517) 339-1935, BA 84 MI St Univ; MA 87 MI St Univ; 87–Sp-Lang Path, Tamarack Inc, **SLP**

Billeaud, Mrs Frances P 306 Vital Street, Lafayette, LA 70506, (318) 984-4691, BA 57 Univ of Southwestern LA; MA 65 LA St Univ - Baton Rouge; 83–Dir Sp-Lang Path, Univ Southwestern Louisiana, **SLP**

Billens-Ivory, Dr Susan 5113 Academy Drive, Metairie, LA 70003, (504) 588-5661, BA 75 Univ of CA - Santa Barbara; MA 77 Univ of MN - Minneap-St Paul; PH 83 (NS) Univ of KS; Sp-Lang Path, Tulane Med Ctr, **SLP**

Biller, Ann Elizabeth 2212 Girard Avenue South, #306, Minneapolis, MN 55405, (612) 347-8550, BS 85 Univ of MN - Minneap-St Paul; MS 86 Univ of MI - Ann Arbor; Sp-Lang Path, Hennepin Co Med Center, **SLP**

Biller, Maysoon Ibrahim 113 Violet Drive, Madison, AL 35758, (205) 772-9982, BA 82 Univ of OK - Norman; MA 84 Univ of KS; Sp-Lang Path, Madison Co Schs, **SLP**

Billet, Jacqueline Maria 1 East Main Street #4, Cortland, NY 13045, (607) 257-0777, **SLP**

Billetdeaux, Mrs Laura E 417 Territorial, Manchester, MI 48158, (313) 428-8265, BA 80 Univ of MI - Ann Arbor; MS 81 Univ of MI - Ann Arbor; Superv/Aphasia Cl, U of MI, **SLP**

Billharz, Constance 467 Munroe Avenue, North Tarrytown, NY 10591, **SLP**

Billheimer, Kenneth D 4466 Black Avenue Suite C, Pleasanton, CA 94566, (415) 484-3507, BA 74 CA St Univ - Fresno; MA 76 CA St Univ - Fresno; Aud, Hearing Services, **A**

Billik, Cheryl W 16911 Summer Creek Circle, San Antonio, TX 78248, (512) 492-1674, BS 72 Univ of North TX; MS 74 Univ of North TX; 86–Sp-Lang Path, Associated Healthfocus, **SLP**

Billings, Bradley L Audiology Center Of Redlands, 245 Terracina Boulevard, Suite 101, Redlands, CA 92373, (714) 793-2631, BA 67 CA St Univ - Los Angeles; MA 69 CA St Univ - Los Angeles; PH 72 (NS) Univ of OK Medical Center; Dir/Aud Sers, Aud Cen of Redlands, **A**

Billings, Mrs Catherine A 4621 7th Avenue North, St Petersburg, FL 33713, (813) 327-2152, MS 82 Univ of South FL; 87–SLP, Lashley & Associates Inc, **SLP**

Billingsley, Mrs Marilyn M V 3033 Herman Street, Honolulu, HI 96816, (808) 922-8458, MS 81 Portland St Univ; Sp-Lang Path, Dept of Educ-Honolulu Dist, **SLP**

Billington, Carla Jill 2010 North Mohawk, Chicago, IL 60614, (312) 266-4822, BS 75 Murray St Univ; MA 78 Ball St Univ; Reg Sls Mgr, ITI, **SLP**

Billman, Mrs Kimberly Smith 6166 Del Cerro Boulevard, San Diego, CA 92120, (619) 286-4061, BA 79 San Diego St Univ; MA 86 San Diego St Univ; 81–Sp-Lang Path, San Diego USD, **SLP**

Bills, Jennifer Lynn 8372 S W Mohwak Street, Tualatin, OR 97062, (503) 694-2884, Sp-Lang Path, Good Samaritan Hosp, **SLP**

Billups-Morgan, Barbara A 901 West Duncannon Avenue, Philadelphia, PA 19141, (215) 665-5071, BA 77 Univ of Pittsburgh - Pittsburgh; MA 79 Univ of Pittsburgh - Pittsburgh; Sp-Lang Path, Magee Rehab Hosp, **SLP**

Bilton, Regina R 127A North State Street, Dover, DE 19901, (302) 734-4700, BA 73 Univ of DE; MA 81 West Chester Univ of PA; Sp/Lang Path, Kent General Hospital, **SLP**

Bilyeu, Connie L 4800 Reinhardt Drive, Shawnee, KS 66205, (913) 722-5543, BS 66 Univ of KS; MA 68 Univ of KS; Sp-Lang Path, Bethany Med Cen, **SLP**

Bilyeu, Delores Lena 13875 Ella Blvd, Apartment 1106, Houston, TX 77014, (713) 449-1011, MS 83 Central MO St Univ; Aldine School District, **SLP**

Bilyeu, Mrs Katherine Michele Route 2 Box 196, Peru, NY 12972, (518) 643-8684, **SLP**

Binder, Margaret Dunn 10781 S W 128th Street, Miami, FL 33176, BS 62 Bowling Green St Univ; MS 86 Nova Univ; **SLP**

Binder, Mrs Marilyn R 9231 Snowshoe Lane, Columbia, MD 21045, (301) 992-9436, BS 70 Boston Univ; ME 71 Univ of VA - Charlottesville; Sp-Lang Path, Balt Co Pub Sch, **SLP**

Binderoff, Randy 3435 Milburn Avenue, Baldwin, NY 11510-5150, (212) 598-1345, BA 76 Queens Coll; MS 78 CUNY - Brooklyn Coll; Chief Aud, NY Eye & Ear Inf, **A**

Bindert, CarolLynn 13556 Deerwater Drive, Germantown, MD 20874, (301) 253-7004, MA 83 Long Island U - CW Post Ctr; Sp-Lang Path, Montgomery Co Pub Sch, **SLP**

Binford, Kimberly Sue 905-201 Summit Walk Drive, Charlotte, NC 28226, (704) 364-3001, BA 85 Marshall Univ; MA 87 Marshall Univ; Sp-Lang Path, Charlotte-Mecklenburg Schs, **SLP**

Bingaman, Mrs Donna Mitchell 27 Deerfield Road, Waterford, CT 06385, BS 78 IN St Univ - Terre Haute; MS 79 IN St Univ - Terre Haute; Sp/Lang Path, Lisbon Sch Dist, **SLP**

Bingaman, Mrs Sharon P 115 Monocacy Hill Road, Birdsboro, PA 19508, (215) 582-0907, BS 80 Bloomsburg Univ of PA; MS 81 Bloomsburg Univ of PA; Sp-Lang Path, Hamburg Cen, **SLP**

Bingea, Rebecca L 155 Nova Albion Way #15, San Rafael, CA 94903, (415) 499-2331, BA 72 Doane Coll; MA 82 Univ of MT; 83–Audiologist, Kaiser Permanente Med Ctr, **A ACE**

Binger, Mrs Annette T 6104 Stannye Drive, Louisville, KY 40222, (502) 361-2301, BS 57 Marquette Univ; MS 83 Fontbonne Coll; Sp-Lang Path, Hazelwood Icf Facility, **SLP**

Bingham, Mrs Carol Cole 3100 Shore Drive Apartment #919, Virginia Beach, VA 23451, (804) 496-1439, BS 29 Univ of WI - Madison; MA 37 Columbia Univ Teachers Coll; **SLP LM**

Bingham, Dale S R R 2 Box 173, North Liberty, IA 52317, (319) 353-4825, BA Univ of IA; MA 51 Univ of IA; Sp-Lang Path, Special Child Health Services, **SLP F**

Bingham, Donna G 2306 Stanley Street, New Britain, CT 06053, (203) 223-8294, BS 61 Eastern MI Univ; SLP, New Britain Pub Sch, **SLP**

Bingham, Mrs Lisa W 16320 Dearborn Drive, Stilwell, KS 66085, (913) 897-5740, BA 76 Univ of AR - Fayetteville; MA 77 Univ of AR - Fayetteville; 87–Sp-Lang Path, Blue Valley PS, **SLP**

Bingham, Mrs Marcia Roles 6801 Incas Drive, North Little Rock, AR 72116, (501) 835-9651, **SLP**

Bingham, Pam 5511 Tipton Drive, Austin, TX 78723, (512) 458-6123, BS 74; MA 76; 88–Asst Chief of MR Svcs, Texas Dept of Health, **SLP**

Bingham, Mrs Virginia W 1805 Longview, Eugene, OR 97403, (503) 686-7085, BA 52; MS 67; 67–Sp-Lang Path, Eugene Hrng & Sp Cen, **SLP ACE**

Bingle, Janice M 440 Richmond Park East, Apartment 212C, Richmond Heights, OH 44143, (216) 444-6303, BA 78 Fontbonne Coll; MS 80 Purdue Univ - West Lafayette; 80–Aud, Cleveland Clinic Foundation, **A**

Bingler, Mrs Julie Lentz 11534 Waterflower Lane, Charlotte, NC 28213, (704) 867-9021, BS 84 Western Carolina Univ; MA 85 Western Carolina Univ; **SLP**

Bingley, Mrs Katherine 1306 Aloha, St Louis, MO 63126, (314) 644-2902, MA 81 Univ of IL - Urbana; BA 80 Augustana Coll; Sp-Lang Path, St Louis Co Spec Sch Dist, **SLP**

Binkow, Mrs Nancy H 6915 Castleton Drive, Atlanta, GA 30328, (404) 256-2489, BS 75 Emory Univ; MS 76 Vanderbilt Univ; Coord Outpatient Serv, Northside Hosp, **SLP**

Binney, Mrs Janet Jarrell 231 Clarksville Road, PO Box 218, Princeton Junction, NJ 08550-0218, (609) 799-3935, BS 62 Purdue Univ - West Lafayette; MA 72 Trenton St Coll; Vice President, The Speech Bin Inc, **SLP**

Binnie, Dr Carl A Dept Of Audiology & Speech Sci, Purdue University, Heavilon Hall, Lafayette, IN 47907, (317) 494-3797, BA 62 Northern IL Univ - De Kalb; MS 63 Univ of Denver; PH 70 (NS) Univ of Denver; Professor, Audiology, Purdue Univ, **A F**

Binnie, Mrs Doreen 5033 Fenn Road, Medina, OH 44256, (216) 236-5020, BS 76 Kent St Univ; MA 78 Cleveland St Univ; Sp/Lang Path, Columbia Local Schs, **SLP**

Binotti, Mrs Nancy Lea Wester 12735 S Westport Drive, Palos Park, IL 60464, BA 77 Saint Xavier Coll; MA 79 Northern IL Univ - De Kalb; Sp-Lang Path, Southwest Cook Co Coop, **SLP**

Bins-Hattaway, Alice Taylor P O Box 1525, Sanford, NC 27330-3953, (919) 774-6846, BA 74 Univ of NC - Chapel Hill; MS 78 Univ of NC - Chapel Hill; Sp-Lang Path, Communications One, **SLP**

Binstock, Eve Renee 4624 Torley Street, Pittsburgh, PA 15224-1532, **SLP**

Bintz, Mrs Sally H 2118 Evans Road, Flossmoor, IL 60422, (219) 933-0361, BA 74 Marshall Univ; MA 75 Marshall Univ; Sp-Lang Path, Speech Plus Inc, **SLP**

Binus, Gale Z 32 Glenwood Avenue, Newton Center, MA 02159-2503, (617) 965-7479, **SLP**

Binzer, Susan M Washington University School Of Medicine, 517 South Euclid Avenue, St Louis, MO 63110, (314) 362-7245, BS 81 Univ of Cincinnati; MA 84 Univ of Cincinnati; 84–Coord Cochlear Implant Program, Washington Univ Sch of Med, **A**

Biondi, Gina 631 Savin Avenue, West Haven, CT 06516, (203) 933-7867, BA 86 Southern CT St Univ; MA 88 Southern CT St Univ; 88–Sp-Lang Path, West Haven Bd of Educ

Biondo, Barbara J P O Box 6064, Reno, NV 89513, (702) 348-0200, BS 82 Univ of NV - Reno; MS 84 Univ of NV - Reno; SLP, Washoe County School District, **SLP**

Bir, Mrs Margaret F 2173 Lyndway, Beachwood, OH 44122, (313) 423-8678, BA 75 Univ of MI - Ann Arbor; MS 76 Univ of MI - Ann Arbor; **SLP**

Birbeck, Dr Herbert E Mankato State University, Mankato, MN 56001, (507) 389-1122, BA 50 Tarkio Coll; MA 54 Univ of MO - Columbia; PH 60 (NS) Univ of IA

Birch, Bruce J 9521 Bedford, Omaha, NE 68134, (402) 559-3463, BS 69 Brigham Young Univ; MS 71 Brigham Young Univ; Aud, Bishop Clarkson Mem Hosp, **A**

Birch, Mrs Susan J 3141 Woodward Avenue, Burlington, ON, Canada L7N 2M3, (416) 639-8832, 87 Univ of Toronto - Ontario

Bird, Allan K University Affiliated Center, 200 Treadway Plaza, Dallas, TX 75235-5408, (214) 904-2217, BA 67 Univ of UT; MA 68 Univ of UT; PH 72 (NS) MI St Univ; Sp-Lang Path, Univ Affilated Cen, **SLP**

Bird, Mrs Ann L 300 Raritan Avenue, Middlesex, NJ 08846, (201) 464-1717, BA 78 Rutger's St Univ - Douglas Coll; MS 81 Rutgers St Univ -N Brunswick; Sp-Lang Path, Berkeley Heights Bd of Ed, **SLP**

Bird, Mrs Ann Olsen 7303 Western Avenue, Omaha, NE 68114, (402) 471-2471, BS 69 Univ of NE - Lincoln; MA 75 Univ of NE - Lincoln; State Consult Sp-Lang Prog, NE Dept of Ed

Bird, Ann Thomas 4717 Oakvale Circle, Knoxville, TN 37920, (615) 577-3227, BS 64 Univ of TN - Chattanooga; MA 84 Univ of TN - Knoxville; Sp-Lang Path, Knox Co Sch Sys, **SLP**

Bird, Mrs Carolyn T 2938 Canterbury Road, Westlake, OH 44145, BS 64 Kent St Univ; ME 65 Univ of AZ; Sp-Lang Path, North Olmsted City Schools, **SLP A**

Bird, Elisabeth Grace 1452 Letitia Street, Baton Rouge, LA 70808, (504) 381-6520, BS 81 LA St Univ - Baton Rouge; MA 83 LA St Univ - Baton Rouge; Sp-Lang Path, Baton Rouge Gen Med Ctr, **SLP**

Bird, Joyce Elaine Box 384, Carlsbad, NM 88221, (505) 887-2902, BA 82 Wichita St Univ; MA 84 Wichita St Univ; 84–Sp-Lang Path, Carlsbad Municipal Schs, **SLP**

Bird, Mrs Linda Gray 5410 Woodhill Circle, Tuscaloosa, AL 35405, (205) 553-3760, BA 75 Western WA Univ; MS 79 Univ of WY; Sp-Lang Path, VA Med Cen, **SLP**

Bird, Linda J 990 Broadmeadow Drive, Pittsburgh, PA 15237-4151, (313) 937-2530, BA 78 MI St Univ; MA 79 MI St Univ; Sp-Lang Path, Wayne Co ISD, **SLP**

Bird, Mrs Luann L 9820 S W 69th, Auburn, KS 66402, (913) 671-2527, BS 76 KS St Univ; MA 77 KS St Univ; Sp-Lang Path, Private Practice, **SLP**

Bird, Marilyn R 2458 Neville Drive, San Jose, CA 95130, (408) 379-0245, BA 74 Univ of CA - Santa Barbara; MS 75 Western OR St Coll; Sp-Lang Path, Private Practice, **SLP**

Bird, Raymond J HCR 1 Box 160, Sparrow Bush, NY 12780, (914) 858-8367, BS 82 Elmira Coll; MS 84 Bloomsburg Univ of PA; Sp-Lang Path, Head Inj Rec Ctr, **SLP**

Bird, Richard Albert 2938 Canterbury Road, Westlake, OH 44145, (216) 826-1987, BA 65 Univ of AZ; MS 67 Gallaudet Coll; Aud, ENT Serv/Cleve Aud Serv, **A**

Birdsall, Marian P 137 West 3rd Street, Frederick, MD 21701, (904) 771-1458, BA 77 Univ of North FL; ME 83 Univ of North FL; Sp-Lang Path, InSpeech Inc, **SLP ACE**

Birdsell, Denise Lasnier 8250 Sharptown Road, Stuyvesant, NY 12173, (518) 445-4526, BS 73 Boston Univ; MA 76 Univ of CT; Sp-Lang Path, Albany Med Cen Hosp, **SLP**

Birk, Angela C 3685 Ridgeway Road, Dayton, OH 45419, BS 78 TX Christian Univ; MA 81 Univ of MO - Columbia; Sp-Lang Path, Fulton St Hosp, **SLP**

Birk, Janice Thompson RR2 Box 1080, Union, ME 04862, (207) 236-8381, BS 76 Bloomsburg Univ of PA; MS 79 Bloomsburg Univ of PA; **SLP**

Birkenruth, Mrs Honore H 81 Ball Hill Road, Storrs, CT 06268, (203) 928-2718, BA 57 Emerson Coll; Sp-Lang Path, Bolton Ct Pub Sch, **SLP**

Birkenstock, Nora Karla/Holl 3801 Regent Road, Sacramento, CA 95821, (916) 481-8585, BA 81 CA St Univ - Sacramento; MA 84 CA St Univ - Sacramento; 86–Aud, Sacramento Hrng Svcs Ctr, **A**

Birkle, Mrs Lydia S 1901 Leyden Street, Denver, CO 80220, (303) 322-1871, BA 27 Univ of Denver; MA 59 Univ of Denver; **A**

Birkmann, Mrs Mildred Harnett 19 Burbank Street #1-A, Yonkers, NY 10710, (914) 793-0196, BA 72 CUNY - Lehman Coll; MA 76 CUNY - Lehman Coll; SLP, **SLP**

Birky, Nanette Rummel P O Box 41, 515 West Exchange, Danvers, IL 61732, BS 78 IL St Univ - Normal; MS 80 IL St Univ - Normal; Sp-Lang Path, Deer Creek School District 701, **SLP**

Birleffi, Mrs Judith A 1414 Green Oak Terrace Court, Suite 200, Kingwood, TX 77339, (713) 358-2314, BS 85; MA 86 Univ of Northern CO; 87–Aud, Kingwood ENT Ctr, **A**

Birman, Marina 64 Welland Road, Brookline, MA 02146, (617) 573-3266, BS 83 CA St Univ - Hayward; MS 85 San Francisco St Univ; Aud, MA Eye & Ear Inf, **A**

Birmingham, Barbara Ann 5604 Beaver Court, Greendale, WI 53129, (414) 449-2422, BS 70 Univ of WI - Milwaukee; MS 84 Univ of WI - Milwaukee; 70–Sp-Lang Path, Milwaukee Pub Sch, **SLP ACE**

Birmingham, Debra A 15531 South Long Avenue, Oak Forest, IL 60452, (312) 687-0900, BS 78 IL St Univ - Normal; MS 79 IL St Univ - Normal; Sp/Lang Path, S W Case, **SLP**

Birmingham, Mrs Elizabeth A 29411 4th Avenue South, Federal Way, WA 98003, (206) 839-3196, BS 77 Univ of OR; MA 79 CA St Univ - Northridge; Sp-Lang Path, Kent School District, **SLP ACE**

Birmingham, Mrs Ingrid B 16048 Callahan, Sepulveda, CA 91343, (213) 993-0255, BA 61 Univ of CA - Santa Barbara; MA 62 Purdue Univ - West Lafayette; Sp-Lang Path, LA City Sch, **SLP**

Birmingham, Marie Kay 700 Cypress Avenue, Marshfield, WI 54449, (715) 223-3939, BS 67 Univ of WI - Stevens Point; MS 69 Univ of WI - Stevens Point; Sp-Lang Path, Colby School District, **SLP**

Birmingham, Mrs Shirley 710 West Airwood, East Alton, IL 62024, (618) 259-7415, BS 58 IL St Univ - Normal; MS 72 Southern IL Univ-Edwardsvill; Sp/Lang Path, E Alton Elem Dist, **SLP**

Birnbaum, Lisa V 2809 5th Street SW #2, Minot, ND 58701, BA 86 SUNY - Center at Buffalo; BA 86 SUNY - Center at Buffalo; MS 88 CUNY - Hunter Coll; 88–Aud, NY League for hard Hearing

Birnbaum, Michele J 1035 Park Avenue, New York, NY 10028, (212) 427-8250, BA 64 CUNY - Brooklyn Coll; MS 67 CUNY - Brooklyn Coll; **SLP**

Birr, Sydney R 1207 Bly Court, Eustis, FL 32726-7104, BS 69 OH Univ - Athens; MA 72 Univ of Houston - Univ Park; Sp/Lang Path, Private Practice, **SLP**

Birrenkott, Mrs Jan Marianne 3965 Syme Drive, Carlsbad, CA 92008, (619) 434-1954, BA 72 CA St Univ - Long Beach; MA 86 San Diego St Univ

Birtcil, Mrs Susan Alice 199 East 2nd Avenue, Chico, CA 95926, (916) 244-4600, MS 79 CA St Univ - Chico; 81–Sp-Lang Path, Shasta Co Office of Educ, **SLP**

Bisang, Sharon J 9529 West 78th Street, Overland Park, KS 66204, (913) 281-8947, OB 84 Univ of KS; MA 86 Wichita St Univ; Sp-Lang Path, Bethany Medical Ctr, **SLP**

Bisantz, Jane L Bay Boulevard, East Hampton, CT 06424, BA 69 Univ of CT; MA 72 Univ of CT; Sp-Lang Path, Hartford Board of Education, **SLP**

Bisbano, Mrs Carol W 11 Fairways Drive, Mount Kisco, NY 10549-3609, (914) 666-0061, BS 73 Ithaca Coll; MS 75 Southern CT St Univ; Sp-Lang Path, Bedford Cntrl Sch Dist, **SLP**

Bisbee, Donna Joy 10 Milton Avenue, Sanford, ME 04073, (207) 324-1550, BS 78 Syracuse Univ; MA 86 Univ of MA - Amherst; 86–Sp-Lang Path, York Co Counseling Svcs, **SLP**

Bisbee, Julie Kathleen P O Box 263, Sebastopol, CA 95473-0263, (707) 823-2283, BS 72 SUNY - Coll at Fredonia; MA 75 AZ St Univ; Sp-Lang Path, Sebastopol Union Sch Dist, **SLP**

Bischof, Ellen Marie 311 Colfax Avenue #C, Michigan City, IN 46360, (219) 874-0734, BS 85 Purdue Univ - West Lafayette; MS 87 Purdue Univ - West Lafayette; 87–Sp-Lang Path, Argabright Communications, **SLP**

Bischof, Mrs Katharyn Worthingto 5710 Sherman Avenue, Downers Grove, IL 60516, (312) 515-9413, BA 83 SUNY - Coll at Plattsburgh; MS 85 Ithaca Coll; 88–Sp-Lang Path, Regional Educ Svc Agency, **SLP**

Bischoff, Deborah Cohen 2512 Dundee Drive, Tallahassee, FL 32308, (904) 386-4987, BA 81 Univ of FL; MS 85 FL St Univ; **SLP**

Bischoff, Joanne R 2159-A South Mound Street, Milwaukee, WI 53207, BS 76 Univ of WI - Milwaukee; MS 77 Univ of WI - Milwaukee; Sp-Lang Path, Milwaukee Pub Sch, **SLP**

Bischofshausen, Dr Sharon 314 Costa Del Oro, Victoria, TX 77904, **SLP**

Biscow, Gail M 1392 President Street, Brooklyn, NY 11213, **A**

Bise, Penny S 2319 East Avenue, Gulfport, MS 39501, (601) 388-5541, BA 78 Univ of MS; MS 79 Univ of MS; Sp-Lang Path, VA Med Ctr, **SLP**

Bisek, Thorice S 1195 Rancho Road, Ojai, CA 93023-1628, (805) 646-4455, BS 69 Old Dominion Univ; MA 73 Trenton St Coll; Dir Esl, Tabuk Internat'l Sch Saudi Ar, **SLP**

Bisel, Mrs Sheila Dehaas P O Box 64, Ames, OK 73718, (405) 753-4213, BS 84 Northwestern OK St Univ; MA 85 OK St Univ

Bishoff, Tracey Jeanne 169 South Los Feliz Drive, Chandler, AZ 85226, (602) 239-4577, BS 81 Univ of WY; MS 83 Univ of WY; Aud, Good Samaritan Medical Center, **A**

Bishop, Candace H P O Box 126, Mansfield, CT 06250, (203) 423-3641, BA 73 Univ of CT; MS 74 Univ of ME - Orono; SLP, Bozrah Bd of Ed, **SLP**

Bishop, Doris Lynn Route 3 Box 252, Baldwyn, MS 38824, (601) 355-4818, BS 74 MS Univ for Women; MS 75 MS Univ for Women; Sp-Lang Path, Jackson Mun Sch Dist, **SLP**

Bishop, Mrs Elaine Legler 3650 Wilshire Avenue, Cincinnati, OH 45208, (513) 871-6239, BS 71 Nazareth Coll of Rochester; MS 72 Univ of VT; Sp-Path Superv, Drake Mem Hosp, **SLP**

Bishop, Dr Judith Hidding 2031 Lyttleton Street, Camden, SC 29020, (803) 777-4813, BA 60 Northwestern Univ; MA 61 Northwestern Univ; PH 87 (Sp Path) Univ of SC - Columbia; 87–Research Asst Prof, U of SC, **SLP**

Bishop, Lewis D N E Iowa Rehabilitation Agency, R R 1 Box 166, West Union, IA 52175, (319) 422-5082, BA 60 Univ of Northern IA; MA 68 Univ of MN - Minneap-St Paul; Administrator, NE Iowa Rehabilitation Agency, **SLP A**

Bishop, Libby K 10201 Breconshire Road, Ellicott City, MD 21043, (301) 465-4433, BA 77 Univ of MD - College Park; MA 79 Univ of MD - College Park; Sp/Lang Path, Howard Co Pub Schs, **SLP**

Bishop, Mrs Lilli Ann 924 South Second Street, De Kalb, IL 60115, (815) 753-6527, BS 82 Northern IL Univ - De Kalb; MA 83 Northern IL Univ - De Kalb; SLP, Northern IL Univ Spch Clinic, **SLP**

Bishop, Linda H 9550 Coolbrook, San Antonio, TX 78250, (512) 522-1965, MS 78 TX Tech Univ; Dir Sp-Lang Path & E Chldhd In, Easter Seal Rehab Center, **SLP**

Bishop, Mrs Mary Greene Post Office Box 1188, Box Elder, SD 57719, (605) 923-3273, BS 86 East Carolina Univ; OM 87 Univ of NC - Greensboro; 87–Sp-Lang Path/Aud, Douglas Sch Sys

Bishop, Mrs Patricia Lee 151 Southgate Drive, Hyannis, MA 02601, (617) 775-0959, BS 75 SUNY - Center at Albany; OM 83 LA St Univ - N O Medical Ctr; Aud, Cape & Islands Hrng Ctr, **A**

Bishop, Sandra G 6701 North Charles Street, Baltimore, MD 21204, (301) 828-2087, MS 72 Southern Methodist Univ; Chief Sp-Lang Path, Mj Dance Rehab Center - Gbmc, **SLP**

Bishop, Mrs Sumie 1634 Makiki Street #1102, Honolulu, HI 96822, (808) 941-8315, OB 54 Univ of HI - Manoa; MA 59 Univ of HI - Manoa; **SLP**

Bishop, Mrs Susan A 55 Leuckel Avenue, Trenton, NJ 08619, BA 80 Rutger's St Univ - Douglas Coll; MA 81 Trenton St Coll; Sp-Lang Path, Hamilton Twp Brd of Educ, **SLP**

Bishop, Thomas Everett 1110 Peppertree Circle, St Helena, CA 94574, (707) 963-2468, BS 84 Loma Linda Univ - Riverside; MS 86 Loma Linda Univ - Riverside; **SLP**

Bishop-St Clair, Mrs Cynthia M 12138 Eastglen Street, San Diego, CA 92131, BS 65 SUNY - Coll at Brockport; MS 67 Univ of IL - Urbana; SLP/Aud, La Mesa Spring Valley Sch Dist, **SLP**

Biskup, Charlotte Lou 474 West 238th Street, Apartment 4D, Riverdale, NY 10463, MS 78 Central MI Univ; Aud, New York Hosp, **A ACE**

Bisset, Dr Janet D 1743 Capouse Avenue, Scranton, PA 18509, (717) 348-1118, BA 71 MI St Univ; MA 77 MI St Univ; PH 82 (NS) Memphis St Univ; 84–Assoc Prof, Marywood Coll, **SLP**

Bissinger, Kathy M 505 East 8th Street, Mesa, AZ 85203, (602) 839-7375, BS 75 Northwest MO St Univ; MS 77 Central MO St Univ; 85–Aud, Tempe Sch Dist 3, **A**

Bissonette, Mrs Linda L 15600 Nursery Drive, Minnetonka, MN 55345, (612) 874-6219, BS 72 Univ of MN - Minneap-St Paul; MA 75 Univ of MN - Minneap-St Paul; Sp-Lang Path, Minneapolis Childrens Med Ctr, **SLP**

Bistany-Brown, Robin A 4101 Branding Place, Allison Park, PA 15101, (312) 968-9421, BS 76 IN Univ - Bloomington; MA 78 IN Univ - Bloomington; SLP, Sch Assc Spec Ed Dupage, **SLP**

Bittel, Cynthia S 324 Raritan Avenue, Middlesex, NJ 08846, BS 79 Bloomsburg Univ of PA; MA 80 Bloomsburg Univ of PA; Sp-Lang Path, Midland Sch, **SLP**

Bittel, Dr Peter J Valley Rehabilitation Inc, 16 Center Street Suite 325, Northampton, MA 01060, (413) 586-7145, ED 81 Univ of MA - Amherst; MA 74 Univ of MA - Amherst; MA 72 Univ of MA - Amherst; Dir, Valley Rehab Inc, **SLP**

Bittner, Carol J 605 East 3970 South, Salt Lake City, UT 84107, (801) 262-7688, BS 70 Brigham Young Univ; OM 72 Brigham Young Univ; Prin, Alpine Sch Dist, **SLP**

Bittner, Mrs Colleen Creason 20911 33rd Avenue S E, Bothell, WA 98021, (206) 672-9323, BA 84 Univ of WA; MS 85 Univ of MI - Ann Arbor; Sp-Lang Path, New Medico-CRS-WA, **SLP**

Bitton, Sidena Gardner 170 Ranch Drive, Pocatello, ID 83204, (208) 232-1603, BS 79 ID St Univ; MS 84 ID St Univ; SLP, Pocatello Regional Medical Ctr, **SLP**

Bivens, Cathy Ann 1784 Jameston Drive, Charlotte, NC 28209, (704) 376-1377, BS 83 Appalachian St Univ; MA 86 Appalachian St Univ; 87–Sp-Lang Path, LOGOS, **SLP**

Bivens, Cheryl Jean 616 South Barrett, Sedalia, MO 65301-3929, (816) 826-5538, **SLP**

Bivens, Kathleen McCarty 16661 Wanderer Lane, Huntington Beach, CA 92649, (714) 846-4812, **SLP**

Bivins, Cynthia F 3534 Warner Avenue, Louisville, KY 40207-3728, (502) 636-2084, BS 79 Brescia Coll; MA 81 Univ of IA; 87–Sp-Lang Path, Louisville Deaf Oral School, **SLP**

Bivins, Mrs Linda M 5513 Estrellita Del Norte, Albuquerque, NM 87111, (505) 823-9264, **SLP**

Bivona, Mrs Theresa G P O Box 24, Centerport, NY 11721, (516) 271-5419, BA 64 Saint Mary-of-the-Woods Coll; MA 73 Northwestern Univ; Sp-Lang Path, Commack Pub Sch, **SLP**

Bixenmann, Mrs Carolyn Faulder 2120 West Charles, Grand Island, NE 68801, (402) 463-5611, BA 81 Kearney St Coll; MS 82 Kearney St Coll; Sp-Lang Path, Educ Svc Unit #9, **SLP**

Bixler, Ralph W 36674 Melton, Westland, MI 48185, **SLP**

Bizoza, Bonnie H 14144 Dickens #104, Sherman Oaks, CA 91423, **SLP**

Bizoza, Stuart Lee 985 Dartmouth Lane, Woodmere, NY 11598, (212) 330-9360, BA 66 CUNY - Brooklyn Coll; MS 67 Univ of WI - Madison; SLP, NYC Bd of Ed, **SLP**

Bjekich, Karen Hauber 2115 Van Ness Drive, Roseville, CA 95661-4934, (916) 786-3602, BA 76 Northern IL Univ - De Kalb; MA 79 Univ of Denver; Sp-Lang Path, Private Practice, **SLP**

Bjella, Michele Angrisano 1160 Holbrook Road, Homewood, IL 60430, (312) 799-3979, BS 77 SUNY - Coll at Buffalo; MA 82 Northern MI Univ; Sp-Lang Path, Ctr for Commun Dis, **SLP**

Bjork, Jean Anne W 8460 Williamsburg Drive, Colorado Springs, CO 80920, (719) 598-9552, BS 75 CO St Univ; MS 77 CO St Univ; Sp-Lang Path, Sch Dist 11 Colo Sprngs Co, **SLP**

Bjork, Melanie 8211 Corliss Avenue N, Seattle, WA 98103, (206) 743-0616, BS 82 Univ of WA; MS 84 Univ of WA; **SLP**

Bjorkfelt, Christine Marie 267 Lamoka Place, West Islip, NY 11795, (516) 543-5100, BS 84 Elmira Coll; MA 86 Hofstra Univ; Sp-Lang Path, UCP, **SLP**

Bjork-Hilsinger, Cristine A 33 Via Farallon, Orinda, CA 94563, (415) 254-8255, BA 76 CA St Univ - Chico; MA 78 CA St Univ - Chico; 85–Sp-Lang Path, Private Practice, **SLP**

Bjorklund, Janet V 2015 41st Avenue E, Seattle, WA 98112, (206) 325-5642, BA 69 Pacific Univ; MA 77 San Francisco St Univ; Sp-Lang Path, Everett Sch Dist #2, **SLP A ACE**

Bjorklund, Mrs Joylyn Louise 1025 Columbia Road, Madison, WI 53705, (608) 849-8191, BS 77 Univ of WI - Madison; MS 79 Univ of WI - Madison; Sp-Lang Path, Waunakee Elem Sch, **SLP**

Bjorklund, Kristen B 118 Parkwood Drive, Redlands, CA 92373, (619) 323-6175, BA 77 CA St Univ - Chico; MS 78 Univ of Redlands; Sp-Lang Path, Desert Hosp, **SLP**

Bjorklund, Tamy F P O Box 74, Hales Corners, WI 53130, (414) 529-2801, BA 83 Univ of MO - Columbia; OM 87 Univ of MO - Columbia; **SLP**

Bjorkman, Karen D 120 North 33rd Avenue East, Duluth, MN 55804, (218) 727-0900, BA 73 Univ of MN - Duluth; MA 74 Univ of MN - Duluth; Sp-Lang Path, Polinsky Medical Rehab Center, **SLP**

Bjornberg, Vianne Larson 8601 Democracy Road N E, Albuquerque, NM 87109, (505) 821-9393, BA 84 Univ of NM; MS 86 Univ of NM; **SLP**

Bjornson, Mrs Jean N 53-615 Kamehameha Highway, Punaluu Oahu, HI 96717, (808) 239-6164, OB 63 Univ of HI - Manoa; SLP, Dept of Ed, **SLP**

Bjornsti, Patricia Hill 19107 Cherry Bend Drive, Germantown, MD 20874, (202) 745-5600, BA 79 SUNY - Coll at Cortland; MA 81 Univ of MD - College Park; Aud, Childrens Hosp National Med Ctr, **A**

Blache, Dr Stephen E Dept Communication Dis & Sic, Southern Illinois Univ, Carbondale, IL 62901, (618) 684-4498, BA 64 Univ of MA - Amherst; MA 67 Univ of MA - Amherst; PH 70 (NS) OH Univ - Athens; Assoc Prof, Southern IL U-Carbondale

Blachman, Lynn 1215 Claremont Avenue, Richmond, VA 23227, (804) 266-1642, BS 69 Northwestern Univ; ME 70 PA St Univ - Univ Park; OM 85 5579; 79–Sp-Lang Path, Henrico Co PS, **SLP**

Black, Brenda Joyce 317 Oakwood Avenue, State College, PA 16803-1610, (814) 231-1076, BA 76 PA St Univ - Univ Park; MS 88 PA St Univ - Univ Park; 88–Sp-Lang Path, St Coll Area Sch Dist, **SLP ACE**

Black, Carol B North Hills Hearing Aid Center, 1100½ Center Avenue, Pittsburgh, PA 15229, (412) 931-9290, BS 73 Univ of Pittsburgh - Pittsburgh; MS 76 Univ of Pittsburgh - Pittsburgh; 86–Owner, North Hills Hrng Aid Ctr, **A**

Black, Mrs Cheryl Sexton 230 Bethel Drive, Salisbury, NC 28144, (704) 636-6750, **SLP**

Black, Dana B 619 North Stratford Road, Wichita, KS 67206, **SLP**

Black, Denise Marie 2818 Melony Drive, Salt Lake City, UT 84124, (801) 350-4880, BS 67 Indiana Univ of PA; MS 72 Univ of UT; In Patient Coord, Quinney Rehab-Holy Cross Hosp, **SLP**

Black, Jennifer Marrer Carle Clinic Association, 602 W University Avenue, Urbana, IL 61801, (217) 337-3130, MA 84 Northwestern Univ; BS 82 Purdue Univ - West Lafayette; 87–Sp-Lang Path, Carle Clinic Association, **A**

Black, Mrs Joyce Elizabeth 8024 Westburg Avenue, San Diego, CA 92126, (503) 479-2676, BS 73 AZ St Univ; MS 83 Northern AZ Univ; Sp/Lang Path, Granada De Santa Fe Nurs Hm, **SLP**

Black, Judith W 2312 N W 52th, Oklahoma City, OK 73112, (405) 271-4214, BS 72 Phillips Univ; MS 74 Univ of OK Medical Center; Asst Prof-Dept of Commun Dis, U of OK, **SLP ACE**

Black, Mrs Judy K 616 Dodge Street, West Lafayette, IN 47906, (219) 253-6663, BA 69 CA St Univ - Chico; MA 74 CA St Univ - Fresno; Sp-Lang Path, Logansport Pub Sch, **SLP**

Black, Mrs Karen Schroeder 15028 Cherrydale Drive, Dale City, VA 22193, BS 83 Radford Univ; MS 84 Baylor Univ; SLP, Keystone Rehabilitation, **SLP**

Black, Katherine 1812 West Freeman Street, Carbondale, IL 62901, **SLP**

Black, Lillian M 2405 Tunlaw Road N W, Washington, DC 20007, (202) 333-8312, BS 76 SUNY - Center at Albany; MS 78 NY Univ; **SLP**

Black, Linda S P O Box 14601, Augusta, GA 30919, (404) 724-5116, BS 85 Univ of GA; ME 86 Univ of GA; Aud, VA Hosp, **A**

Black, Margaret A 4438 North 21st Place, Phoenix, AZ 85016, (602) 275-7821, BA 74 Creighton Univ; MS 75 Syracuse Univ; SLP, St of AZ-Dept Dev Dis, **SLP ACE**

Black, Margaret J 873 Greenway Court, Derby, KS 67037, (316) 788-5067, MS 75 Wichita St Univ; 78–Sp-Lang Path, USD 261, **SLP**

Black, Mrs Marjorie Blass 83 Arthur Court, Port Chester, NY 10573, (914) 937-2056, BS 78 Univ of MA - Amherst; ME 80 Northeastern Univ; Sp-Lang Path, Private Practice, **SLP**

Black, Mrs Muriel K 4820 East Earl Drive, Phoenix, AZ 85018, (602) 840-2602, BA 43 Cornell Coll; MS 67 AZ St Univ; **SLP**

Black, Mrs Nancy Jane 17 Parsonage Street, Newville, PA 17241, (717) 737-6728, BS 67 Indiana Univ of PA; ME 75 Shippensburg Univ of PA; 88–Supvr Sp-Lang Path, Capital Area Intermediate Unit, **SLP**

Black, Mrs Nancy Strainic 5207 Whiteville, Mount Pleasant, MI 48858, (517) 772-0120, **SLP**

Black, Mrs Natalye S 5050 Barranca Parkway, Irvine, CA 92714, (714) 651-0444, BA 74 CA St Univ - Fullerton; MA 76 CA St Univ - Fullerton; 80–Prog Spec, Irvine USD, **SLP**

Black, Peggy S 3140 Clay Street #5, San Francisco, CA 94115, BA 72 Univ of CA - Berkeley; MA 76 Univ of MN - Minneap-St Paul; Sp/Lang Path, Chldn Hosp Med Cen/N Ca, **SLP**

Black, S K 3931 N W Fairway Lane, Bremerton, WA 98312, (206) 692-1344, BA 75 WA St Univ; MA 77 Western WA Univ; 88–Sp-Lang Path, N Mason Sch Dist, **SLP ACE**

Black, Sandra M 21 Dawes Road, Lexington, MA 02173, (617) 354-2275, BS 61 Simmons Coll; ME 75 Northeastern Univ; 87–Co-Dir Consultation Prog, Cambridge Guidance Ctr, **SLP ACE**

Black, Susan G 2206 N W 55th, Oklahoma City, OK 73112, (405) 752-2377, BS 73 OK St Univ; MA 75 OK St Univ; Sp-Lang Path/Stud Intern Coord, Tulsa Rehab Cen, **SLP**

Black, Mrs Susan K G 203 Lynn Way, Grove City, PA 16127, (412) 458-6700, BA 70 Geneva Coll; MA 72 Univ of AL- Tuscaloosa; **SLP**

Black, Thomas S 370 Alumni Circle, Wilmington, OH 45177, (513) 393-1904, BA 75 OH Wesleyan Univ; MS 76 Vanderbilt Univ; 86–Aud, Hopewell Spec Educ Reg Res Ctr, **A**

Black, Virgil L 607 19th Avenue South, Fargo, ND 58103, (701) 232-1389, BA 58; MS 61 ND St Univ; **SLP**

Blackadar, Sue Helen 12265 Arrow Point Drive, Bainbridge Island, WA 98110, (206) 842-6432, BS 74 CO St Univ; MS 80 ID St Univ; Sp-Lang Path, Bainbridge Hrng & Sp Ctr, **SLP**

Blackard, Mrs Cornelia Nelms Route 2 Box 79, Irvington, AL 36544, (205) 957-2857, BS 82 Auburn Univ - Auburn; OM 84 Auburn Univ - Auburn; Sp-Lang Path, InSpeech Inc, **SLP**

Blackbourn, Mrs Betty N 502 Meadowview Drive, Starkville, MS 39759, (601) 323-2451, BS 70 MS Univ for Women; MS 71 Central MO St Univ; OD 75 (NS) Univ of MS; Aud/Sp-Lang Path, Starkville Mun Sep Sch, **SLP A**

Blackbourn, Jennifer W 2908 West Deborah, Monroe, LA 71201-2070, **SLP**

Blackburn, Mrs Karen D 490 Highland Drive, Mountville, PA 17554, (717) 285-5921, BS 82 Bloomsburg St Coll; MS 83 Bloomsburg St Coll; 87–Sp-Lang Path, Lancaster-Lebanon IU, **SLP**

Blackburn, Mrs Lennis Rebecca 7113 Skylark Lane, Oklahoma City, OK 73132, (405) 789-7913, MA 83 Central St Univ; **SLP**

Blackburn, Mrs Phyllis G P O Box 163, Southworth, WA 98386, (206) 478-4762, BA 70 Univ of WA; MA 79 Univ of WA; SLP, Bremerton Sch Dist, **SLP**

Blackburn, Mrs Sharon L The Mitchell House, 200 East Mason, Cadillac, MI 49601, (616) 775-9398, BA 77 Boston Coll; MA 79 Central MI Univ; Aud, Aud Svcs of Cadillac Inc, **A**

Blackburn, Mrs Starla Lucido 545 North 500 East, American Fork, UT 84003, (801) 756-2072, BS 76 Brigham Young Univ; OM 87 Brigham Young Univ; **SLP**

Blackburn, Mrs Susan Marjorie 17000 West Highway, Rocheport, MO 65279, (314) 698-4345, OB 85 Univ of MO - Columbia; OM 86 Univ of MO - Columbia; **SLP**

Blackburn, Mrs Vita Bava 108 Railroad Street, Bentleyville, PA 15314, BS 71 CA Univ of PA; ME 72 CA Univ of PA; SLP, Intermediate Unit I, **SLP**

Blackford, Mrs Connie L 607 Hillcrest, Newburgh, IN 47630, (812) 853-2432, BS 71 IN Univ - Bloomington; MA 72 IN Univ - Bloomington; SLP, Res-Care Commun Altern, **SLP**

Blackford, Michele A 2300 South Rancho Drive, Suite 214, Las Vegas, NV 89102, (304) 384-9393, BA 78; MA 79; Sp-Lang Path, NV Sp & Hrng Meaning Consult, **SLP**

Blackford, Mrs Susan H Route 6 Box 178-D, Murray, KY 42071, (502) 753-9972, BS 73 Murray St Univ; MS 75 Murray St Univ; Sp-Lang Path, Calloway Co Sch Syst, **SLP**

Black-Lawson, Virginia L 16585 Blanco Road #708, San Antonio, TX 78232, (512) 493-8643, BS 83 Southwest TX St Univ; ME 85 Southwest TX St Univ; **SLP**

Blackledge, Mrs Hilda A 211 Ferrill Avenue, Quitman, MS 39355, (601) 776-2003, BS 62 Univ Southern MS-Hattiesburg; MS 63 Univ Southern MS-Hattiesburg; 63–Sp-Lang Path, Quitman Consolidated Sch, **SLP A**

Blackley, Mrs Lynn G 9021 Holly Springs Road, Apex, NC 27502, (919) 362-0335, BS 78 Appalachian St Univ; MA 80 Appalachian St Univ; 87–Sp-Lang Path, LOGOS Inc, **SLP**

Blacklin, Mrs Jerrie Schmalzer 349 Park Street N W, Vienna, VA 22180, (703) 255-0515, MS 75 Towson St Univ; 88–Sp-Lang Path, Private Practice, **SLP**

Blackman, Ellen D 4750 Bedford Avenue, Brooklyn, NY 11235, (212) 891-1107, BA 74 CUNY - Hunter Coll; MA 75 NY Univ; **SLP**

Blackman, Jasmin 4404 Marble Hall Road, Apartment #304, Baltimore, MD 21218, (301) 435-4182, BA 83 Rutgers St Univ -N Brunswick; MS 86 Syracuse Univ; 88–Sp-Lang Path, MD Inst for EMS Sys, **SLP**

Blackman, Lisa Hearing Speech Hearing Aid Services, 1900 Rittenhouse Square C-1, Philadelphia, PA 19103, (215) 985-4964, BA 73 CUNY - Queens Coll; MA 75 CUNY - Queens Coll; Dir, Private Practice, **A**

Blackman, Mrs Ruth Rose 26 Jacamar Drive, Voorhees, NJ 08043, (609) 662-8500, BS 80 West Chester Univ of PA; MA 85 Trenton St Coll; 88–Sp-Lang Path, Robin Muller & Assoc, **SLP**

Blackman, Mrs Sylvia B 2056 81st Street, Brooklyn, NY 11214, (212) 780-5225, MA 44 Washington Univ; BA 43 Univ of IA; Assoc Prof, CUNY-Brooklyn

Blackmer, Kathryn M 3760 Texas Street, Apartment 19, San Diego, CA 92104, (619) 294-8753, BA 73 Univ of Northern IA; MA 75 Northern MI Univ; Sp/Lang Path, InSpeech Inc, **SLP ACE**

Blackmon, Dr Robert C 9 Trinity Lane, Chico, CA 95926, (916) 895-6421, BA 71 Montclair St Coll; MA 72 OH Univ - Athens; PH 76 OH Univ - Athens; CA St U Chico, **A**

Blackmon, Shirley Renee 3827 East 3rd Street #81, Tucson, AZ 85716, (602) 745-5588, BS 85 Univ of WI - Milwaukee; MS 87 Univ of AZ; 88–Sp-Lang Path, Dept of Dev Dis Tucson AZ, **SLP**

Blackmore, Denise A 178-A Kenville Road, Cheektowaga, NY 14215, (716) 838-6487, BA 84 SUNY - Center at Buffalo; MA 87 SUNY - Center at Buffalo; **A**

Blackshare, Cynthia McDonald 118 Cabana, Victoria, TX 77901, (512) 573-6143, BS 84 AR St Univ; OM 85 AR St Univ; 88–Sp-Lang Path, Bloomington ISD

Blackshear, Mrs Angela Denise 807 B Longacrea Drive, St Louis, MO 63132, (314) 993-3914, BS 78 Saint Louis Univ; MA 80 Saint Louis Univ; Rehabilitation Supervisor, Deaconess Home Health Services, **SLP**

Blackstone, Barbara 2810 Rochester Road, Zelienople, PA 16063, (412) 794-7105, Assistant Professor, Slippery Rock University, **SLP**

Blackstone, Lynn Gibbons 6700 Roswell Road #18-B, Atlanta, GA 30328, (404) 255-5734, BA 84 Albright Coll; MA 87 Temple Univ; Sp-Lang Path, Atlanta Rehab Inst, **SLP**

Blackstone, Dr Sarah W 1 Surf Way #215, Monterey, CA 93940, (408) 649-3050, BS 69 Univ of Pittsburgh - Pittsburgh; MS 75 Univ of Pittsburgh - Pittsburgh; PH 80 (NS) Univ of Pittsburgh - Pittsburgh; Editor, Private Practice, **SLP ACE**

Blackstone, Sylvia Renee 6332 Meadow Ridge Road, Baltimore, MD 21227, (202) 675-5171, **SLP**

Blackwelder, Mrs E Diane 3022 Tilden, Houston, TX 77025, (713) 668-2861, BA 74 George Washington Univ; MA 75 George Washington Univ; 88–Dir of Client Svc, American Med Commun, **SLP**

Blackwelder, Mrs Joan B 317 Cranewater Dr, Columbia, SC 29212, (803) 732-2694, **SLP**

Blackwell, Mrs Dabney Woolford 167-C Tracy Place, Hackensack, NJ 07601, (201) 441-2165, BS 83 Miami Univ - Oxford; MS 86 Boston Univ; 86–Sp-Lang Path, Hackensack Med Ctr-Inst for Child Dev, **SLP**

Blackwell, Joyce R 2100 High, Beatrice, NE 68310, (402) 223-5065, MS 71 Univ of OK - Norman; SLP, Beatrice Public Schools, **SLP**

Blackwell, Lisa Freeman 2227 Elizabeth Drive, Brandon, FL 33511, (813) 626-8156, BS 82 Delta St Univ; MS 84 Univ Southern MS-Hattiesburg; 88–Aud, Occupational Health Conservation, **A**

Blackwell, Pat B 1400 Woodland, West Lafayette, IN 47906, (317) 494-0771, BS MS Coll; MA LA St Univ - Baton Rouge; 88–Research Associate, Purdue University, **SLP**

Blackwell, Suzanne R Ni W31097 Wildwood Trail, Waukesha, WI 53188, (414) 259-1414, BA 73 Univ of MI - Ann Arbor; MS 75 Univ of MI - Ann Arbor; 87–Prog Dir, Curative Rehab Ctr, **SLP**

Blackwood, Christina Newgarden 29 Gilbert Street Box 595, Rushville, NY 14544, (716) 394-6060, MA 83 SUNY - Coll at Geneseo; Sp-Lang Path, Canandaigua City Sch District, **SLP**

Blackwood, Linda Carol 324A Main Street, Easthampton, MA 01027, (617) 662-2784, BA 82 Univ of MA - Boston; MS 87 Northeastern Univ; 88–Sp-Lang Path, Easthampton PS, **SLP**

Blackwood, Mrs Sherry Lane 4126 Maryland Avenue, Shreveport, LA 71106, (318) 636-0210, BA 70 Centenary Coll of LA; OM 86 LA St Univ - Shreveport; **SLP**

Blackwood, Mrs Toni W 227 Riverside North, Elkhart, IN 46514, BS 80 Purdue Univ - West Lafayette; MS 81 Purdue Univ - West Lafayette; Sp-Lang Path, Private Practice, **SLP**

Blades, Mrs Janet Hamby 210 Bedford Avenue, Morganton, NC 28655, (704) 433-2763, BS 78 Appalachian St Univ; MA 79 Appalachian St Univ; 83–Clinical Manager, Wn Carolina Cen, **SLP**

Bladow, Catherine Mary 12848 West Iliff Avenue, Lakewood, CO 80228, BA 81 ND St Univ; MS 83 Univ of WI - Stevens Point; Sp-Lang Path, Learning Svcs Corp-Bear Creek Comm Re-Entry Prog, **SLP**

Blaemire, Mrs Robin L 3505 Coxcomb Mews, Woodbridge, VA 22193, (301) 796-8256, BS 78 Univ of WI - Stevens Point; MA 79 George Washington Univ; **SLP**

Blaesing, Basille Evelyn P O Box 2513, Sandusky, OH 44870, (419) 627-1868, BS 79 Ball St Univ; MS 82 SUNY - Center at Buffalo; **SLP**

Blaesing, Dr Leslie L 12841 Jones Road Ste 101, Houston, TX 77070, (713) 469-7811, BS 64 Univ of IL - Urbana; MA 66 Bradley Univ; PH 78 (NS) Univ of NC - Chapel Hill; Sole Proprietor, The Sp-Lang-Learning Center, **SLP**

Blaesing, Martha E 3483 Bridgeporte Place, Boise, ID 83706, (208) 345-8220, BS 75 Western IL Univ; MA 81 Northwestern Univ; 88–Aud, VA Med Ctr, **A**

Blagden, Carolyn M c/o Linguisystems Inc, 716 17th Street, Moline, IL 61265, (309) 762-5112, BA 66 Grove City Coll; MS 80 Univ of San Francisco; Sp-Lang Path, LinguiSystems Inc, **SLP ACE**

Blager, Dr Florence B 2338 South Jasmine Place, Denver, CO 80222, (303) 270-8826, BA 50 OH Univ - Athens; MA 66 Univ of Denver; PH 70 (Sp Path) Univ of Denver; 78–Assoc Prof, Otolaryngology Univ of CO Health Sci Ctr, **SLP**

Blahut, Donald C 5 North 886 Castle Drive, St Charles, IL 60175, (312) 742-7458, BS 72 Northern IL Univ - De Kalb; MA 79 Northern IL Univ - De Kalb; **A**

Blahut, Mrs Ingrid 5 North 886 Castle Drive, St Charles, IL 60175, (312) 377-6545, BS 77 Western IL Univ; MA 79 Northern IL Univ - De Kalb; Aud, Northwestern Il Assoc, **A**

Blaige, Judith Frances 207 Regency Drive #149, Bloomingdale, IL 60108, (312) 307-0596, BS 85 IL St Univ - Normal; MS 87 IL St Univ - Normal; Sp-Lang Path, New Medico Rehab Srvs of Chic, **SLP**

Blaine, Mrs Maryanne 50 Livermore Avenue, Staten Island, NY 10302, (718) 448-6413, BS 62 SUNY - Coll at Geneseo; MA 65 NY Univ; Sp-Lang Path, NYC Bd of Ed Speech Serv Ut, **SLP**

Blair, Bruce Bennett 8820 Salisbury Road, Monclova, OH 43542, (419) 865-0251, MA 83 Bowling Green St Univ; 87–Sp-Lang Path, Sunshine Community Services, **SLP**

Blair, Mrs Carol Ann 2194 Hobblebush Lane, Lake View, NY 14085, (716) 992-3413, BS 81 SUNY - Coll at Fredonia; MS 83 2825; Sp-Lang Path, Erie Cattaraugus BOCES 2, **SLP**

Blair, Cathleen Ann Box 492, West Falmouth, MA 02574, (508) 548-0411, BA 76 PA St Univ - Univ Park; MS 83 PA St Univ - Univ Park; Sp-Lang Path, Visit Nursing Upper Cape Cod, **SLP**

Blair, Cristine Ann 361 Crockett, Seattle, WA 98109, (206) 258-7304, BA 71 Southern Methodist Univ; MA 72 Univ of AL- Tuscaloosa; Sp-Lang Path, Providence Hosp-Everett, **SLP**

Blair, Greta B 2014 Margaret Avenue, Las Vegas, NV 89101, BS 63 Univ of NV - Reno; ME 64 Univ of NV - Reno; Sp-Lang Path, Clark County School District, **SLP LM**

Blair, Dr James Carson 1563 East 1455 North, Logan, UT 84321, (801) 750-1375, BS 66 Univ of UT; MS 69 UT St Univ; PH 76 (NS) Northwestern Univ; Prof, Utah State Univ, **A**

Blair, Mrs Jo Ann 15732 Dawson Lane, Huntington Beach, CA 92647, (714) 893-6571, BA 62 Univ of FL; MA 80 CA St Univ - Fullerton; Sp-Lang Path, Huntington Beach Un Hs Dist, **SLP**

Blair, Jolynn Hopkins 4600 Willmington Pike #102, Dayton, OH 45440, (614) 962-2470, BS 84 OH Univ - Athens; MA 86 OH Univ - Athens; **A**

Blair, Julie Ann 4102 East Ray Road #1198, Phoenix, AZ 85044, (602) 759-0251, BA 79 Univ of CO - Boulder; OM 84 AR St Univ; Sp-Lang Path, Arizona State Univ, **SLP**

Blair, Mrs Kim M Box 211146, Auke Bay, AK 99821, (907) 789-3556, BA 76 Univ of FL; MA 77 Univ of FL; Sp-Lang Path/Owner, Sp Path Svcs, **SLP**

Blair, Mrs Lillian Kurtz 3 Pleasant Place, Rockaway, NJ 07866, (201) 347-0008, BA 72 William Paterson Coll; MS 82 William Paterson Coll; Sp/Lang Path, Stanhope Pub Sch, **SLP**

Blair, Mrs Lisa Annette 44 Mariner Street, Buffalo, NY 14201, (716) 882-3541, BA 81 SUNY - Center at Buffalo; MA 83 SUNY - Center at Buffalo; 83–Sp/Lang Path, The Lang Dev Prog of Wn NY, **SLP ACE**

Blair, Mrs Pamela Sue 8314 Plum Lk, Houston, TX 77095, (217) 347-7761, BS 72 Eastern IL Univ; MS 73 Eastern IL Univ; Sp-Lang Path, Cypress Fairbanks ISD, **SLP**

Blair, Mrs Patricia M 101 Colony Lane, Trinity, NC 27370, (919) 431-6772, BA 72; ME 73; **SLP**

Blair, Rebecca Lucille 21109 Northline Road, Taylor, MI 48180, (313) 287-3823, BS 82 Western MI Univ; MA 84 Western MI Univ; 87–Aud, George M Iwanow Hrng Aid Ctr, **A**

Blair, Mrs Sara Beth 30 Dorset Court, Edwardsville, IL 62025, (618) 377-7200, MS 83 Southern IL Univ-Edwardsvill; Sp-Lang Path, Special Ed Region III, **SLP**

Blair, Mrs Shirley L 530 Tomichi Trail, Gunnison, CO 81230, (303) 641-2083, BS 65 CO St Univ; MA 72 AZ St Univ; Sp-Lang Path, Gunnison PS, **SLP ACE**

Blaising, Mrs Janice C 124 Oakland Place, Battle Creek, MI 49015, (616) 963-8203, BA 67 Marygove Coll; MA 77 Western MI Univ; Sp-Lang Path, Cisd Vns of Calhoun Co, **SLP**

Blaisus, Jacqueline Treichler PSS Special Education, Saipan, Mariana Islands 96950, (670) 322-3875, BS 77 Univ of MN - Duluth; MS 80 Univ of WI - Milwaukee; Sp-Lang Path, PSS Special Educ, **SLP**

Blake, Mrs Barbara A 5 Coleman Place, Londonderry, NH 03053, (603) 434-8411, BA 76 Bridgewater St Coll; MA 77 Edinboro Univ of PA; 78–Sp-Lang Path, Londonderry School District, **SLP**

Blake, Bonnie Marie 8241 Chinook Place #3-A, Worthington, OH 43085, (614) 383-7801, BA 77 Ashland Coll; MA 85 Cleveland St Univ; 86–Sp-Lang Path, Med Center Hosp, **SLP**

Blake, Mrs Donna M 2000 Forest Dale Drive, Silver Spring, MD 20903, (301) 434-6928, BS 75 Brigham Young Univ; MA 76 Brigham Young Univ; Sp-Lang Path, Private Practice, **SLP**

Blake, Mrs Elaine B 30 Wentworth Avenue, Lowell, MA 01852, (617) 459-6186, BA 70 Univ of NH; MA 71 Bowling Green St Univ; Sp-Lang Path, Dracut Pub Sch, **SLP**

Blake, Dr Irwin H 143 Elmer Street, Westfield, NJ 07090, (201) 232-2900, BS 57 Rutgers St Univ - Newark; MA 64 NY Univ; PH 74 (NS) NY Univ; Owner, Hearing & Sp Consults, **SLP**

Blake, Mrs Jane G 7601 Coquina Drive, North Bay Village, FL 33141, (305) 757-6894, OB 65 Univ of Miami; ME 75 Univ of Miami; Sp-Lang Path, Dade Co Pub Sch-Narea, **SLP**

Blake, Dr Joan B P O Box 862, Chestnut Station, Union, NJ 07083, (201) 527-3141, BA 63 Kean Coll of NJ; MA 67 Kean Coll of NJ; PH 78 (Sp Path) NY Univ; Asst Prof, Kean Coll of New Jersey, **SLP**

Blake, Mrs Linda Miller 314 North Division, Cleveland, OK 74020, (918) 245-5911, BS 79 OK St Univ; MA 81 OK St Univ; Sp-Lang Path, The Hissom Memorial Center, **SLP**

Blake, Lizanne P 1203 12th Way, West Palm Beach, FL 33407, (305) 471-9693, BA 78 MI St Univ; MS 80 Purdue Univ - West Lafayette; Private Practice, **SLP**

Blake, Lynn Ann 3310 33rd Street, San Diego, CA 92104, (619) 541-3088, BS 81 Northern IL Univ - De Kalb; MA 83 Univ of IA; Sp-Lang Path, Children's Hosp and Health Ctr, **SLP**

Blake, Marilu W 7013 East 124th Terrace, Grandview, MO 64030, (816) 229-3869, OB 69 Central MO St Univ; MS 76 Central MO St Univ; Dir/SLP, Rainbow Cen for Commun Dis, **SLP**

Blake, Patricia Celina 65 Elm Street #16, Worcester, MA 01609, (617) 765-9771, BA 76 Coll of the Holy Cross; MA 80 Saint Louis Univ; Sp-Lang Path, Hahnemann Rehabilitation Cen, **SLP ACE**

Blake, Patricia E 2300 Ashwood Drive #A, Nashville, TN 37212-4915, (615) 297-8502, MS 76 Univ of South FL; Aud, **A**

Blake, Mrs Rhoda S 1126 Colonial Way, Bridgewater, NJ 08807, (201) 658-4064, BA 58 Boston Univ; Sp-Lang Path, Dunellen Pub Schs, **SLP**

Blake, Mrs Sandra Leona 3857 Pine Cone Circle, Waldorf, MD 20601, (301) 843-5725, BA 75 Rutgers Coll; MA 76 Univ of MD - College Park; Aud, **A**

Blake, Mrs Susan C 1823 South August, Stillwater, OK 74074, (405) 743-0010, BS 68 Central St Univ; MA 81 OK St Univ; 88–Sp/Lang Path, Stillwater PS, **SLP**

Blake, Susan Emily 84 North Third Street, Campbell, CA 95008, (408) 866-0942, BA 80 San Jose St Univ; MA 86 San Jose St Univ; 88–Sp-Lang Path, Pine Hill Sch

Blake, Susan L Special Education Services, 1208 Magnolia Avenue, Gardena, CA 90247, (213) 515-3015, BA 82 Univ of Northern CO; MA 84 Univ of Northern CO; **A**

Blakeley, Janet C 1418 Luisa, Suite 4, Santa Fe, NM 87501, (505) 982-4547, BA 77 Univ of NM; MS 80 Univ of AZ; Sp-Lang Path, Speech-Language Path Consult, **SLP**

Blakeley, Dr Robert W 3181 S W Sam Jackson Pk Rd, Portland, OR 97201, (503) 279-8356, BA 51 Univ of CA - Santa Barbara; MS 52 Univ of OR; PH 58 (NS) Univ of MI - Ann Arbor; Prof & Dir SLP/Aud Sect, Or Hlth Sci U Crpld Chldn Div, **SLP A F**

Blakely, Mrs Patricia Smith 60 Chestnut Street, Newark, OH 43055, (614) 687-6666, BA 77 OH St Univ; MA 79 OH St Univ; 82–Dir Sp-Lang Path, Professional Rehab Assoc Inc, **SLP**

Blakely, Thomas L 1423 S E 17th Street, Portland, OR 97214, (503) 661-6226, BS 84 Pacific Univ; MS 86 Eastern WA Univ; 86–Sp-Lang Path, Gresham Sch Dist, **SLP**

Blakeman, Anita Dela Garza 204 Englewood, Oak Ridge, TN 37830, (615) 482-2189, BS 70 Univ of TN - Knoxville; MA 73 Univ of TN - Knoxville; **SLP**

Blakemore, Mrs Susan K 945 Deschutes Road, Palo Cedro, CA 96073, (916) 222-1333, BS 61 Univ of WI - Madison; MA 72 San Francisco St Univ; Sp-Lang Path, Enterprise Sch Dist, **SLP**

Blakeney, Mrs Rachel Joan 6926 Faculty Circle #D, Buena Park, CA 90621, (714) 447-3091, BS 85 CA St Univ - Hayward; MS 87 CA St Univ - Hayward; 88–Sp-Lang Path, Rancho Los Amigos Med Ctr, **SLP**

Blaker, Howard Michael 408 East State Street, Doylestown, PA 18901-4708, (215) 345-7590, MA 88 Hahnemann Univ Grad Sch

Blaker, Mrs Renee G Blaker Associates, 62 West State Street, Doylestown, PA 18901, (215) 345-8682, BA 68 George Washington Univ; MA 78 Trenton St Coll; 79–Sp-Lang Path, Blaker Assoc, **SLP ACE**

Blaker, Mrs Sandra Weinberger 3 King Canute Court, Owings Mills, MD 21117, (301) 356-9064, Sp-Lang Path, Private Practice, **SLP**

Blakesley, Kathryn Lucier 1727 Hodge Lake Lane, Sugar Land, TX 77478, BA 71 LA St Univ - Baton Rouge; MA 72 LA St Univ - Baton Rouge; Sp-Lang Path, Assoc Speech & Lang Services, **SLP**

Blakey, Barbara Hackett 28 Winslow Place, Liberty, NY 12754, (914) 292-0082, BS 77 Nazareth Coll of Rochester; MS 82 Coll of Saint Rose; 86–Training Spec, Sullvian Spec Educ Training & Resource Ctr, **SLP**

Blalock, Dr Jane Wade Atlanta Speech School, 3160 Northside Parkway N W, Atlanta, GA 30327, (312) 492-3183, OB 61 Univ of FL; MS 62 Vanderbilt Univ; PH 77 (Learning Disabilities) Northwestern Univ; 85–Dir Pro Serv, Atlanta Sp Sch, **SLP**

Blalock, Philip D North Carolina Baptist Hosp, Speech And Hearing, Winston-Salem, NC 27103, (919) 748-3103, BS 70 East Carolina Univ; MA 72 East Carolina Univ; Sp-Lang Path, Nc Baptist Hosp, **SLP**

Blanar, Mrs Carol Braman 203 Johnson Road, Wadsworth, OH 44281, (216) 239-2712, BA 81 Univ of Akron; MA 87 Univ of Akron

Blanc, Julie Kay 1320 West Columbia Avenue #303, Chicago, IL 60626, (312) 743-0543, MS 88 Univ of WI - Madison; 88–Sp-Lang Path, South Metropolitan Assoc

Blanchard, Deborah Jeanne 11432 Cimarron Circle, Largo, FL 34644, (813) 462-9641, MS 83 SUNY - Coll at Buffalo; 87–SLP, Pinellas Co Brd of Educ, **SLP**

Blanchard, Mrs Diane Tooke 1209 Fairlee Street, Lakeland, FL 33803, MS 81 Univ of South FL; 87–Prog Dir, Central FL Sp & Hrng, **SLP**

Blanchard, Jane Maxwell Medical College Of VA, Box 150 McV Station, Richmond, VA 23298, (804) 359-6778, BA 78 Univ of NC - Chapel Hill; ME 86 Univ of VA - Charlottesville; **A**

Blanchard, Mrs Laurie J 11566 Wokingham Drive, Mishawaka, IN 46545, (219) 259-3763, BS 76 Univ of WI - Madison; MA 77 Western MI Univ; SLP, Sch City of Mishawaka, **SLP**

Blanchard, Shirley A 200 S W Noel #L, Lee's Summit, MO 64063, (515) 782-6211, BS 85 Southeast MO St Univ; MA 87 Southeast MO St Univ; **SLP**

Blanchard, Dr Sumner L 1226 Trestle Glen Road, Oakland, CA 94610, (415) 667-7676, MS 69 Univ of Southern CA; MA 72 Univ of Denver; PH 77 (Sp-Lang Path) Univ of Denver; 86–Sp-Lang Path & Aud, Fairmont Hosp, **SLP**

Blanchette, Jacqueline Anne 503 El Dorado Boulevard #907, Webster, TX 77598, (409) 948-2521, BA 81 Univ of TX - El Paso; ME 84 Stephen F Austin St Univ; Sp-Lang Path, Texas City ISD, **SLP**

Blanck, Mrs Cathy Pryatel 10908 Black Mountain Road, Apartment 1, San Diego, CA 92126, (619) 586-1734, BA 76 San Diego St Univ; MA 78 Saint Louis Univ; SLP, San Diego USD, **SLP**

Blanco, Felicia 2100 College Drive #123, Baton Rouge, LA 70808, (504) 927-2933, MA 86 Univ of Southwestern LA

Blanco, Mrs Lorraine R 301 Shropshire Drive, West Chester, PA 19382, (215) 431-9510, BA 74 Temple Univ; MA 76 Temple Univ; 88–Aud, J R Anncaglia MD, **A**

Blanco, Patricia M 7 Bambi Lane, Commack, NY 11725, (516) 864-2796, BA 74 SUNY - Coll at Buffalo; MS 78 Columbia Univ Teachers Coll; Coord Sp-Lang Serv, Sch for Lang & Commun Dev, **SLP**

Bland, Mrs Cheryl Ready 5125 South Kipling #205, Littleton, CO 80127, (303) 971-0411, BA 77 Andrews Univ; MS 79 CO St Univ; 85–Director/Sp-Lang Path, Ctr for Chldrn Sp-Lang Dis Inc, **SLP**

Bland, Lauren Elaine 2101 Algonquin Parkway #3, Louisville, KY 40210, (502) 776-4620, BS 79 Murray St Univ; MS 82 Univ of Louisville; Sp-Lang Path, Jefferson County Public Schs, **SLP**

Bland, Linda Marie 9737 Mt Pisgah Road #1001, Silver Spring, MD 20903, (301) 434-0269, BA 83 Univ of Pittsburgh - Pittsburgh; MA 85 Univ of Pittsburgh - Pittsburgh; 85–Sp-Lang Path, Treatment & Learning Centers, **SLP**

Bland, Ruth Anne Route 1 Box 105-B, Dunmore, WV 24934, (304) 799-4505, BS 83 CA Univ of PA; MS 86 CA Univ of PA; 83–Sp-Lang Path, Pocahontas Co Bd of Educ

Blanda, Denise J 6901 Tobik Trail, Parma Heights, OH 44130, (216) 574-8514, BS 74 Bowling Green St Univ; MA 77 Cleveland St Univ; SLP, Cleveland Pub Schs, **SLP**

Blando, Barbara Owens 18911 East 44th Place, Denver, CO 80249, (303) 741-7828, BS Northern St Coll; MS Univ of WY; 87–Sp-Lang Path, Cherry Creek Sch Dist, **SLP**

Blane, Mrs Ann D 7030 Hunters Knoll, Atlanta, GA 30328, (404) 668-0335, BS 77 Auburn Univ - Auburn; ME 78 Univ of GA; **SLP**

Blane, Kathleen F 8616 Camille Drive, Potomac, MD 20854, (201) 299-3008, BS 70 Towson St Univ; MS 72 Gallaudet Coll; Aud, Feldman Otol Assoc, **A**

Blank, Candace Rose 1211 Homestead #E, La Grange Park, IL 60525, (312) 799-5520, BS 82 Northern IL Univ - De Kalb; MA 85 Northern IL Univ - De Kalb; **A**

Blank, Catherine 2625 149th Street Court E, Tacoma, WA 98445, (206) 967-7933, BS 78 OH Univ - Athens; OM 80 Univ of WA; Sp/Lang Path, Madigan Army Med Ctr, **SLP**

Blank, Janet Louise 4390 Johnsborough Ct #10, Winston-Salem, NC 27104, (919) 748-3103, BA 80 Lenoir-Rhyne Coll; MA 85 Univ of NC - Greensboro; Audiologist, N Carolina Baptist Hospital, **A**

Blank, Karen W 50 Highgate Road, Olivette, MO 63132, (314) 454-7759, BA 71 Univ of AL- Tuscaloosa; MA 72 Univ of AL- Tuscaloosa; SLP, Jewish Hosp of St Louis, **SLP**

Blank, Lillian Lurie 4214 Mary Ridge Drive, Randallstown, MD 21133, (301) 764-6482, BA 79 Univ of MD - College Park; MA 80 George Washington Univ; Sp-Lang Path, P'Tach of Baltimore, **SLP**

Blank, Linda Rodgers 445 Tupelo Drive, Naperville, IL 60540, (312) 416-8746, SLP, Sased, **SLP**

Blank, Marcia Smith 3731 Stocker Street, Suite 211, Los Angeles, CA 90008, (213) 290-1051, BS 79 Univ of IA; MA 80 Univ of IA; Aud, Private Practice, **A**

Blank, Mrs Meryl c/o Lewis, Lewis 98 Villard Avenue, Hastings on Hudson, NY 10706, MS 69 Adelphi Univ; Workshop Consultant, Communication Skill Builders, **SLP**

Blankenship, Mrs Jacquelyn Sue Box 32 Route 1, West Hamlin, WV 25571, (304) 824-7238, MA 73 Marshall Univ; 84–Sp-Lang Path, Lincoln Co Bd of Educ, **SLP**

Blankenship, Mrs Sally Warner 3039 Catalpa Court #C, Redding, CA 96002, (916) 244-3260, BA 82 CA St Univ - Chico; MA 84 CA St Univ - Chico; Sp-Lang-Hrng Spec, Fresno Co Dept of Ed, **SLP**

Blankenship, Sue A 116 Prospect Road #M-135, Bloomington, IL 61704, (309) 359-4321, BS 86 IL St Univ - Normal; MS 87 IL St Univ - Normal; 88–Sp-Lang Path, Deer Creek-Mackinaw Comm U Dist #701

Blankenship, Mrs Terre Kay 659 South Yale, Wichita, KS 67218, (316) 755-2321, BA 82 Wichita St Univ; MA 83 Wichita St Univ; Sp-Lang Path, Sedwick Co Area Ed Ser, **SLP**

Blankinship, Mrs Becky Tomlinson 13319 Canaan Bridge Drive, Houston, TX 77041, (713) 447-0311, BA 75 Sam Houston St Univ; MA 81 Univ of Houston - Univ Park; Sp/Lang Path, Klein ISD, **SLP**

Blankinship, Mrs Mary C 24604 Marlboro Drive, Damascus, MD 20872, (301) 869-2423, BS 67 PA St Univ - Univ Park; MA 71 Univ of MD - College Park; Sp-Lang Path, Frederick Co Pub Sch, **SLP**

Blanning, Linda C 800 Custer Avenue #2-H, Evanston, IL 60202, (312) 491-4171, BA 78 Univ of Central FL; ME 80 Univ of NC - Greensboro; **SLP**

Blanski, Mrs Sheree L 1717 New Holland Road, Kenhorst, PA 19607, (215) 777-2104, BS 79 Kutztown Univ of PA; MA 87 West Chester Univ of PA; 80–Sp-Lang Path, Berks Co Intermediate Unit, **SLP**

Blanton, Mrs Mary Jacqueline 708 Prairieview Drive, Columbia, MO 65202, (314) 882-6988, MA 78 Univ of MO - Columbia; OM 84 Univ of MO - Columbia; 84–Sp-Lang Path, Univ of Missouri Hosp & Clinic, **SLP ACE**

Blare, Lindy Elizabeth 169 North Wake Forest, Ventura, CA 93003, (805) 648-5391, BA 72 Univ of CA - Santa Barbara; MA 73 Univ of the Pacific; SLP, Ventura USD, **SLP**

Blascoe, Marcia O 1257 Barberry Lane, Belvidere, IL 61008, (815) 966-3770, BS 74 Southern IL Univ -Carbondale; MA 75 Northern IL Univ - De Kalb; Sp-Lang Path, Rockford Sch Dist #205, **SLP**

Blasdel, Mary McKay 15 Moss View Court, Catonsville, MD 21228, (301) 744-1461, BA 75 Loyola Coll; MA 76 Saint Louis Univ; SLP, Anne Arundel County Pub Sch, **SLP**

Blase, Mrs Jane Z 6207 Pine Needles, San Antonio, TX 78244, (512) 659-1223, BS 74 Eastern MI Univ; ME 75 Bloomsburg Univ of PA; Admin-Owner, Crossroads Testing Service, **SLP**

Blaser, Joy O 1401 5th Street N W, Austin, MN 55912, (507) 281-6063, BS 70 Univ of WI - Eau Claire; MS 79 Saint Cloud St Univ; Sp-Lang Path, School District #492, **SLP**

Blasier, Mrs Marcia W 403 Feather Rock Drive, Rockville, MD 20850, (301) 279-5868, BA 70 Rollins Coll; MA 72 Univ of MD - College Park; SLP, Glenbrook Day School, **SLP**

Blasier, Mrs Martha H 5904 Mt Eagle Drive, Apt #1414, Alexandria, VA 22303, (703) 960-9293, BA 45 Univ of IL - Urbana; MS 69 Univ of Pittsburgh - Pittsburgh; Member State Licensure Brd, St of PA, **SLP**

Blasing, Mrs Carolyn Jo 6210 S W 21st Terrace, Topeka, KS 66614, (913) 272-2217, BA 76 Fort Hays St Univ; MS 77 Fort Hays St Univ; Sp-Lang Path, USD #501, **SLP**

Blasingame, Mrs Kelly 606 Glenbrooke #17305, Pontiac, MI 48054, (313) 683-7416, BA 85 Harding Univ; MS 87 Univ of MI - Ann Arbor; SLP, Sch Dist of Pontiac, **SLP**

Blasting, Tami H 622 Mercer Street, Albany, NY 12208, (518) 664-5066, ME 88 Coll of Saint Rose; 87–Sp-Lang Path, Helping Hands Sch, **SLP**

Blatchford, Katheryn Dean 240 South 40th Street, Boulder, CO 80303, (303) 494-9171, BA 83 MI St Univ; MA 86 MI St Univ; 88–Mgr/Aud, The Hrng & Sp Ctr, **A**

Blatchley-Hibbard, Mary Lynn 2641 Hawk Circle, Corona, CA 91720, (714) 351-9336, BA 82 Univ of CA - Santa Barbara; MA 85 IN Univ - Bloomington; SLP, Alvord USD, **SLP**

Blatt, Arlene L 70-25 Yellowstone Blvd, Forest Hills, NY 11375, (212) 546-4565, BS 73 SUNY - Center at Albany; MS 74 Univ of WI - Madison; OM 82 Northeastern Univ; 86–Group Research Mgr, Bristol-Myers Co, **SLP**

Blatt, Beverly Mara 5 Swamp Road Box 231, Whately, MA 01093, (413) 772-0211, BA 74 SUNY - Coll at Geneseo; MA 86 Univ of MA - Amherst; **SLP**

Blatt, Clayton L 2131 Via Tomas, Camarillo, CA 93010, (805) 484-3661, MA 75 Case Western Reserve Univ; Dir/Aud, Camarillo St Hosp, **A**

Blatt, Mrs Pamela Ptacek 2131 Via Tomas, Camarillo, CA 93010, BS 70 OH Univ - Athens; MA 71 Case Western Reserve Univ; SLP, Private Practice, **SLP**

Blatt, Susan Lori 81 Marlborough Street #4, Boston, MA 02116, (617) 267-5179, BA 83 Univ of VT; MS 85 Emerson Coll; 88–Sp-Lang Path, Dorchester Early Inter Prog, **SLP**

Blatt, Mrs Susan R 1520 San Vicente Boulevard, Santa Monica, CA 90402, (213) 394-8890, BS 65 Univ of IA; MA 66 Northwestern Univ; Tchr, LA USD, **SLP**

Blattstein, Mrs Barbara M 31 Southpark Drive, Garnerville, NY 10923, (914) 634-4648, BS 64 CUNY - City College; MA 81 CUNY - Lehman Coll; Audiologist, Rockland Co Assn-Phys Hndcpd, **A**

Blau, Andrea F 4901 Henry Hudson Parkway, Riverdale, NY 10471, (212) 796-5890, MS 76 CUNY - Brooklyn Coll; OM 82 CUNY - Grad Sch & Univ Cntr; PH 86 (Sp & Hrng Sciences) CUNY - Grad Sch & Univ Cntr; Consultant, Private Practice, **SLP**

Blau, Chava 12 Charles Lane, Spring Valley, NY 10977, (212) 387-2613, BA 75 CUNY - City College; MA 76 CUNY - City College; **SLP**

Blau, Deborah A 964 Lydia Place, Baldwin Harbor, NY 11510, (516) 379-9679, BA 77 SUNY - Center at Buffalo; MA 79 CUNY - Queens Coll; 87–Sp-Lang Path, Develop Ther Consult, **SLP**

Blauel, Susan B Brevard Interdisciplinary Clinic, Atlantis Professional Center #208, 2194 Highway A1A, Indian Harbor Beach, FL 32937, (407) 777-1373, BS 74 SUNY - Center at Albany; MA 78 Univ of IA; Aud, Private Practice, **A**

Blauert, Mrs Gladys Gleason 3 Candlewood, Buena Park, CA 90621, (714) 821-3620, BA 65 CA St Univ - Long Beach; MA 68 Univ of CA - Los Angeles; Asst Dir, Sp & Lang Dev Cen, **SLP**

Blauner, Mrs Betty Jo Bass 3782 East Antisdale Road, South Euclid, OH 44118, (216) 932-8765, BA 69 Univ of Denver; MS 70 Univ of MI - Ann Arbor; Sp-Lang Path, Private Practice, **SLP ACE**

Blaus, Mrs Jane Hamrick 269-B Sidney School Road, Annandale, NJ 08801, (201) 544-9394, BA 72 Randolph-Macon Woman's Coll; MA 83 Kean Coll of NJ; Sp-Lang Path, The Harbor School, **SLP**

Blaustein, June H 2000 South Tamiami Trail, Sarasota, FL 34239, (813) 365-6575, BA 69 FL Atlantic Univ; MS 71 Univ of South FL; Dir SLP, Private Practice, **SLP**

Blaustein, Steven 512 Arbuckle Avenue, Cedarhurst, NY 11516, (212) 650-6153, BA 72 SUNY - Coll at New Paltz; MS 73 PA St Univ - Univ Park; OM 78 CUNY - Grad Sch & Univ Cntr; Sp-Lang Path, Mt Sinai Med Cen, **SLP**

Blaxley, Lynn R 51 Swanwick Avenue, Toronto, ON, Canada M4E 1Z4, (416) 979-2437, BS 78 Univ of Western Ontario; MS 80 Univ of Western Ontario; Sp-Lang Path, Sp Found of Ont, **SLP**

Blayer, Nancy O 1132 West George, Chicago, IL 60657, BS 73 Univ of IL - Urbana; MA 74 Northwestern Univ; Sp-Lang Path, Chicago Bd of Ed, **SLP**

Blaz, Margaret G P O Box 573, Agana, GU 96910, (671) 734-2951, BA 77 Univ of Denver; MA 78 Univ of Denver; 79–Sp-Lang Path/Supvr, Dept of Pub Hlth & Soc Svcs, **SLP**

Blazek, Barbara Lynn 2881 Oakmont Drive, San Bruno, CA 94066, (415) 761-3347, BA 79 San Francisco St Univ; MS 81 San Francisco St Univ; Aud, VA Medical Center, **A**

Bleakney, Mary E 239 Bay 41st Street Apt 2, Brooklyn, NY 11214, (718) 449-9212, BA 78 CUNY - Brooklyn Coll; MA 80 Univ of MD - College Park; Aud, Li Coll Hosp, **A**

Blecker, Rose W Polyclinic Medical Center, Speech & Hearing Center, 3rd And Radnor Streets, Harrisburg, PA 17110, (717) 782-4350, BA 55 Univ of PA; MA 56 Columbia Univ Teachers Coll; 77–Coordinator Sp-Lang Services, Polyclinic Medical Center, **SLP ACE**

Bledsoe, Faith Elizabeth 3728 North Commercial, Portland, OR 97227, (503) 280-4400, BS 83 KS St Univ; MA 85 KS St Univ; 86–Sp-Lang Path, Emanuel Hospital & Health Ctr, **SLP**

Bledsoe, Mrs Irma M 610 Baker Street, Longmont, CO 80501, (303) 776-9366, BA 32 Univ of Northern CO; MA 46 Univ of Northern CO; MA 59 Univ of Denver; Homebound/Tutor, St Vrain Valley Sd/Private Practice, **SLP LM**

Bledsoe, Mrs Vicki Lynn 8647 Barncliff Road, Charlotte, NC 28212, (704) 372-7790, MA 83 Kent St Univ; Sp-Lang Path, Center for Human Development, **SLP**

Bleiberg, Dr Aaron H 372 Central Park West, New York, NY 10025, (212) 650-7143, OB 53; MA 56 Columbia Univ Teachers Coll; ED 68 (Speech Pathology) Columbia Univ Teachers Coll; Sp-Lang Path, Private Practice, **SLP LM**

Bleicher, Patti P 45 Oak Hill Drive, Wayne, NJ 07470-5548, (201) 633-5312, BA 74 Univ of MI - Ann Arbor; MS 77 Columbia Univ Teachers Coll; **A**

Bleichfeld, Sharla R 246 Robin Hill, Williamsville, NY 14221, (716) 688-5296, BA 75 Tulane Univ; OM 77 LA St Univ - N O Medical Ctr; **SLP**

Bleigh, Mrs Marjorie Eady 5888 Dugan, La Mesa, CA 92042, (619) 463-1111, BA 64 San Diego St Univ; MA 72 LA Tech Univ; SLP, Chula Vista Elementry Sch Dist, **SLP**

Bleil, Mrs Theresa R 953 Old Hickory Road, Pittsburgh, PA 15243, (412) 394-5815, BS 70 Indiana Univ of PA; MA 72 Bowling Green St Univ; Sp-Lang Path, Allegheny Inter Ut, **SLP**

Bleile, Dr Kenneth Mitchell 3100 St Paul #501, Baltimore, MD 21218, (301) 522-2100, BA 79 San Francisco St Univ; MS 82 Univ of OR; PH 87 (NS) Univ of IA; 87–Sp-Lang Path, Johns Hopkins Sch of Med, **SLP**

Blenderman, Phyllis Ruth 120 Hillside Avenue, Waterloo, IA 50701, (319) 273-2542, BA 83 Univ of Northern IA; MA 84 Univ of Northern IA; 88–Clin Supvr, Univ of Northern Iowa, **SLP**

Blenkarn, Mary M Cherokee County Health Dept, 912 South College, Tahlequah, OK 74464, (918) 456-8828, BA 75 Brown Univ; MA 77 Northwestern Univ; Sp-Lang Path, Cherokee Co Guid Cen, **SLP**

Bless, Dr Diane McQueen University Of Wisconsin-Madison, WCMR Room 485, 1500 Highland Avenue, Madison, WI 53705, (608) 263-8913, BA 64 San Diego St Univ; MS 65 Univ of Redlands; PH 71 (NS) Univ of WI - Madison; 86–Prof, U of WI, **SLP**

Blessing, Mrs Elizabeth Armstrong Box 569, APO New York, NY 09132, BA 83 TX Tech Univ; MS 84 Univ of SC - Columbia; 87–Sp-Lang Path, Bitburg USAF Hosp

Blessington, Therese Eileen 57 Academy Road, Albany, NY 12208, Aud, Community Health Plan, **A**

Blevins, Mrs Michelle Hampton 6917 Poplar Ridge Road, Lewisville, NC 27023, (704) 872-8931, BS 80 Edinboro Univ of PA; ME 85 Univ of NC - Greensboro; **SLP**

Blevis, Lisa S K-W Rotary Children's Centre, 828 King Street West, Kitchener, ON, Canada N2M 5B8, (519) 579-3850, BA 85 York Univ - Ontario; MS 87 Syracuse Univ; 87–Sp-Lang Path, K-W Rotary Children's Ctr

Blewett, Mrs Jana L 4981 West Charleston Street, Glendale, AZ 85308, (602) 978-6518, BS 85 Baylor Univ; MS 86 Univ of TX - Dallas; 88–Sp-Lang Path, Good Samaritan Med Ctr, **SLP**

Blews, Mrs Deborah Lyle Route 2 Box 160 A, College Grove, TN 37046, (615) 361-6450, MS 84 FL St Univ; 85–Sp-Lang Path, Professional Health Services, **SLP ACE**

Blick, Judith M 3100 Grant Avenue #E-43, Philadelphia, PA 19114-2540, **SLP**

Blickhan, Janice P 131 Windsor Drive, De Kalb, IL 60115, (815) 756-4471, MS 68 Northeast MO St Univ; 88–Prog Coord, DeKalb County Spec Educ Assoc, **SLP**

Blickle, Jennifer 470 St Andrews, Akron, OH 44303, (216) 864-1194, BA 73 Univ of Akron; MA 75 Kent St Univ; Aud, Audie Inc, **A**

Bligh, Mrs Sally B 319 Erie Street, Oak Park, IL 60302, (312) 530-8551, BA 62 Northwestern Univ; MA 64 Univ of OK Medical Center; Co-Dir, Cen for Sp & Lang Dis, **SLP**

Bliler, Dr Robert L 1221 Essex #12, San Diego, CA 92103, (714) 560-7662, BA 59 Millikin Univ; MS 60 Univ of TN - Knoxville; ED 73 (NS) Univ of Northern CO; Resource Tchr, San Diego City Schs, **SLP**

Blinderman, Michael 155 Maxine Court, Oceanside, NY 11572, (516) 536-4062, BS 60 CUNY - Brooklyn Coll; MA 61 CUNY - Brooklyn Coll; Sp-Lang Path, Mb Creative Communications, **SLP**

Blinkinsop, Paula H 2331 East 33rd Street, Davenport, IA 52807, (319) 359-1371, BS 74 Northeast MO St Univ; MA 75 Northeast MO St Univ; 75–Sp-Lang Path, MS Bend AEA, **SLP**

Blinn, James F Orange County Dept Education, South Orange County Selpa, 24701 San Doval Drive, Mission Viejo, CA 92691, (714) 859-0331, BA 73 CA St Univ - Long Beach; MA 75 CA St Univ - Long Beach; Sp-Lang Path, Orange County Dept Education, **SLP**

Blinson, Mrs Sharon Moore 30 Olde Towne Wynd North, Leland, NC 28451, BS 82 Appalachian St Univ; MS 84 East Carolina Univ; Sp-Lang Path, Comprehensive Home Health Care, **SLP**

Blischak, Doreen M Hopewell Special Education, Regional Resource Center, 5799 West New Market Road, Hillsboro, OH 45133, (513) 393-1904, BA 79 Univ of Akron; MA 81 OH Univ - Athens; Commun Consult, Hopewell Sp Ed Reg Reg Res, **SLP**

Bliss, Beverly B Box 919, Clarkdale, AZ 86324, BA 77 Univ of Southern CA; MA 79 Northwestern Univ; Sp-Lang Path, Private Practice, **SLP**

Bliss, Bonnie J Hospital For Sick Children, Aud Dept 6th Flr Em Wing, 555 University Avenue, Toronto, ON, Canada M5G 1X8, (416) 598-6770, BA 72 Univ of Toledo; MA 81 Univ of TX - Austin; Aud, Hosp for Sick Children, **A**

Bliss, Mrs Dorothy A 22424 Lake Shore Drive, Richton Park, IL 60471, (312) 748-2242, BS 68 De Paul Univ; MA 69 De Paul Univ; Sp-Lang Path, Crete Monee Sch Dist 201 U, **SLP**

Bliss, Joanne M P O Box 85, Milford, NY 13807, (607) 432-8200, BS 72 SUNY - Coll at Geneseo; MS 76 SUNY - Center at Albany; SLP, Otsego Nn Catskills BOCES, **SLP**

Bliss, Lynn S 1313 Nicolet Place, Detroit, MI 48207, (313) 577-3337, BA 61 Univ of WI - Madison; MA 66 Columbia Univ Teachers Coll; PH 71 (NS) Univ of MI - Ann Arbor; Assoc Prof, Wayne State U, **SLP**

Blitzer, Mrs Sheree B 43 Highview Drive, Woodbridge, NJ 07095, (201) 268-8140, BA 64 Adelphi Univ; MS 79 Rutger's St Univ - Douglas Coll; Sp/Lang Path, Utd Hosp Hrng/Sp Cen, **SLP**

Blitz-Noel, Elyse 5430 Baltimore Drive, Apartment 23, La Mesa, CA 92041, (619) 449-8141, BA 78 San Diego St Univ; MA 84 San Diego St Univ; SLP, Santee School District, **SLP**

Blitz-Weisz, Mrs Sally 11671 Amigo Avenue, Northridge, CA 91326, BA 76 SUNY - Center at Buffalo; MA 78 SUNY - Center at Buffalo; Sp-Lang Path, Pasadena USD, **SLP**

Blizard, Dorothy E 3738 North Abby, Fresno, CA 93726, (209) 229-9389, BA 34 CA St Univ - Fresno; MA 56 CA St Univ - Fresno; **SLP LM**

Bloch, Carole S 250 East 87th Street #28F, New York, NY 10128, (212) 439-3385, BA 63 Univ of MN - Minneap-St Paul; MA 64 Columbia Univ Teachers Coll; Chief Sp-Lang Path Svc, Lenox Hill Hosp Cen Commun Dis, **SLP ACE**

Bloch, Gerald A 418 Silver Meadows Blvd, Kent, OH 44240, (216) 467-4246, MA 78 Univ of TN - Knoxville; BA 76 Cleveland St Univ; 88–Dir of Auditory Research, Harmony Hearing Aids, **A**

Bloch, Mrs Joy P O Box 81, Vaucluse Sydney, New South Wales, Australia 2030, BA 58; **SLP**

Bloch, Joyce Katinka 16 Sachem Street, East Rockaway, NY 11518, (516) 593-2144, BA 54 Univ of Bridgeport; MA 55 Columbia Univ Teachers Coll; Sp-Lang Path, Private Practice, **SLP**

Bloch, Mrs Nancy Masnado 22440 Overlake Drive, St Clair Shores, MI 48080, (313) 465-5501, BS 80 Univ of WI - Oshkosh; MA 82 MI St Univ; SLP, Total Therapy Management, **SLP**

Bloch, Patricia J 13602 South Village Drive, Apartment 109, Tampa, FL 33624, (813) 236-5589, BA 58 Univ of Miami; MS 62 FL St Univ; Sp-Lang Path, Er Sl Cen, **SLP ACE**

Bloch, Sharon Ruth/Cohen Speech & Language Enrichment, 1015 Gayley Avenue Suite 338, Los Angeles, CA 90024, (213) 271-8613, BS 67 Northwestern Univ; MS 68 Univ of MI - Ann Arbor; Sp-Lang Path, Speech & Language Enrichment, **SLP**

Block, Alyse Glaser 511 Princeton Terrace, Paramus, NJ 07652, (212) 591-7599, BA 79 CUNY - Queens Coll; MA 80 Hofstra Univ; PH 84 (NS) CUNY - Queens Coll; 87–Supvr, NYC Bd of Educ, **SLP**

Block, Mrs Beverly S 12027 Candlewyck Lane, Jacksonville, FL 32225, (904) 641-1020, MA 76 MI St Univ; 82–Sp-Lang Path, School District, **SLP**

Block, Ellen Patricia 2342 North 56th Street, Milwaukee, WI 53210, (414) 384-2000, MS 84; 85–Aud, VA, **A**

Block, Evelyn S W 2718 West Greenleaf, Chicago, IL 60645, BA 75 CUNY - Brooklyn Coll; MS 77 Loyola Coll; SLP, **SLP**

Block, Mrs Frances K 1034 North Lasalle Street, Chicago, IL 60610, (312) 491-5012, BS 68 Northwestern Univ; MA 69 Northwestern Univ; Sch & Cl Superv/Lect, Northwestern U, **SLP F ACE**

Block, Ina Levine 804 Hillaire Drive, Pittsburgh, PA 15243, (412) 276-2865, MS 75 Univ of Pittsburgh - Pittsburgh; MA 82 Univ of Pittsburgh - Pittsburgh; Sp-Lang Path, Michael Gerard Rehab Inc, **SLP**

Block, Joanne K 309 7th Avenue East, Shakopee, MN 55379, (612) 445-4884, BS 74 Univ of WI - Milwaukee; MS 79 Univ of WI - Eau Claire; Sp-Lang Path, ISD #720, **SLP**

Block, Mrs Linda D 4000 Leighton Court, Winston-Salem, NC 27104, (919) 760-0077, BA 74 Witwatersrand Univ S Africa; MA 78 Univ of Denver; 84–Aud, Nc Baptist Hospitals Inc, **A ACE**

Block, Lisa Joan Route 1 Box 852, Evington, VA 24550, (804) 528-6956, BA 84 MI St Univ; MA 85 MI St Univ; 87–Sp-Lang Path, Ctr for Rehab & Dev Inc, **SLP**

Block, Margery E 2222 Fuller #712A, Ann Arbor, MI 48105, (313) 665-0353, BA 73 IN Univ - Bloomington; MS 74 Univ of MI - Ann Arbor; **SLP ACE**

Block, Marie K 27726 Cummins Drive, Laguna Niguel, CA 92656, (714) 492-3060, BA 81 Univ of the Pacific; BA 81 Univ of the Pacific; MA 83 Univ of CA - Santa Barbara; 87–Sp-Lang Path, Capistrano USD, **SLP**

Block, Dr Michael G Rochester Institute Of Technology/NTID, One Lomb Memorial Drive, PO Box 9887, Rochester, NY 14623-0887, (716) 475-6869, BA 69 Univ of South FL; MS 71 Univ of South FL; PH 75 (NS) Northwestern Univ; 88–Chair-Dept of Aud, Rochester Inst of Tech/NTID, **A**

Block, Mrs Wendy Heller 618 Treaty Road, Norristown, PA 19401, (215) 233-9559, MS 82 PA St Univ - Univ Park; SLP, Montgomery Co Intermed Unit, **SLP**

Block, Wendy Jayne 812 Haverford Avenue, Pacific Palisades, CA 90272, (213) 825-0067, **SLP**

Blockberger, Susan J 18-4350 Valley Drive, Vancouver, BC, Canada V6L 3B5, (604) 271-6934, **SLP**

Blockcolsky, Valeda N 673 Fordham Drive, Fairbanks, AK 99709, (907) 479-6901, BS 62 KS St Univ; MS 63 Southern IL Univ -Carbondale; Sp-Lang Path, North Star Borough School Dist, **SLP**

Block-Miller, Joyce A 4041 Via Solano, Palos Verdes Estates, CA 90274, BA 48 Univ of MI - Ann Arbor; MA 75 CA St Univ - Long Beach; Sp-Lang Path, Daniel Freeman Hosp, **SLP**

Block-Selwyn, Rochelle 34 Bannister Road, Andover, MA 01810, BS 77 SUNY - Center at Albany; MA 79 IN Univ - Bloomington; SLP, Shaughnessy Rehabilitatn Hosp, **SLP**

Blodgett, Dr Elizabeth 1636 Main Street, Murray, KY 42071, (502) 762-6810, MA 66 Auburn Univ - Auburn; MA 71 Univ of AL- Tuscaloosa; ED 85 (Special Ed/Sp-Lang Path) Univ of AL- Tuscaloosa; 88–Chair-Dept of Spec Educ, Murray State Univ, **SLP**

Blodgett, Lori Ruth 6521 Telia Drive, Pinson, AL 35126, (205) 868-2248, BS 85 Murray St Univ; MS 86 Univ of AL-Tuscaloosa; SLP, Lakeshore Rehab Hosp, **SLP**

Blodgett, Mary Jo Box 915, Rota, Mariana Islands 96951, (671) 532-9502, BA 73 Univ of WI - Eau Claire; MS 75 Univ of WI - Eau Claire; 88–Sp-Lang Path, PS Sys CNMI, **SLP**

Blodgett, Mrs Nancy H 1907 Crossgate Lane, Louisville, KY 40222, (502) 454-8240, BS 63 Univ of MO - Columbia; MA 68 Emory Univ; Sp-Lang Path, Jefferson Co Pub Sch, **SLP**

Bloechle, Mrs Lisa M 16 Edward Court, Lake Ronkonkoma, NY 11779, (516) 737-2113, BS SUNY - Coll at Brockport; MS 87 Hofstra Univ; **SLP**

Bloeser, Mrs Rubye H 4315 East Thunderbird #225, Phoenix, AZ 85032, (602) 867-3890, BA 60 Abilene Christian Univ; MA 67 Univ of NM; 87–SLP, Easter Seals Soc, **SLP**

Blohm, Mrs Elizabeth J 1620 East Northshore Drive, Tempe, AZ 85283, (602) 839-8268, AZ St Univ

Blom, Mrs Annem G 1902 North Himount Blvd, Milwaukee, WI 53208, (414) 425-4000, BS 71 Marquette Univ; MS 79 Marquette Univ; Sp-Lang Path, Whitnall Area Sch, **SLP**

Blom, Dr Eric D Head & Neck Surgery Associates, Suite 780 Medical Tower, 1633 North Capitol Avenue, Indianapolis, IN 46202, (317) 926-1056, BS 66 Miami Univ - Oxford; MA 67 Ball St Univ; PH 72 (Sp-Lang Path) Univ of MD - College Park; Sp-Lang Path, Head & Neck Surgery Associates, **SLP**

Blomberg, Mrs Barbara A 1706 Glenwood Drive, Fort Collins, CO 80526, (303) 669-3940, BS 80 CO St Univ; MS 82 CO St Univ; Sp-Lang Path, Thompson Sch Dist R2J, **SLP**

Blomberg, Karen R 12004 Rushworth Terrace, Germantown, MD 20874, (301) 497-7902, BA 79 MI St Univ; MA 81 George Washington Univ; 84–Sp-Lang Path/VP, Commun Therapy Inc, **SLP**

Blond, Mrs Marylouise Ann 30 Martin Place, Syosset, NY 11791, (516) 937-0475, BA 79 SUNY - Center at Binghamton; MS 81 Adelphi Univ; 86–Sp-Lang Path, Private Practice, **SLP**

Blonigen, Mrs Julie A 1882 Kilian Boulevard, St Cloud, MN 56304, (612) 253-0506, BA 71 Saint Cloud St Univ; MS 72 Saint Cloud St Univ; Sp-Lang Path, School District 47, **SLP**

Blood, Dr Gordon W 649 Devonshire Drive, State College, PA 16803, (513) 529-2326, BS 74 SUNY - Coll at Buffalo; MA 76 Bowling Green St Univ; PH 78 (NS) Bowling Green St Univ; Assoc Prof, PA State U, **SLP**

Blood, Dr Ingrid M U 649 Devonshire Drive, State College, PA 16803, BA 74 Montclair St Coll; MA 75 Bowling Green St Univ; PH 78 (NS) Bowling Green St Univ; Assoc Prof, PA State U, **A**

Blood, Marie Anne 4286 A Reed Road, Livonia, NY 14487, (716) 346-6967, MS 88 Nazareth Coll of Rochester; 86–Sp-Lang Path, Sch of the Holy Childhood

Bloodstein, Dr Oliver Department Of Speech, Brooklyn College, Brooklyn, NY 11210, (718) 780-5186, BA 41 CUNY - City College; MA 42 Univ of IA; PH 48 (Speech Pathology) Univ of IA; Prof/Sp-Lang Path, Brooklyn Coll, **SLP F LM**

Bloodworth, Freida Dale 161 Lingold Road Northwest, Milledgeville, GA 31061, (912) 452-0578, OM 74 Univ of MS; 86–Sp-Lang Path, Freida Bloodworth CCC-SLP, **SLP**

Bloom, Andrea 124 Blake Street, New Haven, CT 06511, (203) 387-7793, **SLP**

Bloom, Anita R 800 High School Road, Philadelphia, PA 19117-2647, (215) 663-1121, MA 80 Temple Univ; BA 78 Temple Univ; Aud, Drs Wilf Silberman Hampel, **A**

Bloom, Annette Faye 702-A Ferndale Avenue, Johnstown, PA 15905, (814) 535-5508, BS 83 Indiana Univ of PA; MS 87 Indiana Univ of PA; Sp-Lang Path, Easter Seal Soc

Bloom, Barbara J 388 Clarkson, Denver, CO 80218, (303) 629-4459, **SLP**

Bloom, Barbara M 2214 Ramsey Road, Monroeville, PA 15146, (412) 372-1080, BS 75 Univ of WI - Madison; MS 77 AZ St Univ; Sp/Lang Path, Mary Jo Truschel, **SLP**

Bloom, Bryna Schoffel 2847 Clubhouse Road, Merrick, NY 11566, (516) 543-5400, BS 73 Ithaca Coll; MA 83 Hofstra Univ; **SLP**

Bloom, Dr Charleen Marie College Of St Rose, 482 Western Avenue, Albany, NY 12203, (518) 454-5122, BS 57 Coll of Saint Rose; MA 67 Catholic Univ of America; PH 71 (NS) Univ of IL - Urbana; Admin Consult-NSSLHA, Coll of St Rose, **SLP ACE**

Bloom, Mrs Deborah B 205 Sabina Court, Danville, CA 94526, (415) 820-7664, BS 70 Boston Univ; MS 73 Univ of CO - Boulder; Sp-Lang Path, Private Practice, **SLP**

Bloom, Diane L 520 High Street, West Medford, MA 02155, (617) 488-3929, BS 73 SUNY - Coll at Buffalo; MS 74 Univ of MI - Ann Arbor; Reg VP, Nat Rehab Management Group, **SLP**

Bloom, Mrs Elaine Shapiro 1159 Shady Avenue, Pittsburgh, PA 15232, (412) 362-9175, BS 62 Emerson Coll; MS 69 Emerson Coll; Dir, Commun Dis, McKeesport Hosp, **SLP**

Bloom, Harriet Debra 125 Blanchard Boulevard, Braintree, MA 02184, (617) 935-5050, BS 83 Univ of MA - Amherst; MS 85 Boston Univ; **SLP**

Bloom, Joanne A 83 Spur Road, Dover, NH 03820, MS 74 Our Lady Lake Univ-San Anton; **SLP**

Bloom, Lawrence A 1159 Shady Avenue, Pittsburgh, PA 15232, (412) 362-8142, OB 55 Carnegie-Mellon Univ; MS 63 Univ of Pittsburgh - Pittsburgh; PH 74 (Sp-Lang Path) Univ of Pittsburgh - Pittsburgh; Family & Children's Svc, **SLP**

Bloom, Dr Lois Columbia University, Teachers College Box 5, 525 West 120th Street, New York, NY 10027, (212) 678-3888, BA 56 PA St Univ - Univ Park; MA 58 Univ of MD - College Park; PH 68 (NS) Columbia Univ Teachers Coll; Prof, Teac Coll Columbia U, **SLP F**

Bloom, Lucy 4419 Fulton Avenue #12, Sherman Oaks, CA 91423, (213) 825-5579, BA 82 CA St Univ - Los Angeles; MA 87 CA St Univ - Los Angeles; SLP, UCLA

Bloom, Mrs Nancy L R R 1 Box 59, Farmingdale, NJ 07727, (201) 938-5220, MS 76 Purdue Univ - West Lafayette; Riding Instructor & Trainer, **SLP**

Bloom, Dr Richard M 6274 Fairbrook Court, West Bloomfield, MI 48033, (313) 494-1643, BS 69 Wayne St Univ; ME 72 Wayne St Univ; ED 80 (NS) Wayne St Univ; Sp-Lang Path, Detroit Bd of Ed, **SLP**

Bloom, Ronald L 63 Main Street, Irvington, NY 10533, (914) 591-6028, BS 76 SUNY - Coll at Buffalo; MA 77 Univ of ME - Orono; Assoc Dir, Ccny Sp & Hrng Cen, **SLP**

Bloom, Mrs Thea I 13170 Hunters Brook, San Antonio, TX 78230, (512) 492-8214, BS 77 Miami Univ - Oxford; MS 78 Miami Univ - Oxford; Consultant, Cresthaven Children's Ctr, **SLP**

Bloomberg, Mrs Ruth M 15409 Vineyard Lane, Chesterfield, MO 63017, (314) 447-1151, BS 76 Univ of IL - Urbana; MS 77 Univ of IL - Urbana; Sp-Lang Path, Francis Howell Sch Dist, **SLP**

Bloomer, Dr H Harlan 708 Broadway, Normal, IL 61761, (309) 452-6638, BA 30 Univ of IL - Urbana; MA 33 Univ of MI - Ann Arbor; PH 35 (Sp (Experimental Phonetics)) Univ of MI - Ann Arbor; 88–Adjunct Prof, IL State Univ, **SLP F H LM**

Bloomfield, Barbara C 106 Stoneybrook Road, Wilmington, NC 28405, (919) 762-1744, BS 71 East TN St Univ; MA 73 East TN St Univ; Sp-Lang Path, Dev Eval Cen, **SLP**

Blose, Connie 903 Pheasant Lane, Lawton, OK 73501, (405) 248-5300, BA 70 Univ of OK - Norman; MA 71 Wichita St Univ; Sp-Lang Path, Sp/Lang Services, **SLP**

Blosser, Dr Jean L Department Of Communicative Disorders, The University Of Akron, Akron, OH 44325, (216) 375-7883, BS 69 OH Univ - Athens; MA 74 Kent St Univ; ED 86 (Higher Education Administration) Univ of Akron; 79–Assoc Prof Dir Sp/Hrng Ctr, U Akron Dept Commun Dis, **SLP ACE**

Blott, Mrs Judith P 1157 Oakland Avenue, Grandview Heights, OH 43212, (614) 486-8763, BS 71 OH St Univ; MA 73 OH St Univ; 86–Sp-Lang Path, First Choice Home Health Services Inc, **SLP**

Blouin, Mrs Carolyn K Route 1 Box 12, Ethel, LA 70730, (504) 683-8137, BA 73 LA St Univ - Baton Rouge; MA 87 LA St Univ - Baton Rouge; 79–Sp-Lang Path, E Feliciana Parish Sch Bd, **SLP**

Blouin, Martha Jo 116 Stone Lake Court, Tabb, VA 23602, (804) 865-8615, BS 64 LA St Univ - Baton Rouge; **SLP**

Blount, Mrs Adella H 3020 Berkshire Road, Cleveland Heights, OH 44118, (216) 268-6685, BA 65 Case Western Reserve Univ; MA 67 Case Western Reserve Univ; 78–Supervisor Special Education, East Cleveland Board of Educ, **SLP**

Blount, Hal Russell 1452 White Cross Drive, Baton Rouge, LA 70810, (504) 769-1659, BS 76 Edinboro Univ of PA; MA 83 Edinboro Univ of PA; 83–Sp/Lang Path, Private Practice, **SLP**

Blount, Dr Mary Ann Records 52557 Heatherfield Dr, South Bend, IN 46637, (219) 277-9397, BS 70 OH Univ - Athens; MA 74 Western MI Univ; PH 82 (NS) Univ of MN - Minneap-St Paul; Sp-Lang Path, Self Employed, **SLP**

Blount, Mary Lucille 1515 East Swan Circle, Brentwood, MO 63144, (314) 454-6213, BS 78 Northeast MO St Univ; MA 79 Northeast MO St Univ; Sp-Lang Path, Childrens Hosp-Washington Univ, **SLP**

Blount, Sharon Alexis P O Box 45089, Oak Park, MI 48237, (313) 861-0910, **SLP ACE**

Blount, Mrs Shirley M P O Box 880293, San Diego, CA 92108, (619) 574-0797, BA 50 MI St Univ; Sp-Lang Path, Private Sp & Hrng Serv, **SLP**

Bloustine, Mrs Karen S 4808 Royal Cpurt, Sioux City, IA 51104, (712) 239-2475, BS 65 Northwestern Univ; MA 66 Northwestern Univ; 88–Sp-Lang Path, Mid-Step Svcs, **SLP ACE**

Blow, Georgia W 2334 S Silver Oak Circle, Shreveport, LA 71107, (318) 424-6090, BA 76 LA Tech Univ; MS 77 LA Tech Univ; MA 80 LA Tech Univ; 78–Chief of Aud & SLP Svc, Overton Brooks/VA Med Ctr, **SLP A**

Bloxom, Mrs Katie Riddle 4024 Boyd Avenue, Fort Worth, TX 76109, (817) 926-4189, BS 83 TX Christian Univ; MS 85 Univ of TX - Dallas; Audiologist - Center Manager, Freedom Hearing Aid Center, **A**

Bloxsom, Mrs Jan L PO Box 181, Clancy, MT 59634, (406) 933-5674, BS 69 Univ of UT; MS 71 Purdue Univ - West Lafayette; 88–Sp-Lang Path, Helena Speech & Lang Coop, **SLP**

Bloyer, Cynthia J 9427 East University #42, Mesa, AZ 85207, (602) 820-6001, BS 79 Univ of WI - Stevens Point; MS 80 Univ of WI - Stevens Point; Aud, US Hearing Centers, **A**

Blue, Dr Carl M 180 Plantation Drive, Athens, GA 30605, (404) 542-1685, BS 50 Southwest MO St Univ; MA 51 LA St Univ - Baton Rouge; PH 62 (Sp Ed/Sp Path) G Peabody Coll-Vanderbilt U; Prof, U of Georgia, **SLP**

Blue, Samual, Jr 40 Morningside Avenue #53, New York, NY 10026, (212) 749-7209, **SLP**

Bluestone, Judith B 4724 Wilshire Drive, Whitefish Bay, WI 53211, (414) 963-8664, MA 85 Montclair St Coll; 86–Sp-Lang Path, St Francis Childrens Ctr, **SLP**

Bluestone, Ruth 49 Kent Street, Somerville, MA 02143, (617) 720-6726, BA 79 Witwatersrand Univ S Africa; MA 85 OH Univ - Athens; 85–Sp-Lang Path, Spaulding Rehab Hosp, **SLP**

Blugerman, Mrs Denise F 23830 Beacon, Farmington Hills, MI 48024, (313) 347-0370, BS 76 Eastern MI Univ; MA 77 Eastern MI Univ; Sp-Lang Path, Haggerty Ctr, **SLP**

Bluhm, Mrs Sharon B 406 Anderson Street, Manhattan Beach, CA 90266, (213) 379-1153, MA 88 CA St Univ - Northridge

Blum, Arthur M Columbia Pacific University, 1415 3rd Street, San Rafael, CA 94901, (415) 459-1650, BA 56 Univ of PA; MS 58 Univ of Pittsburgh - Pittsburgh; Dean, Columbia Pacific U, **SLP**

Blum, Mrs Dana J 2551 West Miami Trail, Marion, IN 46952, (317) 664-9416, BS 72 AZ St Univ; MS 73 AZ St Univ; **SLP**

Blum, Jacqueline Marci 76 Arrowwood Drive North, Winnipeg, MB, Canada R2V 2R1, BA 81 Univ of Manitoba - Winnipeg; MS 84 Univ of ND; **SLP**

Blum, Mrs Joanne Amodeo 422 North Gladstone Avenue, Margate, NJ 08402, (609) 823-4110, **SLP**

Blum, Patricia L 7032 Newton Avenue South, Richfield, MN 55423, (612) 869-0987, BS 67 Univ of NE - Lincoln; MA 68 Univ of NE - Lincoln; 80–Sp/Lang Path, United & Childrens Hosp, **SLP**

Blum, Mrs Stephanie Shaw 172 17-Mile Drive, Pacific Grove, CA 93950, (415) 728-5185, BA 76 CA St Univ - Chico; MA 80 CA St Univ - Chico; SLP, San Francisco USD, **SLP**

Blum, Mrs Wendy Beth 12 Jones Falls Terrace, Baltimore, MD 21209, (301) 396-0882, **SLP**

Bluma, Susan Marie 1659 Short Street, Berkeley, CA 94702, (415) 527-6835, BS 71 Univ of WI - Madison; MS 76 Univ of WI - Madison; 88–Sp-Lang Path, Spectrum Ctr

Blumberg, Mrs Beverly G 402 Midland Avenue, Wayne, PA 19087, (215) 527-8557, BS 73 West Chester Univ of PA; BA 77 Trenton St Coll; Co-Dir, Sp & Lrng Assoc, **SLP**

Blumberg, Mrs Ina S 8604 Timber Hill Lane, Potomac, MD 20854, **SLP**

Blumberg, Mrs Joan L 12 Old Lyme Road, Lutherville, MD 21093-3718, (301) 667-4565, BS 70 Towson St Univ; MS 71 PA St Univ - Univ Park; Aud, Carroll Co Hlth Dept, **A**

Blumberg, Mrs L B 7015 Catalonia Avenue, Jacksonville, FL 32217, (904) 725-5211, BS 76 PA St Univ - Univ Park; MS 77 Bloomsburg Univ of PA; 80–Sp-Lang Path, Duval Co Sch Bd, **SLP**

Blumberg, Mrs Lisa Stein 6705 Laurelwood Avenue, Baltimore, MD 21209, (301) 484-6989, **SLP**

Blumberg, Pamela P 7408 Tomcris Court, Springfield, VA 22153, **SLP**

Blume, Mrs Annette Harris 414 Waring Street, Philadelphia, PA 19116, (215) 677-4165, BS 61 Temple Univ; ME 83 Trenton St Coll; Teacher, School Dist of Philadelphia, **SLP**

Blumenfeld, Amy Elizabeth 123 South Broadway, White Plains, NY 10605, (203) 325-1544, BA 84 CT Coll; MS 88 Columbia Univ Teachers Coll; 88–Sp-Lang Path, Easter Seal Rehab Ctr

Blumenfeld, Mrs Brenda C 9015 North King Road, Bayside, WI 53217, (414) 352-7535, BS 81 Univ of WI - Madison; MS 83 Univ of WI - Madison; 88–Coord of Clin Svcs, Univ of Wisconsin-Milwaukee, **SLP**

Blumenfeld, Mrs Sandra Alswang 6 Wood Drive, Morris Plains, NJ 07950, (201) 540-1222, BA 68 William Paterson Coll; MS 85 William Paterson Coll; **SLP**

Blumenfeld, Mrs Vera G 69-35 173rd Street, Flushing, NY 11365, BA 59 CUNY - Brooklyn Coll; MS 61 PA St Univ - Univ Park; Sp-Lang Path, New York City Board of Educ, **SLP**

Blumenthal, Elizabeth Georgia 2708 Hillcroft Drive, Chesterfield, MO 63017, (314) 227-5140, BA 73 Loyola Coll; MS 85 Univ of AR - Fayetteville; Sp-Lang Path, Private Practice, **SLP**

Blumenthal, Ida L 136 Rosedale Circle, Winston-Salem, NC 27106, (919) 924-9309, BA 77 OH Wesleyan Univ; MA 79 Memphis St Univ; SLP, Northwest Ministry Dev Day Sch, **SLP**

Blumenthal, Reeva S 3046-B Jackson Street, San Francisco, CA 94115, (415) 563-6541, MA 88 Northwestern Univ; 88–Sp-Lang Path, Alameda County Ofc of Educ

Blumer, Janet G 4035 Woodland Creek Dr S E, Apartment 202, Kentwood, MI 49508, (616) 949-6060, BA 70 Alma Coll; ME 72 PA St Univ - Univ Park; MA 74 Northwestern Univ; Sp-Lang Path, Mary Free Bed Hospital & Rehab Ctr, **SLP**

Blumhagen-Gill, Anne L 4930 Pine Cone Drive, Durham, NC 27707, (919) 966-3325, BS 80 IA St Univ; MA 81 Northeast MO St Univ; Sp-Lang Path, Nc Mem Hosp, **SLP**

Blumke, Shelby Poindexter 430 East Park Ridge Lane, Winston-Salem, NC 27104, (704) 249-9880, BA 84 Univ of NC - Greensboro; ME 86 Univ of NC - Greensboro; 86–Sp-Lang Path, Davidson Co Schs, **SLP**

Blumling, Mrs Rochelle Cullen 3 Folger Lane, Dix Hills, NY 11746-5805, (516) 549-2634, BS 75 Ithaca Coll; MA 77 CUNY - Queens Coll; Sp-Lang Path, W Islip Pub Sch, **SLP**

Blumofe, Amy Wulf 5031 West Lunt, Skokie, IL 60077, BS 62 Northwestern Univ; MA 76 Univ of Cincinnati; Sp/Lang Path, Chicago Board of Education, **SLP**

Blumsack, Dr Judith T 2003 Chuli Nene, Tallahassee, FL 32301, (904) 656-9350, **A**

Blumstein, Linda H 979-A East 27th Street, Brooklyn, NY 11210, (212) 636-4573, BA 74 CUNY - Brooklyn Coll; MS 77 CUNY - Brooklyn Coll; Sp-Lang Path, NYC Boe, **SLP**

Blumstein, Penny R 9 Stanley Place, Edison, NJ 08817, (201) 494-5755, BA 80 SUNY - Center at Buffalo; MS 82 Columbia Univ Teachers Coll; Sp-Lang Path, Private Practice, **SLP**

Blumstein, Vivian H 65 Wilson Road, Valley Stream, NY 11581, (516) 872-0061, BA 74 CUNY - Hunter Coll; MS 76 Southern CT St Univ; **SLP**

Blundon, Patricia L H 11603 76th Avenue, Edmonton, AB, Canada T6G 0K9, (403) 437-5439, BA 78 Mount Allison Univ - Nb; MS 80 Dalhousie Univ - Nova Scotia; Sp-Lang Path, Glenrose Rehabilitation Hosp, **SLP**

Blunk, Sheila L 7878 North Wilding Dr #64, Spokane, WA 99208, (509) 299-3111, BA 75 Gonzaga Univ; MS 79 Eastern WA Univ; Sp-Lang Path, DSHS-Interlake Sch, **SLP**

Blust, Mrs Cynthia Boyd P O Box 188, Blowing Rock, NC 28605, (704) 652-6811, BS 80 Appalachian St Univ; MA 82 Appalachian St Univ; Sp-Lang Rehabilitation Spec, Private Practice, **SLP**

Bluth, Yvonne F 1914 Sioux Court, Burnsville, MN 55337, **SLP**

Blythe, Mrs Debra Lorraine 6370 Pemberton Way, Colorado Springs, CO 80919, (719) 475-5422, BA 83 NM St Univ; MA 85 NM St Univ; Sp-Lang Path, Memorial Hosp, **SLP**

Blythe, Michael E Sudbury Audiology Clinic, 845 Regent Street South, Suite 103, Sudbury, ON, Canada P3E 4T3, (705) 673-2885, BS 74 Univ of North TX; MA 77 Univ of TX - Austin; Cl Dir, Sudbury Aud Cl, **A**

Boals, Mrs Carol Martini 125 Sherbrook Road, Mansfield, OH 44907, (419) 756-1197, BS 77 OH Univ - Athens; MA 79 Kent St Univ; Sp/Lang Path, Private Practice, **SLP**

Boardley, Lorraine P 1300 Fayette Street, 26 Franklin, Conshohocken, PA 19428, (215) 828-6190, BS 78 Hampton Univ; MA 80 Univ of FL; 88–Mktg Assoc, New Medico Head Injury Sys, **SLP**

Boardman, Mrs Francine Presser 504 Rhode Island Avenue, Cherry Hill, NJ 08002, (609) 667-0981, BS 73 Emerson Coll; MA 75 Trenton St Coll; SLP, Lawnside Publ Sch, **SLP**

Boardman, Laura Jo 19444 Via Madronas Court, Saratoga, CA 95070, (408) 867-4903, BA 83 San Jose St Univ; MA 86 San Jose St Univ; 88–SLP, San Jose USD, **SLP**

Boas, Beverly S 112 South Magnolia, Tampa, FL 33606, (813) 254-8255, BS 70 Univ of MI - Ann Arbor; MS 83 Univ of South FL; Sp-Lang Path, Boas and Gildar, **SLP ACE**

Boatfield, Mary Elizabeth P O Box 503, Brockport, NY 14420-0503, (716) 663-7291, **SLP**

Boatright, Mrs Deborah S 225 Carlisle Street, Platteville, WI 53818, (608) 348-4524, BS 75 Univ of IA; MA 76 Univ of IA; 87–Sp-Lang Path, Darlington Comm Sch, **SLP**

Boatz, Mrs Donna Sheryl McDonough District Hospital, 525 East Grant Street, Macomb, IL 61455, (309) 833-4101, BS 79 IL St Univ - Normal; MS 80 IL St Univ - Normal; 87–Aud, McDonough District Hospital, **A**

Boaz, Mrs Paula H Speech Pathology Services, 222 North Pine, Magnolia, AR 71753, (501) 234-4020, BA 74 Southern AR Univ; MS 78 Univ of AR - Little Rock; Sp-Lang Path, Sp Path Serv, **SLP**

Bobbish, Mrs Ruth E 1137 South Mulberry, Ottawa, KS 66067, (913) 242-3012, BA 53 Georgetown Coll; MA 54 Univ of MO - Columbia; 79–Sp-Lang Path, USD 290 Ottawa Sch Dist, **SLP**

Bobbitt, Mildred B 912 Timber Branch Parkway, Alexandria, VA 22302, ME; **SLP**

Bober, Sally Bradburn 4416 Rebel Lane, Marshall, TX 75670, (214) 935-2725, BA 68 Univ of North TX; MA 70 Univ of North TX; Sp-Lang Path, Private Practice, **SLP**

Boberg, Dr Einer Dept Of Speech Pathology, University Of Alberta, Edmonton, AB, Canada T6G 2G4, (403) 432-5990, BA 61 Univ of IA; MA 63 Univ of IA; PH 68 (Stuttering: Sp Path) Univ of MN - Minneap-St Paul; 71–Prof, U of Alberta, **SLP**

Boboltz-Kitchen, Janice K Alpena Public Schools, 2373 Gordon Road, Alpena, MI 49707, (517) 356-6161, BA 72 Central MI Univ; MS 77 MI St Univ; Sp/Lang Path, Alpena Public Schools, **SLP**

Bobowicz, Mrs Karen Harper 6514 West Vancey Drive, Brook Park, OH 44142, (216) 937-5565, BA 79 Cleveland St Univ; MA 82 Cleveland St Univ; Sp-Lang Path, Parma Comm Gen Hosp, **SLP**

Bobowiec, Mrs Mary Suzanne 11000 Lolo Creek Road, Lolo, MT 59847, (406) 728-4000, BA 69 Univ of MT; Sp-Lang Path, Missoula Sch Dist #1, **SLP ACE**

Bobrick, Mrs Jane A 1742 North Larrabee, Chicago, IL 60614, (312) 492-5012, BS 74 Boston Univ; MA 76 Northwestern Univ; **SLP**

Bobrowsky, Dr Gerrian M 205 Trotwood Drive, Pittsburgh, PA 15241-2227, (412) 561-2121, BS 71; MS 72 2921; PH 77 (NS) 2921; Psychologist & Sp-Lang Path, Psychological & Commun Service, **SLP**

Bobruk, Toni S 2002 Avenue O, Huntsville, TX 77340, (409) 295-2263, BA 70 Sam Houston St Univ; MA 71 Univ of MO - Columbia; Sp/Lang Path, Private Practice, **SLP**

Bobry, Mrs Doris R 898 Eastbrooke Lane, Rochester, NY 14618, (716) 442-2538, MS 85 Nazareth Coll of Rochester; 88–Sp-Lang Path, BOCES Rochester, **SLP**

Boch, Mrs Caryl L 2208 Lake Hills Drive, Vandalia, IL 62471, BS 71 Southern IL Univ-Edwardsvill; MS 73 Washington Univ; Sp-Lang Path, Private Practice, **SLP**

Bochbot, Mrs Deborah Robin 1348 East 86th Street, Brooklyn, NY 11236, (718) 763-0734, BA 81 CUNY - Brooklyn Coll; MS 84 CUNY - Brooklyn Coll; Sp-Lang Path, Hebrew Academy for Spec Childn, **SLP**

Bochek, Dawn 2642 Central Drive Apartment GN, Flossmoor, IL 60422, (312) 798-1180, BS 78 Univ of WI - Madison; BA 78 Univ of WI - Madison; MS 81 Univ of WI - Stevens Point; Sp-Lang Path, **SLP**

Bochner, Laurie Flamm 2904 Lincoln Street, Alameda, CA 94501, (415) 848-4724, BA 74 Univ of MA - Amherst; MS 76 Univ of MA - Amherst; Dir, Sp Lang & Lrng Servs of E Bay, **SLP**

Bochnovich, Elaine 307 Woodhill Drive, Goshen, NY 10924, (914) 294-8806, BS 75 PA St Univ - Univ Park; MA 76 Univ of TN - Knoxville; Dept Head Audiologist, Orange Co Cerebral Palsy Assoc, **A**

Bochynski, Cathy K 47 Mirador Drive, Irvine, CA 92715, (714) 833-3644, BS 72 SUNY - Coll at Buffalo; MA 75 Kent St Univ; Sp-Lang Path, Irvine USD, **SLP**

Bocian, Mark A 84 Flint Drive, Lake Barrington, IL 60010, (312) 381-5049, BA 80 Augustana Coll; MA 81 Western MI Univ; SLP, Therapeutic Systems, **SLP**

Bock, Bonna Dee 1952 Lizanne Drive, Yuba City, CA 95991, (916) 877-9361, **SLP**

Bock, Chuck E R R Box 1350, Great Falls, MT 59404, (406) 761-1200, BS 71 Saint Cloud St Univ; MA 75 NM St Univ; Sp/Lang Path, Mt Deaconess Med Cen, **SLP**

Bock, Julie M 1210 Valence Street, New Orleans, LA 70115, (504) 893-4323, BA 72 Univ of Southwestern LA; OM 80 LA St Univ - N O Medical Ctr; Sp-Lang Path, Jefferson Parish Sch Bd, **SLP**

Bock, Lynn Annette 4122 Exeter, St Louis, MO 63119, (314) 535-8627, OB 83 Univ of MO - Columbia; MS 84 Fontbonne Coll; 86–Sp-Lang Path, Good Shepherd Sch for Chldn, **SLP**

Bock, Mrs Margaret Buckridge 49 Seaside Avenue, Westbrook, CT 06498, (203) 399-9273, BS 62 Central CT St Univ; MS 66 Southern CT St Univ; OM 72 Univ of CT; **SLP LM**

Bock, Mrs Martha R 3321 N W 27th Terrace, Gainesville, FL 32605, (904) 376-2419, BA 66 Univ of FL; MA 68 Univ of FL; SLP, Alachua Co Sch Bd, **SLP**

Bock, Ruth Elizabeth R R 1 Gr 21 Box 8, Headingly, MB, Canada R0H 0J0, BA 81 Univ of Winnipeg - Manitoba; MS 85 Univ of ND; **SLP**

Bockhaus, Nancy Jean 104 Cowdray Park, Columbia, SC 29223, (803) 788-3853, BA 59 Univ of Denver; MA 60 Univ of Denver; **SLP**

Bocko, Elizabeth Ann 925A Julia Lane, Lafayette, IN 47905, (317) 494-3792, BS 84 Univ of NH; MS 86 Purdue Univ - West Lafayette; 88–Sp-Lang Path, Purdue Univ, **SLP**

Bockover, Mrs Donna Louise 311 Massachusetts, Riverside, CA 92507, (714) 788-7114, BS 61 Ball St Univ; MS 84 CA St Coll - San Bernardino; Prog Spec-Ed, Riverside USD, **SLP**

Bockus, Sherry Lee 302 Nemeiben Road, Saskatoon, SK, Canada S7J 4S7, (306) 934-0208, BA 81 Minot St Univ; MS 82 Minot St Univ; 85–Dir Commun Dis, City Hosp

Bockway, Nancy C 749 12th Avenue, Huntington, WV 25701, **A**

Boczko, Mrs Faerella E 100 Overlook Road, New Rochelle, NY 10804, (914) 632-0535, BA 72 CUNY - Brooklyn Coll; MS 74 Columbia Univ Teachers Coll; Sp-Lang Path, Jewish Home & Hospital, **SLP**

Boddie, Geraldine P O Box 423, Waverly Hall, GA 31831, (404) 361-8650, **SLP**

Bodding, Heidi L 4323 Meridian North, Seattle, WA 98103, (206) 433-2557, BA 80 Univ of WA; MS 82 Univ of WA; Sp-Lang Path, Highline Sch Dist #401, **SLP**

Bode, Janet L 3911 Redding Road, Muncie, IN 47304, (317) 288-6384, BS 81 Ball St Univ; MA 82 Ball St Univ; 83–Sp-Lang Path, Randolph Co Schs, **SLP**

Bode, Mary G 960 Hesper Avenue, Metairie, LA 70005, (504) 888-6807, BA 71 Nicholls St Univ; MS 73 Univ of OK Medical Center; Sp-Lang Path, Jefferson Parish Pub Sch Syst, **SLP**

Bodek, Mrs Laurie J P O Box 839, 20 East Huckleberry Road, Lynnfield, MA 01940-0839, (617) 334-3794, **SLP**

Bodem, John Anthony 2 Blackberry Run, Centralia, IL 62801, (618) 532-1811, BS 67 FL St Univ; MS 68 FL St Univ; 68–Aud, Warren G Murray Dev Ctr, **A**

Boden, Kimberly 10306 Plains Court, Anchorage, KY 40223, MS 73 IN Univ - Bloomington; Sp-Lang Path, Jefferson Co Schools, **SLP**

Boden, Laura Canter 9757 Clearwater Drive, Knoxville, TN 37923, (513) 457-5400, BS 84 Miami Univ - Oxford; MA 85 Miami Univ - Oxford; 86–Sp-Lang Path, Anderson County Schs, **SLP**

Bodenhamer, Judy H 3821 Oakdale Forest Rd, Edmond, OK 73013, (405) 478-7851, BA 75 Univ of OK - Norman; MS 76 Univ of OK Medical Center; Aud, VA, **A**

Bodenhemier, Dr Wayne G 4280 Hale Parkway, Denver, CO 80220, (303) 322-1871, BA 68 Univ of Pittsburgh - Pittsburgh; MS 70 Univ of Pittsburgh - Pittsburgh; PH 77 (Aud) Univ of Pittsburgh - Pittsburgh; Exec Dir, Cen for Hrng Sp & Lang, **A**

Bodensteiner, Carole Julia 1601 West 75th Street #1-H, Richfield, MN 55423, (612) 469-4461, BA 82 Univ of IA; MA 84 Univ of IA; 86–Sp-Lang Path, Lakeville Sch Dist, **SLP**

Bodet, Glen P 120 Goode Street, Thibodaux, LA 70301, (504) 446-5079, MS 86 FL St Univ; **A**

Bodily, Noralee 6418 1/2 Woodlawn Avenue Nort, Seattle, WA 98103, (206) 524-7946, BS 81 Brigham Young Univ; MS 83 Brigham Young Univ; Sp-Lang Path, South Central Sch Dist, **SLP**

Bodily, Sherlene Ann 1325 South 400 East, Salt Lake City, UT 84115, (801) 565-7100, BS 83 Univ of UT; BA 84 Univ of UT; MS 86 Univ of UT; 87–Sp-Lang Path, Jordan Sch Dist

Bodine, Cathy Sue 8301 Elizabeth Drive, Lincoln, NE 68505, (816) 741-6470, BS 83 Southeast MO St Univ; MA 85 Southeast MO St Univ; SLP, Department of Mental Health, **SLP**

Bodkin, Donna Kay 4814½ West Southgate Road, Enid, OK 73703, (405) 237-1027, BS 82 OK St Univ; MS 86 Univ of OK Medical Center; 86–Sp-Lang Path, Dept of Human Svcs, **SLP**

Bodle, Mrs Carol Ann 21639 Carriage Lane, South Bend, IN 46614, (219) 282-4128, BS 65 Ball St Univ; MA 68 Ball St Univ; SLP, South Bend Community Sch Corp, **SLP**

Bodnar, Andrew 2442 Cherry, Dubuque, IA 52001, **SLP**

Bodnar, Bonnie M 52 Walhalla Road, Columbus, OH 43202, (614) 263-7497, MS; **SLP**

Bodnar, Mrs Kathleen Ann 117 Burke Drive, Monroeville, PA 15146, (412) 856-5826, BS 76 Indiana Univ of PA; MS 81 Indiana Univ of PA; SLP, Westmoreland Intermediate Unit, **SLP**

Bodner, Mrs Ellen F 12 Beech Road, West Orange, NJ 07052, (201) 736-0422, BA 70 Rutgers St Univ - Newark; MS 72 William Paterson Coll; **SLP**

Bodolay, Deborah L 1255 N Sandburg Terrace, Apartment 611, Chicago, IL 60610, (312) 894-9200, BS 77 Western IL Univ; MA 78 Western IL Univ; OM 84 Loyola Univ of Chicago; Sp-Lang Path, Bloomingdale Sch Dist #13, **SLP**

Bodolay, Kerry Broussard 1826 Creekbend Drive, Lakeland, FL 33811, (813) 647-2173, BA 84 Univ of Central FL; MA 85 Univ of Central FL; SLP, Polk Co Schl Bd, **SLP**

Bodrock-Raksi, Mrs Mary Katherine 9005 Memphis Villas Blvd, Brooklyn, OH 44144, (216) 749-4859, MA 84 Central St Univ; **A**

Bodtke, Mrs Liana Shreve 7401 West G Avenue, Kalamazoo, MI 49009, (616) 375-9244, BA 82 Valparaiso Univ; MA 83 Western MI Univ; Sp-Lang Path, **SLP**

Bodvig, Merrilee Jane R R Box 89-A, Tappen, ND 58487, (701) 754-2244, BS 83 Univ of SD - Springfield; MS 84 Minot St Univ; Sp-Lang Path, South Central Prairie Spec Ed, **SLP**

Body, Carmen Renee 6505 Marsol #324, Mayfield Heights, OH 44124, (216) 371-7230, BS 84 Kent St Univ; MA 84 Kent St Univ; Sp-Lang Path, Cleveland Heights City Schools, **SLP**

Bodziony, Mrs Beverly Bucell 3857 Surfside Circle, Reminderville, OH 44202-9025, (216) 562-7874, MS 85 Miami Univ - Oxford; 86–Sp-Lang Path, Portage Co Bd of MR, **SLP**

Boe, Debra J 401 Dulin, Madisonville, KY 42431, (502) 825-7388, **SLP**

Boechler, Julie A 2115-D Millbrook Court, Jefferson City, MO 65101, (314) 635-3201, BS 79 Univ of MO - Columbia; MA 80 Univ of MO - Columbia; **SLP**

Boeder, Jess Seymour 244 Sandra Lane, Eagle, ID 83616, (208) 939-0835, BS 74 CO St Univ; MS 76 CO St Univ; SLP, St Lukes Regional Medical Ctr, **SLP**

Boehlert, Lenora Therese 1261 Crane Street, Schenectady, NY 12303, (518) 456-9064, BA 79 SUNY - Coll at Cortland; MS 84 Coll of Saint Rose; Sp-Lang Path, Sas BOCES, **SLP**

Boehm, Mrs Kathleen Ann W Rd 2 8 Phillips Court, Sussex, NJ 07461, (201) 337-6106, BA 78 Kean Coll of NJ; MA 80 Montclair St Coll; Sp-Lang Path, Oakland Bd of Ed, **SLP**

Boehm, Mrs Marian B 30 Clinton Street, Sea Cliff, NY 11579, (516) 922-4100, BA 76 SUNY - Center at Binghamton; MS 78 Adelphi Univ; Sp-Lang Path, Mill Neck Manor Sch for Deaf, **SLP**

Boehmer, Janet Nabozny 301 Kensington Drive, Biloxi, MS 39530, (601) 863-0583, BA 74 Univ of MA - Amherst; MS 79 Univ of WI - Madison; Sp-Lang Path, Harrison Co Trng Cen, **SLP**

Boehmler, Dr Richard M 3125 Old Pond Road, Missoula, MT 59802, (406) 549-3421, BA 50 Univ of IA; MA 51 Univ of IA; PH 53 (NS) Univ of IA; 58–Prof Emeritus, U of Montana, **SLP F**

Boehne, Le Ann F 2508 Towne House Drive N E, Cedar Rapids, IA 52402, (319) 398-2169, BS 75 Eastern IL Univ; MS 76 Eastern IL Univ; SLP, Grant Wood AEA, **SLP**

Boehringer, Hans Walter 6011 Castleton Drive, San Diego, CA 92117, (619) 292-1180, BA 60 Albion Coll; MA 63 Univ of MI - Ann Arbor; SLP, San Diego USD, **SLP**

Boehringer, Mrs Marilyn 6011 Castleton Drive, San Diego, CA 92117, (619) 691-5536, BA 57 Central MI Univ; MA 59 OH St Univ; SLP, Sweetwater Un Hs Dist, **A**

Boeldt, Elmer A 4808 W Shore Drive, McHenry, IL 60050-3636, (815) 385-0640, BS 59 Northwestern Univ; MA 67 Northern IL Univ - De Kalb; MS 74 Northern IL Univ - De Kalb; Sp-Lang Path, McHenry Elem Sch Dist 15, **SLP**

Boeninger, Mrs Frances R 1103 Panorama Drive, Chattanooga, TN 37421, (615) 892-0286, BA 40 MS Univ for Women; MA 54 Univ Southern MS-Hattiesburg; Retired, Chattanooga Cty Sch Sys, **SLP**

Boentgen, Mrs Rae 293 Dupont Street, Long Lake, MN 55356, (612) 473-7301, BA 78 Univ of ND; MS 80 Saint Cloud St Univ; SLP, Orono Sch Dist, **SLP**

Boersma, Mrs Susan K P O Box 6, Richland, MI 49083, (616) 387-8050, BS 66 Northern IL Univ - De Kalb; MA 67 Western MI Univ; Assistant Professor, West Michigan U Dept Sp Path & Aud, **A ACE**

Boeshart, Linda R West Texas Rehab Center, 4601 Hartford, Abilene, TX 79605, (915) 691-7300, BS 74 Hardin-Simmons Univ; MS 75 TX Tech Univ; Ch, Sp-Lang Path Serv, W Tx Rehab Cen, **SLP**

Boesing, Mrs Marguerite T Dague 58 Brad Court, Floyds Knobs, IN 47119, (812) 923-7245, BS 83 Purdue Univ - West Lafayette; MA 85 IN Univ - Bloomington; 85–Sp-Lang Path, Easter Seal Hrng & Sp Ctr, **SLP**

Boettcher, Mrs Terry Latham 4881 Glenwhite Drive N W, Duluth, GA 30136, (404) 446-1998, BS 78 Univ of TN - Knoxville; MA 79 Univ of TN - Knoxville; Sp-Lang Path, Metro Area Sp Lang Serv, **SLP**

Boettger, Mrs Jill Hodgett 697 Wilford Avenue, Salt Lake City, UT 84107, (801) 521-1685, BA 79 Univ of CA - Santa Barbara; MS 82 UT St Univ; Aud-Sp-Lang Path, UT State Dept of Hlth, **SLP A**

Boettger, Mrs Lynn S 24 Pheasant Walk, Ithaca, NY 14850, (716) 243-5747, BA 76 SUNY - Coll at Cortland; MA 79 SUNY - Coll at Geneseo; SLP, Dansville Cen Sch, **SLP**

Boettger, Robert Joseph 259 West Johnson St #C-4, Philadelphia, PA 19144, (215) 596-8058, BA 82 Temple Univ; MA 84 Temple Univ; Sp-Lang Path, Self Employed, **SLP**

Boever, Anne E 8025 Upton Circle North, Brooklyn Park, MN 55444, (612) 420-7002, BS 80 Univ of MN - Minneap-St Paul; MA 82 Univ of MN - Minneap-St Paul; Sp-Lang Path, North Mem Med Ctr, **SLP**

Bofenkamp, Stewart P 2804 South Garfield Avenue, Sioux Falls, SD 57105, (605) 331-3225, BS 74 ND St Univ; MA 76 Ball St Univ; Audiologist, Central Plains Clinic, Ltd, **A**

Bogardus, Ann Olson 4-D Northwood Lake, Northport, AL 35476, (205) 759-1211, MS 83 Univ of AL- Tuscaloosa; Sp-Lang Path, Loie P Sears, **SLP**

Bogarosh, Mrs Lorna Y 12112 North Washington, Spokane, WA 99218, (509) 466-4320, BA 68 Saint Cloud St Univ; MS 69 Univ of OK Medical Center; **A**

Bogart, Lynn M 3263 Hartford Avenue, Fairfield, CA 94533, **SLP**

Bogatch, Mrs Amy R 26 Clair Street, Great Neck, NY 11021, (516) 829-8259, BS 74 Syracuse Univ; MS 75 Syracuse Univ; Sp-Lang Path, Private Practice, **SLP**

Bogdanoff, Mrs Eleanor L 684 Cliffside Drive, Akron, OH 44313, (216) 484-2547, BS 78 West Chester Univ of PA; MS 80 Loyola Coll; 81–Sp-Lang Path, Stark Co Bd Ment Ret/Dev Disab, **SLP**

Bogdanow, Janet R 1114-1/2 North Durkee St, Appleton, WI 54911, (414) 734-1808, BS 84 Univ of WI - Madison; MS 86 Univ of WI - Eau Claire; **SLP**

Boger, Janice Arlene 360 6th Street South, St Petersburg, FL 33701, (813) 821-4784, MS 76 Univ of South FL; Aud, Private Practice, **A**

Boger, Jennie L 51 Edgewood Avenue, A-8, Concord, NC 28025, (704) 788-6472, **SLP**

Bogert, Penny Smith Rural Delivery 2 Box 469, 29 East Road, Voorheesville, NY 12186, (518) 370-7582, BS 78 SUNY - Center at Albany; MS 80 Coll of Saint Rose; Sp-Lang Path, O D Heck Dev Cen, **SLP**

Boggan, Mrs Deborah A Route 2 Box 210-C, Decatur, MS 39327, (601) 635-2825, OB 78 Univ of MS; MS 80 Univ Southern MS-Hattiesburg; Sp-Lang Path, Newton Co Pub Sch Syst, **SLP**

Boggess, Dr G Jean Audiology And Speech Sciences, Purdue University, West Lafayette, IN 47907, (317) 494-3814, BS 68 Purdue Univ - West Lafayette; MA 70 Univ of IA; PH 81 (NS) Kent St Univ; Asst Prof-Aud, Purdue University, **A**

Boggia, Mrs Susan Bucalo Friends Lake, Chestertown, NY 12817, (518) 494-2768, BA 72 SUNY - Coll at Oneonta; MS 73 Adelphi Univ; 88–Dir, Glens Falls Hosp, **A**

Boggis, Ivy Marie 72 Oaks Street #1, Dover, NH 03820, (603) 692-4411, BS 81 Univ of NH; MS 84 Univ of NH; 88–Sp-Lang Path, Strafford Learning Center, **SLP**

Boggs, James R 1419 West Division, Grand Island, NE 68801, (308) 381-5931, BA 72 Kearney St Coll; MS 80 Kearney St Coll; Sp-Lang Path, Grand Island Pub Sch, **SLP**

Boggs, Margaret J 475 Bowerman Road, Scottsville, NY 14546, (716) 889-1717, BA 71 Allegheny Coll; ME 75 Clarion Univ of PA; SLP, Rochester Cty Sch Dist, **SLP**

Boggs, Teresa Ann 6242 Warner Avenue #28-H, Huntington Beach, CA 92647, (714) 847-6163, BA 82 Univ of KY; MS 84 Univ of KY; **SLP**

Bogin, Esther 44 Old Brook Road, Dix Hills, NY 11746, (516) 242-2663, MS 70 CUNY - Brooklyn Coll; Sp-Lang Path, Private Practice, **SLP**

Bogle, Janice T 2500 81st Avenue SE, Mercer Island, WA 98040, (206) 326-3483, BS 73 Vanderbilt Univ; MA 74 Vanderbilt Univ; Sp-Lang Path, Group Hlth Coop, **SLP A ACE**

Bogner, Mrs Frayne A 210 Moss Stone Way, Roswell, GA 30075, (404) 998-3048, BA 68 CUNY - City College; MA 70 Columbia Univ Teachers Coll; Sp-Lang Path, Private Practice, **SLP ACE**

Bogner, Laura Ann 129 Buckeye Street, Westerville, OH 43081, (614) 891-4532, BA 85 Lycoming Coll; MA 87 Lycoming Coll; **SLP**

Bogner, Mrs Phyllis M 120 Dunwoody, Athens, GA 30605, (404) 548-3550, BS 43 Western MI Univ; OM 70 IN Univ - Bloomington; **SLP LM**

Bognet, Dr Lea Andreuzzi 155 Coxe Street, Hazleton, PA 18201, (717) 454-3368, BS 74 Bloomsburg Univ of PA; MA 75 Seton Hall Univ; PH 83 (NS) PA St Univ - Univ Park; Sp/Lang Path, Luzerne Iu #18, **SLP**

Bogue, Dr John Phillip, Sr 1168 Drennan Park, Fort Campbell, KY 42223, (502) 798-3582, BS 64 Univ of Toledo; OD 75 Univ of MO - KS City; DD 68 (NS) Loyola Univ of Chicago; Chief of Orthodontic Serv, United States Army Ft Benning

Bogus, Janet Carol 2750 Laurel Street Suite 203, Columbia, SC 29204, (803) 256-7076, MA 84 Univ of NC - Greensboro; BS 82 Univ of NC - Greensboro; 85–Aud, Drs Haile Warder & Paysinger PA, **A**

Bogush, Laurie J 628 Erhardt Avenue, Beverly, NJ 08010, (201) 244-3100, BS 87 Syracuse Univ; ME 87 Univ of VA - Charlottesville; SLP, Deborah Tomaino, **SLP**

Bohac, Mrs Carol A 7010 Mike Lane, Panama City, FL 32404, (904) 785-0264, BS 80 FL St Univ; MS 81 FL St Univ; Superv Cl Sp-Lang Path, ABC Rehab Serv Inc, **SLP**

Bohan, Mrs Eileen Finnegan 18 Pheasant Way, Florham Park, NJ 07932, (201) 277-3353, BA 64 Marymount Coll; MA 70 CUNY - Hunter Coll

Bohaning, Teresa Lynn 207 Michelle Run, Elizabethtown, KY 42701, (502) 737-0284, BA 83 Univ of KY; MS 84 Univ of Louisville; Sp-Lang Path, Communicare Inc, **SLP**

Bohannon, Donald Lee 291 Avant Drive, Hazelwood, MO 63042, (314) 831-3658, MS 86 Southern IL Univ-Edwardsvill; 87–Sp-Lang Path, Spec Sch Dist of St Louis Co, **SLP**

Bohannon, Dorothy E 916 West 6th, Joplin, MO 64801, MS; **LM**

Bohannon, Edgar Robin 1511 Anthony Road, Augusta, GA 30904, (404) 738-7726, BS 72; MS 73; Aud, Private Practice, **A**

Bohannon, Mrs Melisa Wilcox 291 Avant, Hazelwood, MO 63042, (314) 831-3658, BS 86 Southern IL Univ-Edwardsvill; MS 87 Southern IL Univ-Edwardsvill; 88–Sp-Lang Path, Alton Catholic Children's Home, **SLP**

Bohan-Shults, Mrs Jill 235 Old Tree Trace, Roswell, GA 30075, (804) 256-2489, BA 76 Randolph-Macon Coll; MS 80 Emory Univ; Sp-Lang Path, Northside Hospital, **SLP**

Bohleen-Ferguson, Ellen Elizabeth 21828 Belshire #1, Hawaiian Gardens, CA 90716, BA 78 CA St Univ - Long Beach; MA 81 CA St Univ - Long Beach; SLP, Anaheim Un Hs Dist, **SLP**

Bohlen, Holly Heiser 16 Viking Drive, Englewood, CO 80110-7053, (901) 761-9720, BS 82 CO St Univ; MA 85 Memphis St Univ; **A**

Bohling, Ellen Roslyn 3816 Cattail Marsh Court, Apartment 253, Palm Harbor, FL 34684, (303) 425-2425, MA 84 Univ of Northern CO; 86–Sp/Lang Path Supvr, St Joseph's Hosp, **SLP**

Bohlman, Mrs Patricia A 5122 West Bluemound Road, Milwaukee, WI 53208, (414) 257-4198, BS 78 Marquette Univ; MS 80 Marquette Univ; 80–Sp-Lang Path, Milwaukee Public Schools, **SLP**

Bohman, Mrs Renee J 916 Sbragia Way, Sparks, NV 89431, (702) 358-1505, BS 74 Univ of NV - Reno; MS 82 Univ of NV - Reno; SLP, Washoe Cty Sch Syst, **SLP**

Bohn, Alexis Jane 3148 Brookwood Drive #A, Macon, GA 31204-2302, (912) 745-5497, BA 84 Univ of KY; MS 86 PA St Univ - Univ Park; 87–Sp-Lang Path, Central GA Sp & Hrng Center, **SLP**

Bohn, Eileen Hunziker 816 Memorial Drive, Sturgeon Bay, WI 54235, (414) 825-1242, BS 57 Univ of WI - Madison; MS 60 Univ of WI - Madison; 75–Sp-Lang Path, Southern Door Schs, **SLP**

Bohn, Jane E 4001 Treasure Island, Waco, TX 76705, (817) 755-2567, BS 78 Baylor Univ; MS 82 Southern IL Univ-Edwardsvill; Clin Super, Baylor U, **SLP ACE**

Bohn, Mrs Lilah M 4700 Krueger, Wichita, KS 67220, (316) 283-5011, MA 70 Wichita St Univ; Sp-Lang Path, Harvey Co Spec Ed Coop-USD 373, **SLP**

Bohn, Patti Claire 831 Barland Street, Eau Claire, WI 54701, (715) 839-4502, BS 81 Univ of MN - Duluth; MA 83 Univ of MN - Duluth; 88–Sp-Lang Path, Sacred Heart Hosp, **SLP**

Bohne, Michele Beth 5100 West 100th Street, Oak Lawn, IL 60453-3923, (312) 636-4160, BS 81 IL St Univ - Normal; MS 82 IL St Univ - Normal; Sp-Lang Path, Columbus Hosp, **SLP**

Bohne, Susan K 353 East 83rd Street #16A, New York, NY 10028, **SLP**

Bohnenblust, Brenda Diane Route 3 Box 172, Clay Center, KS 67432, (913) 485-2327, BS 84 KS St Univ; MA 85 KS St Univ; 88–Sp-Lang Path, Clay Co Hosp, **SLP**

Bohnhoff, Mrs Cathy I 7926 203rd Street SW, Edmonds, WA 98020, (206) 281-6796, BA 81 Eastern WA Univ; OM 83 Univ of WA; Aud, Seattle PS, **A**

Bohning, Susan A 1420 1/2 Gilmer Drive, Salt Lake City, UT 84105, (801) 521-1680, BS 81 Univ of UT; MS 84 Univ of UT; Aud, Prim Chldns Med Cen, **A**

Bohntinsky, Mrs Dorothy J 25890 Fairview Avenue, Hayward, CA 94541, (415) 577-1579, BS 74 CA St Univ - Hayward; MA 76 San Jose St Univ; Chief/Sp-Path & Aud, Fairmont Hosp, **SLP**

Bohon, Mrs Marian Vandenoven P O Box 2858, Roswell, NM 88201, (505) 623-0940, BA 58 Univ of WI - Madison; MS 65 Univ of WI - Madison; Sp-Lang Path, Roswell ISD, **SLP**

Bohrman, Sandra A 1809 East Cumberland Blvd, Milwaukee, WI 53211, BS 69 Univ of WI - Milwaukee; MS 73 Univ of WI - Milwaukee; Sp-Lang Path, Milwaukee Public Schools, **SLP**

Boisen, Mrs Sandra K 3203 Mission Drive, Santa Ynez, CA 93460, (805) 688-3715, BA 65 San Jose St Univ; MS 81 Adelphi Univ; Tchr, College Sch Dist, **SLP**

Boisselle, Mrs Dolores Crichlow 137 Manhattan Avenue, Teaneck, NJ 07666, (201) 881-6210, **A**

Bokelmann, Dorothy T 4604 Carriage Lane, Las Vegas, NV 89119, (702) 799-7437, BS 43 Univ of WI - Madison; ME 67 Univ of NV - Las Vegas; Coord of Sp-Lang Therapy Svcs, Clark Co Sch Dist, **SLP**

Bol, Susan Hanson 5008 14th Avenue, Minneapolis, MN 55417, (612) 448-2854, BA 77 Univ of WI - Eau Claire; MS 78 Univ of WI - River Falls; Sp-Lang Path, Chaska Pub Sch, **SLP**

Bolan, Mrs Margaret Ellen 5536 Gingerclove Way, Columbus, OH 43213, (614) 864-6035, **SLP**

Boland, Barbara A 54 Briar Lane, Basking Ridge, NJ 07920, BS 74 Seton Hall Univ; MA 80 Seton Hall Univ; Sp-Lang Path, Hunterdon Central High Sch, **SLP**

Boland, Dr John L, Jr 1113 N W 50th Street, Oklahoma City, OK 73118, (405) 842-4435, BA 38 Univ of Louisville; MA 49 Univ of MI - Ann Arbor; PH 52 (NS) Univ of MI - Ann Arbor; Sp-Lang Path &Cl Psychol, Private Practice, **SLP F LM**

Boland, Mrs Linda B 4 Nassau Circle, Flying Hills, Reading, PA 19607, (215) 775-5816, BS 75 PA St Univ - Univ Park; ME 76 Bloomsburg Univ of PA; Sp-Lang Path, Private Practice, **SLP ACE**

Boland, Lynne Marie 201 Norwood Avenue Apt 1, Buffalo, NY 14222, (716) 681-2380, BS 76 SUNY - Coll at Fredonia; MS 78 SUNY - Coll at Buffalo; **SLP**

Boland, Sr M 85 Bethany Road, Framingham, MA 01701, (508) 879-0971, 47 3793; ME 54 Case Western Reserve Univ; Retired, Bethany Hill Sch, **LM**

Bolch, Tammie M 2324 Cox Street, Port Arthur, TX 77640, (713) 985-4336, BS 79 Lamar Univ; MS 81 Lamar Univ; SLP, Port Arthur ISD, **SLP**

Boldt, Winifred F 330 Jeffrey Drive, Lincoln, NE 68505, (402) 466-9766, **SLP**

Bole, Mrs Patricia L P T And Rehab Specialists, 6917 New York Avenue, Des Moines, IA 50322, (515) 270-9376, BS 78 IA St Univ; MA 79 Univ of NE - Lincoln; Sp-Lang Path, P T and Rehab Specialists, **SLP**

Bole, Rosalie G 6260 South Jamestown, Tulsa, OK 74136, (918) 245-4491, BS 63 CO St Univ; MA 66 Stanford Univ; Sp/Lang Path, Sand Springs PS, **SLP**

Bolea, Mary Kathleen 1132 1st Avenue, Coraopolis, PA 15108, (412) 264-0565, BS 80 PA St Univ - Univ Park; MA 82 Memphis St Univ; 87–Sp-Lang Path, Diagnostic Sp and Hrng Clinic, **SLP**

Boles, Mrs Joy Liebman 973 California Street, Chico, CA 95928, (916) 538-7116, BA 79 Univ of RI; MS 81 Univ of WI - Madison

Boles, Larry A 4 Sunset Drive, Essex Junction, VT 05452, (802) 878-7653, BA 78 San Francisco St Univ; MS 82 San Francisco St Univ; 88–Sp-Lang Path, Essex Ctr Sch Dist, **SLP**

Boles, Mrs Susan P 10322 Ross, Irving, TX 75061, (214) 579-7174, BA 70 Univ of North TX; MA 71 Univ of North TX; Diag Tchr, Irving ISD, **SLP**

Bolesta, Mary Melinda 9140 Desmond Drive, St Louis, MO 63126, (314) 842-1449, OB 83 Univ of MO - Columbia; MS 85 Purdue Univ - West Lafayette; Sp-Lang Path, Head Injury Resource Ctr, **SLP**

Boley, Mrs Delesa Fox Route 1 Box 54-B, Osseo, WI 54758, (715) 597-2353, MS 83 Univ of WI - Eau Claire; SLP, Whitehall Pub Sch, **SLP**

Bolger, Beth-Lynn 2305 Ridgeway, Evanston, IL 60201, (312) 339-6227, **SLP**

Bolie-Costello, Shila R 4905 277th Avenue N E, Redmond, WA 98052, **SLP**

Bolig, Loyola Leveroni 38039 Vallejo Street, Fremont, CA 94536, (415) 790-6226, BA 63 San Francisco St Univ; MS 82 San Francisco St Univ; Aud, Agnew's Developmental Center, **A**

Bolin, Julianne C 1634 North Chambers, Wichita, KS 67212-6919, (316) 722-0114, BA 80 Wichita St Univ; MA 81 Wichita St Univ; **SLP**

Bolin, Theresa Richburg 6309 Shoal Creek Boulevard, Austin, TX 78757, (512) 323-2414, BA 82 Univ of AL-Tuscaloosa; MA 87 Univ of TX - Austin; 86–Sp-Lang Path, Austin MHMR-Infant-Parent Prog, **SLP**

Boling, Mrs Patricia V 2229 Stafford Lane, Mesquite, TX 75150, (214) 270-3594, BS 76 Univ of TX - Dallas; MS 79 Univ of TX - Dallas; 78–Sp-Lang Path, Mesquite ISD, **SLP**

Bollard, Dr Priscilla Eaves 2428 Long Ridge Road, Stamford, CT 06903, (914) 634-4648, BS 52 Columbia Univ Teachers Coll; MA 66 Columbia Univ Teachers Coll; ED 72 (NS) Columbia Univ Teachers Coll; Assoc Dir of Clinical Serv, Rockland Co Cen/Phys Hndcpd, **SLP A**

Bollerer, Susan Puryear 10826 Holly Spring, Houston, TX 77042, (713) 493-1070, BA 64 OH Univ - Athens; Sp-Lang Path, Briarwood Sch, **SLP**

Bolles, Tamara S 1212 1/2 Goodrich Avenue, Olean, NY 14760, (716) 372-7768, BS 85 SUNY - Coll at Fredonia; MS 86 SUNY - Coll at Fredonia; 86–Sp-Lang Path, Cattaraugus-Allegany County BOCES, **SLP**

Bollier, Betty J 5501 Canyonside Road, La Crescenta, CA 91214, (213) 225-6187, BA 73 CA St Univ - Northridge; MA 74 CA St Univ - Northridge; MA 88 CA St Univ - Northridge; Diag Follow-Up Coord, CA St Dept of Educ-Diag Sch, **SLP**

Bollin, Katherine M 3 Hawthorne Avenue, Albany, NY 12203-2112, (518) 370-7582, BS 79 Coll of Saint Rose; MS 83 Coll of Saint Rose; 87–SLP, O D Heck Developmental Ctr, **SLP**

Bolling, Mrs Julie F 2623 Clays Mill Road, Lexington, KY 40503, (606) 622-4442, BS 70 East TN St Univ; MA 71 Univ of KY; 72–Assistant Professor, Eastern Kentucky University, **SLP**

Bollinger, Dr Rick L ASP Service, Miami Veterans Administration Medical Center, 1201 NW 16th Street, Miami, FL 33125, (305) 324-3148, BA 66 San Francisco St Univ; MA 67 San Francisco St Univ; PH 70 (Sp) Univ of WA; 87–Chief-Aud & Sp-Lang Path Svcs, Miami VA Med Cen, **SLP F**

Bollinger-McNall, Mrs Sondra Kay 7319 B Badger Court, Indianapolis, IN 46260, (317) 259-8105, BS 85 Purdue Univ - West Lafayette; OM 87 IN Univ - Bloomington; 87–Sp-Lang Path, Indianapolis Sp & Hrng Ctr, **SLP**

Bollingmo, Susan Spivak 29632 Colebrook Drive, Laguna Niguel, CA 92677, (714) 831-2224, BA 83 CA St Univ - Fullerton; MA 86 CA St Univ - Fullerton; **SLP**

Bolson, Mrs Virginia A 1304 Seafarer Street, Ventura, CA 93001, (213) 880-4200, BA 65 CA St Univ - Northridge; MA 75 CA Lutheran Coll; Sp-Lang Path, Las Vigenes USD, **SLP LM**

Bolt, Winifred Fitzgerald 613 Dogwood Street, Amherst, VA 24521, (804) 846-8437, BS 77 James Madison Univ; MS 84 James Madison Univ; Sp-Lang Path, InSpeech Inc, **SLP**

Boltik, Mrs Kathleen L 2462 Raleigh Drive, Lancaster, PA 17601-2950, (717) 560-0747, BS 75 Marquette Univ; MS 77 Univ of WI - Madison; SLP, **SLP**

Boltjes, Mrs Connie Lee 14614 East 17th -Veradale, Spokane, WA 99037-9456, (509) 926-7320, BA 78 Eastern WA Univ; MS 82 UT St Univ; 86–Sp-Lang Path, Holy Family Hosp, **SLP**

Bolton, Mrs Debra Jean 370 Gloria Street, Shreveport, LA 71105, (318) 868-5902, BA 81 LA St Univ - Shreveport; OM 86 LA St Univ - N O Medical Ctr; 82–Sp-Lang Path, Caddo Parish Sch Bd, **SLP**

Bolton, Mrs Elizabeth Ann 302 Rowland Drive, Lynchburg, VA 24503, (804) 847-8080, BS 81 SUNY - Coll at Fredonia; ME 83 Univ of VA - Charlottesville; Sp/Lang Path, Central VA Community Services, **SLP**

Bolton, Mrs Judith Murphy Route 1 Box 284, Highland, IL 62249, (618) 644-5746, BA 72 Southern IL Univ-Edwardsvill; MS 77 Southern IL Univ-Edwardsvill; SLP, Bond Co Schs, **SLP**

Bolton, Kathleen 68 Morris Street, Hamden, CT 06517, (203) 366-7551, BS 77 Univ of NH; MA 79 Northwestern Univ; 80–Sp-Lang Path, Rehab Ctr of Fairfield Co, **SLP**

Bolton, Kathy C 4502 Keswick Road, Baltimore, MD 21210-2515, **SLP**

Bolton, Mrs Margaret G 96 Moore Street, Princeton, NJ 08540, (609) 588-8500, BA 56 Rutgers St Univ -N Brunswick; MS 74 Rutgers St Univ -N Brunswick; Sp-Lang Path, Mercer Co Spec Serv Sch Dist, **SLP**

Bolton, Maureen Talbot 3037 Clawson Avenue, Royal Oak, MI 48073, (313) 573-5545, BA 85 MI St Univ; MA 86 Northwestern Univ; 87–Sp-Lang Path, Macomb Hosp Ctr, **SLP**

Bolton-Hunt, Lisa Clark 2110 Harding, Lansing, MI 48910, (517) 337-1646, **SLP**

Bolton-Koppenhaver, Mrs Mary L 901 Vassar N E, Albuquerque, NM 87131, (505) 277-4453, BS 68 Univ of KS; MA 69 Univ of KS; Asst Prof, U of NM/Dept of Commun Dis, **SLP ACE**

Boltz, Irene M 1977 Ascot Drive, Moraga, CA 94556, (415) 376-3527, ME 77 Holy Names Coll; MA 82 Univ of San Francisco; 87–Branch Dir, Olsten Health Care Svcs, **SLP**

Boman, Tel S Ogden Speech And Hearing, 3293 Harrison Boulevard, Suite 213, Ogden, UT 84403, (801) 399-5601, BS 76 UT St Univ; MS 78 UT St Univ; Aud, Ogden Sp & Hrng Cen, **A**

Bombara, Tracy Anne 205 Vanneman Avenue, Apartment E, Swedesboro, NJ 08085, (609) 629-2400, BA 85 Univ of DE; MS 87 PA St Univ - Univ Park; **SLP**

Bombard, Mrs Linda Ann 9003 New Britain Circle, Manassas, VA 22110, (703) 361-7919, BS 82 Univ of HI - Manoa; MA 84 Univ of HI - Manoa; **SLP**

Bomberger, Victoria E 1630 2nd Avenue, York, PA 17403, (414) 632-8778, BA 74 Edinboro Univ of PA; MA 79 Northern IL Univ - De Kalb; Sp/Lang Path, Racine USD, **SLP**

Bombicino, James T Audiologist-Austine Hrng Ctr, 120 Maple Street, Brattleboro, VT 05301, (802) 254-4571, BA 75 Univ of MA - Amherst; MA 77 Univ of MA - Amherst; Aud, Austine Sch for the Deaf, **A**

Bombick, Dianne L 9101 29th Street, Brookfield, IL 60513, (312) 485-2608, BS 78 Univ of IL - Urbana; MS 79 Univ of IL - Urbana; 80–Sp-Lang Path, Arlington Hts Pub Sch, **SLP**

Bonadies, Mrs Pamela Ryan 9935 3rd Avenue, Apartment E4, Brooklyn, NY 11209, (718) 238-3142, BA 84 Providence Coll; MS 87 Southern CT St Univ; 87–Sp-Lang Path, The Child Study Ctr of NY, **SLP**

Bonadio, Mary Susan 1704 Monroe Avenue, Dunmore, PA 18509, (717) 342-5796, MS 79 Bloomsburg Univ of PA; SLP, Neiu #19

Bonagura-Grehl, Mrs Debra Rose 37 Foxwood Road, West Nyack, NY 10994, (914) 358-8348, BA 80 SUNY - Coll at Plattsburgh; MS 82 Adelphi Univ; Sp/Lang Path, Nyack Hospital, **SLP**

Bonander, Lynn A 45A Kilsyth Road, Brookline, MA 02146, (617) 731-5974, BA 69 Skidmore Coll; ME 73 Boston Univ; Sp-Lang Path, North Shore Consortium, **SLP**

Bonanni, Christine Marie 1918 Route 65, Honeoye Falls, NY 14472, (716) 924-3252, BS 84 Nazareth Coll of Rochester; MS 85 Nazareth Coll of Rochester; **SLP**

Bonanno, Amy 9734 Lochwood Road, Philadelphia, PA 19115, (215) 221-3661, BA 84 Temple Univ-Tyler Sch of Art; MA 86 Temple Univ-Tyler Sch of Art; 88–Aud, Temple Univ Health Sci, **A**

Bonanno, Mrs Diane Hope 24720 Rouge River Drive, Dearborn Heights, MI 48127, (313) 592-3342, BS 81 Eastern MI Univ; MA 82 Eastern MI Univ; Sp-Lang Path, Redford Un Sch, **SLP**

Bonastia, Mrs Lou Rita 7092 Markim Drive, Bartlett, TN 38133, (901) 528-6511, ME 84; Sp-Lang Path, Univ of Tenn Ctr for Dev Disab, **SLP**

Bonato, Mary M 7494 Vinewood Court, Maple Grove, MN 55369, (612) 682-5200, BS 79 Saint Cloud St Univ; MS 80 Univ of WI - River Falls; Sp-Lang Path, Buffalo Public School #877, **SLP**

Bonavich, Mrs Louise F 236 La Quinta Drive, Glendora, CA 91740, (714) 383-3537, BA 82 Univ of LA Verne; MS 83 Univ of LA Verne; **SLP**

Bonavico, Joni Cristine 8730 North Himes Avenue, Apartment 109, Tampa, FL 33614, (813) 931-3929, MS 86 Univ of South FL; **A**

Boncher, JoAnne B 10131 Pinnacle Lane, La Mesa, CA 92041, (619) 447-2138, BA 60 Whittier Coll; MA 86 San Diego St Univ; 88–Sp-Lang Path, Private Practice, **SLP**

Bond, Beth B 3010 Pines Road, Shreveport, LA 71119, **SLP**

Bond, Christine M 4 Peabody Road, Stoneham, MA 02180, (617) 438-8371, BS 80 Boston Univ; MA 83 Univ of MA - Amherst; 86–Aud, Head & Neck Surgical Assoc, **A**

Bond, Flavia Michelle 325 Day Street, San Francisco, CA 94131, (415) 648-8985, BS 73 Univ of OR; MA 84 San Jose St Univ; **SLP**

Bond, Mrs Jean M 1617 Lafayette Drive N E, Albuquerque, NM 87106, BS; **SLP LM**

Bond, Mrs Jennifer L Route 1, Eldon, MO 65026, (314) 392-4588, BS 73 Univ of MO - Columbia; MA 74 Univ of MO - Columbia; **SLP**

Bond, Jennifer L 796 Locust Circle, Arnold, MD 21012, (301) 729-6331, BS 80 Towson St Univ; MS 81 Loyola Coll; Sp-Lang Path, I for Hndcpd Chldn, **SLP**

Bond, Judith Louise 58 Keewatin Avenue, Toronto, ON, Canada M4P 1Z8, (416) 486-7622, BA 75 Carleton Univ - Ontario; OM 83 Univ of Toronto - Ontario; 88–Sp-Lang Path, Clarke Inst of Psychiatry, **SLP**

Bond, Karen S P O Box 343, Alliance, NE 69301, (308) 762-8926, BA 76 Univ of WY; MA 87 Univ of CO - Boulder; **SLP**

Bond, Linda Chepponis 3306 Antler Drive, Gibsonia, PA 15044, (412) 647-5580, BA 80 Univ of Pittsburgh - Pittsburgh; MS 82 Purdue Univ - West Lafayette; Sp/Lang Path, Chldns Hosp of Pgh, **SLP**

Bond, Loretta A 1017-B Old Drennan Park, Fort Campbell, KY 42223, (513) 299-6872, BS 76 Northern MI Univ; MA 79 KS St Univ; Audiologist, 121 Evacuation Hosp, **A**

Bond, Marcia D 2105 Walshview Terrace 302, Silver Spring, MD 20902, (202) 576-1677, BA 60 Univ of IA; MA 70 Univ of IA; Sp-Lang Path, Walter Reed Army Med Cen, **SLP ACE**

Bond, Mrs Nona 8072 Counselor Road, Manassas, VA 22111, (703) 347-2927, OB 57 Eastern IL Univ; MS 70 Univ Southern MS-Hattiesburg; SLP, Private Practice, **SLP**

Bond, Sandra Lynn 5649 Maurice Bell, El Paso, TX 79932, (915) 544-0139, **SLP**

Bond, Mrs Suzanne B 11746 Dixfield Drive, Dallas, TX 75218, (214) 340-1316, BS 80 Univ of VA - Charlottesville; ME 82 Univ of VA - Charlottesville; **SLP**

Bond, Dr Zinny I Linguistics, Ohio University, Athens, OH 45701, (614) 594-6364, BA 62 Univ of Akron; MA 67 OH St Univ; PH 71 (NS) OH St Univ; Prof, Ohio University

Bonderow, Mrs Helene R 2311 Borbeck Avenue, Philadelphia, PA 19152, (215) 351-7036, BA 55 Temple Univ; ME 59 Temple Univ; 56–Sp-Lang Path, Sch Dist of Phila, **SLP ACE**

Bondesson, Mrs Kelly Froning 1657 Hill Top Lane, Encinitas, CA 92024, (619) 632-9676, BS 83 Univ of IA; MA 86 Univ of Northern IA; 88–Sp-Lang Path, TriCity Med Ctr, **SLP**

Bondi, Mrs Carole Turner 1614 Elderwood Circle, Middleton, WI 53562, (608) 836-1728, BA 61 Univ of IA; **SLP**

Bondi, Marcel M 2247 Lake Spur Road, Seneca Falls, NY 13148, (315) 568-5747, BS 83 SUNY - Coll at Geneseo; MS 88 Nazareth Coll of Rochester; Sp-Lang Path, WFL BOCES, **SLP**

Bondi, Terry M 5731 North Withrop, Chicago, IL 60660, (309) 367-2388, BS 78 IL St Univ - Normal; MS 80 IL St Univ - Normal; Sp-Lang Path, Chicago Board of Education, **SLP ACE**

Bond-Moore, Sharon A Box 201, Bredenbury, SK, Canada S0A 0H0, (306) 786-1600, BS 71 Lamar Univ; MS 72 Lamar Univ; Sp/Lang Path, Yorkton-Melville Hlth Reg, **SLP**

Bonds, Elisabeth Via 651 Probasco Street, Cincinnati, OH 45220, (513) 923-4000, Aud, Ear Nose Throat Cl, **A**

Bonds-Baird, Joy 5511 Ashland Way, Sacramento, CA 95822, (916) 451-5279, BA 78 San Francisco St Univ; MS 80 San Francisco St Univ; Sp-Lang Path, Sacramento Co Office Ed, **SLP**

Bondurant, Lynn Swain 1015 Culver Road, Rochester, NY 14609, (716) 243-5470, BA 82 SUNY - Coll at Potsdam; MA 84 Nazareth Coll of Rochester; 85–Sp-Lang Path, Livingst-Steuben-Wy Co BOCES, **SLP**

Bondy, Alice 3353 Dumaine Street, New Orleans, LA 70119, (504) 486-4262, BA 60 Tulane Univ; OM 82 Tulane Univ; Sp-Lang Path, Jefferson Parish School System, **SLP**

Bondy, Pamela S 1842 West Barry, Chicago, IL 60657-2041, (312) 281-2466, BS 78 Univ of AZ; MS 80 Univ of WI - Madison; Sp-Lang Path, Il Masonic Med Cen, **SLP**

Boneberg, Joan Marie 10 Elderberry Lane, Liverpool, NY 13090, BS 83 SUNY - Coll at Buffalo; MS 84 SUNY - Coll at Buffalo; SLP, Baldwinsville Central Schools, **SLP**

Bonenberger, Pamela L Box 483, Kadoka, SD 57543, (605) 837-2371, MA 76 Univ of SD - Vermillion; Sp/Lang Path, Kadoka Sch, **SLP**

Boner, Mrs Maureen Maney 4411 Forest Walk Drive, Greensboro, NC 27408, (919) 621-0631, BA 81 Univ of NC - Chapel Hill; MS 82 Univ of NC - Chapel Hill; Sp-Lang Path, Greensboro PS, **SLP**

Bonerbo-Marino, Mrs Marie Louise Unit 410 Drew Lane, Carmel, NY 10512, (914) 278-7435, BA 83 Marymount Coll; MS 85 Columbia Univ Teachers Coll; 86–Aud, St Josephs Sch for Deaf, **A**

Bonet, Mrs Jeanne Spinoso 18 West 141 Holly, Westmont, IL 60559, (312) 834-4541, MS 80 IL St Univ - Normal; Sp-Lang Path, Elmhurst Dist 205 Elmhurst Il, **SLP**

Bonewitz, Mrs Karen S 309 East 1st, Newton, KS 67114, (316) 283-5011, BA 75 KS St Univ; MS 76 KS St Univ; 86–Sp-Lang Path, USD #373, **SLP**

Boney, Stephen J Dept Communication Disorders, University Of Nebraska, 253 Barkley Memorial Ctr, Lincoln, NE 68583, (402) 472-2071, BA 72 Kent St Univ; MA 74 Kent St Univ; PH 86 (Aud) Vanderbilt Univ; 86–Asst Prof, Univ of Nebraska, **A**

Bonfante, Laurie Ann 67 Norwalk Avenue, Buffalo, NY 14216, (716) 894-0427, BA 85 SUNY - Center at Buffalo; MS 86 SUNY - Coll at Buffalo; **SLP**

Bonfanti, Dr Barbara H 335 National Pike East, Brownsville, PA 15417, (412) 664-5018, BS 67 Indiana Univ of PA; ME 69 CA Univ of PA; PH 76 Univ of Pittsburgh - Pittsburgh; Man SLP/Aud, South Hills Hlth Sys, **SLP**

Bonfanti, Richard T 803 Ashcroft Avenue, Cresson, PA 16630, (814) 472-7350, BS 67 Clarion Univ of PA; MS 79 Univ of Pittsburgh - Pittsburgh; ME 69 CA Univ of PA; Mental Retired Unit Mgr, Ebensburg Center, **SLP A**

Bonfield, Mrs Marianne Chapas 818 Jefferson Drive, Pittsburgh, PA 15229, (412) 665-4985, BS 73 Edinboro Univ of PA; MA 81 Univ of Pittsburgh - Pittsburgh; Sp-Lang Path, Pittsburgh Pub Sch, **SLP**

Bong, Joanne L 12515 S E 15th Street, Vancouver, WA 98684, (503) 635-0372, BS 69 Univ of WI - Eau Claire; MS 70 Univ of WI - Madison; Sp-Lang Path, Lake Oswego Pub Sch, **SLP**

Bongers, Libewij F 30526 Laramie, Redlands, CA 92374, (714) 794-7743, BA 84; MS 86 Univ of Redlands; **SLP**

Bongfeldt, Mary L T 1533 Atlanta Drive, Irving, TX 75062, (214) 255-8572, BS 77 Univ of North TX; MS 79 Univ of North TX; Sp-Lang Path, Irving ISD, **SLP**

Bongiorno, Joseph A 90 Bay Road, Huntington, NY 11743, (516) 781-8000, BA 58 Adelphi Univ; MS 64 Adelphi Univ; Sp-Lang Path, Wantagh PS, **SLP**

Bonhag-Hansen, Mrs Elizabeth 1726 Belmont Avenue, South Belmar, NJ 07719, (201) 775-5319, BS 79 SUNY - Coll at New Paltz; MS 81 PA St Univ - Univ Park; 84–Sp-Lang Path, Neptune City School System, **SLP**

Bonham, Mrs Carlene Snider 7801 Dartmouth Road, Indianapolis, IN 46260, (317) 253-2645, BS 78 Ball St Univ; MA 79 Ball St Univ; 88–Sp-Lang Path, Avon Community Sch Corp, **SLP**

Bonicatto, Mrs Corinne H Route 9, Hayward, WI 54843, (715) 634-8463, BS 66 Univ of MN - Duluth; MA 68 Univ of AZ; SLP, Hayward Commun Sch, **SLP**

Bonich, Diane Scarcelli 168 Nassau Boulevard, Garden City, NY 11530, (516) 221-4700, BA 80 Long Island U - CW Post Ctr; MA 82 Hofstra Univ; 81–Sp-Lang Path, Assoc for Children w Down Syn, **SLP**

Boniciolli, Lori Marie 37 Euclid Avenue, Dix Hills, NY 11746, (516) 924-6008, BA 80 Long Island U - Southampton; MA 86 Hofstra Univ; **SLP**

Bonifant, Debra Croft 1337 Excaliber Lane, Sandy Spring, MD 20860, (301) 570-4057, BS 78 James Madison Univ; MS 80 James Madison Univ; Sp-Lang Path, Montgomery Co Pub Sch, **SLP**

Bonin, Betsy Jean 1110 McArthur Avenue, Colorado Springs, CO 80909, (719) 475-5292, BA 71 Keuka Coll; MA 81 Univ of CO - Boulder; Sp-Lang Path, Mem Hosp, **SLP**

Bonine, Louann Marie 601 Glencoe Street N E, Fridley, MN 55432, (612) 263-2911, BS 84 Saint Cloud St Univ; MA 85 Univ of MN - Duluth; **SLP**

Bonino, Joanne O 52 Robbins Avenue, Newington, CT 06111, (203) 521-5849, BS 77 Univ of CT; MS 80 Southern CT St Univ; Sp-Lang Path, Bristol Bd of Ed, **SLP**

Bonitati, Mrs Carolyn L 602 North May Unit 110, Mesa, AZ 85201, (602) 481-4887, BA 85 Western KY Univ; MA 87 Univ of CO - Boulder; 87–Sp-Lang Path, Lee Silverman Ctr for Parkinsons, **SLP**

Bonk, Mary Shannon 2600 New Concorde Court, Herndon, VA 22071, (703) 522-2777, BS 81 Marquette Univ; MS 82 Marquette Univ; Sp-Lang Path, Easter Seal Society, **SLP**

Bonko, Mrs Julie Anne 3720 Washington Pike Blvd, Newburg Heights, OH 44105, (216) 641-4752, BA 85 Cleveland St Univ; MA 87 Cleveland St Univ

Bonnell-Corcoran, Mrs Catherine 408 Yoder Road, Harleysville, PA 19438, BA 81 Glassboro St Coll; MS 83 PA St Univ - Univ Park; Sp-Lang Path, Montgomery Cnty Intermed Unit, **SLP**

Bonnell-Farmer, Mrs Cathy Ann R R 5 Box 45, Ottumwa, IA 52501-9203, (515) 684-4265, BS 78 Northeast MO St Univ; MA 79 Northeast MO St Univ; SLP, Sn Prairie AEA, **SLP**

Bonnema, Mrs Christine Monticello 2220 Estelle S E, Grand Rapids, MI 49506, (616) 242-0425, BA 85 MI St Univ; MA 87 Eastern MI Univ; Sp-Lang Path, Mary Freebed Rehab Ctr & Hosp, **SLP**

Bonner, Mrs Jerri Lynn P O Box 536, Pollock, LA 71467, (318) 445-5111, BA 84 LA St Univ - Shreveport; MS 87 Univ of Southwestern LA; 88–Sp-Lang Path, Psy Cog Associates Inc

Bonner, Katherine Ann Star Route Box 245-I, Tijeras, NM 87059, (505) 821-2211, BS 82 Univ of MN - Duluth; MA 83 Univ of MN - Duluth; Sp/Lang Path, Private Practice, **SLP**

Bonner, Marilou P 619 Pinehaven, Houston, TX 77024, **SLP**

Bonner, Mrs Norma T City Estates, R R 1 Box 65, Sweetwater, TX 79556, (915) 235-8982, BA 70 Univ of North TX; MA 73 Univ of North TX; **SLP**

Bonner, Mrs Regina 10515 Sagewick, Houston, TX 77089, (713) 751-8463, BS 79 Eastern IL Univ; MA 83 Univ of Houston - Univ Park; Sp-Lang Path, Baylor College of Medicine, **SLP**

Bonner, Sheri Nelson 912 North Elem Street, Greensboro, NC 27401, (919) 275-2400, BA 71 Catawba Coll; ME 74 Univ of NC - Greensboro; ME 82 Univ of NC - Greensboro; Sp-Lang Path, Private Practice, **SLP**

Bonner, Sue J R R 1 Box 83, South Lyndeboro, NH 03082-9501, **SLP**

Bonness, Sheryll Lynn Calle Italia 2006, Ocean Park, Santurce, PR 00911, (809) 728-5440, BS 85 Ball St Univ; MA 87 Ball St Univ; 87–Aud, Sp & Hearing Ctr of San Juan, **A**

Bonnett, Mrs Marilyn Via Route 1 Box 462-3, St Albans, WV 25177, (304) 722-0224, BA 79 Marshall Univ; MA 80 Marshall Univ; 80–Sp-Lang Path, Kanawha Co Bd of Ed

Bonney, Mrs Carol L North 703 Monroe, Spokane, WA 99201, BA 78 Central WA Univ; MS 79 Eastern WA Univ; 84–Sp-Lang Path, Lakeland Village Sch, **SLP**

Bonney, Susan D 953 Kains Avenue, Albany, CA 94706, (415) 222-2161, BA 71 Austin Coll; MA 74 Our Lady Lake Univ-San Anton; 79–Sp-Lang Path, Richmond USD, **SLP**

Bonno-King, Carmelita M 3029 Huntington Drive, Arlington Heights, IL 60004, (312) 253-4841, BA 79 Elmhurst Coll; MA 81 CA St Univ - Long Beach; Sp-Lang Path, Shaumburg Comm Consol Sch 54, **SLP**

Bono, Joan 80 Austin Drive #74, Burlington, VT 05401, (802) 524-3613, BS 82 Bloomsburg Univ of PA; MS 83 Bloomsburg Univ of PA; Sp-Lang Path, Franklin Cen Supervisory Union, **SLP**

Bonomo, Dorothy Hughes 20 Grace Avenue, Lynbrook, NY 11563, BA 76 Marymount Coll; MA 80 CUNY - Queens Coll; Aud, Wilks Hrng Ctr, **A**

Bonsangue, Nancy J 17432 Walnut Street, Yorba Linda, CA 92686, (213) 698-9531, BA 79 CA St Univ - Fullerton; MA 81 CA St Univ - Fullerton; 88–Sp-Lang Path, Whittier City Sch Dist, **SLP**

Bonslett, Merrylee M 2306 Imran Dr, Sacramento, CA 95825, (916) 920-8957, BA 76 CA St Univ - Sacramento; OM 79 Univ of WA; 87–Aud, Univ of CA Davis Med Ctr, **A**

Bonus, Katherine A 14 Cheyenne Circle, Madison, WI 53705, **SLP**

Bonvillian, John D Department Of Psychology, Gilmer Hall, University Of Virginia, Charlottesville, VA 22903, (804) 924-0646, BA 70 Johns Hopkins Univ; PH 74 (NS) Stanford Univ; Assoc Prof, U VA

Boo, Meredith L 274 2nd Street, Excelsior, MN 55331, (612) 881-5883, OB 77 Univ of MN - Duluth; MA 78 Mankato St Univ; Sp-Lang Path, ISD #271, **SLP**

Boochever, Mrs Kathleen R 2910 Hermosa View Drive, Hermosa Beach, CA 90254, (213) 379-9981, BA 70 Stanford Univ; MA 76 Univ of CA - Santa Barbara; SLP, Los Angeles Co Office of Educ, **SLP**

Booher, Deborah E 446 Stoney Hill Court East, Langhorne, PA 19047, (215) 539-8550, BS 76 West Chester Univ of PA; MA 79 West Chester Univ of PA; Sp-Lang Path, Montg Co Interm Unit, **SLP ACE**

Booher, Kenneth 1008 East Jean Street, Tampa, FL 33604, (813) 870-3560, MS 80 Univ of South FL; Director Aud, Tampa Speech and Hearing Ctr, **A**

Booher, Sheryl Anne 2707 Walbrook Avenue, Cleveland, OH 44109, (216) 331-3602, BA 80 Cleveland St Univ; MA 84 Cleveland St Univ; Aud, ENT Group of Cleveland Inc, **A**

Book, Sandra Lynn 11219 Northeast 10th Avenue, Vancouver, WA 98685, (503) 222-9221, MA 87 Western WA Univ; **A**

Book, Susan Fields 9602 Shadow Oak Drive, Gaithersburg, MD 20879, (301) 572-5301, BA 70 George Washington Univ; MA 72 Howard Univ; 70–Sp-Lang Path, Prince George's Co Pub Schls, **SLP**

Book, Terrel D 4490 Reservoir Road, Geneseo, NY 14454, (716) 245-5333, BS 60 Kent St Univ; MA 81 SUNY - Coll at Geneseo; 88–Instr, SUNY at Geneseo, **SLP**

Bookbinder, Julia Dwyer 1617 Sturbridge Court, Cheshire, CT 06410-3751, (203) 272-0889, BA 80 Brown Univ; MA 84 Univ of CT; Sp-Lang Path, **SLP**

Bookbinder, Mrs Marlene R 1937 Briarcliff Avenue, Meadowbrook, PA 19046, BS 55 Univ of PA; MA 70 Temple Univ; MA 70 Temple Univ; Sp-Lang Path, Sch Dist of Phila, **SLP**

Booker, Denise M 86 Wayland Street, North Haven, CT 06473, (203) 248-9255, BA 74 Univ of CT; MS 75 Southern CT St Univ; Sp-Lang Path, North Haven Bd of Ed, **SLP**

Booker, Patricia E 2936 Virginia Road, Birmingham, AL 35213, (205) 871-5317, **SLP**

Bookshester, Dr Joyce C 1468 W Grace, Chicago, IL 60613, (312) 908-7285, BA 70 Univ of IL - Urbana; MA 71 Univ of IL - Urbana; OD 86 (Clinical Psychology) IL Sch of Professional Psychology; Clin Psych, Private Practice, **SLP**

Bookstein, Mrs Ellen W 2530 Farringdon Road, Baltimore, MD 21209, (301) 321-3099, BA 77 Montclair St Coll; MA 80 Univ of MD - College Park; Aud, Towson State University, **A**

Boomsliter, Dr Paul C 8 Lawnridge Avenue, Albany, NY 12208, (518) 462-6222, BA 35 WV Univ; MA 38 Univ of IA; PH 42 (NS) Univ of WI - Madison; Dir of Prof Serv, Capital Area Speech Center Inc, **SLP F LM**

Boone, Mrs Carol A 401 Locust Street, Indiana, PA 15701, (412) 463-7019, BS 75 Indiana Univ of PA; MS 76 PA St Univ - Univ Park; Sp-Lang Path, Visiting Nurse Association, **SLP**

Boone, Cyndi Cuba 1701 Cliffside Drive, Wichita Falls, TX 76302, (817) 723-5294, BS 74 Midwestern St Univ; MS 76 Univ of North TX; Sp-Lang Path, Commun Dis Clinic, **SLP**

Boone, Dr Daniel R 5715 North Genematas Drive, Tucson, AZ 85704, (602) 888-0427, BA 51 Univ of Redlands; MA 54 Case Western Reserve Univ; PH 58 (NS) Case Western Reserve Univ; 88, Private Practice, **SLP F H**

Boone, Mrs Elaine Marie 27 Dale Avenue, Toronto, ON, Canada M4W 1K2, (416) 393-0644, BA 65; ME 66 PA St Univ - Univ Park; 71–Sp-Lang Path, Toronto Bd of Ed, **SLP**

Boone, Kathleen M 3711 Hunters Circle, San Antonio, TX 78230, (512) 696-2444, BS 74 IL St Univ - Normal; MS 77 Univ of North TX; Audiologist, Self Employed, **A**

Boone, Mrs Linda Ann 9590 Lott Road, Durham, CA 95938, (916) 891-6629, BA 80 CA St Univ - Chico; MA 82 CA St Univ - Chico; 84–Sp-Lang Path, Co Lusa Co Supt of Schs, **SLP**

Boone, Mary J G 1653 Fairfax, Denver, CO 80220, (303) 388-2762, BA 74 Univ of WA; MA 75 Univ of WA; **SLP**

Boone, Shirley Reynolds 520 Venezia Park, Venice, FL 33595, (813) 493-1979, BA 81 Univ of FL; ME 82 Univ of FL; SLP, Sarasota Co Sch, **SLP**

Boone, Susan Michelle H-7 Villager Apartment, Sunset Avenue, Rocky Mount, NC 27804, (919) 443-5578, BS 85 East Carolina Univ; MS 86 East Carolina Univ; **SLP**

Boone, Mrs Theresa Lynn Rd 1 Mardon Drive Box 3, Pennsburg, PA 18073, (215) 679-4151, BS 82 Bloomsburg Univ of PA; MS 83 Bloomsburg Univ of PA; Sp-Lang Path, Montgomery Cnty Intermed Unit, **SLP**

Boonin, Mrs Joan M 2219 Copley, Ann Arbor, MI 48104-4535, (313) 769-4218, **SLP**

Boos, Bette A 3845 Vineywar Avenue #G, Pleasanton, CA 94566, (314) 863-1920, BS 84 Fontbonne Coll; MS 86 Fontbonne Coll; **SLP**

Boos, Mrs Kay Turbett 323 North Holland Street, Blue Earth, MN 56013, (509) 526-3215, BS 84 Saint Cloud St Univ; MA 85 Univ of MN - Duluth; Sp-Lang Path, Blue Earth Com Schls, **SLP**

Boose, Martha Anne 1445 S Ellis, Wichita, KS 67211, (316) 689-3240, BS 74; MA 79; MA 84; **SLP**

Booth, Beneature Sander Route 6 Box 230, Conway, SC 29526, (803) 248-2206, BA 74 SC St Coll; MA 77 SC St Coll

Booth, Denise S P O Box 571, Plains, MT 59859, (406) 826-5642, BA 70 CA St Univ - Fresno; MA 73 Univ of KS; Sp-Lang Path, Private Practice, **SLP**

Booth, Frank D Sono-Tex, 4020 Junius, Dallas, TX 75246, (214) 823-3082, BA 71 Baylor Univ; MS 76 Southern Methodist Univ; President, Sono-Tex, **A**

Booth, Janette A 1007 Northpine Drive, Conroe, TX 77301, (409) 539-4325, BA 74 Univ of Northern CO; MA 75 Univ of Northern CO; **SLP**

Booth, Judith A 312 Gabrielle Way, Redlands, CA 92374, (714) 788-7377, BS 67 Univ of Akron; MS 79 Univ of Redlands; Sp-Lang Path, Riverside USD, **SLP**

Booth, Mrs Margaret L 3439 Douglas Street, Sioux City, IA 51104-2645, (402) 287-2061, BA 69 Univ of SD - Vermillion; MA 75 Univ of SD - Vermillion; Coord of Sp-Lang-Hrng Serv, Ed Serv Ut One, **SLP**

Booth, Mary J Y 963 East Dunedin, Columbus, OH 43224, (614) 263-3908, BS 64 MS Univ for Women; OM 78 LA St Univ - N O Medical Ctr; 84–Sp-Lang Path, Northwest LA St Sch, **SLP**

Booth, Patricia S 9848 Broken Bow, Dallas, TX 75238, MS; **A**

Booth, Mrs Sara A 247 Fairway Drive, Harrisonburg, VA 22801, (703) 434-0259, **SLP**

Booth, Thomas P O Box 430, Plains, MT 59859, (406) 728-8753, BA 67 Univ of CA - Santa Barbara; MS 68 FL St Univ; Sp-Lang Path, Private Practice, **SLP**

Boothe, Tamara Jan Adkins P O Box 56, Indianola, IA 50125, (515) 281-3176, BA 73 Univ of IA; MA 75 Univ of IA; 87–Consult, Iowa Dept of Educ, **A**

Boothroyd, Arthur City University Of New York, 33 West 42nd Street, New York, NY 10036, (212) 642-2351, BS 57; PH 68 (NS); Prof, City University of New York, **A F**

Booton, Barbara Lynne 8142 Marty, Overland Park, KS 66204, (913) 621-3073, OB 84 Univ of KS; MA 86 Wichita St Univ; 86–Sp-Lang Path, Wyandotte Spec Educ Cooperative, **SLP**

Boots, Mrs Myra Ruth 1912 Pleasant Drive, Cedar Falls, IA 50613, (319) 273-2577, BA 50 Grinnell Coll; MA 65 Univ of Northern IA; Asst Prof, U of N IA, **SLP**

Bootsma, Jan Rasmusson 5500-A Pompano Drive, Minnetonka, MN 55343, (612) 938-9054, BS 78 Univ of MN - Duluth; MS 83 Univ of WI - River Falls; **SLP**

Booziotis, Kathy Kelly 811 South Liberty Lane, Carbondale, IL 62901, (618) 457-8348, BS 81 Southern IL Univ -Carbondale; MS 83 Southern IL Univ -Carbondale; Sp-Lang Path, Unity Point School Dist 140, **SLP**

Bopanna, Dr Ballachanda Belliappa Department Audiology & Speech Sciences, Purdue University, West Lafayette, IN 47907, (317) 494-3804, MS 82 Univ of TX - Dallas; PH 88 (Comm Disorders) Univ of TX - Dallas; 88–Asst Prof, Purdue Univ, **A**

Borack, Mrs Sheila 46 Willow Way, Berkeley Heights, NJ 07922, (201) 464-2519, BA 59 CUNY - Brooklyn Coll; MA 69 CUNY - Brooklyn Coll; Res Assoc, Bell Commun Res Inc, **SLP**

Boragina, Annette 2620 East Fairfield, Mesa, AZ 85203, (602) 833-5152, MS 88 Northern AZ Univ

Borawski, Karen S P O Box 71, Stittville, NY 13469, (315) 724-5101, BS 85 Nazareth Coll of Rochester; MA 86 SUNY - Coll at Plattsburgh; 86–Aud, Children's Hosp & Rehab Ctr, **A**

Borbely, Steven J 719 North Kickapoo, Lincoln, IL 62656, (217) 788-2800, BS 66 Northern IL Univ - De Kalb; MA 69 Western IL Univ; Staff Rep, Amer Fed St-Co-Mun Emp Coun 31, **SLP**

Borchardt, Mrs Debra Ann 148 Hillock Court, Appleton, WI 54914, (414) 735-9977, BS 79 Univ of WI - Stevens Point; MA 81 Northwestern Univ; **SLP**

Borchelt, Janet Katherine 3000 Hillsboro Road, #120, Nashville, TN 37215, (615) 292-9917, BS 82 Western KY Univ; MS 83 Murray St Univ; Sp-Lang Path, Rebound Inc, **SLP**

Borchers, Mrs Alice D 1315 Locust Place, Davis, CA 95616, (304) 345-6565, BA 74 Marshall Univ; MA 75 Marshall Univ; SLP, Private Practice, **SLP ACE**

Borchert, Cynthia Ruth 2820 North Park Drive Lane, Apt 11, Appleton, WI 54911, (414) 494-1060, BA 82 Univ of WI - Eau Claire; OM 86 Univ of WI - River Falls; **A**

Bordeaux, Marcy Annice 3125 N W 18th, Oklahoma City, OK 73107, BS 69 TX Tech Univ; MS 83 Univ of UT; 88–Sp-Lang Path, Oklahoma City PS, **SLP ACE**

Borden, Dr Gloria Jones 160 Hodge Road, Princeton, NJ 08540, (215) 787-8407, BA 52 CT Coll; MA 55 Columbia Univ Teachers Coll; PH 72 (NS) CUNY - Grad Sch & Univ Cntr; Professor of Speech, Temple University, **SLP**

Bordenick, Roy M 500 Sunlight Road, Reisterstown, MD 21136, (301) 944-3100, BA 72 Park Coll; MS 76 Columbia Univ Teachers Coll; Vp, Aud Assoc Inc, **A**

Borders, Jennifer Carole 320 Deepwood Drive, Elizabethtown, KY 42701, (502) 765-7703, BS 84 Spalding Coll; MS 85 Univ of Louisville; 86–Aud, KY Commission for Handicapped Children, **A**

Borders, Mrs Mary Sue 34 Martin Circle, Paducah, KY 42001-5410, (502) 554-1542, BA 68 Bellarmine Coll; MS 74 Murray St Univ; **SLP**

Bordman, Martin Park Towne North Suite 405, 2200 Ben Franklin Parkway, Philadelphia, PA 19130, (215) 564-5429, BS 40 Temple Univ-Tyler Sch of Art; ME 41 Temple Univ-Tyler Sch of Art; SLP, Private Practice, **SLP LM**

Bordogna, Marianne 108 St Jean Court, Danville, CA 94526, (415) 823-2874, BS 75 Edinboro Univ of PA; MA 76 Edinboro Univ of PA; Engrg Mgr, Pacific Bell, **SLP**

Bordok, Barbara Coons 3 Willowgrove, Irvine, CA 92714, BA 68 Univ of Redlands; MA 69 Univ of Redlands; Sp-Lang Path, Tustin USD, **SLP**

Borel, Denise A 275 North Kalorama #305, Ventura, CA 93001, (805) 643-4264, BA 79 LA Tech Univ; OM 85 LA St Univ - N O Medical Ctr; Pre School Spec, Ventura Unified School Dstr, **SLP**

Borelli, Nancy R 974 Ranch House Road, Westlake Village, CA 91361, (805) 497-4408, BS 68 Northwestern Univ; MA 69 Northwestern Univ; Sp-Lang Path, Private Practice, **SLP**

Boren, Grace Daly 15 Three Village Lane, Setauket, NY 11733, (516) 751-3188, BS 70 Nazareth Coll of Rochester; MS 71 SUNY - Center at Albany; OM 82 Long Island U - CW Post Ctr; Chairperson of Itinerant Serv, Middle County Central Schools, **SLP**

Borengasser, Sara Lynn 10801 West Estates Drive, Cupertino, CA 95014, (408) 255-3822, BS 76 Univ of AR - Fayetteville; MA 77 Univ of AR - Fayetteville; Cupertino Union Sch Dist, **SLP**

Bores, Mrs Joyce Anne Costello 614 Paramus Road, Paramus, NJ 07652, (201) 731-3600, BA 77 CUNY - Queens Coll; MS 81 William Paterson Coll; Sp-Lang Path, Kessler Inst for Rehab, **SLP**

Borg, Carmel Eleno Dennis Ville, Hompesch Road, Fgura, Malta, BA 74; MA 84; Sp-Lang Path, Communications Outstation

Borg, Nancy E 551 Poplar Street, Roslindale, MA 02131, BS 77 Univ of Southern ME; MS 84 Boston Univ; 86–Sp-Lang Path, Private Practice, **SLP**

Borga, Gerri Beth 2400 Calle Los Altos, Tucson, AZ 85715, (602) 299-1369, BS 82 Univ of AZ; MS 85 Northern AZ Univ; **SLP**

Borgatti, Mrs Juliana Zimmer 1720 Hill Drive, South Pasadena, CA 91030, (213) 258-5050, BA 80 San Jose St Univ; MA 85 CA St Univ - Los Angeles; 85–Sp-Lang Path, Hear Ctr, **SLP**

Borgeas, Mrs Serita B 2127 West San Miguel, Phoenix, AZ 85015, (602) 246-7112, MS 73 AZ St Univ; 86–Sp-Lang Path, Phoenix Union HS Dist, **SLP**

Borgemenke, Mrs Jana Kay 3261 Greenwich Drive, Fairfield, OH 45014, (513) 242-3933, BS 85 Miami Univ - Oxford; MS 86 Miami Univ - Oxford; SLP, **SLP**

Borger, Harry L 118 Newman Road, Orrtanna, PA 17353, (717) 624-4616, BS 70 Murray St Univ; ME 74 Clarion Univ of PA; 71–Sp-Lang Path, Lincoln Inter Ut #12, **SLP**

Borger, Mrs Linda A 4 On-The-Boulevard, Cornwall, NY 12518, (914) 534-2483, BA 71 SUNY - Coll at Geneseo; MS 73 Southern CT St Univ; 87–Sp-Lang Path, Cornwall Central Schs, **SLP**

Borger, Mrs Michele Strauss 2550 Independence Avenue, Apartment 2-U, Bronx, NY 10705, (212) 796-4233, BS 79 SUNY - Coll at Oneonta; MS 81 Purdue Univ - West Lafayette; 85–Sp-Lang Path, NYU Med Ctr-Rusk Inst of Rehab, **SLP**

Borgeson, Kathleen Ann 2301 Via River, Palos Verdes Estates, CA 90274, (213) 377-3849, MS 86 Boston Univ; 88–SLP, Switzer Center, **SLP**

Borghi, Mrs Mary Jo Borghi & Borghi Associates, 101 South Barranca, Suite 210, Covina, CA 91723, (818) 331-4949, BS 66 Memphis St Univ; MA 68 Memphis St Univ; Sp-Lang Path, Borghi & Borghi Assoc, **SLP**

Borghi, Dr Robert W Borghi & Borghi Associates, 101 South Barranca Avenue, Suite 210, Covina, CA 91723, (213) 331-4949, BA 54 Univ of Redlands; MA 56 Univ of Redlands; PH 68 (Communicative Disorders) Univ of Southern CA; 80–Sp-Lang Path, Borghi & Borghi Associates, **SLP**

Borgia, Roberta L 312 Billington Street, Plymouth, MA 02360-3580, (617) 747-0327, BS 69 Kent St Univ; MA 70 Kent St Univ; Sp-Lang Path, Private Practice, **SLP**

Borglund, Patricia 202 Candler, San Antonio, TX 78210, (512) 533-1041, BA 73 Our Lady Lake Univ-San Anton; MA 74 Our Lady Lake Univ-San Anton; **SLP**

Borgmeyer, Ann P 2 Williamsburg Court, St Charles, MO 63301, (314) 447-4232, MS 79 Southern IL Univ-Edwardsvill; Sp/Lang Path, Francis Howell Sch Dist, **SLP**

Borgreen, Julia A 3238 3rd Avenue South, Great Falls, MT 59405, (406) 727-3333, BA 72 Univ of Denver; MA 73 Univ of Denver; 88–Sp-Lang Path, Columbus Hosp, **SLP ACE**

Borgsmiller, Paul T 2871 Radnor, St Charles, MO 63301, (314) 577-5671, BS 74 Southeast MO St Univ; MS 76 Southern IL Univ -Carbondale; Dir-Aud Dept, Cardnl Glennon Child Hosp, **A**

Boria, Carolyn A 19 Crowningshield Drive, Paxton, MA 01612, (508) 757-7803, BS 76 Emerson Coll; MS 79 Catholic Univ of America; **SLP**

Boring, Mrs Melinda Lee 1517 Hess Street, Columbus, OH 43212, (614) 263-5151, BS 83 Miami Univ - Oxford; MA 85 OH St Univ; Sp-Lang Path, Columbus Speech & Hearing Ctr, **SLP**

Borinsky, Janet S 1075 E 10th Street, Brooklyn, NY 11230, (718) 946-9700, Brooklyn Schl for Spec Chldrn, **SLP**

Boris, Carol Jean 2005 78th Street, Kenosha, WI 53140, **SLP**

Boris, Mrs Linda T 11737 Devilwood Drive, Potomac, MD 20854, (301) 340-8090, BA 61 Univ of MD - College Park; MA 63 Univ of IA; Sp-Lang Path, Private Practice, **SLP**

Boriskin, Mrs Ellen Goldman 35 Foxglove Drive, Cranston, RI 02920, (401) 943-0033, **SLP**

Bork, Debra A B 108 Bishop Quarter Lane, Oak Park, IL 60302, (312) 524-3070, BA 73 Augustana Coll; MS 75 Eastern IL Univ; Sp/Lang Path, Oak Park Elem Sch Dist 97, **SLP**

Bork, Dr Norma K The Norma Bork Associates, 4220 Silverado Trail, Napa, CA 94558-1117, (707) 965-2455, BS 54 Kean Coll of NJ; MS 65 CA St Univ - Los Angeles; PH 67 (NS) Univ of CA - Los Angeles; Pres/Ceo, Private Practice, **SLP**

Borkenhagen, Mrs Anne M 5635 Holland Street, Vancouver, BC, Canada V6N 2A7, (604) 263-4285, BS 68 McGill Univ - Quebec; MS 70 McGill Univ - Quebec; MS 74 McGill Univ - Quebec; Sp-Lang Path, Private Practice, **SLP**

Borkman, Nancy L 226 Douglas Avenue, Waukegan, IL 60085, (312) 336-5390, BA 83 Rutger's St Univ - Douglas Coll; MS 86 Rush Univ; 86–Sp-Lang Path, Woodstock Health Care Ctr, **SLP**

Borkowski, Mrs Linda L 1011 Kansas, Longmont, CO 80501, (303) 772-7700, BA 72 SUNY - Coll at Buffalo; MA 74 Univ of FL; Sp/Lang Path, St Vrain Valley Sch Dist, **SLP**

Borland, Laurie James 1002 Turtle Lake Drive, Leeds, AL 35094, (205) 991-7802, BS 85 Auburn Univ - Auburn; MS 86 Univ of AL- Tuscaloosa; 88–Sp-Lang Path, Jefferson County Bd of Educ, **SLP**

Borland, Mrs Susan 318 Greenfield Avenue #7, Box 565, Maugansville, MD 21767, (301) 791-2993, BS 84 CA Univ of PA; MS 85 CA Univ of PA; 85–Sp-Lang Path, Bd of Educ of Washington Co

Borman, Deborah Lynn 505 W Baseline Rd #1057, Tempe, AZ 85283, (602) 833-6483, BA 83 Morningside Coll; MS 86 Univ of NE - Lincoln; 87–SLP, Mesa USD, **SLP**

Bormann, Nelson H 670 Shryock Avenue, Indiana, PA 15701, (412) 357-2486, BS 62 Southwest TX St Univ; MA 65 Western MI Univ; 67–Assoc Prof, IN Univ of Pa, **SLP ACE**

Born, Lori Ann RR1 Box 14-A, Lovington, IL 61937, (217) 424-3000, MS 88 Eastern IL Univ

Born, Rebecca A 736 South Stuart, Palatine, IL 60067, (312) 359-7746, BS 74 Western IL Univ; MA 75 Western IL Univ; Sp-Lang Path, Ccsd #15 Palatine, **SLP**

Borneman-Eckels, Dr Janice B P O Box 321, Forest Hill, MD 21050, (301) 642-2411, BA 72 Wake Forest Univ; MA 79 Univ of MN - Minneap-St Paul; PH 81 (NS) Univ of MN - Minneap-St Paul; SLP, VA Med Cen, **SLP**

Borning-Cordova, Katherine Ellan 4721-B La Villa Marina, Marina Del Rey, CA 90292, (213) 837-5236, BA 75 Scripps Coll; MA 86 CA St Univ - Northridge; 87–SLP, LA USD, **SLP**

Bornstein, Byrna Arron 85 Sexton Avenue, Westwood, MA 02090, (617) 461-0806, BA 78 George Washington Univ; MA 80 Temple Univ; 86–Clinical Supervisor Sp-Lang, Private Practice, **SLP**

Bornstein, Mrs Carolyn S P O Box 95, Pittsford, NY 14534, (716) 482-4836, BS 65 Bowling Green St Univ; MA 66 Wayne St Univ; 66–Sp-Lang Path, Rochester City Sch Dist, **SLP ACE**

Bornstein, Margaret Burn P O Box 251, Wayne, ME 04284, (207) 685-4171, BS 75 CO St Univ; MS 76 Univ of OR; Sp-Lang Path, Sch Union #42, **SLP**

Bornstein, Pamela S 513 Wellfleet Road, Cinnaminson, NJ 08077, (609) 829-3515, BA 70 CUNY - Queens Coll; MA 72 Univ of Cincinnati; Sp/Lang Path, Private Practice, **SLP**

Bornstein, Steven P W 39 Ethelbert Place, Ridgewood, NJ 07450, **A**

Borofka, Debbie Marie 2825 East Palo Alto, Fresno, CA 93710, (209) 225-3000, BS 79 Lewis-Clark St Coll; MS 82 Univ of AL- Tuscaloosa; Sp-Lang Path, Valley Chldn Hosp, **SLP**

Boroughs, Kathleen 1336 Lakeview Boulevard, E #2, Seattle, WA 98102, (206) 364-0500, BA 76 Univ of HI - Manoa; BS 76 Univ of HI - Manoa; MS 80 Univ of HI - Manoa; SLP, Northwest Hosp Sp & Hrng Cen, **SLP**

Borowitz, Mrs Kathleen C Rt 2 Box 166, Earlysville, VA 22936, (804) 924-8241, BA 79 Hollins Coll; MS 81 Vanderbilt Univ; Sp-Lang Path, Univ of VA Children's Rehab Ctr, **SLP**

Borowski, Mrs Marilyn McCormick 38 Colonial Circle, Thornton, PA 19373, (215) 637-9070, BS 82 West Chester Univ of PA; MA 87 West Chester Univ of PA; 82 Sp Lang Path, Sch Dist of Phila

Borrero, Aixa 71 Rossmore Road, Apartment 6, Jamaica Plain, MA 02130, (617) 522-7045, MS 86 Boston Univ; 88–Sp-Lang Path, Martha Eliot Health Ctr-Child's Hosp, **SLP**

Borsari, Mrs Carol Hintz 30 Strawberry Hill, Wallingford, CT 06492, (203) 584-7709, BA 76 Univ of CT; MS 78 Southern CT St Univ; Sp-Lang Path, Bristol Board of Education, **SLP**

Borsch, Jennifer Kay Rt 12 Box 201, Morgantown, WV 26505, (304) 594-1490, BA 82 Glenville St Coll; MS 84 WV Univ; 85–Sp-Lang Path, Monongalia County Bd of Educ, **SLP**

Borsh, Mrs Frances L 2352 East Lake Road, Skaneateles, NY 13152, (315) 685-8235, BA 65 Montclair St Coll; MA 69 William Paterson Coll; **SLP**

Borson, Carol Ann 6918 Cathedral, Birmingham, MI 48010, (313) 424-3907, BA 76 Univ of CO - Boulder; MA 77 Wayne St Coll; Sp/Lang Path, Providence Hosp, **SLP**

Borst, Mrs Noreen Nelson 67 East Main Street, Fredonia, NY 14063, (716) 672-4371, OB 74 SUNY - Coll at Fredonia; OM 80 SUNY - Coll at Fredonia; Sp-Lang Path, Chautauqua Co BOCES, **SLP**

Borten, Mrs Norma T 2671 Covered Bridge Road, Merrick, NY 11566, (516) 868-7275, BA 73 Hofstra Univ; MS 75 Adelphi Univ; Sp-Lang Path, **SLP**

Borthick, William Arnold PO Drawer 2227, Palm Springs, CA 92263, (619) 323-4559, BA 57 Univ of Tulsa; MA 59 Univ of Tulsa; OM 62 Univ of Tulsa; Sp-Lang Path, Riverside County Ofc of Educ, **SLP**

Bortnick, Mrs Rosalie M 9812 Mainsail Drive, Gaithersburg, MD 20879, (301) 926-4538, BS 75 Southern CT St Univ; MA 80 Southern CT St Univ; Sp/Lang Path, Frederick Co Bd of Ed, **SLP**

Bortnyik, Mrs Mary M 107 Valleyview Drive, Mars, PA 16046, (412) 776-2409, BS 76 Univ of KY; MS 80 Univ of Louisville; SLP, Assoc for Retarded Citizens, **SLP**

Borton, Mary Kealey Pineywood Trace, Birmingham, AL 35242, (205) 991-2623, BS 68 Univ of IA; MA 70 Northern IL Univ - De Kalb; 87–Sp-Lang Path, Shelby County Bd of Educ, **SLP**

Borton, Dr Thomas E, III Dept Of Surgery/Otolaryngology, Univ Of Al At Birmingham, 1501 5th Avenue South, Birmingham, AL 35233, (205) 934-9766, BA 66 Univ of IL - Urbana; MA 68 Univ of IL - Urbana; PH 73 (Aud) Univ of IL - Urbana; 86–Assoc Prof of Surgery (Otol), Univ of Alabama at Birmingham, **A**

Borts, Mary Wilcox Route 14 Box 59, Columbia, MO 65202, (314) 443-5270, BA 77 Univ of Northern IA; MA 78 Univ of Northern IA; Sp-Lang Path, Mid-Missouri Mental Health Cen, **SLP**

Borucki, Donna Kay 1416 Elmwood Apt #203, Greenville, MI 48838, (616) 754-7301, BA 84 MI St Univ; MA 85 MI St Univ; Sp-Lang Path, Montcalm Area ISD, **SLP**

Boruff, Diane C 702 Belvin Street, San Marcos, TX 78666, (501) 594-5341, BS 75 Univ of North TX; ME 80 Southwest TX St Univ; Clinical Dir, Communicorp, **SLP**

Boruff, Mrs Susan Flynn 3000 Queens Court, Norcross, GA 30071, (404) 257-2075, BA 83 Columbia Coll; MS 84 Univ of SC - Columbia; 86–Sp-Lang Path, Scottish Rite Children's Hosp, **SLP**

Borus, Dr Judith F 297 Clearview Avenue, Worthington, OH 43085, (614) 228-2287, BA 59 Univ of CT; MA 61 Univ of CT; PH 70 (NS) MI St Univ; Executive Director, Ohio Conference-Am Assn U Prof, **SLP A**

Bosack, Linda B 6410 West 127th Street, Palos Heights, IL 60463, (312) 388-4499, BA 75 Loyola Univ of Chicago; MS 77 Bradley Univ; Aud, Private Practice, **A**

Bosboom, Lisa Beth 15 Beach Road #3F, Great Neck, NY 11023, (516) 560-8843, BA 82 Long Island U - CW Post Ctr; MA 83 Hofstra Univ; 85–Sp-Lang Path, Brookhaven Beach HRF/SNF, **SLP**

Boscamp, Patricia Ann 350 Sharon Park Drive, Apartment S-1, Menlo Park, CA 94025, (415) 854-2330, BA 79 SUNY - Coll at Cortland; MS 81 Columbia Univ Teachers Coll; **SLP**

Boscardin, Dr Mary Lynn 22 Goldenrod Circle, Amherst, MA 01002, (413) 253-3687, BS 75 Univ of IL - Urbana; MS 76 Univ of WI - Milwaukee; PH 84 (NS) Univ of IL - Urbana; Asst Prof, U of MA, **SLP**

Boschen, Mrs Sara Lou 8928 Judith Lane, St Louis, MO 63123, (314) 569-8100, BS 80 Univ of MO - Columbia; MS 85 Fontbonne Coll; 85–Sp-Lang Path, Spec Sch Dist of St Louis Co, **SLP**

Boschma, Mrs Wendy R F 16049 Calahan Street, Sepulveda, CA 91343, (818) 894-2711, BA 74 CA St Univ - Northridge; MA 75 CA St Univ - Northridge; Sp-Lang Path, LA USD, **SLP**

Boscia, Mrs Cathy A P O Box 196, Danville, PA 18038, (215) 252-3461, BS 78 Bloomsburg Univ of PA; MS 79 Bloomsburg Univ of PA; Sp-Lang Path, Helen Beebe Sp & Hrng Ctr, **SLP**

Bose, Nancy DuBois 539 Valleyview Street, Kent, OH 44240, (216) 745-1611, BS 83 PA St Univ - Univ Park; MA 85 Kent St Univ; 86–Dir of Comm Disorders, Barberton Citizens Hosp, **SLP**

Boser, Jody G 1122 Hawthorn, Red Wing, MN 55066, (612) 388-1464, BS 75 Univ of ND; MS 77 Univ of WI - River Falls; Sp-Lang Path, Red Wing School #256, **SLP**

Boser, Sheryl L L 2610 Westbrook Lane, Madison, WI 53711, (608) 271-3411, BS 75 Univ of WI - Madison; MS 76 Univ of WI - Milwaukee; **SLP**

Boshart, Charlotte 600 Central Avenue #398, Riverside, CA 92507, (714) 783-1415, BA 71 Loma Linda Univ - Riverside; MA 74 Western MI Univ; Sp-Lang Path, Colton USD, **SLP**

Boshnack, Arlene B 108 Surrey Commons, Lynbrook, NY 11563, (516) 593-5816, BS 75 SUNY - Coll at Geneseo; MS 76 Ithaca Coll; Sp-Lang Path, Private Practice, **SLP**

Boshoven, Margaret M 17719 Old U S 12, Chelsea, MI 48118, **SLP**

Bosin, Mrs Debra Isaacman 503 South 9th Street, Philadelphia, PA 19147, (215) 329-5715, BS 82 PA St Univ - Univ Park; MA 84 Northwestern Univ; 87–Sp-Lang Path, The Graduate Hosp, **SLP**

Bosin, Mrs Elizabeth W 1300 Valley Forge Road, Bloomington, IN 47401, BA 67 De Paul Univ; OM 71 IN Univ - Bloomington; **SLP**

Boske, Mrs Laurie J S 11 Summer Street #B, Portland, CT 06480, (203) 342-2824, BA 78 Southern CT St Univ; MA 80 Univ of MA - Amherst; Sp-Lang Path, Middletown Bd of Ed, **SLP**

Bosko, Carmela Sansone 220 South Lucerne Blvd, Los Angeles, CA 90004, (213) 936-5534, BA 63 Stanford Univ; MA 62 Stanford Univ; **SLP**

Bosler, Mrs Jenine 210 West 89th Street, New York, NY 10024, (212) 688-9400, BA 68 CUNY - Hunter Coll; MA 71 Columbia Univ Teachers Coll; Chief, Communicative Dis Serv, New York Med Coll, **SLP**

Bosler, Michelle 1911 Sussex Drive, Carrollton, TX 75007, (214) 323-6695, BS 74 Univ of North TX; MS 76 Univ of TX - Dallas; Sp-Lang Path, Carrolton Branch Indep Sch Dis, **SLP**

Bosler, Sharon A 6225 S E Belmont Street, Portland, OR 97215-1939, (503) 233-4844, BA 70 Univ of CA - Santa Barbara; MA 72 Univ of CA - Santa Barbara; SLP, Clackamas Esd, **SLP**

Bosley, Mrs Elizabeth C Box 1, Cascade, CO 80809, (719) 684-9108, BA 33 Friends Univ; MA 35 Univ of KS; Retired, **SLP LM**

Bosner, Mrs Cynthia R 5 Everly Street, Old Bridge, NJ 08857, (201) 679-2321, BA 68 Kean Coll of NJ; MA 69 Kean Coll of NJ; Retired, Old Bridge Twsp Bd of Ed, **SLP**

Bosnjak, Vesna 1330 Foothills Blvd #203, Prince George, BC, Canada V2M 6V8, (604) 562-3768, MA 87 Western IL Univ; **SLP**

Bosone, Dr Zilpha T 930 Fairway Drive N E, Vienna, VA 22180, (202) 745-8270, BA 51 Trinity Coll; MA 67 Catholic Univ of America; PH 74 (Sp Path) Univ of KS; 78–Sp-Lang Path, Veterans Administration, **SLP**

Boso-Suggs, Rhonda Lynn 802 Old English Court, Apt 1C, Bel Air, MD 21014, (301) 838-3524, BA 84 WV Univ; MS 86 WV Univ; Sp-Lang Path, **SLP**

Boss, Peggy Hawbecker 16223 Lower Colfax, Grass Valley, CA 95945, (916) 265-2487, BA 62 Carlow Coll; MS 63 Univ of WI - Madison; SLP, Nevada City Sch Dist, **SLP**

Bosse, Mrs Julie K 2742 Gladhaven Drive, Oregon, OH 43616, (419) 472-0061, BS 77 Miami Univ - Oxford; MA 78 Kent St Univ; Multihndcpd Tchr, Lucas Co Off of Ed, **SLP**

Bosse, Mrs Virginia Horne 1454 Briarmeadow Drive, Worthington, OH 43085, (614) 369-3650, BA 61 OH Univ - Athens; MA 81 OH St Univ; Sp-Lang Path, Private Practice, **SLP**

Bossenberry, Julie 1732 Dixwell Avenue #5-E, Hamden, CT 06514, (203) 288-3108, BA 82 Central MI Univ; MA 84 Central MI Univ; 86–Aud, The Hearing Laboratory Inc, **A**

Bosshart, Mrs Carole 10 Monteray Drive, Kincheloe, MI 49788, (906) 495-5246, BS 63 Univ of MI - Ann Arbor; MS 67 Univ of MI - Ann Arbor; Pre-Prim Class Tchr, Sault Area PS, **SLP**

Bossier, Mrs Ida J 1260 Masters Lane, Anaheim, CA 92804, (213) 324-6668, BA 59 Southern Univ - Baton Rouge; MA 72 CA St Univ - Los Angeles; Prin, Los Angeles USD, **SLP**

Bosso, Yu-Wen Shih 1137 South Sierra Vista Avenue, Alhambra, CA 91801, (818) 796-3043, MA 83 CA St Univ - Los Angeles; **A**

Bossuyt, Colette M 1650 South Arizona Avenue, Apartment 240, Chandler, AZ 85224, (602) 963-7356, BS 79 AZ St Univ; MS 83 AZ St Univ; SLP, Chandler Public Schools, **SLP**

Bost, Dianne M 3915 R Street S E, Washington, DC 20020, (301) 243-3800, BA 77 Catholic Univ of America; MS 80 Univ of the DC; SLP, Hrng and Sp Agcy, **SLP**

Bost, Mrs Katherine Route 1 Box 323, Woodleaf, NC 27054, (704) 278-2892, ME 56 Univ of NC - Chapel Hill; BA 38 Winthrop Coll; **SLP LM**

Bost, Sheila P 360 24th, Santa Monica, CA 90402, **SLP**

Boster, Gail Brook 11622 Foxclove Road, Reston, VA 22091, (703) 860-9102, BA 71 Univ of AZ; MA 72 Univ of AZ; Sp-Lang Path, Prince Wm Co Sch, **SLP**

Bostick-Morgan, Oreather J 2825 Arlington Road, East Point, GA 30344, (404) 624-2097, BS 74 TN St Univ; MS 77 TN St Univ; Sp-Lang Path, Atlanta PS, **SLP**

Bostow, Vicki V W 1304 3rd Avenue S W, Minot, ND 58701, (701) 857-4410, BS 79 Minot St Univ; MS 80 Minot St Univ; Sp-Lang Path, Souris Valley Spec Serv, **SLP**

Bostrom, Debra Withers 1912 South River Drive, Tempe, AZ 85281-6118, (602) 967-6473, BS 72 MS Univ for Women; MS 73 MS Univ for Women; Priv Prac, Bethany Sp/Path Serv, **SLP**

Boswell, Mrs Deborah Byrd 1321 Sequoia Trail, Alabaster, AL 35007, (205) 663-7011, MS 87 Univ of Montevallo; 85–Sp-Lang Path, Shelby Co Bd of Educ, **SLP**

Boswell, Gary Lee Rural Route 1, Davis City, IA 50065, (515) 782-8443, BS 69 Univ of Science & Arts of OK; MA 71 Univ of Tulsa; Superv-Hrng Conserv/Ed, Green Valley AEA #14, **A**

Boswell, Joanne Elizabeth 3 Williamsburg Briarcrest, Gardens, Hershey, PA 17033, (207) 582-2571, MA 85 Univ of Denver; **SLP**

Boswell, Mrs Nancy Jane Rural Route 1, Davis City, IA 50065, (515) 442-3655, BS 78 Central MO St Univ; MA 79 Central MO St Univ; **SLP**

Boswell, Teresa Clay Hr 70 Box 530, Van Lear, KY 41265, BA 75 Marshall Univ; MA 76 Marshall Univ; Sp/Lang Path, Private Practice, **SLP**

Bosworth, Cathy Lynn 1121 Garfield Street, McMechen, WV 26040, (614) 633-3751, BS 85 WV Univ; MS 86 WV Univ; 87–Aud, Eastern Ohio Sp & Hearing Ctr, **A**

Bosworth, Mary Ann 4016 67th Street N W, Albuquerque, NM 87120, (505) 839-9422, BA 74 SUNY - Center at Buffalo; MA 76 SUNY - Center at Buffalo; Sp-Lang Path, Bur of Indian Affairs, **SLP ACE**

Bosy, Anne Elizabeth 3106 Seaway Court #202, Tampa, FL 33629, (813) 831-2053, MS 86 Univ of South FL; 87–Aud, Univ of S FL Med Ctr, **A**

Botchis, Mrs Gloria 8 Cherry Hill Road, Norwich, CT 06360, (203) 887-2988, BA 54 Univ of Hartford; MS 57 Boston Univ; **SLP**

Botelho, Jeannie S 3822 Northeast 66th Avenue, Portland, OR 97213-4451, (503) 760-4070, BS 77 Portland St Univ; MS 86 Portland St Univ; 84–Sp-Lang Path, Centennial Sch Dist, **SLP**

Both, Linda Elise 73-30 53rd Avenue, Maspeth, NY 11378, (212) 598-6154, BA 78 CUNY - Queens Coll; MA 80 NY Univ; Sp-Lang Path, Orthopaedic -Cndd, **SLP**

Bothell, Raymond C Hearing Aid Sales & Service, 4444 South Harvard #100, Tulsa, OK 74135, (918) 744-1390, BA 66 Northeastern OK St Univ; MA 70 Univ of Tulsa; Aud, Ear Nose & Throat Clinic Tulsa, **A**

Bothwell-Blanchet, Mrs Kathleen A 6766 Nicolett Street, Riverside, CA 92504, (714) 686-7709, BA 78 Univ of CA - Santa Barbara; MS 81 FL St Univ; Sp-Lang Path, **SLP**

Botstein, Laurie K 3026 Cravey Trail, Atlanta, GA 30345, (404) 939-9986, BA 71 CUNY - Brooklyn Coll; MS 76 CUNY - Brooklyn Coll; Sp-Lang Path, Private Practice, **SLP ACE**

Bott, Mrs Diane E Z 200 Bret Harte Road, San Rafael, CA 94901, (415) 897-4691, BA 74 San Francisco St Univ; MA 76 San Francisco St Univ; SLP, Novato USD, **SLP**

Bottari, Mrs Cynthia L 9 Red Coach Lane, Holmdel, NJ 07733, (201) 244-3595, BA 75 Rutger's St Univ - Douglas Coll; MS 77 Howard Univ; **SLP**

Bottenberg, Dr Donna J 1712 33rd Avenue, Greeley, CO 80631, (303) 353-1578, BA 72 Univ of Northern CO; MA 72 Univ of Northern CO; PH 87 (Comm Dis & Sp Science) Univ of CO - Boulder; Assoc Prof, U of No CO, **SLP**

Botti, Mrs Christine Pingree 318 Homer Drive, Turtle Creek, PA 15145, (412) 829-1061, BS 80 PA St Univ - Univ Park; MA 85 Univ of Pittsburgh - Pittsburgh; **SLP**

Botto, Michelle 61 S Village Green, Budd Lake, NJ 07828, (201) 533-5786, BS 85 Bloomsburg Univ of PA; MS 87 Bloomsburg Univ of PA; **SLP**

Bottom, Mrs Harriette O 2200 N W 114th, Oklahoma City, OK 73120, (405) 752-2752, BA 74 Univ of IL - Urbana; MS 78 WA St Univ; Sp-Lang Path, Mustang Publ Schs, **SLP**

Bottorf, Barrie O 3251 Ninety Road, Ashtabula, OH 44004, (216) 998-0222, BS 56 Bowling Green St Univ; MA 59 OH St Univ; SLP, Ashtabula Area Cty Schs, **SLP**

Bottorf, Lucinda E 1426 North Freeman, Santa Ana, CA 92706, (714) 673-8701, BA 75 Univ of CA - Santa Barbara; MS 77 Univ of WA; Sp-Lang Path, Providence Sp and Hearing Ctr, **SLP**

Botts, Mrs Dawn Cultra 801 Race Street, Rolling Fork, MS 39159, (601) 873-2342, BS 80 MS Univ for Women; MA 82 Univ of Tulsa; Sp-Lang Path, Private Practice, **SLP**

Botts, Lucia Marian 6604 Carolina Court, Mobile, AL 36695, (205) 639-9274, BS 75 Univ of TX - Austin; MA 83 Univ of North TX; **A**

Botts-Penrod, Mrs Elizabeth 306 Michigan Avenue, Monticello, KY 42633, (606) 348-9108, BS 77 Eastern KY Univ; MS 80 Univ of KY; Sp-Lang Path, Wayne County Schools, **SLP**

Botuck, Deborah Ann 8370 Uxbridge Court, Springfield, VA 22151, (703) 764-2895, BS 83 Univ of VA - Charlottesville; MS 85 James Madison Univ; 87–Sp-Lang Path, Sp & Lang Svcs of McLean Inc, **SLP**

Bouchard, Mrs Anne B RR1 Box 434-C, Westview Lane, Lebanon, NH 03766, (603) 448-2297, **SLP**

Bouchard, Ellen 5821 Tupelo Turn, Wilmington, DE 19808, BS 77 Wayne St Univ; MA 78 Wayne St Univ; Sp-Lang Path, Prof Home Hlth Care Agcy, **SLP**

Bouchard, Mrs Kathie A 141 Central Avenue, North Scituate, RI 02857, (401) 785-0400, BA 71 RI Coll; MS 77 Univ of RI; Sp-Lang Path, Cranston Public Schools, **SLP**

Bouchard, Dr Kenneth R 7169 Edinborough, West Bloomfield, MI 48322, (313) 476-4622, BA 68 Wayne St Univ; MA 75 Wayne St Univ; PH 81 (Aud) Wayne St Univ - Sch of Med; Dir Aud, Michigan Ear Inst, **A**

Bouck, Janis K 16430 Emory Lane, Rockville, MD 20853, (301) 651-5000, BA 70 Univ of TX - Austin; MA 73 Univ of TX - El Paso; Doctoral Stud & Asst, Gallaudet College, **SLP**

Bouck, Joanne King 33931 Calle Conejo, San Juan Capistrano, CA 92675, (714) 240-8138, **SLP**

Boudreaux, Cynthia Leigh 5401 Chimney Rock, #433, Houston, TX 77081, (713) 757-1000, OM 87 LA St Univ - N O Medical Ctr; 88–Sp-Lang Path, St Joseph Hosp, **SLP**

Boudreaux, Mrs Ellen F 3118 Cheverly Avenue, Cheverly, MD 20785, (301) 535-1700, MA 78 CA St Univ - Los Angeles; Sp-Lang Path, Prince Georges PS, **SLP**

Boudreaux, Dr Jean Rose Route 1 Box 1070, Covington, LA 70433, (504) 892-0765, BA 54 Univ of Southwestern LA; MA 57 WV Univ; PH 60 (Sp-Lang Path) Case Western Reserve Univ; 88–Consultant & President, Target Blue Enterprises, **SLP**

Bouillon, Mrs Rita Wetzstein 640 Lund Lane, Moscow, ID 83843-9550, (208) 882-1120, BS 80 Eastern IL Univ; MS 81 Eastern IL Univ; Sp-Lang Path, Moscow Sch Dstr, **SLP**

Boulange, Mrs Linda A 104 Round Trail, West Seneca, NY 14218, (716) 674-5300, BS 73 SUNY - Coll at Buffalo; MS 76 SUNY - Coll at Buffalo; Sp-Lang Path, Wseneca Ctrl Sch Dist, **SLP**

Boulanger, Mrs Sue P 1400 E Bayou Parkway #7-B, Lafayette, LA 70508, (318) 989-1343, BA 69 Northeastern OK St Univ; OB 71 Northeastern OK St Univ; MA 76 Univ of Tulsa; Sp/Lang Path, **SLP**

Boulette, Donna M 105 Smith Avenue, Nampa, ID 83651, (208) 466-9255, BS 79 Univ of WY; MS 80 Univ of WY; Aud, ID State Hospital Sch, **A**

Boulter, Mrs Kathryn 601 Sun Manor, Flushing, MI 48433, (313) 762-7500, BA 77 Univ of VT; MA 79 Western MI Univ; Sp/Lang Path, Bay Valley Home Hlth Serv Inc, **SLP**

Boultinghouse, Mrs Sherry Arlene 106 Williams Street, Girard, KS 66743, (316) 231-3870, BS 82 Univ of KS; MA 84 Univ of KS; Sp-Lang Path, Sek Special Ed Coop, **SLP**

Bouman, Joan 2920 6th Avenue North, Great Falls, MT 59401, (406) 452-1974, BS 80 Univ of WI - Stevens Point; MS 82 Univ of WI - Stevens Point; Aud, Great Falls Pub Sch Sys, **A**

Bounds, Mrs Angelique Harrison 317 Oakland Street, Decatur, GA 30030, (404) 233-5332, BA 78 OH Wesleyan Univ; ME 80 Univ of VA - Charlottesville; Sp-Lang Path/Aud, Atlanta Sp Sch, **SLP A**

Bounds, Mrs Cynthia Green Route 1 Box 282, Oxford, MS 38655, (601) 234-3497, BA 72 Univ of MS; OM 75 Univ of MS; Sp-Lang Path, Oxford Elementary School, **SLP**

Bounds, Dawn Leigh 4 Bonnie Ridge Court #201, Baltimore, MD 21209-1709, (301) 653-2850, BS 84 Towson St Univ; MS 86 Towson St Univ; 87–Sp-Lang Path, Sinai Hosp of Baltimore, **SLP**

Bounds, Mrs Suzanne L 120 Lakeview Drive, Grand Rapids, MN 55744, (218) 326-0826, BS 50 Univ of Tulsa; MS 55 Univ of IL - Urbana; Sp-Lang Path, Private Practice, **SLP**

Bountress, Mrs Martha G 1017 Manchester Avenue, Norfolk, VA 23508, (804) 683-4117, BS 70 Univ of North TX; MS 72 Univ of North TX; 76–Sp-Lang Path, Old Dominion U, **SLP A ACE**

Bountress, Dr Nicholas G 1017 Manchester, Norfolk, VA 23508, (804) 683-4117, BS 66 Central CT St Univ; MS 69 Southern CT St Univ; ED 73 (NS) Univ of North TX; Prog Dir, Old Dominion U, **SLP**

Bourassa, Diane 26 Parkwood, Laguna Hills, CA 92656, (714) 957-5147, BA 76 CA St Univ - Fullerton; MA 79 CA St Univ - Northridge; Sp-Lang Path, Fairview Developmental Ctr, **SLP**

Bourbouse, Janet M 911-D South Casitas Drive, Tempe, AZ 85281, (602) 968-6461, BS 67 CA Univ of PA; MA 71 Univ of Pittsburgh - Pittsburgh; SLP, Children's Rehab Svcs, **SLP**

Bourdon, Donna L Erlanger Med Ctr Sp/Path Dept, 975 East 3rd Street, Chattanooga, TN 37403, (615) 778-7916, BS 79 Univ of TN - Knoxville; MA 80 Univ of TN - Knoxville; 85–Sp-Lang Path, Erlanger Medical Center, **SLP ACE**

Bourgault, Rachel M 2186 Highway 14, Banner, WY 82832, (307) 737-2274, BS 70 Black Hills St Coll; MS 73 Univ of OR; 75–Sp-Lang Path, Sch Dist 1 West Ranchester, **SLP**

Bourgeois, Debra Ann 1465 East Willow Lake Dr, Apartment E, Atlanta, GA 30329-2804, (404) 636-4202, BA 78 Northeast LA Univ; OM 81 Auburn Univ - Auburn; Sp-Lang Path, Dekalb Co Schs, **SLP**

Bourgeois, Mrs Lynne L 171 Bayou Vista Drive, Thibodaux, LA 70301, (504) 447-5119, BA 74 Nicholls St Univ; OM 78 LA St Univ - N O Medical Ctr; Sp-Lang Path, Lafourche Parish School System, **SLP**

Bourgeois, Michelle Suzanne 3102 Beechwood Blvd, Pittsburgh, PA 15217, (412) 363-4900, BS 76 Georgetown Univ; MS 78 Univ of WA; PH 88 (Communication Disorders) Univ of Pittsburgh-Johnstown; 88–Sp-Lang Path, Eye & Ear Institute, **SLP**

Bourgeois, Pamela Chevreaux Queen Of The Valley Hospital, 1115 South Sunset Avenue, West Covina, CA 91790, BA 77 Univ of Denver; MA 79 Univ of Denver; VP, Queen of the Vlly Hosp, **SLP**

Bourne, Jenny 2925 Susan Carol, Fayetteville, AR 72703-3953, (501) 521-4631, BS 74 Henderson St Univ; MS 77 Univ of OK Medical Center; Sp-Lang Path, Springdale Schools, **SLP**

Bourne, Mrs Lynne M Rt 1 Lake Oshawno, Carbondale, KS 66414, (913) 232-0551, BS 74 KS St Univ; MA 75 KS St Univ; Sp/Lang Path, Topeka Pub Sch, **SLP**

Bourne, Mrs Victoria L 613 Pearl Street, Bluefield, WV 24701, (304) 325-3745, BS 74 WV Univ; MS 75 Vanderbilt Univ; Sp-Lang Path, Private Practice, **SLP**

Bourque-Ardoin, Deborah 419 East Norwood Drive, Jennings, LA 70546, (318) 734-2351, BA 75 Univ of Southwestern LA; MS 76 Univ of Southwestern LA; Sp-Lang Path, Jeff Davis Parish Sch Syst, **SLP**

Boutte, Donna Maria 1606 Kimberly, Amarillo, TX 79111-1328, (806) 359-7681, BA 85 George Mason Univ; MA 87 Wichita St Univ; 87–Sp-Lang Path/Aud, Amarillo Sp Hrng & Lang Ctr

Boutte-Chambers, Mrs Janice S 251 Livermore Drive, Fayetteville, NC 28304, (919) 864-0092, BS 73 Univ of Cincinnati; MA 75 Univ of Cincinnati; 83–Sp-Lang Path, Cumberland County Pub Schools, **SLP**

Boutwell, Mrs Margaret 1636 Pineford Court, Stone Mountain, GA 30088, (404) 987-4935, BS 68 IL St Univ - Normal; MA 74 Wichita St Univ; 88–Sp-Lang Path, Hearing & Sp Ctr Inc, **SLP**

Bouvier, Mrs Maryann Janet 122 Sawyer, Grand Blanc, MI 48439, (319) 556-1040, BS 78 Univ of WI - Oshkosh; MA 80 Northeast MO St Univ; SLP, Brandon Schs, **SLP**

Bouwes, Nona G 740 West Avenue, Brockport, NY 14420, (716) 352-2440, BS 74 Nazareth Coll of Rochester; MA 78 SUNY - Coll at Geneseo; Sp-Lang Path, Monroe #2-Orleans BOCES, **SLP**

Bouyer, Penelope 1 Man Of War Drive, Media, PA 19063, (215) 565-4650, BS 85 West Chester Univ of PA; MS 87 Loyola Coll; 87–Sp-Lang Path, Devereux Foundation, **SLP**

Bova, Lisa Gross 343-B South Fig, Escondido, CA 92025, **SLP**

Bove, Celeste F 2339 Holly Spring Drive, Silver Spring, MD 20904, (301) 427-8185, BA 70 Memphis St Univ; MA 71 Memphis St Univ; 87–Aud, Food & Drug Admin, **A**

Bove, Mrs Doreen Quiry 673 Franklin Street #101-A, Worcester, MA 01604, (617) 568-8316, BS 80 Anna Maria Coll; MS 85 Worcester St Coll; Sp-Lang Path, Hudson Ps, **SLP**

Bove, Lydia Jean 22 Haynes Street, Worcester, MA 01603, (617) 765-9771, SLP, Harrington Mem Hosp, **SLP**

Bowden, Dr Ann E RR 3, Blenheim, ON, Canada N0P 1A0, (416) 965-4945, BA 71 York Univ - Ontario; MA 73 Univ of MT; PH 80 (NS) Univ of KS; 88–Policy Analyst, Ministry of Comm & Soc Svcs, **SLP**

Bowden, Brenda Jones 7306 Donnell Place #B-8, Forestville, MD 20747, (301) 894-0320, MS 83 Univ of NC - Chapel Hill; Sp-Lang Path, Prince Georges Co Sch, **SLP**

Bowden, Mrs Debra J 6849 Almada Street, Long Beach, CA 90815, (213) 496-2424, BS 75 PA St Univ - Univ Park; MS 76 Univ of MI - Ann Arbor; Sp-Lang Path, Bowden & Darringer Rehab Assoc, **SLP**

Bowden, Pamela S 110 Nanna Court, Santa Cruz, CA 95060, (408) 426-6479, BA 77 CA St Univ - Stanislaus; MA 79 CA St Univ - Stanislaus; Sp/Lang Path, Santa Cruz Cty Sch Dist, **SLP**

Bowe, Angela J 107 Simmons Terrace, Syracuse, NY 13219, (315) 487-5469, BS 41 Syracuse Univ; MS 51 Syracuse Univ; Sp-Lang Path, Syracuse Pub Schs, **SLP LM**

Bowe, Teresa Gunter 1024 Medfield Road, Lugoff, SC 29078, (803) 438-4815, BA 83 Columbia Coll; MS 84 Univ of SC - Columbia; 86–Director Speech Pathology Dept, Kershaw County Mem Hosp, **SLP**

Bowen, Mrs Barbara M 1025 St Peter Street, New Orleans, LA 70116, (504) 861-2545, BA 66 Albion Coll; MA 67 OH St Univ; Sp-Lang Path, New Orleans Pub Sch, **SLP**

Bowen, Beverly A 35 Silver Birch Lane, Clinton, CT 06413, (203) 669-1055, BA 80 Southern CT St Univ; MS 82 Southern CT St Univ; 88–SLP, Madison PS, **SLP**

Bowen, Brigitta P Route 2 Box 182-C, Houston, MS 38851, (601) 456-5552, BA 86 Univ of MS; MS 88 Univ of Southwestern LA

Bowen, Carol Marie 1373 Tomlee Drive, Berkeley, CA 94702, (415) 794-3666, OB 61 Washington Univ; Aud, CA Sch for the Deaf, **A**

Bowen, Deborah Trent Route 7 Box 779-B, Fort Payne, AL 35967, (205) 638-4131, BA 75 Marshall Univ; MA 86 Marshall Univ; 87–Sp-Lang Path, Dekalb Co Bd of Educ

Bowen, Jeanie Gurney 760 Ashland Avenue, Buffalo, NY 14222, (716) 686-2000, BS 84 SUNY - Coll at Buffalo; MS 86 SUNY - Coll at Buffalo

Bowen, Mrs Judy W P O Box 794, Washington, GA 30673, (404) 678-7132, BA 61 Mercer Univ - Macon; ME 64 Emory Univ; Sp-Lang Path, Wilkes County Board of Educ, **SLP**

Bowen, Katherine Ricchetti 2723 Hyde Park Street, Sarasota, FL 34239, (813) 954-3491, BS 74 Kent St Univ; MS 78 Univ of South FL; 75–SLP, Sch Bd of Sarasota Co FL, **SLP**

Bowen, Kathryn H Route 2 Box 8, Bible Hill Road, Claremont, NH 03743, (603) 927-4261, BA 75 Tufts Univ; MS 78 Boston Univ; Sp-Lang Path, SAU #43, **SLP**

Bowen, Mrs Lynn Wehrenberg 3427 Elwood Drive, Fort Wayne, IN 46815, (219) 425-7463, Sp-Lang Path, Ft Wayne Comm Sch, **SLP**

Bowen, Mary B R R 1 Box 104, Palisades, NY 10964, (914) 634-7385, BS 74 SUNY - Center at Albany; MA 79 Kent St Univ; **SLP**

Bowen, Nancy Marie Audiology Clinic, 411 N E 87th Avenue, Suite B, Vancouver, WA 98664, (206) 892-9367, BS 79 Portland St Univ; MS 82 Portland St Univ; Audiologist, Audiology Clinic, **A**

Bowen, Pamela A 3031 S Second St 2nd Fl, Whitehall, PA 18052, (215) 266-6128, BS 85 Kutztown Univ of PA; MA 87 OH Univ - Athens; 88–Sp-Lang Path, Sacred Heart Hosp, **SLP**

Bowen, Mrs Paula Poirier 41-B Nipmuc Trail, North Providence, RI 02904, (401) 739-2700, BS 83 Univ of NH; MS 85 Boston Univ; 86–Sp-Lang Path, South Kingstown Sch Dept, **SLP**

Bowen, Mrs Terry T 132 Bailey Drive, Grafton, VA 23692, (804) 398-7003, BA 74 Univ of CA - Santa Barbara; MA 80 CA St Univ - Los Angeles; 87–Aud, Naval Hosp, **A**

Bowen-Pearson, Patricia 1465 East 4230 South, Salt Lake City, UT 84124, (801) 272-3409, MS 86; Sp/Lang Path, Jordan Sch Dist, **SLP**

Bowens, Sandra Felecia 664 4th Avenue #4R, Brooklyn, NY 11232, BS 79 SUNY - Coll at Buffalo; MS 86 Adelphi Univ; 88–Sp-Lang Path, Small Stuf Inc, **SLP**

Bowens, Virginia Nmn P O Box 163, Cambridge, NY 12816, (518) 793-7721, BS 74 FL A & M Univ; MS 75 FL St Univ; 84–Sp-Lang Path, So Adirondack Educ Ctr, **SLP ACE**

Bower, Mrs Deborah R UCLA Audiology Clinic, UCLA Medical School, Chs 62-202, Los Angeles, CA 90024, (213) 825-5721, BS 58 Northwestern Univ; MS 60 Univ of PA; Aud, UCLA Med Sch Aud Cl, **A**

Bower, Dr Glenda Gay 224 N W Circle, Topeka, KS 66606, (913) 272-1944, BA 65 Fort Hays St Univ; MS 66 Fort Hays St Univ; ED 74 (NS) Univ of CA - Los Angeles; Sp-Lang Path, Presch Intervent Proj USD 501, **SLP**

Bower, Mrs Julie Ann 1022A Julia Lane, Lafayette, IN 47905, (317) 783-8321, MS 82 Purdue Univ - West Lafayette; Aud, St Francis Cen, **A**

Bower, Loren J 129 Sunset Drive, Montoursville, PA 17754, (717) 328-8441, BS 59 Bloomsburg Univ of PA; ME 65 PA St Univ - Univ Park; Superv/Sp Lang Hrng, Blast-I U #17, **SLP**

Bower, Marcia Louise 1100-A Glade Hill Drive, Knoxville, TN 37909, (615) 694-5951, MS 83 Univ of WI - River Falls; Aud, Knox County Sch Spec Services, **A**

Bower, Robert D 1607 Acorn Place, Clementon, NJ 08021, (609) 346-9292, BS 55 IL St Univ - Normal; Sp-Lang Path, Private Practice, **SLP**

Bower, Wendy Anne 524 Theo, Lansing, MI 48917, (517) 321-6146, BS 79 Wayne St Univ; MA 86 Eastern MI Univ; 87–Sp-Lang Path, Charlotte PS, **SLP**

Bower, Mrs Wendy Obourn Village Park Apts #15-104, North Avenue, Pleasant Valley, NY 12569, (203) 797-7597, BS 82 Marywood Coll; MS 84 Univ of WI - Madison; Sp-Lang Path, Danbury Hosp, **SLP ACE**

Bowers, Mrs Betty N 2305 Ridge View Drive, Wausau, WI 54401-2460, (715) 845-7035, BA 50 Univ of SD - Vermillion; MS 70 Univ of WI - Stevens Point; OM 80 Univ of WI - Stout; Psychol, N Ctrl Tech I, **SLP**

Bowers, Mrs Brenda R 2011 Madrid Court, Riverside, CA 92506, (714) 351-9336, BA 64 Univ of the Pacific; MS 82 Univ of Redlands; Sp-Lang Path, Alvord USD, **SLP**

Bowers, Mrs Jane P Route 3 Box 44, Monroe, GA 30655, (404) 267-6574, BS 50 Case Western Reserve Univ; ME 69 Univ of GA; OD 69 (NS) Univ of GA; Sp-Lang Path, Walton Co Bd of Ed, **SLP**

Bowers, Mrs Linda G 344 Helena Drive, Newport News, VA 23602, (804) 599-2094, BS 71 WV Univ; MS 72 WV Univ; Aud, Riverside Reg Med Cen, **A**

Bowers, Mrs Linda Sandusky P O Box 2364, Cullowhee, NC 28723, (704) 227-7251, BA 70 FL Southern Coll; MS 75 Auburn Univ - Auburn; Sp-Lang Path, Wn Carolina U, **SLP**

Bowers, Mrs Louise E 30 Rocky Ridge Road, Dillsburg, PA 17019, (717) 432-8305, **SLP**

Bowers, Marilyn Darcel 5913 Overhill Drive #3, Los Angeles, CA 90043, (213) 625-6000, BA 77 Univ of CA - Santa Barbara

Bowers, Mary Ellen 903 Redfield Road, Bel Air, MD 21014, (301) 363-0300, BS 78 Towson St Univ; ME 79 Clarion Univ of PA; Sp-Lang Path, ACC/Villa Maria Sch, **SLP**

Bowersock, Mrs Lisa A 2857 Sherwood Road #A, Columbus, OH 43209, (614) 263-5151, 1988; MS 87 Bowling Green St Univ; Sp-Lang Path, Columbus Sp Hrng Ctr

Bowes, Alice H S 28 Hampshire Road, Portsmouth, NH 03801, **SLP**

Bowes, Ann Jeane 7734 37th Avenue N E, Seattle, WA 98115, (206) 523-0738, **SLP**

Bowes, Mrs Miriam E D 341 Meadowbrook Road, North Wales, PA 19454, (215) 539-8550, BS 73 Indiana Univ of PA; MA 76 Trenton St Coll; SLP, Montgomery Co I U, **SLP**

Bowes, Nancy Jane 708 South 200 West, Crawfordsville, IN 47933, (317) 339-7262, BS 74 Purdue Univ - West Lafayette; MS 85 IN St Univ - Terre Haute; **SLP**

Bowhers, Mrs Wendy 612 Berkley Place, Virginia Beach, VA 23452, (804) 431-0228, BS 82 Clarion Univ of PA; MA 84 Univ of MD - College Park; Sp-Lang Path, Hampton Rds Easter Seal Soc, **SLP**

Bowie, Rosemary Chandler 220 St Stephens East, Irmo, SC 29063, (803) 252-2538, BA 78 Columbia Coll; MA 79 Univ of TN - Knoxville; Sp/Lang Path, Sp Path Assocs, **SLP**

Bowlen, James H 364 Morgantown Street, Uniontown, PA 15401, (412) 437-0402, BA 31 WV Univ; MA 46 Columbia Univ Teachers Coll; **SLP LM**

Bowler, Dr Ned W HC 60 Box 1155, Bliss, ID 83314, (208) 837-4590, BA 46 Univ of ID; MA 47 NY Univ; PH 57 (Sp Path & Aud) Stanford Univ; Retired, **SLP LM**

Bowles, Marion D 2000 Bunker Street, Anchorage, AK 99501, **SLP**

Bowles, Martha A Bi-State Speech & Lang Clinic, 1895 Middle Road, Suite 1, Bettendorf, IA 52722, (319) 359-5867, BS 80 Phillips Univ; MA 81 Northeast MO St Univ; Dir / Owner, Private Practice, **SLP**

Bowles, Pamela Elizabeth 400 Maynard Street #1007, Ann Arbor, MI 48104-2438, (313) 663-1867, MS 88 Univ of MI - Ann Arbor

Bowles, Mrs Patsy H 1208 Elmwood Road, Bloomington, IL 61701, (309) 827-6654, BS 69 IL St Univ - Normal; MS 71 IL St Univ - Normal; 87–Sp-Lang Path, Bloomington PS Dist #87, **SLP**

Bowlin, Tina M McLean 411 E Mason Street, Polo, IL 61064, (815) 625-0400, OB 84 Univ of MO - Columbia; OM 86 Univ of MO - Columbia; SLP, Com Gen Hosp, **SLP**

Bowline, Mrs Wilma L 1104 Crestline Drive, Lawrence, KS 66044, (913) 864-4690, BA 53 Ottawa Univ; MA 71 Univ of KS; 73–Sp-Lang Path, U Ks, **SLP**

Bowling, Dr Evelyn B 7806 Madison Avenue #D-107, Fair Oaks, CA 95628, (916) 961-8549, BA 58 Univ of CA - Los Angeles; MA 73 CA St Univ - Sacramento; PH 85 (NS) 0; Dir, Sunrise Lang Sp Inc, **SLP**

Bowling, Mrs Karin Ann 1542 Fairhill Drive, Ashland, KY 41101, (606) 739-4141, BA 76 Marshall Univ; MA 81 Marshall Univ; **SLP**

Bowling, Dr Lloyd S Route 1 Box 231, Charlotte Hall, MD 20622, (202) 994-7166, BA 54 Univ of MD - College Park; MA 57 Univ of MD - College Park; ED 64 (NS) Univ of MD - College Park; Prof, Geo Washington U, **A F**

Bowling, Mary Arrington 3513 Louis Drive, Plano, TX 75023, (214) 618-1122, BS 72 Purdue Univ - West Lafayette; MS 77 Miami Univ - Oxford; Sp/Lang Path, **SLP**

Bowling, Stephen Dale 2401 Salutaris, Apartment A-3, Cincinnati, OH 45206, (513) 923-4446, BS 82 Univ of Cincinnati; Audiologist, Ear Nose and Throat Clinic, **A**

Bowlin-Johnson, Jo Anna P O Box 336, Deer Park, WA 99006, (509) 276-2939, BA 83 WA St Univ; MA 86 WA St Univ; 88–Aud/Store Mgr, Dees Park Pharmacy & Hrng Ctr, **A**

Bowlus, Janet Mae 345 Southwood Drive, Perrysburg, OH 43551, (419) 874-0886, BS 72 Bowling Green St Univ; MA 85 Bowling Green St Univ; 87–Sp-Lang Path-Rehab Svcs, Med Coll of Ohio, **SLP**

Bowlus, Rebecca Ann Highline Hospital Sp-Hrng, 14245 Ambaum Blvd S W, Seattle, WA 98166, (206) 246-8677, BS 75 Bowling Green St Univ; BS 80 Univ of WA; OM 82 Univ of WA; Aud, Highline Commun Hosp, **A**

Bowman, Alison Faith Special Childrens Center, 211 Wilkens Road, Ithaca, NY 14850, (607) 272-5891, MS 84 Ithaca Coll; BA 83 SUNY - Coll at Cortland; Sp-Lang Path, Special Childrens Center, **SLP**

Bowman, Ann S Box 16, Hood, VA 22723, (804) 985-2460, BS 74 Longwood Coll; ME 75 Univ of VA - Charlottesville; **SLP**

Bowman, Brooks A 230 Lower Magothy Beach Rd, Severna Park, MD 21146, (301) 396-0503, BA 74 Towson St Univ; MS 80 Univ of South FL; **SLP**

Bowman, Mrs Carol J 1348 Plum Creek Drive, Bourbonnais, IL 60914-1565, (815) 933-0720, BS 76 IL St Univ - Normal; MS 78 IL St Univ - Normal; Sp-Lang Path, Kaukakee Sch Dist #111, **SLP**

Bowman, Dr Clarence A Dept Speech Path & Audiology, Illinois State University, Normal, IL 61761, (309) 438-5704, BA 75 Augustana Coll; MS 76 Eastern IL Univ; PH 79 (Sp Path) Univ of IL - Urbana; 78–Assoc Prof, Il St U, **SLP**

Bowman, Jan M 10 Timberidge Court, Ringgold, GA 30736, (615) 855-2605, BS 69 PA St Univ - Univ Park; ME 71 Indiana Univ of PA; SLP, Chattanooga Cty Schs, **SLP**

Bowman, Judith K 616 Walnut Street, Tipp City, OH 45371, (513) 335-5624, BS 84 Univ of Cincinnati; MA 86 OH Univ - Athens; **SLP**

Bowman, Julia Beeson 1515 Holcombe, M D Anderson Cancer Center, Box 69, Houston, TX 77030, (713) 792-6565, BA 69 Converse Coll; MA 73 Univ of TN - Knoxville; 83–Sp-Lang Path, MD Anderson Cancer Ctr, **SLP**

Bowman, Katie Monty 999 Quincy Circle, Anaheim Hills, CA 92807, (714) 637-7923, BA 78 CA St Univ - Long Beach; MS 85 Chapman Coll; Sp-Lang Path, Orange Sp & Lang Ctr, **SLP**

Bowman, Linda Susan 44 Chiswick Circle, Bloomington, IL 61704, (309) 663-5082, BS 81 IL St Univ - Normal; MS 83 IL St Univ - Normal; 86–Sp-Lang Path, Illinois State Univ, **SLP**

Bowman, Melinda Vice 5615 Chateau Way, Fairfield, OH 45014, (419) 227-6001, BS 84 Ball St Univ; MA 85 Ball St Univ; **SLP**

Bowman, Rick G 4805 South Powerline, Nampa, ID 83651, (208) 376-3591, BS 71 ID St Univ; MS 72 ID St Univ; 76–Aud, Boise Sp/Hrng Cl, **A**

Bowman, Mrs Sally Ann 8111 Rumford Road, Indianapolis, IN 46219, (317) 264-8868, BS 51 Western MI Univ; MS 65 Butler Univ; Assoc Prof of SLP, Indiana Univ Sch of Medicine, **SLP**

Bowman, Mrs Susan Cherry Mednet/Euclid Clinic, Audiology Department, 18599 Lake Shore Blvd, Euclid, OH 44119, (216) 383-5913, BA 82 OH Wesleyan Univ; MA 84 Case Western Reserve Univ; Aud, Euclid Clinic Foundation, **A**

Bowman, Susan E 2208 East Divide Avenue #1, Bismarck, ND 58501, (701) 839-3031, BA 84 Univ of ND; MS 86 Minot St Univ; **SLP**

Bowman, Mrs Sylvia Ann 52-701 Avenida Navarro, La Quinta, CA 92253, (619) 327-1553, BA 64 San Jose St Univ; Classroom Teacher, Palm Springs USD, **SLP**

Bowman, Tamara Replogle 107 Oak Park Court, Athens, GA 30605, (404) 546-9261, BS 74 Purdue Univ - West Lafayette; MA 84 Univ of IL - Urbana; **SLP**

Bowman, Zeph M 3209 Bristol Highway, Johnson City, TN 37601, (615) 282-3311, BS 52 LA St Univ - Baton Rouge; MS 62 Univ of TN - Knoxville; 77–Sp-Lang Path, Pro Health Svcs, **SLP A**

Bowman-Nance, Kay L 369 Piney Forest Road, Danville, VA 24541, (804) 792-5299, Dir, Commun Cl for Sp-Lang/Hrng Dis, **SLP**

Bowman-Sorine, Marilyn L P O Box 1213, Morgantown, WV 26507, (304) 296-7880, BS 73 WV Univ; MS 74 WV Univ; Sp/Lang Path, Self Employed, **SLP**

Bown, Dr Jesse Clinton, Jr 657 16th Avenue, Salt Lake City, UT 84103, BS 59 Brigham Young Univ; MS 60 Brigham Young Univ; PH 69 (NS) Univ of UT; Sp-Lang Path, **SLP A**

Bowron, Mrs Dawn Ann 1125 East Nelson Avenue, Indianapolis, IN 46203, (317) 357-3666, BS 82 Purdue Univ - West Lafayette; MS 85 Purdue Univ - West Lafayette; Aud, Hrng Ctr Inc, **A**

Bowser, Barbara M 1234 Triviz Drive, Las Cruces, NM 88001, MA 80 NM St Univ; Las Cruces Pub Sch, **SLP**

Bowser, Janice Pivik 206 Hill Avenue, Cheswick, PA 15024, (412) 941-4434, MS 84 Clarion Univ of PA; BS 83 Clarion Univ of PA; Sp-Lang Path, Harmarville Rehab Ctr, **SLP**

Bowser, Terri Louise 89 Lewis Bay Road, Hyannis, MA 02601, (617) 771-0612, BA 81 Thiel Coll; MS 85 Indiana Univ of PA; **SLP ACE**

Bowsher, Robert B 2807 Harlan Street #308, Edgewater, CO 80214, (303) 758-3415, BA 83 Univ of Northern CO; MA 85 Univ of Northern CO; **SLP**

Bowz, Renee D 28 Woodley, Watertown, MA 02172-3550, (617) 924-2635, **SLP**

Box, Mrs Jane D 8718 East Wilderness, Shreveport, LA 71106, (318) 686-0383, BA 65 LA Tech Univ; OM 77 LA St Univ - N O Medical Ctr; 88–Consult-Sp-Lang Path, Clin Comm Ctr, **SLP ACE**

Boxbaum, Allen H 15 Pond Valley Circle, Penfield, NY 14526, (716) 271-0680, BS 77 SUNY - Coll at Geneseo; MS 78 Syracuse Univ; Mgr of Mobile Serv, Hrng & Sp Cen of Rochester, **A**

Boxbaum, Michele Cerio 15 Pond Valley Circle, Penfield, NY 14526, (716) 546-3550, BS 78 SUNY - Coll at Geneseo; MA 79 SUNY - Coll at Geneseo; Sp-Lang Path, Monroe Dev Cen, **SLP**

Boyarsky, Marcia J 802 Birchview Drive, Encinitas, CA 92024, (619) 753-0126, MA 85 San Diego St Univ; **SLP**

Boyce, Maureen A 1610 West 227th Street #3, Torrance, CA 90502, (213) 540-4327, BA 85 Univ of Redlands; MA 87 San Diego St Univ

Boyce, Mrs Susan H 5425 Brenner Road N W, Olympia, WA 98502, (206) 866-6399, BS 68 George Washington Univ; MS 70 Univ of MI - Ann Arbor; Sp-Lang Path, Providence Hosp, **SLP**

Boychuk, Mrs Carol A 101 Glentworth Road, Willowdale, ON, Canada M2J 2E7, (416) 756-6359, BA 77 Rutger's St Univ - Douglas Coll; MS 79 Columbia Univ Teachers Coll; 87–Aud, North York Gen Hosp, **A**

Boyd, Mrs Carole G 548 32nd Street, West Des Moines, IA 50265, (515) 225-7391, MS; **SLP**

Boyd, Carolyn J 1434 McMullen Lane, Laurel, MT 59044, (406) 628-8860, BA 69 Univ of Puget Sound; MA 71 Univ of WA; Sp-Lang Path, Yellowstone County Head Start, **SLP**

Boyd, Christina A 694 Mull Avenue Apt #1-A, Akron, OH 44313, (714) 788-7305, BA 78 Univ of Redlands; MS 80 Univ of Redlands; SLP, Riverside USD, **SLP**

Boyd, Diane K 18520 Azalea Drive, Derwood, MD 20855, (202) 877-6717, BA 77 Montclair St Coll; MS 79 Columbia Univ Teachers Coll; Aud, Washington Hosp Cen, **A**

Boyd, Evelyn G 1330 Waters Lane, Sandy, UT 84093, (801) 571-8736, BA 78 Andrews Univ; MA 80 Northern MI Univ; 83–Sp-Lang Path, Private Practice, **SLP**

Boyd, Mrs Jacqueline Compere Rt 7 Box 445, Burleson, TX 76028, (817) 295-8108, BA 54 Baylor Univ; MA 69 TX Christian Univ; Burleson ISD, **SLP**

Boyd, Janet L 5809 South 76th E Avenue, Tulsa, OK 74145, (918) 743-7767, BS 81 Univ of Tulsa; MA 82 Univ of Tulsa; Sp/Lang Path, Town & Country Sch, **SLP**

Boyd, Jean 2730 Camino Chueco, Santa Fe, NM 87505, (505) 989-5483, BS 74 Univ of Houston - Univ Park; MA 75 Univ of Houston - Univ Park; Sp-Lang Path, Santa Fe Pub Sch, **SLP**

Boyd, Dr John 941 Dalkeith Avenue, London, ON, Canada N5X 1S0, PH; **SLP**

Boyd, Judith M 5236 North Sydenham Street, Philadelphia, PA 19141, **SLP**

Boyd, Mrs Kimberly Ann 711 Spruce, Wamego, KS 66547, (913) 456-7271, **SLP**

Boyd, Lynda Ann RFD #6, 50 Perkins Drive, Laconia, NH 03246, (603) 524-5907, BA 70 Univ of NH; MS 85 Univ of NH

Boyd, Marjorie L 100 Windy Lane, Edinboro, PA 16412, (814) 455-6711, MA 78 Edinboro Univ of PA; Chief SLP, Hamot Med Cen, **SLP**

Boyd, Mrs Mary Jane 131 Foxtail Drive, St Charles, MO 63303, (314) 521-6776, BS 71 Univ of MO - Columbia; MS 82 Fontbonne Coll; SLP, Spec Sch Dist of St Louis Co, **SLP**

Boyd, Miriam R 110 Locust Lane, Pittsburgh, PA 15241, (412) 464-6221, BS 69 Carnegie-Mellon Univ; MA 81 Univ of Pittsburgh - Pittsburgh; Sp-Lang Path, S Hills Hlth Sys Home Care, **SLP**

Boyd, Mrs Pamela Dianne W 1111 Navajo, Carrollton, TX 75007, (214) 323-6603, BS 79 Univ of North TX; MS 80 Univ of North TX; Sp/Lang Path, Carrollton-Farmers Branch ISD, **SLP**

Boyd, Mrs Patricia T 2300 West Michigan Suite 8, Midland, TX 79701, (915) 684-4345, BA 70 Southern Methodist Univ; MS 71 TX Tech Univ; Sp-Lang Path, Midland Sp Hrng Lang Ctr, **SLP**

Boyd, Ronald D 1308 Brindwood Lane S E, Decatur, AL 35601, (205) 355-8430, BA 72 Univ of Montevallo; MS 74 Univ of Montevallo; 86-Sp-Lang Path, Private Practice, **SLP**

Boyd, Suzanne C 160 Butman Road, Lowell, MA 01850, (617) 957-4633, BS 69 Boston Univ; ME 73 Boston Univ; Chpers/Core Eval Team, Dracut Pub Sch, **SLP**

Boyd, Mrs Sylvia Sturz 5806 Fairbrook Street, Long Beach, CA 90815, (213) 602-6930, BS 66 CA St Univ - Long Beach; BA 50 San Diego St Univ; Sp-Lang Path, Paramount USD, **SLP**

Boyd, Thomas C 548 32nd Street, West Des Moines, IA 50265-3106, (319) 753-6561, BS 74 Univ of IA; MA 76 Univ of IA; **A**

Boyden, Mariln Fay Department Of Audiology, Hospital For Sick Children, 6th Floor Elm Wing, 555 University Avenue, Toronto, ON, Canada, (416) 598-6558, BA 69 Univ of NE - Lincoln; MA 72 Univ of NE - Lincoln; Dir of Aud, Hospital for Sick Children, **A**

Boydston, Mrs Anne Elizabeth 3169 Cowden, Memphis, TN 38111, (901) 323-9008, BS 85 Univ of GA; MA 86 Memphis St Univ; 87-Sp-Lang Path, Mid-South Sp Path Group, **SLP**

Boydstun, Mrs Sherry Bechard 431 N W 33rd Avenue, Gainesville, FL 32601, (904) 377-4126, BA 76 Univ of FL; ME 78 Univ of FL; **SLP**

Boyd-Whitley, Robert Forrest 4060 207th Street, Langley, BC, Canada V3A 2E1, (604) 534-4931, OB 74 Univ of Saskatchewan Sask; MA 82 Univ of CA - Santa Barbara; 88-Sp-Lang Path, Sch Dist #35 Langley BC, **SLP**

Boyea, Mrs Jill Ann 326 Evergreen Blvd, Browns Mills, NJ 08015, (609) 893-1400, BA 83 SUNY - Coll at Plattsburgh; MA 84 SUNY - Coll at Plattsburgh; Sp-Lang Path, Pemberton Twnshp P S, **SLP**

Boyer, Barbara M 3523 Shannon Road, Albany, GA 31707, (912) 759-2966, BA 51 Univ of KY; MA 66 Our Lady Lake Univ-San Anton; Dir, Tlw Shared Ser, **SLP**

Boyer, Debra A 301 North 25th Avenue, Hattiesburg, MS 39401, (601) 268-5131, BA 73 Southeastern LA Univ; MS 75 Univ Southern MS-Hattiesburg; Aud, ENT & Facial Plas Surg, **A**

Boyer, Mrs Gail S 5712 Woodlyn Road, Frederick, MD 21701, (301) 371-9485, BA 78 Boston Coll; MA 80 Univ of MD - College Park; 85-Sp-Lang Path, Private Practice, **SLP**

Boyer, Kathryn K 19350 Gainsborough, Detroit, MI 48223, **SLP**

Boyer, Pauline M 420 Lockville Road, Pickerington, OH 43147, (614) 877-4345, **A**

Boyer, Regina U 663 Denise Road, Rochester, NY 14616, (716) 621-3452, BS 81 SUNY - Coll at Geneseo; MA 82 SUNY - Coll at Geneseo; 86-SLP, Monroe #2-Orleans Co BOCES, **SLP**

Boyer, Mrs Rosemary Teresa 362 Wellesley Street East, Toronto, ON, Canada M4X 1H4, (416) 890-1221, BS 81 Univ of Western Ontario; OM 84 Univ of Western Ontario; 84-Sp-Lang Path, Dufferin Peel Cath Sch Bd, **SLP**

Boyer, Tracey Dianne 1567 Southwest Boulevard, Apartment 2-L, Tulsa, OK 74107-1804, (918) 455-3535, BA 85 Wichita St Univ; MA 86 Wichita St Univ; 88-Sp-Lang Path, Broken Arrow Med Ctr, **SLP**

Boykin, Mrs Estelle V 4216 Bucknell Drive, Decatur, GA 30034, (404) 292-7272, BS 62 Morgan St Univ; MS 64 PA St Univ - Univ Park; Sp/Lang Path, Dekalb Co Sch Syst, **SLP**

Boykin, Lesley L 318 Kerby Road, Grosse Pointe, MI 48236, (313) 881-4296, BA 72; OM 74 6982; Private Practice, **SLP**

Boykin, Pamela T 1281 Balmoral, Detroit, MI 48203, (313) 927-7640, BA 70 Catholic Univ of America; ME 71 Northeastern Univ; Sp-Lang Path, Mount Carmel Mercy Hospital, **SLP ACE**

Boyko, Mrs Janice Carter 27 Church Street, Gorham, ME 04038, (207) 839-2126, BA 76 Univ of RI; ME 78 Northeastern Univ; Sp-Lang Path, Private Practice, **SLP**

Boyko, Nora Ann 1749 Chester Road Apartment 8, Bethlehem, PA 18017, (215) 759-7600, BS 73 Edinboro Univ of PA; MS 81 Bloomsburg Univ of PA; Sp-Lang Path, Col N Hampton Intermediate Ut, **SLP**

Boyko, Robin K 18 Little Oak Lane, Rocky Hill, CT 06067, (203) 527-2631, BA 75 Hofstra Univ; MA 76 Univ of IL - Urbana; 76-Sp-Lang Path, Hartford Pub Sch, **SLP**

Boylan, Donna M 308 Polonia Street, Menasha, WI 54952-2723, (414) 738-2045, BS 79 Univ of WI - Oshkosh; MS 81 Univ of WI - Madison; 85-Sp-Lang Path, St Elizabeth Hospital, **SLP**

Boylan, James E 32 Gail Drive, Ellington, CT 06029-9771, (203) 872-9077, BA 68 Univ of VT; MA 69 Western MI Univ; Sp-Lang Path, Windham Pub Sch, **SLP**

Boylan, John A, Jr Rd 3 6N, Edinboro, PA 16412, (814) 732-2431, BA 63 WV Wesleyan Coll; ME 69 Clarion Univ of PA; Prof Sp-Lang Path, Edinboro U, **SLP**

Boylan, Linda Carol 7898 Pavillion Drive, Severn, MD 21144, (301) 551-4943, BA 82 Allegheny Coll; MA 86 Univ of TX - Austin; 87-Aud, Hrng & Sp Agency of Metro Baltimore Inc, **A**

Boylan, Mary F 4154 Summit Drive, Columbus, OH 43224, (215) 631-9300, BA 85 Coll of Mount Saint Joseph; MS 86 Univ of Louisville; **SLP**

Boyle, Katherine 249 Alpine Street #40, Pasadena, CA 91106, (213) 625-4183, BS 72 Univ of WI - Madison; MS 73 Univ of WI - Madison; Sp-Lang Path, Los Angeles Cty Sch, **SLP**

Boyle, Mrs Lakshmi Joshi R R 2 Box 27H, Jericho, VT 05465-9402, (617) 345-0146, Prof Assoc, InSpeech Inc, **SLP**

Boyle, Dr Mary Dept Speech & Comm Sciences, St John's University, Grand Cntrl & Utopia Pkwys, Jamaica, NY 11439, (312) 570-4171, BS 77 Univ of MA - Amherst; MA 79 Northwestern Univ; PH 85 (Communication Sciences & Dis) Northwestern Univ; 85-Assistant Professor, St John's Univ, **SLP**

Boyle, Mary Catherine 51 Kenwood Avenue, Wakefield, RI 02879, (401) 294-4561, BS 79 Bloomsburg Univ of PA; MS 80 Bloomsburg Univ of PA; Sp-Lang Path, State of RI, **SLP ACE**

Boyle, Mary Christina #7 Shawnee Hills, Wheeling, WV 26003, (304) 277-2977, BA 85 Marshall Univ; MA 86 Marshall Univ; **SLP**

Boyle, Susan Stark Audiology Associates, 1793 East 71st Street, Tulsa, OK 74136-5108, (918) 495-1650, BA 70 William Jewell Coll; MA 77 Univ of Tulsa; Aud, Aud Assoc, **A**

Boyle, Dr Thomas 43 Sharon Street, Bloomfield, CT 06002, (203) 289-7187, BS 70 Bradley Univ; MS 71 Bradley Univ; PH 78 (Aud) Univ of Denver; Aud, East Hartford Hrng Cen, **A**

Boyle, Timothy A 2905 East 84th Street, Tulsa, OK 74137, BS 71 Clarion Univ of PA; MA 77 Tulane Univ; **A**

Boyle, Mrs Virginia Galvin 4520 Iberville Street, New Orleans, LA 70119, (504) 567-3111, BA 82 Univ of Southwestern LA; MA 84 LA St Univ - N O Medical Ctr; Aud, Hearing Instruments Inc, **A**

Boylin, Catherine 334 Arbutus Street, Durham, CT 06422, (203) 238-6058, MA 79 NY Univ; SLP, Altobello Youth Cen, **SLP**

Boylston, Eula W 2714 Cypress Street, Columbia, SC 29205, (803) 734-5040, BA 70 Columbia Coll; ME 71 Univ of SC - Columbia; SLP, Sc Dept of Hlth & Env Control, **SLP**

Boyne, Rita B Route 1 Box 143-G, Ville Platte, LA 70586, (318) 948-3011, BS 75 LA St Univ - Baton Rouge; MA 77 LA St Univ - Baton Rouge; 81-Sp-Lang Path, Opelousas Gen Hosp, **SLP**

Boyne, Sandra Olsson 13 Kimberlin Lane, Belleville, IL 62221, (618) 277-0629, BA 81 McKendree Coll; MS 86 Southern IL Univ-Edwardsvill; 86-Sp-Lang Path, Christian Hospital NE, **SLP**

Boysen, Dr Allen E Veterans Administration (126), 810 Vermont Avenue NW, Washington, DC 20420, (202) 745-8578, BA 62 Univ of IA; MS 65 CO St Univ; PH 70 (Communication Disorders) Univ of OK Medical Center; 88-Dir Aud Sp-Lang Path, Veterans Administration, **SLP**

Boysen, Dona Hudson 307 Trapper Circle, Windsor, CT 06095, (203) 242-2274, BA 79 Univ of KY; MA 80 Ball St Univ; Superv of SLP, Rehab Cen, **SLP**

Bozarth, Gloria A M Audiology & Speech Pathology, VA Hospital, 921 N E 13th, Oklahoma City, OK 73104, (405) 272-9876, BS 68 Western IL Univ; MS 70 Univ of OK Medical Center; Aud, VA Med Cen, **A**

Braasch, Thomas J 3813 West 24th Avenue, Vancouver, BC, Canada V6S 1L8, (604) 224-1331, BS 84 CA St Univ - Hayward; MS 86 Gallaudet Coll; 86-Aud, B C Ministry of Health, **A**

Braat, Mrs Dortha Buchtel 14989 Barton Road, Vicksburg, MI 49097, (616) 467-9745, BS 75 Western MI Univ; MA 87 Western MI Univ

Brace, Terri L 509 5th Avenue West, Kirkland, WA 98033, (206) 827-1110, MA 88 Western WA Univ

Bracey, Ann M 5050 South Lake Shore Drive, #2505, Chicago, IL 60621, (312) 947-0579, BA 77 Mundelein Coll; MS 79 Bradley Univ; Sp-Lang Path, Chicago Bd of Ed, **SLP ACE**

Brach-Bonkowski, Mrs Valerie 44 Knollwood Drive, Westfield, MA 01085, (413) 562-4131, BA 79 Bridgewater St Coll; MS 80 Emerson Coll; Director Commun Disorders, Western Massachusetts Hospital, **SLP ACE**

Brachfeld, Jill Robin 25-43 32nd Street, Astoria, NY 11102, (212) 320-0123, BA 84 SUNY - Center at Buffalo; MA 87 CUNY - Hunter Coll; **SLP**

Brack, Barbara Anne 114 Hillside Avenue, Chatham, NJ 07928, (201) 879-6004, BA 78 Augustana Coll; MA 84 Montclair St Coll; Sp-Lang Path, Chester Twp Board of Education, **SLP**

Bracken, Annamarie Mariani 12204 Parkstream Terrace, Herndon, VA 22070, (703) 437-6842, BS 83 PA St Univ - Univ Park; MA 84 Univ of Pittsburgh - Pittsburgh; 87-Sp-Lang Path, Loudoun Hosp Ctr, **SLP**

Bracken, Maryann P 2309 Terrell Road, Greenville, TX 75401, BA 56 Emmanuel Coll; MS 80 East TX St Univ - Commerce; Sp/Lang Path, Greenville ISD, **SLP**

Brackett, Mrs April Anne P O Box 890822, Houston, TX 77289-0822, (409) 761-2331, Bellvel ISD, **SLP**

Brackett, Diane 313 West 88th Street #1B, New York, NY 10024, (212) 741-7698, BS 67 Univ of CT; MA 69 Univ of CT; PH 78 (NS) Univ of CT; Dir Commun Therapies, NY League/Hard of Hrng, **SLP**

Brackett, Dr Isaac P Route 4, Carbondale, IL 62901, (618) 453-4301, BS 38 Northwestern Univ; MS 40 Northwestern Univ; PH 47 (NS) Northwestern Univ; **SLP F LM**

Brackett, Katherine P O Box 5911, Tuscaloosa, AL 35405, (800) 223-2614, Aud, **A**

Brackett, Vanessa 10 Shadywood Circle, Asheville, NC 28803, (704) 274-2400, BS 80 Eastern MI Univ; MA 81 Eastern MI Univ; 88-Sp-Lang Path, Thoms Rehab Hosp, **SLP**

Brackey, Mrs Pamela L S 55 Julia Ann Drive N W, Cedar Rapids, IA 52405, BA 78 Univ of Northern IA; MA 79 Univ of Northern IA; 88-Sp-Lang Path, St Luke's Hosp, **SLP**

Brackin, Cheryl A 120 East 55th Street #1, Savannah, GA 31405, (912) 355-4601, BS 69 GA Southern Coll; ME 74 Univ of GA; SLP, Savannah Sp-Hrng Cen, **SLP**

Brackney, Mrs Teresa Marie 32 Hilltop Drive #5, West Lafayette, IN 47906, (317) 497-3053, BS 83 Ball St Univ; MA 85 Ball St Univ; **SLP**

Bracy, Mrs Connie Lynn 3811 Compton, Little Rock, AR 72205, (501) 224-2350, BS 83 Univ of AR - Little Rock; MS 86 Univ of AR - Little Rock; **SLP**

Bradburn-Oates, Ann 8628-B West Howard, Milwaukee, WI 53228, (414) 541-6694, BS 80 Univ of WI - Stevens Point; MS 81 Univ of WI - Eau Claire; Sp-Lang Path, St Lukes Hospital, **SLP**

Bradbury, Rebekah Ann 2861 Patterson Drive, Aliquippa, PA 15001, (412) 378-0144, BA 84 Geneva Coll; MS 86 Boston Univ; **SLP**

Bradbury, Rosanne B 606 David Street, Winter Springs, FL 32708, (305) 327-0624, BS 67 Univ of GA; ME 71 Univ of GA; SLP, Orange Co Pub Sch, **SLP**

Bradbury, Steven H Newton Hearing Aid & Aud Ser, 607 West 1st Street, Newton, KS 67114, (316) 283-0908, BA 76 Wichita St Univ; MA 74 Wichita St Univ; Aud, USD #373, **A**

Brade, Mrs Vivian A 3718 Mukilteo Boulevard, Everett, WA 98203, (206) 653-0662, BA 78 Univ of WA; OM 80 Univ of WA; Sp-Lang Path, Marysville Sch Dist #25, **SLP**

Braden, Mrs Linda F 1101 West Charles, Champaign, IL 61821, (217) 398-0738, BS 73 Univ of WI - Madison; MS 74 Univ of WI - Madison; 87-Sp-Lang Path, Champaign Unit 4, **SLP**

Braden, Marcia M 2903 South Vaughn Way, Aurora, CO 80014, (303) 751-5910, BS 76 CO St Univ; MA 78 Univ of Denver; **SLP**

Braden, Mrs Pamela King 9334 State Route 44, Mantua, OH 44255, (216) 274-2598, BS 76 Bowling Green St Univ; MA 85 Kent St Univ; 79-Sp-Lang Path, Crestwood Schs, **SLP**

Braden, Mrs Vicki Hillis 1106 South 7th, Ponca City, OK 74601-6711, (405) 363-4175, BS 81 Central St Univ; MA 84 OK St Univ; 81-Sp-Lang Path, Blackwell Pub Schs, **SLP**

Bradfield, Mrs Karen S 7945 Acuff Lane, Lenexa, KS 66215, (816) 942-5885, BS 69 Univ of KS; MA 71 Univ of KS; Sp-Lang Path, Ctr Sch Dist 58, **SLP**

Bradfield, Lisa C 521 North 32nd, Waco, TX 76707-3223, (817) 752-3451, BS 76 Baylor Univ; MS 80 Baylor Univ; Sp-Lang Path, Heart Texas Reg Mental Health, **SLP**

Bradfield, Patricia Annette 1022 South Longwood Avenue, Los Angeles, CA 90019, (818) 308-2419, BA 62 CA St Univ - Los Angeles; MA 76 CA St Univ - Los Angeles; MS 78 Pepperdine Univ - Los Angele; 65-SLP, Alhambra City Schs, **SLP**

Bradford, Debra Bukwaz 1221 Bernath Parkway, Toledo, OH 43615, (419) 866-1060, **SLP**

Bradford, Judith Ann 854 Massachusetts Avenue, Apartment 6, Cambridge, MA 02139-3024, (617) 581-9200, ME Northeastern Univ; SLP, Atlanticare Medical Center, **SLP**

Bradford, Mrs Karen Ann 717 Loop Road, Monroe, LA 71201, (318) 342-3052, MA 84 LA Tech Univ; Clinical Super, NE LA U, **SLP**

Bradford, Dr Larry J 1809 Webster Avenue, Topeka, KS 66604, (913) 233-5033, BA 51 Stanford Univ; MA 63 Univ of KS; PH 65 (NS) Univ of KS; Dir/Cen for Comm Dis, Menninger Found, **SLP A F**

Bradford, Mrs Mary James 1228 North 16th Street, Bismarck, ND 58501, (701) 663-5796, BS 81 Minot St Univ; MS 82 Minot St Univ; 88-Sp-Lang Path, Mandan PS Dist, **SLP**

Bradford, Pamela Walker 1015 Brandywine Road, Tuscaloosa, AL 35406, (205) 349-5669, **SLP**

Bradford, Sheryl Ann 21428 Hickory Branch Trail, Strongsville, OH 44136, (216) 238-4977, BS 84 Bowling Green St Univ; MA 85 Bowling Green St Univ; Sp-Lang Path, Deaconess Hosp of Cleveland, **SLP**

Bradford, Susan C P O Box 95, Birch Point Shores, Oxford, MA 01540, (617) 987-8390, MS 83 Worcester St Coll; 87-Sp-Lang Path, Putnam PS, **SLP**

Bradford-Amrhein, Mrs Denise 5846 Woods Edge Road, Madison, WI 53711, BA 78 Univ of VT; MS 79 Univ of VT; SLP, **SLP**

Brading, Mrs Christine Ann 2218 Basston Drive, St Louis, MO 63146, (314) 925-0205, BS 81 Southeast MO St Univ; MA 83 Southeast MO St Univ; SLP, United Services F/T Handicap, **SLP**

Bradley, Alana K 16934 S E 325th Place, Auburn, WA 98002, (206) 735-2482, BS 73 Univ of OR; MS 76 Portland St Univ; Sp-Lang Path, **SLP**

Bradley, Betty 411 Green Street, Alexandria, VA 22214, (703) 360-8000, BS 73 Univ of MD - College Park; MS 74 Loyola Coll; Sp-Lang Path, Brown Schools Ranch Treat Ctr, **SLP**

Bradley, Mrs Catherine 308 Broad, De Ridder, LA 70634, (318) 463-8465, BS 74 LA St Univ - Baton Rouge; MS 75 Vanderbilt Univ; Sp-Lang Path, Beauregard Parish Sch Bd, **SLP**

Bradley, Mrs Claire Ledden 49 Driftwood Drive, Port Washington, NY 11050, (516) 767-1843, 84–Sp-Lang Path, Glen Cove City Schs, **SLP**

Bradley, Clifford R 1730 East Woodland, Sapulpa, OK 74066, (918) 832-8782, BA 58 Wichita St Univ; MA 65 Wichita St Univ; Sp-Lang Path, Private Practice, **SLP**

Bradley, Denita Hyler 1302 Davis Lane, Knoxville, TN 37923, (615) 691-5536, BS 78 Univ of MO - Columbia; MS 80 Vanderbilt Univ; 87–Sp-Lang Path, Prof Hlth Svcs, **SLP**

Bradley, Dr Doris Parker Univ Of Southern Mississippi, Dept Speech & Hearing Sci, P O Box 5092 Southern Sta, Hattiesburg, MS 39401, (601) 266-5216, BS 53 Univ Southern MS-Hattiesburg; MA 57 Univ of FL; PH 63 (NS) Univ of Pittsburgh - Pittsburgh; 88–Prof, Univ of Southern Mississippi, **SLP F**

Bradley, Emilie S 4976 Pearce Street, Huntington Beach, CA 92649-3582, (714) 846-5505, BA 77 CA St Univ - Fullerton; MA 82 CA St Univ - Fullerton; 88–Sp-Lang Path, Private Practice, **SLP**

Bradley, Gary Kent 1912 West 48th Street, Westwood, KS 66205, (816) 891-4965, BS 82 Univ of MO - KS City; MA 84 Univ of KS; Aud, Twa

Bradley, Gerri A 3825 14th Avenue, Oakland, CA 94602, (415) 848-1741, BA 65 Coll of New Rochelle; MA 67 Columbia Univ Teachers Coll; Private Practice, **SLP**

Bradley, Mrs Janet Cheryl 5166 Harriett Circle, Riverside, CA 92505, (714) 788-7460, MS 81 Loma Linda Univ - Riverside; BS 75 Loma Linda Univ - Riverside; SLP, Rvrsd Unif Sch Dist, **SLP**

Bradley, Mrs Janice Marie 1402 Walnut Street Apartment 3, Hollidaysburg, PA 16648, (814) 695-7371, BS 79 Indiana Univ of PA; MS 84 Indiana Univ of PA; 87–Reg Consult, Prentke Romich Co, **SLP**

Bradley, Jean C 1408 Kearney Street, Laramie, WY 82070, (307) 766-6426, BS 74 PA St Univ - Univ Park; MS 76 PA St Univ - Univ Park; Sp-Lang Path, U of WY, **SLP**

Bradley, Kathy Cobbs 5050 South Lakeshore Dr, Apartment 3608-S, Chicago, IL 60615, (312) 793-4393, MA 83 Univ of IL - Urbana; Regional Consultant, Illinois Dept of Public Health, **A**

Bradley, Leslie Ann Guy F Gardner MD, 220 Doctors Park Bldg, Little Rock, AR 72205, (501) 221-0086, BA 80 Univ of AR - Little Rock; MS 83 Univ of AR - Little Rock; 87–Aud, Guy F Gardner MD, **A**

Bradley, Marcia E F Memorial Hospital, 8 Prospect Street, Nashua, NH 03061, (603) 883-5521, BA 75 Univ of MA - Amherst; MS 76 Marquette Univ; Superv Sp-Lang Path, Nashua Mem Hosp, **SLP**

Bradley, Margaret T Route 2 Box 6360, Wheatfield, IN 46392, (219) 866-5441, BS 72 Purdue Univ - West Lafayette; MS 72 Purdue Univ - West Lafayette; Sp-Lang Path, Rensselaer Ctrl Sch Corp, **SLP**

Bradley, Mrs Mary Catherine 183 Hoover Road, Rochester, NY 14617-3641, (716) 544-4976, BS 83 SUNY - Coll at Fredonia; MA 84 Bowling Green St Univ; 86–Sp-Lang Path, Mary Cariola Children's Center, **SLP**

Bradley, Mary Katherine 2352 South Seamans Road, Seaford, NY 11783, (212) 305-2961, BA 84 SUNY - Coll at Plattsburgh; MA 86 Hofstra Univ; **A**

Bradley, Nancy Wilson 18-C Country Club Lane, Milford, MA 01757, (203) 561-2458, BA 82 Univ of CT; MA 85 Univ of CT; Sp-Lang Path, Bristol Public Schools, **SLP**

Bradley, Mrs Roberta Lynn 3340 W Mulberry Drive, Mequon, WI 53092, (414) 242-0099, BA 70 Univ of WI - Madison; MS 79 Marquette Univ; 87–Sp-Lang Path, Prt Washington-Saukville Sch Dist, **SLP**

Bradley, Rose Oswald 1841 Douglass Boulevard, Louisville, KY 40205, (502) 454-4129, BA 78 Bellarmine Coll; MS 85 Univ of Louisville; 81–Sp-Lang Path, Jefferson Co PS, **SLP**

Bradley, Sarah E 2716 East Towers Drive #6, Cincinnati, OH 45238, (513) 541-4214, MA 87 Univ of Cincinnati

Bradley, Dr Scott T Department Of Communication Disorders, Box 86, Minot State University, Minot, ND 58701, (701) 857-3058, BA 74 Univ of WI - Milwaukee; MA 76 OH Univ - Athens; PH 84 (Hrng and Sp Sciences) Vanderbilt Univ; Asst Prof, Minot State Univ, **A**

Bradley, Susan Kay 2604 Palo Duro Drive #148, San Angelo, TX 76904, (915) 465-4391, BS 82 Univ of WY; MS 84 Univ of WY; Aud, San Angelo State School, **A**

Bradley, Willie B 842 Putnam Avenue, Brooklyn, NY 11221, (212) 574-2408, BA 73 CUNY - Brooklyn Coll; SLP, Speech Services Unit-Bd of Ed, **SLP**

Bradley-Boggi, Mrs Jayne Anne 1207 Ballard Street, Silver Spring, MD 20910, (301) 589-4158, BS 80 PA St Univ - Univ Park; MS 83 PA St Univ - Univ Park; Sp-Lang Path, National Rehabilitation Hosp, **SLP**

Bradshaw, Clive Robert 8317 Rhode Island Drive, Brooklyn Park, MN 55445, (612) 425-4131

Bradshaw, Denise 915 21st Street, San Diego, CA 92102, (619) 291-2506, MA 76 Univ of CA - Los Angeles; Director, Scottish Rite Clinic, **SLP**

Bradshaw, Janice F 5972 Baxter Drive, Jackson, MS 39211, (601) 957-3575, **A**

Bradshaw, Mrs Kelli Diane 2807 N E Bel Aire Circle, Lawton, OK 73501, (405) 353-0334, BS 83 OK St Univ; MS 85 Univ of OK - OK City; Sp-Lang Path, Lawton Pub Schs, **SLP**

Bradshaw, Mary H 1226 Bellevue Avenue #1-E, Richmond Heights, MO 63117, (314) 647-5358, OB 85 Univ of MO - Columbia; MA 87 Saint Louis Univ; 87–Sp-Lang Path, Spec Sch Dist of St Louis Co, **SLP**

Bradtke, Farral J 1005 West Bluff #2, Marquette, MI 49855, (906) 227-2125, BA 73 Univ of MI - Ann Arbor; MA 80 Northern MI Univ; 86–Asst Prof, Northern Michigan Univ, **SLP**

Bradway, Dr Lauren M 2519 Northwest 42nd, Oklahoma City, OK 73112, (405) 840-1864, BA 68 MO Valley Coll; MS 71 Central MO St Univ; PH 74 (NS) Univ of OK Medical Center; Sp-Lang Path, Private Practice, **SLP**

Brady, Arnell A 11542 South Laflin, Chicago, IL 60643, (312) 493-0900, BA 82 Saint Xavier Coll; MA 84 Northwestern Univ; Sp-Lang Path, Private Practice, **SLP**

Brady, Barbara Ann 411 Peterson Apt 11, Iowa City, IA 52240, (319) 356-7365, BS 82 Univ of SD - Vermillion; MA 84 Univ of SD - Vermillion; Aud, Univ of Iowa Hosp, **A**

Brady, Bonnie B 4402 Beulah Drive, La Canada, CA 91011, (213) 960-3802, BA 65; MA 76; SLP, LA Co Supt Sch, **SLP**

Brady, Carolyn C 2133 South Shore, Apartment 201, Kentwood, MI 49508, (616) 242-0425, MA 87 Case Western Reserve Univ

Brady, Debbie E 112 Deer Glade Run, Lexington, SC 29072, (803) 786-3845, BA 74 Columbia Coll; ME 75 Univ of GA; 79–Asst Prof, Columbia Coll, **SLP ACE**

Brady, Deborah H 934 Cheyenne Boulevard, Colorado Springs, CO 80906, (719) 578-1130, MS 75; Dir Cl Serv, Private Practice, **SLP**

Brady, Granville Y, Jr P O Box 68, Bound Brook, NJ 08805, (201) 231-0621, BA 67 Montclair St Coll; MA 68 Montclair St Coll; Owner, Private Practice, **SLP A**

Brady, Judith W 1294 Lavall Drive, Davidsonville, MD 21035, (301) 261-0533, BS 68 Carlow Coll; MA 77 Catholic Univ of America; Sp/Lang Path, Anne Arundel Co Publ Sch, **SLP**

Brady, Laura Loraine 1031 Kirts Boulevard #150, Troy, MI 48084, (313) 362-4628, BS 83 OH Univ - Athens; MA 86 Kent St Univ; 88–Aud, Children's Hosp of MI, **A**

Brady, Litha K Airsouth Box 112, FPO New York, NY 09524, BS 68 Univ of OK - Norman; MS 69 CO St Univ; **SLP**

Brady, Mrs Margaret S Rural Delivery 1, 974 Harris Hill Manor, Elmira, NY 14903, (607) 734-2301, BS 50 Shippensburg Univ of PA; MA 64 Ball St Univ; **SLP LM**

Brady, Nancy Caroline 2708 Wilson, Parsons, KS 67357, (612) 755-4110, MA 84 Univ of MN - Minneap-St Paul; Research Asst, Univ KS Bureau Child Rsch, **SLP**

Brady, Mrs Nancylee Emerson 217 Dickens Drive, Delran, NJ 08075, (609) 890-3717, BS 80 Trenton St Coll; MA 82 Trenton St Coll

Brady, Mrs Patricia A 286 Pepperwood Street, Hercules, CA 94547, (707) 257-2820, BA 79 San Francisco St Univ; MS 82 San Francisco St Univ; Dir Clin Svcs, Team Rehab, **SLP**

Brady, Patricia E O'Rourke 7 Emerald Road, Kendall Park, NJ 08824, BS 75 Trenton St Coll; MA 80 Kean Coll of NJ; SLP, Elizabeth Bd of Ed, **SLP**

Brady, Patricia Eileen 646 South Grand Street #E, Orange, CA 92666, (714) 532-5596, BA 82 CA St Univ - Fullerton; MA 86 CA St Univ - Fullerton; 87–Sp-Lang Path, Children's Ctr of Riverside, **SLP**

Brady, Mrs Rebecca Mills Northeast Georgia Speech Ctr, P O Box 1482, Gainesville, GA 30503, (404) 534-5141, BS 78 Western Carolina Univ; MS 82 Univ of GA; Sp-Lang Path, Northeast Georgia Speech Cen, **SLP**

Brady, Mrs Ricki I 5 Lackland Circle, Wichita Falls, TX 76306, (817) 720-3116, BA 74 Univ of TX - Arlington; MS 81 TX Tech Univ; 88–Sp-Lang Path, Wichita Falls ISD, **SLP**

Brady, Dr William A 4521 Washington Square #2, Youngstown, OH 44515, (216) 726-8155, BS 66 Clarion Univ of PA; ME 67 PA St Univ - Univ Park; PH 78 (NS) Kent St Univ; 86–Sp-Lang Path, Private Practice, **SLP**

Brady, William P, Jr 531 Fairfield Avenue, Ridgewood, NJ 07450, (201) 445-5350, BA 72 William Paterson Coll; MA 78 Montclair St Coll; MA 78 Montclair St Coll; Sp/Lang Path, Midland Pk Bd of Ed, **SLP**

Braeges, Judy L 18 Southland Drive, Rochester, NY 14623, (716) 427-7762, BS 71 Cleveland St Univ; MS 72 SUNY - Coll at Geneseo; Research Asst, NTID, **SLP**

Braff, Dr Reba G 711 West Montecito Avenue, Sierra Madre, CA 91024, (213) 651-1711, MA 67 Univ of Southern CA; PH 71 Univ of Southern CA; PH 82 (NS) United States Int'l Univ; Clinical Psychologist, Private Practice, **SLP**

Brafman, Alicia H L 2658 East 64th Street, Brooklyn, NY 11234, (718) 495-9600, MS 75 CUNY - Brooklyn Coll; 85–Asst Chairperson, Comm on Spec Educ

Braga, Mrs Danielle B R R 3 Box 425, Valley Farm Road, Millbrook, NY 12545, (914) 677-9348, BA 67 Adelphi Univ; MA 68 Columbia Univ Teachers Coll; **SLP**

Bragen, Deborah E 16 Fairmount Terrace, Jersey City, NJ 07306, (201) 433-5214, BA 78 Jersey City St Coll; MA 80 CUNY - Hunter Coll; 83–Sp-Lang Path, Private Practice, **SLP ACE**

Bragg, Dr Vernon C Oak Hills Medical Bldg, 7711 Louis Pasteur Drive, Suite 203, San Antonio, TX 78229, (512) 690-8941, BS 50 Northwestern Univ; MA 50 Northwestern Univ; PH 58 (Aud) Northwestern Univ; Pres, Private Practice, **A LM**

Bragg, Mrs Virginia D 115 Montclair Court, Macon, GA 31210, (912) 474-8790, BS 76 Univ of GA; ME 77 Univ of GA; SLP, Central State Hosp, **SLP**

Bragman, Mrs Janet Strawgate 735 Beneuento Avenue, Coral Gables, FL 33146-2012, (305) 667-1614, BS 79 FL St Univ; MS 80 FL St Univ; Sp-Lang Path, Private Practice, **SLP**

Brahm, Jill L 703 5th Street, New Cumberland, PA 17070, (717) 657-3373, BS 74 Kent St Univ; MA 75 Kent St Univ; Master Itin SLP, Capital Area Inter Ut, **SLP ACE**

Braidwood, Lynne A 611 Wadsworth, Traverse City, MI 49684, (616) 929-1653, BA 85 MI St Univ; MA 87 Eastern MI Univ; **SLP**

Brainin, Mrs Blanche M 16133 Meadowcrest Road, Sherman Oaks, CA 91403, (213) 997-2357, BA 45 Univ of IL - Urbana; 70 CA St Univ - Northridge; Sp-Lang Path, Los Angeles USD, **SLP**

Braithwaite, Beverley Ann 8517 Carroll Avenue, Silver Spring, MD 20903, (301) 445-4694

Brak, Mrs Sheila M Peoria ENT Group, 2627 North Knoxville Avenue, Peoria, IL 61604, (309) 686-5900, BA 62 Mundelein Coll; MS 64 Purdue Univ - West Lafayette; 80–Aud, Peoria ENT Group Sc, **SLP A**

Brake, Kristy Lunt 2020 Greenglen Drive #303, Kirkwood, MO 63122, (712) 322-7354, BA 82 Brigham Young Univ; OM 84 Brigham Young Univ; **A**

Braley, Karen Kathleen 126 Tera Manor, Wintersville, OH 43952, (614) 283-3674, BA 86 Baldwin-Wallace Coll; MS 87 Clarion Univ of PA; 88–SLP, Eastern OH Sp/Hrg Ctr Inc

Bralley, Dr Ralph C University Of Virginia, P O Box 9022, Charlottesville, VA 22906-9022, (804) 924-7107, BA 50; ME 59 Univ of VA - Charlottesville; ED 64 (NS) Univ of VA - Charlottesville; Assoc Prof, Comm Disorders Prog, **SLP F**

Bramble, Mrs Margaret W Box 964, Gunnison, CO 81230, (303) 641-2088, BS 51 MI St Univ; MA 68 MI St Univ; **SLP**

Bramblett, Dixon A 1 Ford Court, Sicklerville, NJ 08081, (609) 728-1486, BA 73 Auburn Univ - Auburn; MA 76 Temple Univ; MA 88; 86–Grad Stu, Temple Univ-Psychology Dept, **A**

Bramer, Jean M P O Box 5408, Ventura, CA 93003, (805) 658-8125, BA 76 San Francisco St Univ; MA 81 Univ of CA - Santa Barbara; Infant Specialist, Santa Barbara County Schools, **SLP**

Brammer, Mrs Brenda G 210 Adair Avenue, Shelbyville, KY 40065, (502) 633-0031, BS 73 Murray St Univ; MS 80 Univ of Louisville; SLP, Shelby Co Board of Ed, **SLP**

Brammer, Melanie Ann Speech And Hearing Center, 8001 Frost Street, San Diego, CA 92123, (619) 576-5845, BS 81 CO St Univ; MS 83 Univ of AZ; Aud, Hrng & Sp Ctr, **A**

Bramschreiber, Mrs Joy A Southern Prairie Area Ed Agny, Ottumwa Industrial Airport, Route 5 Box 55, Ottumwa, IA 52501, (515) 682-8591, BS 72 Northeast MO St Univ; MA 73 Northeast MO St Univ; Superv of Sp/Lang Depart, Sn Prairie AEA, **SLP**

Branan, Georgiana 515 Mossy Vale Way, Atlanta, GA 30328, (404) 292-7272, BS 69 Univ of GA; ME 71 Univ of GA; Sp/Lang Path, Dekolp Co Bd Ed, **SLP**

Brancato, Elizabeth Ann c/o Dr J Moss, 310 Dyer St Apt T-A, New Haven, CT 06515-9999, (203) 789-3362, MS 85 3362; BA 81 3195; **SLP**

Branch, Mrs Carol 4153 Del Mar Trails Road, San Diego, CA 92130, (619) 576-5838, MA 81 Univ of San Diego; 83–Aud, Chldn Hosp & Hlth Ctr, **A**

Branch, Judith B Route 4 Box 1760, Tifton, GA 31794, (912) 386-5005, BS 74 Univ of GA; ME 86 Valdosta St Coll; 83–Sp-Lang Path, Tift County Bd of Educ, **SLP**

Branch, Mrs Judith L 9611 Ottewell Road, Edmonton, AB, Canada T6B 2E3, (403) 432-8858, BA 66 Univ of KS; MA 68 Univ of KS; 73–Sp-Lang Path, Univ of Alberta Hospitals, **SLP**

Brand, Mrs Bobbye Rennae 2203 Timberwood, Carrollton, TX 75006, (214) 387-9315, BS 73 Univ of OK - Norman; MS 84 Univ of TX - Dallas; **A**

Brand, Helene Ann 304 Dickinson Street, Philadelphia, PA 19147, (215) 887-5266, BS 77 PA St Univ - Univ Park; MA 81 Temple Univ; 84–Sp-Lang Path, Speech Pathology Consultants, **SLP ACE**

Brand, Kathleen Ann 10802 W Hillsborough Avenue, Apartment 2102, Tampa, FL 33615, (813) 933-8930, MS 86 Univ of South FL; 87–Sp-Lang Path, Hillsborough Co Sch Sys, **SLP**

Brand, Madeline 135 Clairemont Circle, El Paso, TX 79912, (915) 584-0474, BA 45 Univ of Toronto - Ontario; MA 47 Columbia Univ Teachers Coll; Retired, University of Texas-El Paso, **SLP LM**

Brandeland, Mrs Marilyn A 1028 Cummings Avenue, Eau Claire, WI 54701, (715) 836-4186, BS 76 Mankato St Univ; MA 79 Univ of MN - Duluth; **SLP**

Brandell, Mary E 619 Chippewa, Mount Pleasant, MI 48858, (517) 774-3471, BS 55 Central MI Univ; BA 55 Central MI Univ; ES 84 Central MI Univ; 88–Dir Sp-Lang Path, Central Mich U, **SLP**

Brandenburg, Mrs April Dawn 429 Partridge, De Soto, TX 75115, (214) 223-0904, BS 82 Baylor Univ; MS 84 Univ of TX - Dallas; **SLP**

Brandenburg, Mrs Louise A 414 Monaco Drive, Warson Woods, MO 63122, (314) 768-8946, MS 80 Fontbonne Coll; Director Sp-Lang Path, Ssm Rehab Ins, **SLP**

Brandenburg, Sara A 6726 Bowman Lane N E, Cedar Rapids, IA 52402, (319) 373-1313, BS 72 Northwestern Univ; MA 73 Northwestern Univ; Dir Info & Commun Devel Prog, Trace Cen U of WI, **SLP**

Brandenburger, Nancy 8656 Head Harbour, Pasadena, MD 21122, (301) 355-0100, **SLP**

Branderbit, Pamela Lynne 204 Newport Court, Fords, NJ 08863, (201) 634-8411, BA 82 Rutger's St Univ - Douglas Coll; MA 84 Hahnemann Univ Grad Sch; 86–Custom Prod Spec, Slemens Hearing Instruments, **A**

Brandes, Mrs Polly P 5022 Henke Road, Milton, WI 53563, (608) 868-7664, BA 64 Univ of WI - Madison; MS 65 Stanford Univ; 79–Sp-Lang Path, Milton Area Schs, **SLP ACE**

Brandes-Meyerfeld, Mrs Holly 2263 East 27th Street, Brooklyn, NY 11229, (212) 683-6970, BA 75 CUNY - Brooklyn Coll; MS 83 CUNY - Brooklyn Coll

Brandl, Lynne PO Box 3559, St Croix, VI 00841, (809) 772-1412, BA 79 Univ of WI - Eau Claire; MS 81 Univ of WI - Stevens Point; Sp-Lang Path, US Virgin Island Government, **SLP**

Brandmeyer, Mrs Georgina Cagas 5244G Salinas Valley, St Louis, MO 63128, (314) 991-5035, BA 28 Southern IL Univ-Edwardsvill; MS 84 FL St Univ; 86–Sp-Lang Path, Spec Sch Dist of St Louis Co, **SLP**

Brandner, Susan Miller 508 Madison Drive, East Windsor, NJ 08520, (609) 655-4586, BA 64 CUNY - Hunter Coll; MS 70 CUNY - Brooklyn Coll; Aud, Medical Center at Princeton, **A**

Brandner, Mrs Tamara Dee 7150 Olivia Road, Baltimore, MD 21220, (301) 396-9125, MS 84 Loyola Coll; 84–Sp-Lang Path, Balt Cty-PS, **SLP**

Brandon, Andrew E 788 Central Avenue, Dover, NH 03820, (603) 749-2447, BA 69 TX Tech Univ; MS 70 TX Tech Univ; Aud, Prof Hrng Servs, **A**

Brandon, Dickey L Anderson-Oconee Sp & Hrng Serv, 106 Dostak Drive, Anderson, SC 29621, (803) 226-2477, BA 78 TX Tech Univ; MA 80 Univ of North TX; Aud, Anderson-Oconee Sp & Hrng Serv, **A**

Brandon, Judith K 320 Fields Road, Dansville, MI 48819, BS 80; MA 82 Eastern MI Univ; **SLP**

Brandreth, Shirley Elizabeth 101 Baldwin Road, Warwick, RI 02886, (617) 695-2561, **SLP**

Brandriet, Stanley E 5550 North 41st Street, Milwaukee, WI 53209, (414) 272-1466, BA 64 Hamline Univ; MA 66 Univ of ND; Dir Aud Svcs, Wisconsin Hrng Aid Ctrs, **SLP**

Brandt, Mrs Antoinette 25466 Wareham, Huntington Woods, MI 48070, (313) 541-0764, BA 70 Wayne St Univ; ME 73 Wayne St Univ; SLP, Detroit Pub Sch, **SLP**

Brandt, Betty C Willistown Woods, 3105 Stoneham Drive, West Chester, PA 19382, MA 64 Columbia Univ Teachers Coll; Sp-Lang Path, Delaware County Intermed Unit, **SLP**

Brandt, David A 1925 Glenbarr Court, Bakersfield, CA 93309, (805) 397-6703, BA 67 San Jose St Univ; MA 69 San Jose St Univ; Sp-Lang Path, Kern County Supt of Schools, **SLP**

Brandt, Dr Grace Emery Children's Therapy Center, 1371 Del Norte Road, Camarillo, CA 93010, (805) 988-9815, BA 67 Beloit Coll; MA 71 Univ of CA - Santa Barbara; PH 85 (Lang Dev & Reading Prog within Educ Psy) Univ of CA - Santa Barbara; Dir or Research, Children's Therapy Center, **SLP**

Brandt, Jane Ann 5252 44th Avenue South, Minneapolis, MN 55417, (612) 627-2732, BS 78 Moorhead St Univ; MS 83 Saint Cloud St Univ; Sp-Lang Path, Minneapolis Pub Schs, **SLP**

Brandt, Dr John F Dept Speech - Language - Hearing, University Of Kansas, 290 Haworth Hall, Lawrence, KS 66045, (913) 864-4570, BA 60 Univ of IA; MA 63 Univ of IA; PH 65 (Sp/Hrng Science) Univ of IA; Professor, University of Kansas, **F**

Brandt, Lynne Marie 227 Austin, Park Ridge, IL 60068, **SLP**

Brandt, Mela B 1249 East 82nd Street, Brooklyn, NY 11236, (718) 495-9600, BA 73 CUNY - Brooklyn Coll; MS 75 PA St Univ - Univ Park; Sp-Lang Path, Bd of Ed of NYC, **SLP**

Brandt, Dr Sara Dale 2624 Bardith Court, Lawrence, KS 66046, (913) 588-5937, BA 63 Univ of IA; MA 64 Univ of IA; PH 87 (Sp-Lang Path/Aud) Univ of KS; 87–Supvr, KU Med Ctr, **SLP ACE**

Brandt, Tina C 1 Highland Terrace, Pleasantville, NY 10570, (914) 528-0600, BS 65 Adelphi Univ; MA 78 Adelphi Univ; Sp-Lang Path, Lakeland Sch Dist, **SLP**

Brandt-Guckes, Deborah 1840 Argosy Court, Bloomfield Hills, MI 48013, BS 78 Northwestern Univ; MS 80 Univ of WI - Madison; Sp-Lang Path, Wm Beaumont Med Ctr, **SLP**

Brandy, Dr William T Audiology Speech Pathology Ser, VA Hospital, 1900 East Main Street, Danville, IL 61832, (217) 442-8000, BA 59 Heidelberg Coll; MS 62 Univ of Pittsburgh - Pittsburgh; PH 69 (NS) Univ of OK Medical Center; Chief, Aud SLP, VA Med Cen, **A**

Branfman, Dorrise 64-25-A 186th Lane, Fresh Meadows, NY 11365, (718) 454-9839, BA 72 Long Island U - CW Post Ctr; MS 73 Adelphi Univ; Sp-Lang Path, Private Practice, **SLP**

Branham, Charlotte Bandi 1201 West Siglo Place, Tucson, AZ 85705, BA 85 WA St Univ; MA 86 WA St Univ; **SLP**

Branham, Mrs Nancy G J 6413 Amundson Street, Tampa, FL 33614, (813) 425-3362, MS 79 Univ of South FL; Sp-Lang Path, Polk Co Sch Bd, **SLP**

Branker, Mrs Cheryl R 8329 Old Deer Trail, Raleigh, NC 27615, (919) 848-1503, BA 77 Univ of NC - Greensboro; MA 79 CUNY - Queens Coll; Sp-Lang Path, Wake Co Pub Sch Syst, **SLP**

Brankey, Mrs Fern T P O Box 117, Kooskia, ID 83539, (208) 983-0400, BA 45 Univ of IL - Urbana; MS 49 Univ of IL - Urbana; 83–Sp-Lang Path, Sch Dist, **SLP**

Brann, Eileen 821 Lake Street #1-N, Oak Park, IL 60302, (312) 848-9511, BS 75 IL St Univ - Normal; MS 76 IL St Univ - Normal; Sp/Lang Path, Gottleib Mem Hosp, **SLP**

Brannen, Mrs Ann Marie 1234 Shelton Way, Lawrenceville, GA 30245, (615) 477-4878, BS 82 Univ of GA; ME 85 Univ of GA; **SLP**

Brannen, Kimberly Jean 1912 Green Mountain Drive, Apartment #245-P, Little Rock, AR 72211, (501) 224-6067, BS 86 Univ of AR - Little Rock; MS 88 Univ of AR - Little Rock; 88–Sp-Lang Path, UCP

Brannen, Susan J 474 Benson Road, Victor, NY 14564, (716) 475-6554, BA 72 Marist Coll; MA 79 SUNY - Coll at Geneseo; Audiologist, Monroe-Orleans BOCES 2, **A**

Brannock, Mrs Betty B 2529 Albert Rasche Drive, Cape Girardeau, MO 63701, (315) 335-1251, BS 73 Southeast MO St Univ; ME 74 Southeast MO St Univ; Sp & Hrng Dept Superv, St Francis Med Cen, **SLP**

Brannon, Cindy Sue 1942 A Virginia, Homestead AFB, FL 33039, BA 82 Univ of CO - Boulder; MS 85 TX Tech Univ; Sp-Lang Path, Crosbyton Independent Sch Dist, **SLP**

Brannon, Dr John B, Jr 119 Manlyn Drive, Kirkwood, MO 63122, PH; Sch Psyc, St Louis Schs, **A**

Brannon, Mrs Laurie 5574 Riviera Walk, Long Beach, CA 90803, (213) 439-4554, BA 75 Univ of the Pacific; MA 76 Univ of the Pacific; SLP, ABC USD, **SLP**

Brannon, Patricia C 11715 Whisper Dew, San Antonio, TX 78230, (512) 492-0592, BA 74 Univ of AR - Fayetteville; MS 76 Univ of TX - Dallas; Sp-Lang Path, Northside ISD, **SLP**

Branscum, Mrs Dixie C 708 North 3rd, Augusta, AR 72006, (501) 347-2432, BS 74 AR St Univ; MA 75 Univ of MS; Sp-Lang Path, Augusta Pub Sch, **SLP**

Branson, Mrs Ann 619 N Franklin, Cuba, MO 65453, (314) 885-3208, BS 72 Central MO St Univ; MS 73 Central MO St Univ; Sp-Lang Path, Crawford R-II Sch, **SLP**

Branson, Cynthia W 736 N Stadium Way, Tacoma, WA 98403, (206) 545-2529, BA 68 Denison Univ; MA 70 Northwestern Univ; 74–Lecturer-Sp & Hrng Sci Dept, Univ of WA, **SLP**

Branson, Page Strickland 1004 S E 14th Avenue, Ocala, FL 32671, (904) 351-5871, BS 84 FL St Univ; MS 85 FL St Univ; Sp-Lang Path, Marion County School Board, **SLP**

Branson, Renee D 8013 East Morris, Wichita, KS 67207, (316) 683-4011, BS 77 Friends Univ; MA 82 Wichita St Univ; SLP, Wichita Pub Schs USD #259, **SLP**

Branson, Dr Virginia M P O Box 314, Williamstown, WV 26187, (304) 375-3699, OM 71 Smith Coll; MA 55 OH Univ - Athens; PH 61 (NS) OH Univ - Athens; Retired, **SLP LM**

Brant, Mrs Lynne M 40 Bow Road, Wayland, MA 01778, (617) 358-7074, BA 70 George Washington Univ; ME 73 Boston Univ; Sp-Lang Path, Wellesley Pub Schs, **SLP**

Brant, Paula Rae 8297 West Chestnut Avenue, Littleton, CO 80123, (303) 973-2355, BS 73 CO St Univ; MS 75 Univ of OK Medical Center; 86–Sp-Lang Path, Southwest Ped Habilitation Ctr, **SLP**

Brantingham, Bruce F 5007 East 67th Street, Indianapolis, IN 46220, (317) 872-8811, BS 56 Univ of IL - Urbana; MS 68 Loma Linda Univ - Loma Linda; 87–Dept Head-Sp-Lang Path, North Willow Ctr, **SLP**

Brantley, Denise S 111 Crowell Street, Hempstead, NY 11550, (718) 963-8319, BS 76 Northwestern Univ; MS 78 Vanderbilt Univ; OM 87 2162; 84–Assoc Dir, Med Assoc of Woodhill PC, **A**

Brantley, Maxie C 329 11th Street, Atlantic Beach, FL 32233, **SLP**

Brantley, Mrs Susan Lee 222 East Mc Elroy, Morganfield, KY 42437, (502) 389-1694, BS 76 Murray St Univ; MS 85 Murray St Univ; 77–Sp-Lang Path, Union County Bd of Educ, **SLP**

Branum, Mrs Anne Chandler 6811 Charis Court, Eden Prairie, MN 55346, (612) 934-3648, BA 82 Valparaiso Univ; MS 83 Marquette Univ; 88–Sp-Lang Path, Bloomington ISD 271, **SLP**

Branum, Mrs Cynthia Pinewood Springs, Lyons, CO 80540, (303) 823-5004, BS 72 CO St Univ; MS 73 CO St Univ; **SLP**

Brasch, Marilyn L 213 14th Avenue S Apt 2, Great Falls, MT 59405, (406) 453-4728, BA 71 Univ of Northern IA; MA 72 Univ of Northern IA; 87–Sp-Lang Path, Montana Sch for the Deaf and Blind, **SLP**

Brashears, Margaret M 14421 N W 13 Court, Miami, FL 33167-1106, (212) 749-2435, BA 70 Univ of Miami; MS 74 Columbia Univ Teachers Coll; SLP, Private Practice, **SLP**

Brashier, Ronda E Route 2 Box 530, Burleson, TX 76028, (817) 295-5879, BS 87 Baylor Univ; MS 88 Baylor Univ

Braskamp, Frederick 900 Oxford Lane, Wilmette, IL 60091, BA 79 Elmhurst Coll; MA 81 Western IL Univ; SLP, Chicago Public Schools, **SLP**

Braslau, Cynthia Gay 226 Tower Drive #7, Beverly Hills, CA 90211, (213) 651-2541, BS 82 Univ of TX - Austin; MA 85 TX Woman's Univ; 88–Sp-Lang Path, Naomi Heller & Assoc, **SLP**

Braslaw, Mrs Michele D 21223 Harvard Road, Southfield, MI 48076, (313) 355-5379, MA 88 Wayne St Univ; 88–Sp-Lang Path, Saratoga Comm Hosp

Brass, Mrs Edna M 101 Wildwood Lane, Joliet, IL 60433, (815) 727-6758, BS 75 Western IL Univ; MA 75 Western IL Univ; Sp/Lang Path, Joliet Twsp Hs Dist 204, **SLP**

Brass, Mrs Raye Simon 8868 Cavalier Drive, Cincinnati, OH 45231, (513) 742-2200, BS 67 Ithaca Coll; MA 69 Case Western Reserve Univ; Sp-Lang Path, Hamilton Co Offi of Ed, **SLP**

Brassard, Mrs Tracy Blevins 206 Dutch Lane, Lutz, FL 33549, (813) 949-8638, BS 84 Purdue Univ - West Lafayette; MA 85 Memphis St Univ; 88–Sp-Lang Path, Dist Sch Bd of Pasco County, **SLP**

Brassell, Mrs Esther G 105 Wedgwood Drive, Morganton, NC 28655, (704) 433-2919, BA 67 Mercer Univ - Macon; MA 69 Auburn Univ - Auburn; SLP, North Carolina School for Deaf, **SLP A**

Brassem, Maureen Joy 37 Bedford Crescent, Bramalea, ON, Canada L6T 1R5, (416) 793-6245, OM 87 Univ of Western Ontario

Brasser, Barbara Aylward 650 Pickford Street, Madison, WI 53711, (608) 266-6150, BS 77 Univ of WI - Madison; MS 79 Univ of WI - Madison; Aud, Madison Metropolitan Sch Dist, **A**

Brasseur, Dr Judith A #1 Kent Court, Chico, CA 95926, (916) 895-5871, BS 72 IN St Univ - Terre Haute; MS 75 IN St Univ - Terre Haute; PH 80 (NS) IN Univ - Bloomington; Assoc Prof, CA St U-Chico, **SLP**

Brasted, Sandra C Rd 1 Box 326, Kutztown, PA 19530, (215) 683-8275, MS 87 Rutgers St Univ -N Brunswick; 88–Sp-Lang Path, Easton Hosp, **SLP**

Bratcher, Carole Ann 2035 Deerwood, Murfreesboro, TN 37130-5772, (615) 865-2373, BS 84 Univ of IA; MA 85 Univ of TN - Knoxville; 88–Sp-Lang Path, Tennessee Christian Med Ctr, **SLP**

Braterman, Francine 2779 Clubhouse Road, Merrick, NY 11566, (516) 747-5400, BA 69 Adelphi Univ; MA 73 Hofstra Univ; Sp-Lang Path, Human Resources Sch, **SLP**

Brathwaite, Mrs Charlotte Denise 406 Goldfinch Drive, Augusta, GA 30907, (404) 737-7310, BS 79 Univ of GA; ME 81 Univ of GA; **SLP**

Bratt, Gene W Audiology & Speech Path (126), VA Medical Center, 1310 24th Avenue South, Nashville, TN 37203, (615) 327-5325, BA 69 Calvin Coll; MA 75 MI St Univ; PH 80 (NS) Vanderbilt Univ; Chief/Aud & SLP, VA, **A**

Bratten, Julie Ann 545 South Warren Sp #12, Monmouth, OR 97361, (503) 838-3001, **A**

Brault, Judith C 1366 Michelle Drive, Palatine, IL 60067, (312) 577-9943, BS 64 De Paul Univ; MA 66 De Paul Univ; 85–Sp-Lang Path, NSSEO, **SLP**

Brault, Mrs Mary Ann Scavotto 398 Sheridan Street, Chicopee, MA 01020, (413) 592-4302, BA 83 Elms Coll; MS 86 Worcester St Coll; **SLP**

Braun, Janet M 762 Somerset Drive, Janesville, WI 53545, (608) 868-2880, BS 72 Univ of WI - Milwaukee; MS 75 Moorhead St Univ; Sp-Lang Path, Milton Sch Dist, **SLP**

Braun, Jeri Brynildson 15820 Oak Ridge Road, Eden Prairie, MN 55344, (612) 949-2929, BS 80 Saint Cloud St Univ; MS 81 Univ of WI - Eau Claire; SLP, Minnetonka Public Schools, **SLP**

Braun, Mrs June E B 100 Angell Street, Bakersfield, CA 93309, (805) 831-4400, BS 74 Univ of Southwestern LA; MS 81 Univ of Southwestern LA; 87–Sp-Lang Path, Kern Co Schools, **SLP ACE**

Braun, Lori A 1898 Revere Lane, Elk Grove Village, IL 60007-2744, (312) 857-4050, BA 85 Univ of Denver; MS 87 Rush Univ; 88–Aud, Family Hearing Ctr

Braun, Mrs Marianne L 90 Dwinell Street, West Roxbury, MA 02132, (617) 359-4352, BA 71 Univ of Stockholm - Sweden; MS 79 Univ of RI; Sp-Lang Path, Medfield Pub Sch, **SLP ACE**

Braun, Mary Beth 896 Brookfield Drive #4, Mansfield, OH 44907, (419) 756-1133, BS Northwestern Univ; MA 85 Northwestern Univ; 88–Sp-Lang Path, Rehab Svc of Ohio, **SLP**

Braun, Mrs Mary Strzelczyk 5860 Riverside Drive, Fredonia, WI 53021, (414) 692-2124, BS 81 Marquette Univ; MS 82 Marquette Univ; Associate Administrator, Rehabilitation Associates Inc, **SLP ACE**

Braun, Mrs Susan W 65 Easton Lane, Moreland Hills, OH 44022, (216) 574-8512, BS 59 Univ of Miami; MS 73 John Carroll Univ; Asst Superv Offi Sp/Lang, Cleveland B of Ed

Braunagel, Becky J 7433 Mallard Court, Indianapolis, IN 46260, BS 78 Miami Univ - Oxford; MS 79 IN Univ - Bloomington; SLP, Lebanon Comm Sch, **SLP**

Braunfeld, Giselle H 100 Bennett Avenue, New York, NY 10033, (212) 923-0797, BA 82 CUNY - City College; MA 86 CUNY - City College; 88–Sp-Lang Path, Private Practice, **SLP**

Braunsky, Mrs Susan B 625 South Jackson Street, Batavia, IL 60510, (312) 879-8536, BA 85 Augustana Coll; MA 87 Northern IL Univ - De Kalb

Braunstein, Carol S 167 Springtime Lane, Levittown, NY 11756, **SLP**

Braunstein, Joan J 10204 Counselman Road, Potomac, MD 20854, **SLP**

Braunstein, Mrs M Sue 11217 Fall River Court, Potomac, MD 20854, (301) 299-6678, BS 68 Miami Univ - Oxford; MA 69 Bowling Green St Univ; Sp-Lang Path, Private Practice, **SLP**

Braunstein, Mrs Pamela R 52 Parkview Drive, Succasunna, NJ 07876, (201) 584-4312, BA 78 CUNY - Queens Coll; MA 80 CUNY - Queens Coll; **SLP**

Braverman, Devida Michelle 3615 Central Road, Apartment 203, Glenview, IL 60025, (312) 729-6965, BS 85 Univ of IL - Urbana; MA 87 Northwestern Univ; 87–Sp-Lang Path, Therapeutic Systems, **SLP**

Braverman, Mrs Janet M East Surburban Sp & Lang Clinic, 3950 Orangewood Drive, Cleveland, OH 44122, (216) 292-3530, BA 72 Boston Univ; MA 74 Case Western Reserve Univ; Sp/Lang Path, East Suburban Sp/Lang Cl, **SLP**

Braverman, Kathleen M 1038 Hatch Street, Cincinnati, OH 45202, (513) 651-1157, BS 68 Kent St Univ; MS 70 Emerson Coll; 85–Stu Lecturer in SLP, Univ of Cincinnati, **SLP**

Braverman, Leonard 504 Constitution Avenue N E, Washington, DC 20002, (202) 543-6135, BA 75 CUNY - Brooklyn Coll; MA 76 George Washington Univ; SLP, Montg Co Pub Schls, **SLP**

Braverman, Mrs Meryl Spector 9611 N W 49th Court, Sunrise, FL 33351, (305) 985-3200, BA 77 Hofstra Univ; MA 78 Hofstra Univ; SLP, Broward Co Schl Sys, **SLP**

Braverman, Mrs Sharon G 6426 Spear Street, San Diego, CA 92120, BA 79 Univ of CA - Santa Barbara; MS 81 Columbia Univ Teachers Coll; SLP, Grossmont District Hospital, **SLP**

Bravos, Christine Speech-Language Pathology, 9201 Sunset Boulevard, Suite 310, Los Angeles, CA 90069, (213) 273-4952, BA 73 Univ of Southern CA; MS 75 Loma Linda Univ - Loma Linda; Owner, Bravos-Miller Sp-Lang Path, **SLP**

Bravstein, Mrs Linda L B 59 Crest Hollow Lane, Searingtown, NY 11507, (516) 625-1725, BA 73 CUNY - Brooklyn Coll; MA 74 Trenton St Coll; PH (Sp Path) Adelphi Univ; 84–Sp-Lang Path, Private Practice, **SLP**

Brawley, Mary C 425 Park Avenue, Burlington, WI 53105, (414) 763-7795, BA 75 Coll of Saint Teresa; MA 77 Governors St Univ; 86–Sp-Lang Path, Private Practice, **SLP**

Brawner, Christine Marie 537 Gum Street, Vandenberg AFB, CA 93437, (805) 734-1796, BA 84 Univ of MI - Ann Arbor; MS 86 Univ of MI - Ann Arbor; 86–Sp-Lang Path, Private Practice, **SLP**

Braxton, Mrs Patricia Lynn 1730 Sunnypark Lane, Redlands, CA 92374, (714) 924-9811, BA 81 San Diego St Univ; MS 82 Univ of Redlands; **SLP**

Bray, Mrs Deborah Rea 1106-2 North Harlem Avenue, River Forest, IL 60305, (312) 470-0434, BA 75 Case Western Reserve Univ; MA 77 Northwestern Univ; Sp/Lang Path, Niles Twnsp Dept Spec Ed, **SLP**

Bray, Deirdre 128 Meadow Glade Circle, Kingsport, TN 37663, (615) 239-7115, BA 75 Southern CT St Univ; MS 78 FL St Univ; Knox Co Head Start, **SLP**

Bray, Mrs Jacque Neilson 4450 Peach Street, Salt Lake City, UT 84117, (801) 272-0838, BA 72 Brigham Young Univ; MS 85 Univ of UT; Sp-Lang Path, Granite School District, **SLP**

Bray, Mrs Katherine J 4206 37th Street, Lubbock, TX 79413-2128, (806) 799-5705, BA 74 Metropolitan St Coll; MA 75 Univ of TX - El Paso; **SLP**

Bray, Mrs Mary K 6901 94 Avenue S E, Mercer Island, WA 98040, (206) 232-9370, BS 81 Univ of WA; MS 84 Univ of WA; Aud, Herbert C Thomas MD, **A**

Bray, Mary Petrea 1216 Corral Creek Avenue #3, Paso Robles, CA 93446, (805) 239-9661, BA 83 Univ of the Pacific; MA 84 Univ of the Pacific; 84–Sp-Lang Path, Newport Lang Sp Audio Ctr, **SLP**

Bray, Mrs Robin J 11 Reading Terrace, Fair Lawn, NJ 07410, (201) 688-5150, BS 82 Stockton St Coll; MA 84 CUNY - Queens Coll; Aud, Seimans, **A**

Bray, Victor H, Jr 801 Forest Glen Cove, Round Rock, TX 78664, (512) 471-3841, BS 76 Univ of GA; OM 80 Auburn Univ - Auburn; **A**

Brayer, Mary Ann 690 Mentor Road, Akron, OH 44303, (216) 867-7212, BS 77 Bowling Green St Univ; MS 82 Southern IL Univ -Carbondale; Sp-Lang Path, **SLP**

Braytenbah, Mrs Marlene 524 Glenmeadow Road, Midlothian, VA 23113, (804) 379-3561, BA 74 CUNY - City College; MA 79 James Madison Univ; 84–Sp-Lang Path, Johnston-Willis Hospital, **SLP**

Brayton, Dr Evelyn R 7 Merion Avenue, Clifton Park, NY 12065, (518) 445-4526, BS 55 SUNY - Coll at Plattsburgh; MS 71 Syracuse Univ; PH 75 (NS) Syracuse Univ; Dir Commun Dis Cen, Albany Med Cen Hosp, **SLP**

Brayton-Gerratt, Shaun Daniel Freeman Memorial Hosp, 333 North Praire Avenue, Inglewood, CA 90301, (213) 674-7050, BS 76 Univ of MA - Amherst; MA 78 Univ of MA - Amherst; Cl Spec/Sp-Lang Path, Freeman Mem Hosp, **SLP**

Brazda-Witters, Jorja M 4142 Sheridan Blvd, Lincoln, NE 68506, (402) 483-5748, BA 83 Univ of NE - Lincoln; MS 86 Univ of NE - Lincoln; SLP, Lincoln Ps, **SLP**

Brazier, Mrs Susan H 5415 N E 55th, Seattle, WA 98105, (206) 524-6153, BA 41 Univ of WA; **SLP**

Breakey, Mrs Angela Raphael 1002 Metfield Road, Baltimore, MD 21204, (301) 838-7300, MS 86 Towson St Univ; 86–Sp-Lang Path, Bd of Educ of Harford Co, **SLP**

Breakey, Lisa K 2444 Moor Park Avenue, Suite 300, San Jose, CA 95128, (408) 297-9740, BA 67 Univ of CA - Santa Barbara; MA 75; 76–Sp/Lang Path, Private Practice, **SLP ACE**

Breakey, Margaret R 1220 Bellevue Avenue #8, Burlingame, CA 94010, (415) 344-8327, BA 37 Univ of CA - Berkeley; MS 48 Washington Univ; **A LM**

Breakstone, Mrs Beth Ellen 335 Woodland Avenue, Westfield, NJ 07090, (201) 232-9028, BA 77 Brown Univ; MS 79 Columbia Univ Teachers Coll; ME 79 Columbia Univ Teachers Coll; **SLP**

Breaud, Mrs Jane Maness 226 Pike Drive, Gretna, LA 70053, (504) 361-4782, BA 82 Nicholls St Univ; OM 87 LA St Univ - N O Medical Ctr; Sp-Lang Path, **SLP**

Breault, Leslie M 5923 Cavalleri Road, Malibu, CA 90265, (805) 484-3661, BA 65 Univ of CA - Los Angeles; MA 80 CA St Univ - Northridge; Sp-Lang Path, Camarillo State Hospital, **SLP**

Breazeale, Mrs Karen Lynn 423 North Main Street, Collierville, TN 38017, (901) 767-8831, BA 83 Univ of TN - Knoxville; MA 84 Memphis St Univ; **SLP**

Breazeale, Theresa Faye 34 Williams Street, Watertown, MA 02172, (617) 923-4673

Brecher, Adelyn R 2169 Lincoln Drive, Huntingdon Valley, PA 19006, BS 74 PA St Univ - Univ Park; MS 75 Vanderbilt Univ; Sp-Lang Path, Private Practice, **SLP**

Breckenridge, Cora S 54653 Briarwood Drive, Elkhart, IN 46514, (219) 264-5675, BS 59 IN Univ - Bloomington; MS 63 IN Univ - Bloomington; Sp-Lang Path, Elkhart Community Schools, **SLP**

Brecker, Rona Carol 2590 Albatross Road #C, Delray Beach, FL 33444, (407) 243-1762, BS 85 FL St Univ; MA 86 Northwestern Univ; **SLP**

Breckwoldt, Dr Gerhard H Platessa, 3430 Illinois Avenue, St Louis, MO 63118, (314) 664-9200, PH 44 (NS); Professor Emeritus, Was St Louis University, **LM**

Bredemeier, Mrs Nancy Sorn 11510 Olde Gate Drive Apartment C, Cincinnati, OH 45246, (513) 771-4028, MA 87 Miami Univ - Oxford; 87–Sp-Lang Path, Butler Co Bd of Educ, **SLP**

Bredes, Diane E 22 Monroe Street, Honeoye Falls, NY 14472, MS 78 2335; Sp-Lang Path, UCP, **SLP**

Bredt, Polly W 40 Adair Lane, Portola Valley, CA 94025, (415) 851-1755, BA 63 Univ of MI - Ann Arbor; MA 66 Seton Hall Univ; Chief-SLP, Private Practice, **SLP**

Bree, Loris G 4304 Brigadoon Drive, St Paul, MN 55126, BA 70 Univ of MN - Minneap-St Paul; MS 77 Univ of MN - Minneap-St Paul; 71–Sp-Lang Path, Roseville Area Schls, **SLP**

Breeden, Nancy D 6748 Chapel Hill Road, Indianapolis, IN 46214, (317) 241-3507, BA 58 IN Univ - Bloomington; OM 66 IN Univ - Bloomington; 61–Sp-Lang Path, MSD Wayne Township, **SLP**

Breeding, Albert G 57 Shadyknoll Drive, Longmeadow, MA 01106-3082, **A**

Breeding, Brenda Sue 5508 Pony Farm Drive, Richmond, VA 23227, BS 80 Univ of VA - Charlottesville; ME 82 Univ of VA - Charlottesville; Sp-Lang Path, McV Hosp, **SLP**

Breeding, Malesa Smith 3817 Mark Court, Abilene, TX 79606, (915) 698-0735, BS 80 Abilene Christian Univ; MA 86 Abilene Christian Univ; 80–Sp-Lang Path, Abilene ISD, **SLP**

Breeding, Marcia Keller 1600 Pine Street, Rolla, MO 65401, (314) 364-7954, BS 80 Eastern IL Univ; MA 81 Univ of IL - Urbana; Sp-Lang Path, Steelville R 3 School, **SLP**

Breedlove, Vickey 2217-12 Stofehenge Drive, Raleigh, NC 27615, (919) 575-7373, BS 77 Appalachian St Univ; MA 78 Appalachian St Univ; Sp-Path, Murdoch Center, **SLP**

Breeland, Mrs Nancy S 2727 Wilkes Avenue, Biloxi, MS 39530, (601) 432-1571, BS 54 Univ Southern MS-Hattiesburg; MA 54 Univ Southern MS-Hattiesburg; Dir Pub Rel/Patient Rel, Biloxi Reg Med Cen, **SLP**

Breen, Mrs Elise S 2521 Hudson Place, New Orleans, LA 70114, (504) 394-4869, BA 73 Southeastern LA Univ; MA 78 Tulane Univ; SLP, Jefferson Parish School Board, **SLP**

Breen, Mrs Jennifer Gates 1454 Cedar Lane, Lemoore, CA 93245, (209) 924-7991, BA 80 Univ of the Pacific; MS 82 James Madison Univ; Sp/Lang Path, Hanford Speech & Hearing Ctr, **SLP**

Breen, Katherine A 6865 West 51st Terrace #1C, Shawnee Mission, KS 66202, (913) 236-8140, BS 70 Northwestern Univ; MA 71 Univ of MO - Columbia; 73–Sp-Lang Path, Shawnee Mission Pub Sch, **SLP**

Breen, Melissa Anne 16704 Clifton Boulevard, Lakewood, OH 44107, (216) 231-8787, BS 83 OH Univ - Athens; MA 86 Univ of Cincinnati; 86–SLP, The Cleveland Hr & Sp Ctr, **SLP**

Breen, Mrs Phyllis O 3250 Hardisty Avenue, Cincinnati, OH 45208, (513) 871-3827, BS 64 Phillips Univ; MA 65 Western MI Univ; 83–Clin Supvr, U of Cincinnati, **SLP**

Breese, Mrs Judith 18 East Street, Walton, NY 13856, (607) 865-6343, BA 71 Hartwick Coll; MA 73 Univ of Northern IA; Sp-Lang Path, Private Practice, **SLP**

Breese, Kathleen Munroe Rd #2 Box 12 Zimmer Road, Newark Valley, NY 13811, (607) 770-6276, BS 86 Ithaca Coll; MS 88 Ithaca Coll; 88–Sp-Lang Path, United Hlth Svcs-Wilson Hosp

Breeze, Christine 401 Mount Sanford Road, Cheshire, CT 06410, (203) 271-1258, BA 79 WA St Univ; MA 83 WA St Univ; 88–Sp-Lang Path, Gaylord Hosp, **SLP**

Bregstone, Mrs Andrea P 2607 Central Avenue, Alexandria, VA 22302, (703) 765-6900, BS 67 OH St Univ; MS 69 Univ of MI - Ann Arbor; Sp-Lang Path, Fairfax Co Pub Sch, **SLP**

Brehm, Mrs Catharine M 6104 Williams, Lawton, OK 73505, BA 73 Univ of TX - El Paso; MA 74 Univ of TX - El Paso; Sp-Lang Path, Dod-Depend Schs

Brehm, Mrs Elaine 41 Bloomingdale Avenue, East Greenbush, NY 12061, BA 67 SUNY - Coll at Fredonia; MS 71 Coll of Saint Rose; Sp-Lang Path, BOCES of Rensselaer County, **SLP**

Brehmer, Ann Kathryn Box 184, 820 3rd Avenue, Madison, MN 56256, (612) 598-7556, BS 79 Mankato St Univ; MS 83 Univ of WI - River Falls; Aud, Madison Hosp, **A**

Breidenbach, Mrs Lynda M 15806 Wilderness Parkway, San Antonio, TX 78232-4839, BS 65 OK St Univ; MS 69 Univ of OK Medical Center; Sp/Lang Path, Abilene ISD, **SLP**

Breiding, Philip R 1404 West Brown Street, Arlington Heights, IL 60004, (312) 259-9640, BS 50 Carthage Coll; MS 58 Univ of IL - Urbana; SLP, Township High School Dist 214, **SLP**

Breier, Mrs Martha Helen 6509 Hellner, Ann Arbor, MI 48105, (313) 348-1390, BS 82 Eastern MI Univ; MA 83 Eastern MI Univ; 87–Sp-Lang Path, South Lyon Comm Schs, **SLP**

Breighner, Sr M Wilma 3105 Lexington Road, Louisville, KY 40206, (502) 897-1811, BA 43 Ursuline Coll; MS 70 Marquette Univ; SLP, Ursuline Sp Cl, **SLP**

Breines, Gail L 30242 Belmont Court, Agoura Hills, CA 91301-4611, (818) 707-3167, **SLP**

Breit, Mrs Miriam C 841 Dorncliff, Buffalo Grove, IL 60089, (312) 541-9601, BS 76 IL St Univ - Normal; MS 77 IL St Univ - Normal; SLP, Spec Educ Dist of Lake County, **SLP**

Breitbach, Idelle J 14720 West Honey Lane, New Berlin, WI 53151, (414) 425-3230, BS 76 Univ of WI - Milwaukee; MS 78 Univ of WI - Milwaukee; 78–Sp-Lang Path, Franklin PS, **SLP**

Breitenfeldt, Dr Dorvan H Eastern Washington University, Speech Bldg, Cheney, WA 99004, (509) 359-2301, BS 55 Univ of MN - Minneap-St Paul; MA 57 Univ of MN - Minneap-St Paul; PH 62 (NS) Southern IL Univ -Carbondale; Dir Speech & Hearing Clinic, Eastern Washington University, **SLP**

Breiter, Mrs Ronni F 19 Tanglewood Road, West Hartford, CT 06117, (203) 233-3459, BA 70 IN Univ - Bloomington; ME 73 Boston Univ; Sp/Lang Path, Private Practice, **SLP**

Breithaupt, Douglas H Otolaryngology Associates Pc, 8316 Arlington Boulevard, Fairfax, VA 22031, (703) 573-7606, BS 72 Ithaca Coll; MS 73 Ithaca Coll; Aud, Otolaryneology Assoc Pc, **A**

Breitler, Mrs Elaine K 1009 Arcola Avenue, Silver Spring, MD 20902, (301) 649-5031, BA 62 Univ of MD - College Park; MA 65 Univ of MD - College Park; 86–Sp-Lang Path, Maxwell-Barbour & Assoc, **SLP**

Breitzke, Mrs Juanita L W150 S6957 Cornell Circle, Muskego, WI 53150, (414) 384-2000, BA 70 Univ of WI - Milwaukee; MA 71 Univ of WI - Milwaukee; Sp-Lang Path, VA Med Cen, **SLP**

Breitzman, Julie J 814 Fourth Street #1, Menomonie, WI 54751, (414) 241-5530, BA Univ of WI - Eau Claire; MS 85 Univ of WI - Eau Claire; **SLP**

Brekke, Jody Ann 3061 La Selva #C-202, San Mateo, CA 94403, (415) 723-6818, BS 83 Univ of WI - Stevens Point; MS 85 Univ of WI - Stevens Point; **A**

Breland, Kristi J 2121 Line Avenue, Shreveport, LA 71104, (318) 226-9441, BS 72 Univ of NE - Lincoln; MS 76 Univ Southern MS-Hattiesburg; Aud, Drs Pou,Quinn,Watkins,Thorton, **A**

Brelinsky, Mrs Sandra Kaplan 725 South Highlands Drive, Hollywood, FL 33021, (305) 891-8850, BS 75 FL St Univ; MS 76 FL St Univ; SLP, Bon Secours Hosp, **SLP**

Brelsford, Jacalyn Lee 247 East Lullwood, San Antonio, TX 78212, (512) 824-0579, BS 75 PA St Univ - Univ Park; OM 77 Univ of WA; 78–Aud, Sunshine Cottage, **A ACE**

Bremer, Mrs Barbara Waaland 317 Pinewood Road, Greenville, NC 27858, (919) 756-7974, BS 64 Duke Univ; MS 83 East Carolina Univ; Sp-Lang Path, **SLP ACE**

Brems, Stephen C 1309 Hill Road, Geneva, IL 60134, (312) 888-0663, BS 75 Northern IL Univ - De Kalb; MA 77 Northern IL Univ - De Kalb; Aud, Dr David S Hemmer, **A**

Breneman, Alyce I 406 2nd Avenue N W, Box 40, Byron, MN 55920, (507) 775-2687, BS 70 Mankato St Univ; MA 76 Univ of MN - Minneap-St Paul; 86–Aud, Region 10 Spec Educ Proj, **A ACE**

Breneman, Mrs Nancy Palmieri N4 W29717 Blodwen Drive, Waukesha, WI 53188, (414) 646-8291, BS 73 Univ of WI - Milwaukee; MS 74 Univ of WI - Milwaukee; 74–Sp-Lang Path, Milwaukee Pub Sch, **SLP**

Brener, Dr Rosemary Young Linguistics Department, SUNY At Stony Brook, Stony Brook, NY 11794, (516) 632-7774, BA 66 Univ of TN - Knoxville; MS 69 Univ of TN - Knoxville; PH 86 (Devel Psycholinguistics) Univ of Hull - Yorkshire, England; 88–Sp-Lang Path, Suffolk Child Dev Ctr, **SLP**

Brengman, Mrs Christine Janet 9190 Springborn, Anchorville, MI 48004, (313) 754-2230, **A**

Brennan, Anne E 1304 Airfield Lane, Midland, MI 48640, (517) 832-0728, BS 85 PA St Univ - Univ Park; MS 87 PA St Univ - Univ Park; 87–Sp-Lang Path, Head Inj Therapy Svcs Inc, **SLP ACE**

Brennan, Anne M 132 T Street, Salt Lake City, UT 84103, (801) 266-3100, SLP, Primary Childrens, **SLP**

Brennan, Mrs Carol Resch 2239 Highbury, Troy, MI 48098, (313) 286-7625, BS 78 Wayne St Univ; MA 79 Western MI Univ; OM 81 Oakland Univ; Sp-Lang Path, Chippewa Valley Schools, **SLP**

Brennan, Mrs Colleen Curcillo 439 Brookwood Drive, Webster, NY 14580, (716) 671-8953, BA 85 Univ of CT; MA 87 Univ of MA - Amherst; Sp-Lang Path, Rochester Gen Hosp, **SLP**

Brennan, Dr Donald G 15 Country Fair Lane, St Louis, MO 63141, (314) 658-2939, BS 67 Saint Louis Univ; MA 69 Saint Louis Univ; PH 74 (NS) Univ of OK Medical Center; Chair-Assoc Prof, St Louis U, **SLP**

Brennan, Mrs Elizabeth Long 101 Rosewood Drive, Hagerstown, MD 21740, (301) 582-0935, BA 82 Allegheny Coll; MA 84 SUNY - Coll at Geneseo; Sp-Lang Path, Allegany Co Bd of Ed, **SLP**

Brennan, Florence A 67 Innsbruck, Belleville, IL 62221, BS 60 Saint Louis Univ; MS 66 Southern IL Univ -Carbondale; SLP, Belleville Sch Dist #118, **SLP**

Brennan, Frances M 67 Innsbruck, Belleville, IL 62221, (618) 397-0312, BS 60 Saint Louis Univ; MS 66 Southern IL Univ-Edwardsvill; SLP, Grant Sch Dist #110, **SLP**

Brennan, Gayle C J 4536 South 100 East, Lafayette, IN 47905, (317) 448-8000, BA 61 Univ of Denver; MS 66 Washington Univ; 85–Dir Sp-Lang Path Dept, Arnett Clinic, **SLP A**

Brennan, Henry Patrick 2546 West 115th Street, Chicago, IL 60655, (312) 779-9297, BS 83 IL St Univ - Normal; OM 86 Governors St Univ; **SLP**

Brennan, Mrs Jacalyn M R R 8 5068 Middle Line Road, Ballston Spa, NY 12020-9807, (518) 885-0656, BA 78 SUNY - Coll at Plattsburgh; MS 79 Coll of Saint Rose; Sp-Lang Path, Saratoga BOCES, **SLP**

Brennan, Joan K 2212 Washington Avenue, Apartment 103A, Silver Spring, MD 20910, **SLP**

Brennan, Mrs Josephine 58 Darcey Avenue, Staten Island, NY 10314, (718) 984-9800, BS 76 CUNY - Coll of Staten Island; MA 80 Kean Coll of NJ; 79–SLP, NYC Bd of Ed Sp Serv Ut, **SLP**

Brennan, Judy Ann 2800 North Pine Grove #5-E, Chicago, IL 60614, (312) 751-4345, **SLP**

Brennan, Martha K 15 Country Fair Lane, St Louis, MO 63141, (314) 658-2939, BA 69 Univ of TN - Knoxville; MA 70 Univ of IL - Urbana; Lecturer, St Louis U, **SLP ACE**

Brennan, Mary K 112 Orchard Lane, De Kalb, IL 60115, (815) 758-1229, BS 77 IL St Univ - Normal; MS 79 IL St Univ - Normal; Sp-Lang Path, DeKalb Co Spec Educ Assoc, **SLP**

Brennan, Mary Margaret 101 Shady Lane, Lexington, KY 40503, (513) 221-3946, **SLP**

Brennan, Mrs Mary Schindler 2703 E Towers Drive #409, Cincinnati, OH 45238, (513) 922-6960, BS 79 Brescia Coll; MS 80 Univ of WI - Stevens Point; Sp-Lang Path, Private Practice, **SLP**

Brennan, Michael E 824 Liberty Street Ext, Warren, PA 16365, (814) 723-3930, BS 68 Edinboro Univ of PA; MS 72 PA St Univ - Univ Park; Prog Super, Northwest Tri Co Iu #5, **SLP**

Brennan, Michelle R 4 Physicians Park, Frankfort, KY 40601, (502) 223-8400, BA 78 Univ of KY; MS 79 Univ of KY; 81–Sp-Lang Path, Private Practice, **SLP**

Brennan, Mrs Nancy Ann 1017 Valley Creek, Plano, TX 75075, (214) 423-7660, BA 61 Wheaton Coll; MA 64 Univ of OK - Norman; 82–Sp-Lang Path, PISD Head Start, **SLP**

Brennan, Tom Post Office Box 4544 SFA, Nacogdoches, TX 75962, (409) 569-1187, BS 81 Stephen F Austin St Univ; ME 84 Stephen F Austin St Univ; 87–Sp-Lang Path, Private Practice

Brennan, William P 5503 108th Street, Edmonton, AB, Canada T6H 2Y87, **A**

Brennan-Kania, Blanche Frances 66-10 Grand Avenue #3C, Maspeth, NY 11378, (718) 857-9177, MS 86 CUNY - Brooklyn Coll; 86–Sp-Lang Path, Brooklyn Childhood Ctr, **SLP**

Brenneman, Mrs Mary A T 8949 Autumngate Lane, Huber Heights, OH 45424, (513) 226-7877, BA 79 OH St Univ; MA 81 OH St Univ; Aud, Aud and Speech Assoc, **A**

Brenner, Mrs Ann C 8555 East Via DE Risa, Scottsdale, AZ 85258, (602) 941-1653, BS 59 SUNY - Center at Buffalo; MS 79 AZ St Univ; Sp-Lang Path, Scottsdale Pub Sch, **SLP**

Brenner, Mrs Arlene O 365 South Main Street, New City, NY 10956, (914) 634-2900, BA 67 CUNY - City College; MA 68 Columbia Univ Teachers Coll; Sp/Lang Path, Private Practice, **SLP**

Brenner, Clyde J 525 Powell Avenue, Exeter, CA 93221, (209) 733-6333, BA 63 Jamestown Coll; MA 70 Univ of NE - Lincoln; Sp-Lang Path, Farmersville School District, **SLP**

Brenner, Eve H 2327 West Silverlake Drive, Los Angeles, CA 90039, (213) 661-7688, BA 70 CA St Univ - Los Angeles; MA 76 CA St Univ - Los Angeles; Sp-Lang Path, Heller Inc, **SLP**

Brenner, Faith Anne 601 Solon Court, Dunbar, WV 25064, (304) 768-4570, BS 82 IL St Univ - Normal; MS 83 IL St Univ - Normal; Aud/Sp-Lang Path, InSpeech Inc, **SLP A**

Brenner, Mrs Jan 1866 Sheridan Road, Highland Park, IL 60035, (312) 433-1331, BA 69 SUNY - Coll at Cortland; MA 70 Case Western Reserve Univ; Sp-Lang Path, Jan Brenner, **SLP**

Brenner, Mrs Joann F 1810 Tunbridge Drive, Richmond, VA 23233, (804) 747-6337, BS 75 Univ of VA - Charlottesville; ME 77 Univ of VA - Charlottesville; **SLP**

Brenner, Josephine 4113K Beechwood Lane, Harrisburg, PA 17112, (717) 736-6728, BS 55 PA St Univ - Univ Park; MS 60 PA St Univ - Univ Park; Sp-Lang Path, Capital Area Intermed Unit 15, **SLP**

Brenner, Karen F 25 Sherwood Lane, Cedarhurst, NY 11516, (516) 223-8100, BA 79 SUNY - Coll at Brockport; MS 80 Adelphi Univ; Sp-Lang Path, Baldwin Un Free Sch Dist, **SLP**

Brenner, Lory L 3325 Green Street, Harrisburg, PA 17110, (717) 234-8290, BA 69 Temple Univ-Tyler Sch of Art; MA 71 Temple Univ-Tyler Sch of Art; Aud, Private Practice, **A**

Brenner, Merle Joan 29 Barberry Lane, Williamsville, NY 14221, (716) 835-6009, BA 71 Univ of PA; MA 73 Temple Univ-Tyler Sch of Art; Sp-Lang Path, Buffalo Hearing & Speech Ctr, **SLP**

Brenner, Michelle Gowen 33 Coventry Lane, Laguna Hills, CA 92656, (213) 394-3244, BA 83 Univ of CA - Santa Barbara; MA 85 San Diego St Univ; SLP, Lincoln Ctr Speech Pathology, **SLP**

Brenner, Sheila K 19 Winchester Street #812, Brookline, MA 02146, BS 71 Univ of GA; ME 73 Boston Univ; Real Estate Broker, Ellen Biren Assoc, **SLP**

Brenner-Yborra, Linda S 109 Iona Avenue, Narberth, PA 19072, (215) 667-4410, BA 67 Temple Univ-Tyler Sch of Art; MA 69 Temple Univ-Tyler Sch of Art; Sp-Lang Path, Private Practice, **SLP**

Brenn-White, Bonnie M 901 North Oak Park, Oak Park, IL 60302, MS

Brent, Mrs Elizabeth Rabalais 2600 Belle Chase Highway Suite 208, Gretna, LA 70056, (504) 392-0172, BS 80 Saint Mary's Dominican Coll; MA 82 Memphis St Univ; Dir/Sp-Lang Path, Ther Assoc of La Inc, **SLP**

Brent, Susan A 395 Revere Beach Parkway, Apartment 2C, Revere, MA 02151, (617) 286-2422, BA 84 SUNY - Center at Buffalo; MA 86 SUNY - Center at Buffalo; 87–Sp-Lang Path, Youville Hosp & Rehab Ctr, **SLP**

Brentan, Anne G 2223 Crestview Lane, Wilmette, IL 60091, **SLP**

Breon, Mrs Nanine C 108 Red Fox Lane, Spartanburg, SC 29301, MS 73 PA St Univ - Univ Park; SLP, Spartanburg District 6, **A**

Brescher, Sherri A 1 Merion Avenue, Clifton Park, NY 12065-1111, (518) 399-9119, MS 78 Univ of South FL; Sp-Lang Path, Newmeadow Pre Sch, **SLP**

Brescia, Pamela Annette 557 Pelham Road, Philadelphia, PA 19119, (215) 877-7708, BS 81 PA St Univ - Univ Park; MA 83 Temple Univ; **SLP**

Breshike, Kevin John 121 Evac Hospital, Box 12, Apo, San Francisco, CA 96301-5000, (808) 671-3523, **A**

Breslau, Carol 680 Lukens Ln, King of Prussia, PA 19406, (302) 856-5213, BS 79 James Madison Univ; ME 81 James Madison Univ; Aud, De Div of Pub Hlth, **A**

Breslau, Lewis B 2408 Logue Street, North Bellmore, NY 11710, (516) 826-3850, BS 84 SUNY - Coll at Plattsburgh; MA 86 Hofstra Univ; **A**

Breslau, Susan R Z 60 Haylin Drive, Vernon, CT 06066, (203) 649-4547, BS 68 Univ of WI - Madison; MA 70 Univ of CT; **SLP**

Breslouf, Lynne Diane 17-A Read Street, Salem, MA 01970-2817, (508) 745-9000, ME 83 Northwestern Univ; 86–Asst Dir, Shaughnessy-Kaplan Rehab Hosp, **SLP**

Breslow, Ellen N c/o Fdlrs, 1400 N E 6th Street, Pompano Beach, FL 33060, (305) 786-7701, BA 75 Univ of FL; ME 77 Univ of GA; Sp-Lang Path, FL Diag & Lrng Resources Syst, **SLP ACE**

Breslow, Karen Ann 13264 Rhoda Drive, Los Altos, CA 94022, MS; **SLP**

Breslow, Mrs Roberta K 5329 Winter Moss Court, Columbia, MD 21045, (301) 997-0679, BA 76 Univ of MD - College Park; MA 77 Univ of MD - College Park; Sp-Lang Path, Howard County Public Schools, **SLP**

Bresnock, Sr Catherine L 2734 West 52nd Street, Chicago, IL 60632, (312) 434-5036, BS 60 Marquette Univ; MA 69 Cardinal Stritch Coll; Princ, St Simon the Apostle Sch, **SLP**

Bressi, Susan Ann 180 Main Parkway West, Plainview, NY 11803, (516) 663-1003, **A**

Bressler, Mrs Emily Gordon 14026 Saddle River Drive, Gaithersburg, MD 20878, (301) 897-8100, BS 82 Univ of MD - College Park; MS 84 Boston Univ; Sp-Lang Path, Rehab Serv Inc, **SLP**

Bresticker, Mrs Carol Marie 822 Glenwood Avenue, Williamsport, PA 17701, BS 83 Marywood Coll; MA 85 Univ of Pittsburgh - Pittsburgh; 88–Sp-Lang Path, Geisinger Med Ctr, **SLP**

Bretney, Louise E 19731 Verona Lane, Yorba Linda, CA 92686, BA 68 CA St Univ - Los Angeles; MA 81 CA St Univ - Long Beach; SLP, Fulleton Joint Un Sch Dist, **SLP**

Breton, Janice G RFD 2 Box 2870, Dexter, ME 04930, (207) 924-5571, BA 71 Univ of ME - Orono; MA 73 Univ of ME - Orono; Sp-Lang Path & Dir Spec Serv, Sch Admin Dist #46, **SLP**

Brett, Richard J 616 4th Street, Waukegan, IL 60085, (312) 360-5643, OB 43 Northern IL Univ - De Kalb; MS 47 Univ of IL - Urbana; 46–Sp-Lang Path, Waukegan Pub Sch, **SLP F**

Brett, Rory C 307 Heathfield Lane, Annapolis, MD 21403, (301) 386-4242, BA 71 SUNY - Coll at Oneonta; MS 76 Adelphi Univ; Exec Dir, Rehab Opportunities Inc, **SLP**

Bretz, Mrs Barbara A B 4063 Larkspur Drive, Springfield, IL 62707-9248, (217) 544-6464, BS 80 Miami Univ - Oxford; MS 80 Miami Univ - Oxford; Sp-Lang Path, St John's Hosp, **SLP**

Breuer, Wanda R 9 Laurel Glen, Huntington, CT 06484, (203) 261-3607, BA 76 Hofstra Univ; MA 77 Hofstra Univ; Sp-Lang Path, Easton PS, **SLP**

Brevda, Mrs Shelley Newman 35-11 85th Street, Jackson Heights, NY 11372, (718) 507-5200, BA 71 CUNY - Queens Coll; MA 73 Hofstra Univ; Dir Sp & Hrng, Gouverneur Hosp, **SLP**

Brevda, Yale 35-11 85th Street #8K, Jackson Heights, NY 11372, (718) 507-5200, BA 71 Hofstra Univ; MA 73 Hofstra Univ; 88–Dir Aud/Owner, Hrng Technologies Ctr, **A**

Brevoort, Sarah Hines 2506 North 10th Street, Phoenix, AZ 85006, (602) 255-3448, **SLP**

Brewer, Mrs Andrea Polley 1205 New Hampshire Lane, Downingtown, PA 19335, (215) 431-8112, BS 77 Purdue Univ - West Lafayette; OM 79 IN Univ - Bloomington; 87–Sp-Lang Path, Devereux Foundation, **SLP**

Brewer, Dr Carmen C 4409 Van Buren Street, University Park, MD 20782, (202) 877-6717, BA 72 Rutger's St Univ - Douglas Coll; MA 74 Univ of MD - College Park; PH 81 (Hrng Science/Aud) Univ of MD - College Park; 74–Asst Dir, Hrng & Sp Cen Wash Hos Cen, **A**

Brewer, Mrs Claudia Stagner 1231 West Hull, Denison, TX 75020, (214) 465-2313, BA 68; MS 69; SLP, Texoma Med Cen, **SLP**

Brewer, Mrs Debra Burnett 316 22nd Avenue North, Nashville, TN 37203, (615) 327-1383, BS 84 IL St Univ - Normal; MS 87 IL St Univ - Normal; 86–Aud, Crook Downey & Witherspoon, **A**

Brewer, Diane M 4312 Warren Street N W, Washington, DC 20016, (202) 676-7167, BA 64 Univ of IA; MA 65 Univ of IA; Assoc Prof, Geo Wash U, **A F**

Brewer, Ellen Jane 48 Grove Street, Great Barrington, MA 01230, (413) 243-4611, BA 77 Fairfield Univ; BS Univ of NH; MS 84 Emerson Coll; **SLP**

Brewer, Mrs Gwendolyn Harland 4931 Xanadu, Denver, CO 80239, (303) 447-1010, BA 75 Univ of CT; MA 77 Univ of Denver; Sp-Lang Path, Boulder V Pub Sch, **SLP**

Brewer, Mrs Karen M 839 North Elm Street, Greenville, IL 62246, (618) 664-3117, BS 53 Eastern IL Univ; Sp-Lang Path, Bond Co Comm Ut #2, **SLP**

Brewer, Kathryn A ENT Clinic F4/214, Clinical Science Center, 600 Highland Avenue, Madison, WI 53792, (608) 263-6197, BS 74 Univ of WI - Madison; MS 77 Univ of WI - Madison; Clinical & Rehab Audiologist, Holy Cross Hospital, **A**

Brewer, Kelly Scannell Our Lady Of Compassion Care Center, 4900 Eagle Street, Anchorage, AK 99503, (907) 562-2281, BS 81 UT St Univ; MS 83 Univ of OR; 85–Sp-Lang Path, Our Lady Compassion Care Ctr, **SLP**

Brewer, Mrs Mary L M High Point Regional Hospital, P O Box Hp-5, High Point, NC 27261, (919) 884-2206, BA 77 Univ of NC - Greensboro; ME 79 Univ of NC - Greensboro; Sp-Lang Path, Private Practice, **SLP**

Brewer, Mrs Sharon C 38 Locust Avenue #3-E, New Rochelle, NY 10805, (914) 632-9000, BS 69 Univ of IL - Urbana; ME 71 PA St Univ - Univ Park; Sp-Lang Path, Cty Sch Dist/New Rochelle, **SLP**

Brewington, Mrs Theresa K 204 Grace Street, Mount Airy, NC 27030, (919) 786-7501, BS 70 WV Univ; OM 76 Univ of SC - Columbia; Sp-Lang Path, Yadkin Valley Headstart, **SLP**

Brewster, Cynthia Constance Route 6 Box 501, Carbondale, IL 62901, (618) 529-1382, BS 79 IL St Univ - Normal

Brewster, Elaine M 1609 Sleepy Hollow Circle, Olathe, KS 66062, (913) 829-4299, BA 69 OH St Univ; MA 71 Columbia Univ Teachers Coll; **SLP**

Brewster, Maureen C 230 Hazel Avenue, Westfield, NJ 07090, (201) 245-7245, BA 74 Montclair St Coll; MA 75 Montclair St Coll; Learning Dis Tchr-Consultant, Roselle Bd of Ed, **SLP**

Brey, Dr Robert H Brigham Young University, 138 John Taylor Bldg, Provo, UT 84602, (801) 378-4319, BA 67 Univ of UT; MA 68 Univ of UT; PH 72 (NS) Wayne St Univ - Sch of Med; Prof, Brigham Young U, **A**

Breza, Constance M 1963 Decatur Avenue, Wheeling, WV 26003, (304) 243-0030, OB 73 WV Univ; MS 76 WV Univ; Sp-Lang Path, Ohio County Public Schools, **SLP**

Brezner, Mrs Diane J L 5610 Jasen, Houston, TX 77096, (713) 774-7879, BS 65 Northwestern Univ; MA 79 Univ of Houston - Univ Park; Sp-Lang Path, Houston ISD, **SLP**

Brezner, Ellen L 88 Keene Street, Brockton, MA 02401, (508) 339-9561, BA 75 Univ of MA - Amherst; MS 82 Univ of RI; 86–Sp-Lang Path, Mansfield PS, **SLP**

Brezsny, Mrs Felice J 1401 Sterling Road, Redlands, CA 92373, (714) 793-2301, BA 43 MI St Univ; MS 82 Univ of Redlands; Sp-Lang Path, Redlands CA Unified Sch, **SLP**

Brian, Mrs Jody D 711 Valencia Unit #1, Coral Gables, FL 33134, (305) 987-2000, BS 73 Eastern IL Univ; MS 83 FL St Univ; 88–Sp/Lang Path, Memorial Hosp of Hollywood, **SLP**

Briand, Claire Marie Chelmsford High School, Richardson Road, Chelmsford, MA 01863, (617) 251-8792, **SLP**

Briant, June E 58 Flintlock Road, Morris Plains, NJ 07950, **SLP**

Bricault, Melody Natl Tech Inst For The Deaf, One Lomb Memorial Drive, Rochester, NY 14623, (716) 475-6870, BS 77 Univ of IL - Urbana; MA 79 Univ of IL - Urbana; Aud, NTID, **A**

Bricca, Barry Steven P O Box 146, Wrightwood, CA 92397, (714) 829-5950, Aud, So Ca Permanente Med Group, **A**

Brice, Alexander Emris 301-13 Diamond Village, Gainesville, FL 32603, (904) 373-0347, BA 80 Univ of FL; MA 84 Univ of FL; 87–Sp-Lang Path, Sch Bd of Alachua County FL

Brice, Caroline B Diamond Village #301-13, Gainesville, FL 32603, (904) 336-2841, BA 79 Univ of FL; MA 81 Univ of FL; 86–Sp-Lang Path, Sch Bd of Alachua Co, **SLP**

Brick, Mrs Mara Green 7510 Coddle Harbor Lane, Potomac, MD 20854, (301) 983-8752, BA 79 Hofstra Univ; OM 83 Emory Univ; Sp/Lang Path, The Glenbrook Day School, **SLP**

Brickell, Mrs Nancy A 6 Wilmette Drive, Normal, IL 61761, (309) 438-5308, BA 63 CA St Univ - Fresno; MS 80 IL St Univ - Normal; Instr/SLP, Il St U, **SLP**

Brick-Goodman, Nancy G P O Box 12476, Reno, NV 89510, (702) 785-4394, BA 78 CA St Univ - Fullerton; MA 81 CA St Univ - Fullerton; Sp/Lang Path, NV Commun Dis Serv, **SLP**

Brickner-Hoath, Sheri 6089 Ropes Drive, Cincinnati, OH 45244, **SLP**

Brideweser, Mrs Darlene R 10229 Bourbon Street, Newburgh, IN 47630, (812) 853-6504, BS 86 Bowling Green St Univ; MA 87 Kent St Univ; 87–Sp-Lang Path, Deaconess Service Corp, **SLP**

Bridgeford, Ethel B Route 1 Box 3100, Rapid City, SD 57702, (605) 342-6425, BA 37 Humboldt St Univ; MA 47 Univ of IA; Private Practice, **SLP F LM**

Bridges, Annette K 7761 Matterhorn Court, Rancho Cucamonga, CA 91730, (714) 989-6257, BS 78 Southwest TX St Univ; ME 79 Southwest TX St Univ; Resource Teacher Jr High, Alamo Heights Jr High Sch, **SLP**

Bridges, Mrs Dickie L 400 College Avenue, Jackson, AL 36545, (205) 246-9301, BS 73 Univ of Montevallo; MS 75 Univ of Montevallo; Sp-Lang Path, Clarke Co Bd of Ed, **SLP**

Bridges, Jean Ellen 501 Garden Court, Atlanta, GA 30328, (404) 392-9794, OB 82 Univ of GA; ME 83 Univ of GA; Sp-Lang Path, The Davison Sch, **SLP**

Bridges, Monte L 4236 Baker Avenue N W, Seattle, WA 98107, (206) 782-2777, BA 78 Univ of WA; OM 79 Univ of WA; MA 86 Seattle Univ; SLP, Edmonds Sch Dist #15, **SLP**

Bridges, Sheila J Spartan Village #1520-F, Michigan State University, East Lansing, MI 48823, (517) 353-9206, BS 77 Univ of MA - Amherst; MA 79 Bowling Green St Univ; **SLP**

Bridges, Mrs Susan K 818 Robin Road, Muscatine, IA 52761, (319) 263-8476, BA 69 Univ of Northern IA; MA 70 Univ of Northern IA; Sp-Lang Path, MS Bend AEA, **SLP**

Bridgewater, Mrs Barbara Gilford 611 Wake Robin Lane, San Rafael, CA 94903-2420, (415) 499-5807, BA 63 Univ of Denver; Sp-Lang Path, Marin Co Off of Ed, **SLP**

Bridgman, Connie Marie 521 South Charvers, West Covina, CA 91791, (818) 332-0269, BA 84 CA St Univ - Fullerton; MA 87 CA St Univ - Fullerton; 87–Sp-Lang Path, Ontario Montclair Sch Dist, **SLP**

Bridwell, Mrs Carol Pearce R R 7 Box 9267, Hanover, PA 17331, (717) 632-2001, MS 84 Loyola Coll; 86–Sp-Lang Path, UCP of So Central PA, **SLP**

Brief, Mrs Caryl Alterbaum 205 West End Avenue #3N, New York, NY 10023, (201) 877-8710, BS 67 Boston Univ; MA 68 Columbia Univ Teachers Coll; Dir, Private Practice, **SLP**

Brierly, Anne Carolyn 1648 Upland Drive, Yuba City, CA 95991-1920, (619) 463-1590, BA 83 Univ of CA - Santa Barbara; MA 86 San Diego St Univ; **SLP**

Briery-Leon, Debra J Route 5 Box 133, Fredericksburg, TX 78624, (512) 997-8551, BS 73 KS St Univ; MA 75 KS St Univ; 86–Aud, R Gordon Delaney MD, **A**

Briese, Mrs Anne D 1532 Founders Drive, Bogalusa, LA 70427, (504) 735-1392, BS 73 LA St Univ - Baton Rouge; MA 74 LA St Univ - Baton Rouge; Child Search Coord, Bogalusa Cty Sch, **SLP**

Briesemeister, Mrs Karen Ruth 617 Rice Creek Terrace, Minneapolis, MN 55432, (612) 789-8831, BS 62 Univ of MN - Minneap-St Paul; MA 67 Univ of MN - Minneap-St Paul; Sp Lang Cl, Moundsview Pub Sch, **SLP**

Brigante, Marie 99 Sussex Avenue, Morristown, NJ 07960, (201) 538-7899, BA 74 Seton Hall Univ; MA 76 Seton Hall Univ; Sp-Lang Path, Morris School District, **SLP**

Briganti, Lisa Marie 14 Hudson Street, Quincy, MA 02169, (617) 471-6543, BA 85; MS 88 Univ of RI; 88–Sp-Lang Path, Braintree Hosp, **F**

Briggie, Ann M H 811 30th Street Drive S E, Cedar Rapids, IA 52403, (319) 369-7491, BA 71 Univ of IA; MA 72 Univ of IA; **SLP**

Briggs, Mrs Beverly M 1820 Fairway Circle, Las Cruces, NM 88001, (505) 437-3505, BS 51 Univ of WI - Madison; MS 52 Univ of WI - Madison; 73–Sp/Lang Path, NM Sch for Vis Hndcpd, **SLP**

Briggs, Connie D 1410 32nd Street, Vienna, WV 26105, (304) 485-3569, BA 72 Harding Univ; OM 73 Univ of MS; Dir/SLP, OH Vlly Coll Sp Cl, **SLP**

Briggs, Mrs Joanne S 1812 Huntington Street, Huntington Beach, CA 92648, (714) 960-3262, BS 66 Kent St Univ; MA 74 CA St Univ - Long Beach; **SLP**

Briggs, Kim Varoutsos 1 Seneca Road, Woburn, MA 01801, (617) 662-2000

Briggs, Linda Jean The Consortium, P O Box 17, Phanat Nikhom, Chonburi, Thailand 20140, BA 80 Univ of MT; MA 84 Univ of MT; 88–Tchr/Consult, The Consortium, **SLP**

Briggs, Dr Margaret H Culhane Briggs & Associates, 735 West Duarte Rd Suite 206, Arcadia, CA 91006, (818) 445-3102, BS 69 SUNY - Center at Buffalo; MA 72 SUNY - Coll at Geneseo; PH 84 (NS) Univ of CA - Los Angeles; 88–Exec Dir, Culhane Briggs & Associates, **SLP**

Briggs, Milton M 2516 Winsford Lane, Carmichael, CA 95608, **SLP**

Briggs, Noreen V 3560 West 99th Street, Evergreen Park, IL 60642, **SLP**

Briggs, Robert E W 9712 Champion Ln, Cheney, WA 99004-9613, (509) 456-0950, BA 66 Whitworth Coll; ME 70 Eastern WA Univ; 78–Sp-Lang Path, Ed Serv Dist #101, **SLP**

Briggs, Dr Sandra Lee 949 Ferry Street, Marshfield, MA 02050, (617) 697-1200, BS 61 Lewis-Clark St Coll; MS 66 Western OR St Coll; PH 72 (Aud) Univ of KS; Assoc Prof/Cl Dir, Bridgewater St Coll, **A**

Briggs, Stephanie C 4324 Village Street, Erie, PA 16506, (814) 459-2755, BA 69 SUNY - Coll at Plattsburgh; MA 87 Edinboro Univ of PA; 87–Sp-Lang Path, Erie Cty Crippled Chldn Soc, **SLP**

Briggs, Mrs Susan Anderson 201 East Wabasha, Winona, MN 55987, (608) 785-0530, BS 63 Northwestern Univ; MA 66 Univ of IA; Sp-Lang Path, Lutheran Hsop/Gundersen Cl, **SLP ACE**

Briggs-Whittaker, Janice 39 Intervale Terrace, Reading, MA 01867-2022, (617) 275-7500, BS 67 Univ of CT; MS 73 Univ of OK Medical Center; Chief/Aud & SLP, Bedford VA Hosp, **SLP**

Brigham, Ellen Taer 98 Pollard Street, Marshfield, MA 02050, (508) 697-1200, BA 75 SUNY - Center at Binghamton; MS 77 Syracuse Univ; 87–Instr/Clin Supvr, Bridgewater State Coll, **SLP ACE**

Brigham Do, Fleda M 491 Costa Mesa Street, Costa Mesa, CA 92627-2320, MD; **SLP LM**

Bright, Donna Marie 1454 St Francis Drive, Santa Fe, NM 87501, (505) 988-9818, BA 85 NM St Univ; MA 87 Univ of CO - Boulder; Aud, Santa Fe Ctr for Aud, **A**

Bright, Florence D 8923 Kasteel Way, Indianapolis, IN 46250, (317) 266-4521, BA 65 Hampton Univ; MS 72 Old Dominion Univ; Sp-Lang Path, Indianapolis Pub Schs, **SLP**

Bright, Janice L 428-A Mission Street, South Pasadena, CA 91030, (213) 688-3850, **SLP**

Bright, Robbie Yesilonis 817 Lincoln Avenue, Pine Beach, NJ 08741, (201) 286-7672, BS 85 Indiana Univ of PA; MS 86 Univ of NC - Chapel Hill; **A**

Brightenback, Andrea Rural Free Delivery, Hardwick, VT 05843, (802) 472-6279, BA 71 Rutger's St Univ - Douglas Coll; MS 74 Rutgers St Univ - Newark; SLP-Dir, Orleans S W Sch Dist, **SLP**

Brightman, William P 730 Roanoke Avenue Suite A-2, Roanoke Rapids, NC 27870, (919) 537-5687, BA 78 Univ of Denver; MA 80 Univ of TN - Knoxville; 85–Sp-Lang Path, Private Practice, **SLP**

Brightmire, Mrs Janet Dee 3816 South Trenton, Tulsa, OK 74105-3325, (918) 585-2992, BS 82 OK St Univ; ME 83 Southwest TX St Univ; Sp-Lang Path, Warm Springs Rehab Hosp, **SLP**

Brightwell, Dr Mary A Rd 3 Box 280, Belle Vernon, PA 15012, (412) 872-5877, BS 72 WV Univ; ME 74 CA Univ of PA; ED 85 (Educational Administration) WV Univ; Sp-Lang Path, Westmoreland Iu #7, **SLP**

Bril, Mrs Mary R 506 Center Street, Decorah, IA 52101, (319) 382-9506, BS 77 Univ of IA; MA 78 Univ of IA; **SLP**

Brill, Mrs Barbara F 6144 Agail Place, Columbia, MD 21045, (301) 997-8030, BA 58 PA St Univ - Univ Park; MS 61 PA St Univ - Univ Park; Sp-Lang Path, Private Practice, **SLP ACE**

Brill, Mrs Cynthia Lawson 7707 Harshmanville Road, Dayton, OH 45404, (513) 236-5397, BS 83 Bowling Green St Univ; MA 84 Bowling Green St Univ; Coordinator Sp-Pathology Serv, Greene County Comb Health Dist, **SLP**

Brill, Linda P 108 Genesee Avenue, Staten Island, NY 10308-1331, (718) 273-1548, MS 75 Columbia Univ Teachers Coll; BA 69 SUNY - Center at Buffalo; **SLP**

Brill, Mrs Marilyn 6914 East 64th Place, Tulsa, OK 74133, (918) 299-4411, BS 72 Univ of Tulsa; MA 74 Univ of Tulsa; Sp-Lang Path, Jenks Pub Sch, **SLP**

Brilliant, Mrs Cynthia Gitelman 6/8 Rehov Schwartz, Raanana, Israel 43370, (301) 585-3103, BA 69 CUNY - Hunter Coll; MA 71 NY Univ; Sp-Lang Path, Private Practice, **SLP**

Brimacombe, Judith A Cochlear Corporation, 61 Inverness Drive East, Suite 200, Englewood, CO 80112, (303) 790-9010, BA 77; MA 81; 87–Dir of Clin Svcs, Cochlear Corporation, **A**

Brimberry, Alexis C 300 City View Drive, Fort Lauderdale, FL 33311-9159, (305) 561-5559, BS 70 IN St Univ - Terre Haute; MS 71 IN St Univ - Terre Haute; Director of Operations, Covenant House

Brimigion, Mrs Barbara Joan 6519 Monroe Avenue, Sykesville, MD 21784, (301) 781-7328, MS 86 Towson St Univ

Brind, Myrna K 236 South 3rd Street, Philadelphia, PA 19106, **SLP**

Brindle, Barbara R Central Virginia Training Cen, P O Box 1098, Lynchburg, VA 24505, (804) 947-2132, BS 75 Carlow Coll; MA 76 Univ of IA; Sp-Lang Path, Central VA Training Ctr, **SLP**

Brine, Mrs Lou Ann 5242 Obispo Avenue, Lakewood, CA 90712-3101, (213) 692-0615, BA 72 Univ of MN - Duluth; MA 77 Univ of MN - Duluth; SLP, Los Nietos Sch Dist, **SLP ACE**

Brinegar, Dr Kimberly Park 1585 Wedgewood Way, Upland, CA 91786, (714) 624-9041, BA 74 Univ of LA Verne; MS 76 Univ of LA Verne; ED 88 (Education) Univ of LA Verne; Prog Spec, Claremont USD, **SLP**

Bringman, Norman A 21732 Lorain Road, Fairview Park, OH 44126, (216) 333-0606, BA 76 Cleveland St Univ; MA 78 Cleveland St Univ; Aud, Private Practice, **A**

Brink, Lynnette K 4015 Angelina Drive, Plano, TX 75074, (214) 423-6543, 67; BA 69 Univ of MI - Ann Arbor; MA 74 Eastern MI Univ; Sp/Lang Path, Kanawha Co Schs, **SLP**

Brinker, Mrs Debra S 17319 Sandy Knoll Drive, Olney, MD 20832, (301) 774-7424, BS 76 Eastern MI Univ; MA 77 Eastern MI Univ; 88–Sp-Lang Path, MD Sch for the Deaf

Brinkerhoff, Diane Sue 5500 Windmill Lane, Raleigh, NC 27606, (919) 828-6756, BA 74 IN Univ - Bloomington; MS 81 Univ of NC - Chapel Hill; SLP, Wake County Schools, **SLP**

Brinkley, Mary L 3009 Longhorn Drive, Lawrence, KS 66044, (913) 842-7676, BA 68 Fort Hays St Univ; MA 71 Univ of SD - Vermillion; **SLP**

Brinkman, Mrs Rosemary Patricia 905 Holyrood, Midland, MI 48640, (517) 781-4911, BS 83 Central MI Univ; MA 85 Central MI Univ; **SLP**

Brinkmann, Mrs Dawn Cross 548 South Ruby Lane, Fairview Heights, IL 62208, (618) 398-7500, BS 85 Southern IL Univ-Edwardsvill; MS 87 Southern IL Univ-Edwardsvill; **SLP**

Brinser, Mrs Chryl C 12525 Little Pond Lane, Midlothian, VA 23113, (804) 556-5321, BS 78 James Madison Univ; ME 79 Univ of VA - Charlottesville; Sp-Lang Path, Goochland Co Pub Sch, **SLP**

Brinsko, Mrs Kit Evans 2337 Northwest 54th Place, Gainesville, FL 32606, (904) 392-2041, BS 79 FL St Univ; MS 80 FL St Univ; Sp-Lang Path, Univ of FL, **SLP**

Brinson, Joann 11305 51st Street #A-13, Tampa, FL 33617, (813) 985-9334, MS 87 Univ of South FL

Brinton, Dr Bonnie Parsons Research Center, P O Box 738, Parsons, KS 67357, (316) 421-6550, BA 75 Univ of UT; MA 77 San Jose St Univ; PH 81 (Sp Path & Aud) Univ of UT; Assoc Sci, Univ of Kan Bureau of Child Res, **SLP**

Brinza, Tamera Ann 809 Merchants Bank Bldg, Terre Haute, IN 47807, (812) 232-8172, BS 83 IN St Univ - Terre Haute; MA 85 Ball St Univ; Aud, Beltone Hearing Aid Center, **A**

Briody, Rickey Donnetta 5101 Longbranch Lane, Edmond, OK 73034, (405) 341-1429, BA 74 OK St Univ; MS 75 Lamar Univ; Sp-Lang Path, Edmond Guidance Clinic, **SLP**

Brion, Jennifer Smith 6 Red Wing Road, Enfield, CT 06082, (517) 834-7722, BS 80 Elmira Coll; MA 82 Univ of Pittsburgh - Pittsburgh; Sp-Lang Path, St Coletta's Day Sch, **SLP**

Brisbane, Sr Arlene Silver Lake College, 2406 South Alverno Road, Manitowoc, WI 54220, (414) 684-6691, BA 50; MA 60 Marquette Univ; 85–Prof, Pres of Silver Lake College, **SLP LM**

Brisbane, Glenda 1861 N Van Ness Avenue #102, Hollywood, CA 90028-4371, (216) 669-2137, BS 79 Hampton Univ; MS 82 PA St Univ - Univ Park; Aud, Childrens Hosp of La, **A**

Brisbois, Susan G 9 Greenfield, Irvine, CA 92714, (714) 760-3259, BA 79 CA St Univ - Long Beach; MA 82 CA St Univ - Long Beach; Sp-Lang Path, Newport Mesa USD, **SLP**

Briscoe, Anthony C PO Box 88, Fort Fairfield, ME 04742, (207) 768-4739, BA 80 GA St Univ; ME 83 GA St Univ; ES 86 Univ of GA; 88–Sp-Lang Path & Admin, Northern Maine Sp-Lang Path Svc Inc, **SLP ACE**

Briscoe, Mrs Valerie C 9461 Spring Branch, Dallas, TX 75238, (214) 238-8111, BA 78 TX Tech Univ; MA 79 Univ of North TX; Sp/Lang Path, Richardson ISD, **SLP**

Briscoe-Hamilton, Patricia Lynn 1903 Corona Avenue, Jasper, AL 35501, (205) 221-4342, BS 77 Auburn Univ - Auburn; MS 82 Auburn Univ - Auburn; 84–Aud, Private Practice, **A**

Brisendine, Maria K 1704 Kathryn Drive, Tallahassee, FL 32308, (904) 877-6158, BS 77 FL St Univ; MS 78 FL St Univ; SLP, Private Practice, **A**

Brisimitzakis, Mrs Joan G 67 Bellmore Drive, Pittsfield, MA 01201, (413) 442-8446, BS 80 NY Univ; MA 82 NY Univ; 80–Sp-Lang Path, Bd of Ed, **SLP**

Briskey, Robert J 370 Ardmore Road, Des Plaines, IL 60016, (312) 296-5720, MA 49 Wayne St Univ; BA 47 Wayne St Univ; 75–Aud, Beltone Electronics, **SLP A**

Briskin, Dr Ilene Hearn Childrens Facial Rehab Center, 3825 Greenspring Avenue, Baltimore, MD 21211, (301) 462-6861, BA 69 Case Western Reserve Univ; MS 71 Case Western Reserve Univ; OD 85 (Health Serv Admin) Johns Hopkins Univ; 86–Aud, Children's Hospital, **A**

Brislin, Helen Ann 6263 South 153rd Street, Tukwila, WA 98188, (206) 246-1075, BS 80 Univ of South AL; MS 82 Univ of South AL; Aud, Auburn ENT Clinic, **A**

Brister, Dr Frank Lutz, Jr Communication Disorders Center, East Texas State Univ, Commerce, TX 75428, (214) 886-5910, BA 60 MS Coll; MS 65 Univ Southern MS-Hattiesburg; PH 79 (Aud) Univ Southern MS-Hattiesburg; Dir Commun Dis Cen, East Texas State University, **A**

Brister, Mrs Gloria R Route 1 Box 20-H, Highway 8 West, Cleveland, MS 38732, (601) 846-1876, BS 76 Delta St Univ; MS 77 Univ Southern MS-Hattiesburg; Instr, Delta St U, **SLP**

Bristow, Diane C Dept Communication Disorders, 1900 Gravier Street, L S U Medical Center, New Orleans, LA 70112, (504) 582-5379, BS 78 Old Dominion Univ; MS 80 Purdue Univ - West Lafayette; Instructor, LA St U/New Orleans Med Cen, **SLP ACE**

Brito, Cynthia Kojima Maui District Liaison, P O Box 920, Kaunakakai, HI 96748, (808) 553-3787, BS 81 Univ of CA - Santa Barbara; MA 83 Humboldt St Univ; Sp-Lang Path, Maui Dist Dept of Ed, **SLP**

Britt, Mrs Colleen D 25 Mallard Lane, Dadeville, AL 36853, (205) 825-8818, BS 73 FL St Univ; MS 74 FL St Univ; Sp-Lang Path, Tallapoosa Co Sch Syst, **SLP**

Britt, Debbie Lynne 334 West Dickens, Chicago, IL 60614, (312) 929-4367, BA 85 MI St Univ; MA 86 MI St Univ; SLP, InSpeech Inc, **SLP ACE**

Britt, Dr Eulalia Evelyn 11510 Gramercy Place, Riverside, CA 92505, (714) 785-2157, BS 57 CA St Univ - Los Angeles; OD 63 (NS) Johns Hopkins Univ; **A**

Brittain, Mrs Gwen Frutchey Qtrs 2662-A, Fort Lewis, WA 98433, (206) 964-5860, BS 69 Ithaca Coll; MS 81 Western OR St Coll; SLP, **SLP**

Brittain, Mary Jean 1747 Mulberry Avenue, Upland, CA 91786, (714) 987-2541, BS 64 Univ of ND; MA 68 CA St Univ - Los Angeles; Sp-Lang Path, Central School District, **SLP**

Britten, Dr Frederick 3317 Willow, Hays, KS 67601, (913) 628-5366, BA 72 Univ of AR - Fayetteville; MS 73 Univ of WY; PH 81 (Aural Rehab with Older Adults) Wichita St Univ; Assoc Prof/Coord Aud Serv, Fort Hays St U, **A ACE**

Britten, Mrs Karin Elisabeth 1611 Valley Road #E-2, Champaign, IL 61820, (217) 359-8941, BS 85 Univ of OK - Norman; MS 87 Univ of OK Medical Center; 87–Sp-Lang Path, Rehab Ctr Mercy Hosp, **SLP**

Brittin, Dr Marie E 1220 7th Avenue SW, Puyallup, WA 98371-6759, (206) 845-0088, BS Northwestern Univ; MA Univ of IA; PH (NS) Northwestern Univ; Assoc Prof, **SLP F LM ACE**

Brittingham, Lisa W 423 Walnut Street #314, Harrisburg, PA 17101, (717) 234-5662, BS 83 PA St Univ - Univ Park; MA 87 West Chester Univ of PA; SLP, Elwyn Inst, **SLP**

Britton, Barbara D 3431 Yuma Street N W #102, Washington, DC 20008, (301) 598-6000, BA 73 Univ of Pittsburgh - Pittsburgh; MS 75 Indiana Univ of PA; Sp/Lang Path, Visiting Nurse Asso, **SLP**

Britton, Mrs Barbara L 104 West Upper Ferry Road, West Trenton, NJ 08628, (609) 394-4020, BS 71 Trenton St Coll; ME 72 Trenton St Coll; MA 80 Rider Coll; VP, Mercer Med Cen

Britton, Jane Natalie P O Box 827, Pacific Grove, CA 93950, (408) 373-5441, BA 67 Univ of Redlands; MA 68 Univ of Redlands

Britton, Jean M 17685 S W Richmond Way, Beaverton, OR 97006, MS; **LM**

Britton, Joal H 16 Crest Drive, Colts Neck, NJ 07722, (201) 842-1597, BS 63 William Paterson Coll; ME 78 William Paterson Coll; **SLP**

Britton, Karen Ann 9 Admiral Lane, Hicksville, NY 11801, (516) 625-0960, BA 80 Univ of WY; MS 82 Univ of WY; 87–Asst Dir, Assn Children W/Learning Disab, **SLP**

Britton, Michelle A 1650 Schweitzer Basin Road, Sandpoint, ID 83864, (208) 263-6663, BS 75 Univ of KS; MA 77 Univ of KS; Sp-Lang Path, Adult/Child Dev Cen, **SLP**

Britton, Shelia Ann Greene P O Box 735, Waynesboro, MS 39367, (601) 735-3811, BS 83 Univ Southern MS-Hattiesburg; MS 84 Univ Southern MS-Hattiesburg; Sp-Lang Path, Wayne County Schools, **SLP**

Brix, Tina G 9631 Donna Avenue, Northridge, CA 91324, (818) 993-4663, BA 65 Univ of CA - Los Angeles; MA 85 CA St Univ - Northridge; 86–Sp-Lang Path, Los Angeles USD, **SLP**

Brixey, Nancy L 4361 58th Street, Sacramento, CA 95820, (916) 733-6820, BA 73 San Francisco St Univ; MA 75 San Francisco St Univ; Aud, Private Practice, **A ACE**

Broad, Audrey Fern 28303 Delaire Landing Road, Philadelphia, PA 19114, (215) 281-1500, BS 81 Boston Univ; OM 83 Hahneman Medical Coll; Sp-Lang Path, Moss Rehab Svcs, **SLP**

Broadbent, Josephine M 86 Coolidge Street, Lawrence, MA 01843, (508) 686-6376, BS 57 Emerson Coll; 52–Retired, **SLP A**

Broadhead, Mrs Sandra Lee 2511 West 20th Place, Yuma, AZ 85364, (505) 334-8934, Sp-Lang Path, Crane School District

Broadus, Sheila C 1124 Downlook Avenue, Pittsburgh, PA 15201, **SLP**

Broadwell, Mrs Josephine Ann 611 North Aurora Street, Ithaca, NY 14850, (607) 257-6374, BS 59 Bowling Green St Univ; MA 87 Ithaca Coll; 87–Sp-Lang Path, Groton Elem Sch, **SLP**

Brobeck, Teresa Carol 2040 9th Street #64, Coralville, IA 52241, BS 81 IN Univ - Bloomington; MA 83 IN Univ - Bloomington; Sp-Lang Path, University of Iowa, **SLP**

Brobst, Mrs Glenda A 7315 Scarlet Oak Court, Fairfax Station, VA 22039, (704) 554-8384, BS 77 Univ of North TX; MS 79 Univ of North TX; **SLP**

Brock, Angela 1690 Dunn Avenue #722, Daytona Beach, FL 32014, (904) 253-1051, BS 85 Ball St Univ; MA 87 Ball St Univ

Brock, Mrs Gaby 13325 Valley Vista Blvd, Sherman Oaks, CA 91423-4362, (818) 784-3099, BA 70 Sir George Univ - Quebec; MS 74 McGill Univ - Quebec; Sp/Lang Path, Private Practice, **SLP**

Brock, Karen Elizabeth 1848 Columbia Road N W #45, Washington, DC 20009, (202) 462-4108, **A**

Brock, Lala Suzanne PO Box 1737, Park City, UT 84060, (801) 649-4971, BS 77 Auburn Univ - Auburn; MS 79 Auburn Univ - Auburn; **SLP**

Brock, Mrs Linda J 16 Country Club Lane, Fort Madison, IA 52627, (319) 372-8515, BS 73 Northeast MO St Univ; MA 80 Northeast MO St Univ; 85–Sp-Lang Path, Great River AEA, **SLP**

Brock, Miriam B 5205 Scenic View Drive, Austin, TX 78746, (512) 454-4731, BA 72 Univ of MS; OM 76 Univ of MS; Sp/Lang Path, Austin State School, **SLP ACE**

Brock, Miriam S 21509 4th Avenue West, Apartment A-22, Bothell, WA 98021, (206) 486-7867, BA 75 Univ of CA - Los Angeles; MA 79 CA St Univ - Northridge; Program Director, Evergreen Head Injury Ctr, **SLP**

Brock, Mrs Sharon F 1116 Townsview Place, Wooster, OH 44691, (615) 525-8277, BS 78 Auburn Univ - Auburn; MS 80 Auburn Univ - Auburn; Sp/Lang Path, Knox Co Sch, **SLP**

Brock, Mrs Sharon L 413 Pecan Lane, Derby, KS 67037, (316) 262-8271, BS 74 Northeast MO St Univ; MA 75 Northeast MO St Univ; SLP, USD #368 Paola Ks, **SLP**

Brockbank, Mrs Linda C 11316 Nancyann Way, Fairfax, VA 22030, (703) 239-1200, BS 70 Indiana Univ of PA; MS 71 PA St Univ - Univ Park; Sp-Lang Path, Fairfax County Public Schools, **SLP**

Brockenborough, Mrs Ann Barrick 10910 Exeter Court, Largo, MD 20772, (301) 350-0592, BS 60 Hampton Univ; MA 66 Temple Univ; 88–Adjunct Fac, Howard Univ, **SLP**

Brockett, Jeff E 1080 Cherry Lane, Pocatello, ID 83201, (208) 238-0020, BS 82 Univ of ID; MS 87 ID St Univ; Aud, Pocatello Hearing Ctr, **A**

Brockett, Mrs Patricia S 8380 Greenboro Drive, Unit 5-805, Mc Lean, VA 22102, (703) 560-2800, BS 77 Baylor Univ; MS 78 Southern Methodist Univ; 87–Sp-Lang Path, Faifrfax Public Schools, **SLP**

Brockevelt, Mrs Susan R 3508 South Glendale Avenue, Sioux Falls, SD 57105, (605) 339-2731, BA 71 Kearney St Coll; MA 78 Univ of ND; Sp-Lang Path, Sioux Falls Sch Dist 49-5, **SLP**

Brockhaus, Rebecca Watson Capital Home Health, 2152 Wisteria Street, Baton Rouge, LA 70806, (504) 923-1140, BA 81 Univ of MD - College Park; MA 84 LA St Univ - Baton Rouge; Sp/Lang Path, Capitol Home Health, **SLP**

Brockman, Janet L H 3195 S W Grace Lane, Portland, OR 97225, (503) 760-7700, BS 73 Lewis & Clark Coll; MS 75 Western OR St Coll; Sp/Lang Path, Oshu Crpld Chldn Div, **SLP**

Brockman, Loreen Rita 590 Baker #1, San Francisco, CA 94117, (415) 346-8904, BA 85 CA St Univ - Stanislaus; MA 87 CA St Univ - Stanislaus; 88–Sp-Lang Path, Easter Seal Soc of San Mateo, **SLP**

Brockman, Mrs Nancy A 26 Loudon Parkway, Loudonville, NY 12211, (518) 463-2583, BS 56 Univ of NE - Lincoln; MA 61 Univ of NE - Lincoln; **SLP A**

Brockman, Mrs Nancy A 9400 Turkey Lake Road, ORMC, Orlando, FL 32819, (407) 351-8574, BS 58 Bowling Green St Univ; MA 82 Univ of Central FL; 87–Prog Dir-Phys Med & Rehab, Orlando Reg Med Cen, **SLP ACE**

Brockmeier, Laura L 1945 South Parfet Drive, Lakewood, CO 80227, (303) 988-0092, BS 68 Univ of NE - Lincoln; MA 71 Univ of NE - Lincoln; **SLP**

Brockmeyer, Mrs Andrea S GPO Box 6269, San Juan, PR 00936, BS 76 IL St Univ - Normal; MA 78 Univ of IL - Urbana; **SLP**

Brockmeyer, Mrs Valerie Ann 2216B Jay Cee Drive, Joppa, MD 21085, (301) 531-6686, BA 81 Loyola Coll; MS 83 Loyola Coll; Sp-Lang Path, Therapy Inc, **SLP**

Brockmiller, Mrs Faye S 5207 Glenwall Drive, Aliquippa, PA 15001, (412) 774-6494, BA 64 Univ of AL- Tuscaloosa; MA 66 Univ of AL- Tuscaloosa; Sp-Lang Path, Crossroads Speech & Hearing Inc, **SLP**

Brockway, Debra Elizabeth 466 East Howard Street, Pasadena, CA 91104, (213) 268-3352, MA 81 CA St Univ - Los Angeles; Audiologist, **A**

Brockway, Mrs Mary Ann 27 Veronica Avenue, Salem, NH 03079, (603) 893-3084, BA 72 MI St Univ; MA 76 MI St Univ; Aud, Adult-Ped Sp & Hrng Assoc, **A**

Brockway, Nancy L 203 31st Avenue E, Tuscaloosa, AL 35404, (205) 759-7305, MS 87 Univ of AL- Tuscaloosa

Brockway, Mrs Susan M Route 2 Box 769, Crandon, WI 54520, (715) 478-3533, BA 79; MS 80 Univ of WI - Eau Claire; 81–Sp/Lang Path, Sch Dist of Crandon, **SLP**

Brockwell, Mrs Celeste Micchelli 154 Pershing Boulevard, Lavallette, NJ 08735, (201) 341-9700, **SLP**

Brodale, Mrs Vicky Ann 1602 Susan Avenue, Cherokee, IA 51012, (712) 225-2568, BA 71 Univ of Northern IA; MA 72 Univ of Northern IA; Sp-Lang Path, Wn Hills AEA 12, **SLP**

Broderick-Backman, Mrs Katherine A 46 Bellingham Road, Blackstone, MA 01504, (617) 384-3116, BS 81 Univ of MA - Amherst; MA 84 Univ of MA - Amherst; 85–Supvr Sp-Lang Path, Wrentham State Sch, **SLP**

Brodersen, Shelach H 136 Evergreen Lane, Berkeley, CA 94705, (415) 276-3692, MS 76 Southern Methodist Univ; SLP, San Lorenzo USD, **SLP**

Brodeur, Mrs Natalie Goodfellow 21015 72nd Avenue S E, Snohomish, WA 98290, BS 81 Univ of WA; OM 84 Univ of WA; 85–Sp-Lang Path, Erikkson House, **SLP**

Brodie, Gail R 3311 Timberlane Drive, Stockton, CA 95209, (209) 944-4262, BA 74 Univ of CA - Santa Barbara; MS 76 Univ of AZ; Tchr, Stockton USD, **SLP**

Brodie, Mrs Janet Elizbeth 1327 North 54th Street, Philadelphia, PA 19131, (215) 299-7000, **SLP**

Brodie, Maureen Nakazawa 1325 Primrose Place, Davis, CA 95616, (916) 752-3184, BA 76 Univ of CA - Santa Barbara; MA 77 Univ of Denver; 87–Dir, Univ of CA-Davis, **SLP**

Brodkey, Mrs Estelle W 1754 Todd Road, Toms River, NJ 08753, (201) 244-3713, Sp-Lang Path, Private Practice, **SLP**

Brodnitz, Dr Friedrich S 157 West 57th Street #1100, New York, NY 10019, (212) 838-9130, MD; Private Practice, **SLP F H LM**

Brodsky, Barbara 420 West Belmont #13-B, Chicago, IL 60657, (312) 348-7978, OM 88 Governors St Univ

Brodsky, Geraldine 9 Cedar Drive, Rhinebeck, NY 12572, (914) 896-7516, BA 60 CUNY - Brooklyn Coll; MA 66 Stanford Univ; Dir, Hudson Valley Sp Cen, **SLP**

Brody, John J 255 Broad Street, Williston Park, NY 11596, (516) 575-2103, BA 76 Long Island U - CW Post Ctr; MS 78 Univ of OK Medical Center; Health Services Manager, Grumman Corp, **A**

Brody, Leslie A 8761 Terrace Drive, Pittsburgh, PA 15237, (412) 364-8650, BA 77 Univ of Pittsburgh - Pittsburgh; MA 79 Univ of Pittsburgh - Pittsburgh; Mercy Hospital, **SLP ACE**

Brody, Philip 853 46th Street, Brooklyn, NY 11220, **SLP A**

Broeg, Charlotte Marie 61 Beech Drive, Edgewood, KY 41017, (606) 824-3323, BA 80 Univ of Cincinnati; MA 82 Univ of Cincinnati; **SLP**

Broege, Barbara Heermeier 70 Redwood, Mansfield, OH 44907, (419) 756-1133, BA 82 Bowling Green St Univ; MA 83 Bowling Green St Univ; Aud, Beltone, **A**

Broen, Dr Patricia A University Of Minnesota, 115 Shevlin Hall, 164 Pillsbury Drive S E, Minneapolis, MN 55455, (612) 624-3322, BS 66 Univ of MN - Minneap-St Paul; MA 70 Univ of MN - Minneap-St Paul; PH 72 (NS) Univ of MN - Minneap-St Paul; Prof, U of MN, **SLP F**

Broeren, Margaret Mary 1934 North 51st Street, Milwaukee, WI 53208, BS 81 Marquette Univ; MS 83 Marquette Univ; 88–Sp-Lang Path, Rehabilitation Associates, **SLP**

Broermann, Elaine S Rural Route 2, Shenandoah, IA 51601, **SLP**

Broesamle, Mrs Katharine Sue 895 Valley High Avenue, Thousand Oaks, CA 91362, (805) 496-4451, BA 64 Univ of the Pacific; MA 84 CA St Univ - Northridge; SLP, Conejo Valley USD, **SLP**

Broffman, Dr Sylvia 49-45 Little Neck Parkway, Little Neck, NY 11362, (516) 686-7557, BA 69 CUNY - Queens Coll; MA 70 NY Univ; PH 81 (Ed Psych) NY Univ; Assoc Prof of Sp, NY I of Tech, **SLP**

Brogden, Mrs Sharon L W P O Box 51683, Raleigh, NC 27609, (919) 575-7406, BA 68 East Carolina Univ; ME 78 Univ of NC - Greensboro; SLP, John Omstead Hosp, **SLP**

Broghammer, Mrs Jane A Northern Trails AEA, Box M, Clear Lake, IA 50428, (515) 357-6125, BA 67 Univ of IA; MA 69 Univ of IA; Aud, Nn Trails AEA, **A**

Broida, Dr Helen 5362-0 Algarrobo, Laguna Hills, CA 92653, BS 38 WA St Univ; MS 59; PH 62 (NS); **SLP LM**

Brokaw, Mrs Sonia P 2553 Mercedes Drive NE, Atlanta, GA 30345, (404) 728-1047, BS 62 OH St Univ; MA 63 OH St Univ; Sp-Lang Path, DeKalb Co Sch Sys, **SLP**

Broker, Carol A 15 Barnes Road, Hingham, MA 02043, (617) 749-3788, BS 62 SUNY - Coll at Buffalo; MA 69 Univ of MO - Columbia; **SLP ACE**

Brom, Carole Ann 1831 Pheasant Hill Drive, Loveland, OH 45140, (513) 683-3984, BS 58 Univ of WI - Madison; MA 68 Univ of NE - Lincoln; Sp-Lang Path, Private Practice, **SLP**

Bromberg, Mrs Betsy 85-16 122nd Street, Kew Gardens, NY 11415, (718) 441-2167, BA 85 CUNY - Queens Coll; MA 87 CUNY - Hunter Coll; Aud, Elmhurst Hosp, **A**

Bromberg, Mrs Elinor J 30 Lincoln Circle, Andover, MA 01810, (508) 475-7677, BA 63 Univ of CT; MA 67 Univ of CT; Sp-Lang Path, N Andover Pub Sch, **SLP**

Bromer, Mrs Denise Helene 437 Trappe Lane, Langhorne, PA 19047, (215) 757-7665, BS 75 LA St Univ - Baton Rouge; MA 76 Memphis St Univ; **SLP**

Bromley, Maryellen 1630 Worster Road #522-C, Framingham, MA 01701, (617) 820-1149, MA 87 MI St Univ

Bromm, Mary 327 Calle Cuervo, San Clemente, CA 92672, **SLP**

Bromstrup-Garrity, Mrs Kathleen F 438 Bernadette, Batavia, IL 60510, (312) 879-6707, BS 73 Eastern IL Univ; MS 78 Governors St Univ; 85–Sp-Lang Path, Aurora West Sch Dist, **SLP**

Brondel, Florence Box 412 Knob Hill Road, Stanfordville, NY 12581-0412, (914) 758-3421, BA 79 SUNY - Coll at New Paltz; MS 81 Columbia Univ Teachers Coll; Sp-Lang Path, Private Practice, **SLP**

Brondyke, Vicki L P O Box 458, Clinton, SC 29325, (803) 984-3067, BS 72 Univ of MO - Columbia; MA 74 Univ of MO - Columbia; Sp-Lang Path, Laurens Sch Dist #55, **SLP**

Broner, Judy 7791 East Osorn Road #280, Scottsdale, AZ 85251, **SLP**

Bronk, Mrs Maxine M 3740 School Drive, Morris, IL 60450, (815) 942-5766, BS 73 Univ of WI - Stevens Point; MS 74 Univ of WI - Stevens Point; Sp-Lang Path, Grundy Co Spec Ed Coop, **SLP**

Bronnert, Lois Marie 660 Green Hedge Drive, Fenton, MO 63026, (314) 225-3822, BS 64 IN St Univ - Terre Haute; MS 66 IN St Univ - Terre Haute; Sp-Lang Path, St Louis Co Spec Sch Dist, **SLP**

Bronson, Kathryn Thelen 16766 Bernardo Center Drive, Suite 111A, San Diego, CA 92128, (619) 485-8490, BS 85 Marquette Univ; MS 87 Univ of AZ; 87–Sp-Lang Path, Chldn Hosp & Hlth Ctr

Bronson, Peggy J P O Box #206, Elkader, IA 52043, (319) 245-1480, BA 63 Saint Cloud St Univ; MA 77 Northeast MO St Univ; Sp-Lang Path, Keystone AEA, **SLP**

Bronstein, Dr Arthur J 975 Underhills Road, Oakland, CA 94610, (415) 763-6216, BA 34 CUNY - City College; MA 36 Columbia Univ Teachers Coll; PH 49 (NS) NY Univ; 55–Prof Emeritus, The Grad Sch City Univ of NY, **SLP F LM**

Brook, Mrs Jane J 8138 Prince Charming Lane, Roscoe, IL 61073, (608) 755-3530, BS 75 IL St Univ - Normal; MS 76 IL St Univ - Normal; Aud, P H McDonald MD, **A**

Brook, Janet Vallese 1217 Gabaldon Road, Belen, NM 87002, (505) 864-0561, BA 79 RI Coll; MS 85 Univ of NM; 88–Sp-Lang Path, Private Practice, **SLP**

Brooke, Donna 107 Cavalry Road, Westport, CT 06880, **SLP**

Brooker, Mrs Gayle E 1980 White Oak, Springfield, MO 65804, BS 73 KS St Univ; MA 74 Memphis St Univ; Sp-Lang Path, Private Practice, **SLP**

Brookner, Christine Labenski 515 West 59th Street, New York, NY 10019, (212) 554-7581, BS 73 Boston Univ; MA 75 CUNY - Hunter Coll; Aud, Roosevelt Hosp, **A**

Brookner-Stein, Mrs Sheryl P 990 North Lake Shore Drive, Apartment 18-C, Chicago, IL 60611, (312) 337-1079, BS 70 Northwestern Univ; MS 71 Univ of MI - Ann Arbor; Sp-Lang Path, Private Practice, **SLP**

Brooks, Mrs Alta Fann 1925 Cypress Point West, Austin, TX 78746, PH; **SLP**

Brooks, Mrs Andrea S 5361 N W 66th Avenue, Coral Springs, FL 33067, (305) 753-6725, BA 75 Univ of MD - College Park; MA 76 Montclair St Coll; 82–Aud, Palm Beach Med Gp, **A**

Brooks, Mrs Barbara A 2111 Michie Drive #25, Charlottesville, VA 22901, (804) 979-1367, BS 77 Univ of IA; MA 79 Univ of IA; Aud, Univ of VA Health Sci Ctr, **A**

Brooks, Beverly Ann 148 Springside Drive, Timonium, MD 21093, (301) 252-8054, BS 85 WV Univ; OM 86 Univ of SC - Columbia; **A**

Brooks, Mrs Bonnie H Route 2 Box 29-P, Cabot, AR 72023, (501) 552-3261, BA 75 Univ of AR - Little Rock; MS 80 Univ of AR - Little Rock; Sp-Lang Path, Carlisle Pub Sch, **SLP**

Brooks, Carla Ann 10306 Fischer Place N E, Seattle, WA 98125-7732, (206) 543-9078, BA 72 Univ of CA - Santa Barbara; MA 75 Univ of CA - Santa Barbara; 83–Lecturer/Supervisor, University of Washington, **SLP**

Brooks, Mrs Cecelia A 1741 Live Oak Lane, Atlantic Beach, FL 32233, (904) 241-1840, BA 76 Univ of FL; ME 77 Univ of FL; Sp-Lang Path, Private Practice, **SLP**

Brooks, Cherylan 12 Fern Avenue, Toronto, ON, Canada M6R 1K1, (416) 578-1683, BS 76 Boston Univ; MS 79 Columbia Univ Teachers Coll; Aud, Brooks Audiology, **A**

Brooks, David H 8 Whitney Court, Brick, NJ 08724, (201) 840-4163, BS 54 Glassboro St Coll; MA 58 Columbia Univ Teachers Coll; **SLP**

Brooks, Donna Kay Route 3 Box 367-C, Brooks Road, Montgomery, AL 36110, (205) 263-5871, **SLP**

Brooks, Elizabeth Alicia 502 Broadleaf Circle, Raleigh, NC 27613, (919) 787-3661, MS 87 Univ of NC - Chapel Hill; Sp-Lang Path, MedVisit Inc, **SLP**

Brooks, Francis D 743 Montecito Way, Salinas, CA 93901, (408) 422-8381, BA 33 Pacific Univ; ME 54 Univ of OR; **SLP A LM**

Brooks, Mrs Jacqueline E 7825 Lakeview, Lexington, MI 48450, (313) 359-7564, MA 83 MI St Univ; Asst Dir, C & C Hlth Care Asso, **SLP**

Brooks, Jacqueline Marie 320 West Valencia-Mesa #14, Fullerton, CA 92635, (714) 787-0204, BA 85 CA St Univ - Fullerton; MA 87 CA St Univ - Fullerton; Sp-Lang Path, Rehab Alliance

Brooks, Mrs Jami Harris 2919 Post Oak Drive, Euless, TX 76039, (817) 429-2059, BS 86 Baylor Univ; MS 87 Baylor Univ; 88–Sp-Lang Path/Aud, Meadowbrook Hrng & Sp Ctr

Brooks, Mrs Jean Naeye 6277 Pfafflin Lake Blvd, Newburgh, IN 47630, (812) 853-2250, BS 79 Ashland Coll; MA 80 SUNY - Coll at Geneseo; Supervisor, InSpeech Inc, **SLP ACE**

Brooks, Jill 3800 Crawford Avenue, Coconut Grove, FL 33133, (305) 549-6397, BS 74 Northwestern Univ; MS 75 Univ of WI - Madison; Ch Dept Sp-Lang Path, Jackson Mem Hosp/U Miami, **SLP**

Brooks, Mrs Jill Elaine 1620 Beck, Cody, WY 82414, (303) 778-5817, OM 86 Univ of MT; 88–Sp-Lang Path, Big Horn County Sch Dist #1, **A**

Brooks, Joyce McCurley Speech And Hearing Clinic, Glenwood State Hosp School, Glenwood, IA 51534, (712) 527-4811, BS 62 Univ of IL - Urbana; MA 64 Univ of IL - Urbana; Sp-Lang Path, Glenwood St Hosp-Sch, **SLP**

Brooks, Mrs Julie Ann Missoula School District Number 1, 215 South 6th Street West, Missoula, MT 59801, (406) 542-4020, BA 81 Univ of MT; OM 84 Univ of MT; Sp-Lang Path, Missoula Sch Dist #1, **SLP**

Brooks, Karen Bruns 4319 N E Arbort Road, Kansas City, MO 64117-1616, (816) 459-7152, BA 82 Univ of MO - KS City; MS 85 Central MO St Univ; **SLP**

Brooks, Mrs Kathy Marie 11 Diana Drive, Fairmont, WV 26554, (304) 366-2070, BS 73 WV Univ; MS 75 WV Univ; Sp-Lang Path, Marion County Bd of Education, **SLP**

Brooks, Mrs Lee Ann 104 Abundance Court, Lafayette, LA 70506-6607, (713) 578-3050, **SLP**

Brooks, Leonard L 9976 East Sagebrush Drive, Prescott Valley, AZ 86314, (602) 772-8026, PH; **SLP A**

Brooks, Lisa Colette 1401 Blair Mill Road #1711, Silver Spring, MD 20910, BA 82 Univ of MD - College Park; MA 85 Univ of MD - College Park; 88–Sp-Lang Path, Childrens Hosp Natl Med Ctr, **SLP**

Brooks, Martha Wisly 18 Kingston Court, Merrimack, NH 03054, (603) 673-7234, BA 79 Univ of CT; ME 83 Northeastern Univ; Sp-Lang Path, Regional Spec Educ Consortium, **SLP**

Brooks, Mary M 12406 King, Overland Park, KS 66213, BA 71 KS St Univ; MA 72 Univ of KS; **SLP**

Brooks, Mira J 2319 Oren Avenue, Flint, MI 48505, (313) 232-8855, MA 88 Western MI Univ

Brooks, Nadine R 1406 Holman View, Wyoming, OH 45215, MS; **SLP**

Brooks, Nondi Carol 2278 Fairway Circle N E, Atlanta, GA 30319, (404) 786-2636, ME 85 GA St Univ

Brooks, Mrs Patricia Shaw 9413 Emmett Road, Glen Allen, VA 23060, BS 71 Hampton Univ; ME 74 Univ of VA - Charlottesville; Sp-Lang Path, Henrico Co Pub Sch, **SLP**

Brooks, Penny McClard 6296 Old Alba, Gaylord, MI 49735, (616) 584-3464, BA 84 Ouachita Baptist Univ; MS 86 Univ of OK Medical Center; 88–Sp-Lang Path, Northern Speech Services, **SLP**

Brooks, Rebecca P University Of Alabama, Box 870242, Tuscaloosa, AL 35487-0242, (205) 348-7131, BS 74 East TN St Univ; MA 76 Univ of TN - Knoxville; Coord of Aud Svcs, U of AL, **A**

Brooks, Rebecca S 17 Oak Knoll Road, Williston, VT 05495, (802) 658-9044, BA 69 Univ of WI - Madison; MA 73 CUNY - Hunter Coll; Sp-Lang Path, South Burlington Sch Dist, **SLP**

Brooks, Dr Robert S Mankato State University, Dept Of Commun Disorders, 103-K Armstrong Hall, Mankato, MN 56001, (507) 389-1415, BA 52 Ottawa Univ; MS 54 Univ of KS; PH 64 (Sp Path & Aud) Univ of KS; Prof, Mankato St Univ, **SLP**

Brooks, Roberta L 17 Thames Street, Norwalk, CT 06851, (203) 787-9941, BA 75 Univ of MO - KS City; MA 78 Univ of KS; 88–Sp-Lang Path, Jill Cohn Ctr for Head Injury Rehab, **SLP**

Brooks, Mrs Ruth Ann 10095 Bunker Woods Court, Burke, VA 22015, (703) 455-6500, BS 75 Old Dominion Univ; ME 81 Univ of VA - Charlottesville; 84–Sp/Lang Path, Fairfax Co Pub Sch, **SLP**

Brooks, Sandra D 400 Thames Parkway #1-A, Park Ridge, IL 60068, (312) 318-0452, BA 70 Univ of IL - Chicago; MA 72 NY Univ; Training Mgr, Texas Instruments Inc, **SLP**

Brooks, Stanley M 4 Marty Close, Glenmoore, PA 19343, (215) 383-3883, BS 73 PA St Univ - Univ Park; MA 75 Western MI Univ; Sp-Lang Path-Aud, Chester Co Inter Ut, **SLP A**

Brooks, Mrs Stephanie B 4407 Rondo Place, Wilmington, NC 28403, (919) 799-1258, BA 76 Univ of NC - Chapel Hill; MS 77 Univ of NC - Chapel Hill; Sp-Lang Path, Self Employed, **SLP**

Brooks, Susan Katz 3 Babbitt Lane, Harvard, MA 01451, (508) 772-2544, BS 65 Boston Univ; MA 67 Stanford Univ; 84–Sp/Lang Path, Private Practice, **SLP**

Brooks, Valerie L 18 Ramblewood Court, Schenectady, NY 12309, (518) 382-0282, BS 74 Syracuse Univ; MS 75 Syracuse Univ; Sp/Lang Path, Valerie Brooks, **SLP**

Brooks, Wendell M 7 White Terrace, Cornwall on Hudson, NY 12520, (914) 782-8215, BS 63 SUNY - Coll at Geneseo; MS 68 CUNY - Queens Coll; Sp-Lang Path, Monroe Woodbury Ctrl Sch Dist, **SLP**

Brookshaw, Neddy R 1301 Pebble Creek, Memphis, TN 38119, **SLP**

Brookshire, Bonnie 9115 Kapri, Houston, TX 77025, (713) 665-6297, MA 75 Univ of Houston - Univ Park; 88–Research Asst, M D Anderson Science Ctr, **SLP**

Brookshire, Dr Robert H P O Box 17036, Minneapolis, MN 55417, (612) 725-2000, BA 61 Huron Coll; MA 64 Univ of MN - Minneap-St Paul; PH 65 (NS) Univ of MN - Minneap-St Paul; Ch SLP Sec, VA, **SLP F**

Brooks-James, Ossie 1128 Sheridan Avenue North, Minneapolis, MN 55411, (612) 721-5508, BS 68 Memphis St Univ; MA 75 Memphis St Univ; Sp-Lang Path, Special Sch Dist #1, **SLP**

Brooks-King, Kimberly Diann 24455 Lake Shore Boulevard #1807, Euclid, OH 44123, (216) 731-6013, BA 86 Baldwin-Wallace Coll; MS 87 Clarion Univ of PA; 88–Sp-Lang Path, InSpeech Inc

Brooks Ma Ccc, Gerard B Poughkeepsie Sp & Lang Assoc, 229 All Angels Road, Wappingers Falls, NY 12590, (914) 298-0020, BA 78 SUNY - Coll at New Paltz; MA 79 Central MI Univ; Sp-Lang Path, Private Practice, **SLP**

Brooks-Miller, Mrs Susan Lynne 6814 Ravenscroft, St Louis, MO 63123, (314) 362-1443, BS 83 Southwest MO St Univ; MA 85 Saint Louis Univ; **SLP**

Broom, Donna Raye 6632 Calle DE San Alberto, Tucson, AZ 85710, (602) 296-3211, BA 64 Univ of AZ; MS 67 AZ St Univ; Dept Head, Private Practice, **SLP**

Broom, Mrs Stacey P 7153 Secretariat Drive, Columbus, GA 31909-1851, (404) 568-6306, BS 86 Columbus Coll; ME 87 Columbus Coll; 88–Sp-Lang Path, Muscogee County Sch Dist, **SLP**

Broome, Mrs Maxine A B 28 Mildred Place, East Rockaway, NY 11563, (516) 599-8185, BA 77 Hofstra Univ; MA 79 Hofstra Univ; Sp-Lang Path, Private Practice, **SLP**

Broomer, Mrs Mona S 27 Lyon Lane, Franklin Park, NJ 08823-4505, (201) 821-5664, BA 78 CUNY - Queens Coll; MA 80 Hofstra Univ; Sp-Lang Path, Sp Serv UT/NYC Bd of Ed, **SLP**

Brophy, Mrs Kathryn Kuykendall 4043 Burning Tree Lane, Augusta, GA 30906, (404) 790-2464, BA 79 Univ of TX - El Paso; MA 80 Univ of TX - El Paso; **SLP**

Brophy, Dr Nancy Hovorka South 5208 Magnolia, Spokane, WA 99223, BS Eastern MI Univ; MA Wayne St Univ; ED 87 (Learning Disabilities) Univ of MO - Columbia; **SLP**

Brorson, Kent Robert 132-5103 35th Avenue S W, Calgary, AB, Canada T3E 6L9, (403) 246-0570, BS 81 ND St Univ; MS 83 Ithaca Coll; Sp/Lang Path, Alberta Children Hospital, **SLP**

Brosh, Mrs Lee Ann P O Box 21716, Little Rock, AR 72221, (501) 223-8810, OB 79 AR St Univ; MA 82 Memphis St Univ; Sp-Lang Path, W Memphis Pub Sch, **SLP**

Brosius, Michele 6622 Glacier Avenue, Reynoldsburg, OH 43068, (614) 475-0564, BS 75 Clarion Univ of PA; MA 77 Kent St Univ; SLP, Franklin County Bd Ment Retrdn, **SLP A**

Brosius, Mrs Valerie Ann 4705 48th Street A, Moline, IL 61265, (309) 793-2009, BA 78 Augustana Coll; MA 79 Univ of IL - Urbana; Sp-Path, Franciscan Rehab Cen, **SLP**

Brosnan-Maddox, Susan 3460 Capital Circle NW, Tallahassee, FL 32303, (904) 562-2750, BS 79 FL St Univ; MS 81 FL St Univ; 81–Sp-Lang Path, Leon Co Schs Ruediger Elem, **SLP**

Bross, Mrs Caryn H 1802 Country Club Drive, Cherry Hill, NJ 08003, (609) 795-9607, BA 76 Rutger's St Univ - Douglas Coll; MS 78 Columbia Univ Teachers Coll; 88–Aud, Haddonfield Sp & Hrng Ctr, **A**

Bross, Mrs Maureen Patrick 519 E Liberty Street, Hubbard, OH 44425, (216) 755-3354, BS 81 Kent St Univ; MA 81 Kent St Univ; Sp-Lang Path, Struthers City Schs, **SLP**

Brossard, Debra Flood 2282 Bootmaker Drive, Beloit, WI 53511, (608) 364-6080, MS 84 Univ of WI - Stevens Point; Sp-Lang Path, School District of Beloit, **SLP**

Brossart, Carol Marie 604 East Divide Avenue, Bismarck, ND 58501-3553, (701) 221-3490, BS 81 ND St Univ; MS 84 Minot St Univ; Sp-Lang Path, Bismarck P S, **SLP**

Brossia, Mrs Martha Burrell 3455 Oleander Drive, Highland, CA 92346, (714) 862-3891, BA 66 MI St Univ; MS 87 Univ of Redlands

Brothers, Mrs Nancy P S 429 Woodbridge Drive, Chesapeake, VA 23320, (804) 473-5023, BS 70 Clarion Univ of PA; MS 75 Old Dominion Univ; Sp-Lang Path, VA Beach Pub Schs, **SLP**

Brotherton, Gary James 1320 Buena Vista, Amarillo, TX 79106, (806) 353-2820, BS 85 Hardin-Simmons Univ; MA 87 TX Woman's Univ; 87–Sp-Lang Path, High Plains Baptist Hosp

Brotman-Domoracki, Sandra R 7657 Blackford Drive, Chagrin Falls, OH 44022, (216) 372-2200, BS 76 Univ of Cincinnati; MA 77 OH St Univ; Coord/Aud Servs, Trumbull Co Bd of Ed, **A**

Brou, Sharon Elizabeth 5757 West Hefner Road, Apartment 1017, Oklahoma City, OK 73132, (405) 720-6306, BS 85 OK St Univ; MS 87 Univ of OK - OK City; **SLP**

Brough, Nancy Carroll 408 Rustic Drive, Los Angeles, CA 90065, (213) 742-5568, BA 81 CA St Univ - Northridge; MA 85 CA St Univ - Northridge; 87–Sp-Lang Path, Carondelet Rehab Ctrs of America, **SLP**

Broughton, Mrs Ann L 303 East North Street, Durand, IL 61024, (815) 248-4540, MA; 86–Aud, Freeport ENT Assoc Ltd, **A**

Broughton, Mrs Carol Kittrell 3800 Highway 104, Fairhope, AL 36532, BA 79 Univ of AL- Tuscaloosa; MS 80 Univ of AL- Tuscaloosa; Sp/Lang Path, Baldwin County Pub Sch, **SLP**

Broughton, Mrs Janette Marie 3098 Lodgewood Street, Newbury Park, CA 91320, (805) 498-4099, BA CA St Univ - Los Angeles; MA 84 CA St Univ - Los Angeles; Sp-Lang Path, **SLP**

Broughton, Jennifer Lee 129 North Cherry, Centralia, IL 62801, (618) 533-5628, MS 86 Eastern IL Univ; 88–Sp-Lang Path, St Mary's Hosp, **SLP**

Broughton, Jill Glass 11 April Avenue, Carmi, IL 62821, (618) 382-5608, BS 84 IA St Univ; MA 86 Univ of IA; 87–Sp-Lang Path, Wabash OH Valley Spec Educ Dist, **SLP**

Broussard, Mrs Mary Margaret 609 Greenbriar Drive, Brandon, FL 33511, (813) 654-3664, BS 70 Nazareth Coll of Rochester; MS 81 Univ of Southwestern LA; 86–Sp-Lang Path, Bay Area Rehab, **SLP**

Broussard, Mrs MaryJo L 2220 Thomas Road, Beaumont, TX 77706, (409) 892-2212, BS 55 Lamar Univ; ME 56 Univ of Houston - Univ Park; Sp-Lang Path, **SLP**

Broussard, Robin Elizabeth 563 Ashlawn Drive, Harahan, LA 70123, (504) 367-3120, **SLP**

Brouwers, Simone Elisabeth 2309 Shelley Avenue, San Jose, CA 95124, (408) 371-8293, MA 82 San Jose St Univ; 82–Instr, W Valley/Mission Coll Dist, **SLP**

Brower, Catherine J 2104 North Jefferson St, Arlington, VA 22205, (703) 321-7979, BA 72 Univ of AL- Tuscaloosa; MA 75 Memphis St Univ; Sp-Lang Path, Comp Home Hlth Serv, **SLP**

Brower, Diane M 4244 Fuller Road, Talmo, GA 30575, (404) 534-5141, BA 73 Brenau Coll; ME 75 Univ of GA; Dir, NE Georgia Speech Center Inc, **SLP ACE**

Brower, Mrs Joan 4709 Berrywood Court, Virginia Beach, VA 23464, (203) 354-2786, BS 79 Eastern MI Univ; MA 80 Eastern MI Univ; Sp-Lang Path, Greater Atlanta Sp & Lang Ser, **SLP**

Brown, Alexandra P O Box 3504, Arcadia, CA 91006, (818) 445-4441, BS 76 Pomona (Polytechnic) Coll; MA 80 CA St Univ - Los Angeles; Sp-Lang Path/Owner, A Brown & Assoc Sp Path Serv, **SLP**

Brown, Alice B 4909 N Rock Spring Road, Arlington, VA 22207, (703) 532-7718, BS 67 Univ of WI - Madison; MS 66 Miami Univ - Oxford; 88–ESL Tchr, Arlington Pub Sch, **SLP**

Brown, Mrs Alice F University Of Pittsburgh, 313 Salk Hall, Pittsburgh, PA 15261, (412) 648-8400, BA 51 Pomona Coll; Coord, Spec Serv, Cleft Palate Cen - U Pittsburg, **SLP**

Brown, Mrs Alison Kyro 333 Melrose Avenue, Toronto, ON, Canada M5M 1Z5, (416) 784-1306, BA 78 Univ of Western Ontario; OM 82 Univ of Western Ontario; Sp-Lang Path, Private Practice, **SLP**

Brown, Anita Gibson 1220 Grand Avenue, San Diego, CA 92109, (619) 298-8120, **SLP**

Brown, Mrs Anita J 293 North Poplar, Manteno, IL 60950, (815) 468-3934, BS 84 KS St Univ; MA 85 Wichita St Univ; 86–Sp-Lang Path, South Metropolitan Assoc, **SLP**

Brown, Ann Thompson 20 Sharmont, Hattiesburg, MS 39402-1950, (601) 544-5600, BS 74 LA St Univ - Baton Rouge; MA 86 Univ of IL - Urbana; **SLP**

Brown, Mrs Anna S 613 Walnut Avenue, Colonial Heights, VA 23834, BS 35 Syracuse Univ; MS 37 Syracuse Univ; **SLP**

Brown, Antigone Howick 1690 Northwest 136th Avenue, Portland, OR 97229, (503) 641-7224, BS 80 Univ of OR

Brown, Arlene Stredler 3882 Bosque Court, Boulder, CO 80301, (303) 444-1314, MA 83 Univ of Denver; Sp-Lang Path, Private Practice, **SLP**

Brown, Dr Arthur P O Box 412, Ahoskie, NC 27910, (919) 358-1761, MA 65 Western Carolina Univ; ES 75 East Carolina Univ; ED 78 (NS) Nova Univ; Assoc Supt, Hertford Co Schs, **SLP**

Brown, B Evelyn 1460 N Sandburg Terrace, Apartment 2302, Chicago, IL 60610, (312) 791-2920, BA 60 Vanderbilt Univ; MA 64 Northwestern Univ; Aud, Siegel I Michael Reese Hosp, **A**

Brown, Barbara 1462 Tubbs Lane, Calistoga, CA 94515, (707) 257-8622, **SLP**

Brown, Mrs Barbara Lynn 4332 Division Road, West Lafayette, IN 47906, (317) 494-3817, BS 82 Purdue Univ - West Lafayette; MS 84 Purdue Univ - West Lafayette; 87–Sp-Lang Path, Purdue Univ, **SLP**

Brown, Mrs Belinda R 1300 7th Street N W, Altoona, IA 50009, (515) 964-2550, BS 75 IA St Univ; MA 76 Northeast MO St Univ; Sp-Lang Path, Heartland AEA 11, **SLP**

Brown, Mrs Beth A 1949 Forest Street, Wauwatosa, WI 53213, (414) 774-4017, BA 81 Univ of WI - Eau Claire; MS 82 Univ of WI - Eau Claire; SLP, Waukesha Pub Sch, **SLP**

Brown, Beth Ann New Medico CRS Of Lynn, 162 Boston Street, Lynn, MA 01904, (617) 595-1840, BS 82 Univ of TX - Austin; MA 88 Univ of TX - Austin; 88–Sp-Lang Path, New Medico Comm Re-Entry Svcs, **SLP**

Brown, Mrs Betsy Shulkin 68 Sevland Road, Newton Center, MA 02159, (617) 969-5000, BS 75 Univ of Miami; MS 76 Loyola Coll; Sp-Lang Path, Newton Pub Schs, **SLP**

Brown, Mrs Betty L Hearing Clinic, Michigan Sch For The Deaf, Flint, MI 48502, (313) 238-4621, BA 71 Univ of MI - Ann Arbor; MA 73 Univ of MI - Ann Arbor; Aud, MI Sch for Deaf, **A**

Brown, Beverly Elizabeth P O Box 1301, Euless, TX 76039-1301, (214) 454-3082, BS 80 East TX St Univ - Commerce; MS 85 East TX St Univ - Commerce; 86–Sp-Lang Path, Early Childhood Intervention Ft Worth State Sch, **SLP**

Brown, Mrs Beverly J 2525 Erie Street, Bellingham, WA 98226, (206) 676-6514, BS 76 Univ of WI - Oshkosh; MS 78 Univ of WI - Madison; 88–Sp-Lang Path, Bellingham Sch Dist, **SLP**

Brown, Beverly P 1648 Farrier Trail, Clearwater, FL 34625, (813) 796-2734, MS 72 Univ of South FL; **SLP**

Brown, Mrs Bonnie Kositzky c/o The Sydney Ross Co Y, Cia (Ltda), Casilla 163-D, Santiago, Chile, BA 64 Univ of MT; MA 70 Univ of MT; **SLP**

Brown, C Rebecca 3737 Atlantic Avenue #607A, Long Beach, CA 90807, BS 36 Drake Univ; **LM**

Brown, Carol A 225 Coffee Road #14D, Lynchburg, VA 24503, (804) 846-4626, BS 76 Univ of the DC; MS 83 Howard Univ; PH 88 (NS) Univ of VA - Charlottesville; Sp-Lang Path, Express Yourself, **SLP ACE**

Brown, Mrs Carol A 1704 Lincoln Street, Camp Hill, PA 17011, (717) 737-6728, BA 78 Towson St Univ; MS 79 Towson St Univ; SLP, Capital Area Intermediate Unit, **SLP**

Brown, Carol Anne 3235 S 14th Street #4, Lincoln, NE 68502, (402) 489-7102, BS 84 Univ of NE - Lincoln; MS 86 Univ of TX - Dallas; SLP, Madonna Centers, **SLP**

Brown, Carol D 3475 Brokenhill Street, Newbury Park, CA 91320, **SLP**

Brown, Carol Jean 7254 Paul Street, Pigeon, MI 48755, (517) 269-9274, BS 80 Northwest MO St Univ; MS 81 Northwest MO St Univ; Preprimary Imp Tchr, Huron ISD, **SLP**

Brown, Carol Lynn 5960 Dixie Lane, Alexandria, LA 71301-2426, MA 80 Northwestern St Univ; **SLP**

Brown, Mrs Carol T 2673 Ashley Court, Tremont, IL 61568, (309) 925-5650, BS 66 Univ of IL - Urbana; MA 70 Univ of IL - Urbana; **SLP**

Brown, Dr Carolyn J 1135 Melrose Avenue, Iowa City, IA 52240, (319) 353-4304, BS 76 Eastern NM Univ; MS 77 Eastern NM Univ; PH 81 (NS) Univ of IA; Reserach Sci, Univ of Iowa, **SLP**

Brown, Carolyn Marie 8511 22nd Avenue #18, Kenosha, WI 53140, (414) 694-8087, BS 84 Univ of WI - Oshkosh; MS 86 Univ of WI - Oshkosh; Sp-Lang Path, Kenosha USD, **SLP**

Brown, Dr Catherine S 1075 Lewisville Clemmons Road, Lewisville, NC 27023, (919) 760-5770, BA 69 Univ of SD - Vermillion; MA 72 Univ of OK Medical Center; PH 79 (Communication Disorders) Univ of OK Medical Center; 87–Dept Head of Sp-Lang Path, John C Whitaker Reg Rehab Ctr, **SLP**

Brown, Cheryl Ann Audiology Associates, 2 Wellman Avenue, Nashua, NH 03060, (603) 880-4499, BA 84 SUNY - Coll at Plattsburgh; MA 85 SUNY - Coll at Plattsburgh; Owner, Aud Assoc, **A**

Brown, Cheryl Annette Route 4 Box 129, Summerville, GA 30747, (404) 226-4623, OM 85 Auburn Univ - Auburn; **SLP**

Brown, Christina M 9717 Chapala N E, Albuquerque, NM 87111, (505) 296-5693, BA 78 IN Univ - Bloomington; MA 81 Northwestern Univ; Sp-Lang Path, Private Practice-Christina M Brown, **SLP**

Brown, Mrs Christine 215 Hembree Road, Roswell, GA 30075, BS 74 FL St Univ; MS 75 FL St Univ; Sp-Lang Path, Fulton Co Bd of Ed, **SLP**

Brown, Mrs Claire E 4026 Flandre Cove Court, Florissant, MO 63034, (314) 921-7853, BS 70 Univ of KS; MA 72 Univ of KS; **SLP**

Brown, Colleen Kenny 10930 Sahler Street, Omaha, NE 68164, (402) 551-3528, BS 73 Univ of NE - Omaha; MS 75 Univ of NE - Omaha; Sp-Lang Path, U NE/Omaha, **SLP**

Brown, Mrs Cynthia Roberson 366 Jefferson, Natchitoches, LA 71457, (318) 352-4098, **SLP**

Brown, David Kenneth Assistant Director-Audiology, University Of Alberta Hospital, 8440-112th Street, Edmonton, AB, Canada T6G 2B7, (403) 432-8859, BA 81 Western WA Univ; MA 84 Western WA Univ; 88–Aud, Univ of Alberta Hosp, **A**

Brown, David Russell P O Box 1302, Santa Teresa, NM 88008, (505) 589-1570, SLP, Regional 19 County Coop, **SLP**

Brown, Mrs Deborah Landry 2501 West Pearl Drive, Marrero, LA 70072, (504) 340-0417, **SLP**

Brown, Mrs Deborah M 2913 Salford Drive, Abingdon, MD 21009, (301) 668-3300, BS 75 SUNY - Center at Albany; MS 77 SUNY - Center at Albany; Sp/Lang Path, Charles Hickey Jr Sch, **SLP**

Brown, Debra A Walnut Valley Unified Sch Dist, 880 South Lemon, Walnut, CA 91789, (714) 595-1261, BA 73 CA St Univ - Chico; MA 75 Whittier Coll; Prog Spec, Walnut Valley USD, **SLP**

Brown, Debra J 8600 East Alameda, Bldg 20 #206, Denver, CO 80231, (303) 861-0504, BA 72 CUNY - Hunter Coll; MS 74 Columbia Univ Teachers Coll; Sp-Lang Path, Spalding Rehabilitation Hosp, **SLP**

Brown, Mrs Debra L 2110 Ridge Drive #23, St Louis Park, MN 55416, (612) 593-1180, BA 80 Univ of RI; MS 82 Univ of WI - Madison; SLP, Anoka-Hennedin Sch Dist, **SLP**

Brown, Mrs Debra Mines 929 Maplecrest Drive, North Bellmore, NY 11710, (301) 341-6448, BS 76 PA St Univ - Univ Park; MA 77 George Washington Univ; Rehab Coord, Private Pracome Care Serv, **SLP**

Brown, Debra V 1125 St Christopher Drive, Apartment 60, Russell, KY 41169-1559, (606) 324-0465, BA 84 Univ of Louisville; MS 87 Univ of Louisville; 87–Sp-Lang Path, Geiger Easter Seal Sp & Hrng Ctr

Brown, Dr Denice P 2633 Arbuckle, Houston, TX 77005, (713) 797-4194, BS 75 TX Tech Univ; MS 76 TX Tech Univ; PH 83 (Aud) Baylor Coll of Medicine; Aud, Hermann Hosp, **A ACE**

Brown, Diane D 4650 175th Avenue S E, Issaquah, WA 98027, (800) 343-1238, BS 71 WV Univ; MS 73 WV Univ; Reg Mgr, New Medico Head Injury System, **SLP**

Brown, Diane L Audiology (117), VA Medical Center, South Lincoln Avenue, Lebanon, PA 17042, (717) 272-6621, BS 69 Western IL Univ; MA 70 Western IL Univ; Aud, VA Med Cen, **A**

Brown, Mrs Diane Lynn 6500 Gray Fox Curve, Chanhassen, MN 55317, (612) 339-0304, BS 80 Univ of IA; MA 81 Univ of IA; Aud, ENT Prof Assoc Ltd, **A**

Brown, Donna Glaser 70 Rock Street, Norwood, MA 02062-4244, (617) 344-0600, BS 80 Ithaca Coll; MS 83 Emerson Coll; Sp/Lang Path, New England Sinai Hosp, **SLP**

Brown, Mrs Donna J R 2408 Lawndale Drive, Greensboro, NC 27408, (919) 288-7964, BS 78 Auburn Univ - Auburn; OM 79 Auburn Univ - Auburn; 87–Sp-Lang Path, Michael Gerard Inc, **SLP**

Brown, Donna M 1420 11th Street Drive N W, #14, Hickory, NC 28601, (704) 322-1975, BS 73 WV Univ; MS 75 Univ of Southwestern LA; Sp-Lang Path/Team Leader, N C St Div of Hlth Serv, **SLP**

Brown, Mrs Donna S Box 6237, Vero Beach, FL 32961, (305) 562-7752, BA 74 Univ of CT; MA 77 Hofstra Univ; Sp-Lang Path, Private Practice, **SLP ACE**

Brown, Donna U Route 3 Box 3950, Holts Summit, MO 65043, **SLP**

Brown, Douglas G St Josephs Hospital Acu, 301 Prospect Avenue, Syracuse, NY 13203, (315) 448-5500, BA 73 SUNY - Coll at Plattsburgh; ME 74 Syracuse Univ; Owner, Private Practice, **A**

Brown, Earl J 11516 Bedfordshire Avenue, Potomac, MD 20854, (202) 295-4665, BS 57 Kent St Univ; MA 68 Univ of MD - College Park; 72–Chief Audiology Division, Bethesda Naval Hosp/Dept Otol, **SLP A ACE**

Brown, Mrs Elizabeth PO Box 62, Mandeville, LA 70470-0062, (504) 626-7269, BA 71 Southeastern LA Univ; OM 75 LA St Univ - N O Medical Ctr; **SLP**

Brown, Elizabeth A 3223 Westport Road, Peoria, IL 61615, (309) 672-6340, BS 77 IL St Univ - Normal; MS 78 Univ of MI - Ann Arbor; 82–Sp-Lang Path, UCP Central IL, **SLP**

Brown, Elizabeth A H 4033 Sunset Boulevard, Los Angeles, CA 90029, (818) 840-7908, BS 75; MS 79 CA St Univ - Los Angeles; 86–Sp-Lang Path, St Joseph Med Ctr, **SLP**

Brown, Ellen R 2054 Legion Street, Bellmore, NY 11710, (516) 544-2237, BA 82 Adelphi Univ; MS 84 Adelphi Univ; Sp-Lang Path, Kings Prk Psych Cen, **SLP**

Brown, Eloise Furiga 706 Glen Allen Drive, Baltimore, MD 21229, (301) 325-7015, BS 72 WV Univ; MA 74 Central MI Univ; Aud, Baltimore Co Bd of Ed, **A**

Brown, Mrs Frances T 6152 Shamrock Drive S E, Covington, GA 30209, (404) 483-8713, BS 73 Univ of GA; ME 74 Univ of GA; 81–Sp-Lang Path, Rockdale Co Bd of Ed, **SLP**

Brown, Gail Ann 679 West 239th Street, Bronx, NY 10463, (212) 884-6861, BA 68 CUNY - City College; MA 70 CUNY - City College; Cl Assoc, Private Practice, **SLP**

Brown, Mrs Gail Berger 40 Raily Court, Staten Island, NY 10312, (212) 683-6970, BA 80 CUNY - Brooklyn Coll; MS 85 CUNY - Brooklyn Coll; 81–Sp-Lang Path, NYC Bd of Educ Speech Svcs

Brown, Gail F 1909 Livingston, Evanston, IL 60201, (312) 492-1754, BA 72 MI St Univ; MA 73 Univ of FL; Aud, **A**

Brown, Gale M 118 Pecan, Buda, TX 78610, (512) 268-1110, BS 72 NM St Univ; MA 74 NM St Univ; 86–Sp-Lang Path, Hays-Blanco Spec Educ Coop, **SLP**

Brown, George D 5700 Carbon Canyon Road, Space 124, Brea, CA 92621, (714) 983-9501, OB 55; BA 49 Chapman Coll; BA 72 CA St Univ - Los Angeles; Sp-Lang Path, Ontario-Montclair Sch Dist, **SLP**

Brown, Georgia C 4972 Rue Le Mans, San Jose, CA 95136-3380, (408) 289-8909, BS 77 Coll of Saint Rose; MS 78 Coll of Saint Rose; Sp/Lang Path, Private Practice, **SLP**

Brown, Geraldine Harris 7821 Camino Tranquilo, San Diego, CA 92122, (619) 293-8158, **SLP**

Brown, Mrs Ginger Hargis 2640 Solon Drive, Nashville, TN 37206, (615) 259-8702, BS 74 Middle TN St Univ; MA 79 Memphis St Univ; Sp-Lang Path, Metropolitan Nashville Schools, **SLP**

Brown, Gwen T 806 Maple Street, Spartanburg, SC 29302, (803) 582-1802, BA 75 Univ of SC - Columbia; MS 79 Univ of SC - Columbia; Sp-Lang Path, Spartanburg Cty Publ Schs, **SLP**

Brown, Harriet Patricia 2731 Blairstone Road #124, Tallahassee, FL 32301, (904) 656-7996, BS 71 Hampton Univ; MA 73 Case Western Reserve Univ; OD 88 (JD-Law) Tulane Univ; 88–Law Clerk, Advocacy Center Inc, **SLP**

Brown, Heather L 3205 Royal Huntsman Court, South Bend, IN 46637, (219) 234-3136, BS 73 Purdue Univ - West Lafayette; MS 76 Purdue Univ - West Lafayette; Program Director, Hrng & Sp Ctr of St Joseph Co, **SLP**

Brown, Mrs Helen E D 2330 Ashland Avenue, Santa Monica, CA 90405, (213) 967-2806, BA 73 CA St Univ - Northridge; MA 75 CA St Univ - Northridge; SLP, Los Angeles Co Supt of Sch, **SLP LM**

Brown, Jack B 11 Elderberry Lane, Valley Stream, Long Island, NY 11580, (212) 240-6441, BA 61 CUNY - Brooklyn Coll; MA 68 CUNY - Brooklyn Coll; Dir:, Ctr for Improved Comm, **SLP A**

Brown, Mrs Jacqueline Anita 2402 Parliament Drive, Abingdon, MD 21009, (301) 838-7300, BS 84 Towson St Univ; MS 86 Towson St Univ; **SLP**

Brown, Jacqueline M 2237 N W 61st, Seattle, WA 98107, (206) 324-6293, **SLP**

Brown, Jan Rutledge 2532 Via Avenida, Carrollton, TX 75006, (214) 245-4206, BA 76 Our Lady Lake Univ-San Anton; MS 79 0897; Aud, W R Kirkham MD & Assoc, **A**

Brown, Jane A 104 Atwood Avenue, Newtonville, MA 02160, (617) 289-9200, BS 52 Boston Univ; MS 69 Boston Univ; OM 80 Boston Univ; Revere Pub Sch, **SLP ACE**

Brown, Mrs Jane Hughes 610 Cranfield Court, Katy, TX 77450, (405) 341-7927, BS 72 Northern IL Univ - De Kalb; MA 73 Northern IL Univ - De Kalb; **SLP**

Brown, Jane L Wommack Rt 10 Box 85, Asheboro, NC 27203, (919) 626-0342, BA 73 Randolph-Macon Woman's Coll; ME 81 Univ of NC - Greensboro; **SLP**

Brown, Janet Ann 1005 S E 40th Street #7, Cape Coral, FL 33904, (813) 549-6230, BA 81 Bethel Coll; MA 85 Northeast MO St Univ; **SLP**

Brown, Janet Barnett 205 Lancashire Drive, Bossier City, LA 71111, (318) 221-1712, **SLP**

Brown, Janet E 1732 Baldwin Drive, Mc Lean, VA 22101, (202) 745-8270, BA 74; MA 78 Catholic Univ of America; Res Sp-Lang Path, VA Med Cen, **SLP**

Brown, Dr Jean B Vocal Point Therapies Inc, 3900 Juan Tabo N E, Suite 17, Albuquerque, NM 87111, (505) 275-2079, BA 73 Memphis St Univ; MA 74 Memphis St Univ; PH 81 (NS) Memphis St Univ; Dir-Priv Prac, Vocal Point Therapies Inc, **SLP A ACE**

Brown, Jean C 505 West Baseline Rd #2032, Tempe, AZ 85283, (602) 831-1695, BS 77 Univ of TN - Knoxville; MA 79 Univ of Montevallo; Sp-Lang Path, Gulf Coast Ment Hlth Cen, **SLP**

Brown, Mrs Jean Puppe Route 7 Box 62-E, Lynchburg, VA 24503, BS 60 Univ of NE - Lincoln; MA 65 Univ of NE - Lincoln; Sp-Lang Path, Lynchburg Cty Sch, **SLP**

Brown, Jeffrey L Rd 1 Box 66B, Sigel, PA 15860, (814) 782-3011, BS 76 Clarion Univ of PA; ME 77 Clarion Univ of PA; Sp-Lang Path, Clarion Manor Intermed Unit 6, **SLP**

Brown, Jennifer L 2930 International Drive, Apartment 217-B, Ypsilanti, MI 48197, (313) 572-2744, BA 76 Univ of MI - Ann Arbor; MA 77 Eastern MI Univ; Sp-Lang Path, St Joseph Mercy Hosp, **SLP**

Brown, Dr Jerome D 3077 S E 100th Street, Runnells, IA 50237, (515) 281-3176, BA 63 Kearney St Coll; MA 68 Univ of NE - Lincoln; PH 78 (NS) IA St Univ; 71–Consult-Spec Educ Admin Svcs, IA Dept of Educ, **A F**

Brown, Joan C 140-26 Asch Loop, Bronx, NY 10475, (212) 320-0619, BA 57 CUNY - Hunter Coll; MA 68 CUNY - Brooklyn Coll; Sp-Lang Path, New York City Board of Educ, **SLP**

Brown, Mrs Joan M 20973 Alpine Avenue, Port Charlotte, FL 33952, (813) 343-9731, BS 70 Purdue Univ - West Lafayette; MA 72 CA St Univ - Long Beach; 85–Sp-Lang Path, Assoc Rehab Serv, **SLP**

Brown, Mrs Joan Moede 6125 Beard Avenue, Edina, MN 55410, (612) 348-8412, BA 52 Grinnell Coll; MA 62 Univ of MN - Minneap-St Paul; SLP, Minneapolis Public Schools, **SLP**

Brown, Mrs Joanne M 11301 Alms House Court, Fairfax Station, VA 22039, (703) 246-7120, BA 64 WA St Univ; MA 81 George Washington Univ; Sp-Lang Path, Fairfax County Health Dept, **SLP**

Brown, Dr Jonathan R 234 Ridgewood Road, Shippenville, PA 16254-0065, (814) 782-3011, BS 73 Edinboro Univ of PA; MA 74 Kent St Univ; PH 85 (NS) PA St Univ - Univ Park; Asst Professor of Audiology, State University of New York, **A**

Brown, Mrs Judith Ann 121 Clarendon Terrace, Newington, CT 06111, (203) 666-4687, BA 61 MacMurray Coll; MA 63 Univ of CT; 64–Sp-Lang Path, Newington Ct Sch Sys, **SLP**

Brown, Judith Ann Route 1 Box 376-H, Farmington, MO 63640, (314) 756-1113, BS 74 Southwest MO St Univ; MS 83 Southern IL Univ -Carbondale; SLP, Farmington R-Vii Schs, **SLP**

Brown, Mrs Judy Anne 223 Strickler Avenue, Waynesboro, PA 17268, (301) 582-2266, BS 80 East Stroudsburg Univ of PA; MS 84 Bloomsburg Univ of PA; Sp-Lang Path, Wash Co Boe, **SLP**

Brown, Judy H 538 Madison Street, New Orleans, LA 70116, (504) 522-0162, BA 56 Agnes Scott Coll; ME 57 Emory Univ; **SLP**

Brown, Mrs Julie Anne 3332-A South 12th Street, Milwaukee, WI 53215, (414) 259-1414, BS 83 Univ of WI - Milwaukee; MS 85 Univ of WI - Milwaukee; **SLP**

Brown, Mrs Karen Clinton University Of Texas, Callier Center, 1966 Inwood Road, Dallas, TX 75235, (214) 905-3008, BA 76 Univ Southern MS-Hattiesburg; MA 78 Univ of TX - Dallas; Proj Supvr, Univ of Texas of Dallas, **A**

Brown, Karen D 22854 Calvert Street, Woodland Hills, CA 91367-5024, (805) 497-3516, BA 78 Univ of CA - Santa Barbara; MA 81 CA St Univ - Northridge; SLP, Conejo Valley USD, **SLP**

Brown, Karen Elman 22 Jenny Lane, Jackson, NJ 08527, (201) 363-0698, BS 80 Trenton St Coll; MA 83 Trenton St Coll; Sp-Lang Path, Monmouth Cnty Day Training Cen, **SLP**

Brown, Karen J 284 Hickory Boulevard, Des Moines, IA 50317, (515) 262-3197, BA 69 Mary Washington Coll; ME 70 Univ of VA - Charlottesville; 80–Sp-Lang Path, Heartland AEA, **SLP**

Brown, Mrs Karen J 22 Winterberry Court, Peekskill, NY 10566, BA 80 Russell Sage Coll; MA 86 CUNY - Lehman Coll; **SLP**

Brown, Mrs Karissa Taylor 10021 Joel Avenue, River Ridge, LA 70123, (504) 822-9316, BS 83 Univ Southern MS-Hattiesburg; MS 84 Univ Southern MS-Hattiesburg; Sp-Lang Path, Jefferson Sp & Lang Ctr, **SLP**

Brown, Mrs Kathleen Cross 124 Shirley Street, Route 15, Kingsport, TN 37660, (615) 378-3566, BA 78 Univ of MT; MA 81 Temple Univ; 87–Sp-Lang Path, Mountain Region Sp & Hrng Ctr, **SLP**

Brown, Kathleen H 1236 Glencove Road North, Syracuse, NY 13206, (315) 656-7222, BS 70 Nazareth Coll of Rochester; MS 77 Ithaca Coll; Sp/Lang Path, E Syracuse Minoa Ctrl Schs, **SLP**

Brown, Mrs Kathleen R RR 31 Box 758, Terre Haute, IN 47803, (812) 894-2557, BS 85 IN St Univ - Terre Haute; MS 86 IN St Univ - Terre Haute; Sp-Lang Path, Union Hosp, **SLP**

Brown, Mrs Kathleen Wright 2805 Hollymead Drive, Charlottesville, VA 22901, (804) 973-9322, ME 84 Univ of VA - Charlottesville; **SLP**

Brown, Mrs Kathy Taylor 12143 Old Country Road, Wellington, FL 33414, (407) 798-6217, BS 69 Ithaca Coll; MA 71 NY Univ; 88–Tchr, Assoc for Retarded Citizens-Wellington Pre-Sch

Brown, Keith O Marion Esd, 3400 Portland Road N E, Salem, OR 97303, (503) 588-5124, BA 66 Central WA Univ; MS 70 Univ of WY; Coord, Marion Ed Serv Dist, **SLP**

Brown, Kimberly Ann 2 Sherman Terrace, Apartment 5, Madison, WI 53704, (608) 255-7878, BS 83 Univ of WI - Madison; MS 85 Univ of WI - Madison; **A**

Brown, Mrs Kimberly Demary 1732 Orrington Avenue #3W, Evanston, IL 60201, (312) 346-1136, BS 83 Marquette Univ; MA 85 Northwestern Univ; Aud, Charles A Lowe & Assoc, **A**

Brown, Laurel Jean 1210 South Highland, Tacoma, WA 98465, (206) 472-6454, BS 72 Portland St Univ; MS 73 Portland St Univ; 83–Sp-Lang Path, Private Practice, **SLP**

Brown, Laurel O Murray-Cottonwood Sp & Lang, 5311 Lucky Clover Lane, Murray, UT 84123, (801) 261-4221, BS 75 Brigham Young Univ; OM 76 Brigham Young Univ; Sp-Lang Path, Murray-Cottonwood Spec & Lang, **SLP**

Brown, Lauren Krimsky 1220 Michael Hughes N E, Albuquerque, NM 87112, (405) 224-2022, BS 80 Univ of AZ; MS 82 Univ of OK Medical Center; Sp-Lang Path, Grady Co Guidance Ctr, **SLP ACE**

Brown, Lauretha V 1370 Nash, Ypsilanti, MI 48198, (313) 485-3384, BS 86 Eastern MI Univ; MA 88 Eastern MI Univ

Brown, Mrs Laurie McPhillips 1867 Loyola Court, Chula Vista, CA 92013, (619) 421-7740, BA 76 CA St Univ - Los Angeles; MS 84 Univ of LA Verne; **SLP**

Brown, Mrs Lavergne B 4663 Cordoba Way, Ocean Hills, CA 92056, (818) 896-7402, BA 68 CA St Univ - Northridge; MA 71 CA St Univ - Northridge; Prog Spec, Los Angeles Co Office of Ed, **SLP**

Brown, Mrs Lavonda L 507 Briarcliff, Garland, TX 75043, (214) 681-7457, BS 82 Baylor Univ; MS 83 Baylor Univ; Sp-Lang Path, Private Practice, **SLP**

Brown, Mrs Lenora Harden 4926 W Butler, Chandler, AZ 85224, (602) 961-3345, BA 73 Lake Erie Coll; MA 80 Cleveland St Univ; SLP, Mesa USD, **SLP**

Brown, Mrs Linda Bell Tri-County Hearing Service, 22 North Evans Street, Pottstown, PA 19464, (215) 970-3277, BS 69 Bloomsburg Univ of PA; MA 73 Temple Univ-Tyler Sch of Art; 88–Aud, Tri County Hearing Svc, **A ACE**

Brown, Linda L 37 Gleneagles Court, Dover, DE 19901, **A**

Brown, Lisa C c/o Tribbett, 741 West Gordon Terrace, Chicago, IL 60613-2224, (312) 281-4958, BS 76 Northwestern Univ; MA 78 Northwestern Univ; **SLP**

Brown, Mrs Logan L 6417 Cherrywood, Portage, MI 49081, (616) 674-8091, BS 66 Western MI Univ; MA 71 Western MI Univ; Sp-Lang Path, Van Buren ISD, **SLP**

Brown, Lois A 129 Oak Forest Circle, Charlottesville, VA 22901, (804) 296-5885, BS 60 Northern IL Univ - De Kalb; MS 64 Univ of KS; Sp-Lang-Hrng Spec, Albermarle Co Sch, **SLP**

Brown, Lorena Ann 134 Timberline Drive, Savannah, GA 31404, (912) 354-0927, BS 77 SUNY - Coll at Buffalo; ME 86 Armstrong St Coll; 83–Sp-Lang Path, Savannah-Chatham Bd of Educ, **SLP**

Brown, Dr Loretta G 1419 Clermont Drive, Birmingham, AL 35209, (205) 665-6720, BA 47 Birmingham-Southern Coll; MA 55 Univ of AL- Tuscaloosa; ED 71 (NS) Univ of AL-Tuscaloosa; Sp-Lang Path, Univ of Montevallo, **SLP F**

Brown, Mrs Louise G Route 3 Box 38H, Columbus, MS 39429, (601) 736-2216, BS 72 Univ Southern MS-Hattiesburg; MS 73 Univ Southern MS-Hattiesburg; Sp-Lang Path, Columbia City School System, **SLP**

Brown, Luann 3158-80 Berry Lane S W, Roanoke, VA 24018, (703) 989-9432, BS 83 CA Univ of PA; MS 84 CA Univ of PA; **SLP**

Brown, Mrs Lynne M 1235 Seminole Drive, Richardson, TX 75080, MS 77 CO St Univ; 87–Sp-Lang Path, UTN-Callier Ctr, **SLP**

Brown, Mrs Madeline G Ctrl Florida Clinic For Rehab, 1315 North Van Nortwick Road, Lecanto, FL 32661, (904) 795-1033, BA 73 Univ of MS; OM 74 Univ of MS; Admin/Sp/Lang Path, Ctrl FL Cl for Rehab, **SLP**

Brown, Marcia Jean 2238 Logan Street, Murphysboro, IL 62966, (318) 687-2510, BS 77 Fontbonne Coll; ME 81 Southeast MO St Univ; Graduate Fellowship, Southern Illinois University, **SLP**

Brown, Marcia Linda 1334 Fort Stevens Drive N W, Apartment 302, Washington, DC 20011, (301) 496-4733, BA 76 Univ of MD - College Park; MA 79 Hampton Univ; Sp-Lang Path, NIH, **SLP**

Brown, Marcie V 22698 Essex Way, Southfield, MI 48034, (813) 858-8111, BS 76 Wayne St Univ; MA 80 Wayne St Univ; Aud, Private Practice, **A**

Brown, Marianne Kathryn 5842 Marshall Drive, Huntington Beach, CA 92649, (213) 337-1820, BS 85 Bloomsburg Univ of PA; MS 86 Bloomsburg Univ of PA; Sp-Lang Path, InSpeech Inc, **SLP**

Brown, Mrs Marilyn K 21300 Almar Drive, Shaker Heights, OH 44122, (216) 561-2714, BA 69 OH Wesleyan Univ; MA 72 Case Western Reserve Univ; Sp-Lang Path, Private Practice, **SLP**

Brown, Marsha P O Box 1001, Cleveland, TN 37364-1001, (615) 472-5521, BS 77 Univ of TN - Knoxville; MS 81 Univ of TN - Knoxville; Self Employed, **SLP**

Brown, Mrs Marsha A 25930 Narbonne Avenue #110, Lomita, CA 90717, (213) 326-6755, OB 77 Univ of MN - Duluth; MA 78 Univ of MN - Duluth; Sp-Lang Path, Los Angeles Office of Educ, **SLP**

Brown, Martha B 304 Pritchard Avenue, Chapel Hill, NC 27516, (919) 929-6914, BA 70 Greensboro Coll; ME 71 Univ of SC - Columbia; Sp-Lang Path, Private Practice, **SLP**

Brown, Mary Beth P O Box 386, Norway, SC 29113, (803) 534-8081, BA 76 Columbia Coll; MS 77 Univ of SC - Columbia; Sp-Lang Path, Edisto District Schools #4, **SLP**

Brown, Mrs Mary E 6518 East Indigo Street, Mesa, AZ 85205, (602) 985-2842, BS 85 AZ St Univ; MS 87 AZ St Univ; 88–Aud, Aud & Hrng Aid Ctr Ltd, **A**

Brown, Mrs Mary Ellen 219 Westridge Drive, Tallahassee, FL 32304, (904) 893-8743, MS 86 FL St Univ; **SLP**

Brown, Mary J S 3 Shellwood Drive, Rochester, NY 14618, (315) 923-2881, BA 55 Univ of MI - Ann Arbor; MS 77 SUNY - Coll at Geneseo; 70–Sp-Lang Path, Wayne-Finger Lakes BOCES, **SLP**

Brown, Melba V 5439 Ocean View Boulevard, La Canada, CA 91011, (213) 248-7912, BS 38 Los Angeles CO Med Ctr; PH 62 Univ of CA - Los Angeles; MA 61 CA St Univ - Los Angeles; **A LM**

Brown, Mrs Melissa Bengtson 636 16th, Clarkston, WA 99403, (208) 743-6421, BS 82 Brigham Young Univ; MA 84 WA St Univ; 88–Sp-Lang Path, Lewiston PS Dist, **SLP**

Brown, Michael J 635 Leslie Lane, Schaumburg, IL 60194, (312) 885-7316, BS 65 De Paul Univ; MA 68 De Paul Univ; Sp-Lang Path, School District 54, **SLP**

Brown, Michael Patrick ENT Department, 101 West University, Champaign, IL 61820, (216) 351-1243, MS 82 Purdue Univ - West Lafayette; Director of Aud, Christie Clinic, **A**

Brown, Michele G 371 North Lincoln Avenue, Villa Park, IL 60181, (312) 677-9600, BS 83 Northern IL Univ - De Kalb; MA 86 IL St Univ - Normal; **A**

Brown, Muriel Ronee 1122 South 60th Street, Philadelphia, PA 19143, (215) 567-4675, BA 79 Temple Univ-Tyler Sch of Art; MA 81 Temple Univ-Tyler Sch of Art; Aud, ENT Prof Assoc/De Valley, **A**

Brown, Mrs Pamela H 3108 Northeast Colonial Dr, Lawton, OK 73507, (405) 355-4871, BS 75 Southwest TX St Univ; ME 76 Southwest TX St Univ; Owner-Cl, Private Practice, **SLP**

Brown, Pamela I 6549 Quiet Hours #102, Columbia, MD 21045, (301) 596-4856

Brown, Mrs Patricia A 2904 Twickingham, Muncie, IN 47304, (317) 747-5437, BS 76 Ball St Univ; MA 80 Ball St Univ; Sp-Lang Path, Muncie Comm Schs, **SLP**

Brown, Patricia Benson 1222 Northwestern Street, Perryton, TX 79070, (806) 435-5762, BS 72 West TX St Univ; MA 75 West TX St Univ; 75–Sp-Lang Path, Perryton ISD, **SLP**

Brown, Patricia S 15700 Lexington Boulevard, Apartment #1502, Sugar Land, TX 77478-4172, (409) 886-5920, BS 50 Muskingum Coll; MS 78 Lamar Univ; Sp/Lang Path, West Orange Cove ISD, **SLP**

Brown, Paula Christine 6197 Michael Kenny Lane, Dublin, OH 43017, (614) 457-1548, BS 21 Ashland Coll; MS 86 Rutgers St Univ - Newark; SLP, Afiliated Aud & S/P, **SLP**

Brown, Dr Paula M 40 Coral Way, Rochester, NY 14618, (716) 475-6262, BA 72 Univ of MO - Columbia; MA 74 Kent St Univ; PH 85 (NS) Univ of Rochester; SLP, Rochester I of Tech, **SLP**

Brown, Penny B 598 Woodland Drive, Rich Creek, VA 24147, (703) 921-2711, BA 77 Marshall Univ; MA 78 Marshall Univ; Sp-Lang Path, Mercer Co Bd of Ed, **SLP**

Brown, Phyllis Franke 52897 Timberland Drive, Granger, IN 46530, (219) 272-3957, BA 38 Univ of IA; MA 39 Univ of IA; Retired, **SLP LM**

Brown, Ralph Elton c/o Swaziland Desk Officer, Peace Corps, 806 Connecticut Avenue N W, Washington, DC 20526, BA 74 GA Southern Coll; ME 83 Univ of GA; Sp-Lang Path, Private Practice, **SLP**

Brown, Mrs Rebecca Rhodes 11471 South Douglas Avenue, Jenks, OK 74037, (918) 622-7064, BS 80 OK St Univ; MA 82 Univ of Tulsa; Sp-Lang Path, Assoc Sp & Hrng Services, **SLP**

Brown, Rhea Strauss 8944 Nottingham Place, La Jolla, CA 92037, (619) 221-3753, BS 69 Univ of IL - Urbana; MA 80 Univ of Cincinnati; 88–Sp-Lang Path, Sharp Cabrillo Hosp, **SLP**

Brown, Rhomas Jacqueline 42 Brinkerhoff Street, Jersey City, NJ 07304, **SLP**

Brown, Richard K 416 Van Buren Avenue South, Edina, MN 55343, (612) 933-6616, BA 68 CA St Univ - Long Beach; MA 69 CA St Univ - Long Beach; 88–Aud, Automated Comm Inc, **A**

Brown, Dr Robert A Associated Rehabilitative Services, 2495 Caring Way Suite C, Port Charlotte, FL 33952, (813) 629-1814, BS 68 Miami Univ - Oxford; MA 73 CA St Univ - Long Beach; PH 76 (NS) OH Univ - Athens; Admin, Assoc Rehab Serv, **SLP**

Brown, Mrs Robyn A 19 Murray, Waltham, MA 02154, (617) 647-4230, BS 81 Univ of MA - Amherst; MS 83 Boston Univ; Sp-Lang Path, Private Practice, **SLP**

Brown, Mrs Rose M 8304 Cedar Road, Elkins Park, PA 19117, (215) 332-9666, MA 71 Temple Univ-Tyler Sch of Art; **SLP**

Brown, Russell Cooper 3585 Broken Arrow, Silver City, NM 88061, (505) 546-6568, BS 75 TX Christian Univ; MS 76 TX Christian Univ; Sp-Lang Path, Deming Public Schools, **SLP**

Brown, Ruth Elizabeth 2225-F Prior Road, Wilmington, DE 19809, (302) 764-6120, BA 79 Univ of TN - Knoxville; MA 82 Univ of TN - Knoxville; 86–Aud, Riverside Hospital, **A**

Brown, Mrs Sandra A 5811 West 89th Terr, Overland Park, KS 66207, (816) 531-7373, BS 72 KS St Univ; MA 73 KS St Univ; 81–Aud, Otologic Center Inc, **A**

Brown, Mrs Sandra E 245 Fox Run Drive, Northbrook, IL 60062, (312) 673-1222, BS 68 Northwestern Univ; MA 75 Northwestern Univ; **SLP**

Brown, Mrs Sandra L 2621 North 4th Street, Columbus, OH 43202, (614) 262-4678, OB 80 Baylor Univ; MS 82 Univ of AR - Little Rock; **SLP**

Brown, Mrs Sandra Stiles 63 East Washington Street, Jamestown, OH 45335, **SLP**

Brown, Sarah Z 513 N W 39th, Oklahoma City, OK 73118, (405) 521-9590, BA 73 LA St Univ - Baton Rouge; MS 75 Univ of OK Medical Center; **SLP**

Brown, Sharon A 8154 1/2 Troost #66, Kansas City, MO 64131, (816) 276-4023, BS 79 Lincoln Univ; MA 80 OH St Univ; **SLP**

Brown, Sharon Maxine 852 Wright #3, Oshkosh, WI 54901, (414) 236-2230, MS 83 Univ of WI - Oshkosh; 85–Sp-Lang Path, Mercy Medical Center, **SLP**

Brown, Sharon Miller 2907-E South Woodstock St, Arlington, VA 22206, (703) 525-1898, BS 82 Univ of VA - Charlottesville; MS 85 Gallaudet Coll; 85–Aud, Arlington Hearing Center, **A**

Brown, Shelli L Andrews Road, La Grangeville, NY 12540, (914) 223-7227, BA 85 SUNY - Coll at Plattsburgh; MS 86 Bowling Green St Univ; Sp-Lang Path, BOCES Putnam/Northern West, **SLP**

Brown, Sherry B c/o Devel Disabilities Agency, Dept Of Education, P O Box 2565, Saipan, Mariana Islands 96950, (602) 285-3282, BA 78 Univ of Northern CO; MA 79 Univ of Northern CO; Aud, St Joseph's Hosp Barrow Neur I, **A**

Brown, Mrs Shirley R 6 Sisson Terrace, Tenafly, NJ 07670, (201) 894-3286, MA 58 CUNY - Brooklyn Coll; Dir SLP Dept, Englewood Hospital, **SLP ACE**

Brown, Mrs Shirley W 419 Carol Villa Drive, Montgomery, AL 36109, (205) 272-5611, BA 48 Kent St Univ; **SLP**

Brown, Steven L Semo Otolaryngolgy, 17 Doctors Park, Cape Girardeau, MO 63701, (314) 335-4448, BS 78 Univ of North TX; MS 79 Univ of North TX; Aud, Semo Otol, **A**

Brown, Sue Ann 113 North Gleneagles Drive, Wichita, KS 67212, (316) 722-9630, MA 75 Wichita St Univ; BA 73 Wichita St Univ; Sp-Lang Path, Private Practice, **SLP**

Brown, Sue Anne 11925 New Country Lane, Columbia, MD 21044, (301) 992-0500, BS 66 Eastern MI Univ; MA 74 Univ of MD - College Park; Supvr of Sp Lang Hrng Svcs, Howard Co Pub Sch Sys, **SLP**

Brown, Sue Ellen 1999 Nottingham Lane, Wheaton, IL 60187, (312) 469-5220, BS 77 IL St Univ - Normal; MS 79 IL St Univ - Normal; Sp/Lang Path, Glen Ellyn Elem Sch Dist 89, **SLP**

Brown, Mrs Susan Mathews 32811 David Circle, Dana Point, CA 92629, (714) 956-6650, BA 79 Univ of CA - Santa Barbara; MA CA St Univ - Fullerton; Sp-Lang Path, Capistrano USD, **SLP**

Brown, Suzanne 2237 Village Green Parkway, Chesterfield, MO 63017, (314) 432-1108, BS 52 Purdue Univ - West Lafayette; MS 63 Purdue Univ - West Lafayette; SLP, Spec Sch Dist of St Louis Co, **SLP**

Brown, Suzanne Greening 56 Arbor Street, Lunenburg, MA 01462, (508) 772-0200, BA 78 MI St Univ; MS 80 Purdue Univ - West Lafayette; 87–Aud, The Nashoba Comm Hosp, **A**

Brown, Suzanne Logan 1113 Ellis, Fort Collins, CO 80524, OB 68 American Univ; MS 81 Univ of AZ; Consult-Ther, Lang Systems, **SLP**

Brown, Suzanne Redmond 12203 Belaire Place, Maryland Heights, MO 63043, MS 76 Central MO St Univ; Sp-Lang Path, Special School District, **SLP**

Brown, Mrs Suzanne Reid Rd 1 Box 150, Meadow Street, Otego, NY 13825, (607) 865-4116, BA 75 SUNY - Coll at Cortland; MS 78 Ithaca Coll; Sp-Lang Path, Walton Ctl Sch, **SLP**

Brown, Mrs Therian N 119 Ronald Road, Lakewood, NJ 08701, (201) 363-7987, BA 76 Univ of MI - Ann Arbor; MA 80 Wayne St Univ; Audiologist, Riverview Medical Center, **A**

Brown, Thomas Rodger 508 Cedar Forest Court, Nashville, TN 37221-1203, (615) 356-3956, BS 70 Kent St Univ; MA 72 Cleveland St Univ; Major, US Army, **A**

Brown, Tonya Graham 1509-B White Drive, Lee's Summit, MO 64063, (816) 524-6479, BA 85 Southeast MO St Univ; MA 87 Southeast MO St Univ; 87–Sp-Lang Path, Grain Valley R-5 Sch Dist, **SLP**

Brown, Mrs Valerie Leon 106 South Humphrey Avenue, Oak Park, IL 60302, (312) 929-8200, BS 76 Hampton Univ; MA 79 Hampton Univ; 84–Sp-Lang Path, Ctr for Rehab and Trng of Persons with Disab, **SLP**

Brown, Vicki C 100 Beechpoint Drive, Oxford, OH 45056, (513) 523-0396, BA 81 Univ of Southwestern LA; MS 85 Univ of Southwestern LA; Sp-Lang Path, **SLP**

Brown, Vicki Lynn 4669 Walford Road #20, Warrensville Heights, OH 44128, (216) 231-0961, BS 73 OH Univ - Athens; MA 78 Cleveland St Univ; Sp-Lang Path, Cleveland Public Schools, **SLP**

Brown, Mrs Vivian J 1002 Martinez Lane, Colton, CA 92324-6252, (714) 874-4195, BS 78 Trenton St Coll; MS 80 Rutger's St Univ - Douglas Coll; Sp-Lang Path, InSpeech Inc, **SLP**

Brown, Wendi Dempsey HCRS 272A, New Salem, MA 01355, (508) 544-2542, BS 85 Univ of MA - Amherst; MA 87 Univ of MA - Amherst; 87–Sp-Lang Path, Ralph C Mahar Reg Sch, **SLP**

Brown, Dr William J 550 Medical Towers South, Louisville, KY 40202, (502) 583-0189, BS 49 Wilmington Coll; MA 51 Kent St Univ; PH 58 (NS) Syracuse Univ; Aud, Private Practice, **SLP A**

Brown, Dr William S, Jr 1517 N W 19th Street, Gainesville, FL 32605, (904) 392-2046, BS 62 Edinboro Univ of PA; MA 67 SUNY - Center at Buffalo; PH 69 (Sp Science) SUNY - Center at Buffalo; Prof/Sp & Linguistics, U of FL, **F**

Browne, Alan, Jr 210 Fairway Avenue, Belleville, NJ 07109, (201) 266-4325, BA 69 Rutgers St Univ - Newark; MA 75 Seton Hall Univ; Sp-Lang Path, Orange Bd of Ed, **SLP ACE**

Browne, Kelly Dolores 431 Pleasant Ridge Drive, Grand Junction, CO 81503, (605) 472-2400, BA 83 Univ of SD - Vermillion; MA 85 Univ of SD - Vermillion; **SLP**

Browne, Marilyn K 227 South Lark Lane, Wichita, KS 67209, (316) 268-5246, BA 74 Wichita St Univ; MA 76 LA St Univ - Baton Rouge; Sp-Lang Path, St Francis Reg Med Ctr, **SLP**

Browne, Mrs Mary Anne Turner 1785 Providence Farms Lane, Alpharetta, GA 30201, (404) 442-5747, BS 82 Univ of GA; ME 83 Univ of GA; Sp-Lang Path, **SLP**

Browne, Maureen Therese 12648 East Kansas Place, Aurora, CO 80012, (303) 368-7389, BS 85 CO St Univ; MS 86 CO St Univ; 87–Aud, Assoc of Otolaryngology, **A**

Browne, Mrs Nancy P 12110 Waterford Way Place, Richmond, VA 23233, (804) 740-1930, BS 83 Univ Southern MS-Hattiesburg; MS 85 Univ Southern MS-Hattiesburg; Aud, Sheltering Arms Rehab Hosp, **A**

Browne, Tomi Thibodeaux 3260 Wilson Boulevard, Arlington, VA 22201, (703) 525-1898, BS 75 Univ of VA - Charlottesville; ME 76 Univ of VA - Charlottesville; Owner, Arlington Hearing Cen, **A**

Brownell, Mrs Karen J L 804 Eagle Road, Weddington, NC 28173, (704) 843-4125, BS 62 OH Univ - Athens; MA 64 IN Univ - Bloomington; SLP, Total Care Inc, **SLP**

Brownfield, Mrs Janet S 516 North Douglas, Shelbyville, IL 62565, (217) 774-2620, BS 80 IL St Univ - Normal; MS 82 IL St Univ - Normal; 88–Sp-Lang Path, St Mary's Hosp, **SLP**

Brown-Grant, Mrs Elaine L 449 Woodland Road, Highland Park, IL 60035, (312) 433-4868, BS 46 Northwestern Univ; MA 61 Northwestern Univ; Prof Emeritus, Nwn U, **SLP F ACE**

Brown-Herman, Catherine 18 Howard Avenue #1, Tilton, NH 03276, (603) 524-5373, BS 83 SUNY - Coll at Geneseo; MS 87 Univ of NH; 87–Sp-Lang Path, Laconia Dev Svcs, **SLP**

Browning, Ann L Rochester Pediatrics, 224 Peters Road, Knoxville, TN 37923, (615) 693-5016, BS 70; MA 72; Sp-Lang Path, Blount Hrng & Sp Serv, **SLP**

Browning, Mrs Cheryl Virginia 619 West Lee Avenue, Kingsville, TX 78363-4331, (512) 595-3401, BS 74 Univ of North TX; MS 75 Univ of North TX; 87–Dir/Instr-Comm Dis Dept, Texas A&I Univ, **SLP**

Browning, Mrs Denise Dotts 7710 East Brainerd Road, Apartment 314, Chattanooga, TN 37421, (615) 892-3941, BA 81 Univ of Central FL; OM 83 Auburn Univ - Auburn; SLP, Comm Clinic, **SLP ACE**

Browning, Denise Joy 1000 Pine Gate Drive #B-23, Spartanburg, SC 29303-9364, (803) 269-9239, **SLP**

Browning, Dorothea J 26435 West 90th, Lenexa, KS 66227, (913) 441-2115, MA 84 Univ of KS; Sp-Lang Path, Bethany Medical Center, **SLP**

Browning, Janice L 816 27th Street, Cairo, IL 62914, (618) 734-3326, BS 73 Southern IL Univ -Carbondale; ME 81 Southeast MO St Univ; Sp-Lang Path, Cairo Pub Sch, **SLP**

Browning, Julia Elizabeth 2401 N W 122nd #21, Oklahoma City, OK 73120, (405) 752-2025, MS 88 9033

Browning, Mrs Krista B 150 Southampton Drive, Harrisonburg, VA 22801, (703) 433-2479, BS 71 WV Univ; MS 73 WV Univ; 86–SLP Supvr, Woodrow Wilson Rehab Ctr, **SLP**

Browning, Marla Anne P O Box 2325, Conway, NH 03818, (603) 447-3885, BS 82 Bradley Univ; MS 86 Univ of VT; **SLP**

Browning, Michael Box 561, Gilbert, WV 25621, **SLP**

Browning, Mrs Patricia Ann 6115 Johnson Chapel, Brentwood, TN 37027, (314) 443-8709, BS 73 Auburn Univ - Auburn; MS 83 Univ of MO - Columbia; **SLP**

Browning, Tammy Kim 2405 Dulaire Road, Greensboro, NC 27407, (919) 292-4489, MA 88 Appalachian St Univ; 88–Sp-Lang Path, Greensboro PS

Brownlee, Lavinia Joyce 148 West 112th Place, Floor 2, Chicago, IL 60628, (312) 890-8366, BA 72 MI St Univ; MA 81 Wayne St Univ; Sp-Lang Path, Chicago Bd of Ed, **SLP**

Brown-Martin, Mrs Penny I 6717 Hilltop Drive, Brookhaven, PA 19015, (215) 876-7795, BS 74 James Madison Univ; MS 78 James Madison Univ; Sp-Lang Path, Crozer - Chester Med Cen, **SLP**

Brown-Myers, Stephanie 33 Ocho Rios Place, Danville, CA 94526, (415) 820-6815, BA 73 Univ of CA - Santa Barbara; MA 74 CA St Univ - Chico; Sp-Lang Path, San Ramon Valley USD, **SLP**

Brownsberger, Susan L 27 Deerfield Avenue, Milford, CT 06460, (203) 878-1257, BS 83 Western MI Univ; MA 85 Western MI Univ; **SLP**

Brownson, Mariam Allen P O Box 345, Little River, CA 95456, (415) 692-1988, BA 63 Stanford Univ; MA 64 Stanford Univ; Tchr, San Mateo Co Spec Ed Div, **A**

Brownstein, R Dede North Side Audiology Group, 5015 North Paulina Suite 330, Chicago, IL 60640, (312) 784-3277, BA 76 Beloit Coll; MA 85 Northwestern Univ; 86–Aud, North Side Audiology Group, **A**

Brownstein, Shelley L 272 Paxson Lane, Langhorne, PA 19047, (609) 394-4177, BS 76 Trenton St Coll; MS 78 Hahneman Medical Coll; Sp/Lang Path, Mercer Medical Center, **SLP**

Brown-Sweeney, Sharon G 2325 Wood Drive, Northbrook, IL 60062, (312) 272-7935, BA 80 Northwestern Univ; MS 82 Northwestern Univ; Sp/Lang Path, Private Practice, **SLP**

Brown-Young, Kay M 708 West Warren Street, Shelby, NC 28150, **A**

Broy, Mrs Kathleen I 35492 Kenneth Drive, Lake Villa, IL 60046, (312) 362-2900, BS 77 IL St Univ - Normal; MS 79 IL St Univ - Normal; 82–Sp-Lang Path Dir, Broy Sp-Path Assoc, **SLP ACE**

Broyard, Jennifer Bernadette 1930 Annette Street, New Orleans, LA 70116, (504) 527-0400, OM 79 6388; Aud/Sp-Lang Path, Orleans Parish School Board, **SLP A**

Brozgal, Ruth 1501 Hampshire West Court, Apartment 9, Silver Spring, MD 20903, (202) 832-4400, **SLP**

Brozka, Thomas William 4266 West Pioneer #2036, Irving, TX 75061, (214) 570-7400, Sp-Lang Path, Centre for Neuro Skills, **SLP**

Brubacher, Margaret 17 Centre Street #5-C, Mount Vernon, NY 10552, **A**

Brubaker, B J P O Box 900, Aspen, CO 81612, (303) 923-2511, MA 71 OH Univ - Athens; Dir, Aspen Camp Sch for the Deaf, **SLP**

Brubaker, Judith Jones 1920 Lanesboro, Oklahoma City, OK 73120-3928, (405) 755-5375, BS 83 Central St Univ; ME 86 Central St Univ; **SLP**

Brubaker, Lynne E 2870 Manor Road, Coatesville, PA 19320, (215) 486-0800, BS 71 Millersville Univ of PA; ME 75 Bloomsburg Univ of PA; SLP, Commonwealth of PA, **SLP**

Brubaker, Mrs Mary Booth Route 2 Box 231, Crawford, GA 30630, (404) 783-2797, BS 73 Univ of GA; ME 83 Univ of GA; Sp-Lang Path, Madison Co Pub Sch Syst

Brubaker, Susan Howell 2157 Dorchester, Birmingham, MI 48009, (313) 258-1090, BS 72 Saint Lawrence Univ; MS 73 Ithaca Coll; Asst Dept Director, William Beaumont Hospital, **SLP**

Brubaker, Susan L 1424 Fulton Road N W #2, Canton, OH 44703, (216) 455-0726, SLP, Miami Valley Hosp, **SLP**

Bruce, Alice Thompson 4146 Britts Gate Lane, Tucker, GA 30084, (404) 432-9384, BA 80 Emory Univ; BS 80 Emory Univ; OM 82 Emory Univ; Sp/Lang Path, Georgia Baptist Medical Center, **SLP**

Bruce, Alton J, Jr P O Box 1018, Caribou, ME 04736, (207) 498-6431, BA 68 Univ of ME - Orono; MA 73 Univ of ME - Orono; Dir Sp& Hrng, Aroostook Ment Hlth Cen, **SLP**

Bruce, Arden G N W 715 Darrow, Pullman, WA 99163, (509) 456-7086, BA 56 WA St Univ; MA 78 WA St Univ; Sp-Lang Path, Ed Serv Dist 101, **SLP**

Bruce, Mrs Carla Jo 1229 Wenlock Road, Knoxville, TN 37922, (615) 966-5848, **SLP**

Bruce, Mrs Carolyn Walker 2725 Dalkeith Drive, Richmond, VA 23233, (804) 740-3554, BS 75 Vanderbilt Univ; MS 76 Vanderbilt Univ; Sp-Lang Path, **SLP**

Bruce, Christina 500 Bay Green Court, Arnold, MD 21012, (301) 647-3773, **SLP**

Bruce, Clifford E 35 Arbor Drive, Glens Falls, NY 12801, (518) 793-6776, BS 63 IN Univ - Bloomington; MS 66 Saint Joseph's Coll; Owner-Manager, Village Booksmith, **SLP**

Bruce, Mrs Dara A P O Box 14, Junction City, KS 66441, (913) 762-3350, BS 72 KS St Univ; MA 73 KS St Univ; Sp-Lang Path, Junction Cty Sp & Lang Cl, **SLP**

Bruce, Mrs Elvy 1566 Spartan Village #D, East Lansing, MI 48823-5811, (616) 473-2600, BA 71 SC St Coll; MS 72 PA St Univ - Univ Park; Graduate Asst/Aud & Speech Dep, Michigan State University, **SLP**

Bruce, Mrs Helen B 6209 Mineral Point Road, Madison, WI 53705, (608) 233-1002, BA 25 Univ of WI - Madison; **SLP LM**

Bruce, Kaye S 5 Alta Vista, Batesville, AR 72501, (501) 793-6406, BA 67 Univ of AR - Fayetteville; MA 69 Univ of AR - Fayetteville

Bruce, Mary Katherine 2525 East Belleview Place #4, Milwaukee, WI 53211, (414) 527-5109, BS 82 Marquette Univ; MS 84 Marquette Univ; Sp-Lang Path, St Michael Hosp, **SLP**

Bruce, Melissa C 5232 Memorial Drive, Houston, TX 77007, (713) 749-2547, BA 72 Henderson St Univ; MS 74 Purdue Univ - West Lafayette; Coor, U Houston Commun Disorders Prg, **SLP**

Bruce, Nancy Van P O Box 83, Randolph, VT 05060-0083, (802) 728-3397, BA 81 SUNY - Center at Buffalo; MA 84 SUNY - Center at Buffalo; Sp-Lang Path, Inter-Disciplinary Educ Assoc, **SLP**

Bruce, Peter I VA Medical Center, Audiology (126), 135 East 38th Street, Erie, PA 16501, (814) 868-8661, BS 74 Ithaca Coll; MS 75 Ithaca Coll; Chief/Aud & SLP, VA Med Cen, **SLP A**

Bruch, Mrs Rosemary B 193 Crosswicks, Chesterfield Road, Trenton, NJ 08620, (609) 298-3234, BA 69 Rutger's St Univ - Douglas Coll; MS 71 Univ of Pittsburgh - Pittsburgh; Dispensing Audiologist, Penta Hearing Care, **A**

Bruchas, Dr Joan K 3000 Weslayan, Suite 255, Houston, TX 77027, (713) 523-0816, BS 67 Saint Louis Univ; MS 68 Univ of WI - Madison; PH 77 (NS) Univ of Pittsburgh - Pittsburgh; Psychother/Dev Spec, Psychotherapy Consultants, **SLP**

Bruckhart, Mrs Margaret Nissley 9315 Electra Lane, Richmond, VA 23228, (804) 266-3985, BS 63 Millersville Univ of PA; ME 84 Univ of VA - Charlottesville; Sp/Lang Path, Henrico Co Publ Schs, **SLP**

Bruckner, Kristy Sue 1100 Northview Drive #16B, Hillsboro, OH 45133, (513) 393-4234, BS 83 Bowling Green St Univ; MA 84 Bowling Green St Univ; Sp-Lang Path, Hillsboro Sp & Hrng Aid Ctr, **SLP**

Brucks, Jane Ann 3718 Charleston Square, Memphis, TN 38122, (901) 523-8990, BS 76 Central MO St Univ; MS 77 Central MO St Univ; Aud, VA Medical Center, **A**

Brueggemann, David J 234 East 15th Avenue #402, Anchorage, AK 99501, (615) 246-4600, BA 76 Humboldt St Univ; MS 78 Univ of OK Medical Center; Aud, US Publ Hlth Serv, **A ACE**

Bruemmer, Mrs Susan M 4740 Mallard Court, West Richland, WA 99352, (509) 967-3525, BS 75 IL St Univ - Normal; MS 76 Univ of IL - Urbana; Sp-Lang Path, Certified Speech-Lang Services, **SLP**

Bruening, Dr Robert A John Carroll University, University Heights, OH 44118, (216) 491-4378, MA 57 John Carroll Univ; MA 61 Case Western Reserve Univ; PH 72 (NS) Case Western Reserve Univ; Associate Prof Communications, John Carroll University, **SLP**

Bruhn, Mrs Margaret L 11520 Newton, Overland Park, KS 66212, (913) 661-9373, BS 77 Univ of MO - Columbia; MA 78 Univ of MO - Columbia; Sp-Lang Path, Private Practice, **SLP**

Bruhy, Sharon S Bruhy & Associates, Box 238, Hailey, ID 83333, (208) 788-4181, BS 65 Marquette Univ; MS 75 Marquette Univ; Sp-Lang Path, Private Practice, **SLP**

Brukoff, Mrs Bonnie L 3364 Bloomfield Shores Dr, Orchard Lake, MI 48033, (313) 626-6556, BA 62 Barnard Coll; MA 63 Columbia Univ Teachers Coll; Sp-Lang Path, Detroit Pub Sch, **SLP**

Brumbaugh, Mrs Brenda J 8209 Willowhurst Circle N W, North Canton, OH 44720, (216) 833-8497, BS 79 Kent St Univ; MA 80 Kent St Univ; Sp-Lang Path, Perry Local Schs, **SLP**

Brumfield, Mrs Katharine 209 Buford Road, Williamsburg, VA 23185, (804) 565-0977, BA 69 Coll of William & Mary; ME 72 Univ of VA - Charlottesville; Tchr, Sunrise Montessori Sch, **SLP**

Brumfield, Dr Shannon 4333 Loveland, Metairie, LA 70002, (504) 455-5441, BA 68 LA St Univ - Baton Rouge; MA 70 Temple Univ-Tyler Sch of Art; PH 78 (NS) Univ of FL; Sp/Lang Path, Private Practice, **SLP**

Brumm, Robin Ann 1300 South Border Avenue Apartment 2, Inverness, FL 32652, (904) 637-4603, MS 88 Mankato St Univ; 88–Sp-Lang Path, Citrus County PS

Brummer, Mrs Candice L P O Box 429, Corrales, NM 87048, (505) 898-1160, BA 66 Jersey City St Coll; MA 67 Syracuse Univ; **SLP**

Brummett, Mrs Theresa A 335 St Lawrence, Buffalo, NY 14216, (716) 837-2441, BA 78 SUNY - Center at Buffalo; MA 80 SUNY - Center at Buffalo; 87–Coord Preschool Satellites, Language Development Program, **SLP**

Bruneau-Ritterman, Mrs Sharen Forensic Communication Assoc, 181 Ellerbee Road, Wesley Chapel, FL 34249-4202, (813) 973-0504, MS 72 Univ of South FL; Administrator, Forensic Communication Assoc, **A**

Brunelle, Louise 368 DE Lepee Avenue, Montreal, PQ, Canada H2V 3T6, **A**

Brunell-Nelson, Mrs Sheyla Loren 31521 Ganado Road, San Juan Capistrano, CA 92675, (714) 661-1995, BA 77 Chapman Coll; MS 83 Chapman Coll; Sp-Lang Path, New Port Mesa USD, **SLP**

Bruner, Mrs Barbara J Escambia County Schools, 30 East Texar Drive, Pensacola, FL 32503, (904) 432-6121, BS 65 Auburn Univ - Auburn; MS 67 FL St Univ; Coord Sp Lang Imp, Escambia Co Sch Bd, **SLP ACE**

Bruner, Mrs Diane Lynn 10 South Millward Road, Savannah, GA 31410, (912) 355-4601, BA 81 Wichita St Univ; MA 84 Wichita St Univ; Sp-Lang Path, Savannah Speech-Hearing Center, **SLP**

Bruner, Kathryn Ann 3338 E Rotamer Road, Janesville, WI 53545, (414) 241-5530, BS 85 Univ of WI - Whitewater; MS 87 Univ of WI - Whitewater

Bruner, Mrs Marianne 2483 Rebecca Lynn Way, Santa Clara, CA 95050, (408) 265-0353, BA 81 Rutger's St Univ - Douglas Coll; MS 83 Rutgers St Univ -N Brunswick; **SLP**

Bruner, Mrs Thelma J 2635 East 22nd Street, Tulsa, OK 74114, (918) 743-2947, BA 56 Univ of Tulsa; **SLP LM**

Brunette, Gerald Wayne Rt 1 Box 571, Mexia, TX 76667-9745, (817) 562-2821, BS 74 Southwest TX St Univ; MS 76 Gallaudet Coll; 86–Sp-Lang Path, Mexia State Sch, **A**

Brunette, Mrs Kim Garrett 1931 Windsor, Duncan, OK 73533, (405) 255-7326, BS 77 Univ of North TX; MS 82 Univ of OK Medical Center; 88–Sp-Lang Path, Stephens County Guidance Ctr, **SLP**

Brunetti, Mrs Vicki Catherine 3-01 Lyncrest Avenue, Fair Lawn, NJ 07410, (201) 478-2242, BA 73 Rutger's St Univ - Douglas Coll; MS 84 William Paterson Coll; SLP, Garfield Brd of Educ, **SLP**

Brungard, Dr Maude O 136 Cambridge Street, Indiana, PA 15701, (412) 465-2083, BS 35 Lock Haven St Coll; ME 51 PA St Univ - Univ Park; ED 61 (NS) PA St Univ - Univ Park; **SLP A LM**

Brungardt, Mrs Kristie Rae 2103 North Robin Avenue, Duluth, MN 55811, (218) 879-1283, BA 84 Univ of ND; MA 85 Univ of MN - Duluth; Sp-Lang Path, Cloquet Spec Educ Coop, **SLP**

Bruni, Cheryl A 112 Meadow Lane, Kersey, PA 15846, (814) 834-7052, BA 80 Edinboro Univ of PA; MA 84 Marshall Univ; 86–Sp-Lang Path, Elk County Soc For Spec Svcs, **SLP**

Bruning, Mrs Annette Cavalli 1923 Seabrook Drive, Duncanville, TX 75137, (214) 298-3934, MA 77 Our Lady Lake Univ-San Anton; 88–Sp-Lang Path, Private Practice, **SLP**

Brunk, Sakina T 1400 Smokeywood Drive #610, Pittsburgh, PA 15218, (412) 647-5575, BS 76 CA St Univ - Fresno; MS 78 Univ of IL - Urbana; Sp-Lang Path, Chldn Hosp of Pittsburgh, **SLP A**

Brunken, Mrs Cynthia Diane 1230 Wells Court #16, Lincoln, NE 68505, (402) 464-8917, BA 82 Univ of NE - Lincoln; MS 83 Univ of NE - Lincoln; Sp-Lang Path, Lincoln PS, **SLP**

Brunkhardt, Melinda Sue Route #3, Sterling, CO 80751, (303) 522-0996, BA 86 Univ of Northern CO; BA 86 Univ of Northern CO; MA 87 Univ of Northern CO; 87–Sp-Lang Path, RE-1 Valley Sch Dist

Brunner, Barbara Jarboe 33 Bryant Street N E, Washington, DC 20002, (202) 651-5328, BA 82 Univ of MD - College Park; MS 84 Gallaudet Coll; Aud, Gallaudet Univ, **A**

Brunner, Joseph L 5404 Laurelwood Place, Sarasota, FL 34232, (813) 377-6907, BS 70; MA 78; Sp/Lang Path, Brunner Sp Lang Cog Inc, **SLP ACE**

Brunner, Mrs Karen Hoppman 802 Blue Gate Lane, Sinking Spring, PA 19608, (215) 378-6694, BS 81 PA St Univ - Univ Park; MS 83 PA St Univ - Univ Park; 84–Sp-Lang Path, The Reading Hosp and Med Ctr, **SLP**

Brunner, Kathleen Louise 101 Emerson Avenue, Pittsburgh, PA 15215, (412) 782-1131, BS 73 Indiana Univ of PA; ME 76 Indiana Univ of PA; Dir-Sp-Lang Path, Comp Ther Serv, **SLP ACE**

Brunner, Mrs Patty J Rt 5 Box 1060, Rapid City, SD 57701-9311, (605) 393-2577, MA 76 Univ of SD - Vermillion; Sp-Lang Path, Rapid City Sch, **SLP**

Bruno, Mrs Alexandra H 18 Cleary Avenue, Butler, NJ 07405, BA 62 Hofstra Univ; MS 82 William Paterson Coll; Sp-Lang Path, Newark Board of Education, **SLP**

Bruno, Concetta 1925 N E 117th Road, North Miami, FL 33181, (305) 654-5077, BA 74 Univ of FL; MA 75 Univ of FL; Sp-Lang Path, Parkway Regional Medical Ctr, **SLP ACE**

Bruno, J Joan 1120 Hedgecliff Drive, Wooster, OH 44691, (800) 642-8255, BA 73 Marywood Coll; MS 74 PA St Univ - Univ Park; PH 88 (Sp-Lang Path) Temple Univ; 88–Research Assoc, Prentke Romich Co, **SLP**

Bruno, Mrs Janet Kay 9 Lakeview Drive, Lansing, NY 14882, (607) 533-4183, BS 79 SUNY - Coll at Geneseo; MS 82 Ithaca Coll; Sp/Lang Path, Lansing Central Sch, **SLP**

Bruno, Mrs Janet S 51 Alta Mesa Circle, Monterey, CA 93940, BA 59; MA 60; Sp/Lang Path, Montoroy Unif Sch, **SLP**

Bruno, Leonard 1013 Beech Street, East Lansing, MI 48823, (319) 354-5780, **A**

Bruno, Mrs Lorraine Schultz 6 Sylvan Road, Smithtown, NY 11787, (516) 543-5100, BA 78 SUNY - Coll at Cortland; MA 79 Hofstra Univ; Sp-Lang Path, UCP of Suffolk County, **SLP**

Bruno, Mrs Patricia S 1300 S W 17th Street, Fort Lauderdale, FL 33315, (305) 763-2300, BA 59 Fairmont St Coll; MS 68 WV Univ; Sp-Lang Path, ARC of Broward Inc, **SLP**

Bruns, Janet M M 2135 Briarwood, Fayetteville, AR 72703, **SLP**

Brunson, Mrs Alance 1120 Pine Grove Pointe Dr, Roswell, GA 30075, (404) 329-7790, BA 56 Randolph-Macon Woman's Coll; MS 62 Vanderbilt Univ; Sr Assoc/Superv SLP, Emory U Med Sch Prg Commun Dis, **SLP**

Brunson, Nancy M 22321 Evalyn Avenue, Torrance, CA 90505, (213) 375-3785, BS 76 SUNY - Coll at Geneseo; MA 78 Kent St Univ; SLP, San Pedro Peninsula Hospital, **SLP**

Brunt, Dr Michael A Dept Speech Path & Audiology, Illinois State University, 204 Fairchild Hall, Normal, IL 61761, (309) 438-8643, BA 62 Allegheny Coll; MS 65 Univ of Pittsburgh - Pittsburgh; PH 69 (NS) Univ of KS; Assoc Prof, IL St U, **A**

Bruntzel, Melvin D 1852 N W Carlson Road, Topeka, KS 66615-9603, (913) 296-4942, BA 64 Bethany Coll; MS 56 Fort Hays St Univ; Sp-Lang Path, State of KS, **SLP**

Brunz, Mrs Janice J 745 N W 36th Street, Fort Lauderdale, FL 33309, (305) 426-6648, BS 65 CO St Univ; MA 67 Univ of NM; ES 84 (NS) Nova Univ; Ed Spec, Broward Co Sch Bd, **SLP**

Brunz, Mrs Susan B 2218 Shari Lane, Garland, TX 75043, (214) 240-0608, BS 73 Univ of NE - Lincoln; ME 76 Stephen F Austin St Univ; Spec Ed Consult, Garland ISD

Brupbacher, Mrs Nancy Aldrich 1749 Grey Friars Chase, Virginia Beach, VA 23456, (804) 471-4457, BA 71 Pacific Union Coll; MS 75 Loma Linda Univ - Riverside; **A**

Brusegaard, Mrs Leann M 2722 First Street, St Paul, MN 55110-2415, (612) 429-5391, BS 74 Moorhead St Univ; MS 78 Moorhead St Univ; Coor Sp-Lang Path Serv, White Bear Lake Ar Sch, **SLP**

Brush, Debra Irene 635 Holly Lane, Griffith, IN 46319, (312) 596-2220, BS 83 Clarion Univ of PA; MA 85 Kent St Univ; **SLP**

Brush, Mrs Eleanor L 142 Tracy Circle, Amherst, MA 01002, (413) 549-3690, BA 58 Univ of MA - Amherst; MA 59 Mount Holyoke Coll; Dir of Pupil Pers Svcs, Amherst-Pelham Regional Schs, **SLP**

Brush-Lorey, Patricia M 3953 Forsythe Drive, Lexington, KY 40503, (606) 254-5701, BA 73 Univ of MO - Columbia; MA 75 Univ of MO - Columbia; Dir, Dept of Sp/Lang Path, Cardinal Hill Hosp, **SLP**

Brusniak, Mrs Rosario R 8518 Bacardi Drive, Dallas, TX 75238-4924, (817) 898-2025, BA 72 Our Lady Lake Univ-San Anton; MA 73 Our Lady Lake Univ-San Anton; Adjunct Instr, Texas Woman's Univ, **SLP**

Brust, Suzanne E 1520 Raymond, St Paul, MN 55108, (612) 421-9172, BA 76 Univ of MN - Minneap-St Paul; MA 78 Mankato St Univ; SLP, Anoka-Henn ISD #11, **SLP**

Bruton, Mrs Cynthia Lee 1131 Bryson City Road, Franklin, NC 28734, (704) 369-6600, MS 82 Univ of NC - Chapel Hill; Sp-Lang Path, Rabun Co Bd of Ed, **SLP**

Bruton, Debbie S 2030 Markham Drive, Chapel Hill, NC 27514, (617) 665-1740, BS 77 East Carolina Univ; MA 82 OH St Univ; Aud, Duke U Med Cen, **A**

Bruton, Peggy B 641 Burnham Road, Philadelphia, PA 19119, (215) 527-5090, BA 57 Mount Holyoke Coll; ME 59 Boston Univ; MA 76 Temple Univ; Sp-Lang Path, Chld Study Inst Bryn Mawr Coll, **SLP**

Brutten, Dr Gene J Chairman, Department Communication Disorders & Sciences, Southern Illinois University, Carbondale, IL 62901, (618) 453-4301, BA 50 Kent St Univ; MA 52 CUNY - Brooklyn Coll; PH 57 (NS) Univ of IL - Urbana; Research Prof/Chmn, Southern IL U, **SLP A F**

Brutz, Mrs Loretta R Box 1923, Window Rock, AZ 86515, (602) 755-3436, BA 75 Univ of AZ; ME 79 Univ of AZ; MS 81 Univ of AZ; Sp-Lang Path, Gando USD #20, **SLP**

Bruxvoort, Evelyn Jo 1406 Clementine Court, Fort Collins, CO 80526, (303) 229-9474, BS 84 Univ of North TX; MS 86 CO St Univ; 86–Sp-Lang Path, Poudre Valley Hosp, **SLP**

Brya, Mrs Catherine Anne 9205 Avenida DE La Luna, N E, Albuquerque, NM 87111, (505) 821-4170, BA 64 Frostburg St Coll; MS 86 Univ of NM; 88–Sp-Lang Path, Albuquerque PS, **SLP**

Bryan, Catherine 35572 Reymouth Drive, Newark, CA 94560, (415) 791-7088, BA 62 Univ of UT; MS 61 Stanford Univ; **SLP**

Bryan, Mrs Cecelia Davidson 124 Vista Place, Mount Vernon, NY 10550, (212) 585-9052, MS 85 Adelphi Univ; 87–Coord, NYC Bd of Educ Comm Sch Dist 7, **SLP**

Bryan, Debbie A 3400 Treeline Court, Apt 1503, Birmingham, AL 35216, (205) 979-7024, BS 86 Univ of Montovallo; MS 87 Univ of Montevallo; Sp-Lang Path, InSpeech Inc, **SLP**

Bryan, Dr George A 1105 N E 55th Street, Oklahoma City, OK 73111, (405) 272-9876, BA 50 Abilene Christian Univ; MA 60 Univ of OK Medical Center; PH 63 (NS) Univ of OK Medical Center; Sp-Lang Path, VA Hosp, **SLP**

Bryan, Gerald E Oklahoma School For The Deaf, East 10th & Tahlequah Sts, Sulphur, OK 73086, BS 66 Univ of CO - Boulder; MS 68 CO St Univ; Sp-Lang Path, OK Sch for the Deaf, **SLP ACE**

Bryan, Janie C 1355-C Bear Mountain Drive, Boulder, CO 80303, (303) 466-7391, BA 73 Auburn Univ - Auburn; MA 80 Univ of CO - Boulder; SLP, Wallace Village for Chldn, **SLP**

Bryan, Mrs Joanne Salay 1022 N E 181st #4-B, Portland, OR 97230, (503) 669-8024, BA 80 Univ of OR; MA 87 Univ of OR; Sp-Lang Path, Reynolds Sch Dist, **SLP**

Bryan, Mrs Linda D 710 East Tenth Street, Centralia, IL 62801, (618) 532-1811, **SLP**

Bryan, Marjorie N 899 East King Street, Franklin, IN 46131, (317) 738-3258, BA 67 Muskingum Coll; MA 69 Northwestern Univ; SLP, Regency Place Home Health Serv, **SLP**

Bryant, Antoinette 29819 Cottonwood Court, Farmington Hills, MI 48018-7609, **SLP**

Bryant, Barbara A 541 King Road, Petaluma, CA 94952, (707) 763-6419, BA 72 CA St Univ - Chico; MS 74 Univ of NM; Sp-Lang Path, Sp Lang Svcs of Marin-Sonoma, **SLP**

Bryant, Mrs Barbara L 3403 Eden Park Drive, Carmel, IN 46032, (317) 845-9241, BS 69 IN Univ - Bloomington; MA 69 IN Univ - Bloomington; **SLP**

Bryant, Beverly J 3927 Shade Tree Lane, Bessemer, AL 35023, (804) 398-7914, BA 73 Univ of AL- Tuscaloosa; MA 74 Univ of AL- Tuscaloosa; Retired, Naval Hosp-Aud Cl, **A**

Bryant, Diane Marie S Route 1, 10759 North Cove, Hernando, MS 38632, **SLP**

Bryant, Dr Douglas F 3921 Wakefield Road, Richmond, VA 23235, (804) 358-6704, BS 75 Univ of NH; ME 78 Univ of VA - Charlottesville; PH 82 (NS) Univ of VA - Charlottesville; Dir of Aud, Dodd & Meeks Inc, **A**

Bryant, Gretchen R 40 Elmhurst Avenue, Stratford, CT 06497, (203) 378-8135, BA 72 Geneva Coll; MA 74 Bowling Green St Univ; Dir SLP, Wightman Health Cntr, **SLP**

Bryant, Mrs Jacqueline F 2135 Lincolnshire Drive SE, Cedar Rapids, IA 52403, (319) 398-2174, BS 56 SUNY - Coll at Fredonia; MA 60 Univ of IA; Sp-Lang Path, Grant Wood AEA, **SLP**

Bryant, Jane Elizabeth P O Box 42808 Department T, Houston, TX 77242, (409) 849-2447, BS 78 Univ of WY; MA 88 Univ of ND

Bryant, Jonathan D Valley Childrens Hospital, 3151 North Millbrook, Fresno, CA 93703, (209) 225-0148, BA 76 CA St Univ - Fresno; MA 78 CA St Univ - Fresno; Aud, Northwest Speech & Hearing Ctr, **A**

Bryant, Judith M 11182 Seabeck Highway N W, Seabeck, WA 98380, (206) 830-9139, BA 75 San Jose St Univ; MA 76 San Jose St Univ; Sp-Lang Path, **SLP**

Bryant, Mrs Karen Theresa 10787 North 103rd Way, Scottsdale, AZ 85260, (602) 952-6100, BS 77 Univ of WI - Whitewater; MS 78 Univ of WI - Whitewater; **SLP**

Bryant, Mrs Kim Christman 3921 Wakefield Road, Richmond, VA 23235, (804) 272-1414, BS 81 Univ of VA - Charlottesville; ME 83 Univ of VA - Charlottesville; Aud, VA Otolaryngology, **A**

Bryant, Leslie A 27 O'Moore, Maynard, MA 01754, (617) 897-6086, BS 75 Worcester St Coll; MA 78 SUNY - Center at Buffalo; **SLP**

Bryant, Leslie Bond 326 Bryan Avenue, Salt Lake City, UT 84115, (801) 484-3763, BA 75 Univ of New Orleans; MS 83 Univ of NM; **SLP**

Bryant, Dr Lynda C 7937 Royal Lane #124, Dallas, TX 75230, (214) 358-5261, OB 61 TX Christian Univ; MA 62 TX Woman's Univ; PH 76 (Spec Ed Sp-Lang Path & Aud) TX Woman's Univ; Dir-Comm Dept, Dallas Easter Soc for Children, **SLP A ACE**

Bryant, Marcella Lynn 1720 A Justin Lane, Austin, TX 78757, (512) 467-9049, BA 80 East TX St Univ - Commerce; MA 84 Univ of TX - Austin; Sp-Lang Path, **SLP**

Bryant, Marilyn Louise Rd Box 373, East Shore Road, South Hero, VT 05486, (802) 524-6763, BA 71 Univ of VT; MS 73 Univ of VT; 84–Mng Broker, L S Realty Inc, **SLP**

Bryant, Mrs Mary Kay 4100 Lexington Avenue South #201, Eagan, MN 55123, (612) 688-8130, BS 85 Univ of SD - Vermillion; MA 86 Univ of SD - Vermillion; 88–Sp-Lang Path, InSpeech Inc, **SLP**

Bryant, Maureen Ann 580 South Pear Orchard #1017, Ridgeland, MS 39157, (601) 856-9189, BS 85 Univ Southern MS-Hattiesburg; MS 87 Univ Southern MS-Hattiesburg; 87–Sp-Lang Path, Dogwood Sch for Children, **SLP**

Bryant, Mrs Nancy Jackson 9009 East 28TYH Street, Tulsa, OK 74129, (918) 451-2345, BA 81 Northeastern OK St Univ; MS 83 Univ of OK Medical Center; Sp-Lang Path, Tuttle Pub Sch, **SLP**

Bryant, Mrs Patricia A 2803 South Surrey Drive, Carrollton, TX 75006, (416) 416-0321, BA 73 Univ of MI - Ann Arbor; MS 75 Univ of OK Medical Center; 78–Sp-Lang Path, Irving ISD, **SLP**

Bryant, Stephanie 6611 Folsom-Auburn Road, Suite K, Folsom, CA 95630, (916) 988-7955, BA 75 CA St Univ - Sacramento; MA 77 CA St Univ - Sacramento; Aud, James Yee MD, **A**

Bryant, Susan McPhail 403 Smith, Lansing, MI 48910-9035, (517) 353-8780, BA 72 NC St Univ at Raleigh; MA 82 Univ of TN - Knoxville; 84–Cl Superv-Aud, Michigan St U, **A**

Bryant, Virginia Anne 2019 Chelsea Lane, State College, PA 16803, (814) 234-2469, BA 83 Rutgers St Univ - Newark; MS 85 PA St Univ - Univ Park; Sp-Lang Path, Rehab Hosp of Nittany Valley, **SLP**

Bryant-Landry, Mrs Linda M 7923 Jahncke Road, New Orleans, LA 70128, (504) 483-6483, BS 73 Saint Mary's Dominican Coll; OM 78 LA St Univ - N O Medical Ctr; 88–Spec Educ Coord, New Orleans Public Schools, **SLP**

Bryant-Sawyers, Carol Y 670 Honeycreek Road, Conyers, GA 30208, **SLP**

Bryde, Regina L 127 Washington Street #5, Hoboken, NJ 07030-4613, (315) 428-0016, BS 74 Ithaca Coll; MA 78 SUNY - Center at Buffalo; Syracuse University, **A**

Brynelsen, Charles Allen 639 Alger Street S E, Grand Rapids, MI 49507-3528, **SLP**

Bryson, Elizabeth Ann 1030 Frank Avenue, Albert Lea, MN 56007, (507) 373-6455, MA 86 Univ of MN - Duluth; 86–Sp-Lang Path, Achievement Rehab Corp, **SLP**

Bryson, Frances Rebecca 207 Jennings Avenue, Greenwood, SC 29646-2209, (803) 223-3944, BA 84 Univ of SC - Columbia; OM 86 Univ of SC - Columbia; **SLP**

Bryson, Mrs Marilyn Scott 138 Shannon Lee, San Antonio, TX 78216, (512) 622-3436, BA 59 Univ of AL-Tuscaloosa; OM 61 Univ of OK - Norman; MA 87 Our Lady Lake Univ-San Anton; 86–Sp-Lang Path, Southwest ISD, **SLP**

Brzenk, Donna Blankenshi 2397 Traci Drive, Pittsburgh, PA 15237, BA 68 Southern IL Univ-Edwardsvill; MS 86 Fontbonne Coll; **SLP**

Brzuszek, Melissa Gibb 9279 Kingcrest Parkway, Baton Rouge, LA 70810, (504) 295-4402, BA 83 MI St Univ; MA 84 MI St Univ; Sp-Lang Path, Ochsner Clinic, **SLP**

Bucci, Linda Ann Yorktown 1A Sentry Place, Scarsdale, NY 10538, (914) 937-3800, BS 83 SUNY - Coll at Geneseo; MS 86 Coll of Saint Rose; SLP, UCP, **SLP**

Buccola, Mrs Susan Mary 2268 Beechwood Place, Scotch Plains, NJ 07076, (201) 889-8184, BA 75 Kean Coll of NJ; MA 82 Kean Coll of NJ; 84–Sp-Lang Path, Scotch Plains/Fanwood Bd of Educ, **SLP**

Bucek, Valerie McCann 1625 Orchlee Street, Pittsburgh, PA 15212, (412) 369-2116, BA 84 Duquesne Univ; MA 86 Univ of Pittsburgh - Pittsburgh; **SLP**

Buchalter, Laurie 2605 Gregory Street, Madison, WI 53711, (608) 238-1133, BA 72 George Washington Univ; MS 73 Univ of WI - Madison; SLP, Madison Metro Sch Dist, **SLP**

Buchalter-Levitan, Esther 4172 Elizabeth Lane, Annandale, VA 22003, (703) 323-6729, BS 75 SUNY - Center at Albany; MA 78 San Diego St Univ; Sp-Lang Path, Fairfax Co Pub Sch, **SLP**

Buchanan, Mrs Christine Mary 19195 Shoreline Drive, #6, Huntington Beach, CA 92648, (703) 364-1515, BS 82 Univ of VA - Charlottesville; ME 84 Univ of VA - Charlottesville; SLP, **SLP**

Buchanan, Denise M 4571 24th Avenue #4, Port Huron, MI 48060-8414, (313) 987-5000, BA 85 Central MI Univ; MA 87 Wayne St Univ; **SLP**

Buchanan, Sr Dorothea Fontbonne College, 6800 Wydown Boulevard, St Louis, MO 63105, (314) 652-3600, BA 47 Fontbonne Coll; MA 57 Catholic Univ of America; Resident Liason Person, Cardinal Ritter I, **SLP LM**

Buchanan, Judith Sutherland 23 Fieldstone Circle, North Attleboro, MA 02760, (508) 695-3886, MS 83 Univ of RI; Sp-Lang Path, **SLP**

Buchanan, Julia N 7932 S W 146th Avenue, Miami, FL 33183, (305) 235-6811, BA 67 Univ of NC - Chapel Hill; MS 86 Nova Univ; 86–Sp-Lang Path, Dade Co Sch Bd, **SLP**

Buchanan, Lena Faye 2819 West 113th, Jenks, OK 74037, **SLP**

Buchanan, Dr Leo H Audiology Department, Shriver Center University Affiliated Program, 200 Trapelo Road, Waltham, MA 02254, (617) 642-0222, BA 64 Howard Univ; MS 71 Univ of WI - Madison; PH 77 (Comm Dis (Aud)) Univ of WI - Madison; 72–Aud, Shriver Ctr UAP, **A**

Buchanan, Mrs Mary Anne 8216 Tomahawk Road, Prairie Village, KS 66208, (913) 341-2644, BS 76 Central MO St Univ; MS 84 Central MO St Univ; **SLP**

Buchanan, Maureen J 2 Kiowa Court, Coram, NY 11727, (516) 929-8500, BS 76 SUNY - Coll at Geneseo; MS 77 SUNY - Coll at Buffalo; Tchr, Shoreham-Wading River Ctrl Sch, **SLP**

Buchanan, Michael S 200 West Hereford Street, Gladstone, OR 97027, (406) 365-5446, BS 73 Portland St Univ; MS 78 Western OR St Coll; Sp-Lang Path, Gladstone Sch Dist, **SLP**

Buchanan, Patricia K 6258 Branch Beech, Columbia, MD 21044, BA 64 Our Lady Lake Univ-San Anton; MA 69 Our Lady Lake Univ-San Anton; Sp-Lang Path, Nellingen Elem Sch, **SLP**

Buchanan, Robert J 9 Overlook Avenue, Gloucester, MA 01930, (617) 956-5300, BA 74 SUNY - Coll at Potsdam; MA 76 SUNY - Center at Buffalo; 76–Aud, New England Med Ctr Hosp, **A**

Buchanan, Sharon Elizabeth 143 West South Street, Mooresville, IN 46158, (317) 362-4988, BS 81 Ball St Univ; MA 82 Ball St Univ; Sp-Lang Path, Central Convalescent Services, **SLP**

Buchanan, Mrs Susan H 703 Carlton, Springdale, AR 72764, (501) 751-5534, BA 77 Univ of AR - Fayetteville; MA 79 Univ of AR - Fayetteville; 88–Spec Prog Dir, Pea Ridge Decatur Gravette PS, **SLP**

Buchanan, Mrs Susanna W 904 Oakwood Court, New Albany, IN 47150, (812) 944-9869, BS 60 IN Univ - Bloomington; ME 78 Univ of Louisville; Sp-Lang Path, Greater Clark County Schools, **SLP**

Buchanan, Virginia 500 Rogers Court, New Bern, NC 28562, (919) 633-2501, BA 70 Univ of MI - Ann Arbor; MA 78 Western WA Univ; Sp-Lang Path, Private Practice, **SLP**

Buchaniec, Mary Elisabeth 7901 College Drive, Palos Park, IL 60464, (312) 841-2508, BA 80 Saint Xavier Coll; MS 82 Governors St Univ; Sp-Lang Path, Flossmoor Sch Dist 161, **SLP**

Bucher, Doris A 3264 Henderson Creek Road, Atlanta, GA 30341, **SLP**

Bucher, Mrs Irene R 9122 Linder, Morton Grove, IL 60053, (312) 492-6476, BS 77 Northwestern Univ; MA 79 Northwestern Univ; Dir Sp-Lang Path, Evanston Hosp, **SLP ACE**

Bucher, Nancy A 2137 Lillie Avenue, Davenport, IA 52806-2040, (319) 322-7899, BA 78 Temple Univ-Tyler Sch of Art; MA 80 Temple Univ-Tyler Sch of Art; SLP, Comm Hlth Care Inc, **SLP**

Bucher, Nancy Pomeroy 1561 Balboa Street, Eugene, OR 97401, (503) 484-5216, BA 71 CA St Univ - Chico; MS 86 Univ of OR; 87–Sp-Lang Path, Springfield Sch Dist, **SLP**

Bucher, Pamela M 228 1/2 Cocoa Avenue, Hershey, PA 17033, (717) 533-8720, BS 85 East Stroudsburg Univ of PA; MS 86 Bloomsburg Univ of PA; 88–Sp-Lang Path, The Good Samaritan Hosp, **SLP ACE**

Buchler, Mrs Deborah Tribou 11030 South Hardy Street, New Orleans, LA 70127, (504) 947-2444, BS 69 Saint Mary's Dominican Coll; OM 82 LA St Univ - N O Medical Ctr; Aud, Private Practice, **A**

Bucholtz, Mrs Joan Goldberg 575 Trotwood Ridge Road, Pittsburgh, PA 15241-2042, (412) 429-9251, BS 76 Ithaca Coll; MA 77 Case Western Reserve Univ; Sp/Lang Path Senior, Beth Israel Med Cen, **SLP**

Buchwald, Gerald J Severson Werson Et Al, 1 Embarcadero Center 25 Fl, San Francisco, CA 94111, (415) 398-3344, BS 70 Northwestern Univ; OD 73 (NS) Northwestern Univ; Attorney at Law, Severson Werson Berke & Melchior

Buchwald, Mrs Janet S 20 Live Oak Lane, Hillsborough, CA 94010, (415) 344-5079, BS 69 Northwestern Univ; MA 70 Northwestern Univ; Sp/Lang Path, Private Practice, **SLP**

Buck, Mrs Barbara H 300 East 40th Street, Norfolk, VA 23504, (804) 722-9961, BS 54 VA Commonwealth Univ; MS 71 Old Dominion Univ; Aud, VA Medical Center, **A ACE**

Buck, Mrs Beverly Douglas 1184 Greenbriar Avenue, San Jose, CA 95128, (408) 243-8156, BA 78 San Jose St Univ; MA 82 San Jose St Univ; Sp/Lang Path, Private Practice, **SLP**

Buck, Caroline M 9745 Old Lincoln Trail, Fairview Heights, IL 62208, (618) 259-0411, BS 56 IL St Univ - Normal; MA 61 Univ of IL - Urbana; 85–Aud, TENCO/SIRSEA, **A**

Buck, Christine Wahler 1920 Newburyport Road, Chesterfield, MO 63017-4728, (314) 821-0008, BS 79 Univ of MO - Columbia; MS 81 Fontbonne Coll; Sp-Lang Path, Professional Rehab Center Inc, **SLP**

Buck, Mrs Deborah Cockrell 10277 Bay Hills Drive North, Largo, FL 34644, (813) 596-5003, BS 74 Univ of TX - Austin; MA 75 Univ of TX - Austin; 87–Sp-Lang Path, Pinellas County Schs, **SLP**

Buck, Garry Earl 369 Marrell, Gallatin, TN 37066, (615) 451-2408, BS 78 Lambuth Coll; MA 85 Memphis St Univ; 87–Sp-Lang Path, Cedarbrook Rebound Inc, **SLP**

Buck, Jeanne L 3479 Vivian Avenue, Shoreview, MN 55126, **SLP**

Buck, Dr Joyce F 311 West 24th Street, New York, NY 10011, (212) 643-8598, BA 48 CUNY - Hunter Coll; MA 49 Univ of WI - Madison; PH 72 (NS) CUNY - Grad Sch & Univ Cntr; Prof/Sp, NYC Tech Coll, **SLP**

Buck, Julie Rene' 2045 South Arlington, Indianapolis, IN 46203, (317) 356-6051, BA 85 Wichita St Univ; MS 86 Univ of KY; 87–Sp-Lang Path, Visiting Nurse Svcs, **SLP**

Buck, Paula King 12982 Green Chapel Road, Johnstown, OH 43031, (614) 967-5043, MS 81 FL St Univ; Aud, East Hearing Ctr, **A**

Buck, Robert J P O Box 424, St Marys, WV 26170, **SLP A**

Buck, Sandra L 8286 North Calaveras, Fresno, CA 93711, (209) 432-9171, BA 70 CA St Univ - Fresno; SLP, Fresno USD, **SLP**

Buck, Mrs Susan M 4155 West Alvina Avenue, Greenfield, WI 53221, (414) 768-6295, BS 77 Univ of WI - Milwaukee; MS 78 Univ of WI - Milwaukee; Sp-Lang Path, Oak Creek Franklin Sch Dist, **SLP**

Buck, Virginia R 17 Clay Street, Dansville, NY 14437, **SLP**

Buckberry, Emily S 683 Beechwood Estates, Athens, OH 45701, (614) 593-1419, BA 64 Marshall Univ; MA 69 OH Univ - Athens; Asst Prof/Cl Superv, OH U Sch of Hrng & Sp Sci, **SLP**

Buckels, Marcia K 301 Cheshire Drive #189, Knoxville, TN 37919, (615) 588-9058, BS 81 Univ of South AL; MS 83 Univ of South AL; Sp-Lang Path, First Rehab, **SLP**

Buckendorf, Glen R 660 SE Baseline Suite B, Hillsboro, OR 97123, (503) 640-6065, BS 71 Coll of ID; MS 75 ID St Univ; Sp-Lang Path, Private Practice, **SLP**

Buck-Gordon, Susan 119 Nalisty Drive, Vallejo, CA 94590, (707) 557-8677, BA 72 Univ of CA - Santa Barbara; MS 74 Western OR St Coll; MA 80 Mills Coll; 80–Sp-Lang Path, Vallejo USD, **SLP**

Buckham, Mrs Barbara A 58 Lakewood, St Charles, IL 60174, MS 73 Northwestern Univ; Director of Services, The Therapy Center, **SLP**

Buckingham, Dr Hugh W, Jr Louisiana State University, Program In Linguistics, 136B Coates Hall, Baton Rouge, LA 70803, (504) 388-6682, BA 64 American Univ; MA 68 American Univ; PH 74 (NS) Univ of Rochester; Dir Intdept Prog/Linguistics, Louisiana State Univ

Buckler, Mrs Georgiana S 10790 Rosalie Drive, Northglenn, CO 80233, (303) 287-0181, BS 72 Univ of MN - Minneap-St Paul; MS 73 Univ of WI - Eau Claire; 87–Sp-Lang Path, Adams Co Schs, **SLP**

Buckler, Mrs Jennifer Margaret 15213 North 62nd Drive, Glendale, AZ 85306, (602) 878-1010, MS 87 AZ St Univ; Sp-Lang Path, Peoria USD

Buckler, Dr Joyce 2900 Marshall Avenue, St Louis, MO 63143, (314) 647-0318, BA 56 Fontbonne Coll; MA 65 Northwestern Univ; ED 77 (NS) Columbia Univ Teachers Coll; Prin, St Josephs I, **A**

Buckles, Krista M 10 Braeburn Court, San Ramon, CA 94583, (415) 577-1579, BA 75 Bowling Green St Univ; MA 77 Central MI Univ; Audiologist, Fairmont Hospital, **A**

Buckles, Patricia Kay 1540 208th Street, Bayside, NY 11360, (914) 666-9553, BS 84 Walla Walla Coll; MS 87 Adelphi Univ

Buckles, Theresa Ann 505 West White Oak Avenue, Porterville, CA 93257, (209) 784-2000, BA 80 CA St Univ - Fresno; MA 83 CA St Univ - Fresno; Sp/Lang Path, St of CA Dept of Dev Serv, **SLP**

Buckley, Anne H 841 West Truesdell Street, Wilmington, OH 45177, (513) 382-8348, BA 71 Lawrence Univ; MS 74 Univ of MI - Ann Arbor; **SLP**

Buckley, Mrs Emily Susan 17841 Pond Road, Ashton, MD 20861, BA 78 Univ of MD - College Park; MA 80 Univ of MD - College Park; Aud, Balto Cty Pub Schs, **A**

Buckley, Gloria L 1521 Northwest Highway, Garland, TX 75041, (214) 271-0516, BS 76 Univ of North TX; MS 77 Univ of North TX; Director Hearing & Speech Div, Ear Nose Throat Med Centrs Tx, **A**

Buckley, John E 1885 Lake Avenue, Scotch Plains, NJ 07076, BA 61 Seton Hall Univ; MA 64 Seton Hall Univ; Dir Sp & Hrng, Aud & Hrng Aid Disp of Nj, **SLP A**

Buckley, Mrs Katherine Gregory 5155C Overland Drive, Roanoke, VA 24014, BA 82 Univ of FL; MS 84 FL St Univ; 87–Sp/Lang Path, Roanoke City Sch Bd/Hurt Park, **SLP**

Buckley, Mary E 500 Santa Barbara Avenue, Fullerton, CA 92635, MA 76 5489; 79–Sp-Lang Path, Kaiser Permanente, **SLP**

Buckley, Mary Maria 1162-F Desert Willow Lane, Corona, CA 91720, (714) 734-4810, BS 80 CA St Univ - Stanislaus; Sp-Lang Path, Sch Dist-Riverside City Dist, **SLP**

Buckley, Mrs Maureen Cahill R R 1 Box 212, Tuxedo Park, NY 10987, (914) 477-2491, BA 80 Dominican Coll of Blauvelt; MS 83 William Paterson Coll; Sp-Lang Path, Greenwood Lake Un Free Sc Dist, **SLP**

Buckley, Regina 1804 Myrtle Road, Silver Spring, MD 20902, **SLP**

Buckley, Mrs Vicki Annette PO Box 30245, Pensacola, FL 32503, MA 77 Univ of Tulsa; 88–Sp-Lang Path, Escambia County Sch Sys, **SLP**

Buckman, Gerald F, Jr Buckman & Medland Inc, 1009 Maitland Ctr Commons, Suite 200-A, Maitland, FL 32751, (407) 660-2936, BS 65 Bradley Univ; MS 67 IL St Univ - Normal; Sp/Lang Path, Private Practice, **SLP**

Buckman, Mrs Gwenda P 4208 Browning Drive, St Joseph, MI 49085, (616) 471-1836, BS 77 Western MI Univ; MA 78 Western MI Univ; Sp-Lang Path, Berrien Spgs Publ Schs, **SLP**

Buckner, Mrs Rebecca Ray One Bunker Hill, Richardson, TX 75080, (214) 699-1217, BS 79 Baylor Univ; MS 80 Baylor Univ; Pres/Sp-Lang Path, Private Practice, **SLP**

Bucks, Mrs Patricia J R R 1 Box 100, Star City, IN 46985, (219) 643-2255, BS 76 Ball St Univ; MA 78 Ball St Univ; 77–Sp-Lang Path, Logansport Comm Sch Corp, **SLP**

Bucquet, Susan Reed 220 Palo Alto Avenue #301, Palo Alto, CA 94301, (415) 326-5530, BA 75 Univ of the Pacific; ME 77 Univ of AZ; MS 84 San Francisco St Univ; SLP, Childrens Health Council, **SLP**

Buczynski, Mary Frances 1 Harris Street, Wilkes-Barre, PA 18702, (717) 822-7764, BS 76 PA St Univ - Univ Park; MS 85 Bloomsburg Univ of PA

Budacki, Robert M 225 West 25th Street, Suite 207, Erie, PA 16502, (814) 456-7866, BS 77 IN Univ - Bloomington; MA 78 IN Univ - Bloomington; Aud, S Lipman MD/R Guelcher MD Inc, **SLP A**

Budde, Betty Ion N83 W13696, Fond Du Lac Avenue, Menomonee Falls, WI 53051, (414) 251-6279, BS 84 Clarion Univ of PA; MS 86 Clarion Univ of PA; 87–Sp-Lang Path, InSpeech Inc, **SLP**

Budde, Mark J 111 3rd Avenue #9-A, New York, NY 10003, (212) 982-7085, BS 74 Moorhead St Univ; MS 75 Univ of WI - Stevens Point; 87–Sp-Lang Path/Supvr, The Shield Inst, **SLP**

Budgar, Laurie Beth 2234 East 27th Street, Brooklyn, NY 11229, (201) 321-7764, BA 85 SUNY - Center at Buffalo; MS 87 Boston Univ; 88–Sp-Lang Path, JFK Med Ctr, **SLP**

Budinger, Ann Calkins Audiology Service, 34th General Hospital, APO New York, NY 09178-3311, BS 84 Univ of VA - Charlottesville; MS 86 Vanderbilt Univ; 88–Aud, 34th Gen Hosp-US Army, **A**

Budney, Mrs Elizabeth Allison 30 N Michigan Avenue Ste 824, Chicago, IL 60602, (312) 782-0025, Aud, Telex Hrng Aid Inc, **A**

Budney, Seth Martin 30 North Michigan #824, Chicago, IL 60602, (312) 782-0025, BS 79 IN Univ - Bloomington; MS 83 Rush Univ; Aud, Telex Hearing Aids Inc, **A**

Budney, Sheryl Edwards 419 Triphammer Road, Ithaca, NY 14850, BA 77 Univ of RI; MA 79 SUNY - Coll at Geneseo; 87–Sp-Lang Path, Spec Child Ctr Inc, **SLP**

Budnick, Amy S Memorial Sloan Kettering Cancer Center, 1275 York Avenue, New York, NY 10021, (212) 794-5856, BS 74 Boston Univ; ME 75 Univ of VA - Charlottesville; OM 84 Columbia Univ Sch of Gen St; 86–Dir of Aud, Memorial Sloan Kettering, **A**

Budnick, Bonnie M 3332 Highgate Lane, St Charles, MO 63301, (314) 447-8697, BA 76 Univ of MO - Columbia; MA 77 Univ of IL - Urbana; **SLP**

Budovitch, Mrs Rona L Dupont Company, Legal Department, 1007 Market Street, Wilmington, DE 19898, (215) 665-5203, BS 74 Ithaca Coll; MA 76 Case Western Reserve Univ; **SLP**

Budrzysky, Julie Ann 1935 West Morten Avenue #30, Phoenix, AZ 85021, (602) 973-3314, BS 83 Central MI Univ; MA 85 MI St Univ; 85–Sp-Lang Path, Deer Valley USD #79, **SLP**

Budweiser, Mrs Judith D 420 Limestone Road, Ridgefield, CT 06877, (203) 438-0747, BA 66 CUNY - Hunter Coll; MA 71 CUNY - Lehman Coll; Admin, Westchester Ddso, **SLP**

Budzenski, Mrs Donna E B Route 1, Arthur Road, New Era, MI 49446, (616) 725-7100, BS 79 Eastern MI Univ; MA 80 Eastern MI Univ; Sp-Lang Path, Muskegan PS, **SLP**

Buechler, Mrs Carolyn C 6 North Candlewood Path, Dix Hills, NY 11746, (516) 499-7254, BA 69 Marymount Coll; MA 72 CUNY - Queens Coll; Sp-Lang Path, Cold Spring Harbor Sch Dist, **SLP**

Bueermann, Donald William 1500 S Highland Avenue, #A, Fullerton, CA 92632, (714) 680-4265, BA 83 CA St Univ - Fullerton; MA 85 Northwestern Univ; Aud, Newport Language & Aud, **A**

Buehler, Sandra A R Valley Road, Oriskany, NY 13424, **SLP**

Bueker, Susan Elizabeth 2120 Fairfax Avenue #6, Nashville, TN 37212, (615) 329-5841, BS 81 Western KY Univ; MA 85 Univ of Northern CO; **SLP**

Buell, Barbara Sutton 1474 Nesbitt Lane, Madison, TN 37115, (615) 860-1767, Coor SLP, Rebound Inc, **SLP**

Buell-Chittenden, Mrs Claudia 14 Underhill, Mill Valley, CA 94941, (415) 388-9205, BA 69 MI St Univ; MA 74 George Washington Univ; Dir Sp-Lang Path, La Mel Childrens Cen, **SLP**

Buen, Patricia Marie 3433-B 33rd Avenue, Nashville, TN 37212, (615) 329-5283, BS 81 Boston Univ; MA 83 Univ of CA - Santa Barbara; Sp-Lang Path, Baptist Rehabilitation Center, **SLP**

Buerkli-Halevy, Ora Phonak Ag, Laubisruetistr 28 Ch 8712, Staefa, Switzerland, (01) 928-01-01, BA 77 CUNY - Hunter Coll; MS 79 Univ of San Francisco; 84–Dir of Aud Svcs, Phonak AG, **A**

Buesking, Susan M 925 West Balboa Blvd, Apt B, Balboa, CA 92661, (714) 723-0373, BS 84 Eastern IL Univ; MS 86 TX Tech Univ; Lynn McInally and Assoc, **SLP**

Buethe, Diane D R R 27 Box 252, Terre Haute, IN 47802, (812) 237-2805, BA 53 Univ of NE - Lincoln; MS 54 Syracuse Univ; MA 64 Univ of NE - Lincoln; Assoc Prof Communicatn Disord, Indiana State University, **SLP**

Buettemeier, Cheryl Ann 7517 145th Avenue N E, Redmond, WA 98052, (206) 462-7800, **SLP**

Buff, Mrs Judith S 3 Bridgestone Lane, Avon, CT 06001, (518) 371-6471, BS 72 SUNY - Coll at Buffalo; MS 73 SUNY - Coll at Buffalo; 86–Sp-Lang Path, Capital Region Educ Council, **SLP**

Buffa, Phyllis M 40 Wedgewood Drive, Woodbridge, CT 06525, **SLP**

Buffardi, Jean R 9903 Wood Actor Court, Burke, VA 22015, (703) 876-5244, BS 69 KS St Univ; MS 73 Univ of Pittsburgh - Pittsburgh; Sp-Lang Path, Fairfax Co PS, **SLP**

Buffie, Mrs Sandra Merritt 7831 Winterset Drive, Matthews, NC 28105, (812) 988-6601, BS 81 PA St Univ - Univ Park; MS 82 Western MI Univ; Sp-Lang Path, Child and Family Development, **SLP**

Buffington, Jenny Lin 1719 Woodcliff Court N E, Atlanta, GA 30329, (404) 321-1906, BS 85 Univ of GA; ME 86 Univ of GA; SLP, Dekalb Co Schools, **SLP**

Buffington, Kimberly Marie 12 Carlmark Street, Apt #3, Quincy, MA 02169, (617) 787-3390, BS 85 Towson St Univ; MS 86 Loyola Coll; SLP, The Greenery, **SLP**

Buffman, Mrs Julie Kay 90 Highland Street, South Easton, MA 02375, (508) 238-5347, BS 81 IA St Univ; MA 82 Northeast MO St Univ; 87–Sp-Lang Path, Wareham PS, **SLP**

Buffon, Katherine Prince 8947 McCloud Road, Ventura, CA 93004, (805) 648-5391, BA 77 Humboldt St Univ; MA 82 Humboldt St Univ; Sp-Lang Path, Ventura USD, **SLP**

Bufi, Doreen Elizabeth 145 Harrison Avenue, Harrison, NY 10528, (914) 381-2006, BA 84 SUNY - Coll at Cortland; MS 85 Nazareth Coll of Rochester; **SLP**

Buford, Mrs Jennifer Perry P O Box 1201, Cordele, GA 31015, (912) 874-5875, BS 83 GA Southwestern Coll; ME 85 Univ of GA; **SLP**

Bugbee, Judith K 6191 Turkey Run Court, Manassas, VA 22111, (703) 369-8194, BA 77 Mary Washington Coll; MA 79 San Diego St Univ; Coord Sp-Lang Path, Prince Wm Hosp, **SLP ACE**

Bugh, Judith R 38W118 Hawkins Lane, St Charles, IL 60175, (312) 893-7995, BA 64 Capital Univ; MA 66 Northern IL Univ - De Kalb; 86–Clin Dir, Comm Therapy Svcs, **SLP**

Buglewicz, Mrs Ellen Theresa 1005 Kingston Avenue, Bellevue, NE 68005, (402) 292-1733, BA 83 Univ of NE - Lincoln; MS 85 Univ of NE - Lincoln; 87–Sp-Lang Path, Bellevue Ps, **SLP**

Bugli, Mrs Terri Lynn 38934 Westchester Road, Sterling Heights, MI 48077, (313) 353-0310, MA 84 MI St Univ; Sp-Lang Path, Speech Language Rehab Serv Inc, **SLP**

Bugman, Laura Marie 335 Bird Avenue, Buffalo, NY 14213, (716) 835-6009, BS 84 SUNY - Coll at Buffalo; MS 86 SUNY - Coll at Buffalo; 87–Sp-Lang Path, Buffalo Hearing and Speech Ctr, **SLP**

Buhler, Helen C 12 Degarmo Place, Poughkeepsie, NY 12601, (914) 485-2211, BS 71 Duquesne Univ; MA 74 Long Island U - CW Post Ctr; SLP, Gerard B Brooks & Assoc, **SLP**

Buhler, Jill L Indiana Veterans Home, 3851 North River Road, West Lafayette, IN 47906-8699, (317) 497-8672, BS 84 Purdue Univ - West Lafayette; MS 86 Purdue Univ - West Lafayette; 87–Sp-Lang Path, IN Veterans Home, **SLP**

Buhler, Mrs Rita G RD #1 Box 530A, Germantown, NY 12526, (518) 537-4032, BS 82 Univ of AZ; MS 86 Univ of AZ; **A**

Buhr, Barbara Ann 36 Kittredge Terrace, San Francisco, CA 94118, (415) 386-2524, BS 52 Saint Cloud St Univ; OM 61 San Francisco St Univ; Retired, San Francisco USD, **SLP**

Buhr, Joann Coleen 324 Birch Lane, Lawrence, KS 66044, (913) 842-0960, BA 82 Univ of Northern IA; MS 84 Univ of WY; **SLP**

Buhrke, Mrs Cheryl K 1400 North 24th Avenue #6, Melrose Park, IL 60160, (312) 622-5400, BA 83 Univ of MN - Duluth; MA 84 Univ of MN - Duluth; Sp-Lang Path, Shriner's Hosp, **SLP**

Buianowski, Eileen M 147 Cedar Street #3L, Somerville, MA 02143, (617) 628-7606, BA 74 Univ of MA - Boston; ME 76 Northeastern Univ; Sp/Lang Path, Boston Pub Sch, **SLP ACE**

Buin, Susan M 109 Richard Drive, Hackettstown, NJ 07840, (201) 234-0011, Matheny School, **SLP**

Bukantz, Mrs Carol I 47 Filmore Avenue, Livingston, NJ 07039, (201) 533-1845, BS 79 West Chester Univ of PA; MS 81 Columbia Univ Teachers Coll; **A**

Bukaty, Carolyn N 8909 Colton #92, Spokane, WA 99218, (509) 928-2602, BS 84 Central MO St Univ; MS 87 Central MO St Univ

Bukauskas, Cynthia Louise 3903 Mountain Rose Lane, Houston, TX 77043, (713) 466-3429, MA 87 Univ of Houston - Univ Park; **SLP**

Bukowski, Mrs Darlene Collins 6158 Bridlewood Drive, Fairview, PA 16415, (814) 833-3724, BS 73 Clarion Univ of PA; ME 75 Clarion Univ of PA; Director Neurosensory Center, St Vincent Health Center, **SLP**

Bukowski, Gene W 3231 Ben Hogan Lane, Billings, MT 59106, (406) 652-5325, BS 74 Univ of WI - Madison; MS 75 Univ of WI - Madison; Aud, Private Practice, **A**

Bukowski, Mary Davis 327 Park Avenue #A, New Castle, PA 16101, (412) 658-5566, BS 76 Clarion Univ of PA; MS 78 Indiana Univ of PA; 81–Sp-Lang Path, Shenango Area Sch Dist, **SLP**

Bulakites, Mrs Debra L 53 Christopher Lane, Guilford, CT 06437, (203) 453-1961, BS 78 Univ of MA - Amherst; MA 80 Univ of CT; SLP, Middletown Public Schools, **SLP**

Buldas, Nancy M 8600 S W 184th Lane, Miami, FL 33157, (305) 221-8212, BS 77 SUNY - Coll at Buffalo; MA 80 Univ of Miami; Sp-Lang Path, Dade Co Pub Sch-S Ctrl Area, **SLP**

Bulgaris, Valerie A 39 Maxim Street, Brockton, MA 02401, (508) 559-9697, BA 75 Bridgewater St Coll; ME 77 Northeastern Univ; Sp-Lang Path, Abington Pub Sch, **SLP**

Bulich, Brenda L 1637 Forest Hill Court, Crofton, MD 21114, (301) 721-2463, BA 76 Univ of Akron; MA 80 Univ of Cincinnati; 88–Sp-Lang Path, Private Practice, **SLP**

Bulka, Nancy Ann 5128 West 105th Place, Oak Lawn, IL 60453, (312) 687-7200, MS 87 Rush Univ; 87–Sp-Lang Path, Oak Forest Hosp

Bull, Dr Glen L University Of Virginia, Curry School Of Education, 405 Emmet Street Room 278, Charlottesville, VA 22903, (804) 924-7471, BA 73 Western KY Univ; MA 75 OH St Univ; PH 76 (NS) OH St Univ; U of VA, **SLP**

Bull, Marilyn E 3620 N E 141st Court, Edmond, OK 73013, (405) 478-4103, BS 78 Central St Univ; ME 87 Central St Univ

Bulla, Pat O Div Of Communication Disorders, North Texas State Univ, P O Box 5008, Denton, TX 76203, (817) 565-2262, BS 63 East TX St Univ - Commerce; OM 69 Univ of OK Medical Center; Faculty, North Texas St U, **SLP ACE**

Bullard, Mrs Billie H Route 3 Box 150-E, Farmersville, TX 75031, (214) 475-3380, BS 74 East TX St Univ - Commerce; MS 78 East TX St Univ - Commerce; Sp-Lang Path, Garland ISD, **SLP**

Bullard, Mrs Irene W 705 East Lake Drive, Edwardsville, IL 62025, (618) 398-2800, BS 67 Mary Manse Coll; MS 77 Southern IL Univ-Edwardsvill; Sp-Lang Path, Visiting Nurse Assn, **SLP**

Bullard, Joann B 202 West Ercoupe Drive, Midwest City, OK 73110, (405) 848-0431, BA 70 Univ of OK - Norman; MA 71 Univ of OK - Norman; Owner Sp-Lang Path, Private Practice, **SLP**

Bullard, Lynn T Route 15 Box 180, Statesville, NC 28677, (704) 873-7354, BS 76 East Carolina Univ; MS 77 East Carolina Univ; Sp-Lang Path, Statesville City Sch, **SLP**

Bullard, Shirley P Larrabee's Point, Shoreham, VT 05770, (802) 897-8255, BS 63 Syracuse Univ; MS 72 Univ of VT; Sp-Lang Path, Private Practice, **SLP ACE**

Buller, Leisa Joy P O Box 163, Florence, MS 39073-0163, (601) 845-8249, **SLP**

Bullett, John J 88 Durland Avenue, Elmira, NY 14905, (607) 734-2081, BS 72 Univ of UT; MS 75 Univ of UT; Dir-Prog Svcs, UCP Chemung Co, **SLP**

Bullett, Maryann Shelton 88 Durland Avenue, Elmira, NY 14905, (607) 733-6541, BA 76 Southern CT St Univ; MS 77 Univ of WY; 86–Dir of Aud Svcs, St Joseph's Hosp, **A**

Bulley, Kathleen Ann Scripps Memorial Hospital, Dept Of Audiology, 9888 Genesee Avenue, La Jolla, CA 92037, (619) 457-6394, BA 80 San Diego St Univ; MA 84 San Diego St Univ; Aud, Scripps Memorial Hospital, **A**

Bulloch, Mrs Kathleen L 466 Westridge Circle, Anaheim, CA 92807, (714) 974-0684, BA 71 Paterson St Coll; MA 72 Montclair St Coll; OM 82; Sp-Lang Path, Riverside Co Supt of Sch, **SLP**

Bullock, Mrs Charlene 300 Swallow Drive, Brandon, MS 39042, (601) 992-2483, BA 63 Univ of MS; OM 71 Univ of MS; **SLP**

Bullock, Craig W 18020 Belview Trail, Faribault, MN 55021, (507) 334-7577, BS 77 Moorhead St Univ; MS 79 Moorhead St Univ; SLP, Faribault Regional Center, **SLP**

Bullock, Mrs Elizabeth Johnson P O Box 5227, Charlottesville, VA 22905, (804) 293-7037, BS 60 Longwood Coll; MS 68 Vanderbilt Univ; Pres, American Retirement Homes Inc, **SLP**

Bullock, Gwynetta Y 7150 North Terrace Vista Dr, Apartment 402, Peoria, IL 61614-1308, (309) 685-6731, BS 75 Bradley Univ; MS 77 Bradley Univ; 78–Sp-Lang Path, The Children's Home Assoc of IL, **SLP**

Bullock, Keith Eldon P O Box 296, New Richland, MN 56072, (218) 847-5611, BA 71 Dakota Wesleyan Univ; OM 74; MS 79 Moorhead St Univ; Sp-Lang Path, Mankato Rehabilitaion Center, **SLP**

Bullock, Mary Beth 1124 High Street, Marquette, MI 49855, (906) 225-0372, BS 68 Northern MI Univ; MA 75 Northern MI Univ; Sp-Lang Path, Marquette Alger Inter Sch Dist, **SLP**

Bullock, Michele Koenig Route 3 Box 27 F, Chadbourn, NC 28431, (919) 642-4119, BS 78 Bloomsburg Univ of PA; MA 82 Univ of Pittsburgh - Pittsburgh; **SLP**

Bullock-McConnell, Janna Lu 6030 Kenwood, Kansas City, MO 64110, (816) 363-1414, MS 84 Central MO St Univ; 87–Sp-Lang Path, Gillis Ctr, **SLP**

Bultas-Ryba, Mrs Karen Marie 639 Lombard, Lombard, IL 60148, (312) 837-2430, BS 78 Northern IL Univ - De Kalb; MS 80 IL St Univ - Normal; Spch-Lang Path, Schaumburg Dist 54 Elem Schls, **SLP**

Bultemeyer, Christine Denise 851 Cotton Bay Drive West, Apartment 714, West Palm Beach, FL 33406-9053, (407) 482-8075, BA 84 Valparaiso Univ; MA 85 Saint Louis Univ; 86–Sp-Lang Path, Palm Beach Co Schs, **SLP**

Bultmann, Mrs Carole Sweeney Route 1 Box 198, Henley, MO 65040, (314) 636-7171, BS 75 Univ of MO - Columbia; MA 76 Univ of MO - Columbia; Sp-Lang Path, Jefferson Cty Pub Sch, **SLP**

Bumb, Mrs Chrys C 8 Pebble Ridge Court, St Peters, MO 63376, (314) 278-8096, BS 75 Ithaca Coll; MS 78 Miami Univ - Oxford; Sp-Lang Path, Pt Services, **SLP**

Bumbry, Linda Leanna 132 Bayview Drive, St. Louis, MO 63136, (314) 521-6185, BS 81 Univ of Montevallo; MS 83 Univ of South AL; **SLP**

Bumford, Deborah D 770 Pennsylvania Avenue, Southampton, PA 18966, (215) 757-0227, BS 74 East Stroudsburg Univ of PA; MS 76 PA St Univ - Univ Park; Sp-Lang Path, Bucks Co Inter Ut, **SLP**

Bumpus, Mrs Mary C 2003 11th Street, Charleston, IL 61920, (217) 348-7943, BS 80 Western IL Univ; MA 81 Northern IL Univ - De Kalb; Sp-Lang Path, Lincoln Hlth Cen, **SLP**

Bunce, Dr Betty H 853 Broadview Drive, Lawrence, KS 66044, (913) 864-4690, BS 66 Univ of CO - Boulder; MA 71 Temple Univ-Tyler Sch of Art; PH 86 (Child Language) Univ of KS; 88–Asst Prof, Univ of Kansas, **SLP**

Bunch, Mrs Barbara Jean 1021 Roselawn Way, Bowling Green, KY 42101, (502) 782-7770, SLP, Clover Bottom Develop Center, **SLP**

Bunch, Carolyn O P O Box 350, Ark, VA 23003-0350, (804) 722-9961, BS 70 Univ of HI - Manoa; MS 72 CO St Univ; 73–Sp-Lang Path, VA Med Cen, **SLP ACE**

Buncher, Robert Martin 880 Park Lake Circle, Maitland, FL 32751, (305) 574-2742, MA 83 Univ of FL; Audiologist, Central Florida Ear Hearing Cl, **A**

Bunderson, Karin 4512 Mayflower Lane, Las Vegas, NV 89107, (702) 878-2243, BS 80 Brigham Young Univ; OM 82 Brigham Young Univ; 88–Aud, Paradise Valley Sp & Hearing, **A**

Bundrick, Mrs Judy S 7822 Millicent Circle, Shreveport, LA 71105, (318) 798-0786, BA 85 LA Tech Univ; MS 87 Univ of TX - Dallas; **SLP**

Bungard, Mrs Elizabeth Ann 7238 Ortega Hills Drive, Jacksonville, FL 32244, (904) 390-2079, BS 77 Univ of ME - Farmington; ME 84 TX A & I Univ; ME 87 Univ of North FL; 84–Sp-Lang Path, Duval Co Sch Bd, **SLP**

Bunge, Mrs Cindy Whisler 5312 Twana Drive, Des Moines, IA 50310, (515) 964-2550, BA 77 Univ of Northern IA; MA 78 Univ of Northern IA; Sp-Lang Path, Heartland AEA, **SLP**

Bunker, Mrs Rosemary O 6 Maryland Avenue, Towson, MD 21204, (301) 363-0300, BA 73 Loyola Coll; MS 74 Loyola Coll; Sp-Lang Path, Baltimore Co Pub Sch, **SLP**

Bunker, Vanessa Jow Route 2 Box 466, Beaverton, OR 97007, (503) 645-4242, BA 75 Pacific Univ; MS 79 Portland St Univ; Assist Coordinator of Spec Ed, Washington Co Ed Serv Dist, **SLP**

Bunn, Deidra L 4177 Lake Mist Drive, Kennesaw, GA 30144, (404) 432-0177, BA 74 Newberry Coll; OM 80 Emory Univ; Sp-Lang Path, Cobb County Bd of Ed, **SLP**

Bunn, Thomas T 60 Greenfield Court, Winter Haven, FL 33884, (813) 299-1251, BA 74 Univ of Central FL; MA 75 Univ of Central FL; Aud, Hearing Consultants Inc, **A**

Bunnell, Joyce Brown 2613 Mimi Circle, Philadelphia, PA 19131, (215) 878-7574, BA 79 East Carolina Univ; MS 86 East Carolina Univ; **A**

Bunnell, Mrs Maryann Riesland 540 Sunset, St Anthony, ID 83445, (208) 624-7427, BS 76 Walla Walla Coll; MS 78 Loma Linda Univ - Riverside; 88–Sp-Lang Path, Fremont Tri Dist Spec Svcs, **SLP**

Bunni, Maureen Bridget 90 Park Villa Court, Dayton, OH 45459-4724, (513) 835-5624, **SLP**

Bunselmeier, Karen Baxter 2803 Owens Street, Fairfield, CA 94533, BA 80 Humboldt St Univ; MA 83 Humboldt St Univ; SLP, Fairfield-Susan USD, **SLP**

Buntin, Bonnie P 95 North Street, Hurando, MS 38632, **SLP**

Bunting, Bonita M 2740 Woodley Place N W, Washington, DC 20008, (202) 462-0482, MA 87 George Washington Univ; **SLP**

Bunting, Glenn W 22 Pondview Circle, Sharon, MA 02067, (508) 273-8955, BA 78 Univ of ME - Orono; MS 80 Boston Univ; 86–Sp-Lang Path, Lahey Clinic Med Ctr, **SLP**

Bunting, Mrs Janet Lanfranco 6341 North Lead, Fresno, CA 93711, (209) 441-3328, BA 78 Univ of the Pacific; MA 79 Univ of the Pacific; SLP, Fresno USD, **SLP**

Bunting, Susan P O Box 122, Sitka, AK 99835, (907) 966-8320, BA 79 Univ of MT; MA 82 Univ of MT; SE Regional Aud, State of Alaska Commun Dis Prg, **A**

Buntzman, Louise B 2557 Morning Glory Drive, Bowling Green, KY 42101, **SLP**

Bunyard, Mrs Susan M G 109 Oakhurst Drive, Madison, AL 35758, (205) 895-0010, BS 78 Baylor Univ; MS 80 Phillips Univ; Sp-Lang Path, Center for Sp-Lang Path, **SLP**

Bunzendahl, Vivianne Wilson Box 10391, APO New York, NY 09012, (501) 834-2734, BA 82 Auburn Univ - Montgomery; ME 85 Univ of VA - Charlottesville; **SLP**

Buonaguro, Dr Antonia J 308 Casino Avenue, Cranford, NJ 07016, (212) 340-6025, BS 70 Seton Hall Univ; MA 71 Seton Hall Univ; ED 80 (NS) Rutgers St Univ -N Brunswick; Asst Res Sci/Sp-Lang Path, NYU Med Ctr/Rusk I Rehab Med, **SLP**

Buonpane, Sharyn L E 52 Agawam Drive, Wayne, NJ 07470, (201) 633-5262, BS 70 William Paterson Coll; MS 74 William Paterson Coll; Sp-Lang Path, Franklin Lakes Bd of Ed, **SLP**

Buoscio, Ronald M 1910 East 173rd Place, South Holland, IL 60473, **SLP**

Bupp, Mrs Chandler M 7321 Outhaul Lane, Burke, VA 22015, (703) 455-7180, BS 77 Central MO St Univ; MS 78 Central MO St Univ; **SLP**

Buppert, Mary Blair 17 Bellclare Circle, Sparks, MD 21152, (301) 529-4275, BS 80 Towson St Univ; MS 82 Towson St Univ; Sp-Lang Path, Balto Co Pub Sch, **SLP**

Bura, Marilyn B 232 Baldwin, Birmingham, MI 48009, (313) 682-2280, BA 52 Univ of MI - Ann Arbor; MA 76 Wayne St Univ; SLP, Waterford Sch, **SLP**

Burak-Bertram, Virginia 4 Windy Woods Circle, Newtown, CT 06470, (203) 426-1126, BA 72 Univ of CT; MS 73 Columbia Univ Teachers Coll; OM 80 Western CT St Univ; SLP, Commun Center, **SLP**

Burba, Linda Ann R P O Box 2994, Glen Ellyn, IL 60138, (312) 469-9200, BS 80 Purdue Univ - West Lafayette; MS 81 Purdue Univ - West Lafayette; Aud, Glen Ellyn Cl, **A**

Burbach, Cathy Ann 912 25th Avenue N W, Minot, ND 58701, BS 84 Minot St Univ; MS 85 Minot St Univ; **SLP**

Burberry, Jacqueline 68 Dutcher Street, Hopedale, MA 01747, (508) 478-8333, BS 75 SUNY - Coll at Brockport; MA 77 SUNY - Coll at Geneseo; Sp-Lang Path, Brookline PS, **SLP**

Burbey-Flingos, Mrs Jill 1160 Heron Avenue, Miami Springs, FL 33166, (305) 887-7786, BA 82 Univ of FL; ME 84 Univ of FL; Sp-Lang Path, Dade County PS, **SLP**

Burbridge, Mrs Sherry L 2200 South 14th, Blue Springs, MO 64015, (816) 224-3644, BS 78 Northeast MO St Univ; MA 80 Northeast MO St Univ; Sp-Lang Path, **SLP**

Burce, Carrie Alma 464 East Nevada, St Paul, MN 55101, (612) 771-7710, BA 83 Valparaiso Univ; MS 84 Univ of WI - Eau Claire; 85–Sp-Lang Path, St Paul PS, **SLP**

Burch, Donna 444 North Cedar Street, Florence, AL 35630, (205) 766-6686, BS 76 MS St Univ - MS State; MS 80 MS Univ for Women; Sp-Lang Path, Private Practice, **SLP**

Burch, Mrs Gloria Haynes P O Box 632, High Rolls, NM 88325, (505) 434-6200, MA 84 NM St Univ; Sp-Lang Path, Digame Sp-Lang Consultants, **SLP**

Burch, Mary Danko 101 Kerwood Place, Palestine, TX 75801, (214) 764-2615, BS 75 Southwest TX St Univ; MS 76 Univ of North TX; Aud, Dr Melinoa Duncan, **A**

Burch, Nancy Louise 535 Country Club Lane, San Bernardino, CA 92404, (714) 883-0129, BA 86 CA St Univ - Northridge; MA 88 CA St Univ - Northridge; 88–Sp-Lang Path, San Bernardino School District

Burch, Teresa S 203 38th Street East, Tuscaloosa, AL 35405-3011, (904) 682-9033, **A**

Burchett, Julie Lynn 1281 Village Drive #C-11, Lexington, KY 40504, (606) 254-6654, BA 86 Univ of KY; MS 87 Univ of KY; 88–Sp-Lang Path, Excepticon-Lexington Campus

Burchfiel, Michele F 1288 University Avenue, San Jose, CA 95126, BA 71 Univ of CA - Santa Barbara; MA 72 Univ of the Pacific; **SLP**

Burchfield, Mrs Bella Parro 302 Jacobs Street, Berwick, LA 70342, (504) 385-1983, BS 79 LA St Univ - Baton Rouge; OM 80 LA St Univ - N O Medical Ctr; Sp-Lang Path, Lakewood Hosp, **SLP**

Burchfield, Samuel B University Of Tennessee, Hearing Center Annex, 444 South Stadium Hall, Knoxville, TN 37916, (615) 974-5453, BS 65 East TN St Univ; MA 66 Univ of TN - Knoxville; PH 70 (NS) MI St Univ; Associate Professor, University of Tennessee, **A**

Burchyett, Shane Mulias 208 Southwest 83rd Way, Pembroke Pines, FL 33025, **SLP**

Burd, Laurie Lee 1312 Barton Avenue, Point Pleasant, NJ 08742, (201) 892-1559, BS 83 East Stroudsburg Univ of PA; MA 87 Trenton St Coll; 85–Sp-Lang Path, Freehold Twp Bd of Educ

Burda, Pamela Kay 204 N Mt Rushmore, Cedar Park, TX 78613, (512) 346-5562, BS 82 Univ of TX - Austin; MA 87 Univ of TX - Austin; **A**

Burden, Cynthia J 800 Stamford Drive, Neptune, NJ 07753, (201) 229-4089, BA 74 Rutger's St Univ - Douglas Coll; MS 76 Kean Coll of NJ; 81–Sp-Lang Path, Neptune Township Bd of Educ, **SLP**

Burdette, Regina L 171 Golden Gate Point #2, Sarasota, FL 33577, (813) 488-6880, BS 76 Univ of Montevallo; MS 81 Univ of Montevallo; Director/Sp-Lang Patology, Doctors Hospital of Sarasota, **SLP**

Burdick, Mrs Edythe O 64 Five Fields Road, Madison, CT 06443, (203) 245-7345, BS 54 Univ of CT; MS 72 Southern CT St Univ; Sp-Lang Path, Madison Bd of Ed, **SLP**

Burdick, Eleanor W 5529 Vernon Avenue South, Minneapolis, MN 55436, **A**

Burdick, Eve C 235 Prince Drive, Leesburg, FL 32748, (904) 728-3245, BS 43 Western MI Univ; MS 52 Univ of MI - Ann Arbor; **SLP LM**

Burdick, Dr Jeanne H PO Drawer 3320 Ess, Tuscaloosa, AL 35404, (205) 553-5500, BA 47 Andrews Univ; MA 52 Univ of Southern CA; PH 77 (NS) KS St Univ; Sp-Lang Path, Medtherapy, **SLP**

Burdine, Gayle Janeane 13839 Beckwith, Houston, TX 77014, (713) 872-8737, BS 76 Lamar Univ; MS 78 Lamar Univ; 88–Sp-Lang Path, River Oaks Tutor Lab, **SLP**

Burdine, Mrs Judy Crisp 4903 Sanderson Lane, Texarkana, AR 75502, (501) 774-9691, BS 78 Univ of Central AR; MA 86 LA Tech Univ

Burdine, Mrs Martha Jane Mt Region Speech & Hearing Ctr, 330 Broad Street, Kingsport, TN 37660, (615) 246-4600, BS 79 East TN St Univ; MS 82 East TN St Univ; Sp/Lang Path, Mt Reg Sp & Hrng Cen, **SLP**

Burdinie, Mrs Heather Turner P O Box 7303, Hilton Head, SC 29938, (803) 686-2273, BA 76 Loyola Univ of Chicago; MA 80 Northwestern Univ; 88–Director Sp-Lang Path, Special Care Therapy Assoc Inc, **SLP ACE**

Burditt, Gayle J L 11006 N E 37th Court, Bellevue, WA 98004, (206) 822-1365, BA 70; MA 71 Univ of the Pacific; Sp-Path Consul, Private Practice, **SLP**

Burdulis, Miriam M 42 Robinson Road, Woburn, MA 01801, (617) 334-5545, BS 65 Fitchburg St Coll; MA 70 Univ of MA - Amherst; Sp-Lang Path, Lynnfield Pub School System, **SLP ACE**

Burford, Ann Elaine 610 Nelson Circle, Noblesville, IN 46060, (317) 646-8171, BS 82 Purdue Univ - West Lafayette; MS 84 Purdue Univ - West Lafayette; 87–Sp-Lang Path, Saint John's Med Ctr, **SLP**

Burford, Mrs Nancy Grubbs 12122 Wembley, Houston, TX 77031, (713) 981-5713, BA 70 Marshall Univ; MA 71 Marshall Univ; Sp-Lang Path, Neuro-Dev Assoc of Houston, **SLP**

Burford, Sandra I 3222 1st Road North, Arlington, VA 22201, (703) 354-3940, BA 74 Portland St Univ; MS 76 Portland St Univ; 79–Sp-Lang Path, Fairfax Co Pub Sch, **SLP**

Burg, Mrs Linda Sue Department Of Otolaryngology, Med College Of Wisconsin, 8700 West Wisconsin Avenue, Milwaukee, WI 53226, (414) 257-5866, BS 82 Univ of WI - Whitewater; MS 84 Univ of WI - Stevens Point; 86–Aud, Med Coll of WI, **A**

Burgan, Mrs Rebecca Sieck 1016 Tracy Court, Cincinnati, OH 45245, (513) 671-7446, BS 82 Univ of Cincinnati; MA 84 OH Univ - Athens; Sp-Lang Path, Tri-Co Speech Assoc Inc, **SLP**

Burgard, Theresa C 1235 South Lincoln, Kankakee, IL 60901, (815) 932-4539, BS 80 Southern IL Univ -Carbondale; MA 81 Univ of IL - Urbana; Sp-Lang Path, Kankakee Sch Dist #111, **SLP**

Burgdorf, Sherrill Arlene 5000 Belmont, Apartment 124, Dallas, TX 75206, (214) 821-2511, BA 80 LA St Univ - Baton Rouge; MA 82 Univ of Houston - Univ Park; Prog Coord, ReEntry at Baylor, **SLP**

Burge, Heather Lois 90 Greenville Avenue, Clarion, PA 16214, (814) 226-4376, MS 88 Clarion Univ of PA

Burge, Nancy L 8401 Willows Road NE, Apartment GG 2116, Redmond, WA 98052, (206) 881-6494, BS 77 Purdue Univ - West Lafayette; MS 81 Univ of WI - Madison; 88–Sp-Lang Path, Univ of Washington, **SLP ACE**

Burgei, Thomas J 2439 Dolphin Drive, San Jose, CA 95124, MS 76 San Jose St Univ; Junior High School Principal, Oak Grove School District, **SLP**

Burger, Hannah J 29 Seward Lane, Stony Brook, NY 11790, **SLP LM**

Burger, Mrs Linda H PO Box 31161, Walnut Creek, CA 94598, (415) 934-8932, MA 80 Univ of CA - Santa Barbara; Sp/Lang Path, Private Practice, **SLP**

Burger, Lori Lee Route 2 Box 241, Clovis, NM 88101, (505) 762-0547, BS 83 Eastern NM Univ; MS 85 Northern AZ Univ; **SLP**

Burger, Robin R 10815 67th Avenue, Flushing, NY 11375, (212) 793-5799, BA 74 CUNY - Lehman Coll; MA 77 CUNY - Hunter Coll; Aud, HMO, **A**

Burger, Mrs Teresa A 174 Overbrook Road, West Hartford, CT 06107, BA 78 Boston Coll; MS 81 Southern CT St Univ; Sp-Lang Path, Southington Pub Sch, **SLP**

Burgeson, Marilee Burnett 167 Via La Paz, San Marcos, CA 92069, (619) 741-7369, BA 76 Univ of CO - Boulder; MA 78 Univ of CO - Boulder; SLP, San Diego County Office of Ed, **SLP**

Burgess, Mrs Anne D D 44038 Parkside, Canton, MI 48187, (313) 758-2819, BA 74 MI St Univ; MA 75 MI St Univ; SLP, Metro Home Hlthcare Serv Inc, **SLP**

Burgess, Sr Augusta Ann St Josephs Provincial House, 385 Watervliet-Shaker Road, Latham, NY 12110, (518) 785-4632, BS 67 Coll of Saint Rose; MA 75 Coll of Saint Rose; 75–Sp/Lang Path, Carondelet Ed Cen, **SLP**

Burgess, Barbara B 535 7th Avenue N E, Tuscaloosa, AL 35405, (205) 348-7131, BA 81 Univ of AL- Tuscaloosa; MS 82 Univ of AL- Tuscaloosa; 87–Supvr-Head Start Prog, Univ of AL Speech & Hearing Ctr, **SLP**

Burgess, Mrs Bethany J 9188 Fletcher Trace, Memphis, TN 38134, (901) 388-0113, BS 80 IN St Univ - Terre Haute; MA 82 OH Univ - Athens; 83–Aud, ENT Consultants of Memphis, **A**

Burgess, Mrs Carla Dodd 1736 Pine Street, New Orleans, LA 70118, (504) 861-4625, BA 31 6839; MS 65 6839; **SLP LM**

Burgess, Cynthia A 2747 North Wilderness Ct, Wichita, KS 67226-2109, (316) 681-0474, BS 73 Univ of KS; MA 75 Univ of KS; **SLP**

Burgess, Mrs Dawn Thompson 611 Payton Drive, Fredericksburg, VA 22405-2252, (703) 373-5569, BA 81 Mary Washington Coll; MS 83 Miami Univ - Oxford; **SLP**

Burgess, Mrs Eleanor H 114 Troup Street, Rochester, NY 14608, BA 51 Albion Coll; MA 61 MI St Univ; Retired, **SLP F LM**

Burgess, Kathleen 41 Danby Street, Providence, RI 02904, (401) 831-2474, BA 82 Univ of RI; MS 86 Emerson Coll; 86–Sp-Lang Path, Rhode Island Hosp, **SLP**

Burgess, Mrs Laura Frances 4141 W City Court #71, El Paso, TX 79902, BA 84 Univ of TX - El Paso; MS 86 Univ of TX - El Paso; **SLP**

Burgess, Lucinda Anne 8540 Citation Drive #121, Richmond, BC, Canada V8A 2Z1, (604) 946-1221, BA 82 Univ of WA; MA 84 IN Univ - Bloomington; Sp-Lang Path, Ministry of Health, **SLP ACE**

Burgess, Mrs Mary Ann A 12421 23rd Avenue N E, Seattle, WA 98125, (206) 367-1111, BA 76 Univ of WA; OM 78 Univ of WA; SLP, Shoreline Public Schools, **SLP**

Burgess, Mrs Nancy Gallier 1647 West Lindberg, Springfield, MO 65807-2223, (417) 869-8878, **SLP**

Burgess, Paul D, Jr 42 East 63rd #1B, New York, NY 10021, (212) 678-5360, OB 53; BA 50 WA St Univ; MA 60 Columbia Univ Teachers Coll; Dir-SLP/Aud, Sydenham Nfcc Dev Eval Ut, **SLP A**

Burgess, Dr Ruth Vassar Southwest Missouri State Univ, 901 South National, Springfield, MO 65804, (417) 836-5593, BS 60 TX Tech Univ; MA 68 Univ of MO - Columbia; PH 79 (NS) Univ of MO - Columbia; Assoc Prof, SW Mo St U, **SLP**

Burgess, Stephanie Dawn Route 5 Box 29, Bardstown, KY 40004, (502) 348-6848, MS 86 Western KY Univ; **SLP**

Burgess, Mrs Valerie Ann 2206 Lee Lane, Aston, PA 19014, (215) 494-4474, BS 81 Bloomsburg Univ of PA; MS 82 Bloomsburg Univ of PA; Sp-Lang Path, Private Practice, **SLP**

Burgess, Mrs Vicky L 1940 Skyline Vista, La Habra, CA 90631, (213) 691-1131, BA 70 Holy Names Coll; OM 73 Univ of WA; **SLP**

Burgess-Hall, Mrs Nancy Dyer 1405 Edgewater Road, Daytona Beach, FL 32014, (904) 255-0377, BS 77 West Chester Univ of PA; MA 83 Univ of FL; 86–Sp/Lang Path, Volusia Co Sch Bd, **SLP**

Burgett, Sally A 5029 18th Street North, St Petersburg, FL 33714, (813) 522-0993, MS 77 Univ of South FL; SLP, Burgett Rehabilitation Therapy, **SLP**

Burggraaf, Cynthia Lieberg 643 East Palm Drive, Glendora, CA 91740, Assoc Prof / Clinical Superv, U of Redlands, **SLP**

Burgi, Dr Ernest J Rd 2 Box 291-A, Cheswick, PA 15024, (412) 624-6751, BA 50 AZ St Univ; MA 51 Univ of Denver; PH 57 (Aud) Univ of Pittsburgh - Pittsburgh; Retired, U of Pittsburgh, **SLP A F**

Burgin, Marilyn R 1718 47th Street, Pennsauken, NJ 08110, (609) 779-1125, BS 74 Bloomsburg Univ of PA; MA 77 Trenton St Coll; Sp-Lang Path, Maple Shade Bd of Ed, **SLP**

Burgraff, Dr Roger I P O Box 909, Redlands, CA 92373, (714) 793-1283, BA 63 De Paul Univ; MA 65 De Paul Univ; PH 70 (NS) Univ of Denver; Sp-Lang Path, Pettis Mem VA Hosp, **SLP**

Burhans, Mrs Denise Strickler 1491 Grace Avenue, Lakewood, OH 44107, (216) 221-2930, BS 76 WV Univ; MS 77 WV Univ; **A**

Burhans-Ross, Wendy Ann St Marys Hospital For Children, 29-01 216th Street, Bayside, NY 11360, (718) 990-8883, BA 79 SUNY - Coll at Cortland; MS 82 Columbia Univ Teachers Coll; Sp-Lang Path, St Mary's Hosp for Chldn, **SLP**

Burica, Cathleen Sue 14430 East Mulberry Drive, Apartment 233, Whittier, CA 90604, BS 81 Miami Univ - Oxford; MS 83 Rush Univ; Sp-Lang Path, Newport Lang Sp Aud Ctr Inc, **SLP**

Burigo, Janice R 11 Hyatt Lane, Westport, CT 06880, (203) 762-3374, BA 72 Boston Univ; MA 73 Northeastern Univ; SLP, Wilton Public Schools, **SLP**

Burik, Christine E RD #1, Jacksonville Road, Burlington, NJ 08016, (201) 613-6815, BA 72 Rutger's St Univ - Douglas Coll; MS 78 Rutgers St Univ - Camdem; Sp-Lang Path, E Brunswick Bd of Ed, **SLP**

Burk, Mrs Anita Manning Route #6 Wheeler Drive, Lenoir City, TN 37771, (615) 986-2936, BS 75 Univ of TN - Knoxville; MA 86 Univ of TN - Knoxville; 86–Sp-Lang Path, Knox Co Sch Sys, **SLP**

Burk, Cathy Guinty 2002 South Parkwood Lane, Wichita, KS 67218, (316) 262-8271, BA 77 Wichita St Univ; MA 79 Wichita St Univ; 88–Sp-Lang Path, HCA Wesley Med Ctr, **SLP**

Burk, Mrs Cindy 11022 West Crimson Lane, Phoenix, AZ 85039, BS 73 AZ St Univ; MS 75 AZ St Univ; 75–Sp-Lang Path, Avondale Sch Dist/Union Sch Dist, **SLP**

Burk, Dr Kenneth W 2002 South Parkwood Lane, Wichita, KS 67218, (316) 689-3240, BA 53 Univ of IA; MA 55 Univ of KY; PH 62 (NS) Purdue Univ - West Lafayette; Professor, Wichita State University, **SLP F**

Burk, Mrs Sherri Nell Box 50, Chicota, TX 75425, (214) 785-7539, **SLP**

Burka, Barbara N P O Box 16, Great Falls, VA 22066, **SLP A**

Burkard, Amy Brown 1406 Acton Street, Berkeley, CA 94702, (415) 652-0234, MS 86 San Francisco St Univ

Burkard, Robert F Dept Of Communication Disorders, Boston University, 48 Cummington Street, Boston, MA 02215, (617) 353-5640, BA 76 SUNY - Coll at Buffalo; MS 78 Univ of WI - Madison; PH 83 (Aud) Univ of WI - Madison; 85–Asst Prof, Boston Univ, **A**

Burke, Mrs Alice W 902 Parkview Drive, New Iberia, LA 70560, (318) 365-4506, BS 71 Saint Mary's Dominican Coll; MS 74 Tulane Univ; Sp-Lang Path, Private Practice, **SLP**

Burke, Barbara R 8023 Spottswood Road, Richmond, VA 23229, (804) 270-6647, BA 72 Mary Baldwin Coll; ME 75 Univ of VA - Charlottesville; SLP, Henrico Co Publ Sch, **SLP**

Burke, Bonnie F 412 Ole Dominion Road, Bristol, VA 24201, (703) 669-7422, BA 73 Wayne St Coll; MA 78 Univ of NE - Lincoln; Sp-Lang Path, Private Practice, **SLP**

Burke, Cabell R 12600 Foxstone Court, Midlothian, VA 23113-2279, (804) 794-4152, BA 74 Randolph-Macon Woman's Coll; MA 75 Vanderbilt Univ; Sp-Lang Path, Chesterfield Co PS, **SLP**

Burke, Mrs Catherine Anne 222 Prospect Street, Midland Park, NJ 07432, (201) 567-7292, BA 81 Coll of Mount Saint Vincent; MA 84 Seton Hall Univ; Sp-Lang Path, American International School

Burke, Catherine Anne 1111 Thornwood Drive, Birmingham, AL 35209, (205) 879-2640, BS 82 Univ of South AL; MS 84 Univ of Montevallo; Sp-Lang Path, Sparks Cen Fr Devlp & Lrng Dis, **SLP**

Burke, Mrs Christie Lynn 2645 Hickory Lawn, Rochester Hills, MI 48063, (313) 852-5681, BS 85 Central MI Univ; MS 86 Central MI Univ; 86–Sp-Lang Path, Total Rehab, **SLP**

Burke, Deborah M 14 Lefebvre Lane, Williston, VT 05495, (802) 893-1188, MS 76 Univ of VT; BA 74 Univ of VT; Sp-Lang Path, Milton Graded Sch Dist, **SLP**

Burke, Mrs Deborah Stirrat 3238 Reeve Drive West, Bethlehem Township, PA 18017, (215) 868-3284, BS 75 Northeastern Univ; MA 77 Seton Hall Univ; Sp-Lang Path, Providence Hospital, **SLP**

Burke, Mrs Diane R 2315 Houston Avenue, Norman, OK 73071, (405) 325-3111, BA 75 Univ of OK - Norman; MS 77 Univ of OK Medical Center; Sp-Lang Path, Private Practice, **SLP**

Burke, Mrs Elaine Brown 1021 Blueberry Hill, Mount Vernon, IL 62864, (618) 242-4600, BS 76 Central MO St Univ; MS 77 Central MO St Univ; Aud, Good Samaritan Hosp, **A**

Burke, Mrs Elizabeth H F 410 North Booth, Dubuque, IA 52001, (319) 588-1530, BS 72 Univ of WI - Madison; MS 73 Univ of WI - Madison; 88–Sp-Lang Path, Med Assoc Clinic, **SLP**

Burke, Grace M 665 Hope Street, Providence, RI 02906, (401) 421-7284, BS 80 West Chester Univ of PA; MS 84 Univ of RI; Sp-Lang Path, Bradley Hosp, **SLP**

Burke, John J Computer Speech Systems, 17 Rosemont Road, Oak Ridge, NJ 07438, (201) 584-8145, BA 72 Fordham Univ; MA 81 Montclair St Coll; Sp-Lang Path, Computer Speech Systems, **SLP**

Burke, John R P O Box 770042, Steamboat Springs, CO 80477, (303) 879-7286, BA 78 San Diego St Univ; MA 82 San Diego St Univ; Aud, Northwest Speech & Hearing Ser, **SLP A**

Burke, Kathleen F P O Box 57, Cocoa Beach, FL 32931, (305) 783-2382, BA 68 Oakland Univ; MA 77 Western MI Univ; Sp-Lang Path, Private Practice, **SLP**

Burke, Mrs Kathleen McVicar 10440 Marion Street, Northglenn, CO 80233, (303) 798-1309, BS 82 CO St Univ; MS 85 Univ of OK Medical Center; **A**

Burke, Kathleen Smith 20 West Meadow Drive, Albany, NY 12203, (518) 442-5385, BA 73 SUNY - Coll at Plattsburgh; ME 82 Coll of Saint Rose; Sp-Lang Path, Res Found Sunya Prekndgrn, **SLP**

Burke, Mrs Leslie Croft 15 Carolyn Drive, Westborough, MA 01581, (508) 460-3507, BS 77 Univ of NH; MS 83 Worcester St Coll; Sp-Lang Path, Marlborough Pub Sch, **SLP**

Burke, Linda Dunneage 903 Martins Creek Blvd, Summerville, SC 29483, (803) 871-7398, **SLP**

Burke, Mrs Linda M 16021 Diagonal Road, Lagrange, OH 44050, (216) 355-6965, BA 74 SUNY - Coll at Oswego; MA 76 Kent St Univ; Sp/Lang Path, Private Practice, **SLP**

Burke, Lois E 82 Honeysuckle Drive, Chicopee, MA 01020, (413) 781-9100, BA 74 Univ of NH; MS 77 ID St Univ; Audiology Coor, Mercy Hospital, **A**

Burke, Margaret C Baltimore Gas & Electric Co, Attn Medical Department, P O Box 1475 Charles Center, Baltimore, MD 21203, (301) 234-6433, BS 77 WV Univ; MS 79 WV Univ; Aud, Balto Gas & Elec Co, **A ACE**

Burke, Margaret Noel 1025 Avenue C Apartment 113, Bayonne, NJ 07002, BA 80 Kean Coll of NJ; MA 81 Kean Coll of NJ; 88–Aud, Elizabeth Bd of Educ, **A**

Burke, Marlene W 4009 Avenue B, Scottsbluff, NE 69361, (308) 635-3155, BS 86 CO St Univ; MS 88 CO St Univ; 88–Aud, Western ENT Assoc

Burke, Mrs Mary Anne 312 Belanger, Grosse Pointe Farms, MI 48236, (313) 341-1353, BA 78 MI St Univ; MA 80 Wayne St Univ; Sp-Lang Path, Warren Woods Pub Sch, **SLP**

Burke, Mary Eileen S 7 Gardner Avenue, Middletown, NY 10940, (914) 294-8806, BS 79 SUNY - Coll at Geneseo; MS 81 Columbia Univ Teachers Coll; Sp/Lang Path, Orange Co Cpa, **SLP**

Burke, Nancy M 6131 North 16th St #B-101, Phoenix, AZ 85015, **SLP**

Burke, Mrs Patricia E 19 Split Tree Drive, Wappingers Falls, NY 12590, (914) 342-7205, BS 78; MS 79; 88–Sp-Lang Path, Horton Mem Hosp, **SLP**

Burke, Mrs Sharon Lynn 610 S Camino Saguaro, Apache Junction, AZ 85219, (602) 982-4562, BS 82 AZ St Univ; BS 84 AZ St Univ; OM 87 AZ St Univ; 87–Sp-Lang Path, Chandler USD, **SLP**

Burke, Sheila Burnett 1234 Divisadero Street, San Francisco, CA 94115, (415) 921-7658, BA 85 0583; MS 87 San Francisco St Univ; **A**

Burke, Sherri S 1209 W 16th Street S #104, Newton, IA 50208, BS 84 IA St Univ; MS 87 Univ of NE - Lincoln; **SLP**

Burke, Susan 153 Cole Court, Buchanan, NY 10511, (914) 739-2855, BA 75 Marymount Coll; MS 76 Columbia Univ Teachers Coll; 86–Sp-Lang Path, Early Intervention Svcs PARC, **SLP**

Burke, Terry L 1905 Blake Avenue Ste 201, Glenwood Springs, CO 81601, (303) 945-8989, BS 70 Southeast MO St Univ; MA 74 Memphis St Univ; Owner, Hrng & Sp Assoc, **A**

Burke, Veronica A 2470 Charms Road, Milford, MI 48042, (313) 685-1869, BA 74 Western MI Univ; MA 79 Eastern MI Univ; Sp-Lang Path, Private Practice, **SLP**

Burke-Constantineau, Eileen M North Scituate Elementary School, Institute Lane, North Scituate, RI 02857, (401) 647-5926, BS 76 SUNY - Coll at New Paltz; MA 77 SUNY - Coll at Geneseo; 88–Sp-Lang Path, No Scituate Elem Sch, **SLP**

Burke-Daoust, Jeanette Eileen 8676 Yukon #302-F, Arvada, CO 80005, (303) 424-4704, MA 88 Univ of CO - Boulder

Burke-Martin, Laura Ann 113 Peach Lane, Ames, IA 50010, BS 85 Northern IL Univ - De Kalb; MA 87 Northern IL Univ - De Kalb; Aud, Heartland AEA, **A**

Burke-Peterson, Mary D Childrens Memorial Hospital, Communicative Disorders, 2300 Childrens Plaza, Chicago, IL 60614, (312) 880-4530, BS 73 Univ of Cincinnati; MA 75 Northwestern Univ; 79–Aud, Chldn's Mem Hosp, **A**

Burkes, Mrs Susan C 1560 Lee Drive, Clarksdale, MS 38614, (601) 627-5247, BA 78 Univ of MS; OM 80 Univ of MS; Sp-Path, Clarksdale Separate Schools, **SLP**

Burke-Thompson, Maureen 2140 Elm Tree Road, Elm Grove, WI 53122-1118, (414) 782-2614, BA 74 Rutger's St Univ - Douglas Coll; MS 81 Univ of WI - Milwaukee; Sp-Lang Path, Private Practice, **SLP**

Burkett, Argyra Marie 3307 North 63th Place, Scottsdale, AZ 85251, (602) 947-0332, BA; 87–Aud, Audiology Associates, **A**

Burkett, Sidney Wright 988 Oak Ridge Turnpike, Suite L-10, Oak Ridge, TN 37830, (615) 482-4727, BA 83 Auburn Univ - Montgomery; OM 84 Auburn Univ - Auburn; 86–Sp-Lang Path, Oak Ridge Speech Center, **SLP**

Burkhard, Beth A 7876 Spring Avenue, Park Spring Manor #3F, Elkins Park, PA 19117, (215) 928-7445, BA 80 MI St Univ; MS 82 Univ of WI - Madison; Sp-Lang Path, Thomas Jefferson Univ Hosp, **SLP**

Burkhardt, Linda Mae 1205 South 12th Avenue, Yakima, WA 98902, (509) 248-2360, BA 74 Central WA Univ; ME 81 Western WA Univ; SLP, Moxee Sch Dist #90, **SLP**

Burkhart, Brian Paul 5715 Jurgella Lane, Stevens Point, WI 54481, (715) 345-5454, MS 85 Univ of WI - Stevens Point; 88–Sp-Lang Path, Stevens Point PS, **SLP ACE**

Burkhart, Elizabeth Hohl 8 Madary Road, Severna Park, MD 21146, (301) 262-5550, BA 79 Ball St Univ; MA 81 Ball St Univ; Sp-Lang Path, Kilby Easter Seal Ctr, **SLP**

Burkhart, John N 165 Slatewood Court, Bethel Park, PA 15102, (412) 873-3489, BS 68 CA Univ of PA; ME 70 CA Univ of PA; Coord-Dept Comm Dev, Western Center, **SLP**

Burkhart, Mrs Nancy Ellen 53 Loyola Avenue, Ventura, CA 93003-2313, (805) 527-2462, BS 78 IL St Univ - Normal; MA 83 Northern IL Univ - De Kalb; 86–Sp-Lang Path, Simi Valley Adventist Hosp, **SLP**

Burkhart, Nancy L 533 Fieldstone Drive, Amherst, OH 44001, (216) 984-2416, BS 76 SUNY - Coll at Brockport; MA 78 Bowling Green St Univ; Aud, Rehab Cen Lorain Co Inc, **A**

Burkholder, Joann E 64 East College Avenue, Westerville, OH 43081, BS 71 OH St Univ; MA 76 Kent St Univ; Sp-Lang Path, De Co Pub Sch, **SLP**

Burkholz, Robin Aimee 374 Palos Verdes Blvd, Redondo Beach, CA 90277, (213) 674-7050, BS 79 Emerson Coll; MA 81 Univ of Pittsburgh - Pittsburgh; Sp-Lang Path, Daniel Freeman Mem Hosp, **SLP**

Burkink, Denise Wyman 3635 Landers Lane, Arlington, TX 76014, (817) 292-9723, BS 84 Univ of SD - Vermillion; MA 86 Univ of SD - Vermillion; 86–Sp-Lang Path, Erly Chldn Inter/Ft Worth State Sch, **SLP**

Burkland, Mrs Marjorie B 1020 Grove Street, Evanston, IL 60201, (312) 328-4328, BA 41 Augustana Coll; MA 42 Northwestern Univ; Sp-Lang Path, Evanston Township Hgh Sch, **SLP F LM ACE**

Burklund, Lee Marie 10409 South Menard #107, Oak Lawn, IL 60453, (312) 754-3537, BA 77 Valparaiso Univ; OM 84 Governors St Univ; Sp-Lang Path, South Metro Assoc, **SLP**

Burkowsky, Dr Mitchell R Speech And Hearing Clinic, State University College, Fredonia, NY 14063, BA 52 SUNY - Center at Albany; PH 60 (Sp) Wayne St Univ; Prof SLP/Aud, SUNY/Fredonia, **SLP ACE**

Burks, Cheryl Lynn 3840 Mizell Road #F, Greensboro, NC 27405, (919) 621-5081, BS 82 Radford Univ; MS 83 Radford Univ; Sp-Lang Path, MedTherapy Rehab Svcs, **SLP**

Burks, Dan A Route 1 Box 710, Lakeview, AR 72642, (501) 435-6655, BS 76 AR St Univ; MS 77 AR St Univ; Sp-Lang Path, Cotler Pub Sch, **SLP**

Burks, Gregory L Mid-Valley Speech & Hrng Ctr, 950 S W 29th Street, Albany, OR 97321, (503) 926-8092, BS 71 ID St Univ; MS 72 ID St Univ; Sp-Lang Path, Mid Valley Sp/Hrng Cen, **SLP**

Burks, Dr Sheila S Rt 4 Box 51, Terrell, TX 75160, BA 61 Univ of North TX; MA 65 TX Woman's Univ; PH 80 (NS) Univ of MO - Columbia; 88–Dir Sp-Lang Path, Terrell State Hosp, **SLP**

Burl, Nola T 1505 West 55th, North Little Rock, AR 72118, (501) 450-3176, BS 77 Univ of AR - Little Rock; MS 79; Memphis St Univ; 88–Sp-Lang Path, Univ of Central Arkansas, **SLP**

Burleigh, Andrew J 5219 McMurray Drive, Fort Collins, CO 80525-5525, (303) 226-0829, BS 78 CO St Univ; MS 79 CO St Univ; **A**

Burleigh, Mrs Joan M 5219 McMurray Drive, Fort Collins, CO 80525, (303) 226-0829, BS 71 Univ of Tulsa; MA 73 Northwestern Univ; Asst Dir Central Aud Research, Co St U, **SLP A**

Burleigh, Sally 601 East Micheltorena, Santa Barbara, CA 93103, (805) 962-7661, BA 70 Univ of CA - Santa Barbara; MA 72 CA St Univ - Fullerton; Dir, Private Practice, **SLP**

Burleson, Paula Deyon 1211 Lanier Boulevard, Atlanta, GA 30306, (404) 325-3011, BS 77 Univ of GA; ME 79 GA St Univ; Sp-Lang Path, Dekalb County Board of Educ, **SLP**

Burleson, Paula L P O Box 579, Houlton, ME 04730, (207) 532-7130, MA 87 Univ of ME - Orono; 87–Sp-Lang Path, Aroostook Mental Health Center, **SLP**

Burley, Kathryn L 6191 County Road 33 RD 3, Canandaigua, NY 14424, (315) 789-6828, BS 83 SUNY - Coll at Geneseo; MA 85 OH Univ - Athens; Sp-Lang Path, Finger Lakes UCP, **SLP**

Burley, Mrs Rachel S Asa Wood School, 700 Idaho Avenue, Libby, MT 59923, (406) 293-8881, BS 73 Univ of TN - Knoxville; MS 81 Eastern WA Univ; 75–Sp/Lang Path, Libby Pub Sch, **SLP**

Burley, Dr Robert M Burley And Associates, 5012 Liberty Avenue, Vermillion, OH 44089, (216) 967-4267, BA 74 Kent St Univ; MA 76 Kent St Univ; OD 82 (NS) IL Coll of Optometry; Ch Exec Officer, Burley & Assoc, **A**

Burlingame, Tammy L Rolling Oaks Apts #9-A, 8th Street North, Clanton, AL 35045, (205) 755-1807, 87 Univ of Montevallo

Burman, Barbara E Box 1121, Soldotna, AK 99669, (907) 262-9006, BS 74 CO St Univ; MS 76 CO St Univ; Sp-Lang Path, Kenai Penins Bor Sch, **SLP**

Burman, Mrs Brenda J 21229 Alexander Drive, St Clair Shores, MI 48081, (313) 772-8863, BS 63 Emerson Coll; Sp-Lang Path, Private Practice, **SLP**

Burman, Mrs Julia Ann 5909 Chalmers Drive, Knoxville, TN 37920, (615) 577-5970, BS 78 Univ of TN - Knoxville; MA 80 Univ of TN - Knoxville; 80–Sp-Lang Path, Sevier County Board of Educ, **SLP**

Burman, Laurie E 6805 Mayfield Road #1507, Mayfield Heights, OH 44124, (216) 231-8787, BA 83 SUNY - Center at Buffalo; MA 85 Univ of CT; 86–Coor of Aud, Cleveland Hrng & Sp Ctr, **A**

Burmeister, Patricia B 288 Kehoe, Randle, WA 98377-9207, (206) 694-4469, BA 76 Univ of Northern CO; MA 77 Univ of Northern CO; Aud, Vancouver Hearing & Sp Cen, **A**

Burmesch, Julianna Fisher 1101 Hickory Drive, Stevens Point, WI 54481, (715) 341-6464, BS 82 Univ of WI - Stevens Point; MS 84 Univ of WI - Stevens Point; Sp-Lang Path, Dc Everest Schools, **SLP**

Burmester, Mrs Barbara Bridges Route 6 Box 41, Decatur, AL 35603, (205) 355-4549, BS 79 Auburn Univ - Auburn; MS 80 Univ of AL- Tuscaloosa; Sp-Lang Path, Private Practice, **SLP**

Burn, Mrs Lois Murphy 29 Ellen Street, Bethpage, NY 11714, (516) 922-4100, BS 74 SUNY - Coll at Geneseo; MA 78 Hofstra Univ; 77–Sp-Lang Path, Mill Neck Manor Sch for Deaf, **SLP**

Burnell, Christine Switzer 2811 East Katella Avenue, Suite 204, Orange, CA 92667-5234, (714) 997-7459, BA 75 Univ of MT; MA 77 Univ of MT; Sp-Lang Path, Private Practice, **SLP**

Burnell, Mrs Marilyn K 111 North Brook Forest, Derby, KS 67037, (316) 682-9383, BA 69 Wichita St Univ; MA 70 Wichita St Univ; **SLP**

Burneo, Dr Cesar A Catholic Univ Of Ecuador, P O Box 2184, Quito, Ecuador, OB 67; MS 77 PA St Univ - Univ Park; ED 78 (NS); Professor, Catholic U of Ecuador

Burnett, Ardyce Elaine 2800 Lexington Place N E, Apartment 37, Albuquerque, NM 87112, (505) 299-6023, BA 83 Univ of NM; MS 86 Univ of North TX; 88–Sp-Lang Path, Albuquerque PS, **SLP**

Burnett, Arlene E 207 Dogwood Lane, Berkeley Heights, NJ 07922, (201) 665-9075, BA 73 Univ of Rochester; MA 75 Northwestern Univ; Sp/Lang Path, Overlook Hosp, **SLP**

Burnett, Catherine Patricia 377 Main Street, Owego, NY 13827, (607) 722-5308, BA 50 Coll of Saint Rose; MS 73 Ithaca Coll; Dir Sp/Hrng Dept, Rehab Serv Inc, **SLP**

Burnett, Mrs Judy C 3138 Stratford, Arlington Heights, IL 60004, (312) 870-0622, BS 75 Univ of IL - Urbana; MS 76 Univ of IL - Urbana; **SLP**

Burnett, Mrs Kathleen Smith 20604 Ehle Road, Route 1, Woodburn, IN 46797, (219) 632-5966, BA 78 Bowling Green St Univ; MA 82 IN Univ - Bloomington; **SLP**

Burnett, Lynn M 102 Olde Springs Road, Columbia, SC 29223, (803) 736-8268, BS 72 Univ of GA; ME 73 Univ of GA; ME 87 Univ of SC - Columbia; Educ Prog Spec, Sumpter District 2 Schools, **SLP A**

Burnett, Marsha K R R 2 Lot 39, Idlewood Drive, Bloomington, IL 61701, (217) 648-2731, MS 81 IL St Univ - Normal; Sp-Lang Path, Illinois St Univ Lab School, **SLP**

Burnett, Melodi Anne 2800 Northeast 14th Street, Apartment 208, Pompano Beach, FL 33062, (305) 393-9150, MA 84 Univ of FL; Aud, Ear Nose Throat Assc S Florida, **A**

Burnett, Patricia Ann Oklahoma City Clinic/Audiology, 701 N E 10th Street, Oklahoma City, OK 73104, (405) 271-2791, BS 74 PA St Univ - Univ Park; MS 81 Univ of WA; Aud, OK City Clinic, **A**

Burnett, Mrs Sherilyn Powell 8 Chapel Street, Summit, NJ 07901, (201) 273-3560, BA 83 OH St Univ; MA 85 OH St Univ; 88–Sp-Lang Path, Children's Specialized Hosp, **SLP**

Burnette, Jacqueline Tiongson 3560 Hughes Avenue, Apt 109, Los Angeles, CA 90034, (213) 839-1530, BS 83 Vanderbilt Univ; MA 86 Northwestern Univ; **SLP**

Burney, Ellen V 18934 East Gunnison Place, Aurora, CO 80017, (303) 428-1405, BA 76 Univ of Denver; MA 77 Univ of Denver; SLP, Dist 50 Pub Shc, **SLP**

Burney, Phillip A Desert Hearing Consultants Inc, 555 Tachevah, Bldg 2E Suite 107, Palm Springs, CA 92262, (619) 323-5645, BA 67 CA St Univ - Long Beach; MA 71 CA St Univ - Long Beach; Aud, Desert Hrng Consultants Inc, **A**

Burnham, Mrs Margaret G 13218 Agarita Lane, Houston, TX 77083, (713) 498-8110, BA 75 Baylor Univ; MA 80 Univ of Houston - Univ Park; Sp-Lang Path, Alief ISD, **SLP**

Burnham, Nora Eileen P O Box 167, Calistoga, CA 94515, (707) 253-6865, BA 77 CA St Univ - Chico; MA 82 CA St Univ - Chico; Sp-Lang Path, Napa Co Ofs of Ed, **SLP**

Burns, Angele W P O Box 642, Madison, MS 39110, (601) 856-3955, BS 73 Univ Southern MS-Hattiesburg; MS 81 Univ of MS; Sp-Lang Path, Pearl Municip Separate Sch Dis, **SLP**

Burns, Arlene G 145 Hewett Road, Wyncote, PA 19095, (215) 663-6063, BA 73 Princeton Univ; MS 75 Columbia Univ Teachers Coll; Sp-Lang Path, Private Practice, **SLP**

Burns, Mrs Bethany A 100 North Wolf, Apt 2W, Wheeling, IL 60090-2959, (312) 541-2454, BS 82 Central MI Univ; MA 84 Central MI Univ; Sp-Lang Path, Northwest Educational Coop, **SLP**

Burns, Mrs Carol J 45 Park Avenue, Delaware, OH 43015, (614) 363-0965, BS 82 OH Univ - Athens; MA 87 Kent St Univ; 88–Prog Dir of Aud, DE Sp and Hrng Ctr, **A**

Burns, Mrs Catherine Pelham 15110 West 131st Street, Olathe, KS 66062, (913) 780-4117, BA 86 Depauw Univ; MA 88 Univ of KS; 88–Sp-Lang Path, Communi Care

Burns, Mrs Cinda S C 13 Doolin Drive, Williamstown, WV 26187, (304) 420-9544, BS 75 WV Univ; MA 80 OH Univ - Athens; Sp-Lang Path, Wood Co Bd of Ed, **SLP**

Burns, Mrs Danielle S 1220 Arthur, Davis, CA 95616, BA 75 CA St Univ - Long Beach; MA 79 CA St Univ - Long Beach; Spec Day Class Tchr, Joint Unified Schools, **SLP**

Burns, Deborah H 5255 Camden Avenue #12, San Jose, CA 95124, (408) 842-8234, BS 79 Univ of CA - Santa Barbara; MS 81 Univ of OR; SLP, Gilroy USD, **SLP**

Burns, Mrs Debra J 7201 Mildred Court, Machesney Park, IL 61111, (608) 364-5203, BS 81 Northern IL Univ - De Kalb; MA 83 Northern IL Univ - De Kalb; Sp-Lang Path, Beloit Memorial Hosp, **SLP**

Burns, Edward M Univ Of WA, M/S JG-15, 1417 NE 42nd Street, Seattle, WA 98195, (206) 543-7979, BS 62 Univ of Notre Dame; MS 66 Univ of AZ; PH 77 (NS) Univ of MN - Minneap-St Paul; Assoc Prof, Univ of WA

Burns, Frank R MDPH No Reg Div, 3500 N Logan, Lansing, MI 48909, (906) 226-3519, BS 67 Northern MI Univ; MA 69 Western MI Univ; Consult, Mich Dept of Pub Hlth, **A**

Burns, Gail Ann 2240 Vermilion Road, Duluth, MN 55803, (218) 723-4150, BS 68 Bowling Green St Univ; MA 85 Univ of MN - Duluth; **SLP**

Burns, Janet Pasteris 21 Deer Run, Plantsville, CT 06479-1303, (203) 276-0206, BA 73 Coll of Saint Francis; MA 77 Governors St Univ; **SLP**

Burns, Janet Zickfield 1216 Owens Road, Auburn, AL 36830, (205) 821-8336, BS 70 Southeast MO St Univ; MA 72 IN Univ - Bloomington; Sp-Lang Path, Al Council/Head Start, **SLP**

Burns, Joan C Eastern Oklahoma Ear Nose & Throat, 5020 East 68 Street, Tulsa, OK 74136, (918) 492-5140, BS 77 Univ of UT; MA 79 CA St Univ - Los Angeles; Aud, Ea Ok ENT Inc, **A**

Burns, Mrs Joyce Shahan 21844 Michale Street, Canoga Park, CA 91304, (818) 347-5050, BA 77 CA St Univ - Northridge; MA 79 CA St Univ - Northridge; Sp-Lang Path, Glendale Adventist Med Cen, **SLP**

Burns, Judith M 1880 Brady Creek Drive, Sandy, UT 84092, (801) 278-2609, BS 73 Univ of UT; MS 74 Univ of UT; Sp/Lang Path, Granite Sch Dist, **SLP**

Burns, Mrs Julianne Zielaski 13100 Bangor, Garfield Heights, OH 44125, (216) 587-1061, BS 76 Bowling Green St Univ; MA 82 Cleveland St Univ; Sp-Lang Path, Shaker Hts Bd of Educ, **SLP**

Burns, Mrs Karen Billeter 5406 Shady Gardens, Kingwood, TX 77339, (713) 360-4813, BA 82 LA Tech Univ; MA 85 Univ of Houston - Univ Park; Sp-Lang Path, Houston Sch for Deaf Chldrn, **SLP**

Burns, Kathleen Ruth 3408 Hollygreen Drive, Apartment 202, Virginia Beach, VA 23452, (804) 340-8458, BS 84 WV Univ; MS 86 WV Univ; SLP, Wood Co Bd of Ed, **SLP**

Burns, Kathryn L 3560 Washington Avenue #8, Cincinnati, OH 45229, (513) 961-7559

Burns, Mrs Lisa Anne 2012 Simsbury Court, Thousand Oaks, CA 91360, (805) 495-3318, BA 81 CA St Univ - Northridge; MA 83 CA St Univ - Northridge; Admin/Sp-Lang Path, CA Sp & Rehab Inc, **SLP**

Burns, Lisa Maria 1325 East Beaufort Street, Laramie, WY 82070, (307) 742-0074, BS 82 Univ of WY; MS 84 Univ of WY; SLP, Albany Cty Sch District, **SLP**

Burns, Lisa Puckett 805 Branchwood Court, Norman, OK 73072, BS 82 OK St Univ; MS 85 Univ of OK Medical Center; 87–Sp-Lang Path, Oklahoma City PS, **SLP**

Burns, Marcia Smith 4909 Rocky Spring Lane, Bowie, MD 20715, (303) 493-8915, BS 73 CO St Univ; MA 74 Memphis St Univ; Internship, Gw Univ, **SLP**

Burns, Margaret C Route 13 Box 289, Gray, TN 37615, (615) 246-4600, BS 76 Old Dominion Univ; MS 86 East TN St Univ; Aud, Mt Region Sp & Hrng Ctr, **A**

Burns, Dr Martha S 2706 Lincoln, Evanston, IL 60201, (312) 328-5180, PH 75 (NS) Northwestern Univ; Sp-Lang Path, Private Practice, **SLP ACE**

Burns, Patricia J Yurko 2274 Sherman Avenue, North Merrick, NY 11566, (516) 223-8100, BA 77 Hofstra Univ; MA 78 Hofstra Univ; MS 83 Adelphi Univ; Sp-Lang Path, Baldwin Pub Sch, **SLP**

Burns, Regina Coeli Ochsner Clinic, 1514 Jefferson Highway, New Orleans, LA 70121, (504) 838-3900, BS; MS; 86–Sp-Lang Path, Ochsner Clinic, **SLP**

Burns, Mrs Rosealee L 508 East Highland, Hinsdale, IL 60521, (312) 654-2811, BA 58 Northwestern Univ; **SLP**

Burns, Sarah E 10818 134th Street, Edmonton, AB, Canada T5M 1H8, (403) 473-5616, BS 74 Northern MI Univ; MS 78 Univ of WI - Stevens Point; Aud, Edmonton Pub Sch Bd, **A**

Burns, Mrs Sharon 606 East Church Street, Kewanee, IL 61443, (309) 852-2449, BS 64 IL St Univ - Normal; MS 70 IL St Univ - Normal; 64–Sp-Lang Path, Henry-Stark Special Education, **SLP**

Burns, Susan Walsh 360 1st Avenue #8B, New York, NY 10010, (212) 782-6800, BA; MS; 87–Sp-Lang Path, American Nursing Home, **SLP**

Burns, Thomas D Acousticon Of Texarkana, P O Box 1993, 214 West 3rd, Texarkana, TX 75504, (214) 793-2177, BS 76 Baylor Univ; MS 83 East TX St Univ - Commerce; Acousticon of Texarkana, **A**

Burns, Wendy Duguid 1212 Priscilla Lane, Alexandria, VA 22308, (703) 780-3204, BS 67 Boston Univ; ME 69 Boston Univ; Sp-Lang Path, Fairfax Co Pub Sch, **SLP**

Burns, William Joseph 6776 Chicago Avenue, Pensacola, FL 32506, (904) 434-2355, BA 81 John Carroll Univ; MS 88 Lamar Univ; 88, InSpeech Inc

Burns, William W 312 Boardman Avenue, Bay St Louis, MS 39520, (601) 865-1070, BA 66 Old Dominion Univ; MA 73 Memphis St Univ; 84–Sp-Lang Path, VA Med Ctr, **SLP**

Burns Daniels, Mrs Debora A 15808 West 147th Street, Olathe, KS 66062, (816) 276-4023, BS 75 Univ of KS; MA 78 Univ of KS; 86–Ped Coord, Research Med Ctr, **SLP**

Burnside, Patricia S 5409 Lane Place, Downers Grove, IL 60515, (312) 969-6494, BS 76 Northern IL Univ - De Kalb; MA 78 Northern IL Univ - De Kalb; Sp-Lang Path, Woodridge Sch Dist 68, **SLP**

Burnstad, Evelyn G 8372 Oak Knoll Drive, Roseville, CA 95611, (916) 791-1679, BA 42 Univ of CA - Berkeley; MS 67 Minot St Univ; **SLP LM**

Buro, Mrs Jeanne R 34 Lafayette Drive, New City, NY 10956, (914) 634-6448, BA 73 CUNY - Brooklyn Coll; MS 75 CUNY - Brooklyn Coll; Sp-Lang Path, Private Practice, **SLP ACE**

Burough, Leallan L 4618 Emory Oak Woods, San Antonio, TX 78249, (907) 552-3361, BA 70 Univ of WY; MS 78 Univ of WY; Chief of Aud Serv, USAF Hosp Elmendorf AFB Ak, **A ACE**

Burr, Dr Helen Gunderson Carrsgrove, Stribling Avenue, Charlottesville, VA 22903, (804) 293-5419, BA 37 Stanford Univ; MA 40 Univ of Southern CA; PH 49 (Communication Disorders) Columbia Univ Teachers Coll; 84–Prof Emeritus, U of VA, **SLP F LM**

Burradell, Amy Lee 1337 Woodfield #202, South Bend, IN 46615, (219) 234-3136, BA 85 MI St Univ; MA 87 Western MI Univ; 88–Sp-Lang Path, United Health Svcs

Burrell, Mrs Sandra Cozad 1321 Ohio Avenue, York, NE 68467, (402) 362-2024, BS 82 Southwest MO St Univ; MS 87 Univ of NE - Lincoln; **SLP**

Burrell-Griffin, Jane Route 1 Box 83-J, Franklinton, NC 27525, (919) 575-7618, BS 73 East Carolina Univ; MS 75 East Carolina Univ; Sp-Lang Path, Franklin County Public Schools, **SLP**

Burres, Pamela Zoe 7004 N E 44th Circle, Apartment A, Vancouver, WA 98661, (206) 696-7256, BA 81 WA St Univ; MA 82 WA St Univ; SLP, Vancouver School District, **SLP**

Burress, Bruce E Duluth Clinic, 400 East 3rd Street, Duluth, MN 55805, (218) 722-8364, BS 72 Univ of WI - Stevens Point; MS 73 Univ of WI - Stevens Point; Aud, Duluth Cl Ltd, **A**

Burress, Kathleen J 4631 Otsego Street, Duluth, MN 55804-1537, (218) 722-3775, BS 71 Univ of WI - Stevens Point; MS 73 Univ of WI - Stevens Point; 86–Sp-Lang Path, ISD #709, **SLP**

Burris, Laura Ann 8633 Datapoint Drive #216, San Antonio, TX 78229-3253, (512) 670-5430, BA 84 Fort Hays St Univ; MA 86 Wichita St Univ; **A**

Burriss, Mrs Catherine Dandl 4809 Northwind Drive, Chattanooga, TN 37416, (615) 629-1451, BA 79 Univ of TN - Knoxville; MA 81 Univ of TN - Knoxville; SLP, Orange Grove Cen Inc, **SLP**

Burriss, Mrs Pamela W 27 Distillery Road, Warwick, NY 10990, (914) 357-8315, BA 75 Mary Washington Coll; ME 76 Univ of VA - Charlottesville; Sp-Lang Path, Ramapo Ctrl Sch Dist, **SLP**

Burritt, Grace Aletha 220 Fellows Avenue, Syracuse, NY 13210, (315) 479-7744, BA 81 SUNY - Coll at Buffalo; MA 84 SUNY - Coll at Buffalo; 83–Sp-Lang Path, Jowonio Sch, **SLP**

Burroughs, Mrs Beverly W 3675 Oak Lake Lane, Memphis, TN 38118, (901) 761-1500, BA 72 Univ of South AL; MA 75 Memphis St Univ; SLP, Memphis City Sch, **SLP**

Burroughs, Dr Elizabeth Irene Department Of Communication Disorders, Bowling Green State University, Bowling Green, OH 43403, (419) 372-7191, BS 76 Purdue Univ - West Lafayette; MA 80 Univ of IA; PH 84 (Sp Path) Univ of IA; 86–Asst Prof, Bowling Green State Univ, **SLP**

Burroughs, Dr Glenn R 1811 20th Street, Bakersfield, CA 93301, (213) 378-4966, BA 52 Univ of CA - Berkeley; MA 64 4252; PH 79 (NS) Univ of Southern CA; Teacher, Palos Verdes Pen Unif Sch Dist, **SLP**

Burroughs, H D Rob, Jr 416 Stone Ridge Drive, Hixson, TN 37343, (615) 624-0393, BA 76 Univ of Central FL; MS 82 Western KY Univ; Sp-Lang Path, Chattanooga Pub Sch, **SLP**

Burroughs, Jill A 3001 Pheasant Run Road, #187, Norman, OK 73072, (501) 225-3766, BA 82 Harding Univ; MS 86 Univ of AR - Little Rock; **SLP**

Burroughs, Kathleen Walker 824 S W 81st, Oklahoma City, OK 73139, (405) 632-4769, BA 73 Univ of OK - Norman; MA 76 Northwestern Univ; Sp-Lang Path, Hillcrest Hlth Ctr, **SLP**

Burroughs, Mrs Peggy Ann 2109 Halsey Drive, Des Plaines, IL 60016, (312) 827-5383, BS 83 Univ of IL - Urbana; MA 85 Northwestern Univ; 85–Sp-Lang Path, Northwestern U, **SLP**

Burrow, Cathy Lynn Kaywood Garden Apartment, 4207 Russel Avenue #3, Mount Rainier, MD 20822, (202) 234-4836, MS 88 Howard Univ

Burrow, Mrs Pamela Lee 1205 South Culberhouse, Jonesboro, AR 72401, (501) 935-2841, BS 79 AR St Univ; MS 87 AR St Univ; 82–Sp-Lang Path, Jonesboro PS, **SLP**

Burrow, Sandra C 509 Ashley Downs, Anderson, SC 29621, (803) 260-5000, BA 69 Univ of KS; MA 71 Univ of KS; 84–Sp-Lang Path, Anderson Sch Dist 5, **SLP ACE**

Burrows, Cashwell L 201 East Hughes, Glendive, MT 59330, **SLP**

Burrows, Clydeena Gaye 7 West Creek, McAlester, OK 74501, (918) 548-3864, MS 85 Univ of OK Medical Center; **SLP**

Burrows, Dr Dennis Lee 412 Meadow Drive, Macomb, IL 61455, (309) 298-1955, BS 80 Western IL Univ; MA 80 Western IL Univ; PH 87 (Aud) Univ of OK - Norman; 87–Asst Prof & Dir, Western Illinois Univ, **A ACE**

Burrows, Evelyn H P O Box 35912, Fayetteville, NC 28303, PH; **SLP**

Burrows, Heidi Olson 29920 43rd Avenue South, Auburn, WA 98001, (206) 854-5660, BA 82 Western WA Univ; MA 84 Western WA Univ; **SLP**

Burrows, Mrs Judith A 412 Meadow Drive, Macomb, IL 61455-9321, (309) 298-1955, BS 74 Western IL Univ; MA 75 Western IL Univ; 87–Asst Prof, Western Illinois Univ, **SLP ACE**

Burrows, Mrs Kimberly Ann 2549 Lynn Lake Circle S, St Petersburg, FL 33712, (813) 773-2857, BS 85 Mankato St Univ; MS 87 FL St Univ; Sp-Lang Path, New Medico Rehab Ctr of Florida

Burrus, Mrs Jennifer Ann 1309 Autumn Ridge Drive, Columbus, GA 31904, (404) 322-1336, BA 82 Columbus Coll; ME 85 Columbus Coll; 83–Sp-Lang Path, Muscogee County Sch Dist, **SLP**

Burruss, Patricia J 2486 South 1500 East, Salt Lake City, UT 84106, (801) 484-7806, BA 77 Univ of CA - Santa Barbara; MS 81 UT St Univ; 81–Sp-Lang Path, Jordan Sch Dist, **SLP**

Burson, Laura 3783 Meyers Road, San Bernardino, CA 92407, (714) 593-7521, BA 79 Whittier Coll; MA 84 Whittier Coll; Sp-Lang Path, Casa Colina Hospitall, **SLP**

Burson, Susan L 45-546 Aladdin B107, Indio, CA 92201, (619) 347-8631, BS 82 SUNY - Coll at Geneseo; MS 85 San Diego St Univ; 86–Sp-Lang Path, Desert Sands USD

Burstein, Caryn L S 1096 Kent Avenue, Highland Park, IL 60035-1314, (312) 432-2441, BS 78 Univ of IL - Urbana; MS 79 Univ of IL - Urbana; 88–Sp/Lang Path, Sch Dist 34, **SLP**

Burstein, Susan A 2210 Nassau Drive, Holiday Hill, Wilmington, DE 19810, **SLP**

Burt, Mrs Cheryl D 29300 Cambridge Court, Augoura Hills, CA 91301, (818) 889-5202, BA 69 CA St Univ - Northridge; MA 71 CA St Univ - Northridge; Self Employed, **SLP**

Burt, Darla H 426 Austin, Rockwell City, IA 50579, (712) 297-7942, BA 74 Univ of Northern IA; MS 75 Univ of WI - Stevens Point; 85–SLP, InSpeech Inc, **SLP**

Burt, Mrs Frances Corine 624 Termino Avenue, Long Beach, CA 90814, (213) 438-1509, BA 84 Chapman Coll; MA 86 Whittier Coll; 84–Sp-Lang Path, Villa Serena, **SLP**

Burt, Mrs Linda R 66 Dogwood Circle, Woodbridge, CT 06525, (203) 393-3881, BA 64 Bryn Mawr Coll; BS 82 Southern CT St Univ; Sp-Lang Path, Private Practice, **SLP**

Burt, Mrs Phyllis J 105 Alden Avenue, Rohnert Park, CA 94928, (707) 763-3161, BA 68 SUNY - Center at Buffalo; MA 70 Univ of CA - Santa Barbara; 85–Aud, Park Place Hearing Aids, **A**

Burt, Mrs Susan M 67 Washington Avenue, Needham, MA 02192, (617) 444-7041, MS 70 Univ of WI - Madison; **SLP**

Burtch, Mrs Roberta F 2615 Dartmouth Woods Road, Wilmington, DE 19810, (302) 475-1588, BS 75 Miami Univ - Oxford; MA 76 Bowling Green St Univ; **SLP**

Burtis, Mrs Barbara D 7 Felton Place, Bloomington, IL 61701, (309) 699-1322, OB 73 IL St Univ - Normal; MA 75 Univ of IL - Urbana; Sp/Lang Path, E Peoria Sch Dist #86, **SLP ACE**

Burtis, Marguerite Burtis Speech-Language Center, 5925 Forest Lane, Suite 517, Dallas, TX 75230, (214) 661-5157, BS 70 Stephen F Austin St Univ; MS 76 East TX St Univ - Commerce; Sp/Lang Path, Burtis Speech-Language Center, **SLP**

Burtis, Mary I Burtis Speech/Language Center, 5925 Forest Lane, Suite 517, Dallas, TX 75230, (214) 661-5157, BS 67 Stephen F Austin St Univ; MS 76 East TX St Univ - Commerce; Sp-Lang Path, Burtis Speech/Language Center, **SLP**

Burtka, Mary Jo 29555 Briarton, Farmington Hills, MI 48018, (313) 876-3280, BS 82 Western MI Univ; MA 84 Western MI Univ; 85–Audiologist, Henry Ford Hospital, **A ACE**

Burtness, Carol Diffenbaugh 734 East 4th Avenue, Denver, CO 80207, (303) 399-6227, BA 78 IN Univ - Bloomington; MA 87 Univ of CO - Boulder; 88–Sp-Lang Path, Adams County SD #12, **SLP**

Burtnett, Mrs Pamela L 907 Brookhill Road, Louisville, KY 40223, BA 75 Univ of Northern CO; MS 78 Univ of AR - Little Rock; 80–Sp-Lang Path, Jefferson Co PS, **SLP ACE**

Burton, Annette A 933 Pearl Harbor Street, Bridgeport, CT 06610, (203) 366-1504, BA 82 Univ of CT; MA 84 Univ of CT; Aud, ENT Assoc of Waterbury, **A**

Burton, Cynthia Jane 4534 Sinclair Avenue, #8-203, Midland, TX 79707, (915) 267-3806, BA 81 OK Baptist Univ; MS 84 Univ of North TX; Sp-Lang Path, Dora Roberts Rehab Center, **SLP**

Burton, Ellen Howard 2633 Rathbone Road, Lincoln, NE 68502, (402) 483-6105, BA 76 Univ of FL; MA 83 Univ of FL; 85–Aud, Lincoln PS, **A**

Burton, Kathleen Lynn 118 Burke Drive, Monroeville, PA 15146, (412) 281-7244, BA 76 Duquesne Univ; MA 79 Kent St Univ; Sp/Lang Path, Er Sl So, **SLP**

Burton, Pamela Y 834 Lancaster Drive, Claremont, CA 91711, (714) 599-6787, BS 73 Univ of Redlands; MS 74 Univ of Redlands; SLP, Bonita USD, **SLP**

Burton, Patricia H 5239 Graham Street, Kalamazoo, MI 49002, (616) 323-3051, BA 75 SUNY - Center at Buffalo; MA 77 SUNY - Center at Buffalo; Sp-Lang Path, Upjohn Hlthcare Ser, **SLP**

Burton, Mrs Pearl B 101 Wild Rose Drive, Andover, MA 01810, (508) 475-8209, BA 72 CUNY - Brooklyn Coll; MS 75 Boston Univ; Sp/Lang Path, Private Practice, **SLP**

Burton, Mrs Thea Koenig Box 478, Wolfville, NS, Canada B0P 1X0, (902) 423-7354, BS 84 Northwestern Univ; MA 86 Northwestern Univ; 88–Sp-Lang Path, King's County Schs, **SLP**

Burton, Wendy Elizabeth 3717 East Second Street, Apartment 5, Long Beach, CA 90803, (213) 434-6213, OB 84 Stanford Univ; MA 86 Univ of CA - Santa Barbara; Sp-Lang Path, Rancho Los Amigos Med Cntr, **SLP**

Burton-Tihen, Mrs Deborah L 3531 S E 3rd Avenue, Cape Coral, FL 33904, (813) 334-1102, BA 76 IN Univ - Bloomington; MA 77 IN Univ - Bloomington; Sp-Lang Path, Lee Co Sch Syst, **SLP**

Burwell, Cynthia L 1736 Seaton Drive, Virginia Beach, VA 23464, (804) 486-7876, **SLP**

Burwell, Mrs Donna 1302 North Willis, Champaign, IL 61821, (217) 356-9176, BA 69 Augustana Coll; MA 70 Univ of IL - Urbana; 74–Sp-Lang Path, Developmental Ser Cen, **SLP ACE**

Burwell, Mrs Linda June 1214 West Ross Avenue, Tahlequah, OK 74464, (918) 456-5980, BS 80 OK St Univ; MS 82 Univ of OK Medical Center; Sp/Lang Path, Choctaw Sch Syst, **SLP**

Burysek-Cherry, Mrs Denita J 783 Raymond Kent Court #1, Louisville, KY 40217, (812) 945-5287, MS 87 Western KY Univ; 87–Sp-Lang Path, Silvercrest Chldn's Dev Ctr, **SLP**

Busacco, Dr Debra Ann 955 S Columbus St #617, Arlington, VA 22204-3448, (703) 651-5328, BA 80 Marywood Coll; MS 81 Columbia Univ Teachers Coll; PH 88 (Aud) Columbia Univ Sch of Gen St; 88–Asst Prof, Loyola Coll, **A**

Busalacchi, Mrs Gail Marie 2754 South 63rd Street, Milwaukee, WI 53219, (414) 541-8080, BA 78 Univ of WI - Eau Claire; MS 80 Univ of WI - Stevens Point; SLP, W Allis - W Milwaukee Pub Sch, **SLP**

Busard-Cates, Susan 15112 Stars Pride Court, Carmel, IN 46032, (216) 943-0320, BS 78 IN Univ - Bloomington; OM 79 IN Univ - Bloomington; Sp-Lang Path, Wickliffe City Sch, **SLP**

Busbee, Jane B School Board Of Orange County, 520 Selkirk Drive, Winter Park, FL 32792, (407) 423-9293, BA 69 Univ of AL- Tuscaloosa; MA 73 Univ of Montevallo; 88–Admin Sp/Lang & Presch Hndcpd, School Board of Orange Cty, **SLP**

Busby, Robert A 1 Pandora, Irvine, CA 92714, (714) 559-1171, BA 63 CA St Univ - Long Beach; MA 65 CA St Univ - Long Beach; Sp-Lang Path, Sp-Lang Dev Cen, **SLP**

Buscema, Michele Marie 13 Haddonfield Avenue, Lavallette, NJ 08735, (201) 793-6736, BA 76 Montclair St Coll; MA 81 Montclair St Coll; 88–Sp-Lang Path, Mcoss Nursing Services Inc, **SLP**

Busch, Cynthia R 203 Exeter Place, St Paul, MN 55104, (612) 722-7988, BA 71 Northwestern Univ; MS 73 Univ of MI - Ann Arbor; MS 73 Univ of MI - Ann Arbor; SLP Consult, Medicare Minn, **SLP**

Buschbacher, Pamelazita Wilbur 10103 Crosier Lane, Cincinnati, OH 45242, BS 74 Univ of Cincinnati; MA 78 Univ of Cincinnati; 86–Sp-Lang Path, Hamilton Co Ofc of Educ, **SLP**

Buschini, Gail M 370 Santa Margarita, Menlo Park, CA 94025, (415) 321-7828, BS 67 Stanford Univ; MA 68 Stanford Univ; 2nd & 3rd Grade Teacher, Peninsula School, **SLP**

Buse, Mrs Maria Christina 7414 Seton Lake Drive, Houston, TX 77086, (713) 479-2831, **SLP**

Bush, Mrs Catherine W 6033 East Wilshire Drive, Scottsdale, AZ 85257, (602) 994-1383, BA 56 AZ St Univ; MA 66 Univ of NM; 75–Sp-Lang Path, Scottsdale PS, **SLP**

Bush, Gregory Alan Route 1 Box 1708A, Grayling, MI 49738, (517) 366-8550, BA 80 Univ of MI - Ann Arbor; MA 84 Central MI Univ; 87–Prog Dir, N Ctrl Comm Ment Hlth Serv Bd, **SLP**

Bush, Janie P 81 Washington Avenue, Streamwood, IL 60103, (312) 259-5503, BS 83 Univ of KY; MS 84 Univ of Louisville; 88–Sp-Lang Path, NW Sp Path & Assoc, **SLP**

Bush, Katheryn B 974 Veltre Circle S W, Atlanta, GA 30311, MS; **SLP**

Bush, Linda Southwick Route 3 Box 152, Brush Creek Road, Kingston Springs, TN 37082, (615) 797-2715, BS 79 OH Univ - Athens; MA 82 Univ of Cincinnati; SLP, Mid-Cumberland Headstart, **SLP**

Bush, Mrs Lisa L P O Box 333, Calhoun, LA 71225, (318) 388-2541, BA 83 Southeastern LA Univ; MS 85 Univ of Southwestern LA; SLP, Ouachita Parish School System, **SLP**

Bush, Dr Marcia A Xerox Palo Alto Research Center, Systems Sciences Lab, 3333 Coyote Hill Road, Palo Alto, CA 94304, (415) 494-4391, BS 79 PA St Univ - Univ Park; MS 77 MA Inst of Tech; PH 81 (NS) MA Inst of Tech; Researcher, Xerox Palo Alto Research Ctr

Bush, Marcia Frances 1247 Fillmore Street, Hollywood, FL 33019, (305) 534-3676, BS 81 Auburn Univ - Auburn; OM 86 Auburn Univ - Auburn; **SLP**

Bush, Margaret S 38 Fairmont Avenue, Stamford, CT 06906, (203) 348-0817, BA 68 Marymount Coll; MA 69 NY Univ; 86–Sp/Lang Path, Greenwich PS, **SLP**

Bush, Martha 7804 High Oaks Circle, Dallas, TX 75231, (214) 987-4114, MS 87 Washington Univ; Aud, Deborah Price

Bush, Nancy Marguerite 12019 Lincolnshire Drive, Austin, TX 78758, (512) 835-1763, BS 79 Univ of TX - Austin; MA 83 Univ of TX - Austin; Sp-Lang Path, Speech Services for Children, **SLP**

Bush, Patricia Mullin P O Box 1609, Phenix City, AL 36867, (404) 327-2213, BA 75 Columbus Coll; MA 78 Univ of TN - Knoxville; Sp-Lang Path, Sp Path Ser, **SLP**

Bush, Mrs Yolanda R Ike Nobel Drive #9-D, Canton, NY 13617, (315) 344-2414, BS 78 SUNY - Coll at New Paltz; MS 83 Coll of Saint Rose; **SLP**

Bushey, Marylou R 6501 Geneseo, Plano, TX 75023, (214) 596-4738, BS 69 Concordia Teachers Coll; MS 75 Univ of North TX; Sp-Lang Path, Plano Coop Presch, **SLP**

Bushey, Philip A 234 North Wood Street, East Canton, OH 44730, (216) 455-0022, BA 70 Malone Coll; MA 74 Kent St Univ; Cl Supev, Bes-Mont Sp/Lang Cen, **SLP**

Bushey, Mrs Tahirih Rose 300 21st Avenue North, Hopkins, MN 55343, (612) 935-5094, MA 87 Univ of MN - Minneap-St Paul

Bushfield, Dr Martee R 4911 South Belmont, Grand Forks, ND 58201, BA Univ of SD - Vermillion; MA 79 Univ of ND; PH 80 (NS) Harvard Univ; Dir/Research-Curriculum-Devel, Univ North Dakota Medical Sch, **SLP**

Bushman, Nancy Jeanne 248 Oxford Street Apartment 7, Rochester, NY 14607, (716) 442-2234, BA 85 Valparaiso Univ; MA 87 OH Univ - Athens; 87–Sp-Lang Path, UCP Association

Bushmann, Mrs Maureen Murphy 4464 Mohegan, St Louis, MO 63123-6666, (314) 776-1128, BS 81 Saint Louis Univ; MA 82 Saint Louis Univ; SLP, Iwj Washington U, **SLP**

Bushnell, Dale R 1019 Agate St #F, San Diego, CA 92109, (619) 488-9161, MA 88 San Diego St Univ

Bushong, Mrs Laurel Lynn 2707 Inlet Court, Route 1, Wheelersburg, OH 45694, (614) 776-2468, BA 84 Univ of Toledo; MA 85 Bowling Green St Univ; 88–Sp-Lang Path, Private Practice, **SLP**

Busi, Susan Elizabeth Valley View Apartment, Watervliet, NY 12189, (518) 438-8785, BA 76 CUNY - Lehman Coll; MA 78 CUNY - Lehman Coll; Sp-Lang Path, Easter Seals Society, **SLP**

Busija, Nancy Barrett 4152 Barfield Road, Memphis, TN 38117, **SLP**

Busillo, Mrs Judith E 5 Wendover Drive, Mount Laurel, NJ 08054, (609) 778-4287, BA 78 Univ of Rochester; MA 81 Case Western Reserve Univ; 87–Sp-Lang Path, Speech Pathology Consultants, **SLP**

Busko, Mrs Sally C 818 East Morningside Drive, Atlanta, GA 30324, OB 70 GA St Univ; ME 76 GA St Univ; Sp-Lang Path, **SLP**

Buss, Denise P 24 Cherry Tree Road, Loudonville, NY 12211, (518) 272-5000, BS 70 Long Island U - CW Post Ctr; MS 77 Coll of Saint Rose; Dir, St Mary's Hosp Sp/Hrng Cl, **SLP**

Bussa, Denise Wetherille 1123 Mississippi Avenue, Duluth, MN 55811, (218) 724-4146, MS 77 Univ of WI - Eau Claire; 86–Clinical Supvr, Univ of Minnesota, **SLP**

Bussard, Mrs Susan Hill 520 Cherry Road N E, Massillon, OH 44640, (216) 454-2510, BA 79 Univ of Akron; MA 87 Univ of Akron; **A**

Busse, David J 3932 Lantern Drive, Wheaton, MD 20902, (301) 946-5260, BS 70 Saint Louis Univ; MA 71 Saint Louis Univ; Sp-Lang Path, Montgy Co Pub Sch, **SLP**

Busse, Lu Ann 1805 Donna Street, Arlington, TX 76013, (817) 795-1638, BA 75 Univ of Central FL; MA 77 Northwestern Univ; 85–Aud, Cochlear Corporation, **A**

Busse, Mrs Mary S 3932 Lantern Drive, Wheaton, MD 20902, BS 70 Saint Louis Univ; MA 71 Saint Louis Univ; Sp-Lang Path, Montgomery Co Pub Sch, **SLP**

Bussiere, Mrs Deborah Joline 10 Aron Dr Apt 4, Auburn, ME 04210-6109, (207) 782-9460, Aud, Central Maine Medical Center, **A**

Busta, Mrs Julie I 1556 11th Avenue SE, St Cloud, MN 56304, (612) 259-8004, BS 82 Saint Cloud St Univ; MS 87 Univ of NE - Lincoln; **SLP**

Busta-Kolick, Kathleen A 20686 Wildwood Lane, Strongsville, OH 44136, (216) 572-3535, BS 77 Univ of Cincinnati; MA 79 Univ of Cincinnati; 79–Sp-Lang Path, Parma Cty Sch Dist, **SLP**

Bustaque, Mrs Patricia G 285 Willow Dell Lane, Leola, PA 17540, (717) 656-6335, BS 73 PA St Univ - Univ Park; MA 76 West Chester Univ of PA; Sp-Lang Path, Private Practice, **SLP**

Bustillo, Maria C Calle 10-A 863 Montecarlo, Rio Piedras, PR 00924, (809) 752-3040, BA 80 Univ of PR - Rio Piedras; MS 82 Univ of PR - Rio Piedras; SLP, Head Start Arzobispado San Jua, **SLP**

Butcher, Mrs Barbara Kaufman Rt 3 Box 168, Pequot Lakes, MN 56472, (218) 587-4447, BA 68 Univ of Denver; ME 71 Boston Univ; 74–Sp-Lang Path, Pine River Pub Sch, **SLP**

Butcher, Dennis James Route 3 Box 183, Elizabeth, WV 26143, (304) 420-1300, **SLP**

Butcher, Dr Jaynee A Rush-Presby-St Lukes Med Ctr, Sect Of Communicative Dis, 1753 West Congress Parkway, Chicago, IL 60612, (312) 942-5332, BA 76 Univ of MI - Ann Arbor; MA 80 Univ of KS; PH 83 (NS) Univ of KS; Aud / Asst Prof, Rush Presby St Lukes Med Ctr, **A**

Butcher, Joanie Siverston 111 North Marion Drive, Goldsboro, NC 27530-3390, (919) 731-3590, BS Minot St Univ; MS 85 Minot St Univ; **SLP**

Buteau, Mrs Carol Liddiard 10430 Loma Rancho Drive, Spring Valley, CA 92077, (619) 463-1922, MA 85 San Diego St Univ; BA 81 San Diego St Univ; Sp-Lang Path, Kaiser Permanente, **SLP**

Butensky, Mrs Jane E 99 Sun Valley Road, Toms River, NJ 08753, (201) 341-6281, BS 69 Adelphi Univ; MA 83 Kean Coll of NJ; SLP, Private Practice, **SLP ACE**

Butera, Mrs Judith C 936 Lilac Lane, Naperville, IL 60540, (312) 717-1962, BA 71 Univ of MD - College Park; MA 73 Univ of MD - College Park; 87–Aud, Edward Hosp Hearing Ctr, **A**

Buth, Mrs Lisa L 2438 Oakwood Drive, Grand Rapids, MI 49506, BA 80 MI St Univ; MA 81 MI St Univ; Sp-Lang Path, Mary Free Bed Rehab Ctr, **SLP**

Buthman, Joanne 3535 Apollo Drive #K-221, Metairie, LA 70003, (504) 891-7891, BS 83 Western IL Univ; MA 84 Western IL Univ; SLP, LA Cen for Cp and Dev Disabil, **SLP**

Butler, Barbara Ann 59 Colton Road, Somers, CT 06071, (203) 684-4211, BA 63 Univ of Denver; MS 86 Worcester St Coll; 86–Sp-Lang Path, Stafford PS, **SLP**

Butler, Mrs Barbara J 325 Magnolia, Everett, WA 98203, (206) 339-4335, BA 78 Univ of WA; MS 79 Univ of WA; 80–Sp-Lang Path, Everett Sch Dist, **SLP**

Butler, Mrs Carol Reedy 7224 Old Clinton Highway, Apartment C, Knoxville, TN 37921, (615) 938-3516, BA 82 Univ of TN - Knoxville; MA 86 Univ of TN - Knoxville; **A**

Butler, Chana L 1653 Dahill Road, Brooklyn, NY 11223, **SLP**

Butler, Charles Eugene 3501 1st Street, Brownwood, TX 76801, (915) 643-6130, BS 82 Univ of TX - Austin; MA 84 Univ of TX - Austin; Head Dept SLP and Aud, Howard Payne U, **A**

Butler, Daniel J 44 Glenn Terrace, Vineland, NJ 08360-4815, (609) 691-4162, BS 78 Seton Hall Univ; MA 80 Univ of FL; 88–Southern NJ Svc Coord, Miracle Ear, **A**

Butler, Mrs Debra Kay 1450 Dixie Drive, Rockford, IL 61108, (309) 274-5438, **SLP**

Butler, Estella Denise 503 Lyons Lane, Chapel Hill, NC 27514, (919) 596-2189, BA 84 Univ of NC - Chapel Hill; MS 86 Univ of NC - Chapel Hill; 87–Sp-Lang Path, Durham Co Schs, **SLP**

Butler, Glenda C 2218 Rolling Meadows, Kingwood, TX 77339, (713) 358-0577, BS 67 Univ of Houston - Univ Park; MS 81 Lamar Univ; Sp-Lang Path, Kingwood Speech Pathology, **SLP**

Butler, Mrs Ida Canady 521 Stadium Road, Goldsboro, NC 27530, (919) 735-2544, BS 44; MA 50 Univ of MI - Ann Arbor

Butler, Mrs Janice Good 2050 Ann Avenue, St Louis, MO 63104, (317) 772-2820, BS 84 Purdue Univ - West Lafayette; MS 87 Purdue Univ - West Lafayette; **SLP**

Butler, Janice Merrial P O Box 2128, Wise, VA 24293, (703) 328-8017, BS 80 East TN St Univ; OM 85 Univ of SC - Columbia; **SLP**

Butler, Mrs Jill Cosby 320 North Shumway, Taylorville, IL 62568, (217) 287-7424, BS 84 Southern IL Univ -Carbondale; MS 87 Southern IL Univ -Carbondale; 88–Sp-Lang Path, Private Practice, **SLP**

Butler, Judith V 7615 Brashear Street, Pittsburgh, PA 15221, (412) 281-7244, BA 79 Brown Univ; MA 81 Univ of CT; Sp-Lang Path, Er Sl So-Allegheny Co, **SLP**

Butler, Karen L 1918 Montana Avenue, Santa Monica, CA 90403, **SLP**

Butler, Dr Katharine Gorrell 5165 Skyline Drive, Syracuse, NY 13215, (315) 443-1121, BA 50 Western MI Univ; MA 53 Western MI Univ; PH 67 (NS) MI St Univ; Dir-Cen for Res, Syracuse U, **SLP F H**

Butler, Mrs Kathy Jean 155 Mary Street, Stonwall, LA 71078, (318) 826-3393, BS 81 Southeast MO St Univ; MA 82 Southeast MO St Univ; Sp-Lang Path, Desoto Parish School Board, **SLP**

Butler, Kevin William 1150 North El Dorado Place, Apartment 115, Tucson, AZ 85715-4616, (602) 296-6582, BA 71 Univ of Denver; MA 72 Univ of Denver; Sp/Lang Path, Private Practice, **SLP**

Butler, Mrs Kim-Ellen Schombert 168 Hayden Road, Hollis, NH 03049, (203) 237-7835, BA 80 SUNY - Coll at Cortland; MA 82 Univ of MA - Amherst; Sp/Lang Path, St Josephs Hosp, **SLP**

Butler, Linda Bartron 2319 Irene Street, Boise, ID 83702, (303) 861-6800, BA 71 Univ of OR; MS 73 CO St Univ; Sp-Lang Path, Denver Childrens Hospital, **SLP**

Butler, Mrs Linda C 355 Edenwood Lane, Jackson, TN 38301, (901) 664-3118, BA 73 Southwestern at Memphis; MA 75 Vanderbilt Univ; **SLP**

Butler, Lori Lee 1357 Crestwood Drive, San Jose, CA 95118, (408) 266-3453, BA 85 Univ of CA - Santa Barbara; MS 87 AZ St Univ; 87–Sp-Lang Path, Speech & Learning Services

Butler, Lucy E 510 Vivian Road, Sumter, SC 29150, (803) 773-2002, BS 76 Appalachian St Univ; MS 77 East Carolina Univ; Sp-Lang Path, National Health Care

Butler, Mrs Lynne L 4112 Stonewick Drive, Arlington, TX 76016, (817) 654-4280, BA 70 Auburn Univ - Auburn; MS 73 Auburn Univ - Auburn; Aud, Dallas VA Med Cen, **SLP A**

Butler, Marcia T M 3541 Nakoma Road, Madison, WI 53711, (608) 835-3161, BS 74 Univ of WI - Madison; MS 76 Univ of WI - Madison; Sp-Lang Path/Chap I Tchr, Or Sch Dist, **SLP**

Butler, Mrs Margaret Smith 1420 Trails End, Clinton, OH 44216, (216) 882-3891, BA 85 Univ of Akron; MA 87 Univ of Akron; 87–Sp-Lang Path, Stow Learning Ctr

Butler, Mrs Mary A G 3235 Reisor Road, Shreveport, LA 71118-2925, (318) 872-1286, BA 76 LA St Univ - Shreveport; OM 77 LA St Univ - N O Medical Ctr; Sp-Lang Path, De Soto Parish Sch Board, **SLP**

Butler, Mrs Maureen O'Neill 115 Foss Street, Biddeford, ME 04005, (207) 676-9811, BA 83 Regis Coll; MA 86 Univ of ME - Orono

Butler, Dr Myrtice R 17843 North 45th Avenue, Glendale, AZ 85308, (602) 876-5349, BS 61 Univ of CO - Boulder; MS 70 Univ of CO - Boulder; PH 72 (NS) Univ of CO - Boulder; SLP, Maricopa Med Ctr, **SLP**

Butler, Nancy Elizabeth 1120 Parkview Lane, Largo, FL 33540, (404) 321-0111, BA 84 Univ of FL; MA 87 Univ of FL; **A**

Butler, Patricia Ann 11207 Rocky Valley Drive, Little Rock, AR 72212, (501) 224-9940, BA 69 Univ of AR - Fayetteville; OM 85 AR St Univ; 87–Sp-Lang Path, Sp Ther Svcs, **SLP**

Butler, Mrs Rebecca 1 Live Oak, Irvine, CA 92714, (714) 857-1914, BA 72 Univ of CA - Los Angeles; MA 75 Catholic Univ of America; Sp-Lang Path, Private Practice, **SLP**

Butler, Mrs Roseann Walker Route 1 Box 2369, Taylors Mill Road, Fort Valley, GA 31030, (912) 825-8893, BS 80 SUNY - Coll at Geneseo; ME 83 Columbus Coll; 88–Sp-Lang Path, Peach County Sch Sys, **SLP**

Butler, Mrs Sharon S Route 1 Box 223-A, Queenstown, MD 21658, MA 71 Univ of MD - College Park; **SLP**

Butler, Sheila Ann Veterans Administration, Audio/Speech Path Service, Suite 126, Bay Pines, FL 33504, (813) 398-5123, BA 62 Marymount Coll; MA 70 CUNY - Hunter Coll; **SLP A**

Butler, Stephanie Alice 17906 Villamoura, Poway, CA 92064, (619) 789-6734, **SLP**

Butler, Terrence Robert 622 Kings Lane S W, Winter Haven, FL 33880, (813) 967-8535, BS 76 CA Univ of PA; MS 86 CA Univ of PA; SLP, Polk Cty Sch Board, **SLP**

Butler, Mrs Toni Marie 11204 Lakeridge Run, Oklahoma City, OK 73170-2452, (405) 848-7603, BS 81 Murray St Univ; MS 84 Murray St Univ; Sp-Lang Path, Crawford Memorial Hospital, **SLP**

Butler-Rybicki, Anne E 637 Grandview Avenue, Olean, NY 14760, (716) 373-0530, BS 79 Nazareth Coll of Rochester; MA 81 SUNY - Coll at Geneseo; Sp-Lang Path, Private Practice, **SLP**

Butt, Dolores S 5120 Sunningdale Avenue N E, Albuquerque, NM 87110, **SLP**

Butt, Francis V 4411 Tophill, Irving, TX 75038, (214) 438-9313, BA 57 Southern Methodist Univ; ME 64 Univ of North TX; MS 69 Univ of North TX; Sp-Lang Path, Irving ISD, **SLP**

Butterfield, Mrs Ann Fickes 95 Knollwood Road, Farmington, CT 06032, (203) 673-0475, BA 73 Emory Univ; ME 77 GA St Univ; Sp-Lang Path, CT PS, **SLP**

Butterfield, Mrs Lisa Bennett 2960 Canyon Crest Drive, Apartment #1, Riverside, CA 92507, (714) 781-9957, BA 81 CA St Univ - Long Beach; MA 84 CA St Univ - Long Beach; 84–Sp-Lang Path, Moreno Valley USD, **SLP**

Butterfield, Sally D 14 Park Terrace, Cambridge, England CB1 1JH, BS 75 Georgetown Univ; OM 79; MA 81 Northwestern Univ; Research Assistant, Medical Research Council

Butterly, Beth 2871 South Locust Street, Denver, CO 80222, BS 78 CO St Univ; MA 80 Univ of Denver; Exec Dir, ARC/Aurora, **A**

Butterworth, Mrs Kathleen Marie 146 Strephen Drive, Stonington, CT 06378, (203) 887-1654, MS 84 Univ of WI - Madison; SLP, Ledyard Sch Sys, **SLP**

Buttner, Patricia E 9172 E Highland Pines Blvd, Palm Beach Gardens, FL 33410, (305) 842-3252, OB 79 SUNY - Coll at Fredonia; ME 83 Valdosta St Coll; **SLP**

Button, Mrs Arlys S Noyac Harbor Road, R R 1 Box 719, Sag Harbor, NY 11963, (516) 725-3668, BA 55 Univ of MI - Ann Arbor; MS 74 Columbia Univ Teachers Coll; 84–Sp-Lang Path, Suffolk Co Dept of Hlth Serv, **SLP**

Button, Marjorie A Rural Route 1, Kinburn, ON, Canada K0A 2H0, (613) 722-6521, BA 74 Carleton Univ - Ontario; MS 77 Syracuse Univ; Sp-Lang Path, Royal Ottawa Hosp, **SLP**

Buttrill, Judith C 1417 Parkinson, Palo Alto, CA 94301, (415) 855-8296, BA 68 Stanford Univ; MA 72 Univ of MN - Minneap-St Paul; Resource Spec, Palo Alto USD, **SLP**

Buttross-Brinegar, Margaret 315 South 17th Avenue, Hattiesburg, MS 39401, (601) 266-5232, BS 74 Univ Southern MS-Hattiesburg; MS 76 Univ of NC - Chapel Hill; 78–Asst Dir Presch Lang Prog, U of Sn MS, **SLP**

Butts, Catherine P 1161 Baltic Lane, Winter Springs, FL 32708, (305) 695-8289, MS 77 Univ of South FL; Sp-Lang Path, Orange County PS, **SLP**

Butts, Mrs Deborah Banks 110 Hedgecock Avenue #4, Winston-Salem, NC 27104, (919) 768-6551, ME 88 Univ of NC - Greensboro

Butts, Dr Frank M Medical College Of Virginia, Audiology Service, P O Box 150 McV Station, Richmond, VA 23298, (804) 786-0431, BS 70 WV Univ; ME 71 Univ of VA - Charlottesville; PH 84 (NS) Univ of VA - Charlottesville; Assoc Prof, Med Coll of VA-Vcu, **A**

Butts, Mrs Sandra Dysart 3902 Montego, Baytown, TX 77521, (713) 428-7039, BS 79 Baylor Univ; MA 85 Univ of Houston - Univ Park; Sp-Lang Path, Patricia Johnson & Assoc PC, **SLP**

Butzen-Murdock, Mrs Rita A 714 Dekalb Street, Wausau, WI 54401, (715) 842-1132, BA 74 Saint Xavier Coll; MA 76 Northwestern Univ; **SLP**

Butzen-Sheridan, Mrs Joanne M 1549 North 2650th Road, Ottawa, IL 61350, (815) 223-1629, BA 73 Saint Xavier Coll; MS 78 Southern IL Univ -Carbondale; Sp-Lang Path, Lasalle Pub Elem Sch, **SLP**

Butzer, Mrs Jan Renner 5933 Wadsworth Road, Orrville, OH 44667, (216) 683-5347, BS 84 Miami Univ - Oxford; MS 85 Miami Univ - Oxford; Sp-Lang Path, Wayne Co Ofc of Educ, **SLP**

Buurma, Kathleen A 829 Northlawn N E, Grand Rapids, MI 49505, (616) 364-6756, BA 64 Western MI Univ; MA 72 Eastern MI Univ; MA 84 Western MI Univ; Sp/Lang Path, Grand Rapids Publ Sch, **SLP**

Buus, Dr Soren 9 Tower Drive, Dover, MA 02030, (617) 437-5196, MS 76; MA 79 Northeastern Univ; PH 80 (Psychoacoustics) Northeastern Univ; Asst Prof, Nthen Univ

Buyok, Gloria Mascarenas 5250 Hickory Avenue, Farmington, NM 87401, (503) 327-1418, BS 82 Eastern NM Univ; MS 85 Univ of NM; **SLP**

Buyok, Nancy Elizabeth 1700 Cliffside Drive #302, Farmington, NM 87401, (505) 368-4984, BS 82 Eastern NM Univ; MS 85 Northern AZ Univ; **SLP**

Buysse, Mrs Miriam Swedberg 12714 Braewood Glen, Houston, TX 77072, (713) 491-7100, BS 72 Western IL Univ; MA 83 Univ of Houston - Univ Park; 83–Sp-Lang Path, Fort Bend ISD, **SLP**

Buzash, Mrs Lola M 65 Colonial Avenue, Pitman, NJ 08071, (609) 589-2966, BS 44 Slippery Rock Univ of PA; ME 58 PA St Univ - Univ Park; **SLP LM**

Buzby, Janet R 159 West Summit Street, Somerville, NJ 08876, (201) 231-0069, SLP, The Cerebral Palsy Assoc, **SLP**

Buzolich, Dr Marilyn J 443-7 Green Ridge Drive, Daly City, CA 94014, (415) 992-7039, MS 77 Univ of South FL; PH 83 (NS) Univ of CA - San Francisco; Sp-Lang Path, Private Practice, **SLP**

Buzynski, Mrs Kathleen S 1134 Leona Avenue, Waterloo, IA 50702, (319) 273-8250, BA 78 Univ of Northern IA; MA 79 Univ of Northern IA; Sp-Lang Path, AEA 7, **SLP**

Buzzard, Mrs Christine Ann 8608 South Marion, Tulsa, OK 74137, (918) 743-9636, BA 69 Univ of WI - Madison; MA 83 Univ of Tulsa; Sp/Lang Path, Caney Valley Schs, **SLP**

Byarlay, Mrs Diane Lynn 15009 Peppermill, Olathe, KS 66062, (816) 234-3392, BS 80 KS St Univ; MA 81 KS St Univ; 85–Sp-Lang Path, Crippled Childrens Nursery Sch, **SLP**

Byars, Susan W 1889 Winchester Trail, Atlanta, GA 30341, (404) 457-9689, MS 73 FL St Univ; BS 72 Univ of GA; Sp-Lang Path, Dekalb Co Bd of Ed, **SLP**

Bycraft, Mrs Helen B 5555 Sheridan Road #911, Chicago, IL 60640, (312) 878-0248, OB 25 Northwestern Univ; **SLP LM**

Byer, Annette Ellen Cherokee Forest, Route 4, Covington, VA 24426, (703) 962-1073, BS 80 James Madison Univ; ME 84 James Madison Univ

Byerly, Mary Ann 602 North May Street #68, Mesa, AZ 85201, (602) 267-1755, **SLP ACE**

Byerly, Susan Jane 2881 Bellaire Road, Silver Lake, OH 44224, **A**

Byers, Candace Lafferty P O Box 547, Dunlevy, PA 15432, **SLP**

Byers, Deborah Kay 1100 Oaktree Avenue #N-7, Norman, OK 73072, (405) 947-7989, BA 79 Northeastern OK St Univ; MS 87 Univ of OK - OK City; 88–Sp-Lang Path, Easter Seals Agency

Byers, Mrs Judith Braud 1825 Gamwich, Baton Rouge, LA 70810, (504) 292-5407, BA 82 LA Tech Univ; MA 84 LA St Univ - Baton Rouge; **SLP**

Byers, Katherine Merchlinsk 541 East Indian Spring Dr, Silver Spring, MD 20901, (301) 588-6726, BA 84 Univ of MD - College Park; MA 87 Univ of MD - College Park; Slp, Natl Rehab Hosp, **SLP**

Byers, Mrs Patricia Ann 61 Bonifant Rd, Silver Spring, MD 20904, (301) 384-0502, BS 80 Indiana Univ of PA; MS 82 PA St Univ - Univ Park; **SLP**

Byers, Mrs Shirley D P O Box 603, Nassau, NY 12123, (518) 325-4471, MS 71 SUNY - Center at Albany; BA 68 SUNY - Center at Albany; Retired, **SLP**

Byers, Mrs Suzanne K 529 North Lombard, Oak Park, IL 60302, (312) 848-4478, BA 76 Duquesne Univ; MS 78 Univ of WI - Milwaukee; **SLP**

Byers, Dr Vincent W Dept Of Communication Disorder, 1900 Gravier Street, New Orleans, LA 70112, BS 55 Univ of KY; MA 56 Univ of KY; PH 61 (NS) Univ of Pittsburgh - Pittsburgh; Prof, LSU Med Ctr, **A F**

Bykowski, Kathleen Adam 11642 West Edgerton Avenue, Hales Corners, WI 53130, (612) 934-0465, BA 83 Univ of SD - Vermillion; MA 86 Univ of MN - Minneap-St Paul; **SLP**

Byle, Larry J 134 West University Drive, Suite 312, Rochester, MI 48063, (313) 651-5051, BS 68 Central MI Univ; MA 71 Wayne St Univ - Sch of Med; Aud, Michael S Menge MD Pc, **A**

Bylo, Marianne G 16 Winchester Road, Livingston, NJ 07039, MS Loyola Coll; 77–Sp-Lang Path, Lake Drive Sch for Hrng Impaired Chldn, **SLP**

Bylotas, Mrs Cynthia L 619 Charles Road, Dauphin, PA 17018, (717) 782-4350, BS 75 Bloomsburg Univ of PA; MS 78 Bloomsburg Univ of PA; 78–Sp/Lang Path, Polyclinic Med Ctr, **SLP**

Bylsma, Bruce Alan 4743 East Meadows S E, Grand Rapids, MI 49506, BS 81 Central MI Univ; MA 83 Central MI Univ; Aud, Burns Cl Med Cen, **A**

Bymers, Susan 66 Pinnacle Road, Ellington, CT 06029, (203) 872-6039, BS 68 Univ of WI - Oshkosh; MA 71 Univ of WI - Madison; SLP, Susan Bymers, **SLP**

Bynum, Donald F 132 Shasta Lane, Charlotte, NC 28211, (704) 372-7170, BS 55 Appalachian St Univ; ME 59 Univ of Pittsburgh - Pittsburgh; VP-Organizational Dev, United Way of Cent Carolinas Inc, **A F**

Bynum-Welfare, Mrs Harriett Lettitia 137 Kimberly Avenue, New Haven, CT 06519, (203) 787-8986, BS 79 Elizabeth City St Univ; MS 83 Southern CT St Univ; 86–Sp-Lang Path, New Haven PS, **SLP**

Byrd, Anna Christina 6220 Shallowford Road #99, Chattanooga, TN 37421, BA 84 David Lipscomb Coll; MA 86 Univ of TN - Knoxville; 87–Sp-Lang Path, Comm Cl, **SLP**

Byrd, Christina E 212 Emerald Lane, Wallingford, PA 19086, (215) 566-3938, MA 88 OH Univ - Athens

Byrd, Faythe S 2035 Dartmouth Avenue, Boulder, CO 80303, (303) 499-5414, BA 73 Univ of MD - College Park; MS 77 Towson St Univ; Sp-Lang Path, Private Practice, **SLP**

Byrd, Mrs Gwendolyn Everhart Rt 1, Box 152B, Harrisburg, AR 72432, (501) 578-5871, BS 83 AR St Univ; MS 86 AR St Univ; 83–Sp-Lang Path, Harrisburg PS, **SLP**

Byrd, Juliane Federico 1637 Biloxi Court, Orlando, FL 32818-9047, (407) 298-2044, BS 82 CA St Univ - Hayward; MS 85 Univ of NV - Reno; 87–Sp-Lang Path, InSpeech Inc, **SLP**

Byrd, Kathryn P O Box 1326, 84 Riverdale, Tuscaloosa, AL 35403-1326, (205) 758-2137, BA 69 Grinnell Coll; MA 71 Univ of TX - Austin; MS 87 Univ of AL- Tuscaloosa; **SLP**

Byrd, Mrs Lisa J Rural Route 2, Greentop, MO 63546, (816) 665-1694, BS 79 Northeast MO St Univ; MA 87 Northeast MO St Univ; 80–Sp-Lang Path, Schuyler R-1 Sch Dist, **SLP**

Byrd, M Rita 3500 Warwick Drive #36, Lexington, KY 40502, (502) 564-4970, BS 69 Murray St Univ; MS 72 Murray St Univ; OM 79 GA St Univ; Consult, Ky Dept of Ed, **SLP**

Byrd, Mrs Mary Delamar 6879 South Prince Way, Littleton, CO 80120, (303) 791-1115, BS 82 Baylor Univ; MS 83 Baylor Univ; Sp-Lang Path, Douglas County Sch Dist, **SLP**

Byrd, Mrs Nancy Sorrentino 726 W Hopkins Street, San Marcos, TX 78666, (512) 353-6790, BS 82 Southwest TX St Univ; ME 84 Southwest TX St Univ; Sp-Lang Path, San Marcos ISD, **SLP**

Byrd, Susan Marie 7548 Charmant Drive, #1425, San Diego, CA 92122, (619) 455-7724, Aud, Aud & Hrng Aid Assoc, **A**

Byrd, William H, Jr Route 1, Lynnwood Lane, Rockford, TN 37853, (615) 982-8557, BA 60 David Lipscomb Coll; MS 61 Univ of TN - Knoxville; Aud, Blount Hrng & Sp Serv, **A**

Byrne, Maj Clyde D 109 Darwin Drive, Snyder, NY 14226, (716) 839-5359, BA 71 Angelo St Univ; MA 75 Univ of North TX; Aud, US Army, **A**

Byrne, 1Lt David C Reynolds Army Comm Hospital, Audiology, Box 38, Fort Sill, OK 73503, (405) 351-5509, BA 84 Univ of Pittsburgh - Pittsburgh; MS 87 PA St Univ - Univ Park; 88–Aud, US Army

Byrne, Mrs Debra D Wyllie Road, Norfolk, MA 02056, (617) 528-4094, BA 74 Univ of RI; ME 76 Northeastern Univ; Sp-Lang Path, Franklin Pub Sch, **SLP**

Byrne, Lisa 2 Beach Street, Beverly Farms, MA 01915, (617) 894-4600, MS 88 Northeastern Univ; 88–Sp-Lang Path, Middlesex County Hosp

Byrne, Marie E 1303 West 27th Street, Apt 9, Hays, KS 67601, (913) 628-4108, BS 73 East Stroudsburg Univ of PA; MA 79 Trenton St Coll; Cl Superv, **SLP**

Byrne, Mary Lou C 45727 27th St, Mattawan, MI 49071, (616) 674-8091, BA 70 MI St Univ; MA 75 MI St Univ; MA 82 Western MI Univ; SLP, Van Buren Inter Sch Dist, **SLP**

Byrne, Patricia A 21 Colonial Circle, Fairport, NY 14450, (716) 265-4057, BS 68 Nazareth Coll of Rochester; MS 74 SUNY - Coll at Geneseo; Principal, Monroe BOCES 1, **SLP**

Byrne, Polly 176 Caldecott Lane #209, Oakland, CA 94618, (415) 228-6800, BA 80 Univ of the Pacific; MA 82 Univ of Northern CO; 85–Aud, Veterans Administration, **A**

Byrne, Sharon Fandrey 16984 Saddlewood Trail, Minnetonka, MN 55345-2678, (612) 932-5486, MS 71 Saint Cloud St Univ; **SLP**

Byrne, Susan C 11953 Glen Alden Road, Fairfax, VA 22030, (703) 361-4811, BS 78 Marquette Univ; MA 79 SUNY - Coll at Geneseo; SLP, Prince William Co Pub Sch, **SLP**

Byrne, Suzanne M 425 34th Street, Lindenhurst, NY 11757-3250, (516) 226-3569, BS 83 SUNY - Coll at Oneonta; MA 85 CUNY - Queens Coll; 87–Sp-Lang Path, North Shore Univ Hosp, **SLP**

Byrne-Hamilton, Mrs Karen Lyn 705 Symphony Woods Drive, Silver Spring, MD 20901, (301) 593-7535, BS 81 SUNY - Coll at Geneseo; MA 83 Univ of MD - College Park; Sp-Lang Path, Private Practice, **SLP**

Byrnes, Mrs Arlene 11 Danville Court, New Castle, DE 19720, (302) 323-9112, BS 83 Worcester St Coll; 87 Worcester St Coll; 87–Sp-Lang Path, Delaware Curative Workshop, **SLP**

Byrnes, Mrs Cathy Hicks 5954 Crittenden Drive, Cincinnati, OH 45244, (404) 963-7174, BS 80 Miami Univ - Oxford; MS 81 Miami Univ - Oxford; Sp-Lang Path, Cincinnati Pub Schs, **SLP**

Byrnes, Nona Jane 1184 Leisure World, Mesa, AZ 85206-3065, MS; **SLP LM**

Byrns, Glenda E 5918 Theall, Houston, TX 77066, (918) 258-0152, **SLP**

Byron, Michael K 1117 Stolp Avenue, Syracuse, NY 13207, (315) 487-1178, BA 75 SUNY - Coll at Oswego; MS 80 Syracuse Univ; Sp-Lang Path, Onondaga/Mad BOCES Pro for Dea, **SLP**

Bystrom, Susan Kay Route 5 Woodridge Drive, River Falls, WI 54022, (608) 647-6106, BS 82 Univ of WI - River Falls; OM 83 Univ of WI - River Falls; **SLP**

Bywaters, Mrs Eleanor B 430 Mutton Creek Drive, Seymour, IN 47274, (812) 522-7979, BS 44 IN St Univ - Terre Haute; MA 66 IN Univ - Bloomington; Retired, **SLP LM**

Bzdula, Paula A P O Box 452, Winchester, MA 01890, BS 68 Univ of MA - Amherst; MS 77 Lesley Coll; **SLP**

Bzoch, Dr Kenneth R Dept Communication Disorders, University Of Florida, Box J-174, Gainesville, FL 32610, (904) 392-2636, BA 51 De Paul Univ; MA 52 Northwestern Univ; PH 56 (NS) Northwestern Univ; Prof & Chmn, U of FL, **SLP A F**

C

Caba, Mrs Mary W 626 Chapel Street, Ottawa, IL 61350, (815) 357-8744, BA 78 Augustana Coll; MS 80 IL St Univ - Normal; 81–Sp-Lang Path, Seneca Grade Sch, **SLP**

Caballero-Somawang, Julieta 46-318 Haiku Road #79, Kaneohe, HI 96744, (808) 262-5115, BA 79 Univ of the Pacific; MA 80 Univ of the Pacific; SLP, Windard Oahu School Dist, **SLP**

Cabanting, Erlinda 242 Marquette Street, Park Forest, IL 60466, (312) 747-8100, SLP, Elizabeth Ludeman Devel/Ctr, **SLP**

Cabe, Donna J 6754 Dicenza Way, San Diego, CA 92119, (619) 442-2501, BA 75 Univ of CA - San Diego; MA 80 San Diego St Univ; Aud, Kaiser Permanente Medical Gp, **A**

Cabe, Patricia M 96 Jack Cabe Road, Franklin, NC 28734, ES 71 Univ of GA; Sp-Lang Path, Macon County Schs, **SLP**

Cabello, Arturo 3036 Juniper Street #3, San Diego, CA 92104, (619) 284-7276, BA 83 San Diego St Univ; MA 86 San Diego St Univ; **SLP**

Cabeza, Mrs Constance H L 409 Mercy Professional Bldg, 3661 South Miami Avenue, Miami, FL 33133, (305) 854-8171, BS 68 Univ of TN - Knoxville; MS 69 Univ of TN - Knoxville; Dir, Miami Hrng & Sp Cen, **A**

Cable, Della Jane 610 Ahtanum, Wapato, WA 98951, (509) 575-3308, BA 64 Central WA Univ; ME 68 Central WA Univ; SLP, Yakima Sch Dist #7, **SLP ACE**

Cable, Jetta L 2329 Addison, Wichita, KS 67226, (316) 684-5892, BA 76 Wichita St Univ; MA 78 Wichita St Univ; Sp-Lang Path, Private Practice, **SLP**

Cable, Mrs Virginia Evans Route 2 Box 118-1, Bastrop, LA 71220, (318) 283-2857, BA 77 Northeast LA Univ; MA 87 Northeast LA Univ; 85–Sp-Lang Path, Morehouse Parish Schs, **SLP**

Cabral, Claudia Jean 3324 Perisburg Lane, Ceres, CA 95307, (209) 545-1732, BA 84 CA St Univ - Stanislaus; MA 86 CA St Univ - Stanislaus; 86–Sp-Lang Path, Stanislaus Co Dept of Educ, **SLP**

Cabral, Mrs Donna M 314 Hope Street, Bristol, RI 02809, (401) 254-0462, BA 82 RI Coll; MS 86 Emerson Coll; 86–Sp-Lang Path, Morton Hosp & Med Ctr Inc, **SLP**

Cacace, Anthony T Rd 2 Box 229, Voorheesville, NY 12186, **A**

Caccamise, Dr Frank C National Technical Institute For The Deaf, PO Box 9887, Rochester, NY 14623-0887, (716) 475-6420, BA 66 Saint John Fisher Coll; MS 68 Gallaudet Coll; PH 73 (Aud) Univ of WA; 74–Res Assoc, Rochester I of Tech, **A**

Caccamo, Dr James M School Dist Of Independence, 1231 South Windsor, Independence, MO 64055, (816) 833-3433, BS 66 Saint Louis Univ; MA 68 Saint Louis Univ; PH 71 (NS) Saint Louis Univ; Dir/Spec Prog, Sch Dist of Independence, **SLP**

Caccavo, Dr Mary T 2315 South Street, Lafayette, IN 47904, (317) 448-6226, BS 77 Purdue Univ - West Lafayette; MA 79 Univ of Northern CO; PH 85 (NS) Purdue Univ - West Lafayette; Aud, Lafayette Hrng Ctr, **A**

Caceres, Milagros Ong 3240 W Juneau Avenue, Milwaukee, WI 53208, (414) 931-8071, BA 75 Univ of Philippines; MA 80 IN Univ - Bloomington; 80–Sp-Lang Path, Milwaukee PS, **SLP**

Cadaret, Mrs Sally Joan 22869 North Nunneley #204, Mount Clemens, MI 48043, (313) 985-1372, BS 83 Eastern MI Univ; MA 85 Eastern MI Univ; SLP, Mercy Hosp, **SLP**

Caddy, Charna B Garden City Medical Center, 520 Franklin Avenue, Garden City, NY 11530, (516) 741-1390, MS 77 Southern Methodist Univ; Sp-Lang Path, Private Practice, **SLP**

Cade, Elisabeth L 2842 Old Dixwell Avenue #B, Hamden, CT 06518, (203) 288-4831, BA 86 Univ of CT; MA 88 Univ of CT; 88–Sp-Lang Path, Rehabilitation Associates Inc

Cadley, Donald K 925 Center Street, Ashland, OH 44805, **SLP**

Cadogan, Dr Paula M 6206 East 77th Street, Tulsa, OK 74136, (918) 492-8310, BS 73 Northwestern Univ; MS 76 Univ of CT; ME 85 Harvard Univ; Asst Prof Commun Disorders, U of Tulsa, **SLP**

Cady, Dr Barbara B 2013 Joseph Circle, Huntsville, AL 35811, (205) 859-7367, BA 65 Auburn Univ - Auburn; MA 68 Univ of AL- Tuscaloosa; PH 81 (Sp Path & Aud) Univ of KS; Chairperson Dept Special Educ, Alabama A&M University, **SLP**

Cady, Candace A 8200 Walnut Hill Lane, Dallas, TX 75231, (214) 696-7984, BS 74 Southern Methodist Univ; MS 76 Southern Methodist Univ; Sp-Lang Path, Presby Hosp Dallas, **SLP**

Cady, Mrs Patricia Nash 18 Southridge Drive, Glendale, MO 63122, (314) 961-8742, BS 83 Fontbonne Coll; MS 84 Fontbonne Coll; 87–Sp-Lang Path, Sisters of St Mary Rehab Inst, **SLP**

Cady, Mrs Susan Lynn 30628 Winston Drive, Bay Village, OH 44140, (216) 324-7500, BS 80 Bowling Green St Univ; MA 85 Cleveland St Univ; **SLP**

Caell, Teresa A 4228 Tennyson, Houston, TX 77005-4920, MS 70 Univ of GA; **SLP**

Cafarelli-Dees, Denise L The Baechus, High Street, West Meon, England GU3 21JL, (447) 308-6334, BA 74 Adelphi Univ; MS 75 Syracuse Univ; Coord Aural Rehab Cen, Cleveland Cl Fndtn, **A**

Caffarella, Janice M Edward Hospital Hearing Center, 801 South Washington Avenue, Naperville, IL 60566, (312) 355-0450, BS 84 IL St Univ - Normal; MS 85 IL St Univ - Normal; 86–Audiologist, Edward Hosp Hearing Ctr, **A**

Cafmeyer, April M Hammond Clinic, 7905 Calumet Avenue, Munster, IN 46321, (219) 836-5800, BA 79 Kalamazoo Coll; MS 81 Washington Univ; Aud, Hammond Clinic, **A ACE**

Caforio, Mrs Judith Mae-England 10647 El Adelante, Fountain Valley, CA 92708, (714) 964-6088, BA 71 CA St Univ - Fullerton; MA 76 CA St Univ - Fullerton; Sp-Lang Path, Fountain Vy Sch Dist, **SLP**

Cafritz, Donna M 12033 Montrose Village Ter, Rockville, MD 20852, (301) 424-5200, BA 80 Univ of MD - College Park; MA 81 Hofstra Univ; Aud, Treatment & Lrng Ctr, **A**

Cage, Mrs Janiece Lynn 250 Maryland Avenue, Portsmouth, VA 23707, (804) 393-7714, BS 83 Old Dominion Univ; MS 85 Old Dominion Univ; 88–Sp-Lang Path, Private Practice, **SLP**

Cage, Johnnye Annzanetta 839 Flora Lane, Baton Rouge, LA 70810, (504) 766-3544, BA 83 Northwestern St Univ; MS 85 Univ Southern MS-Hattiesburg; **SLP**

Cagle, Daphne 4941 Brownstone Court, Elk Grove, CA 95624, (916) 454-8183, BS 75 Univ of Southwestern LA; MS 79 Univ of Southwestern LA; Sp-Lang Path, Sacramento City USD, **SLP ACE**

Cagle, Lonna Faye Forsyth Head & Neck Associates, 1420 Plaza Drive, Winston-Salem, NC 27103, (919) 765-4922, BA 78 Univ of NC - Greensboro; MA 79 Univ of NC - Greensboro; Aud, Forsyth Head & Neck Assoc, **A**

Cagle, Mrs Lotus M 1539 John Drive, Lake Charles, LA 70605, (318) 478-4469, BA 63; MA 69; Sp-Lang Path, **SLP**

Caha, Anne Margaret 713 Midland Boulevard, Union, NJ 07083, (201) 539-9630, BA 84 Kean Coll of NJ; MA 85 Kean Coll of NJ; Sp-Lang Path, Reg Day Sch at Morris

Cahill, Mrs Ellen Rauchway 44 Iroquois Road, Richboro, PA 18954, (215) 757-7667, BS 76 Trenton St Coll; MA 77 Trenton St Coll; Sp-Lang Path/Proj Mgr, Rehab Mgmt Grp, **SLP**

Cahill, Mrs Judy G 71 Green Avenue, Lawrenceville, NJ 08648, (609) 895-0239, MA 76 CUNY - Queens Coll; Aud, ENT & Facial Plastic Assn, **A**

Cahill-Norton, Mrs Kelly 32 Middlesex Road, Topsham, ME 04086, (207) 729-3899, BA 81 CA St Univ - Fresno; MA 83 Univ of the Pacific; Sp-Lang Path, Pine Tree Society, **SLP**

Cahoon-Simon, Mrs Sandra 1820 Samish Lane, Bellingham, WA 98226, (206) 675-5811, BA 75 Univ of WA; MA 79 Univ of WA; Esd 189, **SLP**

Caiaccio, Mrs Marjorie V 2132 Academy Drive, Clearwater, FL 34624, (813) 446-4525, MS 85 Univ of South FL; 88–Sp-Lang Path, Communi-Care, **SLP**

Caiella, Mrs Josephine Shuman 6048 Jerusalem Drive, Clay, NY 13041, (315) 963-7251, BS 79 SUNY - Coll at Geneseo; MA 82 SUNY - Coll at Geneseo; Sp-Lang Path, Oswego Co BOCES, **SLP**

Cain, Debra Hubley Route 1 Box 1770, Cornelia, GA 30531, (404) 778-9608, BS 84 FL St Univ; MS 85 FL St Univ; **SLP**

Cain, Mrs Elizabeth Houseman 1023 Fairwood Court, Acworth, GA 30101, (404) 427-7726, BS 85 Auburn Univ - Auburn; MS 87 Auburn Univ - Auburn; **SLP**

Cain, James V 10743 Stark Avenue, Kansas City, MO 64134, (816) 763-1169, **A**

Cain, Mrs Jean Beauloc 1595 Manzanita Avenue, Apartment 27, Chico, CA 95926, (916) 893-5698, MA 87 CA St Univ - Chico

Cain, Mrs Kay Conway 3405 Markwell Avenue, Bethany, OK 73008, (405) 787-8142, BS 80 OK St Univ; MS 82 Univ of OK Medical Center; Sp-Lang Path, Putnam City Sch, **SLP**

Caine, Joyce Barker 700 Broken Dollar Court, Odessa, MO 64076, (816) 625-4156

Cains, Lynne G 170 Highland Street #306, Taunton, MA 02780, (617) 824-5881, BA 74 CUNY - Brooklyn Coll; MA 75 MI St Univ; Dir/Sp-Hrng Ser, Paul A Dever State Sch, **SLP**

Cairella, Cynthia A 2570 South Dayton Way, Apartment F-210, Denver, CO 80231, (303) 287-8086, BA 77 Southern CT St Univ; MS 79 CO St Univ; 80–Sp-Lang Path, Adams Co Sch Dist #12, **SLP**

Caisse, Mrs Karen Lynne 201 Meng Road, Schwenksville, PA 19473, (215) 256-4211, BS 72 Trenton St Coll; MA 76 Trenton St Coll; 87–Sp-Lang Path, Easter Seal Society, **SLP**

Caissie, Rachel Audiology Department, Ottawa Civic Hospital, 1053 Carling Avenue, Ottawa, ON, Canada K1Y 4E9, (613) 725-4087, OB 81 Universite DE Moncton - New Brunswick; MS 83 McGill Univ - Quebec; 88–Aud, Ottawa Civic Hosp, **A**

Calabresa-Echelard, Mrs Maria Louise 15748 West Ridge Road, New Berlin, WI 53151, (414) 796-0587, BS 82 Univ of WI - Milwaukee; MS 84 Univ of WI - Milwaukee; 88–Sp-Lang Path, Self Employed, **SLP**

Calabrese, Barbara J 1408 West Berwyn, Chicago, IL 60640, (312) 878-0186, MS 75 Univ of IL - Urbana; Asst Dir Research Admin, Il Inst of Tech, **SLP**

Calamaras, Dr Peter 142 Hackensack Street, Woodridge, NJ 07075, (201) 939-6294, BA 50 CUNY - Brooklyn Coll; MA 52 CUNY - Brooklyn Coll; PH 64 (NS) NY Univ; Retired, **SLP A LM**

Calams, Timothy J 23425 Glenridge Drive, Newhall, CA 91321-3956, (805) 942-8111, MS; **A**

Calavano, Mrs Joycelyn R 415 North San Mateo Drive, Suite 6, San Mateo, CA 94401, (415) 343-2779, OM 68 San Francisco St Univ; OM 68 San Francisco St Univ; Dir/Cl Activities, Center Four, **SLP A**

Calbazana, Maya Victoria 314 Catherine Street #104, Philadelphia, PA 19147-3202, (215) 427-5590, BA 83 Loyola Coll; MS 84 Loyola Coll; 88–Sp-Lang Path, Philadelphia Early Childhood Evaluation Ctr, **SLP**

Calbos, Eleni T EFMS 130th Station Hosp, APO New York, NY 09102, BS 80 Western IL Univ; MA 82 Western IL Univ; Sp-Lang Path, Gov Service Program, **SLP**

Calculator, Mrs Jean M 160 Maple Street Ext, Somersworth, NH 03878, (603) 692-2544, BA 74 Univ of MA - Amherst; MA 76 SUNY - Coll at Geneseo; Sp-Lang Path, Somersworth Sch Dept, **SLP**

Calculator, Dr Stephen 160 Maple Street Ext, Somersworth, NH 03878, (603) 862-2110, BA 74 SUNY - Coll at Oswego; MS 75 SUNY - Coll at Geneseo; PH 80 (NS) Univ of WI - Madison; Assoc Prof of Commun Dis, Univ of New Hampshire, **SLP**

Caldarera, Mrs Dana M 879 Storer Avenue #3, Fayetteville, AR 72701, (501) 521-7923, BS 86 Univ of Central AR; MS 87 Univ of Central AR; 87–Sp-Lang Path, Springdale Sch Dist, **SLP**

Calder, Dr H B 2779 Georgetown Boulevard, Ann Arbor, MI 48105, (313) 662-0312, BS 71 UT St Univ; MS 72 9857; PH 76 (Aud) Northwestern Univ; Pres, Biotronic, **A**

Calder, Mrs Pat E 13127 Archwood Street, North Hollywood, CA 91606, (818) 781-1200, BA 76 CA St Univ - Northridge; MA 78 CA St Univ - Northridge; Prof, LA Comm Coll Dist, **SLP**

Calderon, Mrs Judith Roman 207 Dana Drive, Salisbury, NC 28144, (704) 633-8282, BA 78 Catawba Coll; ME 81 Univ of NC - Greensboro; Sp-Lang Path, Rowan Co Sch, **SLP**

Calderon-Dworetzky, Dianne L 3923 Sea Wind Place, Woodland Hills, CA 91364, (818) 712-9349, BA 76; MA 80 NY Univ; SLP, **SLP**

Calderone, Mrs M Lynn 802 Jamie Lane, Macomb, IL 61455, (309) 655-2630, BS 78 Northern IL Univ - De Kalb; MA 79 Northern IL Univ - De Kalb; Aud, St Francis Med Cen, **A**

Calderone, Susan C 208 Harmony Lane, Elk Grove Village, IL 60007, (312) 228-9813, BA 81 MI St Univ; MA 82 Univ of IL - Urbana; 83–Sp-Lang Path-Early Childhood Prog, Schaumburg Sch Dist #54, **SLP**

Calderone, Mrs Tancine W 145 West Union Avenue, Bound Brook, NJ 08805, (201) 757-7464, BA 73 Montclair St Coll; MS 75 IL St Univ - Normal; Sp-Lang Path, Warren Twp Board of Education, **SLP**

Calderon-Rogers, Mrs Esperanza G 1033 Piedmont Drive, Abilene, TX 79601, (915) 676-9568, BA 74 Univ of North TX; MA 76 Univ of North TX; Sp-Lang Path, **SLP**

Calderwood, Rebecca W 505 West Highland Avenue, Wooster, OH 44691-1359, (216) 698-2411, BS 79 Kent St Univ; MA 81 Kent St Univ; SLP, Apple Creek Dev Cen, **SLP**

Caldwell, Carol A Medical Ctr Hrng-Balance Diag, 2660 Main Street Suite 317, Bridgeport, CT 06606, (203) 334-6012, BA 77 Univ of CT; MA 78 Univ of CT; Director, Medical Cen Hrng-Balance Diag, **A**

Caldwell, Carol S 2406 South 9th Street, Sheboygan, WI 53081, (414) 459-3886, MS 78 Univ of WI - Madison; Sp-Lang Path, Handicapped Chdrns Ed Bd, **SLP**

Caldwell, Catherine Lynne 817 Westminster Ct N E, Lacey, WA 98506, (206) 748-3384, BS 83 Southwest TX St Univ; MA 86 WA St Univ

Caldwell, Mrs Credonna L 708 Greenhill Road, Benton, AR 72015, (501) 776-0371, MS 88 Univ of AR - Little Rock; 88–Aud, The Ear Nose & Throat Clinic, **F**

Caldwell, Ethlyn D 1807 North 20th Avenue, Pensacola, FL 32503-5760, (904) 432-2275, BS 72 Auburn Univ - Auburn; MA 75 Univ of AL- Tuscaloosa; SLP, Escambia County Bd of Ed, **SLP**

Caldwell, Gail Olive 1814 No 46th, Seattle, WA 98103, (206) 543-4011, BA 78 Univ of AZ; BA 84 Univ of WA; MS 86 Univ of WA; Sp-Lang Path, Univ of WA

Caldwell, Helen M 1613 Brookridge Drive, Elizabeth City, NC 27909, MS; **SLP**

Caldwell, Mrs Janine Ann Rd #1 Box 375, Harmony, PA 16037, (412) 452-5999, BS 82 PA St Univ - Univ Park; MS 83 Clarion Univ of PA; Sp-Lang Path, Boardman Local Schs, **SLP**

Caldwell, Mrs Katy E Route 1 Box 102-A, Glade Valley, NC 28627, (919) 372-5641, BS 74 Appalachian St Univ; MA 75 Appalachian St Univ; Sp-Lang Path, Appalachian Dist Hlth Dept, **SLP**

Caldwell, Keith C 79 Village Parkway, Napa, CA 94558, (707) 944-4427, **A**

Caldwell, Lacey J S 7306 Cart Gate Drive, Houston, TX 77095, MS; **SLP**

Caldwell, Margo L 127 Turtle Creek Road #6, Charlottesville, VA 22901, (804) 286-2441, BA 70 Allegheny Coll; ME 74 Univ of VA - Charlottesville; OM 84 James Madison Univ; Sp-Lang Path, Albemarle Co Pub Sch Syst, **SLP**

Caldwell, Mary A Hixson Hall Room 921, 820 18th Street South, Birmingham, AL 35256, (205) 934-4897, BS 86 Western Carolina Univ; MA 87 Western Carolina Univ

Caldwell, Mary D P O Box 146, Chalk Hill, PA 15421, (412) 439-0559, MS 88 CA Univ of PA

Caldwell, Nancy A 2591 Goodenough Road, Fillmore, CA 93015, (805) 524-2569, BA 82 Univ of Southern CA; MS 87 Emerson Coll

Caldwell, Sherrie Delores Route 3 Box 1, Canton, NC 28716, (704) 264-0566, MA 87 Western Carolina Univ

Caldwell, Mrs Susan Aguzin 625 East Central Parkway, Lake Charles, LA 70605, (318) 775-7570, BS 74 Saint Mary's Dominican Coll; MS 78 Univ Southern MS-Hattiesburg; Sp-Lang Path, Cameron Parish Sch Bd, **SLP**

Caleffe-Schenck, Nancy S 32458 Little Cub Road, Evergreen, CO 80439, (303) 670-0029, OB 74 Indiana Univ of PA; ME 79 PA St Univ - Univ Park; Auditory-Verbal Consult, Auditory-Verbal Services, **A**

Calhoun, Mrs Cindy C 1020 Rose Road, Albertville, AL 35950, (205) 878-1183, BS 82 Auburn Univ - Auburn; OM 84 Auburn Univ - Auburn; **SLP**

Calhoun, Janna K 733 Channing Drive N W, Atlanta, GA 30318, (404) 352-3909, BA 68 TX Tech Univ; MA 69 TX Tech Univ; 83–Pres, Calhoun & Assoc, **SLP**

Calhoun, Marian Hope P O Box 732, Mansfield, LA 71052, (318) 872-0286, BS 84 Baylor Univ; MS 86 Baylor Univ; **SLP**

Calhoun, Melissa Hotto #4 Juanita Place, Belleville, IL 62223-2330, (314) 839-3800, BA 84 Southern IL Univ-Edwardsvill; MS 85 Southern IL Univ-Edwardsvill; **SLP**

Calhoun, Sarah Ann 410 Park Ridge Lane #V, Winston-Salem, NC 27104, (919) 725-0222, BA 82 LA Tech Univ; MA 85 LA St Univ - Baton Rouge; Assoc Dir, SPEECHCENTER, **SLP**

Calhoun-Peters, Mrs Susan N 2131 Kinridge Road N E, Marietta, GA 30062, (404) 973-1935, MA 78 San Jose St Univ; 86–Sp-Lang Path, Private Practice, **SLP**

Cali, Thomas F 33000 Fredoom Road, Farmington Hills, MI 48024, (313) 477-3700, BS 66 Eastern MI Univ; MA 68 Eastern MI Univ; Sp-Lang Path, Farmington Public Schools, **SLP**

Califf, Elizabeth Kimberly 13746 Kingsridge Lane, Houston, TX 77079, (713) 984-0217, BA 77 Univ of OK - Norman; MS 80 Univ of OK Medical Center; 88–Aud, Katy ISD, **A**

Calio, Victoria Anne 13109 Bustleton Avenue, Apartment A-35, Philadelphia, PA 19116, (215) 671-5202, BS 84 Albright Coll; MA 87 Temple Univ; 88–Sp-Lang Path, Temple Univ-Woodhaven Ctr, **SLP**

Calkins, Dr Janice Lockhart 10709 N W 31st Place, Gainesville, FL 32606-4949, (904) 375-3845, BS 75 OH Univ - Athens; ME 76 Univ of FL; PH 83 (NS) Univ of FL; Sp-Lang Path, Alachua County Public Schools, **SLP**

Calkins, Lynnell Flynn 2113-B Vanderbilt Lane, Redondo Beach, CA 90278, (213) 372-8613, BA 74 Northeast LA Univ; MA 75 Memphis St Univ; MA 80 CA St Univ - Los Angeles; 76–Sp-Lang Path, LA Co Office of Ed, **SLP**

Call, Janell 246 Palmer Street, Middleport, OH 45760, (614) 992-5538, MA 78 Marshall Univ; OM 86 OH Univ - Athens; PH 88 (Health Svcs Admin/Health Comm) OH Univ - Athens; 82–Sp-Lang Path, Private Practice, **SLP**

Call, Janice Merlo 7392 Stream Way, Springfield, VA 22152, (703) 866-0753, BS 78 ID St Univ; MS 84 Governors St Univ; Sp-Lang Path, Accotink Academy, **SLP**

Call, Timothy A 6394 Twin Lakes Road, Boulder, CO 80301, (303) 772-7700, BA 71 Univ of MI - Ann Arbor; MS 76 CO St Univ; Sp-Lang Path, St Vrain Valley Sch Dis, **SLP**

Call, Wendy M W 1943 East Diamond, Tempe, AZ 85283, (602) 831-6783, BS 74 AZ St Univ; MS 79 AZ St Univ; 88–Sp-Lang Path, East Valley Sp Path Assoc, **SLP**

Callaghan, Carol A 2586 19th Avenue, San Francisco, CA 94116, BA 78 CA St Univ - Long Beach; MA 84 Univ of San Francisco; SLP, San Francisco USD, **SLP**

Callaghan, Janet Turansky 89 High Street, Armonk, NY 10504, (914) 273-9227, BA 79 CUNY - Queens Coll; MA 82 CUNY - Hunter Coll; Sp-Lang Path, BOCES #2, **SLP**

Callaghan, Kathy Lynn 4334 Downs Square, Belcamp, MD 21017, (301) 444-5000, BA 80 Loyola Coll; MS 82 Loyola Coll; Sp-Lang Path, MD Sch for the Blind, **SLP**

Callaghan, Sheelagh A 202 Edith Boulevard S E, Albuquerque, NM 87102, BS 79 Univ of Alberta - Alberta; MS 81 Univ of NM; Sp/Lang Path, Educational Assessment Systems Inc, **SLP**

Callaghan, Mrs Wendy M 415 Orangewood Drive, Lemoore, CA 93245, (619) 446-5547, BA 72 Ashland Coll; MA 73 OH Univ - Athens; SLP, Kings Co Supt of Sch, **SLP**

Callaham, Marilyn Llewellyn 610 South Third Avenue #E, Arcadia, CA 91006, BA 70 Univ of Redlands; MA 86 CA St Univ - Los Angeles; 87–Sp-Lang Path, Claremont USD, **SLP**

Callahan, Angela Marie 1608 Enterprise Lane, Sun Prairie, WI 53590, (414) 648-2338, BS 84 IA St Univ; MS 86 Univ of WI - Whitewater; 88–Sp-Lang Path, Lake Mills Area Sch Dist, **SLP**

Callahan, Barbara Heinz 1200 South Torrey Pines Dr, Apartment 36, Las Vegas, NV 89102, (702) 383-2385, MS 80 Univ of South FL; 81–Sp-Lang Path, Univ Med Ctr of So NV, **SLP**

Callahan, Mrs Barbara M 1228 Glade Street, Winston-Salem, NC 27101, (919) 723-2655, BS 72 WV Univ; ME 74 Univ of NC - Greensboro; SLP, Winston-Salem Forsythe Co Sch, **SLP**

Callahan, Edith E Corley 105 Lyman Court, Morganton, NC 28655, (704) 433-2754, BS 84 Appalachian St Univ; MS 85 East Carolina Univ; SLP, Western Carolina Center, **SLP**

Callahan, Dr Joan B 33 Arbor Lane, Roslyn Heights, NY 11577, (516) 294-8700, BA 60 Adelphi Univ; MA 61 Columbia Univ Teachers Coll; OD 82 (NS) Adelphi Univ; Coord of Deaf Ed, Adelphi U, **SLP A**

Callahan, Mrs Kim Bauer 25 Kuchenski Drive, Dickinson, ND 58601, (701) 227-0728, BS 76; MS 79 UT St Univ; Aud/Reg Dir, Private Practice, **A**

Callahan, Margaret J 4561 Lake Washington Blvd, N E #203, Kirkland, WA 98033, (206) 828-0934, BS 72 Univ of OR; MS 74 Portland St Univ; **SLP**

Callahan, Mrs Patricia 203 St Lawrence Avenue West, P O Box 548, Brownville, NY 13615, (315) 785-8208, BS 70 SUNY - Coll at Buffalo; MS 74 SUNY - Coll at Buffalo; 83–Sp/Lang Path, Jefferson Lewis BOCES, **SLP**

Callahan, Robert Ross 2753 Ceres Avenue, Chico, CA 95926, (916) 534-4277, BA 75 CA St Univ - Chico; MA 81 CA St Univ - Chico; **SLP**

Callahan, Rosemary E 1139 River Bank Road, Stamford, CT 06903, (203) 625-7496, MS 78 Adelphi Univ; **SLP**

Callahan, Ruth A 563 Rock Springs Road N E, Atlanta, GA 30324, (404) 542-4561, BS 72 Kent St Univ; MA 74 Kent St Univ; ED 88 (Educational Administration) Univ of GA; 85–Research Coord, U of GA, **SLP**

Callahan, Mrs Susan Finegan 999 Oakland Lane, Aurora, IL 60504-2904, (312) 820-0829, MA 84 Northern IL Univ - De Kalb; BS 82 Northern IL Univ - De Kalb; **SLP**

Callahan-Smerdzinaki, Judith 308 Elrino Street, Baltimore, MD 21224, (301) 838-1122, BS 75 Towson St Univ; MS 78 Loyola Coll; Sp-Lang Path, Harford Co Bd of Ed, **SLP**

Callaway, Deborah 4851 Sheridan Drive, Jackson, MS 39206-4820, (601) 362-4156, BA 72 Delta St Univ; OM 73 Univ of MS; SLP, Jackson Muncpl Separ Sch Dist, **SLP**

Callaway, Elizabeth Veterans Administration Medical Center, Ann Arbor, MI 48104, (313) 769-7100, MS 83 Univ of MI - Ann Arbor; 87–Sp-Lang Path, VA Med Ctr, **SLP**

Callaway, Mrs Mary Ann 113 Blue Heron Drive, Savannah, GA 31410, (912) 897-6753, BS 79 Univ of GA; ME 83 Univ of GA; Sp-Lang Path, Savannah Sp & Hearing Ctr, **SLP**

Callaway, Noah Mae Route 6 Box 7, Blanchard, OK 73010, (405) 527-3325, BA 77 San Diego St Univ; ME 81 Univ of OK - Norman; **SLP**

Callen, Douglas N 967 Cherry Lane, Apollo, PA 15613, (412) 548-4455, BS 68 Clarion Univ of PA; ME 70 Clarion Univ of PA; MS 81 Clarion Univ of PA; Aud/ Sp-Lang Path, Armstrong Sp & Hrng Aid Cen, **SLP A**

Callen, John R 338 22nd Place, Clinton, IA 52732, (309) 344-3400, BS 80 Eastern IL Univ; MS 82 Eastern IL Univ; Sp-Lang Path, Community General Hospital, **SLP**

Callender, Mrs Martha M 5217 Lake Shore Road, Virginia Beach, VA 23455, (804) 440-4117, BA 68 Longwood Coll; ME 69 Univ of VA - Charlottesville; Superv Cl Practicum, Old Dominion U, **SLP ACE**

Callery, Mrs Donna L S 77 Parker Road, Plainsboro, NJ 08536, (201) 799-9670, BS 74 Emerson Coll; MS 78 Rutgers St Univ - Newark; **SLP**

Callery, Ingrid Margot 3081 North Main Street #4, Walnut Creek, CA 94596, (415) 944-9352, MA 88 San Diego St Univ

Callia, Ramona Leydecker 131 Elaine Avenue, Harahan, LA 70123, (504) 738-1615, BA 81 Southeastern LA Univ; OM 84 LA St Univ - N O Medical Ctr; 81–Sp-Lang Path, Jefferson Parish PS Sys, **SLP**

Callis, Lisa A 2525 St Christopher #2022, League City, TX 77573, (409) 938-5419, BS 85 Univ of Central AR; MA 87 Univ of Houston - Univ Park; 87–Sp-Lang Path, Mainland Center Hosp, **SLP**

Callner, Lisa Beth 17040 El Camino Real, Suite 102, Houston, TX 77058, (713) 488-7221, MA 76 Univ of CO - Boulder; Sp-Lang Path, Private Practice, **SLP**

Callow, Mrs Mary M 33 Newbridge Circle, Cheshire, CT 06410, (615) 472-6269, BS 69 WV Univ; MS 70 WV Univ; Sp-Lang Path, Cheshire Boe, **SLP**

Calloway, Mrs Kristal Smith 2420 Green Acres Drive, Visalia, CA 93291, (207) 733-5222, BA 79 San Diego St Univ; MA 82 San Diego St Univ; Audiologist, Visalia Medical Center, **A**

Calloway, Mary Lee C 655 Atkinson Road S W, Christiansburg, VA 24073, (703) 731-5204, BS 72 AR St Univ; MA 73 Univ of TN - Knoxville; Asst Prof/Commun Dis, Radford Univ, **SLP**

Calmels, Mrs Anne Trautmann 67 Laurel Hill Road, Brookfield, CT 06804, (203) 775-6343, MS 84 Southern CT St Univ; Sp-Lang Path, Brookfield Boe, **SLP**

Calnan, Jeanne Zellner P O Box 2, East Pembrooke, NY 14056, (716) 762-8481, MS 86 SUNY - Coll at Buffalo; **SLP**

Calogrides, Cynthia 3061 Belmont Street, Mobile, AL 36606, (205) 479-0471, BS 79 Univ of South AL; MS 80 Univ of South AL; Sp-Lang Path, Private Practice, **SLP**

Calvanico, Donna Marie 27 Millridge Road, Secaucus, NJ 07094, (201) 865-8168, BA 84 Kean Coll of NJ; MA 85 Kean Coll of NJ

Calvert, Dr Anne S 4317 Timberglen, Dallas, TX 75287, (214) 352-3923, BS 68 Fort Hays St Univ; MA 71 Univ of KS; PH 76 (NS) Univ of KS; 88–Aud, Miracle-Ear Hearing Aid Ctr, **A**

Calvert, Mrs Brenda Plourde 16 Ranch Drive, Fayetteville, AR 72703, (501) 442-6052, BS 80 Coll of Saint Rose; MS 81 Univ of AR - Fayetteville; SLP, Fayetteville PS, **SLP**

Calvert, Dr Donald Raymond 804 Lake Oak Court, Sacramento, CA 95864, (916) 487-2963, BA 52 Univ of CA - Berkeley; MS 54 Washington Univ; PH 61 (Sp Path and Aud) Stanford Univ; Private Practice, **A F**

Calvert, Elizabeth Mary 8 Canterbury Woods, Glens Falls, NY 12801, (518) 583-2810, BS 71 OH Univ - Athens; MS 76 SUNY - Center at Albany; Sp-Lang Path, Wilton Dev Disabilities Svc, **SLP**

Calvert, Marianne Jordan 10614 Sycamore Court, Louisville, KY 40223, BS 71 LA Tech Univ; MS 81 Univ of Louisville; SLP, Univ Louisville Child Eval Cen, **SLP**

Calvert, Mrs Mary Balfour 118 Wolfe Street, Alexandria, VA 22314, (703) 549-3929, MS 75 Univ of the Pacific; Sp-Lang Path, Private Practice, **SLP**

Calvert-Noble, Mrs Elizabeth Lynn RFD 1 Box 28-A, Pittsford, VT 05763, (802) 775-2395, MA 81 Univ of NE - Lincoln; Sp-Lang Path, Vermont Achievement Center, **SLP**

Calvetti, Gwyneth J 702 East Garland, West Salem, WI 54669, (608) 785-0803, BA 76 Univ of MN - Minneap-St Paul; MS 80 Univ of WI - Stevens Point; Sp-Lang Path, Sch Dist of Lacrosse, **SLP**

Calvillo, M Kimberly Box 324, Niobrara, NE 68760, MA 77 Univ of Northern IA; **SLP**

Calvin, Julie Marie 3801 Lindlavista Way, Des Moines, IA 50310, (515) 278-0195, BA 82 Univ of Northern IA; MA 84 Univ of Northern CO; **SLP**

Calvin, Mrs Sarah Ellis 7413 East Turquoise, Scottsdale, AZ 85258, (602) 952-6110, BS 68 CO St Univ; MA 82 AZ St Univ; Sp-Lang Path, Scottsdale Pub Schs, **SLP**

Calvo, Raymond J 14 Sunset Road West, North Branford, CT 06471, (203) 484-9772, BS 40 Univ of ME - Orono; MS 61 Southern CT St Univ; SLP, Milford Bd of Ed, **SLP**

Camara, Mrs Ann Marie Heffron 2462 F Cochran St McAs, Kailua, HI 96734, (808) 254-2898, BS 81 Appalachian St Univ; MA 82 Appalachian St Univ; SLP, Caldwell Co Sch, **SLP**

Camarata, Mrs Phyllis Ann 11827 Sawmill Stream, Houston, TX 77067, (713) 893-5655, BA 80 Univ of Houston - Univ Park; MA 86 Univ of Houston - Univ Park; 86–Sp-Lang Path, Aldine ISD, **SLP**

Camarata, Dr Stephen M Department Of Speech & Hearing Sciences, University Of California, Santa Barbara, CA 93106, (805) 961-2164, BA 79 San Diego St Univ; MA 81 San Diego St Univ; PH 84 (NS) Purdue Univ - West Lafayette; Assistant Prof, Univ of CA, **SLP**

Camardo, Mrs Joan L 47 Park Circle East, Rochester, NY 14623, (716) 424-4526, BA 43 Univ of IL - Urbana; ME 65 SUNY - Coll at Geneseo; **SLP LM**

Camastro, Mrs Theresa Seeber 40 Elm Street, Glenview, IL 60025, (312) 724-9489, **SLP**

Cambon, Marjorie Burwell Ulm American School, APO New York, NY 09035-0509, (504) 866-4161, BA 76 0500; MA 81 Tulane Univ; **SLP**

Camden, Mrs Rebecca Rankin 9848 Mosswood Road, Richmond, VA 23236, (804) 254-6154, OB 77 Lenoir-Rhyne Coll; BA 77 Queens Coll; ME 81 Univ of VA - Charlottesville; Aud, Shelter Arms Rehab Hosp, **A**

Camenzuli, Dr Lorraine F 4011 Idaho Street #6, San Diego, CA 92104, (619) 295-0571, BA 70 Long Island U - Brooklyn Ctr; MA 77 Univ of CO - Boulder; PH 87 (Cl Psychology) CA Sch of Professional Psychology; Sp-Lang Path, Private Practice, **SLP**

Cameron, Mrs Carol B 7434 South Sherman Drive, Indianapolis, IN 46237, (317) 888-5377, BS 63 Ball St Univ; MA 64 Ball St Univ; Sp-Lang Path, Americana Healthcare, **SLP**

Cameron, Darcey A R 19 Pleasant Bay, Winnipeg, MB, Canada R2K 0C9, (204) 477-4424, OB 80 Univ of Manitoba - Winnipeg; MA 82 Univ of MN - Duluth; Sp-Lang Path, Chld Guid Cl of Gtr Winnipeg, **SLP**

Cameron, Mrs Joy Diane 2517 Cherokee Hills Place, Bartlesville, OK 74006, (918) 335-3674, BS 75 Phillips Univ; MS Univ of OK - Norman; **SLP**

Cameron, Kristine S 1400 Solano N E, Albuquerque, NM 87110, (505) 292-4635, BA 73 Univ of WI - Eau Claire; MS 74 Univ of WI - Eau Claire; Sp-Lang Path, Designs for Lrng Diff Sch, **SLP**

Cameron, Dr Thomas H 116 West Queen Street, Hillsborough, NC 27278, (919) 966-5171, BS 63 NC St Univ at Raleigh; MS 75 Univ of NC - Chapel Hill; PH 85 (Special Ed) Univ of NC - Chapel Hill; 76–Aud, Center for Development and Learning, **A**

Cameron, Yolanda V 8502 South 65th East Place, Tulsa, OK 74133, (918) 495-3735, BA 71 Univ of AR - Fayetteville; MA 72 Univ of Tulsa; Dir Sp & Hrng, Tulsa Rehab Cen, **SLP**

Camfield, Pamela Jean 9025 N W Fir Ridge Place, Corvallis, OR 97330, (503) 757-5984, BA 77 WA St Univ; MA 78 WA St Univ; Sp-Lang Path, Corvallis Sch Dist 509J, **SLP**

Camiener, Mrs Michele Schwartz 4891 Farnhurst Road, Lyndhurst, OH 44124, (216) 524-3000, BS 83 Univ of Cincinnati; MA 86 Cleveland St Univ

Camilleri, Kathryn C 1223 Sarah Drive, Semmes, AL 36575, (205) 649-2828, BS 80 Univ of South AL; MS 85 Univ of South AL; 88–Sp-Lang Path, Mobile County PS, **SLP**

Camins, Mrs Judith P 321 West Allens Lane, Philadelphia, PA 19119, (215) CH8-2108, BA 56 Temple Univ; MA 60 Temple Univ; SLP, Sch Dist of Phila, **SLP**

Cammarata, Mrs Ann M 8033 North Lorel Avenue, Skokie, IL 60077, (312) 676-9380, BS 48 Northwestern Univ; MA 49 Northwestern Univ; SLP, Sch Dist 68, **SLP**

Cammarata, Jerry F 185 Maryland Avenue, Staten Island, NY 10305, **SLP**

Cammisa, Elaine 34 Hawthorne Avenue, Delmar, NY 12054, (518) 489-8336, BS 73 SUNY - Coll at Fredonia; ME 77 Coll of Saint Rose; Chief SLP, C P Cen for the Disabled, **SLP**

Camnitz, Amy S 9021 No Skokie Blvd, Apartment 1-N, Skokie, IL 60077, (312) 676-0846, BA 80 CUNY - Queens Coll; MA 85 Northwestern Univ; **SLP**

Camp, Mrs Cheryl Ann 11017 Sedlak Lane, Indianapolis, IN 46229, (317) 894-8502, BS 84 Ball St Univ; MA 85 Ball St Univ; 85–Sp-Lang Path, Rehab Health Svcs, **SLP**

Camp, Kathy Vaughn 11 Linview Drive, Paragould, AR 72450, (501) 236-6369, OB 75 AR St Univ; OM 79 AR St Univ; SLP, Northeast Arkansas District, **SLP**

Camp, Kelly MacLeod 2301 Rouse Road, Kinston, NC 28501, (919) 559-5371, BA 82 OH St Univ; MA 83 Bowling Green St Univ; 83–Aud, Caswell Center, **A**

Camp, Marcia Winecoff 1 Phillips Trail, Paris Point, Greenville, SC 29609, (803) 233-5243, BS 78 Appalachian St Univ; MA 81 Univ of TN - Knoxville; Aud, Hrng Cen, **A**

Camp, Marita J 8825 Raven Oaks Drive, Omaha, NE 68152-1752, (402) 572-2380, BA 55 Southern AR Univ; MS 70 Univ of NE - Omaha; 83–Sp-Lang Path, Immanuel Med Ctr Rehab, **SLP**

Camp, Mrs Nancy W Route 4 Box 19, Aberdeen, MS 39730, (601) 369-2022, BS 76 MS Univ for Women; MS 77 MS Univ for Women; 77–Sp-Lang Path, Monroe Co Sch Dist, **SLP**

Camp, Mrs Polly N 38 North Main Street, Orono, ME 04473, (207) 941-6260, BA 56 Wellesley Coll; MA 78 Univ of ME - Orono; Sp-Lang Path, Bangor Sch Dept, **SLP**

Camp, Mrs Susan E 124 Montreal Street, Playa Del Rey, CA 90291, (213) 823-6411, BS 77 OH Univ - Athens; MS 81 Bloomsburg Univ of PA; Sp-Lang Path, Private Practice, **SLP**

Campa, Connie L 2407 El Burlon Circle, Rancho Cordova, CA 95670, (916) 362-5529, BA 83 CA St Univ - Sacramento; MS 85 CA St Univ - Sacramento; **A**

Campagna, Barbara A 14 Eldridge Place, Westwood, MA 02090-3708, (617) 326-6871, BS 73 Northeastern Univ; MA 74 MI St Univ; Sp-Lang Path, Trenton School District, **SLP**

Campagna, Laurie S 47 North East Street #2, Carlisle, PA 17013, (717) 243-0777, BS Bloomsburg Univ of PA; MS 85 Bloomsburg Univ of PA; **SLP**

Campain, Robert F P O Box 36, Mad River, CA 95552-0036, (707) 574-6574, BS 63 Northern MI Univ; MA 66 Western MI Univ; PH 70 (Sp Path and Aud) Univ of Denver; Sp-Lang Path, Trinity Cty Dept of Educ, **SLP**

Campanelli, Mrs Angela L 760-A Gordon Drive, Charleston, WV 25303, (301) 528-2419, BS 80 WV Univ; MS 81 WV Univ; Sp-Lang Path, Charleston Area Med Ctr, **SLP**

Campanelli, Dr Peter A 1502 North Ivanhoe Street, Arlington, VA 22205, (202) 343-3498, MA 53 Univ of MD - College Park; OM 77 Univ of Southern CA; ED 67 (NS) Univ of MD - College Park; 74–Procurement Analyst, US Dept of Interior, **SLP A**

Campanile, Mrs Joyce Lynn Rd L Box 334A, Pittstown, NJ 08867, (201) 735-7097, BS 72 Trenton St Coll; MS 73 PA St Univ - Univ Park; Tchr, Robert Hunter School, **A**

Campbell, Alice L 1601 South Lewis Place, Tulsa, OK 74104, (918) 744-1825, BA 44 CO Coll; MA 58 Wichita St Univ; Sp-Lang Path, Alice Lou Campbell, **SLP LM**

Campbell, Ann M 310 North Burghley Avenue, Ventnor, NJ 08406, **SLP**

Campbell, Mrs Bambi Lynn Route 1 Box 190, Chesapeake, OH 45619, (614) 894-7418, **SLP**

Campbell, Bertha M 16434 Haven Park Drive, Houston, TX 77059, MS; **SLP**

Campbell, Carol D 180 Bryant Street, Buffalo, NY 14222, **SLP**

Campbell, Carola R 5528 Big Oak Drive, San Jose, CA 95129, **SLP**

Campbell, Catherine Edwards 920 Beau Drive, Des Plaines, IL 60016, (312) 455-3143, BS 73 Univ of SD - Vermillion; MA 76 Univ of SD - Vermillion; Sp-Lang Path, Leyden Area Spec Ed Coop, **SLP**

Campbell, Cheryl A 192 Pine Valley Plantation, Belchertown, MA 01007, (413) 323-7092, MA 84 Univ of MA - Amherst; Sp-Lang Path, Baroco Corp, **SLP**

Campbell, Mrs Cynthia G Route 8 Box 175, New Braunfels, TX 78130, (512) 245-0234, BS 70 Southwest TX St Univ; ME 71 Southwest TX St Univ; Clinic Director Sp-Lang-Hearng, Southwest Texas State Univ, **SLP**

Campbell, Deborah L Taegu American School, PO Box 2612, APO San Francisco, CA 96218, BA 76 Univ of OK - Norman; MS 78 Univ of OK Medical Center; 84–Sp/Lang Path, Dept of Defense Dependents Schs, **SLP**

Campbell, Diane 22961 Austin Street, Woodland Hills, CA 91364, (818) 997-2357, BA 85 CA St Univ - Fresno; MA 87 CA St Univ - Northridge; 87–Sp-Lang Path, Los Angeles USD, **SLP**

Campbell, Mrs Diane Sciullo 37 Graystone Road, Ambler, PA 19002, (215) 456-7110, BA 82 Temple Univ; MA 84 Temple Univ; 87–Sp-Lang Path, Albert Einstein Med Ctr, **SLP**

Campbell, Doris R 888 Intracoastal Drive, Apartment 5-G, Fort Lauderdale, FL 33304, (305) 566-8361, BS 48 Northwestern Univ; MA 53 Northwestern Univ; SLP, Sch Bd of Broward Co, **SLP**

Campbell, Ellen Jane 5801 Eubank Boulevard N E, Apartment 6, Albuquerque, NM 87111, (505) 884-8282, BA 84 Univ of NM; MS 85 Univ of NM; SLP, Easi, **SLP**

Campbell, Evelyn C 2260 West Rialto Street, Apartment 52, San Bernardino, CA 92410, (818) 761-7319, BA 42 Univ of Southern CA; BS 53 Univ of Southern CA; MS 54 Univ of Southern CA; **SLP**

Campbell, Jane Siever 1200 West Radio Lane, Arkansas City, KS 67005, (316) 441-0630, BA 80 Wichita St Univ; MA 81 Wichita St Univ; 86–Aud, Cowley Co Spec Svcs Coop, **A**

Campbell, Mrs Jeanne P 5 Ruben Duren Way, Bedford, MA 01730, (617) 275-0326, BA 70 Univ of MA - Amherst; ME 75 Northeastern Univ; **SLP**

Campbell, Joan H Box 318, Saxtons River, VT 05154, (802) 869-2797, MS 88 Univ of VT

Campbell, John C USAF Medical Center Elmendorf, Audiology Clinic, Elmendorf AFB, AK 99506, (907) 752-2651, BA 69 Univ of Akron; MA 72 Cleveland St Univ; Chief of Audiology, USAF Medical Center Elmendorf, **A**

Campbell, Mrs Judith R 739 Scottish Mill Run, Marietta, GA 30067-2772, (714) 778-3700, BA 77 CA St Univ - Fullerton; MA 79 CA St Univ - Fullerton; **SLP**

Campbell, Judy Lynn 116 Vets Club Road, Butler, PA 16001, (412) 482-2042, BS 80 Clarion Univ of PA; MS 85 Clarion Univ of PA; **SLP**

Campbell, June Haerle 619 Forest Avenue, Wilmette, IL 60091, (312) 492-5012, BS 66 Univ of WI - Madison; MA 73 Northwestern Univ; Lect-Cl Superv, Nwn U, **SLP**

Campbell, Kathleen C Murphey Department Of Otolaryngology, University Of Iowa Hosp, Iowa City, IA 52242, (319) 356-2222, BA 73 SD St Univ; MA 77 6158; Aud, Dept of Otolaryngology, **A**

Campbell, Kathleen Haunani 1091 Alahaki Street, Kailua, HI 96734, (808) 948-8279, OB 73 Univ of WA; MS 81 Univ of HI - Manoa; Instr, U of HI, **A**

Campbell, Kathryn M 12999 Regent Circle, Carmel, IN 46032, (317) 842-4757, BA 75 IN Univ - Bloomington; MA 76 IN Univ - Bloomington; Aud, Ear Institute of Indiana, **A**

Campbell, Kay 519 Hemphill Drive, San Marcos, CA 92069-1876, (619) 471-1135, BS 72 Northern MI Univ; MA 74 Western MI Univ; Sp/Lang Path, **SLP**

Campbell, Kelli Sue 5020 94th Street S W #25-F, Mukilteo, WA 98275, (206) 353-4899, BA 85 WA St Univ; MA 87 WA St Univ; 87–Sp-Lang Path, Marysville Sch Dist #25, **SLP**

Campbell, Kristen E 56 A Willard Street, Hartford, CT 06105, (203) 522-0184, BS 84 SUNY - Coll at Geneseo; MA 86 Univ of CT; 88–Sp-Lang Path, Hartford Bd of Educ, **SLP**

Campbell, Mrs Lauralee F 1528 Croston, Plano, TX 75075, (214) 422-4117, BA 72 Univ of NM; MA 73 Univ of Denver; Sp-Lang Path, Private Practice, **SLP**

Campbell, Leslie M L 496 Alvarado, San Francisco, CA 94114-1059, (415) 349-9922, BA 75 Univ of CA - Santa Barbara; MA 78 Univ of CO - Boulder; SLP, San Mateo City Schools, **SLP ACE**

Campbell, Mrs Lisa M Box 271, Dighton, KS 67839, (316) 397-5319, BA 71 Wichita St Univ; MA 72 Wichita St Univ; Sp-Lang Path, SW Ks Area Coop Dist 613, **SLP**

Campbell, Mrs Louise M 73 North Street, Mattapoisett, MA 02739, (617) 758-6924, BS 68 Boston Univ; ME 73 Northeastern Univ; Sp-Lang Path, Twn of Marion Sippican Sch, **SLP**

Campbell, Lynda R 1260 Queen Street, Halifax, NS, Canada B3J 2H4, (902) 423-7354, BA 72 Univ of MI - Ann Arbor; MS 73 Univ of MI - Ann Arbor; Superv SLP Div, Nova Scotia Hrng & Sp Cl, **SLP**

Campbell, Dr Lynda R Southern University, P O Box 11565, Baton Rouge, LA 70813, (504) 771-3950, BA 78 Univ of MS; MS 79 Univ of MS; PH 85 (NS) Howard Univ; Asst Prof, Southern University, **SLP**

Campbell, Mrs Marcia 4012 East Whittier, Tucson, AZ 85711, MS; **SLP LM**

Campbell, Mrs Margaret Anne 1012 Hillwood S W, Decatur, AL 36501, (205) 350-6189, **SLP**

Campbell, Mrs Marian Fagin 812 Fair Meadow Drive, Webster City, IA 50595, (515) 832-2077, BS 32 OH St Univ; MS 64 Fort Hays St Univ; **SLP LM**

Campbell, Martha I 148 Clearview Avenue, State College, PA 16803, (814) 234-5223, MS; PH 80 (Commun Dis) PA St Univ - Univ Park; **SLP**

Campbell, Mrs Mary Alesia 2712 Olive, Texarkana, TX 75503, (214) 792-1907, BS 83 Univ of Central AR; MS 85 Univ of North TX; Sp-Lang Path, Liberty-Eylau ISD, **SLP**

Campbell, Dr Mary E 3161 Lewis Avenue, Ida, MI 48140, (313) 269-3875, BS 53 Eastern MI Univ; MA 54 Columbia Univ Teachers Coll; PH 78 (NS) Univ of MI - Ann Arbor; Supverv Hi Prog, Ida Public Sch, **A**

Campbell, Mary G 6416 Windsong, Dallas, TX 75252, **SLP**

Campbell, Mary Lee 309 East Dixon, Charlevoix, MI 49720, (616) 547-2478, BA 69 MI St Univ; MA 70 MI St Univ; **SLP**

Campbell, Mary Lucia 212 West Alice # E, Mount Vernon, MO 65712, (417) 466-3711, OB 78 Central MO St Univ; MS 85 Central MO St Univ; **SLP**

Campbell, Michael Frank 6 Foltz Place, Muskogee, OK 74403, (918) 683-6428, BS 76 Phillips Univ; MS 82 Univ of AR - Fayetteville; Sp-Lang Path, VA Medical Center, **SLP**

Campbell, Nancy Jane 4707 Chestnut Street, Bethesda, MD 20814, (202) 362-5500, BA 85 Augustana Coll; MA 86 Western MI Univ; 86–Prof Assoc, InSpeech Inc, **SLP**

Campbell, Nausha C 3023 Washington Boulevard, Huntington, WV 25705, (606) 325-0465, BA 68 Marshall Univ; MA 71 Marshall Univ; Sp-Lang Path, Wayne Co Boe, **SLP**

Campbell, Mrs Patricia A 632 Bridgewater Circle, Danville, CA 94526, (415) 820-6815, BA 58 Marygove Coll; MA 63 Univ of MI - Ann Arbor; SLP, San Ramon Valley USD, **SLP**

Campbell, Mrs Peggy E 3211 Ridge Green Drive, Kingwood, TX 77345, (305) 255-8319, BA 74 Saint Olaf Coll; MS 75 Rutgers St Univ -N Brunswick; **SLP**

Campbell, Dr Richard A State University Of New York, 109 Park Hall, Buffalo, NY 14260, (716) 834-3400, BA 56; MA 58; PH 62 (Sp-Lang Path & Aud)

Campbell, Robert L 301 Mill Street, Coudersport, PA 16915, (814) 274-7761, BS 78 Edinboro Univ of PA; MA 79 Bowling Green St Univ; Aud, ME Nurbhai MD, **A**

Campbell, Rosolyn C 3730 Brentwood Court, Melbourne, FL 32935-4570, (305) 254-7261, **SLP**

Campbell, Mrs Ruby P 4 Laurelwood Drive, Fairfield, CT 06812, (203) 746-5240, BA 61 TX Southern Univ; MS 78 Governors St Univ; Sp-Lang Path, New Milford PS, **SLP**

Campbell, Mrs Sarabeth Jung 20161 Viking Crest Drive, Apartment 5-202, Poulsbo, WA 98310, (206) 697-3709, BA 83 Univ of WA; MS 85 Univ of WA; **SLP**

Campbell, Mrs Sharon T 120 Clearbrook Road, Matthews, NC 28105, (803) 855-2411, OB 72 Univ of GA; ME 77 Univ of NC - Greensboro; Aud, Charlotte-Mecklenburg Schs, **A**

Campbell, Susan P 200 West South Orange, South Orange, NJ 07079, BA 60 Rutger's St Univ - Douglas Coll; MA 65 Kean Coll of NJ; Super/Cl Servs, Mt Carmel Guild, **SLP**

Campbell, Sylvia L 7714 Rowan Court, Annandale, VA 22003, (703) 642-1867, MS 74 Univ of NC - Chapel Hill; Dir, Private Practice, **SLP**

Campbell, Sylvia Marie 10 Fisk Circle, Annapolis, MD 21401, (301) 396-1207, BS 85 Howard Univ; MA 87 Univ of Pittsburgh - Pittsburgh; 87–Sp-Lang Path, Baltimore City PS, **SLP**

Campbell, Terri Lynn 5637 Hankins Road, Middletown, OH 45044, (513) 539-8880, MA 88 Univ of Cincinnati; 88–Sp-Lang Path, Ft Hamilton Hughes Mem Hosp

Campbell, Dr Thomas Franklin Children's Hospital Of Pittsburgh, 200 Meyran Avenue, Pittsburgh, PA 15213, (412) 647-5571, BA 74 Univ of NE - Lincoln; MA 75 Univ of NE - Lincoln; PH 82 (Communication Disorders) Univ of WI - Madison; Dir-Dept of Comm Disorders, Children's Hosp of Pittsburgh, **SLP**

Campbell, Virginia A 351 Oakview Drive, San Carlos, CA 94070, (415) 591-6490, BA 80 San Francisco St Univ; MS 82 San Francisco St Univ; SLP, San Mateo City Sch Dist, **SLP**

Campbell, Vlacia Z 928 Suellen Drive, Whitford Hill, Reading, PA 19605, (215) 929-0918, BS 76 PA St Univ - Univ Park; MS 78 Bloomsburg Univ of PA; Sp-Lang Path, Berks Co Interm Unit, **SLP**

Campbell, William J 5396 Peach Drive, Gibsonia, PA 15044, (412) 282-1737, BA 73 Univ of Pittsburgh - Pittsburgh; MS 75 Univ of Pittsburgh - Pittsburgh; Aud, Private Practice, **A**

Campbell-Evans, Mrs Carolyn L 984 N E 9th Street, Grants Pass, OR 97526, **SLP**

Camper, Tina Karen 631 West Church Street, Ahoskie, NC 27910, (919) 332-5190, BS 85 East Carolina Univ; MS 86 East Carolina Univ; 87–Sp-Lang Path, Roanoke Chowan Hospital, **SLP**

Campion, Mrs Lori Ann 35332 Malibu, Sterling Heights, MI 48077, (313) 573-5123, **SLP**

Campo, Angene M 800 Martin Berhman, Apartment #102, Metairie, LA 70005, (504) 363-2368, BA 82 Univ of New Orleans; OM 85 LA St Univ - N O Medical Ctr; Sp-Lang Path, F Edward Hebert Hospital, **SLP**

Camponovo, Mrs Trudie G 5407 West Cheryl Drive, Glendale, AZ 85302, (805) 258-6597, BA 75 SUNY - Center at Buffalo; MA 76 George Washington Univ; **SLP**

Campos, Chris Timothy Xomed Ind, 6743 Southpoint Drive N, Jacksonville, FL 32216, (904) 737-7900, BA 75 Univ of Northern CO; MA 76 Univ of Northern CO; Clinical Specialist, Xomed, **A**

Campos, Debra Sue 808 Meadow Place, Roswell, NM 88201-1968, (505) 623-8171, BA 84 Grand Canyon Coll; MS 86 Eastern NM Univ; **SLP**

Campos, Susan A 7 Carnation Place, Lawrenceville, NJ 08648, (609) 882-4820, BS 79 Trenton St Coll; MA 81 Trenton St Coll; **SLP**

Canada, Mrs Conna Route 12 Box 1941, Cullman, AL 35055, (205) 739-5660, BS 72 Purdue Univ - West Lafayette; MS 78 Purdue Univ - West Lafayette; Owner, Private Practice / Miracle Ear Ctr, **A**

Canaday, Mary Jo Department Speech-Language Pathology And Audiology, Andrews University, Berrien Springs, MI 49104, (616) 471-3468, BA 69 Walla Walla Coll; MS 71 Univ of OR; 88–Assoc Prof, Andrews University, **SLP A**

Canadeo, Lisa Cady Vista School, 10010 Duane Court, Caledonia, WI 53108, (414) 835-2811, BS 82 Univ of WI - Madison; MS 84 Univ of WI - Milwaukee; Sp-Lang Path, Racine USD, **SLP**

Canady, Mrs Pamela Cooper 62 Matthews Lane, Washingtonville, NY 10992, (914) 359-3400, BS 78 Ithaca Coll; MS 82 CUNY - Lehman Coll; **SLP**

Canahl, Sue E Basore Audiology, VA Medical Center, 1670 Clairmont Road, Decatur, GA 30033, (404) 321-6111, BS 72 OK St Univ; MS 73 Univ of OK Medical Center; Aud, VA, **A**

Canale-Hess, Jane Ellen 503 Aberdeen Avenue, Hamilton, ON, Canada L8P 2S6, (416) 524-1255, BA 79 Saint Louis Univ; MA 82 Memphis St Univ; 87–Sp-Lang Path, C Hess and Associates, **SLP**

Canales, Mrs Betty H 3030 Merrill Drive #34, Torrance, CA 90503, (213) 320-3419, BS 51 Northwestern Univ; ME 62 Univ of Southern CA; **SLP LM**

Canaley, James R 32 Clinton Avenue, Kearny, NJ 07032, (201) 997-3434, MA 61 Seton Hall Univ; **SLP**

Canar, Nelly Teresa 5305 Tyler Boulevard #7, Temple City, CA 93780, **SLP**

Canavan, Maria Rose 501 North Avenue # B-3, Elizabeth, NJ 07208, (201) 688-0100, BS 83 Purdue Univ - West Lafayette; MS 86 Purdue Univ - West Lafayette; 86–Aud, Hearing Lab Inc, **A**

Cancel, Dr Cruz A Box 40623 Minillas Station, San Juan, PR 00940, (809) 892-4902, MS 51 Univ of MI - Ann Arbor; PH 57 (NS) OH St Univ; Professor, Interamerican University, **SLP A F**

Cancio, Mrs Jane Elizabeth Rt 147 Box 5516, Galway, NY 12074, (518) 882-9223, BS 74 SUNY - Coll at Geneseo; MS 79 Coll of Saint Rose; Sp-Lang Path, Gloversville Sch Dist, **SLP**

Cancro, Mrs Janice Hinsley 6 Avon Court, East Brunswick, NJ 08816, (201) 251-6800, BA 74 Rutger's St Univ - Douglas Coll; MA 78 Montclair St Coll; 77–Sp-Lang Path, Spotswood Bd of Educ

Cancro-Welling, Deborah Regina 90 Midland Avenue #45, Kearny, NJ 07032, (201) 596-3931, BA 80 Hofstra Univ; MA 82 CUNY - Queens Coll; 85–Supervisor of Aud, Mount Carmel Guild, **A**

Candido, Mrs Anna Rodriguez 42-61 79th Street, Elmhurst, NY 11373, (718) 453-4511, BA 81 CUNY - City College; MA 85 CUNY - City College; 87–Sp-Lang Path, NYC Bd Educ Comm on Spec Educ

Candiotte, Elayne 201 North 3rd Street, Bethpage, NY 11714, (516) 938-9341, BA 80 Hofstra Univ; MA 86 Long Island U - CW Post Ctr; **SLP**

Candito, Carol Landers 8 Sheridan Drive, Plymouth, MA 02360, (617) 746-5883, BA 74 Bridgewater St Coll; ME 75 Northeastern Univ; Sp-Lang Path, Plymouth Public Schools, **SLP**

Candor-Kennedy, Peggy A 2658 Oakshire Avenue, Berkley, MI 48072, (313) 542-2252, BA 76 MI St Univ; MA 78 Central MI Univ; 87–Sp-Lang Path, Harper Woods School District, **SLP**

Cane, Paula B 1404 Pass-A-Grille Way, St Petersburg Beach, FL 33706, (813) 263-3890, **SLP**

Canel, Mrs Judith Forman 344 Surfside Place, Glencoe, IL 60022, (312) 835-0422, OB 67 Nat'l Coll of Ed - Evanston; MA 87 Northwestern Univ; 87–Sp-Lang Path, Evanston-Skokie Consolidated Sch Dist 65

Canetta, Dr Robert 1344 West Lunt, Chicago, IL 60626, (312) 848-9750, **SLP**

Canetti, Mrs Marianne 1244 West 15th Street, San Pedro, CA 90731, (213) 514-3057, BS 73 Univ of CA - Los Angeles; MA 77 CA St Univ - Los Angeles; SLP, LA Co Supt of Sch, **SLP**

Canfield, Dana W 512 Cedar Avenue #5, Tillamook, OR 97141, (503) 842-7921, BA 41 CA St Univ - Chico; ME 52 Univ of OR; **SLP LM**

Canfield, Elizabeth Cecilia 2146 East 61st Apartment H, Tulsa, OK 74136, (918) 745-9179, BA 81 6456; MA 82; 87–Sp-Lang Path, Tulsa PS, **SLP**

Canfield, Helen Jean 1463 Chelmsford, St Paul, MN 55108, (612) 646-6436, BA 77 Univ of MN - Minneap-St Paul; MA 79 Univ of MN - Duluth; SLP, Roseville School District 623, **SLP**

Canfield, Karen Lyn West Gibson Street, Canadaigua Elementary, Canandaigua, NY 14424, (716) 394-2626, BS 86 SUNY - Coll at Geneseo; MS 87 SUNY - Coll at Fredonia; **SLP**

Canfield, Dr Kenneth L Wellsville Central School, Wash Intermediate Bldg, Wellsville, NY 14895, (716) 593-1035, BS 58 SUNY - Coll at Fredonia; MS 65 SUNY - Coll at Geneseo; PH 73 (Speech Communication) SUNY - Center at Buffalo; Dir of Pupil Pers Serv, Wellsville Cen Sch, **SLP**

Canfield, Mrs Marilyn A 8706 140th Court Northeast, Redmond, WA 98052, (509) 489-7850, BA 72 San Diego St Univ; MS 77 Eastern WA Univ; SLP, Mead Sch Dist #354, **SLP**

Canfield, Dr Norton P O Box 1383, Miami, FL 33133, (305) 666-1631, BS 25 Dartmouth Coll; MD 29 (NS) Univ of MI - Ann Arbor; Aud Consult, Private Practice, **A F LM**

Canfield, Dr William H 16 East 84th Street, New York, NY 10028, (212) 628-4344, BS 42 Northwestern Univ; MA 50 Columbia Univ Teachers Coll; ED 59 (NS) Columbia Univ Teachers Coll; Prof Emeritus, Adelphi U, **SLP A F LM**

Cangelosi, Natalie Joan 28536 Elmira, Livonia, MI 48150, (313) 849-3701, ME 76 Wayne St Univ; 69–SLP, Detroit Bd of Educ, **SLP**

Caniglia, Christine Ann 23 1/2 South Rodney, Helena, MT 59601, (406) 442-5677, BS 84 Univ of NE - Lincoln; MA 87 Univ of OR; 87–Sp-Lang Path, Mary Anne Molineux Sp & Lang Cl, **SLP**

Caniglia, Dr Joseph A 4256 Douglass, Omaha, NE 68131, BA 61 Univ of NE - Omaha; MS 76 Univ of NE - Omaha; PH 76 (NS) Univ of NE - Lincoln; Sp-Lang Path, Lab of Sp & Lang, **SLP ACE**

Canil, Amy Jean 1015 Old Post Road #2-N, Mamaroneck, NY 10543, (914) 967-6100, BA 81 SUNY - Coll at Cortland; MS 82 Ithaca Coll; Sp-Lang Path, Rye City Sch Dist, **SLP**

Cann, Mrs Anne Garside 181 Mill Lane, Amherst, MA 01002, (413) 549-3975, BA 64 Univ of MA - Amherst; MA 66 Univ of MA - Amherst; Sp-Lang Path, Amherst-Pelham Reg Sch Dist, **SLP**

Cannarella, Mrs Beverly Tedards P O Box 1557, Hartsville, SC 29550, (803) 383-6895, BA 77 Columbia Coll; MS 78 Univ of SC - Columbia; Sp-Lang Path, Private Practice, **SLP**

Cannito, Dr Michael P Univ Of Texas At Austin, Commun Disorders Program, Dept Of Speech Comm, Austin, TX 78712-1089, (214) 783-3049, BA 75 Lamar Univ; MS 81 Lamar Univ; Rsrch Asst, U of TX-Dallas, **SLP**

Cannon, Audrey S 12 Grace Court, Troy, NY 12180, (518) 584-3110, MS 86 Coll of Saint Rose; SLP, Wilton Dev Ctr, **SLP**

Cannon, Carol L 1251 Marks Avenue, Jackson, MS 39213, (601) 355-6000, BS 85 Univ Southern MS-Hattiesburg; MS 87 Univ Southern MS-Hattiesburg

Cannon, Charlotte Perala 3250 Hurst Road, North Pole, AK 99705, (907) 456-2640, BA 80 Univ of WI - Eau Claire; MS 84 Univ of AK - Fairbanks; Sp-Lang Path, Project Teach, **SLP**

Cannon, Mrs Claire Wynn Rd 2 Box 239, Pleasant Valley Road, Titusville, NJ 08560, (609) 393-8228, BA 54 Univ of AL- Tuscaloosa; MA 72 Trenton St Coll; Sp-Lang Path & Aud, Ej Constance, Jr & Assoc, **SLP A ACE**

Cannon, Mrs Janet A 5256 Holladay Boulevard, Salt Lake City, UT 84117, (801) 272-3750, BA 70 Univ of UT; MA 71 Univ of UT; **SLP**

Cannon, Mrs Karen Ann 133 Devonwood Drive, Calhoun, GA 30701, (404) 629-8323, BS 74 Middle TN St Univ; ME 85 West GA Coll; 81–Sp-Lang Path, Calhoun City Schs, **SLP**

Cannon, Linda Ann 873 Knollwood Court, Stillwater, MN 55082, BA 80 Univ of MN - Duluth; MS 81 Saint Cloud St Univ; 88–Sp-Lang Path, No St Paul Schs, **SLP**

Cannon, Linda Carol 1514 Hurley Circle, Macon, GA 31206, (912) 781-5199, **SLP**

Cannon, Mrs Loretta Frances 5812 Mango Drive, St Louis, MO 63129, (314) 937-3633, Sp-Lang Path, Spec Sch Dist, **SLP**

Cannon-Kramer, Mrs Kathleen A 6818 Deer Hollow Place, San Diego, CA 92120, (619) 582-7017, BA 76 Univ of CA - Santa Barbara; MA 79 Univ of FL; Lecturer, San Diego State Univ, **SLP**

Cannupp, Mrs Kathryn E 95 Kings Court, Hickory, NC 28602, (704) 284-2581, BA 80 Univ of NC - Chapel Hill; MS 82 Univ of NC - Chapel Hill; Sp-Lang Path, Catawba Co Schs, **SLP**

Canny, Rickie Ann P O Box 232, Guilford, CT 06437, (203) 453-6246, BA 66 Davis & Elkins Coll; MA 70 OH Univ - Athens; Dir Sp-Lang Path, The Soundings Pre-Sch, **SLP**

Canode, Melanie E 415 Rock Creek Road, Gold Hill, OR 97525, (503) 776-8552, BS 74 Univ of AZ; MS 77 Univ of AZ; SLP, Jackson Co Ed Serv Dist, **SLP**

Canon, Eleanor K 950 South Foster Drive #42, Baton Rouge, LA 70806, (504) 346-8598, OB 77 Univ of MS; OM 78 Univ of MS; Sp-Lang Path, East Baton Rouge Parish Sch Bd, **SLP**

Canright, Lynnette Jo 5600 Sandalwood Blvd, Columbus, OH 43229, (614) 293-8065, BA 84 OH St Univ; MA 86 OH St Univ; 88–Aud, OSU Aud, **A**

Cantele, Mrs Susan Marie 519 Magnolia Drive, Woodstock, GA 30188, (404) 924-0008, **SLP**

Canter, Dr Gerald J Northwestern University, Communication Sciences, 2299 Sheridan Road, Evanston, IL 60201, BA 55 Montclair St Coll; MA 56 Bowling Green St Univ; PH 61 (NS) Northwestern Univ; Prof, Nwn U, **SLP A F**

Canter, Janet C C 19274 Berclair Lane, Tarzana, CA 91356, (213) 343-7167, BA 66 Univ of CA - Berkeley; MA 68 Univ of Southern CA; **SLP**

Canter, Mrs Susan M 3151 Harrison Street, Evanston, IL 60201, (312) 835-2238, BS 66 Northwestern Univ; MA 67 Northwestern Univ; Sp/Lang Path, Nssed, **SLP**

Canterbury, Dr David Richard 5311 Tudortop Circle, Anchorage, AK 99507, (907) 562-2675, BA 65 Univ of Northern CO; MA 66 Univ of Northern CO; ED 73 (NS) Univ of Northern CO; Chief of Commun Dis, Commun Dis Prog St of Ak, **A F**

Cantor, Mrs Gail B 23 Hoover Lane, New City, NY 10956, (914) 354-9070, BS 73 SUNY - Coll at New Paltz; MS 76 Adelphi Univ; Sp-Lang Path, Private Practice, **SLP**

Cantor, Mrs Hedia M D 3130 North 49th Avenue, Hollywood, FL 33021, BA 68 Univ of VT; MS 70 Adelphi Univ; Private Practice, **SLP**

Cantor, Mrs Linda L 4912 Melrow Court, Tampa, FL 33624, (813) 884-2923, BS 65 Kent St Univ; MS 72 FL St Univ; 83–Sp-Lang Path, Hillsborough Co Sch, **SLP ACE**

Cantor, Mark Mitchell 458 Edith Avenue #4, Salt Lake City, UT 84111, (801) 565-7100, BA 77 Humboldt St Univ; MS 86 Univ of ID; **SLP**

Cantor, Paul E Wellesley Theraputic Services, 422 Worcester Street, Suite 303, Wellesley, MA 02181, (617) 237-1769, BA 76 Univ of NM; MS 78 Ithaca Coll; Director, Wellesley Therapeutic Services, **SLP**

Cantor, Susan Helene 61 Bay Street, Bronx, NY 10464, (212) 299-7600, BA 79 CUNY - Lehman Coll; MA 83 CUNY - Lehman Coll; **SLP**

Cantor-Apfel, Debra E 21 Nautilus Avenue, Plainview, NY 11803, (212) 923-6435, BA 81 Montclair St Coll; MS 82 Adelphi Univ; 87–Dir Sp-Lang Path, Floral Park Ctr for Rehab, **SLP**

Cantrell, Connie Stephens 107 Willow Branch Drive, Simpsonville, SC 29681, (803) 963-4040, BA 78 Columbia Coll; MS 80 Univ of SC - Columbia; Sp/Lang Path, Sch Dist of Greenville Co, **SLP**

Cantrell, Dr James C 4960 Candlewyck Lane, Greenville, SC 29615-3618, (803) 242-7713, MA 75 Marshall Univ; MA 77 Marshall Univ; PH 86 (NS) OH Univ - Athens; Sp-Lang Path, Speech Hearing & Learning Cen, **SLP**

Cantrell, Mrs Judy Eileen 6350 Cape Cod Drive, Columbus, GA 31904, (404) 324-5661, **SLP**

Cantrell, Mrs Susan Kay 831 Northh Taft Hill #2, Fort Collins, CO 80521, (303) 482-6455, BS 86 Miami Univ - Oxford; MS 87 Miami Univ - Oxford

Cantrill, Craig E 3735 West Yucca, Phoenix, AZ 85029, (602) 843-6913, BA 73 Wichita St Univ; MA 75 Wichita St Univ; Sp-Lang Path, Boswell Mem Hosp, **SLP ACE**

Cantrill, Mrs Vicki C 3735 West Yucca, Phoenix, AZ 85029, (602) 843-6913, BS 72 Univ of KS; MA 74 Wichita St Univ; 87–Sp-Lang Path, Deer Valley USD, **SLP**

Cantu, Evangeline 4015 Glen Rock, San Antonio, TX 78240, (512) 670-5420, BS 65 Southwest TX St Univ; ME 72 Southwest TX St Univ; Asst Chief Sp Pathology, Wilford Hall Med Cen, **SLP ACE**

Cantwell, Marilyn M 1615 East Sussex Road N E, Atlanta, GA 30306, **SLP**

Canty, Mrs Pamela Sue R R 1 Box 4B O'Fallon Drive, Caseyville, IL 62232, (618) 398-5794, BS 79 Southern IL Univ-Edwardsvill; MS 80 Southern IL Univ-Edwardsvill; Sp/Lang Path, Collinsville Comm Unit #10, **SLP**

Canubida, Mrs Carolyn E 98-947 Kahapili Street, Aiea, HI 96701, (808) 735-2978, BA 64 Univ of HI - Manoa; MA 66 Univ of HI - Manoa; Sp-Lang Path, Famy Hlth Serv Div, **SLP**

Capano, Dr Richard F 1560 University Avenue, San Jose, CA 95126, (408) 924-3665, BA 56 Univ of Miami; MA 57 Univ of MI - Ann Arbor; PH 62 (NS) Univ of MI - Ann Arbor; Prof, San Jose St U, **A F**

Capano, Sharon A 10 Forest Drive, Florham Park, NJ 07932, **SLP**

Capazzi, Amy November 25 Villas Circle, Melville, NY 11747, (516) 348-5037, MA 84 Hofstra Univ; Sp-Lang Path, Central Islip Schools, **SLP**

Capellari, Mrs Reva K 12 Laurel Wood Drive, Worcester, MA 01605, (508) 856-9928, BS 75 Boston Univ; MS 77 Purdue Univ - West Lafayette; **A**

Capelli, Robin Maria 2809 North Delno, Fresno, CA 93705, (209) 225-0148, MA 85 CA St Univ - Fresno; BA 83 CA St Univ - Fresno; Sp-Lang Path, Northwest Sp & Hrng Cen, **SLP**

Capezza, Lenora M B 90 Horizon Drive, Edison, NJ 08817, (201) 985-1102, BA 69 Newark St Coll; MA 76 Kean Coll of NJ; SLP, Pub Sch of Edison Twp, **SLP**

Capezzuto, Vincent A 301 Raymond Street, Pittsburgh, PA 15218, (412) 242-0260, BS 70 Indiana Univ of PA; MA 78 Univ of Pittsburgh - Pittsburgh; Sp-Lang Path, McKeesport Area Sch Dist, **SLP**

Capitena, Mrs Vickie Wallace 1068 W Camino Real, Boca Raton, FL 33486, (407) 393-4684, MA 78 Bowling Green St Univ; 86–Sp-Lang Path, Boca Speech Ctr, **SLP**

Caplan, Bonnie Jean 2705 DE Bouchel Boulevard, Meraux, LA 70075, (504) 682-0223, BS 82 Univ of NV - Reno; MS 85 Univ of NV - Reno; **SLP**

Caplan, Cheryl Lynn 3577 Pleasant Hollow Drive, Apartment 94, Memphis, TN 38115, (901) 362-3483, OB Univ of TN - Knoxville; OM 86 Univ of TN - Knoxville; Aud, Arnolds Hrng Aid Co, **A**

Caplan, Mrs Elizabeth A 15-19 Silvestri Circle, Derry, NH 03038, (603) 893-7059, BS 79 Univ of MA - Amherst; MA 81 Univ of MA - Amherst; Sp-Lang Path, Salem Sch Dist, **SLP**

Caplan, Mrs Elyse Spatz 182 Wildflower Drive, Plymouth Meeting, PA 19462, (215) 834-1536, BA 79 Univ of Miami; MA 80 Montclair St Coll; Sp-Lang Path, Private Practice, **SLP**

Caplan, Frances A 468 Central Avenue, Needham, MA 02194, (617) 924-3434, BA 75 Univ of MA - Amherst; MA 77 Univ of MA - Amherst; Sp-Lang Path, Perkins Sch for Blind, **SLP**

Caplan, Mrs Sharon Freeman 7047 Concord Road, Baltimore, MD 21208, BA 80 Univ of MD - College Park; MS 82 Boston Univ; Sp-Lang Path, Francis Scott Key Med Ctr, **SLP**

Caples-Price, Mrs Sherrie D 1736 North Glen Avenue, Pasadena, CA 91103, (213) 603-4836, BA 80 Univ of Redlands; MA 82 CA St Univ - Los Angeles; Aud, King/Drew Med Ctr, **A**

Capobianco, Maria Carrescia Walter Reed Army Medical Center, Army Audiology And Speech Center, Washington, DC 20307-5001, (202) 576-1649, BA 82 Univ of MD - College Park; MA 85 Univ of MD - College Park; 85–Aud, Army Aud & Sp Ctr, **A**

Capobianco, Mrs Martha L 25 Westcott Street, Inwood, NY 11696, (718) 945-7100, BA 86 SUNY - Center at Buffalo; MA 88 CUNY - Queens Coll; 88–Sp-Lang Path, Peninsula Hosp Ctr

Capocciama, John A 312 Summit Way, Clairton, PA 15025, (412) 394-5700, BS 71 CA Univ of PA; ME 74 CA Univ of PA; SLP, Allegheny Intermediate Unit, **SLP**

Capoferi, Laurie Kyle 14315 Brookings Drive, Sterling Heights, MI 48078, (313) 286-7611, BS 78 Central MI Univ; MA 85 Eastern MI Univ; **SLP**

Capone, Mrs Lorraine Schulz 15 Bailey Street, Foxboro, MA 02035, (508) 543-7052, BS 78 Worcester St Coll; MS 84 Worcester St Coll; Sp-Lang Path, **SLP**

Caponi, Karen 202 Bayberry Hill Lane, Leominster, MA 01453, (617) 792-9293, BS 84 Univ of MA - Amherst; MS 86 Northeastern Univ; Aud, Aud Assocof Worcester, **A**

Capossela, Mrs Cynthia L R R 1 Box 1192, Fairfax, VT 05454, (802) 878-2117, BS 76 Indiana Univ of PA; MA 77 Western MI Univ; Sp-Lang Path, Colchester Public Schools, **SLP**

Capozzelli, Mary G 323 Northern Parkway, Ridgewood, NJ 07450, (201) 447-1883, BS 69 Coll Misericordia; MS 74 Boston Univ; 86–Aud, Workmens Cir Home for the Aged, **A**

Capozzi-Lombard, Mrs Lisa Marie 121 Quarry Village, Cheshire, CT 06410, (203) 271-1109, BS 83 Fairfield Univ; MS 86 Southern CT St Univ; 86–Sp-Lang Path, Milford Bd of Educ, **SLP**

Capozzoli, Annette T 1336 Pesavento Drive, Bridgeville, PA 15017, (412) 429-0700, BA 77 Univ of Pittsburgh - Pittsburgh; MA 80 Univ of Pittsburgh - Pittsburgh; Home Care Sp-Lang Path, South Hills Hlth Syst, **SLP ACE**

Capozzoli, Mrs Kathleen R 2 Woodhaven Wood Court, The Woodlands, TX 77380, BS 76 Northeastern Univ; MA 80 CUNY - Hunter Coll; **SLP**

Cappellano, Joseph G 129-02 Sutter Avenue, South Ozone Park, NY 11420, (718) 380-3000, BA 83 Saint John's Univ - Jamaica; MS 86 Adelphi Univ; **SLP**

Cappello, Mrs Domenica Vitale 6592 Edwards Street, Mentor, OH 44060, (216) 475-8100, MA 84 Cleveland St Univ; BA 82 John Carroll Univ; Sp-Lang Path, Garfield Hgts Bd of Ed, **SLP**

Capps, Mrs Ruby Ann Route 1 Box 38, Graham, NC 27253, (919) 226-3329, BA 75 Appalachian St Univ; MA 76 Appalachian St Univ; Qual Ment Retired Prof, Ralph Scott Gp Homes Inc, **SLP**

Capps, Mrs Sunshine Williamson P O Box 86, Palmer, TX 75152, (214) 544-3212, BS 83 Univ of TX - Dallas; MS 85 Univ of TX - Dallas; 85–Sp-Lang Path, Ferris ISD, **SLP**

Capri, Linda Susan 13 Lane Crest Avenue, New Rochelle, NY 10805, (914) 235-9497, BA 81 Long Island U - CW Post Ctr; MA 86 Long Island U - CW Post Ctr; SLP, BOCES

Caprioli, Corinne Seltzer Rd 4 Box 4850, East Stroudsburg, PA 18301, (201) 989-3122, BS 76 Kutztown Univ of PA; MA 83 Montclair St Coll; 88–Sp-Lang Path, Dover Gen Hosp & Med Ctr, **SLP ACE**

Capuano, Mrs Dale W 5 Olde Woode Road, Salem, NH 03079, (603) 898-5468, MS 84 Univ of NH; Sp-Lang Path, Whittier Vo-Tech High School, **SLP**

Caputa, Antoinette Marie 4330 Colonial Circle A, Bradenton, FL 34208, (904) 575-9346, MA 87 FL St Univ

Caputo, Karen L 4538 McBeth Court, Moorpark, CA 93021-3217, (818) 885-5330, BA 80 Univ of AL- Tuscaloosa; MS 81 Univ of AL- Tuscaloosa; Sp-Lang Path, Northridge Hosp, **SLP**

Caputo, Linda A 105 Yellowstone Avenue #1, Billings, MT 59101-1811, (406) 252-9858, BA 72 Bucknell Univ; MA 77 Univ of CO - Boulder; Sp-Lang Path, Private Practice, **SLP**

Caputo, Susan Marie 17236 South Ridgeland #432, Tinley Park, IL 60477, (312) 862-6484, BS 85 Northern IL Univ - De Kalb; MA 86 Northern IL Univ - De Kalb; **SLP**

Caputo, Valorie K Green Valley Area Educ Agy #14, Green Valley Road, Creston, IA 50801, (515) 782-8443, BS 79 Northern IL Univ - De Kalb; MA 80 Northern IL Univ - De Kalb; Aud, Gr Vlly Ar Ed Agcy 14, **A**

Caputo-Giancola, Mary J 202 Old Forge Road, Jamesburg, NJ 08831, MS; **SLP**

Caputo-Schwarz, Carol A 59 Shadow Lane, Rochester, NY 14606, (716) 482-9614, BS 73 SUNY - Coll at Geneseo; MA 75 SUNY - Coll at Geneseo; Sp-Lang Path, Rochester City Schl Dstr, **SLP**

Carabetta, Mrs Denise Donovan 44 Lepage Drive, Southington, CT 06489, (203) 584-7754, BA 76 Univ of CT; MS 77 PA St Univ - Univ Park; 86–Supvr-Pupil Pers Svcs, Bristol Bd of Ed, **SLP**

Caracciolo, Dr Gerard L 10 Yale Terrace, Montclair, NJ 07042, (201) 893-4226, BA 56 Montclair St Coll; MA 61 Montclair St Coll; ED 76 (NS) Columbia Univ Teachers Coll; 63–Prof Commun Sci & Dis, Montclair State College, **SLP ACE**

Caracciolo, Laurie Ann 37A Sutton Street #6, Brooklyn, NY 11222, (718) 389-6397, MA 87 CUNY - Queens Coll; 88–Aud, Arigo ENT Ctr

Caramagno, Mrs Leslie Marie 28801 Armanda, Warren, MI 48093, (313) 569-1500, BA 80 Wayne St Univ; MA 81 Wayne St Univ; Dir/Sp-Lang Path, Southfield Rehab Hosp, **SLP ACE**

Caranasos, Dr Constance 2606 N W 27th Terrace, Gainesville, FL 32605, (904) 378-2069, BS 55 Univ of WI - Milwaukee; MS 67 Univ of WI - Milwaukee; PH 76 (Sp Path) Univ of FL; **SLP**

Caravella, Mrs Yvonne L 3 Olde Salem Drive, Somers, CT 06071, (203) 763-1749, BA 77 Univ of CT; MS 80 Southern CT St Univ; **SLP**

Caravello, Cecelia LeAnn 532 Parish Point, Mary Esther, FL 32569, (904) 581-2080, BA 72 CA St Univ - Sacramento; MA 73 Univ of the Pacific; Sp-Lang Path, Private Practice, **SLP ACE**

Caraway, Mrs Teresa Heim 401 Outwest Trail, Yukon, OK 73099, (405) 272-5545, **SLP**

Carberry, Patricia C 3 Dellcrest Garth, Lutherville, MD 21093-5730, (301) 435-4775, BA 71 9302; MS 72 Loyola Coll; **SLP**

Carbone, Olga Cordero 65-10 Utopia Parkway, Fresh Meadows, NY 11365, (212) 430-3280, BA 80 Pace U -NY City; MA 82 NY Univ; Sp-Lang Path, Albert Einstein Hospital, **SLP**

Carbone, Mrs Susan P 2337 Rattlesnake Court #B, Grand Junction, CO 81503, BA 74 Augustana Coll; MA 75 Univ of IL - Urbana; Sp/Lang Path, Mesa Co Vall Sch Dist 51, **SLP**

Carcich, Mariann 46 Grantwood Road, Delmar, NY 12054, **SLP**

Card, Deborah L PO Box 702, Santa Teresa, NM 88008, (915) 593-8841, BA 79 Univ of TX - El Paso; MS 86 Univ of TX - El Paso; 79–Sp-Lang Path, Ysleta ISD, **SLP**

Card, Georgia Therese 14686 North Olympic Way, Fountain Hills, AZ 85268, (602) 837-7039, BA 78 Univ of CA - Santa Barbara; MA 80 CA St Univ - Northridge; Sp/Lang Path, Scottsdale Sch, **SLP**

Card, Mrs Helen W 12536 Hatteras Street, North Hollywood, CA 91607, (818) 795-6987, BA 70 Univ of Southern CA; MA 72 Univ of Southern CA; SLP, Pasadena USD, **SLP**

Card, Mrs Yolonda Baker 2302-3A Hickory Creek Circle, Richmond, VA 23229, (804) 346-9751, MS 84 Univ of South FL; Sp-Lang Path, **SLP**

Carden, Denise Gregson 127 La Fontenay Drive, Louisville, KY 40223, (502) 583-8303, MS 82 Miami Univ - Oxford; MS 85 Univ of Louisville; 84–Sp-Lang Path, Univ Sp Path Assoc, **SLP**

Cardenas-Hagan, Elsa 7100 Almeda #1402, Houston, TX 77054, (713) 796-9109, BS 82 Univ of TX - Austin; MA 85 Univ of Houston - Univ Park; 87–Team Supvr-Head Injury Prog, Del Oro Inst for Rehab, **SLP**

Cardenuto, Nancy Jeanne 6401 Julian Street, Springfield, VA 22150, (309) 526-3386, BA 83 SUNY - Coll at Cortland; MA 85 Western IL Univ; Sp-Lang Path, Northern Virginia Training Ctr, **SLP**

Cardillo, Mrs Kathleena 657 Fairview Place, Utica, NY 13502, BS 74 SUNY - Coll at Buffalo; MS 77 Syracuse Univ; Instr, New York St Sch for the Deaf, **SLP**

Cardinale, Carol M 317 Judy Drive, Winchester, VA 22601, (703) 662-1745, BS 85 Univ of VA - Charlottesville; MA 87 Univ of MA - Amherst; Sp-Lang Path, Easter Seal Society of Virginia, **SLP**

Cardwell, Barbara Ann 350 Valley View Drive, Carlyle, IL 62231, (618) 532-1811, BA 80 Coll of Saint Francis; MS 82 Southern IL Univ-Edwardsvill; 86–Sp-Lang Path, W G Murray Developmental Ctr, **SLP**

Cardwell, Cindy L 7200 Pirates Cove Rd #2029, Las Vegas, NV 89128, (702) 363-5981, BS 79 Appalachian St Univ; MA 80 Appalachian St Univ; SLP, Clark Co School District, **SLP**

Cardwell, Elizabeth M 4845 Transit Road #B12, Depew, NY 14043, (716) 282-1836, BA 84 SUNY - Center at Buffalo; MA 86 SUNY - Center at Buffalo; 86–Sp-Lang Path, Niagara Co Sp Hrng and Lang Ctr, **SLP**

Cardwell, Mrs Janet Bush 8871 Applegate Lane, Dunwoody, GA 30350, (404) 355-2146, BS 82 Auburn Univ - Auburn; OM 83 Auburn Univ - Auburn; Sp/Lang Path, Chambers Co Bd of Ed, **SLP**

Carefoot, Mrs Nancy J 137 Riel Avenue, Winnipeg, MB, Canada R2M 2M7, (204) 787-2326, BA 78 WA St Univ; MA 80 WA St Univ; Sp/Lang Path, Health Science Centre, **SLP ACE**

Carey, Ann Grace P O Box 668, Guthrie, OK 73044, (405) 282-5080, BS 71 Eastern MI Univ; MA 72 Eastern MI Univ; 86–Sp-Lang Path, Logan County Guidance Clinic, **SLP**

Carey, Dr Ann Lee 33 Estates View Drive, Fairview Heights, IL 62208, (618) 692-3672, BA 50 Southern IL Univ -Carbondale; MS 59 Southern IL Univ -Carbondale; PH 69 (Sp Path & Aud) Saint Louis Univ; 64–Sp-Lang Path/Aud, So IL Univ at Edwardsville, **SLP A F**

Carey, Mrs Barbara Chicola 584 Polytech Drive, Baton Rouge, LA 70808, BA 68 LA St Univ - Baton Rouge; MA 71 LA St Univ - Baton Rouge; Dir of Sp Serv, Assoc III, **SLP**

Carey, Barbara Jocelyn P O Box 493, Cape Neddick, ME 03902, (207) 363-5842, BS 83 Univ of NH; MS 86 Univ of NH; **SLP**

Carey, Barbara L 2025 South Adams, Denver, CO 80210, (303) 986-4448, BA 72 Univ of Southern CA; MA 73 Univ of Denver; Sp-Lang Path, Jefferson Co Sch, **SLP**

Carey, Mrs Diane Turecamo 1677 Tarleton Way, Crofton, MD 21114, (301) 721-7218, BA 65 Loyola Coll; MA 67 NY Univ; **SLP**

Carey, Linda R 108 Hedgehog Lane, West Simsbury, CT 06092, (203) 658-2251, BA 77 Southern CT St Univ; MA 81 Univ of CT; Sp/Lang Path, Simsbury PS, **SLP**

Carey, Mrs Mary F 811 Prospect Avenue, Winnetka, IL 60093, (312) 441-7449, BA 61 MI St Univ; MA 62 MI St Univ; Sp-Lang Path, **SLP**

Carey, Sarah Jane 1245 North Prairie, Galesburg, IL 61401, (309) 644-1000, BA 80 Univ of IA; BS 81 Univ of IA; MA 82 Western IL Univ; Aud, The Galesburg Cl Assn, **A**

Carey, Sharon L 1540 44th Avenue Court, Greeley, CO 80634, (303) 356-6428, BS 79 Univ of NE - Lincoln; MA 80 Univ of NE - Lincoln; Sp-Lang Path, No CO Med Ctr, **SLP**

Carey, Susan W P O Box 505, Mountain View, HI 96771, (808) 961-3081, BS 73 Univ of HI - Manoa; MS 75 Univ of HI - Manoa; Program Director Sp/Lang Path, Er Sl So-Hilo, **SLP**

Carey, Vanessa Aliesa 25 Lafayette Avenue #6F, Brooklyn, NY 11217, (212) 523-2387, SLP, Bd of Ed, **SLP**

Carfagna, Mrs Freda 2962 Deen Street, Oceanside, NY 11572, (718) 636-4573, BA 76 CUNY - Queens Coll; MA 78 Hofstra Univ; Sp-Lang Path, St Francis De Sales Sch Deaf, **SLP**

Cargill, Sharon A 230 Colewood Way N W, Atlanta, GA 30328, (404) 252-6869, **SLP**

Cargill, Susannah Halpern P O Box 1263, North Conway, NH 03860, (603) 356-2665, BS 82 Univ of MA - Amherst; MA 84 Univ of CT; 87–Sp-Lang Path, Conway Sch Dist, **SLP**

Cargo, Elizabeth A Usafa Hospital, SGHSE, USAF Academy, CO 80840-5308, BS 72 IN Univ - Bloomington; MS 77 Southern Methodist Univ; Asst Chief Aud/Sp Services, USAF, **A**

Carignan, Mrs Karen Linda 5 Hemlock Street, Rochester, NH 03867, (603) 332-1987, BS 75 Univ of NH; MS 82 Univ of NH; 86–Sp-Lang Path, Rochester Sch Dept, **SLP**

Cariker, Mrs Teresa J 7005 Trenton Road, Oklahoma City, OK 73116, (405) 842-3185, BS 78 Univ of North TX; MS 79 Univ of North TX; Sp-Lang Path, Private Practice, **SLP**

Carin, Sandy 12400 Montecito Road #308, Seal Beach, CA 90740-2735, (213) 922-7687, BA 84 Univ of MD - College Park; MS 86 Univ of MI - Ann Arbor; **SLP**

Carini, Mrs Patricia Kane 11286 Edgemoor Court, Woodbridge, VA 22192, (703) 791-3152, BA 71 Mary Washington Coll; ME 72 Univ of VA - Charlottesville; 79–Sp-Lang Path, Prince William Co Pub Sch, **SLP**

Carino, Mrs Mary H 9405 Eagleton Lane, Gaithersburg, MD 20879, (301) 869-7486, BS 69 Ithaca Coll; MS 72 Ithaca Coll; **SLP**

Cariola, John W 1046 Shermer Road, Northbrook, IL 60062, (312) 685-9202, **A**

Cariri, Benjamin A 1 West Hill Road, Stamford, CT 06902, (203) 324-6865, BA 50 Wichita St Univ; MA 55 Wichita St Univ; Sp-Lang Path, Private Practice, **SLP**

Cariri, Mrs Marilyn W 1 West Hill Road, Stamford, CT 06902, (203) 324-6865, BA 47 Wichita St Univ; SLP, Westport Bd of Ed, **SLP**

Cariski, Denise M 473 Sweetbriar Drive, Harrisburg, PA 17111, (717) 561-0651, BS 74 Univ of MD - College Park; MS 76 Univ of WI - Madison; 84–Sp-Lang Path/Aud, Rehab Hosp-Mechanicsburg, **SLP A**

Carl, Maureen Ellen 3455 South West 18th Place, Ocala, FL 32674-2841, (904) 595-3500, BS 81 OK St Univ; MA 83 OK St Univ; Sp-Lang Path, National Spch & Hring Services, **SLP**

Carl, Mrs Rada B 638 Maxine N E, Albuquerque, NM 87123, (505) 881-8313, BA 75 NM St Univ; MA 76 NM St Univ; Sp-Lang Path, Albuquerque Pub Sch, **SLP**

Carl, Mrs Suzanne C 765 Lower Colonial Drive, Mendota Heights, MN 55118, (612) 455-4102, BS 73 CO St Univ; MS 75 CO St Univ; Sp-Lang Path, St Paul PS Sys, **SLP**

Carlaw, Caren Elizabeth 7497 116th Street, North Delta, BC, Canada V4C 5T1, (604) 321-2661, BA 83 Western WA Univ; MA 85 Western WA Univ; **SLP**

Carlberg, Karen S 11620 Audelia Road #125, Dallas, TX 75243, (214) 690-9270, BS 73 Western IL Univ; MA 74 Western IL Univ; Coordinator, Oklahoma State Dept of Educ, **A**

Carlberg, Mike Oscar 14316 Sunswept Park Court, Apartment 206, Florissant, MO 63033, (314) 388-8000, **SLP**

Carlbery, Carol Fitzgerald 14316 Sunswept Park Ct, Apartment 206, St Louis, MO 63033, (314) 351-4658, BS 84 Saint Louis Univ; MA 86 Saint Louis Univ; **SLP**

Carle, Timothy D 2092 Forest Lakes Boulevard, Charleston, SC 29414, (803) 745-7150, BS 72 Syracuse Univ; ME 74 Syracuse Univ; 74–Sp-Lang Path, Charleston County Schools, **SLP**

Carlesimo, Mrs Patricia B 4 Marie Street, Highlands, NJ 07732, (201) 291-5450, BA 75 Skidmore Coll; MA 79 NY Univ; Transdisciplinary Coord, UCP Inc, **SLP**

Carleton, Linda Diane Rural Route 8, 6407-A Mary Ann Circle, Columbia, MO 65202, (314) 443-5913, BS 84 Central MO St Univ; MS 86 Central MO St Univ; **A**

Carlevale, Jean Karen 39 Fairfield Street, Watertown, MA 02172, BS 81 Northeastern Univ; MS 82 Emerson Coll; 82–Sp-Lang Path, Boston PS, **SLP**

Carley, Linda L M 8 Halsey Avenue, Laguna Niguel, CA 92656, BA 70 Univ of CO - Boulder; MA 73 Univ of CO - Boulder; Sp-Lang Path, **SLP**

Carley, Marvin E 85 Williams Road, Cheshire, CT 06410, BS 65 Southwest TX St Univ; ME 68 Southwest TX St Univ; 88–Sp-Lang Path, Meriden PS, **SLP**

Carlile, Mrs Jill Ann 1221 Queen Street, Bellingham, WA 98226, (206) 592-5174, BA 75 Western WA Univ; MA 76 Western WA Univ; 78–Sp-Lang Path, Mt Baker Sch Dist #507, **SLP**

Carlin, Mrs Jerri C 3431 Bonview Drive, Erie, PA 16506, (814) 454-8485, BS 75 Edinboro Univ of PA; MA 77 Edinboro Univ of PA; **SLP**

Carlin, Judith Ann 3861 East Antisdale, South Euclid, OH 44118, (216) 381-7375, BA 74 OH St Univ; MA 76 Case Western Reserve Univ; Aud, Stephen D Schreibman MD Inc, **A**

Carlin, Kathleen C P O Box 112, 33 Meetinghouse Road, Sterling, MA 01564, (617) 264-4700, BS 74 Boston Univ; ME 76 Northeastern Univ; SLP, Acton-Boxborough Reg Sch Dist, **SLP**

Carlin, Dr Margaret F 827 Johnson Avenue, Hattiesburg, MS 39401, (601) 266-5224, BA 61 Cornell Univ; MS 64 Univ of Pittsburgh - Pittsburgh; PH 79 (NS) Wichita St Univ; Associate Professor, Univ of Southern Mississippi, **SLP A ACE**

Carlin, Dr T Walter P O Box 162290, Austin, TX 78716-2290, (512) 473-8751, BS 54 Ithaca Coll; PH 65 (NS) Manchester Bus Sch - England; Pres, Hrng Mgmt, **SLP A**

Carlins, Mrs Nancy Walsh 48 Sceneridge Avenue #2, Pittsburgh, PA 15227, (412) 885-3551, BA 85 Duquesne Univ; MA 87 Univ of Pittsburgh - Pittsburgh; 88–Sp-Lang Path, St Francis Med Ctr, **SLP**

Carlis, Mrs Kimberly 2916 North Marietta Avenue, Milwaukee, WI 53211, (414) 962-4059, BS 81 Purdue Univ - West Lafayette; MS 83 Univ of WI - Milwaukee; Sp-Lang Path, Sacred Heart Rehab, **SLP**

Carlisle, Ellen W 45 Tremont Street, Winchester, MA 01890, (617) 721-2420, BA 78 Univ of ME - Orono; MS 80 Emerson Coll; Aud, Boston University, **SLP A**

Carlisle, Margaret A 6620 Eastridge #221, Dallas, TX 75231, (214) 688-2143, OB 77 Baylor Univ; MS 86 Univ of TX - Dallas; 87–Sp-Lang Path, Univ of Texas at Dallas-Callier Ctr, **SLP**

Carll, Marcia Marie 69 Gibson Street, North East, PA 16428, (814) 453-5602, BS 84 CA Univ of PA; MA 85 Edinboro Univ of PA; **SLP**

Carlock, Jenifer Lee 8210 Walnut Hill Lane, Suite 402, Dallas, TX 75231, (214) 691-7367, BS 82 Baylor Univ; MS 85 Univ of TX - Dallas; Aud, Dallas Hrng & Balance Lab, **A**

Carlow, Mrs Patricia J 87 Risebrough Avenue, Willowdale, ON, Canada M2M 2E2, (416) 626-4360, BA 50 Cornell Univ; MS 51 Univ of Pittsburgh - Pittsburgh; Sp-Lang Path, Etobicoke Bd Ed, **SLP**

Carlsen, Alice F 4317 Jenning Court, Plano, TX 75075, **A**

Carlsen, Mrs Susan G S 1605 Camino Rio, Farmington, NM 87401, (505) 327-0301, MS 67 San Francisco St Univ; Sp-Lang Path, San Juan Home Health Care, **SLP A**

Carlsen, Mrs Vause S 612 Shawnesee, Flushing, MI 48433, (313) 257-9326, BA 54 Marshall Univ; MA 55 OH Univ - Athens; 73–Mgr Sp-Lang Path, Hurley Med Cen, **SLP**

Carlsgaard, Rowena Mazzei 812 West 23rd Street, Merced, CA 95340, (209) 394-8031, BA 75 CA St Univ - Stanislaus; MA 77 CA St Univ - Stanislaus; Sp-Lang Path, Speech Lang & Hrng Ctr, **SLP**

Carlson, Mrs Barbara H 71 Sloping Hills Cove, Grand Forks, ND 58201, (701) 775-6529, BA 71 San Jose St Univ; MA 75 Univ of ND; Sp/Lang Path, Grand Forks Pub Sch, **SLP**

Carlson, Bertha K 3605 North Monitor Circle, Stockton, CA 95205, BA 75 Univ of the Pacific; MA 76 Univ of the Pacific; Sp-Lang Path, Stockton USD, **SLP**

Carlson, Beverly Kay 1456 Edmund Avenue, St Paul, MN 55104, BA 76 Univ of MN - Minneap-St Paul; MA 86 Univ of MN - Minneap-St Paul; **SLP**

Carlson, Carol H 6621 Cornelia Dr, Edina, MN 55424, (612) 922-2565, SLP, **SLP**

Carlson, Charlotte E P O Box 9151, Waltham, MA 02254-9151, (617) 894-4600, BS 67 Boston Univ; MS 72 Emerson Coll; OM 86 Framingham St Coll; Dir of Commun Dis, Middlesex Co Hosp, **SLP ACE**

Carlson, Claudia Ann 1640 Edgewood Drive N W, Cedar Rapids, IA 52405, (319) 399-6853, BA 74 Fort Hays St Univ; MA 75 Fort Hays St Univ; Sp/Lang Path, Grant Wood AEA, **SLP**

Carlson, Connie C 14232 Huntington, Riverview, MI 48192, (313) 282-7879, BS 84 Western MI Univ; MA 86 Western MI Univ; 88–Instr, Western Michigan Univ, **A**

Carlson, Dr Deborah Lynn VA Medical Center, Audiology & Sp Path (126), 1201 N W 16th Street, Miami, FL 33125, (305) 324-3148, BA 80 Augustana Coll; MS 82 Southern IL Univ -Carbondale; PH 86 (Communication Disorders & Sciences (Discipline-Aud)) Southern IL Univ -Carbondale; 87–Aud, VA Med Ctr, **A**

Carlson, Diane B 6 Chesham Way, Fairport, NY 14450, (716) 425-3731, SLP, Pennfield Central Schools, **SLP**

Carlson, Mrs Diane J R R 3 Box 11-L, Cumberland, WI 54829, (715) 822-3628, OB 81 Univ of MN - Duluth; MA 82 Univ of MN - Duluth; **SLP**

Carlson, Dianne Coy 907 Oak Street, Lake Oswego, OR 97034, (503) 229-7239, BA 62 Univ of OR; MS 63 Univ of OR; Sp-Lang Path, Good Samaritan Hosp, **SLP**

Carlson, Donna M 7350 South Wasatch Blvd, Salt Lake City, UT 84121, BA 69 Univ of Northern IA; MA 70 Univ of Northern IA; SLP, St Joseph Hospital, **SLP**

Carlson, Mrs Elaine C 70 Stillman Road, North Stonington, CT 06359, (203) 599-4266, BA 73 Univ of RI; MS 75 Univ of RI; 80–Aud, Woodworth Med Assoc, **A**

Carlson, Elizabeth Ann 689 Trapping Brook Rd #108, Genesee Village, Wellsville, NY 14895, (716) 593-5504, BS 83 SUNY - Coll at Fredonia; MA 84 Kent St Univ; 85–Sp-Lang Path, Wellsville Cen Schs, **SLP**

Carlson, Elizabeth Cranford 1608 Sierra Drive, Baytown, TX 77521, (713) 422-3475, **SLP**

Carlson, Faith 314 Overdale Road, Pittsburgh, PA 15221, BA 64 Wichita St Univ; MA 68 Central MI Univ; 85–Sp/Lang Path, Rehab Inst of Pittsburgh, **SLP**

Carlson, Gerald A St Cloud Hospital, St Cloud, MN 56301, (612) 255-5678, BA 63 Augustana Coll; MA 66 Univ of IA; 69–Sp-Lang Path, St Cloud Hosp, **SLP**

Carlson, Joan M 71 Townsend Drive, Florham Park, NJ 07932, (201) 354-5800, BA 58 Montclair St Coll; MA 79 Kean Coll of NJ; Sp-Lang Path, UCP Cen, **SLP**

Carlson, Judith Hammerlind 6 Edmond Circle, Warwick, RI 02886, (401) 438-9500, MS 81 Univ of RI; 82–Sp-Lang Path, Meeting St Sch/Eas Seal RI, **SLP**

Carlson, Mrs Judith Marie 420 Tulane S E, Albuquerque, NM 87106, (505) 827-6712, **A**

Carlson, Judith Marie 6010 Shaker Woods Circle, Apartment B206, Tamarac, FL 33319, (305) 726-5391, BA 69 Saint Xavier Coll; MS 85 Nova Univ; **SLP**

Carlson, Kathleen Sue P O Box 203, Hotchkiss, CO 81419, BS 82 CO St Univ; MS 84 CO St Univ; Sp-Lang Path, Delta Co Sch Dist 50-J, **SLP**

Carlson, Laurette L P O Box 386, Orono, ME 04473, (207) 827-8567, ME 76 Northeastern Univ; Sp-Lang Path, Devel Services Stafford County, **SLP**

Carlson, Linda K 2616 Belfast S E, Grand Rapids, MI 49507, (616) 364-6756, BA 77 Western MI Univ; MA 82 Western MI Univ; Sp-Lang Path, Grand Rapids Public Schools, **SLP**

Carlson, Mrs Margo Elaine 1203 Tilden Street, Holdrege, NE 68949, (308) 995-6814, BA 64 Univ of Northern CO; MS 85 Kearney St Coll; 86–Sp-Lang Path, Good Samaritan Hosp, **SLP**

Carlson, Mrs Mary Ginder 117 Bridle Path, North Andover, MA 01845, (508) 685-8499, BA 69 Rutger's St Univ - Douglas Coll; ME 70 PA St Univ - Univ Park; Sp-Lang Path, **SLP**

Carlson, Norrene L 330 Maryland N E, Grand Rapids, MI 49503, **SLP**

Carlson, Rebekah L 18807 Tournament Trail, Tampa, FL 33647, (813) 974-2006, BS 60 IL St Univ - Normal; MS 70 Univ of South FL; Clinical Supvr, U of S FL, Dpt of Commun, **SLP ACE**

Carlson, Mrs Susan Ellen 20311 N Larkmoor, Southfield, MI 48076, (313) 356-3449, BS 79 OH Univ - Athens; MA 84 Eastern MI Univ; **SLP**

Carlson, Susan Mae 19 West Center Street, Florence, MA 01060, (413) 584-6540, BA 79 CT Coll; MS 81 Boston Univ; Sp-Lang Path, **SLP**

Carlson, Mrs Teresa H HHC Ist Armor Division, APO New York, NY 09326, (502) 624-6750, BS 86 Western KY Univ; MS 87 Western KY Univ; **SLP**

Carlson, Terry E 12021 South Wilmington Avenue, Los Angeles, CA 90059, (213) 603-4836, MS 76 Univ of VA - Charlottesville; 86–Sp-Lang Path, King/Drew Med Ctr, **SLP**

Carlson, Mrs Vicki Lynn Rd 2 Box 335-A, Sinclairville, NY 14782-9611, (716) 532-5522, BS 83 Nazareth Coll of Rochester; MS 85 SUNY - Coll at Fredonia; SLP, Jn Adam Developmental Ctr, **SLP**

Carlson, Wendy Allen 1327 Superior Street, Sandpoint, ID 83864, (208) 263-1843, BA 72 Univ of WA; MS 75 Univ of NM; **SLP**

Carlson-Geer, Mrs Susan L 8406 Hardwick Ct, Upper Marlboro, MD 20772, **A**

Carlstrom, Jane E 116 Shevlin Hall, University Of Minnesota, Minneapolis, MN 55455, (612) 624-3322, BA 71 Bennington Coll; MA 76 Univ of IA; Cl Superv, U of MN, **A**

Carlton, Janet C Route 10 Box 519-A, Winston-Salem, NC 27127, (919) 760-5770, BA 76 Univ of NC - Charlotte; ME 80 Univ of NC - Greensboro; 86–Sp-Lang Path, Carolina Medicorp ENT, **SLP**

Carlyle, Irene Varcados Whittier College, PO Box 634, Whittier, CA 90608, (213) 693-0771, MA 84 Whittier Coll; Instructor/ Clinical Suprv, Whittier College, **SLP**

Carmack, Mrs Brooke Alene 581 Harvard Avenue, Santa Clara, CA 95051, (408) 246-5498, BS 83 Brigham Young Univ; OM 84 Brigham Young Univ; 88–Aud, Ear Med Clinic, **A**

Carmack, Dr Fairy 415 Lakeshore, Monroe, LA 71201, (318) 343-2340, BA 65 LA Tech Univ; MA 69 LA Tech Univ; ED 76 (NS) Northeast LA Univ; Coord/Sp & Hrng Servs, Private Practice, **SLP**

Carman, Carol K 118 Windsor Avenue, Kensington, CA 94708, (415) 476-5101, BS 56 Saint Louis Univ; MS 59 Univ of Pittsburgh - Pittsburgh; 70–Aud, Aud & Sp Clinic Univ of Cal, **A**

Carmel, Mrs Barbara R 79 Orchard Road, Dalton, MA 01226, (413) 655-8035, BS 58 Emerson Coll; Sp-Lang Path, Ctrl Berkshire Reg Sch Dist, **SLP**

Carmel, Norman Hirsch 1961 Floyd Street, Suite A, Sarasota, FL 34239, (813) 366-9222, BA 59 OH St Univ; MA 62 OH St Univ; 74–Aud, Hearing & Balalce Clinic, **SLP A ACE**

Carmel, Norman R Burlingame Hill Road, Adams, MA 01220, (413) 743-1201, BS 59 Emerson Coll; MA 64 Univ of MA - Amherst; Dir Spec Ed, Ctrl Berkshire Sch Dist, **SLP**

Carmeli, Sara 84-10 120st, Queens, NY 11415, (718) 805-0136, MA 86 Temple Univ-Tyler Sch of Art; **SLP**

Carmen, Mrs Elizabeth M 73 Concord Road, Lebanon, NJ 08833, (201) 236-9143, BA 72 Rutger's St Univ - Douglas Coll; MA 73 NY Univ; Sp-Lang Path, Private Practice, **SLP**

Carmen, Richard E P O Box 2828, Los Angeles, CA 90078, (818) 990-5320, BA 68 SUNY - Center at Buffalo; MA 73 CA St Univ - Los Angeles; Aud, Private Practice, **A**

Carmichael, Carol L 909 30th Street South Apartment 13, Birmingham, AL 35205, (205) 251-7169, OB 78 Auburn Univ - Auburn; OM 79 Auburn Univ - Auburn; Dir of Aud, Pappas Ear Clinic PC, **A**

Carmichael, Dorothy Harry 11319 Williamsburg Drive, Houston, TX 77024, (713) 785-8260, BS 70 Univ of GA; ME 74 Univ of GA; Sp-Lang Path, Spring Branch Indepen Sch Dist, **SLP**

Carmichael, Mrs Jennifer J R R 1 Box 631, Selma, IN 47383, BS Ball St Univ; MA Ball St Univ; **SLP**

Carmichael, Joyce K 2351 North Forest Drive, Marietta, GA 30062, (404) 998-8125, **SLP**

Carmichael, Linda Ann 889 Bond Street, Sarnia, ON, Canada N7S 3C4, (519) 337-8415, BS 74 Wayne St Univ; MA 78 Wayne St Univ; Sp-Lang Path, Lambton County Board of Educ, **SLP**

Carmichael, Mrs Virginia 3841 Cherry Hill Lane, Memphis, TN 38134-1435, (901) 794-6151, BS 68 Univ of NE - Lincoln; MS 75 Univ Southern MS-Hattiesburg; SLP, Memphis City Schools, **SLP**

Carmichael, Mrs Wendy A 2103 Ridge Avenue, Evanston, IL 60201, (312) 432-4260, BS 73 Bowling Green St Univ; MS 78 Miami Univ - Oxford; Sp-Lang Path, Highland Park Sch Dist #108, **SLP**

Carmon, Mrs Sharon Marie Bolling Air Force Base, 324 Vandenberg Street, Washington, DC 20336-3660, (202) 562-2251, BS Univ of AZ; MA George Washington Univ; Sp-Lang Path, Private Practice, **SLP**

Carmouche, Margaret A 927 Ontario Street, Shreveport, LA 71106, **SLP**

Carnahan, Cheryl F 6228 Dawn Day Drive, Columbia, MD 21045, (301) 997-2542, BS 73 Towson St Univ; MS 75 Towson St Univ; SLP, Howard Co Bd of Ed, **SLP**

Carne, Maureen E P O Box 434, 4 Merrill Street, West Newbury, MA 01985, (508) 363-2279, BS 70 Emerson Coll; ME 71 Northeastern Univ; Sp-Lang Path, Newburyport PS, **SLP**

Carnell, Dr Claude M, Jr 2444 Birkenhead Drive, Charleston, SC 29407, (803) 577-5410, BA 56 Furman Univ; MA 58 Univ of AL- Tuscaloosa; PH 72 (Sp Path) LA St Univ - Baton Rouge; 64–Executive Director, Charleston Speech/Hearing Ctr, **SLP F**

Carneol, Susan Oliff 11343 North Linnwood Lane, Mequon, WI 53092, (414) 931-4065, BS 75 IL St Univ - Normal; MS 77 IL St Univ - Normal; Sp-Lang Path, Childrens Hosp of Wisconsin, **SLP ACE**

Carner, Mrs Linda D 315 West Allens Lane, Philadelphia, PA 19119, (215) 242-1696, BA 64 Univ of PA; MA 67 Temple Univ; 85–Dir Sp-Lang Path, Multicon Rehab Sgency Inc, **SLP**

Carner, Mrs Teresa Jo 3020 South 104th, Fort Smith, AR 72903-5355, (501) 758-2501, BS 81 Southwest MO St Univ; MS 84 Univ of AR - Little Rock; Sp-Lang Path, Ft Smith PS, **SLP**

Carnes, Patricia B 549 Cypress Trace Drive, Fayetteville, NC 28304, (919) 485-5145, BS 81 Univ of Cincinnati; MA 83 Univ of Cincinnati; Sp-Path, Sen Sp/Hrng Serv of Nc Inc, **SLP**

Carnes, Robert C 30 Onderdonk Place, Pleasantville, NY 10570, (914) 769-8259, BA 73 CUNY - City College; MA 74 NY Univ; Sp/Lang Path, Waterview Hills Nursing Cen, **SLP**

Carnesi, Karyn Ann 133 Autumn Drive, Hauppauge, NY 11788, (516) 783-7523, BS 86 SUNY - Coll at Geneseo; MS 88 Adelphi Univ

Carnevale, Susan C 80 Alder Brook Drive, Cranston, RI 02920, (401) 737-7000, BA 77 Univ of RI; MA 79 NY Univ; Sp-Lang Path, Kent Cty Mem Hosp, **SLP**

Carney, Dr Arlene E Boys Town National Institute, 555 North 30th Street, Omaha, NE 68131, (402) 498-6692, BS 69 Saint John's Univ - Jamaica; MA 73 Univ of MA - Amherst; PH 77 (NS) Univ of MN - Minneap-St Paul; 88–Dir-Ctr for Childhood Deafness, Boys Town National Institute, **A**

Carney, Mrs Jeanne Arnell 6230 Hunter Road, Corcoran, MN 55340-9637, (612) 478-9438, MS 83 Saint Cloud St Univ; 86–Sp-Lang Path, Anoka-Hennepin Sch Dist #11, **SLP**

Carney, Kathleen M 82 Chamberlin Drive, Buffalo, NY 14210, (716) 887-4635, BS 79 SUNY - Coll at Fredonia; MS 80 FL St Univ; Sp-Lang Path, Millard Filmore Hosp, **SLP**

Carney, Kathleen Mary University Of Rochester Medical Center, Department Of Speech Pathology & Audiology, 601 Elmwood Avenue, Rochester, NY 14642, (716) 275-2501, BS 82 SUNY - Coll at Geneseo; MA 83 SUNY - Coll at Geneseo; Aud, Univ of Rochester Medical Ctr, **A**

Carney, Marilyn Jean 1722 North 47th #C, Seattle, WA 98103, (206) 547-4802, BS 83 Univ of WA; MS 86 Univ of WA; 87–Sp-Lang Path, Univ Hosp, **SLP**

Carney, Mary S 423 South Scoville #3N, Oak Park, IL 60302, (312) 383-1203, BS 78 Marquette Univ; MS 79 Marquette Univ; Sp-Lang Path, Willett Easter Seal Society, **SLP**

Carney, Patricia Ann 7670 West 131st Street, Palos Heights, IL 60463, (312) 597-3155, BS 83 Northern IL Univ - De Kalb; OM 86 Governors St Univ; Sp-Lang Path, Kirby Sch Dist 140, **SLP**

Carney, Dr Patrick J Dept Audiology & Speech Path, University Of Tennessee, Knoxville, TN 37996, (615) 974-5019, BA 58 Wichita St Univ; MA 65 Wichita St Univ; PH 69 (Sp-Lang Path) Univ of IA; Prof, U of TN- Knoxville, **SLP F ACE**

Carney, R John 1724 Holly Hill Drive, West Columbia, SC 29169, (803) 796-3648, BS 53 Univ of Houston - Univ Park; ME 54 Univ of Houston - Univ Park; Consult, Private Practice, **SLP LM**

Carney, Mrs Sharon Sonnek 12900 Twinbrook Parkway, Rockville, MD 20851, (301) 468-1421

Carney-Jankoviak, Cathy Marie 925 Canterbury, Madison Heights, MI 48071, BA 84 Wayne St Univ; MA 86 Wayne St Univ; 88–Sp-Lang Path, Media-Speech Service Inc, **SLP**

Carnicom, Mrs Ruth C 10706 Villa Lea Lane, Houston, TX 77071, (713) 783-6220, BA 52 OH Wesleyan Univ; MA 71 Univ of Tulsa; 80–SLP, Houston ISD, **SLP**

Carns, Carol Louise 11270 Deborah Drive, Parma, OH 44130, (216) 886-4849, BS 85 Bowling Green St Univ; MA 87 Cleveland St Univ; **SLP**

Carolan, Mrs Louise W 129 McFadden, Brownsville, TX 78520, (512) 423-5077, BS 65 Boston Univ; BS 64 Boston Univ; MD (NS); Dir of SLP, Rio Grande St Cen Mhmr, **SLP**

Caron, Alfred L R265 Herrick Road, Blandford, MA 01008, (617) 939-2161, BA 64 Univ of MA - Amherst; MA 66 Univ of MA - Amherst; Superv Sp & Hrng, Fernald St Sch, **SLP ACE**

Caron, Mrs Debra Lynne 340 Cole Street, Seekonk, MA 02771, (617) 695-7525, BA 76 Coll of the Holy Cross; MS 84 Univ of RI; 86–Sp-Lang Path, North Attleboro Sch Dept, **SLP**

Caron, Mrs Susan Pagluica P O Box 336, Wells, ME 04090, (207) 324-1550, BA 81 Univ of CT; MS 83 PA St Univ - Univ Park; Sp-Lang Path, York Co Counseling Serv, **SLP ACE**

Carothers, Patrice Orosz Cleveland Hearing & Speech Ctr, 11206 Euclid Avenue, Cleveland, OH 44106, (216) 231-8787, BS 74 Ithaca Coll; MS 78 Ithaca Coll; Coord Sp Prod Dis, Hrng/Sp Cen, **SLP**

Carotta, Mrs Catherine Cronin 15711 Western Avenue, Omaha, NE 68118, (402) 493-8355, SLP, Boys Town Natl Institute, **SLP**

Carozza, Linda S 255 West 84th Street, New York, NY 10024, (212) 220-3158, BA 71 CUNY - City College; MA 72 CUNY - City College; Dir-Fordham Dev Dis Cl, Flower Hosp, **SLP**

Carp, Mrs Jane R 984 Singleton Avenue, Woodmere, NY 11598, (516) 569-6392, BA 71 CUNY - Queens Coll; MA 73 CUNY - Queens Coll; **SLP**

Carpender-Robin, Debra K 2052 Southridge Drive, Coralville, IA 52241, (319) 354-7648, BA 76 San Diego St Univ; MS 81 Univ of Redlands; Sp-Lang Path, Grantwood AEA, **SLP**

Carpenter, Mrs Barbara Kay 1400 51st Avenue S W, Minot, ND 58701, (701) 857-4595, OB 80 Minot St Univ; MS 82 Minot St Univ; Sp-Lang Path, Minot Public Schools, **SLP**

Carpenter, Mrs Barbara L 230 South Krameria, Denver, CO 80224, (303) 388-8960, BS 64 Emerson Coll; MA 67 Univ of Denver; **SLP**

Carpenter, Dorothy Jan 871 Captain Shore Drive, Shreveport, LA 71105, (318) 478-0185, **SLP**

Carpenter, Eileen M P O Box 284, Silverton, ID 83867, (208) 556-1531, BA 73 WA St Univ; MA 74 WA St Univ; **SLP**

Carpenter, Gaye H 5319 Rimwood Drive, San Jose, CA 95118, (408) 395-6610, BA 71 San Jose St Univ; SLP, Los Gatos Elem Sch Dist, **SLP**

Carpenter, Dr Jane M 2759 Lancaster Circle, Boise, ID 83702, (208) 344-3123, BS 70 ID St Univ; MS 72 ID St Univ; PH 79 (Lang Development) Univ of UT; Sp/Lang Path, Intermountain Institute, **SLP**

Carpenter, Mrs Janice Grissom 2315 South 7th Street, Terre Haute, IN 47802, (812) 234-0185, BA 81 IN St Univ - Terre Haute; MS 87 Univ of TN - Knoxville

Carpenter, Mrs Janice Lynn 2077 Chalet Drive, Rochester, MI 48309, (313) 375-2064, BS 81 Central MI Univ; MA 82 Central MI Univ; Sp-Lang Path, Rochester Community Schools, **SLP**

Carpenter, Mrs Jessie Lou 103 Reynolds Road, Boone, NC 28607, (704) 264-3014, BA 47 Depauw Univ; MS 49 Purdue Univ - West Lafayette; Retired, **SLP**

Carpenter, Mrs Judy D P O Box 721, Cedar Crest, NM 87008-0721, (505) 281-1667, BS 76 Univ of NM; MA 78 Univ of NM; Sp/Lang Path, Albuquerque Pub Schs, **SLP**

Carpenter, Kyle M PO Box 310, 33 Mitchell Avenue, Binghamton, NY 13902, (607) 754-7148, BS 79 SUNY - Coll at Geneseo; MA 81 Western MI Univ; Aud, Rehab Serv Inc, **A**

Carpenter, Laurence John 1412 3rd Avenue, Sterling, IL 61081, (815) 625-1308, BA 81 Chadron St Coll; MS 84 Univ of WI - Oshkosh; Audiologist, Comm General Hosp, **A**

Carpenter, Dr Linda J 409 Summit Avenue, Eau Claire, WI 54701, BA 69 George Washington Univ; MS 70 Univ of MI - Ann Arbor; PH 86 (Special Education) Univ of CA - Los Angeles; 88–Asst Prof, Univ of Wisconsin-Eau Claire, **SLP**

Carpenter, Mrs Margaret J 1135 N East Avenue, Oak Park, IL 60302, (312) 848-4969, BS 73 Marquette Univ; MA 78 Governors St Univ; **SLP**

Carpenter, Mrs Marilyn S Route 6 Box 535-A, Staunton, VA 24401, (703) 885-8430, BS 73 James Madison Univ; MS 84 James Madison Univ; Sp-Lang Path, Western Hospital, **SLP ACE**

Carpenter, Mary 25955 Akins Road, Columbia Station, OH 44028, (216) 282-9171, BS Kent St Univ; MA 85 Kent St Univ; **SLP**

Carpenter, Mary Ann Hearing And Speech Department, Univ Of Kansas Medical Ctr, 39th & Rainbow Boulevard, Kansas City, KS 66103, (913) 588-5937, BA 63 Saint Mary's Coll; MA 66 Univ of IA; PH 69 (Sp Path) Univ of IA; Assoc Prof/Cl Coord Sp, U of KS, **SLP**

Carpenter, Michele D The Hear Center, 1971 Port St Lucie Blvd, Port St Lucie, FL 34952, (407) 335-3455, MA 73 Univ of FL; Aud/Owner, The Hear Center, **A**

Carpenter, Nancy M 48 Winthrop New Road, Aurora, IL 60504, (312) 466-7902, OB 69 OH Univ - Athens; MS 74 Cleveland St Univ; **SLP**

Carpenter, Neil E 750 Ransom Road, Valparaiso, IN 46383, (219) 464-9607, BS 54 Ball St Univ; MA 55 Ball St Univ; Superv/Commun Hndcp, Porter Co Spec Ed Coop, **SLP**

Carpenter, Mrs Patricia B 3903 Beacon Trace, Marietta, GA 30062, (404) 565-2324, BA 76 Univ of Pittsburgh - Pittsburgh; MA 77 Univ of Pittsburgh - Pittsburgh; SLP, **SLP**

Carpenter, Paul E 428 Villa Road, Newberg, OR 97132, (503) 538-3197, MS Portland St Univ; ME Univ of OR; BS Portland St Univ; Sp-Lang Path, Private Practice, **SLP**

Carpenter, Regina M 1229 North Inlynnview Road, Virginia Beach, VA 23454, (804) 441-2743, BA 72 CUNY - Queens Coll; MA 74 Cleveland St Univ; 86–Supvr-Sp & Sensory Pgms, Norfolk Pub Sch, **SLP**

Carpenter, Dr Robert L 10026 46th Place N E, Seattle, WA 98125, (206) 545-2188, BA 64 Augustana Coll; MA 65 Northwestern Univ; PH 68 (NS) Northwestern Univ; Assoc Prof, U of WA/Dept Sp & Hrng Sci, **SLP**

Carpenter, Stephen J 2368 Aldine NE, Keizer, OR 97303, (503) 390-5422, BS 86 Univ of OR; MS 87 Western OR St Coll; 88, Salem Sp & Lang Ctr

Carpenter, Susan Annette 607 Hess Road, Concord, NC 28025, (704) 376-1342, BS 85 Univ of NC - Greensboro; MA 86 Univ of NC - Greensboro; SLP, Charlotte Sp & Hrng Ctr, **SLP**

Carpenter, Mrs Susan Carroll 504 East 24th Street, Cheyenne, WY 82001, (307) 634-5545, BS 80 Univ of WY; MS 82 Univ of WY; 82–Sp-Lang Path Prog Dir, Stride Lrng Cen, **SLP**

Carpenter, Susan K Mary Bridge Speech And Hearing Center, 1220 Division, Tacoma, WA 98403, (206) 572-5252, BS 64 Syracuse Univ; MS 65 Univ of WI - Madison; Mgr Sp & Hrng Serv, Multicare Med Cen, **SLP A**

Carpenter, Susan S 1120 Fenley Avenue, Louisville, KY 40222, (502) 426-1656, BA 74 Univ of MS; MA 77 Memphis St Univ; Sp-Lang Path, Private Practice, **SLP**

Carper, Kelly Anne 7580 Sunny Ridge Coop, East Highland, CA 92346, (818) 349-2440, MA 88 CA St Univ - Northridge

Carpi, Mary Wibbert 1913 South 16th Street, Las Vegas, NV 89104, (702) 732-7700, BA 75 Chapman Coll; MA 76 CA St Univ - Fullerton; 80–Aud, Spec Chlrn Cl, **A**

Carr, Ann B 1781 Sanchez, San Francisco, CA 94131, (916) 921-0531, BA 75 John Carroll Univ; MS 77 Vanderbilt Univ; 88–Coord, Pers Dev for Infant/Preschool, **SLP**

Carr, Mrs Camille Slavin 1772 Campbell Avenue, Thousand Oaks, CA 91360, (805) 495-2842, BA 75 Univ of Redlands; MA 83 CA St Univ - Northridge; 85–Sp-Lang Path, Private Practice, **SLP**

Carr, Charlene A P O Box 247, 164 Woodward Avenue, Springville, NY 14141, (716) 827-9737, BS 85 SUNY - Coll at Buffalo; MS 86 SUNY - Coll at Buffalo; 86–Sp-Lang Path, Baker Hall, **SLP**

Carr, Christopher George 13833 East 28th Street, Tulsa, OK 74134, (918) 744-6591, BA 74 OK St Univ; MA 78 OK St Univ; 87–Sp-Lang Path, Private Practice, **SLP**

Carr, Cynthia D 4601 North 102nd Avenue, Unit 1189, Phoenix, AZ 85039, (602) 967-8036, BS 82 AZ St Univ; OM 86 AZ St Univ; **SLP**

Carr, Mrs Ellen S 2761 Mandalay Beach Road, Wantagh, NY 11793, BA 72 Pace U -NY City; MS 76 CUNY - Brooklyn Coll; SLP, Bd of Ed NYC Bur for Sp Imp, **SLP**

Carr, Mrs Faith Casey 14 Tall Meadow, Painted Post, NY 14870, (607) 962-7529, BS 80 SUNY - Coll at Geneseo; MS 82 Syracuse Univ; Sp-Lang Path, Monroe Co Assoc for Ret Citiz, **SLP**

Carr, Mrs Georgette Lincoln Intermediate Unit, Box 70, New Oxford, PA 17350, (717) 624-4616, BA 74 Loyola Coll; MS 79 Loyola Coll; 87–SLP, Lincoln Inter Ut, **SLP**

Carr, Jacquelyn Carney 2727 Snow Lane, Redding, CA 96003, (916) 244-9280, BA 79 Humboldt St Univ; MA 81 Humboldt St Univ; Sp-Lang Path, Redding Sch Dist, **SLP**

Carr, Mrs Lisa A 1615 Woodbrook Drive #105, East Lansing, MI 48823-7601, (517) 337-7258, **SLP**

Carr, Mrs Margaret Diane 1821 Webster Avenue, Topeka, KS 66604, (913) 272-3111, BA 70 Univ of MO - Columbia; MA 71 Univ of MO - Columbia; Sp-Lang Path, Colmery-O'Neil V Hosp, **SLP**

Carr, Mary E 7819 Marion Lane, Bethesda, MD 20814, (301) 654-5195, BS 73 Marquette Univ; MA 74 Central MI Univ; 88–Dir, Mary E Carr & Associates PA, **SLP**

Carr, Nancy Goodman 3952 Merganser Drive, Liverpool, NY 13090, (315) 652-7472, BS 85 SUNY - Coll at Fredonia; MS 86 SUNY - Coll at Fredonia; **SLP**

Carr, Mrs Patricia Etten W-295 F-10937 Honeywell Dr, Mukwonago, WI 53149, BS 74 Univ of WI - Madison; MS 75 Univ of WI - Eau Claire; Sp-Lang Path, West Allis Pub Sch, **SLP**

Carr, Mrs Patricia Irene 4013 Forecast Drive, Brandon, FL 33511, (813) 684-7458, BA 77 Univ of CT; ME 79 Northeastern Univ; **A**

Carr, Peggy 1307 Greene Acres Ct O V, Cheyenne, WY 82001, **SLP**

Carr, Mrs Rebecca Ritchie 6004 Elk River Road, North Little Rock, AR 72116-5723, (501) 834-5402, **SLP**

Carr, Sherrean Marie 7511 Dowdy Street, Gilroy, CA 95020-5721, **SLP**

Carr, Mrs Susan A 11 Dale Lane, Malvern, PA 19355, (215) 696-8800, BA 74 Temple Univ; MA 76 Temple Univ; **A**

Carrara-O'Brien, Catherine Lynn 8329 N Galena Road, Peoria, IL 61615, (309) 673-2341, BA 82 Creighton Univ; MS 84 Bradley Univ; **SLP**

Carrasquillo, Mrs Ann Jabsen 3812 Hidden Acres Circle N W, North Fort Myers, FL 33903, (813) 546-6543, BA 68 Our Lady Lake Univ-San Anton; MA 69 IL St Univ - Normal; **SLP**

Carraway, Mrs Bobbye A W Speech Language Learning Services, 2300 Oakwood Drive, Biloxi, MS 39531, (601) 388-5978, BS 74 Univ Southern MS-Hattiesburg; MS 75 Univ Southern MS-Hattiesburg; Private Practice, **SLP**

Carraway, Mrs Tonda Pierce 3913 St Andrews Church Rd, Sanford, NC 27330, (919) 774-6829, BS 81 East Carolina Univ; MS 83 East Carolina Univ; Aud, Central Carolina ENT Assoc, **A**

Carrell, Mrs Marilyn F 7612 Nall Avenue, Prairie Village, KS 66208, (816) 753-5663, BA 68 Southwest MO St Univ; MA 69 Univ of KS; Aud, Midwest Otol Head & Neck Surg, **A**

Carrick, Valerie C 864 West Yale Street, Ontario, CA 91762, (714) 984-2018, BA 74 Univ of CA - Los Angeles; MS 82 Univ of LA Verne; Instr/Oral Lang Hndcpd-Aphas, San Bernardino Co Schs, **SLP**

Carrico, Cheri S 3062-1 Meadowbrook Street, Windsor, ON, Canada N8T 3H4, (519) 344-3944, BS 80 Northern MI Univ; MA 81 Western MI Univ; Sp/Lang Path, Sarnia-Lambton Cen, **SLP**

Carrico, Mrs Denise Marie 1310 J South Monaco Parkway, Denver, CO 80224, (303) 355-7337, MA 88 Univ of IL - Urbana; 88–Sp-Lang Path, UCP Assn of Denver

Carrico, Mrs Dianna Arlene 609 Ridge Park Drive, Beckley, WV 25801, (304) 252-0254, BA 79 Marshall Univ; MA 80 Marshall Univ; **SLP**

Carrier, Mrs Elizabeth P O Box 185, Bluff City, TN 37618, BA 61 East TN St Univ; MA 74 East TN St Univ; SLP, Sullivan Co Sch Syst, **SLP**

Carrier, Jackie M 513 Jena Beth Drive, Elizabethton, TN 37643, (703) 669-6331, BS 77 East TN St Univ; MS 78 East TN St Univ; Aud, Bristol Regional Sp-Hrng Ctr, **A**

Carriere, Diane Renee 1625 20th Avenue South #310, Grand Forks, ND 58201, (701) 780-2447, BS 79 ND St Univ; MS 81 Minot St Univ; 86–Sp-Lang Path, Med Ctr Rehab Hosp, **SLP**

Carrieri, Laura Jean 4982 South Ulster Parkway, Apartment 513, Denver, CO 80237, (303) 695-2644, Elizabeth A Fry, **SLP**

Carrig, Edward James 321 North Chestnut Street, Butler, PA 16001, (412) 282-2234, BS 82 Clarion Univ of PA; MS 84 Clarion Univ of PA; Aud, Hrng & Sp Assoc, **A**

Carrig, Mrs Faye 321 North Chestnut Street, Butler, PA 16001, (412) 282-2234, BS 83 Clarion Univ of PA; MS 85 Indiana Univ of PA; SLP, Hrng & Sp Assoc, **SLP**

Carrigan, Mrs Norma L 4710 Lynton Court, Indianapolis, IN 46254, (317) 266-4267, BA 68 Bellarmine Coll; MA 77 Western KY Univ; 80–Sp-Lang Path, Indianapolis PS, **SLP**

Carrigan, Mrs Sharon Route 2 Box 113-K, Caledonia, MS 39740, (601) 356-4936, BA 71 Univ of South AL; MA 72 Univ of AL- Tuscaloosa; 86–Sp-Lang Path, Lowndes Cty Sch Dist, **SLP**

Carrigan, Victoria Ashoff 628 Woodcrest Drive, Pittsburgh, PA 15205, (412) 647-5580, BS 79 Carlow Coll; MA 81 Univ of Pittsburgh - Pittsburgh; Aud, Childrens Hospital Pittsburgh, **A**

Carrigan-Peek, Mrs Mary Ann 46 Van Wie Terrace, Albany, NY 12203, (518) 869-8149, BA 79 SUNY - Coll at Plattsburgh; MS 83 Coll of Saint Rose; 87–Sp-Lang Path, Mohonasen Central Schs, **SLP**

Carrington, Mrs Barbara Brugger 333 Washington Avenue, Bethlehem, PA 18018, (215) 759-7600, BS 77 Indiana Univ of PA; MS 82 PA St Univ - Univ Park; Sp-Lang Path, Colonial Northampton I U #20, **SLP**

Carrington, Terri L Route 1 Box 140-A, Nixa, MO 65714, (417) 725-1629, BS 74 Southwest MO St Univ; MA 75 Univ of MO - Columbia; SLP, Sch Dist of Springfield R-12, **SLP**

Carr-Kraft, Linda Elaine 2430 Vineyard Lane, Crofton, MD 21114, (202) 541-6717, BS 75 FL St Univ; MA 86 Univ of MD - College Park; **A**

Carroad, Pamela 28 Bank Street, Walden, NY 12586, (914) 338-9320, BS 71 Ithaca Coll; MS 73 Ithaca Coll; 78–Director of Clinical Services, UCP/Children's Rehab Ctr, **SLP**

Carroll, Mrs Anita Matthews Route 9 Box 11-B Poplar St, Chapel Hill, NC 27514, (919) 967-5599, **A**

Carroll, Dr Anne W 3941 South Clermont, Englewood, CO 80110, (303) 758-9391, BA 58 Univ of Denver; MA 59 Univ of Denver; PH 65 (NS) Univ of Denver; Prof, U of Denver, **SLP A F**

Carroll, Mrs Carolyn M 9301 Sheffield Circle, Shreveport, LA 71118, (318) 686-1783, OM 84 LA St Univ - Shreveport; 84–Sp-Lang Path, Caddo Parish School Board, **SLP**

Carroll, Charles Randall 2218 Oakhaven Drive, Murfreesboro, TN 37129, (615) 983-1260, **SLP**

Carroll, Christine 97 Freese Road, Ithaca, NY 14850, (607) 277-2084, BS 70 Ithaca Coll; MS 73 Ithaca Coll; **SLP**

Carroll, Dawn Felice 3013 Nash Place S E, Washington, DC 20020, (202) 745-5600, BA 84 CA St Univ - Northridge; MS 87 Howard Univ

Carroll, DeAnne 102 Crestline Drive #807, Clarksdale, MS 38614, (601) 627-3231, BA 84 Univ of MS; MS 86 Univ of MS; 88–Aud, Clarksdale PS, **A**

Carroll, Mrs Deborah Elliott 4601 Whitby Place, Greensboro, NC 27406, (919) 292-5818, BS 77 Appalachian St Univ; MA 83 Univ of NC - Greensboro; Aud, Rheudolph J Wells MD PA, **A ACE**

Carroll, Denise Ann 8130 S Washtenaw, Chicago, IL 60652, (312) 450-2053, BS 85 Eastern IL Univ; MS 86 Eastern IL Univ; **SLP**

Carroll, Mrs Elaine M 279-C, Route 6, Andover, CT 06232, (203) 529-4260, BS 82 Elmira Coll; MS 84 Southern CT St Univ; Audiologist, Crel Hearing Impaired Program, **A**

Carroll, Mrs Hazel Deason 504 South Main, Henderson, TX 75652, (214) 657-8511, BA 51 Southern Methodist Univ; ME 62 Stephen F Austin St Univ; Sp-Lang Path, Henderson ISD, **SLP**

Carroll, Mrs Inez B 3897 Thoroughbred Court, Hilliard, OH 43026, (614) 876-9239, BA 74 Univ of South FL; OM 76 Auburn Univ - Auburn; 88–Aud, **A**

Carroll, Dr Jack Adien 526 South View Court, Thompson, ND 58278, (701) 780-2447, BA 72 OH St Univ; MA 74 Univ of Cincinnati; PH 75 (Aud) Univ of Cincinnati; 75–Asst Admin, Med Ctr Rehab Hosp, **SLP A**

Carroll, Jacqueline D 3504 Creekwood Drive #A, Lexington, KY 40502-3053, (502) 753-6031, **SLP**

Carroll, James R, Jr 2001 Laurel Avenue #Ng-1, Knoxville, TN 37916, (615) 525-0591, BS 73 Univ of TN - Knoxville; MA 77 Univ of TN - Knoxville; Owner, Hrng Conservation Assoc Inc, **A**

Carroll, Jane E 263 Linnmoore Street, Hartford, CT 06106-4339, (203) 722-6790, BA 76 Univ of CT; MA 78 Univ of CT; Sp-Lang Path, City of Hartford, **SLP**

Carroll, Janice Santogrossi 43 La Paloma Drive, Los Alamos, NM 87544, (505) 672-3733, BS 76 IL St Univ - Normal; MS 77 IL St Univ - Normal; **SLP**

Carroll, Kathryn B 620 Long Avenue, Roxboro, NC 27573, (919) 599-7262, BA 64 Catawba Coll; ME 74 Univ of VA - Charlottesville; Sp-Lang Path, Person Co Sch Bd, **SLP**

Carroll, Kathy Lynn 417-B Elizabeth Street, Clinton, NC 28328, (919) 592-1421, BS 82 East Carolina Univ; MS 83 East Carolina Univ; 86–Sp-Lang Path, Home Health & Hospice Care, **SLP**

Carroll, Mark Randolph 2315 Chandawood Drive, Pelham, AL 35124, (205) 934-4467, BA 83 Univ of AL-Tuscaloosa; MS 84 Univ of AL- Tuscaloosa; Coord Hearing Clinic, U of AL, **A**

Carroll, Mary L 12 Woodmont Street, West Springfield, MA 01089, **SLP**

Carroll, Nancy L 125 1/2 N Jefferson Street, Apartment 1, Lancaster, WI 53813, (608) 723-4292, BS 85 Univ of WI - Whitewater; MS 86 Univ of WI - Whitewater; 86–Sp-Lang Path, Lancaster Comm Schs, **SLP**

Carroll, Sara Beth 429 Moraine Street, Brockton, MA 02401, (617) 947-3634, BA 81 Bridgewater St Coll; MA 84 Univ of MA - Amherst; Sp-Lang Path, Reads Collaborative, **SLP**

Carroll, Mrs Susan C D 259 Leo Place, Wayne, NJ 07470, (201) 865-4913, BA 77 Montclair St Coll; MS 80 William Paterson Coll; Sp-Lang Path, Hudson Co Nj Day Trng, **SLP**

Carroll, Susan P 6813 Cowan Mill Road, Winston, GA 30187, (404) 942-4030, BS 81 Appalachian St Univ; MA 82 Appalachian St Univ; Sp-Lang Path, Douglas Co Bd of Ed, **SLP**

Carroll, Valeree S 2115 West 78th, Prairie Village, KS 66208, (816) 221-7565, BS 68 Univ of KS; MA 70 Univ of KS; Spec Education Placement Rep, Sch Dist of Kansas City Mo, **SLP**

Carroll-Kenna, Mrs Mary J 282 Sherbrooke Road, Williamsville, NY 14221, (716) 626-5562, BA 70 Daemen Coll; MA 75 SUNY - Center at Buffalo; 85–Sp-Lang Path, Buffalo Gen Hosp, **SLP ACE**

Carroll-Martini, Jean Frances R R 1 Box 1374, Brunswick, ME 04011, (207) 688-4811, BS 70 OH St Univ; MS 82 Old Dominion Univ; **SLP**

Carroll-Ranieri, Nancy E 807-D Cedar Street, Riverton, NJ 08077, (609) 829-0749, MA 87 Trenton St Coll; 84–Sp-Lang Path, Gloucester Cty Educ, **SLP**

Carrouth, Sharon Stamey Rt 1 Box 25, Loudon, TN 37774, (615) 458-2765, BA 75 Univ of TN - Knoxville; MA 76 Univ of TN - Knoxville; **A**

Carrubba, Mrs Roberta Linda 1942 East 34th Street, Brooklyn, NY 11234, (212) 376-9266, BA 76 CUNY - Brooklyn Coll; MS 82 CUNY - Brooklyn Coll; Sp-Lang Path, Bd of Ed, **SLP**

Carruth, Letricia Louise 6811 Old Canton Road, Apt 1904, Jackson, MS 39211, (601) 957-2888, SLP, The Pearl School System, **SLP**

Carsch, Mrs Deborah Brown 8831 North 85th Place, Scottsdale, AZ 85258, BA 72 Univ of AL- Tuscaloosa; MA 73 Univ of AL- Tuscaloosa; Sp/Lang Path, **SLP**

Carsella, Mrs Janice R 27850 Brandenburg Road, Ingleside, IL 60041, BS 78 Northern IL Univ - De Kalb; MA 80 Northern IL Univ - De Kalb; Sp-Lang Path, Barrington Sch Dist #220, **SLP**

Carson, Kelly Marie 1735 Nemokee Trail #11, Haslett, MI 48840, (517) 676-1051, BS 84 Western MI Univ; MA 86 MI St Univ; **SLP**

Carson, Loretta S 336 South 4th Street, Aurora, IL 60505, (312) 892-8368, OB 36 Northern IL Univ - De Kalb; MA 37 LA St Univ - Baton Rouge; **SLP LM**

Carson, Mary Ellen 717 South West Street, Jacksonville, IL 62650, (217) 245-5141, BA 44 MacMurray Coll; MA 54 MacMurray Coll; Educator, Il Sch F/T Deaf, **A**

Carspecken, Ronald J 121 West Maple, West Union, IA 52175, (319) 245-1480, BA 63 Univ of IA; MA 68 Univ of WY; Super/Cl Sp-Lang Servs, Keystone AEA, **SLP**

Carssow-Robbins, Cynthia 5615 Charlie Chan, San Antonio, TX 78240, (512) 684-4631, MA 86 Our Lady Lake Univ-San Anton; **SLP**

Carstensen, Gustav V 1815 Orchard Avenue #32722, McMinnville, OR 97128, (503) 472-7367, BS 51 Lewis & Clark Coll; ME 62 Univ of OR; **SLP LM**

Carswell, Mrs Jill B 3200 Creighton, Bedford, TX 76021, (817) 571-6734, MS 74 Univ of South FL; **SLP**

Carswell, Mrs Lynn E 564 Bridgewater Avenue, Bridgewater, NJ 08807, (201) 725-2266, BS 81 SUNY - Coll at Geneseo; MA 82 SUNY - Coll at Geneseo; Sp-Lang Path, Somerset Assn for Retarded Cit, **SLP ACE**

Carswell, Sandra G 1102 West 11th Street, Lakeland, FL 33805, (813) 683-1418, MS 78 FL St Univ; **SLP**

Carte, Terry Timberlake 6850-37th N E, Seattle, WA 98115, (206) 587-5150, BA 81 Univ of WA; OM 83 Univ of WA; SLP, Seattle Sch Dist, **SLP**

Carter, Angela N 3304 Castle, Waco, TX 76710, (817) 754-2948, BS 79 Baylor Univ; MS 80 Baylor Univ; Chief SLP, Cntrl Texas Rehabilitation Ctr, **SLP**

Carter, Anna Y P 4606 Highberry Road, Greensboro, NC 27410, MS; **SLP**

Carter, Betsy L Rt 3 Box 115, Saltville, VA 24370, (703) 496-4001, BS 86 Radford Univ; MS 87 Radford Univ; 87–Sp-Lang Path, Mt Reg Sp-Hrng Ctr, **SLP**

Carter, Dr C Dwayne 5806 Cary Drive, Austin, TX 78757-3108, (512) 458-7726, BA 55 TX Tech Univ; MA 64 TX Tech Univ; PH 71 (NS) Southern IL Univ -Carbondale; Coord TX Hrng Aid Loan Prog, TX Dept Hlth, **SLP A**

Carter, Camille Denise 688 Hightower Road, Atlanta, GA 30318, (404) 792-9114, MA 88 Hampton Univ

Carter, Mrs Christine McGregor 3170 17th Street, Boulder, CO 80302, (303) 447-1010, BA 77 Univ of CA - San Diego; MA 85 Univ of CO - Boulder; **SLP**

Carter, Cleo Irene 3842-G 7/10th Road, Route 1, Palisades, CO 81526, (303) 464-5290, BA 32 Southwestern Coll; MA 62 Univ of Denver; Retired, **SLP LM**

Carter, Mrs Cynthia Janelle 1933 Middle Road, Fayetteville, NC 28301, (919) 486-6222, **SLP**

Carter, Mrs Diana M 45278 North Spring Drive, Canton, MI 48187, (313) 459-2971, BS 78 Bowling Green St Univ; MS 83 Univ of MI - Ann Arbor; Sp-Lang Path, Plymouth-Canton Commun Sch, **SLP**

Carter, Mrs Diane Louise 4175 North Locan, Clovis, CA 93612, (209) 299-0436, BA 63 CA St Univ - Fresno; Sp-Lang Path, Clovis USD, **SLP**

Carter, Edmund P 102 Medical Center Bldg, 347 West Berry Street, Fort Wayne, IN 46802, (219) 426-8217, BA 62 Harding Univ; MA 67 Univ of TN - Knoxville; Aud, Prof Aud Ther Inc, **A**

Carter, Elisabeth Young 17150 S W Heritage Court, Apartment 132, Aloha, OR 97006, (503) 642-0922, OB 76 Willamette Univ; MS Portland St Univ; 86–Aud, Portland Ctr for Hrng & Sp, **A**

Carter, Eunice Trask 3333 Queen Ann Lane, Jacksonville, FL 32257, (904) 733-0969, BA 37 FL Southern Coll; MA 55 Univ of FL; 88–Sp-Lang Path, Baptist Med Ctr, **SLP A LM**

Carter, James P 1747 Colquitt, Houston, TX 77098, (713) 798-1960, BA 72 Univ of TN - Knoxville; MA 74 Univ of TN - Knoxville; 77–Tech Dir, Texas Children's Hosp, **SLP ACE**

Carter, Jane Hicks 10136 Barnes Trail, Inver Grove Heights, MN 55075, (612) 725-6767, BS 73 IA St Univ; MA 81 Univ of MN - Minneap-St Paul; Sp-Lang Path, ISD #196, **SLP**

Carter, Jane Royer 257 German Street, Mayville, WI 53050, (414) 387-5740, BA 54 Univ of WI - Madison; Marketing Consultant, **SLP A**

Carter, Jeannie Snodgrass 5910 Oak Flat Avenue, Texarkana, TX 75503, (501) 773-7323, BA 76 Univ of AR - Fayetteville; MA 77 Univ of AR - Fayetteville; SLP, Texarkana Arkansas School Dist, **SLP**

Carter, Dr John Francis 307 North Delaware Avenue, Martinsburg, WV 25401, (304) 263-0811, BS 53 Frostburg St Coll; MA 58 Univ of MD - College Park; PH 69 (Sp & Hrng Science) Univ of MD - College Park; Ch Aud & Sp-Path Serv, VA/Med Cen, **SLP**

Carter, Joyce R 31 Old Post Road, Port Jefferson, NY 11777, (516) 473-1207, ME 63 PA St Univ - Univ Park; BS 61 PA St Univ - Univ Park; 73–Dir/Sp-Lang Path, Longwood Sch Dist, **SLP**

Carter, June Marie 2nd General Hospital, Box 61 - EFMD, APO New York, NY 09180, BA 73 Univ of Tampa; MS 80 FL St Univ; Sp-Lang Path, Dept Army, **SLP ACE**

Carter, Leslie A 95 Madison Avenue, Bergenfield, NJ 07621, (201) 384-8207, BA 80 Trenton St Coll; MA 87 Montclair St Coll; 84–SLP, Spec Svcs Sch Dist of Bergen County, **SLP**

Carter, Linda C F 217 Inner Circle, Maxwell AFB, AL 36113-1201, (203) 288-5999, BS 72 TX Tech Univ; MA 74 TX Tech Univ; 87–Sp-Lang Path, Sp Ther Svcs, **SLP**

Carter, Lisa Kay 704 Monticello Drive #7, Fort Worth, TX 76107, (817) 732-6169, **A**

Carter, Margaret 528 Washington Avenue, Huron, OH 44839, (419) 433-4870, BS 76 Miami Univ - Oxford; MA 85 Kent St Univ; Sp-Lang Path, Huron Cty Sch, **SLP**

Carter, Mrs Margaret Fleming 2107 Brierbrook, Germantown, TN 38138, (501) 886-5737, OM 84 AR St Univ; Sp-Lang Path, E Arkansas Reg Mental Health, **SLP**

Carter, Marilyn J 1068 Owyhee, Kuna, ID 83634, (208) 922-4626, BS 75 IN St Univ - Terre Haute; MS 76 IN St Univ - Terre Haute; Sp-Lang Path, Joint Sch Dist #3, **SLP**

Carter, Mark P 347 West Berry Street, Room 202, Fort Wayne, IN 46802, (219) 426-8217, BA 86 Harding Univ; MA 88 Univ of TN - Knoxville; 88–Aud, Pro Aud Ther Inc

Carter, Michele C 720 Edinburg Road, Trenton, NJ 08619, MS 73 OH St Univ; **SLP**

Carter, Miriam Walker P O Box 25, Oakfield, ME 04763, (207) 532-6523, BA 83 Univ of CA - Santa Barbara; MS 85 Boston Univ; **SLP**

Carter, Mrs Molly Sue R R 1 Box 67, Haslet, TX 76052, (817) 636-2376, BS 84 TX Christian Univ; MS 86 TX Christian Univ; 86–Sp-Lang Path, Birdville ISD, **SLP**

Carter, Nanette E 2150 South Estes, Lakewood, CO 80227, (303) 988-6465, BA 84 Biola Univ; MA 87 Univ of CO - Boulder; **SLP**

Carter, Randall Harrison 4811 E Princess, Mesa, AZ 85205, (602) 994-3443, BA 77 CA St Univ - Long Beach; MS 85 AZ St Univ; Sp-Lang Path, Scottsdale Pub Sch, **SLP**

Carter, Mrs Regilyn W 503 Comfort Lane, Jennings, LA 70546, (318) 824-3522, BA 77 LA Tech Univ; MS 81 Univ of Southwestern LA; Sp-Lang Path, Jefferson Davis Parish Sch Bd, **SLP**

Carter, Mrs Rita Gail 4811 East Princess, Mesa, AZ 85205, (602) 898-7871, BA 77 Chapman Coll; MA 79 Univ of CO - Boulder; Aud, Mesa Pub Sch, **A**

Carter, Roxanne Lanae 1676 East Grand River, Apartment 141, East Lansing, MI 48823, (517) 351-9457, MA 87 MI St Univ

Carter, Sara C 4003 Oak Hill Road, Chapel Hill, NC 27514, (919) 489-5731, MS 79 Univ of NC - Chapel Hill; 88–Sp-Lang Path, Private Practice, **SLP**

Carter, Scott A 4013 W 138th Terrace, Leawood, KS 66224, (816) 276-4023, BA 73 Western WA Univ; MA 76 Univ of KS; 87–Supvr of Aud, Research Medical Center, **A**

Carter, Sherry J 1421 South Bluff Boulevard, Clinton, IA 52732-6551, BA 79 Metropolitan St Coll; MA 80 Univ of Northern CO; Aud, MS Bend AEA #9, **A**

Carter, Mrs Stephanie Ann 65 Copper Glen Drive, Huntington, WV 25701, (304) 762-2522, BS 75 WV Univ; MA 77 Marshall Univ; Sp-Lang Path, Cabell County Bd of Education, **SLP**

Carter, Mrs Susan P 13311 Hathaway Drive, Silver Spring, MD 20906, (301) 649-8056, BS 65 WV Univ; MA 70 WV Univ; Sp-Lang Path, Montgomery Co Pub Sch, **SLP**

Carter, Tammy Lee 4012 Brittany Circle Apt D, Bridgeton, MO 63044, (314) 298-0297, BS 82 Eastern IL Univ; MS 83 Eastern IL Univ; SLP, Spec Sch Dist/St Louis Co, **SLP**

Carter, Mrs Terry T Naples Elementary School #1, Usnsa Box 39 (Pinetamare), APO New York, NY 09521, BA 56 Univ of CA - Santa Barbara; MA 71 AZ St Univ; Sp/Lang Path, Dept of Defense Overseas Sch, **SLP**

Carter, Theresa June 409 West Broadway, Anadarko, OK 73005, (405) 247-3779, BS 78 Univ of Science & Arts of OK; ME 85 Central St Univ

Carter, Thomas J 10655 County Road, Clarence, NY 14031, (716) 887-4763, BA 69 Ottawa Univ; MA 75 SUNY - Center at Buffalo; Director Sp-Lang Path, Millard Fillmore Hospital, **SLP**

Carter, Tracy J 2460 Warwick Road, Melbourne, FL 32935, BS 86 Radford Univ; MS 88 Radford Univ; 88–Sp-Lang Path, InSpeech Inc

Carter, Vicky L 4863 Muirwood Drive SW, Powder Springs, GA 30073, (404) 382-6747, BS 76 Edinboro Univ of PA; MA 79 Memphis St Univ; Sp-Lang Path, Bartow Co Sch, **SLP**

Carter-Forcina, Mrs Greta Mercy Health Center, 4300 West Memorial Road, Oklahoma City, OK 73120, (405) 752-3770, BS 75 OK St Univ; MA 76 Univ of Tulsa; 82–Sp/Lang Path, Mercy Health Ctr, **SLP**

Carter-Jackson, Cynthia A 6742 Jardines Drive, Huntington Beach, CA 92647, (714) 552-5171, BA 77 CA St Univ - Long Beach; MA 79 CA St Univ - Long Beach; Sp-Lang Path, Irvine USD, **SLP**

Cartrite, Celesta F 3910 Old Denton Road #1317, Carrollton, TX 75007, (817) 565-0636, MS 88 Univ of North TX

Cartusciello, Mrs Christine V 189 Muirfield Road, Rockville Centre, NY 11570-2731, (516) 921-7171, BA 79 SUNY - Center at Buffalo; MA 81 Hofstra Univ; Sp-Lang Path, Variety Preschoolers Workshop, **SLP**

Cartusciello, Rosemarie 26 Manistee Lane, East Islip, NY 11730, (516) 783-7523, BA 83 SUNY - Coll at Cortland; MS 84 Adelphi Univ; 84–Sp-Lang Path, Dr Ellenmorris Tiegerman, **SLP**

Cartwright, Barbara A 6659 Manring Court, Reynoldsburg, OH 43068, (614) 866-9339, BS 77 OH Univ - Athens; MA 78 Marshall Univ; Sp-Lang-Hrng Spec, Reynoldsburg Cty Schs, **SLP**

Cartwright, Cathrine 6009 La Chumbre, Somis, CA 93066, (805) 482-2763, BS 69 AZ St Univ; MA 73 Northeast MO St Univ; Prog Spec/Spec Ed, Pleasant Valley Sch Dist, **SLP**

Cartwright, Cynthia Anne 1175 Pineville Road #72, Chattanooga, TN 37405, (404) 861-0863, BA 81 Univ of TN - Knoxville; MA 84 Univ of TN - Knoxville; 85–Sp-Lang Path, Pro Health Svcs, **SLP**

Cartwright, Jane C Minnesota Otolaryngology, 6490 Excelsior Boulevard, Suite W311, St Louis Park, MN 55426, MA 78 Univ of Northern CO; Aud, Minnesota Otolaryngology, **A**

Cartwright, Jenifer M 503 Hessel Boulevard, Champaign, IL 61820, (217) 469-2291, BA 62 Univ of IL - Urbana; MS 78 Univ of IL - Urbana; OM 85 Univ of IL - Urbana; Sp-Lang Path, St Joseph Grade Sch, **SLP**

Cartwright, Lynn Rae Route 4 Box 94, Grafton, WV 26354, (304) 293-4241, BS 71 WV Univ; MS 73 WV Univ; Asst Prof, W VA U, **SLP**

Carucci-Fenyar, Mrs Linda E 40 Burlington Road, Clifton, NJ 07012, (201) 939-9149, BA 71 William Paterson Coll; MA 73 Trenton St Coll; Sp/Lang Path, Lyndhurst Bd of Ed, **SLP ACE**

Caruso, Dr Anthony J NIH SLP Department, Bldg 1O Room 6S -235, Bethesda, MD 20892, (301) 496-4733, BS 72 SUNY - Coll at Geneseo; MA 77 SUNY - Coll at Geneseo; PH 83 (NS) Syracuse Univ; SLP, NIH, **SLP**

Caruso, Mrs Judith Mona 99 Sunrise Lane, Smithtown, NY 11787, (516) 499-1237, **SLP**

Caruso, Mary D 136 Dewey Street, Pittsburgh, PA 15218, (412) 371-7000, MS 62 Univ of Pittsburgh - Pittsburgh; Western PA Sch for the Deaf, **A**

Caruso, Mrs Nancy Sowka 3698 Rawhide Court, Las Vegas, NV 89120, BA 63 Univ of ND; MA 70 CA St Univ - Northridge; 86–Sp-Lang Path, Clark County Sch Dist, **SLP**

Caruso-Davis, Mrs Norma J 2075 North 10th Court, Coos Bay, OR 97420, BA 74 WA St Univ; MA 76 WA St Univ; Sp/Lang Path, Coos Co ESD, **SLP**

Carver, Betty B Route 1 Box 5, Ralph, AL 35480, (205) 348-7131, BA 72 Univ of AL- Tuscaloosa; MA 73 Univ of AL- Tuscaloosa; Coord Children's Lang & Spch, Univ of AL, **SLP**

Carver, Mrs Joanne Y 1500 Clark Court, Chesapeake, VA 23320, (804) 427-4425, BA 71 Norfolk St Univ; MS 74 Adelphi Univ; ES 88 Coll of William & Mary; Instr, VA Beach City Pub Schs, **SLP**

Carver, Mrs Linda Rose 7666 Mission Court, Franklin, WI 53132, (414) 425-2542, **SLP**

Carver, Mrs Phyllis W 3600 Oak Manor Lane #233, Largo, FL 34644, (813) 584-2832, BS 54 Springfield Coll; MA 62 Univ of CT; **SLP LM**

Carver, Mrs Rachelle Lizette 1229 Stemwood Drive, Picayune, MS 39466, (214) 291-1581, MS 86 Univ Southern MS-Hattiesburg; Cedar Hill Indep School Dis, **SLP**

Carver, Mrs RuthAnn D 15114 Yorkpoint, Houston, TX 77084, (713) 550-4723, BS 81 Baylor Univ; MS 82 Baylor Univ; Sp-Lang Path, Assoc In Sp-Lang & Lrng, **SLP**

Carver, Dr William F Auditec Of St Louis, 330 Selma Avenue, St Louis, MO 63119, (314) 962-5890, BA 53 Univ of Southern CA; MA 57 Univ of Southern CA; PH 60 (Aud) Univ of Southern CA; Pres, Auditec of St Louis, **A F**

Carver-Kagy, Deborah L 2508 South Union Road, Cedar Falls, IA 50613, (319) 277-4910, BS 78 Southern IL Univ -Carbondale; MS 79 Southern IL Univ -Carbondale; Sp-Lang Path, Covenant Med Ctr, **SLP**

Carville, Mrs Lynn B 3762 Hundred Oaks Avenue, Baton Rouge, LA 70808, (504) 383-3041, BS 75 LA St Univ - Baton Rouge; OM 76 LA St Univ - N O Medical Ctr; Sp-Lang Path, Private Practice, **SLP**

Cary, Diane Alane 115 North Terrace, Wichita, KS 67208, (316) 684-7060, BA 84 Univ of KS; MA 86 Wichita St Univ; Sp-Lang Path, Rainbows United Inc, **SLP**

Cary, Marilynn 460 Kings Road, Athens, GA 30606, (404) 548-8194, BS 66 Univ of MO - Columbia; MA 72 Univ of NE - Lincoln; **SLP**

Cary, Shelley R 235 Ed Padgett Road, Lakeland, FL 33809, (813) 859-5208, MS 78 Univ of South FL; Sp-Lang Path, Polk Co Sch Bd, **SLP**

Caryl, Carol A 9871 East Amarosa Lane, Tucson, AZ 85748, BA 69 Univ of WA; ME 75 Univ of GA; SLP, San Bernadino Co Schools, **SLP**

Casabonne, Janet Houston 2306 Castle Drive, Twin Falls, ID 83301, (208) 734-1312, BS 79 ID St Univ; MS 81 ID St Univ; Sp-Lang Path, Lenkner Michener and Ass, **SLP**

Casale, Mrs Sandra Eskinzes 10141 N W 21st Street, Pembroke Pines, FL 33026, (305) 437-2836, BS 79 James Madison Univ; MS 81 Old Dominion Univ; Sp-Lang Path, **SLP**

Casali, Janet Louise c/o Country Lane Orchard, R R 3, Campbellville, ON, Canada L0P 1B0, OB 81 Edinboro Univ of PA; MA 82 Edinboro Univ of PA; 87–Sp-Lang Path, E C Drury Sch, **SLP**

Casanova, Mrs Christine Digges 3199 Bentrup Circle North, Chandler, AZ 85224, (602) 496-4694, BS 81 AZ St Univ; MS 85 AZ St Univ; Sp-Lang Path, Kyrene School District 28, **SLP**

Casanova, Ruth G Rural Route 4, 35283 Knox Crescent, Abbotsford, BC, Canada V2S 4N4, (604) 853-5581, BS 76 SD St Univ; MA 77 Univ of SD - Vermillion; 85–Sp-Lang Path, Private Practice, **SLP**

Casarez, Sylvia Ann 5859 Oak Run, San Antonio, TX 78247, (512) 590-2738, MA 87 TX Woman's Univ; 87–Sp-Lang Path, San Antonio ISD

Casas, Melody S V 2108 North 33rd Street, Waco, TX 76708, (817) 753-3707, BA 74 Baylor Univ; MS 75 Baylor Univ; Coord-Stroke/Head Injury Svc, Waco Rehab Inst, **SLP A**

Casassa, Mrs Angela Cassady 14723 Barryknoll #104, Houston, TX 77079, (713) 556-1484, BS 81 Purdue Univ - West Lafayette; MA 83 Univ of Houston - Univ Park; 88–Sp-Lang Path, Katy ISD, **SLP**

Casassa, Arlene J 4 Suzanne Terrace, North Grafton, MA 01536, BS 77 Marywood Coll; MS 78 Ithaca Coll; **SLP**

Casaubon, Kathleen Katka RFD 3 Box 49, Southbridge, MA 01550, BA 75 Univ of MA - Amherst; **SLP**

Casaus, Robin A 3301 Monroe N E #N-141, Albuquerque, NM 87110, BA 68 Univ of Albuquerque; MS 81 Univ of NM; Sp-Lang Path, Pub Sch, **SLP**

Casby, Dr Michael W Audiology And Speech Sciences, Michigan State University, East Lansing, MI 48824, (517) 355-8780, BS 74 Mankato St Univ; MA 76 Mankato St Univ; PH 80 (NS) Univ of KS; Assoc Prof, MI St U, **SLP**

Cascardo, Mrs Debra 1 Fox Run, Armonk, NY 10504, (914) 273-2135, BA 73 CUNY - Hunter Coll; MA 75 CUNY - Hunter Coll; OM 80 NY Univ; Hosp Admin, Hlth Serv, **A**

Cascella, Paul W 146 Silvermine Avenue, Norwalk, CT 06850-1607, (203) 846-9531, BS 85 Marquette Univ; MA 87 SUNY - Center at Buffalo; **SLP**

Casciato, Karen Marie 7703 Queen Street, Wyndmoor, PA 19118, (215) 836-7594, BS 83 West Chester Univ of PA; OM 85 Hahneman Medical Coll; **SLP**

Cascio, Carol F Lowe 3626 Sun Valley Drive, Houston, TX 77025, (713) 621-4874, BS 68 LA St Univ - Baton Rouge; ME 72 LA St Univ - Baton Rouge; OM 78 LA St Univ - N O Medical Ctr; Aud, Houston ISD, **A**

Case, Carol Lynn 608 Rolling Rock, Bloomfield Hills, MI 48013, **SLP**

Case, Elizabeth Fuller 3954 Whittington Drive, Atlanta, GA 30342-4206, (404) 261-7356, BS 76 Univ of VA - Charlottesville; MA 79 Northwestern Univ; Aud, **A**

Case, Dr James L Dept Of Speech & Hearing Sci, Arizona State University, Tempe, AZ 85287, (602) 965-2373, BS 64 Weber St Coll; MS 65 Univ of UT; PH 68 (Sp-Lang Path) Univ of UT; Assoc Prof, Ariz St U, **SLP F**

Case, Linda G D Box 54, Carway, AR 72419, (501) 482-3351, OB 76 AR St Univ; OM 77 AR St Univ; Sp-Lang Path, Riverside PS, **SLP**

Case, Mrs Sally H 1331 Tulane Road, Claremont, CA 91711, (213) 963-1510, BA 62 Univ of MI - Ann Arbor; MA 65 CA St Univ - Los Angeles; SLP, Claremont Schools, **SLP**

Case, Mrs Sandra L Hueneme School District, Port Hueneme, CA 93041, (805) 488-3588, BA 64 San Jose St Univ; MA 69 CA Poly St Univ-San Luis Obi; MA 72 Univ of CA - Santa Barbara; Prog Spec, Hueneme School District, **SLP**

Case, Sue Anne P O Box 263, Brooksville, KY 41004, (606) 735-2523, BS 76 Ball St Univ; MS 84 Univ of KY; 76–Sp-Lang Path, Bracken Co Schs, **SLP**

Casebier, Dr Gabrielle 17808 Buntline Drive, Sun City, AZ 85375, (602) 584-4361, BS 42 Univ of IL - Urbana; MS 42 Univ of IL - Urbana; PH 61 (NS) Univ of WI - Madison; **SLP LM**

Case-Dehaven, Mrs Candace Ann 2114 Dekle Avenue #4, Tampa, FL 33606, (813) 546-9897, MS 86 Univ of South FL; **SLP**

Casel, Mrs Brenda H 313 N Fredricksburg Avenue, Ventnor, NJ 08406, (609) 645-2500, BA 66 Temple Univ; MA 68 Temple Univ; 70–Sp-Lang Path/Aud, Bernard S Casel MD Pa, **SLP A**

Casenave, Mrs Deeann Mari 1381 Calle Christopher, Encinitas, CA 92024, (619) 672-3400, BA 77 San Diego St Univ; MA 80 San Diego St Univ; **SLP**

Caserio, Marcia B 408 Overlook Terrace, Hendersonville, NC 28739, (704) 692-5179, ME 76 Western Carolina Univ; BS 70 Western Carolina Univ; Sp-Lang Path, Marg Pardee Hosp, **SLP**

Casey, Beth M 9853 Kinglet Drive, Baton Rouge, LA 70809, (504) 346-1127, BS 79 LA St Univ - Baton Rouge; OM 80 LA St Univ - N O Medical Ctr; Sp/Lang Path, E Baton Rouge Parish Sch Bd, **SLP**

Casey, Dawnne Margaret 44 South 1000 East, Springville, UT 84663, (801) 489-4636, MS 83 Brigham Young Univ; 83–Sp-Lang Path, Provo Sch Dist, **SLP**

Casey, Edith Nmi 7726 Lemoyne Lane, Springfield, VA 22153, (703) 440-0338, MS 84 Univ of the DC; **SLP**

Casey, Mrs Helen M 47 Indian Hill Road, Milford, CT 06460, (203) 783-3496, BA 51 Univ of CT; MS 74 Southern CT St Univ; Sp-Lang Path, Milford Bd of Ed, **SLP**

Casey, Karen Marie 217 Clayton Road, Durham, NC 27703, (919) 684-6669, BS 82 Kent St Univ; MA 82 Kent St Univ; Sp/Lang Path, Lenox Baker Children's Hosp-Duke Med Ctr, **SLP ACE**

Casey, Kathleen C 134-B Inglewood Avenue, Spartanburg, SC 29302, (803) 585-0322, BA 76 Univ of TN - Knoxville; MA 77 Univ of TN - Knoxville; Sp-Lang Path, Teszler Leaning Adjustment Sch, **SLP**

Casey, Kathleen Ferguson 1610 Claremont Avenue, Richmond, VA 23227, (804) 264-7819, BS 82 James Madison Univ; ME 84 Univ of VA - Charlottesville; Sp-Lang Path, Private Practice, **SLP**

Casey, Margaret M 15 Bogandale Road, West Roxbury, MA 02132, (617) 389-7950, BA 74 Univ of MA - Amherst; ME 76 Northeastern Univ; Aud, Cty of Evenett Sch Dept, **A**

Casey, Dr Maureen T Mid Oregon Regional Program, 3400 Portland Road N E, Salem, OR 97303, (503) 588-6677, MA 74 WA St Univ; MS 78 Western OR St Coll; PH 81 (Psychology) Univ of OR; Coordinator, Marion Ed Serv Dist, **SLP**

Casey, Moira H Box 84, Shasta, CA 96087, MA 79 San Diego St Univ; Special Day Class Teacher, Shasta County Supt of Schools, **SLP**

Casey, Patricia F 1114 19th Avenue South, Nashville, TN 37212, (615) 297-6733, BA 70 Fordham Univ; OM 74 Vanderbilt Univ; MS 76 Vanderbilt Univ; 87–Sp-Lang Path, Pi Beta Phi Rehab Inst, **SLP**

Casey, Dr Patricia Louise 302 East Milwaukee Avenue, Fort Atkinson, WI 53538, (414) 472-1301, BS 69 Univ of WI - Whitewater; MS 72 Univ of WI - Milwaukee; PH 80 (NS) IN Univ - Bloomington; Assoc Prof, U of WI-Whitewater, **SLP**

Casey, Pauline Eilert 7930 South Bemis Street, Littleton, CO 80120-4384, (303) 753-1221, BS 73 Fort Hays St Univ; MS 75 Fort Hays St Univ; Exec Dir, Co Sp-Lang-Hrng Assoc, **SLP**

Casey, Suzanne J Route 1, 13161 Grove Road, Minooka, IL 60447, (815) 475-7315, BA 70 Eastern IL Univ; MS 83 IL St Univ - Normal; Special Education Admin, Oak Park & River Forest HS, **SLP**

Casey, Thomas A, Jr 1610 Claremont Avenue, Richmond, VA 23227, (804) 861-7503, BS 81 Wilkes Coll; MS 84 Bloomsburg Univ of PA; Aud Super, Southside VA Training Ctr, **A**

Casey, Victoria L 241 Calle DE Sereno, Leucadia, CA 92024, (619) 436-7418, BA 82 SUNY - Coll at Cortland; OM 86 AZ St Univ; 88–Sp-Lang Path, Encinitas Union Sch Dist, **SLP**

Casey-Harvey, Deborah G 8423 East 13th Street, Indianapolis, IN 46219, (317) 897-3460, BS 77 Eastern KY Univ, MS 78 Purdue Univ - West Lafayette; Sp-Lang Path, Washington Township Sch Dist, **SLP**

Casey-Wolff, Jeannette 1241 Northeast 28th Avenue, Pompano Beach, FL 33062, (305) 781-3260, BS 77 Western IL Univ; MA 78 Western IL Univ; Sp-Lang Path, Private Practice, **SLP**

Cash, Rebecca A 3527 Springhill Avenue, Mobile, AL 36608, (205) 344-0756, BS 76 Univ of South AL; MS 77 Univ of AL- Tuscaloosa; Sp-Lang Path, Mobile Co Pub Sch, **SLP**

Cash, Wanda M PO Box 914, 1715 Highway 92 West, Woodstock, GA 30188, (404) 926-5522, MA 76; Sp-Lang Path, So Cherokee Aud Svcs, **SLP**

Cashell, Mrs Joyce Mullican Rt 1 Box 466, Mexia, TX 76667-9801, (817) 562-6635, BS 56 TX Woman's Univ; ME 69 East TX St Univ - Commerce; Sp-Lang Path, Mexia ISD, **SLP**

Cashin, Janice M 475 North Harvey, Plymouth, MI 48170, (313) 467-4260, BA 77 Univ of MI - Ann Arbor; MA 79 Western MI Univ; Aud, Annapolis Hosp, **A**

Cashin, Mrs Joan L 3805 West Shaffer, Coleman, MI 48618, (517) 435-9474, BS 71 Central MI Univ; MA 78 Central MI Univ; 71–Sp-Lang Path, Clare-Gladwin ISD, **SLP**

Cashman, Debra A 14 Ashworth Drive, Rochdale, MA 01542, (508) 832-7380, BS 78 Worcester St Coll; ME 81 Northeastern Univ; Sp/Lang Path, Worcester PS, **SLP**

Cashman, Marianne 42 Mason Avenue, Binghamton, NY 13904, (607) 770-0444, BA 85 SUNY - Coll at Cortland; MS 86 Ithaca Coll; 87–Sp-Lang Path, Broome Dev Ctr, **SLP**

Cashman, Marlene Z Sunnybrook Medical Centre, Audiology Unit Room 2010, 2075 Bayview Avenue, Toronto, ON, Canada M4N 3M5, (416) 480-4150, BS 67 McGill Univ - Quebec; MS 69 McGill Univ - Quebec; Ch Aud, Sunnybrook Med Cen, **A**

Casini, Mrs Louann Jo 4748 Knollwood Drive, Las Vegas, NV 89117, (702) 871-4218, BS 83 WV Univ; MS 84 WV Univ; Sp-Lang Path, Clark Co Schl Dstr, **SLP**

Casner, Mrs Mary Witham 11616 Moorestown Place, Gaithersburg, MD 20878, (301) 762-2607, BS 76 Miami Univ - Oxford; MS 77 Miami Univ - Oxford; Sp-Lang Path, Montgy Co Pub Sch, **SLP**

Casper, Dr Janina K SUNY Health Science Center, 766 Irving Avenue, Syracuse, NY 13210, (315) 473-4806, BA 52 Univ of MI - Ann Arbor; MS 54 PA St Univ - Univ Park; PH 83 (Communication Disorders) Syracuse Univ; 77–Asst Prof, St U of NY Health Science Ctr, **SLP ACE**

Casper, Judy R 2727 Navajo Street, Santa Rosa, CA 95401, (707) 527-2271, BA 72 San Francisco St Univ; MA 73 San Francisco St Univ; Sp-Lang Path, Sonoma County Office of Educ, **SLP**

Casper, Marie Anne 621 Park Street, Allentown, PA 18102, (215) 248-5120, BS 85 Marywood Coll; MA 87 PA St Univ - Univ Park; **SLP**

Casper, Marilyn E 14456 Foothill Boulevard, Suite 20, Sylmar, CA 91342, (818) 885-5330, BS 73 Univ of WI - Whitewater; MA 74 Western MI Univ; 85–Sp-Lang Path, Northridge Hosp Med Cen, **SLP**

Casper, Mary Ellen Wycoma Way #31C, Waltham, MA 02154, (617) 647-9970, BS 75 Southern Methodist Univ; MS 77 Univ of TX - Dallas; Ch of Aud, Ctrl TX Rehab Cen, **A**

Casper, Muriel Klein 75 Spruce Street, Roslyn Harbor, NY 11576, (718) 470-8910, BS 55 Kean Coll of NJ; MA 67 Columbia Univ Teachers Coll; Sp-Lang Path, Li Jewish - Hillside Med Cen, **SLP**

Casper, Rosemarie Ann 425 Park Place, Roselle Park, NJ 07204, (201) 241-6205, BA 84 Rutger's St Univ - Douglas Coll; MS 86 PA St Univ - Univ Park; 86–Sp-Lang Path, UCP of North Jersey Inc, **SLP**

Caspi, Mrs Judy H Stanwood Road, Mount Kisco, NY 10549, (914) 241-3796, BA 69 CUNY - City College; MS 70 Rutgers St Univ -N Brunswick; Sp-Lang Path, **SLP**

Cassady, Bonnie Lee Rt 1 Box 121, Buffalo, MN 55313, (612) 682-3285, MS 86 Moorhead St Univ

Cassady, Mrs Debbie D Rural Route 1, Ancona, IL 61311, (815) 672-2909, BS 80 IL St Univ - Normal; MS 82 IL St Univ - Normal; Sp-Lang Path, Woodland Elem, **SLP**

Cassanego, Diane L P 1017 Porto Marino Drive, San Carlos, CA 94070, (415) 592-7379, BA 77 San Francisco St Univ; MS 79 San Francisco St Univ; **SLP**

Cassar, Dorothy A 44 Long Meadow Place, Centereach, NY 11720, (516) 736-3429, BS 70 SUNY - Coll at Buffalo; MA 74 Hofstra Univ; 88–Instr/Consult, St Joseph's Coll/Maryhaven Adult Svcs, **SLP**

Cassatt-Hicks, Linda L 106 Dixie Avenue, Petal, MS 39465, (601) 545-7652, MS 83 Univ Southern MS-Hattiesburg; **SLP**

Cassatt-James, Mrs Edith Lucinda 604 East 34th Street, Baltimore, MD 21218, (301) 338-0959, MS 77 Northwestern Univ; 88–Sp-Lang Path, Johns Hopkins Univ, **SLP**

Casscles, Sheri 95 Jaques Street #2, Somerville, MA 02145, (617) 625-3590, MS 88 Northeastern Univ; 88, Milford Aud Ctr

Cassel, Debbie 2625 Ethel, Waco, TX 76707, (817) 757-1123, BS 79 OK St Univ; MA 81 OK St Univ; Sp/Lang Path, Mexia St Sch, **SLP**

Cassel, Tami S 5119 Williams Fork Trail, #119, Boulder, CO 80301, (303) 772-6363, BS 84 Univ Southern MS-Hattiesburg; MA 86 Univ of CO - Boulder; 87–Sp-Lang Path, St Vrain Valley Sch Dist, **SLP**

Cassell, Mrs Mary Anita 5726 Cricket Lane, Harrisburg, PA 17112, (717) 657-8162, BS 79 Appalachian St Univ; MA 86 Memphis St Univ; 87–Sp-Lang Path, Capital Area Intermediate Unit, **SLP**

Casselman, Sharon H 794 Lincoln Avenue, St Paul, MN 55105, **SLP**

Cassels, Caro M Route 1 Box 26, Trenton, SC 29847, **SLP**

Cassiday, Jacqueline Ann 302 Barrow, Jersey City, NJ 07302, (201) 321-7066, BA 71 Univ of IA; MS 85 Rush Univ; 87–Sp-Lang Path, Johnson Rehab Inst, **SLP**

Cassidy, Deborah Diane 921 Durham Place, Bensalem, PA 19020, SLP, Sch Dist of Phila, **SLP**

Cassidy, Mrs Janet Marsala 14 Partridge Road, Delmar, NY 12054, (518) 439-0688, BS 76 SUNY - Coll at Plattsburgh; MS 79 Coll of Saint Rose; **SLP**

Cassidy, Mrs Karen S 26 Park Lane Circle, Lockport, NY 14094, (716) 434-6744, BS 72 SUNY - Coll at Geneseo; MS 74 SUNY - Coll at Buffalo; Sp-Lang Path, Maryvale School System, **SLP**

Cassidy, Kathleen R 33 Lakewood Place, Troy, NY 12180, (518) 274-6678, BS 80 Coll of Saint Rose; MS 81 Syracuse Univ; Sp-Lang Path, Private Practice, **SLP**

Cassidy, Maureen Somerset Place, 10014 White Bluff Road, Apartment 205, Savannah, GA 31419, BS 84 Purdue Univ - West Lafayette; ME 86 Univ of VA - Charlottesville; **A**

Cassidy, Mrs Renee Marcia 1922 North Atwood Avenue, Tucson, AZ 85745, (602) 743-0431, BS 76 AZ St Univ; MS 79 Univ of AZ; **SLP**

Cassidy, Robert D 2218 Willow, Pekin, IL 61554, **SLP**

Cassidy, Terrence J 524-3 Wood St, West Lafayette, IN 47906, (317) 743-9439, MS 88 Purdue Univ - West Lafayette

Cassidy-Goffnett, Mrs Mary Ellen 324 1/2 West Saginaw, St Louis, MI 48880, (517) 681-4217, MA 80 Central MI Univ; **SLP**

Cassie, Dhyan McCollom PO Box 2155, Eagle Pass, TX 78853, (215) 895-5711, BA 57 Westminster Coll; MA 78 Univ of Pittsburgh - Pittsburgh; Aud, Elwyn Nevil Natl Rehab Cen, **A**

Cassin, Mrs Mary Padula 139 South Highland, Lombard, IL 60148, (312) 654-2188, BS 80 Northern IL Univ - De Kalb; MA 81 Northern IL Univ - De Kalb; Sp-Lang Path, Comm Unit Sch Dist 201, **SLP**

Cassin, Dr Roxanne Marie 208 Greenbriar Estates, Des Peres, MO 63122, (314) 577-5707, MS 77 Saint Louis Univ; ED 83 (NS) Saint Louis Univ; Dir/Pediatric Speech Service, Private Practice, **SLP**

Casso, Thomas, Jr 88 Russell Street, Hamden, CT 06517, (203) 787-8994, BS 53 Univ of CT; MS 61 Southern CT St Univ; MS 75 Southern CT St Univ; 61–Sp-Lang Path, New Haven Board of Education, **SLP**

Castagna, Mrs Christine Marie 216 Rose Street, Massapequa Park, NY 11762, (212) 430-0479, BS 83 SUNY - Coll at Geneseo; MA 85 SUNY - Coll at Geneseo; Sp-Lang Path, Midpoint Assoc Prac, **SLP**

Caste, Debra Fay 1865 Balboa Lane, Clearwater, FL 33516, (813) 442-1171, MS 87 Univ of South FL

Casteel, Dr Robert L 5986 S W Shallowbrook Lane, Beaverton, OR 97007, (503) 649-5193, BA 54 Pacific Univ; MA 60 Univ of WA; PH 69 (NS) Univ of OR; Professor, Portland State University, **SLP F**

Castellan, Susan B 360 Charleston Avenue, Morgantown, WV 26505, (304) 296-0073, BS 72 PA St Univ - Univ Park; ME 73 Boston Univ; **SLP**

Castellani, Mrs Laurelyn Mary 1040 Millview Drive, Batavia, IL 60510, (312) 898-4610, BA 76 Elmhurst Coll; MA 77 Northern IL Univ - De Kalb; SLP, Il Aurora Sch Dist 131, **SLP**

Castellano, Joseph 3049 Ocean Parkway, P O Box 60, Brooklyn, NY 11235, (718) 373-0070, BS 64 Long Island U - Brooklyn Ctr; MA 81 CUNY - City College; Pres, H E A R Inc, **A**

Castellanos, Ana E 1121 S W 122nd Avenue #113, Miami, FL 33184, (305) 553-7461, BA 81 Univ of Miami; MS 83 FL St Univ; 84–Sp-Lang Path, Dade County Schools, **SLP**

Castelli, Beth Ann 100 Bryn Mawr Ct, 101 East, Pittsburgh, PA 15221, (412) 242-8021, BS 84 Edinboro Univ of PA; MA 85 Edinboro Univ of PA; 85–Sp-Lang Path, InSpeech Inc, **SLP**

Casten, Leslie Ann 2078 Arbor Glen Place, Marietta, GA 30066, (404) 565-6849, BS 81 Univ of South AL; OM 83 Auburn Univ - Auburn; 88–Sp-Lang Path, Bartow County Bd of Educ, **SLP**

Casterline, Judy 1070 Delta 77 Drive, Akron, OH 44312, (216) 434-3699, BA 83 Univ of Akron; MA 85 Univ of Akron; Sp-Lang Path, Edwin Shaw Hospital, **SLP**

Castilaw, Karen Ballard P O Box 1872, Vidor, TX 77662, (409) 769-8172, BS 85 Lamar Univ; MS 86 Lamar Univ; **SLP**

Castilla, Carla 1315 Park Ridge Place, Cincinnati, OH 45208-2544, (513) 221-4243, BA 83 OH St Univ; MS 85 Univ of NC - Chapel Hill; Aud, Hearing Speech & Language Inc, **A**

Castilla, Mary Helen 1600 Parkview Lane, San Marcos, TX 78666, (512) 672-7561, BA 84 Our Lady Lake Univ-San Anton; MA 86 Our Lady Lake Univ-San Anton; 88–Sp-Lang Path, Texas Elks Child Diagn Ctr

Castilla-Wilson, Mrs Dora L 11604 Seminole Road, Tacoma, WA 98499, BA 79 Our Lady Lake Univ-San Anton; MA 81 Our Lady Lake Univ-San Anton; 87–Sp-Lang Path, Mary Bridge Sp & Hrng Ctr, **SLP**

Castillo, Mrs Alma Luisa 11729 Tony Tejeda, El Paso, TX 79936-7023, (512) 222-8782, BS Univ of TX - El Paso; MS Univ of Saint Thomas; Sp-Lang Path, Ysleta ISD, **SLP**

Castillo, Elisa Angers 600 Sandman Suite #8, Laredo, TX 78041, (512) 722-1346, BA 73 Our Lady Lake Univ-San Anton; MA 73 Our Lady Lake Univ-San Anton; Sp-Lang Path, Private Practice, **SLP ACE**

Castillo, Kathleen Ann 6024 Salida Del Sol, San Jose, CA 95123, (415) 567-9722, MA 85 San Jose St Univ; SLP, Mtcs, **SLP**

Castle, Dr Diane Sklar 4272 Clover Street, Honeoye Falls, NY 14472, (716) 475-6476, BS 55 Boston Univ; MS 56 Syracuse Univ; PH 67 (NS) Stanford Univ; Audiologist, Rochester Inst of Tech, **A F**

Castle, Mrs Janell Dawn 601 Greenbriar Court, Charleston, IL 61920, (217) 345-2193, BS 82 Eastern IL Univ; MS 83 Eastern IL Univ; Sp-Lang Path, Charleston Comm Ut Schs, **SLP**

Castle, Sandra 5915 Jug Bridge Hill Road, Frederick, MD 21701, (301) 694-0654, BS 65 Old Dominion Univ; ME 67 Univ of VA - Charlottesville; Aud, Hrng Testng Inc, **A**

Castle, Terrina Marie 432 30th Avenue, Moline, IL 61265, (309) 764-6980, BA 84 Augustana Coll; MS 85 IL St Univ - Normal; 86–Sp-Lang Path, Moline PS Dist #40, **SLP**

Castle, Tracy Calpin 2484 Versailles Road, Lexington, KY 40504, (606) 268-4545, BS 82 Kent St Univ; MA 82 Kent St Univ; 86–Sp-Lang Path, Lexington Hrng && Sp Cntr, **SLP**

Castle, Dr William E Rochester Inst Of Technology, One Lomb Memorial Drive, Rochester, NY 14623, (716) 475-6418, BS 51 Northern St Coll; MA 58 Univ of IA; PH 63 (Sp Path & Aud) Stanford Univ; 68–Dir, NTID, **SLP F**

Castleberry, Charlotte J 16 Albert Street, Madawaska, ME 04756, (207) 728-4022, MA 86 CA St Univ - Stanislaus; Sp-Lang Path, Medical Health Center, **SLP**

Castleberry, Mrs Debra J Rt 5 40 Dailey Hills Circle, Ringgold, GA 30736, (615) 344-6044, BS 74 Univ of TN - Knoxville; MA 75 Univ of TN - Knoxville; 82–Sp-Lang Path, Hamilton Co Sch, **SLP**

Castner, Cheryl L 10111 McKenney Avenue #302, Silver Spring, MD 20902, (301) 249-2142, BA 76 Univ of MD - College Park; MS 79 Loyola Coll; Sp/Lang Path, Prince George Co Pub Sch, **SLP**

Castner, Marguerite L 11211 N E Weidler #232, Portland, OR 97220, (503) 252-8088, BS 31 Univ of OR; ME 65 Univ of OR; **SLP LM**

Castor, Devorah L 2431 Barrington Road, Akron, OH 44313-3803, (216) 762-4200, BA 70 Carnegie-Mellon Univ; MA 74 Univ of Akron; Aud, Castor Assoc, **A**

Castrup, Mrs Jacqueline R 1215 Edmunds, Brush, CO 80723, (303) 867-5460, BA 78 Univ of Northern CO; MA 79 Univ of Northern CO; SLP, Fort Morgan Pub Schs, **SLP**

Casuccio, R Christine 7 Lyndhurst Court, Sterling, VA 22170, (704) 430-1992, BA 76 WV Univ; BS 76 WV Univ; MS 77 WV Univ; Aud Superv, **A**

Caswell, Mrs Susan Beth 3107 Graybill Road, Uniontown, OH 44685, (216) 762-6486, BS 84 Kent St Univ; MA 84 Kent St Univ; Inter & Eval Specialist, Kent State U, **SLP**

Cataldie, Mary 2117 Marye Street, Alexandria, LA 71301, (318) 334-5128, BA 82 Northeast LA Univ; MS 85 Univ of Southwestern LA; SLP, Acadia Parish School Board, **SLP**

Cataldo, Mary N 2398 Woodpecker Avenue, Ventura, CA 93003, (805) 525-5603, BA 79 CA St Univ - Chico; MA 81 CA St Univ - Chico; SLP, Fillmore USD, **SLP**

Catanzano, Annemarie 9 Wellstone Drive, Portland, ME 04103, (207) 775-4000, BA 75 Boston Coll; MA 78 OH St Univ; 86–Dir-Comm Dis Dept, New England Rehab Hosp of Portland, **SLP**

Cate, Carol Paulson 16740 Bermuda Street, Granada Hills, CA 91344, (818) 762-4238, BS 74 Portland St Univ; MS 77 Portland St Univ; Sp-Lang Path, St Joseph Med Ctr, **SLP**

Cate, Jeanne Beatrice 3425 Mount Everest, San Diego, CA 92111, (619) 264-0125, BA 74 San Diego St Univ; SLP, San Diego USD, **SLP**

Cater, Mrs Kathleen F R R 1 Box 374, Beacon Heights, North Clarendon, VT 05759, (802) 775-2395, BS 76 SUNY - Coll at Brockport; MS 80 Loyola Coll; Sp/Lang Path, Vermont Achievement Cen, **SLP**

Caterson-Marshall, Mary 50 South Adelaide Avenue, Highland Park, NJ 08904, (201) 548-7610, BS 76 Syracuse Univ; MS 78 Columbia Univ Teachers Coll; Dir, Rock Brook Sch, **SLP**

Cates, Mrs Cheryl A 23361 El Toro Road Suite 112, El Toro, CA 92630, (714) 583-7955, BA 82 Univ of Redlands; MS 84 San Francisco St Univ; 87–Sp-Lang Path/Owner, Saddleback Valley Sp/Lang Ctr, **SLP**

Cates, Mrs Colleen F Route 5 Box 183, Martin, TN 38237, (901) 364-5554, BS 78 Univ Southern MS-Hattiesburg; MA 80 Memphis St Univ; Sp-Lang Path, Weakley Co Sch Syst, **SLP**

Cates, Mrs Laurel B P O Box 1253, Spring, TX 77383, (713) 792-4516, BA 72 CUNY - Queens Coll; MS 74 Boston Univ; **SLP**

Cates, Linda Lee 102-C Newridge Road, Oak Ridge, TN 37830, (615) 482-6515, **SLP**

Cates, Ronald T 9614 Imperial Drive, Ooltewah, TN 37363, (615) 267-5641, BA 75 Auburn Univ - Auburn; MA 77 IN Univ - Bloomington; Audiologist, Chattanooga-Hamilton County, **A**

Cates, Mrs Susan Mary 4808 Refugio Avenue, Carlsbad, CA 92008, (714) 753-1212, **SLP**

Cathell, Kathleen Wimmer RT4 Box 388, Berlin, MD 21811, (302) 856-7364, BS 79 West Chester Univ of PA; MS 81 Loyola Coll; Sp-Path, Worcester Co Board of Ed, **SLP**

Catherall, Paul Glenrose Hosp Com Disorders, 10230 111th Avenue, Edmonton, AB, Canada T5G 0B7, BS 76 Univ of Aston - England; MA 80 Univ of Alberta - Alberta; MS 83 Dalhousie Univ - Nova Scotia; Sp-Lang Path, Glenrose Rehabilitation Hosp, **SLP**

Catherwood, Kay P Greentree Audiology, 2001D Greentree, Executive Campus, Marlton, NJ 08053, (609) 596-8870, BA 72 Univ of DE; MA 74 Temple Univ-Tyler Sch of Art; Aud, Greentree Audiology, **A**

Cathey, Kimberly Dee 2509 Margaret Lynn Lane, Muskogee, OK 74401, BS 84 OK St Univ; MS 86 Univ of OK Medical Center; **SLP**

Catlett, Mrs Margaret E 7533 44th Avenue South, Seattle, WA 98118, (206) 722-8731, MA 88 WA St Univ

Catlin, Dr Francis Irving Department Of Otolaryngology, Texas Childrens Hospital, Box 20269, Houston, TX 77225, (713) 798-1490, 49 Princeton Univ; OD 59 (NS) Johns Hopkins Univ; 72–Prof/Otol, Baylor Coll of Med, **A F**

Cato, Patricia Elizabeth 1074 Noriega Avenue, Sunnyvale, CA 94086, (408) 736-3684, BA 84 Humboldt St Univ; MS 86 San Francisco St Univ; **A**

Caton, Ann 1147 Easton Street, Orlando, FL 32825, (305) 422-3200, BA 75 Univ of Central FL; MA 76 Univ of Central FL; Sp-Lang Path, Orange Co Pub Sch, **SLP**

Caton, Nanette M Speech & Hearing Center, 159 Worcester Court, Falmouth, MA 02540, (617) 540-8600, BS 86 Ithaca Coll; MA 87 Ithaca Coll; Aud, Kathleen M Florance

Catt, Mrs Mary J 414 Western Drive, Danville, IN 46122, (317) 745-6588, BS 72 IN St Univ - Terre Haute; MA 74 IN Univ - Bloomington; **SLP**

Cattaneo, Angela M The Mount Vernon Hospital, 2501 Parker's Lane, Dept P M R, Alexandria, VA 22306, (703) 664-7190, BA 77 Catholic Univ of America; MA 78 Western MI Univ; 88–Coord of Sp-Lang Path, Mt Vernon Hosp, **SLP**

Catterall, Mrs Kathleen A 9917 Scripps Westview Way, Apartment 218, San Diego, CA 92131, (619) 465-0711, BA 75 Univ of the Pacific; MA 76 Univ of the Pacific; Sp-Lang Path, Grossmont District Hospital, **SLP ACE**

Catterall, Nancy S 4556 East Laurel Drive N E, Seattle, WA 98105, (206) 226-1230, BA 80 Univ of WA; MS 82 Univ of WA; Aud, Valley ENT Cl, **A**

Cattey, Tommy J P O Box 45182, Phoenix, AZ 85064, **A**

Cattle, Sally F 1109 2nd Avenue North, Columbus, MS 39701, (601) 329-4750, MA 50 Univ of NE - Lincoln; Assoc Prof Sp-Lang Path, Miss U for Women, **SLP**

Catton, Mrs Barbara Anne 4851 East Alder Drive, San Diego, CA 92116, (619) 283-1067, MA 88 San Diego St Univ

Catts, Dr Hugh W 1706 Indiana Street, Lawrence, KS 66044, (913) 864-4690, BA 74 Univ of FL; MA 76 Univ of FL; PH 79 (NS) Univ of FL; Sp-Lang Path, Univ of Kansas

Catullo, Stephen Joseph 5421 Chestnut Hill, Willoughby, OH 44094, (216) 946-0419, MA 88 Cleveland St Univ

Catz, Mrs Judith C 538 Newton Street, Chestnut Hill, MA 02167, (617) 785-0036, BS 69 Boston Univ; ME 70 Northeastern Univ; Sp-Lang Path, Dover-Sherborn Pub Sch, **SLP**

Caudle, Chris D Denton Hearing Health Care, 4401-A North I-35 #340, Westgate Medical Center, Denton, TX 76201, (817) 387-0550, BS 79 Univ of North TX; MS 80 Univ of North TX; Aud, **A**

Caudle, Mrs Teresa Harrison 810 Willow Oak Drive, Birmingham, AL 35244, (205) 780-7053, BS 78 Troy St Univ - Troy; MS 82 Univ of Montevallo; 88–Aud, Simon-Williamson Clinic, **A**

Caufield, Laurie C 121 Bluffside Drive, Fort Mitchell, KY 41017, (513) 872-2481, BA 71 Cleveland St Univ; ME 73 Univ of VA - Charlottesville; 86–Dir Rehab Cen, Good Samaritan Hosp, **SLP**

Caughey, Mary B 202 Washington Avenue, Kingston, NY 12401-4443, MS; **SLP LM**

Caul, Mrs Linda Doherty 5119 Harthlodge, St Louis, MO 63129, (314) 894-3836, BS 75 Northwestern Univ; MA 77 Northwestern Univ; Sp-Lang Path, Private Practice, **SLP**

Cauley, Mrs Kathleen O'Neill 308 Miracle Strip Parkway, Apartment 36-C, Fort Walton Beach, FL 32548, (904) 664-0719, BS 82 Univ of MA - Amherst; MS 87 Worcester St Coll; 88–Sp-Lang Path, Sp & Hrg Ctr of Ft Walton Beach, **SLP**

Caulfield, Mrs Patricia 23 Backfin Point, Wilmington, NC 28405, (919) 762-5807, BS Loyola Univ of Chicago; MA Catholic Univ of America; SLP/Aud, N Hanover Co Bd of Ed, **SLP ACE**

Causby, Ralph E 300 Woodlawn Avenue, Greensboro, NC 27401, (919) 272-3936, BA 57 Lenoir-Rhyne Coll; MS 63 Univ of TN - Knoxville; Aud/Instr, U of NC-Greensboro, **A**

Causey, Dr G Donald 3504 Dunlop Street, Chevy Chase, MD 20815, (202) 269-4009, BA 50 Univ of MD - College Park; MA 51 Univ of MD - College Park; PH 54 (NS) Purdue Univ - West Lafayette; Research Prof, Cath U of Amer, **SLP A F**

Causey, Susan Jean 1711 South Cleveland Dr, Little Rock, AR 72204, (501) 758-1760, BS 83 Univ of AR - Little Rock; OM 85 Univ of Central AR; **SLP**

Causino, Maryanne 4 Perkins Court, Irvine, CA 92715, (714) 634-5168, BA 77 Coe Coll; MS 85 Emerson Coll; **SLP**

Cavalier, Lynn Ann 1559 11th Street, Trenton, NJ 08638, (609) 989-2600, BS 80 Trenton St Coll; MA 82 Trenton St Coll; 81–Sp-Lang Path, City of Trenton Bd of Educ, **SLP**

Cavalier, Mrs Margaret Grady 46 Elm Drive, Rochester, NY 14609, (716) 482-9290, BS 68 Nazareth Coll of Rochester; MS 73 SUNY - Coll at Geneseo; 70–Sp-Lang Path, Rochester City Sch Dist, **SLP**

Cavalieri, Elizabeth Huckins 8 Watson Street, Dover, NH 03820-4228, (603) 436-8668, BS 81 Univ of NH; MS 83 Univ of WA; Aud, Dana R Fiske, **A**

Cavallo, Dr Stephen A 70 Lasalle Street #11A, New York, NY 10027, (516) 294-8700, BS 75 SUNY - Coll at Oneonta; MS 78 Columbia Univ Teachers Coll; PH 82 (Sp Science) Columbia Univ Teachers Coll; Asst Prof, Adelphi Univ, **SLP**

Cavanagh, Elizabeth 115 Ridge Road, Smithfield, RI 02917, (401) 568-3279, BA 75 Providence Coll; MS 77 Univ of RI; Sp/Lang Path, Glocester Sch Dept, **SLP**

Cavanagh, George J 5012 S W 91st Avenue, Cooper City, FL 33328, (305) 475-6618, BA 61 SUNY - Center at Albany; MA 63 Univ of CT; **SLP LM**

Cavanagh, John M 10800 Paramount 204, Downey, CA 90241, MA 75 CA St Univ - Los Angeles; Aud, John M Cavanagh Inc, **A**

Cavanagh-Bruns, Cynthia R R 1 Box 41, Baldwin, IA 52207, (319) 652-5621, BA 80 Univ of IA; MA 82 Univ of IA; Sp-Lang Path, MS Bend AEA, **SLP**

Cavanah, Mrs Elizabeth 522 Cheshire Avenue, Fort Walton Beach, FL 32548, (904) 244-2161, BA 73 Univ of FL; MS 75 TX Christian Univ; SLP Dept Chairman, Okaloosa Co Sch Board, **SLP**

Cavanaugh, Cathleen Marie 1430 S E 8th Street, Lee's Summit, MO 64063, (816) 525-5470, BA 82 Our Lady Lake Univ-San Anton; MS 83 Southern IL Univ-Edwardsvill; Sp-Lang Path, Deborah A King Assoc Inc, **SLP**

Cavanaugh, Martin Joseph 1005 West La Deney Drive, Ontario, CA 91762, (714) 599-6787, MA 82 CA St Univ - Los Angeles; 86–Spec Educ Mgr, Bonita USD, **SLP**

Cavanaugh-Doud, Crystal 6672 Woodlea, Kalamazoo, MI 49004, (616) 342-5104, BS 79 Western MI Univ; MA 81 Western MI Univ; SLP, Upjohn Healthcare Services, **SLP**

Cave, Cornelia 5410 Netherland Avenue, Apartment A-32, Bronx, NY 10471, (914) 245-4808, BA 75 SUNY - Coll at New Paltz; MA 77 CUNY - City College; MS 84 Bank Street Coll of Educ; SLP, Lakeland Publ Schs, **SLP**

Caverly, Patricia Jean 29732 Mirlon Drive, Farmington Hills, MI 48018, (313) 661-2755, BS 82 Western MI Univ; MA 84 Western MI Univ; Audiologist, Lakeshore ENT, **A**

Caviness, Mrs Rebecca Parker 3580 McGehee Place Drive S, Apartment 901, Montgomery, AL 36111, (205) 284-1870, BS 85 Auburn Univ - Auburn; OM 87 Auburn Univ - Auburn; **A**

Cavitolo, Andrea A 409 South 3rd Street, Philadelphia, PA 19147, (215) 923-1421, BA 75 Saint John's Coll; MA 76 MI St Univ; OD 82 (NS) Villanova Univ; Attorney at Law, Private Practice, **A**

Cawby, Jerry L 3500-399 W Manchester Blvd, Inglewood, CA 90305, (213) 673-3207, BA 72 CA St Univ - Los Angeles; MA 74 CA St Univ - Los Angeles; 72–Sp-Lang Path, LA Co Schs, **SLP**

Cawkwell, Mrs Elizabeth 6221 Fairdel Avenue, Baltimore, MD 21206, (301) 666-0500, BS 72 Towson St Univ; MS 74 Towson St Univ; Sp-Lang Path, Baltimore County Board of Educ, **SLP**

Cawley, Anna P 2019 Ridge, Evanston, IL 60201, (312) 328-2242, MA 73 Univ of IL - Urbana; BS 72 Univ of IL - Urbana; Co-Dir Commun&Behavior Assoc, Evanston Sch Dist 65, **SLP**

Cawn, Mrs Charleyne K 12 Hastings, Highland Park, IL 60035, (312) 432-7936, BS 70 Univ of IL - Urbana; MA 71 Univ of IL - Urbana; Early Chldhood SLP, Sch Dist 108, **SLP**

Cawyer, Mrs S Annette Schaffner 2008 Stradivarius, Carrollton, TX 75007, (214) 931-8304, BS 84 Abilene Christian Univ; MS 86 Univ of TX - Dallas; Sp-Lang Path, Richardson ISD, **SLP**

Cayer, Mrs Nicola Jane 854 24th Street, Brandon, MB, Canada R7B 1Y3, (204) 728-8442, BS 82 Univ of ND; BA 82 Univ of ND; MS 84 Univ of Western Ontario; 86–Sp-Lang Path, Brandon Gen Hosp, **SLP**

Caylor, John E Saco Aud & Hrng Aid Service Inc, 258 Main Street, Saco, ME 04072, (207) 282-5493, BS 69 Univ of WI - Stevens Point; MS 72 Univ of WI - Stevens Point; Aud/Pres, Saco Aud & Hrng Aid Serv Inc, **A**

Cayne, Dr Patricia Denner 510 Park Avenue, New York, NY 10022, (212) 832-1707, BA 60 Univ of PA; MS 84 Columbia Univ Teachers Coll; PH 86 (NS) Columbia Univ Teachers Coll; Private Practice, **SLP**

Cayton, Mrs Georgianne M 4 Cedar Lake Dr, Rt 4, Cordele, GA 31015, (912) 273-0708, BS 74 Huntingdon Coll; MS 76 Auburn Univ - Auburn; Dir & Sp-Lang Path, Cayton Sp & Lang Cen, **SLP**

Caywood, Janet L 1342 West Emerald #386, Mesa, AZ 85202, **SLP**

Cazden, Robert P 207 Peterson Avenue, Louisville, KY 40206, MS 88 Univ of Louisville

Ceballos, Patricia Ann 514 Curie Drive, San Jose, CA 95123, (408) 258-4938, BA 69 Univ of CO - Boulder; MA 72 TX Christian Univ; 83–Sp-Lang Path, Alum Rock Union Elem Sch Dist, **SLP**

Ceccatti, Carol Steffler 14343 Judson Road #206, San Antonio, TX 78233, (512) 493-1415, BS 72 Edinboro Univ of PA; ME 85 Southwest TX St Univ; **SLP**

Cecconi, Christine Rd 4 Box 215-B, North Hunter Lane, Cortland, NY 13045, (607) 272-5891, BA 74 SUNY - Coll at Cortland; MA 75 Bowling Green St Univ; Sp-Lang Path, Special Childrens Center, **SLP**

Cecere, Mrs Debra Lynn 29 Ambassador Drive, Victor, NY 14564, (716) 383-2244, BS 81 SUNY - Coll at Geneseo; MS 82 Ithaca Coll; Sp-Lang Path, Monroe BOCES 1, **SLP**

Cechal, Patricia Jeanne 555 North 89th Street #4, Milwaukee, WI 53226, (414) 259-1414, BS 81 Univ of WI - Madison; MS 84 Univ of WI - Milwaukee; 84–Sp-Lang Path, Curative Rehab Ctr, **SLP**

Cecil, Mrs Elizabeth Ann 5446 Garford Street, Long Beach, CA 90815, (213) 436-7787, MA 83 CA St Univ - Long Beach; Sp-Lang Path, Long Beach Scottish Rite Clin, **SLP**

Cecilsennett, Teresa Marie 411 Winesap Drive, Lafayette, IN 47905, (317) 447-9211, BA 80 Univ of TN - Knoxville; MA 82 Univ of TN - Knoxville; 88–Sp-Lang Path, Rehab Works, **SLP ACE**

Cedar, Ingrid Kristina 730 East McKellips #C-722, Tempe, AZ 85281, (602) 481-9462, **A**

Cegalis, Mrs Nancy Ritchie 142 Dow Road, Hollis, NH 03049, BA 64 SUNY - Coll at Cortland; ME 66 PA St Univ - Univ Park; Sp-Lang Path, Nashua Schs, **SLP**

Cegavske, Beth 14051 Halper Road, Poway, CA 92064, (619) 486-0855, BA 81 SUNY - Center at Binghamton; MS 87 Ithaca Coll; 88–Aud, Hearing Dynamics

Cekada-Kruesel, Mrs Julie A 1130 Sunset Court, Grafton, WI 53024, (414) 673-2100, BS 79 Univ of WI - Milwaukee; MS 81 Univ of WI - Milwaukee; Sp-Lang Path, Hartford Jt Dist #1, **SLP**

Celebre, Mrs Dorothy L 109 Willow Road, Wallingford, PA 19086, (215) 874-8271, BS 71 Purdue Univ - West Lafayette; MA 76 West Chester Univ of PA; Sp-Lang Path, Private Practice, **SLP**

Celentano, Nancy A 1930 Park Avenue, East Meadow, NY 11554, (516) 794-6157, BA 85 IN Univ - Bloomington; MA 87 Univ of CT

Celli, Anita M 125 East Madison Street, Villa Park, IL 60181, (312) 352-1806, BS 78 SUNY - Center at Albany; MS 80 Southern IL Univ -Carbondale; 80–Sp-Lang Path, School District 105, **SLP**

Celotto, Janet 356 Townsend Avenue, New Haven, CT 06512, (203) 467-9249, BA 84 Southern CT St Univ; MS 86 Southern CT St Univ; 86–Sp-Lang Path, New Haven Bd of Educ, **SLP**

Cendejas, Deena L 9807 South Karlov #204-S, Oak Lawn, IL 60453, (312) 599-5550, BS 77 Northern IL Univ - De Kalb; MA 79 Northern IL Univ - De Kalb; 79–Sp-Lang Path, Ridgeland Pub Sch Dist #122, **SLP**

Cendroski, Julie Whiting 2109 Jasmine, Denton, TX 76205, (214) 420-1437, BS 83 Univ of North TX; MS 85 Univ of North TX; 85–Aud, No TX Phys & Surg, **A**

Cenk, Mrs Susan Talavera 1560 Common Drive, El Paso, TX 79936, (915) 895-1622, BA 82 Univ of TX - El Paso; MS 86 Univ of TX - El Paso; 83–Sp-Lang Path, El Paso Independent Sch Dist, **SLP**

Centeno, Jose Gregorio 30-44 29th Street #7-D, Astoria, NY 11102, (212) 238-7870, MA 85 Hofstra Univ; Sp-Lang Path, Gouverneur Hosp, **SLP**

Center, Dr Benjamin 20311 N E 10th Place, North Miami Beach, FL 33179, (305) 836-1940, BS 46 OH St Univ; MA 65 OH St Univ; PH 71 (NS) OH St Univ; Private Practice, **SLP**

Centini, Philippa G 3100 N E 48th Street #315, Fort Lauderdale, FL 33308, (305) 977-2297, BA 68 CUNY - Hunter Coll; MS 71 CUNY - Lehman Coll; MS 86 Nova Univ; 88–Sp-Lang Path, Broward County Sch Bd, **SLP**

Centurioni, Dr Kathleen 615 Stonybrook Drive, Jeffersonville, PA 19401, (215) 539-6600, BS 64 Duquesne Univ; ME 65; PH 72 (NS) Wayne St Univ; Dir of Prof Ser, Chld Devel Cen, **A**

Cepeda, Mrs Bernice Teresa 7 Starlifter Circle, Norton Afb, San Bernardino, CA 92409, (714) 885-2096, BS 80 Univ of OR; MS 86 Univ of Redlands; 86–Tchr, San Bernardino Co Supt Schs, **SLP**

Cepinko, Barbara H 6312 E Santa Ana Canyon Rd, Suite 349, Anaheim Hills, CA 92807, (714) 998-6041, **SLP**

Cera, Nancy M Rt 3 Box 117H, Bridgeville, DE 19933, (302) 284-9611, BA 84 OH St Univ; MA 86 Kent St Univ; SLP, Lake Forest Schools, **SLP**

Cera, Mrs Roselyn M 2152 St Clair Court, Girard, OH 44420, (216) 746-7211, BA 76 Univ of Akron; MA 77 Kent St Univ; Sp-Lang Path, St Elizabeth Hosp Med Cen, **SLP**

Ceragioli, Mrs Joan D 21500 Califa Street #189, Woodland Hills, CA 91367, (213) 348-3395, BA 76 CA St Univ - Northridge; MA 79 CA St Univ - Northridge; SLP, Los Angeles City Schools, **SLP**

Cercone, Judith A 445 Richmond Park West, Richmond Heights, OH 44143, (216) 444-5370, BS 78 Carlow Coll; MA 80 Univ of Pittsburgh - Pittsburgh; Aud, Cleveland Cl Found, **A**

Cereo, Carol A 634 Delmar Place, Syracuse, NY 13208, (315) 425-4570, BS 73 SUNY - Coll at Geneseo; MA 74 Western MI Univ; SLP, Syracuse Cty Sch Dist, **SLP**

Cerf, Dr F Ann 12104 N E 141st, Kirkland, WA 98033, (206) 543-7988, BA 49 WV Univ; MA 50 WV Univ; PH 72 (NS) Univ of WA; Asssistant Professor, Univ of Washington/Dept Speech, **SLP**

Ceriotti, Mary Ann 1234 Divisidero, San Francisco, CA 94115, (415) 921-7658, BS 53 Washington Univ; 63–Dir-Prog for Aphasic Chldn, San Francisco Hrng & Sp Cen, **SLP**

Cerni, Mrs Carol A 1750 Dumont Drive, Mineral Ridge, OH 44440, (216) 758-6689, MA 84 Kent St Univ; Sp-Lang Path, Boardman Local Schools, **SLP**

Cero, Lianne Christine R R 3 Box 250, Milan, IL 61264, BA 80 Augustana Coll; MA 82 Univ of OR; Sp-Lang Path, Easter Seal Fnd, **SLP**

Ceron, Mrs Mildred Viera 250 West 103rd Street, New York, NY 10025, (212) 865-4849, MS 87 Columbia Univ Teachers Coll; 88–Sp-Lang Path, Columbia Presbyterian Med Ctr, **SLP**

Certner-Smith, Marilyn 58 Headley Place, Maplewood, NJ 07040, (201) 731-3600, BS 74 Ithaca Coll; MA 75 Univ of IL - Urbana; Assoc Dir Sp & Aud, Kessler I for Rehab, **SLP**

Cerullo, Mrs Jane K 103 Newman Road, Unit 2, Malden, MA 02148-3945, (617) 397-0372, BA 81 Bridgewater St Coll; MS 83 PA St Univ - Univ Park; 86–Aud, Beverly Hosp, **A**

Cervenka, Mrs Linda Marie 2646 Home Avenue, Berwyn, IL 60402, (312) 795-4470, BS 84 Elmhurst Coll; MA 86 Univ of IL - Urbana; 87–Sp-Lang Path, Proviso Area for Excep Chldn, **SLP**

Cervetti, Carma Call 1616 Coal S E #C, Albuquerque, NM 87106, **SLP**

Cesari, Mrs Belinda Ann 295 Landfall Road, Atlanta, GA 30328, (404) 847-9911, **SLP**

Cesco, Penny Suzanne 9275 White Pine Drive, Loveland, OH 45140-1101, (513) 742-1500, BA 77 Marshall Univ; MA 80 Marshall Univ; **SLP**

Cesnik, Mrs Sharon Doyle 124 Greenmont, Cary, NC 27511, (919) 469-1468, BS 83 Purdue Univ - West Lafayette; MS 84 Purdue Univ - West Lafayette; Sp-Lang Path, **SLP**

Cessaris, Ann Clarke Key Communication, 671 Oak Grove Avenue Suite E, Menlo Park, CA 94025, (415) 321-7936, MA 65 IN Univ - Bloomington; Director, Key Communication, **SLP**

Cessna, Mrs Susan Adams 810 Vance Drive, Lander, WY 82520, (307) 332-4960, BS 76 Moorhead St Univ; MS 84 Moorhead St Univ; **SLP**

Cetak, M J 777 N W 62nd Street #C-105, Miami, FL 33138-4331, (509) 248-3950, BA 75 Central WA Univ; MS 75 Central WA Univ

Cetin, Patricia Davis 2903 Helen Court Apt B, Champaign, IL 61821, (217) 351-3811, BS 82 Univ of IL - Urbana; MS 83 Univ of IL - Urbana; 88–Sp-Lang Path, Champaign USD, **SLP**

Cevasco, Rita Marie 14707 London Lane, Bowie, MD 20715, (301) 652-8997, BS 84 Kent St Univ; MA 84 Kent St Univ; Sp-Lang Path, Private Practice, **SLP**

Cevette, Dr Michael J Mayo Clinic Scottsdale, 13400 East Shea Boulevard, Scottsdale, AZ 85259, (800) 225-2845, BA 72 Univ of NV - Las Vegas; MS 76 UT St Univ; PH 87 (Aud) Univ of UT; Aud, Mayo Clinic Scottsdale, **A**

Chaback, Mrs Laurey W 31 South Pond Circle, Cheshire, CT 06410-0796, (203) 271-2342, BA 76 Hofstra Univ; MA 77 Hofstra Univ; Sp-Lang Path, Cheshire PS, **SLP**

Chabon, Dr Shelly S 1246 River Sound Court, Marietta, GA 30068, MS 72 PA St Univ - Univ Park; MS 76 Towson St Univ; PH 80 (Sp-Lang Path) Univ of Pittsburgh - Pittsburgh; Coord Sp-Lang & Hearing, Atlanta Speech Sch, **SLP**

Chabot, Theresa E 47 Stowell Road, Bedford, NH 03102, (603) 472-5955, BS 75 Keene St Coll; MA 79 Ball St Univ; Sp-Lang Path, Private Practice, **SLP**

Chace, Carmel Joan 5606 Charlotte Way, Livermore, CA 94550, (415) 443-4053, BS 77 CA St Univ - Hayward; MA 82 CA St Univ - Fresno; 87–Sp/Lang Path, Carmel Chace-Sp & Lang Svcs, **SLP**

Chachere, Mrs Arlene Caillier 116 N Tanglewood Drive, Eunice, LA 70535, (318) 457-1250, BS 82 LA St Univ - Baton Rouge; MS 85 Univ of Southwestern LA; 87–Sp-Lang Path, Rehab Svcs Ltd, **SLP**

Chadd, Nancy L 651 Tokay Avenue, Ukiah, CA 95482, (707) 485-8455, BA 79 CA St Univ - Northridge; MA 80 CA St Univ - Northridge; SLP, Mendocino Co Sch, **SLP**

Chadden, Marguerite 2722 West Genesee Street, Lapeer, MI 48446, (313) 664-2951, BS 69 Eastern MI Univ; MA 71 Eastern MI Univ; Sp/Lang Path, Oakdale Reg Cen Dev Dis, **SLP**

Chadwell, Daniel L 2023 South 146th Circle, Omaha, NE 68144, (402) 333-2270, PH 78 (NS) Bowling Green St Univ; Audiologist, Veterans Administration, **A**

Chadwick, Abbie B 25006 Barmby, Spring, TX 77389, (713) 351-1442, BA 75 Univ of MS; MA 77 Memphis St Univ; Sp-Lang Path, Klein ISD, **SLP**

Chadwick, Carol 4465 East County Line Road, Erie, CO 80516, (303) 659-4090, BS 69 Univ of WY; MS 70 CO St Univ; Sp/Lang Path, Private Practice, **SLP**

Chadwick, Donna M 9 Sawmill Drive, Westford, MA 01886, (617) 277-9340, OB 69 Anna Maria Coll; MS 75 Emerson Coll; Chmn Music Dept, Emmanuel Coll, **SLP**

Chadwick, Jean M 824 East Pontiac, Fresno, CA 93704, (209) 935-2088, BA 74 CA St Univ - Fresno; MA 76 CA St Univ - Fresno; Sp-Lang Path, Coalinga Unified School Dis, **SLP**

Chadwick, Julie Carr N Mississippi Retardation Ctr, P O Box 967, Oxford, MS 38655, (601) 234-1476, BA 75 Belhaven Coll; MS 81 Univ of MS; Sp/Lang Path, N MS Retardation Ctr, **SLP**

Chadwick, Marilyn A 201 Lockwood Road, Syracuse, NY 13214, (315) 446-7660, BS 73 Eastern MI Univ; MA 74 Eastern MI Univ; Sp-Lang Path, Syracuse City Sch Dist, **SLP ACE**

Chadwick, Susan G 5305 Landgrave Lane, Springfield, VA 22151, (703) 321-7108, BA 70 George Washington Univ; MA 71 George Washington Univ; **A**

Chaffart, Mrs Lynona Ann P O Box 6179, Porcupine Mall Sub, South Porcupine, ON, Canada P0N 1K0, (705) 235-5307, BS 84 Walla Walla Coll; MS 88 Univ of AZ; 88–Sp-Lang Path, Porcupine Health Unit

Chaffee, Kim A 2941 West Centennial Drive, Apartment F-308, Littleton, CO 80123, BS 84 CO St Univ; MS 86 CO St Univ; **SLP**

Chaffee, Shon M 10685 East Bend Road, Burlington, KY 41005, (513) 721-2611, BS 80 Heidelberg Coll; BS 82 Bowling Green St Univ; MS 86 Univ of MI - Ann Arbor; 86–Aud, Otologists Inc, **A**

Chaffinch-Coyne, Janie Olivia 201 Edgevale #3-B, Baltimore, MD 21210, (814) 865-5414, BS 81 PA St Univ - Univ Park; MS 84 PA St Univ - Univ Park; **A**

Chafin, Mrs Patricia A 112 River Park Circle, Munroe Falls, OH 44262, (216) 688-8201, BS 75 Kent St Univ; MA 77 Kent St Univ; 88–Sp-Lang Path, Green Local Schs, **SLP**

Chafin, Peggy J 3672 Providence Road, Newtown Square, PA 19073, (215) 353-9804, BA 68 Marshall Univ; MA 73 Temple Univ-Tyler Sch of Art; Dir/Aud-Admin/Ent Cl, Elwyn I, **A**

Chagnon, Kathleen J 828B 66th Place S E, Everett, WA 98203, (206) 335-1570, BS 75 Eastern Montana Coll; MS 77 Eastern WA Univ; Sp-Lang Path, Lake Stevens School District, **SLP**

Chagnon, Maryann T 641 West Allenton Road, North Kingstown, RI 02852-6509, (401) 728-2120, BA 69 RI Coll; MS 72 Univ of RI; Sp-Lang Path, Pawtucket Sch Dept, **SLP**

Chaiet, Lori 611 Watertown Street #12, Newton, MA 02160, (617) 527-7927, MS 76 Boston Univ; Sp-Lang Path, Burlington Public Schools, **SLP**

Chaiken, Rita Rosinek 2793B Clairmont Road Suite 2, Atlanta, GA 30329, (404) 634-8781, BS 73 Syracuse Univ; MS 75 Emory Univ; MS 75 Emory Univ; Aud, North Georgia Hearing Serv Inc, **A**

Chaikin, Lauren B 37 Gorham Avenue #1, Brookline, MA 02146, (617) 739-7018, MS 88 Boston Univ

Chaiklin, Dr Joseph B 5113 Belle Drive, Metairie, LA 70006, (504) 589-5566, BA 52 Univ of CT; MA 53 OH St Univ; PH 58 (NS) Stanford Univ; Superv Aud Sect, VA Med Cen - New Orleans, **A F**

Chaitkin, Barbara A 66 Sanders Street, Staten Island, NY 10303, (718) 698-9558, BA 79 Saint Joseph's Coll; MA 81 NY Univ; 87–Sp-Lang Path, Prog for Spec Children, **SLP**

Chakurda, Mrs Diane Ronee 116 Elysian Street, Pittsburgh, PA 15206, (412) 394-5815, BS 77 Univ of Pittsburgh - Pittsburgh; MA 80 Univ of Pittsburgh - Pittsburgh; SLP, Allegheny Inter Ut #3, **SLP**

Chalfant, Gail Ann 5280 North Little Mountain, Apartment H-14, San Bernardino, CA 92407, (714) 887-2335, BA 82 Univ of Redlands; MS 83 Univ of Redlands; Sp-Lang Path, Scottish Rite Clinic, **SLP**

Chalfant, Joyce S 3779 Bakerstown Road, Gibsonia, PA 15044, (412) 443-7740, BS 72 IA St Univ; MS 74 Univ of KS; **SLP**

Chalfin, Mrs Ellen M 5950 Buttonwood Drive, Noblesville, IN 46060-9129, (317) 776-0840, BS 76 Ball St Univ; MA 79 Ball St Univ; SLP, Noblesville Schools, **SLP**

Chalfin-Rosenblum, Roberta 70 Smith Avenue, White Plains, NY 10605, (914) 347-4665, BA 74 CUNY - Brooklyn Coll; MA 77 Columbia Univ Teachers Coll; Aud, Ment Ret I Wcc, **A**

Chalfonte-Evans, Melinda 12032 Cooperwood Lane, Cincinnati, OH 45242-6321, (513) 791-7522, BS 78 Miami Univ - Oxford; MS 79 Miami Univ - Oxford; 84–Sp-Lang Path, Cincinnati Ctr for Dev Disorders, **SLP**

Chaligne, Mrs Carol Grimes 6603 Great Northern Blvd, Austin, TX 78731, (512) 454-8631, BA 77 TX Tech Univ; MA 80 Univ of TX - Austin; Sp-Lang Path, TX Sch for Blind, **SLP**

Challenger, Mrs Sandra S 109 Elk Street, Syracuse, NY 13205-1505, (315) 425-0507, BA 78 Syracuse Univ; MS 87 Syracuse Univ

Chalmers, Crystal L 1050 Gillman Drive, Colma, CA 94015-2001, (415) 346-1723, BA 80 Minot St Univ; MS 81 Minot St Univ; Aud, Aud Serv of San Francisco

Chalmers, Elizabeth 2026 Danville Park Drive, Decatur, AL 35603, (205) 356-9627, MS 75 Univ of South FL; Sp-Lang Path, Dept of Ment Health, **SLP**

Chalmers, Mrs Joyce S 865 Hanlon Way, Benicia, CA 94510, (707) 643-8681, BA 70 CA St Univ - Long Beach; MA 71 CA St Univ - Long Beach; 86–Sp-Lang Path, Vallejo USD, **SLP**

Chalupa, Linda A R 1 Box 142-B, New Lenox, IL 60459, (312) 726-9420, OB 72 Northern IL Univ - De Kalb; MS 74 Northern IL Univ - De Kalb; Sp-Lang Path, Private Practice, **SLP**

Chambelain, Jo Ann K 2219 Coachmans Drive, Germantown, TN 38138, (901) 754-1853, BS 67 Southern IL Univ -Carbondale; MA 75 Memphis St Univ; Dir, Germantown Sp Therapy Cen, **SLP**

Chamberlain, Mrs Catherine P O Box 11022, Lexington, KY 40512, (606) 299-4510, BA 71 Univ of KY; MA 75 Univ of KY; Sp-Lang Path, Fayette County Board of Educ, **SLP**

Chamberlain, Cheryl E 183 South Shore Drive, South Weymouth, MA 02664, (617) 771-0642, BS 85 Elmira Coll; MS 87 Northeastern Univ; **SLP**

Chamberlain, Mrs Karen Shilliday 550 Pacific Avenue, York, PA 17404, (717) 757-1531, BS 84 Kent St Univ; MA 84 Kent St Univ; 85–Sp-Lang Path, Lincoln Intermed Unit #12, **SLP**

Chamberlain, Lisa Lynn 9613-E West Chatfield Avenue, Littleton, CO 80123, BS 83 Northern IL Univ - De Kalb; MA 84 Northern IL Univ - De Kalb; Sp-Lang Path, Porter Memorial Hospital, **SLP**

Chamberlain, Lourdes Marie 8993 Groveside Drive, Strongsville, OH 44136, (216) 234-3565, BS 84 Miami Univ - Oxford; **SLP**

Chamberlain, Martha H Route 7 Box 85, Murray, KY 42071, (901) 642-0961, BS 73 Murray St Univ; MS 76 Murray St Univ; SLP, Paris Sp Sch Dist, **SLP**

Chamberlain, Ruth I 139 N W Gladis, Port Charlotte, FL 33952, (813) 625-5898, BA 29 Drury Coll; MA 67 Univ of AR - Fayetteville; **SLP LM**

Chamberlain, Mrs Sandra L D 105 Western Avenue, Westfield, MA 01085, (203) 745-0938, BA 66 Univ of ME - Orono; MA 68 Univ of CT; Sp-Lang Path, Enfield Pub Sch, **SLP**

Chamberlin, Lynn Louise 1249 N E 168th Street, Seattle, WA 98155, (206) 326-5976, BA 75 Univ of WA; OM 77 Univ of WA; Sp-Lang Path, Providence Med Ctr-Home Care, **SLP**

Chambers, C Lynn 25 South Street, Rockport, MA 01966, (617) 642-0222, BA 72 Thiel Coll; MS 77 Emerson Coll; 88–Sp-Lang Path, EK Shriver Ctr-UAP Cast, **SLP**

Chambers, Carol J 5423 Dale Lane, Orlando, FL 32822, (407) 422-4927, BA 78 SUNY - Center at Buffalo; MA 81 CA St Univ - Los Angeles; Audiologist, John P Taggart MD PA, **A**

Chambers, Mrs Carole Schaffer 222 Wayside Place, Anaheim, CA 92805, (714) 774-3562, BA 81 CA St Univ - Fullerton; MA 82 SUNY - Coll at Geneseo; 87–Sp-Lang Path, Craig & Ford Inc, **SLP**

Chambers, Constance 213 Carlton Lane, North Andover, MA 01845, **SLP**

Chambers, Mrs Dorothy L 2631 9th Street South, Wisconsin Rapids, WI 54494, (602) 974-2457, MS 72 Univ of WI - Stevens Point; BA 44 Univ of MI - Ann Arbor; **SLP LM**

Chambers, Dorothy R 12414 S E Oatfield Road, Milwaukie, OR 97222, (503) 232-2458, BS 64 Marquette Univ; MS 68 Univ of San Francisco; Prog Develop Spec, Portland Pub Sch, **SLP**

Chambers, Mrs Floy Beth 11234 Spring Pine, San Antonio, TX 78249, (512) 299-5500, BA 71 Abilene Christian Univ; MS 75 East TX St Univ - Commerce; SLP, San Antonio ISD, **SLP**

Chambers, Mrs Helen G 3440 Olentangy River Road, Apartment M4, Columbus, OH 43202, (614) 267-6663, BA 32 Case Western Reserve Univ; MA 59 Case Western Reserve Univ; **SLP LM**

Chambers, Mrs Jane C 3915 West Vassar, Visalia, CA 93277, (209) 782-2692, OB 71 Univ of OK - Norman; MA 75 Univ of OK - Norman; OM 85 CA St Coll - Bakersfield; 79–Sp-Lang Path, Porterville Dev Ctr, **SLP**

Chambers, Katherine E 2615 East Randolph, Enid, OK 73701, (405) 234-3734, BA 72 Phillips Univ; MS 77 Phillips Univ; 79–Sp-Lang Path, Hedges Comm Sp & Hrng Ctr, **SLP**

Chambers, Lisa Young 746 Fairmont Pike, Wheeling, WV 26003, (304) 242-1390, BS 82 WV Univ; MS 83 WV Univ; Sp-Lang Path, Easter Seals Wheeling, **SLP**

Chambers, Nancy C 4545 Centerview Drive #180, San Antonio, TX 78228, (512) 735-9505, BA 60 Our Lady Lake Univ-San Anton; ME 62 Our Lady Lake Univ-San Anton; Director, San Antonio Spch,Lang,Hrng Ser, **SLP**

Chambers, Nancy C 750 D Street, Madras, OR 97741, (503) 553-1161, BA 71 WA St Univ; MA 73 WA St Univ; Sp-Lang Path, Jefferson County Esd, **SLP**

Chambers, Patricia L P O Box 557, Half Moon Bay, CA 94019, (415) 476-6896, BS 73 Univ of HI - Manoa; MS 74 Univ of HI - Manoa; Research Asst, Univ of CA, **SLP**

Chambers, Patricia Rodney 4377 South Ceylon Street, Aurora, CO 80015, BA 74 Elmira Coll; MS 77 Coll of Saint Rose; Sp-Lang Path, **SLP**

Chambers, Dr Ron D Dept Speech & Hearing Sciences, University Of Illinois, 901 South 6th Street, Champaign, IL 61820, (217) 333-2230, BA 73 TX Tech Univ; MS 76 TX Tech Univ; PH 83 (Aud) Purdue Univ - West Lafayette; 84–Asst Prof, Univ of IL, **A**

Chambers, Dr Ronald Dean Communicative Disorders & Sci, Wichita State University, Box 75, Wichita, KS 67208, (316) 689-3240, BA 64 Wichita St Univ; MA 68 Wichita St Univ; PH 79 (NS) Wichita St Univ; Asst Prof, Wichita St U, **SLP**

Chambers, Mrs Toni Furman R R 4 Box 197, Charleston, IL 61920, (217) 258-2568, BS 80 Eastern IL Univ; MS 81 Eastern IL Univ; SLP, Sarah Bush Lincoln Health Cen, **SLP**

Chamblee, Mrs Barbara Fowler 304 Ashland Lane, Birmingham, AL 35226, (205) 674-6481, BA 80 Univ of AL-Tuscaloosa; MS 81 Univ of AL- Tuscaloosa; SLP, Jefferson Co Bd of Ed, **SLP**

Chamblin, Diana Lynne 1713 West Highway 50 #75, O'Fallon, IL 62269, (618) 465-0105, BS 82 Southern IL Univ-Edwardsvill; MS 85 Southern IL Univ-Edwardsvill; **SLP**

Chambliss, Mrs Colleen M 202 Cleveland Road, Sebring, FL 33870, (813) 385-5448, BA 66; MA 68; Sp-Lang Path, **SLP**

Chambliss, Marcia J 2207 Meadow Gardens Drive, Houston, TX 77062-4713, (713) 332-8538, BS 72 Univ of TX - Austin; MA 73 Univ of Houston - Univ Park; Ed Diagnostician, Clear Crk ISD, **SLP**

Chamoun, Vivian Louise 829 Oakhurst Avenue, Clarksdale, MS 38614, (601) 624-5247, BS 79 Univ Southern MS-Hattiesburg; MS 83 Univ Southern MS-Hattiesburg; Sp-Lang Path, Coahoma Co Sch Dist, **SLP**

Champ, Carmela L 645 Flmwood Drive, Winter Springs, FL 32708, MS 79 FL St Univ; Self Contained Lang Disorders, Seminole County Schools Bd, **SLP**

Champagne, Jodie Richard 4537 East Meadow Lane, Lake Charles, LA 70605, (318) 436-3277, BA 81 Univ of Southwestern LA; MS 86 Univ of Southwestern LA; 88–Sp-Lang Path, Acadian Hearing-Sp Services, **SLP**

Champagne, Mrs Virginia Greeley 62 Yeomans Avenue, Medford, MA 02155, (617) 395-5372, BA 76 Boston Coll; MS 78 Univ of Southwestern LA; Sp-Lang Path, Andover Public Schools, **SLP**

Champion, Cynthia Carter 2261 Crescent Hill Drive, Mebane, NC 27302, (919) 946-8131, BA 82 Univ of NC - Chapel Hill; MS 85 Univ of NC - Chapel Hill; **SLP**

Champion, Tempii Bridgene 334 Eastern Parkway, Apt #5H, Brooklyn, NY 11225, (718) 953-9131, BS 83 Northeastern Univ; MA 86 Hampton Univ; Sp-Lang Path, Private Practice, **SLP**

Champion, William N 1956 Coral Gardens Drive, Fort Lauderdale, FL 33306, MS; **SLP LM**

Champlain, Mary Catherine Middlesex Garden Apartment, Apartment 6-F, Ferdonia, NY 14063, (716) 679-4234, BS 86 SUNY - Coll at Geneseo; MA 87 SUNY - Coll at Geneseo

Champley, Mrs Jill Leslie 2365 South Cypress, Wichita, KS 67207, (316) 689-4820, BS 83 KS St Univ; MS 85 Univ of OK - OK City; Sp-Lang Path, St Joseph Med Ctr, **SLP**

Champlin, Dr Craig A Department Of Psychology, University Of Texas, Austin, TX 78712, (512) 471-1704, BA 78; MA 82 Univ of KS; Aud, Univ Kan, **A**

Champlin, Jeanne M 5675 Whimsical Drive, Colorado Springs, CO 80917, (303) 596-7275, BS 54; MS 80; Sp-Lang Path, Spec Sch Dist St Louis Co, **SLP**

Champlin, Lisa D 6405 Roe Street, Cincinnati, OH 45227, (513) 272-0033, BS 76 Univ of Cincinnati; MA 78 Univ of Cincinnati; SLP, United Home Care, **SLP**

Champoux, Dr Ronald Roland Dept Communication Disorders, Bloomsburg State College, Bloomsburg, PA 17815, (717) 389-4443, MA 71 Univ of MI - Ann Arbor; MS 73 Univ of MI - Ann Arbor; PH 81 (NS) Univ of MI - Ann Arbor; Assoc Prof, Bloomsburg U, **SLP ACE**

Chan, Mrs Brenda Miu-Ying 2837 Henderson Street, West Lafayette, IN 47906, (317) 497-0655, SLP, **SLP**

Chan, Karen Pui-Lee 16 Ko Shan Village 2nd/F, Cheung Chau Island, Hong Kong, BS 84 IL St Univ - Normal; MS 85 IL St Univ - Normal; 83–Sp-Lang Path, Duch Kent Chldn Hosp at Sandy Bay, **SLP**

Chan, Mrs Nancy T 5601 Merrimac Road, Montreal, PQ, Canada H4W 1S5, (514) 937-6011, BA 57 Denison Univ; MA 60 Univ of MD - College Park; 77–Dir,Dept of Sp-Path and Aud, Montreal Gen Hosp, **SLP**

Chan, Susie 309 West 23rd Place, Chicago, IL 60616, (312) 955-2133, BS 77 Univ of IL - Urbana; MA 78 Northern IL Univ - De Kalb; Sp/Lang Path, Chi Bd of Ed, **SLP**

Chance, Mrs Linda B 636 East Southfield Road, Shreveport, LA 71105, (318) 635-1132, BA 75 LA St Univ - Shreveport; OM 76 Univ of MS; OM 77 Univ of MS; Sp-Lang Path, Caddo Parish Sch Bd, **SLP**

Chancellor, Jana L 1313 West Burnett, Ennis, TX 75119, (214) 875-6688, BS 77 TX Christian Univ; MS 78 TX Christian Univ; **SLP**

Chancey, Mrs Ina M 2407 Tanglewood Drive, New Port Richey, FL 33552, (813) 848-3402, MS 78 Univ of South FL; Superv Sp-Lang Path, Whittley Rehab Assoc, **SLP**

Chandler, Burke 1104 Stanley, Ardmore, OK 73401, (405) 223-3810, MA 75 Univ of Tulsa; Aud, The Hearing Clinic, **A**

Chandler, Cecelia M P O Box 9101, Ketchikan, AK 99901, (907) 225-1594, BS 72 AZ St Univ; MS 75 AZ St Univ; **SLP**

Chandler, David W 2 Athey Court, Burtonsville, MD 20866, (202) 576-1646, Audiologist, Walter Reed Army Hospital, **A**

Chandler, Elizabeth Frances 5330 North 20th Street, Phoenix, AZ 85016, (602) 263-0463, **SLP**

Chandler, Emily D 137 Shooting Star, Foster City, CA 94404, (415) 345-3033, BA 64; MA 71; SLP, Private Practice, **SLP**

Chandler, Mrs Jill Porter Route 3 Scenic Drive, Lenoir City, TN 37771, (615) 986-3262, BS 83 Univ of TN - Knoxville; MA 85 Univ of TN - Knoxville; **SLP**

Chandler, Jill S 2314 Meadowmont, San Jose, CA 95133, (408) 977-4557, BA 74 San Jose St Univ; MA 76 San Jose St Univ; Director Sp-Lang Path, San Jose Med Ctr, **SLP ACE**

Chandler, Julie Scharff 1435 Sycamore Lane, Northbrook, IL 60062, (312) 272-8829, BA 83 Univ of CO - Boulder; MA 86 Northern IL Univ - De Kalb; Sp-Lang Path, District 36, **SLP**

Chandler, Mrs Mary Kay W 8518 Sugarman Drive, La Jolla, CA 92037, (619) 277-3411, BS 67 Purdue Univ - West Lafayette; MS 68 CO St Univ; Tchr, San Diego USD, **SLP**

Chandler, Mrs Yolande V 2483 Valleydale Road, Stow, OH 44224, (216) 297-7605, BA 74; MS 76 Kent St Univ; Sp-Lang Path, Aurora Pub Sch, **SLP**

Chandler-Rosenblatt, Cheryl Gay 1409 Pennsylvania Avenue N, Minneapolis, MN 55427, (612) 588-5344, **SLP**

Chaney, Amy M 124 Chatham Woods Drive, Cary, NC 27511, BA 84 Univ of NC - Chapel Hill; MS 86 Univ of NC - Chapel Hill; **SLP**

Chaney, Dr Carolyn 313 Lakeview Way, Redwood City, CA 94062, (415) 338-1195, BS 67 PA St Univ - Univ Park; MS 68 Univ of MI - Ann Arbor; ED 77 (Applied Psycholinguistics) Boston Univ; 84–Assoc Prof of Sp Commun, San Francisco State Univ, **SLP**

Chaney, Mrs Gayle Lynn 1445 Grant Circle, Spartanburg, SC 29302, (803) 585-7711, BS 76 IN Univ - Bloomington; MA 84 Ball St Univ; Hd of Aud Dept, Sc Schl for Deaf & Blind, **A**

Chaney, Mrs Jeanine Schmidt 2051 Townhill Drive, Cincinnati, OH 45238, (513) 742-2200, **SLP**

Chaney, Joyce Marie 2415 Dawson Road #B-7, Albany, GA 31707, (912) 883-1425, BS 82 Univ of GA; ME 83 Univ of GA; 88–Sp-Lang Path, Dougherty Co Bd of Educ, **SLP**

Chaney, Dr Robert B, Jr Speech And Hearing Clinic, University Of Montana, Missoula, MT 59801, (406) 243-4131, BA 58 Univ of MT; MA 60 Univ of MT; PH 65 (NS) Stanford Univ; Prof of Aud, University of Montana, **A**

Chaney, Mrs Sarah Lanier 3411 Winding Lane, Haines City, FL 33844, (813) 422-1389, BA 70 Southeastern Coll; ME 73 Rollins Coll; MA 82 Univ of Central FL; Sp/Lang Path, Polk Co Sch Bd, **SLP**

Chaney, Victoria Lea 6254 Woodland Drive, Dallas, TX 75225, (214) 348-1240, BS 76 Southern Methodist Univ; MS 77 Southern Methodist Univ; **SLP**

Chang, Mrs Laura Gethard 1559 Everglade Circle, Placentia, CA 92670-4007, (714) 879-5050, BA Whittier Coll; MA 84 Whittier Coll; Sp-Lang Path, Fullerton School District, **SLP**

Chang, Robert K 2402 California Avenue, Apartment 308, San Francisco, CA 94115, (415) 433-7945, BA 67; MA 71 Univ of MO - Columbia; Owner, Sino American Hearing Aid Cen, **A**

Channell, Dr Ron W Brigham Young University, 128 Tlrb, Provo, UT 84602, (801) 378-6457, BS 77 Brigham Young Univ; MS 79 Brigham Young Univ; PH 83 (Sp-Lang Path) Univ of UT; 83–Asst Prof, Brigham Young Univ, **SLP**

Channell, Mrs Sandy S 719 North 945 West, Orem, UT 84057, (801) 225-1526, BS 78 Brigham Young Univ; OM 87 Brigham Young Univ; 87–Sp-Lang Path, Nebo Sch Dist, **SLP**

Channon, Mrs Lisa Kerstin 5885 Forest View Road #630, Lisle, IL 60532, (312) 971-8951, MA 88 Univ of IL - Urbana; 88–Sp-Lang Path, Aurora Sch Dist #131

Chao, I-Na 3908 Morrison Circle, Norman, OK 73072, (405) 238-6401, BS 71 Nat'l Cheng Kung Univ - Tawian; MS 80 Phillips Univ; Aud Serv Superv, Pauls Valley State Sch, **A**

Chapa, Mrs Mary Anne P O Box 20163, Columbus, OH 43220, (614) 459-0319, BA 74 Univ of Akron; MA 77 OH St Univ; **SLP**

Chapa, Virginia Fiastro 543 Rutile Drive, Ponte Vedra Beach, FL 32082, (904) 390-1143, BS 78 Towson St Univ; MS 79 Loyola Coll; Superv Sp-Lang Path, Baptist Med Cen, **SLP**

Chapell, Patti E 6706 New Hope Drive, Springfield, VA 22151, **SLP**

Chapey, Dr Geraldine 243 Beach 135th Street, Belle Harbor, NY 11694, (718) 447-4343, MA 62 CUNY - Brooklyn Coll; ED 75 (NS) Fordham Univ; Prof, St Johns Univ, **SLP**

Chapey, Dr Roberta Department Of Speech, Brooklyn College, Brooklyn, NY 11210, (212) 988-4541, BA 64 Marymount Coll; MA 65 NY Univ; ED 75 (NS) Columbia Univ Teachers Coll; Professor, Brooklyn Coll-CUNY, **SLP**

Chaplick, Susan C 770 South 6th Street, Philadelphia, PA 19147, (215) 427-5488, BS 79 East Stroudsburg Univ of PA; MS 83 Boston Univ; 88–Sp-Lang Path, St Christophers Hosp for Chldr, **SLP**

Chaplin, Mrs Beulah Mae 1039 North 8th Street, Rochelle, IL 61068, BS 64 Eastern IL Univ; MA 70 Northern IL Univ - De Kalb; SLP, Sch Dist #231, **SLP**

Chaplin, Mrs Beverly Fagen 1960 Lombardy Drive, La Canada, CA 91011, BA 72 SUNY - Center at Buffalo; MA 82 CA St Univ - Los Angeles; 85–Aud, Assoc Specialists In Hearing, **A**

Chaplin, Mrs Cathy M 54 Poplar Drive, Tuscola, IL 61953, (217) 253-2712, BA 76 Eastern IL Univ; MA 77 Eastern IL Univ; Speech-Language Pathologist, Tuscola Public Schools, **SLP**

Chaplin, Robert G Indiana Univ Sch Of Medicine, Riley Hospital #A-56, 702 Barnhill Drive, Indianapolis, IN 46223, (317) 274-8868, BS 52 Northwestern Univ; MA 53 Northwestern Univ; Aud, IN U Sch of Med, **A**

Chaplin, Mrs Ruth T C-101 Spanish Arms, 800 South Main Street, Salisbury, NC 28144, (704) 637-0942, BA 35 Colby Coll; MS 65 VA Commonwealth Univ; ME 69 Univ of VA - Charlottesville; 85–Sp-Lang Path, Total Care-Home Hlth, **SLP LM**

Chapman, Ann Yager 906 Copperas Drive, Caldwell, TX 77836, (409) 567-7521, BA 80 Southern Methodist Univ; BS 80 Southern Methodist Univ; MS 81 Southern Methodist Univ; Sp/Lang Path, Office at Burleson County Hosp, **SLP**

Chapman, Mrs Beth Ellen 148 Fenway Avenue, Winslow Township, NJ 08004, (609) 429-0010, BS 85 Indiana Univ of PA; MS 86 Adelphi Univ; 88–Sp-Lang Path, The Bancroft Sch, **SLP**

Chapman, Cathy A 314 Shady Lane, Marlton, NJ 08053, (609) 795-0061, BS 73 Glassboro St Coll; MS 78 Rutgers St Univ - Newark; Sp/Lang Path, New Jersey Sp Consultants, **SLP ACE**

Chapman, Darwin Lee 103 Asbury Drive, Wilmore, KY 40390, PH; **SLP**

Chapman, Mrs Diane H 4308 Necker Avenue, Baltimore, MD 21236, (301) 444-5000, BA 80 Towson St Univ; MS 82 Towson St Univ; Sp-Lang Path, MD Sch for the Blind, **SLP**

Chapman, Mrs Francine L RD 5 Box 134-C2, Dover, DE 19901, (302) 653-8825, BA 72 SUNY - Center at Buffalo; MA 73 Hofstra Univ; 79–Sp-Lang Path, Smyrna Sch Dist, **SLP**

Chapman, Iva M 235 Carta Road #M-2, Knoxville, TN 37914, (601) 643-2221, BS 69 Univ Southern MS-Hattiesburg; MS 83 Univ Southern MS-Hattiesburg; Clinical Instructor, U of Tennessee Hrng & Sp Cen, **SLP**

Chapman, Janet L 610 North Prairie, Hamilton, MO 64644, (816) 645-2284, BS 77 Northeast MO St Univ; MS 88 Central MO St Univ

Chapman, Mrs Janet Sidmon Route 7 Box 302D, Springfield, MO 65802, (417) 885-3282, **SLP**

Chapman, Dr Kathy L Case-Western Reserve Univ, Dept Communication Sciences, Cleveland, OH 44106, BS 74 TX Tech Univ; MS 75 TX Tech Univ; PH 84 (NS) Purdue Univ - West Lafayette; Assistant Professor, Case-Western Reserve Univ, **SLP**

Chapman, Mrs Kristen M 3722 Grennoch Lane, Houston, TX 77025, (713) 791-4298, BA 78 IN Univ - Bloomington; MA 80 Univ of Houston - Univ Park; Sp/Lang Path, St Lukes/Texas Chldn Hosps, **SLP**

Chapman, Mrs Kyle Anne 11474 Floyd #107, Overland Park, KS 66210-2696, (913) 383-3400, BA 77 Univ of MO - Saint Louis; MS 81 Southern IL Univ-Edwardsvill; 86–Aud, Timbre Hearing & Speech Ctrs Inc, **A**

Chapman, Mrs M Janet 2209 Auina Place, Kihei, HI 96753, (808) 244-4458, BS 66 Purdue Univ - West Lafayette; MS 74 Univ of HI - Manoa; 86–Aud, Hawaii Dept of Hlth, **SLP A ACE**

Chapman, Marian Rose 3220 Virginia Way, Longview, WA 98632, (206) 577-9136, MS 83 Univ of WI - Stevens Point; Assoc for SLP, Orthel and Assoc, **SLP**

Chapman, Maureen Ann 1901 North 66th Street, Scottsdale, AZ 85257, (602) 947-8720, OM 88 AZ St Univ

Chapman, Michele D 231 Glentay Road, Lansdowne, PA 19050, (215) 284-8570, BA 72 Holy Family Coll; MA 82 Temple Univ; Aud, Delaware Co Memorial Hospital, **SLP A ACE**

Chapman, Dr Robin S Dept Communicative Disorders, University Of Wisconsin, 1975 Willow Drive, Madison, WI 53706, (608) 262-3951, BA 64 Swarthmore Coll; PH 67 (NS) Univ of CA - Berkeley; Prof of Commun Dis, U of WI

Chapman, Mrs Robin W 4315 Cedar Valley Drive, Kingwood, TX 77345, (713) 360-5939, BA 78 Univ of Houston - Univ Park; MA 80 Univ of Houston - Univ Park; Sp-Lang Path, Fort Bend ISD, **SLP**

Chapman, Dr Sandra Bond 9230 Meadowbrook, Dallas, TX 75220, (214) 368-4121, BA 73 Univ of North TX; MA 74 Univ of North TX; PH 86 (Communication Disorders) Univ of TX - Dallas; 86–Research Sci, Univ of Texas at Dallas, **SLP**

Chapman, Mrs Tina H 303 South Howard Circle, Tarboro, NC 27886, (919) 823-7393, BS 84 East Carolina Univ; MS 85 East Carolina Univ; Sp-Lang Path, Nash General Hospital, **SLP**

Chapman, Mrs Verna Jean 224 Elder Avenue, Chula Vista, CA 92010, (619) 420-3603, BS 53 Univ of NE - Omaha; MA 61 Northwestern Univ; **SLP LM**

Chappel, Mrs Jan Marie 316 Hamby Avenue, Dawson Springs, KY 42408, (502) 797-2991, BS 75 Murray St Univ; MS 83 Murray St Univ; Sp-Lang Path, Dawson Springs Indep Schools, **SLP**

Chappell, Cheryl R 2201 South 85th Avenue, Omaha, NE 68124, (402) 397-9771, BS 72 Univ of NE - Lincoln; OM 83 Univ of NE - Omaha; MS 77 Univ of NE - Omaha; **SLP**

Chappell, Mrs Elizabeth Hamm 2117 Inverness Drive, Lawrence, KS 66046, (913) 272-3811, OB 84 Univ of KS; MA 87 Univ of KS; 87–Sp-Lang Path, USD #501 Shawnee Co Coop, **SLP**

Chappell, Gerald E 2409 Prais Street, Stevens Point, WI 54481, (715) 346-2250, PH 68 (Communicative Disorders) Univ of WI - Madison; 62–Prof, Univ of WI, **SLP**

Chappell, Jennifer Leah 550 Techno Lane #303, Memphis, TN 38105, (901) 527-5733, MA 88 Memphis St Univ

Chappell, Mrs Linda J 2127 Landis Valley Road, Lancaster, PA 17601, (717) 396-9131, BS 70 Indiana Univ of PA; MS 74 Indiana Univ of PA; 86–Sp-Lang Path, Lancaster-Lebanon IU #13, **SLP**

Chappell, Pamela A 2113 Wright Avenue, Greensboro, NC 27403, (919) 282-1100, BA 72 Mercer Univ - Macon; ME 74 Univ of FL; SLP, Dev Eval Cen, **SLP**

Chappelle, Mrs Eva Ulrich 6101 River Road #14, Columbus, GA 31904, (912) 838-4280, BA 66 Wake Forest Univ; ME 83 Columbus Coll; Sp-Lang Path, Stewart Co Bd of Ed, **SLP ACE**

Chappen, Pamela Lee Rd #5 Box 339, Danville, PA 17821, (412) 941-4434

Chapple, Persis M 1516 Little Court, Carmichael, CA 95608, (916) 922-3496, BA 64 CA St Univ - Sacramento; MA 72 CA St Univ - Sacramento; SLP, Grant Jt Union Hs Dist, **SLP**

Chappotin, Laura Pierce 3004 Rollins Street, Melbourne, FL 32901, (407) 724-2718, BS 84 FL St Univ; MS 85 FL St Univ; 87–Aud, ENT Health & Surgical Ctr, **A**

Chaput, Patricia Ann 29 Woodwood Heights, Pleasant Ridge, MI 48069, BS 70 Central MI Univ; MA 77 Eastern MI Univ; 87–Sp-Lang Path, MI Ctr for Dev Dis, **SLP**

Charan, Dr Kirti Kumar 1266 Pine Avenue West, Beatty Hall, Montreal, PQ, Canada H3G 1A8, (514) 398-5000, MA 52; MA 56 Washington Univ; PH 70 (NS) McGill Univ - Quebec; Assoc Prof, McGill Univ, **A**

Charchian, Martha M 4715 Tipton, Troy, MI 48098, (313) 641-0001, BA 63 Western MI Univ; MA 68 Western MI Univ; Sp-Lang Path, Private Practice, **SLP**

Chard, Jan Bryggmanh RR1 Box 370, Custer, SD 57730, (605) 673-2371, BA 79 Univ of CA - Santa Barbara; MA 81 Univ of MT; Sp/Lang Path, Helena Sch Dist #1, **SLP**

Charest, Mrs Linda R Dutton Road, P O Box 537, New Hartford, CT 06057, (203) 582-6046, BS 75 SUNY - Center at Albany; MA 77 Hofstra Univ; Sp-Lang Path, Plymouth Bd of Educ, **SLP**

Charette, Mrs Lori Wills 11A North Elm Street, Wallingford, CT 06492, (203) 284-2880, BS 81 Univ of NH; MS 83 Vanderbilt Univ; Aud, Gaylord Hosp, **A**

Chargo, Steven J 6911 West 23rd Street, St Louis Park, MN 55426, (612) 941-6401, BS 79 Univ of MN - Minneap-St Paul; MA 81 Univ of MN - Minneap-St Paul; Marketing Director, Starkey Lab Inc, **A**

Chari, Dr Nallan C A Altamonte Hearing Clinic, Fro Bldg, 101 Wymore Road #326, Altamonte Springs, FL 32714, (407) 682-3130, MS 66 8145; MA 71 Washington Univ; PH 75 (NS) Bowling Green St Univ; Owner, Altamonte Hearing Clinic, **A**

Charlebois, Linda Marie Indiana School For The Deaf, 1200 East 42nd Street, Indianapolis, IN 46205, (317) 924-4374, BA 75 Depauw Univ; MS 78 Purdue Univ - West Lafayette; Aud, Indiana Sch for the Deaf, **A**

Charles, Linda Kathryn 1015 Porter Lane, Normal, IL 61761, BS 70 Indiana Univ of PA; MS 85 IL St Univ - Normal; **SLP**

Charles, Malusha Marie 5 Hufton Court, Ajax, ON, Canada L1T 2R3, (416) 576-8711, BA 82 Univ of Toronto - Ontario; MA 85 SUNY - Center at Buffalo; 86–Sp-Lang Path, Oshawa Gen Hosp, **SLP**

Charles, Mrs Patricia D 1606 Pine Shadow Court, Richmond, VA 23233, (804) 780-7809, BS 74 Univ of VA - Charlottesville; ME 75 Univ of VA - Charlottesville; Sp-Lang Path, Richmond Public Schools, **SLP**

Charlesworth, Barbara S 20222 North 21st Drive, Phoenix, AZ 85027, (602) 876-5349, BS 70 Kent St Univ; MA 76 Kent St Univ; Sp-Lang Path, Walter O Boswell Memorial Hosp, **SLP**

Charley, Mrs Linda Kay 2827 Belhaven Place, Davis, CA 95616, (916) 454-8387, BA 80 CA St Univ - Northridge; MA 83 CA St Univ - Sacramento; Sp-Lang Path, Sacramento USD, **SLP**

Charlip, Dr Walter S Audie L Murphy Mem VA Hospital, 7400 Merton Minter Blvd, San Antonio, TX 78284, (512) 694-5209, BA 63 Hofstra Univ; MS 65 Purdue Univ - West Lafayette; PH 68 (NS) Purdue Univ - West Lafayette; Aud, Audie L Murphy Mem Hosp, **A**

Charlson, Mrs Teresa Jean 2042 1st Street, Brookings, SD 57006, (605) 783-3409, **SLP**

Charlton, Ella M 2831 Midland Street, Pittsburgh, PA 15226, (412) 561-4848, ME 57 Duquesne Univ; 57–Aud, De Paul Institute

Charlton, Georgina 709 7th Street N W, Jamestown, ND 58401, (701) 252-3850, BS 61 Minot St Univ; MS 69 Minot St Univ; 65–Sp-Lang Path, Anne Carlsen Sch, **SLP**

Charlton, Judith S 9 Clark Subdivision, Northport, AL 35476, (205) 553-4550, BA 76 Univ of AL- Tuscaloosa; MS 78 Univ of AL- Tuscaloosa; 78–Quality Assurance Dir, Partlow State Sch & Hosp, **A**

Charlton, Steve R 921 3rd Avenue East #104, Tuscaloosa, AL 35401, (205) 758-9041, BS 63 Univ of Montevallo; MA 71 Univ of AL- Tuscaloosa; Dir, Al Hrng & Sp Cl, **A**

Charney, Elaine Ann 6663 Jackson Street, Taylor, MI 48180, **SLP**

Charnov, Mrs Ellen Klinenberg 709 N Sierra Drive, Beverly Hills, CA 90210, (213) 278-7597, BS 85 Boston Univ; MS 87 San Francisco St Univ; 88–Sp-Lang Path, Methodist Hosp, **SLP**

Charpentier, Cynthia A 3030 Polk Street #2, San Francisco, CA 94109, (415) 922-9514, BA 74 Univ of MA - Amherst; MS 77 Univ of WY; Sp-Lang Path/Coord of Chldn, I of Lang & Path, **SLP**

Charrier, Sheila Crosby P O Box 615, Boyce, LA 71409, (318) 443-0579, BA 79 Northwestern St Univ; MA 80 Northwestern St Univ; Sp-Lang Path, Rapides Parish Sch Bd, **SLP**

Charron, Deanne M 21144 Le Fever, Warren, MI 48091, (313) 757-2794, MA 87 MI St Univ

Charron, Dechantal Marie 1038 Braeview Drive, Howell, MI 48843, (312) 890-8752, MA 85 Eastern MI Univ; 86–Sp-Lang Path, Livingston ISD, **SLP**

Charron-Shea, Maureen H P O Box 575, Waitsfield, VT 05673, (802) 583-2469, BA 76 Univ of VT; MS 78 Univ of VT; Sp-Lang Path, Montpelier Pub Sch, **SLP**

Charters, Dr Nancy 531 South Ventura Street, Ojai, CA 93023, (805) 646-2728, BA 60 Pomona Coll; MA 61 San Francisco St Univ; PH 72 (NS) Univ of Southern CA; Sp-Lang Path, St John's Reg Med Ctr Rehab Unit, **SLP**

Charuhas, Peter A 2126 N E Stanton, Portland, OR 97212, (503) 228-6479, BA 73 Western WA Univ; MA 75 Western WA Univ; 78–Director Audiology Services, Portland Cen Hrng Sp, **A**

Charuhas, Sally J T 2126 N E Stanton, Portland, OR 97212, (503) 280-4505, BA 73 Western WA Univ; MA 74 Western WA Univ; 88–Clin Coord, Emanuel Hosp & Health Ctr, **SLP**

Chase, Caren Ann 7527-C Pitch Pine Circle, Tampa, FL 33617-8519, (813) 988-7040, MS 85 Univ of South FL; 88–Sp-Lang Path, Professional Health Services, **SLP**

Chase, Mrs Carole J 4975 Dalton Drive, Columbia, MD 21045, (301) 455-0857, BS 56 Ball St Univ; MS 80 Towson St Univ; Sp/Lang Path, Baltimore Co Bd of Ed, **SLP**

Chase, Christina Cheryl 19840 Fort Street #204, Riverview, MI 48192, (313) 479-1861, BA 84 Wayne St Univ; MA 86 Wayne St Univ; **SLP**

Chase, Deborah A 4113 Eastern Avenue North, Seattle, WA 98103, MS 78 Univ of WA; Sp-Lang Path, Private Practice, **SLP**

Chase, Judith A 7 Militia Lane, Scarborough, ME 04074, (207) 883-6638, BA 73 Rutger's St Univ - Douglas Coll; MA 75 Montclair St Coll; Sp-Lang Path, Scarborough PS, **SLP**

Chase, Mrs Julie Rhodes 2337 Costa Verde Boulevard, Apartment 302, Jacksonville, FL 32250, (904) 246-0426, BS 80 Univ of FL; MA 86 SC St Coll; **SLP**

Chase, Mrs Karen Nailling Greenery Rehab Center, 3100 Erwin Road, Durham, NC 27705, (919) 383-1546, BS 74 FL St Univ; MS 75 FL St Univ; 87–Dir Sp-Lang Path, Greenery Rehab Center, **SLP**

Chase, Kathy K Department Of Oto, 5323 Harry Hines, Dallas, TX 75235, (214) 688-3458, BA 83 MI St Univ; MS 86 Univ of North TX; 88–Aud, Univ TX Southwestern Med Ctr, **A**

Chase, Mardi 5844 Noon Road, Bellingham, WA 98226, (206) 336-2178, MA 85 Western WA Univ; Audiologist, Skagit Surgery Center, **A**

Chase, Mrs Maribeth D , Ida Grove, IA 51445, (712) 662-4339, BA 51 Univ of IA; MS 72 Univ of NE - Omaha; Sp-Lang Path, Arrowhead AEA, **SLP**

Chase, Michele 5222-F Penrith Drive, Durham, NC 27713, (919) 544-4642, BA 81 Humboldt St Univ; MA 83 WA St Univ; Sp-Lang Path, Private Practice, **SLP ACE**

Chase, Susan Leeper Box 305 B Rd #1, Natrona Heights, PA 15065, (412) 828-1300, BA 77 Allegheny Coll; MA 79 Univ of Pittsburgh - Pittsburgh; 88–Coord of Staff Educ, Harmarville Rehab Ctr, **SLP**

Chase, Tamara K 1324 14th Avenue, Greeley, CO 80631, (303) 356-2787, MS 87 Kearney St Coll

Chase, Tara C 9833 Halifax, Ventura, CA 93004, (805) 644-2154, BA 75 Univ of CA - Santa Barbara; MA 77 CA St Univ - Stanislaus; SLP, Ventura USD, **SLP**

Chasin, Judith G Brookline Hearing Services, 115 Marion Street, Brookline, MA 02146, BA 59 Univ of MI - Ann Arbor; MA 61 Case Western Reserve Univ; Aud, Brookline Hrng Serv Inc, **A**

Chasin, Mrs Rachel L 5001 Paseo Dali, Irvine, CA 92715, MA 61 Temple Univ; Sp-Lang Path, Irvine USD, **A**

Chassen, Mrs Deborah 167 Paine Avenue, New Rochelle, NY 10804, (914) 576-2729, BS 71 SUNY - Center at Albany; ME 74 Northeastern Univ; Private Practice, **SLP**

Chassin, Beryl 22 Longbow Drive, Englishtown, NJ 07726, (201) 870-5067, BA 63 Boston Univ; MA 76 Kean Coll of NJ; Aud, Monmouth Med Cen, **A**

Chastain, Mrs Alice Veach 1901 Independence Road, Greensboro, NC 27408, (704) 249-8182, BA 76 Univ of NC - Greensboro; MA 78 Univ of NC - Greensboro; Aud, Davidson Co Schs, **A**

Chastain, Pamela J P O Box 68, Wetumka, OK 74883, (405) 452-3756, BA 73 OK St Univ; MA 75 OK St Univ; **SLP**

Chastel, Penny Jean 140 Fowler Hill Road #2, Wellsburg, WV 26070, (304) 737-3515, BS 80 Edinboro Univ of PA; MS 83 CA Univ of PA; 83–Sp-Lang Path, Brooke Co Bd of Educ

Chatfield, Mrs Janet Leutel 643 4th Street, Encinitas, CA 92024, (619) 942-5346, BA 73 San Jose St Univ; MA 77 San Diego St Univ; SLP, Solana Beach School District, **SLP**

Chatham, Barry Gene 708 Brewer Place, Greenwood, IN 46142, (317) 881-5823, BS 64 IN St Univ - Terre Haute; MS 68 IN Univ - Bloomington; Executive Vice President, Rehabilitative Health Services

Chatterton, Bruce Kerr 20362 West Rue Crevier, Apartment 601, Canyon Country, CA 91351, (213) 977-1215, BA 80 San Diego St Univ; MA 82 CA St Univ - Los Angeles; Audiologist, Auditory Vestibular Center, **A**

Chatterton, Mrs Suzanne V R R 1 Box 145A, Avon, IL 61415, (309) 465-7471, BS 68 Western IL Univ; MA 71 Western IL Univ; Sp-Lang Path, Knox Warren Spec Ed Coop, **SLP**

Chattler, Mrs Lisa Kalisher 217 Harvard Lane, Seal Beach, CA 90740, (213) 430-6280, BA 76 CA St Univ - Long Beach; MA 78 CA St Univ - Long Beach; 82–Sp-Lang Path, Private Practice, **SLP**

Chaudoin, Barbara Ann 2415 Bradley Avenue, Louisville, KY 40217, (502) 636-2084, BS 76 Western KY Univ; MS 80 Univ of Louisville; Aud, Louisville Deaf Oral Presch, **A**

Chaudron, Donna Dellinger 86 Sunline Drive, Brandon, MS 39042-2147, (601) 922-5530, BA 84 Univ of AL- Tuscaloosa; MS 85 Univ of AL- Tuscaloosa; **SLP**

Chaumont, Beverly Ann P O Box 229, Edmond, OK 73083, (405) 277-3264, BA 70 Univ of Southwestern LA; ME 85 Central St Univ; **SLP**

Chauvin, Mrs Cathy Schroder P O Box 65, Port Sulphur, LA 70083, (504) 657-9435, BA 79 Nicholls St Univ; OM 83 LA St Univ - N O Medical Ctr; SLP, Plaquemines Parish Sch Bd, **SLP**

Chauvin, Mrs Leslie Ann 111 Langride Drive, Belle Chasse, LA 70037, BA Southeastern LA Univ; ME 85 Southeastern LA Univ; **SLP**

Chavez, Mrs Juli Ann Church 8000 Waters Avenue, Apartment #187, Savannah, GA 31406, (912) 351-9554, BS 80 Northern AZ Univ; MS 81 Northern AZ Univ; OM 81 Northern AZ Univ; 88–Sp-Lang Path, Liberty County PS, **SLP**

Chavez, Mrs Marian A P O Box 14043, Albuquerque, NM 87191, BS 59 Case Western Reserve Univ; MA 50 OH St Univ; OM 62 Case Western Reserve Univ; 86–Sp-Lang Path, Albuquerque PS, **SLP**

Chavez-Law, Mrs Rita 1003 N Crescent Heights, Los Angeles, CA 90046, (213) 656-3031, MS 55 Univ of CA - Los Angeles; Los Angeles Commun College Dis, **SLP**

Chavira, Mrs Diane Noel 3660 West San Jose #109, Fresno, CA 93711, (209) 276-1970, BS 84 Longwood Coll; ME 86 Univ of VA - Charlottesville; 86–Sp-Lang Path, Comm Hosp of Central CA, **SLP**

Chavis, Mrs Marlene Cecilia 4601 Chaney Lane, Bakersfield, CA 93311, (805) 398-2248, BS 75 SUNY - Center at Buffalo; MA 79 SUNY - Coll at Buffalo; SLP, Office of Kern Co Sup of Schls

Chavoor-Pardes, Mrs Claude Mv 5803 Chain Bldg Forest Ct, Arlington, VA 22207, (703) 538-7030, BS 82 George Washington Univ; MS 87 Univ of the DC; 88–Sp-Lang Path, Child Ctr, **SLP**

Chawkin, Phyllis Thorne 303 West 66th Street #13GE, New York, NY 10023, (212) 523-6810, BA 57 CUNY - Brooklyn Coll; MA 65 Columbia Univ Teachers Coll; Dir, St Lukes-Roosevelt Hosp Ctr, **SLP A**

Chayt, Mrs Meryl B 3317 Thornhill Road S W, Winter Haven, FL 33880, (813) 294-6976, BA 76 CA St Univ - Northridge; MA 79 CA St Univ - Northridge; SLP, Polk Co Sch Bd, **SLP**

Chazen, Patricia B 227 Sudbrook Lane, Baltimore, MD 21208, **SLP**

Cheatham, Mrs Melinda M 600 Aspen, Gainesville, TX 76240, (817) 668-7009, BS 69 TX Tech Univ; MA 70 TX Christian Univ; Sp-Lang Path, Cooke Co Spec Educ Coop, **SLP**

Checchi, Anne M 24 Cleveland Street, Apartment 1, Valhalla, NY 10595, BA 73 Vassar Coll; MS 80 Columbia Univ Teachers Coll; 86–Sp-Lang Path, Blythedale Children's Hosp, **SLP**

Check, Christine Ann 2419 Heatherwood Court, Escondido, CA 92026, (916) 740-0636, BA 85 CA St Univ - Chico; MA 86 CA St Univ - Chico; 87–Tchr, Cajon Valley Sch Dist, **SLP**

Check-Tapler, Maureen Lynn 40 North Lake Avenue, Troy, NY 12180, (518) 489-8336, BA 82 SUNY - Coll at Cortland; MS 83 Ithaca Coll; Sp-Lang Path, Cerebral Palsy Cen for Dis, **SLP**

Cheek, Mrs Diane Jones 9632 Windsor, Leawood, KS 66206, BS 75 Univ of Tulsa; MA 82 Univ of KS; Sp-Lang Path, Private Practice, **SLP**

Cheek, Ellen Berry 1952 W Record Street, Tucson, AZ 85705, (602) 298-4358, BS 83 Univ of AZ; MS 85 Univ of AZ; 88–Aud, Tucson ENT Assoc, **A**

Cheek, Linda T 5909 Montford Drive, Colleyville, TX 76034, **SLP**

Cheek, Mrs Sharon G 720 South 8th, Oxford, MS 38655, (601) 234-1476, BA 84 Univ of MS; MS 85 Univ of MS; 86–Dir of Interdisciplinary Prog, North MS Retardation Ctr, **SLP**

Cheeseman, Nancy E K 6100 Pleasant, Des Moines, IA 50312, (515) 277-6238, BS 73 IA St Univ; MA 75 Univ of Northern IA; Sp-Lang Path, Des Moines Pub Sch, **SLP**

Cheeseman-Foulk, Sara 5221 North Tigua, Tucson, AZ 85704, BS 81 Univ of AZ; MS 82 Univ of AZ; 86–Sp-Lang Path, Amphitheater PS, **SLP**

Cheesman, Margaret Fern 119 Wychwood Park, London, ON, Canada N6G 1R8, (519) 472-3198, BA 77 Univ of Ottawa - Ontario; BS 80 Univ of Calgary - Alberta; MA 85 Univ of Calgary - Alberta; 88–Lecturer, Univ of Western Ontario

Cheifetz, Mrs Myrna Fox 82 Townsend Drive, Freehold, NJ 07728, (718) 351-5454, BA 63 CUNY - Brooklyn Coll; MS 70 CUNY - Brooklyn Coll; 80–Sp-Lang Path, NY City Bd of Ed, **SLP**

Chelius, Mrs Leah Marlene 1906 North Mississippi Avenue, Roswell, NM 88201, (505) 622-7521, Sp-Lang Path, Southeastern NM Sp & Hrng Cl, **SLP**

Chelius, Stephen Michael 1906 N Mississippi, Roswell, NM 88201, (505) 623-8474, BS 82 Brigham Young Univ; OM 84 Brigham Young Univ; 86–Aud, SE NM Sp/Hrng Cl Inc, **A**

Chellappa, Mariam 3362 Kreitler Road, Forest Hill, MD 21050, (301) 557-7884, MS 87 Towson St Univ

Chelminiak, Mrs Diane K 5 Knights Bridge Court, Baltimore, MD 21236, (301) 272-1470, BA 78 Coll of Notre Dame of MD; MS 79 Loyola Coll; Sp/Lang Path, Harford Cty Publ Schs, **SLP**

Chelst, Dr Tamy S 22536 North Bellwood Dr, Southfield, MI 48034, (313) 548-2908, BA 70 Barnard Coll; MA 73 CUNY - Hunter Coll; PH 85 (NS) Univ of MI - Ann Arbor; **SLP A**

Chemelli, Melanie P Rd 3 Box 282, Kittanning, PA 16201, (412) 548-4098, BA 85 Indiana Univ of PA; MS 86 Clarion Univ of PA

Chen, Diana N G Beverly Oaklawn Hrng Aid Ser, 4923 West 95th Street, Oak Lawn, IL 60453, (312) 424-0143, BS 75; MS 78 Purdue Univ - West Lafayette; Aud, Beverly Oaklawn Hrng A Serv, **A**

Chen, Hsiao-Chuan 1611 Laurel Avenue #1408, Knoxville, TN 37916, (615) 524-8901, BS 78 Nat'l Taiwan Normal Univ; MA 83 Univ of TN - Knoxville; Aud, Univ of TN, **A**

Chen, Josephine P O Box 171, Cos Cob, CT 06807, (914) 947-3000, BA 71; MS 77 Univ of NM; Sp-Lang Path, Helen Hayes Hosp, **SLP ACE**

Chen, Rose Jenman 16571 Tripp Circle, Huntington Beach, CA 92647, BS 84 Northwestern Univ; MS 86 Univ of Redlands; 88–Sp-Lang Path, Memorial Med Ctr of Long Beach, **SLP**

Chenet, Patricia P O Box 305, Hopkinton, MA 01748, (617) 435-5595, BS 71 Western MI Univ; MS 74 Western MI Univ; **SLP**

Cheney, Mrs Audrey P Kamnarsvagen 3 C237, Lund, Sweden 222-46, BA 78 Western WA Univ; OM 81 Univ of WA; Sp-Lang Path, **SLP**

Cheney, Mrs Caron 106 Edgewater Drive, Hull, MA 02045, (617) 925-5539, BA 79 CUNY - Brooklyn Coll; MS 81 Columbia Univ Teachers Coll; **A**

Cheng, Joan Elizabeth 1915 Maple Avenue #1017-2, Englehart Hall, Evanston, IL 60201-3194, (312) 328-6179, BS 84 Univ of GA; ME 85 Univ of GA; **SLP**

Cheng, Dr Li-Rong L 4954 Maynard Street, San Diego, CA 92122, (619) 563-3619, MA 69 Southern IL Univ -Carbondale; MA 73 MI St Univ; PH 82 (NS) Claremont Graduate Sch; Asst Prof, San Diego State U, **SLP**

Cheng, Mei-Kuan C/15 Hanley House, 68-80 Canton Road, Kowloon, Hong Kong, BA 82 Nat'l Taiwan Normal Univ; MA 86 Univ of TN - Knoxville; 88–Sp-Lang Path, Watchdog Early Learning & Dev Ctr, **SLP**

Chen-Hall, Mrs I-Fan M 60 Wadsworth Street #11-A, Cambridge, MA 02142, (617) 494-8203, BS 83 Univ of TX - Dallas; MS 87 Emerson Coll; **SLP**

Chennault, Mrs Yanira Caparros 11328 Conch Court, Jacksonville, FL 32223, (904) 268-6062, BA 82 Univ of PR - Rio Piedras; MS 84 Univ of PR - San Juan; 86–Sp-Lang Path, Duval Co Sch Bd, **SLP**

Chenoweth, Mrs Marybeth Keith 356 S Prospectors Road, Apartment 83, Diamond Bar, CA 91765, (714) 861-1219, BA 83 Univ of CO - Boulder; MA 85 San Diego St Univ; **SLP**

Chenoweth, Robin 5367 North Franklin Road, Merced, CA 95348, (209) 723-3327, BA 73 CA St Univ - Chico; BA 77 CA St Univ - Fresno; MA 79 CA St Univ - Fresno; 88–SLP, Merced City Schools, **SLP**

Chenoweth, Wayne L 1334 Carter Way, Redding, CA 96002, (916) 223-6440, BA 84 CA St Univ - Chico; MA 87 CA St Univ - Chico; 86–Sp-Lang Path, Susan Whitaker, **SLP**

Chenoy, Sohrab Y 1169 Huff Street, Rialto, CA 92376, (619) 339-6428, BA 75 Univ of UT; MS 82 UT St Univ; Sp-Lang-Hrng Spec, Imperial Co Office of Ed, **SLP**

Cheple, Mark A 973 Nebraska Avenue W, St Paul, MN 55117, (612) 339-2836, OB 77 Univ of MN - Duluth; MS 78 Univ of WI - Stevens Point; Dir of Aud, MN Ear Head & Neck Clinic, **A**

Cheraso, Samuel C Gov Baxter School, Box 799, Portland, ME 04101, (207) 781-3165, BS 53 Kent St Univ; MS 57 Syracuse Univ; Aud, Gov Baxter Sch, **SLP A**

Cherchio, Noella A Llewellyn Park, West Orange, NJ 07052, (201) 268-8140, BA 79 Kean Coll of NJ; MA 80 Kean Coll of NJ; Sp-Lang Path, Utd Hosp Med Ctr, **SLP**

Cherecwich, Mrs Barbara J 314 Commonwealth Avenue, Attleboro Falls, MA 02763, (617) 824-6911, BS 79 Worcester St Coll; MA 81 Univ of MA - Amherst; Aud, Morton Hosp Inc, **A ACE**

Cherepski, Mary Ann 12 Nottingham #5, Little Rock, AR 72205, (501) 660-2581, BS 81 AR St Univ; MS 83 Univ of AR - Little Rock; Sp/Lang Path, St Vincent Infirmary, **SLP**

Cherewka, Mrs Michele R 64 Little Run Road, Camp Hill, PA 17011, (717) 737-6728, BS 79 Bloomsburg Univ of PA; MS 80 Bloomsburg Univ of PA; Sp-Lang Path, Capital Area Inter Ut, **SLP ACE**

Cherf, Mrs Laura Ericsen 11616 West Walnut Road, Wauwatosa, WI 53226, (414) 548-0560, BS 85 Univ of WI - Stevens Point; MS 86 Marquette Univ; 86–Sp-Lang Path, Waukesha PS, **SLP**

Cherkas, Mrs Anne Blumenthal 17 North Riding Drive, Cherry Hill, NJ 08003, (609) 428-6099, BA 71 Hofstra Univ; OM 74 Trenton St Coll

Chermak, Dr Gail D Department Of Speech & Hearing Sciences, Washington State Univ, Pullman, WA 99164, (509) 335-8368, BA 72 SUNY - Center at Buffalo; MA 73 OH St Univ; PH 75 (Hrng Science) OH St Univ; Assoc Prof, WA St U, **A**

Cherney, Leora Reiff 8248 Springfield Avenue, Skokie, IL 60076, (312) 908-6134, BS 78 Univ of Capetown - S Africa; MA 80 Northwestern Univ; 85–Sp-Lang Path, Rehab I of Chicago, **SLP ACE**

Cherniak, Gary B 5913 Open Sky N W, Albuquerque, NM 87120, (505) 344-4412, BA 74 Oakland Univ; MA 80 Wayne St Univ; Sp/Lang Path, Albuquerque Pub Sch, **SLP**

Chernikoff, Leslie R 4317 Sangamore Rd, Bethesda, MD 20816, (301) 229-2069, OB 72 Univ of Miami; MA 74 OH St Univ; 87–Sp-Lang Path, The Lab Sch of Washington, **SLP**

Chernin, Florence P O Box 201, St Johns, St Johns, Antigua, BA 52 Rutgers St Univ - Newark; MA 70 Kean Coll of NJ; Dir of the English Prog, J F Kennedy Sch Queretaro Mx, **SLP**

Cherniss, Mrs Suzan Marie 8430 Hidden Meadow, San Antonio, TX 78230, (512) 534-6951, BS 78 Southwest TX St Univ; ME 79 Southwest TX St Univ; Sp-Lang Path, San Antonio ISD, **SLP**

Cherno-Matievich, Mrs Joan 681 Deerhunter Lane, Camarillo, CA 93010, (805) 484-2811, BA 79 CA St Univ - Northridge; MA 81 CA St Univ - Northridge; 80–Sp-Lang Path, Pleasant Valley School Dist, **SLP**

Cherof, Mrs Ruby C 620 S E 10th Street, Pompano Beach, FL 33060, (305) 765-6644, BS 76 SUNY - Center at Albany; MA 79 Univ of Houston - Univ Park; Sp-Lang Path, **SLP**

Cherow, Evelyn 5805 Melvern Drive, Bethesda, MD 20817, (301) 897-5700, BA 67 Rutger's St Univ - Douglas Coll; MA 68 Northwestern Univ; Dir Aud Liaison Branch, ASHA, **A**

Cherpillod, Deborah Lee 13101 Morning Star Drive, North Royalton, OH 44133, (216) 459-3213, BA 82 Cleveland St Univ; MA 84 Cleveland St Univ; 84–Aud, Cleveland Metro Gen Hosp, **A**

Cherry, Mrs Barbara Waterman 8821 Ivey Road, Jacksonville, FL 32216, (904) 725-6113, BS 72 Univ of FL; MA 82 Univ of FL; Sp-Lang Path, Duval Co Sch Sys, **SLP**

Cherry, Ellen Lee 6702 Gold Moss Cove, Austin, TX 78745, (512) 440-5427, BS 79 Purdue Univ - West Lafayette; ME 84 Southwest TX St Univ; Sp-Lang Path, Texas Sch for the Deaf, **SLP**

Cherry, Jay D 6 Norva Avenue, Frederick, MD 21701, (301) 662-4159, BS 73 IN Univ - Bloomington; MA 75 Ball St Univ; Aud, Maryland School for the Deaf, **A**

Cherry, Mrs Maureen M 6335 Phillips, Pittsburgh, PA 15217, BA 71 Univ of Pittsburgh - Pittsburgh; MA 72 Univ of Pittsburgh - Pittsburgh; Sp-Lang Path, Er Sl So of Clearfield Co, **SLP**

Cherry, Mrs Nancy C 6 Norva Avenue, Frederick, MD 21701, BS 73 IN Univ - Bloomington; MA 75 IN Univ - Bloomington; Sp-Lang Path, Maryland School for the Deaf, **SLP**

Cherry, Mrs Peggy R 8244 Perry, Shawnee Mission, KS 66204, BS 77 Southwest TX St Univ; ME 78 Southwest TX St Univ; Sp-Lang Path, Univ of Kansas Med Ctr, **SLP**

Cherry, Dr Rochelle S 1675 Glenwood Road, Brooklyn, NY 11230, (212) 780-5186, BS 68 Ithaca Coll; MA 70 Case Western Reserve Univ; ED 79 (NS) Columbia Univ Teachers Coll; 80–Assoc Prof/Head Aud, Brooklyn Coll, **SLP A**

Cherry-Cruz, Mrs Teresa Ann 56 Camp Place, Bridgeport, CT 06606, (203) 372-7083, BA 77 Temple Univ; MS 86 Southern CT St Univ; 86–Sp-Lang Path, Dept of Mental Retardation, **SLP**

Chertoff, Keyna Klein 409 North Eau Claire #220, Madison, WI 53705, (608) 274-0686, BS 79 SUNY - Coll at Buffalo; MA 84 SUNY - Coll at Buffalo; 85–Aud, Nicolet Instruments, **A**

Chertoff, Mark E 409 North Eau Claire #220, Madison, WI 53705, (608) 274-0686, BS 81 SUNY - Center at Buffalo; MA 84 SUNY - Center at Buffalo; **A**

Chertok, Susan Gail 4127 West 192nd Place, Country Club Hills, IL 60477, (312) 957-4228, BA 64 Boston Univ; ME 66 Boston Univ; Sp-Lang Path, Professional Rehab Assoc, **SLP**

Chery, Pamela L 2456 West Kiva Avenue, Mesa, AZ 85202, (602) 820-8899, MA 69 Saint Louis Univ; Sp-Lang Path, InSpeech Inc, **SLP**

Cheshier, Mrs Suzanne Smith 1628 Eagle Nest Drive, Norman, OK 73071, (405) 238-7346, BS 85 Baylor Univ; MS 86 Univ of TX - Dallas; **SLP**

Cheshire, Mrs Anne M 22 Poliquin Drive, Nashua, NH 03062, (603) 891-1146, BA 73 Loyola Coll; ME 74 Univ of VA - Charlottesville; Sp-Lang Path, NASH, **SLP**

Cheshire, Mrs Margie G 100 East Northwood Street, Greensboro, NC 27401, (919) 373-8239, BS 75 Western Carolina Univ; ME 79 Univ of NC - Greensboro; SLP, Private Practice, **SLP**

Cheskin, Mrs Adele 7286 Huntington Lane, Bldg 25 Apartment 302, Delray Beach, FL 33446, (407) 499-8764, BS 61 SUNY - Coll at Buffalo; MS 64 SUNY - Coll at Buffalo; Sp-Lang Path, **SLP LM**

Cheskin, Mrs Arlene C 106 Stevens Avenue, Cedar Grove, NJ 07009, (201) 299-0166, BA 77 Montclair St Coll; MA 79 Montclair St Coll; Sp/Lang Path, Lake Dr Sch for Hrng Imp Chldn, **SLP**

Chesley, Mrs Mary Kay 1217 Fir Avenue, Rifle, CO 81650, (303) 625-2438, BS 74 Univ of NE - Lincoln; MA 76 Univ of NE - Lincoln; Sp-Lang Path, Mtn Bd of Coop Educ Svcs, **SLP**

Cheslik, Paula C 505 West Baseline #1052, Tempe, AZ 85283, (602) 820-9167, BS 80 TX Christian Univ; MA 82 Memphis St Univ; 87–Sp-Lang Path, St Joseph's Hosp, **SLP**

Cheslow, Martha Frimer 25 Cambridge Road, Freehold, NJ 07728, (201) 462-9610, BS 74 Emerson Coll; MS 75 Rutgers St Univ -N Brunswick; Sp-Lang Path, Private Practice, **SLP**

Chesner, Mrs Kathleen Everson 6756-B Trail Lake Drive, Fort Worth, TX 76133, (817) 534-5731, BA 77 SUNY - Coll at Cortland; MS 78 PA St Univ - Univ Park; Aud, Ft Worth ISD, **A**

Chesnick, Dr Marie A 10 Village Green Lane #16, Natick, MA 01760, (617) 578-8730, BS 77 SUNY - Coll at Buffalo; MS 79 Emerson Coll; ED 88 (Applied Psycholinguistics) Bennington Coll; 84–Sp-Lang Path, Emerson College, **SLP**

Chess, Tiffany Felts 11613 Rushmore, Oklahoma City, OK 73162, (405) 348-2720, BA 84 Univ of OK - Norman; MS 86 Univ of OK Medical Center; Sp-Lang Path, Edmond Ps, **SLP**

Chesser, Beverly J Great Rivers Educational Cooperative, PO Box 2837, West Helena, AR 72390, (501) 338-6461, BS 81 Univ of AR - Fayetteville; MS 84 Univ of AR - Little Rock; 86–Aud, Arkansas Sch for the Deaf, **A**

Chesser, Mrs Jody Edwards 6027 Walnut Grove Road, Suite 411, Memphis, TN 38119, (901) 767-7750, BS 79 Univ of South AL; MA 81 Memphis St Univ; Aud, Shea Otologic Cp, **A**

Chessher, Mrs Rita Ann 4100 Vista #214, Pasadena, TX 77504, (713) 946-6638, BS 84 Lamar Univ; MS 85 Lamar Univ; Sp-Lang Path, Speech and Language Associates, **SLP**

Chester, Mrs Christine Dallam 3131 Meetinghouse Road, Apartment A-16, Boothwyn, PA 19061, (302) 995-8676, BS 83 Bloomsburg Univ of PA; MS 82 Bloomsburg Univ of PA; 87–Sp-Lang Path, Delaware Div of Pub Health, **SLP**

Chester, Mrs Enda Elaine 1225 Stiles Landing Road, Paducah, KY 42003, (502) 898-7757, MS 82 Murray St Univ; Sp-Lang Path Consultant, Charlene D Cummings, **SLP**

Chester, Mrs Joyce Rhodes 4018 Cabin Creek Court, Hopewell, VA 23860, (804) 458-1144, BS 85 Central MI Univ; MA 86 Central MI Univ; 87–Sp-Lang Path, Southside VA Training Ctr, **SLP**

Chester, Kathleen Arvidson 7546-L Cutters Edge Court, Dublin, OH 43017, (614) 261-5364, BA 81 Univ of Northern CO; MA 83 Univ of Northern CO; Sp-Lang Path, Riverside Methodist Hospital, **SLP**

Chester, Mrs Mary Louise 3034 Steven Martin Drive, Fairfax, VA 22031, (202) 255-9884, BA 69 MI St Univ; MA 71 MI St Univ; Sp-Lang Path, City & Burrough Juneau Sch Dis, **SLP**

Chester, Roberta L 9926 N Valley Hill Drive, Mequon, WI 53092, **SLP**

Chester, Sondra Lee 6376 Burchfield Avenue, Pittsburgh, PA 15217, MS; U of Pittsburgh, **SLP**

Chesterley, Victoria L 30 Ledgewood Hills Drive, Apartment 205, Nashua, NH 03062, (603) 882-2314, BA 72 Brown Univ; MS 75 Boston Univ; 88–Closing Coord Mort Dept, Bank of New Hampshire, **SLP**

Chevis, Mrs Mary Melanie Route 1 Box 218X14, Opelousas, LA 70570, (318) 942-7234, MS 88 Univ of Southwestern LA

Chevrette, William 1253 Laurel, Whitewater, WI 53190, (414) 472-1301, BA 69 Northern MI Univ; MS 70 Univ of Denver; PH 73 (NS) Univ of Denver; Assoc Prof, U of WI-Whitewater, **A**

Chew, Elizabeth P 382 Highland Road, Tiverton, RI 02878, (401) 274-6310, BA 77 Bates Coll; MS 82 Boston Univ; Sp-Lang Path, The Groden Ctr Inc, **SLP ACE**

Chezik, Kathryn H Marshall University, 148 Smith Hall, Huntington, WV 25701, (304) 696-2979, BA 67 IN Univ - Bloomington; MA 69 IN Univ - Bloomington; Prog Dir SLP/Aud, Marshall U, **SLP**

Chial, Dr Michael R Univ Of Wisconsin Madison, Dept Of Comm Disorders, 1975 Willow Drive, Madison, WI 53706, (608) 262-3951, MA 68 Univ of WI - Madison; MS 68 Univ of WI - Madison; PH 73 (Experimental Aud) Univ of WI - Madison; 88–Prof, Univ of Wisc-Madison, **F**

Chiapello, Dennis Albert 1125 West Pasadena Avenue, Apartment #2, Phoenix, AZ 85013, (602) 285-3473, MS 84 AZ St Univ; 87–Sp-Lang Path, Barrow Neurological Institute, **SLP**

Chiappinelli, Mrs Margo Ann 65 Laurel Avenue, Providence, RI 02906, (401) 944-6510, BA 61 Univ of RI; ME 75 RI Coll; MS 84 Univ of RI; 84–Aud, Anthony J Barone MD, **A**

Chiarello, Alice G 118 South Stiles Street, Linden, NJ 07036, (201) 558-3001, BA 70 Montclair St Coll; MA 76 Montclair St Coll; Sp/Lang Path, Elizabeth Bd of Ed, **SLP**

Chiarello, Joseph P 325 Whittaker Street, Riverside, NJ 08075, (215) 735-0205, BS 80 Murray St Univ; MA 81 Univ of TN - Knoxville; 87–Aud, Hrng Conservation Noise Control, **A**

Chiaromonte, Leatrice Auzenne 12721 Bauro #H, Garden Grove, CA 92640, (714) 553-9225, BA 83 CA St Univ - Long Beach; MS 85 Univ of AZ; **SLP**

Chichester, Donna J 9607 Bonair Drive, Manassas, VA 22110, (703) 361-0625, **SLP**

Chickedantz, Lise A 6532 Via Siena, Rancho Palos Verdes, CA 90274, (213) 328-3100, MS 72 CO St Univ; SLP, LA USD, **SLP**

Chickey, Janet Hagan 710 Ardmore Terrace, Libertyville, IL 60048, (312) 362-1798, BS 76 Univ of WI - Oshkosh; MS 77 Marquette Univ; **SLP**

Chicouris, Cynthia Lynn PO Box 482, Redlands, CA 92373, (714) 793-2121, BS 80 IN Univ - Bloomington; MS 82 Univ of WI - Madison; Asst Prof, Univ of Redlands, **SLP**

Chicvara, Joann M 17268 South 71st Court, Apartment 10, Tinley Park, IL 60477, (801) 469-4450, MA 80 Univ of IL - Urbana; BA 79 Mundelein Coll; SLP, S Metro Assoc/Hndcpd, **SLP**

Chien, Mrs Patricia Anne 6232 Calle Vera Cruz, La Jolla, CA 92037, (619) 453-0428, MS 83 Univ of TX - Dallas; Sp-Lang Path, Private Practice, **SLP**

Chien, Patricia S 2219 North Avenue, Westfield, NJ 07090, (201) 582-7580, MS 88 CUNY - Queens Coll

Chi-Fishman, Mrs Gloria 10644 Muirfield Drive, Potomac, MD 20854, (202) 576-1676, BA 68 Fu Jen Catholic Univ -Taiwan; MA 71 Kent St Univ; Dir/Sp-Lang Path, Intl Ctr for Accent Imprvmnt, **SLP ACE**

Chilcutt, Virginia Wozniak 14243 Meadowview Court, Orland Park, IL 60462, (312) 799-7520, BS 74 Northern IL Univ - De Kalb; MA 75 Northern IL Univ - De Kalb; Co-Dir, Cen for Commun Dis Ltd, **SLP ACE**

Child, Dee R Utah State University, Dept Of Commun Disorders, Umc 1000, Logan, UT 84322, (801) 750-1375, BS 76 UT St Univ; MS 78 UT St Univ; Cl Super, UT St U Dept of Commun Dis, **SLP**

Childers, Mrs Blake Brasel 3220 Wroxton, Fayetteville, AR 72703, (501) 442-2742, BA 80 Univ of AR - Fayetteville; MA 81 Univ of AR - Fayetteville; Sp-Lang Path, Fayetteville Piblic School, **SLP**

Childers, Dr Donald G Dept Of Elec Engineering, 405 CSE, Univ Of Florida, Gainesville, FL 32611, (904) 335-8428, BS 58 Univ of Southern CA; MS 59 Univ of Southern CA; PH 64 (NS) Univ of Southern CA; Prof, U of FL

Childers, Dr Robert L 6762 North Camino Abbey, Tucson, AZ 85718, (602) 792-1450, BA 65 Northeastern OK St Univ; MA 68 Univ of CO - Boulder; PH 74 (Aud) Univ of CO - Boulder; Chief/Aud & Sp-Path Service, VA Medical Center, **A**

Childress, Gloria G 3713 Douterive Drive, Chalmette, LA 70043, (504) 271-6553, BA 72 Univ of Southwestern LA; OM 76 LA St Univ - N O Medical Ctr; Sp/Lang Path, St Bernard Parish Sch Bd, **SLP**

Childress, Mrs Margaret W 16 Homewood Drive, Kirkwood, MO 63122, (314) 821-4327, BS 72 Saint Louis Univ; MA 74 Saint Louis Univ; **SLP**

Childress, Marian M S 70 Hobson Street, San Jose, CA 95110, **SLP**

Childs, Mrs Barbara L 5290 South Joliet Way, Englewood, CO 80111, (303) 796-7140, BA 65 Univ of Denver; MA 67 Univ of Denver; **SLP**

Childs, Carol Ann 1632 Mason Valley Road, Town & Country, MO 63131, (314) 993-1207, BA 83 Wichita St Univ; MA 85 Wichita St Univ; 87–Sp-Lang Path, Ranken Jordan Extended Pediatric Care, **SLP**

Childs, Deborah H Bardwells Ferry Road, Conway, MA 01341, (413) 584-8271, MS 77 SUNY - Center at Albany; SLP, Pioneer Valley Hd Injury Cntr, **SLP**

Childs, Mrs Lynne B 142 Northwoods Drive N E, Milledgeville, GA 31061-8767, (912) 453-3238, BS 77 Univ of GA; ME 78 Univ of GA; Sp-Lang Path, Private Practice, **SLP**

Childs, Mrs Phyllis 550 Harrow Court, Rochester Hills, MI 48063, (313) 852-9242, BA 57 Univ of MI - Ann Arbor; MS 60 Univ of MI - Ann Arbor; 77–Tchr, Warren Woods Pub Sch, **SLP A ACE**

Chiles, Joleen A 310 Washington Street #B, Findlay, OH 45840, (419) 354-3200, BS 86 Ashland Coll; MS 87 Bowling Green St Univ

Chiles, Mrs Michaela B 103 Steiner Boulevard, Barboursville, WV 25504, (304) 736-5099, BA 76 Marshall Univ; MA 77 Marshall Univ; Sp-Lang Path Diagnostician, Sp Path Servs, **SLP**

Chilia-Hodges, Susan 106 Hiscott Drive, Pittsburgh, PA 15241, (412) 854-0825, BA 77; MA 78 Univ of Pittsburgh - Pittsburgh; Aud, S Hills ENT Assn, **A**

Chilsen, Mrs Jody Marie 36536 Lawrence Drive, Lake Villa, IL 60046, MS 83 Univ of South FL; Aud, Hrng Assoc, **A**

Chilson, Mrs Ruth F 3 Agawam Point Road, Bourne, MA 02532, (508) 759-6659, BS 74 Ithaca Coll; MA 80 Univ of RI; SLP, PS of Mashpee, **SLP**

Chilton, Mrs Shelley Kermeen 13610 Lytton Way, Tampa, FL 33624, (813) 972-8449, BS 81 Univ of MN - Duluth; MA 85 Univ of MN - Duluth; 88–Sp-Lang Path, Moffitt Cancer Hosp & Research Ctr, **SLP**

Chin, Amy K 24962 Woolwich Street, Laguna Hills, CA 92653, **SLP**

Chin, Mrs Charlotte Y c/o Chemical Bank, PO Box 142, Makati Metro, Manila, Philippines 1299, BA 71 IN Univ - Bloomington; MS 79 Columbia Univ Teachers Coll; Clssrm Tchr, Seoul Amer Elem Sch Dods, **SLP**

Chin, Jeanie 37 Mountain Street, Woburn, MA 01801, (617) 933-8028, BA 83 Boston Coll; MS 86 Northeastern Univ; **SLP**

Chin, Linda Chang 2844 Floral Drive, Northbrook, IL 60062, (312) 480-7092, BS 77 Univ of IL - Urbana; MA 79 Univ of IL - Urbana; Sp-Lang Path, Private Practice, **SLP**

Chin, Margaret Wai-Yee 110-61 63rd Road, Forest Hills, NY 11375, (212) 904-2677, BA 85 Chinese Univ of Hong Kong; MA 87 Univ of IA; Aud, Albert Einstein Coll of Med

Chin, Dr May Elizabeth 230 North Nicholson Avenue, Condo B, Monterey Park, CA 91754, (213) 343-4695, BS 54 OH St Univ; MA 66 CA St Univ - Long Beach; PH 73 (Aud) Northwestern Univ; Aud, CA St U/La, **A**

Chinen, Mrs Verna Mae Kn 1128 Ala Napu Nani #1108, Honolulu, HI 96818, (808) 423-2477, BS 77 Univ of WA; MS 79 IL St Univ - Normal; Sp-Lang Path, Dept of Ed, **SLP**

Ching, Shannon Y 22-A Coelho Way, Honolulu, HI 96817, (808) 537-5456, BS 72 Univ of OR, OM 74 Univ of WA; 84–Aud, Hi Prof Aud, **A**

Chinitz, Shari K 54 Northfield Road, New Rochelle, NY 10804, (914) 576-2768, BA 73 Boston Univ; MS 75 Boston Univ; **SLP**

Chinn, Andrea 743 South Magnolia #10, El Cajon, CA 92020, (714) 447-0625, **SLP**

Chinn, Mrs Deborah Lee 8907 West 77th Street, Overland Park, KS 66204, (913) 341-9892, BS 79 Univ of MO - Columbia; MA 81 Univ of KS; Sp-Lang Path, Children's Therapy Group, **SLP**

Chinn, Mrs Gaye Sasaki 2024-D S W 318th Place, Federal Way, WA 98023, (206) 874-6500, BS 82 Univ of WA; MS 85 Univ of WA; 85–Aud, Glenn J Kietzer MD Inc PS, **A**

Chinn, Roxanne M 2140 Sepulveda Avenue, Milpitas, CA 95035, (408) 258-4923, BA 78 San Francisco St Univ; MA 81 CA St Univ - Long Beach; Sp-Lang Path, Alum Rock Union Sch Dist, **SLP**

Chinnick, Phyllis S 2073 Skimmer Court #225, Clearwater, FL 34622, BA 74 SUNY - Center at Buffalo; ME 75 Univ of FL; 82–Sp-Lang Path, Pinellas Co Sch, **SLP**

Chiocca, Barbara J 9 Lindsay Circle, North Granby, CT 06060, (413) 499-4537, BS 75 Trenton St Coll; MA 76 Western MI Univ; Sp-Lang Path, Pediatric Dev Cen, **SLP**

Chiodini, Valerie J 910 West Granite, Butte, MT 59701, (406) 782-8045, BS 75 Eastern IL Univ; MS 76 Eastern IL Univ; Sp-Lang Path, Anaconda School District, **SLP**

Chiodo, Denise Margaret 37 Woodbridge Park, Weirton, WV 26062, (614) 288-3674, BS 85 WV Univ; MS 87 WV Univ; Sp-Lang Path, Eastern Ohio Sp & Hearing Ctr, **SLP**

Chipelo, Mrs Helena Maria 1264 Miriam Place, Hillside, NJ 07205, (201) 596-3930, BA 80 Rutger's St Univ - Douglas Coll; MS 82 William Paterson Coll; Sp-Lang Path, Mount Carmel Guild, **SLP**

Chipkin, Mrs Linda B 3 Hawthorne Terrace, Branford, CT 06405, (203) 488-5000, BA 59 CUNY - Brooklyn Coll; MS 78 Southern CT St Univ; 78–Sp-Lang Path, Branford Bd of Ed, **SLP**

Chipman, Elizabeth Anne 12824 East 49th Terrace, Independence, MO 64055, (816) 756-2250, BS 82 AZ St Univ; MA 85 KS St Univ; 88–Sp-Lang Path, Rehab Inst, **SLP**

Chirichetti, Joann M 29 Marshall Avenue, Malden, MA 02148, (508) 937-7662, BS 74 Boston Univ; ME 78 Northeastern Univ; 74–Sp-Lang Path, Lowell Pub Sch, **SLP**

Chirico, Jo Ann T 143 Ridge Street, Pearl River, NY 10965, (914) 359-7400, BS 68 SUNY - Coll at Buffalo; MA 70 Coll of Saint Rose; 76–SLP & Aud Prog Coor, Rockland Chldn Psych Cen, **SLP**

Chisholm, Barbara B 240 West Meadowland, Sterling, VA 22170, (703) 430-0193, BA 74 Univ of MI - Ann Arbor; MS 76 Univ of MI - Ann Arbor; 88–Sp-Lang Path, Loudon County, **SLP ACE**

Chisholm, Genie L 1005 Chillum Road #207, Hyattsville, MD 20782, (703) 691-2751, BA 79 Duquesne Univ; MA 80 George Washington Univ; SLP, Fairfax Co Hlth Dept, **SLP**

Chisholm, Mrs Katrina E 4301 13th Way NE, St Petersburg, FL 33703, BS 76 SUNY - Coll at Potsdam; MS 77 Ithaca Coll; 87–Aud, Pinellas Co Schs, **A**

Chisholm, Mary C 1841 North Halstead, Unit A, Chicago, IL 60614, (312) 392-2250, BA 74 Univ of IL - Urbana; MA 75 Univ of IL - Urbana; Dir, NW Sp & Hrng Cen, **A**

Chisholm, Mrs Rebecca Wise 616 Twin Oak Drive, Raceland, LA 70394-2828, (504) 537-7345, BS 77 LA St Univ - Baton Rouge; MA 79 LA St Univ - Baton Rouge; Sp-Lang Path - Elem Sch, St Charles Parish Sch Bd, **SLP**

Chisholm, Mrs Sally Ann Ruehr 2917 Macona Lane, Billings, MT 59102, (406) 255-3882, BA 83 CO St Univ; MA 85 Univ of MT; 87–Sp-Lang Path, Billings Sch Dist #2, **SLP**

Chisum, Mrs Linda H 200 West Hermosa Drive, Fullerton, CA 92635, (714) 779-2111, BA 63 OK St Univ; MA 66 Univ of KS; SLP, Yorba Linda School District, **SLP**

Ch'iu, Julie M 23724 Gamma Street, Moreno Valley, CA 92388, (714) 681-4533, BA 60 Nat'l Tawian Univ - Taipei, Tawian; MA 65 Univ of TX - Austin; Sp-Lang Path, Riverside Co Ofc of Educ, **SLP**

Chiusano, Roseann Atkin 39 Glidden Street, Beverly, MA 01915, (617) 927-4387, BA 68 Case Western Reserve Univ; MS 72 Univ of Southern CA; Sp-Lang Path, Private Practice, **SLP ACE**

Chivetta, Antoninett 2345-F Sandalwood Creek Court, Glencoe, MO 63038, (314) 458-0625, BS 67 Univ of MO - Columbia; MA 69 Saint Louis Univ; Sp-Lang Path, Sp Sch Dist, **SLP**

Chizner, Mrs Susan 4900 North Hills Drive, Hollywood, FL 33021, (305) 989-7664, BA 73 CUNY - Brooklyn Coll; MS 74 Columbia Univ Teachers Coll; SLP, Private Practice, **SLP**

Chizzik, Stacey G 34 Newkirk Avenue, East Rockaway, NY 11518, **SLP**

Chlarson, Leann 335 West 500 North, Brigham City, UT 84302, (801) 451-1169, BS 82 Univ of UT; MS 85 Univ of UT; 88–Sp-Lang Path, McKay Dee Hosp, **SLP**

Chlipala, M Linda Route 5, 31 Rolling Hills, Sherman, TX 75090, (214) 893-7457, BS 77 Univ of North TX; MA 82 TX Woman's Univ, Sp/Lang Path, Grayson County Ctr, **SLP**

Chlopan, Lesley Carol 58 Academy Park Road, Regina, SK, Canada S4S 4T7, (306) 966-2434, BS 85 Minot St Univ; MS 86 Minot St Univ; 88–Sp-Lang Path, Univ Hosp Sasktoon, **SLP**

Chmiel, Rose A 8902 Ilona Street #8, Houston, TX 77025-3636, (713) 661-3228, BS 80 Purdue Univ - West Lafayette; MS 83 Purdue Univ - West Lafayette; Res Asst, Baylor Coll of Med, **A**

Chmiola, Mrs Mary Ann 602 16th Street, New Cumberland, PA 17070, (717) 774-2716, BS 76 Bloomsburg Univ of PA; MS 77 PA St Univ - Univ Park; Sp-Lang Path, **SLP**

Choate, Mrs Jane G T 1002 Summerbrook Place, Jacksonville, NC 28540, (919) 347-2808, BS 71 East Carolina Univ; MA 75 Univ of NC - Greensboro; 78–Sp-Lang Path, Onslow Co Sch, **SLP**

Choate, Rosmyr L, Jr Route 2 Box 407, Dardanelle, AR 72834, (501) 968-6493, BA 73 Univ of NE - Omaha; MS 74 Univ of NE - Omaha; Coord/Hndcpd, AR Riv Valley Area Council, **SLP**

Chobor, Karen Lynn 515 East 88th Street, Apartment 3-A, New York, NY 10128, (212) 628-2665, MS; 85–Research Clinician, Inst/Res-Behav Neurosci, **SLP**

Chochinov, Mrs Michelle Ann 59 Sandalwood Crescent, Winnipeg, MB, Canada R2V 3V6, (204) 786-7841, BA 79; MS 82 Univ of ND; Sp/Lang Path, Chld Guid Cl, **SLP**

Chodikoff, Karen Ann 44 St Joseph Street #1207, Toronto, ON, Canada M4Y 2W4, (416) 530-2215, OB 85 York Univ - Ontario; MS 87 Boston Univ; 87–Sp-Lang Path, Queen Elizabeth Hosp

Chodorow, Mrs Rowena B 4000 Brandi Court, Austin, TX 78759, (512) 451-2514, BS 70 Univ of TX - Austin; ME 75 Southwest TX St Univ; Sp-Lang Path, Aisd, **SLP**

Chodos, Lynn E 18 Lake Louise Road, Morganville, NJ 07751, **SLP**

Chohanin, John P 1704 Sedgewick Drive, Knoxville, TN 37922, (615) 745-4210, BA 69 Salem Coll; MA 78 Univ of TN - Knoxville; Sp-Lang Path, Athens Cty Sch, **SLP**

Cholakian, Cathy M P O Box 171, Fowler, CA 93625, **SLP**

Chomak, Joan E 1528 Channing Way, Berkeley, CA 94703, (415) 682-6330, BA 70 SUNY - Center at Binghamton; MS 82 San Francisco St Univ; SLP, Herrick Hosp, **SLP**

Chong, Sandra G H 3016 Date Street #2, Honolulu, HI 96816, **SLP**

Chonzena-Clark, Lareen K 3717 South Taft Hill Road, Apartment 262, Fort Collins, CO 80526, (307) 632-6411, BA 79 San Jose St Univ; MS 83 CO St Univ; 87–Sp-Lang Path, Heritage Rehab Ctr, **SLP**

Chopek, Dr Elena D 68 West Pierrepont Avenue, Rutherford, NJ 07070, (201) 595-2209, BA 56 Montclair St Coll; MA 65 Columbia Univ Teachers Coll; ED 71 (Sp Path) Columbia Univ Teachers Coll; Assoc Prof Commun Dis, William Paterson Coll of Nj, **SLP**

Chorney, Craig A 817 Scott Street, Stroudsburg, PA 18360, (717) 476-3440, BS 75 SUNY - Coll at Brockport; MS 80 PA St Univ - Univ Park; Ch of Aud, Pocono Med Ctr, **A**

Chou, Michele Ann 94 30 50 Avenue, Elmhurst, NY 11373, (516) 434-7957, BS 84 SUNY - Coll at Geneseo; MA 85 Bowling Green St Univ; **SLP**

Chouard, Jeanne Campbell 1321 S Beck, Tempe, AZ 85281, (602) 239-4755, BS 83 Southwest MO St Univ; MS 86 AZ St Univ; 88–Sp-Lang Path, Good Samaritan Med Ctr, **SLP**

Chouinard, David R 100 South Hunter Avenue, Joliet, IL 60436, **SLP**

Chow, Margaret K 4124 Staulo Crescent, Vancouver, BC, Canada V6N 3S2, (604) 434-1331, BS 75 IN Univ - Bloomington; MA 76 IN Univ - Bloomington; Sp-Lang Path, Sunny Hill Hosp for Chldrn, **SLP**

Chow-Hoy, Mrs Diane M S 98-844 Ainanui Loop, Aiea, HI 96701, (808) 488-1314, BA 67 Pacific Univ; MS 69 Univ of HI - Manoa; Sp-Lang Path, Department of Education, **SLP**

Choy, Ines P O Box 1633, San Ysidro, CA 92073, (706) 685-1474, BA 84 San Diego St Univ; MA 88 San Diego St Univ

Choy, Sharon Rose 914 Wind Drift Drive, Carlsbad, CA 92009, (619) 434-0607, BA 81 San Diego St Univ; MA 84 San Diego St Univ; 86–Sp-Lang Path, Carlsbad USD, **SLP**

Choyce, John C 104 Via Collado, Los Gatos, CA 95030, (408) 374-6225, BA 56 Bradley Univ; MA 63 Stanford Univ; Aud, Private Practice, **SLP A**

Christ, Linda Townsend 6612 110th Street, Kenosha, WI 53142, (414) 681-0300, BS 73 Marquette Univ; MS 75 Marquette Univ; Coord-Sp-Lang Path Dept, Racine USD, **SLP**

Christ, Marlene N 17625 Hawthorne Drive, Country Club Hills, IL 60477, (312) 687-0900, BA 60 Coll of Saint Francis; MS 81 Governors St Univ; Sp-Lang Path, SW Cook Co Coop Assn/Spec Ed, **SLP ACE**

Christ, Mrs Paula J 2 Ramblewood Drive, Chatham, IL 62629, (217) 483-5024, BA 71 Augustana Coll; MA 75 Western IL Univ; State of IL, **SLP**

Christen, Mrs Marjorie Trainor 839 Brae Burn Lane, Rockford, IL 61107, (815) 877-7001, BS 76 Northeastern Univ; OM 79 IN Univ - Bloomington; Sp-Lang Path, Milestone Inc, **SLP**

Christensen, Mrs Alyson Aycock 131 South 860 East, Orem, UT 84058, (801) 225-7465, BS 70 Brigham Young Univ; MA 85 Brigham Young Univ; 85–Sp-Lang Path, Alpine Sch Dist, **SLP**

Christensen, Mrs Ann Oddy 1024 Taft Road, Chesapeake, VA 23322, (804) 489-7068, BS 76 Nazareth Coll of Rochester; MS 86 Old Dominion Univ; **SLP**

Christensen, Dr Arden H 4341 West 58th Place, Los Angeles, CA 90043, (213) 292-5757, BA 34 Univ of IA; ME 37 Univ of Southern CA; PH 51 (NS) Univ of Southern CA; **SLP LM**

Christensen, Barbara Michele 1201 57th Street, West Des Moines, IA 50265, (515) 224-0979, BS 84 IA St Univ; MA 86 Northeast MO St Univ; Sp-Lang Path, Central Sp Rehab, **SLP**

Christensen, Carol S 8401 Spain Road N E #7A, Albuquerque, NM 87111, (505) 255-7571, BS 66 Univ of WI - Madison; MS 68 Univ of WI - Madison; 82–Pres, Jennings Hunt & Christenson PA, **SLP**

Christensen, Mrs Connie Kay 450 North Mathilda Avenue, Apartment S-204, Sunnyvale, CA 94086, (408) 773-9920, BS 85 Univ of UT; MS 87 Univ of UT

Christensen, Mrs Diana M B 6048 East 129th Street, Grandview, MO 64030, (816) 331-3945, BA 77 Univ of MO - KS City; BA 77 Univ of MO - KS City; MS 79 Central MO St Univ; Sp/Lang Path, Belton Sch Dist, **SLP**

Christensen, Mrs Donna Y 3748 Jordan Lane, Stevens Point, WI 54481-2380, (715) 346-4517, BS 76 Univ of WI - Madison; MA 77 Western MI Univ; 87–Clin Asst Prof, Univ of WI, **SLP**

Christensen, Gordon V 5316 South 750 East, Ogden, UT 84403, (801) 479-4485, BS 60 Brigham Young Univ; MS 61 Brigham Young Univ; Head Counselor, Weber Basin Job Corps, **SLP**

Christensen, Holli J 1911 Browne Avenue, Yakima, WA 98902, (509) 575-1000, BA 81 Univ of MT; MA 85 Univ of MT; Aud, ENT Assoc, **A**

Christensen, Mrs Janet Z 3155 Rambling Road, Bettendorf, IA 52722, (319) 332-7234, BA 61 Univ of IA; MA 62 Univ of IA; **SLP**

Christensen, Jean C 17 Sycamore Street, Melville, NY 11747, (516) 549-4900, BA 77 Hofstra Univ; MA 79 Hofstra Univ; Sp-Lang Path, BOCES III, **SLP**

Christensen, Dr John Eric 15805 Capitol Avenue, Omaha, NE 68137, (402) 554-2203, BS 71 Dana Coll; MS 74 Univ of NE - Omaha; PH 80 (Sp Path) Univ of KS; 80–Chrperson-Spec Educ/Comm Disorders, Univ Nebraska at Omaha, **SLP**

Christensen, Dr John M Dept Communicative Disorders, University Of Tulsa, 600 Couth College Avenue, Tulsa, OK 74104, (918) 631-2897, BS 66 Brigham Young Univ; MS 67 Brigham Young Univ; PH 75 (NS) Purdue Univ - West Lafayette; Assoc Prof, U of Tulsa, **SLP ACE**

Christensen, Judith Eileen 1853 Randolph Avenue, Apartment #204, St Paul, MN 55105, (612) 627-2732, BS 81 Moorhead St Univ; MS 84 Univ of WI - Madison; SLP, Minneapolis Public Schools, **SLP**

Christensen, Karen T 500 South Green, Toledo, IA 52342, (515) 752-1578, BS 69 Univ of IA; MA 70 Univ of IA; 75–Super/Sp-Lang Path Svcs, AEA 6, **SLP**

Christensen, Dr Kathee Ann 5283 Countryside Drive, San Diego, CA 92115, (619) 265-6139

Christensen, Mrs Margaret S 2072 Atkin Avenue, Salt Lake City, UT 84109, (801) 485-3681, BA 48 Univ of UT; MS 77 Univ of UT; SLP, Davis Co Sch Dist, **SLP**

Christensen, Mrs Marlene N 3842 West Elwood Way, West Jordan, UT 84084, (801) 569-2013, BS 74 UT St Univ; MS 76 UT St Univ; Sp-Lang Path, Jordan School District, **SLP**

Christensen, Mary V 5488 Oleta Street, Long Beach, CA 90815, (213) 603-1511, 73 Univ of CA - Santa Barbara; MA 86 CA St Univ - Los Angeles; Sp-Lang Path, Los Angeles Office of Educ, **SLP**

Christensen, Michelle K 1786 Neale Street, San Diego, CA 92103, (619) 299-5515, BA 73 Loyola Coll; MA 75 Catholic Univ of America; SLP, San Diego USD, **SLP**

Christensen, Nancy 8265 West 2700 South, Salt Lake City, UT 84044, (801) 250-8400, BS 78 ID St Univ; MS 80 Purdue Univ - West Lafayette; 88–Dir-Mktg, Villa Serena, **SLP**

Christensen, Dr Ned Jay University Of Oregon, 354 Clinical Services Bldg, Eugene, OR 97403, (503) 686-3591, BA 54 Brigham Young Univ; MA 55 Brigham Young Univ; PH 59 (NS) PA St Univ - Univ Park; Prof/Dir SLP Prog, U of OR, **SLP A F**

Christensen, Patricia 3708 Glen Canyon N E, Albuquerque, NM 87111, (505) 345-9021, BS 67 Brigham Young Univ; MS 69 Brigham Young Univ; Chpers/Spec Ed Dept, Albuquerque Pub Sch, **SLP**

Christensen, Sally A 7630 E Warren Circle #7-208, Denver, CO 80231, (303) 745-5617, BS 85 Univ of MN - Duluth; MA 86 Univ of MN - Duluth; SLP, InSpeech Inc, **SLP**

Christensen, Mrs Susan Hoster 1130 Cedar Branch Court, Marietta, GA 30064, (404) 426-3328, OB 78 Univ of GA; ME 82 Univ of GA; Sp-Lang Path/Prog Coord, Cobb Co Pub Schools, **SLP**

Christensen, Mrs Susan S 704 Printz Road, Arroyo Grande, CA 93420, (805) 543-2010, BA 72 Univ of Redlands; MS 73 Univ of Redlands; Sp-Lang Path, San Luis Coastal USD, **SLP**

Christenson, Merilyn J 3872 Chapman Place, Riverside, CA 92506, (714) 683-8140, BA 67 Loma Linda Univ - Riverside; MA 68 Univ of Redlands; Diagnostic Teacher, CA Sch for the Deaf, **SLP**

Christenson, Russell L 300 South Water, Clinton, MO 64735, (816) 885-5511, BS 68 Mankato St Univ; MA 75 OK St Univ; SLP, Golden Vlly Mem Hosp, **SLP**

Christiaansen, Mrs Ellen 3224 Whip-Poor-Will Lane, Appleton, WI 54915, (414) 738-2582, BS 73 SUNY - Center at Albany; MA 74 Kent St Univ; Sp/Lang Path, St Elizabeth Hosp, **SLP**

Christian, Beverly A 415 South Chelsea Road, White Plains, NY 10603, (914) 422-2320, BA 73 Brown Univ; MS 76 Teachers Coll - Boston; 77–Sp-Lang Path, White Plains PS, **SLP**

Christian, Mrs Carolyn Brovold 2340 15th Street, Eau Claire, WI 54703, (715) 839-9119, BS 77 Univ of WI - River Falls; MS 78 Univ of WI - River Falls; SLP, Private Practice, **SLP**

Christian, Mrs Debra A 11026 Ingram, Livonia, MI 48150, (313) 421-1115, BS 78 Eastern MI Univ; MA 78 Eastern MI Univ; SLP, Garden City Schs - Burger Ctr, **SLP**

Christian, Jana Lee 1001 Iloxi Drive #1107, Ennis, TX 75119, (817) 755-2567, BS 85 Baylor Univ; MS 86 Baylor Univ; SLP, Ennis ISD, **SLP**

Christian, Kathryn Farnen 293 11th Street, Brooklyn, NY 11215, (718) 768-2723, BA 76 Univ of MO - Columbia; MA 77 Univ of IA; 86–Sp-Lang Path, NY League for Early Learning, **SLP**

Christian, Sara Schultz 2721 West Princeton Avenue, Eau Claire, WI 54703, (715) 723-5542, BA 84 Univ of WI - Eau Claire; MS 85 Univ of WI - Eau Claire; 85–Sp-Lang Path, Northern Wisconsin Center for the Developmentally Disabled, **SLP**

Christiana, Diana Grana 2514 Glen Haven Lane, Richmond, TX 77469, (713) 342-7154, BS 81 SUNY - Coll at Fredonia; MA 82 IN Univ - Bloomington; Sp-Lang Path, Private Practice, **SLP**

Christiansen, Diana J 314 West 5th, Carson City, NV 89701, (702) 882-2565, BA 67 Univ of Northern IA; MA 68 Univ of Northern IA; Sp-Lang Path, Private Practice, **SLP ACE**

Christiansen, Kay 1049 Shell Blvd #10, Foster City, CA 94404, (415) 578-1642, BA 86 Univ of CA - Santa Barbara; MA 87 Univ of the Pacific; 87–Sp-Lang Path, Agnews Dev Ctr, **SLP**

Christiansen, Loretta M 529 South Chestnut Street, Kewanee, IL 61443, **SLP**

Christianson, Mary Lou 1103 Prospect Place, Vista, CA 92083, (619) 724-7799, BA 66 CA St Univ - Long Beach; MA 68 CA St Univ - Long Beach; SLP, Los Angeles Co Supt of Schools, **SLP**

Christianson, Mrs Pamela Paguia Box 647, Barrow, AK 99723, (907) 852-5308, MS 87 Portland St Univ

Christie, Carol Schramm 3325 East Monument Street, Baltimore, MD 21205, (904) 734-3320, BA 74 Loyola Coll; MS 75 Loyola Coll; Dept Hd Sp & Hrng, W Volusia Mem Hosp, **SLP**

Christie, Mrs Judith Ann P O Box 3060 Upb, Las Cruces, NM 88003, (505) 382-7472, BS 83 Grand Canyon Coll; MA 85 Grand Canyon Coll; **SLP**

Christie, M Michele 2512 Avenue K, Bay City, TX 77414, (409) 245-6318, BS 84 Western Carolina Univ; MS 86 Western Carolina Univ; **SLP**

Christina, Mrs Margaret 3035 Greenwood, Rochester Hills, MI 48309, (313) 547-7608, BS 63 Bloomsburg Univ of PA; ME 74 Wayne St Univ; Sp-Lang Path, Cty of Ferndale Pub Sch, **SLP**

Christison, Lori Sue 6409 West 101st Street, Overland Park, KS 66212, (913) 224-0201, BS 82 Bradley Univ; OM 84 AZ St Univ; **SLP**

Christman, Josephine E 1909 Mosher Drive #C, Enid, OK 73701, (405) 234-3734, BA 38 Wichita St Univ; Sp-Lang Path, Comm Sp & Hrng Cen, **SLP LM**

Christman, Mary Ann 1693 Peony Lane, San Jose, CA 95124, (408) 270-6447, BS 66 Univ of ND; OM 71 Univ of WA; 79–Sp-Lang Path, San Jose Comm Coll Dist, **SLP ACE**

Christman, Mrs Sarah Slack 110 Hermitage Avenue, Maurice, LA 70555-9422, (504) 549-2214, BS 80 IL St Univ - Normal; MA 82 LA St Univ - Baton Rouge; Instuctor, SE LA U, **SLP**

Christoffel, Mrs Elizabeth Faith 1834 Amity Drive, Lancaster, PA 17601-6204, (717) 569-5422, BS 78 Kutztown Univ of PA; MA 84 West Chester Univ of PA; S June Smith Center, **SLP**

Christon, Mrs Michele PO Box 611, Burnsville, NC 28714, BA 71 Univ of MA - Amherst; MA 72 Univ of MA - Amherst; 87–Reg Consult, LOGOS, **SLP**

Christopher, Mrs Dana E 2034 Ames Street, Los Angeles, CA 90027-6009, (213) 661-6222, BA 73 CA St Univ - Los Angeles; MA 78 CA St Univ - Northridge; Sp-Lang Path, Private Practice, **SLP**

Christopher, Dr Judith L 222 Martling Avenue, Tarrytown, NY 10591, (914) 693-4500, BS 68 Boston Univ; MA 70 Columbia Univ Teachers Coll; PH 79 (NS) Columbia Univ Teachers Coll; Chrp Dept of Sp, Mercy Coll, **SLP**

Christopher, Mrs Lynn Rankin Box 102, Hiller, PA 15444, (412) 439-1444, MS 87 CA Univ of PA; 87–Sp-Lang Path, SG Speech Associates, **SLP**

Christopher, Patricia A 7955 Rock Hill Road, St Louis, MO 63123, (314) 344-6460, BS 79 Fontbonne Coll; MS 80 Southern IL Univ-Edwardsvill; Supervisor, Depaul Health Center, **SLP**

Christopherson, Sharon 3454 Cornell Place, Cincinnati, OH 45220, (513) 559-1054, BA 68 SUNY - Center at Albany; MA 74 IN Univ - Bloomington; Aud, Cincinnati Ctr for Imp Comm, **A**

Christos, Mrs Sandra Shuman 1426 Old West Chester Pike, West Chester, PA 19382, (215) 692-5816, BS 82 Old Dominion Univ; MS 87 Old Dominion Univ; 87–Sp-Lang Path, Team Rehab Inc, **SLP**

Christy, Mrs Darlene Marie 501 Florence Avenue, Pittsburgh, PA 15202, (412) 761-6062, **SLP**

Christy, Dianne P O Box 7046, Opelousas, LA 70570-7046, (318) 948-9472, BA 76 Univ of Southwestern LA; ME 87 Southern Univ - Baton Rouge; **SLP**

Christy, Felicia Ann 43 Clay Street #5, Fairburn, GA 30213, (404) 664-6818, BS 78 CA Univ of PA; ME 80 CA Univ of PA; Sp/Lang Path, Communicare, **SLP**

Christy, Mrs Janis Lynn 101 Rivergate Place, Lodi, CA 95240, (209) 368-3503, BA 82 CA St Univ - Sacramento; Sp-Lang Path, Lodi USD, **SLP**

Christy, Lloyd Wayne 2400 Chestnut Street #1702, Philadelphia, PA 19103, (215) 596-9125, BS 70 IN St Univ - Evansville; MA 73 Temple Univ; Dir-Sp-Lang Path/Aud, Cooper Hosp/Univ Med Ctr, **A**

Christy, Mary Ellen 88 Congress St, #304, Saratoga Springs, NY 12866, (518) 584-6337, BS 82 Coll of Saint Rose; MS 84 Ithaca Coll; 85–Supvr-Comm Dis, Amsterdam Memorial Hosp, **A**

Chrusciel, Judy Beth 1163 Sumner Avenue, Upper Schnectady, NY 12309, (518) 377-2879, BS 82 Univ of MA - Amherst; MS 86 SUNY - Coll at Buffalo; **SLP**

Chrystal, Jean L University Of Illinois Eye & Ear, 1855 West Taylor, Audiology Section Room B46, Chicago, IL 60012, (312) 996-6520, BS 86 Univ of IL - Urbana; MA 88 Univ of IL - Urbana; 88–Aud, Univ of IL Eye & Ear Infirmary

Chu, Diane Elizabeth 7200 Mariner Drive #5, Racine, WI 53406-3836, (713) 792-4500, BS 83 Univ of IA; MA 85 Univ of IA; **SLP**

Chubrich, Robert 2346 East Lajolla Drive, Tempe, AZ 85282, (602) 839-7156, BS 63 OK St Univ; MA 65 IN Univ - Bloomington; Sp-Lang Path, Tempe Elem Dist #3, **SLP**

Chubrich, Mrs Ronda C 2346 East Lajolla Drive, Tempe, AZ 85282, MS; **SLP**

Chucales, Katherine Anne 2785 Brady Lane, Bloomfield Hills, MI 48013, (313) 343-3728, BA 80 Univ of MI - Ann Arbor; MS 82 Univ of MI - Ann Arbor; 87–Sp-Lang Path, Lakeshore ENT Cen, **SLP**

Chuchas, James G 3320 Ben Lomond Drive, Sacramento, CA 95821, **SLP**

Chud, Mrs Randi L R 2050 Butternut Drive, Huntingdon Valley, PA 19006, (215) 539-8550, BS 77 PA St Univ - Univ Park; MA 79 Trenton St Coll; Sp-Lang Path, Montgomery County Indepen Unit, **SLP**

Chudej, Mrs Mary M 2608 Galpin #209, Royal Oak, MI 48073, (313) 452-8509, BS 77 Northern MI Univ; MS 82 Univ of WI - Eau Claire; 85–Sp-Lang Path, MacOmb-Oakland Regional Center, **SLP**

Chudik, Eileen M 329 Douglas Drive, Bloomingdale, IL 60108, (312) 351-2941, BS 79 Northern IL Univ - De Kalb; MS 81 Univ of IL - Urbana; Sp-Lang Path, Horizons Sp-Lang Path Consult Inc, **SLP**

Chudy-Hesselberg, Mrs Barbara Ann 332 Folsom Street, Columbus, WI 53925, (414) 623-2225, BS 83 Univ of WI - Madison; MS 85 Marquette Univ

Chuk, Ann E Chaplin Village, Chaplin, CT 06235, (203) 455-9593, BA 69 SUNY - Center at Buffalo; MA 71 Univ of CT; Sp/Lang Path, Windham Bd of Ed, **SLP**

Chumley, Audrey Santa Fe Center For Audiology, 1454 St Francis, Santa Fe, NM 87501, (505) 988-9818, BA 72 LA Tech Univ; MS 74 Univ of NM; Aud, Santa Fe Center for Aud, **A**

Chun, Darleen G 1088 Bishop Street #3007, Honolulu, HI 96813, **SLP**

Chun, Mrs Jan E Arakaki 2384 Makanani Drive, Honolulu, HI 96817, (808) 845-4319, BS 76 Univ of HI - Manoa; MS 78 Univ of HI - Manoa; Sp-Lang Pathologist, State of HI Dept of Education, **SLP**

Chun, Raquel Ortiz 21 Lakewood Drive, South Windsor, CT 06074, (203) 549-6371, BA 83 Univ of PR - Rio Piedras; MS 85 Univ of PR - San Juan; **SLP**

Chung, Mrs Jane Ellyn 9607 West Hampton Avenue, Wauwatosa, WI 53225, (414) 462-4199, BS 86 Univ of WI - Milwaukee; MS 88 Marquette Univ

Chunn, Patricia C Communicology Inc, 8220 Naab Road, Suite 311, Indianapolis, IN 46260, (317) 872-3131, BS 72 G Peabody Coll-Vanderbilt U; MS 73 Vanderbilt Univ; Dir, Communicology Inc, **SLP ACE**

Churan, Cynthia S P O Box 207, West Park, NY 12493, (914) 338-9320, **SLP**

Church, Mrs Debra L 890 Poplar Church Road #405, Camp Hill, PA 17011, (717) 761-6794, BS 77 WV Univ; MS 78 WV Univ; 87–Sp-Lang Path, Private Practice, **SLP**

Church, Dr Gerald T Dept Communication Disorders, Central Michigan Univ, 452 Moore Hall, Mount Pleasant, MI 48859, (517) 774-7301, BS 73 Saint Lawrence Univ; MS 75 Syracuse Univ; PH 81 (NS) Syracuse Univ; Assoc Prof of Aud, Cen Mich Univ, **A**

Church, Mrs K L Church Estates Road, P O Box 2069 Otto Branch, Imperial, MO 63052, (314) 942-3823, OB William Jewell Coll; MA 64 Saint Louis Univ; Private Practice, **SLP**

Church, Marie Ahern 205 Cherry Lane, Pearisburg, VA 24134, (703) 552-6641, BA 85 Univ of Akron; MS 86 Radford Univ; 86–Aud, The Hearing & Sp Ctr, **A**

Church, Rose May 1315 Hillcrest Nisbet, Sarnia, ON, Canada N7S 4T4, MS; **LM**

Churchill, Mrs Faye M 2031-E Canyon Road, Birmingham, AL 35216, (205) 822-8560, BA 62 Univ of Montevallo; MA 66 Auburn Univ - Auburn; Owner/Dir/Pres, Hrng Sp Cl/Indus Ttng Assoc, **SLP A**

Churchill, Santi Jane 348 East Peach Drive, Shreveport, LA 71106, (318) 632-4889, BA 83 LA St Univ - Shreveport; OM 85 LA St Univ - N O Medical Ctr; **SLP**

Churich, Mrs Jan M 1267 Sunrise Way, Milpitas, CA 95035, (408) 985-1050, BA 64 San Jose St Univ; MA 71 San Jose St Univ; SLP, Santa Clara USD, **SLP**

Chute, Mrs Patricia Molinelli 210 East 64th Street, New York, NY 10021, (212) 605-3793, BA 72 CUNY - Hunter Coll; MA 74 CUNY - Hunter Coll; Dir, Manhttn Eye ENT Hosp, **A**

Chute, Mrs Sharon M 1701 Easy Lane, Charlottesville, VA 22901-7418, (804) 973-1253, BS 77 Marywood Coll; MA 80 OH Univ - Athens; Sp-Lang Path, Albemarle Co, **SLP**

Chute, Wendy Wenker Cincinnati Speech & Hearing Ct, 3021 Vernon Place, Cincinnati, OH 45219, (513) 221-0527, BS 85 Miami Univ - Oxford; MS 86 Bowling Green St Univ; **A**

Chuzi, Ken Martin 3239 N Christmas Avenue, Tucson, AZ 85716, (602) 626-7222, MS 86 Univ of AZ; 88–Sp-Lang Path, Univ Med Ctr, **SLP**

Chvatal, Mrs Sarah Curtis 1007 Mira Vista Road, Huntsville, AL 35802, (205) 532-4718, BS 71 Auburn Univ - Auburn; MS 73 Vanderbilt Univ; Sp-Lang Path, Huntsville Cty Schs-Ctr for Devel Learn, **SLP ACE**

Chvotkin, Mrs Lynn Simmons 14002 North Commons Way, Potomac, MD 20854, (301) 279-7847, BA 69 Univ of FL; MA 71 Univ of CT; **SLP**

Chwalek, Maryann C P O Box 495, La Honda, CA 94020, (415) 747-0984, BA 74 Univ of MA - Amherst; MS 80 San Francisco St Univ; SLP, **SLP**

Chwang, Mrs Karen Malick 5515 Plymouth Road, Baltimore, MD 21214, (301) 396-3100, **SLP**

Chwat, Sam E 250 West 103rd Street, Apartment 5-A, New York, NY 10025, (212) 242-8435, BA 74 Sarah Lawrence Coll; MS 77 Columbia Univ Teachers Coll; Dir, Speakup Inc, **SLP**

Chwierut, Barbara J 6146 South Kolmar, Chicago, IL 60629, (312) 767-3562, BA 76 Governors St Univ; MS 79 Governors St Univ; Sp-Lang Path, Aero Spec Ed Co-Op, **SLP**

Ciaccia-Woskey, Mrs Kathleen 2011 Hilltop Road, Whiting, NJ 08759, (201) 849-4127, BA 81 Kean Coll of NJ; MA 84 Montclair St Coll; 87–Sp-Lang Path, Early Intervention Prog of Monmouth & Ocean Co Inc, **SLP**

Ciamarra, Cheryl Ringuette 3820 Cromwell Drive, Mountain Brook, AL 35243, (205) 871-2495, BS 79 Univ of Southwestern LA; OM 80 LA St Univ - N O Medical Ctr; Sp-Lang Path, Private Practice, **SLP**

Ciambrone, Gary Sp & L Services Of Gr Boston, 212 Ashmont Street, Dorchester, MA 02124-3829, (617) 265-0280, BS 74 Trenton St Coll; MS 79 Purdue Univ - West Lafayette; Dir Sp-Lang Path, Sp-Lang Serv of Greater Boston, **SLP**

Ciambrone, Sarah W 10 Adanac Terrace, Dorchester, MA 02124, (617) 265-0280, MS 79 Purdue Univ - West Lafayette; Sp/Lang Path, Massachusetts Gen Hosp, **SLP**

Ciampa, Elaine N Box 503, Weston, MA 02193, (617) 237-4885, BA 68 Boston Coll; ME 69 Boston Univ; SLP/Cl Super, Commun Hlth Care Assoc, **SLP**

Ciampaglio, Mrs Susan N A 208 Regent Drive, Bel Air, MD 21014, (301) 879-5123, BS 76 Towson St Univ; MS 77 Towson St Univ; **SLP**

Ciampi, Mrs Valerie Marie 6318 35th Way S E, Auburn, WA 98002, (206) 833-9196, BA 81 San Jose St Univ; MA 84 San Jose St Univ; Sp-Lang Path, Rainer Sch, **SLP**

Cianci, Ann Marie 23 Maple Avenue, Harrison, NY 10528, (718) 793-9629, BA 73 Iona Coll; MS 79 Columbia Univ Teachers Coll; 87–Aud, Sawtech Communications Inc, **A**

Cianci, Susan Williamson 790 Prescott Place, West Babylon, NY 11704, (516) 321-4010, BA 84 SUNY - Coll at Plattsburgh; MS 86 Adelphi Univ; **SLP**

Cianciolo, Alison Grace 23 Wedgewood Drive, Watertown, CT 06795, (203) 574-8109, BS 84 East Stroudsburg Univ of PA; MA 85 Kean Coll of NJ; 85–Sp-Lang Path, Waterbury Bd of Educ, **SLP**

Ciaranello, Mrs Nancy J R 996 Wing Place, Stanford, CA 94305, (415) 855-8419, BS 65 Purdue Univ - West Lafayette; MA 66 Stanford Univ; SLP, Palo Alto USD, **SLP A**

Ciarlo, Debra A JC Speech Pathology Clinic, 210 Methow, Wenatchee, WA 98801, (509) 662-3762, BS 74 CO St Univ; MS 76 Univ of WA; Dir-Sp-Lang Path, Jc Sp Path Cl, **SLP**

Ciavarella, Carol 118 South Dory Road, North Palm Beach, FL 33408, (305) 626-5248, MS 83 FL St Univ; Sp-Lang Path, **SLP**

Ciccariello, Mrs Mary P 520 West Gray Street, Elmira, NY 14905, (607) 734-0308, BS 87 Elmira Coll; MS 87 Ithaca Coll; 87–Sp-Lang Path, Addison Sch Dist, **SLP**

Cicci, Dr Regina L 4000 North Charles Street, Apartment 1403, Baltimore, MD 21218-1737, (301) 328-5948, BS 60 Kent St Univ; MA 61 Northwestern Univ; PH 78 (NS) Northwestern Univ; Assistant Professor, Univ of Maryland Hospital, **SLP**

Ciccone, Catherine 3177 Ashlyn Street, Pittsburgh, PA 15204, MS 79 Univ of Pittsburgh - Pittsburgh; Sp-Lang Path, Pittsburgh Board of Pub Educ, **SLP**

Cicero, Carol Ann 2220 Ocheltree, Olathe, KS 66061, BS 77 PA St Univ - Univ Park; MS 81 Univ of HI - Manoa; Sp-Lang Path, Providence-St Margaret Hlth Cn, **SLP**

Cicholski, Mrs Barbara A 812 Timberwood Drive, Mars, PA 16046, (412) 829-7082, BA 79 Univ of Pittsburgh - Pittsburgh; MA 81 Univ of Pittsburgh - Pittsburgh; **SLP**

Cichowitz, Mrs Deborah J 7216 Aspen Glen Lane, Colorado Springs, CO 80919, (303) 688-3187, BA 80 Univ of Northern CO; MA 81 Univ of Northern CO; SLP, Colo School for Deaf & Blind, **SLP**

Cicolello, Beverly 133 St Louis Avenue, Rockford, IL 61104-1518, (815) 734-6071, BA 79 Adelphi Univ; MA 82 Univ of IL - Urbana; Sp-Lang Path, Ogle Co Ed Coop, **SLP**

Cicotello, Christine 5383 Leicester Court, Virginia Beach, VA 23462, (804) 490-1951, ME 88 Old Dominion Univ; 88–Sp-Lang Path, VA Beach PS

Cicotte, Mrs Carol Alvord 10281 Grayfox Drive, San Diego, CA 92131, (619) 292-9931, BA 80 San Diego St Univ; MA 85 San Diego St Univ; 88–Sp-Lang Path, San Diego Sp & Rehab Svcs

Cieliczka, David J Aud & Hrng Instruments Of Nh, 194 Pleasant Street, Suite 2, Concord, NH 03301, (603) 224-3346, BS 68 Northern MI Univ; MA 71 Central MI Univ; Aud/Owner, Aud & Hrng Inst of Nh, **A**

Ciely, Paula M 1800 North Andrews Avenue, Apartment #7-D, Fort Lauderdale, FL 33311, (305) 928-1540, BA 76 Montclair St Coll; MA 77 Bowling Green St Univ; Aud-Except Stud Ed, Broward Co Sch Bd, **A ACE**

Ciepiela, Mrs Lisa Marie 11 South Irwinwood Road, Lancaster, NY 14086, (716) 684-3547, BS 84 SUNY - Coll at Buffalo; MS 86 SUNY - Coll at Buffalo; **SLP**

Cieplinski, Mrs Nancy 4 Litchfield Crescent, Halifax, NS, Canada B3P 2N2, (902) 477-1515, BS 66 Dalhousie Univ - Nova Scotia; ME 68 Boston Univ; **SLP**

Ciesielski, Teresa M 2902 Elm Street, Parkersburg, WV 26101, (304) 428-6277, BA 85 IN Univ - Bloomington; MA 86 IN Univ - Bloomington; 86–Sp-Lang Path, Wood Co Bd of Educ, **SLP**

Cilek, Toni D University Of Iowa, Speech & Hearing Clinic, Iowa City, IA 52242, (319) 335-8744, BA 75 Univ of IA; MA 76 Univ of IA; Supervisor, University of Iowa, **SLP**

Cilella-Meyer, Mrs Janet Mary 1948 North Burling, Chicago, IL 60614, (312) 333-7812, BS 81 IL St Univ - Normal; MS 83 IL St Univ - Normal; Sp-Lang Path, S Metro Assoc, **SLP**

Ciliax, Dr Donald R 1112 Hendrix Court, Bel Air, MD 21014, (202) 693-5460, BA 65 Univ of CA - Santa Barbara; MS 66 CO St Univ; PH 73 (Aud) MI St Univ; Aud, U S Army, **A**

Cimino, Mary F Fox Chapel Arms #105, 265 Freeport Road, Pittsburgh, PA 15238, (412) 429-0280, BS 68 Clarion Univ of PA; ME 69 Clarion Univ of PA; Sp-Lang Path, Vna-Allegheny Co, **SLP**

Cinciripini, Mrs Doreen Dora 2303 Colleen Drive, Pearland, TX 77581, (713) 438-0260, MS Auburn Univ - Auburn; 88–Sp-Lang Path, Fort Bend ISD, **SLP**

Cincotta, Martha F 15-B Troy Drive, Springfield, NJ 07081, (201) 994-1550, OB 50 Northwestern Univ; BA 69 Kean Coll of NJ; Sp-Lang Path, Livingston Bd of Ed, **SLP ACE**

Ciocci, Sandra R 8 Melikian Drive, Wilbraham, MA 01095, BS 78 Univ of MA - Amherst; ME 80 Northeastern Univ; 80–Sp-Lang Path, Willie Ross Sch for the Deaf, **SLP**

Cioffi, Lisa M Rd 1 Box 370, Averill Park, NY 12018, (518) 674-2502, MS 87 Coll of Saint Rose

Cioffi, Mrs Maribeth Matthews 1 Myrtle Avenue, Troy, NY 12180, (518) 270-2517, **SLP**

Ciolli, Lois Gregory 8006 Sharpcrest, Houston, TX 77036, (713) 995-6745, BS 80 Univ of Houston - Univ Park; MA 84 Our Lady Lake Univ-San Anton; Sp-Lang Path, Alief, **SLP**

Cipolletti, Michael W 510 Vance Avenue, Wyckoff, NJ 07481, (212) 584-9000, BA 71 William Paterson Coll, MS 74 William Paterson Coll; Sp-Lang Path, VA Med Cen, **SLP**

Cire, George E 309 Maplewood Drive, Victoria, TX 77901, (512) 573-4832, BA 77 LA Tech Univ; OM 78 LA St Univ - N O Medical Ctr; 82–Aud, Victoria Regional Hearing Center, **A**

Cirelli, Richard A 21 Lunn Avenue, Bergenfield, NJ 07621, (201) 384-9789, BA 64 Univ of Miami; MA 78 Montclair St Coll; 64–Dir of Rdng & Sp Serv, Bergenfield Pub Sch, **SLP**

Cirigliano, Paulette 112 Sylvan Drive, Lower Burrell, PA 15068, (412) 281-1375, BS 72 Carlow Coll; MA 74 Catholic Univ of America; Sp-Lang Path, Pittsburgh Hrng,Spch & Deaf Sv, **SLP**

Cirilli, Patti J 5964 North Bay Ridge Avenue, Whitefish Bay, WI 53217, (414) 931-4065, BS 76 Univ of WI - Stevens Point; MS 78 Univ of WI - River Falls; Sp-Lang Path, Chldn Hosp, **SLP**

Cirillo, Mrs Lisa A 301 Linden Street, Mahwah, NJ 07430, (201) 529-5287, BA 80 Kean Coll of NJ; MA 82 Montclair St Coll; Sp-Lang Path, Paul-Davis Regional Center, **SLP**

Cirillo, Richard R 162-25 Laburnum Avenue, Flushing, NY 11358, (516) 731-9076, BA 76 CUNY - Queens Coll; MA 79 Hofstra Univ; PH 84 (NS) Long Island U - CW Post Ctr; Sp-Lang Path, Levitown Bd of Educ, **SLP**

Cirka, Nancy A 16 Bay Avenue, Barrington, RI 02806, (201) 245-5762, BS 79 Emerson Coll; MS 80 Emerson Coll; 88–Sp-Lang Path, Private Practice, **SLP**

Cirkiel-Naftel, Karen 2206 Holland Avenue, Bronx, NY 10467, BA 78 CUNY - City College; MS 80 Columbia Univ Teachers Coll; Indep Aud Consultant, Consult to Dr Felix Sniffman, **A**

Cirmo, Mrs Nancy L 1279 Highview Terrace, Cheshire, CT 06410, (203) 272-4290, BA 74 Univ of CT; MA 76 Univ of CT; 81–Sp-Lang Path, Bristol CT PS, **SLP**

Ciro, Linda A B 10310 Windriver Drive, Houston, TX 77070, **SLP**

Cirrin, Dr Frank M Minneapolis Public Schools, Special Education Services Center, 254 Upton Avenue South, Minneapolis, MN 55403, (612) 627-3085, BA 72 SUNY - Coll at Plattsburgh; MS 75 SUNY - Center at Albany; PH 80 (NS) Univ of IA; Asst Prof Sp-Lang Path, Idaho St U -Dept Sp-Path & Aud, **SLP**

Cislo, Mrs Heidi M 114 South 3rd Street, Harrison, NJ 07029, (201) 441-2165, SLP, Hackensack Med Centr, **SLP**

Cistone, Mary Padula 2123 20th Street, Cuyahoga Falls, OH 44223, (216) 762-5425, MA 85 2839; 87–Sp-Lang Path, Bliek Clinic Inc, **SLP**

Citron, Dr David, III South Shore Hearing Center, 825 Main Street, P O Box 134, South Weymouth, MA 02190, (617) 337-6860, BA 71 Northern IL Univ - De Kalb; MS 72 Univ of OK Medical Center; PH 79 (NS) Purdue Univ - West Lafayette; Dir, S Shore Hrng Cen, **A ACE**

Citron, Louise G 11 Locksley Road, Newton Center, MA 02159, (617) 337-6860, BS 73 Boston Univ; MA 71 Univ of CT; Dir, Bay Colony Hearing Instruments, **A**

Ciuberkis, Arunas Jonas 40 West 18th Street #4, New York, NY 10011, (212) 741-0107, BA 75 Cleveland St Univ; MA 77 Kent St Univ; Sp-Lang Path, Visiting Nurse Service, **SLP**

Ciucci, Mrs Rebecca Lee 107 Marleybone Court, Goose Creek, SC 29445, (803) 553-1906, BS 81 PA St Univ - Univ Park; MS 83 PA St Univ - Univ Park; Aud, **A**

Ciurczak, Judith G 6 Riverside Drive, Denville, NJ 07834, (201) 299-0166, BA 67 Rutger's St Univ - Douglas Coll; MA 68 Newark St Coll; SLP, Lake Drive Sch Hrng Imp Childn, **SLP**

Civils, Mrs Carol Ann 714 North Allyson Drive, Baton Rouge, LA 70815, (504) 923-2630, BA 66 CA St Univ - Fullerton; MA 82 LA St Univ - Baton Rouge; Sp/Lang Path, East Baton Rouge Parish Sch Bd, **SLP ACE**

Claassen, Mary 6404 Glenwood Road, Omaha, NE 68132, (402) 553-0917, BA 56 Univ of NE - Omaha; MA 84 Univ of NE - Omaha; Sp-Lang Path, Omaha Public Scools, **SLP**

Clabo, Mrs Pamela A 851 Maple Road, Williamsville, NY 14221, (716) 631-4866, BS 79 SUNY - Coll at Buffalo; MS 82 SUNY - Coll at Buffalo; Sp-Lang Path, Williamsville Central Sch Dist, **SLP**

Clabuesch, Rebecca P 2652 Eastern Avenue S E, Grand Rapids, MI 49507, (616) 455-5000, OM 85 Wayne St Univ; SLP, Pine Rest Christian Hospital, **SLP**

Claeys, Polly E F 923 W Hayes, Charleston, IL 61920, (217) 258-2568, BA 77 Augustana Coll; MS 78 Eastern IL Univ; Asst Dir/Sp-Lang-Hrng Ser, Sarah Bush Lincoln Hlth Cen, **SLP**

Claeys, Wanda M 450 Laurel Circle, Cookeville, TN 38501, **SLP LM**

Claflin, Donna L W 6826 Arbor Lane, Cedar Rapids, IA 52402, (319) 399-6700, BA 79 Univ of Northern IA; MA 80 Univ of Northern IA; SLP, Grant Wood AEA, **SLP**

Clair, Mrs Margaret Goss 4515 Oakcreek Street, Apartment 105, Orlando, FL 32811, (407) 299-2060, BS 82 Univ of NC - Chapel Hill; MS 83 Univ of NC - Chapel Hill; 84–Sp-Lang Path, **SLP**

Clamp, Mrs Jana Poynor Speech Pathology Department, Queen's Medical Center, 1301 Punchbowl, Honolulu, HI 96813, (808) 547-4277, BS 86 Baylor Univ; MS 87 Baylor Univ; 88–Sp-Path & Aud, The Queens Med Ctr

Clanahan, Karen J 420 East Clark Trail #1, Herrin, IL 62948, (618) 993-2138, BS 74 Southern IL Univ -Carbondale; MS 75 Southern IL Univ -Carbondale; Sp-Lang Path, Williamson Co Spec Educ Dist, **SLP**

Clancy, Ann Marie 14243 Cape Horn Place, Florissant, MO 63034, (314) 261-0527, BS 82 Southern IL Univ-Edwardsvill; MS 83 Southern IL Univ-Edwardsvill; Sp/Lang Path, Spec Sch Dist/St Louis Co, **SLP**

Clancy, Mrs Annemarie Bock 4 Rosedown Drive, Destrehan, LA 70047, (504) 887-7593, BA 76 Kean Coll of NJ; MA 77 Kean Coll of NJ; Sp-Lang Path, Rehab Ctr-East Jefferson Hosp, **SLP**

Clancy, Donnamae Fitz 6 Delta Court, North Brunswick, NJ 08902, (201) 821-4885, BS 83 Univ of ME - Farmington; MS 85 Columbia Univ Teachers Coll; Sp-Lang Path, **SLP**

Clancy, Pamela H 356-D Willowbrook Drive, Jeffersonville, PA 19403, (215) 539-3581, BS 82 James Madison Univ; MA 84 Univ of CO - Boulder; Sp-Lang Path, Abington Memorial Hosp, **SLP**

Clanfield, Kathleen Kiehl 304 Sixth Street #A4, Coralville, IA 52241, (319) 338-6556, BS 82 Univ of IL - Urbana; MS 83 Univ of IL - Urbana; **SLP**

Clanton, Andrea Doris 441 Montgomery Ferry Drive, Apartment 1, Atlanta, GA 30309, (404) 257-2075, BS 85 Univ of GA; ME 87 Univ of GA

Clapper, Mrs Karen Maria RD #6 Box 101, Indiana, PA 15701, (412) 349-5070, BA 84 Univ of Pittsburgh - Pittsburgh; MS 85 Indiana Univ of PA; 88–Sp-Lang Path, Aud and Sp Assoc Inc, **SLP**

Clapper, Mrs Nanette Doran 4768 Four Seasons Drive, Liverpool, NY 13088, (315) 451-1898, BS 77 SUNY - Coll at Cortland; MS 83 Coll of Saint Rose; **SLP**

Clare, Laurel Ann P O Box 375, 616 Cedar Street #1, Chelan, WA 98816-0375, (509) 682-5792, BA 82 WA St Univ; MA 83 WA St Univ; 87–Sp-Lang Path, Omak Sch Dist No 19, **SLP**

Clarizio, Mrs Katharine Rutherford P O Box 515, Pawnee, IL 62558, (217) 625-2231, BS 72 Western IL Univ; MA 76 Western IL Univ; Sp-Lang Path, Sangaman Area Spec Educ Dist, **SLP**

Clark, Mrs Amy R G 355 Fairview Street, Danville, CA 94526, (415) 838-4194, BS 76 Univ of WI - Madison; MS 78 Univ of WI - Madison; 83–Sp-Lang Path, San Jose Hosp, **SLP**

Clark, Ann L 730 Oakes Boulevard, San Leandro, CA 94577, (408) 243-7861, BA 80 Holy Names Coll; MA 81 Univ of the Pacific; Sp/Lang Path, Crippled Chldns Soc, **SLP**

Clark, Barbara A 1315 Hauser, Helena, MT 59601, BA 70 Northern MI Univ; MA 74 Northern MI Univ; Sp-Lang Path, Southwestern Montana Educ Coop, **SLP ACE**

Clark, Barbara J P O Box 1121, South Lancaster, MA 01561, (508) 343-5005, BA 76 Univ of VT; MS 81 Univ of VT; 86–Aud, Burbank Hosp, **A**

Clark, Mrs Barbara S 5727 Carriage Barn Lane, Montgomery, AL 36116-5000, BS 67 Whittier Coll; MS 75 Univ of WY; **SLP**

Clark, Dr Bertha Smith Middle Tn State University, Dept Of Speech & Theatre, Box 309, Murfreesboro, TN 37132, (615) 898-2661, BS 64 TN St Univ; MA 65 G Peabody Coll-Vanderbilt U; PH 82 (Early Childhood Education) Vanderbilt Univ; Asst Prof, Middle TN St Univ, **SLP ACE**

Clark, Mrs Betty Jean 6727 Blessing Drive, Dallas, TX 75214, (214) 490-8701, BS 57 Univ of TX - Austin; MA 61 Univ of TX - Austin; Sp-Lang Path, Dallas ISD, **SLP**

Clark, Beverly Anne P O Box 157, Deep Gap, NC 28618, (919) 877-3387, BS 74 Appalachian St Univ; MA 77 Appalachian St Univ; Sp-Lang Path, Ashe Co Schs, **SLP**

Clark, Mrs Beverly L 4516 Westward, Wichita Falls, TX 76308, (817) 692-2426, BS 75 OK St Univ; MA 76 OK St Univ; Sp-Lang Path, **SLP**

Clark, Bonita L 911 Bethany Court, Annapolis, MD 21403, (301) 761-7196, BS 68 Indiana Univ of PA; MS 70 WV Univ; Sp-Lang Path, Anne Arundel Co Bd of Ed, **SLP**

Clark, Mrs Bonita P Route 4 Box 345, Chesapeake, OH 45619, (614) 867-3448, BA 74 Marshall Univ; MA 75 Marshall Univ; Sp-Lang Path, Chesapeake University, **SLP**

Clark, Mrs Carol Kopp 821 East Broadway, Newton, KS 67114, (316) 283-2355, BS 57 Eastern OR St Coll; MS 61 Syracuse Univ; Director-Owner, Helping Hands Presch-Day Care, **SLP A**

Clark, Catherine Celeste 291 West Squire Drive #3, Rochester, NY 14623, (716) 475-6354, **A**

Clark, Mrs Charlene E 11320 S W Foothill Drive, Portland, OR 97225, (503) 292-9778, BS 74 Portland St Univ; MS 79 Portland St Univ; Sp/Lang Path, Private Practice, **SLP ACE**

Clark, Mrs Cheryl P O Box 739, Verdi, NV 89439, (702) 358-6363, BA 69 Univ of Redlands; MS 77 Univ of NV - Reno; Sp-Lang Path, Washoe Co Sch Dist, **SLP**

Clark, Cheryl Louise Route 1, Balsam Lake, WI 54810, **SLP**

Clark, Mrs Christine M 5625 Wheatsheaf Court, Virginia Beach, VA 23464, (804) 479-0230, BS 72 SUNY - Coll at Geneseo; OM 79 Univ of MS; Sp-Lang Path, Private Practice, **SLP**

Clark, David Paul West Brook Hills Apartment, Bldg 22 #3, Syracuse, NY 13215, (315) 457-3508, BA 83 SUNY - Coll at Plattsburgh; MA 84 SUNY - Coll at Plattsburgh; **SLP**

Clark, Mrs Dawn M 670 Franklin Avenue, North Muskegon, MI 49445, (616) 429-6131, BS 71 Central MI Univ; MS 77 Western MI Univ; Coord Preprimary Impaired, Reeths Puffer Public Schools, **SLP**

Clark, Mrs Deanna M 3201 Wallace Street, Clovis, NM 88101, BS 77 Eastern NM Univ; MS 79 Eastern NM Univ; Sp-Lang Path, Clovis Municipal Schools, **SLP**

Clark, Diann G RR #1 Box 2435, Birch Hill Road, Westford, VT 05494, (802) 527-0565, BA 80 Univ of VT; MS 81 Univ of VT; ME 88 Saint Michael's Coll; Sp-Lang Path, St Albans Cty Elem Sch, **SLP**

Clark, Donald I Clark Hearing Aids & Audiology, 2720 West Jackson Street, Muncie, IN 47303, (317) 284-4224, BA 52 Harvard Univ; MA 78 Ball St Univ; Aud, Clark Hrng Aids & Aud, **A**

Clark, Donna C 36 Westwood Drive, Waldorf, MD 20601, (301) 645-4882, BA 71 KY Wesleyan Coll; MS 80 Murray St Univ; Sp-Lang Path, Chesapeake Sp-Lang-Hrng Ctr, **SLP**

Clark, Mrs Dorothy W Route 2 Box 411, Mount Crawford, VA 22841, (703) 434-3449, BA 34 Western MI Univ; MA 36 Univ of MI - Ann Arbor; **SLP LM**

Clark, Elizabeth 1910 Route 70 East, Suite 5, Cherry Hill, NJ 08003, (609) 424-9084, BS 74 Marquette Univ; MA 75 Temple Univ; Dir Sp-Lang Path, Atrium Hrng and Sp Cen Inc, **SLP**

Clark, Elizabeth Moore 2619 N E Lake Avenue, Lawton, OK 73507, (405) 351-5509, **A**

Clark, Dr Frances L Research Learning Disabities, University Of Kansas, Lawrence, KS 66045, (913) 864-4780, BA 66 Southwestern Coll; MS 71 Univ of KS; PH 81 (NS) Univ of KS; Coordinator of Training, Inst for Research In Learn Dis

Clark, Frank E 4 Honeysuckle Hill, Hampton, VA 23669, (804) 446-5934, BS 73 WV Univ; MA 74 OH Univ - Athens; Sp/Lang Path, Cen for Commun Dis, **SLP**

Clark, Geraldine 2501 Lake Avenue, Wilmette, IL 60091, (312) 441-9212, BA 64 Saint Xavier Coll; MA 67 Northwestern Univ; Sp-Lang Path, Private Practice, **SLP**

Clark, Mrs Hollie- Quillayne 11400 Cochiti Road S E, Space C-1, Albuquerque, NM 87123, (505) 294-7571, BA 52 George Washington Univ; MA 55 Univ of Southern CA; Sp-Lang Path, Moriarty Municipal Sch, **SLP ACE**

Clark, Ione A 3435 Mayfair Drive South, Fresno, CA 93703, BS; **SLP LM**

Clark, Ira B Route 1 Box 307, Greenwood, FL 32443, BS 85 FL St Univ; MS 86 FL St Univ

Clark, Jackie Phelps 5038 Creekwood Drive, Flower Mound, TX 75028, (214) 539-8558, BS 75 CO St Univ; MS 87 Univ of TX - Dallas; 88–Aud, Private Practice, **A**

Clark, Jacqueline Cindy 508 Wallace Way, Lexington, SC 29072-8071, (803) 794-6724, OM 86 Univ of SC - Columbia; 88–Sp-Lang Path, SCDMR, **SLP**

Clark, Mrs Jacquelyn 5400 N W Walden Drive, Kansas City, MO 64151, (913) 682-3721, BS 73 Univ of KS; MS 77 Univ of NE - Omaha; Prog Liaison, Meadowbrook Neurocare Hosp, **SLP**

Clark, Mrs Janet Maurine 37 Sandalwood Court, Oviedo, FL 32765, (407) 366-0393, MS 88 Univ of South FL; 88–Sp-Lang Path, Winter Springs Elem Seminole Co Sch

Clark, Mrs Janice Burnett 10751 Frank Daniels Way, San Diego, CA 92131, (619) 566-8146, BS 82 AZ St Univ; MS 84 Univ of Redlands; 85–Sp-Lang Path, Chula Vista City Sch Dist, **SLP**

Clark, Janice Z 3 Paisano Lane, Rockport, TX 78382, (512) 729-9347, BS 65 Bradley Univ; **SLP**

Clark, Jeanne Paquette 2326 East Clarendon, Phoenix, AZ 85016, (602) 955-6077, BA 37 Cornell Univ; MA 60 AZ St Univ; Consult/Sp-Lang Path, Private Practice, **SLP LM**

Clark, Jenny Sue 2011 South Fannin, Amarillo, TX 79109, (806) 358-9716, BA 72 East TX St Univ - Commerce; MA 79 Abilene Christian Univ; 88–Sp-Lang Path, Bivins Rehab Ctr, **SLP**

Clark, Mrs Jo Ann 2555 Wending Drive, Glendale, WI 53209, (414) 352-6230, BA 72 Univ of NC - Greensboro; MA 74 Univ of NC - Greensboro; 88–Sp-Lang Path, Marquette Univ, **SLP**

Clark, Jo-Anna P 5520 Wescott Place, Durham, NC 27712, (919) 688-5541, BS 75 East Carolina Univ; MS 77 East Carolina Univ; Sp-Lang Path, Headstart/OBT, **SLP**

Clark, Joan 416 East 23rd Street, Owensboro, KY 42301, (502) 684-2181, BA 75 Brescia Coll; MA 79 Western KY Univ; Tchr, Owensboro Pub Sch, **SLP**

Clark, Mrs Joan H 6386 Puupilo Road, Kapaa, HI 96746, (808) 822-7374, MA 78 Univ of CO - Boulder; Tutor, Kauai Community College, **SLP**

Clark, John D 959 Torrence Drive, Springfield, OH 45503, (513) 328-2102, BS 68 Bowling Green St Univ; MA 75 Univ of Cincinnati; 72–Sp/Lang Path, Springfield Cty Sch, **SLP**

Clark, Dr John Greer 3316 Werk Road, Cincinnati, OH 45211, (513) 661-4327, BS 75 Purdue Univ - West Lafayette; MA 77 Univ of TX - Austin; PH 82 (Aud & Sp) Univ of Cincinnati; 82–Dir, Cincinnati Ctr Imprv Commun, **SLP A**

Clark, John R, Jr 7811 Cobden Road, Laverock, PA 19118, BS 73 PA St Univ - Univ Park; MS 74 Univ of the DC; SLP, Sch Dist of Phila, **SLP**

Clark, John Richard 314 South 10th Street, Quakertown, PA 18951, (215) 536-5147, BS 66 PA St Univ - Univ Park; MA 72 Temple Univ; 66–Sp-Lang Path Consult, Bucks Co Sch Iu #22, **SLP**

Clark, Joyce Fretz Route 4 Box 799, Palatka, FL 32077, (904) 328-5763, OB 74 Univ of FL; ME 76 Univ of FL; Sp Prog & Stffng Spec, Putnam Co Sch, **SLP**

Clark, Mrs Judith A K 169 North 77th Street, Milwaukee, WI 53213, (414) 645-4466, BS 76 Univ of WI - Milwaukee; MS 77 Univ of WI - Milwaukee; Sp-Lang Path, Milwaukee Pub Sch, **SLP**

Clark, Mrs Judith G 7722 Pella Drive, Houston, TX 77036, (713) 523-3633, BA 79 Univ of Houston - Univ Park; MA 81 Univ of Houston - Univ Park; 82–Sp-Lang Path, Houston Sch for Deaf Chldn, **SLP ACE**

Clark, Mrs Judith M P O Box 247, Eastport, MI 49627, (616) 599-2197, BS 66 Eastern MI Univ; MS 77 Eastern MI Univ; Sp-Lang Path, Charlevoix-Emmet ISD, **SLP**

Clark, Julie M 531 South Depeyster Street, Kent, OH 44240, (814) 724-3946, MA 88 Kent St Univ

Clark, Mrs Karen Whipple S920 West Villa Maria Dr, Phoenix, AZ 85023, BA 81 Univ of TX - El Paso; MA 83 Univ of TX - El Paso; Sp-Lang Path, **SLP**

Clark, Katherine Gail Rd #3 Box 213, Brattleboro, VT 05301, (802) 254-9661, BA 72 Univ of NH; MA 83 Univ of MA - Amherst; **SLP**

Clark, Kathleen Laurane c/o W R Arms, 1008 West Fremont, Selah, WA 98942, (509) 697-4941, BA 81 Univ of WA; MA 83 Univ of WA; **A**

Clark, Mrs L Genie 6624 Centerton Drive, Fort Wayne, IN 46815, (219) 493-4696, BS 78 Purdue Univ - West Lafayette; MA 80 Ball St Univ; 88–Sp-Lang Path, Parkview Regional Outreach, **SLP ACE**

Clark, Lamont L 403 Ridgeland, Elmhurst, IL 60126, (312) 279-2259, BS 70 Eastern IL Univ; MA 71 Northwestern Univ; Sp-Lang Path, Lincolnwood Sch, **SLP**

Clark, Mrs Laurie Jane 53 Oak Street, Oakland, ME 04963, (207) 453-7173, BS 79 Univ of ME - Farmington; MA 81 Univ of ME - Orono; Sp-Lang Path, SAD #49, **SLP**

Clark, Mrs Lillian N 456 North 200 East, Provo, UT 84601, (801) 373-1746, BA 84 Brigham Young Univ; MA 86 Brigham Young Univ; SLP/Aud, Alpine School Dstr, **SLP**

Clark, Mrs Linda C 209 Dilling Lake Drive, Monroe, LA 71201, (318) 323-2237, BS 69 Southern IL Univ -Carbondale; MA 71 Univ of FL; Teacher Deaf Hearing Impaired, Monroe City Schools, **SLP**

Clark, Linda Jean 2660 Hornblend Street #P, San Diego, CA 92109-4843, (619) 581-1735, BA 82 Western WA Univ; MA 84 Univ of Denver; Sp-Lang Path, Center for Hearing-Speech-Lang, **SLP**

Clark, Lisa Michelle 11 Elizabeth, Calumet City, IL 60409, (312) 333-8687, BS 84 IL St Univ - Normal; MS 86 IL St Univ - Normal; **SLP**

Clark, Lois Diane Box 225, Booker, TX 79005, (806) 435-4412, **SLP**

Clark, Mrs Lynn 2035 Cliff Road, North Bend, OH 45052, (513) 574-2372, BS 86 Miami Univ - Oxford; MS 87 Miami Univ - Oxford; Sp-Lang Path, Hamilton Co Bd of Mr, **SLP**

Clark, Dr Lynne W 261 South Boulevard, Nyack, NY 10960, (914) 358-1847, BS 69 Elmira Coll; MS 72 Columbia Univ Teachers Coll; PH 84 (NS) CUNY - Grad Sch & Univ Cntr; Asst Prof/Prog Dir, Hunter College-CUNY, **SLP**

Clark, Lynnette 125 11th Avenue S W, Birmingham, AL 35211, (205) 591-7167, BS 80 Univ of GA; MS 82 Univ of AL- Tuscaloosa; Aud, Sertoma Intnatl Cen Commun Dis, **A**

Clark, Marilyn Louise 3044-D Monticello Lane, Chico, CA 95926, (916) 673-6110, **SLP**

Clark, Marion B 1363 Lillian Avenue, Sunnyvale, CA 94087, (415) 856-0660, BA 53 MI St Univ; MA 65 Bradley Univ; Co-Dir Lang Prog, Stanbridge Acad, **SLP**

Clark, Mark Charles 64 Laurelwood Drive, Stoughton, MA 02072, (617) 821-4120, **SLP**

Clark, Mark E Commonwealth Ear Nose & Throat, Dupont Medical Center Suite 220, 4004 Dupont Circle, Louisville, KY 40207, (502) 893-0159, BS 76 Brescia Coll; MS 77 Univ of Louisville; Aud, Commonwealth Ear Nose & Throat, **A**

Clark, Mary Ann B 9 Via Verde, Wichita, KS 67230, (316) 833-3550, BA 80 Wichita St Univ; MA 81 Wichita St Univ; Sp-Lang Path, USD 259, **SLP**

Clark, Mrs Mary Beth Boos Route 3 Box 193, Chippewa Falls, WI 54729, (715) 923-9341, **SLP**

Clark, Marybeth G 8 Marilyn Drive, Canton, MA 02021, BA 69 Univ of NH; ME 79 Northeastern Univ; Sp-Lang Path, Early Beginning Ctr-Early Intervention, **SLP**

Clark, Dr Michael J Dept Speech Path & Audiology, Western Michigan Univ, Kalamazoo, MI 49008, (616) 387-8065, BA 64 Oberlin Coll; MA 65 Univ of MI - Ann Arbor; PH 71 (Speech) Univ of MI - Ann Arbor; Assoc Prof, Wn MI U, **SLP**

Clark, Michele Marie 19920 Bartell, Gregory, MI 48197, (313) 295-5258, BA 84 MI St Univ; MA 87 Eastern MI Univ, 87–Sp-Lang Path, Heritage Hosp, **SLP**

Clark, Mrs Michele Mary 1909½ Warfield Avenue, Redondo Beach, CA 90278, (213) 603-6050, BA 64 Coll of Saint Catherine; MA 81 CA St Univ - Long Beach; 84–Sp-Lang Path, St Francis Med Cen, **SLP**

Clark, Mrs Mona Lisa 2117 9th Street, Port Neches, TX 77651, (409) 722-5237, BS 85 Lamar Univ; MS 87 Lamar Univ; **SLP**

Clark, Mona M 2001 Court Street, Pueblo, CO 81003, (303) 542-2147, BA 67 Univ of Denver; MA 68 Univ of Denver; **SLP**

Clark, Nancy T P O Box 1033, Hockessin, DE 19707-5033, (302) 239-1413, BS 70 Univ of KS; MA 72 Univ of KS; **SLP**

Clark, Mrs Nila M F 419 Geiger Street, Huntingburg, IN 47542, (812) 683-2531, BS 73 IN St Univ - Terre Haute; MS 75 IN St Univ - Terre Haute; 88–Sp-Lang Path, Private Practice, **SLP**

Clark, Mrs Olivia A 14127 Meyersville, Houston, TX 77049, (713) 521-9584, BA 70 OK Christian Coll; MS 72 Univ of OK Medical Center; 83–Supvr Infant Prog, Men Hlth/Ret of Harris Co, **SLP**

Clark, Pamela S 555 North 30th Street, Omaha, NE 68131, (402) 498-6666, BS 79 Northwestern Univ; MS 82 Univ of WI - Madison; Sp-Lang Path, Boys Town Nat Instit, **SLP**

Clark, Mrs Patricia H Route 1 Box 90, Santee, SC 29142, (803) 854-2758, BA 73 Columbia Coll; OM 74 Univ of SC - Columbia; Sp-Lang Path, Elloree High Sch, **SLP**

Clark, Patricia Marie 176 Candia Street, East Weymouth, MA 02189, (617) 331-9545, BS 73 Marywood Coll; MS 75 PA St Univ - Univ Park; **SLP**

Clark, Paula Jurnak Providence Medical Center, Rehabilitation Department, 500 17th Avenue, Seattle, WA 98122, (206) 326-5701, BA 77 SUNY - Coll at Plattsburgh; MA 82 Univ of MT; Sp-Lang Path, Providence Med Cen, **SLP**

Clark, Mrs Pearl Mary 2151 Highland Oaks Drive, Arcadia, CA 91006, (818) 355-1165, BA 40 WA St Univ; OB 41 WA St Univ; MA 49 Columbia Univ Teachers Coll; 83–Retired, Los Angeles USD, **SLP LM**

Clark, R Jeanne 1625 Mowry Square, Richland, WA 99352, (509) 946-2231, BA 68 Univ of WA; OM 79 Univ of WA; Sp-Lang Path, Certified Sp-Lang Svcs Inc, **SLP**

Clark, Mrs Raynell Brown 25281 Lois Lane Drive, Southfield, MI 48075, (313) 499-4560, BS 76 Wayne St Univ; MA 78 Eastern MI Univ; 88–Sp-Lang Path, Detroit Riverview Hosp, **SLP**

Clark, Mrs Sara H Audiological Services Of La Mesa, 8415 Grant Street, La Mesa, CA 92041, (619) 462-8784, BA 77 Univ of IA; MA 78 Univ of IA; 86–Aud, Private Practice, **A**

Clark, Sharon H 7533 Wrenview Drive, Springfield, OH 45502, **SLP**

Clark, Mrs Sharon Mitchell 4943 Emmet, Omaha, NE 68104, (402) 330-2770, BA 65 Univ of Northern CO; MS 84 Univ of NE - Omaha; **SLP**

Clark, Sheri E 710 West Price River Drive, Price, UT 84501-2404, (801) 637-8900, MA 83 Univ of UT; 88–Aud/Sp-Lang Path, Clark Sp and Hrng Clinic, **SLP A**

Clark, Susan M Kilgore 215 South Edgewood, La Grange, IL 60525, (312) 482-3640, BA 81 Bradley Univ; MS 83 Purdue Univ - West Lafayette; Sp-Lang Path, LADSE LaGrange Ar Dept of Spec Educ, **SLP**

Clark, Sylvia Yvonne 3273 Hillwood Lane, Augusta, GA 30909, (404) 790-2101, MA 81 SC St Coll; BA 79 Augusta Coll; Sp-Lang Path, Gracewood State School & Hosp, **SLP**

Clark, Mrs Tamara L 3400 Shore Drive, Browns Lake, Burlington, WI 53105-9163, BA 84 Univ of WI - Eau Claire; MS 85 Univ of WI - Eau Claire; 88–Sp-Lang Path, Kenosha USD, **SLP**

Clark, Mrs Teresa Marie 2580 Diamond Street, San Francisco, CA 94131, (415) 469-8824, **A**

Clarke, Dr Christina 1153 Churchill Street, St Paul, MN 55103, (715) 425-3801, MS 68 Gallaudet Coll; OM 82 Coll of William & Mary; PH 86 (Aud) Univ of Cincinnati; Asst Prof, Univ of Wisc-River Falls, **A**

Clarke, Debbie W 287 Edinburgh Lane, Orange Park, FL 32073-4231, (904) 388-8756, MS 75 Univ of South FL; Sp-Lang Path, Sp & Lang Consultants, **SLP**

Clarke, Mrs Donna M 2649 East Louise, Phoenix, AZ 85032, BA 77 SUNY - Coll at Buffalo; MS 78 Adelphi Univ; Sp-Lang Path, Sun Rehab Agcy, **SLP**

Clarke, Mrs Ellen V 93 Trieste Street, Iselin, NJ 08830, (201) 231-1022, BA 76 Rutger's St Univ - Douglas Coll; MA 77 Trenton St Coll; Sp-Lang Path, Bridgewater Board of Education, **SLP**

Clarke, Gay Jean 100 Patrick Drive, Biloxi, MS 39531, **SLP**

Clarke, Mrs Gloria Lynn 1336 West Market Street, Akron, OH 44313, (216) 867-2353, BA 72 SUNY - Coll at New Paltz; MA 85 Univ of Akron; Aud, Childrens Hospital of Akron, **A**

Clarke, Jane C 29 1/2 Old Arroyo Chamiso, Santa Fe, NM 87501, (505) 986-0831, **SLP**

Clarke, Judith Ann 311 Bayswater, Andalusia, PA 19020-7710, (215) 244-1725, BS 83 Indiana Univ of PA; MA 80 Univ of CO Boulder; **A**

Clarke, Justine L 107 Highland Drive, Warner Robins, GA 31088, (912) 929-7809, OB 74 Valdosta St Coll; ME 76 Univ of GA; ME 81 Valdosta St Coll; SLP, Houston Co Bd of Ed, **SLP**

Clarke, Kim Spina 41 Floral Avenue, Bethpage, NY 11714, (516) 724-3635, BS 83 AZ St Univ; MA 85 Hofstra Univ; 86–Aud, Long Isl Ctr for Aud, **A**

Clarke, Leanne Liden P O Box 707, Tesuque, NM 87574, (505) 989-5480, BA 84 Univ of CA - Santa Barbara; MS 86 UT St Univ; SLP, Santa Fe P S, **SLP**

Clarke, Mrs Marianne McKenna 1879 Crompond Road #B-1, Peekskill, NY 10566, BA 80 CUNY - Lehman Coll; MA 84 CUNY - Lehman Coll

Clarke, Mary A 809 W Lill #1-W, Chicago, IL 60614, (312) 472-4034, BA 76 Univ of MO - Columbia; MS 77 Fontbonne Coll; SLP, Chicago PS, **SLP**

Clarke, Michael J 1412 Landon Avenue, Winthrop Harbor, IL 60096-1844, (312) 872-4817, MA 77 Northern IL Univ - De Kalb; SLP, Er Sl So-Lake Co, **SLP**

Clarke, Pamela Yvonne 7815 S W 88th Street #E-227, Miami, FL 33156, (305) 666-6511, OB 84 FL St Univ; OM 85 FL St Univ; SLP, Miami Childrens Hospital, **SLP**

Clarke, Mrs Patricia McGinley 2617 South 272nd St #12, Kent, WA 98032, (206) 941-4679, BA 83 Univ of CA - Santa Barbara; OM 85 San Diego St Univ; **SLP**

Clarke, Ronnie M 10926 Autillo Way, San Diego, CA 92127, (303) 329-0630, BS 73 OH St Univ; MA 71 Univ of Denver; **A**

Clarke, Sharon Janette P O Box SS 6886, Nassau, Bahamas, BS 80 Elmira Coll; MA 86 Wayne St Univ - Sch of Med; 80–Sp-Lang Path, Ministry of Education, **SLP**

Clarke, Shawn Sawyer 91 West 100 South, American Fork, UT 84003, (801) 756-5214, MA 86 WA St Univ; SLP, Alpine School District, **SLP**

Clarke, Stacey Lynn William Beaumont Hospital, 3601 West 13 Mile Road, Speech Pathology Department, Royal Oak, MI 48072, (313) 288-2728, BS 82 Western MI Univ; MS 84 Univ of MI - Ann Arbor; 84–Sp-Lang Path, William Beaumont Hosp, **SLP**

Clarke, Mrs Susan M 314 Sturges Road, Fairfield, CT 06430, (203) 762-8526, BA 75 Univ of RI; MS 78 Southern CT St Univ; Aud, CES, **A**

Clarke, Susan M 344 Prospect Street, Apartment C, La Jolla, CA 92037, (619) 456-9211, BS 76 CA Poly St Univ-San Luis Obi; MS 79 Univ of IL - Urbana; Sp-Lang Path, **SLP**

Clark-Hahn, Jannet Eileen PO Box 101, Kirkland, WA 98083, (206) 368-1736, OB 75 Central WA Univ; MA 83 Western WA Univ; Dir/Hrng & Sp, Seaside Gen Hosp, **A**

Clark-Hill, Mrs Lesley M 11 South Shore Drive, Galveston, TX 77550, (409) 761-2711, BA 76 Univ of Denver; MA 77 Univ of Denver; Asst Director Speech Pathology, Univ of TX Med Branch, **SLP**

Clark-Lewis, Sandra 337 Payne Street, Auburn, AL 36830, (205) 821-6165, BS 72 Auburn Univ - Auburn; OM 74 Auburn Univ - Auburn; Cl Instr, Auburn U, **A**

Clark-McGowan, Mrs Jill M N85 W15650 Ridge Road #301, Menomonee Falls, WI 53051, (414) 255-4548, MS 83 Univ of WI - Stevens Point; Sp-Lang Path, Elmbrook Sch Dist, **SLP**

Clarkson, Sandra Lynne 1628 Vicksburg Drive, Bedford, TX 76021, (817) 654-9218, BS 70 CO St Univ; MA 71 Southern Methodist Univ; Pres, Aud Consults Inc, **A**

Clarkston, Mrs Jane Marshall 6 Lemontree, Edwardsville, IL 62025, (618) 877-6864, BS 83 Southern IL Univ-Edwardsvill; MS 84 Southern IL Univ-Edwardsvill; **SLP**

Clark-Thomas, Mrs Eleanor M State Department Of Education, Special Educ Suite 1014, 601 West 5th Street, Los Angeles, CA 90071, (213) 620-4244, BS 60 Kent St Univ; MA 73 CA St Univ - Sacramento; Consult, CA St Dept of Ed, **SLP A**

Clasgens, Mrs Pamela Sue P O Box 26262, Phoenix, AZ 85068, (602) 395-0652, BA 83 Univ of MS; MA 85 Memphis St Univ; Audiologist, Shea Clinic, **A**

Clasing, Anita T 8701 South Baker Avenue, Baltimore, MD 21234, **SLP**

Class, Lois Wunker 379 Buffalo S E, Albuquerque, NM 87123, (505) 766-3880

Clateman, Mrs Joyce Z 140 East 81st Street, New York, NY 10028, (212) 988-9409, BA 59 CUNY - City College; MA 62 Columbia Univ Teachers Coll; **SLP**

Claus, Russell S Psc #1 Box 1567, Apo, San Francisco, CA 96286, BA 75 KS St Univ; MS 77 Towson St Univ; Sp-Lang Path, Dod Depend Schs, **SLP**

Claus, Mrs Theresa A Psc 31 Box 1567, Apo, San Francisco, CA 96286, BS 75 Towson St Univ; MS 77 Towson St Univ; Compensatory Ed Teacher, Dod Dependent Schs, **SLP**

Clausen, Carol L 4064 West 115th #411, Chicago, IL 60655, (312) 779-2699, BA 76 Mundelein Coll; MA 77 Western MI Univ; Sp-Lang Path, Private Practice, **SLP**

Clausen, Helen Kay 456 South State Street, Elgin, IL 60120, (312) 695-5512, BS 65 Univ of IA; MA 67 Univ of IA; 85–Sp/Lang Path, Comm Consolidated Sch Dist 54, **SLP**

Clausen, Larry E 508 West 6th Street, Muscatine, IA 52761, (319) 263-8476, BA 78 IL St Univ - Normal; MS 80 IL St Univ - Normal; SLP, Mississippi Bend AEA, **SLP**

Clausen, Margaret A 1510 Thoroughbred Lane, Florissant, MO 63033, (314) 388-1026, BS 76 Univ of MO - Columbia; MS 77 Southern IL Univ-Edwardsvill; 77–Sp/Lang Path, St Louis Co Spec Sch Dist, **SLP**

Clausen, Roseanne P 4014 Rickover Road, Silver Spring, MD 20902, (301) 279-4955, BA 61 Queens Coll; MA 68 Univ of MD - College Park; Secondary Prog Liason, Montg Co MD Sch, **SLP**

Clauser, Mrs Patricia S P O Box 1006, Corrales, NM 87048, (505) 897-0070, BS 61 Simmons Coll; MS 82 Univ of NM; Sp-Lang Path, Albuquerque Public Schools, **SLP ACE**

Clawson, Bonnie E Box 414, Black Lick, PA 15716, (412) 248-3529, BS 70 Indiana Univ of PA; MS 74 Indiana Univ of PA; 84–Supvr of Spec Educ, Arin Inter Ut, **SLP**

Clawson, Coy L 3336 Larchmont Drive, Salt Lake City, UT 84109, (801) 487-8105, BA 80 Univ of UT; MS 84 Univ of UT; Tchr, Utah School for the Blind, **SLP**

Clay, Mrs Cynthia C 8817 West Herbert Avenue, Milwaukee, WI 53225, (414) 462-5081, BS 78 Univ of WI - Milwaukee; MS 79 Univ of WI - Milwaukee; Sp-Lang Path, We Care Nursing Service Inc, **SLP**

Clay, Marcy Dumoch HHD USMCA, Box 149, APO New York, NY 09176-0006, 011-49-7131-582340, BA 80 Rutger's St Univ - Douglas Coll; MA 83 Trenton St Coll; 86–Sp-Lang Path, **SLP**

Clay, Mrs Molly Quin 331 West Porter, Ridgeland, MS 39157, (601) 922-6522, BA 80 Univ of MS; MS 81 Univ of MS; Sp/Lang Path, Starkville Lrng Resource Cen, **SLP**

Clay, Teresa H 509 Lanny Drive, Winchester, VA 22601, **SLP**

Claybaugh, Gloria Petitclair 8232 Bernard Drive North, Millersville, MD 21108, (301) 462-6800, BS 67 Towson St Univ; ME 70 Loyola Coll; OM 82 Johns Hopkins Univ; Sp-Lang Path, Johns Hopkins Univ Sch Med, **SLP**

Clayburn, Alisa Boykin 1441 Front Street, East Meadow, NY 11554, (516) 483-3926, BS 84 East Carolina Univ; MS 85 East Carolina Univ; 86–Sp-Lang Path, Suffolk Child Dev Ctr, **SLP**

Clayton, Mrs Elizabeth Patterson 910 Constitution Drive, Apartment 808, Durham, NC 27705, (919) 489-2361, BS 84 Appalachian St Univ; MS 85 Univ of NC - Chapel Hill; Sp-Lang Path, InSpeech Inc, **SLP**

Clayton, Katherine J 524 South Grand Avenue #1, Fort Thomas, KY 41075, (606) 441-0822, BS 84 Eastern KY Univ; MS 86 Univ of Louisville; **A**

Clayton, Lawrence G 435 North Mulford Road, Ten Village Square, Rockford, IL 61107, (815) 399-5279, BA 66 Northern IL Univ - De Kalb; MA 68 Northern IL Univ - De Kalb; Aud, Private Practice, **A**

Clayton, Mary K 4500 Hudgins Drive, Virginia Beach, VA 23455, **SLP**

Clayton, Sue K 512 South Oak Knoll #4, Pasadena, CA 91101, (818) 790-9100, BS 80 Brigham Young Univ; OM 81 Brigham Young Univ; SLP, La Canada USD, **SLP**

Clearman, Patsy Thomas 513 Haisten Drive, Dothan, AL 36301, (205) 794-9225, BA 70 Auburn Univ - Auburn; MA 71 Auburn Univ - Auburn; MA 72 Auburn Univ - Auburn; Sp-Lang Path, Private Practice, **SLP**

Cleary, Mrs Anne M 12911 Harney Street, Omaha, NE 68154, (402) 333-8432, BA 77 Creighton Univ; MS 78 Univ of NE - Omaha; Sp-Lang Path, Private Practice, **SLP**

Cleary, Carol Sue 6904 Manatee Avenue West #13C, Bradenton, FL 34209-0613, **SLP**

Cleary, Mrs Christine Fowler 10131 Huntersdell Lane, Richmond, VA 23235, (804) 272-4170, BS 80 James Madison Univ; MS 82 James Madison Univ; Sp/Lang Path, Chesterfield Co Pub Sch, **SLP**

Cleary, Denise Elizabeth 160 Riviera Drive, Bricktown, NJ 08724, (201) 840-0876, BS 78 Marywood Coll; MA 82 Montclair St Coll; Sp-Lang Path, Wall Township Bd of Educ, **SLP**

Cleary, Mary Ellen 134 West End Avenue, Somerville, NJ 08876, (201) 218-4117, BA 83 Rutger's St Univ - Douglas Coll; MS 86 Rutgers St Univ -N Brunswick; 83–Sp-Lang Path, Somerville PS, **SLP**

Cleave, Doris C 2247 Paddock CO9URT, Geneva, IL 60134, (312) 232-9553, BS 74 Northern IL Univ - De Kalb; MA 75 Northern IL Univ - De Kalb; **SLP**

Cleave, Patricia Lynn 73 Bruce Street, Unit 7, London, ON, Canada N6C 1G7, (519) 679-2111, BA 82 0936; OM 85 Univ of Western Ontario; 87–Research Assoc, Univ of Western Ontario, **SLP**

Cleaver, Mrs Patricia Quigley 64 Swift Street, Auburn, NY 13021, (315) 255-2746, BS 72 SUNY - Coll at Geneseo; MA 75 SUNY - Coll at Geneseo; Sp-Lang Path, E John Gavras Cen, **SLP**

Cleek, Thyra J 4503 Clifton Avenue, El Paso, TX 79903, (915) 565-3016, BS 68 Abilene Christian Univ; MA 72 NM St Univ; Aud, El Paso Pub Schs, **A**

Cleeland, Linda K 1001 43rd Avenue #44, Greeley, CO 80634, (303) 351-2012, BS 69 CO St Univ; MA 74 Univ of Northern CO; ME 87 CO St Univ; 74–Asst Prof, Univ of Northern Colorado, **A**

Clees, Patricia B 4212 North 16th Street, Phoenix, AZ 85016, (602) 263-1200, BA 71 Univ of Northern CO; MA 72 Univ of Northern CO; Aud, Phoenix Indian Medical Center, **A**

Clegg, Stanley J Atlanta Audiology Clinic Inc, 2910 N Druid Hill Road N E, Suite I, Atlanta, GA 30329, (404) 634-2445, BA 60 Valdosta St Coll; ME 63 Emory Univ; 77–President/Audiologist, Atlanta Audiology Clinic Inc, **A**

Clegg, Mrs Tina Carter 2539 Willard Dairy Road, High Point, NC 27260, (919) 454-2211, BA 80 Univ of NC - Greensboro; ME 85 Univ of NC - Greensboro; Sp-Lang Path, Guilford Co Schs, **SLP**

Cleland, Mrs Michele Tripp 208 Michele Drive, New Bern, NC 28560, (919) 633-1340, BS 84 East Carolina Univ; **A**

Cleland, Sally B 1038 73rd Avenue North, Brooklyn Park, MN 55444, (612) 295-5185, BS 75 Saint Cloud St Univ; MS 80 Saint Cloud St Univ; Sp-Lang Path-Coord, Monticello Pub Sch, **SLP**

Clem, Mrs Jane M 4100 South Cathy, Sioux Falls, SD 57106, (605) 361-6504, BA 80 Univ of SD - Vermillion; MA 81 Univ of SD - Vermillion; Sp-Lang Path, Beverly Home Health, **SLP**

Clem, Mrs Karen L 5994 Palencia Drive, Riverside, CA 92509, (714) 788-7441, BA 74 Univ of MT; MA 76 Univ of MT; Sp-Lang Path, Riverside USD, **SLP**

Clem, Roger Fair Lamar University, P O Box 10076, Beaumont, TX 77710, (409) 880-8179, BS 76 Lincoln Univ; MS 82 Lincoln Univ; Clinical Supervisor/Instructor, Lamar University, **A**

Clemens, Denise Leslie 2155 N W Flanders #11, Portland, OR 97210, (503) 224-9224, BA 84 Western WA Univ; 88–Sp-Lang Path, Portland Adventist Med Ctr, **SLP**

Clemens, Karen L 1626 East 7th Street, Olympia, WA 98501, (206) 352-4272, BS 71 IA St Univ; BA 76 Univ of MT; MS 78 Univ of MT; SLP, Head Start, **SLP**

Clement, Mrs Ann Morrison 2223 South Madison Street, Denver, CO 80210, (303) 795-7007, BS 69 CO St Univ; MA 71 Univ of CO - Boulder; OM 76 Univ of Northern CO; Resource Specialist, Littleton Public Schools, **SLP**

Clement, Maj Augustus T Psc 2 Box 593, APO New York, NY 09220, MA 75 CA St Univ - Los Angeles; Chief Sp-Path Service, USAF, **SLP ACE**

Clement, Diane E 4403 Woodpoint Court, Dayton, OH 45424, (513) 226-7877, BS 77 KS St Univ; MA 78 Wichita St Univ; 82–Aud, Aud & Sp Assoc, **A**

Clemente, Mrs Dorothy Anne 25 North Lake Avenue, Troy, NY 12180, (518) 271-1179, BS 82 SUNY - Coll at Geneseo; MS 87 Coll of Saint Rose; **SLP**

Clements, Charmaine 132 West Claiborne Square, Chalmette, LA 70043, **SLP**

Clements, Cheryl Marie 3301 S W 13th Street #D-140, Gainesville, FL 32608, (904) 335-6604, MA 84 Central MI Univ; Sp-Lang Path, InSpeech Inc, **SLP**

Clements, Darlene C P O Box 1239, Wrightwood, CA 92397, (619) 249-6337, BS 76 Loma Linda Univ - Riverside; MS 77 Loma Linda Univ - Loma Linda; Sp-Lang Path, San Bernardino Co Schls, **SLP**

Clements, Denise A 10509 South Hamilton, Chicago, IL 60643, (312) 520-9850, BA 76 Univ of MI - Ann Arbor; MA 77 Western MI Univ; Sp-Lang Path Supervisor, Excellcare Rehabilitation, **SLP**

Clements, Sr Elizabeth 634 New Scotland Avenue, Albany, NY 12208, (518) 489-8341, BA 50 9091; MA 72 SUNY - Coll at Geneseo; **SLP LM**

Clements, Gail Anne 760 Berkshire Drive #88, London, ON, Canada N6J 4A5, (519) 471-3510, BS 77 Univ of Western Ontario; MS 79 Univ of Western Ontario; 79–Sp-Lang Path, Mdsex Co Bd Ed, **SLP**

Clements, Mrs Gracie Thoman 1105 Georgia Street, Shreveport, LA 71104, (404) 424-6090, BA 82 Columbus Coll; MA 87 LA Tech Univ; 88–Aud, Overton Brooks VA Med Ctr, **A**

Clements, Mrs Linda W 8634 Manitoba Drive, Cincinnati, OH 45230, (513) 474-3272, BA 77 Marshall Univ; MA 78 Marshall Univ; Sp-Lang Path, Private Practice, **SLP**

Clemmens, Mrs Jan M 2305 Butler Road, Butler, MD 21023, (301) 866-3313, BA 76 Loyola Coll; MS 77 Loyola Coll; Sp-Lang Path, Baltimore Co Bd of Ed, **SLP**

Clemons, Bobbie Jo 325 West 54th Street South, Wichita, KS 67217-5537, (918) 272-0240, BA 74 KS St Univ; MA 75 KS St Univ; Sp-Lang Path, Tri-Quad Special Services Coop, **SLP**

Clemons, Mrs Jeanette W Route 2 Box 217-J, Jones, OK 73049, (405) 771-5338, BS 75 OK St Univ; MA 76 OK St Univ; Sp-Lang Path & Dir, Guthrie Scot Rite Chldh Aph Cl, **SLP**

Clemons, Mrs M Elaine 3853 West 14th Avenue, Vancouver, BC, Canada V6R 2X1, (604) 224-0394, BA 39 Samford Univ; MA 64; Sp/Lang Path, Private Practice, **SLP LM**

Clemons, Sara Jayne 2678 Trader Court, Bldg 20, South Bend, IN 46628-3634, (215) 631-9300, BS 82 Northern IL Univ - De Kalb; MA 86 Western IL Univ; **SLP**

Clemons, Mrs Sue Ellen 3251 Jasper Street, West Lafayette, IN 47906, (317) 463-5222, BS 80 Purdue Univ - West Lafayette; MS 81 Purdue Univ - West Lafayette; **SLP**

Clenseur, Mrs Jane MacLeod 1519 Oriole Place, Greensboro, NC 27408, (919) 274-3144, BA 54 Vanderbilt Univ; MA 72 Univ of NC - Greensboro; Sp-Lang Path, Greensboro Cty Sch, **SLP**

Clerkson, Marion 3613 Seahorn Circle, San Diego, CA 92130, **SLP**

Clery, Mrs Carolsue Harr 342 West Windsor, Lombard, IL 60148, (312) 620-3700, BA 64 Univ of IL - Urbana; MS 67 Univ of MI - Ann Arbor; MS 83 Purdue Univ - Calumet; Sp-Lang Path, Villa Park Sch Dist #45, **SLP**

Cleveland, Karla P 2435 South Kevin Lane, Sapulpa, OK 74066, (918) 224-1492, MA 81 Univ of Tulsa; Sp/Lang Path, Sapulpa Public Schools, **SLP**

Cleveland, Mrs Lea Niblett 458 Sunset Drive, Spartanburg, SC 29302, (803) 576-4212, BS 76 Univ of TX - Austin; MS 77 TX Christian Univ; Sp-Lang Path, District 6 Schools, **SLP**

Cleveland, Sandra S 48 Babcock Street #1, Brookline, MA 02146, (617) 254-3800, BS 72 SUNY - Coll at Geneseo; ME 83 Northeastern Univ; Aud, Childrens Hospital, **A**

Clevenger, Mary F 4817 Montcalm Court, Fort Wayne, IN 46815, (219) 485-1062, BA 75 Our Lady Lake Univ-San Anton; MA 76 Our Lady Lake Univ-San Anton; **SLP**

Cleworth, Mrs Janice E 1179 Kodiak, Fairbanks, AK 99709, BA 75 Univ of AK - Fairbanks; MS 78 Eastern WA Univ; Sp-Lang Path, Fairbanks N Star Bor Sch Dist, **SLP**

Clezy, Mrs Gillian M Speech Language Department, Primary Children's Medical Center, 320 12th Avenue, Salt Lake City, UT 84103, (801) 521-1680, OB 75 Lincoln Inst Hlth- Australia; 86–Sp-Lang Path, Primary Child Med Ctr, **SLP**

Click, Marilyn J 2046 East Aspen, Tempe, AZ 85282, (602) 966-5220, BS 59 OK Baptist Univ; MA 65 Central St Univ; SLP, Private Practice, **SLP**

Cliff, Mrs Susie Elaine 33 El Monte Way, Davis, CA 95616, (916) 758-3939, MA 86 Univ of CA - Santa Barbara; 88–Sp-Lang Path, Sacramento City USD, **SLP**

Cliffe, Mollie D Rural Route 2, Lansdowne, ON, Canada K0E 1L0, (613) 382-4194, BS 67 Russell Sage Coll; MS 69 Syracuse Univ; **SLP**

Clifford, Clare 21 Linden Street, #319, Quincy, MA 02169, (715) 369-2177, BA 80 Univ of MN - Minneap-St Paul; MS 85 Univ of WI - Stevens Point; **SLP**

Clifford, Mrs Lois J 7 Pheasant Court, Wesley Park Townhouses, Mechanicsburg, PA 17055, (717) 737-6728, BA 62 CUNY - Hunter Coll; MA 68 Bloomsburg Univ of PA; Sp-Lang Path, Capital Area Intermed Ut #15, **SLP ACE**

Clifford, Lucinda A Route 8 Box 399-D, Morganton, NC 28655, **SLP**

Clifford, Mrs Martha Susan 374 Charles River Road, Watertown, MA 02172-2738, (201) 441-2165, **SLP**

Clifford, Maureen Louise Sir Francis Motel Rt 131, 140 Main Street #8, Sturbridge, MA 01566, (508) 764-7035, BS 83 Worcester St Coll; MS 85 Univ of HI - Manoa; Sp-Lang Path, Southbridge Public Schools, **SLP**

Clifford, Dr Sylvester 424 East Main Street, Vermillion, SD 57069, (605) 677-5474, BA 51 Northwestern OK St Univ; MA 57 Univ of Denver; PH 59 (NS) Univ of Denver; Prof, U of SD Sp & Hrng Cen, **SLP A F ACE**

Clifford, Virginia Varner 1111 Hillcrest, Chapel Hill, NC 27514, (919) 929-2206, BA 65 Greensboro Coll; MS 73 Univ of NC - Chapel Hill; Sp-Lang Path, Chapel Hill-Carrboro Cty Sch, **SLP**

Clift, Mildred Ann 751 Loretto Avenue, Louisville, KY 40211, (502) 772-3161, BA 35 IN Univ - Bloomington; ME 38 IN Univ - Bloomington; MA 41 IN Univ - Bloomington; **SLP LM**

Clift, Tamra Ann 2720 Belaire Drive, Lansing, MI 48911-1619, (517) 772-5317, BS 84 Central MI Univ; MA 85 Central MI Univ; **SLP**

Clifton, Mrs Carrie Campbell 1903 Fairlane Road, Tallahassee, FL 32303, (904) 385-5523, BS 84 Valdosta St Coll; ME 85 Valdosta St Coll; 87–Sp-Lang Path, Rose Sp & Acad Ctr

Clifton, Gina Anne 6590 Royal Gorge Court, San Diego, CA 92119-1136, (619) 287-1087, BS 83 Brigham Young Univ; OM 85 Brigham Young Univ; 87–Sp-Lang Path, Lakeside Union Sch Dist, **SLP**

Clifton, Noel F 6822 Rochelle, Amarillo, TX 79109, (806) 376-5521, BA 68 TX Tech Univ; MA 71 TX Tech Univ; Sp-Lang Path Rel Serv Team, Region Xvi Educ Services Ctr, **SLP**

Clifton, Mrs Sharon Jo 3445 Mountain Avenue, San Bernardino, CA 92324, (714) 825-9453, BS 79 SD St Univ; MA 81 Univ of Redlands; **SLP**

Clinard, Donna Masters 3336 Glenside Avenue, Erie, PA 16508, (814) 456-9157, BA 85 Edinboro Univ of PA; MA 87 Edinboro Univ of PA; **SLP**

Cline, Mrs Claire McDaniel 263 Albert Court, Charlottesville, VA 22901, (804) 973-7840, BS 80 Coll of William & Mary; MA 82 Univ of TN - Knoxville; SLP, Albemarle County Schools, **SLP**

Cline, Debbie Nilwon 3450 Palencia Drive #1820, Tampa, FL 33618, BA 77 Univ of South FL; 87–Aud, Central FL Sp and Hearing Ctr, **A**

Cline, Janna M 24171 Hollyoak #D, Laguna Hills, CA 92656, (714) 643-0905, BA 83 Univ of CA - Santa Barbara; MS 84 Univ of North TX; Audiologist, Cigna, **A**

Cline, Jennifer Marie P O Box 462, Holt, MI 48842, (517) 487-2251, **SLP**

Cline, Mrs Joan A P O Box 13351, Clearwater, FL 34621, (813) 462-9641, MS 77 Univ of South FL; Sp-Lang Path, Pinellas Co Sch Bd, **SLP**

Cline, Mrs Lezlie H 3227 Maxwell Street, Tallahassee, FL 32301, (904) 877-3397, BS 78 FL St Univ; MS 79 FL St Univ; Sp-Lang Path, Leon Co Sch Syst, **SLP**

Cline, Mrs Roberta Mae 1112 Avalon, Olathe, KS 66062, (913) 764-2303, BS 57 Northeastern OK St Univ; MS 67 Univ of KS; Coord of Sp-Lang Serv, Olathe USD #233, **SLP**

Cline, Sue Ellen Route 2 Box 84A, Little Hocking, OH 45742, (304) 422-7243, BS 83 OH Univ - Athens; MA 85 OH Univ - Athens; Sp-Lang Path, Easter Seal Society, **SLP**

Clines, Sharon Marie P O Box 414, Englewood, FL 34295, (813) 366-4703, BA 74 Univ of Akron; MS 77 FL St Univ; Sp-Lang Path, Private Practice, **SLP ACE**

Clingerman, Mrs Judith Jump 2235 Ellen Avenue, Baltimore, MD 21234, (301) 665-3810, BS 79 SUNY - Coll at Geneseo; MA 82 SUNY - Center at Buffalo; Sp-Lang Path, Easter Seal Society, **SLP**

Clingmon, Ilene C 3247 Rubio Canyon Road, Altadena, CA 91001, (818) 795-6981, BA 74 Chapman Coll; MA 84 Point Loma Nazarene Coll; 87–Prog Coord-Spec Educ, Pasadena USD, **SLP**

Clink, Mrs Pamela J 13131 Ebbtide Circle, North Royalton, OH 44133, (216) 630-3042, BA 74 Cleveland St Univ; MA 76 Cleveland St Univ; 77–SLP, Co of Summit Bd of Ment Ret, **SLP**

Clinker-Farquhar, Margo S Communication Rehabilitation Services, 47 Provincial Park Road, PO Box 239, Moonbeam, ON, Canada P0L 1V0, (705) 367-2787, BS 78 Univ of Western Ontario; MS 80 Univ of Western Ontario; 85–Sp-Lang Path, Private Practice, **SLP**

Clinton, Arlene M 1719 Sheffield Drive, Ypsilanti, MI 48198, **A**

Clinton, Kathy Lunstrum 29954 Paint Brush Drive, Evergreen, CO 80439-8527, (303) 674-6767, BA 80 Metropolitan St Coll; MA 82 Univ of Denver; Sp-Lang Path, Jefferson County R-1 SERS, **SLP**

Clobridge, Carol Ann 1384 Greenwood Drive, Dunedin, FL 33528, (813) 446-6833, MS 74 Univ of South FL; Aud, Chas L Dykstra MD, **A**

Clodfelter-Cartier, Mrs Carla 7011 North Janmar Drive, Dallas, TX 75230, (214) 494-8377, BS 76 Southern Methodist Univ; MS 77 Southern Methodist Univ; Sp/Lang Path, Garland ISD, **SLP**

Clodius, Anne Patricia 1606 Williamsburg Drive, Hendersonville, TN 37075, (615) 822-1476, BA 81 Eastern WA Univ; MS 82 Eastern WA Univ; SLP, Rebound Inc, **SLP**

Clompus, Edie Merle 96 South Main Street Apartment 7, Waterbury, VT 05676, (802) 476-6617, BS 72 PA St Univ - Univ Park; MA 75 Western MI Univ; 88–Sp-Lang Path, Barre Town Elem Sch, **SLP**

Clonan, Ann F 110 Ellingwood Drive, Rochester, NY 14618, (608) 831-1699, BS 76 Ithaca Coll; ME 79 Northeastern Univ; SLP Suprv, Ucptorative Care Assoc, **SLP**

Clontz, Mrs Connie Rae 3916 Ayscough Road, Charlotte, NC 28211, (704) 364-0507, BS 75 Western Carolina Univ; MS 77 Univ of SC - Columbia; Audiologist/SLP, George E Newsome MD, **SLP A**

Clontz, Kimberly B 2807-D Cottage Place, Greensboro, NC 27405, (704) 282-6830, MA 88 Univ of NC - Greensboro

Clopper, Dr Donald L 2118 Marin Avenue, Berkeley, CA 94707, (415) 827-0949, BS 54 Shippensburg Univ of PA; ME 58 PA St Univ - Univ Park; ED 66 (NS) PA St Univ - Univ Park; 86–SELPA Dir, Contra Costa SELPA, **SLP**

Clore, Susan Christensen Route 2 Box 50-K, Culpeper, VA 22701, (703) 825-5448, BA 85 Mary Washington Coll; ME 87 Univ of VA - Charlottesville; 87–Sp-Lang Path, Culpeper County Sch Sys, **SLP**

Clore-Phillips, Sandra Kay 5576 Gleason, Shawnee Mission, KS 66226, (913) 422-5113, BS 81 KS St Univ; MA 83 KS St Univ; Sp-Lang Path, Kansas City KS USD #500, **SLP**

Close, Nancy C 6001 North Classen Blvd, Oklahoma City, OK 73118, (405) 848-3515, BS 75 OK St Univ; MA 76 OK St Univ; Sp-Lang Path, Private Practice, **SLP**

Close, Terry Annn Box 2260, North Ferrisburg, VT 05473, (802) 388-9712, BS 73 Saint Lawrence Univ; MS 88 Univ of VT; 87–Sp-Lang Path, Addison Cen Supervisory Union

Clote, Mrs Cynthia Ann 22 Hammel Street, Webster Groves, MO 63119, (314) 968-7247, BS 84 Fontbonne Coll; MS 86 Fontbonne Coll; Sp-Lang Path, St Louis Assoc for Retarded Ct, **SLP**

Cloud, Steven J 804-E Parker Drive, Florence, SC 29501, (803) 669-8891, BS 82 Western Carolina Univ; OM 85 Univ of SC - Columbia; SLP, Health So Rehab Cntr, **SLP**

Cloud, Mrs Zletta K 4407 Mesa Verde Drive, St Cloud, FL 32769, (305) 892-8424, BA 54 Univ of Science & Arts of OK; BS 55 Univ of Science & Arts of OK; **SLP A LM**

Clougherty, Mrs Melinda E 8 Shepard Court, Sharon, MA 02067, (617) 769-0593, BS 81 Emerson Coll; MS 83 Emerson Coll; **SLP**

Clouse, Mrs Patricia Lynn Spokane ENT Clinic, 104 West 5th Avenue Suite 340 W, Spokane, WA 99204, (509) 624-2326, BA 72 Univ of Portland; MA 86 WA St Univ; 86–Aud, Spokane ENT Clinic, **A**

Clouser, Richard A 148 Clearview Avenue, State College, PA 16803, (814) 234-5223, PH (Aud); **A**

Clover-Mallory, Mrs Jill 20361 Yosemite Boulevard, Waterford, CA 95386, (209) 576-4155, **SLP**

Clowe, Gail G 717 Ridgemont, San Antonio, TX 78209, **SLP**

Clower, Laura Ruth 950 North Pleasant #4, Amherst, MA 01002, (413) 549-4899, BA 82 Brown Univ; MS 85 Boston Univ; **SLP**

Cluff, Dr Gordon L Speech And Hearing Science, Arizona State University, Tempe, AZ 85287-0102, (602) 965-2373, BA 59 AZ St Univ; MS 62 Southern IL Univ -Carbondale; PH 66 (NS) Southern IL Univ -Carbondale; Prof of Aud, Arizona State U, **SLP A**

Clugston, Deidra K W 610 University Drive, East Lansing, MI 48823, (517) 353-8780, BS 73 Eastern MI Univ; MA 76 MI St Univ; Sp-Lang Path, East Lansing PS, **SLP**

Clulee, Carol K Rt 1 Box 27A, La Vale, MD 21502, (301) 759-4555, BS 65 Indiana Univ of PA; ME 66 PA St Univ - Univ Park; Aud-Sp-Lang Path, Allegany Hrng & Sp Assoc, **SLP A**

Clumeck, Dr Harold V 1198 Dolores Street, San Francisco, CA 94110, (415) 493-5000, BA 70 Univ of CA - Berkeley; MA 82 Northwestern Univ; PH 78 (Linguistics) Univ of CA - Berkeley; Sp-Lang Path, VA Med Cen, **SLP**

Clumeck, Mary Annetta 4115 Brooklyn Avenue N E, Apartment #412, Seattle, WA 98105, (206) 764-2404, BA 83 CA St Univ - Fullerton; MS 85 Univ of WA; **SLP**

Clupny, Carol A P O Box 607, Stanfield, OR 97875, (503) 276-6616, BA 79 Eastern WA Univ; MS 80 Eastern WA Univ; Sp-Lang Path, Umatilla Ed Serv Dist, **SLP**

Clupny, Charles Edward P O Box 607, Stanfield, OR 97875, (503) 276-6616, BA 75 Linfield Coll; MS 78 Western OR St Coll; 78–Sp-Lang Path, Umatilla County ESD, **SLP**

Clute, Jan Hayes 320 College Boulevard, Mount Vernon, IA 52314-1027, (319) 927-2143, MA 72 Clark Univ; MA 75 Univ of Northern IA; MA 78 Univ of Chicago; SLP, Keystone AEA, **SLP**

Cluver, Dr Elizabeth 4401 Morehouse Terrace, Chesterfield, VA 23832, (804) 225-2873, BS 75 Univ of VA - Charlottesville; ME 76 Univ of VA - Charlottesville; PH 82 (NS) Univ of VA - Charlottesville; 86–Assoc Dir Spec Educ, VA Dept of Educ, **SLP A**

Cluxton, Kelly Jo 4412 Anvil Drive, Colorado Springs, CO 80925, (719) 520-2000, BS 85 CO St Univ; MS 87 CO St Univ; **SLP**

Clyde, Mrs Connie Marie 3400 N Timberwood Drive, Traverse City, MI 49684, (616) 938-2707, BA 77 MI St Univ; MA 82 MI St Univ; 88–Sp-Lang Path, Gary L Nederveld & Assoc

Clymer, Mrs Beryl F 85 Stonybrook Drive, Rochester, NY 14618, (716) 328-0120, BS 73 Long Island U - CW Post Ctr; MS 74 Ithaca Coll; Sp-Lang Path, Rochester City School District, **SLP**

Clynes, Mrs Deborah Dewey 38 Davis Street, Glens Falls, NY 12801, (518) 793-7721, BA 78 SUNY - Coll at Cortland; MS 83 Coll of Saint Rose; Sp-Lang Path, Washington Warren Bd Coop Ed Serv, **SLP**

Coachbuilder, Dr Deenaz P 8225 Baldwin Avenue, Riverside, CA 92509, PH 70 (NS) Brigham Young Univ; Coord Communicatively Handicpd, San Bernardino City Schools, **SLP**

Coachman, Lin Box 40424, Albuquerque, NM 87196, BA 78 Univ of MN - Minneap-St Paul; MA 82 Univ of MN - Minneap-St Paul; Sp/Lang Path, Private Practice, **SLP**

Coachman, Valerie Leah S 11210 Evans Trail #103, Beltsville, MD 20705, (301) 529-7600, **SLP**

Coakley, Mrs Frieda Truman N8 W33843 Forest Ridge Dr, Delafield, WI 53018, (414) 646-4359, BS 81 Baylor Univ; MS 82 Marquette Univ; Chief Sp-Path, Columbia Hosp, **SLP**

Coakley, Mrs Mabel W 4472 Rebel Valley View, Atlanta, GA 30339, (404) 352-8444, BA 54 Univ of AZ; MS 79 Univ of NE - Omaha; **SLP ACE**

Coale, Sharon Ann 1752 Staimford Drive, West Palm Beach, FL 33414, (407) 936-0108, BS 81 Univ of MD - College Park; MS 83 Vanderbilt Univ; Sp-Lang Path, RehabWorks Inc, **SLP**

Coale, Mrs Sharon Smithey 9208 Cypress Avenue, Bethesda, MD 20814, (301) 897-5474, BA 71 OH Wesleyan Univ; ME 75 Western MD Coll; MS 84 Univ of the DC; 88–Sp-Lang Path, Private Practice, **SLP**

Coan, Susan Lee 7303 Feyhurst Drive, Louisville, KY 40258, (502) 585-9911, BS 85 Spalding Coll; MS 86 Univ of Louisville; SLP, Spalding, **SLP**

Coate, Melanie Lynn 2911 Southern, Parsons, KS 67357, (316) 421-6550, BS 78 Univ of TX - Dallas; MS 81 Univ of TX - Dallas; SLP, Parsons St Hosp & Trng Ctr, **SLP ACE**

Coates, Charles J, Jr 7 Lemon Lane, Mifflinburg, PA 17844, (717) 922-5206, BS 72 PA St Univ - Univ Park; MS 74 PA St Univ - Univ Park; Unit Mgr, Laurelton Cen, **SLP**

Coates, Kathleen M 1720 West La Palma, Suite B, Anaheim, CA 92801, BA 72 Univ of Denver; MA 74 Univ of Denver; Aud, Private Practice, **A**

Coates, Mrs Nadine H 1960 Rocky Ridge Road, Morgan Hill, CA 95037, (408) 268-1411, BA 47 Univ of Southern CA; MA 49 Univ of Southern CA; Dir-Assessment & Cnsl, Los Gatos Christian Church, **SLP F LM**

Coates, Suzanne Lake 704 Schenley Road, Knoxville, TN 37923, (615) 691-3576, BA 77 Univ of VA - Charlottesville; ME 79 Univ of VA - Charlottesville; 87–Sp-Lang Path, Professional Health Services, **SLP**

Coats, Mrs Jo Anne J Star Route 1, Box 1104, Branson, MO 65616, (417) 338-2978, BS 57 Univ of MN - Minneap-St Paul; MA 74 Southeast MO St Univ; Sp-Lang Path, **SLP**

Coats, Mrs Sherry L 9 East Ridge Road, Laurel, MS 39440, (601) 426-2315, BS 77 Univ Southern MS-Hattiesburg; MS 78 Univ Southern MS-Hattiesburg; 86–Sp-Lang Path, Jones Cty Sch, **SLP**

Coats-Garrett, Mrs Paula C 2314 Akron Road, Caro, MI 48723, (517) 673-7573, BA 77 MI St Univ; MA 80 Central MI Univ; Sp-Lang Path, Caro Regional Center, **SLP**

Coaxum, Barbara Ann 5501 Willows Avenue, Philadelphia, PA 19143, (215) 747-5243, BA 81 Clarion Univ of PA; MA 85 West Chester Univ of PA; **SLP**

Cobb, Mrs Christine 6207 Driftwood Drive, Midland, TX 79707, (915) 697-2355, BS 68 Marquette Univ; MS 69 Univ of WI - Stevens Point; 86–Sp-Lang Path, Midland Memorial Hosp, **SLP**

Cobb, Dr Frederick Edmund Audiology Speech Pathology Ser, VA Medical Center, Salem, VA 24153, **A**

Cobb, Jane Emily P O Box 363, Burlington, MA 01803, (617) 935-5050, Sp-Lang Path, New England Rehab Hospital, **SLP**

Cobb, Mrs Jayne Staler 11903 Plum Brook Drive, Houston, TX 77099, (713) 780-5857, BA 79 Univ of Dallas; MA 87 Univ of Houston - Univ Park; 88–Sp-Lang Path, Rosewood Med Ctr

Cobb, John C 11803 South Freeway, Suite 205 P O Box 6426, Fort Worth, TX 76115, (817) 551-1010, BA 73 Univ of AZ; MS 75 Univ of AZ; Aud, Shea Ear Nose & Throat Clinic, **A**

Cobb, Mrs Julia Trainum 580 Pear Orchard Road #223, Ridgeland, MS 39157, (601) 939-0541, BA 85 Univ of MS; MS 87 Univ of MS; Aud, Head & Neck Surgical Group, **A**

Cobb, Justine C Northside Readiness School, 4300 Northside Drive N W, Atlanta, GA 30327, (404) 261-3838, BA 70 G Peabody Coll-Vanderbilt U; MA 74 CUNY - Hunter Coll; Dir/Founder, Therapeut Presch of Atlanta, **SLP**

Cobb, Karen L 333 Prestonwood Drive, Apartment #702, Richardson, TX 75081, (214) 907-0306, BA 78; MS 80; 80–Special Education Lead Teacher, Plano ISD, **SLP**

Cobb, Leslie Louise 19230 Riverside Drive, Sonoma, CA 95476-6126, (707) 938-6822, **SLP**

Cobb, Mary Dawn Rt 5 Box 548, La Grange, NC 28551, (919) 566-9181, **SLP**

Cobb, Pamela Patrice 1550 Terrell Mill Road, Apartment 1-E, Marietta, GA 30067, (404) 971-0838, BS 83 Purdue Univ - West Lafayette; MS 85 Purdue Univ - West Lafayette; **SLP**

Cobb-Cooper, Julie 20406 52nd Avenue West, Lynnwood, WA 98036, (206) 670-7212, BS 78 Univ of KS; MS 81 Univ of WA; 87–Sp-Lang Path, Edmonds Sch Dist, **SLP**

Cobbs, Karen D 1843 Candlelight Drive, Chesapeake, VA 23325, (804) 427-6500, BA 73 Norfolk St Univ; ME 74 Univ of VA - Charlottesville; Sp-Lang Path, VA Beach City PS, **SLP**

Cobbs, Marlene H 399 Primrose Circle, Chesterton, IN 46304, (219) 926-6711, BS 71 Purdue Univ - West Lafayette; MA 73 Purdue Univ - West Lafayette; 85–Sp-Lang Path, Speech Dynamics, **SLP**

Coble, Teresa Goldman 436 Naughright Road, Long Valley, NJ 07853, (201) 342-1121, BS 77 Old Dominion Univ; MA 79 Univ of TN - Knoxville; 86–Sp-Lang Path, Spectrum for Living Inc, **SLP**

Coblentz, Hope M 105 Park Street, Apt #1, North Attleboro, MA 02760, (508) 384-3114, BS 83 Univ of MA - Amherst; MS 85 Indiana Univ of PA; Sp-Lang Path, Wrentham State School, **SLP**

Cobos, Mrs Anne S 3313 Dublin, El Paso, TX 79925, (915) 532-6281, BA 70 Univ of NM; MS 75 AZ St Univ; Sp-Lang Path, Vista Hills Med Ctr, **SLP**

Coburn, Lisa Marie 85 Kirman Avenue #403, Reno, NV 89502, (702) 348-8555, BS 85 Univ of NV - Reno; MS 86 FL St Univ; 87–Aud, William Trimmer MD, **A**

Coburn, Mrs Pamela Lee 175 Todd Road, Wolcott, CT 06716, BS 62 Eastern MI Univ; MA 83 Eastern MI Univ; Sp-Lang Path, Waterbury Pub Schs, **SLP**

Coccaro, Mrs Lynda R 45 Etna Place, Nanuet, NY 10954, (914) 627-2374, BA 76 CUNY - Queens Coll; MA 78 Univ of Pittsburgh - Pittsburgh; Sp-Lang Path, Private Practice, **SLP**

Coccoluto-Davidson, Donna M 91 North Street, Danvers, MA 01923, (617) 482-3370, BA 78 Boston Coll; ME 80 Northeastern Univ; 87–Sp-Lang Path, Mass Easter Seal Society, **SLP**

Cochran, Amy Lynn 4700 South Stewart, Springfield, MO 65807-6272, (816) 587-9541, BS 79 Southwest MO St Univ; MA 84 TX Woman's Univ; Sp-Lang Path, Dallas ISD, **SLP**

Cochran, Mrs Averil C C 4215 Pony Express Road, Kearney, NE 68847, (308) 234-9997, BS 50 UT St Univ; MS 64 Eastern NM Univ; MS 77 Kearney St Coll; Retired, NE Diag Resou Cen, **SLP**

Cochran, Dr Corydon E 1005 Mary Lee Lane, Edmond, OK 73034, (405) 341-2980, BA 54 Univ of OK - Norman; ME 59 Univ of OK - Norman; ED 69 (NS) OK St Univ; Assoc Prof, Ctrl St U, **SLP**

Cochran, Cynthia E 3351 Franklin Avenue, Miami, FL 33133, (305) 445-3699, BS 71 FL A & M Univ; MS 73 FL St Univ; 79–Sp/Lang Path, Private Practice, **SLP**

Cochran, Mrs Debra Jo 1708 Carlsbad Drive, Lafayette, IN 47905, (317) 447-8352, BS 75 Southern IL Univ -Carbondale; MS 83 Purdue Univ - West Lafayette; Aide, McCutcheon High Sch, **SLP**

Cochran, Mrs Evelyn C 225 11th Street, Huntington Beach, CA 92648, (714) 536-7650, BA 64 CA St Univ - Long Beach; MA 71 CA St Univ - Long Beach; **SLP LM**

Cochran, Ione M Box 224, Dinuba, CA 93618, (209) 591-1934, BA 30 Occidental Coll; **SLP LM**

Cochran, Jane Doak 2728 Overbrook Road, Cuyahoga Falls, OH 44221, (216) 928-8903, BS 45 Kent St Univ; Retired, Cwyahoga Falls City Sch Dist, **SLP LM**

Cochran, Dr John R 4215 Pony Express Road, Kearney, NE 68847, (308) 234-9997, BS 49 UT St Univ; MS 50 UT St Univ; PH 59 (Comm Disorders) Univ of UT; Retired, Kearney St Coll, **SLP**

Cochran, Dr Paula S Northeast Missouri State Univ, Dept/Communication Dis, Violette Hall 161, Kirksville, MO 63501, (816) 785-4669, OM 77 Univ of Cambridge - England; MA 78 OH Univ - Athens; PH 86 (Communication Disorders) Univ of VA - Charlottesville; Asst Prof, Northeast Missouri State Univ, **SLP**

Cochran, Mrs Teresa Walton 1036 Keith Street, Hurst, TX 76053, (817) 283-3191, BS 81 West TX St Univ; MS 83 TX Tech Univ; Sp-Lang Path, Callier Speech-Hearing Clinic, **SLP**

Cochrane, Lorelei A 1313 13th Avenue North, Fort Dodge, IA 50501-7529, (515) 955-1405, BA 80 Univ of Northern IA; MA 81 Univ of Northern IA; SLP, Grant Wood AEA, **SLP**

Cochrane, Mrs Mary Ellen 357 Wood Duck Lane, Newport News, VA 23602, (804) 877-8061, BA 63 Mary Washington Coll; ME 68 Univ of VA - Charlottesville; 86–Sp-Lang Path, Newport News PS, **SLP**

Cochrane, Dr Rosalind McCrae Center For Continuing Development, 64 Mountain Street, Sharon, MA 02067, (617) 784-8453, BA 63 Harvard Univ; MA 75 Univ of CT; PH 77 (Language Learning) Univ of CT; Associate Director, Cen for Continuing Development, **SLP**

Cochrane, Susan Mary P O Box 147, Honeoye, NY 14471, (716) 229-2112, BS 82 Nazareth Coll of Rochester; MA 86 Nazareth Coll of Rochester; 88–Sp-Lang Path, Rochester City Schs, **SLP**

Cocke, Mrs Carol B 828 Burdette Street, New Orleans, LA 70118, (504) 527-0303, BS 60 Univ of AL- Tuscaloosa; MA 76 Tulane Univ; Aud, Orleans Parish Sch Bd, **A**

Cocke, Carol B 819 Olive Street, Florence, AL 35630, (205) 974-1146, BA 68 Maryville Coll; MA 73 Memphis St Univ; Sp-Lang Path, Professional Health Services, **SLP**

Cocke, Robin Page 611 Oakhurst, Clarksdale, MS 38614, (601) 624-4967, BA 69 Longwood Coll; ME 71 Univ of VA - Charlottesville; Sp-Lang Path, Private Practice, **SLP**

Cockey, Mrs Elizabeth Ann Route 1 Box 593, Frostburg, MD 21532, (301) 689-6872, BS 77 Clarion Univ of PA; MA 80 Edinboro Univ of PA; Sp-Lang Path, Allegany Co Board of Ed, **SLP**

Cockin, Mrs Margaret A 160 Moulton Road, Brooksville, FL 34610, (813) 868-3376, MA 71 Univ of South FL; Sp-Lang Path, Private Practice, **SLP**

Cocklin, LuAnn J P O Box 1540, Florence, SC 29503, (803) 662-7802, BA 77 York Coll of PA; ME 81 Clarion Univ of PA; Sp-Lang Path, Pee Dee Sp & Hrng Cen, **SLP ACE**

Cockram, Mrs Shannon Smith Route 1 Box 228, Woolwine, VA 24185, (703) 650-3838, BS 83 Radford Univ; MS 84 Radford Univ; **SLP**

Cockrell-Santee, Mrs Trena Route 1 Box 181, Lawrence, KS 66044, (913) 841-5715, BS 79 West TX St Univ; MS 81 Univ of North TX; Sp-Lang Path, Visiting Nurses Association, **SLP**

Cockrum, Mrs Emily S 2804 West 40th Street, Pine Bluff, AR 71603, (501) 534-6822, BA 57 Univ of AR - Fayetteville; MA 75 Univ of AR - Fayetteville; Sp-Lang Path, Jenkins Mem Cen, **SLP**

Coco, Mrs Bernadette Maria Y Rd 4 Box 30-H, Clarks Summit, PA 18411, (717) 587-4542, BS 77 Marywood Coll; MS 81 Bloomsburg Univ of PA; 77–Sp-Lang Path, N E I U #19 Lackawanna Co, **SLP**

Cocran, Cynthia Diane Route 21 Box 265, Highway 11, Slidell, LA 70458, (504) 863-5069, ME 88 Southeastern LA Univ; 88–Sp-Lang Path, St Tammany Parish Sch Bd

Codd, Dorothy S 51 Lakeshore Drive, Oakland, NJ 07436, **SLP**

Coddington, Colleen T Rosewood Center, Leo Kanner Speech & Hearing Center, Owings Mills, MD 21117, (301) 363-2758, BS 83 PA St Univ - Univ Park; MS 85 PA St Univ - Univ Park; Aud, Rosewood Ctr, **A**

Coddington, Jane H 4659 Winterset Drive, Columbus, OH 43220, (614) 293-3818, BS 48 Dickinson Coll; MA 74 OH St Univ; Dir SLP Serv, OH St U Hosp, **SLP**

Coddington, Robert K 3383 Woodrun Trail, Marietta, GA 30062, **SLP**

Codeghini, Donna M 450 Ferry Boulevard #3A, Stratford, CT 06497, (203) 852-9611, BA 75 Southern CT St Univ; MS 78 Southern CT St Univ; OM 81 Fairfield Univ; Sp-Lang Path, Norwalk Pub Sch, **SLP**

Coderre, Mrs Louise University DE Montreal, Ecole D'Orthophonie Et, Case Postale 6128, Montreal, PQ, Canada H3C 3J7, MA 59; Dir, U Montreal

Coderre, Maryann 38 Moraine Street, Jamaica Plain, MA 02130, (617) 232-9500, BS 77 Univ of MA - Amherst; MA 80 Northwestern Univ; Aud, Boston VA Hosp, **A**

Coderre, Mrs Tina R 5 Ponnakin Hill Road, Charlton, MA 01507, (508) 792-8500, BS 79 Worcester St Coll; MA 81 Univ of MA - Amherst; Aud, Hahnemann Rehab Cen, **A**

Codwise, L Jody Mitchell Route 1 Box 394, Tellico Road, Canton, GA 30114, (404) 928-4796, BS 69 SUNY - Coll at Fredonia; MS 74 SUNY - Center at Albany; Sp/Lang Path, Cobb Co Pub Sch, **SLP**

Cody, Janet Patricia P O Box 2607, Salmon Arm, BC, Canada V0E 2T0, (403) 432-8859, BA 82 Western WA Univ; MA 85 Univ of TX - Austin; **A**

Cody, Kathleen Maloney Rd #1 Box 336-A, Baptist Church Road, Hampton, NJ 08827, (201) 735-9175, BS 84 Coll of Saint Rose; MS 87 Southern CT St Univ; Sp-Lang Path, Private Practice, **SLP**

Cody, Mary M All Ears Hearing Center, 131 Court Street, PO Box 3135, Plymouth, MA 02361, (508) 747-4055, BA 75 Bridgewater St Coll; ME 79 Northeastern Univ; Director, All Ears Hrng Cen, **A ACE**

Cody, Mary Teresa 189 Farrington Street, Wollaston, MA 02170, (617) 471-3907, BA 81 Boston Coll; ME 83 Northeastern Univ; Sp-Lang Path, Boston Pub Sch, **SLP**

Cody, Patsy Davis P O Box 1364, Banner Elk, NC 28604, (704) 898-5458, BS 83 Appalachian St Univ; MA 88 Appalachian St Univ; Sp-Lang Path, Private Practice

Cody, Robert Charles Speech And Hearing Clinic, Wvu Medical Center, Morgantown, WV 26506, (304) 293-4250, BA 56 Univ of Northern IA; MA 63 Univ of IA; Prof/Ch Sp & Hrng Cl, WV U Med Cen, **A**

Cody, Shirley R 1607 West Austin Road, Decatur, GA 30032, MS 74 Univ of MI - Ann Arbor; 76–Sp-Lang Path, Fulton Co Bd of Educ, **SLP**

Coe, Carolyn M 2740 Scarborough Drive, Anchorage, AK 99504, (907) 274-4582, BS 73 Bowling Green St Univ; MA 76 Kent St Univ; Supervisor, Anchorage School District, **SLP**

Coe, Sandra L 1121 Walker, Suite 1900, Houston, TX 77002, (713) 225-4327, BA 78 Univ of Northern CO; MA 83 Univ of North TX; Aud, Hearing Inc, **A**

Coe, Thomas E P O Box 32634, Oklahoma City, OK 73123, (405) 842-0469, BS 78 Northern AZ Univ; MS 80 Univ of OK - OK City; Sp-Lang Path, Private Practice, **SLP**

Coelho, Dr Carl A 306 Cedar Lane, Cheshire, CT 06410, (203) 284-2880, BA 74 MI St Univ; MS 76 Univ of AZ; PH 82 (NS) Univ of CT; Director Commun Disorders Dept, The Gaylord Hospital, **SLP**

Coen, Donald P 509 Belleview Boulevard, Steubenville, OH 43952, (614) 283-3674, BA 67 West Liberty St Coll; ME 70 Kent St Univ; Exec Dir, En OH Sp and Hrng Cen In, **SLP**

Coen, Mrs Laura E P O Box 471, Effingham, IL 62401, (217) 347-7457, BS 79 Eastern IL Univ; MS 80 Eastern IL Univ; Sp-Lang Path, Effingham School District #40, **SLP**

Coen-Cummings, Martha Carol 5315 Fenwick Avenue, Cincinnati, OH 45212-1609, (606) 491-1171, BS 84 Miami Univ - Oxford; MS 85 Miami Univ - Oxford; Sp-Lang Path, Northern KY Easter Seal Cen, **SLP**

Cofer, Mrs Sandra K 16091 Sharon Lane, Salinas, CA 93908, (408) 455-1332, BA 68 Eastern WA Univ; MS 71 Eastern WA Univ; **SLP**

Cofey, Carol J 9616 Nonquitt Drive, Fairfax, VA 22031, (703) 241-7600, BA 44 Augustana Coll; MA 59 Northwestern Univ; Sp-Lang Path, Falls Church Sch Brd, **SLP F**

Coffee, Mrs Lauren K 3352 Taleen Court, Annandale, VA 22003, (703) 356-0700, BS 68 Univ of VA - Charlottesville; ME 70 Univ of VA - Charlottesville; Sp-Lang Path, Fairfax County Public Schools, **SLP**

Coffey, Christine Beth 17 Johnson Road, Latham, NY 12110, (518) 664-5066, MA 83 Univ of FL; Sp-Lang Path, Helping Hands School, **SLP**

Coffey, Cynthia 1630 Summer Run, Florissant, MO 63033, (314) 569-8311, MA 77 Northeast MO St Univ; 87–Sp-Lang Path, Special Sch Dist of St Louis Co, **SLP**

Coffey, Elizabeth R R 1 Box 496-H, Monticello, KY 42633, (606) 348-7757, Sp-Lang Path, Lake Cumberland Home Health, **SLP**

Coffey, Geneva J 123 Morehead Street, Morganton, NC 28655, (704) 437-4191, BA 71 Univ of NC - Greensboro; MS 76 Univ of NC - Chapel Hill; Sp-Lang Path, Morganton Sp & Lang Serv, **SLP**

Coffey, Jacqueline 191 Stirling Court, West Chester, PA 19380, BS 72 West Chester Univ of PA; MA 77 West Chester Univ of PA; **SLP**

Coffey, Mrs Jill Renee 811 A East 32nd Terrace, Hutchinson, KS 67502, (316) 665-5694, BA 86 Wichita St Univ; MA 87 Wichita St Univ; **SLP**

Coffey, M Alexandra Lennox Apts 250 South, 13th Street #5D, Philadelphia, PA 19107, **A**

Coffey, Mrs Mary Elisabeth P O Box 204, Bent Mountain, VA 24059-0204, (703) 343-2753, BA 80 Marshall Univ; MS 82 James Madison Univ; Sp-Lang Path, Ctr for Rehab & Dev, **SLP**

Coffey, Thomas S 123 Morehead Street, Morganton, NC 28655, (704) 433-2443, BA 72 Univ of NC - Chapel Hill; MS 76 Univ of NC - Chapel Hill; Aud, West Carolina Cen, **A**

Coffie, Mrs Lucie Callaway 230 Broadland Road N W, Atlanta, GA 30342, (404) 237-7121, BA 63 Agnes Scott Coll; OM 87 Emory Univ; 87–Psychiatric Soc Wkr, Kennestone Hosp, **A**

Coffield, Eleanor 1718 South Garrison, Carthage, MO 64836, (417) 358-2980, BS 48 Central MO St Univ; MA 60 Univ of Denver; Retired, Carthage R-9 Sch, **SLP LM**

Coffield, Phyllis Reel 2900 Moss Road N W, Huntsville, AL 35810, (205) 859-7368, BS 51 Northwestern Univ; MS 71 Vanderbilt Univ; Dir Sp-Lang-Hrng Cl, Al A & M U, **SLP**

Coffin, Mrs Jo Ann B 41122 Buttternut Ridge, Elyria, OH 44035, (216) 458-6093, BS 70 OH St Univ; MA 74 Bowling Green St Univ; Aud, Kenwood Aud Sers, **A**

Coffman, Mrs Angela Weston 1717 Northwest Drive N W, Cullman, AL 35055, (205) 269-3809, BA 78 Auburn Univ - Montgomery; MS 80 Univ of AL- Tuscaloosa; Sp-Lang Path, Montgomery Public Schools, **SLP**

Coffman, James M 3316 Prairie Avenue, Mattoon, IL 61938, (217) 235-5446, BS 69 Eastern IL Univ; MS 75 Eastern IL Univ; Sp-Lang Path, Mattoon Commun, **SLP**

Coffman, Mary Beth 97 Oak Drive, Millsboro, DE 19966, (302) 856-5213, BS 76 James Madison Univ; MS 78 James Madison Univ; **SLP**

Coffman, Mrs Robbin K 120 Runaway Bay Drive #303, Virginia Beach, VA 23452, (804) 481-4004, BS 86 Southern IL Univ-Edwardsvill; MS 87 Southern IL Univ-Edwardsvill

Coffman, Mrs Susan V 8100 Glenmore Springs Road, Bethesda, MD 20817, (202) 337-5220, BS 64 OH Univ - Athens; MA 68 Univ of MD - College Park; Dir-Pro Prog & Svcs, A Graham Bell Assn for Deaf, **SLP**

Cofoni, Mrs Diane Elizabeth 14 Hampton Court, Slanders, NJ 07836, (201) 691-1085, BA 71 Univ of RI; MS 81 Univ of RI; **SLP**

Cofrancesco, Mrs Deborah T 4315 Winchester, Vicksburg, MS 39180-9780, (601) 636-0176, BS 72 Univ Southern MS-Hattiesburg; MS 73 Univ Southern MS-Hattiesburg; 81–Sp-Lang Path, Vicksburg Warren Sch Dist, **SLP**

Cogen, Lynn C 160 Crane Drive, San Anselmo, CA 94960-1014, (213) 454-5046, BS 65 PA St Univ - Univ Park; ME 69 PA St Univ - Univ Park; **SLP**

Coger, Patricia Johnson 1517 Murner Rd, Gaylord, MI 49735, (517) 732-6292, BS 79 Central MI Univ; MA 82 Central MI Univ; 87–Sp-Lang Path, Northern MI Comm Men Health, **SLP**

Coggins, Mrs Kathleen Bryan 19825 32nd N E, Seattle, WA 98155, MS 74 Univ of WI - Madison; Lecturer, University of Washington, **SLP**

Coggins, Dr Truman E 19825 32nd N E, Seattle, WA 98155, (206) 545-2999, BA 70 Univ of Redlands; MS 71 Univ of Redlands; PH 76 Univ of WA; Assoc Prof, U of WA, **SLP**

Coggins-Stoltz, Carolyn 5905 Reservoir Heights Avenue, Alexandria, VA 22311, (703) 379-0274, BA 72 Univ of KY; MS 74 Purdue Univ - West Lafayette; 76–Sp-Lang Path, Alexandria City Sch, **SLP**

Coghlan, Mrs Catherine H 8 West 5th Street, Port Reading, NJ 07064, (201) 634-4571, BA 70 Rutger's St Univ - Douglas Coll; MA 72 Montclair St Coll; 88–SLP, Woodbridge Twp Sch Dist, **SLP**

Coghlan, Mrs Patricia M 9956 South Campbell, Chicago, IL 60642, BS 78 Univ of IL - Urbana; OM 80 Governors St Univ; **SLP**

Cogley, Wallace H 3105 169th S W, Lynnwood, WA 98037, (206) 281-6866, BA 62 WA St Univ; MS 68 Univ of WA; Sp-Lang Path, Seattle Pub Sch, **SLP**

Cogswell, Annastacia Rural Route 1, Padgett Road, Powell River, BC, Canada V8A 4Z2, (604) 485-2440, BA; MA; **SLP**

Cogswell, Cynthia Church 131 Fairfield Place, Moraga, CA 94556, (415) 376-1917, BA 77 Univ of the Pacific; MA 78 Univ of the Pacific; Sp-Lang Path, Private Practice, **SLP**

Cogswell, Mrs Pamela E 3618 N E Couch Street, Portland, OR 97232, (503) 233-6748, MS 88 Portland St Univ

Cohagan, Amelia A 4102 Stratton, Midland, TX 79707, (915) 694-2741, BA 80 Univ of Denver; MA 82 Univ of Denver; 84–Sp-Lang Path, **SLP**

Cohan, Donnajo A P O Box 166, Winslow, NJ 08095, (609) 561-1700, MS 80 PA St Univ - Univ Park; Sp-Lang Path, Ancora Hospital, **SLP**

Cohan, Joan Strandberg 1628 Monroe Street, Evanston, IL 60202, (312) 256-2450, BS 81 Northwestern Univ; MA 82 Northwestern Univ; Sp-Lang Path, Wilmette Public Schools, **SLP**

Cohen, Alan 841 North Leh Street, Allentown, PA 18104, (215) 435-7755, OB 66 OH Univ - Athens; MA 67 Western MI Univ; Aud/Sp-Lang Path, Allentown Audiology & Speech Assoc, **SLP A**

Cohen, Dr Alan H 47 Emerald Lane, Willingboro, NJ 08046, (609) 652-1776, BS 64 PA St Univ - Univ Park; MA 67 Temple Univ-Tyler Sch of Art; PH (NS) Temple Univ-Tyler Sch of Art; Associate Professor, Stockton State College, **SLP**

Cohen, Mrs Amy J 117 Stephenville Parkway, Edison, NJ 08820, (201) 548-3883, BS 75 Boston Univ; MA 77 SUNY - Center at Buffalo; **SLP**

Cohen, Dr Anna B Communication Disorders Dept, Worcester State College, Worcester, MA 01602, (617) 793-8055, BA 64 Newark St Coll; MA 65 Univ of WI - Madison; ED 75 (NS) Columbia Univ Teachers Coll; Prof, Worcester St Coll, **SLP**

Cohen, Barbara A 330 3rd Avenue #14-K, New York, NY 10010, (212) 689-8717, BA 70 CUNY - City College; MA 76 NY Univ; 86–Sp-Lang Path, Consultant/Private Practice, **SLP**

Cohen, Beth D 11 Bridges Avenue, Newtonville, MA 02160, **SLP**

Cohen, Betsy Jane 323 South Union Avenue, Havre de Grace, MD 21078, (301) 939-2030, BA 82 Univ of MD - College Park; MA 84 Hofstra Univ; 87–Aud, Hearing Associates Inc, **A**

Cohen, Beverly Rose 2255 Braeswood Park Drive, # 314, Houston, TX 77030, (212) 678-4539, BS 83 Montclair St Coll; MS 85 Columbia Univ Teachers Coll; SLP, Univ of Texas, **SLP**

Cohen, Brenda P P O Box 32, Rutland, VT 05701, (802) 775-7111, BA 64 Univ of AL- Tuscaloosa; MA 67 Case Western Reserve Univ; SLP, Rutland Reg Med Cen, **SLP**

Cohen, Mrs Carol Berman 171 West Poplar Avenue, San Mateo, CA 94402, BS 68 Univ of Rochester; MA 74 SUNY - Center at Buffalo; Sp-Lang Path, San Mateo Co Offi of Ed, **SLP**

Cohen, Carol G 110 Thomas Road, De Witt, NY 13214, (315) 446-0371, BS 71 Syracuse Univ; MS 72 Syracuse Univ; Dir, Enable/Schneier Comm Unit, **SLP F**

Cohen, Mrs Debra LeShay 617 Weadley Road, Strafford, PA 19087, (215) 587-3142, BA 72 PA St Univ - Univ Park; MA 74 George Washington Univ; Asst Dir/Sp-Lang Path, Magee Rehabilitation Hospital, **SLP**

Cohen, Mrs Diane H 139 Fearing Drive, Westwood, MA 02090, (617) 327-4358, BA 63 Syracuse Univ; MA 67 Emerson Coll; **SLP A**

Cohen, Dianne E 21 Eagle Street, Chestnut Ridge, NY 10977, (215) 657-6534, BA 75 SUNY - Center at Binghamton; MS 79 Boston Univ; SLP, **SLP**

Cohen, Eileen F 37 Hamlet Drive, Owings Mills, MD 21117, (301) 225-5581, BA 67 Univ of MD - College Park; MA 68 Univ of WI - Milwaukee; Sp-Lang Path, MD St Dept of HI&H Ment Hyg, **SLP**

Cohen, Mrs Elisa Susan 4601 Henry Hudson Parkway, Riverdale, NY 10471, (212) 671-6373, MS 83 Adelphi Univ; Sp-Lang Path, Morris Park Dental Association, **SLP**

Cohen, Elisha Beth 516 Hillside Avenue, Westfield, NJ 07090, (201) 233-1553, MA 87 Hofstra Univ

Cohen, Mrs Elizabeth P O Box 16542, West Palm Beach, FL 33416, (407) 967-1060, BS 71 Marquette Univ; MA 74 Marshall Univ; SLP, Dakota Inc, **SLP**

Cohen, Mrs Elizabeth P 1804-B Soloman Road, Charlottesville, VA 22901, (804) 979-4190, ME 88 Univ of VA - Charlottesville

Cohen, Ellyn M Northside Plaza, Rt 45, Pomona, NY 10970, (914) 354-6772, BS 70 Syracuse Univ; MS 71 Columbia Univ Teachers Coll; Sp/Lang Path, Private Practice, **SLP**

Cohen, Mrs Erica A 2 Hartland, Emerson, NJ 07630, (201) 592-1234, BA 68; MA 69; Sp-Lang Path, Emerson Bd of Ed, **SLP**

Cohen, Dr Frederick 421 Carroll Avenue, Mamaroneck, NY 10543, (201) 595-2209, BS 48 CUNY - City College; MA 49 Columbia Univ Teachers Coll; ED 61 (Sp-Lang Path) Columbia Univ Teachers Coll; 68–Prof Sp-Lang Path, Wm Paterson Coll, **SLP A ACE**

Cohen, Gail E Frankfort American High School, Box 30, APO New York, NY 09710, **SLP**

Cohen, Gail Katz 4201 Silsby, Cleveland, OH 44118, **SLP**

Cohen, Garland J 35 East 40th Avenue, Vancouver, BC, Canada V5W 1L3, MS; **SLP LM**

Cohen, Dr Gary S 8909 North Port Wash Road, Suite 206, Bayside, WI 53217, (414) 352-2900, BA 68 Univ of Charleston; MS 74 Univ of Pittsburgh - Pittsburgh; PH 78 (Sp-Path) Memphis St Univ; Sp/Lang Path, Private Practice, **SLP**

Cohen, Mrs Harriet B 2806 Seabreeze Drive South, Gulfport, FL 33707, (813) 321-4000, BA 66 Montclair St Coll; ME 69 Univ of VA - Charlottesville; Private Practice, **SLP ACE**

Cohen, Harriet R 82-07 259th Street, Floral Park, NY 11004, (718) 347-6187, BA 73 CUNY - Queens Coll; MA 75 CUNY - Queens Coll; Sp-Lang Path, NY Cty Bd of Ed, **SLP**

Cohen, Helene Janis 192 Willowbreeze, Tonawanda, NY 14223, (716) 835-6009, MA 87 SUNY - Center at Buffalo; 87–Sp-Lang Path, Buffalo Hearing & Speech Ctr, **SLP**

Cohen, Ivan J Audiology & Hearing Aid Assoc, 5470 La Jolla Boulevard, La Jolla, CA 92037, (619) 454-1309, BA 72 Univ of San Diego; MA 75 Univ of San Diego; Owner Aud, Aud & Hrng Aid Assoc, **A**

Cohen, Jane S 15 Vista Avenue, Piedmont, CA 94611, (415) 653-6522, BA 67 CUNY - Hunter Coll; MA 69 San Francisco St Univ; Sp-Lang Path, Piedmont USD, **SLP**

Cohen, Mrs Janet Kabakoff 3933 East 58th Place, Tulsa, OK 74135, (918) 742-8118, BA 52; MA 71 Univ of Tulsa; Sp-Lang Path, Private Practice, **SLP**

Cohen, Jerome M Hearing Unlimited Inc, 301 5th Avenue, Bldg Suite 1305, Pittsburgh, PA 15222, (412) 281-1122, BS 49 CUNY - City College; MA 82 Univ of Pittsburgh - Pittsburgh; Aud, Hrng Unlimited Inc, **A**

Cohen, Mrs Joy B 1960 N W 25th Street, Boca Raton, FL 33431-6376, (407) 997-7223, BS 67 Univ of WI - Madison; MA 69 Case Western Reserve Univ; Sp-Lang Path, Private Practice, **SLP**

Cohen, Judith L 454 Truman, Bowling Green, OH 43402, (419) 354-1331, BA 71 Univ of MI - Ann Arbor; MA 75 Univ of NE - Lincoln; Cl Superv, Bowling Green St U, **SLP**

Cohen, Mrs Judith Marks 645 Flagstaff Drive, Cincinnati, OH 45215, (513) 742-2200, BS 77 Miami Univ - Oxford; MA 78 MI St Univ; Sp-Lang Path, Hamilton Co Offi of Ed, **SLP**

Cohen, Karen E 2016 Locksley Lane, Denton, TX 76201, (214) 241-4111, BS 77 KS St Univ; MS 79 Univ of TX - Dallas; 87–Sp-Lang Path, Special Care & Career Ctr, **SLP**

Cohen, Mrs Karen Hope 882 Stockton Road, Valley Cottage, NY 10989, (212) 436-7600, BA 80 SUNY - Coll at Cortland; MA 82 Hofstra Univ; Sp/Lang Path, UCP of NY, **SLP**

Cohen, Mrs Karen R 56 Levering Circle, Bala-Cynwyd, PA 19004, (215) 221-3636, BA 77 Univ of MD - College Park; OM 79 Hahneman Medical Coll; 86–Sp-Lang Path, Private Practice, **SLP**

Cohen, Mrs Kathy J 14423 White Birch Valley, Chesterfield, MO 63017, (314) 532-8284, BS 77 Univ of TX - Austin; MS 79 Baylor Univ; Aud, Pediatric Otol Inc, **A**

Cohen, Kenneth D 2434 Wismer, Overland, MO 63114, (314) 423-0622, BS 73 Northeast MO St Univ; MA 75 Saint Louis Univ; Sp-Lang Path, Sp Sch Dist of St Louis Co, **SLP**

Cohen, Lauren Stephanie 149-30 88th Street #4-K, Howard Beach, NY 11414, (718) 837-5866, BA 86 CUNY - Queens Coll; MS 87 Adelphi Univ; 88–Sp-Lang Path, Milestone Sch for Child Dev

Cohen, Lenore W 72 Fairway Avenue, Verona, NJ 07044, (201) 857-1698, BA 49 Upsala Coll; OM 69 Seton Hall Univ; 82–Sp-Lang Path, Private Practice, **SLP**

Cohen, Mrs Lillian K 4013 Basswood Road, Minneapolis, MN 55416, (612) 926-1882, BA 38 Univ of Manitoba - Winnipeg; MA 39 Columbia Univ Teachers Coll; **SLP LM**

Cohen, Linda E 1115 Limekiln Pike, Maple Glen, PA 19002, (215) 643-6669, BS 66 PA St Univ - Univ Park; MA 79 Temple Univ; Sp-Lang Path, Sch Dist of Phila, **SLP**

Cohen, Lindy S 524 General Lafayette Road, Merion, PA 19066, (215) 668-1836, BA 77 Univ of MD - College Park; MA 79 Univ of MD - College Park; 84–Grad Progr Coord, Hahnemann Univ, **SLP**

Cohen, Lisa Rachelle 526 North 19th Street, Philadelphia, PA 19130, (302) 733-1000, BS 83 Knoxville Coll; MA 85 TN Temple Univ; **SLP**

Cohen, Lucy L 11609 Magruder Lane, Rockville, MD 20852, (301) 984-9481, BS 68 Boston Univ; MS 71 Univ of NC - Chapel Hill; Aud, Hndcpd Inf Interven Prog, **A**

Cohen, Dr Marion F Dept Of Communication Science, University Of Connecticut, Storrs, CT 06268, (203) 486-3166, BS 61 Emerson Coll; MA 63 IN Univ - Bloomington; PH 75 (NS) Stanford Univ; Assoc Prof, Univ of CT, **A**

Cohen, Mrs Marjorie H College Street, Hamilton, NY 13346, (315) 824-2834, MS 76 Syracuse Univ; Aud, M L Delmonico MD, **A**

Cohen, Marla S 8119 Fairview Road, Elkins Park, PA 19117, BS 76 Ithaca Coll; MA 79 Temple Univ-Tyler Sch of Art; Audiologist, Yale-New Haven Hospital, **A**

Cohen, Marsha S 119 Carpenter Avenue #A4, Mount Kisco, NY 10549, (914) 669-5804, BA 75 Case Western Reserve Univ; MA 77 Case Western Reserve Univ; Sp-Lang Path, Westchester Develop Serv, **SLP**

Cohen, Martin 661 Rutland Avenue, Teaneck, NJ 07666, (201) 836-1360, BA 47 CUNY - Brooklyn Coll; MA 49 Columbia Univ Teachers Coll; Aud, Private Practice, **SLP A LM**

Cohen, Mrs Melissa R 420 Breakwater Ridge, Atlanta, GA 30328, (404) 457-6303, BS 74 Univ of GA; ME 75 Univ of GA; Aud, GA Head Neck&Facial Plas Surg, **A**

Cohen, Dr Melvin S Cedars-Sinai Medical Center, Department Of Physical Medicine & Rehabilitation, 8700 Beverly Boulevard SCH 215, Los Angeles, CA 90048-0750, (213) 855-6265, OM 87 Loma Linda Univ - Riverside; MA 71 Univ of the Pacific; PH 73 (Sp Path & Aud) Univ of UT; 88–Chief Sp-Lang Path, Cedars-Sinai Med Ctr, **SLP ACE**

Cohen, Mrs Minda J 1513 Hillhaven Drive, Marietta, GA 30062, (404) 977-7906, BS 79 Univ of GA; ME 80 Univ of GA; Sp-Lang Path, Speech Pathology Services Inc, **SLP ACE**

Cohen, Mrs Nancy Fell 214 White Branch Court, Buffalo Grove, IL 60089, (312) 729-8800, BA 81 Univ of WI - Madison; MS 83 Univ of WI - Madison; Sp-Lang Path, Il Therapeutics Assoc Ltd, **SLP**

Cohen, Nancy L Lahey Clinic Medical Center, 41 Mall Road, Burlington, MA 01805, (617) 273-8452, BS 80 Elmira Coll; MA 82 Kent St Univ; Aud, Lahey Clinic, **A**

Cohen, Nathan M 14 Sturbridge Court, Nanuet, NY 10954, (212) 992-9265, BA 72 CUNY - Lehman Coll; MS 75 CUNY - Brooklyn Coll; Sp-Lang Path, Montefiore Chcc, **SLP**

Cohen, Mrs Noemi F 333 Marlborough Road, Englewood, NJ 07631, (201) 569-2104, MS 78 Boston Univ; Dir, Gldn Hill Hd Injry Comm Prog, **SLP**

Cohen, Mrs Patricia A 554 Seaman Avenue, Baldwin, NY 11510, (516) 482-8778, BA 77 CUNY - Queens Coll; MA 79 CUNY - Queens Coll; Aud, N Shore Otor Assoc, **A**

Cohen, Mrs Penny Lynn 12743 Texana Street, San Diego, CA 92129, (619) 484-2888, BA 82 McGill Univ - Quebec; MA 85 San Diego St Univ; 88–Sp-Lang Path, Penny Cohen, **SLP**

Cohen, Phyllis Plastic Surgical ENT Associate, 181 Woodhill Lane, Media, PA 19063, (215) 566-7671, BA 72 MI St Univ; MA 73 MI St Univ; 88–Aud, Plastic Surg ENT Assoc, **A**

Cohen, Rhoda T 10 Sugar Maple Drive, Roslyn, NY 11576, (212) 381-6454, BA 54 Adelphi Univ; MA 74 Adelphi Univ; OM 82 Long Island U - CW Post Ctr; Chairperson Commit On Hndcpd, NYC Bd of Ed, **SLP**

Cohen, Mrs Rita U 11902 Blue February Way, Columbia, MD 21044, (301) 649-8046, BA 74 CUNY - Queens Coll; MA 75 CUNY - Queens Coll; Sp-Lang Path, Mont Co Pub Sch/Sp-Lang Prog, **SLP ACE**

Cohen, Robert A Pelham Audiology Association, 1931 Williamsbridge Road, Bronx, NY 10461, (212) 822-4100, BA 73 CUNY - Lehman Coll; MS 74 PA St Univ - Univ Park; Owner/Manager, Pelham Aud Assoc, **A**

Cohen, Mrs Roberta S 34 Country Drive, Plainview, NY 11803, (516) 566-5774, BA 72 CUNY - Queens Coll; MA 73 Hofstra Univ; Dir of Aud, A Holly Patterson Home, **A**

Cohen, Mrs Robin B 8 Keswick Drive, Voorhees, NJ 08043, (609) 654-7284, **SLP**

Cohen, Dr Ronald Lee 5354 Palisades Drive, Cincinnati, OH 45238, (606) 292-4021, BS 70 Univ of Cincinnati; MA 71 Univ of Cincinnati; PH 75 (NS) Univ of Cincinnati; Priv Pract, **A**

Cohen, Mrs Ronnie D 84 McCulloch Drive, Dix Hills, NY 11746, (516) 499-3476, BA 69 Hofstra Univ; MA 72 Gettysburg Coll; **SLP**

Cohen, Ronnie K 2051 Arbor Drive, Linwood, NJ 08221, (609) 926-1166, BA 75 Rutger's St Univ - Douglas Coll; MA 78 Catholic Univ of America; Sp-Lang Path, Atlantic Speech Therapy, **SLP**

Cohen, Mrs Sharon F 69 Devonshire Road, Cedar Grove, NJ 07009, (201) 256-1700, BA 73 CUNY - Queens Coll; MA 76 Case Western Reserve Univ; Aud Dir, Nrth Jersey Devel Cen, **A**

Cohen, Shelley Robin 200 East 15th Street #10-E, New York, NY 10003, (212) 677-7400, BA 79 Southern CT St Univ; MA 81 NY Univ; Sp/Lang Path, UCP of NYC Inc, **SLP**

Cohen, Mrs Shirley A 45 Colonial Terrace, Springfield, NJ 07081, (201) 533-5788, BS 52 SUNY - Coll at Geneseo; MS 57 SUNY - Center at Buffalo; Coord Craniofacil Cen, St Barnaba's Med Cen, **SLP**

Cohen, Siri Ilene 4427 Woodman Avenue #15, Sherman Oaks, CA 91423, (818) 995-6049, BA 85 SUNY - Center at Buffalo; MS 87 Adelphi Univ; **SLP**

Cohen, Stuart L 1132 Culpepper Circle, Charleston, SC 29407, (803) 577-5410, BS 71 Univ of SC - Columbia; MA 74 Univ of SC - Columbia; Ch Aud, Charleston Sp & Hrng Cen, **A**

Cohen, Susan 10 Mallard Road, Acton, MA 01720, MS 75 Trenton St Coll; Sp-Lang Path, Private Practice, **SLP**

Cohen, Susan Reincke 4814 Grand Bend Drive, Catonsville, MD 21228, (301) 252-4000, BA 79 Loyola Coll; MS 80 Loyola Coll; Sp-Lang Path, UCP Cen MD, **SLP**

Cohen, Mrs Susan Wynn 11 Evergreen Drive, Bldg 5 Unit 56, Clifton, NJ 07013, (718) 498-2500, BA 80 Washington Univ; MA 82 Northwestern Univ; Sp/Lang Path, The League Sch, **SLP**

Cohen, Mrs Terri Baltier 141 Sycamore Circle, Stony Brook, NY 11790, BA 78 Hofstra Univ; MA 81 Trenton St Coll; **SLP**

Cohen, Mrs Terri Haskins 116 Jamestown Road, Basking Ridge, NJ 07920, (201) 580-9217, BA 86 Univ of MD - College Park; MS 88 Rutger's St Univ - Douglas Coll; 88–Sp-Lang Path, Sp & Hrng Assoc

Cohen, Mrs Vicki C 6942 Salamanca Avenue, Jacksonville, FL 32217, (904) 733-7674, BA 64 Univ of FL; MS 77 FL St Univ; Sp-Lang Path, Private Practice, **SLP**

Cohen, Wendy Joy 816 Densmore Road, Philadelphia, PA 19116, (215) 934-6174, BS 76 Temple Univ-Tyler Sch of Art; MA 81 Trenton St Coll

Cohen-Essig, Shary I 13411 Killion Street, Van Nuys, CA 91401-5339, (818) 780-6202, BA 75 Univ of MN - Minneap-St Paul; MS 77 Saint Cloud St Univ; 88–Sp-Lang Path, Private Practice, **SLP**

Cohenour-Sexson, Suzanne M 3712 Chapala Drive N E, Albuquerque, NM 87111, (505) 821-9393, MS 84 Univ of NM; **SLP**

Cohill, Kathleen A 121 South Highland Avenue Apartment 4G, Ossining, NY 10562, (914) 245-2700, BA 77 Loyola Coll; MS 78 Loyola Coll; Sp/Lang Path, Putnam/N Westchester BOCES, **SLP**

Cohill, Mary B 1720 Chilhowie Circle, Virginia Beach, VA 23464, (804) 467-3548, BA 73 Loyola Coll; MS 74 Loyola Coll; 86–Sp-Lang Path, Chesapeake Infant Inter Prog, **SLP**

Cohlberg, Nancy K 402 Pembroke Road, Bala-Cynwyd, PA 19004, **SLP**

Cohn, Anita Lynne 192 Jackson Court, Burlington, VT 05401, (802) 656-3861, MS 85 Univ of VT; Grant Coord, Univ of VT, **SLP**

Cohn, Dr Ellen Rassas 5436 Northumberland Avenue, Pittsburgh, PA 15217, (412) 682-4550, BS 74 Rutger's St Univ - Douglas Coll; MA 76 Vanderbilt Univ; PH 81 (Sp-Lang Path) Univ of Pittsburgh - Pittsburgh; Clinical Assistant Professor, University of Pittsburgh, **SLP**

Cohn, Gail Cartenuto 2269 Willoway Street, Yorktown Heights, NY 10598, (212) TY2-3710, **SLP**

Cohn, Helene T 108 Valentine Street, Highland Park, NJ 08904, (801) 249-8292, SLP, **SLP**

Cohn, Laurie E 1 Horseshoe Drive, Hyde Park, NY 12538, (914) 229-8262, BS 71 Emerson Coll; MA 73 Case Western Reserve Univ; 75–Supvr Sp-Lang Path, St Francis Hosp, **SLP**

Cohn, Mrs R Phyllis 20 Wendell Street, Hempstead, NY 11550, (516) 328-4652, BA 63 CUNY - Brooklyn Coll; MS 67 CUNY - Brooklyn Coll; SLP, Sewanhaka Ctrl Hs Dist, **SLP**

Cohn, Susan G 3055 Quinalt Court SW, Issaquah, WA 98027-4414, (206) 462-7800, BA 71 IN Univ - Bloomington; OM 73 IN Univ - Bloomington; 83–Director/Sp-Lang Path, Hope Clinic, **SLP**

Cohn, Mrs Susan Greenberg 776 Asbury Street, New Milford, NJ 07646, (201) 977-6606, BS 66 Univ of WI - Milwaukee; MA 86 Montclair St Coll; **SLP**

Cohon, Mrs Robin Y 90 Atwell Lane, Monticello, NY 12701, (914) 794-8113, BS 68 Emerson Coll; MA 69 Western MI Univ; **SLP**

Coie, John Paul Audiology, Naval Hospital, Portsmouth, VA 23708, (804) 398-5873, MA 67 Univ of Denver; Naval Hosp, **A**

Coiner, Juanita L 601 North Wall, Joplin, MO 64801, (918) 592-6000, BS 66 Univ of Tulsa; MA 69 Univ of Tulsa; Coord of Cl Serv, U of Tulsa, **SLP**

Cokely, Jeffrey A 805 Eddington Court, Bloomington, IN 47401, (812) 335-2602, Asst Prof, IN Univ, **A**

Coker, Mrs Jena Davis 843 Deanna Court, Radcliff, KY 40160, (502) 624-7449, BA 71 Murray St Univ; MS 72 Murray St Univ; **SLP**

Coker, William B, Jr 187 Melmore St, Tiffen, OH 44883, (419) 448-8718, BA 79 Asbury Coll; MA 81 MI St Univ; 87–Dir, St Francis Rehab Hosp & Nursing Home, **SLP**

Colang, Cheryl M 4210 Christy Way, Reno, NV 89509, (702) 747-6269, BA 71 Albertus Magnus Coll; MS 78 Univ of NV - Reno; Sp-Lang Path, Washoe Co Sch Dist, **SLP**

Cola-Schuh, Ann L 11 West Thrid Avenue, Columbus, OH 43228, (614) 291-9486, BS 83 Bowling Green St Univ; MA 85 MI St Univ; Aud, West Cen Ohio Hearing/Spch Ctr, **A**

Colberg, Mrs Carlota M 1889 Cracovia, Ext College Park, Rio Piedras, PR 00921, (809) 751-7737, BS 74 Chestnut Hill Coll; MS 76 Univ of PR - Rio Piedras; SLP, Private Practice, **SLP**

Colbert, Lisa Carol 603 Tyler Avenue, Oxford, MS 38655, (601) 234-1496, BS 80 Delta St Univ; OM 81 Univ of MS; Sp-Lang Path, N Mississippi Retardation Ctr, **SLP**

Colbert, Martha S 808 Sao Jorge Way, Sacramento, CA 95831, (916) 424-4886, BA 75 Univ of Northern CO; MA 77 Univ of TX - Austin; SLP, Rio Linda Union Sch Dist, **SLP**

Colburn, Dr Norma M 83 Sayre Drive, Princeton, NJ 08540, (201) 390-6611, BA 64 Rutgers St Univ -N Brunswick; MA 67 Columbia Univ Teachers Coll; PH 79 (Sp Development Disfluency) Columbia Univ Teachers Coll; Sp-Lang Path, Private Practice, **SLP ACE**

Colby, Mrs Eileen R 11325 West Willow Lane, Phoenix, AZ 85039, BA 77 CUNY - Lehman Coll; MS 79 Emerson Coll; 87–Sp-Lang Path, Peoria USD, **SLP**

Colby, Mrs Jane Campion 167 Knob Road, Chatham, MA 02633, (617) 896-5933, BS 51 Fordham Univ; MA 52 Northwestern Univ; Sp-Lang Path, Brewster Ma Bd of Ed, **SLP**

Colby, Janet Catherine 5757 South Troy, Chicago, IL 60629, (312) 947-3000, BA 80 Saint Xavier Coll; MA 84 Northern IL Univ - De Kalb; Aud, Chicago Osteopathic Med Ctr, **A ACE**

Colby, Susan L 1005 Crowley Road, Arlington, TX 76012-2812, **SLP**

Colby-Coveney, Mrs Marianne 12 Old Maple Avenue, Fulton, NY 13069, (315) 593-8608, BA 77 Boston Coll; MA 79 Univ of CT; Sp-Lang Path, Oswego County BOCES, **SLP**

Colcord, Mrs Donna Jo 22 Georgetown Drive, Bowling Green, OH 43402, (419) 321-2981, BS 74 Purdue Univ - West Lafayette; MS 76 Purdue Univ - West Lafayette; Sp/Lang Path, St Vincent Medical Cen, **SLP**

Colcord, Dr Roger D Bowling Green University, Communication Disorders, Bowling Green, OH 43403, (419) 372-7184, BS 74 Purdue Univ - West Lafayette; MS 76 Purdue Univ - West Lafayette; PH 84 (Sp-Lang Path) Northwestern Univ; 82–Assoc Prof, Bowling Green St U, **SLP**

Cole, Mrs Babette W 20 High Ridge Road, Plainview, NY 11803, (516) 938-5838, BS 81 Syracuse Univ; MA 83 NY Univ; Speech-Language Pathologist, The Herbert G Birch Early Ch C, **SLP**

Cole, Mrs Barbara Dolf 4024 Jacoby Creek Road, Bayside, CA 95524, (707) 822-3885, BA 57 Humboldt St Univ; MA 69 Humboldt St Univ; Retired, Arcata Elem Sch Dist, **SLP**

Cole, Mrs Barbara K 1719 Stonebridge Road, Alexandria, VA 22304, (703) 379-3535, BA 72 Univ of RI; MA 74 Catholic Univ of America; Sp-Lang Path, The Alexandria Hospital, **SLP**

Cole, Carole Stimac 1384 Rosemary Lane, Concord, CA 94518, (415) 685-0734, BS 82 Eastern MI Univ; MA 83 Eastern MI Univ; Sp-Lang Path, Private Practice, **SLP**

Cole, Mrs Catherine D 5312 Forest Heights Road, Huntington, WV 25705, **SLP**

Cole, Diane M 105 Cherokee, Lake Winnebago, MO 64034, (816) 537-7174, **A**

Cole, Donna Ann 32133 45th Place S W #F-8, Federal Way, WA 98023-3259, (206) 874-1186, BA 83 Univ of CO - Boulder; MS 87 Univ of WA; **SLP**

Cole, Mrs Donna I P O Box 2822, Joplin, MO 64803, (417) 782-2315, BS 65 Univ of MO - Columbia; MA 69 Univ of MO - Columbia; Superv Sp-Lang Path Dept, St Johns Reg Med Cen, **SLP**

Cole, Dorothy C 2622 Toddville Road, Charlotte, NC 28214, (704) 393-8474, BS 56 Univ of North TX; **SLP**

Cole, Dr Elizabeth B 1266 Pine Avenue West, Montreal, PQ, Canada H3G 1A8, (503) 235-6551, MA 73 Univ of KY; MA 79 Univ of Cincinnati; ED 80 (Spec Ed) Univ of Cincinnati; 80–Assoc Prof, McGill University, **A**

Cole, Emily M 523 Broad Street #D, Mount Airy, NC 27030, (919) 789-9046, BA 75 Univ of NC - Greensboro; ME 77 Univ of NC - Greensboro; 78–Sp-Lang Path, Mt Airy City Sch, **SLP**

Cole, Mrs Evelyn Brown 721 Walker Springs Road, Apartment M-3, Knoxville, TN 37923, (615) 453-4671, SLP, Fort Sanders Regional Med Ctr, **SLP**

Cole, Mrs Georgeanne P O Box 2160, Wise, VA 24293, (703) 328-6623, BS 74 Univ of VA - Charlottesville; ME 75 Univ of VA - Charlottesville; Sp-Lang Path, Norton City Schs, **SLP**

Cole, Mrs Irma J New Britain Cons School Dist, 27 Hillside Place, New Britain, CT 06050, (203) 827-2263, BA 58 OH Univ - Athens; MS 68 Central CT St Univ; Dist Coord/Sp-Lang-Hrng Srvcs, New Britain Consol School Dist, **SLP**

Cole, Janice Kuioka 2120B Tennessee Circle, Loring AFB, ME 04751, (207) 764-0134, BA 80 Univ of WA; MA 84 Univ of IA; Sp-Lang Path, Aroostook Mental Hlth Ctr, **SLP**

Cole, Mrs Jody L W 4777 N Hollywood Avenue, Whitefish Bay, WI 53211, (414) 332-9901, BS 76 Bradley Univ; MA 78 Ball St Univ; **A**

Cole, Mrs Julie Spangler RR 1 Box 18E, Moran, KS 66755, (316) 237-4347, BA 83 Fort Hays St Univ; MS 85 Fort Hays St Univ; 88–Sp-Lang Path, ANW Spec Educ Coop, **SLP**

Cole, Kimberlee 920 Winesap Drive, Beaver Creek, OH 45385, Dayton Hearing and Speech, **SLP**

Cole, Mrs Laura Stokes 1807 McArthur Drive, Philadelphia, MS 39350, (601) 324-4059, BS 81 Univ of GA; MS 82 MS Univ for Women; 88–Sp-Lang Path, Starkville PS, **SLP**

Cole, Mrs Libbie Sisto 5313 North Charles, Wichita, KS 67204, (316) 838-2490, BA 80 Wichita St Univ; MA 87 Wichita St Univ; Sp-Lang Path, Wichita PS Sys

Cole, Dr Lorraine T ASHA, 10801 Rockville Pike, Rockville, MD 20852, (301) 897-5700, BS 71 Northern IL Univ - De Kalb; MA 72 Northern IL Univ - De Kalb; PH 80 (Communicative Disorders) Northwestern Univ; Dir Minority Concerns, ASHA Natl Office, **SLP F**

Cole, Mrs Lynn Charlton P O Box 389, Primghar, IA 51245, (712) 722-4374, BA 81 Univ of Northern IA; MA 82 Univ of Northern IA; SLP, AEA #4, **SLP**

Cole, Madeleine Burch L Lyman Street, The Willows, Westborough, MA 01581, (508) 366-0970, BA 30 Syracuse Univ; ME 61 Boston Univ; **SLP LM**

Cole, Mary H 2408 Monarch Drive, Austin, TX 78748, BA 64 Carlow Coll; MS 66 Wichita St Univ; Special Education Specialist, Texas Education Agency, **SLP**

Cole, Mary Jo 121 Pine Ridge Drive, Newark, NY 14513, (315) 331-1700, BA 80 SUNY - Coll at Plattsburgh; MS 86 SUNY - Coll at Geneseo; Sp-Lang Path, Newark Dev Ctr, **SLP**

Cole, Pamela J 704 Tanglewood, Arlington, TX 76012, **SLP**

Cole, Pamela Sue 65 East Scott #10-A, Chicago, IL 60610-2357, (312) 943-6594, BA 82 MI St Univ; MA 84 Wayne St Univ; Sp-Lang Path, Rehabilitation Inst of Chicago, **SLP**

Cole, Patricia A 1110 Fidler Lane # 1006, Silver Spring, MD 20910, (202) 636-6990, BA 77 Tougaloo Coll; MS 79 Univ of MS; PH 86 (Sp-Lang Path) Howard Univ, 88–Asst Prof, Howard Univ, **SLP**

Cole, Dr Patricia R 1300 Guadalupe #108, Austin, TX 78701, (512) 477-7704, BS 63 Univ of TX - Austin; MA 66 Univ of TX - Austin; PH 76 (NS) Univ of TX - Austin; Consult, **SLP F**

Cole, Dr Richard M 2190 Golfview Drive #102, Troy, MI 48084, (313) 446-1908, BA 52 Univ of NH; MA 58 Northwestern Univ; PH 65 (NS) Northwestern Univ; 74–Dir of Orthodontic Res, U of Detroit Dent Sch

Cole, Dr Robert C Comm Handicapped Programs, 3401 Clairmont Drive #17, San Diego, CA 92117, (619) 272-9023, PH 72 (NS) Univ of Southern CA; SLP, San Diego Sch Dist, **SLP**

Cole, Roselyn R 7482 Meridian Hills Court, Apartment A, Indianapolis, IN 46260-5403, (219) 287-7245, BA 60 IN Univ - Bloomington; MA 67 Saint Mary's Coll; Principal, South Bend Community Sch Corp, **SLP**

Cole, Mrs Sarah 925 Forest Road, New Haven, CT 06515, (203) 787-8981, BA 49 Fisk Univ; MS 72 Southern CT St Univ; MA 80 Southern CT St Univ; 88–Fac, Southern Connecticut State Univ, **SLP**

Cole, Susan Jeanette 245 Hot Springs Road, Santa Barbara, CA 93108-2442, (805) 964-0529, BS 78 Univ of CA - Santa Barbara; MS 81 AZ St Univ; Sp-Lang Path Lecturer & Superv, University of California, **SLP**

Cole, Tanya Elizabeth 115 Ontario Street, Georgetown, ON, Canada L7G 3L2, (416) 243-4128, MA 83 SUNY - Center at Buffalo; **SLP**

Cole, Terrilynn 821 9th Avenue, Kingsburg, CA 93631-2309, (209) 897-2653, BA 81 CA St Univ - Fresno; MA 83 CA St Univ - Fresno; SLP, Kings Cxanyon USD, **SLP**

Cole-Crawford, Nancy 8749 Mud Creek Road, Indianapolis, IN 46256, (317) 924-3251, BS 73 Univ of MO - Columbia; MS 74 Southern IL Univ -Carbondale; Mgr/Dept-SLP & Aud, Crossroads Rehab Cen, **SLP**

Colegrove, Katherine A 6540 Seapearl Lane, Columbia, MD 21045, (301) 730-6577, BA 77 Bellarmine Coll; MS 85 Towson St Univ

Coleman, Mrs Ann Marie 511 Southeast 33rd Terrace, Cape Coral, FL 33904, (813) 334-8367, BS 75 Worcester St Coll; MS 86 Northeastern Univ; 88–Sp-Lang Path, Lee County Sch Bd, **SLP**

Coleman, Betty D 1817 River Shore Drive, Knoxville, TN 37914, (615) 974-4123, BA 64 Montclair St Coll; MA 66 CUNY - Hunter Coll; Assoc Coord & Cl Superv, Dept Aud & Sp Path U TN, **SLP ACE**

Coleman, Mrs Carole J 915 Neal, Navasota, TX 77868, (409) 825-3949, BS 61 Univ of TX - Austin; MA 66 Univ of TX - Austin; **SLP**

Coleman, Dr Colette L Dept Speech Path & Audiology, California State Univ, 6000 J Street, Sacramento, CA 95819, (916) 278-6601, BA 60 Univ of Denver; MA 62 Univ of Denver; PH 74 (NS) Univ of WA; Prof, CA St U-Sacramento, **SLP**

Coleman, Mrs Cynthia E North 10510 Russett Drive, Spokane, WA 99208, (509) 838-7258, BA 80 Gonzaga Univ; MS 82 Eastern WA Univ; 86–Sp-Lang Path, St Lukes Mem Hosp, **SLP**

Coleman, Cynthia Lynn 2391 Crestcliff Drive, Tucker, GA 30084, (404) 354-8555, BS 85 Univ of GA; ME 86 Univ of GA; **SLP**

Coleman, Deborah Z 17111 Carriage Dale Court, Spring, TX 77379, (713) 376-7251, BS 76 TX Christian Univ; MS 77 TX Christian Univ

Coleman, Mrs Diana Blachly 17 Nutmeg Lane, New Canaan, CT 06840, (203) 966-3940, BA 80 CA St Univ - Chico; Sp-Lang Path, CT Rehab & Nutrition Svcs, **SLP**

Coleman, Mrs Diane L 6220 Patagonia S E, Grand Rapids, MI 49506, BA 77 MI St Univ; MA 79 Central MI Univ; Sp-Lang Path, **SLP**

Coleman, Dr Gerry Watson 500 Wenwood Road #1323, Greenville, SC 29607, (803) 288-9506, BA 73 SC St Coll; MS 74 Univ of IL - Urbana; PH 81 (Sp and Hrng Science) Univ of IL - Urbana; 83–Sp-Lang Path, Greenville Co Sch Dist

Coleman, Mrs Heidi J 456 Irving Avenue, Dayton, OH 45409, (513) 268-6511, BS 76 Miami Univ - Oxford; MS 77 Miami Univ - Oxford; Sp-Lang Path, VA Med Cen, **SLP**

Coleman, Mrs Jeanne F 14813 West 91st Street, Shawnee Mission, KS 66215, (913) 888-8387, BA 63 Univ of NE - Lincoln; MS 83 Univ of KS; Special Needs Preschool, Olathe School District 233, **SLP**

Coleman, Jeanne Marie 3306 Mulberry Hill Lane, Houston, TX 77084, (713) 498-8110, BS 80 Purdue Univ - West Lafayette; MA 85 Univ of Houston - Univ Park; **SLP**

Coleman, Joanne P Box 554, Balsam Lake, WI 54810, **SLP**

Coleman, John R Otologic Medical Group, 2122 West 3rd, Los Angeles, CA 90057, (213) 483-9930, BA 75 CA St Univ - Fullerton; MA 79 CA St Univ - Fullerton; Aud, Otologic Medical Group, **A**

Coleman, Judy F Harmon 49 Fernwood, Texarkana, TX 75503-1651, (214) 794-0626, BS 75 Univ of AR - Fayetteville; MA 76 Memphis St Univ; Priv Pract, **A**

Coleman, Mrs Julia W 3607 Cloverfield Road, Harrisburg, PA 17109, (717) 545-1886, BS 80 2641; MS 81 Bloomsburg Univ of PA; Sp-Lang Path, Private Practice, **SLP ACE**

Coleman, Julie Marie 3203 York Lane, Cincinnati, OH 45215, (513) 229-6081, BA 85 Coll of Mount Saint Joseph; MS 86 Univ of Louisville; 87–Sp-Lang Path, St Elizabeth Med Ctr, **SLP**

Coleman, Mrs Kathy L 3111 South Dayton, Springfield, MO 65807, (417) 831-3814, BS 75; MA 76 Univ of AR - Fayetteville; 83–Sp-Lang Path, Springfield R-12 PS, **SLP**

Coleman, Mrs Linda G Sp-Path Serv Of Brevard Inc, P O Box 4002, Indialantic, FL 32903, (407) 724-6761, BA 68 Auburn Univ - Auburn; MS 76 Southern IL Univ-Edwardsvill; Pres, Sp Path Sers of Brevard, **SLP**

Coleman, Lynne 42897 Swan Lake Drive, Northville, MI 48167, (313) 246-6051, BA 76 MI St Univ; MA 77 MI St Univ; 88–Aud, Wyandotte Hosp & Med Ctr, **A**

Coleman, Lynne G 814 East Avenue, Tallmadge, OH 44278, (216) 672-2672, BS 72 OH St Univ; MA 77 Kent St Univ; Supervisor, Kent State University, **SLP**

Coleman, Mrs Marcella Bell 2139 Young Street S E #101, Washington, DC 20020, BS 68 Univ of the DC; OM 78 Trinity Coll; MS 85 Univ of the DC; 87–Sp-Lang Path, DC PS Sys, **SLP**

Coleman, Maryann 176 Plantation Court, East Amherst, NY 14051, (716) 694-4500, BA 74 SUNY - Center at Buffalo; MA 76 SUNY - Center at Buffalo; Dir Sp-Lang Path Dept, Degraff Mem Hosp, **SLP**

Coleman, Mattie B 77 Mistletoe Drive, Niles, OH 44446, (216) 652-5811, BA 73 Adrian Coll; MA 75 OH Univ - Athens; SLP, Fairhaven Schl, **SLP**

Coleman, Mrs Patricia A Route 1 Box 739, Hattiesburg, MS 39401, (601) 584-9303, BS 78 Univ Southern MS-Hattiesburg; MS 80 Univ Southern MS-Hattiesburg; SLP, Forrest County Schools, **SLP**

Coleman, Patricia A R R 1, Box 165, Lathrop, MO 64465, (816) 296-3310, BS 84 Central MO St Univ; MS 87 Central MO St Univ; **SLP**

Coleman, Patsy Pierce 1808 Bentwood Drive, Graham, NC 27253, (919) 966-5171, BA 81 Univ of NC - Greensboro; MS 82 Univ of NC - Chapel Hill; 87–Sp-Lang Path, UNC-Chapel Hill, **SLP**

Coleman, Dr Ralph O 2923 S E Tolman, Portland, OR 97202, (503) 225-8356, BS 54 OR St Univ; MS 60 Univ of OR; PH 63 (NS) Northwestern Univ; Assoc Prof, Or Hlth Sci U, **SLP A F**

Coleman, Dr Robert F Box 1980, 825 Fairfax Avenue, Norfolk, VA 23501, (804) 446-5923, BA 59 Georgetown Coll; MS 60 Vanderbilt Univ; PH 65 (Speech Science) Univ of MN - Minneap-St Paul; Dir Cen Commun Dis, Med Coll of Hampton Roads, **SLP F**

Coleman, Mrs Roseann Fasi 2233 Woodfield Circle, Waukesha, WI 53188, (414) 549-1659, BS 83 Marquette Univ; MS 84 Marquette Univ; 86–Sp-Lang Path, Rehabilitation Associates, **SLP**

Coleman, Mrs Susan E 3006 Paladin Terrace, Olney, MD 20832, (301) 460-0096, BA 82 SUNY - Center at Binghamton; MA 84 Univ of TN - Knoxville; 88–Aud, Bruce S Bloom MD FACS PA, **A**

Coleman, Dr Thalia J 713 Cherry Lane, Orangeburg, SC 29115, (803) 539-8075, BA 70 SC St Coll; MS 71 PA St Univ - Univ Park; PH 88 (Sp Path) 3812; 88–Assoc Prof, South Carolina St Coll, **SLP**

Coleman, Thomas D Bari Manor #52-B, Croton on Hudson, NY 10520, (914) 941-7700, BS 51 Boston Univ; MA 55 Boston Univ; Retired, Bd of Ed Ossining NY, **SLP**

Coleman, Trudy H 7710 Twisted Oaks Circle, Dallas, TX 75231, (214) 348-5440, BS 74 Southern Methodist Univ; MS 76 Southern Methodist Univ; MS 79 Univ of TX - Dallas; **A**

Coleman, Victoria Linder 316 Cambridge Street, Prattville, AL 36067, (904) 478-9195, 77; BA 80 Auburn Univ - Auburn; MS 81 Auburn Univ - Auburn; Sp/Lang Path, Rehab In of West Florida, **SLP**

Coleman, Yvette St Martin 1701 Ellerslie, La Place, LA 70068, (504) 652-1804, BS 83 LA St Univ - Baton Rouge; MA 86 LA St Univ - Baton Rouge; **SLP**

Colen, Robin D 12 Kirkfield Court, Rockville, MD 20850, (301) 279-4955, BS 62 Syracuse Univ; MA 67 Syracuse Univ; Sp-Lang Path, Montgomery County Pub Schools, **SLP**

Coles, Margaret R 8927 Ravenna Avenue N E, Seattle, WA 98115, (206) 583-8613, BA 75 Univ of CA - Santa Cruz; MA 80 Univ of MN - Minneap-St Paul; 88–Microcomputer Analyst, Perkins Coie, **SLP**

Coles, Pamela L W 5120 Silver Reef Drive, Fremont, CA 94538, (415) 770-0414, BA 76 San Diego St Univ; MA 79 San Diego St Univ; Aud, **A**

Coletta, Mrs Deborah J 96 Green Meadow Court, Pittsburgh, PA 15239, (412) 795-8416, BA 77 Duquesne Univ; MA 78 Central MI Univ; Sp-Lang Path, W Pa Sch for Blind Chldn, **SLP A**

Coley, Karen E 101 Margaret Lane, Suite C, Grass Valley, CA 95945, (916) 272-2247, BA 69 Stanford Univ; MA 74 CA St Univ - Long Beach; Aud, Aud Assoc Hrng Ser Cen, **A**

Coley, Mrs Sherrill Quinn 403 Bridle Lane, Birmingham, AL 35243, (205) 969-2590, BS 82 Univ Southern MS-Hattiesburg; MS 83 Univ Southern MS-Hattiesburg; Aud, Robert L Baldwin MD, **A**

Coley-Donohue, Mrs Lisa Katherine 11704 Primrose Drive, Vernon, BC, Canada V1B 2E9, (604) 542-3180, BA 81 Univ of ND; MS 83 Univ of ND; 87–Sp-Lang Path, Sch Dist #24, **SLP**

Colfelt, Mrs Gail S 642 Llewlyn Road, Berwyn, PA 19312, (215) 539-8550, BA 63 Dickinson Coll; ME 64 PA St Univ - Univ Park; SLP, Montgomery Co Inter Unit, **SLP**

Colflesh, Marie A 2180 New Rodgers Road #1912, Levittown, PA 19056, (215) 824-2730, BS 73 East TN St Univ; MA 75 East TN St Univ; Aud, Private Practice, **A**

Colgan, Mrs Ellen H 850 Thomas Road, Beaumont, TX 77706, (409) 892-4558, BS 77 Univ of WI - Madison; OM 79 Emory Univ; **SLP**

Colgan, Karen Koudal 37 Pamela Avenue, Groton, CT 06340, (203) 446-0750, BA 80 2588; MS 85 Northeastern Univ; SLP, **SLP**

Colgan, Linda T 547 Richard Place, Wyckoff, NJ 07481, (201) 891-6321, MS 80 William Paterson Coll; 88–Sp-Lang Path, Private Practice, **SLP**

Colick-Hapner, Edie R 317 Ronnie Drive, Buffalo Grove, IL 60089, (312) 634-9398, BS 80 Univ of MO - Columbia; MS 81 Fontbonne Coll; Sp-Lang Path, Northwest Sp Path Assoc, **SLP**

Collard, Mary E Cleveland Clinic Foundation, 9500 Euclid Avenue, Desk A-71, Cleveland, OH 44106, (216) 444-5370, BS 58 Marquette Univ; MA 75 Case Western Reserve Univ; 75–Aud, Cleveland Cl Found, **A ACE**

Collazo, Nilda 17 Iris Ct #31, Tinton Falls, NJ 07724, (617) 437-2492, BS 75; MS 77; Cl Instr/Superv, Northeastern Univ, **SLP**

Colle, Mrs Josephine Speech Pathology Services, P O Box 4377, Alexandria, LA 71301, (318) 443-0559, MS 66 LA St Univ - Baton Rouge; BS 64 MS Univ for Women; SLP Owner-Dir, Sp Path Serv, **SLP**

Colleran, Eileen Marie 1213 West 10th Place, Tempe, AZ 85281, (602) 968-3816, BS 81 AZ St Univ; MS 84 AZ St Univ; Aud/Hrng Consult, AZ Dept of Hlth, **A**

Colleran, Michael J Mountain Plains Audiology, 1909 Mt Rushmore Road, Rapid City, SD 57701, (605) 341-1288, BA 74 Univ of SD - Vermillion; MA 76 Univ of SD - Vermillion; Aud Co Owner Admin, Mnt Plains Audiology Assoc, **A**

Collett, Holly Marjorie Kingman Elementary District Four, 3033 McDonald, Kingman, AZ 86401, (602) 753-5678, MA 59 Univ of MN - Minneap-St Paul; 88–Sp-Lang Path, **SLP**

Colletta, Marsha A 195 Seabury Lane, Bolingbrook, IL 60439, **SLP**

Colletti, Laurel Jean 601 Allison Avenue S W #B, Roanoke, VA 24016-4518, (507) 288-1818, **SLP**

Colley, Mrs Carol A 7202 Pinetree Place, Tyler, TX 75703, (214) 597-1351, BA 79 Stephen F Austin St Univ; MS 80 Baylor Univ; Sp-Lang Path, MHMR, **SLP**

Collier, Mrs Alice L P O Box 546, Beaverton, OR 97075, (503) 591-4518, BS 53 Bowling Green St Univ; MS 55 Western NM Univ; 62–Sp-Lang Path, Beaverton Sch Dist #48, **SLP**

Collier, Mrs Cheryl W 2941 Coral Strip Parkway, Gulf Breeze, FL 32561, (904) 932-1853, BS 80 Univ of South AL; MS 82 Univ of South AL; Aud, **A**

Collier, Cynthia Janese 3847 Timberglen Apt#3322, Dallas, TX 75252, (214) 881-8100, BS 81 Univ Southern MS-Hattiesburg; MS 84 Univ Southern MS-Hattiesburg

Collier, Pamela Lesak 1811 Crescent Avenue, Fort Wayne, IN 46805, (219) 426-4025, BS 84 Northern IL Univ - De Kalb; MA 86 Wichita St Univ; **SLP**

Colligan, Mrs Helen Claire 334 Colfax Avenue, Clifton, NJ 07011, (201) 471-8436, BA 63 Montclair St Coll; MA 86 Montclair St Coll; 81–Sp-Lang Path, Paramus Bd of Educ

Colligan, Mrs Margaret Raby 8354 Datum Lane, Baldwinsville, NY 13027, (315) 341-5940, BS 85 Ithaca Coll; MS 86 Ithaca Coll

Colligan-Kovarik, Michelle K 607 Glen Crossing Road, Glen Carbon, IL 62034, (618) 288-9894, BS 85 Southern IL Univ-Edwardsvill; MS 86 Southern IL Univ-Edwardsvill; 87–Sp-Lang Path, Madison Co Assn for Retarded Citizens, **SLP**

Collignon, Margaret Melton 8124 Cloverland Drive, Nashville, TN 37211, (615) 297-9040, BS 73 Univ of TN - Knoxville; MS 74 Vanderbilt Univ; SLP Consult, Private Practice, **SLP ACE**

Colling, Mrs Maryellen D 1353 Eggert Road, Amherst, NY 14226, (716) 838-5938, **SLP**

Collings, James Everett 913 East Boise Avenue, Boise, ID 83706, (208) 343-2583, BA 75 Northern St Coll; MA 78 Univ of SD - Vermillion; Sp-Lang Path, Idaho Elks Rehabilitation Hosp, **SLP**

Collins, Alicia J 308 Riley Road, Niceville, FL 32578, (904) 678-8930, BA 86 Univ of FL; MS 88 Gallaudet Coll

Collins, Beth Salvin 256 Frederick Road, Havertown, PA 19083, (215) 446-1305, BA 78 Univ of PA; ME 83 Temple Univ

Collins, Dr Bill M P O Box 295, Kinston, NC 28501, (901) 644-9920, BS 61 Southeast MO St Univ; MA 67 Univ of MO - Columbia; PH 70 (NS) Univ of MO - Columbia; Ch of Lab Serv, The Neurodiagnostic Cen, **SLP**

Collins, Carol Diane 1822 Barker Cypress Road, #1423, Houston, TX 77084, (713) 466-4128, BS 84 Ball St Univ; MA 85 Ball St Univ; **SLP**

Collins, Carol L 8511 Pine Run Court, Ellicott City, MD 21043, (301) 730-4140, BS 74 Univ of MD - College Park; MS 76 Loyola Coll; Sp-Lang Path, Howard County Public Schools, **SLP**

Collins, Dr Carolyn S Memorial 300, Western Illinois University, Macomb, IL 61455, (309) 298-1507, BS 63 Western IL Univ; MA 67 Western IL Univ; PH 74 (NS) Univ of IL - Urbana; Assoc Prof, Western Ill U, **SLP**

Collins, Mrs Constance R 546 East Second Street, Bloomsburg, PA 17815, (717) 784-1251, MS 74 IN Univ - Bloomington; Sp-Lang Path, Inter Unt 16, **SLP**

Collins, David E 612 Petaluma Boulevard South, Petaluma, CA 94952, BA 59 San Francisco St Univ; MA 69 San Francisco St Univ; Sp-Lang Path, Private Practice, **SLP**

Collins, Mrs Deborah Taylor 2216 Old Niles Ferry Road, Maryville, TN 37801, (615) 983-6343, BA 83 Dickinson Coll; MA 85 Univ of TN - Knoxville; Sp-Lang Path, Sevier County Schs, **SLP**

Collins, Mrs Dorla Durr 2211 Landau Lane, Bossier City, LA 71111, (318) 949-2279, BA 75 LA St Univ - Shreveport; OM 83 LA St Univ - N O Medical Ctr; Sp/Lang Path, Bossier Parish Sch Bd, **SLP**

Collins, Elizabeth A 770 Ashley Lane, Orlando, FL 32825, (407) 423-9293, BS 75 Bowling Green St Univ; MA 80 Bowling Green St Univ; Sp-Lang Path, Orange Co Pub Sch, **SLP ACE**

Collins, Emilie S 220 North Highland, Sherman, TX 75090, (214) 868-2650, OB 79; BS 76 Stephen F Austin St Univ; MS 80 Univ of North TX; Aud-Owner, Private Practice, **A**

Collins, Mrs Georgia B 3225 Willowbrook Road, Oklahoma City, OK 73120, (405) 755-0887, BS 51 Univ of IL - Urbana; **SLP**

Collins, Jacqueline 15174 Cavour, Livonia, MI 48154, **SLP**

Collins, Janis K 400 36th Avenue, Seattle, WA 98122, (206) 329-3367, BA 69 Univ of WA; MA 71 Univ of WA; 75–Sp-Lang Path, Private Practice, **SLP**

Collins, Mrs Jean Tallyn 4120 Dijon Drive, Orlando, FL 32808, (407) 290-3107, BS 81 James Madison Univ; MS 82 Univ of SC - Columbia; 88–Sp-Lang Path, Florida Hosp, **SLP ACE**

Collins, Joan Pratt 1607 North Hale, Fullerton, CA 92631, BS 62 Univ of IL - Urbana; MA 68 San Jose St Univ; Sp-Lang Path, Montebello USD, **SLP**

Collins, Judith W 316 Locust, Boise, ID 83712, (208) 365-5971, BS 64 ID St Univ; ME 68 ID St Univ; SLP, Boise Sch Dist, **SLP**

Collins, Mrs Junelle M 5533 North Clinton, Fort Wayne, IN 46825-2216, (219) 425-7463, BA Paine Coll; MA Northwestern Univ; MA 77 CA St Coll - Bakersfield; Sp-Lang Path, Fort Wayne Community Schools, **SLP**

Collins, Kevin P Route 171, Woodstock Valley, CT 06282, **SLP**

Collins, Linda B 23 Oakwood, Athens, OH 45701, (614) 594-4235, BA 68 OH Univ - Athens; MA 76 OH Univ - Athens; Sp-Lang Path Superv, Seoh Sp Ed Reg Res Ctr, **SLP**

Collins, Linda G 1514 Hillridge, Ann Arbor, MI 48103, (313) 662-8306, BA 61 Univ of TX - El Paso; MA 67 Univ of CO - Boulder; SLP, St Joe Mercy Hosp, **SLP**

Collins, Linda Marie 1212 Rebecca Court, Oakdale, PA 15071, (412) 787-0967, BS 82 Edinboro Univ of PA; MA 88 Univ of Pittsburgh - Pittsburgh; 88–Sp-Lang Path, The Med Ctr of Beaver PA Inc

Collins, Loralyn Perry 143 Stoneridge Drive #B7, Columbia, SC 29210, (803) 256-1482, BA 84 Columbia Coll; OM 86 Univ of SC - Columbia; **SLP**

Collins, Lula Mae Twin Pines Nursing Home, 3301 Mockingbird, Victoria, TX 77901, (512) 573-6480, MA 55 Univ of Houston - Univ Park; BS 54 Univ of Houston - Univ Park; **SLP LM**

Collins, M Jane Communication Disorders, Music Dramatic Arts Bldg, Louisiana State Univ, Baton Rouge, LA 70803, (319) 353-3545, BA 61 Vanderbilt Univ; MS 63 Vanderbilt Univ; PH 70 (Hrng Science) Univ of IA; 85–Assoc Prof, LA State U, **A F**

Collins, Martha B Route 4 Box 391, Mount Pleasant, TX 75455, (214) 572-8553, BS 71 East TX St Univ - Commerce; MS 74 East TX St Univ - Commerce; 77–Dir of Instructional Svcs, Reg Viii Ed Serv Cen, **SLP**

Collins, Mary L 612 N E 154th Street, Vancouver, WA 98685, (206) 574-8808, BA 70 Univ of CO - Boulder; MA 71 Univ of Denver; 88–Sp-Lang Path, Portland Adventist Med Ctr, **SLP**

Collins, Dr Michael James Department Of Speech And Language Pathology, Dean Medical Center, 1313 Fish Hatchery Road, Madison, WI 53705, (608) 252 8349, BA 69; MA 72; PH 74 (Sp Path) Univ of CO - Boulder; 88–Dir Sp-Lang Path, Dean Med Ctr, **SLP**

Collins, Patricia J 504 Tideway Drive, Alameda, CA 94501, BS 60 Univ of OR; MS 72 Portland St Univ; 88–Publisher, Bristol Publishing Enterprises, **SLP**

Collins, Robert P 32 Ashton Court, Vallejo, CA 94591, (707) 643-7641, BA 72 San Jose St Univ; MA 74 San Jose St Univ; 77–Sp-Lang Path, Vallejo County USD, **SLP**

Collins, Mrs Sally A 2 Ferrous Court, Chester, NJ 07930, (201) 879-7828, BS 76 Trenton St Coll; MS 80 Rutger's St Univ - Douglas Coll; **SLP**

Collins, Sharon K 11442 Lippelman Road, Cincinnati, OH 45246, (513) 771-7655, BS 78 Miami Univ - Oxford; MS 79 Miami Univ - Oxford; Sp-Lang Path, Cincinnati Ctr for Imprv Comm, **SLP**

Collins, Shelley Kay 1315 26th Avenue North, St Petersburg, FL 33704, (813) 576-5471, **SLP**

Collins, Sherryl Jeannine 130 Second Street, Neenah, WI 54956, (414) 892-2661, MS 85 Univ of WI - Milwaukee; 87–Coord of Speech Pathology, Theda Clark Reg Med Ctr, **SLP**

Collins, Sonia G 2770 Springer Road #36, Galesburg, IL 61401, (309) 343-8131, BA 79 Augustana Coll; MA 80 Northeast MO St Univ; SLP Serv Superv, Galesburg Cottage Hosp, **SLP**

Collins, Mrs Susan H P O Box 1975, Cullowhee, NC 28723, (704) 586-2819, BS 78 Western Carolina Univ; MA 79 Western Carolina Univ; Sp-Lang Path, Jackson County PS, **SLP**

Collins, Teresa Kay 7030 Remington, Woodridge, IL 60517, BS 74 Ball St Univ; MA 85 Ball St Univ; 88–Sp-Lang Path, Sch Assn for Spec Educ DuPage Co, **SLP**

Collins, Virginia Betts Rural Delivery 1, P O Box 288 Christian Ridge, South Paris, ME 04281, (207) 743-8541, MS 83; SLP, Maine School District 17, **SLP**

Collins, Virginia Rose 3321 Zillah Street, Tallahassee, FL 32301, (904) 878-1826, **A**

Collins-Byrne, M 1410 N W 196th Street, Seattle, WA 98177, (206) 325-8500, BS 69 SUNY - Coll at New Paltz; MA 70 Univ of WA; OM 80 Univ of WA; Admin, Eye Clinic of Seattle, **SLP**

Collins-Lu, Catherine 11780 S W Terrace Linda, Beaverton, OR 97005, (503) 774-8871, BS 65 Washington Univ; MS 75 Portland St Univ; Tchr, Tucker-Maxon Oral Sch, **SLP**

Colliton, Kathleen Ann Apartment 54B Cherry Street, Milford, CT 06460, (203) 783-1638, BA 84 Univ of SD - Vermillion; MA 85 Bowling Green St Univ; 88–Sp-Lang Path, UCP Spec Needs Ctr, **SLP**

Collop, Kathy Marie 1311 Elm Street, Plymouth, MI 48170, (313) 459-5741, BS 78 Northeast MO St Univ; MA 79 Eastern MI Univ

Colman, Joan C B 6442 Riggs Place, Los Angeles, CA 90045, (213) 370-5705, BA 67 CA St Univ - Northridge; MA 76 Whittier Coll; SLP, Lacny Office of Ed, **SLP**

Colo, Denise Marie 24700 Lorain Road Suite 306, North Olmsted, OH 44070, (216) 779-0301, BA 81 Cleveland St Univ; MA 83 Cleveland St Univ; 87–Aud, Westside Hearing and Speech, **A**

Colodzin, Louise M 11829 Hunting Ridge Court, Potomac, MD 20854, (301) 762-2093, BS 59 George Washington Univ; MA 62 Univ of MD - College Park; OM 80 Loyola Coll; 73–Aud Coord, Montgomery Co Pub Sch, **A**

Colomaio, Robert James 4 West Washington Blvd, Apartment 2, Bath, NY 14810, (607) 776-7919, BS 85 SUNY - Coll at Fredonia; MS 86 SUNY - Coll at Fredonia; **SLP**

Colombo, Mrs Christine E Rural Delivery 1, 3 Belle Lane, Lee, NH 03857, (603) 659-2692, BA 82 Hofstra Univ; MS 84 Adelphi Univ; Sp/Lang Path, Dover Sch Dist, **SLP ACE**

Colombo, Joanne Marie Children's Hospital Of Wisconsin, 1700 West Wisconsin, Milwaukee, WI 53201, BA 73 MI St Univ; MA 80 Wayne St Univ; Aud, Children's Hosp of WI, **A**

Colombo, Patricia M 3336 Avalon Road, Shaker Heights, OH 44120, (216) 241-8230, BA 70 Loyola Univ of Chicago; MS 72 Univ of MI - Ann Arbor; Superv of Sp-Lang Path Serv, Cuyahoga Co Bd of Ment Ret, **SLP**

Colon, Joann Sposini 2449 Huckleberry Road, Lakehurst, NJ 08733, (201) 349-4442, BS 73 Trenton St Coll; MS 75 Trenton St Coll; Supervisor of Education, Ocean Day Training, **SLP**

Colon, Mrs Marieclaud Ganthier 119 Wendy Dr, Holtsville, NY 11742, (516) 758-4936, **SLP**

Colonna, Alexandria 420 Bronxville Road, Bronxville, NY 10708, (914) 337-7267, BA 78 Iona Coll; MS 79 Adelphi Univ; Audiologist, Private Practice, **A**

Colonno, Cynthia 2427 Dwight Avenue, Point Pleasant, NJ 08742, (201) 899-5661, BA Kean Coll of NJ; MA 86 Kean Coll of NJ; **SLP**

Colosimo, Mrs Ruth A G 18972 Ironwood Lane, Santa Ana, CA 92705, BA 75 Towson St Univ; MA 78 Temple Univ-Tyler Sch of Art; **SLP**

Colpoys, Brian P Broome Developmental Center, Glenwood Road, Binghamton, NY 13905, (607) 770-0211, BS 63 SUNY - Coll at Buffalo; MS 68 SUNY - Coll at Buffalo; Chief, Broome Dev Cen, **SLP**

Colson, Connie J 5113 S W 20th Terrace, Topeka, KS 66604, (913) 273-8363, BS 78 KS St Univ; MA 81 KS St Univ; Sp-Lang Path, Topeka USD 501, **SLP**

Colson, Karen A 906 Benton Drive #33, Iowa City, IA 52240, (319) 353-3859, BS 78 Middle TN St Univ; MA 79 Univ of TN - Knoxville; Graduate, U of IA, **SLP**

Coltharp, Loretta J Professional Audiology Service, 6057 Executive Centre Dr, Suite 3, Bartlett, TN 38134, (901) 372-0040, BS 79 Univ of TN - Knoxville; MA 81 Memphis St Univ; 83–Exec Dir, Prof Aud Serv, **A**

Coltharp, Mary Beth 19 North Front Street, Richmond, ME 04357, (207) 782-1680, BS 81 Clarion Univ of PA; MS 82 IN St Univ - Terre Haute; 85–Sp/Lang Path, Griffiths-Larrabee Inc, **SLP**

Colton, Mrs Carolyn Mensh 158 Salisbury Road, Brookline, MA 02146, (617) 325-8000, BA 59 George Washington Univ; ME 71 Boston Univ; Chief Audiologist, Hebrew Rehab Cen Aged, **A**

Colton, Kathleen Cook 2601 Zika Avenue N W, Cedar Rapids, IA 52405, (319) 399-6700, BA 82 Univ of Northern IA; MA 84 Univ of IA; 87–Sp-Lang Path, Grant Wood AEA, **SLP**

Colton, Dr Raymond H Department Of Otolaryngology & Communication Sciences, SUNY Health Science Center At Syracuse, 750 East Adams Street, Syracuse, NY 13210, (315) 473-5573, BS 63 Central CT St Univ; MA 66 Univ of CT; PH 69 (Communication Sciences) Univ of FL; Assoc Prof, St Univ of NY, **F**

Colton, Sophia S 9091 Lime Bay Boulevard, Tamarac, FL 33321, (305) 722-0675, BA 31 CUNY - Hunter Coll; MA 38 Columbia Univ Teachers Coll; **SLP LM**

Coltrane, Connie Jo 4178 Cass Apartment C, Omaha, NE 68131, (402) 556-7325, BA 77 Univ of Northern IA; MA 79 Univ of Northern IA; Sp-Lang Path, Boys Town Institute/Comm Dis, **SLP**

Colucci, Mrs Maryann M 132 Wilson Avenue, Long Beach, NY 11561, (516) 431-7176, BA 75 CUNY - Brooklyn Coll; MS 77 CUNY - Brooklyn Coll; Sp-Lang Path, City of Long Beach PS, **SLP**

Colussi, Jane Marie 3811 Fox Run Drive #1119, Cincinnati, OH 45236-1150, (513) 791-8467, BS 83 Ball St Univ; MA 84 Ball St Univ; Sp-Lang Path, Porter Co Spec Ed Coop, **SLP**

Colville, Mrs Mary B 200 Long Branch Road, Cullowhee, NC 28723, (704) 293-5651, BS 37 Western Carolina Univ; ME 51 Univ of NC - Chapel Hill; **SLP LM**

Colvin, Mrs Lyn M 1820 North Terry Street, Portland, OR 97217, (503) 285-3193, BS 74 Univ of OR; MS 75 Univ of OR; Sp-Lang Path, Portland Public Schools, **SLP**

Colwell, Andrea Thompson 4005 Golf Creek Drive, Champaign, IL 61821, (217) 351-3555, MA 86 Univ of IL - Urbana; 86–Sp-Lang Path, ABL Unit 6 Schs, **SLP**

Colwell, Teresa B P O Box 1168, Blairsville, GA 30512, **SLP**

Colwell, Mrs Wanda Ward 630 Central Avenue #G-13, Lexington, KY 40502, (606) 623-1380, BA 73 Univ of KY; MA 80 Eastern KY Univ; Sp-Lang Path, Richmond Independent Schools, **SLP**

Colyar, Terry C 7622 North 48th Drive, Glendale, AZ 85301, (602) 934-4186, BS 76 AZ St Univ; MS 77 ID St Univ; 79–Sp-Lang Path, Peoria USD, **SLP**

Coman, J Michael, II PO Box 749, Cascade, CO 80809, (219) 239-7735, BS 79 Southwest TX St Univ; ME 81 Southwest TX St Univ; Sp-Lang Path, **SLP**

Coman, Mary Judson 424 Fayette Park, Lexington, KY 40508, (606) 255-0953, MS 88 Univ of KY

Combs, Barbara Sue Route 2 Box 283, Hazard, KY 41701, (606) 785-3153, BA 81 Univ of KY; MS 83 Univ of KY; Sp-Lang Path, Knott County Board of Educ, **SLP**

Combs, Deadra Havens 3739 Lima Drive, Indianapolis, IN 46227, (317) 736-8495, BS 77 IN Univ - Bloomington; MA 78 IN Univ - Bloomington; Sp-Lang Path, Johnson Co Spec Serv, **SLP**

Combs, Mrs Deborah Jean Rural Delivery 6, Old River Road, Norwich, CT 06360, (203) 572-0541, BA 76 SUNY - Coll at Geneseo; MS 77 Ithaca Coll; Sp-Lang Path, Seaside Regional Center

Combs, Diana Sue 1606 Bunker Hill, Pueblo, CO 81001, (303) 564-4800, BS 78 UT St Univ; MS 81 UT St Univ; Aud, J Valentine Cichon MD PC, **A**

Combs, Mrs Jami Baker Mid Cities Speech & Hearing Clinic, 1701 West Euless Boulevard Suite 210, Euless, TX 76040, (817) 283-3191, BS 83 OK St Univ; MA 85 OK St Univ; Sp-Lang Path, Mid Cities Sp & Hearing Clin, **SLP**

Combs, Mrs Judith A 4911 Millsprings Court, Arlington, TX 76017, (817) 465-8700, BS 73 Univ of TX - Austin; MS 74 Univ of North TX; Sp-Lang Path, Arlington ISD, **SLP**

Combs, Margaret R 1600 Smithville Road, Havre, MT 59501, (406) 357-2269, 74 San Francisco St Univ; MA 77 San Francisco St Univ; 88–Sp-Lang Path/Supvr, Bear Paw Spec Educ Cooperative, **SLP**

Combs, Mary Elizabeth 8235 Lakeshore Trail East, #134, Indianapolis, IN 46250, (317) 577-8134, MS 87 Purdue Univ - West Lafayette; Sp-Lang Path, InSpeech Inc, **SLP**

Combs, Raymond B 4911 Millsprings Court, Arlington, TX 76017, (214) 372-7013, BS 73 Univ of North TX; MS 75 Univ of North TX; Aud, VA Med Cen Dallas, **A**

Combs-Denavs, Debra K 1845 D Street, Lincoln, NE 68508, (402) 477-9940, BS 75 Univ of NE - Lincoln; MA 78 Univ of NE - Lincoln; Aud, US Hearing Centers, **A**

Comeau, Betty Lynn Speech & Hearing Department, Sunmount Dev Center, Tupper Lake, NY 12986, (315) 262-2323, BA 76 SUNY - Coll at Plattsburgh; MA 83 SUNY - Coll at Plattsburgh; Sp/Lang Path, St Lawrence Co BOCES, **SLP**

Comer, Carmen Melinda 6724 #6 East 91st Street S, Tulsa, OK 74133, BS 86 TX Christian Univ; OM 87 Univ of Central AR; **SLP**

Comer, Cynthia J 3967 Albany Street, Schenectady, NY 12304, (518) 438-8785, BA 81 Allegheny Coll; MA 83 Montclair St Coll; Sp-Lang Path, Easter Seal Soc, **SLP**

Comer, Mrs Elaine K 2019 Pine Street, Philadelphia, PA 19103, (215) 221-3661, BA 59 Univ of PA; MA 73 Temple Univ-Tyler Sch of Art; Aud, Temple Univ Med Sch, **A**

Comer, Mrs Judith W 126 Holly Court, Prattville, AL 36067-4904, (205) 365-5709, MS 71 Auburn Univ - Auburn; **SLP ACE**

Comer, Pamela J 3202 18th Street N W, Washington, DC 20010, (301) 654-5264, BS 70 Bowling Green St Univ; MA 73 Bowling Green St Univ; Spec Ed Tchr, Montgy Co Pub Sch, **SLP**

Comer, Mrs Patricia Fabiola 29922 Rainbow Crest Drive, Agoura Hills, CA 91301, (818) 706-1215, BA 82 CA St Univ - Northridge; MA 84 CA St Univ - Northridge; Sp-Lang Path, Los Angeles USD, **SLP**

Comer, Sally D 129 West Park Drive, Raleigh, NC 27605, (919) 832-7285, **SLP**

Comer, Sherry L 8400-65 Olde Colony Trail, Knoxville, TN 37923, (615) 971-1349, BS 76 James Madison Univ; MS 80 James Madison Univ; 88–Sp-Lang Path, Ft Sanders Reg Med Ctr, **SLP**

Comerchero, Sherry R 1264 E Granada Street, Mesa, AZ 85203, (602) 827-1838, BA 74 SUNY - Coll at New Paltz; MS 76 SUNY - Coll at Buffalo; Sp/Lang Path, Camelback Comm Center, **SLP**

Comerford, Michael A 1148 Moreland Place S E, Atlanta, GA 30316-1834, (404) 952-3222, BS 77 Northwestern Univ; MS 81 Emory Univ; Aud, Cobb ENT Assoc Pc, **A**

Comfort, Mrs Carolyn 5 Rue DE Sontay 75116, Paris, France, BA 71 Smith Coll; MA 76 George Washington Univ; Sp-Lang Path, Marymount Sch, **SLP**

Comin, Mrs Amy Cyphers 207 Darlington Road, Beaver Falls, PA 15010, (412) 846-3725, BA 85 Geneva Coll; MS 86 WV Univ; 88–Sp-Lang Path, Easter Seal Society of Beaver Co, **SLP**

Comiter, Mrs Marilyn T 9540 S W 6th Court, Pembroke Pines, FL 33025, (305) 432-6631, BA 77 Univ of FL; MA 78 Univ of Miami; Sp-Lang Path, Dade Co Pub Sch, **SLP**

Comkowycz, Sharon M 134 Audubon Road, Winter Haven, FL 33884, (813) 534-2833, BA 75 Southern CT St Univ; MS 77 Southern CT St Univ; Prog Supvr Sp-Lang, Polk Co Sch, **SLP**

Commers, Barbara Elaine 37 Boyinton Road, Clear Lake, MN 55319, BS 73 Saint Cloud St Univ; MS 79 Saint Cloud St Univ; MS 79 Saint Cloud St Univ; SLP, Dodds-Ger-Ed Res Cen, **SLP**

Commodore, Robert W 9901 81st Street, Fort Saskatchewan, AB, Canada T8L 3K6, (403) 478-0522, BA 74 Univ of Alberta - Alberta; MS 77 Univ of AL-Tuscaloosa; SLP, Edmonton Pub Sch, **SLP**

Commons, Susan D 9320 Parkwest Boulevard, Suite 100, Knoxville, TN 37923, (615) 690-7531, BA 74 Univ of MD - College Park; MA 77 Univ of TN - Knoxville; 80–Sp-Lang Path, Susan D Commons Ma Ccc Sp, **SLP**

Compagnone, Angela R 73 Congress Street, Milford, MA 01757, (508) 473-9131, BS 80 Boston Univ; MS 81 Univ of MI - Ann Arbor; 82–Sp-Lang Path, Bellingham Pub Sch Syst, **SLP**

Compton, Dr Arthur J Institute Of Child Language & Phonology, 450 Mission Street, Suite 504, San Francisco, CA 94105, (415) 777-2334, BS 58 OH St Univ; MA 61 OH St Univ; PH 65 (NS) OH St Univ; Dir, I of Lang & Phonology

Compton, Carol A Donald Reed Speech Center, c/o Phelps Memorial Hosp, North Tarrytown, NY 10591, (914) 631-6711, BS SUNY - Coll at Geneseo; MA Bowling Green St Univ; Dir, Donald R Reed Sp Cen, **SLP**

Compton, Cynthia L Audiology Department, Gallaudet University, 7th & Florida Avenue N E, Washington, DC 20002, (202) 651-5328, BA 73 Rutger's St Univ - Douglas Coll; MS 74 Vanderbilt Univ; Dir-Assistive Devices Ctr, Gallaudet Univ, **A**

Compton, Gayle Renee Route 10 Box 451, Morganton, NC 28655, (704) 433-2794, MS 84 Univ of NC - Chapel Hill; Sp/Lang Path, Western Carolina Center, **SLP**

Compton, Mrs Gladys B Aud Services & Hearing Aids Inc, 1050 East Southern Avenue Suite F1, Tempe, AZ 85282, BS 70 AZ St Univ; MS 73 AZ St Univ; Pres, Aud Serv & Hrng Aids Inc, **A**

Compton, Judith G 4027 Old Federal Hill Road, Jarrettsville, MD 21084, (301) 357-4313, **SLP**

Compton, Kathy S 300 Polk, Charleston, IL 61920, (217) 345-4287, MS 88 Eastern IL Univ

Compton, Mary V 5117-B Lawndale Drive, Greensboro, NC 27405, BA 67 Greensboro Coll; ME 68 Univ of NC - Greensboro; OM 75 Smith Coll; Asst Prof, Univ of Nc-Greensboro, **SLP ACE**

Compton, Roger Lee Audiology Clinic, P O Box 369, 845 North Limestone Street, Gaffney, SC 29342, (803) 487-7207, BS 68 East TN St Univ; MA 71 Univ of TN - Knoxville; Owner, Aud Cl, **A**

Comroe, Mrs Judith S 6348 Rhea, Reseda, CA 91335, (818) 997-2357, BA 66 Univ of CA - Los Angeles; MA 74 CA St Univ - Northridge; SLP, Los Angeles USD, **SLP**

Comstock, Cathryn Lynn West Texas Rehab Center, 3001 Jackson, San Angelo, TX 76904, (915) 949-9535, BS 78 TX Tech Univ; MA 83 Univ of TX - Austin; Chief Aud Sers, W Tx Rehab Cen, **A**

Comstock, Mrs Diane Reichert 3639 Salem Walk #A-1, Northbrook, IL 60062, BS 81 Marquette Univ; MS 82 Marquette Univ; SLP, InSpeech Inc, **SLP ACE**

Comstock, Judith K 1660 Cedarwood #241, Westlake, OH 44145, (216) 871-3672, BA 85 OH St Univ; MA 87 Cleveland St Univ; **SLP**

Comstock-Reid, Ann K 1800 Hatcher, Ann Arbor, MI 48103, (313) 936-8070, BS 78 Western MI Univ; MS 82 CO St Univ; Sp-Lang Path, Univ of MI Hosp, **SLP**

Conae, Francine D 3436 West Paul, Fresno, CA 93711, BA 70 Univ of Denver; MA 71 CA St Univ - Los Angeles; Sp-Lang Path, Fresno USD, **SLP**

Conahan, Helen P 7 Woodland Drive, Coatesville, PA 19320, (215) 383-3862, BS 74 West Chester Univ of PA; MA 78 West Chester Univ of PA; Sp-Lang Path, Chester County Interme Unit 24, **SLP**

Conan, Mrs Eileen T 2915 Cottonwood #11, Orange, CA 92665, (714) 637-8532, BA 68 Loyola Marymount Univ; MA 74 CA St Univ - Fullerton; SLP, Fullerton USD, **SLP**

Conant, Janet Lynn 9941 Brier Lane, Santa Ana, CA 92705, (714) 639-4990, BA 78 Humboldt St Univ; MS 85 CA St Univ - Sacramento; **A**

Conaway, Jo Adele 259 Walhalla, Columbia Station, OH 43202, (614) 225-5070, BA 66 OH Univ - Athens; MA 85 OH St Univ; **SLP**

Conaway, Karen B 115 Walker Road, Kelso, WA 98626, (503) 556-3722, BS 77 Univ of OR; MS 78 Univ of OR; Sp-Lang Path, Columbia Co 13 Sch Dist, **SLP**

Conaway, Patrick Kelly 655 West Erving Park Road, Apartment 5115, Chicago, IL 60613, (312) 935-9538, MA 86 San Jose St Univ; 88–Aud, Mount Sinai Hosp Med Ctr, **A**

Conboy, Elizabeth A 1313 Gilpin Avenue #4, Wilmington, DE 19806, (302) 651-6054, BS 79 West Chester St Coll; MS 87 Indiana Univ of PA; **SLP**

Conboy, Mrs Joan Carver 727 Meadowcreek Court, Garland, TX 75043, (214) 494-8382, BS 81 East TX St Univ - Commerce; MS 83 East TX St Univ - Commerce; Sp-Lang Path, Garland ISD

Conca, Mrs Cindy R 33-33 149 Place, Flushing, NY 11354, (718) 353-5698, BA 84 CUNY - Queens Coll; MA 87 CUNY - Hunter Coll; Sp-Lang Path, First Step Early Childhood Ctr, **SLP**

Concannon, Julia Ann 101 Casey Street, Norwood, MA 02062, (617) 242-2565, BS 82 Univ of ME - Farmington; MS 84 Northeastern Univ; Sp-Lang Path, Boston Pub Schs, **SLP**

Conde, Rebecca Hart 1509 22nd Street, Galveston, TX 77550, (409) 763-3462, BS 76 Lamar Univ; MS 79 Lamar Univ; Sp-Lang Path, Galveston Independent Sch Dist, **SLP**

Conder, Eileen 730 DE Witt Street, Linden, NJ 07036, (212) 929-1551, MA 88 CUNY - Hunter Coll

Condevaux-Dahlberg, Annie 1055 Seascape Court, Rodeo, CA 94572, (707) 425-6775, BS 77 CA St Univ - Hayward; MA 79 CA St Univ - Sacramento; Sp-Lang Path, Fairfield-Suisun USD, **SLP**

Condie, Ronda K W 2570 East 10000 South, Sandy, UT 84092, (801) 943-2332, BS 75 UT St Univ; MS 77 UT St Univ; Aud, **A**

Condit, Linda Christine 1310 2nd Street, Manhattan Beach, CA 90266, (805) 964-8076, MA 87 Univ of CA - Santa Barbara; 87–Sp-Lang Path, Rancho Los Amigos Med Ctr

Condoluci, Mrs Patricia W 124 Avon Terrace, Moorestown, NJ 08057, BS 72 Nazareth Coll of Rochester; MA 76 West Chester Univ of PA; Sp-Lang Path, Private Practice, **SLP**

Condon, Karen S Callier Center, 1966 Inwood Road, Dallas, TX 75235, (214) 783-3046, BS 77 Southern Methodist Univ; MS 78 Southern Methodist Univ; Audiologist, Callier Center, **SLP A**

Condon, Marilyn T Murray State University, Dept Of Spec Education, Murray, KY 42071, (502) 762-2446, BS 66 Ithaca Coll; MS 68 Univ of WI - Madison; ED 78 (NS) Univ of AL- Tuscaloosa; Assoc Prof, Murray St U, **A**

Condon, Mrs Mary Z 437 Brookwood Drive, Downingtown, PA 19335-1646, (215) 328-5287, BA 75 Marywood Coll; MA 80 Temple Univ; Sp/Lang Path, Private Practice, **SLP**

Condon, Mrs Shelley J 218 East Kavaney Drive, Bismarck, ND 58501, (701) 224-1346, BS 84 Minot St Univ; MS 85 Minot St Univ; Sp-Lang Path, Bismarck Spec Svcs, **SLP**

Condrin, Mrs Susan Loen 2421 Edgeview Lane, Midlothian, VA 23113, (804) 379-9672, BA 80 Univ of MD - College Park; MA 82 Ball St Univ; Sp-Lang Path, Fairfax County Pub School Sys, **SLP**

Condron, Mrs Ellen W 6012 West 90th Terrace, Shawnee Mission, KS 66207, (913) 642-6200, BS 75 Univ of MO - Columbia; MA 76 Univ of MO - Columbia; Sp-Lang Path, Shawnee Mission Kansas Sch Dis, **SLP**

Condry, Mrs Sherrill R P O Box 1413, Burney, CA 96013, (916) 335-4139, BA 72 Augustana Coll; MA 73 Northwestern Univ; **SLP ACE**

Cone, Charlene Pease 3525 Singapore Circle N E, Albuquerque, NM 87111, MS 86 Southern IL Univ-Edwardsvill; **SLP**

Cone, Martha A 810 Parkcenter Drive #54, Santa Ana, CA 92705, (714) 547-0640, BA 70 CA St Univ - Fullerton; MA 72 CA St Univ - Fullerton; Sp-Lang Path, St Jude Hosp and Rehab Ctr, **SLP**

Cone, Sarah W 1130 Salisbury Drive, Cincinnati, OH 45226, (513) 321-4874, BA 79 Miami Univ - Oxford; MA 80 Bowling Green St Univ; **SLP**

Conetta, Elizabeth Hannaberry 53 Chester Court, Peekskill, NY 10566, (914) 739-1933, BA 74 Iona Coll; MA 86 CUNY - Lehman Coll; 87–Sp-Lang Path, Putnam Valley Cent Sch Dist, **SLP**

Cone-Wesson, Dr Barbara K 7122 Knowlton Place, Los Angeles, CA 90045, (213) 226-5073, BA 73 Univ of CA - Santa Barbara; MA 75 Univ of CA - Santa Barbara; PH 79 (Communication Disorders) Univ of TX - Dallas; Asst Prof/Chief of Aud, USC Med Ctr, **A**

Congdon, Christina Margaret 1306 A Blue Lake Way, Bowling Green, KY 42101, (502) 782-7960, BA 80 Univ of KY; BS 80 Univ of KY; MS 82 Murray St Univ; Sp-Lang Path, InSpeech Inc, **SLP**

Conger, Mrs Jane J Route 5, Fayetteville, TN 37334, (615) 577-8664, BS 74 Univ of GA; MS 78 Univ of GA; Sp-Lang Path, Maryville City Sch, **SLP**

Conger, Sharon J 42 Hoerle Boulevard, Torrington, CT 06790, (203) 379-0852, BS 68 WV Univ; MS 71 Northwestern Univ; Sp-Lang Path, Winchester Pub Sch, **SLP**

Conkey, Dr Harlan D 2255 N E 194th Avenue, Portland, OR 97230, (503) 754-2461, ED 64 (NS) Univ of Tulsa; **SLP A**

Conklin, Caroline 2032 32nd Street South, Great Falls, MT 59405, (406) 791-2270, BA 57 Radcliffe Coll; MA 71 Univ of MT; SLP, Sch Dist #1, **SLP**

Conklin, Gloria Jean 32 Parkway Manor, 100 Parkway Blvd, Kingston, PA 18704, (717) 826-3766, BS 85 SUNY - Coll at Geneseo; MS 86 Bloomsburg Univ of PA; 86–Sp-Lang Path, John Heinz Inst of Rehab Med, **SLP**

Conklin, Jane S 11 Brookview Avenue, Delmar, NY 12054, (518) 439-3529, BS 70 PA St Univ - Univ Park; ME 74 Bloomsburg Univ of PA; **SLP**

Conklin, John M 21 Wadsworth Street, Geneseo, NY 14454, MS 75 SUNY - Coll at Geneseo; Sp-Lang Path, Rochester Inst of Tech, **SLP**

Conlan, Maureen T 171 Aldershot Lane, Manhasset, NY 11030, (516) 365-8344, BA 79 Saint John's Univ - Jamaica; MA 81 Hofstra Univ; 85–Sp-Lang Path, Maryhaven Ctr of Hope, **SLP**

Conley, Deangela Box 955, Chapmanville, WV 25508, (304) 529-0598, MA 86 Marshall Univ; **SLP**

Conley, Kathleen 1044 East 35th Place, Tulsa, OK 74105, (918) 749-6018, BS 75 OK St Univ; MA 76 OK St Univ; 88–Sp-Lang Path, New Medico Head Injury Sys, **SLP**

Conley, Kathleen Scherbick 100 Fifth Avenue Bldg Suite 1208, Pittsburgh, PA 15222, (412) 471-4352, BS 80 WV Univ; MS 81 WV Univ; 86–Pres, Maico Hrng Serv of Pgh, **A**

Conley, Lynne J 277 Suffolk Street, #3-R, Holyoke, MA 01040, (413) 538-9906, BA 83 Univ of WI - Green Bay; MA 88 Univ of MA - Amherst; 88–Sp-Lang Path, Communication Therapy Inc

Conley, Mrs Mary Jane Giovengo 1391 Old Meadow Road, Pittsburgh, PA 15241, (412) 221-6270, BA 71 CA Univ of PA; MA 73 Coll of Saint Rose; 87–Sp-Lang Path, Pittsburgh Mt Oliver IU, **SLP A**

Conley, Patricia Tautfest 7255 East McKinley, Scottsdale, AZ 85257, (602) 946-2552, **SLP**

Conley, Paul W 920 Carolyn Avenue, Modesto, CA 95350, (209) 575-1771, MA 72 CA St Univ - Fresno; 72–Dir, Manor Investment Co Inc

Conlin, Leah T Simon Fraser Health Unit, 80A 6th Street, New Westminster, BC, Canada V3L 5B3, (604) 660-8819, BA 79 LA St Univ - Baton Rouge; OM 80 LA St Univ - N O Medical Ctr; Aud, Bc Ministry of Hlth, **A**

Conlon, Dr Sara E 430 M Street SW #N505, Washington, DC 20024, (202) 732-1157, BA 47 Univ of MD - College Park; MA 50 Univ of IA; PH 65 (Sp Path) Univ of FL; 84–Education Program Specialist, US Department of Education, **SLP F**

Conlon-Johnson, Mrs Ann 1601-B Chaffee Court, Patexent River, MD 20670, (301) 862-9792, BS 81 Towson St Univ; MS 82 FL St Univ; **SLP**

Conn, Mrs Julie W G 42112 Cherry Hill, Novi, MI 48050, (313) 684-8278, BS 75 Western MI Univ; MA 77 Eastern MI Univ; Sp-Lang Path, Huron Valley Schools, **SLP**

Connard, Sheryl Johanson P O Box 164, Wycombe, PA 18980, (215) 598-3183, BS 78 Univ of GA; ME 80 Univ of VA - Charlottesville; Aud, Private Practice, **A**

Connare, Lynn Puliafico 182 Anderson Place, Buffalo, NY 14222-1804, (716) 898-3212, BA 76 SUNY - Coll at Buffalo; MS 85 SUNY - Coll at Buffalo; **SLP**

Connaughton, Kathryn Bernice 8798 North State Road, St Louis, MI 48880, (517) 875-5101, BA 76 Central MI Univ; MA 77 Central MI Univ; SLP, Gratiot-Isabella ISD, **SLP**

Connell, Mrs OARY S 20 Rodline Road, Danbury, CT 06811, (203) 746-3486, BA 77 SUNY - Coll at Potsdam; MA 78 Ithaca Coll; Sp-Lang Path, Danbury School System, **SLP**

Connell, Jane S 2828 Green Street, San Francisco, CA 94123, MD; **LM**

Connell, Kathleen Patricia 4230 Morris Road, Hatboro, PA 19040, (215) 674-3035, BA 84 Univ of Pittsburgh - Pittsburgh; MA 86 Temple Univ; 88–Sp-Lang Path, Montgomery Co Intermediate Unit, **SLP**

Connell, Nancy J 4605 Arnica, Missoula, MT 59803, (406) 549-0352, BA 74 Univ of CA - Santa Barbara; MA 76 Univ of MT; **SLP A**

Connell, Phil J 376 South Leslie Lane, Wheeling, IL 60090, (312) 492-5073, BA 72 Univ of ME - Orono; MA 73 Univ of ME - Orono; PH 76 (Sp-Lang Path & Aud) Univ of KS; Northwestern Univ, **SLP**

Connell, Mrs Sharon Marie 3304 Vanquil Trail, Dayton, OH 45449, (513) 436-2843, BS 84 Miami Univ - Oxford; MS 85 Miami Univ - Oxford; Sp-Lang Path, Franklin City Schools, **SLP**

Connell, Sheila M 1055 West Baseline #1071, Mesa, AZ 85210, (602) 898-7871, BS 76 Northwest MO St Univ; MS 81 AZ St Univ; Aud, Mesa Public Schools, **A**

Connelly, Mrs Corliss Ann 7509 South Pitkin Court, Aurora, CO 80016, (303) 699-8539, BA 76 Marygove Coll; MS 77 Univ of MI - Ann Arbor; 88–Sp-Lang Path, Havern Center, **SLP**

Connelly, Diane Schwarz 9545 South Trumbull, Evergreen Park, IL 60642, (312) 636-9796, BA 77 Valparaiso Univ; MA 78 Western MI Univ; Sp-Lang Path, SW Cook Co Coop Assn Spec Ed, **SLP**

Connelly, Mrs Elva A P O Box 3812, Estes Park, CO 80517, (303) 586-9451, BS 65 Univ of Houston - Univ Park; MA 66 Univ of Houston - Univ Park; Retired, Houston ISD, **SLP**

Connelly, Gail J 321 Eugenie Street, Chicago, IL 60614, (312) 787-0820, BA 71 Ripon Coll; MS 73 Univ of IL - Urbana; Tchr/English-Study Skills, The Latin School of Chi, **SLP**

Connelly, Sr Helen L DE Paul Institute, Castlegate Avenue, Pittsburgh, PA 15226, (412) 561-4848, BS 46; ME 54 Univ of Pittsburgh - Pittsburgh; Tchr, De Paul I, **LM**

Connelly, Jane Elizabeth 430 Wildwood Avenue, White Bear Lake, MN 55110, (612) 426-7658, BS 80 Moorhead St Univ; MA 85 Univ of MN - Minneap-St Paul; 84–Aud, St Paul PS, **A**

Connelly, Dr Patricia E 33 Garden Street, Ramsey, NJ 07446, (201) 934-6048, BA 74 Rutger's St Univ - Douglas Coll; MA 76 Wayne St Univ - Sch of Med; PH 83 (NS) MI St Univ; Aud, Private Practice, **A**

Connelly, Robert J Audiometric Inc, 2500 West Higgins Road, Suite 580, Hoffman Estates, IL 60195, (312) 519-0666, BA 60 De Paul Univ; MA 63 Northern IL Univ - De Kalb; 73–Aud, Audiometrics Inc, **A**

Conner, Cathy I Callier Ctr For Comm Disorders, 1966 Inwood, Dallas, TX 75235, (214) 905-3134, BS 79 Stephen F Austin St Univ; MS 81 Univ of TX - Dallas; Sp-Lang Path, Callier Cen for Commun Dis, **SLP**

Conner, Mrs Deborah Boyd 6410 Banockburn Lane, Rural Hall, NC 27045, BA 79 Univ of NC - Greensboro; MS 81 East Carolina Univ; Sp/Lang Path, Western Rockingham Cty Schools, **SLP**

Conner, Dennis E 10547 Copperfield Drive, St Louis, MO 63123, (314) 865-3333, BS 70 CO St Univ; MA 74 Western IL Univ; Dir Sp & Hrng Dept, Alexian Brothers Hosp, **A**

Conner, Eleanor Sophia 1127 Seminole East #27-D, Jupiter, FL 33477, (305) 744-4826, BS 84 James Madison Univ; MS 86 James Madison Univ

Conner, Mrs Janis Nunnally 6238 Cricket Lane, Columbus, GA 31909, (404) 324-6112, BA 75 Univ of NC - Greensboro; ME 77 Univ of NC - Greensboro; 87–Sp-Lang Path, Columbus Sp & Lang Ctr, **SLP**

Conner, Mrs Joanne Kathleen 5523 Mavis Avenue, Whittier, CA 90601, (818) 445-3102, BA 81 CA St Univ - Los Angeles; MA 84 CA St Univ - Los Angeles; 88–Sp-Lang Path, Culhane Briggs & Assoc, **SLP**

Conner, Mrs Kelly E 3025 East Boulevard #7, Bethlehem, PA 18017, (215) 866-3697, BA 82 KS St Univ; MA 84 KS St Univ; 88–Sp-Lang Path, Carbon lehigh IU, **SLP**

Conner, Mrs Patricia Ann 7123 Willow Brook Way, Columbia, MD 21046, (301) 381-9181, BS 77 Purdue Univ - West Lafayette; MS 83 Towson St Univ; 80–Sp-Lang Path, Baltimore City Schs, **SLP**

Conner, Peggy S c/o W B Conner, 28 Dapp Lane, Mechanicsburg, PA 17055, (717) 766-9244, BS 78 Ithaca Coll; MS 81 Univ of WI - Madison; Sp-Lang Path, Internationl Cen for Disabled, **SLP**

Conner, Dr Thomas N 7031 Flint Hill Road, Owings Mills, MD 20736, (301) 224-5482, BS 70 Towson St Univ; MS 72 Towson St Univ; ED 85 (Special Education) George Washington Univ; Sp-Lang Path, Anne Arundel Co Pub Sch, **SLP**

Conners, Mrs Cindy L 47 Pleasant Acres Community, Hammond Lane, Plattsburgh, NY 12901, (518) 562-0412, BS 80 SUNY - Coll at Plattsburgh; MS 85 SUNY - Coll at Plattsburgh; 88–Sp-Lang Path/Instr, SUNY-Coll at Plattsburgh, **SLP**

Conners, D Elizabeth 4002-D Linkwood Road, Baltimore, MD 21210, BS 75 Boston Univ; MA 77 Case Western Reserve Univ; Sp-Lang Path, **SLP**

Conners, Marjory A 50 Lakeland Drive #F-8, Atlanta, GA 30305, (404) 426-3328, BS 73 Univ of GA; ME 74 Univ of GA; 80–Prog Coord, Cobb Co Pub Sch, **SLP**

Connery, Ellen Gallagher 25 Saltaire Avenue, Narragansett, RI 02882, (401) 792-9682, BA 80 Univ of RI; MS 82 Univ of RI; Sp-Lang Path, South Kingstown Sch Dept, **SLP**

Connery, Patricia K 10428 Michael Todd Terrace, Glenview, IL 60025, **A**

Connett, Mrs Nancy R 14 Dos Rios, Greeley, CO 80634, (303) 330-8939, BS 71 Southern IL Univ -Carbondale; MS 73 Univ of OK Medical Center; SLP, New Life Center, **SLP**

Connolly, Mrs Loretta DeCrou 37 Bull Run, Holden, MA 01520, (508) 829-9817, BS 76 Bowling Green St Univ; MA 78 Kent St Univ; Sp-Lang Path, Darso Inc, **SLP**

Connolly, Mary Ann S 1505 Eagles Landing, Rehoboth Beach, DE 19971, (302) 645-4505, BS 80 PA St Univ - Univ Park; MA 87 Temple Univ; Sp-Lang Path, Paul E Howard MD, **A**

Connolly, Susan B 182 East 95th Street, #14-G, New York, NY 10128, (718) 390-9470, MA 87 NY Univ; **SLP**

Connor, Adrienne G 7209 Maple Avenue, Chevy Chase, MD 20815, (301) 657-4374, MA 87 George Washington Univ

Connor, Catherine John P O Box 817, Cheshire, CT 06410, (203) 628-0331, BA 68 MI St Univ; MA 69 MI St Univ; Sp-Lang Path, Southington Board of Education, **SLP**

Connor, Jacqueline 65 Essex Street #1, Beverly, MA 01915, **A**

Connor, Karla Kae 5-8 Woodlake Road, Albany, NY 12203, (518) 452-0797, BA 84 Coll of Wooster; MS 85 Univ of NC - Chapel Hill; Sp-Lang Path, Easter Seal Soc, **SLP**

Connor, Mrs Kathleen S 464 South Nectar Avenue, Absecon, NJ 08201, (609) 645-3550, BS 69 Indiana Univ of PA; MA 81 Trenton St Coll; Sp-Lang Path, Egg Harbor Twsp Bd Ed, **SLP**

Connor, Lisa Rae 659 Avant Lane North, Memphis, TN 38105, (901) 529-0233, BS 85 Oakwood Coll; MS 87 AL A & M Univ

Connor, Mrs Margaret M 511 Broadacres, Penn Valley, PA 19072, (215) 668-1850, BS 63 LA Tech Univ; ME 66 Univ of VA - Charlottesville; Aud, Head & Neck Assoc of SE PA, **A**

Connor, Nadine P University Of Wisconsin, Waisman Center, 1500 Highland Avenue, Madison, WI 53705-2280, (608) 263-5726, BA 79 Univ of MD - College Park; MA 82 Univ of MD - College Park; 86–Proj Asst, Speech & Motor Control Labs, **SLP**

Connors, Elizabeth C Dept Of Communicative Disorder, University Of Rhode Island, Kingston, RI 02881, (401) 792-4741, BS 79 Northern MI Univ; MA 81 Northern MI Univ; 86–Clin Coord, Univ of Rhode Island, **SLP**

Connors, Janet Marie 7051 S W 111th Place, Miami, FL 33173, (305) 649-2811, BS 79 Univ of WI - Madison; MS 81 Univ of WI - Madison; Sp-Lang Path, Dade Co Pub Sch, **SLP**

Connors, Mrs Ronnie Marolf 321 Edward J, Clinton, MI 49236, (313) 994-8111, BS 71 SUNY - Center at Albany; MS 72 Syracuse Univ; 84–Sp-Lang Path, Washtenaw ISD-High Point Ctr, **SLP**

Connors, William A Allegheny Speech & Hearing Ctr, 9104 Babcock Boulevard, Suite 5109, Pittsburgh, PA 15237, (412) 367-1402, BA 71 Univ of Pittsburgh - Pittsburgh; MA 75 Univ of Pittsburgh - Pittsburgh; Admin, Allegheny Sp&Hrng Cen, **SLP**

Connors Miller, Mrs M Chris 602 Western Avenue, Joliet, IL 60435, (815) 723-2156, BS 77 IL St Univ - Normal; MS 78 IL St Univ - Normal; Sp/Lang Path, Lockport Area Sp Ed Coop, **SLP**

Conolly, Mrs Elizabeth A Srsic 1910 Woodlyn Drive, Apartment 202, Fredericksburg, VA 22401, (703) 373-9353, BA 85 Mary Washington Coll; ME 87 Univ of VA - Charlottesville; 88–Sp-Lang Path, Orange Co PS, **SLP**

Conover, Elizabeth 9 Ridge Hill Road, Norwell, MA 02061, (617) 878-0213, BS 57 East TN St Univ; BS 57 East TN St Univ; Sp-Lang Path, W Bridgewater PS, **SLP A**

Conover, Helen B Speech And Hearing, Lindley Hall, Ohio University, Athens, OH 45701, (614) 593-1417, BA 56 Grinnell Coll; MA 71 OH Univ - Athens; Cl Coord, Ohio University, **SLP**

Conover, Kathleen D 1465 Hayes Street, San Francisco, CA 94117-1425, (415) 469-0448, BS 74 Univ of OR; MS 75 Portland St Univ; 85–Sp-Lang Path, San Francisco USD, **SLP**

Conrad, Mrs Barbara Jean 120 Roshon Drive, Medina, OH 44256, (216) 948-2500, BA 80 Univ of Akron; MA 85 Univ of Akron; Sp-Lang Path, Cloverleaf Loc Sch, **SLP**

Conrad, Mrs Beverly Lazaroff 10212 Pumphrey Court, Fairfax, VA 22032, (202) 784-3690, BA 75 Univ of RI; MA 77 Univ of TN - Knoxville; 87–Sp-Lang Path, Georgetown Univ Hosp, **SLP**

Conrad, Brenda K 7574 Ohaver Drive, Loomis, CA 95650, (916) 652-5106, MA 87 Univ of the Pacific

Conrad, Dr Carolyn Thera Office Of Academic Affairs, University Park, IL 60466, (312) 534-5000, BA 63 Roosevelt Univ; MA 75 Governors St Univ; PH 85 (NS) Northwestern Univ; 88–Assoc VP-Acad Aff, Governors State U, **SLP**

Conrad, Christie A 1705 Pinetree Drive, Pittsburgh, PA 15241, (412) 831-6362, BA 73 Allegheny Coll; MA 75 CA Univ of PA; 81–Director/President, Crossroads Sp & Hrng, Inc, **SLP**

Conrad, Mrs Diane F Rt 3 Box 169 Downey Drive, Lancaster, SC 29720, (803) 286-1492, BS 70 Southern IL Univ -Carbondale; MS 71 Southern IL Univ -Carbondale; 87–Sp-Lang Path, Rebound Inc, **SLP**

Conrad, Mrs Faith F 9 Arlington Avenue, Beverly, MA 01915, (508) 468-2312, BA 52 Univ of MA - Amherst; MA 66 Emerson Coll; 63–Sp/Lang Path, Hamilton-Wenham Sch Dist, **SLP**

Conrad, G Beth 220 Park Avenue, Southport, NC 28461, (919) 457-9588, BS 70 OH Univ - Athens; ME 77 GA St Univ; SLP, Dosher Mem Hosp, **SLP**

Conrad, Mrs Janet Bohling 220 Penhurst Way, Roswell, GA 30076, (404) 475-2097, BS 68 Southeast MO St Univ; MA 69 Univ of IL - Urbana; **SLP**

Conrad, Marybeth S 6217 Amber Mist Lane, Charlotte, NC 28211, (704) 364-9085, BS 81 East Carolina Univ; MS 83 East Carolina Univ; **A**

Conrad, Susan J 10786 Missouri Avenue #7, Los Angeles, CA 90025, (213) 474-5251, BA 84 American Univ; MA 87 George Washington Univ; 87–Aud, Otolgic Med Group Inc, **A**

Conradt, Mark Nicolet Clinic, 411 Lincoln Street, Neenah, WI 54956, (414) 727-4327, BS 84 Univ of WI - Oshkosh; MS 85 Univ of WI - Oshkosh; Audiologist, Nicolet Clinic, **A**

Conran, Mrs Kathleen S 734 Lombard Road, Addison, IL 60101, (312) 543-7633, BA 78 Elmhurst Coll; MS 79 IL St Univ - Normal; **SLP**

Conrick-Gaborek, Maryann 475 Lyman, Des Plaines, IL 60016, (312) 681-3000, BS 81 Northern IL Univ - De Kalb; MA 84 Northern IL Univ - De Kalb; 87–Aud, Westlake Comm Hosp, **A**

Conrod, Mrs Jo Ann Bisignano 5 Village Street, Bristol, CT 06010, (203) 582-7643, BA 78 Elms Coll; MS 83 Southern CT St Univ; Sp-Lang Path, Simsbury Pub Sch Syst, **SLP**

Conroy, Barbara B 1646 Temple Terrace, North Fort Myers, FL 33903, **SLP**

Conroy, Mrs Sally Joan 1611 Windy View Drive #8, Garden City, KS 67846, (316) 276-4428, BA 85 Univ of WI - Eau Claire; MS 87 Univ of WI - Eau Claire; 87–Sp-Lang Path, USD #457, **SLP**

Conroy-Peckham, Kay Marie 1309 North Wisconsin Avenue, Apartment 2, Rice Lake, WI 54868, (715) 234-2170, BA 78 Univ of WI - Eau Claire; OM 83 Univ of WI - River Falls; **SLP**

Conry, Christine Patricia 226 Eureka Street, San Francisco, CA 94114, (413) 456-9680, BA 74 Emmanuel Coll; MS 82 San Francisco St Univ; SLP, Kentfield Medical Hospital, **SLP**

Considine, Kathleen A 222 Twin Oaks Road #31, Akron, OH 44313, (216) 379-8264, BA 76 Univ of Akron; MA 78 OH Univ - Athens; 80–Sp-Lang Path, Chldn Hosp Med Cen-Akron, **SLP**

Consolini, Mrs Mary Therese Valdosta Speech And Hearing Clinic, Valdosta State College, Valdosta, GA 31698, (912) 333-5931, BS 83 Univ Southern MS-Hattiesburg; MS 84 Univ Southern MS-Hattiesburg; Audiologist, Valdosta State College, **A**

Constable, Anne Parnell 4050 Kelly Drive, Durham, NC 27707, (919) 684-3859, **SLP**

Constable, Catherine M 8/1 Woods Brook Terrace, Ossining, NY 10562-1327, (914) 967-1740, ME 76 Bloomsburg Univ of PA; 84–Sp-Lang Path, Private Practice, **SLP**

Constable, Constance 1209 Charlotte Street, Pekin, IL 61554, (309) 346-1186, BS 73 IL St Univ - Normal; MS 75 IL St Univ - Normal; Sp/Lang Path, Tazwell-Mason Co-Sped Assn, **SLP**

Constad, Mrs Ann B 845 Sherwood Road, Bridgewater, NJ 08807, (201) 526-2445, BA 76 Rutger's St Univ - Douglas Coll; MA 77 Montclair St Coll; 88–Sp-Lang Path, Private Practice, **SLP**

Constance, Eugene J, Jr 976 Bear Tavern Road, Trenton, NJ 08628, (609) 393-8228, BA 70 Trenton St Coll; MA 72 Trenton St Coll; Director/Speech & Hearing Ctr, Trenton State College, **SLP ACE**

Constance, Jane R1 116CE The Cedars, Augusta, KS 67010, (316) 775-1181, BA 74 Univ of WI - Whitewater; MS 77 Wichita St Univ; 88–Sp-Lang Path/Consult, Private Practice, **SLP**

Constantino, Mrs Kimberli Rumburg 700 Albermarle, Bluefield, WV 24701, (304) 325-2228, BA 73 Marshall Univ; MA 74 Western MI Univ; Dept Dir, Bluefield Comm Hosp, **SLP**

Constantz, Mrs Grace A 2704 Grandview Place, Endicott, NY 13760, (607) 785-8636, BS 75 Elmira Coll; MS 77 Emerson Coll; Sp-Lang Path, Broome-Tiroga BOCES, **SLP**

Constanza, Mrs Kathleen M 343 Western Boulevard, Bayville, NJ 08721, (201) 321-7063, **SLP**

Constanzo, Cindy A 14030 Tree Crossing, San Antonio, TX 78247, (512) 340-3814, BS 79 Southwest TX St Univ; MA 80 Southwest TX St Univ; Sp-Lang Path, Nuernberg Ed Resource Cen, **SLP**

Conston, Marcia E 751 Righters Mill Road, Penn Valley, PA 19072, (215) 667-6298, BA 77 MI St Univ; MA 78 MI St Univ; **SLP**

Contastin, Francoise M 1738 Jeanne Circle, Martinez, CA 94553, (415) 372-7984, BA 77 Univ of San Francisco; MA 81 CA St Univ - Chico; Sp-Lang Path, Private Practice, **SLP**

Conte, Beverly M 137 Sumner Street, Quincy, MA 02169, (617) 821-5070, BS 72 Emerson Coll; MS 74 Emerson Coll; ME 77 Northeastern Univ; Sp-Lang Path, Canton Pub Sch, **SLP**

Conte, Rosemarie 111 Sherwood Avenue, Yonkers, NY 10704, (914) 937-5426, MS 88 CUNY - Hunter Coll

Contento, Kathryn Ann 1616 Ohm Avenue, Bronx, NY 10465, 21-251-6352, BS 84 Saint John's Univ - Jamaica; MS 86 Adelphi Univ; **SLP**

Conter, Joanne Born Physicians Hearing Clinic, Pinebrook Regional Medical Center, 14540 Cortez Boulevard Suite 100, Brooksville, FL 34613, (904) 596-7208, BS 81 Western Carolina Univ; MS 85 Univ of South FL; 85–Aud, Physicians' Hearing Clinic, **A**

Conti, Donna Marie 1009 Oakland Avenue, Akron, OH 44310, (216) 836-3734, BA 84 Univ of Akron; MA 86 Univ of Akron; 86–Sp-Lang Path, Our Lady of the Elms Spec Educ Sch, **SLP**

Conti, Mrs Judith R 40 Harris Mountain Road, Amherst, MA 01002, (413) 253-2001, OB 76 Univ of KY; MS 78 Univ of KY; ED 86 (Psycholinguistics) Univ of MA - Amherst; 88–Sp-Lang Path, Hampshire Educ Collaborative, **SLP**

Contieri-Pease, Mrs Carol F 230 28th Street, Hermosa Beach, CA 90254, (213) 857-2518, BS 78 SUNY - Coll at Brockport; MS 81 Boston Univ; Aud, Kaiser Permanente, **A**

Contino, Karen Carmela 244 Betsy Ross Drive, Orangeburg, NY 10962, (914) 358-5700, BA 80 Dominican Coll of Blauvelt; MS 86 William Paterson Coll; 80–Sp-Lang Path, Nyack PS, **SLP**

Conti-Ramsden, Dr Gina Maria 17 Suffolk Road, Wellesley, MA 02181, (617) 237-2195, MS 81 Univ of Dallas; OM 78 Univ of Cambridge - England; PH 82 (NS) Univ of Dallas; University Lecturer, University of Manchester, **SLP**

Conture, Dr Edward G Department Communication Sciences & Disorders, 805 South Crouse Avenue, Syracuse, NY 13244-2280, (315) 443-9660, BS 67 Emerson Coll; MA 68 Northwestern Univ; PH 72 (NS) Univ of IA; Professor, Syracuse Univ, **SLP**

Conture, Mrs Shelley Smith 400 Scott Avenue, Syracuse, NY 13224, (315) 487-1178, BA 64 Swarthmore Coll; MA 68 Emerson Coll; Sp/Lang Path, Onondaga-Mad BOCES, **SLP**

Converse, Marilyn V 501 Post, San Francisco, CA 94102, (415) 346-4096, BA 62 East TX St Univ - Commerce; OM 77 Pittsburg St Univ; MA 66 Baylor Univ; SLP, Self Employed, **SLP**

Conway, Mrs Eileen Lyons 306 Brighton Avenue, Hawthore, NY 10532, (914) 769-1322, BA 83 SUNY - Coll at Cortland; MS 84 Univ of NC - Chapel Hill; **SLP**

Conway, Elizabeth Law 2368 North 64th Street, Wauwatosa, WI 53213, (414) 258-5091, BS 85 Marquette Univ; MS 87 Univ of WI - Madison

Conway, Mrs Jane Parker 4771 Hillsboro Circle, Santa Rosa, CA 95405, BA 73 Univ of the Pacific; MA 74 Univ of the Pacific; **SLP**

Conway, Joan Marie 57 Troy Drive, Springfield, NJ 07081, (201) 273-6658, MA 54 Columbia Univ Teachers Coll; MA 71 Coll of Saint Rose; MA 73 Fairleigh Dickinson U-Madisn; SLP, Summit Board of Education

Conway, Kathleen M 1061 West Oakland Park Boulevard, Fort Lauderdale, FL 33311, (305) 565-8374, BS 80 Stockton St Coll; MS 86 Nova Univ; 88–Sp-Lang Path, Private Practice, **SLP**

Conway, Mrs Kathleen R P O Box 49, Boones Mill, VA 24065, (703) 334-1210, BA 78 Univ of FL; MS 80 Univ of South FL; SLP, Sp & Com Ctr, **SLP**

Conway, Loretta A 2859 College Drive, Allentown, PA 18104, (215) 437-2918, BA 72 Creighton Univ; MS 79 Bloomsburg Univ of PA; Dir-Sp-Lang Servs, Er SI So-Lebanon Co, **SLP ACE**

Conway, Marjorie J 135 Crocker Neck Road, Cotuit, MA 02635, **SLP**

Conway, Mary Patricia 82 Pilgrim Road, Springfield, MA 01118, (413) 782-3930, BA 75 Boston Coll; MS 84 Worcester St Coll; 75–Sp-Lang Path, Springfield Sch Dept, **SLP**

Conway, Mrs Nancy A 3702 Holden Circle, Los Alamitos, CA 90720-2216, (213) 430-1734, BA 72 CA St Univ - Long Beach; MA 78 CA St Univ - Long Beach; **SLP**

Conway, Nancy Ann 3266 North 53rd, Milwaukee, WI 53216-3245, (414) 445-9376, **SLP**

Conway, Peggy Ann 3660 North Lake Shore, Drive Apartment 601, Chicago, IL 60613, (312) 883-2154, **SLP**

Conway, Mrs Rosemary Morse 11 Mary Agnes Road, Framingham, MA 01701, (617) 877-9028, BA 77 Univ of RI; MS 80 Boston Univ; Sp-Lang Path, Framingham Sp & Lang Clinic, **SLP**

Conway, Mrs Valerie Hilliard Box 6053, APO New York, NY 09179-5420, (0638) 522536, BS 80 West Chester Univ of PA; OM 82 Hahnemann Univ Grad Sch; 87–Sp-Lang Path, DOD, **SLP**

Conyers, Mrs Annette Wilson 1040 Security Road, Hagerstown, MD 21740, (301) 791-4000, BA 77 SC St Coll; MA 78 SC St Coll; **SLP**

Conyers, Olivia Wallace 655 Lafayette Avenue, Hawthorne, NJ 07506-1664, BS 84 Northeastern Univ; MA Kent St Univ; **A**

Coody, Mrs Kaylin M 11529 South Mingo, Bixby, OK 74008, (918) 369-3633, BA 77 Univ of OK - Norman; MA 79 Univ of Tulsa; Sp-Lang Path, Private Practice, **SLP**

Cook, Ann G 12417 Bailey Bridge Road, Midlothian, VA 23113, (804) 786-0431, **A**

Cook, Anne Mary 14422 NE 10th Place, Bellevue, WA 98007, (206) 764-2404, BS 83 Univ of WA; MA 86 Univ of MT; Aud, Seattle VA Med Ctr, **A**

Cook, Annette Lajean 2620 North Belt, St Joseph, MO 64506, (816) 232-4327, OB 82 Central MO St Univ; MS 83 Central MO St Univ; Aud, Ashland Hearing Serv, **A**

Cook, Mrs Barbara G 2502 Jerusalem Road, Joppa, MD 21085, (913) 776-3322, BA 67 Wichita St Univ; MA 68 Wichita St Univ; Sp/Lang Path, Private Practice, **SLP**

Cook, Barbara L 209 Roswell #4, Long Beach, CA 90803, (213) 439-3966, MA 87 Temple Univ; **SLP**

Cook, Barbara S Speech Pathology (126), VA Hospital, Hines, IL 60141, (312) 343-7200, BS 77 Purdue Univ - West Lafayette; MS 79 Purdue Univ - West Lafayette; 83–Sp-Lang Path, Hines VA Hosp, **SLP ACE**

Cook, Mrs Brenda L Route 2 Box 415, Chateaugay, NY 12920, (518) 497-6230, BA 83 SUNY - Coll at Plattsburgh; MA 84 SUNY - Coll at Plattsburgh; **A**

Cook, Carolee B 4607 Bulova Street, Torrance, CA 90503, (213) 371-2706, OB 63 OH Univ - Athens; MS 65 PA St Univ - Univ Park; **SLP**

Cook, Catherine 614 West Adams, Greenwood, MS 38930, (601) 453-4231, BS 76 MS Univ for Women; MS 77 MS Univ for Women; Assistant Director of Spec Ed, Greenwood Municipal Sep Sch Di, **SLP**

Cook, Mrs Christine A 532 Kathryn Court, Merced, CA 95340, (209) 722-2840, BA 75 CA St Univ - Stanislaus; MA 79 CA St Univ - Stanislaus; Sp-Lang Path, Merced City Schs, **SLP**

Cook, Connie S 5236 Tendilla Avenue, Woodland Hills, CA 91364, (818) 993-9311, MA 85 CA St Univ - Northridge; Sp-Lang Path, Sfv Child Guidance Clinic, **SLP**

Cook, Dr Darrell R 2253 Maplewood Road, Cleveland, OH 44118-2815, (216) 932-3443, OM 81 Case Western Reserve Univ; MS 65 Univ of UT; PH 72 (NS) Case Western Reserve Univ; Coord Soc Serv, Cleveland Hrng & Sp Cen, **SLP**

Cook, Deborah C 424 Main Street, Wilbraham, MA 01095, **SLP**

Cook, Deborah Knowles 700 South 4th #412, Waco, TX 76706, BS 85 Baylor Univ; MS 86 Baylor Univ; **SLP**

Cook, Dewanda 11169 Luther Avenue South, Seattle, WA 98178, (206) 721-5877

Cook, Donna Walker 708 Clifton Road, Pittsburgh, PA 15102, (412) 281-7244, BS 80 WV Univ; MS 81 WV Univ; Sp-Lang Path, Er Sl So-Allegheny Co, **SLP**

Cook, Mrs Elaine Harris Star Route#1, Box 43A, Fleischmanns, NY 12430, (914) 586-2651, BA 66 Univ of GA; ME 67 Univ of GA; Sp-Lang Path, Broome Dev Svcs, **SLP**

Cook, Mrs Elizabeth Batson 1521 Longcreek Drive #1224, Columbia, SC 29210, (803) 772-2965, BS 85 Univ of South AL; MS 87 Univ of South AL; 88–Sp-Lang Path, Lexington County Sch Dist 1, **SLP**

Cook, Gayle W 6244 Westover Drive, Fort Worth, TX 76107, (817) 732-6730, BS 57 TX Tech Univ; ME 70 TX Christian Univ; Sp-Lang Path, Fort Worth ISD, **SLP**

Cook, George R, Jr Health & Hygiene Inc, 4605 E Dundas Dr, Greensboro, NC 27407, (919) 854-2303, BS 65 VA Commonwealth Univ; ME 70 Univ of VA - Charlottesville; 84–VP, Health & Hygiene Inc, **A**

Cook, Harriet Sacks 66 Amherst Road, Newton, MA 02168, **SLP**

Cook, Irita Diane 4049 Lakeland Hills Drive, Douglasville, GA 30134, (404) 832-3568, OB 71 West GA Coll; ME 85 GA St Univ; **SLP**

Cook, Jeannie Marie 500 110th Avenue North, Apt #1008, St Petersburg, FL 33716, (813) 398-0123, MS 83 Univ of South FL; 88–Sp-Lang Path, Rahab Works of Florida, **SLP**

Cook, Jill Ann 29 Eldorado Street, Toms River, NJ 08757, (201) 370-1150, BS 83 Kean Coll of NJ; MA 84 Kean Coll of NJ; **SLP**

Cook, Juanita W Rd 1 Box 411, Sunset Hill, Pownal, VT 05261, (802) 442-5502, BA 59 SUNY - Center at Buffalo; MS 67 Univ of VT; SLP, Private Practice, **SLP**

Cook, Mrs Julie Alderman Georgia Baptist Medical Center, 300 Boulevard NE, Atlanta, GA 30312, (404) 653-4700, BA 83 Univ of TN - Knoxville; MA 85 Memphis St Univ; Sp-Lang Path, GA Baptist Med Ctr, **SLP**

Cook, Mrs Katherine 221 East Seminary, Wheaton, IL 60187, (312) 858-8981, BA 66 Mundelein Coll; MS 67 Univ of WI - Madison; Dir, Commun Dis Cen, **SLP**

Cook, Mrs Katherine D Route 1 Box 462, Vinita, OK 74301, (918) 256-5529, BS 74 OK St Univ; MA 75 OK St Univ; Dir, Spec Serv, Craig Co Ed Coop Vinita Lea, **SLP**

Cook, Mrs Kathryn H 126 Aztec, Los Alamos, NM 87544, (505) 672-9380, BS 64 CO St Univ; MA 80 Adams St Coll; Sp-Lang Path, Los Alamos PS, **SLP**

Cook, Mrs Kathy Elaine 256 Deerfield Lane, Martinez, GA 30907, (404) 860-6969, BS 79 Purdue Univ - West Lafayette; MA 84 CA St Univ - Long Beach; 85–Aud, VA Hosp, **A**

Cook, Leslie Ann 540 West 41st Street, Shadyside, OH 43947, (304) 243-3275, BS 81 WV Univ; MS 83 WV Univ; Sp-Lang Path, Wheeling Hosp Med Pk, **SLP**

Cook, Mrs Linda G 2559 N W 31st Street, Boca Raton, FL 33434, (305) 482-2026, BS 73 SUNY - Coll at Buffalo; MS 76 SUNY - Center at Albany; Sp-Lang Path, Private Practice, **SLP**

Cook, Linden S Box 1402, Humboldt, SK, Canada S0K 2A0, (306) 682-5765, BA 76 Univ of Saskatchewan - Sask; MS 83 Univ of OR; 87–Sp-Lang Path, Region V Central Shared Svcs, **SLP**

Cook, Lois B Speech & Comm Professionals, 344 Main Street, Suite 408, Mount Kisco, NY, (914) 245-0211, BS 56 Syracuse Univ; MS 57 Columbia Univ Teachers Coll; Sp-Lang Path, Speech & Comm Prof, **SLP ACE**

Cook, Lynn E 6623 Greenvale Parkway, Riverdale, MD 20737, (301) 295-1202, BS 77 Univ of VA - Charlottesville; ME 79 Univ of VA - Charlottesville; 87–Aud, Bethesda Naval Hosp, **A**

Cook, Mrs Madelyn K 2410 Happy Hollow Road, Apartment A-17, West Lafayette, IN 47906, (317) 463-0297, Sp-Lang Path, Home Hosp, **SLP**

Cook, Mrs Marcia L 5527 Hamilton Avenue, Cincinnati, OH 45224, (513) 681-1299, BS 74 Univ of Cincinnati; MA 76 Univ of Cincinnati; SLP, Hamilton Co Board of Ment Ret, **SLP**

Cook, Mary Ann 12658 Torrey Bluff Drive, Apartment 274, San Diego, CA 92130, (619) 541-3088, BS 82 Central MI Univ; MA 83 Central MI Univ; Manager Sharp Rehab Ctr, Childrens Sp H & Neurosensory, **SLP**

Cook, Mary S 423 Vale Avenue North, Rockford, IL 61107, (815) 654-4501, BA 76 Augustana Coll; MA 77 Univ of IL - Urbana; Sp-Lang Path, Harlem Consol Sch Syst, **SLP**

Cook, Michelle Ann 4220 Irish Hills Drive, Apartment 2-B, South Bend, IN 46614-3093, (219) 546-2392, BS 85 Ball St Univ; MA 86 Ball St Univ; **SLP**

Cook, Mrs Mildred B 7 Random Road, Princeton, NJ 08540, (609) 924-3578, BS 68 Trenton St Coll; MS 71 Rutgers St Univ - Newark; **SLP LM**

Cook, Mrs Nancy W 150 Carriage Station Circle, Roswell, GA 30075, (404) 351-7776, OM 84 Auburn Univ - Auburn; Aud, Aud Consultants of Atlanta

Cook, Nicholas J 7381 Coho Drive #203, Huntington Beach, CA 92648, (213) 224-8090, BA 76 Chapman Coll; MS 82 Chapman Coll; Sp-Lang Path, CA State Diagnostic Ctr, **SLP**

Cook, Mrs Pamela R Route 2 Box 629, Sumrall, MS 39482, (601) 731-2318, BS 80 Univ Southern MS-Hattiesburg; MS 82 Univ Southern MS-Hattiesburg; 87–Sp-Lang Path, Columbia Speech Clinic, **SLP**

Cook, Mrs Patricia M 5979 East Livingston Avenue, Columbus, OH 43232, (614) 868-9993, BS 74 Miami Univ - Oxford; MA 75 OH St Univ; Sp-Lang Path, Cook and Northrup, **SLP**

Cook, Patsy Ruth 241 Shady Lane, Lexington, KY 40503, (502) 695-4035, BS 77 Univ of KY; ME 83 Eastern KY Univ; 88–Elem Level Sp/Lang Path, Franklin Co Schs, **SLP**

Cook, Mrs Phyllis Newell 13063 Brookside Drive, Omaha, NE 68123, (402) 293-9013, BS 73 Univ of NE - Omaha; MA 85 KS St Univ; ME 76 Boston Coll; 86–Aud, Loess Hills AEA 13

Cook, Mrs Rita Spiller 21174 Greenview, Southfield, MI 48075, (313) 862-8000, BA 75 Univ of MI - Ann Arbor; MA 79 Northern IL Univ - De Kalb; SLP, Private Practice, **SLP**

Cook, Sally J 17640 S F Mission Blvd, Granada Hills, CA 91344, (213) 732-1976, BA 62 Univ of CA - Los Angeles; MA 79 CA St Univ - Northridge; 79–Sp-Lang Path, Los Angles USD, **SLP**

Cook, Sandra 185 North Whitney, Hartford, CT 06105, (203) 548-5443, BS 80 Boston Univ; MS 82 Univ of WI - Madison; SLP, St Francis Hospital & Med Ctr, **SLP**

Cook, Sharon Lynne 8675 Dubonnet Street, San Diego, CA 92123, BA 80 Univ of ND; MS 83 Univ of ND; SLP, Bay Hosp & Med Cen, **SLP**

Cook, Mrs Sherri B 219 Willow Street, Hohenwald, TN 38462, (615) 446-8046, BA 80 Univ of TN - Knoxville; MA 81 Univ of TN - Knoxville; 84–Sp-Lang Path, Prof Hlth Sevs Corp, **SLP**

Cook, Mrs Sheryce Lynn 725 N E 18th Avenue, Aberdeen, SD 57401, (605) 622-2621, BS 82 Morehead St Univ; MS 83 Morehead St Univ; 85–Dir/Sp-Lang Path, St Luke's Midland Reg Med Ctr, **SLP**

Cook, Mrs Suzanne M 3D Heather Court, Lansdale, PA 19446, (215) 368-0315, BA 71 Univ of NH; MA 75 Kent St Univ; Sp-Lang Path, Montgy Co Inter Unit #23, **SLP**

Cook, Theresa M 18 Macy Place, Mobile, AL 36604-1212, (205) 476-4736, BS 76 Univ of South AL; MS 78 Univ of South AL; Sp/Lang Path, Private Practice, **SLP**

Cook, Timothy G 1242 N Crescent Heights, Apartment 14, Los Angeles, CA 90046, (213) 650-0667, BS 72 Kent St Univ; MA 73 Kent St Univ; Aud, Sheldon N Klausner MD Inc, **A**

Cook, Timothy Paul 25184 Hoover Road #302, Warren, MI 48089, (313) 755-3617, BS 81 Central MI Univ; MS 83 Univ of MI - Ann Arbor

Cook, Yvette Marie 1329 Littleton Road, Morris Plains, NJ 07950, (201) 267-8555, MA 87 Central MI Univ; Speech and Hrng Assoc

Cooke, Amy Lou 3814 Selden Cove, Memphis, TN 38128, (901) 357-9269, BS 81 Coll of Saint Rose; MS 83 Ithaca Coll; SLP, Shelby County Schools, **SLP**

Cooke, Betty B 554 Lindsay, Fort Sill, OK 73503, **SLP**

Cooke, Mrs Judith W P O Box 37, Collegeville, PA 19426, (215) 489-4805, BS 71 West Chester Univ of PA; MA 76 West Chester Univ of PA; 87–Dir Sp/Hrng Svcs, Valley Forge Plastic Surgery, **SLP**

Cooke, Patricia Ann 309 West Division Street, Dover, DE 19901-3228, (302) 674-5808, BA 80 Loyola Coll; MS 82 Loyola Coll; Sp-Lang Path, Capital School District, **SLP**

Cooke, Dr Paul Alan 1910 Navaho Trail, Okemos, MI 48864, (517) 353-7175, BS 72 MI St Univ; MS 74 Purdue Univ - West Lafayette; PH 80 (Sp Sciences) Purdue Univ - West Lafayette; 77–Assoc Prof, Michigan State Univ, **SLP**

Cooke, Dr Stan S 1649 Chestnut Street, Bowling Green, KY 42101, (502) 842-0094, BA 60 Millsaps Coll; MS 63 Univ Southern MS-Hattiesburg; ED 74 (Language Disabilities) Univ of VA - Charlottesville; 75–Dir Comm Dis Prof, Western KY U, **SLP**

Cookerly, Karen Marie 9 West Weir Street #2, Taunton, MA 02780, (617) 822-7074, BS 75 Bridgewater St Coll; MA 85 George Washington Univ; **SLP**

Cook-Westfall, Deborah A Box 2438, Salmon, ID 83467, (208) 756-3663, BS 74 ND St Univ; MA 80 Univ of MT; Sp-Lang Path, Sch Dist #291, **SLP**

Cool, Marie Hale 1542 Highcrest Drive, Medford, OR 97504, (503) 779-7630, BA 84 Univ of Redlands; MS 85 Univ of Redlands; 88–Sp-Lang Path, Providence Hosp, **SLP**

Cooler, Sarah J 12421 S Oneida Court, Phoenix, AZ 85044, (602) 251-8100, BA 74 Univ of TN - Knoxville; MA 76 Univ of TN - Knoxville; 83–Sp-Lang Path, St Lukes Med Ctr, **SLP**

Cooley, Mrs Carol Durkin 3175 Cocoplum Circle, Coconut Creek, FL 33063, (305) 928-1540, BA 77 Univ of FL; MS 79 FL St Univ; 82–Sp-Lang Path, Broward Co Pub Sch, **SLP ACE**

Cooley, Debra Ann 6750 Phelan Blvd #141C, Beaumont, TX 77706, MA 85 SUNY - Center at Buffalo; Aud, Capland Cntr for Com Dis, **A**

Cooley, Kathleen Shannon 857-B Liriope Lane, Mount Pleasant, SC 29464, (803) 884-5179, BS 85 West Chester Univ of PA; MS 86 Loyola Coll; 88–Sp-Lang Path, ACRA, **SLP**

Cooley, Leslie Lynne 912 Northfield Court, Modesto, CA 95350, (209) 526-5023, BA 80 Humboldt St Univ; MA 81 Univ of the Pacific; 81–Sp-Lang Path, Stanislaus Cty Dept of Ed, **SLP**

Cooley, Mary Josephine 25 West 33rd Street, Apartment 301, Minneapolis, MN 55408, (612) 824-6782, BA 81 Univ of IA; MA 84 Univ of IA; Audiologist, **SLP A**

Cooley, Sara Ann Route 1 Box 102, Bigelow, AR 72016, (501) 370-6651, BA 61 Memphis St Univ; MA 63 Univ of AL- Tuscaloosa; SLP, VA Medical Center, **SLP**

Coombes, Susan S 17029 South Outlook Road, Oregon City, OR 97045, (503) 280-4403, BA 73 OR St Univ; MA 75 Univ of Denver; Sp-Lang Path, Emanuel Hosp, **SLP**

Coomer-Rothman, GloryAnn M 601 SW 42nd Street, Gainesville, FL 32607, (904) 378-4622, BA 76 Univ of FL; MA 79 Univ of FL; Sp-Lang Path, Alachua County School Board, **SLP**

Coomes, Barbara Lynn 12594 West Dakota #203, Lakewood, CO 80228-2535, (303) 987-3521, MA 87 Univ of CO - Boulder

Coomes, Mrs Carla Rae 1661 Inca Drive, Laramie, WY 82070, (307) 745-7791, BS 66 UT St Univ; MS 67 UT St Univ; Sp-Lang Path, Albany County Sch District, **SLP**

Coon, Diana Lynne 1626 Satinwood Circle, Springfield, OH 45504, (513) 324-4620, BS 85 Miami Univ - Oxford; MS 86 Miami Univ - Oxford; SLP, West Milton Schools, **SLP**

Coon, Mrs Jeannie Rose 1010 Calle Del Encanto, Las Cruces, NM 88001, (505) 882-4551, BS 84 NM St Univ; MS 87 NM St Univ; 87–Sp-Lang Path, Gadsden ISD #16

Coon, Merriel C 14920 91st Street West, Taylor Ridge, IL 61284, (301) 798-2536, BA 50 Univ of IA; MA 68 Univ of MD - College Park; Sp-Lang Path, **SLP**

Coon, Shonna Stanfill 530 South 400 East #2206, Salt Lake City, UT 84111, (801) 561-3415, MS 72 UT St Univ; Sp-Lang Path, Jordan Sch Dist, **SLP**

Coonce, Gayle S 10375 Spruce Grove, San Diego, CA 92131-2218, (619) 578-3043, BA 69 Univ of CA - Riverside; MA 82 San Diego St Univ; Sp-Lang Path, San Diego USD, **SLP**

Coone, Mrs Lori K 1917 Adams Boulevard, Saginaw, MI 48602, BS 74 Central MI Univ; MA 75 Central MI Univ; 83–Sp-Lang Path, VNA of Saginaw, **SLP**

Cooney, Cheryl Staruk P O Box 333, Leicester, MA 01524, (617) 892-3131, BS 78 Worcester St Coll; MS 85 Worcester St Coll; Sp-Lang Path, Leicester Sch Dept, **SLP**

Cooney, Mrs Kathryn Mack 6629 Tampa Avenue, Reseda, CA 91335, (818) 781-0360, BA 82 Univ of OR; MA 84 Univ of OR; 87–Chief/Sp-Lang Path, Los Angeles Ctr For Therapy & Educ, **SLP**

Cooney, Mrs Marion K 17 Moody Place, Staten Island, NY 10310, (718) 447-1741, BS 54 Fordham Univ; MS 57 Wagner Coll; MA 77 Kean Coll of NJ; Sp-Lang Path, Private Practice, **SLP**

Cooney-Eickelman, Margaret Peggy 705 East Myrtlewood Court, Highlands Ranch, CO 80126, (303) 688-3195, BA 78 Univ of CO - Boulder; MS 80 CO St Univ; Sp-Lang Path & Lrng Dis, Douglas Co Sch, **SLP**

Coons, Mrs Donna M 516 Overcrest Road, Baltimore, MD 21204, (301) 396-0839, BS 69 Univ of TN - Knoxville; MS 78 Loyola Coll; Sp-Lang Path, Baltimore City Pub Sch, **SLP**

Coons, Ellen E 1109 North Washington, Nevada, MO 64772, (417) 667-7833, BA 79 Wichita St Univ; MA 80 Wichita St Univ; Sp-Lang Path, Nevada Hab Cen, **SLP**

Coons, Mrs Lynn Westlake 1035 12th Avenue #1, Havre, MT 59501, (406) 265-4356, BA 77 Univ of MT; MS 79 Univ of MT; Sp-Lang Path, Havre PS, **SLP**

Coons, Mrs Pamela Johnson 2914 West 95th, Lubbock, TX 79423, (806) 747-2641, BS 77 Hardin-Simmons Univ; MS 80 TX Tech Univ; Sp-Lang Path, Lubbock ISD, **SLP**

Coons, Sandra La Verne 46245 Auhi Nani Place, Kaneohe, HI 96744-4052, **SLP**

Coope, Mrs Beverly Ray 42 West Marlette Avenue, Phoenix, AZ 85013, BA 52 Univ of Rochester; MA 56 Stanford Univ; **SLP**

Cooper, Allyn D 10 Trombley Drive, Livingston, NJ 07039, (201) 535-8110, BS 63 Univ of PA; MA 74 Kean Coll of NJ; Sp/Lang Path, Livingston Bd of Educ, **SLP**

Cooper, Amy Marie 2732 White Oak Lane, Kannapolis, NC 28081, BS 83 Appalachian St Univ; MS 84 Univ of NC - Chapel Hill; Aud, Charlotte Mecklenberg Schools, **A**

Cooper, Andrea S 13 Robertson Road, East Windsor, NJ 08520, (609) 448-5129, BA 77 Hofstra Univ; MA 79 Hofstra Univ; MA 82 Kean Coll of NJ; 88–Sp-Lang Path, Private Practice, **SLP**

Cooper, Mrs Anna Wagg 1119 Raton, Manhattan, KS 66502-5139, (913) 539-3660, BA 85 Fort Hays St Univ; MS 87 Fort Hays St Univ; 87–Sp-Lang Path, Holton Spec Educ Coop, **SLP**

Cooper, Mrs Avis P 11142 West Oregon Place, Lakewood, CO 80226, (303) 797-0851, BS 57 ND St Univ; MA 79 Univ of CO - Boulder; SLP, Jefferson Co R-1 Sch, **SLP**

Cooper, Christophr 6070 Highway 93 South, Whitefish, MT 59937, (406) 892-4321, MS 77 Central MI Univ; Sp-Lang Path, School District 6, **SLP ACE**

Cooper, Mrs Cindy Rosenberg 1249 Park Avenue #9E, Manhattan, NY 10029, (212) 996-0081, MA 82 Hofstra Univ; SLP, **SLP**

Cooper, Mrs Crystal S 4919 Woodland Forrest Dr, Tuscaloosa, AL 35405, (205) 553-2030, BA 64 CUNY - Hunter Coll; MS 66 PA St Univ - Univ Park; 70–Curr Assoc/Sp-Lang Path, Tuscaloosa Cty Sch, **SLP**

Cooper, Deborah Lynn 1813 Indian Woods Drive, Neptune Beach, FL 32233, (904) 725-8972, BA 85 Univ of North FL; ME 87 Univ of North FL; 88–Sp-Lang Path, A Smith Clinic

Cooper, Debra H Parent-Infant Prog Hrng Imprd, Thomas Claggett Elem Sch, 2001 Addisson Road South, District Heights-Forestville, MD 20747, (301) 499-2357, BA 77 Univ of MD - College Park; MS 79 Gallaudet Coll; Aud, Prince Georges Co Pub Sch, **A**

Cooper, Debra Huther 21 Green Street, Newbury, MA 01951, (508) 462-8277, BS 80 Purdue Univ - West Lafayette; MS 82 Southern CT St Univ; Director Sp-Lang Path Services, Private Practice, **SLP**

Cooper, Mrs Denise L 16187 Reedmere, Birmingham, MI 48009, (313) 433-1761, BA 78 MI St Univ; MA 79 Northwestern Univ; **SLP**

Cooper, Mrs Diana L B 4127 Yale Avenue, Arlington Heights, IL 60004, (312) 307-2155, BS 77 Eastern IL Univ; MA 79 Univ of KS; 79–Sp-Lang Path, Commun Cons Sch Dist 54, **SLP**

Cooper, Mrs Diane Hirschbeck 30 Palmdale Drive, Williamsville, NY 14221, (716) 636-6470, MA 87 SUNY - Center at Buffalo; 87–Sp-Lang Path, Erie I BOCES, **SLP**

Cooper, Dr Donald Stewart Univ Of S Ca Sch Of Medicine, Dept Of Otolaryngology, 903 Hoffman 2025 Zonal Avenue, Los Angeles, CA 90033, (213) 224-7984, BA 62 Harvard Univ; MA 81 Univ of IA; PH 71 (Linguistics) Harvard Univ; 84–Asst Prof, USC

Cooper, Dr Donna J 24948 Jim Bridger Road, Hidden Hills, CA 91302, (213) 271-6956, BA 66 Univ of CA - Los Angeles; MA 70 Univ of Southern CA; PH 72 (NS) Univ of Southern CA; **SLP**

Cooper, Mrs Eleanor A 532 Cherry Tree Lane, Smoke Rise, Kinnelon, NJ 07405, (201) 838-4405, BA 77 CUNY - Lehman Coll; BA 77 CUNY - Lehman Coll; MA 79 CUNY - Lehman Coll; Aud, Private Practice, **A**

Cooper, Ellen D 215 Coachman Place East, Muttontown, NY 11791, (516) 681-9039, BS 76 SUNY - Center at Albany; MA 77 Hofstra Univ; Sp/Lang Path, Private Practice, **SLP**

Cooper, Dr Eugene B 4919 Woodland Forrest Dr, Tuscaloosa, AL 35405, (205) 348-7131, BS 55 SUNY - Coll at Geneseo; ME 57 PA St Univ - Univ Park; ED 62 (NS) PA St Univ - Univ Park; Chmn Dept of Commun Dis, U of AL, **SLP F**

Cooper, Dr Franklin S 270 Crown Street, New Haven, CT 06511, BS 31 Univ of IL - Urbana; PH 36 (NS); Assoc Res Dir, Haskins Lab, **H**

Cooper, Gary J 1965 Verner, Grosse Pointe Woods, MI 48236, PH; **SLP**

Cooper, Mrs Georgia T 1209 Gregory Street, Ojai, CA 93023, BA 26 Univ of WA; MA 33 Mills Coll; **SLP LM**

Cooper, Heather A Box 1630, Morden, MB, Canada R0G 1J0, (204) 822-4429, MS 87 Univ of ND; 87–Sp-Lang Path, Govt of Manitoba Dept of Educ

Cooper, Mrs Iris P 2406 Halcyon Avenue, Baltimore, MD 21214, (301) 789-1881, BS 70 Towson St Univ; MS 76 Johns Hopkins Univ; Sp/Lang Path, Anne Arundel Co Bd of Ed, **SLP**

Cooper, J C, Jr HC Route 1, Box 19293, Bulverde, TX 78163, (512) 567-5655, BS 57 Auburn Univ - Auburn; MS 65 Wayne St Univ; PH 68 (Aud) Wayne St Univ; 69–Prof, U of TX Hlth Sci Cen, **A**

Cooper, Mrs Janet M 117 Camille Lane, East Patchogue, NY 11772, (516) 724-1717, BS 81 Bradley Univ; MS 83 Adelphi Univ; Sp-Lang Path, Suffolk Child Dev Cen, **SLP**

Cooper, Joyce E Box 116, Prosperity, PA 15329, (717) 374-2911, BA 70 CA Univ of PA; ME 74 Clarion Univ of PA; Unit Manager, Western Center, **SLP**

Cooper, Dr Judith Ann Federal Bldg Room 1C-06, 7550 Wisconsin Avenue, Bethesda, MD 20892, (301) 496-5061, OB 71 Southern Methodist Univ; MS 72 Vanderbilt Univ; PH 82 (NS) Univ of WA; Sp-Lang Path, NIH/NINCDS, **SLP**

Cooper, Judith K 26 South Main Street, Assonet, MA 02702, (401) 847-2100, BA 76 Univ of CT; MS 79 Univ of RI; Sp-Lang Path, Newport Publ Schs, **SLP**

Cooper, Judith Schiller 1059 Old Ford Road, Huntingdon Valley, PA 19006, (215) 643-4142, BA 62 Temple Univ-Tyler Sch of Art; MA 76 Temple Univ-Tyler Sch of Art; Dir, Play and Learn Inc, **SLP**

Cooper, Dr June M VP Faculty & Staff Relations, 1250 Bellflower Boulevard, Long Beach, CA 90840, (213) 985-5157, BA 54 CUNY - Queens Coll; MA 56 CUNY - Brooklyn Coll; PH 64 (NS) NY Univ; Vp-Faculty & Staff Rel, CA St U-Long Bch, **SLP**

Cooper, Karen Jacobs Sacred Heart Hospital, 1430 DeKalb Pike, Norristown, PA 19401, (215) 278-8360, BA 73 Univ of MA - Amherst; MA 75 Temple Univ-Tyler Sch of Art; 78–Aud, Sacred Heart Hosp, **A**

Cooper, Katherine 225 Arch Street, Apartment 52 Mulberry Ct, Philadelphia, PA 19106, BA 67 PA St Univ - Univ Park; MA 70 Temple Univ-Tyler Sch of Art; Aud, ENT Professional Associates, **A**

Cooper, Mrs Kimberley P O Box 1081, North Platte, NE 69101, (308) 532-3300, BA 76 Kearney St Coll; MS 80 Kearney St Coll; Sp-Lang Path, N Platte Pub Sch, **SLP**

Cooper, Kimberly Hanna 180 Dean Street, Brooklyn, NY 11217, BS 79 Univ of MO - Columbia; MA 80 Univ of MO - Columbia; Sp-Lang Path, St Francis De Sales Sch Deaf, **SLP**

Cooper, Mrs Kimberly Sturgis 2918 Hydrangea Place, Wilmington, NC 28403, (919) 343-7218, BA 78 Univ of MS; MA 81 Memphis St Univ; Sp-Lang Path, New Hanover Mem Hosp, **SLP**

Cooper, Larry M 4637 East Wood, Phoenix, AZ 85040, (602) 967-6473, BA 76 Univ of IA; MA 78 Univ of IA; Administrator, Sun Rehabilitation Agency, **SLP**

Cooper, Mrs Linda C 10289 East Sahuaro Drive, Scottsdale, AZ 85260, (602) 833-4246, BS 71 Southern IL Univ-Edwardsvill; MA 76 Southern IL Univ-Edwardsvill; SLP, Mesa Pub Sch, **SLP**

Cooper, Mrs Marcia Hartung 10921 Wilshire Boulevard, Suite 401, Los Angeles, CA 90024, BS 58 IN Univ - Bloomington; MA 60 Stanford Univ; **SLP**

Cooper, Marie D 2100 Parkridge Lane, 1000-105 Nicholwood Drive, Raleigh, NC 27605, (919) 839-2117

Cooper, Marsha M 6840 Hatillo Avenue #D, Canoga Park, CA 91306, (805) 252-8590, BA 71 CA St Univ - Northridge; MA 76 CA St Univ - Northridge; MA 83 CA St Univ - Los Angeles; SLP, Las Virgenes USD, **SLP**

Cooper, Martha A 2509 Thomas Avenue South, Minneapolis, MN 55405, (612) 627-3085, MA 87 Univ of MN - Minneap-St Paul; 87–Sp-Lang Path, Minneapolis PS, **SLP**

Cooper, Mary B 2219 College Green Drive, Houston, TX 77058, (713) 482-0022, BA 68 Mundelein Coll; ME 69 PA St Univ - Univ Park; Sp-Lang Path, Clear Crk ISD, **SLP**

Cooper, Mrs Mary C 1013 Burgundy, Manchester, MO 63011, (314) 227-4853, BS 75 Saint Louis Univ; MA 76 Saint Louis Univ; 76–Sp-Lang Path, Cardinal Glennon Chldn Hosp, **SLP**

Cooper, Mrs Mona R 19 8th Avenue SW, Cairo, GA 31728, (912) 377-9716, ME 88 Valdosta St Coll; 88–Sp-Lang Path, Grady County Bd of Educ Southside Elem Sch

Cooper, Dr Morton 10921 Wilshire Boulevard, Suite 401, Los Angeles, CA 90024, (213) 208-6047, BA 52 CUNY - Brooklyn Coll; MA 57 IN Univ - Bloomington; PH 64 (NS) Univ of CA - Los Angeles; **SLP**

Cooper, Mrs Nancy H 1055 West Walworth, Whitewater, WI 53190, (414) 473-2878, BS 58 Wheelock Coll; MS 80 Univ of WI - Whitewater; Sp-Lang Path, Whitewater USD, **SLP**

Cooper, Pauline Anne 826 Glendover Circle, Lexington, KY 40502, (502) 839-3406, BA 82 Univ of KY; MS 84 Univ of KY; 84–Sp-Lang Path, Anderson Co PS, **SLP**

Cooper, Reuben 1443 Bayville Street, Norfolk, VA 23503, (804) 583-9323, BS 33 CUNY - City College; MS 47 CUNY - City College; Prof Emeritus, Old Dominion Univ, **SLP LM**

Cooper, Sandra Gail 200 Bentree Lane #E-9, Florence, SC 29501, **SLP**

Cooper, Mrs Sheilah Auderer 3537 Kings Drive, Chalmette, LA 70043, (504) 279-3106, MS 84 LA St Univ - N O Medical Ctr; 87–Sp-Lang Path, Private Practice, **SLP ACE**

Cooper, Mrs Sherrie J 21424 N E 165th St, Woodinville, WA 98072, (206) 788-0827, BS 78 Univ of OR; MS 81 Adelphi Univ; Self Employed, **SLP**

Cooper, Mrs Shirley A 13931 Tyler, Sylmar, CA 91342, BA 79 CA St Univ - Northridge; MA 80 CA St Univ - Northridge; Sp-Lang Path, California Comm Coll, **SLP**

Cooper, Susan J Impact Hearing Conservation, 406 West 34th Street, Suite 410, Kansas City, MO 64111, (816) 531-4847, MA Univ of KS; Mgr of Client Serv, Impact Hrng Conservation Inc, **A**

Cooper, Teresa Ann 2411 Bramblewood, Wichita, KS 67226-1016, (316) 685-1099, BA 74 Wichita St Univ; MA 76 Wichita St Univ; MA 78 Wichita St Univ; Sp-Lang Path/Aud, Winfield State Hosp & Trng Ctr, **A**

Cooper, Victoria A 1203 East 9th Street, Winfield, KS 67156, (316) 221-7021, BA 76 Wichita St Univ; MA 77 Wichita St Univ; PH 87 (Commun Dis) Wichita St Univ; 83–Dir, Cowley County Spec Serv Coop, **SLP**

Cooper, Dr William A, Jr Dept Communicative Disorders, Univ Of South Carolina, Columbia, SC 29208, (807) 777-4813, BS 57 Wayne St Univ; PH 64 (Aud) Univ of OK - Norman; Prof, Univ of SC, **A F**

Cooperman, Dr Donna Klur 12 Cosgrove Drive, Glen Cove, NY 11542, (516) 759-1555, BA 66 CUNY - Queens Coll; MS 68 CUNY - Queens Coll; OD 86 (Communication Disorders) Adelphi Univ; 88–Asst Prof, The Coll of Saint Rose, **SLP ACE**

Cooperman, Estelle B 16-40 200th Street, Bayside, NY 11360, (516) 842-4000, BA 76 CUNY - Queens Coll; MA 78 Hofstra Univ; SLP, Copiague Union Free Sch Dist, **SLP**

Cooperman, Susan N 14612 Village Glen Circle, Tampa, FL 33624, (813) 960-8657, SLP, **SLP**

Coorpender, Linda M T 3206 Rigolette Road, Pineville, LA 71360, (318) 473-0010, BA 68 Northwestern St Univ; MS 72 Northwestern St Univ; 88–Sp-Lang Path, VA Med Ctr, **SLP**

Coover, Mrs Amy Cohen 564 Woodberry Drive, Arnold, MD 21012, (301) 267-8717, BA 77 CUNY - Queens Coll; MA 78 Univ of MD - College Park; Sp-Lang Path, Anne Arundel Co Pub Sch, **SLP**

Coover, Mauri J 423 Potomac Avenue, Buffalo, NY 14213, (716) 882-6380, ME 87 SUNY - Coll at Buffalo

Cope, Sharon Leah 316 West 7th Street, Traverse City, MI 49684, (616) 922-6200, BA 61 San Diego St Univ; MA 72 Northern MI Univ; Sp/Lang Path, Traverse Bay Area ISD, **SLP**

Copeland, Dr Alfred Beryl 5505 Saddleback Road, Garland, TX 75043, (214) 248-7975, BA 58 Univ of Redlands; MA 60 Univ of Redlands; PH 64 (NS) Univ of WA; Dir/Aud Consult, Better Hrng Aid Cen, **A**

Copeland, Mrs Barbara R 2846 North Three Springs Drive, Westlake Village, CA 91361, BS 76 Marywood Coll; MS 77 Ithaca Coll; Sp-Lang Path, Santa Monica-Malibu USD, **SLP**

Copeland, Janet E 6 West 14th Street, Frederick, MD 21701, (301) 698-3370, BA 74 Earlham Coll; MA 77 Univ of MD - College Park; Sp-Lang Path, Frederick Memorial Hosp, **SLP**

Copeland, Mrs Judith L 8734 Delcris Drive, Gaithersburg, MD 20879, BS 78 PA St Univ - Univ Park; ME 81 Northeastern Univ; Sp/Lang Path, Palatine Sch Dist #15, **SLP**

Copeland, Mrs Katherine Eby 6427 Glenrose Court, Dallas, TX 75214, (214) 827-5962, BA 70 Wichita St Univ; MA 71 Wichita St Univ; **SLP**

Copeland, Lisa Kay Center For Sp-Lang Pathology, 3807 G Morrison Place, Monroe, LA 71201, (205) 536-3364, BS 83 Auburn Univ - Auburn; OM 85 Auburn Univ - Auburn; Sp-Lang Path, Center for Sp-Lang Pathology, **SLP**

Copeland, Sr Marie Estelle DE Paul Institute, Castlegate Avenue, Pittsburgh, PA 15226, (412) 561-4848, BS 48 Univ of Pittsburgh - Pittsburgh; MA 55 Northwestern Univ; 55–Sch Aud, De Paul I, **A LM**

Copeland, Mrs Mary Hammond 8 Hyatt Street #5, Norwalk, CT 06850, (203) 259-7106, BA 83 Univ of CT; MA 85 Univ of CT; Sp-Lang Path, Rehab Assoc of Ct, **SLP**

Copeland, Mrs Pauline B 2012 Sherwood Drive #132, Johnson City, TN 37601, (615) 929-1312, BA 50; MA 52 East TN St Univ; **SLP A LM**

Copeland, Terrilyn Denise 1658 Brownstone Boulevard, Apartment 134, Toledo, OH 43614, (419) 867-0717, BS 76 Kent St Univ; MA 80 Bowling Green St Univ; 86–Sp/Lang Path, St Francis Rehabilitation Hosp, **SLP**

Copithorne, Nancy Adelle 311 Belmont Avenue, North Babylon, NY 11703, (516) 366-2900, BA 86 Univ of Central FL; MA 87 Univ of Central FL; Sp-Lang Path, Suffolk County Dev Center

Copley, Mrs Marilyn J 6200 North Avon Avenue, San Gabriel, CA 91775, BA 69 CA St Univ - Los Angeles; MA 73 CA St Univ - Los Angeles; Sp-Lang Path, LA Co Supt of Sch, **SLP**

Coplin, Mrs Robin S 8 Darnley Greene, Delmar, NY 12054, (518) 475-1175, BS 76 SUNY - Center at Albany; MS 77 SUNY - Center at Albany; Instr/SLP, NTID, **SLP**

Copmann, Dr Kathryn S 11860 Blue February Way, Columbia, MD 21044, (301) 730-4689, BA 74 Elmira Coll; MA 76 Kent St Univ; PH 88 (Special Educ/Deaf Educ/Aud) Kent St Univ; 85–Asst Prof, Loyola Coll, **A ACE**

Copp, Leslie M P O Box 134, Bracey, VA 23919, ME 73 Univ of VA - Charlottesville; Sp-Lang Path, Warren County Health Departmnt, **SLP**

Copp, Mrs Martha Lamb ENT Audiology Association, 515 East Garden Street, Lakeland, FL 33805, (813) 683-5454, MS 80 Univ of South FL; Aud, Lakeland ENT Assoc, **A**

Coppedge, Mrs Lynn F 227 Beverly Road, Asheville, NC 28805, (704) 298-2351, BS 75 East Carolina Univ; MA 76 Univ of TN - Knoxville; Sp-Lang Path, Private Practice, **SLP**

Coppel, Marcia E 3900 Tunlaw Road N W #505, Washington, DC 20007, **SLP**

Coppel, Miriam L 3162 Wharton Drive, Yorktown Heights, NY 10598, (914) 962-9021, BS 71 Univ of Cincinnati; MA 72 Univ of Cincinnati; **A**

Coppin, Mrs Rachel Irene 807 8th Avenue SE, Jamestown, ND 58401, (701) 252-1392, BS 83 Moorhead St Univ; MS 85 Moorhead St Univ; 85–Sp-Lang Path, Anne Carlsen Sch For Handicapped, **SLP**

Copple, Mrs Karen Sue 8013 Chicago Avenue, Lubbock, TX 79424, (806) 794-0121, ME 82 6407; 86–Sp-Lang Path, Lubbock ISD, **SLP**

Coppola, Anthony 82 Pineaire Avenue, Farmingville, NY 11738, (516) 732-4924, BA 79 Hofstra Univ; MA 80 Hofstra Univ; 81–SLP, Hempstead Public Schools, **SLP**

Coppola, Lisa 699 W Magee #8201, Tucson, AZ 85704, (602) 745-3006, BS 82 Univ of AZ; MS 85 Univ of AZ; **SLP**

Coppola, Michael J 23 Sherwood Place, Wayne, NJ 07470, BA 69 Newark St Coll; MA 74 Newark St Coll; Sp-Lang Path, Rutherford Bd of Ed, **SLP**

Coppola, Valarie A 90 Concord Street, New Haven, CT 06512, BA 76 Southern CT St Univ; MA 79 Univ of IL - Urbana; Sp-Lang Path, Milford Bb Ed, **SLP**

Corazza, Antoinette Mignano 149-01 84th Street, Howard Beach, NY 11414, (718) 835-4182, BA 84 CUNY - Queens Coll; MA 87 CUNY - Queens Coll; **SLP**

Corazza, Janice A 501 Slaters Lane #301, Alexandria, VA 22314, (703) 454-5989, BS 76 Bloomsburg Univ of PA; ME 75 Bloomsburg Univ of PA; **SLP**

Corbaley, John L, II 5714 McGee Street, Kansas City, MO 64113, (816) 932-3262, MS 75 Vanderbilt Univ; SLP, St Lukes Hospital, **SLP**

Corbe, Grace Ann Rd 5 Box 313-A, Towanda, PA 18848, (717) 265-8273, BS 86 Bloomsburg Univ of PA; MS 87 Bloomsburg Univ of PA; 88–Sp-Lang Path, BLaST IU #17, **F**

Corbeil, Mary Kay 236 Magnolia, Coppell, TX 75019, (214) 462-9322, MA 84 Univ of IA; BA 82 Augustana Coll; Sp-Lang Path, Dallas Rehab Inst, **SLP**

Corbello, Mrs Patricia B P O Box 98, Sunset, LA 70584, (318) 942-9426, BA 71 Univ of Southwestern LA; MS 79 Univ of Southwestern LA; Sp/Lang Path, St Landry Parish Sch Bd, **SLP**

Corbett, Mrs Ann Leslie 3619 Dover Road, Youngstown, OH 44511, (216) 424-7787, BS 81 Kent St Univ; MA 83 Kent St Univ; 88–Sp-Lang Path, Robert Bycroft Sch, **SLP**

Corbett, Gioia M 7822 Twin Hills, Houston, TX 77071, (713) 792-4500, BS 85 Univ of Houston - Univ Park; MS 88 Univ of TX - Dallas; 88, Sp & Hrng Inst

Corbett, Jodi G 7941 North Kedvale, Skokie, IL 60076, (312) 982-9116, BS 78 Southern IL Univ -Carbondale; MA 80 Northern IL Univ - De Kalb; Admin, Jodi Golembo-Corbett, **SLP**

Corbin, Elizabeth 3700 Flagler Avenue, Key West, FL 33040, **SLP**

Corbin, Hollis J Audiology Department 7EN, Toronto Gerneral Hospital, 200 Elizabeth Street, Toronto, ON, Canada M5G 1L7, (416) 595-3667, BA 71; MA 72 Wichita St Univ; Cl Superv, Toronto General Hosp, **A**

Corbin, Mrs Kathleen K 710 Green Meadow Drive, Greenwood, IN 46143, BS 81 Ball St Univ; MA 82 Ball St Univ; Aud, Methodist Hosp of Indiana, **A**

Corbin, Mrs Kim Caffey 3323 Whippoorwill Lane, Oxford, MS 38655, (601) 236-1676, BS 76 Delta St Univ; OM 81 Univ of MS; Sp-Lang Path, North Mississippi Retardatn Cn, **SLP**

Corbin, Kim M 2351 Allied Drive #135, Madison, WI 53711, (608) 262-6478, BA 79 Loyola Coll; MS 80 Loyola Coll; SLP, University of Wisconsin, **SLP**

Corcione, Mrs Sarah W 32 Mountainview Avenue, Albany, NY 12208, (518) 482-6195, BS 73 SUNY - Center at Albany; MS 74 Syracuse Univ; Sp-Lang Path, Albany Med Cen, **SLP**

Corcoran, Donna M 210 Monmore Road, London, ON, Canada N6G 3A6, (519) 679-6465, BS 76 Univ of Western Ontario; OM 78 Univ of Western Ontario; Coordinator Aud Services, U of Western Ontario, **A**

Corcoran, John Allen Rural Free Delivery 2, Winsted, CT 06098, **SLP**

Corcoran, Dr Joseph A, Jr University Of Western Ontario, Program In Comm Disorders, London, ON, Canada N6G 1H1, (519) 679-2111, BA 60 Univ of Notre Dame; MA 69 IN Univ - Bloomington; PH 71 (Sp Path) IN Univ - Bloomington; Asst Prof, U of Wn On, **SLP**

Corcoran, Mrs Judith Allison 9328 So 53rd Court, Oak Lawn, IL 60453, (312) 423-8519, BA 83 Saint Xavier Coll; OM 85 Governors St Univ; **SLP**

Corcoran, Kathie A 42 Shady Lane, East Hartford, CT 06118, (203) 228-9465, BA 78 Southern CT St Univ; MS 80 Southern CT St Univ; Sp-Lang Path, Hebron Elem Sch, **SLP**

Corcoran, Kathleen Ann 1817 North 117th Street, Wauwatosa, WI 53226, (414) 257-6720, BS 86 Marquette Univ; MS 87 Marquette Univ; 87–Sp-Lang Path, Curative Rehabilitation Ctr, **SLP**

Corcoran, Mrs Maureen Patricia 44 King Phillips Path, Marshfield, MA 02050, (617) 834-8221, BA 75 Catholic Univ of America; MA 77 Ball St Univ; SLP, Cardinal Cushing Sch

Corcoran, Susan Evans 2200 Richland #C, Metairie, LA 70001-1644, BS 82 Southwest MO St Univ; MA 85 Southwest MO St Univ; **SLP**

Cord, Mary T 3850 Tunlaw Road N W #709, Washington, DC 20007, (202) 576-4062, BA 79 Augustana Coll; MA 80 Univ of IL - Champaign; MA 85 Northern IL Univ - De Kalb; Aud/Sp-Lang Path, Walter Reed Army Medical Ctr, **SLP A**

Corder, Mrs Barbara L 12220 Fairway, Leawood, KS 66209, BS 70 Central MO St Univ; MS 74 Central MO St Univ; SLP, Shawnee Mission Pub Sch D #512, **SLP**

Corder, Mrs Betty L 30900 68th N W, Stanwood, WA 98292, BA 44; MA 82; Sp-Lang Path, SPARC Devel Sch, **SLP**

Cordero, Mrs M Suzanne 4233 Econlockhatchee Trail, Orlando, FL 32817, (407) 657-4412, BA 63 Greensboro Coll; MA 65 NY Univ; **SLP**

Cordes, Mrs Claudia A 275 North 119th Street, Omaha, NE 68154, (402) 334-1136, BS 71 Univ of NE - Lincoln; MS 76 Univ of NE - Omaha; **SLP**

Cordes, Mrs Dede Gerke 36 Lake Drive, Woodville, TX 75979, (409) 283-3698, BS 62 TX Christian Univ; Sp-Lang Path, Private Practice, **SLP**

Cordier, Mrs Charlene L Box 1551, Columbia Falls, MT 59912, (406) 862-3509, BA 77 Univ of MT; Sp/Lang Path, Whitefish Pub Sch, **SLP ACE**

Cording, Joanne C Algozzino 9696 Walnut Street #1516, Dallas, TX 75243, (214) 235-7512, BA 71 Univ of North TX; MA 74 Univ of North TX; Sp-Lang Path, Richardson ISD, **SLP**

Cordio, Sally Lynn S 220 South Taft Street, Whitewater, WI 53190, **SLP**

Cordova-Voron, Mrs Cecilia 6507 South Hardy Drive #255, Tempe, AZ 85283, (602) 730-6798, MA 88 Univ of TX - Austin

Core, Mrs Coleen Shank 215 Valirey Drive, Hampton, VA 23669, (804) 229-3232, BS 82 ID St Univ; MS 84 ID St Univ; 87–Sp-Lang Path, Williamsburg Comm Hosp, **SLP**

Core, Nancy Reighley Route 66 Box 102, Cullowhee, NC 28723, (704) 293-9455, BA 72 Mount Holyoke Coll; MA 78 Vanderbilt Univ; Aud, Wcu Speech & Hearing Ctr, **A**

Corey, Mrs Suzanne Kincaid 2109 Concord, Muncie, IN 47304, (317) 759-8113, BS 80 Ball St Univ; MA 83 Ball St Univ; Sp-Lang Path, Delaware Community School Corp, **SLP**

Coreys, Mrs Esther 919 Bromton Drive, Westbury, NY 11590, BA 66 CUNY - Brooklyn Coll; MS 68 Adelphi Univ; Supervisor, Adelphi University, **SLP LM ACE**

Corfariu, Mrs Manuela 2001 North Deerpark Drive, Apartment 733, Fullerton, CA 92631, (714) 961-0814, MA 88 CA St Univ - Fullerton

Corfield, Joan 121 South Wilson Avenue, Unit 105, Pasadena, CA 91106, (818) 796-5309, BA 51 Whittier Coll; MA 53 Whittier Coll; **SLP**

Corinblit, Barbara 247 25th Avenue #2, San Francisco, CA 94121, (415) 221-4119, BA 75 San Francisco St Univ; MS 79 Univ of WI - Madison; Sp-Lang Path, Mt Zion Hospital & Medical Ctr, **SLP**

Corker, Mrs Susan Chase 1001 West Sycamore, Carbondale, IL 62901, (618) 833-4541, BS 82 Southern IL Univ -Carbondale; MS 84 Southern IL Univ -Carbondale; **A**

Corlew, Dr Marilyn M 15445 Woodbridge Road, Brookfield, WI 53005, (414) 384-2000, BA 67 Vanderbilt Univ; MA 69 Case Western Reserve Univ; PH 71 (NS) Case Western Reserve Univ; 74–Ch-Aud & Sp-Lang Path Serv, VA Med Cen, **SLP ACE**

Corley, Cecelia Elizabeth Route 7 Box 116, Malvern, AR 72104, (501) 246-8011, BS 71 Kent St Univ; MS 83 Univ of AR - Little Rock; 84–Sp-Lang Path, Arkadelphia Human Dev Ctr, **SLP ACE**

Corley, Ellen C Route 1 Box 82, St Johns Road, Irmo, SC 29063, (803) 781-1591, BA 73 Columbia Coll; OM 77 Univ of SC - Columbia; Owner/Director, Private Practice, **SLP**

Corley, Mrs Terry N 1601 McIntyre Drive, Mobile, AL 36618, (205) 343-2415, BA 76 Univ of FL; MA 78 Univ of FL; Sp-Lang Path, Private Practice, **SLP**

Corley, Virginia M 30 Moise Drive, Sumter, SC 29150, (803) 778-1514, BS 75 Durham Univ - England; OM 80 Univ of SC - Columbia; Aud, Sumter Hrng Cl, **A**

Corliss, Mrs Edith L R Forest Hills Laboratory, 2955 Albemarle Street N W, Washington, DC 20008, (202) 362-6085, BS 41 MA Inst of Tech; MS 41 MA Inst of Tech; Physicist, Forest Hills Lab

Cormack, Barbara Jean 16 Martin Close, Red Deer, AB, Canada T4N 0H1, (403) 343-1405, BS 74 Univ of Alberta - Alberta; MA 83 Univ of MT; 75–Sp-Lang Path, Red Deer Public Sch Dist #104, **SLP**

Cormier, Carolann Marie 589 Maple Avenue, Hartford, CT 06114, (203) 241-8186, BA 82 George Washington Univ; MS 84 Boston Univ; Sp-Lang Path, Capital Region Educ Council, **SLP**

Corn, Pamela Leisa 10 Charlton Road, Rome, GA 30161, (404) 777-3322, BS 82 Univ of GA; ME 83 Univ of GA; Aud, Georgia Sch for the Deaf, **A**

Corn, Richard K P O Box 597, Oxford, KS 67119-0597, (316) 221-1200, BS 82 Lamar Univ; MS 84 Lamar Univ; MS 84 Lamar Univ

Corn, Sharon K Route 1 Box 124-B, Clayton Road, Arden, NC 28704, (704) 684-6181, BS 79 Western Carolina Univ; ME 80 Univ of NC - Greensboro; 80–Sp-Lang Path, Buncombe Co Pub Sch, **SLP**

Cornack, Julianna Holme 814 Glendale Court, Evans City, PA 16033, (412) 452-4390, BA 82 Wayne St Univ; MA 86 OH St Univ; 86–Sp-Lang Path, St Francis Med Ctr, **SLP**

Corneau, Janette B 4302 Gunn Highway, Tampa, FL 33624, (813) 238-1743, BS 77 Northwestern Univ; MA 79 Northwestern Univ; Sp Lang Cl, Hillsborough Co Pub Sch, **SLP**

Cornelia, Barbara Jane 8438 Chadwood Lane East Drive, Apartment 2B, Indianapolis, IN 46268, (317) 482-2700, MS 84 Purdue Univ - West Lafayette; 87–Dir of Aud, Witham Mem Hosp, **A**

Cornelius, Cathleen Adele 16830 Kingsbury Street, #246, Granada Hills, CA 91344, BA 83 Univ of CA - Los Angeles; MA 86 CA St Univ - Northridge; 87–Sp-Lang Path, LA County Office of Educ, **SLP**

Cornelius, Donna Bean 330 Main Street #H-177, Gardendale, AL 35071, (205) 631-8874, MS 87 Univ of Montevallo

Cornelius, Jodie L 5813 Northhills Drive, Fort Worth, TX 76117, (817) 831-0951, BS 83 TX Christian Univ; MS 85 TX Christian Univ; **SLP**

Cornelius, Judith Marie 10900 Pebble Run Drive, Silver Spring, MD 20902, (703) 698-3788, BA 82 Loyola Coll; ME 84 Univ of VA - Charlottesville; Sp-Lang Path, Fairfax Hosp, **SLP**

Cornelius, Suzanne 236 1/2 First Street #1, Jersey City, NJ 07302, (212) 947-5770, BA 68 Univ of TX - Austin; MA 74 Univ of TX - Austin; **SLP**

Cornelius-Randt, Mrs Tamara J 6728 Fescue, Portage, MI 49002, (616) 342-7412, BS 78 Western MI Univ; MA 80 Western MI Univ; Sp-Lang Path, Parchment Sch Dist, **SLP**

Cornell, Jolynn Ann 16 N W Cottage, Newport, OR 97365, (503) 485-8521, MS 83 Univ of OR; 88–Sp-Lang Path, Private Practice, **SLP**

Cornell, Mrs Marcia 10 Arnold Drive, Bloomfield, CT 06002, (203) 278-4256, MA 72 Univ of CT; Aud, Priv Pract, **A**

Cornell, Mrs MaryAnn 3691 Cumberland Lane, Hamburg, NY 14075, (716) 649-6818, BS 72 SUNY - Coll at Fredonia; MS 76 SUNY - Coll at Buffalo; 72–Sp-Lang Path, Buffalo Bd of Educ, **SLP**

Cornell, Mrs Pamela Pope 119A Plains Road, Wallkill, NY 12589, (914) 564-1780, BA 81 SUNY - Coll at New Paltz; MS 86 SUNY - Coll at New Paltz; 82–Sp-Lang Path, Wallkill Sch Dist, **SLP**

Cornell, Dr Rhonda Holmes 15 Country Club Road, Shalimar, FL 32579, (904) 651-0768, BS 72 Univ of AL-Tuscaloosa; MA 86 Univ of AL- Tuscaloosa; PH 88 (Psychology) Heed Univ; 86–Sp-Lang Path, Private Practice, **SLP**

Cornell, Dr Richard A 3420 Old Dobbin Road, Montgomery, AL 36116, (205) 271-9408, BA 55 OH Univ - Athens; MS 61 Vanderbilt Univ; PH 74 (NS) Northwestern Univ; Assoc Prof & Dir of SLP, Auburn U of Montgy, **A**

Cornett, Dr Becky Sutherland 472 College Parkway #203, Rockville, MD 20850, (301) 897-5700, MA 76 Northwestern Univ; MA 80 Western MI Univ; PH 88 (Communication Disorders) Univ of Pittsburgh - Pittsburgh; Asst Dir Priv Programs Ins, ASHA, **SLP ACE**

Cornett, Mrs Daphne S 52 Tidewater Road, Hattiesburg, MS 39402, (601) 264-6201, BS 78 Univ Southern MS-Hattiesburg; MS 81 Univ Southern MS-Hattiesburg; Sp-Lang Path, Univ of Srthn MS, **SLP**

Cornett, Mrs Lona Ghent R R 1 Box 383, Manchester, KY 40962, (606) 598-2168, BS 78 Eastern KY Univ; MA 82 Eastern KY Univ; **SLP**

Cornett, Lynn H 1514 Ridge Street, Cullman, AL 35055, **SLP**

Cornetta, Eileen Marie 1313 Oakwell Farms Lane, Hermitage, TN 37076, (615) 444-6500, BS 85 Marywood Coll; MS 87 Vanderbilt Univ

Cornforth, Mrs Marilyn Voth Route 3, Jamestown, ND 58401, (701) 252-8449, BA 64 Loma Linda Univ - Riverside; MA 65 Univ of Denver; **SLP**

Cornicelli, Mildred H 2293 Parkwood Drive N W, Warren, OH 44485, **SLP**

Cornuelle, Robert Keith 1104 Holz Avenue, Cincinnati, OH 45230, (513) 231-3045, MA 88 Univ of Cincinnati; 88–Aud, ENT Assoc of Cincinnati

Cornwall, Mrs Judith A 18209 167 Avenue N E, Woodinville, WA 98072, (206) 486-7096, BA 59 WA St Univ; MA 61 Univ of Denver; **SLP**

Cornwell, D Jeanne 665 Mendocina #4, Florissant, MO 63031, (314) 447-4232, BS 81 Southwest MO St Univ; MS 84 Central MO St Univ; 83–Sp-Lang Path, Francis Howell Sch Dist, **SLP**

Cornyn, Aprel L F 206 Sandalwood Drive, Lafayette, LA 70507, **SLP**

Corona, Mrs Diana Marie 908 Lipan Drive, New Braunfels, TX 78130, (512) 629-7726, BS 83 Univ of North TX; MS 87 Southwest TX St Univ; SLP, InSpeech Inc, **SLP**

Coronado, Marcia Chur 1031 Maunaihi Place #802, Honolulu, HI 96822, (808) 433-6488, BS 73 Univ of HI - Manoa; MS 75 Univ of HI - Manoa; Sp-Lang Path, Tripler Army Med Cen, **SLP**

Coroneos, Judith Cann 1227 Westminster, Duncanville, TX 75137, (214) 298-0664, BA 62 Univ of CO - Boulder; MS 86 Univ of TX - Dallas; 86–Sp-Lang Path, Duncanville ISD, **SLP**

Corr, Jill Ziegler St Johns Mercy Medical Center, Dept Of Rehabilitation, 615 South New Ballas Road, St Louis, MO 63141, (314) 569-6175, BS 72 Saint Louis Univ; MA 74 Saint Louis Univ; Dir of Aud, St Johns Med Cen, **A**

Corra, Mrs Norabelle Shuman 1222 20th Street #1, Parkersburg, WV 26101, (304) 420-9554, BS 71 WV Univ; MA 73 OH Univ - Athens; MA 81 WV Univ; 73–Sp-Lang Path, Wood Co Bd of Ed, **SLP**

Corradi, Mrs Barbara Jean 130 Andrew Lane, Lansdale, PA 19446, (215) 997-1261, BS 69 PA St Univ - Univ Park; MS 71 Tulane Univ; Doctoral, Temple Univ, **SLP**

Corradini, Mrs Carol A 5805 S W 113th Street, Miami, FL 33156, (305) 643-5780, BA 63 Montclair St Coll; MA 68 Seton Hall Univ; Sp-Lang Path, Dade Co Pub Sch, **SLP**

Correa, Alma Morales 307 Lyric Drive, San Antonio, TX 78223, (512) 532-4095, BS 54 Southwest TX St Univ; ME 60 Southwest TX St Univ; Sp-Lang Path, Correa Sp-Lang Path Serv, **SLP**

Correll, Judith T 7373 Meridian Hills Court, Apartment C, Indianapolis, IN 46260, (317) 646-8411, BS 78 Ball St Univ; MA 81 Ball St Univ; **A**

Corrigan, Mrs Cynthia Marie 110 Beachview Avenue #224, Bridgeport, CT 06605, (203) 877-0371, BA 80 Univ of CT; MA 81 Univ of CT; Sp-Lang Path, New Medico Assoc, **SLP**

Corrigan, Gayle 4775 Taft, Beaumont, TX 77706, **SLP**

Corrigan, Mrs Judy A 3326 Hampton, Corpus Christi, TX 78414, (512) 991-2814, BS 76 Towson St Univ; OM 74; OM 77 LA St Univ - N O Medical Ctr; Aud, **A**

Corseri, Susan G Newport County Regional Special Education Program, Glen Road, Portsmouth, RI 02871, (401) 683-3570, BA 78 Univ of RI; MA 81 Univ of MA - Amherst; 81–Sp-Lang Path, Newport Co Reg Spec Ed Prog, **SLP**

Corsi-Fraundorf, Laura J N84 W18406 Seneca Drive, Menomonee Falls, WI 53051, (414) 673-6011, BS 77 Old Dominion Univ; MS 79 Marquette Univ; Sp-Lang Path, Dist of Hartford Joint #1, **SLP**

Cort, Mrs Vianne K 1722 South Durango Avenue, Los Angeles, CA 90035, (213) 515-3008, MA 87 CA St Univ - Northridge

Cortazzo, Mary A P O Box 326, Moscow, PA 18444, (717) 842-7222, BS 67 Univ of IA; MS 70 Bloomsburg Univ of PA; SLP, Scranton Sch Dist, **SLP**

Cortelezzi, Mrs Deborah A 9626 Brimfield Dr, Mentor, OH 44060, (216) 882-4133, BS 80 Kent St Univ; MA 80 Kent St Univ; Sp-Lang Path, Manchester Local Sch, **SLP**

Cortese, Emma E 206 High Street, Nutley, NJ 07110, BA 74 Wagner Coll; MA 77 Montclair St Coll; Sp-Lang Path, Sp & Lang Assoc, **SLP**

Cortez, Richard A 28-08 202nd Street, Bayside, NY 11360, (212) 365-5353, BA 73 CUNY - Queens Coll; MS 75 Columbia Univ Teachers Coll; Pres, Mr Otometrics Inc, **A**

Corth, Susan B 331 Quincest, Salt Lake City, UT 84103, (801) 566-1291, BS 79 Univ of UT; MS 81 Univ of UT; Aud, Jordan Sch Dist, **A**

Cortinas, Rochelle M 2821 Trinity Oaks Drive, #352, Arlington, TX 76006, (214) 328-4308, BS 83 TX Christian Univ; MS 85 TX Christian Univ; **SLP**

Cortright, Mrs Joan E M 28760 Norwood, Warren, MI 48092, (313) 264-6080, BA 66 MI St Univ; MA 82 Wayne St Univ; Sp-Lang Path, Warren Consol Sch, **SLP ACE**

Corum, Mrs Susan Smith 4508 Oriole Drive, Knoxville, TN 37918, (615) 521-7476, BS 80 Univ of TN - Knoxville; MA 81 Univ of TN - Knoxville; 88–Sp-Lang Path, Knox County Schs, **SLP**

Corvini, Mrs Joann D 2 Arbor Lane, St James, NY 11780, OB 64 Univ of Miami; MS 69 Adelphi Univ; 75–Sp-Lang Path, BOCES 2, **SLP**

Corwin, Mrs Bonnie Layerle 1160 Willow Avenue, Napa, CA 94559, (707) 253-6865, BA 72 LA St Univ - Baton Rouge; MA 74 LA St Univ - Baton Rouge; SLP, Napa Val USD, **SLP**

Corwin, Carole Route 1 Box 110-B, Fremont, NC 27830, (919) 559-5371, BS 62 Syracuse Univ; MA 65 Syracuse Univ; Sp-Lang Path, Caswell Center, **SLP**

Corwin, Jan R 68 Templar Place, Oakland, CA 94618-2659, (415) 540-4415, BA 81 Univ of MI - Ann Arbor; MS 82 Univ of MI - Ann Arbor; Sp-Lang Path, Alta Bates Herrick Hosp, **SLP**

Corwin-Gotimer, Maria 65 Swift Street, Providence, RI 02904, (617) 528-1266, BA 80 SUNY - Coll at Cortland; MS 81 Syracuse Univ; Sp-Lang Path, Norfolk Public Schools, **SLP**

Cory, Mrs Martha W 3211 7th Street, Boulder, CO 80302-2108, (303) 444-3865, MS 68 Wichita St Univ; 88–Sp-Lang Path, Memorial Hosp-Boulder, **SLP**

Cory, Mrs Miriam E 8346 Isleton Court, Cottage Grove, MN 55016, (612) 487-1445, BS 57 Ball St Univ; SLP, Spec Inter Sch Dist 916, **SLP**

Cory, Thomas L 4780 Logana Plaza, Yorba Linda, CA 92686, BA 73 CA St Univ - Los Angeles; MA 74 CA St Univ - Los Angeles; Resource Spec, Orange USD, **SLP**

Cosaro, Mrs Janet A 75 Flint Lock Lane, Bell Canyon, CA 91307, (818) 347-8316, BA 74 CA St Univ - Northridge; MA 75 CA St Univ - Northridge; Sp-Lang Path, Las Virgenes Sch Dist, **SLP**

Cosart, Mrs Anne Rattray 330 Riverview Drive, Oroville, CA 95966, BA 41 SUNY - Center at Albany; MA 67 CA St Univ - Chico; **SLP LM**

Cosby, Sancha Sharon 2051 Hessian Court, Stone Mountain, GA 30087, (404) 466-2271, **SLP**

Coscarelli-Buchanan, Janet E Tennessee Dept Of Hlth & Envir, Speech & Hearing Services, 100 9th Avenue N Bldg 5405, Nashville, TN 37219, (615) 741-7353, BA 64 OH Univ - Athens; MS 68 Vanderbilt Univ; St Dir Sp & Hrng Serv, St of TN-TN Dept of Hlth-Envir, **SLP A**

Coscia, Mary Ellen 579 Tacoma Avenue, Buffalo, NY 14216, (716) 835-8122, BS 77 SUNY - Coll at Buffalo; MS 81 SUNY - Coll at Buffalo; SLP, Bd of Ed Buffalo, **SLP**

Cosentine, Mrs Brenda H 1445 St Johns Avenue, Highland Park, IL 60035, (312) 432-7180, BA 61 Miami Univ - Oxford; MS 62 Univ of WI - Madison; Sp-Lang Path & Aud, Private Practice, **SLP A**

Cosentino, Cathy A 19530 Shadowoods Drive, Roseville, MI 48066, (313) 293-6157, MA 88 MI St Univ

Cosentino, Mary J 9814 Presidential Drive, Apartment 305, Allison Park, PA 15101, (412) 224-0300, BS 77 Indiana Univ of PA; MS 82 PA St Univ - Univ Park; 87–Sp-Lang Path, Allegheny Intermediate Unit, **SLP**

Coseo, Jane Melanie 120 Maynard Street, Northboro, MA 01532, (508) 393-9509, BS 80 Saint Joseph's Coll; MS 86 Worcester St Coll; 87–Sp-Lang Path, Harrington Memorial Hosp, **SLP**

Cosgray, Nancy D 705 Enderby Drive, Alexandria, VA 22302, **SLP**

Cosgrove, Dawn Michele 7948 North Hayden Road, #E203, Scottsdale, AZ 85258, (602) 951-8681, BA 83 Univ of Northern IA; MA 86 Univ of KS; Sp-Lang Path, **SLP**

Cosgrove, Joan N 120 Deer Point Drive, #14-B, Hendersonville, TN 37075, BS 58 Wayne St Univ; MS 69 Univ of MS; 88–Owner Sp-Lang Path, Commun Skills Enhancement Ctr, **SLP ACE**

Cosgrove, Sarilla B 208 Sweetbriar Road, Greenville, SC 29615, (803) 268-7498, OB 73 Univ of FL; OM 75 Emory Univ; **SLP**

Cosgrove, Mrs Sheree H Rt 3 Box 21, Auburn, AL 36830, (205) 821-4065, OB 76 Univ of FL; MS 77 Auburn Univ - Auburn; 88–Coord-Proj AIM, Auburn Univ, **SLP**

Cosgrove, Yvonne Beth 3 Forest Street, Merrimac, MA 01860, (617) 346-8061, **SLP**

Cosoleto, Catherine Elizabeth Rd 2 Box 134, Millville, PA 17846, (717) 323-8441, MS 84 Bloomsburg Univ of PA; **SLP**

Costa, Carol A 222 South Park Street, Willimantic, CT 06226, (203) 442-0711, BS 74 Northeastern Univ; MA 80 Univ of CT; Aud, Lawrence & Mem Hosp, **A**

Costa, Victoria M 93 Chestnut Avenue, Floral Park, NY 11001, (516) 783-7523, BA 85 Hofstra Univ; MS 87 Adelphi Univ; 88–Sp-Lang Path, Sch for Lang & Communication Development

Costa, Vivian Camille Route 3 Box 418, Pikeville, NC 27863, (919) 731-2234, BA 80 Univ of NC - Greensboro; MS 85 East Carolina Univ; **SLP**

Costa-Natario, Karen Lee 3 Felton Lane, West Newbury, MA 01985, (617) 935-5050, BS 79 Boston Univ; MA 80 Univ of FL; 84–Sp-Lang Path, New England Rehabil Hospital, **SLP**

Costantino, Evelyn Suib 100 Old Farmers Road, Long Valley, NJ 07853, (201) 876-3649, BS 67 OK St Univ; MA 69 OK St Univ; Instr & Cl Superv, U of MS Dept of Commun Dis, **SLP**

Costanzo, Marcia Office Of Speech Language Hearing, Tallman Bldg, 3000 Newport Gap Pike, Wilmington, DE 19808, BS 75 Bowling Green St Univ; MS 81 Miami Univ - Oxford; Sp-Lang Path, Sp Lang Hrng DE Div-Pub Hlth, **SLP**

Costello, Colleen Austin 4945 Dahlia Circle, Liverpool, NY 13088, (315) 470-3223, BS 83 SUNY - Coll at Fredonia; MS 86 Syracuse Univ

Costello, Elizabeth M 604 West Washington Street, Bradford, PA 16701, (814) 368-4545, BS 77 Brescia Coll; MS 78 Univ of WI - Stevens Point; Sp/Lang Path, Private Practice, **SLP**

Costello, Jacalyn Rose 12 Providence Road, Mendon, MA 01756, (508) 478-3147, BS 74 Univ of MA - Amherst; ME 75 Boston Univ; 75–Sp-Lang Path, Town of Milford, **SLP**

Costello, Mrs Jean F O 3224 Kimberly Road, Shingle Springs, CA 95682, (916) 622-7130, BA 76 CA St Univ - Sacramento; MA 78 CA St Univ - Sacramento; SLP, El Dorado Co Off of Ed, **SLP**

Costello, John Michael 132 Arlington Street, Brighton, MA 02135, (617) 782-6305, BA 83 Boston Coll; MA 85 Univ of MA - Amherst; **SLP**

Costello, Margaret Neary 910 North Irving Avenue, Scranton, PA 18510, (717) 586-2511, BA 70 Marywood Coll; ME 75 Bloomsburg Univ of PA; Sp-Lang Path, Northeastern Intermediate Unit

Costello, Dr Mary R 5210 Tangerine South, Gulfport, FL 33707, BS 39 Washington Univ; MA 46 Northwestern Univ; PH 57 (NS) Northwestern Univ; **SLP A F LM**

Costello, Mrs Nancy L 1308 South Halliburton, Kirksville, MO 63501, (816) 665-2326, MA 88 Northeast MO St Univ; 87–SLP, Kirksville R-III Sch Dist

Costello, Thomas J Rd 1 Box 219-C, Ligonier, PA 15658, (412) 836-2460, BS 62 Indiana Univ of PA; MS 66 Univ of MI - Ann Arbor; **SLP**

Costenero, Mrs Joan M 1N043 Papworth, Wheaton, IL 60187, (312) 620-3780, BS 81 Ball St Univ; MA 82 Western IL Univ; Sp-Lang Path, Lombard Sch Dist #44, **SLP**

Coster, Mrs Judianne Longfield Ews Bushy Hill Road, Simsbury, CT 06070, (203) 658-2690, BS 76 Bowling Green St Univ; MA 87 Univ of CT

Coster, Mrs Judy L 3298 Essex, Troy, MI 48084, (313) 661-9400, 88–Sp-Lang Path, Communication Disorders Inc, **SLP ACE**

Costigan, Mrs Carter Rainsford 225 Knox Avenue, Aiken, SC 29801, (803) 649-9811, BA 74 Hollins Coll; OM 75 Auburn Univ - Auburn; Sp-Lang Path, Private Practice, **SLP**

Costigan, Linda D 516 Bailey Road #102, Naperville, IL 60565, (312) 355-8358, BS 78 SUNY - Coll at New Paltz; MA 83 Hofstra Univ; Sp-Lang Path, BOCES II, **SLP**

Costigan, Sharon L 178 Purchase Street, Milford, MA 01757, (603) 742-4731, MS 88 Univ of NH

Costin, Gail 904 Cheryl Lane, Wilmington, NC 28405, **SLP**

Costin, Karen S 4206 West Orchard Drive, Bloomfield Hills, MI 48013, (313) 642-8805, BS 64 Bowling Green St Univ; **SLP**

Costlow, Linda Ann 8513 Evangeline N E, Albuquerque, NM 87111, (505) 298-0572

Coston, Mrs Carol C University Of South Carolina, 1601 St Julian Place, Columbia, SC 29204, (803) 777-2614, BA 67 Columbia Coll; MS 69 Vanderbilt Univ; 73–Sp-Lang Path, U So Carolina Sp & Hrng Clinic, **SLP**

Coston, Dr Gale Norman Dept Communicative Disorders, Univ Of South Carolina, Columbia, SC 29208, (803) 777-4813, BA 65 Univ of GA; MS 66 Univ of GA; ED 69 (NS) Univ of GA; Prof Dir Cleft Palate Lab, Univ of SC, **SLP F**

Coston, Mrs Susan Steinour 220 Ewell Avenue, Gettysburg, PA 17325, (717) 334-8756, MS 77 Loyola Coll; Sp-Lang Path, Private Practice, **SLP**

Cote, Mrs Donna Jane 2 Sharon Drive, Bow, NH 03301-6759, (603) 224-8446, BS 76 Univ of NH; ME 81 Northwestern Univ; 86–Sp-Lang Path, NH Sch Dept, **SLP**

Cote, Mrs Isabelle 932 Payant, Ville Lasalle, PQ, Canada M8R 3Y9, (514) 363-2819, OM 88 McGill Univ - Quebec

Cote, Mrs Janet Marion 488 Bushy Hill Road, Simsbury, CT 06070, (203) 651-4741, **SLP**

Cote, Mary Particia 612 Orion Road #221, Lake Orion, MI 48035, (313) 656-8380, BS 84 MI St Univ; MA 88 Central MI Univ; 85–Aud, Professional Consultant, **A**

Cote-Akerley, Stephanie P O Box 2173, Lewiston, ME 04240-0042, (207) 795-6117, BS 84 Univ of ME - Farmington; MS 86 Syracuse Univ; 86–Sp-Lang Path, NE Hearing & Speech Ctr Inc, **SLP**

Cotter, Mrs Debora Joyce 726 South El Molino, Pasadena, CA 91106, (213) 224-0100, BA 79 NM St Univ; MS 83 AZ St Univ; Sp-Lang Path, State Diagnostic School, **SLP**

Cotter, Nancy Brennan 2 Tremont Street, Charlestown, MA 02129, (617) 242-9024, BA 81 Bridgewater St Coll; MS 87 Emerson Coll; 87–Sp-Lang Path, Boston City Schs

Cotter, Pricilla M 395 Freedom Road, Freedom, PA 15042, (412) 787-2350, BA 79 Univ of Pittsburgh - Pittsburgh; MA 81 Univ of Pittsburgh - Pittsburgh; Coordinator SLP & Aud, Robinson Developmental Ctr, **SLP**

Cotter, Tracy Lynn 40 Collinwood Drive, Pittsburgh, PA 15215, (215) 631-9300, BA 2605; MA 86 2605; **SLP**

Cotterell, Mrs Kathy L 222 East North Avenue, Sumner, IL 62466, MS 78 Eastern IL Univ; **SLP**

Cotterell, Patricia A 13 Plum Street #B, New Brunswick, NJ 08901, (201) 937-8655, BS 79 PA St Univ - Univ Park; MA 81 Univ of TN - Knoxville; 88–Asst Dir-Sp & Hrng Dept, Robert Wood Johnson University Hosp, **A**

Cottier, Cynthia A 7006 Shinning Avenue, San Gabriel, CA 91775, (818) 285-2525, BA 76 Univ of Southern CA; MA 80 CA St Univ - Long Beach; Sp-Lang Path, Los Angeles USD, **SLP**

Cottingham, Linda M 5870 East Illinois, Fresno, CA 93727, (209) 638-6976, BA 76 CA St Univ - Fresno; MA 78 CA St Univ - Fresno; Sp-Lang Path, Kings Canyon USD, **SLP**

Cottle, Cheri Colleen 117A East Biddle Street, West Chester, PA 19380, (215) 431-7123, BS 84 PA St Univ - Univ Park; MS 87 PA St Univ - Univ Park; 88–Aud, Team Rehabilitation Inc, **A**

Cottone, Debra Ann 10250 Caenen, Lenexa, KS 66215, (816) 276-4027, BS 84 Central MO St Univ; MS 87 Central MO St Univ; Aud, Research Medical Center, **A**

Cottor, Mary Kappel 2124 Yorkshire Road, Sacramento, CA 95815, **SLP**

Cottrell, Gary T 1773 State Route 59 #7, Kent, OH 44240, (216) 678-5839, BA 80 MI St Univ; MA 82 Central MI Univ; **A**

Cottrell, Dr Mary M 3411 San Felipe Drive, Baton Rouge, LA 70809, (504) 769-5664, BS 69 WV Univ; MS 73 WV Univ; PH 77 (NS) Univ of UT; SLP, Cl Affiliates Inc, **SLP**

Couch, Mrs Gibbs Daniel 1007 Felton Lane, Auburn, AL 36830, (205) 887-2100, BS 59 Univ of Montevallo; MA 70 Auburn Univ - Auburn; Sp/Lang Path, Auburn City Schools, **SLP**

Couch, Marla Floy P O Box # 1, Grand Island, NY 14072, (716) 773-3198, BS 85 SUNY - Coll at Buffalo; MS 86 SUNY - Coll at Buffalo; 88–Sp-Lang Path, The Rehabilitation Ctr, **SLP**

Couch, Meredith Ellen 147 Alpine Knoll, Fairport, NY 14450, (716) 425-1180, BS 86 SUNY - Coll at Geneseo; MA 87 SUNY - Coll at Geneseo; 87–Sp-Lang Path, Monroe #1 BOCES, **SLP**

Couch, Teri C 1905 Rosewood, Pocahontas, AR 72455, (501) 886-5737, BS 72 AR St Univ; MS 79 AR St Univ; Sp-Lang Path, Hoxie Pub Sch, **SLP**

Couchenour, Laurie Ann 34255 Coastal Drive, Sterling Heights, MI 48310, (313) 280-8400, OB 84 Geneva Coll; MA 86 Wayne St Univ; **SLP**

Couey, Mrs Catherine W 105 Nelson, NBU 44G, Fort Huachuca, AZ 85613, (602) 459-4751, BS 74 Vanderbilt Univ; MA 78 TN Tech Univ; Sp-Lang Path, **SLP**

Coufal, Kathy L 16642 Dorcas Circle, Omaha, NE 68130, (402) 330-3858, BS 72 Univ of NE - Lincoln; MA 73 Univ of NE - Lincoln; Sp-Lang Path, **SLP ACE**

Coughlin, Bobette Marie 122 Rue Du Jardin, Lafayette, LA 70507, (318) 237-6470, BA 86 Univ of Southwestern LA; MS 86 Univ of Southwestern LA; 88–Sp-Lang Path, St Landry Parish Sch Bd, **SLP**

Coughlin, Mrs Bonita G 13652 North 69th Drive, Peoria, AZ 85345, (602) 938-7218, BS 73 Univ of IL - Urbana; MS 74 Univ of IL - Urbana; 79–Sp-Lanq Path, Deer Valley USD, **SLP**

Coughlin, Mrs Jane R 315 Meadowcroft Lane, Lutherville, MD 21093, (301) 321-1304, BA 74 Univ of Rochester; MA 77 Northwestern Univ; Sp-Lang Path, Private Practice, **SLP**

Coughlin, Mrs Janel McKinney Route 8 Box 525, 309 Walnut Drive, Paducah, KY 42001, (502) 444-7017, BS 74 Murray St Univ; MS 81 Murray St Univ; Sp-Lang Path, Paducah Public Schools, **SLP**

Coughlin, Joanne Perdzock 2455 South Main Street, Ann Arbor, MI 48103, (313) 572-3816, BS 77 Miami Univ - Oxford; MA 82 Kent St Univ; Audiologist, Catherine McAuley Health Cen, **A**

Coughlin, Mary Therese 7807 West 82nd Place, Bridgeview, IL 60455, (312) 731-1161, **SLP**

Coughlin, Patrick M Aberdeen Prof Hearing Service, 310 8th Avenue N W, P O Box 1916, Aberdeen, SD 57401, (605) 229-3688, BS 72 Minot St Univ; MS 74 Minot St Univ; Audiologist, Aberdeen Prof Hearing Service, **A**

Coughlin, Mrs Sheryl Thomas 5 Terron Court, Baltimore, MD 21234, (301) 522-5700, BA 83 Loyola Coll; MS 84 Loyola Coll; 85–Sp-Lang Path, Kennedy Inst, **SLP**

Coughlin, Susan S 727 Cummings Avenue, Kenilworth, IL 60043, BA 64 Univ of KY; MA 65 Univ of KY; **SLP**

Coughlin, Suzanne Sobaski 1427 North Mission Road, Mount Pleasant, MI 48858, (517) 774-7290, BS 74 Central MI Univ; MA 76 Central MI Univ; MA 85 Central MI Univ; Dir Summer Remedial Clin, Central MI U, **SLP ACE**

Coughlin, Dr William A 204 Audubon Road, Fayetteville, NY 13066, (315) 476-7461, ME 66 Boston St Coll; MA 69 Univ of MA - Amherst; PH 80 (NS) SUNY - Center at Buffalo; Sp-Lang Path, VA Medical Center, **SLP**

Coulles, Mrs Linda C 8719 Cobblecreek Drive, Dayton, OH 45458, (513) 435-1234, BS 71 Miami Univ - Oxford; MS 72 Miami Univ - Oxford; 73–SLP, West Carrollton City Schs, **SLP**

Coulon, Ellen L 192 Bay 47th, Brooklyn, NY 11214, (212) 390-9470, BS 79 Ithaca Coll; MA 80 George Washington Univ; Sp-Lang Path, Staten Island Hosp, **SLP**

Coulson, Tamara E A 21327 52nd Avenue S E, Woodinville, WA 98072, (206) 526-2104, BS 84 Univ of WA; MS 86 Univ of WA; **SLP**

Coulter, Jody Katt 13971 La Maida Street, Sherman Oaks, CA 91423, MA 72 Univ of Southern CA; SLP, LA Cty USD, **SLP**

Coulter, Leanne McJunkin 119 Dorsey Street, Cincinnati, OH 45210, (606) 581-6391, BS 80 Miami Univ - Oxford; MA 82 Marshall Univ; Sp-Lang Path, Hamilton County Office of Educ, **SLP**

Coulter, Linda W 1975 Red House Road, Richmond, KY 40475, (606) 254-5701, BS 84 Eastern KY Univ; MA 85 Eastern KY Univ; 87–Sp-Lang Path, Child Dev Ctrs, **SLP**

Coulter, Mrs Lisa Tateoka 12550 South 2700 West, Riverton, UT 84065, (801) 254-7840, MS 87 UT St Univ

Coulter, Lisa Tateoka 12550 So 2700 West, Riverton, UT 84065, (801) 254-7840, BS 83 UT St Univ; **SLP**

Coulter, Mary Elise 4454 Cardiff, Fort Worth, TX 76133, (817) 294-4730, BS 67 Univ of KS; MA 74 KS St Univ; 88–Sp-Lang Path, InSpeech Inc, **SLP**

Coulter, Mrs Susan Green 9245 Seawind Court, Columbia, MD 21045, (301) 964-8302, BA 75 Mary Baldwin Coll; ME 79 Univ of NC - Greensboro; 87–Sp-Lang Path, St Agnes Hosp, **SLP**

Councill, Cheryl Anne 1210 Canberwell Road, Catonsville, MD 21228, (301) 381-9700, BA 81 Loyola Coll; MS 82 Loyola Coll; Clin Supvr, Loyola Coll, **SLP**

Counihan, Dr Donald T Univ Of Oklahoma Medical Ctr, 825 N E 14th, Oklahoma City, OK 73104, (405) 271-4214, BS 49 Northwestern Univ; MA 51 Northwestern Univ; PH 56 (NS) Northwestern Univ; Prof & Chair, U of OK Hlth Sci Cen, **SLP F**

Counihan, Mrs Marylin A 10701 Eastlake Circle, Oklahoma City, OK 73132, (405) 721-6199, MA 52; BA 51; Sp/Lang Path, Private Practice, **SLP**

Counter, S Allen Biological Laboratories, Harvard University, 16 Divinity Avenue, Cambridge, MA 02138, **A**

Counters, Thomas A 13212 Elm Lane, Burnsville, MN 55337, (612) 890-0420, BS 66 Univ of MN - Minneap-St Paul; MA 71 Univ of MN - Minneap-St Paul; Supvr, Dist 917, **A**

Countryman, Cora A 2345 Northumberland, Orange, CA 92665, (714) 847-8571, **SLP**

Countryman, Darlene M 33266 Ocean Bright, Dana Point, CA 92629, BS 84 SD St Univ; MS 86 Univ of WI - River Falls

Counts, Dr Alfred B 6402 Route 32, Clarksville, MD 21029, (301) 854-0084, BA 50 Pepperdine Univ - Los Angele; MA 56 Univ of Southern CA; PH 72 (NS) Univ of MD - College Park; Psychol & SLP Consult, Their Inc, **SLP**

Counts, Clarice R 6402 Route 32, Clarksville, MD 21029, (301) 531-6686, BA 43 Univ of MD - College Park; MA 56 Univ of Southern CA; Pres, Care Inc, **SLP**

Counts, Lou H 6869 Circle Creek Drive, Pinellas Park, FL 34665, (813) 544-3021, MS 72 Univ of South FL; Aud, Private Practice, **A**

Coursen, Judith Denenberg 20260 Brookshire, Southfield, MI 48076, (313) 557-3650, BA 81 MI St Univ; MA 82 MI St Univ; Aud, Rontal Rontal & Jacob, **A**

Coursey, Mrs Susan Route 1 Box 112, Dexter, KY 42036, (502) 437-4253, BS 75 Murray St Univ; MS 81 Murray St Univ; Sp-Lang Path, Marshall County Board of Educ, **SLP**

Courter, Teresa Marie 2100-325 Paces Forest Court, Raleigh, NC 27612, (919) 787-7159, BS 81 Indiana Univ of PA; MS 86 James Madison Univ; Sp-Lang Path, Wake Co PS, **SLP**

Courtney, Anne Sheffield 612 South Courtland, Park Ridge, IL 60068, (312) 823-6131, BA 63 Univ of UT; MS 65 Univ of UT; Sp-Lang Path, Spec Ed Dept Cicero Pub Schls, **SLP**

Courtney, Deborah P 2375 Tudor Drive, Cleveland Heights, OH 44106, (216) 459-3161, BA 53 Univ of CO - Boulder; MA 74 Case Western Reserve Univ; Sp-Lang Path, Clev Gen Hosp-Dept-Commun Dis, **SLP**

Courtney, Mrs E LaWanda DoDDS-Kaiserslautern DSO, APO New York, NY 09094-0005, BS 61 Southwest TX St Univ; MA 62 Southwest TX St Univ; Special Educ Specialist, DoDDS, **SLP**

Courtney, Joan Bedford 16506 Bridge End Road, Miami Lakes, FL 33014, (305) 376-1290, BA 68 Barry Univ; MS 76 Barry Univ; MS 87 Nova Univ; **SLP**

Courtney, Julia A 41 Ballard Street, Jamaica Plain, MA 02130, (617) 522-4532, BS 84 Univ of MA - Amherst; MS 86 Northeastern Univ; **SLP**

Courtney, Margie Lynn 138-C Kellogg Road, Cortland, NY 13045, (607) 722-5308, BS 80 OH Univ - Athens; MS 86 Ithaca Coll; SLP, Rehab Srvs Inc, **SLP**

Courtney, Thomas W 43531 37th Street West, Lancaster, CA 93536, (805) 943-7630, **SLP**

Courtright, Illene C 4 Fairvalley Court, Newark, DE 19711, (302) 738-9188, BS 72 Univ of IA; MS 73 Univ of IA; 86–Sp-Lang Path, Christina Sch Dist, **SLP**

Courville, Adele R L 11110 Whiteside Road, New Orleans, LA 70128, **SLP**

Cousino, Mrs Mary E 4429 North Haven Avenue, Toledo, OH 43612, (419) 278-3050, MA 83 Bowling Green St Univ; Sp-Lang Path, Toledo Hospital, **SLP**

Cousino, Pamela H 5372 River Oaks Court, Sylvania, OH 43560, (419) 321-2981, BS 80 Clarion Univ of PA; MS 81 Clarion Univ of PA; Sp-Lang Path, St Vincent Med Ctr, **SLP**

Cousins, Mrs Becky R Afelm Nato Awacs Box 1524, APO New York, NY 09104, MS 71 IN Univ - Bloomington; Tchr, DODDS-Germany, **SLP**

Cousins, Mrs Gayle R R R 2 Box 9, Deerwood, MN 56444, (218) 546-6941, BA 74 Univ of OR; MS 76 CO St Univ; 88–Aud, Central Lakes Hrng Svcs, **A**

Couts, Nancy 21 Woodbridge Street, Cambridge, MA 02140, (617) 499-5061, BS 75 Kent St Univ; MA 77 Kent St Univ; Sp-Lang Path, Mount Auburn Hosp, **SLP**

Coutts, Marylou Mt Developmental Center, Box 87, Boulder, MT 59632, (406) 225-3311, BS 76 Marywood Coll; MS 78 Bloomsburg Univ of PA; 85–Supervisor Communication Dept, Montana Developmental Center, **SLP**

Covell, Mrs Jane Scory 881 North River Road, Coventry, CT 06238, (203) 647-3313, BA 56 Tufts Univ; ME 59 Boston Univ; Sp-Lang Path, Manchester Co Bd of Ed, **SLP**

Cover, Mrs Suzanne Britt 2232-B Bonaparte Boulevard, Montgomery, AL 36116, (205) 284-5470, BS 80 East Carolina Univ; MS 81 Univ of NC - Chapel Hill; Aud, Hrng Aid Cen/Panama Cty Inc, **A**

Coverman, Mrs Gail B 593 Whisper Wood Drive, Longwood, FL 32779, BA 72 Univ of Miami; ME 73 Univ of Miami; Sp-Lang Path, **SLP**

Covert, Mrs Kathleen Windy Hill Professional Center, 2050 Garber Road, Box 16, Winchester, VA 22601, (703) 667-0100, BS 69 OH Univ - Athens; MA 72 Marshall Univ; Dir Sp-Lang Path Serv, Private Practice, **SLP**

Covert, Kathleen Gillin 401 Ultimo Avenue, Long Beach, CA 90814-2044, (805) 489-1351, BA 69 San Francisco St Univ; MA 71 San Francisco St Univ; SLP, Lucia Mar USD, **SLP**

Covey, Lee Ellen 301 Oak Street, Carterville, IL 62918, (618) 997-5311, BS 84 Northern IL Univ - De Kalb; MS 86 Univ of AR - Little Rock; 88–Sp-Lang Path, VA Med Ctr, **SLP**

Covey-McKeage, Mrs Jennifer Lu 1160 Main Street, Vestal, NY 13850, (607) 798-7117, BS 76 SUNY - Coll at Geneseo; MS 80 PA St Univ - Univ Park; Sp-Lang Path, United Health Services, **SLP**

Covin, Regina R 54 Seneca Drive, Noank, CT 06340, (203) 536-0550, BA 72 SUNY - Coll at Plattsburgh; MS 75 Ithaca Coll; Sp-Lang Path, Ledyard Pub Sch, **SLP**

Covington, Dr Ann J 1936 West Boston Boulevard, Tougaloo College, Detroit, MI 48206, (313) 883-6417, BA 52 Eastern MI Univ; MS 54 Milligan Coll; PH 72 (NS) Univ of Pittsburgh - Pittsburgh; Academic Dean, Tougaloo College, **SLP A F**

Covington, Mrs Jan R MSU Speech And Hearing Center, 807 Jefferson Avenue, Memphis, TN 38105, BS 69 Memphis St Univ; MA 71 Memphis St Univ; Clinical Instructor, Memphis State University, **SLP**

Covington, Mrs Kathy Lynn Route 2 Box 11, Meridian, MS 39305, (601) 681-8195

Covington, Sheryl J S 13600 Woodmont, Detroit, MI 48227, (313) 455-8880, BA 80 MI St Univ; MA 81 MI St Univ; 85–Sp-Lang Path, MI Dept Mental Health, **SLP**

Covington, Zenara Walthea 3878 17th Street, Ecorse, MI 48229, (313) 745-9721, BS 85 Univ of MI - Ann Arbor; MS 87 PA St Univ - Univ Park; 87–Sp-Lang Path, Rehab Institute Inc, **SLP**

Cowan, Beth Ann 8205 Raintree Circle, Culver City, CA 90230, (213) 396-5343, BS 77 SUNY - Coll at Buffalo; ME 79 Northeastern Univ; **SLP**

Cowan, Bonnie Weinberg 13817 Congress Drive, Rockville, MD 20853-2632, (301) 460-0220, BA 78 Univ of MO - Columbia; MA 81 Memphis St Univ; Sp-Lang Path, Private Practice, **SLP**

Cowan, Mrs Dorothy R 320 Oakhurst Lane, Colorado Springs, CO 80906, (719) 576-2177, BA 57 Univ of MT; MA 63 Univ of MN - Minneap-St Paul; **SLP**

Cowan, Heather E 534-Chelsea Avenue, Winnipeg, MB, Canada R2K 1A3, (204) 787-2740, BA 77; MS 79 Minot St Univ; Aud, Hlth Sci Cen, **A**

Cowan, Katherine Elizabeth Sullivan School, Box 96, FPO Seattle, WA 98762, 81-468-26-1911, BA 83 Mary Washington Coll; MS 87 Univ of KY; 87–Sp-Lang Path, Dept of Def Dep Schs, **SLP**

Cowan, Dr Nancy S 10400 Gatewood Terrace, Silver Spring, MD 20903, (202) 651-5466, BA 54 Depauw Univ; MA 74 WV Coll of Graduate Studies; PH 80 (Human Dev) Univ of MD - College Park; 75–Sp-Lang Path, Gallaudet Univ, **SLP**

Cowan, Pamela R 519 Elizabeth Street, Elmira, NY 14901, (607) 734-3911, BS 74 Syracuse Univ; MS 75 Syracuse Univ; Cl Superv/SLP, Elmira College, **SLP**

Cowand, Paula Joan 4444 South Rio Grande #802, Orlando, FL 32809, (813) 972-7259, BA 84 Univ of Central FL; MS 87 Univ of South FL; **A**

Cowan-Oberbeck, Catherine 1663 Painter Street S E, Palm Bay, FL 32909, (407) 676-2353, BA 77 Univ of South FL; MA 81 Univ of Central FL; Aud, Private Practice, **A**

Cowart, Gwendolyn 2413 Ellingham, Wichita Falls, TX 76308, (817) 692-6611, BS 47 TX Tech Univ; ME 64 West TX St Univ; MA 70 Univ of North TX; Program Director, Midwestern State University, **SLP**

Cowart, Mrs Rosa Cash 990 Central Avenue, Apartment 157, Riverside, CA 92507, (714) 784-1838, BS 38 West TX St Univ; MA 67 West TX St Univ; **SLP LM**

Cowder, W Wayne Rd 1 Box 213, Lindside, WV 24951, (304) 753-4328, BA 66 Trenton St Coll; MS 71 Rutger's St Univ - Douglas Coll; Sp-Lang Path, Monroe Co BOCES, **SLP**

Cowen, Alexandra Lee 353 Kenilworth Drive, Akron, OH 44313, (216) 867-2172, BS 84 Northwestern Univ; MA 85 Northwestern Univ; Sp-Lang Path, Childrens Hospital/Med Ctr/Ak, **SLP**

Cowen, Mrs Roberta Polgar 1044 Erin Drive, El Cajon, CA 92020, (619) 589-2045, BA 78 Univ of the Pacific; MA 81 San Diego St Univ; Sp-Lang Path, Lakeside Union Sch Dist, **SLP**

Cowgill, Mrs Susan P 2260 23rd Street, Beaumont, TX 77706, (409) 886-2253, BA 74 Univ of MS; MA 75 Univ of TN - Knoxville; Aud, Private Practice, **A**

Cowherd, Mrs Ruth Karen 326 Crown Point, Columbia, MO 65203, (314) 696-2282, BS 75 Central MO St Univ; MS 79 Central MO St Univ; Sp-Lang Path, Boone Co Riv Schs, **SLP**

Cowin, Eileen Cotovsky 1588 Chapel Court, Northbrook, IL 60062, (312) 480-3035, BS 73 Southern IL Univ -Carbondale; MA 74 Univ of IL - Urbana; SLP, Hs Dist 214, **SLP**

Cowley, Debra 2129 North Towne Court N E, Apartment 8, Cedar Rapids, IA 52402-1959, (605) 624-6723, BA 82 Augustana Coll; MA 87 Univ of SD - Vermillion; **A**

Cowling-Reed, Dr Karen M 1003 Briarhill Court, New Bern, NC 28560, (904) 638-3994, BS 76 Bloomsburg Univ of PA; MS 77 Bloomsburg Univ of PA; ED 82 (Educ Psych) WV Univ; 87–Sp-Lang Path, Private Practice, **SLP**

Cowper, Mrs Ellen Elizabeth 25 Buxton Road, Cherry Hill, NJ 08003, (609) 424-3483, OB 37 Univ of Akron; BA 37 Univ of Akron; MA 43 Univ of MI - Ann Arbor; 88–Sp-Lang Path, Private Practice, **SLP**

Cox, Mrs Barbara M 448 Bentleyville Road, Chagrin Falls, OH 44022, (216) 564-2282, MA 57 Univ of MI - Ann Arbor; SLP, Newbury Local Schs, **SLP**

Cox, Benton W, III 1423 Hawkdrest Cove North, Cordova, TN 38018-2911, (901) 682-1529, BA 76 Memphis St Univ; MA 78 Memphis St Univ; Aud, Cox Hearing Serv, **A**

Cox, Dr Bernard P 9005 Wandering Trail Drive, Potomac, MD 20854, (202) 651-5328, BA 63 George Washington Univ; MS 66 Univ of Pittsburgh - Pittsburgh; PH 69 (NS) Univ of Pittsburgh - Pittsburgh; Dir Cl Serv/Assis Prof of Aud, Gallaudet College, **A**

Cox, Beth P 36 Lakeview Drive S E, Lindale, GA 30147, **SLP**

Cox, Mrs Betty T 105 Brookwood Drive, Thomasville, GA 31792, (912) 225-2600, BS 51 Univ of GA; ME 70 FL St Univ; Spec Ed Dir, Thomasville Cty Bd of Ed, **SLP**

Cox, Billie P 2955 Pineridge Avenue, Cincinnati, OH 45208, (513) 321-2629, BA 47 Drury Coll; MS 50 Univ of MI - Ann Arbor; SLP, **SLP**

Cox, Cynthia A 1109 Lakeway, Kalamazoo, MI 49001, (616) 382-1216, BS 67 Western MI Univ; MA 77 Western MI Univ; Sp-Lang Path, Kalamazoo Pub Sch, **SLP**

Cox, Deborah A P O Box 265, Wethersfield, CT 06109, (203) 342-3131, BS 72 WV Univ; MS 74 WV Univ; Sp-Lang Path, Glastonbury CT PS, **SLP**

Cox, Edith Lynne 8421 Rustwood Place, Charlotte, NC 28212, (704) 333-6634, BA 81 Univ of TN - Knoxville; MA 82 Univ of TN - Knoxville; Aud, Charlotte Rehab Hosp, **A**

Cox, Dr Geraldine P O Box 307, Summersville, WV 26651, (803) 798-3978, BS 64 WV Univ; ME 66 Univ of VA - Charlottesville; ED 74 (NS) Univ of VA - Charlottesville; **SLP**

Cox, Mrs Geraline Hinton 2156 Millville Road, Chesapeake, VA 23323, (804) 393-8751, BS 69 Hampton Univ; MA 79 Hampton Univ; **SLP**

Cox, Herbert A, III 5711 Gardner Court Drive, Tampa, FL 33604, (813) 879-8045, MS 72 Univ of South FL; Aud, Tampa ENT Cl, **A**

Cox, Dr James R P O Box 307, Summersville, WV 26651, (803) 777-4813, BS 64 WV Univ; ME 66 Univ of VA - Charlottesville; PH 74 (NS) Univ of VA - Charlottesville; Assoc Prof of Aud, Univ of S Carolina, **A**

Cox, Mrs Juanita Z 1309 Fountain, Ann Arbor, MI 48103, (313) 994-8111, BS 64 Eastern MI Univ; MA 72 Eastern MI Univ; Sp-Lang Path, Washtenaw ISD, **SLP**

Cox, Mrs Karen L 3345 North 50 East, Greenfield, IN 46140, (317) 462-5265, BS 81 Ball St Univ; MA 82 Ball St Univ; Sp-Lang Path, Indianapolis Pub Sch, **SLP**

Cox, Mrs Kathleen M 1904 East Oakland Avenue, Bloomington, IL 61701, (309) 663-7154, BS 77 Ball St Univ; MA 78 Univ of IL - Urbana; SLP, Private Practice, **SLP**

Cox, L Clarke 720 Harrison Avenue, Suite 601, Boston, MA 02118, (617) 536-3220, BS 72 UT St Univ; MS 73 UT St Univ; PH 75 (NS) Bowling Green St Univ; Aud, Boston Univ Sch of Med, **A**

Cox, Leslie Wooddy 22 Faith Court, Damascus, MD 20872, (301) 253-1331, MA 84 Univ of Houston - Univ Park; Sp-Lang Path, Montgomery County Pub Schools, **SLP**

Cox, Linda Ruth Pasco County Public Schools, Audiology Department, 1500 Parkway Boulevard, Land O'Lakes, FL 34639, (813) 996-3600, BS 80 Minot St Univ; MA 86 5518; 87–Aud/Tchr, Dist Sch Bd of Pasco Co, **A**

Cox, Mrs Lisa Thurman 5929 Ridgewood Road, Knoxville, TN 37918, (515) 637-4935, BA 80 Univ of TN - Knoxville; MA 81 Univ of TN - Knoxville; Sp-Lang Path, Pediatric Language Clinic, **SLP**

Cox, Mrs Marielise Kress 34-B Locust Drive, Jamesburg, NJ 08831, (201) 521-2145, BA 78 Rutger's St Univ - Douglas Coll; MS 81 Rutgers St Univ -N Brunswick; Sp-Lang Path, Middlesex Cnty Ed Serv Comm, **SLP**

Cox, Mary Steele 206 West Stayton, Victoria, TX 77901, (512) 576-3003, BS 72 Univ of TX - Austin; ME 76 Trinity Univ; OM 80 Univ of TX - Austin; **SLP**

Cox, Mrs Michelle Elizabeth 200 Millwood Circle Apartment 721, Maumelle, AR 72118, (501) 223-7558, BA 83 Ouachita Baptist Univ; MS 85 Univ of AR - Little Rock; 88–Sp-Lang Path, Arkansas Rehab Inst, **SLP**

Cox, Mrs Nancy L 211 Shadow Wood Drive, Hattiesburg, MS 39401, (601) 266-5223, OB 69 Univ of NE - Lincoln; MS 85 Univ Southern MS-Hattiesburg; **SLP**

Cox, Mrs Robbie Rice 119 Clancy Circle, Cary, NC 27511, (919) 467-5661, BA 79 Univ of NC - Greensboro; ME 82 Univ of NC - Greensboro; Sp-Lang Path, **SLP**

Cox, Dr Robyn M Memphis Speech & Hearing Ctr, 807 Jefferson Avenue, Memphis, TN 38105, (901) 525-2682, BS 69 Ball St Univ; MA 71 Ball St Univ; PH 74 (NS) IN Univ - Bloomington; Prof, Memphis St U, **A**

Cox, Ronald S 123 San Leon #123, Irvine, CA 92714, (714) 261-6569, BA 81 Biola Univ; MA 83 CA St Univ - Fullerton; Sp-Lang Path, Marina Prof Serv, **SLP**

Cox, Sandy K 6911 50th Terrace #140, Mission, KS 66202, (913) 588-5730, BS 84 ID St Univ; MS 86 Univ of UT; Aud, Ku Med Ctr, **A**

Cox, Mrs Sharon O 1187 Culligan Lane, St Paul, MN 55118, (612) 228-3627, BA 58 Univ of IA; MA 64 Univ of IA; Asst Dir-Curr Instr-Sp Ed, St Paul Pub Sch, **SLP**

Cox, Susan E 3907 East 27th Street, Des Moines, IA 50317, **SLP**

Cox, Mrs Teresa J P O Box 3674 Crs, Johnson City, TN 37602, (615) 538-5793, BS 75 East TN St Univ; MA 77 East TN St Univ; Sp-Lang Path, Private Practice, **SLP**

Cox-Andrews, Helen Kaye 8 Sandon Circle, Asheville, NC 28804, (704) 255-5001, BS 75 Univ of VA - Charlottesville; ME 76 Univ of VA - Charlottesville; Sp-Lang Path, Asheville City Schs, **SLP**

Cox-Willms, Carol C 217 Arabian Court, Loveland, CO 80537, (303) 584-7087, BA 74 San Diego St Univ; MA 76 San Diego St Univ; **A**

Coyle, Carol Ann 1907 Woodland Drive, Yardley, PA 19067, (215) 757-0227, BS 69 East Stroudsburg Univ of PA; ME 73 Trenton St Coll; Sp-Lang Path, Bucks Co Inter Ut 22, **SLP**

Coyle, Mrs Jane Cannon 271-M Signs Road, Staten Island, NY 10314, (212) 596-3545, BA 68 SUNY - Coll at Oneonta; MS 70 SUNY - Coll at Geneseo; Supervisor of Speech, New York City Board of Educ, **SLP**

Coyle, Jane N 3304 Rollingwood Drive, Woodbridge, VA 22192, (703) 866-3070, BS 76 Univ of IL - Urbana; MS 77 Univ of IL - Urbana; **SLP**

Coyle, Mrs Kathryn M 1205 Adeline, Dubuque, IA 52001, (319) 556-3591, BS 70 Univ of IA; MA 71 Univ of IA; 87–Sp-Lang Path, Medical Associates Clinic PC, **SLP**

Coyne, Lesley Bracken 31 Berkwood Place, Fonthill, ON, Canada L0S 1E0, (416) 892-6927, BS 84 Univ of Western Ontario; MA 86 SUNY - Center at Buffalo; 87–Sp-Lang Path, Niagara Peninsula Rehab Ctr, **SLP**

Coyne, Linda Borgmann 1402 Misty Lane, Indianapolis, IN 46260, (317) 736-3399, BS 82 Purdue Univ - West Lafayette; MA 85 Butler Univ; **SLP**

Coyner, Marilyn R 4210 26th Avenue, Rock Island, IL 61201, (309) 795-0131, BA 56 Augustana Coll; MS 68 Univ of IL - Urbana; MS 68 Southern IL Univ -Carbondale; SLP, Rock Isl Pub Sch, **SLP**

Cozad, Mrs Betty Berry 1513 Bella Vista Court, Redlands, CA 92373, (714) 882-8597, BS 53 Univ of KS; MA 57 Northwestern Univ; Sp-Lang Path, San Bernardino Cty USD, **SLP ACE**

Cozad, Dr Robert L 1513 Bella Vista Court, Redlands, CA 92373, (714) 825-7084, BS 57 Southern IL Univ -Carbondale; MS 59 Southern IL Univ -Carbondale; PH 68 (NS) Univ of KS; Audiologist, VA, **SLP A**

Cozakos, Nick G 1713 Princeton Avenue, Salt Lake City, UT 84108, (801) 582-0103, BA 50 Univ of UT; MS 66 Univ of UT; Retired, Utah Dept Hlth, **SLP A**

Coze, Elizabeth Alexandra 6201 West Olive Avenue, Apartment 3118, Glendale, AZ 85302, (602) 255-3448, BS 82 Northern AZ Univ; MS 84 Northern AZ Univ; SLP, Phx Day Sch for the Deaf, **SLP**

Cozean, Mrs Jeanne Marie 7 Canner Street, New Haven, CT 06511, (203) 630-4226, BS 84 Bowling Green St Univ; MA 85 Bowling Green St Univ; 85–Sp-Lang Path, City of Meriden, **SLP**

Cozzette, Rose M D 925 North 5th, Canon City, CO 81212, (719) 275-8826, BA 81 Adams St Coll; MA 82 Adams St Coll; 86–Sp-Lang Path, RMC Speech Therapy, **SLP ACE**

Cozzi, Angela 7056 Sunnyslope Avenue, Van Nuys, CA 91405, (213) 625-4183, BA 84 CA St Univ - Northridge; MA 85 CA St Univ - Northridge; **SLP**

Crabb, Mrs Carol S 1811 Birmingham Avenue, Durham, NC 27704, (919) 544-1721, BS 80 Univ of IL - Urbana; MS 81 Univ of IL - Urbana; Sp-Lang Path, Durham Co Sch, **SLP**

Crabtree, Beverly Anne 724 Lafayette Avenue, Buffalo, NY 14222, (716) 845-2201, BS 77; OB 78 Brock Univ - Ontario; MA 82 SUNY - Center at Buffalo; Sp-Lang Path, Buffalo General Hospital, **SLP**

Crabtree, Chris Tina 225 Monte Vista Avenue, Healdsburg, CA 95448, (707) 433-6711, MA 76 Humboldt St Univ; **SLP**

Crabtree, Dr Margaret 127 Bridgewater, Midland, TX 79707, (503) 535-6850, BA 31 TX Tech Univ; MS 38 Univ of MI - Ann Arbor; ED 58 (NS) Univ of Houston - Univ Park; **SLP LM**

Crabtree, Rebecca Denise 2305 70th Street Apt 441, Lubbock, TX 79412, (806) 745-0593, BS 84 TX Tech Univ; MS 86 TX Tech Univ; 86–Sp-Lang Path, Sp-Lang Hrng Ctr of Lubbock, **SLP**

Crabtree, Mrs Tammy Hudson Eye Ear Nose And Throat Hospital, 2626 Napoleon Avenue, New Orleans, LA 70115, (504) 896-1171, OM 85 LA St Univ - N O Medical Ctr; Dept Head, Eye Ear Nose & Throat Hosp, **A**

Crackel, Carol S 916 McCormick Boulevard, Clifton Forge, VA 24422, (703) 862-1935, BA 72 Univ of VA - Charlottesville; MA 73 George Washington Univ; 88, **SLP**

Cracknell, Meredith E 1818 Jackson Drive, Voorhees, NJ 08043-2625, (215) 222-1300, MA 81 Montclair St Coll; BS 79 East Stroudsburg Univ of PA; 87–Sp/Lang Path, HMS Sch for Cerebral Palsy, **SLP**

Cradic, Mrs Pamela Sue 1000 Beechwood Drive, Johnson City, TN 37604, (615) 929-5661, BS 65 East TN St Univ; MA 68 Univ of TN - Knoxville; Sp-Lang Path, Washington County School Syst, **SLP**

Crafton, Marilyn P 122 Nautilus Drive, Madison, WI 53705, (203) 269-3344, BA 69 Univ of MI - Ann Arbor; MA 71 Univ of IA; **SLP**

Cragin, Mrs Elizabeth Papiro 10 Burgundy Hill Lane, Middletown, CT 06457, (203) 632-0709, BS 85 West Chester Univ of PA; MS 87 Bloomsburg Univ of PA; 88

Cragin, Mrs Karen Ann 13110 Creekview Drive, # 204, Garden Grove, CA 92644, (714) 556-3482, BA 82 CA St Univ - Fullerton; MA 85 CA St Univ - Fullerton; **SLP**

Cragwall, Mrs Kathryn D 935 Santa Barbara Drive S E, Grand Rapids, MI 49506, (616) 241-2531, BA 75 MI St Univ; MA 76 MI St Univ; **SLP**

Craig, Ava Brodie 1303 Old Spanish Trail, Bay St Louis, MS 39520, (601) 255-9681, BA 83 MS Coll; ME 86 Southeastern LA Univ; 88–Sp-Lang Path, Pass Christian PS, **SLP**

Craig, Mrs Becky Ann P O Box 707, Kingston, OK 73439, BS 71 Univ of OK - Norman; ME 86 Central St Univ; SLP, **SLP**

Craig, Mrs Betty C 2024 Rebel Road, Lexington, KY 40503, (616) 254-6353, BA 68 Univ of KY; MA 75 Univ of KY; SLP, Fayette Cty Schs, **SLP**

Craig, Cathleen C 2800 Jeanetta #1804, Houston, TX 77063, (713) 498-8110, MS 80 Baylor Univ; Sp-Lang Path, Alief ISD, **SLP**

Craig, Dr Chie Higuchi University Of Wisconsin-Milwaukee, Speech Pathology & Aud, P O Box 413, Milwaukee, WI 53201, (414) 229-4263, BA 72 Univ of WI - Madison; MA 76 Univ of KS; PH 83 (NS) PA St Univ - Univ Park, Asst Prof, U of WI, **A**

Craig, Mrs Constance 309 Trinity Lane, Oak Brook, IL 60521-2564, (312) 920-9640, BA 61 Elmhurst Coll; MA 71 Northeastern IL Univ; Sp-Lang Path, River Forest Public Schools, **SLP**

Craig, Denise 402 Dunedin Avenue, Temple Terrace, FL 33617, (813) 272-4533, BS 72 NY Univ; ME 74 Northeastern Univ; SLP, Hillsborough Co Schs, **SLP**

Craig, Mrs Emily D 4415 Kennedy Street, Chino, CA 91710, (818) 964-6409, BS 78 Univ of CA - Santa Barbara; MA 81 CA St Univ - Fullerton; Sp-Lang Path, Rowland USD, **SLP**

Craig, Dr Holly K University Of Michigan, 1111 East Catherine Street, Ann Arbor, MI 48109-2054, (313) 764-8441, BA 70; MA 72 Northwestern Univ; PH 79 (NS) Univ of MI - Ann Arbor; Assoc Prof, U Mich, **SLP**

Craig, Dr J Marvin 429 North 3rd Street, Cheney, WA 99004, (509) 359-6623, BA 58 Occidental Coll; MS 59 Purdue Univ - West Lafayette; PH 68 (NS) Univ of WA; Prof of Aud, En Washington U, **SLP A**

Craig, Mrs Jenise Palermo 48 Hillcrest Avenue, Port Jefferson, NY 11777, (203) 287-1781, BA 76 Adelphi Univ; MS 77 Adelphi Univ; Sp-Lang Path, Private Practice, **SLP**

Craig, Mrs Karen Louise 226 Muller #2, Nacogdoches, TX 75961, (409) 829-3100, BS 83 Stephen F Austin St Univ; ME 86 Stephen F Austin St Univ

Craig, Mrs Kathryn C 113 Brockhampton Court, Goodlettsville, TN 37072, (615) 859-7084, BA 75 Univ of NC - Greensboro; MA 76 Memphis St Univ; Dir-Sp-Lang Path, Craig Lang & Sp Svcs, **SLP**

Craig, Laurie Mandly 108 Laurel Hill Drive, Starkville, MS 39759, (601) 522-3051, BS 82 MS St Univ - MS State; MA 84 Memphis St Univ; Sp-Lang Path, Mississippi State Dept of Educ, **SLP**

Craig, Leslie D 3549 Curry Lane #2611, Abilene, TX 79606, (915) 695-6437, MA 88 Abilene Christian Univ; 88–Sp-Lang Path, Abilene State Sch (CFY)

Craig, Dr Lillian M Hearing And Speech Associates, 300 East Main, Carbondale, IL 62901, (618) 529-3652, BA 60 Shorter Coll; OM 62 Duke Univ; PH 72 (NS) Southern IL Univ -Carbondale; Director, Hearing and Speech Associates, **SLP A**

Craig, Mary Helen 25932 Palomar Court, San Bernardino, CA 92404, (714) 829-6461, **SLP**

Craig, Mrs Mary L 255 San Joaquin Drive, Red Bluff, CA 96080, (916) 527-3140, BA 71 Holy Names Coll; OM 73 Univ of WA; SLP, Tehama Co Dept of Ed, **SLP**

Craig, Mrs Mary S 4911 Woodlawn, Pineville, LA 71360, (318) 640-4221, BA 59 Univ of Northern CO; MA 70 Northwestern St Univ; Sp-Lang Path, St Mary's Residential Sch, **SLP**

Craig, Michelle S 24 Festoon Lane, Chico, CA 95926, (916) 896-5381, BS 74 Syracuse Univ; MS 76 Univ of NM; SLP, Chico Comm Hospital, **SLP**

Craig, Pamela J 302 South Coquillard, South Bend, IN 46617, (219) 282-4129, BS 67 Ball St Univ; MA 72 Ball St Univ; Sp-Lang Path, S Bend Comm Sch Corp, **SLP**

Craig, Mrs Peri M 1410 Yorkshire, Grosse Pointe Pk, MI 48230, (313) 881-7162, BS 78 Wayne St Univ; MA 79 Western MI Univ; Sp-Lang Path, Self Employed, **SLP**

Craig, Dr Rebecca Sue 29 Spears Avenue, Asheville, NC 28801, (704) 253-7543, BA 31 Asbury Coll; MA 40 Northwestern Univ; PH 51 (NS) Northwestern Univ; Sp-Lang Path, Private Practice, **SLP LM**

Craig, Dr Richard K 302 South Coquillard, South Bend, IN 46617, (219) 271-0000, BS 68 Ball St Univ; MA 71 Ball St Univ; PH 78 (Aud) Kent St Univ; Aud, Professional Hearing Service PC, **A**

Craig, Roberta May 14 Park Street, Oxford, MA 01540, (617) 765-9771, BS 80 Worcester St Coll; MS 84 Univ of VT; Sp-Lang Path, Harrington Mem Hosp, **SLP**

Craig, Mrs Roberta Preston 478 Thames Street, Newport, RI 02840, (401) 849-9955, BS 68 Purdue Univ - West Lafayette; MS 69 Purdue Univ - West Lafayette; Superv SLP, Purdue Univ, **SLP**

Craig, Robin Lee 31 Moraine Street, Jamaica Plain, MA 02130, (617) 573-3266, BA 82 IN Univ - Bloomington; MS 87 Gallaudet Coll; 87–Aud, Eye & Ear Infirmary, **A**

Craig, Sam B Western Pennsylvania School, For The Deaf, Pittsburgh, PA 15218, MS; **LM**

Craig, Sarah Culver 308 Lockhouse Road, Westfield, MA 01085, (413) 562-4131, BS 79 Coll of Saint Rose; ME 80 Coll of Saint Rose; Sp-Lang Path, Western Mass Hosp, **SLP**

Craig, Sherry Annette 33 High Trail Drive, Maumelle, AR 72118, (501) 329-6851, BS 82 AR St Univ; OM 83 AR St Univ; **SLP**

Craig, Dr William N Western Pa School For The Deaf, 300 Swissvale Avenue, Pittsburgh, PA 15218, (412) 371-7000, BA 55; MS 58 Gallaudet Coll; PH 62 (NS) Univ of Pittsburgh - Pittsburgh; Aud, Wn Pa Sch for Deaf, **A**

Craiger, Dr Pamela A 1023 Main Suite 3, Woodward, OK 73801, (405) 256-1439, BA 64 6241; OM 65 Univ of OK Medical Center; PH 70 (NS) Univ of OK Medical Center; Aud, Private Practice, **A**

Crain, Mrs Cherie L 12901 Dale Street #10, Garden Grove, CA 92641, (714) 638-4677, BS 58 CA St Univ - Long Beach; 88–Tchr, Cypress ISD, **SLP**

Crain, Lydia H 97 Dale Drive, Keene, NH 03431, (603) 357-9769, BS 72 Univ of IL - Urbana; MA 73 Univ of IL - Urbana; Sp/Lang Path, **SLP**

Crain, Rebecca Andes 5720 West 86th Street, Overland Park, KS 66207, (913) 642-9592, BS 73 Univ of KS; MA 75 Univ of KS; Sp-Lang Path, Shwanee Mission Pub Sch, **SLP**

Crain, Rene A 1026 Heap Avenue, Prescott, AZ 86303, (602) 778-4752, BS 76 Univ of TX - Austin; MS 78 Univ of WI - Madison; SLP, Prescott Unified School, **SLP**

Crain, Sharon Sapp 329 Faulkner Drive, Lancaster, PA 17601, BA 81 Univ of AL- Tuscaloosa; MS 82 Univ of AL- Tuscaloosa; Sp-Lang Path, UCP, **SLP**

Crain, Mrs Sheila F 2005 Croydon, Springfield, IL 62703, (217) 529-4511, BS 66 Northwestern Univ; MS 67 Univ of OK Medical Center; Sp-Lang Path, Little Flower Sch, **SLP**

Crain, Sheri L 379 Becket Apartment 6, Brighton, MI 48116, (313) 229-2324, BS 85 Univ of IL - Urbana; MS 86 Southern IL Univ-Edwardsvill; Sp-Lang Path, Okemos PS, **SLP**

Crain, Thomas R 592 Ottawa Avenue, St Paul, MN 55107, (612) 227-0029, BS 85 Univ of MN - Minneap-St Paul; MA 88 Univ of MN - Minneap-St Paul; 85–Research Asst, Univ of MN

Craine, Teri 32255 Northwestern Highway, Suite 182, Farmington Hills, MI 48018, (313) 737-2272, BS 71 Wayne St Univ; MA 73 Wayne St Univ; OD 85 (NS) Wayne St Univ; Pres, Commun Dis Inc, **SLP**

Crais, Dr Elizabeth R Division Of Speech & Hearing, CB #7190 Wing D Medical School, University Of North Carolina, Chapel Hill, NC 27599, (919) 966-1006, BS 72 Univ of AL- Tuscaloosa; MS 74 Vanderbilt Univ; PH 87 (Commun Dis) Univ of WI - Madison; 87–Asst Prof, Univ of NC at Chapel Hill, **SLP**

Crall, Brenda M 66 Hunter Street, Glens Falls, NY 12801, (518) 792-3560, BA 85 SUNY - Coll at Plattsburgh; MA 87 SUNY - Coll at Plattsburgh; Sp-Lang Path, UCP Assoc of the Tri-Co Inc, **SLP**

Cram, Janet Ellen 84-17 94th Street, Woodhaven, NY 11421, (212) 750-6786, BA 84 CT Coll; MS 86 Columbia Univ Teachers Coll; Sp-Lang Path, New York Univ Med Ctr, **SLP ACE**

Cramb, Debbie A 38 Thatcher Avenue, Scarborough, ON, Canada M1M 2M2, (416) 261-5029, OM 87 Univ of Western Ontario; 87–Aud, Centenary Hosp, **A**

Cramer, Cathleen L 13143 Margate Street, Van Nuys, CA 91401, (213) 761-6147, BA 74 CA St Univ - Northridge; MA 81 CA St Univ - Northridge; SLP, LA USD, **SLP**

Cramer, Mrs Debra Lynn 649 Foxtree Circle #8, Burlington, WI 53105, (414) 537-2211, BA 84 Univ of WI - Eau Claire; MS 86 Univ of WI - Eau Claire; Sp-Lang Path, CES #2, **SLP**

Cramer, Mrs Judy C 301 Drake Court, Benicia, CA 94510, (707) 746-7739, BS 75 Univ of WI - Stevens Point; MA 87 Southwest MO St Univ; **SLP**

Cramer, Mrs Sandra Kay 162 Vineyard Road, Avon Lake, OH 44012, (216) 933-3529, MS 84 WV Univ; BS 83 WV Univ; Aud, **A**

Cramer, Sue Rae 1204 Knollhaven #G, Manchester, MO 63021, (314) 256-4938, MS 84 Central MO St Univ; SLP, Special School District, **SLP**

Cramer-Richards, Janet P O Box 277, APO New York, NY 09164, 011-06205-17734, BS 77 Portland St Univ; MS 79 Western OR St Coll; Sp-Lang Path, Dept of Defense Schs, **SLP**

Cramp, Carolyn A Rural Delivery 1, Wernersville, PA 19565, **SLP**

Crampton, Joann M Wildflecken Am School, APO New York, NY 09026-0005, BA 73 Creighton Univ; MA 75 Univ of NE - Lincoln; SLP, Dept of Defense Dept Sch, **SLP**

Cranberg, Mrs Norma A 427 51st Street, Des Moines, IA 50312, (515) 255-6551, BA 46 Univ of IA; MA 48 Univ of IA; Owner & Dir, Private Practice, **SLP**

Crancer, Michele 611 Greenville, Rector, AR 72461, (501) 595-3248, **SLP**

Crandall, Cynthia D 25007 Davidson Street, San Bernardino, CA 92408, MA 82 CA St Univ - Northridge; 87–Sp-Lang Path, San Bernardino City USD, **SLP**

Crandall, James R 1110 North School, Santa Maria, CA 93454, **SLP**

Crandall, Dr Kathleen Eilers Ntid-Rit, Ome Lomb Memorial Drive, P O Box 9887, Rochester, NY 14623, (716) 475-5111, BA 69 CA St Univ - Fresno; MA 70 CA St Univ - Fresno; PH 74 (Communication Disorders) Northwestern Univ; Assoc Prof, Rochester I of Tech

Crandall, Nancy M 14 Douglas Parkway, Wichita, KS 67206, (316) 268-5246, BA 60 Univ of Southwestern LA; MA 71 Wichita St Univ; Director, St Francis Regional Med Ctr, **SLP**

Crandall, Tracy Teal 5795 Sr 656, Sunbury, OH 43074, (614) 261-5843, BS 83 Miami Univ - Oxford; MS 84 Miami Univ - Oxford; Sp-Lang Path, Riverside Methodist Hospital, **SLP**

Crandell, Carl C 515 Basswood, P-143 Rock Harbor, Nashville, TN 37209-1659, (814) 234-7237, **A**

Crane, Mrs Bonnie F S 240-07 65th Avenue, Douglaston, NY 11362, (718) 224-0245, BS 75 Ithaca Coll; MA 76 Hofstra Univ; SLP, NYC Bd of Ed, **SLP**

Crane, Jane Pack 625 S W 19th Street, Fort Lauderdale, FL 33315, (305) 836-2820, MS 78 Univ of South FL; Sp-Lang Path, Dade Co Sch Syst, **SLP**

Crane, Mary F 741 West Belden Avenue, Chicago, IL 60614, (312) 945-9660, BA 77 Western WA Univ; MA 82 Northwestern Univ; Sp-Lang Path, N Suburban Sp Ed Dist, **SLP**

Crane, Mrs Patricia Anne c/o Lt J A Crane, Comsubron, Twenty Two, FPO New York, NY 09501, BA 82 0500; MS 85 Univ of VT; **SLP**

Crane, Phyllis Taillon 408 South Paula Avenue, Fullerton, CA 92633, (714) 992-5245, BA 71 Univ of Southern CA; MA 72 Univ of Southern CA; PH 87 (Educational Psychology) Univ of Southern CA; 85–Educ Consult, Los Angeles County Sch of Nursing, **SLP**

Crane, Robin Snedeker 1442 Pontiac Trail, Ann Arbor, MI 48105, (313) 996-4217, BA 79 MI St Univ; MA 82 Central MI Univ; Sp-Lang Path, Ann Arbor Pub Schs, **SLP**

Crane, Susan Lake 245 Symphony, Shreveport, LA 71105-4207, (318) 424-8263, BS 79 LA St Univ - Baton Rouge; MS 80 Univ of AL- Tuscaloosa; Sp-Lang Path, Caddo Parish Sch Bd, **SLP**

Crane, Mrs Suzanne A 14 River Cove Circle #5, Williston, VT 05495, (802) 878-3702, BA 76 Bates Coll; MS 78 Univ of VT; Tchr, Trinity Christian Sch, **SLP**

Crane, Terrence L 415 W North, Geneseo, IL 61254, (309) 786-7793, BA 62 Univ of Northern IA; MA 70 Northern IL Univ - De Kalb; Asst Principal, Alleman High Sch, **SLP**

Crane-McCall, Debra Ann 8 High Gate Trail #5, Fairport, NY 14450, (716) 248-3220, BA 82 SUNY - Center at Buffalo; MA 84 Kent St Univ; Sp-Lang Path, Penfield School District, **SLP**

Crane-Riley, Catherine 172 Vanderbilt Avenue, Brentwood, NY 11717, (516) 867-7738, **SLP**

Cranfill, Tamara B 610 Dale Morrison Road, Glensfork, KY 42741, (502) 384-5621, BA 79 Univ of KY; MA 86 Eastern KY Univ; 88–Sp-Lang Path, Somerset Cty Schs, **SLP**

Cranford, Dr Jerry Lynn Dept Comm Disorders & Sci, Wichita State University, Wichita, KS 67208, (316) 689-3240, MA 68 Vanderbilt Univ; PH 69 Vanderbilt Univ; OM 84 LA St Univ - N O Medical Ctr; Assoc Prof Aud, Wichita State U, **A**

Cranny, Constance Joan 3035 18th Avenue, Marion, IA 52302, (319) 245-1480, MA 85 Univ of IA; **SLP**

Cranston, Cathi 2320-C Springhouse Lane, Martinez, GA 30907, (404) 868-8175, BS 83 Univ of AR - Fayetteville; MS 85 Univ of AR - Fayetteville; 87–Sp-Lang Path, InSpeech Inc, **SLP**

Cranston, John E 1037 Phay Avenue, Canon City, CO 81212, (719) 275-0331, BS 71 Humboldt St Univ; OM 73 Phillips Univ; MS 73 Phillips Univ; SLP, South Central Bd Coop Ed Serv, **SLP A**

Crary, Delores F 1708 Mimosa Place, Fullerton, CA 92635, (213) 336-5061, BA 63 Univ of KS; MA 65 Univ of KS; Tchr, LA Co Supt of Schools, **SLP**

Crary, Margaret A 306 Grafhill Drive, Mobile, AL 36606, (205) 479-3863, OB 49; MA 52 Univ Southern MS-Hattiesburg; MS 61 Vanderbilt Univ; Aud, **SLP A LM**

Crary, Dr Michael A Dept Communicative Disorders, University Of Florida, Box J-174 Jhmhc, Gainesville, FL 32610, (618) 453-4301, BA 74 SUNY - Coll at Plattsburgh; MA 76 OH Univ - Athens; PH 78 (NS) OH Univ - Athens; Assoc Prof, University of Florida 84, **SLP**

Crary, Sharon Kay 745 Kenilworth Parkway, Baton Rouge, LA 70808, (504) 766-9365, BS 61 Bowling Green St Univ; MA 69 Univ of Southern CA; **SLP**

Crary, Suzan B 3130 Rolling Wood Loop, Colorado Springs, CO 80918, (719) 590-7120, **SLP**

Cratcha, Stanley G 6820 Melridge Street, Painesville, OH 44077, **SLP**

Craun-Carey, Mrs Kelly Vivian 838 Paul Street, Staunton, VA 24401, (703) 885-7147, BS 81 James Madison Univ; MA 82 Univ of TN - Knoxville; 86–Sp-Lang Path, DeJarnette Ctr for Children, **SLP**

Craven, Candida M 208 Montclair Avenue, Pittsburgh, PA 15229, BS 75 PA St Univ - Univ Park; MA 78 Univ of Pittsburgh - Pittsburgh; 85–Sp-Lang Path, Allegheny Intermediate Unit, **SLP**

Craven, Mrs Dorothy D 4921 WAA Street, Honolulu, HI 96821, (808) 948-8279, BS 45 Southeast MO St Univ; MA 48 Univ of IA; 70–Assoc Prof, John Burns Sch Med U of Hawaii, **SLP A F**

Craven, Dr Duane C California State University, Department Of Cdo, 1250 Bellflower Boulevard, Long Beach, CA 90840, (213) 602-1541, BA 55 Pepperdine Univ - Los Angele; MA 58 Pepperdine Univ - Los Angele; PH 72 (NS) Univ of Southern CA; Associate Professor, California State U Long Beach, **SLP**

Craven, Lisanne Simms 2028 Strathmoor Boulevard, Louisville, KY 40205, (502) 561-3349, BS 80 Western KY Univ; MS 81 Univ of Louisville; Sp-Lang Path, Private Practice, **SLP ACE**

Craven, Roberta L 3256 Hammond Avenue, Waterloo, IA 50702, (319) 233-2048, MA 69 Univ of MN - Minneap-St Paul; BA 68 Univ of Northern IA; Clinical Supervisor/Instructor, University of Northern Iowa, **SLP**

Cravens-Matheson, Mrs Catherine 3326 Sawtelle Boulevard, Apartment 26, Los Angeles, CA 90066, (213) 391-9620, BA 78 Univ of NM; MS 80 Univ of NM; 88–Res Asst, UCLA Grad Sch of Educ, **SLP**

Crawford, Mrs Arleen B 5432 Peggy Circle, Virginia Beach, VA 23464, (804) 473-5029, BS 77 Bloomsburg Univ of PA; MS 78 Bloomsburg Univ of PA; Sp-Lang Path, VA Beach Pub Sch Sys, **SLP**

Crawford, Mrs Barbara P 3106 East 27th Street, Tulsa, OK 74114, (918) 663-3646, BA 72 Northeastern OK St Univ; MA 74 Univ of Tulsa; Speech-Language Pathologist, Union Public Schools, **SLP**

Crawford, Mrs Beth P O Box 468, Louisville, MS 39339, (601) 773-2521, BS 74 Univ Southern MS-Hattiesburg; MS 75 Univ Southern MS-Hattiesburg; **SLP**

Crawford, Cheryle Saunders 1246 General Bragg, San Antonio, TX 78245, (512) 675-4708, BA 71 Howard Univ; MA 73 Howard Univ; Sp-Lang Path, San Antonio ISD, **SLP**

Crawford, Cynthia L 28221 Somerset, Mission Viejo, CA 92692, (714) 830-4163, BA 77 Univ of CA - Santa Barbara; MA 80 Univ of Northern CO; Sp-Lang Path, Newport Lang Sp&Aud Cen Inc, **SLP**

Crawford, Mrs Cynthia L 1723 Rosslare Court, Manchester, MO 63021, (314) 227-7501, BS 80 Eastern MI Univ; MA 81 Eastern MI Univ; Sp-Lang Path, Private Practice, **SLP**

Crawford, Mrs Deanna M R R 3 Box 198-P, Augusta, KS 67010, (316) 262-8271, MA 78 Wichita St Univ; 88–Sp-Lang Path, Private Practice, **SLP**

Crawford, Mrs Gladys H 3305 Robinhood Road, Tallahassee, FL 32312, (904) 385-3291, BA 36 Northwestern Univ; MS 55 Washington Univ; **SLP LM**

Crawford, Jean Verleny 1960 Tremont Road, Columbus, OH 43212, (614) 836-3946, BS 79 Miami Univ - Oxford; MS 81 East Carolina Univ; SLP, Franklin Co Bd of Mr/Dd, **SLP**

Crawford, Joan L 10435 South Sandusky, Tulsa, OK 74137, **SLP**

Crawford, John W 1515 6th Place, Port Hueneme, CA 93041, (805) 486-4777, BA 50 Univ of Pittsburgh - Pittsburgh; ME 51 Boston Univ; Sp-Lang Path, Oxnard Union Hs Dist, **SLP**

Crawford, Lorri Couch 1600 Pullen Road, Apartment 2-E, Tallahassee, FL 32303, (904) 385-6738, BS 86 FL St Univ; MS 87 FL St Univ; 87–Sp-Lang Path, InSpeech Inc, **SLP**

Crawford, Lynn J 141 Timber Lane, Antioch, IL 60002, (312) 395-1550, BS 81 Northern IL Univ - De Kalb; MA 82 Northern IL Univ - De Kalb; 83–Sp-Lang Path, Grass Lake Sch Dist #36, **SLP**

Crawford, Margie Renee 2091 Cabana Circle South, #2, Memphis, TN 38107, (901) 525-2682, BA 82 Cleveland St Univ; MA 86 Cleveland St Univ; 88–Aud, Drs Schlesinger & Weems, **A**

Crawford, Mary B 1519 Locust Avenue #11, Marshfield, WI 54449, BS 77 Univ of WI - Eau Claire; MS 79 Univ of WI - River Falls; Sp-Lang Path, Granton Area Schools, **SLP**

Crawford, Mary Schmalz 2519 Shades Crest Road, Birmingham, AL 35216, (205) 591-7167, BA 74 Auburn Univ - Auburn; MS 75 Auburn Univ - Auburn; Executive Director, Speech Pathology Services, **SLP**

Crawford, Nancy C 15 Robert Lennox Drive, Northport, NY 11768, (617) 765-9771, BA 71 Middlebury Coll; MS 79 San Francisco St Univ; Sp-Lang Path, Suffolk Child Development Cen, **SLP**

Crawford, Nancy P 2513 St Michel Court, Ponte Vedra Beach, FL 32082-9622, (904) 285-1098, BS 76 Univ of KS; MA 77 Wichita St Univ; 87–Sp-Lang Path, Private Practice, **SLP**

Crawford, Nannette 2850 Old Meadville Road Box 86, Mill Village, PA 16427, (814) 453-5602, BS 71 Edinboro Univ of PA; MA 77 Edinboro Univ of PA; Sp-Lang Path/Dir, Lake Erie I of Rehab, **SLP**

Crawford, Patricia Lee 707 North Larkfield Circle, Hartsville, SC 29550, (803) 383-3127, OM 80 Univ of SC - Columbia; Sp-Lang Path, Darlington County School Dist, **SLP**

Crawford, Sandra G 9531 Dartridge Circle, Dallas, TX 75238, (214) 349-3978, BS 73 Southern Methodist Univ; MS 74 Southern Methodist Univ; **SLP**

Crawford, Sandra V 59 West Mission Plaza Dr, Ventura, CA 93001, (805) 643-6039, BA 72 Occidental Coll; MA 81 Univ of CA - Santa Barbara; SLP, Pleasant Valley Sch Dist, **SLP**

Crawford, Suzanne F 30 Nichols Road, Fitchburg, MA 01420, (503) 343-5005, BS 84 Worcester St Coll; MS 85 Univ of VT; 85–Sp-Lang Path, Burbank Hosp Sp/Hrng Ctr, **SLP**

Crawford, Mrs Valerie Y 18228 Steel Street, Detroit, MI 48235, (517) 393-4072, BS 72 Univ of WI - Milwaukee; OM 73 Univ of WA; 74–Sp-Lang Path, Lansing Sch Dist, **SLP**

Crawford, Mrs Wendy A W 3463 196-A Street, Langley, BC, Canada V3A 7X2, (604) 534-8936, BS 74 Univ of Western Ontario; MS 75 Univ of Western Ontario; Sp-Lang Path, **SLP**

Crawley, Brenda J 3751 S W 20th Avenue #145, Gainesville, FL 32607, (904) 335-2954, MA 88 Univ of FL

Crawley, Kathryn 4 Stearns Road, Belmont, MA 02178, (617) 484-3810, **SLP**

Crawley, Mrs Kennie J 6603 East 89th Place, Tulsa, OK 74133, **SLP**

Crawley, Mrs Linda Pendleton 3 Canterbury Lane, Arkadelphia, AR 71923, (501) 777-4501, BS 76 Henderson St Univ; MS 82 Univ of AR - Little Rock; Sp-Lang Path, Sp Path Serv, **SLP**

Crawley, Mrs Lois Freeman 6906 West Park Drive, Hyattsville, MD 20783, (301) 422-7645, BA 81 Univ of the DC; MS 86 Univ of the DC; **SLP**

Craycraft, Constance Taylor 5951 Waters Edge Drive, Fayetteville, NC 28304-1728, (804) 420-5687, **SLP**

Craycroft, Jessica T 1847 North Newmark, Sanger, CA 93657, **A**

Crea, Raymond John 7411 Sunny Beach Road, Grand Rapids, MN 55744, (218) 326-3213, BS 76 Univ of ND; MS 84 Moorhead St Univ; Sp-Lang Path, ISD 318, **SLP**

Creager, Mrs Carol F 1821 Southwood Lane, Dayton, OH 45419, (513) 222-5597, BS 53 Bowling Green St Univ; Sp-Lang Path, Hearing and Speech Center, **SLP**

Creager, Mrs Joan E 1820 West Lamont Avenue, Peoria, IL 61614, BA 69 Augustana Coll; MS 70 Univ of WI - Madison; Sp-Lang Path, Private Practice, **SLP**

Creaghead, Dr Nancy Acra 4 East Interwood Place, Cincinnati, OH 45220, BA 65 Denison Univ; MS 66 Purdue Univ - West Lafayette; PH 78 (NS) Univ of Cincinnati; Prof, University of Cincinnati, **SLP F**

Creamer, Mrs Wendy K 1409 Hollywood Drive, Lancaster, PA 17601, (717) 291-1955, BA 75 Dickinson Coll; MS 78 PA St Univ - Univ Park; **SLP**

Crean, Mrs Joanne Ziegler 1567 Edgewood, Redding, CA 96001-9293, (916) 365-0083, MS 79 CA St Univ - Long Beach; 80–SLP, Shasta Co Sch Dist, **SLP**

Creasey, Kay W 100 Seven Oaks Park, Muscatine, IA 52761, (319) 263-8476, BA 74 Univ of IA; MA 76 Univ of IA; Sp-Lang Path, MS Bend AEA, **SLP**

Crecine, Mrs Kathleen B 1916 Gordon, Lansing, MI 48910, (517) 485-4215, BA 68 MI St Univ; MA 74 MI St Univ; Sp-Lang Path, Jackson Pub Schs, **SLP**

Creech, Dr Henry B 5903 Harbourwood Place, Midlothian, VA 23113, (804) 230-1326, BS 58 East Carolina Univ; MA 59 OH St Univ; PH 62 (NS) OH St Univ; Ch Aud & SLP Serv, VA Admin Med Cen Richmond VA, **SLP A**

Creed, Judith S 355 Valley Road, Merion Station, PA 19066, (215) 664-6440, BA 65 Temple Univ; MA 67 Temple Univ; Dir Sp/Lang Cen, Cora, **SLP**

Creedon, Francine Locastro 24205 61st Avenue, Flushing, NY 11362, (516) 922-4100, BA 79 SUNY - Coll at New Paltz; MS 85 Adelphi Univ; **SLP**

Creegan, Elizabeth 2861 West International Airport Road E-102, Anchorage, AK 99502, (907) 274-4582, MS 79 NM St Univ; 88–Sp-Lang Path, Anchorage Public Schools, **SLP**

Creekmore, Mrs Susan A 862 London Green Way, Colorado Springs, CO 80906, (303) 576-8563, BS 85 Univ of Montevallo; MS 86 Univ of Montevallo; SLP, **SLP**

Creel, Lynn P Browne-McHardy Clinic, 4315 Houma Boulevard, Metairie, LA 70006-2981, (504) 887-5500, BA 76 Univ of MS; OM 77 Univ of MS; Aud, Browne-McHardy Cl, **A**

Creen, Mrs Gloria F T 1317 25th Avenue, Moline, IL 61265, (309) 792-0639, BS 72 Univ of ND; MS 77 Western IL Univ; Sp-Lang Path, Silvis Pub Sch Dist #34, **SLP**

Creger, Mrs Alexandra Joan 1027 Loyalist Court, Mount Pleasant, SC 29464, (803) 884-7590, BA 81 Univ of the Pacific; MA 82 Univ of the Pacific; Sp-Lang Path, Charleston Co Sch, **SLP**

Cregg, Mrs Leesa Suddath 718 Herrick Court, Katy, TX 77450-2104, BA 76 Tulane Univ; MS 77 FL St Univ; **A**

Crehan, Sheila Mary 106-64 Finch Drive, Sarnia, ON, Canada N7S 4T7, (519) 332-5935, BS 85 Western IL Univ; MA 87 Western IL Univ; **A**

Creighton, Mrs Barbara B Marina High School, 15871 Springdale Street, Huntington Beach, CA 92648, (714) 893-6571, BA 70 Univ of Redlands; MS 71 Vanderbilt Univ; Rsrc Spec/Ch, Huntington Beach Uhsd, **SLP**

Cremeans, Mrs Lura Thern 3639 Skyview Drive, Huntington, WV 25701, BA 81 Marshall Univ; MA 82 Marshall Univ; 86–Sp-Lang Path, Developmental Therapy Ctr, **SLP**

Cremeens, Penny R 2407 26th Street, Lubbock, TX 79411, (806) 766-1198, BS 79 Southern IL Univ -Carbondale; MS 81 TX Tech Univ; Sp-Lang Path, Lubbock ISD, **SLP**

Cremen, Mrs Lynn K 15 Crescent Drive, Las Vegas, NV 89102, (702) 383-2385, BA 70 Mansfield Univ of PA; MA 73 Univ of Pittsburgh - Pittsburgh; Supvr SLP & Aud, Univ Med Ctr of Southern NV, **SLP**

Crennen, Cynthia L 799 Dahlia #403, Denver, CO 80220, (303) 355-6218, BA 76 Univ of MT; MS 79 CO St Univ; Sp-Lang Path, Littleton Public Schools, **SLP**

Crenshaw, Fredda W P O Box 160345, Mobile, AL 36616, (205) 343-0703, MA 67 3000; Sp-Lang Path, Private Practice, **SLP**

Crenshaw, Mrs Nancy L Star Route Box 551, Winston, OR 97496, BA 74 WA St Univ; MA 75 WA St Univ; SLP, Douglas Esd, **SLP**

Crescenzo, Warren Lewis 77 South Valley Avenue, Vineland, NJ 08360, (609) 692-3798, BS 71 Glassboro St Coll; OM 78 Glassboro St Coll; MA 83 Trenton St Coll; Sp-Lang Path, Vineland Pub Schs, **SLP ACE**

Crespo, Patricia 91 East 17th Street, Huntington Station, NY 11746, MA 80 NY Univ; Sp-Lang Path, Long Island Developmental Ctr, **SLP ACE**

Crespy, Marilyn Steinberg 1008 Maple Avenue, Piscataway, NJ 08854, **SLP**

Cress, Pamela S 204 North Island View Avenue, Long Beach, MS 39560, (601) 864-4114, BA 78 Wichita St Univ; MA 79 Wichita St Univ; Sp/Lang Path, Private Practice, **SLP**

Cress, Sharon T 10 Windcreek, Friendswood, TX 77546, (713) 482-1201, BA 66 Univ of Science & Arts of OK; MA 70 Univ of Houston - Univ Park; 86–Sp-Lang Path, Friendswood ISD, **SLP**

Cress-Bush, Louise B 828 Serramonte Drive, Marietta, GA 30068, (404) 926-4453, BS 78 Eastern KY Univ; MA 80 Univ of TN - Knoxville; Sp-Lang Path, Cobb Co Bd of Ed Pub Sch, **SLP**

Cresswell, Nancy S 4315 N E Lavrelhurst Place, Portland, OR 97213, **SLP**

Cresta, Mrs Debra Roberts 262 Goodwin Road, Eliot, ME 03903, (603) 778-7311, BS 79 Univ of NH; MS 82 Univ of NH; Mgr/Sp-Lang Path, Exeter Hos, **SLP**

Creticos, Ruth Morton 15003 Lavale Road, Monkton, MD 21111, (301) 628-6390, BA 72 Columbia Coll; MS 82 Towson St Univ; Sp-Lang Path, Harford County Schools, **SLP**

Crettol, Elaine L T Psc Box 1002, APO New York, NY 09057-5363, (512) 774-4651, BS 79 Northern IL Univ - De Kalb; MA 80 Northern IL Univ - De Kalb; Dir of Rehab Serv, Visiting Nurses of Del Rio Inc, **SLP**

Creveling, Regina C 7000 Louisiana N E #410, Albuquerque, NM 87109, BS 83 Eastern NM Univ; MS 85 Northern AZ Univ; 85–Sp-Lang Path, Albuquerque PS, **SLP**

Crew, Mrs Deanna H 7906 East North Lane, Scottsdale, AZ 85258, (602) 991-3872, BS 73 Whittier Coll; MS 75 Ithaca Coll; **SLP**

Crews, Mrs Debbie 2623 Pennington Circle, Madison, WI 53711, (608) 273-1709, BS 77 Western IL Univ; MA 78 Western IL Univ; 88–SLP, Verona Area Sch Dist, **SLP**

Crews, Linda Johnston 23 Orange Blossom, Irvine, CA 92720, (714) 962-4408, BS 71 Ball St Univ; MA 80 CA St Univ - Fullerton; SLP, Fountain Valley Sch Dist

Crews, Lynette Marlowe Route 9 Box 458, Johnson City, TN 37601, (615) 639-2131, BS 79 Campbell Univ; OM 85 Univ of SC - Columbia; 85–Aud, Greene Valley Dev Ctr, **SLP A**

Crews, Patricia Lynn 3105 Danny Park, Metairie, LA 70002, (504) 588-5661, BA 78 Univ of MS; MA 79 Univ of MS; **A**

Crews, Richelle Webster 200 Twin Lake Avenue, Opelika, AL 36801, (205) 749-6543, BS 81 Auburn Univ - Auburn; OM 83 Auburn Univ - Auburn; Adjunct Instructor, Auburn University, **SLP**

Cribbs, Mrs Janet L 9159 Scenic Lake Drive, Laingsburg, MI 48848, (517) 743-3471, BA 73 MI St Univ; MA 74 MI St Univ; Sp/Lang Path, Shiawassee ISD, **SLP**

Cribbs-Heenan, Lee Ann 47 Mill Street, Easton, MA 02356, (617) 238-8103, BA 73 Univ of Denver; ME 74 Northeastern Univ; Cl Superv, Sp-Lang-Hrng Assoc, **SLP**

Crichton, Mrs Linda Jaine Corfton Manor, Lower Corfton, Craven Arms, Shropshire, England SY7 9LD, OB 73; MS 81 William Paterson Coll; **SLP**

Crickmay, Marie C Gorge Road Hospital, Speech Pathology Department, 63 Gorge Road East, Victoria, BC, Canada V9A 1L2, (604) 386-2464, OB; MS; **SLP LM**

Cridland, Mrs Charlotte Woolley 2938 S W Fairmount Blvd, Portland, OR 97201, (503) 241-5442, BS 50 Northwestern Univ; MA 69 De Paul Univ; Sp-Lang Path, Private Practice, **SLP**

Crigger, Mrs Kathryn H P O Box 1366, Paintsville, KY 41240-5366, (606) 297-5137, BA 74 Marshall Univ; MA 75 Marshall Univ; Owner, Private Practice, **SLP**

Crim, Mrs Sidney A 1207 Hampshire #107, Richardson, TX 75080, (214) 231-4639, BS 72 Univ of TX - Austin; MA 73 Univ of TX - Austin; Dir/Sp-Lang Path, Richardson Sp & Lang Cl, **SLP**

Crimi, Mrs Cynthia Squillace 1019 South Ninth Street, Philadelphia, PA 19147, (215) 922-5349, MA 87 Temple Univ

Crimmins, Diana C 20 Ware Road, Auburndale, MA 02166, (617) 884-8300, BA 77 Boston Coll; MA 79 Univ of CT; 82–Sp-Lang Path, MA Gen Hosp, **SLP ACE**

Cripe, Dr Antje E 10835 East Wesley Place, Aurora, CO 80014, (303) 771-4393, BA 60 Grinnell Coll; MS 63 Purdue Univ - West Lafayette; PH 66 (NS) Purdue Univ - West Lafayette; Pre-Acad Instr, Cherry Creek Sch Dist #5, **SLP**

Cripe, Juliann J Center on Human Development, University Of Oregon, 901 E 18th Street, Eugene, OR 97403, (503) 686-3568, BA 73 Univ of Northern IA; MA 74 Univ of Northern IA; Research Asst, U of OR, **SLP**

Cripe, Mrs Kimberly A 3751 Appian Way #172, Lexington, KY 40502, (606) 254-5701, BS 86 Eastern KY Univ; MA 87 Eastern KY Univ; **SLP**

Cripps, Mrs Gina Nation 1725 Thistle Court, Owensboro, KY 42301, (502) 685-6006, BS 83 Brescia Coll; MS 85 Western KY Univ; 83–Sp-Lang Path, Owensboro PS, **SLP**

Cripps, Mrs Susan B 9798 Peatwood Drive, Ladson, SC 29456, (803) 873-5750, BS 74 WV Univ; MS 76 WV Univ; 76–Sp-Lang Path, Sc Dept Mental Retardation, **SLP**

Criscione, Regina Barbieri 2 Elmwood Park Drive #316, Staten Island, NY 10314, (212) 420-2760, BA 81 Marymount Coll; MS 83 Columbia Univ Teachers Coll; Aud, Beth Israel Med Ctr, **A**

Crislip, Debra Ann Baptist Memorial Hosp East, 6019 Walnut Grove, Memphis, TN 38119, (901) 766-5145, OB 79 Memphis St Univ; MA 81 Memphis St Univ; Sp-Lang Path, Ped Sp Th Ctr-Baptist East, **SLP**

Crisman, Mrs Diane R P O Box D, Fremont, IN 46737, (219) 495-9803, BS 74 IN Univ - Bloomington; OM 75 IN Univ - Bloomington; 83–Sp-Lang Path, Steuben Cnty Comm Shelt Wrkshp, **SLP**

Crispin, Bonnie Lynn 3888 North Butler #8, Farmington, NM 87401, (505) 325-5011, BA 81 CA St Univ - Los Angeles; MS 85 Univ of Redlands; 87–Sp-Lang Path, San Juan Regional Med Ctr, **SLP**

Criss, Mrs Carol C 190 Huckleberry Road, Macedon, NY 14502, (716) 265-4030, ME 75 Univ of Rochester; 88–SETRC Training Coord, Monroe BOCES #1

Criss, Judith O 12204 Blaketon Street, Upper Marlboro, MD 20772, (301) 262-9560, BS 64 WV Univ; MA 78 Gallaudet Coll; Sp-Lang Path, Pr Geo Co Bd of Ed, **SLP**

Crissey, Joan Florence 115 Cynthia Drive, Chapel Hill, NC 27514, (919) 575-7565, BA 74 Univ of CO - Boulder; MA 84 Central MI Univ; Sp/Lang Path, Murdoch, **SLP**

Crissup, Larry A Rd 1 Box 250, Reading, PA 19607, (215) 856-7438, BA 61 Wichita St Univ; MA 67 Columbia Univ Teachers Coll; VP-Clin Svcs, Reading Rehab Hosp, **SLP**

Cristan, Monica Suzanne 5501 Lakeview Drive, Greendale, WI 53129, (414) 352-1580, BS 82 Marquette Univ; MS 84 Marquette Univ; SLP, North Shore Rehab Assoc Inc, **SLP**

Cristiano, Patricia Airyn Eastern Oklahoma ENT, 5020 East 68th Street, Tulsa, OK 74136, (918) 492-3636, BA 71 Univ of OK - Norman; MA 72 Univ of OK - Norman; MS 84 Univ of OK - OK City; Aud, Eastern Oklahoma Ear Nose & Throat Inc, **A**

Criswell, Martha S 2330 Penmar Avenue #A, Venice, CA 90291, (213) 398-0419, BA 66 OK St Univ; MA 75 CA St Univ - Los Angeles; Sp-Lang Path, Los Angeles City Sch, **SLP**

Criswell, Wendy 1700 N W North River Drive, Apt #302, Miami, FL 33125, (305) 545-8942, Regional Director, InSpeech Inc, **SLP**

Criswell-Baird, Mrs Barbara A 1332 Franklin, Edwardsville, IL 62025-2418, (815) 933-1711, BS 77 Southern IL Univ-Edwardsvill; MS 78 Southern IL Univ-Edwardsvill; Private Practice, **SLP**

Critcher, Dr C Robert 817 Ontario, Shreveport, LA 71106, (318) 797-5081, BA 71 Univ of Houston - Univ Park; MA 72 Univ of Houston - Univ Park; PH 78 (NS) Univ of IA; 82–Assoc Prof, LSU-Shreveport, **SLP**

Critcher, Carolyn G 921 Kenesaw Avenue, Knoxville, TN 37919, (615) 525-1917, BS 71 OK St Univ; OM 73 Univ of WA; Sp-Lang Path, Little TN Valley Ed Coop, **SLP**

Critchfield-Schultz, Mary L 9107 Wedgewood Street S W, Tacoma, WA 98498, (206) 581-7219, BA 85 Eastern WA Univ; MS 86 Eastern WA Univ; Sp-Lang Path, Clover Park Sch Dist, **SLP**

Critelli, Gloria Ellen 2100 West Palmyra Avenue, Apartment 66, Orange, CA 92668, (714) 556-9520, BS 82 SUNY - Coll at Buffalo; MS 84 Univ of WI - Madison; **SLP**

Crites, Laura S 4247 Minnesota, St Louis, MO 63111, (314) 832-6773, BA 83 Saint Louis Univ; MA 86 Saint Louis Univ; 88–Sp-Lang Path, Card Glennon Children's Hosp, **SLP**

Crittenden, Mrs Constance P O Box 249, Mathews, VA 23109, (804) 725-2471, BS 70 Longwood Coll; ME 74 Univ of VA - Charlottesville; Sp-Lang Path, Matthews Co Sch Bd, **SLP**

Crittendon, Anne Marie C 2332 Woodridge Way #1-A, Ypsilanti, MI 48197, (313) 434-5883, MA 88 Eastern MI Univ

Croak, Tammy Schlim 5939 Norham Drive, Alexandria, VA 22310, (703) 922-1723, BS 84 James Madison Univ; MS 85 Boston Univ; 88–Sp-Lang Path, Fairfax Co PS, **SLP**

Croasdale, Helen Lee 340 Crescent Avenue, Buffalo, NY 14214, (716) 878-7371, BS 84 SUNY - Coll at Geneseo; MS 85 SUNY - Coll at Buffalo; **SLP**

Croasmun, Mrs Patricia A 1958 Robincrest Lane, Glenview, IL 60025, (312) 491-3183, BA 75 Case Western Reserve Univ; MA 75 Case Western Reserve Univ; PH 86 (Learning Disabilities) Northwestern Univ; Clin Supvr, Nwn U Prog In Lrng Disabl, **SLP**

Crock, Janet Lynn 2316 East 121st Street, Burnsville, MN 55337, (612) 895-9490, BA 81 Univ of IA; MA 83 Univ of IA; 87–Aud, 3M Med Dept, **A**

Crock, Mary Louise 609 South 5th Street, Youngwood, PA 15697, BS 84 Clarion Univ of PA; MS 86 Clarion Univ of PA; **A**

Crocker, Mrs Kathleen Ann Route 4 Box 286, Monticello, MN 55362, (612) 295-2093, MS 87 Saint Cloud St Univ; 87–Sp-Lang Path, ISD 728

Crockett, Emily Cary 622 Rain Forest #D, Knoxville, TN 37923, (615) 544-0332, BS 86 Univ of TN - Knoxville; MA 88 Univ of TN - Knoxville

Crockett, Dr Karen E 4218 Meadow Hill Drive, Tampa, FL 33624, (813) 969-1339, BS 71 CA Univ of PA; ME 73 CA Univ of PA; PH 83 (Sp-Lang Path) Univ of Pittsburgh - Pittsburgh; Chief-Speech & Aud, Tampa General Hosp, **SLP ACE**

Crockett, Lawrence O 303 Watkins Road, Belleair, FL 34616, (813) 397-5426, MS 80 Univ of South FL; Aud, West Florida Hearing & Speech Inc, **A**

Croft, Heather K 7314 Winter Valley Court, Riverdale, GA 30274, (404) 366-4940, BS 76 Univ of GA; ME 77 Univ of GA; Sp/Lang Path, Clayton County Board of Ed, **SLP**

Croix, Mrs Patricia J 915 Pheasant Drive, Bradley, IL 60915, (815) 937-2082, BS 76 Eastern IL Univ; MA 79 Northern IL Univ - De Kalb; Aud, St Mary's Hosp, **A**

Croly, Richard L 101 North Grape Street, Medford, OR 97501, (503) 776-8587, BA 63 ID St Univ; MS 68 CO St Univ; Aud, Jackson Ed Serv Dist, **A**

Cromer, Patricia A Speech And Hearing Center, Indiana University, Bloomington, IN 47405, (812) 335-6251, BS 51 IN Univ - Bloomington; MA 61 IN Univ - Bloomington; Clin Fac, Indiana Univ Dept Sp-Hrng Sci, **SLP**

Cromley, Elisabeth 2591 Gilbert Street, Broomall, PA 19003, (215) 656-6400, MA 84 West Chester Univ of PA; Sp/Lang Path, Lisa Blackmanb Keonig & Assoc, **SLP**

Cromwell, Kenalyn Morrow 971 Finchwood Lane, Las Vegas, NV 89110, (702) 438-3117, BS 81 MS Univ for Women; MS 85 AZ St Univ; **SLP**

Cromwell, Mrs McCraw Duncan 3908 Glengarry Drive, Austin, TX 78731, (512) 459-5826, BA 78 Univ of NC - Chapel Hill; MA 80 Univ of TX - Austin; Private Practice, **SLP**

Cromwell, Prudence A 8039 14th Avenue NE, Seattle, WA 98115, (206) 527-9105, BA 76 Univ of MT; MA 85 Univ of MT; **SLP**

Cron, Deborah A 21-42 45th Avenue #3, Long Island, NY 11101, (212) 947-5770, BS 75 Southwest MO St Univ; ME 81 Univ of GA; SLP, UCP Assn-Nyst, **SLP**

Cron, Mrs Marla Coulton 3729 Horton Avenue S E, Wyoming, MI 49508, (616) 772-9050, BS 81 PA St Univ - Univ Park; MA 82 MI St Univ; Sp/Lang Path, West Ottawa Pub Schs, **SLP**

Cronan-Polhemus, Anne 325 Erie Avenue, Midland Park, NJ 07432, (914) 623-0897, BA 80 SUNY - Coll at Cortland; MS 82 William Paterson Coll; SLP, Letchworth Vlg Dev Cen, **SLP**

Cronen, Myrna P 45 Hunter Hill Circle, Amherst, MA 01002, (413) 253-3687, BA 66 Tulane Univ; MA 68 Univ of IL - Urbana; Cl Superv, U of MA/Commun Dis Cl, **SLP**

Cronin, Denise Lynn 712 East Sesame Street, Tempe, AZ 85283, (602) 820-0591, BS 85 AZ St Univ; OM 87 AZ St Univ; 88–Sp-Lang Path, Mesa PS, **SLP**

Cronin, Diana Lynn 9555 North Central, Indianapolis, IN 46240, (317) 846-7967, BS 84 Ball St Univ; MA 85 Ball St Univ; 86–Sp-Lang Path, Eagle Union Community Schools, **SLP**

Cronin, Mrs Nadine Merrihew 46 Lawrence Lane, Bristol, CT 06010, (203) 583-6138, BA 81 Northeast LA Univ; MS 83 Univ of North TX; Sp-Lang Path, Naugatuck Public Schools, **SLP**

Cronk, Mrs Rebecca A 30 Alexander Street, Babylon, NY 11702, (516) 422-4295, MA 88 CUNY - Queens Coll

Cronshaw, Mrs Kayla E D 63 Wycliffe Place, Kitchener, ON, Canada N2M 5J7, (216) 929-6634, OB 75 Univ of Saskatchewan - Sask; MA 83 Univ of Akron; Aud, Kitchener/Waterloo Hospital, **A**

Crook, Carol M 1299 East Crestwood Drive, Memphis, TN 38119-5015, **SLP**

Crook, Dalise Taylor 1175 Nancy Lee Way, Decatur, GA 30035-1049, (404) 653-4700, **SLP**

Crook, Margaret Blackwell 1242 Raleigh Circle, Lawrenceville, GA 30245, (404) 925-7833, BA 80 Univ of Central FL; ME 82 GA St Univ; **SLP**

Crook, Mrs Randi Richter 6017 Avery Road, Amlin, OH 43002, (614) 761-9176, BS 82 OH Univ - Athens; MA 87 OH St Univ; 88–Sp-Lang Path, Hilliard City Schs

Crooks, Cynthia M 329 Boundary Avenue, Hanover, PA 17331, **SLP**

Crooks, Deborah Jo 2922 Middle Road, Davenport, IA 52803, (319) 355-7244, **SLP**

Crookston, Garr J Pocatello Hearing Center, 4155 Yellow Stone Hwy, Pine Ridge Mall, Chubbuck, ID 83202, (208) 238-0020, BA 70 UT St Univ; MS 71 UT St Univ; Aud, Pocatello Hrng Cen, **A**

Cropley, Robert W 5149 South Findlay Street, Seattle, WA 98118, (206) 725-6813, BA 70 Univ of WA; MA 72 Univ of WA; Sole Proprietor, Advanced Acoustics, **A**

Crosby, Mrs Brenda Weiland 6435 Michelson Street, Lakewood, CA 90713, (213) 920-2382, BA 84 Univ of CA - Santa Barbara; MA 86 CA St Univ - Long Beach; 87–Tchr, Hunt Beach City Sch Dist, **SLP**

Crosby, Cynthia Pamela 1900 Charleston Place, Apartment 1-D, Charlotte, NC 28212-7803, BA 75 Univ of NC - Charlotte; MS 79 Winthrop Coll; Sp/Lang Path, Charlotte Mecklenburg Sch, **SLP**

Crosby, Donna Jane 40 Grape Lane, Hicksville, NY 11801, (516) 265-3727, BA 84 SUNY - Coll at Plattsburgh; MA 85 SUNY - Coll at Plattsburgh; Aud, Huntington Hearing & Sp Ctr, **A**

Crosby, Janis L 37 Proctor Street, Worcester, MA 01606, (508) 248-7774, BA 65 Emerson Coll; MS 79 Worcester St Coll; 79–Sp-Lang Path, Dudley Charlton Reg Sch Dist, **SLP ACE**

Crosby, Lisa T 6144 Robbins Circle North, Jacksonville, FL 32211, (904) 724-4814, BS 75 FL St Univ; MS 76 FL St Univ; Sp-Lang Path, Morning Star Sch, **SLP**

Crosby, Nancy P 657 Oakland Avenue, Oakland, CA 94611, **SLP**

Crosby, Paula Critz 4417 Englewood Road, Helena, AL 35080, (205) 985-0809, MA 87 Univ of AL- Tuscaloosa

Crose, Elizabeth 4727 Canterbury Court, Ashland, KY 41101, (606) 739-4141, BA 72 Univ of KY; MA 76 Marshall Univ; Sp-Lang Path, Boyd Co Sch Sys, **SLP**

Croshier, Barbara B 4001 Aguila Street #E, Carlsbad, CA 92008, (619) 583-0007, BA 65 Miami Univ - Oxford; MA 66 MI St Univ; Sp-Lang Path, Eloise R Johnston & Assoc, **SLP**

Croskey, Cheryl S 226 Woodridge Road, Tallmadge, OH 44278, (216) 633-5427, BS 66 Kent St Univ; MA 68 Kent St Univ; Sp-Lang Path, Tallmadge Bd of Ed, **SLP**

Crosland-Real, Marybeth 15 Dumbarton Oaks, Stratham, NH 03885, (603) 772-7627, MS 72 PA St Univ - Univ Park; 88–Sp-Lang Path, Private Practice, **SLP**

Crosley, Mrs Pamela Ann 3726 Bartons Lane, Sugar Land, TX 77479, (713) 522-1051, BA 86 Univ of Houston - Univ Park; MA 87 Univ of Houston - Univ Park; 88–Sp-Lang Path, Children's Ctr for Dev Therapy

Cross, A Donald 1024 Greenwich Street, San Francisco, CA 94133, (415) 673-6479, BA 48 Univ of the Pacific; MA 63 San Francisco St Univ; MA 61 Univ of the Pacific; **SLP**

Cross, Donald M Rural Route 3, 1109 Westview Drive, Creston, IA 50801, MS; **SLP**

Cross, Dr Douglas E Speech Pathology & Audiology, Ithaca College, Ithaca, NY 14850, (607) 274-3248, BS 72 Univ of AL- Tuscaloosa; MA 74 Univ of AL- Tuscaloosa; PH 78 (NS) Univ of TN - Knoxville; Assoc Prof, Ithaca Coll/Dept Sp Path, **SLP**

Cross, Mrs Gloria J 22284 Carta Blanca Street, Cupertino, CA 95014, (407) 738-2242, BS 48 Northwestern Univ; MA 50 Northwestern Univ; **SLP**

Cross, Janet Ann 10327 Western Avenue #B, Downey, CA 90241, (818) 917-3403, **SLP**

Cross, Judith Patricia 5619 S E Hacienda, Hillsboro, OR 97123, (503) 649-2565, BS 81 Portland St Univ; MS 86 Portland St Univ; 88–Sp-Lang Path, Reedville Sch Dist, **SLP**

Cross, Kathleen R Rural Route 3, 1109 Westview Drive, Creston, IA 50801, **SLP**

Cross, Mrs Laura S Cross Ctr For Speech Disorders, 191 West Burton Mesa Blvd, Suite B, Lompoc, CA 93436, (805) 733-1622, BA 67 Univ of CA - Riverside; MA 74 Univ of CA - Santa Barbara; Sp-Lang Path, Private Practice, **SLP**

Cross, Lesley V 1900 S Eads Street #631, Arlington, VA 22202, (202) 745-5600, MS 87 Univ of WI - Madison; 88–Sp-Lang Path, Children's Hosp Natl Med Ctr, **A**

Cross, M Stephanie 273 Genesee Park Drive, Syracuse, NY 13224, (315) 652-1262, BA 77 SUNY - Coll at Plattsburgh; MS 83 Purdue Univ - West Lafayette; Sp-Lang Path, Liverpool Sch Dist, **SLP**

Cross, Mrs Sharon Thomas 8799 Burning Tree Road, Pensacola, FL 32514, (904) 478-0448, MS 84 Univ of South AL; 84–Sp-Lang Path, Escambia County Sch Dist, **SLP**

Cross, Mrs Sherrie Nesmith 5655 N 9th Avenue #J-111, Pensacola, FL 32504, (904) 477-8889, BS 81 Univ Southern MS-Hattiesburg; MS 83 Univ Southern MS-Hattiesburg; Sp-Lang Path, Santa Rosa Co, **SLP**

Crossen, Marcia M 4480 Pheasant Run, Reading, PA 19606, (717) 323-8441, BS 56 Syracuse Univ; MS 57 Syracuse Univ; Superv Presch Spec Ed, Bciu 14, **SLP**

Crossley, Marilyn Rivkin 1101 North Fountain Avenue, Springfield, OH 45504, (513) 324-3395, BA 74 SUNY - Coll at Cortland; MA 75 Western MI Univ; 78–Sp-Lang Path, Private Practice, **SLP**

Crossmier, Mrs Judith Lynn 630 Stanford Drive, Altamonte Springs, FL 32714, (305) 788-8598, BS 60 Bowling Green St Univ; MA 84 Univ of Central FL; Sp-Lang Path, Orange Co Schs, **SLP**

Crosswhite, Mrs Cynthia Lynn R 12915 Tosca, Houston, TX 77024, (713) 461-0339, BS 77 Southwest TX St Univ; ME 78 Southwest TX St Univ; Sp-Lang Path, **SLP**

Crotteau, Mary Catherine 46221 Bloomcrest Drive, Northville, MI 48167, (313) 349-1492, BS 65 Marquette Univ; MA 66 MI St Univ; 85–Sp-Lang Path, Wayne County Intermed SD, **SLP**

Crotteau, Nancy R 722 Stafford Court, Alamogordo, NM 88310, (505) 437-1244, BS 76 Univ of WI - Stevens Point; MS 79 MS Univ for Women; Sp-Lang Path, Alamogordo Pub Schs, **SLP**

Crotty, Dr Carol M 880 North Lake Shore Drive, Apartment 5, Chicago, IL 60600, (312) 642-9134, MA 52 De Paul Univ; MS 54 Northwestern Univ; PH 65 (NS) Northwestern Univ; Instr & Conslt, Private Practice, **SLP F LM**

Crouch, Mrs Diane Powell 2007 Avenue B, Council Bluffs, IA 51501-2364, (712) 328-7274, BA 80 Univ of Northern IA; MA 81 Univ of Northern IA; Sp-Lang Path, Loess Hills AEA #13, **SLP**

Crouch, Georgia E 2236 Redwood Road, Ceres, CA 95307, BA 82 CA St Univ - Stanislaus; MA 81 CA St Univ - Stanislaus; SLP, Monteca USD, **SLP**

Crouch, Mrs Starline R RT1 Box 294D, 13N841 Thornton Dr, Kingston, IL 60145, (815) 784-2448, BS 77 Northern IL Univ - De Kalb; MA 81 Northern IL Univ - De Kalb; Sp-Lang Path, Genoa-Kingston Comm Ut DIST424, **SLP**

Crouse, Beverly T 703 3rd Street, Radford, VA 24141, (703) 831-5453, BA 72 Wake Forest Univ; ME 78 Univ of VA - Charlottesville; 84–Dir of Clin Svcs, Radford University, **SLP**

Crouse, Mrs Marjorie K 876 Euclid Avenue, Atlanta, GA 30307, (404) 564-2076, BS 76 Ithaca Coll; MA 78 George Washington Univ; Sp-Lang Path, North Metro Psychoed Prog, **SLP**

Crouse, Mrs Mary Ann B 3 Albro Lane, White Plains, NY 10603, (914) 428-5240, BA 71 CUNY - Lehman Coll; ME 72 Boston Univ; 86–Sp-Lang Path, BOCES, **SLP**

Crouse, Mrs Mary Ellen 4 St Marys Drive, Allegany, NY 14706, (716) 372-8909, BA 58 Baldwin-Wallace Coll; MA 60 Case Western Reserve Univ; Sp-Lang Path, Rehab Cen Cattaraugus Co NY, **SLP ACE**

Crouse, Maureen Elizabeth Ludwigsburg Middle School, APO New York, NY 09279, (202) 325-0885, BS 79 PA St Univ - Univ Park; ME 85 Southeastern LA Univ; Sp-Lang Path, Dept Defense Dependents Schs, **SLP**

Croutch, Carl A 400 Parnassus Avenue #705A, San Francisco, CA 94143, (415) 476-5101, BA 74 CA St Univ - Sacramento; MS 76 UT St Univ; Aud, Univ of Calif, **A**

Crowder, Elaine Mayhall 57 Pierce Road, Watertown, MA 02172, (617) 259-9291, BA 75 Pomona Coll; MS 80 Emerson Coll; Sp-Lang Path, Private Practice, **SLP**

Crowder, Joy Lynn 1119 Cherokee Road, Louisville, KY 40204-1268, (502) 893-0255, BS 84 IN St Univ - Terre Haute; MA 85 Ball St Univ; **SLP**

Crowder-Wile, Marilyn Theresa 100 Park Avenue #E, Morris, IL 60450-8823, (815) 942-0929, BA 83 Augustana Coll; MS 85 Eastern IL Univ; SLP, Northern Trails AEA, **SLP**

Crowe, Dr Barbara J Valdosta State College, Department Of Special Education, Education Center, Valdosta, GA 31698, (912) 333-5932, BS 66 Purdue Univ - West Lafayette; MS 67 Purdue Univ - West Lafayette; PH 87 (Sp-Lang Path) OH St Univ; 87–Asst Prof, Valdosta State Col, **SLP**

Crowe, Mrs Beth Ann 4515 Cambridge Court, Bloomington, IN 47401, (812) 988-6601, BS 80 Purdue Univ - West Lafayette; OM 84 IN Univ - Bloomington; **SLP**

Crowe, Mrs Carol 911 Poplar, Royal Oak, MI 48073, (313) 651-6210, BS 66 Eastern MI Univ; MA 77 Eastern MI Univ; Sp-Lang Path, Rochester Community Schools, **SLP**

Crowe, Cheryl A 6069 Jacques Drive, San Jose, CA 95123, (408) 281-0452, BS 70 TX Christian Univ; MA 71 TX Christian Univ; **SLP**

Crowe, Linda Kay Route 1 Box 49, Raymond, NE 68428, (402) 783-2803, BS 78 Southeast MO St Univ; MS 86 Univ of NE - Lincoln; **SLP**

Crowe, Mary R 1018 Alpine Ridge Mo, Manchester, MO 63021, (314) 447-4965, BS 78 Univ of MO - Columbia; MA 79 Univ of MO - Columbia; SLP, Francis Howell School District, **SLP**

Crowe, Mrs Suzanne S Henderson Falls Road, Toccoa, GA 30577, **SLP**

Crowe, Dr Thomas A Dept Communicative Disorders, University Of Mississippi, University, MS 38677, (601) 232-7271, BA 73 Univ of AL- Tuscaloosa; MA 75 Univ of AL- Tuscaloosa; PH 80 (Sp Path/Psychology) LA St Univ - Baton Rouge; 87–Chmn/Assoc Prof, University of Mississippi, **SLP**

Crowell, Mrs Susan Marto 9029 Siletz Drive, Tualatin, OR 97062, (503) 692-0539, BA 80 Pacific Univ; 88–Sp-Lang Path, Lake Oswego Sch Dist, **SLP**

Crowell, Tama S 4725 Pinecrest Terrace, Eden, NY 14057, (716) 662-0135, BS 74 Syracuse Univ; MS 76 SUNY - Coll at Buffalo; Sp-Lang Path, Bd Coop Ed Serv #2, **SLP**

Crowl, Mrs Kathy W 7794 East Linden Lane, Parma, OH 44130, (216) 476-7104, BS 79 Kent St Univ; MA 79 Kent St Univ; Sp-Lang Path, Fairview Gen Hosp, **SLP**

Crowley, Albert Brian 4125 N W 19th Plce, Gainesville, FL 32605-3527, (904) 395-1793, **A**

Crowley, Alice L Liebfrauenstrasse 95 D-6100, Darmstadt, West Germany, BS 72 SUNY - Coll at Buffalo; MS 78 San Francisco St Univ; 86–Aud, Hoergeraete Bonsel, **A**

Crowley, Donna J Florida State University, Speech & Hearing Clinic, Tallahassee, FL 32306, (904) 644-2238, BA 66 Univ of FL; MA 68 Univ of FL; Assoc Prof, FL St U, **SLP**

Crowley, Mrs Ellen C 201 Vanderpool #97, Houston, TX 77024, (713) 794-2526, BS 72 Marquette Univ; MS 73 Marquette Univ; Sp-Lang Path, Baylor Coll of Med, **SLP**

Crowley, Mrs Grett Doneen 5422 Forest Oaks Dr South, Mobile, AL 36618, (205) 343-8015, BS 84 Talladega Coll; MS 86 Talladega Coll; **SLP A**

Crowley, Joanne M 2108 Salisbury Road, Silver Spring, MD 20910, (202) 576-1646, BS 76 Emerson Coll; MA 78 Univ of MD - College Park; Aud, Army Aud & Sp Cen, **A**

Crowley, John Francis Route 1 Box 137-B, Salmon, ID 83467, (208) 756-2016, **SLP**

Crowley, Kathleen Moynahan 4102 East St Joseph Way, Phoenix, AZ 85018, (602) 998-0894, BS 71 Northern AZ Univ; MS 83 AZ St Univ; Sp-Lang Path, Scottsdale USD, **SLP**

Crowley, Margaret Stanton 4125 N W 19th Place, Gainesville, FL 32605-3527, (904) 373-5507, BA 78 Univ of Central FL; MS 80 Rutger's St Univ - Douglas Coll; Sp-Lang Path, Spec Commun, **SLP**

Crowley, Melissa Ann 25607 Ridgebrook, Spring, TX 77380, (713) 586-1100, BS 83 Univ of Houston - Univ Park; MA 86 Univ of Houston - Univ Park; 86–Sp-Lang Path, Spring ISD, **SLP**

Crowley, Paula Wilson 210 Annetta Circle, Trussville, AL 35173, (205) 251-3246, BA 76 Auburn Univ - Auburn; OM 78 Auburn Univ - Auburn; Sp-Lang Path, Echo Foundation/Allancott Sch, **SLP**

Crowley, Mrs Therese M 21829 Grant Avenue, Torrance, CA 90503, (213) 533-4519, BA 73 CA St Univ - Long Beach; MA 76 CA St Univ - Long Beach; Sp-Lang Path, LACOE Supt of Schs, **SLP**

Crowl-Gallagher, Renee 925 South Clinton Street, Baltimore, MD 21224-5025, (301) 675-8192, MS 82 Loyola Coll; 88–Sp-Lang Path, Easter Seals Soc of MD, **SLP**

Crown, Mrs Kathleen M 4408 Kellia Lane N E, Albuquerque, NM 87111, (505) 247-4224, BA 81 Catholic Univ of America; MS 83 Univ of MI - Ann Arbor; Sp-Lang Path, Albuquerque Hrng & Sp Cen, **SLP**

Croyle, Mrs Denise A F 1050 Wade Lane, Oakmont, PA 15139, (412) 828-8871, BS 75 Indiana Univ of PA; MA 79 Univ of Pittsburgh - Pittsburgh; Sp-Lang Path, Allegheny Intermediate Unit, **SLP**

Croyle, Mrs Edana C 5425 Lake Killarney, Waco, TX 76710, (817) 772-9200, BA 70 Univ of Houston - Univ Park; MA 74 Univ of Houston - Univ Park; **SLP**

Crudo, Lynn Hilley Route 1 Box 137, Vashon, WA 98070, (206) 582-8900, BA 79 Univ of FL; ME 80 Univ of FL; SLP, Western State Hosp, **SLP**

Cruickshank, Teresa Lee 4084 Stardust Road, Lompoc, CA 93436, (805) 733-4542, BS 85 Univ of WY; MS 87 Univ of WY; Sp-Lang Path, Cross Sp & Hrng, **SLP**

Cruise, Mrs Susan Karpe 50 Overlook Road, Narragansett, RI 02882, (401) 783-8578, BA 84 Univ of RI; MS 86 PA St Univ - Univ Park; 88–Sp-Lang Path, Rhode Island Hosp, **SLP**

Crujido, Mrs Lisa Payne 2945 Marjorie Place, Cambria, CA 93428-5033, (805) 546-7693, MS 79 IL St Univ - Normal; 86–Sp-Lang Path, Private Practice, **SLP**

Crull, Mrs Sharon I D 22 Keepataw Court, Lemont, IL 60439, (312) 257-2297, BS 75 Eastern IL Univ; MS 76 Eastern IL Univ; Sp-Lang Path, SW Cook Co Coop Assn Spec Ed, **SLP**

Crum, Marian 4860 Ivanhoe Avenue, Sheffield Lake, OH 44054, (216) 949-5979, BA 83 Bowling Green St Univ; MA 87 Cleveland St Univ

Crum, Dr Michael A VA Medical Center (126), 2100 Ridgecrest Drive S E, Albuquerque, NM 87108, (505) 265-1711, BS 64 Ball St Univ; MA 68 Univ of TN - Knoxville; PH 74 (NS) Northwestern Univ; Aud, VA Med Cen, **A**

Crum, Robyn L 6490 Landover Road Suite E, Landover, MD 20785, (301) 772-0990, BA 77 Univ of MD - College Park; MA 79 Univ of MD - College Park; Asst Chief, Pg Co Hlth Dept, **A**

Crump, Elizabeth S 713 Manor Drive, Iowa City, IA 52246, (319) 351-1048, BS 78 Univ of MN - Minneap-St Paul; MA 80 Univ of MN - Minneap-St Paul; 87–Aud, The Univ of IA Hosp & Clinics, **A**

Crumpler, Mrs Gloria T 9107 7th Avenue, Inglewood, CA 90305, (213) 515-3084, BA 53 TN St Univ; MA 57 TN St Univ; Sp-Lang Path, L A USD, **SLP**

Crumpler, Linda S 1222 South Pierce, Little Rock, AR 72204, (501) 371-1949, OB 77 Univ of Central AR; MS 79 Univ of AR - Little Rock; Sp-Lang Path, Ark Schl for the Deaf, **SLP**

Crumpton, Teresa B 1027 Homecrest, Kalamazoo, MI 49001, BA 78 MI St Univ; MA 80 Western MI Univ; 88–Aud, Constance Brown Ctr, **A**

Crum-Sweely, Lori L 1190 Ramblewood Drive, Annapolis, MD 21401, (301) 266-1396, BS 82 Bloomsburg Univ of PA; MS 83 Bloomsburg Univ of PA; 87–Sp-Lang Path, Private Practice, **SLP**

Crunk, Mrs Anne M Knoxville Convalescent Center, 809 Emerald Avenue, Knoxville, TN 37917, (615) 524-7366, BA 75 Hofstra Univ; MS 76 PA St Univ - Univ Park; Sp-Lang Path, Prof Hlth Serv, **SLP**

Cruse, Caroline M 2803 Bonita, Great Bend, KS 67530, (316) 792-4087, BS 76 Univ of WI - Stevens Point; MA 79 Wichita St Univ; 83–Sp-Lang Path, Jim Johnson, **SLP**

Crutcher, Damaris W 7777 Forest Lane A-103, Dallas, TX 75230, **SLP A**

Crutcher, Deborah G 4640 Lucerene Lakes Blvd, Apartment 404, Lake Worth, FL 33463, (407) 737-7733, BS 74 Murray St Univ; MS 78 Murray St Univ; Sp-Lang Path, Bethesda Memorial Hosp, **SLP**

Crutchfield, Dr Verna Mae Box 569, Comfort, TX 78013, (512) 634-2218, BA 41 Howard Payne Univ; MA 50 Hardin-Simmons Univ; ED 64 (NS) Univ of Denver; **SLP LM**

Cruthirds-Meyers, Mrs Lynda Lee Hq Usmca-Gsn Box 328, APO New York, NY 09169-1610, BS 82 Univ Southern MS-Hattiesburg; MS 83 Univ Southern MS-Hattiesburg; 87–Sp-Lang Path, US Army-Excep Family Mem Prog, **SLP**

Cruthis, Mrs Quinta Lockhart 429 Lone Wolf Road, Cave City, AR 72521, (501) 283-5738, OB 78 AR St Univ; OM 81 AR St Univ; Sp-Lang Path, Northcentral Ar Dev Council, **SLP**

Cruz, Dr Angel R C L-32 5th Street, Hnas Davila, Bayamon, PR 00619, BS 74 Univ of PR - Rio Piedras; MS 76 Univ of PR - Rio Piedras; MD 81 (NS) 0171; **A**

Cruz, Eduardo 6527 Deane Hill Drive #35, Knoxville, TN 37919, (615) 588-7745, BS 76 Univ of North TX; MS 78 Univ of North TX; Faculty Assoc Otor, Univ of Texas-Health Sci Ctr, **A**

Cruz, Mrs Eneida Maldonado 401 Lafayette Boulevard, Bowling Green, OH 43402, (419) 352-5115, BS 80 SUNY - Coll at Geneseo; MA 81 Bowling Green St Univ; 83–Sp-Lang Path, Wood Co Bd of Men Ret/Dev Dis, **SLP**

Cruz, Mayra 6 Berglund Avenue, Staten Island, NY 10314, (718) 442-8588, BA 81; MS 83 Univ of PR - San Juan; **SLP**

Cruzan, Mrs Margaret K 1597 Clark Drive, Yardley, PA 19067, (609) 896-9500, BA 67 Temple Univ; ME 81 Trenton St Coll; Sp-Lang Path, St Lawrence Rehab Cen, **SLP**

Cruzen, Linda Louise 3325 West Hillsdale Drive, Apartment C, Visalia, CA 93291, (209) 625-6500, 82 CA St Univ - Sacramento; 84 CA St Univ - Sacramento; 84–Sp-Lang Path, Visalia USD, **SLP**

Cryder, Ellen Gail 790 Greenridge Drive, La Canada, CA 91011, (818) 790-6066, BA 76 Occidental Coll; MA 83 CA St Univ - Northridge; Sp-Lang Path, Pasadena USD, **SLP**

Csargo, Georganne Marie 12714 East Asbury Circle, Apartment V-202, Aurora, CO 80014, (303) 752-3613, BA 84 Univ of MN - Duluth; MA 86 Univ of Denver; 86–Sp-Lang Path, Aurora PS, **SLP**

Csatari, Marjorie Pizer 11 Tarrytown Road, Englishtown, NJ 07726, (609) 443-7820, BA 67 Trenton St Coll; MS 86 Rutgers St Univ - Newark

Csicsay, Mrs Katalin M Central Speech-Language Pathology PC, 33 Fort Hill Road, Yonkers, NY 10710, (914) 337-3500, BA 81 Hofstra Univ; MS 86 Columbia Univ Teachers Coll; 88–Sp-Lang Path, Central Speech-Lang Path, **SLP**

Cubert, Mrs Catherine L 1231 DE La Guerra Road, Santa Barbara, CA 93103, (805) 966-9086, BS 46 Nat'l Coll of Ed - Evanston; MA 52 Nat'l Coll of Ed - Evanston; **A LM**

Cuccaro, Mrs Joann Valentine 2 Rainbow Terrace, West Orange, NJ 07052, (201) 299-0166, BA 81 Montclair St Coll; MS 83 Columbia Univ Teachers Coll; Sp-Lang Path, Mountain Lakes Bd of Educ, **SLP**

Cuda, Mrs Rae A 901 Loch Lommond Drive, Hutchinson, KS 67502, (316) 662-8566, BA 74 Wichita St Univ; MA 76 Wichita St Univ; Sp-Lang Path, USD 308, **SLP**

Cudahy, Dr Edward A Lexington Speech &Hearing Ctr, 30th Avenue &75th Street, Jackson Heights, NY 11370, (718) 899-8800, BA 68 Stanford Univ; PH 74 (NS) AZ St Univ; Dir Aud Resrch

Cudworth, Hilary F 123 Bridge Street, Salem, MA 01970, (617) 745-9743, BS 79 Univ of VA - Charlottesville; MA 86 Northeastern Univ; Speech-Language Pathologist, UCP Program, **SLP**

Cuff, Martin Daniel 6 South Boulevard #2, Richmond, VA 23220, (800) 368-3472, MA 87 Kent St Univ; Reg Consultant, Prentke-Romich Co

Cuffia, Mrs Deborah Anne 5621 McCulloch, Temple City, CA 91780, (818) 285-2111, BA 81 CA St Univ - Los Angeles; MA 85 CA St Univ - Los Angeles; Sp-Lang Path, Temple Cty USD, **SLP**

Cugin, Janet Melissa 864 Sunset Blvd, #13, Kenner, LA 70065, (504) 464-1654, ME 88 Southeastern LA Univ

Cujino, Joan E 10439 Willowbrae Avenue, Chatsworth, CA 91311, BS 68 SUNY - Coll at Fredonia; MS 72 CUNY - Brooklyn Coll; **SLP**

Culatta, Dr Barbara E University Of Rhode Island, Adams Hall, Kingston, RI 02881, (401) 792-5969, BS 69 CA Univ of PA; MS 70 Univ of Pittsburgh - Pittsburgh; PH 75 (NS) Univ of Pittsburgh - Pittsburgh; Assoc Prof, U of RI, **SLP**

Culatta, Janet D 3272 Hunters Point Drive, Lexington, KY 40502, (502) 863-1170, BS 78 Miami Univ - Oxford; MS 79 Univ of KY; Sp-Lang Path, Scott Co Sch, **SLP**

Culatta, Dr Richard A Department Of Language Reading & Exceptionalities, Appalachian State University, Boone, NC 28608, (704) 262-6064, BA 64 CUNY - Brooklyn Coll; MS 66 CUNY - Brooklyn Coll; PH 71 (Sp Path & Aud) Univ of Pittsburgh - Pittsburgh; Prof, Appalachian State Univ, **SLP F**

Culberson, Carole Lynne 424 Oakland Street #4, Morgantown, WV 26505, (304) 599-3400, 88 WV Univ

Culbertson, Cheryl Ellen 5237 Horton, Mission, KS 66202, (816) 833-2088, BA 82 Univ of MO - KS City; MS 85 Central MO St Univ; 87–Sp-Lang Path, Sunshine Ctr Inc, **SLP**

Culbertson, Mrs Patricia Marie 8609 West Oklahoma Avenue, Milwaukee, WI 53227, BS 73 Univ of WI - Oshkosh; MS 79 Univ of WI - Milwaukee; Sp/Lang Path, Sch Dist of West Allis, **SLP**

Culbertson, Mrs Patti F 628 Oak Marsh Drive, Mount Pleasant, SC 29464, (803) 881-8820, BA 70 Univ of SC - Columbia; MS 76 Univ of SC - Columbia; Contract SLP, South Carolina Health Dept, **SLP**

Culbertson, Dr William R, III P O Box 66, Cartersville, VA 23027, (804) 264-1447, BA 70 Univ of Richmond; MS 75 Old Dominion Univ; PH 81 (Aud/Sp Sciences) MI St Univ; 81–Sp-Lang Path, Private Practice, **SLP**

Culbertson-Egan, Maurine A 4 Risingwood, Bow, NH 03301, (603) 774-3803, BS 80 Northeastern Univ; ME 82 Northeastern Univ; Aud, Private Practice, **A**

Culhane, Colleen Ann 9108 35th Avenue North, New Hope, MN 55427, (612) 546-2894, **SLP**

Culhane, Karen D 13034 Woodrose Way, Grass Valley, CA 95945, (916) 273-8026, MS 72 Univ of Redlands; BA 71 Univ of Redlands; Sp/Lang Path, Karen D Culhane & Associates, **SLP**

Culibrk, Janine P O Box 1544, Sunset Beach, CA 90742-1544, (213) 592-4767, MA 81 CA St Univ - Long Beach; SLP, Long Beach USD, **SLP**

Culkin, Mary La Rue 13 Parklane North, Mountain Top, PA 18707, BA 72 Univ of Denver; MS 83 Bloomsburg Univ of PA; 86–Sp-Lang Path, Wyoming Valley Children's Assoc, **SLP**

Cullar, Ann 20 South Bankers Lane, Indianapolis, IN 46201, (317) 264-1422, BS 83 IN Univ - Bloomington; MA 87 Ball St Univ

Cullen, Mrs Barbara Ellen 5746 Georgetown Drive, Erie, PA 16509, (814) 864-6608, OB 76 Edinboro Univ of PA; BS 74 Carlow Coll; MA 81 Edinboro Univ of PA; Sch Dist of the City Erie, **SLP**

Cullen, Mrs Gail F 8 Homestead Lane, Stoneham, MA 02180, (617) 438-8167, BS 76 Northeastern Univ; ME 79 Northeastern Univ; **SLP**

Cullen, Mrs Louise W 824 Pinecrest Drive, Mc Keesport, PA 15135, (412) 394-5744, BS 51 Indiana Univ of PA; OM 78 Univ of Pittsburgh - Pittsburgh; Sp-Lang Path, Allg Inter Ut, **SLP**

Cullen, Margaret 204 South Macarthur, Springfield, IL 62704, (217) 738-3767, BA 65 Mundelein Coll; MA 70 De Paul Univ; Sp-Lang Path, Mem Med Cen, **SLP**

Cullen, Monica L 1220 Treefern Drive, Virginia Beach, VA 23451, (804) 481-4003, BS 80 Old Dominion Univ; OM 82 Univ of SC - Columbia; Aud, VA Aud Assoc, **A**

Cullen, Patrick Edward P O Box 920, Barnstable, MA 02630, (617) 255-4421, BA 69 Southern IL Univ -Carbondale; MS 71 Southern IL Univ -Carbondale; Owner, Cape & Islands Hear Serv, **SLP A**

Culler, Ted A Charlotte-Mecklenburg Schools, P O Box 30035, Charlotte, NC 28230, (704) 379-7120, BA 70 Univ of NC - Chapel Hill; ME 72 Univ of NC - Chapel Hill; SLP, Charlotte-Mecklenburg Schools, **SLP**

Culleton, Ruth S 194 Grand Avenue, Rochester, NY 14609, (716) 288-3306, BS 77 Stockton St Coll; MA 80 Central MI Univ; Sp-Lang Path, City Sch Dist of Rochester, **SLP**

Cullinan, Denise Graziano Box 439-C, Cooperhill Road, Northwood, NH 03261, (617) 453-1797, BS 82 Elmira Coll; MS 84 Emerson Coll; 84–Sp-Lang Path, Dracut Pub Schs, **SLP**

Cullinan, Mrs Elnora T 3412 Windsor Avenue, Oklahoma City, OK 73122, (405) 789-1711, BA 52 OH Univ - Athens; MA 59 Univ of IA; SLP, Putnam Cty Sch Dist, **SLP**

Cullinan, Maureen Ann 100 Woodshire Drive, Pittsburgh, PA 15215, (412) 624-2324, BS 78 PA St Univ - Univ Park; MS 80 Vanderbilt Univ; Sp-Lang Path, Western Psych I & Cl, **SLP**

Cullinan, Timothy B Fircrest School Pat 1 DSHS, 15230 15th Avenue N E, B17-31, Seattle, WA 98155, (206) 364-0300, BA 75 SUNY - Center at Buffalo; BA 75 SUNY - Center at Buffalo; MS 77 Univ of WA; 86–Sp-Lang Path, Dept of Soc/Hlth Serv Fircrest, **SLP**

Cullinan, Dr Walter L Keys Speech & Hearing Center, Health Sci Ctr Univ Of Ok, P O Box 26901, Oklahoma City, OK 73190, (405) 271-4214, BA 53 Boston Coll; MA 60 Univ of IA, PH 61 (NS) Univ of IA; Prof Commun Dis, U Ok Hlth Sc Cen, **SLP F**

Cullinane, Mrs Ruth Ann 20 Rochester Street, Somersworth, NH 03878, **SLP**

Cullison, Bonita L 2917 McGee Way, Olney, MD 20832, (301) 493-8342, BA 76 Univ of MD - College Park; MA 78 Univ of MD - College Park; Sp-Lang Path, Montgomery Co Public Schools, **SLP**

Cullop, Joann Robertson Frankfurt American High School, APO New York, NY 09039, **SLP**

Culp, Ann E 168 Somershire Drive, Rochester, NY 14617, (716) 338-3562, BS 85 Ithaca Coll; MS 87 Syracuse Univ

Culp, Deidra Beth Route 2 Box 410, Presque Isle, ME 04769, (214) 635-9130, BS 85 Baylor Univ; MS 87 Baylor Univ

Culp, Delva Mae 4124 Amherst, Dallas, TX 75225, (214) 783-3137, BS 74 Northwestern Univ; MA 75 Northwestern Univ; Sp-Lang Path, Callier Cen-U of Tx at Dallas, **SLP**

Culpepper, N Brandt 3652 Phinney Avenue North, Apartment 3, Seattle, WA 98103, (206) 547-3049, BS 82 Univ of GA; ME 83 Univ of GA; 88–Research Asst, Univ of Washington, **A**

Culton, Dr Gerald Lee The University Of Alabama, P O Box 1903, Tuscaloosa, AL 35487, (205) 348-7131, BA 60 Univ of NE - Omaha; MA 62 KS St Univ; PH 68 (Sp Path) Univ of Denver; Prof of Commun Dis, The Univ of Alabama, **SLP**

Culver, Mrs Margaret A 5510 North 33rd Street, Milwaukee, WI 53209, (414) 272-1344, BS 80 Univ of WI - Madison; MS 81 Univ of WI - Milwaukee; Sp-Lang Path, Milwaukee Pub Schs, **SLP**

Cumbie, Mrs Janet 3002 Encino Avenue, Bay City, TX 77414, (409) 245-1145, BS 73 Baylor Univ; ME 75 Southwest TX St Univ; Private Practice, **SLP ACE**

Cumby, Polly B 4244 Garden Avenue, Western Springs, IL 60558, (312) 246-8912, BA 70 Elmhurst Coll; MA 71 Northern IL Univ - De Kalb; Sp/Lang Path, Aero Spec Ed Coop, **SLP**

Cumiskey, Sr Marian 545 Broadway, Dobbs Ferry, NY 10522, (914) 693-4500, BS 61 Fordham Univ; MA 69 Coll of Saint Rose; Asst Prof, Mercy Coll, **SLP**

Cumisky, Mrs Joan Gavitt 190 East Shore Drive, Massapequa, NY 11758, (516) 795-8854, BA 76 Long Island U - CW Post Ctr; MA 82 Long Island U - CW Post Ctr; SLP, BOCES II, **SLP**

Cumley, Gary D 205 Canyon Way, Arroyo Grande, CA 93420, (805) 543-6940, BS 69 CO St Univ; MS 70 Univ of OR; Sp-Lang Path, Office County Supt of Schools, **SLP**

Cummard, Mrs Kathryn Anne 715 North Orange Circle, Mesa, AZ 85201, (601) 892-2022, BS 70 Brigham Young Univ; OM 71 Brigham Young Univ; Sp-Lang Path, Gilbert School District, **SLP**

Cumming, Mrs Kelley Lawson 5366 S W Red Leaf Street, Lake Oswego, OR 97034, (503) 280-6527, BS 81 Univ of AZ; MA 85 San Jose St Univ; 85–Sp-Lang Path, Portland PS, **SLP**

Cummings, Betty J 2112 Independence, Fort Smith, AR 72901, (501) 474-8084, BA 73 Univ of AR - Fayetteville; MA 73 Univ of AR - Fayetteville; Sp-Lang Path, Wn AR Counsel & Guid Cen, **SLP**

Cummings, Charlene D 3800 South Beltline, Paducah, KY 42001, (502) 443-7541, MS 79 Murray St Univ; Sp-Lang Path, Paducah Pub Sch, **SLP**

Cummings, Janet L 1755 CY Court, Vienna, VA 22180, (703) 281-9566, BS 72 Brigham Young Univ; MA 81 Univ of MD - College Park; Sp-Lang Path, Fairfax Co Pub Sch, **SLP**

Cummings, Mrs Jolie E 185 Edgewater Drive, Coral Gables, FL 33133, (305) 235-6811, BA 77 Tulane Univ; MS 78 Boston Univ; Sp-Lang Path, Dade Co Pub Sch, **SLP**

Cummings, Mrs Laura 213 West Park, Wheaton, IL 60187, (312) 790-2474, BS 78 Southern IL Univ -Carbondale; MA 79 Northern IL Univ - De Kalb; Sp-Lang Path, Il Deaf-Blind Sch, **SLP**

Cummings, Mrs Lori A 6362 Townsend Road, Jacksonville, FL 32244, (904) 771-7050, BA 84 Western MI Univ; MA 85 Western MI Univ; 87–Aud, Robert K Middlekauff MD PA, **A**

Cummings, Marjorie D 1700 Glendon Avenue, Los Angeles, CA 90024, MS; **SLP LM**

Cummings, Mrs Marlene Rayner 314 West 4th Street, Rochester, MI 48063, (313) 739-0400, BS 77 Central MI Univ; MS 78 Univ of WI - Stevens Point; Spec Ed Preprimary Tchr, Utica Comm Sch, **SLP**

Cummings, Mary A 135 Jason Street, Arlington, MA 02174, (617) 641-0954, BA 70 Fordham Univ; MS 73 Emerson Coll; Sp-Lang Path, Choate-Symmes Hlth Serv, **SLP**

Cummings, Patricia Ann Moore 1034 Imhoff, Norman, OK 73072, (405) 527-5506, BA 62 Univ of Tulsa; MS 77 Univ of OK Medical Center; Sp-Lang Path, Purcell Pub Sch& Can Val Co-Op, **SLP**

Cummings, Robinson 6362 Townsend Road, Jacksonville, FL 32244, (904) 771-7050, BS 80 Grand Valley St Coll; MA 85 Western MI Univ; 88–Aud, Speech & Hearing Center Inc, **A**

Cummings, Tara T 2011-A Calumet Drive, New Holstein, WI 53061-1009, (414) 898-0083, BA 81 Univ of WI - Eau Claire; MS 86 Univ of WI - Whitewater; 86–Sp-Lang Path, New Holstein PS, **SLP**

Cummings-Ingram, Peggy Jean 2810 Jefferson Avenue, Yuba City, CA 95991, (916) 673-8152, BA 74 CA St Univ - Chico; Sp-Lang Path, Sutter County Superintendent, **SLP**

Cummins, Christine Ellen 3631 E Sunnyside Drive, Phoenix, AZ 85028, (602) 263-9002, BS 85 Northern AZ Univ; MS 87 Univ of TX - Dallas; 88–Aud, Cigna Health Plans, **A**

Cummins, Mrs Diane M 172 South Columbia Avenue, Columbus, OH 43209, (614) 252-3148, BS 59 OH St Univ

Cummins, Lori Gealer 28339 Green Willow, Farmington Hills, MI 48018, (313) 326-7443, **SLP**

Cummins, Margaret M 1900 Everest Avenue, Coos Bay, OR 97420, (503) 269-1611, BS 77 IN Univ - Bloomington; MA 79 IN Univ - Bloomington; 79–Sp-Lang Path, Coos Co Ed Ser Dist, **SLP**

Cummins, Mrs Melissa Grier 128 Brandon Road, Baltimore, MD 21212, (301) 396-8207, MS 84 Loyola Coll; SLP, Baltimore City Schools, **SLP**

Cummons, Gail Ann 237 East Main Street #B-3, Moorestown, NJ 08057-2982, (609) 424-9084, BS 75 Bloomsburg Univ of PA; MA 83 Temple Univ; 88–Aud/Dir, Atrium Hrng & Sp Ctr, **A**

Cumpata, Joellen Frere Massachusetts General Hospital, Speech-Lang Pathology Dept, Acc Suite 637, Boston, MA 02114, (617) 726-2763, BA 76 MI St Univ; MA 77 MI St Univ; 84–Assistant Director, Massachusetts General Hospital, **SLP**

Cundiff, Phyllis Mae Roanoke City Schools, P O Box 13145, Roanoke, VA 24031, (703) 989-1024, BS 78 Radford Univ; MS 82 Radford Univ; Sp-Lang Path, Roanoke City Public Schools, **SLP**

Cuneo, Margaret Elaine 20 McAlee Avenue, Framingham, MA 01701, (617) 588-5034, BS 83 Worcester St Coll; MA 85 Univ of CT; **A**

Cunico, Lucille A 16063 6th Street North, Lakeland, MN 55043, (612) 690-2497, BA 67 Univ of Northern CO; MS 78 Univ of WI - River Falls; SLP, Horace Mann St Paul Pub Sch, **SLP**

Cunningham, Barbara C Route 4 Box 91, Crowley, LA 70526, (318) 824-6250, BA 73 Northwestern St Univ; MA 75 Northwestern St Univ; 77–Sp-Lang Path, SW La St Sch & Reg Cen, **SLP**

Cunningham, Clare F 119 Ayers Court #J3, Teaneck, NJ 07666, (201) 441-2161, BA 80 Rutger's St Univ - Douglas Coll; MS 82 Univ of WI - Madison; 84–Aud, Hackensack Medical Center, **A**

Cunningham, Mrs Colette Adele Box 63, Lansford, ND 58750, (701) 784-5489, BS 84 ND St Univ; MS 85 Minot St Univ; 85–Sp-Lang Path, Glenburn PS

Cunningham, Dr David Robert Div Of Comm Dis Dept Of Srgy, Myers Hall Health Sci Ctr, U Of Louisville Sch Of Med, Louisville, KY 40292, (502) 588-5274, BA 69 Geneva Coll; MA 70 Univ of KS; PH 72 (Aud) Univ of KS; Prof Dir, Div of Commun Dis U of Louisv, **A**

Cunningham, Mrs Elizabeth Anne 5-D Parris Meadow Drive, Newburgh, NY 12550-1120, (914) 562-4947, BS 84 Ithaca Coll; MA 85 Bowling Green St Univ; 87–Sp-Lang Path, Newburgh Dev Learning Ctr, **SLP**

Cunningham, Dr Everlene Giles 11048 Swansfield Road, Columbia, MD 21044, (202) 363-0990, BS 62 Hampton Univ; MS 63 Gallaudet Coll; PH 80 (NS) Univ of MD - College Park; 87–Coord Clin Svcs, Assoc Univ Consultants Inc, **A**

Cunningham, Gail Grace 11729 S W Windmill Drive, Beaverton, OR 97005, (503) 641-5881, BS 81 Univ of OR; MS 83 Portland St Univ; Sp-Lang Path, Portland Public Schools, **SLP**

Cunningham, Gary W 8 Sudden Valley, Bellingham, WA 98226-4819, (503) 620-6076, BA 65 Eastern WA Univ; ME 71 Univ of the Pacific; Pres, Cc Publications Inc, **SLP**

Cunningham, Jane Tubbs 2028 South Adams, Spokane, WA 99203, (509) 455-4060, BA 51 MI St Univ; MS 71 Eastern WA Univ; Retired, Spokane Sch Dist #81, **SLP**

Cunningham, Jeannette 1731 Guilford Lane, Oklahoma City, OK 73120, (405) 843-5121, BS 85 OK St Univ; MS 87 Univ of OK - OK City

Cunningham, Mrs Judith Harber 3521 Cherry Hill Drive, Greensboro, NC 27410, (919) 668-4185, BA 83 Univ of NC - Chapel Hill; MS 85 Univ of NC - Chapel Hill; 88–Sp-Lang Path, Margie Cheshire MED CCC-SLP, **SLP**

Cunningham, Judith Rees 1820 Fulton Street, Palo Alto, CA 94303, (415) 967-7235, MA 84 San Jose St Univ; Sp-Lang Path, Whisman Sch Dist, **SLP**

Cunningham, Mrs Linda G 8-B Paris Avenue, Worcester, MA 01603, (617) 765-9771, BA 76 Univ of VT; MA 78 Univ of CT; Aud, Harrington Memorial Hospital, **A**

Cunningham, Mrs Marcia Dzaman 120 Desmarais Street, Cumberland, RI 02864, (401) 765-2444, MA 83 Univ of MA - Amherst; Sp-Lang Path, Blackstone-Millville Sch Dept, **SLP**

Cunningham, Monyette W 216 11th Avenue S W, Birmingham, AL 35211, (205) 323-5057, BS 77 TN St Univ; MS 78 Univ of Montevallo; SLP, Jefferson County Board of Educ, **SLP**

Cunningham, Mrs Nancy 724 Eldorado Drive, Omaha, NE 68154, (402) 493-2799, BA 59 Saint Louis Univ; MA 72 Lindenwood Coll; **SLP**

Cunningham, Mrs Nancy M 748 Bayou Shores, Monroe, LA 71203, (318) 343-0853, BA 65 Univ of Southwestern LA; MA 66 LA St Univ - Baton Rouge; 87–Sp-Lang Path, Ouachita Parish Sch Bd, **SLP**

Cunningham, Peter Douglas The Audiology Group, 1032 Luke Street, Fort Collins, CO 80524, (303) 482-5700, BS 78 CO St Univ; MS 82 CO St Univ; 84–Aud, Audiology Group, **A**

Cunningham, Rosemary A J 700 Hidden Valley Court, Fairborn, OH 45324, (513) 255-5227, BS 76 FL St Univ; MS 78 FL St Univ; 87–Exec Ofcr, Armstrong Aerospace Med Res Lab (AAMRL), **A**

Cunningham, Virginia 152 Wood Acres, Amherst, NY 14051, **SLP**

Cunningham-Egan, Mrs Jacqueline 206 Whiting Street, Hanover, MA 02339, (617) 878-0679, BA 79 Simmons Coll; MS 85 Emerson Coll; Sp-Lang Path, N River Collab Early Chdhd Ctr, **SLP**

Cunningham-Grant, Mrs Jean D S 1861 Edwards Avenue, Wooster, OH 44691, (216) 345-7506, MA 72 SUNY - Center at Buffalo; 72–Sp-Lang Path, Private Practice, **SLP**

Cunningham-Wong, Patricia Ann 4035 Plateau Road, Reno, NV 89509, (619) 340-4566, **A**

Cupini, Mrs Mariellen 23 Park Square Lane, Pittsford, NY 14534, (716) 586-6820, BS 74 Nazareth Coll of Rochester; MS 76 Nazareth Coll of Rochester; 79–Sp-Lang Path, Private Practice, **SLP**

Cupples, Joseph K 517 Brookline Boulevard, Pittsburgh, PA 15226, (412) 665-4975, BA 72 Univ of Pittsburgh - Pittsburgh; ME 76 Univ of Pittsburgh - Pittsburgh; MA 73 Univ of Pittsburgh - Pittsburgh; SLP, Pittsburgh - Mt Oliver Iu #2, **SLP**

Cupples, Dr Willie P, Jr 403 Five Farms Lane, Timonium, MD 21093, (202) 994-7357, BA 71 Baylor Univ; MA 72 Western IL Univ; PH 78 (Sp-Lang Path) Northwestern Univ; 88–Assoc Clin Prof, George Washington U, **SLP**

Cuquet, Mrs Elizabeth Atkinson 305 Whitehall Drive, Manchester, MO 63011, (314) 631-7800, BS 82 Fontbonne Coll; MS 82 Fontbonne Coll; SLP, St Mary On the Mt Hosp, **SLP**

Curatolo, Jill Maloney 100 Bellingham Street, Chelsea Memorial Health Center-MGH, Chelsea, MA 02150, (617) 884-8300, BA 80 Wellesley Coll; MS 82 Vanderbilt Univ; Sp-Lang Path, Mass Gen Hosp, **SLP ACE**

Curel, Julia Akimi 4421 Ashworth Street, Lakewood, CA 90712-1153, (714) 628-2407, BA 83 Whittier Coll; MA 84 Whittier Coll; Sp-Lang Path, Assoc Sp and Lang Svcs, **SLP**

Curfman, Mrs Susan Margaret 7400 East Woodsboro Avenue, Anaheim, CA 92807-2428, (714) 779-0871, BA 80 CA St Univ - Fullerton; MA 82 CA St Univ - Fullerton; Sp-Lang Path, Private Practice, **SLP**

Curl, Mrs Mary Reid 10063 Haddington Drive, Houston, TX 77080, (713) 493-2494, OB 67 OH Univ - Athens; MA 83 Univ of Houston - Univ Park; Sp-Lang Path, The Briarwood Sch, **SLP**

Curlee, Mrs Deborah L 9516 Briarwood Drive, Knoxville, TN 37923, (615) 693-9408, BA 77 Smith Coll; MA 79 Univ of CT; Sp-Lang Path, Private Practice, **SLP ACE**

Curlee, Dr Richard F 4881 North Camino DE Oeste, Tucson, AZ 85745, (602) 621-1644, BA 61 Wake Forest Univ; MA 65 Univ of Southern CA; PH 67 (NS) Univ of Southern CA; Prof, U of AZ, **SLP F**

Curley, Mrs Janet 35 Meadowbrook Lane, Barrington, RI 02806, (401) 245-4976, MS 80 Northwestern Univ; SLP, Meeting Street Sch, **SLP**

Curley, Mrs Judy R 8809 East 134th Street So, Bixby, OK 74008, (918) 369-1045, BA 77 Univ of OK - Norman; MS 79 Univ of OK - OK City; **SLP**

Curley, Kathleen Mary 268 Timber Point Road, East Islip, NY 11730, (516) 581-1600, BA 79 SUNY - Coll at Cortland; MS 82 Adelphi Univ; Sp-Lang Path, East Islip Pub Sch, **SLP**

Curley, Margaret M 1037 West Barry #1, Chicago, IL 60657, (312) 471-5633, BS 79 Marquette Univ; MS 80 Marquette Univ; Sp-Lang Path, Holy Cross Hosp-Chicago, **SLP**

Curlin, Elizabeth Kramer 530 Sdouth Westlawn, Decatur, IL 62522, (217) 428-7163, BS 85 Eastern IL Univ; MS 86 Eastern IL Univ; **SLP**

Curnett, Jeffrey C 98 Cobble Hill Road, Warwick, RI 02886, (401) 737-3300, BA 75 Univ of RI; MS 77 Univ of RI; Sp-Lang Path, Warwick Sch Syst, **SLP**

Curphey, Mrs Kathleen Theresa 718 Second Street S E, Independence, IA 50644, (319) 334-6639, BA 83 Univ of Northern IA; MA 84 Northern IL Univ - De Kalb; SLP, AEA 7, **SLP**

Curran, Catherine Elizabeth 1510 20th Street #206, Boulder, CO 80302, (303) 789-9217, BA 80 Trinity Univ; MS 84 Univ of NM; Sp-Lang Path, **SLP**

Curran, Mrs Jean L 3865 Alice Lane, Las Vegas, NV 89103, (702) 876-8648, BA 71 Univ of MN - Minneap-St Paul; MS 75 Univ of NV - Reno; Sp-Lang Path, Private Practice, **SLP**

Curran, Mrs Joan Donovan 46 Royal Crest Estates #9, North Andover, MA 01845, (508) 975-8740, MS 84 Boston Univ; Sp-Lang Path, Private Practice, **SLP**

Curran, Mrs Kathryn Lambros 84 Turney Road, Fairfield, CT 06430-6952, (203) 255-3797, BA 77 SUNY - Coll at Cortland; MS 82 East Carolina Univ; SLP, Rehabilitation Consultants, **SLP**

Curran, Lynn M 245 Mohawk, Dearborn, MI 48124, **SLP**

Curran, Dr Michael F 36 Christine Terrace, South Weymouth, MA 02190, (617) 935-2500, BA 70 Boston Coll; MA 72 Bowling Green St Univ; PH 74 (NS) Bowling Green St Univ; President, Advantage Health Corp, **SLP**

Curran, Nancy Voegeli 2891 Tucker Lane, Los Alamitos, CA 90720, (206) 696-4282, BA 78 CA St Univ - Long Beach; MA 82 Humboldt St Univ; 88–Sp-Lang Path, Bowden & Derringer Rehab Assoc, **SLP**

Curran-Zahra, Pamela E 14719 Waterway Drive, Rockville, MD 20853, (301) 460-7452, BA 73 Univ of MD - College Park; MA 79 Univ of MD - College Park; **SLP**

Current, Mrs Jeanne Louise 1681 Lundren, New Carlisle, OH 45344, (513) 921-1750, Sp-Lang Path, Parkview Memorial Hospital, **SLP**

Currey, Lindsay A 18051 Wakefield Lane #103, Huntington Beach, CA 92649, (213) 438-9781, BA 77 Univ of CA - Santa Barbara; MA 79 CA St Univ - Northridge; Sp-Lang Path, Villa Serena Trans Living Ctr, **SLP**

Currie, Cathleen Marie 508 Stewart Avenue, Staten Island, NY 10314, (718) 448-9775, BS 77 Long Island U - CW Post Ctr; MS 79 Adelphi Univ; Sp/Lang Path, Staten Island Ment Hlth, **SLP**

Currie, Kathleen M 714 Lincoln Avenue #2, Port Huron, MI 48060, (313) 987-5000, BA 84 MI St Univ; MA 86 Eastern MI Univ; **SLP**

Currie, Paula Sue 433 Metairie Road, Suite 115, Metairie, LA 70005, (504) 834-4744, BS 74 LA St Univ - Baton Rouge; OM 76 LA St Univ - N O Medical Ctr; PH 86 (Sp Ed Habilative Svc) Univ of New Orleans; 81–Sp-Lang Path, Private Practice, **SLP**

Currie, Sally Jo 2465 Loring Street, San Diego, CA 92109, (619) 272-0621, MS 84 UT St Univ; Sp-Lang Path, South Bay Union Sch Dis, **SLP**

Currie, Yolanda K 217 Webster, Yazoo City, MS 39194, (601) 746-6522, BS 78 Univ of MS; ME MS Coll; MS 81 Univ Southern MS-Hattiesburg; 81–Sp-Lang Path, Private Practice, **SLP**

Currie-Crowell, Joanne 4122 Oak Hollow Road, Calabasas, CA 91302, (818) 888-5887, BA 65 Mount St Mary's Coll; MA 87 CA St Univ - Northridge

Currie-Heytens, Mrs Desiree Ann 13 White Birch Drive, Superior, WI 54880, (715) 392-2853, BA 86 Univ of WI - Eau Claire; MA 87 Univ of MN - Duluth; Sp-Lang Path, Sandstone Ps Dstr, **SLP**

Currier, Mrs Laura Chesler 8701 East Lincoln Drive, Scottsdale, AZ 85253, (602) 843-3400, BS 79 Bradley Univ; OM 83 AZ St Univ; Sp/Lang Path, Cave Creek Public Schools, **SLP**

Curry, Mrs Dawn Denise 6073 South Lake Drive, Cudahy, WI 53110, (414) 769-0599, BS 84 Univ of WI - Madison; MS 87 Marquette Univ; 87–Sp-Lang Path, S Milwaukee PS Sys, **SLP**

Curry, E Thayer 6249 49th Court East, Tuscaloosa, AL 35401, PH (NS); **SLP A F LM**

Curry, Genevieve Marie 1189 East Long Place, Littleton, CO 80122, (303) 337-5846, BA 81 Univ of CO - Boulder; MA 83 Univ of Northern CO; SLP, Douglas County School District, **SLP**

Curry, Joan E 419 West Reynolds, Pontiac, IL 61764, (815) 842-2944, BS 75 IL St Univ - Normal; MS 76 IL St Univ - Normal; Sp/Lang Path, Pontiac Elem Sch Dist, **SLP**

Curry, Joseph J 2929 Old Gettysburg Road, Camp Hill, PA 17011, (717) 737-6728, BA 71 King's Coll; ME 75 Bloomsburg Univ of PA; Audiologist, Capital Area Intermediate Unit, **A**

Curry, Mrs Kerin Cunning 3035 Commodore Drive, Colorado Springs, CO 80920, BS 78 CO St Univ; MS 80 Univ of AZ; SLP, Pikes Peak Bd of Coop Serv, **SLP**

Curry, Laura Ann 191 Fernwood Terrace, Stewart Manor, NY 11530, (718) 441-5333, BA 82 Adelphi Univ; MS 83 Adelphi Univ; 85–Sp-Lang Path, First Step Early Childhood Cen, **SLP**

Curry, Patricia Zellner 17 Greenbriar Lane, Danville, PA 17821, (717) 275-8531, BA 79 4070; MA 80 4070; **A**

Curry-Carter, Mrs Elena Maria 4875 North Backer Avenue, Apartment 129, Fresno, CA 93726-7502, BA 81; MS 83 Southern CT St Univ; Sp-Lang Path, Fresno USD, **SLP**

Curtin, Sr Rose 227 Stone Street, Watertown, NY 13601, (315) 782-7400, BS 70 Ithaca Coll; MS 71 SUNY - Center at Albany; **SLP A**

Curtis, Dr Ann P RFD 2 Box 7280, Welchs Point, Winthrop, ME 04364, (207) 395-4549, BA 71 Univ of ME - Orono; MA 72 OH Univ - Athens; PH 78 (NS) OH Univ - Athens; Sp/Lang Path, Private Practice, **SLP**

Curtis, Mrs Christine 438 Chelan Drive, Vacaville, CA 95688, (707) 448-0108, BA 72 CA St Univ - Chico; MA 74 CA St Univ - Chico; SLP, Solano Co Supt of Sch Offi, **SLP**

Curtis, Mrs Gale H 4235 Gundry Avenue, Long Beach, CA 90807, (213) 595-8923, BS 77 Univ of Southern CA; MA 81 Whittier Coll; 85–Sp-Lang Path, Private Practice, **SLP**

Curtis, Glen W Rural Route 1, Bryan, OH 43506, (419) 636-7409, BS 56 Eastern IL Univ; MS 66 IN Univ - Bloomington; Sp & Hrng Path, Williams Co Schs, **SLP**

Curtis, Hillary 111 Fox Hill Lane, Enfield, CT 06082, (413) 781-9100

Curtis, James F 9650 Grant Creek Road, Missoula, MT 59802, (406) 543-3644, BA 35 Univ of Northern IA; MA 40 Univ of IA; PH 42 (NS) Univ of IA; **A F H LM**

Curtis, Janet S 8632 Sargent Creek Lane, Indianapolis, IN 46256, (317) 226-4299, BS 74 IN Univ - Bloomington; MA 75 IN Univ - Bloomington; 78–Sp-Lang Path, Indianapolis Pub Sch, **SLP**

Curtis, Mrs Kerry H P O Box 100, Levant, ME 04456, (207) 884-7651, BA 71 Univ of ME - Orono; MA 74 Univ of ME - Orono; Sp-Lang Path, Brewer School Department, **SLP**

Curtis, Kim Ann 152 Country Wood Circle, Nashville, TN 37214, (615) 865-7400, BS 84 Southern IL Univ -Carbondale; MA 85 Saint Louis Univ; SLP, Com Hlth Services, **SLP**

Curtis, Mrs Nancy Wildstein 25 Ford Place, Murray Hill, NJ 07974, (201) 464-2763, BS 62 Emerson Coll; MA 63 Stanford Univ; Sp-Lang Path, Early Chldhd Lrng Ctr, **A**

Curtis, Nathan Holbrook RFD 1 Box 456, Belfast, ME 04915, (207) 548-6351, **SLP**

Curtis, Patricia Lou G 10012 Autumnview Lane, Ellicott City, MD 21043, **SLP**

Curtis, Ruth 912 Shore Club Drive, St Clair Shores, MI 48080, MS; **SLP LM**

Curtis, Sandra D 1334 West Xyler, Tulsa, OK 74127, (918) 245-2774, BS 68 Univ of VA - Charlottesville; MA 72 Eastern MI Univ; Sp-Lang Path, Sand Springs PS, **SLP**

Curtis, Mrs Sandra S 6884 Greenleaf Drive, North Richland Hills, TX 76180, (817) 898-2025, BS 71 East Carolina Univ; MA 73 Univ of AL- Tuscaloosa; 87–Sp-Lang Path, Texas Woman University, **SLP**

Curtis, Sue Ellen 1763 Appleton Road, Menasha, WI 54952, (414) 735-9977, BS 84 Univ of WI - Stevens Point; MS 86 Univ of WI - Stevens Point; 86–Sp-Lang Path, Gmeiner Clinic, **SLP**

Curtis, Sue Llewellyn 45 South Childrens Home Rd, Troy, OH 45373, (513) 233-8108, BS 76 Miami Univ - Oxford; MA 78 Miami Univ - Oxford; Prog Dir, Montgomery Decelopmental Cen, **SLP**

Curtis, Dr W Scott University Of Georgia, 570 Aderhold Hall, Athens, GA 30601, (404) 542-1685, BS 54 Northwestern Univ; MA 58 Western MI Univ; PH 60 (Speech Pathology) Purdue Univ - West Lafayette; Prof, U of GA, **SLP**

Curtiss, James Willard 107 Seminole Drive, Springfield, IL 62704, (217) 546-4188, PH 70 (NS) Univ of Denver; 75–Pres PCRI, Private Practice, **SLP**

Curtsinger, Barbara Gayle Star Route Box 221, Airport Trailer Park, Hager Hill, KY 41222, (606) 789-1863, BS 82 Eastern KY Univ; MA 83 Eastern KY Univ; 83–Sp-Lang Path, Eastern KY Sp & Hearing Clinic, **SLP**

Curwen, Mrs Vicki E 4504 Rita Street, La Mesa, CA 92041-5757, (619) 588-3187, MA 88 San Diego St Univ; 86–Sp-Lang Path, Cajon Valley Union Sch Dist

Curylo, Caroline Patricia 43 Tumblebrook Lane, West Hartford, CT 06117, (203) 232-3997, BA 84 Elms Coll; MS 86 Boston Univ; **SLP**

Cush, Gina 386 Jackson Avenue, Washington Township, NJ 07675, (914) 947-1000, BA 80 Paterson St Coll; MS 81 Paterson St Coll; SLP, Letchworth Dev Servs, **SLP**

Cushman, Mrs Betty B 1812 Village Road, Glenshaw, PA 15116, Univ of Pittsburgh - Pittsburgh; MS; 86–Sp-Lang Path, Allegheny Intermdiate Unit, **SLP**

Cushman, Melissa J 15 East Street, Fairport, NY 14450, (716) 334-8788, BS 84 Nazareth Coll of Rochester; MA 86 SUNY - Coll at Geneseo; **A**

Cusick, Joanne Pine View Apartment #6, Harmony, PA 16037, BS 74 Indiana Univ of PA; MS 79 Indiana Univ of PA; 87 Slippery Rock Univ of PA; 74–Sp-Lang Path, Seneca Valley Sch Dist, **SLP**

Cusimano, Barbara Walker Hamiter Professional Bldg, 801 Gaines Avenue, Suite 305, Gadsden, AL 35903, (205) 547-6550, BA 67 Univ of AL- Tuscaloosa; MA 68 Univ of AL- Tuscaloosa; Dir Sp-Lang Path, Sp-Lang Pathology Associates, **SLP**

Custer, H Dean Amberlands #16-R, Croton on Hudson, NY 10520, **SLP**

Custer, Kathryn K 3708 139th Avenue N W, Andover, MN 55304, (612) 421-6187, BS 84 Univ of MN - Minneap-St Paul; MS 85 Saint Cloud St Univ; **SLP**

Custis, Mrs Wendy Lu 2626 14th Street, Lincoln, IL 62656, (217) 732-4131, BS 78 IL St Univ - Normal; MS 79 IL St Univ - Normal; Sp-Lang Path, Lincoln Comm Hgh Sch, **SLP**

Cusumano, Mrs Marilyn T 6 Washington Avenue, Elmwood Park, NJ 07407, (201) 797-8621, BA 76 Montclair St Coll; MA 81 Montclair St Coll; Sp-Lang Path, Allendale Bd/Ed, **SLP**

Cutchen, Mrs Judy Lee 140 Gillon Drive, Birmingham, AL 35209, (205) 983-1085, BS 81 Delta St Univ; MS 84 Auburn Univ - Auburn

Cuthbertson, David Alan 24 Gould Street, Reading, MA 01867-0060, (617) 944-1119, BS 79 Purdue Univ - West Lafayette; MA 81 Univ of CT; Aud, Solo Palt Hrng Cen, **A**

Cutler, Cheryl Ellen 110 Hesse Road, Hamden, CT 06517, (203) 366-7551, BA 82 Univ of CT; MA 84 Univ of CT; Sp-Lang Path, Rehab Ctr of Ffld Co, **SLP**

Cutler, Ellen S 2131 Century Park Lane#213, Los Angeles, CA 90067, (213) 277-1149, BA 71 Univ of CA - Los Angeles; MS 76 Mount St Mary's Coll; MA 78 CA St Univ - Northridge; Sp-Lang Path, Santa Monica Coll, **SLP**

Cutler, Mrs Gayle Moyer 2606 Alabama Avenue South, St Louis Park, MN 55416, (612) 922-5426, BA 84 Univ of MI - Ann Arbor; MS 86 Univ of MI - Ann Arbor; 87–Sp-Lang Path, Sp-Lang-Hrng Clinic, **SLP**

Cutler, Mark Jay 14254 McCormick Street, Van Nuys, CA 91401, (818) 789-2142, BA 80 CA St Univ - Northridge; MA 83 CA St Univ - Northridge; Sp-Lang Path, LA USD, **SLP**

Cutler, Michelle J 904 Wheelers Farms Road, Milford, CT 06460, **SLP**

Cutler, Mrs Rae S 17 Scarlet Oak Drive, Lafayette Hill, PA 19444, (215) 825-4462, BA 66 Temple Univ; MA 68 Temple Univ; Sp-Lang Path, Sch Dist of Phila, **SLP**

Cutler, S James 106 Beauregard Avenue, Highland Springs, VA 23075, (804) 737-1150, BS 41 Temple Univ; OM 58 Coll of William & Mary; MS 68 VA Commonwealth Univ; Consultant, Private Practice, **A LM**

Cutler, Dr William H VA Hospital, Gainesville, FL 32601, (904) 376-1611, BA 53 FL St Univ; MS 58 IL St Univ - Normal; PH 69 (NS) Univ of Southern CA; Ch Aud & Sp-Path, Veterans Administrations, **SLP A**

Cutler-Held, Dr Marcia 2107 Bridgewood Drive, Boca Raton, FL 33434, MS; SLP, **SLP**

Cutrer, Mrs Cathryn Sue 10901 Catthorn Cove, Austin, TX 78759, (512) 388-4184, BS 73 Southwest TX St Univ; ME 74 Southwest TX St Univ; 86–Sp-Lang Path, Round Rock ISD, **SLP**

Cutright, Mrs Jayne F P O Box 152, APO New York, NY 09056, BS 75 WV Univ; MS 77 WV Univ; 87–Sp-Lang Path, Dept of Defense Depend Sch, **SLP**

Cutrone, Linda R 218-37 94th Road, Queens Village, NY 11428, (516) 378-2000, BA 72 CUNY - Queens Coll; MA 74 CUNY - Queens Coll; Dir Sp-Lang Serv, Utd Cp Treat/Rehab Cen Inc, **SLP**

Cutshall, Susan Kennedy 3872 McGarry Drive, Lexington, KY 40514, (606) 223-4618, BS 76 Purdue Univ - West Lafayette; MS 80 Univ of KY; Sp-Lang Path, Woodford County Schools, **SLP**

Cutsinger, Linda K Arizona Speech And Rehab, 3634 West Danburh Drive, Phoenix, AZ 85029, (602) 375-0390, BS 71 Univ of Tulsa; MA 72 Univ of Tulsa; Dir, AZ Sp Path & Rehab Assocs, **SLP**

Cuttie, Vallarie Smith 455 Vista Grande, Greenbrae, CA 94904, (415) 461-8851, BA 75 San Jose St Univ; MA 77 San Jose St Univ; Aud, US Army, **A**

Cutting, Michael W Acadia Hearing Center, 700 Mount Hope Avenue, Office #4-East, Bangor, ME 04401, (207) 947-4970, BS 74 OK St Univ; MS 76 Purdue Univ - West Lafayette; Dir of Aud, Bangor Ear Nose & Throat PA, **A**

Cuttner, Nancy Kratzer 301 East Avenue, Norwalk, CT 06855, (904) 289-0121, BS 76 Univ of GA; ME 77 Univ of GA; Sp-Lang Path, Norwalk Boe, **SLP**

Cutts, Mrs Betty Powell 7711 Broadway #28-C, San Antonio, TX 78209, (512) 732-3000, **A**

Cutts, Elaine Valerie 10 Lebel Road, Lynn, MA 01904, (617) 837-1311, BS 80 Worcester St Coll; MS 84 Emerson Coll; **SLP**

Cuyjet, Carol L 3804 Sunflower Circle, Mitchellville, MD 20716, (301) 454-6913, BS 68 Northern IL Univ - De Kalb; MA 71 Northern IL Univ - De Kalb; OM 78 Northern IL Univ - De Kalb; 87–Sp-Lang Path, U of Maryland-College Park, **SLP**

Cuyler, Juliana S 36505 N E Washougal River R, Washougal, WA 98671-9549, (503) 344-5863, MS 87 Univ of OR

Cwiklinski, Mrs Karen A RD #2 Box 27, Fillmore, NY 14735, (716) 476-2234, BS 81 SUNY - Coll at Geneseo; MA 83 SUNY - Coll at Geneseo; 83–Sp-Lang Path, Keshequa Central School, **SLP**

Cych, Susan Jeanette 90 Laurentian Drive, Cheektowaga, NY 14225, (716) 686-2000, BS 79 SUNY - Coll at Buffalo; MS 84 SUNY - Coll at Buffalo; 88–Sp-Lang Path, Erie #1 BOCES, **SLP**

Cygnarowicz, Mrs Teresa Marie 4600 Morningwood Drive, Olney, MD 20832-2013, (301) 570-4364, BA 83 MI St Univ; MA 84 MI St Univ; 86–Aud, Aud Washington Co Inc, **A**

Cymbal, Edith Wickli 37643 2nd Street, Willoughby, OH 44094-6124, (216) 951-6063, **SLP**

Cymerman, Shmuel 5609 15th Avenue, Suite 6A, Brooklyn, NY 11219, (212) 854-6244, BS 74 Northeastern Univ; ME 82 Northeastern Univ; Audiologist, Audiological Prescriptions, **A**

Cyphers, Mrs Nancy W 3066-A West 107th Place, Westminster, CO 80030, (303) 428-3511, BS 79 CO St Univ; MS 80 CO St Univ; Aud, Adams County School District, **A**

Cypress, Marian Amanda Route 2 Box 510, Smithfield, VA 23430, (804) 229-8051, BS 82 Hampton Univ; MA 84 Hampton Univ; Sp-Lang Path, Williamsburg/James City Co PS, **SLP**

Cyr, Dr David G Boys Town National Institute, 555 North 30th Street, Omaha, NE 68131, (402) 498-6520, BA 70 San Jose St Univ; MA 71 Univ of IL - Urbana; PH 83 (NS) Univ of NE - Lincoln; Coord Cl Vestibular Serv, Boys Town Nat'l Inst, **A**

Cyrus, Sandra A 1626 Bane Avenue, Henderson, NC 27536, **SLP**

Czaplewski, Mrs Cathleen Marie 84 Green Meadow Drive, Glendale Heights, IL 60139, (312) 668-6872, BA 81 Elmhurst Coll; MS 84 Governors St Univ; Sp-Lang Path, Sase D, **SLP**

Czarnecki, Tama D 317 7th Street Extension, New Kensington, PA 15068, (412) 335-9414, BS 80 WV Univ; MS 82 Univ of NM; Sp-Lang Path, National Rehabilitation Hosp, **SLP**

Czarnik, Karen A 7906 West 97th Place, Hickory Hills, IL 60457, (312) 333-0300, BA 82 Saint Xavier Coll; OM 84 Governors St Univ; Sp-Lang Path, Harvey Pub Sch, **SLP**

Czarnota, Annemarie 241 Broadway Road #58, Dracut, MA 01826, (617) 454-7593, BS 82 Univ of MA - Amherst; MS 86 Northeastern Univ; 86–Aud, Audio Hearing Ctr, **A**

Czerwinski, Mrs Charlene Stringer 8615 Stonewall Drive, Indianapolis, IN 46231-2562, (317) 248-9328, Sp-Lang Path, New Hope of Indiana Inc, **SLP**

Czesak, Beth A 24 Bonn Place, Weehawken, NJ 07087, (201) 997-0500, BS 73 William Paterson Coll; MS 75 William Paterson Coll; Sp-Lang Path, Kearny Bd of Ed, **SLP**

Czuchna, Paul E 550 Rhods Avenue, Mansfield, OH 44906, (616) 383-0963, Wmu Kolamazoo Mi, **SLP**

Czuleger, Mrs Collette Moulton 2809 Verde Vista, Santa Barbara, CA 93105, (805) 569-1061, MS 83 AZ St Univ; Sp-Lang Path, Sharon Wilcox & Assoc, **SLP**

Czuzak, Mrs Alicia Mitter 714 North Howard #E, Glendale, CA 91206, (818) 843-5111, BA 83 CA St Univ - Northridge; MA 85 CA St Univ - Northridge; Aud, Med Diagnostic Ctr, **A**

Czvik, Mrs Patsy Smith 1138 East 24th Street, San Bernardino, CA 92404, (714) 887-6333, BA 57 Stanford Univ; MA 59 Stanford Univ; Dir Dept Sp/Lang Path, R T Ballard Cen Rehab, **SLP ACE**

Czyzewski, Mrs Helen J 6550 South Komensky, Chicago, IL 60629, (312) 767-6226, BA 72 Saint Xavier Coll; MS 81 Governors St Univ; Sp-Lang Path, Chicago Bd of Ed, **SLP**

D

Daane, Tami Jo 2909 South Martha, Sioux City, IA 51106-3321, (408) 394-3916, BA 84 Univ of SD - Vermillion; MA 85 Univ of SD - Vermillion; **SLP**

Dabbs, Terri Anne 12007 Colin Road, Silver Spring, MD 20906, (301) 946-9250, BS 84 Towson St Univ; MS 86 Towson St Univ

Dabel, Mrs Debora Klein RFD 5 Box 236, Old Standish Road, Gorham, ME 04038, (207) 871-2463, BS 80 Univ of WI - Stevens Point; MS 81 Univ of WI - Stevens Point; Sp-Lang Path, ME Med Ctr, **SLP**

Dabney, Marsha Jo 3105 West 27th Street #31, Los Angeles, CA 90018, (213) 515-3008, BA 76 CA St Univ - Los Angeles

Dabrow, Mrs Lori Michelle 621 Heather Lane, Bryn Mawr, PA 19010, (215) 527-6228, BS 81 PA St Univ - Univ Park; MA 82 George Washington Univ; Sp-Lang Path, UCP Head Start Clinic Team, **SLP**

Dabrowski, Mrs Patricia Anne 7 Woodhill Road, Newtown Square, PA 19073, (215) 874-5366, BS 82 East Stroudsburg Univ of PA; MA 84 Hahnemann Univ Grad Sch; Aud, Plastic Surgical ENT Assoc, **A**

Dabrowski, Patricia Duffy 1140 East Bywater Lane, Fox Point, WI 53217-3955, (414) 351-6702, **SLP**

Dabul, Dr Barbara L 3033 East Valley Boulevard Space 7, West Covina, CA 91792, (818) 289-5454, BA 65 Univ of Southern CA; MA 67 Univ of Southern CA; PH 70 (Communicative Disorders) Univ of Southern CA; 85–Director of Speech Services, San Gabriel Valley Med Ctr, **SLP**

Dacey, Deborah A 1082 Kimberly Lane, Milford, OH 45150, (513) 559-4601, BS 74 Univ of Cincinnati; MA 80 Univ of Cincinnati; 87–AAC Proj Coord, Cerebral Palsy Services Center, **SLP**

Dachauer, Mrs Joyce Susan 2421 E Washington, Bloomington, IL 61701, (309) 727-1241, BS 83 IL St Univ - Normal; MS 84 IL St Univ - Normal; **SLP**

Dachtera, Linda Byrne 1592 Merrill Street, St Paul, MN 55108, (612) 439-5160, BS 71 Univ of MN - Minneap-St Paul; MS 74 Univ of WI - Eau Claire; Sp-Lang Path, ISD 834 Stillwater, **SLP**

Dacres, Joan L 4532 NE 94th Street, Seattle, WA 98115, (206) 455-6077, BS 74 CO St Univ; MS 76 CO St Univ; Sp-Lang Path, Bellevue PS, **SLP**

Dadabo, Michele Marie Rd #7 Barrett Hill Road, Lake Carmel, NY 10512, (914) 225-5650, MS 85 FL St Univ; **SLP**

Daddario, Mrs Cynthia Carol 306 Orchard Avenue, Cuyahoga Falls, OH 44221, (216) 379-8350, BA 81 Univ of Akron; MA 83 Univ of Akron; Aud, Chldn's Hosp Med Ctr of Akron, **A**

D'Addario, Mary Ann 16 Blueberry Hill Road, Woburn, MA 01801, (617) 251-4071, MA 82 Univ of MA - Amherst; MS 85 Wheelock Coll; SLP, North Middlesex Reg Sch Dist, **SLP**

Daddiego, Randi S 43-36 Robinson Street, Flushing, NY 11355, MA 76 NY Univ; Sp-Lang Path, Nn Westchester Ctr Sp Dis, **SLP**

Daddio, Mary McLellan 820 Bali Court, Danville, CA 94526, (818) 716-9866, BA 80 William Paterson Coll; MA 83 Univ of CO - Boulder; Sp-Lang-Path, Cherry Creek Schools, **SLP**

Daddura, Mrs Rosalie E 1002 Meriweather Drive, Fallston, MD 21047, (301) 661-2400, BA 74 Loyola Coll; MS 75 Loyola Coll; Sp-Lang Path, Baltimore County Board of Educ, **SLP**

Dadon, Angela Russo 2073 East 67th Street, Brooklyn, NY 11234, (718) 531-4964, BA 76 Pace U -NY City; MA 77 NY Univ; Super Sp-Lang Path, Private Practice, **SLP**

Dae, Donna 7982 Cavalli Way, Fair Oaks, CA 95628, (916) 965-9115, BA 65 CA St Univ - Fresno; MA 73 San Francisco St Univ; 87–Sp-Lang Path, Burger Rehab & Therapy Agency, **SLP**

Daes, Evelyn I 16141 Blatt Boulevard #203, Fort Lauderdale, FL 33326, (305) 389-4313, BA 83 Univ of NC - Greensboro; MS 88 Nova Univ; 88–Sp-Lang Path, Ambi-Lingual Assoc

Dafforn, Rhonda M B 2512 126th Avenue N E, Bellevue, WA 98005, (206) 325-8477, BA 75 Univ of WA; MA 76 Univ of WA; Parent Infant Specialist, Hearing Speech Deafness Ctr, **SLP**

Daffron, Margaret D 178 Huntinton Place, Northport, AL 35476, (205) 339-9370, **SLP**

Dagate, Robin Ann 605 June Drive, Houma, LA 70360, BS 83 Nicholls St Univ; OM 85 LA St Univ - N O Medical Ctr; MA 88 Southwest MO St Univ; Tchr, Lafayette Parish Sch Bd, **A**

Dagenais, Donna Jo Mid Peninsula Sp & Lang Clinic, 445 East Charleston Road, Palo Alto, CA 94306, (415) 493-8111, **SLP**

Dagenais, Dr Paul A Univ Of Alabama At Birmingham, Dept Of Biocommunication, UAB Station, Birmingham, AL 35294, (205) 934-4814, BS 76 Univ of Ottawa - Ontario; MA 83 Northern MI Univ; PH 87 (Speech and Hearing Science) Univ of TN - Knoxville; 87–Research Asst Prof, Univ of AL at Birmingham, **SLP**

Daggett, Mrs Helen C 14200 Pt Cabrillo Drive, Mendocino, CA 95460, BA 24 Univ of MN - Minneap-St Paul; MA 54 San Francisco St Univ; **SLP LM**

Daggett, Mary D 1101 Salisbury #2, Cincinnati, OH 45226, (513) 751-1716, MA 80 Western MI Univ; Aud, ENT Assoc of Cincinnati Inc, **A**

Dagle, Kathleen Minna 909 Clinton Street, Hoboken, NJ 07030, (201) 963-4024, BA 77 Montclair St Coll; MA 85 Montclair St Coll; 79–Sp-Lang Path, Union City Bd of Educ, **SLP**

Dagley, Mrs Glenna M 960 Roslyn Road, Glen Ellyn, IL 60137, (312) 790-2474, BS 72 Univ of IL - Urbana; MA 73 Univ of IL - Urbana; Coord, Il Deaf-Blind Ser Cen & Sch, **A**

D'Agostino, Mrs Ann M One Taft Street, Milford, MA 01757, (617) 478-4462, BS 76 Emerson Coll; ME 78 Northeastern Univ; Sp-Lang Path, **SLP**

D'Agostino, Christine L 6019 10th Place, Hyattsville, MD 20782, (301) 439-4330, BA 86 Loyola Coll; MS 88 Loyola Coll; 88–Sp-Lang Path, Centers for the Handicapped Inc

D'Agostino, Eliza D Box 303, Chesterfield, MA 01012, (413) 296-4387, MA 86 Univ of MA - Amherst; **SLP**

Dahill, Carol Ann 103 Thaxter Street, Hingham, MA 02043, **SLP**

Dahl, Mrs Beverly Anne 335 Penryn Crescent, Saskatoon, SK, Canada S7H 5G7, (306) 934-2203, OB 67; MS 83 Minot St Univ; Sp-Lang Path, Saskatoon Pub Sch Div, **SLP**

Dahl, Cecilia W 505 East San Juan, Phoenix, AZ 85012, (602) 265-6742, BS 76 AZ St Univ; MS 79 AZ St Univ; Sp-Lang Path, Creighton Spec Educ, **SLP**

Dahl, Mrs Sherry Gail 26311 Bendickson Drive, Wind Lake, WI 53185, (414) 281-7200, BS 86 Univ of WI - Milwaukee; MS 88 Marquette Univ; 88–Dir of Sp-Lang Path, Mt Carmel Care Ctr

Dahlberg, Cynthia A 10725 West Berry Drive, Littleton, CO 80127, (303) 789-8228, BA 71 Univ of Denver; MA 72 Univ of Denver; 80–Dir Dept of Sp-Lang Path, Craig Hosp, **SLP**

Dahle, Alice L 1502 26th S E, Cedar Rapids, IA 52403, (319) 399-6818, BA 70 Univ of Northern IA; MA 71 Univ of Northern IA; MA 80 Univ of IA; Sp-Lang Path, Grant Wood AEA, **SLP**

Dahle, Dr Arthur J Ctr For Develop & Learning Dis, University Of Alabama, Birmingham, AL 35233, (205) 934-5448, BS 61 Saint Cloud St Univ; MS 65 PA St Univ - Univ Park; PH 68 (NS) PA St Univ - Univ Park; Dir-Div of Sp & Hrng, U of AL-Birmingham, **SLP A F**

Dahlem, Mrs Laura Theil 324 Paddock Drive West, Savoy, IL 61874, (217) 337-2482, BA 82; MA 83 OH St Univ; 84–Sp-Lang Path, Rehab Ctr of Mercy Hosp, **SLP**

Dahlen, Elizabeth 20 East Peru Street #3, Princeton, IL 61356, (815) 699-2251, BA 75 Augustana Coll; MS 76 Eastern IL Univ; **SLP**

Dahler, Mrs Mary F Z 1645 Clarence Avenue, Lakewood, OH 44107, (216) 574-8514, BA 73 Bellarmine Coll; MA 77 Cleveland St Univ; Sp-Lang Path, Cleveland Bd of Ed, **SLP**

Dahlgren, Karen B 6013 Plumthicket Road, Oklahoma City, OK 73132, **SLP**

Dahlgren, Phyllis O 5942 Colhurst, Dallas, TX 75230-5022, (214) 692-1439, BS 73 Southern Methodist Univ; MS 74 Southern Methodist Univ; **SLP**

Dahlke, Joan M 5970 Leonard Avenue, Idaho Falls, ID 83402, (208) 529-3837, BA 59 Stanford Univ; MA 71 OR St Univ; **SLP**

Dahlke, Michael G Ear Nose & Throat Associates, 425 Pine Ridge Boulevard, Suite 305, Wausau, WI 54401, (715) 845-9634, BS 73 Univ of WI - Stevens Point; MS 74 Univ of WI - Stevens Point; Dir Aud Ser, ENT Assos, **A**

Dahlke, Mrs Nanette Carlmark 60 Coventry Cove, Lake Villa, IL 60046, (312) 420-6335, BA 79 Augustana Coll; MS 81 Northern IL Univ - De Kalb; 88–Sp-Lang Path, Antioch Sch Dist 34, **SLP**

Dahlquist, Lois H 4821 Fremont Avenue South, Minneapolis, MN 55409, (612) 377-8900, BA 70 Grinnell Coll; MA 71 Univ of Denver; Sp-Lang Path, Spec Sch Dist #1 - Minneapolis, **SLP**

Dahlquist, Mrs Marcia E 3385 Chandler Road, Shoreview, MN 55126, BA 74 Univ of SD - Vermillion; MA 75 Univ of MO - Columbia; Sp-Lang Path, White Bear Lake Sch Dist, **SLP**

Dahlstrand, Mrs Cheryl A 3634 Bernay, Northbrook, IL 60062, (517) 372-6725, BS 71 Northwestern Univ; MA 72 Northwestern Univ; Coord of Sp Serv, Audio Vestibular Test Cen, **SLP**

Dahm, Barbara Lee 27 Einstein Street, Raanana, Israel 43272, BS 68 Boston Univ; ME 71 Boston Univ; 88–Sp-Lang Path, SET Speech Ctr, **SLP**

Dahmer, Susan McVaney 417-A Rossell Loop, Fort Belvoir, VA 22060-1908, (703) 781-8839, BS 84 Armstrong St Coll; ME 86 Armstrong St Coll; **SLP**

Dahn, Barbara Gordon 1563 South Oxalis Avenue, Orlando, FL 32807, (407) 277-5866, BA 82 Univ of Central FL; MA 84 Univ of Central FL; Sp-Lang Path, Orange Co Pub Schs, **SLP**

Daigle, Mrs Teresa A R R 1 Box 380, Ashby, MA 01431, (617) 386-7140, BS 82 Coll of Saint Rose; MA 84 Univ of MA - Amherst; **SLP**

Daigle, Theresa Kay 330 Feu Follet #166, Lafayette, LA 70508, (318) 235-1301, BA 77 Univ of Southwestern LA; MS 87 Univ of Southwestern LA

Dailey, Ann Madsen 10 Mill Street #N, Maynard, MA 01754, (508) 829-4766, BA 45 Baylor Univ; MA 47 Univ of MI - Ann Arbor; Cl Super/Coord Lang Prog, Town of Holden Ma, **SLP**

Dailey, Daniel J Audiology Department, Western Hills AEA12, 1520 Morningside Avenue, Sioux City, IA 51106, (712) 274-6023, BA 71 Western IL Univ; MA 74 Western IL Univ; Aud, Western Hills AEA 12, **A**

Dailey, Mrs Janis A 6830 Hampton Wood Circle, Hixson, TN 37343, (615) 842-5054, BA 74 Auburn Univ - Auburn; MS 76 Auburn Univ - Auburn; Aud/Presch Hrng Imp Coord, Chattanooga Sp & Hrng Ctr, **A**

Dailey, Kathleen Ft Hamilton Hughes Hospital, Physical Med & Rehab, Hamilton, OH 45013, (513) 867-2000, BS 75 OH Univ - Athens; MA 76 Central MI Univ; Sp/Lang Path, Ft Hamilton Hughes Hospital, **SLP**

Dailey, Kimberly K 1028 Bay Road, Webster, NY 14580, (716) 671-3499, BS 80 Nazareth Coll of Rochester; MS 82 Nazareth Coll of Rochester; 82–Sp-Lang Path, Mary Cariola Children's Ctr, **SLP**

Dailey, Mary B P O Box 165, Dellslow, WV 26531-0165, (304) 292-8019, BS 83 Stockton St Coll; MS 85 WV Univ; **SLP**

Dailey, Mrs Vicki C Nash General Hospital, Speech & Hearing Services, Curtis Ellis Drive, Rocky Mount, NC 27801, (919) 443-8048, BS 74 East Carolina Univ; MS 75 East Carolina Univ; Super/SLP, Nash Gen Hosp-Sp & Hrng Serv, **SLP**

Daily, Kathryn Ann 2514 22nd, Lubbock, TX 79410, (806) 766-1198, BA 84 Abilene Christian Univ; MS 86 Univ of OK Medical Center; 86–Sp-Lang Path, Lubbock ISD, **SLP**

Daily, Linda Jennings 28 Meadowgrass, Irvine, CA 92714, (714) 581-2800, BS 79 Univ of OR; MA 82 CA St Univ - Long Beach; 82–Aud, Newport Lang Sp Aud Ctr Inc, **A**

Daily, Mrs Mary S 355 Green Acres Drive, Valparaiso, IN 46383, (219) 464-9607, **SLP**

Daines, Mrs Nancy C 2657 Warwick, Bloomfield Hills, MI 48013, (313) 338-8996, BA 53 Univ of MI - Ann Arbor; MA 55 Univ of MI - Ann Arbor; MA 78 Wayne St Univ; 86–Dir-Dept Hrng Sp Lang, Kenny MICH Rehab Fndtn, **SLP ACE**

Daitch, Wendy L 59 East Bonita Drive, Simi Valley, CA 93065, (805) 583-5436, BA 80 CA St Univ - Northridge; MA 82 CA St Univ - Northridge; SLP Supvr, Comm Sp and Hrng Cen, **SLP**

Daitch-Dell, Suzanne Beth 26640 East Carnegie Park Drive, Southfield, MI 48034, (313) 353-3283, BA 84 Univ of MI - Ann Arbor; MS 86 Univ of MI - Ann Arbor; **SLP**

Daiy, Kelly Ann 4550 Queen Elizabeth Court, Apartment 279, Alexandria, LA 71303, (318) 487-2022, BA 82 LA Tech Univ; MA 83 LA Tech Univ; Sp-Lang Path, Rapides General Hospital, **SLP**

Dalack-Ellias, Laila Marie 5611 Clearview Drive, Sylvania, OH 43560, (419) 885-4914, BA 82 Smith Coll; MS 84 Columbia Univ Teachers Coll; SLP, The League School, **SLP**

D'Alberto, Cindy Jane 343 County Road 75, Mechanicville, NY 12118, (518) 664-4450, **SLP**

Dalby, Mrs Pamela 1807 Wingate Lane, Wheaton, IL 60187, (312) 665-6352, BA 69 Univ of MI - Ann Arbor; MS 70 Univ of MI - Ann Arbor; **SLP**

Dale, Mrs Beverly H 627 Williamsburg Drive, Broomall, PA 19008, (215) 356-6635, BA 78 Coll of Wooster; MA 81 Temple Univ; Sp-Lang Path, Magee Rehabilitation Hosp, **SLP**

Dale, Duane A 10 Grantham Place, St Albert, AB, Canada T8N 0W8, (403) 488-4826, BS 68 Moorhead St Univ; MS 74 Univ of ND; 88–Dir Sp-Lang Svcs Div, Edmonton Bd of Health, **SLP**

Dale, Elizabeth c/o Assoc Speech Hearing Services, 3478 Gaviot, Long Beach, CA 90807, (213) 426-3795, Dir Aud, Assoc Sp & Hrng, **A**

Dale, Mrs Margaret Olga R 10 Grantham Place, St Albert, AB, Canada T8N 0W8, (403) 459-6671, BS 70 Moorhead St Univ; MS 80 Univ of ND; 88–Sp-Lang Path, Sturgeon Health Unit, **SLP**

Dale, Dr Paulette 17705 S W 83rd Court, Miami, FL 33157, (305) 385-4910, BA 72 CUNY - Queens Coll; MS 73 Univ of South FL; PH 80 (NS) Univ of FL; Assoc Prof/Dir Sp&Hrng Cl, Miami Dade Community College, **SLP**

Dale, Dr Phillip S University Of Washington Ni-25, Psychology Department, Seattle, WA 98195, (206) 543-4329, BS 63 Univ of Chicago; MA 66 Univ of MI - Ann Arbor; PH 68 (Communication Sciences) Univ of MI - Ann Arbor; 68–Assoc Prof, Univ of Washington

Dale, Mrs Sharon R P O Box 441491, Aurora, CO 80044-1491, (303) 371-3780, BS 77 SUNY - Coll at Buffalo; MS 80 SUNY - Coll at Buffalo; 87–Sp-Lang Path, Denver PS, **SLP**

Dalene, Mrs L Juli 1906 Stratford Drive, Champaign, IL 61821, (217) 359-0092, BS 79 Evangel Coll; MS 80 Central MO St Univ; **SLP**

D'Alessandro, Mrs Joan Valevas Tri-County Hearing Service, 22 North Evans Street, Pottstown, PA 19464, (215) 970-3277, MA 78 Temple Univ; Aud, Private Practice, **A**

D'Alessandro, JoAnn Marie 909 Millridge Road, Highland Heights, OH 44143, (216) 942-6424, BS 85 Univ of Cincinnati; MA 87 Case Western Reserve Univ; Sp-Lang Path, Heather Hill Inc

D'Alessio, Linda J 670 Mix Avenue #5A, Hamden, CT 06514, **A**

D'Alessio-Caniza, Prudence Dianne 3046 North Cramer Street, Milwaukee, WI 53211, (414) 963-9074, MS 84 Univ of WI - Milwaukee; 85–Sp-Lang Path, Milwaukee Public Schools, **SLP**

Daley, Mrs Elysse B 51 Linden Avenue, Bethpage, NY 11714, (516) 420-5238, BA 71 Adelphi Univ; MA 74 Hofstra Univ; Sp-Lang Path, Nassau Co Dept of Health, **SLP**

Daley, Linda A 6 Geer Avenue, Utica, NY 13501, BA 74 Univ of CT; MS 77 Syracuse Univ; 80–Sp-Lang Path, Oneida Co BOCES, **SLP**

Daley, Mrs Sue Ann Kenlee 4223 Toronto Street, Ames, IA 50010, (515) 296-2416, BA 83 Univ of Northern IA; MA 85 Univ of Northern IA; 88–Sp-Lang Path, Hrng and Sp Svcs of Iowa, **SLP**

Daley, Dr William T 1012 Taussig Place N E, Washington, DC 20017, (301) 535-3569, BA 50 Catholic Univ of America; MA 51 Catholic Univ of America; PH 76 (Educational Psychology) Catholic Univ of America; 80–Sp-Lang Path, Calvert Co Pub Sch, **SLP**

Dalfonso, David L 705 Parkway Avenue, Salisbury, MD 21801, (301) 742-5128, BS 63 CA Univ of PA; MS 69 WV Univ; Sp-Lang Path, Wicomico Co Bd of Ed, **SLP**

D'Alfonso, Patricia H 95 Paddock Drive, Warwick, RI 02886-6602, (401) 884-3341, BS 77 Univ of RI; MS 79 Southern CT St Univ; Sp-Lang Path, W Warwick Sch Dept, **SLP**

Dalfonso, Raymond J 1161 Eagle Street, Wescosville, PA 18106, (215) 683-4293, BA 68 Marshall Univ; ME 75 Salisbury St Coll; MS 79 Towson St Univ; Assoc Prof, Kutztown Univ, **SLP ACE**

Dalimonte, Mrs Cynthia W Via Dante Da Castiglione, 33/24 50125, Florence, Italy, 5-522-9268, BA 71 Depauw Univ; MA 73 Northwestern Univ; **SLP**

Dalin, Galen E 505 9th Street S W, Pipestone, MN 56164, (507) 825-5424, BS 54 Mankato St Univ; MS 55 Mankato St Univ; Sp-Lang Path, Pipestone Pub Sch, **SLP**

Dalin, Stephen Raymond 251 East 3rd North, St Anthony, ID 83445, (208) 624-3744, Dev Spec Snr, St of ID Dept of Health, **SLP**

Dalin, Mrs Tamora Mueller 2901 Chapel Lane, Rapid City, SD 57702, (605) 343-4301, BS 82 Univ of SD - Vermillion; MA 84 Univ of SD - Vermillion; SLP, Julia Hobbs, **SLP**

Dalkey, Sharon Lee P O Box 5364, Carmel, CA 93921, (408) 755-0339, BA 63 San Jose St Univ; MA 68 San Jose St Univ; Sp-Lang Path, Spec Ed Local Planning Area, **SLP**

Dallal, Mrs Rhonda G 5 Cypress Avenue, Great Neck, NY 11024, (516) 487-8956, BA 76 Univ of Miami; MA 78 Hofstra Univ; Sp-Lang Path, Private Practice, **SLP**

Dallos, Peter Northwestern University, 2299 Sheridan Road, Evanston, IL 60201, (312) 492-3175, BS 58 IL Inst of Tech; MS 59 Northwestern Univ; PH 62 (NS) Northwestern Univ; Prof, Northwestern U

Dally, Mrs Anne E 1050 Wintergreen Terrace, Rockville, MD 20850, (301) 340-8048, BS 54 Univ of WI - Madison; MA 58 Northwestern Univ; Sp-Lang Path, Montgy Co Pub Sch, **SLP**

Daloise, Mrs Shelley L RD 1 Box 422-B, Saxonburg Road, Natrona Heights, PA 15065, (412) 226-3867, BS 74 Indiana Univ of PA; MS 80 Indiana Univ of PA; 75–Sp-Lang Path, Westmoreland Inter Ut #7, **SLP**

Dalston, Eileen T 100 Hunters Ridge Road, Chapel Hill, NC 27514, (919) 966-5290, BS 64 Bowling Green St Univ; MA 65 Northwestern Univ; 86–Sp-Lang Path, Univ of NC-Chapel Hill, **SLP**

Dalston, Dr Rodger M Oral-Facial & Comm Disorders, Univ Of North Carolina, 52 Dental Clinic Bldg CB#7450, Chapel Hill, NC 27514, (919) 933-0553, BA 64 Cornell Univ; MA 66 Northwestern Univ; PH 72 (NS) Northwestern Univ; Dir Sp-Lang Path, U-Chapel Hill, **SLP F**

Dalton, Beth Marie 7219 Crisp, Raytown, MO 64133, (816) 234-3677, BA 84 KS St Univ; MA 86 KS St Univ; Sp-Lang Path, Childrens Mercy Hosp, **SLP**

Dalton, Mrs Donna Anne 9040 South Claremont, Chicago, IL 60620, (312) 233-1753, BA 73 Saint Xavier Coll; MS 78 Governors St Univ; 88–Pvt Practice, **SLP**

Dalton, Kathleen B 200 North Cornell Avenue, Fullerton, CA 92631, (714) 599-6787, BS 72 CO St Univ; MS 74 CO St Univ; 88–Sp-Lang Path, Bonita USD, **SLP**

Dalton, Dr Leslie W, Jr 755 Tleshore #102-C, Las Cruces, NM 88001, (505) 522-2073, BS 60 Univ of VA - Charlottesville; MS 65 FL St Univ; PH 68 (NS) FL St Univ; Sp-Lang Path/Aud, Private Practice, **SLP A**

Dalton, Marilyn G 7102 Blanchard Drive, Derwood, MD 20855, (301) 474-7209, BS 67 Kent St Univ; MA 72 Kent St Univ; 86–Sp-Lang Path, Private Practice, **SLP**

Dalton, Maureen Lisbeth 5, 155 White Street, 2nd Floor, Belmont, MA 02178, (617) 893-8050, BA 70 Emmanuel Coll; ME 84 Northeastern Univ; **SLP**

Dalton, Penny M Summers 215 Horrocks Drive, Blackfoot, ID 83221, (208) 785-5826, BS 74 ID St Univ; MS 76 ID St Univ; SLP, State of Idaho Hlth & Welfare, **SLP**

Dalton, Wendy R 4329 Phinney Avenue North, Seattle, WA 98103, (206) 587-5150, BA 82 Western WA Univ; MA 85 Western WA Univ; **A**

Dalton, Mrs Wilma K 16 New Meadow Road, Lynnfield, MA 01940, (617) 334-4837, BS 69 PA St Univ - Univ Park; MS 70 Vanderbilt Univ; 87–Sp-Lang Path, Melrose PS, **SLP**

Daly, Mrs Barbara Balboni 391 Reservoir Street, Norton, MA 02766-1424, (617) 643-3700, BS 84 Northeastern Univ; MS 87 Southern CT St Univ; Aud, Boston Guild for Hard of Hrng, **A**

Daly, Bobbie D Ac York Vamc #126, 3400 Lebanon, Murfreesboro, TN 37130, (615) 893-1360, BA 78 Univ of MS; MA 79 Univ of MS; Aud, Murfreesboro VA Med Cen, **A**

Daly, Cynthia 25025 Sunset Place East, Laguna Hills, CA 92653, (714) 586-1234, BS 47 Univ of WI - Madison; MS 49 Univ of WI - Madison; Retired, Saddleback Valley USD, **SLP LM**

Daly, Dr David A Director Comm Disorders Clinic, University Of Michigan, 1111 East Catherine Street, Ann Arbor, MI 48109, (313) 764-8440, BA 63 Central MI Univ; MA 64 OH Univ - Athens; ED 68 (NS) PA St Univ - Univ Park; Assoc Prof, University of Michigan, **SLP F**

Daly, Deborah S 136 Heritage Drive, Whittinsville, MA 01588, (617) 588-8034, BS 83 Univ of MA - Amherst; MA 85 Univ of CA - Santa Barbara; **A**

Daly, Eleanor Mary 89 Mt Auburn Street, Watertown, MA 02172, (617) 298-0785, MS 85 Northeastern Univ; **SLP**

Daly, Mary Patricia 4014 S E Ash Street, Portland, OR 97214, (503) 280-3923, BS 80 Portland St Univ; MS 83 Univ of WA; 85–Sp-Lang Path, Emanuel Hosp, **SLP**

Daly-Daysden, Julianne 4400 Marcourt Lane, West Des Moines, IA 50265, (515) 225-0666, **SLP**

Dalzell, Larry E 175 Glenhill Drive, Rochester, NY 14618, (716) 275-4852, BA 71 ND St Univ; MA 72 Northwestern Univ; PH 78 (Aud) Univ of IA; 78–Dir Dept/Aud/Sp-Lang Path, U of Rochester Med Ctr, **A**

Dalzell, Mrs Mary Ellen 44562 Mayberry Avenue, Hemet, CA 92343, (714) 652-8511, BA 80 Univ of Redlands; MS 82 Univ of Redlands; Sp-Lang Path, Wg Dalzell MD Inc, **SLP**

Dalzell, Mrs Sheila M 175 Glenhill Drive, Rochester, NY 14618, (716) 461-9192, BS 71 ND St Univ; MA 74 NM St Univ; Dir, The Hearing Center Inc, **A**

Damalt, Mrs Nancy Lisano 8 Orchard Avenue, Auburn, NY 13021, (315) 255-2746, BS 75 SUNY - Coll at Geneseo; MS 76 SUNY - Coll at Buffalo; Sp-Lang Path, E John Gavras Cen, **SLP**

Dameron, Mrs Hannah H 3625 Litchfield Drive, Rocky Mount, NC 27801, (919) 291-7001, BS 74 East Carolina Univ; MS 75 East Carolina Univ; Aud, Wilson Cl Pa, **A**

Damian, Judith Abriol 62 Bay State Road #6, Boston, MA 02215-1903, (617) 581-2400, BS 84 Univ of Philippines; MS 87 Boston Univ; **SLP**

Damiano, Laura Marie Westlake Hearing & Speech Clinic, 29101 Health Campus Drive, Room 290, Westlake, OH 44145, (216) 835-6160, BA 81 Cleveland St Univ; MA 83 Cleveland St Univ; Aud, W Lake Hrng & Sp Cl Inc, **A**

Damico, Mrs Gem E 15227 Cone Road, Maybee, MI 48159, (313) 439-2350, BS 79 Northeast MO St Univ; MS 81 Eastern NM Univ; **SLP**

Damico, Dr Jack S Speech Comm Theatre & Comm Dis, Louisiana State University, Speech And Hearing Clinic, Baton Rouge, LA 70803, (504) 388-2545, BA 74 Northwestern St Univ; MS 76 Univ of OK Medical Center; PH 85 (Linguistics) Univ of NM; Asst Prof, Louisiana St U, **SLP**

D'Amico, Josephine 47 Elinor Place, Yonkers, NY 10705, BA 71 CUNY - Lehman Coll; MA 73 Univ of MA - Amherst; 74–Sp-Lang Path, Yonkers Bd of Ed, **SLP**

Damico, Mrs Sandra K 1150 Wylie Drive, Baton Rouge, LA 70808, (504) 388-2545, MA 80 Univ of KS; Instructor/Clin Super, LA State U, **SLP**

Dammann, Dr Elly 2375 S Dogwood Terrace, Cornelius, OR 97113, (503) 648-8881, BS 62 Northern IL Univ - De Kalb; MS 72 Univ of OR; PH 76 (NS) Univ of OR; 88–DD Prog Mgr, Washington County Dept of Hlth & Hrng Svcs, **SLP**

Dammeyer, Mrs Denise L RR 2 Box 189, St Mary's, OH 45885, (513) 498-2131, MA 88 OH St Univ; 88–Sp-Lang Path, Sidney City Schs

Damon, Mrs Kristine E 27016 Azul, Capistrano Beach, CA 92624, (714) 496-9804, BS 70 IN Univ - Bloomington; MA 78 CA St Univ - Fullerton; SLP, Fountian Valley School Dist, **SLP**

Damon, Sheryl A 399 North Main Street, Suffield, CT 06078, (203) 242-0791, BA 75 Univ of CT; MS 77 Southern CT St Univ; Sp-Lang Path, Bloomfield Pub Schls, **SLP**

D'Amore, Donald D #25 12511 Clifton, Lakewood, OH 44107, (216) 741-4957, BA 84 John Carroll Univ; MA 86 Cleveland St Univ; **SLP**

Damore, Gina Marie 2233 Michael SW #6, Wyoming, MI 49509, (616) 245-0794, BA 85 MI St Univ; MA 87 0896; 88–Aud, McDonald Aud & Hrng Aid Hlth Care

Damron, Nancy Ann 42611 Northville Place Dr, Apartment 1004, Northville, MI 48167-3176, (313) 745-8903, BA 84 MI St Univ; MA 87 MI St Univ; Aud, Health Alliance Plan, **A**

Damron-Belote, Mrs Dawne A 409 Jackson Street, Martin, TN 38237, (901) 587-9059, MS 88 Murray St Univ; 88–Sp-Lang Path, Obion Co Sch Sys

Dana, Mrs Amy Thompson 529 Cambridge Drive, Greensburg, PA 15601, (412) 523-6593, BS 80 Clarion St Coll; MS 84 Indiana Univ of PA; 88–Sp-Lang Path, Family Home Health Svcs Inc, **SLP**

Dana, Diane Sniegoski P O Box 202, New Boston, NH 03070-3908, (603) 886-2710, OB 80 Northeastern Univ; ME 82 Northeastern Univ; Dir SLP, New England Rehab Cntr, **SLP**

Dance, Dr Frank E X 99 South Emerson, Denver, CO 80209, (303) 722-4800, BS 51 Fordham Univ; MA 53 Northwestern Univ; PH 59 (NS) Northwestern Univ; Professor, University of Denver

Dance, Joan L 56 Woodland Hills Drive, Apartment 1, Southgate, KY 41071, (606) 781-7846, MS 85 Univ of Louisville; **A**

Dancek, Mrs Laura F P 3067 Tamiami Trail, Suite 10, Port Charlotte, FL 33952, (813) 625-8800, BS 81 Andrews Univ; MA 82 Western MI Univ; Owner/Sp-Lang Path, All Speech, **SLP**

Dancer, Dr Jesse E Department Communication Disorders, University Of Arkansas At Little Rock, 2801 South University, Little Rock, AR 72204, (501) 569-3155, BS 63 Univ of Central AR; MS 66 Southern IL Univ -Carbondale; ED 75 (NS) Columbia Univ Teachers Coll; Prof, U of AR-Little Rock, **A**

Dancewicz, Susan Pulli 14 Newcastle Road, Peabody, MA 01960, (617) 531-6108, BS 79 Northeastern Univ; MS 81 Columbia Univ Teachers Coll; SLP, Dr J R Shaughnessy Rehab Hosp, **SLP**

Dancu, Mrs Rose Defazio 1265 Lakevue Drive, Butler, PA 16001, (412) 458-6700, BS 63 Indiana Univ of PA; MS 85 Clarion Univ of PA; Sp-Lang Path, Southwest Butler School Dist, **SLP**

Dancull, Denise Marie 832 Washington Street 1E, Evanston, IL 60202, (312) 491-5012, BS 86 Northwestern Univ; MA 87 Northwestern Univ; 88–Supvr-Sp-Lang Path, Northwestern Univ, **SLP**

D'Andrea, Gerald Arthur 1001 Sweet Briar Court, Monmouth Junction, NJ 08852, (201) 547-3024, BA 56 Long Island U - Brooklyn Ctr; MA 57 Columbia Univ Sch of Gen St; Assoc Prof-Spec Ed, Jersey City State Coll, **SLP A**

D'Andrea, Linda 135 Post Avenue #2G, Westbury, NY 11590, (516) 361-2613, BS 72 Saint John's Univ - Jamaica; MA 74 CUNY - Queens Coll; Sp/Lang Path, Smithtown Ctrl Sch Dist, **SLP**

Dandy, Mrs Annemarie P 284 Dewey Street, West Springfield, MA 01089, (413) 737-5743, BS 77 Worcester St Coll; MA 82 Univ of MA - Amherst; Sp-Lang Path, W Springfield Pub Sch, **SLP**

Danekas, Andrea Nicholas 511 South Pine, Arlington Heights, IL 60005, (312) 824-1136, BS 81 Northern IL Univ - De Kalb; MA 82 Northern IL Univ - De Kalb; Sp/Lang Path, Sch Dist 62 of Des Plaines, **SLP**

Danenberg, Mary A 119 Four Mile River Road, Old Lyme, CT 06371, (203) 434-5982, BA 68 Wellesley Coll; MS 86 Southern CT St Univ; 86–Sp-Lang Path, Montville Bd of Educ, **SLP**

Danford, Daniel Ernest HC 87 Box 167, Ermine, KY 41815, (606) 633-2211, **SLP**

Danford, Roy, Jr 3126 Manila Drive, San Antonio, TX 78217, (512) 536-2177, BA 57 Univ of TX - Austin; MA 70 Our Lady Lake Univ-San Anton; Aud, USAF Sch of Aerospace Med, **A ACE**

Danforth, Patricia Martin 4499 Juneberry Court, Concord, CA 94521, (415) 282-2551, BA 80 San Francisco St Univ; MA Univ of San Francisco; **SLP**

Danforth-Dargie, Mrs Anita Louise 449 Brights Lane, Penllyn, PA 19422, (215) 542-0622, BA 75 Boston Univ; MS 77 Emerson Coll; Sp-Lang Path, UCP Assoc, **SLP**

Dang, Celeste B 6750 5th N W, Seattle, WA 98117, (206) 361-4238, BA 76 Univ of Northern CO; MA 78 Univ of WA; Sp-Lang Path, Shoreline Sch Dist, **SLP**

D'Angelo-Carley, Mrs Kathleen 86 Deer Run, Burlington, CT 06013, (203) 673-9847, BA 75 Southern CT St Univ; MS 78 Univ of RI; Sp/Lang Path, Berlin PS Sys, **SLP**

Danhauer, Dr Jeffrey L Department Of Speech & Hearing Sciences, University Of California, Santa Barbara, CA 93106, (805) 961-2684, BA 70 OH St Univ; MA 72 OH Univ - Athens; PH 74 (Aud) OH Univ - Athens; 79–Prof/Aud, Univ of CA Santa Barbara, **A**

Daniel, David Aubrey 11445 Dawson Springs Road, Crofton, KY 42217, (502) 821-5564, BS 85 Murray St Univ; MS 87 Murray St Univ; 88–Sp-Lang Path, Pro Health Svcs, **SLP**

Daniel, Mrs Julie Ann 9256 Bird Street, Santee, CA 92071, (619) 258-1454, BA 84 Point Loma Nazarene Coll; MA 87 San Diego St Univ

Daniel, Linda L 8405 East Hampden #16J, Denver, CO 80231, (303) 695-9109, BS 73 Univ of IA; MA 74 Univ of Denver; MA 74 Univ of Denver; Habilatative/Diag Aud, Aud/Verbal Consult, **A**

Daniel, Lynn Mutual At Omaha Bldg, 7602 Lee Highway, Suite 2, Chattanooga, TN 37412, (615) 894-5220, BA 50 Univ of TN - Chattanooga; MA 57 G Peabody Coll-Vanderbilt U; Dir Sp-Lang Path, Cl of Sp Path, **SLP**

Daniel, Margaret Ellen Methodist Hospital Of Memphis, 1265 Union Avenue, Memphis, TN 38104, (901) 726-7684, OB 82; MA 86; 87–Sp-Lang Path, Methodist Hospitals of Memphis, **SLP**

Daniel, Marilyn J 103 Hilltop Road, Silver Spring, MD 20910, BA 70 Western KY Univ; MS 74 Vanderbilt Univ; 88–Sp-Lang Path, Private Practice, **SLP**

Daniel, Martha Hardin 11445 Dawson Springs Road, Crofton, KY 42217, (502) 424-5310, BS 85 Western KY Univ; MS 87 Murray St Univ; 88–Sp-Lang Path, Pennyroyal Ctr, **SLP**

Daniel, Mrs Nina MacAulay 1150 Chestnut Street, Escondido, CA 92025, (619) 741-5158, BA 75 CA St Univ - Fullerton; MA 78 CA St Univ - Fullerton; **SLP**

Daniel, Sarah Weller 5200 Abedul, El Paso, TX 79932, (915) 581-5947, BA 72 Univ of TX - Austin; MA 76 Univ of TX - Austin; 87–Aud, Private Practice, **A**

D'Aniello, Anthony J 15603 Gulf Freeway, Apartment 1323, Webster, TX 77598, (713) 484-8187, BA 68 Boston Univ; MS 73 Univ of RI; Aud, **A**

Daniels, Betty J Route 1 Box 54, Hazlehurst, MS 39083, (601) 987-3555, BS 77 Jackson St Univ; MS 79 MS Univ for Women; Sp-Lang Path, Jackson Pub Sch Syst, **SLP**

Daniels, Charleen Mary 44C Gillis Street, Nashua, NH 03060, (603) 595-2446, BA 70 Lynchburg Coll; MS 84 Univ of NH; Sp-Lang Path, St Joseph's Hospital, **SLP**

Daniels, Cynthia Krug 11802 Mackey, Overland Park, KS 66210, (913) 621-5155, BS 80 Univ of MO - Columbia; MA 83 Univ of KS; Sp/Lang Path, Ks Cty Ks Sch Dist #500, **SLP**

Daniels, Elizabeth Anne 2826 North 41st Street, Milwaukee, WI 53210, BS 73 Univ of WI - Milwaukee; MS 79 Marquette Univ; Sp/Lang Path, Milwaukee Pub Sch, **SLP**

Daniels, Joyce Sak 1 Thorman Lane, Huntington, NY 11743, (516) 361-2612, BA 59 CUNY - Brooklyn Coll; MA 61 CUNY - Brooklyn Coll; Sp-Lang Path, Smithtown Ctrl Sch Dist, **SLP**

Daniels, Karen Jeanne 488 Perkins Avenue, Bldg 1 Unit 1, Waterbury, CT 06704-1978, (203) 236-1919, BA 85 Elms Coll; MS 87 Emerson Coll; 86–Sp-Lang Path, **SLP**

Daniels, Katherine A PO Box 56, Moline, KS 67353, (316) 647-8127, BS 72 Portland St Univ; MS 79 Western OR St Coll; Sp-Lang Path, Elk & Chautauqua Co Spec Educ Coop, **SLP**

Daniels, Mrs Kathy Colene 6407 West North Lane, Glendale, AZ 85302-1116, (602) 973-3314, MS 84 Northern AZ Univ; Sp-Lang Path, Arizona Speech Pathology, **SLP**

Daniels, Mrs Kay Ileene 1533 Swenson Street, Abilene, TX 79603, (915) 677-2103, **SLP**

Daniels, Kelly Lee 217 East Bowie, Luling, TX 78648, (512) 379-2003, BS 82 Southwest TX St Univ; ME 84 Southwest TX St Univ; 84–Sp-Lang Path, Seguin ISD, **SLP**

Daniels, Kurt R 343 North Edinburgh Lane, Frankfort, IL 60423, (312) 532-7000, BS 76 Eastern IL Univ; MS 77 Eastern IL Univ; Sp-Lang Path, W A Howe Dev Cen St of Il, **SLP**

Daniels, Larose S 402 Dogwood Trail, Goldsboro, NC 27530, (919) 735-8450, BS 76 East Carolina Univ; MS 78 East Carolina Univ; Exec Dir, En Assoc Sp & Lang Serv, Inc, **SLP ACE**

Daniels, Lisa G 43-20 163rd Street, Flushing, NY 11358, (718) 359-0236, BA 83 CUNY - Queens Coll; MA 87 CUNY - Queens Coll

Daniels, Mrs Lynn Ann 2422 11th Avenue East, Hibbing, MN 55746, (218) 262-5704, BA 66 Augustana Coll; MA 68 Northwestern Univ; **SLP**

Daniels, Marjorie C 2147 South Hurds Corner Rd, Caro, MI 48723, (517) 673-5671, BA 67 Eastern MI Univ; MA 71 CA St Univ - Northridge; Dir Dept Commun Trng & Lang De, Caro Reg Cen, **SLP**

Daniels, Mary Rose Turley 36 Callender Court, Laguna Niguel, CA 92677, (714) 496-7358, BS 78 CA St Univ - Long Beach; MS 86 Chapman Coll; **SLP**

Daniels, Paulette Gerard 3505 Prairie, Berkley, MI 48072, (313) 543-7591, BA 82 MI St Univ; MA 84 Wayne St Univ - Sch of Med; 86–Aud, Michigan Ear Institute, **A**

Daniels, Sheila J R R 4 Box 139-C, Kirksville, MO 63501, (816) 665-7505, BS 77 Northeast MO St Univ; MA 78 Northeast MO St Univ; Sp-Lang Path, Private Practice, **SLP**

Daniels, Stephanie Kay 735 Exposition Blvd #A, New Orleans, LA 70118, (504) 838-3900, BS 83 East TX St Univ - Commerce; MS 85 Univ of TX - Dallas; Sp-Lang Path, Ochsner Clinic, **SLP**

Daniels, Teri Joseph 5 Lord Nelson Court, Columbia, SC 29209, (803) 776-5959, **SLP**

Daniels, Wendy Louise 914 St Johns Wood Drive, Richmond, VA 23225, (804) 320-3900, BS 84 James Madison Univ; MS 86 James Madison Univ; **SLP**

Daniels-Miller, Dr Lenore 46 Central Avenue, Newton, MA 02160, (617) 956-5300, BA 58 CUNY - Brooklyn Coll; MA 61 CUNY - Brooklyn Coll; OD 83 (Communication Disorders) Boston Univ; 68–Dir Sp-Lang Path, New England Med Cen Hosp, **SLP ACE**

Danielson, Holly L RFD 1 Box 60, Pomfret Center, CT 06259, (203) 928-2640, MA 87 Univ of CT; 87–Sp-Lang Path, CT Region 3 John Dempsey Ctr, **SLP**

Danielson, Mrs Jan M 10041 Bradbury Drive, Indianapolis, IN 46231, **SLP**

Danielson, Mrs Nenita P 145 Carmel Riviera Drive, Carmel, CA 93923, (619) 481-0566, BA 71 Univ of CA - Santa Barbara; MA 73 San Diego St Univ; Sp-Lang Path, **SLP**

Danielson, Priscilla Mary 4626 Muggleton Road, Wilmington, DE 19808, (302) 428-2286, BA 77 Emory & Henry Coll; MA 80 Memphis St Univ; 87–Sp-Lang Path, Private Practice, **SLP**

Danielson, Maj Richard W Madigan Army Medical Center, Box 262 Audiology, Tacoma, WA 98431, (206) 967-6496, BS 73 ND St Univ; MS 74 Minot St Univ; PH 87 (Human Develop & Comm Sciences) Univ of TX - Dallas; Chief Aud, US Army, **A**

Danielson, Sarah J 2025 South Humboldt, Denver, CO 80210, (303) 861-6800, BA 74 Univ of Denver; MA 77 Univ of Denver; Sp-Lang Path, Chldns Hosp, **SLP**

Daniloff, Raymond Louisiana State University, Speech And Hearing Clinic, 163 MDA Bldg, Baton Rouge, LA 70803-2606, (504) 388-2545, BS 61 CA Univ of PA; MA 63 Harvard Univ; PH 67 (NS) Univ of IA; Dir-Comm Disorders, Louisiana State University, **F**

Danjelic, Erica 4 Las Casas Drive, San Rafael, CA 94901, (415) 921-7658, BA 64 Marymount Coll; MA 74 Catholic Univ of America; 76–Sp-Lang Path, San Francisco Hearing/Spch Ctr, **SLP**

Dank, Seth 894 Melvin Drive, North Bellmore, NY 11710, (516) 354-6882, BA 76 CUNY - Queens Coll; MA 77 Hofstra Univ; Aud, Private Practice, **A**

Danko, Mrs Angela N 6725 Orchard Boulevard, Parma Heights, OH 44130, (216) 843-6596, BS; Retired, **SLP LM**

Dankovich, Jacqueline 1060 Bank Street, Bridgeville, PA 15017, (412) 429-3116, BS 70 CA Univ of PA; ME 82 CA Univ of PA; Coord/SLP-Aud, Allegheny Co Inst Dist, **SLP**

Dankowski, Mrs M Korine 1234 Pondoray Circle, Salt Lake City, UT 84117, (801) 531-7022, BS 60 Univ of WY; MS 83 Univ of UT; Aud, Symbion Inc, **A**

Dankowski, Margaret Mary 10636 Woodley #25, Granada Hills, CA 91344, (818) 506-0183, BS 85 East TN St Univ; MA 87 George Washington Univ; SLP, Synergos Neuro Ctr, **SLP**

Danley, Mrs Judy Harris 11209 Slippery Elm Trail, Austin, TX 78750, BA 74 Abilene Christian Univ; MA 79 TX Christian Univ; Sp-Lanq Path, Private Practice, **SLP**

Danna, Victoria Lee 4215 Avenue R, Galveston, TX 77550, (409) 765-8787, BS 81 SUNY - Coll at Oneonta; MA 88 Univ of TX - Austin; **A**

Dannheisser, Karen S 737 Nagel Drive, Pensacola, FL 32503, (904) 433-4198, BA 78 Univ of FL; MA 80 Univ of FL; Audiologist, Roger Earl Bowie MD, **A**

D'Annibale, Marisa G 74 East Bridge Street, Morrisville, PA 19067, (609) 896-9500, BS 76 Marywood Coll; MA 81 OH Univ - Athens; 86–Sp-Lang Path, St Lawrence Rehab Ctr, **SLP**

Dans, Dr Jimmie C 1603 Furman, Ruston, LA 71270, (318) 357-4169, BA 61 LA Tech Univ; MA 65 Univ of AL-Tuscaloosa; PH 85 (Sp-Lang Path) Memphis St Univ; Assoc Prof, LA Tech U, **SLP**

Dansak, Denise Ann 56 N Starr Apt #301, Pittsburgh, PA 15202, (412) 232-7788, Sp-Lang Path, Mercy Hospital of Pittsburgh, **SLP**

Danse, Mrs Marian Burnett 6141 S W 85th Street, Miami, FL 33143-8145, (716) 473-4080, BS 78 Univ of VA - Charlottesville; ME 79 Univ of VA - Charlottesville; Slp, Monroe Community Hospital, **SLP**

Dante, Joanne H 825 Robinhood Lane, La Grange Park, IL 60525, (312) 277-7755, BS 69 Kent St Univ; MA 71 Kent St Univ; Sp-Lang Path, Chicago Bd of Ed, **SLP**

Danto, Dr Joseph 214 Engle Street, Englewood, NJ 07631, (201) 567-8408, BA 67 CUNY - Brooklyn Coll; MS 69 CUNY - Brooklyn Coll; PH 71 (Aud) CUNY - Grad Sch & Univ Cntr; Assoc Prof, CUNY-Cty Coll, **A**

D'Antoni, Maria L 12 Greenway Plaza, Suite 1100, Houston, TX 77046, (713) 840-8390, BS 69 LA St Univ - Baton Rouge; MA 70 Univ of MD - College Park; Sp-Lang Path, Private Practice, **SLP ACE**

D'Antonio, Mrs Cynthia Cinderella 19 Coolidge Avenue, Totowa, NJ 07512, (201) 697-1700, BA 84 William Paterson Coll; MS 87 William Paterson Coll

D'Antonio, Dr Linda L Providence Sp And Hearing Ctr, 1301 Providence Avenue, Orange, CA 92668, (714) 639-4990, BA 75 Univ of CA - Berkeley; PH 82 (NS) San Francisco St Univ; 87–Coord-Craniofacial & Voice Prog, Providence Sp and Hrng Ctr, **SLP**

Danwitz, Sr M Winifred 39 Willow Drive, New Rochelle, NY 10801, (212) 584-7679, PH 70 (Sp-Lang Path) CUNY - Grad Sch & Univ Cntr; Admin, Mount St Ursula Speech Ctr, **SLP F**

Danz, Dr Alan D 290 N W 165th Street, Plaza 250, Miami, FL 33169, (305) 944-8378, BA 77 CUNY - Queens Coll; MA 78 Univ of MD - College Park; PH 83 (NS) Purdue Univ - West Lafayette; Aud, Family Hearing Center, **A**

Danzeisen, Nancy B 506 Mill Cove Court, Fayetteville, NC 28304, (919) 867-3469, BS 76 Univ of VA - Charlottesville; MS 84 James Madison Univ; Chief/SLP Services, Center for Speech, **SLP**

Danzer, Virginia A 4202 S W 44th Avenue, Portland, OR 97221, (503) 280-5757, BA 55 Saint Louis Univ; ME 56 Saint Louis Univ; Superv Assesment Cen, Portland Publ Schs, **SLP**

Dapkus, Mrs Kathy Heil 519 Letcher Avenue, Richmond, KY 40475, (606) 623-1777, BS 77 Eastern KY Univ; ME 80 Eastern KY Univ; SLP, Stanford Elem, **SLP**

Dapollonio, Joann 490 Mount Hope Avenue, Cincinnati, OH 45204, (606) 331-0880, BS 84 OH Univ - Athens; MA 86 OH Univ - Athens; Sp-Lang Path, Redwood School, **SLP**

Da Pra, Denise M 2899 S W 22nd Circle #43-B, Delray Beach, FL 33445, (407) 393-4071, MA 81 Univ of FL; 84–Supvr of Sp-Lang Path, Boca Raton Comm Hosp, **SLP ACE**

Dapuzzo, Theresa 1510 45th Street, North Bergen, NJ 07047, (201) 533-5786, BA 83 Rutger's St Univ - Douglas Coll; MS 85 Rutgers St Univ - Newark; Sp-Lang Path, St Barnabas Medical Center, **SLP ACE**

D'Aquisto, Maureen 24 Beverly Court, Fort Salonga, NY 11768, **SLP**

Darah, Mrs Linda Sue 7736 Grenlock Drive, Sylvania, OH 43560-3631, (419) 352-3576, BS 80 Univ of Toledo; BA 80 Univ of Toledo; MA 84 Eastern MI Univ; 88–Sp-Lang Path, Toledo PS, **SLP**

Darata, Mrs Carrie E 241 Brookway Road, Dayton, OH 45459, (513) 433-0253, BS 84 Brigham Young Univ; OM 86 Brigham Young Univ; **A**

Darby, Mrs Ann M 611 Overlook Drive, Beckley, WV 25801, (304) 256-4555, BA 74; MA 75 Marshall Univ; Sp/Lang Path, Raleigh Co Schs, **SLP**

Darby, John L Hrng Soc For The Bay Area Inc, 20 10th Street 2nd Floor, San Francisco, CA 94103, (415) 863-4710, BA 50 Stanford Univ; Exec Dir, Hrng Soc for the Bay Area, **F**

Darby, Jon A Rwsir Box 328, Warm Springs, GA 31830, (404) 655-2016, BS 72 Univ of GA; ME 75 Univ of GA; 77–Dir Sp-Lang Path & Aud Dept, Roosevelt Warm Spr I for Rehab, **SLP**

Darby, Kathe Shannon 2000 Haverford Road, Ardmore, PA 19003, (215) 649-1025, BS 78 Central CT St Univ; MA 86 Univ of CO - Boulder; 86–Sp-Lang Path, Private Practice, **SLP**

Darcey, Mrs Molly Mitchell 2266 Cottonwood Circle, Salt Lake City, UT 84117, (213) 208-4938, BS 66 Miami Univ - Oxford; MA 67 Univ of WI - Madison; Stewardess, Pan Am World Airways, **SLP**

Darcy-Campbell, Karen 2416 N Fairview Lane, Rochester Hills, MI 48064, (313) 652-3318, BA 78 Boston Coll; ME 80 Northeastern Univ; Sp-Lang Path, **SLP**

Dardas Rn, Mrs Kathryn D 6404 21st Avenue West, #M-214, Bradenton, FL 33529, MS; **SLP A LM**

Darden, Celia Parker 511-B Boxwood Lane, Goldsboro, NC 27530, BS 85 East Carolina Univ; MS 86 East Carolina Univ; 88–Sp-Lang Path, LOGOS Inc, **SLP**

Dardick, Leila R 760 Mix Avenue, Hamden, CT 06514, (203) 729-6819, BA 40 CUNY - Brooklyn Coll; MA 60 Columbia Univ Teachers Coll; **SLP LM**

Dardis, Mrs Linda L 2900 West Oklahoma, Milwaukee, WI 53215, (414) 649-6400, BA 71 Univ of WI - Milwaukee; MS 80 Univ of WI - Milwaukee; Sp-Lang Path, St Luke's Hosp, **SLP**

Dargan, Margaret A 921 South Laflin, Chicago, IL 60607, (312) 829-5016, BS 84 Fontbonne Coll; MS 86 Fontbonne Coll; **SLP**

Darian, Rosemary B 3350 Burbank, Ann Arbor, MI 48105, (313) 747-9333, BA 76 Univ of MI - Ann Arbor; MA 79 Eastern MI Univ; Sp-Lang Path, Redford Union Schools, **SLP**

Darley, Dr Frederic L 1007 17th Street N E, Rochester, MN 55904, (507) 289-0694, BA 39 NM St Teachers Coll; MA 40 Univ of IA; PH 50 (Sp Path) Univ of IA; 83–Prof, Mayo Clinic, **SLP F H LM**

Darling, Angela Kay 6309 Hilly Way, Cary, IL 60013, (312) 639-8771, BS 85 Purdue Univ - West Lafayette; MS 87 Purdue Univ - West Lafayette; 88–Aud, Audiometrics Inc

Darling, Mrs Christine Petkovsek 6880 Marshall Place, Beaumont, TX 77706, (409) 899-4099, BS 85 Lamar Univ; MS 87 Lamar Univ; 87–Sp-Lang Path, Sp & Lang Assoc Inc, **SLP**

Darling, Linda Joy 2950 South Mooney Blvd, Suite E, Visalia, CA 93277, (209) 733-3818, BA 77 CA St Univ - Fresno; MA 80 CA St Univ - Fresno; Dir, Sierra Sp & Hrng, **SLP ACE**

Darling, Mrs Nancy H 2503 Buckingham Road, Wilson, NC 27893, (919) 291-7001, BS 76 Univ of Montevallo; MS 78 Univ of Montevallo; Sp-Lang Path, CRF Sp & Lang Assoc, **SLP**

Darling, Dr Rieko Marie Dept Of Comm Disorders, 1199 Haley Center, Auburn University, Auburn, AL 36849-5232, (205) 826-5545, BS 82 FL St Univ; MS 83 FL St Univ; PH 87 (Aud) FL St Univ; 88–Asst Prof of Aud, Auburn Univ, **A**

Darlow, Mrs Mary S 630 Commons Drive, Sacramento, CA 95825, (916) 454-8387, BA 57 Univ of AZ; Sp-Lang Path, Sacramento Cty USD, **SLP**

D'Armi, Mrs Patricia Cipoletti 24 Dunham Loop, Berlin, NJ 08009, (609) 767-5795, BA 80 Rutger's St Univ - Douglas Coll; MS 85 William Paterson Coll; 82–Sp-Lang Path, West Deptford Bd of Educ, **SLP**

Darnell, Mrs Suzanne H 3523 Carnoustie, Augusta, GA 30907, (404) 722-1957, BS 63 Purdue Univ - West Lafayette; Sp-Lang Path, Hrng&Sp Cen/Augusta & E Ctrl G, **SLP**

Darnton, Sue Wilder 916 Raymond Court, Ann Arbor, MI 48103, **SLP**

Darr, Christine 1289 West New Britton Dr, Hoffman Estates, IL 60195, (312) 358-9068, BS 73 Univ of WI - Stevens Point; MA 76 Northern IL Univ - De Kalb; **SLP**

Darr, Claudia E 3613-15 Colony Road, Charlotte, NC 28211, (704) 372-3300, BS 85 James Madison Univ; ME 87 Univ of VA - Charlottesville; 87–Aud, Charlotte Eye ENT Assoc, **A**

Darragh, Mrs Staci Haines 211 Laurel Drive, Peekskill, NY 10566, (914) 245-2700, BS 83 Univ of IL - Urbana; MS 84 Univ of IL - Urbana; Sp-Lang Path, N Westchester/Putnam Co BOCES, **SLP**

Darrow, Mrs Marianne D Rd 7 Box 97, Kingston, NY 12401, (914) 331-6885, BA 46 SUNY - Center at Albany; MA 52 2162; 88–Sp-Lang Path, Childrens Annex, **SLP**

Darrow, Mrs Mary Ann M 7 Yellow Orange Circle, Middletown, CT 06457, (201) 347-5624, BS 64 SUNY - Coll at Geneseo; MA 65 Univ of CT; SLP, Middletown Bd of Ed, **SLP**

Darrow, Will T 8833 West 32nd Place, Wheat Ridge, CO 80033-5859, **SLP**

Dart, Cheryl Bennett 7507 South Trenton Court, Englewood, CO 80112, (303) 629-4459, BS 75 NE Wesleyan Univ; MS 82 Univ of CO - Boulder; 84–Supvr, St Anthony Hosp Sys, **SLP**

Dart, Dawn Marie 112 Philadelphia Street, Apartment 1, Saratoga Springs, NY 12866, (518) 583-3266, BA 81 Univ of Pittsburgh - Pittsburgh; MS 85 Coll of Saint Rose; 86–Sp-Lang Path, Wilton Dev Ctr, **SLP**

D'Artista, Diane F 5 Park Street #3, Brookline, MA 02146, (617) 566-3609, BS 78 Northeastern Univ; MS 79 Rutgers St Univ - Newark; **SLP**

Darville, Mrs Lesa Ward 1129 W Main #6, Franklin, TN 37064, (615) 791-5058, BA 78 Univ of AR - Fayetteville; MS 81 East Carolina Univ; Sp-Lang Path, **SLP**

Daryoush, Mehrdad Samimi 27155 Chardon Road #203, Richmond Heights, OH 44143, (216) 943-1626, BA 78 Case Western Reserve Univ; MA 80 Cleveland St Univ; Aud, Jalal Afnan MD

D'Asaro, Dr Lois N 4319 Redwood Avenue #3, Marina Del Rey, CA 90292, (213) 474-7216, BS 46 Ball St Univ; MA 48 Univ of NE - Lincoln; PH 73 (Psychology); Sp-Lang Path, Private Practice, **SLP**

D'Asaro, Dr Michael J 2901 Wilshire Boulevard, Suite 319, Santa Monica, CA 90403, (213) 474-7216, BA 45 Bowling Green St Univ; MA 52 Univ of Southern CA; PH 55 (Sp) Univ of Southern CA; Sp-Lang Path, Private Practice, **SLP F LM**

Dashefsky, Mrs Lisa Kowall 825 Sherbrook Street, Winnipeg, MB, Canada R3A 1M5, (204) 786-5601, BA 82 Univ of ND; OM 85 Univ of Western Ontario; 85–Sp-Lang Path, Soc For Manitobans & Dis Inc, **SLP**

Dashefsky, Mrs Randy L 15618 North Hanna Maui Dr, Phoenix, AZ 85022, (602) 866-9606, BA 75 McGill Univ - Quebec; MS 76 Univ of VT; Sp-Lang Path, Private Practice, **SLP**

Dashiell, Mrs Judith G 1069 Monserate, Chula Vista, CA 92011, (619) 421-3500, BS 60 Auburn Univ - Auburn; MS 61 Vanderbilt Univ; Sp-Lang Path, Chula Vista Elem Schs, **SLP**

Dashiell, Mrs Lynn Purnell 6025 Eastwood Terrace, Norfolk, VA 23508, (804) 827-1545, ME 82 James Madison Univ; **A**

Dashiell, Mrs Pamela B 11339 Hemlock, Overland Park, KS 66210, (913) 661-9308, BA 62 Univ of AR - Fayetteville; MA 75 Univ of Tulsa; SLP, North Fulton Med Ctr, **SLP**

Dashiell, Sallie E 143 Greenfield, Irvine, CA 92714, (714) 786-6731, BS 74 Georgetown Univ; MA 76 George Washington Univ; Sp-Lang Path, Huntington Beach Union Hs Dist, **SLP**

Da Silva, Mrs Maria M P 6044 Wingedfoot Ct, Indianapolis, IN 46254, (317) 298-8019, MA 88 Butler Univ

Da Silva, Mrs Virginia G 5403 Rogers Highway, Tecumseh, MI 49286, (517) 423-6657, BA 75 Univ of MN - Duluth; MA 77 Northern MI Univ; 83–Sp-Lang Path, Dexter Comm Schs, **SLP**

Daskin, Barbara J 3700 S W 59th Terrace, Davie, FL 33314, (305) 797-0124, BA 67 Hofstra Univ; MS 68 Univ of OK Medical Center; SLP, Holly Cross Hosp, **SLP**

Dasovich, Dr Mary O St Louis University, Department Of Education, 221 North Grand Boulevard, St Louis, MO 63103, (314) 658-2510, BS 64 Saint Louis Univ; MA 65 Saint Louis Univ; PH 71 (NS) Saint Louis Univ; Prof, St Louis U, **SLP**

Dasso, Mrs Sandra Sandstrom 1699 Cypress Street, Orange City, FL 32763, (904) 775-3090, **SLP**

Datel, Tanya Marie Audiphone Of Maryland, 4235 28th Avenue Suite 109A, Marlow Heights, MD 20748, (301) 899-2050, BA 82 McGill Univ - Quebec; MS 84 Columbia Univ Sch of Gen St; 88–Aud, Audiphone Washington Co Inc, **A**

Datino, Nancy Louise 323 Wagner Avenue, Mamaroneck, NY 10543, (212) 741-7677, BA 79 Dominican Coll of Blauvelt; MS 81 Columbia Univ Teachers Coll; Aud, NY League of Hard of Hrng, **A**

Dato, Dr Daniel P 13902 Shippers Lane, Rockville, MD 20853, (301) 871-7477, PH 59 (NS) Cornell Univ; Assoc Prof of Ling, Georgetown U, **SLP**

Datres, Glen Phillip 105 West Wiley Street, Maybrook, NY 12543, (914) 285-8186, Aud, Westchester Cty Medical Ctr, **A**

Datsko, Mrs Margaret L 108 Rider Drive, Beckley, WV 25801, (304) 252-2704, BS 76 Clarion Univ of PA; MA 77 OH Univ - Athens; Sp-Lang Path, Raleigh Co Bd of Ed, **SLP**

Dattilo, Carol Langford 1379 Westminster Lane, Bourbonnais, IL 60914, (815) 939-8244, MA 83 Ball St Univ; Sp-Lang Path, Bourbonnais Schools, **SLP**

Dattilo, Mrs Joan L 4224 Rudy Lane, Louisville, KY 40207, (502) 893-5092, BA 64 George Washington Univ; ME 75 Univ of Louisville; **SLP**

Datwyler, Bonita Brooks 7073 Stabulis Road, Linden, CA 95236, (209) 786-2597, **SLP**

Daubenspeck, Deborah 443 Richmond Park West, Apartment 322D, Richmond Heights, OH 44143, (216) 721-5400, SLP, Health Hill Hospital, **SLP**

Daucsavage, Janet Lee 22033 Stormy Lane, Bend, OR 97701, (503) 389-1754, BA 74 Univ of ND; Sp-Lang Path, Private Practice, **SLP**

Daudistel, Mrs Sandra 6733 Mariposa Drive, El Paso, TX 79912, BA 70 Univ of CA - Santa Barbara; MA 76 Univ of TX - El Paso; Sp-Path, El Paso ISD, **SLP**

Dauenhauer, Sandra G 507 Ookpik Way, Fairbanks, AK 99709, (907) 456-4884, BA 64 Memphis St Univ; BA 74; OM 82 Univ of MO - Columbia; Sp-Lang Path, Alaska Crpld Chldn & Adults, **SLP**

Dauer, Kathleen E 1154 Norbert Lane, St Paul, MN 55116, (612) 298-8288, MS 84 Mankato St Univ; Sp-Lang Path, United Childrens Hosp, **SLP**

Dauer, Theresa Mae 1279 E Beaver Road, Kawkawlin, MI 48631, (517) 686-4410, BS 83 Western MI Univ; MA 85 Western MI Univ; Sp-Lang Path, Bay-Arenac Int Schl Dstr, **SLP**

Daugherty, Dale E 1619 North Greenwood, Suite 309, Pueblo, CO 81003, (719) 544-7115, BA 75 Kearney St Coll; MA 76 Univ of SD - Vermillion; 85–Dir-Aud Svcs, Charles H Bedard MD PC, **A**

Daugherty, Jamey A K 2671 Lookout Circle, Ann Arbor, MI 48104, (301) 926-7537, **A**

Daugherty, Mrs Kathleen Gaydos 4808 Turtle Creek, Ruston, LA 71270, (318) 644-5842, BA 79 LA Tech Univ; MA 82 LA Tech Univ; Sp-Lang Path, Ouachita Parish Sch Bd, **SLP**

Daugherty, Marybeth 15 Holbrook Avenue, North Attleboro, MA 02760-2326, (319) 399-6874, OB 82 Western MI Univ; OM 83 Central MI Univ; **SLP**

Daugherty, Mrs Saundra H 260 Pine Tree Lane, Ballwin, MO 63011, MA 78 Univ of TN - Knoxville; Sp-Lang Path, Ctrl Inst for Deaf, **SLP**

Daughtry, Dr Ginger H Route 1 Box 203, Holly Ridge, NC 28445, (919) 347-2738, BA 71 Univ of NC - Greensboro; ME 72 Univ of NC - Greensboro; PH 78 (NS) Univ of TN - Knoxville; Sp-Lang Path, Onslow County Public Schools, **SLP**

Daughtry, Mrs Susan Carreker Route 1, Americus, GA 31709, (912) 924-6949, BS 86 Auburn Univ - Auburn; OM 87 Auburn Univ - Auburn; Sp-Lang Path, Sumter Co Bd of Ed, **SLP**

Daulton, Mrs Donna S 6381 Buckeye Lane, Roseville, CA 95661, (916) 791-1115, BA 71 Univ of CA - Santa Barbara; MA 73 Univ of CA - Santa Barbara; SLP, Placer Co Office of Ed, **SLP**

Daum, Katherine Kuhn 482F Dewdrop Circle, Forest Park, OH 45240, (513) 733-1661, BA 86 IN Univ - Bloomington; MA 88 OH Univ - Athens; 88–Aud, The Ear Center

D'Aurio, Mrs Gale M 19 Garrison Drive, Spring Valley, NY 10977, NY Univ; SLP, S Orangetown School District, **SLP**

Dausman, Rebecca Carroll 10401 Florian, Louisville, KY 40223-3444, (502) 584-9781, BS 70 Univ of KY; MS 85 Univ of Louisville; **SLP**

Davalos, Lancey H 2135 Cedar Run, San Antonio, TX 78245, (512) 670-5967, BA 63 Univ of Saint Thomas; MA 73 Our Lady Lake Univ-San Anton; Sp-Lang Path, Wilford Hall Med Cen, **SLP**

Davee, Veralyn T 1416 Stonetree, Troy, MI 48083, (313) 689-7124, BS 71 SUNY - Coll at Oneonta; ME 73 Univ of AZ; MA 85 Wayne St Univ; **A**

Davenport, Beverly W 305 Diana, Converse, TX 78109, **SLP**

Davenport, Florence E West Point Pepperell, Medical Department, P O Box 71, West Point, GA 31833, (404) 645-4429, BS 80 MS Univ for Women; MA 82 Univ of MS; 88–Aud, West Point Pepperell, **A**

Davenport, Dr Richard W 724 Spruce North, Gunnison, CO 81230, (303) 641-0201, BS 67 Kearney St Coll; MS 69 CO St Univ; PH 77 (NS) IA St Univ; Chmn/Dept of Commun Disorders, College of St Theresa, **SLP**

Davenport, Wanda A 4616 Telestar, St Louis, MO 63128, (314) 464-5866, BA 70 Southeast MO St Univ; MA 73 Southeast MO St Univ; **SLP**

Daves, Mrs Rita Rome 487 Broad Street, Windsor, CT 06095, (203) 688-1066, Sp-Lang Path, Vernon Park Schs, **SLP**

Davey, Mrs Joan L 4121 Clement, Saginaw, MI 48603, (517) 793-7160, MS 80 Central MI Univ; 86–Sp-Lang Path, Saginaw PS, **SLP**

Davey, Mrs Karen M 7820 Long Avenue, Morton Grove, IL 60053, (312) 965-1409, BA 76 Southern IL Univ-Edwardsvill; MS 77 Southern IL Univ-Edwardsvill; Sp-Lang Path, The Evanston Hosp, **SLP**

Davey, Mrs Terry Kay 38 Hickory Street, Norwich, CT 06360, (203) 442-0711, BS 85 Eastern IL Univ; MA 87 Univ of CT; Sp-Lang Path, Lawrence & Memorial Hosp, **SLP**

David, Cleone F 5313 Water Wood Drive, Gainesville, GA 30506-9809, (404) 233-4238, BS 58 Univ of GA; ME 59 Univ of GA; Sp-Lang Path, Atlanta Bd of Ed, **SLP**

David, Deborah J 3914 Fairwood Drive, Sylvania, OH 43560, (419) 841-5527, BA 78 Univ of Redlands; MS 80 Univ of WI - Madison; Sp-Lang Path, Med Coll Hosp, **SLP**

David, Joan E R R 4 Box 260, Paris, IL 61944, (217) 662-6981, BS 84 Eastern IL Univ; MS 86 Eastern IL Univ; SLP, Georgetown Com Unit Dis #3, **SLP**

David, Mrs Karen S Rd 3, 40 Salem Drive, Greensburg, PA 15601, (412) 668-2337, BS 72 Indiana Univ of PA; MS 77 Indiana Univ of PA; **SLP**

David, Lisa K 4862 Matilija Avenue, Sherman Oaks, CA 91423, (818) 997-2357, BA 79 CA St Univ - Northridge; MA 81 CA St Univ - Northridge; Sp-Lang Path, LA USD, **SLP**

Davidoff, Marsha N 1001 Kenfield Avenue, Los Angeles, CA 90049, **SLP**

Davidoff-Adelson, Mrs Rita C 8 Farmingdale Road, Latham, NY 12110-5106, (518) 445-4526, BS 74 SUNY - Coll at Buffalo; MA 75 SUNY - Coll at Geneseo; Sp-Lang Path, Albany Med Cen Hosp Commun Dis, **SLP**

Davidow, Mrs Diana Sue 1721 Carlyle Avenue, Santa Monica, CA 90402, (213) 394-7559, BA 66 CUNY - Brooklyn Coll; MS 71 CUNY - Brooklyn Coll; Private Practice, **SLP**

Davids, Mrs Francine Elissa 3214 West Morrow Drive, Phoenix, AZ 85027, (602) 869-7038, BA 75 Adelphi Univ; MS 83 AZ St Univ; SLP, Washington Public School 6, **SLP**

Davidson, Anne D P O Box 1455, Stillwater, OK 74074, **SLP**

Davidson, Mrs Anne Massenburg 925 Old Cutler Road, Virginia Beach, VA 23454, (804) 496-9635, BS 78 James Madison Univ; OM 83 Old Dominion Univ; Sp-Lang Path, Los Angeles USD, **SLP**

Davidson, Barbara 41 North Court Street, Westminster, MD 21157, (301) 848-8698, **SLP**

Davidson, Barbara Sara 82 Beacon Hill Road, Port Washington, NY 11050, (516) 883-7823, BA 83 SUNY - Coll at Cortland; MA 87 Hofstra Univ

Davidson, Ben N 200 South Pecos, Fort Stockton, TX 79735, (915) 336-6409, BS 64 Abilene Christian Univ; MA 69 CA St Univ - Long Beach; Sp-Lang Path, Ft Stockton PS, **SLP**

Davidson, Deborah L 302-2450 Cornwall Avenue, Vancouver, BC, Canada V6K 1B8, (604) 731-9297, BA 78 Carleton Univ - Ontario; MS 80 Syracuse Univ; 88–Sp-Lang Path, Children's Hosp, **SLP**

Davidson, Mrs Deborah S 7027 Summer Place, Charlotte, NC 28213, (704) 376-1342, BA 76 Coll of William & Mary; MA 80 Univ of FL; 80–Sp-Lang Path, Charlotte Sp & Hrng Ctr, **SLP**

Davidson, Mrs Dora L 229 West Upsal Street #215, Philadelphia, PA 19119, MS; **SLP LM**

Davidson, Gayle A 7121 Members Place, Baton Rouge, LA 70817, (504) 383-5055, OB 73 Central MO St Univ; MS 75 Central MO St Univ; Dir of Sp, Renaissance Rehab Ctr, **SLP**

Davidson, Mrs Irene E 4962 Corinthia Way, Ocean Hills, CA 92056, (619) 940-4205, BA 40 CUNY - Brooklyn Coll; MA 65 Univ of CA - Los Angeles; **SLP**

Davidson, Mrs Jacqueline 5605 N W Pondosa Drive, Portland, OR 97229, (503) 645-1611, BA 70 Westmont Coll; MS 81 Portland St Univ; SLP, **SLP**

Davidson, James V 615 West Grove, El Dorado, AR 71730, (501) 862-5339, BA 74 CA St Univ - Los Angeles; MA 76 CA St Univ - Los Angeles; Aud, Audiology Resources LTD, **A**

Davidson, Jane B 4527 Briardale, San Antonio, TX 78217, (512) 434-6711, BS 67 Univ of TX - Austin; MS 70 Univ of TX - Austin; Dir, Harry Jersig Cen, **SLP**

Davidson, Mrs Jane R 103 Farmingdale Drive, Wexford, PA 15090, (412) 935-4381, BS 64 Indiana Univ of PA; MA 65 Western MI Univ; **SLP**

Davidson, K Rochelle 3120 Albemarle Road, Wilmington, DE 19808, (302) 454-2312, BS 64 Bloomsburg Univ of PA; MA 67 Temple Univ-Tyler Sch of Art; Sp-Lang Path, Christina Sch Dist, **SLP**

Davidson, Kathryn Pohlit 590 Thames Drive, Colorado Springs, CO 80906, (617) 698-6259, BA 75 Univ of CO - Boulder; MA 81 Saint Louis Univ; **SLP**

Davidson, Mrs Keiko Y 19102 Ruble Drive, Houston, TX 77084, (713) 391-2184, BA 76 Univ of MI - Ann Arbor; MS 77 Univ of MI - Ann Arbor; 84–Sp-Lang Path, Katy ISD, **SLP**

Davidson, Keith C Dept Speech Path & Audiology, Illinois State University, Normal, IL 61761, (309) 438-3960, OB 42 IL St Univ - Normal; MS 50 Columbia Univ Teachers Coll; **SLP**

Davidson, Mrs Lanita Whitten 7717 Belmont Avenue, Birmingham, AL 35206, (205) 838-1072, BA 85 Univ of AL-Tuscaloosa; MS 87 Univ of Montevallo

Davidson, Mrs Laura Krieger 114 Timberbrook, St Peters, MO 63376, (314) 895-4148, BS 77 Fontbonne Coll; MS 78 Southern IL Univ-Edwardsvill; Sp-Lang Path, St Josephs Health Center, **SLP**

Davidson, Mrs Leah Adler 4619 Lowell Avenue, Tampa, FL 33629, (813) 837-4788, BS 70 Univ of FL; MS 72 Univ of South FL; Sp-Lang Path, Private Practice, **SLP**

Davidson, Mrs Leslie Ann 5213 Pond Lake, San Antonio, TX 78244-2042, (512) 434-6711, BS 68 Univ of TX - Austin; MA 70 Univ of TX - Austin; 85–Sp-Lang Path, Harry Jersig Center, **SLP**

Davidson, Mrs Linda Fox 1814 N W 31st Terrace, Gainesville, FL 32605, (904) 378-0401, BA 69 OH St Univ; MA 74 Case Western Reserve Univ; **SLP**

Davidson, Mrs Lisa Surber 10617 Lochess Court, St Louis, MO 63141, (314) 991-2471, MS 87 Washington Univ; **A**

Davidson, Lloyd E 1232 West, Emporia, KS 66801, (316) 343-3218, BA 57 Fort Hays St Univ; MS 63 Fort Hays St Univ; Sp-Lang Path, USD #253, **SLP**

Davidson, Mrs Margaret 10312 76th Street, Edmonton, AB, Canada T6A 3A7, (403) 477-6784, BS 69 KS St Univ; MA 71 KS St Univ; Sp/Lang Path, Edmonton Publ Sch Bd, **SLP**

Davidson, Marjorie E 127 West 86th Street #8, New York, NY 10024, (212) 722-0610, BA 73 Hofstra Univ; MA 75 Long Island U - CW Post Ctr; Sp-Lang Path, The Churchill School, **SLP**

Davidson, Roseanna C 5221 28th Street, Lubbock, TX 79407, MS

Davidson, Salley Barton 35 Legare Street, Charleston, SC 29401, MA 76; **SLP A**

Davidson, Sandra Bushey 2015 North 56th Street, Omaha, NE 68104, (402) 553-4375, BS 81 Univ of NE Lincoln; MS 85 Univ of NE - Lincoln; Sp-Lang Path, Millard Ps, **SLP**

Davidson, Sharee Graddy P O Box 1028, Greenwood, AR 72936, (501) 996-4249, BS 78 Univ of AR - Little Rock; MS 85 Univ of Central AR; SLP, Greenwood Public Schools, **SLP**

Davidson, Stephanie Ann 1691 Rome Corners Road, Galena, OH 43021, (614) 292-8207, BA 80 MI St Univ; MA 82 OH St Univ; PH 85 (Aud) OH St Univ; 88–Asst Prof, The Ohio State Univ, **A**

Davidson, Thomas Oferrell P O Box 13799, Tallahassee, FL 32317, (800) 526-3921, BS 64 Univ of TN - Knoxville; MA 65 Univ of TN - Knoxville; Terr Mark Man, Oticon Corp, **A**

Davie, Mrs Cynthia C S 603 Glenview, Carbondale, IL 62901, (618) 549-6811, BS 78 Southeast MO St Univ; MS 81 Southern IL Univ -Carbondale; Sp-Lang Path/Prog Coord, Cen for Comp Ser, **SLP**

Davied, Leah Anne 1994 Rule, Maryland Heights, MO 63043, (314) 581-3065, MA 85 Wichita St Univ; SLP, State of Missouri, **SLP**

Davies, Cheryl Delight 3504 Myrtle Street, Evans, CO 80620, (303) 352-1543, BA 82 Univ of Northern CO; MA 85 Univ of Northern CO; 86–Sp-Lang Path, Weld Dist #6-Greeley, **SLP**

Davies, Darlene Gould 2265 Pine Street, San Diego, CA 92103, BA 62 San Diego St Univ; MA 65 San Diego St Univ; ES 85 Point Loma Nazarene Coll; 76–Asst Prof, San Diego State Univ, **SLP**

Davies, Jacquelyn R D 1839 Cavell, Highland Park, IL 60035, (312) 725-1572, BS 74 Northern IL Univ - De Kalb; MA 75 Northern IL Univ - De Kalb; OM 82 Univ of IL - Chicago; Sp/Lang Path, Chicago Bd of Ed, **SLP**

Davies, Janet Barbara 15052 Inbrook, Plymouth, MI 48170, (313) 981-6644, BA 83 MI St Univ; MA 85 Wayne St Univ; 85–Sp-Lang Path, Catherine McAuley Health Ctr, **SLP**

Davies, Dr Jeffrey W Tripler Army Medical Center, Box 744, Audiology & Speech, Honolulu, HI 96859, (808) 433-5334, BA 71 Harding Univ; MA 76 Univ of Cincinnati; PH 77 (NS) Univ of Cincinnati; Aud, Tripler Army Med Ctr, **A ACE**

Davies, Jenny Frances 815 Hickory Street, Martins Ferry, OH 43935, (813) 321-2627, BS 84 Kent St Univ; **A**

Davies, Judy E 53 Oakville Street, Staten Island, NY 10314, (718) 494-1106, BA 74 CUNY - Brooklyn Coll; MS 76 CUNY - Brooklyn Coll; 86–Sp-Lang Path, Staten Island Aid Inc, **SLP**

Davies, Laurel James 2100 South 29th Street, Apartment 304, Grand Forks, ND 58201, (704) 780-2447, BA 85 San Jose St Univ; MA 87 San Jose St Univ; 87–Aud, Univ of North Dakota, **A**

Davies, Lorene Catherine 32-230 West 14th Street, North Vancouver, BC, Canada V7M 1P3, (403) 229-7060, **SLP**

Davis, Mrs Abbe Denise 2145 South 50th, Lincoln, NE 68506, (402) 483-4953, MS 87 Univ of NE - Lincoln

Davis, Albert L 2216 West Magnolia, Fort Worth, TX 76110, **A**

Davis, Alice-Jean 1101 East Ventura Blvd, Space 149, Oxnard, CA 93030, MA 60 Columbia Univ Teachers Coll; MS 57 Univ of WI - Madison; Tchr, Simi Valley USD, **SLP A**

Davis, Alicia M P O Box 784, Wheatland, WY 82201, (307) 322-5480, BA 81 Univ of Northern CO; MS 83 CO St Univ; 88–Sp/Lang Path, Platte Co Sch Dist R-1, **SLP ACE**

Davis, Alvin J Constance Brown Hrng & Sp Ctr, 1521 Gull Road, Kalamazoo, MI 49001, (616) 343-2601, BS 56 Bloomsburg Univ of PA; MS 58 PA St Univ - Univ Park; Director, Constance Brown Hrng & Sp Ctr, **SLP A**

Davis, Mrs Amy Paul 141 Leisure Lane, Pine Mountain, GA 31822, (404) 663-2599, BA 79 Univ of GA; ME 86 Columbus Coll; 88–Sp-Lang Path, Private Practice, **SLP**

Davis, Mrs Anita C Reading Road #4-H, Edison, NJ 08817, (201) 544-9394, MS 84 James Madison Univ; Sp-Lang Path, Rks Assoc, **SLP**

Davis, Mrs Ann M 5612 Brookview Avenue, Edina, MN 55424, (612) 927-4986, BS 65 Univ of WI - Madison; MA 67 Univ of MN - Minneap-St Paul; 67–Sp-Lang Path, Minneapolis Pub Sch Spec Ed, **SLP**

Davis, Ann M 11647 Avenida Sivrita, San Diego, CA 92128-3383, BA 73 Univ of RI; MS 77 Univ of RI; Sp-Lang-Hrng Spec, San Diego City Sch, **SLP**

Davis, Mrs Ann W 6769 Lancaster Pike, Hockessin, DE 19707, (302) 454-2142, BA 68 Elmira Coll; MS 70 Syracuse Univ; Sp-Lang Path, Christina School District, **SLP ACE**

Davis, Anne Varner 460 West 57th Street #5S, New York, NY 10019-3051, (203) 334-2118, **SLP**

Davis, Barbara J 565 Captain Dement Drive, Waldorf, MD 20601, (301) 753-6220, BA 78 Univ of MD - College Park; MA 80 Univ of MD - College Park; Sp-Lang Path, Charles Co Bd of Ed, **SLP**

Davis, Barbara L 101 West 33rd Street, Austin, TX 78705, (512) 471-3841, BA 68 Univ of TX - Austin; MS 70 Univ of TX - Austin; PH 86 (Sp Path) Univ of TX - Austin; 87–Sp-Lang Path, Private Practice, **SLP**

Davis, Beth A 1015 Washington Avenue #C, New Orleans, LA 70130, (504) 363-2271, BA 76 Wake Forest Univ; MA 79 OH Univ - Athens; OM 83 Baylor Univ; Supervisor, F Edward Hebert Hospital Nme, **SLP ACE**

Davis, Mrs Betty J 5865 North Mina Vista, Tucson, AZ 85718, (602) 742-8086, BA 67 SUNY - Center at Albany; MA 68 Columbia Univ Teachers Coll; Head Dept Speech & Hearing, Amphitheater Public Schools, **A**

Davis, Carol Ann 13511 Westwood Lane, Omaha, NE 68144, (402) 333-6684, BA 81 Univ of NE - Lincoln; MS 82 Univ of NE - Lincoln; Sp Lang/Path, Omaha Pub Sch, **SLP**

Davis, Carol Williams 16603 21st Avenue S W, Seattle, WA 98166, (206) 848-6661, MS 87 Univ of WA; 87–Sp-Lang Path, Good Samaritan Hosp, **SLP**

Davis, Carole A 21 Ground Pine Court, Dix Hills, NY 11746, (516) 673-7094, BA 68 Long Island U - Brooklyn Ctr; MS 72 CUNY - Brooklyn Coll; OD 84 (Educational Admin) Hofstra Univ; 88–Sp-Lang Path, Half Hollow Hills Cen Sch Dist, **SLP**

Davis, Mrs Catherine C 718 Murph Road, Pauline, SC 29374, (803) 833-2733, BS 80 Univ of VA - Charlottesville; ME 82 James Madison Univ; 86–Aud, S C Dept of Mental Retardation, **A**

Davis, Catherine D 100 W Berkshire Lane, Mount Prospect, IL 60056, (312) 392-2474, BA 79 MI St Univ; MA 85 MI St Univ; 87–Sp-Lang Path, Marianjoy Rehab Ctr, **SLP**

Davis, Cathy Ann 9504 Ravenel Lane, Knoxville, TN 37922, (615) 693-5939, BA 82 Univ of TN - Knoxville; MA 83 Univ of TN - Knoxville; **A**

Davis, Charlotte A 6211 Cobblers Drive, East Lansing, MI 48823, (517) 337-2353, BS 64 Eastern MI Univ; MA 72 MI St Univ; SLP, Lansing School District, **SLP**

Davis, Christine 1205 Old Barn Lane, Mesquite, TX 75149, (214) 391-2143, OB 76 Sam Houston St Univ; MS 78 Univ of North TX; Sp-Lang Path, Dallas ISD, **SLP**

Davis, Christine Herrick 4100 Folsom Boulevard #2-C, Sacramento, CA 95819, (916) 457-3624, BA 78 CA St Univ - Chico; MA 79 CA St Univ - Chico; 88–Chief: Sp-Lang Path, Univ of Davis Med Ctr, **SLP**

Davis, Connee S 414 Bay Road, Menlo Park, CA 94025, (415) 365-1550, BA 60 Univ of the Pacific; MA 63 Tulane Univ; MS 79 Univ of KY; Sp-Lang Path, Redwood Cty Sch Dist, **SLP**

Davis, Connie L 1610 Shands Drive, Tupelo, MS 38801, (601) 842-1891, BA 73 Univ of MS; OM 75 Univ of MS; Dir Commun Dis Dept, Regl Rehabn Cen Inc, **SLP**

Davis, Corieta J Route 3 Box 603-A, Hazard, KY 41701, (606) 439-1331, BS 82 LA St Univ - Baton Rouge; MA 85 LA St Univ - Baton Rouge; Sp-Lang Path, Appalachian Reg Hosp, **SLP**

Davis, Deanna Sue P 800 North Lindbergh Blvd, Apartment Mz 5295, St Louis, MO 63167, **SLP**

Davis, Deborah 11794 Northeast, 72nd Street, Bondurant, IA 50035, (515) 270-9030, BS 72 Mankato St Univ; MA 74 Mankato St Univ; 76–Sp-Lang Path, Heartland AEA #11, **SLP**

Davis, Deborah 4778 Jack Tone Road, Stockton, CA 95205, (209) 931-1516, BA 74 Southern CT St Univ; MA 76 Univ of the Pacific; Tchr-Severe Oral Lang Hndcpd, Lodi USD, **SLP**

Davis, Deborah J 213 Meadowbrook Lane, Hinsdale, IL 60521-5085, **SLP**

Davis, Debra Marie 630 Smithfield Road Apartment 413, North Providence, RI 02904, (401) 725-5798, MA 87 Univ of CT; Sp-Lang Path, Hrng Sp & L Services, **SLP**

Davis, Debra Moon 6479 Sunset Terrace, Des Moines, IA 50311, (515) 277-8756, BA 74 Univ of IA; MA 75 Univ of IA; **A**

Davis, Deidre Marie 87 Rutland Road, Brooklyn, NY 11225, (212) 284-6821, MS 84 Columbia Univ Teachers Coll; Sp-Lang Path, New York State, **SLP**

Davis, Mrs Delores F 7815 Hayfield Road, Alexandria, VA 22310, MA 66 Northern IL Univ - De Kalb; SLP, Fairfax County Public Schools, **SLP**

Davis, DeMaris A 1211 McGee, Kansas City, MO 64106, (816) 374-0410, BA 64 William Jewell Coll; MA 65 Univ of KS; Coord Early Childhood Dev, Sch Dist Ks Cty, **SLP**

Davis, Denise Homes 6512 Hollins Way, Centerville, OH 45459, (513) 376-3314, BS 79 Bowling Green St Univ; MA 80 Bowling Green St Univ; 82–Sp/Lang Path, Greene Co Bd Ed, **SLP**

Davis, Diane A 2401 Stanford Road #805, Panama City, FL 32405, (904) 785-9991, **SLP**

Davis, Diane Dorothy 3012 59th Street Court W, Bradenton, FL 34209, (813) 792-6611, BS 84 AZ St Univ; OM 86 AZ St Univ; **SLP**

Davis, Mrs Diane Marsh 28 Kool Place, Port Jefferson Station, NY 11776, (516) 473-2800, BS 83 WV Univ; MA 84 Univ of TN - Knoxville; Aud, St Charles Hospital, **A**

Davis, Dr Diane Vennessa 16 Elm Court, Calumet City, IL 60409, (312) 841-3952, BS 76 Northwestern Univ; MS 79 Governors St Univ; ED 85 (NS) G Peabody Coll-Vanderbilt U; 86–Sp-Lang Path, Chicago PS, **SLP**

Davis, Dianne Lynn 116 Brookwood Avenue, Santa Rosa, CA 95404, (707) 544-9146, MA 82 CA St Univ - Chico; Sp-Lang Path, Private Practice, **SLP**

Davis, Mrs Dianne S 72 Hiwon, Conroe, TX 77301, (409) 856-5637, BA 74 Wichita St Univ; MA 76 Wichita St Univ; **SLP**

Davis, Dr Donald C 3450 24th Street, Rock Island, IL 61201, (309) 788-6890, BA 47 Augustana Coll; MA 49 Northwestern Univ; PH 51 (NS) Northwestern Univ; Retired, Augustana Coll, **SLP F LM**

Davis, Doreen P O Box 39, Balboa Island, CA 92662, (213) 825-3691, BA 71 CA St Univ - Northridge; MA 74 CA St Univ - Northridge; **SLP**

Davis, Mrs Dorinne S 4 Musconetcong Avenue, Stanhope, NJ 07874, (201) 838-9383, BA 71 Montclair St Coll; MA 73 Montclair St Coll; Aud, Kinnelon Bd of Ed, **A**

Davis, Edward T 175 Verde Mesa Drive, Danville, CA 94526, **SLP**

Davis, Ellen E 1100 Skyland Drive, 0-5 Riverhill Condos, Columbia, SC 29210, (803) 737-7508, BS 69 OH Univ - Athens; MA 70 OH Univ - Athens; Admin Health Prog, Dept Ment Ret Midlands Reg Cen, **SLP**

Davis, Mrs Emily H 2906 Sunbird Drive, Fairfield, CA 94533, (707) 425-8451, BA 58 Allegheny Coll; MA 69 San Jose St Univ; Dir of Serv, Fairfield-Suisun USD, **SLP**

Davis, Emily H 1380 Monterey Boulevard N E, St Petersburg, FL 33704, (813) 746-5111, BA 72 Maryville Coll; MS 77 Univ of South FL; Dir-Sp Svcs, Manatee Memorial Hosp, **SLP**

Davis, Mrs F Teresa Runzo 165 Joseph Drive, Tonawanda, NY 14150, (716) 691-6992, BS 74 SUNY - Coll at Buffalo; MS 75 SUNY - Coll at Buffalo; SLP, Sweet Home School District, **SLP**

Davis, Dr G Albyn Dept Communication Disorders, Univ Of Massachusetts, Arnold House, Amherst, MA 01003, (413) 545-0131, BA 68 Stanford Univ; PH 72 (NS) OH Univ - Athens; Assoc Prof, U of MA, **SLP**

Davis, Gehl M 128 Glen Summer Road, Pasadena, CA 91105, **SLP**

Davis, Dr George D Dept Communicative Disorders, The University Of Akron, Akron, OH 44325, (216) 375-6119, BS 49 Kent St Univ; MA 59 OH St Univ; PH 68 (NS) OH St Univ; Hd-Dept Commun Dis, U of Akron, **SLP A**

Davis, Helen Handley Route 8 Box 117, Granbury, TX 76048, (817) 573-3684, BS 62 Abilene Christian Univ; MS 82 TX Christian Univ; SLP, Granbury Speech Lang Serv, **SLP**

Davis, Helen S 61 Madison Avenue, New Providence, NJ 07974, (201) 558-3001, **SLP**

Davis, Mrs Ivey Jean 404 S Mlk Drive, Thomasville, GA 31792, BS 82 Univ of GA; ME 83 Univ of GA; 88–Sp-Lang Path, Thomasville City Bd of Educ, **SLP**

Davis, Jacqueline Bryant 1105 St Joseph Street #19, Dallas, TX 75204, (214) 824-1620, BA 85 Marshall Univ; MA 86 Marshall Univ; **SLP**

Davis, Jacqueline Denise 201 9th Street, Vienna, GA 31092, (912) 268-4761, BS 83 AL A & M Univ; ME 87 Valdosta St Coll

Davis, Jacquelyn Irene 501 Contentnea Street, Greenville, NC 27834, (919) 731-3520, MS 86 Univ of NC - Chapel Hill; **SLP**

Davis, Dr James Dept Communication Disorders, Northern Michigan Univ, Marquette, MI 49855, (906) 227-2125, BA 66 San Jose St Univ; OM 70 Univ of WA; PH 74 (NS) Univ of Cincinnati; Prof/Head, Nn MI U, **A**

Davis, Mrs Jane B P O Box 28, Spirit Lake, IA 51360, (712) 336-4494, MA 69 Univ of South FL; Sp-Lang Path, Private Practice, **SLP ACE**

Davis, Janet B 5644 Ravenspur Drive #301, Rancho Palos Verdes, CA 90274, (213) 832-3311, Sp-Lang Path, San Pedro Pensula Hosp, **SLP**

Davis, Mrs Janet Van Orsdel 6730 Muirfield Court S E, Grand Rapids, MI 49506, (616) 676-1738, BA 64 Kent St Univ; MA 65 Univ of MI - Ann Arbor; **SLP**

Davis, Janice A 2905 Sheffield Lane, Modesto, CA 95350, BA 74 CA St Univ - Stanislaus; MA 76 CA St Univ - Stanislaus; Sp-Lang Path, Modesto Cty Schs, **SLP**

Davis, Janice M 133 Linseed Road, West Hatfield, MA 01088, (413) 247-5866, BA 80 Univ of RI; MA 85 Univ of MD - College Park; Sp-Lang Path, Private Practice, **SLP**

Davis, Jay P Park Central Institute, 6125 Clayton Avenue #430, St Louis, MO 63139, (314) 768-3222, BA 68 Univ of Toledo; MA 72 Univ of FL; 87–Dir-Aud, Park Central Institute, **A**

Davis, Mrs Jeanine K 143 Green Acres Estates, Hurricane, WV 25526, (304) 757-8908, BA 75 Marshall Univ; MA 76 Marshall Univ; Sp-Lang Path, **SLP**

Davis, Jill S P O Box 1059, Rutherfordton, NC 28139-1059, (704) 286-2781, BS 78 Univ of GA; MA 80 Univ of TN - Knoxville; 86–Sp-Lang Path, Shelby City Schs, **SLP**

Davis, Mrs Joan Marie 2909 Woodbridge Creek Drive, St Louis, MO 63109, (314) 454-7759, BS 84 Saint Louis Univ; MA 85 Saint Louis Univ; 88–Sp-Lang Path, St Mary's Rehab Inst, **SLP**

Davis, Johnetta G 519 Brummel Court N W, Washington, DC 20012, (202) 636-7469, BS 61 Univ of the DC; MA 69 George Washington Univ; PH 76 (NS) Howard Univ; Assoc Dean / Grad Prof, Howard U, **SLP**

Davis, Mrs Judith J 15770 Queensferry Drive, Fort Myers, FL 33912, (813) 768-3867, BS 64 Saint Louis Univ; MA 65 Saint Louis Univ; Sp-Lang Path, Lee Co Schl Brd, **SLP**

Davis, Dr Julia M 3325 Cheviot Drive, Tampa, FL 33618, (813) 974-2503, BA 51 Northwestern St Univ; MS 65 Univ Southern MS-Hattiesburg; PH 66 (NS) Univ Southern MS-Hattiesburg; 87–Prof & Dean, Univ of South Florida, **A F**

Davis, Mrs Karen Moreno 13311 South Chester Road, Chester, VA 23831, (804) 732-8000, BS 76 Longwood Coll; MS 78 James Madison Univ; Sp/Lang Path, Chesapeake Pub Sch, **SLP**

Davis, Karen Sue 10513 Steve Court, Fredericksburg, VA 22401, (703) 373-7458, BS 80 James Madison Univ; MS 82 James Madison Univ; Sp-Lang Path, Stafford Co PS, **SLP**

Davis, Mrs Karla Frost 211 East 35 Street, Apartment 7-C, New York, NY 10016, (212) 689-8808, BS 86 Northwestern Univ; MA 87 Northwestern Univ; 87–Sp-Lang Path, UCP of NYC Inc, **SLP**

Davis, Karlyn H 7860 Skyline Drive, San Diego, CA 92114, (619) 267-1973, BS 74 Columbia Union Coll; MS 75 Univ of MA - Amherst; 88–Sp-Lang Path, Southwood Psyciatric Ctrs, **SLP**

Davis, Mrs Kathleen Duffy Good Samaritan Medical Center, Speech Pathology Dept, 1111 East McDowell Road, Phoenix, AZ 85062, (602) 239-4755, BA 76 Univ of Southern CA; MS 81 AZ St Univ; Sp-Lang Path, Good Samaritan Medical Center, **SLP ACE**

Davis, Kathleen V 53 Robinwood Avenue, Jamaica Plain, MA 02130, (617) 522-7333, MA 78 Kent St Univ; 88–Prog Coord, Anne Sullivan Ctr, **SLP**

Davis, Mrs Kay D 4157 Beaune Drive, Kenner, LA 70065, (504) 482-3901, BA 73 LA St Univ - Baton Rouge; MA 75 OK St Univ; Sp-Lang Path, Private Practice, **SLP ACE**

Davis, Kelley Marie 4006 Saint Andrews Circle 2C, Mishawaka, IN 46545, (219) 294-2621, BS 85 Central MI Univ; MA 86 Central MI Univ; 88–Sp-Lang Path, Elkhart General Hosp, **SLP**

Davis, Kelly J 1038 North Calvert Street, Apartment 1, Baltimore, MD 21202-3833, (301) 576-9514, BA 85 Loyola Coll; MS 87 Loyola Coll; 87–Sp-Lang Path, Sinai Hosp, **SLP**

Davis, Kelly Jo 8895 Monument Drive, Grants Pass, OR 97526, (503) 479-0088, BS 83 Portland St Univ; Sp-Lang Path, Grants Pass Dstr 7

Davis, Mrs Khris Mumby 711 East Colfax, South Bend, IN 46617, (219) 234-3136, BS 80 Ball St Univ; MA 83 Saint Louis Univ; Sp-Lang Path, Hearing and Speech Center, **SLP**

Davis, Kimberly M 6201 Harwin Lane, Austin, TX 78745, (512) 444-9561, BA 82 Univ of Southwestern LA; ME 85 Southwest TX St Univ; 88–Sp-Lang Path, The Oaks Treatment Ctr, **SLP**

Davis, Laura S 601 Mountain View Drive, Bozeman, MT 59715, (406) 587-8257, BS 73 Minot St Univ; MS 74 Minot St Univ; Aud, Private Practice, **A**

Davis, Lauren A 1091-B Bridgeway Circle, Columbus, OH 43220, (614) 276-8231, BA 85 Cleveland St Univ; MA 87 Cleveland St Univ; 88–Sp-Lang Path, Franklin Co Bd of Mental Retard & Dev Disa, **SLP**

Davis, Leslie Faye 41 Lafayette Place, Woodmere, NY 11598, (516) 374-4992, BS 68 SUNY - Coll at Fredonia; MS 70 SUNY - Coll at Fredonia; 80–Dir, Leslie Faye Davis Consult Inc, **SLP**

Davis, Mrs Linda Prince 202 Mill Crossing, Hampton, VA 23666, (804) 766-1075, BS 69; MS 76; **SLP**

Davis, Mrs Linda W 2214 West 21st Avenue, Emporia, KS 66801, (316) 343-2302, BA 69 Univ of Northern IA; MA 70 Univ of Northern IA; 81–Sp-Lang Path, Flint Hills Spec Educ Coop, **SLP**

Davis, Lisa Ann 1628 West 9th Street, Pomona, CA 91766, (714) 622-0186, BS 82 Loma Linda Univ - Riverside; MS Loma Linda Univ - Riverside; **SLP**

Davis, Lisa D P O Box 39, Coldwater, MS 38618, (214) 255-6862, MS 88 Univ of TX - Dallas

Davis, Lisa E 401 3rd #207, Des Moines, IA 50309, (515) 283-2609, **SLP A**

Davis, Lois-Anne W 139 Stillwater Circle, Jupiter, FL 33458, (407) 744-1570, BS 78 FL St Univ; MA 81 Univ of FL; 86–Sp-Lang Path, Private Practice, **SLP**

Davis, Mrs Lynn A 8886 Meadow Drive, Mason, OH 45040, (513) 677-0817, BA 78 MI St Univ; MA 79 MI St Univ; 84–Sp-Lang Path, Lakota Local Schs, **SLP**

Davis, Lynn C 7233 Mallard Drive, West Chester, OH 45069, BS 74 SUNY - Coll at Geneseo; MS 77 Coll of Saint Rose; **SLP**

Davis, Lynne A 5945 Meadowsglen Drive, Dublin, OH 43017-1846, (614) 292-6251, BS 78 PA St Univ - Univ Park; MA 80 Univ of IA; 81–Coord of Aud, Ohio St U, **A**

Davis, Mrs Lynne D Box 236, Milan, IN 47031, (812) 689-4001, BA 70 Morehead St Univ; MS 73 IN St Univ - Terre Haute; Sp-Lang Path/Spec Ed, Jac-Cen-Del Comm Sch, **SLP**

Davis, M Sue 105 Pilgrim's Point Road, Greenville, SC 29615, BS 71 Univ Southern MS-Hattiesburg; MS 72 Univ Southern MS-Hattiesburg; **SLP**

Davis, Margaret Alsworth 200 Jerry Street, Lafayette, LA 70503, BS 76 Univ Southern MS-Hattiesburg; MS 77 Univ Southern MS-Hattiesburg; Sp-Lang Path, Vermilion Parish Sch Bd, **SLP**

Davis, Mrs Margaret B 1716 Delaney Street, Virginia Beach, VA 23464, (804) 623-8072, BA 52 Shaw Univ; MA 57 Case Western Reserve Univ; Asst Prof / Sp Commun, Norfolk State U, **SLP**

Davis, Mrs Margaret W 870 Park Avenue #101, Capitola, CA 95010, (408) 462-1808, BA 31 Univ of CA - Santa Barbara; **A LM**

Davis, Mrs Marie Talarico 7050 Harbour Village Court, Apartment T1, Annapolis, MD 21403, (301) 280-2068, BA 84 Temple Univ; MA 85 George Washington Univ; 87–Sp-Lang Path, Fairfax Hosp Sys, **SLP**

Davis, Mrs Marie W P O Box 57, Conesus, NY 14435, (716) 243-5480, MA 75 SUNY - Coll at Geneseo; SLP, Craig Ddso, **SLP**

Davis, Marilyn J 822 Simmons, Kirkwood, MO 63122, (314) 569-8100, BA 69 Northeastern OK St Univ; MA 71 Saint Louis Univ; Diagn Chprs, St Louis Co Spec Sch Dist, **SLP**

Davis, Mrs Marjorie Lee 107 Windblown Court, Baltimore, MD 21209, (301) 356-0762, BS 69 Towson St Univ; MS 74 Loyola Coll; Sp/Lang Path, Baltimore Co Publ Schs, **SLP**

Davis, Marjorie Renee 10901 Meadowglen Lane, Apartment 80, Houston, TX 77042, (713) 795-4411, MS 84 Univ of MS; Audiologist, Houston VA Hospital, **A**

Davis, Mrs Mary Kay 16 Greenbriar, New Madrid, MO 63869, (314) 688-2161, BS 72 Univ of MS; MA 73 Univ of MO - Columbia; Special Programs Staff, New Madrid Co R-1 Enlarged, **SLP**

Davis, Mary Lynn 3219 Park St N, St Petersburg, FL 33710, (904) 344-9611, MS 84 Univ of South FL; **SLP**

Davis, Melinda M 808 South Lawrence Street, Montgomery, AL 36104, (205) 834-2002, BS 77 Univ of AL- Tuscaloosa; MS 81 Univ of AL- Tuscaloosa; Aud, Auburn U Mont, **A**

Davis, Dr Michael J Dept Of Speech Communication, California State University-Fullerton, Fullerton, CA 92634, (714) 773-3617, BS 74 UT St Univ; MS 76 UT St Univ; PH 79 (NS) Wayne St Univ - Sch of Med; Assoc Prof, CA St U-Fullerton, **A**

Davis, Michelle 770 Schenectady Avenue, Brooklyn, NY 11203, (718) 735-6251, BA 82 CUNY - Brooklyn Coll; MS 84 Columbia Univ Teachers Coll; 83–Sp-Lang Path, NYC Bd of Educ-Clin Svcs Unit, **SLP**

Davis, Nancy L 13016 N E 87th, Kirkland, WA 98033, (206) 822-9588, BA 70 Univ of WA; MS 75 Western OR St Coll; SLP, Lake Washington School Dist, **SLP**

Davis, Mrs Naomi W 3214 Nerak Road, Baltimore, MD 21208, (301) 486-2540, BA 78 Univ of MD - College Park; MS 80 Univ of Louisville; Sp-Lang Path, Annandale Fluency Cl, **SLP**

Davis, Mrs Pamela K 15922 Wyndover Road, Tampa, FL 33647, (813) 977-9844, BA 79 Univ of South FL; MS 82 Univ of South FL; **SLP**

Davis, Mrs Patricia A 62 Stoneywood Drive, Niantic, CT 06357, (203) 739-6754, BS 79 IL St Univ - Normal; MS 80 IL St Univ - Normal; 88–Sp/Lang Path, Project Learn, **SLP**

Davis, Patricia Jane 15 Gray Avenue, Apartment 302, Toronto, ON, Canada M6N 4S5, (416) 243-4128, BS 83 Univ of Western Ontario; MA 84 MI St Univ; **A**

Davis, Mrs Patricia R 10135 S W 135th, Beaverton, OR 97005, (503) 645-4242, BS 82 Portland St Univ; MS 84 Portland St Univ; Sp-Lang Path, Washington County Esd, **SLP**

Davis, Mrs Phyllis K 228 Farnham Road, Havertown, PA 19083, (215) 789-4306, BA 71 Cornell Univ; ME 74 Temple Univ; MA 88 Temple Univ; 88–Sp-Lang Path, Delaware Co Intermediate Unit

Davis, Polly Welty 16250 North County Rd #25E, Loveland, CO 80537, (303) 226-2345, BA 64 Marshall Univ; MA 72 Univ of ND; 78–Dir of Therapies, Foothills Gateway Rehab Center Inc, **SLP**

Davis, Mrs Pota J 399 North Broadway #3GW, Yonkers, NY 10701, (914) 423-7079, MA 86; Sp-Lang Path, Pocantico Hills Board of Educ, **SLP**

Davis, Mrs Rebecca A 2912 Longfellow, Denton, TX 76201, (817) 566-5353, BS 76 Howard Payne Univ; MS 77 Univ of North TX; 88–Grad Supvr, Univ of North Texas, **A**

Davis, Rebecca M Springer Clinic, 6160 South Yale, Tulsa, OK 74136, (918) 492-7200, BS 76 Univ of OK - Norman; MS 78 Univ of OK Medical Center; Audiologist, Springer Clinic, **A**

Davis, Regina Lloyd 5545 Hill Avenue, Toledo, OH 43615, (419) 537-9143, BA 79 MI St Univ; MA 80 MI St Univ; Sp-Lang Path, Lucas Co Bd of Ment Ret, **SLP**

Davis, Regina Lynne 1909 Prospect Road, Lawrenceville, GA 30245, (404) 321-6111, BS 84 Univ of GA; ME 85 Univ of GA; **A**

Davis, Robert W Midwest Rehabilitation Center, 20 East Gregory, Kansas City, MO 64114, (816) 363-1411, BA 44 Wichita St Univ; MA 55 Wichita St Univ; **SLP**

Davis, Dr Robin L Eaton Peabody Laboratory, Massachusetts Eye & Ear Infirmary, 243 Charles Street, Boston, MA 02114, (617) 573-3156, BS 73 PA St Univ - Univ Park; MA 78 Univ of San Diego; PH 87 (Neurobiology) Stanford Univ; 87–Researcher, MA Eye & Ear Inf, **A**

Davis, Mrs Ronda L 5535 South Danube Way, Aurora, CO 80015, (303) 693-1635, BA 70 Univ of Northern CO; MA 71 Our Lady Lake Univ-San Anton; Sp-Lang Path, Cherry Creek HS-CCSD #5, **SLP**

Davis, Rose Marie 29951 Happy Sparrow Lane, Laguna Niguel, CA 92677, **SLP**

Davis, Mrs Rosemary B 929 Remington Road, Wynnewood, PA 19096, (513) 221-0527, BA 69 Catholic Univ of America; MS 72 Gallaudet Coll; Coor of Aud Serv, Clnci Sp-Hrng Cen, **A**

Davis, Russell E 201 Range Street, Manistique, MI 49854-1560, BA 64 Moorhead St Univ; MS 65 Vanderbilt Univ; Assoc Prof, Northern MI U, **SLP**

Davis, Ruth Norene 5850 Beltline Road, Apt #1005, Dallas, TX 75240-7780, (214) 960-2318, BS 79 Univ of TX - Austin; ME 82 Southwest TX St Univ; 87–Sp-Lang Path, InSpeech Inc, **SLP**

Davis, Mrs Sharon 5727 Winslow Court, Ypsilanti, MI 48197, (313) 484-0688, BA 73 Univ of MI - Ann Arbor; MS 75 Univ of MI - Ann Arbor; Sp-Lang Path, St Joseph Mercy Hosp, **SLP**

Davis, Sharon M 1402 Bancroft Way, Berkeley, CA 94702, (415) 644-3632, BA 73 Whittier Coll; MA 78 San Diego St Univ; Sp-Lang Path, Private Practice, **SLP ACE**

Davis, Sharon W 702 Thorpe Drive, Louisville, KY 40243, **SLP**

Davis, Sheila Lane 114 Auburn Street, Cranston, RI 02910, (401) 434-3400, BS 81 Radford Univ; MS 83 Southern IL Univ -Carbondale; Sp-Lang Path, Emma Pendleton Bradley Hosp, **SLP**

Davis, Sherri Allred 321 West Wendover Avenue, Greensboro, NC 27408, (919) 379-9445, ME 86 Univ of NC - Greensboro; 86–Aud, Greensboro Head & Neck Surg Assoc, **A**

Davis, Sherry Renee 6079 Youngstown Conneaut R, Kinsman, OH 44428-9751, (216) 772-3809, BS 85 Kent St Univ; MA 85 Kent St Univ; **SLP**

Davis, Mrs Shirley C 1476 Alta Vista Court, Seaside, CA 93955, (408) 646-6545, BS 75 Southwest TX St Univ; ME 78 Southwest TX St Univ; Sp-Lang Path, Pacific Grove USD, **SLP**

Davis, Shirley J 3301 Westminister Drive, Pearland, TX 77581, (713) 485-3203, BS 64 Univ of Houston - Univ Park; MS 78 Univ of Houston - Univ Park; SLP, Pearland ISD, **SLP**

Davis, Sue E Anderson 5615 Mateo Drive, Fort Wayne, IN 46835, (219) 458-2244, BS 76 Ball St Univ; MA 77 Ball St Univ; Mgr Dept of Commun Dis, Lutheran Hosp, **SLP**

Davis, Susan Edge Tabby Lane Unit G-3, Bull River Shoals, Savannah, GA 31410, (912) 355-7313, ME 84 Armstrong St Coll; Sp-Lang Path, Private Practice, **SLP**

Davis, Susan Elaine 924 Lake Nora South Drive, Apartment B, Indianapolis, IN 46240, (317) 848-9392, BA 84 IN Univ - Bloomington; MA 86 IN Univ - Bloomington; **A**

Davis, Mrs Susan J Route 2 Box 461, Deer Park, WA 99006, (509) 455-6656, BA 69 WA St Univ; MA 70 WA St Univ; Sp-Lang Path, Sp-Lang & Lrng Cen, **SLP**

Davis, Dr Sylvia M Dept Communication Disorders, LSU Medical Center, 1900 Gravier Street, New Orleans, LA 70112, (504) 568-4348, BS 72 Lamar Univ; MS 73 Lamar Univ; PH 76 (NS) Wichita St Univ; Prof, LSU Med Cen, **SLP**

Davis, Teresa Martinelli 10549 Winding Way, Harrison, OH 45030, (513) 367-9122, BS 78 Miami Univ - Oxford; MS 79 Miami Univ - Oxford; SLP, Private Practice, **SLP**

Davis, Traci Karlene 4480 Banner Drive, Apt #4, Long Beach, CA 90807, (213) 426-9262, BA 85 Univ of CA - Santa Barbara; MA 87 Univ of CA - Santa Barbara; 87–Sp-Lang Path, Dr Bernard Landes and Assoc, **SLP**

Davis, Mrs Virginia L 49 Redfield Road, Island Park, NY 11558, (516) 889-2000, BA 64 WA St Univ; MA 66 Columbia Univ Teachers Coll; Tchr, Long Beach Pub Sch, **SLP**

Davis, William A 15 Hallowell Lane, Coram, NY 11727, (516) 520-5266, BA 74 Hofstra Univ; MA 76 Hofstra Univ; SLP, Levittown Sch Dist, **SLP**

Davis, Yondle Climer 2626 North Boulevard #8, Houston, TX 77098, (713) 523-4299, BS 64 Southwest TX St Univ; ME 75 TX Southern Univ; 78–Asst Dir Spec Ed, Pasadena ISD, **SLP**

Davis-Dansky, Mrs Ellen J 588 Harpeth Trace Drive, Nashville, TN 37221, (615) 320-5353, BA 74 Northwestern Univ; MA 75 Northwestern Univ; Sp-Lang Path, Bill Wilkerson Hrng & Sp Cen, **SLP**

Davis-Drake, Mrs Lisa J 9811 Cobblestone, Stockton, CA 95209, (209) 944-4953, BA 77 CA St Univ - Chico; MA 79 CA St Univ - Fresno; Sp-Lang-Hrng Spec, Stockton USD, **SLP**

Davis-Lary, Andrea S c/o Pee Dee Speech & Hrng Ctr, P O Box 1756, Myrtle Beach, SC 29577, (803) 448-2913, BA 77 Berry Coll; MS 80 Emory Univ; 88–Sp-Lang Path, Pee Dee Speech & Hrng Ctr, **SLP A**

Davison, Mrs Janet Clark 402 West Central, Missoula, MT 59801, (406) 721-6096, MS 73 Univ of OK Medical Center; Sp-Lang Path, Bitter Root Speech Center, **SLP**

Davison, Mrs Linda Lesnick Spring Park, St Clairsville, OH 43950, (304) 232-4352, BS 75 OH St Univ; MA 76 OH St Univ; Audiologist, M Merrick & Associates Inc, **A**

Davison, Louise D 3750 Peachtree Road N E, Apartment 410, Atlanta, GA 30319, BS; **SLP F LM**

Davison, Michelle M 1830 Grace Avenue #7, Hollywood, CA 90028, **SLP**

Davis-Pedrle, Mrs Denise 1260 Big Valley Drive, Colorado Springs, CO 80919, (719) 593-1301, BA 76 Univ of Northern CO; BA 76 Univ of Northern CO; MA 77 Univ of Northern CO; Early Intervention Specialist, Colorado Springs School Dist, **SLP**

Dawe, Mary J 26 Rice Avenue, Northboro, MA 01532, (508) 393-9889, BA 77 Univ of CT; MA 79 Northern IL Univ - De Kalb; Sp-Lang Path, Valley Child Develop Center, **SLP**

Dawes, Michele Lynn 3321 Carriage Lane, Plano, TX 75023, (214) 985-8933, BA 84 MI St Univ; MA 85 MI St Univ; **SLP**

Dawes, Patricia Jann 2895 Wilson Avenue, Redding, CA 96002, (209) 627-4855, BA 84 CA St Univ - Fresno; MA 87 CA St Univ - Fresno; **SLP**

Dawgert, Mrs Grace F 1006 Woodland Way, Clarks Summit, PA 18411, (717) 587-5437, BA 68 Marywood Coll; MA 69 Univ of IL - Urbana; Sp-Lang Path, Private Practice, **SLP**

Dawkins, Avis Wheeler P O Box 10001, Marina Del Rey, CA 90291, (213) 870-0466, BA 75 Winthrop Coll; MS 79 Univ of SC - Columbia; Sp-Lang Path, Private Practice, **SLP**

Dawkins, Patricia Harper 5232 Clairmont Avenue, Birmingham, AL 35222, (205) 595-1818, BS 84 Univ of Montevallo; MS 85 Univ of Montevallo

Dawn-Kosteva, Laura Ann 41105 Northwind Drive, Canton, MI 48188, (313) 593-7725, MS 84 Univ of MI - Ann Arbor; Sp-Lang Path, Oakwood Hosp, **SLP**

Dawsey, Ben W 410 East Henry Street, Spartanburg, SC 29302, (803) 583-7644, BS 70 East TN St Univ; MA 74 East TN St Univ; Aud, Aud Assoc of Spartanburg Pa, **A**

Dawsey-Brown, Mrs Deborah 4058 Shell Point Road, Beaufort, SC 29902, (803) 524-2065, BS 75 MS St Univ - MS State; MS 77 MS Univ for Women; Sp-Lang Path, Beaufort Co Pub Sch, **SLP**

Dawson, Clara Virginia 10391 S W 198th Street, Miami, FL 33157, (305) 253-3969, BA 85 Univ of TN - Knoxville; MS 86 TX Christian Univ; **SLP**

Dawson, Debby M Route 1 Box 450-16, Muskogee, OK 74401, (918) 456-5511, BS 80 Central MO St Univ; OM 81 Central MO St Univ; MS 85 Central MO St Univ; **SLP**

Dawson, Deborah Ann 1120 Longfellow Drive, Beaumont, TX 77708, (409) 898-7847, BS 76 Lamar Univ; MS 82 Lamar Univ; 88–Sp/Lang Path, Private Practice, **SLP**

Dawson, Gerald J 306 Seabreeze Court, League City, TX 77573, (713) 332-4575, BS 69 Saint Cloud St Univ; MS 73 Phillips Univ; Owner, Bay Area Aud & Hrng Aids, **A**

Dawson, Joanne H P O Box 2530, New Liskeard, ON, Canada P0J 1P0, (705) 647-4305, BS 68 Univ of GA; MS 72 Univ of GA; 87–Aud, Timiskaming Health Unit, **A**

Dawson, Kathryn E 37 Alberta Road, Chestnut Hill, MA 02167, (617) 552-3460, **SLP**

Dawson, Mary Ridgeway 35 Eisenhower Drive, East Quogue, NY 11942, (516) 728-9154, BA 67 IN Univ - Bloomington; MA 83 Hofstra Univ; 76–Sp-Lang Path, Hampton Bays Sch Dist, **SLP**

Dawson, Ronald E 6021 Midas, El Paso, TX 79924, **SLP**

Dawson, Sue A Blount Hrng & Speech Sci Inc, 404 Church Avenue, Suite 1, Maryville, TN 37801, (615) 982-8557, BA 69 Maryville Coll; ME 77 Univ of VA - Charlottesville; Sp/Lang Path, Blount Hrng & Sp Serv, **A**

Dawson, Mrs Susan H 2595 Quail Street, Lakewood, CO 80215, (303) 771-1353, BA 77 Univ of CO - Boulder; MA 79 Univ of CO - Boulder; Sp-Lang Path, Arapahoe Co Sch Dist 6, **SLP**

Dawson, Mrs Theresa Sheahen 29317 Lincoln Road, Bay Village, OH 44140, (216) 521-4200, BA 58 Marygove Coll; MA 60 Case Western Reserve Univ; Dir Sp-Lang Path, Lakewood Hosp, **SLP**

Dawson, Mrs Theresa T 1915 Morgan Lane #A, Redondo Beach, CA 90278, (213) 434-8421, BS 81 Univ of Cincinnati; MS 83 Vanderbilt Univ; 88–Prog Case Mgr, NeuroCare, **SLP**

Dawson, Dr Warren R 2148 North 115th Street, Seattle, WA 98133, BS 49 Univ of WA; MA 50 Univ of WA; PH 56 (NS) Stanford Univ; Aud/SLP, Mason Cl, **SLP A LM**

Dawson, Wendy R 9840 89th Avenue, Edmonton, AB, Canada T6E 2S4, (403) 471-2262, BS 77 Univ of Alberta - Alberta; MA 78 Univ of MN - Minneap-St Paul; Sp-Lang Path, Glenrose Hosp, **SLP**

Day, Mrs Antoinette Debner 3014 East Cortez Court, Irving, TX 75062-4606, (214) 255-2285, BS 79 Univ of North TX; MA 81 Our Lady Lake Univ-San Anton; **SLP**

Day, Beverly Elaine 411 West Third Avenue, Redfield, SD 57469, (605) 352-4109, BS 80 Edinboro Univ of PA; MA 84 Univ of SD - Vermillion; 87–Sp-Lang Path, Huron PS Dist, **SLP**

Day, Carol Sue 2096 West Halifax Drive, Daytona Beach, FL 32014, (904) 255-1034, **SLP**

Day, Charles E 3505 Valley Road #6, Bonita, CA 92002, (619) 470-2505, BA 79 Univ of Redlands; BA 79 Univ of Redlands; MS 81 Univ of Redlands; Dir, San Diego Scottish Rite I, **SLP**

Day, Dana Louise P O Box 4944, Scottsdale, AZ 85261, (602) 264-1008, BS 82 AZ St Univ; MS 85 CO St Univ; **A**

Day, David R 3908 Connecticut, St Louis, MO 63116, (314) 961-5757, BA 73 Depauw Univ; MS 78 Southern IL Univ-Edwardsvill; Sp-Lang Path, Spec Sch Dist of St Louis Co, **SLP**

Day, Janice Eisma 116 South Division Street, Northfield, MN 55057, (507) 663-7849, BA 79 Univ of Northern IA; MA 80 Univ of Northern IA; Sp-Lang Path, **SLP**

Day, Karen Loly 22655 Brookhaven, El Toro, CA 92630, (714) 458-7446, BA 82 CA St Univ - Long Beach; MA 84 CA St Univ - Long Beach; 85–Sp-Lang Path, Huntington Beach City Sch Dist, **SLP**

Day, Mrs Kim Martin 660 Liberty Street, Dansville, NY 14437, (716) 335-2464, BS 84 SUNY - Coll at Geneseo; MA 87 SUNY - Coll at Geneseo

Day, L Karen Carter 6203 Hatfield Circle, Amarillo, TX 79109, (806) 359-7681, MA 84; **SLP**

Day, Linda Susan 915 West Stewart Road, Columbia, MO 65203, (314) 882-8408, BS 71 Southwest MO St Univ; MA 74 Univ of MO - Columbia; MA 77 Univ of MO - Columbia; Clinic Director, U of MO Sp/Hrng Cl, **SLP**

Day, Margaret C Pecora 914 Jade Avenue, Lancaster, PA 17601, (717) 285-4275, BS 81 WV Univ; MS 81 WV Univ; 83–Sp-Lang Path, Private Practice, **SLP**

Day, Mrs Mary P 685 Cherry Road, Eland, WI 54427, (715) 346-3588, BA 77 Coll of Saint Teresa; MS 79 Univ of WI - Madison; 83–Supvr, University of Wisconsin, **SLP ACE**

Day, Mrs Marylou M 2407 Lyndhurst, Champaign, IL 61820, (217) 351-3884, BS 75 IL St Univ - Normal; MS 77 IL St Univ - Normal; Sp-Lang Path, Champaign Sch Dist #4, **SLP**

Day, Dr Pat Spencer 10118 Ashburton Lane, Bethesda, MD 20817, (202) 651-5206

Day, Patsy W 3075 Grace Street, West Melbourne, FL 32904, (407) 631-1911, BS 57 East TN St Univ; MS 58 Vanderbilt Univ; Tchr, Brevard Co Sch Bd, **A**

Day, Mrs Susan M B 6001 Salida Del Sol, San Jose, CA 95123, (408) 356-1400, BS 76 Saint Mary's Dominican Coll; MS 78 Univ of NC - Chapel Hill; Sp/Lang Path, Private Practice, **SLP**

Dayne, Mrs Margaret N 636 Crestglen Road, Glendora, CA 91740, (818) 963-8754, BS 69 Clarion Univ of PA; MA 71 CA St Univ - Los Angeles; SLP, Private Practice, **SLP**

Day-Register, Mrs Patricia 11924 Mayfield Avenue #5, Los Angeles, CA 90049, (213) 820-2050, BS 77 IA St Univ; MA 79 Univ of IA; Sp-Lang Path, LA Co Supt of Sch, **SLP**

Day-Shockey, Mrs Diane 1611 Cathedral Avenue, Hagerstown, MD 21740, MS 80 WV Univ; Director/Audiologist, Washington County Health Dept, **A**

Deacy, Denise Bauman 4266 South Honey Creek Dr, Milwaukee, WI 53220, (414) 649-3900, BS 83 Univ of WI - Oshkosh; MS 85 Univ of WI - Oshkosh; **A**

Deadrick, Mrs Dana Lynn 1771 Wooden Rail Lane, Jacksonville, FL 32225, (904) 737-7900, BS 80 Radford Univ; ME 84 James Madison Univ; Aud, Xomed, **A**

Deahl, Mrs Susan K 6735 East Mockingbird, Dallas, TX 75214, (214) 827-4849, BA 76 Northeast LA Univ; OM 78 LA St Univ - N O Medical Ctr; Aud/Dept Head, Chldn Med Cen of Dalls, **A**

Deakin, Carol Stephens 902 Cindy Drive, Carbondale, IL 62901, (618) 549-0801, MS 87 Southern IL Univ -Carbondale

Deal, Donald Bryan 310 North Bryant, Sherman, TX 75090, (214) 868-9595, BA 81 Univ of OK - Norman; MS 83 Univ of OK Medical Center; 84–Aud, Texoma Head & Neck Surgery Clin, **A**

Deal, Jane E 1505 Oak Bluff Circle N W, Massillon, OH 44646, (216) 438-2551, OB 73 Kent St Univ; MA 78 Univ of Akron; Sp-Lang Path, Canton Cty Sch, **SLP**

Deal, Dr Jon L VA Medcial Center, 30th And Euclid, Des Moines, IA 50310, (515) 271-5691, BS 67 Univ Southern MS-Hattiesburg; MS 69 Univ Southern MS-Hattiesburg; PH 70 (NS) Univ Southern MS-Hattiesburg; Chief Audiology/Sp-Path Serv, VA Medical Center, **SLP**

Deal, Dr Leo V 5966 Patriots Way, East Lansing, MI 48823, (517) 353-7892, BA 51 Depauw Univ; MA 58 OH St Univ; PH 65 (NS) MI St Univ; Professor, Michigan State University, **SLP A F**

Deal, Margaret Elizabeth Rural Route 1 Box 57, Bleeker Road, Vernon Center, NY 13477, (315) 363-8000, BS 80 SUNY - Coll at Geneseo; MS 84 Syracuse Univ; **SLP**

Deal, Dr Randolph E Southwest Missouri State Univ, Dept Of Com Dis, 900 So National, Springfield, MO 65804-0095, (417) 836-5275, BA 66 OK St Univ; MS 67 Univ of OK Medical Center; PH 71 (NS) Univ of OK Medical Center; Prof, SW Mo State Univ, **SLP**

Deal, Vicki R 6005 Cherrywood Court, Apartment 302, Greenbelt, MD 20770, (301) 897-5700, BS 81 Northwestern Univ; MA 82 Northwestern Univ; 86–Asst Dir Minority Concerns, American Sp-Lang-Hearing Assoc, **SLP ACE**

Deal-Tackett, Laurie K 817 North Church Street, Redlands, CA 92374, (714) 788-7300, 69; BA 77 Univ of LA Verne; MS 78 Univ of Redlands; Sp-Lang Path, Riverside USD, **SLP**

Dean, Carol Kaliebe 6715 Farmleigh Drive, Indianapolis, IN 46220, (317) 842-2001, BS 64 Univ of WI - Milwaukee; MA 85 Butler Univ; **SLP A**

Dean, Carolyn A 127 Olive Street, Huntington, WV 25705-1516, (304) 344-7227, **A**

Dean, Charlene 30 Bradstreet Road #12, Centerville, OH 45459, (513) 228-7083, BS 76 Miami Univ - Oxford; MS 79 Miami Univ - Oxford; Sp-Lang Path, Total Living Care, **SLP**

Dean, Charles R 487 Estates Drive, Athens, OH 45701, (614) 593-1412, BS 60 OH Univ - Athens; MA 64 OH Univ - Athens; PH 80 (NS) Stanford Univ; Asst Prof, Ohio Univ, **SLP**

Dean, Mrs Cheryl C 3848 Gardner Avenue, Cincinnati, OH 45236, (513) 745-0615, BS 85 Miami Univ - Oxford; MS 86 Miami Univ - Oxford; 86–SLP, Hamilton Co Bd of Mental Retard Dev Disabilities, **SLP**

Dean, Curtis Lawrence Star Route 17D, Poca, WV 25159, (304) 776-7316, BS 82 WV Univ; MS 83 WV Univ; Sp-Lang Path, Putnam County Board of Educ, **SLP**

Dean, Mrs Diana C 3422 47th Street Ct N W, Gig Harbor, WA 98335, (206) 851-6922, BS 68 Univ of NE - Lincoln; MA 69 Univ of NE - Lincoln; Sp-Lang Path, Jamie H Stevens, **SLP**

Dean, James 205 Silver Road, Bangor, ME 04401, (207) 581-2006, BA 77 Univ of MA - Amherst; MS 83 Univ of WI - Madison; 85–Dir/Aud, Bangor/Ellsworth Hearing Ctrs, **A**

Dean, Janet Therese 4704 E Paradise Village Pk, Apartment 119, Phoenix, AZ 85032, (306) 848-0114, BS 85 Minot St Univ; BS 85 Minot St Univ; MS 86 Minot St Univ; **SLP**

Dean, Jeffery Lynn 940 Hancock #2, West Hollywood, CA 90069, (213) 657-8569, MA 85 San Diego St Univ; **A**

Dean, Julia Ann 10270 Fleming Road, Lynchburg, OH 45142, (513) 987-2600, BS 84 Miami Univ - Oxford; MS 85 Miami Univ - Oxford; 87–Sp-Lang Path, Highland Co Schs, **SLP**

Dean, Karen J 10 North Elmhurst Road, Prospect Heights, IL 60070, (312) 939-6888, BA 84 MacMurray Coll; MS 87 Rush Univ; **A**

Dean, Karen Louise 29005 Aranel Street, Farmington Hills, MI 48018-3629, (313) 489-5920, MA 87 Edinboro Univ of PA

Dean, Kathryn N 2015 Anacapa Street, Santa Barbara, CA 93105, (805) 964-4711, BA 70 4935; MS 75 Univ of CA - Santa Barbara; 73–Sp-Lang Path, Santa Barbara Co Schs, **SLP**

Dean, Dr Linda May 13914 Riverbirch Trace Rd, Midlothian, VA 23113, (804) 744-3087, BA 64 Univ of VT; MA 67 Syracuse Univ; PH 74 (NA) Syracuse Univ; Aud, Pratt Med Cen Ltd/J Shim MD, **A**

Dean, Mrs Manita B P O Box 143, Bishop, GA 30621, (404) 769-6977, BA 55 Wesleyan Coll; MS 65 Purdue Univ - West Lafayette; Sp-Lang Path, St Mary's Hosp Rehab Svc, **SLP**

Dean, Marcia Southwell 291 Lincoln Street, Suite 203, Worcester, MA 01605, (617) 792-9293, BS 72 Boston Univ; MA 74 Univ of CT; Dir, Aud Assoc of Worcester, Inc, **A ACE**

Dean, Marla Rae 301 14th Avenue S W #2, Minot, ND 58701, (701) 857-3030, BS 78 Minot St Univ; MS 81 Minot St Univ; Sp-Lang Path, Minot State Univ, **SLP**

Dean, Mary A 4854 Forestglade Circle, Stone Mountain, GA 30087, (404) 934-5924, BA 72 Agnes Scott Coll; MS 74 Emory Univ; **SLP ACE**

Dean, Mary Pat 5607 Riverview Court, Stevens Point, WI 54481, (715) 346-2021, BS 70 Univ of IL - Urbana; MA 73 Univ of IL - Urbana; Sp-Lang Path, Stevens Point Area Schs, **SLP**

Dean, Nadine Salacone 7826 Arlington Drive, Boulder, CO 80303, (303) 447-1010, BA 68 San Jose St Univ; MA 84 Univ of CO - Boulder; Sp-Lang Path, Boulder Valley Pub Sch, **SLP**

Dean, Renee 1736 Rose Briar Lane, Stroudsburg, PA 18360, (717) 421-5123, BS 74 East Stroudsburg Univ of PA; MS 79 PA St Univ - Univ Park; Clinical Supervisor, Logopedic Associates Inc, **SLP**

Dean, Ronald J R R 1 Box 176, Hennepin, IL 61327, (815) 925-7098, **SLP**

Dean, Mrs Sheila A 1003 Heathwood Drive, Englewood, OH 45322, (513) 832-0668, BS 86 OH Univ - Athens; MS 87 Miami Univ - Oxford; **SLP**

Dean, Mrs Susan Ann 6429 Clough Pike #2, Cincinnati, OH 45244, BS 76 Trenton St Coll; MA 78 Univ of Cincinnati; 88–Aud, **A**

Deane, Barbara G Rt 7 Box 303, Bedford, VA 24523, (703) 586-1180, BS 68 Old Dominion Univ; ME 74 Univ of VA - Charlottesville; 86–Mgr-Empl & Comm Rel, Golden West Foods McCormick, **SLP**

Deane, Janis Hartsfield 6502 Betts Avenue, Cincinnati, OH 45239, (513) 369-4736, ME 84 Univ of NC - Greensboro; Sp-Lang Path, Cincinnati Public Schools, **SLP**

Deaner, Eileen L Kallarekroken 31, Lund, Sweden 222 47, BS 71 Univ of MN - Minneap-St Paul; MA 75 Univ of MN - Minneap-St Paul; 86–Sp-Lang Path, Lund County PS, **SLP**

Deane-Watson, Edie Hope 1103 77th Street Court N W, Bradenton, FL 33529, (813) 792-2876, MS 84 FL St Univ; **A**

Dean-Floridis, Dorothy 5142 Woodmark Drive, Fort Wayne, IN 46815, (219) 637-3166, BA 58 Lake Erie Coll; MA 61 Case Western Reserve Univ; Sp-Lang Path, Byr, **SLP**

De Angelis, Cynthia Stone 57 Bellemonte Avenue, Lakeside Park, KY 41017, (513) 369-2474, BA 68 Univ of Dayton; MA 85 Univ of Cincinnati; Sp-Lang Path, The Christ Hospital, **SLP**

Deangelis, Deborah Ann 124 West Thomas Road, PO Box 34970, Phoenix, AZ 85067, (602) 263-7138, BS 82 AZ St Univ; MA 84 CA St Univ - Los Angeles; Sp-Lang Path, St Joseph's Hosp, **SLP**

De Angelis, Mrs Nadine W 25 Riverside Drive, Florham Park, NJ 07932, MA 78 Kean Coll of NJ; SLP, Florham Park Schools, **SLP**

De Angelo, Mrs Maryann P 35 Salem Drive, Greensburg, PA 15601, (412) 836-2460, BS 63 OH Univ - Athens; SLP, Westmoreland I U #7, **SLP**

Dean-Myrda, Mrs Nancy E 5853 North St Louis, Chicago, IL 60659, (312) 588-8978, BS 79 Bradley Univ; MA 83 Western IL Univ; SLP, Chicago Board of Education, **SLP**

Deans, Mary Frances 1576 N Valley Road, Apache Junction, AZ 85220, (602) 496-4730, BA 84 Univ of CA - Santa Barbara; OM 86 AZ St Univ; SLP, Kyrene Schl Dstr, **SLP**

Deans, Nancy C 3819 Westbury Drive, Eagan, MN 55122, (612) 463-4671, BS 71 Mankato St Univ; MA 76 Univ of MN - Duluth; SLP, Lakeville Sch Dist #194, **SLP**

Dear, Mrs Rickly Neiman 969 East 7th Street, Brooklyn, NY 11230, (212) 338-3333, BA 75 CUNY - Brooklyn Coll; MS 80 CUNY - Brooklyn Coll; **SLP**

Dearchs, Mrs Marianne Jackson 1403 Malvern Avenue, Ruxton, MD 21204, (301) 296-6574, BA 78 Loyola Coll; MS 79 Loyola Coll; 79–Sp-Lang Path, Carroll County PS, **SLP**

Deardeuff, Mrs Linda Route 2 Box 670, Rolla, MO 65401, (314) 364-0809, BS 73 Univ of MO - Columbia; MA 75 Univ of MO - Columbia; Sp-Lang Path, Meremac Home Hlth Agcy, **SLP**

Dearholt, Janice Lange 2135 Thomas Drive, Las Cruces, NM 88001, (505) 882-4561, BA 78 NM St Univ; MA 81 NM St Univ; Sp-Lang Path, Gadsden ISD, **SLP**

Dearing, Carol F 2624 Andrea Lane, Dallas, TX 75228, (214) 343-2344, MS 67 Eastern IL Univ; Managing Consult, Sp Commun Consult, **SLP A**

Dearinger, Patricia McCombs 1429 Foothill Road, Ojai, CA 93023, BA 77 Univ of CA - Santa Barbara; MA 78 CA St Univ - Los Angeles; Audiologist, Private Practice, **A**

Deasy, Mrs Laurie Noriega 1221 Longview Drive, Diamond Bar, CA 91765, (818) 446-0131, BA 80 Univ of Southern CA; MA 82 CA St Univ - Long Beach; SLP, Arcadia USD, **SLP**

Deatherage, Violet M 101 Southbrookside Drive, Apt 2002, Dallas, TX 75214, (214) 821-6836, BA 83 Univ of OK - Norman; MS 85 Univ of OK Medical Center; 87–Sp-Lang Path, Dallas ISD, **SLP**

Deavours, Dr George M Valdosta Speech&Hearing Clinic, Valdosta State College, Education Center Room 107, Valdosta, GA 31698, (912) 333-5931, BA 65 Valdosta St Coll; MA 71 NM St Univ; PH 78 (Sp & Hrng Science) Univ Southern MS-Hattiesburg; Prof/Dir Sp-Hrng Clinic, Valdosta State College, **A**

Deavours, Mrs Ross S 7371 Smithfield Road, Mobile, AL 36695, (205) 633-0241, BS 76 Univ Southern MS-Hattiesburg; OM 77 Auburn Univ - Auburn; Aud, Mobile Co Pub Sch Syst, **A**

Debano-Burns, Dee Ann 4023 Cranberry, Wichita, KS 67226, (316) 688-7269, BA 82 Univ of KS; MA 84 Univ of KS; 88–Sp-Lang Path, Wesley Med Ctr, **SLP**

Debelius, Sarah Costlow 20634 Hazelnut Court, Germantown, MD 20874, (301) 253-3736, BA 76 Univ of MD - College Park; MS 78 Univ of AL- Tuscaloosa; Dir Sp Lang Serv, Self Employed, **SLP**

De Benedetto, Jane R 23 Sea Bridge Road, Alameda, CA 94501, (415) 523-7355, BS 70 Southwest TX St Univ; ME 72 Southwest TX St Univ; Sp-Lang Path, Utd Testng Ser, **SLP**

Deberardinis, Carol S Box 301 Orchard Drive RD1, Chadds Ford, PA 19317, (302) 368-6790, BS 78 Clarion Univ of PA; MS 79 Univ of NC - Chapel Hill; Sp-Lang Path, Div of Pub Hlth/De, **SLP**

Debertin, Mrs Phyllis L 1903 Norma Road N E, Tacoma, WA 98422, (206) 839-8264, BA 66 Univ of MT; OM 68 Univ of MT; Prog Mgr, Multicare Med Cen, **SLP**

Debes, Phyllis R 1414 Brown Hills Road, Rockford, IL 61107, **SLP**

De Blander, Mrs Marjorie Ann 274 Mt Vernon Circle, Bensalem, PA 19020-4057, (215) 639-4589, MS 84 PA St Univ - Univ Park; Sp-Lang Path, Desa Inc, **SLP**

Deboard, Mrs Cheryl J 3965 Riverview Drive, Columbus, OH 43026, (614) 833-2011, BA 77 OH St Univ; MA 79 OH St Univ; SLP, Groveport Madison Loc Schools, **SLP**

Deboer, Bonnie L 4974 Long Acre Drive, Syracuse, NY 13215, (315) 473-6905, BS 75 SUNY - Coll at Geneseo; MS 77 Marquette Univ; SLP, Syracuse Dev Cen, **SLP**

Deboer, Carolyn 751 Quailwood Drive, Loveland, OH 45140, (513) 683-1586, BA 68 Kean Coll of NJ; MA 72 Univ of CT; Sp-Lang Path, Hamilton County Office of Educ, **SLP**

Deboer, Debbie Diann 215 East Arbor Avenue, Apartment 302-A, Bismarck, ND 58504, (701) 223-4459, BS 85 Moorhead St Univ; MS 86 Moorhead St Univ

Deboer, Jack A 924 Reynard S E, Grand Rapids, MI 49507, (616) 246-5104, BS 75 Calvin Coll; MA 77 MI St Univ; Aud, Grand Rapids Pub Sch, **A**

Debois, Michelle E 14331 North Pennsylvania, Apartment E, Oklahoma City, OK 73134-6034, BS 83 OK St Univ; MS 86 Univ of OK Medical Center; **SLP**

DeBole, S Mario 1515 Huth Road, Grand Island, NY 14072, (716) 884-4327, BS 53 SUNY - Coll at Geneseo; ME 57 PA St Univ - Univ Park; Aud, Private Practice, **SLP A**

deBondt, Susan Maynard 6346 Emberwood Drive, Dublin, OH 43017, (614) 267-0570, MS 80 Univ of South FL; Aud, Riverside Hearing Svcs Inc, **A**

De Bonis, David A Sunnyview Hospital & Rehab Ctr, 1270 Belmont Avenue, Schenectady, NY 12308, (518) 382-4500, BA 79 Coll of Saint Rose; MS 80 PA St Univ - Univ Park; Aud, Sunneyview Hosp & Rehab Ctr, **A**

Deboth, Renee Marie 41 Goemble Avenue, Buffalo, NY 14211, (416) 521-2100, BA 86 SUNY - Center at Buffalo; MA 88 SUNY - Center at Buffalo

Debrincat, Mrs Geraldine 5934 Shaun, West Bloomfield, MI 48322, **SLP**

de Brueys, Mrs Mary T Communication & Learning Ctr, 433 Metairie Road, Suite 115, Metairie, LA 70005, (504) 834-4744, BS 76 LA St Univ - Baton Rouge; OM 77 LA St Univ - N O Medical Ctr; Director of Devel Speech-Lang, Commun & Lrng Cen, **SLP**

De Bruin, Mrs Mary Noren 439 Green Street, Seymour, WI 54165, (414) 497-3889, BA 75 Univ of MN - Duluth; MA 76 Univ of MN - Duluth; Sp-Lang Path, Green Bay Area Pub Schs, **SLP**

De Carlo, Mrs Susannah Mathis 200 Mainsail Drive, Grayslake, IL 60030, (312) 662-1877, BS 70 Bradley Univ; MS 71 Bradley Univ; Parent-Infant Sp/Lang Path, Lake McHenry Reg Prog, **SLP**

Decarlo-Erickson, Mrs Ginny 420 Cambridge Way, Bolingbrook, IL 60439, (312) 567-2160, BS 84 Saint Xavier Coll; MS 87 Rush Univ; Sp-Lang Path, Mercy Hosp, **SLP**

De Castro, Mrs Jennifer Louise Virginia Mason Clinic G2-AU, 1100 9th Avenue, P O Box 900, Seattle, WA 98111, (206) 223-6393, BS 79 Univ of Capetown - S Africa; MA 83 Univ of WA; Aud, Virginia Mason Clinic, **A**

Dececco, Mrs E Patricia Becker 39 Elwood Road, Box 306, Slingerlands, NY 12159, (518) 459-2803, BS 59 Coll of Saint Rose; MA 63 Coll of Saint Rose; Sp-Lang Path, S Colonie Central Schs, **SLP**

Decere, Mrs Genevieve 48 Nelson Avenue, Harrison, NY 10528, (914) 835-0703, BS 62 Adelphi Univ; MS 73 CUNY - Lehman Coll; Sp/Lang Path, City Sch Dist of New Rochelle, **SLP**

De Cesari, Rico 5601 North Sheridan, Apartment 18E, Chicago, IL 60660, (312) 275-0734, BA 83 CA St Univ - Fresno; MA 85 CA St Univ - Fresno; Sp-Lang Path, St Joseph Hosp, **SLP**

Dechant, Joseph Michael 3726 Sarasota Court, Orlando, FL 32812, (407) 282-1897, BS 80 Kent St Univ; MA 82 Kent St Univ; Aud, Naval Hospital, **A ACE**

Dechant, Susan B 1003 Lincoln Drive East, West Bend, WI 53095, (414) 338-5480, BS 74 Univ of WI - Stevens Point; MS 75 Univ of WI - Stevens Point; Sp-Lang Path, Joint School District 1, **SLP**

De Chicchis, Dr Albert R 820 St Sebastian Way, Suite 4-D, Augusta, GA 30910, (404) 724-0668, BA 73 Univ of Southwestern LA; MA 75 Central MI Univ; PH 81 (NS) Memphis St Univ; Coord Aud Serv, VA Med Cen/Augusta GA, **A**

De Ciccio, Maria 28-32 44th Street, Astoria, NY 11103, (212) 481-0316, BA 79 Long Island U - CW Post Ctr; MS 84 Columbia Univ Teachers Coll; Sp-Lang Path, Staten Island Hospital, **SLP**

Decicco, Barbara A 460 Ovington Avenue #2-B, Brooklyn, NY 11209-1516, (718) 238-3899, BA 76 SUNY - Coll at New Paltz; MA 79 CUNY - Hunter Coll; Sp-Lang Path, Mt Sinai Med Cen, **SLP**

Deck, Christie Reichert 701 Fox Drive, Great Falls, MT 59404, (406) 791-2270, BS 72 Univ of ND; MA 76 KS St Univ; 88–Coord/Empl Ben & Trng, Great Falls Pub Sch, **SLP**

Deck, Mrs Janette H 3537 Aspenwood, Sioux City, IA 51104, (712) 546-4192, BA 76 Univ of NE - Lincoln; MA 78 Univ of NE - Lincoln; Sp-Lang Path, Western Hills AEA 12, **SLP**

Deck, John W P O Box 28, Catlin, IL 61817, (217) 442-8000, BS 69 IN St Univ - Terre Haute; MA 70 Univ of IL - Urbana; Sp-Lang Path, VA, **SLP**

Decker, Mrs Amy K 814 Church Street, Hollidaysburg, PA 16648, (814) 695-5643, BS 76 Indiana Univ of PA; MS 78 PA St Univ - Univ Park; 85–Sp-Lang Path, Appalachia Intermediate Unit 8, **SLP**

Decker, Cathy J S 1339 Friar Creek, Houston, TX 77055, **SLP**

Decker, David I 291 Coyne Street, Bourbonnais, IL 60914, (815) 939-8751, BS 74 Northern MI Univ; MA 75 Western MI Univ; Men Hlth Admin/Unit Dir, Shapiro Dev Cen, **SLP**

Decker, Deborah Jean #F 6911 Society Drive, Tampa, FL 33617, BA 82 SUNY - Center at Buffalo; MS 85 Univ of South FL; **SLP A**

Decker, Mrs Hilary McAllister 3023 Linda Lane, Sinking Spring, PA 19608, (215) 678-4184, BS 71 Bradley Univ; MS 73 PA St Univ - Univ Park; Sp-Lang Path, Berks County Head Start, **SLP**

Decker, Mrs Joann A 1029 Linden Avenue #2, Wilmette, IL 60091, (312) 446-9400, BS 75 TX Tech Univ; MA 79 Our Lady Lake Univ-San Anton; Sp-Lang Path, Winnetka Sch Dist 36, **SLP**

Decker, Margaret L 2909 Woodhaven, Carrollton, TX 75006, (214) 238-0324, BS 68 Hardin-Simmons Univ; MA 70 Our Lady Lake Univ-San Anton; Spec Ed Consult, Richardson ISD, **SLP**

Decker, Marie N RD #9 Box 9340, Newton, NJ 07860, (201) 383-1487, BA 65 Newark St Coll; MS 85 William Paterson Coll; 79–Sp-Lang Path, Kittatinny Reg HS Bd of Educ, **SLP**

Decker, Mrs Patricia Alice 115 S Montgomery Street, Walden, NY 12586, (914) 431-8801, **SLP**

Decker, Mrs Synnove E 237 Thimbleberry Road, Ballston Spa, NY 12020, (518) 785-9971, BS 64 Northwestern Univ; MA 65 Northwestern Univ; Sp-Lang Path, N Colonie Cen Sch Dist, **SLP**

Decker, Dr T Newell Department Special Education & Communication Disorders, 253 Barkley Memorial Center, University Of Nebraska-Lincoln, Lincoln, NE 68583-0731, (402) 472-5456, BA 66 Univ of WA; ME 69 Eastern WA Univ; PH 75 (NS) Univ of WA; Assoc Prof of Aud, U of NE-Lincoln, **A**

Deckert, Mrs Linda Koehler 14170 Forest Crest Drive, Chesterfield, MO 63017, (314) 434-8845, BS 72 Fontbonne Coll; MA 73 Memphis St Univ; Sp-Lang Path, Special School District, **SLP**

Deckinger, Mrs Gloria May 221 Albemarle Road, White Plains, NY 10605, (212) 655-0261, MS 75 CUNY - Brooklyn Coll; SLP, New York Board of Education, **SLP**

De Clark, Janet Louise 571 Turnabout Road, Orange, CA 92669, (714) 581-2800, **SLP**

De Clerck, Mrs Ingrid Gundersen 425 Thrushwood Lane, Rochester, NY 14580, (716) 671-9216, BS 82 SUNY - Coll at Geneseo; MS 85 Nazareth Coll of Rochester; 85–Sp-Lang Path, W Irondequoit Sch Dist, **SLP**

De Cola-Samoylo, Mrs Debi Patricia P O Box 577 Carl Ann Lane, Valley Cottage, NY 10989, (914) 634-7510, BA 80 Dominican Coll of Blauvelt; MS 85 William Paterson Coll; 80–Sp-Lang Path, Clarkstown Central Schools, **SLP**

Deconde-Johnson, Dr Cheryl 2109 44th Avenue, Greeley, CO 80634, (303) 351-2261, BA 75 Univ of CA - Santa Barbara; MA 76 Univ of Northern CO; ED 82 (NS) Univ of Northern CO; 76–Aud, Weld County Sch Dist 6, **A**

Deconna, Mrs Susan McCue Sp & Lang Ctr Of Palm Beaches, 1012 Clearwater Place, West Palm Beach, FL 33402, (305) 833-6630, BS 76 FL St Univ; MS 77 FL St Univ; Pres, Sp & Lang Cen of Palm Beaches, **SLP**

De Corso, Jill Buelow 10770 Mortons Crossing, Alpharetta, GA 30201, (404) 594-8229, BS 80 Loma Linda Univ - Riverside; MS 85 UT St Univ; **SLP**

De Costa, Mrs Linda Anne 9350 Skillman Street #3717, Dallas, TX 75243, (214) 340-5327, BS 85 WV Univ; MS 86 Univ of SC - Columbia; 87–Sp-Lang Path, Dallas ISD, **SLP**

De Costa, Virginia Nell 4100 Gregory Street, Oakland, CA 94619, (415) 456-9680, BS 80 CA St Univ - Hayward; MS 86 CA St Univ - Hayward; SLP, Kentfield Rehab Hospital, **SLP**

De Cotiis, Ellen H R R 3 Box 155, Gorham, ME 04038, (207) 874-8100, BS 73 Montclair St Coll; MS 74 Univ of VT; Sp-Lang Path, Portland PS, **SLP ACE**

Dediminicantanio, Susan Paige 2809 New Castle Way, Carlsbad, CA 92008, (619) 726-2170, BA 83 Univ of CA - Santa Barbara; MA 85 CA St Univ - Chico

Dedinas, Anthony S 7159 Ward Eagle North, West Bloomfield, MI 48033, (313) 737-0036, BS 73 Worcester St Coll; MS 75 Univ of NM; **A**

Dedinsky, Karen Children's Hospital Medical Center Of Akron, 281 Locust, Akron, OH 44308, 88–Sp-Lang Path, Children's Hosp Med Ctr of Akron, **SLP**

Dedmond, Cindy Lynn 308 Azalea Boulevard, Douglas, GA 31533, (912) 384-7014, ME 82 Univ of GA; Sp-Lang Path, Appling County Schools, **SLP**

Dedo-Bailey, Vesna M 30 Lathrop Lane, Leamington, ON, Canada N8H 4B4, (519) 252-7281, BA 81 Univ of Western Ontario; MA 83 Wayne St Univ - Sch of Med; 86–Sp-Lang Path, The Children's Rehab Ctr, **SLP**

Dedrick, Marsha Lee 1908 Calhoun, Chillicothe, MO 64601, (816) 646-1480, BS 74 Fontbonne Coll; MA 75 Saint Louis Univ; Sp-Lang Path, Meadville R-4 Sch Dist, **SLP**

Dee, Anita D 45 Georgian Court, Elizabeth, NJ 07208, (201) 964-5155, BA 72 Newark St Coll; MA 74 Newark St Coll; Early-Intervent Couns, Private Practice, **SLP**

Deeb, Barbara M 9031 Fort Hamilton Parkway, Brooklyn, NY 11209, (718) 854-3737, BA 77 Long Island U - Brooklyn Ctr; MA 79 NY Univ; Sp/Lang Path, NY Chldhd Ctr, **SLP**

Deegan, Marywin 604 Amador St, Richmond, CA 94805, (415) 234-6200, BA 66 Marymount Coll; MS 73 Southern CT St Univ; Sp-Lang Path, Richmond USD, **SLP**

Deegan, Mrs Shelley A 9 Blue Forest Drive, Grimsby, ON, Canada L3M 4R4, (416) 945-5884, BA 75 0222; MA 77 SUNY - Coll at Buffalo; Sp/Lang Path, Chedoke-McMaster Hosp, **SLP**

Deem, Jodelle F Div Of Comm Disorders, Department Of Special Education, Murray State University, Murray, KY 42071, (502) 762-2855, BS 69 WV Univ; MS 71 WV Univ; PH 88 (Sp-Lang Path) Memphis St Univ; 88–Dir-Div of Comm Dis, Murray State University, **SLP ACE**

De Erdmann, Mrs Georgina R Ap Postal 59, Blvd 53140, Edo De, Mexico, (915) 572-0360, BS 60 Washington Univ; MA 80; Coord Spec Ed for Commun Dis, Universidad De Las Americas, **SLP A**

Deering, Mrs Kathleen Mary 936 West Bath Road, Cuyahoga Falls, OH 44223, (216) 666-6501, MA 84 Univ of Akron; Sp-Lang Path, Copley-Fairlawn City Schools, **SLP**

Deering, Rosemary M 22 Deerwood Drive, New City, NY 10956, **SLP**

Deery, Debra Joines 1121 Salsbury Avenue, Cody, WY 82414, (307) 587-4275, BS 74 Trenton St Coll; MS 78 Saint Cloud St Univ; 88–Sp-Lang Path, Cody Sch Dist, **SLP**

Dees, Sharon E P O Box 904, Gilbert, AZ 85234, (602) 892-3150, MS 88 Northern AZ Univ

Deeter, Arlyce K 4776 Sundown Trail, Ravenna, OH 44266, (216) 325-1601, BS 76 Kent St Univ; MA 77 Kent St Univ; 87–Sp-Lang Path, County of Summit Board of MR, **SLP**

Deetz, Debbie M 333 Springer Drive, Redding, CA 96003, (916) 244-4600, BA 78 Humboldt St Univ; MA 85 Humboldt St Univ; Sp/Lang Path, Shasta Co Off of Educ, **SLP**

Deetz, Mrs Janis Lee 13711 Nob Avenue, Del Mar, CA 92014, (612) 432-1186, MA 78 Univ of MN - Duluth; **SLP**

Defazio, Dr Jean Levin 1468 Hillbrook SE, North Canton, OH 44709, (216) 499-7090, BA 73 Baldwin-Wallace Coll; MA 74 Kent St Univ; PH 82 (NS) Kent St Univ; Asst Prof/Coord-Spec Educ, Walsh Coll, **SLP**

De Fehr, Mrs Melanie Garner 1501 Timbercreek Drive, Weatherford, OK 73096-3427, (405) 774-1031, BA 83 Univ of OK - OK City; MS 85 Univ of OK - OK City; **SLP**

Defendi, Christel C 55 Greenacres Avenue, Scarsdale, NY 10583, **SLP**

DeFeo, Anthony B University Of Arizona, Department Of Speech & Hearing Sciences, University Way, Tucson, AZ 85721, (602) 621-1826, BA 70 Montclair St Coll; MA 71 Northwestern Univ; PH 77 (Sp-Lang Path) Northwestern Univ; 81–Dir of Sp Lang Cl, Univ of AZ, **SLP**

Deffley, Monica Ann 14 Pamela Court, Broad Brook, CT 06016, Sp-Lang Path, Manchester Bd of Ed, **SLP**

De Filippo, Dr Carol L NTID Rochester Inst Of Tech, One Lomb Memorial Drive, Rochester, NY 14623, (716) 475-6456, MS 71 Purdue Univ - West Lafayette; MS 72 Washington Univ; PH 80 (Communication Sciences) Washington Univ; 81–Res Assoc, NTID, **A**

Defoor, Mrs Joy C 113 Dennis Place, Clovis, NM 88101, (505) 762-2737, BS 80 Eastern NM Univ; MS 81 Eastern NM Univ; Sp-Lang Path, Clovis Municipal Sch, **SLP**

Defoor-Hill, Lori A 1638-A North Mohawk, Chicago, IL 60614, (312) 942-5332, BS 80 Western KY Univ; MS 81 Western KY Univ; Sp-Lang Path, Rush-Presb-St Luke's Med Ctr, **SLP**

Deford, Sheila Andrea 385 Castleton Avenue, Staten Island, NY 10301, (718) 345-5219, BS 83 WV Univ; MS 85 Loyola Coll; 86–Sp-Lang Path, Human Comm Svcs Inc, **SLP**

De Fosse, Dr Carlton O 841 Wylie Avenue, Toledo, OH 43609, (419) 537-2184, BS 71 Western IL Univ; MA 72 Western IL Univ; PH 78 (NS) Univ of Toledo; Assoc Prof, U of Toledo, **SLP A**

DeFrance, Mrs Dorothy Wells 2001 Dennison Place N W, Canton, OH 44709, (216) 492-5450, BS 59 Kent St Univ; ME 64 Kent St Univ; **SLP**

De France, Mrs Nancy L R 1366 Balfour, Grosse Pointe, MI 48230, (216) 228-6629, BS 75 OH Univ - Athens; MA 77 Cleveland St Univ; Outside Cen Serv-Consult, Cleveland Hearing & Speech Ctr, **SLP**

Defrancesco, Mrs Joyce M 4 Kerr Farm Road, Simsbury, CT 06070, (203) 658-4197, BA 73 Univ of CT; MS 74 Southern CT St Univ; Sp-Lang Path, Avon PS, **SLP**

Defrancesco, Marisa 85 Thompson Avenue, Toronto, ON, Canada M8Z 3T5, (416) 848-7281, BS 81 Univ of Western Ontario; OM 85 Univ of Western Ontario; 85–Aud, The Mississauga Hosp, **A**

Defrancesco, Miki P 3744 Lankenau Road, Philadelphia, PA 19131, (215) 424-8234, BS 75 West Chester Univ of PA; MA 80 Trenton St Coll; Sp-Lang Path, Sch Dist of Phil, **SLP**

De Franco, Mrs Kathleen D 21 Berkshire, Belleville, IL 62223, (618) 234-6876, BS 83 Southern IL Univ-Edwardsvill; MS 84 Fontbonne Coll; **SLP**

Defranco, Sharon A 10811 Via Solida, Yuma, AZ 85634, (602) 324-1317, BS 71 Edinboro Univ of PA; MS 73 SUNY - Coll at Fredonia; Sp-Lang Path, Yuma Union HS Dist, **SLP**

Defrank, Lois Young 1-01 Morlot Avenue, Fair Lawn, NJ 07410, (201) 427-1300, BS 56 SUNY - Center at Buffalo; MA 67 Montclair St Coll; Sp-Lang Path, Hawthorne Board of Education, **SLP**

Defrantz, Dr Anita P 500 Los Palmos, San Francisco, CA 94127, (415) 334-4455, BA 55 IN Univ - Bloomington; MA 65 IN Univ - Bloomington; PH 75 (NS) Univ of Pittsburgh - Pittsburgh; **SLP**

Deftos, Mrs Linda H 225 Torrey Pines Terr, Del Mar, CA 92014, (619) 274-9871, BA 63 Univ of VT; MA 66 Columbia Univ Teachers Coll; 79–Sp-Lang Path, San Diego USD, **SLP**

Degeeter, Judith W Tall Oaks Court, Franklin Lakes, NJ 07417, (201) 891-1802, BS 67 Univ of DE; MS 72 Paterson St Coll; **SLP**

Degen, Mrs Elizabeth Crosswait 1430 West Jackson, Spearfish, SD 57783, (605) 642-7476, BS 76 Black Hills St Coll; MS 86 Univ of NE - Omaha

Degennaro, Andrea T 5774 Green Road, Haslett, MI 48840, **SLP**

Degirolamo, Dale A 311 Crestview Drive, Elyria, OH 44035, (216) 775-2786, BS 69 Kent St Univ; MA 72 Kent St Univ; Dir, Nn OH Spec Ed Reg Resource Cen, **SLP**

Degnan, Deborah W 6130 North Berkeley Blvd, Whitefish Bay, WI 53217-4315, (414) 332-3764, BS 72 Plymouth St Coll; MS 74 Emerson Coll; **SLP**

Degolier, Mrs Elinor J 1217 Carrie Avenue, Rochelle, IL 61068, (815) 562-6665, BS 70 Univ of WI - Whitewater; MA 75 Northern IL Univ - De Kalb; Sp-Lang Path, Rochelle Elem Sch, **SLP**

De Gomez, Elizabeth A M 475 Bronx River Road #2F, Yonkers, NY 10704, **SLP**

Degraauw, Mrs Claudette 215 3rd Street, Abbeville, LA 70510, (318) 265-5322, BS 75 Saint Mary's Dominican Coll; MA 77 LA St Univ - Baton Rouge; 77–Sp-Lang Path, LA Div Hlth & Human Res, **SLP**

Degraff, Mrs Sheila Norton 29 Camborne Circle, Fairport, NY 14450, (716) 377-0781, BS 75 Nazareth Coll of Rochester; MS 76 Nazareth Coll of Rochester; 84–SLP, Private Practice, **SLP**

Degraffenried, Dr Helen Lee 803 Monroe Drive, Elizabethtown, KY 42701, (502) 588-5049, BS 56 Brigham Young Univ; MS 68 Brigham Young Univ; PH 76 (NS) Brigham Young Univ; Dir/Psychological Services, Hazelwood Icf/Mr, **SLP A**

De Gregorio, Emmy K 9 Dinell Drive, Pittsburgh, PA 15221, (412) 371-9853, BA 74 Niagara Univ; ME 76 Clarion Univ of PA; Sp/Lang Path, Allegheny Sp/Hrng Cen, **SLP**

De Haan, Mrs Shellee Cates 11805 West 71st Terrace, Shawnee, KS 66203, (816) 276-7352, BS 82 Northeast MO St Univ; MA 84 Northeast MO St Univ; Sp-Lang Path, Baptist Med Ctr, **SLP**

Dehaan-Hill, Julie Mae 4518 Cheyenne Blvd, Sioux City, IA 51104-4017, (712) 258-6046, BA 80 Univ of SD - Vermillion; MA 81 Univ of SD - Vermillion; SLP, Siouxland Easter Seal Soc, **SLP**

Dehart, Mrs Nancy Nunley 3345 Clearview Street, Knoxville, TN 37917-2706, (615) 546-2888, BA 85 Univ of TN - Knoxville; MA 87 Univ of TN - Knoxville; 87–Aud, Francisco G Moreno MD, **A**

Dehaus-Mattson, Mrs Mary Carol 1588 Southlawn, Jenison, MI 49428, (616) 457-1417, BS 83 Western MI Univ; MA 85 Western MI Univ; Sp-Lang Path, Holland Public Schools, **SLP**

Dehem, Cynthia S 4059 Gatesford Circle, Troy, MI 48098, (313) 263-8754, BS 75 Eastern MI Univ; MA 76 Eastern MI Univ; Supervisor Sp-Lang Path Dept, MacOmb Oakland Regional Ctr, **SLP**

De Hirsch, Katrina 33 East 70th Street, New York, NY 10021, PH (NS); **SLP F LM**

Deibele, Denise Ristow 20329 Rockville Road, Kiel, WI 53042, (414) 894-3630, BS 79 Marquette Univ; MS 81 Marquette Univ; Sp/Lang Path, Homecare Hlth Serv Inc, **SLP**

Deibert, Beverly Diane 710 Heritage Lane Apartment D, Bel Air, MD 21014, BS 84 Kutztown Univ of PA; MS 86 WV Univ; 88–Sp-Lang Path, Harford County Pub Sch, **SLP**

Deicas, Wendy Marie Grant County Schools, Petersburg, WV 26847, (304) 257-1011, ME 81 2697; 82–Sp-Lang Path, Grant Co Bd of Ed, **SLP**

Deierlein, Therese Marie 40 Overpeck Avenue, Ridgefield Park, NJ 07660, (212) 319-0770, MS 83 Columbia Univ Teachers Coll; 88–Aud, Manhattan Aud Svc, **A**

Deifel, Gayle R 3000 Singing Hills Drive, Bakersfield, CA 93306, **SLP**

Deighton, Mrs Karen McQuade 30774 Beechwood Street, Apartment 44201, Wixom, MI 48096-9312, (313) 455-2286, **SLP**

Deily, Dr Ann Beth S Rural Delivery 3 Box 360, Merwin Road, Valatie, NY 12184, (518) 454-5205, MA 71 Vanderbilt Univ; MS 72 Vanderbilt Univ; PH 77 (NS) SUNY - Center at Albany; Prof, The College of Saint Rose, **SLP ACE**

Deines, Rick Raymond 630 6th Street, Wakeeney, KS 67672, (913) 462-8282, **A ACE**

De Innocentes, Maryann Rose 1415 Broad Ripple Avenue, Indianapolis, IN 46220, (317) 259-8105, **SLP A**

Deisenroth, Mrs Patricia L 3102 South Harvard #83, Tulsa, OK 74135, (918) 743-3036, BS 66 Univ of Tulsa; MA 71 Univ of Tulsa; Sp-Lang Path, Private Practice, **SLP**

Deitch, Susan Anne 2001 Delancy Place, Philadelphia, PA 19103, (302) 658-8860, BS 82 PA St Univ - Univ Park; MA 85 CUNY - Queens Coll; **A**

Deitchman, Pamela Susan 7445 Del Mar, Second Floor, University City, MO 63130, (314) 727-6862, MS 80; Sp-Lang Path, De Paul Hlth Cen, **SLP**

Deitz, Laura F 313 South 10th Street, West Helena, AR 72390, (501) 572-3437, BA 53 Univ of AR - Fayetteville; ME 73 Univ of VA - Charlottesville; Sp-Lang Path, Helena-W Helena Public Schools, **SLP**

Deja, Patricia Ann 6304 Boone Avenue North, Brooklyn Park, MN 55428, (612) 295-5191, MS 84 Univ of WI - River Falls; SLP, Montecello Schl Sys, **SLP**

De Jarnette, Dr Glenda East Tennessee St University, Dept Of Communication Dis, Box 21790A, Johnson City, TN 37614, (619) 929-4272, BA 78 Allegheny Coll; MA 80 Cleveland St Univ; PH 84 (NS) Bowling Green St Univ; Assistant Professor, East Tennessee State U, **SLP ACE**

Dejean, Jeanne V 150 Lily Lane, Opelousas, LA 70570, (318) 264-5610, BA 71 Univ of Southwestern LA; MA 73 LA St Univ - Baton Rouge; Adult Prog Coord, Offi of Mental Ret, **SLP**

Dejesus, Maria M 992 Calle Manila, Urb Santa Rita, Rio Piedras, PR 00921, (407) 697-3018, BA 75 Inter American Univ; MS 79 Univ of PR - Rio Piedras; 88–Sp-Lang Path, New Medico Rehab, **SLP**

Dejmal, Nancy L Veterans Admin Medical Center, Audiology 126, 1660 South Columbian Way, Seattle, WA 98108, MS 77 Univ of NE - Lincoln; Sp-Lang Path, Dade Co Pub Sch, **SLP**

Dejonge, Mrs Linda B 35 Timberline, Warrensburg, MO 64093, (816) 747-6687, BS 73 Univ of IL - Urbana; MS 74 Univ of IL - Urbana; Sp-Lang Path, Central MO State U, **SLP**

Dejonge, Dr Robert R, Jr Dept Speech Path & Audiology, Central Missouri St Univ, Warrensburg, MO 64093, (816) 429-4918, BS 72 Univ of IL - Urbana; MA 75 Univ of IL - Urbana; PH 76 (NS) Univ of IL - Urbana; 76–Prof Aud, Ctrl MO St U, **A**

DeJoy, Dr Daniel A 8804 Royalwood Court, Raleigh, NC 27613, (919) 737-3204, BA 70 Westminster Coll; MA 72 Northwestern Univ; PH 75 (Sp-Lang Path) Northwestern Univ; Assoc Prof-Dept of Sp Comm, North Carolina State Univ, **SLP**

De Julius, Bernadette Picardi 2435 North 77th Court, Unit 3-East, Elmwood Park, IL 60635, (312) 908-6134, BA 83 Elmhurst Coll; MA 85 Univ of IL - Urbana; 86–Sp-Lang Path, Rehab Inst of Chicago, **SLP**

Dekas-Marafiote, Elizabeth 2977 South Genoa Street, Aurora, CO 80013, (303) 690-1845, BS 79 CA St Univ - Hayward; MA 81 Univ of Denver; 84–Sp/Lang Path, Saint Joseph Hosp, **SLP**

De Kemel, Kathryn Patrice 4290 San Remo, New Orleans, LA 70129, (504) 277-8144, BA 82 LA St Univ - Baton Rouge; MA 85 LA St Univ - Baton Rouge; 87–Sp-Lang Path, St Bernard Parish Sch, **SLP**

Dekrey, Silvia 1343 9th Street South, Fargo, ND 58103, (701) 241-4800, MA 80 Moorhead St Univ; SLP, Fargo Pub Schs, **SLP**

De La Cruz, Angel F 8450 Cambridge Street, Apt#2152, Houston, TX 77054, (713) 797-9246, BA 83 Univ of VT; OM 86 LA St Univ - N O Medical Ctr; **A**

De La Cruz, Mrs Maritza Lucia 27935 North Park Meadow Dr, Canyon Country, CA 91351, (805) 251-0069, BA 83 CA St Univ - Northridge; MA 85 CA St Univ - Northridge; **SLP**

De La Cruz, Mrs Omayda G P O Box 52-1223, Miami, FL 33152-1223, (305) 325-0470, MS 87 Univ of South FL; 88–Sp-Lang Path, Easter Seal Soc Dade Co

Delacy, Hester S 1924-1/2 Lake Shore Avenue, Los Angeles, CA 90039, (213) 662-7343, BA 24 Univ of MN - Minneap-St Paul; MA 65 Univ of CA - Los Angeles; **SLP LM**

Delafuente, Jose R P O Box 580, La Salle, CO 80645, (303) 352-1876, BA 74 Univ of Northern CO; BA 74 Univ of Northern CO; MA 76 Univ of Northern CO; 75–Sp/Lang Path, Weld Co Sch Dist 6, **SLP**

Delagrange, Teryl N 321 West Wendover Avenue, Greensboro, NC 27408, (919) 379-9445, BS 69 Univ of Akron; MA 71 Univ of Akron; Aud, Greensboro Head & Neck Surg PA, **A**

Delahanty, Mrs Katherine Dannettel 11 Miller Drive, Avondale, PA 19311, (609) 678-7548, BS 81 Towson St Univ; MS 83 Loyola Coll; Sp-Lang Path, Norwalk Hospital, **SLP**

Delahoyde, Mrs Charlene B 2635 Raven Circle, Corona, CA 91720, (714) 735-4431, OB 68 Univ of Redlands; MA 70 Univ of Redlands; MS 80 Univ of Redlands; SLP, Corona-Norco USD, **SLP**

De La Mar, Mrs Melody A 1611 Harrington Drive, Champaign, IL 61821, (217) 333-4892, BS 67 Univ of IL - Urbana; MA 72 Univ of IL - Urbana; 88–Sp-Lang Path, Univ of IL Spectrum, **SLP**

Deland, Mrs Nancy E 5 Cedar Place, Ossining, NY 10562, (914) 941-5622, BS 51 PA St Univ - Univ Park; MS 57 PA St Univ - Univ Park; Sp-Lang Path, Private Practice, **SLP**

Delaney, Mrs Kathleen Ann Rd 5 Box 5581, Potters Road, Newton, NJ 07860, (201) 579-6097, BA 82 Kean Coll of NJ; MA 84 Ball St Univ; Aud, Dr B Skobel, **A**

Delaney, Kathleen Anne 664 Lotus Avenue, Oradell, NJ 07649, (201) 548-7610, BA 83 Univ of CT; MS 84 Ithaca Coll; **SLP**

Delaney, Mrs Laura Robbins 7150 Wynter Way, Indianapolis, IN 46250, (317) 773-8781, BA 81 IN Univ - Bloomington; MA 82 Ball St Univ; Sp-Lang Path, Janus Dev Serv Inc, **SLP**

Delaney, Patricia Marie 349 Academy Avenue, Providence, RI 02908, (617) 856-2398, BS 82 Elmira Coll; MA 85 SUNY - Coll at Geneseo; SLP, U of MA Medical Ctr, **SLP**

Delange, Mrs Sonya B 150 Morningside Lane, Redlands, CA 92374, (714) 797-9163, BS 74 Pacific Union Coll; MS 75 Loma Linda Univ - Riverside; Sp-Lang Path, San Bernardino Co Schs, **SLP**

De La Paz, Alina 10585 SW 109 Ct Suite 207, Miami, FL 33176, (305) 274-8348, BA 82 Univ of IL - Urbana; BS 82 Univ of IL - Urbana; MS 83 Univ of IL - Urbana; 88–Dir-Sp-Lang Path, Ctr Bilingual Sp & Lang Dis, **SLP**

Delapenha, Sandra Elaine 1128 Brooklyn Avenue, Brooklyn, NY 11203, (718) 821-2062, BA 80 CUNY - Hunter Coll; MA 85 CUNY - Hunter Coll; **A**

De La Rosa, Mrs Elly M 50 Adriano Gonzalez Street, Arecibo, PR 00612, (809) 878-1809, BA 73; MA 74 NY Univ; MS 82 Univ of PR - Rio Piedras; Sp-Lang Path, Pediatric Crippled Center H D, **SLP**

De La Torre, Mrs Jodi Tice 7960 N W 4th Street, Plantation, FL 33324, BA 80 Univ of FL; MA 82 Univ of FL; Sp-Lang Path, Dade Co Pub Schs, **SLP**

de Laubenfels, Prof Richard J 609 Stewart Avenue #D, Englewood, FL 34223, MS; **SLP LM**

Delaune, Mrs Pamela L 754 Magnolia Woods Avenue, Baton Rouge, LA 70808, (504) 346-8342, BS 68 LA St Univ - Baton Rouge; MA 73 LA St Univ - Baton Rouge; Spec Ed Coord, E Baton Rouge Parish Sch Bd, **SLP**

De La Vallee, Dolores Meola 5204 Beachcomber Street, Oxnard Shores, CA 93035, (805) 985-8494, BS 50; MA 52; Sp-Lang Path, Los Angeles USD, **SLP**

De Laveaga, Mrs Sharon Ruth 168 North Manila, Fresno, CA 93727, (209) 297-4000, **SLP**

Del Calzo, Dr Primo V 2505 River Road, Willoughby, OH 44094, (216) 687-3807, BS 61 Case Western Reserve Univ; MA 68 Case Western Reserve Univ; PH 73 (NS) Case Western Reserve Univ; Cl Asst Prof, Cleveland St Univ, **SLP**

Delconte, Laurie Ann 35-D Brookwood Drive, Rocky Hill, CT 06067, (203) 563-7095, BS 84 Northeastern Univ; MS 86 Gallaudet Coll; 87–Dist Mgr-Northeast US, Unitron Industries Inc

Del Coro, Paula Sosulski 40 Briar Lane, Basking Ridge, NJ 07920, (201) 522-2215, SLP, Overlook Hospital, **SLP**

Deleo, Mrs Barbara Marie 3108 Ginger Lane, Nampa, ID 83651, (208) 888-1381, BS 70 CO St Univ; MA 84 Northeast MO St Univ; **SLP**

Deleo, Monica Rose 523 Harrow Road, Richmond, VA 23225, (804) 320-3822, BS 84 Univ of WI - Madison; MS 86 Univ of WI - Madison; **SLP**

De Leon, Carmen M 5223-2 Cedarbend Drive, Fort Myers, FL 33919, (813) 939-4114, BA 77 Univ of FL; MA 79 Univ of FL; Sp-Lang Path, Assoc In Sp Path, **SLP**

Delf, Debra Susan 1444 West River Road #L, Elyria, OH 44035, (216) 324-5514, OB 86 Univ of Toledo; MS 87 Bowling Green St Univ; 87–Sp-Lang Path, Lorain Co Bd of Mental Retardation & Dev Dis, **SLP**

Delfino, Gregory Daniel 1934 Pelham Road, Bethlehem, PA 18018, (215) 694-9123, BA 77 Seton Hall Univ; MA 85 Montclair St Coll; Aud, United Hospital, **A**

Delfosse, Mrs Anne L 12 Circle Hill, Laguna Niguel, CA 92677-5902, (714) 974-1697, BS 79 Chapman Coll; MS 81 Chapman Coll; SLP, Anaheim Union High Sch Dist, **SLP**

Delfosse, Michael L 12 Circle Hill, Laguna Niguel, CA 92677-5902, (714) 558-1615, BA 75 CA St Univ - Chico; MA 77 CA St Univ - Chico; Sp/Lang Path, Irvine Ther Serv, **SLP**

Delgado, Lupe L 13932 Eastridge Drive, Whittier, CA 90602, (213) 922-6201, MA 81; 80–Sp-Lang Path, Los Angeles Co of Educ, **SLP**

Delgado, Mrs Pollie Johnson 7757 Inca, El Paso, TX 79912, (505) 882-4561, BA 75 Univ of TX - El Paso; MA 82 Univ of TX - El Paso; Sp/Lang Path, Gadsen Inde Sch Dist, **SLP**

Delgado-Gaitan, Margaret 8927 Rich Trace, San Antonio, TX 78251, (512) 532-9610, BA 76 Our Lady Lake Univ-San Anton; MA 78 Our Lady Lake Univ-San Anton; Coordinator Speech-Hearing, San Antonio State SCHOOL63894, **SLP**

Delgado-Vilches, Mrs Gloria 5500 North Braeswood #244, Houston, TX 77096, (713) 790-5913, BS 83; MS 86 Purdue Univ - West Lafayette; 86–Aud, The Methodist Hosp, **A**

Del Grosso, Mrs Gail Anne P O Box 283, Glenwood, NJ 07418, BS 79 FL St Univ; MS 80 FL St Univ; SLP, Vernon Board of Education

Del Guidice, Mary D 6 Slocum Heights #B-28, Syracuse, NY 13210, (315) 488-2951, BS 81 John Carroll Univ; MA 84 Kent St Univ; **SLP**

Delhommer, Jan M Route 4 Box 4330, St Martinville, LA 70582, (318) 981-6458, BA 82 Univ of Southwestern LA; MS 86 Univ of Southwestern LA; **A**

Delhommer, Mrs Janet A 10613 Willowgrove, Houston, TX 77035, MS 62; Sp-Lang Path, Alief ISD, **SLP**

Delhorne, Lorraine Anne MIT 50 Vassar Street, Rle 36-730, Cambridge, MA 02139, (617) 253-8134, MS 82 Washington Univ; 82–Research Spec, MIT

Delicati, Dawn G 4326 Atlin Street, Vancouver, BC, Canada V5R 2C2, (604) 875-2345, BA 67; MS 76 McGill Univ - Quebec; Aud, Bc Chldns Hosp, **A**

Deliema, Mrs Kathy Ledeen 26245 Buscador, Mission Viejo, CA 92692, (714) 643-0797, BA 72 Univ of Southern CA; MA 74 CA St Univ - Fullerton; **SLP**

Delisa, Diana C Rd 6 Box 1, Bill Hill Road, Lyme, CT 06371, (203) 434-8388, BA 79 Univ of CT; MA 81 Univ of CT; Dir of Aud, Private Practice, **A**

Delisa, Lauren R 38 Miracle Lane, Loudonville, NY 12211, (518) 449-2475, BA 69; MS 71 SUNY - Center at Albany; Sp-Lang Path, E Greenbush Sch Dist, **SLP**

Delisa, Mrs Sally T 163 King Phillips Pathe, Marshfield, MA 02050, (617) 934-6528, BA 64 MI St Univ; MS 78 Southern CT St Univ; 85–Sp-Lang Path, Duxbury PS, **SLP**

Delisi, Adele O 4805 134th Place S E, Bellevue, WA 98006, (206) 747-3341, BS 66 PA St Univ - Univ Park; MS 67 Univ of MI - Ann Arbor; 87–Sp-Lang Path, Lake Washington Sch Dist, **SLP**

Delisle, Anita L Box 408, Portageville, MO 63873, (314) 569-8311, BS 59 Marquette Univ; MA 67 Saint Louis Univ; Sp/Lang Path, Spec Sch Dist-St Louis Co, **SLP**

Delisle, Colleen Ann 34281 Coastal Drive #121, Sterling Heights, MI 48310, (313) 557-3650, BA 83 MI St Univ; MA 84 MI St Univ; **A**

Delisle, Dorothy M 2143 University Avenue, Apartment 2, Madison, WI 53705, (608) 233-0435, BS 78 Univ of WI - Madison; MS 80 Univ of WI - Madison; Sp-Lang Path, **SLP**

Delisle, Shirley H 104 Hampton, Gulf Breeze, FL 32561, (904) 932-9160, OB 69 Univ of AR - Fayetteville; MA 72 Memphis St Univ; Sp-Lang Path Consultant, Northview Community, **SLP**

Dell, Beverly D 1418 D Street S W, Ephrata, WA 98823, (509) 754-3538, BA 59 Univ of WA; MS 63 Univ of MI - Ann Arbor; Aud, Ephrata Public School 165, **SLP A**

Dell, Dr Carl W, Jr Eastern Illinois University, Speech Pathology & Aud, Charleston, IL 61920, (217) 581-2712, BA 67 Hope Coll; MA 74 Western MI Univ; PH 85 (Stuttering Sp) Bowling Green St Univ; Asst Prof, Eastern IL U, **SLP**

Dell, Elise Louise 1083 Michigan Drive #A, Harrisburg, PA 17111, (717) 737-6728, BA 82 Towson St Univ; MS 83 Towson St Univ; Sp-Lang Path, Capitol Area Inter Unit, **SLP**

Dell, Katherine 51 Chestnut Hill Road, Norwalk, CT 06851, (203) 847-5085, MS 78 Univ of MI - Ann Arbor; SLP, Norwalk Board of Education, **SLP**

Dell, Mrs Lynn Ann 318 Helen Drive, Chillicothe, IL 61523, (309) 672-6863, BS 80 Univ of IL - Urbana; MS 81 IL St Univ - Normal; Sp/Lang Path, Peoria Pub Sch & Dev Cen, **SLP**

Dell, Mrs Naomi R 1200 Gerrads Cross, Webster, NY 14580, BA 53 SUNY - Center at Buffalo; MS 74 SUNY - Coll at Geneseo; Sp-Lang Path, BOCES #1, **SLP**

Della Cava, Andrea 1427 Oneida Street #E-5, Utica, NY 13501, (315) 733-7957, BA 84 SUNY - Center at Binghamton; MS 86 Syracuse Univ; 88–Sp-Lang Path, Faxton-Children's Hosp & Rehab Ctr, **SLP**

Dell'Aira, Angel L 9 East Lakeshore Drive #22, Cincinnati, OH 45237, (513) 831-8487, BA 85 Univ of Cincinnati; MA 87 Univ of Cincinnati; Sp-Lang Path, Providence Hosp, **SLP**

Dell'Angelo, Denise Dominique P O Box 362, Waterford, CT 06385, (203) 447-0301, **SLP**

Dellapenna, Loren A 94 Homestead Avenue, Amityville, NY 11701, (516) 598-2668, MS 86 Adelphi Univ

Dellaria, Nancy Broadhurst 190 Waverly Court, Athens, GA 30606, (404) 534-5141, BS 82 Univ of GA; ME 84 Univ of GA; SLP, Northeast Georgia Speech Ctr, **SLP**

Dell'Aringa, Judith E 1420 Aber, Iowa City, IA 52240, (319) 335-8716, BS 81 Univ of IL - Urbana; MS 82 Univ of IL - Urbana; Clin Supvr, Univ of Iowa, **SLP**

Della Sala, Eugenia Valeria 12 Sebring Round, Belle Mead, NJ 08502, (201) 735-4031, MA 76 Seton Hall Univ; 78–Sp-Lang Path, Hunterdon Developmental Center, **SLP ACE**

Dellasanta, Mrs Marcia L 11532 Soda Springs Way, Gold River, CA 95670, (916) 631-0218, BA 77 CA St Univ - Sacramento; MA 81 CA St Univ - Sacramento; Sdl Teacher, Elk Grove USD, **SLP**

Dellecker, Cynthia M 83 Altadena Drive, Pittsburgh, PA 15228, (412) 647-5580, BS 79 PA St Univ - Univ Park; MS 80 PA St Univ - Univ Park; Aud, Chldrn's Hosp of Pitts, **A**

Dellegrotto, John T 1703 Kathryn Street, New Cumberland, PA 17070, (717) 737-6728, BS 72 Bloomsburg Univ of PA; ME 73 Bloomsburg Univ of PA; Instr Supvr, Capital Area Inter Unit, **SLP ACE**

Dellegrotto, Mrs Mary Anne 1703 Kathryn Street, New Cumberland, PA 17070, (717) 737-6728, BA 73 SUNY - Coll at Fredonia; MA 74 SUNY - Coll at Fredonia; Sp-Lang Path, Capital Area Iu, **SLP**

Dellenback, Cynthia H 4402 Vance Jackson, Suite 206, San Antonio, TX 78230, (512) 344-8179, BS 80 Univ of TX - Austin; MA 82 Univ of KS; Sp/Lang Path, Communication Associates, **SLP**

Dellibovi, Regina Marino 500-1C Auten Road, Hillsborough, NJ 08876

Dellicarpini, Mrs Carla J 24 Lee Avenue, Rockville Centre, NY 11570, (516) 321-3138, BA 75 SUNY - Coll at New Paltz; MS 76 Adelphi Univ; Sp-Lang Path, W Babylon Pub Sch, **SLP**

Dellinger, David H 8526 Storch Woods Drive, Apartment 2-C, Savage, MD 20763, (301) 498-8082, BA 79 Univ of MD - College Park; MA 81 Univ of MD - College Park; 81–Audiologist, US Army, **A**

Dellit, Pamela M 218 North 18th Street, Clinton, IA 52732, (319) 242-6454, BS 75 Univ of WI - Whitewater; OM 76 Univ of WI - Whitewater; 77–Sp-Lang Path, Mississippi Bend AEA, **SLP**

Delmonico, Rosslyn Jean 33267 Shelley Avenue, Abbotsford, BC, Canada V2S 1A6, (604) 853-0574, BA 80 Western WA Univ; MA 87 Western WA Univ; 88–Sp-Lang Path, Abbotsford Sch Dist

Delmonico, Mrs Terri A R 538 Miller Road, Wyckoff, NJ 07481, (201) 891-3476, BA 73 Montclair St Coll; MA 77 Montclair St Coll; SLP, Bergen County Special Services, **SLP**

De Loach, Betty Ann 6516 Longbrook #8, Memphis, TN 38134, (901) 761-1220, BS 83 Delta St Univ; MS 85 Univ of MS; Audiologist, Ear Nose & Throat Group Inc, **A**

Deloach, Michelle Logensie 5900 Culzean Drive, Apt 208, Dayton, OH 45426, (513) 376-8217, BS 85 Jackson St Univ; MA 87 OH St Univ; SLP, InSpeech Inc

De Long, Mrs Joan Nelson 7804 Kincardine Court, Alexandria, VA 22310, (703) 922-8433, BS 64 Eastern IL Univ; MS 65 IL St Univ - Normal; Sp-Lang Path, Fairfax County PS, **SLP**

Delong, Mrs Lisa F Route 4, Whitemans Gully Road, Dansville, NY 14437, (607) 776-2777, Sp-Lang Path, Stuben Allegany BOCES, **SLP**

Delong, Mrs Sally Ann 2130 Curran, Troy, MI 48098, (313) 476-4622, **A**

De Longa, Mary P 5105 Ravensworth Road, Annandale, VA 22003-5557, **SLP ACE**

Delongchamp, Mrs Kerri Joanne 5956 McKinley Drive, Garden Valley, CA 95633, (916) 333-2304, BA 83 CA St Univ - Chico; MA 85 CA St Univ - Chico

Delorenzis, Anne M 18521 Embury Drive, Santa Ana, CA 92705, (714) 558-5501, BA CA St Univ - Fullerton; MA 85 CA St Univ - Fullerton; **SLP**

DeLorenzo-Guinn, Mrs Therese 9205 Clendenen Way, Sacramento, CA 95826, (916) 454-8183, BA 75 Univ of the Pacific; MA 76 Univ of the Pacific; Sp-Lang Path, Sacramento City USD, **SLP**

Deloria, Anne Frances 1839 Springvale Drive, Crown Point, IN 46307, (312) 957-7100, BS 86 Western MI Univ; MA 87 Western MI Univ; 87–Sp-Lang Path, South Metropolitan Assoc, **SLP**

Delorier, Joseph R Speech And Hearing Clinic, Northern Illinois Univ, De Kalb, IL 60115, (815) 753-1481, BS 70 Northern IL Univ - De Kalb; MA 72 Northern IL Univ - De Kalb; Aud, Dept Commun Dis-Nn Il U, **A**

Delotto, Antoinette 921 East Crenshaw Street, Tampa, FL 33604, **SLP**

Delp, JoAnn Thomas 10892 Yakima Valley Highway, Zillah, WA 98953, (509) 865-4555, BA 83 Eastern WA Univ; MS 85 Eastern WA Univ; 87–Sp-Lang Path, Toppenish Sch Dist #202, **SLP**

Delplain, Robert C 15522 S E 49th Street, Bellevue, WA 98006, (206) 747-2279, BS 67 Brigham Young Univ; MS 69 Brigham Young Univ; Aud, Private Practice, **SLP A**

Del Polito, Dr Gene A 1919 Brightleaf Court, Silver Spring, MD 20902, (202) 347-0055, BA 68 Montclair St Coll; MS 70 Purdue Univ - West Lafayette; PH 72 (NS) Purdue Univ - West Lafayette; Exec Dir, Third Class Mail Assoc, **A**

Del Rosso, Darlene Kay 103 Heritage Road #1, Guilderland, NY 12084, (518) 869-6045, BS 82 Univ of WI - Madison; MS 84 Univ of WI - Madison; Sp-Lang Path, Sunnyview Hosp & Rehab Ctr, **SLP**

Delsack, Barbara Stern Rural Delivery 1, 2 Brown Court, Annandale, NJ 08801, (201) 725-4000, BA 78 Univ of MD - College Park; OM 80 Hahneman Medical Coll; 87–Sp-Lang Path, Mandel Speech Pathology Assoc, **SLP**

Del Toro, Janice Feagin 3320 Wall Boulevard #5-106, Gretna, LA 70056, (504) 361-4469, BA 81 Univ of FL; MA 87 Univ of FL; 87–Sp-Lang Path, Jefferson Parish PS Sys, **SLP**

Deltoro, Mrs Karalynne Pope 85 Davis Road, Chicopee, MA 01022, (413) 593-1016, BS 81 Northern AZ Univ; MS 83 ID St Univ; **SLP**

Deltuva, Mrs Janet M 16 Vern Lane, Buffalo, NY 14227, (716) 891-6433, BA 79 SUNY - Center at Buffalo; MA 81 SUNY - Center at Buffalo; Sp-Lang Path, Cheektowaga Sloan Sch Dist, **SLP ACE**

Deluca, Joseph A 43 Woolsey Street, Huntington, NY 11743, (516) 427-2258, BS 48 Southern CT St Univ; MA 56 Columbia Univ Teachers Coll; Sp-Lang Path, Private Practice, **SLP LM**

De Luca, Kathleen 149-09 Centreville Street, Ozone Park, NY 11417, (212) 847-4370, BA 74 CUNY - Queens Coll; MA 78 NY Univ; Sp/Lang Path, First Step Early Chldhood Cen, **SLP**

De Luca, Mrs Paula D 635A Country Lane, First Floor, Morton, PA 19070, (215) 237-4388, BS 75 IL St Univ - Normal; MS 76 Eastern IL Univ; 88–Dir, Mercy Catholic Med Ctr, **SLP**

De Luca, Renee Marie 1 Lisa Drive, Budd Lake, NJ 07828, (201) 876-3616, BA 81 Montclair St Coll; MA 86 Montclair St Coll; **SLP**

Deluca-Braccio, Virginia A 13033 La Mancha Street, La Mirada, CA 90638, (213) 868-0431, BS 73 SUNY - Center at Albany; MA 75 NY Univ; Sp-Lang Path, Norwalk-La Mirada Sch Dist, **SLP**

De Lucenay, Mrs Cynthia Darlene 1317 Fishermans Road, Norfolk, VA 23503, (919) 232-2223, BS 81 Old Dominion Univ; MS 83 Old Dominion Univ; 84–Sp-Lang Path, Currituck Co Pub Sch, **SLP**

Delude, Mrs Nancy L 10 Winterberry Lane, Seekonk, MA 02771, (617) 675-2785, BS 77 Worcester St Coll; ME 83 Northeastern Univ; 78–Sp-Lang Path, Somerset Sch Dept, **SLP**

De Lullo, Dianne Marie 540 1/2 E King Street, Chambersburg, PA 17201, (717) 267-7720, BS 85 Edinboro Univ of PA; MA 86 Edinboro Univ of PA; SLP, Chambersburg Hosp, **SLP**

Del Val, Erica 6001 Auburn Street #147, Bakersfield, CA 93306, (805) 398-3799, BA 80 Pacific Univ; MS 81 Univ of WI - Eau Claire; Sp-Lang Path, Kern Co Supt of Sch, **SLP**

Del Vecchio, Ruth Bretan 89-50 56th Avenue #3-K, Elmhurst, NY 11373, (212) 429-1682, BS 70 Emerson Coll; MA 71 NY Univ; **SLP**

Demaio, Mrs Diane Dunhoff 2901-A South Woodstock St, Arlington, VA 22206, (202) 475-4440, BA 67 Boston Univ; MA 68 Columbia Univ Teachers Coll; Admin / Prog Dir, United Testing Svc, **SLP**

DeMaio, Dr Louis J 801 South 6th Street, Fargo, ND 58103, (218) 236-4643, BS 68 Brescia Coll; MA 72 Montclair St Coll; PH 80 (NS) Southern IL Univ -Carbondale; Assoc Prof, Moorhead St U, **SLP**

Demakis, Marianne McDonald 243 Larchmont Lane, Hanover, MA 02339, (617) 588-2088, **SLP**

Deman, Jill Susan 3522 Hunter, Royal Oak, MI 48073, (313) 286-8800, BS 83 Wayne St Univ; MA 86 Wayne St Univ; **SLP**

Demarco, Mrs Ann W 168 Sergeantsville Road, Flemington, NJ 08822, (609) 394-4177, BS 79 Bloomsburg Univ of PA; MS 80 Bloomsburg Univ of PA; Sp/Lang Path, Mercer Med Cen, **SLP**

Demarco, Mrs Kathy Clarkson 49 Plymouth Dr, Tonawanda, NY 14150, (716) 837-2441, BS 84 SUNY - Coll at Geneseo; MS 87 SUNY - Coll at Buffalo

Demarco, Salvatore 622 South Elm Street, Greenville, NC 27834, **SLP**

Demaree, Gina L 2801 Shanmor, Cincinnati, OH 45212-4037, (513) 351-7878, BS 82 Univ of Cincinnati; MA 84 Univ of Cincinnati; 86–Sp-Lang Path, SpeechPath, **SLP**

Demaris, Mrs Terri M West 10410 Granger Road, Nine Mile Falls, WA 99026-9627, (509) 353-3796, BA 72 Eastern WA Univ; MS 73 Eastern WA Univ; 81–Sp-Lang Path, Spokane PS Dist #81, **SLP**

Demars, Sally S P O Box 493, Storrs, CT 06268, (203) 429-1682, BA 70 Univ of MA - Amherst; MS 73 Univ of RI; **SLP**

Demars, Virginia Ella 5038 West Jupiter Way, Chandler, AZ 85226, MS 82 Univ of WI - River Falls; Sp-Lang Path, Private Practice, **SLP**

De Martino, Edna M R 2270 North Avenue, Westfield, NJ 07090, **SLP**

DeMartino, Karen A 114 Martin Road, Rd #9, Hopewell Junction, NY 12533, (914) 831-3500, BS 84 Ithaca Coll; MS 85 Bloomsburg Univ of PA; 86–Sp-Lang Path, St Francis Hosp, **SLP**

De Masi, Cheryl Drumheiser 117 South Woodstock Drive, Cherry Hill, NJ 08034, (609) 795-8531, MS 87 PA St Univ - Univ Park; SLP, Sunny Day School Treatment Ctr

De Matteo, Mrs Annette P 4575 Clearview Drive, Canfield, OH 44406, (216) 744-7324, BS 73 Carlow Coll; MA 80 Kent St Univ; 77–Sp-Lang Path, Youngstown Cty Sch, **SLP**

Demb, Nancy L 4611 Morgan Drive, Chevy Chase, MD 20815, (301) 654-1984, BA 77 IN Univ - Bloomington; MA 78 IN Univ - Bloomington; Sp/Lang Path, Montgy Co Pub Sch, **SLP**

Dembeck, Pamela Mary PSC #1 Box 21846, APO San Francisco, CA 96230, BA 82 MI St Univ; MA 84 MI St Univ; 88 Sp-Lang Path, Dept of Defense Dependents Sch, **SLP ACE**

Dembner, Mrs Elissa C 53 Hartshore Way, Parlin, NJ 08859, BS 76 Eastern MI Univ; MA 77 Eastern MI Univ; Sp-Lang Path, New Hyde Park-O School Dist, **SLP**

Demby, Linda Ann 5 Lyric Court, Sicklerville, NJ 08081, (609) 768-1473, BA 72 Long Island U - CW Post Ctr; MS 73 Columbia Univ Teachers Coll

Demchak, Mary Ann Perry 52 Rittenhouse Court, Wayne, PA 19087, (215) 889-0499, **SLP**

Demchuk, Mrs Marcia Karen 296 Torresdale Avenue #18, Willowdale, ON, Canada M2R 3N3, (416) 663-1142, BA 70 982; MS 72 982; 87–Sp-Lang Path, Private Practice, **SLP**

Demello, Mrs Corazon Nievera 94-1479 Waipio Uka Blvd, F-103, Waipahu, HI 96797, (808) 677-0435, BS 81 Univ of HI - Manoa; MS 82 Univ of HI - Manoa; Sp-Lang Path, Central Oahu Dept of Ed, **SLP**

Demello, Mrs Sharon L 8713 Falkstone Lane, Alexandria, VA 22309, (703) 360-7928, BS 70 Boston St Coll; MS 72 Syracuse Univ; Tchr & Sp Consult, Mt Vernon Weekday Sch, **SLP**

DeMers, Mrs Gayle Hare 5017 Mayview Road, Minnetonka, MN 55345, (612) 347-2675, BS 75 Miami Univ - Oxford; MA 77 Memphis St Univ; 86–Sp-Lang Path, Henn Co Med Ctr, **SLP**

Demers, Margaret Hoey 12 Oakdale Drive, R R #1 Box 104, Peru, NY 12972, (518) 562-1614, BA 71 Univ of MD - College Park; MS 83 Univ of NH

Demetras, Dr Martha Jo-Ann University Of Arizona, Division Of Spec Ed/Rehab, College Of Education, Tucson, AZ 85721, (602) 621-5890, BS 75 Univ of UT; MS 79 Univ of AZ; **SLP**

Demetrion-Boatright, Helen 3694 Meyers Road, San Bernardino, CA 92404, (714) 988-5560, BA 78 Univ of LA Verne; MS 82 Univ of Redlands; Sp-Lang Path, Hk Demetrion Boatright, **SLP**

Demetros, Mrs Cheryl Irene 2 East Willow Street, Beacon, NY 12508, (914) 831-6370, BA 79 Univ of CT; MA 82 Univ of CT; **SLP**

De Micco, Lisa Jane 27 Huntington Circle #2-G, Peekskill, NY 10566, (914) 736-7214, BA 83 CUNY - Lehman Coll; MA 85 CUNY - Lehman Coll; Sp-Lang Path, Blythedale Chldrns Hosp, **SLP**

Deming, Mrs Jeanne Marie 44 Center Grove Road #L-38, Randolph, NJ 07869, (201) 989-0397, BA 83 Rutger's St Univ - Douglas Coll; MS 85 PA St Univ - Univ Park; Sp-Lang Path, Kessler Inst for Rehabilitatn, **SLP**

deMink-LeDuc, Julaine Elizabeth 1400 White Street, Ann Arbor, MI 48104, (313) 769-9453, BA 80 Univ of MI - Ann Arbor; MS 82 Univ of MI - Ann Arbor; Sp-Lang Path, St Joseph Mercy Hosp, **SLP**

Deminoff, Anne Louise One Mill Street, Mailbox #019, Dover, NH 03820, (603) 749-0116, BA 78 Grinnell Coll; MA 88 Univ of IL - Urbana

Demko, Karen L 2170 Village West Dr North, Lapeer, MI 48446, **SLP**

Demko, Sharon R 2120 Queens Drive #B-2, Harrisburg, PA 17110, (717) 737-6728, BS 83 Bloomsburg Univ of PA; MS 84 Bloomsburg Univ of PA; Sp-Lang Path, Polyclinic Med Ctr, **SLP**

Demler, Jane W M 1638 Hawthorne Lane, Glenview, IL 60025, (312) 998-9373, BA 76 Miami Univ - Oxford; MA 77 Kent St Univ; Sp/Lang Path, W Northfield Sch Dist #31, **SLP**

Demler, Mrs Mary McDermott 105 East Cypress, Redlands, CA 92373, (714) 793-7680, MS 88 Univ of Redlands

Demmert, Karen R 7257 N E 158th, Bothell, WA 98011, (206) 488-0597, BS 81 Univ of WA; MA 83 Western WA Univ; SLP, Edmonds Sch Dist #15, **SLP**

Demo-Anderson, Laura 1864 North Winds Drive, Winston-Salem, NC 27107, (919) 773-3779, BS 81 Univ of TN - Knoxville; MA 83 Univ of TN - Knoxville; Sp-Lang Path, Forsythe Memorial Hospital, **SLP**

Demond, Elizabeth Lambert 410 Orchard Road, Newark, DE 19711, (302) 454-2142, BS 72 PA St Univ - Univ Park; MA 75 Univ of MD - College Park; SLP, Christina School District, **SLP ACE**

Demore, Janice Elaine 1049 3rd Street, Hermosa Beach, CA 90254, (213) 318-2060, **SLP**

Demorest, Dr Marilyn Elizabeth Department Of Psychology UMBC, 5401 Wilkens Avenue, Catonsville, MD 21228, (301) 455-2364, BA 65 Trinity Coll; MA 67 Johns Hopkins Univ; PH 69 (Psychology) Johns Hopkins Univ; Assoc Prof, U of MD

Demoss, Mrs Wendelyn L 3105 Shadybrook, Midwest City, OK 73110, (405) 272-5594, BA 85 Univ of OK - Norman; MS 85 Univ of OK Medical Center; **SLP**

Demott, Anne 1000 Elmwood Avenue, Rochester, NY 14620, (716) 271-0680, MS 79 PA St Univ - Univ Park; Aud, Hrng & Sp Ctr, **A**

Demott, Dr Lois E 45 Ackerman Avenue, Oradell, NJ 07649, (201) 499-5751, BA 67 William Paterson Coll; MA 69 Seton Hall Univ; PH 78 (Comm and Severely Retarded) Temple Univ; Dir of Spec Educ, Woodbridge Dev Ctr, **SLP**

Dempesy-Hart, Deborah 55 Cliff Avenue 2nd Floor, Winthrop, MA 02152, (617) 735-3171, BA 74 Beloit Coll; MA 82 Northwestern Univ; Aud, Beth Israel Hosp, **A**

Demps, Mrs Karen Nelson 5447 New Park Road, White Hall, MD 21161, (301) 398-0400, BS 77 Indiana Univ of PA; MS 82 IN St Univ - Terre Haute; Sp-Lang Path, Cecil Co Pub Sch, **SLP ACE**

Dempsey, Dr James J 6 Willowtree Place, South Huntington, NY 11746, (516) 673-7244, BA 77 CUNY - Queens Coll; MS 78 PA St Univ - Univ Park; PH 82 (NS) Univ of CT; Asst Prof/Dept/Sp/Comm/Theatre, St John's Univ, **A**

Dempsey, Mrs June M 66 Gevers Deynootwet, Le Hague, Netherlands 2586, BA 73 Univ of TX - El Paso; MA 75 Univ of Houston - Univ Park; **SLP**

Dempsey, Mrs Stacy P 687 Bocage Lane, Mandeville, LA 70448, (504) 831-9706, BA 69 Our Lady Lake Univ-San Anton; MA 70 Our Lady Lake Univ-San Anton; Sp-Lang Path, Private Practice, **SLP**

Dempster, Mrs Del O 498 Hollydale Drive, Pittsburgh, PA 15241, (412) 394-5744, BS 75 Bowling Green St Univ; MS 79 Univ of Pittsburgh - Pittsburgh; Sp-Lang Path, Allegheny Inter Ut, **SLP**

Demuniz, Karen Anne 5215 Ben Avenue #3, North Hollywood, CA 91607, (213) 222-0148, BA 80 CA St Univ - Northridge; MA 86 CA St Univ - Northridge; **SLP**

De Narie, Mrs Mary Young 1609 Fairhill Place, Clementon, NJ 08021, (609) 783-1140, BS 78 Trenton St Coll; MA 80 Trenton St Coll; 85–Sp-Lang Path, Gibbsboro Sch Dist, **SLP**

Dendinger, Marcia Lynn 9525 Oak Stream Court, Fairfax Station, VA 22039, (703) 690-7453, BA 77 Boston Coll; MS 79 Emerson Coll; SLP, **SLP**

Dendiu, Paula D ENT Head & Neck Surgeons Inc, 3545 Olentangy River Road, Suite 525, Columbus, OH 43214, (614) 267-2587, BA 74 OH St Univ; MA 76 Kent St Univ; Aud, ENT Head & Neck Surgeons Inc, **A**

Denekas, Mrs Susan W 15 Kingswood Drive, Belle Mead, NJ 08502, (201) 359-2185, BA 68 CUNY - Brooklyn Coll; MA 70 Univ of Southern CA; Sp-Lang Path, Private Practice, **SLP**

Denenberg, Mary E E 1275 Montgomery Avenue, Wynnewood, PA 19096, (215) 339-4276, BS 77 East Stroudsburg Univ of PA; MS 79 Hahneman Medical Coll; **SLP**

Dengerink, Joan E Washington State University, 213 Daggy Hall, Pullman, WA 99163, BA 64 Calvin Coll; MA 76 WA St Univ; Asst Prof, WA St U, **SLP A**

Dengler, Judith 1 East River Road #527, Tucson, AZ 85704, (602) 293-8364, BA 65 Univ of Northern IA; MS 68 CO St Univ; Tchr, Saddleback Valley USD, **SLP**

Denham, Linda 527 South Crossley, Detroit, MI 48209, **A**

Denham, Patricia Gail 30 King Arthur Road, North Easton, MA 02356, (617) 775-6240, BS 77 SUNY - Coll at Buffalo; ME 82 Northeastern Univ; Sp-Lang Path, Cape Cod Chld Dev Prog Inc, **SLP**

De Nicola, Mrs Barbara Catherine 93 Cherry Lane, Hecksville, NY 11801, (516) 797-7346, BA 80 SUNY - Coll at Cortland; MS 85 Adelphi Univ; **SLP**

De Nil, Luc F 41B University Houses, Madison, WI 53705, (618) 549-0568, MS 88 Southern IL Univ -Carbondale

De Ninno, Joanne Patricia 42 Westgate Road, Massapequa Park, NY 11762, (516) 799-2922, BS 72 SUNY - Coll at Fredonia; MS 74 CUNY - Brooklyn Coll; Sp/Lang Path, Massapequa Public Schools, **SLP**

Denison, Dr Joyce 2600 Kentucky Avenue, Salt Lake City, UT 84117, (801) 581-2260, BA 50 Univ of MI - Ann Arbor; MA 55 Univ of MI - Ann Arbor; PH 71 (NS) Univ of UT; SLP/Aud, U of UT Med Cen, **SLP A**

Denison, Marsha Figg 503 East Street, Chelsea, MI 48118, (313) 482-8710, BS 74 Western MI Univ; MA 79 Eastern MI Univ; SLP, Lincoln Consolidated Sch, **SLP**

Denison, Peter B 356 Kaufman Road, Somerset, MA 02726, (617) 252-3311, BA 50 Yale Univ; MA 53 Northwestern Univ; Sp-Lang Path, Rehoboth Sch Dept, **SLP ACE**

Denk, Mrs Renee Ritchie 5706 Piping Rock Road, Madison, WI 53711, (608) 271-1323, BA 81 Univ of WI - Eau Claire; MS 83 Univ of WI - Eau Claire; SLP, Dakota Inc, **SLP**

Denker, Nancy B 410 Richmond Place N E, Albuquerque, NM 87106, (505) 256-3264, BA 73 Univ of MA - Amherst; MS 80 Univ of NM; SLP, Private Practice, **SLP**

Denkinger, Sandra G 3915 Laro Court, Fairfax, VA 22031, (703) 978-5838, OB 63 Univ of FL; MS 66 Univ of MI - Ann Arbor; **SLP**

Denman, Mrs Edna A 2516 Harvey, Mc Allen, TX 78501, (512) 686-4871, BA 74 Univ of Houston - Univ Park; MA 75 Univ of Houston - Univ Park; Sp-Lang Path, McAllen ISD, **SLP**

Denmeade, Patti Buell Rd 2 Box 282, Cincinnatus, NY 13040, (607) 756-7668, BA 85 SUNY - Coll at Cortland; MS 86 Ithaca Coll; **SLP**

Denne, Mrs Claire M 109 Hutchinson Drive, North East, PA 16428, (814) 870-7070, BA 80 Allegheny Coll; MS 81 Clarion Univ of PA; Sp-Lang Path, Community Rehab Specialist,Inc, **SLP**

Dennehy, Mrs Jane G 8 Signal Court, Dayton, NJ 08810, (201) 329-6460, MS 83 Columbia Univ Teachers Coll; Sp-Lang Path, Staten Island Hosp, **SLP**

Denneny, Rebecca Jane 260 Cricklewood Circle, Lansdale, PA 19446, (215) 822-3076, BA 83 Temple Univ; MA 85 Temple Univ; 88–Sp-Lang Path, North Penn Hosp, **SLP**

Denney, Janet M 1191 High Street, Eugene, OR 97401, (503) 342-1155, BA 75 CA Poly St Univ-San Luis Obi; BS 79 CA St Univ - Hayward; MS 81 Univ of San Francisco; SLP, Private Practice, **SLP**

Dennie, Mrs Helen Marcopoulos 130 Tidal Drive, Newport News, VA 23606, (804) 727-7168, BS 80 Univ of VA - Charlottesville; ME 82 Univ of VA - Charlottesville; 86–Aud, Sentara Hampton Gen Hosp, **A**

Dennin, Rebecca Ann 126 Cedar Street, Carlisle, PA 17013, (717) 737-6728, BS 82 Bloomsburg Univ of PA; MS 83 Bloomsburg Univ of PA; Sp-Lang Path, Capital Area Intermediate Unit, **SLP**

Denning, Jacqueline Ann 2321 Geneva Street, Racine, WI 53402, (414) 632-8778, BS 84 Univ of WI - Stevens Point; MS 87 Univ of WI - Whitewater; 88–Sp-Lang Path, Racine USD

Denning, Mrs Susan Whitener 4600 Lancashire Drive, Raleigh, NC 27612, (919) 755-6980, BS 74 Appalachian St Univ; MS 76 East Carolina Univ; SLP, Wake Co Pub Sch, **SLP**

Dennis, Mrs Cassandra Chavez 1006-A Crockett, Lockhart, TX 78644-3208, (512) 672-6592, BA 86 Abilene Christian Univ; MS 88 TX Christian Univ; 88–Sp-Lang Path, Warm Springs Rehab Hosp, **F**

Dennis, Elaine A 11137 Black Forest Way, Gaithersburg, MD 20879, (301) 443-2512, MS 77; Sp-Lang Path, US Public Health Service, **SLP**

Dennis, Dr J Michael 3424 Hemlock Lane, Oklahoma City, OK 73120, (405) 271-8046, BA 65 ID St Univ; MS 66 CO St Univ; PH 72 Univ of OK Medical Center; Vice Head Dept Orl, Dept Orl Ouhsc, **A**

Dennis, Janet B 580 S E Corliss Avenue, Corvallis, OR 97333, (503) 753-1322, BA 74 OR St Univ; MA 75 OR St Univ; SLP, Philomath Sch Dist 17J, **SLP**

Dennis, Joanne Mary 1122 East Sylvan Avenue, Whitefish Bay, WI 53217, (414) 383-4490, BS 62 Univ of WI - Milwaukee; MS 67 Univ of WI - Milwaukee; OM 78 (NS) Univ of WI - Milwaukee; 86–Mgr Dept of SLP, Sacred Heart Rehab Hosp, **SLP**

Dennis, Mrs Judith W 3424 Hemlock Lane, Oklahoma City, OK 73120, (405) 755-3893, BS 65 CO St Univ; MS 66 CO St Univ; Sp-Lang Path, Private Practice, **SLP**

Dennis, Dr Kyle C VA Westside Medical Center, Audiology & Sp Path Service (126), PO Box 8195, Chicago, IL 60680, (312) 633-2169, BA 74 Tulane Univ; MS 77 Tulane Univ; PH 87 (Aud) Northwestern Univ; Aud, VA Westside Med Ctr, **A**

Dennis, Mrs Laura Godbold 6040 Camelot Court, Montgomery, AL 36117, (205) 279-0625, BS 85 Auburn Univ - Auburn; MS 87 Univ of Montevallo; SLP, Montgomery Public School Sys

Dennis, Mary E 3820 St Charles Avenue #F, New Orleans, LA 70115, (504) 835-2561, BS 75 Saint Mary's Dominican Coll; OM 77 LA St Univ - N O Medical Ctr; Sp-Lang Path, Jefferson Parish Pub Sch Syst, **SLP**

Dennis, Richard A 11268 Signal Ridge Drive, El Paso, TX 79936-1222, (915) 569-2065, BA 70 Eastern NM Univ; MA 72 Univ of NM; Dir, U S Army, **A**

Dennis, Susan Elizabeth 400 North Emerald Road, Apartment #D-2, Greenwood, SC 29646-3063, (803) 223-4862, BA 83 Auburn Univ - Montgomery; MA 84 Univ of TN - Knoxville; 85–Aud, St Nicholas Speech & Hearing Ctr, **A**

Dennis, Susan Gay RFD 8 Box 286-C, Concord, NH 03301, (603) 267-6025, **SLP**

Dennis, Mrs Suzanne Garcia 912 North Guadalupe Street, Carlsbad, NM 88220, (505) 887-2821, BS 77 Bloomsburg Univ of PA; MS 78 Bloomsburg Univ of PA; Sp-Lang Path, Carlsbad Mun Schs, **SLP ACE**

Dennis, Mrs Teresa Agnew 20 Ferndale Avenue, Ferndale, MD 21061, (301) 760-1297, BS 78 James Madison Univ; MS 80 Towson St Univ; Sp-Lang Path, Anne Arundel County Schools, **SLP**

Dennison, Beth Ann 4783 Norstar Boulevard, Bldg 3 #315, Liverpool, NY 13088, (315) 445-0709, BS 76 Elmira Coll; MA 77 Ball St Univ; 81–Sp-Lang Path, Onondaga-Cortland-Madison BOCES, **SLP**

Dennison, Mrs Kelly Hamilton Rural Route 1 Box 170, Albers, IL 62215, BS 84 Southern IL Univ-Edwardsvill; MS 85 Southern IL Univ-Edwardsvill; Sp-Lang Path, Spec Sch Dist of St Louis Co, **SLP**

Dennison, Laura L Las Colinas Office Center, 5525 Macarthur Boulevard, Suite 600, Irving, TX 75038, BS 68 Univ of NM; MA 72 Emerson Coll; OM 78 Univ of Miami; SLP, Private Practice, **SLP**

Dennler, Mrs Debra J 1602 Darby Road, Goldsboro, NC 27530, (509) 458-6203, BS 76 IA St Univ; MA 78 Saint Louis Univ; Assistant Professor, Eastern Washington U, **SLP**

Denny, Joan Marie 1451 Fairhaven Boulevard, Elm Grove, WI 53122, (414) 782-8454, BS 84 Marquette Univ; MA 85 Western MI Univ; **SLP**

Denny, Marcia C 286 Anita Terrace Court #205, Antioch, IL 60002, (312) 395-4631, BS 85 IL St Univ - Normal; MA 86 Northern IL Univ - De Kalb; 86–Sp-Lang Path, Spec Educ Dist of Lake County, **SLP**

Denny, Mrs Martha Q 18-13 Minami-Senju, Arakawa Ku, Tokyo, Japan 116, MS; **SLP LM**

Denny, Mary L S 5017 Harvey, Western Springs, IL 60558, (312) 246-9023, BS 73 Univ of MO - Columbia; MS 79 Central MO St Univ; Sp-Lang Path, Dist 102, **SLP**

Densmore, Ann 9 Roanoke Road, Wellesley, MA 02181, (617) 235-6974, BS 63 Univ of CA - Los Angeles; MA 74 CA St Univ - Northridge; Aud/Sp-Lang Path, Private Practice, **SLP A**

Densmore, Ann E 2293 Winding Brook Court, Bloomington, IN 47401, (812) 335-6251, BS 66 Univ of WI - Oshkosh; MA 71 Northern IL Univ - De Kalb; Dir, IN U, **SLP**

Densmore, Cynthia George 2488 South Wisner Road, Fremont, MI 49412, (616) 757-3716, BA 81 MI St Univ; MA 82 MI St Univ; Sp-Lang Path, Mason-Lake Indep School Dist, **SLP**

Denson, Anna Haines 4333 Rebecca Avenue, Charlotte, NC 28208-6728, (704) 343-6815, BS 82 Appalachian St Univ; MA 84 Appalachian St Univ; 84–Sp-Lang Path, Charlotte/Mecklenburg Sch Sys, **SLP**

Dent, Dr Ruth I 3568 Palmerston Road, Shaker Heights, OH 44122, (212) 681-3810, BS 66 Wayne St Univ; MS 68 Wayne St Univ; PH 74 (NS) Wayne St Univ; Director, Cleveland City School District, **SLP**

Dentino, Monica Dixon 64 Claremont Avenue, Tonawanda, NY 14223, (716) 885-8318, MA 85 Kent St Univ; Aud, Buffalo Hearing and Speech, **A**

Denton, Mrs Carolyn Jo 4649 South Jewell, Springfield, MO 65807, (417) 864-3607, **SLP**

Denton, David R 37 Trenridge Road, Lincoln, NE 68505, (402) 466-2109, OB 73 Univ of Miami; MA 75 Our Lady Lake Univ-San Anton; Sp-Lang Path, VA Med Cen, **SLP**

Denton, Mrs Elisabeth 1037 Pinon Lane, Carlsbad, NM 88220, BS 45 Univ of IL - Urbana; MA 56 Univ of IL - Urbana; Sp-Lang Path, Carlsbad Schs, **SLP**

Denton, Elizabeth Muddiman 311 23rd Avenue North, Nashville, TN 37203, (615) 327-9313, BS 83 Univ of VA - Charlottesville; MS 85 Vanderbilt Univ; 88–Sp-Lang Path, Metropolitan Health Dept, **SLP**

Denton, Rebecca Bennert 1134 Conlon S E, Grand Rapids, MI 49506, (616) 957-5971, BS 79 Central MI Univ; MA 81 Central MI Univ; **SLP**

Denton, Sandra Sue 1175 Albion Street, Apartment 113, Denver, CO 80220, (303) 377-8530, BS 85 CO St Univ; MS 87 Univ of North TX; Aud, Center for Hearing Speech & L, **A**

Denton, Mrs Susan F 4749 Idlewild Road, Salt Lake City, UT 84124, (801) 273-2065, BA 67 Western WA Univ; MA 70 Western WA Univ; Prin, Granite Sch Dist, **SLP**

Deolalikar, Padmaja Anil 2030-G South Street, Philadelphia, PA 19146, (215) 732-7999, BS 80 Bombay Univ - India; MS 83 Univ of OK - OK City; 88–Aud, Culotta & Gallagher ENT, **A**

Depalma, Mrs Janet 138-B Woodstock Street, Crystal Lake, IL 60014, (815) 459-2559, BS 79 Northern IL Univ - De Kalb; MA 80 Northern IL Univ - De Kalb; Aud, Nwm Il Assn, **A**

De Paolo, Kathleen M 16-G Cedar Court, East Haven, CT 06513, (203) 783-3527, BS 70 Central CT St Univ; MS 75 Southern CT St Univ; Sp-Lang Path, Milford Bd of Ed, **SLP**

Depape, Donna J Communication Aids Sys Clinic, 1500 Highland Avenue, Room S 120, Madison, WI 53706, (608) 263-7726, BA 71 Univ of Manitoba - Winnipeg; MS 73 Univ of WI - Madison; Clinic Head, Univ of WI-Hospital & Clinic, **SLP**

Depasquale, Mrs Jessie Devlin 3054 South Abingdon Street, Arlington, VA 22206-1615, (703) 931-0940, BS 67 Towson St Univ; ME 69 Univ of VA - Charlottesville; **SLP**

Depasquale, Maria C 98 Lafayette Avenue, Brooklyn, NY 11237, (212) 879-8157, BS 84 Syracuse Univ; MS 87 CUNY - Brooklyn Coll; **SLP**

Depaul, Roxanne 1508 Capital Avenue, Madison, WI 53705, (414) 472-5203, BA 74 CUNY - Brooklyn Coll; MS 77 Columbia Univ Teachers Coll; Instr, Univ of Wisconsin-Whitewater, **SLP**

De Paz, Brunilda Gomzalez 709 N W 84th Street, Gainesville, FL 32607, (904) 332-6765, MA 87 Univ of FL

Deperno, Denise 35 Oak Street #B1, Brewster, NY 10509, (203) 355-3793, BS 77 Elmira Coll; MS 79 Columbia Univ Teachers Coll; Sp-Lang Path, Sherman Sch, **SLP**

Depetro, William A Box 127, Kandiyohi, MN 56251, (612) 235-4613, BS 67 Peru St Coll; MS 68 Univ of NE - Omaha; Sp-Lang Path, W Ctrl Comm Serv Cen, **SLP**

De Pew, Mrs Teresa J Route 2 Box 253, Kennett, MO 63857, (314) 792-3550, OB 76 AR St Univ; MS 80 AR St Univ; 76–Sp/Lang Path, Holcomb R-3 Sch, **SLP**

De Pola, Mrs Adeline S 15418 Peach Orchard Road, Silver Spring, MD 20904, (301) 384-9191, BA 69 Univ of FL; MA 72 Univ of CT; Sp-Lang Path, Montgomery County Pub Schools, **SLP**

Depola, John J 15418 Peach Orchard Road, Silver Spring, MD 20904, (301) 649-6400, BA 70 SUNY - Center at Albany; MA 72 Univ of CT; Comptr Prog, Bd of Ed-Montgy Co, **SLP**

De Pompei, Galvin John 3840 Kent Road, Stow, OH 44224, ME 70 Kent St Univ; SLP, Cuyahoga Falls City Schools, **SLP**

De Pompei, Mrs Roberta F 3840 Kent Road, Stow, OH 44224, (216) 375-7884, BS 64 Kent St Univ; MA 69 Kent St Univ; Assoc Prof, U of Akron, **SLP A ACE**

De Poto, Mrs June M 580 Middletown Avenue, North Haven, CT 06473, (203) 239-5545, BA 66 Muhlenberg Coll; MS 68 Syracuse Univ; Aud, Zenith Hrng Aid Cen, **A**

Deppe, Janet A 1646 10th Avenue, San Francisco, CA 94122, (415) 759-0665, BS 76 Univ of MO - Columbia; MS 78 Southern IL Univ-Edwardsvill; Prgm Director Spec Infant Svcs, San Francisco State Univ, **SLP**

Deppensmith, Kathryn McDonald 131 Kinross, San Antonio, TX 78209, (512) 221-5773, BA Univ of San Francisco; MS 80 Univ of San Francisco; **A**

Deppler-Smith, Dr Doreen D 1740 Willow Creek Road, Paso Robles, CA 93446, (805) 543-7732, BS 52 Univ of CA - Santa Barbara; MA 72 Univ of CA - Santa Barbara; ED 82 (NS) Brigham Young Univ; Coord/Curriculum & Instruc, San Luis Obispo Co Supt's Offi, **SLP**

De Priest, Donald Lee 855 Smith Avenue, Marshfield, MO 65706, (417) 468-3326, BA 62 Coll of the Ozarks; MA 87 Southwest MO St Univ; **SLP**

Depriest, June M 302 Longwood Drive, Clinton, MS 39056

Deptula, Patrick M 700 East Brighton Avenue, Syracuse, NY 13205, (315) 469-5561, BS 72 Syracuse Univ; MS 73 Syracuse Univ; Exec VP, Loretto Geriatric Cen, **A**

Depue, Mrs Deborah Guidry 11705 Mercy Blvd, Savannah, GA 31419, (912) 927-5490, BA 77 Univ of Southwestern LA; MA 78 Bowling Green St Univ; 81–Sp-Lang Path, St Josephs Hosp, **SLP**

Deputy, Dr Paul N Dept Speech Path & Audiology, Idaho State University, Box 8116, Pocatello, ID 83209, (208) 236-3495, BA 71 CA St Univ - Fullerton; MA 72 CA St Univ - Fullerton; PH 78 (Sp Path Phonology) MI St Univ; 82–Assoc Prof, Idaho State Univ, **SLP**

Depuy, Mrs Mabel B 580 Hunt Avenue, Red Bluff, CA 96080, (916) 527-2307, BA 73 CA St Univ - Chico; MA 74 CA St Univ - Chico; Sp-Lang Path, Colusa County Supt of Schools, **SLP**

Dera, Dawn C 13139 New Parkland Drive, Herndon, VA 22071-2675, (703) 378-8674, BS 80 SUNY - Coll at Geneseo; MS 81 Syracuse Univ; Sp-Lang Path, Fairfax County Public Schools, **SLP**

Deranger, Mrs Cynthia A 311 West Tennis Street, Opelousas, LA 70570, (318) 942-4892, BA 74 Northeast LA Univ; MS 78 Univ of Southwestern LA; SLP, St Landry Parish Sch Bd, **SLP**

Deranleau, Madeleine T 54 Webster Court, Newington, CT 06111, (203) 563-8181, BA 63 Saint Joseph Coll; MS 74 Southern CT St Univ; Sp-Lang Path, Wethersfield Bd of Ed, **SLP**

Deranleau-Urban, Lisa Catherine 2014 Ivy Lane, Mount Prospect, IL 60056, (312) 438-6319, BS 86 Marquette Univ; MS 87 Marquette Univ

Derenzo, Adrianne C 18 Grant Lane, Wayne, PA 19087, (215) 964-8489, BA 70 CUNY - Queens Coll; MA 71 CUNY - Queens Coll; Dir, Speech Pathology Serv, **SLP**

Derga, Kathleen E 256 Broken Fence Drive, Medina, OH 44256, (216) 835-6160, BS 78 Bowling Green St Univ; MA 79 Kent St Univ; Sp-Lang Path, Westlake Hearing & Speech Clinic, **SLP**

Derkacz-Bolen, Mrs Mary Ann 31242 West Rutland, Birmingham, MI 48009, (313) 646-3521, BS 83 Central MI Univ; MA 85 Wayne St Univ; Sp-Lang Path, William Beaumont Hosp-Children's Svcs, **SLP**

Derk-Gans, Dr Karen 2005 Skyview Lane, Kent, OH 44240, (216) 673-6524, BS 73 Kent St Univ; MA 75 Kent St Univ; PH 83 (Special Education) Kent St Univ; 83–Dir, Kent Behavioral Studies & Res, **SLP**

Derks, Jane A 8581 Camp Awana Road, Fredonia, WI 53021, (414) 692-2554, BS 66 Univ of WI - Stevens Point; MA 75 Univ of WI - Milwaukee; Sp-Lang Path, West Bend Pub Sch, **SLP**

Derleth, Mrs Denyce A 516 Sweetbriar Lane, Watertown, WI 53094, (414) 261-4461, BS 85 Univ of WI - Whitewater; MS 87 Univ of WI - Whitewater

Derman, Sheila K 3340 Maple Leaf, Glenview, IL 60025, (312) 878-8200, BA 63 Univ of MI - Ann Arbor; MS 64 Univ of MI - Ann Arbor; Sp-Lang Path, Swedish Covenant Hosp, **SLP**

Dermody, Mrs Joan A 34572 Camino Capistrano, Capistrano Beach, CA 92624, (714) 581-2800, BA 60 Univ of Redlands; MA 70 CA St Univ - Fullerton; Dir of SLP, Newport Lang-Sp & Aud Cen, **SLP**

Dermody, Lynn Ann 203 Dianne Place, St Rose, LA 70087, (504) 469-6070, BS 84 Saint Mary's Dominican Coll; ME 87 Southeastern LA Univ; **SLP**

Dermody, Rebecca Lynn 3018 Bunker Hill Drive, Louisville, KY 40205, (502) 584-9781, MS 88 Murray St Univ

De Roche, Jane Frances 148 Farrwood Drive, Bradford, MA 01835, (603) 883-5521, BS 82 Univ of MA - Amherst; MS 84 WV Univ; Sp-Lang Path, Nashua Memorial Hosp Sp & Hrng Ctr, **SLP**

De Roche, Lisa Anne 13 Venus Road, South Amboy, NJ 08879, (201) 727-1017, BA 83 Montclair St Coll; MA 86 Montclair St Coll; **A**

Deroche, Maija A P O Box 571, 233 South Genesee Street, Montour Falls, NY 14865, (607) 734-6135, BA 70 SUNY - Coll at Oswego; MA 78 SUNY - Coll at Geneseo; Treat Team Leader, Craig Dev Cen, **SLP**

De Roia, Mrs Marielaine Dicillo 15408 Ramage, Maple Heights, OH 44137, (216) 663-6334, BA 80 John Carroll Univ; MA 83 Cleveland St Univ; Sp-Lang Path, Private Practice, **SLP**

deRoos, Diane Elizabeth Rd 1 Box 60-A, Union Springs, NY 13160, (315) 255-2746, BS 82 SUNY - Coll at Geneseo; MS 83 Syracuse Univ; Sp-Lang Path, E John Gavras Cen, **SLP**

Deroo-Wagman, Carolyn J 18964 Brasilia, Northridge, CA 91326, (818) 363-4805, MA 83 CA St Univ - Long Beach; Sp-Lang Path, Northridge Hosp Med Ctr, **SLP ACE**

De Rosa, Kimberly Marie 534 Smiley Avenue, Cincinnati, OH 45246, (812) 346-4401, BA 78 OH St Univ; MS 81 IN St Univ - Terre Haute; Sp-Lang Path, Butler Co Dept MRDD, **SLP**

De Rosa-Lukach, Patricia Ann 221 Margaret Drive, South Windsor, CT 06074, (203) 563-9638, BA 79 Univ of CT; MS 82 Southern CT St Univ; SLP, Wethersfield Bd of Education, **SLP**

DeRose, Joseph 2287 Long Road, Grand Island, NY 14072, (716) 878-5429, BS 58 Bloomsburg Univ of PA; MS 63 PA St Univ - Univ Park; **SLP**

Derosier, Paula E S 253 North Street, Williamstown, MA 01267, **SLP**

DeRoss, Mrs Sandy S 1232 Lantern Court, Sacramento, CA 95864, (916) 924-3502, BA 73 CA St Univ - Sacramento; MA 75 CA St Univ - Sacramento; 85–Program Specialist, North Sacramento School Dist, **SLP**

Derowitsch, Mrs Marlene P 1780 Glen Creek N W, Salem, OR 97304, BA 76 Western OR St Coll; MS 78 Western OR St Coll; **SLP**

Derr, Ann C Nelson 1742 Portland, St Paul, MN 55104, (612) 293-8647, BA 72 MacAlster Coll; MA 79 Univ of MN - Minneap-St Paul; 85–Sp-Lang Path, St Paul Public Schools, **SLP**

Derr, Mrs Martha Pool 88 East Main Street, Newville, PA 17241, (717) 243-2345, OB 76 Univ of FL; MA 78 Univ of TN - Knoxville; Aud, Private Practice, **A**

Derrenbacher, Carol Cooke 8013 North Bridgewater Ct, Raleigh, NC 27615, (919) 790-2500, BA 65 Coll of New Rochelle; ME 81 GA St Univ; 88–Sp-Lang Path, Wake Co Pub Sch, **SLP**

Derrick, Betty K 11459 North 28th Drive, #1113, Phoenix, AZ 85029, (817) 795-2124, BS 73 East Carolina Univ; MS 75 East Carolina Univ; Aud, Alhambre Ele Sch Dist, **A**

Derrick, Kathryn G 1841 Birch Road, Northbrook, IL 60062, **SLP**

Derrick, Mrs Virginia J Star Route, Peru, NY 12972, (518) 561-2000, BS 50 Univ of MN - Minneap-St Paul; MS 56 Univ of IL - Urbana; Sp/Lang Path, Champlain Valley Phys Hosp, **SLP**

D'Errico, Irene 36 Birch Terrace, Parlin, NJ 08859, (201) 354-5800, BA 79 Montclair St Coll; MA 83 Montclair St Coll; SLP, UCP League, **SLP**

Derringer, Ann R Route 2 Box 192-A, Danville, KY 40422, (606) 854-3956, BA 75 Univ of KY; MA 80 Eastern KY Univ; SLP, Boyle Co Bd of Ed, **SLP**

Derris, Sandy J 104 Cannonade Drive East, Marlboro, NJ 07746, MS 72 CUNY - Brooklyn Coll; Aud, Private Practice, **SLP**

Derry, Andrea Rebecca Box 5620 RFD 2, Oxford, ME 04270, (207) 998-2180, **SLP**

Derse, Christine Louise 15 Warwick Road, Belmont, MA 02178, (617) 894-3600, ME 83 Univ of VA - Charlottesville; Sp-Lang Path, W E Fernald State Sch, **SLP**

Dersh, Laurie M 330 South Almont Drive, Apartment A-3, Los Angeles, CA 90048, (714) 957-5147, BA 77 Univ of CA - Santa Barbara; MA 80 CA St Univ - Los Angeles; 84–Sp-Lang Path, CA Lanterman St Hosp, **A**

Deruy, Debora G 941 Crane Street, Foster City, CA 94404, **SLP**

DeRuyter, Dr Frank Communication Disorders Dept, Rancho Los Amigos Med Ctr, 7601 East Imperial Highway, Downey, CA 90242, (213) 940-7682, BA 72 Univ of the Pacific; MA 73 Univ of the Pacific; PH 78 (Sp & Hrng) Univ of WA; 81–Sp-Lang Path, Rancho Los Amigos Med Ctr, **SLP ACE**

Derx, Mrs Corinne Houlis 6123 Donegal West, Lakeland, FL 33803, (813) 533-2279, BS 75 FL St Univ; MS 76 FL St Univ; ED 84 (NS) Rollins Coll; Staffing Specialist, Polk District Schools Ese Dept, **SLP**

Desai, Mrs Nivedita N 6517 Stair Street, Downers Grove, IL 60516, (312) 964-3504, ME 71 Marygove Coll; Sp-Lang Path, Marianjoy Rehab Ctr, **SLP**

De Salle, Jean Marie 1906 North 38th Street, Killeen, TX 76543, (817) 526-9506, BA 54 Univ of Northern CO; MA 71 NM St Univ; Superv/Deaf & Sp Ed, Killeen ISD

De Sante, Mrs Mary Ann 21 Treaty Drive, Wayne, PA 19087, (215) 233-9559, BA 76 Univ of KY; MA 84 Cleveland St Univ; 88–Sp-Lang Path, Montgomery Co Interm Unit, **SLP**

Desanti, Susan M 105 15th Avenue, Sea Cliff, NY 11579, (212) 464-7500, BA 78 CUNY - Queens Coll; MS 79 Adelphi Univ; Sp-Lang Path, Creedmoor Psych Cen, **SLP**

De Santis, Brenda R 2400 Johnson Avenue #4-H, Riverdale, NY 10463, (212) 549-6659, BA 69 CUNY - Brooklyn Coll; MS 71 CUNY - Brooklyn Coll; 86–Sp-Lang Path, Self Employed, **SLP**

Desaulniers, Renee Michelle 5 Autum Leaf Drive, Apartment 10, Nashua, NH 03060, (603) 434-6681, MS 86 Northeastern Univ; **SLP**

Deschenes-Desmond, Mrs Anita Star Route, New Hartford, CT 06057, (203) 522-0166, BA 74 Univ of NH; MS 78 Southern CT St Univ; Sp-Lang Path, Hartford Board of Education, **SLP**

Desell-Lund, Paulette Marie Rd 2 Box 1180, Johnson, VT 05656, (802) 644-2620, BS 76 Nazareth Coll of Rochester; MA 77 SUNY - Coll at Geneseo; SLP, Lamemorial In Vt, **SLP**

Deshaw, Mrs Donna 1215 North Adams Street, Carroll, IA 51401, (712) 792-1265, BA 66 Univ of Northern IA; MA 74 Univ of Northern IA; Sp-Lang Path, Private Practice, **SLP ACE**

Deshayes, Irvin L Barkley Memorial Cetr Unl CMPS, 42nd And Holdrege, Lincoln, NE 68583-0731, (402) 472-5455, BA 64 NE Wesleyan Univ; MA 66 Univ of NE - Lincoln; 66–Asst Prof, U of NE - Lincoln, **A**

Deshpande, Kamal D 245 West 63rd Avenue, Vancouver, BC, Canada V5X 2H9, (604) 875-2112, BS 58; MA 63 CUNY - Brooklyn Coll; Aud & Sp/Lang Path, Chldns Hosp, **SLP A**

De Silva-Elich, Elaine Theresa 136 Weston Road, Rochester, NY 14612, (716) 325-7828, BS 80 Nazareth Coll of Rochester; MS 84 Nazareth Coll of Rochester; 81–Sp-Lang Path, Rochester City Sch Dist, **SLP**

Des Jardins, Jane S Mercy Hospital, Rehabilitation Center, 1400 West Park, Urbana, IL 61801, (217) 337-2109, BS 73 Northern MI Univ; MA 77 Univ of IL - Urbana; Sp-Lnag Path, Mercy Hosp Rehab Ctr, **SLP**

Des Lauriers, Dione Marie 7337 Franklin Circle, Eden Prairie, MN 55346, (612) 933-9160, BS 83 Univ of MN - Minneap-St Paul; MS 85 Univ of MN - Minneap-St Paul; 85–Sp-Lang Path, Hopkins Dist #270, **SLP**

Desmet, Ann Lahr 2159 Meade, North Bend, OR 97459, (503) 269-1611, BS 64 Northwestern Univ; MS 76 Univ of OR; Coord Regional Sp Serv, Coos Co Ed Serv Dist, **SLP**

Desmond, Alan Louis 19 Medical Arts Clinic, Princeton, WV 24740, (304) 487-2487, MS 80 Radford Univ; Owner-Manager, Princeton Aud-Sp-Lang Path Cl, **A**

Desmond, Deborah Jean 85 Golden Hind Passage, Corte Madera, CA 94925, (415) 558-3386, BS 82 Univ of CA - Santa Barbara; MS 84 Vanderbilt Univ; Aud, San Francisco Dept Pub Health, **A**

Desmond, Patricia K 4780 North Idlewild Avenue, Whitefish Bay, WI 53211, (414) 962-8168, BS 66 Saint Louis Univ; MS 80 Univ of WI - Milwaukee; 86–Sp-Lang Path, Children's Hosp of Wisconsin, **SLP**

Desmone, Linda Few P O Box 34, Andover, CT 06232, (203) 742-7341, BS 68 Univ of KS; MA 70 Univ of KS; SLP, Coventry Pub Sch, **SLP**

Desnoyers, Anne M 41 Paula Avenue, Pittsfield, MA 01201, (413) 443-4298, MS 88 Boston Univ

Desola, Deborah M 1014 Rottkamp Street, Apartment 3, Valley Stream, NY 11580, (718) 377-5040, BS 76 NY Univ; MS 78 Columbia Univ Teachers Coll; 87–Sp-Lang Path, VTA Management Svcs, **SLP**

Desormeaux, Mrs Linda B 103 Denette Drive, Duson, LA 70529, (318) 873-3781, MA 87 Univ of Southwestern LA

De Soto, Jane Everhardt 1840 North Gate Drive, Beloit, WI 53511, (608) 756-8323, BS 68 Univ of WI - Madison; MS 70 Univ of WI - Stevens Point; Sp-Lang Path, Sch Dist of Janesville, **SLP**

Desousa, Rhonda Ann 22978 Inlet Circle, Boca Raton, FL 33428, (305) 483-9421, OB 84

Despain, Mrs Susan Christine 14 West Goldfinch Court, Savannah, GA 31419, (912) 927-2997, BS 83 Univ of WY; MS 85 Univ of WY; **A**

Desporte, Edward J Covington Audiological Service, 620 West 13th Avenue, Covington, LA 70433, (504) 892-3992, BA 73 Univ of New Orleans; MS 77 Univ of TX - Dallas; Prop/Aud, Covington Aud Servs, **A**

Desrochers, Chet M Glenrose Rehabilitation Hospital, 10230-111 Avenue, Edmonton, AB, Canada T5G 0B7, (403) 471-7970, BS 68 Univ of WI - Madison; MS 73 Univ of WI - Madison; 85–Dir-Dept of Aud, Glenrose Rehab Hosp, **A**

Dessen, Mrs Mimi Lynne 2 Melby Lane, East Hills, NY 11576, (516) 484-6133, BA 62 CUNY - Brooklyn Coll; MS 85 CUNY - Brooklyn Coll; 87–Tchr, NYC Bd of Educ, **SLP**

Desser, Mrs Linda 231 Greenleaf, Wilmette, IL 60091, (312) 675-3040, MS 61 Univ of Chicago; Private Practice, **SLP**

Dess-Schwender, Mrs Amy Lynn 1375 Anderson Road #2, Pittsburgh, PA 15209, (412) 487-0832, BS 85 Indiana Univ of PA; MS 87 WV Univ; 87–Aud, Pittsburgh Otological Assoc, **A**

De Stafney, Jan Elisabeth 285 East Burgess Road, Pensacola, FL 32503, (904) 476-1249, **A**

Destefano, Carla Haymaker 207 Tappan Avenue, Hampton, VA 23664, (804) 826-8746, BS 72 Western IL Univ; MA 75 Western IL Univ; Sp-Lang Path, Commonwealth Health Care, **SLP**

De Stefano, Cheryl Cheroki 1322 Wickerham Drive, Monongahela, PA 15063, (412) 837-2070, **SLP**

Destefano, Lori McNamara 2 Ladd Road, Sturbridge, MA 01566, (617) 792-8500, BA 79 Boston Coll; MA 81 George Washington Univ; Sp-Lang Path, Hahnemann Rehab Cen, **SLP**

Destro, Diane R 31524 Ronald Drive, Willowick, OH 44094, (216) 944-5859, BA 86 Cleveland St Univ; MA 87 Cleveland St Univ; 87–Sp-Lang Path, Chardon Local Schs, **SLP**

Deters, Mrs Christina Flynn 587 Washington Boulevard, Union Lake, MI 48085-3034, (313) 698-4056, **SLP**

Dethlefs, Mrs Kathleen 8906 West 97th Street, Overland Park, KS 66212, (913) 381-5650, BA 73 Southern IL Univ-Edwardsvill; MA 74 Univ of NE - Lincoln; 83–Sp-Lang Path, Chldn Ther Grp, **SLP**

Dethlefs, Richard D 8906 West 97th Street, Overland Park, KS 66212, (913) 888-5228, BS 72 Univ of NE - Lincoln; MA 74 Univ of NE - Lincoln; SLP, Shawnee Mission U S D 512, **SLP**

Dethmers, Anna Ayers 11164 West Fremont Place, Littleton, CO 80127, (303) 399-0603, BA 83 Hofstra Univ; MA 87 Hofstra Univ; 87–Sp-Lang Path, Child Opportunity Prog Inc

Detorie, Deborah La Mesa Elementary, 7500 Copper N E, Albuquerque, NM 87108, (505) 262-1581, BA 72 NM St Univ; MA 74 NM St Univ; Sp-Lang Path, La Mesa Elementary School, **SLP**

Detour, Christine C 395 Davit Street, Jamestown, RI 02835, (401) 789-3950, BA 73 Univ of CT; MS 76 Univ of RI; Sp/Lang Path, Cranston Cen for Ret Citizens, **SLP**

Dettelbach, Mrs Joan A 2770 Chesterton Road, Shaker Heights, OH 44122, BS Case Western Reserve Univ; MS 80 Case Western Reserve Univ; Consultant Sp-Lang Path, Sunny Acres Skilld Nursing Fac, **SLP**

Dettlaff, Krystina 6N578 Pine, Bensenville, IL 60106, (312) 595-7459, BS 74 Northern IL Univ - De Kalb; MA 75 Northern IL Univ - De Kalb; SLP, Sherman Hospital, **SLP**

Dettloff, Mrs Julie Greenop 2770 - 5 Woodlake Road, Wyoming, MI 49509, (616) 455-7300, BA 84 MI St Univ; MA 85 Central MI Univ; SLP, Mary Free Bed Hospital & Rehab, **SLP**

Dettman, Kim Annette 6635 Spring Flower Drive, Apartment 13, New Port Richey, FL 34653, (813) 841-8091, 1988; MS 87 Univ of WI - Eau Claire; Sp-Lang Path, Dist Sch Bd of Pasco Co, **SLP**

Dettman, Mary Jane 2979 Meadow Lane, Cleveland, OH 44145, PH (NS); **SLP**

Dettore, Marlene G 225 Parkway Drive, Pittsburgh, PA 15228, (412) 563-2396, BS 69 Carlow Coll; ME 70 PA St Univ - Univ Park; Sp-Lang Path, Comprehensive Therapy Services, **SLP**

Detweiler, Lynda G 1665 Juniper Hill, Encinitas, CA 92024, **SLP**

Detwiler, Mrs Cathleen A 1860 Northview Drive, Colorado Springs, CO 80909, (303) 635-5467, BA 80 Univ of CO - Boulder; MA 82 Univ of Denver; Sp-Lang Path, Child Dev Ctr of Colorado Springs, **SLP**

Deuermeyer, Mrs Sally P 3000 Jennifer, College Station, TX 77840, (409) 696-8655, BA 74 Univ of MN - Duluth; MS 78 Purdue Univ - West Lafayette; Sp-Lang Path, Coll Station ISD, **SLP**

DeuPree, Dr Robert M 2625 West Huckleberry Road, Santa Ana, CA 92706, (714) 554-3666, BA 62 CA St Univ - Fullerton; MA 63 CA St Univ - Long Beach; DD 88 (Medicine Theology); 81–Med Dir, Area US Pub Health Svc, **LM**

Deus, Julia B 2100 Sawmill Road 10A-203, Harahan, LA 70123, (504) 482-3901, BA 86 LA St Univ - Baton Rouge; MA 87 LA St Univ - Baton Rouge; 87–Sp-Lang Path, Remedial Spec, **SLP**

Deuter, Carol Breckley 15 E Katharine Avenue, Seaville, Ocean View, NJ 08230, (609) 465-2721, BS 70 Univ of MO - Columbia; MA 84 Trenton St Coll; **SLP**

Deutsch, Andrea Sachs 12 Knight Lane, Kings Park, NY 11754, (516) 585-0100, BA 80 MI St Univ; MA 81 MI St Univ; Aud, Assoc for Ret Chldn Inc, **A**

Deutsch, Karen G Box 429-F Route 15, Indianapolis, IN 46259, (317) 232-4353, BS 76 Purdue Univ - West Lafayette; MS 77 Purdue Univ - West Lafayette; Sp-Lang Path Consult, Indiana Medicaid Prog, **SLP**

Deutsch, Dr Lawrence 55-28 Main Street, Flushing, NY 11355, (718) 445-1400, BA 63 CUNY - City College; PH 68 (NS) CUNY - Grad Sch & Univ Cntr; Owner, Lawrence Deutsch PhD & Assoc, **A**

Deutsch, Shirley M L 8451 Clarkdale, Huntington Beach, CA 92646, **SLP**

Deutsch, Dr Steven E 3972 San Bonito Avenue, Los Alamitos, CA 90720, (213) 494-5415, BA 69 CUNY - Brooklyn Coll; MS 72 CUNY - Brooklyn Coll; PH 76 (NS) Univ of IA; SLP, VA Med Cen-Long Beach, **SLP**

Deutsch, Steven M 7034 Heather Road, Macungie, PA 18062, (215) 866-5915, BA 80 Bradley Univ; MA 82 Memphis St Univ; Sp/Lang Path, UCP of Lehigh Valley, **SLP**

Deutsch, Mrs Sylvie R 11738 Baird Avenue, Northridge, CA 91326, (818) 368-1224, BA 73 Univ of CA - Los Angeles; MA 77 CA St Univ - Los Angeles; Director, Private Practice, **SLP**

Devan, Mrs Sheila Ann 1 Woodcrest, Searcy, AR 72143, (501) 268-5823, BS 82 Univ of Central AR; MS 84 AR St Univ; Sp-Lang Path, Kensett Pub Sch, **SLP**

Devane, Gladys F Speech And Hearing Center, Indiana University, Bloomington, IN 47401, (812) 335-3797, BS 63 OK St Univ; MS 65 IN Univ - Bloomington; Clinical Instructor, Indiana University, **SLP**

Devane, Margaret Edwards 22124 Belle Street, Castro Valley, CA 94546, (415) 881-7725, BA 82 San Jose St Univ; MS 86 San Francisco St Univ; 87–Aud, Holt's Hrng Aid Ctr, **A**

Devane, Susan Mary 1158 Palermo Court, Franklin Square, NY 11010, (516) 338-4204, **SLP**

Devaney, Eileen M 50 School Street, East Williston, NY 11596, (516) 742-7826, BA 75 CUNY - Hunter Coll; MS 80 Adelphi Univ; 81–Sp-Lang Path, Private Practice, **SLP**

Devaney, Mrs Jane M 174 Roughing It Road, Dayton, NV 89403, (702) 246-5000, BS 64 Eastern MI Univ; BS 64 8201; **SLP**

Devaney, Janet Shaw 423 Lawrenceville Road, Apartment 108, Lawrenceville, NJ 08648, (609) 396-4380, BS 75 Trenton St Coll; MA 78 Trenton St Coll; Sp-Lang Path, E Windsor Reg Sch Dist, **SLP**

Devens, Dr John S Valdez Hearing & Speech Serv, P O Box 730, Valdez, AK 99686, (907) 835-2421, BS 64 Belmont Coll; ME 66 Emory Univ; PH 75 (NS) Wichita St Univ; President, Pr William Sound Commun Coll, **SLP A**

Dever, Deen A Mandana Farms, Victor, WV 25938, (304) 872-4649, BA 74 WV Inst of Tech; MA 76 Marshall Univ; Sp-Lang Path, Nicholas Co Bd of Ed, **SLP**

Devillier, Mrs Wanda Normand 1320 East Laurel Avenue, Eunice, LA 70535, (318) 457-2380, SLP, St Landry Parish School Board, **SLP**

Devine, Mrs Jeanne Canty 8344 Tidewater Court, Cincinnati, OH 45255, (513) 232-2299, BS 82 Univ of IA; MA 84 Northwestern Univ; Aud, Hearing Care Professionals, **A**

Devine, Mrs Laura Elizabeth P O Box 362, 505 Elm, Fowler, KS 67844, (316) 227-8002, BA 80 Fort Hays St Univ; MS 81 Fort Hays St Univ; Sp-Lang Path, SW Kansas Area Coop District, **SLP**

Devine, Mary Ellen 8615 South Kenton Avenue, Chicago, IL 60652, (312) 596-3200, BA 82 Saint Xavier Coll; MA 84 IL St Univ - Normal; **SLP**

Devine, Nancy F 1414 Brunson Court, Cary, NC 27511, (919) 467-3432, BS 70 PA St Univ - Univ Park; MS 71 PA St Univ - Univ Park; Sp-Lang Path, Private Practice, **SLP ACE**

Devine, Mrs Patricia B 1735 South Wagner, Ann Arbor, MI 48106, (313) 994-8111, BS 76 Eastern MI Univ; MA 77 Eastern MI Univ; Sp-Lang Path, Washtenaw ISD-High Point Ctr, **SLP**

Devita, Ann Marisa DCH Professional Bldg, Suite 310, 606 Wilson Creek Road, Lawrenceburg, IN 47025, (812) 537-8166, BS 78 Univ of Cincinnati; MA 85 Univ of Cincinnati; 88–Dir Sp-Lang Path, Dearborn County Hosp, **SLP**

DeVito, Teresa 21896 River Oaks Drive #C2, Rocky River, OH 44116, (216) 459-3178, MA 82 Cleveland St Univ; Sp-Lang Path, Cleveland Metro General Hosp, **SLP**

Devitt, Elizabeth Ann West 1800 Nelson #151, West Covina, CA 91792, BS 84 Univ of IA; MA 86 Univ of IA; **SLP**

Devlin, Brigitte Margaret 15 Grove Lane, Levittown, NY 11756, (516) 673-1670, BS 79 SUNY - Coll at Fredonia; MS 82 Adelphi Univ; Sp-Lang Path, South Huntington Sch Dist, **SLP**

Devlin, David Lawrence Acoustic Arts Lab, 315 Nokomis Avenue South, Venice, FL 34285, (813) 488-4980, MS 76 Univ of South FL; Aud, Acoustic Arts Labs, **A**

Devlin, Judith C 4628 Keswick Road, Baltimore, MD 21210, (301) 665-0040, BS 77 Towson St Univ; MS 79 Towson St Univ; Sp-Lang Path, Private Practice, **SLP**

Devlin, Kim R 4740 Trevins Avenue, Las Vegas, NV 89103-4355, BA 77 SUNY - Center at Buffalo; MS 79 Univ of IL - Urbana; **SLP**

Devlin, Lisa C 13659 Cedar Creek Lane, Silver Spring, MD 20904, (202) 651-5328, BS 77 Northeastern Univ; MS 79 Gallaudet Coll; Aud, Gallaudet College, **A**

Devlin, Sr M St Josephs Provincial House, 385 Watervliet-Shaker Road, Latham, NY 12110, (518) 785-4632, BS 58 Coll of Saint Rose; MA 65 Coll of Saint Rose; 64–Sp-Lang Path, Carondelet Ed Cen, **SLP**

Devlin, Mrs Robin W 315 Nokomis Avenue So, Venice, FL 34285, (813) 488-4980, MS 78 Univ of South FL; Aud, Aud & Hearing Aid Ctr, **A**

Devlin, Susan M 6123 Kara's Walk, Elkridge, MD 21227, BA 77 Loyola Coll; MS 78 Loyola Coll; Sp-Lang Path, Board of Educ Frederick County, **SLP**

Devlin-De Lisle, Kathleen 52 Nonotuck Street, Holyoke, MA 01040, (413) 536-5599, BS 80 Emerson Coll; MA 86 Univ of MA - Amherst; Sp-Lang Path, Pioneer Dev Ctr, **SLP**

De Voe, Anne S Pomperaug Woods #137, 80 Heritage Road, Southbury, CT 06488, (203) 264-8518, MA 36 Columbia Univ Teachers Coll; **SLP A LM**

Devoe, Merle F 3504 Gold Dust Drive #41, Helena, MT 59601, (406) 444-3114, BS 62 Western MT Coll; MS 67 Western OR St Coll; Coord-Hear Cons Prog, Ofc of Pub Inst, **A**

Devoe, Shirley J 418 Butler, Helena, MT 59601, (406) 442-6440, BS 67 Western OR St Coll; MS 68 Western OR St Coll; Coop Coord, Helena Pub Schs, **SLP**

De Voll-Dahl, Tracy Lynn RR 1 Box 66, Gackle, ND 58442, (701) 252-4100, BA 81 Univ of WI - Eau Claire; MS 84 UT St Univ; Aud, Sp and Hrng Svcs, **A**

Devon-Frank, Mrs Gloria 1349 Encinitas Boulevard, Encinitas, CA 92024, (619) 944-6381, BA 82 Univ of MI - Ann Arbor; MS 84 Univ of Redlands; **A**

Devore, Mrs Estra Joy 112 Alberts Way, Langhorne, PA 19047, (609) 394-4177, BA 72 Rutgers St Univ -N Brunswick; ME 84 Trenton St Coll; 87–Sp-Lang Path, Mercer Med Ctr, **SLP**

Devost, Mrs Pamela Conway 18 Imperial Drive, South Burlington, VT 05401, (802) 656-3970, BA 77 Univ of VT; MS 78 Univ of VT; Sp-Lang Path, VT Med Cent Hosp/Dis Commun, **SLP ACE**

DeVreugd, Paul E 869 Ironstone Drive, Rochester Hills, MI 48309, (313) 362-4299, BS 78 MI St Univ; MA 82 Wayne St Univ; Cl Dir, Medi-Sp Ser Inc, **SLP**

Devries, Donna A 2530 South Wallis Smith, Springfield, MO 65804, **SLP**

De Vries, Karen Leigh PO Draw 1648, Lufkin, TX 75902-1648, (409) 634-3353, BS 77 Murray St Univ; MS 79 Murray St Univ; Aud, TDMHMR-Lufkin State Sch, **A**

Devries, Luanne K 2411 Lalkwood Drive, Midland, MI 48460, **SLP**

De Vries, Mrs Sherri Marie 2901 Tennyson Street, Lincoln, NE 68516, (402) 464-8385, BS 85 Univ of NE - Lincoln; MS 87 Univ of NE - Lincoln; 88–Aud, Great Plains ENT Head Inst, **A**

De Vuyst, Mrs Anita Comfort 3162 Benton Boulevard, Pace, FL 32571, (904) 994-0300, BS 82 Auburn Univ - Auburn; MS 83 FL St Univ; 85–Sp-Lang Path, Escambia County Schools, **SLP ACE**

Dewald, Patricia A 306 Depew Street, Dumont, NJ 07628, (201) 768-6060, BA 75 William Paterson Coll; MS 78 William Paterson Coll; Sp-Lang Path, Demarest Pub Schs Nj, **SLP**

Dewar, Mrs Sally Rule VA Hospital, 2300 Ramsey Street, Fayetteville, NC 28306, (919) 488-2120, BA 74 Univ of NC - Greensboro; ME 76 Univ of NC - Greensboro; Sp-Lang Path, VA Hosp, **SLP**

DeWeese, Mrs Barbara P 2146 Motor Avenue, Kingman, AZ 86401, (602) 753-6307, BA 50 Miami Univ - Oxford; MA 52 Case Western Reserve Univ; 80–Sp-Lang Path, Kingman Elem Sch Dist, **SLP**

Deweese, Mrs Pamela D 320 Rudgate Drive, Plainfield, IN 46168, BA 75 IN Univ - Bloomington; MA 76 IN Univ - Bloomington; Mental Retardatn Professional, Private Practice, **SLP**

Deweese, Thomas E 1302 Port Arthur, Mena, AR 71953, (501) 394-5277, BS 74 Delta St Univ; OM 76 Univ of MS; 76–Sp-Lang Path, W AR Counsel & Guidance Ctr, **SLP**

Dewey, Charlene M 1 Ridgewood Drive, Plattsburgh, NY 12901, (518) 563-8321, BS 69 SUNY - Coll at Fredonia; MS 73 SUNY - Center at Albany; SLP, Beekmantown Ctrl Sch, **SLP**

Dewey, Mrs Claire C 17 Wainwright Street, Dorchester, MA 02124, (617) 542-1384, BS 74 Taylor Univ; MS 80 Boston Univ; Sp-Lang Path, Visiting Nurse Association, **SLP**

Dewey, Ellen Gano 828 North Rockford Avenue, Rockford, IL 61107, **SLP**

Dewey, Jody A 8033 12th Avenue N E, Seattle, WA 98115, (206) 526-0634, BA 75 Univ of VT; MA 78 Emerson Coll; Unemploy, **SLP**

Dewey, Mrs Martha N 612 Meadow Ridge Road, Baltimore, MD 21204, (301) 243-3800, BA 75 Saint Lawrence Univ; MS 80 Emerson Coll; Sp-Lang Path, Hrng & Sp Agcy of Metro Balt, **SLP**

Dewey, Susan Jean 319 E 56th Street, Long Beach, CA 90805, (213) 861-2891, **SLP**

Dewhirst, Susan Watts 332 Hampton Drive, Feasterville, PA 19047, BS 73 Northeastern Univ; MA 76 Trenton St Coll; **SLP**

Dewine, Laurie J 886 Woodlyn Drive South, Cincinnati, OH 45230, (606) 331-8416, BS 77 Univ of Cincinnati; MA 79 OH St Univ; Aud, Drs Haas Mayer Hausladen, **A**

Dewire, Nancy Kirn 14317 Aldengate Road, Midlothian, VA 23113, (804) 748-1691, BS 77 East Carolina Univ; MS 81 James Madison Univ; Sp-Lang Path, Chesterfield Co Inf Prog/Arc, **SLP**

Dewitt, Mrs Carolyn Dankowski 547 King Street, Redwood City, CA 94062, (415) 589-5900, BA 80 Creighton Univ

Dewitt, Linda Marie Route 6 Box 72 C, Fairmont, WV 26554, (304) 367-1431, BS 84 WV Univ; MS 85 WV Univ; **A**

Dewitt, Mrs Mary Catherine The Dewitt Clinic, 117 South Johnson, Alvin, TX 77511, (713) 331-5153, BA 55 Incarnate Word Coll; MA 80 Univ of Houston - Univ Park; Sp-Lang Path, Speech-Lang & Learning Srvices, **SLP**

Dewitt, Rich B 1547 N W Lake, Newport, OR 97365, (503) 336-2299, BA 72; MS 74 Univ of NE - Omaha; Sp-Lang Path, Private Practice-Lincoln Sch, **SLP**

Dexter, Mark Edward 1661 Park Road N W #103, Washington, DC 20010, (301) 279-8490, BA 82 Eastern MI Univ; MA 84 Eastern MI Univ; Sp-Lang Path, Montgomery Co PS, **SLP**

Dextraze, Kelly Mulrooney 64 Wilber Avenue #A, Arlington, MA 02174-5739, (617) 641-3316, BA 82 Univ of CA - Santa Barbara; MS 83 Emerson Coll; Sp-Lang Path, Brockton Early Intervention, **SLP**

Dey, Vanda Lee 14190 East Temple Drive, Apartment #O-9, Aurora, CO 80015, (303) 688-9510, BA 83 Univ of Denver; MA 86 Univ of Denver; SLP, Douglas Co Ps, **SLP**

Deyoung, Mrs Barbara J 12 Grimsby Gate, Fairport, NY 14450, (716) 223-3547, BS 73 Univ of WI - Madison; MS 74 Univ of WI - Madison; Cadre Teacher Spec Ed, Cty Sch Dist NY, **SLP**

Deyoung, Bonnie Marie 5489 Ravine Road, Kalamazoo, MI 49009, (616) 349-4760, BA 82 Hope Coll; MS 85 Univ of WI - Madison; SLP, Mary Free Bed Rehab Center, **SLP**

Deyoung, Linda S 424 Cypress, Laguna Beach, CA 92651, (714) 581-2800, BA 75 Univ of VT; MS 76 Adelphi Univ; MS 77 Univ of WI - Madison; Assoc Executive Director, Newport Lang Speech Aud, **SLP A**

Dey-Sigman, Susan 3901 Amherst Street, Houston, TX 77005-2831, (713) 795-7492, BA 73 Tufts Univ; MS 77 Southern CT St Univ; Aud, VAMC Houston, **A**

De Zelar, Lynne M 1675 Beam Avenue Suite 200, St Paul, MN 55109, (612) 770-1105, BS 84 Univ of MN - Minneap-St Paul; MS 86 Univ of WI - River Falls; 86–Aud, ENT Head & Neck Surgery PA, **A**

DeZwaan, Mrs Janet 3609 Old Colony Road, Kalamazoo, MI 49008, BS 73 IL St Univ - Normal; MA 74 Univ of IL - Urbana; **SLP**

Dezzutti, Ida L 3460 Sardis Road, Murrysville, PA 15668, **SLP**

D'Huy, Kathy Ann 687 Ocean Avenue, New London, CT 06320, (203) 572-0541, BS 80 PA St Univ - Univ Park; MS 82 Vanderbilt Univ; Icf/Mr Sp-Lang Path, Seaside Reg Cen, **SLP**

Diachok, Kathleen M 10005 Greenbrier Road, Apartment 313, Minnetonka, MN 55343, (612) 546-7554, BA 80 Univ of MN - Duluth; MA 81 Univ of MN - Duluth; Sp-Lang Path, Eden Prairie ISD 272, **SLP**

Diacono, Lori Kay 11736 Columbia, Redford, MI 48239, (313) 420-9015, **SLP**

Diak, Mrs Kathryn R 908 Chancellor, Edwardsville, IL 62025, (618) 262-7125, MS 80 IL St Univ - Normal; SLP, Professional Rehabil Center, **SLP**

Dial, Bill Dean 803 Meadow Lawn, Geneseo, IL 61254, (309) 944-3000, BS 56 IL St Univ - Normal; MS 70 Northern IL Univ - De Kalb; Sp-Lang Path, Private Practice, **SLP**

Diamantes, Helen 302 Monatona Street, Paramus, NJ 07652, (201) 977-2136, BA 80 Rutger's St Univ - Douglas Coll; MS 81 Columbia Univ Teachers Coll; SLP, St Joseph Hospital Medical Cen, **SLP**

Diament, Mrs Cynthia J 3520 St Susan Place, Los Angeles, CA 90066, (213) 670-1643, BS 70 Univ of WI - Madison; MS 71 Univ of WI - Madison; **SLP**

Diament, Mrs Deborah S 3 Opatut Court, Edison, NJ 08817, (201) 572-3540, BA 76 CUNY - Brooklyn Coll; MS 78 Columbia Univ Teachers Coll; Sp-Lang Path, Private Practice, **SLP**

Diament, Mrs Elise Trader 931 Independence Street, New Orleans, LA 70117, (504) 361-4469, BS 72 Saint Mary's Dominican Coll; OM 76 LA St Univ - N O Medical Ctr; 72–Asst Coord of Sp Hrng & Lang Svcs, Jefferson Parish Pub Sch Syst, **SLP**

Diamond, Barbara S 2513 La Golondrina Street, Carlsbad, CA 92008, (619) 438-7847, OB 71 Univ of Miami; MA 74 Univ of CA - San Diego; **SLP**

Diamond, Barry S 9900 President Street, Philadelphia, PA 19115, (215) 671-4108, BA 64 Rider Coll; MA 67 Temple Univ-Tyler Sch of Art; SLP, Philadelphia State Hospital, **SLP**

Diamond, Mrs Beverly A 1010 Westwind Way, Newport Beach, CA 92660, (714) 642-5338, BA 64 Univ of CA - Berkeley; MA 79 CA St Univ - Northridge; **SLP**

Diamond, Judie Arbess 5709 Smart Avenue, Cote St Luc, PQ, Canada H4W 2M6, (514) 482-0500, BS 63 McGill Univ - Quebec; MA 66 Univ of Southern CA; SLP, MacKay Center, **SLP**

Diamond, Laura A P O Box 4543, Davis, CA 95617, (916) 753-8731, MA 79 CA St Univ - Northridge; 88–SLP, Folsom-Cordova USD, **SLP**

Diamond, Linda 6460 Chapman Field Drive, Miami, FL 33156, (305) 661-1946, BS 74 Univ of UT; MS 76 Univ of MI - Ann Arbor; Sp-Lang Path, Hrng & Sp Cen FL Inc, **SLP**

Diamond, Linda Feldsott 6441 Moore Drive, Los Angeles, CA 90048, (213) 855-3145, BS 72 Univ of RI; MS 73 Univ of VT; Sp-Lang Path, Private Practice, **SLP**

Diamond, Matthew 3091 North Course Drive, Bldg 49 #105, Pompano Beach, FL 33060, (305) 979-0268, PH (NS); **SLP LM**

Diamond, Mrs Mona Foster 28 Fanshawe Drive, Richmond Hill, ON, Canada L4B 1P5, (416) 764-6336, BA 82 York Univ - Ontario; MA 85 SUNY - Center at Buffalo; **SLP**

Diamond, Shari R 32 Arcadia Avenue, Dedham, MA 02026, (617) 326-3202, BS 86 Syracuse Univ; MS 88 Emerson Coll; 88–Sp-Lang Path, Mass Hospital School

Diamond, Susan S 473 West End Avenue, New York, NY 10024, **SLP**

Diamonstein, Beth A 1117 Buckingham, Norfolk, VA 23508, (804) 440-8342, MS 80 Auburn Univ - Auburn; Sp-Lang Path, **SLP**

Dias, Molly M 10459 Courthouse Drive, Fairfax, VA 22030, (703) 777-5050, BA 68 Western MI Univ; MA 73 MI St Univ; Aud, Blue Ridge Sp & Hrng Ctr, **A**

Diaz, Elizabeth Ann 8345 Mercier, Kansas City, MO 64114, (913) 334-2005, BA 81 Univ of MO - KS City; MS 83 Central MO St Univ; Sp-Lang Path, Deborah A King & Associates, **SLP**

Diaz, Karen L 5096 Tortuga Drive #105, Huntington Beach, CA 92649, (213) 926-5566, **SLP**

Diaz, Maria-Hele 632 Charles St Avenue, Towson, MD 21204, (301) 825-3552, BS 84 Towson St Univ; MS 87 Univ of NC - Chapel Hill

Diaz, Suzanne Gail 255 Frost Court, Riverside, CA 92507, MA 83 CA St Univ - Fullerton; Sp-Lang Path, Riverside USD, **SLP**

Diaz-Plaja, Dr Ruth R 6927-E Donachie Road, Baltimore, MD 21239, (301) 337-3862, BA 61 Huntingdon Coll; MA 63 Univ of AL- Tuscaloosa; OD 73 (NS) Johns Hopkins Univ; SLP, Baltimore County Board of Educ, **SLP A**

Diaz-Torres, Mrs Bonnie 396 Autumn Lane, Anniston, AL 36206, (205) 235-8965, BA 75 Univ of PR - Rio Piedras; MS 79 Univ of PR - Rio Piedras; Sp-Lang Path, Private Practice, **SLP**

Dibartolomeo, Dr Joseph R 2420 Castillo Street Suite 100, Santa Barbara, CA 93105-4302, (805) 563-1111, BS 59 Saint John's Univ - Jamaica; MD 63 (NS) Georgetown Univ; Otolaryngologist, Private Practice

Dibble, Lawrence M Michigan Dept Of Public Health, 9th Floor North Tower, MI Plaza Bldg 1200 6th St, Detroit, MI 48226, (313) 256-3613, BA 64 Univ of AZ; MA 67 Univ of AZ; Hrng & Sp Con, Michigan Dept of Pub Hlth, **SLP A**

Dibble, Mrs Linda Crandall 3546 River Pines Drive, Ann Arbor, MI 48103, (313) 994-2646, BA 65 Univ of MI - Ann Arbor; MS 68 Univ of MI - Ann Arbor; Sp-Lang Path, Washtenaw ISD-High Pt Cen, **SLP**

Dibble, Peggy C 1107 East Courtland Place, Whitefish Bay, WI 53211, (414) 332-3374, BA 58 Univ of CO - Boulder; MA 59 Stanford Univ; **A**

DiBenedetto, Donna J 14 Stone Avenue, Somerville, MA 02143, (617) 876-4344, **SLP**

Dibrell, Jayne W 2107 Griswold Lane, Austin, TX 78703, (512) 478-3078, BA 51 Univ of TX - Austin; MA 78 Univ of TX - Austin; Sp-Lang Path, Private Practice, **SLP**

Dicairano, Nancy Louise 153 Meadow Lane, Apartment 2 C, New Rochelle, NY 10805, (914) 235-2592, BA 81 Iona Coll; MS 86 Emerson Coll; SLP, Reese School, **SLP**

Dicarlo, Louis M 9413 Route 46, Westernville, NY 13486, (315) 827-4479, BA 32 Union Coll; MS 37 Univ of MA - Amherst; ED 48 (Aud-Sp Path) Columbia Univ Sch of Gen St; Aud/Sp-Lang Path, **SLP A F H LM**

Di Carlo, Susan M 5331 Curtis Road, Hemlock, NY 14466, BA 76 SUNY - Center at Buffalo; MA 79 SUNY - Center at Buffalo; Sp-Lang Path, Cont Developmental Svcs, **SLP**

Dicarlo-Kramer, Annette Marie 6332 Sutherland Avenue, St Louis, MO 63109, (314) 569-6040, BS 84 Fontbonne Coll; MS 85 Fontbonne Coll; 86–Sp-Lang Path, St John's Mercy Med Ctr, **SLP**

Dicarrado, Mrs Connie P Angola Road, Cornwall, NY 12518, BA 72 CUNY - Lehman Coll; MA 74 CUNY - Lehman Coll; **SLP**

Dicasimirro, Donna M 508 New Boston, Mahanoy City, PA 17948, (717) 787-1848, BS 76 Marywood Coll; MA 77 Univ of FL; 87–Mental Retardation Prog Spec, PA Dept of Pub Welfare, **A**

Di Cecca, Charles Louis RFD 1 Box 99-P, Center Harbor, NH 03226, (603) 279-5913, BS 80 Northeastern Univ; ME 82 Northeastern Univ; 85, Private Practice, **SLP**

Dicesare, Jeanette M 46 Tobin Drive, Rochester, NY 14615, (716) 392-5225, BS 81 SUNY - Coll at Geneseo; MA 83 SUNY - Coll at Geneseo; Sp-Lang Path, BOCES 2 Monroe/Orleans Co, **SLP**

Dichmann, Mrs Karla Louise 2616 Micarta Drive, Plano, TX 75023, BA 83 Univ of KY; OM 83 IN Univ - Bloomington; SLP, Richardson ISD, **SLP**

Dichter, Mrs Carol A 230 East 52nd Street, New York, NY 10022, (212) 751-5162, BA 65; MS 76 Boston Univ; Sp-Lang Path, City of New Rochelle, **SLP**

Dicioccio, Mrs Patricia B 6825 Gates Mills Boulevard, Gates Mills, OH 44040, (216) 464-9500, BS 65 Miami Univ - Oxford; MA 67 Case Western Reserve Univ; Sp-Lang Path, Sunny Acres Skilled Nurs Fac, **SLP**

Dick, Nancy Lee 27 William Street, St Thomas, ON, Canada N5R 1H1, (519) 631-2020, BA 83 Brandon Univ - Manitoba; MS 85 Minot St Univ; MS 86 Univ of London - England

Dick, Dr William K 230 South 50 West, Orem, UT 84058, (801) 373-7850, BA 77 ID St Univ; OM 80 Brigham Young Univ; PH 88 (Aud) Brigham Young Univ; 83–Dir Sp/Hrng, UT Valley Reg Med Cen, **A**

Dickard, Mrs Elizabeth Bentley 101 Springbrook, Tuscaloosa, AL 35405, (205) 759-7305, BS 84 Auburn Univ - Auburn; MA 86 Memphis St Univ; 88–Sp-Lang Path, DCH Sp & Hrng Clinic, **SLP**

Dickens, Patsy Hill 6612 Kingswood Drive, Fort Worth, TX 76133-5215, (817) 346-7959, BA 70 Ouachita Baptist Univ; MA 71 Southern Methodist Univ; Sp/Lang Path, Huguley Home Health Agency, **SLP**

Dickenson, Leslie Ann 5112 Ravenna Avenue N E #21, Seattle, WA 98105, (213) 273-8480, BS 83 Univ of WA; MS 85 Univ of OK Medical Center

Dickenson, Priscilla 1006 Shelley Avenue, Austin, TX 78703, (512) 482-0205, BA 75 Univ of Houston - Univ Park; MA 76 Univ of Houston - Univ Park; Sp-Lang Path, Priscilla Dickenson, **SLP**

Dickerhoof, Richard Gary 4016 Mesa Circle N W, Massillon, OH 44646, (216) 454-9152, BS 68 Kent St Univ; MA 73 Kent St Univ; Aud, Joseph P Yut MD, **A**

Dickerson, Mrs Bertha M 19193 Monica Street, Detroit, MI 48221, (313) 494-1643, BS 67 Wayne St Univ; ME 78 Wayne St Univ; 66–Sp-Lang Path, Detroit Bd of Ed, **SLP**

Dickerson, Mrs Debra Oakley 1824 Georgia Street N E, Albuquerque, NM 87110, (505) 268-4259, MS 85 Western KY Univ; **SLP**

Dickerson, Jan Marie 5975 Meadowsglen Drive, Dublin, OH 43017, (614) 761-2513, BA 84 OH St Univ; MA 87 OH St Univ; **SLP**

Dickerson, Mrs Janet L 4505 Clayborne Court, Kalamazoo, MI 49009, (616) 649-2321, BA 86 Ball St Univ; MA 88 Ball St Univ; SLP, Constance Brown Hrng & Sp Ctr

Dickerson, Janice V 423 Ridgewood, Monroe, NC 28110, (704) 283-9104, BA 72 Univ of NC - Greensboro; ME 75 Univ of NC - Greensboro; Sp/Lang Path, **SLP**

Dickerson, Linda H 7500 San Felipe, Suite 460, Houston, TX 77063, (713) 785-6760, BS 67 Univ of Houston - Univ Park; MA 72 Univ of MD - College Park; Co Director, Sp & Lang Remediation Cen Inc, **SLP**

Dickerson, Linda L Route 2 Box 41-G, North Vernon, IN 47265, (812) 458-6911, BA 72; MS 79 Univ of KY; Sp-Lang Path, Madison Area Spec Ser Ut, **SLP**

Dickerson, Dr Mary V Dearstone 2781 Tahoe Drive, Livermore, CA 94550, (408) 924-3675, BS 55 East TN St Univ; MA 56 Univ of AL- Tuscaloosa; PH 71 (NS) FL St Univ; 72–Professor of SLP & Aud, San Jose State University, **SLP F**

Dickerson, Mrs Nancy Jo 107 Bison Trail, Longview, TX 75601, (214) 758-0571, BS 79 East TX St Univ - Commerce; ME 86 Stephen F Austin St Univ; 88–Sp-Lang Path, Longview ISD, **SLP**

Dickert, Mrs Karen B 3625 Pond Branch Road, Leesville, SC 29070, (803) 532-2619, BS 77 Western Carolina Univ; MS 78 Univ of SC - Columbia; 83–Sp-Lang Path, Lexington Co Sch Dist, **SLP**

Dickey, Mrs Claire W 7056 Styers Ferry Road, Clemmons, NC 27012, (919) 722-8173, BA 63 Hollins Coll; ME 64 Univ of VA - Charlottesville; Education Supervisor, Family Services Inc, **SLP A**

Dickey, Mrs Lynette Case 2235 Starr Drive, Lodi, CA 95242, (209) 331-7087, BA 78 CA St Univ - Sacramento; MA 80 CA St Univ - Sacramento; Sp-Lang Path, Lodi USD, **SLP**

Dickey, Mrs Margaret Keck 601 Peters Road #E-7, Knoxville, TN 37922, (615) 690-6186, BS 77 James Madison Univ; MA 79 Univ of TN - Knoxville; Sp-Lang Path, St Marys Med Ctr, **SLP**

Dickey, Nancy 1801 Earthstone Drive, Valparaiso, IN 46383, (219) 464-9580, BA 81 IN Univ - Bloomington; MA 82 IN Univ - Bloomington; Aud, Prof Hrng Management Inc, **A**

Dickey, Mrs Sally R 2624 Rebecca Drive, Springfield, OH 45503-2256, (513) 390-1114, BS 59 Boston Univ; **SLP**

Dickey, Sarah K B 5198 South Memphis Court, Aurora, CO 80015, (303) 289-3154, BS 71 Univ of WY; MA 78 Univ of CO - Boulder; 78–Sp-Lang Path, Adams Co Sch Dist #14, **SLP**

Dickinson, Barbara 2306-A North Grand, Roswell, NM 88201, BS 68 Minot St Univ; MS 69 Minot St Univ; Sp-Lang Path, Roswell ISD, **SLP LM**

Dickinson, Mrs Cheryl L 960 West Orange Grove, Arcadia, CA 91006, (818) 355-0294, BS 70 CO St Univ; MA 75 Univ of CO - Boulder; **SLP**

Dickinson, David L 304 Gray Fox Square, Taylors, SC 29687, (803) 292-3151, BS 74 Kent St Univ; MA 76 Kent St Univ; **A**

Dickinson, Lynn M 4944 Sherwood Forest Blvd, Apartment 172, Baton Rouge, LA 70816, (504) 292-6259, BA 74 LA St Univ - Baton Rouge; MA 76 LA St Univ - Baton Rouge; Sp/Lang Path, E Baton Rouge Parish Sch Bd, **SLP**

Dickinson, Mrs Muriel E 5478 Rudy Drive, San Jose, CA 95124, (408) 378-3405, BA 72 San Jose St Univ; MA 74 San Jose St Univ; SLP, Campbell USD, **SLP**

Dickinson, Pamela J 147 Conover Road, Pittsburgh, PA 15208, BA Syracuse Univ; MS 70 Univ of Pittsburgh - Pittsburgh; 82–Aud, Univ Otolaryngology, **A**

Dickinson, Dr Sandra 345 West 55th Street #1A, New York, NY 10019, (718) 626-5082, MA 74 Univ of Rochester; MS 77 Emerson Coll; PH 84 (NS) NY Univ; Asst Prof, City Univ of New York, **SLP**

Dickinson, Mrs Stella C 3960 Coronado Avenue, San Diego, CA 92107, (714) 421-6700, BA 63 San Diego St Univ; MA 65 San Diego St Univ; **SLP**

Dickman, Donna M 2623 O Street N W, Washington, DC 20007, (202) 337-5220, MA 64 Mary Washington Coll; ME 65 Univ of VA - Charlottesville; PH 74 (NS) Univ of MD - College Park; 86–Exec Dir, Alex Graham Bell Assn, **SLP A**

Dickman, Mrs Harriet B 511 Heather Drive, Virginia Beach, VA 23462, (804) 499-7663, BS 60 Boston Univ; MA 65 Montclair St Coll; Director, Private Practice, **SLP**

Dickman, Jahnett L 1953 Lawrence Drive, Fort Mitchell, KY 41011, (606) 727-1488, BS 76 Univ of Cincinnati; MA 78 Univ of Cincinnati; Erlanger/Elsmere Boed, **SLP**

Dickson, Catherine A 2005 S E 22nd Avenue, Mineral Wells, TX 76067, (817) 325-6806, BS 77 TX Christian Univ; MA 86 TX Woman's Univ; **SLP**

Dickson, Mrs Christine Box 1914, Marathon, ON, Canada P0T 2E0, (807) 229-1820, BA 73 CA St Univ - Northridge; MA 74 CA St Univ - Northridge; 88–Sp/Lang Path, Thunder Bay Dist Health Unit, **SLP**

Dickson, Mrs Dana Javo 34 Noble Glen Drive, Savannah, GA 31406, (912) 355-4311, BS 76 Univ of GA; MS 77 Winthrop Coll; 87–Sp-Lang Path, Beaufort Co Schs, **SLP**

Dickson, Dr David Ross Mailman Ctr Child Devel (D820), University Of Miami, P O Box 016820, Miami, FL 33101, (305) 547-6123, BA 53 Grinnell Coll; MA 54 Northwestern Univ; PH 61 (NS) Northwestern Univ; Prof of Pediatrics, Univ of Miami, **SLP F**

Dickson, Jacqueline T 103 Central Avenue, Stirling, NJ 07980, (201) 647-5177, BA 61 Univ of Denver; SLP, Passaic Township Pub Schools, **SLP**

Dickson, Jean 416 South Loomis Street, Fort Collins, CO 80521, (303) 330-2138, BA 77 CO St Univ; MA 80 Univ of Northern CO; SLP, Weld Co Sch Dist Six, **SLP**

Dickson, Mrs Kathleen L P O Box 165, Russellton, PA 15076, (412) 658-3511, BS 72 Edinboro Univ of PA; MA 75 Western IL Univ; Sp-Lang Path, Speac-Aid Ltdn Dis, **SLP**

Dickson, Mrs Linda G Bradham 19401 Hubbard Drive, Audiology Department, Dearborn, MI 48126, (313) 593-8172, BA 76 Univ of MI - Ann Arbor; MA 77 MI St Univ; 85–Aud, Henry Ford Hospital, **A**

Dickson, Mrs Lori Sue 3650 Pennyroyal Lane, Colorado Springs, CO 80906, (719) 579-0874, BS 82 Brigham Young Univ; MS 83 Brigham Young Univ; 87–Co-Owner/, As They Grow Inc, **SLP**

Dickson, Maribeth 15316 Pond Woods Drive E, Tampa, FL 33618, (813) 264-1083, BS 85 Univ of AR - Fayetteville; MA 87 Memphis St Univ

Dickson, Mark T P O Box 165, Russellton, PA 15076, (216) 782-4183, BS 71 Edinboro Univ of PA; MA 75 Western IL Univ; Indust & Priv Aud Consult, Speac-Aid, **A**

Dickson, Dr Stanley 34 Park Lane Court, Williamsville, NY 14221, (716) 878-5319, BA 50 CUNY - Brooklyn Coll; MA 54 CUNY - Brooklyn Coll; ED 60 (NS) SUNY - Center at Buffalo; 56–Prof Commun Disorders, State University of New York, **SLP A F**

Dickson-Dutrow, Mrs Deborah A RD 2 Box 862, New Columbia, PA 17856, (717) 568-0237, BS 77 Clarion Univ of PA; MA 79 Kent St Univ; Aud, Dr Wm Bruce ENT Phys, **A**

Dickson-Loreti, Mrs Linda K RFD 4 Box 267, Leavenworth, KS 66048, (913) 651-5041, BS 76 KS St Univ; MA 77 KS St Univ; Sp-Lang Path, Leavenworth Special Educ Coop, **SLP**

Dickson-Serenita, Kerrin 3 Longacre Drive, Huntington, NY 11743, (516) 543-0458, BS 82 NY Univ; MS 87 Adelphi Univ; **SLP**

Dickstein, Lisa Zucker 54 Mulberry Circle, Staten Island, NY 10314, (718) 645-2852, BS 81 SUNY - Coll at Oneonta; MS 84 CUNY - Brooklyn Coll; **SLP**

Dickter, Ann Ellen Delaware Co Memorial Hospital, Hearing & Speech Center, 501 North Lansdowne Avenue, Drexel Hill, PA 19026, (215) 284-8570, BA 70 CUNY - Brooklyn Coll; MS 73 Southern IL Univ -Carbondale; Dir Hrng & Sp Cen, DE Co Memorial Hosp, **A**

Dickter, Mrs Farryl Suplin 14245 Ventura Boulevard, Suite 212, Sherman Oaks, CA 91423, (818) 501-1129, BA 68 Univ of CA - Berkeley; MA 70 Boston Univ; 88–Dir, Farryl Dickter MA & Assoc, **SLP**

Dickun, Patricia A 1118 Camp Nancy Road, Apollo, PA 15613, (412) 335-9860, BA 79 Univ of Pittsburgh - Pittsburgh; MA 81 Univ of Pittsburgh - Pittsburgh; Sp-Lang Path, Parents Lgue for Emotional Adj, **SLP**

Di Cola, George A 1112 Village Oak Drive, Winston-Salem, NC 27106, MS 77 WV Univ; SLP, Forsythe Memorial Hospital, **SLP**

Di Cristofalo, Mrs Karen Margaret 9057 Beach Road, Spring Hill, FL 34606, (904) 688-0530, BS 81 Elmira Coll; MA 83 Hofstra Univ; 87–Sp-Lang Path, Citrus County Sch Bd, **SLP**

Dictor, Mrs Rona S 2905 Piedmont Street, El Paso, TX 79902, (915) 533-0034, BA 73 Univ of TX - El Paso; MA 77 Univ of TX - El Paso; Sp-Lang Path, Canutillo ISD, **SLP**

Dictus, Kristine Ann 1430 Seville Drive #8, Green Bay, WI 54302, (414) 494-5627, BS 80 Univ of WI - Milwaukee; MS 83 Univ of WI - Milwaukee; Sp-Lang Path, Cerebral Palsy Inc, **SLP**

Didech, Marleen S 1044 Cumberland Place, San Jose, CA 95125, (408) 723-2452, BS 73 Univ of IL - Urbana; MA 74 Northwestern Univ; Teacher, Sinai Nursery School, **SLP**

Di Donato, Roberta M 8621 Cedardale, Houston, TX 77055, (714) 871-3280, BA 80 Rutgers St Univ - Camdem; OM 82 Hahnemann Univ Grad Sch; SLP, Methodist Hospital, **SLP**

Didow, Sharon M 117 Springhill Forest, Chapel Hill, NC 27514, (919) 684-3859, MS 73 Univ of NC - Chapel Hill; BA 71 Univ of NC - Chapel Hill; Sp/Lang Path, Duke U Med Cen, **SLP**

Didun, Lisa DeAngelo 340 Morris Avenue, Trenton, NJ 08611, (609) 989-9285, BA 82 Kean Coll of NJ; MA 84 Trenton St Coll; Sp-Lang Path, Mercer County Special Services, **SLP**

Dieball, Linda Kaye S 505 Arbor Lane, Austin, TX 78745, (512) 327-7420, BS 67 OK St Univ; MA 78 Univ of TX - Austin; Sp-Lang Path, Eanes ISD, **SLP**

Diebold, Dr Martin H Auburn University, Dept Rehabilitation/Sp Ed, Auburn, AL 36849, (205) 826-5943, MA 69 Univ of South FL; ED 75 (Sp Path) Univ of GA; Assoc Prof, Auburn University, **SLP**

Diebold, Rene 514 7th Street, Granite Falls, MN 56241, MS 73 Univ of MN - Minneap-St Paul; The Language Lab, **SLP**

Diederich, Jane B 1583 East Nichols Drive, Littleton, CO 80122, (303) 794-2205, BA 69 Elmhurst Coll; MA 74 Northern IL Univ - De Kalb; Sp-Lang Path, **SLP**

Diederich, Nancy Ann 2310 Tulip Road, San Jose, CA 95128, (408) 252-3000, BA 61 San Jose St Univ; MA 63 Stanford Univ; Sp-Lang Path, Cupertino Un Sch Dist, **SLP**

Diedrich, Joan Marie P O Box 825, Indian Hills, CO 80454, (303) 761-7050, MS 73 Marquette Univ; BS 60 Marquette Univ; Coord of Spec Edu, Englewood Sch, **SLP**

Diedrich, Julie L 403 N Green Street, McHenry, IL 60050, (815) 385-0645, BS 86 Eastern IL Univ; MS 87 Eastern IL Univ; **SLP**

Diedrich, William M Hearing And Speech Department, Univ Of Kansas Medical Ctr, 39th & Rainbow Boulevard, Kansas City, KS 66103, (913) 588-5937, BS 50 Rutgers St Univ -N Brunswick; MS 52 NM Highlands Univ; PH 58 (Sp-Lang Path) Case Western Reserve Univ; 55–Prof, U of KS Med Cen, **SLP F**

Diefendorf, Dr Allan O University Of Tennessee, South Stadium Hall, Stadium Drive, Knoxville, TN 37996, (615) 974-5017, BS 72 OR St Univ; MS 74 Vanderbilt Univ; PH 80 (Hrng & Sp Science) Univ of WA; Associate Professor, University of Tennessee, **A ACE**

Diehl, Mrs Adeline E 4480 East Colorado Avenue, Denver, CO 80222, (303) 756-8489, BA 55 Univ of Denver; MA 56 Univ of Denver; Retired, Denver Pub Sch, **SLP**

Diehl, Alicia S 531 North Fir, Jenks, OK 74037, (918) 299-3970, BS 76 OK St Univ; MA 78 OK St Univ; Self Employed, Diehl Aero-Nautical, **SLP**

Diehlmann, Tonia Marie 6919-I Victoria Drive, Alexandria, VA 22310, (703) 385-2810, BA 81 George Washington Univ; MS 83 Towson St Univ; **A**

Diekelman, Mrs Suzanne M 5481 La Cumbre Lane, Rockford, IL 61107-3776, (815) 966-3141, BS 66 Drake Univ; MA 84 Northern IL Univ - De Kalb; 85–Sp-Lang Path, Rockford Bd of Educ, **SLP**

Diekmann, Sharon B 16107 Springbank, Houston, TX 77095, (713) 462-5351, BS 71 Spalding Coll; MS 72 Murray St Univ; Sp-Lang Path, Cypress-Fairbanks ISD, **SLP**

Diekmann, Teri Lynn 9156 North Swan Circle, Brentwood, MO 63144, (314) 768-5337, BA 83 Univ of MO - Columbia; MA 87 Fontbonne Coll; Sp-Lang Path, SSM Rehab Inst, **SLP**

Diel, Mrs Dorothy L 18650 Pacific, Rockaway, OR 97136, (503) 355-2666, BS 51 Univ of OR; ME 61 Univ of OR; **SLP LM**

Dielmann, Sharon M 9110 Powhatan, San Antonio, TX 78230, (512) 221-2507, BA 66 Our Lady Lake Univ-San Anton; MA 69 Our Lady Lake Univ-San Anton; 87–Sp-Lang Path, Brooke Army Med Ctr, **SLP**

Diemer, Barbara K 11 Somerset Court, Bloomington, IL 61701, (815) 945-2971, BS 70 IL St Univ - Normal; MS 71 IL St Univ - Normal; Sp/Lang Path, Chenoa Comm Unit Dist 9, **SLP**

Diemer, Mrs Marlane J 4604 Wildwood Place, Las Cruces, NM 88001, (505) 526-6663, BS 72 IA St Univ; MS 74 CO St Univ; Sp-Lang Path, Las Cruces Pub Sch, **SLP ACE**

Diener, Bethany L 6212 Lakeview Drive #40, Indianapolis, IN 46224, (317) 297-2273, MS 87 Purdue Univ - West Lafayette; 87–Sp-Lang Path, Rehab Works Inc

Diener, Mrs Rhonda Ash 86 Virginia Avenue, Plainview, NY 11803, (718) 380-3000, BA 72 CUNY - Queens Coll; MA 74 Hofstra Univ; 86–Sp-Lang Path, UCP of Queens, **SLP**

Diener, Dr Stuart 3405 Old Forest Road, Baltimore, MD 21208, (301) 642-2411, BA 66 Univ of VA - Charlottesville; ME 68 Univ of VA - Charlottesville; PH 73 (NS) Univ of MD - College Park; 82–Dir Aud/Sp-Path, Perry Point MD, **SLP A**

Diener, Mrs Wendy P 3405 Old Forest Road, Baltimore, MD 21208, (301) 653-9194, BA 71 Univ of MD - College Park; MS 73 Loyola Coll; 73–Sp-Lang Path, Anne Arundel Co Board of Educ, **SLP**

Dienhart, Susan E 11912 East Louisiana Avenue, Aurora, CO 80012, (303) 360-3049, BS 75 Southeast MO St Univ; MS 78 AZ St Univ; 87–Sp-Lang Path Superv, Columbine Therapies Inc, **SLP**

Dierking, Mrs Patricia Elizabeth R R 2 Box 21, Grand Pass, MO 65339, (816) 493-2763, MS 88 Central MO St Univ

Dierksen, Carol A 4606 Detelemark Drive, Dundas, MN 55019, (507) 645-9742, BA 65 Augustana Coll; MA 68 Northwestern Univ; Elem Prin Grades K-8, MN State Acad for the Deaf, **SLP**

Diestler, Mrs Kathryn E 5301 Benton Avenue, Downers Grove, IL 60515, BS 73 Univ of UT; MS 74 Univ of UT; 78–Aud, DuPage-West Cook Reg Spec Educ Assoc, **A**

Dietch, Ellen L 1993 Heathcliff Drive #2B, Columbus, OH 43209, (614) 294-6403, BS 76 OH Univ - Athens; MA 78 OH St Univ; Sp/Lang Path, Columbus Sp/Hrng Cen, **SLP**

Dieter, Mrs Wendy Kay 501 33rd Street S W, Rochester, MN 55902-1225, BS 82 Kearney St Coll; MS 84 Univ of NE - Omaha; **SLP**

Dieterle, Francis R 503 8th Avenue, Salt Lake City, UT 84103, (801) 355-1830, BS 55 Univ of UT; MS 65 Univ of UT; Owner, Private Practice, **SLP**

Dieterle, Joanne M 5038 Carlyn Drive, Pittsburgh, PA 15236, (412) 884-9357, MS 87 Clarion Univ of PA; **SLP**

Dietert-Carnes, Denise 4101 South Alameda, Corpus Christi, TX 78411, (512) 857-6161, BA 76 Our Lady Lake Univ-San Anton; MA 77 Our Lady Lake Univ-San Anton; 88–Prog Coord, South Texas Area Rehab Ctr, **SLP**

Dietiker, Terri A 642 Via Los Miradores, Redondo Beach, CA 90277, BA 83 San Jose St Univ; MA 86 San Jose St Univ; 86–Aud, Parker Hrng & Sp Inst, **A**

Dietlein, Mrs Dona Lopez 109 Lietmeyer Street, New Iberia, LA 70560, (318) 364-3609, BA 80 Univ of Southwestern LA; MS 86 Univ of Southwestern LA; **SLP**

Dietrich, Mrs Cecelia A 3024 North 10th Street, Wausau, WI 54401, (715) 848-2062, BS 75 Marquette Univ; MS 76 Marquette Univ; Sp-Lang Path, Wausau Hosp Ctr, **SLP**

Dietrich, Frances Harag 3409 Winterberry Court S E, Grand Rapids, MI 49506, (616) 957-4326, BA 77 MI St Univ; MA 78 MI St Univ; Sp-Lang Path, Mary Free Bed Hosp & Rehab Cen, **SLP**

Dietrich, Mrs Jill Molock 1515 Huddersfield Court, San Jose, CA 95126, (408) 998-8447, BS 84 Univ of AR - Little Rock; MA 86 George Washington Univ; Sp-Lang Path, Casa Serena Hospital, **SLP**

Dietrich, Joan M 2415 Erin Lane, Nashville, TN 37221, (615) 352-3367, BS 84 Univ of WI - Madison; MS 86 Univ of WI - Madison; 88–Sp-Lang Path, Vanderbilt Univ Hosp & Cl, **SLP**

Dietrich, Susan 3114 North Kentucky, Oklahoma City, OK 73118, (405) 521-0261, **SLP**

Dietrich, Mrs Virginia Joyce 11791 Onyx Street, Garden Grove, CA 92645, (213) 926-5566, BA 82 CA St Univ - Long Beach; MA 86 CA St Univ - Fullerton; 86–Sp-Lang Path, ABC USD, **SLP**

Dietz, Mrs Judith 8845 East Phillips Place, Englewood, CO 80112, (303) 790-0789, BS 69 OH St Univ; OM 72 IN Univ - Bloomington; Sp-Lang Path, Private Practice, **SLP**

Diewald, Lisa Ann 251 Richard Drive, Palatine, IL 60067, (309) 452-2247, BS 84 Northern IL Univ - De Kalb; MS 86 IL St Univ - Normal; **A**

Diffley, Mary M 129 Hardwick Avenue, Westfield, NJ 07090, (212) 447-8205, BS 77 SUNY - Coll at Fredonia; MA 79 Hofstra Univ; SLP, Ucpassn-NYS, **SLP**

DiFilippo, Mrs Marla A 14530 Madison Avenue, Lakewood, OH 44107, (216) 521-2252, BS Kent St Univ; MA 87 Kent St Univ; 88–Sp-Lang Path, Berea City Sch Dist, **SLP**

Difilippo, Mrs Suzanne D 43 Pinetree, Seymour, IL 61875, (217) 687-2860, BA 71 Univ of Winnipeg - Manitoba; MS 73 Southern IL Univ -Carbondale; **SLP**

DiFilippo-Angelo, Renee E Tryon Circle, Peekskill, NY 10566, BS 84 SUNY - Coll at New Paltz; MS 86 Columbia Univ Teachers Coll; 87–Aud, Audiology & Speech Assoc, **A**

Difoggio, Jacy Doumas 3925 Thundercloud Drive, Colorado Springs, CO 80920, (303) 599-5826, **SLP**

Digaudio, Mrs Anna B 41 Whittier Avenue, Pittsfield, MA 01201, (413) 664-4541, BS 67 2441; MA 69 Bowling Green St Univ; Sp/Lang Path, Pittsfield Public Schools, **SLP**

Digby, Matthew J P O Box 154, Cromberg, CA 96103, (916) 836-2450, BA 53 San Diego St Univ; MS 65 Loma Linda Univ - Loma Linda; **SLP LM**

Dige, Janet L T 1390 Amstel Drive, Colorado Springs, CO 80907-4083, (303) 630-5204, MA Univ of MT; Sp/Lang Path, Penrose Hospital, **SLP**

Digeorgio, Mrs Karen M 11 Bakers Drive, Washington Crossing, PA 18977, BA 70 Adelphi Univ; MS 72 Adelphi Univ; **SLP**

Diggs, Dr Charles C, Jr American Speech - Language - Hearing Association, 10801 Rockville Pike, Rockville, MD 20852, (301) 897-5700, BA 69 Loyola Coll; MS 72 Purdue Univ - West Lafayette; PH 73 (NS) Purdue Univ - West Lafayette; 88–Dir-Consumer Info, ASHA, **SLP**

Diggs, Jayne Carithers 10821 Green View Way, Columbia, MD 21044, (301) 730-7818, BS 72 Purdue Univ - West Lafayette; MA 82 Univ of MD - College Park; **SLP**

Di Giantonio, Heidi A Hathaway- 3420 Culver Drive N W, Canton, OH 44709, (216) 493-3255, BS 75 Kent St Univ; MA 80 Kent St Univ; Sp-Lang Path, Human Dev & Cnsl Assoc Inc, **SLP**

Digilio, Mrs Carolyn A 517 Riverdale Avenue #2-E, Yonkers, NY 10705, (914) 965-9168, BS 77 9409; MS 79 9905; **SLP**

Digiovanni, Mrs Kathleen Marie 6302 14th Avenue, Brooklyn, NY 11219, BS 85 Carlow Coll; MA 87 Univ of Pittsburgh - Pittsburgh; **A**

Di Girolamo, Mrs Linda A 106 Wyoming Street, Westfield, NJ 07090, (201) 277-3875, BA 76 Rutger's St Univ - Douglas Coll; ME 77 Univ of VA - Charlottesville; Aud, Stephen Freifeld MD, **A ACE**

Dignam, Francis X 414 Summer Street, North Andover, MA 01845, (508) 681-0433, BA 65 Saint Alphonsus Coll; MS 73 Columbia Univ Teachers Coll; **SLP**

Dignan, Mrs C Louise 401-9 Avenue South, Fargo, ND 58103, (701) 241-9490, BS 69 Minot St Univ; MS 70 Minot St Univ; 86–Sp-Lang Path, Sheyenne Valley Spec Educ Unit, **SLP**

Digrande, Adriana Jole 219 Lynn Fells Parkway, Apartment 4, Melrose, MA 02176, (617) 979-0242, BA 76 SUNY - Coll at New Paltz; MS 79 Coll of Saint Rose; 82–Dir Precision Fluency Shaping, New England Rehab Hosp, **SLP**

Dikeman, Karen Joyce 132 Horton Street #2D, City Island, NY 10464, (212) 750-6940, MA 84 CUNY - Queens Coll; SLP, Goldwater Memorial Hospital, **SLP ACE**

Dikengil, Angela Tipton 6A Yacenda Drive, Morris Plains, NJ 07950, (201) 984-0523, MS 86 William Paterson Coll; 86–Sp-Lang Path, Kessler Inst for Rehab, **SLP**

Dilallo, Mary D 17599 Dartmoor Drive, Grayslake, IL 60030-1981, (312) 367-4300, BS 78 Northwestern Univ; MA 79 Northwestern Univ; 88–Sp-Lang Path, Lake-McHenry Reg Prog, **SLP**

Dilapo, Deborah Lagodna 8715 Cole Road, Colden, NY 14033, **SLP**

Dildine, Mrs Mary Sue Route 1, Patterson, MO 63956, (314) 856-4621, BS 73 Southern IL Univ -Carbondale; ME 75 Southeast MO St Univ; Sp-Lang Path, Clearwater R-1 Sch, **SLP ACE**

Dileo, Mrs Elizabeth Kirby 11019 Oregon Avenue, Bloomington, MN 55438-2463, (612) 338-3378, BS 73 Southern Methodist Univ; MS 74 Vanderbilt Univ; 87–Aud, Northstar Audiology, **A**

Dilgard, Susan S 1760 Taunton, Birmingham, MI 48009, (313) 258-3780, BA 72 Denison Univ; MA 75 Northwestern Univ; Sp-Lang Path, Wm Beaumont Hosp Barnum Hlth Ctr, **SLP**

Di Lillo, Michelle Anne 33 Colonial Street, East Northport, NY 11731, (516) 462-1495, BS 85 Long Island U - CW Post Ctr; MS 86 Adelphi Univ; 87–Sp-Lang Path, East Northport UFSD, **SLP**

Dill, Ann Lawrence 349 Fillmore Street #104, San Francisco, CA 94117, (415) 861-4832, BA 81 Mary Washington Coll; ME 84 Univ of VA - Charlottesville; Sp-Lang Path, Transitions-Berkeley, **SLP**

Dillaplain, Jeanne L 208 Pierce Boulevard, O'Fallon, IL 62269, (618) 632-4239, BS 86 Southern IL Univ-Edwardsvill; MS 87 Southern IL Univ-Edwardsvill; 87–Sp-Lang Path, St Louis Co Spec Sch Dist, **SLP**

Dillard, Cindy A 12601 South Green Drive, Apartment 1708, Houston, TX 77034, (713) 484-6639, ME 83 Southwest TX St Univ; Sp-Lang Path, Pat J Johnson PhD & Assoc PC, **SLP**

Dillard, Elizabeth Marie 1200 E Main Street, P O Box 557, Green Forest, AR 72638, (501) 438-5421, BS 83 AR St Univ; MS 84 AR St Univ; Sp-Lang Path, Green Forest Pub Schs, **SLP**

Dille, Marilyn F VA Medical Center, 1660 South Columbian Way, Seattle, WA 98108, (206) 764-2404, BA 72 Central WA Univ; OM 77 Univ of WA; Aud, VA Med Cen, **A**

Dillen, Sue Ann 810 Washington Avenue #318, Memphis, TN 38105, (901) 522-5199, BS 82 PA St Univ - Univ Park; MS 84 Vanderbilt Univ; 88–Sp-Lang Path, Baptist Memorial Hosp, **SLP**

Diller, Mrs Tomi-Tara K R3 Box 257-A, Hickory Harbor Drive, Gallatin, TN 37066, (615) 325-3233, BA 63 FL St Univ; MS 80 Western KY Univ; Sp/Lang Path, Sumner Co Sch Sys, **SLP**

Dilleshaw, Susan L 1606-C Oak Creek Lane, Bedford, TX 76021, (817) 284-5502, BS 79 Elmhurst Coll; MA 81 Univ of North TX; Sp-Lang Path, Hurst-Euless-Bedford Ism, **SLP**

Dillingham, Mrs Nancy T 3607 Locust Circle East, Prospect, KY 40059, (502) 228-0223, BS 72 Murray St Univ; MS 74 Murray St Univ; Sp-Lang Path, Oldham County School System, **SLP**

Dillman, Mary Kathryn 153 Bay Wood, Houston, TX 77571, (713) 471-1530, BS 69 OH St Univ; MS 86 Univ of Houston - Clear Lake; 86–Consult, Prentke Romich Co

Dillon, Ann Smith 3706 N W 25th Avenue, Gainesville, FL 32605, (904) 373-2999, BA 72 Transylvania Univ; MS 82 Univ of NC - Chapel Hill; Substitute Tchr, Alachua Cty Schs

Dillon, Debra Dawn 148 East Coral Gables, Phoenix, AZ 85022, (602) 866-8892, BS 80 Univ of AZ; MA 82 OK St Univ; 87–Sp-Lang Path, Mesa PS, **SLP**

Dillon, Diane Lynn 117 Sequoia Drive, San Anselmo, CA 94960, BS 84 Edinboro Univ of PA; MA 85 Edinboro Univ of PA; Sp-Lang Path, Novato USD, **SLP**

Dillon, Mrs Donna Witerski 313 Cornell Road, Bryans Road, MD 20616, (301) 283-2249, BS 83 SUNY - Coll at Buffalo; MA 87 Univ of Houston - Univ Park; 87–Sp-Lang Path, Charles County Bd of Educ, **SLP**

Dillon, Eileen A 6957 Spruce Pine Drive, Columbus, OH 43235, (614) 263-5151, BS 69 Bowling Green St Univ; MS 78 Univ of WI - Whitewater; Sp-Lang Path, Columbus Sp & Hrng Ctr, **SLP ACE**

Dillon, James Anthony 24 National Street, Salinas, CA 93901, (408) 424-8072, MS 86 San Francisco St Univ; 87–SLP, Casa Serena Rehab, **SLP**

Dillon, Lexa L 1786 Crofton Parkway, Crofton, MD 21114, (301) 952-6348, BA 67 Univ of MD - College Park; MA 69 Northwestern Univ; SLP, Prince Georges County Pub Sch, **SLP**

Dillon, Lorie Houston 9 Tulip Street, Cos Cob, CT 06807, (914) 948-0050, BS 80 PA St Univ - Univ Park; MS 83 PA St Univ - Univ Park; 85–Coord, Burke Rehabilitation Ctr, **SLP**

Dillon, Mary Ellen 1655 North Gladstone St, Suite E, Columbus, IN 47201, (812) 376-3071, BA 81 IN Univ - Bloomington; MS 83 Purdue Univ - West Lafayette; 84–Aud, Southern Indiana ENT, **A**

Dillon, Terese Marie 774 Pacific, Plymouth, MI 48170, (313) 451-6610, **SLP**

Dillon, Willard H 734 Highland Avenue, Latrobe, PA 15650, (412) 539-7451, BS 64 CA Univ of PA; ME 79 Indiana Univ of PA; Teacher, Westmoreland Inter, **SLP**

Dilthey-Griggss, Mary Jean 7327 Badger Court #D, Indianapolis, IN 46260, (317) 872-0710, BS 81 IN Univ - Bloomington; ME 84 IN Univ - Bloomington; 87–Sp-Lang Path, Hancock-S Madison Joint Svcs, **SLP**

Di Luzio, Angela Maria 34 Keenan Street, Watertown, MA 02172, BS 84 Northeastern Univ; MS 86 Boston Univ; 87–SLP, Jewish Mem Hosp, **SLP**

Di Luzio, Janice Marie 2420 Filmore Avenue #3, Erie, PA 16506, (814) 453-5602, BS 75 Boston Univ; MA 86 Edinboro Univ of PA; **SLP**

Dilworth, Robin Powers 628 North 5th Avenue, Tucson, AZ 85705, (602) 621-1969, BS 72 Kent St Univ; MA 73 Kent St Univ; Prog Coord, U of AZ, **SLP**

Dimambro, Mrs Laurie Anne 17449 Cedar Lake Circle, Northville, MI 48167, (313) 762-2123, BS 82 Worcester St Coll; MS 87 Univ of MI - Ann Arbor; 88–Sp-Lang Path, McHaven Gen Hosp

Dimarco, Mrs Carol Fruchtman 73-82 Springfield Blvd, Bayside, NY 11364, (718) 357-4650, BA 81 SUNY - Coll at New Paltz; MA 83 SUNY - Center at Buffalo; Sp-Lang Path, NYC Brd of Educ, **SLP**

Di Mare, Mrs Mateja J 421 Sandhurst Drive, Highland Heights, OH 44143, (216) 442-1718, BA 79 Cleveland St Univ; MA 81 Cleveland St Univ; 80–Aud, EENT Associates Inc, **A**

Di Martino, Marie J G 18 Wood Street, 3rd Floor, Providence, RI 02909, (401) 456-9330, BA 75 Univ of RI; MS 77 Univ of RI; Sp-Lang Path, Providence Sch Dist, **SLP**

Di Matteo, June S 8 Greenbriar Drive, Barrington, RI 02806, (401) 245-0521, BA 77 CUNY - Hunter Coll; MA 79 Temple Univ-Tyler Sch of Art; Aud, Cranston Aud Labs & Srv, **A**

Dimatteo, Pamela Kay 157 Aldershot Lane, Carlisle, MA 01741, (617) 369-3697, BS 71 Univ of TX - Austin; ME 73 Boston Univ; Sp-Lang Path, Chelmsford Pub Sch Syst, **SLP**

DiMatteo, Rhonda Lynn 803 Cattell Street, Easton, PA 18042, (215) 559-0981, BS 83 Trenton St Coll; MA 85 Hahneman Medical Coll; Dir of Sp-Lang Path, Warren Hills Regional Bd/Ed

Di Mauro, Judith A 81-5 Church Street, Lodi, NJ 07644, (201) 262-7181, BA 74 Montclair St Coll; MA 75 Montclair St Coll; 88–SLP, Paramus PS, **SLP ACE**

Di Meglio, Angela 117 Laredo Avenue, Staten Island, NY 10312, (718) 448-9775, BS 77 East Stroudsburg Univ of PA; MS 80 Columbia Univ Teachers Coll; Sp-Lang Path, Staten Island Mental Health, **SLP**

Dimeglio, Angela 21-B Stadium Way, Kentfield, CA 94904, (415) 457-8102, BA 78 CUNY - Hunter Coll; MS 81 PA St Univ - Univ Park; Sp-Lang Path, Private Practice, **SLP**

Di Meglio, Mrs Susan Anne 602 Paxson Avenue, Hamilton Township, Trenton, NJ 08619, (609) 586-1979, **SLP**

Dimenna, Mrs Deborah G 14520 Castleford Drive, Midlothian, VA 23113, (804) 379-9187, **SLP**

Dimiceli, Michele A 2911 Charlotte Avenue, Easton, PA 18042, (215) 253-9866, MA 82 Trenton St Coll; Sp-Lang Path, Hunterdon Dev Ctr, **SLP**

Diminuco, Frank G 455 Wilkinson Street, Syracuse, NY 13204, (315) 422-4372, BS 59 SUNY - Coll at Fredonia; MS 62 Syracuse Univ; Special Education Teacher, Syracuse Board of Education, **SLP**

Dimmitt, Mrs Sandra C 1304 South Maple, Fairfield, IA 52556, (515) 472-6118, BA 72 Kearney St Coll; MA 73 Northeast MO St Univ; Sp-Lang Path, Sn Prairie AEA 15, **SLP**

Dimon, Mrs Elise Bolen 2300 Lyman, Lansing, MI 48912, (517) 372-9924, BS 72 SUNY - Center at Albany; MS 74 Purdue Univ - West Lafayette; 88–Hearing Consult, MI Dept of Pub Health Ctr, **A**

Dimusto, Mrs Lisa 1642 Orchard Drive, Canton, MI 48188, (313) 728-1535, MA 88 Eastern MI Univ

Dinan, Christine Anderson 816 Alton Woods Drive, Concord, NH 03301, BS 76 SUNY - Coll at Geneseo; MS 79 Univ of UT; 88–Sp-Lang Path, Concord School District, **SLP**

Dinan, Mrs Shelley 74 Lakeview Avenue, New Canaan, CT 06840, (203) 966-9575, BA 65 Montclair St Coll; MA 67 Columbia Univ Teachers Coll; MA 83 Fairfield Univ; Sp-Lang Path, Private Practice, **SLP**

Dinapoli, Joseph M 16 Shepard Street, Cambridge, MA 02138, (617) 281-3174, BS 77 Emerson Coll; MS 78 Columbia Univ Teachers Coll; Sp-Lang Path, Private Practice, **SLP**

Dincher, Barbara Jean 5020 West Avenue, Ocean City, NJ 08226, (609) 398-1668, BA 80 West Chester Univ of PA; MS 82 Bloomsburg Univ of PA; SLP, Helmbold Ed Cen, **SLP**

Dineen, Mary Goes 6828 Grand Parkway, Wauwatosa, WI 53213, (414) 224-3377, BS 74 Marquette Univ; MS 75 Marquette Univ; Clin Supvr, Marquette Univ, **SLP**

Dinenna, Mrs Doreen S 4621 Ashberry Drive, Sarasota, FL 33580, (813) 955-0271, BS 75 PA St Univ - Univ Park; MS 78 Bloomsburg Univ of PA; SLP, School Board of Sarasota Co

Dinger, Mrs Nancy A 7841 South Scepter Drive #24, Franklin, WI 53132, (414) 529-4268, MA 88 San Diego St Univ

Dinges, Dr Maureen McGarvey 2080 Pine Forest Drive N E, Atlanta, GA 30345, (404) 524-2883

Dingess, Mrs Cheryl Ratliff Route 2, Box 132, Harts, WV 25524, (304) 855-3173, BA 75 Marshall Univ; MS 86 Marshall Univ; 87–Sp-Lang Path, Lincoln Co Bd of Educ, **SLP**

Dingle, Mrs Ann E R R 1 Box 164B, Charlton, MA 01507, (617) 248-6517, BS 78 Univ of MA - Amherst; MA 80 Univ of MA - Amherst; **SLP**

Dingwall, Louise L 9789 Springwood Drive, Kalamazoo, MI 49009, (616) 385-0887, BA 75 Univ of CT; MA 77 Western MI Univ; SLP, Kalamazoo Pub Sch, **SLP**

Dingwall, William O 6511 Wilson Lane, Bethesda, MD 20817

Dinielli, Marion L P O Box 1514, Danville, KY 40422, (606) 528-7782, BS 80 Univ of MD - College Park; MS 82 Gallaudet Coll; Aud, Eastern KY Sp-Hrng Clinic, **A**

Dininny, Dr Donald H 302 Wood Street, Clarion, PA 16214, (814) 226-2148, BS 62 Clarion Univ of PA; ME 63 PA St Univ - Univ Park; PH 69 (NS) OH Univ - Athens; Prof of SLP and Sp Sci, Clarion Univ of Pa, **SLP**

Dinner, Dr M Bernice 4001 South Magnolia Way, Denver, CO 80237, (303) 393-5821, BA 71 Univ of Denver; MA 73 Univ of Denver; PH 81 (NS) Univ of CO - Boulder; 88–Pres, Hear Now, **A**

D'Innocenzo, Mrs Maureen M 41 Queen Avenue, Enola, PA 17025, (717) 732-4839, MS 85 Bloomsburg Univ of PA; SLP, Capitol Area Int Unit, **SLP**

Dinnsen, Daniel A Indiana University, Department Of Linguistics, Lindley Hall 401B, Bloomington, IN 47405, (812) 336-4987

Dinsdale, Mrs Dawn L S 803 Elm Hurst Drive, Omaha, NE 68128, (402) 331-0499, BS 76 Univ of NE - Lincoln; MA 77 Univ of NE - Lincoln; **A**

Dinsmoor, Joyce H 5647 Phelps Luck Drive, Columbia, MD 21045, MS; **SLP**

Dinsmore, Cassandra Elizabeth 5070 River Glen Drive #396, Las Vegas, NV 89103, (702) 799-7123, BS 84 Northeast MO St Univ; MA 85 Northeast MO St Univ; Sp-Lang Path, Clark County Sch Dist, **SLP**

Dinucci, Linda Miller 20367 Ljepava Drive, Saratoga, CA 95070, BA 84 San Jose St Univ; MA 86 San Jose St Univ; **SLP**

Dinwoodie, Mrs Cheryl Klobnak 14011 Pinerock, Houston, TX 77079-2661, (713) 880-7199, BA 79 Southern IL Univ-Edwardsvill; MS 80 Southern IL Univ-Edwardsvill; 85–Sp-Lang Path, Memorial Northwest Hospital, **SLP**

Dionigi, Cynthia Marie 3254 West 41st Avenue, Denver, CO 80211, (303) 287-0181, BA 73 Univ of CO - Boulder; MA 78 Univ of CO - Boulder; Sp-Lang Path, Adams Co Sch Dist #12, **SLP**

Dionne, Carole S 206 Baxter Blvd, Apt #4, Portland, ME 04101, (207) 774-0314, BS 75 Univ of ME - Farmington; MA 80 Univ of ME - Orono; SLP, Woodfords Educational Ctr, **SLP**

Di Orazio, Nicholas 2909 Avenue E, Holmes Beach, FL 34217, (813) 778-4212, BA 69 SUNY - Center at Buffalo; MA 72 SUNY - Center at Buffalo; SLP, The Center at Manatee Springs, **SLP**

Dipalma, Mrs Ann Marie 1315 9th Street N W, Calgary, AB, Canada T2M 3L1, (403) 229-7022, BA 78 Univ of ND; MS 79 Univ of WI - Stevens Point; Sp/Lang Path, Alberta Chld Hosp, **SLP**

DiPalma, Felix M 14 East Macon Avenue, Staten Island, NY 10308, (718) 948-7381, BA 74 CUNY - Brooklyn Coll; MS 76 CUNY - Brooklyn Coll; 81–Sp-Lang Path, Private Practice, **SLP ACE**

DiPaola, Phyllis A 261 Westminster Road, Rochester, NY 14607, (716) 461-0343, BS 73 Nazareth Coll of Rochester; MS 74 SUNY - Coll at Geneseo; Sp-Lang Path, Mary Cariola Childrens Cen, **SLP**

DiPasquale, Mrs Priscilla R 11708 Slater, Overland Park, KS 66210-3169, (913) 451-2958, MA 78 Univ of KS; BS 75 Univ of KS; Sp-Lang Path, USD 229, **SLP**

Dipetta, Mrs Mary Ann 1554 Maple Avenue, Elmira, NY 14901, (607) 734-0124, **SLP**

DiPlacidi, Mrs Barbara M 12631 Heritage Farm Lane, Herndon, VA 22071, (703) 476-1534, BS 71 SUNY - Coll at Geneseo; MA 74 Montclair St Coll; Sp-Lang Path, Fairfax Co Sch Sys, **SLP**

Dipple, Annette Lynn 154 Tolman Street, Westbrook, ME 04092, (207) 854-1620, BA 83 Univ of MI - Ann Arbor; MS 85 Univ of MI - Ann Arbor; Sp-Lang Path, Scarborough PS, **SLP**

Dipzinski, Christine Ann 198 Arora #2908, Orange Park, FL 32073, (904) 272-1394, BS 84 Central MI Univ; MA 85 Central MI Univ; Sp-Lang Path, Clay Co Sch Bd, **SLP**

Diraimo, Laura Wisniewski 277 Brandon Road, Rochester, NY 14622, (716) 271-6423, BS 80 SUNY - Coll at Geneseo; MA 82 OH Univ - Athens; 85–Sp-Lang Path, UCP, **SLP**

Dirando, Mrs Maria 2645 Northwood, Toledo, OH 43606, (419) 241-6219, BS 85 John Carroll Univ; MS 87 Bowling Green St Univ; Sp-Lang Path, Toledo Hearing & Speech Ctr, **SLP**

Director, Larry 720 Arapaho Trail, Maitland, FL 32751, (305) 628-0770, BA 63 Univ of FL; MS 66 FL St Univ; Sp/Lang Path, Orange County Sch, **SLP**

Diresta, Diane 198 Ward Avenue, Staten Island, NY 10304, (718) 273-7199, BA 74 CUNY - Brooklyn Coll; MS 77 Columbia Univ Teachers Coll; SLP, NY Bd of Ed Sp Serv Ut, **SLP**

Dirks, Dr Donald D University Of California, Room 62-129 Chs, Los Angeles, CA 90024, (213) 825-6147, BS 55 Saint Louis Univ; MS 59 Univ of KS; PH 62 (NS) Univ of CA - Los Angeles; Professor, University of California, **SLP A F**

Dirks, Thomas Jay 20 Wingfield Way, Benicia, CA 94510, (707) 644-8921, 73 San Jose St Univ; 80 San Jose St Univ; 74–Sp-Lang Path, Vallejo USD, **SLP**

Diroll, Mrs Debbie J 2401 Eilers Lane #303, Lodi, CA 95240, (209) 944-4235, BA 80 Univ of the Pacific; MA 81 Univ of the Pacific; SLP, Stockton USD, **SLP**

Dirr, Susan PO Box 197, Deep Gap, NC 28607, (704) 264-5989, BS 68 Lamar Univ; MA 75 Univ of Houston - Univ Park; Dir-Oper Support, CommuniCare Inc, **SLP ACE**

Di Russo, Mrs Irma B 15 Locke Lane, Lexington, MA 02173, OB 39 Emerson Coll; MS 59 Emerson Coll; **SLP LM**

Dirvonas, Mrs Deborah F 8417 Westchester, Canton, MI 48187, (313) 459-6682, BS 78 Indiana Univ of PA; MS 79 Indiana Univ of PA; **SLP**

DiSalvo, Mrs Maureen Foster 17 Meadowbrook Drive, Hadley, MA 01035, (413) 549-6026, MA 87 Univ of MA - Amherst; 87–Sp-Lang Path, Children's Lang Inst, **SLP**

Disanti, Mrs Catherine A 7933 Tower Court Road, Severn, MD 21144, (301) 474-0430, BS 84 SUNY - Coll at Fredonia; MA 86 Univ of MD - College Park; 87–Aud, The Hearing Lab, **A**

Di Santo, Susan M 1651 16th Street, Santa Monica, CA 90404, (213) 450-8338, BA 70 Marygove Coll; MA 72 Eastern MI Univ; Spec Educ Prog Spec, Santa Mon-Malibu USD, **SLP**

Disarno, Neil J Regional Rehabilitation Center, Florida State University, Tallahassee, FL 32306, (904) 644-2238, BA 75 SUNY - Center at Buffalo; MS 76 FL St Univ; Aud, **A**

Dischiav, Kristine Marie 288 North Goodman Street, Apartment 12, Rochester, NY 14607, (716) 442-0745, BS 86 SUNY - Coll at Geneseo; MS 87 SUNY - Coll at Fredonia; **SLP**

Discount, Mrs Kathy Debra 14 Snowball Court, Mount Laurel, NJ 08054, (609) 235-3004, BA 80 Temple Univ; ME 81 Trenton St Coll; Sp-Lang Path, Mt Laurel Bd of Educ, **SLP**

Disharoon, Sandra B 1112 Heather Court, Fort Worth, TX 76126, (615) 472-1553, BS 74 Univ of TN - Knoxville; MA 76 Univ of TN - Knoxville; Sp/Lang Path, Fort Worth ISD, **SLP**

Disher-Hobeika, Linda Marie 30 Prospect Avenue, Hackensack, NJ 07601, (201) 441-2165, BA 81 0500; OM 84 Univ of Western Ontario; Speech Language Pathologist, Hackensack Medical Center, **SLP**

Disibio, Diane L 280 Park Avenue South #16-M, New York, NY 10010, (212) 230-7711, BA 75 Saint John's Univ - Jamaica; MS 77 CUNY - Brooklyn Coll; Admin Ed Services, Metropolitan Hospital, **SLP**

Di Simoni, Dr Frank G Grouse Hill Road, RD 1 Box 359, Dalton, PA 18414, (717) 969-8000, BS 63 East Stroudsburg Univ of PA; MA 66 Temple Univ-Tyler Sch of Art; PH 72 (Sp Science) Temple Univ-Tyler Sch of Art; Sp-Lang Path, The Speech Therapists, **SLP**

Di Simoni, Rosemary 278 Wilbraham Road, Hampden, MA 01036, MA 75 Univ of MA - Amherst; Supervisor Sp-Lang Path, Mercy Hosp, **SLP**

Diskind, Mrs Faiga 1004 Lexington Avenue, Lakewood, NJ 08701, (201) 367-8577, BA 73 CUNY - Hunter Coll; MA 75 CUNY - Hunter Coll; Dir, Ctrl Jersey Sp & Hrng Cen, **SLP**

Dismuke, Ruth P Therapeutic Horsemanship Of Nm, P O Box 30, North Highway 14, Sandia Park, NM 87047, (505) 281-1811, BA 79 Univ of NM; MS 80 Univ of NM; Dir, Ther Horsemanship of Nm, **SLP**

Disney, Sarah Thompson 8911 Symmes Trace Court, Cincinnati, OH 45140, (513) 742-2200, BS 70 Miami Univ - Oxford; MS 77 Miami Univ - Oxford; Consult Supvr, Hamilton Co Off Ed, **SLP**

DiSogra, Robert M Regency Bldg, 31 Schanck Road Suite D, Freehold, NJ 07728, (201) 462-1413, BS 75 Saint John's Univ - Jamaica; MA 76 Hofstra Univ; 85–Aud, Private Practice, **A ACE**

Dispensa, Mrs Kristine Mary 8008 S Pulaski #3-North, Chicago, IL 60652, (312) 585-8924, BA 83 Saint Xavier Coll; MS 86 Rush Univ; **SLP**

Diss, Mrs Nancy Muscato 3615 West Granada, Tampa, FL 33629, (817) 926-0488, BS 76 Ball St Univ; MA 79 Ball St Univ; Audiologist, Hillsborough County Schools, **A**

Di-Stasio, Mrs Linda C 257 Carbondale Road #219, Waymart, PA 18472, (717) 278-1106, MS 78 Bloomsburg Univ of PA; 79–Sp-Lang Path, Elk Lake Sch Dist, **SLP**

Distin, Viki Linneman 4750 East Sunrise, Phoenix, AZ 85044, (602) 830-0994, BS 82 IL Wesleyan Univ; MS 84 IL St Univ - Normal; Aud, **A**

Di Thomas, Mary B Drawer 888, Weston, WV 26452, (304) 269-4585, ME 78 Clarion Univ of PA; BS 75 Clarion Univ of PA; Sp-Lang Path, Lewis Co Bd of Ed, **SLP**

Ditmanson, AnnaDell 4018 West Hillsdale Drive, Visalia, CA 93291, (209) 732-3808, BA 80 CA St Univ - Stanislaus; MA 78 CA St Univ - Stanislaus; Sp-Lang Path, Visalia Unif Sch Dist, **SLP**

Dittman, Mrs Kim Elias Northwest Ohio Sp Education, Regional Resource Center, 10142 Dowling Road, Bowling Green, OH 43402, (419) 833-6761, BS 77 Edinboro Univ of PA; MA 78 Bowling Green St Univ; Sp-Lang Path, NW Oh Sp Ed Reg Resource Cen, **SLP**

Dittmer, Judy 72-B Halaulani Street, Hilo, HI 96720, (808) 961-3081, BA 69 Kalamazoo Coll; MS 72 Univ of MI - Ann Arbor; Sp-Lang Path, Easter Seal Society, **SLP**

Dittrick, Ginger Lee 24341 Gessner Road, North Olmsted, OH 44070-1549, (216) 282-4683, BA 77 Kent St Univ; MA 83 Univ of TN - Knoxville; Sp-Lang Path, Lorain Comm Hosp, **SLP**

Ditty, Karen Markuson 2021 General Mouton, Baton Rouge, LA 70810, (504) 769-1040, BA 78 Univ of Houston - Univ Park; MS 80 Lamar Univ; Aud, Baton Rouge ENT Clinic, **A**

Ditusa, Mrs Mildred M 178 Belvoir Road, Williamsville, NY 14221, (716) 689-7178, BA 60 SUNY - Center at Buffalo; MS 73 SUNY - Coll at Buffalo; SLP, Williamsville Central Schools, **SLP ACE**

Divenyi, Dr Pierre L Speech & Hearing Research 151, VA Medical Center, Martinez, CA 94553, (415) 228-6800, OM 65; MA 67 Univ of WA; PH 70 (NS) Univ of WA; 79–Ch Sp Hrng Res, VA Med Cen

Diver, Kathleen Joan 9960 Racquet Club Lane, Apartment #2A, Glen Allen, VA 23060, (804) 273-1683, BS 84 Purdue Univ - West Lafayette; ME 86 Univ of VA - Charlottesville; 88–Sp-Lang Path, Medical Coll of Virginia, **SLP**

Divizio, Gail Ellen 1418 Newell Road, Oakhurst Manor, Richmond, VA 23225, (804) 264-2446, BS 74 Radford Univ; MA 79 OH Univ - Athens; Sp/Lang Path, Chldn's Hosp, **SLP**

Dix, Beth Ann 10150 St Joe Road, Fort Wayne, IN 46835, (219) 493-1685, BS 85 IN St Univ - Terre Haute; MA 87 Ball St Univ; 87–Sp-Lang Path, Ft Wayne St Dev Center

Dix, Mrs Cheryl Herman 22 Sandburg Drive, Morganville, NJ 07751, (212) 464-2900, BS 75 SUNY - Coll at Geneseo; MA 77 SUNY - Coll at Geneseo; Sp/Lang Path, Child Study Center of New York, **SLP**

Dix, Cynthia A 10206 Hickory Ridge Rd, #202, Columbia, MD 21044, (301) 995-1852, BA 80 Loyola Coll; MS 81 Loyola Coll; 81–Sp-Lang Path, Howard Co Pub Sch, **SLP**

Dix, Patricia Elizabeth 137 West Sunset Road, San Antonio, TX 78209-2632, (512) 829-1745, MA 85 Our Lady Lake Univ-San Anton; Vice President, Speech Associates Inc, **SLP**

Dixon, Mrs Beverly J 16007 N E Siskiyou, Portland, OR 97230, (503) 257-5350, MS 68 Portland St Univ; BS 61 Univ of Northern CO; Sp-Lang Path, Parkrose Pub Sch, **SLP**

Dixon, Carmen C 194 G Street, Chula Vista, CA 92010, (619) 425-9600, MA 46 IA St Univ; BS 43 Bradley Univ; 54–Retired, Chula Vista City Schs, **SLP LM**

Dixon, Carol H 284 Highland Street, Dedham, MA 02026, (617) 461-0522, BA 76 SUNY - Coll at Plattsburgh; MS 77 Univ of WI - Stevens Point; Sp-Lang Path, Dedham Pub Sch, **SLP**

Dixon, Carol Zimmerman P O Box 111, Liberty, MS 39645, (601) 657-8583, BS 81 LA St Univ - Baton Rouge; MA 85 LA St Univ - Baton Rouge; 85–Sp-Lang Path, Amite County School Board, **SLP**

Dixon, Carolyn 147 Stonewall #10, Memphis, TN 38104, (901) 272-1487, BA 76 Univ of MS; MA 87 Memphis St Univ; 88–SLP, Baptist Memorial Hosp, **SLP**

Dixon, Cynthia Anderson 601 Napa Valley #312, Little Rock, AR 72211, (501) 376-1559, BS 82 Univ of Central AR; MS 86 Univ of Central AR; 88–Sp-Lang Path, Ark Ped Facility, **SLP**

Dixon, Emily H 112 Jackson Road, Mount Airy, NC 27030, (919) 789-9171, **SLP**

Dixon, Henry P Rd 2 Box 196, Centre Hall, PA 16828, (717) 922-3311, BS 72 PA St Univ - Univ Park; MS 74 PA St Univ - Univ Park; Dir Sp & Hrng Dept, PA Dept/Pub Welfare-Laurelton, **SLP A**

Dixon, Dr James D 13471 Stuart Court, Broomfield, CO 80020, (303) 837-2135, BS 58 Brigham Young Univ; MA 60 Univ of MD - College Park; PH 67 (NS) Univ of WA; Reg Rehab Spec, US Dept Ed/Off of Rehab Serv, **A**

Dixon, Mrs Jennifer L Psc #2, P O Box 1015, APO New York, NY 09405, (602) 571-1220, BA 81 CA St Univ - Fresno; MS 87 Univ of AZ

Dixon, Karen Sue 66900 Ironwood Drive, #1610, Desert Hot Springs, CA 92240, (619) 323-6175, BA 83 CA St Univ - Sacramento; MS 86 CA St Univ - Sacramento; SLP, Desert Hospital, **SLP**

Dixon, Kristen Lynn 901 West Main, Apartment 101, Puyallup, WA 98371, (206) 840-0386, MS 88 Univ of WA

Dixon, Leeann Hanson 2310 Jasmine, Denver, CO 80207-3422, (303) 320-6114, BS 78 AZ St Univ; MS 80 AZ St Univ; Sp-Lang Path, Sp & Lang Assocs, **SLP**

Dixon, Marilyn Marie 802 Ashville, Slidell, LA 70458, (504) 448-0644, MS 88 Univ of AR - Little Rock; 88–Aud, Therapy Associates of LA Inc

Dixon, Mrs Martha M 115 Blacksmith Lane, Greenville, NC 27834, (919) 757-4448, BA 75 Mary Washington Coll; MS 77 East Carolina Univ; Dept Mgr/Sp-Lang Path & Aud, Pitt Co Mem Hosp/Reg Rehab Ctr, **SLP**

Dixon, Melinda S 2310 Carlmont Drive #4, Belmont, CA 94002, (415) 877-8738, BA 84 Univ of CA - Santa Barbara; MS 87 San Francisco St Univ; 87–Sp-Lang Path, So SF USD, **SLP**

Dixon, Michelle Marie 2540 Severn Drive, Reno, NV 89503-2146, (503) 378-0723, BS 84 Univ of NV - Reno; MS 86 Univ of NV - Reno; **SLP**

Dixon, Nancee L 20 Plaza Olas Altos N E, Villa Encantada, Albuquerque, NM 87109, (505) 841-5385, BS 79 CA St Univ - Fresno; MS 82 Univ of HI - Manoa; 88–Dir-Sp-Lang Path/Aud, Los Lunas Hosp and Training Sch, **SLP ACE**

Dixon, Patricia Eilene 485 Whitman St South, Monmouth, OR 97361, (305) 838-4016, BA 73 OH St Univ; MA 80; Sp-Lang Path, Salem-Keizer PS, **SLP**

Dixon, Patricia Lynch 1566 Del Rio Avenue, Fort Myers, FL 33901, (813) 337-1951, BA 76 Univ of AR - Fayetteville; MA 77 Univ of AR - Fayetteville; Sp-Lang Path, Private Practice, **SLP**

Dixon, Rhoda Thomas 422 Thomas Avenue, Ferguson, MO 63135, (314) 569-8100, BS 82 MS Univ for Women; MS 84 Southern IL Univ-Edwardsvill; **SLP**

Dixon, Mrs Richard E 619 Princeton-Lawrencevill, Princeton, NJ 08540, (609) 921-6264, BS 63 Baylor Univ; MS 66 Vanderbilt Univ; **SLP**

Dixon, Dr Richard F University Of North Carolina, As 300, Greensboro, NC 27412, (919) 379-5184, BA 51 SUNY - Center at Binghamton; MA 53 Syracuse Univ; PH 55 (NS) Syracuse Univ; Dir Commun Dis, U Greensboro, **SLP A F**

Dixon, Sharon B 705 Toms Creek Road, Hopkins, SC 29061, BA 78 Columbia Coll; OM 79 Univ of SC - Columbia; Sp-Lang Path, Richland County School Dist, **SLP**

Dixon, Susan D 1600 Strickland, Martinsville, IN 46151-9314, (317) 349-1353, BS 77 Univ of WI - Madison; MA 79 Western IL Univ; Sp-Lang Path, Private Practice, **SLP**

Dixon-Ernst, Christine Alcoa, 1501 Alcoa Bldg, Pittsburgh, PA 15219, (412) 553-3612, BS 75 Chatham Coll; MS 78 Univ of Pittsburgh - Pittsburgh; MA 85 Univ of Pittsburgh - Pittsburgh; 86–Admin, Alcoa, **A**

Dixson, JoAnne Alma 512 Breezy Point Drive, Apt 4, Clinton, IA 52732, (319) 242-6454, BA 81 Univ of Northern IA; MA 82 Univ of SD - Vermillion; Sp-Lang Path, Mississippi Bend AEA 9, **SLP**

Dizon, Mary B 1585 Kapiolani Boulevard, Suite 912, Honolulu, HI 96814, (808) 941-8536, BA 65 Univ of HI - Manoa; MS 67 Univ of HI - Manoa; Owner/Sp-Lang Path, Private Practice, **SLP**

Dluhos, Mrs Anna Patricia 909 Preston Road, East Meadow, NY 11514-4535, (516) 489-3810, BA 80 CUNY - Brooklyn Coll; MS 84 CUNY - Brooklyn Coll; **SLP**

Doak, Kathryn M Fikse 630 North Cotner #101A, Lincoln, NE 68505, (402) 466-2331, BS 77 Univ of NE - Lincoln; MA 79 Univ of NE - Lincoln; Aud, Aud Assoc, **A**

Doane, Michele E 471 Acalanes Drive, Apt #35, Sunnyvale, CA 94086, (415) 960-0646, MA 77 Univ of the Pacific; SLP, **SLP**

Doane, Suzanne Catherine 264 Franklin Lane, Ventura, CA 93001-1418, (805) 487-7861, BS 83 Univ of AZ; MS 85 Univ of AZ; **SLP**

Dobash, Cecelia A 46 Benjamin Avenue, Conyngham, PA 18219, MS 75 Bloomsburg Univ of PA; Co-Dir, Wilkes-Barre Sp & Lang Cl, **SLP**

Dobbel-Brown, Mrs Andra L Route 10 Box 336, Columbus, MS 39701, (601) 328-5277, BS 78 MS Univ for Women; MS 79 MS Univ for Women; Sp-Lang Path, Private Practice, **SLP**

Dobbert, Mrs Ruth Rohl 13787 Ishnala Circle, West Palm Beach, FL 33414, (407) 793-6771, OB 65 OH Univ - Athens; MA 67 OH Univ - Athens; **SLP**

Dobbins, Edward Anthony 5757 West Thunderbird, Apartment E251, Glendale, AZ 85306, (602) 584-2100, BA 77 AZ St Univ; MS 82 AZ St Univ; Owner, Dobbins Hrng Serv, **A**

Dobbins, Mrs Patti L 237 Cedar Boulevard, Pittsburgh, PA 15228, (412) 561-0667, MA 75 MI St Univ; **SLP**

Dobeck, Connie Sue 2172 Larch Lane, Tustin, CA 92680, (714) 731-5096, BA 83 Univ of Redlands; MS 85 Univ of WA; 88–Sp-Lang Path, Rancho Los Amigos Med Ctr, **SLP**

Doben-Stevens, Mrs Monica Elaine 8686 Simpson Court, Mason, OH 45040, (513) 398-3776, **SLP**

Dobey, Phyllis Schmidt 2201 Hillmeade Drive, Nashville, TN 37221, (615) 352-8447, BS 74 Murray St Univ; MS 78 Univ of UT; 88–Tchr, Metro-Nashville PS, **SLP**

Dobies, Mrs Sandra C 12513 Streamwood Lane, Potomac, MD 20854, (301) 593-5280, BS 64 Univ of WI - Madison; MA 72 Univ of MD - College Park; Sp/Lang Path, Montgomery Co Publ Schs, **SLP**

Dobkin, Ceil K 181 Greenbiar Drive, Farmington, CT 06032, (915) 581-4373, BA 74 Temple Univ-Tyler Sch of Art; MA 75 Temple Univ-Tyler Sch of Art; **SLP**

Dobkin, Gloria A 4 Red Bark Court, Lafayette, CA 94549, (415) 426-4420, BS 68 Millersville Univ of PA; MA 70 Temple Univ; 88–Sp-Lang Path, Pleasanton USD, **SLP**

Dobkin, Mark S Hearing Enhancement Center, 124 Broadway, Costa Mesa, CA 92627, (714) 645-0886, BA 78 SUNY - Center at Buffalo; MA 83 Univ of CA - Santa Barbara; Aud, The Hrng Enhancement Cen, **A**

Dobkin, Renee Cencel 409 Catalina Drive, Newport Beach, CA 92663-4105, (714) 645-0886, CO St Univ; MS 77; Western Regional Sales Mgr, Qualitone, **A**

Dobkowski, Karen G 65 Parkwood Avenue, Rochester, NY 14620, (716) 244-5221, **SLP**

Dobos, Jennifer 3274 Hampton Ridge Drive, Marietta, GA 30066, (404) 924-2998, MA 75 Ball St Univ; BS 73 Purdue Univ - West Lafayette; **SLP**

Dobran, Esther Mindy 1456 Lagoon #305, Minneapolis, MN 55408-4231, (612) 545-0416, BS 83 Univ of WI - Madison; MS 84 Marquette Univ; 87–Sp-Lang Path, InSpeech Inc, **SLP**

Dobson, Deborah Ruth 77 Bayham Drive, Cincinnati, OH 45218, (513) 851-7541, MA 88 Univ of Cincinnati

Dobson, Mary Iowa Department Of Education, Grimes State Office Bldg, Des Moines, IA 50319, (817) 387-6169, BS 59 Northeastern OK St Univ; MS 65 Univ of OK Medical Center; Asst Prof, Texas Woman's U, **SLP**

Dobson, Patricia T Speech And Language Department, Special Services Center, 288 7th Street S E, Winter Haven, FL 33880, MS; **SLP LM**

Dobson, Robbie Ann 5313 Cecil Avenue, Baltimore, MD 21207, (301) 298-3949, BS 80 Frostburg St Coll; MS 84 Towson St Univ; **SLP**

Dockery, David Ray Route 2 Box 873, Pony Lake Road, Dahlonega, GA 30533, (404) 322-1801, BA 84 Columbus Coll; ME 85 Columbus Coll; Sp-Lang Path, Gainesville City Schs, **SLP**

Dockins, Mrs Sharon F 2810 Fern Drive, Yuma, AZ 85364, (619) 572-0222, BS 59 Eastern IL Univ; MA 74 Ball St Univ; SLP, Imperial Co Supt of Sch, **SLP**

Dockum, Gary D 450 North Eisenhower Avenue, Mason City, IA 50401, (515) 421-5433, BS 69 Mankato St Univ; MA 72 Univ of Northern IA; Audiologist, Surgical Assoc, **A**

Docster, Mrs Lisa D 2633 Princeton Drive, Vestal, NY 13850, (607) 775-0502, BA 78 SUNY - Coll at Cortland; MA 80 Northwestern Univ; **A**

Doctor, Cynthia K 7235 Maples Road, Fort Wayne, IN 46816, (219) 484-6636, BS 83 Purdue Univ - West Lafayette; MS 85 Purdue Univ - West Lafayette; 88–Clin Supvr-SLP, Parkview Memorial Hospital, **SLP**

Dodaro, Dr Robert Raymond 313 Adams Street, Suite 104, North Avington, MA 02351, (617) 878-7100, BS 72 Saint Louis Univ; MA 74 Saint Louis Univ; PH 87 (Sp-Lang Path) Univ of MI - Ann Arbor; Director Sp-Lang Path, The Methodist Hospital, **SLP**

Dodd, Mrs Elizabeth 4527 Harbor Drive, Kingsport, TN 37664, (615) 272-7651, BA 74 Univ of TN - Knoxville; BS 74 Univ of TN - Knoxville; MS 78 East TN St Univ; 88–Sp-Lang Path, Professional Health Services, **SLP**

Dodds, Holly Jo 1012 Saint Julien Drive #A-2, Kenner, LA 70065, (504) 455-3434, BS 80 Univ of MN - Minneap-St Paul; MA 83 Univ of MN - Minneap-St Paul; 88–Aud, Drs Mervin L Trail & Herbert W Marks, **A**

Dodge, Colleen 914 Briarwood, Mexia, TX 76667, (817) 562-2821, BS 76 Univ of TX - Austin; MS 78 Southern Methodist Univ; 78–Dir of Follow-up Svcs, Mexia State Sch, **A**

Dodge, Mrs Diane DiMaio 3923 East Shangrila Road, Phoenix, AZ 85028, (602) 494-9507, BA 74 Murray St Univ; MS 76 IL St Univ - Normal; 78–Sp-Lang Path, Scottsdale Pub Sch, **SLP**

Dodge, Mrs Diane Wood 2197 Bayham S E, Kentwood, MI 49508, BS 76 Western MI Univ; MA 82 Western MI Univ; Sp-Lang Path, Kenowa Hills/Sparta Pub Sch, **SLP**

Dodge, M Cynthia Rt 1 Box 374, Barnstead, NH 03218, (603) 228-1551, SLP, Parent Infant Dev Program, **SLP**

Dodge, Paul 5515 Morris Street, Philadelphia, PA 19144, **A**

Dodge, Mrs Susan Delong 324 Manning Boulevard, Albany, NY 12206, (518) 454-1372, BS 83 Coll of Saint Rose; MS 84 Univ of VT; **A**

Dodge, Susan R 1404 N E 48th Street, Rochester, MN 55904, (507) 289-6371, BA 76 Univ of WI - Eau Claire; MA 77 Univ of MN - Duluth; Sp-Lang Path, ISD #535, **SLP**

Dodgen, Mrs Lana S 11523 Cotillion, Dallas, TX 75228, (214) 279-8094, BS 73 East TX St Univ - Commerce; MS 74 East TX St Univ - Commerce; **SLP**

Dodge-Sipan, Patricia 6595 Caminito Sinecock, La Jolla, CA 92037, (619) 459-1950, BS 73 Pacific Union Coll; MS 74 Loma Linda Univ - Riverside; Director, Private Practice, **SLP**

Dodgson, Mrs Sandra Elizabeth 136 Fenn Avenue, Willowdale, ON, Canada M2P 1X6, (416) 494-2222, BS 76 Univ of Western Ontario; OM 80 Univ of Western Ontario; Sp-Lang Path, Bloorview Chldrens Hospital, **SLP**

Dodson, Betty L Eastern Illinois University, Department Of Communication Disorders & Sciences, Charleston, IL 61920, (217) 581-2712, BA 53 Coll of Wooster; MA 68 Saint Louis Univ; Dir, En IL U, **SLP**

Dodson, Gloria Susan 123 Northmont Court, Danville, VA 24540, (919) 342-4701, BS 83 Radford Univ; MS 84 Radford Univ; Sp-Lang Path, Rockingham County Schools, **SLP**

Dodson, Stephanie Karr Serv In Speech & Lang Disorder, 4120 Rio Bravo, Suite 311, El Paso, TX 79902, (915) 542-0463, BS 72 Emerson Coll; MA 77 Univ of TX - Austin; Owner, Serv In Sp & Lang Dis, **SLP**

Dodson, Susan L 2708 Geraghty, Austin, TX 78757, (512) 465-4668, BA 66 TX Tech Univ; MA 68 TX Tech Univ; Prog Coord, Erly Chldhood Interven - St Tx, **SLP**

Doehring, Donald G 1266 Pine Avenue West, Montreal, PQ, Canada H3G 1A8, (514) 398-4140, BA 49 SUNY - Center at Buffalo; MA 51 Univ of NM; PH 54 (Psychology) IN Univ - Gary; Professor & Research Director, McGill U

Doeksen-Gould, Debra P O Box 181, Newcastle, WY 82701, BS 78 SD St Univ; MA 79 SD St Univ; Sp/Lang Path, Weston Co Sch Dist No 1, **SLP**

Doenges, Donna Ada P O Box 6070, Arnold, CA 95223, (209) 795-2532, MA 75 San Jose St Univ; Sp-Lang Path, Calaveras County Office Educ, **SLP**

Doenges, Mrs Karen Marie Stene 936 N W 41st Street #C-209, Rochester, MN 55901, (507) 288-5296, BA 83 Univ of WI - Eau Claire; MA 85 Univ of IA; Sp-Lang Path, Rochester ISD #535, **SLP**

Doerfler, Dr Leo G 4533 West Barlind Drive, Pittsburgh, PA 15227, (412) 882-7609, BA 39 NY Univ; MS 41 Washington Univ; PH 48 (NS) Northwestern Univ; 76–Aud, L Doerfler Aud Assoc, **A F H LM**

Doerhoff, Mrs Ruth Ann Route 6, Bald Hill Road, Jefferson City, MO 65101, (314) 635-1000, BS 72 Univ of MO - Columbia; MA 73 Univ of MO - Columbia; **SLP**

Doering, Rebecca Elaine 1422 Cloverleaf Drive, Austin, TX 78723, (512) 451-1780, MA 88 Univ of TX - Austin

Doerner, Mrs Sheila Mondino R R 2 Box 382, Mulkeytown, IL 62865, (618) 596-6455, BS 74 Southern IL Univ -Carbondale; MS 75 Southern IL Univ -Carbondale; Sp-Lang Path, Benton Comm Consol Sch Dist 47, **SLP**

Doerpinghaus, Mary Jude 131 Aberdeen Avenue, Dayton, OH 45419, (812) 333-8211, BA 85 Univ of WI - Eau Claire; OM 86 IN Univ - Bloomington; **SLP**

Doerr, Cynthia J 1704 Derrynane Drive, St Louis, MO 63021, (314) 394-9539, MA 84 Saint Louis Univ; Sp-Lang Path, Private Practice, **SLP**

Doerrfeld, Karen Dlugosz P O Box 72, Elliottville, KY 40317, (606) 784-4476, BS 78 Northern IL Univ - De Kalb; MS 81 Univ of OR; Sp-Lang Path, Rowan County Public Schools, **SLP**

Doetzer, Kimberly Ann 6539 Chambersburg Road, Kirkwood Apartment #3, Fayetteville, PA 17222, (717) 267-7719, BS 82 Towson St Univ; MS 84 Towson St Univ; **SLP**

Doffek, Mrs Margaret A 15 Fairview Avenue, Rockville, CT 06066, (203) 872-8571, BA 59 Mount Holyoke Coll; MA 61 Univ of CT; SLP, Vernon Bd of Ed, **SLP**

Doggett, Mrs Andrea Jo Tyler 4015 68th Street, Urbandale, IA 50322, (515) 284-7714, BS 77 Univ of IA; MA 79 SD St Univ; SLP, Des Moines ISD, **SLP**

Dogon, Mrs Sally Sinaiko 75 Maugus Avenue, Wellesley Hills, MA 02181, BS 54 Univ of WI - Madison; ME 56 Boston Univ; **SLP**

Doherty, Mrs Betty 9301 West Hadley, Milwaukee, WI 53222, **SLP**

Doherty, Dr E Thomas Speech Research Lab (126), VA Medical Center, San Francisco, CA 94121, (415) 221-4810

Doherty, Dr Joseph W 318-D Quaker Avenue, Philadelphia, NY 13673, (315) 642-5092, MS; Major, US Army, **SLP A**

Doherty, Karen 11 Cinnamon Springs, South Windsor, CT 06074, (516) 582-9037, BS 85 Univ of RI; MA 87 Univ of CT

Doherty, Patricia M 2705 Poplar Lane, Norman, OK 73072, BS 64 Univ of IL - Urbana; MS 85 Univ of OK - OK City; 86–Sp-Lang Path, Norman PS, **SLP**

Doherty, Mrs Rosalind Tosti 3202 Knollwood Way, Madison, WI 53713, (608) 251-1010, BS 61 Univ of WI - Madison; MS 63 Univ of WI - Madison; SLP, Madison Metro Sch Dist, **SLP**

Doherty, Valerie A 9658 South Ridgeway, Evergreen Park, IL 60642, (312) 636-3619, **SLP**

Doherty-Edlund, Barbara A 309 Washington Street, Hanover, MA 02339, (617) 585-3821, BA 76 Boston Coll; ME 82 Northeastern Univ; Sp-Lang Path, Kingston Pubs Schs, **SLP**

Dohne, Connie Cox 4715 S E Adams #942C, Bartlesville, OK 74006, (918) 333-8910, BS 74 Univ of Science & Arts of OK; BS 75 Univ of Science & Arts of OK; MA 78 Univ of Tulsa; 87–Aud, Dr Robert Craig, **A**

Dohner, Mrs Nancy P 569 Greenwood Avenue, Akron, OH 44320, (216) 836-9741, BS 74 OH St Univ; MA 77 OH St Univ; 87–SLP, Tri-County Easter Seal Society, **SLP**

Dohnt, Debra Williams 12 Akoonah Cl, Donvale, Victoria, Australia 3111, 3 -848-2582, BA 78 CA St Univ - Fresno; MS 81 San Francisco St Univ; SLP, Edmonds Sch Dist, **SLP**

Dohrmann, Mrs Vicki Sue 2415 165th Place N E, Bellevue, WA 98008-2329, (206) 747-9324, BS 83 OR St Univ; MA 86 Western WA Univ; **SLP**

Doi, Mrs Betty S 94-228 Naika Place, Mililani Town, HI 96789, BS 67 Univ of HI - Manoa; MS 69 Univ of HI - Manoa; 70–Sp-Lang Path, Dept of Educ-Cen Oahu Dist, **SLP**

Doidge, Mary C Bayer 65 Peaceable Street, Apt 3, Ridgefield, CT 06877, (203) 431-6251, BA 70 Univ of WI - Madison; MS 71 Univ of WI - Madison; 85–Sp-Lang Path, Datahr, Inc, **SLP**

Doig, Lori C P O Box 772, Cooperstown, NY 13326, (607) 847-6105, BS 77 SUNY - Coll at Geneseo; MS 79 Syracuse Univ; Sp-Lnag Path, Broome Dev Serv, **SLP**

Dokimos, Elizabeth Dept Speech Path & Audiology, California State Univ Sacramento, 6000 J Street, Sacramento, CA 95819, (916) 278-6601, BA 62 CA St Univ - Sacramento; MA 66 CA St Univ - Sacramento; 72–Prof Cl Super, CA St U/Sacramento, **SLP**

Dolan, Ann Goyda 290 Dans Highway, New Canaan, CT 06840, (203) 576-7426, ME 58 PA St Univ - Univ Park; OM 81 Univ of Bridgeport; OM 81 Univ of Bridgeport; Coord Sp-Lang Path, Bd of Ed/Bridgeport Ct, **SLP**

Dolan, Cormack J 32 Dogwood Drive, Ridgefield, CT 06877, (203) 637-9730, BA 53 Stonehill Coll; MS 61 PA St Univ - Univ Park; Sp-Lang Path, Bd of Ed Greenwich, **SLP**

Dolan, Cynthia Jo 1648 Port Drive #2, Baton Rouge, LA 70820, BS 81 LA St Univ - Baton Rouge; MA 85 LA St Univ - Baton Rouge; **SLP**

Dolan, Jean Theresa 808 Lone Tree, Cedar Park, TX 78613, (512) 454-8631, BS 74 Univ of TX - Austin; MA 84 Univ of TX - Austin; **SLP**

Dolan, Mrs Julie Powell 6032 Northland N E, Albuquerque, NM 87109, (505) 842-5967, BA 80 Univ of NM; MS 83 Univ of NM; SLP, Hosp Home Hlth Care, **SLP**

Dolan, Mrs Laurie E 18213 South Morgan #2S, Homewood, IL 60430, (312) 284-0022, BA 80 Mundelein Coll; MA 81 Northern IL Univ - De Kalb; 87–Sp-Lang Path, Trade Winds Rehab Center, **SLP**

Dolan, Leo F 65 Whittier Road, Pawtucket, RI 02861, (401) 728-2120, MA 47 Boston Univ; Consult/Spec Ed, Pawtucket Sch Dept, **SLP LM**

Dolan, Lesley Pinel 4835 Hoyer Drive, Sarasota, FL 34241, (813) 921-3024, BS 71 Boston Univ; MA 73 Univ of CT; Aud, Hearing Care Center, **A**

Dolan, Mrs Marie B 1552 Revere Road, Yardley, PA 19067, BA 75 LA Salle Coll; MA 78 Temple Univ-Tyler Sch of Art; Sp/Lang Path, Private Practice, **SLP**

Dolan, Marie D 2 Sheridan Road, Bedford, MA 01730, (617) 275-7704, MS 88 Northeastern Univ

Dolan, Patricia Eades 6050 Whethersfield #34-E, Birmingham, MI 48010, (313) 745-5111, BS 78 MI St Univ; MA 81 Eastern MI Univ; Sp-Lang Path, Harper Hosp, **SLP**

Dolan, Patricia Susan 99 1/2 Broadway, Salem, MA 01970, (617) 365-5113, BA 82 Salem St Coll; MS 86 Emerson Coll; **SLP**

Dolan, Sally Joan 210 West Main, Beresford, SD 57004, (605) 763-2298, BA 55 Univ of IA; MA 81 Univ of SD - Vermillion; **SLP**

Dolan, Dr Thomas Gordon Dept Of Speech Communication, Portland State University, P O Box 751, Portland, OR 97207, (503) 464-3264, BA 76 Carleton Univ - Ontario; MS 78 McGill Univ - Quebec; PH 83 (NS) Univ of IA; Asst Prof, Portland State Univ, **A**

Dolan, William B Montefiore Hospital Med Ctr, Speech And Hearing, 111 East 210th Street, Bronx, NY 10467, (212) 920-5445, BA 70 CUNY - Hunter Coll; MA 72 OH Univ - Athens; OM 86 New Sch for Social Research; Aud, Montefiore Medical Center, **A ACE**

Dolata, Mrs Cindi L 1016 East San Rafael St, Colorado Springs, CO 80903-2742, (303) 577-9226, BS 77 Central MI Univ; MA 79 Central MI Univ; Sp-Lang Path, Widefield Sch Dist #3, **SLP**

Dole, Barbara R 57 Ketcham Avenue, Patchogue, NY 11772, (516) 654-8520, MA 71 Vanderbilt Univ; 88–Sp-Lang Path, Patchogue-Medford Schs, **A**

Dolence, Mrs Connie A 809 Rodeo Avenue, Cheyenne, WY 82009, (307) 632-0591, BS 76 Univ of WY; MS 77 Univ of WY; Sp-Lang Path, Laramie Co Sch Dist #1, **SLP**

Dolezal, Mrs Laura Kathleen P O Box 786, Mountain View, WY 82939, (307) 782-6220, BS 83 Western IL Univ; MA 84 Western IL Univ; Sp-Lang Path, Lincoln-Uinta Child Dev Assoc, **SLP**

Dolezal, Pamela S 3656 Oak Parkway, Topeka, KS 66614, (913) 232-0551, BS 85 KS St Univ; MA 87 KS St Univ; 88–Sp-Lang Path, Topeka PS #501, **SLP**

Dolk, Michaela L 5704 Independence Avenue, Apt 2-W, Oak Forest, IL 60452, (312) 687-0359, MA 87 Univ of IL - Urbana; 87–Sp-Lang Path, South Metropolitan Assoc, **SLP**

Doll, Julie Burns Box 371, Cummaquid, MA 02637, (508) 771-1800, BS 73 Maryville Coll; MA 76 Saint Louis Univ; Sp-Lang Path, Cape Cod Hospital, **SLP**

Doll, Mrs Lea Daniel 6176 Charring Cross Court, Lavonia, GA 30058, (404) 325-3011, OB 84 Univ of GA; ME 85 Univ of GA; SLP, Dekalb Co Schl Sys, **SLP**

Dollaghan, Dr Christine Ann 718 Cascade Road, Pittsburgh, PA 15221, (412) 624-6573, BA 74 Wesleyan Univ; MA 78 Univ of MT; PH 81 (Communicative Disorders) Univ of WI - Madison; 87–Dir-Sp & Hrng Clinic, Univ of Pittsburgh, **SLP**

Dollinger, Lillian S 25 Melrose Avenue, Livingston, NJ 07039, (201) 992-7205, BA 76 Univ of RI; MA 79 Montclair St Coll; Sp-Lang Path, Private Practice, **SLP**

Dollison, Janet Lynn 2904 Swift Avenue, North Kansas City, MO 64116, (816) 932-3321, BS 83 WV Univ; MA 84 Univ of TN - Knoxville; Aud, St Lukes Hosp, **A**

Dollman, Cynthia 341 Street Louis Avenue, Huntington, WV 25705-1433, (304) 696-6661, BA 80 Marshall Univ; MA 85 Marshall Univ; **SLP**

Dolson, Mrs Kay Marie 430 West 57th Street, Kansas City, MO 64113, (816) 276-4023, BA 63 Univ of MI - Ann Arbor; MA 84 Univ of KS; **SLP**

Domb, Mrs Anik 13125 West Sunset Blvd, Los Angeles, CA 90049, (213) 483-1286, **A**

Domb, Mrs Elona G 1028 Country Club Drive, North Palm Beach, FL 33408, (305) 622-3507, BS 70 Long Island U - Brooklyn Ctr; MS 75 CUNY - Coll of Staten Island; MA 81 Kean Coll of NJ; 87–Aud, Hearx Ltd, **A**

Dombeck, Mrs Monica A 7620 South 70th Street, Franklin, WI 53132, (414) 886-9191, BS 78 Marquette Univ; MS 79 Marquette Univ; Sp-Lang Path, Racine USD, **SLP**

Dombrowski, Mrs Deborah Mary 13 Atlantic Street, Metuchen, NJ 08840, (201) 906-0271, MA 83 Kean Coll of NJ; Sp-Lang Path, Paterson Bd of Ed, **SLP**

Dombrowski, Jane E O 5812 Murray Road, Whitehall, MI 49461, **SLP**

Dome, Andrea Rene 2007 East 21st Street # B, Hays, KS 67601, (913) 483-6180, BA 83 Fort Hays St Univ; MS 84 Fort Hays St Univ; 85–Sp-Lang Path, USD #407 KS, **SLP**

Domenici, Kathy Jo 534 S High Street #8, West Chester, PA 19380, (215) 431-2903, BS 85 Nazareth Coll of Rochester; MS 86 SUNY - Coll at Buffalo; **SLP**

Domenico, Debbie Lee 1319 South Kings Drive, Charlotte, NC 28207, (704) 376-4247, BS 75; MS 78 Univ of OK - OK City; 86–Sp-Lang Path, Private Practice, **SLP**

Domenico, Dr Raymond A 45 Cogan Avenue, Plattsburgh, NY 12901, (518) 564-2186, BA 68 Northeastern Univ; MA 70 Syracuse Univ; PH 74 (NS) Syracuse Univ; Chrmn Assoc Prof/Hrng Sp Sci, State University of New York, **SLP**

Domenie, Deborah Conard 2450 Montgomery Avenue, Cardiff, CA 92007, (619) 691-5536, BA 75 San Diego St Univ; MA 80 San Diego St Univ; SLP, Sweetwater Un Hs Dist, **SLP**

Domers, Hillary S 450 Clothier Road, Wynnewood, PA 19096, **SLP**

Domico, Elizabeth Hutcheson The Shea Clinic, 6133 Poplar Pike At Ridgeway, Memphis, TN 38119, (901) 761-9720, MS 83 Radford Univ; Coord-Cochlear Implant Prog, Shea Clinic Foundation, **A**

Domico, Dr William D 3452 Swanson Cove, Memphis, TN 38118, (901) 726-7684, BS 76 Tulane Univ; MS 78 Tulane Univ; PH 81 (NS) FL St Univ; 86–Dir of Aud, Methodist Hosp, **A**

Domineau, Susanne Breen 261 Franklin Street, Duxbury, MA 02332, (617) 848-4000, **SLP**

Dominello, Anne Marie 7 Baldwin Avenue, Meriden, CT 06450, (203) 634-0198, BS 83 Southern CT St Univ; MS 85 Southern CT St Univ; **SLP**

Dominello, Matthew C, Jr 216 Dogwood Lane, Meriden, CT 06450, **SLP**

Domingo, Robert A 71 Alexander Avenue, Farmingdale, NY 11735, (718) 262-9200, BA 75 SUNY - Coll at Plattsburgh; MS 77 Adelphi Univ; 87–Dir of Sp Svcs, Assn Adv of Blind & Retarded, **SLP**

Dominguez, Mrs Suzanne Marie 325 Fleming Avenue, Placentia, CA 92670, (213) 698-0351, BA 81 CA St Univ - Long Beach; MA 84 CA St Univ - Fullerton; SLP, East Whittier City Sch Dist, **SLP**

Dominick, Mrs Diana Marie 179 Skyline Drive, California, PA 15419, (412) 437-0225, MS 84 CA Univ of PA; Sp-Lang Path, Fayette County Easter Seal Soc, **SLP**

Dominik, Lygia 814 Raymond Drive, Seymour, IN 47274, (812) 522-3340, BA 75 Coll of Saint Francis; MA 77 IN Univ - Bloomington; Sp-Lang Path, Bartholomew Special Serv Coop, **SLP**

Dominique, Patricia Ann 137 Clinton Street, Wauseon, OH 43567, (419) 335-3450, BS 74 Bowling Green St Univ; MA 83 Bowling Green St Univ; Sp-Lang Path, Elmwood Local Schools, **SLP**

Domizio-Pilla, Carmella 1323 Dickinson Street, Philadelphia, PA 19147, BS 76 Temple Univ-Tyler Sch of Art; MS 78 PA St Univ - Univ Park; Sp/Lang Path, Montgomery Co Inter Unit, **SLP**

Domko, Jo Anne Camp 3071 South Bellaire Street, Denver, CO 80222, (303) 756-7181, BS 75 CO St Univ; MA 78 Univ of CO - Boulder; 87–Sp-Lang Path, InSpeech Inc, **SLP**

Domni, Suzanne Halise 2 Lourae Drive, Massapequa Park, NY 11762, (516) 326-5636, BA 85 Montclair St Coll; MS 86 Adelphi Univ; 87–Sp-Lang Path, Long Island Jewish Med Ctr, **SLP**

Domoracki, Dr David 7657 Blackford Drive, Chagrin Falls, OH 44022, (216) 247-6227, BA 76 OH St Univ; MA 78 OH St Univ; PH 87 (Aud-Hrng Sciences) Kent St Univ; 88–Aud, VA Med Ctr, **A**

Domowiczo, Faye Hilary 2359 Rice Avenue, Lake City, PA 16423, (814) 453-5602, MS 83 Indiana Univ of PA; Sp-Lang Path, Lake Erie Institute of Rehab, **SLP**

Domroe, Sandy W 20 Link Court, New City, NY 10956, **SLP**

Domyan, Steve R 523½ North 5th Street, Martins Ferry, OH 43935, (614) 633-2632, BS 71 OH Univ - Athens; MS 75 WV Univ; University Teacher, West Liberty State College, **A**

Don, Eujania B 772 Sapphire Street, San Diego, CA 92109, (619) 541-3088, BA 83 CA St Univ - Fresno; MS 85 Univ of WI - Madison; 86–Sp-Lang Path, Childrens Hosp Sp Hrg Ctr, **SLP**

Donaghey, Mrs Trish A 2929 Potomac Drive, Garland, TX 75042, (214) 494-8389, BA 66 Univ of TX - Austin; MA 71 Univ of TX - Austin; Sp-Lang Path, Garland ISD, **SLP**

Donaghy, Dr William C 2503 Park Avenue, Laramie, WY 82070, (307) 766-6277, MA 64 CA St Univ - Fresno; PH 69 (NS) Northwestern Univ; Professor of Communication, University of Wyoming

Donahoo, Barbara L 4998 Rockaway Beach Dr N E, Bainbridge Island, WA 98110-2161, BS 85 Ithaca Coll; MA 87 George Washington Univ; **SLP**

Donahue, Amy M 705 Irwin Road, Bel Air, MD 21014, (301) 671-3797, BS 78 Middle TN St Univ; MA 79 Univ of TN - Knoxville; PH 85 (Sp & Hrng Science) Univ of TN - Knoxville; 86–Hearing Conservation Consultnt, US Army Envirnmntl Hygiene Agy, **A**

Donahue, Belita A 2800 17th, Great Bend, KS 67530, (316) 792-1321, BA 73 Univ of KS; MA 75 Univ of KS; Dir of Serv, Sunflower Training Cen, **SLP**

Donahue, Blevin M 98 Oakwood Drive, Marion, NC 28752-3460, (404) 778-8026, BS 78 Appalachian St Univ; MA 79 Appalachian St Univ; Sp-Lang Path, Habersham Co Pub Sch, **SLP**

Donahue, Diann F 1377 Stoney Creek Circle, Carmel, IN 46032, (317) 846-1127, BS 74 Purdue Univ - West Lafayette; MA 78 Catholic Univ of America; **SLP**

Donahue, Ellen 60 Haynes Road, Sudbury, MA 01776, (617) 726-2763, BS 80 Boston Univ; MS 82 Univ of WI - Madison; 84–Sp-Lang Path, MA Gen Hosp, **SLP**

Donahue, Jeanne E 637 Hazelwood Terrace, Rochester, NY 14609, (716) 377-4660, BS 83 2551; MS 84 Univ of VT; Sp-Lang Path, BOCES #1 Monroe County, **SLP**

Donahue, Mrs Karen Lee 1266 Redwood View Drive, Pomona, CA 91766, (213) 602-6946, BA 76 SUNY - Coll at Plattsburgh; MA 83 CA St Univ - Fullerton; SLP, Paramount USD, **SLP**

Donahue, Kathryn K 1410 West Ritchie, Enid, OK 73703, (405) 237-6801, BS 77 Northwestern OK St Univ; MS 82 Phillips Univ; Sp-Lang Path, Enid Pub Sch, **SLP**

Donahue, Dr Mavis L University Of Illinois, College Of Education, Box 4348, Chicago, IL 60680, (312) 996-8139

Donahue, Mrs Miriam L 1458 Lakeside Drive, Birmingham, MI 48009, BA 73 MI St Univ; MA 74 MI St Univ; **SLP**

Donahue, Patrice Ann 4 H Street, Reading, MA 01867, (617) 935-5050, MS 83 Boston Univ; Sp-Lang Path, New England Rehab Hosp, **SLP**

Donahue, Phyllis A 730 Valley, Dayton, OH 45404, (513) 222-5597, BA 76 Univ of KY; MS 80 Univ of WY; Sp-Lang Path Supervr, Hrng & Sp Cen for Chldn & Adlt, **SLP**

Donahue-Reese, Mrs Phyllis A 1876 Butler Park, Conshohocken, PA 19428, (215) 825-1859, BA 78 Temple Univ-Tyler Sch of Art; MA 80 Trenton St Coll; Sp/Lang Path, Cascade Aphasia Cen, **SLP**

Donaldson, Anne Chalfin 221 Shore Road, Bourne, MA 02532, (508) 548-7300, BA 84 Univ of CT; MS 87 Northeastern Univ; 87–Sp-Lang Path, Falmouth PS, **SLP**

Donaldson, Mrs Cathy Fay 318 West 31st Street, Cheyenne, WY 82001, (307) 634-4640, BA 78 Northwest Nazarene Coll; MS 82 Central WA Univ; SLP, Nevada Home Health, **SLP**

Donaldson, Mrs Cheryl W 8807 Halford Way, Louisville, KY 40299, (502) 491-9305, ME 76 Univ of Louisville; **SLP**

Donaldson, Mrs Donalyn B 902 East Walnut Avenue, Burbank, CA 91501, (818) 954-9420, BA 73 CA St Univ - Northridge; MA 74 CA St Univ - Northridge; SLP, LA USD, **SLP**

Donaldson, Gail Spaid 105 Marie Place, Charlottesville, VA 22901, (804) 978-1019, BA 73 Duke Univ; ME 82 Univ of VA - Charlottesville; Grad Instr, University of Virginia, **A**

Donaldson, Mrs Gillian K 8319 Morningside Drive, Manassas, VA 22111, (703) 361-8293, BA 68 Catholic Univ of America; MA 71 CA St Univ - Northridge; Sp-Lang Path, Prince Wm Co Parent-Infant Educ Prog, **SLP**

Donaldson, Linda Larson 51-A South Main Street, Centerville, OH 45458, (513) 433-8080, BS 77 ND St Univ; MA 78 Ball St Univ; Aud/Owner, Apple Creek Hrng Aids & Audiol, **A**

Donaldson, Dr Rita Joyce 3214 Lawrence Street, Houston, TX 77018, (713) 861-5069, BS 57 Washington Univ; MA 63 San Francisco St Univ; ED 74 (NS) Univ of KS; **A**

Donalson, Valerie Ann 1820 N E 142 Street, Apartment 8-A, North Miami, FL 33181, (305) 947-9433, Janet Sandler & Associates, **SLP**

Donatelle, Christine Ruth 93 Forest Glen, Highland Park, NJ 08904, (201) 937-8655, BA 84 Rutgers St Univ - Newark; MA 86 Univ of MA - Amherst; Aud, Robert Wood Johnson-Univ Hos, **A**

Donatelli, Deborah Ann One Cold Spring Drive, Bloomfield, CT 06002, (203) 236-6081, BS 76 Univ of CT; MA 84 Univ of CT; Sp-Lang Path, West Hartford Pub Sch, **SLP**

Donatelly, Mrs Maureen Crowley 330 Granite Street, Leominster, MA 01453, (617) 534-5322, BS 77 Univ of MA - Amherst; MS 83 Worcester St Coll; **SLP**

Donati, Stephanie 351 Treasure Lake, Du Bois, PA 15801, (814) 371-0414, ME 79 Indiana Univ of PA; Sp-Lang Path, Transact Health Systems, **SLP**

Donato, Barbara B 5823 Stanton Avenue, Pittsburgh, PA 15206, (412) 622-4484, BS 72 PA St Univ - Univ Park; MS 77 Univ of NC - Chapel Hill; Sp/Lang Path, St Francis Gen Hosp, **SLP**

Donato, Elizabeth Ann 411 Stewart, Woodstock, IL 60098, (815) 338-0538, BS 81 Bradley Univ; MS 83 Bradley Univ; 88–Aud, Robert Stensland & Assoc, **A**

Dondanville, Mrs Karen M 2805 32nd Avenue Drive, Moline, IL 61265, (309) 762-4664, BS 57 Northwestern Univ; MS 58 Vanderbilt Univ; **SLP**

Dondes, Mrs Susan T 21 Firethorn Court, East Brunswick, NJ 08816-2778, (210) 613-8658, BA 78 Univ of MD - College Park; MA 79 Hofstra Univ; 80–Aud, Hearing Lab, **A**

Donewald, Marian 2900 Bellemeade Avenue, Evansville, IN 47714, (812) 476-1561, BA 48 Univ of Evansville; MS 50 Purdue Univ - West Lafayette; **SLP LM**

Dong, Cheryl Diane 2216 N E Everett, Portland, OR 97232, (503) 241-5090, BA 81 Univ of OR; MS 86 Portland St Univ; **SLP**

Dongilli, Paul A, Jr 2200 South 52nd Street, Lincoln, NE 68506, (402) 489-7102, BA 81 Univ of Pittsburgh - Pittsburgh; MA 83 Univ of Pittsburgh - Pittsburgh; Sp-Lang Path, Madonna Centers, **SLP**

Donigan, Margaret 112 Raylinsky Road, Ballston Lake, NY 12019, **SLP**

Donigan, Mary Kellagher The Hearing Clinic Inc, 707 North Michigan Street, Suite 400, South Bend, IN 46601, (219) 232-4040, BS 81 PA St Univ - Univ Park; MA 82 MI St Univ; Aud, The Hrng Cl, **A**

Donigan, Rodney Craig St Josephs Medical Center, 811 East Madison, South Bend, IN 46634, (219) 237-7768, BA 81 MI St Univ; MA 82 MI St Univ; Aud, St Josephs Med Ctr, **A**

Donigian, Christine A Professional Audiology Center, 330 Borthwick Avenue Suite 209, Portsmouth, NH 03801, (603) 436-8668, BS 83 Univ of MA - Amherst; MS 85 PA St Univ - Univ Park; Aud, Professional Audiology Center, **A**

Donkervoort, Janet B 684 Inverness Avenue, London, ON, Canada N6H 3C6, BA 73 MI St Univ; MA 74 MI St Univ; 87–Sp-Lang Path, Bd of Educ for the City of London, **SLP**

Donlan, Mrs Sharon Askew W6467 Birchview Drive, Onalaska, WI 54650, (608) 782-9760, BS 83 ND St Univ; MS 86 Univ of WI - Stevens Point; 86–Aud, Skemp Clinic, **A**

Donlavage-Craft, Sandra L 213 Goundry Street, North Tonawanda, NY 14120, (716) 692-8367, MS 87 SUNY - Coll at Buffalo; 87–Sp-Lang Path, Orleans-Niagara BOCES, **SLP**

Donleavy, Mrs Mary Ella 7 Carriage Hill Drive, Long Valley, NJ 07853, (201) 876-9755, BA 78 Glassboro St Coll; MA 85 Montclair St Coll; 86–Sp-Lang Path, Private Practice, **SLP**

Donley, Debra J 2305 Westbrook Lane, Madison, WI 53711, (608) 845-6451, BS 76 Univ of WI - Madison; MS 77 Univ of WI - Madison; 77–Sp-Lang Path, Verona Area Sch, **SLP**

Donley, Noreen Jean 477 South El Molino #7, Pasadena, CA 91101, (818) 997-2330, BA 82 CA St Univ - Northridge; MA 84 CA St Univ - Northridge; 84–Sp-Lang Path, Los Angeles USD, **SLP**

Donlin-Smith, Colleen M 7 Havenwood Hollow, Fairport, NY 14450, BA 82 OH St Univ; MA 84 Univ of MD - College Park; Supervisor Sp-Lang Path, Woodrow Wilson Rehabil Center, **SLP**

Donlon, Mrs Patricia D Rd 8 Box 155B, Greensburg, PA 15601, BS 65 SUNY - Coll at Cortland; MS 70 Syracuse Univ; Sp-Lang Path, Seton Hill Day Care, Inc, **SLP**

Donlon, Mrs Roswitha Heinicke 8147 Lakeland Drive, Roseville, CA 95661, (916) 961-2154, MS 87 CA St Univ - Sacramento; Aud, Mitchell E Blum MD FACS, **A**

Donn, Jane E 215 Roycroft Road, Syracuse, NY 13214, (315) 463-5406, BS 73 Emerson Coll; MS 74 Syracuse Univ; 88–Dir, NY Therapies Inc, **SLP**

Donnell, Adrienne J 1117 Southwood Court, Lewisville, TX 75067, MS; **SLP**

Donnell, Mrs Betty A 2115 Angela Avenue, Arabi, LA 70032, BS 74 Univ of WY; MA 75 Wichita St Univ; **SLP**

Donnelly, Dr Carole D 9718 Streambrook Drive, Cincinnati, OH 45231, (513) 556-4526, BA 61 Catholic Univ of America; ME 73 Univ of Cincinnati; PH 79 (NS) Univ of Cincinnati; 77–Prof, University of Cincinnati, **SLP**

Donnelly, Mrs Judith A S 2600 Lakeshore Drive, Tavares, FL 32778, (904) 728-8688, MA 72 Univ of MD - College Park; Sp-Lang Path, Private Practice, **SLP A ACE**

Donnelly, Karen L 1211 Lansdowne Drive, Arlington, TX 76012, (817) 336-8611, BS 73 Univ of MA - Amherst; MS 78 Boston Univ; 82–Aud, Child Study Ctr, **A**

Donnelly, Katherine M 1401-1/2 South 22nd Street, Clinton, IA 52732, (319) 242-6454, BA 81 MI St Univ; MA 82 Central MI Univ; Sp-Lang Path, Mississippi Bend AEA 9, **SLP**

Donnelly, Kenneth G Professor Of Audiology, University Of Cincinnati, Mail Lox 379, Cincinnati, OH 45221, (513) 556-4484, BA 60 Catholic Univ of America; MA 61 Catholic Univ of America; PH 64 (NS) Univ of Pittsburgh - Pittsburgh; Prof Aud, Univ of Cincinati, **A F**

Donnelly, Nancy Carver P O Box 704, Boylston, MA 01505-0704, (617) 865-5227, BS 77 Worcester St Coll; ME 80 Northeastern Univ; Sp-Lang Path, Millbury Public Schools, **SLP**

Donnelly, Regina C 34 Revere Street, Holbrook, MA 02343, (617) 767-4548, BA 81 Bridgewater St Coll; MA 83 Northwestern Univ; **A**

Donnelly-Billmeyer, Mary L 2150 Bellenridge Pike, Cape Girardeau, MO 63701-1865, BS 81 Southwest MO St Univ; MS 82 Univ of MO - Columbia; Sp-Lang Path, Jefferson Cty Pub Sch Syst, **SLP**

Donner, Mrs Jean K 5534 S Dorchester Street, Chicago, IL 60637, (312) 241-7896, **SLP**

Dono, Deborah Tobias 709 Silver Court, Hamilton Square, NJ 08690, (609) 586-1597, MA 83 Trenton St Coll; Sp-Lang Path, Mercer Co Special Services, **SLP**

D'Onofrio-Zizzo, Mrs Denise M 85 Scudder Place, Northport, NY 11768, (516) 757-3710, BA 76 Hofstra Univ; MA 77 NY Univ; Sp-Lang Path, BOCES, **SLP**

Donoghue, Kathleen Anne 218 10th Street, Seal Beach, CA 90740, (213) 922-7691, BA 82 CA St Univ - Stanislaus; MA 84 CA St Univ - Stanislaus; SLP, Rancho Los Amigos Medical Ctr, **SLP**

Donohoe, Julia M 58 West Cheltenham Avenue, Philadelphia, PA 19120, (215) 351-7036, BA 69 Temple Univ; MA 71 Temple Univ; SLP, Philadelphia Board of Educ, **SLP**

Donohoe, Robert W Donohoe Audiological Service, 6445 East Ohio Avenue, Suite 300, Denver, CO 80224, (303) 322-0083, BA 66 Univ of Northern CO; MS 68 CO St Univ; Aud, Donahue Aud Serv, **A**

Donohue, Mrs Helen Shay 1414 Whitney Avenue #D-1, Hamden, CT 06517, (203) 248-2346, BS 48 Southern CT St Univ; MA 58 Columbia Univ Teachers Coll; 88–Sp-Lang Path, Private Practice, **SLP LM**

Donohue, Joann S 1137 Northport Drive, Columbus, OH 43235, (614) 292-6251, BS 71 OH St Univ; MA 72 Western MI Univ; 87–Coord of Sp-Lang Path, Sp & Hrng Sci Div Oh St U, **SLP**

Donohue, Mrs Joelen M 10 Alden Place, Bronxville, NY 10708, (914) 238-3911, BA 67 Coll of New Rochelle; MS 79 Columbia Univ Teachers Coll; Sp-Lang Path, Chappaqua Ctrl Sch Dist, **SLP**

Donohue, Sally Jo 1209 Woodchas Lane #A, Chesterfield, MO 63017, (317) 447-1364, BS 81 Purdue Univ - West Lafayette; MS 85 Purdue Univ - West Lafayette; **A**

Donohue, Mrs Susann Islami 159 Alexandria Way, Basking Ridge, NJ 07920, (201) 647-0520, BA 84 Univ of CT; MA 86 Univ of CT; **A**

Donovan, Alice Estelle 64 Hunleigh Circle, Amherst, NY 14226, (716) 358-0171, BA 79 Brock Univ - Ontario; MA 81 SUNY - Coll at Buffalo; 87–Sp-Lang Path, Greater Niagara Gen Hosp, **SLP**

Donovan, Mrs Barbara Ann 12143 Dorset, Cincinnati, OH 45241, (513) 771-8560, BA 58 OH Wesleyan Univ; MS 59 Univ of MI - Ann Arbor; Sp-Lang Path, Princeton City Sch, **SLP**

Donovan, Mrs Beverly G 806 Magnolia Avenue, Inverness, FL 32652, **SLP**

Donovan, Mrs Carol M 5 Washington Drive, Troy, NY 12180, (518) 283-5542, BS 70 SUNY - Coll at Brockport; MS 71 SUNY - Center at Albany; Sp-Lang Path, Geo Wash Sch, **SLP**

Donovan, Mrs Cindy Anne 18 Leah Street, North Providence, RI 02911, (401) 751-3113, BS 79 SUNY - Coll at Geneseo; MA 80 Univ of Northern CO; Sp-Lang Path, Sargent Rehab Ctr, **SLP**

Donovan, Mrs Cori L Route 1 Box 123, Lake Geneva, WI 53147, (414) 741-4118, BS 84 Univ of WI - Milwaukee; MS 86 Univ of WI - Milwaukee; SLP, Walworth Lakeland School, **SLP**

Donovan, Debra Ayleen 191 West Liberty Street, Hernando, FL 32642, (904) 746-9729, MS 78 Univ of South FL; Sp-Lang Path, Citrus Co Sch Sys, **SLP**

Donovan, Donna M 326 Woodbridge Street, Manchester, CT 06040, (203) 529-3273, BA 79 Univ of CT; MS 82 Univ of RI; Sp-Lang Path, Rocky Hill Pub Schls, **SLP**

Donovan, Dorothy R 331 East Lake Avenue, Glenview, IL 60025, **SLP ACE**

Donovan, Kathleen E 33-24 91st Street, Jackson Heights, NY 11372, BA 70 CUNY - City College; MA 73 CUNY - City College; Sp-Lang Path, Menorah Home & Hosp, **SLP**

Donovan, Lori M 485 East Bullard Apt#150, Fresno, CA 93710, (209) 431-2418, BS 85 Southern IL Univ -Carbondale; MA 87 Univ of IA; 88–Sp-Lang Path, Valley Children's Hosp

Donovan, Mrs Noreen Catherine 85 Woodland Road, Montvale, NJ 07645, (914) 354-0214, MA 73 CUNY - Lehman Coll; Sp-Lang Path, Rockland Psychiatric Hospital, **SLP**

Donovan, Mrs Rachael Anne Bad Nauheim Elem School, APO New York, NY 09074, BA 82 Univ of SD - Vermillion; MA 84 Univ of SD - Vermillion; Sp-Lang Path, USA, **SLP**

Doob, Dr Dorothy 1025 5th Avenue #2F-South, New York, NY 10028, (212) 288-3822, BA 32 CUNY - Hunter Coll; MA 34 Univ of CO - Boulder; ED 43 (NS) NY Univ; **SLP LM**

Doody, M Patricia 630 Friscoville Avenue, Arabi, LA 70032, (504) 277-7146, MS 75 Univ of Southwestern LA; Sp-Lang Path, Lsu-Mc, **SLP**

Doolan, Mrs Theresa A 105 Garth Road #1F, Scarsdale, NY 10583, (914) 235-4327, BA 77 CUNY - Queens Coll; MA 78 CUNY - Queens Coll; 84–Aud, Sound Shore Hearing Assoc, **A**

Dooley, Mrs Constance 529 Penllyn Pike, Penllyn, PA 19422, (215) 646-5943, BS 65 Indiana Univ of PA; MA 76 Trenton St Coll; 86–Sp-Lang Path, Elwyn Inc Davidson Sch, **SLP**

Dooley, Mrs Judith R 7207 Augusta Drive, Green Cove Springs, FL 32043, (904) 272-8100, ME 76 Univ of FL; 88–Sp-Lang Path, Clay County School Board, **SLP**

Dooley, Mrs Laurie Jeanne P 6112 Ringsdale Court, Bakersfield, CA 93313, **SLP**

Dooley, Linda Rae 20320 102nd Place S E, Kent, WA 98031, (206) 848-6661, BA 85 WA St Univ; MA 86 WA St Univ; 86–Sp-Lang Path, Good Samaritan Hosp, **SLP**

Dooley, Lizbeth Jean 208 Cambridge Drive, Port Jefferson, NY 11776, (516) 663-1084, BA 83 Adelphi Univ; MS 84 Adelphi Univ; SLP, School for Lang & Commun Disor, **SLP**

Dooley-McLaughlin, Patricia Joan 21 Monroe Drive, Coventry, RI 02816, (401) 727-0150, BA 82 Univ of RI; MS 84 Ithaca Coll; **SLP**

Dooling, Jim Kinston Head & Neck Physicians, Kinston Clinic North, Kinston, NC 28501, (919) 523-0687, BA 72 Creighton Univ; MS 77 Univ of NE - Omaha; 86–Aud, Kinston Head & Neck Physicians, **A**

Doolittle, Dr Jacqueline Baxter 14 Fairview Road, Scarsdale, NY 10583, (914) 681-1114, MA 49 Northwestern Univ; MA 68 Columbia Univ Teachers Coll; PH 82 (Sp-Lang Path) Columbia Univ Teachers Coll; 84–Dir Sp-Lang & Audiology, White Plains Hosp Medical Cen, **SLP**

Doonan, Lesley C S 5 Metropolitan Drive, Warwick, RI 02886, BA 78 Univ of RI; MS 80 Univ of RI; Sp-Lang Path, Cranston Pub Sch, **SLP**

Doose, Alexis 13537 Romany Drive, Pacific Palisades, CA 90272, **SLP**

Dopheide, William R Professor Speech Communication, University Of Maine, 208 East Annex, Orono, ME 04469, (207) 581-2404, BS 52 Western MI Univ; MS 55 PA St Univ - Univ Park; PH 68 (Sp-Lang Path) MI St Univ; Prof Sp Commun, Univ of Maine, **SLP F**

Dopke, Mrs Lynn Constance W3360 Beryl Drive, Watertown, WI 53094, (414) 261-3050, MS 82 Univ of WI - Whitewater; 86–Sp-Lang Path, Speech Pathology Services Inc, **SLP**

Dopp, Shelley R 12119 West 101st Street, Lenexa, KS 66215, (913) 621-5155, BS 80 Univ of KS; MA 82 Univ of KS; Sp-Lang Path, USD 500, **SLP**

Dopson, Deborah R 6801 Rugby Court, New Orleans, LA 70126, MS; **SLP**

Dorais, Mrs Brenda Marcus 3 Libra Lane, Sewell, NJ 08080, (609) 589-8765, BA 79 Rutger's St Univ - Douglas Coll; MA 82 Hahnemann Univ Grad Sch; Sp-Lang Path/Aud, Assoc Aud Consultants, **SLP A**

Doran, Catherine Beam 14 Robertson Avenue, Morrisville, PA 19067, (302) 995-8676, BA 80 Univ of Pittsburgh - Pittsburgh; MA 82 Univ of Pittsburgh - Pittsburgh; SLP, De Div-Pub Hlth, **SLP**

Doran, Mari C 810 Bainbridge Street, Philadelphia, PA 19147, (215) 456-9292, BS 78 Marywood Coll; MA 79 George Washington Univ; Sp-Lang Path, Moss Rehab Hosp, **SLP ACE**

Doran, Paul James 420 Tulane S E, Albuquerque, NM 87106, (505) 255-9924, BS 78 Univ of MT; MS 82 Univ of NM; Sp-Lang Path, Albuquerque Pub Sch, **SLP**

Doran-Quine, Dr MaryEllen 11707 North Shore Drive, Reston, VA 22090, (703) 834-1030, BS 60 Kent St Univ; MS 72 Eastern IL Univ; PH 84 (NS) Kent St Univ; Sp-Lang Path, SpeechWorks Assoc, **SLP**

D'Orazio, Mrs Helene Cecelia 11 Lt John Olsen Lane, St James, NY 11780, (516) 584-9017, MA 79 Hofstra Univ; SLP, BOCES II, **SLP**

D'Orazio, Paula C 11 Primrose Lane, Loudonville, NY 12211, (518) 783-9526, MS 80 Coll of Saint Rose; **SLP**

Dordick, Nancy H 256 Wild Orchid Court, Yardley, PA 19067, (215) 321-0426, BA 78 Univ of MD - College Park; MA 80 Temple Univ-Tyler Sch of Art; MA 80 Temple Univ-Tyler Sch of Art; Aud, Wilf-Silberman-Humpel MD Assoc, **A**

Dorf, Debra S 751 West Brompton, Chicago, IL 60657, (312) 281-0021, BS 74 Univ of IL - Urbana; MA 75 Univ of IL - Urbana; Instr/Sp/Lang Path, U of IL Med Cen, **SLP**

Dorf, Gary R 272 Brentwood, Costa Mesa, CA 92627, (213) 493-3665, MS 76 CUNY - Brooklyn Coll; 79–Owner, Hearing Instrument Consultants, **A**

Dorfman, Cathy 4082 Okalona Road, South Euclid, OH 44121, (216) 381-3515, BS 78 Univ of WI - Madison; MA 80 Case Western Reserve Univ; 80–Sp-Lang Path, Cleveland Bd of Ed, **SLP**

Dorfman, Jodi M 20 Garth Court, Staten Island, NY 10306, (718) 979-8064, BA 80 CUNY - Brooklyn Coll; MS 86 CUNY - Brooklyn Coll; 86–Sp-Lang Path, NY Childhood Ctr, **SLP**

Dorgan, Mrs Barbara G 6202 Canterbury Lane #C, Willowbrook, IL 60514-2920, (312) 323-2086, BA 63 Rockford Coll; MA 65 Univ of WI - Madison; SLP, Maercker School Dist #60, **SLP**

Doring, Mrs Pamela Kodis 51 Wood Lane, Beverly, MA 02151, (518) 922-8611, BS 76 Northeastern Univ; ME 80 Northeastern Univ; **SLP**

Doris, Fran N 2411 Brentwood Road, Beachwood, OH 44122, **SLP**

Doris, Marie J 10 Evans Court, Huntington Station, NY 11746, (516) 549-2538, MS 77 Columbia Univ Teachers Coll; Sp-Lang Path, Queen of Peace, **SLP**

Doris, Stacy A 14908 Notley Road, Silver Spring, MD 20904, (301) 384-8807, MA 88 George Washington Univ

Dormady, Elizabeth P 2155 East Forge Avenue, Mesa, AZ 85204, (602) 926-0956, BA 76 Univ of MD - College Park; MA 78 Univ of NE - Lincoln; 84–Sp-Lang Path, Mesa USD, **SLP**

Dormer, Natalie Ann 230 Fairlawn Drive, Monroeville, PA 15146, (412) 373-1889, BS 82 PA St Univ - Univ Park; MA 86 Univ of Pittsburgh - Pittsburgh; **A**

Dorn, Abigail M 2531 South Cook Street, Denver, CO 80210, (303) 273-6668, BA 84 Univ of Denver; MA 86 Univ of Denver; 88–Sp-Lang Path, Jefferson Co PS, **SLP**

Dorn, Israel Jerome 2400 Shelmire Avenue, Philadelphia, PA 19152, (215) 338-9404, BA 50 CUNY - Brooklyn Coll; ME 60 Temple Univ; Dir, Private Practice, **SLP LM**

Dorn, Kathleen Cecilia 116 Vista Drive, Highland, NY 12528, (914) 877-6821, BA 75 CUNY - Queens Coll; MA 76 Hofstra Univ; Treatment Team Leader, Wassaic Developmental Center, **SLP**

Dorn, Lynne D 21 Rock Street, Whitman, MA 02382, (617) 447-5832, BA 71 Univ of MA - Amherst; MS 72 Univ of WI - Madison; Sp-Lang Path, Holbrook Pub Sch, **SLP**

Dorn, Patricia Ann 3309 Indian Rock Lane, West Lafayette, IN 47906, (317) 463-2760, **A**

Dornbusch, Mrs Deborah Swartz 2109 Killarney Place, Charlotte, NC 28213, (704) 549-1984, BS 83 Miami Univ - Oxford; MA 84 Bowling Green St Univ; Sp-Lang Path, Private Practice, **SLP**

Dorne, Dr William P College Of Education, Florida Atlantic Univ, Boca Raton, FL 33432, PH 59 (NS) Univ of FL; Prof Exceptional Students, FL Atlantic U, **SLP**

Dorney, Diane C 110 Forest Club Drive, Chesterfield, MO 63017, **A**

Doroff, Mrs Judi Anne 656 Ridge, Highland Park, IL 60035, (312) 831-2594, BS 82 Univ of IL - Urbana; MS 83 Univ of IL - Urbana; Sp-Lang Path, Parkside Senior Svcs, **SLP**

Doroff-Johnson, Karen Lynn 223 Arundel Street #5, St Paul, MN 55102-1764, (612) 255-5678, BS 74 Saint Cloud St Univ; MS 77 Univ of WI - River Falls; **SLP**

Dorrell, Cheryl Ann 816 3rd Street N W #1, Minot, ND 58701, (701) 852-1014, **SLP**

Dorrell, Robert M P O Box 487, Frederick, MD 21701, (301) 662-4159, BA 69 Salem Coll; MS 72 Loyola Coll; Dir Aud Serv, Maryland Schl for the Deaf, **SLP A**

Dorr-Hendry, Janis San Juan Hearing Center, 833 East 2nd Avenue, Durango, CO 81301, (303) 247-0808, BS 72 FL St Univ; MS 73 FL St Univ; Aud, San Juan Hearing Center, **A**

Dorris, Mrs Tammy Fox 155 McCormack, Auburn, KY 42206, (502) 542-7668, BS 84 Western KY Univ; ME 87 Univ of GA; 88–Sp-Lang Path, Logon Co Bd of Educ, **SLP**

Dorrow, Mrs Cecilia F 8304 Bells Mill Road, Potomac, MD 20854, (301) 299-7729, BA 69 CUNY - Hunter Coll; MA 70 Univ of MD - College Park; Sp-Lang Path, Montgomery County Board of Ed, **SLP**

Dorsett, Susan G 2295 N W Loop, Stephenville, TX 76401, (817) 968-4174, BS 68 TX Tech Univ; MS 76 TX Tech Univ; Dir, N Ctrl TX Sp & Hrng Cen, **A**

Dorsey, Cynthia Ann 12572 Argyle Drive, Los Alamitos, CA 90720, (213) 926-2365, MA 86 CA St Univ - Long Beach; 86–Sp-Lang Path, Norwalk-La Mirada Uni Sch Dist, **SLP**

Dorsey, Mrs E Peggy 1951 Kerry Creek Drive, Marietta, GA 30066, (404) 767-0505, BS 81 FL St Univ; MS 83 FL St Univ; Sp/Lang Path, VNA Metro Atlanta, **SLP ACE**

Dorsey, Mrs Gillian C 281 Queensberry Court, Longwood, FL 32779, (407) 869-5056, BA 59 Univ of MD - College Park; MS 88 Nova Univ; 88–Sp-Lang Path, Seminole Co Bd of Ed, **SLP ACE**

Dorsey, Mrs Joan J 1900 Mill Lane, Salem, VA 24153, **SLP**

Dorsey, Joseph Earl, Jr 11 Brucester Bridge Court, Catonsville, MD 21228, (301) 374-6135, BA 81 Towson St Univ; MS 83 Towson St Univ; Sp-Lang Path, Carroll County Public Schools, **SLP**

Dorsey, Lisa Gainer 24104 Pecan Grove Lane, Gaithersburg, MD 20879, (804) 792-0650, BS 81 Towson St Univ; MA 82 OH St Univ; Sp-Lang Path, Montgomery County Pub Schools, **SLP**

Dorsey, Lora D B 311 Rowland Drive, Lynchburg, VA 24503, (804) 528-3227, MA 78 Wichita St Univ; Sp-Lang Path/Superv, **SLP**

Dorsey, Pamela Harrington 1903 Springhill Avenue, Mobile, AL 36607, (205) 471-2184, BS 80 Univ of South AL; MS 82 Univ of South AL; SLP, Sp Lang Serv, **SLP**

Dorshorst, Mrs Margie Ann 8286 County Trunk HH, Arpin, WI 54410, (715) 423-4140, BA 83 Univ of WI - Eau Claire; MS 85 Univ of WI - Stevens Point; Sp-Lang Path, Wisconsin Rapids Pub Schools, **SLP**

Dorth, Donna Woodward Rt 3 Box 304-H, Ellijay, GA 30540, (404) 276-4696, BS 83 Western KY Univ; MS 85 Western KY Univ; 88–Sp-Lang Path, Gilmer County Bd of Educ, **SLP**

Dorton, Linda E 709 Battery Place #21, Chattanooga, TN 37403, **SLP**

Dorval, Mrs Bertha Mae P O Box 769, Center Harbor, NH 03226, (603) 253-7662, OB 44 Keene St Coll; OB 59 Boston Univ; 64 Boston Univ; Retired, Gilnanton Elem Sch, **SLP LM**

Dorward, Agnes K 700 Oakwood Lane, Washington, IL 61571, BA 51 Bradley Univ; **SLP LM**

Doscher-Thompson, Mrs Gail K 412 Evelyn Street, Kalamazoo, MI 49001, (616) 385-0591, BS 75 SUNY - Coll at Geneseo; MA 76 Western MI Univ; SLP, Kalamazoo Public Schools, **SLP ACE**

Dosen, Mrs Laura Ann 17156 Hill Creek Court, Orland Park, IL 60462, (815) 469-2415, BS 81 IL St Univ - Normal; MS 83 IL St Univ - Normal; 86–Sp-Lang Path, Lincoln-Way Area Spec Educ Coop, **SLP**

Dosen, Mrs Susan Gail 18421 Highpath Lane, Minnetonka, MN 55345, (612) 445-1194, BS 73 Univ of MN - Minneap-St Paul; MA 75 Univ of MN - Minneap-St Paul; 88–Coord, Minnesota River Valley Sp Educ Coop, **SLP**

Doshier, Mrs Ronita Kay 270 Acorn Drive, Streamwood, IL 60107, (312) 830-3526, BS 83 Univ of Central AR; MS 86 Univ of AR - Little Rock; **A**

Doss, Janet M 18081 Midway Road #2018, Dallas, TX 75287, (214) 323-5954, BA 74 Univ of SD - Vermillion; MA 75 Univ of SD - Vermillion; Sp-Lang Path, Carrollton-Farmers Branch ISD, **SLP**

Doss, Sharon L 4410 Balcones, Austin, TX 78731, (512) 451-7991, BA 71 Southern Methodist Univ; MS 72 Southern Methodist Univ; PH 88 (Figurative language use) Univ of TX - Austin; 79–Sp-Lang Path, Private Practice, **SLP**

Doss-Schliesman, Mrs Patricia Marie 1504 24th Street, Ames, IA 50010, (712) 792-3603, BS 82 Univ of SD - Vermillion; MA 83 Univ of SD - Vermillion; SLP, Heartland AEA, **SLP**

Dostal, Mrs Susan A H 5597 Arbutus Court, Greendale, WI 53129, (414) 421-7347, BS 76 Marquette Univ; MS 78 Marquette Univ; **SLP**

Dostal, Suzanne Marion 58-18 84th Place, Elmhurst, NY 11373, (718) 899-2327, BA 83 CUNY - Hunter Coll; MA 86 CUNY - Hunter Coll; Consultant, **SLP**

Doszak, Arlene L 1100 Hacker Avenue, Joliet, IL 60432, (815) 727-1494, **SLP**

Dotoli, Geraldine A 114 Village Circle, Winslow, NJ 08095, (201) 839-1300, BA 81 Montclair St Coll; MA 84 Seton Hall Univ; **SLP**

Dotson, Debra R 1604 Jefferson Street, Clifton Forge, VA 24422, (703) 862-4719, BS 74 Radford Univ; MS 82 James Madison Univ; Sp-Lang Path, Alleghany Highlands Pub Sch, **SLP**

Dotson, Kimberley Wray 38 Warren Street, Milford, CT 06460, (203) 734-9009, BA 78 Trinity Univ; MS 84 Southern CT St Univ; Aud, The Hrng Laboratory, **A**

Dotson, Nancy J 11403 Hardtner, Wichita, KS 67212-4713, (316) 688-7290, MA 82 Wichita St Univ; Sp-Lang Path, Wesley Med Ctr, **SLP**

Dotterweich, Mrs Margaret Faith 20 El Qaunito Way, Burlingame, CA 94010, (415) 343-3084, BA 79 San Francisco St Univ; MS 82 San Francisco St Univ; Sp/Lang Path, San Francisco USD, **SLP**

Doty, Carolyn Ann 7249 Oak Forest Drive, Clarkston, MI 48016, (313) 625-6425, BS 85 Northern MI Univ; MA 86 Western MI Univ; 87–Sp-Lang Path, William Beaumont Hosp, **SLP**

Doty, Charles L 2220 21st Street N W, Rochester, MN 55901, **SLP**

Doty, Maureen A 9205 Keystone #A, Skokie, IL 60076, (312) 679-0678, BS 80 Northwestern Univ; MA 81 Northwestern Univ; 85–Chief Aud, West Suburban Hosp, **A**

Doubek, Mrs Barbara A 3304 Twin Ridge Lane, Rockford, IL 61109, (815) 874-6419, BS 79 Northern MI Univ; MA 82 Northern IL Univ - De Kalb; **SLP**

Douberley, Joy L 8343 Princeton Square Blvd, Apartment 1202, Jacksonville, FL 32216, (904) 636-0143, BS 85 Auburn Univ - Auburn; MS 86 Univ of Montevallo

Doucette, Susan Marie Good Samaritan Hosp, Department Of Audiology, 1040 NW 22nd, Portland, OR 97210, (503) 229-7860, BS 83 ID St Univ; MS 85 ID St Univ; 86–Aud, Good Samaritan Hosp, **A**

Doudna, Dr Mark E 4702 Guilford Road, College Park, MD 20742, (301) 277-0921, BS 47 OH St Univ; MA 56 OH St Univ; PH 62 (Aud) OH St Univ; 62–Asst Prof, Univ of MD, **A LM**

Dougall, Ronald N 576 Village Green Lane W, Madison, WI 53704, (608) 263-5726, BA 73 San Diego St Univ; MA 80 IN Univ - Bloomington; Research Assistant Doctoral St, U of WI Madison, **SLP**

Dougan, Janet E 3630 East Phillips Avenue, Littleton, CO 80122, (303) 741-0445, BA 73 Univ of CO - Boulder; MS 75 Univ of OK Medical Center; **SLP**

Dougherty, Mrs Barbara B 850 Old State Road, Berwyn, PA 19312, (215) 539-8550, BS 68 Kent St Univ; MA 75 Kent St Univ; Sp-Lang Path, Penn State Univ, **SLP**

Dougherty, Betty Sterling 400 Meadowlark Drive, Greeneville, TN 37743, (615) 638-3380, MS 87 East TN St Univ; 87–Sp-Lang Path, Professional Health Svcs

Dougherty, Mrs Bonnie G 11212 Angus Place, Potomac, MD 20854, (301) 299-5583, BS 72 Ithaca Coll; MA 73 George Washington Univ; 81–Sp/Lang Path, Montgomery Co Pub Sch, **SLP**

Dougherty, Mrs Cynthia Lee 306 West Sunny Hill Blvd, St Peters, MO 63376, (314) 454-7355, BA 75 San Diego St Univ; MA 85 Saint Louis Univ; **SLP**

Dougherty, Mrs Dana Braswell 6700 Holmes Boulevard, Holmes Beach, FL 34218, (813) 778-1997, BS 84 FL St Univ; MS 85 FL St Univ; **SLP**

Dougherty, Mrs Dorothy Marie 31 Gulph Mill Road, Somers Point, NJ 08244, (609) 652-7000, **SLP**

Dougherty, Kathleen Mary 503 Vicnaire, New Iberia, LA 70560, (318) 369-6636, **SLP**

Dougherty, Leona Mae 1620 Minneapolis Avenue, Gladstone, MI 49837, BA 28 Univ of WI - Milwaukee; ME 57 Marquette Univ; Retired, Delta Menominee Hlth Dept, **SLP LM**

Dougherty, Mrs Mary Kathryn Route 1 Box 900, Washington, VA 22747, (703) 987-8259, BA 62 Univ of WA; MS 81 James Madison Univ; Sp-Lang Path, Rappahannock Co Pub Sch, **SLP**

Dougherty, Mrs Susan F 2630 N E WM E Sutton Road, Bremerton, WA 98310, (206) 692-5481, BA 67 Gonzaga Univ; OM 69 Univ of WA; 88–SLP, Central Kitsap Sch Dist, **SLP**

Dougherty Mark, Marie A Chestnutwood Lane, Andalusia, PA 19020, (215) 757-0227, BS 69 Trenton St Coll; MA 76 Trenton St Coll; 73–Sp-Lang Path, Bucks County Intermed Unit 22, **SLP**

Doughman, Sheril L 2621 Colfax Avenue South, Minneapolis, MN 55408, (612) 454-0504, BA 76 Univ of Northern IA; MA 78 Univ of Northern IA; 78–Sp-Lang Path, ISD 196, **SLP**

Doughney, Mrs Sharon Perozzi 157 8th Street, Wood River, IL 62095, (618) 254-8148, BS 71 Western IL Univ; MA 72 Western IL Univ; 88–Sp-Lang Path, Wood Rivr-Hartfrd Sch Dist #15

Doughten, Mrs Barbara Stern 2003 Hillingham Circle, Chadds Ford, PA 19317, (215) 388-7802, BA 63 Grinnell Coll; MA 65 IN Univ - Bloomington; **SLP**

Doughty, Mrs Cecile I 2332 Brennan, Plano, TX 75075, (214) 596-0973, BA 70 Univ of OK - Norman; MA 71 Univ of OK - Norman; **SLP**

Doughty, Patricia Jo 510 Clearview Place, Benton, IL 62812, (618) 378-2131, BS 80 Southern IL Univ -Carbondale; MS 82 Southern IL Univ -Carbondale; 87–Tchr, Wabash OH Valley Spec Educ Dist, **SLP**

Douglas, Ann V 46 Irving Terrace, Buffalo, NY 14223, (716) 937-9116, BA 71 SUNY - Center at Buffalo; MA 74 SUNY - Center at Buffalo; Sp-Lang Path, Alden Central Schools, **SLP**

Douglas, Barbara Jean 35334 Hathaway, Livonia, MI 48150, (313) 779-7610, OB 83 Wayne St Univ; OM 85 Wayne St Univ - Sch of Med; **A**

Douglas, Bettye B 14800 Tyler Street, Miami, FL 33176, (305) 233-2427, BA 55 Univ of CO - Boulder; MA 79 Univ of Miami; SLP, Dade Co Sch, **SLP**

Douglas, Jacqueline B 4906 Painters Street, New Orleans, LA 70122, BS 75 Xavier Univ of LA; OM 77 LA St Univ - N O Medical Ctr; Sp-Lang Path, Jefferson Parish Sch Syst, **SLP**

Douglas, Joan C G 9112 W Lake Highlands Dr, Dallas, TX 75218, (214) 320-3305, **SLP**

Douglas, Judith Ann 65 North Allen #216, Pasadena, CA 91106-2229, (818) 793-7246, MA 85 CA St Univ - Los Angeles; SLP, Los Angeles Co Office of Educ

Douglas, Mrs Kristiann Dept Of Aud & Speech 126/Nlr, VA Medical Center, North Little Rock, AR 72114, (501) 370-6651, BA 74 Northeast LA Univ; MA 76 Memphis St Univ; Aud, VA Med Ctr, **A**

Douglas, Laquita 206-F Union Avenue, Rutherford, NJ 07070, (201) 769-1331, BS 83 Bradley Univ; MA 85 Univ of IL - Chicago; Aud, Hearing Lab, **A**

Douglas, Martha J 2519 Avenue B, Scottsbluff, NE 69361, BA 79 Univ of NH; MA 81 Memphis St Univ; Dir Sp-Lang Path, Natl Therapeutics Assn, **SLP ACE**

Douglas, Priscilla 20 Catherine Street, Burlington, VT 05401, (802) 862-7111, MS 83 Univ of VT; **A**

Douglas-Fee, Elyse 9360 Sessions Road, Sauquoit, NY 13456, (315) 737-9971, BA 80 SUNY - Coll at Brockport; MS 85 Coll of Saint Rose; **SLP**

Douglass, Mrs Lois W 5205 Townsend Avenue, Los Angeles, CA 90041, (818) 795-4091, BA 43 Univ of Redlands; MA 65 CA St Univ - Los Angeles; Sp-Lang Path, Private Practice, **SLP LM**

Douglass, Mrs Rebecca Floyd 111 Bahama Drive, Norwood, MA 02062, (617) 769-4576, **SLP**

Douglass, Dr Robert L 5205 Townsend Avenue, Los Angeles, CA 90041, (818) 795-4091, BA 46 Univ of Redlands; MA 47 Univ of Redlands; PH 51 (NS) Univ of Southern CA; Sp-Lang Path, Private Practice, **SLP F LM**

Dougovito, Mrs Elaine B Route 1 Box 12, L'Anse, MI 49946, (906) 353-7170, BS 68 Central MI Univ; MA 69 OH Univ - Athens; 81–Sp-Lang Path, Baraga Memorial Hosp, **SLP**

Doull, Linda K P O Box 502, Claremont, West Australia, Australia 6010, BA 72 SUNY - Coll at Buffalo; MA 79 Univ of CA - Santa Barbara; Dir Lions Help to Hear Centre, Lions Club International, **A**

Doupe, Mrs Barbara J 2015 Glenwood Drive S W, Calgary, AB, Canada T3E 3Y7, (403) 242-6174, BA 76 Univ of Winnipeg - Manitoba; MA 78 Univ of ND; 86–Sp/Lang Path, Calgary Bd of Educ, **SLP**

Douros, Mrs Angie P 1 50th Street, Weehawken, NJ 07087, (201) 902-9454, BA 84 Kean Coll of NJ; MA 85 Kean Coll of NJ; 86–Sp-Lang Path, Milestone Sch for Child Dev

Douros, Mrs Maria John 380 Mountain Road #803, Union City, NJ 07087, (201) 348-5930, BA 81 Montclair St Coll; MA 85 Montclair St Coll; Sp-Lang Path, Union City Board of Education, **SLP ACE**

Douthett, Mary Beth 1217 Ganado, San Clemente, CA 92672, (714) 492-7739, BA 84 CA St Univ - Fullerton; MA 86 Whittier Coll; 88–Sp-Lang Path, Saddleback Valley USD, **SLP**

Douthit, Lillian 11119 Maykirk, Sugar Land, TX 77478, (713) 734-3426, BS 51 Univ of TX - Austin; ME 52 Univ of TX - Austin; **SLP**

Douville, Rosanne R 3741 Westwind Drive, Beaver Creek, OH 45440, (513) 236-9965, BS 75 Indiana Univ of PA; MA 77 Kent St Univ; Sp-Lang Path/Aud, Miami Vly Reg Cen Hndcpd Chldn, **SLP A ACE**

Dovalina, Norma El Paso Rehabilitation Center, 1101 East Schuster Avenue, El Paso, TX 79902, (905) 566-2956, BA 82 Pan American Univ; MA 85 Univ of TX - Austin; Sp-Lang Path, El Paso Rehabilitation Center, **SLP**

Dovantzis, Mrs Marylou Buckler 16212 Apple Lane #4, Tinley Park, IL 60477, (312) 532-9326, **A**

Dove, Francine Speech Therapy Services, Route 1 Box 93N, Lexington Park, MD 20653, (301) 863-9007, BS 75 Univ of VA - Charlottesville; MS 76 PA St Univ - Univ Park; Consult Sp Lang Therapy, Speech Therapy Services, **SLP**

Dove, Heather M 4506-B Leo Way, Salt Lake City, UT 84117, (801) 581-7514, OB 77 McGill Univ - Quebec; MA 81 Temple Univ; Sp-Lang Path, Univ of Utah Sch of Med, **SLP**

Dove, Hilary 5863 Briarwood Avenue, Sarasota, FL 33581, (813) 923-3343, MS 73 Univ of South FL; Sp-Lang Path, Private Practice, **SLP**

Dover, Mrs Crystal C Route 4, 32 Holly Hill Drive, Asheville, NC 28806, (704) 274-9225, BS 69 Kent St Univ; MA 74 Kent St Univ; Sp-Lang Path, Buncombe Co Sch, **SLP**

Dover, Mrs Pamela Reynolds 3010 Debra, Batesville, AR 72501, (501) 793-2821, OB 81 AR St Univ; OM 84 AR St Univ; Sp-Lang Path, Batesville Sch Dist

Doverspike, Cyd Triche P O Box 159, Larose, LA 70373, (504) 693-3745, BS 80 Univ of Southwestern LA; OM 81 LA St Univ - N O Medical Ctr; Sp-Lang Path, **SLP**

Dow, Mrs Beverly J 571 Rockcliff, Fayetteville, AR 72701, (501) 442-4070, BS 72 Univ of OK - Norman; MS 76 Univ of OK Medical Center; **SLP**

Dow, Mrs Marie L 70 Carolan Avenue, Hampton, NH 03842, (603) 692-3331, BS 51 Tufts Univ; MS 87 Univ of NH; 87–Sp-Lang Path, Sch Admin Unit #56 Somersworth

Dowd, Dorothy Ann 392 Central Park West, Apartment 14-W, New York, NY 10025-5868, (516) 922-4400, BA 78 Long Island U - CW Post Ctr; MS 82 Adelphi Univ; Sp-Lang Path, Beth Israel Medical Center, **SLP**

Dowd, Kathryn R 2230 Sagamore, Charlotte, NC 28209-3346, BA 72 Spalding Coll; ME 78 Univ of Louisville; 86–Aud, Miracle Ear Ctr, **A**

Dowden, Patricia A Rehab Medicine Rj-30, University Hospital, University Of Washington, Seattle, WA 98195, (206) 543-3134, BA 74 SUNY - Center at Binghamton; MS 80 Univ of WA; SLP, University of Washington Hosp, **SLP**

Dowdy, Brenda Hobbs Rt 1 Box 346, Dublin, VA 24084, (703) 731-3359, BA 83 Harding Univ; MS 85 Univ of MS; Sp-Lang Path, **SLP**

Dowdy, Lissa Karen 4450 Ridgemont #2024, Abilene, TX 79606, (915) 691-7250, BS 84 Univ of TX - Austin; MA 86 Univ of TX - Austin; 86–Aud, West TX Rehab Ctr, **A**

Dowell, Bonita Lynne Department Speech Hearing, 901 South 6th Street, Champaign, IL 61820, (217) 344-8667, BA 81 Columbia Coll; MA 84 SC St Coll; 88–Tchg Asst, Univ of IL-Champaign-Urbana, **SLP**

Dower, Nikia Rae Rt 1 Box 6, Arcola, VA 22010, (703) 777-8181, BS 84 James Madison Univ; MS 86 James Madison Univ; SLP, Acre Center, **SLP**

Dowler, Mrs Sharon J M 35 Dos Loma Vista Lane, Portola Valley, CA 94025, (415) 657-2350, BA 65 CUNY - City College; MA 67 Stanford Univ; Sp-Lang Path, Fremont USD, **SLP**

Dowler, Susan 10006 Fairfax Court N W, Albuquerque, NM 87114, (505) 298-6752, BA 65 Univ of Denver; MA 67 Univ of OK Medical Center; Methods and Materials Teacher, Albuquerque Public School, **SLP**

Dowling, Claire J 3823 36th Street #6, San Diego, CA 92104, (518) 445-3713, BS 77 SUNY - Center at Albany; MA 79 SUNY - Center at Buffalo; Aud, Albany Med Cen Hosp, **A**

Dowling, Mrs Ernestine Noferi 591 Stewart Street, Ridgefield, NJ 07657, (201) 438-3070, BA 72 Jersey City St Coll; MS 82 William Paterson Coll; 82–Sp-Lang Path, Woodridge Bd of Ed, **SLP**

Dowling, Mrs Frances R 2015 East Newport #309, North Shore ENT, Milwaukee, WI 53211, (414) 961-1550, BA 69 Univ of WI - Oshkosh; MS 79 Univ of WI - Oshkosh; Aud, North Shore ENT Assoc, **A**

Dowling, Jean Marie 128 Parkside Drive, Suffern, NY 10901, (914) 368-3585, BA 81 SUNY - Center at Binghamton; MA 85 Montclair St Coll; Sp-Lang Path, Private Practice, **SLP**

Dowling, Leslie B 6 Ross Road, Scarsdale, NY 10583-4426, (914) 693-8500, BS 70 OH St Univ; MA 72 CUNY - Hunter Coll; Sp-Lang Path, Chldn Village/Greenburgh, **SLP**

Dowling, Mrs Michelle Micciche 14 Cross Street, Reading, MA 01867, (617) 726-2763, BA 82 Univ of VT; MS 85 Univ of WI - Madison; Sp-Lang Path, Massachusetts General Hosp, **SLP**

Dowling, Mrs Sue Y 502 West Alden Avenue, Valdosta, GA 31602, (912) 247-7483, BS 74 Univ Southern MS-Hattiesburg; MS 75 Univ Southern MS-Hattiesburg; 81–Parent Advr, GA PINES, **SLP A**

Dowling, Dr Susann S 146L SOA-COMD, 4800 Calhoun, University Of Houston, Houston, TX 77204-6611, (713) 749-4553, BA 67 IN Univ - Bloomington; MA 69 IN Univ - Bloomington; PH 76 (Sp-Lang Path-Supervision) IN Univ - Bloomington; 80–Assoc Prof, U of Houston, **SLP**

Downard, Mrs Carol Sue 142 Bristol Court, West Lafayette, IN 47906, (317) 448-8463, BS 85 Purdue Univ - West Lafayette; MS 87 Purdue Univ - West Lafayette; 87–Aud, Arnett Clinic, **A**

Downer, Mrs Margaret L 1818 NW 28th Avenue, Camas, WA 98607, (206) 835-8766, BS 74 Pacific Univ; MA 78 Western KY Univ; Sp-Lang Path, Washougal Schs, **SLP**

Downes, Mrs Charlene S 12664 N E 87th Street, Kirkland, WA 98033, (206) 281-6855, BS 69 Univ of NE - Lincoln; MA 70 Univ of NE - Lincoln; Sp-Lang Path, Seattle School District, **SLP**

Downes, Mrs Meta M 118 Avon Lane, Greenville, NC 27858, (919) 757-6961, BA 58 Bethany Coll; MA 59 Middlebury Coll; ME 74 East Carolina Univ; Assoc Prof/Dir of Cl Experiences, E Carolina U, **SLP ACE**

Downey, Amy Hottes 10934 Little Sparrow Place, Columbia, MD 21044, (301) 997-4646, BS 80 Towson St Univ; MS 81 Towson St Univ; Sp/Lang Path, Howard Co Bd of Ed, **SLP**

Downey, Dr Doris Marie 5325 Kewanee Drive, Boulder, CO 80303, (303) 492-3036, 66 Univ of CO - Boulder; 69 Univ of CO - Boulder; 81 (Communication Disorders) Univ of CO - Boulder; 84–Research Assoc, Univ of Colorado, **SLP**

Downey, Jane Capria 6202 Foundry Road, Guilderland, NY 12084, BS 76; MS 77 Loyola Coll; Sp-Lang Path, Cerebral Palsy Cen for Disabld, **SLP**

Downey, Mrs Jeanne C Neurosensory Center, Saint Vincent Health Center, 232 West 25th Street, Erie, PA 16544, (814) 452-5654, BS 80 Clarion Univ of PA; MS 82 Clarion Univ of PA; 84–Chief/Sp-Lang Path/Aud, St Vincent Hlth Cen, **SLP**

Downey, Marlene G 1105 Alann Drive, Joliet, IL 60435, (815) 939-3651, BA 76 Coll of Saint Francis; OM 81 Governors St Univ; Sp-Lang Path, Kankakee Area Spec Ed Coop, **SLP**

Downey-Barnhardt, Erin Lynn Box 1534, Meadow Lake, SK, Canada S0M 1V0, (306) 845-2310, BA 86 Minot St Univ; MS 87 Minot St Univ

Downie, Mrs Ellen Mary 40 Devonshire Drive, Waterford, CT 06385, (203) 442-9801, BA 81 Rutger's St Univ - Douglas Coll; MS 83 Rutgers St Univ -N Brunswick; 84–Sp-Lang Path, East Lyme Pub Schs, **SLP**

Downie, Mrs Linda K 12 S Buckingham Lane, Buffalo Grove, IL 60089, (312) 392-2250, BS 75 IL St Univ - Normal; MS 76 IL St Univ - Normal; Sp-Lang Path, Northwest Sp & Hrng Cen, **SLP ACE**

Downie, Susan M 45 Willow Street #115, Springfield, MA 01103, (203) 243-9741, BS 78 Univ of MA - Amherst; MA 80 Univ of MA - Amherst; Dir/Traumatic Brain Injury Svcs, The Rehab Ctr, **SLP**

Downing, Carla D 3435 N W 56th Street, Suite 811, Oklahoma City, OK 73112-4402, (405) 945-4255, BS 74 OK St Univ; MA 75 OK St Univ; Owner Sp-Lang Path, Sp-Lang Path, **SLP**

Downing, Mrs Carolyn Butler Route 6, Mayfield, KY 42066, (502) 247-0808, BS 81 Murray St Univ; MS 82 Murray St Univ; Sp-Lang Path, Graves Co Sch Sys, **SLP**

Downing, Mrs Jude M 4414 Fir Lane, Toledo, OH 43613, (419) 885-1444, BA 70; MA 77 Bowling Green St Univ; Sp-Lang Path, Flower Mem/Lake Park Hosp, **SLP**

Downing, Karen Dianne 3524 Lake Heights, Waco, TX 76708, (817) 776-1704, MS 84 Baylor Univ; Sp-Lang Path, Waco Independent School Dist, **SLP**

Downing, Mrs Karla Deane 1838 South Glenview Drive, Mesa, AZ 85204, (602) 839-7157, BA 80 CA St Univ - Fullerton; MA 82 CA St Univ - Fullerton; Sp-Lang Path, Tempe Elementary Sch Dist, **SLP**

Downing, Kenneth N 966 East Gardenia, Madison Heights, MI 48071, (313) 542-3910, BS 54 Central MI Univ; MS 57 Univ of MI - Ann Arbor; Sp-Lang Path, Hazel Park Bd of Ed, **SLP**

Downing-Ball, Mrs Debbie J 336 Village Lane, Eureka, KS 67045, (316) 583-7530, BS 81 KS St Univ; MA 83 Wichita St Univ; Sp-Lang Path, Eureka USD 389, **SLP**

Downs, David W School Of Speech Path,Aud, Kent State University, Kent, OH 44242, (602) 626-2209, BS 75 Univ of NM; MS 77 Univ of NM; PH 82 (Sp & Hrng Sciences) Univ of AZ; 86–Aud, Kent State Univ, **A**

Downs, Mrs Debra B 102 Get A Way Lane, Bahama, NC 27503, (815) 232-2610, BS 74 Univ of KS; MA 75 Univ of KS; Sp-Lang Path, Papillion Public Schools, **SLP**

Downs, Mrs Marion P Box B210 Department Of Otolaryngology, University Of Colorado Health Science Center, 4200 East 9th Avenue, Denver, CO 80262, (303) 322-5461, BA 48 Univ of MN - Minneap-St Paul; MA 51 Univ of Denver; 82–Prof Emerita, U Co Hlth Sc Cen, **A F H LM**

Downs, Mary Patricia 2522 West 39th Place, Chicago, IL 60632, (312) 523-8295, BS 82 Purdue Univ - West Lafayette; MS 84 Univ of IL - Urbana; Sp-Lang Path, SW Cook Co Coop Assoc/Spec Ed, **SLP**

Downs, Mrs Paula c/o Joe Crawford, 325 Highway 299 East, Route 2 Box 213, Burney, CA 96013, (916) 335-2444, **SLP**

Dowsett, Mrs Beth Ann 621 John Street #C, Kalamazoo, MI 49007, (616) 345-6759, BA 83 MI St Univ; MS 85 Univ of MI - Ann Arbor; Speech Language Pathologist, **SLP**

Dowswell, Barbara Spindel 3028 Daybreak Avenue, Coquitlam, BC, Canada V3C 2G2, (604) 939-9261, BS 75 SUNY - Coll at New Paltz; MS 76 Univ of MI - Ann Arbor; Sp/Lang Path, Brit Col Min of Hlth, **SLP**

Doyle, Beth Ann 875 Franklin Road #212, Marietta, GA 30067-7945, (404) 426-1064, BS 86 Univ of GA; MA 87 Memphis St Univ; Sp-Lang Path, Cobb Co Schools

Doyle, Carmela Christine RD 1 Mount Prosper Road, Box 28-A, Wurtsboro, NY 12790, (914) 294-8806, BS 85 SUNY - Coll at Geneseo; MA 87 SUNY - Coll at Geneseo; 87–Sp-Lang Path, Orange Co Cerebral Palsy Assoc Inc, **SLP**

Doyle, Carol Anne 12032 C Royal Birkdale Row, San Diego, CA 92128, (619) 487-3436, BS 80 Pacific Union Coll; MS 82 Univ of Redlands; Sp-Lang Path, Eloise Johnston & Associates, **SLP**

Doyle, Catherine 400 East 70th Street #2204, New York, NY 10021, (515) 964-2550, BS 77 Univ of IA; MA 72 Univ of IA; **SLP**

Doyle, Mrs Debora H 2410 Mohler Drive N W, North Canton, OH 44720, BS 73 Bowling Green St Univ; MA 74 Bowling Green St Univ; SLP, N Canton Cty Sch, **SLP**

Doyle, Deborah S Hearing Resources, 5712 Oakshire Road, Baltimore, MD 21209, (301) 664-0533, BS 76 Northeastern Univ; MS 78 Columbia Univ Teachers Coll; 88–Aud, Hearing Resources, **A**

Doyle, Dolores M 8403 Nunley Drive, Parkville, MD 21234, BS 56 Bloomsburg Univ of PA; MA 61 Loyola Coll; SLP, Bd of Ed of Balt Co, **SLP**

Doyle, Mrs Dorothy G 1600 Quail, Mc Allen, TX 78504, (512) 383-3575, BS 66 Sam Houston St Univ; MS 69 TX Tech Univ; 79–Sp-Lang Path, Edinburg Cons Ind Sch Dist, **SLP**

Doyle, Mrs Harriett E 9666 Springfield Way, Stockton, CA 95212, BA 70 Whittier Coll; MA 73 Univ of the Pacific; SLP, Lodi USD, **SLP**

Doyle, Jane Seymour 43 High Street, Seymour, CT 06483, (203) 334-2118, BS 84 James Madison Univ; MS 86 James Madison Univ; **SLP**

Doyle, Mrs Joann L 120 Pleasant Valley Drive, Daytona Beach, FL 32014, (904) 258-8931, BA 71 Elon Coll; MS 73 FL St Univ; SLP, Valusia Co Sch Syst, **SLP**

Doyle, Joyce Gloeckl 20 Roxbury Road, Pittsburgh, PA 15221-4626, **SLP**

Doyle, Julieanne M 5001 Endolwood Road #0, Charlotte, NC 28215-4184, BS 82 Coll of Saint Rose; MA 85 CUNY - Hunter Coll; **SLP**

Doyle, Mrs Karen Crocker Cedar Ridge Apartment, Flanders Road #6-K, Niantic, CT 06357, (203) 447-0301, MS 88 Southern CT St Univ

Doyle, Kathleen Marie 976 Main Street, #18, Melrose, MA 02176, (617) 665-2661, BA 82 Boston Coll; MA 84 Univ of CT; Sp/Lang Path, Reading Public Schools, **SLP**

Doyle, Mrs Laurie J 5015 Trent Road, Harrisburg, PA 17109, (717) 569-7331, ME 79 Clarion Univ of PA; SLP, Lancaster Lebanon IU13, **SLP**

Doyle, Mrs Linda Ann 5645 Wedgmont Circle, Fort Worth, TX 76133, (817) 737-4231, MA 66 TX Christian Univ; BA 62 TX Christian Univ; Supvr/Spec Educ, Ft Worth ISD, **SLP**

Doyle, Louise Marie 1101 Packers Circle #14, Tustin, CA 92680-3502, (714) 629-4011, BA 79 Univ of Redlands; OM 83 Univ of WA; Sp-Lang Path, Providence Sp & Hrng Cen, **SLP**

Doyle, Lynn Horrigan 5255 North Bay Ridge Avenue, Whitefish Bay, WI 53217, (414) 962-1750, BS 68 Marquette Univ; MS 73 Marquette Univ; SLP, Milwaukee Sch Bd, **SLP**

Doyle, Mrs Margaret Jill 6419 Barkwood Lane, Dallas, TX 75248, (214) 934-0816, BS 71 Univ of KS; MA 83 Univ of Tulsa; Sp/Lang Path, **SLP**

Doyle, Margaret Marie 1900 Abbott Avenue, Alamogordo, NM 88310, (505) 437-3200, BS 77 NM St Univ; BS 80 NM St Univ; MS 83 Eastern NM Univ; Sp-Lang Path, Alamogordo PS, **SLP**

Doyle, Mary M 11122 Claire Avenue, Northridge, CA 91326, (818) 360-7719, BA 84 Univ of CA - Santa Barbara; MS 86 Univ of WA; 88–Sp-Lang Path, Rancho Los Amigos Med Ctr, **SLP**

Doyle, Patrick J 20 Roxbury Drive, Pittsburgh, PA 15221, (412) 363-0451, MS 80 Univ of Pittsburgh - Pittsburgh; PH 87 (Sp Path); Sp-Lang Path, VA Medical Center, **SLP**

Doyle, Dr Philip C Sch Of Human Comm Disorders, Dalhousie University, 5599 Fenwick Street, Halifax, NS, Canada B3H 1R2, (902) 424-7052, BA 79 CA St Univ - Fresno; MA 81 Univ of CA - Santa Barbara; PH 85 (Sp & Hrng Sciences) Univ of CA - San Francisco; 85–Asst Prof, Dalhousie U, **SLP**

Doyle, Mrs Shirley S 4445 Andover Road, Edina, MN 55435, (612) 624-3322, BA 64 Univ of MD - College Park; MA 66 Univ of MD - College Park; 66–Assoc Clin Spec, Univ of Minn, **SLP**

Doyle, Mrs Susan Ann 6042 Oriole Lane, Greendale, WI 53129, (414) 327-6670, BS 82 Univ of WI - Whitewater; MS 84 Murray St Univ; 87–Sp-Lang Path, Physical Ther Svcs Inc, **SLP**

Doyle, Dr Timothy N 4445 Andover Road, Edina, MN 55435, (612) 725-6767, BA 63 Denison Univ; MA 65 Univ of MD - College Park; PH 70 (NS) Univ of MN - Minneap-St Paul; Ch of Aud, VA Admin, **A**

Doyle-Kushner, Mrs Patricia 728 North La Grange Road, La Grange Park, IL 60525, (312) 354-5346, BS 69 Marquette Univ; MS 72 Marquette Univ; Sp-Lang Path, Private Practice, **SLP**

Doyne, Mrs Marcella P 320 Fox Creek Road, Jefferson City, MO 65109, (314) 893-3287, BS 47 Washington Univ; MS 50 Purdue Univ - West Lafayette; 83–Sp-Lang Path, St Mary's Health Ctr, **SLP**

Dozier, Betsy L P O Box 246, Monroeville, AL 36461-0246, (305) 334-8361, **SLP**

Drabyak, Janice Kratz 85 Queens Circle, Chalfont, PA 18914, (215) 348-2940, BS 78 West Chester Univ of PA; MA 80 Trenton St Coll; Sp-Lang Path, Bucks Co Iu #22, **SLP**

Draeger, Mrs Katherine Louise 2184 Yeoman Court, Port Charlotte, FL 33983, (813) 627-0750, BA 68 Univ of CA - Santa Barbara; MA 71 San Francisco St Univ; Sp-Lang Path, Sch Bd of Charlotte Co, **SLP**

Draegert, Margaret E 36 Sherwood Avenue, Madison, NJ 07940, (201) 377-8346, BA 61 Grinnell Coll; Consult, Private Practice, **SLP**

Draewell, Susan K 3715 Bigelow Drive, Louisville, KY 40299, (502) 499-1465, BS 69 Univ of TN - Knoxville; MS 71 Vanderbilt Univ; SLP, Comm Coord Chld Care, **SLP**

Dragavon, Paul 550 Water Street Suite F-4, Santa Cruz, CA 95060, (408) 426-6644, BS 57 Univ of MN - Duluth; MA 62 San Francisco St Univ; Sp-Lang Path, Private Practice, **SLP**

Dragga, Linda C 1221 Westover Street, College Station, TX 77840, (409) 693-9516, BA 74 Colby Coll; MA 77 OH Univ - Athens; **SLP**

Drago, Mrs Jane Cooper 11821 Clay Chester, Des Peres, MO 63131, (314) 344-6460, BA 76 Tulane Univ; MA 78 Vanderbilt Univ; Dir Rehab Medicine, DePaul Health Ctr, **SLP**

Drainville, Mrs Teresa Prusak 5672 Scherff Road, Orchard Park, NY 14127, (716) 492-3154, BS 80 SUNY - Coll at Buffalo; MS 84 SUNY - Coll at Buffalo; SLP, Pioneer Central School Dist, **SLP**

Draizar, Dr Andrea 12280 Southwest, Terrace 104, Miami, FL 33186-3613, (305) 595-4271, BA 73 Case Western Reserve Univ; MA 77 PA St Univ - Univ Park; PH 82 (Linguistics) PA St Univ - Univ Park; Sp-Lang Path, Private Practice, **SLP ACE**

Drake, Barbara N 7600 Wood Hollow Drive, Apartment #204, Austin, TX 78731-2242, (512) 444-4835, BS 75 Southwest TX St Univ; ME 76 Southwest TX St Univ; Dir Serv Consult, Ed Serv Cen-Reg Xvii, **SLP**

Drake, Beverly S Star Route Box 19-A, Addy, WA 99101, (509) 722-6285, BA 70 Univ of MD - College Park; MS 71 Univ of WI - Madison; SLP, Educational Serv Dist 101, **SLP**

Drake, Mrs Diana L 1216 Vista Drive, Fenton, MI 48430, (313) 629-8796, BS 68 Univ of MI - Ann Arbor; MS 70 Univ of MI - Ann Arbor; Sp-Lang Path, Bendle Pub Sch, **SLP**

Drake, Gloria S 1209 East Lawrence Lane, Phoenix, AZ 85020, **SLP**

Drake, Jack 4031 North Creek Road, Palmyra, NY 14522, (315) 597-4593, BA 48 Univ of Akron; MA 59 Univ of IA; **SLP A LM**

Drake, Mrs Janis S 2E Village Of Pine Run, Blackwood, NJ 08012, (609) 435-2789, BS 78 Boston Univ; MS 80 Columbia Univ Teachers Coll; Sp-Lang Path, Our Lady of Lourdes Med Cen, **SLP**

Drake, Karen Lynn 40 Queensberry Street #3, Boston, MA 02215, (617) 732-5601, BS 83 Univ of OR; MA 86 Univ of CA - Santa Barbara; 88–Sp-Lang Path, Brigham & Women's Hosp, **SLP**

Drake, Laurie Ede 3736 Elmhurst Street, Toledo, OH 43613, (419) 474-3041, BS 80 Miami Univ - Oxford; MA 81 Bowling Green St Univ; 87–Aud, Med Coll of Ohio, **A**

Drake, Mrs Lilianne Jacqueline 162 Goldenrod Lane, Rochester, NY 14623-3651, (716) 271-6423, **SLP**

Drake, Lisa Ann 6730 Lincoln Green, Holland, OH 43528, (419) 473-3561, BS 83 Bowling Green St Univ; MA 84 Bowling Green St Univ; 84–Aud, Toledo Clinic Inc, **A**

Drake, Mrs Marion E 18001 Osborne Street, Northridge, CA 91324, BA 42 PA St Univ - Univ Park; MA 70 CA St Univ - Northridge; **SLP LM**

Drake, Marla Colleen 7903 Meadowhaven Blvd, Columbus, OH 43235, (614) 293-3818, BA 83 OH St Univ; MA 85 OH St Univ; Sp-Lang Path, Ohio State Univ Hospitals, **SLP**

Drake, Mrs Patricia A 5189 La Canada Boulevard, La Canada, CA 91011, MA 76 CA St Univ - Northridge; OM 82 CA St Univ - Los Angeles; SLP, Los Angeles County Office Educ, **SLP**

Dranka, Mrs Sydney S 5708 Marquis Court, Mobile, AL 36609, (205) 343-3297, BS 79 Univ of South AL; MA 84 Univ of Houston - Univ Park; 88–Clin Supvr, InSpeech Inc, **SLP**

Dranoff, Carol Beth 770 Parmentier Road, Warminster, PA 18974, (215) 535-0445, BS 65 Temple Univ; MA 81 Trenton St Coll; **SLP**

Drapekin, Mrs Susan Gail 2009 Harrison, Unit #204, Evanston, IL 60201, (314) 527-3359, MS 84 Univ of IL - Urbana; Sp-Lang Path, The Center for Rehab &Trning, **SLP**

Draper, Dr David J 5432 Plaza Lane, Wichita, KS 67208, (316) 685-0400, BA 62 Univ of KS; MA 63 Univ of KS; PH 70 (NS) Univ of KS; 88–Exec Dir, Georgetown Village, **SLP**

Draper, Mrs Eileen S Pine Crest Katakura D, 1-1-13 Minami Azabu, Minato-Ku, Tokyo, Japan 106, (813) 452-3729, BS 65 SUNY - Coll at Geneseo; MA 69 Columbia Univ Teachers Coll; Sp-Lang Path, Private Practice, **SLP**

Draper, John F 530 21st Avenue S E, Puyallup, WA 98371, **SLP**

Draper, Patricia Louise 62 Santa Elena Avenue, Daly City, CA 94015, (415) 756-9169, BS 80 AL A & M Univ; MA 87 Univ of TN - Knoxville

Draper-Parker, Linda Kaye Boot Pond, Plymouth, MA 02360, (617) 746-5883, BS 71 9190; MS 75 Columbia Univ Teachers Coll; Sp-Lang Path, Plymouth Developmental Presch, **SLP**

Draper-Small, Lisa Monique 31 Lockwood Lane, Topsfield, MA 01983, (312) 438-6319, **SLP**

Draves, David William 18 Jefferson Drive, Northfield, MN 55057, (612) 437-6111, BA 76 Saint Olaf Coll; MS 81 Mankato St Univ; Sp-Lang Path, ISD 200, **SLP**

Drawbaugh, Lana Rae 1516 Lanelle Drive, Panama City, FL 32405, (904) 872-4775, BS 77 Indiana Univ of PA; MS 81 Indiana Univ of PA; 78–Sp-Lang Path, Bay County Schls, **SLP ACE**

Drayton, Augusta P 4504 17th Street N W, Washington, DC 20011, **SLP**

Drayton, Mrs Peggy Cardwell 1801 West Rogers Avenue, Baltimore, MD 21209, (301) 396-4906, **SLP**

Drazinski, Lynn Ann 27611 Durazno, Mission Viejo, CA 92692, (714) 458-6777, BS 79 AZ St Univ; MA 84 Univ of KS; **SLP**

Dreasler, Mrs Pauline F 211 South 12th Street, Fort Dodge, IA 50501, (515) 576-7434, BA 60 Northeastern OK St Univ; MA 65 Northeastern OK St Univ; SLP, Arrowhead AEA, **SLP**

Drebin, Mrs Kathleen C 11347 West Woodhaven Court, Boise, ID 83704, (208) 375-4860, BS 78 OR St Univ; MS 81 UT St Univ; Audiologist & Clinical Instr, **A**

Dreifus, Vicky Greenberg 1530 East 19th Street, Brooklyn, NY 11230, (212) 377-5090, **SLP**

Dreiling, Mrs Alica Johnson PO Box 1337, Lawrence, KS 66044, (913) 294-4361, BS 80 Fort Hays St Univ; MA 84 Univ of KS; Sp-Lang Path, USD 497, **SLP**

Dreiling, Mrs Sheryl L 517 West 32nd Street, Hays, KS 67601, (913) 628-1901, MS 72 Fort Hays St Univ; BS 71 Fort Hays St Univ; SLP, USD #489, **SLP**

Dreith-Ratcliffe, Susan 3098 West 39th Avenue, Denver, CO 80908, BS 76 Univ of Northern CO; MS 78 Univ of WY; Aud, **A**

Drennan, Mrs Deborah F 1104 Arrowhead Drive, Brentwood, TN 37027, (615) 333-8989, BS 77 Murray St Univ; MS 79 Vanderbilt Univ; 87–Aud, Eva A Dimitrov MD, **A**

Drennan, Pamela Ann 962 S W Country Commons, Lake Oswego, OR 97034, (503) 635-7468, MA 84 CA St Univ - Fullerton; 85–Sp-Lang Path, Portland PS, **SLP**

Dressler, Mrs Bernice S 1236 Catalina Drive, Monroeville, PA 15146, (412) 648-8384, BS 54 Univ of Pittsburgh - Pittsburgh; MS 58 Univ of Pittsburgh - Pittsburgh; Sp-Lang Path, Cleft Palate Center, **SLP**

Dressler, Diane Peck 1736 Independence Lane, Cherry Hill, NJ 08003, (609) 354-8044, BS 76 SUNY - Center at Albany; MA 77 Univ of FL; Sp-Lang Path, Lower Merion Sch Dist, **SLP**

Dressler, Richard A 3434 Sea Eagle Court, Wilmington, NC 28403, (919) 343-7218, BA 74 Univ of MO - Columbia; MS 80 Central MO St Univ; 86–Sp-Lang Path, New Hanover Mem Hosp, **SLP ACE**

Drevs, Lori Jane R R 2 Box 228, Humboldt, IA 50548, (515) 332-3024, BS 82 IA St Univ; MA 83 Northeast MO St Univ; SLP, Arrowhead AEA, **SLP**

Drew, Barbara Ann R R 2 Box 24, Carbondale, IL 62901, (618) 457-2995, MS 88 Southern IL Univ-Edwardsvill

Drew, Carolyn Ann 59 Newbrook Lane, Springfield, NJ 07081, (201) 376-7323, BS 85 Miami Univ - Oxford; MS 87 PA St Univ - Univ Park; **A**

Drew, Mrs Karin 4415 Harbor Country Drive, Apartment E-3, Gig Harbor, WA 98335-1756, (206) 756-8502, BA 77 Univ of WA; OM 78 Univ of WA; SLP, Clover Park School District, **SLP**

Drew, Nancy Audiology Clinic, Veterans Hospital, 42nd & Clement Street, San Francisco, CA 94121, (415) 221-4810, BA 60 Brown Univ; MA 63 Stanford Univ; Sp-Lang Path, VA, **SLP A**

Drew, Robert P P O Box 68 Airport Road, Bethany, MO 64424, (816) 425-3035, BS 69 Northwest MO St Univ; MS 75 Central MO St Univ; Director, Clinical Spch & Hrng Services, **SLP**

Drew, Ruby Louise 502 Windamer Court, Valparaiso, IN 46383, (219) 462-8482, BS 66 Univ of MN - Duluth; MA 82 Univ of MN - Duluth; Sp-Lang Path, **SLP**

Drewry, Mrs Jane V 5-D University Houses, Madison, WI 53705, (608) 238-0115, BS 80 Univ of WI - Milwaukee; MS 87 Univ of WI - Madison; 87–Aud, Divine Savior Hosp

Drews, Mrs Christine Lutz 546 Harris Hill, Lancaster, NY 14086, (716) 662-0135, BS 76 SUNY - Coll at Buffalo; MA 78 SUNY - Coll at Geneseo; Sp-Lang Path, Erie-Chataugua-Cattaraugus BOCES #2, **SLP**

Drewyer, Mrs Martha B 7315 Pouter, Houston, TX 77083-4854, (713) 498-8110, MS 76 Our Lady Lake Univ-San Anton; 87–Spec Educ Supvr, Alief ISD, **SLP**

Drexler, Allan B 2621 Ogleton Road, Annapolis, MD 21403, (301) 267-7799, PH (NS); **SLP A**

Drexler, Catherine 2621 Ogleton Road, Annapolis, MD 21403, BA 58 Saint Mary-of-the-Woods Coll; MS 61 Univ of Pittsburgh - Pittsburgh; Private Practice, **SLP**

Drexler, Mrs Geraldine Communicology Inc, 8220 Naab Road, Suite 311, Indianapolis, IN 46260, (317) 872-3131, BA 66 Rutger's St Univ - Douglas Coll; MA 68 Newark St Coll; Dir, Comm Inc, **SLP**

Drexler, Dr Hazel G P O Box 857, Livingston, MT 59047, (406) 686-4729, MA 51 PA St Univ - Univ Park; MS 58 Purdue Univ - West Lafayette; PH 61 (NS) Purdue Univ - West Lafayette; **SLP A LM**

Drexler, Mrs Shelley 939 Hewlett Drive, North Woodmere, NY 11581-2728, (718) 854-3737, MA 76 Queens Coll; 84–Coord Sp-Lang Svcs, New York Childhood Ctr, **SLP**

Dreyer, Dr Dorothy E 555 Manoogian Hall, Communication Disorders & Sciences, Wayne State University, Detroit, MI 48202, (313) 577-3337, BS 65 Kent St Univ; MA 66 Kent St Univ; PH 69 (Sp-Lang Path) MI St Univ; Asst Prof, Wayne St U, **SLP F**

Dreyer, Marla Lynn 1885 McKelvey Hill #306, Maryland Heights, MO 63043, (314) 457-8479, BS 77 Southeast MO St Univ; OM 82 Univ of MO - Columbia; 86–Sp-Lang Path, InSpeech Inc, **SLP**

Dreyer, Sharon K 731 South Mississippi, Mason City, IA 50401, (515) 424-7611, BS 80 Northeast MO St Univ; MA 81 Northeast MO St Univ; 81–Dir-SLP, St Joseph Mercy Hosp, **SLP**

Dreyfus, Mrs Barbara Aronow 241 Parkside Avenue, Miller Place, NY 11764, (516) 744-7740, BA 70 Hofstra Univ; MA 72 Hofstra Univ; 87–Aud, Suffolk County Hrng Aid Ctr Inc, **A**

Dreyfus-Landerman, Jamie D 3714-A Savoy Lane, West Palm Beach, FL 33417, BS 81 OH Univ - Athens; ME 82 Univ of Cincinnati; MS 86 Nova Univ; 88–Sp-Lang Path, Wynnebrook Elem Sch, **SLP**

Dreyfuss, Elaine E 661 Guilford Road, Cherry Hill, NJ 08003, (609) 751-1133, BA 76 Temple Univ; MS 79 Columbia Univ Teachers Coll; Sp-Lang Path, Private Practice, **SLP ACE**

Dreyfuss, Nancy Matis 25 Central Park West, New York, NY 10023, (212) 757-3375, BA 76 Barnard Coll; MS 78 Columbia Univ Teachers Coll; 88–Sp-Lang Path, NY League for Early Learning, **SLP**

Drichta, Dr Carl E Metropolitan College, University Of New Orleans, New Orleans, LA 70148, (504) 286-7100, BA 71 Univ of WI - Milwaukee; MA 73 Wichita St Univ; PH 76 (NS) Wichita St Univ; Assistant Dean/Director, University of New Orleans, **SLP**

Dries, Margaret Burton PO Box 111, Tomkins Cove, NY 10986, (914) 942-2700, BS 75 SUNY - Center at Albany; MA 76 OH Univ - Athens; Sp-Lang Path, North Rockland School District, **SLP**

Driggs, Phyllis T 2026 Truett Circle, Thousand Oaks, CA 91360, (805) 493-1498, BA 71 CA St Univ - Northridge; MA 72 CA St Univ - Northridge; Sp-Lang Path, Simi Valley USD, **SLP**

Drikakis, Christine Ann 37 North 27th Street, Battle Creek, MI 49015, (616) 963-5508, MA 82 Western MI Univ; Sp-Lang Path, Lakeview Sch, **SLP**

Drillings, Mrs Flora M Speech And Hearing Center, Brooklyn College, Brooklyn, NY 11210, (212) 780-5186, BA 49 CUNY - Brooklyn Coll; MA 52 CUNY - Brooklyn Coll; Superv/Cl Sers, CUNY-Brooklyn/Sp & Hrng Cen, **SLP**

Drinkwine, Janie 29285 N Poppy Meadow St, Canyon Country, CA 91351, (818) 781-0360, BA 81 Univ of VT; MA 83 IN Univ - Bloomington; Sp-Lang Path, Chldrns Sp & Hrng Ctr, **SLP**

Driscoll, Heather 171 Ashley Avenue, Dept Of Otolaryngology, Charleston, SC 29425, (804) 795-6027, BS 85 Syracuse Univ; ME 87 Univ of VA - Charlottesville; 87–Instr of Aud, Med Univ of SC, **A**

Driscoll, Janene M P O Box 868, Kotzebue, AK 99752, (907) 586-6806, BS 77 Northern IL Univ - De Kalb; MA 79 Northern IL Univ - De Kalb; SLP, SE Reg Res Cen, **SLP**

Driscoll, Julia Ann 770 South 45th Street, Boulder, CO 80303, (303) 440-3050, BA 85 Pacific Univ; MA 87 Univ of CO - Boulder

Driscoll, Karyn Louise 804 East 34th, Spokane, WA 99203, (509) 838-1643, BA 79 WA St Univ; MS 82 CO St Univ; Sp-Lang Path, Spokane Guilds Sch/Neurom Cen, **SLP**

Driscoll, Mark Stephen 1850 West Estes Apartment #1, Chicago, IL 60626, (312) 465-1220, BS 76 James Madison Univ; MA 88 Univ of KS

Driscoll, Patricia Montani 805 South Crouse Avenue, Syracuse, NY 13244, (315) 443-9614, BS 78 SUNY - Coll at Geneseo; MS 79 Syracuse Univ; Sp-Lang Path, Syracuse University, **SLP**

Driscoll, Mrs Therese Ann 213 Sedgwick Street, Syracuse, NY 13203, (315) 488-2951, BS 81 SUNY - Coll at Geneseo; MA 83 Univ of MA - Boston; 83–Sp-Lang Path, St Camillus Hlth & Rehab Ctr, **SLP**

Driscoll-Morgan, Diane 3200 Futura, Roswell, NM 88201, **SLP**

Driskill, Susan W 4754 Roxanne Blvd, Louisville, KY 40218, (502) 583-8303, MS 88 Univ of Louisville; 88–Aud, Univ Surgical Assoc PSC

Dritsas, Jane H 854 Waveland, Chicago, IL 60613, (312) 880-4530, BA 79 MI St Univ; MS 81 Univ of MI - Ann Arbor; Aud, Childrens Memorial Hospital, **A**

Driver, Althea Allison 700 Avenue E N W, Childress, TX 79201, (817) 937-6314, BS 72 Southwest TX St Univ; MA 85 West TX St Univ; 87–Sp-Lang Path, Greenbelt Spec Svcs Coop, **SLP**

Driver, Joyce Eileen 5700 Ming Avenue #66, Bakersfield, CA 93309, BA 79 CA St Univ - Fresno; MA 83 CA St Univ - Fresno; Sp-Lang Path, Bakersfield City Sch Dist, **SLP**

Driver, Lois L 1122 West 56th Street, Indianapolis, IN 46208, (317) 633-8504, BA 57 Wellesley Coll; MS 58 NY Univ; OM 81 IN Univ - Bloomington; SLP, Indiana State Board of Health, **SLP**

Driver, Mrs Lynn E 1109 Spring Street, Ann Arbor, MI 48103, (313) 665-4024, **SLP**

Driver-Gilchrist, Mrs Mary Elizabeth 544 Hollywood Avenue, Salt Lake City, UT 84105, (801) 292-8665, BS 78 CO St Univ; MS 80 CO St Univ; Cl Dir & Sp-Lang Path, Prim Chldrn Med Cen, **SLP**

Droessler, Catherine A 2283 Airport Road, Platteville, WI 53818, (608) 348-9551, BS 78 Univ of WI - Whitewater; MS 79 Univ of WI - Whitewater; Sp-Lang Path, Platteville School District, **SLP**

Droettboom, Mrs M Michelle 1123 Heritage Boulevard, Vancouver, BC, Canada V7J 3G8, (604) 980-9091, BA 69 Univ of WA; MS 72 Univ of NC - Chapel Hill; Sp-Lang Path, Private Practice, **SLP**

Drogin, Mrs Brodea M 4129 Village #4, Camarillo, CA 93010, MS; **SLP LM**

Droho, Mary P O Box 830, Gentry, AR 72734, (501) 736-2076, BS 87 Univ of AR - Fayetteville; 87–SLP, Gentry Sch Dist

Drolet, Cynthia J P O Box 1868, Idyllwild, CA 92349, (714) 659-5905, BS 67 Purdue Univ - West Lafayette; MA 75 CA St Univ - Los Angeles; VP, Imaginart Communication Prod, **SLP**

Drollinger, Jeanne M R R 1 Box 112, Wever, IA 52658, (319) 372-4821, BA 75 Briar Cliff Coll; MA 76 Saint Louis Univ; SLP, Great River AEA #16, **SLP**

Drommond, Ray Earl 9717 S W 48th, Portland, OR 97219, (503) 229-7291, **SLP**

Dronberger, Mrs Elizabeth Anne 831 McDonell Drive, Gahanna, OH 43230, (614) 475-9539, BS 77 Purdue Univ - West Lafayette; MA 86 OH St Univ; **SLP**

Drop, Mrs Judith Waterwash 2622 North Windsor Drive, Apartment 202, Arlington Heights, IL 60004, (312) 255-0120, **SLP**

Drosky, Mrs Ceil Dicerbo 21 Vantassel Lane, Ballston Spa, NY 12020, (518) 584-3453, BS 80 SUNY - Coll at Geneseo; ME 81 Coll of Saint Rose; 87–Sp-Lang Path, Stillwater Central Sch, **SLP**

Drost, Anne Scalise 5263 Wynterhall Way, Atlanta, GA 30338, (404) 396-5569, BS 68 Univ of IL - Urbana; MA 69 Univ of IL - Urbana; Sp-Lang Path, Private Practice, **SLP**

Drost, Hazel Rose Marie 5161 Rice Road #104, Antioch, TN 37013, (615) 327-3011, BS 84 Auburn Univ - Auburn; MS 85 Univ of Montevallo; 87–Sp-Lang Path, Professional Health Svcs, **SLP**

Drost, Kathleen Anderson 21850 Feather Avenue, Yorba Linda, CA 92686, (714) 779-3488, BA 80 CA St Univ - Long Beach; MA 83 CA St Univ - Fullerton; Sp-Lang Path, Jurupa USD, **SLP**

Droste, Mrs Janet M 205 Universal Drive, St Peters, MO 63376, (314) 441-6276, BS 73 Univ of MO - Columbia; MS 74 Southern IL Univ-Edwardsvill; **SLP**

Drower, Mrs Laura Anne 3241 North Panama, Chicago, IL 60634, (312) 589-1510, BA 83 Mundelein Coll; MS 83 Marquette Univ; Sp-Lang Path, Private Practice, **SLP**

Drown, Mrs Carol M 16262 East Whittier Blvd, Suite 1, Whittier, CA 90603, (213) 943-7181, BA 65 Univ of the Pacific; MA 77 CA St Univ - Long Beach; Audiologist, Private Practice, **A**

Drozdowski, Mrs Emily C 36038 Verdant Circle, Apartment 38102, Farmington Hills, MI 48331, (313) 476-0856, MS 83; 87–Sp-Lang Path, Farmington Hills Schools, **SLP**

Drubin, Mrs Susan Wikler 815 Suffolk Road, Rydal, PA 19046, (215) 572-6830, OB 76 Univ of Miami; MA 77 Trenton St Coll; **SLP**

Drucker, Gail S 18911 Jonathan Lane, Homewood, IL 60430, (312) 799-5099, MA 88 Univ of IL - Urbana

Drucker, Mrs Judith C 11325 S W 104th Court, Miami, FL 33176, (305) 324-3148, BS 59 NY Univ; MA 77 Univ of Miami; Aud, VA Med Cen, **A**

Drucker, Lawrence J 3125 Douglas Road, Toledo, OH 43606, (419) 472-1799, BA 72 CUNY - Lehman Coll; MA 76 CUNY - Lehman Coll; Aud, Private Practice, **A**

Drucker, Sharon Stern 14-05 Ellis Avenue, Fair Lawn, NJ 07410, (201) 794-7039, BA 78 CUNY - Queens Coll; MA 80 CUNY - Queens Coll; Sp-Lang Path, Private Practice, **SLP**

Druckman, Mindy Lynn 105 Royal Tark Drive, Apartment 2 F, Oakland Park, FL 33309, (305) 584-8000, OB 81 Salem St Coll; MS 82 Ithaca Coll; Sp-Lang Path, Ann Stork Center, **SLP**

Drudge, Mrs Mary K 3759 Fairwood, Sylvania, OH 43560, **SLP**

Drudge, William Ralph 4751 North Paulina, Chicago, IL 60640, (312) 880-8425, BS 76 MI St Univ; MA 82 Western MI Univ; Sp-Lang Path, Chicago Bd of Ed, **SLP**

Drudy, Michael Edward 90 Conventry At Waterford, York, PA 17402, (205) 933-9110, **SLP ACE**

Druelinger, Nancy Jean 372 Maple Street, East Aurora, NY 14052, (716) 655-0279, MS; 86–Sp-Lang Path, BOCES #2, **SLP**

Drui, Mrs Patricia P O Box 621, Teton Village, WY 83025, (714) 848-4598, BA 81 Univ of SD - Vermillion; MA 82 Univ of SD - Vermillion; Sp-Lang Path, C Bar V Ranch, **SLP**

Drukier, Dr Gale S Trenton State College, Hillwood Lakes CN 4700, Trenton, NJ 08650-4700, (609) 771-2322, BS 72 NY Univ; MS 73 Columbia Univ Teachers Coll; ED 79 (Aud-Middle ear analysis in the Elderly) Columbia Univ Teachers Coll; 78–Asst Prof, Trenton St Coll, **A**

Druliner, Mrs Barbette Carol 1210 Castec Drive, Sacramento, CA 95864, (916) 447-5468, BA 81 CA St Univ - Sacramento; **SLP**

Drum, Markel K 10841 Flat Iron Road, Charlotte, NC 28226, (704) 343-5455, BS 70 Univ of KS; MS 72 Washington Univ; Aud, Charlotte-Mecklenburg Schs, **SLP A**

Drumm, Dr Denise A P O Box 40168, Albuquerque, NM 87196, (505) 883-9116, BA 75 Univ of CT; MS 78 Univ of NM; PH 86 (NS) Univ of NM; Sp-Lang Path, Commun Dis Ut Dist Diag Cen, **SLP**

Drumm, Marcelle Bergeron 560 Stamford Avenue, Baton Rouge, LA 70808, (504) 355-5840, BS 79 LA St Univ - Baton Rouge; OM 80 LA St Univ - N O Medical Ctr; Sp-Lang Path, E Baton Rouge Parish Sch Syst, **SLP**

Drummond, Lori Lee 207 Highland Road, Pittsburgh, PA 15238, (412) 963-6294, BS 84 WV Univ; MS 86 Gallaudet Coll; 86–Aud, OK Otological Assoc, **A**

Drummond, Martha E 168 Beacon Street, Boston, MA 02116, (617) 578-8734, BA 71; ME 73 Univ of AZ; ME 79 Northeastern Univ; Aud/Instruc, Emerson Coll, **A**

Drummond, Dr Sakina S Univ Of Arkansas Medical Sci, Communicative Disorders, 33rd & University Avenue, Little Rock, AR 72204, (501) 661-5591, BS 70 Bombay Univ - India; MA 71 Ball St Univ; PH 78 (NS) Univ of MI - Ann Arbor; Assoc Professor, University of Arkansas, **SLP**

Drumright, Judy D 550 Ridge Road, Lake Forest, IL 60045, (312) 942-5332, BS 83 CO St Univ; MS 85 CO St Univ; Aud, Rush Presb St Lukes Med Ctr, **A**

Drumwright, Mrs Cynthia Dodson 213 West Sturgis Street, St Johns, MI 48879-2542, (517) 224-4673, BS 80 WV Univ; MS 81 WV Univ; Aud, **A**

Drury, Carolyn Ruth 427-3 Amherst Street, CS 2032 Suite 340, Nashua, NH 03061, (603) 883-5521, BS 74 Ithaca Coll; MS 83 Portland St Univ; 88–Aud, Nashua Mem Hosp, **A**

Drury, Mrs JoLynn B 3424 Medical Arts Bldg, 1169 Eastern Parkway, Louisville, KY 40217, (502) 458-4466, BS 75 Vanderbilt Univ; ME 77 Univ of Louisville; Sp-Lang Path, Private Practice, **SLP ACE**

Drury-Young, Roberta F DSCC State Regional Office, 2309 West Main Street, Marion, IL 62959, (618) 997-4371, BS 74 Southern IL Univ -Carbondale; MS 76 Southern IL Univ -Carbondale; 86–Sp Hearing Consult, DSCC Univ of IL, **SLP**

Druse, Mrs Jean Marie 89 Katrina Falls Road, Rock Hill, NY 12775, (914) 794-8830, BS 78 SUNY - Coll at New Paltz; MS 83 Coll of Saint Rose; Sp/Lang Path, Commun Gen Hosp of Sullivan Co, **SLP**

Druziak, Mrs JoAnn Murphy 118 Squirrels Heath Road, Fairport, NY 14450, (716) 223-1797, BS 81 Nazareth Coll of Rochester; MS 84 Nazareth Coll of Rochester; 84–Sp-Lang Path, Monroe BOCES 1, **SLP**

Drvota, Sandra I 2160 Fairmount Avenue, St Paul, MN 55105, (612) 627-2702, BS 72 Coll of Saint Teresa; MA 80 Univ of MN - Minneap-St Paul; Sp-Lang Path, Minneapolis Pub Sch-Spec Ed, **SLP**

Dryburgh, Susan Zabel 740 Tannery Drive, Wayne, PA 19087, (215) 539-8550, BA 75 Dana Coll; OM 81 Hahneman Medical Coll; Sp-Lang Path, Mont Co PA Iu, **SLP**

Dryden, Marianne T 1535 Arroyo View Drive, Pasadena, CA 91103, (213) 795-4797, BA 58 Univ of the Pacific; MA 81 CA St Univ - Los Angeles; 76–Sp-Lang Path, Pasadena USD, **SLP**

Drye, Cynthia A 5921 East Sweetwater Avenue, Scottsdale, AZ 85254, (602) 526-1583, MS 88 Northern AZ Univ

Dryer, Kathleen Mary 207 Institute Street, Valparaiso, IN 46383, (219) 738-2100, BS 80 Purdue Univ - West Lafayette; MS 82 Purdue Univ - West Lafayette; Sp-Lang Path, St Anthonys Hosp, **SLP**

Dryg, Lori Devore 3040 Willow, Bettendorf, IA 52722, (319) 332-5114, BA 84 Augustana Coll; MA 85 Western MI Univ; **SLP**

Dubard, Dr Etoile Box 10035 Southern Station, Hattiesburg, MS 39406, (601) 266-5223, BS 42 Univ of Mary Hardin-Baylor; MA 50 G Peabody Coll-Vanderbilt U; PH 67 (NS) Univ Southern MS-Hattiesburg; 62–Prof Dir Sch Chldn W/Lang Dis, U Southern MS, **SLP A LM**

Dubbs, Patricia J Box 751, Edinboro, PA 16412, (814) 724-0000, BS 70 PA St Univ - Univ Park; MS 71 Univ of OR; Sp-Lang Path, NW Tri-County Intermed Unit, **SLP**

Dube, Mrs Nina K 140-05 Newport Avenue, Belle Harbor, NY 11694, (212) 270-7498, BA 73 Long Island U - Brooklyn Ctr; MS 75 Columbia Univ Teachers Coll; Sp-Lang Path, Maimonides Medical Center, **SLP**

Dubendris, Peter C 60 Oxbow Drive, Wrentham, MA 02093, (617) 384-3116, BA 69 Univ of ME - Orono; MS 75 Boston Univ; Department Director, Wrentham State School, **SLP**

Dubenion, Kimberly Rena 1125 Edgewater #4, Fort Wayne, IN 46805, (219) 484-4175, BS 84 Central MI Univ; MA 86 Central MI Univ; **A**

Dubin, Mrs Carol Kampner 9226 North Pelham Parkway, Milwaukee, WI 53217, (414) 383-4490, BS 57 Univ of WI - Madison; MS 82 Univ of WI - Milwaukee; Sp-Lang Path, Sacred Heart Rehab Hosp, **SLP**

Dubin, Dennis C 9661 West Heather Lane, Miramar, FL 33025, (305) 435-3743, BA 70 Bloomfield Coll; MA 73 Kean Coll of NJ; MA 78 Kean Coll of NJ; Aud, Aud Consult, **A**

Dubin, Erin Hope 1227 West Newport, Chicago, IL 60657, (312) 633-7168, MA 84 Wayne St Univ; BA 82 MI St Univ; **A**

Dubin, Mrs Lillian O P O Box 805, Williamsville, NY 14221, (416) 688-2980, BS 52 Univ of PR - Rio Piedras; MS 55 Johns Hopkins Univ; Dir Aud, Niagara Peninsula Rehab Cen, **SLP A**

Dubin, Madeline S 401 East 74th Street #8J, New York, NY 10021, (212) 780-3231, BA 69 CUNY - Queens Coll; MA 70 SUNY - Center at Buffalo; Sp-Lnag Path, Methodist Hosp of Bklyn, **SLP**

Dublinske, Mrs Leslie H 10033 Dellcastle Road, Gaithersburg, MD 20879, (301) 869-8848, BS 69 Univ of IA; MA 70 Univ of IA; Sp-Lang Path, Montg Co Pub Sch, **SLP**

Dublinske, Dr Stan 10033 Dellcastle Road, Gaithersburg, MD 20879, (301) 897-5700, BA 65 Univ of Northern IA; MA 68 Northeast MO St Univ; ED 81 (NS) Univ of Southern CA; Dir St & Reg Policy, ASHA, **SLP F ACE**

Dubner, Mrs Harriet 449 Beverly Road, Ridgewood, NJ 07450, (201) 652-6987, BA 50 CUNY - Brooklyn Coll; MA 69 Paterson St Coll; **SLP**

Dubner, Mrs Margery M 201 Penn Center Boulevard Suite 555, Pittsburgh, PA 15235, (412) 247-1924, BS 76 Northwestern Univ; MA 78 Univ of Pittsburgh - Pittsburgh; 84–Sp-Lang Path, Private Practice, **SLP**

Dubno, Dr Judy R UCLA School Of Medicine, Div Of Head & Neck Surgery, 31-24 Rehab Center, Los Angeles, CA 90024, (213) 825-3037, BS 72 CUNY - City College; MS 73 Ithaca Coll; PH 78 (Sp and Hrng Sciences) CUNY - Grad Sch & Univ Cntr; 78–Assoc Prof, UCLA Sch of Med, **A**

Duboff, Mindy L 36 Barstow Road, Great Neck, NY 11021, (516) 234-6262, BA 75 CUNY - Queens Coll; MA 77 CUNY - Queens Coll; Aud, Cn Islip Psych Cen, **A**

Dubois, Ann C 781 Cross Road, Stormville, NY 12582, (914) 225-8441, **SLP**

Dubois, Mrs Ann Marie Jepsen 2 Arbroth Street, Dorchester, MA 02122, (617) 651-7113, BS 77 Northeastern Univ; MS 86 Northeastern Univ; 78–Sp-Lang Path, Natick PS, **SLP**

Dubois, Barbara Nuss 162 Maple Avenue, Corry, PA 16407, (814) 664-4641, BS 76 Edinboro Univ of PA; MA 77 Bowling Green St Univ; 84–Sp-Lang Path/Dir, Corry Mem Hosp, **SLP**

Dubois, Cheryl B 423 New London Avenue, Unit 302, Warwick, RI 02893, (401) 722-6000, SLP, Mem Hosp of Ri, **SLP**

Dubois, Mrs Melinda Walsh 52 Oakhill Drive, Oakland, ME 04963, (207) 465-2567, BS 84 Marywood Coll; MA 86 Univ of ME - Orono; **SLP**

Dubosar, Mrs Stacey Meryl 9651 S W 152nd Avenue, Miami, FL 33196, (305) 386-8572, Sp-Lang Path, Hamrock and Gram Pa, **SLP**

Dubrey, Louis Alpine 1444 Crescent Drive, Klamath Falls, OR 97601, (503) 883-3621, MA 88 Western WA Univ

Dubrovner, Mrs Shulamith 16134 Magnolia Boulevard, Encino, CA 91436, (818) 997-2357, BA 57 CA St Univ - Sacramento; MA 62 Univ of CA - Los Angeles; SLP, L A USD, **SLP**

Dubrow, Janine Renee 4145 Saltwater Boulevard, Tampa, FL 33615, (813) 864-3316, MS 79 Univ of South FL; Sp-Lang Path, Paseo Co Sch Syst, **SLP**

Dubrowski, Richard Michael 7381 Richmond Road, Memphis, TN 38125, (901) 522-5651, BA 81 Auburn Univ - Montgomery; MS 83 Univ of TN - Knoxville; Audiologist, Baptist Memorial Hospital, **A**

Duchan, Dr Judith F 130 Jewett Parkway, Buffalo, NY 14214, BA 56 OH St Univ; MS 62 OH St Univ; PH 72 (NS) Univ of IL - Chicago; Prof, State Univ of New York-Buffalo, **SLP F**

Duchan, Mrs Lynn S 21 High Point Road, Westport, CT 06880, (203) 866-8121, BA 72 CUNY - Queens Coll; MA 73 Univ of MD - College Park; Aud, Vaughn Dunn MD, **A**

DuChane, Ann Shaughnessy Good Samaritan Hospital, 5601 Loch Raven Boulevard, Baltimore, MD 21239-2995, (301) 532-3740, BS 77 WV Univ; MS 79 Univ of WI - Madison; 83–Supvr-Dept Sp-Lang Path, Good Samaritan Hospital, **SLP**

Duchene, Charlene A William Beaumont Hospital, Speech/Language Pathology, 3601 West 13 Mile Road, Royal Oak, MI 48072, (313) 288-8086, BS 74 Wayne St Univ; MA 75 Wayne St Univ; Sp-Lang Path, Wm Beaumont Hosp, **SLP ACE**

Duchin, Dr Sandra W 311 Fawn Hill Lane, Penn Valley, PA 19072, (215) 567-3648, MA 64 Seton Hall Univ; ME 83 Columbia Univ Teachers Coll; OM 84 Columbia Univ Teachers Coll; 88–Sp-Lang Path, Private Practice, **SLP ACE**

Duchon, Mrs Rebecca Ann 21712 Santa Pola, Mission Viejo, CA 92692, (714) 628-2407, MS 84 Univ of WI - Madison; Sp-Lang Path, Speech Pathology Services, **SLP**

Duchowny, Reena Julia 145 Marlee Avenue #306, Toronto, ON, Canada M6B 3H3, (416) 782-4317, BA 81 McGill Univ - Quebec; MS 83 Dalhousie Univ - Nova Scotia; 88–Aud, Aud Clinic, **A**

Duciaume, Patricia A 2211 Broadway #10-E, New York, NY 10024, (914) 947-1000, BS 74 SUNY - Coll at Fredonia; MS 81 SUNY - Coll at Fredonia; 81–Sp-Lang Path, Letchworth Village Dev Cen, **SLP**

Duck, Gordon L State Dept Of Education, 721 Capitol Mall, Room 651, Sacramento, CA 95814, BA 56; MA 59; SLP, CA St Dept of Ed, **SLP**

Duckett, Mrs Barbara Ann T 761 Samoa, Crestwood, MO 63126, (314) 965-4053, BS 78 AZ St Univ; MA 81 Saint Louis Univ; Sp-Lang Path, Spec Sch Dist of St Louis Co, **SLP**

Duckett, Kathy 4725 S St Rd 446, Bloomington, IN 47401, (812) 332-6378, BA 81 IN Univ - Bloomington; OM 82 IN Univ - Bloomington; Sp-Lang Path, Monroe Co Comm Sch Corp, **SLP**

Duclos, Deborah A Rd 2 Box 55, Cohocton, NY 14826, (716) 728-2211, BS 77 SUNY - Coll at Geneseo; MA 82 SUNY - Coll at Geneseo; SLP, Wayland Ctrl Sch, **SLP**

Duclos, Mrs Karen Meinert 1270 Prince Avenue, Athens, GA 30606, (404) 353-3575, ME 84 Univ of GA; 88–Dir/Owner, Athens Sp/L Services, **SLP ACE**

Ducombs, Sherry C 12607 Fairhaven Drive, Baton Rouge, LA 70815, (504) 767-7200, BA 73 Southeastern LA Univ; MA 76 LA St Univ - N O Medical Ctr; 86–Aud, Drs Hansbrough & Peters, **A**

Ducombs, Thomas V 12607 Fairhaven, Baton Rouge, LA 70815, (504) 291-7011, BA 69 Southeastern LA Univ; OM 76 LA St Univ - N O Medical Ctr; Audiologist, Private Practice, **A**

Duconge, Jean Ann 4118 Riley Street, Houston, TX 77005, (713) 666-4565, BS 81 Marquette Univ; MS 83 AZ St Univ; Audiologist, Texas Childrens Hospital, **A**

Ducote, Dr Charlotte PO Box 207, Folsom, LA 70437, (504) 796-9232, BA 72 LA St Univ - Baton Rouge; MA 73 Vanderbilt Univ; PH 83 (NS) LA St Univ - Baton Rouge; 82–Dir, New Medico Rehab Ctr LA, **SLP**

Ducote, Dianna Deshotels 105 South Miles, Abbeville, LA 70510, (318) 898-2742, BA 73 Univ of Southwestern LA; MS 76 Univ of Southwestern LA; Sp-Lang Path, Private Practice, **SLP**

Ducote, Mrs Karen B 15807 Mesa Verde Drive, Houston, TX 77059, MS 79 Univ of Houston - Univ Park; Sp-Lang Path, Los Angeles Cnty Office of Ed, **SLP**

Duda, Mrs Karen Borrello 129 Meadow Brook Park, Federalsburg, MD 21632, (301) 754-9054, BA 80 Loyola Coll; MS 81 Loyola Coll; Sp-Lang Path, Caroline Co Bd of Ed, **SLP**

Duddridge, Mary Kathryn 1422 Westwood, Blue Springs, MO 64015, (816) 229-8142, BS 68 Central MO St Univ; MS 85 Central MO St Univ; Sp-Lang Path, Blue Springs Sch Dist, **SLP**

Duddy, Mrs Diane Freiert 4511 Marlboro Court, St Louis, MO 63121, (314) 382-3597, BS 77 Univ of WI - Milwaukee; MS 80 Washington Univ; Consult, Private Practice, **A**

Dudek, Mrs Quincey Marie 26-3 Woodlake Road, Albany, NY 12203, (518) 452-3804, BS 85 Coll of Saint Rose; MS 86 Coll of Saint Rose; 87–Sp-Lang Path, Capital District Beginnings, **SLP**

Dudich, Tim M Otologic Assoc, 7711 Louis Pasteur, Suite 504 Oak Hills Bldg, San Antonio, TX 78229, (512) 691-1046, BS 71 Kent St Univ; MA 74 Univ of Cincinnati; 85–Aud, Otologic Associates, **A**

Dudley, Ann F 2028 S E 44th, Portland, OR 97215, (503) 472-1431, BA 70 Duke Univ; BA 78 Univ of WA; MA 79 Univ of WA; 88, **SLP**

Dudley, Fay J C 1350 River Reach Drive, Apartment 303, Fort Lauderdale, FL 33315, (407) 393-4071, Sp-Lang Path, Boca Raton Community Hospital, **SLP ACE**

Dudley, Jacqueline Hastings 602 North Columbus Street, Alexandria, VA 22314, (703) 548-1753, BA 48 Univ of MD - College Park; MA 65 George Washington Univ; Sp-Lang Path, Private Practice, **SLP**

Dudley, Mary Dipalma 122 Chestnut Street, Apartment 303, Springfield, MA 01103-1872, (413) 256-1783, BA 84 Univ of RI; MA 87 Univ of MA - Amherst; 88–Sp-Lang Path, East Mountain Ctr

Dudley, Mrs Susan M 1817 East Julie Drive, Tempe, AZ 85283, (602) 898-4976, MA 75 Western IL Univ; Sp-Lang Path, Mesa Public Schools, **SLP**

Dudzinski, Mrs Barbara Jean 321 Grant Avenue, Geneva, IL 60134, (312) 208-9147, BS 85 Northwestern Univ; MA 86 Northwestern Univ; **SLP**

Dueber, Mrs Sandee Horton 7610 Montane Drive, Colorado Springs, CO 80920, (513) 222-5597, BS 84 Bowling Green St Univ; MA 85 Bowling Green St Univ; Audiologist, Dayton Hearing & Speech Center, **A**

Duehring, Bonnie R 40 Wakawn Avenue, Fond Du Lac, WI 54935, (414) 921-7357, BS 76; MS 78 Univ of WI - Oshkosh; 85–Sp-Lang Path, Fond du Lac Sch Dist, **SLP**

Duell, Mrs Margaret Green 2619 Colonial Lane, Salina, KS 67401-7717, (913) 827-0208, **SLP**

Duennerman, Mrs Wanda G Route 3 Box 298-A, Grand Island, NE 68801, (308) 946-3057, BS 71 Univ of NE - Lincoln; MS 81 Kearney St Coll; Sp-Lang Path, Ctrl Cty Pub Sch, **SLP**

Duerr, Barbara Mikus Greater Dept Otogic Group, 27555 Middlebelt, Farmington Hills, MI 48018, **A**

Duerr, Mrs Leslie A Rt 4 Box 64C, Shell Road, Delmar, MD 21875, (302) 856-5213, BS 82 Clarion Univ of PA; MS 84 Clarion Univ of PA; 88–Aud, St of DE-Div of Pub Health, **A**

Dufek-Swegarden, Barbara 1345 4th Street North, Fargo, ND 58102, (701) 241-4878, BA 79 Mount Marty Coll; MS 83 Moorhead St Univ; 86–Coord-Sp-Lang-Hrng Svcs, Fargo PS, **SLP**

Duff, Abigail C 49 Oxford Road, Charlton, MA 01507, (508) 248-3797, BS 76 Emerson Coll; MA 78 Kent St Univ; Sp-Lang Path, Massachusetts Easter Seal Soc, **SLP**

Duff, Lynn A Bampton 28 Dickinson Road, Marlborough, CT 06447, (203) 522-0184, BA 78 Univ of CT; MA 81 Univ of CT; 87–Sp-Lang Path, Hartford Bd of Educ, **SLP**

Duff, Margaret A 2103 Wheatland Avenue, Williamsport, PA 17701, (717) 326-8620, BS 70 Ithaca Coll; MA 72 Kent St Univ; 87–Sp-Lang Path, Divine Providence Hosp, **SLP**

Duff, Dr Marigine M 3788 Clubland Drive, Marietta, GA 30067, (404) 329-7790, BA 53 Mary Washington Coll; MA 54 OH St Univ; PH 68 (NS) Northwestern Univ; Assoc Prof Commun Dis, Emory U, **SLP**

Duffee, Mrs Penelope H Rural Route 2, Box 10, Bloomington, IL 61704-9602, (309) 663-2887, BS 64 Miami Univ - Oxford; MA 69 IL St Univ - Normal; **SLP A**

Duffey, Mrs Christine Polito 2489 H Road, Grand Junction, CO 81505, (303) 420-6663, BA 79 Univ of Northern CO; MA 80 Univ of Northern CO; Sp-Lang Path, Mesa Dev Presch, **SLP**

Duffield-Hunthausen, Janice L 14042 College Street, Westminster, CA 92683-3428, (714) 893-6507, BA 71 Miami Univ - Oxford; MS 73 Washington Univ; MA 79 CA St Univ - Los Angeles; Aud, Garden Grove USD, **A**

Duffin, Marybeth 2671 Jenkintown Road, Apt A First Fl, Ardsley, PA 19038, (215) 884-7561, SLP, Mont Co Inter Unit, **SLP**

Duffitt, Deanna V 14 Heath Cres, Gander, NF, Canada A1V 1R1, (709) 256-5458, **SLP**

Duffy, Mrs Darcy P 1635 Graber, Oshkosh, WI 54901, BA 74 Univ of MI - Ann Arbor; MA 75 Eastern MI Univ; **SLP**

Duffy, Denise M 36 Woodway Drive, Shrewsbury, MA 01545, **SLP**

Duffy, Mrs Gloria Beth 247-46 76th Avenue, Bellerose, NY 11426, (718) 347-7508, BA 81 CUNY - Queens Coll; MA 84 Hofstra Univ; SLP, New York City Board of Educ, **SLP**

Duffy, Mrs Janice E P O Box 727, Columbia, CA 95310, (209) 532-4309, BA 59 San Francisco St Univ; Special Day Class Teacher, Tri County Consortium, **SLP**

Duffy, Dr John K 41 Amherst Road, Port Washington, NY 11050, (212) 735-2667, BA 42 Univ of WI - Madison; MA 46 Univ of WI - Madison; PH 49 (NS) Univ of WI - Madison; Dir/Superv Aud, Kings Co Hosp Cen, **SLP A LM**

Duffy, Dr Joseph R Speech Pathology, Department Of Neurology, Mayo Clinic, Rochester, MN 55901, (507) 284-3112, BA 68 Montclair St Coll; MA 71 Univ of CT; PH 74 (Sp Path) Univ of CT; Consult Sp-Path, Mayo Cl, **SLP**

Duffy, Dr Marjorie Richards 2404 Constitution, Fort Collins, CO 80526, (303) 491-6981, BA 52 Univ of Science & Arts of OK; PH 66 (Sp-Lang Path) Univ of OK Medical Center; Retired, **SLP F**

Duffy, Mary Kate 1811 Third, Bay City, MI 48708, (517) 892-5558, BA 85 MI St Univ; MA 86 MI St Univ; **SLP**

Duffy, Mrs Melita Tillery 4620 Avenida Marina, Pensacola, FL 32504, (904) 479-8472, BA 75 Berea Coll; MS 77 Univ of TN - Knoxville; MA 82 Univ of TN - Knoxville; Sp-Lang Path, Private Practice, **SLP**

Duffy, Mrs Nancy Hagle 2100 Pontiac Lake Road, Pontiac, MI 48053, (313) 858-1917, BS 50 MI St Univ; MA 55 MI St Univ; Sp-Lang Path, Oakland Co Inter Dist, **SLP**

Duffy, Nancy Rose 270 Robinson Street, North Tonawanda, NY 14120, (716) 694-6494, BS 82 New York Univ; MA 84 New York Univ; 86–Sp-Lang Path, Orleans-Niagara BOCES, **SLP**

Duffy, Dr Robert J Dept Of Communication Science, University Of Connecticut, Storrs, CT 06268, (203) 486-3187, BA 52 Univ of Notre Dame; MA 57 Univ of IA; PH 58 (NS) Univ of IA; Prof, Univ Ct, **SLP**

Duffy, Theresa Marie P O Box 2019, Vail, CO 81658, (303) 949-7018, OB 85 Univ of KS; MA 87 Univ of Northern CO; Doubletree Hotel

Duffy-Gillespie, Janet 2633 East Larkspur, Phoenix, AZ 85032, (602) 266-9315, BS 80 Univ of IL - Urbana; MS 81 Univ of IL - Urbana; Sp-Lang Path, Judith P Meyer Ccc, **SLP**

Dufkin-Britt, Dawn A RFD 1 Box 600, Orrington, ME 04474, (207) 945-7365, BS 78 Northern AZ Univ; MS 79 Univ of WY; Aud, En ME Med Cen, **A**

Dufon, Margaret A EWC Box 1720, 1777 East West Road, Honolulu, HI 90848, (808) 944-7839, BS 72 Purdue Univ - West Lafayette; MS 73 Univ of WI - Madison; Sp-Lang Path, **SLP**

Dufort, Mrs Mary Margaret 43 Tremblay Avenue, Plattsburgh, NY 12901, (518) 643-9431, MA 83 SUNY - Coll at Plattsburgh; 86–Sp-Lang Path, Peru Central Sch Dist, **SLP**

Du Frane, Mrs Michele McKinnon 931 East Minnesota, Turlock, CA 95380, (209) 526-4500, **SLP**

Dugan, Constance 2136 Agatite, Chicago, IL 60625, (312) 878-9719, BA 71 Wichita St Univ; MA 73 Northwestern Univ; Sp-Lang Path, Professional Home Health Care Inc, **SLP**

Dugan, Mrs Elizabeth M 434 South Clearfield St, Johnstown, PA 15905, (814) 255-6503, BS 69 Indiana Univ of PA; ME 70 PA St Univ - Univ Park; Sp-Lang Path, Westmont Child Dev Ctr, **SLP**

Dugan, Mrs Mary Pavilonis 2137 Hunters Bluff Court, Spring Valley, OH 45370, (513) 885-7320, BS 75 Towson St Univ; MS 78 Towson St Univ; Sp-Lang Path, Private Practice, **SLP**

Dugan, Nancy C P O Box 144, Dover, OH 44622, (216) 343-9415, BS 79 WV Univ; MS 80 WV Univ; Aud, Charleston Co School Distrist, **A**

Dugan, Mrs Patricia J 1137 Granito Drive, Ojai, CA 93023, (805) 646-6898, BA 63 CA St Univ - Long Beach; MA 82 CA St Univ - Northridge; 84–Sp-Lang Path, Oxnard Union Hgh Sch Dist, **SLP**

Dugas, Mrs Anne B 125 Longfellow, Maurice, LA 70555-9413, (318) 989-8315, BS 85 LA St Univ - Baton Rouge; MS 87 Univ of Southwestern LA; Sp-Lang Path, Vermilion Parish Sch Bd, **SLP**

Dugas, Jane Lassalle 119 South Jacqueline Drive, New Iberia, LA 70560, (318) 365-6259, MS 86 Univ of Southwestern LA; **SLP**

Dugas, Mrs Jean Klar 12449 Chelwood Place N E, Albuquerque, NM 87112, (505) 293-4327, MS 83 Univ of North TX; Aud, Family Hearing Ctr, **A ACE**

Duggan, Mrs Elaine Tonarelli Ohio Valley General Hospital, Heckel Road, Mc Kees Rocks, PA 15136, (412) 777-6575, BS 83 WV Univ; MS 84 WV Univ; Aud, Noise/Hearing Consultants Inc, **A**

Duggan, Katherine MacFarlane 527 High Street, Oradell, NJ 07649, (201) 456-4967, BA 78 Rutger's St Univ - Douglas Coll; MS 82 Columbia Univ Teachers Coll; Audiologist, University Hospital, **A**

Duggan, Mrs Marguerite Orlandi 209 Knickerbocker Avenue, Hillsdale, NJ 07642, (201) 358-6080, BA 70 Univ of Hartford; MS 86 William Paterson Coll; 86–Sp-Lang Path, Bronx VA Med Ctr, **SLP**

Dugger, Mrs Nancy Wray 126 Hiler, San Antonio, TX 78209, (512) 732-4741, BS 68 Univ of TX - Austin; MA 70 Univ of North TX; Sp/Lang Path, San Antonio ISD, **SLP**

Duggleby, Mrs Eileen H 21472 Camino Trebol, El Toro, CA 92630, (714) 770-3060, BA 79 Univ of CA - Santa Barbara; MA 80 Univ of the Pacific; Sp-Lang Path, Bay Area Sp & Hrng Clinic, **SLP**

Dugo, Susan M 2338 Sunnyside Avenue, Westchester, IL 60153, (312) 450-2144, BA 83 Elmhurst Coll; MS 84 Eastern IL Univ; **SLP**

Dugolenski, Lynne Giacomino Box 474, Poynette, WI 53955, (608) 635-4131, BS 73 Univ of WI - Oshkosh; MA 77 Univ of MT; Director Sp-Lang Pathology, Divine Savior Hosp & Nurs Home, **SLP**

Dugoni, Marianne C 951 Bedford Street, Fremont, CA 94539, (415) 490-2139, BA 76 Univ of CA - Santa Barbara; MA 77 Univ of the Pacific; SLP, Milpitas USD, **SLP**

Duguay, Douglas M 10 Hummingbird Lane, West Amherst, NY 14228, (716) 689-2099, BA 72 SUNY - Coll at Buffalo; MS 76 SUNY - Coll at Buffalo; Sp-Lang Path, Sweet Home Cent Sch, **SLP**

Duguay, Dr Marshall J 940 Amherst #8, Buffalo, NY 14216, (716) 878-4412, BS 58 SUNY - Coll at Buffalo; MS 61 SUNY - Coll at Buffalo; PH 71 (NS) SUNY - Center at Buffalo; Sp-Lang Path, SUNY-Coll at Buffalo, **SLP F**

Duhl, Mrs Sherrie J 1316 13th Lane, Palm Beach Gardens, FL 33418, (305) 736-3100, BA 79 CUNY - Queens Coll; MS 80 PA St Univ - Univ Park; Sp-Lang Path, Hearing Centers of America, **A**

Duhon, Mrs Andree S 111 Tyrona Street, Lafayette, LA 70507-4829, (318) 237-3274, BA 79 Univ of Southwestern LA; MS 81 Univ of Southwestern LA; Sp-Lang Path, Lafayette Parish Sch Bd, **SLP**

Duhon, Helen Marie S 5024 Marc Drive, Nashville, TN 37211, (615) 361-4528, BA 73 Northeast LA Univ; MS 80 Vanderbilt Univ; Metro-Nashville Davidsn Co Sch, **SLP**

Duhon, Mrs Rosalind Williams 4211 Aralia Road, Altadena, CA 91001, (213) 294-0031, BA 77 Univ of CA - Santa Barbara; MA 83 CA St Univ - Los Angeles; SLP, Los Angeles USD, **SLP**

Duignan, Mrs Sue E 28 Hillview Avenue, Redwood City, CA 94062, (415) 367-1214, BS 67 Marquette Univ; MS 70 IN Univ - Bloomington; Sp-Lang Path, Sequoia Hosp, **SLP**

Duisterhof, Julie K Woodland Creek Apartment, 3311 S Creek Drive #301, Grand Rapids, MI 49508, (616) 343-2601, BS Western MI Univ; MA 87 Univ of IA; **SLP**

Dukas, Marilyn D 6152 Mary Lane Drive, San Diego, CA 92115, (619) 469-6240, BA 56 Univ of MI - Ann Arbor; MA 57 Univ of MI - Ann Arbor; Sp-Lang Path, La Mesa-Sprng Valley Sch Dist, **SLP**

Duke, Carla 201 Hamilton Street, Southbridge, MA 01550-1813, (617) 347-5656, BA 82 Elms Coll; MS 85 Worcester St Coll; Sp-Lang Path, Monson Dev Ctr

Duke, Mrs Judith Ann 3315 Matthews Drive S W, Bremerton, WA 98312, (206) 779-3971, BA 64 Univ of WA; Sp-Lang Path, North Kitsap Sch Dist, **SLP**

Duke, Kathryn 1918 Fox Creek Court, High Point, NC 27260, (919) 621-0631, BA 75 Univ of NC - Greensboro; ME 76 Univ of NC - Greensboro; 88–Sp-Lang Path, Greensboro NC PS, **SLP A**

Duke-Morvant, Deborah A 305 East 15th Street, Covington, LA 70433, (504) 892-6708, BS 75 LA St Univ - N O Medical Ctr; OM 79 LA St Univ - N O Medical Ctr; **SLP**

Duker, Gail S 23000 Edgewood, St Clair Shores, MI 48080, (313) 775-8265, BS 79 Northern MI Univ; MA 80 MI St Univ; Sp-Lang Path, Sinai Hosp of Detroit, **SLP**

Dukes, Linda Zehnder 1026 12th Avenue, Fox Island, WA 98333-9641, (206) 549-2858, BA 77 Univ of WA; OM 79 Univ of WA; SLP, Private Practice, **SLP**

Dukes, Mrs Luann Bashur 2565 Ponsell Lane, Waycross, GA 31501, (912) 283-5822, BS 75 CA Univ of PA; ME 81 Valdosta St Coll; Sp-Lang Path, Ware Co Bd of Ed, **SLP**

Dukes-Mc Mahan, Sandra E 8601 Chaumont Court, Bakersfield, CA 93311, (805) 664-0631, MS 76 NM St Univ; Sp-Lang Path, Kern County Supt of Schools, **SLP**

Duksin, Sherry 75-40 Austin Street #1-F, Forest Hills, NY 11375, (212) 561-3311, BA 72 CUNY - Queens Coll; MA 74 CUNY - Queens Coll; SLP, Bellevue Hosp-Dept Rehab Med, **SLP**

Dulcich, Mrs Donna Mary 780 Alameda, Astoria, OR 97103, (503) 325-2862, BS 51 Univ of OR; MS 72 Western OR St Coll; 64–Superv Sp/Lang/Hrng Prog, Clatsop Ed Serv Dist, **SLP**

Duling, Mrs Leah Obert 26 Schoenbeck Road, Wheeling, IL 60090, (312) 520-2795, BA 56 PA St Univ - Univ Park; ME 58 PA St Univ - Univ Park; Sp-Lang Path, Sch Dist #21, **SLP**

Dulle, Catherine Associated Rehab Services Inc, 104 Jungerman Road, Suite N, St Peters, MO 63376, (314) 441-3035, BA 73 Fontbonne Coll; MA 78 Saint Louis Univ; Pres, Assoc Rehab Servs Inc, **SLP**

Dumaine, Alan J Wethersfield Hearing Center, 935 Silas Deane Highway, Wethersfield, CT 06109, (203) 529-3443, BA 77 MI St Univ; MA 81 Univ of CT; Aud, Wethersfield Hrng Cen, **A ACE**

Dumas, Evelyn Sue 33 Electric Avenue Ste 202, Fitchburg, MA 01420, (508) 343-4788, BA 74 OH St Univ; MA 77 OH St Univ; 86–Aud, Cen Mass Hrng Svcs, **A**

Dumas, Mrs Mary Teresa 139J Marina Drive, Edison, NJ 08817, (201) 572-3948, BA 81 SUNY - Coll at Oneonta; MA 83 Hofstra Univ; 84–Sp-Lang Path, East Brunswick Pub Schs, **SLP**

Dumaux, William E 1626 Loma Crest, Glendale, CA 91205, (213) 337-9513, BA 70 CA St Univ - Los Angeles; MA 71 CA St Univ - Los Angeles; **A**

Dumeer, Betsy H 56 North Lyle Avenue, Tenafly, NJ 07670, BS 49 Univ of NH; MA 74 Univ of MD - College Park; Tchr, NYC Bd of Ed-Citywide Sp Unit, **SLP**

Dumigan, Mrs Lorrie Anne 58 Reddick Lane, Rochester, NY 14624, (716) 594-8693, BS 80 Nazareth Coll of Rochester; MS 84 Nazareth Coll of Rochester; 80–Sp-Lang Path, Monroe-Orleans BOCES II, **SLP**

Dummeyer, Mary Beth 1201 Delaware Boulevard, Madison, WI 53704, (608) 241-4583, BS 79 SUNY - Coll at Buffalo; MS 86 Univ of WI - Madison; 86–Sp-Lang Path, Madison Assoc Rtrded Citizens, **SLP**

Dumoch, Mrs Amy M Bagley Road, Southbury, CT 06488, (203) 264-2214, BA 76 CUNY - Queens Coll; MA 78 Hofstra Univ; 88–Sp-Lang Path, Private Practice, **SLP**

Dumond, Donna Lou 5664 South 88th East Avenue, Tulsa, OK 74145, (918) 592-6000, BS 71 Univ of Tulsa; MA 73 Univ of IA; Director Sp-Lang Services, University of Tulsa, **SLP ACE**

Du Mond, Glenna Colleen 1150 East Tessier Drive, Tarpon Springs, FL 34689, (813) 934-4339, BS 83 Univ of WA; MS 86 Univ of WA

Dumoulin, Lyn Box 96, Irish Settlement Road, Underhill Center, VT 05490, (802) 644-8821, MS 76 Univ of VT; Sp-Lang Path, Milton Sch Dist, **SLP**

Dunan-Vittori, Leslie Richmond 253 5th #C, Seal Beach, CA 90740, (213) 598-9336, BS 85 Univ of Alberta - Alberta; MA 87 Whittier Coll; **SLP**

Dunaway, Claudia L 2746 Nipoma Street, San Diego, CA 92106, **SLP**

Dunaway, Kenneth H P O Box 19, Fawn Grove, PA 17321, **SLP**

Dunbar, Barbara Jean 33 Cuesta Vista Drive, Monterey, CA 93940, BS 58 Northwestern Univ; MA 62 CUNY - Hunter Coll; SLP, Monterey County Office of Educ, **A ACE**

Dunbar, Mrs Fern S 3535 Olive Avenue, Long Beach, CA 90807, (213) 424-2969, BA 78 CA St Univ - Long Beach; MA 80 CA St Univ - Long Beach; Sp-Lang Path, Long Beach USD, **SLP**

Dunbar, James W Walla Walla Clinic, Department Of Audiology, 55 West Tietan, Walla Walla, WA 99362, (509) 525-3720, BA 75 Univ of Northern CO; MA 76 Univ of Northern CO; Aud, Walla Walla Clinic, **A**

Dunbar, Jessica Ann 20225 Grouse Way Apartment B, Sonora, CA 95370, (209) 532-1844, MA 88 CA St Univ - Chico; 88–Sp-Lang Path, Calaveras Co Ofc of Educ

Duncan, Carmen Alcyone Westbury Park #F-8, 1295 Franklin Drive S E, Marietta, GA 30067, (404) 425-0171, BA 69 Walla Walla Coll; MS 83 Adelphi Univ; Self Contained Language Tchr, Cobb County School System, **SLP**

Duncan, Catherine B 1039 North Market Street, Frederick, MD 21701-3076, (301) 694-1453, BA 77 Univ of MD - College Park; MS 79 Loyola Coll; Sp-Lang Path, Frederick Co Bd of Ed, **SLP**

Duncan, Deborah Suzanne 250 Ridge Pike Unit 237-A, Lafayette Hill, PA 19444, (215) 828-7955, MA 85 Kent St Univ; SLP, Holy Redeemer Med Ctr & Hosp, **SLP**

Duncan, Mrs Janice L 3801 West Marseilles, Mequon, WI 53092, (414) 242-5125, BS 73 Marquette Univ; MS 77 Marquette Univ; **SLP**

Duncan, Julia Shirk 3104 South Woodward Blvd, Tulsa, OK 74105, (918) 749-8393, BA 74 Univ of IA; MA 76 Univ of IA; Aud, Assoc ENT of Tulsa Inc, **A**

Duncan, Mrs Julie Ellen 316 La Mirada, El Paso, TX 79932, (915) 584-3504, BS 73 Southern Methodist Univ; BS 80 San Jose St Univ; MA 85 Univ of TX - El Paso; 88–Sp-Lang Path, Gadsden ISD, **SLP**

Duncan, Kathleen P 104 Helen Street, Binghamton, NY 13905, (607) 748-1541, BS 61 Coll of Saint Rose; MA 71 Coll of Saint Rose; Area Supt, Catholic Sch Broome Co, **SLP**

Duncan, Kimberly Ann Akin Medical Center, 2019 State Street, New Albany, IN 47150, (812) 945-3557, BS 81 Ball St Univ; MA 82 Ball St Univ; 83–Aud, Louisville Hearing Aid Ctr Inc, **A**

Duncan, Mrs Marilyn S 15008 Cypress Hills Drive, Dallas, TX 75248, (214) 238-0324, BS 50 Case Western Reserve Univ; MA 69 Southern Methodist Univ; Consultant, Richardson ISD, **SLP**

Duncan, Dr Melba Hurd 1219 La Veta Way, Colorado Springs, CO 80906, (303) 633-9189, BA 27 Univ of MN - Minneap-St Paul; MA 31 Univ of MN - Minneap-St Paul; PH 42 (NS) Univ of MN - Minneap-St Paul; SLP, Private Practice, **SLP LM**

Duncan, Richard A P O Box 874, Augusta, ME 04330, (207) 289-5964, **SLP**

Duncan, Susan Louise 1554 Obispo Avenue, Long Beach, CA 90804, (213) 597-5016, MA 87 CA St Univ - Los Angeles

Duncan, Teresa K 6106 Calle Mariselda, Apartment #304, San Diego, CA 92124-3760, (619) 755-4347, BS 74 Appalachian St Univ; MA 75 Appalachian St Univ; **SLP**

Duncan, Virginia McNamara 105 Sam Snead Circle, Etters, PA 17319, (717) 938-4784, BS 72 Carlow Coll; MA 78 Edinboro Univ of PA; MA 88 Gallaudet Coll; Sp-Lang Path, Private Practice, **SLP**

Dunckel, D Creig Dallas Audiological Services, 8617 N W Plaza Drive, Dallas, TX 75225, (214) 691-5466, MA 72 MI St Univ; Aud, Dallas Aud Serv, **A**

Dundas, Lisa A 6383 San Rafael Court, Rohnert Park, CA 94928, (707) 938-6472, MA 75 San Francisco St Univ; Aud, Sonoma Developmental Center, **A**

Dungan, Dr Ellen Love 157 West 57th Street, Suite 1100, New York, NY 10019, (212) 315-3090, BA 62 Depauw Univ; MA 64 Columbia Univ Teachers Coll; PH 80 (NS) Columbia Univ Teachers Coll; Sp-Lang Path, Private Practice, **SLP**

Dunham, Mrs Angela Harrah 825 Peachers Mill Road, Dale Terrace Apartment 501, Clarksville, TN 37042, (615) 648-8957, BA 86 Marshall Univ; MA 87 Marshall Univ

Dunham, Charles R 679 Oakenwald Avenue, Winnipeg, MB, Canada R3T 1M5, (204) 786-7841, BA 66 Western MI Univ; MA 70 Western MI Univ; SLP, Winnipeg Sch Division #1, **SLP**

Dunham, Elizabeth R R 4 Box 240, Carbondale, IL 62901, (618) 457-7954, BA 73 Univ of ID; MA 76 Univ of SD - Vermillion; **SLP**

Dunham, Mrs Hildy Helene Route 1 Box 309Z, Bealeton, VA 22712, (703) 439-8442, BS 81 Univ of ME - Farmington; MS 84 James Madison Univ; Sp-Lang Path, Fredericksburg Schs-Reg Prog, **SLP**

Dunham, Janet L 74 Pleasant Valley Road, Rd #3, Mansfield Center, CT 06250, (203) 423-8401, BA 72 Univ of CT; MA 73 Western MI Univ; Sp-Lang Path, Windham Pub Sch, **SLP**

Dunham, Judy-Ann Parker 4 Horseshoe Circle, Ware, MA 01082, (413) 283-3411, BA 75 Univ of MA - Amherst; MA 78 Univ of MA - Amherst; 87–Dir-Lang Sp & Hearing Svcs, Monson Developmental Cen, **SLP A ACE**

Dunham, Dr Judy K 22166 Solomon Blvd #152, Novi, MI 48050, (317) 494-7290, PH 85 (Special Education) Purdue Univ - West Lafayette; 88–Asst Prof, Madonna Coll

Dunham, Marilyn J Memphis Speech & Hearing Ctr, 807 Jefferson Avenue, Memphis, TN 38105, (901) 756-5161, BA 77 San Diego St Univ; MA 79 San Diego St Univ; Clinical Supervisor, Memphis State University, **SLP**

Dunham, Ruth J 4031 Oakhaven, San Antonio, TX 78217, (512) 655-7721, MA 64 IN Univ - Bloomington; Tchr, St Marys Hall, **SLP**

Dunhill-Zannoni, Mrs Moreen Ann 2635 Long Leaf Drive #2402, Houston, TX 77088, (713) 498-5152, BA 83 Univ of CO - Boulder; MA 85 Univ of Denver; 88–Sp-Lang Path, Cypress-Fairbanks ISD, **SLP**

Dunhoff, Mrs Tess P Assoc Speech & Lang Services, 5521 Riverside Drive, Chino, CA 91710, (714) 628-2407, BA 74 Whittier Coll; MS 80 Chapman Coll; Sp/Lang Path, Assoc Sp/Lang Hrng Serv, **SLP**

Dunitz, Anne Elizabeth 59 Katrina Falls Road, Rock Hill, NY 12775, (914) 343-2759, BS 83 Marywood Coll; MA 84 SUNY - Coll at Geneseo; Sp-Lang Path, Orange Co Cerebral Palsy Asso, **SLP**

Dunivant, Mrs Janis H 105 Crestwood, Birmingham, AL 35213, (205) 879-7508, BS 76 Univ of TX - Austin; MS 87 Univ of Montevallo; 88–Sp-Lang Path, Pinson Elem Sch, **SLP**

Dunkelberger, Daniel W 264 East Shamokin Street, Trevorton, PA 17881, (717) 374-2911, BS 73 Clarion Univ of PA; ME 74 Bloomsburg Univ of PA; Aud, Comn Wlth of Pa, **A**

Dunkerley, Mrs Nancy B 3430 Hampton Avenue, Nashville, TN 37215, (615) 292-8502, BS 67 Univ of KY; MS 69 Vanderbilt Univ; **SLP**

Dunkle, Karji L 5720 Brentwood Meadow Circle, Brentwood, TN 37027, (615) 859-6600, BA 85 Univ of CA - Santa Barbara; MS 87 Vanderbilt Univ; 87–Sp-Lang Path, Communi-Care Inc, **SLP**

Dunlap, Alice 2324 Ridgeway Road, Memphis, TN 38119, (901) 794-6151, BS 63 Univ of TN - Knoxville; MS 68 Vanderbilt Univ; SLP, Memphis Cty Schools, **SLP**

Dunlap, Alice R 8233 Crown Court Road, Alexandria, VA 22308, (703) 664-7191, BA 69 Univ of KY; MA 73 Univ of MD - College Park; Sp-Lang Path, Mt Vernon Hosp, **SLP**

Dunlap, Mrs D'Lorah Reddell HCR 32 Box 113, Hasty, AR 72640, (501) 429-6814, BS 85 Univ of Central AR; MS 87 Univ of Central AR; 88–Sp-Lang Path, OUR Coop Preschool Project, **SLP**

Dunlap, Mrs Denise Drace 6123 Lupton Drive, Dallas, TX 75225, (214) 750-0919, BS 72 Univ of OK - Norman; MA 74 Univ of OK - Norman; Sp-Lang Path, **SLP**

Dunlap, Kim E 122 - A Lower Stone, Bowling Green, KY 42101, (502) 651-6126, BS 82 Andrews Univ; MS 83 Western KY Univ; SLP, Homewood Health Care Center, **SLP**

Dunlop, Diane L 799 South McLean Boulevard, Elgin, IL 60120, **SLP**

Dunlop, Dr Jeanette M 2606 Redwing Drive, Temple, TX 76502, (817) 774-8418, BS 71 Mankato St Univ; MA 74 Univ of TN - Knoxville; PH 78 (Neurophysiology) Univ of TN - Knoxville; Sp-Lang Path, **SLP**

Dunlop, Dr Robert J Audiology Program (126), Olin E Teaque Veterans Ctr, Temple, TX 76504, (817) 778-4811, BA 70 Mankato St Univ; MA 75 Univ of TN - Knoxville; PH 78 (Sp & Hrng Science) Univ of TN - Knoxville; Aud, VA, **A**

Dunn, Avery E W 184 Nejako Drive, Middletown, CT 06457, (203) 635-5523, BS 56 Bloomsburg Univ of PA; MS 79; SLP, Cromwell Bd of Ed, **SLP**

Dunn, Carla 500 Brookhaven Trail, Austin, TX 78746, (512) 471-3841, BS 70 TX Tech Univ; MS 71 TX Tech Univ; PH 79 (NS) Univ of WA; Assoc Prof, U of TX at Austin, **SLP**

Dunn, Cecilia Ann 5340 Rambo Lane, Toledo, OH 43623, (419) 729-8200, OB 75 Univ of Toledo; MA 86 Eastern MI Univ; 77–Sp-Lang Path, Toledo Bd of Educ

Dunn, Mrs Darlene T 309 Jefferson Street, Kingston Mines, IL 61539, (309) 692-8110, BS 73 Bradley Univ; MS 74 Bradley Univ; Sect Sup SLP, Inst of Phy Med & Rehab, **SLP ACE**

Dunn, David L 1657 James Street, Merrick, NY 11566, **SLP**

Dunn, Deborah A 250 Quail Run, Roswell, GA 30076, (404) 889-1630, BS 74 Univ of GA; ME 83 GA St Univ; Sp-Lang Path, Forsyth Co Board of Ed, **SLP**

Dunn, Mrs Diana Bailey 2105 West Middle Lane, Lecanto, FL 32661, (904) 746-7805, BA 80 Univ of FL; MS 81 FL St Univ; Sp-Lang Path Director, Private Practice, **SLP**

Dunn, Mrs Donna S 4305 Annshire, Louisville, KY 40213, (502) 585-9911, BS 71 Brescia Coll; ME 72 Univ of Louisville; Dir-Commun Dis Prog, Spalding U, **SLP A**

Dunn, Mrs Janice M 2809 Wingren, Irving, TX 75062, (214) 252-3949, BS 67 Abilene Christian Univ; MS 70 Univ of North TX; **SLP**

Dunn, Mrs Jean B 2022 Terre Bonne Avenue, San Dimas, CA 91773, (213) 963-1611, BS 48 Univ of MO - Columbia; MA 79 Azusa Pacific Univ; SLP, Glenoora USD, **SLP**

Dunn, Mrs Joann Hoffmann 21 W 109 Woodview, Itasca, IL 60143, MS 83 IN Univ - Bloomington; Sp-Lang Path, Dupage West Cook Spec Educ Assoc, **SLP**

Dunn, Joanne C 281 Linden Avenue East, East Rochester, NY 14445, (716) 467-7160, BS 80 SUNY - Coll at Geneseo; MA 82 OH Univ - Athens; Sp-Lang Path, Rochester City Sch Dist, **SLP**

Dunn, Mrs Julia E T 501 West 77th Street, Indianapolis, IN 46260, (317) 872-3131, BS 77 Miami Univ - Oxford; MS 78 Miami Univ - Oxford; Sp-Lang Path, Communicology Inc, **SLP**

Dunn, Julie A 750 S W Maplecrest Drive, Portland, OR 97219, (503) 635-0503, BA 77 Univ of OR; MA 82 Univ of OR; Sp-Lang Path, Clackamas Ed Serv Dist, **SLP**

Dunn, Julie Ann 6231 Ellsworth, Dallas, TX 75214, (214) 987-9806, MS 87 Univ of TX - Dallas; **SLP**

Dunn, Kathleen Siobhan 74 Webster Avenue, Manhasset, NY 11030, (516) 549-4999, BA 83 SUNY - Coll at Cortland; MA 86 Long Island U - CW Post Ctr; **SLP**

Dunn, Kristin Kiekhaefer 3810-B Sickle Court, Lafayette, IN 47905, (317) 497-8517, BS 83 Univ of NE - Lincoln; MA 85 Univ of IA; 88–Sp-Lang Path, Indiana Veterans Home, **SLP ACE**

Dunn, Laura Anne 350 24th Street Northwest, #208J, Winter Haven, FL 33880, (813) 294-5180, BA 85 Univ of FL; MA 87 Univ of FL; 88–Sp-Lang Path, Comm Spec Inc, **SLP**

Dunn, Laurie Ann Woodcrest Elementary, 880 N E Osborne Road, Minneapolis, MN 55432, (612) 786-5570, BS 81 Univ of MN - Minneap-St Paul; MA 84 Univ of Northern CO; SLP, Spring Lake Park Public School, **SLP**

Dunn, Lawrence E 1549 San Andreas Road #11, La Selva Beach, CA 95076, (408) 462-5595, BS 79 East TN St Univ; MA 81 Univ of TN - Knoxville; Sp-Lang Path, Samaritan Home Serv, **SLP**

Dunn, Mrs Lisa Baldwin 12539 Brady Place Court, Jacksonville, FL 32223, (904) 262-6890, BS 83 Auburn Univ - Auburn; OM 87 Auburn Univ - Auburn; **SLP**

Dunn, Lisa H 2810 Leanne Drive, Tifton, GA 31794, (912) 382-2691, BS 86 Valdosta St Coll; ME 87 Valdosta St Coll; 87–Sp-Lang Path, Worth County Bd of Educ

Dunn, Lisa Maria 4310-D Appian Way West, Gahanna, OH 43230, (614) 476-0294, BA 85 Hampton Univ; MA 87 OH St Univ; 88–Aud, Ohio Dept of Health, **A**

Dunn, Mrs Luceen J 1009 Robinhood Lane, Norman, OK 73072, (405) 329-0390, BA 65 Univ of CA - Berkeley; MA 67 Univ of NM; MS 80 Univ of OK Medical Center; 83–Aud, Assoc In Aud & Sp Path, **A**

Dunn, Marianne 12352 Chandler Boulevard, Unit E, North Hollywood, CA 91607, (818) 984-2575, BA 45 Univ of AZ; MA 50 Univ of Southern CA; President, Private Practice, **SLP**

Dunn, Marilee G 119 Park Hill Avenue, Columbia, MO 65203, (314) 875-3502, BA 61 PA St Univ - Univ Park; MA 71 Univ of MO - Columbia; Sp-Lang Path, Boone Hospital Center, **SLP**

Dunn, Nancy M 1142 N W Scenic Drive, Albany, OR 97321, (503) 926-8092, BS 69 Hanover Coll; MS 74 Univ of NM; Aud/Sp-Lang Path, Mid-Valley Sp & Hrng Cen, **SLP A**

Dunn, Mrs Nancy Susan 9 Brickton Place, Little Rock, AR 72205-3705, MS 85 Univ of AR - Little Rock; BA 81 Univ of AR - Fayetteville; Sp-Lang Path, Arkansas Easter Seal Society, **SLP**

Dunn, Theresa Ann 228 East Patterson Avenue, Bellefontaine, OH 43311, (513) 592-3449, BS 83 Miami Univ - Oxford; MA 85 Bowling Green St Univ; 85–Sp-Lang Path, Champaign Co Bd of Educ, **SLP ACE**

Dunn, Thomas F 535 West Sandhurst Drive, St Paul, MN 55113-4660, (612) 823-6660, BS 81 Northeastern Univ; MA 84 Univ of Northern CO; **SLP**

Dunn, Thomas M 4305 Annshire, Louisville, KY 40213, (502) 588-4459, BA 70 Brescia Coll; ME 72 Univ of Louisville; 70–Sp-Lang Path, Comm for Handicapped Children, **A**

Dunn, Tracey Michelle 5601 Albany Court, New Orleans, LA 70131, (504) 391-0934, MS 88 LA St Univ - N O Medical Ctr

Dunn, Mrs Valerie Strzalka 701 Wilson Drive, Midland, MI 48640-3037, (517) 773-7921

Dunnan, Judith R 12 Front Street, Exeter, NH 03833, (603) 659-2192, BA 73 Univ of NH; MS 81 Univ of NH; Sp-Lang Path, Newmarket Sch Dist, **SLP**

Dunne, Mrs Judith Gordon 15 The Pines, Roslyn Estates, Long Island, NY 11576, (516) 621-1703, BA 66 CUNY - Queens Coll; MA 78 CUNY - Hunter Coll; Aud, Speech and Hearing Assoc, **A ACE**

Dunne, Lee Anne 16 Houghton Road, Milton, MA 02186-4123, (617) 697-1348, BS 51 Northwestern Univ; MA 65 CUNY - Hunter Coll; 67–Prof, Bridgewater State Coll, **SLP**

Dunne, Mrs Sally A 2425 Hipp Avenue, Brownsville, TX 78520, (512) 541-2812, BS 58 Purdue Univ - West Lafayette; MS 77 Purdue Univ - West Lafayette; Sp-Lang Path, Brownsville ISD, **SLP**

Dunn-Engel, Dr Elaine 1500 Sheridan Road #7-F, Wilmette, IL 60091, (312) 328-5923, BS 45 Univ of WI - Madison; MA 62 Northwestern Univ; PH 64 (Communicative Disorders) Northwestern Univ; 66–Sp-Lang Path, Private Practice, **SLP A ACE**

Dunning, Mrs Cheryl R 105 North Silver Lake Dr, Raytown, MO 64083, (913) 764-4121, BS 77 KS St Univ; MA 79 KS St Univ; Sp/Lang Path, Olathe Dist Schs, **SLP**

Dunning, Dennis P 15523 Arbor Street, Omaha, NE 68144, (402) 346-8800, MS Univ of NE - Omaha; MS Univ of NE - Omaha; OD (Sp Path ScD) Boston Univ; 79–Sp-Lang Path, VA Med Ctr, **SLP**

Dunning, Georgann P O Box 317, Decatur, NE 68020, **SLP**

Dunphy, Diana Gould 33 Sohier Street, Cohasset, MA 02025, (617) 786-8742, BA 68 Kean Coll of NJ; MA 73 Kean Coll of NJ; 84–Sp-Lang Path, Quincy PS, **SLP**

Dunsky, Mrs Patricia Lee 40 Tanglewood Road, Needham, MA 02194, (617) 288-9151, **SLP**

Dunsmore, Caroline E 19 Baker Crescent N W, Calgary, AB, Canada T2L 1R3, (403) 229-7046, BA 66 Univ of Calgary - Alberta; MA 68 Univ of OK - Norman; Dir/Sp-Lang Path Aud, Alberta Chldns Prov Gen Hosp, **SLP**

Dunton, Mrs Sheryl Widen 8701 North Star Grass Drive, Tucson, AZ 85741, (602) 744-0863, BS 80 CA Lutheran Coll; MS 84 Univ of NV - Reno; Sp-Lang Path, Sunnyside School Dist, **SLP**

Dunton, Virginia Jordan 8057 Hermitage Road, Richmond, VA 23228, (804) 266-9666, BS 81 James Madison Univ; ME 83 Univ of VA - Charlottesville; Sp-Lang Path, InSpeech Inc, **SLP ACE**

Dunwoodie, Rosemary T 150 Bidwell Parkway, Buffalo, NY 14222, (716) 835-6009, BS 84 SUNY - Coll at Buffalo; MA 88 SUNY - Center at Buffalo; 88–Sp-Lang Path, Buffalo Hrng & Sp Ctr

Duplantis, Myra B 89 Haroleans Avenue, Harahan, LA 70123, (504) 737-8098, OB 74 Univ of MS; OM 76 LA St Univ - N O Medical Ctr; Sp-Lang Path, Private Practice, **SLP**

Dupre, Gerald F 2665 Meadow Ridge, West Jordan, UT 84088, (801) 250-8400, OM 79 Brigham Young Univ; 88–Dir-Sp Svcs, Villa Serena, **SLP**

Dupre, Michael Joseph 237 West 109th Street #C, New York, NY 10025, (212) 584-9000, BA 80 McGill Univ - Quebec; MS 82 Columbia Univ Teachers Coll; OM 87 CUNY - City College; 82–Sp-Lang Path, VA Med Cen-Bronx, **SLP**

Dupree, Laureen T c/o Lt C A Boenecke, MSC Usnr, Box 18 U S Navy Hospital, FPO New York, NY 09540, (202) 676-7366, BS 74 Northwestern Univ; MS 76 Univ of WI - Madison; **A**

Dupree, Tammy Richelle 101 Laura Lane, C-3 Twin Oaks, Greenville, NC 27834, (919) 291-7001, BS 83 Appalachian St Univ; MS 84 East Carolina Univ; 88–Sp-Lang Path, CRF Sp & Lang Assoc, **SLP**

Dupuis, Jo Ann 6233 Dona Linda Place N W, Albuquerque, NM 87120, (505) 344-1482, BS 78 Central MI Univ; MA 81 Central MI Univ; Sp/Lang Path, Albuquerque Pub Sch, **SLP**

Dupuis, Mrs Robin Deborah 57 Cedar Street, Malone, NY 12953, (518) 483-1697, BA 78 SUNY - Coll at Plattsburgh; MA 85 SUNY - Coll at Plattsburgh; 79–Sp-Lang Path, Franklin Essex Hamilton BOCES, **SLP**

Dupuy, Cheryl Bozik 1910 Holmby #5, Los Angeles, CA 90025, (213) 393-4773, **SLP**

Duques, Wendy Bowden 23 Strawberry Hill Road, Madison, CT 06443, (203) 245-1428, BS 71 OH St Univ; MS 85 Southern CT St Univ; 85–Sp-Lang Path, Guilford PS, **SLP**

Durachta, Mrs Judith A 1334 Duquesne Avenue, Naperville, IL 60565, (312) 749-1264, BS 74 IL St Univ - Normal; MS 77 IL St Univ - Normal; Sp-Lang Path, Sch Dist #100, **SLP**

Durall, Dr Maurice J P O Box 1264, Claremont, CA 91711, (714) 793-2121, BA 60 Fort Hays St Univ; MS 61 Univ of WI - Madison; PH 71 (Communicative Disorders) Univ of WI - Madison; Prof of Commun Dis, U of Redlands, **SLP**

Duran, Margaret Route 10 Box 39A65, New Braunfels, TX 78130, (512) 655-0691, BS 71 TX Tech Univ; MS 73 TX Tech Univ; **SLP**

Duran, Vicki Holbrook 734 Cherry Brook Rd, Canton, CT 06059, MA 80 Bowling Green St Univ; 88–Sp-Lang Path, Farmington PS, **SLP**

Durand, Elizabeth 6106 Twinhill Drive, Arlington, TX 76016-3719, (817) 483-2448, **SLP**

Durand, Paulette Ann 940 Sylvia Lane, St Paul, MN 55126, (612) 483-0369, OB 86 Univ of MN - Duluth; MA 87 Univ of MN - Duluth

Durant, Mrs Linda Godard Route 2 Box 98-1, Granbury, TX 76048, (817) 297-4319, BA 82 Univ of ME - Orono; MS 83 TX Christian Univ; Sp-Lang Path, Crowley ISD, **SLP**

Durante, Mrs Dace Anita 10514 Lady Bug Drive, Houston, TX 77064, (713) 744-3045, BS 77 SUNY - Center at Albany; MA 87 Univ of Houston - Univ Park; 88–Sp-Lang Path, Memorial Cty Rehab Hosp, **SLP**

Durant-Jones, Mrs Lisa Anne P O Box 18686, Rochester, NY 14618-0686, (716) 671-7831, BS 79 Coll of Saint Rose; MS 81 Columbia Univ Teachers Coll; 88–Sp-Lang Path, Univ of Rochester Aud/Sp Dept, **SLP**

Durbach, Miriam H 1034 Clare Street, Victoria, BC, Canada V8S 4B6, **SLP**

Durbin, Christine 1321 East Yndell #C, El Paso, TX 79902, (915) 534-9160, MA 78 Univ of MO - Columbia; Ch of Commun Dis Serv, El Paso Rehab Cen, **SLP**

Durfee, Barbara Lee 23 Stoneleigh Court, Rochester, NY 14618, (716) 377-4660, BA 75 Univ of NH; MS 86 Nazareth Coll of Rochester; 86–Sp-Lang Path, Monroe BOCES #1, **SLP**

Durgin-Clinchard, Mrs Jean 638 North 25th, Lincoln, NE 68503, (402) 473-0278, BS 57 Old Dominion Univ; MA 68 Univ of NE - Omaha; Sp/Lang Path, Lincoln Pub Sch, **SLP**

Durham, Mrs Candace Kaye 332 South East Avenue, Oak Park, IL 60302, (312) 524-3000, BS 84 Southern IL Univ -Carbondale; MA 86 Northern IL Univ - De Kalb; Sp-Lang Path/Orthopedic Prog, Oak Park Dist 97, **SLP**

Durham, Catherine Therese 10115 Castile Road, Richmond, VA 23233, (618) 632-4817, BS 84 Saint Louis Univ; MA 86 Saint Louis Univ

Durham, Glenda Dawn 23 Hiland Place, Benton, AR 72015, (501) 664-2961, BS 82 Univ of AR - Little Rock; MS 86 Univ of AR - Little Rock; 87–Sp-Lang Path, F A Allen Sch for Excep Chldn, **SLP**

Durham, Kathleen E 5219 S Gravenstein Park, Murray, UT 84123, BA 68 Univ of UT; MA 69 Univ of UT; Sp-Lang Path, Salt Lake Bd of Ed, **SLP**

Durham, Kathleen V 340 Sioux Trail, Somerset, KY 42501, (606) 679-4361, BS 74 Saint Louis Univ; MS 75 Vanderbilt Univ; Audiologist, Private Practice, **A**

Durham, Mrs Kimberly Raybuck 3460 Water Oak Drive, Birmingham, AL 35243, (205) 967-4047, MA 87 Univ of AL-Tuscaloosa

Durham, Mary Ellen 5615 Ruthwood Drive, Calabasas, CA 91302, (805) 252-9580, SLP, Saugus Union Sch Dist, **SLP**

Durig, Anthony 776 Hampshire Road, Stow, OH 44224, (216) 923-7119, MA 83 Univ of Akron; Aud, Cleveland Clinic, **A**

Durkee, Mrs Margaret Jill 1114 Coachlight Drive, Houston, TX 77077, (713) 497-1906, BA 79 Univ of Southwestern LA; MS 84 Lamar Univ; 86–Sp-Lang Path, Private Practice, **SLP**

Durkin, Mrs Barbara T 2101 Buckingham, St Joseph, MO 64506, (816) 364-1501, BS 75 Univ of KS; MA 76 Univ of KS; Sp-Lang Path, Family Guidance Cen, **SLP**

Durkin, Teresa K 840 28th Avenue North, St Petersburg, FL 33704, (813) 823-0724, BA 77 Univ of AR - Fayetteville; MS 81 Univ of AR - Fayetteville; Sp-Lang Path, Bost Human Dev Serv, **SLP**

Durkin, Teresa M 146 Grace Court #3, Fort Mitchell, KY 41017, (606) 331-1220, BS 75 Eastern KY Univ; MA 81 Univ of Cincinnati; 81–Sp-Lang Path, Beechwood ISD, **SLP**

Durkin, Teresita Marie 2189 Lincoln Drive, Huntingdon Valley, PA 19006, (215) 539-8550, BS 81 Marywood Coll; MS 83 Univ of MI - Ann Arbor; **SLP**

Durley, Debra L 8451 Carter, Overland Park, KS 66212, **SLP**

Durmon, Mrs Laura Helen 408 West Pine Street, Warren, AR 71671, (501) 735-7303, **SLP**

Durnford, Mrs Susan Elaine 9004 Vance Street #110, Westminster, CO 80020, (303) 467-1266, BA 82 Adams St Coll; MS 84 CO St Univ; Sp-Lang Path, Spalding Rehab Hosp, **SLP**

Durr, Mrs Angela M 2965 Kane Road, Aliquippa, PA 15001, (412) 378-0359, BA 62 CA Univ of PA; ME 74 PA St Univ - Univ Park; 62–Supvr, Beaver Valley Inter Unit #27, **SLP**

Durr, Mrs Karen Breininger 50 Osk Ridge Drive, Meriden, CT 06450, (203) 634-8986, BA 79 Southern CT St Univ; MS 83 Southern CT St Univ; SLP, **SLP**

Durrant, Dr John D Eye & Ear Hospital, Center For Audiology, 230 Lothrop Street, Pittsburgh, PA 15213, (412) 647-2030, OB 67 OH Univ - Athens; MA 68 OH Univ - Athens; PH 72 (NS) Northwestern Univ; 84–Dir of Aud, U of Pittsburgh Med Sch, **A**

Durrette, Wanda G 11010 Hidden Creek Court, Fort Washington, MD 20744, MS; **SLP**

Durst, Brenda Adsit 12511 Blue Spruce Drive, Edinboro, PA 16412, (814) 734-5610, BS 73 Edinboro Univ of PA; MA 77 Edinboro Univ of PA; Sp-Lang Path, NW Tri-Cnty Intermediate Unit, **SLP**

Duryee, Mrs Virginia 262 West Farms Road, Northampton, MA 01060, (413) 527-6000, BS 73 Emerson Coll; MS 75 Columbia Univ Teachers Coll; Sp-Lang Path, E Hampton Pub Sch, **SLP**

Dusckas, Sallie Jeanne 7464 Charrington Court, Indianapolis, IN 46254-9681, (317) 297-CARE, BA 79 Univ of Pittsburgh - Pittsburgh; MA 82 Univ of Pittsburgh - Pittsburgh; Sp-Lang Path, Susan S Rockafellow, **SLP ACE**

Dusenbery, Luanne Kay 205 North Grove Street #A, Bowling Green, OH 43402, (419) 352-3576, BS 78 IL St Univ - Normal; MA 82 Kent St Univ; Sp-Lang Path, Bowling Green City Board of Ed, **SLP**

Duskey, Mrs Janet East 4 Meetinghouse Lane, Durham, NC 27707, (919) 490-5986, BS 80 SUNY - Coll at Geneseo; MA 82 OH Univ - Athens; Sp-Lang Path, Durham Co Schools, **SLP**

Dust, Mrs Donita K 2607 Wing Street, Sedalia, MO 65301, (816) 827-4284, BS 76 Central MO St Univ; MS 79 Central MO St Univ; Sp-Lang Path, Childrens Therapy Center, **SLP**

Dustin, Carla J 6273 Dixie Drive, La Mesa, CA 92041, **SLP**

Dustman, Jami Lynne 103 Mitchell, Greenfield, MO 65661, (417) 637-5777, BS 82 Southwest MO St Univ; MS 83 Southern IL Univ-Edwardsvill; 88–Sp-Lang Path, Barton Dade & Cedar Counties Spec Educ Coop, **SLP**

Dustrude, Stephen R 91274 Donna Road, Springfield, OR 97478, (503) 726-3383, BA 73 Pacific Univ; MS 77 Eastern WA Univ; Sp-Lang Path, Springfield Pub Sch, **SLP ACE**

Dutcher, Pamela S 8380-2 North Hillcrest Dr, Berrien Springs, MI 49103, (616) 471-3468, BS 80 Andrews Univ; MA 81 Central MI Univ; Asst Prof, Andrews University, **SLP**

Duthie, Jill K Communicative Disorders, 1231 Gambell, Anchorage, AK 99501, (907) 276-5354, BA 72 Univ of CA - Santa Barbara; MA 74 CA St Univ - Northridge; Sp/Lang Path, Commun Dis St of Ak, **SLP**

Dutka, Debra A Cleveland Hearing & Speech Ctr, 11206 Euclid Avenue, Cleveland, OH 44106, (216) 231-8787, BS 79 Marywood Coll; MA 81 Case Western Reserve Univ; Sp/Lang Path, Cleveland Hrng & Sp Cen, **SLP**

Dutra, Mrs Leslie R 3442 Zelia Court, Arcata, CA 95521-4861, (707) 822-0838, BA 78 Humboldt St Univ; MA 80 Humboldt St Univ; 79–Sp-Lang Path, Blue Lake Un Elem Sch Dist, **SLP**

Dutra, Maria D F Box 341, North Oxford, MA 01537, (508) 987-0539, BA 75 Boston Coll; MS 77 Emerson Coll; Sp-Lang Path, Private Practice, **SLP**

Dutton, Mrs Ada Mullins Route 3 Box 66, Kingston, TN 37763, (615) 376-2749, MA 76 Univ of TN - Knoxville; 88–Sp-Lang Path, Partners Home Hlth of E TN, **SLP**

Dutton, Donald E, Jr 10251 Stanford Avenue, Garden Grove, CA 92640, (714) 539-2082, BA 81 CA St Univ - Fullerton; MA 84 CA St Univ - Fullerton; Sp-Lang Path, Rancho Santiago Community Col, **SLP**

Dutton, Mrs Susan Marie 4720 W Villa Maria, Glendale, AZ 85308, (602) 439-2275, BS 79 CO St Univ; OM 84 AZ St Univ; **SLP**

Dutton, Mrs Susan R RD #1 Box 326, Glenmoore, PA 19343, (215) 827-9473, BS 75 Bloomsburg Univ of PA; ME 76 Bloomsburg Univ of PA; Sp/Lang Path, Berks County Intermediate Unit, **SLP**

Duval, Chris L 6807 North Sheridan 926, Chicago, IL 60626, (312) 338-8894, BS 77 Mankato St Univ; MS 80 Univ of WI - Stevens Point; Sp/Lang Path, Private Practice, **SLP**

Duval, Mrs Kathryn Mary 4910A 66th Street, Lubbock, TX 79414, (806) 747-2641, BS 84 Purdue Univ - West Lafayette; MS 86 CO St Univ; SLP, Lubbock ISD, **SLP**

Duval, Nicole L 1311 Chicago Avenue #309, Evanston, IL 60201, (312) 491-6819, BS 85 Worcester St Coll; MS 87 PA St Univ - Univ Park; 88–Sp-Lang Path, Lutheran Soc Svcs of Il, **SLP**

Duval, Mrs Sharon Cooper 1814 West Meadow Drive, Houston, TX 77084, (713) 757-1000, BA 79 Marshall Univ; MA 80 Marshall Univ; Sp-Lang Path, St Joseph Hospital, **SLP**

Duvall, Michelle P 1974 South Waldby, Fresno, CA 93727, (209) 255-4821, BA CA St Univ - Fresno; MA 84 CA St Univ - Fresno; 85–Sp-Lang Path, Fresno USD, **SLP**

Duven, Mrs Channa Gae P O Box 88, Almond, NC 28702, (704) 488-2030, **SLP**

Duwell, Lisa Iacobucci 4911 Heuwerth Avenue, Apartment 1, Cincinnati, OH 45238, (513) 921-8798, BS 85 Univ of Cincinnati; **SLP**

Dvoret, Ken R 8519 East Prairie Road, Skokie, IL 60076, (312) 674-4120, **A**

Dvorsky, Mrs Isobel G 2657 Vista Grand Court, San Leandro, CA 94577, (415) 483-0801, BA 49 Univ of IA; **SLP**

Dvosin, Mrs Edna 205 West End Avenue, New York, NY 10023, (212) 724-9451, BA 33 CUNY - Brooklyn Coll; MA 65 CUNY - Hunter Coll; Owner, Edna Dvosin Ma, **A LM**

Dwenger, Mrs Sandra G 51 Journeys End Road, New Canaan, CT 06840, (203) 966-7606, BS 60 Syracuse Univ; MS 71 CUNY - Queens Coll; **SLP**

Dwight, Debra M 1000 Stevens Entry #W114, Peachtree City, GA 30269, (404) 583-2528, BA 73 Univ of South AL; MA 75 Univ of South AL; MA 76 Univ of AL- Tuscaloosa; Cl Supv, U of Alabama, **SLP**

Dwight, Mrs Maria T Campat 24700 Via Pradera, Calabasas, CA 91302-1451, (818) 887-6706, BA 82 Univ of CA - Santa Barbara; MS 84 Univ of AZ; Sp-Lang Path, Brotman Medical Center, **SLP**

Dwinell, Mrs Maureen M P O Box 88, Rockport, MA 01966, (617) 283-8778, BS 64 Syracuse Univ; MA 68 Syracuse Univ; Sp-Lang Path, Private Practice, **SLP**

Dwire, Louis Ian 1647 West Brampton Way, Apartment 303, Salt Lake City, UT 84104-2561, (801) 977-0341, BA 61 Western St Coll of CO; MA 65 Western St Coll of CO; MS 84 Univ of UT; Sp-Lang Path, Salt Lake City Sch Dist, **SLP**

Dworkin, Mrs Doris R R 7300 Valley View Road, Hudson, OH 44236, (216) 656-3957, BA 60 Wayne St Univ; ME 63 Wayne St Univ; Sp-Lang Path, Private Practice, **SLP**

Dworkin, Dr James Paul Transitional Learning Ctr, 1528 Postoffice Street, Galveston, TX 77553, (409) 762-6661, BA 71 CUNY - Brooklyn Coll; MS 73 CUNY - Brooklyn Coll; PH 75 (NS) SUNY - Center at Buffalo; 87–Sp-Lang Path, Transitional Learning Comm, **SLP**

Dworkin, Mona L S 48 Gerardine Place, Spring Valley, NY 10977, (914) 623-2884, BA 73 CUNY - Lehman Coll; MA 77 CUNY - Hunter Coll; Sp-Lang Path, Venture Inn Inc, **SLP**

Dworkin, Nadine Sheri 50 Manchester Lane, Stony Brook, NY 11790, (516) 365-4323, BA 84 SUNY - Coll at Cortland; MA 86 Hofstra Univ; 88–Sp-Lang Path, Transitions of Long Island, **SLP**

Dworkin, Valerie 2740 S Oakland Forest Dr, Apartment 1103, Oakland Park, FL 33309-5634, (305) 484-2128, BA 77 Univ of Miami; MA 78 Univ of Miami; Co-Owner/Sp-Lang Path, Private Practice, **SLP**

Dworkis, Mrs Andrea P 98 Madison Avenue, Island Park, NY 11558, (516) 889-8586, BA 75 CUNY - Brooklyn Coll; MA 76 Hofstra Univ; SLP, BOCES, **SLP**

Dworkis, Audrey Beth 30 South Eckar Street, Irvington, NY 10533, BA 80 CUNY - Queens Coll; MS 82 Columbia Univ Teachers Coll; Sp/Lang Path, Hebrew Hosp-Chronic Sick, **SLP**

Dwyer, Mrs Aurion Louise 3533 Laurel View Court, Laurel, MD 20810, (301) 868-7269, BS 82 Trenton St Coll; MA 86 Univ of MD - College Park; 88–Aud, The Hearing Laboratory, **A**

Dwyer, Bridget M 1776 East 13th Street #3K, Brooklyn, NY 11229, (718) 735-2669, BA 82 CUNY - Brooklyn Coll; MS 84 CUNY - Brooklyn Coll; SLP, Kings County Hospital Center, **SLP**

Dwyer, Cynthia A 9 Rolej Court, Clayton, CA 94517, (415) 938-4722, BA San Francisco St Univ; MS San Francisco St Univ; SLP, Diablo Valley Sp & Lang Cl, **SLP**

Dwyer, Mrs Rosalie RFD 1 Box 41, Presque Isle, ME 04769, (207) 493-3361, BA 77 Southern CT St Univ; MA 79 SUNY - Coll at Geneseo; Sp-Lang Path, Aroostook Ment Hlth Cen, **SLP**

Dwyer, Sharon Patricia 14 Beacon Street, Arlington, MA, (617) 344-1226, BA 85 SUNY - Coll at Cortland; MS 86 Syracuse Univ; W E Fernald State Sch, **SLP**

Dwyer-Urban, Regina 1515 Chauncey Lane, Richmond, VA 23233, (804) 741-1075, BA 76 Montclair St Coll; MA 79 Univ of IA; **SLP**

Dybala, Mrs Ellen Irene 15420 Walnut, Oak Forest, IL 60452, (312) 687-7590, OB 62 Chicago St Univ; MS 84 Governors St Univ; SLP, Chicago Board of Education, **SLP**

Dybka, Dr Michael E Speech Hearing & Lang Center, New England Med Ctr Hosp, 171 Harrison Avenue, Boston, MA 02111, (617) 956-5300, BA 68 San Diego St Univ; MA 69 San Diego St Univ; PH 72 (NS) Univ of WA; 87–Dir Aud Svcs, New England Med Ctr Hosp, **A**

Dyck, Kay Bartel 1814 Cheryl Court, Wichita, KS 67212, (316) 942-4221, BS 83 KS St Univ; MA 86 Wichita St Univ; Sp-Lang Path, ENT Surgical Group, **SLP**

Dyckes-Berke, Diana M 484 West 43rd Street #27-H, New York, NY 10036, (212) 360-3720, BA 86 SUNY - Coll at Cortland; MA 87 Hofstra Univ

Dycus, Mrs Sarah Archer Rt 1 Box 362, Sweetwater, TN 37874, (615) 334-5793, BS 78 TN Tech Univ; MA 82 Univ of TN - Knoxville; 88–Sp-Lang Path, Meigs Co Dept of Educ, **SLP**

Dye, Crisann Louise 5655 Picadilly, Beaumont, TX 77708, BS 84 West TX St Univ; MS 85 West TX St Univ

Dye, Mrs Gaye D P O Box 118, Printer, KY 41655, (606) 432-0123, BA 83 Marshall Univ; MA 84 Univ of TN - Knoxville; Sp-Lang Path, Crigger/Mullins Sp-Lang Lrng Svcs, **SLP**

Dye, Mrs Linda McLean 1921 Royal Oaks, Duarte, CA 91010, (213) 483-4431, BA 81 Univ of CA - Santa Barbara; MA 84 OH Univ - Athens; Aud, House Ear Instit, **A ACE**

Dyer, Anna J 800 Athania Parkway, Metairie, LA 70001, (504) 865-1945, BS 78 Univ of TX - Dallas; MS 80 Univ of MI - Ann Arbor; Sp-Lang Path, Communication & Learning Cen, **SLP**

Dyer, Barbara Jane 3702 Hughes Road, Louisville, KY 40207, (502) 459-3760, BS 72 TN Tech Univ; MA 74 Univ of TN - Knoxville; Aud, Drs Richmond & Pelsel, **A**

Dyer, Erin C 5826 Russett #3, Madison, WI 53711, (608) 273-3588, BS 76 West Chester Univ of PA; MA 78 Saint Louis Univ; Sp/Lang Path, Belleville Sch Dist, **SLP**

Dyer, Mrs Georgia Ann P O Box 315, 115 Edgewood Avenue, Oakdale, NY 11769, (516) 244-2219, BA; MA; 83–Sp-Lang Path, Connetquot Central Sch Dist, **SLP**

Dyer, Mrs Helen A P O Box 1648, Baldwin Park, CA 91706-7648, (818) 960-1344, BS 53; **LM**

Dyer, Mrs Linda King 26 Stanislaus Circle, Sacramento, CA 95831, (916) 453-5409, BA 81 CA St Univ - Sacramento; MA 83 CA St Univ - Sacramento; Aud, U CA Davis Med Cen, **A**

Dyer, Mrs Lynn Carew 1401 W Homestead Drive, Appleton, WI 54914, (414) 729-6985, BS 73 Univ of WI - Stevens Point; MS 74 Univ of WI - Stevens Point; Sp-Lang Path, Neenah Jt Sch Dist, **SLP ACE**

Dyer, Patricia Joan 1025 Michaels Lane, Libertyville, IL 60048, (312) 816-8243, BS 84 Univ of WI - Whitewater; MS 85 Univ of WI - Whitewater; 85–Sp-Lang Path, Round Lake Area Schs, **SLP**

Dyer, Mrs Patricia Lex 5833 Willow Lane, Dallas, TX 75230, (214) 944-8422, MA 72; SLP, Methodist Hosp of Dallas, **SLP**

Dyer, Ruth S 511 Haworth Avenue, Haworth, NJ 07641, BS; **SLP LM**

Dyk, Diane A 906 Avenue F East, Bismarck, ND 58501, (701) 221-3765, BS 77 Augustana Coll; MS 78 Minot St Univ; Sp-Lang Path, Bismarck Pub Sch, **SLP**

Dykas-Fierke, Cheryl M 744 73rd Street, Downers Grove, IL 60516, (312) 599-1050, BA 76 Saint Xavier Coll; MA 78 Northern IL Univ - De Kalb; Sp/Lang Path, Dist 122 Ridgeland PS, **SLP**

Dyke, Carol Lee 10415 West 116th Terrace, Apartment 136, Overland Park, KS 66210, (913) 339-9920, BS 81 Univ of KS; MA 84 Univ of KS; **SLP**

Dykema, Clarice B 1320 North Lasalle Street, Chicago, IL 60610, **A**

Dykes, Sandy Frank 5716 Antioch Boulevard, Baton Rouge, LA 70817, (504) 766-6113, BS 77 Delta St Univ; MS 82 Univ Southern MS-Hattiesburg; 88–Sp-Lang Path, Louisiana Speech & Language Consultants Inc, **SLP**

Dykes, Mrs Sharon H 5716 Antioch Boulevard, Baton Rouge, LA 70817, (504) 292-7736, BS 73 Delta St Univ; MS 79 Univ Southern MS-Hattiesburg; Admin, LA Sp & Lang Consultants Inc, **SLP**

Dykstra, Steven J Box 157, Hardwick, MA 01037, (413) 283-3411, BA 75 SUNY - Center at Buffalo; MS 78 Univ of RI; 86–Dir-Indiv Svc Planning, Monson Devlp Cen, **SLP**

Dynneson, Philip L 5602 Tarry Terrace, Farmington, NM 87401, (505) 325-1741, BS 65 Dana Coll; MA 72 Univ of Northern CO; Aud, Farmington Pub Sch, **A**

Dyrhsen, Mrs Judith C 1380 Delone Drive, Yuba City, CA 95991, (916) 741-5110, BA 62 Coll of Wooster; 64–Sp-Lang Path, Sutter Co Sch Offi, **SLP**

Dysert, Mrs Denise H 11201 Pinewood Court, Richmond, VA 23233, (804) 737-9424, BS 75 Indiana Univ of PA; ME 80 Univ of VA - Charlottesville; Sp-Lang Path, Henrico Co Sch Sys, **SLP**

Dyslin, Mrs Margery M 28 Water Street, Mystic, CT 06355, (203) 536-4957, OB 51 Depauw Univ; MA 70 NY Univ; Sp/Lang Path, Groton Pub Sch Syst, **SLP**

Dyson, Dr Alice Tanner Speech 442 Dauer, University Of Florida, Gainesville, FL 32611, (904) 392-2041, BS 67 Eastern IL Univ; MS 72 Univ of HI - Manoa; PH 79 (Sp-Lang Path/Phonology) Univ of IL - Urbana; Asst Prof, U of FL Dept of Sp, **SLP**

Dzepina, Nada 253 Service Avenue, Sharon, PA 16146, (814) 432-3171, BS 72 Edinboro Univ of PA; MA 74 Case Western Reserve Univ; Audiologist, Polk Center, **A**

Dzewaltowski, Julie Ann 36 Lyman Avenue, Burlington, VT 05401, (802) 656-3970, BA 79 Middlebury Coll; MS 84 Univ of VT; Sp-Lang Path, Med Ctr Hosp of VT, **SLP**

Dziewior, Regina 14818 West 91st Place, Lenexa, KS 66215, (913) 281-8421, MA 76 Northern IL Univ - De Kalb; Aud, Bethany Medical Ctr, **A**

Dzikowski, Kimberly Sue 1215 Lafayette Parkway, Williamsport, PA 17701, (717) 523-1163, BS 84 Bloomsburg Univ of PA; MS 85 Bloomsburg Univ of PA; 85–Aud, Dr William B Bruce ENT, **A**

Dzikowski, Nancy Ann 780 N E Bayberry Lane, Jensen Beach, FL 34957, (904) 355-3403, BA 81 Univ of CA - Santa Barbara; MA 84 Univ of CT; Aud, Geri-Care Inc, **A**

Dzikowski, Richard John 6120 Miller, Detroit, MI 48211, (313) 362-4299, BS 81 Wayne St Univ; MS 85 Minot St Univ; **SLP**

Dzime-Assison, Mrs Venita Gragg 1918 Dana Drive, Adelphi, MD 20783, (301) 651-5018, BS 76 Howard Univ; MS 78 Gallaudet Coll; Aud, Mod Sec Sch for Deaf/Gallaudet, **A**

Dziwulski, Mrs Margery Slosek 15 Maine Avenue, Natick, MA 01760, (508) 788-0288, BS 78 Coll of Saint Rose; MA 79 SUNY - Coll at Geneseo; Sp-Lang Path, Accept Collaborative, **SLP**

Dzombar, Mrs Diane G 5751 Lake Lindero Drive, Agoura Hills, CA 91301-1413, (804) 733-7137, BS 73 WV Univ; MS 75 WV Univ; **SLP**

Dzuba, Selma S Hopkinson House #1616, Washington Square South, Philadelphia, PA 19106, (215) 923-9092, BS 56 Temple Univ; ME 60 Temple Univ; **SLP LM**

E

Eacho, Mrs Caroline Jones 2013 Virginia Dare Place, Raleigh, NC 27610, (919) 934-6854, BA 84 Univ of NC - Chapel Hill; MS 85 Univ of NC - Chapel Hill; 86–Sp-Lang Path, Johnston Co Bd of Educ, **SLP**

Eackles, Jay Donald 921 Seymour Court, Eden, NC 27288, (703) 638-3743, BS 82 James Madison Univ; ME 84 James Madison Univ; Aud, Martinsville Otolaryngology, **A**

Eades, Kristin G 116 Windy Lane #A, Michigan City, IN 46360, (219) 879-2411, BA 76 IN Univ - Bloomington; ME 77 IN Univ - Bloomington; Aud, Michigan City Area Schools, **A**

Eades, Malinda P 16500 Henderson Pass #1002, San Antonio, TX 78232, (512) 657-2881, BS 72 Murray St Univ; ME 76 Univ of Miami; Dept Hd/Stud Resources/SLP, N E ISD

Eades, Sheila N 421 Tupelo Drive, Naperville, IL 60540, (312) 357-8388, BS 80 IN St Univ - Terre Haute; MA 85 Ball St Univ; 85–Sp-Lang Path, AERO Spec Educ Coop, **SLP**

Eady, Mrs Lady Martin 3209 Joliet, Fort Smith, AR 72903, (501) 452-9461, BA 82 Univ of AR - Fayetteville; MS 83 Univ of AR - Fayetteville; Asst Dir-Gen Rehab, Ft Smith Rehab Hosp, **SLP**

Eagans, Karen K 1138 Creekside Lane, Corona, CA 91720, (714) 522-0150, OB 77 Univ of the Pacific; MS 82 Univ of AZ; Sp-Lang Path, La Palma Intercomm Hosp, **SLP**

Eagar, Miriam O 57 Muirfield Lane, Bridgewater, NJ 08807, (914) 962-2462, BA 68 Univ of FL; MA 72 CA St Univ - Northridge; Sp/Lang Path, Lakeland Sch Dist Westchester, **SLP**

Eagen, Mrs Marla L Anderson 2400 13th Avenue N W, Rochester, MN 55901, (507) 324-5786, BS 80 IA St Univ; MA 81 Northeast MO St Univ; Sp/Lang Path, Pine Island Pub Sch #255, **SLP**

Eagen, William H Community Hearing & Speech Ctr, 58 Meadowbrook Drive, Huntington Station, NY 11746, (516) 549-2327, BA 68 Hofstra Univ; MA 70 Hofstra Univ; Aud, Brentwood Publ Schs, **SLP A**

Eager-Kessel, Betsy L 214 Castleair Road, Kennesaw, GA 30144, (404) 928-0186, BS 74 SUNY - Center at Albany; MS 75 Adelphi Univ; 88–Sp-Lang Path, Private Practice, **SLP**

Eaker, Mrs Elisa Colasanto 5121 Hutchins Street, Winston-Salem, NC 27106, (919) 768-9090, BS 80 FL St Univ; MS 81 FL St Univ; 84–Sp-Lang Path, Speech Pathology Associates, **SLP**

Eakes-Frush, Mrs Wendy E 9712 Chaparral Court, Stockton, CA 95209, (209) 477-3979, BA 73 CA St Univ - Chico; MA 74 CA St Univ - Chico; Sp-Lang Path, Lincoln USD, **SLP**

Eakle, Mrs Mary Jo 9707 Dorset Lane, Eden Prairie, MN 55347, (612) 445-4884, BA 69 Univ of WI - Milwaukee; MS 74 Univ of WI - Milwaukee; Sp-Lang Path, Shakopee Pub Sch, **SLP**

Eamon, Diane W 2 Old Westfall Drive, Rochester, NY 14625, BA 77 Univ of AR - Fayetteville; MS 78 Rutger's St Univ - Douglas Coll; **SLP**

Eanes, Martha Robinson 425 Linville Road, Kernersville, NC 27284, (919) 785-0014, BA 78 Univ of NC - Greensboro; ME 85 Univ of NC - Greensboro; 80–Sp-Lang Path, Rockingham County Schs, **SLP**

Eannace, Mrs Mary E 3829 West 81st Place, Chicago, IL 60652, (312) 687-0900, BA 80 Saint Xavier Coll; MA 81 Western IL Univ; Sp/Lang Path, SW Cook Co Coop for Spec Ed, **SLP**

Eardley, Mary Dudek 3903 Kirkshire S E, Grand Rapids, MI 49508, (616) 247-7482, BS 80 Western MI Univ; MA 82 Northwestern Univ; SLP, Mary Freebed Hosp & Rehab Cen, **SLP**

Eareckson, Jane B 102 West 37th Street, Wilmington, DE 19802, (302) 428-2286, BA 72 Temple Univ; MA 81 Temple Univ; Sp-Lang Path, Med Ctr of DE, **SLP ACE**

Earl, Dr Dennis Charles 1349 Armstrong Avenue, Knoxville, TN 37917, (615) 521-8050, BA 79 Univ of AL-Tuscaloosa; MA 83 Univ of TN - Knoxville; PH 87 (Hrng & Sp Science) Univ of TN - Knoxville; Aud, Knoxville Otol & Facial Surg, **A**

Earl, Mrs Linda L 119 Cougar Drive, Mannford, OK 74044, (918) 865-2474, BS 79 OK St Univ; MS 82 Phillips Univ; Sp-Lang Path, Sand Springs P S, **SLP**

Earl, Dr Patricia Wojciak Box U64, UTMCK, 1924 Alcoa Highway, Knoxville, TN 37920, (615) 544-9569, BS 76 PA St Univ - Univ Park; MA 79 Univ of TN - Knoxville; PH 87 (Hrng & Sp Science) Univ of TN - Knoxville; 87–Aud, Univ of TN-Dept Aud-Sp Path, **A**

Earlabaugh, Mrs Susanne 3701 Seascape Drive, Huntington Beach, CA 92649, (714) 730-7381, BS 68 OH St Univ; MA 71 Univ of IL - Urbana; Sp/Lang Path, Tustin USD, **SLP**

Earle, Mrs Cindy Ann 18 Margaret Avenue, Grimsby, ON, Canada L3M 4S1, (416) 521-7951, BS 75 SD St Univ; MA 83 SUNY - Coll at Buffalo; Sp/Lang Path, Chedoke-McMaster Hosp, **SLP**

Earle, Cynthia B 131 McDowell Street, Asheville, NC 28801, (704) 254-3517, BA 77 Univ of NC - Greensboro; OM 79 Univ of SC - Columbia; 81–Dir of Aud, Asheville Head Neck & Ear Surgeons PA, **SLP A**

Earle, Dr Floyd E 911 Monticello Street, Greensboro, NC 27410, (919) 334-5939, BS 53 Kent St Univ; MA 59 Kent St Univ; PH 69 (NS) OH St Univ; Prof, Univ of NC, **SLP**

Earle, Dr Patty A 911 Monticello Street, Greensboro, NC 27410, (919) 294-0555, BA 52 Emerson Coll; MA 58 Kent St Univ; PH 77 (NS) Univ of NC - Greensboro; Dir of SLP Serv, Evergreens Nurs Home, **SLP**

Earley, Mrs Deborah Ann 416 Winston Drive, Norman, OK 73072-3832, (405) 271-7556, MS 82 Univ of OK - OK City; Aud, OK U Hlth Sciences Cen, **A**

Earley, Kenneth W 2214 Bridge Avenue, Northport, AL 35476-3950, (205) 987-2069, BS 75 Univ of Montevallo; ME 83 Univ of Montevallo; MS 76 Univ of Montevallo; Dir Sp & Ser Hrng, Riverchase Sp & Lang Clin, **SLP**

Earley, Marilyn H 4015 North Wappel Drive, Columbia, MO 65203, (314) 445-8293, BS 68 Univ of IA; MA 70 Univ of IA; Sp-Lang Path, Columbia PS, **SLP**

Earls, Mrs Nancy Loree 3908 Sides, Plainview, TX 79072, (806) 293-9980, BS 80 CO St Univ; MS 87 Fort Hays St Univ; 87–Sp-Lang Path, Honda Coop, **SLP**

Early, Elizabeth Ann 19545 Hickory Street, Milan, MI 48160, (313) 439-2568, BA 81 Univ of MI - Ann Arbor; MS 85 Univ of MI - Ann Arbor; **SLP**

Early, Patricia P O Box 1554, Dickinson, TX 77539, (713) 337-4501, BS 74 KS St Univ; MA 76 Univ of Houston - Univ Park; Dir Spec Ed, Dickinson Independent Sch Dist, **SLP**

Earnest, Dr Sue W 1770 Fort Stockton Drive, San Diego, CA 92103, (619) 296-6094, BA 28 San Diego St Univ; MA 38 Univ of Southern CA; PH 47 (NS) Univ of Southern CA; **SLP F LM**

Earnst, Mrs Elizabeth Ann/Holpit 20 Blandford Lane, Fairport, NY 14450, (716) 377-4660, BS 65 SUNY - Coll at Geneseo; MA 77 Nazareth Coll of Rochester; **SLP**

Earp, Christine Joan 3028 Golden Eagle, Modesto, CA 95356-0247, (417) 926-4829, **SLP**

Earp, Rebecca J 6026 Chattanoga Drive, Baton Rouge, LA 70817, (504) 292-3922, **SLP**

Easler, Rochelle L 1817 Castle Court, Flower Mound, TX 75028, (214) 462-1013, BS 80 TX Woman's Univ; MA 84 TX Woman's Univ; Sp-Lang Path, Coppell ISD, **SLP**

Easley, Mrs Cynthia Renee 815 Pinewood Cove, Wynne, AR 72396, (501) 238-2636, BS 82 AR St Univ; MS 84 AR St Univ; 85–Sp-Lang Path, Wynne PS, **SLP**

Easley, Kristin Mueller St Luke's Hospital Of Kansas City, 44th & Wornall Road, Kansas City, MO 64111, (816) 932-3832, MA 87 Univ of KS; Sp-Lang Path, St Luke's Hosp, **SLP**

Eason, Mrs Barbara D 1170 Heather Wood Court, Marietta, GA 30062, (404) 971-7004, BS 74 FL St Univ; MS 75 FL St Univ; Sp-Lang Path, Private Practice, **SLP**

Eason-Sons, Virginia Alberta 1109 Monroe Avenue, Charleston, IL 61920, (217) 348-0682, BS 85 Eastern IL Univ; MS 86 Eastern IL Univ; SLP, Sullivan Community Schools, **SLP**

Easterbrook, Marylou Harrington 34054 N Hampshire, Livonia, MI 48154, (313) 467-4260, MA; SLP, Annapolis Hospital, **SLP**

Easterling, Caryn S C 344 Evergreen Lane, Pewaukee, WI 53072, (414) 257-6720, BS 72 Marquette Univ; MS 75 Marquette Univ; Sp-Lang Path, Curative Rehab Cen/Mil Co Hosp, **SLP**

Easterling, Mrs Cathleen Corbin 236 Shasta Drive, Pittsburgh, PA 15239-2921, (412) 733-2804, BS 85 Miami Univ - Oxford; MS 86 Clarion Univ of PA; 88–Sp-Lang Path, Eye & Ear Hosp of Pittsburgh, **SLP**

Eastes, Mrs Dawn Elizabeth 9016 Chestnut Ridge Road, Fairfax Station, VA 22039, (703) 690-8507, BS 76 Western MI Univ; MA 81 Western MI Univ; 83–Special Agent, FBI, **SLP**

Eastes, Lorene Ellen 19116 Killoch Place, Northridge, CA 91326, (818) 368-8721, BS 81 Purdue Univ - West Lafayette; BA 82 Purdue Univ - West Lafayette; MA 84 CA St Univ - Northridge; Sp-Lang Path, Childrens Hosp of LA, **SLP**

Eastham, Mrs Penelope L P O Box 402, Barker, TX 77413, (713) 492-1502, BS 67 TX Tech Univ; MS 69 TX Tech Univ; Sp/Lang Path, Tulsa Cty Co Hlth Dept, **SLP**

Eastham, Sharon L 3306 Lancelot, Dallas, TX 75229, **SLP**

Eastin, Debra P 1413 West Church, Champaign, IL 61821, (217) 384-3616, MS 76 Univ of IL - Urbana; Sp-Lang Path, Urbana Sch Dist #116, **SLP**

Eastin, Janet S 708 Morning Glory Lane, Bedford, TX 76021, (817) 485-4415, BA 71 Baylor Univ; MA 73 Univ of FL; Sp-Lang Path, All Saints Episcopal Hosp, **SLP**

Eastman, Kimble Manley 4317 Barcelona Street, Tampa, FL 33629, (813) 839-4677, BS 85 Auburn Univ - Auburn; OM 86 Auburn Univ - Auburn; 88–Sp-Lang Path, Tampa Gen Rehab Ctr, **SLP**

Eastman, Sheila J 3100 Tyndale Avenue, Baltimore, MD 21214, (301) 444-4103, BA 72 Rutger's St Univ - Douglas Coll; MS 79 Loyola Coll; **SLP**

Easton, Mrs Celia Elaine Route 2 Box 68, Natchez, MS 39120, (601) 442-0212, BS 81 Univ Southern MS-Hattiesburg; MS 83 Univ Southern MS-Hattiesburg; **SLP**

Easton, Mrs Leslie Ann Route 4 Box 242-D, Charlottesville, VA 22901, (804) 978-2845

Easton, Mrs Patricia Lee 101 Andover Lane, Aberdeen, NJ 07747, (201) 257-7715, BA 80 Univ of RI; MS 82 Univ of RI; Sp-Lang Path, Middlesex Co Voc Tech Hs, **SLP**

Easton, Mrs Sally Jo 19-9 Queens Way, Camillus, NY 13031, MA 82 CA St Univ - Fresno; Sp-Lang-Hrng Spec, Fresno USD, **SLP**

Eaton, Andrea Sinkking 143 Casa Loma Circle, Georgetown, TX 78628, (512) 926-6635, BA 73 Univ of LA Verne; MS 75 Univ of Redlands; 81–Sp-Lang Path, Austin ISD, **SLP**

Eaton, Gail G P O Box 70, Corrales, NM 87048, (505) 883-9116, BA 77 Univ of CA - Santa Barbara; MS 80 Univ of NM; Sp-Lang Path, Albuquerque Public Schools, **SLP**

Eaton, Helen F 5844 Beacon Street, Pittsburgh, PA 15217, (412) 421-5068, BA 47 Carnegie-Mellon Univ; MA 71 Univ of Pittsburgh - Pittsburgh; Sp-Lang Path, Private Practice, **SLP**

Eaton, Janice Kay 410 East Ridge Street, Marquette, MI 49855, (906) 225-1515, BS 81 Northern MI Univ; MA 83 Northern MI Univ; Sp-Lang Path, Marquette County Health Svcs, **SLP**

Eaton, Mrs Jennifer Ann 2771 Pine Trace Drive, Maumee, OH 43537, (419) 865-4887, BS 86 OH Univ - Athens; MA 87 OH Univ - Athens; 88–Sp-Lang Path, Anne Grady Center, **SLP**

Eaton, Mrs Joyce P 1126 Geneva Street, Livermore, CA 94550, (415) 447-9249, BA 64 San Jose St Univ; **SLP**

Eaton, Karen R 1411 St Claire, Ashland, WI 54806, (715) 682-4563, BA 80 Univ of WI - Eau Claire; MS 81 Univ of WI - Eau Claire; Sp/Lang Path, River Ridge Rehab Inc, **SLP**

Eaton, Mrs Mary A 39 Frederick Place, Delmar, NY 12054-2430, (518) 439-0421, BA 71 SUNY - Center at Albany; MS 72 SUNY - Center at Albany; Sp-Lang Path, Sctd-Alby-Scho Cos Coop Ed Ser, **SLP**

Eaton, Sarah Butler 15 River Ridge, Little Rock, AR 72207, (501) 569-3155, BA 61 Baylor Univ; MA 66 TX Woman's Univ; Cl Superv Instructor, Un Ark/Little Rock, **SLP**

Eaton, Mrs Susan Ann 727 Bellis, Newport Beach, CA 92660, (714) 558-5676, BA 65 IN Univ - Bloomington; OM 67 IN Univ - Bloomington; Teacher of Special Day Class, Santa Ana USD, **SLP**

Eaves, Mrs Constance T 5660 S Lakeshore #401, Shreveport, LA 71119, (205) 431-3423, BS 82 Univ of South AL; MS 83 Univ Southern MS-Hattiesburg; Sp/Lang Path, **SLP**

Eaves, Emma L K P O Box 644, Louisville, MS 39339, (601) 773-7962, MS 80 LA St Univ - Baton Rouge; Sp-Lang Path, Private Practice, **SLP**

Ebara, Yukie 205 West 6th Street Box 1693, Roswell, NM 88201, (505) 622-4327, ME 74 TX Tech Univ; MS 77 TX Tech Univ; Aud, Yukie Ebara Hearing Ctr, **A**

Ebaugh, Mrs Elaine Dinst 3611 8th Street North, St Petersburg, FL 33704, (703) 753-8941, BS 81 James Madison Univ; MS 82 James Madison Univ; Sp-Lang Path, Mediplex Rehab-Bradenton, **SLP ACE**

Ebbert, Mrs Janet J 411 Hillcrest Avenue, State College, PA 16801, (412) 247-4801, BS 63 PA St Univ - Univ Park; MS 68 Univ of Pittsburgh - Pittsburgh; **SLP**

Ebbeskotte, Karen A R R 3 Rolling Stone 10, Morganfield, KY 42437, (502) 389-3380, BS 70 IN St Univ - Terre Haute; MA 76 Ball St Univ; Sp-Lang Path, Private Practice, **SLP**

Ebeling, Ann E S 4716 West 66th Terrace, Prairie Village, KS 66208, (913) 831-1476, MA 78 Univ of Tulsa; Sp/Lang Path, Shawnee Mission Pub Sch Dist, **SLP**

Eber, Francine L 208 Miller Avenue, Mill Valley, CA 94941, BA 76 San Francisco St Univ; MS 78 San Francisco St Univ; Sp-Lang-Hrng Spec, Berkeley USD, **SLP**

Eberhardt, Nancy B 502 West Noyes Avenue, Arlington Heights, IL 60005, (312) 424-5236, BS 76 Univ of IL - Urbana; MA 79 Northern IL Univ - De Kalb; Sp/Lang Path, Aero Spec Ed Coop, **SLP**

Eberhart, John L 716 South New Street, West Chester, PA 19382, (215) 436-3447, BS 60 Bloomsburg Univ of PA; MA 64 Syracuse Univ; Ch/Dept of Comm Dis, W Chester Univ, **SLP A**

Eberle, Rebecca Dawn 935 Birnam Woods Trail, Indianapolis, IN 46280, (317) 843-0120, BA 82 IN Univ - Bloomington; MA 84 IN Univ - Bloomington; Sp-Lang Path, Cen Neuropsychological Rehab, **SLP**

Eberle-Brinson, Jane Anne 2209 Glenn Drive, Carson City, NV 89701, (702) 789-0341, BA 82 Univ of Redlands; MS 85 Univ of NV - Reno; 86–Sp-Lang Path, Reno Spec Children's Cl, **SLP**

Eberlein, Nancy J 4719 Jackson #17, Riverside, CA 92503-3713, (714) 788-3208, BA 74 CA St Univ - Fullerton; MA 78 CA St Univ - Fullerton; Sp-Lang Path, Riverside Community Hospital, **SLP**

Eberline, Linda Jean 57 St Luke Court, Danville, CA 94526, (415) 820-6815, BA 58 Univ of IA; MA 63 TX Woman's Univ; Sp-Lang Path, San Ramon Valley USD, **SLP**

Eberly, Mrs Teresa Yengich 7486 South Kendall Blvd, Littleton, CO 80123, (303) 979-1979, BA 75 Univ of Northern CO; MA 76 Univ of Northern CO; Sp-Lang Path, Private Practice, **SLP**

Ebersole, Amy K 15 Keswick Street #3, Boston, MA 02215, (617) 828-2440, BA 81 AZ St Univ; ME 83 Boston Coll; MS 86 Emerson Coll; Sp-Lang Path, MA Hosp Schl, **SLP**

Ebert, Douglas Dwight 6104 18th Street North, St Cloud, MN 56303, (612) 255-1039, MS 83 Moorhead St Univ; Sp-Lang Path, St Cloud Hospital, **SLP**

Ebert, Mrs Pricilla R 105 Forest Drive, Pittsburgh, PA 15238, (412) 963-9826, BS 55 Cornell Univ; MS 68 Univ of Pittsburgh - Pittsburgh; Sp-Lang Path, Private Practice, **SLP**

Eblen, Linda E The Voice Resource, 2611 NE 125th Suite 116, Seattle, WA 98125, (206) 361-4811, BA 67 Univ of GA; MA 69 Univ of CT; Sp-Lang Path, The Voice Resource, **SLP**

Eblen, Roy E 202 North Genevieve, Cedar Falls, IA 50613, (319) 266-8408, BA 41 Williams Coll; MA 44 Wichita St Univ; PH 61 (Sp Path) Univ of IA; Prof Emeritus SLP, U of N IA, **SLP F LM**

Ebner, Mary Jo 17 Winston Place, Rochester, NY 14607, (716) 271-0680, OB 56 Univ of PA; BA 51 Brown Univ; MS 73 Univ of RI; Audiologist, Hrng-Spch Center of Rochester, **A**

Eby, Mrs Janice Read 211 South Ruth Street, Maryville, TN 37801, (615) 546-9221, BA 65 Maryville Coll; MA 81 Univ of TN - Knoxville; 84–Sp-Lang Path, TN Dept of Health & Envir, **A**

Eccleston, Vincent 1416 DE Rose Way, San Jose, CA 95126, (408) 298-8680, BA 72 San Diego St Univ; MS 82 Portland St Univ; 85–Sp/Lang Path, Private Practice, **SLP ACE**

Echelbarger, Clara Dee P O Box 382, Lone Pine, CA 93545, (619) 876-4695, MA 84 CA St Univ - Fullerton; Sp-Lang Path, Private Practice, **SLP**

Echols-Chambers, Lou 2301 Branch Road, Champaign, IL 61821, (217) 337-3130, BA 76 TX Tech Univ; MS 81 Purdue Univ - West Lafayette; Aud, Carle Clinic Assoc, **A**

Eckalbar, Mrs Anne Marie 1039 Marchetti Court, Chico, CA 95926, (916) 343-6791, **SLP**

Eckardt, Judith Borchardt 3409 Chelmsford Drive, Spring Grove, IL 60081, (312) 367-4300, BS 63 Univ of WI - Madison; MS 64 Univ of WI - Madison; Sp/Lang Path, Lake-McHenry Reg Prog, **SLP**

Eckberg MD, Dr Theodore J 12943 Addison Street, Sherman Oaks, CA 91403, MD 58 (NS) Univ of WI - Madison; Chief Otolaryngology, S California Permanente Med Gr

Eckel, Mrs Roberta H 1230 North Palm Avenue, Upland, CA 91786, (818) 967-2841, BA 59 Univ of CA - Santa Barbara; MA 70 Univ of LA Verne; 78–SLP, Los Ang Co Supt of Sch, **SLP**

Eckelmann, Dorathy c/o Harriett J Eckelmann, 1223 Cousin, Cape Girardeau, MO 63701, PH (NS); **SLP F LM**

Eckendorf, Pamela S RR 2 Box 106, Kennedy, NY 14747, (716) 483-4454, BS 80 SUNY - Coll at Fredonia; MA 81 Bowling Green St Univ; Sp-Lang Path, Jamestown PS Sys, **SLP**

Eckenrode, Maribeth Vogel VA Medical Center 566/126, Fort Howard, MD 21052, (301) 687-8852, BA 77 Univ of IA; MA 79 Univ of IA; Aud, VA Med Cen, **A**

Eckerle, Mrs Andrea Rauso 3 Andover Road #4, Yonkers, NY 10710, (914) 337-6294, BS 84 Mercy Coll; MA 87 CUNY - Hunter Coll; 87–Sp-Lang Path, These Our Treasures Inc, **SLP**

Eckert, Anne Marie 2 Quail Drive, Middletown, NJ 07748, (201) 321-7066, BA 78 Montclair St Coll; MA 79 Ball St Univ; 87–Asst Dir Aud, JFK Med Ctr, **A**

Eckert, Celeste F 2521 Whaley Avenue, Pensacola, FL 32503, (904) 432-6121, BS 79 0975; MS 81 Univ of Saskatchewan - Sask; **SLP**

Eckert, Mrs Jill Koch 9534 Woodcrest Road, Pittsburgh, PA 15237, (412) 366-8944, BS 80 Bloomsburg Univ of PA; MS 81 Bloomsburg Univ of PA; Sp-Lang Path, Laughlin Childrens Center, **SLP**

Eckert, Joan A 526 South High Street, Denver, CO 80209-4525, (303) 778-7209, BS 77 CO St Univ; MA 79 Memphis St Univ; President, Multi-Disciplinary Services, **SLP**

Eckhardt, Jenny L Northeast High School, 1717 54th Avenue North, St Petersburg, FL 33714, (813) 864-1909, MS 88 Adelphi Univ; 88–Sp-Lang Path, Pinellas County Sch Bd

Eckhardt, Mrs Lori Rural Route 2, Cedar Hills West, Metamora, IL 61548, MS 84 Eastern IL Univ; Sp-Lang Path, VA, **SLP**

Eckhardt, Virginia Lynne 1424 Kanawha Boulevard #15, Charleston, WV 25301, (304) 343-4371, BS 85 Univ of IA; MA 87 Western MI Univ; 87–Aud, EENT Phys & Surgeons of Charleston, **A**

Eckles, Dennis Edward Rd Box 491, Tobyhanna, PA 18466, (717) 676-9582, BA 76 Ithaca Coll; MS 83 Univ of NV - Reno; Sp-Lang Path, No Warren Regional HS, **SLP**

Eckles, Julie Beth 1324 Vilas Avenue #1, Madison, WI 53715, (608) 255-4689, BA 81 Coll of Wooster; MA 86 Univ of Pittsburgh - Pittsburgh; 87–Sp-Lang Path, Hillhaven Rehab Svcs, **SLP**

Ecklund, Sally Kay 2400 Rhode Island North, Apartment 502, Golden Valley, MN 55427, (612) 347-4332, BS 81 Univ of MN - Minneap-St Paul; MA 84 Univ of MN - Minneap-St Paul; Sp-Lang Path, Metropolitan Med Ctr, **SLP**

Eckstein, Karen Lind 923 Sedgefield Drive, Apt #56, Shelby, NC 28150, BS 83 Longwood Coll; ME 86 Univ of VA - Charlottesville; SLP, Cleveland Home Health Agency, **SLP**

Eckstrom, Carol Ann R R 2 Box 310, Wausa, NE 68786, BS 82 Univ of NE - Lincoln; MS 84 Univ of NE - Lincoln; 85–Sp-Lang Path, Bellevue Public Schools, **SLP**

Eckwall, Randy S 11 Putnam Road, Hyde Park, NY 12538-2331, (914) 229-6041, BS 80 SUNY - Coll at New Paltz; MS 81 IN St Univ - Terre Haute; 86–Sp-Lang Path, Arlington Cen Schl Dstr, **SLP**

Economos, Dorian L 1128 Genesee N E, Warren, OH 44483, (216) 372-6239, BA 84 Univ of Pittsburgh - Pittsburgh; 86–Dir of Aud, Warren Gen Hosp, **A**

Economou, Helen M 505 Sheridan Road, Winnetka, IL 60093, BS; **SLP LM**

Ecung, Mrs Debra Ford 2679 Menlo Avenue, Los Angeles, CA 90007, (213) 731-0019, **SLP**

Edahl, Kristine C 3007 Mountain View Avenue, Schofield, WI 54476, (715) 848-1406, BA 75 Valparaiso Univ; MA 78 Univ of IA; Sp-Lang Path, Vna Home Health Inc, **SLP**

Edbauer, Margaret M 1697 Amherst Street, Buffalo, NY 14214, (716) 874-5400, OB 76 SUNY - Coll at Buffalo; MS 77 Murray St Univ; Sp-Lang Path, Vna Buffalo NY, **SLP**

Edberg, Judith A Douglas Parker Rehabilitation Centre, Tower Road, New Town, Hobart, Tasmania, Australia, (002) 381812, BS 75 Univ of WI - Stevens Point; MS 77 Univ of WI - Whitewater; 88–Sp-Lang Path, Douglas Parker Rehab Centre, **SLP**

Eddington, Mrs Judith Anne 707 Belair, Benton, AR 72015, (501) 847-3506, MA 71 Univ of OR; 86–Sp-Lang Path, State of Arkansas, **SLP**

Eddins, Carolyn L 3300 SW 25th Terrace, Miami, FL 33133, (305) 549-6397, BA 76 Univ of NC - Chapel Hill; MS 85 Univ of NC - Chapel Hill; 86–Sp-Lang Path, **SLP**

Eddy, Debra S 1501 Merchantville Avenue, Pennsauken, NJ 08110, (609) 486-4874, BA 83 Univ of DE; MA 84 Trenton St Coll; Sp-Lang Path, Waterford Pub Schs, **SLP**

Eddy-Lasich, Mrs Mary Ellen 8856 East Gull Lake Road, Augusta, MI 49012, (616) 731-2167, BA 77 MI St Univ; MA 79 Central MI Univ; Aud, **A**

Edelberg, Mrs Ann Rita 1935 West Hayward Avenue, Phoenix, AZ 85021, (602) 255-3448, BS 45 Washington Univ; ME 63 Syracuse Univ; Sp-Lang Superv, Phoenix Day Sch for Deaf, **SLP**

Edelen, Kathleen Gail 7100 Croom Station Road, Upper Marlboro, MD 20772, (301) 952-0615, BA 83 Univ of MD - College Park; MS 84 James Madison Univ; **SLP**

Edelman, Dr Florence 645 Water Street, New York, NY 10002, (212) 481-4464, BA 54 CUNY - Brooklyn Coll; MA 57 CUNY - Brooklyn Coll; PH 70 (Sp Path) NY Univ; Assoc Prof/Clin Dir, Hunter Coll Cuny, **SLP A**

Edelson, Martha 644 Funston, San Francisco, CA 94118, (415) 664-4646, BS 74 Univ of IL - Urbana; MS 76 Bradley Univ; Sp-Lang Path, Scot Rite I/Chldhd Aphasia, **SLP**

Edelstein, Dr Beatrice D 518 Sharon Gardens Court, Woodbridge, NJ 07095, (609) 292-7604, BA 71 OH St Univ; MA 72 Seton Hall Univ; PH 78 (NS) OH St Univ; Consult In Hearing Impair, NJ St Dept of Ed, **SLP**

Edelstein, Brenda F 69 Mullen Drive, Thornhill, ON, Canada L4J 2T6, (416) 425-6220, OM 78 Univ of Toronto - Ontario; 85–Sp-Lang Path, Hugh MacMillian Med Ctr, **SLP**

Edelstein, Esther K 15575 George Washington, Southfield, MI 48075, (313) 494-9721, BA 76 MI St Univ; MA 77 Eastern MI Univ; Sp/Lang Path, Rehab I of Chicago, **SLP**

Edelstein, Mrs Geraldine Ozark 307 North Granby Street, Richmond, VA 23220, (804) 355-5292, BS 76 Edinboro Univ of PA; MS 81 VA Commonwealth Univ; 81–Special Educ Spec, Henrico County PS

Edelstein, Mrs Holly G 1301 Powhatan Trail, Frankfort, KY 40601, (502) 695-3773, MA 80 Univ of KY; Sp-Lang Path, Franklin Co Bd of Ed, **SLP**

Edelstein, Mrs Jacqueline L 300 Winthrop Road, Teaneck, NJ 07666, (201) 977-6613, BA 51 Roosevelt Univ; MS 70 Adelphi Univ; Sp-Lang Path, Barnert Mem Hosp Cen, **SLP**

Edelstein, Karen Feldman 3900 Lake Shore Drive #8-C, Chicago, IL 60613-3464, (612) 627-2702, BS 79 Univ of WI - Madison; MA 82 NY Univ; **SLP**

Edelstein, Mrs Leah L 23 Stevens Drive, Voorhees, NJ 08043, (609) 435-6785, BA 76 CUNY - Brooklyn Coll; MS 79 Rutgers St Univ -N Brunswick; **SLP**

Edenfield, Nikki Anita Route 2 Box 309, Cobbtown, GA 30420, (912) 489-8704, OB 82 Univ of GA; ME 84 Armstrong St Coll; **SLP**

Edens, Kelly A 226-A Columbia Avenue, Lake Waccamaw, NC 28450, (919) 646-3633, BS 76 Miami Univ - Oxford; ME 80 Western Carolina Univ; Sp-Lang Path, Columbus Co Home Hlth, **SLP**

Edens, Mrs Linda Ann 24-A Kingery Quarter #202, Hinsdale, IL 60521, (312) 887-8720, BA 84 Augustana Coll; MA 85 Western MI Univ; Sp-Lang Path, Joliet PS, **SLP**

Ederer, Mrs Tami Duncan 1628 Westminster Drive, Naperville, IL 60540, (312) 357-7737, BA 81 Univ of the Pacific; MA 82 Univ of the Pacific; Sp-Lang Path, **SLP**

Edgar, Mrs Judith Ann 1814 Chestnut Boulevard, Cuyahoga Falls, OH 44223, (216) 929-5697, BS 65 Indiana Univ of PA; MA 69 Temple Univ-Tyler Sch of Art; Sp-Lang Path, Private Practice, **SLP**

Edgar, Julia D 7225 Adams, Forest Park, IL 60130, (312) 908-3341, BA 80 Valparaiso Univ; MA 82 Univ of KS; Clin Supvr, Rehab Institute of Chicago, **SLP**

Edgar, Mrs Nancy R 19336 Hinsdale, Torrance, CA 90503, BA 63 Alma Coll; MA 67 Stanford Univ; Aud, Bay Shores Med Group, **A**

Edgecomb, Pamela Ward 14 Lemay Avenue, Lewiston, ME 04240, (207) 795-2740, BS 82 Univ of ME - Farmington; MA 85 Univ of ME - Orono; 88–Dir of Sp-Lang Path, Central Maine Med Ctr, **SLP**

Edgemon, Mrs Jenny C 410 East Henry Street, Spartanburg, SC 29302, (803) 583-7644, MS 84 Univ of South FL; Aud, Aud Assoc, **A**

Edgerly, Barbara 1306 Ruth Avenue, Cuyahoga Falls, OH 44221, (216) 928-3750, BA 71 Univ of Akron; MA 72 Bowling Green St Univ; Sp-Lang Path, Private Practice, **SLP**

Edgerly, Mrs Gayle A R R 4 Box 62, Logansport, IN 46947, (219) 722-4141, BS 77 Purdue Univ - West Lafayette; MA 78 Univ of IL - Urbana; Aud, Logansport State Hosp, **A**

Edgerton, Judith P 2017 Huntington Circle, Fort Collins, CO 80526, (303) 482-7420, BS 70 CO St Univ; MA 76 Univ of Northern CO; Sp-Lang Path, Poudre R-1 Sch Dist, **SLP**

Edgerton, Katharine M P O Box 2122, Chino, CA 91708, (818) 333-2201, BA 76 Humboldt St Univ; MA 77 Humboldt St Univ; Sp-Lang Path, Hacienda La Puente USD, **SLP**

Edgeworth, Mrs Ann Blazek 1327 Greenwood Avenue, Deerfield, IL 60015, (312) 945-1225, BS 83 Marquette Univ; MA 84 Northwestern Univ; 86–Sp-Lang Path, Private Practice, **SLP**

Edgley, Mrs Edna B 6230 St Anne Forest, Houston, TX 77088, (713) 462-4516, BS 71 Univ of Houston - Univ Park; MA 73 Univ of Houston - Univ Park; Sp-Lang Path, Cypress ISD, **SLP**

Edgmon, Donna M 2700 American Street, Suite D, Springdale, AR 72764, (501) 751-5504, BA 75 Univ of AR - Fayetteville; MA 80 Univ of AR - Fayetteville; 82–Sp-Lang Path, Private Practice, **SLP**

Edgren, Mrs Dawn S P O Box 628, El Granada, CA 94018, (415) 324-0186, BA 72 Univ of CA - Santa Barbara; MA 74 San Diego St Univ; 75–Sp-Lang Path, Menlo Park City Sch Dist, **SLP**

Edick, Mrs Lisa Irby 10 NE Plantation Road #101, Stuart, FL 34996, (407) 225-3120, BS 78 Univ of TX - Austin; MS 80 Univ of TX - Dallas; 88, Private Practice, **SLP**

Edie, Mrs Patricia D 4700 Laudun Street, Metairie, LA 70006, (504) 443-1603, BA 71 Southeastern LA Univ; ME 78 Tulane Univ; Sp-Lang Path, Jefferson Parish Sch Bd, **SLP**

Ediger, Dr Loyal D 2055 West 29th, Eugene, OR 97405, (503) 485-8521, BA 63 Tabor Coll; MS 66 Univ of UT; PH 69 (Aud) Univ of UT; Aud, Eugene Hrng & Sp Cen, **A**

Edinburg, Evelyn Jane 234 South 44th Street, Philadelphia, PA 19104, BA 71 Univ of PA; MA 81 Temple Univ; 85–Sp-Lang Path, Thomas Jefferson Univ Hosp, **SLP**

Edington, Mrs Dian N 12101 Coyle Road, Fort Myers, FL 33905, (813) 693-2473, BS 77 Univ of FL; MS 79 Auburn Univ - Auburn; Sp-Lang Path, Lee Co School Bd, **SLP ACE**

Edler, Elaine I 715 Harvard Road, Burbank, CA 91501, **SLP**

Edler, Mrs Marita 4634 West North Street, Muncie, IN 47304, (317) 282-1101, BS 73 IN Univ - Bloomington; MA 74 IN Univ - Bloomington; 79–Office Mgr, Robert W Edler MD Pc, **SLP**

Edley, Carol D 42-A Prospect Street, Ridgefield, CT 06877, (203) 323-1681, BA 71 Phillips Univ; MS 73 Washington Univ; Sp-Lang Path, Greenwich Hosp Assoc, **SLP**

Edlin, Mrs Vicki M 3316 Hunsinger Lane, Louisville, KY 40220, (502) 451-3997, BS 78 Murray St Univ; MS 80 Univ of Louisville; 80–Sp/Lang Path, Easter Seal Hrng & Sp Cen, **SLP**

Edly, Linda Marie 60 Watervliet Avenue, Dayton, OH 45420, (513) 226-7877, MA 85 Miami Univ - Oxford; 85–Sp-Lang Path, Aud & Sp Assoc, **SLP**

Edmands, Mrs Judith D Kids Connection, 515 Upper Mill Heights, Salina, KS 67401, (913) 825-7664, MA 64 KS St Univ; Sp-Lang Path, Kids Connection USD 305, **SLP**

Edmiston, Karen P 1900 Fine Gold Court, Gold River, CA 95670-3049, **SLP**

Edmond, Mary Beth 3843 Red Bud Lane, Clarkston, MI 48016, (313) 762-2362, BS 84 Central MI Univ; MA 86 Eastern MI Univ; SLP, Mc Laren Gen Hosp, **SLP**

Edmonds, Celestina 9407 Darcy Place, Upper Marlboro, MD 20772, (301) 469-1026, BS 78 Howard Univ; MA 79 George Washington Univ; Sp/Lang Path, Montgomery Co Pub Sch, **SLP**

Edmonds, Henriette 8830 Piney Branch Road, Apartment 405, Silver Spring, MD 20903, **SLP**

Edmonds, Mrs Kaye Louise 1933 North Bowman Avenue, Apartment E, Danville, IL 61832, (217) 443-6557, OB 57 OH Univ - Athens; MA 83 Univ of IL - Urbana; Sp-Lang Path, Danville Comm Cons Sch DIST118, **SLP ACE**

Edmonds, Priscilla E 1838 Auburndale Avenue, Chattanooga, TN 37405, (404) 226-4623, OM 85 Auburn Univ - Auburn; **SLP**

Edmonds, Mrs Rebecca L Route 1 Box 155, Woodlawn, VA 24381, (703) 228-5411, BS 81 James Madison Univ; ME 82 James Madison Univ; Aud, Wythe Co Pub Sch, **A**

Edmonds, Mrs Robin Pennell 536 Northwest 40th Street, Oklahoma City, OK 73118, (405) 521-9860, BS 77 Univ of OK - Norman; MS 79 Univ of OK Medical Center; Sp-Lang Path, Private Practice, **SLP**

Edmonds, Vivian Kaita 2903 Calle DE La Mesa, Pleasanton, CA 94566, (916) 454-8354, BA 73 Univ of CA - Santa Barbara; MA 85 CA St Univ - Sacramento; Sp-Lang Path, Sacramento City USD, **SLP**

Edmonson, Mrs Terry Lynn 4512PROVIDENCE Place, New Orleans, LA 70126, (504) 283-0542, BA 81 Towson St Univ; MS 84 TX Tech Univ; Sp-Lang Path, Jefferson Parish Schools, **SLP**

Edmund, Mrs Elizabeth George 5550 N E Kincaid Road, Topeka, KS 66617, (913) 288-2041, BS 42 Univ of MO - Columbia; MS 68 Fort Hays St Univ; **LM**

Edris, Capt Robert W 300 Botanical Drive, Belleville, IL 62221, (618) 256-7546, BA 70 Catawba Coll; ME 72 Univ of NC - Greensboro; Chief/Aud Ser, U S Air Force, **A**

Edsall, Deborah Gail 155 Rosebury Drive #44, Encinitas, CA 92024, (619) 758-1620, **SLP**

Edscorn, Jane F 2113 Englewood Street, Kannapolis, NC 28081, (704) 933-4793, BA 79 Salem St Coll; MA 81 Univ of TN - Knoxville; Sp/Lang Path, Hogan Reg Cen, **SLP**

Eduardo, JoAnn L 137 Old Farm Road, South Windsor, CT 06074, MA 82 SUNY - Coll at Geneseo; BS 81 SUNY - Coll at Brockport; **SLP**

Edvardsson, Kerstin B 115 West Broadway, New York, NY 10013, (212) 488-1644, BS 76 Univ of WI - Madison; MA 80 Northwestern Univ; 88–Coord, Pace Univ Sp Hrng Ctr, **SLP**

Edward, Donna Marie 779 Rolling View Drive, Annapolis, MD 21401, (301) 757-4748

Edwards, Mrs Anne Bruzzese 4018 Old Mill Cove Trail E, Jacksonville, FL 32211, (904) 390-2075, MA 75 Univ of AL- Tuscaloosa; BA 73 Univ of AL- Tuscaloosa; MA 82 Univ of North FL; Diag Resources Asst, Duval County School Board, **SLP**

Edwards, Barbara B 3737 Moraga Avenue #105, San Diego, CA 92117, (619) 483-2986, BA 72 Univ of MO - KS City; MA 75 Northwestern Univ; 86–Dir Sp-Lang Path, W Coast Sp Lang Cognitive Ctr, **SLP**

Edwards, Mrs Barbara C 1309 Krise Circle, Lynchburg, VA 24503, (804) 522-4520, BS 63 Univ Southern MS-Hattiesburg; MS 66 Univ Southern MS-Hattiesburg; Sp-Lang Path, Ctrl VA Sp & Hrng Cen, Inc, **SLP ACE**

Edwards, Mrs Beverly A 14719 Englewood, Allen Park, MI 48101, (313) 381-4686, BS 77 Eastern MI Univ; MA 78 Eastern MI Univ; 87–Sp-Lang Path, Annapolis Hosp, **SLP**

Edwards, Brian W 7925-A North Oracle, Box 358, Tucson, AZ 85704, (602) 742-5171, BS 71 Eastern MI Univ; MA 72 Eastern MI Univ; Sp-Lang Path, Carondelet Health Svcs, **SLP**

Edwards, Bruce M Geo M Iwanow Hearing Aid Centers, 17800 East Eight Mile Road, Harper Woods, MI 48225, (313) 372-9200, BS 77 Eastern MI Univ; MA 80 Central MI Univ; Dir of Aud, G Iwanow Hearing Aid Centers, **A**

Edwards, Carolyn Anne 83 Watson Avenue, Toronto, ON, Canada M6S 4E2, (416) 346-4745, BS 75 Univ of Western Ontario; MA 76 Univ of Western Ontario; 88–Aud, Private Practice, **A**

Edwards, Mrs Cathleen Pew 1051 Belfast Lane, Ventura, CA 93001, (805) 643-9831, BS 83 Univ of OR; **SLP**

Edwards, Mrs Claudette Route 2 Box 105, Richton, MS 39476, (601) 788-6975, BS 81 Univ Southern MS-Hattiesburg; MS 82 Univ Southern MS-Hattiesburg; Sp-Lang Path, Richton Separate Sch Dist, **SLP**

Edwards, Mrs Colette M 3809 Parkwood Drive, Greensboro, NC 27403, (919) 299-0018, BS 76 Univ of NC - Greensboro; MA 72 Univ of TN - Knoxville; SLP, Private Practice, **SLP**

Edwards, Mrs Diane M 574 Janie Court, Shreveport, LA 71106, (318) 865-7204, BA 73 Northwestern St Univ; MA 74 Northwestern St Univ; Sp-Lang Path, LSU-Shreveport, **SLP**

Edwards, Mrs Dinah Hubbard 2303 34th Avenue South, Seattle, WA 98144, (206) 723-6186, BA 68 OK St Univ; MS 73 IN St Univ - Terre Haute; **SLP**

Edwards, Dr Dorothea B 4401 6th Street S W, Cedar Rapids, IA 52404, (319) 399-6820, BS 41 Univ of MN - Minneap-St Paul; MS 67 Univ of WI - Madison; PH 76 (NS) Univ of WI - Madison; 83–Sp-Lang Path, Grant Wood AEA, **SLP**

Edwards, Dorothy A 2007 46 Street Court East, Bradenton, FL 33508, **SLP**

Edwards, Mrs Dorothy S 4101 Springlake Circle, Buford, GA 30518, (404) 945-5735, BS 73 Univ of GA; ME 74 Univ of GA; ES 87 Univ of GA; Sp-Lang Path, Gwinnett Co Schs, **SLP**

Edwards, Mrs Edith A 9217 West Springs Drive, Knoxville, TN 37922, (615) 690-2923, BS 69 East Carolina Univ; MA 87 Univ of TN - Knoxville; Knox County Schools, **SLP**

Edwards, Mrs Elena G 1211 West 12th Avenue, Escondido, CA 92025, (714) 676-0559, BA 79 San Diego St Univ; MA 87 San Diego St Univ; 88–Sp-Lang Path, Temecula Union Sch Dist, **SLP**

Edwards, Ellen C 2209-D South Jefferson, Roanoke, VA 24014, (703) 344-4769, OB 49 Univ of VA - Charlottesville; MS; **SLP LM**

Edwards, Elsie M Box 323, Dugger, IN 47848, (812) 648-2442, BS 43 IN St Univ - Terre Haute; MS 49 IN St Univ - Terre Haute; ED 56 (NS) Wayne St Univ; **SLP F LM**

Edwards, Ernest Calvin Ctrl VA Speech & Hrng Ctr Inc, Virginia Baptist Hospital, 3300 Rivermont Avenue, Lynchburg, VA 24503, (804) 522-4520, BS 65 Univ Southern MS-Hattiesburg; MS 66 Univ Southern MS-Hattiesburg; Exec Dir, Ctrl Virginia Sp & Hrng Cen, **A**

Edwards, Dr Harold T Communicative Disorders & Sci, Wichita State University, Box 75, Wichita, KS 67208, (316) 689-3240, BA 59 MI St Univ; MA 63 MI St Univ; PH 71 (NS) Univ of WA; Assoc Prof, Wichita St U

Edwards, Mrs Jacque J 1063 Awani Drive, Lodi, CA 95240, (209) 339-8347, BA 77 CA St Univ - Sacramento; MA 79 CA St Univ - Sacramento; Private Practice, **A**

Edwards, Dr Jan Hunter School Of Health Sciences, 425 East 25th Street, New York, NY 10010, (212) 481-5196, PH 85 (NS) CUNY - Grad Sch & Univ Cntr; Asst Prof, Hunter College CUNY, **SLP**

Edwards, Mrs Jane Elizabeth 303 East South Street, Perryville, MO 63775, (314) 651-2495, BS 78 Southeast MO St Univ; ME 83 Southeast MO St Univ; 85–Instr, SE MO St Univ, **SLP**

Edwards, Janet C 4204 Red Bud Lane, Charleston, WV 25313, (304) 744-5623, BS 85 WV Univ; MA 86 Univ of TN - Knoxville; **A**

Edwards, Mrs Jill Dejewski 9727 Softwater Way, Columbia, MD 21046, (301) 356-0766, BS 78 Univ of WI - Milwaukee; MS 79 Univ of WI - Milwaukee; Sp-Lang Path, Baltimore Co Pub Sch Syst, **SLP**

Edwards, Joel Allen 15319 Seward Plaza, Omaha, NE 68154, (402) 390-1324, MA 84 Univ of NE - Lincoln; Aud, Physicians Clinic, **A**

Edwards, Joyce A 7110 Larimer Court, Tampa, FL 33615, **SLP**

Edwards, Joyce M 8058 Abbeyshire Court, Dublin, OH 43017-8999, **SLP**

Edwards, Judith Shoemaker 5729 East Geddes Circle, Englewood, CO 80112-1513, (513) 221-1800, BS 74 OH Univ - Athens; MS 80 Miami Univ - Oxford; 88–Sp-Lang Path, AMI Presbyterian Hosp, **SLP**

Edwards, Julia Ann 1472 Highway 324, Dacula, GA 30211, (404) 962-5929, BS 84 Univ of GA; ME 86 Univ of GA; SLP, Jefferson City Schools, **SLP**

Edwards, Karen 173 West 400 South, Provo, UT 84601, (801) 373-5643, BS 83 Kearney St Coll; OM 87 Brigham Young Univ; 84–Sp-Lang Path, Snow Coll, **SLP**

Edwards, Kathleen 9713 Wendhurst Drive, Glen Allen, VA 23060, (319) 337-9633, BS 76 MI St Univ; MA 78 Univ of IA; SLP, Grant Wood AEA, **SLP**

Edwards, Mrs Kathleen Marie 13422 Lillian Street, Omaha, NE 68138, (402) 896-6035, BA 80 Kearney St Coll; MS 81 Kearney St Coll; Sp/Lang Path, Omaha Pub Schs, **SLP**

Edwards, Laura J 3014 North Louise Drive, Mobile, AL 36606, (205) 433-2564, BS 86 Univ Southern MS-Hattiesburg; MS 87 Univ Southern MS-Hattiesburg; 88–Aud, Dauphin West ENT Spec

Edwards, Linda Kathleen 1008 E Oregon Avenue, Urbana, IL 61801, (714) 381-1160, BA 83 Univ of Redlands; MS 84 Univ of Redlands; **SLP**

Edwards, Linda M 221 Countryhaven, Encinitas, CA 92024, (619) 755-9763, BA 67 Univ of Akron; MS 73 SUNY - Center at Albany; Sp-Lang Path, Del Mar Union Sch Dist, **SLP**

Edwards, Mrs Lurie Ann 1539 Dorgan Street, Jackson, MS 39204, (601) 373-6613, BA 84 MS Coll; MS 87 Univ of MS; 84–Sp-Lang Path, Clinton PS, **SLP**

Edwards, Dr Marcia Sue 3626 Berry Drive, Boise, ID 83703, (208) 384-9262, BA Eastern WA Univ; MS Eastern WA Univ; PH 86 (Special Educ Early Childhood) Univ of ID; 88–Early Childhood Consult, State Dept of Educ, **SLP**

Edwards, Margaret Susan 603 South Waccamaw Avenue, Columbia, SC 29205, (803) 669-3661, BA 81 Univ of SC - Columbia; MS 85 Univ of SC - Columbia; **SLP**

Edwards, Marilyn J 2501 Temple #110, Signal Hill, CA 90806, (213) 424-7039, BA 77 Univ of CA - Santa Barbara; MS 78 Western OR St Coll; 84–Sp-Lang Path, Long Bch Comm Coll Dist, **SLP**

Edwards, Mrs Mary Ann 2600 Algoma Terrace, Waukesha, WI 53188, (414) 544-5053, BS 72 Univ of WI - Madison; MS 73 Univ of WI - Madison; Sp-Lang Path, Med Teams, **SLP**

Edwards, Mary F 122 Susan Drive, Hendersonville, TN 37075, (615) 822-9010, BS 69 OK St Univ; MA 70 Northwestern Univ; Asst VP-Rehab Svcs, Rebound Inc, **SLP**

Edwards, Dr Mary Louise 805 South Crouse Avenue, Syracuse, NY 13224-2280, (315) 443-9645, BA 68 Univ of ME - Orono; MA 70 OH St Univ; PH 79 (Linguistics) Stanford Univ; 79–Assoc Prof/Comm Sci & Disorders, Syracuse U

Edwards, Mrs Mary W 337 Rock Road, Greer, SC 29651, (803) 297-9226, BA 81 Marshall Univ; MA 82 Marshall Univ; Sp-Lang Path, **SLP**

Edwards, Mrs Maura M 49 West Erie Street, Albany, NY 12208, MS 79 Coll of Saint Rose; Sp-Lang Path, CA Ctr for the Disabled, **SLP**

Edwards, Mrs Nancy G 3108 Woodcutter Road, Rock Hill, SC 29730, (803) 329-1520, BS 80 Winthrop Coll; MS 82 Univ of SC - Columbia; 88–Sp-Lang Path, Sp/Hrng Ctr of York & Chester Co, **SLP**

Edwards, Mrs Patricia S 1542 Foothill Boulevard, Santa Ana, CA 92705, (714) 544-3519, BA 50 Occidental Coll; MA 70 CA St Univ - Fullerton; Sp/Lang Path-Consult, Newport Lang-Sp-Aud Cen, **SLP**

Edwards, Rosemary C 429 22nd Street, Belleair Beach, FL 33535, BA 42 Vassar Coll; MA 65 Temple Univ; **SLP LM**

Edwards, Sue J 641 State Highway 603, Chehalis, WA 98532, (206) 748-6259, BA 75 Eastern WA Univ; MS 76 Eastern WA Univ; Sp-Lang Path, Providence Hosp-Centralia, **SLP**

Edwards, Susan J Route 4 Box 204, Sedalia, MO 65301, **SLP**

Edwards, Mrs Susan S 231 Carriage Drive, Glastonbury, CT 06033, (203) 246-4369, BS 68 Indiana Univ of PA; MA 71 Univ of Pittsburgh - Pittsburgh; SLP/Lang Dis Tchr, Hartford Bd of Ed, **SLP**

Edwards, Mrs Suzanne T 6141 Van Alstine Avenue, Carmichael, CA 95608, BA 72 CA St Univ - Sacramento; MA 73 CA St Univ - Sacramento; 88–Sp-Lang Path, Sacramento City USD, **SLP**

Edwards, Thomas Wayne 5269 Rosemont Drive, Madisonville, KY 42431, (502) 825-7377, BA 68 Belmont Coll; OM 71 Southwestern Baptist Theolog; MS 82 Murray St Univ; Director Speech Pathology Dept, Traver Clinic, **SLP**

Edwards-De La Vega, Maureen A 28214 Langside Avenue, Canyon Country, CA 91351, **SLP**

Edwardson, Walter John 436 Sherman Drive, Marshall, MI 49068, (616) 781-1072, BS 78 Calvin Coll; MA 84 Wayne St Univ; SLP, Calhoon Intermed Sch Dist, **SLP**

Eernisse, Claudia C 3000 South Connor Street, Apartment 24, Salt Lake City, UT 84109, (801) 581-3506, BA 74 Univ of NM; MS 75 Univ of NM; Sp-Lang Path, Univ of Utah, **SLP**

Effa-Hill, Catherine Ann 1512 North Kaspar Avenue, Arlington Height, IL 60004-3761, (312) 255-7431, BS 81 Northern IL Univ - De Kalb; MA 83 Northern IL Univ - De Kalb; 83–Aud, JFK Audio Vestibular Lab, **A**

Effenberger, Cynthia Ann 8905 Willmon Way, San Antonio, TX 78239, (512) 659-6775, BA 71 Our Lady Lake Univ-San Anton; MA 72 Our Lady Lake Univ-San Anton; SLP, Judson ISD, **SLP**

Efros, Paul L 1813 Forrest Road, Baltimore, MD 21234, (301) 687-6500, BA 70 Temple Univ; MA 73 Temple Univ; Aud, Balto Co Dept of Hlth, **A**

Eftekhar, Mrs Barbara Lee 23 Hidden Ledge Road, Englewood, NJ 07631, (201) 568-9483, BA 83 Ramapo Coll of NJ; MA 86 Montclair St Coll; SLP, Jawonio, **SLP**

Egan, Christina Marie 23A Lawrence Drive, North White Plains, NY 10603, (914) 128-5451, BS 78 Southern CT St Univ; MA 84 CUNY - Hunter Coll; **SLP**

Egan, Dr James J Director Speech & Hearing Clinic, DC General Hospital, Washington, DC 20003, (202) 675-5225, BS 59 Western MI Univ; BS 59 Western MI Univ; PH 67 (NS) Case Western Reserve Univ; Dir-Sp & Hrng Cl, Dc Gen Hosp, **SLP A**

Egan, James P 1224 Cornwall, Bellingham, WA 98225, (206) 671-0794, BA 38 Univ of IA; MA 39 Univ of IA; PH 47 (NS) Harvard Univ; **A F LM**

Egan, Dr Katherine S 415 16th Street, Bellingham, WA 98225, (206) 671-0794, BA 34 Univ of MO - Columbia; MA 53 IN Univ - Bloomington; PH 60 (Sp Path Aud) IN Univ - Bloomington; Retired, **SLP A F LM**

Egan, Kathleen A 21 Agawam Road South #3D, Yonkers, NY 10704, (914) 592-8440, BS 77 Iona Coll; MS 78 Adelphi Univ; Sp-Lang Path, Elmsford Sch Dist, **SLP**

Egan, Sylvia 2222 Larkin Street, San Francisco, CA 94109, (415) 673-3019, OM 87 Governors St Univ

Egbert, Dr James H 4833 Argosy Lane, Carlsbad, CA 92008, (619) 434-0047, BA 41 WA St Univ; MA 46 Univ of MO - Columbia; PH 55 (NS) Stanford Univ; **SLP LM**

Egbert, Mrs Polly Young 4508 South Aladdin Court, Springfield, MO 65804, (417) 882-2729, BS 73 Miami Univ - Oxford; MA 74 Memphis St Univ; 88-Sp-Lang Path, Sp-Lang Svcs of SW Missouri, **SLP**

Egbert, William S 103 Berkley Place #4, Brooklyn, NY 11217, (212) 636-4573, BS 63 PA St Univ - Univ Park; MA 64 NY Univ; Aud, Francis De Sales Sch for Df, **A**

Egblomasse, Sonja Cosby U S Army Hospital Berlin, Box 4602, APO New York, NY 09742-3366, (301) 656-3616, BS 68 8147; MA CA St Univ - Los Angeles; ED Boston Univ; 84-Sp-Lang Path, Department of the Army, **SLP ACE**

Ege, Diane D 8852 Rooks Mill Lane, Dayton, OH 45458, (513) 293-3574, BA 70 Univ of Dayton; MA 72 OH St Univ; 86-Sp-Lang Path, Kettering Med Ctr, **SLP**

Egeland, Carol S 2317 South Hills Drive, Missoula, MT 59801, **SLP**

Egenberger, Sheila S 308 East 6th, Lexington, NE 68850, (308) 324-4681, BS 63 CO St Univ; Sp-Lang Path, Lexington Pub Sch, **SLP**

Eger, Dr Diane Levy 200 Commerce Court, Pittsburgh, PA 15219, (412) 394-5832, BA 69 Northwestern Univ; MA 71 Univ of Pittsburgh - Pittsburgh; PH 76 (Aud) Univ of Pittsburgh - Pittsburgh; Program Admin/Speech & Lang, Allegheny Intermediate Unit, **SLP A F ACE**

Egert, Allison B 5 Hillcrest Road, Tenafly, NJ 07670, (201) 567-1540, BA 78 CUNY - Brooklyn Coll; MA 80 NY Univ; Private Practice, **SLP**

Egge, Victoria Dreis 2439 North Highland Avenue, Altadena, CA 91001, (818) 798-2602, BS 78 Univ of Redlands; MS 79 Univ of Redlands; Sp-Lang Path, Los Angeles Co Office of Ed, **SLP**

Eggers, Mrs Leslie Jane 810 1/2 Chapin Street, Beloit, WI 53511, (608) 365-8204, BA 84 Univ of WI - Madison; MS 86 Univ of WI - Whitewater; 86-Sp-Lang Path, Beloit Mem Hosp, **SLP**

Eggert, Mrs Christine 428 Lauren Lane, Buffalo Grove, IL 60089, (312) 259-3303, BS 79 Northern IL Univ - De Kalb; MA 80 Northern IL Univ - De Kalb; Sp-Lang Path, River Trails Sch Dist #26, **SLP**

Eggert, Gertrude H 1862 Sherman Avenue #2SW, Evanston, IL 60201, **SLP**

Eggert, Mrs Sandra J 502 West 22nd, Kearney, NE 68847, (308) 234-1335, BA 75 Univ of NE - Lincoln; MA 77 Univ of NE - Lincoln; Sp-Lang Path, Kearney Pub Sch, **SLP**

Eggleston, Mrs Georgena K 306 Hespe Drive, Norfolk, NE 68505, (402) 379-0433, BA Univ of NE - Lincoln; OB 75 Univ of NE - Lincoln; MA 78 Univ of NE - Lincoln; Sp-Lang Path, Dept Head-Educ Svc Unit #8, **SLP ACE**

Eggleston, Mrs Maryann D Mark Mead Road, Cross River, NY 10518, (917) 763-3963, BA 68 Mercy Coll; MA 75 NY Univ; Sp-Lang Path, Yorktown Central Sch Dist, **SLP**

Eggner, Mrs Ruth S 1903 Aladdin, Norman, OK 73069, (405) 521-3571, BA 62 Univ of OK - Norman; OM 65 Univ of OK Medical Center; OM 73 Univ of OK Medical Center; Prog Asst Admin, OK Dep of Human Ser, **SLP**

Egnor, Mrs Debra Frances 1246 South Park Drive, Huntington, WV 25701, (304) 525-9444, BA 75 Marshall Univ; MA 84 Marshall Univ; **SLP**

Egolf, Donald B 307 South Dithridge Street, Apartment 609, Pittsburgh, PA 15213, PH (NS); **SLP**

Egyed-Schultz, Glyce A 1365 Mercy Drive, Muskegon, MI 49444, (616) 739-9095, MA 83 MI St Univ; Aud, West Michigan ENT Pc, **A**

Ehlen, Patrice J 1005 East Miami, McAlester, OK 74501, (918) 426-0240, BS 77 OK St Univ; MA 79 Univ of Tulsa; Aud, McAlester Cl Inc, **A**

Ehlers, Mrs Michele M Saratoga Union School District, Foothill School, 13919 Lynde Avenue, Saratoga, CA 95070, (408) 867-4036, BA 74; SLP, Saratoga Un Sch Dist, **SLP**

Ehlers, Patricia McShane 3308 NE 94th Street, Vancouver, WA 98665, (206) 699-0394, BA 81 Univ of WA; MS 83 ID St Univ; Sp-Lang Path, Clark Coll/Pride Prog, **SLP**

Ehnstrom, Mrs Jane Anne 177 Milk Street, Fitchburg, MA 01420, (617) 342-6609, BS 83 Worcester St Coll; MS 85 Northeastern Univ; Audiologist, Clinton Hospital, **A**

Ehren, Dr Barbara J 15726 S W 7th Place, Sunrise, FL 33326, (305) 393-3288, BA 67 Saint John's Univ - Jamaica; MS 68 Adelphi Univ; ED 81 (NS) FL Atlantic Univ; Faculty, FL Atlantic U, **SLP**

Ehren, Tom C 15726 South West 7th Place, Sunrise, FL 33326, (305) 765-6660, MS 72 Univ of South FL; Curr Superv/Sp-Lang, Broward Co Pub Sch, **SLP**

Ehrenfreund, Joseph 264 Cordial Road, Yorktown Heights, NY 10598, (914) 245-4993, BA 65 CUNY - Hunter Coll; MA 66 CUNY - Hunter Coll; Sp-Lang Path, Private Practice, **SLP LM**

Ehrenkaufer, Louise Pauze 35 Ross Road, Wilmington, DE 19810, (302) 475-0821, BS 67 Central CT St Univ; MA 84 Eastern MI Univ; Sp-Lang Path, Elwyn Institutes, **SLP**

Ehrenpreis, Mrs Elaine R 2900 Atterbein Avenue, Dayton, OH 45406, BA 76 SUNY - Coll at Cortland; MA 78 Northwestern Univ; **SLP**

Ehrens, Gail 1019 North Glenwood Street, Allentown, PA 18104, (215) 437-2513, BA 68 Fairleigh Dickinson U-Teanec; MA 69 Columbia Univ Teachers Coll; Sp-Lang Path, Private Practice, **SLP ACE**

Ehret, Mrs Patricia M 2663 East Fountain Street, Mesa, AZ 85203, (602) 964-5002, BA 76 Elmira Coll; MS 78 Gallaudet Coll; Auderv Aud, Mesa Pub Schls, **A**

Ehrheart, Natalie Anne 360 West 10th Street #4, Erie, PA 16502, (814) 453-7661, BS 85 SUNY - Coll at Fredonia; MS 86 SUNY - Coll at Fredonia; **SLP**

Ehring, Dana Sue 20896 Sailmaker, Huntington Beach, CA 92648-2360, (713) 471-0950, ME 81 Southwest TX St Univ; Early Childhood Teaching, La Porte ISD, **SLP**

Ehritt, Donelle 550 Water Street #B, Santa Cruz, CA 95060, (408) 688-4447, BA 68 Univ of CA - Santa Barbara; Aud-Owner, Hearing Services of Santa Cruz, **A**

Ehrlich, Barbara O 2317 Belvedere Drive, Scotch Plains, NJ 07076, (201) 441-2165, BA 73 CUNY - Hunter Coll; MA 75 Western MI Univ; Sp-Lang Path, Childerns Specialized Hospital, **SLP**

Ehrlich, Beth L Hayward Hearing Aid Center Inc, 22941 Atherton Street, Suite B, Hayward, CA 94541, (415) 537-4211, BA 72 San Diego St Univ; MA 75 San Jose St Univ; Aud, Hayward Hearing Aid Center Inc, **A**

Ehrlich, Carol H 7865 East Mississippi, Apartment 804W, Denver, CO 80231, (303) 320-1437, BA 49 Univ of Denver; MA 61 Univ of Denver; PH 65 (Sp-Lang Path/Aud) Univ of Denver; 84-Aud/Sp-Lang Path, The Children's Hosp Denver, **F**

Ehrlich, Cynthia L 11928 Calle Deposito, El Cajon, CA 92019, (619) 670-0780, BS 74 SUNY - Coll at Fredonia; MS 77 SUNY - Coll at Buffalo; Sp-Lang Path, Sharp Healthcare/Assoc Sp Path, **SLP ACE**

Ehrlich, Jonathan S Long Island College Hospital, 57 Marshall Drive, Edison, NJ 08817, (718) 780-1261, BS 77 Yeshiva Univ; MS 79 Columbia Univ Teachers Coll; Sp-Lang Path, Dept of Cognitive Rehab, **SLP**

Ehrlich, Mrs June W 2353 North 37th Avenue, Hollywood, FL 33021, (305) 534-3676, **SLP**

Ehrlich, Pauline 41 Centre Street #405, Brookline, MA 02146, BS 47 Teachers Coll - Boston; MA 51 Columbia Univ Teachers Coll; **SLP A LM**

Ehrlich, Roberta Elise 111-20 73rd Avenue, Forest Hills, NY 11375, (718) 544-3223, BA CUNY - Queens Coll; MA Columbia Univ Teachers Coll; MA 69 Columbia Univ Teachers Coll; Sp/Lang Path, Private Practice, **SLP**

Ehrlich, Mrs Ruth H 2237 33rd Avenue, San Francisco, CA 94116, (415) 566-3299, BA 76 Brandeis Univ; ME 78 Northeastern Univ; Sp-Lang Path, San Francisco USD, **SLP**

Ehrlich-Herzfeld, Sherry Beth 16 So Dorado Circle #1-B, Hauppauge, NY 11788, (516) 924-0008, MA 86 Hofstra Univ; Sp-Lang Path, Just Kids Early Chld Lrng Ctr, **SLP**

Ehrlickman, Gail S 51 Quaker Ridge Road, Bethel, CT 06801, (813) 962-4322, BA 80 SUNY - Coll at New Paltz; MS 86 Univ of South FL; **SLP**

Ehrman, Mary Hanz 111 Rambler Drive, Sarver, PA 16055, (412) 295-2498, BS 72 Indiana Univ of PA; MA 74 Univ of Akron; 86-Sp-Lang Path, St John Lutheran Care Ctr, **SLP**

Eiban, Mrs Gloria D Route 1 Box 287, Rice, VA 23966, (804) 392-8106, BS 78 Longwood Coll; ME 79 Univ of VA - Charlottesville; Sp-Lang Path, Prince Edward Co Pub Schs, **SLP**

Eiben, Melissa M 1012 Allouez, Marquette, MI 49855, (906) 228-8313, BA 76 Augustana Coll; MA 78 Northern MI Univ; **SLP**

Eichacker, Niclole Elana 1034 Claymark Drive, St Louis, MO 63131, (314) 569-8235, BS 86 Saint Louis Univ; MA 88 Saint Louis Univ

Eichelberg, Debbie Sue 3011 Jane Place NE #259, Albuquerque, NM 87111, (505) 294-4786, MS 88 Univ of AZ

Eichelberger, Mrs Barbara S 524 Cottonwood Drive, Williamsville, NY 14221, (716) 686-2452, BS 59 Marygove Coll; ME 60 SUNY - Center at Buffalo; Sp-Lang Path, Depew Pub Sch, **SLP ACE**

Eichelberger, Mrs Brenda Jones 3706 Greenvale Road, Baltimore, MD 21229, (301) 646-7830, BA 83 Western MD Coll; MA 86 Temple Univ-Tyler Sch of Art; 88-Sp-Lang Path, Baltimore Co PS, **SLP**

Eichelberger, Mrs Diane S 1409 Pythian Avenue, Springfield, OH 45504, BS 72 OH Univ - Athens; MA 73 Bowling Green St Univ; 87-Early Childhood Coord, Town and Country School, **SLP**

Eichenauer, Patricia Louise 2421 E Washington #24-219, Bloomington, IL 61701, (309) 662-5987, BS 81 Southeast MO St Univ; MA 82 Southeast MO St Univ; Sp-Lang Path, Bloomington Ps, **SLP**

Eichenbaum, Roberta Wyffels 1402 Bloomsberry Lane, Waxhaw, NC 28173, (704) 843-5999, BA 85 Univ of CO - Boulder; MA 87 Univ of CO - Boulder; 87-Sp-Lang Path, Charlotte-Mecklenburg PS

Eichenlaub, Diane M RR2 Box 920, East Holden, ME 04429, (207) 843-7245, BA 78 Methodist Coll; MA 84 Univ of ME - Orono; SLP, Private Practice, **SLP**

Eichholz, Mrs Susan Odrezin 100 Stuart Street, Savannah, GA 31405, (912) 927-5479, OB 79 Univ of GA; ME 80 Univ of GA; **A**

Eichhorn, Patricia R 538 Glen View Avenue #2, Oakland, CA 94610, (415) 835-5246, BS 77 Trenton St Coll; MS 84 San Francisco St Univ; **SLP**

Eichler, Mrs Estelle Miller 776 Arbuckle Avenue, Woodmere, NY 11598, (516) 221-4700, BA 81 CUNY - Queens Coll; MS 83 Adelphi Univ; Sp-Lang Path, Acds, **SLP**

Eichler, Kaye B P O Box 80003, Baton Rouge, LA 70898, (504) 342-0173, MS 79 Northwestern St Univ; Superv Sp-Lang Eval, LA Dept of Educ, **SLP**

Eicholtz, Glenn Everett 20414 Reeds Creek Road, Red Bluff, CA 96080, (916) 895-5871, BA 78 CA St Univ - Chico; MA 80 CA St Univ - Chico; Asst Prof, Calif State Univ-Chico, **SLP ACE**

Eicholtz, Helen J 20414 Reeds Creek Road, Red Bluff, CA 96080, (916) 529-3731, BA 79 CA St Univ - Chico; MA 81 CA St Univ - Chico; SLP, Red Bluff Elementary, **SLP**

Eichten, Philip I 2123 Lennox Road, Richmond, VA 23228, (804) 359-3339, BS 75 Univ of VA - Charlottesville; ME 76 Univ of VA - Charlottesville; Private Practice, **SLP**

Eichwald, John Gary Bureau Of Communicative Disord, Utah Department Of Health, 44 Medical Drive, Salt Lake City, UT 84113, (801) 533-6175, BA 74 Univ of MT; MA 78 Univ of UT; Aud, Utah Department of Health, **A**

Eick, Lisa Hill 28412 Farmington Road, Farmington Hills, MI 48018, (313) 489-5407, BA 82 Univ of Northern IA; MA 84 Univ of Northern IA; Sp-Lang Path, Medi Speech Services, **SLP**

Eid, Catherine Nasri 1308 Ross Drive S W, Vienna, VA 22180, (703) 358-6041, BA 83 George Washington Univ; ME 85 Univ of VA - Charlottesville; 88-Sp-Lang Path, Arlington Co Schs, **SLP**

Eide, Mrs Eunice A 2723 Waunona Way, Madison, WI 53713, (803) 271-8551, BA 54 Univ of IA; MS 77 Univ of WI - Madison; SLP, Madison Metropolitan Sch Dist, **SLP**

Eide, Mrs Sandra Kay 1 Windsor Road, Pittsburgh, PA 15239, (412) 856-9330, BS 81 Univ of WI - Stevens Point; MS 83 Univ of WI - Madison; 88-Sp-Lang Path, Rehabilitation Spec, **SLP**

Eidelman, Mrs Jill Finkelstein 6807 Greenspring Avenue, Pikesville, MD 21209, (301) 484-8956, BA 83 Univ of MI - Ann Arbor; OM 85 Emory Univ; 88-Sp-Lang Path, Mount Washington Pediatric Hosp, **SLP**

Eidels, Eleanor R 4170 Lomita Lane, Dallas, TX 75220, (214) 323-5931, BS 77 Univ of Dallas; MS 79 Univ of Dallas; Sp-Lang Path, Priv Pract, **SLP ACE**

Eidenmuller, Kirk J Northwestern Pa Hrng & Sp Ser, 150 Prospect Avenue, Suite 11, Franklin, PA 16323, (814) 437-6848, BA 71 Allegheny Coll; ME 75 Clarion Univ of PA; Sp-Lang Path / Aud, NW Pa Hrng & Sp Serv, **SLP A ACE**

Eidinger, Karen R 515 Chaplin Crescent #506, Toronto, ON, Canada M5N 2N1, (416) 469-6338, BA 78 Univ of VT; MA 80 Western MI Univ; 85-Sp-Lang Path, Toronto East Gen Hosp, **SLP**

Eidson, Sue Ann 118-B Longwood Drive, Charlottesville, VA 22903, (904) 971-8132, BS 76 FL St Univ; MS 81 FL St Univ; Sp/Lang Path, Alachua Co Pub Sch, **SLP**

Eifert, Anna Louise 1345 Southwest 15th Street, Miami, FL 33145, (305) 325-0470, BS 85 Valparaiso Univ; MS 86 FL St Univ; 87-Sp-Lang Path, Easter Seal Soc, **SLP**

Eigenberg, Sigrid R 1726 West 14th, Hastings, NE 68901, **SLP**

Eiger, Jaclyn S 942 Cranford Avenue, North Woodmere, NY 11581, (516) 791-2191, BA 75 SUNY - Center at Buffalo; MS 78 CUNY - Brooklyn Coll; **SLP**

Eikenberg, Mrs Mary Ann Sortore 3720 Font Hill Drive, Ellicott City, MD 21043, (301) 356-0732, BA 79 Loyola Coll; MS 80 Loyola Coll; 80-SLP, Baltimore Co Pub Sch, **SLP**

Eilat, Mrs Laurie W c/o Wolf, 531 East 20th Street, New York, NY 10010, BA 70 Univ of MI - Ann Arbor; MS 73 Univ of MI - Ann Arbor

Eilat, Mrs Rosie N 5850 East 3rd Street, Tucson, AZ 85711, (602) 747-0987, BS 73 Univ of AZ; MS 74 Univ of AZ; 88–Sp-Lang Path, Tucson USD, **SLP**

Eilermann, Denise Ann 7726 Arthur, 1st Floor, St Louis, MO 63117, (405) 272-5545, BS 83 Southwest MO St Univ; MS 85 Univ of OK Medical Center; **SLP**

Eilers, Mrs Gail M 4701 Prince Edward Road, Jacksonville, FL 32210-8117, (904) 272-8100, BA 67 Huntingdon Coll; MA 73 Memphis St Univ; 78–Dir Except Chld Ed, Clay Co Sch Bd, **SLP**

Eilers, Karen R 53 Tomlin Circle, Burr Ridge, IL 60521, (312) 440-1129, **SLP**

Eilers, Dr Rebecca E Mailman Center For Child Development, PO Box 016820, Miami, FL 33101, (305) 547-6350, BS 66 CUNY - Brooklyn Coll; ME 69 Univ of WA; PH 72 (NS) Univ of WA; Prof, University of Miami

Eilts, Judith T 2924 Ormond Avenue, Baton Rouge, LA 70820, (504) 769-2755, BA 76 Univ of MN - Minneap-St Paul; MA 78 Univ of MN - Minneap-St Paul; Sp-Lang Path, E Baton Rouge Parish Schools, **SLP**

Einbinder, Monique Sheryl 7 Sanders Court, West Milford, NJ 07480, (201) 587-8500, BS 83 East Stroudsburg Univ of PA; MS 84 Bloomsburg Univ of PA; Sp-Lang Path, Kessler Inst for Rehab, **SLP**

Einck, Julie Mensing 614 North, Decorah, IA 52101, (319) 382-2870, BA 76 Univ of IA; MA 77 Univ of IA; Sp-Lang Path, Keystone AEA, **SLP**

Einertson, Mrs Janice Loraine 2515 Logan Drive, Loveland, CO 80538, (303) 669-3605, BS 80 CO St Univ; MS 82 CO St Univ; Sp-Lang Path, Thompson R2J Sch Dist, **SLP**

Einhorn, Allan Jack 676 East 86th Street, Brooklyn, NY 11236, (718) 642-6099, **A**

Einhorn, Mrs Elinor S 4 Mohawk Avenue, Rockaway, NJ 07866, (201) 361-3095, BS 60 Emerson Coll; MS 79 Paterson St Coll; SLP, Rockaway Twsp Bd Ed, **SLP**

Einhorn, Ellen A 1129 Coventry Road, Cheltenham, PA 19012, (215) 635-1823, BA 74 Temple Univ; MA 75 Temple Univ; Sp-Lang Path, Private Practice, **SLP**

Einhorn, Rebecca Elizabeth 1750 North Mohawk #203, Chicago, IL 60614, (312) 751-3403, BS 86 Syracuse Univ; MS 88 Emerson Coll; Sp-Lang Path, South Met Assoc

Einhorn, Mrs Robin Dubowe 3220 South Utah Street, Arlington, VA 22206, (703) 777-5050, BS 78 Kent St Univ; MA 82 George Washington Univ; Aud, Blue Ridge Speech & Hrng Cen, **A**

Einolf, Michele M 10601 Glen Hannah Drive, Laurel, MD 20707, (301) 761-6190, BA 78 Loyola Coll; MS 79 Loyola Coll; Sp-Lang Path, Anne Arundel Co Bd of Ed, **SLP**

Einsiedler, Mrs Stephanie L 148 Sea Road, Kennebunk, ME 04043, (207) 985-3631, BA 78 Lesley Coll; MA 82 Univ of Pittsburgh - Pittsburgh; SLP, York Co Couns Serv Sp/Hrng, **SLP**

Eirich, Mrs Mary Sullivan 85 Pine Street, Belmont, MA 02178, (617) 498-9200, BA 71 Salem St Coll; MS 79 Emerson Coll; Sp-Lang Path, Cambridge School Dept, **SLP**

Eisbrener-Hester, Patricia Anne 40056 90th Street West, Leona Valley, CA 93551-9704, (714) 983-0042, **SLP**

Eisele, Dr Wendell A Route 1 Box 276, Jefferson, GA 30549, (404) 367-1133, BS 70 Univ of Central AR; MS 74 Boston Univ; OD 75 (NS) Boston Univ; Retail Manager, Bio-Logic Systems, **A**

Eisen, Dr Audrey H 16 West 16th Street #5H-S, New York, NY 10011, (516) 560-5508, BA 72 CUNY - Queens Coll; MA 75 CUNY - Queens Coll; PH 76 (Sp & Hrng Sciences) CUNY - Grad Sch & Univ Cntr; Asst Prof/Director Ma Program, Hofstra U, **SLP**

Eisen, Mrs Debra S 3008 Ashley Court, Bensalem, PA 19020, (215) 757-6504, BS 81 Boston Univ; MA 82 Temple Univ; 86–Sp-Lang Path, Magee Rehab Hosp, **SLP**

Eisen, Susan H P O Box 1224, Hawthorne, FL 32640-1224, (904) 481-4516, BS 72 Univ of FL; ME 74 Univ of FL; Sp-Lang Path, Ed Ther Ser, **SLP**

Eisenbach, Dr Charles R, II 10447 S W Moratoc Drive, Tualatin, OR 97062, (503) 257-0308, BS 67; MA 74 Univ of FL; PH 83 (Sp-Lang Path) Univ of FL; 88–Dir of Sp-Lang Path, Assoc Health Focus/Portland, **SLP ACE**

Eisenbart, Karen S Box 1715, Homewood, IL 60430, (312) 957-4163, BS 78 Purdue Univ - West Lafayette; MS 80 Purdue Univ - West Lafayette; Sp-Lang Path, Sch Dist 163, **SLP**

Eisenberg, Diane Therapy Associates, 8218 Wisconsin Avenue, Suite 312, Bethesda, MD 20814, (202) 667-2437, BS 66 Emerson Coll; MA 67 NY Univ; **SLP**

Eisenberg, Mrs Hope Sandra 226 Sandringham Road, Cherry Hill, NJ 08003, (609) 267-1404, **SLP**

Eisenberg, Judith Faith 154 Clinton Drive, South Windsor, CT 06074, (203) 286-4627, BA 83 Univ of CT; MA 85 OH St Univ; 88–Sp-Lang Path, Mount Sinai Hosp, **SLP ACE**

Eisenberg, Laurie S House Ear Institute, 256 South Lake Street, Los Angeles, CA 90057, (213) 483-4431, BA 72 CA St Univ - Fresno; MA 76 CA St Univ - Northridge; Aud, **A**

Eisenberg, Mrs Marlene 20979 Olivo Way, Boca Raton, FL 33433, (305) 368-3900, BS 71 Trenton St Coll; MA 75 CUNY - Lehman Coll; Sp-Lang Path, Private Practice, **SLP**

Eisenberg, Richard 1043 Amador Street, Claremont, CA 91711, (714) 621-3405, BA 70 Univ of Charleston; ME 73 Univ of VA - Charlottesville; Sp-Lang Path, Pace Therapy Inc, **SLP**

Eisenberg, Robin Ann 77 Huntley Street #409, Toronto, ON, Canada M4Y 2P3, **SLP**

Eisenberg, Sarita H 39 Dartmouth Road, Mountain Lakes, NJ 07046, (201) 746-3512, BS 74 Emerson Coll; MA 78 Temple Univ-Tyler Sch of Art; 88–Instr, William Paterson Coll, **SLP**

Eisenberg, Mrs Sharon Luber 3324 Bittersweet Court, Herndon, VA 22071, (305) 499-5288, BS 74 Towson St Univ; MS 76 Towson St Univ; **SLP**

Eisenberg, Susan Burde 14 Independence Drive, Roselle, NJ 07203, (201) 241-2749, BA 76 CUNY - Brooklyn Coll; MS 79 CUNY - Brooklyn Coll; 88–Sp-Lang Path, Day Training Ctr of Union Co, **SLP**

Eisenberg-Dorfman, Mrs Melody VA-Opc, Audiology Clinic, 17 Court Street, Boston, MA 02108, (617) 565-9598, BA 76 CUNY - Brooklyn Coll; MS 78 Boston Univ; 79–Aud, VA Outpatient Cl, **A**

Eisengart, Anne Edith 1376 Commonwealth Avenue #A11, Allston, MA 02134, (516) 735-7787, SLP, Boston P S, **SLP**

Eisenhardt, Christine Marie 133 Broadmeadow Road Apartment 10, Marlboro, MA 01752, (508) 791-6351, BA 85 Rutger's St Univ - Douglas Coll; ME 87 Univ of VA - Charlottesville; 88–Sp-Lang Path, Fairlawn Rehabilitation Hosp, **SLP**

Eisenhaure, Dorothy C P O Box 335, Concord, MA 01742, (508) 369-1511, BS 65 Boston Univ; ME 68 Boston Univ; Sp-Lang Path, Lincoln Pub Sch, **SLP**

Eisenlauer, Mrs Ann L 2490 East Crest Avenue, Bettendorf, IA 52722, BS 75 Univ of IA; MA 76 Northeast MO St Univ; SLP, MS Bend AEA, **SLP**

Eisenmenger, Barbara A 2331 Thornhill Road, Louisville, KY 40222, (502) 588-5274, BS 75 Eastern KY Univ; MS 77 Purdue Univ - West Lafayette; Cl Superv, U of Louisville, **A ACE**

Eisen-Siegel, Samantha 2409 Bay Blvd, #3, Indian Rocks Beach, FL 34635, (813) 596-5020, BA 78 Univ of FL; MS 81 Univ of South FL; 88–Sp-Lang Path, Pinellas County Sch System, **SLP**

Eisenson, Dr Jon 82 Pearce Mitchell Place, Stanford, CA 94305, (415) 328-0436, BS 28 CUNY - City College; MA 30 Columbia Univ Teachers Coll; PH 35 (Psychol-Clinical Ed) Columbia Univ Teachers Coll; Sp-Lang Path, Private Practice, **SLP F H LM**

Eisenstadt, Dr Arthur A 40 Oxford Street, Montclair, NJ 07042, (201) 990-6161, BA 38 CUNY - Brooklyn Coll; MA 46 CUNY - Brooklyn Coll; PH 54 (NS) NY Univ; 88–Sp-Lang Path, Private Practice, **SLP F LM**

Eisert, Susan Y St Frances School For The Deaf, 260 Eastern Parkway, Brooklyn, NY 11225, (212) 636-4573, MS; Dir Media, St Francis De Sales Sch Deaf

Eisinger, Mrs Joanne Mary Rd 2 Box 391, Brockway Road, Frankfort, NY 13340, (315) 797-8781, BS 79 SUNY - Coll at Fredonia; BS 83 Syracuse Univ; **SLP**

Eisler, Nancy Ann 8500 Falmouth Avenue #3308, Playa Del Rey, CA 90293, (213) 301-0959, BA 76 Univ of CA - Los Angeles; MA 79 CA St Univ - Northridge; Sp-Lang Path, Private Practice, **SLP**

Eisner, Debra S 6344 Monitor Street, Pittsburgh, PA 15217, (412) 647-2030, BA 77 Univ of MD - College Park; MS 79 Gallaudet Coll; Aud, Eye & Ear Hospital of Pittsbgh, **A**

Eisner, Eileen 421 Quantuck Lane, Westfield, NJ 07090, BA 67 Long Island U - Brooklyn Ctr; ME 68 Northeastern Univ; 86–Demonstration Tchr CH Class, Kean Coll of NJ, **SLP**

Eisnitz, Phyllis Scher Center For Communication Disorders, 101 Old Short Hills Road, Suite 211, West Orange, NJ 07052, 86–Dir of Sp-Lang Path, Ctr for Comm Disorders, **SLP**

Eiten, Leisha R Middlefort Clinic Ltd, 733 West Clairemont Avenue, Eau Claire, WI 54702, (715) 839-6984, BS 83 Univ of IA; MA 86 Univ of IA; **A**

Eitenmiller, Anna Marie Route 1 Box 458, Danville, AR 72833, (501) 967-1460, BS 69 IL St Univ - Normal; MS 71 IL St Univ - Normal; SLP, Russellville Pub Schs, **A**

Eitrheim, Amy Jo 500 17th Street North, Menomonie, WI 54751-2159, (715) 839-4365, BS 81 Univ of MN - Duluth; MA 82 Univ of MN - Duluth; 87–Sp-Lang Path, Sacred Heart Hosp, **SLP**

Ek, Bette J 215 Prospect Hill Road, Horseheads, NY 14845, MS 68 Univ of MA - Amherst; Asst Prof of Sp & Hrng, Elmira College, **SLP**

Ekart, Sally Ann 1316 Ebling Drive, South Bend, IN 46615, (219) 237-7758, BS 74 Purdue Univ - West Lafayette; MA 82 Ball St Univ; Sp-Lang Path, St Joseph Medical Ctr, **SLP**

Ekberg, Judith W 121 South Deframe Way, Golden, CO 80401, (303) 279-2989, BA 70 Univ of Denver; MA 71 Univ of Denver; Sp-Lang Path, **SLP**

Ekegren, Corinne A Fridley Middle School, 6100 West Moore Lake Drive, Fridley, MN 55432, (612) 571-6100, BS 54 Saint Cloud St Univ; MS 79 Univ of WI - River Falls; Sp-Lang Path, Fridley Sch Dist #14, **SLP**

Ekelman, Barbara Lee 3305 Braemar Road, Shaker Heights, OH 44120, (216) 844-3669, BA 80 Case Western Reserve Univ; MS 83 Case Western Reserve Univ; 81–Research Asst, Case Western Reserve Univ, **SLP**

Eklof, Peter 6 Fort Hill Road, Haydenville, MA 01039, (413) 268-3284, BA 66 Tufts Univ; MA 73 Universite DE Grenoble

Eklund, Adele C 3100 West Sheridan Avenue, Milwaukee, WI 53209, (414) 963-4290, BS 76 IL St Univ - Normal; MS 78 IL St Univ - Normal; Proj Spec/Cl Superv, U WI-Milwaukee Dept Sp Path, **SLP**

Eklund, Mrs Michaeleen 103 West Lincoln Way, La Porte, IN 46350, (312) 859-1144, BS 76 Marquette Univ; MA 77 Marquette Univ; **SLP**

Eklund, Mrs Tami Hemby 911 Rocky River Road North, Monroe, NC 28110, (919) 294-4860, BS 81 Appalachian St Univ; MA 82 Appalachian St Univ; SLP, Lancaster County Schools, **SLP ACE**

Ekman, Mrs Dolores Jean 4306 Barry, Klamath Falls, OR 97603, (503) 884-2137, BA 82 CA St Univ - Chico; MA 84 CA St Univ - Chico; **SLP**

Ekren, Wayne K 11716 96th Place North, Seminole, FL 34642, (813) 398-2506, BA 76 Univ of NM; MS 77 Univ of NM; 87–Pres, Rehab Solutions of Florida Inc, **SLP**

Ekren-Cambra, Mrs Susan G 4895 Cobbler Court, Pleasanton, CA 94566, (415) 651-6958, BA 78 CA St Univ - Sacramento; MA 80 CA St Univ - Sacramento; Sp-Lang Path, Fremont USD, **SLP**

Ekstrom, Anita M 6937 Pinkney Street, Omaha, NE 68104, (402) 572-2278, BS 74 Univ of NE - Omaha; BS 75 Univ of NE - Omaha; OM 78 Univ of NE - Omaha; 78–Sp-Lang Path, Immanuel Med Cen, **SLP ACE**

Ekstrom, Barbara I 19 Wales Road, Monson, MA 01057, (413) 283-3411, BA 72 Univ of MA - Amherst; MA 76 Univ of MA - Amherst; Superv Sp & Hrng, Monson Dev Cen, **A ACE**

Ekstrom, Cathy Faeger Violet Road, Rocky Point, NY 11778, BA 79 Adelphi Univ; MS 81 Adelphi Univ; Sp-Lang Path, BOCES II, **SLP**

Elam, David Scott 757 Winding Way, Encinitas, CA 92024, (619) 944-9012, BA 81 Univ of the Pacific; MA 83 Univ of Denver; 84–Sp/Lang Path, Chldn's Hosp & Hlth Cen, **SLP**

Elam, Nancy Revelli 757 Winding Way, Encinitas, CA 92024, (619) 541-3088, BS 80 CA St Univ - Hayward; MA 81 Univ of the Pacific; 85–Sp/Lang Path, Cldn's Hosp and Health Center, **SLP**

Eland, Mrs Marla H 302 Brampton Lane, Lincolnshire Woods, Lake Forest, IL 60045, MA; **SLP**

Elash, Alice I 1805 Belasco Avenue, Pittsburgh, PA 15216, **SLP**

Elash, Mrs Eletah Paula 6362 Farm Hill Way, San Jose, CA 95120-1812, (408) 268-9112, BA 74; MA 80 CA St Univ - Northridge; SLP, Glendale USD, **SLP**

Elassal, Mrs Ruth Marie 2415 S W 122nd, Oklahoma City, OK 73170, (402) 691-0012, MS 85 Univ of WI - Stevens Point; **SLP**

Elaswad, Mary Beth 1696 Cram Circle #8, Ann Arbor, MI 48105, (313) 763-8339, MS 84 Univ of MI - Ann Arbor; SLP, Total Therapy Mgmt, **SLP**

Elbaum, Marjorie 14 Hilltop Drive, Melville, NY 11747, **SLP**

Elbers, Caroline H G 831 Gates Avenue, Norfolk, VA 23517, (804) 547-9627, MS 86 Old Dominion Univ; 88–Sp-Lang Path, Pro Phys Ther & Rehab Inc, **SLP**

Elbert, Mrs Dora L R 3228 Royal Drive, Grand Forks, ND 58201, (701) 594-4441, BS 71 Univ of ND; MS 75 Central MO St Univ; Sp/Lang Path, Grand Forks Pub Schs, **SLP**

Elbert, Dr Mary F 822 South Fess, Bloomington, IN 47401, (812) 337-4864, BA 53 Avila Coll; MA 66 Univ of KS; PH 76 (NS) Univ of KS; **SLP F**

Elder, Frances J 1618 W Arrow Highway #264, Upland, CA 91786, (714) 946-4698, BS 77 Wichita St Univ; MA 78 Wichita St Univ; SLP, Headstart State Preschool, **SLP**

Elder, Sharon Hooper 4101 Prindle Court, Apartment 204, Chesapeake, VA 23321, (804) 465-3407, BS 81 James Madison Univ; ME 85 James Madison Univ; Aud, **A**

Eldis, Dr Frances E Childrens Hospital Of Michigan, 3901 Beaubien, Detroit, MI 48201, (313) 745-8903, BS 60 Wayne St Univ; MA 66 Wayne St Univ; PH 74 (Aud) Wayne St Univ; 71–Dept Head Commun Dis, Chldn Hosp of MI, **SLP A F ACE**

Eldot, Dr Howard L Communication Disorders Prog, Dept Of Special Education, Eastern Kentucky Univ, Richmond, KY 40475, (606) 622-4442, OB 58 Univ of Miami; MS 61 Syracuse Univ; PH 65 (NS) IN Univ - Bloomington; Assoc Prof, Eastern KY U, **A**

Eldredge, Christine 2827 North 84th Street, Milwaukee, WI 53222, BS 77 Marquette Univ; MS 79 Marquette Univ; Sp-Lang Path, Milwaukee Pub Sch, **SLP**

Eldredge, Mrs Patricia Devers 1727 El Vista Circle, Arcadia, CA 91006, (213) 926-5566, MA 75 CA St Univ - Los Angeles; Program Coordinator, ABC USD, **SLP**

Eldrich, Civia Reich 40 Apple Tree Lane, Hamden, CT 06518, Southern CT St Univ; Dept Chairperson SLP, Hamden Pub Sch, **SLP**

Eldridge, Mrs Darby B 1071 Choke Cherry Drive, Winter Springs, FL 32707, (305) 365-5611, BS 74 Univ of VA - Charlottesville; ME 75 Univ of VA - Charlottesville; Sp-Lang Path, Seminole Co Sch Bd, **SLP**

Eldridge, Mrs Doris D 3 Pricewoods Lane, Olivette, MO 63132, (314) 644-9564, BS 56 TN St Univ; MA 69 Saint Louis Univ; 88–Human Resource Dev, St Louis Comm Coll, **SLP**

Eldridge, Mrs Flavia H Route 1 Box 186-B, Jeanerette, LA 70544, (318) 365-2341, BA 68 Our Lady Lake Univ-San Anton; MA 69 Our Lady Lake Univ-San Anton; MA 79 Univ of Southwestern LA; 78–Coord-Sp-Lang Path, Iberia Prsh Sch Bd, **SLP**

Eldridge, Linda Karen 595 North Marengo Avenue, Pasadena, CA 91101, (818) 795-7732, BA 76 San Jose St Univ; MA 80 San Jose St Univ; SLP, San Carlos Sch Dist, **SLP**

Eldridge, Sandra J 3311 Mission Drive, Santa Cruz, CA 95060, **SLP**

Eldringhoff, Judy L 10497 Chardonniere Drive, Ferguson, MO 63135, (314) 569-1503, BA 70 Southern IL Univ-Edwardsvill; MS 74 Southern IL Univ-Edwardsvill; Sp/Lang Path/Erly Chldhd Sp Ed, Spec Sch Dist of St Louis Co, **SLP**

Elenbogen, Janet C 5461 N East River Road, Apartment 209, Chicago, IL 60656, (312) 650-4028, BS 74 Northwestern Univ; MA 75 Northwestern Univ; 84–Sp-Lang Path, Chicago PS, **SLP ACE**

Elensky, Mrs Nancy C P O Box 205, Curwensville, PA 16833, (814) 236-3761, BS 68 Edinboro Univ of PA; ME 73 Clarion Univ of PA; 80–Sp-Lang Path, Private Practice, **SLP**

Eley, Mrs Burnice Bailey 1403 Brierwood, Cleveland, MS 38732, (601) 846-6020, BS 75 Delta St Univ; ME 79 MS St Univ - MS State; MS 85 Univ of MS; Educational Consultant SLP, Educational Remediation Serv, **SLP**

Elfenbein, Dr Jill Libbie Office 125, Wendell Johnson Center, Univ Of Iowa, Iowa City, IA 52242, (319) 335-8726, BS 73 SUNY - Center at Albany; MA 75 Univ of IA; PH 86 (Aud) Univ of IA; 86–Asst Prof, U of IA, **SLP A**

Elftman, Mrs Elizabeth 5959 Beechwood Avenue, Indianapolis, IN 46219, (317) 259-8105, BS 69 CO St Univ; MS 71 CO St Univ; Aud, Indianapolis Sp/Hrng Cen, **A**

Elgaard, Mrs Gina Marie 2323 Hamilton #206, Regina, SK, Canada S4P 3Y5, (306) 569-1053, MA 87 CA St Univ - Long Beach; 88–Sp-Lang Path, Regina Sch Bd, **SLP**

Elgart-Light, Candace 3357 West 97th Avenue, Apart #15, Westminster, CO 80030, **SLP**

Elggren, Barbara Lorille 4387 Cherry Avenue, San Jose, CA 95118, (408) 637-5393, BS 84 Brigham Young Univ; OM 85 Brigham Young Univ

Elgort, Janice Dale 40 Havemeyer Lane, Commack, NY 11725, (516) 027-4780, BA 80 Hofstra Univ; MS 82 Adelphi Univ; SLP, BOCES II, **SLP**

El Halta, Barbara Ellayne 704 North 945 West, Orem, UT 84056, (801) 756-6022, BS 84 Brigham Young Univ; OM 86 Brigham Young Univ

Elias, Katherine M 5 Farm Road, Belmont, MA 02178, (617) 489-5204, BA 71 Univ of MA - Amherst; MA 72 Univ of MA - Amherst; Sp-Lang Path, Belmont Pub Sch, **SLP**

Elias, Mrs Patricia D 4301 West Chester, Waco, TX 76710, (817) 772-6132, BS 56 Marquette Univ; **SLP**

Eliason, Mrs Deborah T HC 1 Box 1629, Pengilly, MN 55775, (218) 262-1000, BS 77 Univ of MN - Duluth; MA 82 Univ of MN - Duluth; Sp-Lang Path, Private Practice, **SLP**

Eliason, Elizabeth St Julien Strasse 2/616, Salzburg, Austria A5020, BS 77 Univ of Redlands; MS 79 Univ of Redlands; Sp-Lang Path, **SLP**

Eliason, Mrs M Jane 2520 Charnelton, Eugene, OR 97405, (503) 726-3380, BA 64 Univ of MN - Minneap-St Paul; MS 82 Univ of OR; 87–Sp-Lang Path, Springfield Sch Dist #19, **SLP**

Elick-Wolyniak, Mrs Katherine L 304 Winchester Drive, South Lyon, MI 48178, BS 73 Eastern MI Univ; MA 74 Eastern MI Univ; Northville Pub Schs, **SLP**

Elieff, Linda M 915 Panorama Drive, Bakersfield, CA 93305, (805) 872-2777, BA 76 CA St Univ - Fresno; MA 79 CA St Univ - Fresno; Sp-Lang Path, Kern Hgh Sch Dist, **SLP**

Eliot, Mrs Joanne 15452 Kippfcrd Court, Miami Lakes, FL 33014, (305) 362-1192, BA 52 Univ of ME - Orono; MA 78 Univ of Miami; Sp-Lang Path, Dade Co Pub Schls, **SLP**

Eliuk, Bonnie E 86-110 Baylor Avenue, Winnipeg, MB, Canada R3T 3K1, (204) 786-7841, BA 77 Univ of Manitoba - Winnipeg; MS 79 Minot St Univ; Sp-Lang Path, Child Guidance Cl of Winnipeg, **SLP**

Elk, Mrs Debby N 54 Olde Carriage Road, Westwood, MA 02090, BA 69 CUNY - Brooklyn Coll; MS 70 Univ of MI - Ann Arbor; Sp-Lang Path, Walpole PS, **SLP**

Elkan, Mrs Mindy C R 111 Dehaven Drive, Yonkers, NY 10703, (914) 963-2259, BS 77 SUNY - Coll at Oswego; MA 78 Hofstra Univ; Sp-Lang Path, Ferncliffe Manor for Retarded, **SLP**

Elkayam, Judith M Regional Hearing Impaired Prog, 1755 South Wolf Road, Des Plaines, IL 60018, (312) 390-9440, BA 71 Univ of MA - Amherst; MA 74 Northwestern Univ; Aud, Reg Hrng Imp Prog, **A**

El Khoury, Mrs Jo-Ellen Oleary 76 Adams Road, Grafton, MA 01536, (617) 839-5025, **SLP**

Elkin, Esther B 9 Orchard Lane, Wayland, MA 01778, (617) 431-7666, BS 63 Baptist Bible Coll; MS 65 Univ of PA; Programmer, Geospace Systems Corp, **A**

Elkins, Mrs Andee Ann 4210 San Augustine, Pasadena, TX 77503, BS 75 Southwest TX St Univ; ME 76 Southwest TX St Univ; **SLP**

Elkins, Dorothy B 3908 Asbury Parker Circle, Birmingham, AL 35243, (205) 491-1002, BS 60 Eastern KY Univ; MA 70 Univ of KY; Sp-Lang Path, Jefferson Co Bd of Ed, **SLP**

Elkins, Dr Earleen 15107 Interlachen Drive, Apartment 511, Silver Spring, MD 20906, (301) 598-3818, BA 54 Univ of MD - College Park; MA 56 Univ of MD - College Park; PH 67 (Hrng & Sp Sciences) Univ of MD - College Park; 87–Chief-Neurosciences, NIAAA, **A**

Elkins, Patricia Anne 8415 Habersham Pointe Circle, Apartment 311, Pineville, NC 28134, (704) 541-6418, BA 81 Univ of NC - Greensboro; ME 82 Univ of NC - Greensboro; Sp-Lang Path, Charlotte-Mecklenburg Sch Syst, **SLP**

Elkins, Mrs Suzanne H 13602 Chatwood, San Antonio, TX 78217, (512) 656-1683, BA 64 Univ of TX - Austin; ME 79 Southwest TX St Univ; Sp-Lang Path, NE ISD, **SLP ACE**

Elledge, Mrs Debra L 16606 Thunderbay, Houston, TX 77062, (713) 471-0954, BS 76 Indiana Univ of PA; MA 80 Ball St Univ; Sp-Lang Path, La Porte Indep Sch Dis, **SLP**

Elledge, Patti L 4618 Idlewilde Lane S E, Albuquerque, NM 87108, (505) 883-0131, BA 74 Univ of OK - Norman; MS 76 Univ of OK Medical Center; 86–Sp-Lang Path, Barnes and Elledge, **SLP**

Elleman, Mrs Charlotte Ann 704 Davidson Street, Raleigh, NC 27609, (919) 737-3767, BA 52 Denison Univ; MA 54 OH St Univ, Lecturer, North Carolina State U, **SLP ACE**

Ellenbogen, Judith Lichtiger 4 Croydon Court, Dix Hills, NY 11746, **SLP**

Ellenbogen, Mrs Nancy Jo 12264 Greenleaf Avenue, Potomac, MD 20854, (301) 251-1716, BS 75 Syracuse Univ; MA 76 George Washington Univ; Sp-Lang Path, Private Practice, **SLP**

Ellender, Mrs Elizabeth 301 San Antonio Boulevard, Houma, LA 70360, (504) 868-7371, BA 64 CUNY - City College; MA 68 LA St Univ - Baton Rouge; **SLP**

Ellenwood, John R R 2 Box 1195, Underhill, VT 05489, (802) 899-3087, OB 57 OH Univ - Athens; MS 63 OH Univ - Athens; Sp/Lang Path, Colchester Sch Dist, **SLP**

Eller, Connie 143 East Circle Drive, Denison, IA 51442, **SLP**

Ellermeyer, Mrs Cynthia Ann Rd 2 Box 139-W, Slippery Rock, PA 16057-8419, (412) 658-3511, BS 80 Clarion Univ of PA; MS 83 Clarion Univ of PA; Sp-Lang Path, Speac-Aid, **SLP**

Eller-Miller, Eileen Faythe 29 Gammons Road, Waban, MA 02168, (617) 522-5434, BA 56 CUNY - City College; MA 57 Columbia Univ Teachers Coll; Director, Language & Cognitive Dev Ctr, **SLP**

Ellett, Mrs Lee Withers 1411 Russell Road, Alexandria, VA 22301, (703) 836-5035, BS 75 Univ of VA - Charlottesville; ME 76 Univ of VA - Charlottesville; 88–Sp-Lang Path, Resurrection Children's Center, **SLP**

Ellibee, Gina Holman 1249 East 2450 North, Layton, UT 84040, (801) 775-0268, BS 82 PA St Univ - Univ Park; MS 85 UT St Univ; 88–Sp-Lang Path, Ogden City Schs, **SLP ACE**

Ellicott, Mrs Barbara A 41 Brookwood Road, Byram Township, NJ 07874, (201) 948-3727, BA 63 Montclair St Coll; MA 67 Montclair St Coll; 88–Sp-Lang Path, Essex County Hosp, **SLP**

Elliehausen, Jennifer Cobb 261 Hackman Road, Ephrata, PA 17522, (717) 569-7331, BS 83 East Stroudsburg Univ of PA; MS 84 Bloomsburg Univ of PA; **SLP**

Elling, Susan Mary P O Box 17515, Boulder, CO 80308, (303) 443-0230, BA 82 Univ of CO - Boulder; MA 86 Univ of CO - Boulder; **SLP**

Ellingsen, Mary Elizabeth 2933 East Exeter Street, Tucson, AZ 85716, (602) 795-2754, MA 76 Univ of AZ; 86–Dir, Ellingsen & Associates Inc, **SLP**

Elliot, Elyse M 527 Pine Street, Leesport, PA 19533, (215) 562-6225, BS 70 Clarion Univ of PA; ME 74 Clarion Univ of PA; Assistant Unit Mananger, Commonwealth of Pennsylvania, **SLP A**

Elliot, Mrs Linda Pighini 2261 El Capitan Drive, Riverside, CA 92506, (714) 784-7027, MS 80 West Chester Univ of PA; SLP, Alvord USD, **SLP**

Elliott, Alicia 1038 Grover Avenue, Glendale, CA 91201, (818) 243-9847, BA 73 CA St Univ - Long Beach; MA 74 CA St Univ - Long Beach; MA 80 CA St Univ - Long Beach; SLP/Educ Consultant, Acad Lang & Behav Inter Serv, **SLP**

Elliott, Ann Driscoll 1220 Glencove Road North, Syracuse, NY 13206, (315) 437-4536, BS 72 SUNY - Coll at Oswego; MS 78 Syracuse Univ; Sp-Lang Path, Onondaga Board Coop Ed Servcs, **SLP**

Elliott, Betty T C-4 Gloucester Court, Lexington Park, MD 20653, (301) 862-2989, BS 82 Indiana Univ of PA; MS 84 WV Univ; Sp-Lang Path, St Mary's County PS, **SLP**

Elliott, Mrs Cathy C 4941 West 129th Terrace, Leawood, KS 66209-1815, (913) 681-3921, BS 78 Univ of MO - Columbia; MA 79 Univ of MO - Columbia; **SLP**

Elliott, Charlene B 25 Mechanic Street, Foxboro, MA 02035-9990, (617) 848-2551, BS 78 Univ of MA - Amherst; MS 80 Univ of OK Medical Center; Sp-Lnag Path, Braintree Hosp, **SLP**

Elliott, Dr Charles R 2049 Pratt Court, Evanston, IL 60201, (312) 328-3964, BA 36 Albion Coll; MA 44 Univ of NC - Chapel Hill; PH 56 (NS) Univ of NC - Chapel Hill; **SLP LM**

Elliott, Mrs Cheryl Walker 5708 Swede Road, Midland, MI 48640, (517) 832-8213, MA 86 Central MI Univ

Elliott, Christine 6208 West Sandra Terrace, Glendale, AZ 85306, (602) 439-3391, BS 74 Univ of Northern CO; MS 76 AZ St Univ; 76–Sp-Lang Path, Private Practice, **SLP**

Elliott, Franklyn 230 Hewlett Avenue, Merrick, NY 11566, (516) 735-0256, MA 51 CUNY - Brooklyn Coll; Psychol, Mineola Pub Sch, **SLP**

Elliott, Jill Louise 632 South 8th Street, La Grange, IL 60525, (312) 579-3584, BS 84 IL St Univ - Normal; MS 85 IL St Univ - Normal; SLP, District 161, **SLP**

Elliott, Dr John W 5715 Meadowbrook Drive, Harrisburg, PA 17112, (717) 787-7666, BS 65 Clarion Univ of PA; MS 67 SUNY - Coll at Buffalo; PH 72 (Speech Pathology) SUNY - Center at Buffalo; 81–Hospital Service Area Manager, Dept of Pub Welfare, **SLP**

Elliott, Mrs Kristine M 114 Peggy Lane, Johnstown, PA 15904, (814) 269-3816, BA 70 Mary Washington Coll; ME 71 Univ of VA - Charlottesville; Chief/Sp-Lang Pathology, Conemaugh Valley Memorial Hosp, **SLP**

Elliott, Linda S 3205 Broken Bow Court, Edmond, OK 73013, (405) 340-7056, BA 69 Univ of OK - Norman; MS 71 Univ of OK Medical Center; 86–Sp-Lang Path, Speech & Hearing Assoc, **SLP**

Elliott, Dr Lois Lawrence Northwestern University, Frances Searle Bldg, 2299 Sheridan Road, Evanston, IL 60201, (312) 491-3161, BA 53 Bryn Mawr Coll; PH 56 (Experimental Psychology) Cornell Univ; 76–Prof, Nwn U

Elliott, Mrs Lori Cross 502 Erich Street, Wernersville, PA 19565, (215) 670-2106, BS 80 OH Univ - Athens; OM 82 Hahneman Medical Coll; SLP/Aud, **SLP A**

Elliott, M Lynn Eugene Hearing And Speech Ctr, P O Box 2087, 1202 Almaden, Eugene, OR 97402, (503) 485-8521, BA 69 Oberlin Coll; MS 71 Washington Univ; Aud, Eugene Hearing & Speech Center, **A**

Elliott, Margaret L 140 East 16th Street, San Bernardino, CA 92404, MS; **SLP LM**

Elliott, Mrs Margaret Tampieri 1 Willow Avenue, Towson, MD 21204, (301) 823-4278, Sp-Lang Path, Harford Co Boe, **SLP**

Elliott, Marian 100 North Dryden, Arlington Heights, IL 60004, OB 40 Northern IL Univ - De Kalb; MA 48 Northwestern Univ; **SLP LM**

Elliott, Mrs Marsha K 12907 Laurel-Bowie Road, Apartment 204, Laurel, MD 20708, (301) 604-2655, BS 79 Northwest MO St Univ; MS 80 Northwest MO St Univ; Sp-Lang Path, Treatment & Learning Centers, **SLP**

Elliott, Mrs Mary-Anne 16011 Fernway Road, Shaker Heights, OH 44120, (216) 531-9000, BS 81 West Chester Univ of PA; MA 83 Case Western Reserve Univ; Sp-Lang Path, Euclid Hosp Rehab Ctr, **SLP ACE**

Elliott, Mrs Mary B 5 Kenstone Court, Florissant, MO 63033, (314) 838-7190, BA 69 Fontbonne Coll; MA 71 Univ of MN - Minneap-St Paul; Sp-Lang Path, Private Practice, **SLP**

Elliott, Norma H 3925 East Camelback Road, Apartment 265, Phoenix, AZ 85018, (602) 468-9744, BS 72 Eastern KY Univ; MS 73 Vanderbilt Univ; 86–Sp-Lang Path, Private Practice, **SLP**

Elliott, Mrs Ovieda Perra 1938 Highland Circle, Eureka, CA 95501, (707) 445-5111, BA 81 Humboldt St Univ; MA 83 Humboldt St Univ; Sp-Lang Path, Gen Hosp Rehab Ctr, **SLP**

Elliott, Mrs Patti Jo 124 South Holbrook, Fort Scott, KS 66701, (316) 223-0360, BA 56 Northeastern OK St Univ; MS 70 Pittsburg St Univ; Sp-Lang Path, USD 234, **SLP**

Elliott, Phyllis R 1118 N Street, Bedford, IN 47421, (812) 275-3555, BA 76 IN Univ - Bloomington; MA 81 IN Univ - Bloomington; Director of Speech Pathology, Dunn Memorial Hospital, **SLP**

Elliott, Rebecca 170 Camelot, Huntington, WV 25701, (304) 529-7764, BS 64 WV Univ; OM 66 Univ of OK Medical Center; **SLP**

Elliott, Samuel B 1101 Colquitt Avenue N E, Atlanta, GA 30307, (494) 957-6601, BA 79 Univ of WA; ME 83 GA St Univ; SLP, Private Practice, **SLP**

Elliott, Mrs Sherry Lynn 3517 Meadow Brook Drive, Midwest City, OK 73110, (405) 787-7886, BS 75 OK St Univ; MA 83 OK St Univ; SLP, Choctaw Nicoma Park Sch Sys, **SLP**

Elliott, Mrs Susan Kay 854 Terrace Trace, Lawrenceville, GA 30244, (404) 963-7624, MS 82 Miami Univ - Oxford; 88–Sp-Lang Path, Private Practice, **SLP**

Elliott, Virginia 124 Keyser Street, Marietta, OH 45750, (614) 373-3781, BA 73 Marietta Coll; MA 74 OH St Univ; Sp-Lang Path, WA Co Bd Men Ret & Dev Disabl, **SLP**

Elliott, Wendy Lee 9601 S W 142nd Avenue #1206, Miami, FL 33186, (305) 251-0710, BA 82 Marshall Univ; MA 83 Marshall Univ; Sp-Lang Path, National Sp & Hrng, **SLP**

Elliott-Blondin, Mrs Robin Ann 400 Manda Lane #203, Wheeling, IL 60090, (312) 215-8405, BS 85 Miami Univ - Oxford; MS 87 Miami Univ - Oxford; 88–Sp-Lang Path, North Chicago Sch Dist #64

Ellis, Charles C Bakersfield Memorial Hospital, Rehabilitation Center, P O Box 1888, Attn SPL Pathology, Bakersfield, CA 93303, (805) 327-1792, BA 76 Univ of Northern IA; MA 78 Univ of Northern IA; Dir Sp-Lang Path, Bakersfield Mem Hosp, **SLP**

Ellis, Mrs Cherrye Hammans 12337 Washington Brice Rd, Fairfax, VA 22033, (703) 620-4912, BA 74 Univ of AR - Fayetteville; MS 76 CO St Univ; **SLP**

Ellis, Christina Ann 1823 Kingsbury Drive, Redlands, CA 92374-1710, (714) 793-1643, MS 84 Univ of Redlands; **SLP**

Ellis, Colette L The Chickasha Clinic, 2222 Iowa Avenue, Chickasha, OK 73018, (405) 224-4853, BS 75 Central St Univ; ME 79 Central St Univ; Sp-Lang Path, Southern Plains Med Ctr, **SLP**

Ellis, Cynthia E 711 Florence Avenue, Astoria, OR 97103, (503) 325-2862, BA 83 Univ of CA - Santa Barbara; MA 85 WA St Univ; Sp-Lang Path, Clatsop Educ Service District, **SLP**

Ellis, Mrs Deborah T 9560 Heatherdale, Dallas, TX 75243, (214) 343-6919, BS 72 East TX St Univ - Commerce; MS 74 East TX St Univ - Commerce; Sp-Lang Path, Mesquite ISD, **SLP**

Ellis, Donna Marie 598 Gleneagles Drive, Kamloops, BC, Canada V2E 1X2, (604) 828-4415, BS 85 ID St Univ; MS 86 ID St Univ; Aud, British Columbia Ministry of Hlth, **A**

Ellis, Elizebeth 5111 Silverwood Court, Great Falls, MT 59401, (805) 734-3686, **SLP**

Ellis, Mrs Ellen K Box 382, North Newton, KS 67117, (316) 283-1562, BA 81 Wichita St Univ; MA 82 Wichita St Univ; 88–Sp-Lang Path, Private Practice, **SLP**

Ellis, Mrs Eva M 1845 Langerdale Boulevard, South Euclid, OH 44121, (216) 421-4481, BS 76 Ashland Coll; MA 81 Case Western Reserve Univ; Sp-Lang Path, Mt Sinai Med Cen, **SLP**

Ellis, Mrs Felinda Trolinder Route 9 Box 195-E, Canyon Lake, TX 78133, (512) 696-1910, BS 85 TX Tech Univ; MA 87 Our Lady Lake Univ-San Anton; 87–Sp-Lang Path, South TX Children's Hab Ctr, **SLP**

Ellis, Gayle J 3344 Dudley Street, Lincoln, NE 68503, (402) 472-5552, BS 76 Univ of NE - Lincoln; MA 78 Univ of NE - Lincoln; Sp-Lang Path, U of NE - Lincoln, **SLP**

Ellis, H Sherrill 7 West Park Avenue, New Haven, CT 06511, (203) 777-7905, ME 72 Univ of VA - Charlottesville; MS 88 Southern CT St Univ; 88–Sp-Lang Path, Stamford PS

Ellis, Mrs Jane M S 633 North 3rd Street, Danville, KY 40422, (606) 236-6157, OB 72 Univ of KY; BA 75 Univ of KY; MA 76 Univ of KY; 76–Sp-Lang Path, Danville Public Schools, **SLP**

Ellis, Joan B 2626 Montrose Avenue, Montrose, CA 91020, (818) 957-7877, BA 68 Univ of CA - Los Angeles; SLP, Los Angeles USD, **SLP**

Ellis, Joan J P O Box 71, Hudson, ME 04449, (207) 924-5571, BS 71 Univ of WI - LA Crosse; MA 81 Univ of ME - Orono; Sp-Lang Path, Msad #46 Dexter Sch Sys, **SLP**

Ellis, Mrs Julia Reiman 742 S E Claremont Court, Lee's Summit, MO 64063, (816) 373-2300, BS 85 IA St Univ; MS 86 Central MO St Univ; **SLP**

Ellis, Julie Heiman 10528 Cortez Circle, Apartment 22, Franklin, WI 53132, **SLP**

Ellis, Mrs Lavonne 14 Creekside Lane, Barrington Hills, IL 60010, (312) 520-2785, BS 73 IL St Univ - Normal; MS 74 IL St Univ - Normal; Sp-Lang Path, Comm Consol Sch Dist #21, **SLP**

Ellis, Lee W 12 Grant Street, The Plains, OH 45780-1241, (614) 797-4023, BA 73 Univ of Southern ME; MA 75 Univ of ME - Orono; Sp-Lang Path, Private Practice, **SLP**

Ellis, Dr Leonard Ministry Of Health Sp & Hrng, Rotherham Place, 1520 Blanshard St 3rd Flr, Victoria, BC, Canada V8W 3C8, (604) 387-2670, BA 59 McGill Univ - Quebec; MA 65 Univ of IA; PH 71 (NS) Univ of IL - Urbana; SLP, Provence of Bc-Minist Hlth, **SLP**

Ellis, Mrs Linda A 123 Melville Street, Cola, SC 29210, (803) 254-2496, BA 75 LA St Univ - Baton Rouge; MA 76 Univ of AL- Tuscaloosa; Sp-Lang Path, Midland Ear Nose Throat Clinic, **SLP**

Ellis, Mrs Lori Klisman 37685 Lancaster Drive, Farmington Hills, MI 48018, (313) 661-9048, BA 81 MI St Univ; MA 82 Eastern MI Univ; Sp-Lang Path, Wayne Co Inter Sch, **SLP**

Ellis, Marian Leigh 748 Yama, Yreka, CA 96097, (916) 842-5751, BS 82 Coll of Charleston; MS 86 Columbia Univ Teachers Coll; 86–Sp-Lang Path, Siskiyou County Ofc of Educ, **SLP**

Ellis, Martha Anne 79 Horatio #1R, New York, NY 10014, (212) 807-1388, BA 75 Univ of CO - Boulder; MS 78 Univ Southern MS-Hattiesburg; **A**

Ellis, Mary Lucena 237 Mortimer Lane, Marina, CA 93933, (408) 384-8673, BS 84 Western IL Univ; MA 85 Western IL Univ; Sp-Lang Path, San Benito Co Ofc of Educ, **SLP**

Ellis, Mary M 1224 Marijon Drive, Chattanooga, TN 37421, (615) 892-3725, BS 46 Univ of TN - Knoxville; MS 54 Univ of TN - Knoxville; Retired, **SLP LM**

Ellis, Mrs Maureen O'Connell 2 Noble Avenue, Barrington, RI 02806, (401) 245-0277, MS 85 Univ of RI; **SLP**

Ellis, Maxine 2420 Castillo Street #100, Santa Barbara, CA 93105, (805) 563-1111, BA 61 CA St Univ - Los Angeles; MA 61 CA St Univ - Los Angeles; Aud, Jr Di Bartolomeo MD Inc, **A**

Ellis, Mrs Nancy A 9643 Treetop Drive, Galesburg, MI 49053, (616) 665-9175, BS 75 Western MI Univ; MA 80 Western MI Univ; Sp-Lang Path, Battle Creek Public Schools, **SLP**

Ellis, Roberta A 35 Bay Terrace, Jamestown, RI 02835, (401) 423-0626, BA 58 RI Coll; MA 67 Northwestern Univ; Sp/Lang Path, West Warwick Sch Dept, **SLP**

Ellis, Mrs Rose M Vasta 22 Orchard Way, Yardley, PA 19067, (215) 493-4451, BA 74 Rutgers St Univ -N Brunswick; MA 75 Trenton St Coll; 85–Sp-Lang Path, Bucks Assn Retarded Citizens, **SLP**

Ellis, Sandra Kase 17617 N E 29th, Redmond, WA 98052, (206) 833-4050, BS 76 Univ of WA; MS 78 Univ of WA; Aud, Green River ENT Cl, **A**

Ellis, Shana 17828 92nd N E, Bothell, WA 98011, **SLP**

Ellis, Susan Kay 2249 East Apple Avenue #12, Muskegon, MI 49442, (616) 777-2581, BS 82 Western MI Univ; MA 83 Western MI Univ; Aud, Muskegon Hearing & Speech Ctr, **A ACE**

Ellis, Mrs Susan L 4035 Prescott, Lincoln, NE 68506, (402) 483-4370, BS 71 Univ of TN - Knoxville; MA 73 Univ of TN - Knoxville; Sp-Lang Path, Tabitha Home Inc, **SLP**

Ellis, Suzanne 61 Prince Way, East Dennis, MA 02641, (617) 540-8600, BA 83 Assumption Coll; MS 86 Worcester St Coll; **SLP**

Ellis, William R 444 North Atlanta Avenue, North Massapequa, NY 11758, (516) 759-0008, BA 82 Hofstra Univ; MA 84 Hofstra Univ; **A**

Ellisen-Doe, Mrs Katherine M 222 Long Court, Appleton, WI 54915, (414) 729-5090, BA 68 Augustana Coll; MS 82 Univ of WI - Oshkosh; Sp-Lang Path, Menasha Public Schools, **SLP**

Ellison, Cynthia L Comprehensive Audiologic Serv, 2566 Woodmeadow Drive S E, Grand Rapids, MI 49506, (616) 942-1660, BS 73 Northern IL Univ - De Kalb; MA 74 Northern IL Univ - De Kalb; Aud, Comprehensive Aud Serv, **A**

Ellison, Mrs Elaine K 404 Ashbourne Road, Elkins Park, PA 19117, (215) 635-1361, BA 57 Temple Univ; MA 73 Temple Univ; Sp/Lang Path, Episcopal Hospital, **SLP ACE**

Ellison, Lisa A 2050 West 10th Avenue, Apt #6-107, Broomfield, CO 80020, (303) 469-5996, BA 85 Univ of CO - Boulder; MA 87 Univ of CO - Boulder; SLP

Ellison, Mrs Marcia F P O Box 27, Anna, IL 62906, (618) 684-2109, BS 63 Southern IL Univ -Carbondale; MS 66 Southern IL Univ -Carbondale; SLP, Tri-Co Spec Ed Dist, **SLP**

Ellner, Scott A 4 Providence Lane, Howell, NJ 07731, (212) 761-2900, BS 73 Long Island U - Brooklyn Ctr; MS 75 Syracuse Univ; Sp-Lang Path, UCP of NY, **SLP**

Ellsworth, Mrs Janet B 3122 East 83rd, Tulsa, OK 74137, (918) 299-4411, BS 71 Univ of OK - Norman; MS 72 Washington Univ; Sp-Lang Path, Jenks Pub Sch, **SLP**

Ellsworth, Mrs Kathleen Marie 2331 Inas Drive, Akron, OH 44321, (216) 848-0482, BS 81 Miami Univ - Oxford; MS 82 Miami Univ - Oxford; Sp-Lang Path, InSpeech Inc, **SLP**

Ellsworth-Severcool, Mrs Rebecca Anne Rd #4 Box 217-C, Montrose, PA 18801, (717) 278-4168, BA 78 SUNY - Coll at Cortland; MS 80 Rutgers St Univ -N Brunswick; Sp-Lang Path, Union-Endicott Cent Sch Dist, **SLP**

Ellwood, Marti Maloney 104 North Prospect Manor Avenue, Mount Prospect, IL 60056-2330, (312) 253-5958, BS 80 Southern IL Univ -Carbondale; MA 82 Northern IL Univ - De Kalb; SLP, Lutheran Gen Hosp, **SLP**

Elman, Roberta J 3996 Lyman Road, Oakland, CA 94602, (415) 228-6800, BA 79 Univ of CA - Santa Barbara; MA 82 Univ of MN - Minneap-St Paul; Sp-Lang Path, VA Hosp, **SLP**

Elmets, Laurie Melamed 3962 White Oak Trail, Orange Village, OH 44122, (216) 831-1576, BS 77 Northwestern Univ; MA 79 Case Western Reserve Univ; **A**

Elmore, Carolyn Grace Rd #1 Box 206, High Falls, NY 12440, (914) 687-9293, BA 83 SUNY - Coll at Cortland; MA 86 Univ of IL - Urbana; Sp-Lang Path, Onteora School District, **SLP**

Elmore, Mrs Janice B 3008 Monarch, Plano, TX 75074, (214) 424-6604, BS 77 KS St Univ; MA 79 KS St Univ; Sp-Lang Path, Plano ISD, **SLP**

Elmore, LtCol John Howard 14639 London Lane, Bowie, MD 20715-0971, (301) 262-2553, BA 68 Adams St Coll; OM 81 OK City Univ; MA 71 Northern IL Univ - De Kalb; Chief Sci/Tech Div, Hqtr USAF Systems Command, **A ACE**

Elmore, Ralph M Gracewood State School & Hosp, Speech & Hearing Clinic, Gracewood, GA 30812, **SLP**

Elmore, Suzanne 2866 South University Dr, #5101, Davie, FL 33328, (305) 475-9610, BS 72 Central St Univ; MA 74 Univ of OK - Norman; 84–Sp-Lang Path Supvr, Mem Hosp of Hollywood, **SLP**

El-Oqlah, Mrs Sherri Michelle 3602 Tyla #4, Memphis, TN 38127, (901) 353-4785, **A**

Elrand, Teri Anita 8038 NE 16th, Seattle, WA 98115, (206) 258-7304, BA 83 Univ of WA; MS 85 Univ of WA; Sp-Lang Path, Providence Hosp, **SLP**

Elrod, Mrs Carol Clingan 2613 Terwilleger Blvd, Tulsa, OK 74114, (918) 743-4168, BS 72 Univ of Tulsa; MA 73 Univ of Tulsa; SLP, Private Practice, **SLP**

Elsaesser, Susan 32 Macmillian Drive, Brunswick, ME 04011, BS 76 Marquette Univ; MA 77 Western MI Univ; 80–Aud, HEAR, **A**

Elsbury, Christine Carol 520 Chinworth Court #B, Warsaw, IN 46580, (219) 267-3823, BA 83 IN Univ - Bloomington; MA 84 Univ of TN - Knoxville; 85–Sp-Lang Path, Cardinal Center Inc, **SLP**

Elsen, Julie Ann 10805 South Le Claire Avenue, Oak Lawn, IL 60453, (312) 423-0782, MA 88 Univ of IL - Urbana; 88, South Metropolitan Association

Elson, Nancy Beth Canyon Woods, 147 Wilcox Ct, Matawan, NJ 07747, (201) 389-0872, BA 83 Southern CT St Univ; MA 86 Univ of MD - College Park; **A**

Elston, Mrs Krista Kile 2519 Summer Tree Lane, Apartment 2059, Arlington, TX 76006, (214) 790-8505, MS 84 IN St Univ - Terre Haute; SLP, Helping Hand Dev Cntr, **SLP**

Elsweiler, Mrs Anne Wolters 166 Preston Avenue, Logan, UT 84321, (801) 752-5368, BS 76 TX Woman's Univ; MA 81 TX Woman's Univ; 88–Sp/Lang Path, Logan City Sch Dist, **SLP**

Elswick, Mrs Nadine B 18625 Delano Street, Reseda, CA 91335, (805) 252-7766, BA 76 CA St Univ - Northridge; MA 78 CA St Univ - Northridge; MA 82 CA St Univ - Los Angeles; Prin, Saugus Union Sch Dist, **SLP**

Elvenstar, McRandon 1251 Armacost Avenue #204, Los Angeles, CA 90025, (213) 474-7216, **SLP**

Elwell, Mrs Mary Margaret 3342 Evergreen Circle, Walworth, NY 14568, (315) 986-9126, BS 75 SUNY - Coll at Geneseo; MA 81 SUNY - Coll at Geneseo; Sp/Lang Path, UCP Assoc, **SLP**

Elwert, Patricia Rita 10 Pearl Street, Montpelier, VT 05602, (802) 223-7989, MS 84 Univ of VT; 86–Sp-Lang Path, Central VT Home Health Agency, **SLP**

Elwinger, Dr Elyda S 6125 Burgundy, Shreveport, LA 71105, (318) 257-2292, BS 48 TX Woman's Univ; MA 68 Our Lady Lake Univ-San Anton; ED 78 (NS) East TX St Univ - Commerce; Assoc Prof, Behav Sci-La Tech U, **SLP**

Elwood, Mrs Joanne F 3404 Shady Hill Circle, Temple, TX 76502, (817) 778-4920, BA 73 Augustana Coll; MS 78 Baylor Univ; Sp-Lang Path, Private Practice, **SLP**

Ely, Amy N 6130 Parkdale Drive, Dallas, TX 75227-3613, (214) 388-9928, BS 74 Southern Methodist Univ; MS 76 Southern Methodist Univ; 87–Sp-Lang Path, Presbyterian Hosp of Dallas, **SLP**

Ely, Carolyn R 2326 North Upton Street, Arlington, VA 22207, (703) 922-7464, BA 70 Univ of MD - College Park; MA 71 Univ of MD - College Park; Sp-Lang Path, Fairfax Co Pub Sch, **SLP**

Ely, Monica 818 South Westwood #234, Mesa, AZ 85202, (602) 954-5866, BA 74 Univ of MN - Minneap-St Paul; MS 75 Saint Cloud St Univ; Stockbroker, Paine Weber Jackson Curtis Inc, **SLP**

Ely, Mrs Nancy Meril 12260 Greenleaf Avenue, Potomac, MD 20854, (301) 552-2270, BA 83 Univ of MD - College Park; OM 85 Emory Univ; 87–Aud, Doctors Hosp Hearing Clinic, **A**

Elzer, Judyth A A 101 Morris Avenue, Summit, NJ 07901, (201) 263-7242, BA 71 Coll of Saint Elizabeth; MA 78 Seton Hall Univ; Sp-Lang Path, Parsippany-Troy Hills Bd of Ed, **SLP**

Emal, Kent Clayton 5204 Avenue K, Kearney, NE 68847, (308) 234-8300, BA 63 Kearney St Coll; MA 67 Univ of Denver; 67–Dir Commun Dis, Kearney St Coll, **SLP**

Emanuel, Dr Floyd W 1113 Glenwood, Oklahoma City, OK 73116, (405) 271-3362, BA 53 Univ of NM; MA 57 Univ of NM; PH 63 (Communication Disorders) Univ of OK Medical Center; Prof of Commun Dis, U of OK Hlth Sci Ctr, **SLP F**

Emanuel, Permelia R 3015 North 6th Street, Harrisburg, PA 17110, (717) 232-6574, BA 26 Lebanon Valley Coll; MA 38 PA St Univ - Middletown; **SLP LM**

Emanuel, Mrs Renee Miller 1639 Willow Bend Way #B, Tallahassee, FL 32301, (912) 225-2611, BS 82 Univ of Montevallo; OM 85 Auburn Univ - Auburn; 86–Sp-Lang Path, Thomasville (GA) City Sch, **SLP**

Emanuele, Diana Dewey 508 Cascade Raod, Forest Hills, PA 15221, (412) 521-9000, BA 78 Coll of Wooster; MA 80 Univ of Pittsburgh - Pittsburgh; 82–Sp-Lang Path, Rehab Inst of Pitts, **SLP**

Emanuel-Regan, Mrs Valerie 3503 S E Harvey Street, Milwaukie, OR 97222, (503) 653-1155, BA 79 Southern CT St Univ; MS 81 Univ of OR; Sp-Lang Path, Irwin Lehroff and Associates, **SLP**

Emberlin, Lety A 287 South College #10, Monmouth, OR 97361, (503) 838-6602, MS 88 Western OR St Coll

Embleton, Arthur C 8-C Rolling Green, Newport, RI 02840, BA 80 Univ of RI; MA 82 Univ of RI; **A**

Embree, Michelle Cordes 9530 England, Overland Park, KS 66212, (816) 363-1411, BS 82 Southern Methodist Univ; MA 84 Univ of KS; Sp-Lang Path, Midwest Rehab Cntr, **SLP**

Embrey, Dr James E 3904 East 32nd Street, Tulsa, OK 74135, (918) 743-1976, BS 52 Pittsburg St Univ; MS 55 Univ of KS; ED 71 (NS) Univ of Tulsa; Aud, Private Practice, **A**

Embrey, Janice K P O Box 2473, Dunedin, FL 34296-2473, (813) 734-2718, MS 76 Univ of North TX; BS 72 Univ of TX - Austin; Process Commun Consult, Kaler Commun Inc, **SLP**

Embry, Cynthia Anne 1013 Hermitage Drive, Owensboro, KY 42301, BS 87 Brescia Coll; MS 88 Univ of KY

Embry, Loretta Hill P O Box 20573, Cleveland, OH 44120, (516) 464-6471, BS 81 Indiana Univ of PA; MA 86 Central St Univ

Emde, Mrs Jennifer Speech And Hearing Clinic, Pacific Union College, Angwin, CA 94508, (707) 965-6437, BS 74 Pacific Union Coll; MA 75 Humboldt St Univ; Asst Professor/Sp Pathology, Pacific Union College, **SLP**

Emer, Robin Burrows 20 Blackhorse Drive, Acton, MA 01720, (617) 453-1761, BA 76 CUNY - Queens Coll; MA 77 Univ of IL - Urbana; 88–Sp-Lang Path, Robin B Emer Private Practice, **SLP**

Emerick, Lon L 224 West Nicolet, Marquette, MI 49855, (906) 227-2125, BA 56 MI St Univ; MA 59 MI St Univ; PH 66 (NS) MI St Univ; Prof, Northern MI U, **SLP**

Emerick, Mary L P O Box 1372, Chehalis, WA 98532, BS 73 IN Univ - Bloomington; MA 76 IN Univ - Bloomington; Sp-Lang Path, St Helen Hospital, **SLP**

Emerick, Mrs Nancy J P O Box 526, Cohoes, NY 12047, (518) 783-5480, BS 80 Coll of Saint Rose; MS 82 Coll of Saint Rose; Sp-Lang Path, Private Practice, **SLP**

Emerling, Lisa Gail 3711 164th St S W #U-282, Lynnwood, WA 98037, (206) 258-7311, BA 85 Univ of CA - Santa Barbara; MS 87 Univ of WA; 88–Sp-Lang Path, Providence Hosp Child Ctr

Emerson, Mrs Delores S 1404 North Harvard, Oklahoma City, OK 73127, (405) 272-5545, BS 64 Univ of OK - Norman; MS 74 Univ of OK Medical Center; SLP, OK Cty Pub Schs, **SLP**

Emerson, Elizabeth W P O Box 1624, Bangor, ME 04401-3916, (207) 843-6169, 88 Univ of ME - Orono; 88–Sp-Lang Path, Bangor Reg Sp & Hrng Ctr

Emerson, Mrs Helen Wagner 595 Willow Knoll Drive, Marietta, GA 30067, (404) 953-0324, BA 67 Univ of WI - Eau Claire; MA 72 Western IL Univ; Consultant, Private Practice, **SLP**

Emerson, Mary Michele 510 W Adams, Taylorville, IL 62568, (217) 287-7929, BS 82 Western IL Univ; MA 83 Western IL Univ; Sp-Lang Path, Hardin Co Sch Dist #1, **SLP**

Emerson, Melanie S 1797 Acreview Drive, Cincinnati, OH 45240, (513) 851-1833, BS 85 Univ of Cincinnati; MA 87 Univ of Cincinnati; **SLP**

Emerson, Nancy Special Childrens Center, 21 Wilkins Road, Ithaca, NY 14850, (607) 272-5891, BS 77 SUNY - Center at Albany; MS 79 Syracuse Univ; Sp-Lang Path, Spec Chldn Cen Inc, **SLP**

Emerson, Robin C 2111 Townsend, Duncan, OK 73533, (405) 255-2012, BA 71 Univ of OK - Norman; MA 74 Univ of OK - Norman; Sp-Lang Path, Duncan PS, **SLP**

Emerson, Mrs Sharon Kay 56572 Via San Giovanni, Elkhart, IN 46516-9781, (219) 295-4491, **SLP**

Emerson, Mrs Sharon S 1830 Valle Vista, Pekin, IL 61554, (309) 347-1151, BA 73 Bradley Univ; MS 74 Bradley Univ; Sp-Lang Path, Inst of Phys Med & Rehab, **SLP**

Emerson-Anderson, Shari Lynne 1200 South Oneida Street, #15-105, Denver, CO 80224-3117, (314) 569-8509, BS 78 Abilene Christian Univ; MS 82 Univ of MO - Columbia; Supvr of Intgrted Svcs, InSpeech Inc, **SLP**

Emery, Mrs Alice Ford Route 2 Box 201, Quincy, FL 32351, (912) 246-0371, BS 86 FL St Univ; MS 87 FL St Univ

Emery, Carol Zwycewicz R R 1 Box 337, Hillview Road, Richmond, VT 05477, (802) 656-3970, BA 73 SUNY - Center at Buffalo; MA 75 SUNY - Center at Buffalo; Sp-Lang Path, Med Cen Hosp of Vt, **SLP**

Emery, James F Granada Square #120, 4253 Montgomery NE, Albuquerque, NM 87109, (505) 889-9000, OB 69 IL St Univ - Normal; MA 77 NM St Univ; Aud, Hearing Evaluation Center, **A**

Emery, Patricia A P O Box 234, Forestdale, MA 02644, (617) 232-9500, BA 81 Bridgewater St Coll; MS 84 Emerson Coll; Research Associate, Boston University Sch of Med, **SLP**

Emery, Mrs Susan S 7105 Old Stage Road, Rockville, MD 20852, (301) 984-5613, BA 65 Hollins Coll; MA 75 George Washington Univ; Sp-Lang Path, Private Practice, **SLP**

Emery, Virginia Joanne 5221 West James Lane, Unit 1507, Crestwood, IL 60445, (312) 385-4990, BS 82 Governors St Univ; MS 84 Governors St Univ; 84–Sp-Lang Path, SW Cook Co Coop for Spec Educ, **SLP**

Emge, Mrs Judith Ann 1232 South Michigan, Bay City, MI 48706, (517) 686-4410, BS 79 Central MI Univ; MA 80 Central MI Univ; Sp-Lang Path, Bay Arenac ISD, **SLP**

Emge, Marie E 6006 Oak Country Way, San Antonio, TX 78247, (512) 654-6552, BA 57 Our Lady Lake Univ-San Anton; MA 58 Univ of IA; Sp-Lang Path, Private Practice, **SLP**

Emlen, Mrs Mary K 5469 South Jasmine, Englewood, CO 80111, (303) 721-8796, BA 68 Stanford Univ; MA 72 San Diego St Univ; **SLP**

Emme, Mrs Patricia C 208 Paula Lynn Drive, Silver Spring, MD 20904, (301) 384-8870, BA 72 Univ of MD - College Park; MA 74 Univ of MD - College Park; SLP, Private Practice, **SLP**

Emmer, DeeAnn 5541 Surrey, Las Vegas, NV 89119, (702) 736-1106, BA 71 Univ of MI - Ann Arbor; MS 74 Univ of MI - Ann Arbor; Sp-Lang Path, Private Practice, **SLP**

Emmerich, Rhoda Susan 209 Mimosa Terrace, Guthrie, OK 73044, (405) 282-5610, BS 79 Central St Univ; ME 82 Central St Univ; Sp/Lang Path, Crescent Pub Schs, **SLP**

Emmerling-Knox, Mrs Lois 2001 Margaret Street, St Paul, MN 55119, (612) 293-8870, BS 77 IL St Univ - Normal; OM 87 Univ of WI - River Falls; 83–Sp-Lang Path, St Paul PS

Emmerman, Mrs Esther P 1635 Eastwood, Highland Park, IL 60035, (312) 831-2488, BS 60 IN Univ - Bloomington; ME 79 Nat'l Coll of Ed - Evanston; Erly Chldn Spec Ed Tchr, Spec Ed Dist of Lake Co, **SLP**

Emond, Judith A P O Box 464, 28 Taft Street, Northbridge, MA 01534, (401) 767-2570, BS 75 Worcester St Coll; MS 80 Worcester St Coll; Sp/Lang Path, Woonsocket Ed Dept, **SLP**

Emonin, Mrs Emily L 506 East Buchanan Avenue, Fairfield, IA 52556, (515) 472-3414, BS 69 Northeast MO St Univ; MA 75 Northeast MO St Univ; SLP, S Prairie AEA #15, **SLP**

Emory-Pacheco, Christine K 3511 Fairview Avenue, Dallas, TX 75223, (214) 783-3030, BS 84 Univ of TX - Austin; MS 87 Univ of TX - Dallas; **SLP**

Empfield, Mrs Dorothy Rae 129-B North 4th Street, Indiana, PA 15701, (412) 354-3111, BS 82 Indiana Univ of PA; MS 85 Indiana Univ of PA; Sp-Lang Path, Arin Intermediate Unit 28, **SLP**

Empie, Kathryn E 6719 Avondale Drive, Oklahoma City, OK 73116, BA 42 Univ of Science & Arts of OK; MS 67 Univ of OK Medical Center; **SLP**

Emrich, Mrs Mary J 827 Franklin Street, Louisville, KY 40206, (502) 582-2231, BS 67 East TN St Univ; MS 69 Purdue Univ - West Lafayette; Sp-Lang Path, Private Practice, **SLP**

Emrick, Mrs Nita P 3225 Ridgelake Drive #C, Metairie, LA 70002, BS 63 OK St Univ; MA 78 LA St Univ - N O Medical Ctr; Sp-Lang Path, Orleans Parish Sch Bd, **SLP**

Emrick, Sandra Catherine 2300 Lincoln Road, Cedar Crest #129, Hattiesburg, MS 39401, (601) 268-6502, BS 76 Southeastern LA Univ; MA 78 Univ Southern MS-Hattiesburg; Sp-Lang Path, Multi Co Home Hlth, **SLP**

Enck, Mrs Carol A 4685 Hitching Post Trail, Atlanta, GA 30342, (404) 843-0176, BA 80 MI St Univ; MA 81 Western MI Univ; Sp-Lang Path, Private Practice, **SLP**

Endebrock, F Andra B 416 Apple Blossom Lane, Hurst, TX 76053, (817) 283-1583, BS 73 Univ of North TX; MS 75 Univ of North TX; 77–Sp/Lang Path, Hurst-Euless-Bedford ISD, **SLP**

Enderle, Elizabeth Elaine 88 Sanford Place, Jersey City, NJ 07307, BA 85 Our Lady Lake Univ-San Anton; MS 88 CUNY - Hunter Coll; **SLP**

Enders, Carolyn Diane 2 Woodcrest Avenue, Burlington, MA 01803, (617) 272-8639, BA 85 Univ of CA - Santa Barbara; MA 88 Univ of MN - Minneap-St Paul

Endersbe, Mikki Kay East 13207 Guthrie Drive, Spokane, WA 99216, (509) 456-7086, BA 82 Eastern WA Univ; MS 84 Eastern WA Univ; Program Director for Cds Serv, Esd #101, **SLP**

Endicott, Dr James E PO Box 909, Lakehills, TX 78063, (512) 694-5209, OB 56 OH Univ - Athens; MA 57 OH Univ - Athens; PH 64 (Aud) Northwestern Univ; 87–Audiologist, U of Texas Health Science Ctr, **A**

Endo, Janet K 501 Magnolia #203, South Pasadena, CA 91030, (818) 799-7661, BA 84 Univ of UT; MS 87 Univ of UT; **A**

Endres, Arlene M 12546 Gracewood Drive, Baltimore, MD 21220, (301) 335-6617, MS 88 Towson St Univ

Eneberg-Farruggia, Karen G 2146 Almond Lane, Glendale Heights, IL 60139, (312) 354-5730, BS Northern IL Univ - De Kalb; MA 85 Northern IL Univ - De Kalb; **SLP**

Enell, Mark William P O Box 8292, Fort Collins, CO 80526-8003, (215) 673-9200, MS 87 CO St Univ

Eneman, Laura Sue 1 Overlook Avenue, Great Neck, NY 11021, (516) 795-9400, BA 59 CUNY - Brooklyn Coll; MS 61 PA St Univ - Univ Park; 62–Sp-Lang Path, Plainedge Pub Sch, **SLP**

Eney, Mrs Stephanie 7005 Arion Avenue, Baltimore, MD 21234, (301) 828-2142, BS 76 Towson St Univ; MS 77 Towson St Univ; 78–Aud, Gtr Balt Med Cen Hrng & Sp Dep, **A**

Eng, Lawrence M 1919 Octavia #1, San Francisco, CA 94109, (415) 852-3251, BA 84 San Francisco St Univ; MS 86 San Francisco St Univ; 88–Aud, VA Med Ctr, **A**

Eng, Marlene 520 West Fairmont, Fresno, CA 93705, (209) 441-3091, BA 79 CA St Univ - Fresno; MA 81 CA St Univ - Fresno; SLP, Fresno USD, **SLP**

Eng, Mrs Pearl Q 2620 Brentwood Circle, Arlington, TX 76013, (214) 790-0706, BS 74 Univ of North TX; MS 75 Univ of North TX; Sp-Lang Path, Grand Prairie ISD, **SLP**

Eng, Mrs Ruth L 12278 Densmore Avenue North, Seattle, WA 98133, (203) 365-0788, BA 82 Univ of WA; OM 84 Univ of WA; SLP, Shoreline School Dist, **SLP**

Engborg, Rebecca J Rd 1 Box 97 Route 57, Washington, NJ 07882, (212) 750-6860, BA 78 Washington Univ; MA 85 NY Univ; 88–Sp-Lang Path, St Luke's Hosp, **SLP**

Engdall, Carol E Albany Speech & Lang Center, P O Box 672, Albany, OR 97321, (503) 370 5486, BS 71 Univ of OR; MS 74 Portland St Univ; Sp-Lang Path, Salem Gen Hosp, **SLP**

Engel, Alida 374 Central Avenue, New Haven, CT 06515, (203) 397-3224, BS 69 Univ of CT; Sp-Lang Path, Private Practice, **SLP ACE**

Engel, Dr Dean C Dept Communication Disorders, University Of North Dakota, Box 8040 Univ Station, Grand Forks, ND 58202, (701) 777-3232, BS 50 Minot St Univ; MA 56 Univ of ND; PH 65 (Sp Path) Univ of MN - Minneap-St Paul; Prof of Commun Dis, U of ND, **SLP F**

Engel, Ellen M 215 East 68th Street #12, New York, NY 10021, **A**

Engel, Heather Lee 1402 East 69th Street, Brooklyn, NY 11234, (718) 436-7600, MS 87 CUNY - Brooklyn Coll; 87–Sp-Lang Path, UCP of NYC, **SLP**

Engel, Mrs Helen L 7149 Springridge Road, West Bloomfield, MI 48322, (313) 626-2941, BS 59 Eastern MI Univ; MA 64 Eastern MI Univ; Sp-Lang Path, Southfield Pub Schls, **SLP**

Engel, Mrs Jean Catherine 3004 Lighthouse Lane, Parlin, NJ 08859, (718) 442-5615, BS 80 SUNY - Coll at Geneseo; MS 83 CUNY - Brooklyn Coll; Sp-Lang Path, UCP-NYC, **SLP**

Engel, Mrs Karen 14 Rafael Drive, San Rafael, CA 94901, (415) 877-8738, BA 71 Wayne St Univ - Sch of Med; MA 73 Wayne St Univ - Sch of Med; MA 82 San Francisco St Univ; Coor/Sp-Lang-Hrng Dept, S San Francisco USD, **SLP**

Engel, Karen W 1315 Crawford Street, Friendswood, TX 77546, (713) 482-0022, BS 69 Univ of TX - Austin; BA 69 Univ of TX - Austin; MA 72 Univ of Houston - Univ Park; Elem Counselor, Clear Creek ISD, **SLP**

Engel, Lisa Gustin 6605 South 88th Street, Omaha, NE 68127, (402) 895-8350, BS 81 Univ of NE - Lincoln; MS 82 Univ of NE - Lincoln; 87–Sp-Lang Path, Millard Pub Schs, **SLP**

Engel, Marcy Eileen 22 R Reading Road, Edison, NJ 08817, (201) 776-4185, **SLP**

Engel, Michelle Lea 8444 Little Road South, Bloomington, MN 55437, (612) 831-6012, BA 85 Univ of WI - Eau Claire; MS 86 Univ of WI - Eau Claire; 88–Sp-Lang Path, Bloomington PS, **SLP**

Engel, Mrs Suzanne Keppel #7 Overland Trail Court, St Charles, MO 63303, (314) 724-5429, BS 77 Fontbonne Coll; MS 78 Fontbonne Coll; Sp-Lang Path, City of St Charles Sch Dist, **SLP**

Engel, Tracy Lynn 11073 Dunklin -A, St Louis, MO 63138, (314) 869-7516, BA 85 IA St Univ; MA 86 Northeast MO St Univ; **SLP**

Engelberg, Dr Marvin W Audiology & Speech Path Serv, VA Hospital, 10701 East Boulevard, Cleveland, OH 44106, (216) 421-3047, BS 52 TX A & M Univ; MA 54 Univ of IL - Urbana; PH 58 (NS) Univ of MI - Ann Arbor; 61–Ch Aud & SLP Service, VA Medical Center, **SLP A**

Engelbrecht, Claire Elizabeth 2119 5th Avenue West, Seattle, WA 98119, (206) 863-2201, MS 85 Univ of WA; 85–Sp-Lang Path, Sumner Sch Dt, **SLP**

Engelhardt, Christine Route 1 Box 210-H, Troy, ID 83871, (208) 882-1120, BA 66 WA St Univ; OM 71 Univ of WA; Sp-Lang Path, Moscow Sch Dist, **SLP**

Engelhardt, Mrs Marian K 21148 Madria Circle, Boca Raton, FL 33433, BA 76 CUNY - Queens Coll; MA 78 Hofstra Univ; SLP, Volz and Amato, **SLP**

Engelman, Mrs Dixie A Rural Route 1, 200 Eastmoor Drive, East Alton, IL 62024, (618) 692-3662, BS 72 Southern IL Univ-Edwardsvill; MS 73 Southern IL Univ-Edwardsvill; Asst Dir, Sn IL U-Edwardsville, **SLP ACE**

Engelman, Mrs Sylvia L 7490 Brompton #169, Houston, TX 77025, (713) 668-1336, BS 70 Miami Univ - Oxford; MA 72 Eastern MI Univ; Sp-Lang Path, **SLP**

Engelmann, Larry R Audiology Clinic, 3330 N W 56th, Oklahoma City, OK 73112, (405) 946-0364, BA 75 Univ of FL; MS 76 Univ of OK Medical Center; Aud, Aud Cl, **A**

Engelmann, Mrs Linda A 8008 Summit, Kansas City, MO 64114, (816) 781-1001, MS 88 Central MO St Univ; 88–Aud, Hearing Specialist Inc

Engel-Rudolph, Robin 18 Heritage Drive, Pleasantville, NY 10570, (212) 430-2677, BA 73 Hofstra Univ; MA 74 Hofstra Univ; Aud, Alber Einstein Coll of Med, **A**

Engels, Laurie E 3231 White Maple Court, South Bend, IN 46628, (219) 284-7312, OB 84 Univ of WI - Whitewater; MS 85 Univ of WI - Whitewater; SLP, Michiana Rehab Ins, **SLP**

Engels, Mrs Tamara Lewis 8302 Christiana Lane, Indianapolis, IN 46256, (317) 841-7191, BS 80 Purdue Univ - West Lafayette; MS 82 Purdue Univ - West Lafayette; 84–Audiologist, Ear Institute of Indiana, **A**

Engel-Sambrana, Mrs Patricia Jeanette 20481 Summer Song Lane, Germantown, MD 20874, (301) 972-9163, BA 82 Baldwin-Wallace Coll; MA 84 SUNY - Coll at Geneseo; 85–Sp-Lang Path, Montgomery Co PS, **SLP**

Engelson, Mrs Henriette R 2260 Nottingham Road, Allentown, PA 18103, (215) 432-0570, BA 35 NY Univ; MA 50 Columbia Univ Teachers Coll; **SLP LM**

Engelstein, Renee Nancy 10-36 Reads Lane, Far Rockaway, NY 11691, (212) 337-5894, BA 84 CUNY - Queens Coll; MA 86 CUNY - Queens Coll; **A**

Engen, Mary Everson 2828 32nd Avenue South, Minneapolis, MN 55406, (612) 348-8965, BS 71 Northern St Coll; MA 75 Univ of MN - Minneap-St Paul; SLP, Minneapolis Pub Sch, **SLP**

Engen, Mrs Sharon A 13650 S W 21st, Beaverton, OR 97005, (503) 646-1805, MS 84 Portland St Univ; Sp-Lang Path, Portland Public Schools, **SLP**

Enger, Janet K Lt 71 Countryside Tr Park, Thief River Falls, MN 56701, **A**

Enger, Mrs Joan Kathleen 5336 Loughborough Avenue, St Louis, MO 63109-3755, (314) 353-8174, BS 84 Marquette Univ; MA 86 Saint Louis Univ; 86–SLP, Spec Sch Dist of St Louis Co, **SLP**

Enger, Nancy Christine 140 Robert Jemison Drive, #206, Birmingham, AL 35209, (205) 939-9149, MS 88 Univ of South AL; 88–Sp-Lang Path, Children's Hosp of Alabama, **SLP**

Engfer, Christine Mary 4383 Heritage Drive, Liverpool, NY 13090, (315) 652-4781, BS 80 Cornell Univ; MS 85 Syracuse Univ; **SLP**

England, Mrs Carol J 403 Malabar, Austin, TX 78734-5513, (512) 261-6572, BA 73 Sam Houston St Univ; MA 76 Univ of Houston - Univ Park; 88–Sp-Lang Path, Georgetown Therapy & Rehab Ctr, **SLP**

England, Christina Ann 710 Taylor Boulevard, Millbrae, CA 94030, (415) 692-7735, BA 78 CA St Univ - Fresno; MA 79 CA St Univ - Fresno; Sp-Lang Path, CA St Dept of Ed, **SLP**

England, Ellen F 7795 Trefeathen Drive, Warren, OH 44484, (216) 856-1458, MA 87 Kent St Univ

England, Dr Juliana E 5436 Diamondhead Drive East, Bay St Louis, MS 39520, (504) 589-5566, MA 69 Univ of MO - KS City; MS 73 Saint Cloud St Univ; PH 86 (Abstr Reasoning) SUNY - Center at Buffalo; Sp-Lang Path, VA Med Ctr New Orleans, **SLP**

England, Kathie Elizabeth 21102 Poolside Lane, Huntington Beach, CA 92648, (714) 832-9200, BA 68 Whittier Coll; MA 84 CA St Univ - Fullerton; Dir-Patient Svcs, Western Neuro Care Center, **SLP**

England, Mrs Kathleen K 806 South Seventh, Ann Arbor, MI 48103, (313) 665-2796, BS 65 Boston Univ; ME 67 Boston Univ; **SLP ACE**

England, Lynne L 3054 Wister Court, Valrico, FL 33594, **SLP A ACE**

England, Mrs Rosemary B 605 South Alton Way #9-A, Denver, CO 80231, (303) 341-4238, BA 74 Univ of Northern CO; MA 78 Univ of Northern CO; Aud, Private Practice, **A**

Englander, Mrs Harriet 10 Crescent Road, Port Washington, NY 11050, (516) 883-4000, BA 56 Alfred Univ; MA 58 Univ of Chicago; MS 72 Columbia Univ Teachers Coll; SLP, Port Washington Public Schools, **SLP**

Engle, Connie L R R 2 Box 255, Richmond, VT 05477, (802) 244-7195, BA 75 Glassboro St Coll; MS 78 Univ of VT; 82–Sp/Lang Path, Waterbury Elem Sch, **SLP**

Engle, Linda A 1513 East Piute Avenue, Phoenix, AZ 85024, (602) 582-0917, BS 75 OH Univ - Athens; MA 76 OH Univ - Athens; Sp-Lang Path, Deer Valley USD #97, **SLP**

Engle, Susan Diane 24 Bradford Street, Apt #7, Charleston, WV 25301, (304) 345-8522, BS 83 WV Univ; MS 84 WV Univ; 84–Aud, Aud & Hrng Aid Svc Inc, **A**

Englehardt, Mrs Alyce C 167 Belgian Drive, Danville, CA 94526, (612) 452-0217, BA 75 Univ of the Pacific; MA 76 Univ of the Pacific; **SLP**

Englehart, Mrs Catherine 1606 Oakstone, Rochester, MI 48309, BS 74 Western MI Univ; MA 78 Western MI Univ; Sp-Lang Path, Richmond Comm Sch, **SLP**

Engleking, Allen F 12504 Surrey Circle Drive, Fort Washington, MD 20744, (301) 839-6060, BA 57 Saint Ambrose Coll; MA 67 Catholic Univ of America; Sp-Path, Prince Geo Co Pub Sch, **SLP**

Engleman, Pearl Ruth 4025 Concord Street, Harrisburg, PA 17109, (717) 652-2464, BA 58 PA St Univ - Univ Park; BA 58 PA St Univ - Univ Park; Prog Dir, Tri-Co Er Sl So, **SLP**

Engler, Robin Janus 9402 Sherwood Trail, Brecksville, OH 44141, (216) 526-5397, BA 75 Univ of Akron; MA 85 Univ of Akron; **SLP**

Engler, Shelley F 3940 Beechmont Trail, Orange Village, OH 44122, **SLP**

Englert, Frances Watson 230 South Sycamore, Los Angeles, CA 90036, BS 78 East Carolina Univ; MS 80 East Carolina Univ; Aud, Dahlberg Electronics, **A**

Englert, Pamela K 1208 Margaret, Peoria, IL 61604, (309) 682-7555, BS 69 Western MI Univ; MS 78 IL St Univ - Normal; Dir Sp-Lang Path, River Valley Sp Assoc, **SLP ACE**

English, Betsy A 1420 West State Street, Janesville, WI 53545, (608) 754-9157, MS 88 Univ of WI - Whitewater

English, Constance Reser 137 North Tecumseh Trail, Tiffin, OH 44883, (419) 447-0087, BS 79 Bowling Green St Univ; MA 81 Bowling Green St Univ; Sp-Lang Path, P T Services Inc, **SLP**

English, Helen Ann 230 East Woodward Blvd, Tulsa, OK 74114-1246, (918) 245-5911, SLP, Hisson Mem Cntr, **SLP**

English, Joy SPEECHCENTER, 100 State Farm Road, Suite B, Boone, NC 28607, (704) 262-1212, BS 76 Appalachian St Univ; MA 82 Appalachian St Univ; Exec Dir, SPEECHCENTER Joy English & Assoc, **SLP**

English, Kristina Marie 1905 Clearbrook Drive, Chula Vista, CA 92013, (619) 461-7930, BA 83 San Diego St Univ; MA 86 San Diego St Univ; Aud, E Co Spec Ed Region, **A**

English, Linda Hammons 7103 Tawny Circle, Austin, TX 78745, (512) 447-1552, **SLP**

English, Mrs Lisa Suzanne 1005 West Maple, Lee's Summit, MO 64063, (816) 525-6892, OB 86 Univ of MO - Columbia; OM 87 Univ of MO - Columbia; 87–Sp-Lang Path, Lee's Summit R-7 Sch Dist, **SLP**

English, Dr Robert H 17825 Southwest Shasta Tr, Tualatin, OR 97062, (503) 229-3534, BA 47 Univ of the Pacific; MA 50 Univ of the Pacific; ED 61 (NS) Univ of OR; 64–Prof Emeritus, Portland St U, **SLP F LM**

English, Mrs Roberta Kent 10 Joanna Way, Summit, NJ 07901, (201) 277-2553, BA 69; MS 87 Rutgers St Univ - Newark; 88–Sp-Lang Path, Kessler Inst for Rehab

English, Sally A D 2803 Pecan Point, Sugar Land, TX 77478, (713) 980-4946, SLP, Houston ISD, **SLP**

English, Susan Hollister Old Colshester Turnpike, Moodus, CT 06469, (203) 873-9533, BA 71 Univ of CT; ME 74 Boston Univ; Sp-Lang Path, East Haddam Bd of Educ, **SLP**

English, Susan M 1535 Powell Tavern Place, Herndon, VA 22070, (703) 860-1030, BS 66 Univ of CO - Boulder; ME 70 Boston Univ; SLP, Fairfax Co Pub Sch, **SLP**

English, Mrs Susan T 6560 Crystal Boulevard, Diamond Springs, CA 95619, (707) 838-4396, BS 72 CO St Univ; MA 75 Univ of CA - Santa Barbara; Director of Spec Ed, El Dorado Co Off of Ed, **SLP**

English, Mrs Wynne Adele 310 South Main Street, Marion, SC 29571, (803) 423-4307, **SLP**

Englund, Bette Visgar 38 Apple Glen Road, Long Lake, MN 55356, (612) 473-6944, BS 75 Univ of WI - Eau Claire; MS 76 Univ of WI - Eau Claire; Sp-Lang Path, Bloomington Public Schools, **SLP**

Engnoth, Dr Gloria 8200 Tally Ho Road, Lutherville, MD 21093, (301) 494-4225, BA 50 Univ of MD - College Park; MA 55 Univ of MD - College Park; PH 74 (NS) Univ of KS; Coord of Sp Ed, Baltimore Co Bd of Ed, **SLP F**

Engstrom-Bauman, Karen Joyce 518 North 2nd Street, Vineland, NJ 08360, (609) 692-8288, BS 85 WV Univ; MA 87 Temple Univ; 87–Aud, ENt Pro Assoc, **A**

Enix, Mrs Candice S 15023 East Floyd, Aurora, CO 80014, (303) 369-9337, BA 78 Univ of CO - Boulder; MS 80 Phillips Univ; Sp-Lang Path, JFK Child Development Center, **SLP**

Enman, Mrs Sharon L 15049 Burbank Boulevard, Apartment 105, Van Nuys, CA 91411, (818) 994-9937, MA 87 CA St Univ - Northridge; 88–Sp-Lang Path, Simi Valley Adventist Hosp, **SLP**

Ennis, Kimberly Ann 957 McKenna Drive, Mountain Home, ID 83647, (208) 587-9702, MA 85 Central MI Univ; Sp-Lang Path, Mount Home School Dist #193, **SLP**

Ennis, Mrs Linda Jo 3115 Citadel Court, Jefferson City, MO 65101, (314) 893-6037, BA 70 Univ of MS; MA 71 Univ of MO - Columbia; 86–Sp-Lang Path, Vogelweid Learning Ctr, **SLP**

Ennis, Sheila Joan 4011 121th Street, Edmonton, AB, Canada T6J 1Y4, (306) 347-8755, BS 81 Univ of Alberta - Alberta; MS 83 Univ of Western Ontario; Sp-Lang Path, Glenrose Hospital, **SLP**

Ennis, Thomas G 113 West Broad Street, Hopewell, NJ 08525, **SLP**

Enns, Mrs Janet M 5878 Avenue 430, Reedley, CA 93654, (209) 638-1165, BA 73 CA St Univ - Fresno; MA 75 CA St Univ - Fresno; **SLP**

Enns, Mrs Joan Y 1650 Hanchett, San Jose, CA 95128, (408) 243-7861, BA 75 San Jose St Univ; MA 77 San Jose St Univ; Director of Speech Pathology, Sp-Hrng Lrng Cen, **SLP**

Enos, Mrs Joann Hiehle 137 Whitehall Road, Amesbury, MA 01913, (508) 683-3139, MS 85 Univ of NH; 86–Sp-Lang Path, MA Cerebral Palsy Assoc, **SLP**

Enright-Stacey, Ellen H 19474 Pollyanna, Livonia, MI 48152, (313) 523-0550, BS 74 Wayne St Univ; MA 75 Wayne St Univ; Sp-Lang Path, Visiting Nurse Association, **SLP**

Enriquez, Mrs Linda Maclas 4000 Horizon Hill #1303, San Antonio, TX 78229, (512) 226-5441, BS 78 TX Woman's Univ; MA 82 Our Lady Lake Univ-San Anton; 82–Sp-Lang Path, San Antonio ISD, **SLP**

Ensign, Patricia Moats 11805 S Coconino, Phoenix, AZ 85044, (602) 277-5551, BS 82 Univ of NV - Reno; MS 87 AZ St Univ

Ensminger, Rosanne M 7824 Kessler Lane, Overland Park, KS 66204, (913) 642-1773, BA 79 Wichita St Univ; MA 80 Wichita St Univ; Sp-Lang Path, **SLP**

Ensminger, Shelly Maxine 520 West 20th Lot B10, Pittsburg, KS 66762, (316) 232-9562, BS 82 Univ of KS; MA 84 Univ of KS; Sp-Lang Path, Sek Spec Ed Coop, **SLP**

Ensminger-Waldman, Mrs Lindi Ann 5243 Somerset Drive, Prairie Village, KS 66207-2235, (913) 649-7131, BS 81 Univ of KS; MA 83 Univ of KS; 88–Sp-Lang Path, Research Med Ctr, **SLP**

Ensrud, Susan Karolyn 845 South First #4, Ann Arbor, MI 48103, BS 76 Miami Univ - Oxford; MA 78 Univ of IA; Sp-Lang Path, Muskegon Public Schs, **SLP**

Ensslen, Mrs Sandra Jadick 105 Cambridge Drive, Mechanicsburg, PA 17055, (717) 766-2894, BS 72 Bloomsburg Univ of PA; ME 73 Bloomsburg Univ of PA; SLP, Capital Area Inter Unit, **SLP**

Ensslin, William R P O Box 41, Swamp Road, Whately, MA 01093, (413) 253-9731, BA 66 Capital Univ; MA 68 OH Univ - Athens; Sp-Lang Path, Amherst Pub Schs, **SLP**

Enstrom, Dr Daly H 67 Colfax Road, Skillman, NJ 08558, (609) 588-3157, BA 60 Emerson Coll; MA 64 Emerson Coll; PH 76 (NS) Univ of Zurich - Switzerland; Administrator, NJ Dept of Human Serv, **SLP**

Enstrom, Mrs Janine C 1016 Brookstone Boulevard, Mount Juliet, TN 37122, (615) 444-6073, BA 71 Birmingham-Southern Coll; MA 74 Univ of AL- Tuscaloosa; Sp-Lang Path, Wilson Co Sch, **SLP**

Ensworth, Mrs Leisa Kathleen 8336 East Ironwood Avenue, Orange, CA 92669, (714) 581-2800, BA 85 CA St Univ - Long Beach; MA 87 CA St Univ - Los Angeles; 87–Aud, Newport Lang Sp & Aud Ctrs Inc, **A**

Entwistle, Mrs Nancy Vogenbergr 37 Pease Road, East Longmeadow, MA 01028, BA 76 SUNY - Coll at New Paltz; MS 81 Worcester St Coll; Sp-Lang Path, Willie Ross School for Deaf, **SLP**

Entzi, Mrs Judith L 253 Grant Avenue, McDonald, OH 44437, (216) 788-2481, BS 75 Kent St Univ; MA 87 Kent St Univ; 75–Sp-Lang Path, Mahoning Co Bd of Educ

Enzenhauer, Mrs Sheila Barrett 5445 Jackson Drive #322, Mounds View, MN 55112, (612) 785-2937, MA 88 Univ of WI - River Falls

Enzer, Susan M 8 Blackstone Boulevard #9, Providence, RI 02906-5450, BA 83 Brandeis Univ; MS 86 Univ of Cincinnati; **A**

Eoannou, Susan A 68 5th Street, Scotia, NY 12302, (716) 877-5831, BA 82 SUNY - Center at Buffalo; MS 83 Syracuse Univ; **SLP**

Eoff, Elizabeth Haaser 2712 South 97th Circle, Fort Smith, AR 72903, (501) 452-7265, BS 83 Univ of AR - Fayetteville; MS 85 Univ of North TX; 86–Sp-Lang Path, Ft Smith PS, **SLP**

Eppeira, Mrs Kathleen Maurer 19 Albano Drive, Hilton, NY 14468, (716) 232-2310, BS 82 Hobart-William Smith Coll; MA 85 SUNY - Center at Buffalo; 85–Sp-Lang Path, Rochester City Sch Dist, **SLP**

Eppel, Mrs Jane Carol 4222-C Carrollton Drive, Bridgeton, MO 63044, (314) 928-7773, BS 84 Ball St Univ; MA 85 Ball St Univ; 87–Aud, **A**

Eppes, Linda F 4 Circle Drive, Teague, TX 75860, **SLP**

Eppler-Kropp, Sheila R Box 321, Ewing, NE 68735, (402) 626-7908, BS 76 Univ of NE - Lincoln; MA 78 Univ of NE - Lincoln; Sp/Lang Path, Ed Serv Unit No 8, **SLP**

Eppley, Kerry Ward Betty Jane Center, 65 Saint Francis Avenue, Tiffin, OH 44883, (419) 447-9811, BS 85 Bowling Green St Univ; MS 86 Bowling Green St Univ; Sp-Lang Path, Betty Jane Memorial Rehab Ctr, **SLP**

Epport, Karen Lynn 4900 South Overland Street, Apartment 259, Culver City, CA 90230, (213) 559-5312, BA 81 CA St Univ - Northridge; MA 82 CA St Univ - Northridge; Staff Research Associate, Univ of Calif-L A/Pediatrics, **SLP**

Epstein, Dr Aubrey 2938 Ramble Road East, Bloomington, IN 47401, (812) 332-9951, BA 47 IN Univ - Bloomington; MS 48 Case Western Reserve Univ; PH 53 (Aud) Univ of IA; 63–Prof Emeritus, Indiana Univ, **A F LM**

Epstein, Carolyn W 3320 East 1st Street, Long Beach, CA 90803, (213) 434-9263, BS 73 Univ of GA; ME 75 Univ of GA; Sp-Lang Path, Private Practice, **SLP**

Epstein, Mrs Caron Shohet P O Box 469, Hewlett, NY 11557, (516) 569-2763, **SLP**

Epstein, Mrs Cheryl S 1136 North Bundy Drive, Los Angeles, CA 90046, **A**

Epstein, Mrs Cynthia S Movement Into Language, 18204 Los Alimos Street, Northridge, CA 91326, (818) 366-4121, BA 69 SUNY - Coll at Buffalo; MS 72 San Francisco St Univ; Sp/Lang Path, Lausd /Private Practice, **SLP**

Epstein, Mrs Elaine G 10 Grouse Lane, Huntington, NY 11743, (516) 549-4080, BA 59 Univ of Louisville; MS 70 CUNY - Brooklyn Coll; MS 80 Adelphi Univ; Sp/Lang Path, Connetquot Pub Sch, **SLP ACE**

Epstein, Ellayne S 410 Avenue X, Brooklyn, NY 11223, (718) 336-8685, BA 82; MS 84 Boston Univ; Sp-Lang Path, Malden Hospital, **SLP ACE**

Epstein, Gloria L 7021-F Lachlan Circle, Baltimore, MD 21239, (301) 529-4278, BA 65 Univ of MD - College Park; MA 70 Univ of MD - College Park; OM 77 Johns Hopkins Univ; Sp-Lang Path, Balt Co Pub Sch, **SLP**

Epstein, Harold 187 Pembroke Street, Brooklyn, NY 11235, **SLP**

Epstein, Mrs Helene Grande 5 Paula Street, Edison, NJ 08820, (201) 548-8386, BA 63 CUNY - Brooklyn Coll; MS 67 CUNY - Brooklyn Coll; 85–Sp-Lang Path, N Brunswick Bd of Educ, **SLP ACE**

Epstein, Mrs Joan Pless 3542 Reign Street, Melbourne, FL 32935, (407) 242-9100, BA 78 Temple Univ; MA 80 Tulane Univ; 87–Sp-Lang Path, Devereux Hosp & Children's Ctr, **SLP**

Epstein, Mrs Lillian C 1929 Blue Ridge, Charlottesville, VA 22901, (804) 977-6411, BA 50 Univ of MI - Ann Arbor; MA 52 Univ of MI - Ann Arbor; **SLP**

Epstein, Lisa Brazel 16 Regent Street, Cambridge, MA 02140, (617) 354-4984, BA 84 Tulane Univ; MA 86 Memphis St Univ; Sp-Lang Path, Boston PS, **SLP**

Epstein, Lynn Ellen 1382 Whitepine Drive, West Palm Beach, FL 33414-5744, (407) 996-4902, MS 86 Univ of South FL; Sp-Lang Path, Palm Bch Co Sch Bd, **SLP**

Epstein, Mark S 2106 Ellerbe Avenue, Louisville, KY 40205, (502) 454-8246, BA 77 IN Univ - Bloomington; MS 78 IN St Univ - Terre Haute; Sp-Lang Path, Jefferson Co Pub Sch, **SLP**

Epstein, Mona R 456 Bridge Road, Walnut Creek, CA 94595, (415) 943-1029, BA 75 Univ of CA - Berkeley; MS 81 San Francisco St Univ; Sp-Lang Path, Children's Hosp Oakland, **SLP**

Epstein, Mrs Ruth Elias 300 West Palmetto Park, Apartment 103-B, Boca Raton, FL 33432, BS 54 Syracuse Univ; MA 81 Appalachian St Univ; 86–Sp-Lang Path, Palmbeach Co Sch, **SLP**

Epstein, Mrs Sherri Joy 898 Oriole Ln, Huntingdon Valley, PA 19006, (215) 947-7707, BS 77 PA St Univ - Univ Park; MA 79 Trenton St Coll; Sp-Lang Path, Phil Sch Dist, **SLP**

Epstein, Dr Stephen The Ear Center, Wheaton Plaza South Annex, 11160 Viers Mill Road, Wheaton, MD 20902, MD 64 (Medicine) Chicago Med Sch; 88–Physician, Private Practice

Epstein-Roberts, Mrs Sharon L 5530 Liverpool Court, Agoura, CA 91301, (213) 452-7074, BA 73 Univ of CA - Los Angeles; MA 76 CA St Univ - Northridge; Aud, **A**

Epstien, Rhona G 7300 Pomander Lane, Chevy Chase, MD 20815, (301) 986-1503, BA 73 NY Univ; MS 75 Ithaca Coll; Sp-Lang Path, Private Practice, **SLP**

Erb, Mrs Linda V 5821 Downey Finch Drive, Anchorage, AK 99516, (907) 337-2525, BS 70 Ball St Univ; MA 75 Ball St Univ; Teacher, AK State Sch for Deaf, **A**

Erb, Margaret Quinn P O Box B-7, Chesterfield, MA 01012, (413) 533-2100, BA 79 Univ of RI; MS 82 Southern CT St Univ; 85–Owner, Communication Therapy Inc, **SLP**

Erber, Dr Norman Phillip Communication Disorders, Lincoln School Of Health Sciences, 625 Swanston Street, Carlton, Victoria, Australia 3053, 3-342-0280, BS 64 Washington Univ; MA 67 Washington Univ; PH 70 (Sp Perception: Hrng Impaired) Washington Univ; 85–Lecturer, Lincoln Sch of Hlth Sci, **A**

Erby, Rosalyn F 6085 Textile, Ypsilanti, MI 48197, (313) 482-2870, **SLP**

Erby, Sheila A 5911 Larchwood Avenue, Philadelphia, PA 19143, (215) 472-0519, MA 73 Temple Univ-Tyler Sch of Art; SLP, Sch Dist of Phila, **SLP**

Erdige-Holz, Susan Route 2 Box 114, Canton, NY 13617, (315) 344-2414, BS 74 SUNY - Coll at Buffalo; MA 77 Kent St Univ; Sp & Hrng Dept Chrpsn, St Lawrence-Lewis Co BOCES, **SLP**

Erdman, Kathleen B 6700 Hill Ridge Drive, Greendale, WI 53572, (414) 529-9597, BS 72 Univ of WI - Madison; MS 74 Univ of WI - Madison; 88–Sp-Lang Path, Milwaukee PS, **SLP**

Erdman, Sue Ann 6261 Cardinal Lane, Columbia, MD 21044, (202) 576-1646, BA 71 OH St Univ; MA 76 OH St Univ; Aud, Army Aud & Sp Cen, **A**

Erdmann, Julie Lynn 1741 West 19th, Apartment 8-B, Lawrence, KS 66044, (913) 842-1586, BA 86 Univ of WI - Eau Claire; MA 88 Univ of KS

Erdmann, Mrs Michele 145 Boone Trail, Richmond, KY 40475, (606) 623-4716, BA 70 OH St Univ; MS 74 Univ of Pittsburgh - Pittsburgh; Sp-Lang Path, Mepco Home Health Agency, **SLP**

Erdos, Mrs Caryl Ann 16 Hancock Street, Winchester, MA 01890, (617) 581-9200, BS 77 Univ of MA - Amherst; MS 78 Ithaca Coll; **SLP**

Erdos, Elaine M 726 Briarwood Lane, San Dimas, CA 91773, (213) 439-6864, BS 74 Bowling Green St Univ; MS 77 Univ of OK Medical Center; Clin Super, Marina Professional Servs, **SLP**

Erdos, Mrs Erda G 549 Fairview Terrace, York, PA 17403, (717) 854-9265, BA 56 Goucher Coll; MA 57 Columbia Univ Teachers Coll; **SLP**

Ereditario, Monica A 7917 St Lawrence Avenue #2, Swissvale, PA 15218, (412) 244-0547, BS 83 WV Univ; MS 85 WV Univ; Audiologist, South Hills ENT, **A**

Erhardt, Sandra Dee Route 4 Box 404, Pittsboro, NC 27312-8431, (618) 235-8641, BS 83 Southern IL Univ-Edwardsvill; MS 86 Southern IL Univ-Edwardsvill

Erhart, Diana Marie 6430 Mountaineer Trail Ct, Reynoldsburg, OH 43068, (614) 864-0800, BS 84 OH Univ - Athens; MA 86 OH St Univ; **SLP**

Erhart, Mrs Louise M 6906 West Haldane Road, Mount Morris, IL 61054, (815) 734-4543, BS 73 Northern IL Univ - De Kalb; MA 75 Northern IL Univ - De Kalb; Sp-Lang Path, Mt Morris Pub Sch, **SLP**

Erich, Mrs Kristen Lea 25720 Lawton Avenue, Loma Linda, CA 92654, (714) 781-1771, BS 85 Loma Linda Univ - Riverside; MS 87 Loma Linda Univ - Riverside; **SLP**

Erichson, Mrs Elaine G 117 Saw Mill Road, Stamford, CT 06903, (203) 329-9432, BA 58 Barnard Coll; MS 78 Columbia Univ Teachers Coll; Sp-Lang Path, Greenwich Pub Sch, **SLP**

Ericksen, Janet L 5 Plover Lane, Hicksville, NY 11801, MA 77 Hofstra Univ; Sp-Lang Path, St Charles Hosp & Rehab Cen, **SLP**

Ericksen, Todd D Box 90AE RR3, Winona, MN 55987, (507) 452-1200, BS 79 Univ of MN - Minneap-St Paul; MA 81 Univ of MN - Minneap-St Paul; Audiologist, Hiawatha Valley Spec Educ Coop, **A**

Erickson, Mrs Alice Marie 43 Hillside Avenue, Westwood, NJ 07675, (201) 664-0880, BA 52 Augustana Coll; **SLP**

Erickson, Mrs Bonnie Rae O 408 Ridge Road, Albert Lea, MN 56007, (507) 377-2125, BS 75 Mankato St Univ; MS 80 Mankato St Univ; SLP, Alden Public Schools, **SLP**

Erickson, Carol Vesta 3320 N Dal Paso #10B, Hobbs, NM 88240, (505) 392-5571, BS 86 Western MI Univ; MA 87 Western MI Univ; 88–Aud, Audio Acoustics Hearing Ctrs

Erickson, Cathy Suzan 29 Redhawk, Irvine, CA 92714, (714) 551-6891, BA 79 Univ of CA - Santa Barbara; MA 83 Univ of TX - Austin; Sp/Lang Path, Oklahoma State Dept of Health, **SLP**

Erickson, Charlotte 410 Day Road North, St Croix Falls, WI 54024, **SLP**

Erickson, Constance Farran 1656 Labrador Drive, Costa Mesa, CA 92626, **SLP**

Erickson, E Joy P O Box 4087, Carson City, NV 89702, (702) 849-0255, BA 69 CA St Univ - Fresno; MS 82 Univ of NV - Reno; 82–Sp-Lang Path, Washoe Co Sch Dist, **SLP**

Erickson, Eleanor R 3701 Severn Avenue, Charlotte, NC 28210, **SLP**

Erickson, Elizabeth R R 2 Box 94, Red Lake Falls, MN 56750, (218) 253-4367, MS; **SLP**

Erickson, Mrs Ellen A 631 Ocean View Avenue, Grover City, CA 93433, BS; **SLP LM**

Erickson, Jane F 3002 North Murray Avenue, Milwaukee, WI 53211, (414) 962-9270, **SLP**

Erickson, Jean M 1810 Hillside Drive N W, Cedar Rapids, IA 52405, (319) 398-2463, MS 71 Minot St Univ; SLP, Cedar Rapids Comm Sch, **SLP**

Erickson, Jill Peterson 513 Fir Street, Shenandoah, IA 51601, BS 79 Southwest St Univ; MA 81 Univ of SD - Vermillion; Sp-Lang Path, AEA 13, **SLP**

Erickson, Dr Joan Good 2204 Brett Drive, Champaign, IL 61821, (217) 333-2230, BS 56 Northern IL Univ - De Kalb; MA 61 Univ of IL - Urbana; PH 77 (NS) Univ of IL - Urbana; Assoc Prof, U of IL Dept of Sp & Hrg Sci, **SLP A**

Erickson, Mrs Kathryn G Box 801, Stanley, ND 58784, (701) 628-2456, BS 78 Minot St Univ; MS 79 Minot St Univ; Sp-Lang Path, Stanley Community Schools, **SLP**

Erickson, Keith D R R 2 Box 94, Red Lake Falls, MN 56750, (218) 253-4367, **SLP**

Erickson, Mrs Laurie Aldrich 2955 Estrellita Brillante NW, Albuquerque, NM 87120, (505) 247-4224, BA 83 Univ of MN - Duluth; MS 85 Univ of WI - Stevens Point; 88–Sp-Lang Path, Albuquerque Hrng & Sp Ctr, **A**

Erickson, Mrs Mary Earl 3024 Round Table Court, Naples, FL 33962, (813) 455-1051, BS 81 Western KY Univ; MS 83 Univ of TN - Knoxville; **SLP**

Erickson, Mrs Nancy A B 1784 Woodland Court, Concord, CA 94521, Sp-Lang Path, Mount Diablo USD, **SLP**

Erickson, Pamela Kaye P O Box 419, Cascade, CO 80809-0419, (303) 630-5208, **SLP**

Erickson, Paula Lois 1950 South Clayton, Denver, CO 80210, BA 60 Univ of Tulsa; MA 76 Univ of Northern CO; SLP, Denver Public Schools, **SLP**

Erickson, Dr Robert L Dept Speech Path & Audiology, Western Michigan Univ, Kalamazoo, MI 49008, (616) 383-0963, BA 55 Univ of NE - Omaha; MA 59 Univ of NE - Lincoln; PH 63 (NS) Univ of IA; Prof/Chmn Dept SLP & Aud, Wn Mich U, **SLP F**

Erickson, Mrs Sarah S 5 Clayton Court, Chadds Ford, PA 19317, (215) 388-1532, BS 66 Miami Univ - Oxford; MS 68 Purdue Univ - West Lafayette; Sp-Lang Path, Brandywine Sch Dist, **SLP**

Erickson, Susan D P O Box 135, Silver Springs, NV 89429, (702) 577-2655, BS 79 SD St Univ; MS 81 Phillips Univ; Sp-Lang Path, Churchill Co Sch Dist, **SLP**

Erickson, Mrs Susan J P O Box 546, La Conner, WA 98257, (206) 424-8110, BA 74 Western WA Univ; MA 75 Western WA Univ; Sp/Lang Path, Isl Sp/Hrng Cl, **SLP**

Erickson, Mrs Terri Louise 5505 Vista Sondia N E, Albuquerque, NM 87111, BA 79 LA St Univ - Shreveport; MA 83 CA St Univ - Stanislaus; Sp-Lang Path, Albuquerque Public Schools, **SLP**

Eriksson, Anne-Guri 2517 North Gordon Court, Milwaukee, WI 53212-3019, (414) 372-3297, BS 68 Univ of MI - Ann Arbor; MS 84 Marquette Univ; 88–Sp-Lang Path, Willowglen Academy, **SLP**

Erkel, Karen L 27532 Lost Trail Drive, Laguna Hills, CA 92653, (714) 643-0949, **SLP**

Erl, Marjorie 3841 Gladman, Lexington, KY 40503, (606) 223-2657, BS 70 Univ of WI - Stevens Point; MS 72 Univ of WI - Stevens Point; **SLP**

Erlandson, Denise Burch 4008 Parkwood Circle, Candlewood Apartment #1-B, Mishawaka, IN 46545, (219) 277-3056, BS 79 Purdue Univ - West Lafayette; MS 87 Saint Cloud St Univ; 88–Sp-Lang Path, InSpeech Inc

Erlbaum, Sheila J 7314 Bryan Street, Philadelphia, PA 19119, (215) 951-4700, BA 76 CUNY - Brooklyn Coll; MA 78 Hofstra Univ; 78–Sp-Lang Path, Penna Sch for the Deaf, **SLP**

Erle, Kerry Denise 1295 Glenora Drive, London, ON, Canada N5X 1T6, (519) 537-5511, BS 82 Univ of Western Ontario; MS 85 Univ of Western Ontario; 88–Sp-Lang Path, Private Practice, **SLP**

Erlebacher, Mrs Marlene 55 Woodland Park Drive, Tenafly, NJ 07670, (212) 249-3792, BS 72 Syracuse Univ; MS 73 Syracuse Univ; Sp-Lang Path, Private Practice, **SLP**

Erlich, Eileen V 1553 Grovania Avenue, Abington, PA 19001, (215) 365-4606, BA 75 Temple Univ-Tyler Sch of Art; ME 78 Trenton St Coll; Audiologist, McMc Eastwick Ohp, **SLP A**

Erlinger, Karen S 644 Wilson Road, Atlanta, GA 30318, (404) 653-4700, **SLP**

Erman, Andrew Allen 12626 Caswell Avenue #4, Los Angeles, CA 90066, (816) 996-7424, MA 87 CA St Univ - Northridge; **SLP**

Ermey, Mary Jean 133 Central Avenue, Glen Rock, NJ 07452, (201) 891-1500, BA 71 William Paterson Coll; MS 72 William Paterson Coll; 72–Sp-Lang Path, Ramapo-Indian Hills Reg H S Di, **SLP**

Ernst, Barbara M 82 Lake Drive, Riviera Beach, FL 33404, **SLP**

Ernst, Mrs Lorraine F 4309 Geislers Court, Birmingham, MI 48010, (313) 423-8696, BA 74 Marygove Coll; MA 79 Wayne St Univ; Sp/Lang Path, Southfield Pub Sch, **SLP**

Ernst, Mrs Marian M 1077 South Gilpin, Denver, CO 80209, (303) 777-0740, BS 52 Univ of NE - Lincoln; MA 54 Univ of NE - Lincoln; Dir, Educ Aud Prog, Inc, **SLP A**

Ernst, Suzanne M 74 Vermont Street, Rochester, NY 14609, (716) 424-5665, BS 70 Nazareth Coll of Rochester; MA 77 SUNY - Coll at Geneseo; Aud, J William Shields MD, **A**

Ernst, Trudy Eileen 8753 East Roundtree Avenue, Englewood, CO 80111-5121, (303) 366-6266, MS 85 Univ of WY; 85–Aud, Aurora Assoc of Otol, **A**

Ernster, Stanley M 530 Helmet Avenue, Waterloo, IA 50703, (319) 277-3330, BA 74 Univ of Northern IA; MA 76 Univ of Northern IA; Sp-Lang Path, AEA Vii, **SLP**

Ernstrom, Vera J P O Box 738, Farmington, UT 84025, (801) 451-5061, BS 76 UT St Univ; MS 79 UT St Univ; SLP, Davis County School District, **SLP**

Ero, Lauren C 19 Leatherwood Court, Burtonsville, MD 20866, (301) 490-1107, MS 84 Gallaudet Coll; Aud, Silver Spring Hrng Aid Spec, **A**

Eron, Brenda Kay 525 Colle, P O Box 119, Luxemburg, WI 54217-0119, (414) 845-2371, BS 85 Univ of WI - Whitewater; MS 86 Univ of WI - Whitewater; 86–Sp-Lang Path, Luxemburg-Casco Sch Dist

Erpen, AnnaMarie 940 Hayne Road, Hillsborough, CA 94010, (415) 579-1336, BA 84 San Francisco St Univ; 88–Sp-Lang Path, Care Point Home Health Care Agency, **SLP**

Erratt, John David 6101 Gundry Avenue, Long Beach, CA 90805, (213) 423-4097, BA 77 Univ of CA - Irvine; MA 84 Univ of CA - Santa Barbara; 82–Aud, Hearing Consultants of Calif, **A**

Errickson, Mrs Christina Ann 3107 Schoolhouse Lane, Harrisburg, PA 17110, BS 83 Trenton St Coll; OM 85 Hahneman Medical Coll; SLP, Easter Seals, **SLP**

Errthum, Joanne Starrett 100 Mercy Drive, Rehabilitation Unit, Dubuque, IA 52001, (319) 589-9074, BS 79 Univ of WI - Whitewater; MS 85 Univ of WI - Whitewater; 87–Sp-Lang Path, Mercy Health Center, **SLP**

Erskine, Barbara J 4603 S E Madison, Portland, OR 97215, OB 81 Univ of Alberta - Alberta; MS 87 Univ of OR; **SLP**

Erskine, Mary Cara Hearing And Speech Clinic, Johns Hopkins Hospital, Carnegie 426, Baltimore, MD 21205, (301) 955-6151, BA 69 9302; ME 70 Loyola Coll; Sp-Lang Path/Aud, Johns Hopkins Hrng/Spch Clinic, **SLP A**

Ertel, Mrs Judith M 780 Garvens Avenue, Brookfield, WI 53005, (414) 521-8833, BS 75 Univ of WI - Stevens Point; MS 76 Univ of WI - Milwaukee; Sp-Lang Path, Waukesha Pub Sch, **SLP**

Ertmer, David 985 Cone Avenue, Canon City, CO 81212, (303) 275-6475, BS 73 Marquette Univ; MS 75 Univ of WI - Milwaukee; Sp-Lang Path, Fremont School District Re-1, **SLP**

Ervin, Dr Jean C 517 Lenoir Street, Morganton, NC 28655, (704) 437-8522, BA 30 Converse Coll; MA 42 Columbia Univ Teachers Coll; PH 50 (NS) Univ of MO - Columbia; **SLP LM**

Erway, Dr Ella A Box 164, East Dover, VT 05341, (203) 397-4569, BA 47 Wheaton Coll; MA 48 Columbia Univ Teachers Coll; ED 66 (NS) Columbia Univ Teachers Coll; Prof of Commun Dis, Sn CT St U, **SLP**

Erwin, Betty J 3500 Broadway, Fort Myers, FL 33901, (813) 936-0721, BA 75 MI St Univ; MS 78 Univ of WY; Aud, ENT Assoc, **A**

Erwin, Mrs Ellen 1903 Park Avenue, Benton, KY 42025, (502) 444-9687, BS 81 Murray St Univ; MA 83 Murray St Univ; Sp-Lang Path, W Ky Er Sl So Cen, **SLP**

Erwin, Mrs Judith L 2866 White Oak Drive, Grand Prairie, TX 75052, (214) 262-4255, BS 78 SUNY - Coll at Geneseo; MA 80 Univ of KS; Sp-Lang Path, Grand Prairie ISD, **SLP**

Erwin, Paul Michael Route 5 Box 474, Malvern, AR 72104, (501) 844-4803, MS 87 Univ of AR - Little Rock; 87–Sp-Lang Path, First Step Sch, **SLP**

Erwin-Miller, Lisa N 774 West Falmouth Hwy, Falmouth, MA 02540, (617) 548-7052, BS 85 Syracuse Univ; MS 87 PA St Univ - Univ Park; SLP, Forest Manor Neuro Center, **SLP**

Esber, Elizabeth C Naples Bath & Tennis Club, 203-B Bobolink Way, Naples, FL 33942, (813) 262-5860, MA 78 PA St Univ - Univ Park; BS 57 PA St Univ - Univ Park; Sp-Lang Path, Private Practice, **SLP LM ACE**

Esch, Barbara E Lansing School District, Everett High School, 3900 Stabler, Lansing, MI 48910, (517) 374-4572, BA 69 Western MI Univ; MA 80 MI St Univ; Sp/Lang Path, Lansing Sch Dist, **SLP**

Eschenbach, Mrs Cheryl D 916 Corn Tassel Trail, Martinsville, VA 24112, (703) 638-8224, BS 73 Univ of WI - Stevens Point; MS 78 Univ of NC - Chapel Hill; Sp-Lang Path, **SLP**

Escher, Mrs Constance 8543 Furrier Drive, Matthews, NC 28105, (704) 847-7310, BA 60 MI St Univ; MA 76 Wayne St Univ; Sp-Lang Path, Private Practice, **SLP**

Escher, Jane Murray 19 Sunnyside Avenue, Reading, MA 01867, MS 82 Univ of KY; Sp-Lang Path, **SLP**

Esch-Johnson, Mrs Geraldine Gerry 2780 South Vance Way, Denver, CO 80227, (303) 985-2765, BS 55 Univ of Denver; MA 58 Univ of Denver; MA 63 Univ of Denver; Retired, Denver Pub Sch, **SLP LM**

Esckelson, Dorothy A The Hollows, 4900 East 5th Street #1405, Tucson, AZ 85711, (602) 798-2699, BA 51 Asbury Coll; MA 60 Univ of MI - Ann Arbor; MA 81 Eastern MI Univ; Sp-Lang Path, Tucson USD, **SLP**

Escott, Judith 2156 Cottage Court, Marietta, GA 30060, BA 68; ME 71 Univ of GA; Sp-Lang Path, Fulton Co Bd Ed, **SLP**

Eshelman, Mrs Chris Winters 10162 Rockwood Drive, San Diego, CA 92131, (619) 588-3170, MA 75 Cleveland St Univ; Resource Specialist, Cajon Valley Union Schools, **SLP**

Eshelman, Mrs Mary P 119 Pass Key Road, Sarasota, FL 34242, (813) 346-2836, BA 43 Univ of IL - Urbana; MS 59 Univ of IL - Urbana; Prof, Wil U, **SLP A F LM**

Eshelman, Mrs Sally L 69 Gilford Avenue, Laconia, NH 03246, (603) 524-7775, BS 68 Emerson Coll; MA 69 Western MI Univ; Sp-Lang Path, Private Practice, **SLP**

Eskelson, Edna Mae Rt 1 Box 148, Colfax, WA 99111, (509) 882-2271, BA 41 WA St Univ; BA 42 WA St Univ; MA 70 WA St Univ; SLP, Grandview School District, **SLP**

Eskew, Mrs Lorraine W 3704 Harrison Street N W, Washington, DC 20015, (202) 363-4557, BA 36 Lawrence Univ; MA 68 George Washington Univ; **SLP LM**

Eskew, Nancy D 214 Echodale Lane, Knoxville, TN 37920, (615) 579-2454, BA 75 Univ of TN - Knoxville; MA 77 Univ of TN - Knoxville; Aud, Tennessee Sch for Deaf, **A**

Eskilson, Mrs Barbara C 216 Wedgewood Drive, Turnersville, NJ 08012, (609) 227-6720, ME 64 PA St Univ - Univ Park; BS 59 Bloomsburg Univ of PA; Sp-Lang Path, Clearview Reg Sch Dist, **SLP**

Eskilson, Jane E 3006 Simas Avenue, Pinole, CA 94564-1135, (707) 643-2501, BS 72 Univ of WI - Madison; MS 73 Univ of WI - Madison; Resource Specialist, Vallejo USD, **SLP**

Eskridge, Marlene 33 Fairview Boulevard, Hempstead, NY 11550, (516) 349-4778, OB 57 OH Univ - Athens; MA 76 Univ of Cincinnati; SLP, Plainview-Old Bethpage Sch Dis, **SLP**

Eskwitt, Dr Donna L 13568 Valleyheart Drive, Sherman Oaks, CA 91423, (213) 483-4431, BS 78 Ithaca Coll; MS 80 Univ of AZ; PH 88 (Deafness Rehabilitation) New York Univ; 84–Aud, House Ear Institute, **A ACE**

Esparza, Cami Lurita 1339 Kansas Circle, Concord, CA 94521, (415) 672-1301, MA 88 San Francisco St Univ

Esparza, Mrs Deborah A 759 Olenhurst Court, West Worthington, OH 43235, (614) 461-3397, BS 73 ND St Univ; MA 79 OH St Univ; Sp-Lang Path Coord, Grant Med Ctr, **SLP**

Espinosa, Melanie K Speech And Language Associates Inc, 4345 Phelan Boulevard, Beaumont, TX 77707, (409) 899-4099, BS 71 LA St Univ - Baton Rouge; MS 79 Lamar Univ; 79–Sp-Lang Path Dir, Sp and Lang Assoc Inc, **SLP ACE**

Espinosa, Mrs Melinda A Box 907, Orofino, ID 83544, (208) 476-5642, BA 75 CA St Univ - Long Beach; MS 77 ID St Univ; Sp-Lang Path, Orofino Sch Dist 171, **SLP**

Espinoza-Varas, Blas Indiana University, Dept Of Speech & Hearing, Bloomington, IN 47405, (812) 335-4156, PH 78 (NS) Washington Univ

Esposito, Andrea S 667 Stratton Street, Logan, WV 25601, (304) 752-6320, BS 76 WV Univ; MS 77 WV Univ; Sp-Lang Path, Logan-Mingo Arca Hlth Inc, **SLP**

Esposito, Catherine 11206 Tast Street, Pembroke Pines, FL 33026, (305) 962-8148, MA 74 Long Island U - CW Post Ctr; Alpha Omega Rdng & Sp Cen, **SLP**

Esposito, Geraldine Anne 93-13 Springfield Blvd, Queens Village, NY 11428, (718) 492-1800, BS 81 Saint John's Univ - Jamaica; MS 84 Adelphi Univ; Sp-Lang Path, East Rockaway Public Schools, **SLP**

Esposito, Josephine Rose 138-49 82nd Drive, Jamaica, NY 11435, (718) 454-6460, BA 84 CUNY - Queens Coll; MA 86 CUNY - Queens Coll; **SLP**

Esposito, Paul R 54 Hollyhock Road, Levittown, NY 11756, (516) 928-0188, BA 76 CUNY - Brooklyn Coll; MA 78 Univ of CT; Aud, North Shore Audiology, **A**

Esposito, Samuel John 1011 New Hope Street #9-A, Norristown, PA 19401, (215) 272-4493, BA 83 East Stroudsburg Univ of PA; MA 85 Temple Univ-Tyler Sch of Art; SLP, Easter Seals of Philadelphia, **SLP**

Esposito Visgitis, Mrs Nina 115 South Pasadena Drive, Pittsburgh, PA 15215, (412) 928-6550, BS 79 Indiana Univ of PA; MS 80 Indiana Univ of PA; Sp-Lang Path, Pittsburgh Pub Sch, **SLP**

Esposto-Franklin, Lesa Fairfield Hearing & Speech Ctr, 1287 Oliver Road, Fairfield, CA 94533, (707) 426-2075, BA 76 San Francisco St Univ; MS 79 San Francisco St Univ; Owner/Sp-Lang Path, Fairfield Hearing & Speech Cen, **SLP**

Espy-Leroy, Roberta 117 Country Close Lane, Lutz, FL 33549, (813) 933-8930, MA 72 Univ of IL - Urbana; Sp-Lang Path, Hillsborough Co Schs, **SLP**

Esral, Naomi T 41-F Westgate Road, Teaneck, NJ 07666, (718) 268-3687, **SLP**

Esry, Mrs Linda J 602 Pennsylvania, Holton, KS 66436, (913) 364-3463, BS 79 KS St Univ; MA 82 KS St Univ; Sp/Lang Path, Holton Spec Ed Coop 336, **SLP**

Ess, Jacqueline S 214 Woodridge, St Louis, MO 63122, (314) 569-8226, BA 60 MI St Univ; MA 64 Wayne St Univ; Area Coord, Spec Sch Dist of St Louis Co, **SLP A**

Essary, Mrs Rebecca Z 28247 Langside Avenue, Cyn Country, CA 91351-3810, (818) 843-4206, BA 81 San Jose St Univ; MA 85 CA St Univ - Los Angeles; **SLP**

Essency, Nadine G 97 Carnation Lane, Waterbury, CT 06704, (203) 754-5141, BS 74 Emerson Coll; MS 76 Southern CT St Univ; 88–Dir of Med Rehab, Easter Seal Rehab Ctr, **SLP**

Essex, Mrs Wanda E 2481 North Nye #318, Fremont, NE 68025, (402) 721-6720, BS 69 Univ of NE - Lincoln; MA 73 Univ of NE - Lincoln; Sp/Lang Path, Fremont Public Schools, **SLP**

Essington, Marianne W 1301 Rahway Avenue, Westfield, NJ 07090, (201) 754-2200, BS 78 WV Univ; MS 79 Rutgers St Univ -N Brunswick; SLP, N Plain Field Bd Ed, **SLP**

Esslinger-Heger, Robin E 3801 E Orchard Road, Littleton, CO 80121, Sp-Lang Path, Denver General Hospital, **SLP**

Estabrook, Mrs Elizabeth T 168 Housatonic Drive, Milford, CT 06460, (203) 576-7426, BA 74 Univ of Northern CO; MS 79 Southern CT St Univ; Sp-Lang Path, Bridgeport Board of Education, **SLP**

Estabrook, Marylin H 4057 Doveville Lane, Fairfax, VA 22032, **SLP**

Estep, Mrs Janet M 26431 Charford Way, El Toro, CA 92630, (714) 760-3505, BA 75 Univ of MO - Columbia; MA 78 Univ of Houston - Univ Park; Sp-Lang Path, Newport-Mesa USD, **SLP**

Esterreicher, Mrs Carol A P O Box 162, Sandy, UT 84091-0162, (801) 565-7500, BS 62 OH Univ - Athens; MA 73 Univ of MD - College Park; ES 81 Univ of UT; 78–Sp/Lang Path, Jordan Sch Dist, **SLP ACE**

Estes, Mrs Patricia T PO Box 506, Ossipee, NH 03864, (603) 875-7500, BS 75 Univ of NH; MS 80 Univ of NH; Sp/Lang Path, Alton School District, **SLP**

Estes, Sandra S 6412 Kenwick, Fort Worth, TX 76116-4409, (817) 732-7332, BA 63 TX Christian Univ; MA 68 TX Christian Univ; Realtor, William Rigg Inc, **SLP**

Estes-Waddell, Anna Gale 7650 Pelbrook Farm Drive, Centerville, OH 45459, (513) 433-2489, BS 76 Eastern KY Univ; MA 78 Univ of IL - Urbana; 88–Sp-Lang Path, Miami Valley Hosp/Rehab of OH, **SLP ACE**

Estomin, Ellen R 333 S Highland Avenue #803, Pittsburgh, PA 15206, (412) 665-4986, BA 68 Montclair St Coll; MA 73 Univ of Pittsburgh - Pittsburgh; Superv Sp/Lang, Pgh Bd of Pub Ed, **SLP**

Estrada, Mrs Sylvia A Route 3 Box 226, Beeville, TX 78102, (512) 358-0130, BS 76 Southwest TX St Univ; ME 77 Southwest TX St Univ; Sp-Lang Path, Beeville ISD, **SLP**

Estrany-Frau, Ingrid P O Box 572, Amherst, MA 01004, (413) 256-0245, BA 78 Univ of PR - Rio Piedras; MA 82 Univ of MA - Amherst; Sp-Lang Path, Holyoke Hosp, **SLP**

Estrem, Theresa Serbus 96 Shasta Circle East, Chanhassen, MN 55317, (612) 427-2200, MA 84 Univ of MN - Minneap-St Paul; Sp-Lang Path, Mercy Medical Center, **SLP**

Eszlinger, Mrs Elizabeth Hall P O Box 6303, Orange, CA 92667, (714) 639-1583, BS 79 CA St Univ - Long Beach; MA 82 CA St Univ - Long Beach; SLP, Newport Ctr for Ed Ther, **SLP**

Etchepare, Teresa Lu 5551 Belgraze Street, Garden Grove, CA 92645, (714) 953-3328, MS; Western Medical Center, **SLP**

Etcheson, Mrs Barbara V P O Box 64, Elnora, IN 47529, (812) 254-2760, BA 60 Syracuse Univ; MA 71 Western MI Univ; Sp/Lang Path, Daviess Cty Hosp, **SLP**

Eterginio, Richard M Myofunctional & Communication, Therapeutics, 411 Payne Drive, Cheshire, CT 06410, (203) 272-7871, MS 69 Southern CT St Univ; Sp-Lang Path, Myofunctional-Comm Therapeutic, **SLP**

Etheridge, Barbara B 26411 Birchfield Avenue, Palos Verdes Peninsula, CA 90274, **SLP**

Etheridge, Carolynn R 643 Northbrook Road, Savannah, GA 31406, **SLP**

Ethier, Mrs Laurel A 308 Oak Street, Warner Robins, GA 31088, BS 73 Univ of WI - Stevens Point; MS 74 Univ of WI - Stevens Point; Sp-Lang Path, Houston Co Bd of Ed, **SLP**

Ethier, Mark E 308 Oak Street, Warner Robins, GA 31093, (912) 929-4968, BS 71 Univ of ND; MS 73 Univ of WI - Stevens Point; Aud, Hrng Aid Cen, **A**

Ethridge, Brenda Revier P O Box 904, Eastman, GA 31023, (912) 374-2027, BS 82 Valdosta St Coll; ME 85 Valdosta St Coll; **SLP**

Ethridge, Nancy L 12518 West 62nd Street, Shawnee, KS 66216, (816) 234-3677, BS 73 CO St Univ; MS 75 CO St Univ; Sp-Lang Path, Childrens Mercy Hospital, **SLP**

Etienne, Joseph E Brescia College Speech & Hearing Clinic, Brescia College, 718 Allen Street, Owensboro, KY 42301, (502) 686-4284, BA 76 IN Univ - Bloomington; MA 77 IN Univ - Bloomington; OM 85 Western KY Univ; Coord of Aud Serv, Brescia Coll Sp-Hrng Cl, **A**

Etish, Mrs Barbara Levin 1013 Swallow Drive, Cherry Hill, NJ 08003, (609) 795-1013, BS 71 Ithaca Coll; MA 83 Trenton St Coll; Sp-Lang Path, P & F Rehab Associates

Etkin, Reuma 2875 Greenwich #102, San Francisco, CA 94123, (415) 567-5967, BA 86 San Francisco St Univ; MS 88 San Francisco St Univ

Etra, Joel L 100 Fanning Avenue, Norwich, CT 06360, (203) 889-3028, BA 72 CUNY - City College; MA 75 Hofstra Univ; Sp-Lang Path, Private Practice, **SLP**

Ettenger, Vicki S 160 Riverside Drive #16C, New York, NY 10024, (212) 517-0576, BA 69 Temple Univ; MA 71 Temple Univ; MA 76 Columbia Univ Teachers Coll; 81–Supvr, Marymount Manhattan Coll, **SLP**

Etter, Brenda F 815 N W 120th Street, Seattle, WA 98177, BA 61 Univ of CT; MS 63 Syracuse Univ; 87–Consult, Private Practice, **SLP A**

Etter, Rhonda R 1419 Broadway, Parsons, KS 67357, (316) 421-2818, BA 84 Univ of Northern IA; MA 86 Univ of Northern IA; Research Assoc, University of Ks, **SLP**

Ettinger, Donna Proctor 4317 Ridgewood Center Dr, Woodbridge, VA 22192, (703) 670-8126, BA 82 Univ of MD - College Park; ME 84 Univ of VA - Charlottesville; Aud, Prince William Sp & Hrng Cen, **A**

Ettman, Susan B S 309 Bolton Road, East Windsor, NJ 08520, (609) 443-9270, BA 78 SUNY - Center at Buffalo; MS 80 Columbia Univ Teachers Coll; Sp-Lang Path, Princeton Educ Res, **SLP**

Etzel, Carmel Dewaal 9753 Deltom Court, Baltimore, MD 21234, (301) 674-2214, BA 83 Loyola Coll; MS 85 Loyola Coll; **SLP**

Etzel, Mrs Tracy L 2015 41st Street NE Apartment E-3, Rochester, MN 55901, (507) 289-4878, MS 88 Purdue Univ - West Lafayette

Eubank, Andrew B Route 2 Box 9, Canadian, TX 79014, (806) 256-2592, BA 60 Univ of North TX; MA 74 Central MI Univ; Sp-Lang Path, Eastern Panhandle Cooperative, **SLP**

Eubank, P Gail 160 Judah Court, Folsom, CA 95630, (916) 989-9762, BS 71 KS St Univ; MA 78 Univ of WI - River Falls; Sp-Lang Path, InSpeech Inc, **SLP**

Eubank, Tammi Jo 1218 Ridgewood, Lindsay, OK 73052, (918) 224-2022, BA 83 Univ of OK - Norman; MS 86 Univ of OK Medical Center; 87–Sp-Lang Path, Grady Co Guidance Ctr, **SLP**

Eubanks, Mrs Cynthia E 1604 Barnstead Drive, Reston, VA 22091, BS 78 Univ of NC - Chapel Hill; MS 80 Univ of NC - Chapel Hill; 87–Elem Tchr, Fairfax Co Pub Sch, **SLP**

Eubanks, Lillie Sharon 1 Raccoon Trail, Conway, AR 72032, (501) 327-0599, BS 81 Univ of AR - Little Rock; MS 85 Univ of AR - Little Rock; 85–Sp-Lang Path, Conway Human Dev Ctr, **SLP**

Eubanks, Mrs Patricia 9593 Burnt Oak Drive, Fairfax Station, VA 22039-2631, (703) 250-8810, BS 74 Southern Methodist Univ; MA 76 George Washington Univ; SLP, Fairfax County Public Schools, **SLP**

Eudaly, Mary J 286 Elmira Place, Atlanta, GA 30307, (404) 294-3776, BS 75 FL St Univ; MS 76 FL St Univ; Aud, Dekalb Co Hlth Dept, **A**

Eugenio, Mrs Carolyn S 8318 Kyle Rote, San Antonio, TX 78240, (512) 680-7794, BS 79 Southwest TX St Univ; ME 80 Southwest TX St Univ; Sp-Lang Path, San Antonio ISD, **SLP**

Eugenio, Elmo E 8318 Kyle Rote, San Antonio, TX 78240, (512) 680-7794, BS 78 Southwest TX St Univ; ME 79 Southwest TX St Univ; Sp-Lang Path, San Antonio ISD, **SLP**

Eugenio-Nahina, Lianne G 2844 East 3rd Street #106, Long Beach, CA 90814, (213) 942-1500, BS 80 Univ of HI - Manoa; MA 85 CA St Univ - Los Angeles; 83–Sp-Lang Path, El Rancho USD, **SLP**

Eule, Mrs Althea Marshall 35 Stewart Street, New Haven, CT 06512, (203) 467-9171, BA 70 Catholic Univ of America; MS 72 George Washington Univ; MA 81 George Washington Univ; Clinical Supervisor, Southern Connestisut State U, **SLP**

Eulenberg, Dr John Bryson 1250 Daisy Lane, East Lansing, MI 48823, (517) 353-6622

Euler, Catherine 900 West Sierra Madre Avenue, Apartment 65, Azusa, CA 91702, (818) 241-3111, BA 76 CA St Univ - Northridge; MA 78 CA St Univ - Northridge; Sp-Lang Path, Glendale USD, **SLP**

Euler, Mrs Pamala D 504 South Dunn, Maryville, MO 64468, (816) 652-3718, BS 78 Univ of MO - KS City; MS 80 Central MO St Univ; Sp/Lang Path, N Andrew S Nod Sch, **SLP**

Eurich, Mrs Kathleen A 2225 Park Ridge Drive, Bloomfield Hills, MI 48013, (313) 540-5712, BS 72 Wayne St Univ; MA 76 Eastern MI Univ; Sp-Lang Path, Bloomfield Hill Sch, **SLP**

Euston, Kathleen 107 T Street, Salt Lake City, UT 84103, (801) 364-7124, BA 64 Brown Univ; MA 67 OH Univ - Athens; **SLP**

Euton, Ruth Marie 2565 West Village Drive, Toledo, OH 43614, (419) 385-0820, OB 76 Univ of Toledo; MA 86 Eastern MI Univ; 76–Sp-Lang Path, Toledo PS, **SLP**

Eva, Michael L 198 Pine Bluffs Road, Roscommon, MI 48653, (517) 275-5137, BS 74 Western MI Univ; MA 80 Central MI Univ; Sp-Lang Path, Coor ISD, **SLP**

Evans, Mrs Adeline L 1628 Hedgefield Court, Tallahassee, FL 32303, (904) 599-3140, BS 60 Grambling St Univ; MA 64 LA St Univ - Baton Rouge; PH 80 (Sp Communication & Path) FL St Univ; 87–Prof of Sp/Lab Coord, Florida A & M University, **SLP**

Evans, Anne Eliza Laconia Clinic, 724 Main Street, Laconia, NH 03246, (603) 524-5151, BA 74 Univ of NH; MS 79 UT St Univ; Aud, Laconia Clinic Inc, **A**

Evans, Mrs Annette B 4380 Cottonwood, Hoffman Estates, IL 60195, (312) 884-3964, BS 65 Bradley Univ; MS 70 Miami Univ - Oxford; **SLP**

Evans, Barbara A 3836 St Paris Pike, Springfield, OH 45504, **SLP**

Evans, Mrs Barbara B 1522 Hermitage Road, Manakin-Sabot, VA 23103, (804) 784-3729, BS 72 Univ of VA - Charlottesville; ME 73 Univ of VA - Charlottesville; 88–Sp-Lang Path, Goochland County PS, **SLP**

Evans, Barbara Liston 3215 33rd Avenue South #2, Minneapolis, MN 55406-2024, **SLP**

Evans, Mrs Becky Seidensticker 9310 Riva Ridge, Shreveport, LA 71115, (318) 632-4889, BA 82 LA Tech Univ; MS 83 Univ of AR - Little Rock; Dir of Sp-Lang Path, Willis Knighton Med Ctr, **SLP**

Evans, Bonita M 16 Harrogate Square, Williamsville, NY 14221, (716) 689-6681, BS 66 Syracuse Univ; MS 78 SUNY - Center at Buffalo; Amherst Presby Cen, **SLP**

Evans, Mrs Brenda E 2900 West Treeline Place, Tucson, AZ 85741, (602) 797-0058, BS 74 Univ of AZ; MS 76 Univ of AZ; Sp/Lang Path, Tucson USD, **SLP**

Evans, Brian J 1 Brewery Square T312, New Haven, CT 06513, (203) 366-7551, BA 78 Boston Univ; MA 81 Univ of MA - Amherst; Sp-Lang Path, Rocky Hill PS, **SLP**

Evans, Mrs Candace M 14105 56th Avenue N W, Gig Harbor, WA 98335, (206) 851-4817, BA 68 WA St Univ; MA 72 WA St Univ; Sp-Lang Path, Peninsula Sch Dist, **SLP**

Evans, Ceanne L c/o Spokane ENT Clinic, 104 West 5th Avenue, Suite 340, Spokane, WA 99204, (509) 624-2326, BS 75 ND St Univ; MS 78 Univ of WY; Aud, Spokane ENT Cl, **A**

Evans, Charlotte Johanna Manitoba School For The Deaf, 500 Shaftesbury Boulevard, Winnipeg, MB, Canada R3P 0M1, (204) 945-8934, OM 85 Univ of Western Ontario; 87–Sp-Lang Path, Manitoba Sch for the Deaf, **SLP**

Evans, Chris Hawrylak 1545 St Paul Street, Rochester, NY 14621, (716) 544-1240, BS 69 East TX St Univ - Commerce; MS 70 CO St Univ; Audiologist, Rochester Sch for the Deaf, **A**

Evans, Christy Robin 2120 Randolph Road #203, Silver Spring, MD 20902, (301) 949-8067, BA 83 Hampton Univ; MS 86 Univ of AR - Little Rock; **SLP**

Evans, Mrs Coletia Brown P O Box 249, Route 3 Box 403-C Shell Rd, Pawleys Island, SC 29585, (803) 237-8591, BA 67 SC St Coll; MA 78 SC St Coll; Instr/Cl Super, Sc St Coll, **SLP**

Evans, Mrs Denise S 207 Chestnut Ridge Road, Bethel, CT 06801, (203) 792-9066, BS 73 SUNY - Coll at Buffalo; MS 74 Columbia Univ Teachers Coll; 88–Sp-Lang Path, Bethel PS, **SLP**

Evans, Diane 3307 Crosswinds Road, Charlotte, NC 28216-6606, (301) 725-1323, **SLP**

Evans, Mrs Dianne Harvey 23 Kendall Lane, Scotts Valley, CA 95066, (408) 439-9523, OB 76; MA 83 CA St Univ - Northridge; SLP, **SLP**

Evans, Mrs Donna J 4 Able View Drive, Butler, PA 16001, (412) 287-4781, BA 69 TX Tech Univ; MA 71 Univ of MD - College Park; SLP, VA, **SLP ACE**

Evans, Mrs Donna S Route 13 Box 67, Bloomington, IL 61701, (309) 663-7002, BS 72 OH St Univ; MA 77 Kent St Univ; Sp-Lang Path, Marc Center Spice Program, **SLP**

Evans, Doreen Ann North 8819 Colton #117, Spokane, WA 99218, (509) 466-0794, MS 85 Univ of TX - Dallas; BA 83 Univ of MT; SLP, Sacred Heart Med Center, **SLP**

Evans, Elizabeth Anne 741 Missouri, Lawrence, KS 66044, (913) 864-3050, BA 68 Univ of UT; MA 73 Univ of CO - Boulder; Sp-Lang Path, Lawrence USD 497, **SLP**

Evans, Dr Evan L 198 East Ackerman, Monmouth, OR 97361, (503) 838-3001, BS 69 Western OR St Coll; MS 69 Western OR St Coll; PH 82 (NS) OR St Univ; Owner/Aud, Willamette Vlly Aud, **A**

Evans, Gail E St Elizabeths Hospital, Speech Path & Aud Branch, Martin Luther King Avenue S E, Washington, DC 20032, (202) 373-7374, BA 75 Univ of MD - College Park; MS 77 Loyola Coll; Sp-Lang Path, St Elizabeths Hosp, **SLP**

Evans, George F Camp Hearing Aid Center, 1100-1/2 36th Street, P O Box 4338, Parkersburg, WV 26104, (304) 422-5611, BS 75 Univ of KY; MA 77 Univ of TN - Knoxville; Owner, Camp Hrng Aid Cen, **A**

Evans, Glenda Kay 3448-I North Druid Hills Road, Rd 1, Decatur, GA 30033-3750, (404) 728-9939, BS 82 LA St Univ - Baton Rouge; MA 84 Memphis St Univ; Sp-Lang Path, Henrietta Egleston Chldn Hosp, **SLP**

Evans, Janet M S 1010 East Montgomery, Knoxville, IA 50138, (515) 842-6640, BA 71 Univ of IA; MA 72 Univ of IA; Sp-Lang Path, Associated Therapy Svcs, **SLP**

Evans, Joan E 329FAIRVIEW Avenue, Ambler, PA 19002, (215) 539-8550, BA 71 Rutger's St Univ - Douglas Coll; ME 72 Rutgers St Univ -N Brunswick; MS 79 Purdue Univ - West Lafayette; Prog Support Spec, Montgomery Co Intermed Unit, **SLP A**

Evans, John R 121 North Broadway, Baltimore, MD 21231, (301) 732-3328, BS 75 Towson St Univ; MS 79 Howard Univ; Sp/Lang Path, Baltimore Cty Pub Schs, **SLP**

Evans, Julia C 812 Wisner Drive, Waterloo, IA 50702, (219) 277-3330, BA 60 Univ of Northern IA; MA 76 Univ of Northern IA; SLP, AEA7, **SLP**

Evans, Julia Lynne 1111 East Catherine, University Of Michigan, Ann Arbor, MI 48109-2054, (303) 764-8440, BA 82 Univ of CO - Boulder; MS 83 Columbia Univ Teachers Coll; 88–Clin Supvr, The Univ of MI, **SLP**

Evans, Mrs Karen E 4603 Andre, Midland, MI 48640, (517) 631-0775, BS 77 Western MI Univ; MA 79 Eastern MI Univ; Sp-Lang Path, **SLP**

Evans, Karen Kathleen 5920 King Charles Court, Clemmons, NC 27012, (919) 760-5770, BS 82 Univ of South AL; MS 83 Univ of South AL; Sp-Lang Path, Forsyth Memorial Hosp, **SLP**

Evans, Kathy 15206 Dewey Avenue, Omaha, NE 68154, (402) 334-7439, BS 86 Univ of NE - Omaha; MS 87 Univ of NE - Omaha

Evans, Laura F 1 Sharpsburg, Irvine, CA 92714, **SLP**

Evans, Marcia Ann Route 3 Box 246, Booneville, AR 72927, (501) 675-2121, BS 82 Univ of AR - Fayetteville; MS 83 Univ of AR - Fayetteville; SLP, Booneville Human Developmt Cen, **SLP**

Evans, Mrs Marilyn G 10735 Pecan Drive, Fairhope, AL 36532, (205) 928-8400, BS 75 Univ of Montevallo; MS 79 Univ of South AL; Sp-Lang Path, Fairhope Primary School, **SLP**

Evans, Marion McTigue 10336 South Georgia Lane, Oak Lawn, IL 60453, (317) 857-7616, OB 63 Chicago St Univ; MS 71 Chicago St Univ; OM 84 Governors St Univ

Evans, Mary Lee 2001 East Vermont, Urbana, IL 61801, (217) 892-2194, BA 65 Univ of IL - Urbana; MA 74 Univ of IL - Urbana; MA 84 Univ of IL - Urbana; Sp-Lang Path, Rantoul City Schools, **SLP**

Evans, Mary P 201 East Ogden, Hinsdale, IL 60521, (312) 323-7970, BA 74 Northern IL Univ - De Kalb; MA 76 Northern IL Univ - De Kalb; 78–Aud, Sound Resources Inc, **A**

Evans, Nancy K 3634 Wyoming S W, Wyoming, MI 49509, (616) 538-4753, BA 73 MI St Univ; MA 81 Western MI Univ; 88–Sp-Lang Path, MI Econ & Human Dev

Evans, Mrs Patricia Ann 3313 Brook Glen, Garland, TX 75042, (214) 939-0593, **SLP**

Evans, Patricia Bryan P O Box 55, Warren, TX 77664, (409) 547-2247, BS 85 Lamar Univ; MS 86 Lamar Univ; **SLP**

Evans, Mrs Paula S H 1413 West Chestnut, Ponca City, OK 74601, (405) 762-2176, BS 74 OK St Univ; MA 76 Univ of Tulsa; Sp-Lang Path, Private Practice, **SLP**

Evans, Randall P 415 2nd Avenue, Manchester, GA 31816, (404) 655-2018, BA 66 San Jose St Univ; MA 67 MI St Univ; Sp-Lang Path, Roosevelt Warm Springs I for R, **SLP**

Evans, Robin Unger 27549 County Road 340, Buena Vista, CO 81211, (719) 395-2491, BS 77 Bowling Green St Univ; MA 79 Bowling Green St Univ; 88–Sp-Lang Path, Chaffee Co Sch Dist R-31, **SLP**

Evans, Roland S 17130 Est Jefferson, Grosse Pointe, MI 48230, (313) 885-8162, BA 56 Wayne St Univ; MA 60 Western MI Univ; Owner/Sp-Lang Path, Private Practice, **SLP**

Evans, Ruth Ellen 6-2204 118th Street, Edmonton, AB, Canada T6J 5K2, (403) 432-8859, BS 78 Dalhousie Univ - Nova Scotia; MS 82 Dalhousie Univ - Nova Scotia; Aud, Glenrose Provincial Gen Hosp, **A**

Evans, Sandra L 718 South Orleans Avenue, Tampa, FL 33606, (813) 251-7737, MA 68 Univ of South FL; Ch of SLP & Aud, Tampa Gen Hosp, **SLP**

Evans, Sandra L P O Box 8946, St Thomas, VI 00801, (809) 774-9982, BA 75 Univ of Pittsburgh - Pittsburgh; MA 77 Univ of Pittsburgh - Pittsburgh; Sp-Lang Path, US Virgin Isl Govt Ed Dept, **SLP**

Evans, Sherri Lynne 1310 McKahan Avenue, Columbus, OH 43232, (614) 868-9256, BS 85 OH Univ - Athens; MA 87 OH Univ - Athens; 87–Sp-Lang Path, InSpeech Inc

Evans, Shirley D 21 McCuthin Drive, Jay, FL 32565, (904) 474-5358, BS 84 Western IL Univ; MA 85 Western IL Univ; Sp-Lang Path, Rehab Institute of Florida, **SLP**

Evans, Susan A Southeastern Sp & Hrng Service, P O Box 50025, Fayetteville, NC 28305, (919) 485-5145, MS 80 Bowling Green St Univ; Aud, Southeastern Sp & Hrng Servive, **A**

Evans, Mrs Susan Ann Holmes 4 Cypress Lane, Winter Park, FL 32789, (305) 628-8957, BA 79 Univ of Central FL; MA 82 Univ of Central FL; SLP, Seminole County Public Schools, **SLP**

Evans, Mrs Susan Lynn 3244 Shelter Creek Lane, San Bruno, CA 94066, (415) 871-0372, BS 71 OH Univ - Athens; MA 72 OH Univ - Athens; Sp-Lang Path, San Mateo Co Bd Ed, **SLP**

Evans, Terrell Riley 7161 Saulsbury Circle, Arvada, CO 80003, (303) 421-4154, BS 73 Kent St Univ; MA 75 Kent St Univ; 86–Sp/Lang Path, Colorado Comm Consultants, **SLP**

Evans, Vicky Sue 1912 Madden Road, Jacksonville, AR 72076-2635, (501) 985-2349, MS 79 Univ of IL - Urbana; **SLP**

Evans, Virginia F 1032 Boughton Street, Watertown, WI 53094, (414) 261-7031, BA 31 Univ of WI - Madison; MA 40 Univ of WI - Madison; Retired, **SLP LM**

Evans, Dr William Bryce Dept Speech Path & Audiology, Coll Of Allied Health Sci, Univ Of South Alabama, Mobile, AL 36688, (205) 460-6327, BS 51 MS Coll; MA 53 Univ Southern MS-Hattiesburg; PH 79; Assoc Professor SLP, University of South Alabama, **SLP**

Evans-Batalucco, Georgianna 805 Barrington, Grosse Pointe Pk, MI 48230, (313) 824-3737, BA 78 Eastern MI Univ; MA 80 Eastern MI Univ; 87–Sp-Lang Path, Private Practice, **SLP**

Evans-McDowell, Mrs Judy K P O Box 1169, Lebec, CA 93243, **SLP**

Evans-Welpe, Mrs Mary C 54 Waverly Street, Potsdam, NY 13676, (315) 265-4642, BA 82 SUNY - Coll at Plattsburgh; MA 84 SUNY - Coll at Plattsburgh; 85–Sp-Lang Path, St Lawrence-Lewis Co BOCES, **SLP**

Evans-Wezel, Mrs Ann Marie Colonial Oaks Drive, Rural Route 4, Oak Ridge, NJ 07438, (201) 697-0437, BA 81 Adelphi Univ; MS 82 Adelphi Univ; 86–Supvr of Sp-Lang Path, Herbert G Birch Early Childhood Ctr, **SLP**

Evasco, Mrs Kathleen M 2330 Stockwell, Lincoln, NE 68502, (402) 464-3749, BS 74 Univ of NE - Lincoln; MA 76 Univ of NE - Lincoln; 77–Sp-Lang Path, Lincoln Pub Sch, **SLP**

Eve, Irwin Leigh 1220 Coast Village Road, Apartment 311, Montecito, CA 93108, (805) 969-9750, BA 80 Univ of CA - Santa Barbara; MA 81 Univ of TN - Knoxville; Director Audiology, PA Hospital, **A**

Eve, Salli Elena 1220 Coast Village Rd #311, Montecito, CA 93108, (805) 969-9750, BA 79 Montclair St Coll; MA 81 Univ of CA - Santa Barbara; Aud, PA Center for Hearing Services, **A**

Evelyn, Karen 146-02 13th Avenue, Whitestone, NY 11357, (718) 767-4106, MA 86 CUNY - Queens Coll; 88–Sp-Lang Path, Long Island Jewish Med Ctr, **SLP**

Even, Mrs Helen H 5844 Little Pine Lane, Rochester, MI 48064, (313) 651-2528, BS 34 Purdue Univ - West Lafayette; ME 56 Wayne St Univ; **SLP LM**

Everding, Mrs Vicki Love 1104 Terrace Drive, St Louis, MO 63117-1335, (314) 849-2000, OB 79 Northeast MO St Univ; MS 84 Fontbonne Coll; 83–Sp-Lang Path, Special Sch Dist, **SLP**

Everett, Darlene Welton 3728 Kaiser Avenue N E, Canton, OH 44705-2718, (216) 492-4925, BS 83 Kent St Univ; Aud, Private Practice, **A**

Everett, Karen Herman 5324 Kester Avenue #3, Van Nuys, CA 91411, (805) 495-7037, BA 75 San Jose St Univ; MA 78 CA St Univ - Northridge; Sp-Lang Path, Conejo Valley USD, **SLP**

Everett, Mary K 825 Rockview Court, Duluth, MN 55804, (218) 722-1431, BA 77 Univ of MN - Duluth; MA 78 Univ of MN - Duluth; SLP, Duluth Pub Sch ISD 709, **SLP**

Everett, Mrs Pamela Joyce 4504 Bridgetown Run, Fort Wayne, IN 46804, (219) 436-6000, BS 70 IN Univ - Bloomington; ME 80 IN Univ - Bloomington; Sp-Lang Path, SW Allen Co Schs, **SLP**

Everett, Mrs Paula L 6212 Glenview Drive #115, North Richland Hills, TX 76180, (817) 485-7624, MS 88 Univ of North TX; Sp-Lang Path, Trucare Rehab Svcs Inc

Everett, Mrs Siri Ann 1510 North Nevada Avenue, Colorado Springs, CO 80907-7433, (617) 924-0590, **SLP**

Everett, Mrs Sue Thayer 13101 Catalpa, Southgate, MI 48195, (313) 285-0738, BS 77 Central MI Univ; MA 82 Central MI Univ; Sp-Lang Path, Visiting Nurse Home Hlth Svcs, **SLP**

Everette, Lisa Sandrolini 829 South Monroe, Hinsdale, IL 60521, (312) 789-8710, BS 80 Univ of IL - Urbana; MS 81 Univ of IL - Urbana; SLP, Dupage-West Cook Association, **SLP**

Everhart, Katherine 110 North Oakland Drive, Mebane, NC 27302, (919) 563-3722, OB 69 Univ of NC - Greensboro; MA 72 Appalachian St Univ; Sp-Lang Path, Alamance Co Pub Sch, **SLP**

Everingham, Neil Mark 4278 Barr Avenue, Memphis, TN 38117-7803, (901) 761-9179, OB 79 Univ of MS; MS 82 Univ of MS; Aud, Memphis City Sch, **A**

Everitt, David Max 5031 Villa Linde Pkwy #20, Flint, MI 48504-6602, (313) 733-1830, BS 80 Brigham Young Univ; OM 81 Brigham Young Univ; 86–Aud, Gerald G Cole MD PC, **A**

Everitt, Wanda Huey 9701 W Ferris Branch Blvd, Apartment 313, Dallas, TX 75243, (214) 340-3018, BS 70 Memphis St Univ; MS 79 Univ Southern MS-Hattiesburg; **SLP**

Everly, Mrs Jaunita A Route 1 Box 64, Grafton, WV 26354, (304) 265-2497, BS 66 WV Univ; MS 73 WV Univ; Sp-Lang Path, Taylos Co Bd of Ed, **SLP**

Evers, Rev Robert T St Marys Seminary & University, 5400 Roland Avenue, Baltimore, MD 21210, (301) 323-3200, OM 58 Saint Marys Seminary & Univ; MA 60 Seton Hall Univ; ED 71 (Sp) Columbia Univ Teachers Coll; Assoc Prof, St Marys Seminary & U, **SLP**

Eversmann, Mrs Jill Grant 1872 Marmande Drive, Kmcas, Kailua, HI 96734, (808) 254-3130, BS 84 James Madison Univ; MS 86 Towson St Univ; Sp-Lang Path, HI Dept of Educ, **SLP**

Eversole, Laura Marie 5982 East McKenzie, Fresno, CA 93727, (209) 439-0282, **SLP**

Everson, Mrs Cheryl Ann 56 Alps Road, Branford, CT 06405, (203) 481-6747, BS 78 Southern CT St Univ; MA 83 CA St Univ - Chico; Sp-Lang Path, Hamden Bd of Ed, **SLP**

Everts, Kathryn W 2111 East Vaughn, Tempe, AZ 85283, BA 74 Univ of UT; BS 74 Univ of UT; MS 75 Univ of UT; Sp-Lang Path, Tempe Elementary School Dist, **SLP**

Every, Donna J 432B Boswell Hill Road, Endicott, NY 13760, Private Practice, **SLP**

Evilsizer, Mrs Marjorie J 8108 Harvest Hills S Blvd, Oklahoma City, OK 73132, (405) 728-2647, BA 83 Univ of OK - Norman; MS 85 Univ of OK - Norman; 87–Sp-Lang Path, Putnam City Schs, **SLP**

Evins, Linda Faye 6401 Eastridge Road #1410, Odessa, TX 79762, (915) 563-0288, **SLP**

Ewanchyshyn, Nadine Elizabeth 108 4th Avenue N E, Dauphin, MB, Canada R7N 0X9, (204) 638-4146, MS 84 Univ of ND; **SLP**

Ewanowski, Dr Stanley J 600 North Highland Avenue, Madison, WI 53792, (608) 263-8412, OB 51 Marquette Univ; MS 60 Univ of WI - Madison; PH 64 (Sp Path) Univ of WI - Madison; 60–Dir of Sp-Lang Path, Univ of Wisconsin Hosp & Clin, **SLP F**

Ewart, Joanne 20 Humming Bird Way, Novato, CA 94949, (707) 526-7920, BA 82 San Francisco St Univ; MS 83 San Francisco St Univ; 85–Aud, Santa Rosa Med Park Aud Ctr, **A**

Ewin, Mrs Carol I 2539 River Road, Modesto, CA 95351, (209) 524-2154, BA 71 CA St Univ - Stanislaus; MA 76 CA St Univ - Stanislaus; Sdl Tchr, Modesto Cty Sch, **SLP**

Ewing, Allison M 109 Beverly Drive, Metairie, LA 70001, **SLP**

Ewing, Elizabeth R 4315 Winterode Way, Baltimore, MD 21236, (301) 256-5194, BA 74 Loyola Coll; MS 75 Loyola Coll; **SLP**

Ewing, Janice Kryski 1311 Whaley Street #602, Columbia, SC 29205, (803) 777-0052, BA 73 Univ of British Columbia; MA 77 WA St Univ; Sp-Lang Path, Univ of SC, **SLP**

Ewing, Janice R P O Box 1825, Gilroy, CA 95021, BA 72 CA St Univ - Chico; Sp-Lang Path, Private Practice, **SLP**

Ewing, Susan A 6225 Worlington, Birmingham, MI 48010, (313) 258-1090, BA 65 Depauw Univ; MA 76 Wayne St Univ; SLP, Wm Beaumont Hosp, **SLP**

Ewing, Mrs Susan E 1836 Hudacsek Drive, Suffield, OH 44260, (216) 628-2929, BS 81 Kent St Univ; MA 81 Kent St Univ; Sp-Lang Path, PSI Affliates Inc, **SLP**

Ewy, Jane Ann Davenport 400 South Santa Fe, Salina, KS 67401, (913) 826-3487, BS 70 Univ of KS; MA 74 Wichita St Univ; Sp-Lang Path, Asbury Hospital, **SLP**

Exas, Mrs Katherine M 2 Steever's Court, Rd #1, Reading, PA 19607, (215) 779-7111, BS 74 SUNY - Coll at Geneseo; ME 75 SUNY - Coll at Geneseo; SLP, Berks Co Iu Spec Ed, **SLP**

Exelbert, Mrs Trudy L 5 Arista Court, Dix Hills, NY 11746, (516) 421-2217, **SLP A**

Exelrod, Iris C 2626 Lakeview #805, Chicago, IL 60614, (312) 248-0244, BS 70 Univ of MI - Ann Arbor; MA 71 George Washington Univ; Coord/SLP, Consol Sch Dist #65, **SLP**

Exnicios, Jill D 275 Glenwood Drive, Metairie, LA 70005, (504) 865-1945, BS 79 LA St Univ - Baton Rouge; OM 80 LA St Univ - N O Medical Ctr; Sp-Lang Path, Communication & Learning Ctr, **SLP**

Exnicios, Sharon Beth 1700 Akron Avenue, Metairie, LA 70003, (504) 733-3459, BA 80 Northeast LA Univ; MA 84 Univ of Northern CO; Sp-Lang Supervisor, Therapy Associates, **SLP**

Exstrom, Mary I 3009 North Tulsa Drive, Oklahoma City, OK 73107, (405) 271-4214, BS 75 Univ of Tulsa; MS 77 Univ of OK Medical Center; Sup/Asst Prof, U of Okla Health Sciences Cen, **SLP**

Eye, Mrs Marcia P 705 St Moritz Court, Switzerland, FL 32043, BS 69 WV Univ; MS 71 WV Univ; Sp-Lang Path, Private Practice, **SLP**

Eyer, Mrs Deborah L 513 Newark Avenue, Bradley Beach, NJ 07720, (201) 755-9058, BS 81 Bradley Univ; MS 83 Bradley Univ; Sp-Lang Path, UCP, **SLP**

Eyer, Dr Julia Dept Of Communication Disorder, Univ Of Ok Hlth Sci Ctr, P O Box 2601, Oklahoma City, OK 73190, (405) 271-4214, BA 77 OK Baptist Univ; MA 79 Univ of KS; PH 88 (Sp Lang Path); 88–Asst Prof, Univ of Ok, **SLP**

Eymann, Kristy A 570 Fairway View Drive #3H, Wheeling, IL 60090, (312) 367-8000, MA 79 Central MI Univ; Sp/Lang Path, Hawthorn School District 73, **SLP**

Eynon, Diane Perras 345 North Court Street, Thunder Bay, ON, Canada P7A 4W8, (807) 345-7560, BA 75 Univ of ND; MA 87 Univ of MN - Minneap-St Paul; 75–Sp-Lang Path, Lakehead Catholic Sch Bd

Ezell, Helen K 643 McCully Street, Pittsburgh, PA 15243, (412) 624-0101, BS 72 WV Univ; MA 73 OH Univ - Athens; **SLP**

Ezell, Robin Ward Ezell Farmstead, PO Box 11, Mont Clare, PA 19453, (215) 935-2923, BA 75 SUNY - Center at Buffalo; MA 76 Northern IL Univ - De Kalb; Sp-Lang Path, Private Practice, **SLP**

Ezelle, Mrs Nancy C N Route 9 Box 352, Martinsville, VA 24112, (703) 638-1022, BS 73 Radford Univ; ME 75 Univ of NC - Greensboro; Sp-Lang Path, Henry Cty Pub Sch, **SLP**

Ezickson, Katherine F 395 Cassatt Road, Berwyn, PA 19312, BA 79 Converse Coll; ME 81 Univ of VA - Charlottesville; Aud, **A**

Ezra, Mrs Cheryl Diane 1101 West Stevens #149, Santa Ana, CA 92707, (714) 540-2469, MS 87 Univ of AZ; 88–Sp-Lang Path, Long Beach Scottish Rite Clin, **SLP**

Ezring, Mrs Barbara M 5030 Northwest 5th Avenue, Boca Raton, FL 33431, BS 73 Univ of IL - Urbana; MS 74 Columbia Univ Teachers Coll; Sp-Lang Path, Private Practice, **SLP**

Ezzat, Mrs Esmat H 32 Pinehurst Road, Holyoke, MA 01040, **SLP**

Ezzell, Debra Demaray 899 Dean Drive N W, Atlanta, GA 30318, (404) 355-6244, BS 74 Vanderbilt Univ; MS 75 Vanderbilt Univ; Sp-Lang Path, Northside Hosp, **SLP**

Ezzell, Lisa Gayle Route 3 Box 421, Whiteville, NC 28472, BS 85 East Carolina Univ; MS 86 East Carolina Univ; 88–Sp-Lang Path, Columbus County Schs, **SLP**

Ezzell-Holdcroft, Melissa 209 W Ingomar Road, Pittsburgh, PA 15237, (412) 828-1300, BS 81 Denison Univ; MA 83 Univ of Pittsburgh - Pittsburgh; Sp-Lang Path, Harmarville Rehab Ctr, **SLP**

F

Faas, Mary Elizabeth Faas Road, Palmyra, NY 14522, (716) 377-4660, BS 82 Nazareth Coll of Rochester; MS 85 Nazareth Coll of Rochester

Faber-Hammond, Gayle 43 Lincoln Road, Barrington, RI 02806, (617) 256-6571, **SLP**

Fabian, Mrs Eulalia W 2403 Cortland Drive, Pittsburgh, PA 15241, (412) 835-7840, BA 41 OH St Univ; BS 41 OH St Univ; MA 42 OH St Univ; **SLP LM**

Fabian, Mrs Frances L 1134 Dodd Road, Mendota Heights, MN 55118, (612) 690-2497, BS 64 Coll of Saint Francis; MS 70 Marquette Univ; Facilitator, St Paul Pub Sch Dist #625, **SLP**

Fabian, Loretta Ann 1519 Gill Hall Road, Clairton, PA 15025, (304) 243-0300, BS 83 CA Univ of PA; MS 85 CA Univ of PA

Fabian, Shari L 51192 E Village 22-203, New Baltimore, MI 48047, (313) 949-3461, BA 83 Augustana Coll; MA 84 Western MI Univ; 88–Sp-Lang Path, Avondale Sch Dist, **SLP**

Fabian, Stephanie Lynne 4434 Silsby Road, University Heights, OH 44118, (216) 382-8374, BA 85 Cleveland St Univ; MA 88 Cleveland St Univ

Fabiano, Mrs Susan Rosa 112 Pinecrest Terrace, Wayne, NJ 07470, (201) 835-5085, BA 83 Montclair St Coll; MA 85 Montclair St Coll; 85–Sp-Lang Path, Cedar Grove Sch Sys, **SLP**

Fabiszak, Dr Angie Jo 4343 North Clarendon #1808, Chicago, IL 60613, (312) 975-1600, BA 71 Northern IL Univ - De Kalb; MA 73 Northern IL Univ - De Kalb; PH 87 (Sp Path (Swallowing)) Northwestern St Univ; Sp-Lang Path, Illinois Masonic Hosp, **SLP**

Fabiszak-Harrison, Mrs Michele K 720 Dalrymple Road, Sunderland, MD 20689, (301) 868-7987, BA 76 Loyola Coll; MS 77 Loyola Coll; 77–Sp/Lang Path, Prince George's Co Pub Sch, **SLP**

Fabricant, Phyllis L 520 East 81st Street, New York, NY 10028, (212) 628-4708, BA 69 CUNY - Queens Coll; MA 70 SUNY - Center at Buffalo; Sp-Lang Path, Private Practice, **SLP**

Fabry, David Alan Research Section, Army Audiology & Speech Center, Walter Reed Army Medical Center, Washington, DC 20307-5001, (202) 576-2413, BA 88; MA 84 Univ of MN - Minneap-St Paul; Aud, US Army, **A**

Facer, M Christina 1538 33rd Avenue, San Francisco, CA 94122, (415) 564-4194, BA 81 San Francisco St Univ; MS 83 San Francisco St Univ; Sp/Lang Path, San Fran USD, **SLP**

Fackler, Mrs Ann G 216 Leawood Drive, Lexington, KY 40502, (606) 278-2444, BS 74 Purdue Univ - West Lafayette; MA 77 WA St Univ; 88–Sp-Lang Path, Swigert & Assoc, **SLP**

Fadden-Herron, Cynthia A Sullivan Diagnostic Treatment Center, Benmosche Road, Harris, NY 12742, (914) 794-1400, BS 84 Marywood Coll; MA 86 Univ of Pittsburgh - Pittsburgh; 88–Aud, Sullivan Diag Treatment Ctr, **A**

Fader, Denise Robin 75-52 199th Street, Flushing, NY 11366, (714) 468-6796, BA 84 SUNY - Center at Buffalo; MA 86 Long Island U - CW Post Ctr; 86–Sp-Lang Path, HTA & Richmond Mem Hosp, **SLP**

Fadness, Mrs Aiko Ruth 445 Stratford Park Court, San Jose, CA 95136, BS 61 Univ of WI - Madison; MS 62 Univ of WI - Madison; 68–Sp-Lang Path, Union Sch Dist, **SLP**

Faems, Mrs Debra H 1302 West Grove Street, Arlington Heights, IL 60005, (312) 394-8021, BA 76 Coll of Saint Teresa; MA 79 Northern IL Univ - De Kalb; SLP, **SLP**

Faermark, Jory 12512 Chandler Boulevard, Apartment 304, North Hollywood, CA 91607, (818) 908-3535, BA 73 Univ of CA - Los Angeles; MS 76 Univ of WI - Madison; Sp/Lang Path, Kaiser Permanente Med Gp, **SLP**

Fagan, Ellen C ASHA, 10801 Rockville Pike, Rockville, MD 20852, (301) 897-5700, BA 76 Columbia Coll; MS 77 Univ of AL- Tuscaloosa; 88–Dir/Continuing Educ Branch, ASHA, **SLP**

Fagan, Leslie Lorraine 4527 Ocana, Lakewood, CA 90713, (213) 926-5566, BS 75 OR St Univ; MA 84 CA St Univ - Long Beach; **SLP**

Fagan, Marcy M 301 North Sappington, Glendale, MO 63122, (314) 822-8663, BS 74 Southern IL Univ -Carbondale; MA 76 Saint Louis Univ; **SLP**

Fagan, Mary K 12430 Schaler Drive, Poway, CA 92064, (619) 489-4856, BA 76 San Diego St Univ; MA 83 San Diego St Univ; 85–Sp-Lang Path, Palomar Med Ctr, **SLP**

Fagan, Mrs Pamela J Hq U S Areur, Box 1762, APO New York, NY 09063, BS 80 Univ of MA - Amherst; MA 82 Univ of MA - Amherst; Sp/Lang Path, Dept Defense Dependents School, **SLP**

Fagan, Paula Louise 19 Lawrence Avenue, Leominster, MA 01453, (617) 534-5604, BA 82 Boston Coll; MA 84 Central MI Univ; Aud, The Lrng Ctr for Deaf Chldn, **A**

Fagan, Roger 985 Forest Avenue, Portland, ME 04103, (207) 797-8738, BS 70 TX Tech Univ; MS 72 Southern IL Univ -Carbondale; Aud, Private Practice, **A**

Fager, Diane Colleen 6944 East 78th Street, Tulsa, OK 74133, (918) 492-9108, BS 83 Univ of Tulsa; MA 85 Univ of Tulsa; **SLP**

Fagg, Susan Gardner 1129 11th Street, Apt #105, West Des Moines, IA 50265, (715) 362-7676, BS 84 Univ of IA; MA 85 Northeast MO St Univ; SLP, Mercy Hospital, **SLP**

Fagin, Kathleen Marie 987 Meadowridge Drive, Kirkwood, MO 63122, (314) 965-6166, BS 84 Saint Louis Univ; MA 85 Saint Louis Univ; 88–Sp-Lang Path, Childhaven, **SLP**

Fagler, Mrs Patricia A 2043 West 153rd Place, Broomfield, CO 80020, (303) 452-3366, BA 69 Univ of Northern CO; MA 76 Univ of Denver; 88–Sp-Lang Path, Adams County Dist #12, **SLP**

Fagrelius, Maryann Bush 2001 Hidden Glen, Farmington, NM 87401, (505) 325-1741, BA 73 MI St Univ; MA 74 Univ of Denver; Consult/Sp-Lang Path, Farmington Pub Sch, **SLP**

Fagre-Springer, Ann L 1127 Tiffany Place #4, Waterloo, IA 50701, (319) 234-3412, BA 81 Augustana Coll; MA 87 Univ of Northern IA; **SLP**

Fagundus, Kay W P O Box 248, Winterville, NC 28590, **A**

Fahan, Linda MacKay 18 Wells Road, Granby, CT 06035, (203) 548-5443, BA 78 SUNY - Coll at Plattsburgh; MA 80 Univ of IL - Urbana; Sp-Lang Path, St Francis Hosp & Med Cntr, **SLP ACE**

Faherty, Amy Susan 1215 Seneca Street #206, Seattle, WA 98101, (206) 526-2104, BS 83 Univ of WA; MS 86 Univ of WA; 86–Sp-Lang Path, Children's Hosp & Med Ctr, **SLP**

Faherty, Darlene N 12 Boutwell Hill Road, Westford, MA 01886, (617) 475-2492, BS 76 Boston Univ; MS 78 Emerson Coll; Sp-Lang Path, Class Inc, **SLP**

Faherty, Monica A 8 Applecross Circle, Apex, NC 27502, (919) 755-6935, BA 74 Duquesne Univ; MS 77 Indiana Univ of PA; MS 84 Washington Univ; 84–Sp-Lang Path, Wake Co Pub Schs, **SLP**

Fahey, Mrs Sheryl Eanet 13376 Meadowsweet Drive, Fairfax, VA 22033, (703) 876-5213, BS 71 Syracuse Univ; MA 72 George Washington Univ; OM 76 Univ of VA - Charlottesville; Educational Diagnostician, Preschool Diag Cen Fairfax Co, **SLP**

Fahle, Jetti Irwin 5316 East 115th Place, Tulsa, OK 74136, (918) 371-6226, **SLP**

Fahlstrom, Merrill S Box 8, Beach, ND 58621, **SLP**

Fahnestock, Kristina Bergland 2021 Thure Avenue, St Paul, MN 55116, (612) 887-7321, BA 82 Univ of WI - Eau Claire; MS 85 Univ of WI - Stevens Point; Sp-Lang Path, Burnsville Pub Sch Dist #191, **SLP**

Fahrenbach, Mrs Patricia E 609 Nelson Road, Johnson City, NY 13790, (607) 770-0211, BS 74 Bloomsburg Univ of PA; ME 76 Bloomsburg Univ of PA; Sp-Lang Path, Broome Dev Serv, **SLP ACE**

Fahrenholz, Kathryn A 999 Mountain Road, West Suffield, CT 06093, (203) 668-4073, MA 76 IN Univ - Bloomington; Sp-Lang Path, Windsor Public School, **SLP**

Fahrlander, Daniel C, Jr 324 E Saint Anne #D, Hobbs, NM 88240, (505) 392-4044, MA 85 Univ of Northern CO; Aud, Hobbs Municipal Schools, **A**

Fahy, Davene S 6 Mechanic Street, Thomaston, ME 04861, (207) 594-8474, BA 59 Temple Univ-Tyler Sch of Art; MA 62 Temple Univ-Tyler Sch of Art; Coord, Mid Coast Children's Svc, **SLP**

Faigen, Janet 2600 West 182nd Street, Redondo Beach, CA 90278, (213) 673-4660, BA 80 Univ of Pittsburgh - Pittsburgh; MA 82 Univ of Pittsburgh - Pittsburgh; Supervsr Communication Disordr, Centinela Hospital Med Center, **SLP**

Faigen, Mrs Rogene M 2811 30th Avenue, Rock Island, IL 61201, (309) 793-5988, BA 55 Univ of IA; MA 78 Western IL Univ; 76–Sp-Lang Path, Rock Island/Milan Sch Dist, **SLP**

Failla, Carl 21216 Harbor Way Bldg 15, Unit 5, North Miami Beach, FL 33180, (305) 868-5000, BS 70 Friends Univ; MA 77 Western MI Univ; Coordinator Sp-Lng Pathology, Miami Rehabilitation Institute, **SLP**

Failla, Peggy P 290 Akiohala Street, Kailua, HI 96734, (808) 261-1758, BS 75 Univ of GA; MA 77 Univ of TN - Knoxville; Aud, Windward ENT/Dr E Dierdorff, **A**

Fain, Dorothy Marie 501 12th Street #1L, Brooklyn, NY 11215, (718) 782-6955, BA 81 Univ of CA - Berkeley; MS 87 San Francisco St Univ; 87–Sp-Lang Path, Blueberry Treatment Ctr, **SLP**

Fain, Mrs Vicki C Route 1 Box 315, Cambridge City, IN 47327, (317) 886-5229, BS 78 Ball St Univ; MA 79 Ball St Univ; Sp-Lang Path, New Castle Commun Sch Corp, **SLP**

Fainberg, Jolie Carin 1114 19th Avenue South, Nashville, TN 37212, (615) 320-5353, BA 81 Univ of CA - Santa Barbara; MA 84 Univ of TN - Knoxville; Aud, Bill Wilkerson Hrng & Sp, **A**

Faine, Susan D 65-61 Saunders Street, Rego Park, NY 11374, (212) 847-1970, **SLP**

Faingold, Mrs Sandra Pribble 1335 South Hudson, Denver, CO 80222, (303) 837-1000, BS 79 Northern AZ Univ; MA 83 Univ of Denver; 83–Sp-Lang Path, Denver Pub Sch, **SLP**

Fairbank, Mrs Carlene Marie 4238 East Saltsage Drive, Phoenix, AZ 85044, (602) 759-0923, BS 77 AZ St Univ; Sp/Lang Path, Scottsdale Sch Dist, **SLP**

Fairbanks, Kelly Ann 10100 Joy Lane, Vienna, VA 22180, (703) 938-1933, BS 83 WV Univ; MA 85 Univ of MD - College Park; Sp-Lang Path, Fairfax County PS, **SLP**

Fairbrother, Ellen J 20268 Beechaven, Southfield, MI 48076, (313) 494-2201, BA 65 Wayne St Univ; MA 71 Wayne St Univ; Sp-Lang Path, Detroit Publ Schs, **SLP ACE**

Fairchild, Janet M 2106 Bonnieview Drive, Royal Oak, MI 48073, (313) 288-1271, MA 79 Wayne St Univ; 79–Supv-Comm Disorders Sec, The Detroit Inst for Chldn, **SLP**

Fairchild, Janice M 604 West Oakdale Drive, Fort Wayne, IN 46807, (219) 425-3053, BS 70 Northwestern Univ; MA 71 Northwestern Univ; Super/SLP, **SLP**

Fairchild, Mrs Leslie P 11313 Bainbridge Avenue, Baton Rouge, LA 70817, (504) 293-0604, BS 84 LA St Univ - Baton Rouge; MA 87 LA St Univ - Baton Rouge; 87–Sp-Lang Path, Ascension Parish Sch Bd

Fairchild, Linda Ann R R 1 Box 276, Center Ossipee, NH 03814, (603) 539-4589, BS 70 Ball St Univ; MA 75 Western MI Univ; Sp-Lang Path, Gov Wentworth Reg Sch Dist, **SLP**

Fairchild, Michael Henry 811 East Burnside, Suite 215, Portland, OR 97214, (503) 238-1514, BS 73 Portland St Univ; MS 80 Portland St Univ; OD 87 (Law) Lewis & Clark Coll; Aud, Private Practice, **A**

Fairchild, Mrs Nancy J 620 North Point Drive, Schaumburg, IL 60193, BS 73 Univ of IL - Urbana; MS 74 Univ of IL - Urbana; **SLP**

Faircloth, Barbara H 4103 N W 13th Place, Gainesville, FL 32605, (904) 336-2709, BA 64 Univ of FL; ME 66 Univ of FL; 80–Sp-Lang Path, Alachua Co Schs, **SLP**

Faircloth, Mrs Betty Y 3555 Lancaster Lane, Montgomery, AL 36106, (205) 271-9409, BA 62 Univ of AL-Tuscaloosa; MA 64 Univ of AL- Tuscaloosa; MA 66 Univ of AL- Tuscaloosa; Regional Director Pip, Alabama I for Deaf & Blind, **SLP**

Faircloth, John William 1709-F Birch Trail Circle, Chesapeake, VA 23320, (804) 545-3541, BS 84 James Madison Univ; MS 84 James Madison Univ; SLP, Chesapeake Public Schools, **SLP**

Faires, Joan W 8126 Robinson Church Road, Charlotte, NC 28215, (704) 537-9228, BA 75 Appalachian St Univ; MA 77 Appalachian St Univ; Sp-Lang Path, Charlotte Mecklenburg Sch, **SLP**

Faires, Dr Wesley L 2933 Porter, Wichita, KS 67204, (316) 689-3241, BA 58 Wichita St Univ; MA 62 Wichita St Univ; PH 65 (NS) Wichita St Univ; Assoc Prof, Wichita St U, **SLP**

Fairfax, Mrs Lyn M 524 West Kaler Drive, Phoenix, AZ 85021, (602) 944-7615, BS 70 Univ of IA; MA 71 Univ of IA; **SLP**

Fairly, Mrs Pamela H 3044 Tidewater Circle, Madison, MS 39110, (601) 856-3204, BS 74 MS Univ for Women; MS 76 Univ Southern MS-Hattiesburg; 88–Sp-Lang Path, Dogwood Sch for Sp/Lang Impr Children, **SLP**

Fairly, Rebecca Ann 41 Alexandra Avenue, Hawthorne, NJ 07506, (201) 427-6712, MS 86 William Paterson Coll

Faith-Peterson, Mrs Carol Ann P O Box 246, Ione, OR 97843, (503) 989-8202, BA 78 Eastern WA Univ; MS 84 Eastern WA Univ; 78–Sp-Lang Path, Morrow Co Sch Dist, **SLP**

Fajoni, Angela Crim 5 Wildwood Circle, Hammond, LA 70401, (504) 345-6194, BA 76 Southeastern LA Univ; ME 80 Southeastern LA Univ; **SLP**

Fakhraie, Mrs Kay Davis 1120 Canyon Road #29, Ogden, UT 84404, (801) 399-3456, BS 73 UT St Univ; MS 75 UT St Univ; Sp-Lang Path, Ogden Cty Sch, **SLP**

Faklis, Mrs Holly Lee 2922 Lebannon Road #A, Donelson, TN 37214, (615) 871-0951, BA 77 CA St Univ - Stanislaus; MA 80 CA St Univ - Stanislaus; **SLP**

Fakoury, Mrs Noura S 230 Carmel Avenue, Piedmont, CA 94611, (415) 658-9697, BA 71 Holy Names Coll; MA 72 San Francisco St Univ; Special Education Teacher, San Lorenzo USD, **SLP**

Falabella, Mrs Linda Q 54 Baldwin Avenue, Point Lookout, NY 11569, BA 70 Hofstra Univ; MA 77 Hofstra Univ; Sp-Lang Path, East Meadow Pub Sch, **SLP**

Falany, Mrs JoEllen H Box 1865, Plant City, FL 34289-1865, (813) 752-9243, BS 69 FL St Univ; MA 70 FL St Univ; Sp-Lang Path, Private Practice, **SLP**

Falat, Mrs Barbara Sovey Orth 93th Street, Milwaukee, WI 53222, (414) 466-5252, BS 80 Marquette Univ; MS 83 Marquette Univ; SLP, Medic-Rehab Assoc, **SLP**

Falcone, Cynthia E 462 Broadway, Providence, RI 02909, (401) 828-6114, BA 79 Boston Coll; MS 82 Univ of RI; Sp-Lang Path, Coventry Sch Sys, **SLP**

Falcone, Mrs Judy Nicholas 209 Valleyvale Drive, Pittsburgh, PA 15209-1203, (702) 737-5207, BS 78 Indiana Univ of PA; MA 82 Univ of Pittsburgh - Pittsburgh; Aud, Audiology Group, **A**

Falcone, Sandra H 629 Cedar Grove Road, Broomall, PA 19008, (215) 763-7666, BA 75 West Chester Univ of PA; MA 81 West Chester Univ of PA; SLP, School Dist of Philadelphia, **SLP**

Falcone-Miller, Judith A 1456 Siver Road, Guilderland, NY 12084, (518) 356-4549, BA 76 Coll of Saint Rose; ME 77 Coll of Saint Rose; 87–Clin Coord, Coll of St Rose, **SLP**

Falconer, Dr George A 7016 Staffordshire, Houston, TX 77030, (713) 795-0546, BS 41 Washington Univ; MS 47 Washington Univ; ED 59 Univ of IL - Urbana; **A F LM**

Falconer, Mrs Kathryn O 1411 West 37th Street, Kearney, NE 68847, (308) 234-8300, BA 60 Middlebury Coll; MA 61 Univ of IA; PH 79 (Communication) Univ of TX - Austin; Assoc Prof, Kearney St Coll, **SLP**

Fales, Mrs Cathy Ann 100 Vincent Avenue, East Providence, RI 02914, (401) 245-7400, BA 81 Univ of RI; MS 84 Univ of RI; **SLP**

Falk, Arlene Sue 10 East 85th Street #2-B, New York, NY 10028, (212) 369-0969, BS 65 Syracuse Univ; MA 66 Columbia Univ Teachers Coll; Sp-Lang Path, Private Practice, **SLP**

Falk, Dr Joy W 626 Bird Bay Drive South, Apartment 209, Venice, FL 33595, BA 65 Hofstra Univ; MS Adelphi Univ; PH 76 (NS) Hofstra Univ; SLP, Uniondale Public Schools, **SLP**

Falk, Dr Mervyn L 34128 Northwick, Farmington Hills, MI 48018, (313) 577-3337, BA 55 WV Univ; MA 56 OH Univ - Athens; PH 64 (Sp-Lang Path) Wayne St Univ; 69–Assoc Prof, Wayne St Univ, **SLP**

Falk, Mrs Terese L R R 2 Box 10, Cuba, IL 61427, (309) 785-5545, BS 83 Western IL Univ; MA 85 Western IL Univ; 86–Sp-Lang Path, Kristy Englert Speech Assoc, **SLP**

Falkavage, Jean A 120 17th Avenue North, South St Paul, MN 55075, (612) 221-3845, BS 76 Univ of WI - Stevens Point; MS 77 Univ of WI - Stevens Point; Aud, St Paul Ramsey Med Cen, **A**

Falkenberg, Inge 1945 North Sheffield #201, Chicago, IL 60614, (312) 281-7870, BA 82 Allegheny Coll; MA 85 Northwestern Univ; SLP, Evanston Township High School, **SLP**

Falkowski, Marilyn K 141 Aubinwood Road, Amherst, MA 01002, (413) 538-5078, BA 71 CUNY - Queens Coll; MA 72 Univ of MA - Amherst; 87–Sp/Lang Path, South Hadley Schs, **SLP**

Falkowski, Sr Mary Felicia Mercy Speech/Lang Hearing Ctr, 243 Steele Road, West Hartford, CT 06117, (203) 236-3503, BS 61 Saint Joseph Coll; MS 68 Southern CT St Univ; Sp/Lang Path, Mercy Sp/Lang/Hrng Cen, **SLP**

Fallat, Claudia J 232 Gould Street, Rochester, NY 14610, (716) 271-7751, BS 79 SUNY - Coll at Geneseo; MS 85 Nazareth Coll of Rochester; 88–Sp-Lang Path, Roosevelt Ctr Preschool, **SLP**

Fallenstein, Judith F 509 West Broadway, Winona, MN 55987, (507) 452-2511, BS 64 Mankato St Univ; MS 71 Univ of WI - Eau Claire; SLP, Dist 861 Winona MN; **SLP**

Fallenstein, Sherry L 2 Ketch #305, Marina Del Rey, CA 90292, (213) 306-1629, BS 78 Southern Methodist Univ; MS 79 Southern Methodist Univ; Dir, Dr Irwin Lehrhoff & Ass Inc, **SLP**

Faller, Jean Marie 16 Tiffany Road #8, Salem, NH 03079, (603) 893-2900, BS 85 Clarion Univ of PA; MS 86 Clarion Univ of PA; SLP, NE Rehab Hosp, **SLP**

Fallico, Peter G 1210 Hermosa Way, San Jose, CA 95125, BA 70 San Jose St Univ; MA 75 San Jose St Univ; Sp-Lang Path, Santa Clara Co Supt of Sch, **SLP**

Fallon, Doris E 1643 Bridge Street, Philadelphia, PA 19124, (215) 533-3871, BA 76 Temple Univ; MA 78 Temple Univ; Aud, Moss Rehabilitation Hospital, **SLP A ACE**

Fallon, Gary E 3205 Powhatan Drive, Linden Hill Village, Wilmington, DE 19808, (302) 428-2286, BS 63 Bloomsburg Univ of PA; MA 67 Temple Univ; 79–Dir, Sp & Hrng Cen, Med Cen of DE, **SLP**

Fallon, John F P O Box 786, Beaufort, SC 29901, (803) 524-2660, BS 74 Saint John's Univ - Jamaica; MA 76 Univ of IL - Urbana; SLP, Beaufort County School Dist, **SLP ACE**

Fallon, Katie Helen 222 Josephine Street Rear, Peckville, PA 18452-2013, (717) 454-4521, BS 83 PA St Univ - Univ Park; MA 84 Univ of Pittsburgh - Pittsburgh; Sp-Lang Path, St Josephs Center, **SLP**

Fallon, Nancy M 119 Gilmore Drive, Pittsburgh, PA 15235, (412) 359-6655, BS 81 CA Univ of PA; MA 83 Bowling Green St Univ; Instr, Duquesne Univ, **SLP**

Falter, Brenda G 348 North Center Street, Statesville, NC 28677, (704) 872-0304, **SLP**

Faltz, Amy E 4279 Piedmont Avenue, Oakland, CA 94611, (415) 654-3381, BA 72 SUNY - Center at Buffalo; MS 74 Univ of MI - Ann Arbor; Sp/Lang Path, Private Practice, **SLP**

Falzarano, Mrs Alisa Lee 5601 North Dixie Highway Suite 101, Fort Lauderdale, FL 33334, (305) 491-4333, BA 82 Univ of FL; MS 85 Univ of TX - Dallas; Aud, Neuro-Otologic Ins Inc, **A**

Falzone-Mangone, Maryellen 147 Mamanasco Road, Ridgefield, CT 06877, (203) 576-7426, BA 81 Iona Coll; MA 82 Hofstra Univ; 82–Sp-Lang Path, Bridgeport Bd of Educ, **SLP**

Famiglietti, Lisa 10810 River Terrace, Austin, TX 78733, (512) 454-4731, BA 75 TX Tech Univ; MS 77 TX Tech Univ; Dir of Aud & Sp-Lang Path, Ctrl TX Aud & Sp Path, **SLP A ACE**

Familant, Mrs Rosalee P 24 Executive Drive, Newport News, VA 23606, (804) 596-3448, BS 65 LA St Univ - Baton Rouge; MA 66 LA St Univ - Baton Rouge; **SLP**

Fancher, Candis R 12908 Eagle Ridge Road, Burnsville, MN 55337, (612) 879-2818, MS 74 Saint Cloud St Univ; SLP, Ebenezer Caroline Cen, **SLP**

Fancher-Cook, Debra 3696 Hyacinth, Memphis, TN 38115, (901) 454-1333, BA 78 Univ of MS; MS 80 FL St Univ; Sp-Lang Path, Methodist Hosp Home Care/Hospc, **SLP**

Fandel, Susan King 2114 Cardinal Drive, Waukesha, WI 53186, (414) 547-1872, BS 69 Univ of WI - Madison; MS 70 Univ of WI - Milwaukee; Sp-Lang Path, Private Practice, **SLP**

Fanelli, Maria Elena 605 Orchard Street, Cranford, NJ 07016, (201) 977-2435, BA 72 Kean Coll of NJ; MA 77 Kean Coll of NJ; Sp-Lang Path, St Josephs Hosp & Med Cen, **SLP**

Fangman, Mrs Margaret White 3597 El Rego Drive, Amelia, OH 45102, (513) 734-4025, BS 79 Univ of Cincinnati; MA 82 Univ of Cincinnati; Sp-Lang Path, Clermont Co Bd of Ed, **SLP**

Fankhauser, Charles E Department Of Otolaryngology, Head & Neck Surgery, Naval Hospital, Oakland, CA 94627, (415) 633-5247, BA 58 OH St Univ; MS 68 Stanford Univ; PH 72 (NS) Univ of WA; Dir-Aud & SLP Serv, Naval Hosp - Oakland, **A**

Fannin, Mrs Annette L 114 East Main Street, Box 260, Addison, MI 49220, (517) 547-7494, BA 75 Univ of MI - Ann Arbor; MS 76 Univ of MI - Ann Arbor; Sp-Lang Path, Lifes Res Inc, **SLP**

Fannin, Virginia L 485 South Highland Avenue #1, Prestonsburg, KY 41653, (606) 886-6069, OM 83 Univ of KY; SLP, Manatte Co Bd of Ed, **SLP**

Fanning, Belinda J 518 B Forney Loop, Fort Belvoir, VA 22060-0811, (703) 781-8609, BS 83 Univ of Montevallo; MS 84 Univ of Montevallo; MS 85 Univ of Montevallo; 87–Sp-Lang Path, St Coletta Sch, **SLP A**

Fanning, Mrs Lucretia 62 Jacques Lane, South Windsor, CT 06074, (203) 289-1769, BA 75 Univ of CT; MA 76 George Washington Univ; Sp-Lang Path, Private Practice, **SLP**

Fanta, Mrs Katherine Ann 404 Emmer Street, Mayville, WI 53050, (414) 485-4423, BS 72 Univ of WI - Stevens Point; MS 82 Univ of WI - Milwaukee; 87–Sp-Lang Path, Horicon PS, **SLP**

Fantry, Timothy J 475 Woodberry Road, Rock Hill, SC 29730, **SLP**

Farabaugh, Kathleen Siobhan 1825 2nd Avenue North, Great Falls, MT 59401-3227, (303) 776-9920, BA 80 Univ of Northern CO; MA 81 Univ of Northern CO; Sp-Lang Path, Mont Deaconness Reg Rehab Cen, **SLP**

Faraguna, Mrs Debra L Smith 501 Echo Lane, Colorado Springs, CO 80904, (303) 392-3831, BA 77 Univ of MT; MA 79 Univ of Northern CO; Sp-Lang Path, Widefield School Dist 3, **SLP**

Faraher-Amidon, Christy A 1765 145th Street, White Rock, BC, Canada V4A 5T2, (604) 946-7601, BA 72 Northern IL Univ - De Kalb; MA 73 Northern IL Univ - De Kalb; Sp-Lang Path, Delta Sch Dist, **SLP**

Farat, Mrs Mary MacDonald 25 Florence Road #23, Branford, CT 06405, (203) 488-7192, MA 83 MI St Univ; Aud, Med Ctr Hrg/Balance Diag, **A**

Farb, Mrs Gwene S 351 La Grande Avenue, Fanwood, NJ 07023, (212) 448-9775, BA 71 CUNY - Queens Coll; MS 75 CUNY - Brooklyn Coll; Asst Director, State Isl Men Hlth Soc, **SLP**

Farber, Mrs Heidi F 19 Lamington Drive, Succasunna, NJ 07876, (201) 697-3606, BA 72 William Paterson Coll; MS 75 William Paterson Coll; Sp/Lang Path, W Milford Twsp Pub Sch, **SLP**

Farber, Mrs Judith S G 21 Glenn Circle, Erdenheim, PA 19118, (215) 351-7036, BA 60 Univ of MI - Ann Arbor; MA 75 Trenton St Coll; 85–Supervisor Sp-Lang Program, Sch Dist of Phila, **SLP**

Farber, Mrs Karen S 10 Muriel Drive, Stamford, CT 06907, (203) 322-4872, BS 78 SUNY - Center at Albany; MA 80 Northwestern Univ; Sp-Lang Path, Private Practice, **SLP ACE**

Farber, Laurie B 382 Thayer Street #2, Providence, RI 02906, (401) 751-3113, BS 78 Univ of NH; MS 80 Univ of WI - Madison; Aud, Beverly Hosp, **A**

Farber, Marilyn E 19 Allen Street, Arlington, MA 02174, (617) 666-1667, **SLP**

Farbstein, Mrs Resa 92 Howe Road, Coram, NY 11727, (516) 698-9897, BA 72 CUNY - Brooklyn Coll; MS 74 Columbia Univ Teachers Coll; 86–Aud/Sp-Lang Path, BOCES 2, **SLP A**

Farenkopf, Doris J 123 Oak Street, Rutland, VT 05701, (802) 773-1917, BS 65 Bloomsburg Univ of PA; BA 82 Trinity Coll; MS 67 Univ of WI - Madison; 88–Spec Educ Admin, Rutland PS, **SLP**

Farhat, Teri Rae 6706 Valley Spring Court, Birmingham, MI 48010, BA 69 Eastern MI Univ; MA 73 Eastern MI Univ; Sp-Lang Path, Pontiac Sch, **SLP**

Faridani, Mrs Samina Ramzan 424 Bellflower #111, Long Beach, CA 90814, (213) 597-6880, MA 83 Univ of KS; Sp-Lang Path, Los Angeles County Education, **SLP**

Farina, Mary Kay 17957 East Berry Drive, Aurora, CO 80015, (303) 861-6800, BS 63 CO St Univ; MS 64 Purdue Univ - West Lafayette; 76–Sp-Lang Path, Chldrns Hosp Denver Co, **SLP**

Fariselli, Mrs Lucille K RFD 6 Box 184, Overlook Drive, Mahopac, NY 10541, (914) 279-2905, BA 76 CUNY - City College; MA 78 CUNY - City College; Sp-Lang Path, Wassaic Dev Dis Svcs Office, **SLP**

Farish, Olivia W 219 North 34th Avenue, Hattiesburg, MS 39401, (601) 266-5223, BS 74 Univ Southern MS-Hattiesburg; MS 75 Univ Southern MS-Hattiesburg; Sp-Lang Path, U So Ms Sch Chldn Lang Dis, **SLP**

Fariss, Mrs Marcia K Marcia Fariss Associates, 2450 Samaritan Drive, San Jose, CA 95124, (408) 356-0404, BS 64 Univ of IL - Urbana; MA 65 Univ of IL - Urbana; Aud, Private Practice, **A**

Farkas, Audrey 6227 Vickijohn, Houston, TX 77096, (713) 479-1668, **SLP**

Farkas, Beth H 24 Sengstacker Drive, Stony Point, NY 10980, BS 78 Coll of Saint Rose; MS 80 Columbia Univ Teachers Coll; Sp-Lang Path, **SLP**

Farley, Mrs Debbie Reiff 5744 Broadway Terrace, Indianapolis, IN 46220, (317) 635-1491, **SLP**

Farley, Mrs Dollie O 122-A Wash Street #5, Leesburg, VA 22075, MS; **SLP LM**

Farley, Mrs Joyce J 11634 Monica Lane, Houston, TX 77024, (713) 467-9457, BA; MA; **SLP A LM**

Farley, Mrs Linda M St Joseph Medical Center, North Church & 9th Streets, Hazleton, PA 18201, (717) 459-4541, BS 78 Marywood Coll; MS 80 Ithaca Coll; Aud, St Joseph Medical Center, **A**

Farley, Mary J 225 Lansdowne Avenue, Wayne, PA 19087, **SLP**

Farley, Nancy Petrus 525 132nd Street S W R-101, Everett, WA 98204, (206) 348-5056, BS 83 SUNY - Coll at Geneseo; MS 87 Ithaca Coll

Farley, Shauna L Martin Luther Hospital Med Ctr, Speech Pathology Services, 1830 West Romneya Drive, Anaheim, CA 92801, (714) 491-5849, BA 68 Chapman Coll; Sp-Lang Path, Sp Path Serv, **SLP**

Farling, Glenn T 827 West Neely Avenue, Muncie, IN 47303, (317) 285-8164, BS 59 Ball St Univ; MA 63 Ball St Univ; Assoc Prof/SLP, Ball St U, **SLP**

Farling, Joyce M 4604 Quarter Charge Drive, Annandale, VA 22003-4620, (301) 567-4877, BA 76 SUNY - Center at Buffalo; MA 78 George Washington Univ; Sp-Lang Path, Prince Geo Co Pub Sch, **SLP**

Farman, Jill Pellerin 2840 Montair Avenue, Long Beach, CA 90815, (818) 963-1611, BA 78 Univ of LA Verne; MS 82 Univ of LA Verne; SLP, Norwalk Lamirada USD, **SLP**

Farmer, Dr Alvirda Speech And Hearing Clinic, San Jose State University, San Jose, CA 95192, (408) 724-1766, PH 72 (NS) Syracuse Univ; Assoc Prof, San Jose State University, **SLP**

Farmer, Mrs Judith L 2015 Gladys Drive, Las Cruces, NM 88001, (505) 646-2631, BS 64 Univ of NE - Lincoln; MS 65 CO St Univ; 76–Coll Asst Prof, New Mexico State U, **SLP**

Farmer, L Judson Communicative Disorders Lab, Univ Mississippi Med Ctr, 2500 North State Street, Jackson, MS 39216-4505, (601) 984-4550, MS 61 Univ of UT; BS 56 Westminster Coll; 72–Aud, Univ of MS Med Ctr, **SLP A**

Farmer, Marian Taylor Route 3 Box 298-B, Newport, NC 28570, BS 70 MS Univ for Women; MA 85 TX Woman's Univ; **SLP**

Farmer, Mrs Paula Ann 454 Meadowlark Lane, Eaton, OH 45320, (513) 456-3313, MS 81; 88–Sp-Lang Path, Darke County Bd of MR/DD, **SLP**

Farmer, Phyllis Allen 601 Northlake Drive, Anderson, SC 29621, (803) 292-5154, BS 83 Univ of GA; ME 85 Univ of GA; **SLP**

Farmer, Dr Stephen S 2015 Gladys Drive, Las Cruces, NM 88001, (505) 646-4339, BA 64 Univ of CO - Boulder; MA 66 Univ of CO - Boulder; PH 83 (NS) Univ of CO - Boulder; Assoc Prof SPED/CD, N Mex St U, **SLP**

Farmer, Mrs Wilma R P O Box 18, Olney, MD 20832, (301) 774-9019, BA 71 Augustana Coll; MS 74 Bradley Univ; Aud Dev Spec, Rock Creek Valley Elem, **SLP**

Farnes, Clyde W 650 Mohican Lane, Pleasant Grove, UT 84062, (801) 756-6022, BS 68 Brigham Young Univ; OM 74 Brigham Young Univ; Sp-Lang Path, Provo Sch Dist, **SLP**

Farnham, Mrs Susan L 883 59th Street S E, Kentwood, MI 49508, (616) 455-7385, BA 74 MI St Univ; MA 75 MI St Univ; **SLP**

Farnham, Todd A 514 Hughes Lane, Ida Grove, ID 51445, (712) 364-2702, BA 84 Univ of SD - Vermillion; MA 86 Univ of SD - Vermillion; Aud, Western Hills AEA 12, **A**

Farnsworth, Mrs Kim Marie 35 Ash Stoker Lane, Horsham, PA 19044, (215) 256-4211, BS 80 West Chester St Coll; MA 84 Univ of Northern CO; 88–Sp-Lang Path, Easter Seals Society, **SLP**

Farnsworth, Page J 2518 Fairfax, Nashville, TN 37212, (901) 794-6151, BA 76 Memphis St Univ; MA 78 Memphis St Univ; SLP, Metropolitan Nashville Schools, **SLP**

Farnum, H Arthur 195 State Street, Montpelier, VT 05602, (802) 888-3142, OB 70 Emerson Coll; MA 71 Case Western Reserve Univ; 85–Asst Supt for Spec Svcs, Lamoille North Supervisory Union, **SLP**

Farnum, Mrs Marcia Ide 73 Ferry Lane, Barrington, RI 02806, (401) 277-5485, MS 84 Worcester St Coll; SLP, Ri Hosp, **SLP**

Farnum, Sandra Duncan 2 Bailey Avenue, Montpelier, VT 05602, (802) 223-6119, **A**

Farny, Mrs Beth N S 4640 Indiana Avenue, Fort Wayne, IN 46807, (219) 744-4668, BS 74 Purdue Univ - West Lafayette; MA 75 Ball St Univ; **SLP**

Farquhar, Mary S 9727 Mt Pisgah Road #1603, Silver Spring, MD 20903, (301) 431-2581, BS 42 Univ of Lowell; ME 50 Boston Univ; ED 58 (NS) Boston Univ; Private Practice, **SLP F LM**

Farr, Lisa Kay 5304 Barouche, Plano, TX 75023, (214) 867-1503, MS 88 Univ of North TX

Farr, Lorraine E 3640 Cleveland Avenue, New Orleans, LA 70119, (504) 830-4424, BA 66 Marywood Coll; MS 69 Tulane Univ; Aud/Sp-Lang Path, Jefferson Parish Public Sch, **SLP A**

Farr, Mrs Rebecca Ray 4181 Westchester Crossing, Roswell, GA 30075, (404) 993-9898, BS 73 G Peabody Coll-Vanderbilt U; MS 76 Vanderbilt Univ; Sp-Lang Path, Marietta City Sch, **SLP**

Farran, Mary Zimmerman 7241 Wilderness Park Dr W, Apartment 302, Westland, MI 48185, (313) 421-9145, BA 84 MI St Univ; MA 85 MI St Univ; 88–Sp-Lang Path, Wayne-Weshand Comm Schs, **SLP**

Farrand, Mrs Diane M 804 M Street, Aurora, NE 68818, (402) 694-6540, BA 73 Kearney St Coll; MS 79 Kearney St Coll; Sp-Lang Path, Educational Services Unit 9, **SLP**

Farrand, Julie Ann 24 Myrtle Avenue, Waterbury, CT 06708, (203) 757-7228, BS 83 Western MI Univ; MA 86 Western MI Univ; 86–Sp-Lang Path, Watertown Bd of Educ, **SLP**

Farrand, Tad 123 West 1st Street, Mesa, AZ 85201, (602) 964-0477, MS 86 Southern IL Univ -Carbondale; **A**

Farrant, Prof R H 27 Princess Road #5, Claremont, West Australia, Australia 6010, (09) 383-3532, BA 42 Univ of Western Australia; MA 59 Northwestern Univ; PH 61 (Lang Disorders & Aud) Northwestern Univ; Prof of Psy Emeritus, Laurentian U, **A LM**

Farrar, Mrs Beverly J Clark 10220 Mapleridge Drive, Dallas, TX 75238, (214) 387-0041, BA 49 Southern Methodist Univ; ME 72 East TX St Univ - Commerce; MA 67 Southern Methodist Univ; 88–Psych Associate, Richardson ISD, **SLP**

Farrar, Dr Cathy Lucile 10008 Richwood Avenue N W, Seattle, WA 98177, (206) 223-6392, BA 66 Univ of WA; ME 71 Univ of VA - Charlottesville; PH 77 (NS) Univ of VA - Charlottesville; Computer Performance Analyst, Boeing Comp Serv

Farrar, Mrs Deborah Schaefer 2371 Le Havre Road, Lexington, KY 40504, (606) 254-2780, MA 77 Univ of KY; ED 81 (NS) GA Southern Coll; 85–Sp-Lang Path, Fayette Co Bd of Educ, **SLP**

Farrar, Karen H 332 1/2 Clinton Terrace, Easton, PA 18042, (215) 253-5374, BA 83 Cleveland St Univ; MA 85 Cleveland St Univ; Aud, Helen Beebe Sp & Hrng Cntr, **A**

Farrar, Mrs Lynne Brew 2912 Hartwood Drive, Fort Worth, TX 76109, (817) 927-2613, BS 76 TX Christian Univ; MS 77 TX Christian Univ; **SLP**

Farrar-Hersch, Julie A Woodrow Wilson Rehab Center, Fishersville, VA 22939, (703) 332-7086, BS 75 Univ of VA - Charlottesville; ME 76 Univ of VA - Charlottesville; Aud, Woodrow Wilson Rehab Cen of VA, **A**

Farrell, Carol A 11704 Melaleuca Way, Cooper City, FL 33026, (305) 435-4846, BA 72 East Carolina Univ; MS 77 Univ of South FL; 82–Sp-Lang Path, Broward County Schs, **SLP**

Farrell, Catherine c/o Sturgeon Bay Pub Schools, 1230 Michigan, Sturgeon Bay, WI 54235, (414) 743-6511, BA 69 Saint Norbert Coll; MS 76 Univ of WI - Madison; SLP, Sturgeon Bay Public Schools, **SLP**

Farrell, Cathleen P 256 Farrington Avenue, North Tarrytown, NY 10591, (718) 899-8800, BA 77 Univ of OR; MA 79 Univ of OR; 85–Sp-Lang Path, Lexington School for the Deaf, **SLP**

Farrell, Cynthia Fangman 4243 East Edgemont Avenue, Phoenix, AZ 85008, (602) 345-2011, OM 83 AZ St Univ; BS 80 KS St Univ; Sp-Lang Path, Arizona Speech Pathology Ltd, **SLP**

Farrell, Mrs Diana Jones 310 Northern Court, Island Lake, IL 60042, (312) 526-1809, BA 79 Univ of CA - Santa Barbara; MS 81 AZ St Univ; **SLP**

Farrell, Dr Dudley E R R 2 Box 27, Council Bluffs, IA 51503, (402) 346-8800, BA 67 Univ of Northern IA; MA 73 Northeast MO St Univ; PH 79 (Aud) Univ of CO - Boulder; 85–Aud, VA Medical Center, **A**

Farrell, Mrs Elizabeth 10428 Rene Drive, Clio, MI 48420, BS 57 Univ of MI - Ann Arbor; MS 60 Univ of MI - Ann Arbor; 86–SLP, Clio Area Schs, **SLP**

Farrell, Gina L 35 Eastview Avenue, 2nd Place, Yonkers, NY 10703, (914) 964-9188, BA 78 SUNY - Coll at Cortland; MA 80 CUNY - Lehman Coll; SLP, St Agnes Childrns Rehabil Ctr, **SLP**

Farrell, Jacqueline 127 Beth Drive, Lansdale, PA 19446, (215) 539-8550, BA 75 SUNY - Coll at Cortland; ME 79 Univ of VA - Charlottesville; SLP, Montgomery Co Inter Unit, **SLP**

Farrell, Jeanne Nicole 33 Willieb Street, Glastonbury, CT 06033, (203) 548-5600, BA 82 Boston Coll; ME 84 Univ of VA - Charlottesville; 87–Aud, St Francis Hosp & Med Ctr, **A**

Farrell, Kathleen Faye P O Box 1233, Sun City, AZ 85372, BS 77 Northern AZ Univ; MS 83 Northern AZ Univ; Sp-Lang Path, Washington Elementary Sch Dist, **SLP**

Farrell, Lesley A 2020 Terrakappa Avenue, Spring Valley, CA 92077, (619) 589-0172, BA 67 CA St Univ - Long Beach; MA 79 CA St Univ - Fresno; Sp-Lang Path, CA-Hi Elks Major Proj, **SLP**

Farrell, Marian E 158 Washington Street, Hanover, MA 02339, (617) 232-2782, BA 71 Catholic Univ of America; ME 73 Northeastern Univ; Commun Consult, Creative Tropism, **SLP**

Farrell, Mrs Martha Domitio 707 Tappan Street, Maumee, OH 43537, (419) 893-2278, OB 83 Univ of Toledo; MA 87 Eastern MI Univ; 83–Sp-Lang Path, Lucas Co Ofc of Educ

Farrell, Nancy I Rural Route 4, Fergus, ON, Canada N1M 2W5, (519) 941-6191, BS 67 Univ of WI - Milwaukee; MS 68 Univ of WI - Milwaukee; **SLP**

Farrell, Mrs Patricia 2504 Osage Drive, Glenview, IL 60025, (312) 564-0935, BA 72 John Carroll Univ; MA 75 Cleveland St Univ; **A**

Farrell, Mrs Susan Torke 2468 North 70th Street, Wauwatosa, WI 53213, (414) 453-0580, BS 60 Miami Univ - Oxford; MS 86 Univ of WI - Milwaukee; 87–Sp-Lang Path, Omni Ther, **SLP**

Farrelly, Mary Walsh 1034 South Euclid Avenue, Oak Park, IL 60304, (312) 524-3080, MS 83 Eastern IL Univ; BS 82 Eastern IL Univ; Sp-Lang Path, Oak Park Elem Sch Dist #97, **SLP**

Farrenkopf, Mrs Linda C 1351 Suncrest, Cincinnati, OH 45208, (513) 369-4790, BA 71 Miami Univ - Oxford; MS 75 Miami Univ - Oxford; Sp-Lang Path, Cincinnati Pub Sch, **SLP**

Farrer, Susan M Childrens Hospital Medical Ctr, Department Of Audiology, Elland & Bethesda Avenue, Cincinnati, OH 45229, (513) 559-4236, BS 75 Univ of Cincinnati; MA 77 Univ of Cincinnati; Dir/Aud, Childrens Hosp Med Cen, **A**

Farrere, Carol A R R 318 Oxbow Road, Hillsdale, NY 12529, (518) 325-3414, BS 78 Coll of Saint Rose; MS 79 Coll of Saint Rose; Sp-Lang Path, Sas BOCES, **SLP**

Farrier, Lynn Dee 5036 15th Avenue N E, Seattle, WA 98105, (206) 543-3134, MA 84 Univ of MT; Sp-Lang Path, Univ of Washington Hosp, **SLP**

Farrimond, Mrs Glenda H 1543 South Ardmore Avenue Apartment F, Villa Park, IL 60181, (312) 833-8833, MS 88 IL St Univ - Normal; 88–Sp-Lang Path, Sch Dist 45

Farrington, Mitzi G 2467 Finlandia Lane #17, Clearwater, FL 34623, (813) 797-2075, BA 34 NY Univ; MA 67 Columbia Univ Teachers Coll; **SLP LM**

Farris, Mrs Kathleen M Rd 4 Station Avenue, Bethlehem, PA 18015, (215) 348-2940, BS 78 West Chester Univ of PA; MA 80 Trenton St Coll; SLP, Bucks Co Inter Un #22, **SLP**

Farris, Kathryn B 30 Wellington Drive, Sugar Land, TX 77478, (713) 491-9404, BS 71 TX Tech Univ; MA 72 Our Lady Lake Univ-San Anton; **SLP**

Farris, Mrs Ruth B 7425 Church Street #90, Yucca Valley, CA 92284, (619) 365-1153, BA 28 Kearney St Coll; MA 42 Southern CA Coll; **LM**

Farrow, Mrs Cheryl Coleman 5030 South Highway 53, Crestwood, KY 40014, (502) 222-1470, BS 81 Baylor Univ; MS 83 Univ of NM; Sp-Lang Path, Private Practice, **SLP**

Farrow, Mrs Judy Little 3105 Carovel Court, Raleigh, NC 27612, (919) 781-8560, BA 73 Meredith Coll; ME 84 Valdosta St Coll; **SLP**

Farr-Petterson, Abigail L 908 East River Terrace, Minneapolis, MN 55414, (612) 642-4030, BA 69 Univ of WI - River Falls; MS 70 Univ of WI - River Falls; Sp-Lang Path, St Paul Pub Sch, **SLP**

Farry, Mrs Corliss C 4 Taylor Road, Matawan, NJ 07747, (201) 583-6773, BA 76 Westminster Coll; MS 78 Adelphi Univ; **SLP**

Farwell, Mrs Dorothy W 500 Aries Drive #4B, Mandeville, LA 70448, (504) 863-5353, BS 58 LA St Univ - Baton Rouge; ME 73 LA St Univ - Baton Rouge; 86–Sp-Lang Path, St Tammany parish Sch Bd, **SLP**

Farzad, Mrs Shapar 38 Bouvant Drive, Princeton, NJ 08540, **SLP**

Farzi, Fred Edward PO Box 264, Louisville, KY 40201, (502) 588-5274, BS 71 Univ of Juudishapoor - Iran; MS 78 OK St Univ

Fash, Mrs Deborah S 27382 Pinuela, Mission Viejo, CA 92691, (714) 364-2633, BA 76 WA St Univ; MA 77 WA St Univ; **SLP**

Faska-Kahana, Eva S 11 Barrie Drive, New Hempstead, NY 10977, (914) 362-1173, BA 83 CUNY - Queens Coll; MA 85 CUNY - Queens Coll; **SLP A**

Faskowitz, Michele B 220 West 71st Street, Suite 42, New York, NY 10023, (212) 496-9510, BA 76 CUNY - Queens Coll; MA 77 Hofstra Univ; SLP, Baskets Ext, **SLP**

Fass, Karen E F 331 Harrison Street, Haworth, NJ 07641, (201) 767-7224, BS 73 Emerson Coll; ME 74 Northeastern Univ; Sp-Lang Path, Nn Valley Reg Hs Sch Dist, **SLP ACE**

Fass, Patricia A 6400 Memorial Drive, Texas City, TX 77591, (409) 938-8466, BS 75 LA St Univ - Baton Rouge; MS 77 Univ of OK Medical Center; Sp/Lang Path, Private Practice, **SLP**

Fast, Carol Martha 722 Linda Vista, Ann Arbor, MI 48103, (519) 966-2211, BA 80 Univ of ND; MS 83 Univ of WA; 88–Sp-Lang Path, The Child's Place

Fast, Mrs Patricia L Delmar Route Box 28, Harrison, AR 72601, MA 71 Northeast MO St Univ; Sp-Lang Path, Harrison Public Schoools, **SLP**

Fastenau, Julianna 4027-O Quail Glen Court, Charlotte, NC 28226, (704) 552-8044, MS 83 Vanderbilt Univ; BS 81 Vanderbilt Univ; Sp-Lang Path, Charlotte Mecklenburg Sch, **SLP**

Fasting, Judith Charlotte Box 2475, Poulsbo, WA 98370, BA 69 Univ of South FL; MA 73 Univ of FL; Sp-Lang Path, Private Practice, **SLP ACE**

Fasulo, Elaine B 2835 SE Skyview Court, Topeka, KS 66605, (913) 232-0551, BA 81 Wichita St Univ; MA 82 Wichita St Univ; 82–Sp/Lang Path, USD #501 Topeka Pub Sch, **SLP**

Fauber, Mrs Lura June Rt 4 Box 103, Lewisburg, WV 24901, (304) 647-4554, BA 71 Marshall Univ; MA 84 Marshall Univ; SLP, Greenbrier County Bd Educ, **SLP**

Faucett, Mrs Ramona Aldridge 2215 Ledgewood Lane, Birmingham, AL 35214, (205) 933-8101, BA 72 Univ of AL- Tuscaloosa; MA 73 Univ of AL- Tuscaloosa; Superv/SLP, VA Med Cen, **SLP**

Faucetta, Mrs Patricia Mary 56 Lennox Avenue, Pompton Lakes, NJ 07442, (201) 839-8334, BA 77 Dominican Coll of Blauvelt; MA 81 Montclair St Coll; **SLP**

Faucette, Mrs Janet E 1938 Woodland Avenue, Burlington, NC 27215, (919) 578-2622, BA 78 Univ of NC - Greensboro; ME 79 Univ of NC - Greensboro; Sp-Lang Path, Alamance Co Sch, **SLP**

Faughnan, Mrs Theresa Joanne 35 Broadway #1B, Pleasantville, NY 10570-1728, (914) 337-1441, **A**

Faught, Carole A 15275 Cascade Drive, Elm Grove, WI 53122, (414) 782-5515, BA 66 MI St Univ; MA 70 MI St Univ; 87–Sp/Lang Path, New Berlin PS, **SLP**

Faugno, Joanne M 5 Anderson Road, Norwalk, CT 06851, (203) 869-4670, BA 78 Southern CT St Univ; MS 81 Southern CT St Univ; 81–Sp/Lang Path, Greenwich Bd of Educ, **SLP**

Faulk, Emily Anne 505 Shenandoah Drive, De Soto, TX 75115, (214) 230-3801, MS 88 Univ of TX - Dallas; 88–Sp-Lang Path, Dallas ISD

Faulk, Jennifer Perkins P O Box 10446, Bakersfield, CA 93389, (805) 398-3799, BS 78 Elmira Coll; MA 79 Bowling Green St Univ; 80–Sp-Lang Path, Kern Co Supt of Sch, **SLP**

Faulk, Mark Steven 4433 North Stanton Apartment 416, El Paso, TX 79902, (915) 533-8788, BS 84 Univ of WA; MS 87 Univ of NM; Aud, Dr Marino Rios MD

Faulkenburg, Kim Rene Audiology Program (126A), Olin E Teague Veterans' Center, Temple, TX 76504, (817) 778-4811, BA 79 IN Univ - Bloomington; MA 86 Univ of TX - Austin; 85–Aud, Olin E Teague Veterans Ctr, **A**

Faulkner, Angela Hammond 167 Lofton Drive, Fayetteville, NC 28311-1410, (919) 323-6093, SLP, Southeastern Rehab Center, **SLP**

Faulkner, Christina Bender Speak Listen And Learn, 7900 Allisonville Road, Indianapolis, IN 46250, (317) 849-2474, BS 74 Purdue Univ - West Lafayette; MA 76 Northwestern Univ; Director, Speak Listen and Learn, **SLP**

Faulkner, Douglas H 4305 Zelar, Tampa, FL 33629, (813) 796-1486, MS 81 Univ of South FL; Dir Prof Serv, Bay Area Hrng Serv, **A**

Faulkner, Mrs Evelyn R 241 Judd Street, Fairfield, CT 06430, (203) 333-0719, OB 72; BA 71 Univ of Montreal - Quebec; MA 74 NY Univ; 79–Sp-Lang Path, Bridgeport Board of Education, **SLP**

Faulkner, Karen Young 15990 Harrison, Livonia, MI 48154, (313) 479-2600, MA 81 Eastern MI Univ; **SLP**

Faulkner, Mrs Marcia J 16 Deborah Drive, South Burlington, VT 05403, (802) 893-1056, BA 63 Univ of RI; MS 83 Univ of VT; Sp-Lang Path, Milton Jr Sr Hs, **SLP**

Faull, Mrs Rosann Wood 1325 South Apollo Blvd, Melbourne, FL 32901, (407) 676-5623, BS 76 Northern IL Univ - De Kalb; MA 77 Northern IL Univ - De Kalb; Pres, Audiology & Hearing Aid Svc Inc, **A**

Faurot, Judith W 4105 Linkwood, Euless, TX 76040, (817) 565-2262, BA 59 Univ of OK - Norman; MA 70 Univ of North TX; Tchr, Univ of North Texas, **SLP ACE**

Faurot, Judy Carol 1010 Cedar Drive, Scott City, KS 67871, (316) 275-0291, MA 86 KS St Univ; 86–Sp-Lang Path, Russell Child Dev Ctr, **SLP**

Fauser, Mrs Janice L S 49 Boothby Drive, Mount Laurel, NJ 08054, (609) 267-8565, BS 73 Trenton St Coll; MA 76 Trenton St Coll; Sp-Lang Path, Sch Dist of Philadelphia, **SLP**

Fausett, Mrs Linda R 4416 South La Corta, Tempe, AZ 85282, (602) 839-3506, BA 72 Loma Linda Univ - Riverside; MS 80 AZ St Univ; Sp-Lang Path, Tempe Elementary Sch Dist #3, **SLP**

Fausone, Beth Anne 2100 Shangri-La, Grand Rapids, MI 49506, (616) 242-0483, **SLP**

Faust, Geralyn Marie 6426 S Mission #14, Mount Pleasant, MI 48858, (517) 772-5576, OB 81 Univ of MI - Ann Arbor; MS 83 Univ of MI - Ann Arbor; **SLP**

Faust, Joan C 200 Locust Street #11-C, Philadelphia, PA 19106, (215) 238-1139, BS 83 PA St Univ - Univ Park; MA 85 Temple Univ-Tyler Sch of Art; **SLP**

Faust, Kathleen Louise 31 Chester Street #3, Mount Vernon, NY 10552, (914) 948-0050, BS 85 West Chester Univ of PA; MS 87 Boston Univ; **SLP**

Faust, Marlene A 8 Horseshoe Lane, Hamilton, MA 01982, (508) 468-5059, BA 79 Univ of MA - Boston; MS 81 Emerson Coll; Sp-Lang Path, Wakefield PS, **SLP**

Faust, Mrs Ruth S 80 South Maple Avenue, Basking Ridge, NJ 07920, BA 31 Rutger's St Univ - Douglas Coll; **SLP LM**

Faux, Cassandra 4126 East 2nd Street, Tucson, AZ 85711, (602) 325-1517, BS 77 Univ of AZ; MS 79 Univ of AZ; Sp-Lang Path, Cp Found/Rehab Assoc Pc, **SLP**

Favaro, Frank J 17 Kansas Road, Lehigh Acres, FL 33936, (813) 936-4656, BS 78 IL St Univ - Normal; MA 79 Central MI Univ; 81–Aud, Hrng Aid Cen of Ft Myers, **A**

Favata, Philip J 359 South Main Street, Jamestown, NY 14701, (716) 664-5401, BS 58 SUNY - Coll at Fredonia; MS 65 SUNY - Coll at Buffalo; Sp-Lang Path, BOCES-NY, **SLP**

Favero, Joe C 17898 S W Pilkington Road, Lake Oswego, OR 97034, (503) 636-7691, BS 59 Eastern Montana Coll; ME 65 OR St Univ; Sp-Lang Path, Lake Oswego Public Dist #7J, **SLP**

Favetta, Fred Joseph 1411 Brookdale Lane, Kent, OH 44240, (216) 678-4646, BA 77; MA 82 Univ of Akron; Aud, Audiological Testing Serv, **A**

Favinger, Mrs Karen Britt 3810 Crestvale Terrace, Baltimore, MD 21236, (301) 665-6505, BS 85 Towson St Univ; MS 87 Towson St Univ; **SLP**

Favors, Dr Aaron 707 Oneida Place N W, Washington, DC 20011, (301) 443-2370, BA 55 Clark Coll; MA 57 Univ of IA; PH 69 (NS) Univ of IA; Aud/Sp-Lang Path, Div of Maternal & Chld Hlth, **SLP A F**

Favors, Vanessa Wilson 707 Oneida Place N W, Washington, DC 20011, (202) 651-5250, BA 76 Temple Univ-Tyler Sch of Art; MS 78 Univ of the DC; SLP, Kendall Demonstration Elem Sch, **SLP A**

Favro, Mary Alice 288 Newton Street, South Hadley, MA 01075, (413) 739-3954, BS 81 Elmira Coll; MA 83 Univ of MA - Amherst; Sp/Lang Path, Valley Infant Dev Serv, **SLP**

Favruzzo, Barbara Shoffner 713 Finsbury Road, Winston-Salem, NC 27104, (919) 760-0997, ME 83 Univ of NC - Greensboro; Sp-Lang Path, Private Practice, **SLP**

Fawkes, Mrs Suzanne A 103 East 4th Street, Cameron, MO 64429, (816) 632-7212, BS 62 Univ of MO - Columbia; MA 63 Univ of MO - Columbia; 72–Sp-Lang Path, Cameron R1 Schs, **SLP**

Fawx, Linda L 1011 F Street, Apt B, Sacramento, CA 95814, (916) 733-3040, BA 76 Univ of CA - Davis; BA 80 CA St Univ - Sacramento; Sp-Lang Path, Sacramento ENT Surg&Med Group, **SLP**

Fax, Mrs Joanne Cantlon 2211 Matterhorn Lane, St Paul, MN 55119, (612) 457-7260, BA 76 Creighton Univ; MS 78 Univ of NE - Omaha; Sp-Lang Path, Inver Grove Heights Schs, **SLP**

Fay, Catherine 348 4th Street, Brooklyn, NY 11215, (212) 768-2188, BA 72 Saint Joseph's Coll; MA 74 NY Univ; **SLP**

Fay, Mrs Kathleen A 143 Foshay Avenue, Pleasantville, NY 10570, (212) 920-9722, **SLP**

Fay, Dr Thomas H Dir Speech Hearing Department, The Presbyterian Hospital, 622 West 168th Street, New York, NY 10032, (212) 305-2961, BA 49 Univ of FL; MA 50 Columbia Univ Teachers Coll; PH 58 (Sp & Hrng Disorders) Univ of IL - Urbana; 71–Dir Sp-Lang Path & Aud, Columbia-Presby Med Cen, **SLP A F ACE**

Fayache, Zina P 22 Rolling Hill Road, Manhasset, NY 11030, (516) 365-7130, BS 63 Syracuse Univ; MA 67 OH Univ - Athens; MS 75 George Washington Univ; Sp-Lang Path, Pt Washington Sp Lang Hrng Cen, **SLP**

Fayad, Donna M 1426 Cambridge Street, Cambridge, MA 02139, (617) 354-2635, BA 75 Bridgewater St Coll; MS 77 Rutgers St Univ - Newark; Dir, Private Practice, **SLP**

Fay-Coelho, Elaine 306 Cedar Lane, Cheshire, CT 06410, (203) 271-0264, BS 74 SUNY - Center at Albany; MS 76 Univ of AZ; Sp-Lang Path, Private Practice, **SLP**

Faye, Mrs Ruth A 2 Condor Road, Sharon, MA 02067, (617) 784-4657, BS 76 Emerson Coll; MS 78 Boston Univ; Owner, Communication & Rehabil Assn, **SLP**

Fazely, Mrs Mondra R 2383-C 46th Street, Los Alamos, NM 87544, (505) 662-2935, BA 78 OH St Univ; MA 79 Kent St Univ; 86–Sp-Lang Path, Private Practice, **SLP**

Fazzio, Mrs Elizabeth Merkel 595 Swain Avenue, Elmhurst, IL 60126, (312) 681-3200, BS 84 Marquette Univ; MA 85 Western MI Univ; 87–Sp-Lang Path, Gottlieb Memorial Hosp, **SLP**

Feakes, Darrel Ray 2803 Richard Drive, Eau Claire, WI 54701, (715) 839-3284, BS 69 Univ of WI - Stevens Point; MS 70 Univ of WI - Stevens Point; Aud, Midelfort Clinic, **A**

Fearman, Eleanor G 125 Via El Chico, Redondo Beach, CA 90277, (213) 540-0629, BA 71 Univ of CA - Los Angeles; MS 73 CA St Univ - Long Beach; Career Ed Tchr, Offi of LA Co Supt Sch, **SLP**

Fearon, Mrs Donna Maria 640 Lanvale Drive, Webster Groves, MO 63119, (314) 961-7938, BS 81 Fontbonne Coll; MS 83 Fontbonne Coll; Sp-Lang Path, St Louis Assn for Ret Citizens, **SLP**

Fears, Anita G P O Box 76, Nassawadox, VA 23413, (804) 442-7119, BS 74 James Madison Univ; ME 76 Univ of VA - Charlottesville; Consultant, Private Practice, **SLP**

Feather-Grozanick, Pamela 304 Coleridge Avenue #1, Altoona, PA 16602, (814) 946-8392, BS 78 Indiana Univ of PA; MS 81 Indiana Univ of PA; Sp-Lang Path, Altoona Area Sch Dist, **SLP**

Featheringill, David Michael 5748 Birch 0 1 St, Gladstone, MI 49837, (906) 786-9301, MA 67 Central MI Univ; MA 76 Northern MI Univ; ES 77 Northern MI Univ; Sp-Lang Path, Delta-Schoolcraft ISD, **SLP**

Feathers, Anne H 2767 Flagstaff Court, Jonesboro, GA 30236, (404) 477-6400, BS 59 Auburn Univ - Auburn; MS 61 Purdue Univ - West Lafayette; **SLP**

Featherston, Mrs Virgianne 139 North Yates, Minden, NE 68959, (308) 832-2460, BS 72 Fort Hays St Univ; MA 76 Univ of NE - Lincoln; 78–Sp/Lang Path, Minden Pub Schls, **SLP**

Feaver, Ann Tisdel 130 Dennison Avenue, Framingham, MA 01701, (617) 376-8773, BA 62 Univ of CA - Santa Barbara; ME 81 Framingham St Coll; Sp-Lang Path, Millis Pub Sch, **SLP**

Febbraro, Catherine A 107 Rosewood Drive, Glenshaw, PA 15116, (412) 487-8082, BA 83 Univ of Pittsburgh - Pittsburgh; MA 85 Univ of Pittsburgh - Pittsburgh; Sp-Lang Path, South Hills Health System, **SLP**

Febo-Rodriguez, Tomas Calle 18 Bldg U-10, Urb Berwind Estates, Rio Piedras, PR 00924, (809) 762-9177, BA 72 Univ of PR - Rio Piedras; MS 76 Univ of PR - Rio Piedras; Sp-Lang Path, Private Practice, **SLP**

Fecek, Ronald J 934 Brown Street, Belle Vernon, PA 15012, (412) 938-3241, BS 73 CA Univ of PA; MA 87 Univ of Pittsburgh - Pittsburgh; **A**

Fechner, Holly Anne 510 West Main, Enterprise, OR 97828, (503) 426-4997, BA 83 Univ of Northern CO; MS 85 CO St Univ; 88–Sp-Lang Path, Wallowa Co Educ Service Dist, **SLP**

Feder, Mrs Karen S 76 Rock Spring Road #A2, Stamford, CT 06906, (203) 327-3874, BA 78 Adelphi Univ; MS 79 Adelphi Univ; Sp/Lang Path, Greenwich Assoc-Retired Ctzn, **SLP**

Feder, Mrs Lee V 12 North Cambridge Avenue, Ventnor, NJ 08406, (609) 823-6097, BA 75 Temple Univ; MA 77 Temple Univ; **A**

Federhar, Lisa Joy 2400 N Lake View Avenue, Apartment 907, Chicago, IL 60614, (312) 427-5464, BS 83 Univ of AZ; MA 85 Northwestern Univ; Prog Coord, Pro Voice Prog-Schwab Rehab Ctr, **SLP**

Federico, Rita Phyllis 37 Pemberton Street, Revere, MA 02151, BA 81 Boston Coll; MA 82 Central MI Univ; SLP, Reads Lang Dev, **SLP**

Federspiel, Marsha J 3216 Sudbury Place, Fort Wayne, IN 46815, (219) 425-7463, BA 75 IN Univ - Bloomington; OM 76 IN Univ - Bloomington; Sp-Lang Path, Ft Wayne Commun Schs, **SLP**

Fedetz, Mrs Sherri Lee 1657 Woodlea Road, Orefield, PA 18069, (717) 386-5900, BS 83 Kent St Univ; MA 84 Kent St Univ; Aud, Private Practice, **A**

Fedge, Marilyn J 67-38 108th Street, Forest Hills, NY 11375, **A**

Fedor, Karen Hardin 2227 Radcliffe Avenue, Charlotte, NC 28207, (704) 377-0486, BA 76 Duke Univ; MS 79 Univ of NC - Chapel Hill; **SLP**

Fedo-Rosvold, Susan M P O Box 415, Marathon, WI 54448, (715) 848-4311, OB 80 Univ of MN - Duluth; MA 81 Univ of MN - Duluth; 88–Sp-Lang Path, N Central Healthcare Fac, **SLP**

Fedrick, Pary K P O Box 2309, Indio, CA 92202-2309, BA 68 Southern IL Univ-Edwardsvill; MA 78 Northeast MO St Univ; SLP, Riverside Co Schools, **SLP**

Fedyniak, Lillian H 5821 North-Cicero, Chicago, IL 60646, (312) 641-4134, **SLP**

Fee, Anne Elizabeth 23-54 27th Street, Astoria, NY 11105, (516) 472-9233, BS 84 King's Coll; MS 85 Baylor Univ; **SLP**

Fee, Barbara P 5511 Landmark Place, Fairfax, VA 22032, **SLP**

Fee, Mrs Christine Diane 6131 Sunfield Avenue, Lakewood, CA 90712, BA 79 CA St Univ - Long Beach; MS 82 Chapman Coll; **SLP**

Feehan, Deborah Anne 69 Westminster Road, Rochester, NY 14607, (716) 271-0680, BS 84 SUNY - Coll at Geneseo; MA 85 SUNY - Coll at Geneseo; **A**

Feehan, Mrs Pamela J 2908 Fifth Street, Rapid City, SD 57701, (605) 348-7706, BS 76 Univ of WY; MA 77 Univ of SD - Vermillion; Aud, Private Practice, **A**

Feehily, Lynne Marie 28-L Brandywine Drive, Shrewsbury, MA 01545, (617) 791-3147, BS 84 Worcester St Coll; ME 86 Univ of VA - Charlottesville; **SLP**

Feeley, John J, Jr 1009 Sigsbee Place N E, Washington, DC 20017, **SLP**

Feely, Rosemary 304 W South College Street, Yellow Springs, OH 45387, (513) 767-9282, BA 71 Leeds Polytechnic - England; MA 82 Univ of Cincinnati; Sp-Lang Path, St Elizabeths Med Ctr, **SLP**

Feemster, Ben David c/o Communication Disorders, PO Box 451, Abilene, TX 79604, (915) 692-4053, BS 78 Southern Methodist Univ; MA 81 Univ of Denver; Dir Comm Dis, Abilene St Sch, **SLP**

Feeney, M Patrick 4107 24th Place S, Seattle, WA 98108, (206) 725-0743, BA 71 Kent St Univ; MA 79 WA St Univ; Aud, **A ACE**

Feeney, Tawn R 199 Peakview Drive, Henrietta, NY 14467, (716) 271-0680, BA 68 Oberlin Coll; MA 72 Univ of MN - Minneap-St Paul; Prog Mgr Daycare Ser, Hrng & Sp Cen of Rochester Inc, **SLP**

Feeney-Grater, Pearl 5 Pine Glen Drive, North Reading, MA 01864, **SLP**

Feenstra, Mrs Catherine B RD 5 Box 5913, Newton, NJ 07860, (201) 383-6460, BS 69 Carlow Coll; MS 76 Paterson St Coll; Sp-Lang Path, Hampton Twp Bd of Educ, **SLP**

Fee-Olsen, Barbara Jean 266 Lena Avenue, Freeport, NY 11520, (516) 867-3645, BA 77 Southern CT St Univ; MA 79 Univ of MA - Amherst; Aud, Suffolk Hrng & Sp Ctr, **A**

Fees, Mrs Margaret Ruffennach 3203 Foothill Street, Woodbridge, VA 22192-1404, (803) 585-0322, MS 84 Indiana Univ of PA; SLP, Sch Dist 7, **SLP**

Fegebank, Mrs Julie A 1029 Bradford Drive, Winter Park, FL 32792, (305) 677-8578, BS 75 Univ of IA; MA 76 Univ of IA; Aud, Semoran Hearing Clinic, **A**

Fehling, Roberta Hill 2306 Birnam Woods Terrace, Midlothian, VA 23112, (804) 744-1101, BS 69 Purdue Univ - West Lafayette; MS 70 Purdue Univ - West Lafayette; 88–Sp-Lang Path, Amelia Co PS, **SLP ACE**

Fehr, Eric M 1007 Woodland Avenue, Winchester, VA 22601, (703) 791-5238, BS 74 VA Commonwealth Univ; ME 79 Univ of VA - Charlottesville; Sp-Lang Path, **SLP**

Fehr, Dr Joann D 4545 North Delco, Wauwatosa, WI 53225, (414) 644-5226, BS 58 Univ of WI - Milwaukee; MS 65 Univ of WI - Milwaukee; PH 71 (NS) Marquette Univ; Dir of Spec Ed, Sch Dist of Slinger, **SLP A**

Fehrs, Kelly Lee P O Box 165991, Irving, TX 75016, (214) 654-5835, **SLP**

Fehst, Dr Christine 12 Loring Road, Hopkins, MN 55343, (612) 373-9837, BS 73 OH St Univ; MA 76 Univ of MN - Minneap-St Paul; PH 79 (NS) Univ of MN - Minneap-St Paul; 88–Dir-Home Start, Self Employed, **SLP**

Feibusch, Arlene W 23 Lawrence Avenue, Lawrence, NY 11559, **SLP**

Feichter, Jill Robbins 6709 Windham Court, Fort Wayne, IN 46835, (703) 522-2777, BA 77 IN Univ - Bloomington; OM 79 IN Univ - Bloomington; Sp/Lang Path, Er Sl So, **SLP**

Feidner, Mrs Mary P P O Box 207, Hinesburg, VT 05461, (802) 658-9060, BS 54 Univ of Dayton; MS 71 Univ of VT; Sp-Lang Path, S Burlington Sch Dist, **SLP**

Feidt, Arlene S 419 Sherry Way, Cherry Hill, NJ 08034, **SLP**

Feigh, Mrs Lori 24 West 668 Parkmeadow, Naperville, IL 60540, (312) 355-5371, BA 79 Coll of Saint Francis; MS 81 IL St Univ - Normal; 86–Sp-Lang Path, Naperville Sch Dist 203, **SLP**

Feigin, Judith G 555 North 30th Street, Omaha, NE 68131, (402) 498-6530, BA 72 Univ of WI - Madison; MS 75 Univ of WI - Madison; Aud, Boys Town Institute, **A**

Fein, Cathy Rochelle 175 Meadowlawn Road, Stratford, CT 06497, (201) 744-7263, **SLP**

Fein, Deborah L 2775 Shore Parkway, Apartment 2-D, Brooklyn, NY 11223, (718) 648-5325, BA 78 CUNY - Brooklyn Coll; MS 80 CUNY - Brooklyn Coll; Sp-Lang Path, Staten Island Aid Inc, **SLP**

Fein, Dr Louis I United Testing Service Incorporated, 9485 Sunset Drive, Suite A-110, Miami, FL 33173, (305) 595-5554, BA 66 Long Island U - Brooklyn Ctr; MS 69 CUNY - Brooklyn Coll; PH 80 (Administration) Elysion Coll; Exec Dir, United Testing Svc, **SLP**

Fein, Rebecca B 12935 S W 108th Place, Miami, FL 33176, (305) 595-5554, BA 75 Univ of FL; ME 76 Univ of FL; **SLP**

Fein, Shelley 3232 Shore Parkway #3-J, Brooklyn, NY 11235, (718) 891-7406, BA 74 CUNY - Brooklyn Coll; MA 82 NY Univ; Sp/Lang Path, Private Practice, **SLP**

Feinberg, Mrs Chantal L 7441 Overhill Road, Melrose Park, PA 19126, (215) 782-1483, BA 72 Temple Univ; MA 73 Temple Univ; 78–Sp-Lang Path, Sch Dist of Phila, **SLP**

Feinberg, Evelyn Maj 4160 Ellenita Avenue, Tarzana, CA 91356, (213) 343-8319, BA 61 Univ of CA - Los Angeles; MA 79 CA St Univ - Northridge; SLP, Conejo Valley USD, **SLP**

Feinberg, Louise S 3400 Greenfield #3, Los Angeles, CA 90034, (213) 837-2460, BA 55 Oberlin Coll; MA 75 CA St Univ - Northridge; Sp-Lang Path, Santa Monica Malibu USD, **SLP**

Feinberg, Regina R K 10828 Tabor Street, Los Angeles, CA 90034, (213) 204-4783, BA 79 Univ of CA - Los Angeles; MA 83 CA St Univ - Northridge; SLP, Montebello USD, **SLP**

Feingold, Mrs Ellen Reisner 1391 Heller Drive, Yardley, PA 19067, (215) 493-0333, BA 66 CUNY - Brooklyn Coll; MS 75 CUNY - Brooklyn Coll; Sp-Lang Path, NYC Bd Ed Committee On Hndcpd, **SLP**

Feingold, Mrs Frances H 3020 North 6th Street, Sheboygan, WI 53081, (414) 458-3798, BS 55 Univ of WI - Madison

Feingold, Robin E 4260 Stirling Road, Hollywood, FL 33021, (305) 987-6165, OB 77 Univ of Miami; MA 79 Univ of Miami; Sp-Lang Path, Sch Bd of Broward Co, **SLP**

Feinholz, Mrs Lori Adrienne 26070 Viento Court, Valencia, CA 91355, (805) 255-8005, BA 83 CA St Univ - Northridge; MA 85 CA St Univ - Northridge; **SLP**

Feinsod, Miriam G P O Box 172, Lee, MA 01238-0172, (516) 825-3193, BA 67 Hofstra Univ; MS 68 Adelphi Univ; Sp/Lang Path, Valley Stream Sch Dist, **SLP LM**

Feinstein, Barry L 1500 Shadyside, Baltimore, MD 21218, **SLP**

Feinstein, Linda S Ore Ledgewood Way Unit #19, Peabody, MA 01960, (508) 745-9000, BS 86 Univ of MA - Amherst; MA 88 Univ of MA - Amherst; 88–Sp-Lang Path, Shaughnessy-Kaplan Rehab Hosp

Feinstein, Marjorie S 2924 Baker Street, San Francisco, CA 94123-1145, (617) 787-3390, BS 81 Ithaca Coll; MS 82 Boston Univ; SLP, Greenery, **SLP ACE**

Feinstein, Mrs Susan C Minneapolis Children's Medical Center, Audiology Clinic, 2525 Chicago Avenue South, Minneapolis, MN 55404, (612) 863-6196, BS 65 Univ of Pittsburgh - Pittsburgh; MA 66 Columbia Univ Teachers Coll; MA 67 Temple Univ; Aud, Minneapolis Children's Med Ctr, **A**

Feiss, Mrs Sarah 7459 North Chadwick Road, Milwaukee, WI 53217, **SLP**

Feiszli, Marianne 1110 Oriole Drive #6, Rapid City, SD 57701, (605) 343-6466, BS 79 Bowling Green St Univ; MA 81 Univ of Akron; 88–Prog Dir, Black Hills Workshop/Comm Trans, **SLP**

Feitel, Mrs Rhonda Rochelle 66-22 Fleet Street #1-L, Forest Hills, NY 11375, (516) 544-2259, BA 78 Hofstra Univ; MA 79 Hofstra Univ; 79–Sp-Lang Path, Kings Park Psychi Hosp, **SLP**

Feiwell Ma, H Aubrey P O Box 751, Bloomfield Hills, MI 48303, (313) 652-5304, BS 50 IN Univ - Bloomington; MA 52 Univ of Denver; 74–Pres, Sp & Lang Path PC, **SLP**

Felckowski, Lynn Marie 6 Stacy Lane, Madison, WI 53716, (608) 252-8414, BS 86 Univ of WI - Stevens Point; MS 88 Univ of WI - Stevens Point; 88–Aud, Jackson Cl-Phys Plus

Feld, Nancy Sue M A 2643 Aspen Street, Philadelphia, PA 19130, (215) 235-6333, BS 63 Emerson Coll; MS 64 Univ of MI - Ann Arbor; Sp-Lang Path, Priv Practice, **SLP**

Feldbaum, Jill M Waterford Apartment #30-C, Cherry Hill, NJ 08034, (609) 354-1182, BA 69 Temple Univ; MA 70 George Washington Univ; 82–Sp-Lang Path, Private Practice, **SLP**

Felder, Lynda J 645 West 239 Street #6-E, Bronx, NY 10463, (212) 652-5303, MS 76 Columbia Univ Teachers Coll; Pres, Spec Commun Ser Inc, **SLP**

Feldherr, Louise B 102 North 8th Street, Philadelphia, PA 19107, (215) 238-6834, BS 79 Northeastern Univ; MS 81 Hahneman Medical Coll; Dir of Aud, Metropolitan Hosp, **SLP A**

Feldman, Dr Alan S 404 University Avenue, Syracuse, NY 13210, (315) 428-0016, BA 49 Syracuse Univ; MS 51 Syracuse Univ; PH 56 (Aud) Syracuse Univ; 81–Aud, Private Practice, **SLP A F**

Feldman, Amy B 6 Bay Avenue, Huntington, NY 11743, (516) 424-2339, BS 77 Boston Univ; MS 79 Columbia Univ Teachers Coll; Private Practice, **SLP**

Feldman, Dr Bernice K 689 Sleepy Hollow Road, Briarcliff Manor, New York, NY 10510, (914) 941-7157, BA 44 CUNY - Hunter Coll; MA 62 Columbia Univ Teachers Coll; PH 79 (Audio-Commun-Disorders) NY Univ; 78–Dir of Prog, Mount St Ursula Sp Ctr, **SLP**

Feldman, Carin Bea 4425 Haverford Drive, Rockville, MD 20853, (301) 949-8070, BA 72 Adelphi Univ; MS 75 CUNY - Brooklyn Coll; Sp-Lang Path, The Hearing Ctr, **SLP**

Feldman, Deborah G 7002 Exeter Road, Bethesda, MD 20814, (202) 523-7065, BS 75 Boston Univ; MS 77 Columbia Univ Teachers Coll; Health Sci, Dept of Labor-OSHA, **A**

Feldman, Eileen Weisen 9 Jefferson Court, Setauket, NY 11733, (516) 987-3093, Sp-Lang Path, Three Village Schools, **SLP**

Feldman, Ellen R Hopkinson House #1208, Washington Square South, Philadelphia, PA 19106, (215) 625-2755, BS 75 Syracuse Univ; MA 77 Northwestern Univ; Sp-Lang Path, Sp Path Consultants, **SLP**

Feldman, Irene R 14695 N E 18th Avenue #3E, North Miami, FL 33181, (305) 945-1946, BS 32 Newark St Coll; MS 40 Newark St Coll; **SLP LM**

Feldman, Janet M 154 William Feather Drive, Voorhees, NJ 08043, (609) 767-5667, BA 72 Univ of MD - College Park; MS 75 Loyola Coll; **SLP**

Feldman, Julie G 6 Stewart Place, Spring Valley, NY 10977, (914) 378-7502, BA 77 CUNY - Queens Coll; MA 79 CUNY - Hunter Coll; ME 88 Columbia Univ Teachers Coll; 88–Asst Dir, St Joseph's Med Ctr, **A ACE**

Feldman, Mrs Linda Morris 2103 Rockefeller Lane #1, Redondo Beach, CA 90278, (213) 376-4142, BS 81 Univ of MD - College Park; MS 82 Loyola Coll; Sp/Lang Path, Casa Colina, **SLP**

Feldman, Louise P 5315 S W Colony Court, Beaverton, OR 97005, (503) 690-5432, BA 51 CUNY - Brooklyn Coll; MA 53 Univ of MI - Ann Arbor; 87–Sp-Lang Path/Aud, Wash Co Educ Svc Dist, **SLP A**

Feldman, Lynn Ann 557 Pelham Road, Philadelphia, PA 19119, (215) 284-8570, BA 81 Univ of Pittsburgh - Pittsburgh; MA 83 Temple Univ; 86–Sp-Lang Path, Delaware Co Mem Hosp, **SLP**

Feldman, Myrna G 5515 Clover Rise Lane, Norcross, GA 30093, (404) 925-2100, BA 71 SUNY - Center at Albany; ME 72 Northeastern Univ; Sp-Lang Path, Gwinnett Co Schs, **SLP**

Feldman, Naida A 89 Eagle Ridge Drive SW, Calgary, AB, Canada T2V 2V6, (403) 229-7065, BA 69 SUNY - Center at Buffalo; MA 72 IN Univ - Bloomington; Sp-Lang Path, Ab Chldn Hosp Sp-Lang Aud Dept, **SLP**

Feldman, Dr R Michael 5709 Elmer Street, Pittsburgh, PA 15232, (412) 938-4389, BA 58 Univ of Pittsburgh - Pittsburgh; MA 61 Univ of IA; PH 64 (NS) Northwestern Univ; Prof, CA U of Pa, **A**

Feldman, Dr Ronald L 6 Stonegate Mall, Roslyn, NY 11576, (516) 294-6661, BA 60 CUNY - Brooklyn Coll; MA 62 CUNY - Brooklyn Coll; PH 71 (NS) NY Univ; Assoc Prof, Brooklyn College, **SLP**

Feldman, Mrs Sharon A 2673 Mangrove Way, Riverside, CA 92506, (714) 788-7203, BA 66 Pacific Lutheran Univ; MS 81 Univ of Redlands; 80–SLP, Riverside USD, **SLP**

Feldman, Mrs Sheree Y 2821 Aspen, Northbrook, IL 60062, (312) 541-8556, BS 76 Tulane Univ; MA 77 Univ of IL - Urbana; Sp-Lang Path, Private Practice, **SLP**

Feldman, Mrs Sheryl N 2 Rainhollow, Houston, TX 77024, (713) 932-7557, MA 79 Univ of Houston - Univ Park; SLP, Private Practice, **SLP**

Feldman, Shirley Charney 20540 Strath-Haven Drive, Gaithersburg, MD 20879, BA 77 Univ of MD - College Park; MA 81 Univ of MD - College Park; Sp-Lang Path, Mont Co Pub Sch, **SLP**

Feldman, Susan L 15 Sheridan Square, New York, NY 10014, (212) 790-8678, BS 76 Syracuse Univ; MA 78 Hofstra Univ; SLP, St Vincents Hosp & Med Cen, **SLP**

Feldman, Wendy K 315 West 70th Street #14-I, New York, NY 10023, **SLP**

Feldmann, M C 1060A #9A Perkins-Jones Road, Apartment 9-B, Warren, OH 44483, (216) 841-3700, BS 76 OH Univ - Athens; MA 77 Kent St Univ; Sp-Lang Path, Hillside Hosp, **SLP**

Feldmann, Mrs Madeline 460 Central Avenue, Milton, MA 02186, (617) 963-8150, BA 59 Regis Coll; ME 65 Boston Univ; Chair Sp & Hrng Dept, Boston Sch for Deaf

Feldner-Pikula, Mrs Janeen M 8425 Orchard Court, Tinley Park, IL 60477, (312) 687-0900, BA 78 Saint Xavier Coll; MA 79 Univ of IL - Urbana; Sp-Lang Path, Southwest Coop/Spec Ed, **SLP**

Felicier, Mrs Maria De Los A Apartado 1406, Rio Grande, PR 00745, (809) 863-8808, BS 82 Univ of PR - San Juan; MS 85 Univ of PR - San Juan; 85–Sp-Lang Path, Dept of Health-Pediatric Ctr, **SLP**

Felins, Mary Angela 36 Patterson Road, Bedford, MA 01730, (617) 274-8017, BS 82 Marywood Coll; MS 84 PA St Univ - Univ Park; 87–Sp-Lang Path, Acton Public School, **SLP**

Felion, Mrs Elizabeth Ann 6600 North Sidney Place, Apartment 205, Glendale, WI 53209, (414) 228-8421, BS 86 Marquette Univ; MS 87 Marquette Univ; 87–Sp-Lang Path, Eisenhower Memorial Cerebral Palsy Work Ctr, **SLP**

Felix, Barbara G 2380 West Placita DE Ramo, Tucson, AZ 85741, (602) 887-7590, BS 73 Eastern MI Univ; MA 74 Eastern MI Univ; Sp-Lang Path, Private Practice, **SLP**

Felix, Mrs Maureen A 257 Central Avenue, West Caldwell, NJ 07006, (201) 226-2649, BA 65 Brandeis Univ; MA 67 Brown Univ; MS 79 William Paterson Coll; Sp-Lang Path, Livingston Boe, **SLP**

Felix, Nancy L 32 Laurie Avenue, Parnell, Auckland, New Zealand, BA 73 Univ of WA; OM 74 Univ of WA; 88–Sp-Lang Path, Private Practice, **SLP**

Felker, Diana Lynn E 1002 East Commercial, Charleston, MO 63834, (314) 335-1251, MA 80 Southeast MO St Univ; Sp-Lang Path, St Francis Med Cen, **SLP**

Felker, Donna Lea 2485 South York, Apt # 103, Denver, CO 80210, (303) 722-2901, BS 82 Univ of AZ; MS 86 UT St Univ; Childrens Hospital, **A**

Felker, Mrs Sharron S Rt 1 Box 112-Y, Rockett Drive, Jackson, MS 39212, (601) 373-6500, BS 74 Univ Southern MS-Hattiesburg; MS 76 Univ Southern MS-Hattiesburg; **A**

Felknor, Gratia Aileen 323 Chimney Rock #1212, Tyler, TX 75703, (214) 531-8190, BS 83 TX Christian Univ; MS 85 Univ of OK Medical Center; Sp-Lang Path, Med Ctr Hosp, **SLP**

Fell, Mrs Alice 2709 Cranbrook, Ann Arbor, MI 48104, (313) 665-8286, MA 71 CA St Univ - Los Angeles; Sp-Lang Path, Ypsilanti Pub Sch, **SLP**

Fell, Mary Adrienne 1712 East 72nd Street, Apartment 1312, Tulsa, OK 74136, (918) 495-3674, BS 83 Univ of Tulsa; MA 85 Univ of Tulsa; **SLP**

Fellendorf, George W 7 Skyview Circle, Keene, NH 03431, BS 46 Union Coll; MS 49 Rensselaer Polytech Inst; ED 74 (NS) Columbia Univ Teachers Coll; President, Fellendorf Associates

Feller, Deborah Tint 320 Green Meadow Lane, Horsham, PA 19044, (215) 675-5774, BA 82 Temple Univ; MA 84 Temple Univ; Sp-Lang Path, Montgomery County Indep Unit, **SLP**

Fellerman, Nanc E 1605 John Street, Fort Lee, NJ 07024, (201) 461-9393, BA 70 Montclair St Coll; MS 72; Sp-Lang Path, Private Practice, **SLP**

Fellin, Mrs Paula S 238 E 11th Avenue #B, Conshohocken, PA 19428, (215) 828-5743, BS 82 PA St Univ - Univ Park; MS 84 PA St Univ - Univ Park; **A**

Felling, Charles R Room 140, Hospital School, University Of Iowa, Iowa City, IA 52242, (319) 353-6125, BA 59 Univ of IA; MA 60 Univ of IA; PH 75 (NS) Univ of IA; Sp-Lang Path, U of IA, **SLP**

Fellman, Mrs Fern D 66 Pine Avenue, Randolph, MA 02368, BS 75 Emerson Coll; MA 76 Hofstra Univ; 87–Sp-Lang Path, Randolph PS, **SLP**

Fellner, Evangeline Estever 6 Zev Court, Monmouth Junction, NJ 08852, (212) 698-7254, BA 76 CUNY - Hunter Coll; MA 79 CUNY - Hunter Coll; Sp-Lang Path, Indep Consit, **SLP**

Fellows, Mrs Alice B 1714 Green Oaks Drive, Irving, TX 75061, (214) 253-0906, BA 50 Univ of TX - Austin; MA 62 Southern Methodist Univ; 66–Sp-Lang Path, Irving ISD, **SLP**

Fellows, Mrs Jane W 4126 Evergreen Drive, Fairfax, VA 22032, (703) 691-1565, BA 61 Univ of ND; **SLP**

Fellows, Judy A 2107 Honor Street Suite D, Monroe, LA 71201, (318) 325-5504, BA 80 SD St Univ; MA 82 OK St Univ; 88–Sp-Lang Path, Fellows SLP Services, **SLP ACE**

Fellows, Steven Arnold 15 John Maddox Drive, Rome, GA 30161, (404) 291-1978, BA 65 Auburn Univ - Auburn; MA 66 Auburn Univ - Auburn; Aud, G D Hoople Hrng & Sp Cen Inc, **A**

Fellows, Thelma M 125 NW 20th Place #507, Portland, OR 97209, (503) 223-5029, BA 64 Univ of MT; MA 67 Univ of UT; MA 85 Univ of ID; Sp-Lang Path, Portland PS, **SLP**

Felmus, Mrs Veta R 6665 Leyland Park Drive, San Jose, CA 95120, (408) 268-9643, BS 57 Univ of IL - Urbana; **SLP**

Felsenfeld, Mark A 28893 Glen Arden, Farmington Hills, MI 48018, (313) 553-4386, BA 77 Univ of MI - Ann Arbor; MA 79 Wayne St Univ; Coord Therapy Serv/Slp, Greenfield Health Sys Corp, **SLP**

Felsenfeld, Susan 2610 Louisa Avenue, Mounds View, MN 55112, (612) 785-1137, BA 77 Univ of CA - Santa Barbara; MA 79 Univ of CA - Santa Barbara; **SLP**

Felsenstein, Dr Bernard 700 Victory Boulevard, Apartment 12-N, Staten Island, NY 10301, (212) 727-7389, BA 31 Long Island U - Brooklyn Ctr; MA 36 Columbia Univ Sch of Gen St; PH 71 (Aphasia) Columbia Univ Teachers Coll; 82–Res Consult, Bklyn VA Med Cen

Felstehausen-White, Susan L 829 15th Street, Moline, IL 61265, (309) 762-7778, BS 84 Eastern IL Univ; MA 86 San Diego St Univ; 86–Aud, Robert Flatley MD, **A**

Felt, Mrs Catherine Renee 217 Boli Lane, Bolingbrook, IL 60439-1520, (312) 524-2978, **SLP**

Felt, Suzanne R 86 Federal Street, Salem, MA 01970, **SLP**

Felterman, Nancy J 126 McGee Dr, Patterson, LA 70392, (318) 861-0750, OM 88 LA St Univ - N O Medical Ctr

Feltes, Mrs Carol Urbanski 1 Airport Road, Ottawa, IL 61350, (815) 433-3761, BS 76 Univ of IL - Urbana; MS 77 Univ of IL - Urbana; Sp-Lang Path, Ottawa Elem Sch Dist #141, **SLP**

Feltman, Arlene J Kessler 343 East 74th Street 9G, New York, NY 10021, (212) 439-1714, MA 67; **SLP**

Felton, Janet Lynn 517 1/2 62nd Street, Oakland, CA 94609, (415) 667-7676, MS 85 San Francisco St Univ; BA 82 CA St Univ - Northridge; Sp-Lang Path, Fairmont Hosp, **SLP**

Felton, Joy E Joy E Felton & Associates, 10041 S W 141st Street, Miami, FL 33176, (305) 251-3313, BA 75 Univ of FL; ME 76 Univ of Miami; 81–Sp-Lang Path, Private Practice, **SLP**

Felton, Karen Kent 3412 Kirby Smith Drive, Wilmington, NC 28403, MS 85 East Carolina Univ; Sp-Lang Path, Murdoch Ctr, **SLP**

Felton, Mrs Louise Black 1422 Larkfield Lane, Charlotte, NC 28210, (704) 553-7428, BS 77 Western Carolina Univ; ME 81 Univ of NC - Greensboro; Tchr for Deaf, Orangeburg Sch Dist #5, **SLP**

Felton-Sheldon, Mrs Melody 109 Clark, Santa Cruz, CA 95060, (408) 475-8081, BA 82 Western WA Univ; Sp-Lang Path, Soquel Elem Sch Dist, **SLP**

Feltz, Mrs Kay Yvonne 1511 Langford Avenue, Albion, IA 50005, (515) 488-2970, BA 81 Univ of Northern IA; MA 82 Univ of Northern IA; Sp-Lang Path, AEA #6, **SLP**

Fendler, Mrs Marla Jacobson 914 Willow Lane, Sleepy Hollow, IL 60118, (815) 385-0600, BA 72 Judson Coll; MA 84 Northern IL Univ - De Kalb; Sp-Lang Path, Pioneer Ctr for the Except, **SLP**

Fendley, Frances M 4913 Branch Mill Circle, Birmingham, AL 35223-1605, (205) 956-7185, **SLP**

Fendrich, Mrs Dale P Euclid Clinic Foundation, 18599 Lakeshore Boulevard, Cleveland, OH 44119, (216) 383-8500, BA 81 Cleveland St Univ; MA 83 Cleveland St Univ; 84–Aud, Euclid Cl Foundations, **A**

Fendrick, Jennifer Elaine 369 Market Square East, Lakeland, FL 33803, (813) 666-1070, BS 82 Univ of South AL; MS 83 Univ of South AL; Sp-Lang Path, Doris Sanders Lrng Cen/Polk Co, **SLP**

Fenichel, Mrs Rita B 2 Tilden Court, Livingston, NJ 07039, (201) 992-0362, BA 49 OH St Univ; BS 49 OH St Univ; MA 70 Montclair St Coll; Sp/Lang Path, Private Practice, **SLP**

Fenick, Blanca V 0-44 Pine Avenue, Fair Lawn, NJ 07410, (201) 791-5643, MS 78 William Paterson Coll; OB 62; Aud, Private Practice, **A ACE**

Fenlason, Catherine D 301 W Broomfield Road #902, Mount Pleasant, MI 48858-4535, (517) 773-4356, BS 74 IA St Univ; MA 80 Western MI Univ; Sp-Lang Path, Stride Inc, **SLP**

Fenley, Hannah L 10016 Noland, Lenexa, KS 66215, (913) 492-4632, BS 75 Univ of KS; MA 78 Univ of KS; 87–Sp-Lang Path, Private Practice, **SLP**

Fennell, Ann M 36 Kenmore Road, Belmont, MA 02178, (617) 935-5050, BA 82 MI St Univ; MS 85 Univ of WI - Madison; Sp-Lang Path, New England Rehab Hosp, **SLP**

Fennell, Mrs Nena C H 427 Patterson Road, Lawrenceville, GA 30245, (404) 769-7791, BS 75 Univ of GA; ME 76 Univ of GA; Sp/Lang Path, Gwinnett Co Schools, **SLP**

Fennimore, Pauline C7 Village Green, Chapel Hill, NC 27514, (919) 787-1374, MS 79 Univ of NC - Chapel Hill; Aud, Capitol ENT, **A**

Fennimore, Rosalind Longley 84-58 159th Street, Jamaica, NY 11432, (718) 990-3832, BA 79 CUNY - Queens Coll; MS 82 Columbia Univ Teachers Coll; 85–Sp-Lang Path, Queens Hosp Ctr/LIJ Affiliation, **SLP**

Fenske, Kay Annette 7845 East River Road #304, Minneapolis, MN 55432, (612) 574-6590, BS 85 Univ of WI - Stevens Point; MA 87 Saint Louis Univ; **SLP**

Fenster, Mrs Joan G 5 Francis Drive, Belle Mead, NJ 08502, (609) 466-2989, BA 72 George Washington Univ; MA 75 Kean Coll of NJ; SLP, Rock Brook Sch, **SLP**

Fenster, Susan Ann 120-23 Erdman Place, Bronx, NY 10475, (212) 320-1575, MA 86 CUNY - Queens Coll; **SLP**

Fenton, Dr Elaine Reiman 36 Sutton Place South, New York, NY 10022, (212) 355-6634, BA 59 Marymount Coll; MA 62 CUNY - Hunter Coll; PH 71 (NS) NY Univ; Dir, Manhat Sp-Lang-Voice Path Serv, **SLP**

Fenton, Mrs Jacqueline Koss 15 Buckingham Circle, Pine Brook, NJ 07058, (201) 515-2424, BA 60 CUNY - Queens Coll; MA 63 CUNY - Brooklyn Coll; 74–Sp-Lang Path, Hanover Twsp Bd of Ed, **SLP**

Fenton-Jones, Jill 24931 Woodridge Drive, Apartment 65101, Farmington Hills, MI 48018, BA 83 MI St Univ; MA 85 Eastern MI Univ; 86–Sp-Lang Path, High Point Ctr Washtenaw ISD, **SLP**

Fentress, Mrs Deborah P 993 Old Northfield Road, Thomaston, CT 06787, (203) 283-0339, BA 79 San Jose St Univ; MA 81 San Jose St Univ; Sp-Lang Path, New Britain Public Schools, **SLP**

Fenyes, Mrs Shelley R T 2324 Buckingham Road, Birmingham, MI 48008, (313) 649-0117, BA 75 CUNY - Queens Coll; MS 76 Univ of MI - Ann Arbor; Sp-Lang Path, **SLP**

Fenzel, Mrs Catherine Curtin 8 Joyce Road, Eastchester, NY 10709, (914) 961-8196, BA 41 CUNY - Hunter Coll; MS 42 Fordham Univ

Ferber-Lerner, Rosanne 2500 Johnson Avenue, Winston Churchill Suite 9C, Riverdale, NY 10463, (212) 796-5721, OB 77 SUNY - Coll at Cortland; MA 78 NY Univ; OM 81 Pace U -Coll of White Plains; Sp-Lang Path, Private Practice, **SLP**

Ferch, Mrs Pamela A 961 S E Brookedge Avenue, Port St Lucie, FL 34983, (305) 879-0193, BS 77 Wayne St Univ; MA 78 Eastern MI Univ; Sp-Lang Path, St Lucie Co Sch Bd, **SLP**

Ferdows, Nazanin 5434 Zelzah Avenue #102, Encino, CA 91316, (818) 344-8405, MS 86 San Francisco St Univ; **SLP**

Ference, Linda A Jones 176 Butterworth Lane, Langhorne, PA 19047, (215) 757-2764, BS 76 Indiana Univ of PA; MA 81 Trenton St Coll; **SLP**

Ference, Terry 6442 Sandstone, Carmichael, CA 95608, (916) 454-8183, BA 73 CA St Univ - Sacramento; MA 75 CA St Univ - Sacramento; 74–Sp-Lang Path, Sacramento Cty USD, **SLP**

Ferencz, Mrs Marla J 1323 Lincoln Avenue South, Highland Park, IL 60035, MA 75 Northern IL Univ - De Kalb; Sp-Lang Path, Private Practice, **SLP**

Ferens, Mrs Donna J 1058 West Maple #2, Plymouth, MI 48170-1557, (313) 451-8298, BS 83 Northern MI Univ; MS 87 Eastern IL Univ

Ferguson, Beth W 287-A Coates Lane, King of Prussia, PA 19406, (215) 272-5151, BS 81 Bloomsburg Univ of PA; MS 82 Bloomsburg Univ of PA; Sp-Lang Path, Montgomery County Ind Unit 23, **SLP**

Ferguson, Betty T 1625 N W 188th Terrace, Miami, FL 33169, MS; **SLP**

Ferguson, Cathleen 1309 Superior Street, Webster City, IA 50595, **SLP**

Ferguson, Mrs Cheryl Lynn 15099 Marl Drive, Linden, MI 48451-9016, BA 84 Univ of Northern IA; MA 86 Univ of Northern IA; **SLP**

Ferguson, Cindy Louise HCR 71, Box 120F, Hustontown, PA 17229, (717) 987-3090, BS 86 Clarion Univ of PA; MS 87 Clarion Univ of PA; **SLP**

Ferguson, Mrs Cynthia Perkins 8820 Reyegate Drive, Knoxville, TN 37922, (615) 632-5899, BS 84 Univ of TN - Knoxville; MA 85 Univ of TN - Knoxville; 88–Sp-Lang Path, E TN Baptist Hospital, **SLP**

Ferguson, Mrs Elizabeth 607 East Lawndale, Peoria, IL 61603-1251, (309) 672-6700, BS 77 IL St Univ - Normal; MS 79 IL St Univ - Normal; Sp-Lang Path, Peoria Pub Sch Dist 150, **SLP**

Ferguson, Mrs Ellen F 4720 Player Drive, Fort Collins, CO 80525, (303) 667-6585, BA 55 IA St Univ; MA 57 IA St Univ; Speech/Language Pathologist, Larimer Co Vna, **SLP**

Ferguson, Hugh D 63 Brandywine Court, Bricktown, NJ 08723, (201) 974-0902, BA 79 Montclair St Coll; MA 81 NY Univ; MA 85 Montclair St Coll; Aud, Hearing Devices Co, **A ACE**

Ferguson, Mrs Jane W 3608 Teakwood, Columbia, MO 65203, (314) 446-1539, BA 73 Southwestern Univ; MA 80 TX Woman's Univ; **SLP**

Ferguson, Judith A North 7316 Colton, Spokane, WA 99208-6511, (509) 466-3060, BA 60 Univ of OR; MA 64 Univ of OR; MS 72 Eastern WA Univ; 72–Sp-Lang Path, Mead Sch Dist, **SLP**

Ferguson, Julie Kathryn 1821 Jefferson Park Avenue #2, Charlottesville, VA 22903, (804) 924-8245, BS 82 Miami Univ - Oxford; ME 88 Univ of VA - Charlottesville; 88–Sp-Lang Path, Univ of Virginia Med Ctr

Ferguson, Mrs Kate Abbott 400 West Pierce Street, Easton, PA 18042, (215) 252-3461, MA 83 West Chester Univ of PA; SLP, Helen Beeve Sp & Hrng Cen, **SLP**

Ferguson, Mrs LaDonna Meeks 7711 Louis Pasteur #504, San Antonio, TX 78229, (512) 691-1046, BA 82 TX Tech Univ; MS 84 TX Tech Univ; 85–Aud, Otologic Associates, **A**

Ferguson, Linda S 14 Harbor Village Drive #1, Middletown, RI 02840-3820, BA 68 Univ of MA - Amherst; MA 72 Ball St Univ; Director, Delaware Speech & Hearing Cen, **A**

Ferguson, Mrs Marian N 32 Washington Square West, New York, NY 10011, (212) 982-3779, BA 53 OH Wesleyan Univ; MA 54 Cornell Univ; **SLP**

Ferguson, Mrs Marie N 244 Ockley Drive, Shreveport, LA 71105, (318) 868-3741, BA 31 LA Coll; **SLP LM**

Ferguson, Mrs Mary A M 3935 Chilton Drive, Winston-Salem, NC 27106, (919) 924-5641, BA 76 Univ of NC - Greensboro; ME 77 Univ of NC - Greensboro; Sp-Lang Path Consultant, Consul-Forsyth Co Men Hlth, **SLP**

Ferguson, Mrs Mary Elizabeth 1500 Arden Vista Court, Arden Hills, MN 55112, (612) 631-1603, BA 66 Augustana Coll; MA 67 Univ of IL - Urbana; Sp-Lang Path, Utd & Childrens Hospital, **SLP**

Ferguson, Mrs Maxine Williams 952 Whispering Lake Drive, Shreveport, LA 71107, (318) 636-0210, MA 88 LA Tech Univ

Ferguson, Monica L 428 Droz Drive, Fairbanks, AK 99701, (907) 488-0134, BA 72 Univ of TX - El Paso; MS 77 Univ of NM; Sp-Lang Path, Fairbanks N Star Borough Sch, **SLP**

Ferguson, Patricia Ann 1254 Ethel Street, Glendale, CA 91207, (818) 246-6225, BA 85 Univ of CA - Santa Barbara; OM 87 AZ St Univ; 88–Sp-Lang Path, Dr Barbara Dabul, **SLP**

Ferguson, Mrs Peggy J 44 Beath Street, West Hill, ON, Canada MIE 3J3, (416) 396-7577, BA 74 Univ of Toronto - Ontario; MS 77 O965; Sp/Lang Path, Scarborough Board of Education, **SLP**

Ferguson, Robert N 2 Chestnut Hill South, Loudonville, NY 12211, (518) 462-3311, BS 63 Howard Univ; MA 66 OH St Univ; Aud, VA Medical Ctr, **A**

Ferguson, Roxann University Of Kansas, 320 Miller Bldg, Dept Hearing & Speech, Kansas City, KS 66103, (913) 588-5905, **A**

Ferguson, Mrs Shirley Gail Speech - Language - Hearing Clinic, Eastern New Mexico Univ, Station 19 Box 19, Portales, NM 88130, (505) 562-2156, BS 64 Eastern NM Univ; MS 65 Eastern NM Univ; Asst Prof/Cocrd-Cl Serv, Eastern New Mexico University, **SLP**

Ferguson, Tracey Marie 1705 East Ash, Enid, OK 73701, (405) 234-3734, BA 82 LA Tech Univ; MS 85 CO St Univ; **A**

Ferguson-Kinney, Mrs Gwendolyn C 9733 Good Luck Road #4, Seabrook, MD 20706, (301) 459-3152, BA 81 NC A & T St Univ; MS 84 Howard Univ; 85–Allocations Prog Analyst III, United Way of the Natl Cap Area

Ferketic, Michelle Mary 5203 Crown Street, Bethesda, MD 20816, (301) 897-5700, BA 80 Univ of Pittsburgh - Pittsburgh; MA 83 Univ of Pittsburgh - Pittsburgh; 87–Sp-Lang Path Tec, ASHA -Professional Practices, **SLP**

Fernandes, Jean Keeffe 26 Bosworth Street, Beverly, MA 01915, BS 78 Salem St Coll; MS 80 Emerson Coll; Sp-Lang Path, Atlanticare Medical Center, **SLP**

Fernandez, Mrs Carol L University Of South Florida, Dept Of Communication Sciences & Disorders, CBA 255, Tampa, FL 33622, (813) 974-2006, BA 67 FL St Univ; MA 70 Univ of South FL; ES 86 Univ of South FL; Sp-Lang Path, Center for Communication Disorders, **SLP**

Fernandez, Mrs Diane Piva 257 Vernon Street #210, Oakland, CA 94610, (415) 863-4710, BA 85 Holy Names Coll; MS 87 San Francisco St Univ; 88–Aud, Burt's Hrng Aid Svc

Fernandez, Gilda Avenue El Bosque-Qta, MI Retiro-La Florida, Caracas, Venezuela 1050, **A**

Fernandez, Mrs Jan-Marie S 2923 Ellenwood Drive, Fairfax, VA 22031, (301) 279-8530, BS 79 Northeastern Univ; MA 81 Temple Univ-Tyler Sch of Art; 85–Aud, Montgomery Co Public Schools, **SLP**

Fernandez, Lisa Ann USF Medical Center Box 16, 12901 Bruce B Downs Boulevard, Tampa, FL 33612, (813) 974-4350, MS 80 Univ of South FL; Chief Aud, USF Med Ctr, **A**

Fernandez, Paula Ann Route 11 #U-1, Kirkwood, NY 13795, (607) 777-2829, BS 81 SUNY - Coll at Geneseo; ME 83 Univ of VA - Charlottesville; Sp-Lang Path, Chld Ut for Treat & Eval, **SLP**

Fernandez-Roque, Natalie 7150 West 15th Court, Hialeah, FL 33014, (305) 854-8171, MA 79 Univ of FL; Audiologist, Miami Hearing & Speech Center, **A**

Fernandez-Soberal, Ana V 8056 Beaverland, Redford, MI 48239, (313) 841-5982, BA 84 Wayne St Univ; MA 87 Wayne St Univ; **SLP**

Fernie, Mrs Rosemary Martino 162 York Street #2, St Catharines, ON, Canada L2R 6E7, (716) 688-5139, MA 87 SUNY - Center at Buffalo

Ferracane, Mrs Barbara J 546 North Country Club Rd, Decatur, IL 62521, (217) 429-5404, BS 79 Fontbonne Coll; MS 80 Fontbonne Coll; Sp-Lang Path, Decatur Public Sch Dist, **SLP**

Ferraioli, Mrs Mary Anne Malone 18 Continental Road, West Milford, NJ 07480, **SLP**

Ferralli, Sharon A 9410 Grandhaven Avenue, Upper Marlboro, MD 20772, (301) 798-1222, BS 75 Towson St Univ; MS 76 PA St Univ - Univ Park; Sp-Lang Path, Anne Arundel Co Bd of Ed, **SLP**

Ferrand, Carole T 12-F Graduate Circle, State College, PA 16801, (814) 863-3118, BA 70; MS 81 PA St Univ - Univ Park; PH 88 (Fluency/Voice) PA St Univ - Univ Park; Instr, Pennsylvania State University, **SLP**

Ferrandino, Regina Mary 8 South Allen Street, Apt #4, Albany, NY 12208, (518) 445-4535, BA 82 Univ of Northern CO; MA 84 SUNY - Center at Buffalo; Audiologist, Albany Medical Center Hospital, **A**

Ferrante, Mrs Marian E 3601 Shaw Circle, Antioch, CA 94509, (415) 439-1051, BA 69 CA St Univ - Sacramento; MA 73 CA St Univ - Sacramento; Sp-Lang Path, Home Hlth & Couns, **SLP ACE**

Ferrara, Kristine Louise 1366 N Plainview Drive, Akron, OH 44321, (216) 535-3101, BS 85 Kent St Univ; MA 88 Univ of Akron

Ferrara, Linda Mizenko 21270 Via Del Lobo, Yorba Linda, CA 92686, (213) 943-6734, BA 80 Rutger's St Univ - Douglas Coll; MS 81 Ithaca Coll; SLP, Placentia USD, **SLP**

Ferrara-Bowler, Mrs Kathleen Monique 54 Spring Street, West Roxbury, MA 02132, (617) 421-5984, BS 82 Saint Louis Univ; MS 85 Northeastern Univ; 88–Sp-Lang Path, Harvard Comm Hlth Plan, **SLP**

Ferrari, Patricia V 756 West Pke Street, Clarksburg, WV 26301, (304) 622-8378, BS 79 WV Univ; MA 80 Marshall Univ; Owner, Sp Lang Serv, **SLP**

Ferraro, Anne M R R 4, Breadalbane, PE, Canada C0A 1E0, (902) 436-7294, BA 78 Univ of VT; MS 81 Syracuse Univ; Sp-Lang Path, Pei Dept of Health & Social SE, **SLP**

Ferraro, Mrs Jamie B 11722 West 101st Terrace, Overland Park, KS 66214, (913) 541-9655, BS 69 Univ of IL - Urbana; MA 70 Univ of IL - Urbana; SLP, Kansas State School for Deaf, **SLP**

Ferraro, Dr John A Dept Of Hearing And Speech, University Of Kansas, Medical Center, Kansas City, KS 66103, (913) 588-5937, BS 68; MS 70 Univ of Denver; PH 72 (Sp & Hrng Sciences) Univ of Denver; Chair Dept Hrng Sp/Assoc Dean, U of KS Med Cen

Ferraro, Judith Ann 4 Alta Vista Circle, Irvington, NY 10533, (914) 591-6091, BS 83 Ithaca Coll; MS 84 Ithaca Coll; 86–Aud, Columbic Presbyterian Hosp, **A**

Ferraro, Judy 28 Winthrop Avenue, Albany, NY 12203, BA 68 SUNY - Coll at New Paltz; MA 70 Northwestern Univ; SLP, Rens-Col-Greene BOCES, **SLP**

Ferraro, Mrs Lynn Marie 17 Harlequin Drive, Smithtown, NY 11787, (516) 724-5575, BA 81 Long Island U - CW Post Ctr; MA 83 CUNY - Hunter Coll; Sp-Lang Path, Brentwood Sch, **SLP**

Ferraro-Saul, Mrs Annette Marie 1231 Rolling Meadow Road, Pittsburgh, PA 15241, (412) 257-3239, BS 81 PA St Univ - Univ Park; MA 82 Univ of Pittsburgh - Pittsburgh; 83–Sp/Lang Path, Easter Seal Soc Allegheny Co, **SLP**

Ferre, Dr Jeanane M 337 South Lombard Avenue, Oak Park, IL 60302, (312) 386-8490, BS 78 IL St Univ - Normal; MS 79 IL St Univ - Normal; PH 84 (NS) Northwestern Univ; 87–Aud, Private Practice, **A**

Ferree, Mrs Ann J Meridian Speech & Hearing Ctr, 2215 15th Street, Meridian, MS 39301, (601) 483-8121, BS 75 Univ of TN - Knoxville; MA 78 Univ of TN - Knoxville; SLP, Meridian Sp & Hrng Cen, **SLP**

Ferree, Mrs Celine M C 5211 8th Avenue, 3rd Floor, Brooklyn, NY 11220, (718) 972-6442, BA 77 Univ of IL - Chicago; MA 79 Wayne St Univ; Sp/Lang Path, Private Practice, **SLP**

Ferreira, Beatriz M 924 Monmouth Street, New Bedford, MA 02745, (617) 679-7026, MA 84 Univ of MA - Amherst; Sp-Lang Path, Charlton Memorial Hospital, **SLP**

Ferrell, Mrs Ann Cooley 208 Hurley Avenue, Newport News, VA 23601, (804) 596-7448, BA 76 Mary Washington Coll; ME 77 Univ of VA - Charlottesville; Sp-Lang Path, Private Practice, **SLP**

Ferrell, Mrs Catherine Ellen 217 Justice Avenue, Logan, WV 25601, (304) 752-7404, BA 83 Marshall Univ; MA 84 Marshall Univ; 84–Sp-Lang Path, Logan Co Boe, **SLP**

Ferrell, Charles J 1516 Westop Trail, Knoxville, TN 37923, (615) 974-5453, BS 66 East TN St Univ; MA 67 Univ of TN - Knoxville; Assoc Dir of Aud Cl Serv, U of TN, Dept of Aud & Sp Path, **A**

Ferrell, Elizabeth Bowman 216 Orange Street, Beaufort, NC 28516, (919) 633-0775, BS 84 East Carolina Univ; MS 85 East Carolina Univ; 86–Sp-Lang Path, Developmental Evaluation Ctr, **SLP**

Ferrell, Judith Y 1516 Westop Trail, Knoxville, TN 37923, (615) 637-0531, BS 67 Univ of TN - Knoxville; MA 69 Univ of TN - Knoxville; Aud, Knoxville ENT Assoc Pa, **A**

Ferrell, Mrs Pamela M Route 17 Box 1266-5, Hattiesburg, MS 39401, (601) 735-2205, BS 81 Univ Southern MS-Hattiesburg; MS 82 Univ Southern MS-Hattiesburg; SLP, Wayne Co Sch Sys, **SLP**

Ferrer, Jami Up Gr Lks Multifunc Res Ctr, 1025 West Johnson Street, Ctr For Ed Research, Madison, WI 53706, (608) 263-3976, BA 68 Univ of CA - Santa Barbara; MA 71 Univ of CA - Santa Barbara; 86–Training & Research Spec, Univ of Wisconsin-Madison, **SLP**

Ferrer, Dr Oscar Apartado DE Chacao 60209, Caracas, Venezuela 1060, MS 66 8144; MD 56 (NS) 8143; 78–Dir, Cen for Human Commun Dis, **SLP A**

Ferrer, Patricia McGowan R R 1 Box 928, Elbert, CO 80106, **SLP**

Ferrer-Vinent, Susan T Audiology Section, Fitzsimons Army Med Center, Aurora, CO 80045-5001, (303) 361-8120, BS 69 Northern IL Univ - De Kalb; MS 70 CO St Univ; Aud, Fitzsimons Army Med Cen, **A**

Ferretti, Arlene V 9008 Kirkdale Road, Bethesda, MD 20817, (301) 832-4400, BS 72 SUNY - Coll at Cortland; MS 78 Emerson Coll; **SLP**

Ferri, Cecelia A 734 Winchester Road, Broomall, PA 19008, (215) 328-1768, BS 85 West Chester Univ of PA; MA 87 Temple Univ; Sp-Lang Path, Moss Rehab Hosp, **SLP**

Ferri, Mrs Deann S 623 1st Avenue North, Surfside, SC 29575, (803) 448-1726, BS 71 Ithaca Coll; ME 73 Bloomsburg Univ of PA; Sp-Lang Path, Horry Co Sch, **SLP**

Ferrie, Adrienne C 438 Driscoll Drive, Bricktown, NJ 08724, (201) 892-1100, BS 76 Univ of GA; ME 77 Univ of GA; Director Sp-Lang Path, Nn Ocean Hosp Syst Inc, **SLP**

Ferrier, Linda J 1475 Massachusetts Avenue, Apartment 464, Lexington, MA 02173-4011, (617) 437-5753, BA 61; BA 63; MS 80 Emerson Coll; Lecturer, Northeastern U, **SLP**

Ferrigno, Sharon J 7519 East Jamison Drive, Englewood, CO 80112, (303) 771-4782, BS 64 SUNY - Coll at Geneseo; MS 77 Ithaca Coll; Sp/Lang Path, Private Practice, **SLP**

Ferris, Mrs Holly E 140 Sanford Street, East Longmeadow, MA 01028, (413) 525-2448, BA 75 Univ of MA - Amherst; MA 77 Univ of MA - Amherst; Sp-Lang Path, Private Practice, **SLP**

Ferris, James M 4132 Van Buren, Sioux City, IA 51108, (712) 722-4374, BA 82 Briar Cliff Coll; MA 83 Univ of SD - Vermillion; 86–Sp-Lang Path, AEA #4, **SLP**

Ferris, Jean B P O Box 315, Ashfield, MA 01330, (413) 536-0718, BS 73 Mary Washington Coll; ME 74 Univ of VA - Charlottesville; **SLP**

Ferris, Karen K 403 East Amin, Vermillion, SD 57069, (605) 624-8051, BA 66 Univ of SD - Vermillion; MA 72 Univ of SD - Vermillion; Sp-Lang Path, Vermillion Pub Sch, **SLP**

Ferris, Linda L 832 Swisher Road, Pocatello, ID 83201, (208) 343-2583, BS 84 ID St Univ; MS 86 ID St Univ; **SLP**

Ferris, Mrs Linda M 27912 Calle Belmonte, San Juan Capistrano, CA 92675, (714) 639-4990, BA 75 Univ of Redlands; MS 76 Univ of Redlands; Sp-Lang Path, Irvine USD, **SLP**

Ferris, Lora M C 8125 Jefferson Highway, Baton Rouge, LA 70809, (504) 927-2477, BS 73 Univ of VA - Charlottesville; MA 79 LA St Univ - Baton Rouge; **SLP**

Ferris, Marilyn M 9408 Trailhill Drive, Dallas, TX 75238, (214) 341-7169, BA 69 George Washington Univ; MA 78 Northwestern Univ; Sp-Lang Path, Richardson Sp-Lang Cl, **SLP**

Ferris, Virginia A 517-A 14th Avenue, San Francisco, CA 94118, (415) 752-7464, BA 79 San Francisco St Univ; MS 81 San Francisco St Univ; 84–Aud, Private Practice, **A**

Ferris-Reid, Gwen 727 South Gay Street, Auburn, AL 36830, (205) 821-3050, BA 70 OH Univ - Athens; BS 81 Auburn Univ - Auburn; MS 82 Auburn Univ - Auburn; Sp-Lang Path, Auburn City Schools, **SLP**

Ferrito, Joseph R 275 Hospital Parkway, Suite 460, San Jose, CA 95119, (408) 225-0688, BA 76 San Jose St Univ; MA 78 San Jose St Univ; Director of Audiology, Private Practice, **A**

Ferro, Deborah A 1696 Treetop Drive #14B, Erie, PA 16509, (814) 453-5602, BA 78 Allegheny Coll; MA 79 Edinboro Univ of PA; 88–Sp-Lang Path, Lake Erie I of Rehab, **SLP**

Ferry, Nancy Ann 21281 Hazelwood Lane, Boca Raton, FL 33428, (305) 973-8642, BA 84 Univ of WI - Eau Claire; MS 85 Univ of WI - Eau Claire; **SLP**

Ferry, Dr Peggy C Dev Neurol Branch/NINCDS NIH, Federal Bldg Room 816, 7550 Wisconsin Avenue, Bethesda, MD 20892, (301) 496-6701, MD 59 (NS) Univ of OR; 79–Prof of Pediatrics & Neuro, U of AZ

Fers, Mrs Therese 89 Hopyard Road, Stafford Springs, CT 06076, (203) 429-6316, BA 74 Rutger's St Univ - Douglas Coll; MS 75 Rutgers St Univ -N Brunswick; 88–Sp-Lang Path, Mansfield PS, **SLP**

Fertig, Kurt Robert Ossd, 999 Locust Northeast, Salem, OR 97303, **A**

Fertig-Friedman, Beth L 2675 Henry Hudson Parkway, Apartment 6E, Bronx, NY 10463, (212) 904-2786, BA 68 CUNY - City College; MA 69 Columbia Univ Teachers Coll; Sp-Lang Path, Albert Einstein Hosp, **SLP**

Fertitta, Mrs Annette T 5137 MacArthur Boulevard, New Orleans, LA 70114-5341, (504) 392-6202, BA 82 Southeastern LA Univ; ME 84 Southeastern LA Univ; 83–Sp-Lang Path, Jefferson Parish Sch Bd, **SLP**

Fertman-Wolff, Dr Joan C 1376 6th Avenue, San Francisco, CA 94122, (415) 665-8344, BA 60 CUNY - Queens Coll; MA 61 Columbia Univ Teachers Coll; PH 71 (NS) Univ of Southern CA; Director, Community Sp Lang & Hrng Serv, **SLP**

Ferullo, Dr Robert J Northeastern University, 360 Huntington Avenue, Boston, MA 02115, BS 58 Boston Univ; ME 61 Boston Univ; ED 61 (NS) Boston Univ; Prof, Northeastern Univ, **SLP A**

Fesenmeyer, Nancy 1736 12th Avenue, Coralville, IA 52241, (319) 338-6220, BA 72 Univ of IA; MA 74 Univ of IA; Sp-Lang Path, Grantwood AEA, **SLP**

Feskanin, Catherine 223 Greenwood Avenue, Jenkintown, PA 19046, (215) 539-8550, BS 80 Bloomsburg Univ of PA; MS 81 Bloomsburg Univ of PA; Sp-Lang Path, Montg Co Iu, **SLP ACE**

Feske, Mrs Susanne R 4314 Appleton Way, Wilmington, NC 28403, (919) 392-1497, BA 72 Univ of Southwestern LA; MS 76 Lamar Univ; Sp-Lang Path, Private Practice, **SLP**

Feskens, Cornelius Jackson Esd, 101 North Grape Street, Medford, OR 97501, (503) 776-8550, BS 63 Western OR St Coll; MS 69 Western OR St Coll; 65–Dir of Spec Ed, Jackson Ed Serv Dist, **SLP**

Festa, Dorothy Colucci 13 Garfield Place, Massapequa, NY 11758, (212) 596-5742, BA 78 CUNY - Brooklyn Coll; MA 85 Long Island U - CW Post Ctr; 83–Sp-Lang Path, NYC Board of Education, **SLP**

Festerling, Jane S 920 Ward Avenue #5G, Honolulu, HI 96814, (808) 737-9730, BS 57 Univ of MO - Columbia; MA 59 Univ of MO - Columbia; Sp-Lang Path, Hawaii State Dept of Ed, **SLP**

Feth, Dr Lawrence L OH State U Sp & Hearing Sci, 324 Derby Hall, 154 North Oval Mall, Columbus, OH 43210, (614) 292-8207, OB 65 OH St Univ; PH 69 (Bio Acoustics) Univ of Pittsburgh - Pittsburgh; 88–Prof, Ohio State Univ

Fetherston, Cynthia Powell 8995 Glen Alder Way, Sacramento, CA 95826-4051, (916) 369-1845, MS 85 CA St Univ - Sacramento; BA 83 CA St Univ - Sacramento; Aud, Kaiser Permenente Hosp, **A**

Fetherston, Gerald J 510 61st Street, Kenosha, WI 53140, **SLP**

Fett, Cynthia Marie 1617 Country Lakes Drive, #103, Naperville, IL 60540, (312) 629-8900, BS 86 Univ of SD - Vermillion; MA 87 Western IL Univ

Fetterer, Mrs Kimberly James P O Box 183, Jacksonville, IL 62650, (217) 243-7428, BS 86 Western MI Univ; MA 87 Western MI Univ; 87–Sp-Lang Path, Fair Rivers Special Educ Dist, **SLP**

Fetterman, Mrs Sally Ann 715 Avondale Road, Erdenheim, PA 19118, (215) 836-9478, BS 81 Bloomsburg Univ of PA; MS 82 Bloomsburg Univ of PA; Sp-Lang Path, **SLP**

Fetters, Mrs Marcia L G 9238 Kingsboro Court, Brentwood, TN 37027, (615) 371-8455, BS 75 Ball St Univ; MA 77 Ball St Univ; **SLP**

Fettinger, Maryfran Camelio 5 Ridgeview Drive, Rochester, NY 14617-4932, (716) 271-0680, BA 72 SUNY - Coll at Geneseo; MA 86 Montclair St Coll; **A**

Fetzer, Mrs Barbara J 13731 Palm Road, Dale City, VA 22193, (703) 590-6983, BS 75 East TN St Univ; MS 76 Minot St Univ

Feudo, Dr Peter, Jr 136 New Bridge Road, Sudbury, MA 01776, (617) 732-5601, **SLP A**

Feuer, Lois Rachel 73 Perham Street, West Roxbury, MA 02132, (617) 323-3925, MS 85 Boston Univ; **SLP**

Feuer, Mrs Shari Lynn 205 Moore Lane, Washingtonville, NY 10992, (914) 496-2925, BA 85 SUNY - Coll at Cortland; MA 87 CUNY - Hunter Coll; 88–Sp-Lang Path, Orange-Ulster Co BOCES, **SLP**

Feuer, Tammy Ebeling 1 Long Bow Drive, Sewell, NJ 08080, (609) 757-3812, BA 80 Trenton St Coll; MA 82 Temple Univ; 86–Dir Sp-Lang Path, Lourdes Reg Rehab Ctr, **SLP ACE**

Feuerberg, Mrs Lydia E 4820 Scale Court, Las Cruces, NM 88001, (915) 542-6561, BS 71 TX Woman's Univ; MA 77 Univ of IA; Sp/Lang Path, Private Practice, **SLP**

Feuerman, Laurie 46 West 75th Street #2, New York, NY 10023, (212) 496-7868, BS 55 CUNY - Brooklyn Coll; MS 70 Adelphi Univ; SLP Consult, Private Practice, **SLP**

Feuerstein, James F 2385 Genesee Street, Piffard, NY 14533, (716) 243-4015, BS 75 SUNY - Coll at Geneseo; MA 77 SUNY - Coll at Geneseo; PH 88 (Aud) SUNY - Center at Buffalo; Prof, SUNY-Geneseo, **A**

Feurstein, Elizabeth 114 Lionsgate, Columbia, SC 29223, (803) 788-5611, BA 68 Furman Univ; ME 73 Univ of SC - Columbia; Sp/Lang Path, Private Practice, **SLP**

Few, Linda J 66 Center Street, Crystal Lake, IL 60014, (815) 385-4421, BS 76 Bloomsburg Univ of PA; MA 77 Western MI Univ; 87–Sp-Lang Path, McHenry Sch Dist #15, **SLP A**

Fey, Daniel William Rt 5 Box 458, Covington, VA 24426, (703) 962-3929, BS 83 Old Dominion Univ; MS 85 Radford Univ; Aud, Alleghany Highlands Hrng & Sp Ctr, **A**

Fey, Dr Marc E Prog In Communication Disorder, Elborn College, Univ Of Western Ontario, London, ON, Canada N6G 1H1, (519) 679-6465, BA 74 Wichita St Univ; ME 75 Univ of GA; PH 81 Purdue Univ - West Lafayette; Associate Professor, University of Western Ontario, **SLP**

Fey, Mrs Sandra H 28 Askin Street, London, ON, Canada N6C 1E3, (519) 679-2111, BA 68 SUNY - Center at Buffalo; ME 74 Univ of GA; Instr, U of Wn On Dept of Commun Dis, **SLP**

Feyerabend, Lucy 235 Melrose Street, Providence, RI 02907, (508) 675-8396, BS 81 Univ of RI; BA 78 Univ of RI; Sp-Lang Path, Fall River PS, **SLP**

Fezette, Mrs Susan Lynn 123 Cypress Avenue, Tiverton, RI 02878, (617) 678-2901, **SLP**

Fiala, Kathleen J 5704 Independence #2-W, Oak Forest, IL 60452, (312) 687-0359, BS 85 Univ of IL - Urbana; MA 88 Univ of IL - Urbana

Fiala, Louise Ann 2236 Electra Avenue, Simi Valley, CA 93065, (209) 227-1671, MA 88 CA St Univ - Fresno; 88–Aud, E Ronn Heiner MD Inc

Fialkoff, Donna Box 623, Shelburne, VT 05482, (803) 985-2985, MS 87 Univ of VT; **SLP**

Fibel, Yvette J 15435 Jeffrey Road, Suite 127, Irvine, CA 92720, **SLP ACE**

Ficca, Mrs Jo-Ann G 21 Benford Drive, Princeton Junction, NJ 08550, (609) 799-2726, BA 68 Marymount Coll; ME 71 PA St Univ - Univ Park; MA 85 Rider Coll; Dir, Associates InSpeech & Lang, **SLP ACE**

Fichman, Mrs Marilyn T 5532 Wolseley Avenue, Cote St Luc, PQ, Canada H4W 2L2, (514) 487-4755, BA 63 McGill Univ - Quebec; MA 68 Univ of Houston - Univ Park; Sp/Lang Path, Lakeshore Sch Bd, **SLP**

Fichtel, Mrs Dina Helene 3170 Arbor Lane, Hollywood, FL 33021, (305) 987-2115, BA 83 Univ of FL; MA 85 Univ of FL; Sp-Lang Path, Stephanie Stryker Ph D, **SLP**

Fichter, Mrs Dana S P O Box 1050, Pine Valley, CA 92062, (619) 473-8339, BS 68 Eastern NM Univ; MS 75 UT St Univ; Tchr, Lakeside Union Sch Dist, **SLP**

Ficken, Mrs Elizabeth Anne 2150 Nad Road #B-13, North Charleston, SC 29418, (803) 723-4627, BA 78 Columbia Coll; MA 85 SC St Coll; **SLP**

Fickenscher, Saundra R 55 Sloping Hills Cove, Grand Forks, ND 58201, (701) 780-5185, ME 74 Univ of OR; MA 78 Univ of ND; Admin Human Resources, Utd Hosp, **SLP**

Ficke-Richtarik, Mrs Karen Lynne 326 North Cherokee, Apartment 2, McCook, NE 69001, (308) 345-2131, BS 86 Univ of NE - Lincoln; MS 87 Univ of NE - Lincoln

Fidler, David B 5239 East Ocean Boulevard, Apartment #5, Long Beach, CA 90803, (213) 861-2891, BS 80 Bowling Green St Univ; MA 81 Bowling Green St Univ; 86–Sp-Lang Path, Los Angeles Co Ofc of Educ, **SLP**

Fidrych-Puzzo, Mrs Holly Fidrych-Communication Consult, 24 Oxford Street, Springfield, MA 01108, (617) 793-8055, BS 75 Worcester St Coll; MS 81 Worcester St Coll; Clinical Director, Worcester State College, **SLP ACE**

Fieber, Deborah Osman 175 Drum Hill Avenue, Wilton, CT 06897, (203) 834-1374, BA 77 Skidmore Coll; MS 79 Univ of NC - Chapel Hill; Sp-Lang Path, Greenwich Public Schools, **SLP**

Fiebert, Janet Diaz RFD 4, Lakewood Drive, Katonah, NY 10536, BA 80 CUNY - Lehman Coll; MA 82 CUNY - Lehman Coll; SLP, N Westchester Cen for Sp Dis

Fiebig, Pamela J Northwestern University Hearing Clinic, 2299 Sheridan Road, Evanston, IL 60208, (312) 491-3165, BA 79 MI St Univ; MA 81 Northwestern Univ; Lecturer Clinical Super, Northwestern U, **A ACE**

Fiedel, Paula L 54 Old Boonton Road, Denville, NJ 07834, (201) 625-1427, BA 56 Montclair St Coll; MS 86 William Paterson Coll; 87–Sp-Lang Path, Paterson Bd of Educ, **SLP**

Fiedler, Dr Irma Gail 3234 North Lake Drive, Milwaukee, WI 53211, (414) 259-9090, BA 57 NY Univ; MA 67 Univ of WI - Milwaukee; PH 81 (Educational Psychology) Univ of WI - Milwaukee; Assoc Chrpn Dept Phy Med&Rehab, Med Coll of WI, **SLP**

Fiedler, Mrs Mary Byrne 1091 Hecker Drive, Elgin, IL 60120, (312) 931-5260, BA 84 Elmhurst Coll; MA 87 Northern IL Univ - De Kalb; 87–Sp-Lang Path, Pioneer Ctr Birth to Three Prog

Fiedler, Rosmarie 1439 Holly Street N W, Washington, DC 20012, (202) 723-3535, BS 84 Univ of the DC; MS 87 Univ of the DC; **SLP**

Fiedler-Fuhrman, Judith Lynn 190 East Big Springs Road, Riverside, CA 92507, (714) 787-0408, MS 86 Univ of Redlands; 87–Sp-Lang Path, Richards Educ Ther Ctr Big Springs Sch, **SLP**

Fiegenbaum, Ilana Reiss 681 Skynob Drive, Ann Arbor, MI 48105, (313) 572-3565, MA 85 Univ of IL - Urbana; **SLP**

Field, David G 2220 Walter Drive, Ann Arbor, MI 48103, **SLP**

Field, Mrs Elizabeth Carol 12341 Well Spring Wy #302B, Lake Ridge, VA 22192, (703) 680-5959, BS 83 SUNY - Coll at Geneseo; MA 84 SUNY - Coll at Geneseo; Aud, **A**

Field, Mrs Elizabeth Ives 189 Norfolk Street, Bangor, ME 04401, (207) 942-3760, BA 70 Univ of NH; ME 71 Boston Univ; SLP, Private Practice, **SLP**

Field, Elizabeth McCracken 154 Louise Lane, San Mateo, CA 94403, (415) 574-4406, BS 83 Univ of OR; MS 86 CA St Univ - Hayward; 87–Sp-Lang Path, Mills-Penninsula Hosp, **SLP**

Field, Mrs Janice Lynn 111 Masters Circle, Lima, OH 45805, (216) 382-7700, MA 82 Cleveland St Univ; **SLP**

Field, Mrs Kathleen J Rd 4 Box 4197A, Stroudsburg, PA 18360, (717) 992-7561, BS 73 East Stroudsburg Univ of PA; MS 78 Bloomsburg Univ of PA; Sp/Lang Path, Blairstown Twp Elem Sch, **SLP**

Field, Terri Lynne 872 Dorchester Circle, Lodi, CA 95240-6634, (209) 467-6345, **SLP**

Field, Dr William G 29 Laurel Hill Drive, Cherry Hill, NJ 08003, (609) 429-1037, BS 47; MD 51 (NS); Pediatrician, Private Practice

Fielder, Mrs Jeanne Holmberg 14720 Borman, Omaha, NE 68138, (402) 978-7074, BA 81 Kearney St Coll; MS 82 Kearney St Coll; SLP, Omaha Pub Sch, **SLP**

Fielder, Kay L G 2904 West Elmlawn, Anaheim, CA 92804, (714) 821-0800, BS 75 IL St Univ - Normal; MA 76 Univ of IL - Urbana; Sp-Lang Path, Gr Anaheim Selpa, **SLP**

Fielder, Mrs Susan B 5182 Yearling Avenue, Irvine, CA 92714, (714) 854-7002, MA 85 CA St Univ - Fullerton; SLP, Anaheim City School District, **SLP**

Fielding, Dolores P 8647 Braddock Avenue, Alexandria, VA 22309, (202) 767-7758, BS 60 Bloomsburg Univ of PA; ME 61 PA St Univ - Univ Park; ME 61 PA St Univ - Univ Park; Cihef/Sp & Hrng Servs, Dc Village, **SLP A**

Fields, Mrs Danell Liberda 2602 Old Humble Road, Humble, TX 77347, (713) 441-2171, MS 82 Univ of North TX; BS 80 Baylor Univ; Sp-Lang Path, Arlington ISD, **SLP**

Fields, Dorothy J 420 Baker Avenue #208, Hazard, KY 41701, (606) 439-4836, MS 88 Univ of OK Medical Center; 88–Sp-Lang Path, Appalachian Reg Med Ctr

Fields, Elaine A 4715 Wakefield Chapel Road, Annandale, VA 22003, BA 61 SC St Coll; ME 71 SC St Coll; ED 81 (NS) Vanderbilt Univ; **SLP**

Fields, Elyse J 32 Beatrice Lane, Old Bethpage, NY 11804, **SLP**

Fields, Mrs Jody Thompson 1115-11th Street, Greeley, CO 80631, (303) 352-5356, BS 79 Phillips Univ; MA 80 Univ of IL - Urbana; Sp-Lang Path, Private Practice, **SLP**

Fields, Mrs Karen A 2588 North Summit, Milwaukee, WI 53211, (414) 425-2554, BS 74 Univ of WI - Milwaukee; MS 76 Univ of WI - Milwaukee; Sp-Lang Path, Franklin Sch Dist #5, **SLP**

Fields, Mrs Kathryn Ann Route 2, Jordan Branch Rd, Mars Hill, NC 28754, BS 81 Radford Univ; MS 82 Radford Univ; Sp-Lang Path, Buncomb Co Pub Sch, **SLP**

Fields, Mrs Marjorie R 95 Harmony Hill Road, Harwinton, CT 06791, (203) 485-1379, MS 87 Southern CT St Univ; 88–Sp-Lang Path, Thomaston Bd of Educ

Fields, Mrs Michelle 2632 Beacon Hill Drive, Apartment 302, Auburn Hills, MI 48057, (313) 373-2974, BA 83 MI St Univ; MA 85 MI St Univ; 88–Sp-Lang Path, William Beaumont Hosp, **SLP**

Fields, Mrs Sondra Kay Box 160, Greenville, TX 75401, (214) 454-3082, BA 69 NM St Univ; MA 70 NM St Univ; Resource Teacher, Lone Oak School, **SLP**

Fields, Mrs Susan E Gould 7220 South Prestwick Place, Miami Lakes, FL 33014, (305) 823-5332, BS 63 Syracuse Univ; ME 64 Boston Univ; **A**

Fields, Dr Thomas A P O Box 160, Greenville, TX 75401, (214) 454-3082, MA 70 TX Tech Univ; MA 71 NM St Univ; PH 74 (NS) Univ of TX - Austin; 86–Owner/Admin, Associated Rehabilitation Svcs Inc, **SLP**

Fields, Tobey Kempler 285 N 100 E Box 31, Wellsville, UT 84339, (801) 752-7162, SLP, Cache Co Schools, **SLP**

Fields, Tracee Lane 1200 Southwest Avenue, Sioux Falls, SD 57105, (605) 339-7501, BA 82 Univ of SD - Vermillion; MA 83 Univ of SD - Vermillion; 86–Chief SLP and Aud, McKennan Hosp & Rehab Ctr, **SLP**

Fields, Mrs Vicki J 3561 Sharon Drive, Eau Claire, WI 54701, (715) 835-5487, BS 70 Univ of WI - Eau Claire; MA 79 Northern IL Univ - De Kalb; **SLP**

Fields, Yolanda Gail 8-04 Deer Creek Drive, Plainsboro, NJ 08536, (609) 799-3951, BS 83 Hampton Univ; MS 87 Univ of the DC; 87–Sp-Lang Path, Med Ctr at Princeton, **SLP**

Fields-Cohen, Mary T 131 East Santa Fe Avenue, Santa Fe, NM 87501, (505) 848-8877, BA 80 Mary Washington Coll; MS 81 Loyola Coll; 87–Inpatient Prog Dir, St Joseph Rehabilitation Ctr, **SLP**

Fields-Kuhn, Mrs Sandra 223 Monmouth Road, West Long Branch, NJ 07764, (201) 229-4089, ME 83 Kean Coll of NJ; Sp & Hrng Cen/W Lng Br Med Pk, **A**

Fife, Pamela B 157 Piedra Loop, Los Alamos, NM 87544, (505) 672-1348, BA 74 NM St Univ; MA 76 NM St Univ; MA 78 NM St Univ; 88–Sp-Lang Path, CES, **A**

Fifer, Mrs Gretchen G 201 Carlisle Avenue, Winnsboro, SC 29180, (803) 635-3225, BS 54 Western MI Univ; OM 79 Univ of SC - Columbia; Sp-Lang Path, Fairfield Co Sch, **SLP**

Fifer, Linda S 217 Dixon Avenue, Missoula, MT 59801-8721, (406) 728-4881, BA 74 Kent St Univ; MS 75 Kent St Univ; Superv-Sp-Path & Aud, Missoula Comm Hosp Rehab Cen, **SLP**

Fifer, Dr Robert C 2610 Southmoor Drive, Champaign, IL 61821, (217) 337-3130, BS 74 Univ of NE - Omaha; MA 76 Central MI Univ; PH 85 (NS) Baylor Coll of Medicine; Chief Audiology & SLP, Carle Clinic Association, **A**

Fifer, Mrs Sara Jane 205 Dover Road, Brownsburg, IN 46112, (317) 852-6576, MS 87 Purdue Univ - West Lafayette; 88–Sp-Lang Path, Old Natl Trail Spec Svcs Coop, **SLP**

Figi-Murzyn, Mrs Denise Ann 1565 Coloma Court, Wheaton, IL 60187, (312) 665-5071, MS 78 Marquette Univ; MS 79 Marquette Univ; Sp-Lang Path, Sch Assoc Spec Ed/Dupage Co, **SLP**

Figueroa, Lorraine 114 Deanza Street, San Gabriel, CA 91775, BS 82 Univ of CT; MS 87 Southern CT St Univ; Sp-Lang Path, Los Angeles USD, **SLP**

Figueroa, Rosario Annette 2105 Brickell Avenue #311, Miami, FL 33129, (305) 856-1651, Sp-Lang Path, Jackson Memorial Hospital, **SLP**

Figula, Diane A 6188 Deer Path Court, Manassas, VA 22111, (703) 978-9315, BS 67 Indiana Univ of PA; MA 70 Catholic Univ of America; 70–Sp-Lang Path, Fairfax Co Pub Schls, **SLP**

Fike, Mrs Barbara C 3823 Harwick Drive, Murrysville, PA 15688, (412) 327-2628, BS 75 Edinboro Univ of PA; MA 79 CA St Univ - Los Angeles; 88–Aud, Pittsburgh Otological Assoc, **A**

Fike, Mrs Suzanne M 4143 Crestmanor Drive, Hamilton, OH 45011, (513) 856-7890, BS 85 Indiana Univ of PA; MS 87 Miami Univ - Oxford; 87–Sp-Lang Path, Butler Co Bd Ment Ret

Fike, Mrs Suzanne R 5084 Greendale, Troy, MI 48098, (313) 528-2305, BA 74 Univ of IA; MA 75 Univ of IA; Sp-Lang Path, Private Practice, **SLP**

Filak, Mrs Marilyn Kimball Box 176, Underhill Center, VT 05490, (802) 863-5885, BS 75 OH Univ - Athens; MA 76 Montclair St Coll; Sp/Lang Path, Burlington Pub Sch, **SLP**

Filak, Mrs Patricia C Rd 1 Box 201 B, Perryopolis, PA 15473, (412) 437-3237, BS 66 CA Univ of PA; ME 71 CA Univ of PA; 66–Instructional Advisor (S/H/L), Intermediate Unit I, **SLP**

Filaseta, Mrs Hope G 38 Glenwood Drive, Hauppauge, NY 11788, (516) 543-0814, BA 74 CUNY - Lehman Coll; MA 75 CUNY - Queens Coll; **SLP ACE**

Filbert, Mrs Susan W 1211 Havenwood Road, Baltimore, MD 21218, (301) 667-0190, BS 74 Bowling Green St Univ; MS 75 Towson St Univ; Sp-Lang Path, Baltimore Co Bd of Ed, **SLP**

Files, Mrs Wendy Welch 1221 Crescendo Drive, Roseville, CA 95678, BA 76 CA St Univ - Chico; MA 78 CA St Univ - Chico; Sp-Lang Path, Vna, **SLP**

Fili, Patricia Iannelli 3124 Levick Street, Philadelphia, PA 19149, (215) 289-8320, BS 80 West Chester Univ of PA; MA 82 Trenton St Coll; 82–Sp-Lang Path, Sch Dist of Philadelphia, **SLP**

Filiberto, Mrs Lisa Ann 9 Carmichael Street, Amsterdam, NY 12010, (518) 370-7505, BS 84 Ithaca Coll; MS 86 Coll of Saint Rose; 87–Sp-Lang Path, New York State Autism Prog, **SLP**

Filice, Lori Demeriez 10330-140 Street, Edmonton, AB, Canada T5N 2L6, (403) 471-2262, BS 85; MS 85 Univ of AZ; 86–Sp-Lang Path, Glenrose Rehab Hosp, **SLP**

Filipek, Kathleen Ready 1254 Lakeland Avenue, Lakewood, OH 44107, (216) 221-5470, BA 74 Cleveland St Univ; MA 80 Cleveland St Univ; **SLP**

Filipiak, Debra Ann 7765 West Oklahoma Avenue, Apartment 8, Milwaukee, WI 53219, (414) 877-3314, BS 80 Marquette Univ; MS 81 Marquette Univ; Sp-Lang Path, Randall Consol Sch, **SLP**

Filkins, Emily 135 Lincoln Drive, Mount Vernon, IA 52314, BS 76 Univ of IA; MA 78 Univ of IA; **SLP ACE**

Fill, Michelle Ridley & Fill Sp & Lang Assoc, 4909 Hampden Lane, Suite One, Bethesda, MD 20814, (202) 233-1969, BS 69 OH Univ - Athens; MS 74 Univ of the DC; Sp/Lang Path, Ridley & Fill Sp & Lang Assocs, **SLP**

Filley, Florence S University Of Wisconsin, 1975 Willow Drive, Room 335, Madison, WI 53706, (608) 262-3951, BA 51 IN Univ - Bloomington; MA 57 IN Univ - Bloomington; 63–Sp-Lang Path, Univ of Wis-Madison, **SLP A**

Fillinger-Kraus, Francine 9 Old Long Ridge Road, Stamford, CT 06903, (203) 977-4560, MA 68 Eastern MI Univ; Sp-Lang Path, Stamford Pub Sch, **SLP**

Fillmore, Mrs Jane M 50-A Embassy Square #5, Tonawanda, NY 14150, (716) 837-2441, BS 84 SUNY - Coll at Buffalo; MS 86 SUNY - Coll at Buffalo; **SLP**

Fillmore, Rebecca Gail 20 Lake Shore Drive, Palm Harbor, FL 34684-1213, (813) 938-3763, BS 82 Auburn Univ - Auburn; OM 83 Auburn Univ - Auburn; 86–Sp-Lang Path, Gulfside Elem, **SLP ACE**

Filosa, Alfred A Vero Audiological Services, 777 37th Street C-101, Vero Beach, FL 32960, (407) 567-1164, BA 69 Hofstra Univ; MA 70 Hofstra Univ; MA 73 SUNY - Center at Buffalo; 77–Aud, Vero Aud Scrv Becker&Stubbs MD, **A**

Fils, Mrs Deborah J 4644 Tobias Avenue, Sherman Oaks, CA 91403-2823, (818) 501-7077, BA 80 Univ of CA - Santa Barbara; OM 82 Univ of WA; Aud, Irwin Lehroff PhD and Associates, **A**

Filson, Kay S Audiology & Speech Pathology (126), Veterans Administration Medical Center, 1660 South Columbian Way, Seattle, WA 98108, (206) 764-2404, BS 73 CO St Univ; MS 76 Univ of WA; 76–Aud, Seattle VA Med Ctr, **A**

Filter, Dr Maynard D 42 East Laurel, Harrisonburg, VA 22801, (703) 433-6630, BA 64 Adrian Coll; MA 66 Bowling Green St Univ; PH 71 (NS) Bowling Green St Univ; Dept Head, James Madison U, **SLP ACE**

Fina, Ruth B 4723 North Hollywood Avenue, Milwaukee, WI 53211, (414) 962-3200, BS 68 Marquette Univ; MS 70 Marquette Univ; Assoc Reg Mktg Mgr, New Medico Head Injury Sys, **SLP ACE**

Finan, Colleen Marie 2624 Rochester Road #8, Royal Oak, MI 48067, (313) 424-8450, BA 84 MI St Univ; MA 86 Wayne St Univ - Sch of Med; Audiologist, Lucas Hearing Aid Service, **A**

Fincher, Cynthia K 14407 Filly Court, Centreville, VA 22020, (703) 378-2598, **SLP**

Finchler, Mrs Michele Salzberg 3 Ennis Drive, Hazlet, NJ 07730, (201) 739-0892, BA 82 CUNY - Brooklyn Coll; MS 84 CUNY - Brooklyn Coll; 85–Sp-Lang Path, Early Intervention Program Inc, **SLP**

Finch-Williams, Dr Amy 267 Princess Street, Apartment #305, Kingston, ON, Canada K7L 1B4, (613) 549-1191, BS 69 CO St Univ; MS 72 CO St Univ; PH 81 (Sp-Lang Path) Univ of KS; 88–Research Assoc, Human Comm Unit Hotel Dieu Hosp, **SLP**

Finck, Carolyn D 307 West Clark, Clarinda, IA 51632, (712) 542-4510, BS 74 Northwest MO St Univ; MS 80 Northwest MO St Univ; SLP, Loess Hills AEA #13, **SLP**

Finck, Mrs Jo Anne M 29600 Franklin Road #4, Southfield, MI 48034-1110, (313) 271-6006, BA 53 Univ of MI - Ann Arbor; MS 78 Univ of MI - Ann Arbor; Aud, Oakwood Audiological Services, **A ACE**

Finck, Sara V 144 Waterman Street, Providence, RI 02906, (401) 351-4770, BA 63 Univ of RI; MA 72 Univ of RI; 69–Sp-Lang Path, Private Practice, **SLP**

Findlay, Cynthia Marie 1317 Highway 52, Antigo, WI 54409, (715) 623-4424, BA 85 Univ of WI - Eau Claire; MS 86 Univ of WI - Eau Claire; Sp-Lang Path, Manitowoc Schl Dstr, **SLP**

Findlay, Laurie Hamilton 45 Felbrigg Avenue, Toronto, ON, Canada M5M 2M2, (416) 489-5381, **SLP**

Findlay, Dr Robert C 611 Woodside Road, Pittsburgh, PA 15221, (412) 624-6762, MA 62 Univ of Aberdeen - Scotland; MA 67 Temple Univ-Tyler Sch of Art; PH 71 (NS) Temple Univ-Tyler Sch of Art; Asst Cl Prof, U of Pitt, **A**

Findley, Mrs Suzy Streamer 7225 La Luna Court, Citrus Heights, CA 95621, (916) 453-3517, BA 84 Univ of the Pacific; MS 85 Univ of Redlands; 87–Sp-Lang Path, UC Davis Med Ctr, **SLP**

Findlow, Julie Gail 1105 San Nicolas Circle, Tucson, AZ 85704, (602) 385-2335, BA 62 Grinnell Coll; MS 82 Univ of AZ; Sp-Lang Path, San Manuel USD #8, **SLP**

Fine, Catherine 7150 San Mateo Blvd #286, Dallas, TX 75223, (214) 327-7223, MS 87 Univ of TX - Dallas; 87–Sp-Lang Path, InSpeech Inc, **SLP**

Fine, Gail P Speech & Hearing Associates, 105 South Bryant, Suite 403, Edmond, OK 73034, (405) 271-4716, BA 65 Emory Univ; MS 67 Vanderbilt Univ; MA 67 G Peabody Coll-Vanderbilt U; Aud, Dept of Otor, **A**

Fine, Mrs Jan Sliger 11020 Farr Drive, Knoxville, TN 37922, (615) 966-8578, BS 81 Univ of TN - Knoxville; MA 82 Univ of TN - Knoxville; Sp-Lang Path, Clinton City Schs, **SLP**

Fine, Janis B 9539 North Lorel, Skokie, IL 60077, (312) 965-3733, BS 75 Univ of IL - Urbana; MS 76 Univ of IL - Urbana; Sp-Lang Path, Chicago Bd of Ed, **SLP**

Fine, Jody E 711 Broadway, Seattle, WA 98122, (206) 324-6264, BA 82 Univ of CO - Boulder; MS 85 Univ of WA; 85–Aud, Ear Associates Inc PS, **A**

Fine, Paula S 330 Rolling Rock Road, Mountainside, NJ 07092, (201) 654-3322, BA 55 Brandeis Univ; MA 56 Northwestern Univ; Sp-Lang Path/Aud, Private Practice, **SLP A**

Fine, Roslyn A 45228 Patrick Drive, Canton, MI 48187, (616) 798-7245, BS 67 Syracuse Univ; MS 69 Univ of MI - Ann Arbor; Sp-Lang Path, Reeths Puffer Bd of Ed, **SLP**

Fine, Susan Kaplan 226 Abilene Lane, Vernon Hills, IL 60061, BS 77 Univ of IL - Urbana; MA 78 Univ of IL - Urbana; Aud, Lake McHenry Reg Prog, **A**

Fineberg, Miriam Sharon 370 Ridelle Avenue #2808, Toronto, ON, Canada M6B 4B4, (416) 964-9595, **A**

Finefrock, Mrs Joan Forney Tinken Mercy Medical Center, 1320 Timken Mercy Drive, Canton, OH 44708, (216) 837-3042, BS 71 Kent St Univ; MA 83 Univ of Akron; Director Sp-Lang Path, Timken Mercy Med Ctr, **SLP**

Finelli, Alexandra 210 Cinnabar Circle, Williamston, MI 48895, **SLP**

Fineman-Singer, Mrs Sharon A 28657 Oak Crest Court, Farmington Hills, MI 48018, (313) 252-4000, BS 58 Wayne St Univ; ME 67 Wayne St Univ; Sp-Lang Path, Detroit Osteopathic Hosp Corp, **SLP**

Fine-Marker, Sandra Bea 40 East 21st Street 7th Floor, New York, NY 10010, (212) 582-9100, BA 83 Hahnemann Univ Grad Sch; MS 71 Temple Univ; Sp-Lang Path, Child Dev Ctr, **SLP**

Finerty, Mrs Mary Ellen 5948 South 94th East Pl, Tulsa, OK 74145-8330, (918) 254-8973, **A**

Finger, Mrs Myrna L 800 5th Avenue, New York, NY 10021, **SLP**

Finger, Sylvia S 4816 Green Acres Court, Metairie, LA 70003, (504) 456-1398, BS 69; OM 78 LA St Univ - N O Medical Ctr; Sp-Lang Path, Private Practice, **SLP**

Fingerhood, Barbara 125 Beacon Hill Drive, Dobbs Ferry, NY 10522, BA 64 CUNY - City College; MA 65 Columbia Univ Teachers Coll; **SLP**

Fingerle, Dr Clarence O 2000 South 9th Street, Salt Lake City, UT 84105, (801) 581-2260, BA 47 Brigham Young Univ; MA 52 Brigham Young Univ; PH 66 (NS) Univ of MI - Ann Arbor; Sp-Lang Path/Aud, U of UT Med Sch, **SLP A**

Finitzo, Dr Terese 4305 Glenleigh Drive, Dallas, TX 75220, (214) 353-9038, BS 69 Northwestern Univ; MA 71 Northwestern Univ; PH 75 (NS) Northwestern Univ; Assoc Prof, U of TX at Dallas, **A**

Fink, Janet L 8555 Fair Oaks Crossing, Unit 406, Dallas, TX 75243, (214) 341-3025, BS 79 Southern Methodist Univ; MS 80 Southern Methodist Univ; TX Area Mktg Mgr, InSpeech Inc, **A**

Fink, Mrs Joan Ann 474 Stony Brook Drive, Bridgewater, NJ 08807, (201) 722-6611, BA 63 Hofstra Univ; ME 88 Trenton St Coll; 88–Sp-Lang Path, Rock Brook Sch

Fink, John J 4711 Hydes Road, Hydes, MD 21082, (301) 828-2142, BA 62 CA St Univ - Los Angeles; MA 63 CA St Univ - Los Angeles; Dir/Hrng & Sp Dept, Greater Baltimore Med Cen, **A**

Fink, Joy Elizabeth 128 Lecline Drive, Concord, NC 28025, (704) 786-1831, MA 88 Appalachian St Univ; 88–Sp-Lang Path, Charlotte Mecklenburg Sch Sys

Fink, Karen Smillie 24854 Winona, Dearborn, MI 48124, (313) 593-7725, BA 71 MI St Univ; MS 72 Univ of MI - Ann Arbor; 86–Dir Phy Med & Rehab, Oakwood Hosp, **SLP**

Fink, Mrs Marsha A Smith 2407 South Kanawha Street, Beckley, WV 25801-9905, (304) 256-4555, BS 76 WV Univ; MS 77 WV Univ; Sp/Lang Path, Raleigh Co Bd of Ed, **SLP**

Fink, Maxine E 2056 N W 55th Boulevard #B6, Gainesville, FL 32606, (904) 395-1578, BA 73 Univ of FL; MS 75 FL St Univ; 85–Sp-Lang Path, Sunland Ctr at Gainesville, **SLP**

Fink, Patricia L 4449 Windsor Oaks Circle N E, Marietta, GA 30066, (603) 424-9427, BA 71 MI St Univ; MA 79 MI St Univ; 82–Sp-Lang Path, Private Practice, **SLP ACE**

Fink, Ruth B 726 Cornelia Place, Philadelphia, PA 19118, (215) 248-2560, BA 67 Montclair St Coll; MA 69 Temple Univ-Tyler Sch of Art; Sp/Lang Path, Ruth Fink, **SLP**

Fink, Dr William H 322 Oak Fern Circle, Ormond Beach, FL 32074, (904) 258-8931, BS 67 CA Univ of PA; MS 71 FL St Univ; PH 77 (NS) FL St Univ; Superv Sp-Hrng & Lang, Sch Bd of Volusia Co, **SLP**

Finkbiner, Nina G 1105 Berkshire, Ann Arbor, MI 48104, (313) 665-5778, SLP, Huron Valley Schools, **SLP**

Finkelstein, Alison Briggs 2 Dewey Road, Cheltenham, PA 19012, (215) 635-1606, MA 86 Univ of MD - College Park; 88–Sp-Lang Path, Bryn Mawr Rehab Hosp, **SLP**

Finkelstein, Mrs Dianne Lynn 7 Quail Mews, North Brunswick, NJ 08902, (609) 466-2989, **SLP**

Finkelstein, Mrs Ellen 134 Baker Hill Road, Great Neck, NY 11023, (516) 773-4160, BA 77 CUNY - Queens Coll; MA 78 CUNY - Queens Coll; Aud, Private Practice, **A**

Finkelstein, Mrs Lorraine Sheila 6557 Lasaine Avenue, Van Nuys, CA 91406, (818) 708-3166, BA 80 CA St Univ - Northridge; MA 82 CA St Univ - Northridge; 86–Sp-Lang Path, ERAS, **SLP**

Finkelstein, Naomi G 316 North Kings Road, Los Angeles, CA 90048, (213) 852-0636, BA 74 CA St Univ - Los Angeles; MA 80 CA St Univ - Los Angeles; **SLP**

Finkelstein, Mrs Patricia Auerbach 116 84th Street, Virginia Beach, VA 23451, (804) 425-6743, BS 75 Old Dominion Univ; MS 77 Old Dominion Univ; Sp-Lang Path, Portsmouth Gen Hosp, **SLP**

Finkelstein, Susan Fay 324 East 81 Street, New York, NY 10028, (212) 861-7059, **SLP**

Finkenstadt, Mrs Susan C 9514 Simpson Road, Brewerton, NY 13029, (315) 473-4806, BS 73 CUNY - Queens Coll; MS 75 Syracuse Univ; Sp/Lang Path, St Univ Hosp Coll Med, **SLP**

Fink-Flam, Vivian C 106 Stratford Place, Lakewood, NJ 08701, (201) 370-2773, BA 78 CUNY - Brooklyn Coll; MS 81 CUNY - Brooklyn Coll; Sp-Lang Path, Ocean County Health Dept, **SLP**

Finley, Adam Lewis 2374 Marlboro Street, East Meadow, NY 11554, (718) 464-7500, BS 86 Nazareth Coll of Rochester; MS 87 Nazareth Coll of Rochester

Finley, Anita Trzobiatow 148 South Kane Street, Burlington, WI 53105, BA 81 Univ of WI - Eau Claire; MS 83 Univ of WI - Madison; Sp-Lang Path, Lakeland Sch, **SLP**

Finley, Deborah A 1633 Belvedere Boulevard, Silver Spring, MD 20902, (301) 681-6981, BA 73; MS 75; PH 87 (Communication Sciences) Howard Univ; 88–Sp-Lang Path, Private Practice, **SLP**

Finley, Mrs Eleanor L 704 Robinhood Lane, Ottawa, IL 61350, (815) 433-1907, BS 48 IL St Univ - Normal; Sp-Lang Path, Ottawa Elem Sch, **SLP**

Finley, Laurene T 1414 11th Street N W, Fayette, AL 35555, (205) 932-4611, BS 62 Bob Jones Univ; MS 63 FL St Univ; Sp-Lang Path, Fayette Co Bd Ed, **SLP**

Finley, Patricia Elaine 925 1/2 N W Charlotte, Pullman, WA 99163, (509) 334-9012, MA 88 WA St Univ

Finn, Debra L 16 Standish Road, Wayland, MA 01778, **SLP**

Finn, Janis Susan 826 Chestnut Ridge Drive, Pittsburgh, PA 15205, (412) 787-5144, BS 83 Ithaca Coll; MA 84 Univ of Pittsburgh - Pittsburgh; 85–Sp-Lang Path, Crossroads Speech & Hearing Inc, **SLP**

Finn, Karen Wimmer 2723 Robina, Berkley, MI 48072, (313) 541-1026, Aud, Outer Drive Hosp, **A**

Finn, Mrs Marilyn S 2511 Kellogg, Ames, IA 50010, (515) 232-7583, BS 71 Univ of IA; MA 72 Univ of IA; SLP, Heartland AEA II, **SLP**

Finn, Mary Cecelia 38 Norma Drive, Nashua, NH 03062, (818) 358-5692, BA 82 CA St Univ - Northridge; MA 84 CA St Univ - Northridge; SLP, Valley Hospital Medical Center, **SLP**

Finn, Dr Myrna W 24 Cochituate Road, Newton Highlands, MA 02161, (617) 527-8533, BA 67 McGill Univ - Quebec; ME 70 Boston Univ; ED 79 (Humanistic & Bahavioral Studies) Boston Univ; 72–Prof, Salem State College, **SLP**

Finnegan, Mrs Carolyn Marie 3 South 010 Sunset Drive, Warrenville, IL 60555, (312) 231-1670, BS 83 Northern IL Univ - De Kalb; MA 84 Northern IL Univ - De Kalb; 85–Sp-Lang Path, West Chicago Elementary School, **SLP**

Finnegan, Dr Denis Edward 136 Brookwood Road, Staunton, VA 24401, (703) 885-6601, BA 69 Univ of Charleston; MS 72 Univ of WI - Madison; PH 76 (NS) Univ of WI - Madison; SLP, Private Practice, **SLP**

Finnegan, Eileen Marquerite 1490 Avon Lane, Apt 1335, North Lauderdale, FL 33068, (305) 978-5189, BS 80 Marquette Univ; MA 82 Univ of IA; 88–Sp-Lang Path, Cleveland Clinic Florida, **SLP ACE**

Finnegan, Mrs Sarah Meffley 1171 E Church Street, Marion, OH 43302, (614) 383-2513, BS 80 Miami Univ - Oxford; MS 81 Miami Univ - Oxford; Sp-Lang Path, Marion Ther Cen, **SLP**

Finnegan, Mrs Teri Lynn 2951 Inverloch Circle, Duluth, GA 30136, (404) 497-8167, BA 84 IN Univ - Bloomington; ME 87 Univ of GA

Finnegan-Kelly, Janet E 277 River Street, Braintree, MA 02184, **SLP**

Finnell, Dee Ann 1922 Baldridge Road, Columbus, OH 43221, (614) 272-0509, BS 77 Bowling Green St Univ; MA 83 OH St Univ; SLP, Franklin Co Bd of Mr/Dd, **SLP**

Finnen, Kathleen Ann 3600 Timberlane Drive, Easton, PA 18042, (215) 776-4799, BS PA St Univ - Univ Park; MS 86 PA St Univ - Univ Park; SLP, Sacred Heart Hosp, **SLP**

Finneran, Mary F 166 Roslindale Avenue, Roslindale, MA 02131, (617) 256-7597, BS 62 Boston St Coll; ME 65 Boston St Coll; ME 75 Northeastern Univ; Sp-Lang Path, Chelmsford Pub Sch, **SLP**

Finnerty, Joan S 35 Ferncroft Road, Shrewsbury, MA 01545, BS 57 Nazareth Coll of Rochester; MA 62 Syracuse Univ; **A**

Finnerty, Patricia Cubells 55 Besemer Road, Ithaca, NY 14850, MS 83 Ithaca Coll; Audiologist, Rehabilitation Services Inc, **A**

Finney, Brenda Jo 509 Dekalb, Princeton, MO 64673, (816) 234-3677, BS 80 Central MO St Univ; MS 81 Central MO St Univ; Sp-Lang Path, Children's Mercy Hosp, **SLP**

Finney, Dollye P 26151 Lakeshore #820, Euclid, OH 44132, (216) 541-3148, MA 88 Cleveland St Univ

Finney, John David 355 South Rose Street, Ishpeming, MI 49849, (906) 485-1542, MA 67 Ball St Univ; Dir of Serv, Aud Serv Group, **A**

Finney, Virginia P 410 Deer Run Road, Auburn, AL 36830, (205) 887-6236, OM 81 Auburn Univ - Auburn; Sp/Lang Path, Valley Haven Sch, **SLP**

Finnigan, Cynthia S 1300 Greenhill Avenue, Wilmington, DE 19809, (302) 454-2202, MA 82 Univ of FL; Sp-Lang Path, Jennie Smith-Autistic Prog, **SLP**

Fino, Mary A 217 Exeter Avenue, West Pittston, PA 18643, (717) 655-2725, BS 86 Marywood Coll; MS 87 Vanderbilt Univ; **A**

Finore, Luanne 132 Mattison Avenue, Ambler, PA 19002, BA 79 Temple Univ; MS 82 William Paterson Coll; Sp/Lang Path, Mercer Med Cen, **SLP**

Finsand, Gail DeeAnn 2701 South 9th Avenue, Sioux Falls, SD 57105, (605) 339-8166, BA 82 Univ of SD - Vermillion; MS 84 Univ of WI - Madison; 86–Sp-Lang Path, McKennan Hosp, **SLP**

Finsley, Kathy M 105 Poplar Avenue, Wheeling, WV 26003, (304) 233-2647, BS 73 WV Univ; MS 75 WV Univ; Sp-Lang Path, WV Dept of Educ, **SLP**

Finsmith, Nancy B Rd 1 P O Box 137, Spring Drive, Yorktown Heights, NY 10598, (914) 245-0988, **SLP**

Finstad, Linette Arloine 1606 Marika Road #4, Fairbanks, AK 99709, BA 78 Depauw Univ; MS 81 CO St Univ; 81–Sp-Lang Path, Fairbanks N Star Bor Sch Dist, **SLP**

Fiore, Mrs Carol B 507 East Franklin Avenue, Edgewater Park, NJ 08010, (609) 871-4384, BA 74 CUNY - Brooklyn Coll; BA 79 CUNY - Brooklyn Coll; MA 82 Trenton St Coll; Sp/Lang Path, Camden City Bd of Ed, **SLP A**

Fiorelli, Maria Tirabasso 8874 Ravine Avenue N W, Pickerington, OH 43147, (614) 263-2448, BS 75 OH Univ - Athens; MA 79 OH St Univ; Sp-Lang Path, Columbus Cty Schools, **SLP**

Fiore-Powell, Joanne P 8 Verka Court, Bayport, NY 11705, (516) 472-5722, BS 72 SUNY - Coll at New Paltz; MA 75 Hofstra Univ; Sp-Lang Path, Suffolk Co Bd Ed Serv, **SLP**

Fiori, Carolyn E 2287 Grouse Way, Union City, CA 94587, (415) 574-6433, BA 72 CA St Univ - Sacramento; MA 75 San Francisco St Univ; 88–Adaptive Comptr Tech Spec, Coll of San Mateo, **SLP**

Firemark, Rosalyn 1633 Chelsea Road, Palos Verdes Estates, CA 90274, (818) 885-2856, BA 62 CUNY - Queens Coll; MA 76 CA St Univ - Los Angeles; Aud, CA St U Northridge, **A**

Firestein, Mrs Laura H 1563 East 91st Street, Brooklyn, NY 11236, (718) 531-6017, BA 76 CUNY - Brooklyn Coll; MS 79 CUNY - Brooklyn Coll; 79–Sp-Lang Path, BOCES-NYC, **SLP**

Firestone, Dr Barbara A 13130 Burbank Boulevard, Van Nuys, CA 91401, (213) 781-0360, BA 70 Rutger's St Univ - Douglas Coll; MA 71 Montclair St Coll; PH 76 (NS) Univ of Southern CA; 75–Pres/CEO, The HELP Group, **SLP**

Firestone, Mrs Denise Dickman 73 Greenbay Drive, Boardman, OH 44512, (216) 726-2923, BA 86 OH Univ - Athens; MS 87 OH Univ - Athens; **SLP**

Firestone, Harvey B 19020 Brewster Road, Aurora, OH 44202, (216) 464-5775, BA 68 John Carroll Univ; MA 73 Cleveland St Univ; Aud, Otiron Corp, **A**

Firestone, Mrs Lynn M 23 Worthington Road, Glastonbury, CT 06033, (203) 633-5001, BA 71 Univ of MA - Amherst; MA 72 MI St Univ; Aud, J B Bae MD Pc, **A**

Firestone, Pamela 101 Wright Street, Apartment B, Frostburg, MD 21532, (304) 636-4120, BS 81 CA Univ of PA; MS 85 CA Univ of PA

Firestone, Mrs Sharon P 4560 Ford Street, Beaumont, TX 77706-7419, (504) 292-3239, MS 74 Univ of AZ; Sp-Lang Path, Conroe ISD, **SLP**

Firey, Trina Diane 3 Wytchwood Court #T-2, Baltimore, MD 21209, (301) 889-8166, BS 82 Towson St Univ; MS 84 Loyola Coll; **SLP**

Firgau, Eileen Mary 83 South Adelaide Avenue, Highland Park, NJ 08904, (201) 389-0313, BS 80 Trenton St Coll; MA 87 Trenton St Coll; 84–Sp-Lang Path, Monmouth Co Educ Svcs Comm

Firling, Mrs Janice D 17 Crown Road, Somerset, NJ 08873, (201) 563-0549, BS 67 KS St Univ; MA 70 KS St Univ; Sp-Lang Path Prog Coord, Ctr for Head Injury, **SLP**

Firszt, Mrs Jill Blair 2006 Mayfair Drive, Champaign, IL 61821-6455, (217) 337-3130, BS 78 Univ of IL - Champaign; MA 82 Univ of IL - Champaign; 85–Coord-Chldrn Cochlear Implant Prog, Carle Clinic Association, **A**

Fischbein, Sylvia G 27 Melrose Road, Dix Hills, NY 11746, (516) 427-3777, BA 68 Hofstra Univ; MA 69 Hofstra Univ; Tchr, Commack Pub Sch, **SLP**

Fischbuch, Tracy Stanford 1506 Hillside, College Station, TX 77840, (409) 693-8667, BS 83 UT St Univ; OM 86 Brigham Young Univ; **SLP**

Fischer, Alecia S 11512 Galt Avenue, Wheaton, MD 20902, (202) 234-6624, BS 82 Southwest MO St Univ; MA 85 Southwest MO St Univ; Sp-Lang Path, Private Practice, **SLP**

Fischer, Allen L R R 1 Box 62A, Bonne Terre, MO 63628, (314) 358-5899, BS 74 Southern IL Univ-Edwardsvill; MS 75 Southern IL Univ-Edwardsvill; Sp-Lang Path, Sp & Lang Services, **SLP**

Fischer, Alva S 11 Singley Court, Great Neck, NY 11021, (516) 487-2222, BA 43 CUNY - Brooklyn Coll; MA 47 NY Univ; **SLP**

Fischer, Mrs Anne W 1740 Lehigh Street, Boulder, CO 80303, (303) 494-2155, BA 62 Muhlenberg Coll; MA 66 Univ of MD - College Park; **SLP**

Fischer, Mrs Cathryn Avallone 4621 West Sumac Place, Milwaukee, WI 53219, (414) 321-8013, BS 83 Marquette Univ; MS 84 Univ of WI - Milwaukee; Sp-Lang Path, Salem Grade School, **SLP**

Fischer, Mrs Clare O 1000 East Buchanan Street, Plainfield, IN 46168, (317) 839-6007, BS 41 IN St Univ - Terre Haute; MS 45 IN St Univ - Terre Haute; **SLP A LM**

Fischer, Mrs Debra Joy 136 Old Buggy Court, St Charles, MO 63303-2814, (314) 928-9153, OB 82 Univ of MO - Columbia; OM 84 Univ of MO - Columbia; 87–Sp-Lang Path, United Services Inc, **SLP**

Fischer, Debra K 501 Edwards Road, 2 Wildaire Condos, Greenville, SC 29615, (803) 233-1652, BA 75 Winthrop Coll; MS 76 Winthrop Coll; Sp-Lang Path, Sch Dist of Greenville Co, **SLP**

Fischer, Jayne M 17861 D Lake Carlton Drive, Lutz, FL 33549, (813) 963-0949, BS 80 Auburn Univ - Auburn; MA 81 Kent St Univ; 83–Sp-Lang Path, Dist Sch Bd of Pasco Co, **SLP ACE**

Fischer, Mrs Kathleen 6653 South Sycamore Street, Littleton, CO 80120, (303) 770-6350, BS 59 Univ of ND; MA 64 Univ of WA; Sp/Lang Path, Littleton Pub Schs, **SLP**

Fischer, Mrs Kayleen Lutts 433 Rosebank Avenue, Baltimore, MD 21212, (301) 628-7330, BA 83 Loyola Coll; MS 84 Loyola Coll; SLP, Mt Washington Pedia Hosp, **SLP**

Fischer, Linda G Stringtown Road, New Hope, KY 40052, (606) 336-7764, BA 70 Bellarmine Coll; MS 75 Murray St Univ; Sp-Lang Path, Washington Co Bd of Ed, **SLP**

Fischer, Mrs Marlowe W 8267 Caminito Modena, La Jolla, CA 92037, (619) 481-0171, BA 67 Univ of the Pacific; MA 68 Univ of the Pacific; Instr Cl Superv, Private Practice, **SLP**

Fischer, Dr Martin A Dept Of Hearing And Speech, Childrens National Medical Center, 111 Michigan Avenue N W, Washington, DC 20010, (202) 745-5600, BA 74 Univ of CA - Santa Barbara; MS 79 Central WA Univ; PH 83 (Sp-Lang Path) Univ of OR; 88–Asst Dir, Chldn Hosp Natl Med Ctr, **SLP**

Fischer, Mary L 34 Walnut Street, New Haven, CT 06511, (203) 787-9655, BA 64 Mundelein Coll; MS 77 Southern CT St Univ; Sp-Lang Path, East Haven Ct PS, **SLP**

Fischer, Mrs Maureen R 1810 West Chicago Road, Coldwater, MI 49036, (517) 278-7524, BA 76 MI St Univ; MA 77 MI St Univ; Sp-Lang Path, Branch Independent School Dist, **SLP**

Fischer, Meredith A 3304 Smoketree Common Dr, Pleasanton, CA 94566, (415) 538-2602, BS 73 CA St Univ - Hayward; MA 75 Humboldt St Univ; SLP, Livermore Unif Sch Dist, **SLP**

Fischer, Michelle Anne 2124 NE 62nd Court, Fort Lauderdale, FL 33308, (305) 491-6761, MS 88 FL St Univ

Fischer, Mrs Nadine S U 320 Whitehorse Avenue, PO Box 8925, Trenton, NJ 08650, (609) 585-0777, BA 64 Montclair St Coll; MA 75 Trenton St Coll; Dir, Nadia Communications, **SLP**

Fischer, Natalie B Rock Run Hollow #165, Rock City, IL 61070, (815) 987-7571, BA 74 MI St Univ; MA 75 MI St Univ; SLP/Aud, Serv for Crpld Childn, **SLP**

Fischer, Patricia Lynn 108 Luther Lane, Forney, TX 75126, (214) 596-4603, BS 81 Univ of North TX; MS 84 Univ of North TX; Aud, David M Rubinstein MD, **A**

Fischer, Roberta J 1405 Brandenburg Way, King of Prussia, PA 19406, (215) 896-3364, BA 75 Washington Univ; MA 79 Saint Louis Univ; Ch Sp/Lang Path, The Bryn Mawr Hosp, **SLP ACE**

Fischer, Shelley Jean Box 105, 334 North Beulah Street, Ellsworth, WI 54011, (715) 388-6721, MS 86 Univ of WI - River Falls; **SLP**

Fischer, Susan D H 2787 Vick Avenue N W, Salem, OR 97304, (503) 585-7937, BA 77 OR St Univ; MS 79 Western OR St Coll; Sp-Lang Path, Salem Pub Schs, **SLP**

Fischetti, Mrs Jill Lorraine 8803 Oxwell Lane, Laurel, MD 20708, (301) 776-8918, BA 84 Univ of MD - College Park; MS 86 Loyola Coll; 86–Sp-Lang Path, Baltimore City PS, **SLP**

Fischi, Mrs Barbara M 2629 DE Paul Drive, Vienna, VA 22180, (703) 573-2078, BA 62 Carlow Coll; ME 65 PA St Univ - Univ Park; 85–Sp-Lang Path, Fairfax County Public Schools, **SLP ACE**

Fischler, Mrs Barbara L 3300 University Drive, Suite 521, Coral Springs, FL 33065, (305) 753-8560, BS 67 NY Univ; MS 68 Univ of WI - Madison; Sp-Lang Path, Private Practice, **SLP ACE**

Fischman, Diana L 3000 St Charles Avenue, Apartment #405, New Orleans, LA 70115, (504) 835-8439, SLP, Jefferson Parish School, **SLP**

Fischman, Ilene Shapiro 1146 Captains Lane, Wheeling, IL 60090, BA 77 MI St Univ; MS 79 Univ of WI - Madison; Aud, Resurrection Hosp, **A**

Fischthal, Mrs Lorraine Buchman 83 Ridge Road, Smithtown, NY 11787, (516) 265-5475, BA 60 Queens Coll; MS 82 Long Island U - CW Post Ctr; 82–Sp-Lang Path, BOCES 2, **SLP**

Fish, Alice McGorman 9200 Madison Avenue #256, Orangevale, CA 95662, (916) 988-3918, BA 79 Hofstra Univ; MA 80 Hofstra Univ; Sp-Lang Path, American River Hosp, **SLP**

Fish, Mrs Brenda S 7357 Granville Road, Mount Vernon, OH 43050, (614) 397-1010, MA 79 OH St Univ; Sp-Lang Path, Mt Vernon Dev Cen, **SLP**

Fish, Mrs Gloria Jane 1226 South 10th, Mount Vernon, WA 98273-5022, (206) 424-8110, **SLP**

Fish, Judith A Rd 3 Box 138, Belle Vernon, PA 15012, (412) 938-3241, BS 71 CA Univ of PA; ME 73 CA Univ of PA; Sp-Lang Path, Inter Ut #1, **SLP**

Fish, Margaret Sidock 1471 Oakwood, Highland Park, IL 60035, (312) 492-5958, **SLP**

Fish, Mrs Marianne MacHala 39644 Byers, Sterling Heights, MI 48311, (313) 977-0866, BA 76 Univ of MI - Ann Arbor; MS 77 Univ of MI - Ann Arbor; Sp-Lang Path, Visiting Nurse Association, **SLP**

Fish, Pamela S Hearing Associates Inc, Georgetown Medical Bldg, 8901 W 74th Street Ste 150, Shawnee Mission, KS 66204, (913) 384-5880, BS 72 Central MO St Univ; MA 73 Central MO St Univ; Aud, Hrng Assoc Inc, **SLP A**

Fishback, Mrs Inez F 816 Cardinal Lane, Huntingdon Valley, PA 19006, (215) 947-0563, BS Univ of PA; MA Columbia Univ Teachers Coll; **SLP**

Fishbein, Gail Sherman Box 296, Fayetteville, NY 13066-0296, (315) 655-3444, BA 81 IN Univ - Bloomington; MS 83 Univ of MI - Ann Arbor; 87–Sp-Lang Path, Cazenovia Central Schs, **SLP**

Fishbein, Mrs Gloria B 51 Concord Park East, Nashville, TN 37205, (615) 383-5340, BS 73 G Peabody Coll-Vanderbilt U; MS 74 Vanderbilt Univ; Sp-Lang Path, **SLP LM**

Fishcer Geldard, Mrs Patricia Von 516 Shorecrest Drive, Clemson, SC 29631, (803) 654-6601, BA 65 Depauw Univ; MA 67 Univ of IL - Urbana; Sp-Lang Path, Anderson-Oconee Sp & Hrng Ser, **SLP**

Fishel, Anne Marlene 1531 Laurel, South Pasadena, CA 91030, (818) 799-9841, BA CA St Univ - Northridge; MA 85 CA St Univ - Northridge; **SLP**

Fisher, Anna P O Box 25008, Houston, TX 77265-5008, (214) 372-7013, BA 83 Univ of TX - Dallas; MS 86 Univ of TX - Dallas

Fisher, Babette Dean 3209 Canterbury Drive, South, Salem, OR 97302, (503) 370-5486, BS 61 Univ of WA; MS 85 Portland St Univ; 86–Sp-Lang Path, Salem Hosp, **SLP ACE**

Fisher, Barbara Cyr 8 Hilltop Terrace, Winchester, VA 22601, (703) 955-2400, BS 82 WV Univ; MS 83 8392; Sp-Lang Path, Grafton Sch, **SLP**

Fisher, Brenda F 412 Trace West, West Monroe, LA 71291, BA 79 Univ of Southwestern LA; OM 80 LA St Univ - N O Medical Ctr; Sp-Lang Path & Aud, St Landry Parish Sch Bd, **A**

Fisher, Mrs Cathy Lane 4332 Chester, El Paso, TX 79903, (915) 544-3399, BS 82 TX Woman's Univ; MS 84 Univ of AZ; Sp-Lang Path, Rio Vista Rehab Hosp, **SLP**

Fisher, Mrs Christine 1214 Winged Foot Drive, Upland, CA 91786, (714) 949-4805, BA 73 Univ of Redlands; MA 75 Univ of Denver; 86–Sp-Lang Path, Alta Loma Sch Dist, **SLP**

Fisher, Dr Cletus G (Raydon) 107 Cynthia Place, De Kalb, IL 60115, (815) 758-6091, BS 49 Kent St Univ; MA 50 Univ of IA; PH 63 (NS) OH St Univ; Prof, Nn IL U, **SLP A F LM**

Fisher, Dayna P 3150 Cobblestone Lane #3, Springfield, IL 62704, (217) 525-3201, MS 87 IL St Univ - Normal

Fisher, Deborah Ann 1110 Llewellyn Avenue, Norfolk, VA 23507-1848, (804) 623-9722, **SLP**

Fisher, Diane Marie 99601 Kahema Place, Aiea, HI 96701, (808) 455-4151, BS 81 Univ of HI - Manoa; MS 83 Univ of HI - Manoa; SLP, Doe Leeward Dist Waipahu,Hi, **SLP**

Fisher, Dorothy 11010 Couger Drive, Granger, IN 46530, (219) 289-0122, BS 68 Western MI Univ; MA 73 Western MI Univ; Sp-Lang Path, Memorial Hospital, **SLP**

Fisher, Frances F 606 Camelot Drive, Bel Air, MD 21014, **SLP**

Fisher, Mrs Francine Kaplan 1211 Carrollton, Baton Rouge, LA 70806, (504) 769-6845, BA 68 Tulane Univ; MS 72 Tulane Univ; Sp-Lang Path, E Baton Rouge Parish Sch Bd, **SLP A**

Fisher, Mrs Gayll A 46 Coolidge Drive, Berkeley Heights, NJ 07922, (201) 665-9319, BA 69 Bowling Green St Univ; MS 79 Rutger's St Univ - Douglas Coll; **SLP**

Fisher, Helen F 1825 S Midvale Avenue 303, Los Angeles, CA 90025, (213) 827-1574, MS 75 Columbia Univ Teachers Coll; Sp-Lang Path, Private Practice, **SLP ACE**

Fisher, Helene Rosman 137 Buckingham Court, Pomona, NY 10970, (914) 354-1980, BS 78 Univ of Cape Town; MA 83 NY Univ; Instr, Long Island Univ, **SLP**

Fisher, Dr Hilda B Dept Communication Science & Disorders, Northwestern University, 2299 Sheridan Road, Evanston, IL 60201, (312) 492-5076, BA Northwestern St Univ; MA LA St Univ - Baton Rouge; PH 49 (NS) LA St Univ - Baton Rouge; Professor Emeritus Sp-Lang Path, Northwestern Univ, **SLP F LM**

Fisher, Mrs Inez Freeney 11805 Bushmills Road, Dallas, TX 75243, (214) 661-7888, **A**

Fisher, James Ernest 1663 Estevan Road, London, ON, Canada N5X 2G8, **SLP**

Fisher, Mrs Jean Marie 1214 North Richmond, Wichita, KS 67203, (316) 946-0867, BA 86 Wichita St Univ; MA 87 Wichita St Univ; 88–Sp-Lang Path, Sedgwick Co Spec Educ Coop

Fisher, Jeanne Hebert 3739 Forest Run Road, Birmingham, AL 35223, (205) 967-7330, BS 73 Northwestern St Univ; MS 74 FL St Univ; 88–Sp-Lang Path, Jefferson County Bd of Educ, **SLP**

Fisher, Mrs Joanne Marie K Rd 2 Box 2120, Effort, PA 18330, (717) 629-3662, BS 77 East Stroudsburg Univ of PA; MS 81 Bloomsburg Univ of PA; Sp-Lang Path, Colonial Northampton IU #20, **SLP**

Fisher, John C 710 Carol Street, Dover, DE 19901, (302) 736-4736, BA 52 Univ of Pittsburgh - Pittsburgh; MS 59 Univ of Pittsburgh - Pittsburgh; Prog Dir, De Div of Pub Hlth, **SLP A**

Fisher, Mrs Joni Jane 3408 Cooper Street, San Diego, CA 92104, (619) 281-0142, BS 84 AZ St Univ; MA 86 San Diego St Univ; **SLP**

Fisher, Karen Elizabeth 551 15th Street, Babylon, NY 11703, (516) 473-2800, BS 84 SUNY - Coll at Plattsburgh; MA 85 SUNY - Coll at Plattsburgh; 87–Aud, St Charles Hosp, **A**

Fisher, Karen Lynn T 25 Cunningham Circle, Taylors, SC 29687, (803) 268-4864, BA 77 Univ of NC - Greensboro; MA 84 OH St Univ; 86–Sp-Lang Path, Greenville Co Schs, **SLP**

Fisher, Lee I 3601 Waville Road N E, Bemidji, MN 56601, (218) 751-9054, BA 60 Univ of IA; MA 67 Univ of IA; Aud/Consult, U S Pub Hlth, **SLP A F**

Fisher, Liliane E 120 Cabrini Boulevard #41, New York, NY 10033, (212) 795-4937, BS 54 CUNY - City College; OM 56 CUNY - Brooklyn Coll; MA 82 Columbia Univ Teachers Coll; Sp-Lang Path, NY Bd of Ed, **SLP**

Fisher, Mrs Maryjo Harlin 4053 Longford Drive, Marietta, GA 30066, (401) 426-3175, BA 82 Univ of MS; MS 83; 87–Sp-Lang Path, Kennestone Hosp, **SLP**

Fisher, Mrs Pamela A 6333 Rolling Glen Drive, Huber Heights, OH 45424, (513) 237-8066, BS 74 Kent St Univ; MA 75 Kent St Univ; Sp-Lang Path, Dayton City Schs, **SLP**

Fisher, Pamela L 4 Henry Drive, Barrington, RI 02806, BS 72 Lesley Coll; MS 75 Univ of VT; SLP, Er SI So of Ri, **SLP**

Fisher, Mrs Patricia K 131 Martha Lane, Fairfield, OH 45014, (513) 829-8634, BS 73 Bowling Green St Univ; MA 79 Bowling Green St Univ; Sp-Lang Path, Tri-Co Sp Assoc, **SLP**

Fisher, Mrs Patricia Trent 2121 Southwest 33rd Street, Topeka, KS 66611-2031, (913) 272-0089, BS 76 Univ of Tulsa; MA 78 OK St Univ; Speech-Language Pathologist, Topeka Public Schools, **SLP**

Fisher, Mrs Randi B 24 Chesham Avenue, London, ON, Canada N6G 3S9, (519) 471-2540, BS 75 Purdue Univ - West Lafayette; MS 77 Purdue Univ - West Lafayette; Clin Supvr, Univ of Western Ontario, **SLP**

Fisher, Mrs Roberta Helene 597 Terrill Road, Fanwood, NJ 07023, (201) 322-4212, BA 74 Kean Coll of NJ; MA 79 Kean Coll of NJ; Sp-Lang Path, Scotch Plains Fanwood Bd of Educ

Fisher, Ronna Labovitz Hearing Health Center, 55 E Washington #1422, Chicago, IL 60602, (312) 263-7171, BA 75 Oglethorpe Univ; MS 77 Univ of Pittsburgh - Pittsburgh; Aud, Hearing Health Center, **A**

Fisher, Susan M 2101 Vera Cruz Drive #113, Modesto, CA 95355, (209) 524-3997, BA 85 San Diego St Univ; MA 87 San Diego St Univ; 87–Sp-Lang Path, InSpeech Inc, **SLP**

Fisher, Teriann 202 Seaton Drive #10, Forrest City, AR 72335, (501) 633-6812, BS 84 Baylor Univ; MS 86 Univ of TX - Dallas; 87–Aud, Arkansas Dept of Health, **A**

Fisher, Mrs Terri Lee 1000 Blueberry Drive, Apollo, PA 15613, (412) 795-0100, BS 79 Indiana Univ of PA; ME 85 Indiana Univ of PA; Sp-Lang Path, Plum Borough Sch Dist, **SLP**

Fisher, Thomas E Ear Nose & Throat Assoc Sc, 425 Pine Ridge Boulevard, Suite 305, Wausau, WI 54401, (715) 845-9634, BS 75 Southern IL Univ -Carbondale; MS 76 Univ of WI - Stevens Point; Aud, ENT Assoc, **A**

Fisher, Valerie Jean P O Box 333, 1205 South Mission, Mount Pleasant, MI 48804-0333, (517) 773-4356, BA 81 Central MI Univ; MA 83 Central MI Univ; Owner, Stride, **SLP**

Fisher, Vicki Ruff Eastern Oklahoma ENT, 5020 East 68th Street, Tulsa, OK 74136, (405) 271-2791, BA 77 Univ of OK - Norman; MS 79 Univ of OK Medical Center; Aud, Eastern Oklahoma ENT Inc, **A**

Fisher, Mrs Virginia E 1519 Sherwood, Bowling Green, KY 42101, (502) 597-2191, BS 83 Western KY Univ; MS 85 Western KY Univ; **SLP**

Fisher-Medina, Julia Ann 587 10th Street, Brooklyn, NY 11215, (718) 240-6431, BA 77 CUNY - Brooklyn Coll; MA 86 CUNY - Hunter Coll; Sp-Lang Path, Brookdale Hosp, **SLP**

Fisher-Minor, Gerri L 125 Harry Truman Drive #22, Largo, MD 20772, (301) 499-4952, BS 82 Ashland Coll; MS 85 Southern CT St Univ; Sp-Lang Path, Med & Rehab Support Svcs, **SLP**

Fishkin, Mrs Debbie S 20 Wayne Drive, Plainview, NY 11803, (516) 433-4920, BA 78 SUNY - Coll at Brockport; MA 80 Long Island U - CW Post Ctr; Sp-Lang Path, Private Practice, **SLP**

Fishkin, Elyse Gustin 158 Winding River Road, Wellesley, MA 02181, (617) 730-2635, BA 73 CUNY - Brooklyn Coll; ME 74 Northeastern Univ; 82–Sp/Lang Path, Brookline Pub Schs, **SLP**

Fishkind-Faber, Mrs Toby G 4240 Savoie Trail, West Bloomfield, MI 48033, (313) 535-2000, BA 63 Central MI Univ; Sp-Lang Path, Redford Un Sch, **SLP**

Fishman, Arlene T 16300 West Nine Mile Road, Apartment 420, Southfield, MI 48075

Fishman, Glenn Sean 144-64 Sanford Avenue #61, Flushing, NY 11355, (718) 539-9444, MS 88 CUNY - Brooklyn Coll

Fishman, Mrs Hedy F 11706 Woodknoll Lane, Houston, TX 77071, (713) 728-5268, BS 70 McGill Univ - Quebec; MS 73 McGill Univ - Quebec; **A**

Fishman, Iris 15 West 72nd Street #10-C, New York, NY 10023, (212) 724-1910, BS 73 NY Univ; MA 78 CUNY - Hunter Coll; Consult, UCP, **SLP**

Fishman, Jane S 9 Tor Terrace, New City, NY 10956, **SLP**

Fishman, Merle A 2143 Sandy Lane, Wilmette, IL 60091, (312) 256-1523, BS 85 Univ of IL - Urbana; MA 87 Univ of IL - Urbana; **A**

Fishman, Robyn Lynn 12385 B Maverick, Maryland Heights, MO 63043, (314) 878-4064, BS 84 Fontbonne Coll; MS 85 Fontbonne Coll; **SLP**

Fishman, Mrs Sally W 139 Dalton Road, Belmont, MA 02178, (617) 484-3785, BA 38 Emerson Coll; **SLP LM**

Fishman, Sheryl L 600 West 107th Street #206, Kansas City, MO 64114-2930, (816) 941-7807, BS 85 Univ of WI - Madison; MA 87 Univ of KS; **SLP**

Fishman, Susan Paula P O Box 1634, Conway, NH 03818, (603) 539-7451, BS 82 Univ of WI - Madison; MS 84 Univ of WI - Madison; **SLP**

Fisk, Susan B 565 St Andrews Road, Vancouver, BC, Canada V7S 1V3, (604) 228-1121, BA 76 Univ of British Columbia; MS 79 Univ of AL- Tuscaloosa; 87–Unit Mgr, Gr Vancouver Men Hlth Svc Soc, **SLP ACE**

Fiske, Dana R Professional Audiology Center, 330 Borthwick Avenue, Suite 209, Portsmouth, NH 03801, (603) 436-8668, BA 71 Univ of NH; MS 72 FL St Univ; Owner, Profes Aud Cen, **A**

Fiskus, Mrs Selwa M 905 York Warwick Drive, Yorktown, VA 23692, (804) 898-0308, BS 60 East TN St Univ; Sp-Lang Path, York Co Pub Sch, **SLP**

Fiss-Zeiger, Ann V 4 Currier Court, Cheshire, CT 06410, (203) 272-8215, BA 64; MS 66 McGill Univ - Quebec; **SLP**

Fistel, Mrs Amy Rena 10 Hampshire Avenue, Sharon, MA 02067, (617) 875-6124, **A**

Fister, Mrs Joy Wallace 503 Essex Rd, Fox River Grove, IL 60021, (815) 338-1133, BS 81 Northern IL Univ - De Kalb; MS 82 Northern IL Univ - De Kalb; 87–Sp-Lang Path, Woodstock Comm Unit Sch Dist 200, **SLP**

Fitch, Mrs Adina Jarvinen 7007 North Sheridan Road, Chicago, IL 60626, (315) 425-7824, BA 85 Syracuse Univ; MS 87 Syracuse Univ; **SLP**

Fitch, Dr James L Speech And Hearing Center, Univ Of South Alabama, Mobile, AL 36688, (205) 460-6327, BS 64 IL St Univ - Normal; MS 68 FL St Univ; PH 69 (NS) FL St Univ; Dir Commun Sci Lab, Dept Sp Path/Aud U S Al, **SLP A F**

Fitch, Jon M 713 Cypress, Bakersfield, CA 93304, (805) 322-5466, BS 49 Central CT St Univ; OB 55 Emerson Coll; MS 64 Purdue Univ - West Lafayette; 86–Aud/Sp-Lang Path, Soc for Crippled Chldn and Ad, **SLP A**

Fitch, Mrs Lucy Ann 2515 Lakeridge Shores West, Reno, NV 89509, (702) 827-2609, BA 70 Saint Mary's Coll; MA 85 Univ of Denver; 88–Sp-Lang Path, Washoe County Sch Dist, **SLP**

Fitch, Ruth Ann L 331 Otero, Santa Fe, NM 87501, (505) 988-9818, MA 65; Sp-Lang Path, Sante Fe Cen for Aud, **SLP**

Fitch, Waring J 5308 Landes Street, Port Townsend, WA 98368, (206) 385-5045, BS 39 Univ of WI - Milwaukee; MS 43 Univ of MI - Ann Arbor; **A LM**

Fitsik, Mrs Lauren B 88 Woodin Road, Clifton Park, NY 12065, (518) 489-8336, BS 80 SUNY - Coll at Fredonia; MA 82 Univ of Denver; Sp-Lang Path, Cpcen for the Dis, **SLP**

Fitton, Mrs Barbara Falese 159 Mariner Circle, Cotuit, MA 02635, (508) 428-5481, BA 74 Regis Coll; MS 81 Boston Univ; Sp-Lang Path, Private Practice, **SLP**

Fitton-Neville, Dr Roxie A 8391 Ranch Estates Road, Clarkston, MI 48016, (313) 391-4921, MA 76 Wayne St Univ; MA 83 Central MI Univ; PH 79 (NS) Wayne St Univ; Engineering Group Manager, General Motors, **A**

Fitz, Mrs Mary L 3927 East Lavender Lane, Phoenix, AZ 85044, (602) 759-9265, BA 76 Bowling Green St Univ; MA 77 Bowling Green St Univ; 86–Sp-Lang Path, Mesa PS, **SLP**

Fitz-Armstrong, Dr Linda C Cascade Sp-Lang Rehab Serv, 817 Commercial Street, P O Box 330, Leavenworth, WA 98826, (509) 548-5815, BA 61 Grinnell Coll; MA 76 WA St Univ; PH 77 (Auditory Processing) WA St Univ; Sp-Lang Path, Private Practice, **SLP**

FitzGerald, Ann E 7745 South Rogers Avenue, Clare, MI 48617, (517) 386-3693, BA 74 Central MI Univ; MA 80 Central MI Univ; **SLP**

Fitzgerald, Mrs Ardell C B 7716 Trail Ridge Road N E, Albuquerque, NM 87109, (505) 255-3702, BA 67 Univ of CO - Boulder; MA 69 Univ of CO - Boulder; Sp-Lang Path, Montezuma Elem Sch, **SLP**

Fitzgerald, Carol Reese 7 Wollaston Road, Wilmington, DE 19810, (215) 447-2044, BA 71 OH St Univ; MA 85 Temple Univ-Tyler Sch of Art; 85–Aud, Crozer-Chester Med Ctr, **A**

Fitzgerald, Debra Adams 209 Hibbert Road, North Wales, PA 19454, (412) 931-3413, BS 78 PA St Univ - Univ Park; MA 81 Univ of Pittsburgh - Pittsburgh; Sp-Lang Path, Private Practice, **SLP**

Fitzgerald, Debra Lyn 51 Nichols Street, Unit 3, Cranston, RI 02920-3914, (401) 943-1476, BS 81 Emerson Coll; MS 83 Boston Univ; Sp-Lang Path, Behavioral Dev Ctr, **SLP**

Fitzgerald, Donna P O Box 781, Nokomis, FL 34274-0781, (813) 485-3290, BS 75 LA St Univ - Baton Rouge; MA 76 LA St Univ - Baton Rouge; 86–Clin Supvr, InSpeech Inc, **SLP**

Fitzgerald, Mrs Glenda Frances R R #4 Box 294-A, Troy, MO 63379, (314) 447-1151, BS 71 Univ of MO - Columbia; MA 82 Northeast MO St Univ; 88–Adjunct Prof, Lindenwood Coll, **SLP**

Fitzgerald, Mrs Karen Ann 8924 West Meadowbrook Avenue, Phoenix, AZ 85037, (602) 849-8137, BA 76 Bellarmine Coll; MS 80 Univ of KY; 83–Sp-Lang Path, Liberty Elementary, **SLP**

Fitzgerald, Margaret Marie 1825 West Ocotillo #150, Phoenix, AZ 85015, (602) 246-5155, MS 85 Moorhead St Univ; **SLP**

Fitzgerald, Mary C 1850 34th Street South, Apartment 317, Grand Forks, ND 58201, (701) 780-2447, BA 77 Concordia Coll - Moorhead; MS 83 Moorhead St Univ; 87–Sp-Lang Path, Univ of North Dakota-Med Ctr Rehab Hosp, **SLP**

Fitzgerald, Mary Jo 2409 Springdale Road #8A, Waukesha, WI 53186, (414) 544-2447, BA 74 Univ of IA; MA 76 Univ of IA; Coord/Sp-Path, Waukesha Mem Hosp, **SLP**

Fitzgerald, Dr Mary T P O Box 150311, Nashville, TN 37215-0311, (615) 292-4741, BA 68 Vanderbilt Univ; MS 69 Vanderbilt Univ; PH 85 (Teaching/Learning) Vanderbilt Univ; Sp-Lang Path/Aud, Private Practice, **SLP A ACE**

Fitzgerald, Michael G Bel Ari Apartment #D-5, Cumberland, MD 21502, (301) 729-2931, BA 76 Loyola Coll; MS 78 Loyola Coll; Sp-Lang Path, Bd of Ed/Allegang Co, **SLP**

Fitzgerald, Mrs Nancy L 118-3C Bluebird Avenue, Hillsborough, NJ 08876, (201) 722-8222, BA 82 Montclair St Coll; MA 86 Montclair St Coll; **SLP**

Fitzgerald, Mrs Patricia De Koning 1137 Ott Lane, North Merrick, NY 11566, (516) 293-0066, BS 83 SUNY - Coll at Geneseo; MS 84 Adelphi Univ; Sp-Lang Path, Nassau Cnty Board Coop Ed Serv, **SLP**

Fitzgerald, Sr Rita A 3333 5th Avenue, Pittsburgh, PA 15213, (578) 615-6225, BS 54 Carlow Coll; MA 57 Northwestern Univ; PH 63 (Sp Path) Northwestern Univ; 56–Prof & Dir SLP Prog, Carlow Coll, **SLP F**

Fitzgerald, Susan Lochren Morse Street School, Freeport, ME 04032, (207) 865-6361, BS 76 SUNY - Coll at Buffalo; MS 77 SUNY - Coll at Buffalo; SLP, Freeport Pub Schs, **SLP**

Fitzgerald, Mrs Susan Swickard 13313 West 112th Terrace, Overland Park, KS 66210, (913) 782-8950, BS 76 Univ of KS; MA 78 Univ of IA; Sp/Lang Path, Olathe USD #233, **SLP**

Fitzgibbons, Dr Peter J 5907 Bryn Mawr Road, College Park, MD 20740, (202) 651-5460, BS 69 Tufts Univ; MS 73 Univ of MA - Amherst; PH 79 (Aud) Northwestern Univ; Research Sci, Gallaudet Univ, **A**

Fitzmaurice, Karen M 200 10th Street N W, Minot, ND 58701, (701) 838-2936, MS 88 Minot St Univ

Fitzmaurice, Kathleen Anne 2915 South 74th Street, Omaha, NE 68124, (913) 621-5155, BA 80 Creighton Univ; MA 82 Univ of KS; SLP, Ops Preschool for Handicapped, **SLP**

Fitzmaurice, Peggy E 3201-A Mariners Island Dr, Canton, OH 44708, (216) 438-2554, BS 67 OH St Univ; ME 72 Kent St Univ; Sp-Lang Path, Canton Cty Sch, **SLP**

Fitzpatrick, Barbara N 12885 S W Havencrest Street, Portland, OR 97225, (503) 251-7433, BA 76 Univ of CA - Santa Barbara; MA 77 Univ of Northern CO; Aud, Multnomah Ed Serv Dist, **A**

Fitzpatrick, Deanne B 191 Deer Field Lane North, Pleasantville, NY 10570, (914) 769-7497, BA 64 OH St Univ; MS 69 Univ of Pittsburgh - Pittsburgh; **A**

Fitzpatrick, Mildred S P O Box 325, Middlebury, VT 05753, (802) 388-2971, BA 71 Middlebury Coll; ME 78 Univ of MT; MA 82 Univ of MT; Sp-Lang Path, Addison Ctrl Spuev Un, **SLP**

Fitzpatrick, Patricia M 19 Perkins Avenue, Reading, MA 01867, **SLP**

Fitz-Patrick, Tijen Beker 109 Pine Street, Franklin, MA 02038, (508) 587-2121, BA 84 Univ of CT; MS 86 Northeastern Univ; 86–Sp-Lang Path, Brockton Visiting Nurse Assoc, **SLP**

Fitzpatrick, Wilma L 2000 West Illinois Avenue, Apartment 316, Aurora, IL 60506, (312) 844-4434, BS 59 IL St Univ - Normal; MA 72 IL St Univ - Normal; Sp-Lang Path, W Aurora Sch Dist 129, **SLP**

Fitzpatrick-Joyce, Maureen 83 Cove Street, Pawtucket, RI 02861, (401) 456-9403, BA 77 Univ of RI; MA 79 Univ of MA - Amherst; 79–Sp-Lang Path, Providence Sch Dept, **SLP**

Fitzpatrick-McKenzie, Susan Wills P O Box 9143, Auburn, CA 95604, (916) 878-2547, MS 84 CA St Univ - Sacramento; SLP, Univ California Davis Med Cen, **SLP**

Fitzsimmons, Laurie Ann 505 Lambert, Fayetteville, NC 28305, (313) 331-0261, BA 80 MI St Univ; MA 84 Wayne St Univ - Sch of Med; Aud, Cape Fear Hosp, **A**

Fitzsimmons, Lori K 3484 West Sunday Court, Tucson, AZ 85741, (602) 881-7100, BA 80 CA St Univ - Northridge; MS 82 Purdue Univ - West Lafayette; Aud, Thomas-Davis Cl, **A**

Fitzsimons, Dr Ruth N 38 Mystic Drive, Warwick, RI 02886, ME Boston Univ; ED (NS) Boston Univ; **SLP F LM**

Fitzwilliam, Mrs Heather M 1 Kitchner Court, Durham, NC 27705, (919) 383-4870, BA 68 Univ of IL - Urbana; ME 70 Univ of NC - Chapel Hill; MS 79 Univ of NC - Chapel Hill; SLP, Durham County Public Schools, **SLP**

Fix, Cynthia C 4 Ashwood, Iowa City, IA 52240, (319) 351-6383, BA 66 IN Univ - Bloomington; MA 72 Univ of IA; Clin Instr, Univ of IA, **SLP**

Fizer, Mrs Claudia Krebs 2209 Lilly Drive, Culloden, WV 25510, (304) 562-3630, BA 70 Marshall Univ; MA 73 Marshall Univ; MA 84 WV Coll of Graduate Studies; 75–Spec Educ Tchr El-SC, Putnam Co Bd of Educ, **SLP**

Fjare, Cheri L P O Box 947, Big Timber, MT 59011, (406) 932-5939, BA 79 WA St Univ; MA 80 WA St Univ; 80–Sp-Lang Path, Big Timber Sch Dist #1, **SLP**

Fjeld, Carol E RD2, Wheeler Road, Brandon, VT 05733, (802) 247-6534, MS 78 Univ of VT; Sp-Lang Path, Rutland NE Supervisory Union, **SLP**

Flaat, Kathryn Gay Rural Route 2, Box 33, Fisher, MN 56723, (701) 777-4144, BA 81 Univ of ND; MS 84 Univ of ND; Sp-Lang Path, North Dakota St Sch for Blind, **SLP**

Flacinski, Ann Frances P O Box 22652, St Petersburg, FL 33742, BA 84 Thiel Coll; MS 85 Ithaca Coll; 87–Sp-Lang Path, Bayfront Med Ctr, **SLP**

Flack, Mrs Marilyn Neder 1900 Lyttonsville Road, Apartment 1318, Silver Spring, MD 20910, (301) 454-6911, BA; MA 79 Univ of MD - College Park; Cl Superv/Instr, U of MD, **A**

Flag, Carol L 660 Wildwood Boulevard SW, #A-15, Issaquah, WA 98027, (206) 392-3748, BA 73 Humboldt St Univ; MA 80 San Diego St Univ; Sp-Lang Path, Tahoma Schl Dstr, **SLP**

Flagg, Mrs Kelly Jo 5827 Montebello Street, Haslett, MI 48840, (517) 339-8841, BA 79 MI St Univ; MA 80 MI St Univ; Sp-Lang Path, Wilkshire Elem, **SLP**

Flagtwet, Katherine Kania 2515 25th Street South, Apartment 301, Fargo, ND 58103, (701) 293-0783, BS 84 Northern St Coll; MS 86 Moorhead St Univ; **SLP**

Flaherty, Mrs Carol 1937 Palacios Drive, San Pedro, CA 90732, (213) 548-8407, BA 65 Univ of MI - Ann Arbor; MA 75 Western MI Univ; OM 84 CA St Univ - Long Beach; 75–Sp-Lang Path, Lausd, **SLP**

Flaherty, James Peter 1621 33rd Street, San Diego, CA 92102, (619) 267-9500, BA 80 CA St Univ - Northridge; MA 82 CA St Univ - Northridge; Sp-Lang Path, Paradise Valley Hosp, **SLP**

Flaherty, Kathleen Anne 4252 North Kedvale, Chicago, IL 60641, (312) 367-4300, BS 83 Marquette Univ; MS 85 Gallaudet Coll; Aud, Lake-McHenry Regional Program, **A**

Flaherty, M Kathleen 6109 Harvard Street, Glen Echo, MD 20812, (301) 762-8335, BS 72 Boston Univ; MS 76 Long Island U - CW Post Ctr; Sp/Lang Path, Mont Co Pub Sch, **SLP**

Flaherty, Mrs Patricia E 76 Old Post Road, East Walpole, MA 02032, (617) 668-6650, BS 72 Suffolk Univ; ME 76 Northeastern Univ

Flaherty, Robin Eileen 16 White Street Place #3, Somerville, MA 02144, (617) 666-1527, BS 85 Boston Univ; MS 86 Boston Univ; 86–Sp-Lang Path, Silverlake Reg Sch Dist, **SLP**

Flaherty, Mrs Sarah M Box 126, Cooksburg, PA 16217, (814) 226-7103, BS 76 Clarion Univ of PA; ME 82 Clarion Univ of PA; 77–Sp-Lang Path, Riverview Intermediate Unit #6, **SLP**

Flahive, Michael J Marywood College, Scranton, PA 18509, (717) 348-6299, OM 73 Western MI Univ; MA 72 Western MI Univ; PH 79 (NS) MI St Univ; Prof & Chmn, Marywood College, **SLP A**

Flair, Mrs Erin M 28692 Rancho Grande, Laguna Niguel, CA 92656, BA 71 CA Poly St Univ-San Luis Obi; MA 80 CA St Univ - Long Beach; Sp-Lang Path, Irvine USD, **SLP**

Flakus, Theresea Marie 2712 Stearns Way, St Cloud, MN 56303, (612) 259-5945, **SLP**

Flam, Madeline 39 Northcote Drive, Melville, NY 11747, (516) 643-8843, BA 63 Adelphi Univ; MS 66 CUNY - Queens Coll; Sp-Lang Path, Private Practice, **SLP**

Flanagan, Mrs Barbara M 223 College Street, Hudson, OH 44236, (216) 650-9741, BS 69 Towson St Univ; ME 83 Harvard Univ; MS 73 Univ of MI - Ann Arbor; Sp-Lang Path, Avon Speech Associates, **SLP**

Flanagan, Dr Bruce C 1005 McClure, Junction City, KS 66441, (913) 532-6879, BS 53 Western MI Univ; MS 58 Southern IL Univ -Carbondale; PH 66 (NS) Univ of FL; Prof of SLP, Kansas St U, **SLP**

Flanagan, Linda B 4998 Dalton Drive, Columbia, MD 21045, (301) 730-0617, BS 72 Univ of UT; MS 75 Univ of UT; Sp-Lang Path, Howard Co Sch Syst, **SLP**

Flanagan, Linda N Box 712, Warren, MA 01083, **SLP**

Flanagan, Maureen Ann 2603 Colonial Road, Accokeek, MD 20607, (703) 691-2751, **SLP**

Flanagan, Sheila Ann Box 5529, APO New York, NY 09123-5378, (312) 450-2100, Proviso Area for Exc Children, **SLP**

Flanagin, Mrs Judy Davis 404 Cottage, Vermillion, SD 57069, (605) 677-5474, BA 64 Univ of NE - Lincoln; MA 75 Univ of SD - Vermillion; Asst Prof, Univ of South Dakota, **SLP ACE**

Flanagin, Mrs Virginia W St Joseph Hospital, 2260 Wrightsboro Road, Augusta, GA 30910, (404) 737-7681, BA 70 Columbia Coll; ME 72 Univ of GA; Dir/Sp-Lang Path, St Joseph Hosp, **SLP**

Flanary, Heather Molly 1135 Murray Court, Santa Rosa, CA 95404, (707) 527-6147, BA 83 CA St Univ - Chico; MA 85 CA St Univ - Chico; Sp-Lang Path, Sonoma Co Office of Educ, **SLP**

Flanders, William E 7 State Circle, Annapolis, MD 21401, (301) 685-4334, BA 79 Univ of MD - College Park; MS 84 Towson St Univ; MD Hrng Aid Serv, **A**

Flanick, Mrs Ann Gilligan 72 Comanche Avenue, Rockaway, NJ 07866, (513) 222-5597, BS 82 Edinboro Univ of PA; MS 84 WV Univ; Sp-Lang Path, Welkind Rehab Hosp, **SLP**

Flanigan, Steve George Middlesboro Community Hospital, Speech Pathology Dept, 3600 West Cumberland Avenue, Middlesboro, KY 40965, (606) 248-3300, BS 81 CO St Univ; MA 82 Univ of TN - Knoxville; 84–Sp-Lang Path, Middlesboro Commun Hosp, **SLP**

Flannery, Donna Kay 10231 Richview Drive, St Louis, MO 63127, (314) 965-0985, BS 83 Southwest MO St Univ; MA 85 Saint Louis Univ; Dir Sp-Lang Path, Med Rehab Ctr of St Louis, **SLP**

Flannigan, William J 305 North 6th, St Marys, KS 66536, (913) 272-1944, BS 71 Emporia St Univ; MA 74 KS St Univ; Coord/Sp-Lang Path, Topeka Pub Sch, **SLP**

Flarity, Jane A 333 E Ontario #3506-B, Chicago, IL 60611, (312) 908-3682, BS 80 Western MI Univ; MA 81 MI St Univ; **SLP**

Flasko, Deborah Jo Rd 3 Box 560-A, Wellsburg, WV 26070, BS 84 WV Univ; MA 86 CUNY - Hunter Coll; **A**

Flater, Mrs Paula Paquette W11590 County Road #D, Holcombe, WI 54745, (715) 595-4241, BA 82 Univ of WI - Eau Claire; MS 83 Univ of WI - Eau Claire; Sp-Lang Path, Lake Holcombe Sch Dist, **SLP**

Flatley, Mrs Susanne Gerace 1726 Larkspur Drive, Placentia, CA 92670, (714) 996-0674, BA 64 Catholic Univ of America; MA 83 CA St Univ - Fullerton; 83–Sp-Lang Path, Placentia USD, **SLP**

Flaton, Rebecca Lynn 3604 Gabriel #124, Parsons, KS 67357, (316) 421-0058, BS 73; MA 74; 88–Sp-Lang Path, Parsons State Hosp & Trng Ctr, **SLP**

Flatte-Hendel, Mrs Daryl F 2401 Halesworth Drive, Potomac, MD 20854, (301) 340-2990, BS 72 Ithaca Coll; MA 73 George Washington Univ; Sp/Lang Path, Montgomery Co Pub Sch, **SLP**

Flax, Dr Judith Fivis 11 Washington Avenue, Short Hills, NJ 07078, (201) 379-7583, BS 71 Trenton St Coll; MA 72 Montclair St Coll; PH 86 (NS) CUNY - City College; Sp-Lang Path, Albert Einstein Coll of Med, **SLP**

Flax, Norma J 330 West Brambleton Avenue, Norfolk, VA 23510, (804) 441-2743, BS 60 Coll of William & Mary; MS 70 Old Dominion Univ; Sp-Lang Path, **SLP**

Flaxman, Sheila Belkin New York Audiology Center Incorporated, Suite 409, 133 East 73rd Street, New York, NY 10021, (212) 861-9000, BS 58 Boston Univ; ME 60 Boston Univ; Dir/Aud & Sp-Lang Path, NY Aud Cen Inc, **SLP A**

Fleckenstein, Mrs Julie Jeanette P O Box 397, Susanville, CA 96130, (916) 257-5161, BA 82 CA St Univ - Chico; MA 84 Humboldt St Univ; 84–Sp-Lang Path, Lassen HS Dist, **SLP**

Fleegal, Mrs Elaine M 148 Blacksmith Road, Camp Hill, PA 17011, (717) 737-2238, BS 66 Emerson Coll; ME 67 PA St Univ - Univ Park

Fleenor, Mrs Diana Lynne 1595 Countryside Drive, Indianapolis, IN 46231, (317) 244-3161, BA 83 IN Univ - Bloomington; OM 84 IN Univ - Bloomington; 88–Sp-Lang Path, Metro Sch Dist of Pike Township, **SLP**

Fleenor, Mrs Elizabeth Gloyeske 2017 Huckleberry Circle, Lexington, KY 40514, (606) 224-9426, BS 78 Purdue Univ - West Lafayette; MA 79 Univ of IL - Urbana; **SLP**

Fleenor, Mary D 9000-A Knight Street, Laughlin AFB, TX 78840, BA 76 Western KY Univ; MA 78 Our Lady Lake Univ-San Anton; **SLP**

Fleenor, Rebecca Ann 208 North 7th, Hiawatha, KS 66434, (913) 742-2798, BS 83 KS St Univ; MA 85 KS St Univ; 87–Sp-Lang Path, Community Therapeutics Inc, **SLP**

Fleet, Audrey Ann 18515 Perkins Oaks Drive, Prairieville, LA 70769, (504) 387-0476, MA 84 LA St Univ - Baton Rouge; Sp-Lang Path, E Baton Rouge Parish Sch Sys, **SLP**

Flege, Dr James Emil Dept Biocommunication-UAB, University Station, Birmingham, AL 35294, (205) 934-9297, MA 75 Univ of FL; MA 77 IN Univ - Bloomington; PH 79 (NS) IN Univ - Bloomington; 82–Assoc Prof, U of AL

Flegel, Cheryl L 74 Oswego Summit, Lake Oswego, OR 97035-1061, (503) 246-5608, BS 78 Univ of WA; MS 80 Univ of WI - Madison; SLP, Providence Med Cen, **SLP**

Fleischer-Hill, Lisa Ann 15 Crook Street, Medway, MA 02053-1321, BA 78 SUNY - Coll at New Paltz; MA 84 CA St Univ - Northridge; SLP, Millis School System, **SLP**

Fleischman, Mrs Stacy Brott 6708 Tusculum Road, Bethesda, MD 20817, (202) 745-5600, BS 81 Boston Univ; MS 83 Univ of WI - Madison; Sp-Lang Path, Children's Hosp, **SLP**

Fleisher, Ada M 1027 Corn Crib Lane, Huntingdon Valley, PA 19006, (215) 947-2429, BA 68 Temple Univ-Tyler Sch of Art; MA 70 Temple Univ-Tyler Sch of Art; **SLP**

Fleishman, Glenda C 323 Lynn Manor Drive, Rockville, MD 20850, BA 77 Univ of CO - Boulder; MA 81 Temple Univ; Sp-Lang Path, Private Practice, **SLP**

Fleisig, Mrs Marsha C 7826 Louis Pasteur #104, San Antonio, TX 78229, (512) 690-9091, BS 70 Univ of Houston - Univ Park; MA 71 Univ of Houston - Univ Park; Sp-Lang Path, Sp Lang & Hearing Assoc, **SLP**

Fleming, Barbara Hoyt 114 Winne Road, Delmar, NY 12054, (518) 273-4782, BS 77 SUNY - Coll at Buffalo; MS 83 SUNY - Coll at Buffalo; Sp-Lang Path, Watervliet City Sch Dist, **SLP**

Fleming, Dr Carol A 2001 Union Street, San Francisco, CA 94123, (415) 346-1555, OB 61 Central WA Univ; MA 63 Northwestern Univ; PH 65 (NS) Northwestern Univ; 80–Sp-Lang Path, Private Practice, **SLP**

Fleming, Mrs Carolyn 204 Chantilly Drive, West Monroe, LA 71291, (318) 325-1507, BA 73 LA Tech Univ; MA 74 LA Tech Univ; SLP, Oua Parish Sch Bd, **SLP**

Fleming, Deodis D 13600 Otter Creek Parkway #121, Little Rock, AR 72209, (501) 864-3487, BS 76 Univ of Central AR; MA 79 Univ of AR - Fayetteville; Sp-Lang Path, New Medico of Arkansas, **SLP**

Fleming, Dorsey A 6527 Colerain Avenue, Cincinnati, OH 45239, (513) 923-4446, BA 73 Coll of Wooster; MA 76 OH St Univ; Aud, E N T Cl Inc, **A**

Fleming, Mrs Geraldine 7 Kimball Street, Chatham, NJ 07928, (201) 635-8115, BS 79 Ithaca Coll; MA 81 Montclair St Coll; Sp-Lang Path, Private Practice, **SLP ACE**

Fleming, Jami Ann 310 E Pierce P O Box 485, Elburn, IL 60119, (312) 438-6319, BA 84 Univ of MI - Ann Arbor; MS 86 Univ of MI - Ann Arbor; Sp-Lang Path, Therapeutic Systems, **SLP**

Fleming, Joanne 3700 West 103rd Street, Chicago, IL 60655, (312) 779-3300, BA 61 Saint Xavier Coll; MA 67 Saint Xavier Coll; MS 70 Marquette Univ; Assoc Prof/Dir Sp-Lang Path, St Xavier Coll, **SLP ACE**

Fleming, Mrs Joyce F 118 May Morning Drive, Lexington, SC 29072, (803) 739-4095, BS 75 Univ of SC - Columbia; OM 77 Univ of SC - Columbia; Sp-Lang Path, Lexington County School Dist, **SLP**

Fleming, Katherine J 10122 River Road Suite 203, Potomac, MD 20854, (301) 299-8666, BA 60 Univ of WA; MA 62 Stanford Univ; Sp-Lang Path, Private Practice, **SLP**

Fleming, Mrs Kimberly O'Hara 2507 N E 17th Court, Jensen Beach, FL 34957, (407) 468-5373, ME 84 Univ of FL; 87–Sp-Lang Path, St Lucie County Schs, **SLP**

Fleming, Lorna J 101 Spray Drive, Munroe Falls, OH 44262, (216) 688-3518, OB 79 Kent St Univ; MA 82 Kent St Univ; SLP, Crestwood Local Sch, **SLP**

Fleming, Lucy Ann 188 North Hanover, Lexington, KY 40502, (606) 266-0887, BA 75 Univ of KY; MS 83 Univ of KY; Sp-Lang Path, Cardinal Hill Hosp, **SLP**

Fleming, Mrs Marcia D 1016 Foxmoor Drive, Clarksville, TN 37042, (615) 645-0354, BS 76 OH Univ - Athens; MA 81 Cleveland St Univ; **SLP**

Fleming, Margaret A 2102 South Hughes, Amarillo, TX 79109, (806) 383-8611, BS 77 Southwest TX St Univ; MS 78 Southwest TX St Univ; SLP, Amarillo ISD, **SLP**

Fleming, Michelle 1761 3rd Avenue #11F, New York, NY 10029, (212) 722-6899, BA 84 Hofstra Univ; MA 86 CUNY - Queens Coll; 86–Aud, Mt Carmel Guild, **A**

Fleming, Mrs Patricia 5700 West State Road 46, Columbus, IN 47201, (812) 376-4415, BS 69 CO St Univ; MS 71 CO St Univ; Sp/Lang Path, Bartholomew Consol Sch Corp, **SLP**

Fleming, Paul L 60 Commonwealth Boulevard, Delaware, DE 19720, BS 64 SUNY - Coll at Geneseo; MS 70 SUNY - Coll at Geneseo; Sp-Lang Path, VA Hosp and Reg Offi, **SLP ACE**

Fleming, Dr Susan G 5952 Royal Ln, Suite 203, Dallas, TX 75230, (214) 696-3690, BA 65 Southern Methodist Univ; MA 67 Southern Methodist Univ; PH 87 (Lang Dev Narrative Dev) Univ of TX - Dallas; 87–Sp-Lang Path, Private Practice, **SLP**

Fleming, Mrs Susan K 4200 Ellington Avenue, Western Springs, IL 60558, (312) 344-7000, BS 74 Univ of IL - Urbana; MS 75 Univ of IL - Urbana; Sp-Lang Path, Proviso Township Hs, **SLP**

Fleming, Dr Susan M Swallowing And Voice Pathology, Harper-Grace Hospital, 4201 St Antoine UHC-5F, Detroit, MI 48201, (313) 745-4098, BA 69 MI St Univ; MA 70 MI St Univ; PH 76 (Speech Science) Wayne St Univ; Assoc Ch Swallow & Voice Path, Harper Hosp, **SLP**

Fleming, Susan Shaw 3807 Rosedale, Memphis, TN 38111, (901) 458-4304, BS 83 Lambuth Coll; MS 86 Univ of MS; **SLP**

Fleming, Terrilyn E 1240 Savoy Street, San Diego, CA 92107-3917, **SLP**

Flemming, Mrs Alison Hedden 5990 Turnbull Drive, Orlando, FL 32822, (813) 439-4017, BS 84 FL St Univ; MS 85 FL St Univ; 86–Sp-Lang Path, Polk County Sch Bd, **SLP**

Flenner, Carolyn Ferrell 596 West Harding Avenue, Coolidge, AZ 85228, (602) 868-4092, BS 64 OH St Univ; MA 71 OH St Univ; 76–Sp/Lang Path, Pinal Co Spec Ed, **SLP**

Flentge, Mrs Margaret Louise 7627 Woodside Drive, Stockton, CA 95207, (707) 374-5335, BA 81 Univ of the Pacific; MA 82 Univ of the Pacific; 82–Sp-Lang Path, Sacramento County Office of Ed, **SLP**

Flesher, Barbara L 1814 Kuser Road #8, Trenton, NJ 08690, (609) 466-0400, BS 75 Trenton St Coll; MA 81 Trenton St Coll; **SLP**

Flessatti, Paula Mary 1757 Bridgecreek Drive, Sacramento, CA 95833, (916) 424-9548, BS 81 CA St Univ - Hayward; OM 83 Univ of WA; 86–Sp-Lang Path, Professional Rehab Assoc, **SLP**

Fletcher, Bonnie Downham 1361 Colony Way, Yardley, PA 19067, (609) 882-1475, BS 77 James Madison Univ; MS 82 Phillips Univ; Sp-Lang Path, Mercer County Sp Serv Sch Dist, **SLP**

Fletcher, Mrs Brenda G 306 Meadow Lea, Austin, TX 78745, (512) 443-4054, BS 71 Univ of TX - Austin; MS 74 East TX St Univ - Commerce; Sp-Lang Path, Austin ISD, **SLP**

Fletcher, Mrs Cornelia H 3171 Northside Parkway N W, Atlanta, GA 30327, (404) 233-5332, BS 73 Central MO St Univ; MS 74 Central MO St Univ; Sp/Lang Path, Atlanta Speech Sch, **SLP**

Fletcher, Deborah G Child Find Coordinator, 811 15th Street, Greeley, CO 80631, (303) 352-1543, BA 71 Univ of Northern CO; MA 72 Univ of Northern CO; Sp-Lang Path, Greeley County School Dist 6, **SLP**

Fletcher, Dorothy Isbell 8925 Stanwood, Dallas, TX 75228, (512) 459-5856, BS 79 Univ of TX - Austin; MS 80 Southern Methodist Univ; Sp-Lang Path, St Michael Sch, **SLP**

Fletcher, Dorothy L 845 Longview Road, Hillsborough, CA 94010, (415) 586-4488, BS 73 Univ of Santa Clara; MS 78 San Francisco St Univ; Sp-Lang Path, S F Unif Sch, **SLP**

Fletcher, Mrs Eileen Rd 5 Box 90, Kingston, NY 12401, (914) 338-4056, BS 69 SUNY - Coll at Buffalo; MA 75 CUNY - Hunter Coll; **SLP**

Fletcher, Elisabeth Cheryl 388 Calle Higuera, Camarillo, CA 93010-1729, (805) 654-3135, BA 68; MA 72 Univ of CA - Santa Barbara; MA 76 Univ of CA - Santa Barbara; Dir Sp-Path/Aud, Ventura Co Med Cen, **SLP**

Fletcher, Gordon L P O Box 944, Hickory, NC 28603-0944, (704) 322-5120, BS 75 Univ of SC - Columbia; OM 78 Univ of SC - Columbia; Viewmont Eent Assoc, **A ACE**

Fletcher, Dr John Lynn Department Of Psychology, Southwest Texas State Univ, San Marcos, TX 78666, (512) 245-2526, BA 50 Univ of AR - Fayetteville; MA 51 Univ of AR - Fayetteville; PH 55 Univ of KY; Lecturer-Psych Dept, SW TX St Univ, **F**

Fletcher, Mrs Margaret I 3950 Black Oak Drive, Santa Rosa, CA 95401, (707) 528-5452, BA 59 Southern Methodist Univ; MA 60 Columbia Univ Teachers Coll; 70–Sp-Lang Path, Sant Rosa Cty Sch, **SLP A**

Fletcher, Pat F 1928 Michel Deloing, Baton Rouge, LA 70810, (504) 644-0230, BS 77 LA Tech Univ; OM 81 LA St Univ - N O Medical Ctr; Tchr of Hearing Impaired, Ascension Parish Sch Bd, **SLP**

Fletcher, Mrs Rose 30 Lynwood Avenue, Ottawa, ON, Canada K1Y 2B3, (613) 728-9859, MS; **SLP LM**

Fletcher, Dr Samuel G Dept Of Biocommunication, University Of Alabama At Birmingham, UAB Station Box 503, Birmingham, AL 35294, (205) 934-4814, BS 51 UT St Univ; MS 56 Univ of UT; PH 57 (NS) Univ of UT; Prof & Chairman, Univ of Alabama at Birmingham, **SLP A F**

Fletcher, Mrs Sharon K L 1420 Coral Tree Road, Colton, CA 92324, (714) 788-7296, BA 64 Univ of Redlands; MA 70 Univ of Redlands; Spec Day Class Tchr, Riverside USD, **SLP**

Fletcher, Wendy J Glenn Devin Condo #45, White Hall Road, Amesbury, MA 01913, (508) 462-9628, MS 87 Ithaca Coll; 88–Aud, North Shore Hearing Ctr

Fletcher-Levasseur, Susan 4265 Mitchell Cresent, Windsor, ON, Canada N9G 2G1, (519) 948-0164, BA 80 Wayne St Univ - Sch of Med; MA 81 Wayne St Univ - Sch of Med; Sp-Lang Path Dept Head, Children's Rehab Ctr of Essex Co, **SLP**

Fletchinger, Sr M Therese 421 Lafourche, Lockport, LA 70374, (504) 532-6412, BS 53 Loyola Univ; MA 61 Ball St Univ; Tchr, Lafourche Parish Sch Bd, **A LM**

Flevaris, Dr Carole A 24315 Hoover Court, Apt #1838, Farmington Hills, MI 48331, (313) 261-7005, BS 71 Eastern MI Univ; ME 73 Wayne St Univ; PH 84 (NS) Wayne St Univ - Sch of Med; Audiologist & Psychologist, VA/Yale University, **A**

Flewelling, Mrs Barbara B 23 Split Rock Road, Pittsford, NY 14534-1834, (716) 586-2886, BA 66 Univ of ME - Orono; ME 67 Boston Univ; **SLP**

Flewelling, Wayne M R R 2 Box 4950, Bennington, VT 05201-9530, BA 77 SUNY - Coll at Plattsburgh; MS 80 SUNY - Coll at Buffalo; Sp/Lang Path, Southwest Vermont Superv Union, **SLP**

Flexer, Dr Carol S 5690 Caranor, Kent, OH 44240, (216) 375-7883, BA 75 Metropolitan St Coll; MA 76 Univ of Denver; PH 82 (NS) Kent St Univ; 82–Assoc Prof, The U of Akron, **A**

Flickinger, Mrs Kimberly L 25722 Whispering Trees Way, Valencia, CA 91355-2437, BA 77 CA St Univ - Northridge; MA 80 CA St Univ - Northridge; 85–Sp-Lang Path, Gardner Manzella & Associates, **SLP**

Flieder, Mrs Sally Willner 1 Pitt Road, East Brunswick, NJ 08816, BS 57 Kean Coll of NJ; MS 84 Rutgers St Univ -N Brunswick; Sp-Lang Path, East Brunswick Bd of Ed, **SLP**

Fliehs, Joan B Box 538, Groton, SD 57445, (605) 622-7192, BA 72 SD St Univ; MS 75 Minot St Univ; Coor Sp/Lang/Hrng Serv, Aberdeen Sch Dist, **SLP**

Flinchum, Mary Brennan 9803 Cahart Place, Silver Spring, MD 20903, (301) 434-8246, BA 82 Univ of MD - College Park; MA 86 Univ of Cincinnati; **A**

Flinn, Mrs Mary Perkins 5308 Southwind Road, Greensboro, NC 27405, (919) 349-5370, BA 79 Univ of NC - Greensboro; MS 81 East Carolina Univ; Sp-Lang Path, Reidsville City Sch, **SLP**

Flinn, Mrs Sally E 205 Banbury Road, Richmond, VA 23221, (804) 353-3026, BA 57 Vanderbilt Univ; MS 61 Vanderbilt Univ; Sp-Lang Path, Private Practice, **SLP**

Flint, V H 3208 Dogwood Lane, Richmond, IN 47374, **SLP**

Flinta, Mrs Andrea J 2248 Cypress Creek Court, Columbus, OH 43228, (614) 761-2811, BS 84 Bowling Green St Univ; MA 87 OH St Univ; 86–Sp-Lang Path, Upper Arlington City Schs, **F**

Flint-Greenberg, Sara 5857 West 74th Street, Los Angeles, CA 90045-1721, BA 78 Univ of CA - Los Angeles; MA 82 CA St Univ - Northridge; 86–Sp-Lang Path, Montebello USD, **SLP**

Flint-Shaw, Mrs Lynn M 7557 Rambler Road #750, Dallas, TX 75231, (214) 373-7557, BS 76 Xavier Univ of LA; OM 77 LA St Univ - N O Medical Ctr; Sp-Lang Path, Private Practice, **SLP**

Flipping, Joette Leslie 8-D Montebello Road, Pueblo, CO 81001, (303) 560-5005, BS 78 CA Univ of PA; MA 82 Adams St Coll; **SLP**

Flitner, Laurene Lukas 3832 East Monterosa, Phoenix, AZ 85018, (602) 898-7854, BS 74 AZ St Univ; MS 77 Univ of AZ; Prog Spec/Commun Disorders, Mesa Pub Schools Special Ed, **SLP ACE**

Floch, Margot Jean 525 Wendell Terrace, Syracuse, NY 13203-1142, (315) 476-7441, BA 78 SUNY - Coll at Cortland; MA 87 SUNY - Center at Buffalo; 87–Supvr Sp-Lang Path, Onondaga Assoc of Ret Citz, **SLP**

Flohr, Mrs Pamela Lampshire 5912 Lemon Avenue, Cypress, CA 90630, (714) 731-7331, BA 83 CA St Univ - Fullerton

Flondarina, Mrs Susan B 8900 Palmer Place N W, Bremerton, WA 98310, (206) 692-1703, BA 80 Univ of SC - Columbia; MS 82 Univ of SC - Columbia; 88–Sp-Lang Path, South Kitsap Sch Dist, **SLP**

Flood, Margaret A 480 3rd Street, East Northport, NY 11731, (516) 924-5583, BS 82 SUNY - Coll at Buffalo; MS 85 SUNY - Coll at Buffalo; **SLP**

Flood, Mary K 1919 North Summit #6A, Milwaukee, WI 53202, **SLP**

Flood, Patricia Anne 1 Victoria Falls Drive, Sparks, MD 21152, (301) 761-1639, BA 85 Loyola Coll; MS 87 Loyola Coll

Florance, Dr Cheri L Communication Disorders Inst, St Anthony Hospital, 1450 Hawthorne Avenue, Columbus, OH 43203, (614) 251-3740, BA 69 Muskingum Coll; MA 70 OH St Univ; PH 75 (NS) OH St Univ; Dir, St Anthony Hosp Commun Dist, **SLP F**

Florance, Kathleen 159 Worcester Court, Falmouth, MA 02540, (508) 540-8600, BA 75 SUNY - Coll at Cortland; MS 76 Ithaca Coll; Dir, Speech & Hearing Ctr, **SLP**

Florence, Diane P 4121 Via Marina #310, Marina Del Rey, CA 90292, (213) 324-7579, BA 72 Univ of CA - Berkeley; MS 75 Boston Univ; SLP, LA Co Supt of Sch, **SLP**

Florence, Mary L 1615 Willoughby Drive, Parkersburg, WV 26101, (304) 485-6513, BS 72 WV Univ; MS 77 WV Univ; **A**

Florensa, Montse 5305 North Tyler #7, Temple City, CA 91780, (818) 268-5000, BS 80 Boston Univ; MS 81 TX Christian Univ; Sp-Lang Path, White Mem Med Cen, **SLP**

Florentine, Dr Mary Dept Of Speech-Lang Path & Aud, Northeastern University, Boston, MA 02115, (617) 437-3084, BA 73 Northeastern Univ; MA 75 Northeastern Univ; PH 78 (NS) Northeastern Univ

Flores, Anita H H 22 Irving Street, Saco, ME 04072, (207) 283-1242, BA 81 Univ of MI - Ann Arbor; MA 84 Univ of ME - Orono; Sp-Lang Path, York County Counseling Svcs, **SLP**

Flores, Grace A 8710 Delmonico Avenue, Canoga Park, CA 91304, MA 78 CA St Univ - Northridge; SLP, Simi Valley USD, **SLP**

Flores, Marsha D 3009 Whiteway Avenue, Louisville, KY 40205, (502) 895-3401, BS 67 IN Univ - Bloomington; MA 69 IN Univ - Bloomington; SLP/Aud, VA Med Cen, **A**

Flores, Mary H 201 Cueva Lane, San Antonio, TX 78232, (512) 494-5948, BA 64 Univ of TX - Austin; MA 70 Univ of NM; Sp-Lang Path, Northeast ISD, **SLP**

Flores, Nancy Martinez 14818 Personality Street, San Antonio, TX 78248, (512) 653-3900, BA 78 Our Lady Lake Univ-San Anton; MA 80 Our Lady Lake Univ-San Anton; Sp-Lang Path, **SLP**

Florick, Wendy M 7634 South Rosemary Circle, Englewood, CO 80112, (303) 740-9663, BS 85 PA St Univ - Univ Park; MA 87 Kent St Univ; 87–Sp-Lang Path, Jeff County Comm Ctr for the Dev Disabled, **SLP**

Florin, Suzanne 505 West University Pkwy, Apartment C-10, Baltimore, MD 21210, **A**

Florio, Mrs Amarilis 6 Hartpence Court, Flemington, NJ 08822, (201) 782-9400, **SLP**

Florman, Mrs Ellen Holly One Watnong Road, Morris Plains, NJ 07950, (201) 267-2596, BA 77 Rutger's St Univ - Douglas Coll; MS 86 Rutger's St Univ - Douglas Coll; 81–Sp-Lang Path, Morris Plains Bd of Educ, **SLP**

Flory, Susan Williamson P O Box 1117, La Motte Professional Bldg, Hilton Head, SC 29925, (803) 681-6070, BA 73 IN Univ - Bloomington; MS 82 Purdue Univ - West Lafayette; Director of Audiology, Hilton Head Hearing Services, **A**

Flory, William C 5051 Flory Drive, Lake Worth, FL 33463, (407) 965-0084, OB 64 Univ of FL; MA 66 Univ of FL; 67–Sp-Lang Path, Speech Pathology, **SLP LM**

Flotten, Marcella S 2233 Inca Lane, New Brighton, MN 55112, (612) 781-3991, BS 62 Univ of MN - Duluth; MA 88 Univ of MN - Minneap-St Paul; 87–Sp-Lang Path, St Paul-Ramsey Med Ctr, **SLP**

Flower, Dr Richard M 34 Seventh Avenue, San Francisco, CA 94118, (415) 751-5865, BA 46 San Jose St Univ; MA 47 Northwestern Univ; PH 53 (Sp Path & Aud) Northwestern Univ; Sp-Lang Path & Aud, U of CA San Francisco, **SLP A F H**

Flower, Susan Lynne 512 Evergreen Drive, Tallmadge, OH 44278, (215) 631-9300, BA 85 Univ of Akron; MA 86 Univ of Akron; **SLP**

Flower, Mrs Wilda M 34 Seventh Avenue, San Francisco, CA 94118, (415) 751-5865, BA 38 Northwestern Univ; MA 41 Northwestern Univ; Sp/Lang Path/Aud, U CA Med Sf, **SLP A F**

Flowers, Arthur 21544 Hickory Wood Drive, Dearborn Heights, MI 48127, (313) 274-5131

Flowers, Dr Charles Ray Mason Clinic Speech Path, 1100 9th Avenue, P O Box 900, Seattle, WA 98111, (206) 223-6618, BA 67 San Francisco St Univ; MA 68 CA St Univ - Los Angeles; PH 72 (NS) Univ of IA; Dir, Virgina Mason Clinic, **SLP**

Flowers, Donna Jean P O Box 3072, Sherman, TX 75090, (214) 893-7457, BS 70 TX Woman's Univ; MA 88 TX Woman's Univ; Sp-Lang Path, Grayson Co Ctr, **SLP**

Flowers, Doris Anita 7-8 Copeley Hill, Charlottesville, VA 22903, BS 80 Univ of the DC; MS 81 Univ of the DC; 86–Dir of Clin Comp Lab, Univ of Virginia, **SLP**

Flowers, Dr Elsie Ann Box 523 McV Station, Richmond, VA 23298, (804) 786-0207, MS 49 Univ of WI - Madison; ED 65 (Sp-Lang Path) Univ of VA - Charlottesville; Assoc Prof Emeritus, Medical College of Virginia, **SLP LM**

Flowers, Mrs Marian H 2405 Forest Bend, Austin, TX 78704, (512) 266-1894, BS 71 Univ of North TX; MS 72 TX Christian Univ; SLP, Lake Travis ISD, **SLP**

Floyd, Karla Jean 2646 Stroschein Road #E-11, Monroeville, PA 15146, (814) 944-5014, **A**

Floyd, Dr Larry R 4601 Crestline Drive, St Louis, MO 63124, (314) 652-4100, BA 69 Univ of MO - KS City; MA 77 Univ of MO - Columbia; PH 83 (NS) Univ of MO - Columbia; SLP, John Cochran Vamc, **SLP**

Fluder, Mary B W 212 Norle Street, State College, PA 16801, (814) 359-3421, BS 73 PA St Univ - Univ Park; MS 80 PA St Univ - Univ Park; 87–Asst Admin, Nittany Valley Rehab Hosp, **SLP**

Flug, Mrs Gail 3 Jamestown Court, East Brunswick, NJ 08816, (201) 246-4255, BS 65 Boston Univ; MA 66 Columbia Univ Teachers Coll; Sp/Lang Path, Univ of Med & Denistry of NJ, **SLP ACE**

Flugrath, Dr James M 1812 McClellan Drive, Johnson City, TN 37601, (615) 926-1171, BA 61 Univ of MI - Ann Arbor; MA 63 Wayne St Univ; PH 65 (NS) Wayne St Univ - Sch of Med; Chief, VA, **SLP A**

Fluharty, George M 4057 South 35th #14, Greenfield, WI 53221, (414) 282-5168, BA 79 Univ of Northern IA; MA 80 Univ of Northern IA; Sp-Lang Path, New Meolico Rehab Center of WI, **SLP**

Fluharty, Mrs Nancy Buono 584 Wirham Place, Cincinnati, OH 45220, (513) 281-5424, BS 69 Carlow Coll; MA 73 Univ of Cincinnati; **SLP**

Flum, Dr Leonard 2798 Shore Drive, Merrick, NY 11566, (516) 623-4048, BA 58 CUNY - Brooklyn Coll; MA 63 CUNY - Brooklyn Coll; PH 74 (NS) CUNY - Grad Sch & Univ Cntr; Director, Private Practice, **SLP A**

Flum, Mary Therese 137 D The Post Road, Springfield, OH 45503, (513) 390-5074, BS 86 Bowling Green St Univ; MS 87 Miami Univ - Oxford

Fly, Mrs Diane T Route 1, Gosely Hill Road, Franklin, TN 37064, (615) 794-8091, BS 80 Univ of WI - Milwaukee; MS 82 Univ of WI - Milwaukee; Sp-Lang Path, Williamson Co Bd of Ed, **SLP**

Flynn, Mrs Barbara Barry 193 Sneden Place West, Spring Valley, NY 10977, (914) 425-2432, BS 77 Mercy Coll; MS 81 William Paterson Coll; Sp-Lang Path, North Rockland Crtl Sch Dist, **SLP**

Flynn, Barbara J White Haven Center, White Haven, PA 18661, BS 74 Univ of WI - Whitewater; ME 76 Bloomsburg Univ of PA; Sp-Lang Path, White Haven Center, **SLP**

Flynn, Barry James 11 Cora Street, New Haven, CT 06512, (203) 397-4650, BA 79 Southern CT St Univ; MS 81 Southern CT St Univ; Sp-Lang Path, New Haven Regional Center, **SLP**

Flynn, Dale T 4219 Latona Avenue N E, Seattle, WA 98105, (206) 775-6651, BA 70 Univ of CA - Berkeley; BS 75 Univ of WA; MA 78 Univ of WA; Aud, Puget Sound Otol Inc Ps, **A**

Flynn, Deanna Colleen 6009 Fountain Pointe #3, Grand Blanc, MI 48439, BA 79 MI St Univ; MA 80 MI St Univ; Sp-Lang Path, Swartz Creek Com Schools, **SLP**

Flynn, Mrs Deborah Ann 5034 52nd Street, Lubbock, TX 79414, (806) 797-4509, BS 81 SD St Univ; MA 82 Univ of SD - Vermillion; Sp-Lang Path, Sp-Lang-Hrng Ctr of Lubbock, **SLP**

Flynn, Diane Marie 113 Valley Street, San Francisco, CA 94131, (415) 540-4415, MS 84 San Francisco St Univ; 85–Sp-Lang Path, Alta Bates-Herrick Hosp, **SLP**

Flynn, Eileen B R 2449 Windermere Road, Windsor, ON, Canada N8W 2T2, (519) 253-4261, BA 79 MI St Univ; MA 80 MI St Univ; Sp-Lang Path, Windsor Western Hosp Cen, **SLP**

Flynn, Janis E 60 Hatherly Road, Scituate, MA 02066, (617) 545-6338, BS 72 Emerson Coll; MS 73 Southern Methodist Univ; Sp-Lang Path, Hanover Pub Sch, **SLP**

Flynn, Karen Anne 320 East 23rd Street #7-C, New York, NY 10010, (212) 362-0449, **SLP**

Flynn, Mrs Linda Denese 3215 East Kaley Avenue, Orlando, FL 32806, (305) 423-9267, **SLP**

Flynn, Linda F 4 Pirates Lane, East Gloucester, MA 01930, (617) 245-2145, BS 66 Univ of MA - Amherst; ME 76 Northeastern Univ; Sp-Lang Path, Wakefield Public Schools, **SLP ACE**

Flynn, Lori D 16417 266th Avenue S E, Issaquah, WA 98027, (206) 591-6763, MA 79 WA St Univ; Director Speech Pathology, St Joseph Hospital, **SLP**

Flynn, Mrs Margaret 27 Yacht Club Cove, Staten Island, NY 10308, (212) 317-9054, BA 60 CUNY - Brooklyn Coll; MA 62 CUNY - Brooklyn Coll; Dept Couns/Lect, CUNY-Brooklyn Coll Dept/Sp, **SLP**

Flynn, Margaret M Meriter Hospital, 202 South Park Street, Madison, WI 53715, (608) 267-6174, BA 67; MA 71 Univ of WI - Madison; MS 77 Univ of WI - Madison; 86–Dir-SLP & Aud, Meriter Hosp-Madison, **SLP**

Flynn, Mary Anne 78 Sunset Avenue, Farmingdale, NY 11735, (516) 378-2000, BA 83 Adelphi Univ; MS 85 Adelphi Univ; **SLP**

Flynn, Patricia Aileen 95 West Columbia Street, Orlando, FL 32806, (407) 422-2200, BA 80 Univ of FL; MA 84 Univ of CA - Santa Barbara; Audiologist, June F Kennedy PhD & Assoc, **A**

Flynn, Paula L I P O Box 294, Newark, AR 72562, (501) 229-3581, BS 72 MS Univ for Women; OM 77 Univ of MS; **SLP**

Flynn, Dr Pauline T 3617 Kirkwood Drive, Fort Wayne, IN 46805, (219) 481-6410, BA 63 Paterson St Coll; MA 66 Seton Hall Univ; PH 70 (Sp Path) Univ of KS; 70–Prof/Chair Aud & Sp Sci, IN U-Prudue Univ at Fort Wayne, **SLP**

Flynn, Perry F 927 Carr Street, Greensboro, NC 27403, (919) 275-6231, ME 86 Univ of NC - Greensboro; **SLP**

Flynn, Mrs Ronda Cain 200 Hiden Creek Lane, Somerset, KY 42501, (606) 678-4713, BA 80 Univ of KY; ME 83 Eastern KY Univ; SLP, Pulaski Co Bd of Ed, **SLP**

Flynn, Mrs Rose Marie 1617 N W Sherwood Street, Bremerton, WA 98310, (206) 692-3152, BA 81 Univ of MT; OM 83 Univ of WA; SLP, Central Kitsap School District, **SLP**

Flynn, Rosemary E 150 Hillside Road, Ashley Hills #A-1, Westfield, MA 01085, (413) 568-1116, BA 75 Boston Coll; MS 80 Univ of RI; Sp/Lang Path, Westfield Pub Sch Syst, **SLP**

Flynn, Teresa F 34 Walnut Street, Shrewsbury, MA 01545, (508) 957-0511, BA 72 Univ of MA - Amherst; MA 73 Univ of MA - Amherst; Aud, Dracut Pub Sch, **A**

Flynn, Vicki H 3010 West Steepbank Circle, Sugar Land, TX 77479, (713) 980-3123, BS 68 Univ Southern MS-Hattiesburg; MS 70 Univ Southern MS-Hattiesburg; Aud, Vhf Aud Serv, **A**

Flynn-Tinsley, Nancy Elaine 205 North Gaylord, Ludington, MI 49431, (517) 773-9403, BA 83 Central MI Univ; MA 87 Central MI Univ; 87–Exec Dir/Sp-Lang Path, Private Practice, **SLP**

Flynt, Cynthia Roberts P O Box 3216, Greenville, NC 27836-3216, (919) 830-1650, BS 81 East Carolina Univ; MS 83 East Carolina Univ; Sp-Lang Path Dir, CRF Sp & Lang Assoc, **SLP**

Foard, Mrs Donna S 390 Mt View Court S E, Concord, NC 28025, (704) 786-4121, BA 67 Catawba Coll; MA 69 Univ of AL- Tuscaloosa; Except Chldn Tchr, Cabarrus Co Sch, **SLP**

Focaracci, Mrs Laura Weiss 1847 Bough Avenue, Apartment C, Clearwater, FL 34620, (813) 539-8034, BA 85 Univ of FL; MS 86 FL St Univ; 88–Sp-Lang Path, Morton Plant Hosp, **SLP**

Focht, Christofer 35 Dolores Terrace, San Francisco, CA 94110, (415) 863-1895, MS 88 San Francisco St Univ

Fockler, Mrs Victoria Gene 133 South Sly Fox Way, Sedalia, CO 80135, (303) 660-0358, BA 67 OH Univ - Athens; MA 72 Univ of Cincinnati; SLP, Littleton Public Schools, **SLP**

Foecking, Ann Leslie 3854 Thyme Dr #1, Rockingford, IL 61111-4873, (217) 223-1200, BS Western IL Univ; MA 85 Western IL Univ; **SLP**

Foerster, Shawn W P O Box 213, High Island, TX 77623, (409) 286-5313, BS Univ of North TX; MS 85 Univ of North TX

Fogarty, Cynthia Ann P O Box 852, Plymouth, FL 32768-0852, (800) 255-4327, MS 85 Univ of South FL; **A**

Fogarty, Mrs M Maurine Speech Pathology Associates, 32 Goldie Road, Youngstown, OH 44505, (216) 759-3636, BS 56 Marquette Univ; MS 58 Univ of KS; Sp-Lang Path, Sp-Path Assoc, **SLP**

Fogel, Deborah Jeanne 447 Route 10 Suite 3, Randolph, NJ 07869, (201) 989-8353, BA 81 SUNY - Coll at Plattsburgh; MS 83 Emory Univ; Aud Manager/Private Practice, Randolph Family Hearing Center, **A**

Fogelson, Mrs Janie Karen 4938 Ledge Avenue, North Hollywood, CA 91601, (213) 839-4361, BA 75 Univ of CA - Santa Barbara; MA 82 CA St Univ - Los Angeles

Fogelstrom, Suzanne S 322 Maryland Avenue N E, Washington, DC 20002, (202) 724-4683, MS; SLP, Dc Publ Schs, **SLP LM**

Fogg, Deborah A 911 Cromwell Avenue, Westchester, IL 60153, (312) 420-6540, BS 79 Elmhurst Coll; MS 81 Northern IL Univ - De Kalb; Sp-Lang Path, Sch Assoc Spec Ed-Dupage Co, **SLP**

Fogg, Patricia Lettko 769 Saint Paul Street, Denver, CO 80206, (303) 837-7021, **SLP**

Fogle, Paul T 3626 Cumberland Court, Stockton, CA 95209, PH (NS); **SLP**

Fogleman, Mrs Jana Dunn 5601 Albany Court, New Orleans, LA 70114, BA 81 Tulane Univ; OM 82 LA St Univ - N O Medical Ctr; Sp-Lang Path, Jefferson Parish Sch Syst, **SLP**

Fogleman, Mrs Karen Hayes 4201 Red Maple Court, Burtonsville, MD 20866, (301) 762-0632, **SLP**

Fokes, Joann Ohio University, Lindley Hall, Athens, OH 45701, (614) 593-1420, BS 49 Univ of TX - Austin; ME 62 Southwest TX St Univ; PH 67 (Hrng & Sp) Purdue Univ - West Lafayette; Prof, Ohio U

Folden, Mrs Julie Sardinha 60 Gulf Boulevard St 104, Indian Rocks Beach, FL 34635, (813) 595-0514, MS 78 Univ of South FL; SLP, Private Practice, **SLP**

Foldvary, Sherry Lee 7760 Jaydee Circle, Tujunga, CA 91042-1260, (818) 353-8848, BS 82 Loma Linda Univ - Riverside; MA 85 CA St Univ - Northridge; SLP, Glendale Adventist Medical Ctr, **SLP**

Foley, Beth E 14A Newton Place, Framingham, MA 01701, (617) 872-4099, BA 75 Univ of MA - Amherst; MA 76 Univ of MA - Amherst; 86–Educ Consult, Private Practice, **SLP**

Foley, Celia 10831 Trails End, Anchorage, AK 99516, (907) 279-9531, BS 70 Saint Louis Univ; MA 71 Case Western Reserve Univ; Sp-Lang Path, Anchorage School District, **SLP**

Foley, Mrs Denise Jennings 10520 N Port Washington Rd, Mequon, WI 53092, (414) 241-8000, BS 82 Marquette Univ; MS 84 Rush Univ; Aud, Milwaukee ENT, **A**

Foley, Eileen Grace 16880 Hubbard Road, Livonia, MI 48154, BA 83 MI St Univ; MA 87 Central MI Univ; **A**

Foley, Elaine H Route 2 Box 155F, Bonner Springs, KS 66012, **SLP**

Foley, Mrs Joyce J 49 Bouchard Drive, Brunswick, ME 04011, (207) 725-4690, BS 70 Appalachian St Univ; MA 71 Appalachian St Univ; Sp-Lang Path, Brunswick School Department, **SLP**

Foley, Mary Josp 768 Galaxy Heights, La Canada, CA 91011, (213) 679-3374, BA 74 CA St Univ - Northridge; MA 75 CA St Univ - Northridge; Admin Asst for Reg Coord, Los Angeles Supt Sch, **SLP**

Foley, Maureen F 5005 Bridgewater Drive, Arlington, TX 76017-2778, (817) 465-5038, MA 76 CUNY - Queens Coll; Sp-Lang Path, Overton Speech & Lang Center, **SLP**

Foley, Michael Joseph 6642 Sunset N E, Bremerton, WA 98310, (206) 478-9214, BA 75 SUNY - Center at Buffalo; MA 77 Hofstra Univ; **A**

Foley, Michele Susan 2820 Crayton Road, Naples, FL 33940, (813) 263-6924, BA 84 Loyola Coll; MS 86 James Madison Univ; 88–Sp-Lang Path, Lee Memorial Hosp, **SLP**

Foley, Rochelle Lynn 2201 Howe Avenue #46, Sacramento, CA 95825-0165, (916) 924-8362, BS 76 Northern St Coll; MA 80 Univ of SD - Vermillion; Sp-Lang Path, Brookings Sch Dist, **SLP**

Foley, Mrs Sheila M 8016 North Gannett Road, Northfield, OH 44067, (216) 526-4370, BA 79 Kent St Univ; MA 80 Kent St Univ; SLP, Brecksvile-Brodvew Hts Bd/Ed, **SLP**

Foley, Theresa Dawn 290 Whisperwood Boulevard, Slidell, LA 70458, (504) 649-6845, BS 81 LA St Univ - Baton Rouge; MA 85 LA St Univ - Baton Rouge; 85–Sp-Lang Path, St Tammcoy Parish Sch Bd, **SLP**

Foley, Veronica D 5901 Unitas Lane N W, Albuquerque, NM 87114, (505) 982-4848, BS 81 Univ of TN - Knoxville; MS 86 Univ of NM; **A**

Folger, Mrs Roscha B 221 North Woodland Drive, Liverpool, NY 13088, (315) 652-1249, BA 56 Univ of CO - Boulder; MS 69 Syracuse Univ; Retired, Liverpool Cen Sch Dist, **SLP**

Folkerts, Mrs Susan Miller 1548 N W 108th Street, Des Moines, IA 50322, BS 75 Univ of NE - Omaha; MA 77 Univ of NE - Omaha; SLP, Heartland AEA, **SLP**

Folkestad, Ann Elizabeth P O Box 531, Sandstone, MN 55072, (612) 245-5281, BS 80 Univ of MN - Minneap-St Paul; MA 84 Univ of Northern IA; 88–Sp-Lang Path, Sandstone Schools, **SLP**

Folkins, Dr John W Dept Speech Path & Audiology, University Of Iowa, Iowa City, IA 52242, (319) 335-8718, BA 70 Univ of Redlands; MS 71 Univ of Redlands; PH 76 (Sp Science) Univ of WA; Prof, Univ Iowa

Follansbee, Lenore 52 Henry Street, Burlington, VT 05401, (802) 863-2006, BA 87 Univ of VT; MS 87 Univ of VT; 86–Sp-Lang Path, Robinson Sch

Follett, Michelle Marie 5899 Keystone Drive, Bethel Park, PA 15102, (412) 854-4592, BS 80 Clarion Univ of PA; ME 82 Slippery Rock Univ of PA; **SLP**

Folse, Mrs Kathleen P 4247 Vincennes Place, New Orleans, LA 70125, (504) 899-9511, BS 77 Saint Mary's Dominican Coll; OM 78 LA St Univ - N O Medical Ctr; 81–Sp-Lang Path, Chldn Hosp of New Orleans, **SLP**

Folsom, Laura Clark 1127 East Butler Drive, Phoenix, AZ 85020, (602) 943-4751, MS 82 Northern AZ Univ; **SLP**

Folsom, Loreen C 442 Kensington, Missoula, MT 59801, (406) 728-2403, BS 65 Univ of MT; OM 69 Univ of MT; Sp-Lang Path, Missoula Co Hs, **SLP ACE**

Folsom, Dr Richard C 4339 N E 56th, Seattle, WA 98105, (206) 545-7425, BA 67 Central WA Univ; MS 70 Portland St Univ; PH 79 (NS) Univ of WA; U of WA, **A**

Folsom, Sarah D 1313 Ivy Lane, Raleigh, NC 27609, (919) 834-3828, BA 75 NC St Univ at Raleigh; ME 80 NC Central Univ; Sp-Lang Path, Private Practice, **SLP**

Foltner, Kathy A Audio-Vestibular Testing Ctr Inc, 1319 East Michigan, Lansing, MI 48912, (517) 372-6725, BS 75 Ithaca Coll; MA 76 MI St Univ; Aud/Pres, Audio-Vestibular Testing Cen, **A ACE**

Foltz, Michael J ENT Department, 2300 North Rockton, Rockford, IL 61103, (815) 968-0051, BS 71 Univ of WI - Whitewater; MA 72 Bowling Green St Univ; Dir of Aud, Rockford Cl Ltd, **A**

Fones, Mrs Susan Plumb 5003 Country Aire Lane, Tampa, FL 33624, (813) 934-4623, MS 85 Univ of South FL; 88–Sp-Lang Path, Pinellas County Sch System-Tarpon Springs Elem, **SLP**

Fong, Carolyn K 3823 N E 23rd Avenue, Portland, OR 97212, (503) 645-4242, **SLP**

Fong, Cheryl Lou 2222 Citron Street #802, Honolulu, HI 96826, BS 69 Univ of HI - Manoa; MS 72 Univ of HI - Manoa; Sp-Lang Path, Dept of Health, **SLP**

Fong, Craig Daniel 820 West 157th Street, Gardena, CA 90247, (213) 324-7087, BA 84 San Francisco St Univ; MS 86 San Francisco St Univ; **A**

Fong, Gwenolyn 16104 Trigate Road, Chester, VA 23831-7337, (512) 599-9326, BA 76 Columbus Coll; ME 78 Univ of GA; Sp-Lang Path, State of HI Spec Serv, **SLP**

Fong, Raymond G 1630 Parkmead Way, Sacramento, CA 95822, (916) 455-5032, BA Stanford Univ; MA CA St Univ - Sacramento; Retired, Sacramento USD, **SLP A**

Fong, Valerie 2116 25th Street, Sacramento, CA 95818, (209) 474-8193, BS 85 CA St Univ - Sacramento; MA 86 Univ of the Pacific

Fonkalsrud, Janice A 4229 East 77th Street, Tulsa, OK 74136, (918) 631-2915, BS 57 Univ of KS; MA 59 Univ of KS; 84–Clin Super, U of Tulsa, **SLP**

Fonssagrives, Dianne 8200 Kroll Way #367, Bakersfield, CA 93311-1120, (805) 398-3793, BA 84 Univ of AR - Little Rock; MS 86 Univ of AR - Medical Sci; 86–Sp-Lang Path, Kern Co Supt of Schs, **SLP**

Fontaine, Lisa M 2030 Georgian Woods Place, Apartment #33, Wheaton, MD 20902, (202) 832-4400, BA 77 Trinity Coll; MA 79 Catholic Univ of America; 81–Sp/Lang Path, Hosp for Sick Chldn, **SLP**

Fontana, Dr Marie 3794 Oatty Court, Bethpage, NY 11714, BA 51 CUNY - Queens Coll; MA 53 CUNY - Queens Coll; ED 72 (Sp/Lang Path) Columbia Univ Teachers Coll; Asst Prof, Queens College, CUNY, **SLP**

Fontanella, Mrs Renee Nancy 1058 Indian Hill Road, Toms River, NJ 08753, (201) 240-6181, **A**

Fontanive, Dr Lynn Oakland Schools, 2100 Pontiac Lake Road, Pontiac, MI 48054, (313) 858-2067, BA Marygove Coll; MA MI St Univ; ED 81 (NS) Wayne St Univ - Sch of Med; Dept Dir, Oakland Sch, **A**

Fontano, Joan Alice 670 Highland Avenue, Waterbury, CT 06708, (203) 753-3325, BA 83 Fairfield Univ; MA 86 Univ of CT; 87–Sp-Lang Path, The Gaylord Hosp, **SLP**

Fontenot, Mrs M Christy 200 Cajun Street, Broussard, LA 70518, (318) 365-2341, BA 79 Univ of Southwestern LA; MS 80 Southern Methodist Univ; Aud, Iberia Parish School Board, **A**

Fontes, Daniel 218 East Sesame Street, Tempe, AZ 85283, (602) 239-4755, BA AZ St Univ; MS 77 AZ St Univ; Sp-Lang Path, Samaritan Hlth Serv, **SLP**

Fontes, Kristine C 218 East Sesame Street, Tempe, AZ 85283, BS 74 PA St Univ - Univ Park; MS 76 AZ St Univ; Sp-Lang Path, Dev Serv Ctr, **SLP**

Fonti, Patti L 2501 Main Street, Stevens Point, WI 54481, (715) 344-4120, BS 85 Univ of WI - Stevens Point; MS 87 Univ of WI - Stevens Point; 87–Aud, Rice Clinic, **A**

Fonville-Mitchell, Mrs Dianne Lyn 105 Country Club Drive, St Clair Shores, MI 48082, (313) 791-6300, BA 84 MI St Univ; MA 85 MI St Univ; Sp-Lang Path, Clintondale Comm Schs, **SLP**

Foos, Rhonda Kaye 915 Camelot Court, Fort Collins, CO 80525, (303) 223-2017, BA 82 Univ of Northern CO; MA 84 Univ of Northern CO; Sp-Lang Path, Poudre Sch Dist R-1, **SLP**

Foose, David B P O Box 7, Mokena, IL 60448, (312) 532-7000, BA 77 Coll of Saint Francis; MS 81 Southern IL Univ-Edwardsvill; 81–Sp-Lang Path, W A Howe Dev Cen, **SLP**

Foote, Mrs Carol Jean 2105 Manchester, Westchester, IL 60153, (312) 865-0963, BA 84 Elmhurst Coll; MS 86 Rush Univ; **SLP**

Foote, Carolyn Elyse 412 E Merrimack Street, Lowell, MA 01852, BS 83 Univ of ME - Farmington; MA 85 Cleveland St Univ; **SLP**

Foote, Martha R 10834 Olde Woods Way, Columbia, MD 21044, (301) 730-9406, BS 68 SUNY - Coll at Fredonia; MS 78 Towson St Univ; Sp-Lang Path, State of MD Rosewood Cent, **SLP**

Footerman, Mrs Gittel G 115 South Adelaide Avenue, Highland Park, NJ 08904, (201) 745-5305, BA 62 Rutger's St Univ - Douglas Coll; MS 83 Rutgers St Univ -N Brunswick; Sp-Lang Path, New Brunswick Bd of Ed, **SLP**

Forbes, Carolin K 301 Kessler Drive, Ben Lomond, CA 95005-1610, (408) 336-2084, BS 72 Saint Cloud St Univ; MS 75 Univ of WI - Eau Claire; 88–Sp-Lang Path, Private Practice, **SLP ACE**

Forbes, Carolyn Elizabeth 11222 Braesridge, #2901, Houston, TX 77071, (713) 777-4417, BS 84 Fontbonne Coll; MS 86 Lamar Univ; **SLP**

Forbes, Gary Richard Rd #2 Hurlbut Road, Mexico, NY 13114, (315) 468-6268, BS 71 Ithaca Coll; MS 78 Syracuse Univ; 88–Aud, Private Practice, **A**

Forbes, Mrs Janice M 5909 Laketon Drive, Indianapolis, IN 46220, (317) 577-1428, BS 73 Purdue Univ - West Lafayette; MA 76 IN Univ - Bloomington; Sp-Lang Path, **SLP**

Forbes, Kevin C 2389 McKinleyville Avenue, McKinleyville, CA 95521, (707) 445-5111, BA 79 Humboldt St Univ; MA 87 Humboldt St Univ; Sp-Lang Path, General Hosp-Eureka Ca, **SLP**

Forbes, Kimball B Box 895, 2995 Crestview Drive, Santa Clara, UT 84765, (801) 628-1107, BS 81 Brigham Young Univ; OM 82 Brigham Young Univ; Coord of Sp & Hrng, Primary Chldrns Hosp, **A**

Forbes, Susan 10003 McKenney Avenue #3, Silver Spring, MD 20902, (301) 854-2075, BS 82 Towson St Univ; MS 86 Univ of NH; **SLP**

Forbes-Garner, Mrs Lynn 547 Woodsong Trail #304, Smyrna, GA 30080-7862, (404) 435-5878, **SLP**

Forbis-Stokes, Nancy K 8026 Bonnie Circle, Abilene, TX 79605, (915) 692-4053, BS 75 Univ of TX - Austin; MA 77 Univ of TX - Austin; Aud, Abilene State School, **A**

Forbord, Mrs Janis L 108 South Dietz, Webberville, MI 48892, (517) 353-8780, BA 71 MI St Univ; MA 72 MI St Univ; Cl Superv Spec, MI St U, **A**

Forbus, Mrs Sandra Sue Route 1 Box 533-A, Mabelvale, AR 72103, (501) 557-2151, MS 87 Univ of AR - Little Rock; **SLP**

Forcello, Juliana C 60 Morgan Street, Eastchester, NY 10709, (203) 454-5815, BS 79 SUNY - Coll at Oneonta; MS 82 Ithaca Coll; 82–Sp-Lang Path, Valhalla Pub Schs, **SLP**

Forcina, Debra L 3600 S W 1st Avenue, Miami, FL 33145, (305) 642-8665, BA 73 Univ of FL; MA 76 Univ of Miami; Sp-Lang Path, Dade Co Pub Sch, **SLP**

Forcucci, Angela K C 2000 West Town Parkway, Apartment 66-C, West Des Moines, IA 50265, (515) 284-7714, BS 74 Northwest MO St Univ; MS 78 Northwest MO St Univ; Sp-Lang Path, Des Moines Pub Sch, **SLP**

Forcucci, Frank R 2000 Westown Parkway #66C, West Des Moines, IA 50265, (515) 225-0042, MS 78 Northwest MO St Univ; BS 75 Northwest MO St Univ; SLP, Des Moines Pub Sch, **SLP**

Forcucci, Dr Richard A 209 North Skytop Drive, Edinboro, PA 16412, (814) 752-2444, BS 64 Edinboro Univ of PA; MA 66 Univ of IL - Urbana; PH 72 (NS) Univ of IL - Urbana; Chrmn Dept Speech Commun, Edinboro U of Pa, **SLP**

Ford, Mrs Alice B 8618 Discovery Boulevard, Walkersville, MD 21793-7841, (301) 694-1485, BA 62 Morgan St Univ; MA 64 Case Western Reserve Univ; Sp-Lang Path, Frederick Co Bd of Ed, **SLP**

Ford, Carolyn S 5839 Porpoise Road N W, Bokeelia, FL 33922, (813) 936-1759, BA 75 Univ of AL- Tuscaloosa; MA 76 Univ of AL- Tuscaloosa; Sp-Lang Path, Lee Co Sch, **SLP**

Ford, Dr Charles N Univ WI - Chs, 600 Highland Avenue, Madison, WI 53792, (608) 263-1223, BA 61 SUNY - Center at Binghamton; MD 65 (NS) Univ of Louisville; Assoc Professor Otolaryncology, University of Wisconsin

Ford, Mrs Cindy C 15114 Bauch Lane, Little Rock, AR 72206, (501) 660-2008, BA 82 Henderson St Univ; MS 87 Univ of AR - Medical Sci; 88–Sp-Lang Path, VA Med Ctr, **SLP**

Ford, Mrs Constance Lynn 5768 Edison Circle, Hanover Park, IL 60103, (312) 289-3273, **SLP**

Ford, Mrs Diane Molitoris 287 4-C Gemini Drive, Somerville, NJ 08876, (201) 281-6897, BA 85 Rutgers St Univ -N Brunswick; MS 86 Rutgers St Univ -N Brunswick; 86–Sp-Lang Path, Tinton Falls Schs, **SLP**

Ford, Donna Lynn 9882 Michigan Avenue, Zion, IL 60099-3851, (312) 623-4360, BS 84 Northern IL Univ - De Kalb; MA 85 Northern IL Univ - De Kalb; **SLP**

Ford, Janna R 1105 Grover Avenue, Lubbock, TX 79416, (806) 797-9017, BS 85 TX Tech Univ; MS 87 TX Tech Univ; **SLP**

Ford, Jean Marie 2109 Westridge Dr, Plano, TX 75075-8314, (214) 422-1869, **SLP**

Ford, Joseph Edward P O Box 339, Columbiana, AL 35051, (205) 933-1857, MS 84 Univ of Montevallo; Aud, VA Medical Center, **A**

Ford, Juilann Marie Box 317, New Carlisle, IN 46552, (219) 326-2395, BS 83 Purdue Univ - West Lafayette; MA 85 Western MI Univ; 87–Sp-Lang Path, LaPorte Hosp, **SLP**

Ford, Karen Gay 114-D Woodway Drive, Jackson, MS 39206, (601) 366-6160, BS 85 MS Univ for Women; MS 86 Univ Southern MS-Hattiesburg; 87–Sp-Lang Path, Miss Methodist Rehab Ctr, **SLP**

Ford, Kathryn Lawson 7823-E Royalty Avenue, Louisville, KY 40222, (502) 425-8604, BS 84 Murray St Univ; MS 85 Univ of Louisville; Sp-Lang Path, InSpeech Inc, **SLP**

Ford, Krista K 111 Cypress Court, Saskatoon, SK, Canada S7K 5C3, (306) 244-2211, BA 80 Univ of Saskatchewan - Sask; MS 82 Minot St Univ; Sp/Lang Path, Saskatoon Bd of Ed, **SLP**

Ford, Mrs Linda L 2338 Rockwood Lane, Norman, OK 73071, (405) 842-8000, BA 83 Univ of OK - Norman; ME 85 Central St Univ; **SLP**

Ford, Marty Suzanne 8208 Rosewood Lane, Prairie Village, KS 66208, (816) 756-2250, BS 83 TX Christian Univ; MA 85 Univ of Denver; Sp-Lang Path, Childrens Mercy Hospital, **SLP**

Ford, Mrs Nanette J 40 Summit Avenue, Webster Groves, MO 63119, (314) 889-1407, BS 75 Saint Louis Univ; MA 76 Saint Louis Univ; 87–Asst Prof/Comm Disorders, Fontbonne College, **SLP**

Ford, Dr Pamela S 3926 Partridge Circle #U, Bettendorf, IA 52722-2291, (319) 332-7488, PH 77 (Sp Path) Univ of IL - Urbana; 88–Sp-Lang Path, Moline PS Dist, **SLP**

Ford, Mrs Patricia H 3160 Isles Road, Marquette, MI 48453, (313) 346-2781, BA 73 MI St Univ; MA 74 MI St Univ; Sp-Lang Path, Brown Cith Schools, **SLP**

Ford, Mrs R Ann 1114 Woodman Drive #F, Worthington, OH 43085, (614) 431-5653, BS 71 Ithaca Coll; MS 72 Univ of WI - Madison; Sp-Lang Path, Private Practice, **SLP**

Ford, R Craig Eugene Hearing & Speech Center, 1500 West 12th, Eugene, OR 97402, (503) 485-8521, BS 80 Brigham Young Univ; OM 81 Brigham Young Univ; Aud, Eugene Hearing & Speech Center, **A**

Ford, Mrs Rebecca L 10806 E Rosewood Circle, Fort Wayne, IN 46845, (219) 637-6291, BA 75 IN St Univ - Terre Haute; MS 76 IN St Univ - Terre Haute; 77–Sp-Lang Path, Presch for the Handicap, **SLP**

Ford, Renee Jarreau 16047 Hidden Acres Drive, Houston, TX 77084, (713) 664-0621, BS 83 LA St Univ - Baton Rouge; MA 86 Univ of Houston - Univ Park; **SLP**

Ford, Mrs Robin Sommer 3420 Clairborne Way, Abingdon, MD 21009, (301) 676-8392, BS 83 Towson St Univ; ME 85 Univ of VA - Charlottesville; Sp-Lang Path, Maryland Sch for the Blind, **SLP**

Ford, Dr Ronald W Chief Audiology & Speech Ser, VA Hospital, Allen Park, MI 48101, (313) 562-6000, BS 60 Kent St Univ; MS 64 Kent St Univ; PH 72 (NS) Univ of MD - College Park; Ch Aud & SLP Serv, VA Med Cen Allen Park Mi, **SLP A**

Ford, Mrs Sue Fillingim 3000 Delcourt Drive, Decatur, GA 30033, (404) 297-5140, BS 82 Auburn Univ - Auburn; MA 85 Univ of TN - Knoxville; 88–Sp-Lang Path, Dekalb General Hosp, **SLP**

Ford, Susette M 2424 North 61st Street, Wauwatosa, WI 53213, (414) 444-5730, BA 76 Univ of WI - Eau Claire; MS 77 Univ of WI - Eau Claire; Sp-Lang Path, Milwaukee Public Schools, **SLP**

Ford, Dr Susie C 2815 Warm Springs Road Suite 1-A, Columbus, GA 31904-5246, (404) 324-6112, OB 64 Univ of GA; MA 65 Univ of TN - Knoxville; PH 75 (Sp & Hrng Science) Univ of TN - Knoxville; 78–Dir, Columbus Sp and Lang Cen, **SLP**

Ford, Teresa Hobbs 110 W 9th Street, Tipton, IA 52772, (319) 339-6700, BS 84 Univ of IA; MA 86 Univ of IA

Ford, Mrs Tresa Ann 412 Palm Avenue, Modesto, CA 95350, (209) 576-4155, MA 84 CA St Univ - Stanislaus; 87–Sp-Lang Path, Modesto City Schs, **SLP**

Ford, Valerie Sarno 7628 Pano Drive, Richmond, VA 23237, BS 78 CA St Univ - Hayward; MS 81 Univ of HI - Manoa; Sp/Lang Path, Cumberland Hosp, **SLP ACE**

Forde, Mrs Doreen Fisher Catholic Medical Center, 33-04 Junction Boulevard, Apartment 6M, Jackson Heights, NY 11372, (718) 657-6800, MA 83 CUNY - Queens Coll; SLP, Catholic Med Cen, **SLP**

Forde, Elizabeth Ann 417 Plainfield Street, Providence, RI 02909, (401) 751-3113, BA 81 RI Coll; MS 83 Boston Univ; Dept Head Sp-Lang/Aud, Sargent Rehab Ctr, **SLP ACE**

Fordon-Abbott, Irene 212 Sandy Lane, Warwick, RI 02889, **A**

Foreman, Dalyn D 6953 Renner Road, Shawnee, KS 66217, (913) 341-9142, BS 82 KS St Univ; MA 85 Univ of KS; Sp-Lang Path, Leavenworth Public Schools, **SLP**

Foreman, Mrs Jan C 105 Dove Circle, Lafayette, LA 70508, (318) 981-2089, BA 71 Southern Methodist Univ; BS 74 Southern Methodist Univ; MS 74 Southern Methodist Univ; **SLP**

Foreman, Joyce Ellen 2301 Bay Street #303, San Francisco, CA 94123, (415) 921-6171, BA 80 San Francisco St Univ; MS 82 San Francisco St Univ; Sp-Lang Path, Garden Sullivan Hosp, **SLP**

Foreman, Mrs Karen Lynne 1721 Division N W, Olympia, WA 98502, (206) 943-3341, BA 76 WA St Univ; MA 86 San Diego St Univ; 88–Sp-Lang Path, St Peters Hosp, **SLP**

Foreman, Lydia Marie 1269 Penfield Road, State College, PA 16801, (812) 238-1008, BA 38 Kearney St Coll; MA 42 TX Woman's Univ; OM 59 Univ of AL- Tuscaloosa; **SLP LM**

Foreman, Paul Michael 700 Friedman Avenue, Las Vegas, NM 87701, (505) 454-1493, MA 80 Univ of MO - Columbia; MS 86 Univ of NM; Sp-Lang Path, N New Mexico Rehab Ctr, **SLP**

Foreman, Tryphena Hyacinth 334 Wilmot Avenue, Bridgeport, CT 06607, (203) 579-6312, BA 81 Southern CT St Univ; MS 84 Southern CT St Univ; 87–Sp-Lang Path, State of CT, **SLP**

Forester, D'Laine 15123 Forest Lodge Drive, Houston, TX 77070, (713) 447-0896, BS 75 Southwest TX St Univ; ME 76 Southwest TX St Univ; Sp/Lang Path, Aldine ISD, **SLP**

Forestieri, Grace 2514 East 19th Street, Brooklyn, NY 11235, (718) 769-1708, BA 85 CUNY - Brooklyn Coll; MS 88 CUNY - Brooklyn Coll; 88–Sp-Lang Path, UCP

Foret, Lois L 105 Templeton Drive, Lafayette, LA 70508, **SLP**

Forget, Karen Aleen 5115 Plymouth Road, Baltimore, MD 21214, (301) 328-2185, MS 84 Loyola Coll; BA 83 Loyola Coll; Sp-Lang Path, Univ of Maryland, **SLP**

Forgione, Angela M 625 Huntington CMS Road, Apartment 411, Mount Prospect, IL 60056, (312) 806-6103, BA 79 Mundelein Coll; MA 83 Northern IL Univ - De Kalb; Sp-Lang Path, New Horizon Cen, **SLP**

Forgione, Mary-Anne 20 Wall Street, Foxboro, MA 02035-2929, (703) 573-5747, BA 83 Boston Coll; ME 85 Univ of VA - Charlottesville; Sp-Lang Path, Wrentham State School, **SLP**

Foristiere, Melonie Y 7918 E Gettysburg Avenue, Clovis, CA 93612, (209) 673-8155, BA 76 CA St Univ - Fresno; MA 78 CA St Univ - Fresno; 86–Resource Spec, Fresno USD, **SLP**

Forkner, Mrs Vera C 1226 Castle Way, Norcross, GA 30093, (404) 296-7032, OB 78 Univ of GA; ME 78 Univ of GA; Sp-Lang Path, Forsyth Co Bd of Ed, **SLP**

Forkosh, Ronna Heidi 11839 Clifton Blvd #107, Lakewood, OH 44107, (216) 221-2762, BA 85 Univ of Pittsburgh - Pittsburgh; MA 87 Univ of Pittsburgh - Pittsburgh; **SLP**

Formaad, Dr William Rua Direita Dafundo, #9-5 Esq, 1495 Dafundo, Lisbon, Portugal, BA 49 New Sch for Social Research; MA 50 Columbia Univ Teachers Coll; ED 65 (NS) Columbia Univ Teachers Coll; Prof Emeritus, Seton Hall U, **SLP A F**

Forman, Mrs Carol Fern 36-08 Bell Boulevard, Bayside, NY 11361, (718) 428-7508, BS 78 Boston Univ; MS 85 Adelphi Univ; **SLP**

Forman, Mrs Joann Querner 110 Griswold Drive, West Hartford, CT 06119, (203) 523-9498, BA 75 Univ of CT; MA 77 Univ of KS; Sp-Lang Path, Private Practice, **SLP**

Forman, Monica N 2230 S E Yamhill #5, Portland, OR 97214, (503) 235-3641, BS 74 ID St Univ; MS 76 ID St Univ; **SLP**

Forman, Ruth L 23061 Mosby Street, Woodland Hills, CA 91364, (818) 710-1962, BS 62 OH St Univ; MA 79 CA St Univ - Northridge; Director, Comm Enhancement Inc, **SLP**

Forman, Mrs Shari G R 154-08 71 Avenue, Apartment 88A, Flushing, NY 11367, BA 75 Hofstra Univ; MA 77 NY Univ; SLP, Private Practice, **SLP**

Forman, Mrs Vernell S 5059 Dog River Road East, Theodore, AL 36582, (205) 690-8379, BS 71 AR St Univ; BS 71 AR St Univ; MA 73 Memphis St Univ; Tchr, Mobile Co Pub Sch, **SLP**

Formanczyk, Karen M 329 Powderhorn Ridge Court, Rochester Hills, MI 48063, (313) 286-8800, BA 75 MI St Univ; MA 76 Wayne St Univ; Sp-Lang Path, MacOmb ISD, **SLP**

Forman-Franco, Bonnie S 120 West Park Avenue Suite 3J, Long Beach, NY 11561, (516) 432-1800, BA 71 Univ of Miami; MA 72 MI St Univ; Exec Dir/Pres, Hrng & Sp Assoc Inc, **A**

Formby, Dr Charles Craig 1841 N W 23rd Terrace, Gainesville, FL 32605-3835, (904) 395-0174, BA 74 Auburn Univ - Auburn; MA 77 Memphis St Univ; PH 82 (Communication Sc) Washington Univ; 88–Assoc Prof, Dept Commun Dis/Neur Uf, **A**

Formby, Ellen S F 8835 Southwestern #2246, Dallas, TX 75206, (214) 783-3130, BA 74 Stephen F Austin St Univ; MA 78 Univ of North TX; Sp-Lang Path, Utd Callier Center, **SLP**

Formentini, Mrs Bonnie J 2634 East Croyden, Tucson, AZ 85716, (602) 573-0031, BS 78 Univ of AZ; MS 80 Univ of AZ; Sp-Lang Path, Sunnyside USD, **SLP**

Formes-Ackerson, Mrs Carol PSC1 Box 5000, McHord AFB, WA 98438, **SLP**

Formica, Deborah N Medical Arts Bldg, 130 Kinderkamac Road, River Edge, NJ 07661, (201) 487-4269, BA 78 Montclair St Coll; MA 80 Montclair St Coll; 84–Sp-Lang Path, Private Practice, **SLP**

Formichella, Katherine 5930 McCommas Boulevard, Dallas, TX 75206, (214) 820-2683, BS 77 Univ of TN - Knoxville; MA 78 Univ of TN - Knoxville; Sp-Lang Path, U of TX Callier Cen/Commun Dis, **SLP**

Fornataro, Lisa Marie Rd 2 Box 4270, Ellwood City, PA 16117, (412) 728-7000, BA 83 Saint Mary's Coll; MA 86 OH St Univ; Sp-Lang Path, Med Cntr of Beaver Co, **SLP**

Forney, Jack L 3900 East Pacific Coast Highway, Suite 310, Long Beach, CA 90804-2013, (213) 597-2196, BA 60 CA St Univ - Sacramento; MA 65 CA St Univ - Los Angeles; Sp-Lang Path, Private Practice, **SLP A**

Foronjy, Eileen M 25 Foster Lane, Westbury, NY 11590, (516) 333-5393, BA 73 CUNY - Lehman Coll; MA 75 CUNY - Hunter Coll; Consultant Sp-Lang Path, Private Practice, **SLP**

Forquer, Brian Durand 1042 Grinnell Drive, Burbank, CA 91501, (818) 994-8927, MS 77 Univ of TX - Dallas; 86–Dir of Aud, Union Aud/Hrng Aid Svc, **A**

Forrest, Mrs Andrea Swenson 930 43rd Avenue #50, Sacramento, CA 95831, (707) 446-6838, BA 79 Univ of WI - Eau Claire; MS 80 Univ of WI - Eau Claire; Sp-Lang Path, Solano Co Offi Ed, **SLP**

Forrest, Diana K 808 So Elm Blvd, Champaign, IL 61820-6404, (217) 351-9870, BA 75 MI St Univ; MA 76 Central MI Univ; Sp-Lang Path, Rantoul High Sch, **SLP**

Forrest, Jean Marie 103 North 11th Street, Charleston, IL 61920, (217) 345-2017, MS 88 Eastern IL Univ; 88–Sp-Lang Path, Eastern Illinois Area of Spec Educ

Forrest, Jeanine Chapman 4277 Vicksburg Court, Riverside, CA 92505, (714) 785-9329, **SLP**

Forrest, Kathleen General Delivery, Wortham, TX 76693-9999, MA 81 Minot St Univ; Sp-Lang Path, Mexia State School, **SLP**

Forrest, Shelley H 232 Valley Street, San Francisco, CA 94131, (415) 573-4026, BS 72 Univ of IL - Urbana; MA 73 Northwestern Univ; MA 81 (NS) San Francisco St Univ; Mgr Severe Disord of Lang Prog, San Mateo Co Off Ed, **SLP**

Forrestel, Mrs Kim H 11730 Spanish Lake Drive, Tampa, FL 33635, (813) 854-2277, BS 77 Eastern KY Univ; MS 78 Purdue Univ - West Lafayette; Sp-Lang Path, **SLP**

Forrester, Mrs Debora A 8 Gipson Court, Columbia, MO 65202, BS 79 Western MI Univ; MA 80 Western MI Univ; ES 83 Univ of GA; Sp-Lang Path, **SLP**

Fors, Karen A 18 Tonetta Circle, Norwalk, CT 06855, (203) 854-4138, BA 73 MI St Univ; MA 74 MI St Univ; 88–Administrator / Suervisor, Norwalk Pub Sch, **SLP**

Fors, Mrs Sarah Drake 112 Timber Ridge, Southington, CT 06489, (203) 621-8818, BS 47 Univ of MI - Ann Arbor; MA 73 Univ of MI - Ann Arbor; Doctoral, U of MI, **SLP**

Forse, Mrs Kathleen H 4142 Willmar Drive, Palo Alto, CA 94306, (415) 363-5477, BS 72 Univ of IL - Urbana; MA 74 Univ of IL - Urbana; Sp-Lang Path, San Mateo Co Off of Ed, **SLP**

Forseter, Annette S 6417 Danville Court, Rockville, MD 20852, (301) 468-7775, BA 68 CUNY - Brooklyn Coll; MA 69 NY Univ; Aud, Dc Dept of Human Serv, **A**

Forst, Ellen G 10 Williams Street #46, Watertown, MA 02172, (617) 455-4000, BS 70 Boston Univ; MA 72 Univ of Southern CA; Sp-Lang Path, Needham Publ Sch, **SLP**

Forst, Mary Canon 520 North Stapley Drive #110, Mesa, AZ 85203, (515) 438-2600, BS 65 Univ of IA; MA 66 Univ of IA; 88–Sp-Lang Path, Gila River Indian Comm, **SLP**

Forstall, Janice M 4952 Marigny Street, New Orleans, LA 70122, (504) 288-1355, BA 79 Univ of New Orleans; OM 81 LA St Univ - N O Medical Ctr; Sp-Lang Path, Orleans Parish Sch Bd, **SLP**

Forster, Mrs Catherine C 7951 Perry Lake Road, Clarkston, MI 48016, (313) 626-1200, MA 83 Western MI Univ; 86–Sp-Lang Path, Farmington PS, **SLP**

Forster, Mrs Charlotte Fich 780 Beach Road, Sanibel, FL 33957, (813) 472-0319, BA 38 CUNY - Hunter Coll; MA 50 Case Western Reserve Univ; **SLP LM**

Forster, Mrs Cynthia Knoll 2800 West County Road 82, Alexandria, MN 56308, (612) 762-2141, BS 82 Moorhead St Univ; MS 83 Moorhead St Univ; Emem Sp-Lang Path, Alexandria School District 206, **SLP**

Forster, Linda Bates 4835 Egypt Road, Canandaigua, NY 14424-9318, (716) 394-6060, BA 77 SUNY - Coll at Cortland; MS 83 Ithaca Coll; Teacher, Canandaigua City Schools

Forster, Thomas Paul 2800 West County Road 82, Alexandria, MN 56308, (612) 763-4909, BA 81 Northern St Coll; MS 83 Moorhead St Univ; SLP, Morris Pub Sch, **SLP**

Forsythe, Mrs Linda A 18801 Deodar Street, Fountain Valley, CA 92708, (714) 897-1009, BA 76 CA St Univ - Long Beach; MA 77 CA St Univ - Long Beach; SLP, Ocean View Sch Dist, **SLP**

Forsythe, Michelle Rene 1904 Eva Road Apt 15, Mosinee, WI 54455, (715) 355-4611, BA 81 Univ of WI - Eau Claire; MS 82 Univ of WI - Eau Claire; **SLP**

Forsythe, Susan I Dept Of Otolaryngolgy & Comm Dis, Cleveland Clinic Foundation, 9500 Euclid Avenue, Cleveland, OH 44106, (216) 444-5370, BS 75 Univ of KS; MA 77 Saint Louis Univ; Sp-Lang Path, Cleveland Cl Found, **SLP**

Fort, Mrs Elizabeth W 13113 Hermitage Road, Savannah, GA 31419, (912) 355-4601, BS 83 Vanderbilt Univ; MS 85 Vanderbilt Univ; 87–Sp-Lang Path, Savannah Sp & Hrng Ctr, **SLP**

Fort, Mary K 8 Grandview Park, Stonington, CT 06378, (203) 739-0557, BS 73 Trenton St Coll; MA 74 Seton Hall Univ; Sp-Lang Path, E Lyme Sch, **SLP**

Fortenberry, Vivian Joyce 515 Westwood Court, Columbus, MS 39429, (601) 736-2216, BS 85 Univ Southern MS-Hattiesburg; MS 86 Univ Southern MS-Hattiesburg; **SLP**

Fortier, Mrs Claire A 5 Gerald Avenue, Coventry, RI 02816, (401) 828-1996, BS 84 Univ of MA - Amherst; MA 85 MI St Univ; **SLP**

Fortier, Julie L 549 Brixton Avenue, St Lambert, PQ, Canada J4P 3A9, (514) 343-7841, BA 72 Univ of Ottawa - Ontario; MS 73 Syracuse Univ; Lecturer, U of Montreal, **SLP**

Fortin, Deborah A 46 School Street, Hopkinton, MA 01748, (617) 435-3067, BS 79 Univ of WA; OM 81 Univ of WA; Sp-Lang Path, Little Peoples Sch, **SLP**

Fortine, Yvonne Marie 2099 Temple Avenue #4, Signal Hill, CA 90806, (213) 924-9581, BA 81 CA St Univ - Long Beach; MA 84 CA St Univ - Long Beach; **SLP**

Fortney, Molly Campbell 912 22nd Avenue South, Moorhead, MN 56560, (218) 236-4940, BS 80 Univ of IA; MA 82 Western IL Univ; Aud, Dr Stephen Asp, **A**

Fortun, Lynn P 107 Sunset Drive, Viroqua, WI 54665, (608) 637-7831, BA 80 Univ of Northern IA; MA 81 Univ of Northern IA; Sp-Lang Path, Tomah Rehab Center Inc, **SLP**

Fortuna-Roy, Mrs Patricia Kay 4785 Hillcrest, Trenton, MI 48183-4513, (313) 676-0168, BS 77 Eastern MI Univ; MA 77 Eastern MI Univ; Sp-Lang Path, Taylor Sch Dist, **SLP**

Fortune-Swartz, Mrs Lynn M 209 Avila Circle, Kansas City, MO 64114-5519, BS 80 Northeast MO St Univ; MA 81 Northeast MO St Univ; Sp-Lang Path /Aud, Private Practice, **SLP A**

Forys, Mrs Donna R 3550 Meadowgate Drive, Murrysville, PA 15668, BS 72 CA Univ of PA; ME 74 CA Univ of PA; Sp-Lang Path, Westmoreland Iu #7, **SLP**

Fosbenner, Kimberly A 338 Green Street, Sellersville, PA 18960, (215) 865-1655, BS 85 Clarion Univ of PA; MS 86 Clarion Univ of PA; 88–Aud, Allen Aud, **A**

Fosnaugh, Steven W 3204 Rolling Road, High Point, NC 27260, (919) 869-6741, BS 79 Wayne St Univ; MA 80 Eastern MI Univ; Dir/SLP, Private Practice, **SLP**

Fosnaught, Lynn M 413 East Fairmont Avenue, Modesto, CA 95354, (209) 525-4925, BS 72 Miami Univ - Oxford; MS 75 OH Univ - Athens; Sp-Lang Path, Stanislaus County Dept of Educ, **SLP**

Fosnot, John D Indian Oven Road, Worthington, MA 01098, (413) 443-3531, Aud, Berkshire Rehab Cen, **A**

Foss, Craig A Grand Island Audiology Clinic, 704 North Alpha Street, Grand Island, NE 68803, (308) 384-2101, BS 76 Brigham Young Univ; OM 77 Brigham Young Univ; Aud, Grand Island Aud Cl, **A**

Foss, Cynthia 1000 Ainsworth #100, Prescott, AZ 86303, (602) 445-1303, BA 71 MI St Univ; MS 72 Univ of MI - Ann Arbor; Sp-Lang Path, Prescoth Speech-Lang Services, **SLP ACE**

Foss, Cynthia Diane 162-A Ledge Street, Nashua, NH 03060, (603) 889-6681, SLP, St Joseph Hosp, **SLP**

Foss, Elizabeth Ann 1102 Jalna Boulevard, Apartment #304, London, ON, Canada N6E 1X8, (519) 686-6085, BS 84 Ithaca Coll; MS 86 PA St Univ - Univ Park; **A**

Foss, Kristy Layne 539 Parkhill Drive, Billings, MT 59102, (406) 256-2500, BA 83 Univ of MT; OM 86 Univ of MT; Aud, The Billings Clinic, **A**

Foss, Michelle Piper 1915A Melrose Drive, Champaign, IL 61820, (217) 351-1243, BS 87 Univ of MN - Minneap-St Paul; OM 87 Univ of WI - River Falls; 88–Aud, Christie Cl

Fossa, Mrs Lorriann Prickett 156 North Main Street, Brewer, ME 04412, (207) 989-1637, BS 83 Univ of ME - Farmington; MS 86 Boston Univ; **SLP**

Fossum, Carol A Peter Woodbury Elementary Sch, Bedford, NH 03102, (603) 622-0431, BA 70 Univ of NH; MA 71 Univ of Northern CO; Sp/Lang Path, Dept Spec Serv, **SLP ACE**

Fossum, Dr Ernest C 2500 Walnut Street, Cedar Falls, IA 50613, PH (NS); **SLP LM**

Foster, Mrs Beverly Cunningham 37944 Rudall Avenue, Palmdale, CA 93550, (805) 947-7191, BA 71 CA St Univ - Long Beach; MA 75 CA St Univ - Long Beach; 85–Sp-Lang Path, Palmdale Sch Dist, **SLP**

Foster, Cecelia P O Box W-29, Blue Anchor, NJ 08037, (609) 567-7858, SLP, Kingsway Learning Ctr, **SLP**

Foster, Debra K 401 North Powder Horn Dr, Anaheim, CA 92807, (714) 974-7180, BA 76 Humboldt St Univ; MA 78 Humboldt St Univ; Sp-Lang Path, Orange USD, **SLP**

Foster, Holly Anne 240 Playa Del Norte, La Jolla, CA 92037, (619) 477-6791, **SLP**

Foster, Holly Krueger 5306 Harvest Ridge Lane, Birmingham, AL 35243, **SLP**

Foster, Isabelle F 14617 Red River Drive, Corpus Christi, TX 78410, (804) 420-7433, BS 76 James Madison Univ; MS 78 Univ of WI - Madison; Sp-Lang Super, **SLP**

Foster, Mrs Jacqueline Star R D1 Box 13-A, Utica, PA 16362, (800) 672-7123, MS 84 Clarion Univ of PA; 79–Sp-Lang Path, Riverview Intermediate Unit, **SLP**

Foster, Dr Jean Rizzo 2801 South College Avenue, Bryan, TX 77801, (409) 822-9186, BA 66 IN Univ - Bloomington; MA 68 IN Univ - Bloomington; PH 75 (NS) Purdue Univ - West Lafayette; Sp/Lang Path, Private Practice, **SLP**

Foster, Joan E 460 Lexington Street, Waltham, MA 02154, **SLP**

Foster, Julie Beard 107 Dinkel Avenue, Bridgewater, VA 22812, (703) 433-3256, BS 78 James Madison Univ; MS 80 James Madison Univ; Hrng Spec, Rockingham Co Pub Sch, **SLP**

Foster, Karen K 9832 Whitecap Drive, Olympia, WA 98502, (206) 458-5731, BA 68 OH Univ - Athens; MA 74 Eastern MI Univ; Sp-Lang Path, Yelm Sch Dist, **SLP**

Foster, Mrs Karen L 3913 Meadowbrook, Troy, MI 48084, (313) 280-8400, BS 77 Wayne St Univ; MA 79 Wayne St Univ; Sp-Lang Path, Wm Beaumont Hosp, **SLP**

Foster, Mrs Karrie Diane 1102 North Buckeye, Iola, KS 66749, (316) 473-2257, **SLP**

Foster, Kathleen D 1835 62nd Terrace South, St Petersburg, FL 33712, **SLP**

Foster, Mrs Kimberly Kay 718 North Sunset, Alva, OK 73717, (405) 327-0515, BS 81 Northwestern OK St Univ; MS 83 Univ of OK Medical Center; 83–Sp-Lang Path, Cherokee PS, **SLP**

Foster, Mrs Leah L 7202 Running Rope Circle, Austin, TX 78731, BA 75 Univ of Southwestern LA; MA 77 LA St Univ - Baton Rouge; Sp-Lang Path, Austin ISD, **SLP**

Foster, Linda D L 865 Fairfield Drive, Marietta, GA 30067, (404) 971-5709, BS 64 Auburn Univ - Auburn; MA 65 Auburn Univ - Auburn; Sp/Lang Path, Sp & Hrng Cl Inc, **SLP**

Foster, Marcia L 16009 E 28th Terrace, Apartment 3118, Independence, MO 64055, (816) 478-4081, BS 84 Northwest MO St Univ; MS 86 Northwest MO St Univ; Sp-Lang Path, Truman Neurological Ctr, **SLP**

Foster, Mrs Michele Marie 2067 Stratford Court, Loveland, OH 45140, (513) 369-4000, BS 81 Indiana Univ of PA; MA 86 Trenton St Coll; 87–Sp-Lang Path, Cincinnati Bd of Educ, **SLP**

Foster, Nyli 2750 Homecrest Avenue #717, Brooklyn, NY 11235, (718) 934-7005, BA 73 CUNY - City College; MA 76 CUNY - City College; Sp-Lang Path, Staten Island Dev Cen, **SLP**

Foster, Mrs Patricia Y Brown 114 Signal Hill Drive #T-1, Statesville, NC 28677, (704) 664-5343, BS 86 Western Carolina Univ; MA 87 Western Carolina Univ; 87–Sp-Lang Path, Mooresville Graded Schs, **SLP**

Foster, Mrs Penny Felix 110 East 25th Street #201, Alliance, NE 69301, (308) 762-4331, BS 83 Clarion Univ of PA; MS 86 Clarion Univ of PA; 83–Sp-Lang Path, Alliance City Schs, **SLP**

Foster, Sharon 4135 West 192nd Place, Country Club Hills, IL 60477, (312) 474-7790, BS 76 IL St Univ - Normal; MS 78 IL St Univ - Normal; 78–Sp-Lang Path, S Metro Assn Hndcpd, **SLP**

Foster, Stephen C 1928 Chicago Avenue, Kingman, AZ 86401, **SLP**

Foster, Susan F 1570 Humboldt Street, Denver, CO 80218, (303) 830-7440, BA 69 Univ of CA - Los Angeles; MA 76 Univ of CO - Boulder; Owner, Private Practice, **SLP A**

Foster, Mrs Suzanne C 9054 Fairglen, Dallas, TX 75231, (214) 494-8329, BS 60 Univ of AR - Fayetteville; MA 63 TX Woman's Univ; SLP, Garland ISD, **SLP**

Foster, Suzanne R 1475 Eloise Avenue, Memphis, TN 38106, **SLP**

Foster, Mrs Teresita Lourdes E M 812 Jefferson Street N W, Apartment 107, Washington, DC 20011, (202) 829-7955, MS 87 Univ of the DC

Foster, Tina L Sobel 2527 Arborwood Drive, Valrico, FL 33594, (813) 251-7701, BA 84 Univ of TN - Knoxville; MA 85 Univ of TN - Knoxville; 86–Sp-Lang Path, Tampa General Hosp, **SLP**

Foster, Wayne A 34 Brookway Drive, Greensboro, NC 27410, (919) 379-4120, BS 76 Univ of SC - Columbia; MS 79 Univ of SC - Columbia; Chief Sp-Lang Path, Moses H Cone Mem Hosp, **SLP A**

Foster, Wesley A VA Medical Center, Audiology (126), 50 Irving Street N W, Washington, DC 20422, BA 81 San Diego St Univ; MA 84 San Diego St Univ; 84–Aud, Veterans Administration, **A**

Foster-Hunter, Mrs Shirley A 2539 Brambleberry Court, Bettendorf, IA 52722, (319) 359-7784, BS 71 Northern IL Univ - De Kalb; MA 72 Northern IL Univ - De Kalb; Sp-Lang Path, Private Practice, **SLP**

Fostvedt, Patricia Ann Box 417, Meckling, SD 57044, (605) 563-2291, BA 82 Univ of SD - Vermillion; MA 84 Univ of SD - Vermillion; **SLP**

Fothergill, Mary E 421 Barber Pond Road, Pownal, VT 05261, (802) 442-5256, BA 77 Univ of VT; MS 82 Worcester St Coll; Sp-Lang Path, Bennington School District Inc, **SLP**

Fotheringham, Lawrence Kent Co Board Of Education, P O Box 1000, Chatham, ON, Canada N7M 5L7, (519) 354-3770, OB 64 Coll of Spch Therapists Eng; MA 72 Western MI Univ; 70–Sp-Lang Path, Kent Co Bd of Ed, **SLP**

Fouchey, Susan Kay 1300 Marywood Drive, Royal Oak, MI 48067, (313) 547-8692, BS 79 Wayne St Univ; MA 80 Wayne St Univ; Sp-Lang Path, Wm Beaumont Hosp, **SLP**

Fountain, Mrs Sandra Elizabeth 2801 Willow Wood Circle, Valdosta, GA 31602-4108, BS 84 Valdosta St Coll; ME 85 Valdosta St Coll

Fountain-Walls, Mrs Karen Lanore P O Box 3814, Bristol, TN 37625, (615) 878-4293, BS 78 East TN St Univ; MA 83 Univ of TN - Knoxville; 88–Sp-Lang Path, Professional Health Services, **SLP**

Fourman, Laura Ann 1017 Grinstead Court, Louisville, KY 40204-2347, (502) 456-4241, BS 86 Ball St Univ; MA 87 Northwestern Univ

Fournier, Mrs Barbara Elizabeth 126 Carriage Hill Road, North Kingstown, RI 02852, (401) 785-0400, BA 80 Univ of RI; MS 83 PA St Univ - Univ Park; Sp-Lang Path, Cranston Sch Syst, **SLP**

Fournier, Denise Ann 6 Craig Road, Framingham, MA 01701-7664, (508) 875-4559, BA 78 Univ of CT; MA 81 Univ of CT; 85–Sp-Lang Path, The Learning Ctr for Deaf Children, **SLP**

Fournier, Steven R 44 Scenic Avenue, Webster, MA 01570, (617) 943-6696, BA 74 Worcester St Coll; MA 76 SUNY - Coll at Geneseo; Dir of Aud, U of MA Med Cen, **A**

Foushee, David R 31388 Crow Road, Coarsegold, CA 93614, (209) 294-2422, BA 69 CA St Univ - Northridge; MA 75 CA St Univ - Fresno; **SLP**

Foushee, Mrs Deborah Dawson 7009 Valley Haven Drive, Charlotte, NC 28211-6160, (704) 333-5491, BS 80 Univ of Montevallo; MS 82 Univ of Montevallo; SLP, Charlotte-Mecklenburg Schools, **SLP**

Foust, Richard W 47 West Long Avenue, Du Bois, PA 15801, (814) 834-7721, BA 68 Bloomsburg Univ of PA; ME 73 Bloomsburg Univ of PA; Aud, Private Practice, **A**

Foust, Robin Ann 440 Wallen Hills Drive #2, Fort Wayne, IN 46825, (219) 489-6232, BS 83 Ball St Univ; MA 85 Ball St Univ; **SLP**

Fouts, Mrs Ann Pierce 948 Cowley Avenue, East Lansing, MI 48823, (517) 332-1226, BS 42 Purdue Univ - West Lafayette; MA 63 MI St Univ; **SLP LM**

Fouts, Mrs Christine Mey 9016D Mahogany Row, Huntsville, AL 35802, (205) 536-3364, BS 77 James Madison Univ; MS 78 AR St Univ; 87–Sp-Lang Path, Ctr for Sp & Lang Pathology, **SLP**

Fowle, Dawn Renee 880 Wesley Circle, Apartment 310, Apopka, FL 32703, (407) 656-4109, BA 79 Univ of FL; MA 87 Univ of FL; 86–Sp-Lang Path, Orange County PS, **SLP**

Fowler, Carolyn Cameron Rt 1 Box 392, Moncure, NC 27559, (919) 258-3828, BS 84 Appalachian St Univ; MA 86 Appalachian St Univ; 86–Sp-Lang Path, Lee Co Bd of Educ, **SLP**

Fowler, Mrs Catherine Route 1 Box 193, Blythe, GA 30805, (404) 554-2265, BS 78 Univ of GA; ME 81 Univ of GA; Sp-Lang Path, Burke Co Bd of Ed, **SLP**

Fowler, Cynthia G Audiology 126, VA Medical Center, 5901 East 7th Street, Long Beach, CA 90822, (213) 494-5414, BA 71 Emory Univ; MA 74 LA St Univ - Baton Rouge; PH 80 (Aud) Northwestern Univ; 80–Aud, VA Med Cen, **A**

Fowler, Diana Teague 37 Towle Farm Road, Unit 23, Hampton, NH 03842, (508) 281-1050, BA 79 Wheaton Coll; MS 81 Columbia Univ Teachers Coll; 81–Aud, Cape Ann Med Ctr, **A**

Fowler, Diane Tumlin 553 Windchase Lane, Stone Mountain, GA 30083, (404) 292-7272, **SLP**

Fowler, Elbert E 407 Old Buncombe Road, Travelers Rest, SC 29690, (803) 834-8539, BA 78 Northwestern St Univ; MA 80 Northwestern St Univ; SLP, Greenville Public School, **SLP**

Fowler, Mrs Janet Sprecher 2525 N Bleckley, Wichita, KS 67220, (316) 684-0622, **SLP**

Fowler, Joyce Lynn Weirton Steel Corp, Audiology Gate 1, Weirton, WV 26062, (304) 797-3616, BS 83 WV Univ; MS 85 WV Univ; 87–Aud, Weirton Steel Corp, **A**

Fowler, K Jean 2189 West 2nd Avenue, Suite 4, Vancouver, BC, Canada V6K 1H7, (604) 731-1131, BS 81 Univ of Alberta - Alberta; OM 84 Univ of Western Ontario; 88–Sp-Lang Path, Vancouver Sch Bd, **SLP**

Fowler, Kathleen S 654 Oakdale, Corte Madera, CA 94925, (415) 924-6461, BA 67 Univ of MD - College Park; MA 69 Univ of MD - College Park; Sp-Lang Path, Home Visiting Sp & Lang Ser, **SLP**

Fowler, Mrs Kathy Edmondson 7680 Ridgewood Drive, Gladstone, OR 97027, (503) 255-1841, BA 76 WA St Univ; MA 81 Western WA Univ; Sp-Lang Path, Multnomah Ed Serv Dist, **SLP**

Fowler, Kymry Hart 28412 Lorente, Mission Viejo, CA 92692, (714) 472-4291, Sp-Lang Path, Easter Seal Rehab Cen, **SLP ACE**

Fowler, Mrs Lavina P S Good Samaritan Hospital, Department Of Audiology, 1040 NW 22nd Avenue, Portland, OR 97210, (503) 229-7860, BA 78 CA St Univ - Long Beach; MA 80 CA St Univ - Long Beach; 83–Aud, Dept of Aud Gd Samaritan Hosp, **A**

Fowler, Marilynn 4571-K Northside Parkway, Atlanta, GA 30339, (404) 952-2342, BS Univ of GA; ME 86 Univ of GA; SLP, Cobb County Public Schools, **SLP**

Fowler, Mrs Martha J 5745-A Canna Lane, San Jose, CA 95124, (408) 448-3430, BA 72 Univ of CA - Santa Barbara; MA 75 Univ of CA - Santa Barbara; SLP, Milpitas USD, **SLP**

Fowler, Mary M 225 Virginia Avenue #2-E, San Mateo, CA 94402-1652, BA 43 CA St Univ - Fresno; BA 43 CA St Univ - Fresno; MA 54 Stanford Univ; **SLP LM**

Fowler, Mrs Patricia Kay 545 Okland Circle, Paducah, KY 42001, (502) 898-2387, OB 74 Murray St Univ; MS 81 Murray St Univ; SLP, Sp Lang Hrng Serv, **SLP**

Fowler, Susan E Route 3 Box 8, Mechanicsville, MD 20659, (301) 475-5636, BS 74 LA St Univ - Baton Rouge; MA 79 George Washington Univ; Sp-Lang Path, St Marys Co Pub Sch, **SLP**

Fowler, Susan M RD 4 Box 424 Corkery Lane, Williamstown, NJ 08094, (215) 596-9122, OB 76 Univ of GA; ME 79 Univ of GA; Sp-Lang Path, Children's Hosp of Phila, **SLP**

Fowler, Suzie 717 Milan Street, New Orleans, LA 70115, **SLP**

Fowlkes, Dr Thomas Eugene 66 West 109th Street, Apt 22, New York, NY 10025, (212) 932-1226, BA 77 Univ of MD - College Park; MA 79 George Washington Univ; PH 85 (NS) OH St Univ; Assistant Professor, **A**

Fox, Bernard J Laureate Learning Systems Inc, 110 East Spring Street, Winooski, VT 05404, (802) 655-4755, BA 76 Univ of MA - Amherst; MS 80 Univ of VT; 82–Vice President, Laureate Learning Systems Inc, **SLP**

Fox, C Brent Audiology Assoc Salt Lake City, 22 South 900th East, Salt Lake City, UT 84102, (801) 364-8692, BS 69 Brigham Young Univ; OM 71 Brigham Young Univ; Aud, Audiology Assoc Salt Lake City, **A**

Fox, Mrs Carol L 1026 Bedford Lane, Ballwin, MO 63011, (314) 569-8311, BA 66 Fontbonne Coll; MA 76 Saint Louis Univ; Dev Sp/Lang Classrm Tchr, St Louis Co Spec Sch Dist, **SLP**

Fox, Carolyn E 6308 Silver Cliff Court, Arlington, TX 76016, (817) 465-4291, BS 71 Abilene Christian Univ; MS 73 Univ of OK - Norman; Sp-Lang Path, Arlington ISD, **SLP**

Fox, Mrs Cydney M Aud Clinic Ctr For Health Science, 10833 Le Conte Avenue, Room 62-202, Los Angeles, CA 90024, (213) 825-5721, BA 72 IN Univ - Bloomington; MA 73 Univ of Denver; Audiologist, UCLA, **A**

Fox, Danette L 190 North Crest Road #4, Chattanooga, TN 37404-1734, (615) 479-9669, OB 78 Univ of FL; MA 80 Univ of TN - Knoxville; Sp-Lang Path, Chattanooga Co Sp&Hrng Cen, **SLP**

Fox, Dr Daphne S 203 First Avenue, Belmar, NJ 07719, (212) 517-0454, BS 54 Northwestern Univ; MA 67 Columbia Univ Teachers Coll; ED 80 (Educ of Hrng Impaired/Aud) Columbia Univ Teachers Coll; Coord Prog, Marymount Manhattan College, **A**

Fox, Mrs Deborah A 4-1B Presidents Drive, Port Jefferson, NY 11777, (516) 331-1440, BS 81 SUNY - Coll at Brockport; MA 87 Hofstra Univ; 81–Sp-Lang Path, East Quoque Sch, **SLP**

Fox, Mrs Donna Marie 6397 Devonshire Lane, Frederick, MD 21701, (301) 694-1401, BS 86 Bloomsburg Univ of PA; MS 87 Bloomsburg Univ of PA; 87–Sp-Lang Path, Frederick Co Bd of Educ

Fox, Dr Donna R University Of Houston, Comm Disorders - 146 Sof, 4800 Calhoun, Houston, TX 77004, (713) 749-2741, BA 48 Univ of WA; MA 49 Univ of IA; PH 65 (NS) Univ of MO - Columbia; Professor, University of Houston, **SLP F ACE**

Fox, Douglas E 3200 Queensland Lane, Plymouth, MN 55447, (612) 520-5614, BA 71 Saint Cloud St Univ; BA 71 Saint Cloud St Univ; MS 72 Saint Cloud St Univ; Dir-Sp-Lang Path, N Mem Med Cen, **SLP**

Fox, Eileen J 7787 North Quivas Street, Denver, CO 80221-4227, (303) 698-0533, **A**

Fox, Frank Lynn, Jr 3815 James Avenue, Huron, OH 44839-2132, (419) 625-7339, BA 73 Baldwin-Wallace Coll; MA 83 Cleveland St Univ; Pres, Sandusky Audiology Inc, **A**

Fox, Gayla DiAnn 220 East 17th, Harper, KS 67058, (316) 896-7932, BA 83 Wichita St Univ; MA 85 Wichita St Univ; 88–Sp-Lang Path, S Central KS Spec Educ Coop

Fox, James M 75 Edgewater Drive, Little Falls, MN 56345, BS 62 Saint Cloud St Univ; **SLP**

Fox, Janet 612 Harmony Road, Rockaway Point, NY 11697, (212) 834-3034, BA 78 CUNY - Brooklyn Coll; MA 79 CUNY - Queens Coll; Aud, Consolidated Edison, **A**

Fox, Mrs Janis A 85 Oak Street, Rd 1, Rensselaer, NY 12144, (518) 286-3206, BA 73 SUNY - Center at Stony Brook; MA 75 Coll of Saint Rose; **SLP**

Fox, Jennifer L 3234 Flag Avenue South, St Louis Park, MN 55426, (612) 931-9144, BS 69 Northwestern Univ; MA 70 Northwestern Univ; Consult, Hearing Care Specialists, **A**

Fox, Joseph P 3432 Clays Mill Road, Lexington, KY 40503, (606) 233-4511, BA 64 Central Methodist Coll; MS 65 Central MO St Univ; PH 70 (Sp-Lang Path) IN Univ - Bloomington; Chief/Audiol & SLP Service, VA Medical Center, **SLP**

Fox, Kathryn M 3050 178th Street #3C, Lansing, IL 60438, (312) 333-7812, BS 80 Purdue Univ - West Lafayette; MA 81 Univ of TN - Knoxville; Sp-Lang Path, S Metro Assoc, **SLP**

Fox, Lisa Latinette 714 East Cherry Street, Columbia, IL 62236-2019, BS 85 Southern IL Univ-Edwardsvill; MS 86 Southern IL Univ-Edwardsvill; **SLP**

Fox, Mrs Lodiana E 49 Marion Street #2-C, Brookline, MA 02146, (617) 361-1101, BA 51 Boston Univ; MA 53 Boston Univ; 78–Sp-Lang Path, Boston Pub Sch, **SLP**

Fox, Lynn Elizabeth 3344 S W Evergreen Terrace, Portland, OR 97201, BA 71 CA St Univ - Long Beach; MA 85 Humboldt St Univ; Sp-Lang Path, Portland VA Med Ctr, **SLP**

Fox, M Elisa Lamb 716 Toulouse Court, Half Moon Bay, CA 94019, (415) 348-8834, MS 74; Sp-Lang Path, San Mateo Un Hgh Sch Dist, **SLP**

Fox, Mrs Madeline F 4513 Dresden Road, Baltimore, MD 21208, (301) 655-0694, BA 66 CUNY - Queens Coll; MS 67 Univ of MI - Ann Arbor; Sp-Lang Path, U of MD Hosp, **SLP**

Fox, Mrs Margaret 1015 Swarthmore Road, New Cumberland, PA 17070, (717) 774-4863, BS 72 Bloomsburg Univ of PA; ME 72 Bloomsburg Univ of PA; SLP, Dept of Commun Dis Caiu, **SLP**

Fox, Mrs Marion Rosenbaum 32 Monroe Street #B-C-P-H, New York, NY 10002, (212) 360-6753, BA 53 CUNY - Hunter Coll; MS 54 Purdue Univ - West Lafayette; Sp-Lang Path, Metropolitan Hosp Cen, **SLP A**

Fox, Mark L 312 J Street, Salt Lake City, UT 84103, (801) 266-8895, MS 88 Univ of UT; 88–Sp-Lang Path, Neuropsychological Consultation Svcs

Fox, Mary E 1709 South Ogden, Denver, CO 80210, (303) 798-8616, BA 72 LA Salle Coll; MS 80 PA St Univ - Univ Park; Sp-Lang Path, Littleton Pub Schls, **SLP**

Fox, Mrs Maura D 41B Howe Road, Lake Lucerne, NY 12846, (518) 696-2030, MS 82 Univ of VT; Sp-Lang Path, UCP Inc of the Tri-Counties, **SLP**

Fox, Maureen Theresa 3412 Kalum Street, Terrace, BC, Canada V8G 2E9, (919) 968-0281, BS 82 Univ of NH; MS Univ of NC - Chapel Hill

Fox, Mrs Nanci Goldsmidt 4700 McKinley Drive, Boulder, CO 80303, (303) 449-4904, BA 61 Univ of WA; MA 88 Univ of CO - Boulder; Sp-Lang Path, **SLP**

Fox, Mrs Nancy Lynn 18 Toppy Lane, Bay Shore, NY 11706, (516) 243-0933, BA 78 SUNY - Coll at Buffalo; MS 87 Long Island U - CW Post Ctr; 87–SLP, BOCES III JEA Melville

Fox, Pamela Debbie 161 W 16th Street #11-G, New York, NY 10011, (718) 833-6633, MS 85 Columbia Univ Teachers Coll; ME 85 Columbia Univ Teachers Coll; **SLP**

Fox, Robert A Ohio State University, 324 Derby Hall, 154 North Oval Mall, Columbus, OH 43210, (614) 292-8207, BA 70 Univ of MD - College Park; MA 78 Univ of Chicago; PH 78 (NS) Univ of Chicago; Assoc Prof, Sp & Hrng Sci Osu

Fox, Robert James 21620 14th Avenue South, Apartment #F101, Seattle, WA 98198, (206) 824-9867, MS 85 IL St Univ - Normal; 87–Aud, NW Hosp Sp & Hearing Ctr, **A**

Fox, Dr Robert L 136 Quail Run, Prattville, AL 36067, (205) 665-6726, BS 68 Southern IL Univ -Carbondale; MS 69 Southern IL Univ -Carbondale; PH 74 Univ of IL - Urbana; Director-Professor Audiology, University of Montevallo, **SLP A**

Fox, Sharon A 136 Quail Run, Prattville, AL 36067, (205) 261-5099, BS 70 Southern IL Univ -Carbondale; MS 74 Univ of IL - Urbana; Educational Specialist, Alabama State Dept of Educ, **SLP**

Fox, Shelly 15 Moss Avenue, Oakland, CA 94610, (415) 671-4540, BS 80 CA St Univ - Hayward; MS 82 San Francisco St Univ; Sp-Lang Path, San Francisco Commun College, **SLP**

Fox, Mrs Susan E 3200 Queensland Lane, Plymouth, MN 55447, (612) 473-1811, BS 79 Marquette Univ; MS 80 Marquette Univ; Sp/Lang Path, On-Call, **SLP**

Fox, Susan M 12009 Running Creek Road, Louisville, KY 40243, (502) 454-8259, BS 73 OH Univ - Athens; MS 79 Univ of Louisville; Sp-Lang Path, Jefferson Co Bd of Ed, **SLP**

Fox, Tina D P O Box 6815, Baltimore, MD 21285-6815, (202) 338-0161, BA 77 George Washington Univ; MA 80 George Washington Univ; Dc Med Soc, **SLP**

Fox, Mrs Vernie R 111 Sharpe, Essexville, MI 48732, (517) 892-6190, MA 51 Univ of MI - Ann Arbor; **SLP LM**

Fox, Virginia R 3706 Columbia Drive, Martinez, GA 30907, (404) 737-7310, BS 75 SUNY - Coll at Geneseo; ME 78 Univ of GA; SLP, Richmond Cty Bd of Ed, **SLP**

Fox, Wendy J 2716 North Upshur Street, Arlington, VA 22207, (703) 527-7448, BS 72 SUNY - Coll at Buffalo; MA 74 Case Western Reserve Univ; Sp/Lang Path, Private Practice, **SLP**

Fox, Wendy Sillick 203-N Springmeadow Drive, Holbrook, NY 11741, (516) 472-6796, BS 81 Ithaca Coll; MS 84 Univ of WI - Madison; 85–Sp-Lang Path, St Charles Hosp & Rehab Ctr, **SLP**

Fox, William J 755 Manomin, St Paul, MN 55107, **A**

Fox, William L 212 Wright Avenue, Ellwood City, PA 16117, **SLP**

Fox-Gleason, Susan A 639 East Glenwood-Lansing, Apartment 2-B, Glenwood, IL 60425, (312) 758-4514, BS 79 Northwestern Univ; MA 81 Univ of IL - Urbana; SLP, S Metro Assn-Birth to Five Div, **SLP**

Fox-Helser, Debra E Route 2 Box 239, Morganton, NC 28655, (704) 397-3491, BS 71 Western Carolina Univ; MA 79 Appalachian St Univ; SLP, Burke Co Sch, **SLP**

Foxman, Carol Ann 140 South University Drive, Suite F, Plantation, FL 33324, (305) 475-3141, BA 68 Temple Univ; MA 71 Temple Univ; 74–Dir-Pres, Image Impact Inc Sp Assoc, **SLP**

Foxman, Mrs Leanne K 6744 Chestnut, Mariemont, OH 45227, BA 75 San Diego St Univ; MA 77 San Diego St Univ; **SLP**

Foy, Kathleen Maureen 1111 Esters Road #2408, Irving, TX 75061, (214) 986-2941, BA 84 Univ of VT; MS 86 Univ of TX - Dallas; **A**

Foy, Mrs Linda P 4096 Sunset Lane, Pebble Beach, CA 93953, (408) 624-8872, OB 62 Washington Univ; BA 66 Univ of the Pacific; MA 68 Univ of CA - Santa Barbara; 88–Sp-Lang Path, Monterey Co, **SLP**

Foye, Mary Dobner 1631 Princeton Avenue, Salt Lake City, UT 84105, (801) 350-4689, BS 75 Univ of WI - Stevens Point; MS 77 Purdue Univ - West Lafayette; 86–Sp-Lang Path, Holy Cross Hosp, **SLP**

Frable, Mrs Kimberly Demara 4998 Battery Lane #307, Bethesda, MD 20814-4959, (301) 951-6319, BS 81 Central MI Univ; MA 82 Central MI Univ; Aud, Washington Hearing & Sp Soc, **A**

Frade, Marilyn Frances 877 West Lill #D-4, Chicago, IL 60614, (312) 456-9094, BA 85 MI St Univ; MA 86 MI St Univ; 88–Sp-Lang Path, Pennoyer Sch Dist #79, **SLP**

Fradette-Sebell, Jeanne 87 Wheelwright Farm, Cohasset, MA 02025, BS 75 Northeastern Univ; ME 78 Northeastern Univ; Sp-Lang Path, Develop Preschool Plymouth PS, **SLP**

Fradkin, David Lawrence 34 Northampton Street, Holyoke, MA 01040, (413) 533-8894, MA 77 Columbia Univ Teachers Coll; MA 83 Univ of MA - Amherst; **A**

Frady, Dr Lynn 2231 Santa Ynez, San Luis Obispo, CA 93401, (805) 546-3149, MA 75 CA Poly St Univ-San Luis Obi; MS 67 Minot St Univ; ED 82 (NS) Brigham Young Univ; Dir/Lrng Skls Serv, Cuesta Coll, **SLP**

Fraher, Arlene L 15 Capri Drive, Framingham, MA 01701, (508) 872-6679, BA 75 Univ of MA - Amherst; MA 76 Univ of MA - Amherst; Aud, Hear Better, **A**

Fraher, Mrs Karen Theresa 6806 Meadow Oak Drive, Bldg #7, Columbus, OH 43235, (614) 792-0267, BS 78 Bradley Univ; MS 79 Bradley Univ; Sp-Lang Path, InSpeech Inc, **SLP**

Frahm, Caren Bernice 1919 Evergreen Park Drive SW #103, Olympia, WA 98502, (206) 352-4167, BS 83 1355; MS 85 ID St Univ; Sp-Lang Path, Olympia Sch Dist, **SLP**

Frail, James H 316 West Lee Street, Charleston, WV 25302, **A**

Frain, Avria Bultz 21-H Colonial Drive #21-H, Little Falls, NJ 07424, (201) 451-9000, BA 81 Univ of Miami; BS 82 FL St Univ; MS 84 FL St Univ; SLP, Jewish Hosp & Rehab Cen of Nj, **SLP**

Fraistat, Judith B 7 Arlington Court, Brookfield, CT 06804, (203) 426-7683, BA 76 Univ of CT; MA 78 Univ of CT; Sp-Lang Path, Newtown Bd of Ed, **SLP**

Fraley, Mrs Marie R 1633 West Street, Wrentham, MA 02093, (401) 456-9330, BA 72 Univ of RI; MS 74 Univ of RI; Sp-Lang Path, Providence School Dept, **SLP**

Frame, Charles Wayne 673 Pearl Street, Oneida, WI 54155, (414) 869-2880, BA 72 Univ of HI - Manoa; MS 76 Washington Univ

Frame, Gloria Dianne 10 Coral Crescent #4, Thompson, MB, Canada R8A 1L1, (204) 778-8993, BS 73 Univ of ND; MS 86 Univ of North TX; 86–Sp-Lang Path, Sch Dist of Mystery Lake #2355, **SLP**

Frame, Rebecca L 826 North 86th Way, Scottsdale, AZ 85257, (602) 239-4755, BS 84 Baylor Univ; MS 86 AZ St Univ; 87–Sp-Lang Path, Good Samaritan Med Ctr, **SLP**

Frame, Mrs Suzanne Parizeau 51 Williams Road, Lexington, MA 02173, (617) 863-5846, BA 81 Univ of VT; MS 82 Univ of VT; **SLP**

Frana, Mrs Julie Dolan 2929 Tama Street S E, Cedar Rapids, IA 52403, (319) 399-6700, BA 74 Coll of Saint Teresa; MS 76 Central MO St Univ; Sp-Lang Path, Grantwood AEA, **SLP**

Frana, Nancy Ann 615 North 39th Street, Apartment D-204, Grand Forks, ND 58201, (701) 352-2140, BS 78 Mankato St Univ; MS 81 Mankato St Univ; Sp-Lang Path Coordinator, Grafton State School, **SLP**

France, Betty Ann/Davis 290 Bentwood Trail, Winterville, GA 30683, (404) 542-8970, BA 77 Univ of KY; MA 84 Univ of KY; **SLP**

France, Mary Colleen 8026 39th Avenue N E, Seattle, WA 98115, (206) 326-5100, BA 81 Univ of MT; MS 83 Univ of WA; 85–Sp-Lang Path, Providence Medical Center, **SLP**

France, Pamela Joyce 111 Winding Creek Trail, Madisonville, KY 42431, (502) 821-6071, BS 75 Miami Univ - Oxford; MS 86 Murray St Univ; 88–Sp-Lang Path, Hopkins County Bd of Educ, **SLP**

Francellini, Dr Anthony J 1231 McKinley Drive, Clairton, PA 15025, (412) 233-7321, BS 63 CA Univ of PA; ME 65 PA St Univ - Univ Park; PH 80 (Cognitive Activities-Lang/Sp Diag) Univ of Pittsburgh - Pittsburgh; Sp-Lang Path, Private Practice, **SLP**

Francer, Mrs Holly Jean 4 Saw Mill Pond Road, Sharon, MA 02067, (203) 584-7709, BS 81 Univ of MA - Amherst; MS 85 Southern CT St Univ; Sp-Lang Path, **SLP**

Franceschini, Thomas G 4195 Washington Avenue, St Joseph, MI 49085, BS 77 IL St Univ - Normal; MS 79 IL St Univ - Normal; **SLP**

Francia, Leonette J 1620 Sweetbriar, San Jose, CA 95125, (408) 295-6115, BA 70 San Jose St Univ; MA 74 San Jose St Univ; Sp/Lang Path, Private Practice, **SLP**

Francione, Cindy Marie 810 Magnolia Drive, Waukesha, WI 53188, (414) 679-1290, BS 79 Univ of WI - Milwaukee; MS 81 Univ of WI - Milwaukee; Sp-Lang Path, Muskego Norway Sch Dist, **SLP**

Francis, Annjala 2773 Wind Swept Drive #108, Lantana, FL 33462, (305) 433-1267, BS 84 FL St Univ; MS 86 FL St Univ; 86–Sp-Lang Path, Palm Beach Co Sch Sys, **SLP**

Francis, Mrs Carolyn J 410 Brockton Lane, Plymouth, MN 55447, (612) 475-3628, BA 69 Augustana Coll; MA 70 Univ of IL - Urbana; **SLP**

Francis, Catherine Moacanin 2441 Beverley Avenue #17, Santa Monica, CA 90405, (213) 396-0097, BA 73 Reed Coll; MA 81 CA St Univ - Los Angeles; SLP, Kaiser Permanente, **SLP**

Francis, Chris 115 Woy Woy Bay Road, Phegans Bay, New South Wales, Australia 2256, BA 70 Syracuse Univ; MS 72 IL St Univ - Normal; Sp-Lang Path, Ctrl Coast Hosp & Area Hlth SE, **SLP**

Francis, Joseph Helbert 7124 Grayfalcon Drive, Norfolk, VA 23518, (804) 853-4274, BS 75 Old Dominion Univ; MS 77 Old Dominion Univ; Sp-Lang Path, Norfolk Pub Sch, **SLP**

Francis, Mrs Marian Forest 218 Davidson, Westby, WI 54667, (608) 634-3101, BA 79 Univ of Northern IA; MA 81 Univ of Northern IA; Sp/Lang Path, Westby Area Sch, **SLP**

Francis, Nancy Spencer 2176 N Beverly Glen Blvd, Los Angeles, CA 90077, (213) 474-3020, BA 70 Univ of CA - Los Angeles; MA 81 CA St Univ - Northridge; Sp-Lang Path, Cedars-Sinai Med Cen Hosp, **SLP**

Francis, Raymond Patrick 108 Fischer Avenue, Pittsburgh, PA 15223, (412) 366-3471, BS 84 WV Univ; MS 86 WV Univ; Aud, Met ENT Assoc, **A**

Francis, Mrs Rosemary Eakes 7124 Grayfalcon Drive, Norfolk, VA 23518, (804) 853-4274, BS 67 Old Dominion Univ; MS 74 Old Dominion Univ; 73–Sp-Lang Path, Norfolk Pub Sch, **SLP**

Francis, Shelley Lynn 725 Maxwell Drive, East Meadow, NY 11554-4008, (516) 565-4552, BS 83 Stephen F Austin St Univ; MS 86 Univ of North TX; Hearing Lab, **A**

Francis, Mrs Shelly 1010 Falls Avenue, Cuyahoga Falls, OH 44221, (216) 929-6634, BA 84 Univ of Akron; MA 85 Univ of Akron; Sp-Lang Path, Barberton City Schools, **SLP**

Francis, Mrs Sherri B 1290 Creeks Edge Drive, Cordova, TN 38018, (901) 377-1993, BS 84 WV Univ; MA 85 Univ of TN - Knoxville; **A**

Francis, Mrs Victoria Tramontano 221 Sage Drive, Lamar, CO 81052, (303) 336-9046, BS 76 SUNY - Coll at Geneseo; MA 79 Univ of Northern CO; Sp-Lang Path, Southeast Col BOCES, **SLP**

Francis, Dr William C 1137 Debbie Lane, Macomb, IL 61455, (309) 298-1585, BS 62 Western MI Univ; MA 65 Central MI Univ; PH 73 (Hearing & Speech Sciences) OH Univ - Athens; Assoc Prof, Western Illinois Univ, **SLP**

Francisco, Arminda 57 Gooding Street, Pawtucket, RI 02860, (401) 723-4930, MS 88 Southern CT St Univ

Francis-Dinstel, Mrs Sharon Box 1646, Colstrip, MT 59323, (406) 748-3840, BS 73 Northeast MO St Univ; MA 76 Northeast MO St Univ; Sp-Lang Path, Colstrip Public Schools, **SLP**

Franck, Mrs Ardath Amond 700 Ghent Road, Akron, OH 44313, (216) 666-1161, BS 46 Kent St Univ; MA 47 Kent St Univ; PH 56 (NS) Case Western Reserve Univ; Dir, Akron Sp & Reading Cen, **SLP**

Franco, Janis W 5049 Northside Drive N W, Atlanta, GA 30327-4421, (404) 257-1688, OB 64 Univ of Miami; **SLP**

Frandle, Kathy Jo 210 El Camino, Scotts Valley, CA 95066, (408) 423-2454, BA 74 WA St Univ; MA 75 WA St Univ; Sp-Lang Path, Scotts Valley USD, **SLP**

Frank, Arthur 325 Queensbury Street, Thousand Oaks, CA 91360, MS 69 CUNY - Brooklyn Coll; SLP, Los Angeles Co Supt Schools, **SLP**

Frank, Mrs Carol L 15 Greenway Plaza #14E, Houston, TX 77046, (713) 993-0413, BS 59 Northwestern Univ; MA 64 Saint Louis Univ; **SLP**

Frank, Cheryl R Audiology And Speech Services, VA Hospital, 4500 South Lancaster Drive, Dallas, TX 75216, (214) 372-7013, BA Fort Hays St Univ; MA Univ of KS; Sp-Lang Path, Dallas VA Med Cen, **SLP**

Frank, Diane Loeb 7531 Graymore Road, Pittsburgh, PA 15221, (412) 647-5580, BA 63 Univ of AZ; ME 64 Univ of AZ; MA 84 Univ of Pittsburgh - Pittsburgh; Aud, Childrenms Hosp, **A**

Frank, Mrs E Stacey 1821 Fort Street #102, Victoria, BC, Canada V8R 1J6, (604) 595-2388, BS 77 Univ of Alberta - Alberta; OM 78 Univ of WA; Aud, Pacific Coast Aud, **A**

Frank, Dr Elaine M 6149 Hampton Ridge Road, Columbia, SC 29209, (803) 776-4000, BS 72 AZ St Univ; MA 76 Univ of SC - Columbia; PH 88 (Sp Lang Path) Univ of SC - Columbia; 81–Sp-Lang Path/Aud, Veterans Administration Hosp, **SLP A ACE**

Frank, Dr Grace W 15036 Killion Street, Van Nuys, CA 91411, (213) 780-4766, BA 65 CA St Univ - Los Angeles; MA 69 CA St Univ - Northridge; ED 85 (NS) Nova Univ; SLP, Simi USD, **SLP**

Frank, Mrs Judith Lein 2477 Kingston, Troy, MI 48084, BS 61 Eastern MI Univ; MS 67 Eastern MI Univ; Sp-Lang Path, Redford Unified Schools, **SLP**

Frank, Mrs Karen E Rd 1 Box 132, Rome, NY 13440, (315) 339-1636, BA 80 SUNY - Coll at Plattsburgh; MA 82 SUNY - Coll at Plattsburgh; Sp-Lang Path, Rome Dev Cen, **SLP**

Frank, Leslie H 607 Azure Hills Drive, Simi Valley, CA 93065, (818) 846-6363, OB 71 Southern Methodist Univ; MA 73 Univ of Southern CA; MS 76 Pepperdine Univ - Los Angele; 86–Prin, Burbank USD, **SLP**

Frank, Lori Mitchell 1431 Blackhawk Drive, Mount Prospect, IL 60056, (312) 392-8400, BS 59 Northern IL Univ - De Kalb; MS 60 Northern IL Univ - De Kalb; Dir Sp-Lang Path, Central Reading/Speech Clinic, **SLP**

Frank, Marla T 5231 Woodstock, Golden Valley, MN 55422, **SLP**

Frank, Mrs Marlene Sharon 502 Kensington Way, Mount Kisco, NY 10549, (914) 241-9439, BA 72 OH St Univ; MS 75 SUNY - Center at Albany; Super of Spec Ed, Byram Schl Dstr, **SLP**

Frank, Mrs Mary A 10094 Lasalle Boulevard, Huntington Woods, MI 48070, (313) 544-9466, OB 77 Emerson Coll; MA 87 Wayne St Univ

Frank, Mrs Mary Elizabeth 307 Central Avenue S W, Glen Burnie, MD 21061, (301) 969-9010, BA 79 Loyola Coll; MS 80 Loyola Coll; Sp-Lang Path, Anne Arundel Co PS, **SLP**

Frank, Mrs Patricia Ann 8209 9th Street West, Rock Island, IL 61201, (319) 359-1371, OB 77 Northeast MO St Univ; MA 83 Northern IL Univ - De Kalb; Aud, Mississippi Bend AEA, **A**

Frank, Patricia R 6257 Hayes Drive, Norcross, GA 30093, (404) 636-1304, BS 75 James Madison Univ; MS 78 GA St Univ; Sp-Lang Path, Dekalb County Schools, **SLP**

Frank, Mrs Phyllis C 5006 Scenic Drive, Yakima, WA 98908, (509) 453-8248, BS 65 Univ of MI - Ann Arbor; MS 66 Univ of MI - Ann Arbor; Sp/Lang Path, Yakima Valley Hrng & Sp Cen, **SLP**

Frank, Phyllis R P O Box 597, Upton, NY 11973, BS 66 Univ of IL - Urbana; MA 67 Univ of IL - Urbana; Sp-Lang Path, Hauppauge Pub Sch, **SLP**

Frank, Ruby Ann Dept Communicative Disorders, San Diego State University, San Diego, CA 92182, (619) 594-2460, BS 67 Univ of IL - Urbana; MA 69 Univ of IL - Urbana; 78–Instr & Supvr, San Diego St U, **SLP**

Frank, Mrs Sharon D 21 Erick Road Unit 35A, Mansfield, MA 02048, (617) 824-6911, BS 80 Univ of WI - Madison; MA 82 Univ of FL; Sp-Lang Path, Morton Hosp Inc, **SLP ACE**

Frank, Sherry Southers 4475 Mayapan Drive, Lamesa, CA 92041, (619) 541-3088, BA 83 San Diego St Univ; MA 84 Univ of the Pacific; Sp-Lang Path, Childrens Hospital Health Ctr, **SLP**

Frank, Susanne O 56 Middle Lane, Jericho, NY 11753, **SLP**

Frank, Dr Thomas Alan Speech And Hearing Clinic, Pennsylvania State Univ, 110 Moore Bldg, University Park, PA 16802, (814) 863-2006, BS 70 Univ of WI - Oshkosh; MS 72 Univ of WI - Madison; PH 75 (NS) Univ of WI - Madison; Prof, Penn St U, **A F**

Frank, Thomas M 11404 Roslyn Road, Fredericksburg, VA 22401, (703) 898-3872, BS 77 James Madison Univ; MS 79 Washington Univ; Aud, Dominion Hearing Services, **A**

Franke, Mrs Cindi Route 2 Box 333-C, Wesport, IN 47283, BA 81 Ball St Univ; MA 82 Ball St Univ; SLP, Decatur Cnty Community Schools, **SLP**

Franke, Gabrielle Ann 2030 North Lake Drive, Milwaukee, WI 53202, (414) 447-2208, BS 79 Marquette Univ; MA 81 Marquette Univ; Sp-Lang Path, Saint Josephs Hosp, **SLP**

Franke, Lauren K 6243 Parima, Long Beach, CA 90803, (312) 431-4530, BA 75 Univ of CA - Santa Barbara; MA 77 CA St Univ - Long Beach; Dir, Long Beach Scottish Rite, **SLP**

Frankeberger, Robert D 6004 Canehill Avenue, Lakewood, CA 90713, (213) 920-2872, BS 77 CA St Univ - Long Beach; MS 79 Univ of Redlands; Sp-Lang Path, Los Angeles County Off of Educ, **SLP**

Frankel, Andrea 18106 Delaire Landing Road, Philadelphia, PA 19114, (215) 877-4135, BS 72 PA St Univ - Univ Park; MS 76 Drexel Univ; ME 82 Trenton St Coll; Sp-Lang Path, Sch Dist of Phila, **SLP**

Frankel, Henny 1654 East 13th Street, Brooklyn, NY 11229, (212) 769-1111, BA 69 CUNY - Brooklyn Coll; MS 74 CUNY - Brooklyn Coll; MS 74 Adelphi Univ; **SLP**

Frankel, Jacqueline A 23 Bellerive Acres, St Louis, MO 63121, (314) 569-6188, BS 77 Fontbonne Coll; MS 78 Fontbonne Coll; Sp-Lang Path, St Johns Mercy Med Ctr, **SLP**

Frankel, Lynn E 1380 Avon Lane #3-15, North Lauderdale, FL 33068, **SLP**

Frankel, Phyllis 50 Euclid Avenue, Hastings on Hudson, NY 10706, (212) 220-8520, MA 86 CUNY - Hunter Coll; 86–Sp-Lang Path, FEGS, **SLP**

Frankel, Mrs Sandra L 134 Monteroy Road, Rochester, NY 14618, (716) 271-0680, BS 63 Tulane Univ; MA 65 Northwestern Univ; Sp/Lang Path, Hrng/Sp Cen of Rochester Nc, **SLP**

Frankel-Freedland, Ellyn 72 Highgrove Crescent, Richmond Hill, ON, Canada L4C 7W6, (416) 883-9895, BA 80 York Univ - Ontario; MA 84 SUNY - Coll at Buffalo; **SLP**

Frankenbach, Mrs Glenda Lynn 208 Tanglewood Drive, Lynchburg, VA 24502, (703) 586-0275, BS 77 Central MO St Univ; MS 81 Southern IL Univ-Edwardsvill; Sp-Lang Path, Bedford Co Schs

Frankenberger, Dr Robert L Speech And Hearing Clinic, Western Illinois Univ, Memorial Hill #116, Macomb, IL 61455, (309) 298-1791, BS 59 OH Univ - Athens; MS 61 Western MI Univ; PH 68 (NS) IN Univ - Bloomington; Sp-Lang Path, Wn Il U, **SLP**

Frankiewicz, Yvonne G 2819 Bernadette Lane, Houston, TX 77043, **SLP**

Frankino, Ellen Connelly 320 Northbrook Drive, Danville, IL 61832, (217) 267-2154, MS 76 IL St Univ - Normal; BS 75 IL St Univ - Normal; Sp-Lang Path, Westville Comm Ut Sch Dist #2, **SLP ACE**

Frankle, Bonnie C 6710 Bonnie Ridge Drive, Apartment 102, Baltimore, MD 21209, (301) 484-9465, BA 80 Univ of MD - College Park; MS 82 Boston Univ; Sp-Lang Path, MD Inst for Emergency Med Serv, **SLP**

Franklin, Dr Barbara 3580 Louis Road, Palo Alto, CA 94303, (415) 338-1161, BA 54 CUNY - Queens Coll; PH 69 (NS) CUNY - Grad Sch & Univ Cntr; Prof, San Francisco St Univ, **A**

Franklin, Barbara S 2521 Julian, Houston, TX 77009, (713) 864-5805, BA 81 Nicholls St Univ; MA 86 Univ of Houston - Univ Park; Sp-Lang Path, Baylor Coll of Med, **SLP**

Franklin, Bruce William Ear Tech, 207-13 Carriage Square, Boone, NC 28607, (704) 262-2184, BA 77 MI St Univ; MA 78 Western MI Univ; Pres, Self Employed, **A**

Franklin, Dana Bendigkeit 1795 Locust, Denver, CO 80220, (303) 986-4587, BS 79 LA St Univ - N O Medical Ctr; OM 79 LA St Univ - N O Medical Ctr; Sp-Lang Path, Havern Center, **SLP**

Franklin, Mrs Deborah R Marshall Habilitation Center, P O Box 190, Marshall, MO 65340, (816) 886-2202, BS 72 Univ of IL - Urbana; MA 73 Univ of MO - Columbia; SLP Coord, Marshall Habilitation Cen, **SLP**

Franklin, Diane Box 85 Star Route, Gouldsboro, PA 18424, (717) 826-6892, BS 78 Marywood Coll; MS 79 Bloomsburg Univ of PA; Aud, Aud Assoc of Wilkes-Barre, **A**

Franklin, Mrs Edith P 1243 Norwood Place, Orlando, FL 32804, MS 75 FL St Univ; Sp-Lang Path, Constance B Rizner MacCc, **SLP**

Franklin, Honor Franklin Sp Lang & Myofun Clin, 5438 Alpha Road, Dallas, TX 75240, BS 74 Univ of TX - Austin; MS 77 Univ of TX - Dallas; PH 82 (Special Education) Columbia Pacific Univ; Director, Private Practice, **SLP ACE**

Franklin, June Marie Route 3 Box 128, Manor, TX 78653, BS 84 Univ of TX - Austin; MA 87 Univ of TX - Austin; **SLP**

Franklin, Kate University Of Nebraska, 317 Barkley Memorial Centr, Lincoln, NE 68583-0732, (402) 472-5418, BA Univ of NE - Lincoln; MS Univ of NE - Lincoln

Franklin, Leslie Diane Rt 1, Hampton, TN 37658, (615) 772-3226, BS 83 East TN St Univ; MS 85 East TN St Univ; 85–Sp-Lang Path, Carter Co TN Schs, **SLP**

Franklin, Leslie Mason 1972 Honey Locust Court, Solvang, CA 93463, (805) 968-2525, BA 79 Univ of MI - Ann Arbor; MA 81 Univ of CA - Santa Barbara; 87–Sp/Lang Path, Santa Barbara County Schs, **SLP**

Franklin, Marcia Reiss 2807 Victoria Drive, Alpine, CA 92001, (619) 445-0210, BS 78 Boston Univ; MA 84 San Diego St Univ; 88–Sp-Lang Path, Private Practice, **SLP**

Franklin, Mrs Sandra S "Coppers", Firfields Cobbetts Hill, Weybridge KT13 OUD, Surrey, England, BA 70 Univ of MD - College Park; MA 72 Univ of MD - College Park; **SLP**

Franklin, Sara Scruggs P O Box 353, Hazelwood, NC 28738, BS 77 Appalachian St Univ; MA 79 Appalachian St Univ; Sp/Lang Path, Haywood Co Hosp, **SLP**

Franklin, Sharon Annette 1329 Lombard Street #302, Philadelphia, PA 19147, (215) 732-4503, BS 77 Villanova Univ; MA 81 Temple Univ-Tyler Sch of Art; **SLP**

Franklin, Susan Cheryl Qtrs 1 English Avenue, Fort Meade, MD 20755, **SLP**

Franklin, Thomas Claiborne 2489-B Wren Hollow Drive, Tallahassee, FL 32303, (904) 386-4623, BA 82 Auburn Univ - Montgomery; OM 84 Auburn Univ - Auburn; **A**

Franklin-Tillman, Vivian C 12657 Biscayne Lake Drive, Jacksonville, FL 32218, **SLP**

Frankoff, Denise J The Greenery Rehabilitation Center, 99 Chestnut Hill Avenue, Boston, MA 02135, (612) 588-0811, BS 76 Northwestern Univ; MA 77 Northwestern Univ; 88–Asst Dir Sp-Lang Path Dept, The Greenery, **SLP**

Frankovich, Mary Jo 3430 Ridgeview Ct #2204, Rochester Hills, MI 48309, (313) 338-1110, BS 76 Northern MI Univ; MA 78 Wayne St Univ - Sch of Med; Aud, Private Practice, **A**

Frankrone, Sr M Dorothy 3115 Lexington Road, Louisville, KY 40206, (502) 897-1811, BA 51 Bellarmine Coll; MS 70 Marquette Univ; Sp-Lang Path, Ursuline Sp Cl, **SLP ACE**

Franks, Mrs Anne 3717 Southeast Lincoln, Portland, OR 97214, (503) 233-1337, BS 77 Univ of OR; MA 79 Western WA Univ; SLP, **SLP**

Franks, Dr Christine H Box 732, Hope, AR 71801, (214) 792-6627, ME 62 Henderson St Univ; MA 70 Southern Methodist Univ; ED 87 (NS) East TX St Univ - Commerce; Owner, Hrng & Sp Cen, **SLP A**

Franks, Daniel Chris APS Stronghurst Complex, 120 Woodland NW, Albuquerque, NM 87107, (505) 345-8531, BS 75 Eastern NM Univ; MS 76 Univ of NM; 80–Aud, Albuquerque P S, **A**

Franks, Harriet Tia 9504 Connell, Overland Park, KS 66212, (213) 378-8388, BS 70 Univ of KS; MA 71 Southern Methodist Univ; SLP, **SLP**

Franks, Dr J Richard 752 Ridgeview Court S E, Pullman, WA 99163, (509) 335-5089, BA 52 Brigham Young Univ; MA 59 Brigham Young Univ; PH 64 (NS) MI St Univ; Prof, WA St U, **A**

Franks, Janice L 21 Norwood Court, Staten Island, NY 10304, (718) 447-4758, BA 67 CUNY - Queens Coll; MA 73 CUNY - Queens Coll; SLP, Private Practice, **SLP**

Franks, Renaee 57 North Somerville #502, Memphis, TN 38104, (501) 534-6822, BS 77 Univ Southern MS-Hattiesburg; MA 78 Memphis St Univ; Aud, Univ Phys Dept Otolaryngology, **A**

Franks, Thomas 1132 Denisonview Street, Pittsburgh, PA 15205, (412) 441-1111, BS 77 Carlow Coll; ME 79 CA Univ of PA; SLP, Pace Sch, **SLP**

Frankwick, Rita 2117 28th Street, Greeley, CO 80631, (303) 352-0683, MA 88 Univ of Northern CO

Franqui, Marisol 845 First Street N W #2, Rochester, MN 55901, (507) 284-2577, MA 84 Univ of CO - Boulder; **A**

Frans, Mrs Noreen P 2312 West Waters Avenue #1, Tampa, FL 33604-2752, (305) 547-6855, MS 79 Univ of South FL; **A**

Frantsov, Marilyn Casaceli 495 New Scotland Avenue, Albany, NY 12208, (518) 482-3600, BA 67 SUNY - Center at Albany; MA 69 Syracuse Univ; Aud, Better Hearing Services, **A**

Frantz, Joy Lee 1751 Riverside Drive, Missoula, MT 59801, (406) 728-4100, BA 77 Univ of Northern CO; MA 78 Univ of Northern CO; Aud, Missoula Comm Hosp Rehab Cen, **A**

Frantz, Marilyn Kay 827 Kearsage, Elmhurst, IL 60126, (312) 971-3344, BS 84 IL St Univ - Normal; MA 86 Univ of IA; 86–Sp-Lang Path, Center Cass Schs Dist #66

Franz, Celia Ann 1310 Lyndon Road, McPherson, KS 67460, (316) 241-2250, BS 65 Fort Hays St Univ; MA 73 Univ of CO - Boulder; 78–Head Sp & Hrng Dept, Memorial Hospital Inc, **SLP A**

Franz, Cheri Nanette 10 Highland Avenue, Catskill, NY 12414, (518) 622-8382, BA 82 SUNY - Coll at Cortland; MS 85 Coll of Saint Rose; 87–Sp-Lang Path, Speech Communications Associates, **SLP**

Franz, Mrs Janet L S 4104 Brooke Drive, Valrico, FL 33594, (813) 685-3320, BA 73 IN Univ - Bloomington; MA 74 IN Univ - Bloomington; Sp-Lang Path, Hillsborough Pub Sch, **SLP**

Franz, Robert J, Jr 319 West Bellview Avenue, Winchester, VA 22601, (703) 662-1745, BS 72 Towson St Univ; ME 73 Univ of VA - Charlottesville; SLP, Er Sl So of VA Inc, **SLP**

Franzblau, Carol G 44 Sturbridge Circle, Wayne, NJ 07470, (201) 694-0836, BS 74 PA St Univ - Univ Park; MS 76 Columbia Univ Teachers Coll; Sp-Lang Path, Private Practice, **SLP ACE**

Franzen, Kathleen A 2400 North Rockton Avenue, Rockford, IL 61103, (815) 968-6861, BS 73 IL St Univ - Normal; MA 86 Northern IL Univ - De Kalb; 84–Sp-Lang Path, Rockford Memorial Hosp, **SLP**

Franzen, Dr Richard Lyle 1402 Skyline Drive, Ellensburg, WA 98926, (509) 962-9841, BA 59 Univ of Puget Sound; MA 65 Univ of WA; PH 70 (NS) Univ of IA; Director/Owner, Mountain View Hrng & Sp Clinic, **A**

Franzke, Debra T 3350 Willow Creek Road, Colgate, WI 53017, (414) 628-1551, MS 76 Univ of WI - Milwaukee; Sp-Lang Path, Milwaukee Public Schools, **SLP**

Franzwa, Agnes B 3538 Arcadian Drive, Castro Valley, CA 94546, (415) 538-6383, BA 67 Holy Names Coll; MS 80 San Francisco St Univ; SLP, San Lorenzo USD, **SLP**

Frarey, Shawn Evans 500 Broton Road, Muskegon, MI 49442, (616) 739-8752, BA 71 Univ of NC - Greensboro; MA 73 Univ of TN - Knoxville; Sp-Lang Path, Sp Path Sers, **SLP**

Frascatore, Beth Bailey 19 Woodcrest Boulevard, Kenmore, NY 14223, (716) 837-2441, BA 64 SUNY - Center at Buffalo; MS 85 SUNY - Coll at Buffalo; 86–Sp-Lang Path, Lang Dev Prog, **SLP**

Fraser, Anita Louise 643 Pierce Street, Port Townsend, WA 98368, (206) 385-2200, BA 76 Western WA Univ; SLP, Jefferson Gen Hosp, **SLP ACE**

Fraser, D Lynn Hospital For Sick Children, Speech Clinic, Toronto, ON, Canada M5G 1X8, (416) 598-6100

Fraser, Janet R 6040 Wilderness Lane, Parma Heights, OH 44130, (216) 231-8787, MA 86 Cleveland St Univ; 86–Aud, Cleveland Hrng & Sp Ctr, **A**

Fraser, Leslie Ann Box PPP-282, Saipan, Mariana Islands 96950, BS 80 Adelphi Univ; MS 84 Kean Coll of NJ; 88–Sp-Lang Path, PS Sys-CNMI, **SLP**

Fraser, Mrs Leslie T 1429 North Isadora Way, Ontario, CA 91764, (714) 992-5701, BA 72 Whittier Coll; MS 74 Univ of IL - Urbana; Sp-Lang Path, InSpeech Inc, **SLP**

Fraser, Malcolm H 177 North Highland #705, Memphis, TN 38111, (901) 452-0995, BS 24 Univ of Pittsburgh - Pittsburgh; Vice Pres/Dir, Speech Foundation of America, **LM**

Fraser, Maryann HCI Box 225, Samsonville, NY 12476, (914) 657-8101, **SLP**

Fraser, Mrs Peggy B Route 6 Box 564, Harriman, TN 37748, (615) 544-5010, BS 57 Univ of TN - Knoxville; MS 77 TN St Univ; 87–Sp-Lang Path, Knox Co Schs, **SLP**

Fraser-Almeida, Sarah B Roberts Road RR1, Frankfort, NY 13340, MA SUNY - Center at Buffalo; Sp-Lang Path, Oneida Co BOCES, **SLP**

Frasier-Lilley, Dixie L Hearing & Speech Services, 2462 Delaney Avenue, Wilmington, NC 28403, (919) 763-1308, BA 73 Univ of MT; MA 75 Univ of MT; Owner, Hearing & Speech Services, **SLP A**

Fratesi, Regina Faye Route 1 Box 544-A, Leland, MS 38756, (601) 335-5678, Sp-Lang Path, National Sp & Hrng Service, **SLP**

Frattali, Dr Carol Marie 4300 North 23rd Road, Arlington, VA 22207, (301) 897-5700, BS 87 Univ of Pittsburgh - Pittsburgh; MA 75 Ithaca Coll; PH 77 (NS) San Francisco St Univ; Asst Dir Reimburse Policy Div, ASHA, **SLP**

Fratzke, Melvin L 106 Forest Acres Drive, Greenville, NC 27834, (919) 551-4448, BA 77 NC St Univ at Raleigh; MS 80 East Carolina Univ; Sp/Lang Path, Pitt County Memorial Hospital, **SLP A ACE**

Fraulo, Marlene K 95 West 1st Street, Clifton, NJ 07011, (201) 261-6230, BA 73 Adams St Coll; MA 73 Adams St Coll; 88–Sp-Lang Path, Bergan Co Day Trng Cen, **SLP**

Frawley, Janis R 1725 Pocatello Street, Sarasota, FL 33581, (813) 485-7188, BA 73 Univ of Miami; MS 82 Univ of South FL; Owner/Sp-Lang Path, Private Practice, **SLP**

Frazee, Mrs Cathy L 4188 Skinner Lake Road, Lapeer, MI 48446, (313) 664-1838, BA 77 Central MI Univ; MA 81 Eastern MI Univ; Sp-Lang Path, Lapeer Co Interm Sch Dist, **SLP**

Frazee, Mrs Cynthia M 25174 Danabirch, Dana Point, CA 92629-3114, (714) 240-9724, BS 78 Loma Linda Univ - Riverside; MS 79 Loma Linda Univ - Riverside; Sp-Lang Path, Capistrano USD, **SLP**

Frazee, Mrs Ellen Frances Route 4 Box 429-A, Laurel Circle, Ringgold, GA 30736, (404) 935-9274, BA 73 Central MI Univ; MA 76 Central MI Univ; 87–Sp-Lang Path, Catossa Co PS, **SLP**

Frazek, Melanie 18615 Ashland Avenue, Homewood, IL 60430, (312) 596-1000, BS 74 Western IL Univ; MA 75 Western IL Univ; 76–Sp-Lang Path, Dist 205, **SLP ACE**

Frazer, Mrs Deborah Seaman 29 Mainview Court, Randallstown, MD 21133, (215) 222-4667, **SLP**

Frazer, Dr Gregory J Auditory-Vestibular Center, 14427 Chase Street, Suite 103, Panorama City, CA 91402, (818) 894-4588, BA 74 CA St Univ - Sacramento; MS 76 Univ of UT; PH 81 (Aud) Wayne St Univ - Sch of Med; Dir, Audiology-Vestibular Ctr, **A**

Frazer, Mrs Joan M 5241 East Calle Ventura, Phoenix, AZ 85018, (602) 468-1880, BA 52 Univ of MI - Ann Arbor; MA 66 AZ St Univ; Pres, Contacts & Connections Inc, **SLP**

Frazer, Mrs Sylvia D 239 Worthen Road East, Lexington, MA 02173, (617) 573-3266, BA 63 McGill Univ - Quebec; MS 65 McGill Univ - Quebec; 68–Aud, MA Eye & Ear Infirmary, **SLP A**

Frazier, Barbara 905 Sherman Street, Danville, IL 61832, MS; **SLP LM**

Frazier, Mrs Herease 1204 East 85th Street, Chicago, IL 60619, (312) 890-8366, BS 69 TX Woman's Univ; MA 75 Governors St Univ; Sp-Lang Path, Chicago Public Schools, **SLP ACE**

Frazier, Mrs Jacqueline Bolders 7892 South Lafayette Way, Littleton, CO 80122, (303) 861-6800, BA 73 CO St Univ; MA 74 Memphis St Univ, Sp-Lang Path, The Chldn Hosp, **SLP**

Frazier, Jamie J 1200 N Cedar #322, Tahlequah, OK 74464, (918) 458-0279, BA 85 Northeastern OK St Univ; MA 87 Univ of SD - Vermillion

Frazier, Julie A 1717 Simpson Street #306, Madison, WI 53713, (608) 267-6174, BS 85 Univ of WI - Madison; MS 87 Univ of WI - Madison; 88–Sp-Lang Path, Meriter/Madison Gen Hosp

Frazier, Mrs Kate Erwin 5223 G Street, Little Rock, AR 72205, (501) 227-5050, MS 84 Univ of MS; Aud, The Ear and Nose-Throat Clinic, **A**

Frazier, Dr Larry A 2100 Pontiac Lake Road, Pontiac, MI 48054, (313) 858-1889, BA 59 Wayne St Univ; MA 64 Wayne St Univ; PH 76 (NS) Wayne St Univ; Aud, Oakland Sch Sp & Hrng Cl, **A**

Frazier, Laura Jane 450 El Dorado Blvd #1006, Webster, TX 77598, (713) 428-2575, BS 85 Baylor Univ; MS 86 Baylor Univ; 88–Sp-Lang Path, Goose Creek CISD, **SLP**

Frazier, Mary E 1204 Broadway #303, Retire Hotel, Lubbock, TX 79401, (803) 965-9331, BS 36 G Peabody Coll-Vanderbilt U; MA 40 G Peabody Coll-Vanderbilt U; **SLP LM**

Frazier, Sally L Madera Cnty Dept Of Education, 28123 Avenue 14, Madera, CA 93637, (209) 673-6051, BA 69 CA St Univ - Stanislaus; MA 71 CA St Univ - Stanislaus; Asst Superintendent Ed Service, Madera Co Dept of Ed, **SLP**

Frazier-Fuemmeler, Mrs Elizabeth Sophia 9410 Fairwood Drive, Kansas City, MO 64138, (816) 763-4198, OB 85 Univ of MO - Columbia; MA 87 Univ of KS; 87–Sp-Lang Path, Children's Therapy Group, **SLP**

Frazzini, Mrs Karen A 1492 Forge Road, San Mateo, CA 94402, (415) 877-5451, BS 65 CO St Univ; MA 69 CA St Univ - Los Angeles; Sdl Tchr, San Mateo Co, **SLP**

Freas, William Erdice, Jr 611 National Highway, La Vale, MD 21502, (301) 759-4555, ME 76 Clarion Univ of PA; Sp/Lang Path, Allegany Hrng & Sp Assoc, **SLP A**

Frechette, Mrs Roberta S 9303 Weathervane Place, Gaithersburg, MD 20879-1414, (301) 990-1320, **SLP**

Freda, Elizabeth L 264 New Street, Belleville, NJ 07109, (201) 473-1153, BA 86 Kean Coll of NJ; MA 87 Kean Coll of NJ; 88–Sp-Lang Path, Lincoln Sch

Frederick, Anne A PO Box 2044, Monterey, CA 93942, (408) 372-6399, BA 75 Wichita St Univ; MA 76 Wichita St Univ; 86–Owner/Exec Dir, Anne Frederick Assoc, **SLP**

Frederick, Julie Anne 622 Anne Street, Oconomowoc, WI 53066, (414) 338-5510, BS 79 Univ of WI - Madison; MS 81 Univ of WI - Madison; 83–Sp-Lang Path, West Bend Jt Sch Dist #1, **SLP**

Frederick, Mrs Lois K Box 9750, 2841 Hermosita Drive, Glendale, CA 91208, (818) 242-8013, BA 44 Univ of IL - Urbana; MA 45 Univ of IL - Urbana; SLP/Sub Tchr, Pub Elem Sch-Ca, **SLP LM**

Frederick, Patricia A 271 Portage Path, Willard, OH 44890, **SLP**

Frederick, Mrs Roan K #5 Vestavia, Northport, AL 35476, (205) 553-4550, BS 72 MS Univ for Women; MS 75 MS Univ for Women; Sp-Lang Path, Partlow State School, **SLP**

Frederick, Shonie Elizabeth 2600 Ontario Street, Bellingham, WA 98226, **A**

Fredericks, Catherine 109 East 1st Street, Clifton, NJ 07011, (201) 546-1179, BS 75 Seton Hall Univ; MA 77 Seton Hall Univ; Sp-Lang Path, The Child Cen, **SLP**

Fredericks-Weber, Jeannette L F Rural Route 1, Box 418, Early, IA 50535, (712) 732-2257, BA 73 Univ of Northern IA; MA 74 Univ of Northern IA; SLP, Arrowhead AEA V, **SLP**

Fredman, Mrs Marion R P O Box 216 Danya, Haifa, Israel 34980, BA 55; MA 70; 75–Sp-Lang Path, Rothschild Hosp/Khoushy Ctr, **SLP**

Fredner, Mrs Marian Swanson New Rochelle Hospital Med Cen, Communication Sciences, 16 Guion Place, New Rochelle, NY 10802, (914) 632-5000, MS 84 Syracuse Univ; 87–Aud, New Rochelle Hosp Med Ctr, **A**

Freeborn, Mrs Carol Hunt P O Box 338, Allamuchy, NJ 07820, (201) 383-2121, BS 81 East Stroudsburg Univ of PA; MA 85 Montclair St Coll; 87–Sp-Lang Path, Newton Memorial Hosp, **SLP**

Freed, Cheryl S 1803 Parnell Avenue, Los Angeles, CA 90025, (213) 854-4045, BS 72 SUNY - Center at Buffalo; MS 75 SUNY - Center at Buffalo; 81–Sp-Lang Path, Private Practice, **SLP**

Freed, Diane Joy 208 Rogers Drive, Lexington Park, MD 20653, (301) 475-8971, BA 83 SUNY - Center at Buffalo; MA 86 Univ of MD - College Park; **SLP**

Freed, Dolores F The Academy At Southgate, Foery Drive #108, Utica, NY 13501, (315) 792-2281, BA 52 CUNY - Brooklyn Coll; MA 55 CUNY - Brooklyn Coll; Admin Spec Ed Instructional, Utica Cty Sch Dist, **SLP ACE**

Freed, Mrs Helene P 73 Coolidge Road, Worcester, MA 01602, (508) 752-4663, BS 68 Boston Univ; ME 70 Boston Univ; Aud, Private Practice, **A**

Freed, Mrs Julienne Marie 308 Franklin Avenue, Beatrice, NE 68310, (402) 228-2601, BS 82 Univ of NE - Lincoln; MS 84 Univ of NE - Lincoln; Sp-Lang Path, Geneva PS, **SLP**

Freed, Marilyn Shosid 2142 Sunstone Drive, Carrollton, TX 75006, (214) 826 3801, BS 79 Univ of TX - Austin; MS 85 Univ of TX - Dallas; Sp-Lang Path, Convalescent Center, **SLP**

Freed, Sharron Eva 99 Tarry Court, Greenwood, IN 46142, (317) 881-0651, **SLP**

Freedman, Mrs Amy Curhan 1409 Commonwealth Avenue, Apartment 205, Boston, MA 02135, (617) 783-5680, BA 84 Univ of MI - Ann Arbor; MS 86 Boston Univ; 86–Sp-Lang Path, New Eng Rehab Hosp, **SLP**

Freedman, Amy Cushner 4249 Bar Harbor Place, Olney, MD 20832, (301) 570-0636, MA 83 George Washington Univ; Sp-Lang Path, Memorial Hospital/ Burlington, **SLP**

Freedman, Mrs Deborah Meckler 1213 Spring Circle Drive, Coral Springs, FL 33071, (607) 753-3599, BS 73 Ithaca Coll; ME 74 Northeastern Univ; Sp-Lang Path, Broward Co Sch Floriad, **SLP**

Freedman, Janie B 111 Beverwyck Drive #8, Guilderland, NY 12084-8676, **SLP**

Freedman, Mrs Judy D 4242 Bushnell Road, University Heights, OH 44118, BS 77 Kent St Univ; MA 80 Cleveland St Univ; SLP, Euclid Public Schools, **SLP**

Freedman, Linda Shepard 111 West South Avenue, Houghton, MI 49931, (906) 482-1525, BA 77 Univ of MD - College Park; BA 80 Univ of MD - College Park; MA 82 Univ of CT; Grad Asst, **SLP**

Freedman, Maurene M 1405 Petronia Street, Key West, FL 33040, (305) 294-0050, BA 71 OH St Univ; MA 72 Univ of IL - Urbana; Sp/Lang Path, Center of Hope, **SLP**

Freedman, Mrs Roni S 558 Tarrington Road, Cherry Hill, NJ 08034, (609) 428-6176, BA 74 NY Univ; MA 75 Hofstra Univ; Sp-Lang Path, Private Practice, **SLP**

Freedman, Sharon Rance 12206 Appleby, Houston, TX 77031, (713) 568-1546, BA 68 CUNY - Queens Coll; MS 71 Univ of WI - Madison; 83–Sp-Lang Path, Alief ISD, **SLP**

Freedman, Mrs Sheryl Beth 24 Ridge Road, Longmeadow, MA 01106-2538, (413) 567-1175, BS 83 Univ of NH; MS 86 Worcester St Coll; 87–Sp-Lang Path, Suffield PS, **SLP**

Freedman-White, Laura B 677 Vine, Highland Park, IL 60035, (312) 237-6394, BS 74 Univ of IL - Urbana; MS 75 Univ of IL - Urbana; Sp-Lang Path, Chicago Bd of Ed, **SLP**

Freeland, Dr E Elaine 4321 Perry Street, Denver, CO 80212, (303) 477-3098, BA 50 Univ of Denver; MA 55 Northwestern Univ; PH 68 (Aud) Wayne St Univ; Exec Dir, **SLP A**

Freeland, Susan M 1010 Lake Adair Boulevard, Orlando, FL 32804, (407) 423-2438, BS 66 Marquette Univ; MA 70 Univ of IA; Sp-Lang Path, Private Practice, **SLP**

Freels, Dale Independence Health Services Pc, 42801 Schoolcraft Road, Plymouth, MI 48170, (313) 420-9015, BS 72 Eastern MI Univ; MA 73 Eastern MI Univ; Aud-Sp-Lang Path, Indep Hlth Serv Pc, **SLP A**

Freels, Deborah A 9662 Bryson Drive, Dallas, TX 75238, (214) 553-8362, BS 77 TX Tech Univ; MS 79 Univ of KS; Sp/Lang Path, Spec Care Sch, **SLP**

Freeman, Dr Algeania W 2407 Stewart Street, Johnson City, TN 37601, (615) 928-1186, BS 70 Fayetteville St Univ; MS 72 Southern IL Univ -Carbondale; PH 77 (NS) OH St Univ; SLP, East Tenn State University, **SLP**

Freeman, Angela Whitehurst Route 1 Box 190-Fw, Crestview, FL 32536, (904) 682-5649, **SLP**

Freeman, Ann Marie 19222 S E 184th Place, Renton, WA 98058, (206) 872-4479, BA 78 Western WA Univ; MA 83 Western WA Univ; SLP, Kent School District, **SLP**

Freeman, Dr Barry A Doctors Bldg, 1731 Memorial Drive, Suite 203, Clarksville, TN 37043, (615) 645-3937, BS 67 Boston Univ; MS 69 Emerson Coll; PH 75 (NS) MI St Univ; Aud, Private Practice, **A**

Freeman, Dr Ben 16542 Ventura Boulevard, Suite 312, Encino, CA 91436, (818) 788-7844, BA 39 Univ of CA - Los Angeles; MA 50 Univ of Southern CA; PH 56 (NS) Univ of Denver; SLP, Private Practice, **SLP LM**

Freeman, Cassie Lynn Route 2 Box 79, Pelahatchie, MS 39145, (601) 854-8792, BS 84 Univ Southern MS-Hattiesburg; MS 85 Univ Southern MS-Hattiesburg; 86–Sp-Lang Path, MS Methodist Rehab Ctr, **SLP**

Freeman, Mrs Cecilia Porter Route 1 Box 330, 2 Travelier Trail, Piedmont, SC 29673, (803) 859-2173, BA 62 TX Tech Univ; MA 63 TX Woman's Univ; Sp-Lang Path, Private Practice, **SLP**

Freeman, Mrs Cheryl H 167 Little John Place, Newport News, VA 23602, (804) 874-7322, BS 73 Hampton Univ; MA 74 George Washington Univ; Clinical Coordinator, Hampton University, **SLP**

Freeman, Clarence J 710 Colonial Drive, Baton Rouge, LA 70806, (504) 927-1019, BA 74 Humboldt St Univ; MA 76 Humboldt St Univ; Dir of Aud, Hearing Sp & Learning Ctr, **A**

Freeman, Douglas C P O Box 489, Rochester, MN 55903, (507) 281-2134, BS 76 Univ of AZ; MS 78 Univ of AZ; Aud, Audiological Enterprises, **A**

Freeman, Eddi-Ann R 4288 Douglas Road, Coconut Grove, FL 33133, (305) 667-8804, OB 74 Univ of Miami; MS 75 Columbia Univ Teachers Coll; Sp-Lang Path, Private Practice, **SLP**

Freeman, Eleanor M 2710 Hopeton, San Antonio, TX 78230, (512) 342-8860, BS 74 Southwest TX St Univ; ME 75 Southwest TX St Univ; Sp-Lang Path, Private Practice, **SLP**

Freeman, Ena Gail 1015 33rd Street N W, Apt 503, Washington, DC 20007, (202) 337-5014, BA 77 Smith Coll; OM 80 Julliard School; MS 82 Adelphi Univ; SLP, **SLP**

Freeman, Mrs Evelyn Veney 207 Mountain View Court, Landover, MD 20785, (301) 336-3796, MS 88 Univ of the DC

Freeman, Francine Carmody 1111 Bryant Drive, Sanford, NC 27330, (919) 774-4384, BA 70 Univ of MA - Amherst; ME 73 Boston Coll; MA 87 Appalachian St Univ; **SLP**

Freeman, Dr Gerald G Sch Of Human & Educational Ser, Oakland University, 526-O Dowd Hall, Rochester, MI 48063, (313) 377-4100, BA 53 Univ of MI - Ann Arbor; MA 54 Univ of MI - Ann Arbor; PH 58 (NS) Univ of MI - Ann Arbor; Prof & Dir Early Chldhd Cen, Oakland Univ, **SLP F**

Freeman, Mrs Gertrude Anne 1905 Manning #102, Los Angeles, CA 90025, (213) 997-2330, BA 73 CA St Univ - Northridge; MA 75 CA St Univ - Northridge; Sp-Lang Path, Los Angeles USD, **SLP LM**

Freeman, Hyman S Speech And Hearing Center, State University College, Plattsburgh, NY 12901, (518) 564-2170, BA 60 Univ of Denver; MA 62 Univ of Denver; Prof, SUNY-Plattsburgh, **SLP A**

Freeman, Janet Gumprich 2700 44th Avenue North, Minneapolis, MN 55412, (612) 786-1127, BS 76 Univ of VA - Charlottesville; ME 78 Univ of VA - Charlottesville; Sp-Lang Path, Achievement Rehab Corp, **SLP**

Freeman, Mrs Jeanne S 4900 Old Mobile Highway, Apartment 53, Pascagoula, MS 39567, (601) 475-8795, BA 84 Univ of MS; MS 86 Univ of MS; Sp-Lang Path, **SLP**

Freeman, Letitia Smith Route 1 Box 155-A7, Paige, TX 78659, (512) 321-7173, BS 84 Univ of TX - Austin; MA 87 Univ of TX - Austin; **SLP**

Freeman, Margaret H 3323-L Circle Brook Dr S W, Roanoke, VA 24014-7283, (703) 981-7928, BA 85 IN Univ - Bloomington; MS 87 IL St Univ - Normal; **SLP**

Freeman, Melissa Lynn 150 West Evergreen #C-1, Philadelphia, PA 19118, (215) 247-8905, BA 82 Coll of Wooster; MA 85 Univ of Pittsburgh - Pittsburgh; **SLP**

Freeman, Mrs Nancy C 8745 Maplewood Road, Seminole, FL 34647, (813) 391-3473, BS 68 Purdue Univ - West Lafayette; MS 71 Univ of South FL; Chief/Sp/Lang Path, Largo Med Cen Hosp, **SLP ACE**

Freeman, Mrs Nancy Lindseth Route 2 Box 113, River Falls, WI 54022, (612) 439-5160, BS 85 Univ of WI - River Falls; OM 87 Univ of WI - River Falls; Sp-Lang Path, ISD 834

Freeman, Patricia A 3024 Aquadale Lane, Cincinnati, OH 45211-8004, (606) 491-2288, BA 78 Portland St Univ; MS 81 Univ of WI - Madison; SLP, Commun Act Cmsn of Cinti Area, **SLP**

Freeman, Patty L 4100 Fulton Street #2, San Francisco, CA 94121, (415) 221-4483, OB 38 Nat'l Coll of Ed - Evanston; **SLP LM**

Freeman, Mrs Rebecca Peterson Box 704, 47 North Hamilton Road FB, Mountain View, WY 82939, (307) 782-6816, MA 84 Univ of SD - Vermillion; Sp-Lang Path, Uinta Co Sch Dist 4, **SLP**

Freeman, Dr Sandra F 535 East 86th Street #10D, New York, NY 10028, (212) 403-1051, BS 50 Syracuse Univ; MA 58 Columbia Univ Teachers Coll; PH 69 (NS) NY Univ; Professor of Speech, Long Island University, **SLP**

Freeman, Mrs Sheila Anne 1392 Cosmos Lane, St Paul, MN 55123, (612) 488-7205, **SLP**

Freeman, Sondra G Jewish Home & Rehab Center, 198 Stevens Avenue, Jersey City, NJ 07305, (201) 451-9000, BA 71 CUNY - Hunter Coll; MA 73 NY Univ; Dir/Sp-Aud Dept, Jewish Home & Rehab Cen, **SLP ACE**

Freeman, Toby Ellen 14 Garrison Drive, Bedford, NH 03102, (603) 472-2529, BA 77 Univ of MI - Ann Arbor; MS 78 Univ of MI - Ann Arbor; Sp-Lang Path, Private Practice, **SLP**

Freeman, William B P O Box 902, Lutz, FL 33549, (813) 949-4052, BA 63 Univ of AL- Tuscaloosa; MA 67; Chief-Aud, VA Hosp, **A**

Freer, Cynthia Anne 544 W 36020 Highway #C, Dousman, WI 53118, (414) 259-1414, BA 81 Univ of Northern CO; MA 84 Northern IL Univ - De Kalb; **SLP**

Freese, Mrs Gail Joan West 1223 Decatur, Spokane, WA 99205, (509) 328-9229, BA 81 Eastern WA Univ; MS 83 Eastern WA Univ; Coordinator, Hearing Impaired Infant Prog, **SLP**

Freese, Paula Rae 2133 South Shore Drive S E, Apartment 201, Kentwood, MI 49508, (616) 242-0425, BS 84 IA St Univ; MA 86 Univ of IA; Sp-Lang Path, Mary Free Bed Hosp & Rehab Ctr, **SLP**

Freiberg, Cathlene J 838 Forest Court #6, Oconomowoc, WI 53066, MS 88 Univ of WI - Madison

Freiberg, Christine L 401 South 36th Avenue, Wausau, WI 54401, (715) 845-1353, BA 72 Univ of WI - Madison; MS 73 Univ of WI - Stevens Point; Sp-Lang Path, Wausau Pub Sch, **SLP**

Freidenberg, Carol J 956 Clayton, San Francisco, CA 94117, (415) 666-5101, BS 65 Univ of MN - Minneap-St Paul; MS 66 Univ of WI - Madison; 71–Sp-Lang Path, UC Med Ctr, **SLP**

Freidman, Helene W 9 Heckamore Avenue, Bala-Cynwyd, PA 19004, (215) 423-1400, BA 69 SUNY - Center at Albany; MA 73 Temple Univ; 88–Supvr/Sp-Lang Svcs, KenCrest Services, **SLP**

Freilinger, Dr J Joseph 8924 Buena Vista Court, Des Moines, IA 50322, (515) 281-3176, BA 55 Univ of Northern CO; MA 60 Univ of Northern CO; PH 73 (Sp-Lang Path/Aud) Univ of KS; 65–Consult, IA St Dept of Educ, **SLP F**

Freiman, Susan 527 25th Street, Santa Monica, CA 90402-3139, (213) 395-7169, BA 74 CUNY - Queens Coll; MA 76 Temple Univ-Tyler Sch of Art; **SLP**

Freimuth, Cynthia Anne 47 Old Wolcott Road, Bristol, CT 06010, (203) 584-7750, BS 76 Central CT St Univ; MS 87 Southern CT St Univ; 88–Sp-Lang Path, Bristol Bd of Educ, **SLP**

Freind, Mrs Deborah B Hearing & Speech Center, The Children's Hospital, 1600 7th Avenue South, Birmingham, AL 35233, (205) 939-9149, BA 78 Auburn Univ - Auburn; OM 79 Auburn Univ - Auburn; 82–Aud, Chldn Hosp of AL, **A**

Freitag, Leonore 9 C Stowe Hill, Thorndon, Wellington 1, New Zealand, MA 72 CUNY - City College; Sp-Lang Path, Hutt Hosp, **SLP**

Freitag, Martha Helen 21 Walbar Street, Rochester, NY 14609, (716) 271-0761, BS 80 Nazareth Coll of Rochester; ME 81 SUNY - Coll at Buffalo; Sp-Lang Path, Mary Cariola Childrens Center, **SLP**

Freitas, Richard Joseph 107 N W 51st Street, Seattle, WA 98107, (206) 789-0671, BA 81 San Jose St Univ; MS 83 Univ of MI - Ann Arbor; Sp/Lang Path, NW Hosp Sp & Hrng Cen, **SLP**

Freiwald, Mrs Julianne Flick P O Box 4790, Miami Lakes, FL 33014, BA 80 Univ of Miami; MS 88 Nova Univ

Fremarek, Mrs Carole M 16501 South 118th Avenue, Orland Park, IL 60462-5832, (312) 460-4832, BA 70 Saint Xavier Coll; OM 87 Governors St Univ; 83–Sp-Lang Path, Lockport Area Spec Educ Coop, **SLP**

French, Amy Ruhl 2187 Kolb Drive, Lancaster, PA 17602, (717) 299-3988, BS 81 Bloomsburg Univ of PA; MS 82 Bloomsburg Univ of PA; Sp-Lang Path, Lincoln Inter Unit #12, **SLP**

French, Mrs Barbara H 1960 South Grandview, Dubuque, IA 52001, (319) 588-0538, BS 59 Longwood Coll; ME 62 Univ of VA - Charlottesville; SLP, Keystone AEA #1, **SLP**

French, Mrs Connie W Route 3, Box 257-F, Blackstone, VA 23824, (804) 292-5300, BA 72 Mary Washington Coll; ME 73 Univ of VA - Charlottesville; Sp-Lang Path, Nottoway Co Pub Schs, **SLP**

French, Mrs Elsie H 4104 Sullivan Road, Knoxville, TN 37921, (615) 689-5978, BS 63 East TN St Univ; MA 66 Univ of TN - Knoxville; Dir/Sp-Lang Path Serv, Home Health Care of East Tenn, **SLP**

French, Mrs Judy Louise 1110 Brentwood, Paris, TN 38242, (901) 642-5891, BS 74 Murray St Univ; MS 78 Murray St Univ; **SLP**

French, Mrs Julie Ann 606 North Emerson Avenue, Indianapolis, IN 46219, BS 84 Purdue Univ - West Lafayette; MS 86 Purdue Univ - West Lafayette; 88–Aud, St Francis Hosp Ctr, **A**

French, Mrs Leigh Ann 5706 Holyoke, Spokane, WA 99208, (509) 327-3550, BA 80 Eastern WA Univ; MS 81 Eastern WA Univ; Sp-Lang Path, Ed Ser Dist 101, **SLP**

French, Louise A R R 1 Box 1030, Rapid City, SD 57702, (605) 348-8140, BA 72 Augustana Coll; MA 82 Univ of SD - Vermillion; MA 86 Univ of Northern CO; Aud, Rapid City Area Schs, **A**

French, Mrs Lydia L 2001 Amesbury, Auburndale, FL 33823, (813) 534-1511, BS 78 FL St Univ; MS 79 FL St Univ; SLP, Polk County Schools, **SLP**

French, Nancy Mangan Town Hill Road, Cuttingsville, VT 05738, (802) 492-3304, MA 80 Univ of FL; Speech/Language Pathologist, Rutland Central Supervisory, **SLP**

French, Mrs Patricia G 3159 Claymore Lane, New Franken, WI 54229, (414) 497-6074, BA 74 Univ of Northern IA; MS 75 Univ of WI - Stevens Point; Sp-Lang Path, Green Bay Pub Sch, **SLP**

French, Richard B 330 West Brambleton Avenue, Norfolk, VA 23510, BS 50 Boston Univ; ME 51 Boston Univ; Retired, **SLP**

French, Mrs Sheryl Salzberg 11319 8th Avenue NE, Apartment 307, Seattle, WA 98125, BS 80 Univ of WA; Sp-Lang Path, Tacoma PS, **SLP ACE**

French, Stephanie M 151 East 62nd Street #4-B, New York, NY 10021, BA 63 Hofstra Univ; MA 64 Syracuse Univ; **SLP**

French, Mrs Wendolyn Houghton 17589 Santa Domingo Circle, Fountain Valley, CA 92708, (714) 842-9726, BA 81 CA St Univ - Long Beach; MA 84 Univ of the Pacific; 86–Sp-Lang Path, Rancho Los Amigos Med Ctr, **SLP**

French-Watts, Mrs Geraldine Anne 15846 West Rosehaven Lane, Canyon Country, CA 91351, (805) 252-9110, BA 77 CA St Univ - Northridge; MA 79 CA St Univ - Northridge; SLP, Los Angeles Co Supt of Sch, **SLP**

Frenkiel, Leah 2615 West Catalpa #303, Chicago, IL 60625, (312) 929-8200, BA 75 IN Univ - Bloomington; ME 76 IN Univ - Bloomington; Sp-Lang Path, Ctr Rehab/Training Persons w/Disabilities, **SLP**

Frerker, Mrs Victoria G 3815 Flad, St Louis, MO 63110, (314) 865-3770, BS 65 Univ of MN - Minneap-St Paul; MA 68 Univ of MN - Minneap-St Paul; Sp-Lang Path, Midtown Habilitation Center, **SLP**

Frese, Donna Essington 1415 Chihuahua Northeast, Albuquerque, NM 87112, (913) 499-6477, BA 77 Univ of KS; MA 81 Wichita St Univ; **SLP**

Fresh, Mrs Jacqueline Finch 27 Carlotia Drive, Jeffersonville, IN 47130, (812) 364-4141, BS 61 IN St Univ - Terre Haute; MS 65 IN Univ - Bloomington; Sp-Lang Path, Dev Ser Inc, **SLP**

Freshley, Nancy L 20 Felix Place, Amity Harbor, NY 11701, (516) 665-7772, BA 61 Bowling Green St Univ; MA 63 Bowling Green St Univ; 72–Cen Dir, Suffolk Hrng & Sp Cen Inc, **SLP**

Freshman, Mrs Roberta Connolly 1 Laurel Street, Peabody, MA 01960, (617) 887-2323, BS 82 Marquette Univ; MA 84 Univ of MA - Amherst; Sp-Lang Path, Masconomet Regional Jr-Sr High, **SLP**

Freshwaters, Karin Jean 2409 39th Street, Des Moines, IA 50310-3914, (319) 232-4578, BS 82 Univ of IA; MA 83 Univ of IA; SLP, Heartland AEA 11, **SLP**

Fressola, Diane R 1702 Woodmore Oaks Drive, Manchester, MO 63021, (314) 569-8229, BS 73 Ithaca Coll; MA 75 Saint Louis Univ; Area Coord, St Louis County Spec Sch Dist, **SLP**

Freudendorf, Karen V 12-4 Pond Way, Manorville, NY 11949, BS 75 Ithaca Coll; MS 77 SUNY - Coll at Buffalo; SLP, BOCES, **SLP**

Freudiger-Grantham, Trish 3524 California Street, Eureka, CA 95501, (707) 445-4119, MA 87 Humboldt St Univ; 87–Sp-Lang Path, Eureka City Schs

Freund, Mrs Anna Daube 111 Delmar Avenue, Glen Rock, NJ 07452, (201) 595-2209, BA 63 William Paterson Coll; MA 64 Columbia Univ Teachers Coll; Retired, William Paterson Coll, **SLP ACE**

Freund, Anne Gustafsson 272 East 7th Street #2-A, New York, NY 10009, (212) 475-6099, MA 87 CUNY - Hunter Coll; 88–Sp-Lang Path, Internatl Ctr for the Disabled, **SLP**

Freund, Mrs Judith Garber 3519 Pine Estates Drive, West Bloomfield, MI 48033, (313) 651-6210, SLP, Rochester Com Schls, **SLP**

Freund, Lise A 4301 South West 15th St, Apt 206, Topeka, KS 66604, (913) 296-5431, BA 85 Wichita St Univ; MA 86 Wichita St Univ; SLP, Kansas Neur Inst, **SLP**

Freund, Nancy Jo 3436 North Central Park, Chicago, IL 60618, BS 74 Northwestern Univ; MA 75 Northwestern Univ; Sp-Lang Path, Evanston Dist #65, **SLP**

Freundlich, Ruth 24 Davis Road, Lakewood, NJ 08701, **SLP**

Freundlich, Susan Gale 929 Fresno Avenue, Berkeley, CA 94707, (415) 893-7343, MA 75 Univ of CO - Denver; 88–Dev Dir, Center for Working Life, **A**

Freundschuh, Laurie Weber 340 Edgewood Avenue, Buffalo, NY 14223-2526, (716) 827-9611, BS 83 Univ of MN - Duluth; OB 83 Univ of MN - Duluth; MA 84 Univ of MN - Duluth; Sp-Lang Path, Our Lady Victory Infant Home, **SLP**

Frevert, Corine T 5051 Camino Esplendora, Tucson, AZ 85718, (602) 299-9669, BA 32 Univ of MN - Minneap-St Paul; MA 33 Univ of MN - Minneap-St Paul; PH 45 (NS) Yale Univ; **SLP LM**

Frey, Barbara S 7 West 14th Street, Apartment 8-L South, New York, NY 10011, (718) 423-7300, BS 77 Syracuse Univ; MA 79 NY Univ; 84–Sp-Lang Path, Steppingstone Day Sch Inc, **SLP**

Frey, Julie Eggleson 5013 Violet Lane, Madison, WI 53714, (608) 267-6174, MS 84 Univ of AZ; BS 81 Univ of WI - Madison; **SLP**

Frey, Marilyn Maclk Northeast Arkansas Speech Pathology Services, 520 Carson, Suite A, Jonesboro, AR 72401, (501) 933-8018, BS 81 Stephen F Austin St Univ; MS 83 Univ of AR - Little Rock; Sp/Lang Path, Northeast Arkansas Sp Path Svcs, **SLP ACE**

Frey, Mrs Marsha 14450 Crest Lane, Plymouth, IN 46563, (219) 936-5963, BA 76 IN Univ - Bloomington; MA 79 IN Univ - Bloomington; SLP, Frey Sp Rehab, **SLP**

Frey, Mrs Regina M 1028 South Braddock Avenue, Pittsburgh, PA 15218, (412) 741-9500, BA 79 Univ of Pittsburgh - Pittsburgh; MA 81 Univ of Pittsburgh - Pittsburgh; 82–Sp-Lang Path, D T Watson Rehab Hosp, **SLP**

Frey, Rosemarie C Illinois Dept Of Public Health, 245 Roosevelt, West Chicago, IL 60185, (312) 293-6840, BA 63 Univ of IA; MA 67 De Paul Univ; Vision & Hrng Consult, Il Dept of Pub Hlth, **SLP**

Frey, Dr William G Central Plains MHMR Center, 2700 Yonkers, Plainview, TX 79072, (806) 293-9391, MA 70 KS St Univ; MA 71 Southern Methodist Univ; ED 83 (NS) Univ of Tulsa; **A**

Freyman, Dr Richard L Dept Communication Disorders, Univ Of Massachusetts, 6 Arnold House, Amherst, MA 01003, (413) 545-0298, BS 76 PA St Univ - Univ Park; MA 78 Temple Univ; PH 84 (Psychoacoustics) Univ of MN - Minneap-St Paul; Assistant Professor, University of Massachusetts, **A**

Frichtl, Mrs Joan Marie 6881 East Fieldstone Lane, Tucson, AZ 85715-2078, (602) 798-2547, BS 59 Marquette Univ; MS 83 Governors St Univ; 87–Sp-Lang Path, Howenstine HS-TUSD, **SLP**

Frick, Dr James V 220 South Corl Street, State College, PA 16801, (814) 237-7752, BS 47 Univ of IA; MA 49 Univ of IA; PH 51 (Sp Path) Univ of IA; 85–Consultant Sp-Lang Path, **SLP F LM**

Frick, Mrs Jill Tiedemann 35 Stoney Drive, Dover, DE 19901, (302) 697-3103, BS 83 Towson St Univ; MS 85 Towson St Univ; Sp-Lang Path, John S Charlton Sch, **SLP**

Frick, Lesa Renee 1805 Roswell Road #40-S, Marietta, GA 30062, (404) 876-7519, BA 83 Univ of KY; MA 86 Univ of IL - Urbana; 88–Aud, AHAS Hearing & Speech, **A**

Frick, Mrs Lisa Faller 2320 Silver Lane #304, New Brighton, MN 55112, BS 84 Indiana Univ of PA; MA 86 Univ of MN - Minneap-St Paul; **SLP**

Frickman, Mrs Gail Adkins 1833 Mount Vernon, Fort Wright, KY 41011, BA 77 Univ of KY; OM 79 Auburn Univ - Auburn; **SLP**

Friday, Mrs Kathleen MacElroy 115 Vine Street, New Britain, CT 06052, (203) 628-0331, BS 56 Boston Univ

Friday, Mrs Lisa T 961 West Monroe #1, Grenada, MS 38901-5043, (601) 226-7175, BA 83 LA St Univ - Shreveport; OM 87 LA St Univ - Shreveport; 87–Sp-Lang Path, Speech Pathology Services, **SLP**

Fridgen, Mrs Marvilyn Kay 3030 14th Avenue South, Moorhead, MN 56560, (218) 236-6400, MS 83 Moorhead St Univ; Sp-Lang Path, Moorhead Public Schools, **SLP**

Fridgen, Mary Jean Route 2 Box 2650, Hager City, WI 54014, (612) 388-8930, BA; MS; 85–Sp-Lang Path, River Ridge Rehabilitation, **SLP**

Fridgen, Michael J East Range Clinics Ltd, 910 6th Avenue North, Virginia, MN 55792, (218) 741-0150, BS 74 ND St Univ; MS 75 Minot St Univ; Aud, East Range Clinics Ltd, **A**

Fridman, Anna 16 Fairholme Avenue, Toronto, ON, Canada M6B 2W5, (416) 259-6671, ME 79 Clarion Univ of PA; Sp-Lang Path, Queensway Gen Hosp, **SLP**

Fridman, Mrs Christine 6304 Fairdel Avenue, Baltimore, MD 21206, (301) 396-6361, BS 64 SUNY - Coll at Fredonia; MS 78 Towson St Univ; SLP, Baltimore City Pub Schs, **SLP**

Frieberger, Mrs Susan M St Johns Mercy Medical Center, 615 South New Ballas Road, St Louis, MO 63141, (314) 569-6040, BS 70 Saint Louis Univ; MA 72 Saint Louis Univ; Aud, St Johns Mercy Med Cen, **A**

Friebus, Mrs Cheryl A 942 Beckman Trail, Elgin, IL 60120, (312) 742-3264, BA 67 Elmhurst Coll; MA 69 Northern IL Univ - De Kalb; Director Early Learning Prog, Easter Seal Rehabilitation Cen, **SLP**

Friebus, Maxine B 6149 East Caley Drive, Englewood, CO 80111, (303) 798-1337, BS 68 Northern IL Univ - De Kalb; MS 74 Univ of UT; Sp-Lang Path, Littleton Public Schools, **SLP**

Fried, Mrs Barbara R 7 Haddonfield Drive, Parsippany, NJ 07054, (201) 335-6762, BA 64 Newark St Coll; MA 67 Newark St Coll; Sp-Lang Path, Montville Bd Ed, **SLP**

Fried, Debra Otolaryngology Associates, 19 East 98th Street, Suite 6A Box 1191, New York, NY 10029, (212) 876-9604, BA 75 SUNY - Center at Buffalo; MS 77 Columbia Univ Teachers Coll; Aud, Mt Sinai Hosp Otol Assoc, **A**

Fried, Mrs Janis E Sattler 5566 Normanhurst, West Bloomfield, MI 48322, (313) 851-0811, BA 76 MI St Univ; MA 77 Eastern MI Univ; Sp-Lang Path, Troy Pub Sch, **SLP**

Fried, Joy Michele 2825 S Drew Avenue, Minneapolis, MN 55416, (612) 927-8015, **SLP**

Fried, Dr Leonard 6225 Coldwater Canyon Avenue, North Hollywood, CA 91606, (818) 769-5484, BS 37 CUNY - City College; ME 48 Duquesne Univ; PH 74 (NS); **SLP LM**

Fried, Marla G 1466 Calle Pajaros, San Dimas, CA 91773, MS; **SLP LM**

Frieda, Linda B 3135 East Redbud, Springfield, MO 65804, (417) 836-0400, BA 74 Univ of CA - Los Angeles; MA 80 CA St Univ - Northridge; Sp/Lang Path, Springfield Reg Cen-Dev Disab, **SLP ACE**

Friedel, Dianne M Rd 1 Box 25, Middle Grove, NY 12850, **SLP**

Friedel, Elane R 2725 Hunter Road, Fort Lauderdale, FL 33331, (305) 389-0555, BS 74 Emory Univ; MS 76 Emory Univ; **A**

Frieder, Mrs Dalia 408 Standish Drive, Syracuse, NY 13224, (315) 446-8876, BA 72 SUNY - Center at Buffalo; MS 79 SUNY - Coll at Buffalo; Clin Supvr/Coord Reduction Prog, Gebbie Speech & Hearing Clinics, **SLP**

Friedl, Christina Ute 26 Pitcher Avenue, West Medford, MA 02155, (617) 862-1004, MS 87 Ithaca Coll

Friedland, Sandra M 107 Briarcrest Drive, Monroeville, PA 15146, BS

Friedlander, Mrs Barbara N 898 Blandford Boulevard, Redwood City, CA 94062, (415) 368-9658, BA 69 Univ of NV - Reno; MS 71 Purdue Univ - West Lafayette; **SLP ACE**

Friedlander, David Gerald, Jr 1341 Read's Run, Traverse City, MI 49684, (616) 922-9000, BA 79 OH St Univ; MA 82 OH St Univ; Home Care Sp-Lang Path, Munion Med Cen, **SLP**

Friedlander, Penney Helene 130 Boylston Street #3, Malden, MA 02148, (617) 535-6197, BA 83 SUNY - Coll at Oneonta; ME 85 Univ of GA; Sp-Lang Path, North Shore Spec Ed Con, **SLP**

Friedlander, Renee S 6423 North Richmond #1-S, Chicago, IL 60645, (312) 973-4712, BS 85 Northwestern Univ; MA 86 Northwestern Univ; **SLP**

Friedlander, Rhonda Lynn P O Box 201, Ronan, MT 59864, (406) 675-0325, BA 84 Gonzaga Univ; MS 86 Eastern WA Univ; 86–Sp-Lang Path, Conf Salish & Kootenai Tribes, **SLP**

Friedley, Mrs Sheridan Coale 4063 Brandon Drive, Delray Beach, FL 33445, (305) 498-8744, BS 76 Univ of TX - Austin; MA 84 Univ of Houston - Univ Park; SLP, Palm Beach County School Dist, **SLP**

Friedlieb, Victoria Josephine 3319 Downing Court, Fort Collins, CO 80526, (303) 669-4640, OB 78 Univ of MN - Duluth; MS 80 CO St Univ; SLP Inreal Spec, McKee Medical Center, **SLP**

Friedman, Mrs Ann D 27 Hearthstone Drive, Riverside, CT 06878, (203) 625-7498, BS 59 Jersey City St Coll; MA 62 Kean Coll of NJ; Sp-Lang Path, Greenwich Board of Education, **SLP**

Friedman, Barbara Jo Univ Of Minnesota Hospital, Audiology Clinic, Box 283 Mayo, Minneapolis, MN 55455, BS 74 Univ of MN - Minneap-St Paul; MS 75 Univ of WI - Madison; Aud, U of MN Hosp, **A**

Friedman, Mrs Carol 18 Brockton Road, Spring Valley, NY 10977, BA 54 CUNY - Queens Coll; Sp-Lang Path, East Ramapo Ctrl Sch Dist, **SLP**

Friedman, Mrs Debbie A 175 Beekman Ln, Neshanic Station, NJ 08853, (201) 281-6330, BA 78 Montclair St Coll; MA 79 Bowling Green St Univ; Sp-Lang Path, JFK Med Ctr, **SLP**

Friedman, Deborah Ann 12 Ridge Road, Shrewsbury, MA 01545, (508) 799-4171, BA 80 CUNY - Queens Coll; MA 82 CUNY - Hunter Coll; Sp-Lang Path, Private Practice, **SLP**

Friedman, Deborah K 12 Quebec Drive, Huntington Station, NY 11746, (516) 883-9292, BA 76 Univ of MD - College Park; MS 78 PA St Univ - Univ Park; Sp/Lang Path, Port Wash Pub Sch, **SLP**

Friedman, Deborah Walker Box 16, OI/C 497 Rtg, APO New York, NY 09457, BS 83 Southwest TX St Univ; ME 84 Southwest TX St Univ; **SLP**

Friedman, Debra Heller 26 Richbourne Lane, Melville, NY 11747, BA 82 Boston Univ; MS 83 Columbia Univ Teachers Coll; Sp-Lang Path, **SLP**

Friedman, Eileen Savage 23 Prospect Avenue, Port Washington, NY 11050-3112, (617) 361-5393, BS 68 Univ of MI - Ann Arbor; MS 77 Emerson Coll; Sp-Lang Path, Private Practice, **SLP**

Friedman, Elaine C 15 Edgebrook Court, New City, NY 10956-2465, MD (NS); **SLP**

Friedman, Ellen Noreen 519 Jeannette Drive, Richmond Heights, OH 44143, (216) 371-2600, BA 78 Cleveland St Univ; MA 79 Cleveland St Univ; Dir-Ctr for Independent Living, Jewish Family Svc Assoc, **SLP**

Friedman, Dr Frances A 44 Fay Lane, Needham, MA 02194, (617) 421-5984, MS 72 Univ of WI - Madison; OD 78 3807; OD 80 (Neuropsychology) Tufts Univ; Dir-Aud, Harvard Comm Hlth Plan, **A**

Friedman, Mrs Francine Rosenzweig 1072 Johnston Avenue, Wantagh, NY 11793, (516) 931-1990, **SLP ACE**

Friedman, Gary 8830 N W 47th Street, Sunrise, FL 33351, (305) 741-3357, BS 78 SUNY - Center at Buffalo; MS 80 Washington Univ; Director, Family Hearing Center, **A**

Friedman, Janice Ruth 183 Henry Street, San Francisco, CA 94114, (415) 861-3154, BA 82 0500; MS 84 Univ of Redlands; 85–Spec Day Class Tchr, San Francisco USD, **SLP**

Friedman, Jerome L 7 Dehon, San Francisco, CA 94114, (415) 863-4710, BS 84 Northeastern Univ; MS 86 Gallaudet Coll; 86–Aud/Dir of Hrng, Hrng Society for the Bay Area Inc, **A**

Friedman, Mrs Joan A 18272 181st Circle So, Boca Raton, FL 33434-8155, (305) 487-1954, BS 76 Miami Univ - Oxford; MA 77 Kent St Univ; Sp-Lang Path, Coral Springs Sp & Lang Ctr, **SLP**

Friedman, Judith Pierce Dean, 204 Wilsey Court, Paramus, NJ 07652, (201) 447-1500, BA 54 Emerson Coll; MA 59 Columbia Univ Teachers Coll; **SLP**

Friedman, Mrs Kathleen Anne 52 Clinton Street, Batavia, NY 14020, (716) 343-1400, BS 74 SUNY - Coll at Brockport; MA 79 SUNY - Coll at Geneseo; **SLP**

Friedman, Kathryn Klein 421 East Ridge, Marquette, MI 49855, (906) 228-6098, BA 86 Univ of WI - Eau Claire; MA 87 Western MI Univ; 88–Sp-Lang Path, Upper Peninsula Home Nursing

Friedman, Lawrence J Communication Disorders Ltd, 2853 Smoke Tree Circle, Stockton, CA 95209, (209) 951-7371, BA 69 CA St Univ - Northridge; MA 71 Univ of the Pacific; Owner-Dir, Commun Dis, **SLP**

Friedman, Lisa Michele 4214 Oakridge Lane, Chevy Chase, MD 20815, (202) 636-2964, BS 86 OH Univ - Athens; MA 88 Univ of Pittsburgh - Pittsburgh; Sp-Lang Path, DCARC

Friedman, Lois Ann 9200 Bustleton Avenue, 204 Alexander Bldg, Philadelphia, PA 19115, (215) 969-3731, BA 77 Rutger's St Univ - Douglas Coll; MA 81 Kean Coll of NJ; 87–Sp-Lang Path, **SLP**

Friedman, Dr Lynne Rosen 445 East 80th Street, New York, NY 10021, (212) 249-0061, MA 68 Columbia Univ Sch of Gen St; OM 76 Columbia Univ Sch of Gen St; PH 80 (Sp Path) Columbia Univ Sch of Gen St; Sp-Lang Path, Private Practice, **SLP**

Friedman, Meryl L 63-25 Saunders Street #3G, Rego Park, NY 11374, (718) 899-8800, BS 76 NY Univ; MS 77 Univ of MI - Ann Arbor; 86–Sp-Lang Path, Lexington Sch for the Deaf, **SLP**

Friedman, Pacy 214 North 23rd Avenue East, Duluth, MN 55812, (218) 724-9205, BS 55 Univ of MN - Duluth; MS 58 Univ of MN - Minneap-St Paul; **SLP A LM**

Friedman, Rachel A 680 Ft Washington Avenue, #6-F, New York, NY 10040, (212) 683-6970, MS 88 Columbia Univ Teachers Coll; 88–Sp-Lang Path, New York City Bd of Educ

Friedman, Mrs Rhonda L 4 Toronto Woods Road, Manalapan, NJ 07726, (201) 780-3167, BA 75 CUNY - Hunter Coll; MA 78 NY Univ; Sp-Lang Path, Manalapan-Englishtown Bd of Educ, **SLP**

Friedman, Rochelle 2289-I Dunwoody Crossing, Atlanta, GA 30338, (404) 451-4271, BS 66 OH St Univ; MA 72 Case Western Reserve Univ; Consultant, Private Practice, **SLP**

Friedman, Rochelle Z 13 Pond Ridge Road, Danbury, CT 06811, (203) 426-7670, BA 60 CUNY - Hunter Coll; MA 70 CUNY - Brooklyn Coll; Sp/Lang Path, Newtown Pub Sch, **SLP**

Friedman, Mrs Ruth F 7053 East McDonald Drive, Scottsdale, AZ 85253, (602) 948-0740, BA 58 Hofstra Univ; MS 61 Adelphi Univ; **SLP LM**

Friedman, Mrs Sandra M 1721 Newman Court, East Meadow, NY 11554, (516) 773-1509, BA 75 Hofstra Univ; MA 76 Hofstra Univ; Sp-Lang Path, Great Neck Pub Sch, **SLP ACE**

Friedman, Shari Arleen 200 East 33rd Street, Apt #16F, New York, NY 10016, (212) 683-2236, BS 84 Boston Univ; MS 85 Boston Univ; 88–Sp-Lang Path, NY Childhood Center-Smalstuf, **SLP**

Friedman, Mrs Susan B 3115 Octavia Street, New Orleans, LA 70125, (504) 897-2606, BS 67 Univ of WI - Madison; MA 68 Univ of Cincinnati; Sp-Lang Path, New Orleans Sp&Hrng Cen, **SLP**

Friedman, Susan E 149 Marine Avenue, Brooklyn, NY 11209, (718) 648-6094, BS 74 CUNY - Brooklyn Coll; MS 76 CUNY - Brooklyn Coll; OM 81 CUNY - Brooklyn Coll; Sp-Lang Path, Bd of Ed Dstr Ofc 22, **SLP**

Friedman-Hanna, Karen Lynn 141 Burt Street #3, Norton, MA 02766-2517, (617) 625-0390, BS 83 Univ of MA - Amherst; MA 85 Univ of CT; 88–Sp-Lang Path, KLK Associates Inc, **SLP**

Friedman-Wilson, Harriet 579 Pelton Avenue, Staten Island, NY 10310, BA 76 CUNY - Hunter Coll; MA 78 Columbia Univ Teachers Coll; 87–Aud, Private Practice, **A**

Fried-Oken, Dr Melanie B 946 Southwest Westwood Dr, Portland, OR 97201, (617) 437-2492, BA 76 Univ of Rochester; MA 78 Northwestern Univ; PH 84 (NS) Boston Univ; Clinical Research Assoc, Rehab Institute of Oregon, **SLP**

Friedrich, Peggy Welsh 608 Sunnycrest Street, Green Bay, WI 54302, (414) 497-3184, BS 74 Univ of WI - Eau Claire; MS 75 Univ of WI - Eau Claire; 77–Sp-Lang Path, Green Bay Area PS, **SLP**

Friel, Eileen Marie 7901 South Kostner, Chicago, IL 60652, (312) 735-4841, 87 Governors St Univ

Friel-Patti, Dr Sandy 5816 Everglade Road, Dallas, TX 75227, (214) 905-3060, BA 67 Catholic Univ of America; MA 69 Catholic Univ of America; PH 78 (NS) Purdue Univ - West Lafayette; 84–Assoc Prof, Univ of TX at Dallas, **SLP**

Friend, Mrs Carolyn Jean 2333 West Solero Drive, Apartment 1003, Tucson, AZ 85741, (602) 577-0953, BS 86 Ball St Univ; MA 87 Ball St Univ

Friend, Connie Marie P O Box 3015, Carbondale, IL 62902-3015, (618) 529-5355, BS 83 Southern IL Univ -Carbondale; MS 86 Southern IL Univ -Carbondale; Sp-Lang Path, InSpeech Inc, **SLP**

Friend, Debra E Route 2 Box 16, Swanton, MD 21561, (301) 334-3452, BS 77 WV Univ; MS 79; PH 88 (Administration & Supervision) 8141; 79–Sp-Lang Path, Garrett Co Bd of Ed, **SLP ACE**

Friend, Helen H 1221 North 3rd Street, Fargo, ND 58102, MS 71 Purdue Univ - West Lafayette; Sp-Lang Path, Moorhead Pub Sch, **SLP**

Friend, Tressa J PO Box 653, Evanston, IL 60204-0653, (312) 491-5073, BS 83 Brigham Young Univ; MA 85 Brigham Young Univ, **SLP**

Frierson, Marsha 146-B Glassboro Road, Woodbury, NJ 08098, (609) 342-7600, Sp-Lang Path, Mediplex Rehab, **SLP**

Fries, Ellen Feinerman 245 West 107 Street #14-B, New York, NY 10025, (212) 830-1016, BA 77 CUNY - Queens Coll; MS 79 Columbia Univ Teachers Coll; Aud, Cty Hosp Cen-Elmhurst, **A**

Friesen, Cheryl V 11 Derby Lane #601, Sarnia, ON, Canada N7T 7V2, (519) 336-2175, MA 87 MI St Univ

Friesen, Ellen A 2236 Mason Lane, Manchester, MO 63011, (314) 821-0008, BS 63 Bradley Univ; MS 79 Fontbonne Coll; Admin, Prof Rehab Cen, **SLP**

Friesenborg, Laurie Ann 1328 Collyer, Longmont, CO 80501, (303) 651-5175, Sp-Lang Path, Spalding Rehab Hosp, **SLP**

Friesenhahn, Mrs Denise Simecki 4111 Stapper Road, St Hedwig, TX 78152, (512) 420-2626, BS 83 Southwest TX St Univ; ME 84 Southwest TX St Univ; Sp-Lang Path, East Central School District, **SLP**

Friess, Susan Sara 36 West 20th Street, 3rd Floor, New York, NY 10011, (212) 675-3003, BA 66 CUNY - Queens Coll; MA 67 Columbia Univ Teachers Coll; 81–Aud, Jewish Home & Hosp for Aged, **A**

Frigo, Mrs Sylvia Alexandra 4520 Grand Avenue, Western Springs, IL 60558, (312) 246-4076, BS 65 Northern IL Univ - De Kalb; OM 85 Governors St Univ; **SLP**

Frimmer, Mrs Barbara 255 Overpeck Avenue, Ridgefield Park, NJ 07660, (201) 440-0806, BA 51 CUNY - Hunter Coll; MA 53 NY Univ; Sp-Lang Path, Ridgefield Park Bd of Ed, **SLP ACE**

Frink, Norman D 3857-16C Wolverine N E, Salem, OR 97305, (503) 588-1039, BS 68 Western OR St Coll; MS 70 Western OR St Coll; Owner-Aud, Salem Aud Cl, **A**

Frisard, Louise M 7501 Munss, PO Box 207, APO New York, NY 09695, MS 75 Univ of South FL; 88–Sp-Lang Path, DODDS-Germany, **SLP**

Frisbie, Kris A 625 South 37th Street #10, Omaha, NE 68105-1209, (913) 621-5155, **A**

Frischman, Anne Weiss 585 Ocean Parkway, Brooklyn, NY 11218, (212) 596-5697, BA CUNY - Brooklyn Coll; ME CUNY - Brooklyn Coll; Sp-Lang Path, NYC Bd of Ed, **SLP**

Frishberg, Debra M 736 McQueen Drive N W, Orangeburg, SC 29115, (803) 536-6355, BA 73 CUNY - Brooklyn Coll; MA 74 Univ of MA - Amherst; Sp-Lang Path, Speech and Language Services, **SLP**

Frisina, Mrs Joann Early Education Center, 40 Park Lane, Highland, NY 12528, (914) 883-5151, BS 73 SUNY - Coll at New Paltz; ME 79 Coll of Saint Rose; Dir, Early Ed Cen, **SLP**

Frissell, Mrs Diane 2834 Stoneleigh Drive, Toledo, OH 43617, (419) 841-4582, BS 70 Bowling Green St Univ; MA 78 Bowling Green St Univ; Sp-Lang Path, Evergreen Bd of Ed, **SLP**

Frist, Eve Judith 5495 Errol Place, Atlanta, GA 30327, (404) 257-1678, BA 72 Univ of MD - College Park; MA 74 Univ of MD - College Park; **SLP**

Fristoe, Dr MacAlyne Dept Of Audiology & Speech Sci, Purdue University, West Lafayette, IN 47907, (317) 494-3795, BA 53 Vanderbilt Univ; MS 60 Vanderbilt Univ; PH 72 (NS) Vanderbilt Univ; Prof, Prudue Univ, **SLP F**

Fritchen, Susan E 6639 West Clarke Street, Wauwatosa, WI 53213, (414) 476-9002, BS 86 Univ of WI - Whitewater; MS 87 Univ of WI - Whitewater; 88–Sp-Lang Path, New Berlin PS

Frith, Mrs Charlotte 1102 Briar Creek Road, Little Rock, AR 72211, (501) 225-0274, BS 64 Auburn Univ - Auburn; MS 81 Univ of AR - Little Rock; Sp-Lang Path, Little Rock Sch Dist, **SLP**

Fritjofson, Mrs Claudia N Box 352, East Barre, VT 05649, (802) 479-0179, BA 77 Univ of VT; MS 78 Univ of VT; Sp/Lang Path, Barre Town Elem Sch, **SLP**

Fritschle, Patricia R R 4 Box 278, Carmi, IL 62821, (618) 382-5542, BS 73 Eastern IL Univ; MS 74 Eastern IL Univ; Sp-Lang Path, Carmi Community University 5, **SLP**

Fritts, Ann Caron 20 Eastside Drive, Lexington, NC 27292, (704) 249-8182, BS 85 Appalachian St Univ; ME 87 Univ of NC - Greensboro; 87–Sp-Lang Path, Davidson Co Schs, **SLP**

Fritz, Barbara A 3416 McKinley Parkway #H-8, Blasdell, NY 14219, (716) 837-2441, BS 79 SUNY - Coll at Buffalo; MS 80 SUNY - Coll at Buffalo; 80–Sp-Lang Path, Lang Dev Prog of W NY, **SLP ACE**

Fritz, Mrs Harriet Cannon 838 Valbrook Court, Lilburn, GA 30247, (404) 767-8259, **SLP**

Fritz, Mrs Lori Snow 2625 Silverado Creek Place, Ontario, CA 91761, (818) 965-3333, BA 82 CA St Univ - Fullerton; MA 85 CA St Univ - Fullerton; **SLP**

Fritz, Mrs Michelle I 6255 106th Avenue North, Pinellas Park, FL 34666, (813) 546-2380, BS 78 FL St Univ; MS 79 FL St Univ; 81–Sp-Lang Path, Pinellas Co Sch Syst, **SLP**

Fritz, Mrs Wendy Anne 324 First Street, Pittsfield, MA 01201, (413) 448-8639, BA 73 Univ of MA - Amherst; MS 74 Syracuse Univ; Sp-Lang Path, Central Berkshire Sch Dist, **SLP**

Fritzell, Dr Bjorn Vastanvagen-4 14600, Tullinge, Sweden, MD 51 Karolinska Inst - Stockholm, Sweden; PH 69 (Phoniatrics) Univ of Goteborg - Sweden; 73–Docent (Assoc Prof), Huddinge University Hospital, **F**

Frobose, Mrs Jane Scaglione 4484 Otha Way, Lilburn, GA 30247, (404) 925-1407, BS 81 Bowling Green St Univ; MA 82 Bowling Green St Univ; Sp-Lang Path, Fulton County School System, **SLP**

Froehlich, Mrs Carole D P O Box 1258, Rehovot, Israel 76112, (972) 034-5147, BS 59 Washington Univ; MS 65 CUNY - Brooklyn Coll; Ed Dir, Micha, **SLP**

Froehlich, Mrs Deborah Sue 142 Woodberry Drive, Athens, GA 30605, (404) 543-4008, MA 83 Eastern MI Univ; Clin Superv, U of GA, **SLP**

Froehlich, Mrs Elaine Mary 2890 Charles Street, Oceanside, NY 11572, (516) 678-4160, BS 83 SUNY - Coll at Cortland; MS 87 Adelphi Univ; 83–Sp-Lang Path, Suffolk BOCES III, **SLP**

Froehlich, Elizabeth O 4901 12th Avenue South, Minneapolis, MN 55417, (612) 827-3007, BA 81 Univ of MN - Duluth; MA 82 Univ of MN - Duluth; Sp-Lang Path, Hennepin Technical Institute, **SLP**

Froehlich, Mrs Judy A 13911 South 36th Street, Omaha, NE 68123, (402) 291-0318, MS 75 Univ of NE - Omaha; **SLP**

Froehlich, Mrs Paula Irene 1220 Meade Lane, Arlington Height, IL 60004, (312) 520-2760, BS 83 Univ of IL - Urbana; MS 85 Univ of IL - Urbana; Sp-Lang Path, Wheeling School District 21, **SLP**

Froehlin, Julia Mary 4992 Sable Pine Circle B-2, West Palm Beach, FL 33417, (305) 622-5506, MA 83 Western MI Univ; Sp-Lang Path, Palm Beach County Sch Dist, **SLP**

Froehling, Mrs Doreen Ann 10423 Dearlove Road #2-B, Glenview, IL 60025, (312) 296-8791, BA 84 IN Univ - Bloomington; OM 86 IN Univ - Bloomington; **SLP**

Froelich, Cathy Dianne 3708-F Mizell Road, Greensboro, NC 27405, (919) 375-7462, BS 85 Appalachian St Univ; ME 87 Univ of NC - Greensboro; 88–Sp-Lang Path, Greensboro PS, **SLP**

Froelich, Thomas M 1521 12th Street N W #2, Minot, ND 58701, (701) 857-3030, BA 74 Minot St Univ; MS 75 Minot St Univ; Asst Prof of Aud, Minot State Coll, **A**

Frohlich, Mrs Laraine Anne 258 Pine Grove Avenue, Rochester, NY 14617, (716) 338-2352, BS 69 Syracuse Univ; MA 70 Syracuse Univ; 87–Dir, NW Hrng & Sp Ctr Inc, **SLP**

Froke, Robert A 515 South Dakota Street, Aberdeen, SD 57401-6033, (605) 226-0003, BS 80 Northern St Coll; MA 82 Univ of SD - Vermillion; **A**

Fromherz, Dr Robin Elizabeth 18620 Oakdale Road, Dallas, OR 97338, (503) 787-3380, (NS)

Fromm, Davida S 1231 Malvern Street, Pittsburgh, PA 15217, (412) 647-5727, BS 79 Univ of MI - Ann Arbor; MS 81 Univ of WI - Madison; PH 88 (Comunication Disorders) Univ of Pittsburgh - Pittsburgh; Sp-Lang Path, Western Psychiatric Inst & Cl, **SLP**

Frommer, Mrs Shelley Berg 178 Canyon Woods, Matawan, NJ 07747, (201) 583-0997, BS 81 Ithaca Coll; MS 82 Ithaca Coll; Sp/Lang Path, Robert Wood Johson Rehab I, **SLP**

Fromowitz, Mrs Betty S 41 Winesap Lane, Monsey, NY 10952, (914) 362-1766, BA 72 CUNY - Brooklyn Coll; MS 74 CUNY - Brooklyn Coll; Sp-Lang Path, East Ramapo Bd of Ed, **SLP**

Fromwiller, Sharon E 14044 Panay Way #231, Marina Del Rey, CA 90292, (213) 825-8551, BA 73 Case Western Reserve Univ; MA 74 Case Western Reserve Univ; Sp/Lang Path, U of CA-La, **SLP**

Fronce, Mrs Marti P 9072 South Sunrise Circle, Sandy, UT 84092, (801) 943-1825, BS 73 Univ of UT; MS 75 Univ of UT; Sp-Lang Path, Private Practice, **SLP**

Fronheiser, Glenn S McLaren Gen Hospital, Speech & Hrng Department, 401 South Ballenger Hwy, Flint, MI 48532-3685, (313) 762-2362, BS 74 PA St Univ - Univ Park; MA 76 Wayne St Univ; Aud, McLaren Gen Hosp Inc, **A**

Front, Rosemary M 14 Walnut Avenue, Woodsdale, Wheeling, WV 26003, (304) 242-1390, BS 66 Southern IL Univ -Carbondale; MA 69 Wayne St Univ; Exec Dir, Easter Seal Rehabilitation Cen, **SLP**

Frontera, Patricia 33 Henry Place Unit A-2, Hackensack, NJ 07601, (201) 835-8355, BA 74 Montclair St Coll; MA 77 Montclair St Coll; Spec Ed Tchr, Pequannock Twsp Bd of Ed, **SLP**

Froslie, Lucille L 1420 Gordon Avenue, Reno, NV 89502, **SLP LM**

Frost, Carol Ann 4255 Humphrey, Apartment 4224, Tampa, FL 33614, (813) 996-3122, BS 85 Univ of VA - Charlottesville; MS 87 Vanderbilt Univ; 88–Sp-Lang Path, Pasco County Sch Dist, **SLP**

Frost, Darcy K 10105 Grand Oak Drive, Austin, TX 78750, BS 78 Baylor Univ; MS 80 Boston Univ; Sp-Lang Path, St David's Comm Hosp, **SLP**

Frost, Don I 810 Joshua Drive, Windsor, CA 95492, (707) 546-7079, BA 53 San Jose St Univ; MA 60 San Francisco St Univ; Sp-Lang Path, Private Practice, **SLP**

Frost, Jamie Ruffatto 4736-1/2 Humble Road, Missoula, MT 59801, (406) 721-2160, BA 82 Carroll Coll; OM 85 Univ of MT; Sp-Lang Path, Hellgate Elementary School, **SLP**

Frost, Miriam B 100 Lincoln Avenue #9A, Mineola, NY 11501, (212) 481-0300, BA 73 Hofstra Univ; MA 75 Hofstra Univ; Sp-Lang Path, NYC Bd of Ed, **SLP**

Frost-Gaffey, Mrs Jill Route 3 Box 564, Durham, CT 06422, (203) 349-8709, BS 75 SUNY - Coll at Geneseo; MA 77 WV Univ; Aud, Hearing Svcs Ctr, **A**

Frostholm, Linda K 4322 S W 67th Terrace, Gainesville, FL 32608, (904) 493-4341, BA 74 Augustana Coll; ME 75 Univ of FL; Sp-Lang Path, Chiefland El & Hs Levy Co Sch, **SLP**

Fruchtman, Amy Beth 2602 Arbor Drive #225, Madison, WI 53711, (414) 241-5530, BS 81 Univ of WI - Madison; MS 84 Univ of WI - Madison; **SLP**

Frueh, Dr Frank Audiology & Speech Path Serv, VA Tampa Hospital, 13000 Bruce B Downs Boulevard, Tampa, FL 33612, (813) 972-7529, BA 49 Marietta Coll; MA 50 Northwestern Univ; PH 55 (Aud) Purdue Univ - West Lafayette; 64–Ch Aud Sp-Lang Path, VA Hosp, **A**

Fruehling, Beverly H 2152 Del Mar Heights Road, Del Mar, CA 92014, **SLP**

Fruehling, Mrs Janet Marlene 1403 Desoto Drive, O'Fallon, IL 62269, (703) 250-0932, BS 75 Purdue Univ - West Lafayette; MA 77 Ball St Univ; **SLP**

Fruge, Karen Kay 103 Westwood # 165, Lafayette, LA 70506, (318) 237-0465, **A**

Frugoli, Pamela Rae 249 N 8th West #1, St Anthony, ID 83445, (208) 359-3315, BA 84 Harding Univ; MS 85 ID St Univ; 88–Sp-Lang Path, Madison Dist #321, **SLP**

Frum, James P Department Of Otolaryngology, Wheeling Clinic, 58 16th Street, Wheeling, WV 26003, (304) 234-2066, BA 61 West Liberty St Coll; MS 66 WV Univ; Aud & Sp-Lang Path/Dir Dept, Wheeling Cl, **SLP A**

Frumkin, Mrs Judith R 4303 Hepatica Hill, Manlius, NY 13104, (315) 455-7591, BA 70 Case Western Reserve Univ; MS 71 Syracuse Univ; Sp-Lang Path, Enable UCP, **SLP**

Frumkin, Neva 605 Glenmoor #3-C, East Lansing, MI 48823, (517) 355-0120, BS 76 Univ of MO - Columbia; MA 77 Univ of MO - Columbia; 87–Research Assoc, MI St Univ, **SLP ACE**

Fruth, Janice K 128 Country Club Lane, Brockton, MA 02401, **SLP**

Fry, Mrs Antoinette Deascenti 15 Wild Rose Lane, Mechanicsburg, PA 17055, (717) 737-6728, BS 79 Indiana Univ of PA; MS 80 WV Univ; 83–Sp-Lang Path, Capital Area Iu, **SLP ACE**

Fry, Carolee 2837 Avenue R Northwest, Winter Haven, FL 33881, (813) 293-6370, BS 80 Eastern IL Univ; MS 81 Eastern IL Univ; 81–Sp-Lang Path, Polk Co Sch, **SLP ACE**

Fry, Debra S 2001 South Stoughton Road, Madison, WI 53704, (608) 271-3333, BS 78 Univ of WI - Stevens Point; MA 79 Central MI Univ; Aud, Nicolet Audiodiagnostics, **A**

Fry, Mrs Elizabeth 8120 South Holly Street, Littleton, CO 80122, BS 67 Nazareth Coll of Rochester; MS 72 Syracuse Univ; Sp-Lang Path, Private Practice, **SLP A**

Fryar, Laura Elizabeth 4603 Holston Hills Road, Knoxville, TN 37914, (615) 971-1349, BS 79 East TN St Univ; MA 85 Memphis St Univ; SLP, Patricia Neal Rehab Ctr, **SLP**

Fryauf-Bertschy, Holly 204 1/2 Park Road, Iowa City, IA 52240, (319) 354-6006, BA 83 Univ of AR - Little Rock; MA 85 Univ of IA; Aud, Univ of IA Hosp, **A**

Frydenberg, Helen R 70-25 Yellowstone Blvd, Apt 12R, Forest Hills, NY 11375, (718) 575-9059, BS 77 Boston Univ; MS 79 Rutgers St Univ -N Brunswick; 86–Sp-Lang Path, Private Practice, **SLP**

Frye, Devona D 2513 Jefferson Avenue, Point Pleasant, WV 25550, (304) 675-6821, BA 73 Marshall Univ; MA 75 Marshall Univ; Sp-Lang Path, Mason Co Bd Educ, **SLP**

Frye, Dorothy A 1716 1/2 Thompson Street, Lafayette, IN 47905, (317) 447-2459, ME 84 Trenton St Coll; SLP, **SLP**

Frye, Jeri Ann 3206A Shenandoah, St Louis, MO 63104, (314) 773-6205, **SLP**

Frye, Mrs Linda Jambor 963 North Saffron, Mesa, AZ 85205, (602) 396-8905, BS 77 Central MO St Univ; MS 80 Central MO St Univ; Sp-Lang Path, Gompers Rehab Ctr, **SLP**

Fryling, Lori Jean Castlewood Apartment #52, Russell, KY 41169, (502) 561-3349, **SLP**

Fryman, M Jeanne P O Box 761, Dulce, NM 87528, (505) 759-3297, **SLP**

Fu, Mrs Mary Claire 1115 Silverstone Road, Holland, MI 49424, (616) 399-2171, BS 70 Marquette Univ; MS 73 Marquette Univ; Sp-Lang Path, Private Practice, **SLP**

Fucci, Dr Donald J 6646 Frum Rd, Athens, OH 45701, (614) 593-1421, BA 62 Univ of Pittsburgh - Pittsburgh; MS 64 Univ of Pittsburgh - Pittsburgh; PH 68 (NS) Purdue Univ - West Lafayette; Prof, Ohio U, **F**

Fucci, Mrs Joan Y 6646 Frum Road, Athens, OH 45701, BA 62 Hiram Coll; MS 67 Univ of Pittsburgh - Pittsburgh; 86–Clinic Coord, OH U, **SLP**

Fuchs, Elizabeth A 162 McSweeney Avenue #16, Moncton, NB, Canada E1C 7E2, (506) 854-8445, BS 83 Northeastern Univ; MS 86 Northeastern Univ; **A**

Fuchs, Mrs Mary D'Amico 124 South 81st Street, Milwaukee, WI 53214, (414) 546-5625, BS 83 Univ of WI - Whitewater; MS 84 Marquette Univ; Sp-Lang Path, Sch Dist of West Allis, **SLP**

Fudala, Dr Janet B Brighton School District 27, 630 South 8th Avenue, Brighton, CO 80601, (303) 659-4820, BA 57 Univ of CA - Riverside; MA 59 Univ of CA - Riverside; PH 73 (NS) Univ of WA; 88–Exec Dir of Curr & Instr, Brighton Sch Dist 27J, **SLP A F**

Fudge, Jerri First National Tower, Suite 939, Las Cruces, NM 88001, (505) 526-2072, BS 77 Eastern NM Univ; MA 80 NM St Univ; Dir, Sp & Lang Path Serv, **SLP**

Fudge, Mrs Linda Marlene Swedish Medical Center, 501 East Hampden Avenue, Englewood, CO 80110-2796, (303) 470-0505, MS 81 Univ of South FL; Aud, **A**

Fudge, Suzanne V 530 Carriage Drive N W, Atlanta, GA 30328, (404) 255-0686, OB 68 Univ of TN - Knoxville; ME 74 Univ of GA; Sp-Lang Path, The New School, **SLP**

Fudickar, Mrs Jane Z 3000 West Deborah Drive, Monroe, LA 71201, (318) 387-4712, BS 77 LA St Univ - Baton Rouge; MS 79 Lamar Univ; Director Sp-Lang Path-Aud, St Francis Medical Center, **SLP**

Fudold, Karen Marie 6851 Guildford Street, Utica, MI 48087, (313) 739-7273, BS 86 Western MI Univ; MA 88 Western MI Univ

Fue, Laurie D 870 East Northlake #31-G, Murray, UT 84107, (801) 268-8818, BS 75 Univ of UT; MS 79 Univ of UT; Sp-Lang Path, Neurology Learn Beh Ctr, **SLP**

Fuehrer, Mrs Patricia McElhinny 562 Crosswinds Drive, Lititz, PA 17543, (717) 627-4226, BS 83 Indiana Univ of PA; MS 84 WV Univ; Sp-Lang Path, Lancaster General Hosp, **SLP**

Fuehrer-Mancl, Joyce Ann 311 Wadleight Street, Stevens Point, WI 54481, (715) 435-3340, BS 85 Univ of WI - Stevens Point; MS 87 Univ of WI - Stevens Point; 88–Sp-Lang Path, Wisconsin Rapids PS

Fuess, Cynthia Jane 21 Bradford Road, Watertown, MA 02172, (617) 926-7783, BS 82 SUNY - Coll at Geneseo; MA 84 SUNY - Coll at Geneseo; 88–Sp-Lang Path, Watertown PS, **SLP**

Fugate, Danna Lisa 916 Valley Brook Road, Decatur, GA 30033, (404) 763-0580, OM 84 Emory Univ; Sp-Lang Path, Fulton Co Sch Sys, **SLP**

Fugate, Mrs Mae Elizabeth 38710 Adkins Road, Willoughby, OH 44094, (216) 942-5603, BA 74 Queens Univ - Ontario; MA 76 Case Western Reserve Univ; Sp-Lang Path, **SLP**

Fugleberg, Ruth Ann 2051 Snowden, Long Beach, CA 90815, (805) 325-2448, BA 83 Univ of MT; MA 85 Univ of MT; Audiologist, Kern Cty ENT Med Clinic, **A**

Fujikawa, Dr Sharon E 10 Goldstone, Irvine, CA 92714, (714) 634-5426, BA 65 Univ of WA; MS 67 Univ of HI - Manoa; PH 76 (NS) Univ of WA; 86–Asst Prof, U of CA, **A**

Fujiki, Dr Martin Parsons Research Center, P O Box 738, Parsons, KS 67357, (316) 421-6550, BS 72 Univ of ID; MS 74 Univ of UT; PH 80 (NS) Univ of UT; Assoc Sci, Bureau of Child Res U of KS, **SLP**

Fujimoto, June Mitsunaga 989 Ashbridge Lane, Harbor City, CA 90710, (213) 530-7730, BA 76 Univ of CA - Los Angeles; SLP, LA USD, **SLP**

Fujioka, Carol A 13660 West Alaska Drive, Lakewood, CO 80228, (303) 422-2334, BS 69 CO St Univ; MS 77 CO St Univ; SLP, Jefferson Co Pub Sch, **SLP**

Fukuhara, Mrs Victoria Lai 202 Shorebird Circle, Redwood City, CA 94065, (415) 299-5617, BA 84 San Francisco St Univ; MS 86 San Francisco St Univ; 87–Sp-Lang Path, Santa Clara Valley Med Ctr, **SLP**

Fukumoto, Paulette Tamie 98-779 Kaamilo Street, Aiea, HI 96701, (808) 941-8536, BS 69 OH Univ - Athens; MS 70 CO St Univ; 86–Sp-Lang Path, Private Practice, **SLP**

Fularz-Sendker, Mrs Kathleen 11400 Fourth Street North, Apartment #1102, St Petersburg, FL 33716, (813) 442-1171, BS 83 SUNY - Coll at Geneseo; MS 86 SUNY - Coll at Buffalo; 88–Sp-Lang Path, Pinellas Co Sch Sys, **SLP**

Fulcher, Starr Reed 1021 Jeffery Drive, Tyler, TX 75703, (214) 597-0351, BS 70 East TX St Univ - Commerce; MA 73 Our Lady Lake Univ-San Anton; Dir, Vaughn Mem Sp & Hrng Cen, **SLP**

Fulcomer, Mrs Lauren Russell P O Box 1024, Patagonia, AZ 85624, (602) 394-2424, BS 80 Univ of AZ; MS 81 Univ of AZ; 87–Sp-Lang Path, Santa Cruz Co Spec Educ Coop, **SLP**

Fulford, Mrs Julie O 2322 Bacon Street Suite 1, Concord, CA 94520, (415) 676-8101, BA 63 Univ of IA; MA 67 De Paul Univ; Aud, Private Practice, **A**

Fulghum, Sandra Casner Naval Hosp, 8750 Mountain Boulevard, Oakland, CA 94627, (415) 633-5271, BA Sweet Briar Coll; MS Vanderbilt Univ; Aud, Naval Hosp, **A**

Fulk, Melissa Anne 807 Harrison Avenue, Greenville, OH 45331, (513) 548-2509, BS 77 Ball St Univ; MA 81 Ball St Univ; Sp/Lang Path, Greenville City Sch Dist, **SLP**

Full, Mariette Helene Star Route, Brighton, UT 84121, (801) 533-8282, BS 74 Univ of UT; MS 77 Univ of UT; Marketing Analyst, Ihc Hospitals, **SLP**

Fullagar, Ann Elise P O Box 286, Rome, NY 13440, (315) 338-3276, MS 80 Ithaca Coll; BS 76 SUNY - Coll at Geneseo; Sp-Lang Path, Rome Cty Sch, **SLP**

Fullam, Mrs Patricia Williams 1715 N Mark Twain Circle, Bethlehem, PA 18017, (215) 866-8092, BA 66 SUNY - Coll at Fredonia; BS 84 East Stroudsburg Univ of PA; MS 87 Rutgers St Univ -N Brunswick

Fuller, Mrs Candice T 313 W 99th St, Kansas City, MO 64114, (816) 941-4741, MA 71 Univ of KS; Sp-Lang Path, St Joseph Hlth Ctr, **SLP**

Fuller, Dr Carl W 919 East 81st Street, Indianapolis, IN 46240, (317) 255-2702, BA 40 Univ of the Pacific; MA 47 Univ of the Pacific; PH 59 (Aud) Northwestern Univ; Retired, **SLP A F LM**

Fuller, Mrs Charlotte 22 Norwood Circle, Route 5, Sherman, TX 75090, (214) 892-9630, OB 68 TX Christian Univ; OM 69 TX Christian Univ; MS 75 TX Christian Univ; 79–Sp-Lang Path, Sherman ISD, **SLP**

Fuller, Mrs Cynthia E 4549 Hunting Hound Lane, Marietta, GA 30062, (404) 956-0474, BS 77 SUNY - Center at Albany; MS 80 Emory Univ; Rehav Coord, N Fulton Med Cen, **SLP A**

Fuller, Dr Dennis P TWJ Rehab Wash Univ Med Sch, 509 South Euclid, Box 8062, St Louis, MO 63110, (314) 362-2355, BS 69 Northeast MO St Univ; MA 74 Saint Louis Univ; PH 82 (NS) Saint Louis Univ; Dir SLP, Washington U Med Sch, **SLP**

Fuller, Diane Michelle 6248 Oram #13, Dallas, TX 75214, (214) 271-0516, BS 79 TX Christian Univ; MS 80 TX Christian Univ; SLP, Otolaryngology Consultants, **SLP**

Fuller, Dr Donald Ray 3060 Pheasant Run Drive, Apartment 1020, Lafayette, IN 47905, (317) 474-6053, OB 82 AR St Univ; OM 83 AR St Univ; Teaching Assistant, Purdue University

Fuller, Mrs Jan H 178 Montvale Avenue, Woburn, MA 01801, (508) 851-0412, BA 76 Univ of VT; MS 77 Univ of VT; Sp-Lang Path, Tewksbury Public Schools, **SLP**

Fuller, Janice S 5260 Williston Road, Minnetonka, MN 55345-4732, MA 79 Univ of MN - Minneap-St Paul; 82–Sp-Lang Path, Hopkins Dist 270, **SLP**

Fuller, Jennifer Kaye 4123 Harrison Avenue, Columbus, GA 31904, (404) 324-5661, BS 79 Univ of Montevallo; ME 83 Columbus Coll; Sp-Lang Path, Muscogee Co Sch Dist, **SLP**

Fuller, Karlene C 6434 West 85th Avenue, Arvada, CO 80003, BA 68 CO St Univ; MA 71 Univ of Northern CO; 85–Sp-Lang Path, VA Med Ctr, **SLP**

Fuller, Linda Kay 7086 Winter Rose Path, Columbia, MD 21045, (301) 298-4179, BA 84 SUNY - Coll at New Paltz; MA 85 George Washington Univ; **A**

Fuller, Paula T 229 Moore Street, Santa Cruz, CA 95060, (408) 429-3900, BA 79 Univ of Santa Clara; MA 82 Univ of MD - College Park; Sp/Lang Path, Santa Cruz Cty Sch, **SLP**

Fuller, Mrs Susan H 3869 Timucua Trail, Jacksonville, FL 32211, (904) 725-5122, BA 70 FL St Univ; MS 71 FL St Univ; SLP, Duval Co Pub Sch, **SLP**

Fuller, Susan T The Asia Foundation, P O Box 3223, San Francisco, CA 94119, (503) 281-4323, BS 80 FL St Univ; MS 82 FL St Univ; **SLP**

Fulling, Thomas M 5 Roland Street, Waterville, ME 04901, (207) 873-0621, BA 69 Catholic Univ of America; MA 73 Catholic Univ of America; SLP, Sad #47 of Oakland Maine, **SLP**

Fullmer, Mrs Sue A D 1812 Crestlyn Road, York, PA 17403, (717) 846-3310, BA 74 Elmira Coll; MA 75 Univ of Denver; Sp-Lang Path, York Hospital, **SLP**

Fullowka McCabe, Mrs Debora Lee 28 Duff Crescent, Chatham, ON, Canada N7L 4X8, (519) 354-5178, BA 81 Univ of ND; MA 83 Univ of KS; 85–Head Sp-Lang Path, Kent Co Roman Catholic Sch Bd, **SLP**

Fullwood, Mrs Joan Horner Route 1, Michie, TN 38357, BS 79 Saint Mary's Dominican Coll; MA 81 Memphis St Univ; SLP, Hardin Co Board of Education, **SLP**

Fulmer, Charles Virgil, Jr Ballard Speech & Hrng Center, 5420-B Barnes N W, Seattle, WA 98107, (203) 525-9002, BA 72 Central WA Univ; MA 80 Western WA Univ; Dir Aud, Ballard Sp/Hrng Cen, **A**

Fulmer, Mrs Janet Elise 6424 Central City Blvd, Apartment 625, Galveston, TX 77551, (409) 761-2711, BS 83 Baylor Univ; MS 85 Univ of TX - Dallas; **A**

Fulmer, Kathy C 254 Wakefield, Memphis, TN 38117, (901) 525-2682, MA 77 Memphis St Univ; 87–Editorial Asst LSHSS, ASHA, **SLP**

Fulp, Angela Morgan 1012 Worth Street, Richmond, VA 23225, (804) 231-2979, BS 83 Longwood Coll; MS 86 James Madison Univ; **SLP**

Fulton, Dr Calvin W 8622 East 25th Place, Tucson, AZ 85710, (313) 487-4413, BA 50 Grinnell Coll; MA 51 Case Western Reserve Univ; PH 61 (Lang Path) Case Western Reserve Univ; 56–Prof Spec Ed Emeritus, En MI U, **SLP A**

Fulton, Mrs Helen L P O Box 632, 1100 Seaeagle Loop, Bodega Bay, CA 94923, (707) 875-2358, BS 42 Univ of MI - Ann Arbor; MS 58 Univ of KS; Aud/SLP, Private Practice, **SLP A LM**

Fulton, Pamela Ann Mager 110 Bartram Lane, Ocean City, NJ 08226, (609) 399-7657, BS 79 West Chester Univ of PA; OM 81 Hahnemann Medical Coll; Sp-Lang Path, Greater Egg Harbor Reg Hs Dist, **SLP**

Fulton, Mrs Patricia H 1307 Kinney Avenue #150, Austin, TX 78704, (512) 441-0353, BA 48 Univ of IA; MA 72 Western IL Univ; Sp-Lang Path, Private Practice, **SLP**

Fulton, Richard M P O Box 561, Sutherlin, OR 97479, (503) 459-9421, BS 60 Western MI Univ; MA 64 MI St Univ; Sp-Lang Path, Douglas Co Ed Serv Dist, **SLP**

Fulton, Mrs Susan Ellison 1100 46th Avenue North, St Petersburg, FL 33703, (813) 892-4141, MS 87 Univ of South FL; 87–Aud, All Children's Hosp, **A**

Fulton, Mrs Terri Browning Rd 3 Box 394L-3, Lake Ariel, PA 18436, (717) 296-9261, BS 82 Marywood Coll; MS 83 Rutgers St Univ -N Brunswick; Director/Sp-Lang Path, Head Injury Recov Cen Hillcrst, **SLP**

Fulton, Timothy P 3308 4th Street, Kenosha, WI 53142, (414) 654-5564, BS 68 CO St Univ; MA 71 Northeast MO St Univ; SLP, Kenosha USD #1, **SLP**

Fung, Debra McDevitt 132 Spruce Avenue, Menlo Park, CA 94025, (415) 325-1756, BA 82 Univ of CA - Santa Barbara; MS 85 San Francisco St Univ; 85–Sp-Lang Path, Santa Clara USD, **SLP**

Fung, Mrs Thelma N 7571 South Race Street, Littleton, CO 80122, (303) 797-1086, BA 66 Univ of the Pacific; MA 68 Univ of the Pacific; Sp-Lang Path, Private Practice, **SLP**

Funk, Carol Lee 16829 Toronto Avenue S E, Apartment 302, Prior Lake, MN 55372, (715) 627-4814

Funk, Dr Harry E Jefferson Co Public Schools, Durrett Education Center, 4409 Prestor Highway, Louisville, KY 40213, BS 64 CA Univ of PA; MA 65 G Peabody Coll-Vanderbilt U; PH 72 (NS) Univ of KS; Prog Speech Hearing Impaired, Jefferson Co Bd of Education, **SLP**

Funk, Janis E 3852 170th Avenue S E, Bellevue, WA 98008, (206) 281-6943, BA 72 CA St Univ - Los Angeles; MA 72 CA St Univ - Los Angeles; Sp-Lang Path, Seattle Pub Sch, **SLP**

Funk, Lisa Kay 6965 Lake Forest Village, Fort Wayne, IN 46815, (219) 493-1031, BA 85 IN Univ - Bloomington; OM 87 IN Univ - Bloomington; 88–Sp-Lang Path, Parkview Memorial Hosp, **SLP**

Funke, Mrs Beth Weisberger Village 2 Tahoe 4, New Hope, PA 18938, (609) 586-1676, BA 59 CUNY - Brooklyn Coll; MA 62 CUNY - Brooklyn Coll; Sp-Lang Path, Mercer Co Spec Serv, **SLP**

Funkhouser, Kristen Dee 3909 Monroe Avenue, Apt #209, San Diego, CA 92116, (619) 576-5836, BA 84 Geneva Coll; MA 85 OH Univ - Athens; Aud, Childrens Hos/Health Ctr, **A**

Fuoco, Vito Nicholas 1150 Berkshire Blvd, Wyomissing, PA 19610, (215) 376-8400, BS 70 West TX St Univ; MA 74 Western MI Univ; Aud, Berks Hearing & Speech Ctr, **A**

Fuoco-McCooley, Barbara 305 South Fairview Street, Riverside, NJ 08075, (609) 461-7498, BS 75 Trenton St Coll; MA 80 Trenton St Coll; Sp-Lang Path Dir, Private Practice, **SLP**

Fuoto, Ellen M 2117 Limewood Drive, Baton Rouge, LA 70816, (504) 923-3420, BA 68 SUNY - Center at Buffalo; MS 71 Tulane Univ; Sp-Lang Path, Cerebral Palsy Center, **SLP**

Fuqua, Stacy G Rt #2 Box 3168, Perry, MO 63462, (314) 565-3105, BS 77 Univ of MO - Columbia; MA 78 Univ of MO - Columbia; Sp-Lang Path, Private Practice, **SLP**

Furbacher, Ellen A 540 Center Street, Walnut Creek, CA 94595, (415) 939-5951, BA 71 Valparaiso Univ; MA 77 San Francisco St Univ; **SLP**

Furby, Robert Leon 4 Wilana Court #7-B, Pikeville, KY 41501, (606) 437-7703, BS 81 Univ of South AL; MS 83 Univ of South AL; Audiologist, Scioto Memorial Hospital, **A**

Furest, Mrs Eileen Kerrigan 22510 Masonic, St Clair Shores, MI 48082, (313) 749-3401, BA 77 MI St Univ; MA 78 MI St Univ; Sp-Lang Path, New Haven Community Schools, **SLP ACE**

Furgason, Kristine Kaiser 1203 La Mesa Avenue, Winter Springs, FL 32708, (407) 699-8909, BA 74 MI St Univ; MA 75 MI St Univ; 88–Sp/Lang Path, Rebound Head Inj Unit/FL Hosp, **SLP**

Furick, Mrs Paula K 950 S W 11th Terrace, Boca Raton, FL 33486, (407) 392-3454, BA 68 Univ of Southern CA; ME 70 Boston Univ; **SLP**

Furio, Ellen D 140 Robert Jemison Drive, #206, Birmingham, AL 35209, (205) 934-5448, BA 85 Birmingham-Southern Coll; MS 88 Univ of AL- Tuscaloosa

Furland, Delores J Pittsford Mills Apartment #2, RR #2 Box 2082, Pittsford, VT 05763, (802) 483-2434, BS 55 Central MI Univ; MA 72 Central MI Univ; Sp-Lang Path, Rutland Central Supervisory Union, **SLP**

Furlano, Deborah Seubert 320 Klein Creek Court, Unit F, Carol Stream, IL 60188, (312) 510-0782, BA 84 Univ of WI - Eau Claire; MS 85 Univ of WI - Eau Claire; Sp-Lang Path, Indian Prarie Comm Uit Sch Dis, **SLP**

Furlette, Deborah Sell P O Box 3411, Ann Arbor, MI 48106-3411, **SLP**

Furlong, Sheila N 1 Harlequin Drive, Smithtown, NY 11787, (516) 883-4000, BA 66 Univ of CT; MA 68 Univ of CT; Sp-Lang Path, Port Washington School Dist, **SLP**

Furlough, Cynthia L P O Box 341, Garner, NC 27529, (919) 782-4184, BS 84 Appalachian St Univ; MA 87 Appalachian St Univ; 87–Sp-Lang Path, Associated Healthfocus Inc, **SLP**

Furman, Mrs Gayle F 101 Nanci Karen Drive, Warwick, RI 02886, (401) 738-5358, BA 79 Univ of RI; MS 81 Univ of RI; 82–Sp-Lang Path, Cranston Pub Sch Dept, **SLP**

Furman, Paul B P O Box 480849, Los Angeles, CA 90048, BA 75 CA St Univ - Northridge; MA 78 CA St Univ - Northridge; Aud, Cigna Hlthplns of Ca, **A**

Furman, Mrs Ruth B 7573 Malvern Avenue, Philadelphia, PA 19151, (215) 473-3371, BS 74 Univ of MD - College Park; MA 76 Univ of MD - College Park; 88–Sp-Lang Path, Sch Dist of Phila, **SLP**

Furman, Mrs Temma 140 Aspinet Drive, Warwick, RI 02888, (401) 737-3300, BA 52 Emerson Coll; SLP, Warwick Sch Dept, **SLP**

Furness, Nancy Anne 1206 Dominion Street, Winnipeg, MB, Canada R3E 2P7, (204) 837-1301, MA 85 Univ of MN - Minneap-St Paul; 85–Sp-Lang Path, Deer Lodge Centre, **SLP**

Furnish-Kollman, Mrs Jean 150 Rivoli, San Francisco, CA 94117, (415) 696-4300, BS 66 Univ of IA; MA 68 Univ of AZ; Sp-Lang Path, Mills Peninsula Hosp, **SLP**

Furst, Mrs Alice Coopersmith 1311 Brewster Court, El Cerrito, CA 94530, (415) 235-8199, BS 53 Tufts Univ; ME 55 Boston Univ; Cnsltnt-Program Design & Eval, Private Practice, **SLP**

Furst, Mrs Dorothy J 8477 Cedarview Drive, Cypress, CA 90630, (714) 760-3222, BA 57 Univ of Denver; MA 65 Univ of Denver; SLP, Newport-Mesa USD, **SLP**

Furst, Mrs Rachel Tova 17 Fort George Hill #3C, New York, NY 10040, (212) 567-0938, BA 84 CUNY - Hunter Coll; MA 85 CUNY - Lehman Coll; **SLP**

Furstenberg, Joan F Medical Center ENT Associates, 6410 Fannin, Suite 1400, Houston, TX 77030, (713) 795-0111, BA 77 Univ of TX - Austin; MA 82 Univ of TX - Austin; Aud, Med Cen ENT Assoc, **A ACE**

Furtado, Stephen J 10 Buist Avenue, Sconticut Neck Road, Fairhaven, MA 02719, (617) 999-5781, BA 68 Univ of MA - Amherst; MS 70 Univ of VT; Sp-Lang Path, Private Practice, **SLP**

Furuheim, Mrs Frances W 859 West Brokaw Road, Camano Island, WA 98292, (206) 387-5485, BA 60 Western WA Univ; **SLP LM**

Furuta, Jennifer Satomi 9652 42nd Avenue N E, Seattle, WA 98115, (206) 524-1565, BS 83 Univ of HI - Manoa; 88–Sp-Lang Path, VA Med Ctr, **SLP**

Furuya, Yoshio J 50 Bellefontaine #308, Pasadena, CA 91105, (818) 795-0679, BA 72 CA St Univ - Los Angeles; MA 74 CA St Univ - Los Angeles; Aud, Pasadena Aud Lab, **A**

Fusco, Mary Lou 219 Davisson Street, Bridgeport, WV 26330, (304) 842-2065, BS 83 WV Univ; MS 84 WV Univ; Sp-Lang Path, Taylor Co Bd of Ed, **SLP**

Fushikoshi, Kellie Ann 45-332 Paewalani Place, Kaneohe, HI 96744, (808) 247-1052, BS 85 Univ of HI - Manoa; MS 87 Univ of HI - Manoa

Fusilier, Betty B 35 Greenbriar Lane, Conway, AR 72032, (501) 450-3176, BA 66 Northwestern St Univ; MA 67 Northwestern St Univ; Instr of SLP, University of Central Arkansas, **SLP**

Fusilier, Freida M 3561 N Street, Sacramento, CA 95816, **SLP**

Fuso-de-Sevilla, Mrs Silvia 14138 Grand Pre Road #42, Silver Spring, MD 20906, (301) 279-4955, MS 85 Univ of WI - Milwaukee; 85–Sp-Lang Path, Montgomery County PS, **SLP**

Fust, Rita Jean Asp Service, 126 JB Veterans Adm Med, St Louis, MO 63125, (314) 894-6675, MA 67 Univ of KS; 67–Sp-Lang Path, VA Med Ctr, **SLP**

Fyfe, Dorothy Grace 319 Franklin Street, Keokuk, IA 52632, (319) 524-7150, BA 51 Wheaton Coll; MA 81 Univ of IA; Aud, Keokuk Hosp, **A**

Fylling, Colleen E 1700 S W 5th Avenue, Minot, ND 58701, **SLP**

G

Gaarder, Marie S 4221 Oakridge Lane, Chevy Chase, MD 20815, (301) 656-0379, BS 57 Univ of IL - Urbana; SLP, Private Practice, **SLP**

Gaasch, Isabel F 2180 Panorama Drive, Arcata, CA 95521, **SLP**

Gabay, Mrs Galina V 512 Main Street, Acton, MA 01720-3933, (617) 862-2219, BA 61 Moscow Pedagogical Inst-Ussr; ME 63 Moscow Pedagogical Inst-Ussr; 83–Sp/Lang Path, Labb, **SLP**

Gabbard, Sandra Abbott Univ Of Co Health Sciences Ctr, 4200 East 9th Avenue, Box B210, Denver, CO 80262, (303) 394-7856, BS 80 Purdue Univ - West Lafayette; MA 81 Univ of Northern CO; Cl Instr, U of CO Hlth Sci Cen, **A**

Gabe, Mrs Deborah Cogan 38874 Country Circle, Farmington Hills, MI 48018, (313) 421-3300, BS 79 MI St Univ; MS 81 Univ of MI - Ann Arbor; Sp/Lang Path, Garden City Hosp, **SLP**

Gabe, Dr Kathleen M 5185 Merritt Road, Ypsilanti, MI 48197, (313) 494-1671, BS 64 Northern IL Univ - De Kalb; MA 65 Smith Coll; PH 73 (NS) Wayne St Univ - Sch of Med; Superv/Special Education, Detroit Board of Education, **A**

Gabel, Michele 317 Martling Avenue, Tarrytown, NY 10591, (914) 963-4567, BA 72 CUNY - Lehman Coll; MA 76 CUNY - Lehman Coll; 86–Sp/Lang Path, Leake-Watts Children's Home, **SLP**

Gabioud, Barbara Harris 1708 Wildwood Lane S W, Albuquerque, NM 87105, (505) 873-3131, BA 73 Univ of MN - Duluth; BS 76 Univ of MN - Duluth; MA 78 NM St Univ; Sp-Lang Path, Albuquerque Pub Sch, **SLP**

Gabler, Mary Jean 4517 Yale Street #D, Metairie, LA 70006, (504) 341-2051, BA 72 Barat Coll; MS 83 Univ of Southwestern LA; Sp-Lang Path, Jefferson Parish Sch Sys, **SLP**

Gabria, Ronald C 2580 Filaree Court, Rocklin, CA 95677, (916) 366-2551, BA 69 Univ of Dayton; OM 83 CA St Univ - Sacramento; MA 73 Univ of IA; Sp-Lang Path, Sacramento Co Office of Ed, **SLP**

Gabriel, Catherine 23-15 Van Delft Drive, South Amboy, NJ 08879, (201) 548-7610, MS 86 Columbia Univ Teachers Coll; Sp-Lang Path, John F Kennedy Medical Ctr, **SLP**

Gabriel, Mrs Chrystal A 506 White Oak Drive, Jasper, GA 30143, (404) 692-5567, BS 73 Univ of GA; ME 74 Univ of GA; Sp-Lang Path, Pickens Co Bd of Ed, **SLP**

Gabriel, Mrs Eileen K 172 West Jefferson, Burlington, WI 53105, (414) 763-7621, BS 74 Marquette Univ; MS 75 Univ of WI - Milwaukee; Sp-Lang Path, Racine Co Sch Off, **SLP**

Gabriel, Mrs Roxanne Marie 4824 West Folley Street, Chandler, AZ 85226, BA 77; MA 80 Ball St Univ; **SLP ACE**

Gabrielse, Patricia Handley St Peter Hospital, 413 North Lilly Road, Olympia, WA 98506, (206) 456-7312, BA 73 Marygove Coll; MS 74 Purdue Univ - West Lafayette; Dir Outpt Rehab Ctr, St Peter Hospital, **SLP**

Gabryel, Mrs Nini W 545 Oaks Lane, Apartment 501, Pompano Beach, FL 33069, (305) 481-5600, BA 75 Univ of FL; ME 77 Univ of FL; SLP, Deerfield Bch High Sch, **SLP**

Gachupin, Rosalind P O Box 117, San Ysidro, NM 87053, BS 73 NM St Univ; Sp-Lang Path, Bureau of Indian Affairs, **SLP**

Gadbury, Mrs Kathryn Miller 1006 Birnam Woods Trail, Indianapolis, IN 46280, (317) 257-9672, BS 79 Ball St Univ; MA 79 Ball St Univ; Sp/Lang Path, Eagle-Union Comm Sch Corp, **SLP**

Gadler, Judi B T 8402 Burwood Park Drive, Spring, TX 77379, (713) 442-1546, BA 77 Univ of TX - El Paso; MA 78 Univ of TX - El Paso; Sp-Lang Path, Aldine Ps, **SLP**

Gadsden-Lopez, Wanda Lenore P O Box 3378, New Haven, CT 06515, (203) 865-8269, MS 87 Southern CT St Univ

Gadson, Pamela Jean 7712 Loudon Drive, Fort Washington, MD 20744, (301) 350-5555, BA 81 Hampton Univ; MS 83 Univ of IL - Urbana; SLP, InSpeech Inc, **SLP ACE**

Gaeddert, Mrs Connie L 1628 Apple Lane, Ottawa, KS 66067, (913) 242-3818, OB 82 Univ of KS; MA 85 Univ of KS; 85–Sp-Lang Path, USD #290, **SLP**

Gaeth, Janice Schaefer 55 North Bompart #G-3-L, Webster Groves, MO 63119, (314) 968-4826, BS 83 Marquette Univ; MS 86 Univ of WI - Madison; **A**

Gaetto, Anita M 15 West 153 Harrison, Elmhurst, IL 60126, (312) 447-9348, BA 83 Elmhurst Coll; MA 85 Univ of IL - Urbana; SLP, Lyons School District 103, **SLP**

Gaffigan, Mrs Hannah Clarke 13127 Musicmaster Drive, Silver Spring, MD 20904, (301) 890-3457, BS 85 Univ of IL - Urbana; MA 87 Univ of IA; 87–Sp-Lang Path, Montgomery Co PS, **SLP**

Gaffney, Ellen P Rd 1 Box 59 Elliot Road, East Greenbush, NY 12061, (518) 489-8336, **SLP**

Gaffney, Lorrie Jeanne 4004 East O'Brien Road, Oak Creek, WI 53154, (414) 762-2087, BA 84 Univ of CO - Boulder; MS 86 Marquette Univ; **SLP**

Gaffney, Mary Susan 24 Old Marlborough Road, East Hampton, CT 06424, (203) 522-0184, BA 81 SUNY - Coll at Potsdam; MA 83 SUNY - Center at Buffalo; SLP, Hartford Bd of Ed, **SLP**

Gaffney, Theresa 5484 Langsworth Drive, St Louis, MO 63129, (314) 894-7789, MA 87 Saint Louis Univ

Gafford, Mrs Susan M 1081 West 2nd Avenue, Columbus, OH 43212, (614) 461-2420, BS 79 Bowling Green St Univ; MA 80 Bowling Green St Univ; Sp/Lang Path, Southwestern City Schs, **SLP**

Gage, Mrs Ann W 455 Old Spanish Trail, Portola Valley, CA 94025, (415) 851-1924, BA 67 Stanford Univ; MA 68 Stanford Univ; **SLP**

Gage, Denise Annette 4300 MacArthur Suite 107, Dallas, TX 75209, (214) 520-2055, BS 80 Bradley Univ; MA 83 Univ of TX - Austin; 86–Sp-Lang Path, Private Practice, **SLP ACE**

Gage, Elizabeth E 228 Pleasant Street, Yellow Springs, OH 45387, (513) 335-5624, BA 64 Millikin Univ; MA 69 Univ of IL - Urbana; MS 73 Univ of IL - Urbana; Dir of SLP, Dettner Hosp, **SLP**

Gage, Mrs La Vada W Herring 2300 North 51st Street, Waco, TX 76710, (817) 772-0742, BS 51 East TX St Univ - Commerce; ME 54 East TX St Univ - Commerce; **SLP LM**

Gage, Mrs Nancy Arden 49 Roger Williams Avenue, Rumford, RI 02916-2811, (401) 438-2730, BA 79 Univ of RI; MS 80 PA St Univ - Univ Park; 85–Sp-Lang Path, East Providence Sch Dept, **SLP**

Gage, Rhea Jacobson 2712 Ashe Street, Durham, NC 27703, (904) 371-6095, BA 80 Univ of Denver; MA 85 Univ of FL; **A**

Gagen, Venisse Theresa 26 Oakcrest Place, Nutley, NJ 07110, (201) 661-2466, BS 76 Trenton St Coll; MA 83 Montclair St Coll; 83–Sp-Lang Path, Hackensack Bd of Educ, **SLP**

Gager, David Wayne R R 1 Box 267, Bennington, VT 05201, (802) 442-6133, MS 86 Univ of VT; Aud, SW VT Supervisory Union, **A**

Gager, Patricia Nimeskern 10417 Rutland Place, Adelphi, MD 20783, (202) 526-7676, BA 75 Univ of MA - Amherst; MA 77 Catholic Univ of America; Sp/Lang Path, St Gertrude's Sch, **SLP**

Gagliardi, Mrs Beverly A 324 Steele Road, Slidell, LA 70461, BS 76 SUNY - Coll at Geneseo; MS 79 SUNY - Coll at Fredonia; Aud, Dr Robert Owens ENT, **A**

Gagliardi, David M Faulkner Hospital, 1153 Centre Street, Boston, MA 02130-2913, (617) 522-5800, BA 79 Salem St Coll; MS 82 Boston Univ; Aud, Faulkner Hospital, **A**

Gagliardo, Mrs Jill Levy 72 Star Route, Woodridge, NY 12789, (914) 434-5403, **SLP**

Gagliotti, Mrs Michelle Eileen 288 Allegheny Street, Meadville, PA 16335, (814) 333-4529, BS 81 Clarion Univ of PA; MA 83 Memphis St Univ; Director of Speech & Heariang, State of Tennessee, **A**

Gagne, Adele Y 153 Centre Street, Milton, MA 02186, (617) 935-5050, **SLP**

Gagne, Dr Jean-Pierre Department Of Communicative Disorders, Elborn College, University Of Western Ontario, London, ON, Canada N6G 1H1, (514) 661-2001, BA 76 Laurentian Univ - Ontario; MS 78 McGill Univ - Quebec; PH 83 (Aud) Washington Univ; 86–Assistant Professor, University of Western Ontario, **A**

Gagnon, Donna Marie 90 Burton Street Apt 4, Watertown, CT 06795, BA 78 Coll of the Holy Cross; MA 82 Saint Joseph's Coll; 80–Sp-Lang Path, Watertown Board of Education, **SLP**

Gagnon, Mrs Rachel F 66 Beach Street, Westerly, RI 02891, (401) 596-6871, BA 83 Univ of RI; MS 87 Univ of RI; **SLP**

Gahagan, Teresa Marie 11604 Cody, Overland Park, KS 66210, (913) 682-3721, BS 80 KS St Univ; MA 82 Univ of KS; 88–Dir-Speech & Hearing Dept, St John Hosp, **SLP**

Gahn, James N Professional Hearing Services, 229 All Angels Hill Road, Wappingers Falls, NY 12590, (914) 473-4777, OB 66 Baldwin-Wallace Coll; MA 75 Kent St Univ; Owner-Admin, Prof Hrng Serv, **A**

Gahre, Teri Lea 411 North Lakeview, Anaheim, CA 92807, (714) 978-4698, BA 80 CA St Univ - Fullerton; MS 83 Univ of LA Verne; Sp-Lang Path, Kaiser Permanente Hospital, **SLP**

Gailey, Clark E 2737 E 8th Street #33, Odessa, TX 79761-4342, (915) 334-6097, BS 83 UT St Univ; MS 87 UT St Univ; **A**

Gailey, Dr Platon G PO Box 12036, 11815 Rock Landing Drive, Newport News, VA 23612-2036, (804) 873-1570, BS 41 Univ of VA - Charlottesville; ME 67 Univ of VA - Charlottesville; PH 75 (Brain Wave Potentials) Case Western Reserve Univ; 76–Exec Dir, Private Practice, **SLP**

Gailey, Terri S 915 East 200 South, Lewiston, UT 84320, (801) 258-5062, BS 80 UT St Univ; MS 82 UT St Univ; **SLP**

Gailliot, Mary L 5734 West Woodland Road, Pittsburgh, PA 15232, (412) 521-2570, BA 64 Carlow Coll; **SLP**

Gaines, Dr Barbara Hartley Alberta Children's Hospital, Speech-Language Pathology Department, 1820 Richmond Road SW, Calgary, AB, Canada T2T 5R7, (403) 229-7060, BA 78 Vassar Coll; MA 81 Univ of CA - Santa Barbara; PH 88 (Lang Behavior) Boston Univ; 86–Sp-Lang Path-Researcher, Alberta Childrens Hosp, **SLP**

Gaines, Mrs Barbara Wayne 50 Beechwood Road, Hartsdale, NY 10530, (914) 967-6100, BA 72 George Washington Univ; MA 73 George Washington Univ; Sp-Lang Path, Rye City Schs, **SLP**

Gaines, Donna S Childrens Speech & Lang Serv, Barcroft Medical Bldg, 939 South Wakefield #101, Arlington, VA 22204, (703) 685-1070, BS 74 Univ of WI - Madison; MA 75 Univ of IL - Urbana; Director, Childrens Sp-Lang Services, **SLP**

Gaines, Donnamarie Basta 2112 Brookhaven Court, Fallston, MD 21047, (301) 285-1914, BA 71 Towson St Univ; MS 76 Towson St Univ; SLP, Baltimore County Board of Educ, **SLP**

Gaines, Ellen Lynn 107 Maplewood Avenue, West Hartford, CT 06119, (203) 635-5523, BA 81 Univ of RI; MA 83 Univ of MD - College Park; Sp-Lang Path, Cromwell Pub Shls

Gaines, Mrs Lynn Susan 14 Cambridge Road, Bedminster, NJ 07921, (201) 267-2642, SLP, Eclc, **SLP**

Gaines, Marilyn D 530 North Shelby, Moweaqua, IL 62550, (217) 424-3035, BS 59 IL St Univ - Normal; MS 62 Millikin Univ; Spec Ed Superv, Macon-Piatt Spec Ed Dist, **SLP**

Gaines, Mrs Merle B Route 3 Box 311, Pittsboro, NC 27312, (919) 776-2722, BA 72 Univ of NC - Greensboro; ME 75 Univ of NC - Greensboro; 87–Sp-Lang Path, Lee County Schs, **SLP**

Gaines, Patricia J Route 2 Box 107-C, Swansboro, NC 28584, (919) 326-4120, BA 74 Univ of NC - Greensboro; MA 78 Univ of NC - Greensboro; Sp/Lang Path, Camp Lejeune Dependent's Sch, **SLP**

Gaines, Mrs Sharon L 1964 Ryons Street, Lincoln, NE 68502, (402) 475-2700, BS 59 Univ of NE - Lincoln; MA 60 Univ of NE - Lincoln; Sp/Lang Path, Lincoln Pub Schs, **SLP**

Gaiser, Mrs Gail H 7 Parkland Avenue, Larchmont, NY 10538, (914) 235-1267, MA 88 CUNY - Lehman Coll

Gaither, Mrs Leslie L 10 Swanson Road, Framingham, MA 01701, (508) 788-0197, BA 78 Our Lady Lake Univ-San Anton; MA 80 Our Lady Lake Univ-San Anton; **SLP**

Gaitros, Mrs Sonita Sue 119 Fidelity St #H4, Village Square, Carrboro, NC 27510, (919) 968-0747, BS 84 Univ of IL - Urbana; MS 85 Univ of IL - Urbana; Sp-Lang Path, Durham Co Schs, **SLP**

Gajewski, Mrs Mary C 49 Mapledale Acres, Barneveld, NY 13304, (315) 736-3301, BS 76 Coll of Saint Rose; MS 78 Coll of Saint Rose; **SLP**

Galambush, Nancy Caswell Center, 2415 West Vernon Avenue, Kinston, NC 28501, (919) 559-5371, BA 74 Elmhurst Coll; MA 76 Case Western Reserve Univ; Dir-Aud Svcs, Caswell Center, **A**

Galant, Kimberly Rae 209 West Lemon Street, Tarpon Springs, FL 34689, (813) 938-3531, MS 82 Univ of South FL; Sp-Lang Path, Private Practice, **SLP**

Galant, Mrs Michelle N 3855 Shamrock Court, San Francisco, CA 94080, (415) 750-5557, BA 60 San Francisco St Univ; MA 64 San Francisco St Univ; SLP, St Mary's Hosp/Sp & Lrng Cen, **SLP**

Galante-Plucenik, Mrs Michelle E R R 2 Box 478, Dayville, CT 06241, (203) 456-4091, **SLP**

Galasso, Laura Ann 12-17 Ravens Crest Drive, Plainsboro, NJ 08536, (718) 390-1480, BA 80 William Paterson Coll; MS 84 William Paterson Coll; 86–Aud, St Vincent's Med Ctr Richmond, **A**

Galbraith, Amy A 4 Prospect Street, Canonsburg, PA 15317-2001, (412) 223-3290, **SLP**

Galbraith, Marla J 2315 Sage Circle, Olathe, KS 66061, **SLP**

Galbreath, Mrs Debbie Dodge 1214 Tabor Avenue, Kettering, OH 45420, (513) 256-8416, BS 84 WV Univ; MS 87 WV Univ; **SLP**

Galbreath, Mrs Jan Kathryn 97th General Hospital, Box 60, APO New York, NY 09757, BS 80 OR Coll of Education; MS 83 Baylor Univ

Galbreath, Kristen Marie Box 1401, Fairview, AB, Canada T0H 1L0, (403) 835-4951, BS 76 ND St Univ; MS 79 Minot St Univ; 79–Supvr Sp-Lang Path, Peace River Health Unit #21, **SLP**

Galbreath, Marilynn Evelyn 804 Northeast 17th #1, Oklahoma City, OK 73105, (405) 528-3127, MS 88 Univ of OK Medical Center

Galchick, Mrs Janis Milligan 915 Exmoor Avenue, Louisville, KY 40223, (502) 245-1890, BS 78 Bowling Green St Univ; ME 82 GA St Univ; Sp-Lang Path, Private Practice, **SLP**

Galdes, Mrs Karen Lee Otter Trail #3, Muscoda, WI 53573, (608) 739-3034, BS 79 Western MI Univ; MA 80 Western MI Univ; Sp-Lang Path, Riverdale Pub Sch, **SLP**

Gale, Carrie G 1 Old Wolomolopoag Street, Sharon, MA 02067, (617) 784-9231, BS 73 Cornell Univ; ME 77 Northeastern Univ; Sp-Lang Path, Spoke, **SLP**

Gale, Christine Annette 1911 Kalanianaole #303, Hilo, HI 96720, (808) 961-7403, BA 81 Central MI Univ; MA 83 Central MI Univ; Sp-Lang Path, Hawaii Department of Education, **SLP**

Gale, Deborah C 8218 Cottage Street, Vienna, VA 22180, (703) 698-5244, BA 78 Swarthmore Coll; MS 81 Emerson Coll; Sp-Lang Path, Fairfax Hosp, **SLP**

Gale, John E 1319 S E 30th Terrace, Cape Coral, FL 33904, **SLP**

Gale, Laura J 32-38 41st Street #3D, Astoria, NY 11103, (212) 924-2912, BA 79 Pace U -NY City; MA 81 NY Univ; Sp/Lang Path, Manhatten Dev Ctr, **SLP**

Gale, Linda C K 3125 Greenbriar Road, Anderson, IN 46011, (317) 649-5324, BS 66 Purdue Univ - West Lafayette; MA 75 Ball St Univ; Director, Anderson Therapy Services, **SLP**

Gale, Mrs Stacy S 2401 S W 86th Avenue, Davie, FL 33324, BA 80 Univ of FL; MA 82 Univ of FL; Sp-Lang Path, Sandler and Associates 85, **SLP**

Galentine, Joy Kimura 111 Maine Street, Dyess AFB, TX 79607-1044, (509) 299-5863, BA 79 Univ of WA; MS 84 Eastern WA Univ; **SLP**

Galeotti, Mrs Lorraine M 2271 Saw Mill River Road, Yorktown Heights, NY 10598, (914) 347-7294, BS 74 SUNY - Coll at Geneseo; MS 77 Columbia Univ Teachers Coll; Aud, Westchester Co Med Cen, **A**

Gales, Charlotte S 6121 E Covey Run Drive, Edmond, OK 73034-9441, (405) 427-8651, BS 74 OK St Univ; MA 76 OK St Univ; Dir, St Dept of Hlth, **SLP ACE**

Gale-Sadler, Cheri 1766 Sunnypark Street, Redlands, CA 92374, (714) 793-2301, BS 75 Loma Linda Univ - Riverside; MS 76 Loma Linda Univ - Loma Linda; Sp-Lang Path, USD, **SLP**

Galetsky, Nancy G 1220 Gemini Drive #L, Annapolis, MD 21403, BA 75 Univ of MD - College Park; MA 78 Univ of MD - College Park; MA 86 Saint John's Coll; 79–Sp-Lang Path, Anne Arundel Co PS, **SLP**

Galiano-Sanders, Mrs Roberta A 811 Hawaiian Drive, Wauchula, FL 33873, (813) 773-2600, MS 82 Univ of South FL; 83–Sp-Lang Path, Hardee Co Sch Bd, **SLP**

Galica, Roxanne Lee 342 Burton Highway, Wilton, NH 03086, (603) 654-2468, BA 81 Univ of CT; MS 85 Univ of NH; 88–Sp-Lang Path, Private Practice, **SLP**

Galimidi, Mrs Robin E 45 Captains Road, North Woodmere, NY 11581, (516) 374-5279, BS 74 NY Univ; MS 75 Columbia Univ Teachers Coll; Sp-Lang Path, Hewlett Woodmere Pub Sch, **SLP**

Galin, Susan Joy 2800 Neilson Way #1416, Santa Monica, CA 90405, (213) 855-6265, BS 66 Univ of WI - Madison; MA 74 Humboldt St Univ; Sp-Lnag Path, Cedars-Sinai Med Cen, **SLP**

Galinsky, Mrs Franci M 520 Highland Grove Drive, Buffalo Grove, IL 60089, (312) 459-6232, BA 77 Univ of IL - Urbana; MS 78 Univ of IL - Urbana; Sp-Lang Path, **SLP**

Galitski, Maureen E 3103 Stevens Street, Madison, WI 53705, (717) 748-2163, MS 87 Univ of NC - Chapel Hill

Galiyas, Mary Jo 114 Herbst Road, Coraopolis, PA 15108, **SLP**

Gall, Michaelann 3201 Scranton Road, Cleveland, OH 44109, (216) 231-8787, BA 81 Cleveland St Univ; MA 82 Cleveland St Univ; Sp-Lang Path, Private Practice, **SLP**

Gallagher, Mrs Ann M 1522 East Boyd Street, Norman, OK 73071, (405) 360-0220, BA 75 Univ of Southwestern LA; OM 76 LA St Univ - N O Medical Ctr; Coord/Speech-Lang Pathology, Norman Public Schools, **SLP**

Gallagher, Dr Betty 196 Crescent Avenue #20E, Buffalo, NY 14214, (716) 834-5233, BS 35 SUNY - Coll at Buffalo; MA 43 Univ of MI - Ann Arbor; PH 60 (NS) Univ of WI - Madison; **SLP LM**

Gallagher, Mrs Beverly Jo 1335 St Francis Road, Bel Air, MD 21014, (301) 396-7463, BA 76 Loyola Coll; MS 77 Loyola Coll; Sp-Lang Path, Baltimore City Schools, **SLP**

Gallagher, Mrs Constance 603 North Maple Bluff Ct, Stevens Point, WI 54481, (303) 226-6485, BA 71 Augustana Coll; MS 73 CO St Univ; **A**

Gallagher, Mrs Debra L 6619 Altama Road, Jacksonville, FL 32216, (904) 725-3627, BA 80 Univ of FL; ME 81 Univ of North FL; ME 86 Univ of North FL; **SLP**

Gallagher, Diane Elmquist 13608 Homestead Avenue, Hugo, MN 55038, BS 75 Univ of MN - Minneap-St Paul; OM 86 Univ of WI - River Falls; **SLP**

Gallagher, Mrs Donna P B 2 Gray Street, Poughkeepsie, NY 12603, (914) 452-0774, BA 72 SUNY - Coll at New Paltz; ME 75 Coll of Saint Rose; Sp-Lang Path, Rehab Prog Inc, **SLP**

Gallagher, Elizabeth Bullard 408 West Blaine, Seattle, WA 98119, (206) 281-9954, BA 83 IN Univ - Bloomington; MA 86 IN Univ - Bloomington; 88–Sp-Lang Path, Little Red School House, **SLP**

Gallagher, Helen F 2704 West Arthur Avenue, Chicago, IL 60645, BA 80 Mundelein Coll; MS 81 Marquette Univ; Sp-Lang Path, Chicago Board of Education, **SLP**

Gallagher, Mrs Helen S 22 Cianchette Avenue, Pittsfield, ME 04967, (207) 487-5575, BS 76 Univ of ME - Farmington; MA 83 Univ of ME - Orono; Sp-Lang Path, Msad #53, **SLP**

Gallagher, Jerry D 52 Days Park, Buffalo, NY 14201-2008, (716) 836-3000, BS 67 SUNY - Coll at Buffalo; MS 71 SUNY - Coll at Buffalo; Sp-Lang Path, Amherst Central Sch, **SLP**

Gallagher, Mrs Katherine 12 Sunderland Road, Denville, NJ 07834-2433, (201) 627-0456, BS 75 Seton Hall Univ; MA 77 Seton Hall Univ; Sp-Lang Path, Private Practice, **SLP ACE**

Gallagher, Kathleen Hennessy 50 Country Corner Lane, Fairport, NY 14450-3032, (716) 223-1436, BS 83 SUNY - Coll at Fredonia; MA 84 Bowling Green St Univ; OM 85 Univ of Rochester; Sp-Lang Path, BOCES Monroe 1, **SLP**

Gallagher, Linda Ann 542 60th Street, Brooklyn, NY 11220, (718) 852-3220, BA 78 Oberlin Coll; MS 84 Columbia Univ Teachers Coll; 85–Sp-Lang Path, The League Ctr, **SLP**

Gallagher, Lynn A Rd 5 Box 247, Troy, NY 12180, (518) 449-4122, BS 81 Coll of Saint Rose; MS 82 Coll of Saint Rose; Rehabilitation Coord, St Peters Hosp-Home Care Dept, **SLP**

Gallagher, Lynn Marie 20656 Elkhart, Harper Woods, MI 48225, (313) 373-3441, BS 84 Central MI Univ; MA 86 Wayne St Univ; **SLP**

Gallagher, Meghan L 61 Madison Street, Huntington, NY 11743, (516) 385-4967, BS 85 Marquette Univ; MS 86 Adelphi Univ; 86–Sp-Lang Path, Huntington Hearing & Sp Ctr, **SLP**

Gallagher, Dr Tanya M School Of Communication Disord, 1266 Pine Avenue West, McGill Univ Beatty Hall, Montreal, PQ, Canada H3G 1A8, (514) 398-4136, BS 67 Univ of IL - Urbana; MA 70 Univ of IL - Urbana; PH 71 (NS) Univ of IL - Urbana; Prof/Dir, McGill Univ, **F**

Gallagher, Mrs Wanda F 19 South Shore Trail, Sparta, NJ 07871, (201) 729-7146, BA 54 Coll Misericordia; MS 79 William Paterson Coll; 85–Sp-Lang Path, Sparta Twsp Sch Dist, **SLP A**

Gallagher-Hornback, Julie G 6608 Azalea Avenue, Bakersfield, CA 93306, (805) 327-3311, **SLP**

Gallagher-Kubat, Mrs Anne Marie 154 Sproul Road, Malvern, PA 19355, (215) 296-4593, BS 83 Indiana Univ of PA; MS 84 Indiana Univ of PA; **SLP**

Gallaher, Dr Alan J 318 West Prospect Avenue, State College, PA 16801, (814) 237-3157, BS 65 Univ of WI - Madison; MA 70 Univ of MN - Minneap-St Paul; PH 79 (Sp-Lang Path) Northwestern Univ; Assistant Professor, PA State Univ, **SLP**

Gallaher, Mrs Carole B 5412 South Martin, Spokane, WA 99223, (509) 466-3060, MS 83 Eastern WA Univ; SLP, Mead Sch Dist, **SLP**

Gallaher, Mrs Wendy J 13212 South Manor Drive, Burnsville, MN 55337, (612) 894-9777, BS 75 IL St Univ - Normal; MS 77 MS Univ for Women; **SLP**

Galland, Elizabeth M 788 Sweeney Street #2, North Tonawanda, NY 14120, (716) 674-6300, OB 81 SUNY - Coll at Buffalo; OM 82 SUNY - Coll at Buffalo; 84–Sp-Lang Path, West Seneca Dev Cen, **SLP**

Gallant, Maureen Victoria 215 Euclid Avenue #305, Long Beach, CA 90803, (213) 439-7533, BS 76 Univ of NH; MA 80 CA St Univ - Long Beach; 87–Sp-Lang Path, Long Beach USD, **SLP**

Gallant, Dr Olivia A 18 Chaundray Lane, Averill Park, NY 12018, (518) 382-4550, BS 69 Univ of TX - Austin; MA 70 Univ of TX - Austin; PH 74 (NS) Univ of CT; Manager/Rehabilitation Center, Sunnyview Hospital, **A**

Gallant, Susan J 1027 Sterling Drive, Rockford, IL 61107, (815) 229-0773, BS 81 Univ of WI - Madison; MS 83 Univ of WI - Madison; Sp-Lang Path, Private Practice, **SLP**

Gallant, Susanne Marie 52 Fourth Street, Fair Haven, VT 05743, (802) 775-2395, BA 76 Univ of ME - Orono; MS 80 IL St Univ - Normal; 87–Sp-Lang Path, Vermont Achievement Ctr, **SLP**

Gallatin, Rhonda Lee 222 East Montclair #3-C, Springfield, MO 65807, (417) 887-5750, BS 81 Southwest Baptist Univ; MS 84 Central MO St Univ; 86–Aud, Reg Ear Nose & Throat Ctr, **A**

Gallegos, Mrs Wendy J 1817 Blume NE, Albuquerque, NM 87112, (505) 293-2548, BA 77 Univ of Denver; MA 79 Univ of Denver; Aud, **A**

Galleher, Jerrold L 43 Overlook Road, Poughkeepsie, NY 12603, (914) 431-8296, BA 60 Heidelberg Coll; MA 63 Case Western Reserve Univ; Aud, St Francis Hospital, **A**

Gallena, Mrs Sally K 509 Moonflower Court, Millersville, MD 21108, (301) 987-9835, BS 77 Towson St Univ; MS 79 Loyola Coll; 86–Sp-Lang Path, Loyola Coll, **SLP**

Gallenberg-Zieve, Felice R 28807 Timberlane Street, Agoura, CA 91301, (818) 706-3101, MA 70 CA St Univ - Los Angeles; Sp-Lang Path, Private Practice, **SLP**

Galley, Mrs Deborah Hager 2717 Westridge, Plano, TX 75075, (214) 352-3923, MS 78 ID St Univ; 88–Aud, Miracle-Ear Ctr, **A**

Galli, Anthony P 310 Francis Street, Manteca, CA 95336, (209) 823-2958, BA 69 CA St Univ - Sacramento; MA 70 CA St Univ - Sacramento; 88–Sp-Lang Path, Manteca USD, **SLP**

Galli, Mrs Claudia S 98 Oakwood, Ypsilanti, MI 48197, (313) 487-4411, BS 67 Eastern MI Univ; MA 70 Eastern MI Univ; Sp-Lang Path, En MI U, **SLP**

Galli, Danny, Jr 98 Oakwood, Ypsilanti, MI 48197, (313) 533-0920, BS 80 Eastern MI Univ; MA 81 Eastern MI Univ; SLP, Detroit Public Schools, **SLP**

Gallier, Mrs Carole Trent 706 Ramblewood Road, Forest, VA 24551, (804) 528-6188, MS 86 Radford Univ; **SLP**

Gallivan, Kerin Mary 32 Eastern Avenue, Haverhill, MA 01830, (617) 665-7740, BA 82 Univ of VT; MS 84 Syracuse Univ; **A**

Gallivan, Paula C Oak Hill Townhouses, 512-C Georgia Avenue, Salisbury, MD 21801, BA 72 Univ of AZ; MS 78 Univ of OR; Sp-Lang Path, Team Rehab, **SLP**

Gallo, Mrs Diane I 1605 East 49th Street, Brooklyn, NY 11234, (212) 763-2510, BA 75 CUNY - Brooklyn Coll; MA 77 NY Univ; SLP, **SLP**

Gallon, Rudolph John P O Box 4103, Star City, WV 26504, (304) 599-0578, OB 78 WV Univ; MA 86 Univ of TN - Knoxville; **SLP**

Galloway, Ann R 9230 East Girard Avenue, Apt #6, Denver, CO 80231, (303) 745-9133, BS 77 Univ of WY; MS 79 CO St Univ; Sp-Lang Path, Spalding Rehab Hosp, **SLP**

Galloway, Camille C 503 Sherwood Drive, Columbus, MS 39701, (601) 494-5900, BS 77 MS Univ for Women; OM 78 Univ of MS; Sp-Lang Path, West Point Mun Separate Sch Dist, **SLP**

Galloway, Cheryl Anne 1352 Aldo Drive North, Mississauga, ON, Canada L5H 3E9, (416) 598-6558, OB 75 Queens Univ - Ontario; 86–Aud, Hosp for Sick Children, **A**

Galloway, Dawn Renee 4695 Lenore Lane, Eagan, MN 55122, (612) 927-7161, BS 83 Univ of WI - Stevens Point; MS 85 Univ of WI - Stevens Point; 86–Aud, Qualitone Hrng Aids & Aud, **A**

Galloway, Mrs Sallye Martin 722 Harpeth Knoll Road, Nashville, TN 37221, (615) 259-8702, BA 64 Vanderbilt Univ; 73–Sp-Lang Path, Metro Pub Sch/Nshvle-Dvdsn Co, **SLP**

Galloway-Curtis, Anne P O Box 10541, Lahaina, HI 96761, (808) 242-6464, BS 63 Univ of Rochester; MS 68 Gallaudet Coll; 82–Aud, Maui Med Group, **A**

Galluzzo, Andrea 24 Harriet Drive, Syosset, NY 11791, (516) 921-5115, BA 84 Adelphi Univ; MS 86 Adelphi Univ; **SLP**

Galper, Marcie R 7463 Duval Drive, Birmingham, MI 48010, (313) 535-7070, BA 76 MI St Univ; MS 78 Univ of WI - Madison; Aud, Redford Union Schs, **A**

Galt, Cynthia F 3311 Mission Drive, Santa Cruz, CA 95065, (408) 476-1333, BA 72 Univ of CA - Santa Cruz; MA 76 San Diego St Univ; Sp-Lang Path, Private Practice, **SLP**

Galt, Sally Ann 330 Mount Vernon Street, Dedham, MA 02026, (617) 326-3432, BS 59 Simmons Coll; ME 60 Boston Univ; Sp-Lang Path, Dedham Pub Sch, **SLP**

Galvan, Minerva M 1141 Corvallis Drive, San Jose, CA 95120, **SLP**

Galvan, Mrs Valerie Ann 416 South 11th Street, Ord, NE 68862, (308) 728-7829, BS 84 Kearney St Coll; MS 85 Kearney St Coll; 85–Sp-Lang Path, Educ Svc Unit 10, **SLP**

Galvin, Mrs Julie Malzone 117 Azalea Circle, Jackson, NJ 08527, (201) 370-8032, BA 80 Montclair St Coll; MA 83 Trenton St Coll; Sp-Lang Path, **SLP**

Galvin, Mrs Michelle Kinley 220 Pintail Lane, Rocky Mount, NC 27804, (919) 758-6646, BS 85 East Carolina Univ; MS 86 East Carolina Univ; **SLP**

Galyean, Barbara B 210 Calle Marina, San Clemente, CA 92672, (714) 731-7331, BA 78 CA St Univ - Los Angeles; MA 85 CA St Univ - Fullerton; 85–Sp-Lang Path, Rileys Speech & Language Inst, **SLP**

Galyen, Mrs Kathryn J 102 Cherokee Drive, Georgetown, IL 61846, (217) 247-2210, BS 78 Eastern IL Univ; MS 78 Eastern IL Univ; Dept Superv SLP, Ridgefarm Pub Sch, **SLP**

Gamache, Gayle Elizabeth 259 West Lexington, Astoria, OR 97103, (503) 325-7535, MA 82 WA St Univ; 86–Sp-Lang Path, Clatsop County ESD, **SLP**

Gamache, Mary E 10916 Ridgecrest Drive, St Ann, MO 63074-3440, (314) 426-4255, BS 76 Southwest MO St Univ; MS 77 Southern IL Univ-Edwardsvill; Sp-Lang Path, Ferguson-Florissant Sch Dist, **SLP**

Gaman, Marthelma Catherine 174 Pasqual Place, San Gabriel, CA 91775, MA 73 CA St Univ - Los Angeles; 73–Sp-Lang Path, Los Angeles County Office of Educ, **SLP**

Gambardella, Mrs Janet Gail 29 Ashwood Court, Staten Island, NY 10308, (718) 891-3600, BA 79 CUNY - Brooklyn Coll; MS 81 CUNY - Brooklyn Coll; SLP, NYC Bd of Ed, **SLP**

Gambee, Mrs Veronica 227 Edgecreek Trail, Rochester, NY 14609, (716) 482-6760, BS 85 Nazareth Coll of Rochester; MS 87 Boston Univ; 88–Sp-Lang Path, Penfield Cen Sch Dist, **SLP**

Gambert, Debby 2014 30th Avenue Apartment 1, San Francisco, CA 94116, (415) 731-9030, BA 85 San Francisco St Univ; MS 87 San Francisco St Univ; 87–Sp-Lang Path, Ther Management Innovations, **SLP**

Gambill, Mrs Kay L 1845 Bobbinray Circle, Florissant, MO 63031, (314) 595-2167, BS 78 Southern IL Univ-Edwardsvill; MA 80 Northern IL Univ - De Kalb; SLP, Spec Sch Dist, **SLP**

Gambino, Mrs Karen 87-27 LL5TH Street, Richmond Hill, NY 11418, (718) 445-0715, BA 79 CUNY - Lehman Coll; MA 81 CUNY - Queens Coll; SLP, Uniondale Pub Sch, **SLP**

Gamble, Mrs Mary Ellen 102 South Home Avenue, Oak Park, IL 60302, (312) 522-2010, BS 84 Ball St Univ; MS 86 TX Christian Univ; 87–Sp-Lang Path, Schwab Rehab Ctr, **SLP**

Gamble, Robert P Prof Hearing Serv Of Fremont, 605 3rd Avenue, Fremont, OH 43420, (419) 334-3879, BS 73 Westminster Coll; MA 79 Univ of IA; Aud, Robert J Mowry MD, **A**

Gambone, Mrs Mary Lynn W 1519 West Lombard Street, Baltimore, MD 21223, (301) 566-2216, BS 82 Bloomsburg Univ of PA; MS 83 Bloomsburg Univ of PA; Sp-Lang Path, American Rehabilitation Inc, **SLP**

Gamby, Mrs Vicki J 935 Houser Road, Fayetteville, PA 17222, (717) 352-3036, BS 80 Bloomsburg Univ of PA; MS 81 Bloomsburg Univ of PA; Sp-Lang Path, Easter Seal Society of Franklin and Adams Counties, **SLP**

Games, Diane C 9614 Otterbein Road, Cincinnati, OH 45241, (513) 733-8395, BA 71 Miami Univ - Oxford; MA 73 IN Univ - Bloomington; Sp-Lang Path, Tri-County Speech Assoc, **SLP**

Gamm, Carrie Beth 619 Sharon Gardens Court, Woodbridge, NJ 07095, (201) 750-4853, BS 82 Wayne St Univ; MS 83 Columbia Univ Teachers Coll; Self Employed, **SLP**

Gamm, Mrs Penelope Ann 1003 Governor Dempsey Drive, Santa Fe, NM 87501, (505) 989-5421, MA 84 CA St Univ - Northridge; 88–Sp-Lang Path, Santa Fe PS, **SLP**

Gammel, Dr Charles L Magnolia Speech School Inc, 733 Flag Chapel Road, Jackson, MS 39209, (601) 922-5530, BA 71 MS Coll; MS 73 Washington Univ; PH 80 (Speech & Hearing) Univ Southern MS-Hattiesburg; 74–Exec Dir, Magnolia Sp Sch Inc, **A**

Gammon, Sarah E 350 East McKinley Avenue, Pomona, CA 91766, (714) 593-7521, BA 72 Stanford Univ; MS 73 Univ of MI - Ann Arbor; Consult, Watermark Group, **SLP**

Gammons, Mrs Roberta Poslusny 97 Bellehurst Drive, Rochester, NY 14617, (716) 254-3110, BS 82 Ithaca Coll; MS 83 Ithaca Coll; 83–Sp-Lang Path, Rochester City Sch Dist, **SLP**

Gamradt, Julie E 6402 Betty's Lane, Madison, WI 53711, (608) 251-2564, BS 82 Saint Cloud St Univ; MS 86 Univ of WI - Madison; Sp-Lang Path, Trace Research & Dev Ctr, **SLP**

Gams-Ehrlich, Alma J 1903 Dennis Avenue, Silver Spring, MD 20902, (301) 593-8760, BA 45 NY Univ; MA 67 Newark St Coll; Sp-Lnag Path, **SLP**

Gamsey, Helen B 600 Ryder Cup Lane, Virginia Beach, VA 23462, (804) 467-1114, BS 70 3935; MS 73 McGill Univ - Quebec; **A**

Gams-Golub, Mrs Stephanie 254 Nome Avenue, Staten Island, NY 10314, (212) 498-2500, BA 75 CUNY - Queens Coll; MA 77 CUNY - Queens Coll; SLP, The League Sch Dist Chld, **SLP**

Gamson, Mrs Joan J 2690 Zorada Drive, Los Angeles, CA 90046, (213) 874-1413, BS 72 NY Univ; MA 74 NY Univ; **SLP**

Gance, Robert A Berks ENT Surgical Assoc, 301 South 7th Avenue, West Reading, PA 19611, (215) 376-9728, BS 70 SUNY - Coll at Geneseo; MA 71 Western MI Univ; Aud, Berks ENT Surgical Associates, **SLP A**

Gancher, Paul D 16-A Dix Avenue, Glens Falls, NY 12801, (518) 792-4994, BA 71 Univ of CT; MS 75 Southern CT St Univ; Aud, Private Practice, **A**

Ganes, Cheryl Proceviat 102 Lloyd Street, Winnipeg, MB, Canada R2H 1Y8, (519) 752-7871, BA 77 Lakehead Univ - Ontario; MA 80 Central MI Univ; Sp-Lang Path, Brantford Gen Hosp, **SLP**

Ganey, Mrs Dorothy Ann 19 Darby Lane, Crystal City, MO 63019, (314) 479-3629, BS 64 De Paul Univ; MS 68 Southern IL Univ -Carbondale; Sp-Lang Path, Chldrns Lrng & Rehab Ctr, **SLP**

Gang, Karen D 198-27 Foothill Terrace, Jamaica, NY 11423, (212) 830-1015, BA 74 SUNY - Center at Buffalo; MS 77 Columbia Univ Teachers Coll; Aud, Mt Sinai Serv at Elmhurst Hosp, **A**

Gang, Mrs Shirley J 1550 Wildwood Lane, Boulder, CO 80303, (303) 422-7052, BA 75 Montclair St Coll; MA 78 Montclair St Coll; 84–Sp-Lang Path, InSpeech Inc, **SLP**

Gangale, Debra Carmela 650 Bougainvillea Lane, Vero Beach, FL 32963, (407) 335-1227, BS 82 Kent St Univ; MA 82 Kent St Univ; Sp-Lang Path, Private Practice, **SLP ACE**

Gangwer, Kathleen Gissoni 11 Driscoll Street, Manville, NJ 08835-2507, (201) 874-4777, BA 78 Paterson St Coll; MS 80 Paterson St Coll; Sp-Lang Path, Hillsborough Township Bd of Ed

Ganis, Mrs Rosemary T 23 Clark Street, Pleasantville, NY 10570, (914) 769-5828, BA 55 Univ of UT; MA 65 Columbia Univ Teachers Coll; Sp-Lang Path, Putnam/Nn Westchester BOCES, **SLP**

Ganjanathavat, Patty S 617 N W 139th, Edmond, OK 73034, **SLP**

Ganley, Dr Peter J 111 Beachview Circle, Long Beach, MS 39560-5829, (601) 388-5541, BA 66 William Paterson Coll; MS 68 SUNY - Coll at Buffalo; OD 76 (Communicative Sciences/Public Health Administration) Johns Hopkins Univ; Chief Aud-SLP Serv, VA Med Cen, **SLP**

Gann, Mrs Patsy J 2905 Watauga Road, Fort Worth, TX 76111, (817) 534-5731, BA 69 Univ of North TX; MA 72 Univ of North TX; Sp-Lang Path, Fort Worth ISD, **SLP**

Gannon, J Kevin 623 Stage Road, Monroe, NY 10950, (914) 294-8806, **SLP**

Gannon, Marlene M 5512 West 75th Place, Arvada, CO 80003, (713) 852-8538, BA 76 Univ of Southwestern LA; MS 80 Univ of Southwestern LA; **SLP**

Gannon, Ruth K 350 Rumsey Road, Toronto, ON, Canada M4G 1R8, (416) 424-3835, MS 70 Purdue Univ - West Lafayette; 74–Dir-Dept Sp-Lang Path & Aud, The Hugh MacMillan Med Ctr, **SLP**

Ganong, Mrs Janice E P O Box 2649, Olympic Valley, CA 95730, (916) 583-3010, BA 72 Univ of OK - Norman; MA 74 CA St Univ - Los Angeles; SLP, Placer Co Office of Education, **SLP**

Gans, Dr Donald P 2005 Skyview Lane, Kent, OH 44240, (216) 672-2672, BS 68 Univ of OR; MA 70 Univ of CO - Boulder; PH 74 (NS) Northwestern Univ; Assoc Prof, Kent State Univ, **A**

Gans, Lynne Golubow 9946 Derbyshire Lane, Bethesda, MD 20817, (301) 365-5931, BA 83 Univ of MI - Ann Arbor; MS 85 PA St Univ - Univ Park; Sp-Lang Path, Mary Carr & Assoc PA, **SLP**

Gans, Dr Richard E 290 N W 165th Street, Plaza 250, Miami, FL 33169, (305) 944-8378, BA 72 Univ of Tampa; MS 78 Univ of South FL; PH 83 (NS) OH St Univ; Director, Family Hearing Center, **A**

Gansen, Christi J Pearson 118 South Jackson Avenue, Jefferson, WI 53549, (414) 674-6864, BS 85 IA St Univ; MA 87 Univ of Northern IA; 87–Sp-Lang Path, Edgerton Comm Sch Dist, **SLP**

Gant, Deborah Elaine 10705 Roger Drive, Apartment E, New Orleans, LA 70127-2827, (504) 568-2837, BS 82 TN St Univ; ME 84 Univ of GA; Dept Hhr Reg 1 Comm Disorders, **A**

Gant, Fiona Robertson 3104 Fieldstone Circle, Birmingham, AL 35215, (205) 841-7541, BS 83 Univ of Montevallo; MS 86 Univ of Montevallo; 84–Sp-Lang Path, Tarrant Sch Sys, **SLP**

Gant, Mrs Leslie Osborne 95 Candy Circle, Winterville, GA 30683, (404) 742-7084, BS 83 East TN St Univ; MA 84 Univ of TN - Knoxville; Audiologist, GA Hearing Cntr, **A**

Gant, Linda R 2749 Jonquil Street, New Orleans, LA 70122-6023, **SLP**

Gant-Johnston, Sheryl S 2072 Lakeway Drive, Holland, MI 49423, (616) 392-5141, BS 71 Univ of MI - Ann Arbor; MS 72 Univ of MI - Ann Arbor; Sp-Lang Path, Holland Comm Hosp, **SLP**

Gantry, Anita Rae 205-13 Newaukum Golf Drive, Chehalis, WA 98532, (206) 748-0151, BA 79 Eastern WA Univ; MS 81 Eastern WA Univ; Private Practice, **SLP**

Gantwerk, Barbara F 196 Mather Avenue, Princeton, NJ 08540, (609) 292-0147, BA 65 CUNY - Brooklyn Coll; MA 67 CUNY - Brooklyn Coll; Plan Assoc, NJ St Dept Ed, **SLP**

Gantz, Mrs Kathryn Snyder 714 Riverview Drive, Logan, UT 84321, (801) 753-8170, BA 81 SUNY - Coll at Cortland; ME 84 Univ of VA - Charlottesville; 87–Sp-Lang Path, Logan Reg Hosp, **SLP**

Ganulin, Mrs Karen Johnson 9532 Zetland Drive, Huntington Beach, CA 92646, (714) 964-1664, OM 82 CA St Univ - Northridge; SLP, Anaheim Union High School Dist, **SLP**

Ganz, Candace K Dept Speech Path & Audiology, Western Washington Univ, Bellingham, WA 98225, (206) 676-3881, BA 70 Univ of KS; MA 72 Univ of KS; Clinical Director Sp-Lang, Western Washington University, **SLP**

Ganz, Mrs Elinor C 18051 Biscayne Boulevard, Apartment 1804, North Miami Beach, FL 33160, BA 55 Univ of PA; MA 57 CUNY - Brooklyn Coll; Co-Director, Florida Speech & Language Ctr, **SLP**

Ganz, Ilene S B 1584 Kew Avenue, Hewlett, NY 11557, (516) 378-2000, BA 79 CUNY - Queens Coll; MA 81 CUNY - Queens Coll; Sp-Lang Path, UCP Assn of Nassau Co, **SLP**

Ganz, Leslie Lapinski 48E Muirfield Drive, Flying Hills, Reading, PA 19607, (215) 775-5918, BS 86 Bloomsburg Univ of PA; MS 87 Bloomsburg Univ of PA; 87–Sp-Lang Path, InSpeech Inc, **SLP**

Ganz, Mrs Sheryl Klein 612 Park Lane, Cedarhurst, NY 11516, (212) 884-1956, BA 78 CUNY - Brooklyn Coll; MS 80 Columbia Univ Teachers Coll; Sp-Lang Path, Private Practice, **SLP**

Ganzman, Ilene P 40 Sandpiper Drive, Voorhees, NJ 08043, (609) 428-2990, BA 77 CUNY - Brooklyn Coll; MS 78 Columbia Univ Teachers Coll; Sp-Lang Path, Voorhees Township PS, **SLP**

Gapa, Rhea M Greer 1830 Carriage House Circle, Apartment 1603, Arlington, TX 76011, (817) 795-7801, BA 74; MA 80 Univ of SD - Vermillion; Sp-Lang Path, Irving ISD, **SLP**

Garabedian, Charlene B Rehabilitation Department, Quincy City Hospital, 114 Whitwell Street, Quincy, MA 02169, (617) 773-6100, BS 75 Univ of VT; MS 76 Univ of MI - Ann Arbor; Dir of Rehabilitation, Quincy City Hosp, **SLP**

Garabedian, Mrs Nancy Anne 72 New Road, Tolland, CT 06084, (203) 872-8571, BS 55 Western MI Univ; MA 63 MI St Univ; 64–Supervisor of Special Educ, Vernon Board of Education, **SLP**

Garas, Mrs Donna M 746 Four Rod Road, Alden, NY 14004, (716) 937-7207, OM 88 SUNY - Coll at Buffalo; 85–Sp-Lang Path, Iroquois Central Schs

Garb, Mrs Hildreth R 7159 South Franklin Way, Littleton, CO 80122, (303) 795-3376, BS 47 PA St Univ - Univ Park; MA 66 Univ of MO - Columbia; Sp/Lang Path, Littleton Pub Sch, **SLP**

Garber, Mrs Betsy L P O Box 621, Wiscasset, ME 04578, (207) 594-7819, BS 58 Southern CT St Univ; MS 81 Southern CT St Univ; Sp/Lang Path, **SLP**

Garber, Mrs Debra Bell 3530 North Wilton #1, Chicago, IL 60657, (312) 528-9351, BS 81 Newcomb Coll Tulane Univ; MA 83 Univ of Denver; Audiologist, Cook County Hospital, **A**

Garber, Gerry Beth Family Survival Project, 458 Waller Street, San Francisco, CA 94117, (415) 493-3662, BA 76 SUNY - Coll at Oswego; MA 80 Univ of Northern IA; Sp-Lang Path, Childrens Hospital Medical Ctr, **SLP**

Garber, Janice Ritsko 1041 Broad Avenue #3, Belle Vernon, PA 15012, (412) 326-8756, **SLP**

Garber, Karen Bentley 6 Tejon, Rancho Santa Margarita, CA 92688, (714) 858-4778, MA 76 CA St Univ - Long Beach; 87–Sp-Lang Path, Private Practice, **SLP**

Garber, Maryann 10 Earich Road, Athens, OH 45701, (614) 385-5393, BA 75 Slippery Rock Univ of PA; MA 77 OH Univ - Athens; Sp-Lang Path, Logan-Hocking Sch Dist, **SLP**

Garber, Dr Norman B Ohio University, 207 Lindley Hall, Athens, OH 45701, (614) 594-5107, BS 66 Southern CT St Univ; MS 68 Southern CT St Univ; PH 71 (Sp-Lang Path) Univ of MO - Columbia; Assoc Prof, OH U, **SLP**

Garber, Sandra L 6193 Village Park Drive, Apartment 202, West Bloomfield, MI 48033-6829, BA 77 MI St Univ; MA 79 Eastern MI Univ; Sp-Lang Path, Speech & Lang Pathology Assn, **SLP**

Garber, Mrs Tammy Brooks 4509 Ale Court, Fayetteville, NC 28304, (919) 323-1250, BS 82 James Madison Univ; MS 85 Univ of NC - Chapel Hill; Aud, Audiology Clinic Inc, **A**

Garbinski, Kimberly Ann 126 North Avenue, Syracuse, NY 13206, (315) 425-4625, BS 83 Ithaca Coll; MS 85 Purdue Univ - West Lafayette; Sp-Lang Path, Syracuse City Sch Dist, **SLP**

Garbose, David Morse P O Box 812, Middlebury, VT 05753, (802) 862-7355, BA 79 Clark Univ; MA 85 Univ of MA - Amherst; **SLP**

Garbowitz, Mrs Barbara H 2348 Troy Road, Schenectady, NY 12309, (518) 439-4921, BA 51 CUNY - Queens Coll; MS 70 SUNY - Center at Binghamton; Sp-Lang Path, BOCES, **SLP**

Garbrecht, Mrs Mary Ellen Ahern 3404 McFarland Road, Tampa, FL 33618, (813) 933-0074, BS 83 Univ of IL - Urbana; MS 85 Rush Univ; 86–Aud, Hillsborough County Sch Sys, **A**

Garbutt, Dr Cameron W 905 Carter Street, Carbondale, IL 62901-2448, (618) 457-6260, BS 27 Northwestern Univ; MA 41 Univ of WA; PH 50 (NS) LA St Univ - Baton Rouge; **SLP LM**

Garcia, Carlos E 315 Salmon, Johnstown, PA 15904, (814) 266-4402, **SLP**

Garcia, Emily Medic 315 Salmon, Johnstown, PA 15904, (814) 266-4402, MS; **SLP**

Garcia, Graciela G 1605 South Shannon Road, Tucson, AZ 85713, **SLP**

Garcia, Guadalupe P O Box 1792, Costa Mesa, CA 92628, (714) 957-5247, **A**

Garcia, Linda Jeannette 353 River Ridge Crescent, Orleans, ON, Canada K1E 3A3, (613) 737-8254, BA 79 McGill Univ - Quebec; MS 81 McGill Univ - Quebec; 81–Sp-Lang Path, Ottawa Gen Hosp, **SLP**

Garcia, Mrs M Erin O'Toole 19812 Venecia Lane, Yorba Linda, CA 92686, (714) 635-6001, BA 78 CA St Univ - Fullerton; MA 81 CA St Univ - Fullerton; Sp-Lang Path, Anaheim Cty Sch Dist, **SLP**

Garcia, Mrs Morrine Moody 115 Northwood Drive #B, Asheboro, NC 27203-3260, (919) 629-2131, BS 82 Central MI Univ; MA 83 Central MI Univ; 88–Sp-Lang Path, Randolph County Schs, **SLP**

Garcia, Priscilla L P O Box 26503, Albuquerque, NM 87125, (505) 277-4453, BS 77 UT St Univ; MS 81 Univ of UT; Sp-Lang Path, Dept Com Dis UNM, **SLP ACE**

Garcia, Renee 940 West Chestnut Street, Washington, PA 15301, (412) 379-6585, MS 87 CA Univ of PA; 87–Sp-Lang Path, SW PA Easter Seal Soc, **SLP**

Garcia, Robert Gene 5464 Quail Run West, Theodore, AL 36582, (402) 559-4069, Univ of NE Med Center, **A**

Garcia, Mrs Suzanne G 14802 54th Way North, Clearwater, FL 34620, (813) 799-3602, MS 80 Univ of South FL; SLP, Pinellas County School Board, **SLP**

Garcia-Giese, Mrs Maria E 6040 Belle Grove, Baton Rouge, LA 70820, (504) 929-5264, BS 79 Carlow Coll; MA 81 LA St Univ - Baton Rouge; Sp-Lang Path, E Baton Rouge Parish Sch, **SLP**

Gard, Mrs Adeline Alderson 1473 Central Conlin Bldg, Dubuque, IA 52001, (319) 588-0538, BA 69 Univ of Northern IA; MA 72 Univ of Northern IA; Sp-Lang Path, Keystone AEA #1, **SLP**

Gardella, Teresa D'Angelo 25-26 33rd Street, Astoria, NY 11102, BA 82 Pace U -NY City; MA 84 CUNY - Hunter Coll; Aud, Brooklyn Audiology Associates, **A**

Gardes, Christy G 4844 Purdue Drive, Metairie, LA 70003, (504) 455-9714, BA 76 Southeastern LA Univ; MA 80 Tulane Univ; Sp-Lang Path, Jefferson Parish Sch Syst, **SLP**

Gardi, Dr John N 325 Parnassus Avenue, San Francisco, CA 94117, (415) 664-5018, BA 73 Univ of CA - Santa Barbara; PH 78 (NS) Univ of CA - San Francisco; Asst Prof Otolaryngology, Univ of CA, **A**

Gardina-Wolfe, Anna M 9S 220 Lake Drive 109, Bldg 16, Clarendon Hills, IL 60514-2553, (312) 462-4220, BS 84 Clarion Univ of PA; MS 85 Clarion Univ of PA; 88–Sp-Lang Path, Marianjoy Rehab Hosp, **SLP**

Gardiner, Holly Jean 10 Sherwood Avenue, Pikesville, MD 21208, (301) 484-4623, MS 84 Loyola Coll; Sp-Lang Path, Baltimore Cty Pub Sch, **SLP**

Gardiner, Maureen M 26822 Sommerset Lane, El Toro, CA 92630, (714) 581-2800, BA 60 Univ of CA - Berkeley; MA 69 San Francisco St Univ; 79–Aud, Newport Lang Sp Aud Cen, **A ACE**

Gardiner, Paula M R 2530 Turkey Oak, San Antonio, TX 78232, **SLP**

Gardiner-Morgan, Mrs Beverly P O Box 3701, Lawrence, KS 66046, (913) 842-1692, BA 68 OK St Univ; MA 70 Univ of KS; Private Practice, **SLP**

Gardner, Mrs Alice L P O Box 172, West Suffield, CT 06093, (203) 566-3767, BA 64; MA 68 Temple Univ; Sp-Lang Path, CT Dept of Hlth, **SLP ACE**

Gardner, Beth Marie Abrahamson 202 11th Street, Hudson, WI 54016-1520, (715) 258-9484, **SLP**

Gardner, Carol B 9609 Heather Court, Cincinnati, OH 45242-6053, (513) 742-2200, **SLP**

Gardner, Cheryl L 14 Payne Street, Winnipeg, MB, Canada R2V 3C2, (204) 338-9159, BA 83 Univ of Winnipeg - Manitoba; MS 86 Univ of ND; **SLP**

Gardner, Daniel P P O Box 1476, Land O'Lakes, FL 34639-1476, (406) 727-6547, **A**

Gardner, Mrs Deborah Bowen 1619 Shady Leaf Drive, Valrico, FL 33594, (813) 681-1742, BS 78 CO St Univ; MS 80 CO St Univ; 88–Sp-Lang Path, Private Practice, **SLP**

Gardner, Mrs Diane G 3913 Jim Robison, Edmond, OK 73034, (405) 755-4327, BA 79 Univ of OK - Norman; MS 81 Univ of OK Medical Center; Aud, OK Hrng Cen, **A**

Gardner, Diane Lynn 211 S Garner, Lawson, MO 64062, BS 82 Central MO St Univ; MS 86 Central MO St Univ; **SLP**

Gardner, Donna H 11501 Gelding Drive, Charlotte, NC 28215, (704) 536-3823, BA 75 George Washington Univ; MS 80 Univ of the DC; Prog Coord, Comm Hlth Alternative Prog, **SLP**

Gardner, Mrs Edna Gadsden 263 Arcadia Boulevard, Springfield, MA 01118, (413) 788-6024, BA 64 SC St Coll; MA 79 Univ of MA - Amherst; 85–Sp-Lang Path, Windsor PS, **SLP**

Gardner, Elizabeth Shepherd 8508 Bargamin Drive, Austin, TX 78736, (512) 392-1224, ME 84 Southwest TX St Univ; SLP, Austin ISD, **SLP**

Gardner, Ellen M 19 Yorkshire Drive, Voorhees, NJ 08043, (609) 667-1790, BA 75 Temple Univ; MA 77 Temple Univ; Sp-Lang Path, Private Practice, **SLP**

Gardner, Mrs Farrell T 5520 Merritt Drive, Concord, CA 94521, BA 72 Univ of the Pacific; MA 73 Univ of the Pacific; 79–Sp-Lang Path, Mt Diablo USD, **SLP**

Gardner, Dr Harvey J Huntington Hearing & Speech, 44 Elm Street, Huntington, NY 11743, (516) 271-6263, BA 53 CUNY - Brooklyn Coll; MA 56 CUNY - Brooklyn Coll; PH 61 (NS) OH St Univ; Dir, Huntington Hrng & Sp Cen, **SLP A**

Gardner, Ingrid Jacqueline 902 N Croft, Los Angeles, CA 90069, (213) 669-2137, OB 82; SLP, Childrens Hospital of Los Ang, **SLP**

Gardner, Jacqui 3923 Huntingdon Drive, Minnetonka, MN 55343, (612) 938-3191, BA 54 Univ of CO - Boulder; **SLP**

Gardner, Janet 9637 68A Street, Edmonton, AB, Canada T6B 1V3, BA 70; MA 71 KS St Univ; Sp/Lang Path, Edmonton Pub Sch Bd, **SLP**

Gardner, Janet Lee 2142 McIntosh Drive, Garland, TX 75040, (214) 271-0516, BA 82 Univ of OK - Norman; MS 84 Univ of OK Medical Center; **A**

Gardner, Judith B Des Moines Public Schools, 1800 Grand Avenue, Des Moines, IA 50309-3382, (515) 242-7714, BS 71 Univ of IA; MA 72 Eastern MI Univ; Superv/Speech-Lang Services, Des Moines Public Schools, **SLP**

Gardner, Dr Julie O 17338 Zola Street, Granada Hills, CA 91344, BA 67 CA St Univ - Northridge; MA 69 Univ of Southern CA; PH 72 (NS) Univ of Southern CA; Prof, CA St U-Northridge, **SLP**

Gardner, Lela Route 3 Box 1350, Harpers Ferry, WV 25425-9721, (304) 535-2520, BS 30 Univ of NE - Lincoln; MS 32 Washington Univ; **SLP LM**

Gardner, Marsha Lee 4635 Clanranald Avenue, Apartment 306, Montreal, PQ, Canada H3X 2R8, (514) 934-8028, BA 68 McGill Univ - Quebec; ME 70 Boston Univ; 70–Chief Aud, Montreal Gen Hosp, **A**

Gardner, Mrs Mary Ellen 705 West 18th Terrace, Russellville, AR 72801, BS 76 Univ of Central AR; MS 86 Univ of Central AR; **SLP**

Gardner, Mrs Nancy Kriz Box 5448 RFD, Long Grove, IL 60047, (312) 272-1934, BS 75 Western IL Univ; MS 76 Bradley Univ; Sp-Lang Path, Highland Park School Dist #108, **SLP**

Gardner, Dr Pamela R 438 13th Avenue, Huntington, WV 25701, (304) 696-3640, BS 64 Syracuse Univ; MA 65 Northwestern Univ; PH 78 (Communication Disorders) CUNY - Grad Sch & Univ Cntr; Assoc Prof, Marshall U, **SLP**

Gardner, Mrs Paula J 929 Chancellor, Edwardsville, IL 62025, (618) 656-0268, BS 77 TX Tech Univ; MS 78 TX Tech Univ; Aud/Deaf-Blind Director, Lubbock State School, **A**

Gardner, Mrs Polly J Speech And Language Services, 1001 Medical Plaza, Suite 140, Woodlands, TX 77380, (713) 367-2035, BA 79 Univ of Houston - Univ Park; MA 80 Univ of Houston - Univ Park; Sp-Lang Path Director, Speech and Language Services, **SLP ACE**

Gardner, Rex 235 West 76th Street #3E, New York, NY 10023, (212) 874-4548, BS 70 OH Univ - Athens; MA 75 OH Univ - Athens; Sp-Lang Path, Private Practice, **SLP**

Gardner, Robert H 24 Birch Street, Saranac Lake, NY 12983, (914) 359-3311, BS 71 SUNY - Coll at Geneseo; MA 73 SUNY - Coll at Geneseo; OM 78 Russell Sage Coll; **SLP**

Gardner, Robin Frances 1883 Fountainview Court, Columbus, OH 43232-3133, (614) 866-7479, BS 83 Northwestern Univ; OM 84 IN Univ - Bloomington; 87–Sp-Lang Path, Good Samaritan Med Ctr, **SLP**

Gardner, Roni Deann 6777 Chaucer Drive, Lawton, OK 73505, (405) 248-5300, BA 80 Univ of OK - Norman; MS 82 Univ of OK Medical Center; Sp-Lang Path, Sp-Lang Services, **SLP**

Gardner-Cyr, Mrs Theresa Marie 3132 B Little Mountain Dr, San Bernardino, CA 92407, (714) 882-8344, BS 83 James Madison Univ; MS 85 James Madison Univ; 87–Dir Clin Svcs, Communication Health Services, **SLP**

Gardner-Reichley, Mrs Elizabeth 4569 Wilson Avenue, San Diego, CA 92116, (619) 563-1410, BA 80 Univ Southern MS-Hattiesburg; MS 83 Univ Southern MS-Hattiesburg; 88–Sp-Lang Path, Private Practice, **SLP**

Gardon, Andrea Marie 3143 South 39th Street, Milwaukee, WI 53215, (506) 855-1600, BS 82 Univ of IL - Urbana; MA 84 Northwestern Univ; Aud, St Lukes Hospital, **A**

Gareau, Ann M 10213 Falconridge Drive, Richmond, VA 23233-3809, (804) 266-4469, SLP, Henrico Co Schools, **SLP**

Gareau, Mrs Kim Marie Summit Road, Gilbertville, MA 01031, (413) 477-6433, BS 82 Univ of MA - Amherst; MA 84 Univ of MA - Amherst; 84–Sp-Lang Path, Monson Developmental Center, **SLP**

Gareau, Maureen E PO Box 281, Almonte, ON, Canada K0A 1A0, (613) 257-2200, BS 74 Emerson Coll; MS 76 Univ of MI - Ann Arbor; Dept Head, Carleton Place & Dist Mem Hosp, **SLP**

Garel, Susan Kathleen 31 Brookford Street #1, Cambridge, MA 02140, (617) 354-7150, **A**

Garfield, Ilene F 4725 Hedgewood Drive, Birmingham, MI 48010, (313) 855-9025, MA 75 Wayne St Univ; Sp-Lang Path, Macomb Hosp Ctr, **SLP**

Garfinkel, Carrie Lyn 2077 Center Avenue #11K, Fort Lee, NJ 07024, (718) 963-8319, BA 76 SUNY - Center at Buffalo; MA 78 NY Univ; Dir Sp-Lang-Hearing, Woodhull Med Cntr, **SLP**

Garfinkel, Janine Boggs 930 Vereda Del Ciervo, Goleta, CA 93117-5304, BA 84 Univ of CA - Santa Barbara; MA 86 CA St Univ - Fresno; **A**

Garfinkel, Mrs Rosalind 2330 Henbird Lane, Lancaster, PA 17601, (717) 757-1531, BA 74 George Washington Univ; MS 75 Vanderbilt Univ; Aud, Lincoln Inter Ut #12, **A**

Gargano, Debra Ann 3238 Lawrence Avenue, Oceanside, NY 11572, (516) 825-4562, BA 84 Saint John's Univ - Jamaica; MS 86 Adelphi Univ; **A**

Gargaro, Janet M 15 Melrose Avenue, Jamestown, RI 02835, (401) 423-1238, BA 73 Salve Regina - Newport Coll; MS 80 Univ of RI; Sp-Lang Path, Early Interventn Prog Fall Rv, **SLP**

Garihee, Laura V 816 Summit N E, Albuquerque, NM 87106, (505) 268-3833, BS 54 IL St Univ - Normal; Sp-Lang Path, Albuquerque Pub Sch, **SLP**

Garis, Mrs Marcine 2927 Indian Hollow, San Antonio, TX 78261-9306, (512) 699-3911, BS 80 East TX St Univ - Commerce; MA 87 Our Lady Lake Univ-San Anton; 88–Sp-Lang Path, Easter Seal, **SLP**

Garito, Mrs Arlene Gold 28 Holland Lane, Colts Neck, NJ 07722, (201) 431-0852, BA 77 Rutger's St Univ - Douglas Coll; MS 81 Rutgers St Univ -N Brunswick; Sp-Lang Path, Colts Neck Twnsp Bd Ed, **SLP**

Garland, Charlene Mary 208 Heatherwood Road, Havertown, PA 19083, (215) 359-4310, BS 76 East Stroudsburg Univ of PA; MA 79 Trenton St Coll; Sp-Lang Path, Marple Newtown Sch Dist, **SLP**

Garland, Cynthia A Hearing Services Of Fremont, 38750 Paseo Padre Parkway #A-4, Fremont, CA 94538, (415) 793-1010, BA 84 San Francisco St Univ; MA 86 Univ of CA - Santa Barbara; 87–Aud, Hearing Services of Fremont, **A**

Garland, Mrs June M 820 Sorolla Avenue, Coral Gables, FL 33134, (305) 633-1424, OB 74 Univ of Miami; ME 78 Univ of Miami; Sp-Lang Path, Dade Co Sch, **SLP**

Garland, Mrs Lori Ann 611 Dew Drop Circle, Apt M, Cincinnati, OH 45240, (513) 891-8700, BS 84 Bowling Green St Univ; MS 86 Bowling Green St Univ; Aud, Montgomery Ear Nose & Throat, **A**

Garland, Mrs Margaret Ann 2704 Redbud Street, Johnson City, TN 37604, (615) 543-3591, BS 80 Western MI Univ; MA 82 Wayne St Univ

Garland, Priscilla 513 Morningside Drive, Louisville, KY 40206, (502) 896-2100, BS 74 WV Univ; MS 75 WV Univ; Aud, **SLP A**

Garland, Sharon Marie 21 Central Park Avenue, Old Orchard Beach, ME 04064-2505, (207) 934-1226, BS 81 Univ of ME - Farmington; MS 85 Univ of NH; 88–Sp-Lang Path, NE Rehab Hosp Portland, **SLP**

Garland, Timothy Robert 558 South Raccoon Road, Apartment H-58, Youngstown, OH 44515, (216) 799-5005, BS 81 Edinboro Univ of PA; MA 83 Edinboro Univ of PA; Sp-Lang Path, Fairhaven Sch-Ment Ret, **SLP**

Garland-Jacobs, Nancy 1744 Sorrel Court, Carlsbad, CA 92009, (619) 258-2390, BA 77 San Diego St Univ; MA 84 San Diego St Univ; **SLP**

Garlich, Mrs Deborah M 308 Basswood Drive, Naperville, IL 60540, (312) 420-0408, BS 71 Purdue Univ - West Lafayette; MS 73 Purdue Univ - West Lafayette; **SLP**

Garlick, Mrs Judith A 20790 Cipres Way, Boca Raton, FL 33433, (305) 488-7166, BS 69 Manhattan Coll; MA 71 Hofstra Univ; **SLP**

Garner, Betty Department Of Audiology, Alaska Native Medical Ctr, PO Box 107741, Anchorage, AK 99510, (907) 279-6661, BA 68 Univ of Science & Arts of OK; MA 73 MI St Univ; Ch of Aud, Indian Health Serv, **A**

Garner, Mrs Carolyn Ball 127 Pinewood Drive, Bloomington, IN 47401, (812) 335-0221, BA 78 Univ of Akron; MA 87 Univ of Akron; **A**

Garner, Donna J 6801 West 70th #40, Shreveport, LA 71129, BA 83 LA Tech Univ; OM 86 LA St Univ - N O Medical Ctr; **SLP**

Garner, Mrs Gloria Donathan 919-B Flythe Drive, Augusta, GA 30904, (404) 733-9899, BS 84 Univ of GA; ME 86 Univ of GA; **A**

Garner, Lynne Marie 4509 86th Street, Apartment 19, Urbandale, IA 50322, (515) 279-9034, BS 85 Univ of IA; MS 87 Marquette Univ; 87–Sp-Lang Path, Des Moines Hrng & Sp Ctr, **SLP**

Garner, Margaret L 423 Clairemont Avenue #7, Decatur, GA 30030, (404) 460-1337, BS 69 Univ of AZ; MS 70 Kent St Univ; **SLP**

Garner, Mrs Marie A 8627 South Melvina, Burbank, IL 60459, (312) 598-6520, BA 78 Elmhurst Coll; MS 79 IL St Univ - Normal; Sp-Lang Path, AERO Spec Educ Coop, **SLP**

Garner, Mrs Mitzie A 1124 Berry Street, Grenada, MS 38901, (601) 226-8900, BA 80 Univ of MS; OM 82 Univ of MS; Sp-Lang Path, Grenada Separate Sch, **SLP**

Garner, Patricia N 5709 Wester Way, Arlington, TX 76013, **SLP**

Garnes, Mrs Willye M 2600 John Ashley Dr #C-107, North Little Rock, AR 72114, (501) 376-7400, BA Ouachita Baptist Univ; MA LA St Univ - Baton Rouge; **SLP A LM**

Garnett, Catherine Mary 16252 Northglen Place, Surrey, BC, Canada V3R 8M9, (604) 588-8394, BS 70 McGill Univ - Quebec; MA 82 Univ of CA - Santa Barbara; 82–Sp/Lang Path, Sch Dist #36 (Surrey), **SLP**

Garnett, Mrs Mary Jane Hq 7 Atc, P O Box 3586, APO New York, NY 09114, BS 71 Univ of NE - Lincoln; MA 73 Univ of KS; **A**

Garn-Nunn, Dr Pamela Dept Communication Disorders, Radford University, Radford, VA 24142, (703) 731-5453, BS 69 OH Univ - Athens; MS 74 Southern IL Univ -Carbondale; PH 82 (NS) Southern IL Univ -Carbondale; Assoc Prof, Radford U-Dept Commun Dis, **SLP**

Garon, Bernard R 1615 Bayard Avenue, St Paul, MN 55116, (612) 227-8471, BS 73 Univ of HI - Manoa; MS 74 Univ of HI - Manoa; SLP, St Paul Rehab Cen, **SLP**

Garosshen, Mrs Cynthia B 32 Gilead Road, Route #2 Box 170, Andover, CT 06232, (203) 667-5320, BA 77 Univ of CT; MS 82 PA St Univ - Univ Park; Sp-Lang Path, Newington Children's Hosp, **SLP**

Garra, John 6611 Burk Road, Lake View, NY 14085, (716) 674-6300, BS 68 SUNY - Coll at Buffalo; MS 73 SUNY - Coll at Buffalo; SLP & Aud Prog Coord II, West Seneca D D S O, **SLP**

Garrahy, Patricia Ellen 133 Timberline Road, Warwick, RI 02886, (401) 885-0571, BA 83 Univ of RI; MS 85 Boston Univ; 88–Sp-Lang Path, Woonsocket Sch Dept, **SLP**

Garrard, Dr Kay Russell 6437 Worchester Drive, Nashville, TN 37221, (615) 898-2661, BS 64 MS Univ for Women; MA 66 Univ of AL- Tuscaloosa; PH 82 (Special Educ) San Francisco St Univ; 83–Assoc Prof, Middle TN St U, **SLP**

Garreffi, Mrs Fern Feinberg 97 Thoreau Drive, Centerville, MA 02632, (617) 548-0151, BS 79 Univ of MA - Amherst; MA 81 Univ of Houston - Univ Park; Sp-Lang Path, Falmouth Pub Sch, **SLP**

Garretson, Dr Carolyn D 2103 Wake Forest Street, Virginia Beach, VA 23451, (804) 481-4004, BA 62 Rutger's St Univ - Douglas Coll; MA 68 Syracuse Univ; ED 82 (NS) Univ of GA; Sp-Lang Path, VA Sp & Lang Associates, **SLP**

Garretson, Lisa Durey 2700 Hanover Drive, Fort Collins, CO 80526, (303) 223-8413, BA 80 Univ of NE - Lincoln; MS 82 CO St Univ; 84–Sp-Lang Path, Thompson R2-J Sch Dist, **SLP**

Garrett, Barbara R B 2511 La Veta Lane, Pueblo, CO 81008, (612) 890-0420, MS 81 CO St Univ; Aud, MN West Metro Aud Services, **A**

Garrett, Bobbie Lee P O Box 520, Atascadero, CA 93423, (805) 922-1025, BA 75 CA St Univ - Sacramento; MA 80 Univ of CA - Santa Barbara; Aud, Private Practice, **A**

Garrett, Carol A 723 Custer Drive, Lynchburg, VA 24502, (804) 239-0850, BS 62 MS Univ for Women; ME 66 Univ of VA - Charlottesville; 62–Sp-Lang Path, Lynchburg City Sch, **SLP**

Garrett, Coy Edwin, Jr 1209 Lake D'Ville Drive, Hendersonville, TN 37075, (615) 822-7516, BS 79 Murray St Univ; MS 80 Murray St Univ; **SLP**

Garrett, Dana Kathryn 10750 Westbrae Parkway, Apartment 2704, Houston, TX 77031, (713) 792-4500, BS 81 Baylor Univ; MA 83 Univ of TN - Knoxville; 88–Sp-Lang Path, Univ of TX Health Sci Ctr, **SLP**

Garrett, Debra M 130 Michigan Avenue N E, Apartment 0-41, Washington, DC 20017, (202) 328-2377, BA 76 Western WA Univ; OM 78 LA St Univ - N O Medical Ctr; ME 85 Tulane Univ; 87–Sp-Lang Path, Montgomery County Pub Schs, **SLP**

Garrett, Mrs Deloris B 5220 Nob Lane, Indianapolis, IN 46226, (317) 545-1768, BS 58 IN St Univ - Terre Haute; MA 61 IN St Univ - Terre Haute; Sp-Lang Path, Indianapolis Pub Sch, **SLP**

Garrett, Dr Edgar Ray P O Box 3534, Las Cruces, NM 88003, (505) 646-4234, BS 42 Western NM Univ; MA 48 Univ of NC - Chapel Hill; PH 54 (NS) Univ of Denver; 48–Dir Comm Disorders, New Mexico St U, **SLP F LM ACE**

Garrett, Mrs Ellen Gordon 25 N W 91st Street, Miami Shores, FL 33150, (305) 751-6648, BS 70 Univ of TN - Knoxville; MA 72 Memphis St Univ; Sp-Lang Path, Private Practice, **SLP**

Garrett, J David University Of Wisconsin, 1975 Willow Drive, Dept Of Communicative Dis, Madison, WI 53706, (608) 262-6481, BA 80 Baylor Univ; MS 81 Baylor Univ; Asst Prof, University of Wisconsin, **SLP**

Garrett, Jill 5678 Highland Terrace, Milford, OH 45150, (513) 948-3647, BS 80 Univ of Cincinnati; MA 83 Univ of Cincinnati; Sp-Lang Path, Millcreek Psych Ctr for Children, **SLP**

Garrett, Joan Route 10 Box 1497, Tyler, TX 75707, (214) 839-2140, BA 73 Baylor Univ; MA 74 Baylor Univ; **SLP**

Garrett, Mrs Joyce Ellen 921 Tyson Place, Syracuse, NY 13206, (315) 488-2951, BA 84 SUNY - Coll at Cortland; MS 85 Syracuse Univ; 86–Sp-Lang Path, St Camillus Health & Rehab Ctr, **SLP**

Garrett, Judith L N 4500 North 19th Road, Arlington, VA 22207, (202) 722-2373, BS 74 SUNY - Coll at Fredonia; MA 75 Univ of TN - Knoxville; Dir of Ear Interv Serv, Natl Chldns Cen, **SLP**

Garrett, Mrs Judith P 2631 Sunset Avenue, Bakersfield, CA 93304, (805) 395-4402, BA 60 CA St Univ - Los Angeles; BA 75 CA St Univ - Northridge; MA 76 CA St Univ - Northridge; Sp-Lang Path, Bakersfield C, **SLP**

Garrett, Kathryn L 1951 D, Lincoln, NE 68502, (402) 489-7102, BS 81 PA St Univ - Univ Park; MS 88 Univ of NE - Lincoln; 87–Sp-Lang Path, Madonna Centers, **SLP**

Garrett, Mrs Lisa Anne 116 Patriots Road, Morris Plains, NJ 07950, BS 80 Ithaca Coll; MA 83 Montclair St Coll; **SLP**

Garrett, Margaret Jean 1500 Arvada Drive, Richardson, TX 75081, (214) 690-9459, BS East TX St Univ - Commerce; MS 82 Univ of TX - Dallas; Sp-Lang Path, Private Practice, **SLP**

Garrett, Mrs Mary F 8877 N W 3rd Court, Coral Springs, FL 33071, (305) 941-3921, BS 64 CO St Univ; MA 77 Univ of Houston - Univ Park; Sp-Lang Path, Broward Co Sch Dist, **SLP**

Garrett, Mrs Mavis W P O Box 843, Smithfield, VA 23430, (804) 599-2094, BS 80 Univ of VA - Charlottesville; ME 82 Univ of VA - Charlottesville; Aud, Riverside Regional Med Ctr, **A**

Garrett, Dr Ruth E C Marshall University, Speech & Hearing Center, Huntington, WV 25701, (304) 696-3640, BS 45 OH Univ - Athens; MA 46 OH Univ - Athens; PH 68 OH Univ - Athens; Prof of Sp, Marshall U, **SLP**

Garrett, Mrs Sharon Ellen 6225 Acorn Street #36, San Diego, CA 92115, (619) 287-7086, BS 82 Univ of IL - Champaign; MS 83 Univ of IL - Champaign; 85–Sp-Lang Path, Children's Hosp-Sp Hrng & Neur Ctr, **SLP**

Garrett, Mrs Susan Casey 64 Archer Avenue, White Plains, NY 10603, (914) 248-8888, BA 75 Mercy Coll; MS 76 Columbia Univ Teachers Coll; Sp-Lang Path, Somers Ctr Sch Dist, **SLP**

Garrick, Mrs Martha Tonos Speech Pathology Services, P O Box 891, 135-1/2 First Street, Grenada, MS 38901, (601) 226-0101, BS 73 MS Univ for Women; MS 85 Univ of MS; SLP, Speech Pathology Service, **SLP**

Garrigan, Kathleen D 224 Wenonah Avenue, Mantua, NJ 08051, (609) 464-0824, BA 73 Newark St Coll; MS 80 San Francisco St Univ; 85–Sp-Lang Path, West Deptford Bd of Educ, **SLP**

Garrigan, Verita M Parker Home, 1421 River Road Room 23, Piscataway, NJ 08854, (201) 545-2228, BS 37; ME 50 Fordham Univ; **SLP LM**

Garrigus, Mrs Rosemary D 11096 47th Road North, West Palm Beach, FL 33411, (305) 965-4712, BA 76 SUNY - Center at Buffalo; MA 77 Hofstra Univ; Sp-Lang Path, School Board of Palm Beach Co, **SLP**

Garrison, James H Box 1298, Bloomington, IN 47402, (812) 333-1900, BA 54 IN Univ - Bloomington; MA 57 Case Western Reserve Univ; Sp-Lang Path, Monroe Co Comm Sch Corp, **SLP**

Garrison, Mrs Lola M Box 532, Jay, OK 74346, (918) 253-8121, BS 62 Northeastern OK St Univ; MS 65 Northeastern OK St Univ; **SLP LM**

Garrison, Maria R 147 Clark's Landing Road, Port Republic, NJ 08241, (609) 628-2701, BS 85 Stockton St Coll; MS 87 Temple Univ; 88–Sp-Lang Path, Toms River Bd of Educ

Garrison, Mrs Mary E M 5442 Newton Avenue South, Minneapolis, MN 55419, (612) 774-6031, BS 77 CO St Univ; MS 79 CO St Univ; Early Ed Sp-Lang Cln, St Paul Public Schools, **SLP**

Garrison, Mrs Mary Jo F Gates Mills Estates Drive, Gates Mills, OH 44040, (216) 442-2200, BS 62 Univ of IL - Urbana; MA 63 Northwestern Univ; Aud, Mayfield Cty Sch Syst, **A**

Garrison, Mrs Patricia M Athena Communications, P O Box 1721, Plainfield, NJ 07061, (201) 757-2407, BA 66 Howard Univ; MS 78 Rutgers St Univ - Newark; Dir, Athena Comm, **SLP ACE**

Garrison, Mrs Sheila Anne P O Box 303, Curtis, NE 69025, (308) 367-4210, Sp-Lang Path, Medicine Valley Pub Sch, **SLP**

Garrison, Sherry Lynne 1603 South 16th Street, Elwood, IN 46036, (317) 552-0181, BS 84 Ball St Univ; MA 85 Ball St Univ; Aud, Comm Hosp Anderson/Madison Co, **A**

Garrity, Mrs Julie Schor 176 Oakwood Lane, Ithaca, NY 14850, (607) 756-5423, BS 69 Ithaca Coll; MS 71 Ithaca Coll; Assistant Professor, State University at Cortland, **SLP**

Garrity, Linda Lee Rd 1 Box 33, Hartwick, NY 13348-9713, (607) 293-6646, **SLP**

Garrity, Rosemary Agnes O 4 Hedgerow, Spring House, PA 19477, (215) 643-1992, BS 77 West Chester Univ of PA; MA 80 West Chester Univ of PA; Sp-Lang Path, Private Practice, **SLP**

Garroway, Mrs Anne Anderson 184 Mount Arlington Blvd, Landing, NJ 07850, (201) 989-3634, BA 84 William Paterson Coll; MA 86 Montclair St Coll; Aud, Dover Gen Hosp, **A**

Garrus, Nancy P 4300 Old Dominion Drive, Apartment 607, Arlington, VA 22207, (703) 522-4651, **A**

Garry, Mrs Elizabeth Philbrick 387 Gladys Avenue, Long Beach, CA 90814, (213) 438-2745, BA 78 Univ of CA - Santa Barbara; MA 81 Univ of CO - Boulder; SLP, Long Beach USD, **SLP**

Garshman, Terry Diane 864 West End Avenue Apartment 3B, New York, NY 10025, (212) 678-3242, BA 83 NY Univ; MA 87 NY Univ; 87–Sp-Lang Path, Columbia Univ, **SLP**

Garson, Blaine A 560 South East Street, Amherst, MA 01002, (413) 253-5447, MS Univ of Pittsburgh - Pittsburgh; Sp-Lang Path, Amherst Pelham Schs, **SLP**

Garson-Selevan, Barbara 83-57 118th Street #3-H, Kew Gardens, NY 11415, (718) 805-4428, MS 87 CUNY - Brooklyn Coll; SLP, Ctr for Child Dev

Garstecki, Dr Dean C Northwestern University-Audiol, Frances Searle Bldg, 2299 Sheridan Road, Evanston, IL 60208, (312) 491-3164, BS 67 Marquette Univ; MS 69 Marquette Univ; PH 74 (Aud) Univ of IL - Urbana; 78–Prog Head Aud & Hrng Imp, Northwestern University, **SLP A F**

Gartenberg, Terri E 6342 North Magnolia, Chicago, IL 60660, (312) 869-6522, BA 75 Univ of CO - Boulder; MS 76 Southern Methodist Univ; Sp-Lang Path, Prentice Women's Hosp, **SLP**

Gartenberg-Fletcher, Mrs Carol 7777 Glen America Drive #221, Dallas, TX 75225, MA 82 Northwestern Univ; Reg Consult, Prentke Romich Co, **SLP**

Garth, Shirley C P O Box 2115, Medford Lakes, NJ 08055, (609) 779-2799, OB 56 Oberlin Coll; MA 76 Trenton St Coll; Sp-Lang Path, Wn Burlington Reg Presch, **SLP**

Gartin, Donna M R Rural Route 3, Haxtun, CO 80731, (303) 774-6152, BS 75 Fort Hays St Univ; MS 76 Fort Hays St Univ; SLP, N E Colo BOCES

Gartlan, Kimberly A 499 Geneva Road, Glen Ellyn, IL 60137, (312) 858-3877, BS 83 IL St Univ - Normal; MA 86 Univ of IL - Urbana; 87–Sp-Lang Path, Marianjoy Rehab Hosp, **SLP**

Gartland, Dr Margaret-Ann D Northern Arizona University, Speech & Hearing Department, Box 15045, Flagstaff, AZ 86011, (602) 523-7436, MS 75 SUNY - Coll at Geneseo; MA 74 SUNY - Coll at Geneseo; PH 83 (NS) Univ of UT; Asst Prof, North Arizona Univ, **SLP ACE**

Gartland, Sandy 12910 West 67th Street, Shawnee, KS 66216, (913) 281-7719, BS 72 Saint Louis Univ; MA 73 Saint Louis Univ; Admin Dir, Bethany Med Cen, **SLP**

Gartley, Linda Ann 537 Arizona Drive, Lower Burrell, PA 15068, (412) 339-7436, BS 79 Clarion Univ of PA; MA 83 Univ of Pittsburgh - Pittsburgh; 85–Sp/Lang Path, Private Practice, **SLP**

Garvalia, Carrie A 5208 N Lovers Lane #4, Milwaukee, WI 53225, (414) 649-6250, BA 86 Univ of WI - Eau Claire; MS 87 Univ of WI - Eau Claire; SLP, St Lukes Ed Ctr

Garver, Mrs Gladis G 708 Wooster Road, Mount Vernon, OH 43050, (614) 393-0697, BS 68 AZ St Univ; MA 81 Bowling Green St Univ; Sp-Path, Providence Hosp, **SLP**

Garvey, Judith P 260 Northampton Road, Amherst, MA 01002, (413) 549-6300, MA 85 Univ of MA - Amherst; **SLP**

Garvey, Lynelle Bailey 112 E Washington, Vicksburg, MI 49097, (616) 649-2913, MA 86 Western MI Univ

Garvin, Mrs Susanne B 13510 Beltway, San Antonio, TX 78217, (512) 653-5293, BA 63 Univ of North TX; MA 70 Univ of North TX; SLP, North East ISD, **SLP**

Garvin, Mrs Virginia Barbara 821 Lizabeth Avenue, Johnson City, TN 37604, BS 74 Univ of TN - Knoxville; MS 84 East TN St Univ; 74–Sp-Lang Path, Johnson City PS, **SLP**

Garvin-Cullen, Allison J 59-40 Queens Boulevard, Apartment 18D, Woodside, NY 11377, (718) 457-9494, BA 80 Saint John's Univ - Jamaica; MA 82 NY Univ; Sp-Lang Path, Private Practice, **SLP ACE**

Garvin-Lease, Mrs Carol A 41 West Canyon, P O Box 57, Hamburg, NY 14075-4737, (716) 837-2441, BS 81 SUNY - Coll at Buffalo; MS 86 SUNY - Coll at Buffalo; **SLP**

Garwood, Dr Victor P 1240 Chautauqua Boulevard, Pacific Palisades, CA 90272, (213) 459-8705, BA 39 Univ of MI - Ann Arbor; MS 48 Univ of MI - Ann Arbor; PH 51 (NS) Univ of MI - Ann Arbor; 88–Prof Emeritus, University Southern California, **SLP A F LM ACE**

Gary, Mrs Caroline Jean 857 Everglades Lane, Livermore, CA 94550, (415) 455-1530, BA 84 Univ of CA - Santa Barbara; MA 85 Univ of the Pacific; 87–Sp-Lang Path, Livermore Valley Unified Schs, **SLP**

Gary, Mrs Leiana Jae 7937 S Evans, Chicago, IL 60619-3906, (312) 542-3400, BS 76 Northern IL Univ - De Kalb; MS 78 Southern IL Univ-Edwardsvill; **SLP**

Gary, Lucinda Boyd Center For Audiology & Speech, Univ Of TX Medical Branch, Galveston, TX 77550, BA 74; MA 76 Baylor Univ; Asst Dir/Aud, U of TX-Med Branch, **A**

Gary, Mrs Mary E 9921 Dolby Avenue, Glenn Dale, MD 20769, BS 64 SUNY - Coll at Geneseo; MS 65 Univ of WI - Madison; Tchr of Deaf, Prince Georges Co Pub Sch, **SLP**

Gary, Sherry J 25703 West Memory Lane, Magnolia, TX 77355, (713) 370-4040, BA 71 Univ of Houston - Univ Park; MA 76 Univ of Houston - Univ Park; Sp-Lang Path, Cypress-Fairbanks ISD, **SLP**

Garza, Anna Belinda 8130 Forest Dawn, San Antonio, TX 78233, (512) 534-2651, BA 77 Our Lady Lake Univ-San Anton; MA 79 Univ of Houston - Univ Park; 86–Sp-Lang Path, San Antonio ISD, **SLP**

Garza, Mrs Frances F 6221 Michaux, Corpus Christi, TX 78414, (512) 994-1827, **SLP**

Gasaway, Jane 1900 East Ocean Boulevard, Apartment 1115, Long Beach, CA 90802, (213) 437-4851, BS 44 IN St Univ - Terre Haute; MA 49 Ball St Univ; SLP, Long Beach USD, **SLP**

Gasch, Mrs Janis Wolfe Arizona Hearing Specialists, 2001 West Orange Grove Rd, Suite 610, Tucson, AZ 85704, (602) 742-2845, BS 73 SUNY - Center at Buffalo; MS 75 Univ of AZ; Owner/Dir, Private Practice, **A**

Gash, Mrs Allyson D 200 Cold Spring Road #B214, Rocky Hill, CT 06067, (203) 563-8181, BA 76 SUNY - Coll at Plattsburgh; MS 77 Adelphi Univ; SLP, Wethersfield Board of Educ, **SLP**

Gaskell, Alice Gail 8415 North Armenia Avenue, Apartment 421, Tampa, FL 33604, (813) 251-7761, BS 83 Purdue Univ - West Lafayette; **A**

Gaskill, Benettee Lee 2502 Royal Lane, Denton, TX 76201, **SLP**

Gaskin, Maura Louise 2673 North Bremen Street #1, Milwaukee, WI 53212, (414) 372-1753, BS 82 Marquette Univ; MS 85 Marquette Univ; Sp-Lang Path, Milwaukee PS, **SLP**

Gasnick, Mary Elizabeth 11265 Evans Street #9, Omaha, NE 68164, (402) 496-0318, BA 80 Kearney St Coll; MS 82 Kearney St Coll; Sp-Lang Path, Omaha Pub Sch/Presch Hndcpd, **SLP**

Gaspelin, Mrs Shirley Mershon 2224 Manor Boulevard North, Clearwater, FL 34625, (813) 796-8438, MS 85 Univ of South FL; **SLP**

Gass, Albert H, Jr 2114 Shreveport Highway, Apartment 273, Pineville, LA 71360, (318) 640-0754, **A**

Gasser, Valerie Katz 11212 Nieman #202, Overland Park, KS 66210, (816) 234-3677, BS 84 Univ of MO - Columbia; MS 85 Boston Univ; **SLP**

Gasson, Linda Dominguez 942 East Cambridge Drive, Burbank, CA 91504, (818) 954-0743, BS 77 Brigham Young Univ; OM 78 Brigham Young Univ; Sp-Lang Path, Olive View Med Ctr, **SLP**

Gast, Linda Sue 1157 Edwards Street, Vassar, MI 48768, (517) 673-3191, BA 81 MI St Univ; MA 82 Western MI Univ; Sp/Lang Path, Ment Health Ctr, **SLP**

Gastel-Pendarvis, Mrs Cristina 21630 Minnehaha Street, Chatsworth, CA 91311, (213) 673-4660, BA 73 Univ of CA - Santa Barbara; MS 76 Univ of AZ; Sp-Lang Path, Centinela Hospital Medical Cen, **SLP**

Gaster, Mrs Lydia Sexton 814-A Cheraw Drive, Florence, SC 29501, (803) 669-8891, ME 84 Univ of GA; Sp-Lang Path, Southeastern Sp & Hrng, **SLP**

Gasthalter, Mrs Margery Atkins 2 Lafayette Road, Larchmont, NY 10538, (914) 834-9386, BA 68 NY Univ; MA 70 NY Univ; Private Practice, **SLP**

Gastwirth-Masone, Judy S Great Neck Audiology Assoc, 525 Northern Boulevard, Room 201, Great Neck, NY 11021, (516) 482-0660, BA 78 CUNY - Brooklyn Coll; MA 82 CUNY - Hunter Coll; Private Practice, **A**

Gasway, Mrs Julie Gay/Hansen 2216 Bever Avenue S E, Cedar Rapids, IA 52403, BS 82 Univ of IA; MA 84 Univ of IA; Sp-Lang Path, St Lukes Hospital, **SLP**

Gatch, Eleanor G Summerville Speech Therapy, P O Box 1181, Summerville, SC 29483, (803) 871-7398, BA 74 Columbia Coll; MA 79 SC St Coll; Sp-Lang Path Admin, Summerville Sp Ther, **SLP**

Gateley, Dr William G 2516 Old Oaks, Waco, TX 76710, (817) 755-2567, BA 51 David Lipscomb Coll; MA 60 Univ of TN - Knoxville; PH 65 (NS) OH Univ - Athens; Chmn Dept Commun Dis, Baylor U, **SLP ACE**

Gatens, Barbara E Dir Oto-Neurology, St Joseph's Hospital, 11705 Mercy Boulevard, Savannah, GA 31420, (912) 927-5479, BA 74 OH Univ - Athens; MA 75 OH Univ - Athens; Dir, St Joseph's Hosp, **A**

Gates, Brenda J 2 Johnny Mercer Boulevard #1313, Savannah, GA 31410, (912) 897-2413, 87 Murray St Univ; **SLP**

Gates, Jane Krohn 15 Thistledown Lane, Kingston, RI 02881, (401) 789-0518, BA 57 Univ of MA - Amherst; MA 65 Univ of CT; Sp-Lang Path, South Kingstown Sch Dept, **SLP**

Gates, Mrs Karen S 31 Pleasant Hill Road, Newtown, CT 06470, (317) 877-6303, BS 74 Southern IL Univ -Carbondale; MS 78 IL St Univ - Normal; **A**

Gates, Kathy Elaine 1C Marian Circle, Mount Holly, NJ 08060, (609) 562-3294, BA 84 SUNY - Coll at Plattsburgh; MA 86 Univ of MD - College Park; **A**

Gates, Mrs Laurie C 6414 East 94th Place, Tulsa, OK 74137, (918) 493-3378, BA 79 Univ of Southern CA; MA 87 Univ of Tulsa; Sp-Lang Path, Saint Francis Hosp, **SLP**

Gates, Rebecca H 114 Bluff Drive, West Monroe, LA 71291, (318) 396-8268, BA 70 LA Tech Univ; MA 76 LA Tech Univ; 88–Sp-Lang Path, Assoc Health Focus, **SLP**

Gates, Valerie Ann 5182 Foxbridge Circle North, Apartment 337, Clearwater, FL 34620, (813) 531-4775, BA 81 SUNY - Center at Buffalo; MA 83 SUNY - Center at Buffalo; 87–Sp-Lang Path, Private Practice, **SLP**

Gatesy, Nancy Matthews 418 Westmoreland, Lansing, MI 48915-1833, **SLP**

Gatgens, Mary Lou 52 Bethany Street, Jackson, TN 38301, (901) 668-4277, BS 68 MS Univ for Women; MS 69 MS Univ for Women; Sp-Lang Path, Private Practice, **SLP**

Gathings, Robert D 517 Chisolm, Denton, TX 76201, (817) 387-3831, BA 65 Univ of North TX; MA 70 Univ of North TX; Aud, Denton State Sch, **SLP A**

Gathman, Mrs Jacqui D 215 Antilla Avenue #1, Coral Gables, FL 33134, (305) 446-2861, BS 85 Evangel Coll; MA 87 Southwest MO St Univ

Gatlin, Kaye L 10022 Antioch Road, Overland Park, KS 66212, **SLP**

Gatlin, Tamara Anne 1814 East 5th Street, Duluth, MN 55812, (218) 724-0146, BS 83 Univ of MN - Duluth; MA 84 Univ of MN - Duluth; Sp-Lang Path, Rehabilitation Specialist Inc, **SLP**

Gatta, Mrs Janice E 1 Anita Drive, Sayville, NY 11782, (516) 467-6010, BS 72 SUNY - Center at Albany; MS 74 SUNY - Center at Albany; SLP, CT Cen Sch, **SLP**

Gatten, Joy Marie 1539 Washington N E, Minneapolis, MN 55413, (715) 425-1039, OM 87 Univ of WI - River Falls; **SLP**

Gatti, Pamela Jean P O Box 2081, Fairfield Glade, TN 38555, (615) 456-2972, BA 83 Univ of OK - Norman; MS 85 Univ of OK Medical Center; 88–Sp-Lang Path, Upper Cumberland Hrng Sp and Lang Ctr, **SLP**

Gattis-McLendon, Mrs Patricia 3867 Laurel Crest Drive, Lithonia, GA 30058, OB 75 Univ of GA; ME 79 Univ of GA; Sp-Lang Path, Gwinnett County Board of Educ, **SLP**

Gatti-Smith, Mrs Filomena 29083 Marilyn Drive, Canyon Country, CA 91351, (805) 297-0166, BA 80 CA St Univ - Northridge; MA 81 CA St Univ - Northridge; Sp-Lang Path, Saugus Union Sch Dist, **SLP**

Gatts, Julie J 414-1/2 Indiana, Lawrence, KS 66044, (913) 295-8045, 0B 85 Univ of KS; MA 87 Univ of KS; 88–Sp-Lang Path, St Francis Hosp & Med Ctr, **SLP**

Gaudin, Diane Shearer 1150 East 83rd Street, Brooklyn, NY 11236, (718) 738-6200, BA 72 CUNY - Brooklyn Coll; MS 78 Columbia Univ Teachers Coll; 88–Coord, Bernard Fineson Dev Ctr, **SLP**

Gaudio, Toni Lynn 446 Sinclair Avenue, Yorkville, OH 43971, (614) 283-3674, BS 80 OH Univ - Athens; MA 86 OH Univ - Athens; 86–Sp-Lang Path, Eastern Ohio Sp & Hearing Ctr, **SLP**

Gaudreau, Jeffrey Norman Route 4 Box 1182, Cushing, OK 74023, (918) 225-6078, BS 81 OK City Univ; ME 84 Central St Univ

Gaudry, Florent P Seven Oaks Hearing Centre, 2300 McPhillips Street, Winnipeg, MB, Canada R2V 3M3, (204) 632-3527, BA 77 Univ of Manitoba - Winnipeg; MA 81 Northern IL Univ - De Kalb; 81–Aud, Manitoba Dept Hlth, **A**

Gauer, Judith L 8701 Holmes, Kansas City, MO 64131, (816) 333-2650, BS 65 Univ of OK - Norman; MA 68 Univ of KS; Sp-Lang Path, Center Sch Dist #58, **SLP**

Gauger, Jaclyn Fritz Road, Worthington, MA 01098, (413) 584-3450, BA 72 Univ of MA - Amherst; MA 74 Northwestern Univ; 88–Aud, Clarke Sch for the Deaf, **A**

Gauger, Mrs Jane E 289 Bingham Circle, Mundelein, IL 60060, (312) 634-3243, BS 82 IL St Univ - Normal; MS 85 IL St Univ - Normal; 85–Sp-Lang Path, CCSD 96 Kilder Sch, **SLP**

Gauger-Crownover, Terry K 4901 Corona Way, Denair, CA 95316, (209) 668-2781, BA 77 Univ of the Pacific; MA 79 CA St Univ - Stanislaus; Tchr, Stanislaus Co Schs, **SLP**

Gaughan, Maureen E 20 Bluff Road, North Weymouth, MA 02191, (617) 340-0413, BS 78 Northeastern Univ; MS 79 Univ of MI - Ann Arbor; SLP, Communication Rehab Specialists Inc, **SLP**

Gaul, Bridget I 1600 Rt 228, Mars, PA 16046, (216) 238-5395, MA 88 Kent St Univ

Gaul, Mrs Roxane Rosy 7337 Bayberry Road, Downers Grove, IL 60516, (312) 969-2177, BS 75 Northern IL Univ - De Kalb; MA 77 Governors St Univ; Sp-Lang Path, Westmont Sch Dist #201, **SLP**

Gaul, Vicki Bridges 702 Idlewood Lane, Knoxville, TN 37923, (615) 482-4081, BS 75 Univ of TN - Knoxville; MA 78 Univ of TN - Knoxville; Sp-Lang Path, Daniel Arthur Rehab Cen, **SLP**

Gaulbon, Mrs Lenore B 7100 Briarstone Lane, Canoga Park, CA 91307, (818) 781-3557, BS 75 Southern IL Univ -Carbondale; MS 76 Southern IL Univ -Carbondale; SLP, Private Practice, **SLP**

Gaulden, Mrs Phyllis Kay B 565 Stoddard, East Lansing, MI 48823, (517) 483-2750, BA 70 Univ of MI - Ann Arbor; MA 79 MI St Univ; SLP, E W Sparrow Hosp, **SLP**

Gaulin, Cynthia A 967 Macon Avenue, Pittsburgh, PA 15218, (412) 647-5575, BA 75 Wellesley Coll; MA 81 Univ of Pittsburgh - Pittsburgh; 88–Sp-Lang Path, Children's Hosp of Pittsburgh, **SLP**

Gault, Jennie 64 Vogel Circle, Arnold, MO 63010, (314) 776-4320, BS 81 Univ of MO - Columbia; OM 82 Univ of MO - Columbia; SLP, Missouri Sch for the Blind, **SLP**

Gault, Lynda M 7801 West 100th Street, Bloomington, MN 55438, (612) 927-0340, BS 72 Univ of the DC; MS 73 Univ of the DC; Coord, MN River Valley Spec Ed Coop, **SLP**

Gault, Sharon Tharp Route 2 Box 345, Jonesville, SC 29353-9644, (803) 427-5624, BS 78 Eastern MI Univ; MA 79 Eastern MI Univ; Sp-Lang Path, Sp Serv/Un Co Sch, **SLP**

Gauman, Lynn Louise 1809 Gait Circle, Warrington, PA 18976, (215) 576-8955, SLP, Abington Memorial Hospital, **SLP**

Gaunt, Mrs Barbara Brown Medical Gardens Hrng Ctr Inc, 111 San Marco Drive, Venice, FL 34285, (813) 485-4592, BA 74 Memphis St Univ; MA 76 Memphis St Univ; Pres, Med Gard Hrng Cen, **A**

Gaunt, Susan M 222 Collins Avenue, Balboa Island, CA 92662, (714) 675-1251, BS 70 Marquette Univ; MS 71 Univ of WI - Milwaukee; Sdc/Ch Tchr, Capistrano USD, **SLP**

Gaur, Mrs Cathryn Lea 401 Church Street #I-7, Hasbrouck Heights, NJ 07604, (201) 393-0169, BS 80 LA St Univ - Baton Rouge; MA 82 LA St Univ - Baton Rouge; 88–Sp-Lang Path, Garfield Bd of Educ, **SLP**

Gaut, Katherine Carol 2614 Artie Street Suite 24, Huntsville, AL 35805, (205) 533-9641, BS 81 Univ of Montevallo; MS 83 Univ of Montevallo; 88–Sp-Lang Path, Speech Care, **SLP**

Gaut, Mrs Snowdrop 706 South McCann, Springfield, MO 65804, (417) 836-5275, BA 62 Baylor Univ; MA 83 Southwest MO St Univ; Instr/Superv, Southwest Missouri State Univ, **SLP**

Gauthier, Mrs Gertrude 7669 Mariner Point, Maple Grove, MN 55369, (612) 627-3085, BS 64 Univ of IL - Urbana; MA 65 Univ of IL - Urbana; Aud, Spec Sch Dist 1, **SLP A**

Gauthier, Mrs Mary O Route 5 Box 65-B, Warrenton, VA 22186, (703) 347-5287, BS 69 SUNY - Coll at Buffalo; MS 75 Univ of RI; Sp-Lang Path, Fauquier Co Sch Bd, **SLP**

Gauthier, Rita Dresp 540 North 4th #7, Seward, NE 68434, BS 84 Kearney St Coll; MS 86 Univ of NE - Lincoln; 88–Sp-Lang Path, Lincoln PS, **SLP**

Gauthier, Sharon V 9750 N E 125th Place, Kirkland, WA 98033, (206) 842-4411, BS 71 SUNY - Center at Albany; MA 73 WA St Univ; SLP, Bainbridge Island Public Schs, **SLP**

Gauvain, Joyce Eileen 251 Big Sur Drive, Goleta, CA 93117, (805) 685-1788, BS 77 Univ of CA - Irvine; MA 84 Univ of CA - Santa Barbara; Sp-Lang Path, Rehab Inst at Santa Barbara, **SLP**

Gauz, Dr Maurice T 65 Roberts Street, Mountain Top, PA 18707, (717) 636-0559, BA 75 Muhlenberg Coll; MA 77 Wayne St Univ - Sch of Med; PH 81 (NS) Wayne St Univ - Sch of Med; Aud, Samuel Rizzo MD, **A**

Gavacs, Nancy M 31 Marne Road, Cheektowaga, NY 14215, (716) 894-2946, BS 85 SUNY - Coll at Buffalo; MS 86 SUNY - Coll at Buffalo; Sp-Lang Path, UCP, **SLP**

Gavarin, Mindy L 141-12 77th Avenue, Flushing, NY 11367, (718) 591-8100, BA 77 CUNY - Queens Coll; MA 78 CUNY - Queens Coll; Sp-Lang Path, Birch Sch for Except Chldn, **SLP**

Gavett, Elizabeth Dept Communication Disorders, Boston University, 48 Cummington Street, Boston, MA 02215, (617) 353-3271, BS 72 Univ of CT; MA 73 Univ of Pittsburgh - Pittsburgh; Clin Assoc Prof, Boston University, **SLP**

Gavin, Beatrice 2 Louis Drive, Melville, NY 11747, BA 84 Hofstra Univ; MS 86 Adelphi Univ; **SLP**

Gavin, Carol P 8415 Knapp Road, West Falls, NY 14170, **SLP**

Gavin, Jo Lynn P O Box 41066, Baton Rouge, LA 70835, (504) 292-9486, **SLP**

Gavin, Dr Kenneth J Marquette University, Speech Path And Audiology, Milwaukee, WI 53233, (414) 224-3428, BA 68 Fordham Univ; MA 72 SUNY - Center at Buffalo; PH 80 (NS) Northwestern Univ; Asst Prof-Commun Dis, Marquette U, **SLP**

Gavin, Linda V 280 Chapalita Drive, Encinitas, CA 92024, (619) 272-9023, BA 70 Saint John's Univ - Jamaica; MA 73 Hofstra Univ; 78–Sp-Lang Path, San Diego Cty Sch, **SLP**

Gavin, Mrs Nancy D 2602 Valencia, Santa Ana, CA 92706, (714) 541-9183, BA 70 Univ of CA - Irvine; MA 76 CA St Univ - Fullerton; Sp-Lang Path, Sp & Lang Dev Ctr, **SLP**

Gavin, Sharon K 28 Kings Grant Way, Scarborough, NY 10510, (914) 631-8777, BS 71 SUNY - Coll at Geneseo; MS 72 PA St Univ - Univ Park; Dir, Private Practice, **A**

Gavinski, Janice Lange 5406 Retana Drive, Madison, WI 53714, (608) 221-6300, BA 76 MI St Univ; MS 78 Univ of WI - Madison; Aud, Madison Metro Sch Dist, **A**

Gavrock, Robbie Angeline 4832 Mallard Nest Drive, Memphis, TN 38115, (601) 895-2256, BA 78 Univ of MS; MA 81 Memphis St Univ; Sp-Lang Path, Olive Branch Elem Sch, **SLP**

Gaw, Mrs Sally A 10908 South Kenneth, Oak Lawn, IL 60453, (312) 448-6520, BS 77 Marquette Univ; MS 78 Marquette Univ; SLP, Lnt J P Kennedy School, **SLP**

Gawey, Susan Kay 3810 South Florence Place, Tulsa, OK 74105, (918) 742-1597, MA 88 Univ of Tulsa

Gawlik, Janice L 2017 Kimball Avenue, Arnold, PA 15068, (412) 282-6806, BS 80 Indiana Univ of PA; MS 81 Indiana Univ of PA; Sp-Lang Path, Visiting Nurse Assn Butler Co, **SLP**

Gawrys, Mrs Elaine E 2702 Homeyer Road, North Tonawanda, NY 14120, (716) 694-3200, BS 73 SUNY - Coll at Fredonia; MS 76 SUNY - Coll at Buffalo; Tchr, N Tonawanda Bd of Ed, **SLP**

Gay, Mrs Bonnie T 1108 South Gary Street, Monahans, TX 79756, (915) 943-2372, BA 69 CUNY - Brooklyn Coll; MA 77 NM St Univ; Educational Diagnostician, Monahans ISD, **SLP**

Gay, Helen Kemp 806 River Drive, Greenville, NC 27834, PH (NS); **SLP**

Gay, Mrs Helen S 3801 Norwood Court, Sarasota, FL 34234, (813) 355-2366, BS 56 Bridgewater St Coll; ME 61 Boston Univ; **SLP LM**

Gay, Mrs Joan M 90 Brookside Drive, West Hartford, CT 06107, (203) 232-9200, BS 64 Univ of IL - Urbana; MS 65 Adelphi Univ; Coord Sp-Lang Path, Town of W Hartford, **SLP ACE**

Gay, Lynn 1552 Clought Street #12, Bowling Green, OH 43402, (419) 354-2979, MA 87 Eastern MI Univ; Sp-Lang Path, Fremont City Schs

Gay, Mary Lee 5831 Winslow Road, Whitehouse, OH 43571, (419) 877-0156, BS 85 Bowling Green St Univ; MA 87 Eastern MI Univ

Gay, Susan Marie 39 Worthington Avenue, Shrewsbury, MA 01545, (617) 485-3176, BS 74 Worcester St Coll; MS 84 Worcester St Coll; **SLP**

Gay, Mrs Yvonne Louise 21290 Woodland Glen #202, Northville, MI 48167, (313) 348-7936, BS 86 Western MI Univ; MA 86 Western MI Univ; **SLP**

Gayan, Lou Ann K 536 Marcy Street, Ottawa, IL 61350, BA 76 Augustana Coll; MS 77 Bradley Univ; 79–Sp/Lang Path, Ottawa Elem Dist 141, **SLP**

Gaydos, William John Country Hill Road #14, Bldg 2, Orwigsburg, PA 17961, (717) 544-4738, ME 72 Bloomsburg Univ of PA; ME 83 Indiana Univ of PA; SLP, Schuylkill Co Iu #29, **SLP**

Gayheart, Tamara Lyn 332 Southeast 29th Street, Portland, OR 97214, MA 84 Bowling Green St Univ; Sp-Lang Path, Providence Med Ctr, **SLP**

Gayler, Barbara C P O Box 703, Llano, TX 78643, (915) 247-3461, MA 73 Univ of the Pacific; Sp-Lang Path, Private Practice, **SLP**

Gayler, Rebecca R 3844 Battleground Avenue, #73, Greensboro, NC 27410, (919) 388-5597, BA 81 NC St Univ at Raleigh; MS 82 East Carolina Univ; Sp-Lang Path, Healthcore, **SLP**

Gaylin, Mrs Rita A 4617 Norwood Drive, Chevy Chase, MD 20815, (301) 656-4367, BA 57 OH St Univ; MA 77 Univ of MD - College Park; Sp-Lang Path, Private Practice, **SLP ACE**

Gaylor, Mrs Minnie Jean 12305 Inletridge Drive, Maryland Heights, MO 63043, (314) 821-0008, BA 72 SC St Coll; MA 73 Univ of IL - Urbana; Dir Commun Dis, Prof Rehab Ctr, **SLP**

Gaylord, Mrs Cathy W 286 Sandhurst Road, Columbia, SC 29210, (803) 798-9606, BS 73 Univ of GA; ME 74 Univ of GA; **SLP**

Gaylord, Donna J 10 Union Street, Keene, NH 03431, (603) 352-6955, BA 78 Allegheny Coll; MS 80 Syracuse Univ; 84–Sp-Lang Path, Sch Admin Unit 38, **SLP**

Gaylord, Mrs Sondra P 5670 Lamplighter Road, Girard, OH 44420, (216) 759-7605, BS 55 IN Univ - Bloomington; ME 77 VA Polytechnic Inst St Univ; 81–Assoc, S F Gaylord MD Inc, **SLP**

Gaynes, Mrs Andrea Sue 555 North Avenue #4V, Fort Lee, NJ 07024, (201) 941-4011, BA 82 Univ of RI; MS 83 Adelphi Univ; 87–Sp-Lang Path, ECLC of New Jersey, **SLP**

Gaynes, Vivien 200 East 33rd Street, Apartment 21 A, New York, NY 10016, (212) 689-1529, **SLP**

Gaynor, Colleen Edith 610 West 110 Street #14B, New York, NY 10025, (212) 683-6975, MS 84 Columbia Univ Teachers Coll; Sp-Lang Path, Montefiore Medical Ctr, **SLP**

Gaynor, Mary Learning Center For The Multiply Handicapped, 411 Waverly Oaks Road, Waltham, MA 02154, (617) 893-6000, BS 76 SUNY - Coll at Geneseo; MA 78 Hofstra Univ; Sp-Lang Path, Protestant Guild for Blind Inc, **SLP**

Gayton, Gidget K RFD Box 7, Shore Drive, Elizaville, NY 12523, **SLP**

Gazaway, Armen 5419 South Osage, Wichita, KS 67217, (316) 529-0669, MA 88 Wichita St Univ; 88–Sp-Lang Path, USD #259 Wichita PS

Gdowski, Becky Sue 1859 North 149th Court, Omaha, NE 68154, (402) 496-1243, BA Univ of NE - Lincoln; MA 85 Univ of NE - Lincoln; **SLP**

Geanious, Gregory Kevin P O Box 224, San Miguel, NM 88058, (505) 233-3475, BS 75 Univ of IL - Urbana; MA 77 Univ of IL - Urbana; MS 85 Univ of IL - Urbana; Sp-Lang Path, Gadsden School District, **SLP**

Gear, Mrs Ann V 21316 W Spruce, Lake Zurich, IL 60047, (312) 367-4300, BS 84 Bradley Univ; MA 85 Northwestern Univ; **A**

Gear, Mrs Nancy H 4 Worth Street, South Burlington, VT 05401, **SLP**

Gear, Mrs Susan Campbell 8000 Five Mile Road, Suite 350, Cincinnati, OH 45230, (513) 232-2299, BS 82 Miami Univ - Oxford; MA 84 Univ of TN - Knoxville; 84–Aud, ENT Surgeons of Cinti Inc, **A**

Geary, Arlene Kopperud 26269 Weld Circle #66, Greeley, CO 80631-9632, (303) 226-2345, BS 75 Saint Cloud St Univ; MS 76 Univ of WI - Madison; Sp/Lang Path, Foothills Gateway Rehab Cen, **SLP**

Geary, Mrs Joan C 942-B 8th Avenue, Honolulu, HI 96816, (808) 737-2258, MS 78 Univ of HI - Manoa; SLP, State of HI Dept of Ed, **SLP**

Geary, Mrs Patricia J 930 Sweetmilk Creek Road, Center Brunswick, NY 12180, (518) 447-5211, BA 72 Hartwick Coll; MS 76 Coll of Saint Rose; Prog Dir,Dev Disabil Prog, Parsons Child & Family Cen, **SLP**

Geary-Cook, Kathleen 312 South Thornwood Drive, Lindenhurst, IL 60046, (312) 367-4300, BS 76 1865; MS 79 Univ of AZ; 81–Sp-Lang Path, Lake McHenry Regional Program, **SLP**

Gebelein, Mary Lynn 4140 North Paulina, Chicago, IL 60613, (312) 491-3165, BA 82 Univ of IA; MA 84 Univ of IA; Audiologist, N Western Univ Hearing Clinic, **A**

Geberin, Mrs Joanne White 640 173rd Street, Hammond, IN 46324, (219) 932-5700, **SLP**

Gebhardt, Dr Carol J 9103 Cinnebar Drive, Indianapolis, IN 46268, (317) 848-3621, BS 67 Purdue Univ - West Lafayette; MS 70 Purdue Univ - West Lafayette; PH 72 (Aud) Purdue Univ - West Lafayette; 83–Aud, Hrng Laboratory Inc, **A**

Gebhardt, Tamara Jayne 1012 North Summit #2-C, Iowa City, IA 52240, (319) 359-1371, BS 84 SD St Univ; MS 86 Fontbonne Coll; Sp-Lang Path, Mississippi Bend AEA, **SLP**

Gebhart, Janice Lou M Route 2 Box 64-P, Rockdale, TX 76567, (512) 446-2501, BS 73 Univ of TX - Austin; ME 80 Southwest TX St Univ; Sp-Lang Path, Rockdale ISD, **SLP**

Gebheim, Mrs Janie Fairchilds Box 766, Pleasanton, TX 78064, (512) 569-3979, BS 65 Univ Southern MS-Hattiesburg; MS 66 Univ Southern MS-Hattiesburg; Aud, **A**

Geclewicz, Mirla 4232 East Cactus #100, Phoenix, AZ 85032, (602) 953-9236, BA 72 Montclair St Coll; ME 75 Seton Hall Univ; Sp-Lang Path, Prof Sp & Lang Serv, **SLP**

Geddes, David Andrew 3170 Bentwood Circle South, Drive #2, Indianapolis, IN 46268-2886, (317) 848-3621, OB 84 Univ of MN - Duluth; BS 84 Univ of MN - Duluth; MA 85 IN Univ - Bloomington; Aud, The Hearing Lab,Inc, **A**

Geddes, Roger Charles 6211 Birchmont Drive, Bemidji, MN 56601, (218) 679-3456, **SLP**

Gee, Erin M Scripps Clinic And Research Foundation, 10666 North Torrey Pines Road, La Jolla, CA 92037, (619) 455-8998, BA 80 San Diego St Univ; MA 81 San Diego St Univ; 85–Aud, Scripps Clinic, **A**

Gee, Zilphia T 4311 23rd Parkway #502, Temple Hills, MD 20748-4464, **SLP ACE**

Geehan, George Ryan R R 2 Box 167, Foster, RI 02825, (401) 277-5485, **A**

Geelan, Mrs Susan Barber 275 Parkside Avenue, Buffalo, NY 14214, (716) 834-8086, BS 81 SUNY - Coll at Buffalo; MS 86 SUNY - Coll at Buffalo

Geen, Judy M 4922 Wallbank, Downers Grove, IL 60515-3402, (312) 620-4433, BA 72 Elmhurst Coll; MA 71 Northern IL Univ - De Kalb; Dir/Sp & Hrng, Dupage Easter Seal Treat Cen, **SLP**

Geer, Mrs Patricia Gartung P O Box 55 5920 Spring St, Mexico, NY 13114, (315) 963-3094, BA 77 SUNY - Coll at Potsdam; MS 83 Nazareth Coll of Rochester; **SLP**

Geers, Dr Ann Elizabeth Central Institute For Deaf, 818 South Euclid, St Louis, MO 63110, (314) 652-3200, BA 65 Washington Univ; MA 67 Washington Univ; PH 77 (NS) Washington Univ; Dir/Cl Sers, Ctrl Inst for the Deaf

Geery, Carol J RR1 Box 1890, West Rutland, VT 05777, (802) 775-3264, BA 73 SUNY - Coll at Plattsburgh; MS 80 Univ of UT; Sp-Lang Path, VT Achievemnt Cen, **SLP**

Geetter, Mrs Ava F 61 Bentwood Road, West Hartford, CT 06107, (203) 561-2902, BA 65 Univ of FL; ME 66 Univ of FL; Sp-Lang Path, Manchester Pub Sch Syst, **SLP**

Geffner, Dr Donna Speech And Hearing Center, St Johns University, Grand Central Parkway, Jamaica, NY 11439, (212) 990-6480, BA 67 CUNY - Brooklyn Coll; MA 68 NY Univ; PH 70 (NS) NY Univ; Ch,Dept Sp Comm-Dir,Sp&Hrng Cr, St Johns Univ, **SLP A F**

Gefroh, Tracy Ann 11 15th Street S E, Minot, ND 58701, (701) 572-6757, BA 84 Univ of ND; MS 85 Minot St Univ; **SLP**

Geglia, Mary-Jo 51 Maxson Street, Rochester, NY 14609, **SLP**

Gehan, Mrs Karen K P O Box 3883, New Hyde Park, NY 11040, Southern CT St Univ; Sp-Lang Path, League School, **SLP**

Gehl, Mrs Ellen Louise 5050 Wardcliff Drive, East Lansing, MI 48823, (517) 676-1051, BA 81 MI St Univ; MA 82 Eastern MI Univ; 87–Sp/Lang Path, Ingham Intermediate Sch Dist, **SLP**

Gehl, Mrs Pamela L 1716 Terrace Drive, Minot, ND 58701, (701) 857-4477, BS 73 Minot St Univ; MS 75 Minot St Univ; Sp-Lang Path, Minot Public Schools, **SLP**

Gehle, Mrs Phyllis D 17 Ridgecrest, Heber Springs, AR 72543, (501) 362-3404, BS 74 Univ of ND; MS 78 Minot St Univ; Sp-Lang Path, Heber Springs School Division, **SLP**

Gehlhausen, Pamela Sue 700 Highland Street, Asheboro, NC 27203, (919) 629-3598, BS 83 Purdue Univ - West Lafayette; MS 85 Purdue Univ - West Lafayette; Sp-Lang Path, Randolph Co Schs, **SLP**

Gehm, John R 12801 Midway Road, Suite 403, Dallas, TX 75244, BS 69 Univ of North TX; MS 72 Univ of North TX; Director of Audiology, Input Hearing Aid Center, **A**

Gehm, Patricia A Audiological Evaluation Serv, 12801 Midway Road #403, Dallas, TX 75234, (214) 484-8851, BS 68 Univ of Tulsa; MS 77 Southern Methodist Univ; Aud, Aud Evaluation Serv, **A**

Gehman, Jane Susan 3919 Gate House Lane, Box 889, Skippack, PA 19474, (215) 675-5005, BA 70 Muhlenberg Coll; MA 86 Temple Univ-Tyler Sch of Art; 86–Sp-Lang Path, InSpeech Inc, **SLP**

Gehringer, Mary Louise 71 West Avenue #60, Brockport, NY 14420, (716) 637-0008, BS 82 Central St Univ; ME 86 Central St Univ; Sp-Lang Path, City Schools of Rochester, **SLP**

Gehrke, Shari L 29820 Wilmot Road #3, Trevor, WI 53179, (312) 395-1440, BS 79 Univ of WI - Oshkosh; MS 81 Southern IL Univ-Edwardsvill; 85–Sp-Lang Path, Antioch Sch Dist #34, **SLP**

Geib, Mrs Gladys Gannon R R 2 Box 10G, Battery Lane, Jamestown, RI 02835, BA 77 Univ of RI; MS 80 Univ of RI; **SLP**

Geib, Mrs Janet R Medical Center Of Delaware, P O Box 6001, 4755 Ogletown-Stanton Road, Newark, DE 19718, (302) 733-1010, BS 76 Trenton St Coll; MS 79 PA St Univ - Univ Park; Sp-Lang Path, Medical Center of Delaware, **SLP ACE**

Geier, John Glover 1711 North Lockhart, Sherman, TX 75090, (214) 893-3114, BA 76 Univ of KS; MA 81 Northeast MO St Univ; Sp-Lang Path, Grayson Co Spec Ed Coop, **SLP**

Geier, Lisa Lyn 3600 Rainbow, Apt 313, Kansas City, KS 66103, (913) 384-9226, OB 83 Univ of KS; **A**

Geiger, Dianne W 5705 Wood Mouse Court, Burke, VA 22015, (703) 451-2238, BA 66 Univ of the Pacific; MA 68 Univ of CA - Santa Barbara; 73–Sp-Lang Path, Fairfax Co Pub Sch, **SLP**

Geiger, Mrs Gail A 686 County Club Road, Holland, MI 49423, (616) 396-8837, BA 63 MI St Univ; MA 69 MI St Univ; **SLP**

Geiger, Judy A 3712 York Lane, Cincinnati, OH 45215, (513) 385-8740, BS 78 Univ of Cincinnati; MS 79 Miami Univ - Oxford; Sp/Lang Path, Hamilton Co Off of Ed, **SLP**

Geiger, Mrs Julia O 4909 Dunn Avenue, Jacksonville, FL 32218, (904) 355-3403, BA 57 Mary Washington Coll; Sp/Lang Path, Sp/Hrng Cen, **SLP**

Geiger, Mrs Kristen L 20 NE Second Street #2105, Minneapolis, MN 55413, (612) 627-2708, BA 81 Univ of Northern IA; MA 82 Univ of Northern IA; Sp-Lang Path, Minneapolis PS, **SLP**

Geiger, Leigh Ellen 2421 North Feathering Road, Media, PA 19063, (215) 566-3263, BS 85 Bucknell Univ; ME 87 Univ of VA - Charlottesville; 87–Aud/Resource Tchr, Penna Sch for the Deaf

Geiger, Patricia 4750 North Elkhart Avenue, Milwaukee, WI 53211, (414) 546-6370, BA 59 Goucher Coll; MA 76 Univ of Denver; Sp-Lang Path, West Allis Memorial Hospital, **SLP ACE**

Geigle, Paula Rae 712 East Capital, Ellensburg, WA 98926, (509) 962-6208, **SLP**

Geile, Suzann M 1234 Divisidero, San Francisco, CA 94115, **SLP**

Geis, Rose Marie 1600 Finch Pl #2, Louisville, KY 40222, (502) 588-5331, MS 85 Purdue Univ - West Lafayette; BS 83 Purdue Univ - West Lafayette; Sp-Lang Path, U of Louisville, **SLP**

Geisen, Helana Sietsma 11706 Williamsburg Drive S, Knoxville, TN 37922, (615) 966-9056, MA 86 Univ of TN - Knoxville; 88–Aud, Knox County Schs, **A**

Geiser, Judith Ann 1145 Roland Lane #3, Green Bay, WI 54303, (414) 846-2834, BS 84 Univ of WI - Madison; MS 86 Univ of WI - Stevens Point; **SLP**

Geisler, Mrs Janice L 12 Meadowbrook Court, Bradford, PA 16701, (814) 368-5560, BA 67 Mercyhurst Coll; MS 72 SUNY - Coll at Buffalo; Sp/Lang Path, Bradford Area Sch Dist, **SLP**

Geisler, Lisa O 4605 Smokey Wreath Way, Ellicott City, MD 21043, BS 77 James Madison Univ; MS 78 Univ of TN - Knoxville; Sp-Lang Path, Howard Co Pub Sch, **SLP**

Geissel, Jean 379 Long Hill Road, Gillette, NJ 07933, BS 85 Bloomsburg Univ of PA; MS 86 Bloomsburg Univ of PA; **SLP**

Geist, Virginia Sefton Rt 8 Box 403, Lebanon, TN 37087, (615) 537-6524, BS 82 TN St Univ; MS 84 TN St Univ; Sp-Lang Path, Commun Skills Consultants Inc, **SLP**

Gelacek, Mrs Mimi Tobias 2054 Atwood Terrace, Coshocton, OH 43812, BS 72 Indiana Univ of PA; ME 74 Indiana Univ of PA; Doctoral, Kent State University, **SLP**

Gelaro, Mrs Glynnis Ann 461 Dela Vina Avenue #207, Monterey, CA 93940, (814) 238-4434, BS 79 PA St Univ - Univ Park; MS 84 PA St Univ - Univ Park; **SLP**

Gelb, Mrs Carol S 20 Old Lane Road, Cheshire, CT 06410, (203) 237-7835, BA 76 Rutger's St Univ - Douglas Coll; MA 78 Montclair St Coll; Aud & Ped Coord, Easter Seal Rehab Ctr, **A**

Gelb, Laura B 66 Gaby Lane, New Rochelle, NY 10804, (914) 636-8535, BA 73 CUNY - Lehman Coll; MA 74 CUNY - Queens Coll; **SLP**

Gelbaugh, Mrs Carole L 4539 Drayton Park, Hamburg, NY 14075, (716) 648-3172, BA 84 Univ of MD - College Park; MA 86 Univ of MD - College Park; 87–Sp-Lang Path, League for the Handicapped, **SLP**

Gelber, Mrs Susan S P O Box 481, Atlantic Highlands, NJ 07716, (201) 291-0266, BA 61 Montclair St Coll; MA 69 Seton Hall Univ; **SLP**

Gelberg, Bernice F 447 Albany Court, Goleta, CA 93117, (805) 967-4331, MA 71 CUNY - Hunter Coll; 88–Sp-Lang Path, Private Practice, **SLP**

Gelbert-Inbornone, Mrs Lisa 408 Driftwood Avenue, Melbourne Beach, FL 32951, (407) 676-1431, BS 81 Auburn Univ - Auburn; OM 84 Auburn Univ - Auburn; Sp-Lang Path, Private Practice, **SLP ACE**

Gelbs, Linda Susan 510 Wright Drive, Massapequa, NY 11758, (516) 541-7980, BA 86 SUNY - Coll at Buffalo; MA 88 SUNY - Center at Buffalo; 88–Sp-Lang Path, Long Island Jewish Med Ctr

Gelbwasser, Mrs Rhonda B 74 Harris Drive, Oceanside, Long Island, NY 11572, (516) 536-3328, BA 71 CUNY - Brooklyn Coll; MA 72 NY Univ; Sp-Lang Path, Private Practice, **SLP**

Gelch, Joan 83 Loring Avenue, Providence, RI 02906, (401) 861-6621, BA 58 Brandeis Univ; MS 77 Emerson Coll; Sp-Lang Path, Providence School Dept, **SLP**

Geldin, Alan M 58 Amberwood Drive, Grand Island, NY 14072, (716) 773-6426, BA 68 SUNY - Coll at Plattsburgh; MA 70 Syracuse Univ; Aud, Private Practice, **A**

Geldin, Irving H 5416 West Laurie Lane, Glendale, AZ 85302, (602) 242-7091, ME 60 Univ of Rochester; BS 52 Univ of Rochester; **SLP LM**

Gelety, Mrs Beverly L 309 Hollywood Boulevard, Steubenville, OH 43952, (614) 283-3764, MS 77 Miami Univ - Oxford; 77–Sp-Lang Path, Eastern Ohio Speech/Hring Ctr, **SLP**

Gelfand, Mrs Dolores E 241 Sabine Drive, Pensacola Beach, FL 32561, (904) 932-1534, BA 66 Case Western Reserve Univ; MA 67 Case Western Reserve Univ; Sp/Lang Path, West FL Reg Med Ctr, **SLP**

Gelfand, Mrs Janice K 101 Wayne Street, Jericho, NY 11753, (516) 933-2036, BA 69 CUNY - Brooklyn Coll; MS 71 Columbia Univ Teachers Coll; Sp-Lang Path, Private Practice, **SLP**

Gelfand, Mrs Shira G 634 Jarvis Avenue, Far Rockaway, NY 11691-5427, (718) 438-9174, BA 84 CUNY - Queens Coll; MS 86 CUNY - Brooklyn Coll; **SLP**

Gelfand, Dr Stanley A 101 Wayne Street, Jericho, NY 11753, (516) 933-2036, BA 70 CUNY - City College; MA 71 CUNY - City College; PH 73 (Sp & Hrng Sciences) CUNY - Grad Sch & Univ Cntr; Chief/Aud & SLP Serv, VA Med Cen, **SLP A F**

Gelfer, Carole E 20 Aberdeen Place, Glen Rock, NJ 07452, (201) 595-2208, BA 71 SUNY - Coll at Cortland; MA 76 CUNY - Hunter Coll; PH 87 (Sp Science) CUNY - Grad Sch & Univ Cntr; 88–Instr, William Paterson Coll, **SLP**

Gelfer, Dr Marylou Pausewang 3503 Dunstan Drive, Bloomington, IN 47401, (812) 855-5407, BS 75 Northwestern Univ; MA 76 Northwestern Univ; PH 84 (NS) Univ of FL; 85–Asst Prof, Indiana University, **SLP**

Gelin, Mrs Devora D 7354 North Braeburn Lane, Milwaukee, WI 53209, (414) 351-7390, BS 61 Univ of WI - Madison; MS 68 Univ of WI - Madison; Learning Disorders Specialist, Maple Dale Schools, **SLP**

Geller, Ann Harding 10614 Genesta Avenue, Granada Hills, CA 91344, (818) 997-2357, BA 77 CA St Univ - Northridge; MA 82 CA St Univ - Northridge; 80–SLP, Los Angeles USD, **SLP**

Geller, Mrs Barbara E 62 Elderwood Drive, Toronto, ON, Canada M5P 1X4, (416) 487-1888, BS 73 Univ of Toronto - Ontario; OM 75 Univ of Toronto - Ontario; Consult Sp-Lang Path, Sandra Henderson, **SLP**

Geller, Barbara J 117 Bedford Lane, Lansdale, PA 19446, **SLP**

Geller, Daniel 4084 Rusty Pine Lane, Liverpool, NY 13090, MS 75 FL St Univ; Aud, Private Practice, **A**

Geller, Elaine Fleisher 801 Union Street #3, Brooklyn, NY 11215, (212) 520-7358, BA 70 CUNY - Queens Coll; MA 72 CUNY - Queens Coll; Lecturer, CUNY-Queens Coll, **SLP**

Geller, Jean A S 312 NW 8th, Pendleton, OR 97801, (503) 276-0802, BA 57 Willamette Univ; MS 65 Univ of OR; Sp-Lang Path, En or Hosp & Trng Cen, **SLP**

Geller, Karla V S 626 Vista Valinda, San Clemente, CA 92672, **SLP**

Geller, Nancy Josephine 526 Glen Oaks Drive, Apartment 2D, Muskegon, MI 49442, BS 85 Western MI Univ; MA 87 Western MI Univ; **SLP**

Geller, Norman P O Box 1283, Lewiston, ME 04240, (207) 483-2400, BA 56 Boston Univ; ME 59 Boston Univ; SLP, St Mary's Gen Hosp, **SLP**

Geller-O'Dwyer, Kathie 5478 N W 79th Way, Parkland, FL 33067, BA 72 Adelphi Univ; MS 73 Adelphi Univ; SLP, Developmental Preschool Center, **SLP**

Geller Vogeli, Mrs Sherry R 2131 Standbridge Avenue, Long Beach, CA 90815, (213) 597-0815, BA 74 Univ of MD - College Park; OM 75 OH Univ - Athens; MA 81 CA St Univ - Los Angeles; SLP, LA Co Supt of Sch, **SLP**

Gellick, Mrs Ramona Rodery 5140 S W 87th Terrace, Cooper City, FL 33328, (305) 386-4413, BA 81 MI St Univ; MS 82 Univ of HI - Manoa; Sp-Lang Path, **SLP**

Gellinger, Susan L 211 Center Street, Whitesboro, TX 76273, (214) 564-6209, BS 70 CA St Univ - Long Beach; MS 71 PA St Univ - Univ Park; **SLP**

Gelman, Irene S 8500 Falmouth #1104, Playa Del Rey, CA 90293, (818) 761-4363, 61 CUNY - Hunter Coll; 80 CA St Univ - Northridge; 80–Sp-Lang Path, Los Angeles USD, **SLP**

Gelman, Mrs Nancy R 19 Darlington Drive, Wayne, NJ 07470, (201) 595-0319, BA 67 McGill Univ - Quebec; MA 69 Northwestern Univ; **SLP**

Gelman-Kukin, Phyllis 181 East 84th Street #16-G, New York, NY 10028, (212) 534-1921, BA 78 CUNY - Hunter Coll; MA 81 NY Univ; **SLP**

Gelmetti, Lisa Winters 401 Route 22 West, Unit 40-C, North Plainfield, NJ 07060, BA 79 Rutger's St Univ - Douglas Coll; OM 81 Hahneman Medical Coll; 87–Sp/Lang Path & Aud, Private Practice, **SLP A ACE**

Gelmon, Reesa Lynn 821 8th Street, New Westminster, BC, Canada V3M 3S9, (604) 522-1631, OB 77 Univ of British Columbia; MS 82 Univ of OR; 84–Sp-Lang Path, New Westminster Sch Bd

Geltman, Carol Lynn 805 Eddington Court, Bloomington, IN 47401, (812) 335-7439, BA 80 CUNY - Queens Coll; MA 82 Northwestern Univ; Aud, IN Univ, **A**

Gelzer-Hill, Brenda Eleanor 243 Wortman Avenue #6-H, Brooklyn, NY 11207, (718) 263-1587, BS 82 NY Univ; MS 84 Columbia Univ Teachers Coll; Sp-Lang Path, Interdis Ctr for Child Develop, **SLP**

Gemberling, Dorothy E 602 Union Street, Marseilles, IL 61341, (815) 795-2428, BS 52 Univ of IL - Urbana; MA 55 Northwestern Univ; 56–Sp-Lang Path, Marseilles Ut Sch Dist 155, **SLP**

Gemler, Marcia J 2011 Cottage Grove, Cleveland Heights, OH 44118, (216) 321-2178, BS 77 Univ of NH; MA 80 Cleveland St Univ; Sp-Lang Path, Cleveland Pub Sch, **SLP**

Gemmell, Terrance G 3922 Clausen Avenue, Western Springs, IL 60558, **A**

Genchur-Lukas, Janet Anne 350 Route 210, Stony Point, NY 10980, (914) 429-0209, BA 75 SUNY - Center at Buffalo; MA 77 SUNY - Center at Buffalo; Aud, Private Practice, **A**

Gendelman, Mrs Evelyn G 11140 Clover Avenue #37, Los Angeles, CA 90034, (213) 479-3144, BS 36 Univ of WI - Madison; MA 59 Univ of Southern CA; Private Practice, **SLP LM**

Gendrou, Mrs Diane Marie 409 Whittier Road, Spencerport, NY 14559, (716) 328-5272, BA 82 SUNY - Center at Buffalo; MA 84 SUNY - Center at Buffalo; Sp-Lang Path, Rochester City School District, **SLP**

Genereux, Jeanne C 285 Taylor Road, Stow, MA 01775, (508) 345-5250, BS 78 Northeastern Univ; ME 80 Northeastern Univ; 83–Sp/Lang Path, FLLAC Collaborative, **SLP**

Genereux, Mrs Kay Swanson 1802 Royal Way, San Luis Obispo, CA 93401, (805) 546-3148, BA 64 Univ of NE - Lincoln; MA 67 Univ of NE - Lincoln; Sp-Lang Path, Cuesta College, **SLP**

Generous, Christine Leigh 711 Ocean Hill Drive, Huntington Beach, CA 92648, (714) 536-8637, BS 84 Southern IL Univ -Carbondale; MS 86 IN St Univ - Terre Haute; SLP, Huntington Bch Cty Schl Dstr, **SLP**

Genet, Mrs Ellen F 14739 S W 54th Terrrace, Miami, FL 33185, (305) 552-5380, OB 77 Univ of FL; MA 79 Memphis St Univ; Sp-Lang Path, Baptist Hosp, **SLP**

Gengel, Roy Werner National Institute Of Standards & Technology, Bldg 225 A216, Gaithersburg, MD 20899, (301) 975-2945, BA 58 Knox Coll; MS 62 Univ of WI - Madison; PH 68 (Aud) Washington Univ; 88–Sp-Lang Path, NIST, **A**

Gengenbach, Mrs Muriel L 2624 Northaven Drive, Gothenburg, NE 69138, (308) 784-4525, BA 80 Kearney St Coll; MS 81 Kearney St Coll; Sp-Lang Path, NE Diagnostic Resource Ctr, **SLP ACE**

Genin, Grace-Ann 2012 Crescent Drive, Las Cruces, NM 88005, (505) 524-3522, BA 59 Univ of London - England; MS 79 Purdue Univ - West Lafayette; 87–Sp-Lang Path, Las Cruces PS Sys, **SLP**

Genkin, Marian Block 18 Levering Circle, Bala-Cynwyd, PA 19004, (215) 664-6852, BS 72 PA St Univ - Univ Park; MA 73 Northwestern Univ; 88–Sp-Lang Path, Private Practice, **SLP**

Genn, Mrs Brenda D S 64 Prospect Avenue, Hewlett, NY 11557, (516) 746-5575, BA 60 CUNY - Brooklyn Coll; MS 63 CUNY - Brooklyn Coll; Dir/Sp-Lang Path, Little Village Sch, **SLP**

Genn, Shari Joy 64 Prospect Avenue, Hewlett, NY 11557, (718) 604-5377, BS 84 Univ of MA - Amherst; MS 85 Columbia Univ Teachers Coll; Sp-Lang Path, Kingsbrook Jewish Med Ctr, **SLP**

Genna, Carolyn Marie 85-40 250th Street, Bellerose, NY 11426, (718) 343-2718, BA 86 Saint John's Univ - Jamaica; MA 88 Saint John's Univ - Jamaica; 88–Aud, Center for Improved Communication

Gennai-Rizzi, Janet L 672 2nd Avenue, San Francisco, CA 94118, (415) 751-5960, BA 72 San Francisco St Univ; MA 76 Northwestern Univ; Sp/Lang Path, Private Practice, **SLP**

Gennicks, Mrs Barbara A 802 South Iron Wood Drive, South Bend, IN 46615, (219) 654-7273, BA 78 IN Univ - Bloomington; MA 79 Ball St Univ; Sp/Lang Path, New Prairie United Sch, **SLP**

Genova, Mrs Wanda K 49 Winding Wood Road, Rye Brook, NY 10573, (914) 934-8986, BA 74 SUNY - Coll at New Paltz; MS 75 Adelphi Univ; Sp-Lang Path, Darien Pub Sch, **SLP**

Genovese, Mary Beth 30 Redwood Terrace, Flemington, NJ 08822, (201) 788-0116, MS 84 Rutgers St Univ -N Brunswick; Sp-Lang Path, Cerebral Palsy Assoc Middlesex, **SLP**

Gens, Dr George W Kean College, Union, NJ 07083, (201) 536-8965, BA 38 Univ of MI - Ann Arbor; MA 39 Univ of MI - Ann Arbor; PH 47 (NS) Univ of MI - Ann Arbor; **SLP F LM**

Gensel, Mrs Donna M 3360 Chichester Avenue, Apartment K-11, Boothwyn, PA 19061, (215) 485-8471, BS 76 James Madison Univ; MA 82 West Chester Univ of PA; SLP, Private Practice, **SLP**

Gensemer, Dr Ira B Geisinger Medical Center, Danville, PA 17822, (717) 271-6419, BS 61 Bloomsburg Univ of PA; ME 64 Temple Univ; ED 68 (Psychology) Temple Univ; 68–Assoc in Neurology, Geisinger Clinic, **SLP**

Genter, Ruth Z 916 Melrose Avenue, Melrose Park, PA 19126, (215) 635-4974, BS 77 Syracuse Univ; MA 80 Temple Univ; 85–Sp-Lang Path, Private Practice, **SLP**

Gentile-Lazarchik, Mrs Christine M 1516 Worcester Drive, Mount Lebanon, PA 15243, (412) 344-2152, BS 82 Indiana Univ of PA; MS 83 Indiana Univ of PA; Sp-Lang Path, Mt Lebanon Sch Dist, **SLP**

Gentner, Debarra S 1636 North Wells #3006, Chicago, IL 60614, (312) 975-5057, **SLP A**

Gentry, Mrs Alice Goldsmith Route 2 Box 52, Earlysville, VA 22936, (703) 832-2922, BA 68 Univ of VA - Charlottesville; MA 70 Univ of MD - College Park; 85–Sp-Lang Path, Orange Co PS, **SLP**

Gentry, Betholyn R 9309 Vanderbilt Drive, Little Rock, AR 72204, (501) 569-3155, BA 75 Univ of AR - Little Rock; MS 77; Asst Prof, U of AR/Little Rock, **SLP ACE**

Gentry, Donna M 34 Wight Place, Tenafly, NJ 07670, (212) 838-0685, BS 71 SUNY - Center at Albany; MA 73 Univ of MA - Amherst; Consult, NY League for HOH, **A**

Gentry, Mrs Joan Arrington 1110 S W 31st, Topeka, KS 66611, (913) 232-0551, BS 63 Univ of OK - Norman; MA 68 Univ of KS; Sp-Lang Path, USD #501, **SLP**

Gentry, Mrs Susan M Holy Family Hospital, North 5633 Lidgerwood, Spokane, WA 99207, (509) 482-0111, BS 71 Central WA Univ; MS 72 Univ of OR; 87–Sp-Lang Path, Holy Family Hosp, **SLP**

Gentry, Mrs Tina Marie 2942 West Yorkshire Street, Tucson, AZ 85741, (602) 887-5500, BA 81 Univ of OK - Norman; MS 83 Univ of AZ; 88–Sp-Lang Path, Amphitheater PS, **SLP**

Gentzel, Melora Jane 6247 East Knoll Drive, Apt #132, Grand Blanc, MI 48439, (313) 762-2362, BA 85 MI St Univ; MA 87 OH St Univ; 87–Sp-Lang Path, McLaren General Hospital

Genuardi, Sharon C 613 North Excelda Avenue, Tampa, FL 33609, **SLP**

Genuit, Christine 722 Fieldston Road, Bellingham, WA 98225, (206) 671-3655, BA 70 Univ of CA - Santa Barbara; MA 71 Univ of the Pacific; Sp-Lang Path, Children's Neuromuscular Prog, **SLP**

Genuth-Fox, April G 6669 Wildwood Way, Houston, TX 77023, (713) 453-8331, BS 78 FL St Univ; MA 80 Univ of Houston - Univ Park; Sp-Lang Path, Galena Park ISD, **SLP**

Genz, Michael G 1215 Pleasant #408, Des Moines, IA 50309, (515) 283-5780, BS 76 Southern IL Univ -Carbondale; MS 78 Southern IL Univ -Carbondale; 84–Dir, Aud Svcs Ltd, **A**

Genzoli, Linda Qualle 5400 South Tegner, Turlock, CA 95380, (209) 668-4606, BA 76 CA St Univ - Stanislaus; SLP, Hilmar USD, **SLP**

Geoffrey, Dr Virginia C 129 North Irving Street, Arlington, VA 22201, (703) 243-7181, BS 66 Purdue Univ - West Lafayette; MS 67 Purdue Univ - West Lafayette; PH 77 Univ of MD - College Park; Expert Consultant, NIH, **SLP ACE**

George, Audrey C 1129 North Jackson Street, Apartment 220C, Milwaukee, WI 53202, **SLP**

George, Mrs Carol P 103 Robert E Lee Boulevard, Vicksburg, MS 39180, (601) 636-4371, BS 73 Univ Southern MS-Hattiesburg; OM 76 Univ of MS; Sp-Lang Path, Vicksburg Warren Sch Dist, **SLP**

George, Catherine 220 S Perkins, Memphis, TN 38117, (901) 683-0424, BS 73 CO St Univ; MA 75 Memphis St Univ; Sp/Lang Path, Private Practice, **SLP**

George, Eleanor M 360 Andover Street, North Andover, MA 01845, (508) 682-6820, BA 52 Wheaton Coll; MA 53 Columbia Univ Teachers Coll; Sp-Lang Path, Dr Fred G Arragg, **SLP**

George, Gail S 13600 Otter Creek Parkway Apartment 115, Little Rock, AR 72209, (501) 455-4964, BS Southern IL Univ -Carbondale; MA 82 KS St Univ; 88–Sp-Lang Path, North Little Rock PS, **SLP**

George, Mrs Helen Gillies 2708 Pelican Bay Court, Plano, TX 75075, (214) 380-8517, BA 65 Univ of CA - Santa Barbara; MA 66 Univ of WA; Sp Ed Prin, Off LA Co Super Sch, **SLP**

George, Jeanne Hegarty 674 Mirandy Place, Reynoldsburg, OH 43068, (614) 866-2495, BA 75 Baldwin-Wallace Coll; MA 85 OH St Univ; 86–Prog Coord, OH St Univ, **SLP**

George, Jill Ann 143 Candle Court, Englewood, OH 45322, (513) 832-3504, MA 85 Univ of Akron; **SLP**

George, Kathryn A 2502 Babcock Road #1611, San Antonio, TX 78229, (512) 696-4541, BS 83 Tulane Univ; MA 85 Univ of TX - Austin; 88–Aud, Med Ctr ENT Associates, **A**

George, Linda Ann 1417 Lexington, Muskegon, MI 49441, (616) 739-4194, MA 79 MI St Univ; **SLP**

George, Linda Louise 2990 Ingalls Way, Eugene, OR 97405, (503) 688-8735, BA 77 WA St Univ; MS 79 Univ of OR; SLP, Bethel Sch Dist, **SLP**

George, Mrs Linda M 7 Carriage Lane, Barboursville, WV 25504, (304) 528-5189, BS 74 Univ of Miami; MA 76 Marshall Univ; Sp-Lang Path, Cabell County Schs, **SLP**

George, Louise Eddy 3605 Earnscliff Place #57, San Diego, CA 92111-4156, BS 75 Lamar Univ; MS 79 Lamar Univ; Aud Superv, Lamar U, **A**

George, Mrs Mary J D Rd 3 Box 229, Leechburg, PA 15656, (412) 845-2801, BS 71 Indiana Univ of PA; MS 74 Indiana Univ of PA; 72–Sp-Lang Path, Allegheny Intermediate Unit, **SLP**

George, Mrs Melba E 512 Highland Woods Drive, Mobile, AL 36608, (205) 476-1365, BA 74 Univ of South AL; MS 79 Univ of South AL; Sp-Lang Path, Rotary Rehab Hosp, **SLP**

George, Mrs Netia Lillian 901 Betz Creek Road, Savannah, GA 31410, (912) 236-4409, BS 84 Armstrong St Coll; ME 86 Armstrong St Coll; **SLP**

George, Patricia R 19029 Stedwick Drive, Gaithersburg, MD 20879, **SLP**

George, Mrs Pauline J 1515 23rd Avenue, Regina, SK, Canada S4S 5Z9, (306) 584-3019, BA 55 973; MA 57 Western MI Univ; 84–Sp-Lang Path, Regina Bd of Educ, **SLP**

George, Mrs Priscilla Hayfield 815 Valley Avenue, Solana Beach, CA 92075, (619) 532-9602, BA 81 Humboldt St Univ; MA 85 CA St Univ - Los Angeles; 85–Aud, Naval Hosp San Diego, **A**

George, William D, Jr 2637 S E 32nd Street, Topeka, KS 66605, (913) 272-3111, BA 71 Univ of AR - Little Rock; MA 73 Univ of AR - Fayetteville; Chief/Aud & Sp-Lang Path, VA Med Ctr-Colmery-O'Neil, **SLP**

Georger, Diane Duggan 8409 Great Lake Lane, Springfield, VA 22153, (703) 690-2919, **SLP**

Georges, Jill B 1940 D Johnson Ferry Road, N E, Atlanta, GA 30319, (404) 728-7624, BA 66 Denison Univ; MS 68 Univ of WI - Madison; Sp-Lang Path, Veterans Administation Hospita, **SLP ACE**

Georgiana, Angela Marie 608 Fox Croft Avenue Apartment 3C, Martinsburg, WV 25401, (304) 263-4267, BS 83 CA Univ of PA; MS 84 CA Univ of PA; 84–Sp-Lang Path, Sg Rehabilitation Agency, **SLP**

Georgiana, Beverly Jean 504 Orchard Avenue Apartment 301, Pittsburgh, PA 15202, (412) 741-9500, BS 83 CA Univ of PA; MS 84 CA Univ of PA; Sp-Lang Path, Watson Rehabilitation Hosp, **SLP**

Gepner, Rebecca S 1500 Brauer Road, Oxford, MI 48051, (313) 628-2100, BA 74 Montclair St Coll; MA 77 Seton Hall Univ; 84–Flint Center Program Director, Total Therapy Management, **SLP**

Geracci, Mrs Jane Marie 2102 Clark Trail, Grand Prairie, TX 75052, (214) 224-5551, BS 76 SUNY - Coll at Buffalo; MS 80 East TX St Univ - Commerce; SLP, Dallas ISD, **SLP**

Geraghty, Sheila Ann Mount Vernon Street, Newport, VT 05855, (802) 334-8090, **SLP**

Geraghty, Susan Green 4529 North Murray, Milwaukee, WI 53211-1226, (414) 632-3706, BS 77 Marquette Univ; MS 78 Marquette Univ; Sp/Lang Path, Racine USD, **SLP**

Gerard, Cheryl Burnett University Of Oregon, Clinical Services 3rd Fl, Eugene, OR 97405, **SLP**

Gerber, Adele J 8317 Childs Road, Wyndmoor, PA 19118, (215) 233-1315, BA 61 Temple Univ; MA 66 Temple Univ-Tyler Sch of Art; Retired, Temple Univ, **SLP F LM**

Gerber, Beth Pressner 8205 West Gulf Boulevard, Sunset Beach, FL 33706, (813) 398-4288, BA 76 SUNY - Center at Buffalo; MA 78 Univ of FL; SLP, Pinellas Co Schs, **SLP**

Gerber, Mrs Christine Grace 601 Lakeside Drive, Vicksburg, MS 39180, (601) 634-1565, BS 78 Clarion Univ of PA; MS 83 CO St Univ; SLP, Warren Co Schools, **SLP**

Gerber, Judy A 475 South Garfield Street, Denver, CO 80209, (303) 757-6201, BS 78 Univ of CA - Davis; BA 79 CA St Univ - Sacramento; MA 82 Univ of Denver; SLP, Cherry Creek Pub Schs, **SLP**

Gerber, Karen Elaine 1177 Norwegian #3, Modesto, CA 95350, (209) 526-4500, BA 83 CA St Univ - Stanislaus; MA 86 CA St Univ - Stanislaus

Gerber, Mrs Lynn Holland 1213 Hinshaw, Rose Hill, KS 67133, BA 80 Univ of OK - Norman; MS 82 Univ of OK - Norman; Sp-Lang Path, USD 259, **SLP**

Gerber, Mrs Marilyn S 5440 East Orchard Lane, Paradise Valley, AZ 85253, (602) 948-3999, BS 64 Syracuse Univ; MS 81 AZ St Univ; Sp/Lang Path, Affiliated Speech Path Serv, **SLP ACE**

Gerber, Dr Sanford E Department Of Speech & Hearing Sciences, University Of California, Santa Barbara, CA 93106, (805) 961-4157, BA 54 Lake Forest Coll; MS 56 Univ of IL - Urbana; PH 62 (NS) Univ of Southern CA; 65–Aud, U of CA, **SLP A F**

Gerber, Dr Sima D 95 Christopher Street, 8J, New York, NY 10014, (212) 255-6319, BA 69 Rutger's St Univ - Douglas Coll; MA 71 CUNY - Queens Coll; PH 87 (Lang Acquisition-Praomatics) CUNY - Grad Sch & Univ Cntr; Asst Prof, Queens Coll, **SLP**

Gerber, Mrs Teresa Ellen 14500 Bellmeade Lane, Darnestown, MD 20874, (301) 869-0996, BA 64 Catholic Univ of America; Sp-Lang Path, The Butler Sch, **SLP**

Gerberding, Mrs Karen E Route 1, Mayfield, KS 67103, (316) 326-3895, BA 72 Wichita St Univ; MA 73 Wichita St Univ; SLP, Sumner Co Spec Ed Sers, **SLP**

Gerber-Weshnak, Mrs Arlene G 6 Wenonah Avenue, White Meadow Lake, NJ 07866, (201) 627-3166, MA 84 Kean Coll of NJ; BA 77 Kean Coll of NJ; Sp-Lang Path, Rockaway Township Public Sch, **SLP**

Gerbino, Thomas C 4415 Metropolitan Parkway, Sterling Heights, MI 48310, (313) 977-8988, BA 72 Univ of MI - Ann Arbor; MA 74 Wayne St Univ - Sch of Med; 75–Aud, Macomb Aud Svcs, **A**

Gerbino-Redick, Mrs Sharlette 9440 West Verde, Las Vegas, NV 89129, (702) 799-7890, BS 75 Kent St Univ; MA 76 Kent St Univ; SLP, Clark Co Sch Dist, **SLP**

Gerdeman, Bernice Smith 1040 Woodmere Road, Columbus, OH 43220, (614) 422-8207, BS 72 OH St Univ; MA 85 OH St Univ; **SLP**

Gerdin, Mrs Meredith A 5663 Matterhorn Drive, Fridley, MN 55432, BA 69 San Diego St Univ; MA 82 Univ of MN - Minneap-St Paul; Sp-Lang Path, U of MN Hosps, **SLP ACE**

Gerdts, Marlin W 745 North Main Street, Blue Earth, MN 56013, (507) 526-3215, BA 54 Gustavus Adolphus Coll; MA 62 Univ of Denver; Sp/Lang Path, Blue Earth Pub Schs, **SLP**

Gereke, Mrs Helene D Speech Therapy Clinic, 139 Masters Drive, Conroe, TX 77304, (409) 856-6880, BA 68 Huntingdon Coll; MA 71 KS St Univ; Sp-Lang Path, Speech Therapy Clinic, **SLP**

Gerety, Martha Blessey 838 West 17th Street, Upland, CA 91786, (818) 967-2841, BS 65 Univ Southern MS-Hattiesburg; MA 67 IN Univ - Bloomington; SLP, Office/LA Co Supt Sch, **SLP**

Gergen, Ann Bauer 6140 Upper 46 Street N, Oakdale, MN 55109, (612) 770-8464, BS 85 Univ of WI - River Falls; MS 86 Univ of WI - River Falls; **SLP**

Gergen, Anne 2485 Fiedler Lane, Madison, WI 53713, BS 75 Univ of WI - Stevens Point; MS 77 Univ of WI - Stevens Point; Aud, Nicolet AudioDiagnostics, **A**

Gergich, Mrs Joyce Andrea R R I Box 480, Hammond Hill Road, Charlton, MA 01507, (508) 791-6351, BS 82 Coll of Saint Rose; MA 84 Univ of MA - Amherst; 88–Sp-Lang Path, Fairlawn Rehab Hosp, **SLP**

Gerhard, Mrs Barbara Foreman 329 Transylvania Avenue, Raleigh, NC 27609, (919) 781-2696, BA 68 Thiel Coll; MS 83 Univ of NC - Chapel Hill; 83–Sp-Lang Path, Wake Co Sch, **SLP**

Gerhardt, Dr Kenneth J 3614 N W 30th Place, Gainesville, FL 32606, (904) 392-2113, BA 70 OH St Univ; MA 73 OH St Univ; PH 76 (NS) OH St Univ; Assoc Prof & Chmn, Univ of Florida, **A**

Gerhardt, Mrs Melissa K 3614 N W 30th Place, Gainesville, FL 32605, (904) 375-4293, BS 78 Univ of FL; MA 80 Univ of FL; Sp-Lang Path, Gainesville Sp and Lang Ctr, **SLP**

Gerhart, Carrie Sue 6707 East 73rd Street, Tulsa, OK 74133, (918) 492-9414, BS 84 OK St Univ; MA 87 OK St Univ; **SLP**

Gericke, Marian Baldacchino 14361 Branham Lane, San Jose, CA 95124, (408) 739-9138, BA 80 San Francisco St Univ; MA 81 Univ of the Pacific; Spec Day Class Tchr, Sunnyvale School Dstr, **SLP**

Gering, Douglas A 217 West Buchanan Rd #138, Pittsburg, CA 94565, MS 78 UT St Univ; SLP, Pittsburg USD, **SLP**

Gerken, Dr George M Callier Center, 1966 Inwood Road, Dallas, TX 75235, (214) 783-3109, BS 55 MA Inst of Tech; PH 59 (Biopsychology) Univ of Chicago; Prof, U TX Dallas

Gerken, Mrs Shelly Lynn 4046 Triangle Road, Mariposa, CA 95338, (209) 966-3779, MA 87 CA St Univ - Fresno; **SLP**

Gerkin, Katherine Pike 4200 East 9th Avenue #B210, Littleton, CO 80262, (303) 394-7856, MA 78 Univ of Denver; Director Newborn Screening, **A**

Gerlach, Janelle 1969 W Mendocino Avenue, Stockton, CA 95204, (209) 931-4514, BA 79 Univ of the Pacific; MA 80 Univ of the Pacific; SLP, San Joaquin Co Office of Ed, **SLP**

Gerlach, Mrs Kirsty E 244 Glendora Avenue, Long Beach, CA 90803, (213) 515-3088, BA 80 CA St Univ - Long Beach; MA 83 CA St Univ - Long Beach; Aud, Los Angeles USD, **A**

Gerlach, Mrs Maureen Kay 6801 Emily Court, Westland, MI 48185, (313) 429-1524, **SLP**

Gerlach, Mrs Melanie L 61 Martinot Avenue, Rochester, NY 14609, (716) 482-0075, BS 84 OH Univ - Athens; MS 86 Nazareth Coll of Rochester; 85–Sp-Lang Path, Roosevelt Ctr

Gerlach-Pastor, Julie Ann 1 Cooper Avenue, Somerset, NJ 08873, (201) 533-5786, BA 83 Rutger's St Univ - Douglas Coll; MS 85 Rutgers St Univ -N Brunswick; 85–Sp-Lang Path, Saint Barnabas Medical Center, **SLP**

Gerling, Dr Irvin J Cleveland State University, Dept Of Speech & Hearing, Cleveland, OH 44115, (216) 687-3808, BS 74 OH St Univ; MA 76 Univ of MD - College Park; PH 83 (Hrng & Brain) Univ of TX - Dallas; 84–Asst Prof, Cleveland State U, **A**

Gerlinger, Mary Jane 634 Salem Heights South, Salem, OR 97302, (503) 588-1478, BS 57 Univ of OR; MA 64 Univ of WA; **SLP**

Gerlt, Elaine A 1803 Village Drive, Blackberry Village, Brewster, NY 10509-1317, (914) 962-2377, BS 75 SUNY - Coll at Geneseo; MS 78 Syracuse Univ; Sp/Lang Path, Putnam-N Westchester BOCES, **SLP**

Germ, Mrs Jane Mary Sutler Hearing And Speech, 2277 Fair Oaks Boulevard, Suite 290, Sacramento, CA 95825, (916) 929-2277, BA 76 Univ of the Pacific; MA 77 Univ of the Pacific; Sp-Lang Path, Folsom-Cordova USD, **SLP**

Germain, Ellen G 5 Kroner Farm Court, Upper Saddle River, NJ 07458, (201) 569-4895, **SLP**

Germaine, Lesley J 100 South Loomis Street, Southwick, MA 01077, (303) 775-2342, Sp-Lang Path, Windham School Department, **SLP**

German, Mrs Cathy McCracken 11430 Covington Road, Fort Wayne, IN 46804, (219) 625-3158, BA 85 Depauw Univ; MA 87 Ball St Univ

German, Janette S 1038 Poplar Street, West Bend, WI 53095, **SLP**

German, Susan B 4901 Staples Avenue, Fort Worth, TX 76133, (817) 534-5731, MS 71 FL St Univ; BS 68 Univ of TX - Austin; Sp-Lang Path, Fort Worth ISD, **SLP**

Germani, Mary Jo 209 North Lincoln Street, Apartment 2, Kent, OH 44240, (216) 678-4177, BS 80 Clarion Univ of PA; MS 84 Clarion Univ of PA; Sp-Lang Path, Kent State University, **SLP**

Germann, Mrs Paula Jo S 4400 Cherrywood Lane, Sioux City, IA 51106, (402) 494-3501, BA 79 Briar Cliff Coll; MA 80 Univ of Northern IA; 87–Sp-Lang Path, Western Hills AEA 12, **SLP**

Germano, Donna M 62 Woodhaven Road, Asheville, NC 28805, (704) 251-6091, BA 74 Cleveland St Univ; MA 79 Cleveland St Univ; Sp-Lang Path, Development Evaluation Cen, **SLP**

Germany, Barbara T 5335 Fox Ridge, Baton Rouge, LA 70817, (504) 292-4138, BA 84 Southeastern LA Univ; MA 86 LA St Univ - Baton Rouge; Sp-Lang Path, Abilities for Speech and Lang, **SLP**

Germany, Nena Maria Rural Route 1 Box 203G, 14 Sage Drive, Riverton, WY 82501, (307) 856-0461, BS 78 CO St Univ; MA 83 Univ of Northern CO; Sp-Lang Path, Private Practice, **SLP**

Germeck, Judith J 917 Stono Trail, Plano, TX 75023, **SLP**

Germinario, Mrs Carol Flagg 4 Foxwood Lane, Medford, NJ 08055, (609) 983-1800, BS 72 Trenton St Coll; MA 75 Trenton St Coll; Sp-Lang Path, Twsp Bd of Ed, **SLP**

Germono, Dr Joseph Frederick Sargant Coll Allied Hlth Prof, Boston University, University Road, Boston, MA 02215, (617) 353-3188, BS 64 1864; MS 65 1864; PH 73 (NS) Univ of MN - Minneap-St Paul; Cl Assoc Prof, Boston U - Dept Commun Dis, **SLP**

Gerofsky, Mrs Deborah Diton 8 Kingston Place, Huntington Station, NY 11746, (516) 385-7147, MA 84 NY Univ; 87–Sp-Lang Path, Commack Ctr for Commun Dis, **SLP**

Geron, Lynda B 2800 Woodley Road N W #113, Washington, DC 20008, (502) 581-4350, BA 68 TX Tech Univ; MS 70 Univ of OK Medical Center; **SLP**

Geronimo, Mrs Kathy Murphy Communication Rehab Inc, 313 Adams Street, Suite 8, North Abington, MA 02351, (617) 878-7100, BS 72 Fontbonne Coll; MA 74 Saint Louis Univ; Pres/Dir, Commun Rehab Specs Inc, **SLP**

Gerovac, Mrs Michelle Marie 134 Thistle Avenue, Tonawanda, NY 14150, (716) 689-7058, BS 76 Purdue Univ - West Lafayette; MA 79 Ball St Univ; Sp-Lang Path, Williamsville Central Schools, **SLP ACE**

Gerratt, Bruce R 4330 Kenyon Avenue, Los Angeles, CA 90066, (213) 824-3100, BA 71 Univ of MA - Amherst; MA 76 Univ of MA - Amherst; PH 80 (NS) Northwestern Univ; Sp-Lath Path, VA Med Cen, **SLP**

Gerraughty, Mrs Mary E C Box 23, Sylvan Drive, Hollidaysburg, PA 16648, (814) 696-0329, BA 68 Univ of MA - Amherst; ME 72 PA St Univ - Univ Park; **SLP**

Gerry, Lorna 1408 South Victoria Avenue, Los Angeles, CA 90019, BA 63 Univ of CA - Los Angeles; MA 75 CA St Univ - Northridge; SLP, Los Angeles USD, **SLP**

Gersen, Robin F 726 Sybilwood Circle, Winter Springs, FL 32708, (305) 699-9953, BA 74 CUNY - Queens Coll; MA 76 CUNY - Queens Coll; Sp-Lang Path, Orange Co PS, **SLP**

Gershbein, Holly Jane 12517 Deer Falls Drive, Austin, TX 78729, (512) 331-8435, BS 71 SUNY - Center at Buffalo; MA 81 Univ of Houston - Univ Park; Sp-Lang Path, Austin ISD, **SLP**

Gershenzon, Mrs Bonnie Esserman 3411 Vantage Lane, Glenview, IL 60025, (312) 327-4012, BA 71 Univ of IL - Urbana; MA 72 Univ of IL - Urbana; Sp-Lang Path, Louis A Weiss Memorial Hosp, **SLP**

Gershkovitch, Mrs Beverly J 1941 Bel-Air Drive, Ottawa, ON, Canada K2C 0X1, (613) 737-2286, BS 61 Boston Univ; 86–Sp-Lang Path, Children's Hosp of E Ontario, **SLP**

Gershman, Jennifer C 11138 Rutledge Drive, Gaithersburg, MD 20878, **SLP**

Gershman, Mrs Linda P 49 Audrey Avenue, Needham, MA 02192, (508) 580-7525, BS 71 Ithaca Coll; ME 72 Univ of GA; Sp-Lang Path, Brockton Public Schools, **SLP**

Gershon, J Casey 7362-2 Woodmoor Lane, Saugerties, NY 12477, BA 78 Univ of VT; MS 79 Univ of VT; 87–Sp-Lang Path, New Medico, **SLP ACE**

Gershwin, Mrs Dolores R 27 Neptune Avenue, Woodmere, NY 11598, (718) 528-7070, BA 71 CUNY - Brooklyn Coll; MA 75 Hofstra Univ; Sp-Lang Path, NY Bd of Educ Dist 28 Queens, **SLP**

Gershwin, Mrs Laynie G 35 Coddington Terrace, Livingston, NJ 07039, (201) 992-8344, BA 73 Kean Coll of NJ; MA 74 Montclair St Coll; Dir, Chldns Sp Serv, **SLP**

Gerson, Barbara Beer 15720 Ventura Boulevard, Suite 602, Encino, CA 91436, (818) 788-2061, BA 70 CA St Univ - Los Angeles; MS 76 CUNY - Brooklyn Coll; Sp-Lang Path, Neighborhood Psychological Srv, **SLP**

Gerson, Deborah E 6924 Ten Timbers Lane, Baltimore, MD 21209, (301) 484-8295, BA 70 Univ of MD - College Park; MA 71 Univ of MD - College Park; **SLP**

Gerson, Lauri D H 29 Leslie Lane, Smithtown, NY 11787, MS; **SLP**

Gerson, Mary 10 Elm Avenue, Wyoming, OH 45215, (513) 369-4000, BA 69 Univ of Cincinnati; MA 72 George Washington Univ; Sp-Lang Path, Cincinnati PS, **SLP**

Gerst, Joy B 2910 Ashebrooke Drive, Marietta, GA 30067, (404) 565-7917, **SLP**

Gerstein, Leonore 18 Varnum Street, Arlington, MA 02174, (616) 385-8535, BA 65 Hebrew Univ; MA 76 Western MI Univ; Sp-Lang Path, Kalamazoo Co Head Start, **SLP ACE**

Gerstenblatt, Deborah S 15 Saxony Drive, Warwick, RI 02886, (401) 739-3529, BA 77 Hofstra Univ; MA 78 Hofstra Univ; Sp-Lang Path, W Warwick Sch Dept, **SLP**

Gerstman, Dr Hubert L 18 Huntington Street, Natick, MA 01760, (617) 956-5300, BS 55 SUNY - Coll at Geneseo; ME 60 PA St Univ - Univ Park; ED 62 (NS) PA St Univ - Univ Park; Chief, Sp Hrng & Lang Cen, **SLP A F**

Gerstner, Mrs Janet C 9804 Wedd, Overland Park, KS 66212, (913) 888-6526, BA 68 Fort Hays St Univ; MA 73 Univ of KS; Sp-Lang Path, Olathe USD 233, **SLP**

Gerteisen, Mrs Rita A Brescia College Speech And Hearing Clinic, Brescia College, 718 Allen Street, Owensboro, KY 42301, (502) 686-4223, BS 83 Brescia Coll; MS 84 Lamar Univ; Aud, Brescia Coll, **A**

Gertge, Lynn Marie 110 Main Street, Fort Morgan, CO 80701, (303) 867-8297, BS 84 CO St Univ; MS 86 CO St Univ; 86–Sp-Lang Path, South Platte Valley BOCES, **SLP**

Gerth, Jean Louise P O Box 1883, Sandpoint, ID 83864, (208) 265-4712, BA 74 Univ of PA; MS 80 Univ of NC - Chapel Hill; 88–Sp-Lang Path, Boundary Sch Dist, **SLP**

Gertler, Mrs Susan Joy 20732 Brookwood Drive, Olympia Fields, IL 60461, (312) 957-7100, MA 84 Northwestern Univ; BS 82 Northern IL Univ - De Kalb; 87–Aud, South Metropolitin Assoc, **A**

Gertner, Alan B 19 Leone Road, Toms River, NJ 08753, (201) 240-2400, BA 72 Univ of Hartford; MA 74 Seton Hall Univ; Dir of Prof Serv, Better Hrng & Sp Ctr, **A**

Gertner, Mrs Jody M 82-07 155th Avenue, Howard Beach, NY 11414, (718) 856-4300, BA 78 CUNY - Queens Coll; MS 80 Columbia Univ Teachers Coll; Sp-Lang Path, Carl Fenichel Comm Sers Inc, **SLP**

Gertsen, Mrs Connie Bard 12 Sunrise Drive, Watertown, SD 57201, (605) 882-3177, BA 75 Univ of SD - Vermillion; MA 77 Univ of SD - Vermillion; Sp-Lang Path, Watertown School District 14, **SLP**

Gertz, Mrs Jil Marie University Medical Center, Department Of Speech Pathology & Audiology, 1800 West Charleston, Las Vegas, NV 89102, (702) 383-2313, BS 78 Wayne St Univ; MA 82 Eastern MI Univ; 83–Sp-Lang Path, Univ Med Ctr, **SLP**

Gertz, Thea-Gail 306 Bangor Road, Bala-Cynwyd, PA 19004, (215) 667-5461, BA 68 Temple Univ; MA 69 Temple Univ; Consult-Hrng/Sp/Indust/Ed, Private Practice, **SLP A**

Gertzulin, Michele 615 Lobos, Pacific Grove, CA 93950, (408) 372-8828, BS 85 Syracuse Univ; MS 87 Univ of AZ

Gertzulin, Rona S 3201 East Fort Lowell Road, Apartment 3028, Tucson, AZ 85716, (602) 621-1826, MS 78 PA St Univ - Univ Park; Clinical Instructor, Univ of AZ Dept of Sp & Hrng, **SLP**

Gervasio, Mrs Anita F 39 Intervale Road, Boonton, NJ 07005, **A**

Gerylo, Kathryn S 189 Whitley Drive, Winnipeg, MB, Canada R2N 1E5, (204) 786-7841, BA 77 Univ of Winnipeg - Manitoba; MS 79 Univ of WI - Madison; 79–Sp/Lang Path, Child Guidance Clinic, **SLP**

Geschke, Kathy M P 108 Woodside Avenue, Narberth, PA 19072, **SLP**

Geschwint, Jill Elizabeth 3032 North Halstead Street, Apartment 2C, Chicago, IL 60657, (312) 829-9115, BS 85 Boston Univ; MS 86 Boston Univ; Sp-Lang Path, Il Masonic Med Ctr, **SLP**

Gesell, Carol Grace 410 San Domingo Way, Los Altos, CA 94022, (415) 493-5000, BA 83 Univ of CA - Santa Barbara; MA 86 San Jose St Univ; 88–Sp-Lang Path, Palo Alto VA Med Ctr, **SLP**

Gessert, Eugene Kelly 603 Presswick, St Charles, MO 63303, (314) 946-7838, BS 83 Southeast MO St Univ; MA 85 Southeast MO St Univ

Gesser-Winter, Mrs Janet S 121 Ramsey Place, Albany, NY 12209, (518) 438-2309, BA 76 CUNY - Brooklyn Coll; MS 78 CUNY - Brooklyn Coll; Superv Sp-Lang Path, Parsons Child & Family Center, **SLP**

Gessini, Lisa J 13085 West Cedar Drive Apt, 210, Lakewood, CO 80228, (303) 988-8990, BS 81 CA St Univ - Hayward; MA 85 Univ of CO - Boulder; **SLP**

Gessner, Barbara Joy 1172 Kirk Drive S E, Grand Rapids, MI 49506, (616) 846-5960, BA 80 MI St Univ; MA 82 MI St Univ; 84–Aud, Drs Vanderveen & Degroot, **A**

Getchell, Sandra D 3127 North Baltimore, Tacoma, WA 98407, (206) 627-1394, BS 76 Univ of WA; OM 79 Univ of WA; Aud, Donald W Shrewsbury MD, **A**

Getlin, Jules P 209 South Detroit Street, Los Angeles, CA 90036, (213) 874-3300, BS 54 Columbia Univ Teachers Coll; MA 58 Univ of Southern CA; Dir Post Stroke Treat, Private Practice, **SLP LM**

Getman, Laura Whipple 1031 Garcia Ranch Road, Martinez, CA 94553, (415) 372-6608, BA 77 Univ of CA - Davis; MA 83 CA St Univ - Sacramento; SLP, U of CA Davis, **SLP**

Getsinger, Ruth H 9214 South California Avenue, Evergreen Park, IL 60642, (312) 425-3654, BS 69 Univ of IL - Urbana; MA 70 Univ of IL - Urbana; Sp-Lang Path, Private Practice, **SLP**

Getta, Mrs Jan P University Of Iowa, Hawkins Drive, Iowa City, IA 52242, (319) 335-8724, BS 78 Univ of IA; MA 80 Univ of IA; 87–Aud Supvr, Wendell Johnson Sp & Hrng Ctr, **A**

Gettelfinger, Mary Beth 33 Interlaken Avenue, New Rochelle, NY 10801, (914) 378-7501, BS 77 Ball St Univ; MA 78 Ball St Univ; 88–Sp-Lang Path, St Joseph Hosp Med Ctr, **SLP**

Gettenberg, Mrs Phyllis C 1600 Parker Avenue, Apartment 25-H, Fort Lee, NJ 07024, (201) 768-8484, BA 66 Hofstra Univ; MA 73 Hofstra Univ; Sp-Lang Path, Northvale Bd of Educ, **SLP ACE**

Gettinger, Daniel P 385 Hamilton Avenue, Hewlett, NY 11557, MA 78 CUNY - Grad Sch & Univ Cntr; **A**

Gettings, Sharon M 647 Chase Avenue, Lyndhurst, NJ 07071, (201) 915-6060, BA 82 Montclair St Coll; MA 86 Montclair St Coll; **SLP**

Gettys, Mrs Jill Marie 364 Bernhardt Drive, Snyder, NY 14226, (716) 837-2441, **SLP**

Gettys, Tina M Rural Delivery 3, Cambridge Springs, PA 16403, (814) 967-3322, MA 75 Edinboro Univ of PA; MA 75 Edinboro Univ of PA; SLP, NW Tri-Co Int Unit #5, **SLP**

Getz, Gail C 122 Wimbish Place, Danville, VA 24541, (804) 799-8620, BA 78 MI St Univ; MA 80 MI St Univ; SLP, **SLP**

Getz, Phyllis Prof Speech & Lang Services, 4232 East Cactus Road, Suite 100, Phoenix, AZ 85032, (602) 953-9236, BA 76 Montclair St Coll; MA 79 CA St Univ - Northridge; Sp-Lang Path, Prof Sp & Lang Serv, **SLP**

Gevaart, Mrs Carol C 101 East Milwaukee Street, Suite 514, Janesville, WI 53545, (608) 868-7658, BS 58 Ball St Univ; ME 60 Smith Coll; Sp-Lang Path, Sp-Lang-Hrng Therapy Assoc, **SLP**

Gevanthor, Peter Greene 1038 West Spruce Street, San Diego, CA 92103, (619) 465-0711, BS 78 PA St Univ - Univ Park; MA 86 San Diego St Univ; Sp-Lang Path, Kaiser Permanente Found Hosp, **SLP**

Geyer, Suzanne T W 331 South 314th Place, Federal Way, WA 98003, (206) 848-6661, BS 81 Northwestern Univ; MA 83 Univ of MN - Minneap-St Paul; Sp-Lang Path, Good Samaritan Hospital, **SLP**

Ghadialy, Fatema Beguwala 20 West Grand Avenue #F, Alhambra, CA 91801, (213) 483-4431, BS 82 Topiwala Nat'l Med Coll Bombay Univ - India; MA 85 CA St Univ - Long Beach; 86–Aud, House Ear Inst, **A**

Ghan, Mary 25642 La Cima, Laguna Niguel, CA 92677, (714) 855-2204, BA 74 Univ of CA - Santa Barbara; MA 80 CA St Univ - Northridge; SLP, Tustin USD, **SLP**

Ghandour, Leila A 54 Gertrude Place #3, Asheville, NC 28801, (704) 258-3005, BS 84 Western Carolina Univ; MS 85 Univ of NC - Chapel Hill; SLP, Thoms Rehab Hosp, **SLP**

Gharky, Mrs Marylou F 4506 Franklin Avenue, Mantua, OH 44255, (216) 673-7232, BA 51 Kent St Univ; MA 58 Kent St Univ; Sp-Lang Path, St Patrick Sch, **SLP**

Gherzi, Barbara M 5450 Kirkwood Drive #B-2, Concord, CA 94521, (415) 672-5281, BS 62 SUNY - Center at Buffalo; MA 76 San Jose St Univ; Sp-Lang-Hrng Spec, Mt Diablo USD, **SLP**

Ghigliotti, Sarah J D 40 Dwight Road, Middletown, NJ 07748, **SLP**

Ghio, Adele Ann 305 St Francis Boulevard, Daly City, CA 94015, (415) 756-9632, MS 87 San Francisco St Univ; **SLP**

Ghio, Mrs Carol Bennett 9335 Wister, La Mesa, CA 92041, (619) 463-0353, BS 75 Univ of MI - Ann Arbor; MA 78 San Diego St Univ; SLP, La Mesa School District, **SLP**

Ghitter, Dr Rosalyn 200 Towsontowne Court #402, Towson, MD 21204, (301) 321-3095, BS 58 Northwestern Univ; MA 70 George Washington Univ; PH 85 (NS) Univ of MD - College Park; Dir Sp-Lang Hrng Cl, Towson State U, **SLP**

Gholson, Mrs Sibyl G The Warrington Suite 9-C, 3831 Turtle Creek Blvd, Dallas, TX 75219, (214) 559-2585, BA 36 Hardin-Simmons Univ; MA 42 Univ of Northern CO; **SLP A F LM**

Ghosh, Constance R 1320 Marley Road, New Lenox, IL 60451, (815) 485-8495, BA 73 Univ of CT; MS 76 Vanderbilt Univ; Sp-Lang Path, Private Practice, **SLP**

Giacalone, Mrs Jeanine Marie 9063 South 27th Street, Franklin, WI 53132, (414) 241-5530, BS 81 Univ of WI - Stevens Point; MS 83 Univ of WI - Stevens Point; Sp-Lang Path, Therapy Assoc, **SLP**

Giacoma, Beth Feeney 2409 Chatham Drive, Wilmington, DE 19803, (302) 478-6491, BA 76 Mary Washington Coll; MS 79 Auburn Univ - Auburn; Sp-Lang Path, Occupation & Phys Therapy Svcs, **SLP**

Giacometti, Mrs Jeanne M B 303 Drake Street, Old Forge, PA 18507, (717) 347-6794, BS 68 Bloomsburg Univ of PA; ME 71 Bloomsburg Univ of PA; **SLP**

Giacone, Mrs Cheryl A 58 Iroquois Road, Arlington, MA 02174, (617) 641-2238, BS 79 Worcester St Coll; MS 84 Worcester St Coll; **SLP**

Giamboi, Lois E 37 Blaine Court, Staten Island, NY 10310-2807, (212) 351-6777, BA 75 Saint Johns Univ - Staten Is; MA 79 Kean Coll of NJ; Sp-Lang Path, Board of Educ Spec Serv Unit

Giammarino, Denise Vega 4501 Cedros Avenue #126, Sherman Oaks, CA 91403, (818) 885-2621, BA 84 CA St Univ - Northridge; MA 86 CA St Univ - Northridge; 86–Sp-Lang Path, Miller & Standel Sp Path Svcs, **SLP**

Giammittorio, Roberta 616 Fort Williams Parkway, Alexandria, VA 22304, (703) 971-0440, BS 74 Ithaca Coll; MA 75 5276; **SLP**

Gianelly, Mrs Cynthia C 38 Concord Road, Longmeadow, MA 01106, **SLP**

Giangrasso, Carol J P O Box 632, Highland, NY 12528, (914) 691-6136, BS 74 Minot St Univ; MA 78 SUNY - Coll at Geneseo; Sp-Lang Path, Ulster Co BOCES, **SLP**

Giannini, Coni J 4308 Charles Gift Court, West River, MD 20778, (301) 761-7196, BS 76 Eastern Nazarene Coll; MS 78 Loyola Coll; Sp-Lang Path, Ann Arundel Co Bd of Ed, **SLP**

Giannone, Toni L 63 Herrmann Lane, Easton, CT 06612-1942, (203) 795-6075, BS 72 Univ of CT; MS 73 Western MI Univ; 76–Co-Dir, The Foundation Sch, **SLP**

Giannoni, Rosa Esther 11875 SW 19th Lane #157, Miami, FL 33175, (305) 949-6156, BS 82 Saint Louis Univ; MA 84 Saint Louis Univ; Sp-Lang Path, Dade County Public Schools, **SLP**

Giardina, Candida 42 Carl Sandburg Drive, Hamilton Square, NJ 08690, (212) 698-7336, BA 76 CUNY - Hunter Coll; MA 78 CUNY - Hunter Coll; Sp-Lang Path, Chld Dev Cen/Coney Is Hosp, **SLP**

Giardino, Dorothy Ann 1651 D Parkline Dr, Pittsburgh, PA 15227, (412) 881-7254

Giattino, Dr Jill Arion 70 East 96th Street, New York, NY 10128, (212) 369-6470, BA 62 CUNY - City College; MA 65 CUNY - Hunter Coll; PH 71 (Sp & Hrng Sciences) CUNY - Grad Sch & Univ Cntr; **SLP**

Gibala, Janice Lynn 3277 Evergreen Circle, Walworth, NY 14568, (315) 331-2086, BS 83 Nazareth Coll of Rochester; MA 84 SUNY - Coll at Geneseo; Sp-Lang Path, Roosevelt Center Preschool, **SLP**

Gibb, Lisa C 110 Lowell Court #2, Princeton, NJ 08540-7018, (201) 322-3899, BS 84 Univ of WI - Stevens Point; MS 86 Univ of WI - Stevens Point; 87–Sp-Lang Path, Med Ctr at Princeton, **SLP ACE**

Gibb, Nancy Jo 1005 North Perry, Tucson, AZ 85705, (602) 628-5357, BS 80 Univ of CO - Boulder; MS 85 Univ of AZ; **SLP**

Gibb, Susan M 452 Oxford Street, Winnipeg, MB, Canada R3M 3J8, MS 74 Univ of WY; 76–Aud, Winnipeg Sch Bd, **A**

Gibbens, Noreen Daly 524 Shady Oaks Lane, Lake Orion, MI 48035, (313) 693-2813, BS 82 Western MI Univ; MS 84 Vanderbilt Univ; 87–Aud, Univ of Mich Hosp, **A**

Gibbens, Theresa Marie 219 Nordbye Lane, Rapid City, SD 57702, (605) 394-4036, BA 82 Univ of ND; MS 84 Univ of ND; **SLP**

Gibbes, Florence W La Motte Professional Bldg, P O Box 1117, Hilton Head, SC 29928, (803) 785-3733, BS 72 Syracuse Univ; ME 73 Univ of GA; Dir, Speech & Lang Professionals, **SLP**

Gibbons, Mrs Ahtoi 2 East River Drive, Willingboro, NJ 08046, (609) 877-3373, ME 87 Trenton St Coll; 88–Sp-Lang Path, Kingsway Learning Ctr

Gibbons, Mrs Carole Curtis 1421 South Potomac Street, Suite 330, Aurora, CO 80012, (303) 369-8449, BS 59 AZ St Univ; MA 60 Stanford Univ; Sp-Lang Path, Private Practice, **SLP**

Gibbons, H Elizabeth 292 Tennessee Drive, Bricktown, NJ 08723, BS 57 Kean Coll of NJ; MS 64 Kean Coll of NJ; **SLP**

Gibbons, Janet M E 7750 West River Road, Baldwinsville, NY 13027, **SLP**

Gibbons, Joan Walker 3167 Beechwood Road, Florence, SC 29501-9523, (803) 393-2572, MA 79 Columbia Coll; OM 85 Univ of SC - Columbia; Aud, Darlington County Schs, **A**

Gibbons, Mrs Marguerite F 15001 Sovereign Drive, Largo, FL 34644, (813) 462-9687, BA 67 Univ of MD - College Park; MA 71 CUNY - Queens Coll; ES 88 Nova Univ; Dir, Advanced Communicators, **SLP**

Gibbons, Patricia Jenkins 7 West Masonic View, Alexandria, VA 22301, (703) 243-2142, **SLP**

Gibbons, Peggy M 1650 South 15th Avenue West, Apartment 11, Newton, IA 50208, (515) 792-3749, BS 83 Univ of IA; MA 85 Univ of IA; **SLP**

Gibbons-Legros, Libby L 1628 Ramboullet, Paso Robles, CA 93446, (805) 541-3061, BA 80 San Francisco St Univ; MS 84 San Francisco St Univ; SLP, Pam Suess and Associates, **SLP**

Gibbs, Angela R 909 Palm Street Apt #A1, Bainbridge, GA 31717, (912) 243-0471, ME 87 Valdosta St Coll; 88–Sp-Lang Path, Bainbridge State Hosp

Gibbs, Mrs Cathy E 722 Eiker Drive, Knoxville, IL 61448, (309) 343-2143, BA 75 Augustana Coll; MS 76 Eastern IL Univ; Sp-Lang Path, Knox-Warren Spec Ed Coop, **SLP**

Gibbs, Dr Denise P 72 Shoshone Drive, Montevallo, AL 35115, (205) 665-6720, BS 74 Univ of Montevallo; MS 75 Univ of Montevallo; ED 85 (Special Ed/Comm Disorders) Univ of AL- Tuscaloosa; 85–Assoc Prof, University of Montevallo, **SLP**

Gibbs, Mrs Inez G 8 Central Lane, Northfield, MN 55057, BS 60 Univ of MN - Minneap-St Paul; **SLP LM**

Gibbs, Kathy L 8518 Birch Drive, Omaha, NE 68128, (402) 346-2716, **SLP**

Gibbs, Marilyn S 82 Wadhams Avenue, Torrington, CT 06790, (203) 379-0852, BS 70 OH St Univ; MS 81 Southern CT St Univ; Sp-Lang Path, Winchester Public Schools, **SLP**

Gibbs, Steven D 72 Shoshone Drove, Montevallo, AL 35115, (205) 665-5335, BS 74 Univ of Montevallo; MS 76 Univ of Montevallo; **A**

Gibel, Rosalind 1909 Rita Court N E, Albuquerque, NM 87106, (505) 268-5078, BA 73 SUNY - Coll at Cortland; MA 77 Southern CT St Univ; **SLP**

Gibert, Ivonne Teresa 7045 Soulier Lane, Fredericksburg, VA 22401, (703) 786-7592, BA 73 Barat Coll; MS 76 Univ of PR - Rio Piedras; 87–Sp-Lang Path/Clin Supvr, Mary Washington Hosp, **SLP ACE**

Gibian, Laura G 3605 Laurel Street, New Orleans, LA 30115, OB 78 Univ of Central AR; MA 81 Memphis St Univ; Sp-Lang Path, Baptist Med Sys Memorial Hosp, **SLP**

Gibler, Anne M 819 Bresslyn Road, Nashville, TN 37205, (615) 353-0327, BA 77 Brown Univ; MS 80 Vanderbilt Univ; **A**

Gibson, Barbara A 5987 Westmere Drive, Knoxville, TN 37909, (615) 521-7476, BS 71 Univ of TN - Knoxville; MA 74 Univ of TN - Knoxville; Sp/Lang Path, Knox Co Sch Syst, **SLP**

Gibson, Barbara A 317 Haines Avenue, Barrington, NJ 08007, (609) 883-5233, BS 80 Trenton St Coll; MA 84 Trenton St Coll; 88–Sp-Lang Path, Robin W Muller & Assoc, **SLP**

Gibson, Mrs Carolyn B 1 Whitney Street, Norwood, NY 13668, (315) 262-2100, BS 75 SUNY - Coll at Geneseo; MS 80 SUNY - Coll at Buffalo; 75–Sp-Lang Path, St Lawrence-Lewis BOCES, **SLP**

Gibson, Mrs Christina Rogers 4065 Lipsey Street #8, New Orleans, LA 70126, (504) 361-4469, OB 83 Hardin-Simmons Univ; OM 87 LA St Univ - N O Medical Ctr

Gibson, Cinda Lou 3298 Devonwood Hills NE, Apartment #A, Grand Rapids, MI 49505, (616) 957-7700, MA 81 MI St Univ; Sp-Lang Path, Grand Rapids PS, **SLP**

Gibson, Deborah Ann 9959 Adleta Boulevard #123, Dallas, TX 75243, (214) 341-8507, BS 81 Baylor Univ; MS 82 Baylor Univ; 84–Tchr, Richardson ISD, **SLP**

Gibson, Eloise J 5308 Kvamme Lane, Madison, WI 53716, (608) 873-7257, BS 73 Univ of WI - Madison; MS 74 Univ of WI - Madison; Early Chld Tchr, Stoughton Area Schs, **SLP**

Gibson, Mrs Frances Lane 618 Catalpa, Clarksdale, MS 38614, (601) 627-5247, BA 74 Univ of MS; OM 75 Univ of MS; Sp-Lang Path, Private Practice, **SLP**

Gibson, Jay Howard 3941 Boston Avenue, Akron, OH 44319-2811, (216) 379-8264, BS 54 Kent St Univ; MA 61 Kent St Univ; Dir-Commun Dis, Chldn Hosp Med Cen, **SLP A**

Gibson, Johanna J 8439 Bluegate, Houston, TX 77025, **SLP**

Gibson, Mrs Kathy W 8 Montclair Drive, Voorhees, NJ 08043, (609) 767-9462, BS 73 Old Dominion Univ; ME 78 Northeastern Univ; SLP, Council for Speech Development, **SLP**

Gibson, Linda Lou 5341 Escover Lane, San Jose, CA 95118, (408) 723-1867, BA 60 San Jose St Univ; MA 63 San Jose St Univ; 87–Adapted Comptr Tech Spec, Evergreen Valley Coll, **SLP**

Gibson, Lynda S 2709 Farnborough Road, Raleigh, NC 27613, (919) 846-2844, BS 71 Univ of VA - Charlottesville; ME 72 Univ of VA - Charlottesville; **SLP**

Gibson, Mrs Mary 3941 Boston Avenue, Akron, OH 44319, (216) 762-8959, BS 59 Kent St Univ; MA 64 Kent St Univ; Sp-Lang Path & Audiology, Private Practice, **SLP A**

Gibson, Mrs Patricia A 1230 Hinton Drive, Huntingtown, MD 20639, (301) 420-7474, BA 79 Univ of MD - College Park; MA 81 George Washington Univ; Sp-Lang Path, Prince George Co Bd of Ed, **SLP**

Gibson, Mrs Peggy Carver 502 West Hubbard, Mineral Wells, TX 76067, (817) 325-7460, BS 85 Lamar Univ; MS 87 Lamar Univ; 88–Sp-Lang Path, Private Practice, **SLP**

Gibson, Peter S 1880 Sodhaven Drive, Erie, PA 16509, (814) 868-1500, BS 77 Edinboro Univ of PA; MA 78 Edinboro Univ of PA; Sp-Lang Path, NW Tri-Co Inter Ut, **SLP**

Gibson, Ruth B Route 4 Box 228, Hutchinson, KS 67501, (316) 662-3584, BS 77 Phillips Univ; MA 78 Wichita St Univ; Sp-Lang Path, Hutchinson Hosp Inc, **SLP**

Gibson, Susan A 4321 South Atchison Circle, Aurora, CO 80015, (303) 788-4028, BA 80 Metropolitan St Coll; MS 82 CO St Univ; 88–Aud, James R Cate MD, **A**

Gibson, Mrs Suzanne Strickland 111 Fennell Drive, Monroe, LA 71203-3923, (318) 345-1037, BA 83 Northeast LA Univ; MA 85 LA St Univ - Baton Rouge; **SLP**

Gibson, Terrie Denise 1703 Cornwallis Road #H, Durham, NC 27713-5703, (919) 683-6470, BS 80 Elizabeth City St Univ; MA 81 Univ of IL - Urbana; Visiting Lecturer, North Carolina Central Univ, **SLP**

Gibson, Mrs Terry Black Rd#5 Sunset Valley Rd, P O Box 582, New Castle, PA 16105, (412) 658-4539, BS 79 Edinboro Univ of PA; MA 84 Kent St Univ; Sp-Lang Path, Lawrence County Rehab Center, **SLP**

Gibson, Valori Norris P O Box 65, Golden, TX 75444, (214) 768-2654, BS 78 Baylor Univ; MS 79 Baylor Univ; 85–Sp-Lang Path, Private Practice, **SLP**

Gibson, Virginia S 5460 Rowley Road #1711, San Antonio, TX 78240, (512) 690-0738, BS 85 Baylor Univ; MS 86 Baylor Univ; **SLP**

Gibson-Dossey, Sandra Jean 2600 Franks Drive, Madison, IN 47250, (812) 265-3448, BS 75 IN St Univ - Terre Haute; MS 84 Univ of Louisville; Sp-Lang Path/Aud, Madison State Hosp, **SLP A**

Gibstine, Mary A S 4717 Briarwood Trace, Carmel, IN 46032, (201) 536-8407, BA 77 Univ of MO - Columbia; MA 78 Univ of MO - Columbia; 87–Sp-Lang Path, St Vincent New Hope, **SLP**

Giddan, Mrs Jane Jaffe Caph Medical College Of Ohio, CS10008, Toledo, OH 43699, (419) 381-3521, BA 62 Cornell Univ; MA 63 Stanford Univ; SLP, Med Coll of OH, **SLP**

Gideon, Mrs Sheila Sered 2450 Cardinal Lane, Wilmette, IL 60091, (312) 256-2411, BS 60; MA 61; Sp-Lang Path, Glencoe Public Schools, **SLP ACE**

Giebel, Mrs Linda Ann 1235 Roosevelt, River Falls, WI 54022, (715) 425-6275, BS 82 Univ of WI - River Falls; MS 83 Univ of WI - River Falls; 85–Sp-Lang Path, Pierce Co Human Serv Dept, **SLP**

Giebink, Lisa Kim 12900 Shaftsburg Road, Apartment A-5, P O Box 192, Shaftsburg, MI 48882-0192, (517) 675-7548, BS 83 Western MI Univ; MS 86 Univ of WI - Madison; 88–Sp-Lang Path, St Lawrence Hosp, **SLP**

Giel, Mrs Janey Carolyn 3403 Glen Avenue, Easton, PA 18042, (215) 250-7133, BA 59 IN Univ - Bloomington; MA 62 Univ of IA; 88–Sp-Lang Path, Windsor SE Sup Union, **SLP**

Giella, Mrs Patricia Main Street, Roxbury, NY 12474, (607) 326-7031, BA 73 CUNY - Lehman Coll; MA 74 CUNY - Lehman Coll; Sp-Lang Path, BOCES, **SLP**

Gienger, Denny L Mountain Plains Audiology Associates, 1909 Mount Rushmore Road, Rapid City, SD 57702, (605) 341-1288, MS 77 Univ of SD - Vermillion; Co-Owner/Aud, Mt Plains Aud Assoc, **A**

Gierke, Mrs Suzanne V 665 Windgrove Road S E, Manetta, GA 30067, (404) 233-5332, BS 78 Auburn Univ - Auburn; MS 80 Univ of WI - Oshkosh; Sp-Lang Path, Atlanta Speech School, **SLP**

Gierut, Dr Judith A Speech And Hearing Sciences, Indiana University, Bloomington, IN 47405, (812) 855-9173, BA 77 Coll of Saint Teresa; MA 79 Univ of KS; PH 85 (Phonology) IN Univ - Bloomington; 88–Research Sci, Indiana University, **SLP**

Giesbrecht, Marilyn P 4760 Montalban Drive N W, Calgary, AB, Canada T3B 1E5, (403) 270-3711, BS Eastern MI Univ; MS 68 Southern IL Univ -Carbondale; 79–Sp-Lang Path, Calgary Bd of Educ, **SLP**

Giesow, Virginia Ellen 474-D Clay Road, Rochester, NY 14623, (716) 461-8554, BS 79 SUNY - Coll at Geneseo; MA 81 SUNY - Coll at Geneseo; 81–Sp-Lang Path, Monroe Dev Cen, **SLP**

Giess, Sallyann 263 Abbington Avenue, Buffalo, NY 14223, (716) 835-7497, MA 88 SUNY - Center at Buffalo

Giess, Suzanne Marie 811 Shawnee Drive, North Augusta, SC 29841, (803) 278-4788, BS 84 Univ of IL - Urbana; MA 86 Univ of IL - Urbana; 88–Aud, Carl M Nechtman MD PC, **A**

Gies-Zaborowski, Jeanne Ellen 3795 East Denton Avenue, Apartment 65, Milwaukee, WI 53207-5582, (414) 769-7980, BS 83 Marquette Univ; MS 86 Marquette Univ; 88–Tchr Asst, Marquette Univ, **SLP**

Gietzen, Deborah D 812 23rd Street N W, Minot, ND 58701, **SLP**

Giffin, Frances E 117 North Street, Hamden, CT 06514-4922, (203) 239-5387, BS 56 OH St Univ; MS 65 Southern CT St Univ; MS 81 Southern CT St Univ; Sp-Lang Path, N Haven Bd of Ed, **SLP**

Gifford, Mrs Catherine 184-51 Hovenden Road, Jamaica, NY 11432, (212) 523-3083, BS 51 Fordham Univ; MA 60 CUNY - Brooklyn Coll; Sp-Lang Path, Dillon Center St Josephs Coll, **SLP**

Gifford, Daniel Mark 248 East Bank Street, Fond Du Lac, WI 54935, (414) 923-1495, BA 72 Univ of WI - Madison; MS 81 Univ of WI - Eau Claire; Sp-Lang Path, St Agnes Hosp, **SLP**

Gifford, Grace M Bee Riddle Farm, Route 8 Box 326, Conway, SC 29526, (803) 248-2206, BS 74 SUNY - Coll at New Paltz; ME 77 Coll of Saint Rose; Sp-Lang Path, Horry Co Sch Dist, **SLP**

Gilabert, Nancy Rehn 106 Calle DE Jardin, Tucson, AZ 85711, (602) 622-5833, BS 66 IL St Univ - Normal; MA 67 Univ of WI - Madison; MS 86 Univ of AZ; **SLP**

Gilbert, Mrs Carol R 44 Knollwood Drive, Morris Township, NJ 07960, (201) 267-1850, BA 76 Elmira Coll; MS 77 Ithaca Coll; Aud, Drs D Peron & D Zenker, **A ACE**

Gilbert, Catherine 2758 Sicklepod Drive, Houston, TX 77084, (713) 578-1001, BA 72 Univ of AL- Tuscaloosa; MA 73 Univ of AL- Tuscaloosa; SLP/Aud, Katy ISD, **A**

Gilbert, Connie Lee 4247 South Highway 89, Apartment 15, Bountiful, UT 84010, (801) 295-0483, BS 85 UT St Univ; MS 87 UT St Univ; **SLP**

Gilbert, Ellen W 309 4th Avenue, San Francisco, CA 94118, (415) 752-7740, BA 80 San Francisco St Univ; MS 83 San Francisco St Univ; Sp/Lang Path, Private Practice, **SLP**

Gilbert, F Meredith 3445 Biegler Lane South, Salem, OR 97302, (503) 364-3131, BS 66 Lewis-Clark St Coll; MA 68 Stanford Univ; **SLP**

Gilbert, Ginger T Route 3 Box 109, Philpot, KY 42366, (502) 686-1120, BS 74 Western KY Univ; MS 75 Vanderbilt Univ; Sp-Lang Path, Owensboro Board of Education, **SLP**

Gilbert, Harvey R Pennsylvania State University, Communication Dis Program, 216 Moore Bldg, University Park, PA 16802, (814) 863-2010, BS 65 Boston Univ; MS 68 Univ of WI - Madison; PH 69 (Comm Disorders) Univ of WI - Madison; Assoc Prof, The Pa St U

Gilbert, Jane Marie 1545 Sleepy Hollow Road, Fort Wright, KY 41011, (513) 875-4893, BA 82 OH St Univ; MA 84 Univ of Cincinnati; **A**

Gilbert, Janet L 702 Redgate Avenue #A, Norfolk, VA 23507, (804) 623-4147, BS 80 Univ of VA - Charlottesville; MS 86 Old Dominion Univ; **SLP**

Gilbert, Mrs Jo Ellen 422 Elizabeth, Albion, MI 49224, (517) 787-2800, BA 79 MI St Univ; MA 80 Western MI Univ; Sp/Lang Path, Jackson ISD, **SLP**

Gilbert, Mrs Kristy K 2301 Ellison Avenue, Omaha, NE 68110, (402) 453-1278, BS 78 Univ of NE - Omaha; MS 79 Univ of NE - Omaha; Sp-Lang/Path, Omaha Pub Sch, **SLP**

Gilbert, Marcia Anne 12520 Bronco Drive, Tampa, FL 33625, (813) 892-4141, MS 85 Univ of South FL; **A**

Gilbert, Margaret B 4308 Goodfellow Drive, Dallas, TX 75229-2816, (214) 688-1995, OB 72 Southern Methodist Univ; MS 73 Southern Methodist Univ; Dir-Child & Adolescent Svcs, Dallas Co Men Hlth/Men Ret, **SLP**

Gilbert, Martha Malone 631 South Pickwick, Springfield, MO 65802, (417) 885-3282, BS 81 Southwest MO St Univ; MS 83 Univ of MO - Columbia; Sp-Lang Path, St Johns Medical Center, **SLP**

Gilbert, Mrs Mary Ann M 1908 South Norma Lane, Anaheim, CA 92802, (213) 698-0582, BA 75 CA St Univ - Fullerton; MA 79 CA St Univ - Fullerton; Aud Consult, Private Practice, **A**

Gilbert, Ramona Jane 6132 Northland N E, Albuquerque, NM 87109, (505) 277-4453, BA 78 Univ of Denver; MS 81 Univ of NM; Aud, Univ of New Mexico, **A**

Gilbert, Sharon Lee 3701 Mossleigh Street, Apartment 23-C, Mobile, AL 36608, (205) 342-6525, BS 86 Univ Southern MS-Hattiesburg; MS 87 Univ Southern MS-Hattiesburg; Sp-Lang Path, Hattiesburg Excep Lrng Center

Gilbert, Shyrle I 30705 Woodside Drive, Franklin, MI 48025, (313) 851-3834, BA 42 Univ of MI - Ann Arbor; ME 63 Wayne St Univ; Consult to Chld Dev Serv, Mt Carmel Mercy Hosp, **SLP**

Gilbert, Susan C EFMD P O Box 60, 97 General Hospital, APO New York, NY 09757, BS 74 East Stroudsburg Univ of PA; MS 80 Bloomsburg Univ of PA; Sp-Lang Path, Madigan Army Med Cen, **SLP**

Gilbertson, Mrs Anne Marie 139 West Union Street, West Chester, PA 19382, (609) 848-9551, BS 83 Towson St Univ; MS 86 PA St Univ - Univ Park; 88–REACH Prog Dir, Manor HealthCare Corp, **SLP ACE**

Gilbertson, Jean Marie 12334 Chandler Blvd Unit E, North Hollywood, CA 91607, (818) 985-1167, BA 81 CA St Univ - Los Angeles; MA 84 CA St Univ - Los Angeles; **SLP**

Gilbertson, Mrs Kim Annette 8354 Skyway, Paradise, CA 95969, (916) 872-2876, BA 84 CA St Univ - Chico; MA 86 CA St Univ - Chico; 86–Sp-Lang Path, Chico Comm Hosp, **SLP**

Gilbertson, Margie Lynn 840 Loeb Street, Memphis, TN 38111, (901) 767-7666, BS 80 Univ of Central AR; MS 85 Univ of Central AR; **SLP**

Gilbery, Mrs Josie Ann PO Box 114, Casselton, ND 58012, (701) 347-4029, BS 85 Moorhead St Univ; MS 86 Moorhead St Univ; SLP, Sheyenne Valley Spec Ed Unit, **SLP**

Gilbreath, Mrs Susan Hollowell 1201 River Ridge, Augusta, GA 30909-2215, (404) 737-7310, BS 80 Augusta Coll; MS 82 Univ of SC - Columbia; Sp-Lang Path, Richmond Co Bd of Ed, **SLP**

Gilchrist, Cheryl O P O Box 6035, Shiprock, NM 87420-8954, (415) 522-1670, BS 77 Univ of Tulsa; MS 79 Vanderbilt Univ; **SLP**

Gilchrist, Diane B Dept Of Speech & Hearing Sci, University Of California, Snidecor Hall Room 1663D, Santa Barbara, CA 93106, (805) 961-3793, BA 69 Univ of CA - Santa Barbara; MA 71 Univ of CA - Santa Barbara; Lect Sp/Lang Path, U of CA, **SLP**

Gilchrist, Florence S 1523 N E 77th Street, Seattle, WA 98115, BA 47; Retired, Seattle PS, **SLP LM**

Gilchrist, Linda A 3107 Morning Trail, San Antonio, TX 78247, (512) 653-1822, BA 75 Our Lady Lake Univ-San Anton; MA 76 Our Lady Lake Univ-San Anton; Sp-Lang Path, Judson ISD-Kirby Elem, **SLP**

Gilchrist, Mrs Shirley B 2808 Hastings Road, Birmingham, AL 35223, (205) 226-6557, BS 64 Auburn Univ - Auburn; MA 67 Auburn Univ - Auburn; SLP, Physn's Phys Ther Servs, **SLP**

Gilda, Dr Barbara Baker Audiology And Speech Center, 129 East Broadway, Louisville, KY 40292, (502) 588-5274, BA 70 Western KY Univ; MS 72 Univ of Louisville; PH 76 Wayne St Univ; Assoc Prof, U of Louisville Med Sch, **SLP**

Gildar, Mrs Enid S 11710 Plumosa Drive, Tampa, FL 33618-3624, (813) 251-0083, BS 66 PA St Univ - Univ Park; MA 72 Temple Univ-Tyler Sch of Art; Sp-Lang Path, Private Practice, **SLP ACE**

Gilday, Mrs Sheila Q 10097 Cedar Ridge, Carmel, IN 46032, (317) 893-7751, BS 57 Marquette Univ; MA 59 Marquette Univ; SLP, Indiana Girls' School, **SLP**

Gilden, Mrs Jan L 3019 Barnhill Lane, Sugar Land, TX 77479, (713) 776-2211, BS 75 Univ of TX - Austin; MA 77 Univ of TX - Austin; Aud, M D Anderson Hospital, **A**

Gilden, Laurie Susanne 5474 Edmonton Avenue, San Diego, CA 92122, (619) 483-6986, BA 84 Univ of CA - Santa Barbara; MA 86 Univ of CO - Boulder; **SLP**

Gildersleeve-Maffitt, Joanna Louise 305 South Howard Street, Fremont, NE 68025, (402) 727-6555, BS 85 Univ of NE - Omaha; MS 86 Univ of NE - Omaha; **SLP**

Gilder-Sloane, Lorie E 1026 Ozone Avenue, Santa Monica, CA 90405, (213) 450-7684, BA 81 CA St Univ - Northridge; MA 83 CA St Univ - Northridge; Sp-Lang Path, Santa Monica-Malibu USD, **SLP**

Gildner, Christy L 1575 Evergreen Place, Elkhart, IN 46514-4766, BS 78 Western MI Univ; MA 79 Western MI Univ; Sp-Lang Path, Elkhart Commun Schs, **SLP**

Gildston, Dr Harold M 2 Hilltop Road, Great Neck, NY 11021, (516) 482-4449, ED 64 (NS) Columbia Univ Teachers Coll; Prof, Cw Post Coll, **SLP A**

Gildston, Dr Phyllis S 2 Hilltop Drive, Great Neck, NY 11021, (516) 482-4444, BA 51 Cornell Univ; MS 59 CUNY - Queens Coll; PH 64 (NS) Columbia Univ Teachers Coll; Prof, Brooklyn Coll/CUNY, **SLP A**

Giles, Gerald L 1331 Grove Way, Concord, CA 94518, (415) 685-2355, BA 42 Univ of IA; MA 65 San Francisco St Univ; **SLP LM**

Giles, Nanette A 550 Rhodes Avenue, Mansfield, OH 44906, **SLP**

Giles, Richard B 602 Moore, Sikeston, MO 63801, (314) 472-2200, BS 61 Southeast MO St Univ; MA 70 Southeast MO St Univ; 78–Elem Admin, Sikeston Pub Sch, **SLP**

Giles, Susan J 932 Maple Drive, Franklin Square, NY 11010, (516) 747-5400, BA 73 Adelphi Univ; MA 75 Hofstra Univ; Sp-Lang Path, Human Resources Sch, **SLP**

Gilewski, Mrs Suzanne Eardley 124 Prospect, Rockford, MI 49341, (616) 887-7359, BS 82 Central MI Univ; MA 87 Central MI Univ; 88–Sp-Lang Path, Sparta Area Sch

Gilfoyle, Mary Nicol 404 Hazel Avenue, Endicott, NY 13760, (607) 773-4255, **SLP**

Gilgannon, Robert E 514 West 8th Street, Hazleton, PA 18201, (717) 454-7208, BA 49 Seton Hall Univ; MA 64 Seton Hall Univ; MS 81 Bloomsburg Univ of PA; Dir, Sp & Hrng Therepy Cl, **SLP A**

Gilhooly, Trudi Patricia 9623 East Valley Ranch, Apartment 1137, Irving, TX 75063, (214) 402-8313, MS 85 Univ of NM; 86–Aud/Sp-Lang Path, Private Practice, **SLP A**

Gililland, Mrs Susan V 110 Thompson Drive, Ada, OK 74820, (405) 332-2323, BA 70 CA St Univ - Fresno; MA 72 CA St Univ - Fresno; Sp-Lang Path, Valley View Reg Hosp, **SLP**

Gilinson, Mrs Pamela F 8 Bisbee Drive, South Salem, NY 10590, (914) 763-9480, BS 69 SUNY - Coll at Buffalo; MS 71 Hofstra Univ; **SLP**

Gill, Dr Alan Jay 52 Beach Road, Fairfield, CT 06430, (203) 255-3533, 57 Syracuse Univ; MS 66 Johns Hopkins Univ; MD 62 (NS) Syracuse Univ; MD, Drs Gill & Levinson PC

Gill, Dr Cynthia B PO Box 906, Greenville, TX 75401, (214) 454-2917, BS 76 Southwest TX St Univ; ME 77 Southwest TX St Univ; ED 86 (Special Education) East TX St Univ - Commerce; Fac, East TX State Univ, **SLP**

Gill, Mrs Cynthia Davis 16 Elm Avenue, Norwich, CT 06360, (203) 536-9710, BS 79 Appalachian St Univ; MA 82 Univ of SC - Columbia; Sp-Lang Path, Greenville City Schools, **SLP**

Gill, Mrs Elizabeth Bryant 3830 Fairfax, Dallas, TX 75209, (901) 761-1500, BA 84 Univ of MS; MA 87 Univ of MS; **A**

Gill, Dr Gary Dee Dept Communicative Disorders, University Of Wisconsin, 1975 Willow Drive, Madison, WI 53706, (608) 262-3951, BS 63 Western MI Univ; MS 67 CO St Univ; PH 75 (NS) Univ of WI - Madison; Fac Assoc, University of Wisconsin, **SLP**

Gill, James M 1115 8th Street, Woodward, OK 73801, (405) 256-5822, MS 88 Univ of OK Medical Center

Gill, Joanne 51 Longfellow Road, Mill Valley, CA 94941, BA 64 Brown Univ; MA 66 Stanford Univ; Prog Evaluator, San Francisco USD, **SLP**

Gill, Mrs Kim Ann 59 Highwater Avenue, Massapequa, NY 11758, BA 79 Hofstra Univ; MA 80 Hofstra Univ; SLP, Massapequa Public Schools, **SLP**

Gill, Lynn Ann 5546 Scranton Road, Raleigh Bldg #11, Hamburg, NY 14075-3759, BS 80 Northern MI Univ; MA 82 SUNY - Center at Buffalo; Sp/Lang Path, Bd Coop Ed Serv II, **SLP**

Gill, Patricia Ann 3540 Southwest 98th Street, Seattle, WA 98126, (206) 364-0300, BA 83 Eastern WA Univ; MS 85 Eastern WA Univ; Sp-Lang Path, Fircrest School, **SLP**

Gill, Terri L F Allied Health Services, 6224 Merger Drive, Holland, OH 43528, (419) 865-6700, BS 76 Bowling Green St Univ; MA 77 Bowling Green St Univ; Sp-Lang Path, Allied Health Services, **SLP**

Gillam, Brenda Gay 1210 Daffodil Lane, Longview, TX 75605-2834, (214) 581-7555, BS 78 Ouachita Baptist Univ; MS 79 Baylor Univ; **SLP**

Gillam, Dr Ronald B Program In Communication Dis, 125 Parker Hall, Columbia, MO 65211, (314) 882-4082, BS 77 CO St Univ; MS 79 CO St Univ; PH 88 (SLP-Child Lang Dis) IN Univ - Bloomington; 88–Assoc Prof, Univ of Missouri-Columbia, **SLP**

Gillam, Suzanne F 78-6920 Alii Drive #140, Kailua Kona, HI 96740, (808) 329-1351, BA 71 San Jose St Univ; MA 76 San Francisco St Univ; **A**

Gillaspie, Prudence Lynn 1764 Brentwood Drive, Mount Sterling, KY 40353, (606) 498-3104, BS 79 Eastern KY Univ; MA 81 Eastern KY Univ; 81–Sp-Lang Path, Mont Co Schs, **SLP**

Gillcash, Mrs Judith Ann Sansone P O Box 42, Windham Center, CT 06280, (207) 537-2371, BS 57 Syracuse Univ; MA 61 Univ of CT; Sp-Lang Path, **SLP**

Gillcrist, Molly M 6234 S E 30th Avenue, Portland, OR 97202, (503) 653-3852, BA 55 Duke Univ; MA 56 Univ of VA - Charlottesville; Sp-Lang Path, N Clackamas Sch Dist #12, **SLP**

Gill-Dorgan, Deborah 220 Winsor Street, Elkhorn, WI 53121, (414) 723-5842, BS 78 Univ of WI - Milwaukee; MS 79 Univ of WI - Milwaukee; **SLP**

Gillen, Carol A 1808 Waunona Way, Madison, WI 53713, (608) 263-8412, BA 70 George Washington Univ; MA 74 George Washington Univ; 88–Sp-Lang Path, Sp Path Dept Univ of WI, **SLP**

Gillespie, Cheryl D 2362 Hickory Creek Court, Apartment 2-A, Richmond, VA 23229, (804) 346-4534, **SLP**

Gillespie, Diane Susan 6923 S W 11th Drive, Portland, OR 97219, BS 77 Univ of WA; MA 80 Univ of Denver; 84–Sp-Lang Path, Good Samaritan Hosp & Med Ctr, **SLP**

Gillespie, Gerry G 1209 Knoll Mist Lane, Gaithersburg, MD 20879, (301) 921-8799, BS 78 Ithaca Coll; MS 81 Gallaudet Coll; Audiologist, Calvary Commission, **A**

Gillespie, Ian Graham 38 Newcroft Road, Winnipeg, MB, Canada R2J 3M8, (204) 787-4212, BS 72 Univ of Manitoba - Winnipeg; MS 83 Minot St Univ; 85–Aud, Health Sciences Cen, **A**

Gillespie, Mrs Janet Vandevelde P O Box 2624, Glen Ellyn, IL 60138, (312) 531-3771, MA 85 Northern IL Univ - De Kalb

Gillespie, Mrs Judith B 3122 Cave Court, Woodbridge, VA 22192-1167, (703) 491-4662, **SLP**

Gillespie, Mrs Karen Denise 9501 Roark #615, Houston, TX 77099-2163, (713) 777-1947, BS 78 MS Univ for Women; MS 79 MS Univ for Women; Sp-Lang Path, Okaloosa County Schs, **SLP**

Gillespie, Mrs M Beth 11629 Camphor Way, Seminole, FL 33542, (312) 896-1961, BA 71 Fontbonne Coll; MA 73 Univ of IL - Urbana; Sp-Lang Path, Morning Star School, **SLP**

Gillespie, Mrs Myrtle E Box 1226, Anderson, SC 29622, (803) 224-6612, BS 60 Univ Southern MS-Hattiesburg; MA 61 OH St Univ; **A**

Gillespie, R David 2229 Mildred Street, Paducah, KY 42001, (502) 444-9687, BS 70 Samford Univ; MA 72 Univ of AL- Tuscaloosa; Aud, W Ky Er Sl Cen, **A**

Gillespie, Dr Robert V Audiology & Speech Pathology, Veterans Administration Medical Center, One Veterans Plaza, San Juan, PR 00927-5800, (809) 758-7575, BS 57 Ball St Univ; MS 59 Case Western Reserve Univ; PH 64 (NS) Univ of IA; Chief Aud & SLP Serv, VA Med Cen, **A**

Gillespie, Teri Evans P O Box 1763, Truth or Consequences, NM 87901, (505) 894-7141, BA 79 NM St Univ; MA 82 NM St Univ; Sp-Lang Path, Truth or Consequences Mun Sch, **SLP**

Gillespie-Rieck, Mrs Eva Marie 1675 Laurel Creek Drive, Troy, OH 45373-9500, (513) 339-3484, BS 79 Edinboro Univ of PA; MA 80 Edinboro Univ of PA; Sp-Lang Path, Troy Board of Education, **SLP**

Gillette, Barbara B 4886 La Gama Way, Santa Barbara, CA 93111, (805) 964-4517, BA 72 Whittier Coll; MA 73 Univ of WA; Sp-Lang Path, Santa Barbara Co Schs, **SLP**

Gillette, Debra H 2 Holiday Avenue, Derry, NH 03038, (603) 437-6945, BS 79 Univ of NH; MS 85 Ithaca Coll; **A**

Gillette, Mrs Kamara Laree 2033 Gloucester, Boise, ID 83706, (208) 343-2583, BS 85 ID St Univ; MS 87 ID St Univ; Sp-Lang Path, Idaho Elks Rehab, **SLP**

Gillette, Yvonne Ohio State University, Nisonger Center, 1580 Cannon Drive, Columbus, OH 43210, (614) 422-9920, OB 71 Univ of Toledo; MA 75 OH St Univ; Coord Res Dev Clin Svc, OH St U/Nisonger Ctr, **SLP**

Gilliam, Lauren S 1344 Old Hickory Road, Tyler, TX 75703, (214) 581-1359, BS 79 Univ of TX - Austin; MA 81 Memphis St Univ; Sp-Lang Path, Vaughn Speech & Hearing Clinic, **SLP**

Gilliam, Pamela P R R 2, Oxford, ME 04270, (207) 743-8652, SLP, Coastal Sp Services, **SLP**

Gillihan, Patricia A 4816 Starflower Drive, Martinez, CA 94553, (415) 933-8462, BA 79 San Francisco St Univ; MS 80 San Francisco St Univ; Aud, Ea Schroff MD-Gg Wilson MD, **A**

Gilliland, Eleanor Lauri 5741 N Via Lozana, Tucson, AZ 85715, (602) 577-8817, BS 68 Univ of MI - Ann Arbor; MS 69 Univ of MI - Ann Arbor; 87–Subacute Coord Restorative Svcs, Tucson Med Ctr, **SLP**

Gilliland, Sharon B 408 North B, Arkansas City, KS 67005, (316) 441-0233, MS 78 Central Methodist Coll; BS 75 Univ of KS; Sp-Lang Path, Special Services Coop, **SLP**

Gilliland, Vickie A 14170 N E Eugene Court, Portland, OR 97230, (503) 241-3488, BS 79 Univ of OR; MS 81 Univ of OR; Sp-Lang Path, Visiting Nurse Assoc, **SLP**

Gillis, Barbara P O Box 117, Skowhegan, ME 04976, (207) 474-5277, BS 78 Emerson Coll; MA 80 Univ of CO - Boulder; Sp/Lang Path, Private Practice, **SLP**

Gillis, Mrs Heather R 2954 West 14th, Vancouver, BC, Canada V6K 2X6, BA 71 Occidental Coll; MS 74 Univ of WA; 86–Occ Saf & Hlth Ofcr, Workers' Compensation Bd of BC, **A**

Gillis, Dr Herbert R 78-57 223rd Street, Bayside, NY 11364, (516) 299-2436, BA 47 Kent St Univ; MA 49 Kent St Univ; PH 58 (Sp Path) Case Western Reserve Univ; Sp-Lang Path, Post Cen/Li U, **SLP**

Gillis, Patricia Sullivan 11 Friar Lane, Cumberland, ME 04021, (207) 781-3988, BS 82 Ithaca Coll; MS 86 Univ of NH

Gillis, Dr Rita J 466 West Crest Drive, Nashville, TN 37211, (615) 320-5353, BA 78 Univ of NC - Chapel Hill; MS 80 East Carolina Univ; PH 86 (Sp-Lang Path) Vanderbilt Univ; 87–Dir Rehab Inst, Bill Wilkerson Hrn & Sp Ctr, **SLP**

Gillis, Roberta Clark Country Club Estates, Rd 1 Box 296-L, Fort Johnson, NY 12070, (518) 829-7731, **SLP**

Gillis, Victoria Joann 4520 Bryan N W, Albuquerque, NM 87114, (505) 831-3301, BA 83 Univ of SD - Vermillion; MA 85 WA St Univ; SLP, Albuquerque Ps, **SLP**

Gillis-Cooper, Paulette Karen 3890 Hoyt Street, Wheatridge, CO 80033, (303) 238-4580, BS 73 Univ of WI - Green Bay; MA 81 Univ of CO - Boulder; SLP, Private Practice, **SLP**

Gillispie, Kathryn P Hampden Hearing Center Inc, 84 Westfield Street, West Springfield, MA 01089, (413) 736-2627, BS 49 Bucknell Univ; MA 65 Temple Univ; Pres, Hampden Hrng Cen Inc, **A**

Gillman, Sherry F 144-36 72nd Drive, Flushing, NY 11367, (212) 268-7216, BA 71 CUNY - Queens Coll; MA 72 CUNY - Queens Coll; OM 79 CUNY - Grad Sch & Univ Cntr; Adj Lect, Touro Coll, **SLP**

Gillon, Laura Ann 601 3rd Street S E, Altoona, IA 50009, (515) 792-4870, BS 84 Univ of IA; MA 85 Univ of IA; Sp-Lang Path, Heartland AEA, **SLP**

Gills, Ann C 351 Hillside Avenue, Elmhurst, IL 60126, **SLP**

Gillum, Charles Jr Lindsey Medical Arts Bldg, Junction City, KS 66441, (913) 238-6633, BS 81 KS St Univ; MA 83 KS St Univ; Aud, Aud Cen, **A**

Gillum, Dr Linda H 3160 Chambord Drive, West Bloomfield, MI 48033, (313) 494-4480, BA 71 MI St Univ; MA 72 Univ of the DC; PH 76 (NS) Univ of MA - Amherst; Asst Prof/Dir Sp/Lang Path, Wayne St U/Detroit Rec Hosp, **SLP**

Gilman, Carol Lynn 5606 West Chapel Hill Road, Douglasville, GA 30135, (404) 949-5768, BS 77 Univ of GA; ME 79 GA St Univ; 88–Sp-Lang Path, Cobb Co Sch Dist, **SLP**

Gilman, Leslea A CSC, 531 SE 14th, Portland, OR 97214, (503) 280-5675, BS 73 Univ of IA; MA 75 Univ of IA; Asst Supvr, Portland Public Schools, **A**

Gilman, Sherri Lynne 135 Mountain Gate Road, Ashland, MA 01721, (617) 369-8798, BS 81 Univ of MA - Amherst; MS 85 Worcester St Coll; 85–Sp-Lang Path, CASE Collaborative, **SLP**

Gilmartin, Ann Speech Pathologist, Mercy Hospital, 1000 North Village Avenue, Rockville Centre, NY 11570, (516) 255-2368, BA 70 CUNY - Hunter Coll; MA 74 Hofstra Univ; MS 79 Adelphi Univ; SLP, Mercy Hosp, **SLP ACE**

Gilmartin, Eva Marie 1759 Crescent Drive, Walnut Creek, CA 94598, (415) 935-0257, BA 38 Seattle Pacific Univ; MA 40 WA St Univ; Consult/Staff Dev, Mt Diablo USD, **SLP LM**

Gilmartin, Kathleen J 11433 Azalea Drive, Pittsburgh, PA 15235, MA 79 Univ of PA; Aud, Eye & Ear Hospital of Pitts, **A**

Gilmartin, Theresa 5644 Netherland Avenue, Riverdale, NY 10471, **SLP**

Gilmer, Mrs Joanna Hudgins 110 Cedar Creek Drive, Asheboro, NC 27203, (919) 626-0334, BS 62 Univ of GA; ME 64 Univ of GA; ES 73 Univ of GA; Sp-Lang Path, Randolph Co Sch Sys, **SLP**

Gilmer, Karen L 527 West Fairmount Avenue, State College, PA 16801, (814) 234-4882, BA 79 Univ of CT; MS 80 Univ of WI - Madison; Sp-Lang Path, Private Practice, **SLP**

Gilmer, Mrs Mary Grace 356 East Yale Loop, Irvine, CA 92714-4641, (213) 438-9781, 83–Sp-Lang Path, Dr Bernard A Landes & Assoc, **SLP**

Gilmore, Christine Anne Memphis Speech & Hearing Cent, 807 Jefferson Avenue, Memphis, TN 38105, (901) 525-2682, BS 82 Boston Univ; MS 84 Columbia Univ Teachers Coll; Doctoral Assistant, Memphis State University, **A**

Gilmore, Dee A 5953 West 67th Avenue, Arvada, CO 80003, (303) 423-8509, MS 79 Univ of NM; **SLP**

Gilmore, Janet Buie Route 6 Box 379-A, Lancaster, SC 29720, (803) 285-8429, BS 68 Central MO St Univ; MS 70 Central MO St Univ; Sp-Lang Path, Private Practice, **SLP**

Gilmore, Joy E M P O Box 354, Hillsboro, OH 45133, (513) 981-2197, BA 77 OH St Univ; MA 80 OH St Univ; Sp-Lang Path, Greenfield Exempt Sch Dist, **SLP**

Gilmore, Keely J 34 Gaynor Place, Winnipeg, MB, Canada R2R 1W5, (204) 786-7841, BS 79 Northern IL Univ - De Kalb; MA 81 Northern IL Univ - De Kalb; Sp-Lang Path, Child Guidance Cl, **SLP**

Gilmore, Lloyd W 14 Stonehenge Circle, Pikesville, MD 21208, (301) 666-0500, BS 56 CA Univ of PA; MS 64 WV Univ; **SLP**

Gilmore, Marian L 516 32nd Street, Beaver Falls, PA 15010, BA 34 Geneva Coll; MA 42 Northwestern Univ; **SLP LM**

Gilmore, Mrs Martha R 102-J Windy Cove, Hampton, VA 23666, (804) 865-8094, BA 85 Univ of TN - Knoxville; MA 87 Univ of TN - Knoxville; **A**

Gilmore, Robert Alan 251 West Central Street, Suite 111, Natick, MA 01760, (508) 655-4049, BA 82 Univ of RI; MS 87 Gallaudet Coll; 87–Aud, Perkins Sch for the Blind, **A**

Gilmore, Sheila Elizabeth 700 Victoria A #1, Costa Mesa, CA 92627, (714) 581-2800, BA 80 Chapman Coll; MS 82 Chapman Coll; Sp-Lang Path, Newport Lang Sp & Aud Inc, **SLP**

Gilmore, Dr Stuart Irby S Australian Coll Advanced Ed, School Of Speech Pathology, Sturt Road, Bedford Park, South Australia, Australia 5042, (08) 275-5310, BA 50 SUNY - Center at Albany; MA 51 SUNY - Center at Albany; PH 62 (NS) Univ of WI - Madison; 87–Lecturer, Sch of Sp Path, **SLP A F**

Gilmore, Mrs Susan E 1904 Edgewater Lane, Edmond, OK 73013, (405) 341-0405, BS 78 OK St Univ; MS 80 Univ of OK Medical Center; Sp-Lang Path, Edmond Pub Schs, **SLP**

Gilmore, Dr Susan L Special Education, 4701 Joaquin Way Rm 24, Sacramento, CA 95822-2190, (916) 454-8387, BA 64 Univ of the Pacific; MA 65 Univ of the Pacific; PH 68 (NS) OH Univ - Athens; Superv Instr/Serv, Sacramento City USD, **SLP**

Gilmore, Virginia Arbuckle 1601 Tamarack Trail, Decatur, GA 30033, (404) 371-4866, BA 56 Univ of MI - Ann Arbor; ME 83 GA St Univ; 79–Sp-Lang Path, Atlanta Pub Sch, **SLP**

Gilmore, Willis C 5400 Orange Avenue #103, Cypress, CA 90630, (714) 827-4650, BA 67 CA St Univ - Long Beach; MA 68 CA St Univ - Long Beach; Sp-Lang Path & Owner, Clark Gilmore Ma Ccc, **SLP**

Gilpin, Mrs Cathy Vanderford 727 State Hwy 11, Laramie, WY 82070, (307) 742-9243, BA 78 Univ of Northern CO; MS 81 Univ of WY; **A**

Gilroy, Mrs Maureen Anne 18 Fairbanks Street, Port Jefferson Station, NY 11776-3206, (516) 435-8564, BS 82 Hofstra Univ; MS 85 Adelphi Univ; **SLP**

Gilson, Abigail Ellen 2713 Lancashire Road, Unit 4, Cleveland Heights, OH 44106, (216) 321-2530, BA 85 Univ of Denver; MA 86 Case Western Reserve Univ; **A**

Gilson, Eileen K 116 Arcadia Drive, Vacaville, CA 95688, (707) 422-3266, BA 73 Chapman Coll; MA 76 Chapman Coll; 78–Sp-Lang Path, Fairfield-Suisun USD, **SLP**

Gilson, Natalie Ellen 182 East 95th Street #29E, New York, NY 10128, (212) 420-4111, BA 83 George Washington Univ; MS 84 Boston Univ; Sp-Lang Path, Beth Isreal Med Ctr- Neuro Beh, **SLP**

Gilson, Mrs Norma Lee 7316 North Seneca Road, Fox Point, WI 53217, (414) 352-2070, BS 70 Univ of WI - Madison; MS 74 Univ of WI - Milwaukee; Sp/Lang Path, Brown Deer Sch Dist, **SLP**

Gilston, Mrs Nancy Siwoff 142 East 27th Street #2-E, New York, NY 10016, MA 87 CUNY - Hunter Coll

Giltner, Elizabeth (Toni) T 1625 Indian Wells Drive, Boulder City, NV 89005, (701) 293-6578, MS 72 Minot St Univ; 88–Sp-Lang Path, Medivisit, **SLP**

Gimbel, Mrs Iris M 4152 Combe Way, San Diego, CA 92122, (619) 452-8994, BS 66 Univ of Cincinnati; MA 67 Northwestern Univ; 86–Dir, Ctr for Language Disorders, **SLP**

Gimbel, Lesley G 9341 North Broadmoor, Bayside, WI 53217, **SLP**

Gimbel, Phyllis 2420 Still Forest Road, Baltimore, MD 21208, (301) 323-8583, **SLP**

Giminaro, Mrs Ruth F 155 Hillside Road, Farmingdale, NY 11735, (516) 794-7694, BS 85 Nazareth Coll of Rochester; MS 86 SUNY - Coll at Fredonia; 87–Sp-Lang Path, Farmingdale PS, **SLP**

Gimlin, Carol L 6225 East 78th Place, Tulsa, OK 74136, (918) 492-3349, BS 73 MI St Univ; MS 74 Purdue Univ - West Lafayette; Aud, Private Practice, **A**

Gimmarro, Patricia Lynora 17401 East 40th Highway, Apartment B-6, Independence, MO 64055, (816) 461-0426, BS 84 Central MO St Univ; MS 87 6096; 88–Sp-Lang Path, Children's Mercy Hosp, **SLP**

Gimpel, Mrs Colleen Marie 24928 New York, Dearborn, MI 48124, (313) 278-4156, BS 83 Western MI Univ; MA 85 Wayne St Univ; 85–Sp-Lang Path, Dearborn Heights PS Dist #7, **SLP**

Ginburg, Mrs Laurie Orkin 4405 Dunmore Road N E, Marietta, GA 30068, (404) 973-2226, BA 79 Tulane Univ; MA 82 Memphis St Univ; 86–Sp-Lang Path/Consult, Private Practice, **SLP**

Ginesi, Linda A M 1180 North Danbury Circle, Medina, OH 44256, (419) 626-5629, **SLP**

Ginest, Mrs Joan H 332 Maybelle, Wichita, KS 67209, (316) 689-4820, BA 62 Wichita St Univ; MA 70 Wichita St Univ; Chief/Sp-Lang Pathology, St Joseph Medical Center, **SLP**

Gingerich, Mrs Peggy Joanne R R 3 Box 82, Iowa City, IA 52240, (319) 683-2715, BS 81 Univ of IA; MA 83 Univ of IA; SLP, Grant Wood AEA, **SLP**

Gingerich, Mrs Rhonda Schoon 4846 Honeysuckle Blvd, Gahanna, OH 43230, (614) 891-7255, BS 82 IL St Univ - Normal; MA 84 Northeastern IL Univ; 87–Sp-Lang Path, Professional Rehab Assoc, **SLP**

Gingold, Iris N 260 Exeter Street, Brooklyn, NY 11235, (212) 743-8723, BA 74 CUNY - Brooklyn Coll; MS 76 CUNY - Brooklyn Coll; Sp-Lang Path, Visiting Ther Assoc, **SLP ACE**

Ginley, Susan Marie 3129 N E 65th Street, Portland, OR 97213, (503) 284-4514, BA 83 Univ of OR; MA 85 Univ of OR; **SLP**

Ginn, Mary E 5 Settlers Drive, Myrtle Beach, SC 29577, (803) 626-8655, BA 67 Winthrop Coll; ME 71 Univ of SC - Columbia; Coor Pf Prgams for Hndcpd, Horry School District, **SLP**

Ginn, Sandra Luenn 5531 South 362nd Street, Auburn, WA 98001, (206) 833-3495, BS 82 Mankato St Univ; MA 83 Univ of SD - Vermillion; Aud, Hearing Health Care Ctr, **A**

Ginocchetti, Darlene Erma 6 East Salor Avenue, Wilkes-Barre, PA 18702, (717) 823-2335, BS 80 Kutztown Univ of PA; MS 85 Bloomsburg Univ of PA; Sp-Lang Path, Wyoming Valley Childrens Assn, **SLP**

Ginsberg, Bernard L Medical Marketing & Management, 12304 Santa Monica Blvd, Suite 300, West Los Angeles, CA 90025, (231) 826-5576, BS 70 Southern IL Univ -Carbondale; MS 74 Wayne St Univ; MA 81 Univ of Southern CA; President, Medical Marketing & Management, **SLP A**

Ginsberg, Esther B 2621 Plaza Del Amo #526, Torrance, CA 90503, (818) 997-2330, BA 66 San Francisco St Univ; MA 80 CA St Univ - Los Angeles; **A**

Ginsberg, Patricia Davis 99 Bank Street #6I, New York, NY 10014, (212) 929-0304, BA 66 CUNY - Hunter Coll; MS 74 Univ of OK Medical Center; Sp-Lang Path, Private Practice, **SLP**

Ginsburg, Sharon Faubel 6 Club Court, Columbia, MO 65201, (314) 882-6988, BA 77 Univ of TN - Knoxville; MA 79 Memphis St Univ; Sp-Lang Path, U of MO Hosp & Cl, **SLP**

Ginsburgh, Dr Laurel Cooper 34 South Main Street #810, Wilkes-Barre, PA 18701, (717) 822-9687, MS 72 Columbia Univ Teachers Coll; OM 76 Columbia Univ Teachers Coll; PH 76 Columbia Univ Teachers Coll; Private Practice, **SLP**

Ginther, Judith A 276 Teague Drive, San Dimas, CA 91773, (818) 967-2841, BA 73 CA St Univ - Northridge; MA 75 CA St Univ - Northridge; SLP, Los Angeles Co Supt of Schs, **SLP**

Ginyard, Cynthia Melissa 12720 Brant Rock Drive, Apartment #202, Houston, TX 77082, (713) 498-8110, BA 80 SC St Coll; MA 81 SC St Coll; Sp-Lang Path, Alief ISD, **SLP**

Gioiello-Meyer, Mrs Jacqueline Jean 8602 Cinnamon Creek #1708, San Antonio, TX 78240, (512) 434-0696, BS 85 Winona St Univ; MA 86 Univ of Northern CO; 87–Sp-Lang Path, Northside ISD, **SLP**

Giolas, Marilyn H 38 Candide Lane, Storrs, CT 06268, (203) 887-1654, BS 57 Purdue Univ - West Lafayette; MS 59 Univ of Pittsburgh - Pittsburgh; 79–Aud, Southeastern Ct Hrng&Sp Ctr, **A**

Giolas, Dr Thomas G 38 Candide Lane, Storrs, CT 06268, (203) 486-3619, BS 54 IN Univ - Bloomington; MA 56 IN Univ - Bloomington; PH 60 (Aud) Univ of Pittsburgh - Pittsburgh; 68–Dean/Graduate School/Professor, U of CT, **A F**

Giordano, Mrs Ellen Angela 3146 Cedar Road, Yorktown Heights, NY 10598, (914) 245-3292, BS 77 Mercy Coll; MS 81 CUNY - Lehman Coll; MA 84 CUNY - Lehman Coll; 86–Sp-Lang Path, Mahopac Central Sch Dist, **SLP**

Giordano, John Joseph 201 South Brady St 2nd Fl, Du Bois, PA 15801, (814) 371-8375, BS 82 Edinboro Univ of PA; MA 84 Edinboro Univ of PA

Giordano, Mrs Lorraine A 19028 North 8th Avenue, Phoenix, AZ 85027, (602) 582-6500, BA 75 Montclair St Coll; MS 76 Columbia Univ Teachers Coll; Sp-Lang Path, Scottsdale Public Schools, **SLP**

Giordano-Olson, Mrs Judy A 225 East Boulevard, Logan, UT 84321, (801) 753-5886, MS 88 UT St Univ; 88–Sp-Lang Path, Logan Sch Dist

Giovanetti, Laura T 219 Deer Run, Huntington, CT 06484, (203) 926-0174, BS 85 Coll of Saint Rose; MS 86 Indiana Univ of PA; 86–Sp-Lang Path, Coop Educ Svcs Dev Learning Ctr, **SLP**

Giovannini-De Renzo, Sheila 319 Coleman Avenue, Elmira, NY 14905, (607) 737-7804, BS 81 Elmira Coll; MA 82 Western MI Univ; 88–Aud, St Joseph's Hosp, **A**

Giovannitti, Mrs Judith B 750 Dogwood Terrace, Boiling Springs, PA 17007, (717) 258-3440, BS 70 Carlow Coll; MA 73 Univ of Pittsburgh - Pittsburgh; Sp-Lang Path, Private Practice, **SLP**

Gipe, Patricia Neal Kapiolani Medical Center For Women & Children, Communication Disorder Clinic, 1319 Punahou Street, Honolulu, HI 96826, (808) 947-8511, BS 81 Brescia Coll; MS 83 Vanderbilt Univ; 84–Audiologist, Kapiolani Med Ctr, **A**

Giraldo, Consuelo Gloria P O Box 280, Reseda, CA 91335, (213) 268-5000, SLP, Whit Mem Hosp, **SLP**

Girard, Andree 350 Winding Pond Road, Londonderry, NH 03053, (603) 437-8237, MS 87 AZ St Univ; 88–Aud, Audio Hearing Centers, **A**

Girard, Mrs Brenda Lindquist P O Box Svl 8157, Victorville, CA 92392, (619) 245-3468, BA 80 CA St Univ - Northridge; MA 82 CA St Univ - Northridge; Sp-Lang Path, Private Practice, **SLP**

Girard, Kathleen Ann P O Box 202, Biscuit City Road, Kenyon, RI 02836, (401) 364-7778, BS 81 SUNY - Center at Albany; MA 84 Univ of RI; Sp-Lang Path, Chariho Regional Sch Dist, **SLP**

Girardot, Karen D 331 South Alvernon #31, Tucson, AZ 85711, (602) 327-4648, BS 81 Eastern MI Univ; MA 82 Eastern MI Univ; 86–Sp-Lang Path, Tucson USD One, **SLP**

Giraudi-Perry, Dr Diane Manlius Hearing Center, 8116 Cazenovia Road, Manlius, NY 13104, (315) 682-2025, BS 74 Syracuse Univ; MA 76 MI St Univ; PH 81 (NS) Syracuse Univ; Aud, Private Practice, **A**

Girdler, Donna M Nuernberg Elementary School, APO New York, NY 09696, BS 78 IL St Univ - Normal; MS 80 IL St Univ - Normal; Preschool Handicapped Tchr, Dept of Defense Depedends Sch, **SLP**

Girdvainis, Cheryl Marie 218 Beach Park Lane, Cape Canaveral, FL 32920, (305) 783-4119, BS 84 Worcester St Coll; MS 87 Worcester St Coll; **SLP**

Girken, Mrs Karen C 4921 Berryhill Circle, Perry Hall, MD 21128, (301) 838-7300, BS 83 Towson St Univ; MS 85 Towson St Univ; **SLP**

Girlando, Lucy M 4127 Bedford Avenue, Brooklyn, NY 11229, BA 73 CUNY - Brooklyn Coll; MS 76 CUNY - Brooklyn Coll; Sp-Lang Path, Kingsbrook Jewish Med Cen, **SLP**

Girmatzion, Mrs Phyllis Jenkins Mill Street Apartment, Apartment A-202, Athens, OH 45701, (614) 592-6493, BS 86 Marywood Coll; MA 88 OH Univ - Athens

Girolametto, Dr Luigi E 135 Bleecker Street #313, Toronto, ON, Canada M4X 1X2, (416) 598-6100, BA 75 McGill Univ - Quebec; MS 78 6935; PH 86 (Special Education) Univ of Toronto - Ontario; 86–Sp-Lang Path, The Hosp for Sick Children, **SLP**

Girolamo, Nanette 23 Woolsey Street, Huntington, NY 11743, (516) 931-1990, BS 75 SUNY - Coll at Fredonia; MS 76 Adelphi Univ; Sp-Lang Path, Bethpage Public Schools, **SLP**

Giroux, Mrs Anne P 59 Benton Avenue, Winslow, ME 04901, (207) 872-4383, BA 72 Univ of ME - Orono; OM 75 Johns Hopkins Univ; Aud, Mid ME Med Cen, **A**

Giroux, Fred A 1221 Sixth Line Road, Oakville, ON, Canada L6H 1X1, (416) 549-6525, OB 52 McGill Univ - Quebec; MS 81 SUNY - Coll at Buffalo; Sp-Lang Path, St Peter's Hosp, **SLP**

Giroux, Lucy A Rd 6 Box 33, Plattsburgh, NY 12901, (518) 563-4826, BA 78 SUNY - Coll at Plattsburgh; MA 81 SUNY - Coll at Plattsburgh; Sp/Lang Path, Beekmantown Ctrl Sch, **SLP**

Girrens, Mrs Ellen Claire 427 South Socora Drive, Wichita, KS 67209, (316) 663-7178, BA 58 Univ of Science & Arts of OK; Sp-Lang Path, Reno County Education Coop, **SLP**

Girson, Mrs Norma R H 1 Jeffrey Lane, Cinnaminson, NJ 08077, (609) 871-9000, BS 77 Trenton St Coll; MA 80 Trenton St Coll; SLP, Willingboro Pub Sch, **SLP**

Girtz, Pamela Sue 638 Glen Park Road, River Falls, WI 54022, BA 73 Saint Cloud St Univ; OM 84 Univ of WI - River Falls; **SLP**

Girvan, Stephanie 7400 Vanalden Avenue, Reseda, CA 91335-2523, (213) 824-3100, BA 76 Univ of Redlands; MA 79 Univ of CA - Los Angeles; Aud, W La VA Med Cen, **A**

Gischia, Mrs Carol Faulkner USNH Box 2764, FPO Seattle, WA 98778, BS 78 Northern AZ Univ; MS 80 Univ of WA; 86–Aud, Dept of Navy-USNH Okinawa, **A**

Gish, Keith D 117 Concordia Drive, Fairbanks, AK 99709, (907) 479-6362, BS 56 Univ of KS; MA 62 CA St Univ - Los Angeles; Retired, St of AK, **A**

Gismondi, Charles A California University Of Pa, College Avenue, California, PA 15419, (412) 938-4388, BS 64 CA Univ of PA; MS 68 WV Univ; Assoc Prof, California Univ Pa, **SLP**

Gisondi, Nancy Eve 1315 Langhorne-Newtown Rd, Langhorne, PA 19047, (215) 547-1070, BA 80 West Chester Univ of PA; MA 84 Trenton St Coll; Sp-Lang Path, Desa Inc, **SLP**

Gissy, Marie Clare 1824 Lynnwood Drive, Charlotte, NC 28209, (803) 585-2231, BS 84 Univ of Cincinnati; MA 85 Kent St Univ; 88–Sp-Lang Path, Charlotte Sp and Hrng Ctr, **SLP**

Gist, Kenneth T P O Box 542, Westport, CT 06881, (203) 397-4574, BA 49 West Liberty St Coll; MA 59 NY Univ; Assoc Prof of Commun Dis, Sn CT St U, **SLP**

Gitin, David L 251 O'Connor Drive, Suite 2, San Jose, CA 95128, (408) 268-7090, BA 62 San Jose St Univ; MA 71 San Jose St Univ; Sp-Lang Path, Blossom Ridge Sp-Myofunct Ctr Inc, **SLP**

Gitin, Eileen B 1608 Guadalajara Court, San Jose, CA 95120, (408) 268-7090, BS 56 CUNY - Brooklyn Coll; MA 82 San Jose St Univ; MA 62 Univ of CA - Los Angeles; Sp-Lang Path, Blossom Ridge Sp & Myo Cen, **SLP**

Gitles, Toni P O Box 910, Winter Park, FL 32790, (407) 831-2555, BA 71 Univ of FL; MA 73 Northwestern Univ; 86–VP of Pro Svc, Electone Inc, **A ACE**

Gitlis, Karyn R 1206 South Ash, Tempe, AZ 85281, (602) 839-7156, BS 70 Univ of IL - Urbana; MA 71 Univ of IL - Urbana; Sp-Lang Path, Tempe Elem Sch, **SLP**

Gitlitz, Shelia R Speech & Hearing Associates, 5 Riverside Drive, Suite 1005, Binghamton, NY 13905, (607) 723-3861, BA 63 Barnard Coll; MA 65 Columbia Univ Teachers Coll; Owner, Sp & Hrng Assoc, **SLP A ACE**

Gitlow, Caryl 10704 Samaga Drive, Oakton, VA 22124, **SLP**

Gitre, Mrs Carol Ann 4491 Hunt Club Drive #1-B, Ypsilanti, MI 48197, (313) 434-5342, MA 87 Eastern MI Univ

Gittelman-Nadeau, Mrs Debbie 2332 Acorn Place, Buffalo Grove, IL 60089, (312) 913-1663, BA 74 Washington Univ; MS 77 Washington Univ; 86–Aud, Dupage West Cook Spec Ed, **A**

Gitter, Beatrice Joan 1168 20th Street, Windom, MN 56101, (612) 489-3147, MS 88 Mankato St Univ

Gitter, Mrs Kelly Jo 7830 W Lisbon Avenue, Apt 5, Milwaukee, WI 53222, (414) 445-8896, BS 83 Univ of WI - Stevens Point; ME 85 James Madison Univ; 87–Aud, Otor Head & Neck Surgery Ltd, **A**

Gitter, Mary Jane 2516 Freedom Lane, Denton, TX 76201, (817) 383-3531, BS 69 OK St Univ; MA 70 OK St Univ; Outreach Dir, Denton St Sch, **SLP**

Gitterman, Dena 2415 19th Street, Boulder, CO 80302, (303) 442-7028, BA 75 SUNY - Center at Binghamton; MA 79 IN Univ - Bloomington; Sp-Lang Path, Student, **SLP**

Gitterman, Susan L 2361 Draper, Ypsilanti, MI 48197, (313) 572-0252, BA 74 Centre Coll of KY; OM 76 Univ of NC - Chapel Hill; MA 80 IN Univ - Bloomington; Audiologist, Apt Health Care Service, **A**

Giudici, Mrs Henrietta Helen 1913 Alford Avenue, Los Altos, CA 94022, (415) 941-4010, BA 58 San Jose St Univ; SLP, Los Altos Sch Dist, **SLP**

Giuliano, Mrs Lynne C 2060 East 65th Street, Brooklyn, NY 11234, (718) 388-4800, BA 84 CUNY - Brooklyn Coll; MS 85 CUNY - Brooklyn Coll; 85–SLP, Spec Serv Unit Board of Educ, **SLP**

Giumento, Angela S 2753 University, Eugene, OR 97403, (503) 344-3565, BS 73 SUNY - Coll at Geneseo; MS 77 SUNY - Coll at Buffalo; SLP, Box Elder Sch Dist, **SLP**

Giunta, Mrs Geralyn B 2706 West Briarcliff, Peoria, IL 61604, (309) 686-1577, BS 76 Univ of IL - Urbana; MS 77 Univ of IL - Urbana; Sp-Lang Path, Creve Coeur Pub Sch Dist #76, **SLP**

Given, Mrs Patricia Lynn 2829 Willow Wood Circle, Valdosta, GA 31602, (912) 244-3945, BS 84 Valdosta St Coll; MA 87 Univ of Central FL; 88–Sp-Lang Path, Lowndes Co Sch Sys, **SLP**

Givens, Alan D 11500 Natrona Cove, Austin, TX 78759, (512) 343-1053, BA 77 TX Tech Univ; MS 79 Univ of TX - Dallas; 82–Sp-Lang Path, Texas Sch for the Deaf, **SLP A**

Givens, Dr Gregg D Dept Speech Language Audiology, East Carolina University, Greenville, NC 27834, (919) 757-6961, BS 70 Ithaca Coll; MS 71 Ithaca Coll; PH 75 (NS) FL St Univ; Prof, E Carolina U, **A**

Givens, Kathleen A 205 Alpine Drive, Lake Zurich, IL 60047, (312) 438-7271, BS 72 Nazareth Coll of Rochester; MS 74 Nazareth Coll of Rochester; 85–Sp-Lang Path, Spec Educ Dist of Lake Co, **SLP**

Givens, Teresa S 1335 Keith, Wichita, KS 67209, (316) 686-4102, BA 76 Wichita St Univ; MA 77 Wichita St Univ; SLP, Starkey Develop Cen, **SLP**

Givler, Mrs Susan Kay 6234 Coachlite Way, Cincinnati, OH 45243, (513) 242-0042, BS 68 Kent St Univ; ME 71 Kent St Univ; Sp-Lang Path, Hamilton County Office of Educ, **SLP**

Givner, Jodi 5901 Oakdale Avenue, Woodland Hills, CA 91367-5619, MA 80 Northwestern Univ; OD 87 (Law) Univ of Southern CA; Attorney, **SLP**

Gjerstad, Marlys Anderson 1211 East Franklin, Indianola, IA 50125, (515) 961-8191, BS 76 Northeast MO St Univ; MA 77 Northeast MO St Univ; SLP, Heartland AEA, **SLP**

Gjording, Linda L 3510 Onyx Place, Eugene, OR 97405, (503) 687-3221, BS 60 Univ of ID; MS 79 Univ of OR; Sp-Lang Path, Eugene School District, **SLP**

Glackman, Margaret E Cloverbottom Developmental Cen, 275 Stewarts Ferry Pike, Nashville, TN 37214, (615) 889-9247, BS 73 Purdue Univ - West Lafayette; MS 74 Univ of WI - Stevens Point; Audiologist, State of Tennessee, **A**

Gladstone, Robin A 8200 Andes, Baltimore, MD 21208, **SLP**

Gladstone, Dr Vic S 8200 Andes Court, Baltimore, MD 21208, (301) 321-2449, BS 68 PA St Univ - Univ Park; MS 69 PA St Univ - Univ Park; PH 77 (Aud) Univ of MD - College Park; Prof/Dir-Aud, Towson State University, **A F**

Gladwin, Helen J Holiday Hearing Aid Center, 1836 U S Hwy 19, Holiday, FL 34691, (813) 934-5559, BA 55 Univ of MN - Minneap-St Paul; MA 68 Univ of MN - Minneap-St Paul; 86–Aud, Private Practice, **A ACE**

Glamb, Mary D 1341 Hepaki Place, Kailua, HI 96734, (808) 261-1698, BA 73 Univ of MI - Ann Arbor; MS 75 Univ of MI - Ann Arbor; SLP, Hi Dept of Ed-Windward Dist, **SLP**

Glance, Steven Eugene 5311 Loyola Avenue, Westminster, CA 92683-2726, (714) 895-2831, BA 77 Univ of CA - Santa Barbara; MS 83 Chapman Coll; Sp-Lang Path, Long Beach USD, **SLP**

Glandon, Mrs Margaret P 2555 East Harley Street, Inverness, FL 32650, (904) 344-1180, MS 79 Univ of South FL; Sp-Lang Path, Citrus County Schools, **SLP**

Glankler, Kathleen C 1321 East 154th Street, Olathe, KS 66062, (913) 782-6727, BS 75 Univ of GA; ME 76 Univ of GA; **SLP**

Glantz, Lisa 4 West Dosoris Lane, Dix Hills, NY 11746, (516) 595-1853, BA 76 CUNY - Queens Coll; MA 78 Hofstra Univ; SLP, Building Blooks Dev Presch, **SLP**

Glantz, Michael J 417-315 Sun Lake Circle, Lake Mary, FL 32746, (800) 432-7483, BA 74 SUNY - Center at Buffalo; MS 78 Boston Univ; 88–Dir of Pro Svcs, Electone Inc, **A**

Glanzman, Adina Rachel 66-40 108th Street Apartment 1G, Forest Hills, NY 11375, (516) 378-2000, MS 83 Adelphi Univ; BA 82 SUNY - Coll at Buffalo; Sp-Lang Path, UCP of Nassau Co, **SLP**

Glascock, Mrs Mary Jane 430 Valley View Court, Jefferson City, MO 65109, (314) 681-5942, MA 74 Southeast MO St Univ; Instructor, Lincoln University, **SLP**

Glascoe, Dr Gary Jay Sch Of Communicative Disorders, University Of Wisconsin, Stevens Point, WI 54481, (715) 346-4513, BS 65 Pacific Univ; MA 66 Western MI Univ; PH 72 (NS) Univ of Denver; Associate Professor, University of Wisconsin, **A**

Glaser, Naomi B 9717 Conestoga Way, Potomac, MD 20854, (301) 983-8311, **SLP**

Glaser, Patricia R Patty Glaser & Associates, 4504 Lorino Street Ste B, SLP Learning Center, Metairie, LA 70006, (504) 887-5780, BS 76 Saint Mary's Dominican Coll; OM 81 LA St Univ - N O Medical Ctr; Sp-Lang Path, Private Practice, **SLP**

Glaser, Mrs Rena H 1972 Norfolk, St Paul, MN 55116, (612) 733-4019, BA 65 Univ of IL - Urbana; MA 66 Univ of IL - Urbana; 71–Hearing Conserv Program Admin, 3M, **A ACE**

Glaser, Dr Robert G Audiology & Speech Associates, 425 Grand Avenue, Suite 1005, Dayton, OH 45405, (513) 226-7877, BS 69 Bowling Green St Univ; MA 72 Kent St Univ; PH 74 (NS) Kent St Univ; President & Aud, Aud & Sp Assoc of Dayton, **A**

Glaser, Mrs Sharon Naomi 1-26 Grunauer Place, Fair Lawn, NJ 07410, (201) 794-3449, BS 82 Boston Univ; MS 85 Columbia Univ Teachers Coll; SLP, Morristown Memorial Hospital, **SLP**

Glaser, Mrs Sherri Lynn 2116 Chelsea Drive, Fort Worth, TX 76134, (817) 731-4931, BS 77 Univ of TX - Austin; MA 85 TX Woman's Univ; 84–Sp-Lang Path, Fort Worth ISD, **SLP**

Glasgow, Kimberly Joanne 8557 Manor Avenue #C, Munster, IN 46321-2232, (219) 932-2300, BS 80 Ball St Univ; MS 84 Rush Univ; 84–Sp-Lang Path, St Margaret Hosp, **SLP**

Glasgow, Susan Haynes 2408 Kentucky Avenue, Baltimore, MD 21213, (301) 243-3800, BS 74 WV Univ; MA 75 Univ of TN - Knoxville; Sp-Lang Path, Baltimore Hrng & Sp Agency, **SLP**

Glasheen, Mrs Marie C 3546 Promontory Street, San Diego, CA 92109, (619) 273-6930, BA 48 Nazareth Coll of Rochester; MA 57 Catholic Univ of America; Sp/Lang Path, San Diego USD, **SLP**

Glasner, Philip J 1190 West Northern Parkway, Apartment 224, Baltimore, MD 21210, (301) 467-0833, BS 37; Asst Prof Psych & Pediatrics, Johns Hopkins U Sch of Med, **SLP F LM**

Glasofer, Mrs Janet T 3010 Sleepy Hollow Drive, Sugar Land, TX 77479, (713) 980-6899, BA 74 Duke Univ; MS 75 Columbia Univ Teachers Coll; SLP, Ft Bend ISD, **SLP**

Glasow, Mrs Georgiana Quest 1734 Broadbridge Avenue, Stratford, CT 06497, (203) 259-7106, MS 82 Univ of South FL; SLP, Rehab Assoc of Ct, **SLP**

Glass, Jeffrey L P O Box 1656, Fort Lee, NJ 07024, **SLP**

Glass, Jodi L Meeting Street School, 667 Waterman Avenue, East Providence, RI 02914, (401) 438-9500, BA 75 SUNY - Center at Buffalo; MA 76 Hofstra Univ; Aud, Meeting St Sch, **A**

Glass, Dr Lillian 435 North Bedford Drive, Suite 209, Beverly Hills, CA 90210, (213) 274-0528, BS 74 Bradley Univ; MS 75 Univ of MI - Ann Arbor; PH 78 (NS) Univ of MN - Minneap-St Paul; Dir, Private Practice, **SLP**

Glass, Mrs Lori Waldo 90 Olson Drive, Southington, CT 06489, (203) 621-9987, MS 84 Southern CT St Univ; Sp-Lang Path, Rocky Hill Board of Education, **SLP**

Glass, Mrs Nancy E 1915 Elmhurst Drive, Germantown, TN 38138, (901) 755-3144, BS 62 Univ of KY; MA 63 Univ of KY; **SLP**

Glass, Dr Rita M 1033 East 49th Street, Chicago, IL 60615, (312) 243-8400, BS 64 Northern IL Univ - De Kalb; MA 67 De Paul Univ; ED 80 (NS) Loyola Univ of Chicago; Sp-Lang Path, Easter Seals, **SLP**

Glass, Sandra D 1756 Cromwell #2, Akron, OH 44313, (216) 836-3163, MA 88 Univ of Akron

Glass, Susan Ruth 1081 Pine Place, Sunset Garden Apts #20K, Kingston, NY 12401, (914) 338-2500, BA 82 SUNY - Coll at Plattsburgh; MA 84 SUNY - Coll at Plattsburgh; **A**

Glassell, William L Box 166, Fontanelle, IA 50846, (515) 745-2291, BA 58 Univ of Northern IA; MA 71 Univ of Northern IA; Teacher, Bridgewater-Fontanelle Com Sch, **SLP**

Glasser-Woolf, Mrs Dorie Ann 23321 El Toro Road Suite C, El Toro, CA 92630, (714) 587-0702, BA 78 Univ of CA - Berkeley; MA 83 Temple Univ; 88–Sp-Lang Path, Private Practice, **SLP**

Glassman, Connie K 103 Timbercreek Road, Laurel Park, NC 28739, (704) 693-4405, BA 71 Univ of FL; MA 72 Montclair St Coll; Sp-Lang Path, Private Practice, **SLP**

Glassman, Mrs Harriet C 909 Lynn Drive, Kinston, NC 28501, (919) 523-9345, BA 72 CUNY - City College; MA 75 CUNY - City College; 86–Sp-Lang Path, Lenoir County Bd of Educ, **SLP**

Glassman, Joel R 909 Lynn Drive, Kinston, NC 28501, (919) 559-5133, BA 71 CUNY - City College; MA 73 CUNY - City College; Sp/Lang Path, Caswell Cen, **SLP**

Glassman-Lee, Mrs Eileen M 6601 Woodlake Avenue, Canoga Park, CA 91307, (818) 882-8673, BA 70 Univ of FL; MA 71 Hofstra Univ; Sp-Lang Path, Private Practice, **SLP**

Glassmann, Deanna M 91 Chichester Road, Huntington, NY 11743, (516) 423-0290, BA 59 CUNY - Brooklyn Coll; MA 67 CUNY - Brooklyn Coll; 78–Sp-Lang Path, Port Washington Pub Sch, **SLP**

Glasson, Dr Chloe C 21187 Byron Road, Shaker Heights, OH 44122, (216) 459-3178, MA 68 Fairfield Univ; MA 70 Case Western Reserve Univ; PH 83 (NS) Kent St Univ; Manager Division of Commun Dis, Cleveland Mentro General, **SLP**

Glatman, Mrs Ilene Sheryl 4 Montrose Dr, Commack, NY 11725, (516) 368-0758, BA 82 SUNY - Center at Buffalo; MA 84 NY Univ; Sp-Lang Path, Private Practice, **SLP**

Glatter, Mrs Marsha R 7589 Calvalry Circle, Manlius, NY 13104, (315) 682-5977, BS 66 SUNY - Coll at Buffalo; MS 68 Syracuse Univ; 87–Sp-Lang Path, Fayetteville Manlius Cen Sch Dist, **SLP**

Glattke, Jean B 120 East Vista Oeste Drive, Tucson, AZ 85704-7024, (602) 622-5833, BA 67 Univ of KS; MA 68 Univ of KS; Dir Sp-Lang Hrng Serv, Carondelet Health Serv, **SLP F ACE**

Glattke, Dr Theodore J Dept Speech & Hearing Science, University Of Arizona, Tucson, AZ 85721, (602) 621-1644, BA 62 Univ of AZ; MA 63 Univ of MI - Ann Arbor; PH 68 (Hrng Science) Univ of IA; Prof, U of AZ, **A F ACE**

Glaub, Susan Ann 805 Turkey Run Road, Mc Lean, VA 22101, (703) 821-8883, BS 74 OH Univ - Athens; MA 76 OH Univ - Athens; Sp-Lang Path, Private Practice, **SLP**

Glay, Mrs Karen Rynish 1219 Sunnyside Lane, Round Lake Beach, IL 60073, (312) 263-1314, BS 81 Marquette Univ; MA 82 Northern IL Univ - De Kalb; 82–Aud, Otologic Prof Assoc, **A**

Glaze, Leslie Ellen 1628 Mayflower Drive, Middleton, WI 53562, (608) 263-6190, BA 79 Scripps Coll; MA 85 Univ of KS; Sp-Lang Path, Univ of WI In Madison, **SLP**

Glaze, Mrs Nancy Humphrey Hunters Glen Med Complex, 5509 Pleasant Valley #90, Plano, TX 75023, (214) 423-7660, BS 70 Univ of TX - Austin; MS 78 Univ of TX - Dallas; 87–Sp-Lang Path, Plano ISD, **SLP**

Glaze, Patricia Lynne 616 Morris Street, Salisbury, MD 21801, (301) 749-4780

Glazebrook, Mrs Evelyn N 7105 Forest Court, Des Moines, IA 50311-1432, (515) 964-2550, OB 49 SUNY - Coll at Oneonta; MA 53 Univ of IA; SLP, AEA II, **SLP**

Glazer, Diane Lynn 3076 Rumsey, Ann Arbor, MI 48105, (313) 996-9589, **A**

Glazer, Ellen S 11 Russell Street, Freeman's Bay, Auckland, New Zealand, BA 62 Sarah Lawrence Coll; MS 65 Univ of MI - Ann Arbor; Sp-Lang Path, Auckland Hospital Board, **SLP**

Glazer, Mrs Jacqueline Gray 111 Dalton Terrace, Cherry Hill, NJ 08003, (609) 428-8848, BA 64 Rutger's St Univ - Douglas Coll; MA 65 OH St Univ; SLP, Cherry Hill Board of Education, **SLP**

Glazer, Shirley L 4100 Cathedral Avenue, Apartment 608, Washington, DC 20016, (202) 745-3636, BS 79 ID St Univ; MS 81 Eastern WA Univ; SLP, PSI Assoc Inc, **SLP**

Glazer-Gordon, Dena Lee 4417 Alexander Drive, Metairie, LA 70003, (504) 830-4424, BA 70 Univ of OK - Norman; MS 72 Univ of OK Medical Center; Sp-Lang Path, Jefferson Parish Sch Syst, **SLP**

Glazewski, Dr Barbara D 226 Highland Drive, Milltown, NJ 08850, (201) 932-9335, BA 67 Rutger's St Univ - Douglas Coll; MS 71 Rutgers St Univ -N Brunswick; ED 88 (Developmental Psychology) Rutgers St Univ -N Brunswick; Asst Prof, Rutgers U/Dept Sp-Lang-Hrng Sc, **SLP**

Glazier, Marijane 1012 Sedwick Drive, Wilmington, DE 19803, (302) 478-2825, BA 79 Chestnut Hill Coll; MS 83 PA St Univ - Univ Park; Sp-Lang Path, Consult, **SLP**

Glazier, Susan Thomas 659 Overlook Drive, Alliance, OH 44601, (216) 823-7096, BA 76 George Washington Univ; MA 78 Marshall Univ; 86–Prog Coord/Chief Sp-Lang Path, Easter Seal Society of Mahoning Trumbull & Columbiana Counties, **SLP**

Gleason, Carol Lyon 7886 Lake View Road, Traverse City, MI 49684, (616) 941-1880, BA 72 MI St Univ; MA 77 Western MI Univ; Tchr, Traverse Bay Area ISD, **SLP**

Gleason, Dawn E 3004 Shady Hill Court, Columbus, OH 43221, (614) 225-1634, BS 79 Denison Univ; MA 82 OH St Univ; Aud, Mt Carmel Health, **A**

Gleason, Mrs Ellen C 14 Lewis Road, Mansfield, MA 02048-1657, (906) 784-3810, BA 75 Stonehill Coll; MS 80 Radford Univ; Sp-Lang Path, Sharon PS, **SLP**

Gleason, Erland W 156 Church Street, Coldwater, MI 49036, (517) 278-3393, BA 69 MI St Univ; MA 74 MI St Univ; 75–Sp-Lang Path, Coldwater Reg Cen, **SLP ACE**

Gleesing, Mrs Cindy K 305 Park Lane, Post Falls, ID 83854, (406) 791-2270, MS 80 Eastern WA Univ; Sp-Lang Path, St Lukes Hosp, **SLP**

Gleeson, Nancy J 6431 Nash, Downers Grove, IL 60516, (312) 852-0400, BS 79 IL St Univ - Normal; MS 81 IL St Univ - Normal; Tchr, Downers Grove North HS, **SLP**

Gleim, Mrs Eileen A 13220 Hanover Avenue, Apple Valley, MN 55124, (612) 432-0485, BS 74 Purdue Univ - West Lafayette; MS 75 Purdue Univ - West Lafayette; 87–Sp-Lang Path, InSpeech Inc, **SLP**

Gleimer, Ellen F 201 East 21st Street #8H, New York, NY 10010, BA 72 Univ of Rochester; MS 73 Univ of MI - Ann Arbor; **SLP**

Gleitman, Ronald Purdue University, Aus Heavilon Hall, West Lafayette, IN 47907, (317) 494-3789, BS 85 Purdue Univ - West Lafayette; MS 87 Purdue Univ - West Lafayette; Grad, Purdue Univ

Glendinning, Shawn Patrice 2910 Hegan Lane, Chico, CA 95928, (916) 345-3198, MA 88 CA St Univ - Chico

Glenn, Mrs Almetta M 5706 East 17th, Wichita, KS 67208, BA 70 Wichita St Univ; MA 77 Wichita St Univ; Retired, Wichita Board of Ed-USD 259, **SLP LM**

Glenn, Mrs Carol Frances 14117 175 Avenue N E, Redmond, WA 98053, (206) 885-0895, BS 79 Western IL Univ; MA 81 Northwestern Univ; **SLP**

Glenn, Cheryl R 358-B Greenwich Street, New York, NY 10013, (212) 608-5005, BA 77 CUNY - City College; MS 78 Adelphi Univ; 87–Sp-Lang Path, Comm on Spec Educ-Dist #1, **SLP**

Glenn, Karin Renee 6710 S Peoria #1311, Tulsa, OK 74136, (918) 245-5911, BS 85 Univ of OK - OK City; MS 87 Univ of North TX; 88–Sp-Lang Path, Dept of Human Services, **SLP**

Glenn, Larry E Department Of Communication Disorders, Southern Connecticut State University, New Haven, CT 06515, (203) 397-4565, BA 66 Chapman Coll; MA 69 CA St Univ - Long Beach; Instr, Sc St Univ/Dept of Comm Dis, **SLP**

Glenn, Marietta G 1765 Applebury Drive, Fayetteville, AR 72701, BS 61 Henderson St Univ; MA 67 Univ of AR - Fayetteville; Sp-Lang Path, Fayetteville Cty Hosp, **SLP**

Glenn, Sharon Murphy 949 South Odgen Street, Denver, CO 80209, BS 77 Ithaca Coll; MS 79 Univ of Denver; SLP, Aurora Public Schools, **SLP**

Glennan-Brethauer, Nancy 14 Blackbird Drive, Bedford, NH 03102-5439, (603) 472-5783, BS 70 Kent St Univ; MA 71 MI St Univ; Sp/Lang Path, Er Sl Rehab Cen, **SLP**

Glennen, Sharon 9720 Basket Ring Road, Columbia, MD 21045, (301) 522-5450, BS 78 Purdue Univ - West Lafayette; MS 80 Purdue Univ - West Lafayette; Aud, Kennedy Institute, **SLP**

Glennon, Kristine 19 Howe Street, Ipswich, MA 01938, (617) 356-0570, BA 73 Univ of MA - Amherst; ME 81 Northeastern Univ; Sp-Lang Path, Masconomet Reg Sch Dist, **SLP**

Glenn-Watson, Althea 14 Covey Court, Hopkins, SC 29180, (803) 758-4849, **A**

Glenz, Susan Marlyn 3501 Roswell Road #A2, Atlanta, GA 30305, (404) 292-7272, **SLP**

Glick, Dr Alan H 6106 Edmondson Avenue, Baltimore, MD 21228, (301) 396-7984, ED 68 (NS) Univ of MD - College Park; **SLP**

Glick, Audrey M 2816 Clover Drive, Grand Forks, ND 58201, (701) 777-3232, BS 61 Univ of ND; MS 74 Univ of ND; Cl Asst Prof, University of North Dakota, **SLP**

Glick, Mrs Bonnie Greenberg 5 Chestnut Ridge Road, Poughkeepsie, NY 12603, (914) 896-5417, BA 76 SUNY - Center at Buffalo; MA 77 Univ of FL; Sp/Lang Path, E Ramapo Cen Sch, **SLP**

Glick, Donna Rochelle 18172 Sweet Elm Drive, Encino, CA 91316, (818) 768-6630, BA 74 CA St Univ - Northridge; MA 75 CA St Univ - Northridge; 85–Aud, Southern CA Hearing Service, **A**

Glick, Freda 222 Cedar Lane, Closter, NJ 07624, (201) 268-5270, BA 72 Univ of Toronto - Ontario; MS 82 William Paterson Coll; 85–Sp-Lang Path, Newark Bd of Ed, **SLP ACE**

Glick, Miriam 240 West 73rd Street #406, New York, NY 10023, (212) 799-6549, BA 80 CUNY - Queens Coll; MS 85 Columbia Univ Teachers Coll; **SLP**

Glick, Robin J 35 Cambria Road, Syosset, NY 11791, (516) 931-0530, BA 79 Adelphi Univ; MS 80 Adelphi Univ; SLP, Nassau BOCES, **SLP**

Glick, Mrs Susan S 1838 North Lincoln Pk West, Chicago, IL 60614-5308, BS 73 Northwestern Univ; MS 74 Univ of IL - Urbana; 80–Sp-Lang Path, Private Practice, **SLP**

Glickenhaus, Mrs Sarah Brody 100 Dorchester Road, Scarsdale, NY 10583, (914) 725-0070, BS 40 Univ of MN - Minneap-St Paul; MS 45 Univ of MN - Minneap-St Paul; **SLP**

Glickman, Lisa Sue 9 Suntop Court Unit T-1, Baltimore, MD 21209, (301) 243-3800, BS 84 Ithaca Coll; ME 86 Univ of VA - Charlottesville; 87–Sp-Lang Path, Hrng and Sp Agency of Baltimore, **SLP**

Glicksberg, Susan P 1101 Collier Road N W #2, Atlanta, GA 30318-8230, (904) 878-4073, **A**

Glickstein, Mrs Donna Rostow 74 Summer Place, Huntingdon Valley, PA 19006-1525, (215) 289-2426, BA 70 Temple Univ; MA 73 Temple Univ; Instr Advisor, Phila Sch Dist, **SLP**

Glickstein, Dr Joan Katz 321 Challen Drive, Pittsburgh, PA 15236, (412) 655-7211, BA 55 CUNY - Brooklyn Coll; MS 57 PA St Univ - Univ Park; PH 79 (NS) Univ of Pittsburgh - Pittsburgh; Consultant, Private Practice, **SLP**

Glickstein, Laurel Chertow 2021 N E 210th Street, North Miami Beach, FL 33179, (305) 932-4444, BS 63 Univ of IL - Urbana; MS 79 Barry Univ; MS 85 Nova Univ; Sp-Lang Path, School Board of Dade County, **SLP**

Glidden, Melissa B 375 Lynn Drive #1, Manteno, IL 60950, (815) 939-3651, BS 86 Eastern IL Univ; MA 87 Northern IL Univ - De Kalb; Sp-Lang Path, Kankakee Area Spec Ed Coop, **SLP**

Glime, Katherine C 245 Monson Turnpike Road, Beaver Lake, Ware, MA 01082, (413) 967-3214, MA 87 Univ of MA - Amherst; 87–Sp-Lang Path, Pioneer Developmental Center, **SLP**

Glines, Lisa Wasick 850 Sawtelle Avenue, San Diego, CA 92114, (619) 463-7133, BA 80 San Diego St Univ; MA 85 San Diego St Univ; **SLP**

Gliniecki, Mrs Karen L 43 Jackson Avenue, Carteret, NJ 07008, (201) 541-4918, BS 83 Bloomsburg Univ of PA; MS 84 Bloomsburg Univ of PA; **SLP**

Glisson-Heffel, Denise L 8486 East Frostwood, Anaheim, CA 92807, (213) 922-7683, BA 78 CA St Univ - Fullerton; MA 83 CA St Univ - Fullerton; SLP, Rancho Los Amigos Hosp, **SLP**

Glista, Sandra O 2324 South Park Street, Kalamazoo, MI 49001, (616) 342-2660, BS 72 Loyola Univ of Chicago; MS 74 Univ of IL - Urbana; Owner/Sp-Lang Path, Kalamazoo Sp & Lang Path Ltd, **SLP ACE**

Gliva, Mrs Denise Panella 722 Eden Lane, Somerdale, NJ 08083, (609) 468-2135, BS 76 West Chester Univ of PA; MA 82 West Chester Univ of PA; Sp-Lang Path, Gloucester Twsp Boe, **SLP**

Globokar, Andrea R 4100 Laclede #208, St Louis, MO 63108, (314) 531-4786, BS 68 Wayne St Univ; MS 71 Univ of MI - Ann Arbor; **SLP**

Glod, David J 19 Halifax Court, Marlton, NJ 08053, (609) 726-1000, BS 74 East Stroudsburg Univ of PA; MS 79 Bloomsburg Univ of PA; **SLP**

Glod, Mrs Linda M 19 Halifax Court, Marlton, NJ 08053, (609) 726-1000, BS 75 East Stroudsburg Univ of PA; MS 79 Bloomsburg Univ of PA; **SLP**

Gloeckler, Karen I Rd 1 Box 78, Feura Bush, NY 12067, (314) 751-4385, BS 77 Univ of MO - Columbia; MA 80 Univ of MO - Columbia; Consultant,Special Education, Mo Dept of Elem & Sec Educ, **SLP**

Glorig, Aram 1 Tornco Road, New Mexico, NM 87505-8810, MD (NS); **A F LM**

Glorioso, Mrs Lisa M 789 Riverside Drive, Arnold, MD 21012, (301) 974-0440, BS 72 Adelphi Univ; MS 77 Loyola Coll; Sp/Lang Path, Private Practice, **SLP**

Gloth, Joanne B 32 Copplestone, Avon, CT 06001, **SLP**

Glotzer, Patti Ann 208 Harris Road #M-6, Bedford Hills, NY 10507-2125, (718) 356-1719, **SLP**

Glover, Mrs Andrea K L 3472 Stallings Island Road, Martinez, GA 30907, (404) 828-2528, BS 74 Univ of GA; ME 75 Univ of GA; **SLP**

Glover, John D 1720 Homan Drive #303, Schererville, IN 46375, (219) 736-6474, BA 79 Wright St Univ; MA 81 Ball St Univ; Supvr Sp-Lang Path, Lake Port Rehab Services Inc, **SLP**

Glover, Mrs Karen A 1941 Franklin Street, Columbus, IN 47201, (812) 376-4447, BS 69 IN Univ - Bloomington; MS 75 IN Univ - Bloomington; Sp-Lang Path, Bartholomew Consol Sch Corp, **SLP**

Glover, Lynn K 4017 Shady Hill, Dallas, TX 75229, (214) 960-6892, BA 72 Northwestern St Univ; MA 74 Northwestern St Univ; **SLP**

Glover, Mrs Margaret 4 Fairview Avenue, Box 626, Henniker, NH 03242, (603) 428-7887, BA 74 Univ of Denver; MA 75 Univ of Denver; Aud, Keene Clinic, Inc, **A**

Glover, Marie E 331 Basalt Springs, Naches, WA 98937, (509) 965-3743, BA 65 San Jose St Univ; MA 80 Eastern MI Univ; MS 83 Emporia St Univ; 88–Tchr, Highland Sch Dist, **SLP**

Glover, Mary Jo P 1413 Arch Street, Pittsburgh, PA 15212, (412) 281-1375, BS 74 WV Univ; MA 75 OH St Univ; Sp-Lang Path, Private Practice, **SLP**

Glover, Mrs Mary Marguerite 416 Amalia Drive, Horizon City, TX 79927, (701) 477-6471, BS 81 Univ of WI - Whitewater; MS 82 Univ of WI - Whitewater; 88–Sp-Lang Path, El Paso ISD

Glover, Sherrie M 14825 Fairway Drive East, Mill Creek, WA 98012-5771, **SLP**

Glover, Mrs Toni A 3018 Edgemoor Drive, Palm Harbor, FL 34685, (813) 787-3221, BS 72 Univ of TN - Knoxville; MA 73 Univ of TN - Knoxville; **SLP**

Glovinsky, Mrs Eleanor B 124 Bellington Lane, Creve Coeur, MO 63141, (314) 469-8981, BS 61 Emerson Coll; President, Promotion -El, **SLP**

Glovinsky, Mrs Marilyn G 800 Kenny Way, Las Vegas, NV 89107, BA 63 CUNY - Brooklyn Coll; **SLP**

Glovsky, Leon 1820 Monarch Lane, Vineland, NJ 08360, (609) 691-7340, BA 59 CUNY - Hunter Coll; MA 63 Temple Univ-Tyler Sch of Art; Sp-Lang Path, Vineland Guid & Sp Cen, **SLP**

Glowacki, Mrs Connie Sangren 1625-148th Lane N E, Ham Lake, MN 55304, (612) 464-4297, BA 84 Univ of MN - Duluth; MS 85 Saint Cloud St Univ; 86–Sp-Lang Path, ISD #831 Forest Lake PS

Gloyer, Carol A 1915 Applewood Drive, Hagerstown, MD 21740, (301) 797-9715, BA 72 PA St Univ - Univ Park; MA 73 Univ of FL; Sp-Lang Path, Easter Seal Society, **SLP**

Gluck, Mrs Dolores Wells 243 Weber Avenue N E, North Canton, OH 44720, (216) 499-3801, BS 66 Univ of Akron; MS 70 Univ of Akron; MA 74 Univ of Akron; Sp/Lang Path, Plain Local Schools, **SLP**

Gluck, Nancy A 18 Plymouth Court, Clinton, CT 06413, (203) 669-0833, BA 78 Salve Regina - Newport Coll; MS 81 Southern CT St Univ; Sp-Lang Path, Regional School Dist 18, **SLP**

Gluck, Shelley S 7 Hughes Avenue, Rye, NY 10580, (914) 835-4433, MA 88; 88–Sp-Lang Path, City Sch Dist New Rochelle, **A**

Gluck, Vivian F 4510 Pinetree Drive, Miami Beach, FL 33140, (305) 673-0866, BA 74 CUNY - Queens Coll; MS 76 Columbia Univ Teachers Coll; **SLP**

Glucksman, Catherine Mary 506 Middle Road, Caledonia, NY 14423-9722, (716) 538-2642, BA 80 SUNY - Center at Stony Brook; MA 84 SUNY - Coll at Geneseo; **A**

Glucksman-Weiss, Vivian 13347 Killion Street, Van Nuys, CA 91407, (818) 902-3848, BA 74 Univ of CA - Los Angeles; MA 76 Saint Louis Univ; Sp-Lang Path, Private Practice, **SLP**

Glus, Mrs Kathleen A 22 Parker Avenue, Cedar Knolls, NJ 07927, (201) 593-3153, BA 73 Rutger's St Univ - Douglas Coll; MA 76 Montclair St Coll; 73–Sp-Lang Path, Madison Bd of Ed, **SLP ACE**

Glynn, Christine Alice 367 West Lismore Road, Duluth, MN 55803, (218) 727-5052, BA 80 Univ of MN - Duluth; MA 81 Univ of MN - Duluth; **SLP**

Glynn, Joni Lee 624 Garfield Avenue, Floor 1, Springfield, IL 62702, (217) 528-6836, MA 83 Northern IL Univ - De Kalb; **SLP**

Glynn, Linda M 10 Corte Granada, Moraga, CA 94556, (415) 283-3646, MA 88 CA St Univ - Hayward

Gmeiner-Heinrich, Ann 1763 Appleton Road, Menasha, WI 54952, MS; **SLP**

Gnewikow, Dr Danny W 743 Main Street, Danville, VA 24541, (804) 799-6288, BA 68 David Lipscomb Coll; MS 72 Vanderbilt Univ; PH 74 (Aud) Vanderbilt Univ; Aud, Private Practice, **A**

Gnotta, Lillian S 974 North Grace Street, Scottsdale, AZ 85257, (602) 967-3197, BA 58 Mount St Mary's Coll; MS 78 Fontbonne Coll; MA 79 Saint Louis Univ; Aud, Aud Consult, **SLP A**

Goates, Dr Wallace A 2419 Stringham Avenue, Salt Lake City, UT 84109, (801) 466-4348, BA 29 Univ of UT; MA 35 Univ of IA; PH 37 Univ of IA; Utah Sp & Hrng Cen, **SLP A F**

Goates-Maughan, Dr Joyce S Intermountain Health Care, Therapy Management, 36 South State Street Floor 10, Salt Lake City, UT 84111, (801) 533-3830, BA 70 Univ of UT; MA 71 Univ of UT; PH 76 (Sp-Lang Path) Univ of UT; Asst Dir, Intermountain Health Care, **SLP**

Gober, Carol A 571 Catherine Court, Wood Dale, IL 60191, (312) 447-5007, BS 74 IL St Univ - Normal; MA 75 Univ of IL - Urbana; 75–Sp/Lang Path, Riverside Pub Sch #96, **SLP**

Gober, Mrs Karen M 123 S E 16th Street, Chehalis, WA 98532, BS 52 Univ of WA; Spec Serv Coop, **SLP**

Gober, Mrs Paula J 200 Crooked Bayou, McGehee, AR 71654, (501) 222-6113, BS 78 Henderson St Univ; MS 87 Univ of AR - Medical Sci; 88–Sp-Lang Path, McGehee PS, **SLP**

Gober, Mrs Ruth H 9426 NW 2nd Street, Coral Springs, FL 33071, (305) 753-7756, BA 74 Univ of Pittsburgh - Pittsburgh; MA 75 George Washington Univ; Sp-Lang Path, Broward Cty Adult Educ, **SLP**

Gober, Mrs Susan L 3514 Eveningside Drive, Topeka, KS 66614, (913) 273-4395, BS 80 Univ of GA; ME 81 Univ of GA; 87–Sp-Lang Path, USD 321 Kaw Valley Spec Svcs, **SLP**

Gobin, Donald D 713 South Spring Street, Nevada, MO 64772, (417) 667-5440, BA 57 Baylor Univ; MA 58 Baylor Univ; 88–Retired, Vernon Co Pub Sch, **SLP**

Goblo, Mrs Linda P P O Box 767, Charleston, IL 61920, (217) 345-6018, BS 82 Eastern IL Univ; MS 83 Eastern IL Univ; Sp-Lang Path, Charleston Community Unit #1, **SLP**

Goble, Tamalyn F P O Box 188, Knox, PA 16232, (814) 782-3011, BS 71 Clarion Univ of PA; ME 76 Clarion Univ of PA; Sp-Lang Path, Riverview Inter Unit #6, **SLP**

Gochnour, Mrs Elizabeth Remedial Specialist Inc, 3221 Behrman Place, Suite 203, New Orleans, LA 70114, BA 61 Univ of IA; MA 65 Univ of IA; Dir, Remedial Spec Inc, **SLP ACE**

Goda, Dr Sidney Harwood Bldg, Scarsdale, NY 10583, (914) 725-5950, BA 48 Univ of Denver; MA 50 Univ of VA - Charlottesville; PH 57 (NS) Univ of MI - Ann Arbor; Sp-Lang Path, Private Practice, **SLP A F**

Godar, Mrs Cheryl Skovsted 829 High Street, Madison, WI 53715, (414) 674-2050, BS 81 Univ of WI - Stevens Point; MS 85 Univ of WI - Eau Claire; Sp-Lang Path, Jefferson Sch Dist, **SLP**

Godar, Marilyn R 823 Brownell, St Louis, MO 63122, (618) 875-8800, BS 70 Saint Louis Univ; MS 79 Southern IL Univ-Edwardsvill; Sp-Lang Path, East St Louis Sch Dist 189, **SLP**

Goddard, David E 8196 Callee Court, Flint, MI 48423, (313) 762-7510, BS 78 Central MI Univ; MA 79 Central MI Univ; Sp-Lang Path Supervisor, Bay Valley Home Health Inc, **SLP**

Goddard, Deborah Crawford 406 Green Acres #19, Sandusky, MI 48471, (313) 648-3290, BA 83 MI St Univ; OM 84 Univ of MO - Columbia; 86–Sp-Lang Path, Sanilac Intermediate Shl Dstr, **SLP**

Goddard, Karla Sargent R R 3 Box 511, Pleasant Valley, NY 12569, (914) 635-2917, BA 84 SUNY - Coll at Cortland; MA 85 SUNY - Coll at Geneseo; **A**

Goddard, Linda Renee 4148-D Knob Oak Lane, Charlotte, NC 28211, BA 83 Univ of CO - Boulder; MA 85 Univ of Denver; **SLP**

Godden, Anne L Department Of Communicative Disorders, University Of Western Ontario, London, ON, Canada N6A 1H1, (519) 661-2021, BA 72; MS 75 McGill Univ - Quebec; Sp-Lang Path Coord, Univ of Western Ontario, **SLP**

Goddu, Mrs Kathleen A RR 1 Box 1025, Bowdoinham, ME 04008, (207) 666-3407, MA 83 Univ of ME - Orono; Sp-Lang Path, Bath Sch Dept Union 47, **SLP**

Godfrey, Mrs Sally C 453 Reed Avenue, Rexburg, ID 83440, (208) 356-4344, BA 68 Brigham Young Univ; MA 70 Brigham Young Univ; SLP, Madison Sch Dist 321, **SLP**

Godfriaux, Mrs Lois D Kennedy Avenue, Rd 2 P O Box 177G, Mertztown, PA 19539, (215) 682-9760, BS 74 Seton Hall Univ; MA 76 Seton Hall Univ; **SLP**

Godine, Frances S 19 Crofton Road, Newton, MA 02168, (617) 552-7680, BA 67 CUNY - Queens Coll; MA 69 Emerson Coll; Sp-Lang Path, Newton Public Schools, **SLP**

Godinez-Chan, Noreen Sycip 1167 Mohave Drive, Colton, CA 92324, (714) 824-8957, **SLP**

Godino, Nancy A 8929 Griffon Avenue, Niagara Falls, NY 14304, (716) 282-1836, BA 82 SUNY - Center at Buffalo; MA 84 SUNY - Center at Buffalo; Sp-Lnag Path, Niagara Co Sp Hrng Lang Cen, **SLP**

Godlewski, Mrs Alyce T P O Box 667, Reed Avenue, Smallwood, NY 12778, (914) 583-7092, BA 85 Marymount Coll; MA 88 CUNY - Hunter Coll

Godlewski-Wise, Karen Ann Box 161 R R 1, Fabius, NY 13063, (315) 852-3321, BS 79 SUNY - Coll at Fredonia; MS 84 Ithaca Coll; 80–Sp-Lang Path, DeRuyter Cen Sch, **SLP**

Godsey, Leslie Ann 21 Lincoln Woods Way #3D, Perry Hall, MD 21128, (301) 444-5000, BA 84 Univ of MD - College Park; MS 87 Towson St Univ; 88–Aud, The Maryland Sch for the Blind, **A**

Godsey-Neubert, Jamie Kathryn 60990 Hillsdale Drive, Montrose, CO 81401, (303) 249-2405, BA 82 Humboldt St Univ; MA 85 Humboldt St Univ; **SLP**

Godshalk, Lori Susan 10214 Dedaker Street, Philadelphia, PA 19116, (215) 675-5005, BA 83 Temple Univ; MA 86 Temple Univ; Sp-Lang Path, Montgomery Co Intermed Unit, **SLP**

Godshall, Laurie C 210 North Locksley, Lafayette, LA 70508, (318) 237-7222, BA 73 Univ of AR - Fayetteville; MS 75 Univ of AR - Little Rock; **SLP**

Godwin, Bernadette Augustine 481 Edwards Drive, Sarasota, FL 34243, (813) 755-2323, BS 75 Western IL Univ; MA 76 Western IL Univ; SLP, Manatee Co Sch Dist, **SLP ACE**

Godwin, Elizabeth 105 Georgiana Circle, Madison, WI 53716, (715) 595-4241, BA 73 Univ of MO - Columbia; MS 75 Univ of WI - Eau Claire; SLP, Lake Holcombe Pub Sch, **SLP**

Goebel, Mrs Elizabeth 1005 Mountain Creek Road, Apartment 503, Chattanooga, TN 37405-1648, MS; **SLP LM**

Goebel, Martha D Annandale Fluency Clinic, 4208 Evergreen Lane, Suite 213, Annandale, VA 22003, (703) 941-8903, BA 61 Univ of IA; BA 79 George Washington Univ; MA 80 George Washington Univ; Cl Dir & Owner, Annandale Fluency Cl, **SLP**

Goehl, Dr Henry 8 Foxglove Road, Levittown, PA 19056, (215) 787-8537, OB 53 Newark St Coll; MA 55 Temple Univ-Tyler Sch of Art; PH 59 Univ of Pittsburgh - Pittsburgh; Prof of Sp, Temple Univ, **SLP**

Goeke, Lorraine A 5755 Longford Drive, Dublin, OH 43017, (614) 263-2448, BA 75 Kean Coll of NJ; MA 77 OH St Univ; Sp-Lang Path, Columbus Pub Sch, **SLP**

Goeler, Mrs Nettie Wagner 111 Woodgate Road, Chittenango, NY 13037, (315) 687-7034, BS 80 SUNY - Coll at Fredonia; MA 81 Bowling Green St Univ; Sp-Lang Path, Camden Ctrl Sch Dist, **SLP**

Goemaat, Jean A Box H, Bennett, IA 52721, (319) 893-6622, MA 77 Western IL Univ; BS 75 6675; SLP, Grant Wood AEA, **SLP**

Goepel, Judy T 1901 17th Avenue N W, New Brighton, MN 55112, (612) 636-7777, BS 71 Marquette Univ; MS 72 Marquette Univ; **SLP**

Goepfert, Mrs Gayle Zimmerman Polyclinic Medical Center, Speech & Hearing Center, North 3rd Street, Harrisburg, PA 17105, (717) 782-4350, BS 79 PA St Univ - Univ Park; MS 81 Purdue Univ - West Lafayette; Sp-Lang Path, Polyclinic Med Cen Sp/Hrng Cen, **SLP**

Goepfert, Mrs Laura Picetti 30 John Street, Chatham, NJ 07928, (201) 635-7567, BA 69 Drew Univ; MA 75 Memphis St Univ; Sp-Lang Path, Private Practice, **SLP**

Goergen, Mrs Joann E 13651 Stonegate Road, Midlothian, VA 23113, (804) 379-4023, BA 75 Longwood Coll; ME 76 Univ of VA - Charlottesville; Sp-Lang Path, **SLP**

Goergen, Sharon Ann 6300 Doron Lane, Edina, MN 55435, (612) 533-2781, MA 85 Univ of MN - Minneap-St Paul; **SLP**

Goering, Mrs Danielle M 3326 North 3rd Avenue, Phoenix, AZ 85013, (602) 264-4834, BS 66 Univ of KS; MS 68 AZ St Univ; Aud, ENT Assoc Ltd, **A ACE**

Goerlitz, Cynthia Jo 1425 Ocean Avenue #3, Del Mar, CA 92014, (619) 259-3139, BA 84 San Diego St Univ; **SLP**

Goerner, Mrs Lisa McHugh 6518 West Wisconsin Avenue, Milwaukee, WI 53213, (414) 529-3215, BA 80 IN Univ - Bloomington; OM 82 IN Univ - Bloomington; 85–Aud, Steven J Miller MD, **A**

Goertel-Breen, Mrs Marilyn Joyce 216 Northwestern Drive, Grand Forks, ND 58201, (701) 775-9933, MS 83 Univ of ND; Sp-Lang Path, Human Commun Assoc Ltd, **SLP**

Goetsch, Melinda K 19418 Holt Street N W, Elk River, MN 55330, (612) 295-2934, BS 75 Saint Cloud St Univ; MS 76 Saint Cloud St Univ; Sp-Lang Path, Monticello Sch Dist #882, **SLP**

Goettee, Mrs Marian S 207 Clear Ridge Road, New Windsor, MD 21776, (301) 323-1010, BA 57 Western MD Coll; MS 82 Loyola Coll; 87–Academic & Clin Fac, Loyola Coll, **SLP**

Goetz, Mrs Celia Drewyer 11855 Peach Grove, Houston, TX 77099, (713) 498-8110, **SLP**

Goetz, Karen Cox 6064 North River Trail Dr, Milwaukee, WI 53225, (414) 352-3100, BS 83 Univ of WI - Stevens Point; MS 85 Univ of WI - Stevens Point; 86–Aud, Milwaukee Medical Clinic, **A**

Goetz, Kathryn Lynn 812 Eastmoor Drive, Iowa City, IA 52240, (319) 338-0121, BS 83 Univ of IA; MA 85 Univ of IA; SLP, **SLP**

Goetz, Dr Norma J 628 Cadmus Court, Teaneck, NJ 07666, (201) 836-6494, BA 59 CUNY - Brooklyn Coll; MA 61 CUNY - Brooklyn Coll; ED 86 (Special Education) Rutgers St Univ - Camdem; 87–Sp-Lang Path, Private Practice, **SLP**

Goetz, Sheila L 525 Pleasant Street, Boulder, CO 80302, (303) 492-3039, BS 74 Univ of Pittsburgh - Pittsburgh; MA 83 Univ of Denver; 86–Instr/Dir-Child Lang Ctr, Univ of Colorado Boulder, **SLP**

Goetz, Mrs Suzanne M 7 Ash Street, Manville, RI 02838, (401) 726-1292, BA 73 Univ of RI; MA 76 Univ of CT; Coord Sp-Lang Serv, Lincoln Sch Dept Stud Serv Off, **SLP**

Goetze, Anne S 447 Bolivar Street, Canton, MA 02021, (617) 828-2440, BA 53 Emerson Coll; MS 77 Emerson Coll; SLP, Town of Canton, **SLP ACE**

Goetzinger, Cornelius Peter 14604 South Chalet Drive, Olathe, KS 66062, (913) 782-3138, MA 44 Gallaudet Coll; MA 50 Univ of CA - Berkeley; PH 55 (NS) Northwestern Univ; **A F H LM**

Goff, Anne M Rogue Valley Medical Center, Child Development Center, 2825 Barnett Road, Medford, OR 97504, (503) 773-4952, BA 80 Univ of MI - Ann Arbor; MS 85 Univ of WA; **SLP**

Goff, Carole L Center For Childhood Aphasia And Apraxia, William Beaumont Hospital, 3601 West 13 Mile Road, Royal Oak, MI 48072, (313) 280-8400, BS 71 Eastern MI Univ; MA 72 Eastern MI Univ; Assistant Director, Wm Beaumont Hosp Sp-Lang Dept, **SLP**

Goff, Mrs Cindy Robinson 1194 Saddle Ridge Road, Moscow, ID 83843, (208) 883-0173, BS 71 Bowling Green St Univ; MA 86 WA St Univ; 86–Sp-Lang Path, Private Practice, **SLP**

Goff, Mrs Gail S 310N 1st Street, Heber Springs, AR 72543, (501) 362-8155, BS 76 Univ of Central AR; MS 79 Univ of AR - Fayetteville; 79–Sp-Lang Path, Home Health/Private Practice, **SLP**

Goff, Jo Ellen Andersen 1767 West 75th Street, Apt #1F, Richfield, MN 55423, (612) 863-4407, BA 82 Saint Cloud St Univ; MS 83 Saint Cloud St Univ; 87–Sp-Lang Path, Sister Kenny Institute, **SLP**

Goff, Stephen William 24865 Lakeland, Farmington Hills, MI 48018, (313) 477-6682, MA 84 Wayne St Univ; Aud, Lucas Hrng Aid Svc, **A**

Goffen, Robin Layle 600 Brandon Avenue #28, Charlottesville, VA 22903, (804) 979-6344, BS 84 Miami Univ - Oxford; OM 85 IN Univ - Bloomington; 86–Sp-Lang Path, Charlottesville City Schs, **SLP**

Goffman, Lisa Alice 1814 West Estef Apt#2, Chicago, IL 60626, (312) 356-6003, BS 82 Purdue Univ - West Lafayette; MS 85 Purdue Univ - West Lafayette; SLP, Lmrp Parent Infant Ctr, **SLP**

Goforth, Mrs Lee S P O Box 433, Manteo, NC 27954, BS 76 Western Carolina Univ; ME 77 Western Carolina Univ; Sp/Lang Path, Albemarle City Sch, **SLP**

Goga, Mrs Judith J 7528 McLellan Drive, Walton Hills, OH 44146, (216) 842-5300, MA 70 Bowling Green St Univ; BS 66 Bowling Green St Univ; SLP, Parma Cty Sch, **SLP ACE**

Gogarty-Gajan, Kathleen R 202 North Main Street, Franklinton, NC 27525, (919) 575-7349, BA 76 Univ of MD - College Park; MA 78 Univ of MA - Amherst; Sp-Lang Path, Franklin Cnty Home Health Agcy, **SLP**

Gogenola-Rothberg, Ann 7029 Lafayette Avenue, Omaha, NE 68132, (402) 556-3334, BS 76 ID St Univ; MS 81 ID St Univ; Sp-Lang Path, Omaha PS, **SLP**

Goggans, Shirley Dale 3248 Brockett Way, Jacksonville, FL 32218, (904) 764-2099, BA 80 Univ of TN - Knoxville; MA 83 Univ of TN - Knoxville; Sp-Lang Path, **SLP**

Goggin, Julie Heide 1301 West 43rd Street, Vancouver, WA 98660, (206) 695-0778, BS 73 Portland St Univ; MS 76 Portland St Univ; 87–SLP, Evergreen Sch Dist #114, **SLP**

Gogolin, Marilyn T 15 Sweetwater, Irvine, CA 92715, (213) 922-6400, BA 67 Univ of LA Verne; MA 68 Univ of Redlands; MS 76 CA St Univ - Fullerton; Asst to Superintendent, Los Angeles County Office Educ, **SLP**

Goh, Annette Wen-Li 258 Barrow Street #2-F, Jersey City, NJ 07302, (201) 795-7156, BS 83 Univ of WI - Madison; MS 84 Marquette Univ; 88–Sp-Lang Path, St Francis Hosp, **SLP**

Gohde, Mrs Sandra E 22 Lakeview Drive, Morris Plains, NJ 07950, (201) 285-9672, BA 72 Montclair St Coll; MA 78 Montclair St Coll; Sp-Lang Path, Parsippany Board of Education, **SLP**

Gohl, Mrs Glenna G 653 Buffalo Bend, Plano, TX 75023, (214) 371-5304, BA 80 TX Tech Univ; MS 82 Univ of TX - Dallas; SLP, Dallas ISD, **SLP**

Goiffon, Joann C 5265 East Lake Beach Court, St Paul, MN 55126, (612) 786-4006, MS 76 Saint Cloud St Univ; SLP, Mounds View Pub Schs, **SLP**

Going, Joan L 140 Main Street #2, Essex Junction, VT 05452, BA 76 Univ of ME - Orono; MS 79 Univ of IL - Urbana; Sp-Lang Path, Chittenden East Sch Dist, **SLP**

Goings, Mrs Regina E 4020 South Arville St #120, Las Vegas, NV 89103, (702) 362-1285, MS 81 Governors St Univ; BS 75 Northern IL Univ - De Kalb; 85–Sp-Lang Path, Clark Co Sch Dist, **SLP**

Goitia, Mrs Lorena Desalvo 41 Belle Grove Drive, Destrehan, LA 70047, (504) 363-2317, OM 84 LA St Univ - N O Medical Ctr; SLP, F Edward Hebert Hosp, **SLP**

Gokan, Lynn Y 224 Kaia Street, Honolulu, HI 96813, (808) 537-6730, MS 88 Univ of HI - Manoa

Gokcen, Jeanne Holloway 3805 Kimberly Pkwy North, Columbus, OH 43232, (614) 461-2420, BS 82 OH Univ - Athens; MA 84 OH Univ - Athens; Sp-Lang Path, Ohio State Univ, **SLP**

Golanka, Janet M 52 Hamilton Blvd, Kenmore, NY 14217, (716) 885-8318, MS 72 SUNY - Center at Buffalo; 86–Exec Dir, Buffalo Hearing & Sp Ctr, **SLP**

Golann, Adria J RFD 1 Box 88, Charlemont, MA 01339, (413) 664-9292, MA 87 Univ of MA - Amherst

Golato, June Ellen 370 Maple Street #G, Burlington, VT 05401, (802) 865-3125, BS 84 Boston Univ; MS 85 Univ of VT; Sp-Lang Path, Bellows Free Academy, **SLP**

Golbabai, Mrs Carolyn J 832 Kennedy Road, Windsor, CT 06095-1927, (203) 983-1027, BS 79 Elmira Coll; MS 81 Purdue Univ - West Lafayette; Sp-Lang Path, Bloomfield Pub Sch, **SLP**

Golberg, Mrs Leslie Levin P O Box 9312, Reno, NV 89507, (702) 784-4887, BA 76 Univ of MD - College Park; MS 77 Univ of NV - Reno; 78–Lect/Cl Coord, U of NV-Reno, **SLP**

Gold, Amy Joy 125 Warner Hill Road #14, Stratford, CT 06497, (203) 375-3770, BA 84 Univ of RI; MS 86 Southern CT St Univ; **SLP**

Gold, Mrs Andrea Just 60 Church Road Street, Morganville, NJ 07751, BA 79 CUNY - Brooklyn Coll; MS 82 CUNY - Brooklyn Coll; SLP, NYC Bd of Ed, **SLP**

Gold, Betsy R 74 Sharon Drive, Richboro, PA 18954, (215) 750-7711, BA 75 Temple Univ; MA 76 Trenton St Coll; 76–Sp-Lang Path, Private Practice, **SLP**

Gold, Jennifer R 835 Richmond Avenue, Buffalo, NY 14222, (716) 882-9516, MS 77 SUNY - Coll at Buffalo; Sp-Lang Path, BOCES I Erie, **SLP**

Gold, Mrs Lynn Dickson 10 Stillwater, Irvine, CA 92715-3426, (714) 854-3417, BA 67 Western WA Univ; MA 69 CA St Univ - Los Angeles; Sp-Lang Path, Private Practice, **SLP ACE**

Gold, Mrs Mindy Rose 74-69 220th Street #B-1, Bayside, NY 11364, BA 79 CUNY - Brooklyn Coll; MS 82 CUNY - Brooklyn Coll; Sp-Lang Path, NYC Boe, **SLP**

Gold, Pennysue 8822 Macon Street, Philadelphia, PA 19152, (215) 698-7457, BS 84 PA St Univ - Univ Park; MA 87 Temple Univ

Gold, Mrs Phyllis G 3023 Central Avenue, Wilmette, IL 60091, **SLP**

Gold, Dr Saralyn 1609 Woodridge Drive, Johnson City, TN 37604, (615) 929-1551, BA 76 SUNY - Coll at New Paltz; MA 79 Kent St Univ; PH 86 (Aud) SUNY - Center at Buffalo; 85–Asst Prof, East Tenn State Univ, **A**

Gold, Sharon J c/o Boston Guild For The Hard Of Hearing, 283 Commonwealth Avenue, Boston, MA 02115, (617) 267-4730, BS 76 Central CT St Univ; MS 86 Northeastern Univ; 87–Aud, Head & Neck Surgical Assoc, **A**

Gold, Mrs Susan J 882 Jamestown Road, East Windsor, NJ 08520, (609) 443-1452, BA 75 SUNY - Center at Buffalo; MS 87 CUNY - Brooklyn Coll; 87–Sp-Lang Path, John F Kennedy Med Ctr, **SLP**

Gold, Mrs Susan L 5065 Stoneboat Row, Columbia, MD 21044, (301) 730-5843, BA 62 Univ of MD - College Park; MA 76 Univ of MD - College Park; 77–Aud, Univ of Maryland Med Sys, **SLP A**

Gold, Wendy M 401 South Narberth Avenue, Apartment 1-A, Narberth, PA 19072, (215) 885-0611, BS 79 PA St Univ - Univ Park; MA 81 Temple Univ; 88–Dir Sp-Lang Path, Universal Rehab Svcs, **SLP**

Goldacker, Frank E Carle Clinic Association, Dept Of Neurology, 602 West University, Urbana, IL 61801, (217) 337-3440, BS 76 Eastern IL Univ; MS 77 Eastern IL Univ; SLP, Carle Clinic Association, **SLP**

Goldaine, John A 4421 Melrose, Erie, PA 16509, (814) 452-5510, BA 79 Duquesne Univ; MS 81 WV Univ; Sp-Lang Path, St Vincent Health Center, **SLP**

Goldbach, Mrs Eileen D 257 Lakeview Avenue, Lynbrook, NY 11563, (516) 887-4196, BA 68 Adelphi Univ; MS 70 Adelphi Univ; SLP, Hewlett-Woodmere Un Fr Sch D, **SLP**

Goldbaum, Mrs Donna D 1332 Stratford, Clovis, NM 88101, (505) 562-2156, BS 78 Eastern NM Univ; MS 79 ID St Univ; Sp-Lang Path, East New Mexico Univ, **A**

Goldberg, Betty L 23 High Point Road, Westport, CT 06880, (203) 795-3505, BA 68 Univ of MI - Ann Arbor; MA 70 Univ of Cincinnati; Sp-Lang Path, Orange Bb of Ed, **SLP**

Goldberg, Christine Riggott 1040 Indian Creek Road, Wynnewood, PA 19151, (215) 829-5253, BA 70 Univ of CT; MS 71 Univ of WI - Madison; Sp-Lang Path, PA Hosp, **SLP**

Goldberg, David H 3554 West Nightflower Pl, Tucson, AZ 85741, (602) 623-8431, BA 68 Univ of MA - Amherst; MS 72 Southern CT St Univ; Sp/Lang Path, Marana AZ PS, **SLP**

Goldberg, Mrs Debra Lynn 81 Tobin Avenue, Great Neck, NY 11021, (212) 596-5698, **SLP**

Goldberg, Mrs Dianne 8020 Prospect Way, La Mesa, CA 92041, (619) 697-6760, BA 67 George Washington Univ; MS 68 Univ of MI - Ann Arbor; Sp-Lang Path, Private Practice, **SLP ACE**

Goldberg, Dr Donald M University Of Connecticut, Department Of Comm Sci, Box U-85, 850 Bolton Road, Storrs, CT 06268, (203) 486-4080, BA 77 Lafayette Coll; MA 79 Univ of FL; PH 85 (NS) Univ of FL; Asst Prof, Univ of Connecticut, **SLP A ACE**

Goldberg, Donald R 346 Woodin Street, Hamden, CT 06514, (203) 977-4523, BA 73 Southern CT St Univ; MS 75 Southern CT St Univ; Sp-Lang Path, Stamford Pub Sch, **SLP**

Goldberg, Mrs Donna 84 Falcon Trail, Pittsford, NY 14534, MS 71 SUNY - Center at Buffalo; Sp-Lang Path, City School District, **SLP**

Goldberg, Donna Lynn 213-49 38th Avenue #3-E, Bayside, NY 11361, (718) 225-6670, **A**

Goldberg, Faye R 142 Washington St, Newton, MA 02158-2250, (617) 969-3376, BS 79 Univ of CT; ME 81 Northeastern Univ; Sp-Lang Path, Mass Easter Seal Society, **SLP**

Goldberg, Mrs Hazel P 10911 Yorkway Lane, Cincinnati, OH 45249, (513) 984-1994, BS 66 Univ of Cincinnati; MA 70 Univ of Cincinnati; 81–Sp-Lang Path, Bethesda Hosp, **SLP**

Goldberg, Joyce S R R 1 Box 8735, 533 Intervale, Sebago Lake, ME 04075, (207) 787-3648, **SLP**

Goldberg, Linda D 13 Raymond Avenue, Spring Valley, NY 10977, (914) 354-0200, BA 66 CUNY - Brooklyn Coll; MS 73 CUNY - Queens Coll; Sp-Lang Path, Rockland Co Hlth Cen, **SLP**

Goldberg, Mrs Linda M 4 Ivy Court, Plainview, NY 11803, (516) 349-0187, BA 78 George Washington Univ; MA 80 NY Univ; Sp-Lang Path, Private Practice, **SLP**

Goldberg, Lori E 2604 North Windsor Drive, Apartment 201, Arlington Heights, IL 60004, (312) 794-3999, BS 72 Northern IL Univ - De Kalb; MA 73 MI St Univ; 75–Aud, IL Dept of Mental Health & Dev Dis, **A**

Goldberg, Mrs Lynette R 5008 Euclid Drive, Kensington, MD 20895, (301) 231-5866, BS 72 Victorian Sch of Speech Science - Australia; MA 75 Western MI Univ; PH 88 (Speech Science) Wayne St Univ; 87–Dir, The Focus Ctr, **SLP**

Goldberg, Mrs Lynn Potashnick 11629 Yeatman Terrace, Silver Spring, MD 20902-3059, (301) 681-9467, BA 84 Univ of MD - College Park; MA 86 George Washington Univ; 88–Aud, Private Practice, **A**

Goldberg, Mary Jane 101 East Edsall Avenue, Apartment B-5, Palisades Park, NJ 07650, (914) 358-6200, BS 80 SUNY - Coll at Buffalo; MS 83 Columbia Univ Teachers Coll; 87–Sp-Lang Path, Nyack Hosp, **SLP**

Goldberg, Mrs Phyllis K 12740 S W 101st Terrace, Miami, FL 33186, (305) 386-2180, BA 70 Univ of FL; MA 77 Univ of Miami; Sp-Lang Path, Dade Co Pub Sch, **SLP**

Goldberg, Rachelle K 23 Lawridge Drive, Rye Brook, NY 10573, **A**

Goldberg, Rhona J 3401 Smith Avenue SE, Apartment #5, Albuquerque, NM 87106, (505) 268-2434, BA 77 Temple Univ; MA 78 Trenton St Coll; 82–Sp-Lang Path, Albuquerque Pub Sch, **SLP**

Goldberg, Robin 19 Skylar Drive, Southborough, MA 01772, (617) 856-2398, BA 74 Adelphi Univ; MS 76 Columbia Univ Teachers Coll; 80–Dir-Sp/Lang Path, Univ of MA Med Ctr, **SLP**

Goldberg, Mrs Rosalyn Berger 6723 Chokeberry Road, Baltimore, MD 21209-1451, (301) 363-0300, **A**

Goldberg, Sandra K 436 West School House Lane, Philadelphia, PA 19144, (215) 849-3635, BA 71 Case Western Reserve Univ; MS 72 Columbia Univ Teachers Coll; **SLP**

Goldberg, Mrs Sara Ann 1905 North 55th Avenue, Hollywood, FL 33021-3937, (305) 961-1163, OB 72 IN Univ - Bloomington; MS 87 Nova Univ

Goldberg, Mrs Sharon G Rural Route 1, Poplar Hills, Princeton, IN 47670, (812) 749-6133, BS 76 IN St Univ - Terre Haute; MS 80 IN St Univ - Terre Haute; Sp-Lang Path, E Gibson School Corporation, **SLP**

Goldberg, Sheila C 48 Abbot Road, Smithtown, NY 11787, (516) 724-9261, BA 60 CUNY - Queens Coll; **SLP**

Goldberg, Dr Stanley A 2695 18th Avenue, San Francisco, CA 94116, (415) 566-3721, BA 67 Univ of Pittsburgh - Pittsburgh; MA 70 Univ of Pittsburgh - Pittsburgh; PH 75 (NS) Univ of Pittsburgh - Pittsburgh; Assoc Prof, San Francisco St U, **SLP**

Goldberg, Sunny Yeddis 502 Orienta Avenue, Mamaroneck, NY 10543, (914) 698-7183, BS 67 Univ of WI - Madison; MS 69 NY Univ; OM 74 Yeshiva Univ; SLP, BOCES - Southern Westchester, **SLP**

Goldberg, Tova R 320 South Linden Drive, Beverly Hills, CA 90212, (213) 660-3530, BA 76 CA St Univ - Northridge; MA 78 CA St Univ - Northridge; Sp-Lang Path Mgr, Hollywood Presby Med Cen, **SLP**

Goldberger, Mrs Joan F 11 Wensley Drive, Great Neck, NY 11021, (516) 437-0090, BA 55 CUNY - Queens Coll; ME 58 Boston Univ; Sp-Lang Path, Jewish Inst for Geriatric Care, **SLP**

Goldberger, Mrs Rhoda S 36 Buff Road, Tenafly, NJ 07670, BS 47 Columbia Univ Teachers Coll; MA 49 Columbia Univ Teachers Coll; **LM**

Goldberg-Stoter, Mrs Gail 17147 Roundhill Drive, Huntington Beach, CA 92649, (714) 840-2005, BS 74 Boston Univ; MS 78 PA St Univ - Univ Park; Sp-Lang Path, Long Beach USD, **SLP**

Goldblatt, Mrs Judith A 156 Thurton Drive, New Canaan, CT 06840, (203) 966-7715, BA 64 Temple Univ; MS 80 Rutgers St Univ -N Brunswick; Sp/Lang Path, Stamford Board of Education, **SLP**

Goldblatt, Mary Anne P O Box 5017, Diamond Bar, CA 91765, (714) 771-1000, BA 71 Univ of CA - Davis; MA 75 CA St Univ - Long Beach; Sp-Lang Path, Cigna, **SLP**

Goldblatt, Ree Ellen Lewen 11 Cannonade Drive, Marlboro, NJ 07746, (201) 370-1150, **SLP**

Goldblatt-Kass, Mrs Mindy Gayle 136 Dawson Lane, Jericho, NY 11753, (516) 924-0008, BS 84 SUNY - Coll at Oneonta; MS 85 Adelphi Univ; **SLP**

Goldblum, Amy Denise 202 East 73rd Street #10-A, New York, NY 10021, (718) 263-1587, BA 85 SUNY - Center at Buffalo; MS 86 Columbia Univ Teachers Coll; **SLP**

Goldblum, Mrs Glenn Binder 14 Herbert Baker Street, Groenkloof, Pretoria, South Africa 0181, MA 84 Univ of CA - Santa Barbara; Lecturer Supervisor, University of Pretoria, **SLP**

Golden, Diane Cordry Route #3 Lake Sundance, 5712 South County Road Kk, Columbia, MO 65203, BS 77 Univ of MO - Columbia; MS 78 Central MO St Univ; Asst Dir Soec Ed, Dept of Ed, **A**

Golden, Mrs Diane W Two Mindy Court, Chico, CA 95928, (916) 891-2793, OB 63 Univ of the Pacific; MA 74 CA St Univ - Chico; 74–Sp-Lang Path, Butte Co Office of Ed, **SLP**

Golden, Ellen Nan 833 North Humboldt #410, San Mateo, CA 94401, (415) 344-6790, MS 88 San Francisco St Univ; 88–Sp-Lang Path, Ctr for Sp Lang Disorders

Golden, Maureen Theresa One Williams Lane, Foster City, CA 94404, (415) 469-6217, BA 80 Univ of Redlands; MS 82 Univ of Redlands; Sp/Lang Path, Diag Ctr for Neuro Hndcap Chldn, **SLP**

Golden, Mrs Sharon R 154 Berkeley Place, Brooklyn, NY 11217, (212) 636-5838, BA 74 CUNY - Brooklyn Coll; MA 76 Hofstra Univ; Sp-Lang Path, Nurs Srs Home Visit Ser, **SLP**

Goldenback, Robin 461 Nassau Boulevard, West Hempstead, NY 11552, (718) 465-8310, BA 79 CUNY - Queens Coll; MA 81 CUNY - Queens Coll; Sp-Lang Path, NYC Bd of Ed-Sp Serv Ut, **SLP**

Goldenberg, Amy 20 Saint Paul Street #6, Brookline, MA 02146, (617) 232-2591, BS 84 Ithaca Coll; MA 86 Boston Univ; Sp-Lang Path, Braintree Hosp, **SLP**

Goldenberg, Barry 1005-1348 Barclay Street, Vancouver, BC, Canada V6E 1H7, (604) 595-3611, BA 72 0222; MA 77 SUNY - Center at Buffalo; **SLP**

Goldenberg, Mrs Jean 17610 N E 7th Place, North Miami Beach, FL 33162, (305) 653-5637, BA 72 CUNY - Queens Coll; MA 74 CUNY - Queens Coll; 88–Sp-Lang Path Supvr, Comm Disorder Ctr-Nova Univ, **SLP ACE**

Goldenberg, Nancy 54 Norwegian Wood Apartment, Tolland, CT 06084, (203) 455-0707, BA 79 Univ of CT; MS 80 PA St Univ - Univ Park; Sp-Lang Path, Eastconn, **SLP**

Goldenziel, Barbara R 603 Gladiola Drive, Clarks Summit, PA 18411, (717) 346-7091, BA 70 PA St Univ - Univ Park; MA 73 Temple Univ-Tyler Sch of Art; Sp-Lang Path, Private Practice, **SLP**

Golder, Kyle A 15 Privateers Lane, Rochester, NY 14624, (716) 232-2310, BS 77 SUNY - Coll at Fredonia; ME 79 Univ of GA; 84–Sp-Lang Path, Rochester City Sch Dist, **SLP**

Goldetsky, Judy M 4860 Saratoga Lane North, Plymouth, MN 55442, (312) 878-8200, BA 73 Univ of MN - Minneap-St Paul; MA 77 Univ of KS; **SLP**

Goldfaden, Mrs Debra Rhonda 41 Belmont Drive, Livingston, NJ 07039, (201) 740-8831, BA 69 CUNY - Queens Coll; MA 71 CUNY - Queens Coll; 79–Sp-Lang Path, West Orange Bd of Educ, **SLP**

Goldfarb, Elizabeth Jane 2131 Columbus Avenue, Duluth, MN 55803, BA 80 Univ of MN - Duluth; MA 84 Univ of MN - Duluth; **SLP**

Goldfarb, Dr Robert M 1160 3rd Avenue, New York, NY 10021, (212) 960-8138, BA 68 CUNY - Brooklyn Coll; MS 72 CUNY - Brooklyn Coll; PH 78 (Sp & Hrng Sciences) CUNY - Grad Sch & Univ Cntr; Assoc Prof and Prgm Dir, Lehman Coll of CUNY, **SLP**

Goldfein, Susan K 37 Riverside Drive, New York, NY 10023, (212) 379-5020, OB 61 CUNY - Bernard M Baruch Coll; MA 72 CUNY - Hunter Coll; ME 83 Columbia Univ Teachers Coll; 87–Clin Supvr/Instr, Teachers Coll-Columbia Univ, **SLP**

Goldhaber, Danna 702 Landmark Two, Cherry Hill, NJ 08034, (215) 338-9600, BS 84 Trenton St Coll; MS 87 Gallaudet Coll; 87–Aud, The Hearing Lab Inc, **A**

Goldhagen, Gregg A 33 Bethal Lane, Commack, NY 11725, (516) 368-3178, BA 84 SUNY - Center at Buffalo; MS 86 Adelphi Univ

Goldhawk-Haag, Mrs Kelly S 42 Crestfield Drive, Rochester, NY 14617, (716) 338-7005, BS 83 SUNY - Coll at Buffalo; MS 84 SUNY - Coll at Buffalo; Sp-Lang Path, Monroe/Orleans BOCES #2, **SLP**

Goldhecht, Debra W 5-D Apple Tree Lane, Old Bridge, NJ 08857, (201) 679-4121, BA 84 CUNY - Brooklyn Coll; MS 86 CUNY - Brooklyn Coll; **SLP**

Goldin, Marci H 46-A Route 303, Valley Cottage, NY 10989, (914) 634-4648, BS 86 SUNY - Coll at Geneseo; MA 88 SUNY - Coll at Geneseo; 88–Sp-Lang Path, Rockland Co Ctr Phys Hndcpd

Goldin, Miriam R 4970 Cleveland Street, Suite 110, Virginia Beach, VA 23462, (804) 467-6400, BS 71 Ithaca Coll; MA 72 Case Western Reserve Univ; Sp-Lang Path, Private Practice, **SLP**

Golding, Mrs Cindy Trotnic P O Box 6985, Brookings, OR 97415, (503) 469-3647, BA 76 Pittsburg St Univ; MA 79 Wichita St Univ; Sp/Lang Path, **SLP**

Golding, Gayla Siegal 11512 Kimbark Court, Gaithersburg, MD 20878, (301) 990-9085, OB 76 Univ of Miami; ME 79 Univ of Miami; MS 84 Univ of RI; Sp-Lang Path, Treatment & Learning Centers, **SLP**

Golding-Kushner, Mrs Karen J Center For Craniofacial Dis, Montefiore Medical Center, 3331 Bainbridge Avenue, Bronx, NY 10467, (212) 920-4781, BS 76 SUNY - Center at Albany; MA 77 Univ of Pittsburgh - Pittsburgh; OM 87 CUNY - Grad Sch & Univ Cntr; 88–Clin Coord, Montefiore Med Ctr, **SLP**

Goldish, Susan R P O Box 1805, Eugene, OR 97440, (503) 345-4978, BS 77 Univ of MN - Duluth; MS 83 Univ of OR; Sp-Lang Path, Ctr for Neuro-Educ Therapies Inc, **SLP**

Goldman, Amy S 203 Nathaniel Avenue, Cherry Hill, NJ 08003, (609) 588-3193, BS 70 Ithaca Coll; MS 71 SUNY - Coll at Buffalo; 85–Coord/Sp-Lang-Path, NJ Office of Educ, **SLP**

Goldman, Bernice Ellen 3775 North Tanuri Drive, Tucson, AZ 85715, (602) 327-4931, BA 78 Univ of AZ; MS 80 Univ of AZ; Aud, U of Arizona, **A**

Goldman, Charles 2651 East 63rd Street, Brooklyn, NY 11234, (718) 498-6902, BA 71 CUNY - Brooklyn Coll; MS 74 CUNY - Brooklyn Coll; Sp-Lang Path, NYC Bd of Ed, **SLP**

Goldman, Clifford S 4504 N E 23rd, Portland, OR 97211, (503) 282-1150, BS 66 Portland St Univ; MA 68 American Univ; MS 79 Portland St Univ; Sp/Lang Path, Portland PS, **SLP**

Goldman, Deborah S 7742 Arcadia, Morton Grove, IL 60053, (312) 966-3735, MA 88 Univ of IL - Urbana; Aud, N Shore Audiovestibular Lab

Goldman, Diane M 121 S W 96th Terrace, Plantation, FL 33324, (305) 741-6220, BS 67 Emerson Coll; MA 68 Columbia Univ Teachers Coll; SLP, Sch Bd of Broward Co, **SLP**

Goldman, Mrs Donna Sue 297 Garfield Place, Brooklyn, NY 11215, (718) 638-3330, BS 82 Ithaca Coll; MS 84 Columbia Univ Teachers Coll; **SLP**

Goldman, Mrs Eileen R 1951 Central Drive North, East Meadow, NY 11554, (516) 541-6600, BA 51 CUNY - Queens Coll; MS 69 Adelphi Univ; Sp-Lang Path, Massapequa Sch Dist 23, **SLP**

Goldman, Gail R 4481 17th Avenue S W, Naples, FL 33999, (813) 455-8918, BA 70 Univ of FL; ME 72 Boston Univ; 88–Sp-Lang Path, Collier Co PS, **SLP**

Goldman, Mrs Karon R 120 Mardan Drive, Reisterstown, MD 21136, (301) 833-9505, BS 72 Towson St Univ; MS 78 Loyola Coll; Sp-Lang Path, Baltimore Co Pub Sch, **SLP**

Goldman, Mrs Laura G Kelso Bldg Suite 202, 10 East Athens Avenue, Ardmore, PA 19003, (215) 642-5070, BS 70 Northwestern Univ; MA 71 Temple Univ; Sp-Lang Path, Private Practice, **SLP**

Goldman, Lisa Mendes 1944 Haight Avenue, Bronx, NY 10461, (212) 597-6817, BS 81 SUNY - Coll at Buffalo; MA 85 CUNY - Lehman Coll; Tchr, NYC Bd of Educ, **SLP**

Goldman, Mrs Marilyn M 275 Orchard Road, Paoli, PA 19301, (215) 647-9330, BA 60 Univ of PA; MA 65 Temple Univ-Tyler Sch of Art; Aud, Valley Forge ENT Assoc, **A ACE**

Goldman, Mrs Mary Ann 34 Edward Drive, Stoughton, MA 02072, (617) 341-2939, BS 63 Ball St Univ; MS 73 Butler Univ; 87–Sp-Lang Path, Town of Braintree, **SLP**

Goldman, Roberta L 9701 Fields Road #2105, Gaithersburg, MD 20878, BS 60 Syracuse Univ; MS 64 Syracuse Univ; Sp-Lang Path, Pg Co Schs, **SLP**

Goldman, Dr Ronald University Of Alabama, 1720 7th Avenue South, Birmingham, AL 35233, BA 55 Birmingham-Southern Coll; MS 57 Univ of Pittsburgh - Pittsburgh; PH 60 (NS) Univ of Pittsburgh - Pittsburgh; 87–Dir of Sp-Lang Path, Univ of AL-Sparks Ctr, **SLP F**

Goldman, Sara B 77-10 171st Street, Flushing, NY 11366, **SLP**

Goldman, Sheila Ochs 4900 Woodman #11, Sherman Oaks, CA 91423, (818) 789-9820, BA 58 Univ of PA; MS 65 Tulane Univ; Sp-Lang Path, Naomi Heller & Associates, **SLP**

Goldman, Stephen Norman 2953 Old Bridgeport Way, San Diego, CA 92111, (619) 294-5700, MA 81 San Diego St Univ; SLP, Ucsd Med Cen, **SLP**

Goldman, Dr Thomas M 5993 Ropes Drive, Cincinnati, OH 45244, (513) 569-2377, BS 77 Univ of Cincinnati; MA 79 Univ of Cincinnati; PH 85 (NS) Univ of Cincinnati; Aud, Jewish Hosp Cincinnati, **A**

Goldman, William H 106 Dostak Drive, Anderson, SC 29621, (803) 226-2477, BS 51 IN St Univ - Terre Haute; MA 59 Northwestern Univ; 72–Director, Anderson-Oconee Sp & Hrng Serv, **SLP A**

Goldman-Gluck, Heryl 300 East 74th Street, New York, NY 10021, **SLP**

Goldmann, Mrs Kathleen M 301 Northridge, Denton, TX 76201, BA 65 Saint Joseph's Coll; MS 70 CUNY - Queens Coll; Sp-Lang Path, Denton ISD, **SLP ACE**

Goldner, Dr Beverly Boling 1721 Flagler Avenue, Key West, FL 33040, (305) 294-6696, BA 72 Columbia Coll; ME 73 Univ of SC - Columbia; PH 83 (Sp) Univ of FL; 85–Sp-Lang Path, Private Practice, **SLP**

Goldner, Mrs Debra L 23728 Rotunda Road, Valencia, CA 91355, (805) 259-5846, BA 77 CA St Univ - Northridge; MA 79 CA St Univ - Northridge; Sp-Lang Path, Los Angles USD, **SLP**

Goldner, Mrs Kathleen M 64-10A 186th Lane, Queens, NY 11365, BS 77 CUNY - Queens Coll; MA 79 CUNY - Queens Coll; Sp-Lang Path, NYC Bd of Ed, **SLP**

Goldojarb, Mrs Muriel F 13934 Chandler Boulevard, Van Nuys, CA 91401, (818) 891-7711, BA 52 CA St Univ - Los Angeles; MA 69 CA St Univ - Northridge; Sp-Lang Path, Vamc Sepulveda, **SLP**

Goldring, Mrs Sondra K Pleasantville Road, New Vernon, NJ 07976, (201) 377-6607, BA 54 Emerson Coll; MA 70 Seton Hall Univ; Sp-Lang Path, Private Practice, **SLP ACE**

Goldsberry, Mrs Gail Edelman 55 Briarwood Drive, Schererville, IN 46375, (219) 322-8285, **A**

Goldsberry, Mrs Shirley W P O Box 1, Meade, KS 67864, (316) 873-2718, BS 76 Fort Hays St Univ; MS 77 Fort Hays St Univ; Sp-Lang Path, Southwest Special Educ Coop, **SLP**

Goldschmid, Mrs Leslie S 17F Putnam Green, Greenwich, CT 06830, (914) 833-3153, BA 68 CUNY - Queens Coll; MA 70 CUNY - Queens Coll; 86–Sp-Lang Path, Mamaroneck Sch Dist, **SLP**

Goldschmidt, Mrs Catherine 27 Woods Grove, Westport, CT 06880, (203) 227-8451, BA 60 Univ of Chicago; BA 61 Univ of Chicago; MA 67 De Paul Univ; SLP, Westport Bd of Ed, **SLP**

Goldsman, Mrs Susanna Klein 311 Byrne Avenue, Staten Island, NY 10314, (718) 983-9187, BA 82 CUNY - Brooklyn Coll; MS 85 CUNY - Brooklyn Coll; SLP, Judi Dobner, **SLP**

Goldsmith, Carole B 110 Tarpon Circle, Winter Springs, FL 32708, (305) 422-3200, BS 66 FL St Univ; MS 67 FL St Univ; SLP, Orange Co Pub Sch-Sp-Lang Imp, **SLP**

Goldsmith, Georgie A 123 Haynie Street, Covington, TN 38019, (901) 867-2921, BA 77 Univ of MS; MA 80 Memphis St Univ; Director/Sp-Lang Pathology, Arlington Developmental Center, **SLP**

Goldsmith, Howard D 19175 Eldridge Lane, Southfield, MI 48076, (313) 433-3871, BS 73 Western MI Univ; MS 74 Univ of WI - Madison; PH 84 (NS) Univ of WA; SLP, Self Employed, **SLP**

Goldsmith, Marian 2407 Jenkins Street, Endwell, NY 13760, (607) 722-5308, BA 74 CUNY - Queens Coll; MS 75 Univ of MI - Ann Arbor; Aud, Rehab Serv Inc, **A**

Goldsmith, Mrs Regina D 21 Hanford Place, Caldwell, NJ 07006, (201) 827-3600, BA 72 William Paterson Coll; MS 74 William Paterson Coll; SLP, Hardyston Townshp Sch, **SLP**

Goldsmith, Dr Sharon C 6 Deerfield Road, Sherborn, MA 01770, (617) 770-7414, MA 69 NY Univ; MA 78 CUNY - Grad Sch & Univ Cntr; PH 81 (Sp and Hrng Sci) CUNY - Grad Sch & Univ Cntr; Dir Bur of Prog Dev & Eval, MA Dept of Educ, **SLP**

Goldsmith, Tessa Ann 46 Msgr Patrick Lydon Way, Dorchester, MA 02124, (617) 638-7370, BA 78 Witwatersrand Univ S Africa; MA 85 Witwatersrand Univ S Africa; 86–Sp-Lang Path, Univ Hosp, **SLP**

Goldsmith, Mrs Therese M 1168 Neptune Place, Annapolis, MD 21401, BS 79 Towson St Univ; MS 81 Towson St Univ; 88–Asst Dir Sp-Lang Path, National Rehab Hosp, **SLP**

Goldstein, Mrs Amy Helene 3007 North Van Buren St, Wilmington, DE 19802, (302) 762-0552, BA 71 Univ of DE; MA 83 West Chester Univ of PA; **SLP**

Goldstein, Amy R G 2515 Williams Court, South Bellmore, NY 11710, **SLP**

Goldstein, Angelyn G 49 Knight Lane, Kings Park, NY 11754, (516) 724-1717, BA 79 Hofstra Univ; MA 81 Hofstra Univ; Sp/Lang Path, Suffolk Child Dev Cen, **SLP**

Goldstein, Mrs Anne L 79 Hill Street, Topsfield, MA 01983, (508) 887-8580, MS 72 Univ of RI; 87–Sp-Lang Path, Private Practice, **SLP**

Goldstein, Dr Barbara A 33 Riverside Drive, New York, NY 10023, (212) 787-3624, BA 63 CUNY - Hunter Coll; MA 68 CUNY - Hunter Coll; PH 80 (NS) CUNY - Grad Sch & Univ Cntr; Aud, Private Practice, **SLP A**

Goldstein, Mrs Barbara Feldman 44 Aventura Court, Randallstown, MD 21133, (301) 848-8280, BA 79 Univ of MD - College Park; MS 81 Loyola Coll; Sp-Lang Path, Carroll Co Bd of Ed, **SLP**

Goldstein, Dr Beverly A 3386 Belvoir Boulevard, Cleveland, OH 44122, (216) 231-8787, BA 68 MI St Univ; MA 72 MI St Univ; PH 82 (NS) Kent St Univ; Dir-Aud, Cleveland Hrng & Sp Cen, **A ACE**

Goldstein, Mrs Beverly Ruth 14 Woodland Drive, Irvine, CA 92714, (714) 667-3397, MA 84 CA St Univ - Fullerton; 88–Sp-Lang Path/Instr, Rancho Santiago Comm Coll, **SLP**

Goldstein, Celia Cohen 2260 Rushmore Drive, Marietta, GA 30062, (404) 426-3175, BS 76 Univ of VA - Charlottesville; MA 78 Vanderbilt Univ; Sp-Lang Path, Kennestone Hosp, **SLP**

Goldstein, Dr David P Department Of Audiology, Purdue University, West Lafayette, IN 47907, (317) 494-3819, BA 59 CUNY - Brooklyn Coll; MA 60 Univ of WI - Madison; PH 63 (NS) Univ of WI - Madison; Prof, Prudue Univ, **A F**

Goldstein, Diann 10 Turell Road, Medford, MA 02155, **SLP**

Goldstein, Mrs Donna Woods 4006 Franklin Court, Chester Springs, PA 19425, BS 76 Wichita St Univ; MA 82 Univ of Tulsa; 88–Sp-Lang Path, Elwyn Inst Developmental Ctr, **SLP**

Goldstein, Mrs Francene C 45 Ten Coat Lane, Shelton, CT 06484, (203) 288-1210, BS 77 Rutger's St Univ - Douglas Coll; MS 78 Columbia Univ Teachers Coll; SLP, Hamden Bd of Ed, **SLP**

Goldstein, Fred 657 Ostemo Place, South Bend, IN 46617, (219) 234-0259, BA 78 Montclair St Coll; MA 79 Western MI Univ; Sp-Lang Path, South Bend Com Schools, **SLP**

Goldstein, Mrs Gail D 2648 Doylesville Road, Richmond, KY 40475, (606) 623-9548, BS 72 Bradley Univ; MA 73 Univ of IL - Urbana; 82–Sp-Lang Path, Private Practice, **SLP ACE**

Goldstein, Gwenn S 279 N W 89th Avenue, Coral Springs, FL 33071, (305) 752-2233, BA 71 CUNY - Lehman Coll; MA 76 CUNY - Lehman Coll; Sp-Lang Path, Private Practice, **SLP**

Goldstein, Helena Deutsch 201 West 70th Street #4J, New York, NY 10023, **SLP**

Goldstein, Howard Department Of Communication, University Of Pittsburgh, Pittsburgh, PA 15260, (412) 624-0101, BA 76 Univ of CA - Santa Barbara; MS 78 Univ of WA; PH 80 (NS) G Peabody Coll-Vanderbilt U; Assoc Prof, U of Pittsburgh, **SLP**

Goldstein, Janet K 2200 East Claybourne Avenue, Salt Lake City, UT 84109, (801) 521-1680, BS 78 Univ of UT; MS 80 Univ of UT; 80–Sp-Lang Path, Prim Childrens Medical Center, **SLP**

Goldstein, Dr Jerod 2070 South Macon Way, Aurora, CO 80014, (303) 695-0362, BA 63 Trenton St Coll; MS 65 PA St Univ - Univ Park; PH 72 (NS) MI St Univ; Chief Aud Aural Rehab, Fitzsimmons Army Medical Cen, **A ACE**

Goldstein, Jill E K 9194 North 103rd Street, Scottsdale, AZ 85258, (602) 860-0671, BA 77 Univ of MI - Ann Arbor; MA 79 SUNY - Center at Buffalo; 88–Sp-Lang Path, Meridian Pt Rehab Hosp, **SLP**

Goldstein, Joan Eagle P O Box 774466, Eagle River, AK 99577, (907) 694-3363, BA 81 Univ of MT; **SLP**

Goldstein, Julie 209 Beaver Road, Southampton, PA 18966, (215) 355-6404, BA 69 Temple Univ; MA 71 Temple Univ; Sp-Lang Path, Comm Home Hlth Serv of Phila, **SLP**

Goldstein, Dr Karen J 10360 S W Hawthorne Lane, Portland, OR 97225, (503) 292-5995, BS 69 Emerson Coll; ME 71 Northeastern Univ; OD 77 (NS) Boston Univ; Sp/Lang Path, Private Practice, **SLP**

Goldstein, Leslie B 6 Saul Place, Plainview, NY 11803, (516) 433-5527, MA 88 CUNY - Queens Coll; 88–Sp-Lang Path, Peninsula Hosp Ctr

Goldstein, Dr Lewis P Audiology & Speech Path (126), VA Medical Center, Gainesville, FL 32602, (904) 376-1611, BA 62 Long Island U - Brooklyn Ctr; MS 67 SUNY - Coll at Buffalo; PH 75 (NS) Univ of KS; SLP, VA Med Cen, **SLP**

Goldstein, Marilyn K 3000 Lee Place, Bellmore, NY 11710, (516) 731-3922, BA 64 Adelphi Univ; MA 65 NY Univ; 79–Sp-Lang Path, Island Trees Pub Sch, **SLP**

Goldstein, Mrs Marilyn Karen 206 Drakes Drum Drive, Bryn Mawr, PA 19010, (215) 438-1194, MA 82 West Chester Univ of PA; Sp-Lang Path, UCP Assoc, **SLP**

Goldstein, Mrs Marion B P O Box 11438, Bainbridge Island, WA 98110, BA Univ of CA - Berkeley; SLP, LA USD, **SLP LM**

Goldstein, Marjorie J 1405 Beacon Street, Brookline, MA 02146, **SLP**

Goldstein, Mrs Merle Ruth 24 Muirfield Road, Rockville Centre, NY 11570, (516) 541-7400, BA Adelphi Univ; MS Adelphi Univ; 83–Sp-Lang Path, Nassau Co BOCES Carman Rd Sch, **SLP**

Goldstein, Michele 1409 Cayuga Avenue, North Bellmore, NY 11710, (516) 795-0950, BA 84 Hofstra Univ; MS 86 Univ of South FL; SLP, Nassau BOCES, **SLP**

Goldstein, Mrs Michele G 6435 Brompton Road, Houston, TX 77005, (713) 776-2211, BA 74 Temple Univ-Tyler Sch of Art; MS 77 Univ of NC - Chapel Hill; 86–Aud, Houston Ear Nose and Throat, **A**

Goldstein, Dr Moise H ECE Department, Johns Hopkins University, Barton Hall, Baltimore, MD 21218, (301) 338-7026, BS 49 Tulane Univ; OM 51 MA Inst of Tech; OD 57 (Electrical Eng) MA Inst of Tech; 63–Prof, Johns Hopkins Univ

Goldstein, Patricia B 3026 Warm Springs Road, Glen Ellen, CA 95442, (707) 996-6774, BS 61 ND St Univ; MS 62 PA St Univ - Univ Park; Sp-Lang Path, Sonoma Valley USD, **SLP**

Goldstein, Phyllis R 5 Lawrence Lane, Lexington, MA 02173, **SLP**

Goldstein, Pia Mindy 242 Branch Avenue, Freeport, NY 11520, (516) 868-0291, BS 83 SUNY - Coll at Buffalo; MA 85 SUNY - Center at Buffalo; 85–Sp-Lang Path, H G Birch Early Child Ctr, **SLP**

Goldstein, Robert Dept Communicative Disorders, University Of Wisconsin, 1975 Willow Drive, Madison, WI 53706, (608) 262-3951, BS 48 PA St Univ - Univ Park; PH 52 (Aud) Washington Univ; 67–Prof of Common Dis, U of WI, **A F H**

Goldstein, Robin Diane 68 Helene Court, Staten Island, NY 10309, BA 77 CUNY - Brooklyn Coll; MA 81 NY Univ; Sp/Lang Path, NYC Bd of Ed/Sp Serv Ut, **SLP ACE**

Goldstein, Sandra D 5149 Dudley Lane, Bethesda, MD 20814-5429, (301) 762-6542, BA 63 Temple Univ-Tyler Sch of Art; MA 67 Temple Univ-Tyler Sch of Art; Sp-Lang Path, Mont Co Pub Sch, **SLP**

Goldstein, Sheila H 20 West 64th Street, New York, NY 10023, **SLP**

Goldstein, Susan L 9 Salem Place, White Plains, NY 10605, (914) 428-1389, BA 66 Univ of IA; MA 68 Univ of MO - Columbia; Computer Spec, Franklin & Joseph Inc, **SLP**

Goldstein, Vicki Morris 15137 East Grand Avenue, Aurora, CO 80015, (412) 244-8800, BA 83 Univ of Pittsburgh - Pittsburgh; MA 85 Univ of Pittsburgh - Pittsburgh; **SLP**

Goldstein-Schneider, Mrs Joy 56 Doyer Avenue #4D, White Plains, NY 10605, (914) 666-9553, BS 85 Syracuse Univ; MS 87 Columbia Univ Teachers Coll

Goldstone, Frances Leigh 340 S Highland Avenue #8-B, Pittsburgh, PA 15206, (412) 661-0216, BA 81 Oberlin Coll; MA 87 Univ of MD - College Park; 87, Western PA Sch for Blind Chldn, **SLP**

Goldsworthy, Dr Candace L 2046 University Park Drive, Sacramento, CA 95825, (916) 278-6601, BA 67 Univ of CA - Los Angeles; MA 71 CA St Univ - Los Angeles; PH 79 (NS) Case Western Reserve Univ; Sp-Lang Path, Goldsworthy & Johnston, **SLP**

Goldwasser, Mrs Marilyn K 724 S Spoede Road, St Louis, MO 63131, (314) 432-5115, BS 62 Washington Univ; MS 79 Fontbonne Coll; Sp-Lang Path, Private Practice, **SLP**

Goldwater, Mrs Joan Mullan 201 East Chestnut Street, Apartment 20F, Chicago, IL 60611, (312) 951-0633, MA 84 Northwestern Univ; **SLP**

Gole, Mrs Lisa 7461 Quail Hollow Street, Apartment F-11, Massillon, OH 44646, (216) 837-3346, MA 87 OH Univ - Athens

Golembieski, June Oster 11274 Southwest 55th Place, Cooper City, FL 33330, (305) 434-3990, BS 72 OH Univ - Athens; MS 73 MI St Univ; SLP, Sch Bd of Broward Co, **SLP**

Golembiewski, Colleen Marie 1360 East Lieg Avenue #6, Shawano, WI 54166, (715) 524-2185, BS 81 Marquette Univ; MS 82 Marquette Univ; Sp-Lang Path, Unif Indust-Shawano, **SLP**

Goleski, Leslie Ann 9725 S 71st E Avenue, Tulsa, OK 74133, (918) 747-9387, BS 81 OK St Univ; MA 87 Univ of TX - Austin; 88–Sp-Lang Path, Tulsa Child Dev/Reg Guid Ctr, **SLP**

Goley, Irene Frances 4 Norwich Court, Gaithersburg, MD 20878, (301) 330-0250, BA 81 Univ of MD - College Park; MA 83 Univ of MD - College Park; Sp-Lang Path, Montgomery County Pub Schools, **SLP**

Golik, Maureen Anne 800 Longview Road Apartment 135, Knoxville, TN 37919, (615) 558-8521, BS 84 East TN St Univ; MA 88 Univ of TN - Knoxville; 88–Sp-Lang Path, University of Tennessee

Goll, Annette Aerts P O Box 1296, Redbud Estate, Manhattan, KS 66502, (402) 472-1590, BA 84 Univ of NE - Lincoln; MS 86 Univ of NE - Lincoln; **SLP**

Goll, Mrs Margaret C 4520 Gladstone Drive, Pensacola, FL 32514, (904) 474-5358, BA 78 Temple Univ; MA 80 Temple Univ; Director of Speech Pathology, Rehabilitation Institute, **SLP ACE**

Golledge, Mrs Joanna P O Box 733, Aumsville, OR 97325, (503) 588-5124, BA 75 Western WA Univ; MA 77 Western WA Univ; Sp-Lang Path, Marion Ed Ser Dist, **SLP**

Gollegly, Karen M Dartmouth-Hitchcock Medical Center, 2 Maynard Street, Hanover, NH 03755, (603) 646-8125, BS 78 Ithaca Coll; MA 80 Northwestern Univ; Aud, Dartmough-Hitchcock Med Ctr, **A**

Goller, Monica C 2503 West Springfield Aven, Apt C9, Champaign, IL 61821, BS 59 Marquette Univ; MA 73 Univ of Northern CO; Aud, Charles W Christie Foundation, **A**

Gollinger, Mrs Deirdre L 686 Apache Lane, Mendota Heights, MN 55120, (612) 454-1254, BS 71 Marquette Univ; MS 87 Univ of WI - River Falls; 87–Sp-Lang Path, ISD #279

Gollinger, Dorothy 8502 Fort Hunt Road, Alexandria, VA 22308, (703) 780-2787, BA 29 Coll of Saint Scholastica; MA 70 Catholic Univ of America

Golliver, Linda M Rt 2 209 Mulberry, Okeene, OK 73763, (405) 822-4769, BS 70 OK St Univ; MA 74 OK St Univ; Sp-Lang Path, Okeene Pub Sch, **SLP**

Golod, Mrs Camille Dedomenico 46 Notch Hill Road, North Branford, CT 06471, (203) 265-2831, BA 75 Univ of CT; MS 78 Southern CT St Univ; 79–Sp/Lang Path, Wallingford Pub Sch, **SLP**

Golos, Neila J 823 Mulvane Suite 255, Topeka, KS 66606, (913) 233-2296, MA 85 Univ of KS; 85–Sp-Lang Path, Speech-Lang Therapy Consult, **SLP**

Golovin, Roselyn W 1714 Friar Tuck Circle, Columbus, MS 39701, (214) 832-5102, BA 55 Coll of William & Mary; ME 65 Northeastern Univ; **SLP**

Golper, Dr Lee Ann C Audiology & Speech Pathology, Portland VA Med Ctr 126-P, 3710 S W Veterans Hosp Rd, Portland, OR 97201, (503) 220-8262, BA 71 IN Univ - Bloomington; MS 76 Portland St Univ; PH 82 (Sp Path) Univ of OR; 81–Asst Prof-Neurology, Ore Health Sci Univ, **SLP F ACE**

Goltz, Nancy Carol 2020 Golf Road #300, Huntsville, AL 35802, (205) 535-2300, BS 84 Univ of Montevallo; MA 86 Univ of TN - Knoxville; **SLP**

Golub, Dr Arnold J 300 East 75th Street, Apartment 12-P, New York, NY 10021, (212) 584-9000, BA 48 Univ of MA - Amherst; MA 51 Univ of IA; PH 52 (Psychology) Univ of IA; 58–Cl Psychol, VA Med Cen, **SLP**

Golub, Latricia Daigle 1040 Waters Edge Drive, Lakeland, FL 33801, (813) 858-3881, BS 81 Univ of Southwestern LA; MA 86 Univ of Southwestern LA; 87–Sp-Lang Path, Polk County Sch Dist, **SLP**

Golub, Shirley L 425 Upper Terrace, San Francisco, CA 94117, (415) 775-4044, BS 68 Boston Univ; ME 70 Boston Univ; Owner, Insta-Tune/Union 76 Station, **SLP**

Golub-Roberts, Mrs Amy B 4091 Tynebourne Circle, San Diego, CA 92130, (619) 579-5855, BA 76 Univ of CA - Los Angeles; MA 80 CA St Univ - Northridge; SLP, Grossmont Un Hs Dist, **SLP**

Golymbieski, Lisa 135 Round Hill Road, Cheshire, CT 06410, (203) 753-8334, BS 77 Southern CT St Univ; MS 79 Southern CT St Univ; Pres, Allid Hlth Care Assoc Pc, **SLP ACE**

Gomberg, Marilyn R 126 Melrose Avenue, Toronto, ON, Canada M5M 1Y7, (416) 229-5800, BA 74 McGill Univ - Quebec; MS 76 Boston Univ; Sp/Lang Path, Home Care Program- Toronto, **SLP**

Gomberg-Hirsch, Beth M 1011 Greenleaf, Wilmette, IL 60091, (312) 869-7736, BS 73 Univ of IL - Urbana; MA 75 Northwestern Univ; Sp/Lang Path, Comm Consol Sch Dist 65, **SLP**

Gomer, Mrs Betty Jean 1818 Fairlawn Way, Anderson, IN 46012, (317) 644-4985, BS 48 Ball St Univ; MA 60 Ball St Univ; **SLP LM**

Gomes, Dr Barbara A 11 Sterling Pk, Braintree, MA 02184, (617) 849-7816, ED 87 (Applied Psycholinguistics) Boston Univ; 88–Proj Coord, Brown Univ, **SLP**

Gomes, Mrs Suellen MacEdonia 9 Arbor Ridge Lane, South Setauket Park, Centereach, NY 11720, (516) 289-2200, BS 77 SUNY - Coll at Geneseo; MS 87 Adelphi Univ; **SLP**

Gomez, Mrs Beverly Hopper 161 South San Mateo Avenue, Ventura, CA 93004, (805) 524-4310, **SLP**

Gomez, Carey C 191 North Avenue, Burlington, VT 05401, BA 75 Univ of VT; MS 76 Univ of VT; Sp/Lang Path, Bellows Free Acad, **SLP**

Gomez, Charlotte Casto P O Box 677, Washington, LA 70589, (504) 342-0018, BA 78 Univ of NM; MS 83 Univ of Southwestern LA; SLP, St Landry Parish School Board, **SLP**

Gomez, Donna Hotra 19202 Tranbarger, Rowland Heights, CA 91748, (714) 595-1221, BA 81 CA St Univ - Long Beach; MA 83 CA St Univ - Fullerton; 83–Sp-Lang Path, Lanterman Developmental Ctr, **SLP**

Gomez, Donna Marie 3306 Stonehall Drive, Beltsville, MD 20705, (301) 572-4943, BA 80 Univ of MD - College Park; MA 83 Univ of MD - College Park; Sp-Lang Path, Kilby Easter Seal Center, **SLP**

Gomez, Malvy Carmen 205 S E 16th Avenue #26-E, Gainesville, FL 32601, (904) 374-4575, MA 88 Univ of FL

Gomeztrejo, Patricia Elena 1707-1/2 Carmelina Street, West Los Angeles, CA 90025, (213) 826-6934, MA 84 CA St Univ - Northridge; SLP, Univ S California Medical Cen, **SLP**

Gomolin, Railey Helen 45 West 81st Street #1009, New York, NY 10024, (212) 289-1755, **A**

Gompers, Mrs Cathleen Callahan 534 Hulton Street, Carnegie, PA 15106, (412) 279-7259, BS 84 Indiana Univ of PA; MS 87 CA Univ of PA; 88–Sp-Lang Path, Crossroads Sp & Hrng Inc

Gomrick, Denise Elaine 37825 Woodridge Drive #105, Westland, MI 48185-5779, (313) 459-4269, BS 83 Indiana Univ of PA; MS 85 Indiana Univ of PA; 86–Sp-Lang Path, Macomb-Oakland Reg Ctr, **SLP**

Gong-Guy, Ellen 9827-F Cedar Street, Bellflower, CA 90706, (818) 448-6196, BA 73 CA St Univ - Long Beach; MA 75 CA St Univ - Long Beach; LA Co Ofc of Educ, **SLP**

Gonik, Andrea Shumaker 5566 Swan Lake Drive, West Bloomfield, MI 48033, (313) 737-9211, BS 76 Wayne St Univ; MA 77 Eastern MI Univ; Dir Sp-Lang Path, Brooke Park Clinic, **SLP**

Gonio-Colaluca, Mrs Lynn Ann 805 Piedmont, Naperville, IL 60565, (312) 961-9010, BS 78 1819; MS 80 IL St Univ - Normal; Sp/Lang Path, Downers Grove N Dstr 99, **SLP**

Gonsalves, Jan M 16806 Algonguin Street, Huntington Beach, CA 92649, (213) 924-1658, BA 77 Univ of the Pacific; MA 78 Univ of the Pacific; SLP, ABC USD, **SLP**

Gonsalves-Wendt, Diana L 7191 S W 152nd Avenue, Beaverton, OR 97007, (503) 644-4887, BA 73 Chaminade Univ of Honolulu; MA 76 Univ of CO - Boulder; Dir Sp/Lang Path, San Juan Reg Med Cen, **SLP ACE**

Gonya, Linda Marie 711 E Main Street #D5, Torrington, CT 06790, (203) 753-8833, BS 83 PA St Univ - Univ Park; MA 88 OH St Univ; 88–Aud, ENT Associates of Waterbury

Gonzales, Jo Ann 246 Pletz Drive, San Antonio, TX 78226, (512) 433-8035, BA 75 Our Lady Lake Univ-San Anton; MA 76 Our Lady Lake Univ-San Anton; Sp/Lang Path, Edgewood ISD, **SLP**

Gonzales, Maria 560 Summer Winds, Rio Rancho, NM 87124, **SLP**

Gonzales, Maria Diana Route 1 Box 42, Donna, TX 78537, (512) 383-0121, BS 81 Univ of TX - Austin; ME 83 Southwest TX St Univ; 84–Sp-Lang Path, Tropical Texas Ctr for MH/MR, **SLP**

Gonzales, Norma 2605 East Plum Street, Laredo, TX 78043, (512) 727-4401, BS 56 Southwest TX St Univ; 78–Sp/Lang Path, Laredo ISD, **SLP**

Gonzales, Victoria Christine 1109 Landman NE, Albuquerque, NM 87112, (505) 848-8695, BA 85 Univ of NM; MS 86 Univ of NM; 87–Sp-Lang Path, St Joseph Hlthcare Corp, **SLP**

Gonzalez, Ana M 1658 Pesqueria Street, Paradise Hills, Rio Piedras, PR 00926, MS; **SLP**

Gonzalez, Carmen L President Ramirez 218, Baldrich, Hato Rey, PR 00918, (809) 751-1693, BA 75 Univ of PR - Rio Piedras; MS 77 Univ of PR - Rio Piedras; Sp-Lang Path, Head Start, **SLP**

Gonzalez, Mrs Julie Gonzalez 6902 S W 88th Street #E-403, Miami, FL 33156, (813) 251-7760, BA 80 Univ of Miami; MA 84 Univ of Central FL; **SLP**

Gonzalez, Mrs Lisa M 2800 Windgate Drive #18, New Braunfels, TX 78130, (817) 759-2859, BS 78 Southwest TX St Univ; ME 80 Southwest TX St Univ; **SLP**

Gonzalez, Lori Stewart Department Of Communication, Disorders & Sciences, Comm 1003 SIU-C, Carbondale, IL 62901, (618) 453-4301, BA 79 Univ of KY; MA 81 Eastern KY Univ; PH (Child Phonology) Univ of FL; 88–Sp-Lang Path, South Ill Univ at Carbondale, **SLP**

Gonzalez, Myrna Doris 82-76 164th Place, Jamaica, NY 11432, (212) 678-5360, BA 80 CUNY - Brooklyn Coll; MA 82 NY Univ; 87–Sp-Lang Path, The Brooklyn Hosp, **SLP**

Gonzalez, Mrs Odette 3913 Sandy Hollow Creek, Corpus Christi, TX 78410, (512) 857-6161, BS 80 TX A & I Univ; MS 81 TX Christian Univ; Sp-Lang Path, S TX Area Rehab Comp Day Ctr, **SLP**

Gonzalez, Mrs Rebecca C 2910 Wyndham Lane, Richardson, TX 75081, (214) 235-2236, BS 73 Univ of North TX; MS 75 Univ of North TX; **SLP ACE**

Gonzalez, Mrs Robin Tapp 12450 W Idaho Drive, Lakewood, CO 80228, (303) 985-0471, MA 84 Univ of Denver; Sp-Lang Path, Wheat Ridge Reg Ctr, **SLP**

Gonzalez, Zulema Perez Box 167, Orange Grove, TX 78372, (512) 384-9351, BS 80 TX A & I Univ; MS 83 TX Christian Univ; **SLP**

Gonzalez-de Paz, Mrs Brunilda 709 N W 84th Street, Gainesville, FL 32607, (904) 371-3218, BA 79 Univ of FL; MA 87 Univ of FL; 88–Sp-Lang Path, Alachua Co Sch Bd, **SLP**

Gonzalez-Rothi, Dr Leslie J Audiology & Speech Pathology, VA Medical Center, Gainesville, FL 32602, (904) 376-1611, BS 71 Northern AZ Univ; MA 74 CA St Univ - Long Beach; PH 78 (NS) Univ of FL; Sp-Lang Path, VA Med Cen, **SLP**

Gonzalez-Sierra, Maria N 5110 Cabin Lake, San Antonio, TX 78244, (512) 662-7005, BA 77 Univ of PR - Rio Piedras; MS 80 FL St Univ; Sp/Lang Path, Judson Ind Schl Dstr, **SLP**

Gonzenbach, Stephen A 570 Calvin Street, Washington Township, NJ 07675, (212) 330-1793, BA 71 William Paterson Coll; MA 75 2502; ME 88 Columbia Univ Teachers Coll; Aud, Brooklyn VA Hosp, **SLP A**

Goo, Shari Yuk Sum 99-969 Lalawai Drive, Aiea, HI 96701, (808) 488-1630, BS 85 Univ of HI - Manoa; MS 87 Univ of HI - Manoa; 88–Sp-Lang Path, Rehab Hosp of the Pacific

Gooch, Gilbert E 1461 Cheyenne Street, Salt Lake City, UT 84104, (801) 972-4611, BS 52 Univ of UT; MS 69 Univ of UT; **SLP LM**

Good, Alison Mary 1032 B Vermont Avenue, San Jose, CA 95126, (408) 998-3212, BA 83 Univ of Redlands; MA 85 Univ of CA - Santa Barbara; **SLP**

Good, Amy L R 205 Aspen St, Liverpool, NY 13088, (315) 451-7474, BS 74 SUNY - Coll at Geneseo; MS 79 Baylor Univ; 79–Sp-Lang Path, North Syracuse Cen Sch, **SLP**

Good, Mrs Elaine R Rural Route 1, Paris, IL 61944, (217) 466-6170, BA 68; MS 70 Southern IL Univ -Carbondale; SLP, Dist 95 Paris II, **SLP**

Good, Mrs Leatrice Faye 505 La Guardia Place, New York, NY 10012, SLP, NY City Boe, **SLP**

Good, Mrs Martia B 173 Allen Drive, Hendersonville, TN 37075, (615) 264-1106, BS 71 G Peabody Coll-Vanderbilt U; MA 76 Univ of RI; Aud, Hitchcock Rehab Ctr, **A**

Good, Mrs Mary J S Route 2 Box 136, Medford, OK 73759, (405) 532-4142, BA 69 Northwestern OK St Univ; MS 75 Phillips Univ; Sp-Lang Path, Pond Creek-Hunter Pub Schools, **SLP**

Good, Susan Brown Rd #2 Box 177, Mineral Point, PA 15942, (814) 269-3315, BS 79 WV Univ; MS 80 WV Univ; Aud / Owner, Johnstown Better Hearing, **A**

Goodban, Dr Marjorie T 425 Prospect, Elmhurst, IL 60126, (312) 279-4100, BA 65 KS St Univ; MA 66 Univ of IL - Urbana; PH 72 (NS) Univ of IL - Urbana; Chair, Elmhurst Coll, **SLP**

Goodding, Dr Patricia Jean 1902 Green Berry Road, Jefferson City, MO 65101, (314) 751-2325, BS 50 Northeast MO St Univ; ME 60 Univ of MO - Columbia; PH 70 (Sp-Lang Path) Univ of MO - Columbia; Sp-Lang Path, Private Practice, **SLP F**

Goode, Carolann 715 Church #2, Ann Arbor, MI 48104, (313) 682-5599, BA 84 Univ of MI - Ann Arbor; MS 86 Univ of MI - Ann Arbor; **SLP**

Goode, Jay M 22641 Imperial Court, Richton Park, IL 60471, (312) 748-0059, BS 72 Southern IL Univ -Carbondale; MA 73 Univ of IL - Urbana; Aud, Private Practice, **A**

Goode, Lisa Lepore 270 East 7th Street Suite 1C, Upland, CA 91786, (714) 981-7616, MS 88 CO St Univ; 88–Aud, Pacific Hearing Services

Goode, Matthew Edward Box 248, Dorchester, MA 02121, (617) 856-4282, BA 61 Emerson Coll; MS 68 Northeastern Univ; Program Coordinator, Fay Spofford & Thorndike Inc, **SLP**

Goode, Mrs Sharon Blackford 225 St John's Square, Sterling, VA 22170, (703) 955-2400, BS 86 AR St Univ; MS 87 AR St Univ; 88–Sp-Lang Path, Grafton Sch Inc

Goodell, Mrs Cynthia A 703 Green Avenue, Bay City, MI 48708, (517) 686-4410, BA 78 MI St Univ; MA 80 MI St Univ; Sp-Lang Path, Bay-Arenac Inter Sch Dist, **SLP**

Goodenough, Sandra E S 3534 Lake Mendota Drive, Shorewood Hills Village, Madison, WI 53705, (608) 767-2251, BA 72 IL St Univ - Normal; MS 75 Univ of IL - Urbana; Sp/Lang Path, Wisconsin Heights Sch Dist, **SLP**

Goodhill, Dr Victor UCLA Medical School, Div Of Head & Neck Surgery, Room 31-24 Rehabilitation, Los Angeles, CA 90024-1794, MD (NS); **F LM**

Goodier, Mrs Brenda M 1810 South Center, Terre Haute, IN 47802, (812) 238-4364, BS 73 IN St Univ - Terre Haute; MS 78 IN St Univ - Terre Haute; Sp/Lang Path, Vigo Co Sch Corp, **SLP**

Goodier, Janet Wall Street, R R 2 Box 806, West Winifield, NY 13491, (315) 736-3042, **SLP**

Goodier, Jay A 1810 South Center, Terre Haute, IN 47802, **SLP**

Goodin, Mrs Gina Lea 3076 Curtis Knoll Drive, Dublin, OH 43017, (614) 761-7011, BS 81 OH Univ - Athens; MA 87 OH St Univ; 88–Sp-Lang Path, Dublin Schs

Goodlett, Donna L 1918 East 22nd Street, Owensboro, KY 42302, (502) 491-8837, BS 84 Spalding Coll; MS 86 Univ of Louisville; **SLP**

Goodling-Beals, Karen M 1980 Carlcliff Drive, Burt, NY 14028, (716) 778-7012, MS 83 SUNY - Coll at Buffalo; 86–Sp-Lang Path, Lockport City Sch Dist, **SLP**

Goodman, Alice N 10400 Great Arbor Drive, Potomac, MD 20854, (301) 279-9040, BA 61 George Washington Univ; MA 70 Univ of MD - College Park; Sp/Lang Path, Mont Ct Pub Sch-Hd Start Prog, **SLP**

Goodman, Dr Allan C 3 Wayne Court, Ardsley, NY 10502, (914) 693-4226, BA 41 CUNY - Brooklyn Coll; MS 49 Univ of MI - Ann Arbor; PH 52 (Sp & Hrng Sciences) Univ of MI - Ann Arbor; Aud Consult, Private Practice, **SLP A F LM**

Goodman, Mrs Anne Ladd 29 Grandview Drive, Radford, VA 24141, (703) 731-3652, BS 82 Radford Univ; MS 83 Radford Univ; Sp-Lang Path, Radford City Public Schools, **SLP**

Goodman, Mrs Barbara Lynne 505 Lindsey Court, Marlton, NJ 08053, (609) 767-5757, BA 81 Rutger's St Univ - Douglas Coll; MA 83 Temple Univ-Tyler Sch of Art; **SLP**

Goodman, Mrs Colette Claire #1 Winterberry Court, Peekskill, NY 10566, (914) 245-2700, BS 80 SUNY - Coll at New Paltz; MA 85 CUNY - Lehman Coll; **SLP**

Goodman, David M P O Box 75, Exeter, RI 02822, (401) 294-4561, BS 77 Univ of MA - Amherst; ME 79 Northeastern Univ; Sp/Lang Path, Laddeen RI, **SLP**

Goodman, Deborah Ann 579 Sagamore Avenue, #119 Tidewatch, Portsmouth, NH 03801, (603) 436-0060, BS 81 Univ of NH; MS 87 Univ of NH; 88–Sp-Lang Path, Portsmouth Sch Dept

Goodman, Mrs Deborah Brown 1676 Redington Lane, Charlottesville, VA 22901, BS 79 Ithaca Coll; ME 81 Univ of VA - Charlottesville; Sp-Lang Path, Little Keswick School, **SLP ACE**

Goodman, Deborah G 7100 Valencia Drive, Boca Raton, FL 33433, (305) 488-2377, BA 75 CUNY - Brooklyn Coll; MA 76 Hofstra Univ; Sp-Lang Path, Private Practice, **SLP**

Goodman, Deborah J 108 Marne Avenue, Fairfield, CT 06432-1754, **SLP**

Goodman, Debra L 3202 East Bellevue #29, Tucson, AZ 85716, (602) 327-3829, MS 88 Univ of AZ

Goodman, Mrs Edith Teper 124 Graymoor Lane, Olympia Fields, IL 60461

Goodman, Elise Sue 221 N Humphrey, Oak Park, IL 60302, (312) 383-3342, **SLP**

Goodman, Mrs Elizabeth Baskervill 500 Cedarbrook, Nolensville, TN 37135, (615) 893-2602, BA 80 Univ of NC - Chapel Hill; MS 82 Univ of NC - Chapel Hill; Sp-Lang Path, Pro Health Svcs, **SLP**

Goodman, Gilbert B, Jr Meadowland Box 25, Millers Creek, NC 28651, (919) 667-2379, BS 72 Appalachian St Univ; MA 73 Appalachian St Univ; Sp-Lang Path, Wilkes County Public Schools, **SLP**

Goodman, Mrs Helene R 26 Piper Drive, Searingtown, NY 11507, (516) 747-4852, BA 53 NY Univ; MS 74 Adelphi Univ; Aud, Private Practice, **A**

Goodman, Mrs Jane Y 2300 Sherman Avenue, Evanston, IL 60201, (312) 864-9085, BA 68 Saint Xavier Coll; MA 70 Northwestern Univ; PH 78 (Ed Psych) Northwestern Univ; Sp-Lang Path, Private Practice, **SLP**

Goodman, Janice K 7100 Constitution N E #16, Albuquerque, NM 87110, (505) 255-4769, BA 51 Univ of MI - Ann Arbor; MA 70 Univ of NM; Sp/Lang Path, Albuquerque Pub Sch, **SLP**

Goodman, Joan Lee 7535 Cadencia Street, La Costa, CA 92009, (619) 944-7741, BA 76 SUNY - Coll at Cortland; MA 79 CUNY - City College; Sp-Lang Path, Vista USD, **SLP**

Goodman, Joanne 89 Pomona Road, Suffern, NY 10901, (212) 260-1918, **SLP**

Goodman, Mrs Julie S 1922 Windingridge Drive, Richmond, VA 23233, (804) 741-6577, BS 77 Univ of VA - Charlottesville; ME 78 Univ of VA - Charlottesville; 82–Sp-Lang Path, Richmond Cerebral Palsy Ctr, **SLP**

Goodman, Karen Totty 7324 Weil Avenue, St Louis, MO 63119, (314) 843-9453, BS 67 Southeast MO St Univ; MA 68 Univ of IL - Urbana; Sp-Lang Path, Spec Sch Dist of St Louis Co, **SLP**

Goodman, Kathy Landau 470 Clothier Road, Wynnewood, PA 19096-2311, (215) 525-7735, BS 77 Syracuse Univ; OM 79 Hahneman Medical Coll; Director, Main Line Aud Consultants, **SLP A**

Goodman, Mrs Linda B 12 Mimosa Circle, Lafayette Hill, PA 19444, **SLP**

Goodman, Mrs Linda T 1795 County Rd #492, Marquette, MI 49855, (906) 226-9591, BS 74 Univ of KS; MA 76 Northern MI Univ; SLP, Marquette Publ Schs, **SLP**

Goodman, Martha V 9629 Weathered Oak Court, Bethesda, MD 20817, (301) 899-9490, BA 71 Beaver Coll; MA 76 Univ of MD - College Park; Sp-Lang Path, Prince Georges County Bd of Ed, **SLP**

Goodman, Mrs Mary Rice 404 South Kenilworth, Elmhurst, IL 60126-3927, (312) 834-9793, BA 69 TX Wesleyan Coll; MS 75 Central MO St Univ; Sp/Lang Path, Judith Pollack Meyer Sp Paths, **SLP**

Goodman, Mrs Mina Silesky 5748 Cross Country Blvd, Baltimore, MD 21209, (301) 381-9700, BA 71 Goucher Coll; ME 73 Loyola Coll; MS 84 Loyola Coll; Clin Superv, Loyola Coll, **SLP**

Goodman, Mrs Mona B 29 Bridle Path Lane, Madison, CT 06443, (203) 421-3676, BS 73 SUNY - Center at Albany; MA 74 NY Univ; Sp-Lang Path, Guilford Public Schools, **SLP**

Goodman, Mrs Nancy Jo 3710 East 87th Place, Tulsa, OK 74137, (918) 491-9200, BS 78 OK St Univ; MS 80 Univ of OR; Sp/Lang Path, Private Practice, **SLP**

Goodman, Mrs Naomi 3531 Broderick Street, San Francisco, CA 94123, (408) 395-8039, BA 73 Montclair St Coll; MA 75 CUNY - Lehman Coll; Lecturer, San Jose State University, **SLP**

Goodman, Pamela F Box 2879, APO New York, NY 09131, **SLP**

Goodman, Pamela Jean Route 4 Box 136, North Wilkesboro, NC 28659, (704) 264-0566, BS 83 Appalachian St Univ; MA 84 Appalachian St Univ; 84–Sp-Lang Path, Pro-Rehab Inc, **SLP**

Goodman, Paula Jodi 150-3 Dreiser Coop, Bronx, NY 10475, (718) 445-1400, **A**

Goodman, Peggy B Route 1 Box 407, Cropwell, AL 35054, **SLP**

Goodman, Mrs Perri Marlene 34528 Princeton Street, Farmington Hills, MI 48331, (313) 553-0577, BA 82 MI St Univ; MA 83 Wayne St Univ; Sp-Lang Path, St Joseph Mercy Hosp, **SLP**

Goodman, Rebecca A 26W055 Sioux Court, Wheaton, IL 60187, (312) 668-9031, BA 76 Muhlenberg Coll; MA 78 Univ of Pittsburgh - Pittsburgh; 85–Dir/Owner, Lang and Comm Assoc, **SLP ACE**

Goodman, Mrs Rona B 6133 Deloache, Dallas, TX 75225, (214) 363-4999, BS 64 OH St Univ; MA 65 OH St Univ; **SLP**

Goodman, Sarah H 2626 North Blvd # 20, Houston, TX 77098-5032, (713) 522-5207, **SLP**

Goodman, Mrs Sharlene 27075 Hidden Trail, Laguna Hills, CA 92653, (714) 544-6043, BA 73 CA St Univ - Long Beach; MA 75 CA St Univ - Long Beach; Exec Dir, Newport Lang Sp & Audio Ctr, **SLP ACE**

Goodman, Susie Lynn #1804 9909 104th Street, Edmonton, AB, Canada T5K 2G5, (403) 471-2262, BA 82 Univ of Western Ontario; MA 86 SUNY - Center at Buffalo; 87–Sp-Lang Path, Glenrose Rehab Hosp, **SLP**

Goodman-Bowden, Jenny Louise Rd #1 Box 474, Middletown, NY 10940, (914) 431-8800, BS 81 NY Univ; MS 85 SUNY - Coll at New Paltz; **SLP**

Goodman-Malamuth, Dr Leo, II Governors State University, University Park, IL 60466, (312) 534-5000, BA 47 Univ of Southern CA; MA 48 Univ of Southern CA; PH 56 (NS) Univ of Southern CA; Pres, Governors St U, **SLP**

Goodman-Saia, Mrs Shari I 4275 Coral Springs Drive, Coral Springs, FL 33065, (305) 749-0300, BA 76 SUNY - Coll at New Paltz; MS 81 Columbia Univ Teachers Coll; Sp-Lang Path, Sunrise Rehab Hosp, **SLP**

Goodman-Schulman, Dr Roberta Department Of Psychology, Johns Hopkins University, Baltimore, MD 21218, (301) 338-6372, BA 79 Clark Univ; MA 83 Univ of MD - College Park; PH 86 (NS) Univ of MD - College Park; Research Assoc, John Hopkins U, **SLP**

Goodreau, May Hoefling 1083 Cornflower Court, Sunnyvale, CA 94086, (408) 244-0877, BA 66 Univ of Santa Clara; MA 87 San Jose St Univ; 88–Sp-Lang Path, Los Gatos Rehab Ctr, **SLP**

Goodrich, Frances H One Maple Lane, Chagrin Falls, OH 44022, (216) 247-7769, MA 82 Kent St Univ; **SLP**

Goodrich, Mrs Marianne L P O Box 556, Saunderstown, RI 02852, BS 76 Univ of RI; MS 79 Univ of RI; **SLP**

Goodrich, Sharon J 13205 Ashvale Drive, Fairfax, VA 22033, (703) 379-6601, BS 64; MA 67 SUNY - Coll at Buffalo; **SLP**

Goodrich, Susan Jean 4925 Virginia Way, Sacramento, CA 95822, (916) 453-5409, BA 77 CA St Univ - Sacramento; MS 84 CA St Univ - Sacramento; 86–Sp-Lang Path, Univ CA-Davis Med Ctr, **SLP**

Goodseal, Wilbur D 12917 Craig Drive, Grandview, MO 64030, (816) 221-7565, BS 53 Univ of KS; MA 62 Univ of KS; Coord Sp/Lang/Hrng Vis, Kansas City Sd, **SLP**

Goodsell, Mrs Kathleen C 1201 Stockbridge Road, Webster, NY 14580, (716) 872-3144, BS 67 SUNY - Coll at Buffalo; MS 71 SUNY - Coll at Geneseo; **SLP**

Goodson, Ginger Lynette 520 Urban Lane, Brookhaven, MS 39601, (601) 835-0099, OB 83 Univ of FL; MS 85 FL St Univ; 88–Aud, Brookhaven Hearing Services, **A**

Goodstein, R Sarah SG Rehabilitation Agency Inc, 136 East Fayette Street, Uniontown, PA 15401, (412) 439-1444, BS 80 CA Univ of PA; ME 81 CA Univ of PA; Dir of Prof Serv, Sg Rehab Agcy Inc, **SLP**

Goodwin, Diana J 29 Front Street, Marblehead, MA 01945, (617) 631-2301, BS 80 Univ of MA - Amherst; MA 82 Univ of CA - Santa Barbara; Sp-Lang Path Consult, Communication Works, **SLP**

Goodwin, Mrs Diana Kay R R 1 Box 151-A, Morrisville, NC 27560, (919) 467-3692, BS 80 Northwestern Univ; MA 81 Northwestern Univ; Sp-Lang Path, Medical Personnel Pool, **SLP**

Goodwin, Emily Apthorp Hurricane Road, Keene, NY 12942, (518) 576-9949, BA 71 Univ of CO - Boulder; MA 74 Sch for Int'l Training; MS 81 Univ of VT; Sp-Lang Path, Private Practice, **SLP**

Goodwin, Harry S 1135 West Genesee Road, Baldwinsville, NY 13027-9657, (315) 473-6914, BS 81 SUNY - Coll at Geneseo; MA 83 SUNY - Coll at Geneseo; Sp-Path, Syracuse Dev Cen, **SLP**

Goodwin, Jane Boutiette 5 Thayer Pond #8, P O Box 434, North Oxford, MA 01537-0434, (508) 791-6351, BA 84 Univ of CT; MA 86 Univ of CT; 88–Sp-Lang Path, Fairlawn Rehab Hosp, **SLP**

Goodwin, Mrs Jeanne M 92 Norway Drive, Rochester, NY 14616, (716) 227-3523, BA 68 Newark St Coll; MS 86 Nazareth Coll of Rochester; 88–Sp-Lang Path, Greece Central Sch Dist, **SLP**

Goodwin, Karen K 22340 Goshen School Road, Gaithersburg, MD 20879, (301) 926-8219, BA 78 SUNY - Coll at Cortland; MS 79 Ithaca Coll; Sp-Lang Path, Private Practice, **SLP ACE**

Goodwin, Mrs Karen Rae 7675 Gibralter Drive, Colorado Springs, CO 80920, (719) 475-5422, OB 77 Northeast MO St Univ; MA 78 Northeast MO St Univ; Sp/Lang Path, Mem Hosp Pediatric Rehab Ctr, **SLP**

Goodwin, Mary Beth 3428 Amherst, Olympia, WA 98051-3929, (503) 469-6643, BA 70 Univ of WA; MS 86 Western OR St Coll

Goodwin, Patricia B 3400 Carter Creek, Bryan, TX 77802, (409) 775-3334, BS 64 Univ of TN - Knoxville; MA 65 Northwestern Univ; Spec Ed Tchr, Byan ISD, **SLP**

Goodwin, Dr Patricia E P O Box 4874, Englewood, CO 80155-4874, (614) 345-9631, BA 54 Univ of FL; MA 55 Stanford Univ; PH 79 Univ of Denver; Research Engineer, Holophane R&D, **A**

Goodwin, Mrs Rebecca Leach 3512 Whirlaway Trail, Tallahassee, FL 32308, (904) 877-6158, BS 66 Memphis St Univ; MA 67 Univ of FL; 79–Sp-Lang Path, Leon Co Pub Sch, **SLP**

Goodwin, Mrs Selma Rabinovitz 721 86th Street, Miami Beach, FL 33141, (305) 865-0158, BA 56 CUNY - Queens Coll; 85–Sp-Lang Path/Aud, VA Med Ctr, **SLP A ACE**

Goodwin, Vicki 2501 Laguna, Emporia, KS 66801, (316) 382-3705, Sp-Lang Path, Marion County Spec Educ Coop, **SLP**

Goold-Caulfield, Jane Evelyn 3349 Brittan Avenue, San Carlos, CA 94070, (415) 839-1513, BA 65 Univ of CO - Boulder; MA 74 San Francisco St Univ; 86–Pvt Practice-Dir, Scottish Rite Clin for Child Lang Dis, **SLP**

Gooldy, William H 2301 East 4th, Tulsa, OK 74104, (918) 592-1100, BA 55 Univ of Tulsa; MA 67 Univ of Tulsa; Sp-Lang Path, Private Practice, **SLP**

Goolsby, Mrs Pamela A 4407 Western Pine Woods, San Antonio, TX 78249-1422, (512) 492-9109, OB 68 Southern Methodist Univ; MA 74 Univ of Tulsa; 85–Sp-Lang Path, Private Practice, **SLP ACE**

Goore, Mrs Deborah S 86 Fountain Avenue, Rockville Centre, NY 11570, (516) 763-1230, BA 59 Adelphi Univ; MS 74 Adelphi Univ; **SLP**

Goossens', Dr Carol A 3492 Wildewood Drive, Pelham, AL 35124, (205) 934-5448, BS 75 Univ of Western Ontario; MS 76 Univ of WI - Madison; PH 83 Purdue Univ - West Lafayette; Sp-Lang Path, U of AL-Birmingham, **SLP**

Goostree, Mary Carol 117 Woodland Drive, Salem, IL 62881, (618) 548-0528, BA 72 Southern IL Univ-Edwardsvill; MS 80 Southern IL Univ-Edwardsvill; 81–Sp-Lang Path, Kaskaskia Spec Ed Dist, **SLP**

Gooze, Dr Edward C 7434 Louis Pasteur #109, San Antonio, TX 78229, (512) 699-1190, BS 65 Wayne St Univ; MA 70 Wayne St Univ; PH 75 (Sp-Lang Path/Sp Science) FL St Univ; Sp-Lang Path, Private Practice, **SLP**

Gooze, Mrs Sally Schneir 6226 Sun Hollow, San Antonio, TX 78238-4539, (512) 342-1776, BS 69 MI St Univ; MS 73 FL St Univ; SLP/Aud, Communication & Learning Serv, **SLP**

Goracke, Mrs Loretta M Route 1 Box 85, Pickrell, NE 68422, (402) 223-2302, BA 74 Univ of KS; MA 76 Wichita St Univ; 80–Dir-Lang Admin, Beatrice St Developmental Cen, **A**

Goran, Kristin A 1500 Rice Creek Drive, Fridley, MN 55432, BA 71; MS 78 Univ of MN - Minneap-St Paul; Sp/Lang Path, Chcg Co Spec Ed Coop, **SLP**

Gorbach, Penelope J 1307 Creek View Drive, Muskegon, MI 49441, (616) 755-4991, MA 71 Western MI Univ; Sp-Lang Path, Montague Area P S, **SLP**

Gorback-Lopez, Nadzia Marie 16 Robinsong, Irvine, CA 92714, (714) 558-5831, MS 83 Chapman Coll; Sp-Lang Path, Santa Ana USD, **SLP**

Gordan, Mrs Wenda L 6093 South Fairfax Court, Littleton, CO 80121, (303) 789-8228, BS 73 Kent St Univ; MA 75 Kent St Univ; 76–Asst Dept Head-Sp-Lang Path, Craig Hospital, **SLP**

Gordon, Mrs Adele B 211 West Lane, Stamford, CT 06905, (203) 323-4217, BS 56 Boston Univ; **SLP**

Gordon, Mrs Anita Shaw 28 McDowell Drive, Wake Forest, NC 27587, (919) 556-6298, BA 81 Univ of NC - Greensboro; ME 82 Univ of NC - Greensboro; 88–Sp-Lang Path, Rehab Svcs of Wake Co, **SLP**

Gordon, Ann E 17 Mills Lane, Long Island, East Setauket, NY 11733, (516) 751-3838, BA 69 CUNY - Brooklyn Coll; MA 72 CUNY - Queens Coll; Director, Ann E Gordon Associates, **SLP ACE**

Gordon, Barbara J 25 Bateson Drive, Andover, MA 01810, (617) 475-2839, BS 72 Univ of MA - Amherst; MS 74 Emerson Coll; Andover Sp Path, **SLP**

Gordon, Mrs Betty J 9613 West 116th Street, Overland Park, KS 66210, (413) 782-8950, BS 76 Univ of KS; MA 78 Univ of KS; Sp-Lang Path, Olathe Ks Sch Dist, **SLP**

Gordon, Mrs Brenda Lee 2729 Schifferdecker, Joplin, MO 64804, (417) 625-2497, BA 82 Univ of OK - Norman; MS 85 Univ of OK Medical Center; 85–Sp-Lang Path, St John's Reg Med Ctr, **SLP**

Gordon, Mrs Candace J 4916 Calle DE Cielo Ct N E, Albuquerque, NM 87111, (313) 288-8085, BA 68 Bradley Univ; MA 71 Univ of IL - Urbana; Coord/Cognitive Retrng Cen, Wm Beaumont Hosp, **SLP**

Gordon, Mrs Carol S 6318 Falling Brook Drive, Burke, VA 22015-4032, (703) 256-7229, BS 70 OH St Univ; MS 74 OH St Univ; Sp-Lang Path, Alexandria City Schools, **SLP**

Gordon, Charlene B 10495 Vernon, Huntington Woods, MI 48070, (313) 424-3392, BA 76 Univ of MI - Ann Arbor; MA 78 Wayne St Univ - Sch of Med; 83–Aud, Providence Hosp Dept of Aud, **A**

Gordon, Debra Ann Long Audiology-Speech Clinic, Box 52, APO New York, NY 09180, BS 80 Northern MI Univ; MS 83 Eastern WA Univ; Sp-Lang Path, Dept of the Army, **SLP**

Gordon, Donna Barclay 13015 Oak Plaza Drive, Cypress, TX 77429, (713) 469-0850, BS 83 Lubbock Christian Coll; MA 85 Abilene Christian Univ; **SLP**

Gordon, Dora N 363 Capron Farm Road, Warwick, RI 02886, (401) 822-0711, BA 75 Univ of RI; MS 77 Univ of RI; 78–Sp-Lang Path, West Warwick Sch Dept, **SLP ACE**

Gordon, Mrs Edith Marie 302 East Joppa Road #1501, Towson, MD 21204, BA 81 Univ of MD - College Park; MA 83 Univ of MD - College Park; **A**

Gordon, Mrs Elaine K 86 Poinciana, Memphis, TN 38119, (901) 685-7240, BA 55 CUNY - Queens Coll; MA 59 Columbia Univ Teachers Coll; Sp-Lang Path, Private Practice, **SLP**

Gordon, Mrs Ellen E 113 Welk Place #B, Charlottesville, VA 22906-4311, (817) 634-5756, BS 79 FL St Univ; MS 80 FL St Univ; SLP, Copperas Cove ISD, **SLP**

Gordon, Dr Ellen J 161 Main Street, Suite 2D, Hackensack, NJ 07601, (201) 342-0154, BA 68 CUNY - Queens Coll; MA 72 Columbia Univ Teachers Coll; PH 85 (Sp-Lang Path) Columbia Univ Teachers Coll; Sp-Lang Path, Communication Disorders Ctr, **SLP**

Gordon, Eric S 659 Pelis Road, Newark, NY 14513, (315) 789-3729, BA 81 SUNY - Center at Buffalo; MA 83 SUNY - Center at Buffalo; Sp-Lang Path, Newark Develop Center, **SLP**

Gordon, Fran Widelitz 7425 N W 52nd Street, Lauderhill, FL 33319, (305) 742-4152, **SLP**

Gordon, Dr Gaile Andrea Bill Wilkerson Hearing And Speech Center, 1114 19th Avenue South, Nashville, TN 37214, (615) 320-5353, BS 72 Univ of Redlands; MS 73 Univ of Redlands; PH 86 (Education) Claremont Graduate Sch; 88–Educ, Bill Wilkerson Hrng/Sp Ctr, **SLP**

Gordon, Mrs Garnet Michelle 2451 Juniper Court, Golden, CO 80401, (303) 526-9428, BA 73 Pacific Union Coll; MS 74 Loma Linda Univ - Riverside; Sp-Lang Path, Exper-Care Homecare/Psl, **SLP**

Gordon, Gloria G 8 Echo Hill Road, Montvale, NJ 07645, (914) 623-3828, BA 77 CUNY - Queens Coll; MS 79 Emerson Coll; Comptr Ctr Coord, Rockland County BOCES, **SLP**

Gordon, Henrietta 1284 Beacon Street, Brookline, MA 02146, MA; **SLP LM**

Gordon, Mrs Jamie Saltrick 208 Briarcliffe East, Elgin, SC 29045, (803) 773-1491, MS 85 WV Univ; OM 86 Univ of SC - Columbia; **SLP**

Gordon, Mrs Jill Suzanne 735 Riverside Avenue #A-8, Lyndhurst, NJ 07071, (718) 981-6020, BA 83 SUNY - Center at Buffalo; MS 85 Columbia Univ Teachers Coll; **A**

Gordon, Mrs Katherine Chism Route 4 Box 246, Lebanon, KY 40033, (502) 692-2989, BS 82 Eastern KY Univ; MA 84 Eastern KY Univ; Sp-Lang Path, Marion County Board of Ed, **SLP**

Gordon, Mrs Kathleen B Educational Service Unit #3, 4224 South 133rd Street, Omaha, NE 68137, (402) 330-2770, BA 54 Grinnell Coll; MS 68 Univ of NE - Omaha; Sp Ed Dir, Ed Serv Unit #3, **SLP**

Gordon, Dr Kathleen Clegg 155 South 2nd, Pocatello, ID 83201, BA 65 OH St Univ; MA 68 OH St Univ; PH 75 (NS) OH St Univ; Sp-Lang Path, Private Practice, **SLP**

Gordon, Linda L 5108 Melvin Avenue, Tarzana, CA 91356, **SLP**

Gordon, Mrs Margaret O 2412 South Holden Road #C, Greensboro, NC 27407, (919) 454-1518, BS 77 Appalachian St Univ; MA 78 Appalachian St Univ; SLP, Guilford Community Schools, **SLP**

Gordon, Martha Elizabeth Cobblestone #G-4, Dublin, GA 31021, (912) 275-3583, BS 82 Univ Southern MS-Hattiesburg; MS 84 Univ Southern MS-Hattiesburg; **SLP**

Gordon, Mary Ellen 2325 S W 21st Avenue, Portland, OR 97201, (503) 464-3533, BS 65 Purdue Univ - West Lafayette; MS 67 Purdue Univ - West Lafayette; Program Dir, Portland St U, **SLP**

Gordon, Mary Jo 101 Wilbourne Blvd, Condo 103, Lafayette, LA 70506, MS 84 Univ of Southwestern LA; Sp-Lang Path, Lafayette Parish Schools, **SLP**

Gordon, Miriam M 203 Marlbrook Lane, Lansdale, PA 19446, (212) 596-5696, BA 64 CUNY - Brooklyn Coll; MA 66 CUNY - Queens Coll; Super Sp-Lang Path, NYC Bd of Ed Sp Serv Ut, **SLP LM**

Gordon, Nancy Halstead Route 1 Box 855, Shepherdstown, WV 25443, (304) 725-9587, BA 76 Marshall Univ; MA 83 Marshall Univ; Sp-Lang Path, Jefferson County Board of Educ, **SLP**

Gordon, Nancy M 314 Adrienne Drive, Apopka, FL 32703, BS 70 Univ of TN - Knoxville; MA 72 Univ of TN - Knoxville; SLP, Seminole Co Sch, **SLP**

Gordon, Pamela J Health Testing Services Inc, 90 Bowdoin Avenue, Waltham, MA 02154-6441, (617) 891-1265, BA 74 Univ of Denver; MS 77 Boston Univ; President, Health Testing Services, **A**

Gordon, Pearl A Department Communication Sciences And Disorders, University Of South Florida, CBA 255, Tampa, FL 33620, (813) 974-2006, BS 70 Murray St Univ; MS 71 Murray St Univ; PH 84 (Hrng & Sp Sci) Univ of TN - Knoxville; Asst Prof, U of So FL, **SLP**

Gordon, Mrs Sharon A 283 Flagstone Terrace, San Rafael, CA 94903, (415) 472-7009, BA 69 San Jose St Univ; MA 73 San Jose St Univ; SLP, Cotati-Rohnert Park USD, **SLP**

Gordon, Mrs Terri Lou 2835 East Eastwood, Springfield, MO 65804, (417) 887-3109, **SLP**

Gordon, Dr Toni Gold 108-56 Jewel Avenue, Forest Hills, NY 11375, (718) 544-1345, BA 69 CUNY - City College; MA 70 CUNY - City College; PH 78 (NS) CUNY - Grad Sch & Univ Cntr; Aud, Arthur Podwall & Assoc, **A**

Gordon, Yvonne C 11724 Negley Drive, San Diego, CA 92131, (619) 693-0083, **SLP**

Gordon-Salant, Dr Sandra M Department Of Hearing And Speech Sciences, University Of Maryland, College Park, MD 20742, (301) 454-4876, BS 74 SUNY - Center at Albany; MA 76 Northwestern Univ; PH 81 (Aud) Northwestern Univ; 87–Assoc Prof, Univ of MD, **A**

Gordon-Siken, Donna 4425 North Alvernon Way, Tucson, AZ 85718, (602) 299-0599, MA 69 Univ of AZ

Gore, Carol N Drs Morton Blumenfeld & Charbo, 1733 Curie Drive, Suite 100, El Paso, TX 79902, (915) 533-5461, BA 73 Univ of TX - El Paso; MA 74 Univ of TX - El Paso; Aud, Morton,Blumenfeld&Charbonneau, **A**

Gore, Mrs Darlene A Speech Pathology Services, 135-1/2 1st Street, P O Box 891, Grenada, MS 38901, (601) 226-0101, OB 74 Univ of MS; OM 76 Univ of MS; Director, Speech Pathology Services, **SLP**

Gore, Donna R Pleasant Hills Condo, Foncine Lane 6-3, South Windsor, CT 06074, (203) 644-4950, BA 77 Southern CT St Univ; MA 80 KS St Univ; **SLP**

Gore, Mrs Donna W 1802 Cedarbrook, Columbia, SC 29212, (803) 781-3827, BA 68 Samford Univ; ME 71 Univ of SC - Spartanburg; Sp-Lang Path, Private Practice, **SLP**

Gore, Dr Larry B P O Box 58025, Fayetteville, NC 28305, (919) 485-5145, BS 71 Old Dominion Univ; ME 74 Univ of VA - Charlottesville; PH 77 (NS) Univ of VA - Charlottesville; Exec Dir, Sen Sp and Hrng Serv, **A**

Gore, Mrs Leah C 1201 Adger Road, Columbia, SC 29205, (803) 779-4155, BA 70 Columbia Coll; ME 72 Univ of SC - Columbia; 88–Sp-Lang Path, Manor Care-Columbia SC, **SLP**

Gore, Linda G 19 Norman Circle, Turners Falls, MA 01376, (413) 863-4009, BA 85 Univ of VT; MA 87 Univ of MA - Amherst; 88–Sp-Lang Path, Gill-Montague Sch Dist, **SLP**

Gore, Marcy 5625 Martel Avenue, Dallas, TX 75206-5619, BS 72 OK St Univ; MS 74 Univ of OK Medical Center; Sp-Lang Path, Richardson ISD, **SLP**

Goren, Mrs Jenine G c/o Glassman, 45 Farnum Drive, Holyoke, MA 01040, BA 78 Northeastern Univ; MA 81 OH St Univ; **SLP**

Gorenflo, Dr Carole Wood 808 Mount Pleasant Avenue, Ann Arbor, MI 48104, (313) 663-3567, BS 76 Purdue Univ - West Lafayette; MS 77 Univ of London - England; PH 86 (Aud & Sp Sciences) MI St Univ; 88–Asst Prof, Eastern Michigan Univ, **SLP**

Gorenko, Alexa Mae 276 Albert Street, 6 Thunderbird Circle, Kingston, ON, Canada K7L 3V6, (613) 547-3190, BA 70 Univ of Saskatchewan - Sask; MS 72 Minot St Univ; 87–Sp-Lang Path, Frontenac Co Bd of Educ, **SLP**

Gorey, Mary E 1077 Saint George Boulevard, Moncton, NB, Canada E1E 4C9, (506) 857-1500, BS 80 Univ of ME - Farmington; MA 87 Univ of ME - Orono; 81–Sp-Lang Path, Sch Dist #15

Gorga, Dr Michael P Boys Town National Institute, 555 North 30th Street, Omaha, NE 68131, (402) 498-6604, BA 72 CUNY - Brooklyn Coll; MS 76 CUNY - Brooklyn Coll; PH 80 (Aud/Hrng Science) Univ of IA; Coord, Cl Sens Physiology Lab, Boys Town Natl Inst, **A**

Gorgone, David John 12 Baldwin Drive, Greenville, RI 02828-6739, BA 78 Univ of RI; MA 80 Univ of MA - Amherst; 88–Chief Sp-Lang Path, St Joseph Hosp, **SLP**

Gorham, William J 1035 West 41st Street, San Bernardino, CA 92407, (714) 882-4517, BA 56 Univ of Notre Dame; MS 58 Purdue Univ - West Lafayette; 87–Sp-Lang Path/Aud, San Bernardino Supt of Schs, **SLP A ACE**

Gorin, Mrs Mary B 2001 Long Knife Court, Louisville, KY 40207, (502) 897-1371, ME; 76–Dir of Therapies, New Hope Svcs, **SLP**

Gorin, Rae I 1032 Pine Street #6, Philadelphia, PA 19107, (215) 546-1800, BA 77 Temple Univ-Tyler Sch of Art; MA 79 Temple Univ-Tyler Sch of Art; Principal, Rae Gorin Communication Assoc, **SLP**

Gorlin, Barbara Helene 4829 Buchanan Street, Hollywood, FL 33021, (305) 945-3215, BA 84 Univ of Central FL; MA 86 Univ of Central FL

Gorlin, Mrs Ruth Annette 6601 Wedgewood Avenue, Davie, FL 33331, (305) 891-8850, BA 83 Univ of FL; MA 85 Univ of Central FL; **SLP**

Gorlin, Todd Nelson 6601 Wedgewood Avenue, Davie, FL 33331, (305) 945-3215, BA 83 Univ of FL; MA 85 Univ of Central FL; **A**

Gormally, Susan Ulness 1519 6th Avenue West, Williston, ND 58801, (701) 572-6757, BS 76 ND St Univ; MS 81 Minot St Univ; SLP, Wilmac Sp Ed, **SLP**

Gorman, Barbara Marie 225 Lamont Drive, Buffalo, NY 14226, (716) 845-2203, BA 81 SUNY - Center at Buffalo; MA 83 SUNY - Center at Buffalo; 88–Dir-Sp-Lang Path, Buffalo Gen Hosp, **SLP**

Gorman, Jacqueline 249 Tuckerman Avenue, Middletown, RI 02840, (401) 849-2124, BA 73 Catholic Univ of America; MA 74 George Washington Univ; Sp/Lang Path, Middletown Pub Schs, **SLP**

Gorman, Nancy Ann 23 Point View Drive, East Greenbush, NY 12061-1813, (518) 489-8336, BS 76 Western MI Univ; MA 80 Univ of TN - Knoxville; 85–Sp-Lang Path, Cp Cen F/T Disabl, **SLP**

Gorman, Dr Pierre Patrick 18 Findon Avenue, Caulfield, Melbourne, Victoria, Australia, BS 49; OB 51; PH 60 (Social Psych of Deafness); Private Practice

Gorman, Stephen J 66900 Ironwood Drive, Apartment 505, Desert Hot Springs, CA 92240, (619) 323-6178, BS 81 Bowling Green St Univ; MS 86 Univ of WI - Madison; SLP, Desert Hospital, **SLP**

Gormley, Patricia Ryland 1625 Vereda Verde, Sarasota, FL 34232, (813) 953-7097, BS 86 FL St Univ; MS 87 FL St Univ

Gormley, Mrs Patricia Teggi 400 Quinnipiac Avenue, North Haven, CT 06473-3754, (203) 358-4390, **SLP**

Gornto, Peggy D 1650 West Carlton Street, Longwood, FL 32750, (305) 834-3060, BS 64 Valdosta St Coll; MA 81 Univ of Central FL; **SLP**

Gorohoff, Mrs Sandra Waters 2005 36th Avenue West, Seattle, WA 98199, (206) 782-2700, BA 63 Baylor Univ; MA 67 Univ of WA; Sp-Lang Path, Ballard Community Hosp, **SLP**

Gorrell, Howard Anthony 403 South Waverly, Dallas, TX 75208, (215) 631-9300, BS 85 Univ of TX - Austin; MS 87 Univ of TX - Dallas; **SLP**

Gorski, Cynthia Frances 761 Panorama Drive, Pismo Beach, CA 93449-3251, (312) 749-2124, **SLP**

Gorski, Cynthia Witt Casilla 15167, Santiago, Chile 11, BA 72 Augustana Coll; MA 73 Northwestern Univ; Sp-Lang Path, Private Practice, **SLP**

Gorski, Janice F 11401 9th Street North, Apartment 1914, St Petersburg, FL 33716, (312) 767-0617, BA 79 Saint Xavier Coll; MA 80 Univ of IL - Urbana; SLP, Chicago Board of Education, **SLP**

Gorski, Mrs Kathleen Mary 5 Aimee Avenue, West Holyoke, MA 01040, (413) 789-1400, BA 77 Elms Coll; MS 85 Worcester St Coll; **SLP**

Gorski, Margaret M 59 Grove Street, Waldwick, NJ 07463, (201) 652-5052, BA 59 Montclair St Coll; MS 72 William Paterson Coll; Hrng Ed, Waldwick Pub Sch, **SLP ACE**

Gorski, Sally Majetich 2917 43rd Avenue South, Minneapolis, MN 55406, (612) 227-8471, BA 79 Univ of MN - Duluth; MA 80 Univ of MN - Duluth; Sp-Lang Path, St Paul Rehab Cen, **SLP**

Gorski, Mrs Therese Marie 1507 N Gulley, Dearborn Heights, MI 48127, (313) 362-4299, SLP, Medi-Sp Service, **SLP**

Gorski, Vincent J 59 Grove Street, Waldwick, NJ 07463, (201) 529-5000, BA 59 Montclair St Coll; MS 61 Montclair St Coll; Tchr, Mahwah Bd of Ed, **SLP**

Gortner, Rebecca Lynn 6157 Ross Road, Fairfield, OH 45014, (513) 874-4831, BS 83 Miami Univ - Oxford; MS 84 Miami Univ - Oxford; **SLP**

Gorzalski, Mrs Janet A 3310 South 8th Street, Milwaukee, WI 53215, (414) 281-5750, BS 73 Univ of WI - River Falls; MS 79 Univ of WI - Milwaukee; Sp/Lang Path, Schl Dist of Greenfield, **SLP**

Goscha, Mrs Rebecca J 5120 Decatur, Omaha, NE 68104, (402) 556-9156, BA 82 Wichita St Univ; MA 83 Wichita St Univ; Sp/Lang Path, Millard PS, **SLP**

Gosche, Bruce Paul 500 South Belcher Road #6, Largo, FL 33541, (813) 985-3173, MS 86 Univ of South FL; **A**

Goset, Frederick 8915 62nd Drive N E, Marysville, WA 98270, (206) 259-0966, BS 73 Walla Walla Coll; MS 76 ID St Univ; Aud, The Everett Clinic, **A**

Goshit, Mrs M Yvonne 642 Morris Park Avenue, Bronx, NY 10460-2525, (212) 863-6905, BA 79 Barnard Coll; MS 83 Columbia Univ Teachers Coll; 85–Sp-Lang Path, NYS Ofc of Men Ret & Dev Dis, **SLP**

Goshorn, Dr Edward L 410 Cleveland Avenue, Long Beach, MS 39560, (601) 864-1077, BS 72 Univ Southern MS-Hattiesburg; MS 73 Univ of NC - Chapel Hill; PH 84 (Aud) Memphis St Univ; Aud, VA Med Ctr, **SLP A**

Gosin-Lynch, Barbara R 111 Five Fields Road, Madison, CT 06443, (203) 245-3802, BA 76 Univ of Northern CO; MA 78 Univ of Northern CO; Sp-Lang Path, Private Practice, **SLP**

Goslin, Mrs Betty 717 Sonya Place, Anaheim, CA 92802, (714) 535-2109, BA 58 CA St Univ - Long Beach; Sp-Lang Path, Anaheim Cty Sch, **SLP**

Gosnell, Mrs Marie Dovre 1516 Dennis Blvd, Moncks Corner, SC 29461, (803) 821-2272, MA 85 SC St Coll; 88–Sp-Lang Path, ACRA, **SLP**

Gospel, Mrs Mary Dragoo 3331 Piccadilly Street, Bloomington, IN 47401, (812) 333-9185, BA 81 IN Univ - Bloomington; MA 82 IN Univ - Bloomington; **SLP**

Goss, Krista Hill 4178 Hemlock Drive, Eagle River, WI 54521-9379, (715) 479-3330, BS 81 Western MI Univ; MA 83 George Washington Univ; Sp/Lang Path, Northwoods Rehab Assoc, **SLP**

Goss, Linda L 9321 Orlando Place N E, Albuquerque, NM 87111, (505) 299-3878, BA 66 Univ of TX - Austin; MS 80 Southern Methodist Univ; **SLP**

Goss, Marilyn Mauck 120 Cheyenne Road, Shelbyville, KY 40065, (502) 633-3246, BA 75 Univ of KY; ME 81 Univ of Louisville; Sp-Lang Path, Shelby Co Schools, **SLP**

Goss, Mrs Monica Lynn 9342-B Jamison Avenue, Philadelphia, PA 19115, (215) 673-8692, BS 82 PA St Univ - Univ Park; MA 84 Trenton St Coll; **SLP**

Goss, Rebecca Singleton Box 1744, Harlan, KY 40831, (606) 573-1400, BS 82 Univ of KY; MA 85 Univ of TN - Knoxville; Sp-Lang Path, Appalachian Reg Hosp, **SLP**

Gossage, Nona Ann 4924 Camino DE Monte N E, Albuquerque, NM 87111-2931, (505) 294-1933, **SLP**

Gosselin, Mrs Lisa A 24 Silverlake Drive, Kingston, MA 02364, (617) 585-8636, BA 79 Bridgewater St Coll; ME 82 Northeastern Univ; **SLP**

Gosselin, Mrs Lisa R 10 Langseth Avenue, Claremont, NH 03743-3320, (603) 543-3720, BA 80 Allegheny Coll; MS 81 Bloomsburg Univ of PA; 81–Aud, Valley Reg Hosp, **A**

Gosselin, Michelle Ann 300 Sulphur Springs Road, Apartment M-6, Greenville, SC 29611, (803) 246-0047, BS 82 Western Carolina Univ; MA 83 Western Carolina Univ; SLP, Schl Dstr of Pickens Co, **SLP**

Gosselin, Patricia M 113 Lincoln Avenue, Saugus, MA 01906, (617) 254-3800, Aud, Kennedy Mem Hosp for Children, **A**

Gosselin-Alfieri, Marcia 19 Glen Street, Malden, MA 02148, (617) 264-4700, BS 79 Providence Coll; MS 81 Boston Univ; SLP, Acton-Boxbourough Reg Sch Dist, **SLP**

Gossman, Mary A 10814 Larimore Avenue, Omaha, NE 68164, (402) 498-6535, BS 73 Univ of NE - Lincoln; MA 78 Univ of NE - Lincoln; Aud, Boys Town Natl Inst, **A**

Gossman, Mrs Sandy Kay 6026 Brighton Meadows #F, Fort Wayne, IN 46804, (219) 426-2644, BS 85 Ball St Univ; MA 86 Ball St Univ; Dir of Aud, Ft Wayne Occupational Hlth Ctr, **A**

Gostow, Terry Lynn 234 West Anapamu #D, Santa Barbara, CA 93101, (805) 564-4816, BA 71 MI St Univ; MA 74 Eastern MI Univ; SLP, Private Practice, **SLP**

Gotaas, Christine Elizabeth #1505 10635 47th Avenue, Edmonton, AB, Canada T5G 0B7, (403) 471-2262, BS 83 Univ of Alberta - Alberta; MA 86 Univ of MN - Minneap-St Paul; **SLP**

Gotlib, Kenneth S 6309 Bengal Circle, Boynton Beach, FL 33437, (407) 499-9596, BA 76 CUNY - Brooklyn Coll; MS 79 CUNY - Brooklyn Coll; 88–Aud, FL Hearing Care Ctrs Inc, **A**

Gotlieb, Mrs Talia F 155 Hazel Street, Clifton, NJ 07015, (201) 772-0193, BA 67 Hebrew Univ-Jerusalem Israel; MA 78 Montclair St Coll; 81–Dir, Randolph Hrng & Sp Cen, **A**

Gotsch, Mrs Donna T 2837 Gateshead Court, Abingdon, MD 21009, (301) 679-0379, BA 67 Elmhurst Coll; MA 68 Bowling Green St Univ; **SLP A**

Gotsch, Mrs Linda Joyce 18027 North 55th Street, Scottsdale, AZ 85254, (602) 493-7958, BA 72 Elmira Coll; MS 74 Southern IL Univ-Edwardsvill

Gotsdiner, Mrs Nancy Shulak Greenpark One Medical Prof Bldg, 7515 South Main, Suite 200, Houston, TX 77030, (713) 795-0922, BA 75 Univ of TX - Austin; MA 76 Univ of Houston - Univ Park; 86–Sp-Lang Path, Private Practice, **SLP**

Gott, Mrs Sylvia Rulff 7815 Terrace Drive, El Cerrito, CA 94530, (415) 525-6169, BA 56 IN Univ - Bloomington; MA 58 IN Univ - Bloomington; Sp-Lang Path, Berkeley USD, **SLP**

Gottardi, Donna L 714 Brougham Road, Fayetteville, NC 28301, (919) 396-5207, BS 72 Indiana Univ of PA; MS 79 Indiana Univ of PA; Sp/Lang Path, Womackarmy Commun Hosp, **SLP**

Gottermeier, Linda G F NTID, 1 Lomb Memorial Drive, Rochester, NY 14623, (716) 475-6429, BS 77 Nazareth Coll of Rochester; MA 81 SUNY - Coll at Geneseo; 81–Aud, NTID, **A**

Gottfred, Dr Catherine H Gottfred Speech Assoc, Northbrook Court Professional Plaza, 1535 Lakecook Road Suite 100, Northbrook, IL 60062, (312) 564-9230, BA 71 Elmhurst Coll; MA 73 Northwestern Univ; PH 79 (Sp-Lang Path) Northwestern Univ; Dir, Gottfred Sp Assco, **SLP**

Gottfried, Linda L Wood 3331 Arlington Avenue, #G-214, Toledo, OH 43614, (413) 381-4012, BS 77 OH Univ - Athens; MA 81 OH Univ - Athens; Sp-Lang Path, Medical College of Ohio, **SLP**

Gottfried, Nancy E P O Box 1088, Stroudsburg, PA 18360, (717) 424-3681, BA 70 Fontbonne Coll; MA 76 Univ of Cincinnati; Sp/Lang Path, St James Assiniboia Dist, **SLP**

Gottfried, Sorel D 1016 Cayuga Heights Road, Ithaca, NY 14850, (607) 753-5028, BA 55 McGill Univ - Quebec; MS 76 Ithaca Coll; 81–Sp-Lang Path, Private Practice, **SLP ACE**

Gotti, Margaret E 401 Hemlock Drive, Lanoka Harbor, NJ 08734, (609) 971-1508, BS 79 Trenton St Coll; MA 82 Trenton St Coll; Sp-Lang Path, Kessler Rehab Hosp, **SLP**

Gottier, Mrs Daryl-Lynne K 37½ B Park Street, Rockville, CT 06066, (203) 871-8594, BS 81 Univ of CT; MA 85 Univ of CT; Sp-Lang Path, South Windsor PS, **SLP**

Gottlieb, Mrs Dvora Posner 5667 North Angela Lane, Memphis, TN 38119, (901) 767-9156, BS 83 Univ of GA; OM 85 Emory Univ; **SLP**

Gottlieb, Mrs Eileen Haber 118 Union Avenue South, Delmar, NY 12054, (518) 439-3327, BA 77 Univ of FL; MS 80 Coll of Saint Rose; **SLP**

Gottlieb, Gayle Pauline 3431 Shaw Avenue #7, Cincinnati, OH 45208, (513) 724-2022, BA 84 OH St Univ; MA 86 OH St Univ; **SLP**

Gottlieb, Kathleen Ann 304 Stockade, Lawrence, KS 66044, (913) 843-8537, BS 78 Univ of WI - Madison; MS 81 Univ of WI - Madison; **SLP**

Gottlieb, Mrs Linda Haas 22 Beechwood Road, Woodbridge, CT 06525, (203) 387-0641, BA 73 SUNY - Center at Buffalo; MA 74 Hofstra Univ; Sp-Lang Path, Private Practice, **SLP**

Gottlieb, Mrs Linda Lehrer P O Box 981, Far Hills, NJ 07931, (201) 234-2648, BA 68 CUNY - Hunter Coll; MS 69 Syracuse Univ; **SLP**

Gottlieb, Sheri Lee 110 Meadors Circle, Morris, IL 60450, (815) 942-3317, BS 81 Eastern IL Univ; MS 83 Eastern IL Univ; Sp-Lang Path, Joliet School System Dist 86, **SLP**

Gottlieb, Dr Sidney Route 1 Box 301-A, Boston, VA 22713, (703) 547-3934, BS 40 Univ of WI - Madison; ME 79 San Jose St Univ; PH 43 (Chemistry) CA Inst of Tech; Dir, Rappahannock Sp and Lrng Cen, **SLP**

Gottlieb, Suzanne Del 16 Trowbridge Street, Apartment 31, Cambridge, MA 02138, (617) 492-2009, MS 85 Columbia Univ Teachers Coll; Sp-Lang Path, Mount St Ursula, **SLP**

Gottlieb-Karp, Beverly N 2947 Greenfield Avenue, Los Angeles, CA 90064, (213) 474-7922, BA 52 Univ of CA - Los Angeles; MA 68 CA St Univ - Long Beach; Sp-Lang Path, Private Practice, **SLP ACE**

Gottsch, Barbara Mayer 2311 South 143 Court, Apartment #7, Omaha, NE 68144, BA 85 Elmhurst Coll; MS 87 IL St Univ - Normal; **SLP**

Gottsch, Mrs Jean Ann Quigley 8 Seaspray Lane, West Islip, NY 11795, (516) 499-1237, BA 69 Molloy Coll; MS 70 Adelphi Univ

Gottschalk, Mrs Becky Rene 218 McCready Avenue, Louisville, KY 40206, (812) 944-7701, BS 79 Eastern KY Univ; MS 81 Univ of Louisville; Sp/Lang Path, Floyd Co Mem Hosp, **SLP**

Gottschalk-Grafman, Carole 1140 #3 South Golden West Avenue, Arcadia, CA 91006, (818) 447-7110, OB 68 Univ of MI - Ann Arbor; BA 68 Univ of MI - Ann Arbor; MS 69 Univ of MI - Ann Arbor; Aud, Private Practice, **A**

Gottsche, Linda L 6028 Christina Drive East, Lakeland, FL 33813, (813) 644-8892, BS 84 Univ of NE - Lincoln; MS 85 Univ of NE - Lincoln; 88–Sp-Lang Path, InSpeech Inc, **SLP**

Gottsleben, Robert H 1176 Rhode Island Street, San Francisco, CA 94107, (415) 664-4646, BS 50 Univ of WI - Madison; MS 54 Univ of WI - Madison; Dir, Scottish Rite Clin Chld Lang Dis, **SLP**

Gottsleben, Sheila Ann Orlando Regional Medical Center, Audiology Department, 1414 South Kyhl Avenue, Orlando, FL 32806, (407) 841-5111, BS 81 SD St Univ; MS 83 Purdue Univ - West Lafayette; Aud, **A**

Gottwald, Sheryl Ridener Rd 1 Box 639, Payne Road, Green Lane, PA 18054, (215) 234-8803, BS 76 Northeastern Univ; MS 77 PA St Univ - Univ Park; Instr, Temple Univ, **SLP**

Goubeaux, Jocelyn H 914 North Kings Road #2, West Hollywood, CA 90069, (213) 656-6440, BS 80 Ball St Univ; MA 82 CA St Univ - Los Angeles; Aud, Kaiser Permanente, **A**

Goud, Ramesh M P O Box 4088, Costa Mesa, CA 92628, (714) 957-5147, BS 69; MA 76 Northern MI Univ; Sp/Lang Path, Fairview, **SLP**

Goud, Mrs Ranjan R P O Box 4088, Costa Mesa, CA 92628, (714) 957-5147, MA 74 Northern MI Univ; Sp/Lang Path, Fairview, **SLP**

Goudie, Janice L 601 East Rosery Road, Apartment 1004, Largo, FL 34640, (813) 462-7030, BS 85 Northern IL Univ - De Kalb; MA 87 Northern IL Univ - De Kalb; 87–Sp-Lang Path, Morton F Plant Hosp, **SLP**

Goudie, Kathryn L Developmental Disabilities Inc, 1018 Atherton, Salt Lake City, UT 84123, (801) 266-3939, BS 76 Univ of UT; BS 77 Univ of UT; MS 81 Univ of UT; Sp/Lang Path, Utah Sch for the Blind, **SLP**

Goudreau, Anne L Boys Town National Institute, 555 North 30th Street, Omaha, NE 68131, (402) 498-6576, BA 83 Univ of MD - College Park; MA 87 Univ of IA; 87–Aud, Boys Town National Inst, **A**

Goudy-Andrew, Sandra 30 Acacia Court, Kentfield, CA 94904, (415) 453-8972, BA 60 Northwestern Univ; MA 65 Northwestern Univ; **SLP**

Gouge, Mrs Cynthia G 1332-E Wicklow Court, Cary, NC 27511, (919) 469-8515, BA 85 NC St Univ at Raleigh; MS 87 Western Carolina Univ; 87–Sp-Lang Path, Logos Inc, **SLP**

Gough, Mrs Karen Frances 2909 Windswept Drive #202, Lantana, FL 33462, (407) 969-2048, MS 87 Minot St Univ; **SLP**

Gough, Dr Kenneth H 4904 124th Street, Edmonton, AB, Canada T6H 3T9, (403) 432-5990, BA 54; MA 57 Univ of IA; PH 67 (NS) Purdue Univ - West Lafayette; Assoc Prof, U Ab Dept Sp Path & Aud, **SLP A**

Gould, Alan B 137 Cheese Spring Road, Wilton, CT 06897, OM 83 Univ of Bridgeport; **SLP**

Gould, Mrs Cecelia A 18 Glen Alpine Road, Phoenix, MD 21131, (301) 592-6713, BA 69 Towson St Univ; MS 87 Towson St Univ; **SLP**

Gould, Elaine Dwyer 405 Wilton Street, Greenville, SC 29609, (803) 242-8040, BS 82 VA Polytechnic Inst St Univ; OM 86 Univ of SC - Columbia; 87–Sp-Lang Path, Meyer Ctr for Spec Children, **SLP**

Gould, Elaine Rose 357 Washington Street, Whitman, MA 02382, (617) 848-5353, **SLP**

Gould, Dr Herbert J Dept Of Audiology, 807 Jefferson Avenue, Memphis, TN 38105, (901) 525-2682, BA 72 MI St Univ; MA 74 Univ of IL - Urbana; PH 75 (Hrng & Sp Science) Univ of IL - Urbana; Assistant Professor, Memphis State University, **A**

Gould, Hope Weinrod 6 Brown Court, Great Neck, NY 11024, (516) 482-8778, BS 77 Ithaca Coll; MS 79 OH Univ - Athens; 88–Aud, Private Practice, **A**

Gould, Mrs Jeanne K 1166 S Fillmore Street, Denver, CO 80210, (303) 722-5326, BS 77 Kent St Univ; MA 77 Kent St Univ; Sp-Lang Path, Private Practice, **SLP**

Gould, Jody Anne 5956 Penfield Avenue, Woodland Hills, CA 91367, (818) 992-5232, BA 79 Univ of CA - Santa Barbara; MA 81 CA St Univ - Los Angeles; Sp-Lang Path, InSpeech Inc, **SLP**

Gould, Judy 9209 East Helen, Tucson, AZ 85715, (602) 745-2113, BS 72 Univ of WI - Madison; MS 73 Univ of WI - Madison; Sp-Lang Path, Tucson USD, **SLP**

Gould, Laura D 114 Birchwood Avenue, Upper Nyack, NY 10960, (914) 353-0139, BS 71 Emerson Coll; MA 78 NY Univ; Sp-Lang Path, Private Practice, **SLP**

Gould, Linda R 1321 Sorolla Avenue, Coral Gables, FL 33134, (305) 444-9638, BS 84 Univ of MA - Amherst; ME 86 Univ of VA - Charlottesville; Audiologist, Modern Health Services, **A**

Gould, Mrs Marsha L 2440 North Bradley Avenue, Claremont, CA 91711, (714) 624-7826, BA 71 Univ of FL; MS 72 Univ of NC - Chapel Hill; 88–Sp-Lang Path, Chino USD, **SLP**

Gould, Mary Devaney 56 Cottage Terrace, Bedford Hills, NY 10507, (914) 666-4160, BA 72 OH St Univ; MA 73 Vanderbilt Univ; Sp-Lang Path, Bedford NY Pub Schs, **SLP**

Gould, Nancy 3643 Upton Street N W, Washington, DC 20008, (301) 762-0632, BA 55 Univ of WI - Madison; MS 58 Stanford Univ; Program Assistant, Montgomery County Pub Schools, **SLP**

Gould, Mrs Rosario G R R #2 10 Fox Run Road, Eastham, MA 02642, (617) 240-0746, MA 78 NY Univ; Aud, **A**

Gould, Susan Hosmer 4854 Constance Street, New Orleans, LA 70115, (504) 271-6553, BA 65 Salve Regina - Newport Coll; MA 83 Univ of RI; SLP, St Bernard Parish, **SLP**

Gould, Trina A 3647 23rd Avenue, Meridian, MS 39301, (601) 483-8121, BA 78 Univ of Miami; MS 81 Univ Southern MS-Hattiesburg; Audiology, Meridian Sp and Hrng Cen, **A**

Goulding, Virginia R 3336 Coleridge Drive, Raleigh, NC 27609, (919) 787-2852, OB 41 Emerson Coll; BA 43 Univ of NC - Chapel Hill; ME 57 Univ of Pittsburgh - Pittsburgh; Retired, Wake Co Pub Sch Syst, **SLP A LM**

Goulding, William P 940 Gunderson, Oak Park, IL 60304, (312) 848-9750, BS 79 IL St Univ - Normal; MS 81 IL St Univ - Normal; Sr Clin Supvr, InSpeech Inc, **SLP**

Gould-MacDonald, Carol L 902 Gainsborough, East Lansing, MI 48823, (517) 887-3227, BA 72 MI St Univ; MA 73 MI St Univ; Sp-Lang Path, Lansing School District, **SLP**

Goulett, Diane M 2609 Robbins Street, Minneapolis, MN 55410, (612) 627-2395, BS 51 Univ of MN - Minneap-St Paul; MA 76 Coll of St Thomas; Sp-Lang Path, Minneapolis Pub Sch, **SLP**

Gousha, Mrs Catherine 707 Christopher Drive, Bloomington, IN 47401, BA 44 OH Univ - Athens; MA 47 OH St Univ; Sp/Lang Path, Richland-Beanblossom Comm Sch, **SLP**

Goutier, Maureen Child Development Centre, 899 North Lahakas Blvd, Kitimat, BC, Canada V8C 1E4, (604) 632-3144, MA 88 Western WA Univ

Gouvier, Rebecca Harrell 13115 Briargrove, Baton Rouge, LA 70810, BS 77 Delta St Univ; MA 80 Memphis St Univ; **SLP**

Gover, Mrs Misha W 3070 Buffalo Trace, Madisonville, KY 42431, Univ of KY; Sp-Lang Path, Hopkins County Bd of Education, **SLP**

Govostes, George J 46 Swanton Street, Winchester, MA 01890, (617) 727-0500, BS 64 Boston Univ; MS 70 Boston Univ; 64–Sp/Lang Path, MA Dept of Educ, **SLP**

Gowan-Baker, Mrs Daralee 17383 Caminito Siega, San Diego, CA 92127-1119, (619) 483-3209, BA 80 Univ of Redlands; MS 81 Univ of Redlands; Sp-Lang Path Indep Contractor, Eloise R Johnston & Assoc, **SLP**

Gowdy, Mrs Shirley P c/o Sam Mattix, Box 1OUTH Barker, Nakorn Phanom, Thailand 48000, **SLP**

Gowens, Pamela A R 3440 Lemmington Road, Pensacola, FL 32504, BS 78 FL St Univ; MS 79 FL St Univ; SLP, Escambia Co Dist Pub Sch, **SLP**

Gower, Kathy J G 1450 100th Avenue N W #205, Minneapolis, MN 55433-5321, (612) 434-5461, **SLP**

Gower-Alba, Mrs Lynne Ellen 6119 Seaside Walk, Long Beach, CA 90803, (213) 328-3611, BA 81 CA St Univ - Long Beach; MA 85 CA St Univ - Long Beach; 85–Dept Supvr-Sp-Lang Path, Switzer Center, **SLP**

Gowin, Jane 910 Lorraine Avenue, Florence, SC 29501, **SLP**

Gowin, Susan Ann Myers 16103 Kent Road, Laurel, MD 20707, **SLP**

Gowling, Mrs Jimmye L 845 Parsons Drive, Beaumont, TX 77706, (409) 385-5286, BS 70 Lamar Univ; MS 71 Lamar Univ; Proj Dir, Silsbee ISD, **SLP**

Gowman, Marilyn 38365 North Lane #G-109, Willoughby, OH 44094, (216) 268-6685, MA 79 Kent St Univ; BS 78 Miami Univ - Oxford; Sp-Lang Path, East Cleveland City Schs, **SLP ACE**

Gownley, Kelly Ann 107 Laurel Lane, Oak Ridge Estates, Mount Carmel, PA 17851, (717) 727-6728, BS 85 Bloomsburg Univ of PA; MS 86 Bloomsburg Univ of PA; **SLP**

Goy, John Michael 8810 Lindsey, Plainwell, MI 49080, (616) 664-4641, BS 77 Western MI Univ; MA 87 Western MI Univ; Aud, Hrng & Sp Ctr-Grand Rapids, **A**

Goy, Mrs Karen Miller 804 Burlington Street, Merdota, IL 61342-1633, (206) 629-3125, **SLP**

Goyings, Mrs Joann S 1208 3rd, Jackson, MI 49203, (517) 787-2800, OB 77 Central MI Univ; MS 78 Univ of MI - Ann Arbor; Sp/Lang Path, Jackon Co Inter Sch Dist, **SLP**

Gozdziewski, Mrs Terry Hausner 71-35 252nd Street, Bellerose, NY 11426, (718) 347-3641, BA 75 Adelphi Univ; MA 76 George Washington Univ; Sp-Lang Path, N Bellmore Un Free Sch Dist, **SLP**

Gozonsky, Mrs Dorothy A 118 Irving Avenue, Providence, RI 02906, (401) 351-1240, BA 52 Brown Univ; OB 62 RI Coll; ME 70 Boston Univ; **SLP**

Graan, Ellen M 5051 West Washington Blvd, Milwaukee, WI 53208, (414) 453-9674, BS 77 Marquette Univ; MS 79 Univ of WI - Madison; Sp-Path, Milwaukee Public Schools, **SLP**

Graban, Mrs Elizabeth A R 659 Maple Drive, Hermitage, PA 16148, (216) 392-4400, BS 68 Edinboro Univ of PA; ME 70 PA St Univ - Univ Park; Assistant Co Superintendent, Trumbull Co Board of Ed, **SLP**

Grabbe, Laura Leigh 1102 South Leslie, Stuttgart, AR 72160, (501) 673-7946, BA 81 Univ of AR - Fayetteville; MS 82 Univ of AR - Fayetteville; Sp/Lang Path, Fayetteville Pub Sch, **SLP**

Graber, Mrs Adele A 13220 Upton Avenue South, Burnsville, MN 55337, (612) 887-7240, MS 82 Mankato St Univ; BS 57 Univ of IA; Sp-Lang Path, Dist 191, **SLP**

Graber, Mrs Barbara R 23 Notch Hill Drive, Livingston, NJ 07039, **SLP**

Graber, Gail Rust 441 South Ham Lane, Suite B, Lodi, CA 95240, (209) 368-9222, BA 77 CA St Univ - Sacramento; MA 79 CA St Univ - Sacramento; Aud, Hrng Serv Cen, **A**

Graber, Kathleen A 5 Heathcliff Road, Rumson, NJ 07760, BS 76 Northwestern Univ; MS 77 Columbia Univ Teachers Coll; Clinic Supervisor, Teachers College Columbia Univ, **SLP**

Graber, Sarah Rachelle 6400 North Sacramento, Apartment 102, Chicago, IL 60645, (312) 338-7448, BA 82 Barnard Coll; MS 84 Columbia Univ Teachers Coll; 87–Sp-Lang Path, **SLP**

Graber, Shannon E 5838 South Pittsburgh, Tulsa, OK 74135, (918) 742-1237, BS 70 Univ of Tulsa; MA 71 Univ of Tulsa; Sp-Lang Path, Union Pub Sch, **SLP**

Grabiak, Susan M 746 West Church Street, Sandersville, GA 31082, (912) 552-6047, BS 75 Auburn Univ - Auburn; ME 80 Univ of GA; Sp-Lang Path, Washington Co Bd of Ed, **SLP**

Grabiec, Mrs Barbara J 332 Colonial Drive, Grand Island, NY 14072, (716) 278-4639, BA 67 D'Youille Coll; MS 74 Univ of Louisville; Sp-Lang Path, Niagara Falls Mem Med Cen, **SLP**

Grable, Mrs Patty Cannon 309 Adams Avenue, Hopkinsville, KY 42240, (502) 886-5163, BS 79 Murray St Univ; MS 80 Murray St Univ; Coord Sp/Hearing Services, Pennyroyal Men Hlth-Men Ret Ct, **SLP**

Grabo, Mrs Diane E E 123 Horstman Drive, Scotia, NY 12302, (518) 374-6617, BS 74 Ithaca Coll; MS 76 Columbia Univ Teachers Coll; Owner/Dir, Sp-Path Serv, **SLP**

Grabow, Mrs Suzan K 1229 Academy Court, Arlington, TX 76013, (714) 529-1620, BA 78 Tulane Univ; MA 80 Northwestern Univ; **A**

Grabowski, Ann J 5 Amherst Place, Parlin, NJ 08859, (201) 571-3975, BA 70 Catholic Univ of America; MA 72 Catholic Univ of America; Sp-Lang Path, Long Branch Pub Sch, **SLP**

Grabowski, Carola Mary Box 326, Dodge, NE 68633, (402) 693-2339, BS 76 Univ of WI - Stevens Point; MS 77 Univ of WI - Stevens Point; 88–Sp-Lang Path, Educational Service Unit #2, **SLP**

Grabowski, Kathleen S 235 North Street, Salem, MA 01970, (617) 745-4812, BA 81 Boston Univ; MS 86 Emerson Coll; **SLP**

Grabowski, Dr Richard R Audiology Services Of Lv, 2895 Hamilton Boulevard, Suite 201, Allentown, PA 18104, (215) 432-5256, BS 54 Bloomsburg Univ of PA; ME 60 Temple Univ-Tyler Sch of Art; PH 76 (NS) NY Univ; Aud Svcs of LV, **SLP A**

Graca, Mrs Lori E 614 East Cronkhite, Knoxville, IA 50138, (515) 842-2719, BS 79 Northwest MO St Univ; MA 81 Northeast MO St Univ; Sp-Lang Path, Heartland AEA, **SLP**

Grace, Ann Wilson Route 3 Box 205, Clinton, TN 37716, (615) 693-9408, BS 82 East TN St Univ; MA 83 Univ of TN - Knoxville; Sp-Lang Path, Private Practice, **SLP**

Grace, Deborah Gorthy P O Box 327, St Francis, KS 67756, (913) 462-8282, BS 74 KS St Univ; MA 76 KS St Univ; Sp/Lang Path, NW Kansas Ed Serv Cen, **SLP**

Grace, Patricia 1918 El Parque #5, Colorado Springs, CO 80907, (818) 718-1397, BS 82 Central MI Univ; MA 83 Wichita St Univ; **SLP**

Gracey, Sally Brown 4339 El Campo, Fort Worth, TX 76107, (817) 732-3919, BS 77 TX Christian Univ; MS 78 TX Christian Univ; 81–Sp-Lang Path, Ft Worth Childrens Hosp, **SLP**

Grachek, Mrs Doris Jeanne 12811 Margo Circle, Omaha, NE 68138, (402) 558-0440, BA 82 Univ of NE - Lincoln; MS 84 Univ of NE - Lincoln; **A**

Grachen, John J 314-B Hermit Street, Philadelphia, PA 19128, (215) 843-1044, BS 67 CA Univ of PA; ME 75 Bloomsburg Univ of PA; Sp-Lang Path, School Dist of Philadelphia, **SLP**

Gracie, Georgie C 131 Sycamore Street, Cary, NC 27511, (919) 469-1848, BA 69 Northwestern St Univ; MA 70 Northwestern St Univ; 86–Sp-Lang Path, Communication Therapy Services, **SLP**

Gradassi, Renee A 5815 N Sheridan Road #706, Chicago, IL 60660, (312) 878-8578, BA 70 Rosary Coll; MA 71 Columbia Univ Teachers Coll; Instructor of Communication, Loyola University, **SLP**

Gradisher, Mrs Myra Summervill 114 North 14th Street, Murray, KY 42071, (502) 236-2050, **SLP**

Grady, Barbara J 3202 West Bell Road #2211, Phoenix, AZ 85023-7515, (602) 995-7178, BS 76 Univ of WI - Stevens Point; MS 77 Univ of WI - Stevens Point; SLP, Deer Valley USD, **SLP**

Grady, Elizabeth 1492 North Avenue #111, Bridgeport, CT 06604-2665, (203) 255-7585, BA 78 Catholic Univ of America; MS 80 Columbia Univ Teachers Coll; Sp-Lang Path, CES, **SLP**

Grady, Ellen Grace 2610 Tunlaw Road Northwest, Apartment 2, Washington, DC 20007, (202) 337-9194, BS 81 Marywood Coll; MA 83 George Washington Univ; Sp-Lang Path, Holy Redeemer Hospital, **SLP**

Grady, Mrs Francine E 5 Clarkes Crossing, Fairport, NY 14450, (716) 377-4660, BS 71 SUNY - Center at Albany; MS 75 Nazareth Coll of Rochester; Sp-Lang Path, BOCES #1 Monroe Co, **SLP**

Grady, Mrs Joan G P O Box 370, La Grangeville, NY 12540-0370, (914) 635-1803, BS 65 SUNY - Coll at New Paltz; MA 67 Columbia Univ Teachers Coll; Sp-Lang Path, Westchester Assn Retarded Citzn, **SLP**

Grady, Mrs Linda D 6001 Harvard Drive, Kokomo, IN 46902, (317) 453-7419, BA 73 Bellarmine Coll; MA 81 Ball St Univ; Sp-Lang Path, Eastern Howard School Corp, **SLP**

Grady, Mrs Lynn B 2118 Lake Bentley Court, Lakeland, FL 33803, BA 68 Rutger's St Univ - Douglas Coll; MA 69 Univ of FL; Coord, FL Diag & Lrng Resource Syst, **SLP**

Graebner, Mrs Corinne M Anderson 2324 N W 95th, Seattle, WA 98117, (206) 783-8277, BA 68 Univ of WA; MS 73 Univ of HI - Manoa; **SLP**

Graef, Mrs Barbara A 314 Scott Drive, Englewood, OH 45322, (513) 836-2631, BA 71 Univ of Akron; MA 74 Univ of Akron; 78–Sp/Lang Path, Northmont City Schools, **SLP**

Graef, Mrs Felicia Harrington 234 South Edgewood, La Grange, IL 60525, BA 77 Mundelein Coll; MA 83 Northern IL Univ - De Kalb; Sp-Lang Path, Good Samaritan Hosp, **SLP**

Graefe, Mrs Joan W 4717 Webb Canyon Road, Claremont, CA 91711, (714) 623-5251, BS 48 IL St Univ - Normal; MA 70 CA St Univ - Los Angeles; Sp-Lang Path, Pomona USD, **SLP**

Graef-Ferman, Denise B 8710 Lincoln, Huntington Woods, MI 48070, (313) 547-4507, BA 79 MI St Univ; MA 80 Central MI Univ; Aud, **A**

Graf, Mrs Ann Jones 2015 Chuli Nene, Tallahassee, FL 32301, (904) 877-8458, BS 76 FL St Univ; MS 77 FL St Univ; **SLP**

Grafenberg, Janice E R R 2 Box 26, West Union, IA 52175, (319) 637-2206, BS 79 Univ of IA; MA 80 Univ of IA; SLP, Keystone AEA, **SLP**

Graff, Mrs Beverly L 2012 Macao Place, Plano, TX 75075, (214) 964-0559, BS 78 Univ of AZ; MS 80 Southern Methodist Univ; Spec/Admin, Prof Sp & Lang Consult, **SLP**

Graff, Cordelia Dahl 131-B Meadowood Street, Greensboro, NC 27409, (919) 373-7568, OB 82 Auburn Univ - Auburn; OM 84 Auburn Univ - Auburn; Sp-Lang Path, Guilford County/Kendau Ctr, **SLP**

Graff, James L Muskego/Norway Schools, P O Box 900, Muskego, WI 53150, (414) 422-1000, BS 69 Marquette Univ; MS 72 Marquette Univ; Dir/Spec Educ, Muskego/Norway Schs, **SLP**

Graff, Lynn L PO Box 627, Essex, CT 06426, (203) 767-8012, BA 77 OH St Univ; MA 79 Kent St Univ; Sp-Lang Path/Mgr, St of CT, **SLP**

Graff, Mary H P O Box 2344, Kalispell, MT 59903, (406) 755-8810, BA 71 Univ of OK - Norman; MA 72 Univ of OK - Norman; SLP, Private Practice, **SLP**

Graff, Nancy J 1136 Robin Lane, Ogallala, NE 69153, **SLP**

Graff, Sharon D Rd 2 Box 17, Stoneboro, PA 16153, (814) 432-3171, BA 77 Univ of Pittsburgh - Pittsburgh; MA 78 Edinboro Univ of PA; SLP, Polk Center, **SLP**

Graff, Shirlee H 1206 Via Montoya, Camarillo, CA 93010, BS 75 CA St Univ - Hayward; MA 77 4648; SLP, Mt Diablo USD, **SLP**

Graff, Mrs Victoria C 3200 Hobcaw Lane, Lexington, KY 40502, (606) 266-2883, BA 69 Univ of KY; MS 71 Vanderbilt Univ; Aud, Dr Richard Smith ENT, **SLP A**

Graham, Dr A Bruce 3236 Lincoln, Dearborn, MI 48124, (313) 565-4856, BA 40 Univ of Northern CO; MA 49 Univ of Denver; PH 53 (Aud/Sp Path) Northwestern Univ; Retired, **A F LM**

Graham, Mrs Alice D 2900 Dresden Road, Zanesville, OH 43701, (614) 455-3869, BA 79 Denison Univ; MA 80 OH St Univ; 84–Sp-Lang Path, Private Practice, **SLP**

Graham, Barbara Bennett 4335 East English, Wichita, KS 67218, (316) 689-3240, BA 54 Univ of MD - College Park; MA 56 Northwestern Univ; Cl Superv, Wichita St Univ, **SLP**

Graham, Barbara J The Forum, 220 Linden Street, Scranton, PA 18503, (717) 961-4676, BS 72 SUNY - Center at Albany; MS 74 Columbia Univ Teachers Coll; Aud, Scranton St Sch Deaf, **A**

Graham, Mrs Brenda Rader c/o Iris Rader, 126 McClintock Drive, Mc Murray, PA 15317, (412) 831-4587, BS 73 Indiana Univ of PA; MA 79 Marshall Univ; Circus Clown, Ringling Bros Circus Blue Unit, **SLP**

Graham, Carol M 903 Franklin, Houghton, MI 49931, (906) 482-7260, BA 78 MI St Univ; MA 79 Central MI Univ; SLP, Copper Country ISD, **SLP**

Graham, Mrs Caryl A 201 Greenbriar Drive, Greenville, NC 27834, (919) 756-9595, OB 72 Univ of FL; MS 75 East Carolina Univ; **A**

Graham, Mrs Edith Elizabeth 577 Lake Mary Road, Flagstaff, AZ 86001, (602) 289-2452, MS 81 Northern AZ Univ; SLP, Flagstaff Pub Sch, **SLP**

Graham, Fatin A 4140 Seminole, Royal Oak, MI 48072, (313) 261-8040, BA 76 MI St Univ; MA 78 Wayne St Univ - Sch of Med; Aud, Dr L T Glinski, **A**

Graham, Frank Richard, Jr 8831 Shaver Drive, Charlotte, NC 28226, (803) 329-1520, BA 79 Univ of NC - Charlotte; MS 85 Winthrop Coll; 85–Sp-Lang Path, The Speech and Hearing Center, **SLP**

Graham, Geneva Louise 9742 52nd Avenue, College Park, MD 20740, (301) 982-3267, BS 83 Walla Walla Coll; ME 86 Univ of VA - Charlottesville; 87–Sp-Lang Path, UCP Wash DC & No VA, **SLP**

Graham, Gwendolyn Henrietta 218 Red And White Street, Sumter, SC 29150, (803) 778-2666, MA 88 SC St Coll

Graham, Harriet J 710 Rebecca Drive, Boulder Creek, CA 95006, (408) 338-4991, BA 36 San Jose St Univ; **SLP LM**

Graham, Dr J Keith Communicative Disorders & Sci, Wichita State University, Wichita, KS 67208, (316) 689-3240, BS 48 Wayne St Univ; MA 51 Wayne St Univ; PH 64 (Sp-Lang Path) Northwestern Univ; Prof & Chair, Wichita St U, **SLP F**

Graham, Jacqueline 12750 Grand Willow, Grand Ledge, MI 48837, (517) 353-8780, BA 71 MI St Univ; MA 73 MI St Univ; 77–Sp-Lang Path, MI St U Sp & Hrng Cl, **SLP ACE**

Graham, Dr James T 1061 Oxford Road N E, Atlanta, GA 30306, (404) 727-5520, BA 52 Stanford Univ; MA 57 Stanford Univ; PH 60 (Aud) Stanford Univ; Prof, Emory Univ, **A F**

Graham, Mrs Joanne Louise P O Box 356, Brant Rock, MA 02020, (617) 294-8064, BA 82 Rollins Coll; MS 84 Vanderbilt Univ; **SLP**

Graham, Mrs Judith Miller 4199 Long Branch Road, Liverpool, NY 13090, (315) 451-6843, BS 83 SUNY - Coll at Geneseo; MA 85 OH Univ - Athens; 85–Sp-Lang Path, Onondago/Cortland/Madison/BOCES

Graham, KaAnn A R R 2 Box 83, Halstead, KS 67056, (316) 663-2671, BA 76 Wichita St Univ; MA 77 Wichita St Univ; Sp-Lang Path, Early Educ Ctr, **SLP**

Graham, Laura Gates 4714 Whispering Rock, Spring, TX 77388, (713) 583-2175, BS 81 Stephen F Austin St Univ; MA 87 Univ of Houston - Univ Park; 87–Sp-Lang Path, Spring ISD, **SLP**

Graham, Mrs Laurie I 1606 Honfleur Dr, Sunnyvale, CA 94087, (408) 739-6265, BS 75 Univ of TX - Austin; MS 77 Southern Methodist Univ; **SLP**

Graham, Linda Ruth 1809 Cleveland, Conway, AR 72032, (501) 329-6851, BS 75 Univ of Central AR; MS 85 Univ of Central AR; **SLP**

Graham, Lisa Fletcher 6349 North 78th Street, Apartment 134, Scottsdale, AZ 85253, (602) 965-6796, BA 81 Stanford Univ; MS 83 AZ St Univ; 88–Proj Asst, Arizona State Univ, **SLP**

Graham, Dr Louella W 1061 Oxford Road N E, Atlanta, GA 30306, (404) 377-6984, BS 62 Minot St Univ; MS 65 Purdue Univ - West Lafayette; PH 69 (Aud) Purdue Univ - West Lafayette; Consultant, Georgia Dept Human Resources, **A**

Graham, Margaret S 41 Wilton Crest, Wilton, CT 06897, (203) 762-1358, MS; **SLP LM**

Graham, Marguerite 4122-A Cove Lane, Glenview, IL 60025, (312) 835-2238, BA 75 Mundelein Coll; MS 76 Marquette Univ; Sp-Lang Path, Nn Sub Spec Ed Dist, **SLP**

Graham, Mrs Marian Vargo 4329 West 145th Street, Cleveland, OH 44135, (216) 251-5036, **SLP**

Graham, Marjorie K Rural Delivery 6, Auburn, NY 13021, **SLP**

Graham, Mrs Marsha G 1204 Major Drive, Jefferson City, MO 65101, (314) 635-4939, BS 68 Univ of MO - Columbia; MA 69 Univ of MO - Columbia; 88–Sp-Lang Path, Jefferson Cty Lrng Ctr, **SLP**

Graham, Melinda A 334 South Franklin Street, Wilkes-Barre, PA 18702, (717) 824-9742, BS 63 Bloomsburg Univ of PA; OM 71 Bloomsburg Univ of PA; MS 67 Temple Univ-Tyler Sch of Art; Consult, Wilkes-Barre Sp-Lang Cl, **SLP**

Graham, Mrs Minnie S 3926 Clay Street, San Francisco, CA 94118, (415) 469-1001, BA 77 Univ of Central FL; MA 78 Univ of Central FL; Lecturer/Cl Superv, San Francisco State University, **SLP**

Graham, Mrs Nancy Dunn 22 Joseph Maurone Drive, Atco, NJ 08004, (609) 767-0997, BS 76 WV Univ; MS 77 WV Univ; 88–Lrng Disabl Tchr Consult, Lower Camden County Reg HS Dist, **SLP ACE**

Graham, Paula Patterson 1133 West Brockett Street, Sherman, TX 75090, (214) 893-7457, BA 59 Univ of North TX; MA 81 TX Woman's Univ; 80–Sp-Lang Path, Grayson Co Ctr, **SLP**

Graham, Mrs Sandra Jean 919 River Rapids Avenue, Brandon, FL 33511, (813) 272-4147, BS 71 Auburn Univ - Auburn; MS 85 Univ of South FL; SLP, Hillsborough Co Sch Sys, **SLP**

Graham, Sandra Kay 114 Arbor Drive, Duluth, GA 30136, (404) 945-7272, BS 84 Univ of GA; ME 85 Univ of GA; 88–Sp-Lang Path, Gwinnett County PS, **SLP**

Graham, Sharon S 8 Racquet Court, Little Rock, AR 72207, (501) 227-5050, BA 67 Southern Methodist Univ; MA 69 Southern Methodist Univ; Dir of Res & Dev, The Ear-Nose-Throat Cl, Pa, **A**

Graham, Susan C M 47 Eastwood Drive, Medford, OR 97501, (503) 773-6281, BS 74 Purdue Univ - West Lafayette; MS 75 Purdue Univ - West Lafayette; 82–Sp-Lang Path, Rogue Valley Med Cen, **SLP**

Graham, Mrs Theoni Savvas 203 Graham Drive, Newport News, VA 23606, (804) 930-0806, MS Radford Univ; 87–Aud, Kelsey-Sebold, **A**

Graham, Dr Victoria S 22 Harper Street, Stamford, NY 12167, (607) 652-3482, ME 76 SUNY - Coll at Oneonta; MS 81 Coll of Saint Rose; PH 84 (Health & Human Serv); 85–Dir, Victoria Graham Assoc, **SLP ACE**

Graham-Hartung, Mrs Jacqueline Ann 230 Foulkrod Boulevard, King of Prussia, PA 19406, (215) 233-9550, BS 78 Marywood Coll; MA 81 Trenton St Coll; 83–Sp-Lang Path, Montgomery Co Intermed Ut #23, **SLP**

Grahamjones, Frances 727 Webster Street, San Francisco, CA 94117, (415) 752-4888, BA 71 Univ of NC - Greensboro; MS 75 Emerson Coll; Sp-Lang Path, San Francisco Easter Seal Soc, **SLP**

Graham-Pool, Leslee Georgia Retardation Center, 4770 North Peachtree Road, Atlanta, GA 30338, (404) 393-7089, BS 75 Univ of VA - Charlottesville; MS 76 Vanderbilt Univ; Aud Dir, GA Retardation Cen, **A**

Grainer, Mrs Kathleen Shpiece 44849 North Hills Drive, Bldg K #154, Northville, MI 48167, (313) 242-7214, BA 80 Wayne St Univ; MA 83 Eastern MI Univ; Sp-Lang Path, Mercy Memorial Hosp, **SLP**

Gral, Elizabeth J 207 Conner Drive, Apartment 3, Chapel Hill, NC 27514, (919) 942-6931, BS 83 Marquette Univ; MS 85 Marquette Univ; **SLP**

Grall, Mrs Mary Bleser P O Box 156, Whitelaw, WI 54247, (414) 459-3661, BS 76 Univ of WI - Stevens Point; MS 78 Univ of WI - Stevens Point; Sp-Lang Path, Sheboygan Pub Schs, **SLP**

Graller, Mrs Lois C 211 Park Avenue, Glencoe, IL 60022, (312) 835-1247, BA 59 IN Univ - Bloomington; Sp-Lang Path, Highland Park Hosp, **SLP**

Gralow, Mrs Sheila M 1494 Siver Road, Guilderland, NY 12084, BS 69 North Adams St Coll; MA 71 Coll of Saint Rose; **SLP**

Gram, Louis E 927 Wheless, Kerrville, TX 78028-3318, (512) 257-2209, BS 79 Southwest TX St Univ; ME 80 Southwest TX St Univ; Sp-Lang Path, Cluster Vii Spec Ed Coop, **SLP**

Gram, Mrs Margaret R R 3 Box 2 Indian Trail, Exeter, NH 03833, BS 72 Kent St Univ; MA 73 Kent St Univ; Co-Administrator, Hamrock & Gram Rehab Cen, **SLP**

Grames, Lynn Marty 1105 Paddock Drive, Florissant, MO 63033, (314) 454-6213, BS 79 Southern IL Univ-Edwardsvill; MA 81 Saint Louis Univ; 86–Sp-Lang Path, IWJ Rehab Inst/Washington Univ, **SLP**

Gramigna, Gary David 85 Arlington Street #2, Watertown, MA 02172, (617) 275-7500, BS 83 Indiana Univ of PA; MS 86 Univ of AZ; 86–Sp-Lang Path, Bedford VA Hosp, **SLP**

Gramling, Susan M S 2430 North Grant Boulevard, Milwaukee, WI 53210, (414) 272-1771, BS 68 Marquette Univ; MS 79 Univ of WI - Milwaukee; 87–Exec Dir, Milwaukee Hearing Society, **SLP**

Gramolini, Mrs Christine Ann 2 Mara Lane, North Smithfield, RI 02895, (401) 739-2700, BA 80 Univ of RI; MS 85 Worcester St Coll; 86–Sp-Lang Path, Bellingham Sch Dept, **SLP**

Granberg, Paula L 21 Sylvan Avenue, West Newton, MA 02165, **SLP**

Grande, Mrs Anne Pinkerton 4136 Highfield Road, Royal Oak, MI 48072, (313) 967-0483, BS 69 Wayne St Univ; ME 74 Wayne St Univ; SLP, Oak Park Sch Dis, **SLP**

Grande, Barbara Sue 5009 North Lake Drive, Milwaukee, WI 53217, (414) 477-2208, BS 60 IN Univ - Bloomington; MS 84 Univ of WI - Milwaukee; Sp-Lang Path, St Josephs Hospital, **SLP**

Grandis, Mrs Joan Eisenson 205 West End Avenue, New York, NY 10023, BA 53 CUNY - Hunter Coll; MA 55 CUNY - Hunter Coll; 84–Consult, New York City Bd of Educ, **SLP**

Grandstaff, Harvey L Speech Clinic, Miami University, Oxford, OH 45056, PH; **SLP**

Grandy, Mrs Victoria V 2023 North 103rd Street, Omaha, NE 68134, (712) 323-3703, BA 67 Marygove Coll; MS 68 Minot St Univ; Elementary School Principal, St Albert School System, **SLP**

Graner, Darlene Hines VA Hospital, Speech Pathology, Route 126, Hines, IL 60141, (312) 343-7200, BS 73 Saint Cloud St Univ; MA 75 Northern IL Univ - De Kalb; Sp-Lang Path, Hines VA Hosp, **SLP**

Graney, Colleen Marie 51 Oregon Trail, Bethel Park, PA 15102, (412) 745-8000, BS 84 CA Univ of PA; MS 85 CA Univ of PA; **SLP**

Granfield, Gretchen Lynn 2261-B Washington Street, Newton Lower Falls, MA 02162, (617) 791-3147, MS 84 Boston Univ; Sp-Lang Path, Heywood Valley Rehab Facility, **SLP**

Granger, Mrs Diana Osik 30 Erie Avenue, Worcester, MA 01605-1608, (617) 365-4531, BS 84 Worcester St Coll; 87–Sp-Lang Path, Clinton Hosp

Granger, Mrs Eileen R 200 Whitethorn Drive, Guilford, CT 06437, (203) 453-6245, BA 62 Marygove Coll; MA 64 Saint Louis Univ; Sp-Lang Path, Guilford Public Schools, **SLP**

Granger, Joyce Deany 843 Dora Place, Bel Air, MD 21014, (301) 893-0386, BS 76 Southern IL Univ -Carbondale; MA 79 Univ of TN - ,Knoxville; 87–Sp-Lang Path, Med Personnel Pool, **SLP**

Granger, Kathleen Theresa 677 Oakdale Avenue, Pottstown, PA 19464, (304) 872-5595, BS 85 Bloomsburg Univ of PA; MS 86 Bloomsburg Univ of PA; **SLP**

Granger, Mardell Moeller 205 Ridge Drive, Chester, IL 62233, (618) 826-2152, BS 85 Southern IL Univ -Carbondale; MS 88 Southern IL Univ -Carbondale; 88–Sp-Lang Path, Chester Mental Health Ctr St of IL

Granger, Misty Leann 1830 West Arrow Route #60, Upland, CA 91786, (213) 337-1820, MS 87 Univ of OK Medical Center; **SLP**

Granitz, Dr David W 5555 Clinton, Beaumont, TX 77706, (409) 892-3616, BS 57 East Carolina Univ; MA 58 OH St Univ; PH 71 (Aud) LA St Univ - Baton Rouge; 70–Owner/Aud, David W Granitz PhD & Assoc Inc, **SLP A**

Granof, Dr Dena H 3605 Arrowhead Drive, Austin, TX 78731, (512) 346-9988, BA 71 Case Western Reserve Univ; MS 72 Univ of MI - Ann Arbor; PH 82 (Communication Disorders) Univ of TX - Austin; Co-Dir, Sp/Lang/Hrng Serv, **SLP**

Granoff, Mrs Rosaline I 243 Hampton Road, Sharon, MA 02067, BS 76 Univ of MA - Amherst; MA 78 NY Univ; Sp-Lang Path, Charmss Collaboratiave, **SLP**

Granson, Marian Kaplan 390 1st Avenue, New York, NY 10010, (212) 561-3564, BS 62 PA St Univ - Univ Park; MA 64 CUNY - Hunter Coll; Aud, Bellevue Hosp Cen, **A**

Grant, Andrea Elaine 657 East Tulare Avenue #D, Visalia, CA 93277, (209) 733-1927, BA 84 Univ of CA - Santa Barbara; MA 86 CA St Univ - Fresno; Sp-Lang Path, Shurson Hearing & Speech Ctr, **SLP**

Grant, Ann M P O Box 2641, Auburn, AL 36831, (205) 826-1287, BS 85 Auburn Univ - Auburn; MS 86 Auburn Univ - Auburn; 86–Sp-Lang Path, Opelika City Schs, **SLP**

Grant, Catherine Shirley 1707 Chimney Vine, Kingwood, TX 77339, (713) 359-7941, MA 86 Univ of Houston - Univ Park

Grant, Cathryn B 12 Ridge Drive, Rome, GA 30161, (404) 235-4411, BS 75 Univ of GA; MA 77 Memphis St Univ; Aud, Hamilton S Dixon MD, **A**

Grant, David Alan 209 Marilyn Avenue, North Syracuse, NY 13212, (315) 457-4024, BS 78 SUNY - Coll at Geneseo; MS 84 Syracuse Univ; 78–Sp-Lang Path, Syracuse City Sch Dist, **SLP**

Grant, Mrs Deborah Lee 827 Kolding Avenue, Solvang, CA 93463, (805) 688-5936, BA 72 CA St Univ - Long Beach; MA 75 CA St Univ - Long Beach; 87–Sp-Lang Path, Cross Sp & Hearing Ctr, **SLP**

Grant, Dr Dorothy E 2201 Archer Trail, Denton, TX 76201, (817) 387-6160, ME 65 Univ of AZ; MS 64 Univ of MI - Ann Arbor; PH 80 (Aud) Univ of MI - Ann Arbor; Asst Prof, TX Woman's U, **SLP A ACE**

Grant, Evelyn Bergh 6515 Halsey, Shawnee, KS 66216, (816) 276-4023, OB 83 Univ of MO - Columbia; MA 85 Univ of IA; Sp-Lang Path, Research Med Ctr, **SLP**

Grant, Felene F 2298 Rose Avenue #104, Signal Hill, CA 90806, (213) 408-2744, BA 77 CA St Univ - Northridge; MA 79 CA St Univ - Northridge; Sp-Lang Path, Private Practice, **SLP**

Grant, G Maura Mason Clinic, Speech Pathology, 100 9th Avenue P O Box 900, Seattle, WA 98111, (206) 223-6618, BA 80 Univ of WA; OM 81 Univ of WA; Sp-Lang Path, The Mason Cl, **SLP**

Grant, Mrs Janet Minner 94 Macon Avenue, Asheville, NC 28801, (704) 254-5518, BS 75 Northern IL Univ - De Kalb; MA 77 Memphis St Univ; Cl Salesperson, Monitor Inc, **A**

Grant, Joan 1919 West 70th Terrace, Shawnee Mission, KS 66208, (913) 621-5155, BA 54 Temple Univ; MA 58 Temple Univ; Coordinator Speech & Hearing, Wyandotte Special Ed Coop, **SLP**

Grant, Dr June Myers 105 Ivy Lane, San Antonio, TX 78209, (512) 736-7501, BS 41 Saint Louis Univ; ME 69 Trinity Univ; PH 75 (NS) Univ of TX - Austin; Prof, Dir Spec Ed, Trinity U

Grant, Karen Eileen 633 Twin River Drive, Forked River, NJ 08731, (412) 283-1010, BS 82 Indiana Univ of PA; MS 83 WV Univ; Super, Butler Co Er Sl So, **SLP**

Grant, Kenneth Wayne MIT Bldg 36-730, Cambridge, MA 02139, (617) 522-4129, BA 76 Washington Univ; MS 80 Univ of WA; PH 86 (NS) Washington Univ

Grant, Lauren 1717 East 18th Street, Brooklyn, NY 11229, BA 66 CUNY - Brooklyn Coll; MS 67 Univ of WI - Madison; Sp-Lang Path, NYC Bd of Ed/Spec Serv Ut, **SLP**

Grant, Dr Leslie Edwina 4303 Mainfield Avenue, Baltimore, MD 21214, (301) 444-5543, BS 72 Boston Univ; OM 78 Univ of WA; DD 86 (Dentistry) Univ of MD - Baltimore CO; 88–Gen Dentist, Wall Street Dental, **SLP**

Grant, Leslie M 398 Cottonwood Court, Fairborn, OH 45324, (523) 878-6646, MS; **SLP**

Grant, Mrs Margie Baucom 3728 Ludgate Drive, Chesapeake, VA 23321, (804) 483-2501, BS 72 East Carolina Univ; MA 78 Old Dominion Univ; Sp-Lang Path, Portsmouth Pub Sch, **SLP**

Grant, Martha Zadrozny 88 Ridgewood Lane, Kensington, CT 06037, (203) 289-7411, BS 76 Marquette Univ; MS 77 Marquette Univ; SLP, E Hartford Bd of Ed, **SLP**

Grant, Mary Thea P O Box 667, Morehouse, MO 63868, (314) 471-0077, BS 82 Southeast MO St Univ; MA 84 Southeast MO St Univ; Sp-Lang Path, New Madrid R-1 Sch Dist, **SLP**

Grant, Mel 3540 Forest Hill Boulevard, Suite 205, West Palm Beach, FL 33406, (407) 969-2001, BS 73 Ithaca Coll; MA 75 Univ of FL; 86–Dir, Aud & Sp/P Inc, **A**

Grant, Michelle L 3688 Sandralin, Cincinnati, OH 45247, (513) 741-3742, BA 78 Univ of KY; MS 80 Purdue Univ - West Lafayette; Audiologist, Hamilton-Fairfield ENT Spec, **A**

Grant, Monica G P O Box 3836, Champaign, IL 61821, (217) 442-8000, BA 77 Univ of the Pacific; MA 80 Univ of IL - Urbana; Aud, VA, **A**

Grant, Naomi M 710 S E Henry Street, Portland, OR 97216, PH (NS); **SLP LM**

Grant, Patricia Jude 555 West Street, Louisville, CO 80027, (303) 441-0437, BA 80 Univ of CA - Santa Barbara; MA 82 Univ of CO - Boulder; Sp-Lang Path, Boulder Mem Hosp, **SLP**

Grant, Mrs Saundra Bone 4583 Jones Road, Macon, GA 31206, (912) 784-9304, BS 84 Univ of GA; ME 85 Univ of GA; SLP, Houston Cty Bd of Education, **SLP**

Grant, Dr Susan R 9233 Dolfield, Owings Mills, MD 21117, (301) 363-3954, BA 70 CO Coll; MS 73 Purdue Univ - West Lafayette; PH 84 (NS) Univ of MD - College Park; Neurolinguist, Private Practice, **SLP**

Grant, Susan V 4139 Greenbush Avenue, Sherman Oaks, CA 91423, (818) 343-8733, SLP, Los Angeles USD, **SLP**

Grant, Mrs Theresa Terry 325 East 8th Street #2, Davis, CA 95616, (916) 757-2143, BS 76 ID St Univ; MS 78 ID St Univ; Consult, Prentke Romich Co, **SLP A ACE**

Grant, Wanda Joyce 10206 Prince Place #T2, Largo, MD 20772, (301) 345-6150, BS 75 Northeastern Univ; ME 78 Northeastern Univ; Sp-Lang Path, Pr Georges Co Pub Sch, **SLP**

Grant, Mrs Wendy Levin 931 Patrick Drive, West Palm Beach, FL 33406, (305) 686-3426, MA 75 Univ of FL; BS 74 Univ of VT; Sp/Lang Path, Private Practice, **SLP**

Grantham, Mrs Charlotte L 200 Amherstdale Road, Snyder, NY 14226, (716) 831-3395, BA 54 Emerson Coll; ME 65 Boston Univ; Cl Asst Prof, SUNY-Buffalo, **A**

Grantham, Leslie Alison 6811 Old Canton Road #2404, Ridgeland, MS 39157, (601) 982-2911, BS 86 Univ Southern MS-Hattiesburg; MS 87 Univ Southern MS-Hattiesburg; **SLP**

Grantham, Mary Linda 200-37 Rollins Drive, Greenville, NC 27834, (919) 355-6349, BS 85 East Carolina Univ; MS 86 East Carolina Univ; 87–Sp-Lang Path, Caswell Center, **SLP**

Grantham, Mrs Regina B 244 Argonne Drive, Kenmore, NY 14217, (716) 878-7371, BS 62 PA St Univ - Univ Park; ME 65 PA St Univ - Univ Park; 67–Assoc Dir, Children's Hosp of Buffalo, **SLP ACE**

Granum, Arline S 635 Wayland Avenue, Kenilworth, IL 60043, (312) 251-7653, BS 42 Univ of WI - Madison; MA 70 Northwestern Univ; Sp-Lang Path, Private Practice, **SLP LM**

Granzo, Mrs Cheryl Marie 6549 Whites Bridge Road, Belding, MI 48809, (517) 831-5261, MA 84 MI St Univ; SLP, Montcalm Independent Sch Dist, **SLP**

Grasberger, Jan E 1465 Granger Avenue, Escondido, CA 92027, (619) 747-7217, BA 78 CA St Univ - Chico; MA 81 CA St Univ - Chico; Sp/Lang Path, San Diego City Schs, **SLP**

Grasel, Theresa C 1904 South Johnson, Mount Pleasant, MI 48858-4407, (313) 327-6141, BA 81 MI St Univ; MA 83 Eastern MI Univ; Sp-Lang Path, Bullock Creek Public Schools, **SLP**

Graser, Mrs Ann Derthick 23 Kennedy Boulevard, Elkton, MD 21921, (301) 398-8229, BA 69 Univ of Puget Sound; ME 71 Western OR St Coll; **SLP**

Graser, Nan Stutzman 1953 Charter Point Drive, Arlington Heights, IL 60004, (312) 298-2608, BA 84 Augustana Coll; MA 86 Northwestern Univ; Sp-Lang Path, Community Consolidated Sch Dist 15, **SLP**

Grasha, Mrs Carol H 1323 Parkridge Place, Cincinnati, OH 45208, (513) 389-5150, BA 64 Carlow Coll; MA 65 Western MI Univ; Sp-Lang Path, St Francis St George Hosp, **SLP**

Grass, Catherine 50 Woodland Drive, South Weymouth, MA 02190, (617) 871-0430, BS 69 Univ of MN - Minneap-St Paul; ME 73 Northeastern Univ; Sp-Lang Path, Abington Public Schools, **SLP**

Grass, Mrs Dorcas E Route 1 Box 1789, St Genevieve, MO 63670, (314) 883-3762, BS 77 Fontbonne Coll; MA 79 Saint Louis Univ; Supervisor Sp-Lang Path, St John's Mercy Med Cen, **SLP**

Grassi, Mrs Susan Marie 38 Burgoyne Road, Saratoga Springs, NY 12866, (518) 793-7721, **SLP**

Grassman, Mrs Joan C 11335 Woodridge Forest, San Antonio, TX 78249, (512) 699-0502, BS 65 Marquette Univ; MS 67 Marquette Univ; **SLP ACE**

Grasso, Susan G 141 Brace Road, West Hartford, CT 06107, **SLP**

Grater, Mrs Melissa J 4617 Sullivan Road, Knoxville, TN 37921, (615) 482-4081, BS 82 Univ of GA; MA 83 Univ of TN - Knoxville; Sp-Lang Path, Daniel Arthur Rehabilitatn Ctr, **SLP**

Grater, Mrs Ruth D 910 West Clark Street, Champaign, IL 61821, (217) 352-9245, BA 70 SUNY - Center at Buffalo; MA 71 NY Univ; **SLP**

Gratto, MaryEthel 1409 Morning Glory Drive, Petaluma, CA 94952, (707) 765-2714, BA 75 CA St Univ - Chico; MA 84 CA St Univ - Chico; 86–Sp-Lang Path, Rincon Valley Union Sch Dist, **SLP**

Gratton, Deborah Rural Free Delivery 2, 16 Holton Circle, Londonderry, NH 03053, **SLP**

Gratton, Michael Anne Hearing Research Lab, 215 Parker SUNY-Buffalo, Buffalo, NY 14260, (716) 831-2001, BS 74 Univ of WI - Milwaukee; MA 76 Univ of Denver; PH 88 (Hrng Science) SUNY - Coll at Buffalo; 88–Research Assoc, SUNY of Buffalo, **A**

Gratzer, Mrs Susan H 114 Croydon Road, Rochester, NY 14610, (716) 352-2400, BS 75 Niagara Univ; MS 85 Nazareth Coll; SLP, BOCES No 2, **SLP**

Grau, Arthur M 10803 Henley Court, Columbia, MD 21044, **SLP**

Grau, Gregory L 4935 King Arthur, Erie, PA 16506, (814) 455-EARS, BS 72 Edinboro Univ of PA; ME 74 Bloomsburg Univ of PA; Aud, Private Practice, **A**

Graunke, Dr W Lloyd 1008 Grace Drive, Johnson City, TN 37604, (615) 282-3247, BA 40 North Central Coll; MA 42 Gallaudet Coll; PH 59 (NS) Northwestern Univ; **A F LM**

Gravani, Eileen H 203 Salem Drive, Ithaca, NY 14850, (607) 753-4204, BS 74 Loyola Univ of Chicago; MA 76 Northwestern Univ; Assistant Professor, SUNY-Cortland, **SLP**

Grave, Mrs Jeanette E Page Box 175, Ottsville, PA 18942, (215) 847-2214, BA 64 Temple Univ; MA 66 Temple Univ; Aud, Private Practice, **A**

Gravel, Jane S 1804 N W 7th Avenue, Gainesville, FL 32603, (904) 371-6887, BA 69 Univ of FL; MA 81 Univ of FL; Sp-Lang Path, J Hillis Miller Hlth Ctr, **SLP**

Gravel, Dr Judith S 128 Orchard Drive, New Canaan, CT 06840, (212) 430-3718, BA 70 Univ of MA - Amherst; MA 71 Univ of MA - Amherst; PH 85 (NS) Vanderbilt Univ; Audiologist, Albert Einstein Col Medicine, **A**

Gravell, Alan W 93 Welfare Avenue, Cranston, RI 02910, (401) 231-6608, BA 72 Providence Coll; MS 76 Univ of RI; Sp-Lang Path, Smithfield Pub Sch, **SLP**

Graver, Constance Marie 335 Barrington Street, Rochester, NY 14607, (716) 244-3445, BA 83 Univ of Rochester; MA 86 Univ of IA; **SLP**

Graves, Elaine E #3 Quail's Nest Court, Defiance, MO 63341, (314) 828-5300, BS 74 6825; MA 75 Univ of MO - Columbia; Sp/Lang Path, Francis Howell Sch Dist, **SLP**

Graves, Mrs Karen B 612 Smithfield Street, Mingo Junction, OH 43938, (614) 283-3674, BS 80 Purdue Univ - West Lafayette; MS 82 Purdue Univ - West Lafayette; Aud, Eastern Oh Sp/Hrng Cen, **A**

Graves, Laurel Nelson Rt 4 Box 117, Northport, AL 35476, (205) 758-2276, BS 79 Purdue Univ - West Lafayette; MS 80 Univ of AL- Tuscaloosa; Sp-Lang Path, Tuscaloosa Co Bd of Educ, **SLP**

Graves, Laury Sanor 1760 Avenida del Mundo #1009, Coronado, CA 92118, (619) 437-1499, BA 76 Univ of Southern CA; MA 78 Whittier Coll; Sp-Lang Path, **SLP**

Graves, Mrs Linda Dawn P 8726 Gopher Lane, Orlando, FL 32825, (305) 293-6252, BS 79 Lambuth Coll; MA 81 Memphis St Univ; SLP, Orange County Schools, **SLP**

Graves, Lynn Leonelli 315 Hemlock, Columbus, MS 39704, (601) 329-4639, BS 84 MS Univ for Women; MS 85 Univ Southern MS-Hattiesburg; Sp-Lang Path, Dyna-Mark Inc, **SLP**

Graves, Martha Taylor 1704 14th, Brownwood, TX 76801, (915) 646-2502, OB 71 Midwestern St Univ; MA 73 Univ of OK - Norman; Asst Prof of SLP, Howard Payne Univ, **SLP**

Graves, Mrs Patricia Lynn 823 East Portland Avenue, Fresno, CA 93710-2133, (209) 627-2882, BA 74 Univ of MN - Minneap-St Paul; MS 78 Saint Cloud St Univ

Graves, Risa Hershman 213 South Third Street, Lompoc, CA 93436, (805) 733-3511, BA 73 Univ of CA - Santa Barbara; MA 75 CA St Univ - Northridge; SLP, Lompoc USD, **SLP**

Graves, Mrs Sharon R 17421 Coronado Lane, Huntington Beach, CA 92647, (714) 581-2800, BS 60 Univ of CA - Los Angeles; MA 80 CA St Univ - Long Beach; Sp/Lang Path, Newport Lang Speech & Aud Ctr, **SLP**

Graves-Rivera, Dr Silvia A P O Box 2221, Orangeburg, SC 29116, (803) 536-8592, BS 72 SC St Coll; MA 73 Ball St Univ; PH 83 (NS) MI St Univ; Assistant Professor Director, South Carolina State Univ, **SLP**

Graville, Mrs Donna Jensen 7600 S W Oleson Road #23, Portland, OR 97223-7463, (503) 245-5623, MS 88 Portland St Univ

Gravino, Mrs Amy W 605 St Charles Court, Charleston, SC 29407, (803) 766-9758, BS 82 Western MI Univ; MA 83 Western MI Univ; **SLP**

Gravkin, Karen Jean 692 Wall Street, Salt Lake City, UT 84103, (801) 566-1291, BS 81 Univ of UT; MS 84 Univ of NV - Reno; **SLP**

Gravley, Patricia M 3612 South Elm-Eugene St, Greensboro, NC 27406, (919) 854-0705, BA 80 Univ of TN - Knoxville; MA 82 Univ of TN - Knoxville; Sp-Lang Path, Carolina Hearing & Sp Svcs Inc, **SLP**

Gravois, Mrs Jean Breaux 10516 Trenton Street, River Ridge, LA 70123, (504) 737-3461, BS 77 Saint Mary's Dominican Coll; MS 78 LA St Univ - N O Medical Ctr; 87–Sp-Lang Path, Patty Glaser & Associates, **SLP**

Gray, Alice Roll 5197 Willowbrook Road, Clarence, NY 14031, (716) 741-3832, MA 86 SUNY - Center at Buffalo; **SLP**

Gray, Ann D 8 Hardwood Hill Road, Pittsford, NY 14534, BS 73 Nazareth Coll of Rochester; MS 74 SUNY - Coll at Geneseo; 88–Instr, Nazareth Coll of Rochester, **SLP**

Gray, Mrs Ann Y 310 North 2nd, Ashdown, AR 71822-2704, (501) 747-3383, OB 72 Univ of AR - Fayetteville; MA 73 Univ of AR - Fayetteville; SLP, Clarendon-Holly Grove Pub Sch, **SLP**

Gray, Barbara Johnson 907 West Cornell, Palatine, IL 60067, (312) 991-2600, BA 80 Valparaiso Univ; MA 81 Northern IL Univ - De Kalb; Sp-Lang Path, Township High School Dist 211, **SLP**

Gray, Barbara M 60 Baltimore Road, Winnipeg, MB, Canada R3L 1G9, (204) 786-7841, BA 76; MA 78 Univ of ND; SLP, Child Guid Cl, **SLP**

Gray, Mrs Beverly K 967 Erica Drive, Sunnyvale, CA 94086, (408) 299-5617, BS 81 Northwestern Univ; MA 83 Northwestern Univ; 85–SLP, Valley Med Cen, **SLP**

Gray, Dr Burl B 1557 Michael Lane, Pacific Palisades, CA 90272, (213) 645-5400, BS 60 Southern IL Univ -Carbondale; MS 61 Southern IL Univ -Carbondale; PH 63 (Sp Path) Southern IL Univ -Carbondale; Sp-Lang Path, Aeroterra, **SLP F**

Gray, Mrs Carol Aimee 837 Princeton Court, Woodland, CA 95695, (707) 425-6855, **SLP**

Gray, Carol Jeanne 5930 Rancho Mission Road, Apartment 102, San Diego, CA 92108, (619) 281-4979, MA 84 Eastern MI Univ

Gray, Mrs Daria Sovyrda 2201 S W Marigold Street, Portland, OR 97219, (503) 229-7239, BS 78 SUNY - Coll at Geneseo; MS 81 Coll of Saint Rose; Sp-Lang Path, Good Samaritan Hosp & Med Cen, **SLP**

Gray, Davon 11917 Knippwood, Houston, TX 77024, (713) 629-8760, BS 70 Univ of TX - Austin; MA 72 Univ of Houston - Univ Park; **SLP**

Gray, Diane W RFD 1 Box 4029, Solon, ME 04979, (207) 635-2727, BS 71 Kent St Univ; MA 87 Univ of MA - Amherst; Sp-Lang Path, Waterville Ps, **SLP**

Gray, Mrs Donna Jean 828 South 100 West, Orem, UT 84058, (801) 225-4733, OM 85 Brigham Young Univ; **SLP**

Gray, Dorothy Davis 2604 South Lane, Birmingham, AL 35223, (205) 687-2550, BA 83 Univ of AL- Tuscaloosa; MA 84 Northwestern Univ; 86–Sp-Lang Path, Spain Rehabilitation Ctr, **SLP**

Gray, Mrs Eliz Gay 13011 Boheme, Houston, TX 77079, (713) 468-5889, BA 70 Southern Methodist Univ; MA 71 Our Lady Lake Univ-San Anton; **SLP**

Gray, Elizabeth Anne P O Box 3257, St Petersburg, FL 33731, (813) 576-2138, BA 75 Bellarmine Coll; MS 83 Univ of Louisville; Sp-Lang Path, Mediplex-Rehab, **SLP ACE**

Gray, Dr Eugene T 4525 Cove Circle #1106, Madeira Beach, FL 33708, (813) 393-9204, BA 50 Union Coll; MA 51 WV Univ; PH 63 (NS) Univ of OK - Norman; 86–Neuropsychiatric Specialties, Private Practice, **SLP**

Gray, Eulalia Rebecca 1203 Reid, Houston, TX 77022, (713) 449-1011, BS 74 Univ of Houston - Univ Park; MA 83 Univ of Houston - Univ Park; 83–Sp-Lang Path, Aldine ISD, **SLP**

Gray, Jennifer L 3549 N E 95th, Seattle, WA 98115, (206) 322-0011, BS 76 Univ of WA; OM 79 Univ of WA; 87–Aud, Pacific Hrng & Sp Svcs, **A**

Gray, Joanne M Route 5 Box 389, Dickson, TN 37055, (615) 896-2300, BS 67 Purdue Univ - West Lafayette; MS 69 Purdue Univ - West Lafayette; Dir, Natl Hlth Corp LP, **SLP**

Gray, Judith M 3308 Prince William Drive, Fairfax, VA 22031, (703) 941-8144, BS 64; MA 67 Case Western Reserve Univ; Hrng/Lang Delay Spec, Fairfax Co Pub Sch, **SLP**

Gray, Mrs Karen C 531 Crestview Road, Kalispell, MT 59901, (406) 752-5300, BA 75 MI St Univ; MA 77 MI St Univ; Sp-Lang Path, Flathead Co Rural Spec Ed Coop, **SLP**

Gray, Karen Rhea 113 W 11th Avenue, Juniata, Altoona, PA 16601, (814) 944-3031, BS 78 Juniata Coll; MS 86 Bloomsburg Univ of PA; 88–Aud, Ramesh K Agarwal MD, **A**

Gray, Katherine A 12152 Allan Drive, Omaha, NE 68137, (402) 895-1062, BS 75 Univ of NE - Omaha; MS 81 Univ of NE - Omaha; Sp-Lang Path, Millard Public Schools, **SLP**

Gray, Mrs Kathryn O 5901 Bellaire, Wichita, KS 67218, (316) 684-3017, BA 71 Wichita St Univ; MA 73 Wichita St Univ; **SLP**

Gray, Mrs Kelley Beth Route 2 #2271, Hillsboro Road, Farmington, MO 63640, (314) 431-3076, MA 85 Wichita St Univ; Sp-Lang Path, St School Severely Hndcpd Chil, **SLP**

Gray, Mrs Lillian W 316 Russett Road, Chestnut Hill, MA 02167, (617) 720-6654, BA 67 William Paterson Coll; MS 70 Emerson Coll; Asst Admin, Spaulding Rehab Hosp, **SLP**

Gray, Mrs Louise K 3316 South 21st, Abilene, TX 79605, (915) 695-2523, BS 71 East TX St Univ - Commerce; MA 75 OH Univ - Athens; Sp-Lang Path, Abilene ISD, **SLP**

Gray, Mrs Margaret H 11606 Primwood Drive, Houston, TX 77070, (701) 376-6090, BA 65 Univ Southern MS-Hattiesburg; MS 66 Univ Southern MS-Hattiesburg; Sp-Lang Path, Cy-Fair ISD, **SLP**

Gray, Mrs Marjorie A 716 Orchard Court, Chambersburg, PA 17201, (319) 359-1371, BS 74 PA St Univ - Univ Park; MS 75 PA St Univ - Univ Park; Sp-Lang Path, Washington Co Brd of Ed, **SLP**

Gray, Marnetta J 33-38 166th Street, Flushing, NY 11358, MS; **SLP LM**

Gray, Mrs Mary Ann D Audiology Associates, Manhattan Medical Center, 1133 College Avenue, Manhattan, KS 66502, (913) 539-7361, BA 66 Univ of Northern IA; MA 67 Univ of Northern IA; Sp-Lang Path, Audiology Associates, **SLP**

Gray, Mary S 3776 Belleau Wood Drive, Lexington, KY 40503, (606) 233-4511, BA 74 Coll of Notre Dame of MD; MS 76 Loyola Coll; Sp-Lang Path, VA Med Cen, **SLP ACE**

Gray, Marybeth 5713 Paiute Road, Virginia Beach, VA 23462, (804) 499-5814, MA 88 Univ of CT

Gray, Mellaney 406 East 7th St, Alton, IL 62002, (314) 868-9855, SLP, Alton Com Schl Dstr 11, **SLP**

Gray, Molly Buckles Baptist Hospital, 1000 W Moreno Street, P O Box 17500, Pensacola, FL 32522, (904) 434-4957, MS 79 Univ Southern MS-Hattiesburg; Aud, Baptist Hosp, **A**

Gray, Pamela Sue 7052 North Burrage, Portland, OR 97217, (503) 220-8262, BS 78 OR St Univ; MA 87 OR St Univ; 88–Aud, VAMC Portland Division, **A**

Gray, Patricia A P O Box 565, North Andover, MA 01845, (508) 682-5117, BS 68 Boston Univ; ME 70 Boston Univ; Sp-Lang Path, Lawrence Sch Dept, **SLP**

Gray, Shareyfah Allyse 3511 Fairview Avenue, Baltimore, MD 21216, (202) 479-6837, MS 88 Howard Univ

Gray, Mrs Sheila Ruth 180 North Hoyt, Lakewood, CO 80226, (505) 445-3017, MS 80 Vanderbilt Univ; SLP, U of CO, **SLP**

Gray, Susan G 515 North Main Street, Apartment 3, Graham, NC 27253, (919) 226-3536, ME 87 Univ of NC - Greensboro

Gray, Dr Susan Gillen 805 Temple Terrace, Los Angeles, CA 90042, (213) 669-2137, BA 66 Marymount Coll; MS 67 SUNY - Coll at Buffalo; PH 79 (NS) Univ of Southern CA; Director Divsn Hearing/Speech, Childrens Hosp of Los Angeles, **SLP**

Gray, Mrs Susan J B 525 Alvarado Lane North, Plymouth, MN 55447, BS 78 IN Univ - Bloomington; MA 79 Ball St Univ; Sp-Lang Path, Cp Serv Cen, **SLP**

Gray, Mrs Susan Nuss 439 South Kelsey Avenue, Evansville, IN 47714, (812) 474-0766, BS 78 Ball St Univ; MA 82 Ball St Univ; 88–Sp-Lang Path, Welborn Baptist Hosp, **SLP**

Gray, Mrs Susan Robinson 4407 West Kimberly Way, Glendale, AZ 85308, (602) 866-5600, **SLP**

Gray, Terri S 4650 South Oak, Wichita, KS 67217, (316) 262-8271, BA 77 Wichita St Univ; MA 79 Wichita St Univ; Sp/Lang Path, Institute of Logopedics, **SLP**

Gray, Dr Thomas F Audiology Associates, 1133 College Avenue, Manhattan, KS 66502, (913) 539-7361, BA 63 Univ of Northern IA; MA 67 Univ of Northern IA; PH 74 (NS) Univ of MN - Minneap-St Paul; Aud, Aud Assoc, **SLP A ACE**

Gray, Mrs Wanda L P O Box 2682, Pinetop, AZ 85935-2682, (602) 368-6281, MS 77 KS St Univ; SLP, The Arrowhead Eval & Intr Ctr, **SLP**

Graybeal, Dr Carolyn M 211 Highland Avenue, West Newton, MA 02165, (617) 332-0139, BA 73 Smith Coll; ED 81 (Applied Psycholinguistics) Boston Univ; Sp-Lang Path, Mainstay-Cen for Chldn, **SLP ACE**

Graybill, Mrs Joanne C 219 North 11th Street, Oakland, MD 21550, (301) 334-4312, BS 66 Bloomsburg Univ of PA; MA 71 Saint Louis Univ; Tchr, Garret Co Board of Education

Graybill, Thomas J 219 North 11th Street, Oakland, MD 21550, (301) 334-1377, BA 64 Univ of Pittsburgh - Pittsburgh; MA 71 Saint Louis Univ; 81–Sp-Lang Path, Garrett County Public Schools, **SLP**

Gray-Hoffman, Mrs Karen 6296 Brookings, Troy, MI 48098, (313) 884-3231, BS 79 Wayne St Univ; MA 80 Wayne St Univ; SLP, Harper Woods Sch Syst, **SLP**

Gray-Richardson, Laurel 654 Phaeton Place, Indianapolis, IN 46227, **A**

Grayson, Mrs Danni Leigh Route 10 Box 222, Waco, TX 76708, (817) 799-1721, BS 79 Baylor Univ; MS 80 Baylor Univ; SLP, La Vega ISD, **SLP**

Grayson, Mrs Lori Savage 2144 Trescott Drive, Tallahassee, FL 32312, (904) 385-5151, BA 77 Emory Univ; OM 79 Emory Univ; Sp/Lang Path, Thomasville City School System, **SLP**

Graziano, Adrienne Lee 1420 Monroe Avenue #5, Rochester, NY 14618-1024, BS 81 Ithaca Coll; MS 87 Nazareth Coll of Rochester

Graziano-Tiso, Mrs Susan 4600 East Overlook Drive, Williamsville, NY 14221, (716) 633-7491, BA 77 SUNY - Center at Buffalo; MA 79 SUNY - Center at Buffalo; Sp-Lang Path, Kenmore-Tonawanda Pub Sch, **SLP**

Greathouse, Susan Renee 434 A Avenue, Coronado, CA 92118, (619) 292-3699, BS 81 Univ of TX - Austin; MA 87 Univ of TX - Austin; 88–SLP, San Diego Co Ofc of Ed, **SLP**

Greb, Kathryn Diana 1780 W 85th Avenue #202, Denver, CO 80221, (303) 428-3511, BA 82 Univ of CO - Boulder; MA 85 Univ of Northern CO; **SLP**

Grecco, Russell 1445 Old Stagecoach Road, Ocean View, NJ 08230, (609) 399-6912, BA 68 Trenton St Coll; MA 71 Univ of CT; OM 75 Univ of CT; Prin/Superv Spec Serv, Hembold Ed Cen, **A**

Greco, Cynthia Micali R R 1 Box 214-A Trolley Rd, Peekskill, NY 10566, (914) 528-9514, BS 80 Mercy Coll; MA 85 CUNY - Hunter Coll; 80–Sp-Lang Path, Putnam Northern West BOCES, **SLP**

Greco, Mrs Mary L 653 Surrey Lane, Algonquin, IL 60102, (312) 658-9030, BS 75 Marquette Univ; MS 77 Southern IL Univ -Carbondale; 88–Sp-Lang Path, Private Practice, **SLP**

Green, Mrs Aleene McKinney P O Box 4123, Beeville, TX 78104, (512) 358-1777, BA 69 Univ of Houston - Univ Park; MA 75 Univ of Houston - Univ Park; 86–Sp-Lang Path, Private Practice, **SLP**

Green, Ann S Box 358, Montrose, BC, Canada V0G 1P0, **SLP**

Green, Barbara Jean 17272 Forbes Lane, Huntington Beach, CA 92649, BA 76 Univ of CA - Santa Barbara; MA 83 CA St Univ - Long Beach; SLP, **SLP**

Green, Billye Marie Mannheim Elementary School, APO New York, NY 09086, **SLP**

Green, Brenda 1032 Vesper Lane, Hillendale West, Fayetteville, NC 28301, (919) 488-6778, BS 84 Shaw Univ; ME 86 AL A & M Univ; Sp-Lang Path, Cumberland County Sch Sys

Green, Brenda M 2330 Forest Glade, Fort Wayne, IN 46845, (219) 637-8615, BS 68 Western MI Univ; MS 77 Coll of Saint Rose; Sp-Lang Path, Private Practice, **SLP ACE**

Green, Carol A 6200 142nd S E, Bellevue, WA 98006, BA 71 Western WA Univ; MA 86 Western WA Univ; 71–Sp-Lang Path, Seattle PS, **SLP**

Green, Carol J 3620 Spring Mountain Road, St Helena, CA 94574, (707) 963-8332, BA 70 CA St Univ - Northridge; MA 72 CA St Univ - Northridge; **SLP**

Green, Mrs Carol Senoyuit Alberta Children's Hospital, 1820 Richmond Road SW, Calgary, AB, Canada T2T 5C7, (403) 229-7061, BS 83 WV Univ; MS 85 WV Univ; 86–Aud, Alberta Children's Hosp

Green, Catherine C 140 Linwood Avenue #E-6, Buffalo, NY 14209, (716) 882-9520, BA 82 SUNY - Center at Buffalo; MS 85 SUNY - Coll at Buffalo; **SLP**

Green, Cynthia 80 Cranberry Street #6F, Brooklyn, NY 11201, (718) 624-3900, BA 66 CUNY - Queens Coll; MS 68 Univ of Pittsburgh - Pittsburgh; Sp/Lang Path, Private Practice, **SLP**

Green, Mrs Cynthia Shealey 10020 Piney Ridge Walk, Alpharetta, GA 30201, (404) 664-9414, BS 83 Univ of GA; ME 85 Armstrong St Coll; 88–Sp-Lang Path, The Davison Sch, **SLP**

Green, Dr David S 33 Queach Road, Branford, CT 06405, (203) 397-4572, BA 50 Syracuse Univ; MA 51 Columbia Univ Teachers Coll; PH 56 (NS) Purdue Univ - West Lafayette; Professor, Southern Connecticut State U, **SLP A**

Green, Deborah Ellen P O Box 5241, Burlington, VT 05402, (802) 985-3468, MS 84 Univ of VT; 87–Aud, Surgical Assoc Foundation Inc, **A**

Green, Diana L G 208 Green Valley Drive, Naperville, IL 60540, (312) 964-9420, BS 70 Western IL Univ; MA 71 Western IL Univ; Sp-Lang Path, Lisle School District 202, **SLP**

Green, Ellen 10313 Dandridge Drive, St Louis, MO 63123, BS 69 OH Univ - Athens; MA 70 OH Univ - Athens; Sp/Lang Path, Spec Sch Dist of St Louis Co, **SLP**

Green, Evelyn M 1008 South 2nd Street, Springfield, IL 62704, (217) 528-3586, BA 31 Cornell Coll; MA 40 Univ of IA; **SLP LM**

Green, Mrs Frances A 2233 Morning Dove Court, Orange Park, FL 32073, (904) 264-3271, BA 75 Univ of FL; ME 76 Univ of FL; **SLP**

Green, Mrs Hanna 17 Druid Road, Warwick, RI 02888, (401) 722-6000, BA 73 Montclair St Coll; MA 76 CUNY - Hunter Coll; Sp-Lang Path, Memorial Hospital, **SLP**

Green, J Michael 100 Gailmoor Drive, Ladson, SC 29456, (803) 553-8568, MA 88 Univ of SC - Columbia; 88–Aud, Health Eval Prog Inc

Green, Jacqueline 15 Dart Drive, Ithaca, NY 14850, (607) 273-6600, BA 72 SUNY - Coll at Oneonta; MS 74 Ithaca Coll; 85–Sp-Lang Path, Empire Rehab Assoc, **SLP ACE**

Green, Jacquelyn 229 West Upsal Street #402, Philadelphia, PA 19119, MS 64 PA St Univ - Univ Park; Sp-Lang Path, Philadelphia School Board, **SLP**

Green, Mrs Jean Y 2432 McKinley Avenue, West Lawn, PA 19609, (215) 775-8337, BS 81 Bloomsburg Univ of PA; MS 82 Bloomsburg Univ of PA; Sp-Lang Path, Reading Rehab Hosp, **SLP**

Green, Mrs Jeanie K 1006 Forest Avenue North, Fort Payne, AL 35967, (205) 845-5135, BS 79 Univ of Montevallo; MS 80 Univ of Montevallo; Sp-Lang Path, Dekalb Co Bd of Ed, **SLP**

Green, Dr Joni Grant 280 Vistalmar Street, Coral Gables, FL 33143, (305) 661-5387, BA 62 CA St Univ - Northridge; MA 68 OH St Univ; PH 73 (NS) OH St Univ; Aud, Private Practice, **SLP**

Green, Mrs Joy R Monte Verde, Argyle, TX 76226, (817) 455-2463, BS 71 Northern IL Univ - De Kalb; MS 79 Univ of KS; Sp-Lang Path, Private Practice, **SLP**

Green, Karen Denise 3813 Sandstone Ct, New Smyrna Beach, FL 32069, (904) 345-3453, BA 79 High Point Coll; ME 83 Univ of NC - Greensboro; Sp-Lang Path, Sch Bd of Volusia Co, **SLP**

Green, Dr Kathleen W State University College, P O Box 2000, Cortland, NY 13045, (607) 753-2702, BA 67 CUNY - Hunter Coll; MA 69 Syracuse Univ; PH 82 (NS) Syracuse Univ; 85–Assoc Dean, St U Coll at Cortland, **SLP A**

Green, Katie W P O Box 12, Bullard Road, Princeton, MA 01541, (617) 485-8100, BA 72 Case Western Reserve Univ; MA 73 Case Western Reserve Univ; Sp-Lang Path, FLLAC Educ Collaborative, **SLP**

Green, Mrs Kelly E 6480 Stone Valley Drive, Reno, NV 89523, (702) 358-3273, BS 81 Univ of WY; MS 83 Univ of WY; Aud, Hearing Plus, **A**

Green, Kelly R 703 Glenda Drive, Longview, TX 75603, (214) 758-9392, BS 75 Stephen F Austin St Univ; MS 77 Univ of North TX; Dir of Aud, Audiometrics Inc, **A**

Green, Laurie 425 Dailey #21, Anchorage, AK 99515, (907) 561-8060, BA 64 Univ of La Verne; MA 68 Univ of Redlands; SLP, Anchorage Prgm for Inf Chldrn, **SLP ACE**

Green, Dr Lawanda 3615 Clifmar Road, Baltimore, MD 21207, (301) 922-5731, MA 72 Univ of Southern CA; MS 76 Harvard Univ; OD 81 (NS) Harvard Univ; Sp-Lang Path, Baltimore City Schs, **SLP**

Green, Mrs Leslie R 979 Chesterfield, Birmingham, MI 48009, (313) 745-8903, BA 73 Albion Coll; MA 76 Wayne St Univ; Sp-Lang Path, Chldn Hosp-Mi, **SLP**

Green, Dr Lois W Elizabeth City State Univ, Box 972, Elizabeth City, NC 27909, (919) 335-3407, BA 64 Spelman Coll; MA 68 Central MI Univ; ED 74 (NS) Univ of GA; 75–Sp-Lang Path, Elizateth City State Univ, **SLP**

Green, Mrs Lori Yates 2753 Windswept Lane, Mesquite, TX 75181, (214) 220-8017, BS 85 TX Woman's Univ; MA 86 TX Woman's Univ; 87–Sp-Lang Path, InSpeech Inc, **SLP**

Green, Marcia H 3611 38th Street N W #405, Washington, DC 20016, (202) 362-8503, **A**

Green, Margaret 323 East Central, Missoula, MT 59801, (406) 258-6021, BS 72 Univ of MN - Minneap-St Paul; MA 75 Univ of MT; Sp-Lang Path, Missowla Area Spec Ed Coop, **SLP**

Green, Margaret E 1B Chilton Manor, Charleston, WV 25314, (304) 348-7760, BS 74 WV Univ; MS 76 WV Univ; Sp/Lang Path, Kanawha Co Bd of Ed, **SLP**

Green, Marilyn S HC 56 Box 1536, Bulverde, TX 78163, (512) 438-3512, BS 65 Purdue Univ - West Lafayette; MS 70 Purdue Univ - West Lafayette; SLP, No East ISD, **SLP**

Green, Martha Hazelwood 5514 Floyd, Amarillo, TX 79106, (806) 353-1987, BA 48 TX Tech Univ; MA 53 TX Tech Univ; 82–SLP, VA Hosp, **SLP LM**

Green, Mrs Marva J 2922 Par 3 Drive #4, Memphis, TN 38115, (901) 761-9517, BA 74 Beloit Coll; MA 76 Memphis St Univ; 86–Aud, Otolaryngol Consult of Memphis, **A**

Green, Mrs Mary Elizabeth 382 Lincoln Street, Bangor, ME 04401, (207) 223-4282, BA 77 Univ of ME - Orono; MA 87 Univ of ME - Orono; 88–Sp-Lang Path, Bangor Sch Dept, **SLP**

Green, Mary R 8101 Laurel Lane, Chagrin Falls, OH 44022, BS 63 OH Northern Univ; MS 72 Rutgers St Univ -N Brunswick; Sp-Lang Path, Sunny Acres Skilled Nursng Fac, **SLP**

Green, Maureen Raedy 138 Greenwood Avenue, San Rafael, CA 94901, (707) 938-6680, BA 83 San Francisco St Univ; MS 85 San Francisco St Univ; 88–Sp-Lang Path, Sonoma Developmental Ctr, **SLP**

Green, Dr Meryl C 33 Lancaster Terrace #101, Brookline, MA 02146, (617) 566-5264, BA 52 CUNY - Brooklyn Coll; MS 53 Purdue Univ - West Lafayette; ED 85 (Psycholinguistics) Boston Univ; 85–Sp-Lang Path, Private Practice, **SLP**

Green, Nancy E 1357 Franklin, Denver, CO 80218, (303) 861-1810, BA 69 Augustana Coll; MA 74 Univ of IL - Urbana; Sp-Lang Path, Private Practice, **SLP**

Green, Mrs Nancy N Communicative Disorders Center, 1731 University Blvd South, Jacksonville, FL 32216, (904) 724-4327, BA 80 FL St Univ; MA 81 FL St Univ; 82–Dir/Ch Aud, Commun Dis Cen, **A ACE**

Green, Mrs Nancy S 13020 S W 69th Avenue, Miami, FL 33156, **SLP**

Green, Mrs Patricia Ann 8545 Bitter Bush Way, Colorado Springs, CO 80918-5729, (303) 528-5782, BS 81 Bowling Green St Univ; MA 82 Bowling Green St Univ; Communication Habilitation Spc, Colorado School Deaf & Blind, **SLP**

Green, Mrs Patricia Mary 4111 Waterford Circle #8, Louisville, KY 40207, (414) 771-1830, BS 86 Marquette Univ; MS 87 Marquette Univ

Green, Patricia W 108 Deer Path Circle, Rural Route 2, Brewster, MA 02631, (508) 255-1901, BS 44 Duke Univ; MA 62 Northwestern Univ; Retired, **SLP**

Green, Patti Lubowitz 73 Heritage Drive, Tewksbury, MA 01876, (617) 858-3965, BS 82 Univ of MA - Amherst; MS 86 Worcester St Coll

Green, Mrs Rhonda M 2026 N W 18th Lane, Gainesville, FL 32605, (904) 377-2022, OB 68 Univ of FL; ME 69 Univ of FL; Sp-Lang Path, Alachua Co Sch Bd, **SLP ACE**

Green, Richard B 2110 East Third Avenue, Vancouver, BC, Canada V5N 1H8, (604) 254-8646, BA 71 Univ of Alberta - Alberta; MA 80 LA St Univ - Baton Rouge; 86–Sp/Lang Path, Private Practice, **SLP**

Green, Dr Robert A Colonial Northampton I U 20, 299 Industrial Park Road, P O Box 179, Nazareth, PA 18064, (215) 759-7600, BS 65 Bloomsburg Univ of PA; MA 70 Temple Univ-Tyler Sch of Art; ED 78 (NS) Nova Univ; Asst Dir Spec Ed, Colonial Northapton Inter Un, **SLP**

Green, Robert Baron 1371 Greenwich Street, San Francisco, CA 94109, (415) 441-4818, BA 83 0500; MA 86 Montclair St Coll; 88–Aud, Childrens Hosp Oakland, **A**

Green, Robin W 6 Wolcott Street, Wakefield, MA 01880, (617) 246-0070, BS 77 Worcester St Coll; MA 78 SUNY - Coll at Geneseo; Sp-Lang Path, Wakefield Public Schools, **SLP**

Green, Dr Rosalind N 15654 Ridge Estates Road, Nevada City, CA 95959, PH (NS); SLP, Nevada City School District, **SLP**

Green, Sharon H 20 Sunnyside Drive, Springfield, IL 62702, (217) 787-4906, BS 73 Bradley Univ; MS 75 Bradley Univ; Aud, Sn IL Head Neck Hrng, **A**

Green, Steven Michael 20323 Damietta, Walnut, CA 91789, (714) 594-1729, MA 85 San Diego St Univ; Dir of Comm Dis, La Palma Comm Hosp, **SLP**

Green, Susan K 2234 Kinbrook Drive, Houston, TX 77077, (713) 496-1420, BA 73 SUNY - Center at Buffalo; OM 75 Emory Univ; SLP, Private Practice, **SLP A**

Green, Suzanne K 1026 West Gregory, Kansas City, MO 64114, (816) 932-1604, BA 75 Univ of NE - Lincoln; MA 77 Univ of NE - Omaha; Sp-Lang Path, Private Practice, **SLP**

Green, Mrs Twhanna J Woodburn Elementary, 3401 Hemlock Drive, Falls Church, VA 22042, (703) 560-2116, BS 76 Howard Univ; MS 79 Univ of the DC; Sp-Lang Path, Fairfax Co PS, **SLP**

Green, Dr Walter B School Of Human Comm Disorders, Dalhousie University, 5599 Finwick Street, Halifax, NS, Canada B3H 1R2, (902) 424-7052, BS 65 Central MI Univ; MA 66 Central MI Univ; PH 71 (Aud) Syracuse Univ; 84–Professor and Director, Dalhousie Univ, **SLP A**

Green, Dr William W 1306 Richmond Road, Lexington, KY 40502, (606) 233-5840, BS 62 Kent St Univ; MA 64 Kent St Univ; PH 70 (Aud) Case Western Reserve Univ; 70–Prof & Dir Neurosen Commun Disor, Dept of Neur/Coll of Med U Ky, **A F ACE**

Green, Yvonne F 2110 East 3rd Street, Vancouver, BC, Canada V5N 1H8, (604) 731-1131, BS 76 Univ of Alberta - Alberta; MA 78 LA St Univ - Baton Rouge; 86–Sp/Lang Path, Vancouver Sch Bd, **SLP**

Greenawald, Mrs Lynn A 2927 Charlotte Avenue, Easton, PA 18042, (201) 735-4031, BS 80 WV Univ; MS 81 WV Univ; Sp-Lang Path, Hunterdon Dev Center, **SLP**

Greenbank, Mrs Debbra A P O Box 1235, El Dorado, KS 67042, (316) 321-1411, BA 81 0884; MA 82 0884; Sp-Lang Path, Private Practice, **SLP**

Green-Barber, Lisa J 126 Holman Street, Laconia, NH 03246, (603) 524-2986, MS 82 UT St Univ; Sp-Lang Path, Private Practice, **SLP**

Greenbaum, Annette 538 Overlake Drive East, Bellevue, WA 98004, (206) 454-0435, MS 88 Univ of WA

Greenbaum, Mrs Bettsie W 35 Haymarket Lane, Bryn Mawr, PA 19010, (215) 527-8299, BS 78 Boston Univ; MA 79 Tulane Univ; **SLP**

Greenbaum, Rochelle I 57B Humphrey Road, Santa Barbara, CA 93108, **SLP**

Greenberg, Dr Bonita R Communication Disorders, Bowling Green State Univ, Bowling Green, OH 43403, (419) 372-7190, BA 66 Adelphi Univ; MS 67 Adelphi Univ; PH 70 (Sp Path) Purdue Univ - West Lafayette; Assoc Prof, Bowling Green St U

Greenberg, Bonnie B 56 Elmore Street, Newton Center, MA 02159, (617) 969-1665, BS 65 Univ of WI - Madison; MS 66 Univ of WI - Madison; 88–Sp-Lang Path, Wellesley PS, **SLP**

Greenberg, Mrs Dawn Jennifer 71 Ray Street, Manchester, NH 03104, (603) 623-7233, BS 84 Univ of NH; MS 85 Univ of NH; 88–Sp-Lang Path, Hooksett Sch Dist SAU #15, **SLP**

Greenberg, Donna C 5042 Los Feliz Boulevard, Los Angeles, CA 90027, BA; MS; **A**

Greenberg, Douglas B 3018 Pickford Road, Victoria, BC, Canada V9B 2K9, (604) 387-2664, BA 74 Univ of WA; MA 75 Univ of WA; Aud, British Columbia Government, **A**

Greenberg, Frederick 10 Old Court Road, Baltimore, MD 21208, (301) 484-2233, BA 48; MA 52 Univ of MD - College Park; Administrator, Private Practice, **SLP**

Greenberg, Dr Frederick R 278 Brookside Terrace, Edmonton, AB, Canada T6H 4J6, (403) 471-7955, BS 58 Univ of MN - Minneap-St Paul; MA 63 Univ of IA; PH 63 (NS) Univ of IA; Asst Exec Dir-Planning, Glenrose Rehab Hosp, **F**

Greenberg, Dr Herbert J Communication Disorders, Bowling Green State Univ, Bowling Green, OH 43403, (419) 372-2515, BS 64 McGill Univ - Quebec; MA 66 Adelphi Univ; PH 69 (NS) Purdue Univ - West Lafayette; Chairman Dept of Commun Dis, Bowling Green State Univ, **A**

Greenberg, Joan 3110 Old Post Drive, Baltimore, MD 21208, (301) 795-5585, BA 79 Univ of MD - College Park; MA 80 George Washington Univ; Sp/Lang Path, Carroll Co Bd of Ed, **SLP**

Greenberg, Joyce M 10 Brook Hill Drive, Worcester, MA 01609, (617) 799-6694, BS 62 Emerson Coll; ME 65 Worcester St Coll; **SLP**

Greenberg, Mrs Lauri I 7 Greenbriar Road, Marmora, NJ 08223, (609) 628-2603, BA 72 CUNY - Queens Coll; MA 74 CUNY - Queens Coll; Sp-Lang Path/Instr Superv, Private Practice, **SLP ACE**

Greenberg, Mrs Lauri R J 7630 Royal Lane, Dallas, TX 75230, (214) 373-3026, MS 81 Tulane Univ; Sp-Lang Path, **SLP**

Greenberg, Mrs Lorraine R 169 High Pond Drive, Jericho, Long Island, NY 11753, (212) 886-5555, BA 62 George Washington Univ; MA 66 Columbia Univ Teachers Coll; SLP, Visting Nurse Service of NY, **SLP**

Greenberg, Mrs Marci Katz 925 Magnolia Avenue, Norfolk, VA 23508, (804) 440-7900, BS 78 Boston Univ; OM 79 LA St Univ - N O Medical Ctr; 87–Sp-Lang Path, Private Practice, **SLP**

Greenberg, Mrs Marilyn B 9 Blue Devil Lane, Mercerville, NJ 08619, (609) 599-5221, BA 72 CUNY - Brooklyn Coll; MA 76 Trenton St Coll; Sp-Lang Path, St Francis Med Cen, **SLP ACE**

Greenberg, Marjorie W 4411 Sentinel Post Road N W, Atlanta, GA 30327, (404) 262-3460, BA 58 Vanderbilt Univ; Sp/Lang Path, **SLP**

Greenberg, Marsha Rhonda 20 LaSalle Place, Oakdale, NY 11769, (516) 473-6321, BA 74 Univ of MA - Amherst; MA 80 Hofstra Univ; 80–Sp-Lang Path, Mt Sinia Sch Dist NY, **SLP ACE**

Greenberg, Stephanie Robin 12 Charles Lane #1-D, Pomona, NY 10970, (914) 942-2700, BS 73 SUNY - Center at Buffalo; MS 74 Columbia Univ Teachers Coll; 88–Sp-Lang Path, North Rockland Central Sch Dist, **SLP**

Greenberg, Dr Sylvia 5636 Phillips Avenue, Pittsburgh, PA 15217, (412) 683-3000, OB 42 Duquesne Univ; ME 47 Univ of Pittsburgh - Pittsburgh; PH 70 (Sp Path) Univ of Pittsburgh - Pittsburgh; 47–Sp-Lang Path, VA, **SLP LM**

Greenberg-Cordero, Barbara Alice 5900 S W 127th Avenue #3305, Miami, FL 33183, (305) 666-6511, BA 77 CUNY - Hunter Coll; MS 80 Southern CT St Univ; 85–Aud, Miami Childrens Hosp, **A**

Greenberger, Mrs Debra Levine 4732 Old Boston Road, Pittsburgh, PA 15227, (412) 261-3950, BA 79 SUNY - Coll at Geneseo; MS 81 Washington Univ; Aud, Head & Neck Surgical Assoc, **A**

Greenberg-Waxman, Faith E 23 Deerfield Lane, St Louis, MO 63146, (314) 569-8100, **SLP**

Greenblatt, Mrs Debra A 2467 Greenhaven Drive, Akron, OH 44313, (216) 666-8815, BA 73 Univ of Akron; MA 75 Univ of Akron; SLP, Co of Summit Bd of Ment Retard, **SLP**

Greenblatt, Nancy L 116 Hennessy Drive, Portland, ME 04103, (207) 797-5519, BA 72 Univ of ME - Orono; ME 73 Northeastern Univ; 88–Sp-Lang Path, First Allied Home Health, **SLP**

Greenday, Mrs Laura Ann 7300 Scarecrow Road, Mechanicsville, VA 23111, (804) 737-9708, **SLP**

Green-Dragony, Jo Allison 2204 North Cherry Lane, Farmington, NM 87499, (505) 325-1741, BS 77 OK St Univ; MA 79 OK St Univ; Sp/Lang Path, Farmington Mun Sch, **SLP**

Greene, Abigail Martha HCR Box 58, Grahamsville, NY 12740, **SLP**

Greene, Mrs Beverly Katz 1638 East Course Drive, Riverwoods, IL 60015, (312) 948-9258, BA 70 IN Univ - Bloomington; MA 72 Northwestern Univ; **A**

Greene, Bonnie M 1224 Seafarer Street, Ventura, CA 93001, (805) 647-1141, MS 76 CA St Univ - Northridge; 86–Dir of Sp Dept, Easter Seal Soc Ventura Co, **SLP**

Greene, Janet D 805 Maley Street, Daytona Beach, FL 32014, (904) 677-3611, BS 63 Hampton Univ; MA 64 MI St Univ; SLP, Volusia Co Sch Bd, **SLP ACE**

Greene, Jill Diamond 23 Flint Ridge Drive, Shillington, PA 19067, (215) 378-0481, BS 75 PA St Univ - Univ Park; ME 76 Bloomsburg Univ of PA; **SLP**

Greene, Louise H 10250 S W Winter Lane, Beaverton, OR 97005, (503) 280-5710, BS 75 Southern OR St Coll; MS 76 Western OR St Coll; Prog Chairperson, Columbia Reg Prog-Special Needs, **SLP**

Greene, Margaret 20 Ashburton Place, Laguna Niguel, CA 92677, MA 54 Temple Univ; **SLP**

Greene, Maribeth 7733 S Rutherford, Burbank, IL 60459, (312) 354-5730, BS 84 Northern IL Univ - De Kalb; OM 86 Governors St Univ; 87–Sp-Lang Path, LADSE, **SLP**

Greene, Martha Julia 1301 Canterbury Lane, Clinton, MS 39056, (601) 924-7261, BA 66 LA Tech Univ; MA 83 Univ of MS; 79–Sp-Lang Path, Clinton PS Dist, **SLP**

Greene, Dr Nancy E 9252 Chesapeake Drive #400, San Diego, CA 92123, (619) 569-1988, ME 71 Boston Univ; MA 75; PH 77 (NS); Sp-Lang Path/Clin Psych, Private Practice, **SLP**

Greene, Patricia D 910 Garfield Street, Denver, CO 80206, (303) 778-5645, BS 75 Ithaca Coll; MS 77 Univ of MI - Ann Arbor; Aud, Porter Memorial Hosp, **A**

Greene, Penny N 201 Northwind Drive, El Paso, TX 79112-3711, (915) 542-6561, BS 76 Univ of TX - Austin; MA 81 Univ of TX - El Paso; Sp-Lang Path Rehab Supervisor, Providence Memorial Hospital, **SLP**

Greene, Renee Y 20-35D W Mosholu Parkway S, Bronx, NY 10468, (212) 750-6789, BA 71 CUNY - City College; MS 74 2605; Superv/Aud, Goldwater Mem Hosnyu Med Cen, **A**

Greene, Sheri Robin 1200 Dale Avenue #46, Mountain View, CA 94040, (415) 964-5546, BA 85 Univ of CA - Santa Barbara; MS 87 Boston Univ; 88–Sp-Lang Path, Alta Bates Corp/Herrick Hosp, **SLP**

Greene, Mrs Soloris J 1828 West 83rd Street, Los Angeles, CA 90047, (818) 288-6681, BA 71 CA St Univ - Los Angeles; MA 73 CA St Univ - Los Angeles; Sp-Lang Path, Offi of LA Co Supt of Sch, **SLP**

Greene-Luba, Mrs Jill A 114 Hampshire Road, Rockville Centre, NY 11570, (516) 825-9130, BS 75 Long Island U - CW Post Ctr; MS 76 Ithaca Coll; SLP, Valley Stream USD #30, **SLP**

Greene-Vaughan, Betty 3051 Kirklevington Drive, Apartment 43, Lexington, KY 40502, **SLP**

Greenfeld, Diane N 9514 Gwyndale Drive, Silver Spring, MD 20910, (301) 587-0213, BS 77 Univ of MN - Minneap-St Paul; MS 79 Tulane Univ; **SLP**

Greenfelder, Mrs Debra Diane 201 Rose Lane S W, Apt 107, North Canton, OH 44720, (216) 497-2841, MA 79 Kent St Univ; SLP, County Board Mental Retardatn, **SLP**

Greenfeld-Furman, Mrs Debra 539 Kensico Court, Suffern, NY 10901, (914) 357-9411, BA 79 CUNY - Queens Coll; MS 80 PA St Univ - Univ Park; Sp-Lang Path, Private Practice, **SLP**

Greenfield, Mrs Deborah Goodman 35 Thornley Road, Eatontown, NJ 07724, (201) 776-2071, MA 62 Columbia Univ Teachers Coll; BA 61 Rutgers St Univ -N Brunswick; 84–Sp-Lang Path, Neptune Township Board of Educ, **SLP**

Greenfield, Donna G 1392 Carling Drive #306, St Paul, MN 55108, (612) 626-5775, BA 78 Univ of CA - Santa Barbara; MS 80 Univ of WI - Madison; Aud, Univ of MN Hosp, **A**

Greenfield, Mrs Ellen Braiman 15 South Goodman Street #2, Rochester, NY 14607, (315) 589-9621, BS 84 Bowling Green St Univ; MS 87 Nazareth Coll of Rochester

Greenfield, Mrs Sharon Jakubowicz 550 J Grand Street, New York, NY 10002, (212) 533-6191, BA 83 CUNY - Brooklyn Coll; MS 85 CUNY - Brooklyn Coll; 86–Sp-Lang Path, New York Childhood Ctr, **SLP**

Greenfield, Susan L R 1168 Besito Avenue, Berkeley, CA 94705, (415) 540-4415, BS 77 SUNY - Center at Albany; MA 79 NY Univ; Sp-Lang Path, Herrick Hospital & Health Cen, **SLP**

Greenhagen, Mrs Pamela Route 4 Box 209-C, Milan, TN 38358, (901) 686-9649, BA 76 Augustana Coll; MS 77 Eastern IL Univ; Sp-Lang Path, **SLP**

Greenhalgh, Mrs Kathy Bouffard 1045 N E 92nd Street, Seattle, WA 98115, (802) 453-3227, MS 82 Univ of VT; Sp/Lang Path, **SLP**

Greenhall, Mrs Irene Leav 7 Nottingham Road, Rockville Centre, NY 11570, (516) 678-5507, BS 56 Syracuse Univ; MS 68 Adelphi Univ; Sp-Lang Path, Private Practice, **SLP**

Greenhill, Ann Hirsh 433 Cabrillo Avenue, Davis, CA 95616, BA 68 Univ of Rochester; MS 71 Southern CT St Univ; Sp-Lang Path, Rehabilitation Health Services, **SLP**

Greenholtz-Carrillo, Mrs Debra Lynn 17845 NW Sedgewick, Beaverton, OR 97006, (503) 648-1126, MS 82 Univ of OR; Sp-Lang Path, Hillsboro Elem Sch, **SLP**

Greenhood, Johanna M 4602 Elsrode Avenue, Baltimore, MD 21214, (301) 647-3890, MS 76 Towson St Univ; Tchr, A A Co Pub Sch, **SLP**

Greening, Marti Netler Rpo Box 480, Reynoldsburg, OH 43068, (614) 864-8295, BS 76 OH St Univ; MA 80 OH St Univ; SLP, Columbus Pub Schs, **SLP**

Greening, Naomi Karen 1786 Crone Avenue, Anaheim, CA 92804, (714) 774-4313, MA 85 CA St Univ - Fullerton; **SLP**

Greenlee, Gloria M D 7104 Tioga Court, Bakersfield, CA 93309, **SLP**

Greenlee, Dr Mary Ellen (Mel) 1780 Franklin Street, Berkeley, CA 94702, (415) 497-0732, BA 67 Catholic Univ of America; MA 73 Univ of CA - Berkeley; PH 78 (NS) Univ of CA - Berkeley; Stanford U

Greenley, Diane Carol 2727 29th Street N W #408, Washington, DC 20008-1802, (202) 483-9146, BA 80 Univ of MI - Ann Arbor; MA 84 Eastern MI Univ; **SLP**

Greenman, Mrs Carol Sellers 97 Brantwood Road, Snyder, NY 14226, (716) 636-3401, BA 72 SUNY - Center at Buffalo; MA 85 SUNY - Center at Buffalo; 86–Clin Asst Prof, SUNY at Buffalo, **SLP ACE**

Greenman, Denise A 26-H Weed Hill Avenue, Stamford, CT 06907, (203) 329-8594, BS 80 Syracuse Univ; MA 82 NY Univ; Sp-Lang Path, UCP, **SLP**

Greensmith, Mrs Jennifer Margaret 35 Pheasant Lane RR #1, Camlachie, ON, Canada N0N 1E0, (519) 336-6121, MS 88 Minot St Univ; 88–Sp-Lang Path, St Joseph's Hosp

Greenspan, Phyllis 11247 Sage Canyon, Houston, TX 77089, (713) 481-3930, BS 78 Eastern NM Univ; MA 80 Univ of Houston - Univ Park; 85–Sp-Lang Path, Private Practice, **SLP**

Greenspan, Wendy Whalen 640 South Humphrey Avenue, Oak Park, IL 60304-1214, (312) 848-4534, BA 80 SUNY - Center at Buffalo; MA 83 SUNY - Center at Buffalo; Sp-Lang Path, Loyola Univ Med Ctr, **SLP**

Greenstate, Mrs Judith Willens 4240 Fulton Avenue #305, Studio City, CA 91604, (818) 997-2357, BA 60 Univ of CA - Los Angeles; MA 77 CA St Univ - Northridge; Sp-Lang Path, LA USD, **SLP ACE**

Greenstein, Arlene T 68 Dennison Avenue, Swampscott, MA 01907, (617) 437-3173, BA 66 SUNY - Center at Buffalo; MS 68 Univ of WI - Madison; PH 74 (Speech Science) Univ of WI - Madison; 85–Assoc Dean, Nen U, **SLP**

Greenstein, Diane B 111 14th Street #8, Hoboken, NJ 07030, (212) 481-0300, BA 78 Northwestern Univ; MA 80 Univ of MN - Minneap-St Paul; Pvt Contractor-SLP, Northern Westchester Ctr for Sp Dis, **SLP**

Greenstein, Mrs Evelyn Beller 1461 East 19th Street, Brooklyn, NY 11230, (718) 627-0060, MS 81 CUNY - Brooklyn Coll; Sp-Lang Path, Childhood Center, **SLP**

Greenstein, Gayle Kaplan 112 Shaw Farm Road, Canton, MA 02021-3435, (617) 878-7100, **SLP**

Greenstein, Katherine Lodenkamp 538 Squire Circle, Clemson, SC 29631, (703) 953-2266, BS 79 Univ of IL - Urbana; MA 80 Univ of IL - Urbana; Sp-Lang Path, Anderson-Oconee Sp-Hrng Serv, **SLP A**

Greenstein, Richard A 1336 East 14th Street, Brooklyn, NY 11230, (212) 375-0673, BS 75 Univ of Bridgeport; MS 79 Columbia Univ Teachers Coll; Sp-Lang Path, Private Practice, **SLP**

Greenstein, Mrs Vicki 74 Broken Tree Road, Newton Center, MA 02159-3449, (617) 964-0447, BS 68 Boston Univ; ME 70 Boston Univ; Aud, VA Outpatient Cl, **A**

Green-Tucknall, Margaret Ann 10 Armstrong Court, Norwalk, CT 06851, (203) 853-9784, MA 88 Southern CT St Univ

Greenwald, Anne L 123-35 82D Road #5F, Kew Gardens, NY 11415, (516) 746-5575, BS 77 SUNY - Center at Albany; MS 78 Adelphi Univ; Sp-Lang Path, Little Village School, **SLP**

Greenwald, Mrs Audrey B 160NW 4th Street, Boca Raton, FL 33432-3826, (305) 391-8444, BS 76 Univ of FL; MS 78 FL St Univ; Sp-Lang Path, Private Practice, **SLP**

Greenwald, Carol A 318 East Nettleton, Jonesboro, AR 72401, (501) 932-4043, BA 63 Univ of North TX; MA 78 Memphis St Univ; 87–Sp-Lang Path Supvr, Jonesboro Human Dev Ctr, **SLP**

Greenwald, Carolyn R CASE-CRC, 51 East Gerty Drive, Champaign, IL 61820, (217) 333-7023, BS 83 IL St Univ - Normal; MS 84 IL St Univ - Normal; Aud, Central Assoc of Special Ed, **A**

Greenwald, Daniel H Otologic Medical Services, 2440 Town Crest Drive, Iowa City, IA 52240, (319) 351-5680, MA 74 Bowling Green St Univ; BA 72 Bowling Green St Univ; Aud, Otologic Med Serv, **A**

Greenwald, Mrs Glenna Griffin 3108 Cypress, Cleveland, OH 44109, (216) 749-3518, BS 74 Bowling Green St Univ; MA 86 Kent St Univ; **SLP**

Greenwald, Jill R 13 Shaded Glen Court, Owings Mills, MD 21117, **SLP**

Greenwald, Judy B 123 North Mansfield Avenue, Los Angeles, CA 90036, **SLP**

Greenwald, Mrs Robin Cassel c/o Larry Greenwald, 235 East 22nd Street #16A, New York, NY 10010, (212) 689-4306, BS 76 SUNY - Center at Albany; MA 82 CUNY - Hunter Coll; 84–Sp/Lang Path, New Rochelle Sch Dist, **SLP**

Greenwalt, Eileen V 311 Bryant, Walla Walla, WA 99362-4141, (509) 529-6032, BS 70 Loma Linda Univ - Riverside; MA 71 CA St Univ - Fullerton; Sp-Lang Path, **SLP**

Greenwell, Mrs Alice R 109 Circle Drive, Shelbina, MO 63468, (314) 588-4609, BS 45 Northeast MO St Univ; MA 73 Northeast MO St Univ; **SLP LM**

Greenwell, Mrs Mary Lorene 7308 NW Anderson Avenue, Vancouver, WA 98665, (206) 696-7256, BA 67 Gonzaga Univ; Sp-Lang Path, Vancouver Sch Dist 37, **SLP**

Greenwood, Becky Zirnstein 1520 North Battin, Wichita, KS 67208, (316) 685-8938, BS 85 OK Christian Coll; MA 86 Wichita St Univ

Greenwood, Mrs Janet Cain 1107 Straight Arrow, San Antonio, TX 78258, (512) 691-0737, BA 80 LA Tech Univ; ME 82 Southwest TX St Univ; Sp-Lang Path, Rehab Inst of San Antonio, **SLP**

Greenwood, Richard Patrick 2502 Woodridge Crescent, Abbotsford, BC, Canada V2S 4E6, (604) 875-2045, BA 80 Western WA Univ; MA 82 Western WA Univ; 82–Aud, Univ Hosp, **A**

Greenwood, Susan Teicher 32 Overlook Drive, Danville, PA 17821, (717) 275-5465, BA 73 CUNY - Brooklyn Coll; MS 86 Bloomsburg Univ of PA; **SLP**

Greenwood, Suzanne 123 South St Louis Street, Lafayette, LA 70506, (318) 988-4120, **SLP**

Greer, Mrs Carol A 25 Alvord Street, Rochester, NY 14609, (716) 461-9192, BS 81 SUNY - Coll at Geneseo; MS 82 Ithaca Coll; Aud, Hearing Center Inc, **A**

Greer, Mrs Deborah Corrine 26425 Springfield Drive, Farmington Hills, MI 48018, (313) 471-2948, SLP, Farmington Schools, **SLP**

Greer, Mrs Lola B R R 1 Box 728, Williamsburg, KY 40769, (606) 549-5092, BS 76 Eastern KY Univ; MA 80 Univ of TN - Knoxville; **SLP**

Greer, Marion P 619 Glen Avenue, Scotia, NY 12302, (518) 377-2988, BA 53 Syracuse Univ; MS 69 Coll of Saint Rose; Sp-Lang Path, Shenendahowa Central Schools, **SLP**

Greer, Phyllis S Fox Pens Road, Shelburne, VT 05482, (802) 985-2838, MS 88 Univ of VT; 88–Sp-Lang Path, Winooski Sch Dist

Greer, Ruth Ellen 5517 Pacific Blvd #4412, Boca Raton, FL 33433, (407) 750-1021, MA 84 CA St Univ - Northridge; BA 78 SUNY - Center at Buffalo; SLP, Broward Co Schools, **SLP**

Greeson, Mrs Patty Dorsett Route 5 Box 208, Chapel Hill, NC 27514, (919) 542-3626, BA 84 Univ of NC - Chapel Hill; MS 85 Univ of NC - Chapel Hill; Sp-Lang Path, Chatham County School System, **SLP**

Greever, Glenna Sue 3030 Bentwood Circle S Dr, Apartment 2-C, Indianapolis, IN 46268, (317) 875-8349, OB 83 Eastern IL Univ; BS 83 Eastern IL Univ; MS 84 Eastern IL Univ; 87–Coord of Speech & Lang Svcs, St Vincent New Hope, **SLP**

Gregg, Ann English 2825 West Spruce Avenue, Fresno, CA 93711, (818) 333-0166, BA 72 CA St Univ - Los Angeles; MA 73 CA St Univ - Los Angeles; LA Co Supt Sch, **SLP**

Gregg, Dr Ellen Meyer University Of Northern Co, McKee Hall #32, Dept Of Comm Disorders, Greeley, CO 80639, (303) 351-1591, BS 74 Northwestern Univ; MA 75 Northwestern Univ; PH 82 (NS) Univ of CO - Boulder; Assistant Professor, Univ of Northern CO, **SLP**

Gregg, Harriette 17 West Lawn Drive, Teaneck, NJ 07666, (212) 694-8032, BA 67 Hampton Univ; MA 68 MI St Univ; **SLP**

Gregg, Mrs Jean Westerman 11 Old Quarry Road, Woodbridge, CT 06525, (203) 397-4830, MA 47 Univ of MI - Ann Arbor; MS 85 Southern CT St Univ; Sp-Lang Path, Amity Regional School Dist #5, **SLP**

Gregg, Rita Ann Cantwell West 1125 22nd Avenue, Spokane, WA 99203, (509) 456-5221, BS 80 West Chester Univ of PA; MS 85 Eastern WA Univ; **SLP**

Gregg-Chlebina, Jerilyn Kay 10428 Sandpiper Road West, Bradenton, FL 33529, (813) 746-5171, MA 84 Memphis St Univ; **SLP**

Gregoire-Koba, Mrs Lucille S 124 Thomas Street, Johnson City, NY 13790, (607) 798-7117, BS 74 Nazareth Coll of Rochester; MS 75 SUNY - Coll at Buffalo; **SLP**

Gregora, April W 17-466 Kenaston Boulevard, Winnipeg, MB, Canada R3N 1Z1, (204) 489-1303, BA 76 Univ of Manitoba - Winnipeg; MA 81 Univ of MN - Minneap-St Paul; Sp-Lang Path, Assiniboine South Sch Div, **SLP**

Gregorash, Charysse M 1109 South Farwell #1, Eau Claire, WI 54701, (715) 832-3622, BA 85 Univ of WI - Eau Claire; MS 87 Univ of WI - Eau Claire; SLP, Sturgeon Bay School District, **SLP**

Gregore, Dale Rebhan 2342 Taggart Court, Wilmington, DE 19810, (215) 793-1212, **SLP**

Gregorio, Mrs Barbara Joan 92-619 Akaula Street, Ewa Beach, HI 96707, BS 63 Univ of Cincinnati; MS 82 Univ of HI - Manoa; SLP, Honolulu Comm Action Prog, **SLP**

Gregorio, Maryann R 812 Robinwood Rd, Washington Township, NJ 07675, (201) 666-3211, BA 72 Montclair St Coll; MA 77 Montclair St Coll; Sp-Lang Path, Secaucus Board of Education, **SLP**

Gregory, Anna Vagin Childrens Health Council, 700 Sand Hills Road, Palo Alto, CA 94304, (415) 326-5530, BA 79 Univ of CA - Santa Barbara; MS 81 Univ of Redlands; Director, St Lukes Hrng & Sp Cen, **SLP**

Gregory, Bonnie R 423 Blackstone Drive, Centerville, OH 45459, (513) 433-6710, BS 65 Bowling Green St Univ; MS 67 Univ of MI - Ann Arbor; Sp-Lang Path, Montgomery Co Bd of Ed, **SLP**

Gregory, Carolyn B 2400 Brown Avenue, Evanston, IL 60201, (312) 328-1460, MA 52 Northwestern Univ; 76–Sp-Lang Path, Private Practice, **SLP ACE**

Gregory, Carrie Frances 9 North Church Street #207, Schenectady, NY 12305-1623, (518) 382-4550, BA 84 SUNY - Coll at Cortland; MS 85 Coll of Saint Rose; SLP, Sunnyview Hosp & Rehab Ctr, **SLP**

Gregory, Charlotte Keane HCR 70 Box 50, Van Lear, KY 41265, (606) 886-8586, BS 83 Western KY Univ; MA 84 Univ of TN - Knoxville; Sp-Lang Path, Crigger-Mullins Sp Lang & Learning Svcs, **SLP**

Gregory, Dr Hugo H 2400 Brown Avenue, Evanston, IL 60201, (312) 491-5073, BS 51 Northwestern Univ; MA 52 Northwestern Univ; PH 59 (Sp-Lang Path) Northwestern Univ; 62–Prof, Northwestern Univ, **SLP F**

Gregory, Janis A 25670 Fountain Park Dr W, Apartment 186, Novi, MI 48050, (313) 344-9443, BA 84 MI St Univ; MA 85 MI St Univ; 87–Dir of Sp-Lang Path, Lakeshore ENT, **SLP**

Gregory, Mrs Judith M 619 Vermont, Dinuba, CA 93618, (209) 528-4751, BA 63 CA St Univ - Fresno; MA 73 CA St Univ - Fresno; SLP, Tulare County Dept Education, **SLP**

Gregory, Karen Sue 35219 Norene, Westland, MI 48185, **SLP**

Gregory, Mrs Marian Frances 311 Chesterfield Avenue, Centerville, MD 21617, (301) 758-1848, BA 76 Loyola Coll; MS 77 Loyola Coll; Sp-Lang Path, Private Practice, **SLP**

Gregory, Mrs Mary PO Drawer 220, Mount Vernon, KY 40456, (606) 256-5431, BS 67 Univ of TN - Knoxville; MA 71 Univ of KY; Sp-Lang Path, Rockcastle Co Bd of Ed, **SLP**

Gregory, Mary L East Tennessee Hearing Center, 605 Hale Street, Johnson City, TN 37601, (615) 928-2885, BS 65 Maryville Coll; MA 67 Univ of TN - Knoxville; 85–Aud, East TN Hrng Ctr, **A**

Gregory, Mrs Roberta A P O Box 424, Louisville, KY 40201, (502) 584-9781, BS 76 Eastern KY Univ; MS 81 Univ of WY; Sp-Lang Path, Harrison County School System, **SLP**

Gregory, Sharon A 14 North Lombardy Street, Richmond, VA 23220, (804) 359-2095, BS 72 Univ of VA - Charlottesville; ME 74 Univ of VA - Charlottesville; ME 81 Univ of VA - Charlottesville; Aud/Sp-Lang Path, Childrens Hosp Richmond, **SLP A**

Gregory, Susan 1709 Holt, Fort Worth, TX 76103, **SLP**

Gregson, Jo Ann 715 20th Street #208, Vero Beach, FL 32960, (305) 567-7465, BS 83 Southern IL Univ-Edwardsvill; MA 85 Univ of IL - Urbana; Clinical Services, Sch Dist of Indian River Co, **SLP**

Greig, Rhonda Banke 1110 North Verdugo Road, Apartment 202, Glendale, CA 91206, (818) 240-8000, BA 80 CA St Univ - Northridge; MA 82 CA St Univ - Northridge; SLP, Glendale Adventist Medical Cen, **SLP**

Greis, Sharon M 833 Twining Road, Dresher, PA 19025, (215) 576-1315, BA 69 Temple Univ; MA 71 Temple Univ; 88–Sp-Lang Path, UCP Assoc, **SLP**

Grekco, Mrs Kathy 400 Front Street, Berea, OH 44017, (216) 459-3166, BS 73 Bowling Green St Univ; MA 80 Univ of Akron; 82–Supervisor Sp-Lang Path, Cleveland Metro General Hosp, **SLP**

Grekin, Terry Rosenblatt 1750 Broadway, San Francisco, CA 94109, (415) 421-1550, BA 70 IN Univ - Bloomington; MS 71 Univ of MI - Ann Arbor; Dir, Union Square Hearing Center, **A**

Gremaud, Janice M 218 S Maryland #6, Conrad, MT 59425, (406) 278-3784, BS 86 Southern IL Univ-Edwardsvill; MS 87 Southern IL Univ-Edwardsvill

Gremillion, Grace P 4201 Saxon Street, Metairie, LA 70002, (504) 888-3316, BA 69 LA St Univ - Baton Rouge; MA 71 LA St Univ - Baton Rouge; Sp-Lang Path/, Jefferson Sp & Lang Cen, **SLP**

Gremillion, Michelle Ann 2705 Pecan Drive, Chalmette, LA 70043, (504) 271-3038, BA 84 Southeastern LA Univ; OM 88 LA St Univ - N O Medical Ctr

Gremillion, Mrs Suzanne B 105 Blouin Street, Raceland, LA 70394, (504) 446-6116, BA 71 LA St Univ - Baton Rouge; MA 73 LA St Univ - Baton Rouge; 86–Sp-Lang Path, Lafourche Parish Schs, **SLP**

Grenier, Mrs Julienne Haro 5640 Read Boulevard, Suite 400, New Orleans, LA 70127, (504) 241-9533, BS 79 Saint Mary's Dominican Coll; MA 80 Memphis St Univ; Aud, Doctor's Hearing Aids, **A**

Grenker, Mrs Harriet A 4 Cory Court, Parsippany, NJ 07054, (201) 263-5896, BA 69 SUNY - Center at Albany; ME 70 Northeastern Univ; SLP, Montville Public Schools, **SLP**

Gresch, Anna M K W266 N7220 Kettle Ridge Ct, Sussex, WI 53089, BS 67 Univ of WI - Madison; MS 73 Bradley Univ; Cl Instr, U of WI - Milwaukee, **SLP**

Grese, Carolyn A 10037 Pallisers Terrace, Charlotte, NC 28210, (904) 241-4635, BS 74 Univ of GA; ME 76 Eastern MI Univ; **SLP**

Gresham, Richard Lee 505 North Columbia Avenue, Sheffield, AL 35660, (205) 386-7040, BS 83 Auburn Univ - Auburn; OM 85 Auburn Univ - Auburn; 86–Aud, F Allen Long MD, **A**

Gresham, Sharon Lea 5 Illoura Street, Wallsend, New South Wales, Australia 2287, BS 77 Mercy Coll; MS 80 Adelphi Univ; Sp-Lang Path, Wallsend Dist Hosp, **SLP**

Gress, Carla Delassus 274 Boston Street, North Andover, MA 01845, (617) 353-5640, BS 77 Saint Louis Univ; MA 78 Saint Louis Univ; 86–Sp-Lang Path, Boston Univ, **SLP**

Gress, Mrs Susan A 723 First Avenue, Antigo, WI 54409, (715) 623-7467, MS 87 Univ of WI - Madison

Greth, Maxine T 855 North Park Road #M-301, Wyomissing, PA 19610, **SLP**

Greve, Mrs Nancy L J 1058 Hackberry Circle, Rochester Hills, MI 48309, (313) 652-0691, BA 69 MI St Univ; MA 73 Eastern MI Univ

Greven, Mrs Carol Maloff 1244 Dartmouth Road, Flossmoor, IL 60422, MS 85 Governors St Univ; Sp-Lang Path, Southwest Coop for Special Ed, **SLP**

Grever, Karl H Grever Hearing Service, Doctors Bldg 500 South Un, Suite 307, Little Rock, AR 72205, (501) 660-1384, BS 73 Univ of AR - Little Rock; MS 79; Aud, Private Practice, **A**

Grey, Dr Howard A 7140 Balboa Boulevard, Van Nuys, CA 91406, (818) 785-2911, BA 57 Univ of CA - Los Angeles; MA 59 Univ of CA - Los Angeles; PH 63 (Sp Path/Aud) Univ of CA - Los Angeles; 69–Dir, Comm Sp & Hrng Ctr, **SLP A**

Grey, Mrs Laura S 15 Tappentown Lane, Brookville, NY 11545, (516) 378-3900, BA 62 CUNY - Brooklyn Coll; MS 63 Purdue Univ - West Lafayette; Sp-Lang Path, Merrick Ufsd, **SLP ACE**

Grey, Linnea R 6400 Pillsbury Avenue South, Richfield, MN 55423, BS 77 CO St Univ; MS 78 Univ of ND; 87–Coord, Minneapolis Children's Med Ctr, **SLP**

Grey, Monica Willoughby 33 Darling Avenue, New Rochelle, NY 10804, **SLP**

Grey, Yona Leigh 41065 Southwind Drive, Canton, MI 48188, (313) 397-8656, BS 83 Old Dominion Univ; MS 85 Univ of MI - Ann Arbor; 86–Sp-Lang Path, Private Practice, **SLP**

Greyerbiehl, Dr Dianne H 9635 Sea Shadow, Columbia, MD 21046, (301) 454-3042, BA 68 Univ of MD - College Park; MA 70 Univ of MD - College Park; PH 80 (Sp Path) Univ of MD - College Park; Assoc Dir, Univ of MD CRMS, **SLP**

Greytak, Sharyn P 4330 Pine Lake Drive, Medina, OH 44256-9031, (216) 723-4330, BA 75 Cleveland St Univ; MS 76 Murray St Univ; Sp/Lang Path, Avon Lake City Sch, **SLP**

Gribben, Dana Jo 1237 Evelyn Avenue, Berkeley, CA 94706, (415) 548-6100, BA 68 TX Christian Univ; MS 70 Purdue Univ - West Lafayette; Consult, Decker Communication, **SLP**

Gribin, Barbara A 63 Cypress Neck Road, Lincroft, NJ 07738, (201) 741-8073, BA 72 CUNY - Queens Coll; MA 74 Montclair St Coll; Sp-Lang Path, Sp Ther Serv, **SLP**

Grice, Rita B Rt 4 Box 264, Forest, MS 39074, (601) 469-4244, OB 73 Univ of MS; OM 75 Univ of MS; MS 81 Univ Southern MS-Hattiesburg; Sp-Lang Path, Forest PS, **SLP A**

Grider, Cathy Belcher P O Box 1852, Waskom, TX 75692-1852, (318) 632-4889, BA 79 Ouachita Baptist Univ; MS 84 Univ of North TX; 87–Sp-Lang Path, Willis-Knighton Med Ctr, **SLP**

Grider, Mrs Elizabeth Callaway 4842 Partridge Run Road, Louisville, KY 40213, (502) 897-2661, BA 83 Univ of KY; MS 85 Univ of Louisville; Sp-Lang Path, Bullitt Co Board of Education, **SLP**

Grider, Mrs Joy Stephens P O Box 267, Russell Springs, KY 42642, (502) 343-4086, BA 68 Univ of KY; MA 78 Western KY Univ; 74–Sp-Lang Path, Russell Co Bd of Educ

Grider, Robert B 341 Southdale Medical Bldg, 6545 France Avenue South, Minneapolis, MN 55435, (612) 926-1867, BA 73 Bob Jones Univ; MS 78 Eastern IL Univ; Sp-Lang Path, Minnesota Voice&Speech Clinic, **SLP**

Gridley, Mrs Katherine L 6700 Lake Charlene Drive, Pensacola, FL 32506, (904) 453-8154, BA 82 Miami Univ - Oxford; MA 83 Bowling Green St Univ; 88–Sp-Lang Path, Natl Hlth Corp, **SLP**

Griebner, Mrs Sandra S 330 South Stadium, Oregon, OH 43616, (419) 691-5444, BS 80 OH Univ - Athens; MA 82 OH Univ - Athens; 87–Sp/Lang Path, St Charles Hosp, **SLP**

Grieco, Jayne Fagan 61 Nyack Street, Watertown, MA 02172, (617) 489-2560, BS 79 Univ of NH; MA 81 Univ of FL; Sp-Lang Path, Private Practice, **SLP**

Grieco, Mrs Nancy Boyd 10 Ivy Glen Lane, Lawrenceville, NJ 08648, BS 63 Northwestern Univ; MA 64 Northwestern Univ; Sp-Lang Path, Princeton Regional Schools, **SLP**

Grieg, Diana H P O Box 610, Isle of Palms, SC 29451, (803) 886-4352, BA 44 CUNY - Hunter Coll; MA 45 Columbia Univ Teachers Coll; PH 85 (Sp-Path) New York Univ; 86–Pvt Practice, Grieg Assoc, **SLP LM**

Griener, Tania D 3520 Roman Street, Metairie, LA 70001, (504) 830-4424, BS 70 LA St Univ - Baton Rouge; MA 72 Tulane Univ; 82–Asst Coord-Sp-Lang-Hrng Svc, Jefferson Parish PS, **SLP**

Griepenburg, Mrs Susan Tanger 35 Hillsdale Road, East Brunswick, NJ 08816, (201) 968-1337, BA 77 Rutger's St Univ - Douglas Coll; MS 79 Rutger's St Univ - Douglas Coll; **SLP**

Grier, Mrs Marla S 400 Southridge, South Sioux City, NE 68776, (402) 494-1917, BA 76 Wichita St Univ; MA 77 Wichita St Univ; 88–Sp-Lang Path, South Sioux City Schs, **SLP**

Grier, Mrs Tose Foote 1342 El Camino Drive, Concord, CA 94521, (415) 672-5059, BS 44 Univ of MN - Minneap-St Paul; MA 81 St Mary's Coll of CA; Retired, **SLP LM**

Griesenauer, Mrs Diane Marie 6607 Kingsway, Affton, MO 63123, (314) 351-9954, BS 77 Northeast MO St Univ; MA 78 Northeast MO St Univ; Sp-Lang Path, Spec Sch Dist/St Louis County, **SLP**

Grieser, Dianne Lynne 422 N E 82nd Street, Seattle, WA 98115, (206) 324-8200, MA 76 Univ of SD - Vermillion; PH 84 (NS) Univ of WA; 88–Sp-Lang Path, Valley Med Ctr, **SLP**

Grieshop, Mrs Cheryl Graves 405 West Blackman Street, Harvard, IL 60033-2327, (815) 943-4380, BS 85 Bradley Univ; MS 86 Marquette Univ; 86–Sp-Lang Path, Spec Educ Dist of McHenry Co, **SLP**

Grieve, Mrs Susan M K 52 Dalewood Drive, Tonawanda, NY 14150-5718, (716) 691-8206, BA 72 SUNY - Coll at Cortland; MA 76 SUNY - Center at Buffalo; Sp-Lang Path, Lang Dev Prgm of NY, **SLP**

Griffall, John 18607 E 18th Terrace N, Independence, MO 64058, (816) 271-7613, BS 76 Central MO St Univ; MS 78 Central MO St Univ; Sp-Lang Path, Heartland Health Systems, **SLP**

Griffer, Mona R 2904 203rd Street, Bayside, NY 11360, (718) 352-4876, BA 79 CUNY - Brooklyn Coll; MS 82 CUNY - Brooklyn Coll; Sp-Lang Path, Birch Early Chldhood Cen, **SLP**

Griffin, Mrs Beverly G 7 Mullaney Road, Greenville, TX 75401, (214) 455-2112, BS 72 East TX St Univ - Commerce; MS 73 East TX St Univ - Commerce; Dir/Sp Ed, Greenville ISD, **SLP**

Griffin, Beverly J 3108 Americano Court, Fairfield, CA 94533, (415) 685-0412, BS 74 CO St Univ; MA 75 Wichita St Univ; Aud, Kaiser Permanente Med Cen, **A**

Griffin, Mrs Candice Burgess 269 Country Club Lane, Paducah, KY 42001, (502) 665-5197, BS 74 Murray St Univ; MS 82 Murray St Univ; Sp-Lang Path, Ballard Co Bd of Ed, **SLP**

Griffin, Cheryl B 135 Kingspoint Blvd, Slidell, LA 70461, (504) 641-2370, BS 80 Univ Southern MS-Hattiesburg; MS 81 Univ Southern MS-Hattiesburg; **SLP**

Griffin, Eileen Leahy 143 South Main Street, Manchester, CT 06040, (203) 649-5198, BA 78 Loyola Coll; MS 79 Loyola Coll; Sp-Lang Path, Manchester Public Schools, **SLP**

Griffin, Elizabeth Barnes 700 Robertsville Road, Oak Ridge, TN 37830, (615) 482-8524, BS 73 Univ of TN - Knoxville; MA 75 Memphis St Univ; Sp/Lang Path, Oak Ridge Schs, **SLP**

Griffin, Mrs Fannie D 3538 Kindling Drive, Augusta, GA 30906, (404) 790-2101, BA 77 SC St Coll; MA 78 SC St Coll; SLP, Gracewood St Sch & Hosp, **SLP**

Griffin, Flavia Ramcharan 745 Boulevard Northeast, Orangeburg, SC 29115, (803) 536-1007, MA 85 SC St Coll; 86–Sp-Lang Path, Dist #5 Schs, **SLP**

Griffin, Mrs Janice Hunter Rt 2 Box 95-C, Valdosta, GA 31601, (912) 242-5276, **SLP**

Griffin, Jeffrey D 1300 28th Street South, Suite 8, Great Falls, MT 59405, (406) 791-2270, BA 72 Univ of ND; MS 75 Gallaudet Coll; Aud, Cascade Audiology Services, **A**

Griffin, Dr Kathleen F 109 Hazel Path, Hendersonville, TN 37077, (615) 822-8430, BS 65 Univ of WI - Madison; MA 66 Stanford Univ; PH 71 (Sp-Lang Path-Aud) Univ of OR; 88–Exec Vice Priesident, Rebound Inc, **SLP A F**

Griffin, Kyle Mark 4815 Darragh, Little Rock, AR 72204, (501) 778-1111, BA 80 Univ of AR - Little Rock; MS 84 Univ of AR - Little Rock; Sp-Lang Path, **SLP**

Griffin, Mrs Margaret Ann Lot 193, Stonegate Trailer Park, Auburn, AL 36830-6607, (205) 272-0171, BS 84 Delta St Univ; OM 85 Auburn Univ - Auburn; **SLP**

Griffin, Margaret Macy 1070 Delta Avenue #2, Cincinnati, OH 45208, (573) 872-2481, BS 83 Univ of Cincinnati; MA 85 Univ of Cincinnati; **SLP**

Griffin, Mary Elizabeth 17 Raynham Drive, Syosset, NY 11791, (516) 921-2008, BA 74 Molloy Coll; MS 76 Adelphi Univ; Sp-Lang Path, Deer Park Pub Schs, **SLP**

Griffin, Mrs Melinda P 2444 Meadow View, Bedford, TX 76021, (817) 283-6448, BS 74 OK St Univ; MS 76 Univ of OK Medical Center; Sp-Lang Path, Arlington ISD, **SLP A**

Griffin, Michael W Michael W Griffin Ma Inc, P O Box 231, 3121 Greenfield, Petoskey, MI 49770, (616) 347-1031, BA 66 MI St Univ; MA 68 MI St Univ; Sp-Lang Path, Private Practice, **SLP**

Griffin, Pamela T 29 Knollwood Road, Reading, MA 01867, (617) 944-0753, BS 86 Univ of MA - Amherst; MA 88 Univ of MA - Amherst; 88–Sp-Lang Path, Reading PS Sys

Griffin, Mrs Ruth Goesele 6599 Happy Valley Road, Anderson, CA 96007, (916) 275-1577, BA 53 CA St Univ - Los Angeles; MA 80 CA St Univ - Chico; 64–Sp-Lang Path, Shasta Lake Union Sch Dist, **SLP ACE**

Griffin, Sarah H 5 Hidden-Brook Lane, Signal Mountain, TN 37377, **SLP**

Griffin, Sharon Louise P O Box 164, Newfields, NH 03856, (603) 778-7311, BS 82 Univ of NH; MA 86 OH Univ - Athens; Sp-Lang Path, Exeter Hosp, **SLP**

Griffin, Stephen J 19 Windermere Road, Dorchester, MA 02125, (617) 745-2100, BA 74 Tufts Univ; MS 79 Emerson Coll; Sp/Lang Path, Brookline Pub Sch, **SLP ACE**

Griffin, Suzanne A Route 12 Box 187, Fayetteville, AR 72703, (501) 443-1929, BS 86 Univ of AR - Fayetteville; MS 87 Univ of AR - Fayetteville; 87–Sp-Lang Path, Ozark Guidance Ctr, **SLP**

Griffin, Theresa M 302 N Saginaw Road, Midland, MI 48640, (517) 631-1100, BS 84 Marquette Univ; MS 86 Marquette Univ; **SLP ACE**

Griffin, Thomas J 510 St Davids Avenue, St Davids, PA 19087, (215) 284-8574, **SLP**

Griffin, Mrs Wendy N 3002 Tonya Drive, Kinston, NC 28501, (919) 527-8649, MS 88 East Carolina Univ; 88–Aud, Audiologic Hearing Ctr

Griffin-Gomez, Rosemary 6 Sunstone Drive, Poughkeepsie, NY 12603, (914) 473-3298, BA 81 Adelphi Univ; MA 83 CUNY - Hunter Coll; Sp-Lang Path, St Francis Hosp, **SLP**

Griffin-Spears, Mrs Dora M 3607 Storm Creek Drive, Houston, TX 77088, (713) 847-1729, BS 78 Univ of North TX; MS 79 Univ of North TX; Sp-Lang Path, Private Practice, **SLP**

Griffin-Ziebart, Mrs Susanne Elizabeth 85 Coulee Road #1, Hudson, WI 54016, (608) 221-8961, BS 84 Univ of WI - River Falls; MS 87 Univ of WI - Madison

Griffith, Amy Marian 453 Pompano, Hitchcock, TX 77563, (409) 935-4526, BS 79 Southwest TX St Univ; MS 80 Univ of North TX; Sp/Lang Path, Gregory Portland ISD, **SLP**

Griffith, Mrs Avis B 907 Somersby Lane, Matthews, NC 28105, (704) 847-7438, OB 76 Univ of GA; OM 81 Univ of SC - Columbia; Sp-Lang Path, Private Practice, **SLP**

Griffith, Mrs Carol Rose 3504 Grooms Street, Austin, TX 78705, (513) 478-8139, BS 81 Baylor Univ; MS 83 Univ of TX - Dallas; Sp-Lang Path, Austin ISD, **SLP**

Griffith, Cheryl Ann 6615 County Road 191, #B, Bellevue, OH 44811, (419) 483-2749, BS 86 Bowling Green St Univ; MS 87 Bowling Green St Univ; **SLP**

Griffith, David L 122 West 200 North, Hyrum, UT 84319, (801) 245-6506, BS 67 Univ of WY; MS 68 Univ of UT; Aud/SLP, Private Practice, **SLP**

Griffith, Mrs Dawn Robertson 1618 Lakeside Drive, Greeley, CO 80631, (601) 327-5367, BS 64 Univ of TN - Knoxville; MA 65 Univ of AL- Tuscaloosa; Sp-Lang Path, Weld County District 6, **SLP**

Griffith, Elizabeth 1334 Queens Road West, Charlotte, NC 28207, (704) 333-5839, BA 60 Converse Coll; ME 74 Univ of SC - Columbia; **SLP**

Griffith, Dr Francis A 1618 Lakeside Drive, Greeley, CO 80631, (601) 329-4750, BA 59 Univ of MD - College Park; MS 61 PA St Univ - Univ Park; PH 65 (NS) PA St Univ - Univ Park; Prof/Chr Dept Commun Dis, U of No CO, **SLP F**

Griffith, Mrs Gail S 55 Dower Road, South Windsor, CT 06074, (203) 528-7544, BA 76 Univ of CT; MS 79 Southern CT St Univ; Sp-Lang Path, Private Practice, **SLP**

Griffith, Jeffrey Samuel 842 Christy Court, Naval Air Station, Pensacola, FL 32508, (904) 456-7494, Branch Med Clinic Long Beach, **A**

Griffith, Dr Jerry Professional Trends, 10833 Farragut Hills Blvd, Knoxville, TN 37922, (615) 675-5100, BS 54 Eastern IL Univ; MS 57 Univ of IL - Urbana; PH 61 (NS) Univ of IL - Urbana; 87–Pres, Professional Trends, **SLP A**

Griffith, Karan Elizabeth 7050 John T White Road, Apartment 1049, Fort Worth, TX 76112, (817) 496-6251, BS 85 Eastern MI Univ; MS 87 Univ of North TX; 88–Sp-Lang Path, Private Practice, **SLP**

Griffith, Patricia M 802 Washington Avenue, Santa Monica, CA 90403, **SLP**

Griffith, Dr Penny L 3580 Adaline Drive, Stow, OH 44224-3956, (216) 686-9836, PH (NS); Associate Professor, Kent State University, **SLP**

Griffith, Sharon Linda Box 2668, Melville, SK, Canada S0A 2P0, (306) 728-4873, MS 87 Minot St Univ; 87–Sp-Lang Path, Southern Shared Services

Griffith, Mrs Susan H 5236 Hialeah Drive, Jackson, MS 39211, (601) 956-3366, BS 72 MS Univ for Women; MA 73 Memphis St Univ; 88–Sp/Lang Path, Covenant Presbyterian Preschool, **SLP**

Griffith, Traci Marie 806 Mountain Valley Drive, Nashville, TN 37209-5111, (615) 356-5754, BS 83 Miami Univ - Oxford; MA 84 Kent St Univ; Speech/Language Pathologist, Rebound Inc, **SLP**

Griffith, Dr Twila E Professional Trends, 10833 Farragut Hills Blvd, Knoxville, TN 37922, (615) 675-5100, BS 67 Eastern IL Univ; MS 69 Eastern IL Univ; PH 75 (NS) Univ of IL - Urbana; Dir of Sp Lang and Hrng Serv, Sarah Bush Lincoln Hlth Cen, **SLP**

Griffiths, Cecilia Marie 427-G Tradewinds Drive, Fayetteville, NC 28304, (919) 323-6151, BS 82 OH St Univ; MA 84 OH Univ - Athens; SLP, St Francis Rehabilitation Hosp, **SLP**

Griffiths, Heather 36 Stoneham, Gardiner, ME 04345, (207) 782-1680, **SLP**

Griffiths, Jana Lee 1900 Solera Drive, Columbus, OH 43229, (614) 864-2406, BS 84 OH Univ - Athens; MA 85 Univ of TN - Knoxville; Sp-Lang Path, Franklin Co Bd of Mental Ret & Dev Disabilities, **SLP**

Griffiths, Mary N W221 N2653 Cherrywood Ct, Waukesha, WI 53186, **SLP**

Griffiths, Scott Keith 2504 1/2 South Anderson, Urbana, IL 61801, (217) 333-2230, BA 81 Univ of Rochester; MA 84 Univ of IL - Urbana; **A**

Griffo, Margaret K 6801 Mac Beth Drive, Anchorage, AK 99516, (907) 346-2483, BS 73 Saint Lawrence Univ; MA 76 Montclair St Coll; Sp-Lang Path, Anchorage Sch Dist, **SLP**

Grigar, Mrs Janice G Route 1 47-C, Medical Lake, WA 99022-9706, (509) 299-7788, BA 74 Southwest TX St Univ; ME 76 Southwest TX St Univ; Eastern WA U, **SLP**

Grigg, Mrs Ann Marie 2601 Nonesuch Road #1405, Abilene, TX 79606, (915) 692-4053, MS 88 Univ of AR - Fayetteville; 88–Sp-Lang Path, Abilene State Sch

Griggs, April S 3139 Casa Loma, Bonita, CA 92002, (619) 470-7332, BA 69 CA St Univ - Fresno; MA 72 CA St Univ - Fresno; Sp/Lang Path, Private Practice, **SLP**

Griglione, Mrs Dolores Bertucco 2718 Park Place, Des Moines, IA 50312, (515) 247-4174, BS 69 Univ of IL - Urbana; MA 72 Northeast MO St Univ; Sp/Lang Path, Mercy Hosp Med Cen, **SLP**

Grigsby, Cynthia L 17531 Chatham Drive, Tustin, CA 92680, (714) 544-7415, BA 80 Univ of CA - Santa Cruz; MA 85 Univ of TN - Knoxville; Sp-Lang Path, Garden Grove USD, **SLP**

Grigsby, Diana Mizell 7692 Timberdale Drive, Columbus, GA 31909, (404) 568-0286, BA 75 Univ of AR - Fayetteville; MA 76 Univ of AR - Fayetteville; Sp-Lang Path, Columbus Speech & Language Cen, **SLP**

Grigson, Mrs Sharon 2436 Hyannis Lane, Crofton, MD 21114, BA 77 Ouachita Baptist Univ; MA 79 Northwestern Univ; **SLP**

Grijalva, Lillian Dolores 1810 Halfmoon Drive, Las Cruces, NM 88005, (505) 877-0400, BA 80 NM St Univ; MA 82 NM St Univ; Sp-Lang Path, Albuquerque Public Schools, **SLP**

Grilley, Mrs Beryl H c/o Steve Taylor, 5317-A W Sylvester, Pasco, WA 99301, (509) 545-6756, MS; **SLP LM**

Grilo, Nanette Renee 720 Spruce, Kansas City, MO 64124, (816) 765-7772, BS 82 Saint Louis Univ; MA 84 Saint Louis Univ; Sp-Lang Path, Timbre Hrng & Sp Ctr, **SLP**

Grim, Mrs Elli 6044 Timberwood Circle, Apartment #227, Fort Myers, FL 33908, (813) 936-0813, BA 81 Ball St Univ; MA 85 Ball St Univ; **SLP**

Grim, Michael Allan 524-3 Wood Street #3, West Lafayette, IN 47906, (317) 743-9439, MS 88 Purdue Univ - West Lafayette

Grim, Virginia S 114 South Laurel, Kutztown, PA 19530-1509, (215) 683-6108, BA 73 Western WA Univ; MA 77 Wichita St Univ; 86–Aud, Private Practice, **A**

Grimard, Dianne D 566 Buckeye Street, Vacaville, CA 95688, (916) 795-4585, BA 73 Univ of MA - Amherst; MA 75 Univ of the Pacific; Resource Specialist, Winters Joint USD, **SLP**

Grimes, Alison M 542-A Presidio Boulevard, San Francisco, CA 94129, (415) 863-4710, BA 72 Humboldt St Univ; MA 73 Humboldt St Univ; MA 74 Univ of Denver; Dir of Aud, Hrng Soc for the Bay Area Inc, **A**

Grimes, Mrs Beth 223 Lazy Hollow Drive, Gaithersburg, MD 20878-2775, BS 81 PA St Univ - Univ Park; MA 82 George Washington Univ; SLP, Ridley and Fill Speech Assoc, **SLP**

Grimes, Dr Charles T SUNY Health Science Center, 766 Irving Avenue, Syracuse, NY 13210, (315) 473-4806, BA 65 Univ of MD - College Park; MA 66 MI St Univ; PH 77 (NS) Syracuse Univ; 82–Aud, SUNY Health Science Ctr, **A**

Grimes, Jan Elaine 502 1st Street Southeast, Waukon, IA 52172, (319) 568-4818, BA 79 Univ of Northern IA; MA 87 Northeast MO St Univ; 87–Sp-Lang Path, Keystone AEA, **SLP**

Grimes, Karen W 1515 Sandy Springs #1903, Houston, TX 77042, (713) 465-4978, BA 69 Southern Methodist Univ; MA 70 Southern Methodist Univ; Sp-Lang Path, Spring Branch ISD, **SLP**

Grimes, Mrs Karin Dale 1814 Rosewood, Benton, AR 72015, (501) 624-4411, BS 81 Henderson St Univ; MS 83 Univ of AR - Little Rock; Sp/Lang Path, Hot Springs Rehab Cen Hosp, **SLP**

Grimes, Mrs Linda L 8350 Zenith Drive, Baldwinsville, NY 13027, BS 73 SUNY - Center at Albany; MS 74 Syracuse Univ; Aud, Syracuse Cty Sch Dist, **A**

Grimes, Mrs Marian M 6 Schoolhouse Road, Dudley, MA 01570, (508) 248-7878, BA 76 Univ of CT; MS 78 Southern CT St Univ; Sp-Lang Path, **SLP**

Grimes, Mrs Marybess V 2451 Angelo Drive, Los Angeles, CA 90077, (805) 252-9580, BA 43 Univ of CO - Boulder; MA 74 CA St Univ - Northridge; Retired, Saugus Union School District, **SLP**

Grimes, Nancy Jensen 3019 Orleans Drive, Grand Island, NE 68801, (308) 381-2350, BS 79 Kearney St Coll; MA 80 Kearney St Coll; Sp-Lang Path, Grand Island Pub Sch, **SLP**

Grimes, Ruth Katherine 340 Mission Hills Way, Colorado Springs, CO 80921, (719) 472-1803, BS 82 Univ of NE - Lincoln; MS 84 Univ of NE - Lincoln; Sp-Lang Path, Academy Sch Dist # 20, **SLP**

Grimley, Mrs Judith L 5 Lakenheath Court, Potomac, MD 20854, (301) 983-0147, BS 61 Boston Univ; MA 82 Univ of MD - College Park; SLP, Montg Co Pub Sch, **SLP**

Grimm, Darryl M Route 5, Canyon Oaks, Claremore, OK 74017, **A**

Grimm, Diann D Children's Health Council, 700 Sand Hill Road, Palo Alto, CA 94304, (415) 326-5530, BS 76 Central MI Univ; MA 77 Univ of ME - Orono; 88–Sp-Lang Path, Children's Health Council, **SLP**

Grimm, Gretchen A 224-5 Selby Ranch Road, Sacramento, CA 95864, (916) 489-9587, BA 71 William Jewell Coll; MA 73 Univ of Tulsa; Self Employed, **A**

Grimm, Mrs Jennifer Herbert 914 Douglas Avenue, Nashville, TN 37204, (615) 320-5353, BS 84 Univ of TN - Knoxville; MS 87 Vanderbilt Univ; 87–Sp-Lang Path, Bill Wilkerson Hrng & Sp Ctr, **SLP**

Grimm, Karen Jane 6426 West Powell Place, Wauwatosa, WI 53213, (414) 567-7639, BS 76 Univ of WI - Stevens Point; MS 77 Univ of WI - Stevens Point; Aud, Hrng Serv Ltd, **A**

Grimm, Mrs Susan S 2545 North 95th Street, Wauwatosa, WI 53226, BS 59 Univ of WI - Milwaukee; MS 81 Univ of WI - Milwaukee; Sp-Lang Path, Pub Schs, **SLP**

Grimm, William A, III 3149 Sylvania Avenue, Toledo, OH 43613, (419) 473-1456, BA 76 OH St Univ; MA 79 OH St Univ; Aud, Beltone Toledo Company, **A F**

Grimmett, Mrs Rachel W 7415 Tetela, Houston, TX 77083, (713) 498-8110, BS 77 Univ of Houston - Univ Park; MA 78 Univ of Houston - Univ Park; Educ Diagn, Lamar Cons ISD, **SLP**

Grimmett, Sharon G 2402 West 47th, Pine Bluff, AR 71603, (501) 535-7467, OM 88 Univ of Central AR

Grinage, Diane M 4555 Pinecrest Heights Dr, Annandale, VA 22003, (703) 941-8143, BS 73 SUNY - Coll at New Paltz; MS 75 PA St Univ - Univ Park; SLP, Fairfax Co Pub Sch, **SLP**

Grindle, Mrs Marsha D 3021 West Dallas, Broken Arrow, OK 74012, (918) 252-1296, BA 76 Univ of OK - Norman; MS 78 Univ of OK Medical Center; **SLP**

Grindstaff, Mrs Barbara D 335 St Edward Lane, Florissant, MO 63033, (314) 569-8100, BS 74 Southeast MO St Univ; MA 76 OH St Univ; SLP, Sp Sch Dist of St Louis Co, **SLP**

Grine, Clifford 110 Lyle Drive, Hermitage, PA 16148, (412) 347-7620, BS 54 PA St Univ - Univ Park; ME 60 PA St Univ - Univ Park; Sp-Lang Path/Aud, Sharon Cty Sch Dist, **SLP A**

Grinsell, Mrs Valerie Ann Box 1361, Lamoille, NV 89828, (702) 753-6820, BA 76 CA St Univ - Sacramento; MA 86 Univ of Northern IA; Sp-Lang Path, Elko Co Sch Dist, **SLP**

Grinstead, Dr Geraldine LaCourt 18750 South Lowrie Loop, Eagle River, AK 99577, (907) 694-7940, BS 78 Univ of WI - Stevens Point; MS 79 Univ of WI - Stevens Point; PH 88 (Aud) OH St Univ; 88–Research Assoc, Drs McGuire & Frost, **A**

Grinstead, M Jennifer 105 Kingwood Drive, McMinnville, OR 97128, BA 72 Miami Univ - Oxford; MA 77 Western WA Univ; Sp/Lang Path, Yamhill Co Esd, **SLP**

Grisham, Robert C Box 2691, Covina, CA 91722, (213) 226-5074, **A**

Grismer, Tamara J 1007 Washington Avenue SE #13, Bemidji, ND 56601, (218) 335-6700, BS 85 Moorhead St Univ; MS 86 Moorhead St Univ; Sp-Lang Path, Bemidji Reg Interdistrict Council, **SLP**

Grispino, Mrs Linda M 21493 Riviera Drive, Fairview Park, OH 44126, BS 67 Kent St Univ; ME 69 Kent St Univ; Sp-Lang Path, Westlake Board of Education, **SLP**

Grissom, Mrs Susan E H 1009 Buckingham Drive, Naperville, IL 60540, BS 80 Northeast MO St Univ; MA 81 Northeast MO St Univ; Sp-Lang Path, W Chicago Elem Sch Dist #33, **SLP**

Grissom, Mrs Susan J H 13585 Elkwood Drive, Apple Valley, MN 55124, (612) 895-7240, BA 75 Univ of MO - KS City; BA 75 Univ of MO - KS City; MS 77 Univ of WI - River Falls; Sp-Lang Path, Burnsville Sch Dist 191, **SLP**

Griswold, Frank Orr 2050 San Antonio Road, Palm Springs, CA 92262, (619) 323-3554, **SLP**

Gritz, Mrs Janet M 200 Kimblewick Drive, Silver Spring, MD 20904, (301) 622-2282, BA 65 George Washington Univ; MA 66 George Washington Univ; Dir/Pres, Private Practice, **SLP ACE**

Gritzan, Mrs Janet Elizabeth 931 Wonderland Road South, Apartment 1010, London, ON, Canada N6K 2X6, (519) 471-6109, OM 88 Univ of Western Ontario

Grix-Kossakoski, Mrs Mary Whelan 311 E Washington Street, Berrien Springs, MI 49103, (616) 471-7724, BS 71 Eastern MI Univ; MA 88 Central MI Univ; 88–Aud, The Hearing Ctr

Grizzell, Mrs Barbara Schwinger 61 Curtis Street, Reading, MA 01867, (617) 745-2100, BA 75 American Univ; MA 77 Hofstra Univ; SLP, North Shore Childrens Hosp, **SLP**

Grobe, Loanne R 2 Elm Creek Drive Apt 203, Elmhurst, IL 60126, (312) 299-9720, BA 79 Briar Cliff Coll; MA 80 Western MI Univ; SLP, NW Suburban Aid for Retarded, **SLP**

Groblewski, Tonjia S 1124 Wembley Drive, Greenville, SC 29607, (803) 297-9667, BA 73 Winthrop Coll; ME 76 Univ of GA; Sp-Lang Path, Sch Dist of Greenville, **SLP**

Groder, Raquel Strauss 129 Essex Drive, Chapel Hill, NC 27514-1682, (919) 929-7555, BA 71 Southern IL Univ -Carbondale; MS 86 Univ of NC - Chapel Hill

Groenewold, Mrs Linda J 2000 St Regis Drive, Apartment A-204, Lombard, IL 60148, (312) 691-1251, BA 80 Univ of Denver; MA 82 Univ of Denver; 87–Sp-Lang Path, Hinsdale Hosp, **SLP**

Groesbeck, Billie J 6616 Lexington Road, Austin, TX 78731, (512) 285-3457, BA 52 Southern Methodist Univ; ME 63 Univ of HI - Manoa; Couns, Elgin Prim & Elem Sch, **SLP A**

Grogan, Susan Lynn 783 South Lincoln Street, Kent, OH 44240, (216) 673-1290, BS 78 Indiana Univ of PA; MS 82 WV Univ; **SLP**

Groginski, Beatrice B 2600 Bellefontaine #12D, Houston, TX 77025, (713) 665-0134, BS 24 Columbia Univ Teachers Coll; MA 60 TX Woman's Univ; **SLP LM**

Groh, Margaret E 531 Bartram Road, Moorestown, NJ 08057, (215) 775-2578, BS 71 Trenton St Coll; MA 73 Trenton St Coll; **SLP**

Groher, Dr Michael E Department Speech & Hearing (126), VA Hospital, 408 1st Avenue, New York, NY 10010, (212) 686-7500, BA 67 Univ of Redlands; MA 68 Univ of Redlands; PH 75 Univ of WA; Supvr Sp-Lang Path, VA, **SLP**

Grolnic, Stephen S 8 Vine Lane, Randolph, MA 02368, (617) 875-9773, BS 76 Univ of MA - Amherst; MS 79 IL St Univ - Normal; Dispensing Aud, Quality Hrng Aid Serv, **A**

Gromack, Gary R Ridgewood Hearing Center, Medical Arts Bldg, 385 South Maple Avenue, Ridgewood, NJ 07450, (201) 447-1090, Audiologist, New York Department of Health, **A**

Groman, Mrs Fern Rogow 5225 Palatine Avenue North, Seattle, WA 98103, (206) 361-1740, BA 75 Univ of British Columbia; MS 77 Univ of TX - Houston; 79–Sp-Lang Path, NW Sp & Hrng Cen, **SLP**

Grombka, Darlene P 2020 West 11th #B, Joplin, MO 64801-3703, (417) 625-2499, BS 83 IL St Univ - Normal; MS 85 IL St Univ - Normal; 85–Sp-Lang Path, St John's Regional Med Ctr, **SLP**

Gromek, Mrs Marilyn M 6604 Fitch Road, Cleveland, OH 44138-1250, (216) 351-3542, BA 74 Cleveland St Univ; MA 76 Cleveland St Univ; **SLP**

Gron, Karen M 2765A Weeping Willow Drive, Lisle, IL 60532, (312) 355-9521, BS 75 Marquette Univ; MS 76 Marquette Univ; **SLP**

Groner, Cathy Sanders Box 548, Charleston, MS 38921, (601) 647-5105, BA 81 Univ of MS; MA 87 Univ of MS

Grong, Linda Stewart 300 Bruce, Marshall, MN 56258, (507) 532-2687, BS 69 Univ of MN - Minneap-St Paul; MA 72 Univ of MN - Minneap-St Paul; Sp-Lang Path, Private Practice, **SLP A ACE**

Gronhovd, Dr K Dale Speech/Language/Hearing Center, Moorhead State University, Moorhead, MN 56560, (218) 236-2286, BS 63 Univ of ND; MS 67 Univ of ND; PH 72 (NS) Univ of OR; Prof, Moorhead St U, **SLP**

Gronhovd, Lee D 329 Brandon West, Bismarck, ND 58501, (701) 222-5397, BS 69 Univ of ND; MS 72 Minot St Univ; Aud, Q & R Clinic, **A**

Groob, Mrs Lisa S 127 Wellington Drive, Farmington, CT 06032, (203) 679-8361, BA 77 Univ of CT; MA 79 Univ of Cincinnati; Sp-Lang Path, State of CT DMR Region 2, **SLP**

Groody, Mrs Maria 9 Ranslow Drive, Wolcott, CT 06716, (203) 584-7828, BA 77 Univ of CT; MS 80 Southern CT St Univ; Sp-Lang Path, Bristol Public Schools, **SLP**

Groom, Mrs Barbara Bogdanoff 5246 Meadowridge Court, Camarillo, CA 93010, (213) 991-3146, BA 77 San Diego St Univ; MA 81 Whittier Coll; SLP, Oak Park USD, **SLP**

Groover, Mrs Beth Broman Central Speech And Hearing Ctr, 300 Rivermont Avenue, Virginia Baptist Hospital, Lynchburg, VA 24503, (804) 522-4520, BS 80 James Madison Univ; ME 82 Northwestern Univ; Sp-Lang Path, Central Virginia Sp-Hrng Cen, **SLP**

Groover, Mrs Nancy D 7523 Red Oak Lane, Charlotte, NC 28226-7246, (704) 541-8518, **SLP**

Gropper, Mrs Nancy R 214 Emmett Place, Ridgewood, NJ 07450, MS 72 NY Univ; Sp-Lang Path, **SLP**

Grosfield, Jane E 720-46th Street South, Great Falls, MT 59405, (406) 791-2270, BA 69 Univ of CA - Riverside; MA 75 Univ of WA; Sp-Lang Path, Great Falls Pub Sch, **SLP**

Gross, LCdr Allan H 508 Saint Charles Court, Charleston, SC 29407, (803) 743-5838, BS 71 Kent St Univ; MA 75 Case Western Reserve Univ; 87–Head/Occupational Med Div, US Naval Hosp, **A**

Gross, Mrs Barbara J 6170 Wellingtom Commons Dr, Alexandria, VA 22310, (703) 922-1933, BS 68 Univ of WI - Oshkosh; MA 87 Univ of NE - Omaha

Gross, Beth C 610 Rutland Avenue, Teaneck, NJ 07666, **SLP**

Gross, Carl David 660 Mix Avenue #4A, Hamden, CT 06514, (203) 248-3221, BS 78 SUNY - Center at Albany; MA 80 Univ of CT; SLP, Hamden Pub Sch, **SLP**

Gross, David I 275 East Walnut Street, Long Beach, NY 11561, (718) 436-7600, BA 77 CUNY - Brooklyn Coll; MS 78 Adelphi Univ; SLP, UCP, **SLP ACE**

Gross, Elizabeth Ann 28158 Danvers, Farmington Hills, MI 48018, (313) 353-0310, BS 84 Western MI Univ; MA 86 Eastern MI Univ; 88–Sp-Lang Path, Rehab Network, **SLP**

Gross, Gail Y 30-123 Sac, Flagstaff, AZ 86001, (602) 523-7911, BA 76 Wayne St Coll; MA 78 Univ of SD - Springfield; Spec Ed Tchr, San Diego USD, **SLP**

Gross, Mrs Georgia H Apartment B-409, Kings Hwy Towers, Maple Shade, NJ 08052, (215) 425-9212, BS 79 Carlow Coll; MS 81 WV Univ; 85–Sp-Lang Path, Co-Mhar, **SLP**

Gross, Gloria R 137 Arthur Avenue S E, Minneapolis, MN 55414, **A**

Gross, Mrs Harriette 6 Bartlett Road, Monsey, NY 10952, (914) 425-2247, BA 72 CUNY - Queens Coll; MA 74 CUNY - Queens Coll; Sp-Lang Path, Private Practice, **SLP**

Gross, Ilene 84 Buckingham Road, Brooklyn, NY 11226, (212) 679-9640, BA 73 CUNY - Brooklyn Coll; MS 76 Columbia Univ Teachers Coll; 83–Aud, Bd of Ed, **A**

Gross, Johanna 713 Thayer Avenue, Silver Spring, MD 20910, (202) 625-7891, BA 72 George Washington Univ; MS 76 Gallaudet Coll; Aud, Georgetown U, **A**

Gross, Leslie Ann 2047B Bedford Drive, Andrews AFB, MD 20335, (301) 770-8700, BS 76 Bloomsburg Univ of PA; MS 77 Bloomsburg Univ of PA; 88–Dir Sp-Lang Path, Pro Rehab Network Inc, **SLP**

Gross, Lynn F 7349 Hosbrook, Cincinnati, OH 45243, **SLP**

Gross, Mark Warren 2040 Cedarbridge Road, Northfield, NJ 08225, (609) 884-3475, BS 71 Univ of Miami; MA 79 Trenton St Coll; Sp-Lang Path, Lower Cape May Reg Bd of Educ, **SLP**

Gross, Melvin K 1251 Nilles Suite #7, Fairfield, OH 45014, (513) 829-7111, BS 72 Univ of Cincinnati; MA 73 Bowling Green St Univ; 87–Aud, Private Practice, **A**

Gross, Michelle Leblanc 17997 East Florida Drive, Aurora, CO 80017, (303) 322-0083, BA 82 Univ of Northern CO; MA 83 Univ of Northern CO; Aud, Donohoe Aud Serv, **A**

Gross, Mrs Nancy T 2330 North 101st Street, Wauwatosa, WI 53226, (414) 259-1414, BA 70 Coe Coll; MS 74 Univ of WI - Milwaukee; Sp-Lang Path, Visiting Nurse Assoc, **SLP**

Gross, Paula Herman 10 Oakwood Road, Newtonville, MA 02160, (617) 969-0477, BA 62 Swarthmore Coll; MS 86 Northeastern Univ; 87–Sp-Lang Path, Div of Sp/Hrng, **SLP**

Gross, Mrs Phyllis 127 Washington Street, Apartment 21, Brighton, MA 02135, MA 68 CUNY - Hunter Coll; SLP, **SLP**

Gross, Robin Ansel 110 Farnum Blvd, Franklin Square, NY 11010, (516) 437-9581, BS 80 Boston Univ; MS 82 Columbia Univ Teachers Coll; Sp-Lang Path, Private Practice, **SLP**

Gross, Mrs Roxann Diez 1300 Deerfield Drive, Monroeville, PA 15146, (412) 828-1300, BA 84 Duquesne Univ; MA 86 Univ of Pittsburgh - Pittsburgh; 86–Sp-Lang Path, Harmarville Rehab Ctr, **SLP**

Gross, Susan K 150 Princeton Heights Town, Princeton Junction, NJ 08550, **SLP**

Grossbard, Mrs Marcia V 4 Chestnut Street, Winchester, MA 01890, (617) 666-5700, 58 Boston Univ; BA 60 Boston Univ; ME 62 Boston Univ; **SLP**

Grossbard, Rebecca J 725 South Barrington Avenue, Apartment 108, Los Angeles, CA 90049, (213) 471-4652, BA 76 SUNY - Center at Binghamton; MS 78 Columbia Univ Teachers Coll; Sp-Lang Path, LA Co Supt of Schs, **SLP**

Gross-Barlow, Lucinda P O Box 973, St Marys, GA 31558, (912) 882-3673, BS 81 Univ of GA; ME 82 Univ of GA; 87–Sp/Lang Path, Hannover Rehab Ctr, **SLP**

Grossbaum, Mrs Dorothy Traub Rehov Hakablan 16 Apt #13, 93874, Jerusalem, Israel, (02) 538439, BA 73 Elmira Coll; MA 74 Hofstra Univ; 87–Supvr of Spec Educ & SLP, The Ctr of Spec Educ, **SLP**

Grossberg, Mrs Donna Sue 44 Mount Pleasant Drive, Morristown, NJ 07960, (201) 366-0591, BS 71 Emerson Coll; MA 73 Seton Hall Univ; 84–Sp-Lang Path, Mine Hill Bd of Educ, **SLP**

Grossberg, Reva Hillary 210 East 15th Street #10-B, New York, NY 10003, (212) 472-2233, BS 81 Boston Univ; MS 83 Boston Univ; SLP, The New York Foundling Hos, **SLP**

Grosse, Mrs Patricia Elizabeth 1655 Live Oak Road Apt #41, Shadow Ridge, Vista, CA 92083, (619) 941-7617, BS 82 Northeastern Univ; MS 86 Worcester St Coll; **SLP**

Grosser, Mrs Abbe C 3720 Independence Avenue, Apartment 5B, Riverdale, NY 10463, SLP, Highland Care Ctr, **SLP**

Gross-Handler, Mrs Iris Beth 632 Warburton Avenue, Apt 6-E, Yonkers, NY 10701, (914) 963-3620, BA 80 SUNY - Center at Binghamton; MS 82 Adelphi Univ; SLP, BOCES of Southern Westchester, **SLP**

Grosshandler, Stacey R 490 North Samuel Drive, Zanesville, OH 43701, (614) 452-3844, BS 76 Univ of Cincinnati; MA 78 OH St Univ; Aud, **A**

Grosshans, Stephanie Garben P O Box 221, Cooperstown, NY 13326, (607) 547-9779, BS 83 SUNY - Coll at Geneseo; MA 85 SUNY - Coll at Geneseo; **SLP**

Grossman, Barbara Ellen Ronald A Hoffman MDPC, 1430 Second Avenue, Suite 110, New York, NY 10021, (212) 535-2298, BA 79 Hofstra Univ; MA 81 Hofstra Univ; Aud, Ronald A Hoffman MDPC, **A**

Grossman, Heather Lynn 2640 Washington Avenue, Oceanside, NY 11572, (516) 764-6122, MA 88 Hofstra Univ

Grossman, James S 230 West Broadway #17, Goldendale, WA 98620, (509) 773-5204, BS 86 Univ of WA; MS 88 Univ of WA; 88–Sp-Lang Path, Educational Service Dist 112

Grossman, Joseph 23 Pika Street, Petach-Tikva, Israel, PH (NS); **A**

Grossman, Mrs Linda S 6996 Claywood Way, San Jose, CA 95120, (408) 268-4053, BA 75 SUNY - Coll at Oswego; MA 76 MI St Univ; 88–Sp/Lang Path, Private Practice, **SLP**

Grossman, Mrs Lynn Shapiro 8 Harold Road, Plainview, NY 11803, (516) 673-1638, BA 80 SUNY - Center at Albany; MA 85 Long Island U - CW Post Ctr; 87–Sp-Lang Path, South Huntington UFSD, **SLP**

Grossman, Mrs Marcia 21 Somerset Road, Tenafly, NJ 07670, (201) 569-4066, BA 57 CUNY - Brooklyn Coll; MS 71 CUNY - Brooklyn Coll; 74–Prof, Bklyn Coll Sp & Hrng Ctr, **SLP**

Grossman, Melvin R 2218 Summitview Drive, Fullerton, CA 92633, (213) 692-0551, BS 52 CA St Univ - Los Angeles; MA 61 CA St Univ - Los Angeles; **SLP**

Grossman, Pearl G 235 Nathan Lane #235, Plymouth, MN 55441, (612) 559-3535, BS 64 Univ of MN - Duluth; MS 66 Washington Univ; Sp-Lang Path, ISD #287, **SLP A**

Grossman, Rhonda K 1370 Vrain Street, Denver, CO 80204, (303) 893-5401, BA 69 McGill Univ - Quebec; MS 77 CUNY - Brooklyn Coll; Sp/Lang Path, Child Oppt Prog, **SLP**

Grossman, Ronald A 827 Blossom Hill Road, San Jose, CA 95123, (408) 578-1625, BA 66 Humboldt St Univ; MA 72 Sonoma St Univ; Sp-Lang Path, Private Practice, **SLP**

Grossman, Susan Leverah 3724 Pikeswood Drive, Randallstown, MD 21133, (301) 396-6506, MS 82 Univ of Redlands; Sp-Lang Path, Baltimore City Pub Sch, **SLP**

Grossman, Wendy S 36-14 165th Street, Flushing, NY 11358, BA 77 SUNY - Center at Buffalo; MA 79 Hofstra Univ; Sp-Lang Path, Glen Cove Pub Schs, **SLP**

Grossmann-Morris, Mrs Therese M 4011 Hillandale #1, Toledo, OH 43606, (419) 244-3321, OB 79 Univ of Toledo; MS 81 Miami Univ - Oxford; Sp/Lang Path, Toledo Bd of Ed, **SLP**

Grosvenor, Mrs Kathleen P 82 McDonough Street, Brooklyn, NY 11216, (212) 789-0033, BA 77 Saint John's Univ - Jamaica; MS 79 Columbia Univ Teachers Coll; **SLP**

Grosvenor, Mrs Terry M 502 Riverside Boulevard, Abilene, TX 79605-2804, (915) 677-2746, BS 76 CO St Univ; MS 78 CO St Univ; Early Childhood Tchr, Abilene ISD, **SLP**

Grote, Barbara Gibbs 7710 Rutgers, Austin, TX 78757, (512) 454-9057, BS 75 Univ of TX - Austin; MA 78 Univ of TX - Austin; Sp-Lang Path, Austin ISD, **SLP**

Grote, Mrs Beth Ann 3803 North Carriage, Lee's Summitt, MO 64063, (816) 836-8100, OB 82 Univ of MO - Columbia; MS 84 Southern IL Univ-Edwardsvill; Sp-Lang Path, Ind Reg Hlth Ctr, **SLP**

Grote, Dr Carole Ann Dir Communicative Disorders, Univ Of Calif Medical Ctr, 3320 3rd Avenue, San Diego, CA 92103, (619) 294-5700, BA 67 San Diego St Univ; MA 69 San Diego St Univ; PH 84 (NS) United States Int'l Univ; Dir-Commun Dis Cen, Ucsd Med Cen, **SLP**

Grotegut, Timothy David RFD 1 Box 59-92, Spanish Fork, UT 84660, (801) 798-8278, BS 84 Brigham Young Univ; MA 85 Brigham Young Univ; **SLP**

Groth, Mrs Jennifer A Lyngborghave 6, 1 Th, Birkerod, Denmark Dk 3460, BA 85 Univ of IA; MA 87 Univ of IA; **SLP**

Groth, Lynn R 106 Breezy Hills Cove, Grand Forks, ND 58201, (701) 777-3232, BS 68 Univ of ND; MS 71 Univ of ND; Asst Prof, U of ND, **SLP**

Groth, Pamela W 137 North 19th Street, Olean, NY 14760, (716) 372-6768, BS 78 SUNY - Coll at Geneseo; MA 80 SUNY - Coll at Geneseo; Sp-Lang Path, Cattaraugus County BOCES, **SLP**

Groth, Mrs Susan F 106 Breezy Hills Cove, Grand Forks, ND 58201, (701) 746-2300, BS 68 ND St Univ; MS 76 Univ of ND; SLP, Grand Forks Pub Sch, **SLP**

Grothaus, Mrs Mary Lou McNickle 12118 Burgoyne Drive, Houston, TX 77077, (713) 556-6937, BS 77 Univ of Cincinnati; MS 79 Univ of OK Medical Center; Sp-Lang Path, Alief ISD, **SLP**

Grothe, Teresa Harrington 9636 206th Street West, Lakeville, MN 55044, OB 85 Univ of MN - Duluth; MA 86 Univ of MN - Duluth; **SLP**

Group, Mrs Joyce Regenbogen 3801 Hudson Manor Terrace, Bronx, NY 10463, (212) 528-5754, BA 79 CUNY - Queens Coll; MA 81 CUNY - Queens Coll; Sp-Lang Path, Herbert G Birch Sch, **SLP**

Grove, Mrs Mary Jo R 7275 Steinmeier Drive, Indianapolis, IN 46250, (317) 226-4000, BS 45 IN St Univ - Terre Haute; MS 48 IN St Univ - Terre Haute; Sp-Lang Path, Indianapolis Pub Sch, **SLP**

Grove, Mrs Tammy Herring Lewis-Gale Hospital, Speech Pathology, 1900 Electric Road, Salem, VA 24153, (703) 989-4261, BS 81 Univ of Montevallo; MS 83 Univ of Montevallo; Supervisor Sp-Lang Pathology, Lewis Gale Hospital, **SLP**

Grover, Christian 4240 Jim Town Road, Helena, MT 59601, (406) 443-6361, BS 71 UT St Univ; MS 73 UT St Univ; Owner/Mngr, Compre Hrng Serv, **A**

Grover, Cynthia Denise 17330 Willowbrook Drive, South Bend, IN 46635, (219) 258-3000, **SLP**

Grover, Marsha J 10213 Norman Avenue N E, Albuquerque, NM 87112, **SLP**

Grover-Gaffney, Mary Corinne 21695 Yucatan Avenue, Woodland Hills, CA 91364, (818) 884-2245, BA 62 Univ of CA - Los Angeles; MA 82 CA St Univ - Los Angeles; Sp/Lang Path, Northridge Hosp Med Ctr, **SLP**

Groves, Alix K 11152 West Meinecke #1, Wauwatosa, WI 53226, (414) 645-1555, BS 75 Marquette Univ; MS 76 Univ of WI - Milwaukee; Sp-Lang Path, Milwaukee Public School System, **SLP**

Groves, Mrs Deborah S 9054 Harvest Court, Wichita, KS 67212, (316) 721-4238, BS 79 Abilene Christian Univ; MA 80 Wichita St Univ; 87–Sp-Lang Path, Private Practice, **SLP**

Groves, Marilyn E 1828 North Dudney, Magnolia, AR 71753, (501) 234-4020, BA 77 LA Tech Univ; MS 79 Univ of AR - Little Rock; Consult, Private Practice, **SLP**

Grow, Mrs Maryann Milich 27 Horseshoe Drive, Northport, NY 11768, BA 75 CUNY - Queens Coll; MA 76 Hofstra Univ; Aud, **A**

Grubaugh, Karen J 124 Southeast 19th Street, Ocala, FL 32671, (904) 876-1452, BA 84 Minot St Univ; MS 85 Minot St Univ; Prof Assoc, InSpeech Inc, **SLP**

Grubb, Mrs Betty F 3811 Emerald Circle, Manhattan, KS 66502, (913) 784-5252, BS 74 KS St Univ; MA 75 KS St Univ; Sp-Lang Path, USD 375 Geary Co Ks, **SLP**

Grubb, Edward N 100 School House Lane, Coatesville, PA 19320, (215) 524-5000, BS 67 Bloomsburg Univ of PA; MA 70 Temple Univ-Tyler Sch of Art; Sp/Lang Path, Chester Co Iu #24, **SLP**

Grubb, Mrs Lynn Marie 2846 72nd Court North, Elmwood Park, IL 60635, (312) 681-3000, BS 82 Northern IL Univ - De Kalb; MA 84 Northern IL Univ - De Kalb; 88–Sp-Lang Path, Westlake Community Hosp, **SLP**

Grubb, Mrs Susan F 500 University Avenue PH 4, Honolulu, HI 96826, (808) 955-1992, MS 74 Univ of South FL; Sp-Lang Path, Variety Club Sch, **SLP**

Grubb, Suzanne Shor 6715 Gold Creek Drive S W, Olympia, WA 98502, (206) 786-6475, BS 70 PA St Univ - Univ Park; MA 71 OH Univ - Athens; Sp-Lang Path, Tumwater Sch Dist #33, **SLP**

Grubbs, Kim Townsdin 12909 Burlingame, Oklahoma City, OK 73120, (405) 755-7347, BS 84 Central St Univ; MS 86 Univ of OK Medical Center; **SLP**

Grubbs, Rosanne 61 Boy Scout Court, Augusta, GA 30909, (404) 738-9287, BA 76 Columbia Coll; MA 81 SC St Coll; SLP, Barnwell Sch Dist #19, **SLP**

Grube, Dr M Marshall PO Box 21 790A, East Tennessee State University, Johnson City, TN 37614, (615) 929-4272, BS 62 OH Univ - Athens; MA 65 Central MI Univ; PH 78 (NS) Univ of MI - Ann Arbor; Asst Prof/Commun, East Tennessee State Univ, **SLP**

Grubel, Mrs Karen B 2327 South Henry, Sioux City, IA 51106, (712) 274-6040, BS 63 Univ of OK - Norman; MS 68 Univ of OK - OK City; 68–Sp-Lang Path, Western Hills AEA, **SLP**

Gruber, Janet L 242 South Hudson Street, Denver, CO 80222, (303) 393-2871, BS 76 Univ of Southern CO; MS 78 Univ of WY; Sp-Lang Path, VAMC-Denver, **SLP**

Gruberger, Carole Ann P O Box 155, Bucksberg Road, Tomkins Cove, NY 10986, **SLP**

Grubman-Black, Dr Stephen D 140 Briarbrook Drive, North Kingstown, RI 02852, (401) 792-5969, BS 67 Temple Univ; MA 69 Temple Univ; PH 72 (NS) SUNY - Center at Buffalo; Assoc Prof Commum Dis, U of RI, **SLP**

Gruen, Andrew Karl 7747 Spencer Drive Road, Glen Burnie, MD 21061, (301) 328-3182, BS 80 Indiana Univ of PA; MS 82 Univ of AZ; 85–Sp-Lang Path/Asst Dir, MIEMSS, **SLP**

Gruen, Karen L 7705 216th Place N E, Redmond, WA 98053-7732, **A**

Gruen, Mrs Lynn S 7747 Spencer Road, Glen Burnie, MD 21061, (301) 955-0225, BS 79 Indiana Univ of PA; MS 80 Indiana Univ of PA; 87–Sp/Lang Path, Private Practice, **SLP**

Gruenewald, Dr Lee John 1109 Waban Hill, Madison, WI 53711, (608) 266-6152, BS 61 Univ of WI - Milwaukee; MS 64 Univ of OR; PH 72 (NS) Univ of WI - Madison; Dir Integrated Stu Serv, Madison Metropolitan Sch Dist, **SLP**

Gruenhagen, Carol Lynn 32 Ridgewood Place, Fort Thomas, KY 41075, (513) 923-4000, **A**

Gruenling, Carol Ann P O Box 2067, Edison, NJ 08818, (201) 321-6800, BA 66 Newark St Coll; MA 67 Newark St Coll; Dir SLP & Aud, Roosevelt Hosp, **SLP ACE**

Gruenwald, Susan M 6230 North Sunny Point Road, Glendale, WI 53217-4170, (414) 332-0525, BS 71 Univ of WI - Milwaukee; MS 85 Univ of WI - Milwaukee; **SLP**

Grueter, Mrs Claire Cuddy 843 Ivy Trace Drive, Manchester, MO 63021, (314) 225-1585, BA 76 Bridgewater St Coll; ME 77 Northeastern Univ; SLP, Ft Wayne Comm Disorders Con, **SLP**

Gruger, Melissa M 2933 North Sheridan Road, Chicago, IL 60657, (312) 795-3130, BA 83 Univ of Cincinnati; MA 84 Northwestern Univ; 85–Sp-Lang Path, MacNeal Hosp, **SLP**

Gruhlke, Mrs Susan Pruitt 109 Fairlane Avenue, Elmhurst, IL 60126, (312) 870-4100, **SLP**

Grulke, Darlyn K 7347 West Greenfield Avenue, West Allis, WI 53214, (414) 259-1414, BS 80 Northeast MO St Univ; MA 81 Northeast MO St Univ; Sp-Lang Path, Curative Reh Ctr, **SLP**

Grumbacher, Mrs Suzanne W 300 Woodland Drive, North Hills, Wilmington, DE 19809, (302) 764-8050, BA 69 Univ of MD - College Park; MA 76 West Chester Univ of PA; Sp-Lang Path, Alloway Twsp Sch-Nj, **SLP**

Grumbine, Mrs Thayer F 2057 Cleveland Street, Greenville, SC 29607, (803) 288-0212, BA 71 Vanderbilt Univ; MA 72 Vanderbilt Univ; 88–Sp-Lang Path, Greenville Co Schs, **SLP**

Grunblatt, Mrs Henna Baila R 1343 East 3rd Street, Brooklyn, NY 11230, (212) 627-4019, BA 77 CUNY - Brooklyn Coll; MS 79 CUNY - Brooklyn Coll; SLP Deaf Prog, St Frances Sch for Deaf, **A**

Grundeman, Mrs Sandra Edson 8808 Dianne Place, Springfield, VA 22152, (703) 451-5425, BS 62 Univ of KS; MA 64 Univ of KS; 88–Sp-Lang Path, Fairfax Co PS, **SLP**

Gruneich, Mrs Mary Pacatte 304 Big Bend Boulevard, Belleville, IL 62221-1844, (618) 277-6189, BS 73 Southern IL Univ-Edwardsvill; MS 74 Southern IL Univ-Edwardsvill; Aud, Southern IL Otolaryngology Ltd, **A**

Gruner, Pamela J B 1233 East Pauline, Appleton, WI 54911, (414) 739-5310, BS 76 Northwestern Univ; MS 78 Univ of WI - Madison; **SLP**

Grunthalt, Laura Lynn 225 New Boston Road, Sturbridge, MA 01566, (203) 928-7793, MA 88 Univ of MA - Amherst; 88–Aud, Hanhemann Rehab Ctr

Grunwald, Eleanor Elizabeth 7808-A Avenue U, Lubbock, TX 79423, (806) 745-4207, BS 84 Murray St Univ; MA 86 Memphis St Univ; **A**

Grupp, Michael G 264 Doyle Avenue, Providence, RI 02906, (401) 272-5341, MS 77 Adelphi Univ; Sp-Lang Path, Private Practice, **SLP**

Grupp, Patricia B 177 Herlong Avenue, San Jose, CA 95123, **A**

Grussendorf, Betty P 4220 Reily Lane, #D-203, Shreveport, LA 71105, (318) 868-4338, OB 83 LA St Univ - Shreveport; OM 86 LA St Univ - N O Medical Ctr; 88–Sp-Lang Path, Clinical Comm Center, **SLP**

Grusy, Ronald E 4031 Thames Way, Rockford, IL 61111, (815) 968-6861, BS 69 Western IL Univ; MS 71 Univ of WI - Stevens Point; 83–Mgr-Comm Disorders, Rockford Mem Hosp, **SLP**

Gruttadauria, Salvatore A 340 West Ferry Street, Buffalo, NY 14213, (716) 883-1372, BA 75 SUNY - Center at Buffalo; MA 76 SUNY - Center at Buffalo; Sp-Lang Path/Owner, Comm Rehab Services, **SLP**

Grutzner-Martell, Heidi Jo 327 Merrimac Trail, Apartment 17-D, Williamsburg, VA 23185, (804) 253-5706, MS 84 Univ of WI - Madison; 88–Sp-Lang Path, Newport News Sch Dist, **SLP**

Grygar, Janet H 472 Wildwood Trails, Lorena, TX 76655, BS 79 Baylor Univ; MS 80 Baylor Univ; Sp/Lang Path, Lavega Elem, **SLP**

Gryniuk, Ronda P 5701 Elmwood Drive N E, Albuquerque, NM 87109, BA 70 Univ of NM; MS 72 Univ of NM; Sp/Lang Path, Albuquerque Pub Sch, **SLP**

Gryzenia, Mrs Sharon S 18601 North Nunley, Mount Clemens, MI 48043, (313) 749-9535, BS 78 Northern MI Univ; MA 80 Northern MI Univ; Sp-Lang Path Teacher, New Haven Community Schools, **SLP**

Guagenti, Virginia M PM&R, 730 West Market, Lima, OH 45801, (419) 226-9019, BS 77 Univ of Cincinnati; MS 78 Miami Univ - Oxford; Supvr Sp-Lang Path, St Ritas Medical Center-PM&R, **SLP**

Gualandi, Rhea Evelyn 70 Rosedale Avenue, 3rd Floor, Hastings, NY 10706, (914) 378-7501, BA 79 SUNY - Coll at New Paltz; MA 83 CUNY - Lehman Coll; 88–Sp-Lnag Path, St Joseph's Med Ctr, **SLP**

Gualdoni, Mrs Valerie Lynn 8236 Greenwich Court, Fort Wayne, IN 46815, (219) 485-6083, BA 76 Univ of MI - Ann Arbor; MA 83 Eastern MI Univ

Gualtieri, Mrs Sherry Ann Alfano 41 Brookshire Drive, Cedar Grove, NJ 07009, (201) 890-7243, BA 82 Kean Coll of NJ; MA 83 Kean Coll of NJ; 84–Sp-Lang Path, Deron Sch

Guardo, Elaine R 8824 7th Avenue, 2nd Floor, Brooklyn, NY 11228, (212) 481-0316, BA 75 CUNY - Queens Coll; MA 77 Long Island U - CW Post Ctr; **SLP**

Guarino, Christine 65 West 96th Street #12H, New York, NY 10025, (212) 865-3754, MA 70 Kean Coll of NJ; OM 81 Columbia Univ Teachers Coll; Sp-Lang Path, Private Practice, **SLP**

Guarnera, Mrs Susan E 9652 Caithness Drive, Huntington Beach, CA 92646, (714) 638-6309, BA 74 CA St Univ - Fullerton; MA 77 CA St Univ - Fullerton; Sp-Lang Path, Garden Grove USD, **SLP**

Guba, Barbara H 1095 Ocean Front, Long Beach, NY 11561, (516) 783-0721, BS 70 SUNY - Coll at Geneseo; MA 75 Hofstra Univ; SLP, Seaford Sch Dist, **SLP**

Gubenski, Mrs Mary Kaye Yeakle 5272 Iroquois Avenue, Ewa Beach, HI 96706, (808) 947-8235, MS 85 Univ of AL-Tuscaloosa; 87–Sp-Lang Path, Kapiolani Med Ctr for Women & Children, **SLP**

Gubernat, Laura A Rural Free Delivery 2, Jacques Road, South Killingly, CT 06239, **SLP**

Gubernick, Mrs Diane P K 1064 Jefferson Court, Warrington, PA 18976, (215) 539-8550, BS 75 Bloomsburg Univ of PA; MA 77 Trenton St Coll; Sp-Lang Path, Mont Co Iu, **SLP**

Guberud, Jane Croce 1490 Balboa Court, Broomfield, CO 80020, (301) 469-7589, BS 77 Univ of WI - Madison; MS 81 Univ of WI - Milwaukee; 87–Sp-Lang Path, St Vrain Valley Sch Dist, **SLP**

Gucwa, Judith Anne 4954 West Barry, Chicago, IL 60641, (312) 862-6484, BA 83 Elmhurst Coll; MA 85 Univ of IL - Urbana; **SLP**

Gude, Stephen Sweeney 1544 44th Street, Des Moines, IA 50311, (515) 285-3156, BA 79 Univ of IA; MA 80 Univ of IA; 88–Sp-Lang Path, Des Moines PS, **SLP**

Guderjohn, Lloyd Marvin 2200 M Avenue, Anacortes, WA 98221, (206) 293-3171, BA 58 ID St Univ; MS 70 Univ of OR; SLP, School Dist #103, **SLP**

Gudis, Sheila Chesnov 7 Tanglewood Court, Randolph, NJ 07869, (201) 361-7282, **SLP**

Gudmundsdottir, Bryndis Sigfusson Haaleitisbraut 20 108, Reykjavik, Iceland, OB 81 Educational Coll of Iceland; MA 86 Univ of TN - Knoxville; Sp-Lang Path, The Deaf Sch in Iceland, **SLP**

Gudmundsen, Gail I Professional Hearing Serv Ltd, 2354 Hassell Road, Hoffman Estates, IL 60195, (312) 490-1670, BA 71 Univ of IA; MA 73 Univ of IA; Dir, Prof Hrng Sers, **A**

Gudmundson, Bonnie S 2497 South 450 East, Bountiful, UT 84010, (801) 292-1822, BS 51 Univ of UT; MA 74 Univ of UT; 75–Sp-Lang Path, Private Practice, **SLP**

Guedet, Mrs Ann F 5485 Gingeridge Lane, Rockford, IL 61111, (815) 966-3141, BS 73 IN St Univ - Terre Haute; MA 79 Northern IL Univ - De Kalb; Sp-Lang Path, Rockford Il Bd of Ed Dist 205, **SLP**

Guendler, Laverne Quadt 113 Jacobs Creek Road, Ewing, NJ 08628, (201) 530-0139, BA 77 Rutgers St Univ -N Brunswick; MS 86 Univ of TX - Dallas; **SLP**

Guenette-Wagner, Barbara Regional Hearing Impaired Prog, 1755 South Wolf Road, Des Plaines, IL 60018, (312) 390-9440, BS 77 Univ of WI - Madison; MS 79 Univ of WI - Madison; Aud, Regional Hrng Impaired Prog, **A**

Guenley, Kay F 11521 Snow Heights N E, Albuquerque, NM 87112, (505) 266-5783, OB 79 Univ of NM; MS 81 Univ of NM; Sp-Lang Path, Private Practice, **SLP**

Guenther, Mrs Claudia Park 960 S Homer Circle, Lafayette, CO 80026, (303) 659-4820, BA 79 Luther Coll; MA 81 Univ of Northern IA; Sp-Lang Path, Adams Co Dist 27J, **SLP**

Guenther, Mrs Megan Marie 9329 Doral Drive, Pittsburgh, PA 15237, (412) 366-6263, BA 73 Univ of Akron; MA 75 Univ of Akron; Sp-Lang Path, Lang Learning Assoc, **SLP**

Guenzel, Cheryl C 7016 53rd N E, Seattle, WA 98115, (206) 527-4493, BA 84 WA St Univ; MA 85 WA St Univ; Sp-Lang Path, Highline Sch Dist

Guerdat, Beverly Lambert 632 Roebuck Circle, Birmingham, AL 35215, (205) 871-8126, BA 73 Univ of AL- Tuscaloosa; MA 75 Univ of AL- Tuscaloosa; Sp-Lang Path, Mt Brook Bd of Ed, **SLP**

Guerette, Jean Ingram R R 2 Box 3027, Bowdoinham, ME 04008, (207) 442-7931, BA 73 WV Univ; MS 80 WV Univ; Sp-Lang Path, St Me Bur Ment Retard, **SLP**

Guerette, Paul R R R 2 Box 3027, Bowdoinham, ME 04008, (207) 879-4270, BS 78 Univ of ME - Farmington; MS 80 Syracuse Univ; Sp-Lang Path, St of ME-Bur of Ment Ret, **SLP**

Guerra, Maria Zoila 2151 N W 13th Street, Miami, FL 33125, (305) 633-1968, MS 66 Recinto DE Ciencias Medices Universidad Puerto Rico; PH 60 (NS) Universidad LA Habana Cuba; **LM**

Guerrero, Janis Mazurek 2822 Village Parkway, San Antonio, TX 78251, (512) 647-2100, BA 83 Our Lady Lake Univ-San Anton; MA 85 Our Lady Lake Univ-San Anton; **SLP**

Guerrero, Oralia Ochoa 5213 Dry Wells Road, Austin, TX 78749, (512) 892-6487, BS 84 Univ of TX - Austin; MS 86 Southwest TX St Univ; **SLP**

Guerriero, John A 18 Foothill Lane, East Northport, NY 11731, (516) 560-5510, BA 52 CUNY - Brooklyn Coll; MA 60 CUNY - Brooklyn Coll; Assistant Professor, Hofstra University, **A**

Guers, Terry K 837 Acacia Avenue, Reading, PA 19605, (215) 683-5422, BS 77 Bloomsburg Univ of PA; MS 78 Bloomsburg Univ of PA; Sp-Lang Path, Berks Co Iu, **SLP**

Guess, Laurie Lee 37 Rainbow Trail, Arnold, MO 63010, (314) 296-5958, MA 87 Southern IL Univ-Edwardsvill

Guess, Lawrence Kevin 2223 North Locust, Denton, TX 76201, (817) 566-7029, MA 87 Univ of North TX

Gugenheim, Susan M 1056 East 19th Avenue, Denver, CO 80218-1088, (303) 837-2580, BS 80 CO St Univ; MS 82 Univ of AZ; 88–Sp-Lang Path, The Children's Hosp, **SLP**

Guggenheimer, Constance 971 Willesley Road, Pittsburgh, PA 15206, BA 73 Univ of Pittsburgh - Pittsburgh; MA 75 Univ of Pittsburgh - Pittsburgh; **SLP**

Guichard, Jeanne Marie 4802 Park Drive South, Metairie, LA 70001, (504) 443-1603, **SLP**

Guidice, Mrs Elaine J 7420 Bellrose N E, Albuquerque, NM 87110, (505) 881-9390, BA 77 Univ of NM; MS 78 Univ of NM; Sp/Lang Path, Albuquerque Pub Sch, **SLP**

Guido, Mrs Mary Krieger 810 Racine Street, Delavan, WI 53115, (414) 728-5093, BS 61 Marquette Univ; **SLP**

Guidry, Annette Marie 12625 Coursey Boulevard #1041, Baton Rouge, LA 70506, (504) 291-5626, MS 87 Univ of Southwestern LA; 88–Sp-Lang Path, Psycog Assoc, **SLP**

Guidry, Mrs Joan Pavur Ravenwood Place, 2100 Sawmill Road #13-103, Harahan, LA 70123, (504) 734-8008, BS 80 Saint Mary's Dominicon Coll; MS 82 Univ of Southwestern LA; Sp-Lang Path, Jefferson Parish Sch Board, **SLP**

Guidry-Marks, Rose 8326 Sycamore Place, New Orleans, LA 70118-2941, (504) 588-3121, BS 77 Tulane Univ; MA 79 LA St Univ - Baton Rouge; Sp-Lang Path, Hotel Dieu Hosp, **SLP**

Guild, Mrs Ann S 28 South Bodin Street, Hinsdale, IL 60521, BA 69 Syracuse Univ; MS 71 Northwestern Univ; Sp-Lang Path, Dupage Easter Seals Ctr, **SLP**

Guild, Jennifer Ann 210 Senate Avenue #320, Camp Hill, PA 17011, (717) 737-5518, BS 82 Bloomsburg Univ of PA; MS 83 Bloomsburg Univ of PA; SLP, Capitol Area Inter Unit, **SLP**

Guilder, Mrs Marcy Leitman 39 Wintergreen Avenue East, Edison, NJ 08820, (201) 272-9100, BA 76 Rutger's St Univ - Douglas Coll; MS 77 Columbia Univ Teachers Coll; 77–Sp/Lang Path, Cranford Public Schools, **SLP**

Guile-Lange, Laurie M 2585 Willow Creek, Prescott, AZ 86301, (602) 776-9762, BS 78 Western MI Univ; MA 80 Central MI Univ; Sp-Lang Path, Small Schs Proj Yavapai Co, **SLP**

Guilford, Dr Arthur University Of South Florida, Dept Of Communicology, Cba-255, Tampa, FL 33620-8150, (813) 974-2006, BA 65 FL St Univ; MA 67 Tulane Univ; PH 70 (NS) Univ of MI - Ann Arbor; Coor Sp-Lang Path, Univ of S FL, **SLP**

Guiliano, Teresa Stehlin 8068 Sagamore Drive, Cincinnati, OH 45236, (513) 369-2474, BS 85 Bowling Green St Univ; MA 87 OH Univ - Athens; 87–Aud, The Christ Hosp, **A**

Guillermo, Carmen R Clinical Audiologist, Woodland Clinic Med Group, 1207 Fairchild Court, Woodland, CA 95695, (916) 666-1631, BA 70 CA St Univ - Sacramento; MA 72 CA St Univ - Sacramento; Aud, Woodland Cl Med Group, **A**

Guillory, Dr Jimmy John Mobile Health Services, P O Box 80008, Lafayette, LA 70598-0008, (318) 233-3955, BS 64 Univ of Southwestern LA; MA 66 LA St Univ - Baton Rouge; PH 84 (NS) AZ St Univ; Aud/Owner, Mobile Health Serv, **SLP A**

Guillory, Joseph A 441 North Walnut, Opelousas, LA 70570, (318) 948-3646, BA 69 Univ of Southwestern LA; MS 73 Univ of Southwestern LA; MS 78 Univ of Southwestern LA; Coord Sp & Hrng, St Landry Parish Sch Bd, **SLP A**

Guillory, Sandra F 4832 Chantilly Drive, New Orleans, LA 70126, (504) 286-2700, BA 68 Xavier Univ of LA; MA 71 LA St Univ - Baton Rouge; SLP, New Orleands Pub Sch Syst, **SLP**

Guinane, Mrs Kathleen Ann 7513 South 135th Street, Omaha, NE 68138, (402) 691-1335, MS 84 Univ of TX - Dallas; BS 82 Kearney St Coll; Sp-Lang Path, Millard Public Schools, **SLP**

Guinn, Gail A 10082 Cynthia Drive, Huntington Beach, CA 92646, MA 80 CA St Univ - Long Beach; SLP, ABC USD, **SLP**

Guinn, Suzanne Y 1438 Dupont Lane, Fairbanks, AK 99709, (907) 479-7539, BS 66 Western MI Univ; MS 67 Univ of WI - Madison; 88–Dir, Communicaid, **SLP**

Guiou, Debra Higgins 145 Milk Street #23, Westborough, MA 01581, BA 84 Univ of ME - Orono; MS 86 Northeastern Univ; 86–Sp-Lang Path, Hahnemann Rehab Ctr, **SLP**

Guiry, Sibyl D PO Box 21912 GMF, Guam, MI 96921, (671) 632-5445, BS 73 Wheelock Coll; MS 76 Boston Univ; Sp-Lang Path, **SLP**

Guis, Amy H 3684 Kings Way, Sacramento, CA 95821, (415) 486-9039, BS 72 Univ of WI - Madison; MS 74 Univ of WI - Eau Claire; **SLP**

Guitar, Dr Barry E University Of Vermont, Department CSD, Allen House, Burlington, VT 05405, (802) 656-3862, BA 66 Dartmouth Coll; MS 67 Western MI Univ; PH 74 (Communicative Disorders) Univ of WI - Madison; 86–Prof, Univ VT, **SLP F**

Gulembo-Plato, Mrs Terri Leah 3909 Larson Road, Fountain, MI 49410, (616) 757-3716, MA 84 Central MI Univ; Sp-Lang Path, Mason-Lake Intermediate School, **SLP**

Gulje, Mrs Kathleen K 3531 Santa Maria Lane, Santa Barbara, CA 93105, (805) 968-2525, BA 73 Univ of CA - Santa Barbara; MA 75 Univ of CA - Santa Barbara; Sp-Lang Path, Devereux Foundation, **SLP**

Gulland, Melinda 5082 Malaga Drive, La Palma, CA 90623, (213) 439-6864, MS 78 Univ of South FL; Vp, Marina Prof Serv, **SLP**

Gullatt, Pamela E 4021 Dolly Ridge Road, Birmingham, AL 35243, (205) 967-5126, BA 85 LA Tech Univ; MS 87 Univ of Montevallo; **SLP**

Gulledge, Kristine Joan 9409 Southmoor Apartment 4, Highland, IN 46322, (219) 922-4458, BS 84 Central MI Univ; MA 85 Central MI Univ; **SLP**

Gulley, Mrs Barbara Ann 577 Coronado Drive, Sedalia, CO 80135, (303) 688-4518, BS 75 CO St Univ; MS 77 Eastern WA Univ; Sp-Lang Path, Douglas Co Sch Dist, **SLP**

Gullickson, Mrs Colleen F R R 2 Box 65, Centerville, SD 57014, (605) 563-2038, BS 79 Univ of SD - Vermillion; MA 81 Univ of SD - Vermillion; SLP, Southeast Coop, **SLP**

Gullickson, Joan Michelle 102 18th Street Northwest, Austin, MN 55912-4648, (507) 451-9513, BS 82 Mankato St Univ; MS 86 Saint Cloud St Univ; **SLP**

Gullo, Mrs Mae Ann 464 Armstrong Road, Mumford, NY 14511, (716) 538-6985, **SLP**

Gully, Ladonna Lea 84 Newbern #3, Medford, MA 02155, (617) 956-5300, BA 82 Univ of CO - Boulder; MS 85 CO St Univ; SLP, New England Med Cntr, **SLP**

Gulotta, Mrs Cynthia T 2904 Kent Avenue, Metairie, LA 70006-6434, (504) 888-3138, BA 77 Univ of Southwestern LA; OM 80 LA St Univ - N O Medical Ctr; Aud, R Daniel Jacob, **A**

Gulyas, Ann E 1913 Paul Spring Parkway, Alexandria, VA 22308, (703) 768-8886, BS 79 Miami Univ - Oxford; MA 80 Kent St Univ; Sp-Lang Path, Mt Vernon Hosp, **SLP ACE**

Gumbel, Gail E S 13 Autumn Street, Windham, NH 03087, **SLP**

Gumbiner, Tracy Ann 416 Norwich Drive, West Hollywood, CA 90048, (213) 652-0424, BA 83 Univ of Southern CA; MA 86 Whittier Coll; **SLP**

Gumeringer, Mrs Antonia Bullinger 609-3rd Avenue NE, Mandan, ND 58554, (701) 663-9554, BS 81 Minot St Univ; MS 82 Minot St Univ; Sp-Lang Path, Private Practice, **SLP**

Gumm, Mrs Carolyn K Route 2 Box 75, Mayville, WI 53050, (414) 334-9487, BS 76 Univ of WI - Stevens Point; MS 77 Marquette Univ; 86–Sp-Lang Path, CESA #6, **SLP**

Gumz, Mrs Lynn M 8707 Bethany Lane, Tinley Park, IL 60477, BS 77 IL St Univ - Normal; MS 78 IL St Univ - Normal; **SLP**

Gundersen, Mrs Debra H 14121 Appalachian Trail, Davie, FL 33325, (305) 741-4135, BS 77 SUNY - Coll at New Paltz; MA 79 Univ of Miami; Sp-Lang Path, Private Practice, **A**

Gundersen, Fredrik 14121 Appalachian Trail, Davie, FL 33325, (305) 741-4135, BS 77 SUNY - Coll at New Paltz; MA 79 Univ of Miami; Aud, VA Out-Patiet Cl, **A**

Gunderson, Duane Nils Box 351, Elgin, NE 68636, (308) 654-3273, BS 71 Northern St Coll; MS 81 Kearney St Coll; Sp-Lang Path, Ed Serv Ut #8, **SLP**

Gunderson, Fiona Walton 820 North Mandan Street, Bismarck, ND 58501, (701) 224-6716, BA 79 Queens Univ - Ontario; MS 82 Univ of ND; Sp-Lang Path, Medcenter One, **SLP**

Gunderson, Gerald D 403 West Channing, Fergus Falls, MN 56537, (218) 736-6987, BS 62 Univ of ND; MS 68 Univ of ND; Sp-Lang Path, Lakeland Men Hlth Cen Inc, **SLP**

Gunderson, Dr Herbert E P O Box 205, Westlake, OR 97493, (503) 997-6935, BA 54; MS 64 Univ of OR; PH 71 (NS) Univ of OR; Prof Emeritus, En WA U, **SLP**

Gunderson, Marsha L House Ear Institute, 256 South Lake Street, Los Angeles, CA 90057, (213) 483-4431, BA 76 Augustana Coll; MA 86 Univ of SD - Vermillion; 88–Research Fellow, House Ear Institute

Gunderson, Mrs Teresa A W 1408 South 13th Street, Blue Springs, MO 64015, (816) 228-7061, BS 76 Central MO St Univ; MS 77 Central MO St Univ; Sp-Lang Path, Blue Springs Riv School Dist, **SLP**

Gunderson-Moses, Cynthea L 2112 Linn Street, Boone, IA 50036-1201, (800) 362-2720, BS 82 Univ of WI - Oshkosh; MS 83 Univ of WI - Oshkosh; Aud, Heartland AEA 11, **A**

Gundlach, Marcia S 7150 County Road #155, Waconia, MN 55387, (612) 442-4316, BS 74 Univ of MO - Columbia; MS 75 Univ of Northern CO; Sp/Lang Path, Private Practice, **SLP**

Gundrum, Gladys R 724 Fairview Avenue #2, Arcadia, CA 91006, BS 67 NY Univ; MA 69 Univ of Southern CA; MA 75 Stanford Univ; Pub Rel Spec, Huntington Mem Hosp, **SLP**

Gunn, Mrs Barbara J Rd 2 Box 117, Orrington, ME 04474, (207) 825-3912, BA 79 Univ of ME - Orono; MA 81 Univ of ME - Orono; Sp-Lang Path, Private Practice, **SLP**

Gunn, Mrs Cynthia 3650 Maxon Road, Paducah, KY 42001, BS 70 Murray St Univ; MS 71 Murray St Univ; Sp-Lang Path, Paducah City Sch, **SLP**

Gunn, Deritha C 1321 Monte Largo Drive N E, Albuquerque, NM 87112, BA 69 Morgan St Univ; OM 71 Oakland Univ; OM 79 Auburn Univ - Auburn; Sp-Lang Path, Albuquerque Pub Sch, **SLP**

Gunn, Kathleen 24 Glenhaven Drive, St Louis, MO 63122, (314) 961-8305, MA 48 Univ of Southern CA; 88–Retired, U of IL-Servs for Crpld Chldn, **SLP LM**

Gunn, Mrs Melanie W Route 2 Box 322, Springfield, TN 37172, (615) 384-8407, BS 71 Univ of TN - Knoxville; MA 72 Univ of TN - Knoxville; Sp-Lang Path, Robertson County Board of Educ, **SLP**

Gunnarson, Dr Adele Delaine Lamar University, P O Box 10076, Beaumont, TX 77710, (409) 880-8170, BS 76 Univ of TX - Austin; MS 81 Univ of TX - Dallas; PH 87 (Hrng) Univ of TX - Dallas; 87–Asst Prof/Dir of Aud, Lamar University, **A**

Gunning, Dr Mary L E Jefferson Family Medicine Department, c/o Jefferson Medical College, Curtis Bldg 1015 Walnut Street Room 401, Philadelphia, PA 19107, (215) 928-7190, BA 75 Marywood Coll; MA 77 George Washington Univ; MD 85 (Medicine) 2336; 88–Physician, Jefferson Medical Coll, **SLP**

Gunnip, Debra 30 Glenwood Avenue, Norwalk, CT 06854, (203) 366-7551, BS 85 Mercy Coll; MS 86 Columbia Univ Teachers Coll; 88–Sp-Lang Path, Bridgeport Reg Ctr, **SLP**

Gunter, Dr Cheryl Darcel Iowa State University, 210 Pearson Hall, Ames, IA 50011, (515) 294-1117, BA 77 Univ of TN - Knoxville; MA 79 Memphis St Univ; PH 87 (Commun Dis Sp Commun) Univ of TX - Austin; Asst Prof, Iowa State U, **SLP**

Gunter, Mrs Kathy Braden P O Box 2382, La Grange, GA 30241, (404) 883-6198, BS 80 Ithaca Coll; MS 82 Univ of AL- Tuscaloosa; Director, Gunter Sp & Lang Ctr, **SLP**

Gunter, Shirley Ann 206 Winter Avenue Box 3, Sallisaw, OK 74955, (918) 775-6201, BA 70 Northeastern OK St Univ; MS 71 TX Tech Univ; Sp/Lang Path, Sequoyah Co Hlth Dept, **SLP**

Guntli, Mrs Janice A P O Box 342, St Peters, MO 63376, (314) 431-1354, BS 79 Saint Louis Univ; MA 80 Saint Louis Univ; SLP, Ctrl R-III Sch Dist, **SLP**

Guntrum, Dwana 10213 Cashel Avenue, Village Petit, Baton Rouge, LA 70815, (504) 923-1140, BA 83 Univ of the South; MA 86 LA St Univ - Baton Rouge; **SLP**

Gupta, Mrs Anne Pottinger 4752 Gabriel Way, La Mesa, CA 92041, (619) 465-7411, BS 72 San Diego St Univ; MA 74 San Diego St Univ; Sp-Lang Path, Private Practice, **SLP**

Gura, Mrs Gloria Antebi 41 Idaho Lane, Aberdeen, NJ 07747, (201) 566-1800, BA 57 Univ of MI - Ann Arbor; MA 81 Kean Coll of NJ; Sp-Lang Path, Matawan Public Schools, **SLP ACE**

Gura, Mrs Randi Paige 68-40 Cloverdale Blvd, Bayside, NY 11364, (718) 428-7507, MS 87 CUNY - Brooklyn Coll

Gura, Rhonda Beth 308 East 80th Street #6, New York, NY 10021, (212) 879-5236, BA 80 SUNY - Center at Stony Brook; MA 84 CUNY - Lehman Coll; 86–Sp-Lang Path, Sr Cecilia Schneider NY Foundling Hosp, **SLP**

Gural-Toth, Virginia J 31 Coleridge Avenue, Yardville, NJ 08620, (609) 779-4821, BS 83 Trenton St Coll; MA 85 CUNY - Hunter Coll; Aud, John F Kennedy Medical Center, **A**

Gurcinas, Birute J P O Box 609, Three Rivers, CA 93271, (213) 828-0509, BA 74 CA St Univ - Los Angeles; MA 77 CA St Univ - Los Angeles; President, Private Practice, **SLP**

Gurdin, Martha H 11 Savoy Drive, Dallas, PA 18612, (717) 288-9386, BS 65 Geneva Coll; MA 67 Bowling Green St Univ; Sp/Lang Path, Scranton City Schs, **SLP**

Gurecki, Rebecca J 200 Maitland Avenue #154, Altamonte Springs, FL 32701, **SLP**

Gureckis, Mrs Kathleen M 7702 Lynn Ann Lane, San Antonio, TX 78240, (512) 520-1150, BS 74 Emerson Coll; ME 75 Trenton St Coll; **SLP**

Gurecky, Cynthia S 1111 Golf View Drive #704, Richmond, TX 77469, (713) 341-3322, BS 80 Southwest TX St Univ; ME 81 Southwest TX St Univ; 81–Sp-Lang Path, Lamar Consol ISD, **SLP**

Gurevich-Uvena, Joyce 1006 Independence Avenue S E, Washington, DC 20003, (202) 544-4181, BS 71 Emerson Coll; MA 72 George Washington Univ; Sp-Lang Path, Walter Reed Army Med Cen, **SLP**

Gurick, Mrs Cathy 620 Virginia Avenue, Martinsburg, WV 25401, (304) 267-4150, BA 75 George Washington Univ; MA 76 George Washington Univ; 88–Sp-Lang Path, Berkeley Co Schs, **SLP**

Gurland, Dr Gail 2425 Kings Highway, Apartment A9, Brooklyn, NY 11229, (718) 780-5186, BA 70 CUNY - Brooklyn Coll; MS 72 CUNY - Brooklyn Coll; PH 79 (NS) CUNY - Grad Sch & Univ Cntr; Assoc Prof, CUNY-Brooklyn Coll, **SLP**

Gurley, Susan A DSOP-DODDS Pacific, APO San Francisco, CA 96274-0005, (63) 392-1110, BA 76 Univ of WA; OM 77 Univ of WA; 88–Spec Educ Coord, Dept of Defense Dep Schs, **SLP**

Gurman, Mrs Martha L 14 Sandie Lane, Marblehead, MA 01945, (617) 631-3210, BS 74 Boston Univ; ME 75 Northeastern Univ; Sp/Lang Path, Winthrop Pub Sch, **SLP**

Gurnick, Ellen B 6647 Cantaloupe Avenue, Van Nuys, CA 91405, (818) 902-1487, BA 77 SUNY - Coll at Brockport; MA 81 CA St Univ - Los Angeles; SLP, Los Angeles USD, **SLP**

Gurolnick, Mrs Joyce W 7921 Wilson Terrace, Morton Grove, IL 60053, (312) 965-0050, BS 52 Univ of IL - Chicago; Sp-Lang Path, E Me Dist #63, **SLP**

Gurr, Linda 324 Montgomery Drive, Belleville, IL 62223, (618) 746-4738, BS 73 Univ of MO - Columbia; MS 81 Southern IL Univ-Edwardsvill; 75–Sp-Lang Path, Mascoutah Comm USD #19, **SLP**

Gurrister, Tom W 2720 South 300 East, Salt Lake City, UT 84115, (801) 565-7100, BS 81 Univ of UT; MS 86 Univ of UT; **SLP**

Gurske-Hladik, Mrs Ellen Speech Plus Inc, 2146 North Old Manor, Wichita, KS 67208, MA 78 Wichita St Univ; Pres/Dir of Speech Pathology, Speech Plus Inc, **SLP**

Gurwitz, Mrs Bailey A 1707 Marigold, Mc Allen, TX 78501, (512) 686-1148, BA 57 Univ of TX - Austin; Sp-Lang Path, McAllen ISD, **SLP**

Guryan, Mrs Barbara M 90-D Pinecroft, Taylors, SC 29687, (803) 244-6841, BS 82 Auburn Univ - Auburn; OM 83 Auburn Univ - Auburn; 86–Sp-Lang Path, The Speech-Hrng-Learning Ctr, **SLP**

Guryan, Stephen Thomas 90-D Pinecroft Drive, Taylors, SC 29687, (803) 235-9689, BS 84 SUNY - Coll at Buffalo; MA 87 2952; 87–Dir of Aud Svcs, Speech Hearing & Learning Ctr, **A**

Gusdal, Sharyn Ann 1114-2080 Pembina Highway, Winnipeg, MB, Canada R3T 2G9, (204) 237-2131, **SLP**

Gusdorf, Mrs Katherine V 1076 Crosspoint Court, San Jose, CA 95120, (408) 268-1266, BA 78 Univ of CA - Santa Barbara; MS 82 San Francisco St Univ; Sp-Lang Path, Oak Grove Sch Dist, **SLP**

Gustafson, Mrs Brigitte Josi 33309 WCR #8, Keenesburg, CO 80643, (303) 424-7791, BA 82 Univ of Northern CO; MA 83 Univ of Northern CO; Sp-Lang Path, Wheatridge Reg Cent, **SLP**

Gustafson, Mrs Kathy Ann Peterson 4920 Otsego, Duluth, MN 55804, (218) 525-1907, BS 70 Univ of MN - Duluth; MA 81 Univ of MN - Duluth; Sp-Lang Path, Duluth ISD 709, **SLP**

Gustafson, Linda Houge 4888 144th Street West, Savage, MN 55378, (612) 447-1953, BA 79 Luther Coll; MA 84 Univ of MN - Minneap-St Paul; Sp-Lang Path, MN River Valley Spec Ed Coop, **SLP**

Gustafson, Margaret Faudree 1120 NW 20th Suite #101, Portland, OR 97209, (503) 227-3668, BS 82 Univ of WA; MS 84 Univ of WA; 86–Aud, Portland Ear Testing Ctr, **A**

Gustafson, Mrs Sharon Elaine 1234 Mohave Drive, Colton, CA 92324, (714) 924-9811, BS 82 Andrews Univ; MS 85 Worcester St Coll

Gustetic, Stanley J, Jr 11980 Oakwood Lane, Chesterland, OH 44026, (216) 729-6135, MA 77 Cleveland St Univ; Director Field Services, Amer Industrial Hrng Services, **A**

Gustetic, Susan M 4812 Spruce Pine Way, North Ridgeville, OH 44039, (216) 327-3068, BA 72 Cleveland St Univ; MA 74 Cleveland St Univ; Sp-Lang Path, Elyria Cty Sch, **SLP**

Gustin, Mrs Nancy Hess 890 Windsor Trail, Roswell, GA 30076, (404) 993-4129, BS 75 Miami Univ - Oxford; ME 86 GA St Univ; 82–Sp-Lang Path, DeKalb Co Schs, **SLP**

Gustine, Mrs Dixie A PO Box 210272, Auke Bay, AK 99821, (907) 789-9290, BS 74 Eastern IL Univ; MS 75 Eastern IL Univ; 88–Sp-Lang Path, Juneau Sch Dist, **SLP ACE**

Gustus, Mrs Christine Hilleary 14373 Appalachian Trail, Chesterfield, MO 63017, (314) 652-3200, BS 73 Purdue Univ - West Lafayette; MS 75 Washington Univ; 86–Sp-Lang Path, Ctrl Institute for the Deaf, **SLP**

Gutekunst, Mrs Cheryl Lee 406 Colony Drive, Lee's Summitt, MO 64063, (816) 842-4644, BS 80 Univ of MO - Columbia; MS 84 Central MO St Univ; Sp-Lang Path, Childrens Therapy Group Inc, **SLP**

Gutenplan, Mrs Lori Mandel 98 Tara Drive, East Hills, NY 11576, (516) 621-0284, BA 74 SUNY - Center at Buffalo; MA 75 Univ of MD - College Park; Aud, Little Village Sch, **A**

Guterson, Mary 27 Springdale Road, New Rochelle, NY 10804, (914) 834-9177, BA 80 Univ of WA; MS 82 Univ of WA; 87–Asst Editor, Venture Magazine, **SLP**

Gutheil, Kathryn R 128 Tyler Street, Buffalo, NY 14214, MS 74 SUNY - Coll at Buffalo; Tchr, Buffalo Bd of Ed, **SLP**

Guthormann, Mrs Deborah M West Newton Hearing Center, 1298 Washington Street, West Newton, MA 02165, (617) 332-7244, BS 74 NY Univ; MA 76 Northwestern Univ; Co-Dir, West Newton Hrng Ctr, **A ACE**

Guthrie, Denise Cornett 3406 Cherry Hill Drive, Fairfield, OH 45014, (513) 874-3761, BS 78 Miami Univ - Oxford; MA 83 Ball St Univ; 83–Sp-Lang Path, Hamilton City Schs, **SLP**

Guthrie, Janet 3721 Sunnyside North, Seattle, WA 98103, (206) 632-0103, BS 84 Univ of WA; MS 86 Univ of WA; **SLP**

Guthrie, Mrs Lynda T 2000 Bishops Bridge Road, Knoxville, TN 37922, (615) 691-2919, BA 78 Univ of KY; MA 79 Univ of TN - Knoxville; **SLP**

Guthrie, Patricia A 7619 Penns Grove Road, Summerfield, NC 27358, **SLP**

Guthrie, Mrs Renee Poteet 2852 Misty Ridge Cove, Cordova, TN 38018, (901) 763-3858, BA 80 Univ of AR - Little Rock; MA 83 Memphis St Univ; 87–Sp-Lang Path, Nancy Wark & Associates, **SLP**

Guthrie, Mrs Roxann A 2486 South Garner Road, Vassar, MI 48768, (517) 823-2018, BA 75 MI St Univ; MA 76 MI St Univ; Sp-Lang Path, Tuscola Independent Sch Dist, **SLP**

Guthrie, Terry M 8215 Mountain Lake, Fort Worth, TX 76179, (817) 335-2583, BS 77 MI St Univ; MS 78 ID St Univ; Aud, Jones Aud & Hrng Aid Ctr, **A**

Gutierrez, Brenda 9853 West Valley Ranch Parkway #1072, Irving, TX 75063, (214) 402-0506, BS 85 Baylor Univ; MS 87 Univ of TX - Dallas; 87–Sp-Lang Path, Dallas Rehab Inst, **SLP**

Gutierrez-Clellen, Vera Florencia 243 West Tulpehocken, Apartment B-408, Philadelphia, PA 19144, (215) 844-0188, MA 76 Universidad Del Museo Social Argentino; Supvr, Temple University, **SLP**

Gutierrez-Mauzy, Regina Anne 7645 Garners Ferry Road, Apartment 1005-A, Columbia, SC 29209, (803) 799-0420, BS 79 Radford Univ; MS 83 James Madison Univ; 88–Sp-Lang Path, Babcock Ctr, **SLP**

Gutkin, Mrs Barbara Arlene 601 Lakewood Drive, Lincoln, NE 68510, (402) 475-1081, BA 68 CUNY - Brooklyn Coll; MS 83 Univ of NE - Lincoln; SLP, Lincoln Public Schools, **SLP**

Gutmann, Sharon Deborah 28675 Franklin #323, Willow Park Apartment, Southfield, MI 48034, (313) 353-6219, BA 84 Univ of MI - Ann Arbor; MA 86 IN Univ - Bloomington; 87–Sp-Lang Path, Hazel Park Pub Schs, **SLP**

Gutnick, Dr Howard N 825 Fairfax Avenue, Norfolk, VA 23507, (804) 446-5934, BA 71 Univ of Chicago; MS 76 Univ of WI - Madison; PH 79 (NS) Univ of WI - Madison; Dir of Aud, Dept of ENT Head & Neck Surg, **A**

Gutowicz, Barbara 10926 Bluffside Drive #9, Studio City, CA 91604, (818) 762-3883, BA 76 Univ of CA - Los Angeles; MA 80 CA St Univ - Northridge; Sp-Lang Path, Private Practice, **SLP**

Gutstein, Mrs Carol F 6233 North Drake Avenue, Chicago, IL 60659, (312) 465-8000, BS 62 Loyola Univ of Chicago; MA 69 De Paul Univ; 88–Sales Assoc, Hallmark & Johnson Prop

Guttenberg, Mrs Hope Stall 300 Community Drive, Manhasset, NY 11030, (516) 562-4600, MS 87 CUNY - Brooklyn Coll; 87–Aud, North Shore Univ Hosp, **A**

Guttman, Mrs Marlene B 326 Chenora Court, Cincinnati, OH 45215, BS 73 Univ of Cincinnati; MA 75 Univ of Cincinnati; Rehab Mgr, United Home Care, **SLP**

Guttman, Dr Newman AT&T Bell Laboratories, Indian Hill Park, 200 Park Plaza, Naperville, IL 60566, (312) 416-7281, BA 49 Univ of MN - Minneap-St Paul; MA 51 Univ of IL - Urbana; PH 54 (Sp) Univ of IL - Urbana; Mem/Tech Staff, AT&T Bell Laboratories, **F**

Guttman, Mrs Sara R 1154 Murray Hill Avenue, Pittsburgh, PA 15217, (412) 362-5959, BA 73 Univ of Pittsburgh - Pittsburgh; MA 74 Univ of Pittsburgh - Pittsburgh; SLP, Private Practice, **SLP**

Guttsman, Mrs Claire 11 Pearl Street, Staten Island, NY 10304, (212) 390-9470, BA 73 CUNY - Brooklyn Coll; MA 75 Univ of CT; SLP, Staten Island Hosp, **SLP**

Gutzwiller, Mary L Loretto Motherhouse, 1873 House, Nerinx, KY 40049, (502) 865-5811, BS 75 Univ of Cincinnati; MA 78 Northwestern Univ; **A**

Guy, Christine 2705 Westwood Drive, Arlington, TX 76012, **SLP**

Guydon, Dr Audrey Sessom 7917 Camelot Road, Fort Worth, TX 76134, (817) 536-7608, BS 60 IN Univ - Bloomington; MA 67 De Paul Univ; PH 77 (Education & Family Environment) IA St Univ; Coordinator, Ft Worth ISD, **SLP**

Guyer, Mrs Deborah Dalin 1739 Tralee Lane, Ballwin, MO 63021, (314) 966-1556, BS 74 Fontbonne Coll; MA 76 Univ of KS; Sp-Lang Path, St Joseph Hosp, **SLP ACE**

Guyer, Mrs Jo 1121 N W 26th Street, Portland, OR 97210, (503) 222-2738, BS 71 Portland St Univ; MS 75 Portland St Univ; Sp-Lang Path, Off-Northrup Sp-Lang Prog, **SLP**

Guyette, Thomas W 6401 Winston, Woodridge, IL 60517, (913) 588-5935, BA 70 Univ of MO - Columbia; MS 76 Univ of WI - Milwaukee; PH 85 (NS) Univ of KS; Asst Prof, Rush Univ, **SLP**

Guyther, Robin E 207 Gaywood Road, Baltimore, MD 21212, BA 79 Loyola Coll; MS 80 Loyola Coll; Sp-Lang Path, Baltimore County Pub Schools, **SLP**

Guzauskas, Ann Helen K 1091 South Green Road, South Euclid, OH 44121, (216) 291-0311, BA 77 Cleveland St Univ; MA 79 Cleveland St Univ; Cl & Dispensing Aud, Eent Associates Inc, **A ACE**

Guzel, Shakeh N 19740 Hatton Street, Canoga Park, CA 91306, (818) 882-1431, BA 73 Whittier Coll; MA 75 CA St Univ - Los Angeles; 81–Sp-Lang Path, Comm Sp & Hearing Ctr, **SLP**

Guzman, Charles R 3660 West Bethany Home Rd, Phoenix, AZ 85019, (602) 973-3314, BA 72; MA 74 Northeast MO St Univ; Dir, Phoenix Ctrl Sp & Lang Cen, **SLP**

Guzman, Luz Rivera P O Box 4930, San Juan, PR 00905, BS 82 Univ of PR - Rio Piedras; MS 85 Univ of PR - San Juan; **SLP**

Guzzardo, Sr Margaret 2957 South Brighton Avenue, Los Angeles, CA 90018, (213) 823-8911, BA 67 Fontbonne Coll; MA 71 Saint Louis Univ; Sp-Lang Path, Daniel Freeman Marina Hosp, **SLP**

Gwin, Barbara Naser 1817 Joseph Circle, Florence, SC 29501, (803) 665-5958, BS 82 CA Univ of PA; MS 84 CA Univ of PA

Gwinn, Mrs Crystal Andrea Stetson Road, Box 61, Levant, ME 04456, (207) 941-6300, BS 65 Univ of ME - Orono; MA 83 Univ of ME - Orono; 85–Sp-Lang Path, Bangor Sch Dept, **SLP**

Gwinn, Mrs Velma Rose PO Box 511, Cottonwood, ID 83522, (208) 962-3036, MS 88 Eastern WA Univ; 88–Sp-Lang Path, Prairie PS

Gwinner, Debra Atkinson 9304 West Iowa Avenue, Lakewood, CO 80226, (303) 757-6201, BA 76 Colby Coll; MA 83 Univ of Denver; **A**

Gwinner, Mrs Nanette Hawks 68 1/2 Rumsey Street, Bath, NY 14810, (607) 776-2111, BS 85 SUNY - Coll at Geneseo; MA 86 SUNY - Coll at Geneseo; **A**

Gwyn, Robert David 905 Sampson Street, Taylor, PA 18517, (717) 961-1520, BS 80 Ithaca Coll; MS 81 Ithaca Coll; Audiologist, Dr A Nalevanko & Dr L Degennar, **A**

Gwyn, Susan E 8706 Ravenglass Way, Gaithersburg, MD 20879, (301) 424-5200, BS 73 Miami Univ - Oxford; MA 74 Univ of IL - Urbana; 88–Dir-Outpatient Cl Svcs, The Treat & Lrng Ctr Inc, **SLP**

Gyant, Mrs Marie Goldson 15888 S W 95th Avenue, Apartment 204, Miami, FL 33157, (305) 255-1045, BS 84 Univ of IA; MA 86 Univ of IA; 86–Sp-Lang Path, InSpeech Inc, **SLP**

Gyory, Mrs Sabina M 8 Glendale Avenue, Somerville, MA 02144, (617) 666-2689, BA 77 Brown Univ; MA 79 Northwestern Univ; Sp-Lang Path, Cambridge School Dept, **SLP**

Gyurek, Deborah Lynn 30 Winchester #18, Mansfield, OH 44907, (419) 756-1133, BA 82 OH St Univ; MA 84 OH Univ - Athens; Sp-Lang Path, Rehab Serv Nc Ohio, **SLP**

H

Haack, Mrs Dean S 220 Lakeview Drive, Auburndale, FL 33823, (813) 534-2111, MS 84 FL St Univ; **SLP**

Haack, Sharon L 4136 Wimbledon Drive, Lawrence, KS 66046, (913) 841-7562, BS 74 Univ of KS; MA 75 Univ of KS; 88–KUAF Sp-Lang Path Coord, Bureau of Child Research-Univ of Kan, **SLP**

Haag, Elizabeth 137-B Woodlawn Avenue, Pittsburgh, PA 15202, (412) 359-3782, **SLP**

Haag, Mrs Joan S 6109 Western Run Drive, Baltimore, MD 21209, (301) 396-6375, BS 51 James Madison Univ; OM 54; MS 73 Towson St Univ; Sp-Lang Path, Balt City Bd of Ed, **SLP**

Haag, Terri L S 16915 Hidden Oak Woods, San Antonio, TX 78248-1404, (512) 674-5231, BA 77 Our Lady Lake Univ-San Anton; MA 78 Our Lady Lake Univ-San Anton; SLP, Northside Sch Dist, **SLP**

Haage, Constance L 318 North D, Herington, KS 67449, (913) 258-3234, BA 69 Wichita St Univ; MA 73 KS St Univ; Sp-Lang Path, Ctrl KS Coop Ed, **SLP**

Haak, Dr Nancy Jeanne 3010 S W 23rd Terrace #86, Gainesville, FL 32608, (904) 377-1014, MS; **SLP**

Haaland, Phil J Route 5 Box 203, Devils Lake, ND 58301, (701) 662-3603, BS 72 Minot St Univ; MS 78 Minot St Univ; SLP/Aud, Lake Reg Spec Ed, **SLP**

Haanen, Donna H 48 Wincrest Drive, Glens Falls, NY 12801, (518) 793-8811, BS 54 Univ of WI - Madison; MA 75 Coll of Saint Rose; Sp-Lang Path, Queensburg Union Free Sch, **SLP**

Haar, Carolyn A 616 Harang Avenue, Metairie, LA 70001, (504) 455-1369, BS 72 Saint Mary's Dominican Coll; MS 75 Tulane Univ; **SLP**

Haarbauer-Krupa, Mrs Juliet K 3172 Wicks Creek Trail, Marietta, GA 30062, (404) 578-9189, BS 77 PA St Univ - Univ Park; MA 80 Univ of Pittsburgh - Pittsburgh; 88–Prog Dev Spec, Atlanta Rehab Inst, **SLP**

Haas, Dr Adelaide Nacamu State Univ Of New York, College At New Paltz, Faculty Tower Room 214, New Paltz, NY 12561, (914) 257-2600, BA 59 PA St Univ - Univ Park; MS 60 Bowling Green St Univ; PH 78 (Sp-Lang Path) Columbia Univ Teachers Coll; Prof, SUNY/Coll New Paltz, **SLP**

Haas, Mrs Carol Ann 155 Narrows Road, Coldwater, MI 49036-9622, (616) 467-9745, BS 79 Western MI Univ; MA 81 Western MI Univ; Sp-Lang Path, St Joseph County ISD, **SLP**

Haas, Mrs Catherine Ann 10 Alpine Road, Binghamton, NY 13903, (607) 722-5308, BS 81 SUNY - Coll at Geneseo; MS 83 SUNY - Coll at Buffalo; 83–Sp-Lang Path, Rehabilitation Services, **SLP**

Haas, Celeste E 8909 Reeder Road #906, Overland Park, KS 66214, (816) 932-3832, BS 84 Univ of KS; MA 87 Univ of KS; Sp-Lang Path, St Lukes Hospital, **SLP**

Haas, Gretchen L 30 Gardner Road #5C, Brookline, MA 02146, (617) 468 2626, BA 76 Univ of CO - Boulder; MA 80 Emerson Coll; **SLP**

Haas, Dr Gustav F The Hearing Center, 1230 Hopkins Avenue, Redwood City, CA 94062, (415) 369-4327, OM 64 Yale Univ; MA 80 Univ of IA; PH 70 (Sensory Systems) Univ of CA - Los Angeles; Dir, Hrng Cen, **A**

Haas, Joann 10177 Goodin Circle, Columbia, MD 21046, (301) 730-5983, OB 77 Univ of Miami; MA 78 Hofstra Univ; Sp-Lang Path, Elwyn I, **SLP**

Haas, Mrs Joanne Ryan 22 West 370 Birchwood Dr, Glen Ellyn, IL 60137, (312) 682-2055, BS 77 Northern IL Univ - De Kalb; MA 78 Western IL Univ; Sp-Lang Path, Dist 200-Wheaton, **SLP**

Haas, Linda Sirianni 414 Sumner Avenue, New Castle, PA 16105, (412) 652-4031, BS 80 CA Univ of PA; ME 82 CA Univ of PA; **SLP**

Haas, Mrs Margot A 26 Rockland Avenue, Larchmont, NY 10538, (914) 834-1315, BS 64 Cornell Univ; MA 66 Columbia Univ Teachers Coll; Sp-Lang Path, Private Practice, **SLP**

Haas, Dr William H Florida State University, 112 RRC Department Com Dis, Tallahassee, FL 32306-2007, (904) 644-2238, BA 53 MI St Univ; MA 60 MI St Univ; PH 70 (NS) MI St Univ; Chair & Assoc Prof, FL St U, **SLP A**

Haas-Belash, Mrs Barbara City Hospital Center At Elmhurst, 79-01 Broadway, Elmhurst, NY 11373, (718) 830-1015, BA 53 Cedar Crest Coll; MA 67 Columbia Univ Teachers Coll; Sp/Lang Path, City Hosp Ctr Elmhurst, **SLP ACE**

Haasch, Kathleen Mary S 504 Warbler Court, Lavalle, WI 53941, (608) 985-8216, MS 84 Rush Univ; Audiologist, Rural Wisconsin Hospital Coop, **A**

Haase, Kathryn S 1416 Lafayette Drive N E, Albuquerque, NM 87106, (505) 299-1937, BS 80 Univ of NM; MS 84 Univ of NM; 84–Sp-Lang Path, Albuquerque Public Schools, **SLP**

Haasis, Mrs Mary A 4935 Nottingham, St Louis, MO 63109, (314) 771-6673, BA 72 Fontbonne Coll; MA 74 Saint Louis Univ; **SLP**

Haave, Mrs Amy Nore 906 South 4th Street, Albion, NE 68620, (402) 395-6882, BS 76 Univ of NE - Lincoln; MA 78 Univ of NE - Lincoln; **SLP**

Haber, Barbara 21 Warwick Avenue, Fort Lee, NJ 07024, (201) 224-9571, BA 72 CUNY - City College; MS 73 Columbia Univ Teachers Coll; PH 80 (NS) Fordham Univ; **SLP**

Haber, Diane Sue 67-15 Dartmouth Street, Forest Hills, Queens, NY 11375, (718) 317-2509, **SLP**

Haber, Dr Lyn Roland Department Of Psychology, University Of Illinois, Chicago, IL 60680, (312) 943-3440, BA 63 Brandeis Univ; MA 65 Univ of CA - Berkeley; PH 70 (NS) Univ of CA - Berkeley; SLP, Chicago Sch, **SLP**

Haber, Mrs Rita Patnoi 19501 Vintage Street, Northridge, CA 91324, (818) 701-0636, BA 64 Univ of CA - Los Angeles; MS 65 Purdue Univ - West Lafayette; 77–Sp-Lang Path, Rita Haber & Assoc, **SLP**

Haber, Sandra K Middlesex County Speech Center, Mini Mall, 499 Ernston Road, Sayreville, NJ 08859, (201) 721-1144, BA 73 Kean Coll of NJ; MA 77 Kean Coll of NJ; Sp-Lang Path / Consult, Private Practice, **SLP**

Haberek, Theresa 29678 High Valley, Farmington Hills, MI 48331, (313) 661-4030, BS 77 Wayne St Univ; MA 79 Wayne St Univ; Sp-Lang Path, Walled Lake Consolidated Schs, **SLP**

Haberman, Mrs Gale Anne 1800 Vine Street, Des Moines, IA 50265, (515) 223-0948, BA 81 Univ of Northern IA; MS 83 Univ of WI - Milwaukee; **SLP**

Habgood, Karen Lynne 13602 North 44th Street, Apt #272, Phoenix, AZ 85032, (602) 953-2942, BA 78 Univ of Redlands; MA 84 CA St Univ - Northridge; **SLP**

Habicht-Grundner, Mrs Marcy J 4059 Bay Park Drive, Liverpool, NY 13090, (315) 622-4071, BS 78 SUNY - Coll at Buffalo; MS 79 SUNY - Coll at Buffalo; 84–Sp-Lang Path, Private Practice, **SLP**

Hacecky, Karla R 2717 Klondike Trail, Sioux Falls, SD 57103-4346, (605) 336-1840, BS 79 Univ of SD - Vermillion; MA 81 Univ of SD - Vermillion; 84–Sp-Lang Path, Crippled Childrn Hosp & School, **SLP**

Hachiya, Janet Schoen 2933 Sea View Parkway, Alameda, CA 94501, (415) 447-8808, MA 84 Univ of San Francisco; Sp-Lang Path, American Speech Pathologists, **SLP**

Hachtel, Mrs Marsha J 908 Dunbarton, Richardson, TX 75081, (214) 235-3665, BS 66 Univ of TX - Austin; MS 80 Southern Methodist Univ; Sp-Lang Path, Foreign Accent Improvement, **SLP**

Hack, Mrs Zarita C 101 Forest Hill Drive, Los Gatos, CA 95032, (408) 358-2170, BS 74 Univ of MD - College Park; MS 79 Washington Univ; **A**

Hacker, Lynne R 105 East 63rd Street, New York, NY 10021, (212) 752-4199, BA 69 CUNY - Brooklyn Coll; MA 71 NY Univ; Sp-Lang Path, Private Practice, **SLP**

Hackett, Mrs Anita C 1834 Palmcroft Drive N E, Phoenix, AZ 85007, (602) 254-8038, BS 65 Columbia Univ Teachers Coll; MA 67 Columbia Univ Teachers Coll; SLP, St Josephs Hospital, **SLP**

Hackl, Mrs Margery B 12001 South 86th Avenue, Palos Park, IL 60464, MS

Hackman, Mrs Lesley J 65 Sarah Bishop Road, Ridgefield, CT 06877, (203) 431-9719, BA 67 Ithaca Coll; ME 69 Boston Univ; Sp-Lang Path, Ridgefield Sch Sys, **SLP**

Hackmeyer, Mrs Linda P 1591 Harbert Avenue, Memphis, TN 38104, (901) 522-6593, BA 71 Southwestern at Memphis; MA 72 Memphis St Univ; Dir SLP Serv, Baptist Mem Hosp, **SLP**

Hackney, Maxine L 4311 San Pedro N E # B 203, Albuquerque, NM 87109, (505) 884-9736, BA 74 Wichita St Univ; MA 75 Wichita St Univ; Sp-Lang Path, Albuquerque Public Schools, **SLP**

Hackworth, Dr Howard Bing Central State University, Edmond, OK 73034, (405) 341-2980, BA 54 Univ of Tulsa; MS 57 Univ of UT; ED 64 (Spec Educ/Sp-Lang Path) Univ of Tulsa; Assoc Prof Sp-Lang Path, Central St U, **SLP**

Hackworth, Maryann 112 Tarpon Drive, Pittsburgh, PA 15212, (412) 361-2801, BS 82 Indiana Univ of PA; MS 83 Clarion Univ of PA; Sp-Lang Path, Craig House Technoma, **SLP**

Hadaway, Mrs Mary Ann Route 1 Box 193-A, Iota, LA 70543, (318) 779-2581, BA 71 Univ of Southwestern LA; MS 77 Univ of Southwestern LA; Sp-Lang Path, Acadia Parish School Board, **SLP**

Hadaway, Mrs Sharon Joy 2051 Huntington, Emporia, KS 66801, (316) 343-2302, BA 64 OK St Univ; MA 69 OK St Univ; SLP, Speech Plus, **SLP**

Haddad, Harriet Jane 904 North 33rd, Monroe, LA 71201, (318) 322-5348, BA 71 LA Tech Univ; MA 73 LA Tech Univ; 84–Sp-Lang Path, Glenwood Reg Med Ctr, **SLP**

Haddad, Layth Nadim 259 Cottonwood Road, Newington, CT 06111, (203) 665-0129, BA 84 Am Univ of Beirut - Lebanon; MA 87 Univ of CO - Boulder; SLP, InSpeech Inc, **SLP**

Haddad, Synthia S 601 Miller Avenue, Norman, OK 73069, (405) 677-8381, BA 77 Univ of OK - Norman; MS 79 Univ of OK Medical Center; SLP, Midwest City-Del City Schl Sys, **SLP**

Haddow, Judith A 1416 South Columbine Street, Denver, CO 80210, (303) 441-0493, BA 79 Univ of CO - Boulder; MA 81 Univ of CO - Boulder; Sp/Lang Path, Boulder Mem Hosp, **SLP**

Hadeed, Nabhan 5057 Woodward, Room Scb 1076, Detroit, MI 48202, MA 75 Wayne St Univ; Sp-Lang Path, Detroit Boe, **SLP**

Haden, Nedah L 1324 Green Gables Court, Fort Collins, CO 80525, (303) 491-7313, BA 60 CA St Univ - Sacramento; MA 74 CA St Univ - Sacramento; Asst to VP of Dev, Southern Methodist U, **SLP**

Haden, Ricole Hayley 6400 Elray Drive #F, Baltimore, MD 21209, (301) 889-6393, MS 88 Univ of AZ; 88–Aud, Michael D Weiss MD PA

Hadjian, Dr Sophia 403 Butterfield Drive, East Lansing, MI 48823, (517) 351-8228, OB 59 OH Univ - Athens; MA 62 IN Univ - Bloomington; PH 72 (Sp-Lang Path Sp Science) SUNY - Center at Buffalo; Sp-Lang Path, Living & Lrng Resource Ctr, **SLP F**

Hadler, Bette L 366 Las Casas, Pacific Palisades, CA 90272, (213) 454-1858, BA 59 Univ of MI - Ann Arbor; MA 61 Temple Univ-Tyler Sch of Art; Sp-Lang Path, Daniel Freeman Mem Hosp, **SLP**

Hadler, Joanne W 437 Woodhaven Drive, Cedarburg, WI 53012, **SLP**

Hadley, Beth Eleanor 173 Hillcrest, Glen Ellyn, IL 60137, (312) 531-3771, BS 65 Univ of MN - Minneap-St Paul; OM 85 Governors St Univ; **SLP**

Hadley, Mrs Beverly B HHC V Corps, Surgeon Office, APO New York, NY 09079, BS 74 MS Univ for Women; MA 76 Univ of AL- Tuscaloosa; **A**

Hadley, Mrs Carin Bridges 2440 Cardington Drive, Columbia, SC 29209, (803) 783-1102, BS 81 Brigham Young Univ; OD 83 (NS) Brigham Young Univ; Sp-Lang Path, **SLP**

Hadley, Debra L 7809 South Spaulding, Chicago, IL 60652, BS 76 UT St Univ; MS 77 Univ of IL - Urbana; **SLP**

Hadley, Sarah Catherine 1831 John Arden Drive #92, Waxahachie, TX 75165, (817) 573-1282, BS 86 Baylor Univ; MS 87 Baylor Univ; Sp-Lang Path, Waxahachie ISD, **SLP**

Hadley, Mrs Shannon Wilder 5227 Tilting Oaks Court, Jacksonville, FL 32258, (904) 260-9354, BS 81 Lambuth Coll; MA 83 Memphis St Univ; 86–Supvr, InSpeech Inc, **SLP ACE**

Hadox, Mrs Bonita Bartlett 302 Bellview Avenue, Fairmont, WV 26554, (304) 366-2070, BS 83 WV Univ; MS 84 WV Univ; Sp-Lang Path, Marion Co Boe, **SLP**

Hadrick, Nancy Z 46-289 Auna Street, Kaneohe, HI 96744, (808) 433-6488, BS 69 Univ of HI - Manoa; MS 71 Univ of HI - Manoa; Sp-Lang Path, Triple Army Med Cen, **SLP**

Hadsell-Brickler, Linda Denise 657 Froome Avenue, Cincinnati, OH 45232, (606) 491-1171, BS 85 Miami Univ - Oxford; MS 88 Miami Univ - Oxford; 88–Sp-Lang Path, No KY Easter Seal Soc

Hadyn-Hawkins, Nancy P 10 Colonial Drive, Snyder, NY 14226, (716) 892-1045, BA 74 SUNY - Coll at Buffalo; MS 75 Purdue Univ - West Lafayette; Sp-Lang Path, Erie-Cattaraugus BOCES II, **SLP**

Hadzima, Susan G 16603 Fischer Rd, Cleveland, OH 44107, (216) 228-2625, BA 82 Univ of Akron; MA 84 Univ of Akron; **A**

Haecker, Ernest E c/o Santa Fe Hearing Center, 227 East Palace Avenue, Kruger Bldg #B, Santa Fe, NM 87501, (505) 982-0085, BA 69 Messiah Coll; MS 71 Washington Univ; 83–Dir/Aud, Santa Fe Hrng Cen, **A ACE**

Haedicke, Susan Phyllis S 14623 River Forest Drive, Houston, TX 77079, (305) 298-6780, BS 78 NY Univ; MA 80 Wayne St Univ; Sp-Lang Path, Orange Co Pub Sch, **SLP**

Haelsig, Mrs Patricia Cahill 1958 N W Mulholland Blvd, Poulsbo, WA 98370, (206) 697-4684, BA 82 WA St Univ; MA 83 WA St Univ; Sp-Lang Path, **SLP**

Haenze, Mrs Karen Crafford 215 South Seymour Avenue, Mundelein, IL 60060, (312) 362-2900, BA 80 San Jose St Univ; MA 83 San Jose St Univ; 88–Sp-Lang Path, Broy Speech Pathology Assoc, **SLP**

Haeusler, Sheryl G 11708 South Penrose Street, Olathe, KS 66061-6629, (913) 894-1709, BS 76 SUNY - Coll at Geneseo; MS 79 Univ of OK - Norman; 88–Sp-Lang Path, Prentke Romich Co, **SLP**

Hafemeister, Mrs Linda V 5860 Bridle Bend Court, Plano, TX 75093, (214) 931-5665, BA 72 Rutger's St Univ - Douglas Coll; MS 73 PA St Univ - Univ Park; 88–Sp-Lang Path, Univ of North Texas, **SLP**

Haffey, Eileen F 14 Christian Lane, Whately, MA 01093, (413) 665-7565, BA 73 Saint John's Univ - Jamaica; MA 80 CA St Univ - Long Beach; **SLP**

Haffner-Spencer, Linda Jean 1534 Bench Road #E-5, Pocatello, ID 83201, (319) 351-6585, BS 84 Univ of IA; MA 86 Univ of IA; **SLP**

Hafitz, Miriam J 515 West 110th Street #12G, New York, NY 10025, (212) 749-0882, MS 79 Columbia Univ Teachers Coll; 88–Sp-Lang Path, H G Birch Early Childhood Ctr, **SLP**

Hafner, Mrs Margaret S 3501 Northview Drive, Joplin, MO 64801, (417) 624-6885, BS 76 Lincoln Univ; MA 77 Univ of MO - Columbia; 86–Sp=Lang Path, Joplin R-8 Sch Dist, **SLP**

Hafner, Mary Beth 121 South Zinnia Way, Lakewood, CO 80228, (303) 989-6820, BA 83 Univ of CO - Boulder; MA 85 Univ of Denver; 88–Sp-Lang Path, Denver PS, **SLP**

Hafner, Mrs Teresa Dreyer 4417 1st Avenue South, Minneapolis, MN 55409, (612) 825-7906, BA 83 Univ of MN - Minneap-St Paul; MS 86 Moorhead St Univ; SLP, **SLP**

Haft, Debra Joy 211-10 73rd Avenue, Apartment 3D, Bayside, NY 11364, (718) 471-9836, BS 85 SUNY - Coll at Plattsburgh; MS 87 CUNY - Brooklyn Coll; 87–Sp-Lang Path, Volz and Amato, **SLP**

Hagan, Adrienne J 2394 Sayre Drive, Grand Junction, CO 81503, (303) 242-6304, BS 72 Eastern NM Univ; MS 74 Univ of North TX; Director / Commun Disorders, Grand Junction Regional Ctr, **SLP**

Hagan, Mrs Debra L 944 Brunswick Circle, Schaumburg, IL 60193, (312) 351-6258, BA 74 Univ of OK - Norman; MS 75 Univ of OK Medical Center; Sp-Lang Path, Addison Pub Sch Dist #4, **SLP**

Hagan, Mrs Donna M 1101 South 74th #12, Belleville, IL 62223, (618) 397-3513, BS 78 Southern IL Univ-Edwardsvill; MS 79 Southern IL Univ-Edwardsvill; SLP, Spec Sch Dist of St Louis Co, **SLP**

Hagan, Mrs Jacquelyn Rural Route 3, Mexico, MO 65265, (314) 581-5268, BA 75 Univ of MO - Columbia; MA 76 Univ of MO - Columbia; Sp-Lang Path, Mexico Pub Sch, **SLP**

Hagan, Marilyn L 1135 Longmeadow Road, Northbrook, IL 60062, MS

Hagan, Rebecca Wilcox 19 Nel Bonney Road, Plympton, MA 02367, (617) 585-2940, BS 79 TX Christian Univ; MS 84 Univ of NC - Chapel Hill; 86–Sp-Lang Path, MA Easter Seal Soc, **SLP**

Hagberg, Eric N 755 Boardman-Canfield Rd, Youngstown, OH 44512, (216) 726-8155, BA 74 SUNY - Center at Buffalo; MA 76 Kent St Univ; Aud-Owner, Neuro-Commun Serv Inc, **A**

Hage, Mrs Luella R T 3406 34th Avenue, Moline, IL 61265, (309) 762-3631, BA 74 Augustana Coll; MA 77 Western IL Univ; Sp-Lang Path, Moline Sch Dist #40, **SLP**

Hage-Brodnansky, Becky 2630 Hartley Road, Lakeport, CA 95453, (707) 263-1949, MA 88 CA Lutheran Coll

Hagedorn, Kay E 1413 Emery Street, Eau Claire, WI 54701, (715) 834-0581, BA 77 Univ of MN - Duluth; MS 78 Univ of WI Eau Claire; Sp-Lang Path, Development & Training Ctr, **SLP**

Hageman, Dr Carlin F 216 Colorado Road, Cedar Falls, IA 50613, (319) 273-2497, BA 73 Univ of CO - Boulder; MA 76 Univ of CO - Boulder; PH 80 (NS) Univ of CO - Boulder; Asst Prof, U of N IA, **SLP**

Hageman, Mrs Cindy 412 South Crestway, Wichita, KS 67218, (316) 683-1559, BS 76 KS St Univ; MA 77 KS St Univ; Sp-Lang Path, Private Practice, **SLP**

Hageman, Mrs Ruth A 6673 Aranda Avenue, La Jolla, CA 92037, BS 57 Univ of Southern CA; SLP, Chula Vista Cty Sch Dist, **SLP LM**

Hagen, Dr Chris 225 Winterhawk Lane, Olivenhain, CA 92024, (619) 576-5837, BA 59 Whittier Coll; MA 62 Univ of Southern CA; PH 64 (NS) Univ of Southern CA; Dir, Sp-Hrng & Neurosensory Cen, **SLP F**

Hagen, Mrs Debra Knauer 15 Charles Street #4-A, New York, NY 10014, (212) 254-7300, BA 75 CUNY - Queens Coll; MA 76 Hofstra Univ; **SLP**

Hagen, Jennifer Lynn 513 North Franklin Avenue, Apartment 2, Madison, WI 53705-3648, (612) 430-1972, BA 84 Univ of WI - Eau Claire; MS 86 Univ of WI - Madison; **SLP**

Hagen, Kathryn J 4603 Drexel Avenue, Edina, MN 55424, (612) 927-7453, BS 74 Northwestern Univ; MA 75 Northwestern Univ; Sp-Lang Path, Anoka-Hennepon Sch Dist, **SLP**

Hagen, Mary E 4003 Idaho Avenue, Crystal, MN 55427, (612) 537-1471, BS 73 Mankato St Univ; MA 76 Mankato St Univ; **SLP**

Hagen, Susan T 1812 North Lincoln Street, Wilmington, DE 19806, (302) 479-1621, BA 68 Marywood Coll; MA 69 Columbia Univ Teachers Coll; Sp-Lang Path, Brandywine Sch Dist, **SLP**

Hagen, Mrs Suzanne G 225 Winterhawk Lane, Olivenhain, CA 92024, (619) 576-5837, BA 59 OH Univ - Athens; MA 65 Univ of Southern CA; Sp/Lang Path, Sp/Hrng/Neur Cen, **SLP**

Hagenbuch, Roxanne R Audiologic Consultants, 1857 Center Street, Camp Hill, PA 17011, (717) 761-7593, BA 77 Bloomsburg Univ of PA; MS 86 Bloomsburg Univ of PA; 88–Aud, Audiologic Consultants, **A**

Hagen-Pilkinton, Karol Lee 1616 Clinch Avenue #4, Knoxville, TN 37916, (615) 523-3093, SLP, Ft Sanders Reg Med Ctr, **SLP**

Hager, Caryn D 240 West 98th Street #10-B, New York, NY 10025, (212) 662-6372, MS 88 Columbia Univ Teachers Coll

Hager, Mrs Nancy S 610 Terrace Lane, Carbondale, IL 62901, BS 57 Univ of IL - Urbana; MS 71 Southern IL Univ -Carbondale; Sp-Lang Path, Carbondale Board Educ Dist 95, **SLP**

Hager, Paul Milton 615 Fleming Street, Eau Claire, WI 54701, (715) 836-4846, BA 80 Univ of WI - Eau Claire; MS 82 Univ of WI - Eau Claire; Lecturer Clin Super, Univ of WI Eau Claire, **SLP**

Hagerman, Ellen C 204 University Avenue, Lexington, KY 40503, (606) 278-0046, BA 77 Univ of KY; MA 79 Univ of Northern CO; Sp/Lang Path, Univ of Kentucky Med Ctr, **SLP**

Hagerman, Evie J Communicative Disorders Dept, Research Medical Center, 2316 East Meyer Boulevard, Kansas City, MO 64132, (816) 276-4023, BS 70 Indiana Univ of PA; MS 71 Vanderbilt Univ; Dir, Research Med Cen, **SLP ACE**

Hagerty, Eileen R 216 Wood Street, Ithaca, NY 14850, (607) 277-4152, BS 75 Ithaca Coll; MS 79 Boston Univ; Sp-Lang Path, Private Practice, **SLP**

Hagerty, Mrs Jane Ellen 525 Glen Ruadh Avenue, Erie, PA 16505, (814) 453-7661, MS 84 Boston Univ; Sp-Lang Path, Dr Gertrude A Barber Center, **SLP**

Hagerty, Mrs Lynette Reville 950 Lois Lane, Titusville, FL 32780, (305) 724-2718, BA 85 Rosary Coll; MA 87 Olivet Nazarene Coll; Aud, ENT Hlth & Surg Ctr

Hagerty, Mary B 1577 Tabor Avenue, Kettering, OH 45420, (513) 254-5637, BS 74 Kent St Univ; MA 75 Kent St Univ; Sp-Lang Path, Montgomery Co Bd of Mr, **SLP**

Haggard, Carolyn S Dos Marinas 1 #709, Fijardo, PR 00648, (716) 878-7371, BA 80 SUNY - Center at Buffalo; MA 82 SUNY - Center at Buffalo; Sp-Lang Path, Children's Hospital, **SLP**

Haggerty, Barbara A 4161 Roxbury Place, Erie, PA 16506, **SLP**

Haggerty, Holly Susan Division Of Otolaryngology, Edwards Bldg Room R-135, Stanford University Medical Center, Stanford, CA 94305, (415) 725-5946, BA 77 Univ of CA - Santa Cruz; MA 84 Univ of CA - Santa Barbara; 88–Sp-Lang Path, Stanford Univ

Haggerty-Paolucci, Mrs Sharla J 4901 Washington, Midland, MI 48640, (517) 631-5420, BS 70 Central MI Univ; MA 72 Central MI Univ; Tchr, Midland Pub Sch, **A**

Hagler, Mrs Marian K 9204 87th Street, Fort Saskatchewan, AB, Canada T8L 2R2, (403) 471-7970, BA 70 Univ of Northern CO; MA 72 Univ of Northern CO; 88–Aud, Glenrose Rehab Hosp, **A**

Hagler, Dr Paul H 9204 87th Street, Fort Saskatchewan, AB, Canada T8L 2R2, (403) 432-5990, BA 70 Wichita St Univ; MA 72 Wichita St Univ; PH (Sp-Lang Path) IN Univ - Bloomington; 74–Assoc Prof, Univ of Alberta, **SLP**

Haglund, Janet M 660 Vine, Denver, CO 80206, (303) 429-4031, BS 68 Univ of CO - Boulder; MS 71 CO St Univ; Owner, Private Practice, **SLP**

Hagness, Dr Don Edward 4 Rutledge Place, Terre Haute, IN 47803, (812) 237-2808, BS 58 Carroll Coll; MS 65 Marquette Univ; PH 69 (Sp Sci & Aud) Univ of IL - Urbana; 69–Prof of Commun Dis, IN St U, **A**

Hagood, Brenda Britton 1982 Cherrywood Street, Vista, CA 92083, (619) 727-0716, BA 82 CA St Univ - Fullerton; MS 85 Loma Linda Univ - Riverside; Sp-Lang Path, Vista USD, **SLP**

Hagood, Linda Wardell 1803 Cannonwood Lane, Austin, TX 78745, (512) 454-8631, BA 77 Univ of TX - Austin; MA 85 Univ of TX - Austin; Speech-Language Pathologist, Texas School for the Blind, **SLP**

Hagood, Mrs Nancy P 402 Pineway Drive, Birmingham, AL 35226, (205) 822-0431, MA 76 Univ of AL- Tuscaloosa; Sp-Lang Path, Midfield City School System, **SLP**

Hagstette, Sharon Murray 3212 Massachusetts Avenue, Kenner, LA 70065, (504) 443-5269, BS 80 Saint Mary's Dominican Coll; OM 81 LA St Univ - N O Medical Ctr; 87–Sp-Lang Path, Private Practice, **SLP**

Hagstrom, Fran W 6 Meadow Lane, Worcester, MA 01602, (617) 797-4268, BA 67 Southwest Baptist Univ; MA 70 Saint Louis Univ; MS 77 Univ of TX - Houston; -Research Asst, Clark Univ, **SLP**

Hague, Kevin W 7929 West Grandridge Boulevard, Kennewick, WA 99336, (509) 735-7461, BS 80 Brigham Young Univ; MA 81 Brigham Young Univ; Aud-Pres, Aud Cen, Inc, **A**

Hahn, Carol Ann 718 South Calumet Avenue, Michigan City, IN 46360, (219) 872-4143, MA 88 Northwestern Univ

Hahn, Mrs Carole Kravec 775 Carr Street, Lakewood, CO 80215-6065, BA 72 IN Univ - Bloomington; MA 73 IN Univ - Bloomington; Sp-Lang Path, Craig Hosp, **SLP**

Hahn, Dr Elise S P O Box 4523, Carmel, CA 93921, (408) 624-1626, BA 32 Univ of CA - Los Angeles; MA 42 Wayne St Univ; PH 47 (Sp Path) Northwestern Univ; Retired, **SLP F H LM**

Hahn, Mary C 4320 Ballaire Drive South, Apartment 213W, Fort Worth, TX 76109, (817) 460-3546, BS 77 Univ of TX - Austin; MA 80 TX Woman's Univ; Sp/Lang Path, Arlington ISD, **SLP**

Hahn, Mrs Milege J 3721 Glenaire Drive, Charlottesville, VA 22901, (804) 977-1431, BA 48 Univ of CO - Boulder; ME 69 Univ of VA - Charlottesville; Aud, Wallenborn/Sydnor/Eastham/Johnson Ltd, **A**

Hahn, Dr Patricia A Eastern Washington University, Communication Disorders, Cheney, WA 99004, (509) 359-2301, BS 54 Univ of NE - Lincoln; MA 59 Northwestern Univ; PH 69 (NS) Univ of OR; Prof Commun Dis, Eastern Washington Univ, **SLP**

Hahn, Patricia M 3360 Marble Terrace, Colorado Springs, CO 80906, (719) 390-8581, BA 71 Univ of NE - Omaha; MS 74 Univ of NE - Omaha; 85–Sp-Lang Path, Widefield Sch Dist, **SLP**

Hahn, Shelly E 626 Haverford Road, Haverford, PA 19041-1102, (215) 649-8255, BS 74 Univ of Pittsburgh - Pittsburgh; OM 82 Temple Univ; MA 75 OH Univ - Athens; Dir, Main Line Sp Consultants, **SLP**

Hahn, Susan E 2918 West Logan Blvd, Chicago, IL 60647-1732, (312) 276-0636, BA 74 Northern IL Univ - De Kalb; MS 76 Eastern IL Univ; Sp-Lang Path, Chicago Bd of Ed, **SLP**

Hahn, Susan Margaret 17020 Patricia Lane, Brookfield, WI 53005, (414) 782-7425, BS 85 Univ of WI - Whitewater; MS 87 Marquette Univ; 88–Sp-Lang Path, Hartford Sch Dist, **SLP**

Hahn, Wilma J 2676 Juniper, Boulder, CO 80302, (303) 449-4717, **SLP**

Hahne, Sharon K 2807 East 600 North, West Lafayette, IN 47906, (314) 884-0310, BS 74 Purdue Univ - West Lafayette; MS 76 Purdue Univ - West Lafayette; Sp-Lang Path, Benton Community Sch Corp, **SLP**

Hahner, Jeffrey C Department Of Speech And Drama, Pace University, Pace Plaza, New York, NY 10038, (212) 488-1311, BA 66 Pace U -NY City; MA 67 NY Univ; 66–Chmn-Dept Sp Comm Studies, Pace University

Haicken, Vivian G 584 Bluffview Drive, Belleair, FL 34640, (813) 581-6740, BA Towson St Univ; MS 72 Loyola Coll; **SLP**

Haid, Mrs Sheila Ann 5853 Greenlawn Road, Hamilton, OH 45011, (513) 894-6261, BS 76 Miami Univ - Oxford; MS 82 Miami Univ - Oxford; Sp-Path, Hamilton City Sch, **SLP**

Haider, Donna M Affiliated Otolaryngologists, 3366 Oakdale Avenue North, Suite 307, Robbinsdale, MN 55422, (612) 588-0851, BS 80 Univ of WI - Stevens Point; MS 82 Univ of WI - Stevens Point; Aud, Affiliated Otolaryngologist, **A**

Haigh, Amy Lee 4035 Camino Real, Sarasota, FL 34231, (813) 923-4535, **SLP**

Haight, Mrs Diane DaveKos 9 Ancient Rubbly, Beverly, MA 01915, (617) 246-6460, BS 81 Emerson Coll; MS 85 Boston Univ; 86–Sp-Lang Path, Wakefield PS, **SLP**

Haight, Patti Lynn 11206 Euclid Avenue, Cleveland, OH 44106, (216) 231-8787, BS 84 Univ of KS; MA 88 Univ of KS; 87–Sp-Lang Path, Cleveland Hearing & Speech Ctr, **SLP**

Hailey, Mrs Ann H W 1205 Knoll Crest Court, Grapevine, TX 76051-5070, (703) 362-9745, BS 77 James Madison Univ; MS 78 James Madison Univ; SLP, Dallas Easter Seal Society, **SLP**

Hailey, Donna R P O Box 61486, Houston, TX 77208-1486, **SLP**

Hailparn, Ellen L 345 East 83rd Street #6-A, New York, NY 10021, (212) 517-9879, BA 78 SUNY - Center at Buffalo; MA 80 Univ of FL; SLP, The Brooklyn Hosp, **SLP**

Haim, Saralyn Polon 1523 18th Street #1, Santa Monica, CA 90404, (818) 997-2330, BA 82 CA St Univ - Northridge; MA 84 CA St Univ - Northridge; Sp-Lang Path, Los Angeles USD, **SLP**

Haimowitz, Audrey R 123 McArthur Avenue, Staten Island, NY 10312, (718) 948-4720, BA 74 CUNY - Brooklyn Coll; MS 79 CUNY - Brooklyn Coll; 75–Sp-Lang Path, NYC Bd of Ed-Sp Serv Ut, **SLP**

Hain, Marsha K 2850 Fairway Drive #33, Las Cruces, NM 88001, (915) 543-6824, BS 84 Millersville Univ of PA; MS 87 PA St Univ - Univ Park; 88–Sp-Lang Path, Rio Vista Rehab Hosp, **SLP**

Hain, Mrs Rosalind J 193 Haddenfield Road, Clifton, NJ 07013, (201) 778-5146, BA 45 Univ of WI - Madison; MA 63 Columbia Univ Teachers Coll; Sp-Lang Path, Private Practice, **SLP**

Haine, Mrs Geraldine 2300 Longfellow Lane, Midland, MI 48640-5723, (517) 631-8138, BA 65 Grinnell Coll; MS 67 Purdue Univ - West Lafayette; **SLP**

Haines, Constance Dee Box 7742, APO New York, NY 09012, BA 81 Eastern WA Univ; MS 82 Eastern WA Univ; Sp-Lang Path, US Army Landstuhl Hospital, **SLP ACE**

Haines, Harold H 829 West Victoria, Santa Barbara, CA 93101, BA 31 WA St Univ; MA 62 Univ of NM; **SLP LM**

Haines, Mrs Karen Barr 114 Horizon Drive, Morgantown, WV 26505, (304) 293-4241, BS 77 WV Univ; MS 78 WV Univ; 87–Asst Prof, West Virginia University, **SLP**

Haines, Marsha Bouchey Route 2 Box 98, Stockton, KS 67669, (913) 425-6887, BA 69 KS St Univ; MS 83 Fort Hays St Univ; Sp-Lang Path, USD 325 & 324, **SLP**

Haines, Sarah Elizabeth 4183 Bloomington Avenue Apartment 201, Arlington Heights, IL 60004, BA 83 Case Western Reserve Univ; MS 85 Univ of MI - Ann Arbor; Sp-Lang Path, Therapeutic Systems, **SLP**

Hainey-Flacke, Martha J 38 Harmon Road, Scotia, NY 12302, (518) 399-2266, BS 79 SUNY - Coll at Geneseo; MA 81 SUNY - Coll at Geneseo; 83–Sp-Lang Path, Southern Adirondack Educ Ctr, **SLP**

Haire, Dr Carol D 1925 Hospital Place, Abilene, TX 79606-5239, (915) 691-5190, BA 70 TX Tech Univ; MA 71 Univ of North TX; ED 76 (NS) TX Tech Univ; 77–Owner/Dir, Haire Sp Lang & Learning Ctr, **SLP**

Hairston, Anne Heinrich Psc 1 P O Box 21588, Apo, San Francisco, CA 96230, BA 75 Univ of CA - Santa Barbara; MS 78 Portland St Univ; Sp-Lang Path, Dod Dep Schs Kadena AFB, **SLP**

Hairston, Karen Jeannine 2728 Peyton Woods TRAIL5, Atlanta, GA 30311, (404) 696-3389, BS 83 Univ of GA; MA 86 Univ of TN - Knoxville; **SLP**

Hairston, Kathryn 8607 South University, Chicago, IL 60619, (312) 962-4765, BA 73 Augustana Coll; MA 75 Northwestern Univ; Sp-Lang Path, Chicago Board of Education, **SLP**

Hairston, Valeri Lyn 2222 Livernois Drive, Howell, MI 48843-8414, (419) 756-1133, BS 81 Univ of Cincinnati; MA 83 Univ of Cincinnati; Sp-Lang Path, Rehab Serv of North Cen Ohio, **SLP**

Haischer, Mrs Lori G N88 W6278 Willowbrook Dr, Cedarburg, WI 53012, (414) 255-2500, MS 84 Univ of WI - Madison; Audiologist, Med Associates Health Center, **A**

Haislup, Linda J 667 Walnut Point Court, Ballwin, MO 63011, (314) 527-3449, BS 74 Purdue Univ - West Lafayette; MA 75 IN Univ - Bloomington; **SLP**

Hajos, Mrs Anita B 182 West E Street, Brawley, CA 92227, (619) 339-6421, BA 65 San Diego St Univ; MA 67 Stanford Univ; 67–Sp-Lang Path, Imperial Co Offi of Ed, **SLP ACE**

Hakala, Mrs Claudia G 1481 Jordan Avenue, Crofton, MD 21114, (301) 262-1110, BA 64 Univ of MD - College Park; MA 72 Univ of MD - College Park; Sp-Lang Path, Prince Georges Co Pub Sch, **SLP**

Hakanson, Kim M 1417 N W Menlo Drive, Corvallis, OR 97330, (503) 757-5048, BS 82 OR St Univ; MS 86 Univ of OR; 87–Sp-Lang Path, Good Samaritan Hosp, **SLP**

Hake, Mrs Ann S 3524 Timberlake Road S W, Knoxville, TN 37920, (615) 577-5970, BA 58 Transylvania Univ; MA 79 Univ of TN - Knoxville; Sp/Lang Path, Sevier Co Sch, **SLP ACE**

Hakel, Mark Edward Madonna Centers, 2200 South 52nd Street, Lincoln, NE 68506, (402) 489-7102, **SLP**

Hakel-Dailey, Mrs Lori J 959 West 8th, Wahoo, NE 68066, (402) 443-4090, BS 86 Univ of NE - Lincoln; MS 88 Univ of NE - Lincoln; 88–Aud, ENT Spec

Halas, Mrs Christine 5880 Edgewood Lane, Willoughby, OH 44094, (216) 256-8483, BS 76 Miami Univ - Oxford; MS 77 Case Western Reserve Univ; Director of Speech Services, Psi Associates Inc, **SLP**

Halayko, Mrs Kathleen A 11614 Springtime Lane, Fairfax Station, VA 22039, (703) 250-2049, BA 69 Boston Coll; MA 71 Coll of Saint Rose; 88–Sp-Lang Path, Falls Church PS, **SLP**

Halbach, Rita Mary 80 Crescent Road, Center City, MN 55012, (612) 257-4836, **SLP**

Halberstam, Feigi Taub 2314 Avenue O, Brooklyn, NY 11210, (212) 377-5090, **A**

Halbert, Mrs Carolyn Cohen 16 Laverack #1, Depew, NY 14043, (716) 683-6425, BS 83 SUNY - Coll at Buffalo; MA 85 SUNY - Center at Buffalo; Sp-Lang Path, Heritage Educ Prog, **SLP ACE**

Halbert, Charlene Georgetti 222 Wellington Rd, De Witt, NY 13214, (315) 445-0997, BS 77 SUNY - Coll at Geneseo; MA 79 Univ of KS; Aud, **A**

Halchishick, Janice Marie 2712 Margate Lane, Augusta, GA 30909, (404) 724-7746, MA 81 Univ of Northern CO; BA 80 Univ of Northern CO; Dir Com Dis, Walton Rehab Hosp, **SLP**

Halcrow, Jeanette Van Camp 9025 Marcella Lane N E, Bemidji, MN 56601, (218) 586-2922, BS 63 Univ of ND; MS 81 Univ of ND; Sp-Lang Path, Bagley Pub Sch, **SLP**

Haldeman, Margaret M 3939 Ellington Road, 2nd Floor, Philadelphia, PA 19131, (215) 877-7708, Dir Sp-Lang Path, Children's Heart Hosp of Phila, **SLP**

Hale, Mrs Bernie A 540 South Avenue C, Kermit, TX 79745, (915) 586-6674, BA 54 TX Christian Univ; MA 71 TX Christian Univ; Kermit ISD, **SLP**

Hale, Mrs Cathy P 455 West Seminole Avenue, Eustis, FL 32726, (904) 589-1944, BA 76 Auburn Univ - Auburn; MS 78 Auburn Univ - Auburn; Dir/Sp-Lang Path, Eustis Sp & Lang Cen Inc, **SLP ACE**

Hale, Diane H 22 Robinhood, Jackson, TN 38305, (901) 658-6113, BA 73 Univ of SC - Columbia; MS 75 Univ of SC - Columbia; SLP, Madison County Schools, **SLP**

Hale, Mrs Dianne Louise Route 1 Box 38-A, Greenville, NC 27834, (919) 758-7140, **SLP**

Hale, Mrs Karen B 14512 Alfalfa Lane, Sand Springs, OK 74063, (918) 245-3640, BA 70 Northeastern OK St Univ; MA 72 OK St Univ; 86–Sp-Lang Path, Lone Star & Allen Bowden Schs, **SLP**

Hale, Dr Lester L 10112 North Magna Carta, Baton Rouge, LA 70815, (504) 927-8431, BA 34 Univ of WI - Madison; MS 35 LA St Univ - Baton Rouge; PH 42 (NS) LA St Univ - Baton Rouge; Presbyterian Church, **SLP F LM**

Hale, Mark Bates 501 Eric Avenue #50, Bowling Green, KY 42101-9293, (800) 331-8840, BS 84 Western KY Univ; MS 85 Western KY Univ

Hale, Mrs Maryjane Bialomizy 3979 Montefrio Court, San Diego, CA 92130, (619) 753-6241, BS 78 SUNY - Coll at Fredonia; MA 86 San Diego St Univ; Tchr, San Dieguito Union HS Dist, **SLP**

Hale, Nancy Tara 1016 1/2 8th Street, Nevada, IA 50201, (515) 239-4480, BS 85 Univ of IA; MS 87 Univ of AZ; Aud, Mc Farland Clinic

Hale, Mrs Sue T 112 Lakeway Drive, Oxford, MS 38655, (601) 232-7271, OB 72 Univ of MS; OM 75 Univ of MS; Sp-Lang Path, Dept Comm Dis U of Ms, **SLP**

Hale, Suzan L Fm 1960 Sp Lang 7 Myofun Thrpy, 15626 Silver Ridge, Suite 107, Houston, TX 77090, (713) 444-3374, BA 77 Univ of Houston - Univ Park; MA 79 Univ of Houston - Univ Park; Owner/Dir, FM1960 Sp-Lang & Ther Cen, **SLP**

Hale, Tammy Schraeder 1504 Laredo, Mesquite, TX 75150, (214) 686-0366, BS 82 Baylor Univ; MA 85 TX Woman's Univ; Sp-Lang Path, Tammy Schraeder Hale, **SLP**

Hale, Mrs Terri Kay 1454 East Keowee Trail, Seneca, SC 29678, MA 84 Towson St Univ; Sp-Lang Path, Oconee Co Sch Dist, **SLP**

Hale, Mrs Wanda Richardson 1700 Little Willeo Road, Marietta, GA 30067, (404) 763-0580, BS 69 Auburn Univ - Auburn; ME 71 Emory Univ; Coord for Staff Serv, Fulton Co Sch Syst, **SLP**

Halegoua, Perla P 1 Crescent Road, Port Jefferson, NY 11777, BA 74 CUNY - Queens Coll; MA 76 Hofstra Univ; **SLP**

Hale-Haniff, Mary 11944 SW 12th Street, Pembroke Pines, FL 33025, (305) 435-3585, MA 79 Univ of MN - Minneap-St Paul; Pres, Catalyst Institute, **SLP**

Halek, Kathleen A 126 Stony Hill Village, Brookfield Center, CT 06805, (203) 797-7504, BA 79 Univ of FL; MS 81 Columbia Univ Teachers Coll; 87–Sp-Lang Path & Aud, Danbury Hospital, **SLP**

Hales, Nancy Burch 78 Chestnut Lane, Newburgh, NY 12550, MS 86 SUNY - Coll at New Paltz; **SLP**

Halevi, Dr Lynne Grossman 1717 Ala Wai Boulevard #2305, Honolulu, HI 96815, (808) 944-4079, BA 64 San Jose St Univ; MA 67 San Jose St Univ; PH 83 (NS) Columbia Pacific Univ; Sp-Lang Path, Halevi Associates, **SLP**

Haley, Ann M 7892 Lakecrest Drive, Greenbelt, MD 20770, (301) 345-6786, BS 77 Emerson Coll; MA 78 George Washington Univ; Sp-Lang Path, Sp-Lang Path Assoc, **SLP**

Haley, Cynthia S 197-C Nashville Road, Saranac, NY 12981, (518) 492-2580, MA 85 SUNY - Coll at Plattsburgh; **SLP**

Haley, Mrs Deena C 1350 Overhill Road, Fairmont, WV 26554, (304) 366-2070, BA 80 Marshall Univ; MA 82 Univ of TN - Knoxville; Sp-Lang Path, Marion County Schools, **SLP**

Haley, Donna Jean 1339 Amherst Place, Dayton, OH 45406, (513) 276-8306, BS 83 Bowling Green St Univ; MA 84 Bowling Green St Univ; 85–Sp-Lang Path Supervisor, Good Samaritan Hospital, **SLP ACE**

Haley, Eileen T 1629 Columbia Road N W, Washington, DC 20009, (202) 223-8400, BA 75 SUNY - Center at Stony Brook; MS 86 Univ of the DC; **SLP**

Haley, Evelyn C 3443 Esplanade Avenue #241, New Orleans, LA 70119, (504) 245-1002, BA 60 Loyola Univ; MS 64 Tulane Univ; Dir Sp-Lang Path, Louise S Davis Dev Cen, **SLP**

Haley, Mrs Judith 1345 Waldheim Road, Chippewa Falls, WI 54729, (715) 723-5753, BA 74 Univ of WI - Eau Claire; MS 75 Univ of WI - Milwaukee; Sp-Lang Path, Private Practice, **SLP**

Haley, Judy 20 Chicory Lane, Riverwoods, IL 60015, (312) 625-3461, BA 72 Univ of MD - College Park; MA 74 Northwestern Univ; SLP, Chicago Pub Schools, **SLP**

Haley, Mrs Susan W 4 Tall Pines Road, Scarborough, ME 04074, (207) 883-5285, BS 77 Univ of ME - Orono; MA 79 Towson St Univ; **SLP**

Haley-Condon, Mrs Lavon 3734 N E Alameda, Portland, OR 97212, (503) 232-4424, BA 67 Mankato St Univ; MA 72 Univ of WA; Dir Spec Instruc, Portland Pub Sch, **SLP**

Halfast, Laurie Ann 4 Hunt Grove Road, Ithaca, NY 14850, (305) 395-8234, BS 82 OK St Univ; MS 85 Univ of OK Medical Center; **SLP**

Halfin, Kimberly Kay 6201 Sneed Cove #1133, Austin, TX 78744, (512) 445-4665, MS 87 Southwest TX St Univ; 88–Sp-Lang Path, Healthcare Rehab Ctr

Halfman, Mrs Patricia J 4745 Apple Valley Drive, Bettendorf, IA 52722, (309) 372-8822, BS 77 Western IL Univ; MA 77 Western IL Univ; Sp-Lang Path, Rockridge School District #300, **SLP**

Halfond, Dr Murray M Department Of Speech-Language Hearing, Temple University, Philadelphia, PA 19122, (215) 787-1872, BA 48 CUNY - Brooklyn Coll; MA 49 Northwestern Univ; PH 52 (NS) Northwestern Univ; Prof of Speech, Temple University, **SLP F**

Halford, Mrs Wilma E 1162 Eastminster Drive, Columbia, SC 29204, (803) 787-3909, BA 48 Univ of GA; ME 50 Emory Univ; Sp-Lang Path, Lexington County School Dist 5, **SLP**

Hall, Alberta W 10756 Cordage Walk, Columbia, MD 21044, (301) 799-7088, BA 69 CUNY - Hunter Coll; BA 69 CUNY - Hunter Coll; SLP, Howard Co Publ Sch Syst, **SLP A**

Hall, Dr Allen Sanders 4243 West Bethany Home Rd, Phoenix, AZ 85019, (602) 841-9151, BS 63 Memphis St Univ; MA 64 Univ of AL- Tuscaloosa; PH 70 (NS) OH St Univ; Director, Glendale Speech & Lang Ctr, **SLP**

Hall, Mrs Ann M M 21 Carnot Avenue, Woodcliff Lake, NJ 07675, (201) 573-1265, BA 76 Univ of CT; MS 77 Univ of MI - Ann Arbor; **SLP**

Hall, Barbara 448 5th Street, Ann Arbor, MI 48103, (313) 764-2148, BA 69 Univ of MI - Ann Arbor; MS 73 Univ of MI - Ann Arbor; Sp-Lang Path, Ann Arbor PS, **SLP**

Hall, Betty F 125 Hwy 101 West, Apartment 5, Port Angeles, WA 98362, (206) 452-3958, BS 73 Middle TN St Univ; OM 74 Univ of MS; Sp-Lang Path, Quillayute Valley Schs, **SLP**

Hall, Mrs Beverly Butler 1004 South Main, Henderson, TX 75652, (214) 657-5800, BS 81 Stephen F Austin St Univ; ME 83 Stephen F Austin St Univ; Sp-Lang Path, Private Practice, **SLP**

Hall, Brenda Bogart 3728 Cannongate Drive, Columbus, OH 43228, (513) 324-2081, BS 84 East Carolina Univ; ME 86 Univ of NC - Greensboro; 86–Aud, W Central Oh Hrng & Sp Cntr, **A**

Hall, Mrs Brenda Bullock 2103 Foxhorn Road, New Bern, NC 28560, (919) 633-2501, BS 77 East Carolina Univ; MS 80 East Carolina Univ; Sp-Lang Path, Private Practice, **SLP**

Hall, C Mike Communicative Services Group, 1479 Ygnacio Valley Road, Walnut Creek, CA 94598, (415) 938-8686, Aud, Csg Hearing Services, **A**

Hall, Mrs Carol Jean 1451 Brookside Drive, High Ridge, MO 63049, (314) 351-9692, BA 81 Central MO St Univ; MA 85 Fontbonne Coll; 87–Sp-Lang Path, St Louis Special Sch Dist, **SLP**

Hall, Carolyn J 13416 East Asbury Drive, Aurora, CO 80014, (303) 861-6800, BS 69 Univ of MN - Minneap-St Paul; MS 67 Univ of OK Medical Center; Sp-Lang Path, Chldrens Hospital, **SLP**

Hall, Mrs Cathleen Thompson 650 Woodbridge Drive, Bloomington, IN 47401, (317) 782-1194, BS 83 FL St Univ; MS 84 FL St Univ; SLP, Indianapolis Spech & Hring Ctr, **SLP**

Hall, Cheryl L 4617 Soho Court, Virginia Beach, VA 23455, (814) 432-3171, BS 69 Indiana Univ of PA; ME 72 Clarion Univ of PA; SLP, Commonwealth of PA, **SLP**

Hall, Cora Belle 2441 West Elizabeth, Fort Collins, CO 80521, (303) 484-7430, BA 38 OK St Univ; MA 49 Northwestern Univ; **SLP LM**

Hall, Deanne Brenda 12531 Coursey Blvd #1103, Baton Rouge, LA 70816, (504) 292-9776, BS 83 Hampton Univ; MS 85 Howard Univ; **A**

Hall, Debra Lee 107 Vernon Street, Dublin, GA 31021, (912) 272-9460, ME 85 Univ of GA; **A**

Hall, Mrs Diane Carey 17926 Elk River Circle, Houston, TX 77090, (713) 550-8132, BS 62 OH Univ - Athens; MA 83 Univ of Houston - Univ Park; 88–Sp-Lang Path, Cypress Fairbanks ISD, **SLP**

Hall, Mrs Diane Hayes 42 Gloucester Road, Hilton Head, SC 29928, (803) 681-3885, BA 75 Shorter Coll; ME 77 Univ of GA; Sp-Lang Path, Private Practice, **SLP**

Hall, Don Raymond 2451 July Street, Baton Rouge, LA 70808, (504) 343-3439, MA 86 LA St Univ - Baton Rouge; **SLP**

Hall, Dr Donald E 638 Orlando Avenue, Akron, OH 44320, (216) 836-6656, BS 61 Indiana Univ of PA; ME 68 Westminster Coll; PH 71 (NS) OH Univ - Athens; Assoc Prof-Commun Dis, The U of Akron, **SLP**

Hall, Dr Edward Pierce 6291 Sylvan, Simi Valley, CA 93063, (818) 885-2858, BS 54 Univ of HI - Manoa; MA 64 Univ of HI - Manoa; PH 71 (NS) Univ of Southern CA; Prof, CA St U, **SLP A**

Hall, Emily L 3609 Cedar Lane S W, Roanoke, VA 24018, (707) 774-4635, ME 88 Univ of VA - Charlottesville

Hall, Flavia Bernado 43 Lincoln Avenue, East Brunswick, NJ 08816, (201) 548-7610, BA 76 CUNY - Hunter Coll; MA 78 CUNY - Queens Coll; SLP, John F Kennedy Medical Center, **SLP**

Hall, Mrs Frances S 2009 Briarwood Drive, Laurel, MS 39440, **SLP**

Hall, Mrs Geraldine A 1247 East 7th Street, Plainfield, NJ 07062, (201) 322-1641, BS 57 Bowling Green St Univ; BA 57 Bowling Green St Univ; MA 60 Univ of Denver; Sp-Lang Path, Union Co Day Trng Cent, **SLP ACE**

Hall, Mrs Gilda E F 3531 N W 27th Street, Gainesville, FL 32605, (904) 371-0214, BA 76 Univ of FL; ME 77 Univ of FL; **SLP**

Hall, Gregory William 1605 Havenwood, Oceanside, CA 92056-2076, (619) 471-1196, MA 83 CA St Univ - Los Angeles; 86–Aud, Private Practice, **A**

Hall, James E 10013 South Saint, Lawrence Avenue, Chicago, IL 60628, (312) 785-1340, BS 74 Western IL Univ; MA 75 Western IL Univ; ME 82 Univ of IL - Chicago; Sp-Lang Path, Chicago Pub Sch, **SLP**

Hall, James Hartmann, Jr University Of Texas Speech And Hearing Institute, 1343 Moursund, Houston, TX 77030, (713) 792-4500, BA 78 Univ of KS; MA 83 Univ of KS; 87–Chief of Aud, Univ of TX Sp & Hearing Inst, **A**

Hall, Dr James W, III Department Of Otolaryngology, School Of Medicine, Vanderbilt University, Nashville, TN 37232-2559, (615) 322-6389, BA 70 Amer Int'l Coll; MA 73 Northwestern Univ; PH 79 (Aud) Baylor Coll of Medicine; 88–Assoc Prof/Dir of Aud, Vanderbilt Univ Sch of Med, **SLP A**

Hall, Mrs Jan McKay 404 South Fourth Street, Amory, MS 38821, (601) 256-4570, BA 77 Univ of MS; OM 78 Univ of MS; **SLP**

Hall, Jane Elizabeth 8050 N 9th Avenue #82, Pensacola, FL 32514, (904) 438-8366, BS 86 FL St Univ; MS 87 FL St Univ; SLP, Escambia Co Schls

Hall, Janet E 2313 Andover Place, Charleston, IL 61920, BS 63 Eastern IL Univ; MA 73 MI St Univ; **SLP**

Hall, Janice 1506-B Philo Road, Urbana, IL 61801, (217) 337-2503, BS 83 IL St Univ - Normal; MS 85 IL St Univ - Normal; 86–Sp-Lang Path, Burnham Hospital, **SLP ACE**

Hall, Jeffrey Lynn 28333 Connie Court, Canyon Country, CA 91351, (805) 251-7398, MA 88 CA St Univ - Los Angeles

Hall, Dr Joseph W Univ Of North Carolina Med Sch, Division Of Otolaryngology, 610 Burnett-Womack Bldg, Chapel Hill, NC 27599, (919) 966-3341, BS 72 Coll of William & Mary; MA 80 Univ of NC - Chapel Hill; PH 76 (Psychology) Univ of NC - Greensboro; 86–Assoc Prof, Univ NC at Chapel Hill, **A**

Hall, Mrs Joyce E 517 E B Street, Moscow, ID 83843, (208) 882-0371, BS 79 Purdue Univ - West Lafayette; MA 81 OH St Univ; **SLP A**

Hall, Mrs Judith K 1302 Bryn Mawr, Lake Wales, FL 33853, (813) 676-8568, BA 71 Univ of Northern IA; MS 79 ID St Univ; Sp-Lang Path, Polk Co Sch Bd, **SLP**

Hall, Julie T 108 Forest Hill Avenue, Jefferson City, MO 65101, (314) 635-4435, BA 64 Univ of AR - Fayetteville; MA 70 Univ of AR - Fayetteville; Chief Sp-Lang Path, Chas E Still Hosp, **SLP**

Hall, Mrs Katherine Marie 6598 Meadow Farm Drive, Hudson, OH 44236, (216) 526-5000, **SLP**

Hall, Kathleen D 14 Valley View Drive, Frewsburg, NY 14738, (716) 664-3893, BS 74 SUNY - Coll at Fredonia; MS 78 SUNY - Coll at Buffalo; Sp-Lang Path, Southwestern Cen Sch, **SLP**

Hall, Kathleen E 610 North Lincoln #204, Addison, IL 60101, (312) 629-7272, BS 73 IL St Univ - Normal; MS 74 IL St Univ - Normal; Sp-Lang Path, S Metro Assoc, **SLP**

Hall, Mrs Kelly Dailey 2008 North Lincoln, Urbana, IL 61801, (817) 244-2561, BS 83 Baylor Univ; MS 84 Baylor Univ; **SLP**

Hall, Kim J 8004 Strong Drive S E, Huntsville, AL 35802, (404) 568-7609, **SLP**

Hall, Mrs Laurie Dees 6411 Fort Scott Court, Plano, TX 75023, (214) 330-5291, BS 81 Univ of South AL; MS 83 Auburn Univ - Auburn; Sp-Lang Path, Dallas ISD, **SLP**

Hall, Mrs Leah Adele 104 West Woodhaven, Ruston, LA 71270, (318) 368-2437, **SLP**

Hall, Mrs Linda C 10 Morrill Avenue, Gorham, ME 04038, (207) 839-3717, BA 70 SUNY - Center at Buffalo; OM 72 IN Univ - Bloomington; SLP, Sch Admin Dist #6, **SLP**

Hall, Lisa Blackburn 302 Lamplighter Circle, Pittsburgh, PA 15212, BA 81 Duquesne Univ; MA 83 Univ of Pittsburgh - Pittsburgh; Sp-Lang Path, Pittsburgh Bd of Ed, **SLP**

Hall, Mrs Malinda M 1479 Ygnacio Valley Road, Apartment 104, Walnut Creek, CA 94598, (415) 938-8686, BS 71 Univ of Tulsa; MA 74 Univ of Tulsa; Csg Hearing Services, **SLP**

Hall, Mrs Martha Nadler Rt 1 Box 399-2, Taylorsville, NC 28681, (704) 495-4578, BS 79 LA St Univ - Baton Rouge; MA 85 LA St Univ - Baton Rouge; Sp-Lang Path, Catawba Co Schs, **SLP**

Hall, Mrs Martha Williams 1016 48th Terrace, Vero Beach, FL 32960, (305) 465-4020, BA 71 OH Univ - Athens; MA 75 Kent St Univ; Preschool Consultant, St Lucie County School Board, **SLP**

Hall, Mrs Mary Ann Langford 184 York Drive, Jackson, MS 39209, (601) 353-1664, **SLP**

Hall, Maura K M 4440 N W Green Hills Place, Topeka, KS 66618-1633, (913) 232-0551, BA 72 Holy Names Coll; MA 76 Univ of CO - Boulder; Sp-Lang Path, USD #501 Dept of Spec Serv, **SLP**

Hall, Maureen Bridget Memorial Medical Center, 2801 Atlantic Avenue, Dept Of Rehabilitation, Long Beach, CA 90801-1428, (213) 595-2411, SLP, Memorial Medical Center, **SLP**

Hall, Melanie G P O Box 49, Mount Holly, VA 22524, (804) 472-2081, BS 76 Howard Univ; MS 80 Univ of the DC; SLP, Westmoreland Co Sch Bd, **SLP**

Hall, Melissa Wiegand New Orleans Sp & H Center, 1636 Toledano Street, New Orleans, LA 70115, (504) 897-2606, BA 81 Northwestern St Univ; OM 83 LA St Univ - N O Medical Ctr; Aud, New Orleans Sp & Hrng Clinic, **A**

Hall, Nancy 812 Victoria Drive #E, Montgomery, IL 60538, (312) 897-6768, BA 79 Augustana Coll; MA 81 Northeast MO St Univ; Sp-Lang Path, Oswego Comm Ut Sch Dist #308, **SLP**

Hall, Nancy Edna 1163 South Green Road, South Euclid, OH 44121, (216) 844-3668, BA 82 Coll of Wooster; MA 85 Case Western Reserve Univ; Research Asst III, Case Western Reserve U, **SLP**

Hall, Nancy L RFD 1 Box 80A, East Burke, VT 05832, (802) 748-4569, BA 78 Blackburn Coll; MA 81 Northwestern Univ; Sp-Lang Path, St Johnsbury Sch Sys, **SLP**

Hall, Patricia 502 Thorn Wood, Euless, TX 76039, (214) 241-2594, BA 79 Univ of North TX; MS 80 Univ of North TX; Sp-Lang Path, Private Practice, **SLP**

Hall, Mrs Patricia Ann 6 Lynda Drive, Denver, PA 17517, BS 75 Indiana Univ of PA; MA 82 SUNY - Coll at Geneseo; **SLP**

Hall, Patricia Hennessy 6160 S E Eastbrook, Milwaukie, OR 97222, (503) 249-8787, MS Bowling Green St Univ; 83–Sp-Lang Path, Private Practice, **SLP**

Hall, Patricia Sanders 5043 South Uravan Court, Aurora, CO 80015-2013, (303) 693-2292, Clinical Director, **SLP**

Hall, Penelope K Wendell Johnson Sp & Hrng Ctr, Dept Of Speech Path & Aud, University Of Iowa, Iowa City, IA 52242, (319) 335-8736, BA 65 Univ of IA; MA 67 Univ of IA; Asst Prof, Dept of Sp Path & Aud-U of IA, **SLP**

Hall, Rachelle Reines 410 Harrison Street, Pueblo, CO 81004, (303) 542-5512, OB 74 Boston Univ; ME 79 Northeastern Univ; SLP, Pub Sch Dist 60, **SLP**

Hall, Raelene A 2525 Minor #402, Seattle, WA 98102, (406) 728-5105, BA 84 Univ of MT; OM 87 Univ of MT; 87–Sp-Lang Path, Providence Med Ctr, **SLP**

Hall, Randy Margaret 5727 35th Northeast, Seattle, WA 98105, (206) 863-2201, MS 84 Univ of WA; Bethel School Dist, **SLP**

Hall, Regina Marie 1317 Bradford Road, Oreland, PA 19075, (215) 242-4200, BA 80 Univ of DE; MA 84 West Chester Univ of PA; Sp-Lang Path, UCP Assn of Philadelphia, **SLP**

Hall, Rita Marie 2419 Sherry Road, Louisville, KY 40217, (812) 945-5287, BS 84 Murray St Univ; MS 85 Univ of Louisville; **SLP**

Hall, Robert E Speech And Hearing Clinic, California State Univ, Chico, CA 95929, (916) 895-6848, BS 67 Brigham Young Univ; OM 70 Brigham Young Univ; Prof/Prog Coord, California State University, **SLP**

Hall, Rubye Maie 733 N E 20th, Oklahoma City, OK 73105, (405) 528-4225, MS; **SLP LM**

Hall, Mrs Ruth L G 3422 Dellwood, Cleveland Heights, OH 44118, (216) 421-7880, BA 56 Western MI Univ; MS 59 Case Western Reserve Univ; Dir of Therapy, Hanna Perkins Sch, **SLP**

Hall, Ruthann 23004 59th Avenue West, Mountlake Terrace, WA 98043, BA 76 OH St Univ; MA 79 OH Univ - Athens; SLP, Group Hlth Coop, **SLP**

Hall, Mrs Sharon C 1970 Michael Drive, Johnson City, TN 37604, (615) 926-9391, MS 87 East TN St Univ; 88–Sp-Lang Path, Communi-Care Inc

Hall, Stacy Alma 1501 North Cherry Street, Apartment 33, Chico, CA 95926, (916) 894-5952, MA 88 CA St Univ - Chico

Hall, Susan 408 B Chapman Court, Lexington, KY 40502, (606) 885-3085, BS 70 OH St Univ; MA 72 OH Univ - Athens; Sp-Lang Path, Jessamine Co SD, **SLP**

Hall, Susan Grasso P O Box 82, Milltown, MT 59851, (406) 728-4100, BS 78 Univ of NE - Omaha; MA 80 Univ of MT; Sp/Lang Path, Community Hosp, **SLP**

Hall, Mrs Susan Larkins 1410 Third Avenue, Fairbanks, AK 99701, (907) 451-6485, BS 79 Ithaca Coll; MA 81 George Washington Univ; **SLP**

Hall, Suzy D 1182 South Shore Road, Newport, WA 99156, (509) 447-2426, BA 85 WA St Univ; MA 87 WA St Univ; 87–Sp-Lang Path, Newport Sch Dist, **SLP**

Hall, Mrs Teresa Lynn 3490 South Forest, Denver, CO 80222, (303) 420-6663, BS 82 CO St Univ; MA 84 Univ of Northern CO; Sp-Lang Path, Jefferson Co Comm Cen, **SLP**

Hall, Terry A 2103 Foxhorn Road, New Bern, NC 28562, (919) 638-2666, BA 78 Univ of MS; MA 80 Univ of MS; Aud, Coastal ENT & Facial Plastic Surgery PA, **A**

Hall, Mrs Valerie Marie P O Box 884, Aquone Road, Andrews, NC 28901, (704) 321-4416, BS 80 Western Carolina Univ; MA 81 Western Carolina Univ; Sp-Lang Path, Cherokee County School System, **SLP**

Hall, Vicki Lynn 203 8th Street #A, St Augustine, FL 32084, (904) 824-1654, BS 78 CA Univ of PA; ME 81 Indiana Univ of PA; Sp-Lang Path, FL Sch for Deaf & Blind, **SLP**

Hall, Vickie L 807 Jefferson Avenue, Memphis, TN 38105, (901) 525-2682, BS 81 Purdue Univ - West Lafayette; MA 82 Memphis St Univ; Supvr/Aud, Memphis State Univ, **A**

Hall, Dr William F 1 Grim Court South, Kirksville, MO 63501, (816) 665-4279, OB 55 Southwest MO St Univ; MA 57 Univ of MO - Columbia; PH 62 (SP) Univ of MO - Columbia; **SLP LM**

Hall, William T 11918 Patroon Circle N W, Canal Fulton, OH 44614, (804) 467-7006, BS 72 James Madison Univ; ME 74 Univ of VA - Charlottesville; OM 86 C B N Univ; **A**

Hallahan, Thomas Jude 222 Beacon Street, Boston, MA 02116, (617) 427-5870, **A**

Hallal, Joseph Daniel 2144 Royalwood, Broadview Heights, OH 44147, (216) 582-3182, BA 79; MA 81 Cleveland St Univ; Aud, Inearset Inc, **A**

Hallam, Jerold J 1237 West El Camino Avenue, Sacramento, CA 95833, (916) 924-1085, BA 59 CA St Univ - Sacramento; MA 64 CA St Univ - Sacramento; Sp-Lang Path, Private Practice, **SLP**

Hallameyer, Mrs Claire M 2657 Ebony Road, Baltimore, MD 21234, (301) 578-5601, BA 80 Loyola Coll; MS 81 Loyola Coll; Sp-Lang Path, Sinai Hospital of Baltimore, **SLP**

Halldorson, Sharon G 255 Horace Street, Winnipeg, MB, Canada R2H 0W7, (204) 786-7841, BA 80 Univ of ND; MS 81 Univ of ND; Sp-Lang Path, Child Guidance Cl, **SLP**

Hallemeier, Kit Maureen 6 Pam Avenue, St Charles, MO 63301, (314) 724-4311, OB 87 Univ of MO - Columbia; OM 88 Univ of MO - Columbia

Hallen, Linda A 1206 11th Avenue West, Ashland, WI 54806, (715) 682-8220, BS 72 Univ of WI - Madison; MS 75 Univ of WI - Eau Claire; Sp-Lang Path, Mellen School Dist, **SLP**

Haller, Dr Raphael M Allied Therapeutic Services, P O Box 2103, Summerville, SC 29484-2103, (803) 873-6935, BA 51 CUNY - City College; MA 52 CUNY - City College; PH 64 (NS) Northwestern Univ; Sp-Lang Path, Private Practice, **SLP**

Haller, Timothy Leonard 61 Mather Avenue, Colonie, Schenectady, NY 12304, (518) 237-9012, BS 82 Coll of Saint Rose; MS 86 Coll of Saint Rose; 87–Sp-Lang Path, Residential Opportunities Inc, **SLP**

Hallett, Mrs Terry Lynn 4840 Westchester #2, Youngstown, OH 44515, (216) 792-7825, BS 74 Kent St Univ; MA 84 Kent St Univ; **SLP**

Hall-Ferchau, Theresa Margaret 6616 West Ridge Drive, Chicago Ridge, IL 60415, (312) 471-5634, BA 81 Northern IL Univ - De Kalb; MA 83 Northern IL Univ - De Kalb; 86–Aud, Holy Cross Hosp, **A**

Halligan, Colene Patricia 36 Abbott Street #3-E, Worcester, MA 01602, (617) 791-3147, BS 85 Univ of NH; MA 87 Univ of Northern CO

Halligan, Pamela L W University Of South Carolina, Speech And Hearing Center, 1601 St Julian Place, Columbia, SC 29204, (803) 777-2614, BA 74 Converse Coll; MS 76 Univ of NC - Chapel Hill; Intructor, University of South Carolina, **A**

Hallihan, Ellen Elizabeth 1203 Bloomfield Street, Hoboken, NJ 07030, (201) 795-7156, BA 83 Rutger's St Univ - Douglas Coll; MA 85 NY Univ; 85–Sp-Lang Path, St Francis Hosp, **SLP**

Halling, Dan C 3006 West Cypress Drive, Muncie, IN 47304, (317) 285-8166, BS 83 UT St Univ; MA 85 Univ of Northern CO; 88–Asst Prof/Aud, Ball State Univ, **A**

Halling, Mrs Shirley Ann 925 Humboldt Road, Brisbane, CA 94005, (415) 664-6768, BS 59 Mankato St Univ; MS 64 Univ of Southern CA; MA 83 Univ of San Francisco; SLP, San Francisco USD, **SLP**

Halliwell, Nancy 8840-219 Villa La Jolla Dr, La Jolla, CA 92037, (619) 457-4670, BA 75 Univ of CA - Santa Barbara; MA 78 Univ of CA - Santa Barbara; 87–Sp-Lang Path, Chula Vista City Sch Dist, **SLP**

Hallman, Mrs Beverly Jean 4127 Cove Drive, Yukon, OK 73099, (405) 495-2219, BA 81 Univ of OK - Norman; MS 83 Univ of OK Medical Center; Sp-Lang Path, Mustang PS, **SLP**

Hallmark, Mary Hulett P O Box 954, APO New York, NY 09057, (512) 925-4166, BA 78 Depauw Univ; MS 79 Univ of MI - Ann Arbor; Aud, Exceptional Family Member Dept, **A ACE**

Hallock, Geraldine P 35-50 78th Street, Jackson Heights, NY 11372, (718) 429-3658, MS 82 Adelphi Univ; **SLP**

Hallock, Keith R 94 Glenbrook Drive, Brownsville, TX 78521, BA 53 Univ of Southern CA; MA 54 Univ of Southern CA; Retired, Brownsville ISD, **SLP**

Hallock, Viola K Box 372, Kansas, IL 61933, MS; **LM**

Hall-Olsen, Kathleen 18 Fox Run Drive, Mount Laurel, NJ 08054, (609) 234-6901, BS 76 Trenton St Coll; MA 78 Temple Univ; SLP, Private Practice, **SLP**

Hallsten, Roger D 520 Washington Street, Las Vegas, NM 87701, (505) 454-1493, BA 83 Univ of CA - Santa Barbara; MS 87 Univ of WA; 88–Sp-Lang Path, Northern NM Rehab Ctr

Halo, Anna M 939 Elk Street, 2nd Floor, Franklin, PA 16323, (814) 432-3171, BS 76 Clarion Univ of PA; MA 79 Kent St Univ; Aud, Polk Center, **A**

Halper, Mrs Anita S 260 East Chestnut Street, Apartment 2901, Chicago, IL 60611, (312) 649-6138, BS 56 Northwestern Univ; MA 59 Northwestern Univ; Dir Dept of Commun Disord, Rehab I of Chicago, **SLP F ACE**

Halper, Betty D 11240 N W 41st Court, Coral Springs, FL 33065, MS 68 Adelphi Univ; SLP, Broward County Public Schools, **SLP**

Halpern, Barbara E 9701 North Dee Road #3L, Des Plaines, IL 60016, (312) 803-8267, BS 81 Northern IL Univ - De Kalb; MS 83 IL St Univ - Normal; Sp-Lang Path, Sased, **SLP**

Halpern, Barbara J 20340 Thornwood, Southfield, MI 48076, (313) 875-5250, ME 65 Wayne St Univ; Detroit Pub Schs-Sp & Hrng Cl, **SLP**

Halpern, Harvey 11 Bellingham Lane, Great Neck, NY 11023, (516) 466-9624, BA 56 CUNY - Brooklyn Coll; MA 58 CUNY - Brooklyn Coll; PH 62 (NS) NY Univ; Professor, Queens College, **SLP F**

Halpern, Mrs Karen T 123 Buckingham Court, Pomona, NY 10970, (914) 947-1000, BA 77 CUNY - Brooklyn Coll; MA 79 NY Univ; Aud, Letchworth Vlg Dev Cen, **A**

Halpern, Mrs Linda D 74 Tara Drive, East Hills, NY 11576, (516) 626-0028, BA 80 Hofstra Univ; MA 82 NY Univ; SLP Superv Consult, Visiting Ther Assoc, **SLP**

Halpern, Mrs Marsha Lommel 3409 South 29th Street, Lincoln, NE 68502, BA 70 Fontbonne Coll; MA 74 Univ of MN - Minneap-St Paul; 83–Sr Vice President, Madonna Ctrs Rehab Hosp, **SLP A**

Halpern, Mrs Mindy Orlow 1719 Ridgeway Road, Havertown, PA 19083, (215) 789-3585, BA 83 Temple Univ-Tyler Sch of Art; MA 85 Temple Univ-Tyler Sch of Art; SLP, Delaware Co Intermediate Unit, **SLP**

Halpert, Helen V 524 Rust Avenue, Big Rapids, MI 49307, (616) 796-2385, BS 41 NY Univ; MA 52 Univ of MD - College Park; **SLP LM**

Halpin, Dr Christopher Francis 50 Concord Street Apartment #4, Malden, MA 02148, (617) 573-3286, BA 77 Univ of VA - Charlottesville; ME 85 Univ of VA - Charlottesville; PH 88 (Aud) Univ of VA - Charlottesville; 88–Clin Assoc, MA Eye & Ear Infirmary, **A**

Halpin, Mrs Kathy S W 10415 Bluejacket Drive, Overland Park, KS 66214-3723, BS 74 Univ of KS; MA 76 Univ of KS; Sp-Lang Path, Shawnee Mission Publ Schs #512, **SLP**

Halsey, Mrs Judith Snyder 3778 Hollybrook Drive, Middletown, OH 45042, (513) 423-0781, BS 78 Miami Univ - Oxford; MS 85 Miami Univ - Oxford; Sp-Lang Path, Middletown City Schools, **SLP**

Halsey, Mrs Karen C P O Box 7000-740, Redondo Beach, CA 90277, (213) 540-5153, BA 79 CA St Univ - Northridge; MA 80 CA St Univ - Northridge; SLP, Los Angeles USD, **SLP**

Halstead, Margaret 3302 Brooklawn Terrace, Chevy Chase, MD 20815-3935, (713) 661-7042, **SLP**

Halstead-Elser, Mrs Sammie 3607 S E 4th Place, Cape Coral, FL 33904, (813) 542-6271, BS 65 East TN St Univ; MA 69 Gallaudet Coll; Consultant, Private Practice, **A**

Halter-Heifetz, Andrea 2713 Raleigh Avenue, St Louis Park, MN 55416, (612) 925-9070, BA 80 Univ of CA - Los Angeles; MA 86 CA St Univ - Northridge

Halterlein, Maria Bernadette 203 St Augustine Drive, Long Beach, MS 39560, (601) 868-1034, MS 86 Univ Southern MS-Hattiesburg; 87–Sp-Lang Path, Harrison Co Ctr-Excep Chldn

Halton, Elizabeth Frances 1330 Pulaski Road, East Northport, NY 11731, (516) 736-4674, **SLP**

Halverson, Joan Marie 135 Madrone Avenue, San Anselmo, CA 94960, (415) 456-0697, BA 69 CA St Univ - Long Beach; MS 84 San Francisco St Univ; SLP, Marin Co Office of Ed, **SLP**

Halverson, Mrs Lisa Anne 1676 68th Avenue N E, Minneapolis, MN 55432, (612) 781-6571, BA 83 Univ of ND; MS 85 IL St Univ - Normal; **SLP**

Halverson, Teresa K 9452 Highway Y, Sauk City, WI 53583-9566, (608) 643-8623, BS 85 Univ of WI - Whitewater; MS 86 Univ of WI - Whitewater; **SLP**

Halvorsen, Jean M 88 Hilltop Avenue, Providence, RI 02908, (401) 831-2205, BS 76 Univ of MA - Amherst; BA 77 Univ of MA - Amherst; MA 79 Univ of MA - Amherst; Sp/Lang Path, Providence Sch Dept, **SLP**

Halvorson, Alice Mae 802 W Third St, Red Wing, MN 55066, (612) 388-9648, BS 64 Univ of MN - Minneap-St Paul; MS 68 Univ of IA; **SLP**

Halvorson, Dr Jerome A University Of Wisconsin, Kleinpell Fine Arts, River Falls, WI 54022, (715) 425-3801, BS 63 Univ of WI - River Falls; MA 65 Univ of IA; PH 68 Univ of MN - Minneap-St Paul; Prof of Commun Dis, U of WI River Falls, **SLP A**

Halvorson, Julia M 4525 18th Avenue South, Minneapolis, MN 55407, (612) 823-6660, BS 77 Purdue Univ - West Lafayette; MA 79 Univ of CO - Boulder; 88–VP-Oper, Sp-Lang Hrng Cl, **SLP**

Halvorson, Kathryn A 785 Mamaroneck Avenue, White Plains, NY 10605, (914) 948-0050, BS 72 Moorhead St Univ; MS 75 Univ of OR; Director of Sp-Lang Path & Aud, Burke Rehabilitation Center, **SLP**

Halvorson, Lori Ann St Mary Of Nazareth Hospital, Audiology Department, 2233 West Division, Chicago, IL 60622, (312) 770-2860, MS 84 Rush Univ; 86–Dir of Aud, St Mary of Nazareth Hosp Ctr, **A**

Ham, Dr Richard E 2938 Foxcroft Drive, Tallahassee, FL 32308-2129, (614) 594-5254, BS 53 Northwestern Univ; MA 54 Western MI Univ; PH 56 (NS) Purdue Univ - West Lafayette; Prof of Commun Dis, FL State U, **SLP F**

Hamada, Cheryl L 1767 W North Shore Avenue, Chicago, IL 60626, (312) 338-7249, BA 75 Northeastern IL Univ; MA 78 Northern IL Univ - De Kalb; Sp/Lang Path, Chicago Board of Ed, **SLP**

Hamalainen, Susan W 85 Hildreth Street, Westford, MA 01886, (617) 667-8300, BS 76 Northeastern Univ; ME 80 Northeastern Univ; Sp-Lang Path, Billerica Pub Sch, **SLP**

Haman-Miller, Karen J 103 North 38th Street, Belleville, IL 62223, (618) 234-6172, BS 79 Southern IL Univ-Edwardsvill; MS 83 Southern IL Univ-Edwardsvill; Sp-Lang Path, **SLP**

Hamann, Mrs Kathryn Louise 1141 Ramsgate Road #5, Flint, MI 48532, (313) 767-5750, BS 82 Carlow Coll; MS 84 Univ of MI - Ann Arbor; 86–Aud, Mott Children's Health Ctr, **A**

Hamano, Pearl Y Tongue River Stage, Miles City, MT 59301, (406) 232-5250, BA 76 Univ of Northern CO; MA 77 Univ of Northern CO; Sp-Lang Path, Miles City USD, **SLP**

Hamant, Mrs Karla Feuchter 9850 Dargate Court, Cincinnati, OH 45231, (513) 825-8635, BS 62 Case Western Reserve Univ; **SLP**

Hamberg, Mrs Mildred S 4215 43rd Avenue, Long Island City, New York, NY 11104, (718) 935-2363, BA 37 CUNY - Hunter Coll; MA 64 NY Univ; 81–Examination Asst, NYC Bd of Educ, **SLP LM**

Hambrecht, Dr Georgia 1306 South 19th, Terre Haute, IN 47803, (812) 237-2806, BS 74 Bowling Green St Univ; MA 75 Western IL Univ; PH 82 (NS) Kent St Univ; 80–Assoc Prof, IN St U, **SLP**

Hamburg, Deborah Susan 403 Willowmere Lane, Ambler, PA 19002, (215) 641-0525, BS 61 Temple Univ-Tyler Sch of Art; MA 64 Temple Univ-Tyler Sch of Art; 86–Consult, Independent Contractor, **SLP**

Hamburg, Ellen M 9006 Abbeydale, Houston, TX 77031, (713) 464-1511, BA 69 CUNY - Brooklyn Coll; MS 73 CUNY - Brooklyn Coll

Hamburger, Mrs Ina 8218 Brattle Road, Baltimore, MD 21208, (301) 922-7332, BA 59 Univ of MD - College Park; MA 67 Univ of MD - College Park; Sp-Lang Path, Baltimore Co Bd of Ed, **SLP**

Hamby, Dr Ellen I 11740 Georgetown Drive, Knoxville, TN 37922, (615) 974-4123, BA 73 Univ of MS; OM 74 Univ of MS; PH 78 (NS) Univ of IA; Asst Prof, Dept of Aud & Sp Path & U TN, **SLP**

Hamel, Catherine Ross 5501 South Everett Avenue, Chicago, IL 60637, (312) 363-7857, BA 84 Univ of WA; MS 86 Univ of WI - Madison; Sp-Lang Path, **SLP**

Hamel, Mrs Cecilia 40 Bessette Lane, Chicopee, MA 01020, (413) 527-6770, BS 76 Univ of MA - Amherst; MA 77 Univ of MA - Amherst; Sp-Lang Path, East Hampton Pub Sch, **SLP**

Hamele, Eileen Skelton 6602 Jacobs Way, Madison, WI 53711, (608) 273-4362, BS 81 Univ of WI - Whitewater; MS 86 Univ of WI - Whitewater; SLP, Therapy Assoc, **SLP**

Hamelin, Mrs Paula Turpack R R 1 Box 107, Douglas Street, Uxbridge, MA 01569, (508) 234-7306, MS 85 Worcester St Coll; Sp-Lang Path, St Camillus & Framingham Rehab Nursing Home, **SLP**

Hamer, Carol Schneck 43 Paula Drive, Long Valley, NJ 07853, (516) 764-7562, BA 85 Hofstra Univ; MA 83 Hofstra Univ; **A**

Hamersky, Daniel Joseph 1226 Del Ray, Green Bay, WI 54304, (414) 468-1161, BA 77 Univ of NE - Lincoln; MA 81 Northern MI Univ; Sp-Lang Path, Curative Rehab Ctr, **SLP**

Hamila, Mrs Debra L 1179 Castleton Road, Cleveland Heights, OH 44121, (216) 461-2431, BA 77 Cleveland St Univ; MA 79 Cleveland St Univ; Audiologist, Charles L Cassady MD Facs Inc, **A**

Hamill, Mrs Pamela L P 1751 Marie Lane, Merced, CA 95340, (209) 384-3163, BS 74 CA St Univ - Fresno; MA 77 CA St Univ - Fresno; Sp-Lang Path, Merced Co Superintendent of Schs, **SLP**

Hamill, Dr Teri Anne Texas Technical University, Speech & Hearing Sciences, Box 4266, Lubbock, TX 79409, (806) 742-1575, BA 82 Univ of Central FL; MS 83 FL St Univ; PH 86 (Aud) FL St Univ; 88–Aud Asst Prof, Texas Tech Univ, **A**

Hamill, Mrs Victoria Reed 30-11 Parsons Boulevard, Apartment 1-A, Flushing, NY 11354, (212) 904-2677, BA 84 Univ of TN - Knoxville; MS 86 Univ of TX - Dallas; **A**

Hamilton, Debra Jo 21 Haven Road, San Angelo, TX 76901, (915) 658-1511, BS 79 Howard Payne Univ; MA 81 Univ of CO - Boulder; Aud, Angelo Cl Assc, **A**

Hamilton, Mrs Dorothy T 8 Blacklog Road, Kentfield, CA 94904, (415) 472-0597, BS 57 Syracuse Univ; ME 79 San Francisco St Univ; Parent-Infant Ed, Marin Co Off of Ed, **A**

Hamilton, Mrs Eilene K East 15714 Valley Way, Veradale, WA 99037, (509) 928-7610, BA 74 Eastern WA Univ; MS 75 Eastern WA Univ; SLP, Central Vly Sch Dist #356, **SLP**

Hamilton, Mrs Elizabeth V 2626 22nd Avenue, San Francisco, CA 94116, (415) 476-5101, MA 78 Univ of CO - Boulder; Aud, U of CA Med Ctr, **A**

Hamilton, Esther I 1620 Weston Avenue, Niagara Falls, NY 14305, (716) 285-1953, BA 69 SUNY - Coll at Buffalo; MA 70 SUNY - Coll at Buffalo; Doctorate Stud, SUNY, **SLP**

Hamilton, Mrs Gerene Moore 921 East Central, Ponca City, OK 74601, (405) 762-2211, BA 76 Phillips Univ; MS 79 Phillips Univ; **SLP A**

Hamilton, Helen Voluckas Box 1079, Bennington, VT 05201, (802) 362-4385, BS 62 Defiance Coll; OM 85 Univ of VT; **SLP**

Hamilton, Jean Wetter Department Of Audiology ASB2-27, Children's Hospital Medical Center, Elland And Bethesda Avenue, Cincinnati, OH 45229, (513) 559-4236, BS 83 Bowling Green St Univ; MS 85 Univ of WI - Madison; 88–Aud, Childrens Hosp Med Ctr, **A**

Hamilton, Jennifer R R 3 Box 385, Lebanon, KY 40033-9403, (213) 696-0085, MA 88 Whittier Coll

Hamilton, Joan M 3700 S Holston Hills Road, Knoxville, TN 37914, BS 60 Western MI Univ; MA 70 Univ of TN - Knoxville; 72–Sp-Lang Path, Univ of Tennessee, **SLP ACE**

Hamilton, Joyce 216 Anna Street, Belleville, IL 62221, (618) 877-6433, BS 80 Southern IL Univ-Edwardsvill; MS 81 Southern IL Univ-Edwardsvill; SLP, Granite City School District, **SLP**

Hamilton, Julie Barfield 2023 Edinburgh Avenue, Baton Rouge, LA 70808, (504) 924-5198, BS 82 LA St Univ - Baton Rouge; OM 83 LA St Univ - N O Medical Ctr; Sp-Lang Path, Private Practice, **SLP**

Hamilton, Kathleen E 1503 Sunrise Lakes Drive, #13-B, Erie, PA 16509, (814) 870-7070, BS 86 Indiana Univ of PA; MA 87 Edinboro Univ of PA; 88–Sp-Lang Path, Community Rehab Specialists Inc, **SLP**

Hamilton, Kimberley Clarice P O Box 49729, Chicago, IL 60649, (815) 725-7133, BS 79 Bradley Univ; MA 85 Univ of Houston - Univ Park; 87–Sp-Lang Path, Saint Joseph Med Ctr, **SLP**

Hamilton, Kurt O Heartland Area Educ Agency, 120 South Hazel Street, Ames, IA 50010, (515) 232-7583, BS 79 Northwest MO St Univ; MS 80 Northwest MO St Univ; SLP, Heartland AEA #11, **SLP**

Hamilton, Lana H 2315 North 12th Street, Coeur d'Alene, ID 83814, (208) 664-1914, BA 76 Univ of Northern CO; MS 80 ID St Univ; Sp-Lang Path, North Idaho Head Start, **SLP**

Hamilton, Laura Hinderer 1674 Riverton Point, Eagan, MN 55122, (612) 642-1264, MS 81 Saint Cloud St Univ; Sp-Lang Path, Rosemount Sch Dist #196, **SLP**

Hamilton, Margaret J 1161-L Frost Road, Streetsboro, OH 44240, (216) 856-4000, BS 83 Kent St Univ; MA 85 Kent St Univ; Aud, Warren Otologic Group, **A**

Hamilton, Marilyn A 2559 Adams Avenue, Baton Rouge, LA 70802, (504) 388-4174, BA 66; OM 71 Univ of WA; PH 81 (NS) Univ of WA; Asst Prof/Sp, LA St U, **SLP**

Hamilton, Mrs Nancy Chase 7707 S W 11th Avenue, Gainesville, FL 32601, (904) 351-3977, BA 82 Univ of FL; MA 84 Univ of FL; Aud, Pro Sp & Hearing Spec, **A ACE**

Hamilton, Mrs Nancy Welsh 928 Lamar Avenue, Gretna, LA 70056, (504) 367-3120, BS 81 Baylor Univ; OM 82 LA St Univ - N O Medical Ctr; SLP, Jefferson Parish Pub Sch Sys, **SLP**

Hamilton, Nora L 6407 Joyce Street, Alexandria, LA 71301, **SLP**

Hamilton, Robert S, Jr 3 Lindsey Avenue, Beverly, MA 01915, (802) 773-1940, BA 72 Univ of CT; MS 73 Univ of VT; 87–Sp-Lang Path, Lynn PS, **SLP**

Hamilton, Ruth G 43 Marcy Street, Edgewood, RI 02905, (401) 461-1351, MA 47 Emerson Coll; ME 42 RI Coll; Consult/Aural Rehab, Francis B Sargent Rehab Cen, **SLP A LM**

Hamilton, Sallie Sederstrom E 1604 11th Avenue, Spokane, WA 99202, (509) 326-1651, BA 76 WA St Univ; MA 79 WA St Univ; 86–Sp-Lang Path, Spokane Sch & Neuromuscular Ctr, **SLP**

Hamilton, Susan L 4719 University Way N E, Suite 210, Seattle, WA 98105, (206) 526-2874, BS 77 Miami Univ - Oxford; MA 78 WA St Univ; 86–Sp-Lang Path, University Way Speech Svcs, **SLP**

Hamilton, Mrs Treva K 1126 Huntington Drive, Fayetteville, AR 72701, (501) 443-9657, BA 69 Northeastern OK St Univ; MA 70 Univ of Tulsa; **SLP**

Hamilton, Victoria Anne 870 Glendale Terrace, Unit 7, Atlanta, GA 30308, (404) 872-5433, ME 83 Univ of GA; MS 80 Univ of GA; Audiologist, Ron Shotts MD, **A**

Hamilton, Mrs Vikki Thompson 25 School Street, Pine Bluff, AR 71602, (501) 535-1816, MS 88 Univ of AR - Little Rock; 87–SLP, Arkansas River Educ Svcs Cooperative

Hamin, Mrs Amy Lynn 1454A CTY JJ, Nekoosa, WI 54457, (715) 384-4747, BS 84 Univ of WI - Stevens Point; MS 85 Univ of WI - Stevens Point; 86–Sp-Lang Path, Sch Dist of Marshfield WI, **SLP**

Hamlet, Elizabeth G 365 Walnut Street, Manchester, NH 03103-3113, (617) 391-1686, BS 77 Univ of NH; MS 82 Emerson Coll; Sp/Lang Path, Bedford NH Pub Sch, **SLP**

Hamlet, Dr Sandra Lee Dept Of Otolaryngology, 5-E University Health Ctr, Wayne State University, Detroit, MI 48201, (313) 745-4178, BA 59 Univ of WI - Madison; MA 67 Univ of WA; PH 70 (NS) Univ of WA; Assoc Prof, Wayne State Univ

Hamlett, Mrs J Ann 1823 Koster, Garden City, KS 67846, (316) 275-0291, BA 76 Wichita St Univ; MA 77 Wichita St Univ; 85–Sp-Lang Path, USD 457, **SLP**

Hamlin, Jeanne F 319 South Gore, Webster Groves, MO 63119, MS 75 Saint Louis Univ; 75–Sp-Lang Path, Jewish Hosp of St Louis, **SLP ACE**

Hamlin, Mrs Juanita Rochelle P O Box 2083, Hammond, IN 46323, (219) 938-3865, BS 79 Clarion Univ of PA; OM 86 Governors St Univ; 79–Sp-Lang Path, Speech Plus Inc, **SLP**

Hamlin, Mary Lee 415 North Bradley Farm Rd, Tomahawk, WI 54487, (715) 362-3465, BS 57 Marquette Univ; Sp-Lang Path, Sch Dist of Rhinelander, **SLP**

Hamlyn, Hugh W 6608 West Avenue, San Antonio, TX 78213, (512) 696-9660, BS 55 Southwest TX St Univ; MA 69 Auburn Univ - Auburn; Aud, Audie L Murphy Mem VA Hosp, **SLP**

Hamm, Mrs Donna Koho 10604 Saber Creek Cove, Austin, TX 78759, (512) 335-8924, BS 75 Abilene Christian Univ; MS 78; **SLP**

Hamm, Marcia G RFD 2 Box 784, Putney, VT 05346, **SLP**

Hamm, Mrs Victoria Lou P O Box 235, Oran, MO 63771, BS 75 Southeast MO St Univ; MA 86 Southeast MO St Univ; 78–Sp-Lang Path, Charleston R-1 Pub Schs, **SLP**

Hammack, Judy F 2215 15th Street, Meridian, MS 39301, (601) 483-8121, BS 69 MS Univ for Women; MS 70 Univ Southern MS-Hattiesburg; Aud, Meridian Sp & Hrng Cen, **A**

Hammack, Mrs Mary Jo 4301 Soundview Lane, Chesterfield, VA 23832, (804) 276-3475, BS 74 Purdue Univ - West Lafayette; MA 79 Ball St Univ; **SLP**

Hammar, Mrs Carolann Corbit 104 Stratford, Naperville, IL 60540, (312) 983-4177, BS 80 Edinboro Univ of PA; MA 81 Kent St Univ; **SLP**

Hammar, Elaine G 5441 East 40th North, Wichita, KS 67220, (316) 733-4114, BA 85 Wichita St Univ; MA 86 Wichita St Univ; 85–Dir Sp-Lang Path, Hillhaven Wichita, **SLP**

Hammatt, Mrs Nancy N 412 East Woodstone Court, Baton Rouge, LA 70808, (504) 346-3142, BA 68 LA St Univ - Baton Rouge; MA 70 LA St Univ - Baton Rouge; **SLP**

Hammel, Diane Roberts Center For Craniofacial Anomalies, University Of Illinois Medical Center, 808 S Wood, Chicago, IL 60612, (312) 996-7546, BS 81 Univ of IL - Urbana; MA 83 Univ of IL - Urbana; Aud, Univ of IL Ctr for Craniofacial Anamolies, **A**

Hammer, Candice Ann 10223 Melrose Street, Overland Park, KS 66214, (913) 676-2454, BS 73 Univ of TN - Knoxville; MA 74 Univ of TN - Knoxville; SLP, Sherry L Wallace and Assoc, **SLP**

Hammer, Carol Scheffner c/o HCRC, PO Box 239 8, Saipan, Mariana Islands 96950, (670) 234-6457, BA 82 Augustana Coll; MA 83 Northwestern Univ; Sp-Lang Path, Dept of Educ-CNMI, **SLP**

Hammer, David W 220 Ligonier Lane, New Kensington, PA 15068, (412) 647-5575, BA 77 Univ of Pittsburgh - Pittsburgh; MA 79 Univ of Pittsburgh - Pittsburgh; Sp/Lang Path, Chldn Hosp Pgh, **SLP**

Hammer, Debra Beth 35 Bell Drive, Westfield, NJ 07090, BA 84 Univ of MD - College Park; MS 86 Rutgers St Univ - Newark; 87–Sp-Lang Path, Children's Specialized Hosp, **SLP**

Hammer, Mrs Jean C 2720 D Street, North Bend, OR 97459, (503) 756-1354, BA 65 IN Univ - Bloomington; MA 67 IN Univ - Bloomington; 84–Sp-Lang Path, Bay Area Hosp, **SLP**

Hammer, Mrs Kay N 533 South 5th Street, Fairbury, IL 61739, (815) 635-3555, BS 60 Eastern IL Univ; MS 70 IL St Univ - Normal; 86–Sp-Lang Path, Prairie Central Schs, **SLP ACE**

Hammer, Larry D 1310 Prentice Drive Suite D, Healdsburg, CA 95448, (707) 431-8244, BA 76 Univ of NE - Lincoln; OM 79 Brigham Young Univ; Sp-Lang Path, Private Practice, **SLP**

Hammer, Dr Lowell Clarke 4909 N W 18th Place, Gainesville, FL 32601, (904) 395-0174, BA 51 Wichita St Univ; PH 65 (Sp Path/Aud) Univ of FL; Prof/Cheif Sp-Lang Path, U of FL Dept of Commun Dis, **SLP F**

Hammer, Mrs Marcia Mary 15618 Sierra Drive, Oak Forest, IL 60452, (815) 740-3196, BS 75 Western IL Univ; MA 77 Governors St Univ; 77–Sp-Lang Path, JFK Diag Cen, **SLP**

Hammer, Mary B P O Box 6264, Louisville, KY 40207, (502) 222-7157, BA 80 John Carroll Univ; MS 82 Vanderbilt Univ; Sp-Path, Easter Seals Clinic, **SLP**

Hammer, Mrs Pamela Smith 700 Sandlewood Lane, Chesapeake, VA 23320, (804) 482-7785, BS 81 Old Dominion Univ; MS 85 Old Dominion Univ; 88–Sp-Lang Path, Private Practice, **SLP**

Hammer, Mrs Ronnie W Gaston Road, Morristown, NJ 07960, (201) 267-2748, BA 60 CUNY - Queens Coll; SLP, Cen for Stress & Dis, **SLP**

Hammer, Sharon Ciccolella P O Box 596, Moorefield, WV 26836, (304) 538-2348, BS 76 WV Univ; MS 77 WV Univ; Sp-Lang Path, Hardy Co Sch, **SLP**

Hammer, Mrs Shirley Jean 8000 Edmonton Road, Summer Shade, KY 42166, (502) 487-5328, BS 77 Murray St Univ; MS 80 Western KY Univ; Sp-Lang Path, Monroe Co BOCES, **SLP**

Hammer, Susan Annette 2050 N Shiloh #202, Garland, TX 75042, (214) 238-8111, BA 82 TX Tech Univ; MS 84 Univ of TX - Dallas; **SLP**

Hammer, Susan F 2 Skyline Drive, Latham, NY 12110, (518) 786-1107, BA 75 Univ of MN - Minneap-St Paul; MA 77 Northwestern Univ; Aud, Cen for the Disabled, **A**

Hammer, Mrs Verla J RR #1 Box 172, Mount Vernon, SD 57363, (605) 996-1349, MA 78 Univ of SD - Vermillion; Sp-Lang Path/Aud, Sp Lang Path Sers, **SLP ACE**

Hammerle, Linda M RD2 Box 359, Ottsville, PA 18942, (800) 362-5341, BS 79 Kutztown Univ of PA; MA 82 Trenton St Coll; Clin Superv, InSpeech Inc, **SLP ACE**

Hammerquist, Teresa L 2808 Glenwood, Billings, MT 59102, BA 75 Univ of SD - Vermillion; MA 77 Univ of IA; SLP, **SLP**

Hammerton, Mrs Cynthia A 14861 Heather Glen Way, San Diego, CA 92128, (312) 649-6134, BA 81 Augustana Coll; MA 82 Western MI Univ; Sp-Lang Path, Sp-Hearing & Neurosensory Cen, **SLP**

Hammes, Barbara Phillips 115 South Drive, Barrington, IL 60010, (312) 223-8223, MS 75 IL St Univ - Normal; OM 81 Nat'l Coll of Ed - Evanston; OM 88 Northwestern Univ; 88–Spec Educ Supvr, Sch Dist 46, **SLP**

Hammesfahr, Judith Ann 23154 S W 59th Avenue, Boca Raton, FL 33428, (407) 483-3057, BA 68 Hofstra Univ; MA 71 Hofstra Univ; ES 87 Nova Univ; Sp/Lang Path, Private Practice, **SLP**

Hammock, Mary E 420 Dunbar Avenue, Ruston, LA 71270, (318) 247-3721, BA 82 LA Tech Univ; MA 88 LA Tech Univ; 88–Sp-Lang Path, Ruston State Sch

Hammock, Mrs Sandra W 6705 Ridgeland Road South, Mobile, AL 36695, (205) 633-8643, BS 70 Auburn Univ - Auburn; ME 71 Univ of GA; **SLP**

Hammond, Brian Reed 1628 Coolidge, Wichita, KS 67203, (316) 835-2241, BS 72 KS St Univ; MA 81 Univ of KS; Aud, The Hertzler Clinic, **A**

Hammond, Mrs Debra Calaway 2200 Heron, El Dorado, AR 71730, (501) 863-5918, BS Univ of Central AR; MA 84 LA St Univ - Baton Rouge; Sp-Lang Path, Commun Disorders Ctr, **SLP**

Hammond, Doylena 202 1/2 East 13th Street, Lumberton, NC 28358, (919) 739-1463, BA 81 Pembroke St Univ; MA 85 Appalachian St Univ; **SLP**

Hammond, Hugh S, Jr 8077 Park Haven Road, Baltimore, MD 21222, (301) 284-8602, **SLP**

Hammond, Joann 211 East 15th, Idaho Falls, ID 83401, (208) 529-6637, BS 79 UT St Univ; MS 81 UT St Univ; SLP, Private Practice, **SLP**

Hammond, Judith G 137 Schrade Road, Briarcliff Manor, NY 10510, (914) 739-2823, BA 60 Univ of VT; MA 61 NY Univ; SLP, Lakeland Schs, **SLP**

Hammond, Mark R 10 Sylvan Avenue, Windham, ME 04062, (207) 871-2463, BA 75 Univ of ME - Orono; MA 77 Univ of ME - Orono; Dir-Commun Dis Div, Maine Med Ctr, **SLP**

Hammond, Mrs Patricia Ann 809 North Country Club Dr, Newark, DE 19711-2750, (302) 454-7242, BS 81 Bloomsburg Univ of PA; MS 82 Bloomsburg Univ of PA; Sp-Lang Path, OPT Services Inc, **SLP**

Hammond, Mrs Rosemary Dupree 140 Orangewood Drive, Lafayette, LA 70503, BS 82 Univ of South AL; MS 84 Univ Southern MS-Hattiesburg; **SLP**

Hammond, Mrs Teresa R Box 67, Burr, NE 68324, (402) 274-4354, BA 81 Kearney St Coll; MS 82 Kearney St Coll; Sp-Lang Path, Ed Serv Ut #4, **SLP**

Hamm-Sickles, Mrs Sharon K 529 Diane Street, Albertville, AL 35950, (205) 878-4904, BA 75 Univ of AL-Tuscaloosa; MA 76 Memphis St Univ; Sp-Lang Path, Guntersville Lrng Cen, **SLP**

Hamner, Constance Elizabeth 3110 Lafayette, Houston, TX 77005-3044, (404) 255-2918, BS 77 Southern Methodist Univ; MS 78 Southern Methodist Univ; Aud, N Sub ENT Cl - Aud Ed Cen, **A**

Hamnett, David 2531 Barkley Memorial Center, University Of Nebraska, Lincoln, NE 68583, (402) 472-5467, BA 50 Monmouth Coll; ME 55 Wayne St Univ; Cl Coord Off Campus Prog, U of Neb-Lincoln, **SLP**

Hamorsky, Lynda 707 Ohio River Boulevard, Apartment 206, Pittsburgh, PA 15202, BA 81 Univ of Pittsburgh - Pittsburgh; MS 83 Clarion Univ of PA; Sp-Lang Path, Robinson Developmental Center, **SLP**

Hampton, Alice W 1108 East Lakeridge Drive, Fayetteville, AR 72703, (501) 521-8378, **SLP**

Hampton, Andrea J B Route 2 Box 266, Sumerduck, VA 22742, (703) 659-4111, BS 78 James Madison Univ; MS 80 James Madison Univ; Sp/Lang Path, Stafford Co Pub Schs, **SLP**

Hampton, Mrs Annie Winchester 5218 Laurel Hall Drive, Indianapolis, IN 46226, (317) 259-5462, BA 81 Butler Univ; MA 83 Butler Univ; **SLP**

Hampton, Dr Dennis C 280 Mamaroneck Avenue, White Plains, NY 10605, (914) 761-4455, BA 69 Univ of CT; MS 73 Columbia Univ Teachers Coll; PH 77 (Aud) Columbia Univ Teachers Coll; Dir, Dennis Hampton PhD and Assoc, **A**

Hampton, Julie Anne 225 Mertz Street, Midland, MI 48640, (517) 839-3537, BA 82 MI St Univ; MA 83 MI St Univ; Sp-Lang Path, Midland Hosp Ctr, **SLP**

Hampton, Mrs Karen H 42 Lamont, Little Rock, AR 72209, (501) 565-1967, BA 77 Univ of AR - Little Rock; MS 78 Univ of AR - Little Rock; Sp-Lang Path, Little Rock Pub Sch, **SLP**

Hampton, Mrs Louise P Box 382, Davidson, NC 28036, (704) 892-7248, BA 53; MA 70; Sp-Lang Path, UCP Dev Cen, **SLP**

Hampton, Susan M 7220 Lake Bluff 19 4 Road, Gladstone, MI 49837-2419, (906) 789-9493, BS 68 Northern MI Univ; MS 70 Univ of WI - Stevens Point; Sp-Lang Path, Delta-Schoolcraft ISD, **SLP**

Hampton, Mrs Suzanne R 1612 Elm Drive, Troy, MI 48098, (313) 689-6000, BA 78 MI St Univ; MA 80 Wayne St Univ; Sp-Lang Path, Troy School District, **SLP**

Hampton, Tama Labreche 12 Sydenham Road, Warren, NJ 07060, (201) 356-5770, BA 78 Univ of CT; MA 80 Temple Univ; Sp-Lang Path, Private Practice, **SLP**

Hampton, Virginia Feldick P O Box 276, Benson, NC 27504, (919) 892-1915, BA 76 Univ of Northern IA; MA 77 Univ of Northern IA; Sp/Lang Path, Med Therapy Rehab Svcs Inc, **SLP**

Hamre, Dr Curtis E Speech And Hearing Sciences, Texas Tech University, Box 4266, Lubbock, TX 79409, (806) 742-3908, BA 64 Moorhead St Univ; MA 66 Univ of WA; PH 68 (Sp-Lang Path) Univ of WA; Assoc Prof, Texas Tech U, **SLP F**

Hamre, Susan Dean 13 Frasco Road, Santa Fe, NM 87505, (505) 827-6738, BA 67 Northern MI Univ; MA 72 Northern MI Univ; Sp-Lang Path, New Mexico Sch for the Deaf, **SLP**

Hamrell, Mrs Recille C Unit D3 Stonehedge, Cedar Glen Drive, South Burlington, VT 05403, (802) 425-3883, BS 60 Univ of IL - Urbana; MS 63 Northwestern Univ; Sp-Lang Path, **SLP**

Hamrick, Mrs Mara C 304 Maryland Street, Spindale, NC 28160, (704) 286-4841, BA 76 Univ of NC - Greensboro; ME 78 Univ of NC - Greensboro; Sp-Lang Path, Private Practice, **SLP**

Hamrock, Marilyn Angela Hamrock-Gram Rehabil Center, 10691 S W 88th Street, Suite 212, Miami, FL 33176, (305) 595-3175, BS 68 Kent St Univ; MA 69 Northwestern Univ; Admin-Owner, Hamrock & Gram Rehab Cen, **SLP**

Hamzik-Mills, Mrs Suzanne 112 Martha Road, Binghamton, NY 13903, (607) 722-5308, BS 74 Nazareth Coll of Rochester; MA 75 MI St Univ; Sp-Lang Path, Rsi, **SLP**

Han, Dr Margaret 1011 Siler Place, Berkeley, CA 94705, (415) 821-8014, BA 67 Chengchi Univ; MA 71 Univ of MO - Columbia; PH 83 (Sp-Lang Path) NY Univ; Sp-Lang Path, San Francisco General Hospital, **SLP**

Hanaford, Mrs Laura Ann 421 Calle Empalme, San Clemente, CA 92672, (714) 492-1796, MA 83; Sp-Lang Path, Garden Grove USD, **SLP**

Hanak, Kathleen C511 McKnight Circle, Pittsburgh, PA 15237, **SLP**

Hananel, Robin J 29 The Oaks, Roslyn Estates, NY 11576, (516) 484-4015, BA 73 Hofstra Univ; MA 74 Hofstra Univ; Sp-Lang Path, Private Practice, **SLP**

Hanasewych, Mrs Marybeth T 1733 Kensington Street, New Kensington, PA 15068, (412) 521-9000, BS 77 CA Univ of PA; MS 81 Indiana Univ of PA; 86–Sp-Lang Path, The Rehab Institute of Pgh, **SLP**

Hanau, Kathleen 7526 Greenly Drive, Oakland, CA 94605, BS 71 Saint Louis Univ; MS 73 Washington Univ; Sp-Lang Path, Private Practice, **SLP**

Hanavan, Perry C 615 South Lake, Sioux Falls, SD 57104, (605) 336-4928, BA 73 Univ of Northern CO; MA 74 Univ of Northern CO; Asst Prof, Augustana Coll, **A**

Hanawalt, Katharine L 11612 Chenault Street #1, Los Angeles, CA 90049, (213) 371-2483, BA 66 Univ of CA - Los Angeles; MA 71 CA St Univ - Northridge; Teacher Specialist, Los Angeles County Supt School, **SLP**

Hanawalt, Mrs Ladonna R 209 Rivendell Lane, Paradise, CA 95969, (916) 877-4127, BA 71 CA St Univ - Fullerton; MA 74 CA St Univ - Fullerton; **SLP**

Hanbery, John G 1 Clifford Terrace, San Francisco, CA 94117, (415) 565-6150, BA 74 Stanford Univ; MS 79 Univ of AZ; Sp-Lang Path, Ralph K Davies Med Cen, **SLP**

Hance, Mrs Ebba Carola Rt 1 Box 139, Deer Isle, ME 04627, (207) 348-2883, MA 84 Univ of ME - Orono; **SLP**

Hance, Mrs Joan Ostlund 1108 8th Street N W, Minot, ND 58701, (201) 628-2990, MS 85 Minot St Univ; **SLP**

Hance, Mrs Susan Ellis 6221 Ballsford Drive, Fairfax Station, VA 22039, (703) 750-8400, OB 79 San Diego St Univ; MS 85 East Carolina Univ; 85–Sp-Lang Path, Fairfax Co Public Schools, **SLP**

Hancock, Mrs Jennifer Kretz 1230 Alder Tree Way, #368, Sacramento, CA 95831, (916) 424-3710, BA 85 Univ of the Pacific; MA 86 Univ of the Pacific; 86–Sp-Lang Path, Olga Ramirez Assoc, **SLP**

Hancock, Mrs Jimelle Rodgers 14222 Dallas Parkway #1025, Dallas, TX 75240, (214) 691-4921, BS 82 Baylor Univ; MS 83 Baylor Univ; Sp-Lang Path, Dallas ISD, **SLP**

Hancock, Mrs Judith Hanson 21 Van Buren Avenue, Castleton, NY 12033, (518) 732-7964, OM 84 SUNY - Coll at Fredonia; **SLP**

Hancock, Kelly Kathleen 3520 Superior Court, Orlando, FL 32810, BA 75 Univ of Central FL; ME 77 Univ of FL; SLP, Orange Co Schools, **SLP**

Hancock, Laura Ellen 707 S W Avens Lane, Port St Lucie, FL 33452, **SLP**

Hancock, Mrs Lydia Ashton 2609 Gillionville Road, Apartment 9-D, Albany, GA 31707, (912) 435-3452, BS 81 Univ of GA; ME 82 Univ of GA; Sp-Lang Path, Walker Co Sch Sys, **SLP**

Hancock, Mrs Melissa Dowse 421 Browns Lane, Louisville, KY 40207, (502) 588-7075, MS; 87–Clin Supvr, Univ of Louisville, **SLP**

Hancock, Pamela K 4726 West 63rd Street, Mission, KS 66208, (816) 276-8225, BA 69 Coe Coll; MA 77 Univ of Northern IA; Sp-Lang Path, Menorah Med Ctr, **SLP**

Hancock, Mrs Sally M 2538 Island Drive N W, Olympia, WA 98502, (206) 866-8038, BA 66 Univ of Portland; MS 71 Portland St Univ; Sp-Lang Path, Private Practice, **SLP**

Hand, Julia W Atlanta Speech School Inc, 3160 Northside Parkway N W, Atlanta, GA 30327, (404) 233-5332, BS 57 LA St Univ - Baton Rouge; ME 63 Emory Univ; Exec Dir, Atlanta Sp Sch Inc, **SLP A**

Handel, Mrs Janice A 714 Bonnie Brae, River Forest, IL 60305, (312) 366-8074, BS 70 Marquette Univ; MA 74 MI St Univ; Aud, Lake-McHenry Reg Prog, **A**

Handel, Julie D 3800 Woodward Suite 202, Detroit, MI 48201, (313) 831-2900, BA 73 Univ of WA; MA 75 Wayne St Univ; 80–Aud, Strong & Johnson MDPC, **A**

Handkins, Jill E 3543 Greystone Drive #1015, Austin, TX 78731-6929, (512) 444-4835, BA 73 Univ of KS; MA 74 Univ of KS; Sp/Lang Path, Brown Sch Ranch Tx Cen, **SLP**

Handley-Thompson, Mrs Louisa B 1516 Shoemaker Court, St Louis, MO 63146, (314) 569-8230, BS 56 Saint Louis Univ; MA 66 Univ of MA - Amherst; Area Coord, Spec Sch Dist of St Louis Co, **SLP**

Handy, Mrs Deborah A 10287 S Ashley Hill Circle, Sandy, UT 84092, (801) 942-5677, BS 76 LA St Univ - Baton Rouge; MS 78 Univ of AL- Tuscaloosa; **SLP**

Handy, Mrs Dianne Janette 5928 Broad Branch Road N W, Washington, DC 20015, (202) 244-0532, BA 72 Univ of MD - College Park; MS 75 Univ of the DC; Cl Superv, U of MD, **SLP**

Handy, Dr Pamela Lucy 712 Bath Avenue, Metairie, LA 70001, (504) 837-5370, BA 63 Saint Mary's Dominican Coll; ME 70 Southeastern LA Univ; ED 74 (NS) Univ Southern MS-Hattiesburg; Sp-Lang Path, Jefferson Parish Pub Sch Syst, **SLP**

Handy, Vickie Kay 4222 Lockfield #507, Houston, TX 77092, (772) 747-8803, BS 78 Univ of Houston - Univ Park; MA 82 Univ of Houston - Univ Park; Sp-Lang Path, Houston ISD, **SLP**

Hanel, Roxanne Bean 2805 South West Marshall, Pendleton, OR 97801, (503) 252-5844, BS 79 Western OR St Coll; MA 82 WA St Univ; Aud, Umatilla Educ Svc District, **A**

Hanes, Dr Madlyn L 844 South New Street, West Chester, PA 19382-5358, (215) 436-6970, PH (NS); **SLP**

Haney, Colleen Ann 4224-D Wagon Wheel Court, Harrisburg, PA 17109, (717) 657-5840, BS 73 CA Univ of PA; ME 77 CA Univ of PA; BS 73 CA Univ of PA; 85–Sp-Lang Path, PA Spec Ed Asstve Device Ctr, **SLP ACE**

Haney, Linda Kay 7800 Pierson #319, Detroit, MI 48228, (313) 455-8880, BA 81 Wayne St Univ; MS 87 Univ of the DC; **SLP**

Haney, Lori Ann Rd #1 Box 242, Franklin, NY 13775, (516) 483-0485, BS 85 SUNY - Coll at Geneseo; MS 86 Adelphi Univ; **SLP**

Haney, Mary R 172 Halls Hill Road, Danielson, CT 06239, (203) 774-5972, 80–Sp-Lang Path, Plainfield PS, **SLP A**

Haney, Nancy Brannon 1655 Blvd Manor, Pensacola Beach, FL 32561, (904) 433-1794, BS 79 Auburn Univ - Auburn; MS 80 Auburn Univ - Auburn; Sp/Lang Path, Escambia Co Sch, **SLP**

Haney, Patricia 13409 North 35th Drive, Phoenix, AZ 85029, (602) 255-1181, BA 75 Creighton Univ; MA 76 Univ of Denver; 88–Health Prog Mgr, AZ Dept of Health Services, **A**

Haney, Patricia L 305 Donna, O'Fallon, IL 62269, (618) 397-7495, BS 75 Southern IL Univ-Edwardsvill; MS 76 Southern IL Univ-Edwardsvill; Aud, Belleville Otol Assoc, **A**

Haney, Dr Russell Route 1 Box 160, Commiskey, IN 47227, (812) 873-6987, BA 46 Univ of CA - Santa Barbara; MA 48 Univ of Southern CA; PH 50 (NS) Univ of Southern CA; SLP and Psychologist, Private Practice, **SLP F**

Haney, Sandra L 302 Hill, Harlan, IA 51537, (712) 755-3896, BS 70 Mankato St Univ; MA 76 Mankato St Univ; SLP, Loess Hills AEA, **SLP**

Haney, Mrs Sheree J 915 North 13th East, Mountain Home, ID 83647, (208) 587-4421, BS 78 Trenton St Coll; MA 80 LA Tech Univ; 88–SLP, Idaho State Sch & Hosp, **SLP**

Hanhold, Diana Tresa Dyky 3882 Windy Trail Cove, Bartlett, TN 38135, (901) 373-6871, BA 83 Allegheny Coll; MA 85 Edinboro Univ of PA; 88–Sp-Lang Path, Baptist Mem Hosp, **SLP**

Hanifin, Cynthia Quackenbus 31 Coney Street, Walpole, MA 02032, (617) 421-5984, BS 83 Northeastern Univ; MS 85 Univ of WI - Madison; Aud, Havard Comm Hlth Plan, **A**

Hanin, Laurie 6601 Burns Street #2D, Rego Park, NY 11374, (212) 642-2352, BA 77 CUNY - Queens Coll; MA 79 CUNY - Queens Coll; PH 88 (Sp & Hrng Sciences) CUNY - Grad Sch & Univ Cntr; 85–Research Assoc, Graduate Ctr of Cuny, **A**

Hanisits, Christine Marie 648 West Vine, Springfield, IL 62704, (217) 753-3231, BS 82 IL St Univ - Normal; MS 86 Southern IL Univ -Carbondale; **A**

Haniu, Yohko 2-11-2 Hamacho 1170, Nihombashi Chu-O-Ku, Tokyo, Japan, BA 74 Univ of HI - Manoa; MS 77 Univ of HI - Manoa; **SLP**

Hankammer, Mrs S Bonnie 943 Finchley Place, Richmond, VA 23225, MS; **SLP LM**

Hanke, Gilbert C Speech & Lang Serv Of East TX, 418 East Main Street, Nacogdoches, TX 75961, (409) 560-2664, BA 72 Lynchburg Coll; ME 77 Southwest TX St Univ; Sp-Lang Path, Sp-Lang Serv of E TX, **SLP**

Hankerson, Jan C 1424 N E 21 #21, Portland, OR 97232, (503) 282-1248, BS 76 ID St Univ; MS 78 ID St Univ; 87–Aud, Private Practice, **A**

Hankey, Mrs Cynthia Mooibroek R R 1 Box 37, Manuel, ND 58256-9758, BA 77; MA 79 Univ of ND; SLP, Bemidji Reg Inter Dist Council, **SLP**

Hankin, Mrs Wendy F 7837 Karakul Lane, Fayetteville, NY 13066, (315) 637-8545, BA 78 CUNY - Queens Coll; MS 79 Ithaca Coll; 84–Sp-Lang Path, Elmcrest Children's Ctr, **SLP**

Hankins, Mrs Joan M 2260 Baywood Drive, Biloxi, MS 39532, (601) 388-5978, BA 56 PA St Univ - Univ Park; ME 57 Harvard Univ; Sp-Lang Path, Sp Lang-Learning Svcs, **SLP**

Hankins, Kathy Dawn 153A Old Denmark Road, Jackson, TN 38301, (901) 424-9200, BS 81 Southern IL Univ -Carbondale; MS 83 Southern IL Univ -Carbondale; 86–Reg Sp & Hearing Dir, TN Dept of Hlth & Environ

Hankins, Ronald Joe 94 Old Goshen Road, Williamsburg, MA 01096, (413) 784-4970, BS 84 Univ of MA - Amherst; MA 87 Univ of MA - Amherst; 88–Sp-Lang Path, Bay State Med Ctr, **SLP**

Hankinson, Anita J 1012 West William, Champaign, IL 61821, BS 74 Univ of IL - Urbana; MS 75 Univ of IL - Urbana; Sp-Lang Path, Champaign Comm Ut Sch Dist #4, **SLP**

Hankinson, Mrs Arline L 2810 Aquaris Avenue, Silver Spring, MD 20906, (301) 390-6323, BA 66 Western MI Univ; MS 72 CUNY - Queens Coll; Sp/Lang Path, Prince Georges Co Bd Ed, **SLP**

Hankinson, Mrs Audrey L 16528 Redlands Road, Rockville, MD 20855, (703) 938-7743, BA 63 FL A & M Univ; MA 76 Catholic Univ of America; Teacher, Fairfax County Board of Educ

Hankla, James W 2611 Winchester Road, Waycross, GA 31501, (912) 283-1875, BA 76 Univ of OK - Norman; MS 78 Univ of OK Medical Center; 78–Aud, Southeast Health Unit, **A**

Hanko, Mrs Joyce M 1010 Greentrail Court, O'Fallon, IL 62269, (618) 624-2891, BS 78 Univ of HI - Manoa; MS 81 AZ St Univ; 88–Aud, Christian Hosp Northeast, **A**

Hanks, Daniel A 748 West Maumee, Adrian, MI 49221, (517) 263-5231, BA 74; MA 75 MI St Univ; Sp-Lang Path, Private Practice, **SLP**

Hanks, Felice A 20 Hillcrest, Lafayette, LA 70507, (318) 234-4032, BA 74 McNeese St Univ; MS 77 Univ of Southwestern LA; SLP, Lafayette Parish Sch Bd, **SLP**

Hanks, Joseph David 2323 North Woodlawn, Apt 104, Wichita, KS 67220, (316) 685-5823, BS 86 Northeast MO St Univ; MA 87 Northeast MO St Univ; **SLP**

Hanks, Julie McShane 1715 14th Avenue, Greeley, CO 80631, (303) 857-2714, BA 82 Univ of CA - Santa Barbara; MA 84 Univ of Northern CO; 86–Sp-Lang Path, Weld Co BOCES, **SLP**

Hanks, Lori Kim P 1230 North 145th Plaza, Omaha, NE 68154, BA 76 6407; MA 80 Univ of NE - Lincoln; 81–Sp-Lang Path, Millard PS, **SLP**

Hanlan, John W Box 2670, Yellowknife, NT, Canada X1A 2P9, (403) 873-3477, OB 72 Univ of Alberta - Alberta; MS 80 Portland St Univ; Sp-Lang Path, Yellowknife Public Schools, **SLP**

Hanley, Mrs Joan C 3037 Deluna Drive, Rancho Palos Verdes, CA 90274, (213) 833-7844, **SLP A**

Hanley, Dr John M 9243 Arrowhead West, Scotts, MI 49088, (616) 383-0963, BA 67 Western MT Coll; MA 73 Univ of MT; PH 80 (NS) Univ of IA; Assoc Prof, Wn MI U, **SLP**

Hanley, Mrs Martha Travis 173 Country Manor Way #4, Webster, NY 14580-3335, (716) 265-4044, MS 83 Nazareth Coll of Rochester; 80–Sp-Lang Path, Wayne Central Schools, **SLP**

Hanley, Sheila Mary Moreland Medical Center, 1111 Delafield Street, Waukesha, WI 53188, (414) 549-5150, BS 84 Purdue Univ - West Lafayette; MS 86 Univ of WI - Madison; 88–Aud, Pro Hearing Svcs Inc, **A**

Hanley, Dr Theodore D 900 Calle de Los Amigos EG 112, Santa Barbara, CA 93105, BA 39 Univ of CA - Santa Barbara; MA 42 Univ of IA; PH 49 (NS) Univ of IA; **SLP F LM**

Hanlon, Joan M 2120 Maleady Drive, Herndon, VA 22070, (703) 670-8126, BA 78 Coll of Saint Benedict; MA 81 Univ of MN - Minneap-St Paul; Sp-Lang Path, Blue Ridge Speech Hearing Cen, **SLP**

Hanna, Mrs Alexis W 112 Finley Circle, Winston-Salem, NC 27127, (919) 727-0617, BS 86 Kent St Univ; MA 86 Kent St Univ; Sp-Lang Path, Family Services Inc, **SLP**

Hanna, Mrs Rhonda Fran 61 Norton Street, Freeport, NY 11520, (516) 379-9057, MS 82 Adelphi Univ; Sp-Lang Path, BOCES, **SLP**

Hanna, Susan Denise 1006 Harvard Street, Rochester, NY 14610, (716) 271-0680, Sp-Lang Path, Hrng & Sp Cntr of Rochester, **SLP**

Hanna, Mrs Sylvia K 401 Jamica Avenue, Pittsburgh, PA 15229, (412) 486-6000, BS 62 Indiana Univ of PA; MS 66 WV Univ; MS 79 Duquesne Univ; 78–Sp-Lang Path, Hampton Sch Dist, **SLP**

Hanna, Mrs Theresa Marie 64 Victoria Lane, Frostburg, MD 21532, (301) 689-9678, BA 79 Carlow Coll; ME 83 CA Univ of PA; Sp-Lang Path, Allegany Co Bd of Ed, **SLP**

Hannafey, Christine A 312 Warde Terrace, Fairfield, CT 06430, (203) 847-0481, BA 78 Southern CT St Univ; MS 81 Southern CT St Univ; SLP, Norwalk Board of Education, **SLP**

Hannah, Dr Elaine P 665 Haverford Avenue, Pacific Palisades, CA 90272, (213) 454-0012, BA 46 SUNY - Center at Buffalo; MA 48 Univ of WI - Madison; PH 56 (NS) IN Univ - Bloomington; Prof, CA St U-Northridge, **SLP ACE**

Hannah, Dr Joan B 626 Old Jasmine Hill Road, Wetumpka, AL 36092, (205) 271-9278, BA 62 Univ of AL- Tuscaloosa; MA 64 Univ of AL- Tuscaloosa; ED 74 (Special Education) Univ of AL- Tuscaloosa; 86–Exec Dir, Mental Hlth Dept, **SLP**

Hannah, Dr Joseph E 626 Old Jasmuine Hill Road, Wetumpka, AL 36092, (205) 567-3821, BS 64 Univ of AL- Tuscaloosa; MA 66 Univ of AL- Tuscaloosa; PH 71 (Aud) LA St Univ - Baton Rouge; 86–Aud, Private Practice, **A**

Hannah, Mrs Kay L 14 Dorset Street Ext, Shelburne, VT 05482, (802) 863-4521, BA 60 Univ of ME - Orono; MS 74 Univ of VT; Sp/Lang Path, Burlington Pub Schs, **SLP**

Hannah, Kevin Allen 10-B Dupuis Avenue, Lewiston, ME 04540, BS 84 WV Univ; MA 86 Univ of SC - Columbia; Aud, Hear Inc, **A**

Hannah, Virginia Ann 1261 Penn Avenue, Pine City, NY 14871, (607) 734-0124, BS 77 Elmira Coll; MS 79 Ithaca Coll; Sp-Lang Path, Elmira Psychiatrtic Center, **SLP**

Hannahan, Mrs Lisa Barbara 27 Gaylord Street #3, Amherst, MA 01002, (413) 253-3886, BS 82 Univ of MA - Amherst; MS 85 Emerson Coll; Sp-Lang Path, Belchertown St Sch, **SLP**

Hanna-Kraus, Mrs Linda Susan 6885 Brighton Drive, Dublin, CA 94568-1729, (415) 833-8714, BA CA St Univ - Chico; MS San Francisco St Univ; Aud, Ear Med Group, **A**

Hannan, Frances D 3740 Metairie Heights Avenue, Metairie, LA 70002, (504) 482-9676, BS 76 Saint Mary's Dominican Coll; OM 79 LA St Univ - N O Medical Ctr; Sp-Lang Path, Private Practice, **SLP**

Hannan, Karen Joan 7524 S W Viewpoint Terrace, Portland, OR 97219, (503) 280-5757, BS 78 Univ of WA; MA 81 Western WA Univ; Sp-Lang Path, Portland Public Schools, **SLP**

Hannan-Merwin, Mrs Mary Frances 1169 South Kings Drive, Charlotte, NC 28207, (704) 333-1357, BA 77 Tulane Univ; MS 80 Univ of NC - Chapel Hill; **SLP**

Hanneman, Launa Kae 311 East National Street, Vermillion, SD 57069, (605) 668-3258, MA 84 Univ of SD - Vermillion; **SLP**

Hanner, Mary Anne P O Box 433, 706 Maple Street, Oakland, IL 61943, (217) 581-2712, BS 72 Eastern IL Univ; MS 74 Eastern IL Univ; Assistant Professor, Eastern Illinois University, **SLP ACE**

Hanners, Dr Barbara A 125 Juanita Street, Columbus, MS 39702, (601) 329-4750, BA 56 Birmingham-Southern Coll; MA 64 Univ of TN - Knoxville; PH 77 (NS) Vanderbilt Univ; 87–Aud, Mississippi Univ for Women, **A**

Hanney, Mrs Elizabeth A 3050 Main Street, P O Box 105, Yorkshire, NY 14173-0105, (716) 492-4012, BA 67 Ithaca Coll; MA 69 MI St Univ; MS 81 SUNY - Coll at Buffalo; Sp-Lang Path, Private Practice, **SLP**

Hannibal, Ruth Renee P O Box 183, Norway, SC 29113, (517) 355-3917, BA 78 SC St Coll; MA 80 SC St Coll; 88–Prof, **SLP ACE**

Hanning, Luella M 1321 East 1st Street, Duluth, MN 55805, BS; **LM**

Hannley, Elizabeth Ann 18525 Snohomish Avenue, Snohomish, WA 98290, (206) 668-3708, **SLP**

Hannon, Mrs Kathleen C 171 Covertry Lane, Newport News, VA 23602, BS 77 Mercy Coll; MS 78 NY Univ

Hanoian-De St Jeor, Mrs Sharon 549 East Mallard Circle, Fresno, CA 93710, (209) 434-4320, BA 70 CA St Univ - Fresno; MA 72 CA St Univ - Fresno; 88, **SLP**

Hanopole, Dr Martin S 197 Kent Street #18, Brookline, MA 02146, BS 60 Rutgers St Univ -N Brunswick; MA 62 Temple Univ-Tyler Sch of Art; PH 78 (NS) Boston Coll; Consultant, Private Practice, **SLP A**

Hanover, Mrs Regina K 8438 Bergen Drive, Cordova, TN 38018, (901) 754-6892, BA 65 Carnegie-Mellon Univ; MA 70 Memphis St Univ; Sp/Lang Path, Mid-S Comp Home Hlth & Hospice, **SLP**

Hanrahan, Donna E 240 Brentwood, Inkster, MI 48141, (313) 295-5575, BS 80 Eastern MI Univ; MA 83 Eastern MI Univ; Sp-Lang Path, Heritage Hosp, **SLP**

Hanrahan, Joan Cirillo 33 Edgar Terrace, Staten Island, NY 10301, (718) 981-0826, BA 72 CUNY - Brooklyn Coll; MS 76 CUNY - Brooklyn Coll; Sp-Lang Path, NYC Bd of Ed/Sp Serv U, **SLP**

Hanrahan, Dr Linda L P O Box 2123, Concord, NH 03301, (617) 437-5424, BA 72 CA St Univ - Long Beach; MA 74 CA St Univ - Long Beach; PH 80 (NS) Univ of OR; Associate Professor, Northeastern University, **SLP**

Hanrahan, Shelley M 3575 Southwest Hillside Dr, Portland, OR 97221, (503) 648-1162, BA 73 Univ of CA - Los Angeles; MA 76 San Diego St Univ; SLP, Reedville Elem School Dist 29, **SLP**

Hans, Jay C 7 Coachman Pike, Ledyard, CT 06339, (203) 446-5372, BS 72 Syracuse Univ; MS 75 Syracuse Univ; Supervisor Hring Conserv & Aud, General Dynamics, **A ACE**

Hans, Mrs Judith L G 8 Sheffield Lane, Pottstown, PA 19464, (215) 233-9559, BS 73 Bloomsburg Univ of PA; MA 76 SUNY - Coll at Geneseo; 85–Sp-Lang Path, Montgomery Co Iu Non Public, **SLP ACE**

Hans, Mrs Patricia G 2909 Bagarry, Amarillo, TX 79103, (806) 359-7681, BA 77 TX Tech Univ; MA 79 Univ of NE - Lincoln; 83–Aud, Amarillo Sp Hrng & Lang Cen, **A**

Hansborough, Mrs Susan Babecki 2800 Old Oaks Drive, Charlottesville, VA 22901, (803) 293-2326, MA 78 Catholic Univ of America; **A**

Hansch, Debra Jean 644 Country Club Road, Bridgewater, NJ 08807, (201) 658-6187, MA 78 Univ of FL; 82–Tech Consult, American Telephone & Telegraph, **SLP**

Hansel, Mrs Susan 4726 Arbor Drive #201, Rolling Meadows, IL 60008, (312) 392-2250, BS 76 Nazareth Coll of Rochester; MS 82 Syracuse Univ; Aud, NW Sp & Hrng Cen, **A**

Hansen, Anne Christine 9077 N Park Plaza Court, Brown Deer, WI 53223, (414) 636-4011, BS 85 Univ of WI - Milwaukee; MS 86 Marquette Univ; **SLP**

Hansen, Dr Barin L Communication Competencies Clinic, 133 County Road, Plympton, MA 02367, (617) 585-6830, BA 51 Harvard Univ; MS 53 Boston Univ; ED 72 (NS) Boston Univ; Dir, Commun Competencies Cl, **SLP**

Hansen, Cassandra 3083 E Granite Meadow Lane, Sandy, UT 84092, (801) 942-2492, BA 76 Univ of UT; MS 78 Univ of UT; 78–Sp/Lang Path, Private Practice, **SLP**

Hansen, Corine S 5476 Kiowa Drive #17, La Mesa, CA 92042, (619) 579-7619, BS 69 Minot St Univ; MS 70 Minot St Univ; Sp-Lang Path, Grossmont USD, **SLP**

Hansen, Daniel L 1012 3rd Avenue West, Oskaloosa, IA 52577, BS 85 Northwest MO St Univ; MS 86 Univ of NE - Lincoln; **A**

Hansen, Mrs Deborah Lessiter 417 North Thompson Drive, Apartment 8, Madison, WI 53714, (608) 246-0551, BS 86 Univ of WI - Madison; MS 87 Marquette Univ

Hansen, Dennis L 603 Colorado Avenue N W, Orange City, IA 51041, (712) 722-4374, BS 65 Mankato St Univ; MA 78 Univ of SD - Vermillion; Aud, AEA 4, **A**

Hansen, Diane Louise 2438 Sapp Road SW, Olympia, WA 98501, (206) 357-4428, BA 81 Univ of WA; MA 84 WA St Univ; **SLP**

Hansen, Donald A 1000 North Oak Street, Marshfield, WI 54449, (715) 387-5371, BS 71 Univ of WI - Stevens Point; MS 72 Univ of WI - Stevens Point; 76–Aud, Marshfield Cl, **A**

Hansen, Ellen A Route 2, Coleman Road, Franklin, TN 37064, **SLP**

Hansen, Ellen Kathryn 525 Downer Street, Westfield, NJ 07091, (201) 233-3720, BA 77 Montclair St Coll; MA 78 Kean Coll of NJ; Aud, Chldn's Specialized Hosp, **A ACE**

Hansen, James E 532 Potter Road, Burlington, WI 53105, MS 70; **SLP A**

Hansen, James J RFD 1 Box 109, New Richland, MN 56072, (507) 465-8618, BS 66 Mankato St Univ; MA 71 Univ of WY; Sp-Lang Path, Private Practice, **SLP**

Hansen, Joan Bode 3023 South 53rd Street, Milwaukee, WI 53219, (414) 545-4672, BS 72 Univ of WI - Oshkosh; MS 78 Univ of WI - Milwaukee; Sp-Lang Path, Wauwatosa Pub Sch, **SLP**

Hansen, John Henry 324 Krattley Lane, Hudson, WI 54016, (715) 386-2917, BA 64 Saint Cloud St Univ; Sp-Lang Path, ISD #197, **SLP**

Hansen, Judith Ann RD #1, Box 626, Titusville, NJ 08560, (201) 788-6424, BA 82 Trenton St Coll; MS 85 Rutgers Coll; 88–Sp-Lang Path, Hunterdon Med Ctr, **SLP**

Hansen, Karen V P O Box 4158, Tubac, AZ 85646, (602) 398-9289, BA 69 Univ of CO - Boulder; MA 75 Univ of Northern CO; Self Employed, **SLP**

Hansen, Kristen Maria 39342 Baroque, Mount Clemens, MI 48044, (313) 263-1378, BS 82 Western MI Univ; MA 84 Central MI Univ; **SLP**

Hansen, Laura Larky 6047 S W Brugger Street, Portland, OR 97219, MA 85 OR St Univ; 86–Sp-Lang Path, Multnomah ESD, **SLP**

Hansen, Lenore Anne 912 Tahoe Drive, Modesto, CA 95350, (209) 667-0637, BA 81 CA St Univ - Sacramento; MS 88 CA St Univ - Sacramento; 88–Sp-Lang Path, Turlock Joint USD, **SLP**

Hansen, Lorraine Hendricks 100 Cannon Court #B, Terre Haute, IN 47803, (812) 877-9187, BS 84 Miami Univ - Oxford; MS 86 Miami Univ - Oxford; 88–Sp-Lang Path, Vigo Co Sch Corp, **SLP**

Hansen, Luann Tietge 3907 Barrelhoop Circle, Sugar Land, TX 77479, (713) 499-9537, BA 83 Univ of Northern IA; MA 84 Univ of Northern IA; Sp-Lang Path, Fort Bend ISD, **SLP**

Hansen, Mrs Lynn M 4947 Perceptive Way, Sacramento, CA 95842, (916) 925-2789, BS 77 SUNY - Coll at Oswego; MA 78 Western MI Univ; Sp-Lang Path, North Sacramento School Dist, **SLP**

Hansen, Mrs Marie Meagher 2217 Cottage Court, Waukesha, WI 53188, (414) 521-1656, BS 78 Marquette Univ; MS 79 Marquette Univ; 80–Sp-Lang Path, Wisconsin Therapy Clinic, **SLP**

Hansen, Mrs Marilynn J 532 Potter Road, Burlington, WI 53105, (414) 763-7669, MS 68 Univ of WI - Milwaukee; 79–Sp-Lang Path, Racine County School Office, **SLP**

Hansen, Mark 13 Stage Street, Suffern, NY 10901, (914) 668-9255, BS 70 SUNY - Coll at Fredonia; MS 74 Columbia Univ Teachers Coll; Audiologist, Westchester Hearing Center, **A**

Hansen, Mark H 2024 Aliso Avenue, Costa Mesa, CA 92627, (714) 760-3506, BA 58 Univ of Redlands; MA 59 Univ of Redlands; Admin-Spec Ed, Newport-Mesa USD, **SLP**

Hansen, Mrs Mary Hedenberg 403 West 3rd Street, Moorestown, NJ 08057, (609) 234-2750, BS 80 Trenton St Coll; MA 82 Trenton St Coll; Sp/Lang Path, Mt Laurel Bd Ed, **SLP**

Hansen, Mary Kathleen P O Box 1962, Gallup, NM 87305, (505) 722-6961, BS 86 Southern IL Univ-Edwardsvill; MS 87 Southern IL Univ-Edwardsvill; SLP, Fort Defiance Agency

Hansen, Nancy L B 110 4th Street, Walnut, IL 61376, (815) 379-2834, BS 63 Bradley Univ; MA 66 Bradley Univ; Sp-Lang Path, Walnut Consol Sch Dist #285, **SLP**

Hansen, Rebecca L 1917 14th Avenue S #10, Great Falls, MT 59405, (406) 761-1200, BA 85 Univ of Northern IA; MA 87 Univ of Northern IA; 87–Sp-Lang Path, Mt Deaconess Med Ctr, **SLP**

Hansen, Roberta H Osteralle 54 8400, Ebeltoft, Denmark, BA 74 Univ of WI - Madison; MA 79 Univ of MO - Columbia; 86–Aud, Aarhus Univ Hosp, **A**

Hansen, Stanley C 162 Union Avenue, Bala-Cynwyd, PA 19004, (215) 878-3400, MA 83 Temple Univ; 87–Sp-Lang Path, Ctr for Autistic Children, **SLP**

Hansen, Susan H 11367 Mason Court, Omaha, NE 68154, (402) 333-5938, BA 68 WA St Univ; MA 69 Northwestern Univ; **SLP**

Hansen, Susan Marie 422 King Street, Houston, MO 65483, (417) 967-4764, OM 85 AR St Univ; Houston School System, **SLP**

Hansen, Mrs Terrilou Craig Hospital, 3425 South Clarkson, Englewood, CO 80110, (303) 788-6366, BA 76 Univ of MT; OM 79 Univ of MT; Sp-Lang Path & Aud, Craig Hospital, **SLP**

Hansen-Emery, Dawn L Learn, 8339 Church Street, Suite 110, Salinas, CA 93907, (408) 462-4080, **SLP**

Hansen-Jones, Karen L 5881 Sinaloa Court, Las Vegas, NV 89103-1229, (702) 799-8181, BA 76 CA St Univ - Fresno; MA 78 CA St Univ - Fresno; Sp-Lang Path, Clark Co Sch Dist, **SLP**

Hanser, Mrs Gladys L Route 5, 62 Kathy Court, Gulfport, MS 39503, (601) 992-5640, BS 74 Univ Southern MS-Hattiesburg; MS 79 Univ Southern MS-Hattiesburg; Sp-Lang Path, Harrison County Sch, **SLP**

Hanses, Sr Carmelia Mundelein College, 6363 Sheridan Road, Chicago, IL 60660, (312) 262-8100, BA 36 Mundelein Coll; MA 47 Univ of IA; **SLP LM**

Hansler, Mrs Barbara Jean 14137 Karl Street, Omaha, NE 68137, (402) 331-6954, **SLP**

Hansmann, Mrs Dawn Monchelle 5741 Autumn Ridge Court #C, Peoria, IL 61615-3043, (309) 691-1000, BS 83 ND St Univ; MS 84 Morehead St Univ; Sp-Lang Path, Inst of Phy Medicine & Rehab, **SLP**

Hanson, Ann V 1302 Ramblewood Road, Baltimore, MD 21239, **SLP**

Hanson, Barbara J HCR 33, P O Box 8426, Rapid City, SD 57701, (605) 342-4412, BA 77 Univ of SD - Vermillion; MA 78 Univ of SD - Vermillion; 86–Sp-Lang Path, Midwest Children's Ctr, **SLP**

Hanson, Bernetta O P O Box 404, Lincoln City, OR 97367, (503) 994-2012, BS 67 Mankato St Univ; MS 79 Western OR St Coll; Sp/Lang Path, Lincoln Co Sch Dist

Hanson, Bruce Roy Moorhead University, P O Box 241, Grier Hall, Moorhead, MN 56560, (218) 236-2286, BS 75 Moorhead St Univ; MS 77 Moorhead St Univ; 79–Instr/Cl Superv, Moorhead St U, **SLP**

Hanson, Connie D 418 3rd Street N W, Le Mars, IA 51031, (712) 546-7114, BS 78; MA 80; SLP, Western Hills AEA 12, **SLP**

Hanson, Dr David G Head And Neck Surgery 112C, Vamc West Los Angeles, Los Angeles, CA 90073, (213) 824-4436, MD 73 (NS) Univ of WA; Chief Head and Neck Surgery, Vamc West Los Angeles

Hanson, Donna M 5439 Camilla Drive, Charlotte, NC 28226, (704) 365-6452, BS 75 Saint Louis Univ; MA 76 Saint Louis Univ; **SLP**

Hanson, Donna M 571 Hudson Street, Apartment #1A, New York, NY 10014, (718) 837-5866, BS 78 Southwest TX St Univ; ME 80 Southwest TX St Univ; Sp-Lang Path-Coord, Milestone Special Preschool, **SLP**

Hanson, Grace Haen 6202 Shadow Valley Drive, Apartment B, Austin, TX 78731, BA 50 Univ of TX - Austin; ME 51 Univ of TX - Austin; Professor, University of Texas, **SLP A**

Hanson, Joanne Alness 116 S E Crestwood, Lee's Summitt, MO 64063-3330, (913) 588-5937, BS 85 SD St Univ; MA 87 Univ of KS; 88–Sp-Lang Path, Kansas Univ Med Ctr, **SLP**

Hanson, Judith J 213 Island Drive, Madison, WI 53705, (608) 238-6678, BS 61 Univ of MN - Duluth; MS 65 Univ of WI - Madison; Sp-Lang Path, Madison Metro Sch Dist, **SLP**

Hanson, Mrs Judith Lynn 1400 East 132 Street, Burnsville, MN 55337, (612) 627-2750, BS 65 Purdue Univ - West Lafayette; MS 84 Univ of WI - River Falls; SLP, Minneapolis Pub Schs, **SLP**

Hanson, Mrs Kathleen O P O Box 1886, Ormond Beach, FL 32075, (904) 673-3643, BS 78 FL St Univ; MS 79 FL St Univ; 82–Sp-Lang Path, Volusia Co Sch Bd, **SLP**

Hanson, Mrs L Lynn Route 8 Box 301, Columbus, MS 39702, (601) 327-4584, BS 75 MS Univ for Women; MS 76 MS Univ for Women; Sp-Lang Path, MS U for Women, **SLP**

Hanson, Mrs Lori Ann H 388 IPAO Road, Tamuning, GU 96911, (671) 646-8881, BS 80 Loma Linda Univ - Riverside; MS 81 Loma Linda Univ - Loma Linda; Sp/Lang Path, Dept Ed, **SLP**

Hanson, Lyle Duane 1359 Parkhill Lane, Escondido, CA 92025, (619) 745-0735, BA 48 Walla Walla Coll; ME 54 OR St Univ; Sp-Lang Path, Private Practice, **SLP LM**

Hanson, Margaret Jean 3107 Village Green Drive, E Loop, Moorhead, MN 56560-5409, BS 82 Moorhead St Univ; MS 84 Moorhead St Univ; **SLP**

Hanson, Dr Marvin L 1201 Behavioral Science, University Of Utah, Salt Lake City, UT 84112, (801) 581-6725, BS 57 Univ of UT; MS 58 Univ of UT; PH 61 (NS) Wayne St Univ; Professor & Department Chmn, University of Utah, **SLP F**

Hanson, Mary Elizabeth P O Box 826, Cave Spring, GA 30124, (404) 777-3778, BA 80 Bryn Mawr Coll; MS 83 Rutgers St Univ - Newark; Teacher of Deaf/Blind, Georgia, **SLP**

Hanson, Maxine R 6700 Emerald Street, Boise, ID 83704-8727, (208) 376-3591, BS 66 UT St Univ; MS 82 UT St Univ; Sp-Lang Path, Boise Sp & Hrng Cl, **SLP**

Hanson, Mrs Pamela Marie 4122 Hallendale Drive, Las Vegas, NV 89117, (702) 362-7689, BS 78 Univ of WI - River Falls; MS 84 Univ of WI - River Falls; Sp-Lnag Path, Clark Co Sch Dist, **SLP**

Hanson, Paul E 711 Cornell Avenue, Rice Lake, WI 54868, (715) 234-9007, BA 71 Univ of WI - Eau Claire; MS 79 Univ of WI - Eau Claire; Sp-Lang Path, Rice Lake Area Sch Dist, **SLP**

Hanson, Rhys E 1207 N W 62nd Street, Vancouver, WA 98663, (206) 693-8955, BA 56 Luther Coll; ME 65 Univ of MT; 88–Aud, Aud Clinic Lab, **SLP A**

Hanson, Ronella V 176 Kennebec Road, Hampden, ME 04444, (207) 866-2350, BA 66 Emmanuel Coll; MA 81 Univ of ME - Orono; 88–Dir Spec Educ, Orono Sch Dept, **SLP**

Hanson, Mrs Shirley S 838 11th Street N E, Mason City, IA 50401, (515) 357-6125, BS 78 Univ of SD - Vermillion; MA 80 Univ of SD - Vermillion; 80–Sp-Lang Path, Nn Trails AEA, **SLP**

Hanson, Dr Wayne R 15341 DE Pauw Street, Pacific Palisades, CA 90272, (818) 891-7711, BA 59 San Jose St Univ; MA 61 San Jose St Univ; PH 70 (Sp Path) Univ of OK Medical Center; 70–Ch/Aud & Sp-Lang Path, VA Med Ctr, **SLP F**

Hanson-Schade, Kathleen M 134 Cow Hill Road, Mystic, CT 06355, (203) 536-4957, BA 72 Univ of MN - Minneap-St Paul; BS 76 Univ of MN - Duluth; MS 78 ID St Univ; Sp-Lang Path, Groton Public School System, **SLP**

Hansson, Marta Jean 44 North Pershing #2, Akron, OH 44313-6239, (216) 666-3781, Aud, L L Miller Inc, **A**

Hanstra, Linda Lee 5014 Lindenwood Drive, South Bend, IN 46637, (219) 277-6504, MS 87 Purdue Univ - West Lafayette; **SLP**

Hansz-Ax, Holly K 2453 Jossman, Holly, MI 48442, (313) 651-6210, BS 76 Oakland Univ; MA 79 Eastern MI Univ; Sp-Lang Path, Rochester Comm Sch, **SLP**

Hanthorne, Gloria D 6079 West Curtice Road, Eaton Rapids, MI 48827, (517) 377-0412, BS 71 Western MI Univ; MA 72 Western MI Univ; Sp/Lang Path, St Lawrence Hosp, **SLP ACE**

Hantman, Mrs Lesli R 80 Peach Drive, Roslyn, NY 11576, (516) 625-0602, BS 79 Boston Univ; MA 81 NY Univ; **SLP**

Hanvey, Sharon B 40 West Greenleaf Drive, Birmingham, AL 35214, (205) 221-4342, BA 81 Univ of AL-Tuscaloosa; MS 82 Univ of AL- Tuscaloosa; Sp-Lang Path, Sp Path Assoc, **SLP**

Hanyak, Robert E Dept Communication Disorders, University Of The Pacific, Stockton, CA 95211, (209) 946-2381, BS 79 Univ of the Pacific; MS 81 Univ of UT; Asst Prof Aud, U of the Pacific, **A**

Hanzman, Mrs Debi K 1200 Cleveland Road, Miami Beach, FL 33141, (305) 864-1915, BS 84 Univ of FL; MA 86 Univ of FL; SLP, Stephanie Stryker and Assoc, **SLP**

Hapala, Mrs Susan B 4904 Long Shadow Terrace, Midlothian, VA 23113, (804) 323-2603, BA 71 Univ of FL; ME 72 Univ of FL; SLP, VA Behavioral Serv Ut, **SLP**

Hapken, Mrs Kim R 40 Woodbridge Lane, Thomaston, CT 06787, (203) 283-5054, BA 78 Univ of CT; MS 80 IL St Univ - Normal; 84–Supervisor, Waterbury Hosp Hlth Cen, **SLP**

Happ, J Yvonne 242 Sand Pine Road, North Indiatlantic, FL 32903, (407) 777-1247, Records, Red Cross, **SLP**

Happ, Karen R 416 East 5th Street, Spring Valley, IL 61362, (815) 664-5448, BS 78 IL St Univ - Normal; MS 80 IL St Univ - Normal; Sp/Lang Path, Commun Assoc, **SLP**

Happas, Diane 18 Knolltop Road, Elmsford, NY 10523, (914) 632-8694, CUNY - Queens Coll; Sp-Lang Path, Private Practice, **SLP**

Haptonstall, Linda C 1312 Willow Glen Circle, Apartment 225, Fort Worth, TX 76134, (817) 883-3587, BS 74 Baylor Univ; MS 75 Baylor Univ; MS 86 Baylor Univ; 88–Early Childhood Tchr, Crowley ISD, **SLP**

Harada, Clark 750 Kaheka Street #407, Honolulu, HI 96814, (808) 947-6014, BS 53 Univ of Southern CA; MA 60 Univ of Southern CA; **SLP LM**

Harano, JoAnn N 5638 N Maplewood, Chicago, IL 60659, (312) 880-4530, BS 79 Northern IL Univ - De Kalb; MA 80 Northern IL Univ - De Kalb; Aud, Children's Memorial Hosp, **A**

Harari-Raful, Michela S 1311 Avenue R, Brooklyn, NY 11229, (718) 339-5810, BA 62 Brandeis Univ; MA 64 Columbia Univ Teachers Coll; Sp-Lang Path, Private Practice, **SLP**

Harayda, Debra Sue 175 Lindbergh Drive, Fairview, PA 16415, (814) 734-5610, BS 83 Edinboro Univ of PA; MA 85 Edinboro Univ of PA; 84–Sp-Lang Path, Northwest Tri-County Intermediate Unit, **SLP**

Harbers, Heidi M 888 Grand Avenue #206, St Paul, MN 55105, (612) 227-8471, BS 80 Marquette Univ; MS 82 Univ of IL - Urbana; Sp-Lang Path, Sprc, **SLP**

Harbert-Joseph, Euna M 4908 Jeanette Drive, Metairie, LA 70003, (504) 589-5566, BS 71 TX Tech Univ; MA 73 Univ of KS; Sp-Lang Path, VA Med Cen, **SLP**

Harbeson, Mrs Cynthia J 6953 Sterling Road, Harrisburg, PA 17112, (717) 737-6728, BS 81 Miami Univ - Oxford; MA 84 Kent St Univ; 83–Sp-Lang Path, Capital Area Intermediate Unit, **SLP ACE**

Harbison, Judith K 2096 Skillman Avenue West, Roseville, MN 55113, **SLP**

Harbour, Anita S H 1903 Thornton N W, Olympia, WA 98502, (206) 754-5817, BA 76 WA St Univ; MA 79 WA St Univ; 87–Sp-Lang Path, Tumwater Sch Dist, **SLP**

Harbour, Anne Marie 314 Friendly Lane, Wilmington, NC 28403, (919) 343-0938, BS 81 East Carolina Univ; MS 83 East Carolina Univ; Sp-Lang Path, Comprehensive Hme Hlth Care, **SLP**

Hard, Vallori K 3921 Calle Andalucia, San Clemente, CA 92672, (714) 788-7117, BA 74 Univ of Redlands; MS 73 Univ of Redlands; SLP, Riverside USD, **SLP**

Hardaway, Mary Beth University Of South Alabama, 64 Humb, Mobile, AL 36688, (205) 460-6327, BA 64 Mercer Univ - Macon; MA 65 Auburn Univ - Auburn; Coord of Sp-Lang Path, U of S Al Dept/Sp Path & Aud, **SLP**

Hardee, Mrs Shirley Jean 2216 64th Street Court E, Bradenton, FL 33508, (813) 494-4222, MA Univ of South FL; **SLP**

Hardee, Terry H 363 Chadwick Place, Fairborn, OH 45324, (513) 879-1834, PH 85 Univ of FL; SLP, **SLP**

Hardee, Dr Weldon P 563 Howard, New Braunfels, TX 78130, (512) 525-9833, BS 76 Southwest TX St Univ; ME 78 Southwest TX St Univ; PH 83 (NS) Northwestern Univ; Director, NE Comm & Lrng Cl, **SLP**

Hardegree, Deborah Kay 6045 Jefferson Rd, Athens, GA 30607, (404) 543-6951, BS 79 Univ of GA; ME 87 Univ of GA; 87–Aud, NE GA Regional Educ Svc Agency, **A**

Hardeman, Christine 346 North Kanan Road, Suite 104, Agoura, CA 91301, (818) 991-9832, MA 74 CA St Univ - Northridge; Sp-Lang Path, Santa Monica USD, **SLP**

Hardeman, Gary T Gary T Hardeman, M A, 346 North Kanan Road, Suite 104, Agoura, CA 91301, (818) 991-9832, MA 77 CA St Univ - Northridge; Sp-Lang Path, Private Practice, **SLP**

Harden, Mrs Jane Eleanor 9516 South Shields #197, Moore, OK 73160, (405) 793-8738, BS 84 Univ of WY; MS 87 Univ of WY; 87–Sp-Lang Path, Moore PS, **SLP**

Harden, Dr R Joyce 6924 Valhalla Road, Fort Worth, TX 76116, (817) 921-7620, BA 49 TX Tech Univ; MA 67 TX Christian Univ; PH 72 (NS) Univ of FL; Assistant Professor, Texas Christian University, **SLP**

Harden, Dr Sheila H 8111 Caminito Mallorca, La Jolla, CA 92037, (619) 452-0261, BA 67 FL St Univ; MS 69 Vanderbilt Univ; PH 86 (NS) United States Int'l Univ; Sp/Lang Path, Private Practice, **SLP**

Harder, Brenda K 2601 Cranbury Circle, Harrisburg, PA 17110, (717) 249-3644, BA 75 SUNY - Center at Buffalo; MA 77 SUNY - Center at Buffalo; 88–Aud, Raymond J Wiss MD, **A**

Harder, Connie B 7517 14th N E, Seattle, WA 98115, (206) 828-3285, BA 76 Univ of WA; MA 78 Univ of WA; SLP, Lake Washington Sch Dist, **SLP**

Hardesty, Dr Patricia E 204 Vennard Avenue, Lafayette, LA 70501, (318) 232-0575, BA 51 Southern Methodist Univ; MA 56 Univ Southern MS-Hattiesburg; PH 75 (NS) Univ Southern MS-Hattiesburg; Director, Lafayette General Med Ctr, **SLP A ACE**

Hardesty-Pittard, Mrs Judith L 414 Wilder Drive, Fayetteville, NC 28304, (919) 486-1605, OB 73 IL St Univ - Normal; MA 75 KS St Univ; Sp/Lang Path, Dev Evaluation Cen, **SLP**

Hardiman, Mrs Carole M 2359 Tour Eiffel Drive, Tallahassee, FL 32308, (904) 644-2238, BS 66 FL St Univ; MS 67 FL St Univ; Sp-Lang Path, Florida State University, **SLP ACE**

Hardiman, Linda Kay 1435 South Emmertson #204, Racine, WI 53406, MS; **SLP**

Hardin, Elisa M 8600 Kings Arus Way, Raleigh, NC 27609, (919) 847-6859, BA 75 Wake Forest Univ; ME 76 Univ of VA - Charlottesville; SLP, Raleigh Lrng & Lang Cl, **SLP**

Hardin, Mrs Janice Marie 9633 Ferris Branch Blvd, Apartment 246, Dallas, TX 75243, (214) 637-1340, BS 84 TX Tech Univ; MS 86 TX Tech Univ; Sp-Lang Path, Dallas ISD, **SLP**

Hardin, Mary A Department Of Communication Sciences, Case Western Reserve University, Cleveland, OH 44106, (216) 368-2470, BS 78 TX Tech Univ; MA 79 TX Tech Univ; PH 84 (Sp Path) Univ of IA; 88–Assistant Professor, Case West Reserve Univ, **SLP**

Hardin, Monte F 1712 East 23rd, Hutchinson, KS 67502, (316) 662-4458, BA 74 Fort Hays St Univ; MA 76 Wichita St Univ; Aud, Drs Pease & Smith, **A**

Hardin, Robin Barnes Audiology, University Of Georgia, 595 Aderhold Hall, Athens, GA 30602, (404) 542-2371, BA 79 Univ of NC - Greensboro; MA 80 Univ of TN - Knoxville; Instr, University of Georgia, **A**

Harding, Mrs Cynthia B 8620 Terrell Drive, North Richland Hills, TX 76180, (817) 281-0493, BS 74 Southern IL Univ -Carbondale; MS 75 Southern IL Univ -Carbondale; **SLP**

Harding, Deborah B 3658 Carmel View Road, San Diego, CA 92130

Harding, Elizabeth Maurer 1613 McCormick Drive, Mechanicsburg, PA 17055, (717) 737-6728, BS 82 Bloomsburg Univ of PA; MS 83 Bloomsburg Univ of PA; SLP, Capitol Area Intr Unit, **SLP**

Harding, Janis Louise 731 East 89th Street, Chicago, IL 60619, (312) 783-1355, BS 77 Saint Louis Univ; MS 80 IL St Univ - Normal; Sp-Lang Path, Slddtc, **SLP**

Harding, Jeanne 523 Bainbrige, Apartment 32, East Lansing, MI 48823, (517) 337-3857, BS 85 Bowling Green St Univ; MS 86 Bowling Green St Univ; 88–Sp-Lang Path, Audio-Vestibular Testing Ctr, **SLP**

Harding, Julie Ann 925 South Pearl Street #4, Denver, CO 80209, (303) 452-1043, BA 78 Metropolitan St Coll; MA 81 Univ of CO - Boulder; Private Practice, **SLP**

Harding, Mrs Julie Diane 5406 N E 63rd Avenue, Vancouver, WA 98661, (206) 694-0156, BA 80 WA St Univ; MA 82 WA St Univ; 82–Sp-Lang Path, Ed Serv Dist #112, **SLP**

Harding, Katherine M 14 Village Way #20, Natick, MA 01760, BS 73 9893; MS 76 Emerson Coll; Aud, Wrentham State Sch, **A**

Harding, Kim Jared 102 West Rawhide, Gilbert, AZ 85234, (505) 425-5437, BS 72; BA 75 Univ of IA; MA 76 Northeast MO St Univ; 88–Sp-Lang Path, Consult Div of Dev Dis, **SLP**

Harding, Marcia A 2025 Brownwood Road, Little Rock, AR 72207, (501) 682-4222, BA 69 Univ of MO - Columbia; MA 70 Univ of MO - Columbia; 85–Admin Compliance St Prog, AR Dept of Educ, **SLP**

Harding, Mrs Mary Jane 698 Crestview Drive, San Jose, CA 95117, (408) 241-9610, BS 52 Northern IL Univ - De Kalb; SLP, Santa Clara Co Office of Educ, **SLP**

Hardman, Mrs Lorraine M 4126 Helena Avenue, Youngstown, OH 44512, BS 75 Bowling Green St Univ; MA 79 Kent St Univ; Sp-Lang Path, Austintown Local Schools, **SLP**

Hardman, Teresa Amuso 804 14th Avenue, Vienna, WV 26105, (304) 295-7841, BS 78 WV Univ; MS 79 WV Univ; Sp/Lang Path, Wood Co Sch, **SLP**

Hardt, Mrs Carol A 749 Harriet Avenue, Campbell, CA 95008, (408) 378-3635, BA 76 San Jose St Univ; MA 81 San Jose St Univ; SLP, Campbell Elem Sch Dist, **SLP**

Hardt, Mrs Marilyn Morgan 322 East New Castle Street, Zelienople, PA 16063, (412) 458-6700, BS 73 Indiana Univ of PA; MS 79 Indiana Univ of PA; SLP, Midwestern Intermediate Unit 4, **SLP**

Hardwick, Martha Anne 1490 St Francis, Santa Fe, NM 87501, (505) 988-3719, BA 72 Univ of NM; MS 76 Univ of NM; MA 75 Univ of NM; Dir Sp & Lang Path Servs, Martha Hardwick & Sp-Lang Path, **SLP**

Hardy, Cynthia L 520 Orange Avenue #20, Altamonte Springs, FL 32701-5665, (407) 834-6338, BA 77 Univ of TN - Knoxville; MA 79 Univ of TN - Knoxville; Sp/Lang Path, Private Practice, **SLP**

Hardy, Mrs Deanna C 1414 East Virginia Avenue, Stillwater, OK 74075, (405) 336-4471, BA 62 Northeastern OK St Univ; ME 68 Northeastern OK St Univ; Sp/Lang Path, Perry Pub Sch, **SLP ACE**

Hardy, Edward Robertson, Jr 14551 Oak Chase Drive, Houston, TX 77062, (409) 763-5301, BS 83 Lamar Univ; MS 84 Lamar Univ; 87–Sp-Lang Path, St Mary's Hosp-Galveston, **SLP**

Hardy, Dr James C Hospital School, University Of Iowa, Iowa City, IA 52242, (319) 353-7007, BS 51 Northeast MO St Univ; MA 57 Univ of IA; PH 61 (Sp Path) Univ of IA; 61–Professor, University of Iowa, **SLP F**

Hardy, Mrs Jocerlyn L 6303 Heather Marie Lane, Panama City, FL 32404, (904) 871-0052, BA 76 SC St Coll; MA 77 SC St Coll; Sp-Lang Path, Brooks Co Sch Syst, **SLP**

Hardy, Mary Lynn Z 2403 Amherst Road, Middleton, WI 53562, (608) 836-5054, **SLP**

Hardy, Maryclare 8302 Bo Jack, Houston, TX 77040, BS 63 SUNY - Coll at Buffalo; MS 67 SUNY - Coll at Buffalo; Ed Diag, Cypress Fairbank ISD, **SLP**

Hardy, Mrs Michelle Crudup 13235 White Cliff Drive, Houston, TX 77065, (713) 783-6220, BS 79 Univ Southern MS-Hattiesburg; MS 81 Univ Southern MS-Hattiesburg; Aud, Houston ISD, **A**

Hardy, Dr Miriam P 2533 Pickwick Road, Baltimore, MD 21207, (301) 448-3327, BA 32 Harris-Stowe St Coll; MA 39 Wayne St Univ; PH 49 (Aud) Northwestern Univ; **SLP A F LM**

Hardy, Mrs Patricia Diemer 17 Wheatland Drive, Coatesville, PA 19320, (205) 383-3853, BS 76 West Chester Univ of PA; MA 79 West Chester Univ of PA; Sp-Lang Path, Chester Co Imtermed Unit #24, **SLP**

Hardy, Richard D 2780 Marsh Drive, San Ramon, CA 94583, (415) 838-9015, BA 66 Univ of Redlands; MA 68 San Francisco St Univ; 81–Sp-Lang Path, Private Practice, **SLP**

Hardy, Robin M 109 Herbst Avenue, Syracuse, NY 13203, (315) 479-8334, BS 78 SUNY - Coll at Geneseo; MA 81 SUNY - Coll at Geneseo; 88–Sp-Lang Path, Syracuse City Schs, **SLP**

Hardy, Ruth Ann D 3634 Windy Court, Tucker, GA 30084, (404) 934-1185, BA 61 OH Univ - Athens; **SLP**

Hardy, Steven Dwight 204 Fort Place, Boise, ID 83701, (208) 343-2583, BS 82 Southern IL Univ-Edwardsvill; MS 83 Southern IL Univ-Edwardsvill; 85–Sp-Lang Path, Idaho Elks Rehabilitation Hosp, **SLP**

Hare, Dr Gary Saginaw Valley Hearing Clinic, 3175 Christy Way, Saginaw, MI 48603, (517) 799-1611, BS 68 Southern IL Univ -Carbondale; MA 70 Western MI Univ; PH 79 (NS) Purdue Univ - West Lafayette; Pres/Owner, Saginaw Valley Hrng Cl, **A**

Hare, Mrs Karla P 4522 West Bonnie Court, Mequon, WI 53092, (414) 242-6395, BS 70 Univ of OR; MS 71 Columbia Univ Teachers Coll; **SLP**

Hare, Timothy R 1509 Winding Way, Anderson, IN 46011, (317) 649-6106, BA 78 Univ of MO - KS City; MS 81 Central MO St Univ; Sp/Lang Path, St Sch for Severely Hndcpd, **SLP**

Hare, Mrs Valerie Arnold 20134 S W Southview, Aloha, OR 97007, (503) 649-5566, BS 79 Auburn Univ - Auburn; MA 85 Univ of TN - Knoxville; 87–Sp-Lang Path, Reedville School District, **SLP ACE**

Harer, Carol J 201 Belle Grove Boulevard, Maurice, LA 70555, (318) 981-3206, BA 83 Nicholls St Univ; MS 86 Univ of Southwestern LA; Sp-Lang Path, Lafayette Parish PS, **SLP**

Harestad, Mrs Carolyn 1373 South 279th, Kent, WA 98032, (206) 939-5636, BA 69 Univ of CA - Santa Barbara; MA 71 Univ of WA; SLP, Auburn Hrng & Sp, **SLP**

Harford, Dr Earl R 3234 Flag Avenue South, St Louis Park, MN 55426, (612) 931-9144, BS 51 FL St Univ; MS 54 Vanderbilt Univ; PH 58 (NS) Northwestern Univ; Aud, Private Practice, **A F**

Hargis, Mrs Janet V 319 Shell Toomer Parkway, Auburn, AL 36830, (205) 825-6811, BS 64 Eastern NM Univ; OM 74 Auburn Univ - Auburn; Sp-Lang Path, Tallapoosa Co Bd of Ed, **SLP**

Hargrave, Mrs Elisabeth K 45 Whispering Oaks, Lebanon, MO 65536, (417) 532-9604, BA 69 East TX St Univ - Commerce; MS 71 East TX St Univ - Commerce; 88–Consult, Private Practice, **SLP**

Hargrave, Mrs Jill Stewart 3213 Southeast 50th Place, Ocala, FL 32671, (904) 629-0461, BS 82 Murray St Univ; MS 84 Murray St Univ; 88–Sp-Lang Path, Munroe Reg Med Ctr, **SLP**

Hargrave, Joan K 14 Maple Street, Arlington, MA 02174-4907, (617) 646-7894, Asst Clinical Professor, Boston University, **SLP**

Hargrave, Rose Kersey 805 West 122nd Avenue, Tampa, FL 33612-4123, (813) 933-4209, MS 84 Univ of South FL; 88–Sp-Lang Path, Easter Seal Rehab Ctr, **SLP**

Hargraves, Mrs Tomma S 5962 Coopers Landing Court, Burke, VA 22015, (703) 644-1033, BA 70 Univ of WA; MS 75 Southern CT St Univ; Sp-Lang Path, Fairfax County Pub Sch, **SLP**

Hargreaves, Joyce M 4336 Bunker Lane, Stow, OH 44224, (216) 673-6939, BS 78 Univ of Akron; MA 79 Bowling Green St Univ; Aud, Professional Hearing Services, **A**

Hargrove, Dr Patricia Marie 117 Mary Circle, North Mankato, MN 56001, (507) 389-1414, BA 70 Adelphi Univ; MA 71 OH St Univ; PH 78 (Sp Path) Kent St Univ; 81–Prof, Mankato State University, **SLP**

Haring, Karen Hardin 2 Peabody Terrace #1904, Cambridge, MA 02138, (617) 720-6735, BA 84 Boston Coll; MA 86 IN Univ - Bloomington; 87–Sp-Lang Path, Spaulding Rehab Hosp, **SLP**

Haring, Linda New England Rehabilitation, 2 Rehabilitation Way, Woburn, MA 01801, (617) 935-5050, BA 76 Elmira Coll; MA 77 OH Univ - Athens; Aud, New England Rehab Hosp, **A ACE**

Harker, Darlene R 1800 Woodland Avenue, Park Ridge, IL 60068, (312) 969-7741, BA 82 Valparaiso Univ; MA 85 Western MI Univ; **SLP**

Harker, Mrs Deborah Burns 507B Maple Avenue, Collingswood, NJ 08108, (609) 854-6523, BS 86 Ithaca Coll; MS 87 Ithaca Coll; **SLP**

Harker, Mrs Eileen Orchard 419 Sixth Street, Idaho Falls, ID 83401, (208) 525-7155, BS 85 ID St Univ; MS 87 ID St Univ; 88–Sp-Lang Path, Eastern Idaho Head Start

Harkin, Brigid C 4127 West 140th, Cleveland, OH 44135-1567, (215) 835-8027, BS 85 Ashland Coll; MS 86 Univ of WI - Eau Claire; **SLP**

Harkin, Mrs Mary Friel 500 Liberty Street, Uniondale, NY 11553, (516) 486-1393, MS 88 Adelphi Univ

Harkins, Barbara L 330 Maryland Avenue, Harrisonburg, VA 22801, (703) 289-9469, BS 77 James Madison Univ; MS 78 James Madison Univ; SLP, Rockingham County Sch, **SLP**

Harkins, Dr Edwina C 7142 Triola, Houston, TX 77074, (713) 498-8110, BA 72 Houston Baptist Univ; MA 75 Univ of Houston - Univ Park; ED 82 (NS) TX Southern Univ; 73–Sp-Lang Path, Alief ISD, **SLP**

Harkson, Janet Snyder 6428 Faith Peak Drive, Las Vegas, NV 89108, (702) 658-1026, BS 80 Univ of WI - Madison; MA 82 Univ of IA; 87–Sp-Lang Path, Private Practice, **SLP**

Harlacher, John C P O Box 1254, Kalaheo, HI 96741, (808) 332-7500, BS 75 Clarion Univ of PA; ME 76 Clarion Univ of PA; Sp-Lang Path, State of Hawaii, **SLP**

Harlan, Dr Carl L, Jr Route 5, Woodland Hills, Warrensburg, MO 64093, (816) 429-4993, BS 67 Univ of UT; BS 70 Univ of UT; PH 73 (NS) Univ of UT; Prof, Ctrl MO St U, **SLP**

Harlan, Mrs Cynthia A 58 Grand Canyon Drive, New Orleans, LA 70131, (504) 392-6380, BS 74 Saint Mary's Dominican Coll; OM 77 LA St Univ - N O Medical Ctr; 83–Sp-Lang Path, Westbank Sp and Lang Cen, **SLP**

Harlan, Glena R 4010 Jasmine Street, Paris, TX 75460, (214) 454-3082, BS 76 LA St Univ - Baton Rouge; MA 78 LA St Univ - Baton Rouge; 87–Sp-Lang Path, Associated Rehabilitation Svcs, **SLP**

Harlan, Mrs Nancy T Landover Professional Bldg, 6490 Landover Road, Suite E, Landover, MD 20785, (301) 772-0990, BA 66 Univ of WY; MA 68 Western MI Univ; 81–Div Chief, Prince Geo Co Hlth Dept, **SLP ACE**

Harlan, Sharon Elizabeth 403 Overholt, Sand Springs, OK 74063, (918) 241-1595, BS 84 Univ of Tulsa; MA 86 Univ of Tulsa; **SLP**

Harless, Dr Edwin L Audiology & Speech Pathology Service (126), VA Medical Center, 1601 Brenner Avenue, Salisbury, NC 28144, (704) 636-2351, BS 66 OK Christian Coll; MS 71 Vanderbilt Univ; PH 76 (Aud) Vanderbilt Univ; 81–Ch Aud & SLP Serv, VA Med Ctr, **A ACE**

Harless, Karen Adams 1934 Hickoryridge Road, Richmond, VA 23233, (804) 740-4153, BS 79 MS Univ for Women; MS 80 Univ of NC - Chapel Hill; Sp-Lang Path, Henrico Co Sch, **SLP**

Harless, Mrs Vivian A 3513 Keebler Court, Clemmons, NC 27012, (919) 766-0778, MS; **SLP A**

Harley, Mrs Elizabeth Keil New Day School Company Bldg 5F, 15-16, 2-Chome, Kokubuncho, Sendai, Japan 980, (404) 252-5325, MS 85 Vanderbilt Univ; Sp-Lang Path, Atlanta Rehab Instit, **SLP**

Harlor, Mark Y 2 Charles Street, Mahoning Meadows, Danville, PA 17821, (717) 271-6379, BS 72 Bloomsburg Univ of PA; ME 73 Bloomsburg Univ of PA; Director/Sp-Lang Path, Geisinger Med Cen, **SLP ACE**

Harlow, Mrs Kathie 825 Pardoners Road, Abilene, TX 79603, (915) 677-6349, BS 75 Abilene Christian Univ; MA 80 Abilene Christian Univ; 87–Sp-Lang Path, Hendrick Med Cen, **SLP**

Harlton, Mrs Kathryn R 61 South Holcomb, Clarkston, MI 48016, (313) 625-7944, BA 71 MI St Univ; MA 72 MI St Univ; Sp-Lang Path, Grand Blanc Comm Schs, **SLP**

Harman, Cynthia J Box 279, Petersburg, WV 26847, (304) 257-1995, BS 74 WV Univ; MS 76 WV Univ; 77–Sp-Lang Path, Grant Co Bd of Ed, **SLP**

Harman, Deborah M 329 Valley Drive, Morganfield, KY 42437, (502) 389-4607, MS 77 WV Univ; 78–Sp-Lang Path, Private Practice, **SLP**

Harman, Mrs Deborah Rae 4323 Saratoga Drive, Bloomington, IN 47401, (812) 988-6601, BA 83 IN Univ - Bloomington; OM 84 IN Univ - Bloomington; 86–Sp-Lang Path, Brown County Sch Corp, **SLP**

Harman, Mrs Jill Brainerd 721 Jenni Lane, Manchester, GA 31816, (404) 672-4810, BS 64; ME 82 Columbus Coll; Sp-Lang Path, Meriwether Co Bd of Ed, **SLP**

Harman, Kathryn T PO Box 219, 756 Central Avenue, Alton, IL 62002, (618) 462-8897, MS 86 Southern IL Univ-Edwardsvill; 87–Sp-Lang Path, Easter Seal Society of Southwestern Illinois, **SLP**

Harman, Marjorie G 206 Mather Street #2, Oakland, CA 94611, **SLP**

Harman, Pamela M 9509 Tuckerman Street, Seabrook, MD 20706, (301) 577-4627, BA 77 Univ of MD - College Park; MA 79 Univ of FL

Harman, Mrs Patricia 1202 Colonial Way, Charleston, WV 25314, (304) 345-3208, BS 73 WV Univ; MS 74 WV Univ; 86–Sp-Lang Path, Kanawha Co Schs, **SLP**

Harmer, Maj S Dean 463 East 8260 South, Sandy, UT 84070, BA 73 Univ of UT; MA 74 Univ of UT; Aud, US Army, **A**

Harmer, Mrs Sandra L 969 Coldspring Court, Northville, MI 48167, (313) 246-6051, BA 71 Univ of Pittsburgh - Pittsburgh; MA 72 Univ of Pittsburgh - Pittsburgh; Dir/Sp-Lang & Aud, Wyandotte Gen Hosp, **SLP ACE**

Harmon, Barbara G 14 West 68th Street, New York, NY 10023, (212) 877-2307, BA 64 Queens Coll; MS 66 Queens Coll; OM 77 Hofstra Univ; Sp/Lang Path, Private Practice, **SLP**

Harmon, Bernard 16 New Street, Huntington, NY 11743, (516) 427-5505, BS 46 NY Univ; MA 48 NY Univ; MA 72 NY Univ; Owner, C D Hearing Labs, **A**

Harmon, Mrs Brenda Carmickle 2607 Gilliom, Houston, TX 77084, (713) 578-8507, BS 79 Univ of North TX; MS 80 Univ of North TX; 85–Sp-Lang Path, Briarwood School, **SLP**

Harmon, Electa M M 414 South Section Street, Fairhope, AL 36532, (205) 928-7369, BS 75 Univ of Montevallo; MA 78 Memphis St Univ; 88–Sp-Lang Path, Private Practice, **SLP**

Harmon, Mrs Gloria W 230 Elysian Fields Drive, Oakland, CA 94605, (415) 540-4415, BA 72 Hampton Univ; MA 75 San Diego St Univ; Dir Sp-Lang Path & Aud, Herrick Hospital/Health Center, **SLP ACE**

Harmon, Harvey S 414 South Section Street, Fairhope, AL 36532, (205) 633-0241, BS 72 Univ of Montevallo; MS 73 Univ of Montevallo; Sp-Lang Path, Mobile County Board Sch Commis, **SLP**

Harmon, Hollie Ward 1135 South Perry Street, Montgomery, AL 36104, (205) 284-7756, BS 84 Auburn Univ - Auburn; OM 85 Auburn Univ - Auburn; SLP, Montgomery Rehab Hosp, **SLP**

Harmon, Mrs Jacqueline Prince 1060 N W 18th Avenue, Delray Beach, FL 33445, (215) 783-6421, BS 48 Boston Univ, MS 62 Boston Univ; Dir SLP & Aud, Eastern St Sch & Hosp, **SLP**

Harmon, Mrs Lucia C 405 Lanewood Lane, Plymouth, MN 55447, (612) 823-6660, BA 72 Manhattanville Coll; MA 74 Case Western Reserve Univ; Sr Supvr, Speech-Language-Hearing Clinic, **SLP**

Harmon, Lynne F Lynne F Harmon MA CCC-SLP & Associates, 6322 Papermill Road Suite 2A, Knoxville, TN 37919, (615) 584-5558, BS 75 Univ of TN - Knoxville; MA 80 Univ of TN - Knoxville; Sp-Lang Path, Private Practice, **SLP**

Harmon, Mary Lou 15910 Harwich Court, Granger, IN 46530, **SLP**

Harmon, Mrs Mertis M 3812 Clark Avenue, Vancouver, WA 98661, **SLP**

Harmon, Mrs Michelle G Mississippi Univ For Women, W-1340, Columbus, MS 39701, (601) 329-7270, BS 72 MS Univ for Women; MS 72 MS Univ for Women; 82–Instructor, Mississippi Univ for Women, **SLP**

Harmony, Leslie Jean 17 Fells Manor Road, Caldwell, NJ 07006, BA 62 Rutger's St Univ - Douglas Coll; MA 64 Middlebury Coll; MS 85 William Paterson Coll; Sp-Lang Path, St Francis Hospital, **SLP**

Harms, Mrs Cheryl Sue 1210 S E 11th Avenue, Spencer, IA 51301, (712) 262-4704, BA 73 Univ of Northern IA; MA 74 Univ of Northern IA; Sp-Lang Path, Lakeland AEA 3, **SLP**

Harms, Christine 101 South Montgomery Avenue, Apartment C, Litchfield, IL 62056, (217) 532-6901, BS 80 Eastern IL Univ; MS 81 Eastern IL Univ; Sp-Lang Path, Hillsboro Sch Dist, **SLP**

Harms, Mrs Eileen Cole 57 West Fourth Street, Dunkirk, NY 14048, (716) 366-8170, BS 80 SUNY - Coll at Fredonia; MS 81 SUNY - Coll at Fredonia; 88–Sp-Lang Path, Erie 2 Chautauqua BOCES, **SLP**

Harms, Gail N 6608 Pony Express Drive, Colorado Springs, CO 80918, (303) 593-2291, BS 83 KS St Univ; MA 84 Wichita St Univ; Sp-Lang Path, Sch District No 11, **SLP**

Harms, Helen L 1704 Johnson Street, La Crosse, WI 54601, (608) 786-1400, BS 49 Univ of MN - Duluth; MS 74 Univ of MN - Minneap-St Paul; Sp-Lang Path, Lakeview Health Center, **SLP**

Harms, Jana Ewart 7202 Harris, Raytown, MO 64133, (816) 356-1277, BS 81 Central MO St Univ; MS 86 Central MO St Univ; **SLP**

Harms, Mrs Karen Lee 18871 Via Sereno, Yorba Linda, CA 92686, MA 79 CA St Univ - Fullerton; Sp-Lang Path, Fullerton Union High Sch Dist, **SLP**

Harms, Sherry S 314 East Woodland, Lake Bluff, IL 60044, **SLP**

Harmuth, Phillip C 3282 Bellevue Road, Victoria, BC, Canada V8X 1C1, (604) 477-1851, BA 74 Univ of San Francisco; MA 77 Univ of Denver; 80–Sp-Lang Path, The Arbutus Society for Children, **SLP**

Harn, Dr William E 5717 89th Street, Lubbock, TX 79424, (806) 794-6852, BS 75 IL St Univ - Normal; MA 77 Northern MI Univ; Doctoral, Southern Illinois University, **SLP**

Harnack, Mrs Carol Susan 490 North Orange, Orange, CA 92666, (714) 558-5591, MS 86 Chapman Coll; **SLP**

Harnden, Mrs Kathie Ann 508 Red Pump Road, Bel Air, MD 21014, (301) 838-9268, OB 82 IL St Univ - Normal; OM 83 IL St Univ - Normal; **SLP**

Harnden, Pamela Sue 2030 Powers Ferry Road, Suite 140, Atlanta, GA 30339, (404) 980-1744, MS 84 Univ of TX - Dallas; Sp-Lang Path, Atlanta Easter Seal Childrens Ctr, **SLP**

Harness, Mrs Denise E 4309 Sugar Cane Avenue, Bakersfield, CA 93309, (915) 684-4345, BS 74 Univ of MN - Duluth; MA 75 Univ of MN - Duluth; Sp/Lang Path, Office of Kern Co Supt Schools, **SLP**

Harnett, Betty W 4201 North Shore Drive, Mound, MN 55364, (612) 472-3435, BA 66 Univ of MN - Minneap-St Paul; BS 67 Univ of MN - Minneap-St Paul; MA 70 Univ of MN - Minneap-St Paul; **SLP**

Harney, Mrs Anne Paris 1525 Sanden Ferry Drive, Decatur, GA 30033, (404) 256-2489, BS 82 Indiana Univ of PA; MS 84 Indiana Univ of PA; 86–Sp-Lang Path, Northside Hosp, **SLP**

Harney, Martha Lynn 3038 N E 85th Street, Seattle, WA 98115, (206) 545-2528, MS 84 Univ of WA; Aud, Univ of Washington, **A**

Harnisch, Mrs Diane L 31255 Stone Gate Court, Farmington Hills, MI 48331, (313) 661-0070, BS 68 Ithaca Coll; ME 69 Wayne St Univ; **SLP**

Harnish, Janet A 2740 Meadow Drive, St Charles, IL 60175, **SLP**

Harnois, Karmen Hanson 906 3rd Avenue NE, Buffalo, MN 55313, (612) 682-6209, MA 88 Univ of SD - Vermillion; 88–Sp-Lang Path, InSpeech Inc

Harold, Mrs Alma H 3433 Green Pine Lane, Virginia Beach, VA 23452-5902, (804) 497-8088, BS 68 Hampton Univ; MA 80 Hampton Univ; SLP, Portsmouth City Pub Schs, **SLP**

Haroldson, Samuel K Univ Minnesota Sp/Hrng Clinic, 15 Shevlin Hall, 164 Pillsbury Drive, Minneapolis, MN 55455, (612) 373-4116, BS 61 Univ of MN - Minneap-St Paul; MA 68 Univ of MN - Minneap-St Paul; Associate Professor, University of Minnesota, **SLP**

Haroun, Mrs Deborah Thorsen 6114 N E 35th Avenue, Portland, OR 97211, (503) 249-2000, 83–Sp-Lang Path, Portland PS, **SLP**

Harp, Bonnie Wilson 214 Riverside Trail, Roanoke Rapids, NC 27870, (919) 537-7508, BS 76 Elizabeth City St Univ; MS 79 East Carolina Univ; Sp-Lang Path, Weldon City Schs, **SLP**

Harpe, Janice N 5460 Skyway Drive N E, Comstock Park, MI 49321, (616) 784-9506, BS 72 Western MI Univ; ME 73 Wayne St Univ; **SLP**

Harper, Arleen R 327 Puritan Road, Tonawanda, NY 14150, (716) 631-4930, BA 66 SUNY - Center at Buffalo; MS 70 SUNY - Coll at Buffalo; Sp-Lang Path, Williamsville Cen Sch, **SLP**

Harper, Mrs Carol P 9001 Copper Oaks Lane, Fort Smith, AR 72903, BA 76 Univ of AR - Fayetteville; MA 77 Univ of AR - Fayetteville; **A**

Harper, Dahlia B S 2710 Grants Lake Boulevard, Apartment C-15, Sugar Land, TX 77479, (713) 797-4213, MA 77 Univ of Houston - Univ Park; MS 79 Univ of TX - Houston; 84–Sp-Lang Path, UT Sp & Hrng Inst, **SLP**

Harper, David E 904 Arkwright, St Paul, MN 55101, (612) 293-7635, BA 72 Earlham Coll; OM 80 Univ of WI - River Falls; SLP, St Paul Pub Sch, **SLP**

Harper, Mrs Diane Michel 96 Norma Street, Belen, NM 87002, (505) 262-7261, **A**

Harper, Dr Edith 332 South Compo Road, Westport, CT 06880, (203) 226-3009, ME; PH 38 (NS); Private Practice, **SLP LM**

Harper, Mrs Elaine D Rt 9 Box 355-M, Sevierville, TN 37862, (615) 436-9494, BA 79 Univ of TN - Knoxville; MA 81 Univ of TN - Knoxville; Sp-Lang Path, Sevier Co Schools, **SLP**

Harper, Mrs Gaye O 1415 Pullen Road #D, Tallahassee, FL 32315, (904) 385-7684, BA 73 Columbia Coll; MS 75 Univ of SC - Columbia; Sp/Lang Path, Consultant Private Practice, **SLP**

Harper, Mrs Jo L 99 Alachua Drive S E, Winter Haven, FL 33880, (813) 324-1004, BA 73 Univ of Akron; MA 74 Western MI Univ; **SLP**

Harper, Mrs Judith S 33 East Broadway, Suite 150, Columbia, MO 65203, OB 68 Univ of GA; MA 70 Memphis St Univ; Sp/Lang Path, Sp Path Ser, **SLP**

Harper, Mrs Judith W Box 272, 1200 8th Street, Peru, NE 68421, MA 69 Univ of NE - Lincoln; Sp-Lang Path, Ed Serv Unit 4, **SLP**

Harper, Mrs Linda Dianne North 5921 Ash, Spokane, WA 99205, (509) 328-6535, BA 66 ID St Univ; MS 80 Eastern WA Univ; **SLP**

Harper, Mary Jan 11660 Mediteranean Court, Reston, VA 22090, **SLP**

Harper, Mary K 11 Macy Avenue, White Plains, NY 10605, **SLP**

Harper, Mrs Nancy Neibert 672 Morningside Drive, Zionsville, IN 46077, (312) 331-0880, BS 79 Eastern IL Univ; MS 80 Eastern IL Univ; Sp-Lang Path, SW Sp Ed Coop, **SLP A**

Harper, Mrs Pandora Slinker 113 Western Hills, Glasgow, KY 42141, (502) 651-8410, BA 72 Western KY Univ; MA 77 Western KY Univ; 77–Sp-Lang Path, Metcalfe Co Bd of Ed, **SLP ACE**

Harper, Sandra Ann 6044 East Desert Cove, Scottsdale, AZ 85254, (602) 277-5551, **A**

Harper, Mrs Sheila Rose 3588 Dogwood Drive South, Salem, OR 97302, (503) 399-3101, BS 69 Ball St Univ; MS 85 Western OR St Coll; 85–Sp-Lang Path, Salem Keizer Schs, **SLP**

Harper, Shelley D 2019 9th Street, Charleston, IL 61920, (217) 348-7605, MS 88 Eastern IL Univ

Harper, Mrs Susan Bowman 1385-D Central Avenue, Harrisonburg, VA 22801, (703) 459-4091, BS 82 James Madison Univ; MS 85 James Madison Univ; 85–Sp-Lang Path, Shenandoah Co PS, **SLP**

Harper, William Frederic, Jr 12801 Indian School N E, Apt #2016, Albuquerque, NM 87112, (505) 864-2215, BS 72 Towson St Univ; MS 77 Towson St Univ; Sp-Lang Path, Belen Consol Sch, **SLP**

Harper-Bundens, Constance 2 North Columbia Street, Woodbury, NJ 08096, (609) 853-1369, BS 76 SUNY - Coll at Buffalo; MS 78 Hahneman Medical Coll; Sp/Lang Path, Private Practice, **SLP**

Harpold, Mrs Karen Shumate 1822 Orangewood Drive, Melbourne, FL 32935, (407) 676-5700, BS 76 WV Univ; MS 78 WV Univ; Sp-Lang Path, Sch Bd of Brevard Co, **SLP A**

Harpole, Susan Lois 9372 Holder Street, Apartment 105, Cypress, CA 90630, (714) 828-5904, BA 80 Univ of CA - Berkeley; MA 85 CA St Univ - Northridge

Harpster, Mrs Diane N 1680 Sunderland Drive, Bethlehem, PA 18015, (215) 821-2661, BS 74 Univ of VA - Charlottesville; ME 75 Univ of VA - Charlottesville; Sp-Lang Path, Sch Dist Cty of Allentown, **SLP**

Harpster-Kazen, Barbara Jean 111 S Pointe Way, Henderson, NV 89015, (702) 383-2385, BS 81 Eastern MI Univ; MA 82 Eastern MI Univ; SLP, Univ Med Ctr of S Nv, **SLP**

Harr, Debra A 2045 Garland, Wichita, KS 67203, (316) 262-8271, BA 77 Wichita St Univ; MA 79 Wichita St Univ; 81–Sp/Lang Path, Inst of Logopedics, **SLP**

Harr, Mrs Karen J 4 Caribou Court, Monterey, CA 93940, (408) 375-9537, BA 66 San Jose St Univ; MA 64 San Jose St Univ; Sp/Lang Path, Monterey Penninsula Vna, **SLP**

Harr, Rhonda Ruth 131 Fairchild Street #1, Babson Park, FL 33827, (813) 638-3443, BA 85 Univ of WI - Eau Claire; MS 86 Univ of WI - Eau Claire; 87–Sp-Lang Path, Polk County Schs, **SLP**

Harrah, Mrs Barbara Bente 7630 Brigham Drive, Dunwoody, GA 30350, (404) 394-1884, ME 88 GA St Univ

Harre, Mrs Swing S 225 South Pitt Street, Alexandria, VA 22314, (703) 548-2142, BS 61 Vanderbilt Univ; Crr Pub Co, **SLP**

Harrell, Diane Ahola 2817 Gwinnett Dr, Macon, GA 31204, (912) 743-3479, BS 82 Univ of GA; ME 83 Univ of GA; 87–Aud, Andrew W Tice MD, **A**

Harrell, Mrs Lisa Bailey 405 Cajawa Drive, Mount Juliet, TN 37122, (615) 865-5530, BS 82 LA St Univ - Baton Rouge; MS 84 Univ of MS; 86–Sp-Lang Path, Clover Bottom Dev Ctr, **SLP**

Harrell, Mrs Ruth Ann 680 Hillcrest, Camarillo, CA 93010-4135, (805) 484-0461, MA 75 Northeast MO St Univ; Sp/Lang Path, Pleasant Valley Sch Dist, **SLP**

Harrell-Cowell, Mrs Carolyn Denise 3504 Irvington Court, Virginia Beach, VA 23456, (804) 481-0385, BS 83 Old Dominion Univ; ME 84 James Madison Univ; **A**

Harrell-Mizerak, Roxanne M 1017-A Wesley Lane, Newport, NC 28570, (919) 728-4583, OB 79 Univ of NC - Greensboro; MS 86 East Carolina Univ; **SLP**

Harrelson, Michael 15360 Lyons Valley Road, Jamul, CA 92035, (619) 789-6711, BS 76 San Diego St Univ; MA 78 San Diego St Univ; Sp/Lang Path, Ramona USD, **SLP**

Harren, Mrs Tami Watson 1400 Mohle, Austin, TX 78703, (512) 328-1416, ME 84 Southwest TX St Univ; Sp-Lang Path, Eanes ISD, **SLP**

Harres, Susan C 3315 West Main Street, Belleville, IL 62221, **SLP**

Harrick, Mrs Elma M 110 Franklin Drive, Mullica Hill, NJ 08062, (609) 582-1989, BS 65 CA Univ of PA; MS 66 WV Univ; SLP, Gloucester Cnty Educ Serv Comn, **SLP**

Harrigan, Christine 56 Shoreland Drive, Madison, CT 06443, (203) 245-9783, BS 45 Univ of MA - Amherst; MS 75 Southern CT St Univ; Sp-Lang Path, Private Practice, **SLP LM**

Harrigan, Mrs Claudia Bakker 4609 Morning Hill Court, Midlothian, VA 23112, BA 59 OH Univ - Athens; MA 62 OH Univ - Athens; Sp/Lang Path, Richmond Pub Sch, **SLP**

Harrigan, Deborah Conley 611-113 Chestnut Oak Circle, Altamonte Springs, FL 32701, (305) 841-5111, MA 84 Univ of Central FL; Sp-Lang Path, Orlando Reg Med Ctr, **SLP**

Harrill, Janet Leigh 811 East Graham Street Ext, Shelby, NC 28150, (704) 262-1212, BA 83 Univ of NC - Chapel Hill; MS 86 Univ of NC - Chapel Hill; **SLP**

Harrington, Dr Don A 1102 Rolling Acres Drive, De Land, FL 32720, (904) 734-5552, BA 42 Wabash Coll; PH 50 (NS) LA St Univ - Baton Rouge; **F**

Harrington, Donna B 17509 Ludlow Street, Granada Hills, CA 91344, **SLP**

Harrington, Mrs Hadley R 1316 Woodbridge Trail, Owensboro, KY 42301, (502) 684-5786, BS 65 G Peabody Coll-Vanderbilt U; MA 80 Western KY Univ; 87–Sp-Lang Path, Ohio County Schs, **SLP**

Harrington, Mrs Jacquelyn Sue 2376 Collins Drive, Worthington, OH 43085, BA 81 MI St Univ; MA 82 OH St Univ; Sp/Lang Path, Mt Carmel Med Ctr, **SLP**

Harrington, Jo Ann 1686 Yorkshire Road, Birmingham, MI 48008, BA 67 Univ of NC - Chapel Hill; MS 69 Univ of IL - Urbana; Sp/Lang Path, Southfield Bd of Ed, **SLP**

Harrington, Judith F Dept Communicative Disorders, Univ Of Northern Iowa, Cedar Falls, IA 50614, (319) 273-2542, BS 59 Boston Univ; MA 65 Univ of IA; Asst Prof, U of N IA, **SLP**

Harrington, Mrs Kathleen A 4240 Pinecrest Circle East, Las Vegas, NV 89121, (702) 435-8748, BS 79 Northeast MO St Univ; MA 81 Northeast MO St Univ; Sp-Lang Path, Clark Cty Sch Dist, **SLP**

Harrington, Mrs Kathleen H 14 Trail Road, Fiskdale, MA 01518, (617) 347-7582, BS 78 Worcester St Coll; MA 79 Case Western Reserve Univ; Sp-Lang Path, Harrington Memorial Hospital, **SLP**

Harrington, Mrs Lana L 4869 North Ardmore Avenue, Whitefish Bay, WI 53217, (414) 332-7307, BS 74 Univ of WI - Milwaukee; MS 75 Univ of WI - Milwaukee; Sp-Lang Path, Shorewood Public Schools, **SLP**

Harrington, Nancy Anne 745 Little East Neckroad, West Babylon, NY 11704, (516) 669-4377, BS 82 SUNY - Coll at Geneseo; MA 83 Hofstra Univ; 87–Sp-Lang Path, LI ACLD Erly Intervention Prog, **SLP**

Harrington, Paul J 1711 Wyoming Avenue, Scranton, PA 18509, (717) 342-8379, BS 80 Marywood Coll; MS 82 PA St Univ - Univ Park; Director of Clinical Services, Marywood College, **SLP**

Harrington, Shirley J 2045-C Alpine Village Apts, Birmingham, AL 35216, (205) 665-1551, BS 76 Auburn Univ - Auburn; MS 78 Univ of Montevallo; Sp-Lang Path, Shelby Co Bd of Ed, **SLP**

Harrington, Suzanne M 4312 Greenmeadow West, Colleyville, TX 76034, (817) 581-1438, BA 70 OH Univ - Athens; MA 71 OH Univ - Athens; **SLP**

Harris, Mrs Amy B 1714 East McLellan Blvd, Phoenix, AZ 85016, (602) 271-2965, BS 58 Miami Univ - Oxford; MA 59 Western MI Univ; Acad Chairpers, Desert Valley Hgh Sch, **SLP**

Harris, Mrs Andrea Pappas 107 Fraternity Drive, Lafayette, LA 70506, (318) 989-1981, BA 85 Univ of Southwestern LA; MS 87 Univ of Southwestern LA; **SLP**

Harris, Mrs Ann Mary 10101 202 Street North, Forest Lake, MN 55025-9731, (612) 433-2323, BS 85 Univ of MN - Minneap-St Paul; MS 86 Univ of WI - River Falls; 87–Sp-Lang Path, White Bear Lake Area Schs Dist #624

Harris, Ann Meador 4606 North Versailles, Dallas, TX 75209, (214) 350-8207, BS 75 Univ of TX - Austin; MS 85 Univ of TX - Dallas; 88–Sp-Lang Path, Shelton Sp Lang & Hearing Clinic, **SLP**

Harris, Ann Sullivan 99 Granby Road, South Hadley, MA 01075, (413) 737-7368, BS 74 Emerson Coll; MA 82 Univ of MA - Amherst; Asst Director, Private Practice, **SLP**

Harris, Audrey Axelrod 1880 Veteran #207, Los Angeles, CA 90025, (213) 473-9888, MA 67 De Paul Univ; **SLP**

Harris, Mrs Barbara C 1175 Park Avenue #5-A, New York, NY 10128, (212) 860-3872, BA 65 IN Univ - Bloomington; MA 76 NY Univ; Sp-Lang Path, Daughters/Jacob Geriatric Ctr, **SLP**

Harris, Barbara E 934 Dolphin, Corpus Christi, TX 78411, (512) 851-8332, BS 68 Southwest TX St Univ; ME 69 Univ of VA - Charlottesville; 69–Sp-Lang Path, S TX Sp Hrng & Lang Cen, **SLP**

Harris, Barbara Jane 2230-195 River Run Drive, San Diego, CA 92108, (619) 465-0711, MA 84 San Diego St Univ; Sp-Lang Path, Grossmont Dist Hospital, **SLP ACE**

Harris, Barbara Zine 260 Circle Hills Drive, Grand Forks, ND 58201, (701) 777-3232, BS 71 ND St Univ; MS 72 Univ of WI - Eau Claire; Clinical Instructor, University of North Dakota, **SLP**

Harris, Mrs Beatrice G 7714 Ridgecrest Drive, Alexandria, VA 22308, MS; **SLP LM**

Harris, Mrs C Denice 3310 Shadowcrest Lane, Spring, TX 77380, BS 74 Southwest TX St Univ; MA 79 Our Lady Lake Univ-San Anton; Sp-Lang Path, Conroe ISD, **SLP**

Harris, Mrs Carolyn M 14 Cambridge Road, Glen Ridge, NJ 07028, (201) 744-4088, BA 75 Montclair St Coll; MS 81 Columbia Univ Teachers Coll; Sp-Lang Path, Montclair St Coll, **SLP**

Harris, Dr Charles Newton 502 Wormwood S E, Salem, OR 97306, (503) 585-2574, BS 41 Univ of ID; MA 45 Univ of Northern CO; ED 60 (NS) Univ of Northern CO; **SLP LM**

Harris, Mrs Cheri Lamont 1409 Candlebrook Drive, Dresher, PA 19025, (215) 646-3577, MA 72 Temple Univ; 72–Sp-Lang Path, Private Practice, **SLP**

Harris, Dr Cheryl 101 Bledsoe Street, Hope Mills, NC 28348, (919) 323-6087, BA 73 Mary Washington Coll; ME 74 Univ of VA - Charlottesville; PH 80 (NS) Univ of VA - Charlottesville; Assoc Admin, Southeastern Reg Rehab Ctr, **SLP ACE**

Harris, Constance B 106 Cheshire Road, Mauldin, SC 29662, (803) 277-2512, BA 72 Agnes Scott Coll; MS 75 Univ of SC - Columbia; Sp-Lang Path, Greenville Co Sch Dist SE Area, **SLP**

Harris, Cristi O'Neal Route 1 Box 116, Cleveland, AR 72030, (904) 390-2060, BS 86 Univ of Central AR; ME 87 Univ of Central AR

Harris, Cynthia Bacon 418 Plymouth, Missoula, MT 59801, (406) 728-4100, BA 81 Univ of MT; Sp-Lang Path, Missoula Comm Med Ctr, **SLP**

Harris, Daniel Preston 2705 Del Rio Drive, Austin, TX 78733, (512) 444-4835, BA 69 CA St Univ - Chico; MA 78 CA St Univ - Chico; PH 85 (NS) OH Univ - Athens; 86–Aud, Healthcare Rehab Ctr, **SLP A**

Harris, Dr Dean A 7121 Fisher Road, Dallas, TX 75214, (214) 823-6867, BS 52 Univ of MI - Ann Arbor; MA 53 Univ of MI - Ann Arbor; PH 61 (NS) Univ of OK Medical Center; Pres, Dean A Harris Assoc Inc, **SLP A F**

Harris, Debby J 1520 Mims, Fort Worth, TX 76112-2629, (817) 496-1900, BS 80 TX Christian Univ; MS 82 Univ of TX - Dallas; Sp-Lang Path, Chld Stdy Cen, **SLP**

Harris, Deborah G 1180 Maryjane, Memphis, TN 38116, (901) 761-1500, BS 69 Memphis St Univ; MA 72 Memphis St Univ; Parent Liaison, Memphis City Schs, **SLP**

Harris, Donald 1830 Monkton Road, Monkton, MD 21111, (301) 396-0770, MS 84 Univ of the DC; **SLP**

Harris, Donald Ray P O Box 493, Ellensburg, WA 98926, (509) 925-2850, BA 78 Central WA Univ; MS 84 Western OR St Coll; Sp-Lang Path, Private Practice, **SLP**

Harris, Mrs Dora Mae 3060 Apollo Drive, Winston-Salem, NC 27101, (919) 727-0108, ME 85 Univ of NC - Greensboro; **SLP**

Harris, Mrs Elizabeth 3917 Pennsylvania Avenue S E, Washington, DC 20020, (212) 971-9203, MA 77 Catholic Univ of America; SLP, Fairfax Co Pub Schs, **SLP**

Harris, Mrs Elizabeth A 4521 Old Village Road, Raleigh, NC 27612, (919) 783-6844, BS 78 Univ of VA - Charlottesville; ME 79 Univ of VA - Charlottesville; 86–SLP, Rehabilitation Services of Wake County, **SLP**

Harris, Mrs Elizabeth H 99 Flanders Road, Woodbury, CT 06798, (203) 263-3511, BS 33 OH St Univ; ME 43 Temple Univ; Private Practice, **SLP LM**

Harris, Mrs Elizabeth T 144 Coventry Lake Drive, Lexington, SC 29072, (803) 754-3419, BA 85 Queens Coll; OM 87 Univ of SC - Columbia; 88–Sp-Lang Path, Richland Sch Dist 2, **SLP**

Harris, Mrs Elizabeth Wheeler 38 Bideford Court, Baltimore, MD 21234, (301) 667-4184, BS 76 Towson St Univ; MS 81 Towson St Univ; Sp-Lang Path Supervisor, Center for Living, **SLP**

Harris, Mrs Eloise Tenney 602 East Race Street, Rolling Fork, MS 39159, (601) 873-4712, MS 88 Univ of MS

Harris, Frances P 605 Forrest Avenue, Griffin, GA 30223, (404) 227-9174, MA 69 Univ of AZ; PH 88 (Hrng Science) Univ of AZ; 88–Sp-Lang Path/Aud, **SLP A**

Harris, Gail A 6765 East Nasumpta Drive, Tucson, AZ 85715, (602) 296-7488, BS 69 Bowling Green St Univ; MS 77 Univ of AZ; **SLP F**

Harris, Dr Gary D 4603 Normar Road, South Charleston, WV 25309, (304) 345-8522, BA 75 Marshall Univ; MA 76 Univ of TN - Knoxville; PH 81 (NS) Univ of TN - Knoxville; Aud, Aud & Hrng Aid Serv Inc, **A**

Harris, Mrs Hannah G 11907 Doncaster Road, Houston, TX 77024, **SLP**

Harris, Mrs Holly F 6125 Chowning Court, Raleigh, NC 27612, (919) 966-1006, BA 72 Duke Univ; MS 73 Univ of NC - Chapel Hill; Sp-Lang Path, U of NC-Chapel Hill, **SLP**

Harris, Howard I 9944 Shoshone Way, Randallstown, MD 21133, (301) 554-2791, OB 76 Bloomsburg Univ of PA; MS 77 Bloomsburg Univ of PA; Aud, Un Mem Hosp, **A**

Harris, Howard R 1109 Wingfield Road, Memphis, TN 38122, (901) 323-6671, MS; **A**

Harris, Jacqueline 809 Ridgewood Drive, Gillette, WY 82716, AZ St Univ; **SLP**

Harris, Jeffrey Paul 531 Coachlight Place, Santa Rosa, CA 95403, (707) 578-0333, **SLP**

Harris, Mrs Jennifer W 7212 Union Avenue, Shreveport, LA 71106, (318) 631-5110, BS 80 Southern Univ - Baton Rouge; OM 85 LA Tech Univ; Sp-Lang Path, Caddo Parish Sch Brd, **SLP**

Harris, Jessica R 12 Webster Court, Amherst, MA 01002-2834, (413) 256-8139, BS 82 Xavier Univ of LA; MS 84 Howard Univ; **SLP**

Harris, Mrs Jodi Kennedy 1115 Whippoorwill Drive, Alabaster, AL 35007, (205) 366-2991, BA 80 Nicholls St Univ; MA 87 Univ of Houston - Univ Park; 88–Sp-Lang Path, Chilton County Bd of Educ

Harris, Jody Lee 641 West Aldine #404, Chicago, IL 60657, (312) 769-2230, BA 83 Univ of CO - Boulder; MS 86 Univ of AZ; SLP, InSpeech Inc, **SLP**

Harris, Joyce L Audie L Murphy Memorial Veterans Hospital, Extended Care Treatment Center, 7400 Merton Minter Boulevard, San Antonio, TX 78284, (512) 696-9660, BA 73 Univ of TX - El Paso; MA 74 Univ of TX - El Paso; 88–Sp-Lang Path, Audie L Murphy Mem Vets Hosp, **SLP**

Harris, Mrs Judith L 1413 S E 7th Place, Lee's Summit, MO 64063-9705, (802) 748-4572, **SLP**

Harris, Julie Ann 5016 #5 Chatterton, Columbus, OH 43232, (614) 225-1634, BS 84 Bowling Green St Univ; MS 86 Murray St Univ; Sp-Lang Path, Mount Carmel Med Ctr, **SLP**

Harris, Dr Katherine City University Of New York, Graduate School, 33 West 42nd Street, New York, NY 10036, (212) 642-2356, BA 47 Radcliffe Coll; PH 54 (Psychology) Harvard Univ; 70–Prof of Sp & Hrng Sci, Grad Sch/CUNY, **F H**

Harris, Katherine Pittenger 3207 Banbury Place, Houston, TX 77027, MS; **SLP LM**

Harris, Laura Lee 2750 North 52nd Street, Milwaukee, WI 53210, (414) 886-0116, BS 83 Univ of WI - Milwaukee; MS 86 Univ of WI - Milwaukee; **SLP**

Harris, Laura R 450 West End Avenue #6B, New York, NY 10024, (212) 584-7679, BA 63 Brandeis Univ; MS 72 Adelphi Univ; SLP, Mt St Ursula Sp Cen, **SLP**

Harris, Lester L Lester L Harris Clinic, Whittier College, Whittier, CA 90608, BA 41 OK Panhandle St Univ; MA 46 Univ of Denver; PH 50 (NS) Univ of Southern CA; **SLP LM**

Harris, Mrs Leta L 132 Pleasant Ridge, Richmond, KY 40475, BS 77 Univ of TX - Austin; MA 78 Univ of North TX; Sp-Lang Path, Madison Co Sch Dist, **SLP**

Harris, Linda Trammell 3812 Abby Court, Doraville, GA 30360, (404) 393-7089, **SLP**

Harris, Dr Lonnie G Dept Of Special Education, Eastern Kentucky University, Richmond, KY 40475-3133, (606) 622-4442, BA 77 TX Tech Univ; MA 78 Univ of North TX; PH 87 (Sp-Lang Path) Univ of SC - Columbia; 87–Asst Prof, Eastern Kentucky Unuversity, **SLP**

Harris, Luetta Pee Dee Speech & Hearing Ctr, 153 North Baroode, Florence, SC 29503, (803) 662-5601, BA 64 Univ of NC - Chapel Hill; ME 72 Univ of SC - Columbia; Dir of Aud Asst Admin Dir, Pee Dee Sp/Hrng Cen, **SLP A**

Harris, Lynn V Garberson Clinic, 2200 Box Elder, Miles City, MT 59301, (406) 232-0790, BA 79 Univ of MT; MA 81 Univ of MT; Aud/Sp/Lang Path, Garberson Clinic, **SLP A**

Harris, Marcia L 53 Clemson Drive, Aiken, SC 29801, (803) 648-8344, BA 69 Catawba Coll; MA 77 Wayne St Univ; Head of Sp-Lang Path/Aud, Hitchcock Rehab Center, **SLP**

Harris, Marilyn Jill 1605 Massachusetts Avenue S E, Washington, DC 20003, (202) 727-3866, BS 81 Towson St Univ; MS 84 Towson St Univ; **SLP**

Harris, Marilyn S P O Box 624, Rusk, TX 75785, **SLP**

Harris, Marilyn Sue 46756 Bartlett Drive, Canton, MI 48187, (313) 459-5687, BA 78 Univ of MI - Ann Arbor; MS 79 Univ of MI - Ann Arbor; Sp-Lang Path, **SLP**

Harris, Marjorie R 2478 Crest View Drive, Los Angeles, CA 90046, (213) 825-5131, BS 64 Cornell Univ; MA 65 OH St Univ; 80–Dir-Comm Outreach Prog, Hope for Hrng Res Found-Ucla, **A**

Harris, Dr Marsha R 316 Nottoway, Pearl River, LA 70452, (508) 863-3682, BA 74 Univ of Houston - Univ Park; MS 75 Southern Methodist Univ; PH 83 (Communication Disorders) Univ of TX - Dallas; Assoc Prof, Louisiana State U - Med Ctr, **SLP**

Harris, Marsha Robin 43 West Blue Ridge Road, Cranston, RI 02920, (508) 226-0091, BA 72 Manhattanville Coll; MS 84 Univ of RI; 85–Aud, Attleboro Hearing Ctr, **A**

Harris, Mrs Mary Helen 71 Doolittle Road, Stamford, CT 06902, (203) 977-4390, BS 71 MS Univ for Women; MS 72 MS Univ for Women; Sp-Lang Path, Stamford Ct Hlth Dept, **SLP**

Harris, MaryJane B 17570 Italy Path, Lakeville, MN 55044, (612) 435-5027, BS 70 Northern IL Univ - De Kalb; MA 71 Northwestern Univ; Sp/Lang Path, Washburn Chld Guid Cen, **SLP**

Harris, Mason Derring 17 Pevalta Avenue, San Francisco, CA 94110, (415) 573-4031, **A**

Harris, Maude M 315 South Sneed, Sedalia, MO 65301, (816) 826-8553, BS 53 Central MO St Univ; **SLP LM**

Harris, Maureen A 108 Lincoln Street, Northboro, MA 01532, (508) 481-5046, BS 77 Univ of MA - Amherst; ME 79 Northeastern Univ; 88–Sp-Lang Path, Assabet Valley Collaborative, **SLP**

Harris, Mrs Meryl K 15 Hart Place, Nyack, NY 10960, (914) 358-5909, BS 74 Northeastern Univ; MS 76 Columbia Univ Teachers Coll; 88–Consult/Sp-Lang Path, Venture Day Treat Ctr, **SLP**

Harris, Michael D 202 1/2 Summit Avenue, P O Box 276, Ellsworth, WI 54011, (715) 273-3886, MS 79 Univ of WI - River Falls; Clinical Supervisor/Instructor, Vw-River Falls, **SLP**

Harris, Mrs Nada E 800 Newport Road, Fort Worth, TX 76112, (817) 838-8622, OM 70 Southwestern Baptist Theolog; BS 74 TX Woman's Univ; MA 76 TX Woman's Univ; 88–Supvr-Spec Educ, Ft Worth ISD, **SLP**

Harris, Mrs Nancy B 3118 N E Colonial Drive, Lawton, OK 73507, (405) 355-8620, BS 76 Southern Methodist Univ; MS 77 Southern Methodist Univ; Sp-Lang Path, Comanche Co Mem Hosp, **SLP**

Harris, Nancy Diane 605 Dellwood Drive, Newport News, VA 23602, (804) 877-9154, BS 84 James Madison Univ; ME 86 James Madison Univ; 87–Aud, Lakeview Med Ctr

Harris, Mrs Nancy Lee 30 South 350 West, Jerome, ID 83338, (208) 324-2443, BS 74 ID St Univ; MS 75 ID St Univ; Sp-Lang Path, Magic Valley Sp & Hrng Cln, **SLP**

Harris, Norma Jane 111A Crescent Court Drive, Decatur, GA 30030, BA 71 George Washington Univ; MA 72 George Washington Univ; Coord-Sp Prog, Morehouse Coll, **SLP**

Harris, Mrs Pamela Elizabeth 906 Parkman Street, Altadena, CA 91001, (213) 684-7887, BA 74 Antioch Coll; MS 76 Howard Univ

Harris, Mrs Pamela Glynn 10958 Barrington Court, Cincinnati, OH 45242, (513) 530-9117, Sp-Lang Path, Learning Comm Ctr, **SLP**

Harris, Mrs Pamela Seamon 6719 Winchester Lane, Helena, AL 35080, (205) 979-3030, BS 76 Auburn Univ - Auburn; OM 77 Auburn Univ - Auburn; Sp-Lang Path, Vestavia Hills Elem-West, **SLP**

Harris, Patricia A P O Box 801, Urbana, IL 61801-0801, (217) 333-2230, BS 74 Northeast MO St Univ; MA 75 Northeast MO St Univ; 87–Grad Asst, Univ of Illinois, **SLP**

Harris, Patricia L 353 Washington Highway, Snyder, NY 14226, (716) 898-3237, BS 66 PA St Univ - Univ Park; MS 68 SUNY - Coll at Buffalo; 86–Coord-Rehab Home Health Care, Erie Co Med Ctr, **SLP**

Harris, Paula Dinkins 8945 North 85th Street, Apartment 204, Milwaukee, WI 53224, (414) 327-6670, BS 84 Marquette Univ; MS 87 Univ of WI - Whitewater

Harris, Dr Richard W Brigham Young University, 131 TLRB, Provo, UT 84601, (801) 378-6460, BS 73 ND St Univ; MS 74 Univ of WI - Stevens Point; PH 78 (NS) Purdue Univ - West Lafayette; Associate Professor, Brigham Young University, **A**

Harris, Dr Robert 41 St James Court, Philadelphia, PA 19106, (609) 771-2322, BA 54 CUNY - Brooklyn Coll; MA 55 CUNY - Brooklyn Coll; PH 62 (Special Educ) Univ of PA; 63–Prof of SLP and Aud, Trenton St Coll, **SLP A**

Harris, Mrs Ruth L 4866 Brewster Avenue, Tarzana, CA 91356, (818) 885-2856, BA 64 Univ of VT; MA 66 OH Univ - Athens; Coord, CA St U - Northridge, **SLP**

Harris, Shelley 802 Woodside Lane East #11, Sacramento, CA 95825, (916) 921-0531, BS 71 Ithaca Coll; MA 82 San Francisco St Univ; MS 72 Univ of WI - Madison; Consult, CA Institute for School Improv, **SLP**

Harris, Sheryl L 1535 Stoneleigh Court, Apartment 2124, Arlington, TX 76011, BS 72 Univ of KS; MS 73 CO St Univ; **SLP**

Harris, Stannye Seay 19 Teardrop, Newbury Park, CA 91320-4243, (213) 664-5035, MA 86 CA St Univ - Los Angeles; **SLP**

Harris, Teresa S 6922 Croyden Circle, Wichita, KS 67226, **SLP**

Harris, Teresa Williamson 3062 Villa Sur Trail, Dallas, TX 75228, (214) 247-1377, BS 81 Univ of TX - Dallas; MS 83 Univ of TX - Dallas; Aud, Input Hearing Systems, **A**

Harris, Dr Timothy B Comprehensive Clinic, Appalachian State Univ, Boone, NC 28608, (704) 262-2185, BA 70 KS St Univ; MS 71 Purdue Univ - West Lafayette; PH 76 (NS) Univ of KS; Coor of Sp Hrng Rdng Ctr, Appalachian St U, **SLP**

Harris, Mrs Veronica M 5531 Estate Drive, Oakland, CA 94618, (415) 652-0234, BA 73 San Francisco St Univ; MA 75 San Francisco St Univ; Sp-Lang Path, Private Practice, **SLP**

Harris, William M 824 Waterview Road, Oklahoma City, OK 73170, (405) 691-4982, BA 70 Coe Coll; MS 80 Univ of OK Medical Center; Sp-Lang Path, Moore Public School, **SLP**

Harris, Willie V 2130 Harrison Street, Cottage 7B, Quincy, IL 62301, (217) 223-3299, BS 26 Central MO St Univ; MA 29 Univ of MO - Columbia; MA 50 Univ of Denver; **SLP LM**

Harrison, Mrs Anne 3185 D Castleton Drive, Bradenton, FL 34208, (813) 745-2306, OB 54 Our Lady Lake Univ-San Anton; MS 65 Vanderbilt Univ; **A LM**

Harrison, Barbara Lynn 1442 Pine Valley, Ann Arbor, MI 48104, (313) 973-8262, BS 65 OH St Univ; MA 70 Miami Univ - Oxford; **SLP**

Harrison, Bartel H 1710 Aliceanna Street, Baltimore, MD 21231, (301) 396-8927, BS 75 Towson St Univ; MS 77 Towson St Univ; 75–Sp-Lang Path, Baltimore City Pub Sch, **SLP**

Harrison, Beverly J Hagen 5 Allen Street, Salem, MA 01970, (617) 526-1908, MS 83 Emerson Coll; Sp-Lang Path, Cape Ann Collab, **SLP**

Harrison, Daniel Paul 14010 Burton Street, Panorama City, CA 91402, (818) 901-8965, MA 84 CA St Univ - Los Angeles; Sp-Lang Path, Southern CA Permanente Med G, **SLP**

Harrison, Mrs Denise Sprouse P O Box 105, Eustis, FL 32726-0105, (904) 589-1891, Sp-Lang Path, Eustis Speech & Language Ctr, **SLP ACE**

Harrison, Diann Micka 205 East Dudley Street, Maumee, OH 43537, (419) 891-1106, OB 84 Univ of Toledo; BA 84 Univ of Toledo; MA 85 Bowling Green St Univ; 87–Aud, Toledo Otolaryngology Group Inc, **A**

Harrison, Francine K 2303 Popkins Lane, Alexandria, VA 22306, (703) 765-0459, MA NY Univ; SLP, Fairfax Co Pub Sch, **SLP**

Harrison, Jan Lanette 4072 Thomas Jefferson Drive, Virginia Beach, VA 23452, (215) 631-9300, BS 84 AR St Univ; OM 86 AR St Univ; 86–Sp-Lang Path, InSpeech Inc, **SLP ACE**

Harrison, Janelle Lee 4400 Clyde, Casper, WY 82609, (307) 234-3287, BS 82 Univ of WY; MA 84 Ball St Univ; Sp-Lang Path, Natrona Co School Dist #1, **SLP**

Harrison, Dr Janet Snyder The Devereux Hospital & Children's Center, 8000 Devereux Drive, Melbourne, FL 32940, (407) 242-9100, BA 76 Marshall Univ; MA 77 Marshall Univ; PH 88 (Sp-Lang Path) Univ of FL; 88–Dir Sp-Lang Path, Devereux Hosp & Chldrns Ctr, **SLP ACE**

Harrison, Jean M R Route 4 Box 53, Edwardsville, IL 62025, (618) 288-3470, BS 73 Eastern IL Univ; MS 74 IL St Univ - Normal; 79–Asst Prof, Sn IL U-Edwardsville, **SLP**

Harrison, Mrs Jean M 624 East Mariposa Drive, Redlands, CA 92373, (714) 792-1212, BA 78 Univ of Redlands; MS 81 Univ of Redlands; Sp-Lang Path, Private Practice, **SLP**

Harrison, Jean M 109 Adkinson Drive, Crestview, FL 32536, (904) 682-2816, BS 82 FL St Univ; MS 84 FL St Univ; 84–Sp-Lang Path, Okaloosa County Sch System, **SLP**

Harrison, John P 213 Indian Lane, Media, PA 19063, (215) 566-5641, BA 47 Univ of PA; MA 51 Univ of PA; **A LM**

Harrison, Kathleen M Odonnell 7398 Presley Avenue, Mentor, OH 44060, (216) 729-1919, BA 82 Cleveland St Univ; MA 84 Cleveland St Univ; Sp-Lang Path, Metzenbaum Shelter, **SLP**

Harrison, Linda D Trumbull County Board Of Ed, 3255 Hommon Avenue, Ravenna, OH 44266, (216) 296-2187, Audiologist, **A**

Harrison, Mary Sue 22011 Silver Lode, Katy, TX 77450, BS 75 Southern Methodist Univ; MS 76 Univ of North TX; **A**

Harrison, Mrs Melinda A 32 Fontaine Drive, Clarksville, AR 72830, (501) 754-7628, **SLP**

Harrison, Melinda K Barrett Outpatient Rehab, Morton Plant Hospital, 430 Pinellas Street, Clearwater, FL 34616, (813) 462-7031, MS 77 Univ of South FL; Aud, Morton F Plant Hosp, **A**

Harrison, Melody F Division Of Speech And Hearing, C3 7190, 78 Wing D Medical School, Chapel Hill, NC 27599-7190, (919) 966-1006, ME 73 Boston Univ; Asst Prof, U Chapel Hill/Sp&Hrng Sct, **SLP**

Harrison, Mrs Nancy Ann Swan Lake Road, Liberty, NY 12754, (914) 292-7500, BS 77 CA Univ of PA; MS 84 Coll of Saint Rose; **SLP**

Harrison, Mrs Norma K 78 Orange Drive, Jericho, NY 11753, (516) 549-6827, BA 53 CUNY - Brooklyn Coll; MA 58 CUNY - Brooklyn Coll; SLP, Half Hollow Hills Sch Dist, **SLP**

Harrison, Mrs Patricia A 3229 McKinley Street, Hollywood, FL 33021, (305) 985-5925, BS 74 Towson St Univ; MS 78 Loyola Coll; Sp-Lang Path, Mem Hosp of Hollywood, **SLP**

Harrison, Patricia S 2051 Wood Hollow Place, Sarasota, FL 34235, (813) 371-2130, BA 70 Univ of MA - Amherst; MA 71 Univ of MA - Amherst; Teacher, School Board of Manatee County, **SLP**

Harrison, Dr Peggy R 6066 Azalea Lane, Dallas, TX 75230, (214) 368-8868, BA 28 Southern Methodist Univ; MA 38 Univ of Southern CA; PH 57 (NS) Univ of Southern CA; **SLP F LM**

Harrison, Rhonda L 213 Captains Way, Bay Shore, NY 11706, **SLP**

Harrison, Robert A 15 Lasalle Street, East Longmeadow, MA 01028-1924, BS 77 Emerson Coll; MS 79 Rutger's St Univ - Douglas Coll; Sp/Lang Path, Self Employed, **SLP**

Harrison, Dr Robert J University Of Miami School Of Medicine, Audiology-Speech Pathology (R-56), PO Box 016960, Miami, FL 33101, (305) 549-6451, BA 51 Wichita St Univ; PH 62 Northwestern Univ; Prof & Ch, Div of Aud-SLP, U of Miami Sch of Med, **SLP A F ACE**

Harrison, Mrs Rosalind 1205 York Road, Suite 29B, Lutherville, MD 21093, (301) 825-9445, BS 65 Purdue Univ - West Lafayette; MA 66 Northwestern Univ; Dir, Assoc Sp-Lang Serv, **SLP ACE**

Harrison, Rosemary S Bitterroot Speech Center, 714 Kensington, Missoula, MT 59801, (406) 721-6096, BA 71 Univ of MT; MS 73 Univ of OK Medical Center; Dir/Owner, Bitterroot Sp Cen, **SLP**

Harrison, Mrs Susan Arnold 3817 San Mateo, Plano, TX 75023, (214) 867-1915, BS 85 Univ of Tulsa; MA 87 Univ of TX - Austin; 88–Sp-Lang Path, Plano ISD, **SLP**

Harrison, Mrs Susan I 25 Rawson Court, Hillsdale, NJ 07642, (201) 664-9144, BS 60; MS 62 Univ of MI - Ann Arbor; Special Education Sp-Lang Path, Montvale Board of Education, **SLP**

Harrison, Mrs Susan Smock 16 Boxwood Lane, Langhorne, PA 19047, MS 82 CO St Univ; Aud, Mercer Med Ctr, **A ACE**

Harrison, Tamara Davis 1237 Kelly Lane, Leeds, AL 35094, (205) 761-3227, BA 83 Auburn Univ - Auburn; MS 85 Univ of Montevallo; 83–Sp-Lang Path, Alabama Inst for Deaf & Blind, **SLP**

Harrison, Wayne L 250 East Strada Patania, Tucson, AZ 85704, (602) 628-5357, BA 78 Grand Canyon Coll; MA 81 Univ of Northern CO; Sp-Lang Path, AZ St Sch for Deaf & Blind, **SLP**

Harrison, Mrs Wendy Cox 394 Millan Court East, Chula Vista, CA 92010, (619) 420-7015, BS 85 Bowling Green St Univ; MS 86 Bowling Green St Univ; 88–Sp-Lang Path, Scottish Rite Clinic, **SLP**

Harris-Ryan, Margaret P O Box 7306, Menlo Park, CA 94026, **SLP**

Harriss, Connie Clinton 866 Sewanee Place, Shreveport, LA 71105, (318) 861-6684, BA 77 Northeast LA Univ; OM 85 LA St Univ - Shreveport; Caddo Parrish Schools, **SLP**

Harriss, Judith C Rt 1 Box 653, Sopchoppy, FL 32358, (904) 962-4561, MS 72 FL St Univ; Sp-Lang Path, Wakulla Co Sch Syst, **SLP**

Harris-Schmidt, Dr Gail P Learning Disabilities Clinic, St Xavier College, 3700 West 103rd Street, Chicago, IL 60655, (312) 779-3300, BA 71 Vanderbilt Univ; MA 72 Vanderbilt Univ; PH 79 (Learning Disabilities) Northwestern Univ; Assoc Prof, Saint Xavier College, **SLP**

Harrod, Mrs Patricia 202 Forest Drive, Quinton, VA 23141-9521, (804) 780-8636, BA 73 CA St Univ - Northridge; MA 74 CA St Univ - Northridge; Sp-Path, Richmond Pub Schs, **SLP**

Harrold, Mrs Starr S 409 Wedgewood Court, Eden, NC 27292, (704) 246-2726, SLP, Lexington City Schools, **SLP**

Harrold, Vickie M 401 Green Street, Apartment 613, Maywood, IL 60153, (312) 681-2183, BS 72 Southern IL Univ -Carbondale; MA 76 Univ of Cincinnati; Audiologist, **A**

Harrold, Mrs Yvonne Rhodes 19731 Ormiston Avenue, Euclid, OH 44119, (216) 531-1776, BS 75 PA St Univ - Univ Park; MA 77 OH Univ - Athens; Sp-Lang Path, Northcoast Rehab Ctr, **SLP**

Harrold Webb, Mrs Mary Lynn Route 1 Box 22, Sergeant Bluff, IA 51054, (712) 943-4529, BA 80 Briar Cliff Coll; MA 81 SD St Univ; SLP, West Hills AEA, **SLP**

Harry, Mary Ellen Bret 12033 Bencrest Place, Dallas, TX 75244, (214) 484-0639, BA 73 Univ of Dallas; MS 86 Univ of TX - Dallas; 88–Sp-Lang Path, Humana-Med City Dallas Hosp, **SLP**

Harryman, Elizabeth 4132 Crosby, Rockford, IL 61107, (815) 229-2840, BA 62 Univ of IL - Urbana; MS 70 Northern IL Univ - De Kalb; Sp-Lang Path, Rockford Bd Ed, **SLP**

Harsany, Mrs Leslie Marcus 2801 Walnut Ridge Estates, Pottstown, PA 19464, (215) 326-4402, BS 84 Univ of South AL; MS 85 Univ of South AL; 87–Sp-Lang Path, Allied Health Specialists, **SLP**

Harsch, Mrs Debra Gallo 21 Fairview Avenue #420, Tuckahoe, NY 10707, (914) 779-6913, BS 79 Mercy Coll; MA 82 CUNY - Hunter Coll; SLP, Lakeland Sch Dist, **A**

Harsh, Betty Anne 1601 Wood Grove Circle, Richmond, VA 23233, (804) 282-1816, BA 68 Univ of WA; BA 76 Univ of WA; OM 78 Univ of WA; Sp-Lang Path, Henrico County PS, **SLP**

Harshbarger, Mrs Kim Batson Rd 6 Parkersville Road, West Chester, PA 19382, (215) 793-2712, BA 77 Univ of Miami; MA 78 Univ of IL - Urbana; 86–Sp-Lang Path, Sp-Lang Services Inc, **SLP**

Hart, Mrs Ann L P O Box 117, Gassaway, WV 26624, (304) 765-5821, **SLP**

Hart, Ann Ross 2350 Cypress Pond Rd #1501, Palm Harbor, FL 33563, (813) 938-9276, OM 85 AR St Univ; SLP, Pinellas Public Schools, **SLP**

Hart, Mrs Deborah L C 20 Estella Drive, Flemington, NJ 08822, (201) 788-8954, BS 77 IL St Univ - Normal; MA 80 Northwestern Univ; **SLP**

Hart, Holly Dixon 27911 Calle Arroyo, San Juan Capistrano, CA 92675, (714) 581-2800, BS 78 CA St Univ - Fullerton; MS 86 Univ of Redlands; **SLP**

Hart, Mrs Janice Schreier 7 Paerdegat 2 Street, Brooklyn, NY 11236, (718) 377-5090, MS 87 CUNY - Brooklyn Coll; **A**

Hart, Karen A 4490 Pawnee Place, Boise, ID 83704-2946, (208) 376-0819, BS 76 Univ of WY; MS 84 Univ of MT; Sp-Lang Path, Meridan Sch Dist 2, **SLP**

Hart, Kathleen Regional Hrg Impaired Prog, 1755 South Wolf Road, Des Plaines, IL 60018, (312) 390-9440, BS 76 Northern IL Univ - De Kalb; MS 78 IL St Univ - Normal; Sp-Lang Path, Reg Hrng Imp Pro, **SLP**

Hart, Kathleen Gibson 4501 Woodfield Road, Kensington, MD 20895, (301) 762-6730, **A**

Hart, Lauana J 8572 Whitesails Circle, Huntington, CA 92646, (714) 536-2514, BA 73 CA St Univ - Long Beach; MA 76 CA St Univ - Long Beach; SLP, Huntington Beach Un Hs Dist, **SLP**

Hart, Mrs Linda Carol 12 Carlyle Court, Ballston Lake, NY 12019, (518) 899-9836, BS 81 Coll of Saint Rose; MS 82 Coll of Saint Rose; **SLP**

Hart, Major Loren Stephen 1836-2 Cherokee Drive, Salinas, CA 93906, (408) 242-3881, MS 76 Western KY Univ; 77–Chief Aud, US Army, **A ACE**

Hart, Mandy Susan 12000 Old Georgetown Road, Apartment #N905, Rockville, MD 20852, (301) 231-9495, BA 83 Towson St Univ; MS 85 Loyola Coll; 87–Sp-Lang Path, Ivymount Sch, **SLP**

Hart, Mrs Margart R 9911 Harford Road, Baltimore, MD 21234, BA 69 9302; ME 70 Loyola Coll; **SLP**

Hart, Merilyn Kay 2435 East Southern Avenue Suite 6, Tempe, AZ 85282, (602) 345-2011, BA 73 Walla Walla Coll; MS 75 Eastern WA Univ; Sp-Lang Path, Arizona Speech Path, **SLP**

Hart, Patricia 4321 Brownfield Highway, Lubbock, TX 79407, (806) 792-6135, BS 83 Northern MI Univ; MA 84 Western MI Univ; 85–Sp-Lang Path, Sp-Lang-Hearing Center, **SLP**

Hart, Mrs Sharon Blodgett 804 Main Street, Murray, KY 42071, (502) 753-5549, BS 83 Murray St Univ; MA 84 Univ of TN - Knoxville; Sp-Lang Path, Henry Co Schools

Hart, Mrs Sharon Elizabeth 4 Tricount Court, Owings Mills, MD 21117, (301) 363-6156, **SLP**

Hart, Stephen Thomas 132 Dake Avenue, Rochester, NY 14617, (716) 266-4130, BS 80 SUNY - Coll at Geneseo; MA 81 SUNY - Coll at Geneseo; Pres, E Ridge Hrng Cen, **A**

Hart, Susan K 49 Stirrup Drive, East Greenbush, NY 12061, (518) 477-8771, BS 65 SUNY - Coll at Fredonia; MA 66 Ball St Univ; SETRC Training Spec, Renslar/Columb/Green Co BOCES, **SLP**

Hart, Terrill L 4670 Woodstock, Carlsbad, CA 92008, (619) 757-0337, BA 76 Univ of MI - Ann Arbor; MA 78 Eastern MI Univ; Sp-Lang Path, Oceanside USD, **SLP**

Hart, Mrs Virginia 8201 Englewood Road, Indianapolis, IN 46240, (317) 255-5584, BS 69 IN Univ - Bloomington; MA 70 IN Univ - Bloomington; Sp-Lang Path, Metro Sch Dist of Lawrence Twp, **SLP**

Hartbauer, Dr Roy Elden Northwest Speech & Hearing Clinics, Delta Triad Bldg Suite 20, 1142 Willagillespie Road, Eugene, OR 97401, (503) 683-1202, OB 50 Walla Walla Coll; MA 61 Univ of Southern CA; PH 67 (NS) MI St Univ; Owner/Dir, NW Sp & Hrng Clinics, **SLP A**

Harte, Barbara A 1205 Germania Drive, Apartment F, Ottawa, IL 61350, (815) 673-1511, BA 75 MI St Univ; MA 76 MI St Univ; 88–SLP, LaSalle Co Educ Alliance/Spec Educ, **SLP**

Hartenbaum, Mrs Susan G 18152 Kingsport Drive, Malibu, CA 90265, (213) 394-3244, BA 76 CA St Univ - Northridge; MA 80 CA St Univ - Northridge; Coord Adult Day Care Comm Prog, Lincoln Cen for Sp Pathology, **SLP**

Hartenstein, Robert W 69 Allen Street, Rutland, VT 05701, (802) 773-8469, BS 75 Syracuse Univ; MS 76 Ithaca Coll; Aud, Private Practice, **A**

Harter, Mrs Diana Jones 616 North Fourth Street, River Falls, WI 54022, (715) 425-0345, BS 82 Univ of WI - River Falls; MS 84 Univ of WI - River Falls

Harter, Mrs Rene Stiteler 57 S High Street, Canal Winchester, OH 43110, (614) 687-7225, BS 84 MS Univ for Women; MS 86 Univ Southern MS-Hattiesburg; 88–Sp-Lang Path, Fairfield Co Bd MRDD, **SLP**

Hartford, Renee S 403 Plymouth Street, Middleboro, MA 02346, (508) 378-3921, BA 73 Univ of MA - Amherst; MA 76 Univ of MA - Amherst; Sp-Lang Path, East Bridgewater Pub Sch, **SLP**

Hartig, Juliana 2200 South Gessner #403, Houston, TX 77063, (713) 776-2211, BA 83 Tulane Univ; MA 85 Univ of TX - Austin; Aud, Houston ENT Clinic, **A**

Hartigan, Mrs Nancy J P O Box 218, Homer, AK 99603, (907) 235-8181, BS 78 Univ of IL - Urbana; MS 79 Univ of IL - Urbana; 88–Sp-Lang Path, Kenai Peninsula Borough Sch Dist, **SLP**

Harting, Mrs Marlene A 2502 Collins, Blue Island, IL 60406, (312) 388-6715, BA 86 Saint Xavier Coll; MA 88 Univ of IL - Urbana; 88–Sp-Lang Path, InSpeech Inc

Hartinger, Joel D 1415 East State Street, Rockford, IL 61104, (815) 962-7800, BS 73 Univ of KS; MS 74 IL St Univ - Normal; 86–Owner, Hartinger Hearing Aid/Aud Ctr, **A**

Hartke, Mrs Susan K 1004 West Shiloh, Effingham, IL 62401, (217) 857-3232, BS 78 Eastern IL Univ; MS 79 Eastern IL Univ; Sp-Lang Path, Teutopolis Elem, **SLP**

Hartke, Susanne 9001 Basher Drive, Anchorage, AK 99507, (907) 338-4914, BA 76 Cleveland St Univ; MA 78 Cleveland St Univ; Director, AK Inst of Lang & Phono, **SLP ACE**

Hartlaub, Alice W 4820 Templeton Park Circle, Apartment 45, Colorado Springs, CO 80917, (303) 473-3475, BS 80 Univ of CA - Irvine; MA 83 Univ of CT; Sp/Lang Path, Rocky Mtn Rehab Ctr, **SLP**

Hartley, Mrs Carol B 924 Marietta Avenue, Lancaster, PA 17603, (717) 393-5797, BS 61 Otterbein Coll; BA 61 Otterbein Coll; MA 78 Temple Univ; Sp/Lang Path, Sch Dist of Lancaster, **SLP**

Hartley, Dr Harold V, Jr Rd 1 Box 60, Cranberry, PA 16319, (814) 226-2452, BS 52 Bloomsburg Univ of PA; ME 58 PA St Univ - Univ Park; PH 72 (Aud) Kent St Univ; Prof, Clarion U, **SLP A ACE**

Hartley, Jack L 9119 W 74th Street Ste 300, Shawnee Mission, KS 66204-2229, (913) 676-2164, BS 59 Univ of Dallas; MA 73 Univ of Southern CA; 85–President, Midwest Management Services, **SLP**

Hartley, Dr Leila L 2311 Ramada Drive, Houston, TX 77062, (409) 762-6661, BA 72 Emory Univ; OM 74 Emory Univ; PH 84 (Sp-Lang Path) Univ of FL; Co-Director, Galveston Inst of Human Comm, **SLP**

Hartman, Adrienne Smith 39 Prospect Street, Norwood, NY 13668, (315) 353-2738, BA 84 SUNY - Coll at Plattsburgh; MA 87 SUNY - Coll at Plattsburgh; 88–Aud, Private Practice, **A**

Hartman, Dr Bernard Thomas Stephen F Austin State Univ, P O Box 13019, Nacogdoches, TX 75962, (409) 569-2906, BA 49 Univ of Denver; MA 51 Univ of Denver; PH 63 (NS) IN Univ - Bloomington; Prof, Stephen F Austin St Univ, **SLP A**

Hartman, Dr David E Sp Path Dept Of Neurology, Gundersen Clinic Ltd, 1836 South Avenue, La Crosse, WI 54601, (608) 782-7300, BS 69 Univ of MN - Duluth; MS 71 Moorhead St Univ; PH 75 (NS) Bowling Green St Univ; Head/Dept SLP Neur, Gunderson Clinic Ltd, **SLP ACE**

Hartman, J L 4642 Nicollet Avenue #3, Minneapolis, MN 55409, (612) 646-2427, BA 84 Univ of Northern IA; MS 86 Univ of NE - Lincoln; Aud, Assoc Hearing Instruments, **A**

Hartman, Jacqueline S Veterans Admin Medical Center, Asp 126 JC, 915 North Grand Boulevard, St Louis, MO 63106, (314) 652-4100, BA 63 Case Western Reserve Univ; MA 65 Washington Univ; Audiologist, VA Medical Center, **SLP A**

Hartman, Mrs Jane D 159 Bowdoinhill, Rochester Hills, MI 48063, (313) 375-2450, BS 59 OH St Univ; MS 78 Univ of WI - Stevens Point; Sp-Lang Path, **SLP**

Hartman, Katherine L 9 Tanglewood Drive, Southern Pines, NC 28387, (919) 947-2342, BS 85 PA St Univ - Univ Park; ME 87 Univ of VA - Charlottesville

Hartman, Kathleen Ann 1135 Fox Hill Drive Apartment 227, Monroeville, PA 15146, (412) 856-6424, BA 81 Univ of Pittsburgh - Pittsburgh; MA 83 Univ of Pittsburgh - Pittsburgh; Sp-Lang Path, Allegheny Intermediate Unit, **SLP**

Hartman, Kathy L 702 West Main, Elizabeth City, NC 27909, (919) 338-4044, BS 75 Western Carolina Univ; ME 81 Western Carolina Univ; Sp-Lang Path, Albemarle Eval & Treatment Ctr, **SLP**

Hartman, Mrs Kerry McGoldrick P O Box 3328 Upb, Las Cruces, NM 88003, (505) 646-3141, BA 79 Beloit Coll; MA 83 NM St Univ; Dir of Aud, New Mexico State Univ, **A**

Hartman, Lisa D 953-D Grayling Court, Port Orange, FL 32019, (904) 756-7953, BS 79 Ithaca Coll; MS 82 CO St Univ; Sp-Lang Path, Easter Seal, **SLP**

Hartman, Mrs Melissa Kay Psc Box 1446, Apo, San Francisco, CA 96293, BS 83 Univ of Houston - Univ Park; MA 85 Univ of Houston - Univ Park; **SLP**

Hartman, Melody Becker Brookside Medical Group, 1215 North Alpine Road, Rockford, IL 61107, (815) 397-0180, MA 79 Northern IL Univ - De Kalb; Audiologist, Brookside Medical Group, **A**

Hartman, Micheal C 430 Davenport Bank Bldg, Davenport, IA 52801, (319) 323-9115, BA 76 Wabash Coll; MA 81 Western IL Univ; Aud, Davenport Hrng Aid Cen Inc, **A**

Hartman, Patricia Joanne 532 North Quanah, Tulsa, OK 74127, (918) 272-1153, **SLP**

Hartman, Dr Paul W 6505 Alvarado Road, Alvarado Medical Center Suite #107, San Diego, CA 92120, (619) 583-7002, BA 58 Univ of CA - Los Angeles; MA 60 CA St Univ - Los Angeles; PH 71 (Communi Disord) Univ of Southern CA; Aud, Private Practice, **A**

Hartman, Robert S 6520 Hollyridge Drive, Riverside, CA 92504, MS 72 FL St Univ; SLP, Riverside USD, **SLP**

Hartman, Mrs Sandra Lee 9309 Vineyard Haven Drive, Gaithersburg, MD 20879, (301) 694-1611, BA 81 Univ of MD - College Park; MA 84 Univ of MD - College Park; 85–Sp-Lang Path, Frederick County Dev Ctr, **SLP**

Hartman, Mrs Susan Deck P O Box 4176, Federal Way, WA 98003, (206) 927-1870, BA 62 WA St Univ; OM 67 Univ of WA; 85–Sp-Lang Path, Oral Surgery Assoc, **SLP**

Hartman, Victoria A 3502 Oakwood Avenue, Elmira Heights, NY 14903, (607) 732-8847, BS 85 SUNY - Coll at Fredonia; MS 87 Ithaca Coll

Hartman-Brockman, M Denise 19893 Pollyanna, Livonia, MI 48152, (313) 478-7940, BA 79 Heidelberg Coll; MA 81 Univ of Cincinnati; Sp-Lang Path, Commun Dis Inc, **SLP**

Hartmann, Barbara Sheehy 44 Avon Road, Kensington, CA 94707, (415) 526-5563, BA 80 Univ of CO - Boulder; MS 85 Univ of WI - Madison; **SLP**

Hartmann, Barbara V 5954 South Sultan Circle, Murray, UT 84107, (801) 581-3506, BA 59 Univ of AZ; MA 60 Stanford Univ; Dir, U of UT, **SLP**

Hartmann, Kathleen G Naval Hospital Naples, P O Box 19, FPO New York, NY 09521-0700, (415) 633-6066, BS 80 Univ of MO - Columbia; MS 82 Central MO St Univ; Operational Aud Officer, Usn, **A**

Hartmann, Lydia Avallone 4 Mike Lane, Smithtown, NY 11787, (516) 744-1600, BA 79 Hofstra Univ; MA 80 Hofstra Univ; 80–SLP, Rocky Pt Pub Sch, **SLP**

Hartmann, Tamila Ann 2913 Wimbledon Way, Madison, WI 53713, (608) 273-4047, BS 84 Univ of WI - Whitewater; MS 86 Univ of WI - Milwaukee; 87–Sp-Lang Path, InSpeech Inc, **SLP**

Hartmann-Kott, Catherine Marie 36920 Clear Creek Road, Saugus, CA 91350-1125, (805) 297-1355, BA 73 Univ of the Pacific; MA 75 Univ of the Pacific; SLP, San Juan USD, **SLP**

Hartmann-Plath, Jane Susan 131 Oak Lane, Becker, MN 55308, (612) 261-4106, BA 82 Saint Cloud St Univ; MS 84 Saint Cloud St Univ; Sp-Lang Path, St Cloud PS, **SLP**

Hartner, Laura L 656 Elliot Court, Somerville, NJ 08876, (201) 218-4117, BA 73 Montclair St Coll; MA 75 Montclair St Coll; Dir-Lafayette Prog, Somerville Board of Education, **SLP**

Hartnett, Debra Scott 1784 Pebblewood, Sacramento, CA 95833, (707) 253-5565, BS 76 Univ of NE - Lincoln; MA 78 CA St Univ - Los Angeles; SLP, Napa St Hosp-Chldrn Prog, **SLP**

Hartnett, Laura Lee 2637 North Frederick #201, Milwaukee, WI 53211, (414) 873-0771, BS 83 Univ of WI - Stevens Point; MS 86 Univ of WI - Milwaukee; SLP, Milwaukee Public Schools, **SLP**

Hartney, Bridget Joan 7250 North 97th Street, Milwaukee, WI 53224-3902, (414) 353-6144, BS 81 Marquette Univ; MS 83 Marquette Univ; **SLP**

Hartom, Jeannine Nappe 122 West Spring Street, Marquette, MI 49855, BS 78 Northern MI Univ; MS 79 Phillips Univ; Sp-Lang Path, Marquette General Hosp, **SLP**

Hartrich, Mrs Debra L 1209 North Morgan, Olney, IL 62450, (618) 392-3754, BS 80 Eastern IL Univ; MS 81 Eastern IL Univ; Sp-Lang Path, E Richland Comm Unit 1 Sch Dis, **SLP ACE**

Harts, Kenneth V 409 8th Street, Sheldon, IA 51201, (712) 722-4374, MA 73 Univ of IA; SLP, AEA 4, **SLP**

Hartsaw, Mrs Lee Ann 5755 Ferstel Road, Newburgh, IN 47630, (812) 853-3076, BS 77 Brescia Coll; MA 81 Ball St Univ; Sp-Lang Path, Rescare, **SLP**

Hartsell, Kimberly Gayle 4050 Stoneview Circle, Stone Mountain, GA 30083, (404) 961-9391, BS 81 Auburn Univ - Auburn; MS 82 Auburn Univ - Auburn; Sp/Lang Path, Heard Co Bd of Ed, **SLP**

Hartsough, Mrs Diane R 552 Gibson Avenue, Hollywood, PA 19111, (215) 663-0915, BS 84 Bloomsburg Univ of PA; MS 85 Bloomsburg Univ of PA; 87–Sp-Lang Path, St Mary Hosp, **SLP**

Hartsough, Kathleen F 920 Emerald Drive, Alexandria, VA 22308, MS; **SLP LM**

Hartstein, Mrs Janice Cooper 2041 Stratford Road, South Charleston, WV 25303, (304) 343-5233, BA 85 Marshall Univ; MA 85 Marshall Univ; Sp-Lang Path, Kanawha County Bd of Educ, **SLP**

Hartung, Barbara A 2066 South Fillmore, Denver, CO 80210, (303) 761-1938, BS 65 CO St Univ; MA 80 Univ of Northern CO; Sp-Lang Path, Cherry Creek School Dist 5, **SLP**

Hartung, Colleen Dzingle 500 8th Street, Red Oak, IA 51566, **SLP**

Hartung, Deedra L St Lukes Hospital, 4400 Wornall Road, Kansas City, MO 64111, (816) 932-3262, BS 67 Univ of KS; MA 69 Univ of KS; Sp-Lang Path, St Lukes Hosp, **SLP**

Hartung, Mrs Mayra Teresita 1178-D Pitusa Court, West Palm Beach, FL 33415, (407) 641-1292, BS 83 PA St Univ - Univ Park; MA 84 Edinboro Univ of PA; 84–Sp-Lang Path, The Sch Bd of Palm Beach Co, **SLP**

Hartwick, Nancy Ann 607 Lincoln Drive, Grand Forks, ND 58201, (701) 772-6463, BS 84 Moorhead St Univ; MS 85 Univ of WI - Eau Claire; **SLP**

Hartwig, Mrs Marguerite 51 Coachwood Place S W, Calgary, AB, Canada T3H 1E1, (403) 270-1110, BS 73 Univ of NE - Lincoln; MA 74 Univ of NE - Lincoln; SLP, Foothillsl Hospital, **SLP**

Harty, Particia E 229 Amherst, St Paul, MN 55105, (612) 293-8630, BS 76 Univ of WI - River Falls; MA 78 Univ of IL - Urbana; Sp-Lang Path, St Paul Public Schools, **SLP**

Hartz, Mrs Julie Diane 1179 Lakedale Way, Sunnyvale, CA 94089, (408) 432-8500, BA 81 San Francisco St Univ; MS 83 San Francisco St Univ; 88–Aud, Agnews Developmental Ctr, **A**

Hartz, Mrs Kathryn S 4752 South Spring #6, St Louis, MO 63116, (712) 546-4192, BA 79 Valparaiso Univ; MA 82 Western MI Univ; SLP, Wn Hills AEA 12, **SLP**

Hartz, Mrs Paula Ann 5744 East Michigan Street, Indianapolis, IN 46219, (317) 356-0091, BS 69 Purdue Univ - West Lafayette; MA 70 Western MI Univ; 87–Sp-Lang Path, Visiting Nurse Svc, **SLP**

Hartzell, Susan Rae 1206 Pine Street, Key West, FL 33040, (305) 296-7541, BA 83 Miami Univ - Oxford; MA 86 Kent St Univ; **SLP**

Hartzer, Mrs Linda Egener Indian Hill Road, Norwalk, CT 06850, (203) 637-0150, BA 67 SUNY - Center at Buffalo; MA 71 CUNY - Hunter Coll; OM 84 Fairfield Univ; Teacher Leader, Greenwich Board of Education, **SLP**

Hartzler, Sharon Busch 3806 Bowen, St Louis, MO 63116, (314) 832-3018, BS 81 Saint Louis Univ; MA 83 Saint Louis Univ; SLP, St John's Mercy Med Cen, **SLP**

Hartzman, Deborah Dosick 5635 Pembroke Court, Santa Barbara, CA 93111, (805) 683-1887, **A**

Hartzog, Melody Althea 1233 South Karlov Avenue, Chicago, IL 60623, (312) 386-0516, BS 80 Northern IL Univ - De Kalb; MA 83 Northern IL Univ - De Kalb; Sp-Lang Path, Southwest Cook County Coop, **SLP ACE**

Harvell, Mrs Priscilla Saffold 4000 Oakhill Road, Oakland, CA 94605, (415) 784-2814, BA 75 CA St Univ - Los Angeles; MA 82 San Jose St Univ; SLP, Hayward USD, **SLP**

Harver, Mrs Nancy Hall 224 Christian Avenue, Stony Brook, NY 11790, (516) 751-5157, BS 80 OH Univ - Athens; MA 83 OH Univ - Athens; Clin Supvr, Hofstra Univ Sp & Hrng Ctr, **SLP**

Harvey, Mrs Barbara C 16 Dolge Court, Oxford, MA 01540, (508) 987-3747, BA 77 IN Univ - Bloomington; MA 78 IN Univ - Bloomington; **SLP**

Harvey, Charlotte M P O Box 1302, Altamonte Springs, FL 32715-1302, (407) 830-8892, BA 70 Elms Coll; MS 77 Southern IL Univ -Carbondale; 81–Sp-Lang Path, Upjohn Healthcare Service, **SLP ACE**

Harvey, David J 107 Vega Place, Chehalis, WA 98532, (206) 748-4862, BA 76 Eastern WA Univ; MS 75 Eastern WA Univ; SLP, Chehalis-Centralia Spec Serv, **SLP**

Harvey, Dr Donald G Audiology Associates Inc, 515 Minor Avenue, Suite 150, Seattle, WA 98104, (206) 622-9916, BS 60 Univ of WA; MA 62 Univ of WA; PH 66 (Aud) Univ of WA; 75–Aud, Aud Assoc Inc, **A**

Harvey, Eileen F 8231 Elizabeth Drive, Lincoln, NE 68505, (402) 464-9423, BA 75 Univ of NE - Lincoln; MA 76 Univ of NE - Lincoln; Sp/Lang Path, Eileen Harvey, **SLP**

Harvey, Mrs Jane Bibeau 1112 Branson, Las Cruces, NM 88001, (505) 267-3076, BS 78 NM St Univ; MA 80 NM St Univ; **SLP**

Harvey, Mrs Jane Hunt 307 Georgetown Drive, Athens, GA 30605, (404) 542-4598, BA 66 FL St Univ; MS 67 FL St Univ; Clin Supvr, Univ of Georgia, **SLP**

Harvey, Janet L 736 River Heights Road, Menomonie, WI 54751, (715) 643-4331, BA 68 Univ of WI - Eau Claire; MS 70 Univ of WI - Eau Claire; SLP, Boyceville Community Schools, **SLP**

Harvey, Mrs Joan L 644 Arlington Avenue, Westfield, NJ 07090, (201) 456-3463, BA 60 Elmhurst Coll; MA 76 Eastern MI Univ; Mgr Sp-Lang Path, Univ Hosp, **SLP**

Harvey, Kathleen 194 Creekside Circle, New Smyrna Beach, FL 32069, (904) 427-1528, BA 74 Univ of FL; MS 77 Univ of South FL; Sp/Lang Path, Volusia Cty, **SLP**

Harvey, Mrs Maresa M 37 Woods Way, Newington, CT 06111, (203) 563-8181, BA 76 Boston Coll; MS 79 Southern CT St Univ; OM 85 Central CT St Univ; 78–Sp-Lang Path, Wethersfield Bd of Ed, **SLP**

Harvey, Pamela Lynn 21 Westerly #3, Wellesley, MA 02181-4666, (617) 237-1864, BS 78 TX Christian Univ; MA 80 Univ of KS; Sp-Lang Path, Private Practice, **SLP**

Harvey, Patricia Lynn 2509 South 25th, Abilene, TX 79605, (915) 670-2134, OB 85 Hardin-Simmons Univ; MS 87 Univ of North TX; 87–Aud, Hendrick Med Ctr, **A**

Harvey, Paul M 16 Dolge Court, Oxford, MA 01540, (617) 987-3747, BS 76 Worcester St Coll; MA 80 IN Univ - Bloomington; Sales Mgr, American Electromatics, **A**

Harville, Mrs Karen C 2176 Wood River Circle, Twin Falls, ID 83301, (503) 298-5563, BS 68 Western WA Univ; MA 71 Western MI Univ; Sp/Lang Path, Lenkner Michener and Assoc, **SLP**

Harward, Richard S Department Of Rehabilitation, 320 12th Avenue, Salt Lake City, UT 84103, (801) 521-1686, BS 74 UT St Univ; MS 78 UT St Univ; 88–Admin Dir Rehab, Primary Childrens Medical Ctr, **A**

Harward, Stephen B Medical Hearing Clinic, 5640 South Wasatch Drive, Ogden, UT 84403, (801) 479-3200, BS 76 UT St Univ; MS 77 UT St Univ; Dir of Aud Serv, Medical Hrng Clinic Inc, **A**

Harwell, Mrs Robin W 5761 Pembrook Drive, New Orleans, LA 70131, (318) 264-1952, BS 76 6376; MA 78 6376; **SLP**

Harwin, Mrs Lisa S 23241 Ventura Boulevard, Suite 207, Woodland Hills, CA 91364, (818) 883-3789, BS 74 Emerson Coll; MA 76 CA St Univ - Northridge; Sp-Lang Path, Wdld Hills-Calbsas Sp/Lang Cen, **SLP**

Harwood, Angela Bartel 19002 Lomond, Cleveland, OH 44122, (216) 991-1268, **SLP**

Harwood, Mrs Monica Anne 7181 Browning Road, Highland, CA 92346, (714) 864-1109, BA 80 Univ of Redlands; MS 83 Univ of Redlands; Sp-Lang Path, Rim of World USD, **SLP**

Harwood, Teresa Carolyn 3120 Richmond Road #603, Lexington, KY 40509, (606) 268-4290, BS 85 Murray St Univ; MS 87 Murray St Univ; **SLP**

Hasan, Mrs Mary Jo 630 Kenwick Circle #202, Casselberry, FL 32707, (407) 830-5320, ME 88 Univ of FL

Hasan, Zahida M 142-25 Pershing Crescent, Apartment 5F, Briarwood, NY 11435, (718) 454-6460, BA 82 CUNY - Queens Coll; MA 87 Saint John's Univ - Jamaica; Sp-Lang Path, Lowell Early Childhood Ctr

Hasbargen, Jerene M 5411 South Cathay Way, Aurora, CO 80015, BA 74 Augustana Coll; MA 75 Univ of IL - Urbana; 87–Sp-Lang Path, Aurora PS, **SLP**

Hasbrouck, Dr Jon M Chief Speech-Lang Rehab Sect, Otolaryngology Service, Fitzsimons Army Medical Ct, Aurora, CO 80045, (303) 361-8120, BA 66 Univ of MT; MA 69 Univ of MT; PH 73 (Sp-Lang Path) Univ of MN - Minneap-St Paul; Ch,Sp-Lang Rehab Sect, Fitzsimons Army Med Cen, **SLP**

Hase, Meredy 2426 North Grandview Boulevard Suite B-1, Waukesha, WI 53188, (414) 547-2227, BS 75 Univ of WI - Oshkosh; MS 76 Univ of WI - Madison; Audiologist, Family Hearing Ctr Inc, **A ACE**

Hasegawa, Mrs Joanne G 1576 Leabrook Lane, Wheaton, IL 60187, (312) 450-2100, BA 68 IN Univ - Bloomington; MA 69 IN Univ - Bloomington; Sp-Lang Path, Proviso Area for Except Chldrn, **SLP**

Hasek, Mrs Carol S 9810 FM 1960 Bypass, Suite 160, Humble, TX 77338, (713) 469-7811, BA 64 Gettysburg Coll; MS 79 Univ of TX - Houston; 88–Dir, Northeast Sp & Lang Ctr, **SLP**

Hasek, Nancy Jane 4506 San Marino Drive, Davis, CA 95616, (916) 666-8710, BA 51 Univ of CA - Los Angeles; MA 76 CA St Univ - Sacramento; **SLP**

Haselhorst, Mrs Susan Santema 406 9th Avenue N W, Byron, MN 55920, (507) 281-6079, BS 82 SD St Univ; MA 83 WA St Univ; Sp-Lang Path, ISD #535, **SLP**

Haseman, Dr Elizabeth Owens 305 Ben Avon Drive, Temple Terrace, FL 33617, (813) 985-9281, BA 72 Univ of FL; MA 73 Univ of FL; PH 79 (NS) Univ of TN - Knoxville; Sp/Lang Path, Private Practice, **SLP**

Hasfjord, Heidi Annette 13718 Janwood, Farmers Branch, TX 75234, (214) 790-8505, BS 82 Baylor Univ; MS 83 Baylor Univ; Sp-Lang Path, Helping Hand Development Cen, **SLP**

Hashi, Michiko CDS Department Siu, Carbondale, IL 62901, (618) 457-5143, MS 88 Southern IL Univ -Carbondale

Hashimoto, Lori A 210 North 115th Street, Seattle, WA 98133, (206) 235-2328, OM 83 Univ of WA; Sp-Lang Path, Renton Sch Dist, **SLP**

Hashimoto, Naomi 3605 4th Avenue, Apartment 10, San Diego, CA 92103, (619) 442-8818, BS 84 Northwestern Univ; MS 86 Univ of WA; 88–Sp-Lang Path, Children's Hosp & Health Ctr, **SLP**

Haske, Dr Susan Claire Dept Speech Path & Audiology, University Of Alberta, 400-11044 82nd Avenue, Edmonton, AB, Canada T6G 0T2, (403) 432-5990, PH 71 (NS) MI St Univ; Prof, U of Alberta, **A**

Haskell, Dr George B Veterans Admin Medical Center, Audiology 126, 1660 South Columbian Way, Seattle, WA 98108, PH 81 Univ of IA; Coord Aud, VA Med Ctr, **A**

Haskell, Dr John A 157 West 57th Street #1100, New York, NY 10019, (212) 315-3090, BA 58 Brandeis Univ; MA 70 Columbia Univ Teachers Coll; ED 76 (NS) Columbia Univ Teachers Coll; Sp-Lang Path, Private Practice, **SLP**

Hasken, Mrs Janet B 4185 Aspen Hills Drive, Bettendorf, IA 52722, (319) 359-1371, BS 76 Univ of WI - Stevens Point; MS 77 Univ of WI - Stevens Point; SLP, MS Bend AEA, **SLP**

Haskins, Mrs Janice H 1090 Colony Park Drive, Lakeland, FL 33813, (813) 646-1182, BA 85 Univ of FL; MA 87 Univ of FL; **SLP**

Haskins, Sherry E 9479 Dunkerrin Way, Elk Grove, CA 95624-4402, (916) 422-5524, BA 68 WA St Univ; MA 72 Univ of MN - Minneap-St Paul; SLP, Sacramento County Office Educ, **SLP**

Haskins-Kobelan, Mrs Christi Lynn 1500 Black Cherry, Cedar Park, TX 78613, (512) 444-9561, BS 81 Baylor Univ; MS 82 Baylor Univ; Superv of Sp Dept, Brown Sch Oaks Treat Cen, **SLP**

Hasko, Joanna Joan 214 Jackson Avenue, Schenectady, NY 12304, (518) 370-7398, BS 78 Coll of Saint Rose; MS 79 Coll of Saint Rose; SLP, E Roosevelt Dev Disabl Serv, **SLP**

Hasler, Lorrie Marie 9325 Cord Avenue, Downey, CA 90240, (213) 216-2600, BA 83 CA St Univ - Fullerton; MA 85 CA St Univ - Fullerton; **SLP**

Haslett, Dr Elizabeth J Children's Hospital & Medical Center, P O Box C-5371, Seattle, WA 98105, (206) 526-2104, MS 56 PA St Univ - Univ Park; MA 63 Case Western Reserve Univ; PH 67 (Aud) Case Western Reserve Univ; Aud, Chldn's Hosp & Med Cen, **A**

Haspiel, Dr George S St Luke's Hearing & Speech Center, 1580 Valencia Street, Suite 508, San Francisco, CA 94110, (415) 282-2551, BA 51 Washington Univ; MA 53 Washington Univ; PH 60 (Aud & Sp Path) PA St Univ - Univ Park; Dir, Private Practice, **SLP A F**

Hass, Mrs Margaret Slough 1906 Northwood Lake, Northport, AL 35476-2506, (205) 339-9825, BS 79 Southwest TX St Univ; MS 87 Univ of AL- Tuscaloosa; 87–Sp-Lang Path, AL Health Related Services, **SLP**

Hass, Pamela Kay 20 Avocado Tree Circle, St Peters, MO 63376, (314) 947-5378, BA 76 Univ of Northern IA; MA 78 Univ of Northern IA; Sp-Lang Path, SSM Rehab Inst, **SLP**

Hass, Mrs Rita L 190 Providence Street, Rehoboth, MA 02769, (401) 245-7649, BA 76 Univ of RI; MS 79 Univ of RI; Sp-Lang Path, Warren Pub Sch, **SLP ACE**

Hasselberger, Warren William 514 North Hoover Street, Los Angeles, CA 90004, (213) 666-7966, BA 74 Fairleigh Dickinson U-Ruther; MA 84 CA St Univ - Los Angeles; **A**

Hassell, M Harden, Jr 1528 Pineywood Drive, McAlester, OK 74501, (918) 426-1445, BS 72 OK St Univ; MA 73 OK St Univ; Sp-Lang Path Dir, Scot Rite Cl for Chldh Lang Di, **SLP**

Hassell, Mrs Mary Cynthia 9830 Cascade Drive, Mobile, AL 36609, (601) 588-6001, BS 82 Talladega Coll; MS 84 Talladega Coll; **SLP**

Hassenstab-Brines, Mrs Catherine Marie P O Box 3081, Chico, CA 95927, (916) 345-2411, **SLP**

Hassett, Kelly Marie 20434 North 30th Drive, Phoenix, AZ 85027, (602) 866-5863, **SLP**

Hassett, Maryclaire T 27 Chadwyck Square, Cohoes, NY 12047, (518) 233-1192, BS 78 Coll of Saint Rose; MS 80 Coll of Saint Rose; 79–Sp-Lang Path, Eleanor Roosevelt Dev Serv, **SLP**

Hassid, Mrs Janis D A 2582 Eileen Road, Oceanside, NY 11572, (516) 678-0138, BA 76 CUNY - Queens Coll; MA 80 Hofstra Univ; 79–Sp-Lang Path, BOCES-Early Child Ctr, **SLP**

Hasson-Axblad, Marcia A P O Box 360, Rosendale, NY 12472, (914) 658-8993, BA 71 SUNY - Coll at New Paltz; ME 79 Coll of Saint Rose; Sp-Lang Path, Private Practice, **SLP**

Hasson-Perakis, Karin Elise 35620 Meyer Court, Fremont, CA 94536, (415) 793-3440, BA 78 San Jose St Univ; MA 83 San Jose St Univ; SLP, Fremont USD, **SLP**

Hastings, Anne Cecile 16836 East Navarro Drive, Aurora, CO 80013, (303) 366-0314, ME 72 Univ of AZ; MS 83 Univ of AZ; Aud, Aurora Public Schools, **A**

Hastings, Eileen 115 Dewey Street, Pittsburgh, PA 15218, (412) 242-3754, MA 59; MA 80; **A**

Hastings, Mrs Kathryn N 8595 Haven Wood Trail, Roswell, GA 30076, (404) 552-0113, BS 76 Univ of TN - Knoxville; MA 79 Univ of TN - Knoxville; SLP, **SLP**

Hastings, Lisa 161 Franklin Corner Road, Apartment C8, Lawrenceville, NJ 08648, (609) 895-0268, MA 85 Trenton St Coll; BA 78 LA Salle Coll; SLP, Medical Center at Princeton, **SLP**

Haston, Judy D Route 3 Box 233, Sparta, TN 38583, (615) 738-2641, MS

Hasty, Sarah A 1204 12th Avenue, Conwayborough Apt 5-D, Conway, SC 29526, (803) 248-7574, **SLP**

Hata, Mrs Susan Sowa P O Box 2078, Kealakekua-Kona, HI 96750, (808) 328-9170, BA 74 Elmhurst Coll; MA 76 Univ of IL - Urbana; **SLP**

Hatala, Mrs Susan Davis 7 Catherine Court, Sicklerville, NJ 08081, (609) 561-7550, BA 73 Rutger's St Univ - Douglas Coll; MA 75 Trenton St Coll; 88–Sp-Lang Path, Winslow Twp Bd of Educ, **SLP**

Hatch, Debora R 229-D Rippling Stream Road, Durham, NC 27704, (919) 966-3244, BS 83 East Carolina Univ; MA 85 OH St Univ; 88–Aud, Univ of NC Mem Hosp, **A**

Hatch, Mrs Janet M 2169 Apple Tree Lane, Schenectady, NY 12309, (518) 785-3211, BS 67 SUNY - Coll at Geneseo; MS 71 Univ of MI - Ann Arbor; Sp/Lang Path, N Colonie Cen Sch, **SLP**

Hatch, Judith E 1170 Hickory Hill Drive, Watkinsville, GA 30677, (404) 548-3550, BA 56 MI St Univ; ME 76 Univ of GA; Sp/Lang Path, Clarke Co Sch Dist, **SLP**

Hatch, Sandra K 2206 Lindell Avenue, Austin, TX 78704-5131, (512) 442-5810, BS 72 Southwest TX St Univ; ME 73 Southwest TX St Univ; Early Chldhd Ed/Hndcpd Tchr, Austin ISD, **SLP**

Hatcher, Candace Ann 137 Rivoli Oaks Circle, Macon, GA 31210-1595, (912) 474-4891, **SLP**

Hatcher, Caro C 1621 East Commonwealth, Fullerton, CA 92631, MS; **SLP LM**

Hatcherson, Mrs Vivianne S 91 Blue Heron Court, East Amherst, NY 14051, (716) 831-3395, **SLP**

Hatfield, Mrs Mary Lou 1578 Sylvan Glen, Okemos, MI 48864, (517) 349-4779, BS 65 IL St Univ - Normal; MA 71 Univ of IL - Urbana; **SLP**

Hathaway, Mrs Carrie Ristow 3611 Maplewood Avenue, Wichita Falls, TX 76308, (515) 244-8152, BS 85 Univ of WI - Stevens Point; MS 87 Univ of WI - Madison; **A**

Hathaway, Tamara F 6613 Eastside Drive N E, Tacoma, WA 98422, (206) 952-3536, MS 88 Univ of WA

Hathcock, Jacquelyn Rae 2428 Michael Drive, Tifton, GA 31794, (912) 386-0301, BS 83 Auburn Univ - Auburn; ME 86 Valdosta St Coll; **SLP**

Hatherill, Betsy Weese 6309 Lime Oak Trails, Abilene, TX 79606, (915) 695-7314, **A**

Hatherill, Dennis L Audiology Department, West Texas Rehab Center, 4601 Hartford Drive, Abilene, TX 79605, (214) 463-1130, BS 69 Point Park Coll; BS 73 Indiana Univ of PA; MS 77 WV Univ; Aud, Texoma Otol Cl, **A ACE**

Hatheway, Mrs Wendy B 729 218th Place N E, Redmond, WA 98053-3738, (206) 828-3200, BA 79 Univ of WA; OM 81 Univ of WA; SLP, Lake Washington Sch Dist, **SLP**

Hathoot, Mary M 514 Blackoak Drive, Michigan City, IN 46360, (219) 879-6531, BA 80 IN Univ - Bloomington; MA 82 IN Univ - Bloomington; Aud, Med Gr of MI Cty, **A**

Hathorne, Dr Howell F 529 Oak Street, Chattanooga, TN 37403, (615) 267-5641, BS 66 Univ Southern MS-Hattiesburg; MS 65 Univ Southern MS-Hattiesburg; Exec Dir, Chattanooga-Hamilton Co Sp Cen, **SLP ACE**

Hatin, Mrs Darcy A PO Box 1148, Fort Valley, GA 31030, (912) 825-3132, BS 80 Auburn Univ - Auburn; MS 82 Purdue Univ - West Lafayette; Sp-Lang Path, Middle Georgia R E S A, **SLP**

Hatt, Shawn Terese P O Box 32575, Juneau, AK 99803, (907) 586-2303, BS 82 Northern St Coll; MA 86 Univ of SD - Vermillion

Hattel, Mrs Susan Carson 3070 Kane Court, Dubuque, IA 52001, (319) 588-0538, BA 70 Univ of Northern IA; MA 72 Univ of Northern IA; Sp-Lang Path, Keystone Ed Agcy, **SLP**

Hatten, Dr John T 2602E 6th Street, Duluth, MN 55812, (218) 726-8205, BS 59 Univ of MN - Duluth; MS 61 Purdue Univ - West Lafayette; PH 65 (NS) Univ of WI - Madison; Professor & Asst Dean Grad Sch, University of Minnesota, **SLP**

Hattis, Mrs Beverly K 71 Westgate Road, Newton, MA 02159, (617) 969-3857, BS 69 Boston Univ; MA 70 Univ of CT; SLP, **SLP**

Hattler, Dr Karl William Hearing Evaluation Center, Granada Square, 4753 Montgomery NE #120, Albuquerque, NM 87109, (505) 889-9000, BA 65 Emerson Coll; MS 68 Univ of OK Medical Center; PH 71 (NS) Univ of OK Medical Center; Dir, Hrng Eval Cen, **A**

Hatton, Nina E 2275 Grassroots Way, Tallahassee, FL 32301, (904) 656-3368, BA 72 FL St Univ; MS 78 FL St Univ; SLP Consult, Private Practice, **SLP**

Hatzkilson, Mrs Jennifer A 5192 Chablis Circle, Irvine, CA 92714, (714) 552-0278, MA 87 CA St Univ - Long Beach; 88–Aud, Head/Neck Assoc of Orange Co

Hauben, Mrs Esther C Grinblat 1757 East 28th Street, Brooklyn, NY 11219, (718) 339-2300, BA 76 CUNY - Brooklyn Coll; MS 78 CUNY - Brooklyn Coll; Aud, Dr Simon H Friedman, **A**

Hauber, Mary D 137-A Greenwood Avenue, Jenkintown, PA 19046, (215) 887-9353, BS 83 PA St Univ - Univ Park; MA 87 Temple Univ; **SLP**

Haubner, Colleen C 4030 North 98th Street, Milwaukee, WI 53222, (414) 645-0106, BS 77 Univ of WI - Milwaukee; MS 78 Univ of WI - Milwaukee; Diag/Prog Support Tchr SLP, Milwaukee Public Schools, **SLP**

Haubner, Mrs Dorothy Bennett 2632 Handley Boulevard, Lakeland, FL 33803, (913) 686-4267, MS 73 Univ of South FL; 88–Sp-Lang Path, New Medico Rehab Ctr of FL, **SLP**

Hauburger, Janice Raineault 14C Tulip Drive, Seymour, CT 06483, (203) 888-7390, BA 83 Central CT St Univ; MS 86 Southern CT St Univ; 88–Sp-Lang Path, Rehab Ctr Eastern Fairfield Co, **SLP**

Hauck, Joan 459 East 4th Street, Bloomsburg, PA 17815, (609) 723-2414, BS 84 Bloomsburg Univ of PA; MS 85 Bloomsburg Univ of PA; **SLP**

Hauck, Mrs Margaret K 3861 Douglas Blvd, Roseville, CA 95661, (916) 663-2096, BS 76 Univ of LA Verne; MS 78 Univ of Redlands; SLP, Placer Co Offi of Ed, **SLP**

Hauff, Eileen K 1209 7th Street North, Fargo, ND 58102, (701) 235-4462, BS 78 Moorhead St Univ; MS 79 Moorhead St Univ; Sp-Lang Path, Dakota Med Ctr, **SLP**

Hauff, Latomah F Box 2722, Sioux City, IA 51106, MA 76 Univ of SD - Vermillion; Sp-Lang Path, Western Hills AEA, **SLP**

Haug, Dr C Olaf P O Box 510, Martindale, TX 78655, (512) 357-6906, BA 47 Univ of WI - Madison; MA 48 Univ of WI - Madison; PH 58 (Aud) Univ of WI - Madison; Retired, Med Cen ENT Assoc/Houston, **A LM**

Haug, Holly T 1011 18th Avenue South, Grand Forks, ND 58201, BA 84 Univ of ND; MS 86 Univ of ND; **SLP**

Haug, Mrs Kathleen Liljemark 2021 West 49th Street, Minneapolis, MN 55409, (612) 627-2050, BS 68 Univ of MN - Minneap-St Paul; MA 85 Univ of MN - Minneap-St Paul; 86–Sp-Lang Path, Minneapolis PS-Spec Sch Dist #1, **SLP**

Haug, Kirsten Marie 10204 38th Court, Plymouth, MN 55441, (612) 823-6660, BS 83 Saint Cloud St Univ; MS 86 Saint Cloud St Univ; **SLP**

Haug, Mrs Laura Ann 10 Hemlock Street, Riverdale, NJ 07457, (201) 772-2600, BS 82 Stockton St Coll; MA 84 OH Univ - Athens; Sp-Lang Path, Bassaic County Elks CP Treat Ctr, **SLP**

Haug, Mrs Mary R 6030 Hollister Drive, Speedway, IN 46224, BS 64 Purdue Univ - West Lafayette; MS 67 Purdue Univ - West Lafayette; 76–Sp-Lang Path, MSD Wayne Sch, **SLP**

Hauge, Mrs Robin Elizabeth 525 Patterson Blvd, Pleasant Hill, CA 94523, (415) 283-6777, BA 80 San Francisco St Univ; MS 82 San Francisco St Univ; Sp-Lang Path, Melmed Reading Cl, **SLP**

Haugen, Dr David M Eastern Washington University, Communication Disorders, Cheney, WA 99004, (509) 359-2301, BA 60 Luther Coll; MA 63 Univ of MN - Minneap-St Paul; PH 69 (NS) Univ of OR; Chr-Prof of Commun Dis, Easter Washington U, **SLP**

Haugen, Kathleen 7118 Halifax Avenue North, Brooklyn Center, MN 55429, (612) 755-8220, BA 75 Saint Cloud St Univ; MS 77 Saint Cloud St Univ; SLP, Anoka-Hennepin ISD, **SLP**

Haugen, Mrs Michelle Ann 1115 N W School Street #31, Elk River, MN 55330, (612) 441-1003, BA 83 Univ of MN - Duluth; MA 84 Univ of MN - Duluth; SLP, ISD 728, **SLP**

Haugen, Rosemary 242 North Algoma Street, Thunder Bay, ON, Canada P7A 5A4, (807) 344-0541, MA 86 Univ of MN - Duluth; 86–Sp-Lang Path, St Joseph's Gen Hosp, **SLP**

Haugen, Stacy Jo Box 99, Pelican Rapids, MN 56572, (218) 739-2947, BS 85 Moorhead St Univ; MS 86 Moorhead St Univ; 86–Sp-Lang Path, Fergus Falls Area Spec Educ Coop

Haugh, Mrs Elise B 7797 Auberry Court, Granite Bay, CA 95661, (916) 791-4312, BA 69 Univ of the Pacific; MA 70 Univ of the Pacific; 88–Sp-Lang Path, Roseville Joint HS Dist, **SLP**

Haugh, Mrs Elizabeth 7767 Westwood Road, Findlay, OH 45840-9542, (419) 424-1393, BS 74 OH Univ - Athens; MA 79 Bowling Green St Univ; Aud, James R Robertson MD Inc, **A**

Haughey, Sr Kathleen 5025 Ilchester Road, Box 813, Ellicott City, MD 21043, (301) 396-9148, BS 62 Trinity Coll; ME 71 Univ of NC - Greensboro; MA 72 Catholic Univ of America; Sp-Lang Path, Balto Cty Pub Sch, **SLP**

Haughton, Norma E 117 DE Haven Drive #145, Yonkers, NY 10703, (212) 828-9000, BA 55 CUNY - Hunter Coll; MA 72 CUNY - Brooklyn Coll; Sp-Lang Path, St Joseph's Sch for the Deaf, **SLP**

Haukenes, Iva Mae 3515 S W Dawson Street, Seattle, WA 98126, (206) 572-5252, BS 76 Univ of WI - River Falls; MS 81 Saint Cloud St Univ; 87–Sp-Lang Path, Mary Bridge Chldn Hosp, **SLP**

Haunreiter, Mrs Rose Kathleen 8012 Mermaid Circle, Huntington Beach, CA 92646, (714) 536-2514, BA 82 WA St Univ; MA 85 CA St Univ - Fullerton; SLP, Huntington Beach Union High Sc, **SLP**

Haupt, Mrs Robin Terry 5151 North 9th Avenue, Pensacola, FL 32504, (904) 474-6148, BS 85 James Madison Univ; MS 87 Univ Southern MS-Hattiesburg; 88–Aud, Sacred Heart Hosp, **A**

Hauptman, Linda K 2529 Whittier Place, Billings, MT 59102, (406) 252-5750, BA 68 Univ of MT; MA 71 Univ of MT; 87–Sp-Lang Path, Yellowstone West Spec Svcs Coop, **SLP**

Haus, Gilda K 4514 Conchita Way, Tarzana, CA 91356, (818) 997-2357, BA 52 Univ of Pittsburgh - Pittsburgh; MA 70 CA St Univ - Northridge; Sp-Lang Path, LA USD, **SLP**

Hauser, Carol A 1140 37th Street, Hudson, WI 54016, (715) 386-9886, BS 68 Saint Cloud St Univ; ME 87 Univ of WI - River Falls

Hauser, Julia A 2512 Starkamp Avenue, Pittsburgh, PA 15226, (412) 647-5580, BA 70 Univ of Pittsburgh - Pittsburgh; MS 75 Univ of Pittsburgh - Pittsburgh; Aud, Chldns Hosp of Pgh, **A**

Hauser, Susan S 1031 North 67th Street, Philadelphia, PA 19151, (215) 242-4200, BA 72 Univ of TX - Austin; MA 79 Univ of TX - Austin; 87–Prog Coord, UCP Assoc, **SLP**

Haushalter, Mrs Phyllis Jayne 1362-B Ceape Avenue, Oshkosh, WI 54901, (414) 756-2166, BS 82 Univ of WI - Oshkosh; MS 84 Univ of WI - Oshkosh; **SLP**

Hausler, Walter E 19901 Elizabeth, St Clair Shores, MI 48080, (313) 445-4325, BS 68 Wayne St Univ; ME 71 Marygove Coll; Sp-Lang Path, South Lake Sch, **SLP**

Hausman, Charles H 6821 Alto Vista Drive, Nashville, TN 37205, (615) 356-7366, MS 74 Vanderbilt Univ; 88–Sp-Lang Path, Metro Nashville Bd of Educ, **SLP**

Hausmann, Joan B 4 St Peters Court, Ledyard, CT 06339, (203) 739-4491, BA 66 Catholic Univ of America; MA 70 CA St Univ - Northridge; Sp-Lang Path, East Lyme Public Schools, **SLP**

Hausmann, Linda P Apartado Del Este 61201, Caracas, Venezuela 1060A, BS 60 OH St Univ; MA 63 Case Western Reserve Univ; Private Practice, **SLP**

Hausserman, Julie L 976 West Grand River, Ionia, MI 48846, BS 70 Western MI Univ; MA 72 MI St Univ; SLP, Lansing Sch Dist, **SLP**

Haut, Mrs Monica Osborne 790 Dutchman Drive, Chippewa Falls, WI 54729, (715) 684-3393, BS 84 Univ of WI - Whitewater; MS 85 Univ of WI - Whitewater; SLP, Midwest Rehab Spec, **SLP**

Hautala, Kelly T 4132 Campana Drive, Palo Alto, CA 94306, (415) 493-7751, BA 83 San Jose St Univ; MA 86 San Jose St Univ; 86–Sp-Lang Path, Menlo Park VA Med Ctr, **SLP**

Havard, Joan L 18531 Ravenwood Drive, Saratoga, CA 95070, BA 71 Salem St Coll; OM 72 Smith Coll; 88–Aud/Tchr of the Deaf, California School of the Deaf, **A**

Havel, Lynn A 58 Radburn Drive, Hauppauge, NY 11788, (516) 366-0073, BA 79 Long Island U - CW Post Ctr; MS 81 Adelphi Univ; SLP, Brentwood Union Fr Sch Dist, **SLP**

Haveman, Jack A Box 343, 334 South Pine Street, Hemlock, MI 48626, (517) 642-2025, BA 68 MI St Univ; MA 73 MI St Univ

Haveman-Kruyf, Susan 2101 Jefferson Drive S E, Grand Rapids, MI 49507-3145, (616) 459-3289, BA 74 Western MT Coll; MA 78 Western MI Univ; Aud, Wn MI Otol Assoc Pc, **A**

Havens, Dr Dolores Route 1 Box 321-B, Columbia, KY 42728, (512) 774-3466, BS 59 Southwest TX St Univ; ME 72 Southwest TX St Univ; PH 75 Univ of WI - Madison; **SLP**

Havens, Judith W 17 Browne Street, Brookline, MA 02146, (617) 739-6519, BA 67 Hofstra Univ; MA 68 NY Univ; **SLP**

Havens, Mrs Laurie A 11701 Dinwiddie Drive, Rockville, MD 20852, (301) 770-8327, BS 72 Univ of IL - Urbana; MA 73 Univ of IL - Urbana; Asst Admin, Hebrew Home of Greater Wash, **SLP**

Havens, Richard M Professional Hearing Services, 9 Haigh Avenue, Niantic, CT 06357, (203) 446-5372, BA 64 OH Univ - Athens; MS 65 PA St Univ - Univ Park; Aud, Gen Dynamics Elec Boat Div, **A**

Haverfield, Mrs Mary 471 N W 101st Avenue, Coral Springs, FL 33071, (305) 977-2215, BA 68 Bellarmine Coll; MA 69 IN Univ - Bloomington; Sp-Lang Path, Brow Ard Co Bd of Ed, **SLP**

Havern, Mrs Amanda Route 2 Box 220-C, El Reno, OK 73036, (405) 262-0440, BS 69 Millersville Univ of PA; MA 74 Univ of OK - Norman; Sp-Lang Path, Banner & Darling Sch, **SLP**

Haverson, Mrs Nancy Ellen 10 Nosband Avenue #5-A, White Plains, NY 10605, (203) 869-6756, BS 76 Boston Univ; MS 78 Columbia Univ Teachers Coll; 81–Sp/Lang Path, Greenwich Pub Schs, **SLP**

Haverstock, Mrs Linda C 16300 Old Oak Ranch Drive, Sonora, CA 95370, (213) 586-2842, BA 67 Loma Linda Univ - Riverside; MA 68 Univ of Redlands; Sp-Lang Path, Vna, **SLP**

Havey, Michele Tousley 61 West Main Street, East Bloomfield, NY 14443, (716) 657-5422, BS 77 SUNY - Coll at Geneseo; ME 78 Univ of VA - Charlottesville; Private Practice, **SLP**

Hawa, Elias M 801 St Mary's Drive, Suite 402, Evansville, IN 47715, (812) 473-6093, BS 69 Brigham Young Univ; MS 70 Brigham Young Univ; 74–Aud, Thomas B Logan Chartered, **A**

Haward, Cynthia P 19 Union Street, Needham Heights, MA 02194-1302, (617) 449-6669, BS 74 Univ of NH; ME 79 Northeastern Univ; 87–Sp-Lang Path, N E Sinai Hosp and Rehab Ctr, **SLP**

Hawes, Kenneth C 454 South 7th Street, Eldridge, IA 52748, (319) 383-1499, BA 71 Univ of WI - Eau Claire; MA 73 Univ of IA; 87–Sp-Lang Path, Mercy Hosp, **SLP**

Hawes, Mary Z 928 School Avenue, Matteson, IL 60443, BA 70 Univ of MN - Minneap-St Paul; OB 84 Governors St Univ; OM 86 Governors St Univ; **SLP**

Hawk, Andrea J NISRO, FPO Box 76, Seattle, WA 98762-2500, BS 77 Indiana Univ of PA; MS 79 Univ of WI - Madison; 86–Sp-Lang Path, Dept of Defense Dependent Schs, **SLP**

Hawk, Dr Ash M 3672 East 3rd Street, Duluth, MN 55804, (218) 726-7974, BS 57 OH St Univ; MA 62 Bowling Green St Univ; PH 67 (NS) Univ of MI - Ann Arbor; Prof and Head, U of MN-Duluth, **SLP**

Hawk, Mrs Cynthia Tabolt 71 Big Tree Street, Box 29, Livonia, NY 14487, (716) 346-3532, BS 84 SUNY - Coll at Geneseo; MS 85 Ithaca Coll; 85–Sp-Lang Path, Livingston-Steuben-WY Co BOCES, **SLP**

Hawk, Del Lynn McPherson Hospital, Audiology Services, 1110 West Main Street, Durham, NC 27701, (919) 682-9341, BS 66 Western MI Univ; MS 67 CO St Univ; 88–Dir Aud Svcs, McPherson Hosp, **A**

Hawk, Dorothy M 312 Grove Avenue, Belle Vernon, PA 15012, (412) 929-4256, BS 62 CA Univ of PA; **A LM**

Hawk, Dr Elizabeth 19671 Surfbreaker Lane, Huntington Beach, CA 92648, (714) 536-0141, BA 27; MA 29 OH Wesleyan Univ; PH 46 (NS) OH St Univ; **SLP LM**

Hawk, Mrs Eloise B 2639 Suffolk Avenue Apartment E, High Point, NC 27260, (919) 883-2240, 33 High Point Coll; ME 51 Stephen F Austin St Univ; MA 66 Western Carolina Univ; **SLP LM**

Hawke, Mrs Carol Ann 214 Stubbs Mills Road, Lebanon, OH 45036, (513) 932-5182, **SLP**

Hawke, Carol J 9210 North Port Court, Bayside, WI 53217, (414) 351-5075, BS 84 Northern IL Univ - De Kalb; MS 87 Univ of WI - Milwaukee

Hawker, Marilyn Evans Marilyn Hawker And Associates, 4700 South McClintock #140, Temple, AZ 85282, BS 69 CO St Univ; MS 70 Univ of WI - Madison; Dir/Owner, Marilyn Hawker & Associates, **SLP**

Hawker, Mrs Pamela Agnes 4875 Monches Road, Colgate, WI 53017, (414) 968-3111, **SLP**

Hawkes, Mrs Cynthia H 1515 W Cornwallis Drive, Suite G-101, Greensboro, NC 27408, (919) 275-5409, MS 80 Memphis St Univ; SLP, Private Practice, **SLP**

Hawkes, Mrs Donna Marie 4821 North 16th Street, Omaha, NE 68110, (402) 453-5250, BS 85 Univ of NE - Omaha; MS 86 Univ of NE - Omaha; 86–Sp-Lang Path, Ralston PS Dist 54, **SLP**

Hawkes, Mrs Kirsten J 8286 Big Springs Court, Huber Heights, OH 45424, (513) 236-5128, BS 82 Mankato St Univ; MS 83 Univ of WI - River Falls; SLP, Tahoma Sch Dist, **SLP**

Hawkes, Mrs Mary H 2410 Shell, Midland, TX 79705, (915) 682-2849, BS 71 TX Tech Univ; MA 75 Our Lady Lake Univ-San Anton; Sp-Lang Path, Midland ISD, **SLP**

Hawkins, Alicia Wylie 1812 Wakeman Court, Wheaton, IL 60187-3741, (312) 393-1787, BS 62 FL St Univ; MS 85 Univ of TX - Dallas; 88–Sp-Lang Path, Wheaton/Warrenville Sch Dist 200, **SLP**

Hawkins, Mrs Carol J 2022 East Frye Road, Chandler, AZ 85225, (602) 899-9219, BA 85 CA St Univ - Fullerton; MA 87 CA St Univ - Los Angeles; 88–Aud, Arizona Hearing Centers, **A**

Hawkins, Cassandra Ann 155 Rosebay #42, Encinitas, CA 92024, (619) 944-9012, BS 85 Stephen F Austin St Univ; MS 87 Univ of TX - Dallas

Hawkins, Mrs Catherine M P O Box 1507, Conway, NH 03818, (603) 447-3989, BS 70 Northwestern Univ; MA 71 Northwestern Univ; Sp-Lang Path, Conway Sch Dist, **SLP**

Hawkins, Dr David B Dept Of Communicative Disorder, Univ Of South Carolina, Columbia, SC 29208, (803) 777-4813, BA 71 Wake Forest Univ; MA 74 Memphis St Univ; PH 77 (NS) Northwestern Univ; 86–Prof, Univ of South Carolina, **A**

Hawkins, Mrs Diana Durham 2 Dark Forest Place, Benton, AR 72015, (501) 227-2118, BA 81 Univ of AR - Little Rock; MS 83 Univ of AR - Medical Sci; Sp-Lang Path, Baptist Med Ctr, **SLP**

Hawkins, Edwina 25840 Croker Road, Valley City, OH 44280, (216) 329-3760, **SLP**

Hawkins, Elizabeth Rae 5419 Dunrobin, Lakewood, CA 90713, (213) 867-4654, **A**

Hawkins, Eloise Rainey 157 Dorado Avenue, Sewell, NJ 08080, (609) 696-6722, BA 76 Rutger's St Univ - Douglas Coll; MS 78 Columbia Univ Teachers Coll; Aud, Vineland Dev Cen, **A**

Hawkins, Mrs Grace Morreale 929 Medora Street, St Ignace, MI 49781, (906) 643-7400, BS 77 Central MI Univ; MA 82 Eastern MI Univ

Hawkins, Howard S 1916 Hopewell Road, Bethlehem, PA 18017, (215) 861-7773, BA 78 Univ of MO - Columbia; MA 79 Univ of MO - Columbia; Audiologist, Cochlear Corp, **A**

Hawkins, Jane A 4905 King Solomon Drive, Annandale, VA 22003, (703) 978-8349, BA 68 Univ of OK - Norman; MA 69 Univ of OK - Norman; **SLP**

Hawkins, Mrs Joyce A 3108 Hamilton Street, West Lafayette, IN 47906, (317) 423-6336, BA 74 Depauw Univ; MS 75 Purdue Univ - West Lafayette; Aud, Arnett Clinic, **A**

Hawkins, Mrs Kaaren O 210 Waverly Street, Winnipeg, MB, Canada R3M 3L2, **SLP**

Hawkins, Kristine J 10924 Girard Circle, Minneapolis, MN 55431, **SLP**

Hawkins, Margaret C 200 South Trotter Street, Dermott, AR 71638, (501) 538-5313, BS 40 PA St Univ - Univ Park; MS 42 PA St Univ - Univ Park; **SLP LM**

Hawkins, Marianne S 1360 Harvard Road N E, Atlanta, GA 30306, (404) 377-7436, BA 62; ME 67 Univ of VA - Charlottesville; Sp/Lang Path, Howard Sch, **SLP**

Hawkins, Mrs Mary E W 2330 Brookside Avenue, Waukegan, IL 60085, (414) 697-2107, BA 73 Henderson St Univ; MS 75 Purdue Univ - West Lafayette; 75–Sp-Lang Path, Kenosha USD #1, **SLP**

Hawkins, Mary F 220 Riley Street, Gadsden, AL 35901, (205) 543-3512, BA 74 Auburn Univ - Auburn; MA 75 Memphis St Univ; Sp-Lang Path, Sp-Lang Path Assoc, **SLP**

Hawkins, Mrs Michele N 6200 N W 84th Place, Oklahoma City, OK 73132, BA 75 Univ of OK - Norman; MS 77 Univ of OK Medical Center; **SLP**

Hawkins, Renae LaJean 2912 Six Gun Trail, Austin, TX 78748-1919, (512) 321-4488, BS 82 Baylor Univ; MA 86 Univ of TX - Austin; 86–Sp-Lang Path, Bastrop Spec Educ Coop, **SLP**

Hawkins, Richard R Roanoke Valley Sp & Hrng Ctr, 2030 Colonial Avenue S W, Roanoke, VA 24015, (703) 343-0165, BA 59 Harding Univ; MA 61 Univ of IA; Exec Dir, Roanoke Valley Sp&Hrng Cen Inc, **A**

Hawkins, Sarah A 287 J Windermere Road, London, ON, Canada N6G 2J7, (416) 898-4125, OM 88 Univ of Western Ontario

Hawkinson, Susan 1133 North Spruce, Bozeman, MT 59715, (406) 587-8897, BS 73 ND St Univ; MS 76 Univ of Northern CO; **SLP**

Hawkinson, Suzanne B 2105 East 46th Street, Davenport, IA 52807, (319) 359-1371, BA 79 Univ of NE - Lincoln; MS 82 Univ of WI - Madison; Sp-Lang Path, Mississippi Bend AEA, **SLP**

Hawkins-Seely, Jennifer 220 Catlin Terrace, Lewisville, TX 75067, (214) 436-8162, BS 76 Baylor Univ; MS 78 Baylor Univ; **A**

Hawkwood, Nielle R Rural Route 2, Cochrane, AB, Canada T0L 0W0, (403) 932-5610, BA 69; MS 72 Univ of OR; **SLP**

Hawley, Claudia D 5641 Zumbra Drive, Excelsior, MN 55331, (612) 474-2305, BA 68 Univ of MA - Amherst; MA 74 Univ of MN - Minneap-St Paul; Sp-Lang Path, West Metro Aud Spec Inc, **A**

Hawley, Connie Vie 127 Dogwood Road, Apt B-2, West Haven, CT 06516, (203) 799-9744, BS 84 Saint Louis Univ; MS 86 Univ of WI - Madison; **SLP**

Hawley-Gunckel, Janet St Marys Hospital, 1601 West St Marys Road, Tucson, AZ 85745, (602) 622-5833, BS 80 Univ of CA - Santa Barbara; MS 82 Univ of AZ; Sp-Lang Path, Carondelet Health Services, **SLP**

Hawn, Mrs Debra Greene 1324 Idlewood Place S W, Lenoir, NC 28645, (704) 758-1378, BS 78 Appalachian St Univ; MA 79 Appalachian St Univ; SLP, Caldwell Co Sch, **SLP**

Haworth, Freda 20 Arland Drive, Pawtucket, RI 02861, (401) 725-2831, BA 72 Univ of RI; MS 75 Univ of RI; **SLP LM**

Hawthorne, Mrs Carole C 620 Spring Valley Lane, Chattanooga, TN 37415, (615) 697-1250, BS 65 Univ of GA; MA 71 Temple Univ-Tyler Sch of Art; Sp-Lang Path, Chattanooga City Schools, **SLP**

Hawthorne, Mrs Maura Lynne PO Box 7332, Fort Myers, FL 33911, (813) 947-3718, BS 84 Univ of GA; MS 85 Univ of GA; **A**

Haxby, Marsha F 4711 South Fairplay Court, Aurora, CO 80015, (303) 680-1913, BS 74 Univ of IL - Urbana; MS 75 Univ of IL - Urbana; Sp-Lang Path, Aurora Pub Sch Assessment Cen, **SLP**

Haxel, Susan Sjoberg 3216 Princess, Bedford, TX 76021, (817) 283-1261, BA 82 Univ of OK - Norman; MS 85 Univ of North TX; 86–Sp-Lang Path, Hurst Euless Bedford ISD, **SLP**

Haxer, Marc J 921 Huntington, Mount Clemens, MI 48043, (313) 332-4410, BS 75 Central MI Univ; MA 78 Central MI Univ; Commun Dis Consult, MacOmb-Oakland Regional Cen, **SLP**

Hay, Mrs Bonnie W 4811 Penn Wyne Drive, Greensboro, NC 27410, (919) 292-8719, ME 82 Univ of NC - Greensboro; Sp-Lang Path, Chatham County Schs, **SLP**

Hay, Karla K 8000 Waters Avenue #166, Savannah, GA 31406, (608) 241-5920, BS 82 Univ of GA; MS 85 Univ of WI - Madison; **SLP**

Hay, Marcella East 2411 35th Avenue, Spokane, WA 99203

Hay, Mary Alice 2215 South Brookfield, South Bend, IN 46613, (219) 288-5928, BS 84 IN St Univ - Terre Haute; MA 86 Ball St Univ; Sp-Lang Path, St Joseph Med Ctr, **SLP**

Hay, Mrs Susan D 109 1st Street, Charleston, IL 61920, (217) 345-7553, BA 76 Augustana Coll; MS 77 Eastern IL Univ; Sp-Lang Path, Charleston Comm Ut #1, **SLP**

Hay, Mrs Veronica W PO Box 114, Rt 22B, Schuyler Falls, NY 12985, (518) 561-0100, BS 84 Nazareth Coll of Rochester; MA 85 SUNY - Coll at Geneseo; Sp-Lang Path, BOCES, **SLP**

Haydek, Cheryl Jean 7407 South Campbell, Chicago, IL 60629, (312) 434-5051, BA 87 Saint Xavier Coll; MA 88 Univ of IL - Urbana; 88–Sp-Lang Path, Cook Co Hosp

Haydel, Tina H 39492 Greg Drive, Prairieville, LA 70769, (504) 622-3224, BS 70 Northern MI Univ; BS 83 LA St Univ - Baton Rouge; MA 86 LA St Univ - Baton Rouge; 84–Sp-Lang Path, LeBlanc Spec Svcs Sch, **SLP**

Hayden, Cecilia Marie The Easter Seals Hearing Assoc, 233 East Broadway, Louisville, KY 40202, (502) 584-9781, BS 79 Brescia Coll; MS 85 Univ of Louisville; 87–Aud, The Easter Seal Society, **A**

Hayden, Elyse Shumway Baycrest Centre For Geriat Car, 3560 Bathurst Street, Toronto, ON, Canada M6A 2E1, (416) 789-5131, BS 77 Univ of VA - Charlottesville; MA 79 Univ of KS; 87–Sp-Lang Path, Baycrest Ctr for Ger Care, **SLP**

Hayden, Heather Lynne 6351 Dunn Street #47, Niagara Falls, ON, Canada L2G 2C8, (416) 688-3550, MS 85 SUNY - Coll at Buffalo; **SLP**

Hayden, Patricia A 39 Rossmore Avenue, Bronxville, NY 10708, (914) 961-7742, BS 77 CUNY - Lehman Coll; MS 78 Columbia Univ Teachers Coll; Sp-Lang Path, **SLP**

Hayden, Paul A Speech & Audiology Department, University Of Wisconsin, River Falls, WI 54022, PH (NS); **SLP**

Hayduk, Roberta Jo 5852 Sundown Circle #824, Orlando, FL 32822, (305) 422-2200, BS 84 Purdue Univ - West Lafayette; MA 86 Memphis St Univ; Aud, June F Kennedy Ph D, **A**

Hayes, Amy Schweigert 46 A Wiley Hill Road, Londonderry, NH 03053, (603) 883-5521, BA 85 SUNY - Coll at Fredonia; MS 86 SUNY - Coll at Fredonia; Sp-Lang Path, Nashua Memorial Hosp, **SLP**

Hayes, Mrs Carol Benjamin 210 Walden Street, West Hartford, CT 06107, (203) 727-1323, Sp-Lang Path, American School for the Deaf, **SLP**

Hayes, Mrs Cheryl Fouts 1612 West Farwell #2D, Chicago, IL 60626, (312) 398-4272, BS 71 De Paul Univ; MA 76 Univ of IL - Urbana; Sp/Lang Path, Arlington Hts Pub Sch #25, **SLP**

Hayes, Dr Claude S 1432 Brampton Cove, Wellington, FL 33414, (407) 790-2727, BS 47 Eastern IL Univ; MA 49 Northwestern Univ; PH 51 (NS) Northwestern Univ; Prof Emeritus Commun Dis, U of WI-Madison, **A F LM**

Hayes, Dr Deborah Childrens Hospital Of Denver, Audiology And Speech, 1056 East 19th Avenue, Denver, CO 80218, (303) 861-6841, BS 71 Northwestern Univ; MA 73 Northwestern Univ; PH 79 (NS) Baylor Coll of Medicine; Dir-Aud/SLP, Children's Hospital-Denver, **A**

Hayes, Deborah A 2122 W Pineview Drive, Muncie, IN 47303, (317) 747-3654, BS 76 Univ of MA - Amherst; MA 77 Univ of MA - Amherst; Sp-Lang Path, Ball Memorial Hosp, **SLP**

Hayes, Deborah Dawn 412 Chester Street, Menlo Park, CA 94025, (415) 326-9558, BA 76 CA St Univ - Chico; MS 82 San Francisco St Univ; 88–Sp-Lang Path, Private Practice, **SLP**

Hayes, Deborah Kay 5924 Goliad, Dallas, TX 75206, (214) 590-8139, BA 76 TX Tech Univ; MA 78 Univ of KS; SLP Dir, Parkland Mem Hosp, **SLP**

Hayes, Mrs Debra H 13851 North 41st Place, Phoenix, AZ 85032, (602) 493-6070, BA 75 Montclair St Coll; MS 77 UT St Univ; Sp/Lang Path, Paradise Valley Sch Dist, **SLP**

Hayes, Donald Edward 528 Lauder Street, Toronto, ON, Canada M6E 3J4, (416) 480-4138, BA 85 SUNY - Center at Buffalo; MA 87 SUNY - Center at Buffalo; 87–Aud, Sunnybrook Med Ctr, **A**

Hayes, Mrs Elizabeth Connors 32 Clifton Road, Hyannis, MA 02601, (617) 775-9609, BA 78 Univ of MI - Ann Arbor; MA 80 Western MI Univ; Consul Sp/Lang Path, Commun Hlth Care Assoc, **SLP**

Hayes, Harriet M Charter House #706, 211 Second Street N W, Rochester, MN 55901, (813) 293-9767, MA Univ of IA; **SLP LM**

Hayes, Hazel Denise 3511 Ridge Knoll, San Antonio, TX 78247, (512) 647-2100, BS 83 Univ of TX - Austin; MA 85 Our Lady Lake Univ-San Anton; **SLP**

Hayes, Sr Janet M House Of Mercy Community, 321 Rosedale Avenue, St Louis, MO 63112, (314) 966-6277, MA 75 Saint Louis Univ; 88–Dir of Comm, Sisters of Mercy-St Louis, **SLP**

Hayes, Mrs Joanne G 10684 Cranks Road, Culver City, CA 90230, (213) 825-8551, BA 57 Univ of MA - Amherst; ME 59 Boston Univ; Sp-Lang Path, Univ Calif Los Angeles Med Cen, **SLP**

Hayes, Mrs Judith Anne 13 Lincolnshire Drive, Bradford, MA 01830, (617) 681-1310, **SLP**

Hayes, Kathleen H 51-B St Andrews Boulevard, Clifton, NJ 07012, (201) 779-4335, BA 72 Bowling Green St Univ; MA 81 Montclair St Coll; 82–Sp-Lang Path, Private Practice, **SLP**

Hayes, Mrs Kathleen Mary 1317 Liberty Street, Oshkosh, WI 54901, (414) 426-3036, MS 88 Univ of WI - Oshkosh; 88–Sp-Lang Path, CES #6

Hayes, Mary Fordyce 604 Chestnut Street #6, Erie, PA 16502, (215) 631-9300, BA 86 Univ of Toledo; MS 87 Bowling Green St Univ

Hayes, Mrs Myra Lynn 1390 Rennet Drive, Naperville, IL 60565-1212, (312) 416-1473, MA 86 Northern IL Univ - De Kalb; 87–Sp-Lang Path, Joliet PS Dist #86, **SLP**

Hayes, Norma H 810 Woodmont Lane, Lakeland, FL 33803, (813) 644-3287, BA 66 Muskingum Coll; MA 68 OH Univ - Athens; SLP, Polk Co Sch, **SLP**

Hayes, Phebe Marie 147 Neco Town Road, New Iberia, LA 70560, (318) 231-6721, **SLP**

Hayes, Robert 45 West Bacon Street, Hillsdale, MI 49242, (517) 437-7208, BS 51 Central MI Univ; MA 57 Eastern MI Univ; 87–Retired, Hillsdale Co ISD, **SLP**

Hayes, Sandra M West Road, Rd 1 Box 377, Pleasant Valley, NY 12569, (914) 561-6373, BS 83 SUNY - Coll at New Paltz; MS 85 SUNY - Coll at New Paltz; **SLP**

Hayes, Tyler S 2319 Birch Drive, P O Box 2038, Running Springs, CA 92382, (714) 867-9427, BA 55 Allegheny Coll; MA 65 Univ of CA - Los Angeles; Principal, Los Angeles USD, **SLP**

Hayes, Victoria S 200 North Redrock Street, Anaheim, CA 92807, (714) 998-5527, BA 75 Univ of San Diego; MS 77 Chapman Coll; Pres, Rehab Alliance, **SLP**

Hayes-Pugh, Christine Ann 293 Linden Avenue Lower, Buffalo, NY 14216, **SLP**

Hayford, Cathy R 3014 Winchester Drive, Valparaiso, IN 46383, (219) 464-9607, BA 70 Univ of Evansville; OM 82 IN Univ - Bloomington; Sp-Lang Path, Porter Co Spec Ed Coop, **SLP**

Hayford, Donna S 16 Sunset Drive, Farmington, CT 06032, (203) 673-6781, BA 74 Univ of Bridgeport; MS 76 Emerson Coll; **SLP**

Hayford, Dr Jane Morris 1524 Hill Avenue, Fort Myers, FL 33901, (813) 995-2258, BS 49 Northwestern Univ; ME 63 Univ of FL; PH 82 (NS) FL St Univ; Sp-Lang Path, Lee Co Sch Bd, **SLP A ACE**

Hayford, Margaret Louise 10617 Spaulding Street, Omaha, NE 68134, (402) 572-2277, **SLP**

Haygood, Mrs Kathy C 12516 Quarterhorse Lane, Woodbridge, VA 22192, (703) 490-0397, BS 76 West TX St Univ; MS 80 Loyola Coll; 87–Dir Sp-Lang Path, Potomac Hosp, **SLP**

Haynes, Charles W 57 Main Street, Boxford, MA 01921, (617) 927-5866, BA 77 Harvard Univ; MS 81 San Francisco St Univ; Head of Sp-Lang Dept, Landmark School, **SLP**

Haynes, Mrs Deborah Gordon 20869 Cricket Lane, Lenexa, KS 66220, (913) 642-9290, BS 71 Univ of TX - Austin; MA 73 Univ of North TX; 73–Sp-Lang Path, Shawnee Mission Sch Dist

Haynes, Elizabeth Jane c/o W S Haynes, General Delivery, Westbank, BC, Canada T2E 0J2, BA 81 Western WA Univ; MA 85 WA St Univ; Sp-Lang Path, **SLP**

Haynes, Glenda Marie 300 Meadowbrook Drive #2, Campbellsville, KY 42718, (502) 465-4097, BA 76 Univ of KY; MS 82 Univ of Louisville; 86–Sp-Lang Path, Lake Cumberland Home Health Agency Inc, **SLP**

Haynes, LeEllen R 3027 West Capital #1, Grand Island, NE 68803, (308) 381-5931, BA 73 Kearney St Coll; MA 77 Univ of Northern IA; Sp-Lang Path, Ctrl NE Support Serv Prog, **SLP**

Haynes, Maria N 35 Parker Street, Lexington, MA 02173, (617) 861-0413, BS 60 Syracuse Univ; MA 63 Stanford Univ; Sp-Lang Path, Lexington Pub Schs, **SLP A**

Haynes, Maureen D 1404 Piedmont, Opelika, AL 36801, MS; **SLP**

Haynes, Sara M Callier Center, 1966 Inwood Road, Dallas, TX 75235, (214) 783-3033, MS 70 FL St Univ; Head Sp-Lang Path, Callier Cen/Commun Dis/Utd, **SLP**

Haynes, Spencer H Route 1 Box 330, Princess Anne, MD 21853, (301) 651-2698, BA 67 OH Univ - Athens; MA 80 Univ of MD - College Park; Sp/Lang Path, Somerset Co Pub Sch, **SLP**

Haynes, Thomas Charles, Jr 420 Hodges Drive N W, Orangeburg, SC 29115, (803) 536-5511, BS 76 Univ of SC - Columbia; OM 77 Univ of SC - Columbia; Aud, Rocco D Cassone MD Pa, **A**

Haynes, William O 1404 Piedmont Avenue, Opelika, AL 36801, PH (NS); **SLP**

Haynie, Mrs Christine Buchholz 1521 Seneca Street, Winston-Salem, NC 27103, (919) 725-7917, BA 84 Univ of NC - Chapel Hill; MS 85 Univ of NC - Chapel Hill; 88–Sp-Lang Path, WSFC Schs/Children's Ctr for Physically Handicapped, **SLP**

Haynie, Jo K 206 West 3rd, Elgin, TX 78621, (512) 883-5559, BA 54 Univ of North TX; MA 70 Univ of North TX; **SLP**

Hays, Mrs Barbara West 3007 Del Sur, Alamogordo, NM 88316, (505) 437-3200, BA 78 CA St Univ - Stanislaus; MS 83 Eastern NM Univ; 87–Sp-Lang Path, Alamogordo PS, **SLP**

Hays, Dr C Lynne 7200 Running Rope, Austin, TX 78731, PH 83 (Aphasia) Univ of TX - Austin; Private Practice, **SLP**

Hays, Debra Engelstein 13601 La Mirada Circle, West Palm Beach, FL 33414, (919) 489-9158, **SLP**

Hays, Mrs Denise B 818 Knightsboro Court, Brentwood, TN 37027, (615) 377-9117, BA 73 Univ of Pittsburgh - Pittsburgh; MS 74 Univ of Pittsburgh - Pittsburgh; **SLP**

Hays, Elizabeth D 20 North Duncan #1, Fayetteville, AR 72701, (501) 443-5968, Sp Service Coor, Ozark Guidance Ctr, **SLP**

Hays, Mrs Jenny G 10406 South 66th East Avenue, Tulsa, OK 74133, (918) 622-8321, OB 71 Univ of AR - Fayetteville; MA 72 Univ of AR - Fayetteville; Sp-Lang Path, Un Sch-Briarglen Elem, **SLP**

Hays, John M 1630 2nd Avenue, York, PA 17403, (414) 681-0300, BA 68 Franklin & Marshall Coll; OM 74 Emory Univ; SLP, Racine USD, **SLP**

Hays, Mrs Lisa Michelle 1334 Dunleith Place, Jackson, MS 39204, (601) 825-4706, BS 83 Delta St Univ; MS 87 Univ of MS; Sp-Lang Path, Rankinco Schl Dstr, **SLP**

Hays, Lynette D South 3206 Sommer Road, Veradale, WA 99037, (509) 456-3948, BA 73 Eastern WA Univ; MS 75 Eastern WA Univ; SLP, Spokane Co Hd Start, **SLP**

Hays, Mrs Susan E RD 1 Box 146, Strattanville, PA 16258, BS 76 Geneva Coll; MS 81 Clarion Univ of PA; Sp-Lang Path, Riverview IU 6, **SLP**

Hays, Sylvia Samples Montclair ENT Associates, 840 Montclair Road, Suite 218, Birmingham, AL 35213, (205) 591-6570, BA 80 Univ of MS; ME 81 LA St Univ - N O Medical Ctr; Aud, ENT Ctr, **A**

Haythorn, Dr Mark M 103 Puma Lane, Chapel Hill, NC 27514, MA 77 Univ of TN - Knoxville; PH 81 (NS) Univ of CA - Davis; Aud, Nc Mem Hosp, **A**

Hayward, Mrs Deborah Carol 2615 Yates Street, Denver, CO 80212, (303) 466-6308, MA 82 Univ of CO - Boulder; 85–Sp-Lang Path, Bal Swan Childrens Center, **SLP**

Hayward, Floanne J 3614 Montrose Boulevard, Apartment 1001, Houston, TX 77006, **SLP**

Haywood, Emily Jo RFD 1 Goffstown, Gorhman Pond Road, Dunbarton, NH 03045, (603) 774-3958, BS 82 Boston Univ; MS 84 Boston Univ; 87–Sp-Lang Path, Pembroke Sch Dist, **SLP**

Haywood, Louise 242 North Russell Street, Troy, NC 27371, (919) 576-6511, BA 54 High Point Coll; MA 62 Western Carolina Univ; Sp/Lang Path, Private Practice, **SLP**

Haywood, Marialys G 8618 Thunderhead Drive, Boulder, CO 80302, (303) 440-3368, BA 69 Mount Holyoke Coll; MS 76 Univ of RI; Agcy Dir, Longmont Tiny Tim Cen, **SLP**

Hazel, William O, II Rural Route 2 Box 109, Harwood, MO 64750, (417) 667-7833, BS 77 Central MO St Univ; MS 79 Central MO St Univ; Sp/Lang Prog Coord, NV Habilitation Cen, **A**

Hazelton, Cathy A RFD 1 Box 1180, West Peru, ME 04290, (207) 364-3721, BS 79 Univ of ME - Farmington; MS 80 Syracuse Univ; 88–Sp-Lang Path, Private Practice, **SLP**

Hazelton, Laura Campbell University Of Texas-El Paso, Speech-Hearing-Lang Disabl, P O Box 639, El Paso, TX 79968, (915) 747-5250, BA 82 Valparaiso Univ; MA 83 Western MI Univ; Sp-Lang Path, University of Texas-El Paso, **SLP**

Hazen, Mrs Carol A K 8021 Sunny Creek, Germantown, TN 38138, (501) 834-1945, BS 77 Univ of Central AR; MS 78 Univ of AR - Little Rock; Sp-Lang Path, Mid South Hosp, **SLP**

Hazen, Jayne L 5298 Cobb Drive, Dayton, OH 45431, BA 78 Wichita St Univ; MA 79 Wichita St Univ; Sp-Lang Path, Mont Cty Bd of Mental Retar, **SLP**

Hazen, Mrs Nancy White 1014 Pinot Noir, Lodi, CA 95240, (209) 368-8404, BA 79 Humboldt St Univ; MA 81 Humboldt St Univ; SLP, Lodi USD, **SLP**

Hazenfield, Mrs Susan L 5457 Stow Road, Stow, OH 44224, (216) 929-2046, BA 77 OH St Univ; MA 79 Case Western Reserve Univ; SLP, Co of Summit Bd of Ment Ret, **SLP**

Hazim, Karolyn 115 Cedar Street, Mount Vernon, NY 10552, (914) 969-4552, BA 85 Marymount Coll; MA 86 Hofstra Univ; SLP, Central Speech Pathology, **SLP**

Hazlett, Mrs Joan M 2659 Sixth Street, Cuyahoga Falls, OH 44221, (216) 923-2555, BA 85 Univ of Akron; MA 87 Univ of Akron; 88–Aud, Southwest Aud, **F**

Hazouri, Patricia A Mill Road, Worcester, VT 05682, (802) 433-6653, BA 74 Univ of FL; ME 76 Univ of FL; **SLP**

Head, Mrs Brenda R 190 Caroline Street South, Hamilton, ON, Canada L8P 3L2, (416) 388-0240, BA 63 Univ of Toronto - Ontario; MA 67 Univ of WI - Madison; Dr Aud, Chedoke-McMaster Hosp, **A**

Head, Mrs Judy H 5537 Morris Street, Philadelphia, PA 19144, (215) 848-9781, BA 83 Earlham Coll; MA 87 Temple Univ; **SLP**

Head, Mrs Pamela G 22702 Crosshill Avenue, Torrance, CA 90505, (213) 419-2540, BS 73 IN Univ - Bloomington; MA 75 Univ of Redlands; Sp-Lang Path, Los Angeles Co Supt of Sch, **SLP**

Headley, Amy B 1052-E Brandywine Boulevard, Zanesville, OH 43701, (614) 453-6866, BS 86 WV Univ; MA 87 OH Univ - Athens; 87–Sp-Lang Path, Good Samaritan Med Ctr

Headley, Mrs Carol McDaniel 3353 East Lakeshore Drive, Tallahassee, FL 32312-1440, (904) 385-0010, **SLP**

Headrick, Mrs Carol Smith Box 1746, Stillwater, OK 74076, (405) 624-6020, BA 64 Baylor Univ; OM 65 Univ of OK Medical Center; 73–Instr-Acad Adv-Cl Superv, OK St U, **SLP**

Heady, Mrs Linda Sue 816 East Adams Street, Muncie, IN 47305, (317) 285-8169, BA 58 Univ of AR - Fayetteville; MA 68 MI St Univ; Asst Prof Sp/Lang Path, Ball State U, **SLP**

Heady-Erickson, Mrs Barbara J Area Educ Agny 11 (Heartland), 120 South Hazel, Ames, IA 50010, (515) 232-7583, BS 72 Northwestern Univ; MA 73 Univ of IA; Sp-Lang Path, AEA 11, **SLP**

Healea, Susan Kay 4400 Ocean Beach Hwy #18, Longview, WA 98632, (206) 636-0520, BA 82 Western WA Univ; MA 84 Western WA Univ; Aud, Longview Hrng & Sp, **A**

Healey, Mrs Barbara N 7350 North Cocoa Boulevard #206, Cocoa, FL 32927, (407) 639-2549, BA 58 Univ of AL-Tuscaloosa; MA 63 Univ of AL- Tuscaloosa; Sp-Lang Path, Brevard Co FL PS, **SLP**

Healey, Daniel K 8 Longview Avenue, Ware, MA 01082, (413) 734-4918, BS 77 Univ of MA - Amherst; ME 79 Northeastern Univ; Aud, Dr Robert Osofsky, **A**

Healey, Dr E Charles 253 Barkley Memorial Center, University Of Nebraska-Lincoln, Lincoln, NE 68583-0731, (402) 472-5459, BA 71 Univ of KY; MA 73 Univ of KY; PH 77 (Sp-Lang Path) Purdue Univ - West Lafayette; Assoc Prof, U of NE-Lincoln, **SLP**

Healey, Grace D 4 2nd Street, North Providence, RI 02911, MS; **SLP LM**

Healey, James Edward 38 Strathmoore Road, Cranston, RI 02905, (401) 781-0909, BA 73 Univ of RI; MS 75 Purdue Univ - West Lafayette; Aud, Sargent Rehab Ctr, **A**

Healey, Mrs Kay Novak 1100 Orchard Avenue, Ogden, UT 84404, (801) 621-1123, MS 85 Univ of UT; Sp-Lang Path, Weber County Sch Dist, **SLP**

Healey, Patricia 148 Westridge Drive, Waterbury, CT 06708, (203) 754-5566, BA 35 Smith Coll; MA 36 Columbia Univ Teachers Coll; Retired, **SLP LM**

Healey, Dr William C Dept Of Special Education & Rehabilitation, College Of Education, University Of Arizona, Tucson, AZ 85721, PH 63 (Sp Path) Univ of MO - Columbia; Adjunct Prof, University of Arizona, **SLP F**

Healey-Dame, Mary 960 Big Sur Court, El Dorado Hills, CA 95630, (916) 366-6181, MS 80 Univ of WY; 87–Sp-Lang Path, Folsom-Cordova USD, **SLP**

Healy, Mrs Carolyn Schmitz 2205 Sanford Avenue, New Lenox, IL 60451, (815) 485-5567, BS 85 Northern IL Univ - De Kalb; MA 86 Northern IL Univ - De Kalb; **SLP**

Healy, Colleen Ellen Grace Warner School, Att: Solh Ii, 3075 Heights Drive, Reno, NV 89504, (702) 423-5187, BS 81 CA St Univ - Hayward; MS 83 CA St Univ - Hayward; SLP, **SLP**

Healy, Maureen Elaine 8123 Begonia Way, Gaithersburg, MD 20879, (301) 774-0074, BA 84 Univ of MD - College Park; MA 85 George Washington Univ; Aud, Dr Hubert Leveque, **A**

Healy, Mrs Sandra K 54718 Country Manor Place, Elkhart, IN 46514, (219) 294-2621, BS 76 IN St Univ - Terre Haute; MS 78 IN St Univ - Terre Haute; Sp-Lang Path, Elkhart Gen Hosp, **SLP**

Heaney, Carol Mary 1935 West 10th Avenue, Vancouver, BC, Canada V6J 2B1, (604) 733-9877, **SLP**

Heaney, Nancy Curchin 651 Applegrove Circle, Webster, NY 14580, (716) 872-5794, **SLP**

Heap, Nancy Jean 2503 Briar Ridge, Houston, TX 77057, (713) 799-1511, BA 73; MA 74 Univ of AR - Fayetteville; 87–Sp-Lang Path, Patricia J Johnson PhD & Assoc, **SLP**

Heaps, Dana C 1410 Bowles Terrace, Forest Hill, MD 21050, **SLP**

Heaps, Mrs Irene S 12 Greenwood Drive, Freehold Township, NJ 07728, (201) 938-5061, BA 72 George Washington Univ; MS 74 Southern CT St Univ; 74–Sp-Lang Path, Brisbane Child Treatment Cen, **SLP**

Heaps, Mrs Nancy I 457 Nevada Street, Paramus, NJ 07652-5621, (212) 588-7000, BA 76 CUNY - Queens Coll; MA 78 OH St Univ; Aud, Bronx Lebanon Hosp, **A**

Heard, Dr Kenneth W 6 Golden Oak Cove, Little Rock, AR 72212, (501) 224-0363, BA 74 Univ of AR - Little Rock; MA 76 Memphis St Univ; PH 87 (Aud) Memphis St Univ; 79–Aud, VA Med Cen, **A**

Heard, Mrs Sheila Trice 920 14th Avenue North, Nashville, TN 37208, (615) 320-1538

Hearn, Mrs Demetria Bilycia 13 Caly Hollow Road, Kennebunk, ME 04043, (207) 985-7910, BA 76 Univ of CT; MA 77 Western MI Univ; Sp-Lang Path, York Co Couns Sers Sp/Hrng Pro, **SLP**

Hearn, Stella B 650 Fairmede Avenue, Palo Alto, CA 94306, (415) 855-8419, BA 60 Univ of the Pacific; MA 64 Stanford Univ; Sp-Lang Path, Palo Alto Sud, **SLP**

Hearns, Virginia M 5 Sea Barn Road, Cape Elizabeth, ME 04107, (207) 799-8176, BA 65 Univ of MA - Amherst; MA 66 Univ of MA - Amherst; Sp/Lang Path, Cape Elizabeth Sch Dept, **SLP**

Hearon, Mrs Betty C 6258 North St Moritz, Mobile, AL 36608, (205) 457-3357, BS 61 MS Univ for Women; MS 77 Univ Southern MS-Hattiesburg; Sp-Lang Path, Mobile Co Schs, **SLP**

Hearst, Mrs Karen Blankenship 808 Smartt's Lane NE, Leesburg, VA 22075, (703) 955-9995, BS 84 Univ of VA - Charlottesville; ME 86 Univ of VA - Charlottesville; Sp-Lang Path, InSpeech Inc, **SLP ACE**

Heary, Mrs Lori J 44 Forest Avenue, Springville, NY 14141, (716) 592-2113, BS 79 SUNY - Coll at Fredonia; MS 82 SUNY - Coll at Fredonia; 88–Sp-Lang Path, Suburban Adult Services Inc, **SLP**

Heasley, Frederick H Box 216, Riverton, CT 06065, **SLP**

Heater, Mrs Cheryl A Sand Fork School, Sand Fork, WV 26430, (304) 462-7386, BS 76 Indiana Univ of PA; MS 77 Indiana Univ of PA; Sp-Lang Path, Gilmer Co Boe, **SLP**

Heater-Lohrman, Mrs Julie Ann Graystone Eye Ear Nose & Throat Center, PO Drawer 2484 Fairgrove Church Road, Hickory, NC 28603, (704) 322-3725, BS 82 Purdue Univ - West Lafayette; MS 84 Purdue Univ - West Lafayette; **A**

Heath, Dianne G 3211 N E 17th, Portland, OR 97212, (503) 223-4959, BA 77 San Francisco St Univ; MS 83 Portland St Univ; Aud, Derek S Lipman MD, **A**

Heath, Jean L RFD 2 Box 1823, Hampden, ME 04444, (207) 947-2716, BS 53 Mount Saint Mary's Coll; MA 74 Univ of ME - Orono; Exec Dir, Bangor Reg Sp & Hrng Cen, **SLP**

Heath, Judith Lynn 185 Scobee Lane, Summerset, NJ 08873, (201) 761-1400, **SLP**

Heath, Linda M 2 Liberty Lane, Bedford, MA 01730, (617) 452-4846, BS 73 SUNY - Coll at Fredonia; MS 77 Long Island U - CW Post Ctr; Sp-Lang Path, **SLP**

Heath, Lynn C 19 Nature Trail, Lutz, FL 33549-5122, (813) 948-1633, BS 74 Purdue Univ - West Lafayette; MS 76 Purdue Univ - West Lafayette; Sp-Lang Path, InSpeech Inc, **SLP**

Heath, Dr Richard G Route 3 Box 64, Pound Ridge, NY 10576, (914) 666-9553, BA 60 Hofstra Univ; MS 65 CUNY - Queens Coll; ED 76 (NS) Columbia Univ Teachers Coll; **SLP**

Heath, Shirley T 585 East Quincy, Fresno, CA 93710, (209) 298-0523, BA 78 CA St Univ - Northridge; MA 80 CA St Univ - Northridge; Sp-Lang Path, Fresno County Dept of Ed, **SLP**

Heath, Mrs Susan Neff Augsburg High School, APO New York, NY 09178, BA 73 Ottawa Univ; MS 77 Central MO St Univ; Sp-Lang Path, Dept of Defense Depend Schs, **SLP**

Heatley, Thomas W 807 North Vista Street, Los Angeles, CA 90046, BA 77 Boston Univ; MS 82 Emerson Coll; 86–Sp-Lang Path, Cedars Sinai Med Ctr, **SLP**

Heaton, Constance 3934-U Partridge Circle, Bettendorf, IA 52722, (319) 359-1371, BA 62 Univ of Northern IA; MA 73 Univ of Northern IA; Sp-Lang Path, MS Bend AEA 9, **SLP**

Heaton, Mrs Elaine M Glenrose Rehabilitation Hosp, 10230 111th Avenue, Edmonton, AB, Canada T5G 0B7, (403) 471-7971, MA 71 Univ of MT; 80–Sp-Lang Path, Glenrose Rehab Hosp, **SLP F**

Heavener, Wren 206 Brookside Circle, Harleysville, PA 19438, (215) 647-3150, BA 75 Univ of TN - Knoxville; MA 78 Univ of TN - Knoxville; Sp-Lang Path, Bryn Mawr Svc Corp, **SLP**

Heavey, Ann E 592 Mitchell Avenue, Elmhurst, IL 60126, (312) 450-2144, BS 75 Marquette Univ; MS 76 Marquette Univ; Sp-Lang Path, Northwest Sub Spec Ed Org, **SLP**

Hebert, Mrs Diane Marie 1560-12 Quail Drive, West Palm Beach, FL 33409, (407) 793-4590, BA 82 Univ of Pittsburgh - Pittsburgh; MS 85 CA Univ of PA; 86–Sp-Lang Path, Palm Beach County Sch Bd

Hebert, Edward C Western Ma Sp & Lang Ser Assoc, 146 Chestnut Street, Springfield, MA 01103, (413) 737-7368, BA 66 Univ of MA - Amherst; MA 72 Univ of MA - Amherst; Cl Dir, Wm MA Sp & Lang Serv Assoc Inc, **SLP**

Hebert, Mrs Lisa Anne 62 Lisa Avenue, Kenner, LA 70065, (504) 443-4962, BS 83 LA St Univ - Baton Rouge; ME 87 Southeastern LA Univ; 83–Sp-Lang Path, Jefferson Parish Sch Bd, **SLP**

Hebert, Mrs Lynne R 805 East First Street, Jennings, LA 70546-5439, (318) 824-8370, BA 75 Univ of Southwestern LA; MS 78 Univ of Southwestern LA; Coordinator Sp-Lang & Hearing, Jefferson Davis Parish Schools, **SLP**

Hebert, Mrs Marianne Lahaye 1021 Auburn Avenue, Lafayette, LA 70503, (318) 232-9177, BS 79 Univ of Southwestern LA; MS 85 Univ of Southwestern LA; **SLP**

Hebert, Michele A Route 131 P O Box 195, Quinebaug, CT 06262, (203) 235-6606, BS 77 Univ of NH; MS 79 Southern CT St Univ; 79–Sp-Lang Path, Meriden Ct Bd of Ed, **SLP**

Hebert, Mrs Pamela Pereira 206 Eastlawn Drive, Hampton, VA 23664, (804) 851-0814, BS 77 James Madison Univ; MS 81 Old Dominion Univ; Sp-Lang Path, Hampton City Schs, **SLP**

Hecht, Kimberly Anne 4203 Kopwood #D, St Louis, MO 63129, (314) 968-5225, MA 85 Southeast MO St Univ; Sp-Lang Path, Miriam Sch, **SLP**

Hecht, Mrs Mindy S 5815 North Winthrop, Chicago, IL 60660, (312) 728-8935, BA 78 CUNY - Queens Coll; MA 80 Northwestern Univ; Sp-Lang Path, Illinois Masonic Medical Ctr, **SLP**

Hecht, Susan Karnes 16 Wagon Wheel Road, Poughkeepsie, NY 12601, (914) 229-0123, BA 79 Univ of Rochester; MS 86 SUNY - Coll at New Paltz; 87–Sp-Lang Path, St Francis Hosp/Presch Prog, **SLP**

Hechtman, Dr Marvin 56 Claradon Lane, Staten Island, NY 10305, (718) 981-0672, BA 54 CUNY - Brooklyn Coll; MA 63 CUNY - Brooklyn Coll; ED 75 (Aud) Columbia Univ Teachers Coll; Aud, Madison Audiology Assoc, **A**

Heck, Bonnie June 18731 Dylan Street, Northridge, CA 91326, (805) 945-8554, BA 80 Univ of CA - Santa Barbara; MS 82 Univ of Redlands; Sp-Lang Path, High Desert Hospital, **SLP**

Heck, Mrs Frances A 2103 Whitewood Court, Indianapolis, IN 46260, (317) 875-9600, BS 62 Univ of KS; MA 66 Univ of KS; **SLP**

Heck, Mrs Kathleen Denise 1803 Longfellow Street, Hyattsville, MD 20782, (202) 722-2463, BS 79 Hampton Univ; MA 83 Hampton Univ; **SLP**

Heck, Mrs Kendee Fawn 1121 Denver, Park City, KS 67219, (316) 744-0549, MA 88 Wichita St Univ

Heck, Sally Beth 7849 South Scepter Drive #8, Franklin, WI 53132, (414) 272-1344, BS 85 Univ of WI - Milwaukee; MS 87 Marquette Univ; 87–Sp-Lang Path, Jewish Vocational Service, **SLP**

Heckel, Mrs Donna M 12146 Harford Road, Glen Arm, MD 21057, (301) 592-6087, MS 84 Towson St Univ; 88–Sp-Lang Path, Private Practice, **SLP**

Hecker, Henry C 12700 McManus Boulevard, Newport News, VA 23602, (804) 874-4665, BA 65 Univ of UT; MA 68 Univ of UT; Aud, Henpa Inc, **A**

Hecker, Dr Michael H L Speech Research Program, SRI International, Menlo Park, CA 94025, (415) 859-4323, BS 59 Northeastern Univ; MS 61 MA Inst of Tech; PH 74 (Sp & Hrng Sci) Stanford Univ; 67–Research Engr, SRI International

Hecker, Mrs Nancy Greenwald 3667 Regent Lane, Wantagh, NY 11793, (516) 796-2966, BA 77 Adelphi Univ; MS 79 Adelphi Univ; Sp/Lang Path, East Rockaway Ufsd, **SLP**

Heckler, Melanie Leigh 46 Ridge Avenue, Telford, PA 18969, (215) 456-9292, BS 85 Bloomsburg Univ of PA; MS 86 Bloomsburg Univ of PA; 88–Sp-Lang Path, Mass Rehab Hosp, **SLP**

Heckman, Maureen Weitzel 27 Heather Hill Road, Weare, NH 03281, (603) 529-7798, BS 72 OH Univ - Athens; MA 73 OH Univ - Athens; Sp-Lang Path, Consult, **SLP**

Heckman, Terri Ellyn 2132 North 118th Street, Wauwatosa, WI 53226, (414) 453-9268, MS 85 Univ of WI - Whitewater; 87–Sp-Lang Path, Rehabilitation Associates, **SLP**

Heckner, Patricia Ann 11711 103 Street, Peace River, AB, Canada T8S 1M1, (403) 624-2889, BS 84 James Madison Univ; ME 86 James Madison Univ; 86–Aud, Peace River Health Unit #21, **A**

Hedberg, Mrs Janet A P O Box 254, Goodland, IN 47948, (815) 432-4931, BA 78 Augustana Coll; MA 79 Saint Louis Univ; Sp-Lang Path, Unit Nine Sch Dist, **SLP**

Hedberg, Karen 1460 N Sandburg Terrace, Apartment 2802, Chicago, IL 60610, (312) 702-1864, BS 65 Univ of IA; MA 66 Northwestern Univ; Aud, U of Chicago Med Cen, **A ACE**

Hedberg, Dr Natalie L University Of Colorado, Box 409, Boulder, CO 80309, (303) 492-6445, BS 52 Syracuse Univ; MA 60 Columbia Univ Teachers Coll; PH 71 (NS) Northwestern Univ; Prof, U of CO, **SLP A**

Hedderig, Charles Theodore 1727 South Grant Street, Marshall, MO 65340, (816) 886-9314, BS 76 Saint Louis Univ; MS 84 Saint Louis Univ; 86–Sp-Lang Path, Marshall Hab Ctr, **SLP**

Hedeen, Mrs Maureen Marie 6128 Cheyenne Court, Sioux Falls, SD 57106, (602) 361-9324, BA 82 Univ of SD - Vermillion; MA 84 Univ of SD - Vermillion; **SLP**

Hedgebeth, Mrs Mary Helen 7335 Kennedy Lane, Cincinnati, OH 45242, (513) 791-2269, BA 78 Bellarmine Coll; MA 83 Univ of Cincinnati; Sp-Lang Path, **SLP**

Hedgecock, Dr Leroy D Mayo Clinic, Rochester, MN 55901, BS 36 WA St Univ; MA 39 Univ of Northern CO; PH 49 (NS); Emeritus Consultant, **SLP A F LM**

Hedges, Ann Mahon 8500 Leatrice, Little Rock, AR 72207, (501) 370-6651, BS 74 OH St Univ; MA 78 Univ of Cincinnati; Aud, VA Med Ctr, **A**

Hedges, Cecelia H 8010 Dustin Drive, Frederick, MD 21701-3304, (301) 845-6703, **SLP**

Hedges, Janet 3451 Kleybolte Avenue #9, Cincinnati, OH 45226, (513) 559-4341, BA 79 Univ of KY; MA 81 Memphis St Univ; Sp-Lang Path, Cincinnati Children's Hosp, **SLP**

Hedges, Joyce Stella 5722 29th Avenue N E, Seattle, WA 98105, (206) 223-3168, BS 79 Univ of WA; OM 81 Univ of WA; Sp-Lang Path, Harborview Med Ctr, **SLP**

Hedges, Mrs MaryAnn 550 West Columbia Street, Schuylkill Haven, PA 17972, (717) 385-0386, MS 88 PA St Univ - Univ Park

Hedges, Susan F 2669 Nottingham, Columbus, OH 43221, (614) 461-2420, BS 78 Miami Univ - Oxford; MA 79 Bowling Green St Univ; SLP, Franklin Co Brd of Mr/Dd, **SLP**

Hedin, Mrs Anne K 62 Spruce Street, Jamestown, NY 14701, (716) 664-7487, BA 72 Elmira Coll; MA 73 Bowling Green St Univ; 79–Aud, Aud Svcs, **A**

Hedin-Peldyak, Kathryn Sue 1706 Avalon Way #102, Hood River, OR 97031, (503) 386-3683, BS 83 Univ of OR; MS 84 Univ of OR; **SLP**

Hedler, Mrs Charlotte Ellen 694 Gravel Road, Seneca Falls, NY 13148, (315) 568-5834, BA 51 Univ of MI - Ann Arbor; MS 77 Nazareth Coll of Rochester; SLP, Seneca Falls Ctrl Sch Dist, **SLP**

Hedlund, Larrain Ann 737 Hinman Avenue #1-E, Evanston, IL 60202, (312) 346-1136, MA 88 Northwestern Univ; 88–Aud, Charles A Lowe & Associates

Hedman, Linda J 4947 West Eddy, Chicago, IL 60641, (312) 333-2300, BS 83 Northern IL Univ - De Kalb; MA 85 Northern IL Univ - De Kalb; Aud, Private Practice, **A**

Hedrick, Dr Dona Lea 21 Village Drive East, Oviedo, FL 32765, (305) 275-2121, BA 54 Univ of IA; MA 60 Univ of IA; PH 67 (NS) Univ of WA; Prof, U of Ctrl FL, **SLP F**

Hedrick, Mark Stephen Route 3 Box S E-3, Troutville, VA 24175, BS 83 WV Wesleyan Coll; ME 86 Univ of VA - Charlottesville

Hedrick, Mrs Tracy L 7804 Stanley Road #164, Powell, TN 37849, (615) 947-3616, BS 82 Univ of TN - Knoxville; MA 86 Univ of TN - Knoxville

Heegel, Mrs Melinda A South Dakota Sch For The Deaf, 1800 East 10th Street, Sioux Falls, SD 57103, (605) 339-6700, BA 78 Univ of OK - Norman; MS 80 Univ of OK Medical Center; Aud, Sd Sch for Deaf, **A**

Heely, Mary Archibald 42 Prospect Street, Norwich, CT 06360, (203) 887-5036, MS 84 Southern CT St Univ; Sp-Lang Path, Norwich Board of Education, **SLP**

Heer, Pamela L 835 El Dorado Drive, Fullerton, CA 92632, (714) 879-9798, BA 83 CA St Univ - Fullerton; MA 86 CA St Univ - Fullerton; **SLP**

Heerboth, Jill K 6805 North Cascade Spring, Tucson, AZ 85718, (602) 325-1571, BA 75 Valparaiso Univ; MS 79 Southern IL Univ -Carbondale; Sp-Lang Path, Crippled Childrens Cl, **SLP**

Heerde, Sally M 15 Wellington Drive, Hudson, MA 01749, (617) 446-6252, BA 74 Univ of NH; ME 77 Northeastern Univ; 84–Sp-Lang Path, Wellesley Public Schools, **SLP**

Heerey, Mary N 4560 Raven Lane, New Berlin, WI 53151, **SLP**

Heery, Mrs Anna R 1309 Greenbriar Lane, Darien, IL 60559, (312) 622-3626, BA 70 Saint Xavier Coll; MA 71 Northwestern Univ; ME 76 Univ of IL - Urbana; Sp-Lang Path, Chicago Bd of Ed, **SLP**

Hefferin, Amy Louise 599 West Washington Street, Grafton, WV 26354, (304) 265-3369, BS 83 WV Univ; MS 84 WV Univ; **SLP**

Heffernan, H Patricia 9730 Wilshire #212, Beverly Hills, CA 90212, (213) 275-9520, BA 60 CA St Univ - Los Angeles; MA 72 CA St Univ - Los Angeles; Aud, Hrng & Lang Spec Inc, **A F**

Heffernan, John W Heffernan Audiology Clinic, 1190 N W 95th Street, Miami, FL 33150, (305) 835-6322, BS 71 FL St Univ; MS 72 FL St Univ; Aud, Private Practice, **A**

Heffinger, Sharon Lynne Raleigh Speech & Hearing Ctr, Route 4 Box 630, Beckley, WV 25801, (304) 255-1337, BS 83 Radford Univ; MS 84 Radford Univ; Aud, Raleigh Speech & Hearing Ctr, **A**

Heffington, Mrs Mary F 4036 Graceland, Memphis, TN 38116, (901) 398-2576, BA 74 Memphis St Univ; MA 76 Memphis St Univ; Sp/Lang Path, Desoto Co Ms Publ Sch, **SLP**

Heffington, Rosalyn E 10831 Swan Glen Drive, Houston, TX 77099, BA 75 FL St Univ; MA 76 FL St Univ; 81–Dir of the Ind Living Prog, Houston ISD, **SLP**

Heffner, Dr David J 5527-C Ea-Lou ln, St Louis, MO 63128, **A**

Heffron, Geralyn M 717 South Mueller Street, Appleton, WI 54914, (414) 735-6256, BS 74 Univ of WI - Madison; MS 75 Univ of WI - Madison; Early Childhood-Een Teacher, Appleton Area Sch Dist, **SLP**

Heflick, Lamonte O 30862 Janet Street, Granger, IN 46530, **SLP**

Heflin, Kay Frances 4151 Liberty Lane, Marietta, GA 30066, BA 69 Univ of North TX; MA 71 Univ of Tulsa; Sp-Lang Path, Portland Pub Sch, **SLP**

Hefner, Pamela Sue 272 9th Avenue #A, San Francisco, CA 94118, (415) 921-7658, BA 84 CA St Univ - Chico; MA 86 CA St Univ - Chico

Heft, Mrs Julee H Leader Nsg And Rehab Ctr, 100 W Queen St, Dallastown, PA 17313, (717) 755-9526, MS 86 Towson St Univ; Dir Speech Therapy Svcs, Manor Care, **SLP**

Heft, Laurel C 655 Glenwyd Road, Bryn Mawr, PA 19010, **A**

Hegde, Dr M N Dept Communicative Disorders, California State Univ, Fresno, CA 93740, (209) 294-3938, BA 60 Univ of Mysore - India; MA 63 Univ of Mysore - India; PH 74 (Sp-Lang Path) Southern IL Univ -Carbondale; 80–Prof of Commun Dis, CA St U-Fresno, **SLP**

Hege, Mrs Gloria S 2702 Abilene Drive, Chevy Chase, MD 20815, (301) 585-5024, BA 70 George Washington Univ; MA 71 George Washington Univ; **SLP**

Hegemier, Lisa Renee 153 Concord Court, Norwalk, OH 44857, (419) 668-8101, BA 85 OH St Univ; MA 87 OH St Univ; 87–Aud, Fisher Titus Med Ctr, **A**

Hegler-Jackle, Cheri L 43415 Devin Drive, Mount Clemens, MI 48044, (313) 463-7336, BS 76 Western MI Univ; MA 81 Western MI Univ; Sp-Lang Path, Chippewa Valley Sch, **SLP**

Hegna, Wendy S 2220 4th Avenue N E #3, Menomonie, WI 54751, BS 83 Univ of WI - Stevens Point; MS 87 Univ of WI - Stevens Point; **SLP**

Hegwood, Mrs Merleen M 5253 Wayneland Drive, Jackson, MS 39211, (601) 981-3711, BS 70 Univ Southern MS-Hattiesburg; MS 71 Univ Southern MS-Hattiesburg; Sp-Lang Path, Speech/Language Therapy Ctr, **SLP**

Heiberger-Hammen, Vicki L 326 N E 54th Street, Seattle, WA 98105, (206) 545-7400, MS; **SLP**

Heide, Veronica 5727 Pembroke Drive, Madison, WI 53711, (608) 252-8219, BS 74 Marshall Univ; MS 77 Univ of WI - Madison; Coord of Aud Serv, Dean Med Cen Sc, **A**

Heidecker, Alan K RR 1 Box 15, Sioux Center, IA 51250, (712) 722-4374, BS 66 Univ of SD - Vermillion; MA 75 Univ of SD - Vermillion; Superv of Hrng & Hlth Serv, AEA 4, **A**

Heidelbach, Cora R R 2 Box 131, Creal Springs, IL 62922, MA 75 Southern IL Univ -Carbondale; 88–Supvr Sp-Lang Path, JAMP Spec Educ Svcs, **SLP**

Heidelberger, Tina E P O Box 401, Pentwater, MI 49449-0401, (201) 256-1700, **SLP**

Heideman, Barbara Smith 1300 North B Street, Indianola, IA 50125, (515) 961-8191, BA 73 Univ of Northern IA; MA 74 Univ of Northern IA; Sp-Lang Path, Heartland AEA, **SLP**

Heideman-Lenz, Diane 704 Montreal Place, De Pere, WI 54115, (414) 497-3886, BS 76 Univ of WI - Stevens Point; MS 78 Univ of WI - Eau Claire; 87–Sp-Lang Path, Green Bay Area PS, **SLP**

Heidemann, Kathleen 1323 Meadow Creek #203, Pewaukee, WI 53072, (414) 965-2414, BS 76 Univ of WI - Madison; MS 78 Univ of WI - Milwaukee; Sp-Lang Path, Kettle Moraine School District, **SLP**

Heiden, Sharon Denise 1961 Parkwild Road #129, Council Bluffs, IA 51501, (712) 322-7354, BS 83 Univ of WY; MS 85 Univ of WY; **A**

Heider, Mrs Katherine Box 2334, Columbia Falls, MT 59912, (406) 892-3130, BA 78 MI St Univ; MA 81 Univ of MT; Sp-Lang Path, Whitefish PS, **SLP**

Heidkamp, Mrs Sada G 6407 Heather Ridge Way, Oakland, CA 94611, (415) 836-8228, BA Wayne St Univ; MA Wayne St Univ; ME 54 Wayne St Univ; SLP, Oakland USD, **SLP**

Heidrich, Mrs Lorraine 49 Lantern Road, Hicksville, NY 11801, (516) 665-7772, BA 74 CUNY - Queens Coll; MA 76 CUNY - Queens Coll; 85–Sp-Lang Path, Suffolk Hearing & Speech Cen, **SLP**

Heidt, Sheryl Lee 45423 10th Street West, Apartment B, Lancaster, CA 93534, (805) 945-3784, BA 82 CA St Univ - Fresno; MA 86 CA St Univ - Fresno; SLP, Selma USD, **SLP**

Heidtman, Cathryn I Speech/Language Therapy Serv, 7863 Broadway Suite 107, Merrillville, IN 46410, (219) 769-8957, BA 75 Valparaiso Univ; MS 77 Purdue Univ - West Lafayette; Sp-Lang Path, Priv Practice, **SLP**

Heien, Marilyn J 3037 South 11th Street, Terre Haute, IN 47802, (317) 235-9891, BS 64 IN St Univ - Terre Haute; MS 68 IN St Univ - Terre Haute; **SLP**

Heighton, Mrs Sharon B P O Box 562, Pictou, NS, Canada B0K 1H0, (902) 755-5360, BS 78 Dalhousie Univ - Nova Scotia; MS 80 Dalhousie Univ - Nova Scotia; Sp-Lang Path, Pictou Dist Sch Bd, **SLP**

Heiko, Mrs Phyllis L 50 West 67th Street, New York, NY 10023, (212) 724-5028, BA 61; MS 70; Sp-Lang Path, Cty Sch Dist of Glen Cove, **SLP**

Heikoff, Raisa Ann 56 Wendy Drive, South Windsor, CT 06074, (203) 528-8428, MA 88 Univ of CT

Heikurinen, Mrs Catherine Tytaneck Chedoke McMaster Hospital, Dept Of Communication Dis, Box 2000, Hamilton, ON, Canada L8N 325, (416) 388-0240, **A**

Heil, Mrs Judith Meyer 1000 Hyland Drive, Stoughton, WI 53589, BS 75 Univ of WI - Stevens Point; MS 77 Univ of WI - Stevens Point; 85–Sp/Lang Path, Edgerton School Dist, **SLP**

Heilig, Barbara McConihe 108 East Jackson Street, Avon Park, FL 33825, (813) 382-1121, BA 49 Grinnell Coll; ME 69 Univ of South FL; 81–Program Specialist, Highlands Co Sch, **SLP**

Heilman, Colette M 132 Baker Street, Gardner, MA 01440, (508) 845-9111, BS 54 Indiana Univ of PA; ME 58 PA St Univ - Univ Park; 88–Sp-Lang Path, Glovin Reg Ctr, **SLP**

Heilman, Mrs Joanne Y 1024 Park Avenue, Pekin, IL 61554, (309) 346-7473, BS 70 Bradley Univ; MS 71 IL St Univ - Normal; Sp/Lang Path, Pekin Pub Sch Dist 108, **SLP**

Heilman, Mrs Susan N 3505 Stobart Road, Milford, MI 48042, (313) 684-8000, BS 63 Central MI Univ; MA 77 Wayne St Univ; SLP, Huron Valley Sch, **SLP**

Heim, Clareen 2651 North El Dorado Place, Chandler, AZ 85224, (602) 821-5008, BS 72 Saint Cloud St Univ; MS 75 Saint Cloud St Univ; 86–Sp-Lang Path, Mesa Pub Sch, **SLP**

Heim, Karen M 654 Bonnie View Drive, Evansville, IN 47715, (812) 473-0651, BS 71; MS 74; Sp/Lang Path, Karen Heim-Baugh Ms Ccc-Sp, **SLP**

Heiman, Sharon K 258 Lowell Avenue, Newtonville, MA 02160, (617) 965-4169, BA 68 Oberlin Coll; ME 71 Boston Univ; Sp-Lang Path, Edco Brookline-Nwton Presc Prog, **SLP**

Heimerle, Becki S 1172 1/2 South Oak Park Avenue, Oak Park, IL 60304, (312) 413-1831, BS 80 Eastern IL Univ; MS 81 Eastern IL Univ; Sp-Lang Path, Illinois Children's Sch Rehab Ctr, **SLP**

Heimrath, Karen 582 Eastbrooke Lane, Brighton, NY 14618, (716) 271-0680, BA 74 CUNY - Queens Coll; MS 76 Adelphi Univ; SLP, Hearing & Speech Center of Roc, **SLP**

Heimrich, Joan Ann 260 Linden Road, Wayne, NJ 07470, (201) 839-3317, BA 82 William Paterson Coll; MS 85 William Paterson Coll; 87–Sp-Lang Path, Bergen-Passac Assoc for Retarded Citizens, **SLP**

Hein, Barbara Phalen 2121 Tunis, Green Bay, WI 54311, (414) 497-3908, BS 75 Univ of WI - Stevens Point; MS 76 Univ of WI - Stevens Point; Sp-Lang Path, Green Bay Bd of Ed, **SLP**

Hein, Caroline Ann 1714 Bluegrass Court, Apartment #3, Owensboro, KY 42302, (502) 684-7454, BS 84 Eastern KY Univ; MS 86 Western KY Univ; **SLP**

Hein, Mrs Diane C 131 Columbus, Wilmington, OH 45177, (513) 382-1500, BS 78 Kent St Univ; MA 78 Kent St Univ; Sp-Lang Path, Private Practice, **SLP**

Hein, Herbert R 4561 Conrad Avenue, San Diego, CA 92117, (619) 576-5837, BA 75 SUNY - Center at Buffalo; OM 77 Emory Univ; SLP, Sp Hrng & Neuro Cen, **SLP**

Hein, Joanne Gerstein 4561 Conrad Avenue, San Diego, CA 92117, (619) 560-0973, BS 74 Ithaca Coll; MS 76 Univ of NC - Chapel Hill; Sp-Lang Path, Private Practice, **SLP**

Hein, Judith Ann 15 Seamist Circle, Newport Beach, CA 92663, **SLP**

Hein, Karen L 5081 Huckleberry N W, North Canton, OH 44720, (216) 499-0683, MA 86 Kent St Univ; 85–Sp-Lang Path, Canton City Schs, **SLP**

Hein, Dr Sally Lee Parkland Memorial Hospital, Educational Services, 5201 Harry Hines Boulevard, Dallas, TX 75235, (817) 565-2262, BS 73 Univ of Cincinnati; MA 74 Vanderbilt Univ; PH 80 (Sp Path) Memphis St Univ; Dir of Ed Serv, Parkland Mem Hosp, **SLP**

Heine, Mrs Kymberly Smith 1916 Bullard Avenue, Metairie, LA 70003, (504) 455-2449, BA 81 Univ of AR - Fayetteville; MS 83 PA St Univ - Univ Park; Sp-Lang Path, Private Practice, **SLP ACE**

Heine, Marilyn K 2852 Smoke Tree Circle, Stockton, CA 95209, (209) 473-5583, BA 75 CA St Univ - Sacramento; MA 77 CA St Univ - Stanislaus; SLP, Lincoln USD, **SLP**

Heineck, Kristine Marie N 5646 Sandpiper Drive, Onalaska, WI 54650, (608) 783-3606, BA 82 Univ of WI - Eau Claire; MS 83 Univ of WI - Eau Claire; Sp-Lang Path, Sch Dist of Slinger, **SLP**

Heino, Jean Marie 1341 Easter Lane, Eagan, MN 55123, (319) 291-3336, BA 78 Univ of IA; MA 83 Univ of IA; Sp-Lang Path, Minneapolis Public Schools, **SLP**

Heino, Pamela Sue 717 C N Irena Avenue, Redondo Beach, CA 90277, (213) 973-1300, BA 71 Univ of CA - Santa Barbara; MA 72 Univ of the Pacific; Coord/Special Education, ABC USD, **SLP**

Heinrich, Ann 146 Murray Street, Portland, ME 04103, (207) 773-3752, BS 78 Univ of WI - River Falls; MS 79 Univ of WI - Eau Claire; Sp/Lang Path, Private Practice, **SLP**

Heinrich, Dixie A 3117 28th, Great Bend, KS 67530, (316) 793-9071, BA 72 Fort Hays St Univ; MS 73 Fort Hays St Univ; Sp-Lang Path, Dixie A Heinrich MS CCC-SLP, **SLP ACE**

Heinrich, Jennifer Anne 7051 S W 8th Court, Plantation, FL 33317, (305) 654-9557, BA 86 Univ of FL; ME 88 Univ of FL

Heinrich, Richard Allen 5608 East Au Gres Avenue, Au Gres, MI 48703, (517) 876-7209, BS 77 Central MI Univ; MA 86 Central MI Univ; 88–Sp-Lang Path, Bay Arenac Inter Sch Dist, **SLP**

Heinrich, Mrs Sharon 48 Pilgrim Lane, Monsey, NY 10952-1518, **SLP**

Heins, Mrs Patricia P Box 998, 605 North Barstow Street, Eau Claire, WI 54701, (715) 839-4365, BS 57 Univ of WI - Madison; MA 81 Univ of Akron; **SLP**

Heinsen-Combs, Alexandra The Brooklyn Hospital, Speech & Hearing Center-OPD III, 121 DE Kalb Avenue, Brooklyn, NY 11201, (718) 403-8431, MA 83 NY Univ; Sp-Lang Path, Brooklyn Hospital, **SLP ACE**

Heintz, Heather Reneee 14612 Tirtle Creek Circle, #307, Lutz, FL 33549, (904) 567-8615, BS 84 Emory Univ; MS 87 Univ of South FL

Heintz, Janet Lynn 4841 North Mohawk #3, Milwaukee, WI 53217, (414) 962-2457, BA 80 Univ of WI - Milwaukee; BS 83 Univ of WI - Milwaukee; MS 85 Univ of WI - Milwaukee; 86–Sp-Lang Path, Rehab Assoc, **SLP**

Heintz, Laurene B P O Box 85, Chaseley, ND 58423, (701) 547-3296, BS 76 ND St Univ; MS 79 Univ of ND; Sp-Lang Path, Fessenden Public School, **SLP**

Heintzelman, Anne Teresa Department Of Communicative Disorders, University Of Wisconsin, 1975 Willow Drive, Madison, WI 53706, (608) 262-3951, BA 76 Washington Univ; MS 82 Univ of WI - Madison; Clin Instr, Univ of Wisc, **SLP**

Heinz, Carolyn Lake 5111 North New England, Chicago, IL 60656, (312) 971-0840, BS 78 Syracuse Univ; MS 80 Emory Univ; 86–Mktg Assoc, NM Head Injury System, **SLP**

Heinz, Dr John M John F Kennedy Institute, 707 North Broadway, Baltimore, MD 21205, (301) 522-5453, BS 55 Univ of SC - Columbia; MS 58 MA Inst of Tech; PH 62 (Communication Acoustics) MA Inst of Tech; 87–Actg Dir-Comm Sci & Disorders, John F Kennedy Institute

Heinz, Mrs Margaret M 13 Little Brook Lane, Jamesburg, NJ 08831, (201) 297-7800, BA 68 Trenton St Coll; MS 69 Rutgers St Univ - Newark; Sp-Lang Path, S Brunswick Township Bd of Ed, **SLP**

Heinze, Mrs Barbara A Augustana College, Bergendoff 64, Rock Island, IL 61201, (309) 794-7583, BA 68 Westminster Coll; MA 70 Northwestern Univ; PH (NS); Instructor & Clinical Superv, Augustana College, **SLP**

Heise, Mrs Cynthia D Hearing Center Of Broward Inc, 3170 North Federal Highway, Suite 208, Lighthouse Point, FL 33064, (305) 943-9020, BA 69 Univ of FL; MS 71 Univ of South FL; Aud/Owner, Hearing Center of Broward Inc, **A**

Heiser, Margaret 2972 Elm Tree Court, Spring Valley, CA 92078, (619) 465-4892, BS 70 Mankato St Univ; MA 75 Northeast MO St Univ; SLP, **SLP**

Heisler-Rapoff, Mrs Valerie A 19 North Ridge, Sherman, IL 62684, (217) 496-2423, BS 79 Univ of MO - Columbia; MA 80 Univ of MO - Columbia; 85–Sp-Lang Path, Springfield Sch Dist #186, **SLP**

Heisley, Nancy R 01616 SW Greenwood Road, Portland, OR 97219, (503) 636-9712, PH (NS); Assoc Prof, U of O Med Sch 66-72, **SLP**

Heisserer, Tina M 6729 North Euclid, Gladstone, MO 64118, (816) 454-2322, BS 84 Saint Louis Univ; OM 85 Univ of SC - Columbia; SLP, Whitehall Schools, **SLP**

Heisterkamp, Jean Christiansen 354 98th Avenue N E, Blaine, MN 55434, (612) 574-6580, BS 77 Univ of MN - Minneap-St Paul; MA 79 Univ of MN - Minneap-St Paul; 79–Sp-Lang Path, Columbia Heights MN Indp Sd 13, **SLP**

Heit, Mrs Barbara S 45 East 89th Street, New York, NY 10128, (212) 945-7100, BA 57 CUNY - Brooklyn Coll; MA 79 NY Univ; Chief Sp/Hrng, Peninsula Hosp Cen, **SLP**

Heitman, Dr Frederick Charlotte Speech & Hearing Ctr, 300 South Caldwell Street, Charlotte, NC 28202, (704) 376-1342, BA 68 Univ of NC - Chapel Hill; MA 74 Univ of FL; PH 80 (NS) Univ of FL; 87–Exec Dir, The Charlotte Sp & Hrng Cen, **SLP**

Heitman, Mrs Robin Marie N 8624 Sally Court, Spokane, WA 99208, (509) 838-2531, BS 82 Univ of TX - Austin; MA 85 Univ of TX - Austin; 87–Aud, Rockwood Clinic PS, **A**

Heitmann, Mrs Marceda Route 2 Box 414-B, Detroit Lakes, MN 56501, (218) 847-9268, BS 67 Minot St Univ; MS 69 Minot St Univ; Sp-Lang Path, Detroit Lakes Pub Sch Dist 22, **SLP**

Heitschmidt, Larry Dean Box 55, Wahkon, MN 56386, (612) 689-2121, BA 57 Fort Hays St Univ; Sp-Lang Path, Cambridge School District 911, **SLP**

Heitz, Ann A S 500 Woodmont Drive, Charlottesville, VA 22901, (804) 295-0144, BA 75 Mary Washington Coll; ME 76 Univ of VA - Charlottesville; SLP, Charlottesville Pub Schs, **SLP**

Heitzman, Mrs Linda J Rd 3 Box 2344, Lafayette, NJ 07848, (201) 579-2031, BS 75 West Chester Univ of PA; MA 79 Seton Hall Univ; Sp/Lang Path, Dover Pub Sch, **SLP**

Heizelman, Mrs Jody Kay Box 65, Buhler, KS 67522, (316) 543-6822, BA 86 Wichita St Univ; MA 87 Wichita St Univ

Hekel, Mrs Marie-Louise Ann 4 Bellaire Court, Beaumaris, Victoria, Australia 3193, (03) 584-8573, BA 68 CUNY - City College; MA 69 Columbia Univ Teachers Coll; 88–Aud, Hrng Diagnostic & Rsch Ctr, **A**

Hekman, Mrs Carol Ann 277 Deacon Haynes Road, Concord, MA 01742, (617) 369-4500, BA 69 William Paterson Coll; MA 70 MI St Univ; Sp-Lang Path, Private Practice, **SLP**

Helbach, Mary T 311 Howe, Seattle, WA 98109, (206) 587-6486, BA 75 Univ of WA; BA 80 Univ of WA; OM 82 Univ of WA; SLP, Seattle Pub Sch, **SLP**

Helbert, Fredia Wise County School Board, Box 1217, Wise, VA 24230, (703) 328-8017, BS 76 King Coll; MS 80 FL St Univ; Aud, Wise Co Sch Bd, **A**

Held, Donald Theodore 3125 Stafford Lane, Florissant, MO 63033, (314) 831-8355, BS 60 Southeast MO St Univ; MS 71 Southern IL Univ-Edwardsvill; Retired, Spec Sch Dist of St Louis Co, **SLP**

Held, Mrs Judith M United Cerebral Palsy Of Nyc, 122 East 23rd Street, New York, NY 10010, (212) 677-7400, BA 51 Univ of MN - Minneap-St Paul; MA 68 Columbia Univ Teachers Coll; Prog Dir, UCP of NYC, **SLP**

Held, Roberta J 30 East Gate Lane, Hamden, CT 06514, (203) 753-8334, BS 75 Ithaca Coll; MA 77 Univ of Denver; Sp-Lang Path, Private Practice, **SLP**

Held, Mrs Stephena D 6548 Kenwater Avenue, Canoga Park, CA 91307, (213) 884-0622, BA 79 CA St Univ - Northridge; MA 81 CA St Univ - Northridge; Super Sp-Lang Path, Commun Sp & Hrng, **SLP**

Heldstab, Mrs Peggy S 1942 Sunflower, Junction City, KS 66441, (913) 238-8859, BS 79 Wayne St Coll; MS 81 Univ of NE - Lincoln; 83–Sp-Lang Path, Geary County USD #475, **SLP**

Heleotis Rn, Joni Lee 901 Interlaken Avenue, Wanamassa, NJ 07712, (201) 531-3351, OM 82 Seton Hall Univ; BS 75 Rutgers St Univ - Newark; MS 80 Univ of PA; **SLP**

Helfenstein, Sheila Darlene 915 9th Street S W, Jamestown, ND 58401, (701) 252-4100, BA 81 Univ of ND; MS 83 Moorhead St Univ; 86–Sp-Lang Path, Speech and Hearing Svcs Inc, **SLP**

Helfer, Karen S Dept Of Communication Disorder, Univ Of Massachusetts, Amherst, MA 01003, (413) 545-2565, BS 82 Boston Univ; MA 83 IN Univ - Bloomington; PH 88 (Aud/Hrng Impairment) Northwestern Univ; 88–Asst Prof, Univ of MA, **A**

Helfer, Dr Thomas M P O Box 1428, Lewisville, TX 75067, (214) 436-8864, BA 69 Univ of TX - Austin; MA 70 Our Lady Lake Univ-San Anton; PH 81 (NS) Univ of TX - Dallas; **A**

Helfman, Mrs Karen Epstein 2087 Ashbury Drive, Harrisburg, PA 17112, (717) 255-1010, BS 80 Ithaca Coll; MS 82 Hahneman Medical Coll; MS 82 Hahnemann Univ Grad Sch; VP, Tri-County United Way-New Markets, **SLP**

Helfrecht, Mrs Paula Jean 1352 Chillem Drive, Batavia, IL 60510, (312) 406-1982, BS 84 Univ of WI - Madison; MS 86 Univ of WI - Milwaukee; 88–Sp-Lang Path, W Aurora Sch Dist #129, **SLP**

Helfrich, Deborah A 6717 Valley Drive, Raleigh, NC 27612, (919) 846-8383, BA 77 Montclair St Coll; MS 81 Univ of HI - Manoa; Sp/Lang Path, **SLP**

Helfrich-Miller, Dr Kathleen R 508 Bellevue Terrace, Pittsburgh, PA 15202, (412) 761-6062, BA 76 Univ of Pittsburgh - Pittsburgh; MS 77 Univ of Pittsburgh - Pittsburgh; PH 83 (Sp Path/Aud) Univ of Pittsburgh - Pittsburgh; Dir, Rehab Spec Inc, **SLP**

Helland, Martha R 1318 Woodstock, Ames, IA 50010, (515) 792-4870, BA 75 Univ of Northern IA; MA 76 Univ of Northern IA; SLP, Heartland AEA, **SLP**

Hellen, Julia Kirwan 5451 Northeast River Road, Apartment 300, Chicago, IL 60656, (312) 687-7200, BS 82 IL St Univ - Normal; MS 84 Eastern IL Univ; **SLP**

Heller, Mrs Audrey B 1120 Nancy Street, Bloomington, IN 47401, (812) 855-5166, BS 54 Boston Univ; MS 59 PA St Univ - Univ Park; Lecturer, IN U Dept of Sp & Hrng Sci, **SLP**

Heller, Francie H 119 Valley Road, New Rochelle, NY 10804, (914) 636-0666, BS 66 Boston Univ; MS 67 Univ of GA; OM 81 Fordham Univ; Director of Special Services, Ossining Sch Dist, **SLP**

Heller, Mrs Gaye G Rd 2 Box 90, Hawes Road, Altamont, NY 12009, (518) 861-6450, BS 80 Coll of Saint Rose; MS 82 Coll of Saint Rose; Sp-Lang Path, Cerebral Palsy Ctr for Disable, **SLP**

Heller, James H 1308 Willow Drive, Chapel Hill, NC 27514, (919) 684-5513, BA 75 Luther Coll; MS 81 Memorial Univ - Newfoundland; MA 79 Univ of MN - Minneap-St Paul; SLP, Lenox Baker Hosp, **SLP**

Heller, Janet Sue N 130 East 18th Street #2A, Manhattan, NY 10003, **SLP**

Heller, Dr Joyce C Dept Speech Path & Audiology, Kean College, Union, NJ 07083, (201) 527-2218, BS 52 Syracuse Univ; MA 54 CUNY - Brooklyn Coll; PH 68 (NS) NY Univ; Prof, Kean Coll of Nj, **SLP F ACE**

Heller, Mrs Judith A 526 Brook Road, Towson, MD 21204, (301) 825-4445, BA 80 Loyola Coll; MS 81 Loyola Coll; 86–Sp-Lang Path, Balto Co PS, **SLP**

Heller, Lisa Lethin 1173 Kent Avenue, Sunnyvale, CA 94087, (408) 243-9502, BA 75 Univ of CA - Berkeley; MS 81 San Francisco St Univ; Sp-Lang Path Consult, Private Practice, **SLP**

Heller, Meryl A 50 Rantoul Street #108 South, Beverly, MA 01915, (617) 745-2100, BA 73 CUNY - Queens Coll; MS 74 Univ of MI - Ann Arbor; 87–Asst Dir, North Shore Childrens Hosp, **SLP**

Heller, Nancy 6020 California Circle, Apt 409, Rockville, MD 20852, (202) 745-5600, BS 85 Syracuse Univ; MA 87 NY Univ; 88–Sp-Lang Path, Children's Hosp Natl Med Ctr, **SLP**

Heller, Naomi C 919 Santa Monica Boulevard, Suite 210, Santa Monica, CA 90401, (213) 393-1503, BA 70; MA 78 CA St Univ - Northridge; Owner Adm, Private Practice, **SLP**

Heller, Mrs Pamela G 182 Gallinson Drive, Murray Hill, NJ 07974, (201) 665-2316, BS 68 OH St Univ; ME 69 Univ of VA - Charlottesville; 88–Sp-Lang Path, Springfield PS-Spec Svcs, **SLP**

Heller, Mrs Susan Goebel ENT & Head & Neck Surgeons Inc, 3545 Olentangy River Road, Suite 525, Columbus, OH 43214, (614) 267-2587, BS 81 OH Univ - Athens; MA 82 OH Univ - Athens; Aud, ENT Head & Neck Surg Inc, **A**

Heller, Tracy Denise c/o Bayer, Rd 5 Box 5435, Fleetwood, PA 19522-9348, BA 84 Kutztown Univ of PA; MA 86 Temple Univ-Tyler Sch of Art; **SLP**

Heller, Mrs Wendy Jacobson 2499 Locust Avenue, North Bellmore, NY 11710-1735, (516) 883-9224, Sp-Lang Path, BOCES, **SLP**

Heller-Ringer, Mrs Donna L 20552 Brian Crescent #1, Bayside, NY 11360, (718) 352-9091, BA 77 CUNY - City College; MS 78 PA St Univ - Univ Park; Sp-Lang Path, Private Practice, **SLP**

Hellesto, Pamela J P O Box 652, Garibaldi, OR 97118-0652, (503) 322-0254, BA 84 WA St Univ; MA 85 WA St Univ, Sp-Lang Path, Tillamok County Esd, **SLP**

Helling, Celeste Rita 400 Timbercreek Drive, Apartment 1106, Richwood, TX 77531, (409) 265-6186, BS 84 Univ of North TX; MA 86 Univ of North TX

Hellinga, Jewel 121 Belvedere Street, Apartment A, San Francisco, CA 94117-3915, (415) 681-3569, BS 82 CA St Univ - Hayward; MS 84 CA St Univ - Hayward; SLP, South San Francisco USD, **SLP**

Hellman, Mrs Hilary 1304 15th Street, Suite 203, Santa Monica, CA 90404, (213) 393-4773, MA 75 San Diego St Univ; Private Practice, **SLP**

Hellman, Laurie Jean 863 East Huber Street, Mesa, AZ 85203, (602) 844-9840, BS 83 Northern AZ Univ; MS 85 Northern AZ Univ; Sp-Lang Path, Mesa Public Schools, **SLP**

Hellman, Rhona Phyllis Northeastern University, Auditory Perception Lab, Dept Of Psychology, Boston, MA 02115, (617) 437-4696, MS; Audiologist, Veterans Administration

Hellmer, Jill F N 522 Dapin Road, Madison, WI 53704, (608) 249-6927, BS 67 Miami Univ - Oxford; MA 69 OH Univ - Athens; **A**

Hellreich, J Miriam Kailua Professional Center Ii, Suite 311, 40 Aulike Street, Kailua, HI 96734, (808) 262-9222, BA 65 Univ of AL- Tuscaloosa; MA 71 Univ of AL- Tuscaloosa; Sp-Lang Path, Sp & Lang Path Svcs, **SLP ACE**

Hellrigel, Diane Patricia 12 Lani Court, Freehold, NJ 07728, (201) 462-4059, MS 88 Rutger's St Univ - Douglas Coll

Hellwege, Eileen W 524 Round Table Drive, Nazareth, PA 18064, (201) 689-6421, BA 75 CUNY - Queens Coll; MA 79 Hofstra Univ; Sp-Lang Path, Norwescap-Headstart, **SLP**

Hellwig, Robin Kay P O Box 402, Limon, CO 80828-0402, (719) 775-9564, BS 86 Univ of SD - Vermillion; MA 87 Univ of SD - Vermillion; 88–Sp-Lang Path, East Central BOCES

Helm, Alexis 836 Stoneman Way, El Dorado Hills, CA 95630, BA 70 CA St Univ - Los Angeles; MA 72 CA St Univ - Los Angeles; SLP, **SLP**

Helm, Mrs Alice M 2302 Stonewall Drive, Macungie, PA 18062, (215) 395-1325, BS 54 Bowling Green St Univ; OM 77 Drew Univ; Sp-Lang Path, Lehigh Val Soc Crip Chldn & Ad, **SLP**

Helm, Barbara J 40 Rabbit Run, Glenmoore, PA 19343, (215) 942-5914, BA 65 Loyola Coll; Sp/Lang Path, Devereux Found, **SLP**

Helm, Mrs Vicki B Lucerne Route Box 302, Thermopolis, WY 82443, (307) 864-2171, BS 76 Univ of WY; MS 77 Univ of WY; Sp-Lang Path, Big Horn Basin Chldn's Cen, **SLP**

Helman, Lori Dee 26100 West 12 Mile Road, Apartment 341, Southfield, MI 48034, (313) 423-8678, BA 81 Univ of MI - Ann Arbor; MS 83 Univ of MI - Ann Arbor; **SLP**

Helman, Sally Eberly 467 East Market Street, Marietta, PA 17547, (717) 771-2380, BS 79 Indiana Univ of PA; MA 81 Adams St Coll; Sp-Lang Path, Ed Assessment Syst Inc, **SLP**

Helmer, Marie C Route 2 Box 12, Yoncalla, OR 97499, (503) 440-4764, BS 69 Univ of OR; MS 77 Univ of OR; SLP, Douglas Co ESD, **SLP**

Helmer, Mrs Penney Lynn 8233 48th Street, Hudsonville, MI 49426, (616) 361-3470, MA 84 Western MI Univ; 85–Sp-Lang Path, Northern PS, **SLP**

Helmers, Donna Lane 738 Brook Hollow Road, Nashville, TN 37205, (615) 386-6671, BA 81 Univ of FL; ME 82 Univ of FL; 88–Sp-Lang Path, St Thomas Hosp, **SLP**

Helm-Estabrooks, Dr Nancy 128 St Marys Street, Boston, MA 02115, (617) 232-9500, BA 62 Univ of MA - Amherst; ME 72 Northeastern Univ; OD 79 (NS) Boston Univ; Ch Aud/Sp-Path, VA Med Cen-Boston, **SLP ACE**

Helmick, Mrs Cynthia J 3031 Glacier, Casper, WY 82604, (307) 235-2888, BS 75 Univ of SD - Vermillion; MA 76 Univ of SD - Vermillion; Sp-Lang Path, Natrona Co Sch Dist No 1, **SLP**

Helmick, Dr Joseph W Miller Speech & Hearing Clinic, Texas Christian University, P O Box 30793, Fort Worth, TX 76129, (817) 921-7621, BA 61 WV Univ; MA 62 WV Univ; PH 68 (Sp-Lang Path) Univ of WA; 88–Assoc Dean, Texas Christian U, **SLP F**

Helminski, Carole A 4610 47th Street N W, Washington, DC 20016, **SLP**

Helmke, Mrs Carla S 5820 Summit, Sylvania, OH 43560, (419) 882-0555, OB 76 Univ of Toledo; BA 76 Univ of Toledo; MA 78 NM St Univ; Sp-Lang Path, Sylvania City Schools, **SLP**

Helms, Dr Beverly P O Box 728, Bonifay, FL 32425, (904) 638-7222, BA 66 FL St Univ; MS 70 FL St Univ; ED 82 (NS) FL St Univ; Dir of Admin Serv, Washington Co Sch Bd, **SLP**

Helms, Deborah D 6019 Hanna Court, Charlotte, NC 28212, (704) 788-5847, BS 79 Appalachian St Univ; MA 80 Univ of TN - Knoxville; Aud, Cabarrus Mem Hosp, **A**

Helms, Mrs Donna Strickland Route 1 Box 172-Bc, Geneva, AL 36340, (205) 684-2294, BS 85 Auburn Univ - Auburn; OM 86 Auburn Univ - Auburn; 87–Sp-Lang Path, Geneva City Schs, **SLP**

Helms, Suzanne B 69 Prospect Street, Portland, ME 04103, (207) 772-2660, BA 70 Univ of ME - Orono; MA 71 Univ of ME - Orono; 83–Sp-Lang Path, Private Practice, **SLP**

Helms, William A 126 South Russell Avenue, Ames, IA 50010, (515) 232-7583, BA 75 Univ of TN - Knoxville; MA 77 Univ of TN - Knoxville; 86–Aud, Heartland AEA, **A**

Helmsing, Theresa Ann 1437 Rustic Drive, Bldg 47 Apartment 9, Ocean, NJ 07712, (201) 774-2208, BA 82 Ball St Univ; MA 84 Ball St Univ; 87–Aud, American Hrng Aid Ctr, **A**

Helpa, David P 19 Heritage Drive, Oxford, MA 01540, (508) 365-4531, BS 77 Worcester St Coll; MS 79 Rutgers St Univ -N Brunswick; 88–Dir of Rehabilitation, Clinton Hosp Sp Lang Hrng Cen, **SLP A**

Helsabeck, Mary R 710 Elberon Avenue, Absecon, NJ 08201, PH 72 (Sp Path Lang Focus) IN Univ - Bloomington; Sp-Lang Path, The Marsh School, **SLP**

Helton, Beverly Gean 2452 Pocahontas Place, St Louis, MO 63144, (314) 962-6824, BS 74 Southeast MO St Univ; MA 82 Univ of MO - Columbia; Sp/Lang Path, St Louis Co Spec Sch Dist, **SLP**

Helton, Mrs Elizabeth Sammer 265 Chimney Top Dr, Antioch, TN 37013, (615) 340-1905, BA 82 IN Univ - Bloomington; MA 84 IN Univ - Bloomington; Sp-Lang Path, Parkview Med Ctr, **SLP**

Helton, John R 608 North Park Avenue, Tifton, GA 31794, (912) 382-0623, BA 71 Univ of KY; MA 74 Univ of TN - Knoxville; Sp-Lang Path, Private Practice, **SLP ACE**

Helton, Mrs Rebecca Elsarelli 1943 Willow Hill Drive, Harrisonburg, VA 22801, (703) 433-1864, BS 81 James Madison Univ; MS 83 James Madison Univ; Sp-Lang Path, Rockingham County PS, **SLP**

Helton, Mrs Sally G 19003 Lowell, Stilwell, KS 66085, (913) 897-3702, OB 75 Univ of KS; MS 78 Southern IL Univ -Carbondale; 84–Sp-Lang Path, Chldrns Mercy Hosp, **SLP**

Helwig, Mrs Mary M K 20128 Lake Chabot Road, Castro Valley, CA 94546, (415) 784-4453, BA 78 CA St Univ - Sacramento; MA 79 CA St Univ - Sacramento; Audiologist, Kaiser Permanente Medical Group, **A**

Hembd, Mrs Bonita M 3108 East Avenue #R-7, Palmdale, CA 93550, (805) 273-5510, BA 74 Eastern WA Univ; MS 75 Eastern WA Univ; **SLP**

Hembree, Mrs Margaret E 2913 Janet Circle, Arlington, TX 76013, (817) 274-4590, BS 60 Univ of UT; MS 61 Univ of UT; **SLP LM**

Hemeyer, Thomas F 3805 Thornburg, Muncie, IN 47302, (317) 285-8175, BA 64 Eastern MI Univ; MA 67 Univ of WA; PH 71 (NS) Univ of MI - Ann Arbor; Coord of Aud, Ball St U Sp/Lang/Hrng Cl, **A**

Heminger-Cowell, Mrs Laurie Jean Community Services, 1 Stranahan Square #342, Toledo, OH 43604, (419) 241-6219, BA 84 OH St Univ; MA 87 Cleveland St Univ; 87–Aud, Toledo Hearing & Speech Ctr, **A**

Hemingway, Karen Louise 500 West Hobbs, Roswell, NM 88201, (612) 255-9923, BS 76 Mankato St Univ; MS 85 Saint Cloud St Univ; Sp-Lang Path, Rowell Independent School Dist, **SLP**

Hemm, Dr Margaret E M 865 Ridgefield Road, Birmingham, AL 35215, (205) 854-5589, BS 79 Univ of Montevallo; MS 80 Univ of Montevallo; ED 87 (Admin & Super of Sp Path & Aud) Univ of AL- Tuscaloosa; 87–Clinical Supervisor, InSpeech Inc, **SLP ACE**

Hemmerlein, Mrs Vicki Diane 31736 Crossbow, Birmingham, MI 48010, (717) 533-5692, **SLP**

Hempe, Deidre Marie 4141 Beard Avenue South, Minneapolis, MN 55410-1012, (612) 535-6171, **SLP**

Hempel, Blanche V 28 Spring Terrace, Greenfield, MA 01301, (413) 743-3242, BA 65 Univ of MA - Boston; MA 64 Univ of MA - Boston; Sp-Lang Path, S P Franklin Rehab Ctr, **SLP**

Hempel, Mrs Nancy J C 122 Sunnybrae Court, Martinez, CA 94553, (415) 370-9707, BS 77 Univ of KS; MA 79 Memphis St Univ; **SLP**

Hemphill, Mrs Maureen Kay 7501 N W 76th Terrace, Kansas City, MO 64152, (816) 741-2100, MA 84 KS St Univ; Sp-Lang Path, Park Hill R-5 School District, **SLP**

Hemphill, Rhonda H 5020 Goddard Avenue, Orlando, FL 32804, (407) 299-1533, OB 75 Univ of FL; MS 76 Vanderbilt Univ; 81–Dir, Cen for Sp Lang, **SLP ACE**

Hemphill, Mrs Sandra J 1505 Hayselton Drive, Jefferson City, MO 65101, (314) 474-5165, BA 79 Univ of MO - KS City; MA 80 Northeast MO St Univ; Sp-Lang Path, Jefferson City Public Schools, **SLP**

Hempstead, Megan P O Box 279, Alameda, CA 94501-9379, (415) 522-6700, BA 65 San Francisco St Univ; BA 79 CA St Univ - Sacramento; MA 82 CA St Univ - Sacramento; Special Day Class Teacher, Alameda USD, **SLP**

Hemsath, Melissa Beth 13431 Byars, Grandview, MO 64030, (816) 942-7200, BA 85 Univ of Northern IA; MA 87 Univ of Northern IA; 87–Aud, Old Westport Med Assoc Inc, **A**

Henagan, Mrs Deanne C 2417 Taylor Drive, Adrian, MI 49221, (517) 263-8931, BA 66 Southern Univ - Baton Rouge; MA 67 Univ of MO - Columbia; Sp-Lang Path, Lenawee ISD, **SLP**

Henaghen, Jill Ann 220-55 46th Avenue, Bayside, NY 11361, (516) 354-5412, BA 62 CUNY - Brooklyn Coll; MA 68 CUNY - Brooklyn Coll; Dir, Sp-Lang-Hrng Cen of Lg Island, **SLP**

Henchey, Cara Elaine 1294 Hadcock Road #103, Brunswick, OH 44212, (216) 225-1657, BS 84 Miami Univ - Oxford; MS 86 Vanderbilt Univ; **SLP**

Hendel, Deborah 201 East 25th Street, New York, NY 10010, (718) 629-2960, **SLP**

Hendelman, Mrs Ruth S 3816 Lands End, Fort Worth, TX 76109, (214) 328-8445, BS 67 Univ of TX - Austin; MA 71 Univ of North TX; Aud, Dr Jerry Sudderth MD/Facs, **A ACE**

Henderlite, Mrs Patricia B 316 Abbotsford Court, Charlotte, NC 28226, BA 69 Univ of NC - Greensboro; ME 72 Univ of NC - Greensboro; Sp-Lang Path, Charlotte Mecklenburg Sch Syst, **SLP**

Henderson, Alice H 102-475 Groves Avenue, Kelowna, BC, Canada V1Y 4Y6, (604) 762-2525, BA 76 Univ of MN - Minneap-St Paul; MS 77 Univ of NM; Owner/Sp-Lang Path, Okanagan Sp & Lang, **SLP**

Henderson, Alicia Box 50 Behr Avenue, San Francisco, CA 94131, (415) 564-0245, BA 79 Humboldt St Univ; MA 80 Humboldt St Univ; Sp-Lang Path, U of CA, **SLP**

Henderson, Amy Kathleen 9527 Tarryton, Whittier, CA 90605, (213) 693-3183, BA 83 Biola Univ; MA 86 CA St Univ - Fullerton; 88, **SLP**

Henderson, Mrs Barbara A 1539 Belmont Avenue, San Carlos, CA 94070, (415) 991-1230, BA 79 CA St Univ - Sacramento; MA 80 Univ of the Pacific; SLP, San Mateo City Sch Dist, **SLP**

Henderson, Dr Barbara C 19525 Normandale Avenue, Cerritos, CA 90701, (213) 402-7951, BA 72 Denison Univ; OD 78 (NS) Johns Hopkins Univ; **A**

Henderson, Carol A 5425 Logan Avenue South, Minneapolis, MN 55419, (612) 929-7035, BA 73 Univ of MN - Minneap-St Paul; MA 75 Univ of MN - Minneap-St Paul; SLP, Minneapolis Pub Sch, **SLP**

Henderson, Carol L 1546 North Shamrock, Upland, CA 91786, **SLP**

Henderson, Carol Williams 348 Ridgecrest, Seguin, TX 78155, (512) 557-6376, BS 84 Southwest TX St Univ; MS 86 Southwest TX St Univ

Henderson, Cathy 765 Stonewall, Memphis, TN 38107, (901) 274-3236, **SLP**

Henderson, Cathy Crow 1013 South Center, Lonoke, AR 72086, (501) 661-5878, BS 69 AR St Univ; MS 80 Univ of AR - Little Rock; Aud, U of AR-Med Sci, **A**

Henderson, Mrs Cathy G 215 Camden Street, Slidell, LA 70461, (504) 641-4752, BS 72 LA St Univ - Baton Rouge; MA 74 LA St Univ - Baton Rouge; 86–Dir/Sp-Lang Path, Children's Sp/Lang/Hrng Ctr, **SLP**

Henderson, Christine D 555 Stanhope Court, Naperville, IL 60565, (312) 983-9708, BS 76 AZ St Univ; OM 80 LA St Univ - N O Medical Ctr; **SLP**

Henderson, Dana Paige 107 Hermit's Trail, Altamonte Springs, FL 32701, (407) 834-9120, BA 84 Univ of FL; MA 86 Univ of Central FL; 88–Aud, Central FL Hrng Ctr, **A**

Henderson, Mrs Diane L 11 Buttermilk Drive, New Windsor, NY 12550, (914) 565-6156, BA 77 CUNY - Lehman Coll; MS 79 Columbia Univ Teachers Coll; 85–Sp/Lang Path, Newburgh Dev Lrng Cen, **SLP**

Henderson, Dr Donald SUNY At Buffalo, Communicative Dis & Sci, 109 Park Hall, Buffalo, NY 14260, (716) 636-3400, BS 62 Western WA Univ; PH 66 (NS) Univ of TX - Austin; Sp-Lang Path, Univ of Buffalo

Henderson, Dorita 63-61 99th Street #F-17, Rego Park, NY 11374, (212) 897-8890, BS 76 CUNY - Queens Coll; MS 78 Columbia Univ Teachers Coll; **SLP**

Henderson, Isabel C R R 2 Box 9 Site 206, St Albert, AB, Canada T8N 1M9, **SLP**

Henderson, Jana L 2105 North 6th St Terrace, Blue Springs, MO 64015, (816) 229-4685, BA 73 Univ of MO - Columbia; MA 74 Univ of MO - Columbia; Dir of Spec Ed, Grain Valley Rv Sch Dist, **SLP**

Henderson, Jennifer Speech Hearing & Language Cntr, Morton Hospital, 88 Washington Street, Taunton, MA 02780, (508) 824-6911, BA 75 OH Wesleyan Univ; MS 77 Univ of MI - Ann Arbor; 86–Dir, Sp-Hrng-Lang Ctr, **SLP**

Henderson, Julie Hallenbeck 109 Pine Court, P O Box 175, Whitewater, KS 67154, (316) 321-2780, BA 75 Wichita St Univ; MA 76 Wichita St Univ; **SLP**

Henderson, Juliet M 12720 Canario Way, Los Altos Hills, CA 94022, (415) 941-8018, BS 68 Purdue Univ - West Lafayette; MA 72 San Francisco St Univ; Sp/Lang Path, Chldn Hosp Stanford Rehab Cen, **SLP**

Henderson, Kathryn Ann 3326 East Overlook, Cleveland Heights, OH 44118, (216) 321-4965, BS 83 Bowling Green St Univ; MS 85 Univ of MI - Ann Arbor; 87–Sp-Lang Path, Cleveland-Univ Heights Sch Dist, **SLP**

Henderson, Leesa Simons 3019 Stearns, Wichita Falls, TX 76308, (817) 322-0771, BA 79 Midwestern St Univ; MA 81 Univ of North TX; Sp-Lang Path, North Texas Easter Seal Center, **SLP**

Henderson, Mrs Leslie Jones 2405 Miller Drive, Niles, MI 49120, (616) 471-2891, BS 66 Ball St Univ; MA 86 Western MI Univ

Henderson, Mrs Linda McRae 2317 Putnam Drive, Clovis, NM 88101, (505) 763-4114, BS 84 FL St Univ; MS 85 FL St Univ; Sp-Lang Path, Orange County Public Schools, **SLP**

Henderson, Lori J 1606 North 17th Street, Apartment 14, Mount Vernon, IL 62864, (618) 242-4998, BA 86 IN Univ - Bloomington; MA 87 Western IL Univ; Southern IL Educ Services Ctr

Henderson, Mari Koda 68 Cuesta Vista Drive, Monterey, CA 93940, (408) 375-6212, BA 86 Univ of CA - Santa Barbara; MA 87 Univ of the Pacific

Henderson, Myrna Longacre Elementary School, 34850 Arundel Road, Farmington Hills, MI 48024, BS 57 Central MI Univ; BA 70 Eastern MI Univ; **SLP**

Henderson, Mrs Nancy Biery 34 Forrest Glade, North Little Rock, AR 72116, MS 83 Univ of AR - Little Rock; SLP, N Little Rock Public Schools, **SLP**

Henderson, Mrs Nancy C 45736 Peck-Wadsworth, Wellington, OH 44090, (216) 647-3636, BA 76 Cleveland St Univ; MA 77 Cleveland St Univ; 77–SLP, Wellington Exempted Village Sch, **SLP ACE**

Henderson, Mrs Pamela Jackson Division Of Speech & Hearing Sciences Clinic, University Of North Carolina, Box 7190, Chapel Hill, NC 27599, (919) 966-1006, BS 73 Univ of TN - Knoxville; MA 74 Univ of TN - Knoxville; 88–Clin Instr, Univ of North Carolina, **SLP**

Henderson, Mrs Patricia 2928 Eastland Avenue, Baton Rouge, LA 70808, (504) 343-4232, BS 69 LA St Univ - Baton Rouge; MA 75 LA St Univ - Baton Rouge; SLP, Baton Rouge Sp/Hrng Foundation, **SLP**

Henderson, Mrs Patricia Callahan 358 Spring Street, West Bridgewater, MA 02379, (617) 584-5347, BS 78 Univ of MA - Amherst; ME 80 Northeastern Univ; Aud, Richard H Fitton MD Inc, **A**

Henderson, Rebecca W 501 80th Street South, Birmingham, AL 35206, (205) 322-1919, BS 62 Univ of Montevallo; 79–Sp-Lang Path, Birmingham Bd of Ed, **SLP**

Henderson, Sandra M 1491 Yonge Street #204, Toronto, ON, Canada M4T 1Z4, (416) 927-9357, BA 60 Univ of Toronto - Ontario; OM 62 Univ of Toronto - Ontario; MA 65 Western MI Univ; Sp-Lang Path, Private Practice, **SLP**

Henderson, Terri Siegel 4734 Boncrest East, Williamsville, NY 14221, (716) 633-4421, BA 71 Univ of WI - Madison; MA 73 Univ of CT; 88–Aud, Lang Dev Prog, **A**

Henderson, Terry L 67 Annawan Road, Waban, MA 02168, **SLP**

Hendler-Lederer, Mrs Susan G 2 Bay Club Drive #17C East, Bayside, NY 11360-2919, (718) 225-5446, BS 79 NY Univ; MA 81 NY Univ; 84–Coord of Therapy Svcs, Stepping Stone Day Sch, **SLP**

Hendren, Mrs Jan Plyler Route 22 Box 4761, Lexington, NC 27292-7856, (919) 764-0360, BS 83 Western Carolina Univ; ME 84 Western Carolina Univ; SLP, Davidson County Schools, **SLP**

Hendrich, Betty G 5624 Candia Court, Mobile, AL 36609, (205) 661-0667, BS 80 Univ of South AL; MS 81 Univ of Montevallo; Sp/Lang Path, Private Practice, **SLP**

Hendrick, Lynn S 3708 Brighton Drive, Bryan, TX 77802, (409) 822-0193, **SLP**

Hendrick, Mrs Nancy A M 151 Ledgewood Circle, Rochester, NY 14615, (716) 225-4120, MS 80 SUNY - Coll at Geneseo; SLP, Greece Cen Sch Dist, **SLP**

Hendricks, Mrs Barbara Rodier 98 Thayer Street RFD #2, Blackstone, MA 01504, (508) 679-7026, BS 77 Univ of MA - Amherst; MA 79 Univ of MA - Amherst; Mgr Dept of Communications Dis, Charlton Memorial Hospital, **SLP**

Hendricks, Betsy A 5789 Arroyo Vista, Rockford, MI 49341, (616) 874-9408, BA 76 MI St Univ; MA 77 MI St Univ; Sp-Lang Path, Mary Free Bed Hosp & Rehab Ctr, **SLP ACE**

Hendricks, Mrs Carolyn G 2466 Indian Tree Circle, Glencoe, MO 63038, (312) 888-5192, BS 66 Northern IL Univ - De Kalb; MA 69 Univ of IL - Urbana; Sp/Lang Path, U-46 Sch Dist, **SLP**

Hendricks, Mrs Donna E 2935 Kirkhaven Drive, Youngstown, OH 44511, (216) 726-8855, BA 80 Bowling Green St Univ; MA 81 Bowling Green St Univ; Sp-Lang Path, Youngstown Hrng & Sp Cen, **SLP**

Hendricks, Jennifer Lynn 1408 8th Avenue, Apt 6, San Francisco, CA 94122, (415) 644-2479, BS 85 TX Christian Univ; MA 87 Univ of KS; 88–Sp-Lang Path, North Coast Rehab Ctr, **SLP**

Hendricks, Kim Marie 2820 Terrace Place #42, Garden City, KS 67846, (316) 356-5577

Hendricks, Mary L 46436 Jonathon Circle West, Bldg 15, Utica, MI 48087, (313) 731-7304, BS 85 Central MI Univ; MA 86 Central MI Univ; 88–Sp-Lang Path, St Johns Hosp-Macomb Ctr, **SLP**

Hendricks, Mrs Rosemary 3006 Darby Street, Baltimore, MD 21211, MS 79 Towson St Univ; Sp-Lang Path, Baltimore City Public Schools, **SLP**

Hendricksen, Mrs Carol B 4013 North North, Peoria, IL 61614, (309) 346-7473, BS 77 IL St Univ - Normal; MS 79 IL St Univ - Normal; Sp-Lang Path, Pekin Pub Sch Dist 108, **SLP**

Hendricksen, Sandra Lee Director Speech Pathology, 934 Center Street, Elgin, IL 60120-9976, (312) 742-9800, BS 82 Bradley Univ; MS 84 Univ of WI - Madison; Sp-Lang Path, Marianjoy Rehabilitation Hosp, **SLP**

Hendricks-Godby, Mrs Beverly J 2009 Ridge Creek, Richardson, TX 75081, (214) 867-6300, BA 73 Wheaton Coll; MS 83 Univ of TX - Dallas; Dispensive Audiologist, Collin County Hearing Aid, **A**

Hendrickson, Mrs Barbara Ann 7730 East Broadway #111, Tucson, AZ 85710, (505) 589-0883, **SLP**

Hendrickson, Joseph G, Jr 1370 Lexington Road, Concord, CA 94520, (415) 685-5945, BS 47 Northwestern Univ; MA 49 Northwestern Univ; Consult, Lafayette Sch Dist, **SLP LM**

Hendrickson, Mrs Susan G 1135 North 17th East, Mountain Home, ID 83647, **SLP**

Hendrickson, Mrs Virginia 456 Margo Lane, Berwyn, PA 19312, (215) 644-5029, BA 74 Elmira Coll; MS 76 PA St Univ - Univ Park; **A**

Hendrickson-Pfeil, Sharon 3433 North Fox, Tucson, AZ 85716, **SLP**

Hendriks, Mary Cavanaugh 2419 Apache Drive, Sioux City, IA 51104, (712) 279-2153, BS 84 Northwest MO St Univ; MA 86 Univ of Northern IA; SLP, Marian Health Center, **SLP**

Hendrix, Jane H 7240 Morrison Drive, Greenbelt, MD 20770, (301) 868-9184, BA 81 George Washington Univ; MS 83 Gallaudet Coll; Aud & Dir, Hrng Balance & Sp Ctr of S MD, **A**

Hendrix-Crommelin, Kathleen F 705 Winter Haven Court, Antioch, TN 37017, (615) 896-5921, BA 79 Univ of GA; ME 86 Univ of GA; 86–Sp-Lang Path, Pro Health Svcs, **SLP**

Hendry, Carl John San Juan Hearing Center, 833 East 2nd Avenue, Suite 100, Durango, CO 81301, (303) 247-0808, BA 63 Univ of WI - Oshkosh; MA 66 Univ of WI - Madison; Aud, San Juan Hrng Cen, **A**

Hendryx, Patricia Mary 806 Robinhood Lane, Redlands, CA 92373, (714) 824-4401, BS 77 Univ of WI - Milwaukee; MS 79 Univ of WI - Milwaukee; PH 87 (Communication Sciences & Disorders) Northwestern Univ; Doctoral Trainee, Vamc Hines, **SLP**

Hendryx, Mrs Rebecca L 1004 North 9th Street, Alpine, TX 79830, (915) 837-3315, BA 76 TX Tech Univ; MA 79 Univ of North TX; Sp-Lang Path, The 588 Ed Co-Op Alpine ISD, **SLP**

Hendryx, Teri L 6425 S W 154th Place, Beaverton, OR 97007, (503) 644-2759, BA 74 OR St Univ; MS 75 Western WA Univ; 83–Sp-Lang Path, Vancouver Children's Ther Ctr, **SLP**

Henegan, Sandra R 6916 Knollwood Drive, Morrow, GA 30260, (404) 227-0632, BA 77 George Washington Univ; MA 78 George Washington Univ; Aud, Griffin Resa, **A**

Hengen, Dr C Garth Asp Inc, 55 Cedar Street, Worcester, MA 01609, (617) 752-4663, BS 61 Univ of NE - Lincoln; MA 64 Syracuse Univ; PH 73 (NS) NY Univ; Aud/Sp-Lang Path, Aud Sp Path Serv, **SLP A**

Hengst, Mrs Judith F 3711 Robin Road, Furlong, PA 18924, (215) 674-2394, BS 75 PA St Univ - Univ Park; MA 78 Trenton St Coll; SLP, Private Practice, **SLP**

Hengst, Julie A 3710 Abbott Avenue North, Robbinsdale, MN 55422, (612) 521-5604, MS 85 Univ of WI - Madison; Sp-Lang Path, North Memorial Hosp, **SLP**

Hengstenberg, Kate 1131 Rockingham Drive #116, Richardson, TX 75080, (214) 783-1823, BA 69 Univ of Miami; MA 70 OH St Univ; Aud, Quality Hearing Ctrs, **SLP A**

Hengtgen, Sharon Wolfram 6142 Hinckley, Union Lake, MI 48085, (313) 360-3254, BS 81 Eastern MI Univ; MA 83 Eastern MI Univ; Sp-Lang Path, St Joseph Mercy Hosp, **SLP**

Henke, Mrs Cornelia J 988 Hawthorne Lane, Cedarburg, WI 53012, (414) 352-1580, MS 79 Marquette Univ; Sp-Lang Path, N Shore Rehab Asso, **SLP**

Henke, Mrs Deborah Barson 4512 Hartford Avenue, Beltsville, MD 20705-2642, (301) 595-2421, BS 82 Purdue Univ - West Lafayette; MA 85 Kent St Univ; Sp-Lang Path, Private Practice, **SLP**

Henke, Mrs Karen 3217 Floridale Lane, Cincinnati, OH 45239, (513) 541-2904, BS 80 Univ of Cincinnati; MA 82 Univ of Cincinnati; 82–Sp-Lang Path, Hamilton Co Bd of Ment Ret, **SLP**

Henkel-Silva, Amy Dodd 2019 Lakeview S W, Albuquerque, NM 87105, (505) 262-1584, BA 72 Purdue Univ - West Lafayette; MS 87 Univ of NM; 87–Sp-Lang Path, Albuquerque PS

Henken, Bernard S 118 Waverly Avenue, Melrose, MA 02176, (617) 665-0408, BS 47 Harvard Univ; MS 50 Purdue Univ - West Lafayette; MS 50 Purdue Univ - West Lafayette; Sp-Lang Path, Private Practice, **SLP**

Henline, Mrs Maureen 2708 Riverview Drive, Riva, MD 21140, (301) 956-4967, BA 81 Univ of MD - College Park; MS 82 Loyola Coll; 88–Sp-Lang Path-Peds, Sinai Rehab Center/Sinai Hosp, **SLP**

Henn, Mrs Teresa A 5814 Oak Pointe, Fort Wayne, IN 46845, (812) 537-8109, BS 77 Univ of Cincinnati; MA 79 Univ of Cincinnati; Sp-Lang Path, Dearborn County Hospital, **SLP**

Henne, Joseph F 526 North Ravine, Sault Sainte Marie, MI 49783, (705) 253-0508, BS 72 Central MI Univ; MA 74 Central MI Univ; Aud, Sault Ste Marie Aud, **A**

Henneberry, Tamara Thompson 1043 Blue Ridge Avenue, Chico, CA 95926, (916) 893-9570, BA 80 CA St Univ - Chico; MA 82 CA St Univ - Chico; **SLP**

Hennessey, Ann-Marie B 53-09 97th Street, Elmhurst, NY 11368, (718) 899-8800, BS 77 Boston Univ; MA 79 NY Univ; Aud, Lexington Hrng & Sp Cen, **A**

Hennessey, Carolyn A 4450 15 Mile Road, Sterling Heights, MI 48310, (313) 245-1317, BS 72 SUNY - Center at Albany; MA 74 Coll of Saint Rose; Ch of Sp & Aud, Saratoga Gen Hosp, **SLP**

Hennessy, Betsy H 325 South Edgewood, La Grange, IL 60525, (312) 279-8024, BS 72 Univ of IL - Urbana; MA 73 Univ of IL - Urbana; **SLP**

Hennessy, Fran Rochelle 737 Scorpio Circle, Colorado Springs, CO 80906, (303) 632-1993, **SLP**

Hennessy, Ruth F 180 West End Avenue #17-P, New York, NY 10023, (212) 595-6254, BS 56 IN Univ - Bloomington; MA 67 Columbia Univ Teachers Coll; **SLP**

Henniges, Marian P 84 Sherwood Place, Greenwich, CT 06830, (914) 682-3503, BA 69 Univ of CT; MA 70 Univ of CT; 83–Sales Rep, Instr Dist Amer, **A**

Henning, Mrs Kay L 311 West Wate Street, Wilton, IA 52778, (319) 732-2023, BA 64 Univ of Northern IA; MA 83 Univ of IA; 84–Sp-Lang Path, Mississippi Bend AEA, **SLP**

Henninger, Mrs Debra R 8905 Avondale Road, Baltimore, MD 21234, (301) 529-4278, BS 75 Towson St Univ; MS 77 Towson St Univ; Sp-Lang Path, Baltimore Co Boe, **SLP**

Hennings, Cheryl Marie 11529 Kemperwoods Drive, Cincinnati, OH 45249, (513) 489-9411, MA 88 Univ of Cincinnati

Henningsen, Mrs Dorothy L 7509 Valley Street, Omaha, NE 68124, BS 70 Univ of NE - Omaha; MS 72 Univ of NE - Omaha; SLP, AEA #13, **SLP**

Henningson-Vanucci, Mrs Marjori A 79-K Fairway Court, Lakewood, NJ 08701, (201) 256-1700, BS 81 Midwestern St Univ; MS 86 Rutgers St Univ -N Brunswick; **SLP**

Henoch, Dr Miriam A 201 South 4th Street #707, San Jose, CA 95112, (415) 852-3251, BA 71 Univ of North TX; MA 72 Univ of North TX; PH 76 (NS) Wayne St Univ - Sch of Med; Aud, VA Medical Center, **A ACE**

Henretig, Max D 8124 S W 199th Terrace, Miami, FL 33189, (305) 253-5193, BS 35 CUNY - City College; **SLP LM**

Henri, Dr Bernard P 15 Tideview Terrace, Kennebunk, ME 04043, BA 68 Boston Coll; ME 69 Boston Univ; PH 73 (NS) Northwestern Univ; Dir, York Co Counseling Serv, **SLP ACE**

Henricks, Mrs Barbara D 142 Garth Road, Scarsdale, NY 10583, (914) 723-5500, BS 58 IN Univ - Bloomington; MA 78 NY Univ; Sp/Lang Path, Scarsdale Pub Sch, **SLP**

Henrickson, Janine Diane 110 Mill Spring Road, Manhasset, NY 11030, (516) 627-3670, BA 84 SUNY - Coll at Cortland; MS 87 Columbia Univ Teachers Coll; **A**

Henrickson, Dr Larry K School Of Human Comm Disorders, Dalhousie University, 5599 Fenwick Street, Halifax, NS, Canada B3H 1R2, (515) 294-6582, OB 70 Univ of MN - Minneap-St Paul; MS 74 CO St Univ; PH 82 (NS) Stanford Univ; Asst Prof Aud, IA St U, **A**

Henriksen, Joellen Jacobs 600 Legacy Drive #2013, Plano, TX 75023, (214) 517-5690, BA 84 Univ of Northern IA; MA 86 Univ of Northern IA; SLP, Wylie Ind School Dstr, **SLP**

Henrikson, Ernest H Dept Communication Disorders, University Of Minnesota, Minneapolis, MN 55455, (612) 722-9614, BA 25 Univ of OR; MA 29 Univ of IA; PH 32 (NS) Univ of IA; Consultant, VA, **SLP F LM**

Henriques, Mrs Jan Heymann 1825 Sessions Walk, Hoffman Estates, IL 60195, (504) 595-6153, BA 83 Univ of Southwestern LA; OM 85 LA St Univ - N O Medical Ctr; **A**

Henry, Andrell W 168-A West Main Street, Sevierville, TN 37862, (615) 453-5529, BS 57 CA St Univ - Los Angeles; MA 66 CA St Univ - Los Angeles; Aud-Sp-Lang Path, Sevier Co Schs, **SLP A LM**

Henry, Mrs Betsy W 5207 West 37th Street, Amarillo, TX 79109, (806) 359-4504, BS 37 TX Tech Univ; ME 53 West TX St Univ; **SLP LM**

Henry, Bonnie S 4131 Pineview Road, Charlotte, NC 28211, (704) 338-4430, BS 72 Appalachian St Univ; MA 73 Appalachian St Univ; Sp-Lang Path, Charlotte Rehab Hosp, **SLP**

Henry, Catherine Seaview Hospital, Audiology Department, 460 Brielle Avenue, Staten Island, NY 10314, (718) 390-8639, **A**

Henry, David F 469 East Elpyco, Wichita, KS 67218, (316) 268-5246, Aud, St Francis Regional Med Center, **A**

Henry, Mrs Deborah A 3601 Arlington, Columbus, IN 47203, (812) 376-5319, BS 75 Murray St Univ; MS 76 Univ of WI - Eau Claire; MA 79 Ball St Univ; Mgr/Sp-Lang Path & Aud, Bartholomew County Hospital, **SLP A**

Henry, Donna Therese 7035 Freemont, Dallas, TX 75231, (214) 341-7536, MS 88 Univ of North TX

Henry, Elaine M 37 Personette Street, Caldwell, NJ 07006, (212) 472-6050, BA 69 Newark St Coll; MA 70 Newark St Coll; Aud, The NY Hosp-Cornell Med Cen, **A**

Henry, Evelyn Carol 1844 Georgiana Drive, Atlanta, GA 30329-3332, (404) 763-0580, MS 84 Auburn Univ - Auburn; BS 82 Auburn Univ - Auburn; SLP, Fulton Cty Schools, **SLP**

Henry, Dr Frances V 2886 Burlington, Ann Arbor, MI 48105, BA 58 Capital Univ; OM 51; PH 57 (Sp Sci Aud) Univ of MI - Ann Arbor; Sp-Lang Path/Aud, Consultant, **SLP A LM**

Henry, Frederick 2604 South 62nd Street, Milwaukee, WI 53219, (414) 543-0715, **SLP**

Henry, Mrs Geri Spencer 175 King George Way, Columbia, SC 29210, (803) 798-3797, MS 83 FL St Univ; 88–Sp-Lang Path, Lexington Dist #1 Schs, **SLP**

Henry, Gretchen B Heritage Professional Bldg, 10 Highland Park Drive, Uniontown, PA 15401, (412) 439-4380, BS 53 PA St Univ - Univ Park; ME 56 PA St Univ - Univ Park; PH 64 (Psychoacoustics) Univ of Pittsburgh - Pittsburgh; Aud, Private Practice, **A**

Henry, James A 14655 S W Forest Place, Beaverton, OR 97007, (503) 220-8262, BS 85 Portland St Univ; MS 87 Portland St Univ; 88–Aud, Portland VA Med Ctr, **A**

Henry, Joan M 5036 Lake Circle West, Columbia, MD 21044, **SLP**

Henry, Mrs Linda Sue 416 Columbia Drive, Rockwall, TX 75087, (214) 788-6236, BS 62 Ball St Univ; 86–Dir-Mktg & PR, Humana Hosp, **SLP**

Henry, Mrs Mary Ann D 6 Schneider Lane, Montville, NJ 07045, (201) 263-9212, BA 74 CUNY - Hunter Coll; MA 77 CUNY - Hunter Coll; SLP, Parsippany-Troy Hills Twsp Sch, **SLP**

Henry, Mary Geralyn 7983 Woodridge Drive #212, Woodridge, IL 60517, (312) 968-9421, BS 82 Marywood Coll; MA 84 Univ of IA; Sp-Lang Path, Sased, **SLP**

Henry, Mrs Melissa Carender 4487 Post Place #83, Nashville, TN 37205, (615) 329-7252, BA 80 Western MI Univ; MA 82 Wayne St Univ; Sp-Lang Path, Baptist Rehab Ctr, **SLP**

Henry, Melissa Morley 2215 Abbott Martin Rd #B-9, Nashville, TN 37215, (615) 868-4016, BS 83 Purdue Univ - West Lafayette; MS 85 Purdue Univ - West Lafayette; 88–Aud, Richard Carlson MD & Robert Willis MD, **A**

Henry, Mrs Patricia Bokan 13 Birmingham Drive, Englishtown, NJ 07726, (609) 734-4616, BA 76 Rutger's St Univ - Douglas Coll; ME 77 Univ of VA - Charlottesville; **SLP**

Henry, Mrs Patricia M 3816 Northview Lane, Dallas, TX 75229, (214) 357-4768, BS 75 Miami Univ - Oxford; MA 76 OH St Univ; **SLP**

Henry, Robert J, Jr P O Box 1206, Belleville, MI 48111, (313) 773-2102, BS 74 Central MI Univ; MA 78 Central MI Univ; Aud, Flint Hrng Serv Inc, **A**

Henry, Sherri Ann 4387 Kathy Lane, Chico, CA 95926, (916) 345-3972, BA 85 CA St Univ - Chico; MA 87 CA St Univ - Chico

Henry, Susan Hogue 14655 S W Forest Place, Beaverton, OR 97007, (503) 279-8510, BA 83 Pacific Univ; MS 88 Portland St Univ; Aud, Oregon Health Sciences Univ, **A**

Henry, Thomas E 2809 Hempstead Lane, Bakersfield, CA 93309, (619) 934-6802, BA 69 Humboldt St Univ; MA 71 Humboldt St Univ; MA 79 CA St Coll - Bakersfield; Supt, Calistoga USD, **SLP**

Henry, Yvonne M 6845 Elm Street, Suite 709, Mc Lean, VA 22101, (703) 821-8883, BA 70 Radford Univ; MS 72 PA St Univ - Univ Park; Sp-Lang Path, Private Practice, **SLP**

Hensel-Cohen, Sharon 516 North Poinsettia Place, Los Angeles, CA 90036, (213) 854-4045, BS 73 SUNY - Coll at Buffalo; MS 74 SUNY - Coll at Buffalo; Proprietor, Private Practice, **SLP**

Henselman, Lynn Wilson 6621 Wakefield Drive #412, Alexandria, VA 22307, (703) 768-2440, BA 79 Univ of OK - Norman; MS 82 Vanderbilt Univ; Aud, US Army, **A**

Hensenne, Janet Louise 749 South 6th Street, Apartment 2, Philadelphia, PA 19147, (215) 922-7432, Speech Language Pathologist, Home of Merciful Saviour, **SLP**

Henslee, Yvonne Annette 7425 Hardy, Raytown, MO 64133, (816) 356-1325

Hensler, Eileen Hansen 69-155 Dinah Shore Drive, #123, Cathedral City, CA 92234, (619) 340-4566, BA 85 Western WA Univ; MA 87 Western WA Univ; 87–Aud, Desert ENT Med Group, **A**

Hensler, Eve Lynn Professional Hrng Services, Box 1357, Watertown, SD 57201, (605) 229-3688, BS 76 Northern St Coll; MS 86 Minot St Univ; **A**

Hensley, Betty Harden 717 Stratfordshire Drive, Matthews, NC 28105, BA 72 Catawba Coll; MS 76 Winthrop Coll; SLP, Charlotte Mecklenburg, **SLP**

Hensley, Carol Ann 2204 Gregory Drive, Forest Hill, MD 21050, (215) 631-9300, BS 84 Loyola Coll; MS 85 Loyola Coll; **SLP**

Hensley, Jan L P O Box 334, Glenwood, IA 51534, (712) 527-4811, BA 84 Univ of Akron; MA 86 Univ of Akron; 86–Aud, Glenwood State Hosp-Sch, **A**

Hensley, Dr Leita Ballew 2536 Timber Lane, Cape Girardeau, MO 63701, (314) 651-2155, BA 52 Hendrix Coll; MA 57 Univ of Denver; PH 81 (NS) Southern IL Univ -Carbondale; Asst Prof of Sp, SE MO St U, **SLP**

Hensley, Mrs Sheila Davis P O Box 11, Clintwood, VA 24228, (703) 926-6312, BA 73 Marshall Univ; MA 76 Marshall Univ; Sp/Lang Path, Private Practice, **SLP**

Henslick, Katharine Haag 7507 3rd Avenue Northwest, Bradenton, FL 33529, (813) 792-7346, BA 80 Univ of FL; MS 81 FL St Univ; Sp-Lang Path, Manatee County Schools, **SLP**

Henson, Claudia Carline P O Box 14, Lumpkin, GA 31815, (912) 838-6166, BA 81 Columbus Coll; ME 85 Columbus Coll; Sp-Lang Path, Chattahoochee Board of Educ, **SLP**

Henson, Mrs Evelyn Bruns 12688 Lawrence Road, Sterling, IL 61081, (815) 626-1169, BA 58 Augustana Coll; MS 61 Northern IL Univ - De Kalb; **SLP LM**

Henson, Mrs Mary Dian 10 Belle Meadow Lane, Little Rock, AR 72210, (501) 445-3154, BS 79 Henderson St Univ; MS 82 AR St Univ; Sp/Lang Path, AR Cldrns Hosp, **SLP**

Henson, Mrs Pamela M 10609 Lowery Drive, Raleigh, NC 27615, (919) 783-8492, BA 80 NC St Univ at Raleigh; MS 82 Univ of NC - Chapel Hill; 82–Sp-Lang Path, MedTherp Rehab Svcs Inc, **SLP**

Henson, Mrs Reeda Ruth 2106 Villawood Lane, Garland, TX 75040-4015, BS 83 Univ of AR - Little Rock; MS 85 Univ of Central AR; **SLP**

Henson, Ruth Annette 1190 Rolling Hills Drive, Bloomfield Hills, MI 48013, (313) 451-6590, BA 65 Univ of MI - Ann Arbor; MS 67 Univ of MI - Ann Arbor; Sp-Lang Path, Plymouth-Canton Comm Sch, **SLP ACE**

Hentz, Kathryn Elizabeth 6935 Stone Ridge Drive #43, Memphis, TN 38115, (901) 522-6593, BS 83 AR St Univ; MS 84 AR St Univ; 88–Sp-Lang Path, Baptist Mem Hosp, **SLP**

Hentzen, Mrs Cheryl W 1618 S Santa Fe, Wichita, KS 67211, (316) 685-1181, BA 86 Wichita St Univ; MA 87 Wichita St Univ; SLP, Natl Sp & Hrng Services, **SLP**

Heob, William G 12301 East Appaloosa Trail, Scottsdale, AZ 85259, BS 79 Univ of AZ; MS 81 Univ of AZ; Aud Consultant, Scottsdale Hrng Ctr, **A**

Hepfner, Mrs Sharon T 5631 Kugler Mill Road, Cincinnati, OH 45236, (513) 872-4241, BA 60 MI St Univ; MA 62 MI St Univ; Aud-Assoc Prof Otol, U of Cincinnati Med Cen, **SLP A**

Hepker, Mrs Sandra Jean Professional Hearing Services, 18 South Howell, Suites 100 & 101, Hillsdale, MI 49242, (517) 439-1610, BA 80 Univ of MI - Ann Arbor; MS 82 Univ of MI - Ann Arbor; Aud, Private Practice, **A**

Hepler, Dr Ernest L, Jr 10th Medical Laboratory, Attn Pm-Ohe, APO New York, NY 09180, BA 71 Univ of FL; MA 72 Univ of FL; PH 84 (NS) Univ of FL; Us Army Aud, **A**

Hepler, Mrs Janet B Box 72, Allison Park, PA 15101, (412) 364-4744, BA 60 Univ of Pittsburgh - Pittsburgh; MS 62 Univ of Pittsburgh - Pittsburgh; Aud, Jerry D Shamblin MD, **A**

Hepner, Mrs Sharon Doane 600 West 123rd Avenue, #3814, Westminster, CO 80234, (303) 451-1561, BA 80 Northeast LA Univ; MA 84 Univ of Northern CO; **SLP**

Hepner-Dion, Susan Meryl 6656 Thornhill Court, Boca Raton, FL 33433, (305) 338-3039, BA 84 Univ of FL; MA 86 Hofstra Univ; **A**

Hepp, Cheryl L 2101 Appleton Lane, Louisville, KY 40216, (502) 454-8247, BA 73 Univ of KY; MA 75 Vanderbilt Univ; Itinerant Computer Insvc Tchr, Jefferson County Board of Educ, **SLP**

Heppe, Jo Anne T 3333 Simms, Wheat Ridge, CO 80033, (303) 232-5735, MA 80 Univ of CO - Boulder; BA 73 Univ of CO - Boulder; Sp-Lang Path, Private Practice, **SLP**

Heppner, Nancee L 3213 Edwards, Alton, IL 62002, BS 75 Southern IL Univ-Edwardsvill; MS 76 Southern IL Univ-Edwardsvill; SLP, Alton Commun Dist #11, **SLP**

Herauf, Mrs Jean L Department Of Speech/Language Pathology, St Josephs Hospital And Health Center, Dickinson, ND 58601, (701) 225-7387, BA 80 Univ of ND; MS 81 Univ of ND; Sp/Lang Path, St Joseph Hosp & Hlth Cen, **SLP**

Herb, Lyman C 3230 Dogwoods, Salem, OR 97302, (503) 399-3300, BA 65 9474; MS 67 9470; **SLP A**

Herbers, Suzanne D Communications Solutions Inc, 8428 Holly Leaf Drive, Mc Lean, VA 22102, (703) 356-1688, BA 73 Catholic Univ of America; MA 75 Catholic Univ of America; Sp-Lang Path, Communications Solutions Inc, **SLP**

Herbert, Mrs Dale Frances 6419 16th Street North, St Petersburg, FL 33702, (813) 391-9723, BS 77 Bloomsburg Univ of PA; MS 78 Bloomsburg Univ of PA; Sp-Lang Path, Pinellas County Schools, **SLP**

Herbert, Mrs Diane Procopio P O Box 141, Dover Plains, NY 12522, (914) 877-6821, BA 74 SUNY - Coll at Geneseo; MA 78 SUNY - Coll at Geneseo; Aud, Wassaic Dev Cen, **A**

Herbert, Esther L 8001 Vicksburg Avenue, Los Angeles, CA 90045, (213) 645-5832, BA 41 CUNY - Brooklyn Coll; MA 42 Univ of IA; **SLP F LM**

Herbert, Mrs Jeanne T P O Box 144, Goshen, NY 10924, (914) 294-8806, BA 77 Saint John's Univ - Jamaica; MS 79 Purdue Univ - West Lafayette; Head Sp-Lang Path, Orange Co C P Assn Inc, **SLP**

Herbert, Judith L 3450 Manchester Road, Wantagh, NY 11793, (516) 785-3136, BA 70 CUNY - Queens Coll; MA 72 Univ of MD - College Park; 88–Sp-Lang Path, Sch for Lang & Commun Dis, **SLP**

Herbert, Mrs Linda May Foster Road, Merrimack, NH 03054, (603) 881-4318, BA 69 Emerson Coll; MS 82 Univ of NH; Sp-Lang Path, Nashua Publ Sch Sys, **SLP**

Herbert, Marybeth 404 Five Farms Lane, Timonium, MD 21093, (201) 688-2750, BS 83 Towson St Univ; MA 87 Towson St Univ

Herbolsheimer, Marla Luella 4520 25th Street, Columbus, NE 68601, (402) 564-0815, **SLP**

Herbst, Mrs Inger A 901 East Jules Street, Arlington Heights, IL 60004, (312) 885-4366, BA 50 Saint Olaf Coll; MS 53 Univ of IA; Sp-Lang Path, Township Hs Dist #211, **SLP**

Herbst, Jean 32 1st Avenue, P O Box 38, Bayville, NY 11709, MA 81 Hofstra Univ; BA 78 Adelphi Univ; Sp-Lang Path, Syosset Sch Dist, **SLP**

Herbst, Nancy Suzanne 10888 North 70th St #215, Scottsdale, AZ 85254, (602) 948-7603, OB 83 LA St Univ - N O Medical Ctr; MA LA Tech Univ; SLP, AZ Sp P Ltd, **SLP**

Herd, Mrs Carol H 130 Lucien Drive, Hamden, CT 06518, (203) 265-2831, BS 67 Univ of WI - Madison; MA 68 Univ of CT; 84–Sp-Lang Path, Wallingford Board of Education, **SLP**

Herder, Julie Christy 7635 Marshall Street, Arvada, CO 80003, (213) 273-8480, MA 86 Univ of Northern IA; **SLP**

Herendeen, Mrs Patricia 1407-A North Harlem, Oak Park, IL 60302, (312) 848-4869, BA 50 Rockford Coll; MA 80 Northeastern IL Univ; Tchr, Chicago Bd of Ed, **SLP**

Herer, Dr Gilbert R 11309 Marcliff Road, Rockville, MD 20852, (202) 745-5600, BS 53 Syracuse Univ; MS 54 Syracuse Univ; PH 64 (Aud) Northwestern Univ; 64–Dir/Chldn Hrng/Sp Cen, Chldn Hosp Natnl Med Cen, **SLP A F**

Hereth, Mrs Kay Carolyn 5594 Dry Ridge Road, Cincinnati, OH 45252, (513) 742-2200, BS 60 Miami Univ - Oxford; ME 68 Miami Univ - Oxford; 81–Sp-Lang Path, Hamilton Co Offi of Ed, **SLP**

Hergenreder, Mrs Patti A 110 Moore Bldg, Pennsylvania State Univ, University Park, PA 16802, (814) 863-2017, BS 77 SD St Univ; MS 79 Univ of WY; Aud Clinical Super, PA St Univ, **A**

Hergert, Mrs Doylene K 1202 Miles Court, North Platte, NE 69101, (308) 532-8502, BS 69 CO St Univ; MS 71 CO St Univ; Sp-Lang Path, North Platte Pub Sch, **SLP ACE**

Herigstad, Mrs Suzanne Jo 2536 Narrows Drive #24, Tacoma, WA 98406, BA 63 Univ of IA; Sp-Lang Path, Tacoma Pub Sch, **SLP**

Hering, Mrs Laurie Works 1539 Lime Drive, Melbourne, FL 32935, (305) 259-9776, BS 81 James Madison Univ; MA 85 Univ of Central FL; Sp-Lang Path, Brevard County Schools, **SLP**

Hering, Mrs Ruth E 428 Bradshaw Avenue, Haddonfield, NJ 08033, (609) 783-2994, BS 51 Univ of PA; **SLP ACE**

Herman, Mrs Anne Hansen 122 North Brainard Avenue, La Grange, IL 60525, (312) 887-2747, BA 82 Univ of WI - Eau Claire; MS 85 Univ of WI - Madison; 88–Dir of SLP, Hinsdale Hosp, **SLP**

Herman, Donna L 7 Karen Drive, Cherry Hill, NJ 08003, (609) 853-0127, MA 76 Trenton St Coll; Sp-Lang Path, Woodbury Public Schools, **SLP**

Herman, Elise K 3330 Yellowstone Drive, Ann Arbor, MI 48105, (313) 426-8983, BA 67 CUNY - Hunter Coll; MS 68 Univ of MI - Ann Arbor; SLP, Dexter Community Sch, **SLP**

Herman, Evelyn M P O Box 532, Goshen, CT 06756, **SLP**

Herman, Mrs Ilana H F 3750 Hudson Manor Terrace, Apartment 2-F East, Bronx, NY 10463, (212) 796-4439, BA 77 CUNY - City College; MA 79 CUNY - City College; SLP, Riverdale Nursing Home, **SLP**

Herman, Mrs Joyce 4289 Cherry Hill, Orchard Lake, MI 48033, (313) 682-7804, BS 74 Eastern MI Univ; MA 75 Eastern MI Univ; **SLP**

Herman, Mrs Lauren W 4939 Arroyo Chamisa N E, Albuquerque, NM 87111-3716, (505) 292-7724, BA 74 CUNY - Lehman Coll; MA 76 CUNY - Lehman Coll; **SLP**

Herman, Leslie E Summit Hearing Aid Center, 75 Summit Avenue, Summit, NJ 07901, (201) 277-6886, BS 72 Syracuse Univ; MS 75 Washington Univ; Aud, Summit Hrng Aid Cen, **A**

Herman, Mrs Louisa M 11610 Wensledale Circle, San Antonio, TX 78251-9637, (512) 523-0760, MS; 87–Sp-Lang Path, San Antonio ISD, **SLP**

Herman, Mrs Maria Luciani 628 Newberry Drive, Elk Grove, IL 60007-2739, (312) 893-0819, BS 83 Western IL Univ; MA 84 Western IL Univ; 84–Sp-Lang Path, HS Dist 211, **SLP**

Herman, Mrs Mary Gage 250 Hillside Avenue, Piedmont, CA 94611, Sp-Lang Path, Childrens Hosp Med Ctr, **SLP**

Herman, Mrs Mary M 1547 Alturas Drive, Burlingame, CA 94010, (415) 574-6433, MA 65 San Francisco St Univ; BA 64 San Francisco St Univ; Sp-Lang Path, College of San Mateo, **SLP ACE**

Herman, Meryl E 710 Powder Mill Lane, Penfield Downs, PA 19151, **SLP**

Herman, Mrs Suzanne Couch 3712 Old Lufkin Road, Nacogdoches, TX 75961, (409) 560-1815, BS 83 Stephen F Austin St Univ; ME 87 Stephen F Austin St Univ; **SLP**

Herman, Mrs Terry S 6209 Innes Trace, Louisville, KY 40222, (502) 425-8017, BA 72 Univ of KY; MA 74 Univ of KY; Sp-Lang Path, Jefferson Co Pub Sch, **SLP**

Hermann, Gregory Paul 112 East Harrie, Newberry, MI 49868, (906) 293-5121, MS 74 Univ of NM; **SLP**

Hermann, Mrs Jennifer S 6278 Co T, Egg Harbor, WI 54209, (414) 868-3284, BS 73 Univ of WI - Stevens Point; MS 74 Univ of WI - Stevens Point; Sp-Lang Path, Gibralter Area Sch, **SLP**

Hermann, Nancy T 2020 19th Street #A, Santa Monica, CA 90404, (216) 392-5939, **SLP**

Hermann-O'Keeffe, Katherine 1959 Georgia, Oshkosh, WI 54901, (414) 235-7305, BS 84 Marquette Univ; MS 86 Univ of WI - Madison; 88–Sp-Lang Path, Neenah PS, **SLP**

Hermanoff, Wendy Sue 2000 North Adams Street, Apartment 401, Arlington, VA 22201, (703) 276-9250, BS 0685; MA 86 Northwestern Univ; **SLP**

Hermanowicz, Carol Jean 1498 Beche Street S E, Palm Bay, FL 32909, (713) 790-8100, BS 82 PA St Univ - Univ Park; MA 85 Univ of Houston - Univ Park; Sp-Lang Path, Medical Ctr Del Oro Hospital, **SLP**

Hermele, Mrs Jean O Echo Lane, Fairfield, CT 06432, (203) 374-3814, BS 69 Northwestern Univ; ME 70 Boston Univ; **SLP**

Hermele, Mrs Lynn Freeman 13 Sylvan Way, Short Hills, NJ 07078, (201) 376-2683, **SLP**

Hermes, Mrs Ellen Valenzi 39 Canter Drive, Sewickley, PA 15143, (412) 741-0308, BS 78 Edinboro Univ of PA; MA 82 Univ of Pittsburgh - Pittsburgh; 86–Sp-Lang Path, Univ of Pittsburgh, **SLP**

Hermes, Estelle L 745 Nevers Road, South Windsor, CT 06074, (203) 644-1313, BA 81 Univ of CT; MA 83 Univ of CT; Sp-Lang Path, South Windsor Board of Educ, **SLP**

Hermsen, Mrs Julie B 27093 Village Drive, Tega Cay, SC 29715, (515) 278-0407, BS 80 Univ of WI - Whitewater; MS 82 Univ of WI - Whitewater; SLP, Des Moines Pub Sch, **SLP**

Hernandez, Aleida M 6821 East Broadway #261, Tucson, AZ 85710, (602) 298-8688, BA 74 Nicholls St Univ; MS 78 LA St Univ - N O Medical Ctr; 88–Sp-Lang Path, Tucson Sch Dist, **SLP**

Hernandez, Denise 9157 S W 72 Avenue #S-7, Miami, FL 33156, (305) 549-6397, BS 84 Univ of Tulsa; MA 85 Univ of Tulsa; **SLP**

Hernandez, Gilbert V 162 West Cheryl Drive, San Antonio, TX 78228, (512) 435-1944, BA 59 Trinity Univ; MA 65 Univ of TX - Austin; Dir SLP, King William Hlth Care Cen, **SLP**

Hernandez, Morene E 907 Purdy Drive, Roswell, NM 88201, BA 84 Grand Canyon Coll; MS 86 Eastern NM Univ; **SLP**

Hernandez, Paloma Izquierdo 45 Verona Avenue, Yonkers, NY 10710, (914) 779-8462, **SLP**

Hernandez, Mrs Stephanie Day 13121 Roberta Place, Garden Grove, CA 92643, (714) 558-5676, BA 75 Univ of Redlands; MS 77 Univ of Redlands; SLP, Santa Ana USD, **SLP**

Hernandez-Grein, Ana Lourdes 95 Oak Street, Floral Park, NY 11001, (516) 352-8759, BA 83 Saint John's Univ - Jamaica; MS 85 Columbia Univ Teachers Coll; Sp-Lang Path, Long Island Jewish Medical Ctr, **SLP**

Herndon, Mrs Claudia K 500 Florida Street, East Alton, IL 62024, (618) 258-1650, BS 77 Southern IL Univ-Edwardsvill; MS 78 Southern IL Univ-Edwardsvill; **SLP**

Herndon, Dr Geneva 213 West 7th, Hays, KS 67601, BS 24 Fort Hays St Univ; MA 30 Univ of CO - Boulder; PH 48 (NS) Northwestern Univ; **SLP LM**

Herndon, Dr George Y 2109 Indian Trails, Jonesboro, AR 72401, (501) 972-3061, BA 48 LA Coll; MA 50 Univ of IA; PH 63 (NS) Univ of OK - Norman; Speak Inc, **SLP**

Herndon, Mrs Kirsten S 3103 Elma, Midland, TX 79707, (915) 694-4345, BS 79 TX Woman's Univ; MA 82 Abilene Christian Univ; 86–Sp-Lang Path, Region 18 Education Svc Ctr, **SLP**

Herndon, Lolita Lorraine Route 1 Box 260, Waycross, GA 31501, (912) 285-8798, ME 87 Valdosta St Coll

Herne, Mrs Robin Mirante 43 High Street, Seymour, CT 06483, (203) 366-7551, BA 80 Boston Coll; MS 88 Southern CT St Univ

Hernes, Mrs Clara G 422 Wingate Road, Huntingdon Valley, PA 19006, (215) 342-7660, BS 57 Univ of PA; MA 78 Temple Univ; Sp-Lang Path, Cora Serv, **SLP**

Herod, Linda R 1387 Sacramento Street, Deltona, FL 32725, (904) 736-9771, MS 77 WV Univ; BS 74 WV Univ; Dir of SLP, Ctrl FL Ear & Hrng Cl, **SLP**

Herold, Joan C P O Box 309, East Aurora, NY 14052, (716) 878-7611, BA 73 2995; MA 76 2995; Sp/Lang Path, Erie-Chautauqua BOCES, **SLP**

Herold, Marcia A 9342 Sibelius Drive, Vienna, VA 22180, (703) 430-7710, BS 74 PA St Univ - Univ Park; MS 76 AZ St Univ; 88–Sp-Lang Path, Loudoun Co Sch, **SLP**

Heron, Mrs Marguerite 4776 Bourke Road, Columbus, OH 43229, (614) 436-1154, BA 70 Temple Univ; MA 73 Temple Univ; Sp-Lang Path, OH St Sch for the Blind, **SLP**

Heron, Michael Jon 3201 Duke Drive, Norman, OK 73071, (405) 360-5279, MS 88 Univ of OK Medical Center

Herr, Mrs Beverly B 31941 Kings Park Court, Westlake Village, CA 91361, BS 55 Shippensburg Univ of PA; MS 60 Univ of IL - Urbana; Sp-Lang Path, Sp Path Associates, **SLP**

Herr, Emma Rose Route 1 Box 30-B, Ruffin, NC 27326, (919) 292-0012, BA 72 Univ of NC - Greensboro; ME 74 Univ of NC - Greensboro; Sp-Lang Path, Caswell Co Sch Sys, **SLP**

Herr, Laura Renee 19 West 36th Street, Minneapolis, MN 55408, (612) 725-2041, MA 86 Univ of MN - Minneap-St Paul; 85–Sp-Lang Path, VA Med Ctr, **A**

Herr, Mrs Leslie C 66970 Solar Road, Montrose, CO 81401, (303) 249-8023, BA 72 Univ of Denver; MA 75 Univ of Denver; Sp-Lang Path, Uncompahgre Valley Speech/Lang, **SLP**

Herr, Patricia Mae E 13033 North 112th Street, Stillwater, MN 55082, (612) 439-7580, BS 60 Univ of MN - Duluth; MS 81 Univ of WI - River Falls; Sp-Lang Path, River Ridge Rehab, **SLP ACE**

Herr, Sally Blanche 124 Linden, Frankfort, KY 40601, (502) 875-2053, BS 70 Purdue Univ - West Lafayette; MA Univ of KY; 79–Sp-Lang Path, Private Practice, **SLP ACE**

Herrbold, Mrs Merrie M 639 Meadowglen, Duncanville, TX 75137, (214) 296-1643, BA 70 Baylor Univ; MS 73 Southern Methodist Univ; **SLP**

Herrboldt, Sydney O 7680 East Broadway #102, Tucson, AZ 85710, (602) 885-8940, BS 76 Northern St Coll; MS 79 Univ of WI - Eau Claire; 86–SLP, Tucson USD, **A**

Herre, Debra L 1555 Savannah Drive, Evansville, IN 47715, (812) 479-1411, BS 77 Purdue Univ - West Lafayette; MS 79 Purdue Univ - West Lafayette; Sp-Lang Path, The Rehab Center, **SLP ACE**

Herrell, Judy 1125 Cummings Court, Eau Claire, WI 54701, (715) 834-4875, BA 70 Univ of MN - Duluth; MS 74 Univ of WI - Eau Claire; SLP, Eau Claire Pub Sch, **SLP**

Herren, Johanna 121 Dover Road, Westwood, MA 02090, (617) 965-5820, BS 85 CA St Univ - Hayward; MS 87 Northeastern Univ; 87–Sp-Lang Path, Learning Prep Sch, **SLP**

Herren, Mrs Shelley Lynn 3224 49th S W, Seattle, WA 98116, (206) 937-5216, BA 79 WA St Univ; MA 86 Western WA Univ; 79–Sp-Lang Path, Puyallup PS, **SLP**

Herrera, Evelyn Catherine 1914 Glenstone Avenue, Hacienda Heights, CA 91745, **SLP**

Herrick, Carol 170 Anton Street #B-6, Bridgeport, CT 06606, (203) 372-5161, BS 80 West Chester Univ of PA; MA 82 Trenton St Coll; SLP, Easton-Redding School District, **SLP**

Herrick, Dr Helen M 723 North 5th Street, Philadelphia, PA 19123, BA 58 Beaver Coll; MA 68 Trenton St Coll; ED 80 (NS) Boston Univ; Hrng Ther, Sch Dist of Phila, **A**

Herrick, Jeryl Lynne 5490 Maple Park Drive #6, Flint, MI 48507, (313) 635-4441, BA 84 MI St Univ; MA 85 MI St Univ; **SLP**

Herrick, Mrs Margaret Hatton 1516 Morris Road, Kent, OH 44240, (216) 673-6251, BA 40 Mount Union Coll; MA 50 Case Western Reserve Univ; **SLP LM**

Herrick, Mrs Stephanie A 5605 N E Skidmore, Portland, OR 97218, (503) 287-1645, BA 71 Univ of WA; MS 87 Portland St Univ; 87–Sp-Lang Path, Portland PS, **SLP**

Herrick, Susan A 1300 Watts Avenue, Rockton, IL 61072, (815) 624-4313, BA 81 Univ of WI - Eau Claire; MS 82 Univ of WI - Eau Claire; **SLP**

Herriges, Catherine Lynn 16120 Smith Drive, Brookfield, WI 53005, (414) 786-4019, BS 83 Univ of WI - Stevens Point; MS 85 Univ of WI - Stevens Point; **A**

Herrin, Debra D 513 Sophia Lane, Shreveport, LA 71115, **SLP**

Herring, Claudia A 2274 Ashley River Road, Apartment 603, Charleston, SC 29407, (803) 797-2721, ME 73 Univ of VA - Charlottesville; Sp-Lang Path, Tri-Co Sp-Path Assoc, **SLP**

Herring, David H 200 East Madison, Yates Center, KS 66783, (316) 724-6281, BA 70 Wichita St Univ; MA 72 Wichita St Univ; 80–Aud, S E KS Reg Serv Cen, **A**

Herring, Mrs Janice Pechter 12205 Guinevere Road, Glenn Dale, MD 20769, (301) 262-6020, BS 76 PA St Univ - Univ Park; MA 77 George Washington Univ; 77–Sp-Lang Path, Private Practice, **SLP**

Herring, June J Route 1 Box 40, Union Grove, NC 28689, (704) 539-5459, BA 73 Univ of NC - Greensboro; ME 74 Univ of NC - Greensboro; Sp-Lang Path & Audiologist, Iredell County Schools, **SLP A**

Herring, Mrs Karen Kissane 25 Edison Street, Bayville, NJ 08721, (201) 793-8744, BS 84 WV Univ; MS 85 FL St Univ; **A**

Herring, Phyllis W 16 Silkgrass, Irvine, CA 92714, MS; **SLP**

Herring, Mrs Rebecca Alleman 4120 27th Street, Des Moines, IA 50310, (515) 277-6023, BS 83 Central MO St Univ; MS 84 Central MO St Univ; Sp-Lang Path, Des Moines Indep Public School, **SLP**

Herrington, Mrs Dominique E Parish 417 Rhett Avenue, Huntsville, AL 35801, (205) 535-2312, BA 85 Univ of AL-Tuscaloosa; MS 86 Univ of Montevallo; Lakeshore North AL Rehab Hosp, **SLP**

Herrington, Mrs Patricia L 70 Orchard Lane, Melrose, MA 02176, ME 79 Northeastern Univ; Sp-Lang Path, Reading Pub Sch, **SLP**

Herrington, Mrs Paula Beckett 3771 West Commadore Way, Seattle, WA 98199, (206) 283-9422, BA 81 Hobart-William Smith Coll; MS 87 Univ of WA; 88–Sp-Lang Path, Edmonds Sch Dist, **SLP**

Herrington-Hall, Barbara Lee 2712 Rhode Island Avenue So, Apt #119, St Louis Park, MN 55426, (612) 293-8715, MA 85 Univ of Cincinnati; BA 78 Saint Olaf Coll; Sp-Lang Path, St Paul Pub Sch, **SLP**

Herrmann, Dr Barbara Sprague 119 Lincoln Road, Walpole, MA 02081, (617) 523-3286, BA 74 Univ of WI - Madison; MS 77 Univ of WI - Madison; PH 81 (Aud) Univ of WI - Madison; 87–Dir-Aud Evoked Resp Lab, MA Eye & Ear Infirmary, **A**

Herrmann, Mrs Colleen Robben Fort Dodge Road, Dodge City, KS 67801, (316) 582-2586, MA 86 Wichita St Univ; **SLP**

Herrmann, Elizabeth 2 Stone Barn Drive, Hockessin, DE 19707, **SLP**

Herrmann, Mrs Martha Ann 350 Agate Way, Redding, CA 96003, (916) 246-3711, BA 75 CA St Univ - Sacramento; MA 80 CA St Univ - Sacramento; 87–Sp/Lang Path, Cascade Union Elem Sch Dist, **SLP**

Herrmann-Brydges, Virginia 6518 29th Avenue, Kenosha, WI 53140, (414) 656-6270, BS 79 Univ of WI - Stevens Point; MS 80 Univ of WI - Stevens Point; Sp-Lang Path, Kenosha USD & Mem Hosp, **SLP**

Herrod, Robin McMahon 13 Sierra Court, North Little Rock, AR 72118, (501) 624-7111, BS 76 OK St Univ; MA 77 Univ of AR - Fayetteville; Sp-Lang Path, Ouchita Reg Ment Hlth Cen, **SLP**

Herron, Dr Edna R 3121 South Heather Court, Springfield, MO 65804, (417) 836-4194, OB 63 Univ of MO - Columbia; MA 64 Univ of MO - Columbia; PH 85 (Child and Family Dev) Univ of MO - Columbia; 86–Assoc Dir, Project ACCESS/SMSU, **SLP**

Herron, Margaret M 519 Groom Street, Perth Amboy, NJ 08861, (201) 705-3951, BS 51 Newark St Coll; MA 54 Columbia Univ Teachers Coll; Vice Prin, Bd of Ed, **SLP A**

Herron, Victoria R 673 North Edgemoor, Wichita, KS 67208, (316) 683-7741, BA 71 Wichita St Univ; MA 72 Wichita St Univ; SLP, USD 259, **SLP**

Hersch, Hariet K 29 Circle Lane, East Hills, NY 11577, **SLP**

Herschberg-Muntner, Mrs Nancy R 23 Orange Drive, Marlboro, NJ 07746, (201) 431-9213, BA 73 CUNY - Brooklyn Coll; MS 74 Univ of MI - Ann Arbor; Sp-Lang Path, Private Practice, **SLP**

Herschfeld, Mrs Michele Waldman 2611 Harris Avenue, Wheaton, MD 20902, (301) 949-2871, BA 83 Univ of MD - College Park; MS 85 Univ of MI - Ann Arbor; 88–Sp-Lang Path, Private Practice, **SLP**

Herscovitz, Toby Lois 1822 Overview Circle, Santa Ana, CA 92705, (714) 731-6955, BA 72 CA St Univ - Northridge; MA 74 CA St Univ - Los Angeles; SLP, Private Practice, **SLP**

Hersey, Martha J 616 West 40th Street, Baltimore, MD 21211, (301) 889-0162, BS 71 Western MI Univ; MA 74 Northern IL Univ - De Kalb; Sp-Lang Path, Private Practice, **SLP**

Hersh, Gene B 145 Heatherstone Road, Amherst, MA 01002, BA 68 IN Univ - Bloomington; ME 69 Boston Univ; Sp-Lang Path, Erving Elem Sch, **SLP**

Hersh, Helen 9 Auerbach Lane, Cedarhurst, NY 11516, **SLP**

Hersh, Julie Dawn 135 Sunnyvale Court, Somerset, NJ 08873, (201) 653-0578, BS 82 Ithaca Coll; MA 84 Montclair St Coll; **SLP**

Hersh, Michelle Zacharia 25-I Arlen Road, Baltimore, MD 21236, (301) 647-3111, BA 84 Univ of MD - College Park; MA 85 George Washington Univ; 86–Sp-Lang Path, Anne Arundel County PS, **SLP**

Hersh, Myra G 48 Ethelridge Road, White Plains, NY 10605, **SLP**

Hersh, Susan B Rehabilitation Institute Of, Pittsburgh, 6301 Northumberland Avenue, Pittsburgh, PA 15217, (412) 521-9000, BA 72 Univ of Pittsburgh - Pittsburgh; MS 76 Univ of Pittsburgh - Pittsburgh; 84–Sp-Lang Path, Rehab I of Pittsburgh, **SLP**

Hershberg, Karen Fran 18 Parkland Road, Needham, MA 02194-2428, (617) 455-9039, BS 81 Emerson Coll; MA 87 Univ of MN - Minneap-St Paul; 86–Sp-Lang Path, Dedham PS, **SLP**

Hershberger, Mrs Patty A 16 Woodland Road, Sapulpa, OK 74066, (918) 224-1416, BS 75 OK St Univ; MA 77 Wichita St Univ; 83–Sp-Lang Path, Private Practice, **SLP**

Hershenfis, Hilda A 18 N Virginia Avenue, Atlantic City, NJ 08401, (609) 344-8978, BA 77 CUNY - Hunter Coll; MA 79 Temple Univ-Tyler Sch of Art; Sp-Lang Path, Private Practice, **SLP**

Hershey, Beverly M 6629 Racquet Club Drive, Lauderhill, FL 33319, (305) 739-4612, BS 68 Ithaca Coll; MA 70 CUNY - Hunter Coll; Sp-Lang Path, Private Practice, **SLP**

Hershey, Wendy Walls 316 Harvest Drive, Lititz, PA 17543, (717) 295-8327, BS 75 Radford Univ; MS 77 Towson St Univ; Sp-Lang Path, Lancaster General Hospital, **SLP**

Hershey-Miller, Mrs Sadelle 75 Henry Street #9G, Brooklyn, NY 11201, (212) 266-5050, BA 73 CUNY - Brooklyn Coll; MS 75 CUNY - Brooklyn Coll; Sp-Lang Path, Jewish Bd/Ihb Treat Cen, **SLP**

Hershfield, Kathy Seigel A-3 Franklin Square, Randolph, MA 02368, (617) 986-8555, MS 84 Boston Univ; 88–Sp-Lang Path, KLK Associates Inc, **SLP**

Hershman, Marsha Jo Speech Pathology Department, Stockton State College, Pomona, NJ 08240, (609) 652-4639, BS 70 OH St Univ; MA 73 Bowling Green St Univ; Dir/Sp-Lang Hrng Cl, Stockton St Coll, **SLP**

Hershon, Roberta Beth 161 Country Club Dr #8, Union, NJ 07083, (201) 686-3411, BS 84 Ithaca Coll; MS 86 Northeastern Univ; **A**

Hersom, Roberta G P O Box 48, Emmetsburg, IA 50536, (712) 424-3720, BS 76 Western IL Univ; MA 77 Western IL Univ; Sp-Lang Path/Supvr, Lakeland AEA 3, **SLP**

Herson, Mrs Andrea 911 White Pine Place, Rockville, MD 20854, (301) 424-5938, BS 72 PA St Univ - Univ Park; MA 74 George Washington Univ; Sp-Lang Path, Montg Co Pub Sch, **SLP**

Hertel, Christina 1042 Redwood Drive, Aptos, CA 95003, (408) 476-7140, BA 63 Univ of CA - Santa Barbara; MA 67 Univ of CA - Santa Barbara; Dir, Santa Cruz Co Office of Educ, **SLP**

Hertig, Mrs Carla Ann 1314 South Albemarle, York, PA 17403, (717) 624-4616, MS 84 Indiana Univ of PA; SLP, Lincoln Intermed Unit 12, **SLP**

Hertrick, Kathy Lynn 994 Weymouth Road, Madina, OH 44256, (216) 723-2524, BS 71 Bowling Green St Univ; MA 84 Cleveland St Univ; 87–Sp-Lang Path, Medina City Schs, **SLP**

Hertz, Mrs Nina R 6 Knoll Lane, Jericho, NY 11753, (516) 681-0204, BS 73 Hofstra Univ; MS 74 Columbia Univ Teachers Coll; Sp-Lang Path, Assoc for Chldn with Down Syndrome, **SLP**

Hertz, Robin L 21 Fruit Street, Worcester, MA 01609, (508) 754-7500, BS 78 Northeastern Univ; MS 80 Univ of RI; Dir of Aud, Fallon Clinic Inc, **A**

Hertzberg, Herman 75-09 169th Street, Flushing, NY 11366, (212) 689-6665, BA 74 CUNY - City College; MA 76 CUNY - City College; Dir of Aud, Park Ave Hrng Serv Ltd, **A**

Hertzfeld, Debra B 1007 Overbrook Road, Wilmington, DE 19807-2235, (302) 654-4485, BS 79 Carlow Coll; MA 81 Univ of Pittsburgh - Pittsburgh; Cl Superv, InSpeech Inc, **SLP**

Hertzler, Donna P 712 Galahad Drive, Newport News, VA 23602, (804) 872-0161, BA 81 Southern IL Univ-Edwardsvill; MS 83 Southern IL Univ-Edwardsvill; 87–Dept Head, Mary Immaculate Hosp, **SLP**

Hertzog, Bonnie B 2814 Heathfield Lane, Richmond, IN 47374, (317) 935-0051, BS 74 SUNY - Coll at Geneseo; MA 77 SUNY - Coll at Geneseo; Sp-Lang Path, Richmond Comm Schs, **SLP**

Hervey, Mrs Terry O'Hair 825 Canterbury Lane, Kissimmee, FL 32741, (305) 846-1840, BS 81 FL St Univ; MS 82 FL St Univ; SLP, Osceola Co Sch Sys, **SLP**

Hervey, Dr Wesley D P O Box 4366, Salem, OR 97302, (503) 378-5130, PH 69 (Sp Path Linguistics) Univ of OR; 85–Sp-Lang Path, State of Oregon, **SLP**

Herx, Dennis A Centre Burlington, Rural Route 1, Hants County, NS, Canada B0N 1E0, MS 77 Gallaudet Coll; Aud Pres, Aud Associates of Nova Scotia, **A**

Herzer, Mrs Michelle Mizell 9810 Shoreview Road, Dallas, TX 75238, (214) 494-8303, MA 87 TX Woman's Univ; 83–Sp-Lang Path, Garland ISD, **SLP**

Herzfeld, Mrs Melanie W 8 Woodhollow Lane, Huntington, NY 11743, (516) 271-3623, BA 71 CUNY - Lehman Coll; MA 75 CUNY - Queens Coll; 84–Aud, Otolaryngology Associates, **A**

Herzler, Stephan Charles 3214 Prange Drive, Cuyahoga Falls, OH 44221, BS 81 Univ of WI - Stevens Point; MS 83 Univ of WI - Stevens Point; Aud, Professional Hrng Services, **A**

Herzog, Eileen Gavin 1803 Georgia Street, Silver City, NM 88061, (505) 388-1591, BA 85 Loyola Coll; MS 86 Loyola Coll; 86–Sp-Lang Path, InSpeech Inc, **SLP**

Herzog, Elizabeth Ellen 134 Durand #5, East Lansing, MI 48823, (616) 459-8277, **A**

Herzog, Glenn L 312 East Hackberry, Fredericksburg, TX 78624, (512) 997-4829, BS 67 Univ of MN - Minneap-St Paul; MA 69 Saint Cloud St Univ; Sp-Lang Path, Fredericksburg ISD, **SLP**

Herzog, Harvey T 745 McKewin Avenue, Baltimore, MD 21218, BA 68 Long Island U - Brooklyn Ctr; MA 74 Kean Coll of NJ; Sp-Lang Path, Wm S Baer Sch, **SLP**

Herzog, Dr Jean Talmage Speech & Hr Institute, University TX Health Sci C, 1343 Moursund, Houston, TX 77030, (713) 792-4500, BA 76 Univ of CA - Los Angeles; MA 79 CA St Univ - Northridge; PH 83 (Neurogenic Communication Disorders) Univ of TX - Austin; 86–Sp-Lang Path, Sp & Hr Institute, **SLP**

Herzog, Mrs Winifred P 4884 Pine Ledge Drive, Clarence, NY 14031, **LM**

Hesketh, Linda J Dept Of Comm Dis-Univ Of WI, 1975 Willow Drive, Madison, WI 53706, (608) 262-3951, BA 79 Univ of WA; MS 83 Univ of WA; 85–Clinical Instructor, University of Wisconsin, **SLP**

Heslin, Susan B 630 Gramatan Avenue #2-I, Mount Vernon, NY 10552, (914) 699-4874, BS 80 SUNY - Coll at Fredonia; MS 87 SUNY - Coll at Fredonia

Heslinga, Mrs Barbara A 704 West Deerbrook Drive, Peoria, IL 61615, (309) 691-4208, BS 76 IL St Univ - Normal; MS 77 IL St Univ - Normal; **SLP**

Hess, Barbara Fabo 1191 Glenside Avenue, Downingtown, PA 19335-3657, (215) 359-4340, MA 79 West Chester Univ of PA; Sp-Lang Path, Marple=Newtown School District, **SLP**

Hess, Mrs Carla Vehling 3684 Chestnut Lake Court, Jonesboro, GA 30236, BA 75 IN Univ - Bloomington; MA 77 IN Univ - Bloomington; 88–Sp-Lang Path, Clayton County GA Bd of Educ, **SLP**

Hess, Dr Carla W Dept Communication Disorders, University Of North Dakota, Grand Forks, ND 58202, (701) 777-3232, BS 62 MT St Univ; MS 67 Univ of ND; PH 71 (NS) OH Univ - Athens; 73–Prof, U of ND, **SLP A F ACE**

Hess, Mrs Carol P 31 Fox Chase Court, Freehold, NJ 07728, (201) 431-1110, BA 67 Hofstra Univ; MA 69 Hofstra Univ; **SLP**

Hess, Carole D 3165 Hunterdon Court, Marietta, GA 30067, BS 65 Univ of IA; MA 66 Univ of IA; **SLP**

Hess, Chad Wilson 503 Aberdeen Avenue, Hamilton, ON, Canada L8P 2S6, (416) 522-0466, BA 80 San Diego St Univ; MA 83 Memphis St Univ; Sp-Lang Path, Private Practice, **SLP**

Hess, Claire Louise 1104 Melody Drive, Metairie, LA 70002, (504) 835-1236, BS 85 Spring Hill Coll; OM 87 LA St Univ - N O Medical Ctr; 87–Aud, Browne-McHardy Clinic, **A**

Hess, Dr Donald A 223 Hennepin Road, Grand Island, NY 14072, (716) 878-5316, BS 42 Clarion Univ of PA; ME 49 PA St Univ - Univ Park; ED 55 (Clinical Speech) PA St Univ - Univ Park; Prof Sp-Lang Path & Aud, St U Coll at Buffalo, **SLP F**

Hess, Mrs Gay S Opelousas Speech & Learning Center Incorporated, PO Box 7085, Opelousas, LA 70571-7085, (318) 942-1100, BA 73 Univ of Southwestern LA; MS 80 Univ of Southwestern LA; Sp-Lang Path, Private Practice, **SLP**

Hess, Gregory R 303 Potter, Bellingham, WA 98225, **A**

Hess, Mrs Janell T 830 N W 135th Way, Sunrise, FL 33325, (305) 473-2483, BS 72 Purdue Univ - West Lafayette; MS 72 Purdue Univ - West Lafayette; SLP, Sch Bd of Broward Co, **SLP**

Hess, Mrs Karen L Route 3 Box 107A, Scott City, KS 67871, (316) 872-3500, BA 79 Wichita St Univ; MA 81 Wichita St Univ; Sp-Lang Path, High Plains Ed Coop, **SLP**

Hess, Linda Kurani 1008 Zephyr Court, Roseville, CA 95678, (916) 929-3669, SLP, North Sacramento School Dist, **SLP**

Hess, Dr Lucille K 3439 Glenhurst Avenue, Fort Wayne, IN 46805, (219) 482-5385, BS 66 Western MI Univ; MA 68 Western MI Univ; PH 84 (Sp-Lang Path) IN Univ - Bloomington; Asst Prof Aud & Sp Sci, In Prudue Univ, **SLP**

Hess, Mrs Lynn Durham 204 Haney Drive, Chattanooga, TN 37411, (615) 698-7043, BS 79 Univ of TN - Knoxville; MA 81 Univ of TN - Knoxville; 84–Sp-Lang Path, Hamilton County Schools, **SLP**

Hess, Mrs Mary Loughney 10 Rosemary Drive, Albany, NY 12211-2326, (518) 664-6396, BS 81 Coll of Saint Rose; ME 83 Coll of Saint Rose; Dir of Clinical Services, Helping Hands Clinic, **SLP**

Hess, Mrs Sandra Lynn 7K Millholland Drive, Fishkill, NY 12524, (914) 336-2616, BA 82 SUNY - Coll at Plattsburgh; MA 84 SUNY - Coll at Plattsburgh; 86–Sp-Lang Path, The Children's Annex, **SLP**

Hess, Sharon A 5801 Eubank Boulevard N E, Apartment 252, Albuquerque, NM 87111, (505) 822-0587, BS 85 Univ of WI - Milwaukee; MS 87 Marquette Univ; 87–Sp-Lang Path, Albuquerque Hrng & Sp Ctr, **SLP**

Hess, Teresa Holdren 1900 S W Arnold Avenue, Topeka, KS 66604, (913) 232-1731, **SLP**

Hess, Mrs Terri Lorene 21 Westminster, Briarcrest Gardens, Hershey, PA 17033, (717) 737-6728, BS 78 Kutztown Univ of PA; MS 85 Bloomsburg Univ of PA; 88–Sp-Lang Path, Cap Area Inter Unit, **SLP**

Hess, Sr Wanda J Northwest Hearing & Speech Clinic, 550 Latona Road, Rochester, NY 14626, (716) 225-1914, BS 72 SUNY - Coll at Geneseo; MA 75 Univ of KS; MA 74 Univ of KS; Director, NW Hearing & Speech, **SLP A**

Hess, Wayne J Central High School, 525 East Avenue, Red Wing, MN 55066, (612) 388-7181, BS 65 Saint Cloud St Univ; MS 75 Univ of MN - Minneap-St Paul; Sp-Lang Path, Red Wing Pub Sch, **SLP**

Hesse, Audrey Lynn 227 North 7th Avenue #3, Twin Falls, ID 83301, (208) 733-5828, BA 83 Eastern WA Univ; MS 84 Eastern WA Univ; Sp-Lang Path, Lenrner Michener & Assoc Inc, **SLP**

Hesse, Mrs Kathleen L 626 West Lawn Avenue, Racine, WI 53405, (414) 637-8654, BS 71 Bradley Univ; MS 87 Marquette Univ; 88–Sp-Lang Path, Racine USD

Hesselblad, Janet Elizabeth 83-11 261st Street, Floral Park, NY 11004, (212) 750-6861, BS 78 SUNY - Center at Albany; MS 83 Columbia Univ Teachers Coll; Aud, Goldwater Mem Hosp, **A**

Hesselroth, Marcia L 14625 Spring Lake Road, Minnetonka, MN 55345, (612) 933-9385, BS 70 Saint Cloud St Univ; MS 79 Univ of WI - River Falls; Sp-Lang Path, Hopkins Pub Schs, **SLP**

Hessenthaler, Mrs Kerry M 1115 Blue Springs Road, Franklin, TN 37064, (615) 791-9877, BS 77 Purdue Univ - West Lafayette; MA 78 Western MI Univ; Sp-Lang Path, Bill Wilkerson Hrng & Sp Ctr, **SLP**

Hessing, Mark 2000 Kings Highway, Brooklyn, NY 11229, (718) 645-6742, MA 80 Hofstra Univ; Director/Founder, Glenwood Sp & Lang Services, **SLP**

Hession, Carol M 2431 Neil Armstrong Blvd, Apartment 1-A, West Lafayette, IN 47906, (317) 494-3789, BS 82 Worcester St Coll; MS 85 Purdue Univ - West Lafayette; **A**

Hession, Lucy Anne 126 West Barre Street, Baltimore, MD 21201-2404, (301) 659-2496, BA 53 Univ of Miami; MA 65 Columbia Univ Teachers Coll; Staff Devel Sp Ed, MD St Dept of Ed, **SLP**

Hessler, Teresa Ann Wetzel Elementary, USMCA-Baumholder, APO New York, NY 09034, (713) 443-1011, BA 83 Univ of WI - Eau Claire; MS 84 Lamar Univ; Sp-Lang Path, DOODS, **SLP**

Hester, Eva J 8623 Hayshed Lane, Columbia, MD 21045, **SLP**

Hester, Joan M Route 2, Salem Road, Greenback, TN 37742, (615) 977-8282, BA 70 Univ of FL; MA 75 Western Carolina Univ; Sp-Lang Path, Private Practice, **SLP**

Hester, Melissa Driskell Post Office Box 1835, Espanola, NM 87532, (505) 753-4539, ME 86 Stephen F Austin St Univ

Heston, Robert E 8987 Root Road, North Ridgeville, OH 44039, (216) 331-3602, BA 69 Univ of Akron; MA 73 Univ of Akron; Aud, ENT Group of Cleveland Inc, **A**

Hestrin, Mrs Marcia K 4694 White Oak Place, Encino, CA 91316, **SLP**

Hethcock, Mrs Laura M 1509 Hamilton, San Marcos, TX 78666, (512) 392-6872, BS 63 Southwest TX St Univ; ME 70 Southwest TX St Univ; Pub Sch Sp/Lang Path, San Marcos Consol ISD, **SLP**

Hetherington, Laurel Jean 418 N 48th Street, Seattle, WA 98103, (206) 258-7304, MS 87 Univ of WA; 88–Sp-Lang Path, Providence Hosp

Hetsko, Richard James 10141 E River Road, Elyria, OH 44035, (216) 775-1651, BS 73 Bloomsburg Univ of PA; ME 74 Bloomsburg Univ of PA; Aud, Oberlin Cl, **A ACE**

Hettinger, Teresa Lynne 600 South Harrison #59, Olathe, KS 66061, (913) 782-0257, BA 86 Wichita St Univ; MA 87 Wichita St Univ

Hettler, Mrs Elizabeth A 3512 Avondale Road, North Little Rock, AR 72116, BA 78 Univ of Puget Sound; MA 80 WA St Univ; **SLP**

Hettrick, Mrs Chrystine M 1101 North Summit, Arkansas City, KS 67005, (316) 686-5899, BA 85 Wichita St Univ; MA 87 Wichita St Univ; 88–Sp-Lang Path, Cowley Co Spec Svcs Coop

Hetzel, Trudy Gordon 971 Thomas Avenue, Baldwin, NY 11510-4142, (718) 642-6099, BA 74 SUNY - Center at Binghamton; MS 78 CUNY - Brooklyn Coll; 87–Aud, Brooklyn Developmental Center, **A**

Hetzler, Mrs Marilyn J 127 Ford Street, Geneva, IL 60134, (312) 844-4490, BA 48 Univ of IA; MA 59 Univ of IA; Teacher of Hearing Impaired, Public School Aurora West II, **SLP**

Heublein, Elizabeth 1315 Centaur Village Court, Lafayette, CO 80026, (303) 492-8727, BA 69 Univ of CO - Boulder; MA 75 Univ of CO - Boulder; PH 85 (NS) Univ of CO - Boulder; Co-Dir, Educ Ctr, **SLP**

Heuer, Deborah Joseph 10 Bistineau Court, Kenner, LA 70065, (504) 367-3120, BS 74 LA St Univ - Baton Rouge; OM 76 LA St Univ - N O Medical Ctr; 78–Sp-Lang Path, Jefferson Parish Pub Sch Syst, **SLP**

Heuer, Dr Reinhardt 930 Oriental Avenue, Collingswood, NJ 08108, (215) 787-8220, BS 58 Univ of WI - Madison; MA 67 CUNY - Brooklyn Coll; PH 70 (Sp Path/Aud) Univ of OR; Assoc Prof, Temple Univ, **SLP**

Heun, Mrs Joanne M 156 Brookfield, Avon Lake, OH 44012, (216) 933-4078, BA 79 Baldwin-Wallace Coll; MS 80 Northwest MO St Univ; Sp-Lang Path, Fairview General Hospital, **SLP**

Heusner, Donna M S 2216 Foothill Drive #G-118, Salt Lake City, UT 84109, (801) 466-8692, BA 74 Russell Sage Coll; MS 81 Univ of VT; Sp/Lang Path, Holy Cross Hosp, **SLP**

Hevezi, Rose Ann 843 S Longmore #2150, Mesa, AZ 85202, (602) 844-5097, BS 80 CO St Univ; MA 83 Univ of Northern CO; Sp-Lang Path, Cigna Hlth Plan, **SLP**

Hevrdeys, Sylvia A 3409 Cottonwood Lane, Omaha, NE 68134-4629, (402) 554-6034, BS 76 Univ of NE - Omaha; MS 77 Univ of NE - Omaha; Sp-Lang Path, Omaha Pub Schs, **SLP**

Hewett, Mrs Jo Murphy 5031 Stanhope Drive, Houston, TX 77084-3032, (713) 855-1937, BS 81 Coll of Charleston; ME 83 Central St Univ; Sp-Lang Path, Memorial City Rehab Hosp, **SLP**

Hewitson, Mrs Deborah Hulbert R R 1 Box 71, Mc Lean, IL 61754-9503, (309) 874-2908, BA 80 IL St Univ - Normal; MS 82 IL St Univ - Normal; Sp-Lang Path, Dist 87 Pub Schs, **SLP**

Hewitt, Cecily T 1674 Wyld Street West, North Bay, ON, Canada P1B 2B7, (705) 472-1641, BA 72 Laurentian Univ - Ontario; OM 74 Univ of Toronto - Ontario; Dir of SLP, St Joseph's Hosp, **SLP**

Hewitt, Mrs Danielle A 16142 E Lake Shore Drive S, Hope, IN 47246, (812) 346-4401, BA 82 IN Univ - Bloomington; MA 83 IN Univ - Bloomington; 87–Aud, Muscatatuck St Dev Ctr, **A**

Hewitt, Joan Glaser 6558 Via Barona, Carlsbad, CA 92009, (619) 280-5444, BA 81 Univ of AZ; ME 83 Smith Coll; 85–Dir, Project TALK, **A**

Hewitt, Joan Tillman 2213 Putnam Street, Antioch, CA 94509, (415) 682-7686, BA 74 Univ of CA - Davis; MA 80 CA St Univ - Northridge; SLP, Mount Diable USD, **SLP**

Hewitt, Mrs Loreen Kay 261 Lancewood Place, Greensburg, PA 15601, (412) 832-1018, BA 80 Univ of South FL; MS 82 Indiana Univ of PA; SLP, **SLP**

Hewitt, Lynne Elizabeth 239 Huntington Avenue, Buffalo, NY 14214, (716) 832-0113, BA 80 Cornell Univ; MA 87 SUNY - Center at Buffalo; 87–Sp-Lang Path, DayTreat Ctr Niagara Co Assoc for Ret Chldn, **SLP**

Hewitt, Pamela Rose P O Box 273, Higganum, CT 06441-0273, (203) 345-4584, BS 83 Southern CT St Univ; MS 85 Southern CT St Univ; Sp-Lang Path, Regional #17 Sch Sys, **SLP**

Hewitt, Veronica G 4079 Millstream Road, Greenwood, IN 46142, **SLP**

Hewkin, Steven Kenneth 1019 S Pearl #J, Tacoma, WA 98465, (206) 491-9733, BA 84 Western WA Univ; MA 88 Western WA Univ; **A**

Hewlett, Catherine Margaret 1032 Palmer Place, Waukegan, IL 60085, (312) 662-6905, BS 82 Southern IL Univ-Edwardsvill; MA 83 Southern IL Univ-Edwardsvill; Sp-Lang Path, Hawthorn Speech/Lang Services, **SLP**

Hewson, Sara A 4 Courtland Street, Pawcatuck, CT 06379, (203) 599-8926, BA 71 Univ of RI; MS 73 Univ of RI; Sp-Lang Path, Ledyard Board of Education, **SLP**

Hey, Mary L 80 Sea Street #4, North Weymouth, MA 02191, (617) 878-3551, BS 75 Univ of RI; MS 81 Syracuse Univ; Sp/Lang Path, So Shore Ed Coolab Hrng Imp, **SLP**

Heyde, Mrs Wendy K 3 Hillbrook Court #303, Timonium, MD 21093, (301) 561-8368, **SLP**

Heydon, Linda Joy 2220-A Almaden Road, San Jose, CA 95125, (408) 378-6131, BA 77 Lewis & Clark Coll; MA 85 San Jose St Univ; SLP, Los Gatos Com Hosp, **SLP**

Heydon, Susan L 5972 Dawson Court, Greendale, WI 53129, (414) 281-7200, BS 83 Univ of WI - Whitewater; MS 84 Univ of WI - Whitewater; SLP, Mount Carmel Health Care Ctr, **SLP**

Heydon-Wrather, Norma Jean Route 1 Box 375, Portageville, MO 63873, (314) 688-2412, OM 84; Consult, Pemiscot Health Systems, **SLP**

Heyen, Donna Louise 4310-D Colonial Circle, Bradenton, FL 33508, (813) 746-0103, BS 84 FL St Univ; MA 86 Univ of KS; **SLP**

Heyer, Judith L 2310 Westminster Road, Cleveland Heights, OH 44118, (216) 687-6984, BS 56 OH St Univ; MA 71 Cleveland St Univ; Asst Cl Prof, Cleveland State Univ, **SLP A ACE**

Heyer, Mrs Mary Haynie 252 Sabal Palm Terrace, Boca Raton, FL 33432, (305) 391-1696, BS 65 Univ of NE - Omaha; MA 68 Univ of South FL; **SLP LM**

Heyl, Donna Shanley 123 High Hill Road, Boulder Creek, CA 95006, (408) 338-4583, BS 65; MS 81; Sp-Lang Path, San Lorenzo Valley Sch Dist, **SLP**

Heyman, Beth Ann 102 Regency Park Drive, Agawam, MA 01001, (413) 534-2508, MA 87 Univ of MA - Amherst; 87–Aud, Holyoke Hosp Sp Hrng Ctr, **A**

Heymann, Mrs Lois K 14 Ballard Place, Fair Lawn, NJ 07410-3610, (201) 797-7068, Bergen Comm Coll, **SLP**

Hiatt, Anne Louise 5434 Spain Avenue, Santa Rosa, CA 95409, (707) 538-5109, BA 73 CA St Univ - Los Angeles; MA 78 CA St Univ - Los Angeles; 87–Sp-Lang Path, Sp & Lang Svcs Inc, **SLP**

Hiatt, Christine L 4377 39th Street #8, San Diego, CA 92105, (619) 295-2835, MA 87 San Diego St Univ

Hiatt, Eloise Bonebright 8400 South 98th, Lincoln, NE 68506, (402) 483-5901, BA 72 Univ of NE - Lincoln; MA 74 Univ of NE - Lincoln; Sp-Lang Path, Lincoln Pub Sch, **SLP**

Hiatt, Joann Marie 120 South Hennepin Avenue, Dixon, IL 61021, (815) 288-4492, BS 78 Northern IL Univ - De Kalb; MS 83 CO St Univ; Aud, Joseph Elie MD, **A**

Hibbard, Mrs Marybeth Kemp 1001 Bullet Hill Road, Southbury, CT 06488, (203) 222-2584, BS 66 Purdue Univ - West Lafayette; MS 71 Cornell Univ; MA 84 CUNY - Hunter Coll; Sp-Lang Path, Weston Board of Education, **SLP**

Hibberd, Mrs Mary G 660 Western Avenue, Glen Ellyn, IL 60137, (312) 790-1827, BA 73 Coll of Saint Francis; MA 74 Northwestern Univ; 85–Sp-Lang Path, Marianjoy Rehabilitation Cen, **SLP**

Hibbett, Jean P 712 Cathy Circle, Gallatin, TN 37066, (615) 452-9704, BS 53 Univ of IL - Urbana; MS 59 Vanderbilt Univ; SLP Coord of Sp Services, Sumner Co Bd of Ed, **SLP**

Hibbs, Melanie June 3225A Emerson Street, Palo Alto, CA 94306, (415) 323-9422, BA 78 Univ of Northern IA; MA 79 Univ of Northern IA; SLP, Ravenswood City School Dist, **SLP**

Hibbs, Mrs Pauline Greve 4710 Duck Creek, Garland, TX 75043, (214) 442-3549, MS 87 Univ of TX - Dallas; **SLP**

Hickcox, Mrs Barbara J 820 6th Avenue, Grafton, WI 53024, (414) 284-7724, BS 77 Univ of WI - Oshkosh; MS 78 Univ of WI - Oshkosh; Sp/Lang Path, Port Washington Sch Dist, **SLP**

Hicken, Susan J 2456 Lyons Boulevard, Poland, OH 44514, (216) 757-8298, BA 74 Univ of NC - Chapel Hill; ME 81 NC Central Univ; **SLP**

Hickerson, A M 347 East 53rd Street, New York, NY 10022, BA 59 Univ of IA; MA 60 Northwestern Univ; MS 72 Columbia Univ Teachers Coll; Sp-Lang Path, NY Hosp, **SLP A**

Hickey, Carla Yim 5411 Sunshine Canyon Drive, Boulder, CO 80302, (303) 444-0105, BA 73 Univ of Denver; MA 74 Univ of Denver; **SLP**

Hickey, Cynthia Spier 4671 N Paseo DE Los Ranch, Tucson, AZ 85745, (602) 620-4927, MS 84 Univ of AZ; SLP, Carondelet Hlth Serv, **SLP**

Hickey, Karen 306 Madison Avenue, Fort Washington, PA 19034, (215) 596-9124, **SLP**

Hickey, Kathleen M 4434 Upton Avenue, Minneapolis, MN 55410, (714) 978-6478, BS 84 Univ of WI - Madison; MS 86 Univ of WI - Madison; Aud, Minneapolis ENT Clinic PA, **A**

Hickey, MaryEllen P O Box 202, South Salem, NY 10590, (914) 681-4660, MA 84 SUNY - Coll at Geneseo; Sp-Lang Path, St Agnes Childrens Ctr, **SLP**

Hickey, Mrs Susan Bell 1603 Greenwood Circle, Conway, AR 72032, (501) 329-8102, OB 82 Univ of Central AR; ME 84 Univ of Central AR; Sp-Lang Path, Faulkner Co Day Sch Inc, **SLP**

Hickey, William 21 Cleveland Street, Greenfield, MA 01301, (413) 863-9311, **SLP**

Hickle, Mrs Polly Ann L 3840 North Calusa Point, Crystal River, FL 32629, (904) 344-8846, BA 75 Univ of MD - College Park; MA 76 Univ of MD - College Park; 82–Sp-Lang Path, Citrus Co Sch, **SLP**

Hickman, Mrs Karen M 3127 Hamilton Street, West Lafayette, IN 47906, (317) 463-2090, BS 75 Purdue Univ - West Lafayette; MA 76 Univ of TN - Knoxville; MS 83 Purdue Univ - West Lafayette; Audiologist, St Elizabeth Hospital, **A**

Hickman, Laurel Anne 1260 Swift Shore Circle, West Linn, OR 97068, (503) 657-2444, BS 81 Portland St Univ; MS 83 Portland St Univ; Sp-Lang Path, Oregon City Public Schools, **SLP**

Hickman, Mrs Pamela Fay R R 1 Box 53, Mound City, KS 66056, (913) 757-4417, MS 84 Central MO St Univ; SLP, East Central Kansas Sp Ed Coop, **SLP**

Hickman-Kamarad, Mrs Bonita M HCR 68 Box 50, Comstock, NE 68828, BS 74 Univ of NE - Lincoln; MA 75 Univ of NE - Lincoln; Sp/Lang Path, Sandhills Ed Serv Coop, **SLP**

Hickox, Sharon Kay P O Box 773, Stockbridge, MI 49285, (517) 851-7447, BS 83 Central MI Univ; MA 84 Central MI Univ; Audiologist, McAuley Clinic, **A**

Hicks, Al Audiology Clinic, 411 N E 87th Avenue, Suite B, Vancouver, WA 98664, (206) 892-9367, BS 70 Portland St Univ; MS 72 Portland St Univ; PH 78 (NS) Univ of WA; Aud, Aud Cl, **A**

Hicks, Mrs Alison F Courtney Square #5-A, Greenville, NC 27858, (919) 756-5265, BA 72 Univ of NC - Chapel Hill; MS 86 East Carolina Univ; 86–Sp-Lang Path, UCP of NC, **SLP**

Hicks, Ann Michelle 503 North 85th Avenue, Omaha, NE 68114, (402) 691-1335, MS 82 Univ of NE - Lincoln; Sp-Lang Path, Millard Pub Schs, **SLP**

Hicks, Charlotte Visniski 1386 South Hale Avenue, Escondido, CA 92025, (619) 743-1050, BA 82 Univ of CA - San Diego; MA 86 San Diego St Univ; 86–Sp-Lang Path, UCP, **SLP**

Hicks, Mrs Cynthia P 103 Gower Road, Spartanburg, SC 29303, (803) 573-9825, BA 79 Univ of NC - Greensboro; ME 81 Univ of NC - Greensboro; 87–Sp-Lang Path, Spartanburg Co Sch Dist #7, **SLP**

Hicks, Dr Douglas M 2130 N W 54th Terrace, Gainesville, FL 32605, (904) 392-2041, BA 71 Coll of Wooster; MA 72 Northwestern Univ; PH 81 (NS) Vanderbilt Univ; Asst Prof/Dept of Sp, U of FL, **SLP**

Hicks, Elaine Robin 807 West High Street, South Hill, VA 23970, (804) 447-3151, BS 85; MS 87 Univ of SC - Columbia; 87–Sp-Lang Path, InSpeech Inc, **SLP**

Hicks, Gayle E 1401 Emerald Avenue, El Cajon, CA 92020, MA 76 San Diego St Univ; Owner, Private Practice, **A**

Hicks, Dr James W, Jr 2421 Brookcrest Drive, Garland, TX 75040, (214) 272-0515, BS 73 Univ of FL; MA 76 Univ of FL; PH 79 (NS) Univ of FL; SLP, E-Systems Inc

Hicks, Mrs Laurie Leslie 2725 Old Jacksonville Road, Tyler, TX 75701, (214) 531-8190, BS 79 Univ of North TX; MS 81 Univ of North TX; Aud, Vaughn Speech & Hearing Center, **A**

Hicks, Loretta A 108 Carriage House Trail, Garner, NC 27529, (919) 254-0211, BS 75 Univ of VA - Charlottesville; MA 77 Univ of MD - College Park; OM 84 Cornell Univ; Information Developer, International Business Machine, **SLP**

Hicks, Naomi Jean 472 Park Street, Tracy, MN 56175, (507) 629-3022, MS 87 Mankato St Univ

Hicks, Patricia Rogers RFD 11 Box 99, Shaker Road, Concord, NH 03301, (603) 224-0161, BA 74 Univ of NH; MS 85 Univ of NH; 85–Sp-Lang Path, Concord Sch Dist, **SLP**

Hicks, Shannon K 1011 Buena Vista Drive SE, Albuquerque, NM 87106, (505) 247-4224, BA 83 Univ of WI - Eau Claire; MA 86 Univ of MN - Minneap-St Paul; Dir Sp-Lang Path, Albuquerque Hear & Speech Ctr, **SLP**

Hicks, Terry C 11590 Old St Charles Rock, Rd, Bridgeton, MO 63044, (314) 569-8100, BS 77 Southwest MO St Univ; MS 78 Southern IL Univ-Edwardsvill; SLP, Spec Sch Dist of St Louis Cnty, **SLP**

Hierlmeier, Debra K 517 South Shore Drive, Land O'Lakes, FL 33539, (813) 996-3877, BS 74 Univ of SD - Vermillion; MA 76 Univ of SD - Vermillion; Dir of Presch, First Utd Methodist Presch, **SLP**

Hiersemann, Ruth L 406 West Regent Street #9, Inglewood, CA 90301, (213) 419-2553, BA 53 Grinnell Coll; MA 61 Northwestern Univ; SLP, Los Angeles Co Supt of Sch, **SLP**

Hietpas, Mrs Kathleen T 4821 South David Street, Casper, WY 82601, (307) 265-3970, BS 75 CO St Univ; MS 77 CO St Univ; Aud, WY Otol, **A**

Higa, Mrs Doreen Yurie 1634 Nuuanu Avenue #405, Honolulu, HI 96817, MS; **SLP**

Higbe, Mrs Jeanette F 6556 Bermuda Green Court, Alexandria, VA 22312, (703) 256-0576, MA 66 Univ of SD - Vermillion; 86–Sp-Lang Path, Fairfax Co PS, **SLP**

Higbee, Nancy L C 21230 Onaknoll Drive, Perris, CA 92370, (714) 780-9237, BA 69 CA St Univ - Fullerton; MA 74 CA St Univ - Fullerton; 83–Sp/Lang Path, CA-Hi Elks Major Proj Inc, **SLP**

Higdon, Lawrence W Audiolabs, 5525 Safari, Corpus Christi, TX 78411, (512) 854-9586, BS 64 Univ of TX - Austin; MS 68 TX A & I Univ; Aud, Pan American Univ, **A F**

Higgerson, Michele M 2223 Winding Way, Davison, MI 48423, (313) 659-0683, BA 78 Univ of MI - Ann Arbor; MS 81 Southern IL Univ -Carbondale; Sp-Lang Path, Flushing Comm Schs, **SLP**

Higginbotham, D Jeffery 108 Highland Avenue, Buffalo, NY 14222-1841, (716) 636-3400, Research Asst Prof, SUNY, **SLP**

Higginbotham, Peggy Virginia 807 Jefferson, Memphis, TN 38105, (901) 525-2682, MS 83 Univ of AL- Tuscaloosa; Cl Superv, Memphis Sp & Hrng, **SLP**

Higginbothan, Susan Long 11408 North Wallace Avenue, Oklahoma City, OK 73132-9640, **SLP**

Higgins, Anne Weise P O Box 152347, Tampa, FL 33684-2347, (813) 870-1652, **SLP**

Higgins, Barbara F 2218 Nova Village Drive, Davie, FL 33317, (305) 475-9358, BA 74 Rutger's St Univ - Douglas Coll; MS 76 Columbia Univ Teachers Coll; Aud, Nova Univer, **A**

Higgins, Mrs Candie L Rd 2 Box 79, John Ringoes Road, Ringoes, NJ 08551-9606, (201) 782-7595, BA 73 Central MI Univ; MA 77 Eastern MI Univ; 83–Sp-Lang Path, Private Practice, **SLP**

Higgins, Cheryl J 704 35th Street West, Bradenton, FL 34205, (813) 747-4815, BA 74 Heidelberg Coll; MA 77 Univ of Akron; Sp-Lang Path, Private Practice, **SLP**

Higgins, Mrs Christine Pauletich 1175 Trestle Glen Road, Oakland, CA 94610, (415) 763-1981, BA 82 Univ of the Pacific; MS 84 Boston Univ; Sp-Lang Path, Faltz Associates, **SLP**

Higgins, Elizabeth Ruth 160 Georgetown Road #3, Charlottesville, VA 22901, (804) 971-1566, BS 81 Bradley Univ; MA 83 Northwestern Univ; Sp/Lang Path, U of VA Med Cen, **SLP ACE**

Higgins, Janice Logg 160 Pasito Terrace #715, Sunnyvale, CA 94086, (415) 493-8111, OB 84 Gonzaga Univ; MA 86 San Jose St Univ; 87–Sp-Lang Path, Mid Peninsula Sp & L Clinic, **SLP**

Higgins, Dr Jerry M Prentke Romich Co, 1022 Heyl Road, Wooster, OH 44691, (800) 642-8255, BA 56 Asbury Coll; MA 65 Univ of IA; PH 71 (NS) MI St Univ; 86–Exec VP, Prentke Romich Co, **SLP**

Higgins, John D 200 West Hoover, Ann Arbor, MI 48103-5433, (313) 994-1934, Aud, **A**

Higgins, Mrs Judy Herold 927 Riverview Road, Rexford, NY 12148, (518) 374-1688, BS 81 SUNY - Coll at Geneseo; MA 83 SUNY - Coll at Geneseo; Instructor Sp/Lang Path, Schonowe Pre-School, **SLP**

Higgins, Mrs June Eden 208 Utah Road, Stevensville, MD 21666, (301) 479-1460, BA 84 Loyola Coll; MS 85 Loyola Coll; **SLP**

Higgins, Mrs Kathleen Kelley 237 Tredwell Avenue, St James, NY 11780, (518) 544-2957, BA 79 SUNY - Coll at Plattsburgh; MA 82 Hofstra Univ; SLP, Kings Park Psych Center, **SLP**

Higgins, Mrs Kelly Call 7826 Maple Brook Lane, Houston, TX 77095, (713) 855-7226, BA 82 Univ of OK - Norman; MS 87 Univ of Southwestern LA

Higgins, Laurie A Watauga Hearing Conserv Pc, 215 East Watauga Avenue, Johnson City, TN 37601, (615) 928-1901, BS 80 East TN St Univ; MS 82 East TN St Univ; Chief Aud-Gen Mgr, Watauga Hearing Conservatn Inc, **A**

Higgins, Dr Mary K 4144 Tenango, Claremont, CA 91711, (714) 624-1631, BA 63 Univ of AZ; MA 64 Univ of AZ; PH 82 (Education) Claremont Graduate Sch; Special Education Principal, Los Angeles Office of Educ, **SLP A F**

Higgins, Maureen B 800 Maryland Avenue, Syracuse, NY 13210, (315) 424-8168, MS 87 Syracuse Univ; 88–Tchg Asst, Syracuse Univ

Higgins, Patricia M 3292-B Highpoint Court, Snellville, GA 30278, (404) 329-5520, BS 76 Marquette Univ; MS 77 FL St Univ; Sp-Lang Path, Emory U-Cen for Rehab Med, **SLP**

Higgins, Patti A 2960 South Magnolia Way, Denver, CO 80224, (303) 759-3958, BS 84 CO St Univ; MS 87 CO St Univ; 88–Sp-Lang Path, Educ Assessment Sys Orate Elem, **SLP**

Higgins, Paul H 4144 Tenango, Claremont, CA 91711, BA 70 CA St Coll - San Bernardino; MA 73 CA St Univ - Los Angeles; **A**

Higgins, Portia R 920 South 47th Street, Louisville, KY 40211, (502) 456-3277, BA 59 Univ of MI - Ann Arbor; MA 65 NY Univ; SLP, Jefferson Co Pub Sch, **SLP**

Higgins, Mrs Teresa Nunn 4181 Floyd Street N E, Covington, GA 30209, (404) 786-7269, BS 80 Univ of GA; MA 81 Univ of TN - Knoxville; Sp-Lang Path, Newton Co Sch Sys, **SLP**

Higgins, Thomas M 13337 Ebell Street, Van Nuys, CA 91402, **A**

High, Jacklyn Joyce 56 Southern Road, Springfield, MA 01129, (413) 739-3954, BS 83 Univ of MA - Amherst; MA 85 Univ of MA - Amherst; **SLP**

High, Linda Marie 434 W Sunbury Road, Apartment 16 Sunbury Estates, Butler, PA 16001, (412) 285-8915, MA 88 Univ of MA - Amherst; 88–Aud, The Hearing Laboratory Inc

High, Mrs Marion L 131 Park Avenue, Swarthmore, PA 19081, (215) 543-1489, BS 71 West Chester Univ of PA; MA 76 West Chester Univ of PA; SLP, Upper Darby Sch Dist, **SLP**

Highfill, Melanie K 4416 East Simsbury Road, Charlotte, NC 28226, (704) 365-8841, MA 88 Univ of NC - Greensboro; 88–Sp-Lang Path, Holy Angels Inc

Highland, Mrs Kristeen H P O Box 517, Yankton, SD 57078, (402) 287-2061, BA 70 Univ of SD - Vermillion; MA 80 Univ of SD - Vermillion; Sp-Lang Path, Yankton Public Schools, **SLP**

Highley, Patricia Ann 140 Booker, Little Rock, AR 72205, (501) 569-3155, BA 73; MS 83 Univ of AR - Medical Sci; 85–Aud, The Ear Nose Throat Clinic PA, **A**

Highnam, Dr Cliff L 2322 Clay Street, Cedar Falls, IA 50613, (319) 233-6884, BA 67 Western WA Univ; MA 69 Univ of WA; PH 75 (NS) Bowling Green St Univ; Assoc Prof, Univ of Northern Iowa, **SLP**

Highnam, Mrs Diane Bell 2322 Clay Street, Cedar Falls, IA 50613, (319) 266-5205, BS 78 IA St Univ; MA 81 Univ of Northern IA; Sp-Lang Path, Private Practice, **SLP**

Highsmith, Mrs Deborah A 56 Leatherman Trail, Hamden, CT 06518-2045, (203) 287-9385, BS 73 East Carolina Univ; MS 76 Southern CT St Univ; Sp-Lang Path, New Haven Board of Education, **SLP**

Hight, Nancy G 134 Lang, Fort Sam Houston, TX 78234-5000, (512) 822-6354, **A**

Hightower, Alicia Diane 1585 Hollywood Drive #C-36, Jackson, TN 38305, (601) 335-5678, BA 81 Univ of MS; MA 83 Memphis St Univ; Sp-Lang Path, West TN Hearing and Speech Ctr, **SLP**

Hightower, Caroline J 135 Avocado Street, Leucadia, CA 92024, **SLP**

Hightower, Mrs Deborah Swank 642 Sunnyfield Road, Belvidere, IL 61008, (815) 332-2495, BS 76 Purdue Univ - West Lafayette; MA 79 Northern IL Univ - De Kalb; Sp-Lang Path, Rockford Pub Sch, **SLP**

Higie, Mrs Pauline G 30 Stone Avenue, Bradford, PA 16701, BS 49 Northwestern Univ; ME 78 Univ of Pittsburgh - Pittsburgh; **SLP**

Higley, Mrs Beulah S 1415 West Smith, Orlando, FL 32804, MS; **SLP LM**

Higman, Barbara J 207 West Williams, Ann Arbor, MI 48103, (517) 546-4126, BA 73 Univ of MI - Ann Arbor; MS 76 Univ of MI - Ann Arbor; 87–Sp-Lang Path, Livingston Co Commun Men Hlth, **SLP**

Hilaire, Francine J 910 Major Sherman Lane, Suite 305, Monterey, CA 93940, (408) 649-5000, BA 75 Boston Coll; MA 78 Univ of Denver; Sp/Lang Path, Speak E-Z Assoc, **SLP**

Hiland, Mrs Kristin J 3695 Cassandra Drive, Troy, OH 45373, (513) 339-2693, BA 76 AZ St Univ; MS 87 Miami Univ - Oxford; **SLP**

Hilber, Mrs Jean S 9360 West Forest Home Avenue, Apartment 5, Greenfield, WI 53228, (414) 425-6035, BA 60 Univ of WI - Milwaukee; MS 70 Marquette Univ; Sp-Lang Path, Wauwatosa Sch Syst of Wisc, **SLP**

Hild, Mrs Patricia J 501 Arthur, Holdrege, NE 68949, (308) 995-6585, BA 72 Kearney St Coll; MS 76 Kearney St Coll; Sp-Lang Path, Ed Serv Ut #11, **SLP**

Hildahl, Barbara B Box 193, Gladbrook, IA 50635, (515) 752-1578, BA 68 Univ of Northern IA; MA 72 Univ of Northern IA; SLP, AEA Six, **SLP**

Hildebrand, Dr Beverly H Audiology & Speech Path 126NLR, VA Medical Center, North Little Rock, AR 72114, (501) 660-2008, BA 68 TX Tech Univ; OM 72 Southern Methodist Univ; PH 76 (Sp Path (Voice Disorders)) Univ of FL; 88–Chief Aud/SLP Svc, VA Med Cen-Little Rock, **SLP**

Hildebrand, Debra Lynn 127-A North Baker Street, Charlottesville, VA 22903, (804) 296-9161, BS 78 Radford Univ; ME 81 Univ of VA - Charlottesville; Audiologist, University of Virginia Hosp, **A**

Hildebrand, Lezlie A 3996 Rollinghills Drive, Bettendorf, IA 52722, (319) 386-6450, BA 72 Univ of Northern IA; MA 76 Univ of Northern IA; Sp-Lang Path, MS Bend AEA, **SLP**

Hildebrand, Mrs Maurine H 1107 St Christopher, Columbia, MO 65203, (314) 445-4403, 58 Univ of MO - Columbia; 73 Univ of MO - Columbia; ES 81 Univ of MO - Columbia; Sp-Lang Path, Columbia PS, **SLP**

Hildebrand, Mrs Pamela Lea 1024 Bourn Avenue, Columbia, MO 65201, (816) 849-2141, BS 74 Southwest MO St Univ; OM 84 Univ of MO - Columbia; **SLP**

Hildebrand, Renee Lynn P O Box 332 Rt 73, Skippack, PA 19474, (215) 584-4877, MS 88 Bloomsburg Univ of PA; 88–Sp-Lang Path, Crozer-Chester Med Ctr

Hildebrand, Susanne Y R R 2 Box 360, Kankakee, IL 60901, (312) 534-5000, BS 68 Northern IL Univ - De Kalb; MS 69 Univ of IL - Urbana; Prof, Governors State U, **SLP**

Hildebrandt, Dr Emery V 3655 N W Highland Drive, Corvallis, OR 97330, (503) 754-2461, BS 50 OR St Univ; MS 56 PA St Univ - Univ Park; PH 70 (Sp Path) Univ of OR; Prof Sp Commun, Or St U, **SLP LM**

Hildebrandt, Jane Kastner 2896 James Avenue S #307, Minneapolis, MN 55408, (612) 566-1814, MA 86 Univ of MN - Minneap-St Paul; **SLP**

Hilden, Rhoda I 713 Custer Street, Dickinson, ND 58601, (701) 225-6767, BA 72 Univ of ND; MA 73 Univ of ND; Sp-Lang Path, Dickinson Pub Schools, **SLP**

Hildick, Dorothy Caccamo 5306 Black Pine Drive, Tampa, FL 33624, (904) 567-3760, MS 84 Univ of South FL; 84–Sp-Lang Path, Pasco County Schools, **SLP**

Hildner, Cynthia 3806 Melstone Drive, Arlington, TX 76016, BA 79 Augustana Coll; MS 81 Univ of WI - Madison; Sp-Lang Path, Excellcare Inc, **SLP**

Hildreth, Mrs Katherine Morton P O Box 158, Richmond, MA 01254, (413) 447-8931, BS 83 SUNY - Coll at Geneseo; MA 85 SUNY - Coll at Geneseo; 88–Sp-Lang Path, Private Practice, **SLP**

Hildreth, Sharon L Box 65-A, Odin, IL 62870, (618) 532-4721, BS Southern IL Univ-Edwardsvill; MS 81 Southern IL Univ-Edwardsvill; Sp/Lang Path, Kaskaskia Spec Ed Dist, **SLP**

Hiles, Marcia M 4133 Tacoma Street, Springfield, OH 45503, (513) 325-9263, BS 76 Fontbonne Coll; MS 78 Fontbonne Coll; SLP, Springview Developmnt Cen, **SLP**

Hiles, Mrs Mary O Greenwich Board Of Education, 290 Greenwich Avenue, Greenwich, CT 06830, (203) 625-7492, BA 56 Univ of CT; MA 57 Univ of CT; Coord of Spec Ed, Greenwich Bd of Ed, **SLP**

Hilger, Mrs Manuela W Route 2, 2199 Pleasant Hill Road, Jefferson City, MO 65109, (314) 496-3882, BS 78 Central MO St Univ; MS 79 Central MO St Univ; Private Practice, **SLP**

Hilger, Sandra I 1633 Tulane, Naperville, IL 60565, (312) 961-3602, BS 76 Northern IL Univ - De Kalb; MA 78 Northwestern Univ; Sp-Lang Path, Private Practice, **SLP**

Hilker, Patricia J 261 Congressional Lane, Apartment 606, Rockville, MD 20852, (301) 424-5088, BA 60 Goucher Coll; ME 69 Univ of VA - Charlottesville; Sp-Lang Path, Montgomery Cty Publ Sch, **SLP**

Hill, Alan R Middletown Hospital Assoc, 105 McKnight Drive, Middletown, OH 45042, **SLP**

Hill, Alice Baer 314 North Wilshire Lane, Arlington Heights, IL 60004, (312) 668-2180, BA 79 Northern IL Univ - De Kalb; MA 81 Northern IL Univ - De Kalb; 81–Aud, Otol-Head & Neck Surgery Ltd, **A**

Hill, Mrs Baird McDonald 1505 Bruner Drive, Greenfield, IN 46140, (317) 898-6133, BA 71 Depauw Univ; MA 73 Univ of AZ; **SLP**

Hill, Barbara Goodman 7406 Midfield Avenue, Los Angeles, CA 90045, (213) 641-1609, BA 67 Univ of MI - Ann Arbor; MA 68 Northwestern Univ; Sp-Lang Path, LA Co Supt Sch, **SLP**

Hill, Mrs Beth S Evaluation Center, 2500 Viking Drive, Bossier City, LA 71111, (318) 746-6890, BA 61 Northwestern St Univ; MA 62 Northwestern St Univ; MA 69 Northwestern St Univ; Dir/Pupil Appraisal Service, Bossier Parish School Board, **SLP**

Hill, Mrs Betsy P 43 East Rose Lane, Phoenix, AZ 85012, BA 72 OH St Univ; MA 80 Appalachian St Univ; **SLP**

Hill, Brent W 5258 Dijon Drive, Baton Rouge, LA 70809, (504) 769-1090, BA 80 Nicholls St Univ; OM 81 LA St Univ - N O Medical Ctr; Aud, ENT Med Ctr, **A**

Hill, Capt Brian J 15030 Breezy Bend, San Antonio, TX 78217-1138, (512) 599-6347, BA 79 Univ of CT; MS 81 Lamar Univ; Ch Aud/Hrng Conserv, Ireland Army Hosp, **A**

Hill, Carol F 11602 Shakespearean Way, Austin, TX 78759, (512) 258-8378, BS 69 Abilene Christian Univ; MS 72 Baylor Univ; Sp/Lang Path, Private Practice, **SLP**

Hill, Carole L 6821 Lyre Lane, Dallas, TX 75214, (214) 368-0664, BS 68 TX Woman's Univ; MS 71 TX Woman's Univ; 87–Exec Dir, Oak Hill Academy, **SLP**

Hill, Carolyn M 1616 Madison Avenue, West Islip, NY 11795, **SLP**

Hill, Mrs Carrie Kae 400 South Bittersweet, Muncie, IN 47304, (317) 747-4258, BS 82 Ball St Univ; MA 84 Ball St Univ; Sp-Lang Path, Ball Memorial Hospital, **SLP**

Hill, Clara V 3513 Brees, Plano, TX 75075, (214) 867-0014, BS 64 Univ of MO - Columbia; **SLP**

Hill, Colleen C 213 Second Street, Ithaca, NY 14850, (607) 272-1913, SLP, Ithaca City Schl Dstr, **SLP**

Hill, Mrs Connie S Rural Route 3, Clarion, IA 50525, (515) 532-2971, BS 69 Mankato St Univ; MA 76 Mankato St Univ; Adlt Bosic Ed Instr, Wright Co Opportunities Inc, **SLP**

Hill, Cynthia L 1338 Barclay Lane, Deerfield, IL 60015, (312) 566-1949, BS 78 IN Univ - Bloomington; MS 79 Univ of IL - Urbana; Sp-Lang Path, Northbrook School District 27, **SLP**

Hill, David 700 Clearview Drive, Glenview, IL 60025, (312) 328-5180, BS 69 Southern IL Univ -Carbondale; MS 70 Southern IL Univ -Carbondale; Dir of Aud Serv, Audio-Vestibular Assoc Ltd, **A**

Hill, David Allan 223 Oakmount Road, Toronto, ON, Canada M6P 3K3, (416) 925-5141, MA 86 SUNY - Center at Buffalo; 88–Coord Comm Therapy & Res Prog, Surrey Place Centre, **SLP**

Hill, Mrs Debbie Robinson P O Box 10603, Springfield, MO 65808, (417) 885-6888, BS 78 Phillips Univ; MS 80 Phillips Univ; Dir of Rehab Svcs, Lester E Cox Medical Center, **SLP**

Hill, Mrs Debra G Route 3 Box 680, Portales, NM 88130, (505) 356-8456, MS 86 Eastern NM Univ; 86–Sp-Lang Path, Portales Municipal Schs, **SLP**

Hill, Debra Nell 5706 Pinewilde, Houston, TX 77066, (713) 893-3332, BS 77 Univ Southern MS-Hattiesburg; OM 85 LA St Univ - Shreveport; **SLP**

Hill, Denzle L 1419 Willow Lane, Bowling Green, KY 42101, (502) 843-5818, BA 62 Southern IL Univ -Carbondale; MS 66 Southern IL Univ -Carbondale; Sp-Lang Path, Comm for Hndcpd Child, **SLP**

Hill, Desdy Joforeka 702 Tamarack Drive #5208, Fayetteville, NC 28311, (919) 822-3751, BA 82 NC St Univ at Raleigh; MA 84 Hampton Univ; Sp-Lang Path, Cumberland Co Schools, **SLP**

Hill, Mrs Diane G Northwestern University, 2299 Sheridan Road, Evanston, IL 60201, (312) 492-5012, BA 66 Augustana Coll; MA 70 Northwestern Univ; Lecturer & Clinical Supervisor, Northwestern University, **SLP**

Hill, Diane Pagnotto 21 Pearl Brook Road, Lunenburg, MA 01462-1224, (508) 343-4064, BS 74 Worcester St Coll; ME 81 Northeastern Univ; Sp-Lang Path, **SLP**

Hill, Dianna Sue 2408 11th Street #2, Emmetsburg, IA 50536, (712) 852-3243, BA 80 Univ of Northern IA; MA 82 Univ of Northern IA; 85–Sp-Lang Path, Lakeland AEA 3, **SLP**

Hill, Mrs Dolores Berry Four Rivers Spec Educ Dist, 936 W Michigan, Jacksonville, IL 62650, (217) 245-7174, BS 59 Eastern IL Univ; MS 69 Univ of IL - Urbana; Sp-Lang Path Supvr, Four Rivers Spec Ed Dist, **SLP**

Hill, Donna Brooks 1104 South 5th Street, Lafayette, IN 47905, MS; **SLP**

Hill, Edeen L 61 Earls Court Road, London, England W8 6EE, 1-937-9372, MS 72 San Diego St Univ; **SLP**

Hill, Edith M P O Box 41860, Santa Barbara, CA 93140-1860, BS 69 Onion Coll; MS 73 Fort Hays St Univ; Real Estate Mgr, Self Employed, **SLP**

Hill, Elaine Maria 1529 Casino Circle, Silver Spring, MD 20906, (301) 424-5200, BS 83 Towson St Univ; BS 83 Towson St Univ; ME 85 Univ of VA - Charlottesville; **SLP**

Hill, Elizabeth Ann 410-8 Wallen Hills Drive, Fort Wayne, IN 46825, (219) 489-6788, BS 85 Purdue Univ - West Lafayette; MA 86 Memphis St Univ; 88–Sp-Lang Path, Allen Co Soc for Crip Chil/Adu, **SLP**

Hill, Ellen M 11 1/2 Damian Road, Wheeling, WV 26003, (304) 242-7714, BS 79 Indiana Univ of PA; MS 80 WV Univ; Sp/Lang Path, Marshall County Schools, **SLP**

Hill, Emmeline Kunde 628 East 5th Street, Tucson, AZ 85705, (602) 622-0031, BS 84 Univ of AZ; MS 86 Univ of AZ; 88–Aud, Children's Rehab Svcs, **A**

Hill, George E, Jr 4201 Victoria Avenue, Los Angeles, CA 90008, PH (NS); **A LM**

Hill, Helen H 457 Pecos Loop, Rio Rancho, NM 87124, **SLP**

Hill, Jo Anne K 40 Lynn Drive, Newark, DE 19711, (312) 658-5205, BA 57 SD St Univ; MS 59 Purdue Univ - West Lafayette; Sp/Lang Path, Visiting Nurse Assoc, **SLP**

Hill, Mrs Joy H 1207 Highland Drive, Picayune, MS 39466, (601) 798-0434, BA 74 Blue Mountain Coll; MS 77 MS Univ for Women; **SLP**

Hill, Mrs Joy Perlove 47C Aspen Hill, Narraticon Apts, Deptford, NJ 08096, (609) 853-1993, BS 80 Eastern MI Univ; MA 81 Eastern MI Univ; 85–SLP, Ai Dupont I, **SLP**

Hill, Mrs Karen L 22005 Linda Drive, Torrance, CA 90503, (213) 540-9837, BA 76 CA St Univ - Long Beach; MA 81 CA St Univ - Long Beach; Director of Speech Pathology, Bay Harbor Rehabilitation Cen, **SLP**

Hill, Mrs Karen S 18000 Ridgewood, Lansing, IL 60438, BS 74 ID St Univ; MS 75 ID St Univ; Sp-Lang Path, Priv Home Prac, **SLP**

Hill, Katharine 5461 Woodlawn Drive PO 446, Edinboro, PA 16412, (814) 734-3223, **SLP**

Hill, Kathy D 7337 South Shore Drive, Apt #802, Chicago, IL 60649, (312) 997-3627, MS 80 Emory Univ; Sp-Lang Path, Chicago Board of Education, **SLP**

Hill, Larry Jay 2850 Kenwood Blvd, Toledo, OH 43606, (419) 472-5563, BS 80 Ball St Univ; MA 84 Ball St Univ; Clin Supvr, InSpeech Inc, **SLP A**

Hill, Mrs Linda C 18 Hillgrass, Irvine, CA 92715, (714) 634-5623, BA 76 Univ of CA - Santa Barbara; MA 78 Northwestern Univ; 87–Sp-Lnag Path, Univ of Calif Irvine Med Ctr, **SLP ACE**

Hill, Lyman M 1743 Via Hermana, San Lorenzo, CA 94580, (415) 577-3056, BA 50 Univ of UT; MA 54 San Francisco St Univ; Sp/Lang Path, San Leandro USD, **SLP**

Hill, Mrs Marcia Claudette 122 Main Street #401, Stoneham, MA 02180, BS 82 Andrews Univ; MA 84 Western MI Univ; 87–Sp-Lang Path, New England Mem Hosp, **SLP**

Hill, Marilyn Taube 10937 Irma Avenue, Tujunga, CA 91042, BA 77 CA St Univ - Los Angeles; MA 79 CA St Univ - Los Angeles; 87–Sp-Lang Path, Glendale USD, **SLP**

Hill, Mrs Mary B 103 Hickory Lane, Talladega, AL 35160, (205) 362-9623, BS 68 Auburn Univ - Auburn; MA 70 Auburn Univ - Auburn; Sp-Lang Path, Talladega Cty Sch Syst, **SLP**

Hill, Mrs Mary Bria P O Box 362, Boomer, WV 25031, (304) 574-1176, BA 73 Marshall Univ; MS 74 Marshall Univ; 88–Sp-Lang Path, Fayette Co Sch Sys, **SLP**

Hill, Mrs Mary E P O Box 263, Geneva, IL 60134, (312) 584-6367, BA 74 Iona Coll; MA 76 Ball St Univ; 87–Sp-Lang Path, St Patricks Sch, **SLP**

Hill, Mrs Mary P 246 Laney Drive, Forrest City, AR 72335, (501) 633-2566, BS 68 IL St Univ - Normal; MS 74 Univ of WI - Milwaukee; SLP, St Francis Area Dev Cen, **SLP**

Hill, Merry G USA-MEDDAC, EFMS Box 293, APO New York, NY 09801, BS 77 Univ of HI - Manoa; MS 79 Univ of HI - Manoa; 85–Sp-Lang Path, USA-MEDDAC Wurzburg, **SLP ACE**

Hill, Michael Lee 2519 Ashton Court, Cincinnati, OH 45244, (513) 621-5360, BA 79 Wright St Univ; MA 82 Univ of Cincinnati; Aud, Private Practice, **A**

Hill, Miriam 9 Denker Place, Staten Island, NY 10314, (718) 494-4194, BA 75 CUNY - Brooklyn Coll; MA 77 CUNY - Queens Coll; Sp-Lang Path, Maimonides Developmental Cen, **SLP**

Hill, Dr Nina M International Ctr For Disabled, 340 East 24th Street, New York, NY 10010, (212) 679-0100, BS 71 Ithaca Coll; MS 72 Columbia Univ Teachers Coll; PH 83 (NS) Columbia Univ Teachers Coll; 83–Dir Cl Serv & Prof Ed, ICD-International Cen for Dis, **SLP**

Hill, Mrs Patricia Vazquez 10 Caton Terrace, Caldwell, NJ 07006, (201) 881-6181, BA 85 Kean Coll of NJ; MA 86 Kean Coll of NJ; 86–Sp-Lang Path, Paterson Bd of Educ, **SLP**

Hill, Paul C 515 Virginia, Ponca City, OK 74601, (405) 762-7561, BS 66 Phillips Univ; MS 69 Phillips Univ; Dir Sp/Lang Path & Aud, Bi-St Men Hlth Found, **SLP**

Hill, Rosemary A 4416-F Simsbury Road, Charlotte, NC 28226, (704) 527-6248, BS 74 Univ of GA; MA 75 Western Carolina Univ; Reg Mgr/VP, Allstates Chemical Corp, **SLP**

Hill, Rowena Resnick 7-11th Avenue S W, Rochester, MN 55902, BA 71 CUNY - Hunter Coll; MA 73 NY Univ; 88–Sp-Lang Path, Stanley Jones & Assoc, **SLP**

Hill, Mrs Ruth E 59 Kinderhook, Chatham, NY 12037, (914) 889-4373, BS 55 SUNY - Coll at Buffalo; MS 64 SUNY - Coll at Buffalo; Sp-Lang Path, Anderson Sch, **SLP**

Hill, Sandra E 919 Amherst Street, Buffalo, NY 14222, (716) 878-4638, BS 72 SUNY - Coll at Buffalo; MS 76 SUNY - Coll at Buffalo; SLP, Buffalo Bd of Ed, **SLP**

Hill, Mrs Sandra L 5145 East Bannock Street, Phoenix, AZ 85044, (602) 893-1791, MS 78 Univ of AZ; Sp-Lang Path, Private Practice, **SLP**

Hill, Sharon Malure 808 East Pine Street, Tarpon Springs, FL 34689, (813) 934-1826, BA 79 Montclair St Coll; MS 82 FL St Univ; Pub Sch SLP, Pasco Co FL Dist Sch Bd, **SLP**

Hill, Mrs Susan Darling 2534 South Evanston, Tulsa, OK 74104, (918) 744-1848, BA 78 Univ of TX - Austin; MA 84 Univ of Tulsa; **SLP**

Hill, Mrs Susan Eileen Route 1 Box 327, Makanda, IL 62958, (618) 833-2545, BS 80 Southeast MO St Univ; MA 85 Southeast MO St Univ; **SLP**

Hill, Susan K 1440 Cherry Laurel, Norman, OK 73072, BA 64 Cornell Coll; MS 80 Univ of OK Medical Center; 80–Sp-Lang Path, Can Valley Coop, **SLP**

Hill, Vanessa Ruth Route 7 Box 1890, Benton, AR 72015, (501) 778-7175, BS 86 Univ of AR - Little Rock; MS 87 Univ of AR - Little Rock; 88–Sp-Lang Path, Bryant Sch Dist, **SLP**

Hill, Dr Wathina Smith 753 Will Scarlet Way, Macon, GA 31210, (912) 477-8683, BS 59 William Paterson Coll; MA 62 Columbia Univ Teachers Coll; ED 69 (NS) Columbia Univ Teachers Coll; Retired, Bronx VA Med Cen, **SLP A LM ACE**

Hill, William Blaine Cheshire Hearing Clinic, 69 Island Street, Keene, NH 03431, (603) 352-6302, MS 71 FL St Univ; MS 74 Gallaudet Coll; Aud, Cheshire Hrng Cl, **A**

Hill, Mrs Winn Warner 3985 Arden Way N E, Atlanta, GA 30342, (404) 237-0345, BS 83 Appalachian St Univ; MA 85 Appalachian St Univ; **SLP**

Hill-Albanowicz, Kerry Lee 774 Jennys Court, Lakewood, NJ 08701, (201) 458-3854, BS 80 Stockton St Coll; MA 83 NY Univ; 88–Sp-Lang Path, Middletown Bd of Educ, **SLP**

Hillard, Sallie Webber 1640 Forrest Avenue, Memphis, TN 38112, (901) 525-2682, BA 69 Vanderbilt Univ; MA 70 Vanderbilt Univ; Cl Superv, Memphis St U, **SLP**

Hill-Brown, Mrs Carolyn J 552 E 7th Street, Beaumont, CA 92223, (213) 483-4431, BS 78 IN St Univ - Evansville; MS 81 IN St Univ - Evansville; Sp-Lang Path, House Ear Institute, **SLP**

Hillenbrand, Kathryn L 4813 Norfolk Circle, Portage, MI 49002, (716) 271-0680, BS 79 Western MI Univ; MA 81 Northwestern Univ; Sp-Lang Path, Hrng &) Sp Cntr of Rochester, **SLP**

Hiller, Jay Felice 8502 Daleview, Austin, TX 78758, (512) 756-2126, BS 84 Univ of TX - Austin; MA 86 Univ of TX - Austin; Sp-Lang Path, Burnet Ps, **SLP**

Hilley, Carol Gourley P O Box 2164, Kirtland, NM 87417, (505) 368-5163, BA 80 NM St Univ; MA 85 NM St Univ; 88–Sp-Lang Path, Cen Consolidated Sch Dist #22, **SLP**

Hilliard, Annette Walser 3005 Stephenson Place N W, Washington, DC 20015, (703) 273-7705, BA 80 Emory Univ; MA 82 George Washington Univ; **SLP**

Hilliard, Clinton Thielens, Jr RFD 1, Mill Pond Road, Durham, NH 03824, BA 51 Muhlenberg Coll; MA 56 Univ of AL- Tuscaloosa; Admin, Hogan Reg Cen, **SLP**

Hilliard, Pamela J 319 North 2nd Street #23, Olean, NY 14760, (716) 375-4740, MS 86 SUNY - Coll at Fredonia; 86–Sp-Lang Path, Rehabilitation Ctr, **SLP**

Hilliard-Franks, Parthenia Evonne 2904 Lynda Place, Decatur, GA 30032, (404) 681-2800, MS; PH 87 (Career Development) GA St Univ; 88–Asst Prof, Morehouse Coll, **SLP**

Hillier, David B Department Of Communications, Ricks College, Rexburg, ID 83440, (208) 356-2929, BA 58 Brigham Young Univ; MA 61 Brigham Young Univ; Prof, Ricks Coll, **SLP**

Hilliker, Allison Marie Box 6 Strong Road, Owego, NY 13827, (607) 733-6541, BS 84 SUNY - Coll at Geneseo; MS 85 Ithaca Coll; Sp-Lang Path, St Josephs Hospital, **SLP**

Hillin, Celeste S Beaumont State Center, P O Box 3846, Beaumont, TX 77704-3846, (409) 833-1485, BS 78 Lamar Univ; MS 81 Lamar Univ; 87–Aud, Beaumont State Center, **A**

Hilling, Mrs Christina A 40 Finisterra, Irvine, CA 92715, (714) 852-1081, BS 72 1974; MA 81 CA St Univ - Long Beach; 80–Sp-Lang Path, Irvine USD, **SLP**

Hillis, Mrs Aimee C 2512 Grist Mill Road, Little Rock, AR 72207, (501) 490-2000, BS 70 FL St Univ; MS 71 FL St Univ; Sp-Lang Path, Pulhski County Spec Sch Dist, **SLP**

Hillis, Ann M 2609 Westover, Austin, TX 78703, (512) 444-4835, BS 80 Baylor Univ; MS 80 Baylor Univ; 86–Sp-Lang Path, HealthCare Rehab Ctr, **SLP**

Hillis, Carolyn Rd 2 Box 463, Oneonta, NY 13820, (607) 652-7821, BA 52 CUNY - Brooklyn Coll; MS 70 SUNY - Coll at Oneonta; SLP, BOCES, **SLP**

Hillis, Dr James W Department Of Speech & Hearing, George Washington Univ, Funger Hall Suite 407, Washington, DC 20052, (202) 994-7208, BS 52 Univ of NE - Lincoln; MA 57 Univ of MD - College Park; PH 63 (NS) OH St Univ; Prof, George Washington U, **SLP A F**

Hill-Latimer, Linda 4160 Jan Jolin Drive, Conley, GA 30027, (404) 351-0351, BS 76 Northwestern Univ; MA 78 Univ of IL - Urbana; SLP, West Paces Ferry Hospital, **SLP**

Hillman, Barbara J P O Box 308, Fort Edward, NY 12828, (518) 793-4150, BS 61 Coll of Saint Rose; MA 70 Coll of Saint Rose; Sp/Lang Path, Warren-Washington-County BOCES, **SLP**

Hillman, Carol E 27 Alan Road, South Hamilton, MA 01982, (617) 922-3000, MS 75 PA St Univ - Univ Park; BS 74 PA St Univ - Univ Park; Admin Dir/Rehabilitation Srvcs, Beverly Hospital, **SLP**

Hillman, Kimberly Ann 245 Broadway #202, South Portland, ME 04106-1610, (413) 534-2508, BS 83 Univ of WA; MS 85 Univ of WA; **SLP**

Hillman, Mrs Pamela R R R 2 Box 12, Syracuse, NE 68446, (402) 873-5561, BS 76 Univ of NE - Lincoln; MA 79 Univ of NE - Lincoln; Sp-Lang Path, Nebraska City Schs, **SLP**

Hillman, Dr Robert E 27 Alan Road, South Hamilton, MA 01982, (617) 353-8965, BS 74 PA St Univ - Univ Park; MS 75 PA St Univ - Univ Park; PH 80 (NS) Purdue Univ - West Lafayette; Assoc Prof, Boston U, **SLP**

Hillman, Sueann N 4658 Elm Street, West Des Moines, IA 50265-2993, (515) 225-1158, BA 67 Augustana Coll; MA 69 Univ of MO - Columbia; 78–Sp/Lang Path Presch Support Tm, Des Moines ISD, **SLP**

Hillner, Mrs Kathleen A 717 Bayside Court, Wheeling, IL 60090, (312) 392-7541, BS 79 Northwestern Univ; MS 81 Univ of WI - Madison; 81–Sp-Lang Path, Commun Consol Sch Dis #54, **SLP**

Hill-Rue, Mary Elizabeth 8401 Pan American Fwy N E, Space #260, Albuquerque, NM 87113, (505) 821-5421, BA 83 Univ of NM; MS 86 Univ of NM; **SLP**

Hills, Mrs Andrea Mary 147 Maywood Court, Decatur, IL 62526, (217) 429-1052, **SLP**

Hills, Mrs Sherrill A Swanson R R 1 Box 108-B, Lynn Center, IL 61262, (309) 529-5011, BA 79 Augustana Coll; MS 80 Eastern IL Univ; Sp-Lang Path, Alwood School District 225, **SLP**

Hilsher, Mrs Eve A S RD 4 Box 134, Montoursville, PA 17754, (717) 433-3121, BS 73 Bloomsburg Univ of PA; ME 75 Bloomsburg Univ of PA; Sp/Lang Path, Blast Inter Unit #17, **SLP**

Hilt, Gary D 20 Sunset Avenue, Bloomfield, NJ 07003, (201) 748-1138, BS 74 William Paterson Coll; MS 77 William Paterson Coll; Sec Chief Aud, Bronx VA Med Ctr, **SLP A**

Hiltenbrand, Marion G 10195 West Glennon Drive, Lakewood, CO 80226, (303) 986-2301, BS 69; MS 70 UT St Univ; Sp/Lang Path, Private Practice, **SLP**

Hiltner, Mrs Rory Anne Musto 2424 Otsego Drive, Fort Wayne, IN 46825-3853, (219) 482-3190, BS 80 Marywood Coll; MA 83 OH Univ - Athens; 87–Sp-Lang Path, Parkview Mem Hosp, **SLP**

Hilton, Mrs Debra Ellen 4806 No Millgrove Road, Akron, NY 14001, (716) 891-6433, BS 81 SUNY - Coll at Buffalo; MS 83 SUNY - Coll at Buffalo; Sp-Lang Path, UCP of Western NY, **SLP**

Hilton, Mrs I Rose W 5599 Fairington Place, Lithonia, GA 30058, (404) 957-3945, MA 72 NY Univ; BS 71 NY Univ; Sp-Lang Path, Henry Co Bd of Educ, **SLP**

Hilton, Judith Ann P O Box 72, Applegate, CA 95703, MA 72 CA St Univ - Sacramento; **SLP**

Hilton, Mrs Judy L 916 N W 3rd, Abilene, KS 67410, (913) 263-1773, BA 64 Wichita St Univ; MA 70 Wichita St Univ; Sp-Lang Path, Ctrl KS Coop In Ed, **SLP**

Hilton, Larry W 1038 Legacy Lane, Lawrenceville, GA 30245-6848, (404) 925-8874, BA 71 SC St Coll; MA 72 Univ of the DC; Sp-Lang Path, Butts Co Bd of Ed, **SLP**

Hilton, Dr Laurence M 671 East 700 North, Orem, UT 84057, (801) 378-6456, BA 69 Univ of UT; MA 70 Univ of UT; PH 73 (NS) Northwestern Univ; Prof-SLP, Brigham Young University, **SLP**

Hiltzik, Linda K 1229 West Laurelton Pkwy, Teaneck, NJ 07666, BS 67 NY Univ; MA 69 Columbia Univ Teachers Coll; **SLP**

Hilyard, Mrs Shelley W 8904 Funston Court, Wichita, KS 67207-5506, (316) 686-0539, BA 75 KS St Univ; MA 76 KS St Univ; SLP, Private Practice, **SLP**

Hilyer, Mrs Tamela Hale 4725 73rd Street North, Birmingham, AL 35206, (205) 491-5310, MS 84 Univ of Montevallo; SLP, Jefferson County Board of Educ, **SLP**

Hilz, Mrs Lani M 1021 Timber Lane, Mc Kinney, TX 75069, MS 75 Univ of North TX; **SLP**

Himelick, Thomas Earl 1708 Sunrise Street, Norman, OK 73071, (405) 949-1906, BS 76 IN Univ - Bloomington; MA 78 IN Univ - Bloomington; Aud, Otologic Medical Clinic Inc, **A**

Himelstein, Emily Zimmer 74 South Randolph Avenue, Poughkeepsie, NY 12601, (914) 229-5703, BA 70 CUNY - Queens Coll; MA 72 Wayne St Univ; Sp-Lang Path, Private Practice, **SLP**

Himes, Mrs Barbara Endle 1501-A Ocean, Seal Beach, CA 90740, (213) 483-9930, BA 68 Heidelberg Coll; MA 82 CA St Univ - Long Beach; Aud, Westmed Sp & Hearing Ctr, **A**

Himes, Mrs Lori A 300 Melmar Drive, Lewisburg, PA 17837, (717) 524-0376, BS 85 Clarion Univ of PA; MS 86 Clarion Univ of PA; Sp-Lang Path, InSpeech Inc, **SLP**

Himes, Terri K 1359 Suncrest Drive, Cincinnati, OH 45208, (513) 871-7901, BS 78 Miami Univ - Oxford; MS 79 Ball St Univ; Sp-Lang-Path-, Sp Path Assoc, **SLP**

Himes, Thomas Alan Crestwood Gardens #F, 108 Depot Street, Georgetown, DE 19947, (302) 934-8031, BS 82 West Chester Univ of PA; MA 85 West Chester Univ of PA; **SLP**

Himler, Mrs Barbara A 230 East 50th Street #5-D, New York, NY 10022, (212) 688-1672, BA 78 Boston Coll; MA 79 Hofstra Univ; Sp-Lang Path, Li Jewish Hill Side Med Cen, **SLP**

Himler, Mrs Linda Edwards Neurotology Unit, Surburban Hospital, Bethesda, MD 20814, (301) 530-3165, BS 84 Boston Univ; MS 86 Univ of WI - Madison; 87–Aud, Suburban Hosp, **A**

Himmel, Jacquelin 261 Prospect Park West, Brooklyn, NY 11215, (718) 965-1986, BS 73 SUNY - Center at Albany; MS 74 Univ of WI - Madison; Sp-Lang Path, Child Dev Ctr JBFCS, **SLP**

Himmelberg, Kebbelin Keith 11208 Crippen Circle, Papillion, NE 68046, (402) 393-4289, BS 83 Univ of NE - Omaha; MS 86 Univ of NE - Omaha; **SLP**

Hincher, Joanne Louise 117 Sandstone Creek Drive, Apartment 9, Grand Ledge, MI 48837, (517) 627-9448, BA 85 MI St Univ; MA 86 MI St Univ; 87–Sp-Lang Path, Portland PS

Hinchey, Carol A R R #1 Box 235-3, Huntington, VT 05462, (802) 878-1384, SLP, Chittenden Cntrl Sup Dis, **SLP ACE**

Hinchliffe, Marie Capozzi 105 Willow Run Road, Pittsburgh, PA 15238, (412) 665-4985, BA 52 Seton Hill Coll; MA 73 Univ of Pittsburgh - Pittsburgh; Instructional Advisor-Sp-Lang Prog, Pittsburgh Bd of Ed, **SLP**

Hinchliffe, Mrs Nancy 22 Hamilton Lane, Huntington, NY 11743, (516) 692-5993, BS 73 SUNY - Coll at Geneseo; MA 78 Univ of Akron; Sp-Lang Path, Port Washington Pub Sch, **SLP**

Hinchman-Giuffre, Mrs Joanne 64 Palisade Avenue, Bogota, NJ 07603-1736, BA 75 Montclair St Coll; MA 78 Montclair St Coll; Sp-Lang Path, Wayne Board of Education, **SLP**

Hinckley, Jacqueline J 3533 Pheasant Run Circle, Apartment 6, Ann Arbor, MI 48108-2474, (313) 936-7080, BA 85 San Diego St Univ; MS 87 Univ of MI - Ann Arbor; 87–Sp-Lang Path, Univ of MI Med Ctr

Hinckley, Penny F 460 Tucson Street, Aurora, CO 80011, **SLP**

Hindenlang, Jane E 162 Lenox Street, New Haven, CT 06513, (203) 397-4567, BA 74 George Washington Univ; MS 76 Columbia Univ Teachers Coll; Clinical Super, Southern CT State U, **SLP**

Hinderer, Jeana 749 Main Apt #6, Boonville, MO 65233, (816) 848-2112, BS 79 Central MO St Univ; MS 80 Central MO St Univ; Sp-Lang Path, New Franklin Sch Dist R-1, **SLP**

Hinderscheit, Linda R Dept Of Comm Disorders, 115 Shevlin Hall, 164 Pillsbury Drive S E, Minneapolis, MN 55455, (612) 624-3322, BA 76 Univ of MN - Minneap-St Paul; MA 78 Univ of MN - Minneap-St Paul; Sp-Lang Path, U of Minnesota, **SLP**

Hindes, Dr Sally K 3 Voorhees Road, New Brunswick, NJ 08901, (201) 545-5328, BA 71 Rutger's St Univ - Douglas Coll; MS 73 Rutgers St Univ -N Brunswick; ED 80 (Learning Disabilities) Rutgers St Univ -N Brunswick; Dir/Consult, Ed Servs Cen, **SLP**

Hindman, Mrs Sandra McGee Route 3 Box 69, Northport, AL 35476, BS 81 MS Univ for Women; MS 82 Univ of AL- Tuscaloosa; Aud, Partlow State School/Hospital, **A**

Hinds, Ronald Van Rt 1 Box 404, Gallipolis Ferry, WV 25515, (304) 675-6200, BS 79 AR St Univ; OM 81 AR St Univ; Sp-Lang Path, Colin Anderson Ctr, **SLP**

Hine, Patricia Lynne 1603 Lozano Drive, Vienna, VA 22130-1947, (703) 534-5353, BA 70 Trinity Univ; MA 72 Our Lady Lake Univ-San Anton; Sp-Lang Path, Chld Dev Cen of Nn VA, **SLP**

Hinerman, Dr Paige 1165 South 700 East, Salt Lake City, UT 84105, (801) 350-4479, BA 73 5579; MS 76 Univ of UT; PH 85 (NS) Univ of UT; Sp/Lang Path, Holy Cross Hosp, **SLP**

Hines, Cathleen Ann 4 New Meadows Road, Winchester, MA 01890, BS 81 Univ of NH; ME 83 Northeastern Univ; Sp-Lang Path, New England Memorial Hospital, **SLP**

Hines, Mrs Elaine L Physicians Hearing Aid Service, P O Box 2180, Tupelo, MS 38803-2180, (601) 844-6513, BA 77 Univ of MS; MA 78 Univ of MS; Aud, Tupelo ENT Surg Cl, **A**

Hines, Janet Lynn 871 Creekside #1, Memphis, TN 38117, (901) 867-2921, BS 84 Univ Southern MS-Hattiesburg; MA 86 Memphis St Univ; SLP, Arlington Dev Cnter, **SLP**

Hines, Joanne L H 318 Wyleswood Drive, Berea, OH 44017, (216) 234-3270, BA 71 Baldwin-Wallace Coll; MA 73 Cleveland St Univ; 86–Sp-Lang Path, PSI Affiliates Inc, **SLP**

Hines, Mrs Lisa Marie 958 North Salem Circle, Mesa, AZ 85205-5539, (602) 892-0545, BA 81 Univ of LA Verne; MS 83 Univ of LA Verne; **SLP**

Hines, Marilyn D 2899 Amy Drive, Library, PA 15129, (412) 835-6485, BS 75 Hampton Univ; MS 76 Univ of MI - Ann Arbor; **SLP**

Hines, Susan D 1012 Alexandria Pike, Fort Thomas, KY 41075, (513) 569-6056, BS 72 Eastern KY Univ; MA 75 Univ of Cincinnati; Director/Sp-Lang Path, Bethesda Hosp, **SLP**

Hiney, Mrs Debra Stanley 36 Jady Hill Avenue, Exeter, NH 03833, (603) 772-3781, BS 81 Purdue Univ - West Lafayette; OM 82 Smith Coll; Sp-Lang Path/Clin Super, Rehab Serv Exeter Hosp, **SLP**

Hing, Julie Diana 1159 Kotenberg Avenue, San Jose, CA 95125, (408) 578-9758, BA 81 San Jose St Univ; MA 84 San Jose St Univ; Sp-Lang Path, Oak Grove Sch Dist, **SLP**

Hinish, Susan Gayle 879 Cotton Bay Drive #1709, West Palm Beach, FL 33406-9046, BS 81 Univ of FL; MS 82 FL St Univ; Sp-Lang Path, Sch Bd of Palm Bch Co, **SLP**

Hinke, Rebecca A 273 Westview Drive #307, West St Paul, MN 55118, (612) 457-0343, OB 78 Univ of WI - Madison; MS 86 Univ of WI - Madison; **SLP**

Hinkle, Jo-Ann M 3840 Oakley, Memphis, TN 38111, (901) 458-2654, Speech-Language Path/Teacher, Les Passees Childrens Rehab, **SLP**

Hinkle, Dr Robert R 40 Southgate Court, Suite 101, Harrisonburg, VA 22801, (703) 434-3977, BS 68 Bloomsburg Univ of PA; ME 72 Bloomsburg Univ of PA; PH 78 (NS) Purdue Univ - West Lafayette; Assoc Prof, JMU, **A**

Hinkle, Dr William G 3840 Oakley, Memphis, TN 38111, PH (NS); Dean/College Allied Health Sci, University of Tennessee, **SLP**

Hinman, Mrs Barbara J 10039 Clearfield Avenue, Vienna, VA 22180, (703) 378-4100, BS 66 San Diego St Univ; MA 76 San Diego St Univ; 77–Sp-Lang Path, Fairfax Co Pub Sch Dist, **SLP**

Hinman, Mrs Marilee Grayce 15447 Southeast Swain Ct, Milwaukie, OR 97267, (503) 255-9037, BA CA St Univ - Fullerton; MA 86 CA St Univ - Fullerton; **SLP**

Hinman, Mrs Mary P 620 Lancaster Street, Fredericksburg, VA 22405, (703) 373-1631, BS 36 Univ Southern MS-Hattiesburg; MA 49 Columbia Univ Teachers Coll; **SLP LM**

Hinman-Dudley, Mrs Narda F 4755 Andalusia Trail, Atlanta, GA 30360, (404) 454-7919, BS 76 Brigham Young Univ; OM 77 Brigham Young Univ; **SLP**

Hinnant, Elizabeth 926 Pine Springs Road, Columbia, SC 29210, MS; **A LM**

Hinnerichs, Mrs Connie K 1523 West County Road #B-2, Roseville, MN 55113, (612) 457-9425, BS 75 Marquette Univ; MS 76 Univ of WI - Eau Claire; Sp/Lang Path, S St Paul Pub Sch Indep Dis #6, **SLP**

Hinshaw, Judith A 1102 South 2nd, Fairfield, IA 52556, (515) 682-8591, BS 70 Northeast MO St Univ; MA 73 Northeast MO St Univ; **SLP**

Hinshaw, Mary C M 7820 Melotte Street, San Diego, CA 92119, (619) 697-8378, BA 71 San Diego St Univ; MA 75 San Diego St Univ; MA 75 San Diego St Univ; Dir, Bilingual Sp Path Ser, **SLP**

Hinson, Carl L 903 South Ashland Avenue, Apartment 1212B, Chicago, IL 60607, (312) 243-8427, BS 66 Southern IL Univ -Carbondale; MS 71 IL St Univ - Normal; Sp-Lang Path, Chicago Board of Education, **SLP**

Hinson, Mrs Mary C Route 2 Box 234, Zebulon, NC 27597, (919) 496-4822, BA 28 Meredith Coll; MA 65 East Carolina Univ; **SLP LM**

Hinson, Susan Ann 655 Hilltop Drive #111, Redding, CA 96003, (916) 244-3740, BS 86 Baylor Univ; MS 87 Baylor Univ; **SLP**

Hinson, Mrs Troye M 5602 Snowy Owl Drive, Fairfax, VA 22032, (703) 425-7180, BS 70 Univ of SC - Columbia; OM 72 Emory Univ; SLP, Gloria B Nelson Assoc, **SLP**

Hintermeier, Ann L 26 Delamere Road, Williamsville, NY 14221, (716) 532-5522, MA 79 SUNY - Center at Buffalo; Aud, J N Adam Dev Disabl Serv Offi, **A**

Hintgen, Thomas L 404 West Fillmore Avenue, Eau Claire, WI 54701, (715) 839-4154, BS 74 Univ of MN - Duluth; MA 75 Western MI Univ; Sp-Lang Path, Sacred Heart Hosp, **SLP**

Hinton, Ann Sullivan 1621 Capouse Avenue, Scranton, PA 18509-1911, (717) 226-0977, BS 81 Bloomsburg Univ of PA; MS 82 Bloomsburg Univ of PA; Sp-Lang Path, Northeast Educ Intermed Unit #19, **SLP**

Hinton, Douglas K 3729 East Main Road, Fredonia, NY 14063, (716) 834-7200, BS 60 SUNY - Coll at Fredonia; ME 61 SUNY - Center at Buffalo; MS 88 Canisius Coll; Aud, St Marys School for the Deaf, **SLP A**

Hinton, Mrs Judy E 800 Penman Road, Neptune Beach, FL 32233, (615) 794-0184, BA 66 Vanderbilt Univ; MS 67 CO St Univ; Sp-Lang Path, Volusia Co Sch, **SLP**

Hinton, Virginia A 9 Highview Knoll, Iowa City, IA 52240, (919) 967-9719, BS 78 Univ of TN - Knoxville; MA 79 Northwestern Univ; Sp-Lang Path/Res Assist, Oral/Facial and Comm Dis Prgm, **SLP**

Hinze, Mrs Dianna Fake 16215 Clay Road #801, Houston, TX 77084, (713) 550-9475, BS 85 Baylor Univ; MS 86 Baylor Univ; **SLP**

Hipp, Donna Lynn 1607 Elizabeth Avenue, Ruston, LA 71270, (318) 255-7834, MA 84 LA Tech Univ; Sp-Lang Path, Speech Pathology Associates, **SLP**

Hippauf, Mrs Lynette Kay 1017 South Fourth, Walla Walla, WA 99362, (509) 527-3000, BA 84 WA St Univ; MS 85 Eastern WA Univ; 85–Sp-Lang Path, Walla Walla Sch Dist #140, **SLP**

Hippert, Mrs Carol Lowrey UCSD Medical Center, 225 Dickinson Street H-660, San Diego, CA 92103, (619) 543-5683, BA 77 San Diego St Univ; MA 81 San Diego St Univ; Aud, Ucsd Med Cen, **A**

Hipskind, Dr Nicholas M Speech And Hearing Center, Indiana University, Bloomington, IN 47405, (812) 335-5144, BS 62 Ball St Univ; MS 63 Ball St Univ; PH 68 (NS) MI St Univ; Assoc Prof & Dir Hrng Cl, IN U - Bloomington, **A**

Hiraki, Cynthia Kathleen 10766 19th Avenue S W, Seattle, WA 98146, (509) 677-3448, BA 82 WA St Univ; MA 84 Univ of MT; SLP, Puyallup School Dist, **SLP**

Hire, Mrs Janeen Mabee 365 Saint Andrews Court, Mansfield, OH 44903, (419) 525-6391, BS 62 Purdue Univ - West Lafayette; Sp-Lang Path, Mansfield Bd of Ed, **SLP**

Hiroo, Vivian F 2201 35th Avenue S E, Puyallup, WA 98374, (206) 475-4611, BA 73 Univ of WA; OM 75 Univ of WA; 82–Sp/Lang Path, Orchard Park Healthcare Ctr, **SLP ACE**

Hirota, Carol S 611 North Central Avenue, Stockton, CA 95204, (209) 948-7553, MA 78 Univ of the Pacific; SLP, **SLP**

Hirsch, Caryl 6051 Allott Avenue, Van Nuys, CA 91401, (213) 825-4821, BA 78 SUNY - Center at Stony Brook; MS 81 Columbia Univ Teachers Coll; SLP, UCLA, **SLP ACE**

Hirsch, Mrs Jodi Sanoff 1852 Sobro Avenue #1, North Valley Stream, NY 11580, (718) 424-1444, BA 83 SUNY - Center at Buffalo; MS 85 Columbia Univ Teachers Coll; Aud, **A**

Hirsch, Judith c/o Dunnder, 440 East 20th Street #9-B, New York, NY 10009, (212) 620-6312, BA 69 Carnegie-Mellon Univ; MA 77 SUNY - Center at Buffalo; Aud, Veterans Administration, **A**

Hirsch, Dr Judith E 1126 East Division, River Falls, WI 54022, (612) 626-5775, BS 61 Univ of WI - Madison; PH 68 (Auditory Neurophysiology) Univ of WI - Madison; Aud, U of MN Hosp-Minneapolis, **A**

Hirsch, Linda M 22 Birchwood Park Crescent, Jericho, NY 11753, (516) 931-6003, BA 73 Rider Coll; MS 74 Adelphi Univ; Aud, Gurwin Jewish Geriatric Ctr, **SLP A**

Hirsch, Mrs Marilyn S 34400 Ada Drive, Solon, OH 44139, (216) 349-0811, BS 75 OH Univ - Athens; MA 79 Cleveland St Univ; Sp-Lang Path, Euclid Pub Sch, **SLP**

Hirsch, Rheta R F 7287 West 90th Street, Los Angeles, CA 90045, PH (NS); **SLP**

Hirsch, Susan 524 Putnam Avenue #14, Cambridge, MA 02139, (617) 498-6267, BA 74 Boston Univ; MS 77 Boston Univ; Sp-Lang Path, Cambridge Sch Sys, **SLP**

Hirschberg, Joyce G 2568 N W 112th Way, Coral Springs, FL 33065, **SLP**

Hirschmann, Mary 6606 Windsor #A1, Berwyn, IL 60402, BA 73 Saint Xavier Coll; MA 75 Notre Dame Coll; **SLP**

Hirsch-Phillips, Lisa 4863 North Cumberland, Whitefish Bay, WI 53217, (414) 259-1414, BS 77 Central MI Univ; MA 79 Univ of IA; Sp-Lang Path, Curative Rehab Cen, **SLP**

Hirsh, Dr Ira J Central Institute For The Deaf, Research Department, 818 South Euclid Avenue, St Louis, MO 63110, (314) 889-6567, BA 42 SUNY - Center at Albany; MA 43 Northwestern Univ; PH 48 (NS) Harvard Univ; Professor, Washington University, **F H LM**

Hirsh, Mrs Vera Anne 10270 S W 109th Street, Miami, FL 33176, (305) 643-5780, OB 64 Univ of Miami; MA 65 Univ of FL; Ed Placement Spec, Dade Co Pub Sch, **SLP**

Hirshburg, Mrs Sandra Tanner Hendersonville Speech And Hearing Services, Route 4 Box 365-C, Hendersonville, NC 28739, (704) 697-2153, BS 71 Marshall Univ; OM 73 Emory Univ; 87–Sp-Lang Path, Private Practice, **SLP A ACE**

Hirshout, Debbie S 2405 Delancey Street, Philadelphia, PA 19103, (215) 581-6094, BS 78 Emerson Coll; OM 80 Hahneman Medical Coll; Audiologist, Phila College Osteopathic Med, **A**

Hiser, Kathy Ann 857-D Ballard Street, Altamonte Springs, FL 32701, (407) 841-5111, BS 83 WV Univ; MA 84 Univ of SC - Columbia; Audiologist, Orlando Regional Med Ctr, **A**

Hiser, Mrs Luann W 443 S R 300, Gibsonburg, OH 43431, (419) 637-7249, BS 75 Bowling Green St Univ; MA 79 Bowling Green St Univ; SLP, Gibsonburg Exempted Vlg Sch, **SLP**

Hiser, Nancy M 545 South Grand Street, Orange, CA 92666-2705, (714) 261-0102, BA 69 Univ of CA - Berkeley; MA 73 CA St Univ - Fullerton; Dir, Sp Commun Assoc, **SLP**

Hiser, Mrs Velma B Rural Route 3, Grinnell, IA 50112, (515) 236-3883, OB 26 Northwestern Univ; MA 38 Univ of IA; Sp/Lang Path, Private Practice, **SLP LM**

Hissong, Christine E 1525 Koehler Court, Green Bay, WI 54311, (414) 469-4790, BA 70 Northern MI Univ; MS 71 Northern MI Univ; Sp-Lang Path, Green Bay Area Pub Sch, **SLP**

Hitchcock, Mrs Barbara Joan 4505 35th Street Cresant, Red Deer, AB, Canada T4N 0P6, (403) 347-7741, BS 79 Univ of Alberta - Alberta; OM 80 Univ of WA; Sp-Lang Path, Red Deer Health Unit, **SLP**

Hitchcock, Virginia M 90 East Padonia Road #303, Timonium, MD 21093, **SLP**

Hite, Deborah Simpson 2200 Sunderland Road #144K, Winston-Salem, NC 27103-6538, (919) 727-2816, BA 75 Univ of NC - Greensboro; OM 84 Univ of SC - Columbia; SLP, Winston-Salem / Forsyth Co Sch, **SLP**

Hite-Hare, Mrs Susan C 104 Wineberry Lane, Ballston Spa, NY 12020, (518) 482-4550, BA 81 Univ of CA - Santa Barbara; MS 84 PA St Univ - Univ Park; Sp-Lang Path, Sunnyview Rehab Hosp, **SLP**

Hitschman, Mrs Hedwig 14 Concord Avenue, Cambridge, MA 02138, BS; **SLP LM**

Hitt, Mrs Toni Leigh 3840-101 Advantage Way So, Memphis, TN 38128, (901) 377-9378, BS 84 WV Univ; MA 86 Univ of Central FL; **SLP**

Hittle, Mrs Susan A 700 West Delavan Avenue, Buffalo, NY 14222, (716) 882-5592, Audiologist, Faxton & Childrens Hospitals, **A**

Hittleman, Warren Lee 269 West Walnut Street, Long Beach, NY 11561, BS 63 SUNY - Coll at Geneseo; MS 66 CUNY - Queens Coll; Dir-Sp-Lang Sers, Seaford Pub Sch, **SLP**

Hittner, Roberta A 688 Clifford Street, Warminster, PA 18974, (215) 672-9484, BS 81 Univ of Cincinnati; OM 85 Hahneman Medical Coll; **SLP**

Hitz, Mrs Loretta O 9511 Ashbourn Drive, Burke, VA 22015, (703) 425-2845, BS 72 Bloomsburg Univ of PA; ME 75 Bloomsburg Univ of PA; Sp-Lang Path, **SLP**

Hively, E Antionette 21 Highland Street #2, Morgantown, WV 26505, (304) 293-4258, BS 82 WV Univ; MS 84 WV Univ; Sp-Lang Path/Instr, WV U Med Ctr, **SLP**

Hlxon, Mrs Cynthia Ellen 5208 Benson Avenue, Arbutus, MD 21227, (301) 247-2404, BA 79 Univ of Pittsburgh - Pittsburgh; ME 83 CA Univ of PA; 80–Sp-Lang Path, Prince George's Co Pub Sch, **SLP**

Hixon, Nancy M 24308 San Juan Road, Carmel, CA 93923, **SLP**

Hixon, Thomas J Department Speech & Hearing Sciences, University Of Arizona, Tucson, AZ 85721, (602) 621-1644, BA 62 CUNY - Brooklyn Coll; MA 63 Univ of IA; PH 65 (Sp-Lang Path) Univ of IA; 76–Prof Sp-Lang Path, Univ of Arizona, **SLP F**

Hixson, Dr Peter K 3820 Burt Street, Omaha, NE 68131, (402) 978-7316, BA 70 Northwestern Univ; MA 71 Northwestern Univ; PH 77 (NS) Purdue Univ - West Lafayette; Asst Superv Sp-Lang-Hrng-Prog, Omaha Pub Schs, **SLP**

Hixson-Robles, Cynthia P O Box 1390, Phoenix, AZ 85001, (602) 254-5725, BA 81 Univ of FL; MA 85 Univ of FL; **A**

Hjelm, Jane D Central Fla Speech Pathologists PA, Jane Hjelm, PO Box 267, Kissimmee, FL 32742-0267, (305) 847-3337, BA 79 Univ of Central FL; MA 77 Univ of Central FL; Sp-Lang Path /President, Central Fla Speech Path, **SLP**

Hjelte, Mrs Phyllis P 8576 E Huntington Drive, San Gabriel, CA 91775, (213) 287-4246, BA 70 CA St Univ - Los Angeles; MA 76 CA St Univ - Los Angeles; 88, State of Calif Cal State LA, **SLP**

Hladek, Glenn 803 Rimrock Road, Billings, MT 59102, (406) 657-6165, BA 69 Fort Hays St Univ; MS 73 Univ of WI - Madison; Aud, Indian Hlth Serv, **A**

Hnath-Chisolm, Theresa E 4502 Montego Bay Court #5, Tampa, FL 33613, (813) 974-2006, PH 87 (Aud) CUNY - Grad Sch & Univ Cntr; 88–Asst Prof, Univ of South Florida, **A**

Hnatiow, Gail Z 31 Mountain View Drive, Westborough, MA 01581, (508) 366-4401, BA 58 Oberlin Coll; MS 62 Univ of Pittsburgh - Pittsburgh; 87–Dir of Sp-Lang Path & Aud, West Borough St Hosp, **SLP A ACE**

Ho, Mrs Esther M 2144 Thayer Avenue, Hayward, CA 94545, (415) 828-1037, BA 52 McPherson Coll; MA 70 Northwestern Univ; Sp-Lang Path, Dublin Sch Dist, **SLP**

Ho, Evelyn Z 1387 Kaweloka Street, Pearl City, HI 96782, BS; **SLP**

Ho, Margaret Lew 2536 Overlook Road, Apartment 202, Cleveland Heights, OH 44106, (216) 932-1436, BA 80 Tufts Univ; MA 85 Case Western Reserve Univ; Sp-Lang Path, Cleveland Hearing & Speech Ctr, **SLP**

Hoadley, Barbara Robertson 703 Dunbarton Circle, Sacramento, CA 95825, (916) 454-6601, BA 57 Univ of Redlands; MA 64 San Francisco St Univ; Prof, Cal St U Sacramento, **SLP**

Hoag, Mrs Diane M 16 Woodhaven Drive, Belchertown, MA 01007, (413) 323-6815, MA 87 Univ of MA - Amherst; 87–Sp-Lang Path, Springfield PS Sys, **SLP**

Hoag, Linda A 225 South Drake Drive, Manhattan, KS 66502, (913) 776-3277, BA 64 Univ of WA; MA 74 Univ of IL - Urbana; PH 79 (NS) Univ of IL - Urbana; 86–Asst Prof, Kansas State Univ, **SLP**

Hoagland, Tina Louise 3285 Canyon Drive #7, Billings, MT 59102-6050, (406) 652-3656, BA 82 Western WA Univ; MA 84 Western WA Univ; 87–Aud, MI Ctr for Hndcpd Children, **A ACE**

Hoar, Colleen J 541 Main Road North, Hampden, ME 04444, (207) 989-7300, BS 79 Univ of MN - Minneap-St Paul; MA 81 Univ of CT; Prog Coord, Head Injury Treatment Ctr-Brewer, **SLP**

Hoar, Rochelle Anne 1420 N Mulberry Street, Mount Vernon, OH 43050, (614) 392-8058, BS 85 Bowling Green St Univ; MS 86 Bowling Green St Univ; Sp-Lang Path, **SLP**

Hoard, Ann 936 West Michigan, Jacksonville, IL 62650, (217) 245-7174, BS 72 Purdue Univ - West Lafayette; MS 75 Purdue Univ - West Lafayette; 80–Aud, Four Rivers Spec Educ Dist, **A**

Hoban, Mrs Ann Marie Birchwood 6E, 27 Crowsnest Lane, Danbury, CT 06810, (203) 743-9748, BS 84 Marywood Coll; MA 85 Univ of Pittsburgh - Pittsburgh; 87–Sp-Lang Path, Danbury Hosp Sp & Hrng Ctr, **SLP**

Hoban, Janet Louise 1151 Floyd, Birmingham, MI 48009, (313) 646-0400, SLP, Detroit Public Schools, **SLP**

Hoban, Mary Angela 2942 West 63rd Street, Chicago, IL 60629, (312) 436-0347, BA 85 Saint Xavier Coll; OM 87 Governors St Univ; 88–Sp-Lang Path, Americana Health Care Ctr, **SLP**

Hobbins, Keith E 21117 Oxford, Farmington Hills, MI 48024, (313) 481-0625, BS 84 Northern MI Univ; MS 86 Wayne St Univ; **SLP**

Hobbs, Brenda Castille 224 Baldwin Street, Breaux Bridge, LA 70517, (318) 332-2844, BS 71 LA St Univ - Baton Rouge; MA 74 LA St Univ - Baton Rouge; Sp-Lang Path, St Martin Parish Sch Bd, **SLP**

Hobbs, Julia Ann 11300 Olympic Boulevard, Apartment 830, Los Angeles, CA 90064-1645, (213) 477-8069, BA 68 Univ of North TX; MA 70 Univ of North TX; Cl Dir, Julia Hobbs Speech Path Inc, **SLP**

Hobbs, Mrs Linda Harrell Roanoke-Chowan Hospital, P O Box 1385, Ahoskie, NC 27910, (919) 332-8121, BS 75 East Carolina Univ; MS 78 East Carolina Univ; Dir of Sp & Hrng Serv, Roanoke-Chowan Hosp, **SLP A**

Hobbs, Linda L Assoc Speech-Lang Pathologists, 580 West 5th Street, Suite 1A, Reno, NV 89503, (702) 329-1075, BS 71 Univ of NV - Reno; MS 81 Univ of NV - Reno; Sp-Lang Path, Private Practice, **SLP**

Hobbs, Lynne W 2813 Oak Avenue, Manhattan Beach, CA 90266, BA 69 Univ of Southern CA; MA 71 Univ of Southern CA; SLP, Santa Monica/Malibu USD, **SLP**

Hobe, Elizabeth A 21696 Oak Bark Trail, Strongsville, OH 44136, (216) 572-1802, MA 88 Kent St Univ

Hoberman, Mrs Fran S 20 Peach Tree Drive, Montville, NJ 07045, (201) 299-1972, BS 75 Emerson Coll; MS 76 Ithaca Coll; Sp-Lang Path, Private Practice, **SLP**

Hoberman, Mrs Joyce B 9 North Five Points Road, West Chester, PA 19380, (215) 696-8800, BA 62 Univ of MI - Ann Arbor; MA 65 Temple Univ; Aud, Chester County Ear-Nose-Throat, **SLP A**

Hoberman, Mrs Shirley E P O Box 241, Hampton Bays, NY 11946, (516) 728-3279, BA 37 CUNY - Hunter Coll; MA 58 Columbia Univ Teachers Coll; Sp-Lang Path/Aud, Private Practice, **SLP A LM**

Hobson, Lisa Brewer 2331 Dana Court, Carlsbad, CA 92008, (619) 720-9952, BA 73 Scripps Coll; MS 84 CA St Univ - Hayward; Sp-Lang Path, **SLP**

Hobson, Sandra Gehling 2100 37th Street, Des Moines, IA 50310-4413, (515) 255-8342, BA 73 Univ of IA; MA 75 Univ of IA; 87–Aud, Univ of Osteopathic Med & Health Sci, **A**

Hobson, Mrs Susan K 6001 Wedgmont Circle N, Fort Worth, TX 76133, (817) 346-6561, BS 74 KS St Univ; MA 77 LA St Univ - Baton Rouge; Sp/Lang Path, Private Practice, **SLP**

Hoch, Mrs Gail Lynn 4187 North Edgemoor, Wichita, KS 67220, (316) 744-2553, BS 83 KS St Univ; MA 84 Wichita St Univ; 86–Sp-Lang Path, Rainbows United Inc, **SLP**

Hoch, Lynn R 102-50 62nd Road, Forest Hills, NY 11375, (212) 430-2786, BA 66 CUNY - Queens Coll; MA 68 NY Univ; Ch Sp-Lang Path, Hosp of A Einstein Coll of Med, **SLP ACE**

Hochberg, Dr Irving City University Of New York, Graduate School, 33 West 42nd Street, New York, NY 10036, (212) 790-4366, BA 55 CUNY - Brooklyn Coll; MA 57 Columbia Univ Teachers Coll; PH 62 (Aud) PA St Univ - Univ Park; 74–Exec Off, CUNY Grad Sch, **A F**

Hochberg, Dr Judith Golden Linguistics Department, Northwestern University, Evanston, IL 60208, (312) 288-2085, BA 82 Harvard Univ; MA 85 Stanford Univ; PH 86 (Linguistics) Stanford Univ; 88–Asst Prof, Northwestern Univ

Hochhalter, Susan M 2504 11th Avenue N W, Mandan, ND 58554, (701) 663-6308, BA 81 Univ of ND; MS 83 Univ of ND; Sp-Lang Path, B I A, **SLP**

Hochman, Mrs Roberta L 22 Hickok Street, Fords, NJ 08863, MS 65 Kean Coll of NJ; Dir Sp & Hrng Dept, Woodbridge Dev Ctr, **SLP**

Hochman, Ruth M 18 Fox Tail Way, Boylston, MA 01505, **SLP**

Hochmuth, Lou A P O Box 1503, Rhinelander, WI 54501, (715) 369-6867, BS 85 Univ of WI - Stevens Point; MS 87 Univ of WI - Stevens Point; 87–Sp-Lang Path, Petersen Health Care of WI, **SLP**

Hochrein, Celeste Renee 5323 A Hasten Court, Chattanooga, TN 37412, (404) 226-3919, BA 80 Univ of Pittsburgh - Pittsburgh; MA 81 Memphis St Univ; ME 88 Univ of TN - Chattanooga; Sp-Lang Path, Whitfield Co Pub Sch, **SLP**

Hochscheid, Mrs Sylvia F 2957 Alexis Drive, Palo Alto, CA 94304, (415) 941-1631, BS 49 Case Western Reserve Univ; MA 54 Columbia Univ Teachers Coll; Instr, Foothill College

Hochstadt, Mrs Mindy S 2 Crosby Circle, Framingham, MA 01701, (617) 894-3600, BS 78 Univ of MA - Amherst; MA 79 Hofstra Univ; Sp Superv, Fernald St Sch, **SLP**

Hockaday, Rebecca Carol P O Box 1084, Boone, NC 28607, (704) 262-0258, BS 83 Appalachian St Univ; MA 85 Appalachian St Univ; 85–Sp-Lang Path, Communicare, **SLP**

Hockenberger, Elaine H PO 542, 506 Main Street, Harmony, PA 16037, (412) 846-5100, BS 78 Bloomsburg Univ of PA; MS 79 Bloomsburg Univ of PA; Coll Instruct, Geneva Coll, **SLP**

Hocker, Mrs Mary Helen 110 Hobbs Street, Arlington, KY 42021, (502) 444-9688, BS 69 Murray St Univ; MS 73 Murray St Univ; Sp-Lang Path, W Ky Er Sl Ctr, **SLP ACE**

Hocker, Mrs Susan G Wilner Road, Somers, NY 10589, **SLP**

Hockersmith, Dr Mary J Route 1 Box 85, Purcellville, VA 22132, (703) 882-3622, BS 61 Henderson St Univ; MA 63 OH St Univ; ED 82 (NS) Georgetown Univ; Part Time Instructor, George Washington University, **SLP A**

Hockett, Mrs Debra Cole 1374 Rice Creek Trail, Shoreview, MN 55126, (612) 786-8270, BA 84 Univ of SD - Vermillion; MS 85 Univ of SD - Vermillion; 88–Sp-Lang Path, St Paul PS Sys, **SLP**

Hoctor, Maria Noe 638 Star Boulevard, Madison, TN 37115, (615) 865-6805, BS 84 Western KY Univ; MS 87 Vanderbilt Univ, **SLP**

Hodapp, Mary E 1215 South Buchanan Street, Arlington, VA 22204, (301) 424-5200, BA 70 Catholic Univ of America; MA 72 Catholic Univ of America; Clin Sup Outpt Speech, Treat & Lrng Ctr Inc, **SLP**

Hodell, Susan F 213 Guaymas, Davis, CA 95616, (916) 756-2906, BA 72 San Jose St Univ; MA 76 Vanderbilt Univ, **A**

Hodes, Mrs Cynthia Blair 1779 2nd Avenue, Walnut Creek, CA 94596, BA 78 CA St Univ - Chico; MA 80 CA St Univ - Chico; SLP, Wasatch Co Sch Dist, **SLP**

Hodgdon, Mrs Linda Q 2928 Hill Drive, Troy, MI 48098, (313) 773-7660, BA 68 Central MI Univ; ME 72 Wayne St Univ; Sp-Lang Path, MacOmb ISD, **SLP**

Hodge, Mrs Betty A 2010 Riverview Drive, Murfreesboro, TN 37130, (501) 893-5812, BS 75 AR St Univ; MS 76 AR St Univ; Sp-Lang Path, Rutherford Co Sch, **SLP**

Hodge, Crystal Camille 13224 South Prairie, Chicago, IL 60627, (219) 738-5147, BS 84 Bradley Univ; MS 86 IL St Univ - Normal; 87–Aud, Sears Hearing Aid Systems, **A**

Hodge, Mrs Laura Fisher 105 Riverside Drive, Spartanburg, SC 29302, (803) 585-0322, BA 84 Columbia Coll; OM 85 Univ of SC - Columbia; Sp-Lang Path, Spartanburg Sch Dist #7, **SLP**

Hodge, Mrs Marilyn Julia 4833 Willow Lane, Dallas, TX 75244, (214) 387-8191, BA 56 Univ of TX - Austin; 88–Dir SLP, Schreiber Methodist Preschool, **SLP**

Hodge, Megan M 11050-80 Avenue, Edmonton, AB, Canada T6G OR3, (403) 432-5990, BS 73 Univ of Alberta - Alberta; MS 79 Univ of AZ; Project Assistant, U of WI-Madison, **SLP**

Hodge, Rickey F 201 Woodlake Circle, Pontotoc, MS 38863, (601) 842-6325, MS 79 Univ of MS; Aud, Beltone Hrng Aid Ctr, **A**

Hodges, Annelle Vaden 942 Rockcreek Road, Charlottesville, VA 22903, (804) 979-2087, BA 75 Coll of William & Mary; MS 77 Univ of AL- Tuscaloosa; **A**

Hodges, Jane P O Box 71, Topsham, ME 04086, (207) 729-1594, MA 87 Univ of ME - Orono

Hodges, Kathleen 3132 Lone Pine Road, Schenectady, NY 12303, (518) 453-1754, BA 63 FL St Univ; MS 70 SUNY - Center at Albany; Sp-Lang Path, E Roosevelt Developmental Serv, **SLP**

Hodges, Monette Gregory 5757 South Staples #3211, Corpus Christi, TX 78413, (512) 241-8158, BS 75 Univ of MO - Columbia; MS 82 Corpus Christi St Univ; Sp-Lang Path, Calallen ISD, **SLP LM**

Hodges, Nancy W 2028 Exeter Road Suite 2, Germantown, TN 38138, (901) 756-4499, BA 76 Univ of MO - Columbia; MA 77 Univ of MO - Columbia; 84–Sp-Lang Path, Private Practice, **SLP**

Hodges, Sue H 1450 Wald Road, Orlando, FL 32806, **SLP**

Hodges-Stillson, Cheryl L 620 West Mishawaka Avenue, Mishawaka, IN 46545, (219) 272-0100, MA 68 Ball St Univ; OM 76 IN Univ - South Bend; 86–Dir Sp-Lang Path, Healthwin Hosp, **SLP**

Hodgson, Margaret Murphy 325 Mission Street, Lodi, CA 95240-5319, (209) 369-6368, BA 80 CA St Univ - Sacramento; MA 83 Humboldt St Univ; Sp-Lang Path, Lodi USD, **SLP**

Hodgson, Dr William R Dept Of Speech & Hearing Sci, University Of Arizona, Tucson, AZ 85721, (602) 621-1266, BS 57 Southeast MO St Univ; MA 59 Univ of AR - Fayetteville; PH 61 OH Univ - Athens; Prof, Univ of Ariz, **A F**

Hodnik, Mrs Janet Ann 9049 South Irwin Avenue, Pittsburgh, PA 15237, (412) 366-5120, BA 78 Univ of Pittsburgh - Pittsburgh; MA 80 Univ of Pittsburgh - Pittsburgh; Sp-Lang Path, Private Practice, **SLP**

Hodous, Mrs Michele McGuire 4137 North Woodburn Street, Shorewood, WI 53211, (414) 962-0676, BS 85 Marquette Univ; MA 86 Northwestern Univ; Aud, Medical Associates, **A**

Hodowal, Mrs Deborah Anne C 3608 North Brick Church Road, Cambridge City, IN 47327-9440, (317) 489-5362, BS 76 IN St Univ - Terre Haute; MA 79 Ball St Univ; Sp-Lang Path, Fayette Co Sch Corp, **SLP**

Hodson, Dr Barbara W Department Of Communicative Disorders & Sciences, The Wichita State University, Wichita, KS 62708-1595, (316) 689-3240, BS 58 Univ of IL - Urbana; MS 60 Univ of IL - Urbana; PH 75 (Phonology) Univ of IL - Urbana; 88–Prof, Wichita State Univ, **SLP F**

Hoedl-Bayer, Mrs Denise M 3324 Quail Lake Road #207, Colorado Springs, CO 80906, (719) 576-6786, OB 85 Tarleton St Univ; MA 87 Univ of Northern CO; 88–Sp-Lang Path, Widefield District No 3, **SLP**

Hoefer, Carol S 450 Wiltshire Lane, Crystal Lake, IL 60014, (815) 455-4182, **SLP**

Hoefer, Julie Ann 5303 West 79 Terrace, Prairie Village, KS 66208, (816) 234-3392, BS 83 Miami Univ - Oxford; MA 85 Univ of KS; **SLP**

Hoefer, Mrs Kathryn O 3820 Nowlin Road, Kennesaw, GA 30144, (404) 426-3175, BS 76 SUNY - Coll at Geneseo; MA 78 IN Univ - Bloomington; Sp-Lang Path, Kennestone Hosp, **SLP**

Hoefer, Mary McCormick 15225 Brookside Circle, Omaha, NE 68144-1955, (402) 978-7079, BS 83 Univ of NE - Omaha; MS 84 Univ of NE - Omaha; Sp-Lang Path, Omaha Public Schools, **SLP**

Hoefer, Sylvia Casper 430 Nelson Circle, Noblesville, IN 46060, (317) 773-4726, BS 79 Ball St Univ; MA 85 Ball St Univ; 86–Aud, Northside ENT Inc, **A**

Hoeft, Mrs Elizabeth 614 Center Street, Elgin, IL 60120, (312) 837-0500, BA 64 Denison Univ; MA 70 Northern IL Univ - De Kalb; SLP, Sch Dist #U-46, **SLP**

Hoehman, Karen J West Fifth Road, RD 7 Box 416, Oswego, NY 13126, (315) 963-3034, BS 86 SUNY - Coll at Geneseo; MS 87 Univ of Louisville; 88–Sp-Lang Path, Oswego County BOCES

Hoehnke, Mrs Valerie Jane 7739 W Grantosa Drive, Milwaukee, WI 53218, (414) 463-6604, BS 81 Univ of WI - Milwaukee; MS 83 Univ of WI - Milwaukee; Sp-Lang Path, Marian Franciscan Home, **SLP**

Hoekstra, Belinda 645 Pacific Avenue #304, Long Beach, CA 90802, (213) 432-7241, **SLP**

Hoekstra, Lowell J 322 East Cherry, Fergus Falls, MN 56537, (218) 739-3052, MS 75 Moorhead St Univ; Sp-Lang Path, Lakeland Mental Health Center, **SLP**

Hoel, Richard L Rural Route 1 Box 128-H, Pequot Lakes, MN 56472, (218) 543-4016, BA 56 Univ of IA; MA 58 Univ of IA; Pres, Lake Region Hearing Ctr, **A**

Hoelscher, Susan G Rd#3 P O Box 139, Williamsport, PA 17701, **SLP**

Hoenig, Mrs Ann S 150 Lapier, Glencoe, IL 60022, (312) 835-5233, BS 62 Univ of WI - Madison; MA 63 Northwestern Univ; Aud, St of IL-O/A Cl, **SLP A**

Hoenk, Megan O 209 East Washington, Lake Bluff, IL 60044, (312) 295-3719, BA 76 Denison Univ; MA 81 Univ of IA; Sp-Lang Path, Antioch Cons Sch Sys, **SLP**

Hoeptner, Mrs Deborah Miller 11767 Fuerte Drive, El Cajon, CA 92020, (619) 466-3259, BA 72 San Diego St Univ; MA 77 San Diego St Univ; Sp-Lang Path, La Mesa Spring Valley Sch Dist, **SLP**

Hoerauf, Pamela D 5136 Cerritos Drive, Orange, CA 92669, (714) 633-7715, BA 79 CA St Univ - Fullerton; MA 82 CA St Univ - Fullerton; **SLP**

Hoernlein, Theresa R 553 Village Drive, Edison, NJ 08817, (201) 819-7862, BA 84 Rutger's St Univ - Douglas Coll; MS 86 Rutgers St Univ -N Brunswick; 87–Sp-Lang Path, JFK Med Ctr, **SLP**

Hoerster, Carol 1239 Parkside Drive East, Seattle, WA 98112, (206) 323-2475, MS 72 Univ of WA; 86–Sp-Lang Path, Childhaven, **SLP**

Hoerstman, Karen Lee 16502 Petro Drive, Mishawaka, IN 46544, (219) 259-5985, MA 87 OH St Univ; **A**

Hoesl, Lori Sue 1725 W Timber Ridge Lane, #6307, Oak Creek, WI 53154, BA 84 MI St Univ; MA 86 MI St Univ; Aud, St Luke's Hospital, **A**

Hoey, Cathy A 663 Rivercrest Drive, Sacramento, CA 95831, BA 69 Holy Names Coll; MA 71 CA St Univ - Sacramento; Sp-Lang Path, Private Practice, **SLP**

Hoey, Mrs Crystal Thornton 15 Lackawanna Avenue, Mount Morris, NY 14510, (716) 658-3797, BA 84 SUNY - Coll at Cortland; MS 85 Ithaca Coll; Sp-Lang Path, Craig Develop Dis Service, **SLP**

Hoey, Mrs Nancy Louise 2555 Delta Street, Orange, CA 92665, (714) 351-9264, BA 80 CA St Univ - Fullerton; MA 82 CA St Univ - Fullerton; 82–SLP, Alvord USD, **SLP**

Hof, Catherine 59 Massari Road, Pueblo, CO 81001, (303) 545-2743, BA 72 Suffolk Univ; MS 73 Adams St Coll; Sp-Lang Path, Private Practice, **SLP**

Hof, Mrs Lenore R 5344 Millwood Drive, Broadview Heights, OH 44147, (216) 838-5939, BA 80 Bowling Green St Univ; MA 81 Bowling Green St Univ; Sp-Lang Path, Parma Community General Hosp, **SLP**

Hofbauer, Carol L 2291 Benning Drive, Powell, OH 43065, (614) 766-8331, BA 73 SUNY - Center at Stony Brook; MS 75 Emerson Coll; Sp-Lang Path, Sp & Lang Assoc, **SLP**

Hofeling, Christine Mary S 12 Cool Creek Circle, Carmel, IN 46032, (317) 872-0710, BS 79 IL St Univ - Normal; MS 80 IL St Univ - Normal; Sp-Lang Path, Cherry Grade Sch, **SLP**

Hoff, Mrs Elaine D 34251 Weld County Road 31, Greeley, CO 80631, (303) 339-5360, BA 77 Univ of Northern CO; MA 79 Univ of Northern CO; 79–Sp-Lang Path, Centennial Developmental Svcs Inc, **SLP**

Hoff, Mrs Janet Kay 1894 Constance Drive, Vermillion, SD 57069, (605) 624-8021, BS 68 Univ of SD - Vermillion; MA 84 Univ of SD - Vermillion; 68–SLP, Vermillion Public Schools, **SLP**

Hoff, Susan L 407 7th Avenue #18, Asbury Park, NJ 07712, (201) 449-5000, BA 80 Montclair St Coll; MA 85 Kent St Univ; 88–Sp-Lang Path, Early Intervention Program, **SLP**

Hoffa, Daniel C, Jr 609 West Ashland, Indianola, IA 50125, (515) 961-2374, BS 75 Univ of IA; MA 76 Northeast MO St Univ; 86–Sp-Lang Path, Private Practice, **SLP**

Hoffa, Esther K 609 West Ashland, Indianola, IA 50125, (515) 961-2374, BA 71 Mankato St Univ; MA 77 Northeast MO St Univ; Sp-Lang Path, Private Practice, **SLP ACE**

Hoffeller, Jill Marie 15324 DE Pauw, Pacific Palisades, CA 90272, (213) 829-6592, BA 81 Creighton Univ; MS 82 Marquette Univ; Sp-Lang Path, St Johns Hosp & Hlth Ctr, **SLP**

Hoffelmeyer, Melissa Guss 10535 Caminito Banyon, San Diego, CA 92131-1710, (619) 549-3299, BA 81 Univ of Southern CA; MS 84 AZ St Univ; Sp-Lang Path, Speech Hrng & Neurosensory Cen, **SLP**

Hoffer, Mrs Dana Lee 13411 S W Chelsealoop, Tigard, OR 97223, (503) 639-1958, BA 80 WA St Univ; MA 81 WA St Univ; SLP, Portland Public Schools, **SLP**

Hoffer, Kathleen R 10604 Noakes Road, La Mesa, CA 92041, (619) 442-6510, BA 71 Univ of CA - San Diego; MA 75 San Diego St Univ; MA 75 San Diego St Univ; Clinical Supervisor, San Diego State U, **SLP**

Hoffer, Kimberly Skarin 231 South Jackson Street, Batavia, IL 60510-4459, (812) 331-2200, BA 78 Augustana Coll; MA 80 Northwestern Univ; SLP, **SLP**

Hoffer, Dr Pamela C 1217 Brooklyn Avenue, Ann Arbor, MI 48104, (313) 662-3435, BA 66 Swarthmore Coll; MS 69 Univ of MI - Ann Arbor; PH 84 (NS) Wayne St Univ; Sp/Lang Path, Private Practice, **SLP**

Hoffer, Sheila Ann 6 Roy Drive, Nesconset, NY 11767, **SLP**

Hoffer, Spencer John 13411 SW Chelsea Loop, Tigard, OR 97223, (503) 639-1958, BS 81 OR St Univ; MS 84 Western OR St Coll; Sp-Lang Path, Portland Public Schools, **SLP**

Hofferber, Mrs Kelly Ann 160 Lincoln Street, Redlands, CA 92374, (714) 882-4972, **A**

Hofflin, Lois E 65-65 Wetherole Street, Rego Park, Queens, NY 11374, (212) 299-7600, BA 76 SUNY - Center at Buffalo; MA 78 NY Univ; Educational Supervisor, Birch Early Childhood Center, **SLP**

Hofflund, Violet Marian 2119 Midway Drive, Rockford, IL 61103, BA 50 Augustana Coll; MA 56 Univ of NM; Retired, **SLP A LM**

Hoffman, Mrs Barbara Carey 17 Venture Terrace, Glenmont, NY 12077, (518) 439-7381, BS 75 SUNY - Center at Albany; MS 77 Columbia Univ Teachers Coll; Sp-Lang Path, Private Practice, **SLP**

Hoffman, Beth Gilbertson 1915 Elm Ridge Drive, Vista, CA 92083, (619) 598-9477, BS 84 IA St Univ; MA 85 Univ of Northern IA; **SLP**

Hoffman, Blair Lynne 5614 Netherland Avenue Apartment 3C, Bronx, NY 10471, (212) 549-4753, BS 81 Cornell Univ; MS 85 Univ of WI - Madison; Sp-Lang Path, H G Birch Early Childhood Ctr, **SLP**

Hoffman, Cheryl P 146 Louise Lane, Athens, OH 45701, (614) 767-2810, BS 80 OH Univ - Athens; MA 82 OH Univ - Athens; 85–Sp/Lang Path, Trimble Local Schools, **SLP**

Hoffman, Mrs Christine 383 Rutgers Lane, Parsippany, NJ 07054, (201) 267-5627, BS 83 Stockton St Coll; MS 86 PA St Univ - Univ Park; **A**

Hoffman, Cindy Sue 4368 West Libby, Glendale, AZ 85308, (602) 939-8682, BA 79 WA St Univ; MA 80 WA St Univ; Sp/Lang Path, Tempe Elementary Dist #3, **SLP**

Hoffman, Denise 102-30 66th Road, Apt 22-A, Forest Hills, NY 11375, (212) 594-6587, BS 73 Syracuse Univ; MA 75 NY Univ

Hoffman, Mrs Florence Eaton 205 West Mennonite Road, Aurora, OH 44202, (603) 524-5373, BS 83 Kent St Univ; MA 83 Kent St Univ; **SLP**

Hoffman, Mrs Harleene S 2010 W Woodbury Lane, Glendale, WI 53209, (414) 461-6110, BS 64 Univ of WI - Milwaukee; **SLP LM**

Hoffman, I Brenda 4700 Bow Mar Drive, Littleton, CO 80123, (303) 798-6995, BA 63 Newark St Coll; MA 65 Temple Univ; SLP, Denver Publ Schs, **SLP**

Hoffman, Janet S 20 Erita Lane, Smithtown, NY 11787, (516) 360-9016, BA 75 CUNY - Queens Coll; MA 77 CUNY - Queens Coll; SLP, Huntington Union Free Sch Dist, **SLP**

Hoffman, Janice Kathryn 13111 West Markham #264, Little Rock, AR 72211, (501) 771-3343, BS 81 TX Christian Univ; MA 83 Memphis St Univ; 88–Sp-Lang Path, Mem Hosp, **SLP**

Hoffman, Dr Jeanette A 4843 Spring Creek Road, Rockford, IL 61111, (815) 877-6629, BA 38 Rockford Coll; MA 40 Univ of WI - Madison; PH 42 (Aphasia) Univ of WI - Madison; 88–Sp-Lang Path, Private Practice, **SLP F LM**

Hoffman, Mrs Jennifer Sue Box 145 Second Street, Mauricetown, NJ 08329-0145, (609) 696-6860, BS 80 Trenton St Coll; MA 86 Trenton St Coll; 81–Sp-Lang Path, Vineland Developmental Ctr

Hoffman, Jeri L 33195 Wagon Wheel, Solon, OH 44139, (216) 248-6206, BS 77 Kent St Univ; MA 80 Kent St Univ; 85–Dir Mktg & Sls, Innocomp Comm Aids, **A**

Hoffman, Mrs Jolene Slocum 8565 West 55th Drive, Arvada, CO 80002, (303) 427-4732, BA 82 Univ of IA; MA 84 Univ of Northern CO; Aud, **A**

Hoffman, Mrs Julie Mae 1512 Valley West Avenue, Yakima, WA 98908, (509) 453-8248, BS 83 Loma Linda Univ - Riverside; MS 86 Loma Linda Univ - Riverside; Sp-Lang Path, Yakima Valley Hrng & Sp Ctr, **SLP**

Hoffman, Kathryn E 818 DE Groff Street, Grand Ledge, MI 48837, (517) 372-6725, BS 79 Univ of Cincinnati; MA 81 Cleveland St Univ; Aud, Audiovestibular Ctr, **A**

Hoffman, Mrs Kathy D 4432 N W 73rd Way, Coral Springs, FL 33065, (305) 344-6309, BS 73 FL St Univ; MS 74 FL St Univ; Sp-Lang Path, Private Practice, **SLP**

Hoffman, Kitty Biven 4438 Camp Street, New Orleans, LA 70115, (504) 895-2206, OB 65 Jacksonville Univ; OM 86 LA St Univ - N O Medical Ctr; **SLP**

Hoffman, Lauren P 1412 St Andrews Drive, Schererville, IN 46375-2916, (219) 322-6512, BS 73 IN Univ - Bloomington; MS 73 IN Univ - Bloomington; Superv Comm Dev Prog, S Metro Assn-Low Inc Hndcpd, **SLP**

Hoffman, Laurie T 434 Michigan, Sturgeon Bay, WI 54235, (414) 825-1212, BS 81 Univ of WI - Stevens Point; MS 83 Univ of WI - Stevens Point; **SLP**

Hoffman, Leah J 1305 Wychwood Road, Charleston, WV 25314, (304) 342-6080, BS 74 WV Univ; MS 75 WV Univ; Dir/Cl Servs, Sp & Lang Therapy Clinic, **SLP**

Hoffman, Lori Ann 1097 Blanche Street #114, Pasadena, CA 91106, (213) 942-1500, MA 84 CA St Univ - Los Angeles; Sp-Lang Path, El Rancho USD, **SLP**

Hoffman, Mrs Madelene 6 Algonquin Place, Elizabeth, NJ 07208, BA 73 CUNY - Brooklyn Coll; MS 75 CUNY - Brooklyn Coll; **SLP A**

Hoffman, Martha-Sue 47 Will Drive Apt #107, Canton, MA 02021, (617) 956-5300, BS 74 Boston Univ; MS 76 Boston Univ; 79–Sp-Lang Path, Tufts N Eng Med Cen, **SLP ACE**

Hoffman, Mrs Mary Elaine 14 Weston Lane, Smithtown, NY 11787, (516) 724-1717, BA 79 Hofstra Univ; MA 80 Hofstra Univ; Sp-Lang Path, Suffold Child Dev Cen, **SLP**

Hoffman, Patricia Diane 2625 Lido Lane, Oakville, MO 63129, (314) 726-1666, BS 85 Univ of NE - Lincoln; MS 86 Univ of NE - Lincoln; Sp-Lang Path, The Sch Dist of Clayton, **SLP**

Hoffman, Paul R 16444 Missionary Ridge, Baton Rouge, LA 70817, (504) 388-2545, BA 73 Univ of MI - Ann Arbor; MA 75 IN Univ - Bloomington; PH 77 (NS) IN Univ - Bloomington; Assoc Prof, Louisiana St U, **SLP**

Hoffman, Mrs Randy A 610 Euclid Court, Highland Park, IL 60035, (415) 366-9857, BS 76 Univ of IL - Urbana; MA 77 Univ of TN - Knoxville; Private Practice, **SLP**

Hoffman, Mrs Robin Menge 924 South Jennie, Visalia, CA 93277, (209) 733-6333, BA 75 Allegheny Coll; MA 78 WA St Univ; Sp-Lang Path, Tulare Co Dept of Ed, **SLP**

Hoffman, Sara G 1017 St Andrews Place, Nashville, TN 37204-4006, (615) 320-5353, BS 77 WV Univ; MS 78 WV Univ; 84–SLP, Bill Wilkerson Hrng & Spch Cen, **SLP**

Hoffman, Mrs Sharon Leitgeb 9 Verdi Boulevard, Latham, NY 12110, (518) 584-7383, BS 76 SUNY - Center at Albany; MS 81 Coll of Saint Rose; SLP, Saratoga Spgs Cty Sch, **SLP**

Hoffman, Sheri R 777 Exmoor, Olympia Fields, IL 60461, (312) 748-6495, BS 70; MA 71; **A**

Hoffman, Teresa E 200 North Phaney Street, Ebensburg, PA 15931, (814) 944-3535, BS 79 CA Univ of PA; ME 81 CA Univ of PA; 87–Dir Sp-Lang Path, The Rehab Hospital of Altoona, **SLP**

Hoffmann, Mrs Dale E 58 127th Street, Lemont, IL 60439, BA 64 Coll of Saint Francis; MS 70 Northern IL Univ - De Kalb; Substitute Tchr, Comm Cons Sch Dist 113, **SLP LM**

Hoffmann, Mrs Ellen L 10908 Beech Creek Drive, Columbia, MD 21045, MA 70 Univ of MD - College Park; SLP, Montgomery County Public Sch, **SLP**

Hoffmann, Kit A 42 Hobbs Road #4, North Hampton, NH 03862, (603) 964-9719, MS 82 Univ of WI - Madison; Sp/Lang Path, York Hosp, **SLP**

Hoffmann, Roger E 2510 South 18th Street, Sheboygan, WI 53081, (414) 459-3766, BA 62 AZ St Univ; MS 69 Marquette Univ; Sp-Lang Path, Sheboygan Co Hndcpd Chld Ed Bd, **SLP**

Hoffmann, Roland Jules, III 2509 Valley Drive, Brenham, TX 77833, (409) 836-5411, MS 84 Lamar Univ; Sp-Lang Path, TX Dept MHMR, **SLP**

Hoffmann, Mrs Susan Kreis 3422 N W 53rd Terrace, Gainesville, FL 32606, (904) 392-5874, BA 79 Univ of FL; MS 81 Univ of MI - Ann Arbor; Sp-Lang Path, U of FL Multidiscip Clasroom, **SLP**

Hoffmeister, Cheryln Kaye 1314 West Cape Rock #75, Cape Girardeau, MO 63701, (314) 243-8424, **SLP**

Hoffnung, Dr Audrey S 3282 Woodward Street, Oceanside, NY 11572, (212) 990-6161, BA 49 CUNY - Brooklyn Coll; MA 50 Columbia Univ Teachers Coll; PH 74 (NS) CUNY - Grad Sch & Univ Cntr; Assoc Prof, St Johns Univ, **SLP**

Hoffnung, Dr Steven Netanya Speech & Hearing Center, 8 Brodetzky Street, Netanya, Israel, (053) 340123, BA 73 CUNY - Brooklyn Coll; MA 74 New York Univ; PH 81 (Sp & Hrng Sciences) New York Univ; 84–Dir, Netanya Sp & Hrng Cen, **A**

Hoffstead, Veronica 1425 East 45th Street, Brooklyn, NY 11234, (718) 253-2523, BA 80 CUNY - Brooklyn Coll; BS 83 CUNY - Brooklyn Coll; **SLP**

Hofman, Mrs Eliza Kubota 7711 Rocio Street, Carlsbad, CA 92009, (619) 471-1198, BA 75 Univ of CA - Los Angeles; MA 84 San Diego St Univ; Sp-Lang Path, Assoc Sp Pathologists, **SLP**

Hofmann, Betty Jane 7401 North Albany Avenue, Tampa, FL 33604, (813) 685-9475, BA 81 Coll of Saint Teresa; OM 83 Univ of WI - Madison; Sp-Lang Path, Lopez Exceptional Center, **SLP**

Hofmann, Mrs Nancy S 420 Walnut Street, Catasauqua, PA 18032, (215) 264-9255, MS 87 Bloomsburg Univ of PA; 88–Sp-Lang Path, Colonial Northampton Interm

Hofmeister, Risa Kay Speech Rehabilitation Serv Pc, 12793 Q Street, Omaha, NE 68137, (402) 895-0387, BS 78 Univ of NE - Omaha; MS 79 Univ of NE - Omaha; 83–Admin, Sp Rehab Serv Pc, **SLP**

Hofstetter, Mrs Lynn D 2014 Clearview Road, Glenshaw, PA 15116, (412) 486-4274, BS 76 Indiana Univ of PA; MA 78 Univ of Pittsburgh - Pittsburgh; **SLP**

Hofstetter, Mrs Lynn P 2718 South Conyer, Visalia, CA 93277, BA 76 Univ of the Pacific; MA 77 Univ of the Pacific; **SLP**

Hogan, Claire Marie 500 N E Chipman Road #17, Lee's Summit, MO 64063, (816) 765-7772, BS 82 Univ of IA; MA 84 Univ of IL - Urbana; Aud, Timbre Hrng & Sp Ctr, **A**

Hogan, Cynthia Ann 3696 Route 14 North, Lyons, NY 14489, BS 81 Clarion Univ of PA; MS 84 PA St Univ - Univ Park; Aud, Park East Hearing Center Inc, **A**

Hogan, Deborah S 1012 Jackson Road, Park Hills, KY 41011, **SLP**

Hogan, Mrs Debra D 521 East 1910 South, Orem, UT 84058, (801) 565-7506, BS 86 Brigham Young Univ; MA 87 Brigham Young Univ; 87–Sp-Lang Path, Jordan Sch Dist, **SLP**

Hogan, Mrs Diane J 7810 61st St Court East, Palmetto, FL 34221, (813) 729-7126, BA 74 Southern CT St Univ; MS 75 Southern CT St Univ; 86–Sp-Lang Path, Rehab Works, **SLP**

Hogan, Diann Davis 323 Country Wood, San Antonio, TX 78216-1610, (512) 490-9583, **SLP**

Hogan, Dolores A 19 Woodland Drive, Irvine, CA 92714, (714) 535-6001, BA 74 Univ of CA - Santa Barbara; MS 75 Western OR St Coll; Sp-Lang Path, Anaheim City Sch Dist, **SLP**

Hogan, Dr Donald D Eastern Airlines Bldg, Office 415, Santurce, PR 00911, (809) 728-3535, BA 60 Univ of AR - Fayetteville; MS 62 Purdue Univ - West Lafayette; PH 66 (NS) Purdue Univ - West Lafayette; Aud, Donald D Hogan PhD, **A**

Hogan, Gerardine Erlangen American Elementary School, APO New York, NY 09066-0005, BS 79 Univ of MA - Amherst; MS 80 Univ of NM; 85–Sp-Lang Path, Dept of Defense Dependent Sch, **SLP**

Hogan, Mrs Kathleen Ann E 628 Roundtable Circle, Spokane, WA 99218, (509) 466-9495, BS 75 Univ of WY; MA 78 WA St Univ; Sp-Lang Path, InSpeech Inc, **SLP ACE**

Hogan, Leigh A P O Box 553, Saugerties, NY 12477, BA 76 Emerson Coll; MA 78 KS St Univ; **SLP**

Hogan, Nicholas 8 Yale Road #A, Storrs, CT 06268, (716) 245-5688, **SLP**

Hogan, Patricia Ellen 319 West Calendar #3-C, La Grange, IL 60525-2306, (312) 246-3210, MS 81 IL St Univ - Normal; SLP, Pleasantdale District 107, **SLP**

Hogan, Robert T 126 Euclid Avenue, Massapequa, NY 11758-4205, (516) 795-4505, BA 64 Saint John's Univ - Jamaica; MA 66 CUNY - Hunter Coll; MA 74 NY Univ; Aud, Rosenbaum Hearing Aid Center, **A**

Hogan, Mrs Susan C 2211 Tennessee Street, Lawrence, KS 66046, (913) 272-3111, BS 82 Univ of KS; MA Univ of KS; **A**

Hogan, Mrs Susan H 619 Alderson Avenue, Billings, MT 59101, (406) 259-5801, BA 74 Univ of VT; MS 76 CO St Univ; Sp-Lang Path, Billings Sch Dist, **SLP**

Hogan, Toni Lea R R 4 Box 202, Coffeyville, KS 67337-9531, (316) 331-6303, BS 84 KS St Univ; MA 86 KS St Univ; 87–Sp-Lang Path, Tri-County Spec Educ Cooperative, **SLP**

Hogan-Henk, Christine J 37624 Adrian, Sterling Heights, MI 48077, (313) 593-7725, BA 78 MI St Univ; MA 80 Wayne St Univ; Sp/Lang Path, Oakwood Hosp, **SLP**

Hoge, Dr Debra Reichert Dept Speech Path & Audiology, Southern Illinois Univ, Box 1776, Edwardsville, IL 62026, (618) 692-3662, BS 74 Southeast MO St Univ; MS 76 Southern IL Univ-Edwardsvill; ED 85 (Lrng & Dev) Southern IL Univ-Edwardsvill; 80–Asst Prof, Southern IL Univ, **SLP**

Hoge, Susan E 775 Chestnut Ridge Manor, Apartment #201, Morgantown, WV 26505, (304) 293-4250, BS 81 WV Univ; MS 83 WV Univ; Aud, W V U Med Ctr, **A**

Hogel, Judith M 5053 Dolores Drive, Pittsburgh, PA 15227, **SLP**

Hogenkamp, Margaret Angelina 4800 University Drive, Apartment 28-H, Durham, NC 27707, (919) 490-2095, BS 84 Mankato St Univ; MS 86 Univ of NC - Chapel Hill; **SLP**

Hogenson Day, Mrs Wendy J 1505 Red Maple Road, Depere, WI 54115, (414) 336-0018, MS 88 Univ of WI - Stevens Point; 88–Sp-Lang Path, Central WI Rehab Assn

Hogg, Mrs Debra F 1172 Washburn Avenue, Idaho Falls, ID 83402, (208) 522-7565, BS 75 ID St Univ; MS 76 ID St Univ; Sp-Lang Path, Idaho Falls Sch Dist #91, **SLP**

Hogg, Jamie Marie 16830 Kingsbury Street, #246, Granada Hills, CA 91344, (818) 894-4588, BA 86 CA St Univ - Northridge; MA 87 CA St Univ - Northridge

Hogg, Mrs Nina Justice 5301 Rice Drive Box 97701, The Colony, TX 75056, (214) 307-8502, MS 84 Univ of South FL; **SLP**

Hogle, Linda S Greer School, 2055 Lambs Road, Charlottesville, VA 22901, (804) 973-8371, BA 74 Sweet Briar Coll; ME 76 Univ of VA - Charlottesville; Sp-Lang Path, Albemarle Co Pub Sch, **SLP**

Hoglin, Mrs Sherrie 11836 Hemlock Street, El Monte, CA 91732, (818) 967-2806, BA 69 CA St Univ - Fullerton; MA 71 Univ of Southern CA; MA 82 CA St Univ - Los Angeles; 77–Aud, Los Angeles County Ofc of Educ, **A**

Hogsett, Denise 5055 West Pea Ridge, Huntington, WV 25705, (606) 324-0465, MA 77 Marshall Univ; Sp-Lang Path, Ky Easter Seal Geiger Cen, **SLP ACE**

Hohman, Mrs Beth Ann 3861 Canterbury Road, Westlake, OH 44145, (216) 666-7373, MS 87 Bowling Green St Univ; 87–Sp-Lang Path, InSpeech Inc, **SLP**

Hohn-Hizal, Mrs Diane Carol 1520 Petree Street Apartment G35, El Cajon, CA 92020, (619) 579-1963, BA 85 CUNY - Queens Coll; MA 87 CUNY - Hunter Coll

Hohorst, Suzanne Marie 15 Adams Street, Pompton Plains, NJ 07444, (201) 533-5786, BA 84 Montclair St Coll; MA 86 Montclair St Coll; 87–Aud, St Bacnabas Med Ctr, **A**

Hoisch, Mrs Ruth Pomeranz 17733 Palora Street, Encino, CA 91316, (213) 997-2357, BA 57 Univ of CA - Los Angeles; MA 84 Univ of LA Verne; SLP, Los Angeles USD, **SLP**

Hoistad, Mrs Kathleen Slick 5151 Gladstone Avenue S, Minneapolis, MN 55419, (612) 825-7709, BA 81 Univ of ND; MA 83 Univ of MN - Duluth; Clin Supvr, InSpeech Inc, **SLP**

Hoit, Dr Jeannette Dept Of Speech & Hearing Sciences, University Of Arizona, Tucson, AZ 85721, (602) 621-7072, BA 75 Univ of CA - Los Angeles; MA 80 San Diego St Univ; PH 86 (NS) Univ of AZ; Asst Research Sci, U of AZ, **SLP**

Hojem, Leslie Eileen San Francisco Audiology, 2100 Webster, Suite 203, San Francisco, CA 94115, (415) 923-3134, BS 79 Western WA Univ; MS 82 San Francisco St Univ; 86–Aud, San Francisco Audiology, **A**

Hokanson, Mrs Joanne Marie 106 Hunt Road, Columbia, CT 06237, (203) 228-0106, **SLP**

Hoke, Mrs Jody Lynn Hilles 5650 Raymar Street, San Diego, CA 92120, BS 81 Ball St Univ; MA 85 Bowling Green St Univ; **SLP**

Hoke, Mrs Sharon A Children's Hospital Medical Center, Elland & Bethesda Avenue, Audiology Department, Cincinnati, OH 45229, (513) 559-4236, BS 86 OH Univ - Athens; MA 87 OH Univ - Athens; 87–Aud, Childrens Hosp Med Ctr, **A**

Holak, Mrs Susan M RFD 4, 5 Garrison Lane, Dover, NH 03820, (603) 749-1619, BA 72 Stonehill Coll; MS 87 Univ of NH; **SLP**

Holas, Marlene Ann 53 Lytton Avenue, Hartsdale, NY 10530, (914) 948-0050, BA 82 Univ of VT; MS 85 Univ of WI - Madison; Sp-Lang Path, Burke Rehab Ctr, **SLP**

Holaway, Mrs Kathy Kubasiak 1067 Scarborough Court 5-G, Chesterton, IN 46304, (219) 763-8090, BA 77 MI St Univ; MA 79 MI St Univ; Sp-Lang Path, Porter Co Coop Ctr

Holbert, Heather Jayne 6833 Roe Avenue, Prairie Village, KS 66208, (913) 362-4499, **SLP**

Holbert, Mrs Susan M 13128 Derbyshire Court, Carmel, IN 46032, (317) 848-7647, BS 70 Purdue Univ - West Lafayette; MS 73 Univ of MI - Ann Arbor; Pres/Sp-Lang Path, Private Practice, **SLP**

Holbrook, Dr Anthony College Of Communication, Florida State University, Tallahassee, FL 32306, (904) 644-5034, BA 51 Univ of CA - Santa Barbara; MA 53 Univ of HI - Manoa; PH 58 FL St Univ; Dir Sp Research Lab, FL St U, **SLP**

Holbrook, Mrs Johanna G Route 2 Box 394, Crawfordville, FL 32327, (904) 926-7155, BS 67 FL St Univ; MS 68 FL St Univ; Sp-Lang Path, Wakulla Co Sch Bd, **SLP**

Holbrook, Sally 88 West 50 South #K-2, P O Box 211, Centerville, UT 84014, (801) 451-1158, BS 75 UT St Univ; MS 77 UT St Univ; SLP, Davis Sch Dist, **SLP**

Holbrook, Mrs Susan Marie 7188 Ridgedale, Lambertville, MI 48144, (313) 856-4018, BA 78 Univ of Toledo; MA 84 Eastern MI Univ; Sp-Lang Path, Lucas Co Office of Education, **SLP**

Holbrook, Wanda Kaye Box 6, Wolfe Creek Road, Rousseau, KY 41366, (606) 666-2373, BS 86 Eastern KY Univ; ME 87 Eastern KY Univ; 87–Sp-Lang Path, Magoffin County Bd of Educ, **F**

Holcman, Mrs Janis F 6226 Laurain Court, West Bloomfield, MI 48322, (313) 661-5798, **SLP**

Holcomb, Barbara J 11614 Symmes Creek Drive, Loveland, OH 45140-9324, (513) 369-2474, BA 78 Univ of Cincinnati; MA 84 Univ of Cincinnati; 86–Sp-Lang Path, The Christ Hosp, **SLP**

Holcomb, Charlie McIlwain, Jr PO Box 8143, Gulfport, MS 39506, (601) 865-1070, BS 79 Univ of MS; MS 84 Univ of MS; Aud, VA Med Ctr, **A**

Holcomb, Tammi A 2121 Green Street #A26, Adel, IA 50003, (515) 270-9030, BA 86 Univ of Northern IA; MA 88 Univ of Northern IA; 88–Sp-Lang Path, Heartland AEA II

Holcombe, Mrs Claire S 141 Main Street, Red Hill, PA 18076, (215) 679-6471, BS 67 Indiana Univ of PA; MS 69 WV Univ; Sp-Lang Path, Mont Co Inter Unit, **SLP**

Holden, Debra Lynn 151 Leicester Street #5D, Auburn, MA 01501, (203) 923-9581, BS 74 Worcester St Coll; MS 80 Worcester St Coll; Sp-Lang Path, Thompson School System, **SLP**

Holden, Mrs Helen Q 530 American Avenue Ext, Dover, DE 19901, (302) 736-5540, BS 65 CO St Univ; MS 66 Vanderbilt Univ; 88–Sp-Lang Path, Capital Sch Dist, **SLP**

Holden, Mrs Kelley A 1140 Cedar Street, San Carlos, CA 94070, (415) 340-9986, Aud, El Camino Hrng Cntr, **A**

Holden, Mary Ann 104 East Bailey #E, Naperville, IL 60565, (312) 983-1810, BA 54 Univ of IL - Champaign; MA 87 Northern IL Univ - De Kalb; 88–Sp-Lang Path, Dist 88-Illinois

Holden-Bryant, Diane 2721 Larkspur Lane, Hazel Crest, IL 60429, (312) 841-7800, BS 70 OH Univ - Athens; MS 72 Univ of MI - Ann Arbor; Coord of Aud, S Metro Assoc, **A**

Holden-Pitt, Lisa Denise 513 Fairhill Drive, Silver Spring, MD 20904, (301) 384-4398

Holder, Elizabeth 7366 South Milwaukee Way, Littleton, CO 80122, (303) 773-0983, BS 74 SUNY - Coll at Brockport; MA 78 Univ of CO - Boulder; SLP, Arapahoe Co Sch Dist #6, **SLP**

Holder, Gregory Marc P O Box D-K, Los Gatos, CA 95031, (408) 379-2580, BS 73 CA St Univ - Hayward; MA 76 San Francisco St Univ; **A**

Holder, Hugh Scott 2116 Cedar Street, Owensboro, KY 42301, (502) 926-3030, MS 85 Western KY Univ; SLP, Owensboro-Daviess County Hosp, **SLP ACE**

Holder, Ronald Lee 640 Evans Street, Missoula, MT 59801, **SLP**

Holder, Mrs Suzanne Wooten 15152 Springview Street, Tampa, FL 33624, (813) 892-4141, BS 82 Univ of GA; ME 83 Univ of GA; 85–Aud Coord, All Chldrns Hosp, **A**

Holderbaum, Flora M 229 West 26th Street #2B, New York, NY 10001, (212) 255-8430, OB 75 SUNY - Coll at Fredonia; MA 77 Univ of KS; Aud, Bellevue Hosp Ctr, **A**

Holderby, Gail G 7318 Elmridge, Dallas, TX 75240, **SLP**

Holdgrafer, Dr Gary E University Of Alberta, Dept Of Speech Path & Aud, 400-11044 82nd Avenue, Edmonton, AB, Canada T6G 0T2, (403) 432-5990, BA 67 Moorhead St Univ; MA 69 Univ of KS; PH 74 (NS) Univ of KS; Professor, University of Alberta, **SLP**

Holdridge, Julie Ann 68161/2 Sultana Avenue, North San Gabriel, CA 91775-1527, (818) 445-3102, OB 81 San Diego St Univ; MA 84 CA St Univ - Stanislaus; **SLP**

Holdsworth, Mrs Joy Lindsey 2118 Robin Hood Drive, Miamisburg, OH 45342, (513) 866-1957, OM 79; Sp-Lang Path, Private Practice, **SLP**

Holdsworth, Mrs Leslie Plowman 926 Spindle Palm Way, Apollo Beach, FL 33570, (813) 971-9506, MS 80 Univ of South FL; Sp-Lang Path, Private Practice, **SLP**

Holdt, Mrs Sarah J 4302 Wolf Hill Drive, Hampstead, MD 21074, (301) 848-3900, BS 70 WV Univ; MS 75 Loyola Coll; 75–Sp/Lang Path, Carroll Co Bd of Ed, **SLP**

Hole, Karen Lynn 16801 Moody Circle #B, Huntington Beach, CA 92649, (213) 926-5566, BA 82 Whittier Coll; MA 83 Whittier Coll; **SLP**

Hole, Mrs Sherri Rae 1519 Laurel Avenue, Hudson, WI 54016, (715) 386-6399, BS 79 Univ of WI - River Falls; MS 81 Univ of WI - River Falls; 88–Sp-Lang Path, Sch Dist of Hudson, **SLP**

Holeman, Deborah A 30 Walnut Street, Enfield, CT 06082, (203) 745-4518, BA 76 Southern CT St Univ; MS 79 Southern CT St Univ; **SLP**

Holeman, Lois J 1011 Altschul Avenue, Menlo Park, CA 94025, (415) 854-1215, BA 51 CO St Univ; MS 55 Univ of OR; Dir Spec Ed, Menlo Park School District, **SLP**

Holen, Deborah 2006 West Summit Place, Chandler, AZ 85224, MS 76 AZ St Univ; **SLP**

Holguin, Mrs Roxanna Ramirez 5435 South Jasmine Way, Tucson, AZ 85706, (505) 898-2663, MS 83 Univ of NM; Sp-Lang Path, Cobre Consolidated Schools, **SLP**

Holguin, Yolanda Garza Alberto T Fernandez Md, 343 West Houston #409, San Antonio, TX 78205, (512) 226-9166, BS 78 TX A & I Univ; MA 81 Univ of Cincinnati; Aud, Alberto T Fernandez MD, **A**

Holian, Mrs Eva Maria 466 Mockingbird Lane, Spartanburg, SC 29302, (803) 579-7913, MA 84 Kent St Univ; Sp-Lang Path, **SLP**

Holifield, Mrs Deborah Wilson Route One Box 184, Soso, MS 39480, (601) 428-1564, BS 83 Univ Southern MS-Hattiesburg; MS 85 Univ Southern MS-Hattiesburg; Sp-Lang Path, Jones County School System, **SLP**

Holifield, Mary M 2924 Pawnee Avenue South, Apartment #5, Birmingham, AL 35205, (205) 348-7131, BS 83 Univ of Montevallo; MS 85 Univ of AL- Tuscaloosa; 88–Aud, VA Med Ctr, **A**

Holiman, Linda Hankins 302 Trailwood Drive, Clinton, MS 39056, (601) 769-5251, **SLP**

Holing, John E 224 Hidden Valley Road, Roseburg, OR 97470, (503) 440-4092, BS 74 Univ of OR; MS 77 Eastern WA Univ; Sp/Lang Path, Roseburg Pub Sch Dist #4, **SLP**

Holker, Nancy L P O Box 1168, Monticello, MN 55362, (612) 295-2057, BS 81 Brigham Young Univ; OM 82 Brigham Young Univ; Dist Aud, Proro Sch Dist, **A**

Holla-Aschenbrenner, Anne Marie Elizabeth RD #8 Box 8853, West Shore Drive, Lake Plymouth, Newton, NJ 07860, (315) 597-2454, BS 85 Marywood Coll; MA 87 OH Univ - Athens

Hollahan, Mrs Kelmie K BEH 255, Department Of Communication Sciences And Disorders, Tampa, FL 33620, (813) 974-2006, BA 50 Univ of AL- Tuscaloosa; MA 69 Univ of South FL; Cl Superv/Sp-Lang Path, Univ of South Florida, **SLP ACE**

Holland, Ange N 816 Leigh, Benton, AR 72015, (501) 794-0263, BA 74 Univ of AR - Little Rock; MS 78 Univ of AR - Little Rock; 80–Sp-Lang Path, Bryant Pub Sch, **SLP**

Holland, Mrs Ann Mitchell 6 Merryman Court, Baltimore, MD 21210, (301) 235-0606, **SLP**

Holland, Dr Audrey L Eye And Ear Institute, 230 Lothrop Street, Pittsburgh, PA 15213, (412) 647-2030, BS 55 Univ of Pittsburgh - Pittsburgh; MS 59 Univ of Pittsburgh - Pittsburgh; PH 61 (NS) Univ of Pittsburgh - Pittsburgh; Prof of Otolaryngology, U of Pittsburgh, **SLP**

Holland, Mrs Betty R 509 Woodcliff Road, Charleston, WV 25314, (304) 345-7311, BA 70 Marshall Univ; MA 71 Marshall Univ; **SLP**

Holland, Mrs Bonnie B 1703 Palace Green, Katy, TX 77449, (713) 391-5431, BS 64 Northwestern Univ; MS 68 East TX St Univ - Commerce; 87–Exec Dir-Stu Support Svcs, Katy ISD, **SLP**

Holland, Carla E 831 Kenwick Road, Columbus, OH 43209-2514, (614) 275-0810, BA 74 OH Univ - Athens; MA 78 OH Univ - Athens; SLP, Ohio Dept of Youth Services, **SLP**

Holland, Mrs Carolyn Allen 20 East Rock Road, Allentown, PA 18103, (215) 791-2424, BS 77 Bloomsburg Univ of PA; MS 78 Bloomsburg Univ of PA; **SLP**

Holland, Mrs Diane Marie/Otte 1529 Davinbrook, Norman, OK 73072, (405) 360-0220, BA 77 Univ of NE - Lincoln; MS 81 Kearney St Coll; 87–Sp-Lang Path, Norman PS, **SLP**

Holland, Donna J 1301 Pennsylvania Avenue, Fort Worth, TX 76104, (817) 882-2045, BS 81 TX Woman's Univ; MA 82 TX Woman's Univ; Dir Sp-Lang Path, Harris Hosp-Meth, **SLP**

Holland, Frances L 307 Romney Road, Akron, OH 44313, (216) 434-3131, BA 60 Wellesley Coll; OM 62 Harvard Univ; MA 70 IN Univ - Bloomington; Sp-Lang Path, Akron Pub Sch, **SLP**

Holland, Dr Francine 14826 Silver Sands, Houston, TX 77095, (713) 462-7708, BA 68 Univ of North TX; MA 70 Univ of North TX; PH 77 (Special Education) Vanderbilt Univ; 88–Prog Dir, Region IV Educ Svc Ctr, **SLP**

Holland, Jay W 4601 Hartford, Abilene, TX 79605, (915) 691-7255, BA 72 TX Tech Univ; MA 74 TX Tech Univ; Ch Aud Serv, W Tx Rehab Cen, **A**

Holland, Joan B 1111 Parkinson Avenue, Palo Alto, CA 94301, **SLP**

Holland, Judi A 115 Byrd Street, Burnsville, NC 28714, (704) 682-6467, MA 87 Appalachian St Univ

Holland, Mrs Judy N 1162 Granito Drive, Laramie, WY 82070, (307) 742-8194, MS 88 Univ of WY

Holland, Mrs Karen E 5628 Glenview Drive, Erie, PA 16509, (814) 864-2725, BA 83 Marshall Univ; MA 84 Marshall Univ; Sp-Lang Path, Gertrude Barber Ctr, **SLP**

Holland, Kathleen 60 Storm Drive, Holtsville, NY 11742, (516) 567-4901, BA 77 Adelphi Univ; MS 79 Rutgers St Univ -N Brunswick; SLP, BOCES II-Suffolk Co, **SLP**

Holland, Leslie Spahr 2432 Traymore Drive, University Heights, OH 44118, (216) 321-1575, BS 81 Univ of MO - Columbia; MA 82 Memphis St Univ; 86–Aud, Evoked Potential Monitoring Svc Inc, **A**

Holland, Mrs Luanne G 3307 Marywood Dr, Durham, NC 27712, (919) 382-2559, BA 79 Univ of NC - Greensboro; ME 81 Univ of NC - Greensboro; 88–Practicum Prog Coord, Murdoch Cen for Ment Ret, **SLP**

Holland, Dr Lynn J Suite 250, P O Box 26800, Albuquerque, NM 87125, (505) 265-1711, BS 55 Northwestern Univ; MA 73 Wayne St Univ; PH 84 (NS) Univ of UT; 86–Sp-Lang Path, Albuquerque VA Med Ctr, **SLP**

Holland, Richard Wayne 762 Tunnel Lane, Westville, CT 06515, **SLP**

Holland, Sue Ann West Texas Rehab Center, 4601 Hartford, Abilene, TX 79605, (915) 692-1633, BS 78 Univ of TX - Austin; MA 80 Univ of TX - Austin; Audiologist, W Tx Rehab Cen, **A**

Holland, Mrs Susan E Route 3 Box 280-B, Lindale, TX 75771, (214) 882-5348, BA 73 Univ of North TX; MA 75 Univ of North TX; Aud, Arlington ISD, **A**

Holland, William H 20122 Lake Chabot Road, Castro Valley, CA 94546, (415) 582-3011, **A**

Hollander, Barbara E 798 Vivian Court, Baldwin, NY 11510, **A**

Hollander, Beverly M 6314 Rio Linda Drive, Rancho Palos Verdes, CA 90274, BA 72 Univ of CA - Riverside; **A**

Hollander, Cynthia S 135 Nottingham Drive, Watchung, NJ 07060, **SLP ACE**

Hollander, Deann Janine 26 Old Fourth Drive, Oak Ridge, NJ 07438, (201) 208-0361, BS 86 Ithaca Coll; MS 87 Ithaca Coll; 87–Sp-Lang Path, Saint Bacnabas Med Ctr, **SLP**

Hollander, Jane G K 25 Crest Hollow Lane, Searingtown, NY 11507, **SLP**

Hollander, Janine Gail 2510 South 6th #B-11, Marshalltown, IA 50158, (515) 753-5159, BA 81 Univ of SD - Vermillion; MA 83 Univ of SD - Vermillion; 86–Sp-Lang Path, AEA #6, **SLP**

Hollander, Jeanne B 1207 Oxford Hill Court #7, St Louis, MO 63146, (314) 569-6040, BA 80 SUNY - Coll at Cortland; MS 82 Boston Univ; 88–Sp-Lang Path, St Johns Mercy Med Ctr, **SLP**

Hollander, Mrs Marilyn R 18 Wren Drive, Roslyn Estates, NY 11576, (516) 626-3624, BA 57 CUNY - Brooklyn Coll; MA 68 CUNY - Brooklyn Coll; Sp-Lang Path, Private Practice, **SLP**

Hollander, Mrs Ruth E H 188 Nogal Drive, Santa Barbara, CA 93110, (805) 964-2562, BA 76 Univ of CA - Santa Barbara; MA 77 Humboldt St Univ; Aud, Sb Co Hlth Dept, **SLP**

Hollback, Jenni Kay Route 6 Box 130, Wheelersburg, OH 45694, (614) 353-7774, BS 86 OH Univ - Athens; MA 87 OH Univ - Athens; 87–Sp-Lang Path, Scioto Mem Hosp, **SLP**

Holle, Jean Louise 442 Rustic Drive, Los Angeles, CA 90065, (213) 824-3100, BA 82 CA St Univ - Los Angeles; MA 86 CA St Univ - Los Angeles; **SLP**

Holle, Peggy J 2350 South 23rd Street, Lot 1087, Manitowoc, WI 54220, (414) 684-1752, **SLP**

Hollenbach, Ann Yazujian RD 5 Box 401, Rocky Valley Road, Quakertown, PA 18951, (215) 282-2301, ME 88 Trenton St Coll; 88–Sp-Lang Path, Robin W Muller & Associates

Hollenback, Mrs Sylvia D 8516 West Entiat Place, Kennewick, WA 99336, (509) 586-0754, BS 82 Brigham Young Univ; OM 83 Brigham Young Univ; Sp-Lang Path, Benton-Franklin Dev Ctr, **SLP**

Hollenbeck, Mrs Judy E 28491 La Falda, Laguna Niguel, CA 92677, (714) 496-1215, BS 76 Central MI Univ; MA 77 Central MI Univ; Sp-Lang Path, Capistrand USD, **SLP**

Hollenkamp, Mrs Teresa A 1619 Beechshire Court, Cincinnati, OH 45255, (513) 474-2339, BS 83 Univ of Cincinnati; MA 85 Univ of Cincinnati; **SLP**

Hollensbe, Mrs Deborah Aumann 2227 Wilkes, Davenport, IA 52804-2344, (319) 359-1371, BA 82 MacMurray Coll; MA 84 Univ of IA; Sp-Lang Path, Miss Bend AEA, **SLP**

Holleran, Laine Mayer 372 Goshen, North Little Rock, AR 72116, (501) 661-2320, BS 83 Univ of Central AR; MS 85 Univ of AR - Little Rock; 85–Aud, Arkansas Dept of Health, **A**

Hollett, Valerie Grace 33 Browning, Toronto, ON, Canada M4K 1V8, (416) 465-6949, 88 Univ of Toronto - Ontario

Hollevoet, Catherine 1203 N W 134th Way, Vancouver, WA 98685, (206) 574-3216, BS 76 Portland St Univ; MS 79 Portland St Univ; Aud/Coord, Educ Serv Dist 112, **A**

Holley, Mrs Bessie L 683 Best Street, Buffalo, NY 14211, MA 82 SUNY - Coll at Buffalo; Sp-Lang Path, Roswell Park Memorial Inst, **SLP**

Holley, Mrs Jamie Sellers 3309 Mockingbird, Oxford, MS 38655, (601) 236-2276, BA 85 Univ of MS; MS 86 Univ of MS; Sp-Lang Path, N MS Retardation Ctr, **SLP**

Holley, Dr Sandra C 215 Stimson Road, New Haven, CT 06511, (203) 865-0454, BA 65 George Washington Univ; MA 66 George Washington Univ; PH 79 (Sp-Lang Path) Univ of CT; 70–Professor, Southern CT State University, **SLP F**

Hollibaugh, Mrs Jennifer Susan 6476 Dwyer Court, San Jose, CA 95120-2845, (408) 847-1328, **SLP**

Holliday, Sarah Ford 3 Wheatland Drive, Hampton, VA 23666, (304) 366-2070, **SLP**

Hollien, Dr Harry University Of Florida, 50 Dauer Hall 1 ASCP, Gainesville, FL 32611, (904) 392-2046, ME 51 Boston Univ; MA 53 Univ of IA; PH 55 (NS) Univ of IA; 62–Prof, Univ of Florida

Hollier, Adrienne K 9511 Wickenburg, Houston, TX 77031, (713) 521-9584, BA 71 Univ of Southwestern LA; MA 72 Univ of Houston - Univ Park; Dir Infant Prog, MHMR of Harris Co, **SLP**

Hollier, Mrs Anne S 10601 Chancelor Drive, Brighton, MI 48116, (517) 546-5550, BS 70 Eastern MI Univ; MA 71 Eastern MI Univ; Sp/Lang Path, Livingston ISD, **SLP**

Hollifield, Laura Jan P O Box 125, Drexel, NC 28619, (704) 584-0762, BS 85 Appalachian St Univ; MA 86 Appalachian St Univ; **SLP**

Hollifield, S Gail 1301 Chestnut Street, Grand Forks, ND 58201, (701) 594-5521, BA 79 Univ of ND; MS 81 Univ of ND; Sp/Lang Path, Grand Forks Pub Sch, **SLP**

Holliman, Dr Doreen G 13518 Lake Magdalene Drive, Tampa, FL 33613, (813) 972-7529, BS 67 FL St Univ; MS 68 FL St Univ; PH 84 (NS) Univ of South FL; Chf SLP Sec, James A Haley VA Hosp, **SLP ACE**

Hollinger, Mrs Dianne S 670 Skyview Drive, York, PA 17402, (717) 846-7745, BS 77 MD Inst Coll of Art; MA 78 Univ of TN - Knoxville; Sp-Lang Path, Lancaster General Hosp, **SLP**

Hollinger, Susan Anne 11231 Route 700, Hiram, OH 44234, (216) 569-3130, BA 83 Hiram Coll; MA 86 Kent St Univ; **SLP**

Hollingham, Mrs Linda Ferraro 19 Stonecliffe Court, Hamilton, ON, Canada L9C 7G5, (416) 388-8192, BS 81 0500; MA 84 SUNY - Coll at Buffalo; **A**

Hollingsworth, Brenda Merritt 1110 Riverside Drive, West Richland, WA 99352-5224, (904) 222-2403, BS 72 FL St Univ; MS 73 FL St Univ; Sp-Path, Tallahassee Sp Path Assoc, **SLP**

Hollingsworth, Mrs Carolyn D 941 Azalea Drive, Costa Mesa, CA 92626, (714) 842-6608, BS 64 Saint Louis Univ; MA 73 CA St Univ - Long Beach; SLP, Ocean View School District, **SLP**

Hollingsworth, Mrs Cheryl Gay 433 Macy, Norman, OK 73071, (405) 321-8882, BS 66 Univ of OK - Norman; OM 67 IN Univ - Bloomington; Sp-Lang Path, Private Practice, **SLP**

Hollingsworth, Mrs Patricia B 37 East Lincoln Avenue, Gettysburg, PA 17325, (717) 624-4616, BS 54 Bloomsburg Univ of PA; ME 65 PA St Univ - Univ Park; Sp-Lang Path, Lincoln Inter Ut 12, **SLP**

Hollingsworth, Rebecca A 402 N W 17th Street #1, Mandan, ND 58554, (701) 663-6200, BS 74 Minot St Univ; MS 80 Minot St Univ; Sp-Lang Path, Mandan Pub Sch, **SLP**

Hollingsworth, Mrs Rita M 708 Pecan Drive, Schertz, TX 78154, **SLP**

Holloman, Angela Law Box 4042, APO New York, NY 09009-5373, BS 83 Univ of Central AR; MS 85 Univ of AR - Little Rock; **SLP**

Hollon, Nancy B 266 Tuthill Lane, Mobile, AL 36608, (205) 343-1570, BA 73 Univ of AL- Tuscaloosa; MA 74 Univ of AL- Tuscaloosa; **SLP**

Holloway, Mrs Cynthia Lee 1409 West 8th Avenue, Eugene, OR 97402, (503) 683-6056, BS 78 Portland St Univ; MS 80 Western OR St Coll; SLP, Lane Co Esd, **SLP**

Holloway, Cynthia Marie 606 Park Lane, Okolona, MS 38860, (601) 447-2073, MS 88 Univ of MS

Holloway, Dr Gordon F 2040 Jennings Avenue, Hot Springs, SD 57747, (605) 745-4101, BS 62 Univ of UT; MS 64 Univ of UT; PH 68 (NS) Southern IL Univ -Carbondale; Chief Aud/Sp-Lang Path, Vamc Hot Springs, **SLP A**

Holloway, Julianne P O Box 1141, McAlester, OK 74502, (918) 426-1445, BA 81 Univ of AR - Fayetteville; MS 82 Univ of AR - Fayetteville; Sp-Lang Path, Scot Rite Cl for Chldrn Lang D, **SLP ACE**

Holloway, Mrs Kathleen R 1489 Rockledge Drive, Rockledge, FL 32955, (305) 631-5150, BS 74 FL St Univ; MS 75 FL St Univ; **SLP**

Holloway, Martha J 3009 Carter Circle, Denver, CO 80222, **SLP**

Holloway, Micki W P O Box 666, Greenwood, AR 72936, (501) 928-4866, BS 76 OK St Univ; MA 77 Univ of AR - Fayetteville; Sp-Lang Path, Mansfield Pub Sch, **SLP**

Holloway, Mrs Shelia Allene Route 1 Box 155, Mayfield, KY 42066, (502) 328-8604, BS 74 Murray St Univ; MS 84 Murray St Univ; 88–Sp-Lang Path, Graves Co Bd Educ, **SLP**

Holloway, Suzanna K 1827 West Crescent, Park Ridge, IL 60068, BA 54 Bowling Green St Univ; BS 54 Bowling Green St Univ; **SLP**

Hollowed, Barbara Lynn 1224 Haase Avenue, Westchester, IL 60153, (309) 828-3045, MS 87 IL St Univ - Normal

Hollowell, Mrs Margaret 15 Orchard Drive, Charleston, IL 61920, (217) 345-2931, BS 55 Northwestern Univ; MS 68 Eastern IL Univ; **SLP**

Holly, Susanna Maniace 1012 Neshaminy Valley Dr, Bensalem, PA 19020, (215) 750-7634, BS 83 Purdue Univ - West Lafayette; MS 85 Purdue Univ - West Lafayette; Sp-Lang Pathologist, Temple Univ, **SLP**

Holm, Ann Czajka 3096 S Coon Creek Drive N W, Andover, MN 55304, (612) 588-0811, BA 83 Univ of MI - Ann Arbor; MS 86 Univ of MI - Ann Arbor; **SLP**

Holm, Marilyn K 11021 S E 182nd Street, Renton, WA 98055, **SLP**

Holman, Eileen S 405 Jennings, Nocona, TX 76255, (817) 894-2011, BA 81 Univ of North TX; MA 87 Univ of North TX

Holman, Mrs Eugenia Turner 7628 Fleming Hills Drive, Huntsville, AL 35802, (205) 859-1151, MA 65 Univ of AL- Tuscaloosa; MS 78 Univ of AL- Tuscaloosa; Aud, Madison Co Bd of Ed, **A**

Holman, Dr Gary Lynn 2323 S E Spyglass Drive, Vancouver, WA 98684, (206) 696-6521, BA 64 ID St Univ; MS 65 Western OR St Coll; PH 74 (Special Education) Univ of Pittsburgh - Pittsburgh; Supt, Wash State Sch for Deaf, **SLP**

Holman, Mrs Lynn S 3918 Turf Lane, Fort Wayne, IN 46804, (219) 436-1965, BS 79 Fontbonne Coll; MS 79 Fontbonne Coll; Sp-Lang Path, Prof Rehab Cen Inc, **SLP**

Holmberg, Mrs Denise Quinn 2090 Whisperwood Glen Lane, Reston, VA 22091, (703) 476-2960, BA 83 Univ of Pittsburgh - Pittsburgh; MA 85 Univ of Pittsburgh - Pittsburgh; Sp-Lang Path, Private Practice, **SLP**

Holmberg, Sandra L 26 Marian Lane, Nashua, NH 03062, (617) 935-5050, BS 83 Northeastern Univ; MS 85 Northeastern Univ; Sp-Lang Path, New England Rehab Hosp, **SLP**

Holmberg, Tristan L Virginia Mason Clinic, Neurotology HRB 2W G2-AU, 1100 9th Avenue, Seattle, WA 98101, (206) 223-6393, BS 74 Univ of MN - Minneap-St Paul; MS 78 Univ of WA; Dir of Aud, Virginia Mason Clinic, **A**

Holmer, Janice A P O Box 454, South Laguna, CA 92677, (714) 494-7928, BA 77 CA St Univ - Fullerton; MA 81 CA St Univ - Fullerton; Sp-Lang Path, Private Practice, **SLP**

Holmes, Dr Alice E Route 3 P O Box 173, Alachua, FL 32615, (904) 392-2041, BS 76 TX Tech Univ; MS 78 ID St Univ; PH 82 (Communication Disorders) PA St Univ - Univ Park; 82–Assoc Prof, U of FL, **A ACE**

Holmes, Mrs Anne S 74 Bunker Hill Road, Lawrence, NJ 08648, (609) 987-0099, MS 81 Rutgers St Univ - Newark; Dir Outreach & Support Ser, Eden Institute, **SLP**

Holmes, Mrs Colleen J 910 Stanton, Iron Mountain, MI 49801, (906) 779-2692, BS 71 Northern MI Univ; MA 72 Northern MI Univ; Sp-Lang Path, Dickinson-Iron ISD, **SLP**

Holmes, Mrs Cynthia Ken P O Box 2462, Winter Haven, FL 33883, (813) 293-6507, **A**

Holmes, Dr David Department Of Communication Disorders, University Of North Texas, PO Box 5008, Denton, TX 76203, (817) 565-2262, BS 64 Ball St Univ; MA 67 Ball St Univ; PH 72 (Aud) Syracuse Univ; Assoc Prof, U North Texas, **A**

Holmes, David A 1450 Iron Springs Rd, Prescott, AZ 86301, (602) 778-5132, BS 79 Northwest MO St Univ; MA 81 Wichita St Univ; 81–Aud, David A Holmes MA, **A**

Holmes, Mrs Dorothy V 1048 Braemoor Drive, Downers Grove, IL 60515-5522, (312) 852-8840, BS 56 IN Univ - Bloomington; MS 63 IN Univ - Bloomington; Sp/Lang Path, **SLP**

Holmes, Elaine J 8302 Shadow Wind, Houston, TX 77040, (713) 466-7405, BS 71 Univ Southern MS-Hattiesburg; MS 83 Univ of South AL; Supervisor, InSpeech Inc, **SLP**

Holmes, Mrs Elizabeth Gossett 3203 Banbury, Houston, TX 77027, (713) 877-1917, BA Univ of TX - Austin; MA Univ of Houston - Univ Park; President, Egh Invest/Man Inc, **SLP**

Holmes, Geraldine A 415 South Windsor Dr, Arlington Height, IL 60004, (312) 577-1475, MA 83 SUNY - Center at Buffalo; Instr/Cl Superv, SUNY at Buffalo, **SLP**

Holmes, Mrs Imogene L 1000 Kings Highway #22, Port Charlotte, FL 33980, (813) 625-5937, MS; **SLP LM**

Holmes, Jane F R R 2 Box 107, Peterborough, NH 03458, (603) 357-1395, BA 73 Univ of FL; MA 75 Univ of FL; Sp-Lang Path, Private Practice, **SLP**

Holmes, Joseph John, Jr 900 N E 19th Street, Cape Coral, FL 33909, (813) 433-0222, BA 80 West Liberty St Coll; MA 83 MI St Univ; 87–Owner, Hearing Care Center, **A**

Holmes, Mrs Judith C 1026 Park Avenue, River Forest, IL 60305, (312) 458-7165, BA 60 Barat Coll; MA 68 Catholic Univ of America; Sp-Lang Path, Aero Spec Ed Coop, **SLP**

Holmes, Judy H 5658 Ridge View Drive, Alexandria, VA 22310, (703) 664-7343, BA 80; MS 81 Southern IL Univ-Edwardsvill; Sp-Lang Path, Mount Vernon Hosp, **SLP**

Holmes, Karol Ann 1539 Allen Drive, Westlake, OH 44145, (216) 835-0016, BA 85 Western WA Univ; MA 87 San Diego St Univ; **SLP**

Holmes, Marian Frances 310 Evans Court, Mount Laurel, NJ 08054, (215) 423-1400, BA 81 Gettysburg Coll; MA 85 West Chester Univ of PA; **SLP**

Holmes, Nancy Rae 141-C Outer Belle Road, Trotwood, OH 45426, (513) 890-3080, BS 83 Purdue Univ - West Lafayette; ME 85 Univ of VA - Charlottesville; **A**

Holmes, Mrs Pamela K 8830 Rendon Drive, Anchorage, AK 99507, (907) 349-2497, MA 84 Univ of IA; 85–Sp-Lang Path, Prog for Infants & Children, **SLP**

Holmes, Richard Woodbury Perham Street Box 1459, Farmington, ME 04938, (207) 778-3501, BA 54 Univ of ME - Orono; MA 63 Syracuse Univ; Sp-Lang Path, Univ of Maine Farmington, **SLP**

Holmes, Mrs Robyn C 2509 Dover Court, Woodbridge, VA 22192, (703) 490-1659, BA 72 Univ of Denver; MA 74 Univ of Denver; 87–Sp-Lang Path, Prince William Co PS, **SLP**

Holmes, Sandra S 1650 Barnes Mill Road, Apartment 2423, Marietta, GA 30062, (404) 421-1082, MS 87 Univ of Montevallo; 88–Sp-Lang Path, Cobb/Douglas Mentl Ret Prog

Holmes, Susan Laurie 6700 Wildridge Circle #4, Memphis, TN 38119, (601) 928-3539, BA 80 Univ of MS; MA 82 Univ of MS; Aud, Drs Teaque and Canale, **A**

Holmskog, Sevia Lynne P O Box 2350, Hesperia, CA 92345, (619) 244-8869, MA 86 Wichita St Univ; SLP, Hesperia Schl Dstr, **SLP**

Holohan, Jeanette M 2210 Hokendauqua Avenue, Northampton, PA 18067, (215) 799-4111, BS 72 Bloomsburg Univ of PA; ME 76 Bloomsburg Univ of PA; Sp-Lang Path, Carbon-Lehigh Inter Unit #21, **SLP**

Holpp, Mrs Maryan M 2913 Alcazar N E, Albuquerque, NM 87110, (505) 884-5129, BA 54 Univ of Denver; MA 56 Univ of NM; 88–Sp-Lang Path, Private Practice, **SLP A**

Holsinger, Mrs Cynthia M P O Box 293, Middletown, VA 22645, (703) 869-4158, MS 88 James Madison Univ

Holsinger, Mrs Esther L 67 East Schreyer, Columbus, OH 43214, (614) 263-5151, BS 77 Clarion Univ of PA; ME 78 Clarion Univ of PA; Asst Prog Dir of SLP, Columbus Sp & Hrng Cen, **SLP**

Holsomback, Barbara Jean P O Box 733, Mannford, OK 74044, (918) 742-7376, BS 81 Univ of Tulsa; MA 82 Univ of Tulsa; Aud, Audiological Consulting Serv, **A**

Holste, Dr Herman M 6861 East Nevada Avenue, Detroit, MI 48234, (313) 368-1220, BS 51 Concordia Teachers Coll; MS 57 Washington Univ; PH 68 (NS) Wayne St Univ; Prin, Lutheran Sch for Deaf, **SLP**

Holstein, Diane Z 6730 121st Avenue North #1, Largo, FL 34643, (813) 531-7370, MS 83 Univ of South FL; Aud, A Center for Speech & Hearing, **A**

Holstein, Janet Laura 6133 N E 28th Avenue, Portland, OR 97211, (503) 649-0471, BS 81 Portland St Univ; Sp-Lang Path, Beaverton School District, **SLP**

Holstine, Mrs Mary Lucile Route 1 Box 56 A, Forest City, MO 64451, (816) 442-5741, BA 56 Tarkio Coll; MS 86 Northwest MO St Univ; 88–Sp-Lang Path, Holt County R-II Sch, **SLP**

Holston, Joseph T 825 Deerfield Drive, Mobile, AL 36608, (205) 460-6327, BS 74 Univ Southern MS-Hattiesburg; MS 75 Univ Southern MS-Hattiesburg; Cl Coor/Aud, Usal Sp/Hrng Cen, **A**

Holt, Barbara A 109 South Faulkner, Pampa, TX 79065, (806) 358-5321, MS 77 Univ of North TX; Sp-Lang Path, Bivines Rehab Center, **SLP**

Holt, Bonnie Riggs 9 Bis Rue DE La Vega 75012, Paris, France, (217) 351-3881, BS 80 Ithaca Coll; MS 81 Bloomsburg Univ of PA; SLP, **SLP**

Holt, Catherine Chun 1137 West Ives Street, Marshfield, WI 54449, BA 75 Univ of MI - Ann Arbor; MA 78 Northwestern Univ; **A**

Holt, Connie Smith 4727 Bay Quarter Court, Virginia Beach, VA 23455, (804) 363-8720, BA 82 NC St Univ at Raleigh; ME 86 Univ of VA - Charlottesville; Aud, Audio Labs, **A**

Holt, Dennis Lavern 2825 Summit Drive N E, Rochester, MN 55904, (507) 285-4626, BS 56 Univ of NE - Lincoln; MA 59 Univ of NE - Lincoln; Sp/Lang Path, Mayo Clinic, **SLP**

Holt, Mrs Janet Clark 118 Melba, Portland, TX 78374, (512) 643-8839, OB 79 Sam Houston St Univ; ME 84 Stephen F Austin St Univ

Holt, Mrs Jo Anne Nyberg 2716 95th N E, Bellevue, WA 98004, (206) 455-4042, BS 65 Univ of OR; MS 66 Univ of OR; Super Adolescent Services, Sp-Lang-Hrng Serv, **SLP**

Holt, Mrs Laurie B 2204 Indian Acres Drive, Hastings, NE 68901, (402) 463-2848, BA 78 Univ of Northern CO; MA 79 Univ of Northern CO; Aud, Ed Serv Ut #9, **A**

Holt, Linda A 30 Troy-Del Way, Williamsville, NY 14221, (716) 831-3395, BA 66 SUNY - Center at Buffalo; MA 71 SUNY - Center at Buffalo; Dir Sp & Hrng Cl, SUNY-Buffalo, **SLP ACE**

Holt, Mrs Lynne Jacobsen 1436 Sinaloa Avenue, Pasadena, CA 91104, (818) 962-3311, BA 80 Univ of CO - Boulder; MS 82 Univ of AZ; 82–Sp/Lang Path, Baldwin Park USD, **SLP**

Holt, Mrs Margaret C Box 623, Alto, NM 88312, (505) 336-7014, BA 59 Marygove Coll; 88–Sp-Lang Path, Ruidoso Sch Sys, **SLP**

Holt, Mrs Margaret H 906 Carol Lane, Fredericksburg, VA 22405, (703) 371-4354, BS 63 Univ of TX - Austin; **SLP**

Holt, Richard L P O Box 314, 114 West 6th Street, Pittsburg, KS 66762, (316) 232-2626, BS 67 Wichita St Univ; MA 69 Wichita St Univ; MS 77 Pittsburg St Univ; R L Holt/Assoc, **SLP**

Holt, Stephanie Virginia 1819 Colonial Medical Ct, Virginia Beach, VA 23454, (804) 496-0100, BS 76 Old Dominion Univ; MS 81 Old Dominion Univ; Sp-Lang Path, Private Practice, **SLP**

Holt, Mrs Virginia R 8 South Michigan #1108, Chicago, IL 60603, (312) 346-1136, BA 77 Univ of Denver; MA 79 Univ of Denver; 87–Pres, Charles A Lowe & Associates, **A**

Holt, William A, Jr P O Box 623, Alto, NM 88312, (505) 336-7014, BS 58 TX Tech Univ; MA 66 Western MI Univ; 87–Sp-Lang Path, Ft Stantn Training Sch & Hosp, **SLP**

Holte, Gayle Arnold Route 1 Box 77A, Elk Mound, WI 54739, (715) 835-6708, BS 76 Univ of WI - River Falls; MS 78 Univ of WI - River Falls; SLP, Mondovi Public Schools, **SLP**

Holte, Lenore A Syracuse University, 805 South Crouse Avenue, Syracuse, NY 13244-2280, (315) 443-9642, BS 77 Univ of MN - Minneap-St Paul; MA 79 Univ of MN - Minneap-St Paul; Instr, Syracuse U, **A**

Holter, Barbara R Rural Route 3, Old Trail Estates, Moorhead, MN 56560, (701) 280-5119, BA 69 Univ of ND; MA 77 Univ of ND; SLP, St Lukes Hospitals, **SLP**

Holterman, Karen Elaine 1509 NE 10th Street #100, Portland, OR 97232, (503) 284-9775, BS 85 ID St Univ; MS 87 ID St Univ; 88–Sp-Lang Path, Mt Hood Head Start, **SLP**

Holtgrewe, Phyllis P 929 W Clinton Street, Elmira, NY 14905, (607) 734-3911, BS 72 Cornell Univ; MS 73 Ithaca Coll; Assoc Prof, Elmira College, **SLP**

Holtz, Mrs Pamela E 6048 West Fair Drive, Littleton, CO 80123, (303) 377-8018, BA 65 Univ of CO - Boulder; ME 66 PA St Univ - Univ Park; 86–Sp-Lang Path, Good Shepherd Sch, **SLP**

Holtz, Mrs Tami Anne 10781 Frank Daniels Way, San Diego, CA 92131, BA 79 San Diego St Univ; MA 85 San Diego St Univ; 85–Sp-Lang Path, South Bay USD, **SLP**

Holtzapple, Pat Ann Audiology Speech Services, VA Hospital, 7th St & Indian School Rd, Phoenix, AZ 85012, (602) 277-5551, BS 63 OK St Univ; MA 65 IN Univ - Bloomington; Sp/Lang Path, Vamc Phoenix, **SLP**

Holtzclaw, Mrs Lisa I S 21781 Eveningside Lane, El Toro, CA 92630, (714) 846-0624, BA 75 CA St Univ - Long Beach; MA 77 CA St Univ - Long Beach; Sp-Lang Path, Private Practice, **SLP**

Holtzclaw, Mrs Margaret S 8636 Winthrop Drive, Alexandria, VA 22308, (202) 244-4420, BS 58 Univ of MO - Columbia; MA 73 George Washington Univ; Dir of Audiology, ENT Medical Group, **A**

Holtzman, Mrs Eleanor Benes 45 Alta Vista Drive, Rochester, NY 14625, (716) 586-8880, BS 74 Nazareth Coll of Rochester; MS 78 Nazareth Coll of Rochester; Sp/Lang Path, Monroe Co BOCES #1, **SLP**

Holtzman, Mrs Naomi S 934 Rollingwood, Highland Park, IL 60035, (312) 880-4530, BA 73 IN Univ - Bloomington; MS 75 Washington Univ; Aud, **A**

Holtzscher, George S 214 Pine Lake Road, Collinsville, IL 62234, (618) 344-6636, MS 66 Southern IL Univ -Carbondale; 75–Aud, Metro-East Aud Svcs, **A**

Holtzscher, Judith M 214 Pine Lake Road, Collinsville, IL 62234, (618) 344-6636, BS 62 Southern IL Univ -Carbondale; MS 65 Southern IL Univ -Carbondale; 66–Sp-Lang Path, Highland Comm Schs, **SLP**

Holub, Carl A 260 Walker Drive, Battle Creek, MI 49017, (616) 965-9773, BA 57 OH Univ - Athens; MA 62 Western MI Univ; Sp-Lang Path, Battle Creek Pub Sch, **SLP**

Holub, Janet Marie 6033 34th Street West, Apt 113, Bradenton, FL 34210, (800) 345-6891, MS 84 Bloomsburg Univ of PA; 88–Sp-Lang Path, Mediplex Rehab, **SLP**

Holub, Karen Dorothy 1 Shoal Court #72, Sacramento, CA 95831, (707) 429-6226, MA 80 Univ of WI - Oshkosh; SLP, Solano Co Supt of Schools, **SLP**

Holub, Mary M 3784 Leonard Road West, Oshkosh, WI 54901, **SLP**

Holzberg, Melanie C 14 Whitman Boulevard, Manalapan, NJ 07726, (201) 446-4282, BA 71 Rutger's St Univ - Douglas Coll; MA 72 Newark St Coll; Aud, Ctr for Sp & Hearing Sciences, **A**

Holzen, Mrs Helen K 393 Wallace Road #202, Nashville, TN 37211, (615) 333-2222, BA 72 Vanderbilt Univ; MA 75 Vanderbilt Univ; Aud, Dr Thomas W Holzen, **A**

Holzhaeuser, Mrs Mary Jo Dewitte 504 11th Street West, Ashland, WI 54806, (715) 682-8417, **SLP**

Holzhaeuser, William Joseph 504 11th Street West, Ashland, WI 54806, (715) 682-9311, BA 82 Univ of WI - Eau Claire; MS 84 Univ of WI - Stevens Point; Aud, ENT Professional Associates, **A**

Holzhausen, Mrs Julie Kay 5623 Kealing Avenue South, Indianapolis, IN 46227, (317) 783-5355, MA 84 Butler Univ; BS 82 IN St Univ - Terre Haute; Sp-Lang Path, Greenfield Central Comm Sch Sy

Holzhauser-Peters, Leslie Susan 1839 Augusta Boulevard, Fairfield, OH 45014, (513) 932-3851, BS 74 Univ of Cincinnati; MS 75 Miami Univ - Oxford; Consult/Superv of Sp-Lang Path, Warren Cty Offi of Ed, **SLP ACE**

Holzhueter, Ann Marie 30 Kevin Court, Walnut Creek, CA 94596, (415) 825-0144, BS 62 Univ of WI - River Falls; MA 64 Univ of SD - Vermillion; SLP, Mt Diablo USD, **SLP**

Holzshu, Nancy Lee 1617 Larch Street, Kodiak, AK 99615, (907) 486-6852, BA 74 Univ of CT; MS 85 Univ of HI - Manoa; 78–Sp-Lang Path, Kodiak Island Borough Sch Dist, **SLP**

Holzworth, Mrs Annamae Box 236, Menahga, MN 56464, (218) 564-4141, BS 75 Moorhead St Univ; MS 77 Univ of WI - Stevens Point; 88–Sp-Lang Path, Menahga PS, **SLP**

Homan, Deborah Ann 3159 Modred Drive, San Jose, CA 95127, (408) 773-0204, MA 83 San Jose St Univ; Aud, Golden State Aud Assoc, **A**

Homann, Dr Hal W University Of Wisconsin, Acc S150, Oshkosh, WI 54901, (414) 424-4415, BS 57 Lawrence Univ; MA 58 Western MI Univ; PH 63 (NS) OH St Univ; Assoc Prof of Sp, U of WI-Oshkosh, **SLP A ACE**

Homer, Emily M 408 East 16th Avenue, Covington, LA 70433, **SLP**

Homer, Gene Wesley 6 La Barre Street, Hancock, NY 13783, (607) 637-2796, BS 67 SUNY - Coll at Fredonia; ME 72 Bloomsburg Univ of PA

Homer, Judy R 16 Willis Road, Bridgewater, MA 02324, (617) 697-3006, BS 71 Northeastern Univ; MS 77 Lesley Coll; 88–Sp-Lang Path, Brockton PS, **SLP**

Homer, Mrs Susan Olivia 3304 Meadowmoor, Fort Worth, TX 76133, (817) 534-5731, MS 82 TX Christian Univ; SLP, Fort Worth ISD, **SLP**

Homiak, Mrs Suzanne MacCallum Veterans Admin Medical Ctr 126, 2100 Ridgecrest Drive S E, Albuquerque, NM 87108, (505) 265-1711, BS 75 Phillips Univ; MS 77 Univ of NM; Sp-Lang Path, VA Med Ctr-Sp Path, **SLP**

Homitz, Susan Lynn 1498 Indiana Avenue, Monaca, PA 15061, (412) 774-8343, MS 88 Gallaudet Coll

Homschek-Grooms, Eileen 200 South Union, Suite B, Roswell, NM 88201, (505) 623-8319, BS 75 Eastern NM Univ; MS 76 Eastern NM Univ; Dir&Owner/Sp-Lang Path Serv, Sen Nm Sp & Hrng Cl, **SLP**

Homuth, Anna K Route 4 Box 67, Owatonna, MN 55060, (507) 451-9513, BA 66 Moorhead St Univ; MA 76 Mankato St Univ; Sp-Lang Path, ISD #761, **SLP**

Homyack, Mrs Elizabeth Baysa 2087 Village Lane, Solvang, CA 93463, (808) 622-2269, BA 81 Creighton Univ; MS 83 CO St Univ; SLP, Santa Maria Elem School Dist, **SLP**

Hon, Mrs Christine Voye 483 Panchita Way, Los Altos, CA 94022, (415) 322-5946, BS 78 Edinboro Univ of PA; MS 85 Indiana Univ of PA; 86–Sp-Lang Path, Palo Alto USD, **SLP**

Hon, Mrs Martha M Rd 4 Box 86, Wheeling, WV 26003, (304) 242-8542, BS 69 Eastern IL Univ; MS 70 Eastern IL Univ; Sp-Lang Path, Easter Seal Rehabilitation Ctr, **SLP**

Honaker, Mrs Jane Griffin 104 Shellywood Lane, Columbia, SC 29212, (803) 732-0540, BS 66 Univ of TN - Knoxville; MS 78 East TN St Univ; Sp-Lang Path, Lexington Sc Sch Dist #5, **SLP ACE**

Honda, Mrs Bedonna J 751 South Fairmont Way, Orange, CA 92669, **SLP**

Honea, Mrs Marilyn Jean 11009 Hansom Lane, Spring Valley, CA 92077, (619) 461-3136, OB 82 San Diego St Univ; MA 87 San Diego St Univ; 82–Sp-Lang Path, Cajon Valley Union Sch Dist, **SLP**

Honey, Patricia 1025 Harvard Avenue, Modesto, CA 95350, (209) 529-2403, BA 54 Univ of the Pacific; MA 64 Univ of the Pacific; Lect Superv of Interns, CA St Coll, **SLP**

Honeycutt, Mrs Carolyn Howlett Route 1 Box 399, Hillsville, VA 24343, (703) 728-3191, BS 74 Appalachian St Univ; MS 82 Radford Univ; Sp-Path/Prog Co-Ord, Carroll County Sch Bd, **SLP**

Honeycutt, Kathy V 5530 Coyote Circle, Lincoln, NE 68516, (402) 473-0278, BS 72 Univ of NE - Lincoln; MA 73 Univ of NE - Lincoln; Sp/Lang Path, Lincoln Pub Schs, **SLP**

Honeycutt, Mrs Phyllis Cole 8 Pontiac Drive, Wayne, NJ 07470, (201) 427-8993, BS 65 Univ of Houston - Univ Park; ME 88 William Paterson Coll; 74–Sp-Lang Path, Wayne Gp/N Haledon Bd Ed, **SLP**

Honeycutt, Theresa 42035 47th Street West, Quartz Hill, CA 93536, (805) 943-7835, MA 77 Humboldt St Univ; SLP, **SLP**

Honeygosky, Robert A 3601 Connecticut Avenue, Apartment 405, Washington, DC 20008, (202) 363-3590, PH 70 (NS) Univ of Southern CA; **SLP**

Honeyman, Susan Jane Rural Route 5, Rockwood, ON, Canada N0B 2K0, (519) 856-9930, BA 74 Queens Univ - Ontario; OB 77 Queens Univ - Ontario; MA 84 SUNY - Coll at Buffalo; **SLP**

Hong, Li-Jane 2550 N Camden Parkway, Houston, TX 77067, (713) 790-8100, BA 76 Fu Jen Catholic Univ -Taiwan; MS 80 TX Tech Univ; Sp-Lang Path, HCA Del Oro Inst for Rehab, **SLP**

Hong-Wang, Mrs Marian Man-Hwei 322-3 University Village South, Gainesville, FL 32603, (904) 371-4859, 88–Sp-Lang Path, Gainesville Sunland Center, **SLP**

Honig, Melissa Rogosin 89 Elm Avenue, San Anselmo, CA 94960, (415) 453-5814, BA 77 Univ of CA - Irvine; MA 83 CA St Univ - Northridge; SLP, Long Beach USD, **SLP**

Honigman, Erica J 211 Winding Way, Merion, PA 19066, (215) 750-4336, BA 86 Univ of Pittsburgh - Pittsburgh; MA 88 Univ of Pittsburgh - Pittsburgh; Sp-Lang Path, Woods Schls

Honigman-Hellman, Mrs Sharon Ann 277 Dwight Street #1, New Haven, CT 06511, (317) 477-6974, MS 88 Purdue Univ - West Lafayette

Honings, Mrs Barbara Entrican 558 South Taylor, Decatur, IL 62522, (217) 429-1309, BS 82 Eastern IL Univ; MS 83 Eastern IL Univ; Sp-Lang Path, District 61 Macon Piatt Co, **SLP**

Honke, Lawrence E 2304 Belmont Avenue, Norfolk, NE 68701, (402) 371-2724, BA 75 Univ of NE - Lincoln; MA 76 Univ of NE - Lincoln; Aud, Norfolk Audiology/Hrng Aid Ctr, **A**

Honken, Mrs Connie Halverson Rural Route 1, Clarinda, IA 51632, (712) 523-2377, SLP, Greenvalley AEA 14, **SLP**

Honochick, Michele Ann Spring Ridge #B-17, Whitehall, PA 18052, (215) 866-8092, MA 83 West Chester Univ of PA; **SLP**

Honowitz, Stacey Rae 15842 Los Alimos Street, Granada Hills, CA 91344, (213) 263-3869, **SLP**

Honsinger, Melissa J Becker Rehabilitation Medicine, Rj-30 University Hospital, Seattle, WA 98195, (206) 543-3134, BA 80 WA St Univ; MA 81 WA St Univ; Sp-Lang Path, Harborview Med Cen, **SLP**

Hood, Amelia Toland 839 Scaleybark Road #8-H, Charlotte, NC 28210, (704) 529-5823, BS 84 Appalachian St Univ; MA 86 Appalachian St Univ; 86–Sp-Lang Path, Communi-Care Inc, **SLP**

Hood, Jack Richard 9531 N E Timber Creek Dr, Bondurant, IA 50035, (515) 279-3873, BS 76 Northwest MO St Univ; MS 82 Northwest MO St Univ; Sp-Lang Path, Des Moines Public Schools, **SLP**

Hood, Dr Linda J Kresge Hearing Research Lab, LSU Medical Center, 2020 Gravier Street, New Orleans, LA 70112, (504) 568-4785, BS 69 Bowling Green St Univ; MA 74 Kent St Univ; PH 83 (Aud) Univ of MD - College Park; 87–Prof, Lsu Med Cen, **A**

Hood, Mrs Louise W 5330 Norgate Drive, New Orleans, LA 70127, BS 68 FL St Univ; MS 69 FL St Univ; Sp/Lang Path, Jefferson Parish Sch Bd, **SLP**

Hood, Michele Ruth 4604 East 80th Street S, Apartment 21-F, Tulsa, OK 74136, (918) 492-5259, **SLP**

Hood, Mrs Patricia Ann 2114 Wythe Avenue, Bluefield, WV 24701, (304) 327-9607, BS 82 WV Univ; MS 83 WV Univ; **A**

Hood, Dr Richard B Dept Communicative Disorders, University Of New Mexico, Albuquerque, NM 87131, (505) 277-4453, BA 54 Duke Univ; MA 62 Syracuse Univ; PH 66 (Aud) Stanford Univ; Chair, U of NM, **A**

Hood, Dr Stephen B 1504 Oak Bend Court, Mobile, AL 36609, (205) 460-6327, BA 64 Denison Univ; MA 66 Univ of WI - Madison; PH 69 (Commun Dis) Univ of WI - Madison; 84–Dir-Sp-Lang Path, Univ of South AL, **SLP F**

Hood, Tamara Andrea 2605 Jackson Avenue, West Memphis, AR 72301, (501) 735-3853, BS 83 AR St Univ; OM 85 AR St Univ; SLP, West Memphis School District

Hood, Valerie Hunsinger 2041 Lockerbie Drive, Columbus, IN 47203, (812) 376-9404, BS 84 Purdue Univ - West Lafayette; MS 85 Purdue Univ - West Lafayette; Sp-Lang Path, Developmental Services Inc, **SLP**

Hoodin, Dr Ronald Bruce 1479 Wisteria, Ann Arbor, MI 48104, (313) 487-4410, BS 67 Miami Univ - Oxford; MS 71 Miami Univ - Oxford; PH 86 (NS) PA St Univ - Univ Park; Assoc Prof, Eastern Michigan Univ, **SLP**

Hoodwin, Marcia L 9805 Mesa Arriba N E, Albuquerque, NM 87111, (505) 296-6687, BS 79 IN Univ - Bloomington; MA 82 San Diego St Univ; Sp-Lang Path, Easi, **SLP**

Hooey, Kimberlee Ann 213 Greystone Lane #29, Rochester, NY 14618, (716) 424-7442, BS 82 Nazareth Coll of Rochester; MA 83 SUNY - Coll at Geneseo; Sp-Lang Path, BOCES No 1 Monroe County, **SLP**

Hoofnagle, Robin E 5817 North 25th Road, Arlington, VA 22207, (703) 534-5347, MS 80 Vanderbilt Univ; BS 78 Univ of VA - Charlottesville; Sp-Lang Path, Fairfax Co Hlth Dept, **SLP**

Hook, Marcia Suzanne 49-E Muirfield Drive, Reading, PA 19607, (215) 775-2077, MA 84 George Washington Univ; Sp-Lang Path, St Joseph Hospital, **SLP**

Hook, Dr Pauline Pepper 3429 South 23rd Street, Chickasha, OK 73018, (405) 224-3140, BA 46 Univ of Montreal - Quebec; MA 73 Wichita St Univ; PH 82 (Special Education) Univ of North TX; 84–Coord - SLP & Aud, Univ of Science & Arts of Ok, **SLP**

Hooker, Margaret A 90 Wallace Road, Memphis, TN 38117, (901) 529-0233, BS 68 Memphis St Univ; MS 69 Vanderbilt Univ; Therapy Coord, Les Passees Children's Rehabilitation Center, **SLP**

Hooker, Polly Ann 1338 Longfellow, South Bend, IN 46615, **SLP**

Hooks, Myra A Route 1 Box 97B, Shorter, AL 36075, **A**

Hool, Mrs Peggy Noroski 7401 Radcliffe Drive, College Park, MD 20740, (301) 345-3934, BS 75 Indiana Univ of PA; MS 79 Bloomsburg Univ of PA; 85–Sp-Lang Path, Associates InSpeech Pathology, **SLP**

Hoole, Caroline E 16036 North 58th Way, Scottsdale, AZ 85254, (602) 241-3284, BA 77 Univ of Denver; MS 79 Univ of AZ; Sp-Lang Path, St Josephs Hosp & Med Cen, **SLP**

Hooper, Arthur D 1610 Cambria Drive, East Lansing, MI 48823, (313) 257-9326, MS; **SLP**

Hooper, Dr Celia R 119 Hudson Wood Road, Pittsboro, NC 27312, (919) 966-1006, BA 73 Wake Forest Univ; MA 74 Univ of NC - Greensboro; PH 79 (NS) Case Western Reserve Univ; 87–Sp-Lang Path, Univ of NC at Chapel Hill, **SLP ACE**

Hooper, Mrs Dorothy W 115 Reba Road, Forney, TX 75126, BA 53 TX Christian Univ; MS 77 Southern Methodist Univ; Sp-Lang Path, Mesquite ISD, **SLP**

Hooper, Franklin E 204 Church Avenue, Follansbee, WV 26037, (304) 748-7676, BA 59 West Liberty St Coll; MA 61 WV Univ; Prin, Brooke Co Bd of Ed, **SLP**

Hooper, Mrs Iris R 2924 Orchard Road, Conyers, GA 30208, (404) 929-8219, BA 70 Univ of SC - Columbia; MS 77 Univ of SC - Columbia; SLP, Newton County Schools, **SLP**

Hooper, Mary U 618 Madison N E, #B, Albuquerque, NM 87110, (505) 255-5773, BA 77 Univ of CA - Santa Barbara; MS 79 Univ of NM; 87–Sp-Lang Path, St Joseph Hospital, **SLP**

Hooper, Mrs Patricia Hamelin 128 Thacher Street, Hornell, NY 14843, (607) 324-1968, BS 76 SUNY - Coll at Geneseo; MA 79 SUNY - Coll at Geneseo

Hooper, Dr Robert Lane 6993 Kimberley Terrace S W, Fort Myers, FL 33907, (813) 549-2313, BS 72 FL St Univ; MS 73 FL St Univ; PH 80 (NS) Walden Univ; Aud, Hearing Cl, **A**

Hooper, Mrs S Michelle Route 3 Box 223, Walters, OK 73572, (405) 353-0350, BA 74 Univ of MO - KS City; MS 75 Central MO St Univ; Aud, Indian Hlth Serv, **A**

Hooper, Mrs Sandra Delberta 312 East Nevada, Walters, OK 73572, (405) 353-0334, BS 73 Univ of Science & Arts of OK; ME 85 Central St Univ; **SLP**

Hoopingarner, Mrs Carla Elaine 18987 Laurel Circle, Cleveland, OH 44136, (216) 238-9314, **SLP**

Hoops, Dr H Ray University Of Mississippi, Academic Affairs, University, MS 38677, (601) 232-5974, BS 62 Eastern IL Univ; MS 64 Purdue Univ - West Lafayette; PH 66 (NS) Purdue Univ - West Lafayette; Vice Chancellor for Academic Aff, Univ of Mississippi, **SLP F**

Hoops, Mrs Helen W Speech And Hearing Clinic, Ball State University, Muncie, IN 47306, (317) 288-1073, BA 57 Univ of IL - Urbana; MS 60 Univ of IL - Urbana; SLP/Aud, Mississinewa Pub Schs, **SLP**

Hoops, Dr Richard A Speech And Hearing Clinic, Ball State University, Muncie, IN 47306, (317) 285-8162, BA 54 Oberlin Coll; MS 56 Univ of IL - Urbana; PH 61 (Aud) Univ of IL - Urbana; Chmn/Dept of Sp-Path & Aud, Ball St U, **SLP A**

Hoorwitz, Marion K 2505 Eastern Parkway, Schenectady, NY 12309, **SLP**

Hoos, Barbara L 55 David Court, Dayton, NJ 08810, (201) 329-8475, BS 56 Syracuse Univ; MS 57 Syracuse Univ; Private Practice, **SLP A**

Hoover, Carla Therese Kentucky School For The Deaf, P O Box 27, Danville, KY 40422, (606) 236-5132, MS 84 Purdue Univ - West Lafayette; Aud, Ky Schl for the Deaf, **A**

Hoover, Hal N 2102 Main Street, Anderson, IN 46016, (317) 643-0128, BS 74 Ball St Univ; MA 78 Ball St Univ; Aud, J C Hoover & Assoc, **A**

Hoover, Julia M 14421 West Everett Road, Lake Forest, IL 60045, (312) 816-1969, BA 82 Univ of WI - Eau Claire; MA 85 Univ of MN - Minneap-St Paul; Sp-Lang Path, Prentke Romich Co, **SLP ACE**

Hoover, Karl M 20 Tacoma Avenue North, Tacoma, WA 98403, (206) 383-5030, BS 78 WA St Univ; MA 80 WA St Univ; Manager, The Hear Center, **A**

Hoover, Lisa 1050 North Farnsworth, Apartment 303, Aurora, IL 60505, (815) 740-3196, MA 81 IL St Univ - Normal; SLP, Private Practice, **SLP**

Hoover, Patti Leigh 6014 North Villa, Oklahoma City, OK 73112, (405) 840-5925, BS 84 OK St Univ; MS 86 Univ of OK Medical Center; 87–Sp-Lang Path, Oklahoma City PS, **SLP**

Hope, Mrs Andrea W Speech And Hearing Center, 820 Charlotte Avenue, Rock Hill, SC 29730, (803) 329-1520, BA 73 Western Carolina Univ; MA 76 Western Carolina Univ; Director SLP, **SLP**

Hope, Donna P O Box 550481, Atlanta, GA 30355, (404) 233-5339, BA 72 Univ of GA; OM 74 Emory Univ; Private Practice, **SLP**

Hope-Bly, Mrs Connie A 38 Country Downs Circle, Fairport, NY 14450, (716) 223-4258, BS 75 SUNY - Coll at Geneseo; MA 76 SUNY - Coll at Geneseo; Sp-Lang Path, Private Practice, **SLP**

Hopf, A Gidget Association For The Blind &, Visually Impaired, 422 Clinton Avenue South, Rochester, NY 14620, (716) 232-1111, BS 72 SUNY - Coll at Geneseo; MA 75 Kean Coll of NJ; Exec Dir, Assoc F/T Blind & Vis Imp, **SLP**

Hopfer, Mrs Adrienne P 32 Canton Road, West Simsbury, CT 06092, (203) 651-9761, BA 72 Univ of CT; MS 74 Southern CT St Univ; **SLP**

Hopkins, Mrs Anita Freeman 2501 Charlestown Lane, Reston, VA 22091, BS 76 Univ of WI - Madison; MA 77 George Washington Univ; **SLP**

Hopkins, Mrs Diana W 3314 Sheffield Drive, Arlington, TX 76013, (817) 460-5724, BS 72 Longwood Coll; ME 73 Univ of VA - Charlottesville; Cl Superv, Univ of North Texas, **SLP**

Hopkins, Dixie G P O Box 659, Murray, KY 42071, (502) 753-3488, BS 69 Murray St Univ; MA 72 Murray St Univ; Sp-Lang Path, Private Practice, **SLP**

Hopkins, Mrs Ethel M 1213 Nixon Avenue, Auburn, AL 36830, (205) 821-4785, BS 75 Univ of KS; MA 79 Univ of KS; Aud, **A**

Hopkins, Gayle L 545 North Milton Drive, San Gabriel, CA 91775-2203, (818) 962-3311, BA 74 Saint Olaf Coll; MA 76 Univ of Denver; MA 80 Univ of Denver; 81–Sp-Lang Path, Baldwin Park Unif Sch, **SLP**

Hopkins, Harley J 1037 N E 131st Place, Portland, OR 97230, (503) 255-2818, BA 62 Seattle Pacific Univ; OM 69 Univ of WA; Sp-Lang Path, Portland Pub Sch, **SLP**

Hopkins, Mrs Harriett F Route 2, Iberia, MO 65486, (314) 793-6267, BS 58 Southwest MO St Univ; MA 71 Univ of MO - Columbia; Sp-Lang Path, Iberia Pub Schs, **SLP**

Hopkins, Jennifer Marie 8656 Lasabre Drive, Maineville, OH 45039, (513) 683-1655, BS 86 Miami Univ - Oxford; MS 87 Bowling Green St Univ; 88–SLP, Hamilton Cty Bd of MR/DD, **SLP**

Hopkins, Judith Anne Psc 7481 Apo, San Francisco, CA 96293-0006, (512) 257-4669, BS 79 Southwest TX St Univ; ME 80 Southwest TX St Univ; SLP, Dept of Defense Schools, **SLP**

Hopkins, Mrs Lori Marie Rt 1 Box 103-T, San Marcos, TX 78666, (512) 396-8348, BA 78 Univ of Redlands; MA 82 CA St Univ - Fullerton; Sp-Lang Path, Homespun Early Childhood Inter, **SLP**

Hopkins, Margot Trushaw 1505 West Waterview, Portland, TX 78374, (512) 853-9977, BA 81 SUNY - Coll at Cortland; ME 85 Southwest TX St Univ; **SLP**

Hopkins, Mrs Mary R 4444 Kirkwood Circle S W, Roanoke, VA 24018-3504, (703) 956-3626, BS 81 James Madison Univ; MS 83 James Madison Univ; Sp-Lang Path, Henry County School System, **SLP**

Hopkins, Rebecca B 1806 Robinson Drive, North Augusta, SC 29841, (404) 736-4834, BA 74 Univ of SC - Columbia; MA 75 Univ of SC - Columbia; Aud, Private Practice, **A**

Hopkins, Sharon Kay 2936 W Via Principal, Tucson, AZ 85741, (602) 327-1756, BA 83 Univ of Northern CO; MA 84 Univ of Northern CO; **A**

Hopkins, Susan G 93 Pinon Heights Road, Sandia Park, NM 87047, (505) 281-4476, **A**

Hopkins, Mrs Wendy B 417 West Garfield, Laurens, IA 50554, (712) 424-3720, MS 76 Central MO St Univ; Sp-Lang Path, Lakeland AEA 3, **SLP**

Hopkins-Acos, Mrs Patty 405 Toro Canyon Road, Carpinteria, CA 93013, (805) 964-4711, BS 69 Mount Marty Coll; MS 70 Saint Cloud St Univ; Sp-Lang Path, Santa Barbara Co Sch, **SLP**

Hopkins-Lorenc, Mrs Cynthia A 12 Hillside Terrace, Jamestown, NY 14701, (716) 484-8374, BS 86 SUNY - Coll at Fredonia; MS 87 SUNY - Coll at Fredonia; 87–Sp-Lang Path, WCA Hosp, **SLP**

Hopkins-Nash, Mrs Andrea Jackson Rd #1 Box 181, Jeffersonville, VT 05464, (802) 827-6639, BA 83 Johnson St Coll; MS 87 Univ of VT; 87–Sp-Lang Path, Fairfield Elem Sch

Hopkinson, Dr Norma T 555-1 South Negley Avenue, Pittsburgh, PA 15232, (412) 361-6485, BA 47 Chatham Coll; MA 49 Northwestern Univ; PH 62 (Aud) Univ of Pittsburgh - Pittsburgh; Retired, **A F**

Hopkins-Rossabi, Theresa Marie 62 Leonardville Road, Leonardo, NJ 07737, (718) 987-9400, BA 82 SUNY - Center at Binghamton; MS 85 Columbia Univ Teachers Coll; 86–Sp-Lang Path, Jersey Shore Med Ctr, **SLP**

Hopman, Mrs Phyllis 150-31 58th Avenue, Flushing, NY 11355, (212) 463-5901, BS 48 Northwestern Univ; MS 67 CUNY - Queens Coll; Sp-Lang Path, NYC Bur for Sp Improve, **SLP**

Hopper, Anna L R R 1 Box 126, Patoka, IL 62875, (618) 432-5435, MS 87 Southern IL Univ-Edwardsvill; 87–Sp-Lang Path, Warren G Murray Dev Ctr, **SLP**

Hopper, Bruce F 2316 Hidalgo Avenue, Los Angeles, CA 90039, (213) 441-2271, BA 60 Univ of AR - Fayetteville; MA 61 Univ of AR - Fayetteville; MA 69 Univ of Southern CA; Teacher, LA Co Supt Sch, **SLP**

Hopper, Dr G Robert Communicative Disorders, Eastern New Mexico University, PO Box 2245, Portales, NM 88130, (505) 562-2654, BA 57 Univ of VA - Charlottesville; MA 58 Univ of VA - Charlottesville; PH 69 (Sp-Lang Path) IN Univ - Bloomington; Asst Prof, Eastern New Mexico University, **SLP**

Hopper, Jenny D 4887 Fenbrook Drive, Stone Mountain, GA 30088, (404) 373-5809, BA 79 Northern IL Univ - De Kalb; MA 81 Northern IL Univ - De Kalb; Sp/Lang Path, City Scools of Decatur, **SLP**

Hopper, Kay Lynn 813 Greenhaven, Richardson, TX 75080, (214) 234-2579, BS 69 TX Tech Univ; MA 74 TX Tech Univ; 83–Sp-Lang Path, Richardson Dev Ctr, **SLP**

Hopper, Nancy C T 1733 N W Sunview, Grants Pass, OR 97526-1173, (503) 476-8427, BA 68 NE Wesleyan Univ; MS 71 Univ of OR; Sp-Lang Path, Jackson County Educ Serv Dist, **SLP**

Hopping, Louise A 9341 Canterchase Drive, Apartment 1-B, Miamisburg, OH 45342-5686, (513) 227-0105, BS 83 Purdue Univ - West Lafayette; MS 85 Purdue Univ - West Lafayette; Aud, Fairview Aud Ctr, **A**

Hopson, Cheryl A 3601 North Greenwood Drive, Victoria, TX 77901, (512) 576-5535, **SLP**

Hopson, Mrs Karen Leslie Kaiser Permanente, ENT Department 6th Floor, 4900 Sunset Boulevard, Los Angeles, CA 90027, (213) 667-7979, BS 73 Ithaca Coll; MS 75 Columbia Univ Teachers Coll; Sp-Lang Path, Kaiser Permanente, **SLP**

Hopwood, Debbie Leigh 656 West Gordon Terrace #2E, Chicago, IL 60613, (312) 234-6114, BS 82 Univ of IL - Urbana; MS 83 Univ of IL - Urbana; Sp-Lang Path, Lake Forest Hosp, **SLP**

Horacek, Shirley M 3307 South Grand, Sedalia, MO 65301, (816) 827-4433, BS 72 Central MO St Univ; MS 74 Central MO St Univ; Aud, G & R Health Assoc Inc, **A**

Horan, Mrs Anne C 5939 Goodwin, Dallas, TX 75206, (214) 339-7128, BS 79 Southern Methodist Univ; MS 80 Southern Methodist Univ; Sp-Lang Path, Dallas ISD, **SLP**

Horan, Janet M 6161 Rosewood Drive, Appleton, WI 54915, **SLP**

Horan, Margaret 2037 South Milwaukee, Denver, CO 80210, (303) 692-0854, BA 69 Univ of CO - Boulder; MA 73 Univ of Denver; **SLP**

Horan, Margaret 3100 Jane Place N E, Apartment T-203, Albuquerque, NM 87111, (813) 296-6522, BS 74 Western IL Univ; MA 75 Western IL Univ; Adlt Prog Coord, UCP-Will Co, **SLP**

Horan, Maryanne Kathleen 43 Briarcliff Road, Westbury, NY 11590, (516) 663-1084, BA 83 Adelphi Univ; MS 84 Adelphi Univ; SLP, Sch for Lang & Commun Dis, **SLP**

Horan, Roseann F 21 High Street, Beacon, NY 12508, (914) 478-1771, BS 79 Coll of Saint Rose; MS 80 Ithaca Coll; Sp-Lang Path, Total Learning Center, **SLP**

Horan-Senechal, Mary Catherine RFD 4, 58 East Bogg Lane, Lebanon, CT 06249, (203) 423-4252, MA 83 Univ of CT; BA 81 Univ of CT; Speech/Language Pathologist, Lawrence Memorial Hospital, **SLP**

Horasanian, Dena 4730 Ben Avenue, North Hollywood, CA 91607, BA 85 Univ of CA - Santa Barbara; MS 87 Univ of AZ; **SLP**

Horbus, Mrs Marilyn 629 Sylvan Place, Batavia, IL 60510, (312) 879-4629, BS 64 Northern IL Univ - De Kalb; MA 71 Northern IL Univ - De Kalb; Sp-Lang Path, Batavia Public School Dist 101, **SLP**

Horchler, Julia W 275 Date Palm Road #206, Vero Beach, FL 32963, (305) 562-7752, BA 72 CUNY - Queens Coll; MS 76 Adelphi Univ; 88–Sp-Lang Path, Donna S Brown & Assoc, **SLP**

Horensten, Mrs Judith Greene 4649 East Via Pimiera Alta, Tucson, AZ 85718, (602) 299-2797, BA 68 Boston Univ; MA 69 NY Univ; ED 76 (NS) Univ of AZ; 88–Sp-Lang Path, Tucson USD, **SLP**

Horewitch, Mrs Laurie Lentz 4158 West Corona Drive, Chandler, AZ 85226, (602) 838-0898, BS 77 Miami Univ - Oxford; MA 78 Kent St Univ; 78–Sp-Lang Path, Murphy Sch Dist, **SLP**

Horgan, Mary C 112 Raylinsky Road, Ballston Lake, NY 12019, **SLP**

Horii, Dr Yoshiyuki 420 22nd Street, Boulder, CO 80302, (303) 492-6445, BA 64 Wichita St Univ; MA 66 Wichita St Univ; PH 69 (NS) Purdue Univ - West Lafayette; 81–Prof, Univ of Colorado

Horkan, Ellen S 8250 North 46th Street, Apartment 236, Brown Deer, WI 53223, (414) 354-4039, BS 76 Univ of WI - Stevens Point; MS 77 Univ of WI - Whitewater; Sp-Lang Path, Milwaukee Pub Sch, **SLP**

Horkans, Sr Lelia Mary 35-50 158th Street, Flushing, NY 11358, (212) 492-1800, BS 58 OH Dominican Coll; ME 62 Duquesne Univ; Sp-Lang Path, Dept Spec Ed Bklyn Diocese, **SLP**

Horkley, Mrs Jeanette S 2359 Richards Avenue, Idaho Falls, ID 83404, (208) 523-7782, MS 87 ID St Univ

Horley, Mrs Mary B 1900 Nobles Mill Road, Darlington, MD 21034, BS 58 Shippensburg Univ of PA; Sp-Lang Path, Baltimore County Head Start, **SLP**

Horn, Mrs Deborah G 129 Park Lane, Deerfield, IL 60015, (312) 945-2695, BS 73 Northern IL Univ - De Kalb; MA 74 Northwestern Univ; **SLP**

Horn, Dr Donna G 3118 Custer Drive, Lexington, KY 40502-4512, (606) 268-8356, MS 77 Univ of KY; MA 81 Univ of KY; PH 85 (Psychology (Cognitive Development)) Univ of KY; Owner, Private Practice, **SLP**

Horn, Mrs Gail Boedeker 5562 South Highland Avenue, Yorba Linda, CA 92686, (714) 528-4830, BA 68 CA St Univ - Fullerton; MA 75 CA St Univ - Fullerton; 71–Sp-Lang Path, Yorba Linda Sch Dist

Horn, Mrs Jane H Sister Kenny Institute, 800 East 28th At Chicago, Minneapolis, MN 55407, (612) 863-4407, BA 62 Phillips Univ; MA 63 Univ of IL - Urbana; Dir Sp-Lang Path, Sister Kenny Institute, **SLP A**

Horn, Mrs Julie Bloom 6753 Tamerlane, West Bloomfield, MI 48322, (313) 626-1537, BA 83 MI St Univ; MA 84 MI St Univ; Sp-Lang Path, Birmingham Public Schools, **SLP**

Horn, Linda Diane P O Box 563, Dauphin Island, AL 36528-0563, (205) 861-4507, BS 78 Univ of South AL; MS 85 Univ of South AL; **SLP**

Horn, Mary Jo Donnelly 6 Yew Court, Baltimore, MD 21221, BA 81 Loyola Coll; MS 83 Loyola Coll; Sp-Lang Path, Brd of Ed Balto Co, **SLP**

Horn, Mrs Melanie 10512 Creekmere, Dallas, TX 75218, (214) 272-9220, BS 78 TX Tech Univ; MA 80 Univ of NE - Lincoln; Director of Hrng & Speech, ENT Med Ctr, **A**

Horn, Monica A 3455 River Path, San Antonio, TX 78230, (512) 492-1463, BA 75 Univ of TX - Austin; MA 76 Univ of Houston - Univ Park; Sp-Lang Path, Speech Pathology Services, **SLP**

Horn, Dr Richard M Childrens Hospital Pittsburgh, 125 Desoto Street, Division Of Audiology, Pittsburgh, PA 15213, (412) 647-5580, MA 73 Wichita St Univ; PH 85 (Administration) Gallaudet Coll; Administrative Director, Childrens Hospital, **SLP**

Horn, Stuart A Horn Hearing Center, 5333 Sepulveda #16, Culver City, CA 90230, (213) 674-5700, BA 75 Univ of CA - Los Angeles; MA 79 CA St Univ - Los Angeles; Aud, Private Practice, **A**

Horn, Sydney G 62-60 108th Street #2F, Forest Hills, NY 11375, (212) 735-2667, BA 71 CUNY - City College; MA 73 CUNY - City College; Aud, NY Med College/Collier Mem Hos, **A**

Hornaday, Nila 599 West Westfield Blvd, Indianapolis, IN 46208, MS; **SLP LM**

Hornback, Mrs Marilyn A P O Box 1382, Murray, KY 42071-1382, (502) 759-9789, BS 70 Murray St Univ; MS 75 Murray St Univ; Clin Superv, Murray State U, **SLP**

Hornbecker, Mrs Renee 4386 South Swadley Court, Morrison, CO 80465, (303) 986-1555, BS 77 CO St Univ; MA 79 Univ of Denver; Sp/Lang Path, Jefferson Co Pub Sch, **SLP**

Hornbostel, Susan Marie 121 Hazelwood Drive, Apartment M-137, Hendersonville, TN 37075, (615) 451-0512, BA 86 Carthage Coll; MS 88 Vanderbilt Univ; 88–Sp-Lang Path, Rebound Inc

Horne, Mrs Laurie Michelle 236 North Servern Circle, Easley, SC 29640, (803) 859-1405, BA 82 Columbia Coll; OM 83 Univ of SC - Columbia; **SLP**

Horne, Mrs Martine Elizabeth 5430 Whispering Spruce Dr, Anchorage, AK 99516, (907) 562-2211, MS 82 Univ of WI - Oshkosh; Sp-Lang Path, Providence Hosp, **SLP**

Horne, Nancy L 19 Hillcrest, Tuscaloosa, AL 35401, (205) 345-3600, BA 67 Univ of WI - Madison; MS 76 Univ of WI - Madison; Sp-Lang Path, Tuscaloosa City Sch, **SLP**

Horner, Mrs Diane S 5723 Mason Bluff Drive, Burke, VA 22015, (703) 239-2418, BS 77 PA St Univ - Univ Park; MA 79 Catholic Univ of America; Sp-Lang Path, Fairfax Co Pub Sch, **SLP**

Horner, Dr Jennifer Duke Univ Medical Center, Box 3887, Durham, NC 27710, (919) 684-3859, BA 71 SUNY - Center at Binghamton; MA 74 Univ of FL; PH 77 (NS) Univ of FL; Asst Prof Sp-Lang Path, Duke U Med Cen Dept of Surg, **SLP**

Horner, Dr John S University Of Virginia, Speech/Language/Hearing Center, Box 9022, Charlottesville, VA 22903, (804) 924-7107, BA 51 Antioch Coll; MA 59 Kent St Univ; PH 64 (Aud) Northwestern Univ; Prof & Dir Commun Disord Prog, University of Virginia, **SLP A**

Horner, Juliette P Route 2 Box 336, Charlottesville, VA 22901, (804) 979-6344, BA 63 Greensboro Coll; ME 69 Univ of VA - Charlottesville; 78–Sp-Lang Path, Charlottesville Pub Sch, **SLP A**

Horner, Nancy S 4310 S W Hamilton Terrace, Portland, OR 97201, (503) 280-5684, BS 74 OR St Univ; MS 75 Univ of WI - Madison; ME 76 Univ of WA; D R A C Supervisor, Portland Public Schools, **A**

Horner, Mrs Nettie K 3944 Johnstown, Montgomery, AL 36109, (205) 277-1355, BS 70 MS Univ for Women; MS 71 MS Univ for Women; **SLP**

Horner, Patricia 3609 Falcon Street, Long Beach, CA 90807, (213) 861-4357, BA 74 CA St Univ - Long Beach; MA 76 CA St Univ - Long Beach; SLP, Los Angeles Office Supt Sch, **SLP**

Horness, Paula Gay 4200 Spanish Bit #E-201, Albuquerque, NM 87111, (505) 884-8282, MA 83 MI St Univ; Sp-Lang Path, Educational Assesment Systems, **SLP**

Horney, Kathryn Ruth 16400 Henderson Pass #234, San Antonio, TX 78232, (512) 491-0542, BS 84 Univ of TX - Austin; MA 86 Our Lady Lake Univ-San Anton; 88–Prog Coord of Sp-Lang Svcs, Rebound Inc, **SLP**

Hornfelt, Lori M 5701 Fleming Terrace, Greensboro, NC 27410, (919) 621-0631, BS 76 Univ of UT; MS 78 Univ of UT; Sp-Lang Path, Gateway Ed Cen, **SLP ACE**

Horning, Judith K 13526 Mora Circle, Poway, CA 92064, (619) 576-5836, BA 69 San Diego St Univ; MA 72 San Diego St Univ; Associate Directory, Sp Hearing & Neurosensory Cen, **A**

Horning, Mrs Ruth S 154 Madison Avenue, Haworth, NJ 07641, (201) 385-1414, BA 72 Paterson St Coll; MA 74 CUNY - City College; SLP, Closter Bd of Ed, **SLP**

Hornlein, Rita H 47 Courtland Hill Street, Stamford, CT 06906, (203) 977-4853, BS 69 Purdue Univ - West Lafayette; MS 74 Columbia Univ Teachers Coll; Sp-Lang Path, Stamford Bd of Ed, **SLP**

Horn-Quarberg, Susan 261 27th Street, Marathon, FL 33050, (305) 743-6551, BA 77 Hofstra Univ; ME 79 Univ of FL; Coord, Guid Cl Middle Keys, **SLP**

Hornsby, Mrs Beth Ann 12 Hunting Horn Circle, Reisterstown, MD 21136, (301) 833-3053, BS 84 Radford Univ; MS 85 Radford Univ; **SLP**

Hornstein, Mrs Cynthia S 43 North Ridge Road, Livingston, NJ 07039, (201) 991-6800, BA 78 Rutger's St Univ - Douglas Coll; MA 81 Montclair St Coll; Sp-Lang Path, North Arlington Board of Educ, **SLP**

Hornstein, Jennifer Lee 413 East Washington, Chagrin Falls, OH 44022, (216) 247-7770, BA 82 OH St Univ; MA 85 Cleveland St Univ; **SLP**

Hornstein, Julie Lynn 2199 Lake Park Drive #I, Smyrna, GA 30080-7603, (404) 435-3444, BS 85 Northwestern Univ; MA 86 Northwestern Univ; 87–Sp-Lang Path, Bartow County Schs, **SLP**

Hornstein, Prof Sara Carol Dowling College, Faculty Speech, Oakdale, NY 11769, (516) 244-3000, BA 51 CUNY - Brooklyn Coll; ME 66 CUNY - Queens Coll; OM 79 CUNY; Assoc Prof Sp, Dowling Coll, **SLP**

Horny, Mrs Anita Louise 11580 Gratiot, Saginaw, MI 48603, (517) 799-3822, BA 80 MI St Univ; MA 84 MI St Univ; **SLP**

Hornyak, Andrew J Dept Speech Path & Audiology, Trenton State College, Trenton, NJ 08650-4700, (609) 771-2322, BA 66 Trenton St Coll; MA 67 Columbia Univ Teachers Coll; Assistant Professor, Trenton State College, **SLP**

Horodezky, Mrs Naomi B 225 Russell Hill Road, Toronto, ON, Canada M4V 2T3, (416) 961-4997, BA 67; MA 68 MI St Univ; **SLP**

Horovitz, Linda J 121 South Broad Street, Norwich, NY 13815, **A**

Horowitz, Alan R 10475 S W Grant Court, Tigard, OR 97223, (503) 538-8361, BA 74 SUNY - Center at Binghamton; MS 79 Portland St Univ; Sp-Lang Path, Newberg Sch Dist 29JT, **SLP**

Horowitz, Christine 227 Davis Avenue, Staten Island, NY 10310, (212) 979-1800, BS 65 WV Univ; MA 67 Univ of IA; Sp-Lang Path, Eger Nursing Home, **SLP**

Horowitz, Eva B 11 Bonaire Circle, Waban, MA 02168, **SLP**

Horowitz, Hilda L 391 Fountain Street, New Haven, CT 06515, BA 48 Univ of CT; MS 72 Southern CT St Univ; **SLP**

Horowitz, Mrs Iris Friedman 8630 N W 52nd Court, Lauderhill, FL 33351, (305) 749-8746, BS 76 Bradley Univ; MA 77 Bowling Green St Univ; MS 86 Nova Univ; Sp-Lang Path, Private Practice, **SLP**

Horowitz, Dr Leola S 80-50 235th Street, Queens Village, NY 11427, (718) 776-4904, BS 41 Univ of NE - Lincoln; MA 43 Univ of NE - Lincoln; PH 54 (NS) Stanford Univ; Assoc Dir, LI Ctr for Comm Disorders, **SLP F LM**

Horowitz, Mrs Louise P Talk To ME Inc, 1634 S E 3rd Court, Deerfield Beach, FL 33441, (305) 755-1456, BS 72 Memphis St Univ; MA 74 Memphis St Univ; SLP, Talk to Me Inc, **SLP**

Horowitz, Mrs Ruth Rappaport 2389 Kenilworth Avenue, Los Angeles, CA 90039, (818) 785-2911, MA 84 CA St Univ - Los Angeles; **SLP**

Horowitz, Sabra 4600 Connecticut Avenue N W, Apartment 524, Washington, DC 20008, (202) 244-6115, MA 88 George Washington Univ; 88–Sp-Lang Path, Ivymount Sch

Horowitz, Susan Goodman 11 Irving Road, Natick, MA 01760, (617) 344-0600, BS 78 Northwestern Univ; MA 79 Northwestern Univ; 83–Sp/Lang Path, New Eng Sinai Hosp, **SLP**

Horowitz, Mrs Tinece L 58 Dortmunder, Manalapan Township, NJ 07726, (201) 446-1136, BA 73 CUNY - Brooklyn Coll; MS 76 CUNY - Brooklyn Coll; **SLP**

Horowitz, Mrs Virginia 2 Tudor City Place, Apartment 5-0 South, New York, NY 10017, (516) 887-7943, BA 59 Saint John's Univ - Jamaica; MA 62 CUNY - Hunter Coll; **SLP**

Horowitz-Moilanen, Nancy 160 West Mendocino, Willits, CA 95490, (707) 459-4454, BA 74 Humboldt St Univ; MA 75 Humboldt St Univ; Dir, Advance Rehab Serv, **SLP**

Horowitz-Ranzi, Karen A 301 East 73rd Street #7B, New York, NY 10021, (212) 860-1616, BA 77 Montclair St Coll; MA 79 NY Univ; Sp-Lang Path, Northside Cen Chld Dev Inc, **SLP**

Horrocks, Barbara L 1722 Merrill Loop, San Jose, CA 95124, (408) 288-3746, BA 72 Univ of CA - Santa Barbara; MA 75 Univ of CA - Santa Barbara; Sp-Lang Path/Co-Dir, Action Rehab Assoc, **SLP**

Horrocks, Mrs Pamela 202 Lewiston Avenue, Willimantic, CT 06226, (203) 429-6410, BA 65 Ithaca Coll; MS 69 Ithaca Coll; Sp-Lang Path, EASTCONN, **SLP**

Horsfall, Dr Geoffrey H USA MEDDAC Nurnberg (EFMS), APO New York, NY 09105, BA 68 Southern Methodist Univ; MA 69 Southern Methodist Univ; PH 72 (NS) Univ of FL; Chf: Sp-Lang Path EFMS Nbg, USA MEDDAC Nurnberg, **SLP A**

Horsfall, Ruth M 1936 North Clark #509, Chicago, IL 60614, (312) 620-4433, BA 75 Catholic Univ of America; MS 77 PA St Univ - Univ Park; Sp-Lang Path, DuPage Easter Seal, **SLP**

Horsfield, Mrs Lisa M C 263 Sugar Hill Road, Tolland, CT 06084, (203) 875-0721, BS 77 Trenton St Coll; MS 80 Southern CT St Univ; Sp-Lang Path, Town of Tolland, **SLP**

Horsley, Beverly Jean M 2927 East San Gabriel, Fresno, CA 93726, (209) 441-3165, BA 72 CA St Univ - Fresno; MA 76 CA St Univ - Fresno; SLP, Fresno USD, **SLP**

Horst, Carol Jo W 3503 Carsinwood Drive, Aberdeen, MD 21001, **SLP**

Horswill, Mrs Lynn A 1904 South Broad Street, Upper Gwynedd, PA 19446, (215) 584-6639, BS 79 Clarion Univ of PA; MA 82 Trenton St Coll; Sp-Lang Path, Delaware County Memorial Hosp, **SLP**

Horton, Ann M 404 Cutlass Road, Knoxville, TN 37922, (615) 745-0434, BS 70 Univ of TN - Knoxville; MA 72 Memphis St Univ; Coord/Communicatn Disordrs Srv, Prof Health Services Corp, **SLP ACE**

Horton, Ann Smyth 8441 7th Way North, St Petersburg, FL 33702, (813) 527-7304, BA 75 Univ of FL; ME 79 Univ of FL; Professional Associate, InSpeech Inc, **SLP**

Horton, Mrs Barbara L 1311 South Edison Way, Denver, CO 80222, **SLP**

Horton, Mrs Betty A 715 East Center, Sheridan, AR 72150, (501) 535-3002, BS 66 Saint Louis Univ; MA 70 Saint Louis Univ; Aud, Pine Bluff ENT Cl PA, **A**

Horton, Mrs Ellen Cowart P O Box 400, Odenville, AL 35120, (205) 251-0165, BS 81 Auburn Univ - Auburn; OM 83 Auburn Univ - Auburn; 87–Sp-Lang Path, UCP of Greater Birmingham, **SLP**

Horton, Mrs Janice A Rt 2 Box 206-A-2, Wynne, AR 72396, (501) 238-8762, OB 86 Univ of Central AR; OM 87 Univ of Central AR; SLP, Arlington Dev Ctr, **SLP**

Horton, Penelope S 3415 Cortina Drive, Colorado Springs, CO 80918, (719) 475-5422, BS 66 Boston Univ; MA 69 Montclair St Coll; Sp-Lang Path, Memorial Hospital, **SLP**

Horton, Sherri H 1204 Wickford Road, Vestavia Hills, AL 35216, (205) 823-4900, BS 77 Univ of Montevallo; MS 81 Univ of Montevallo; Sp-Lang Path, Vestavia Hills Bd of Ed, **SLP**

Horton, Mrs Virginia H 309 Jefferson Street, Natchitoches, LA 71457, (318) 352-2358, BA 63 Tulane Univ; MS 64 Tulane Univ; Coord, Sabine Parish School Board, **SLP A**

Horton-McGinley, Mrs Diane E 970 Hampshire Road, Bay Shore, NY 11706, (516) 422-1440, BS 77 SUNY - Center at Albany; MS 80 Adelphi Univ; Sp-Lang Path, West Islip Pub Sch, **SLP**

Horvath, Anthony 853 18th Street, Des Moines, IA 50314, (515) 279-9034, **A**

Horvath, Ellen M J 14112 Montgomery Drive, Westminster, CA 92683, (714) 891-2660, BA 69 Loyola Marymount Univ; OM 76; MA 75; SLP, LA Co Supt of Schs, **SLP**

Horvath, Mrs Jana Lee M 19582 Arlington Avenue, South Bend, IN 46637, (219) 282-4128, BS 78 Ball St Univ; MA 81 Ball St Univ; Sp-Lang Path, S Bend Comm Sch Corp, **SLP**

Horvath, Mrs Patricia Eileen 8148 Dorothy Court, Racine, WI 53405-3210, BA 81 IN Univ - Bloomington; MA 84 IN Univ - Bloomington; Sp-Lang Path, Racine USD, **SLP**

Horwitz, Dr Betty L 150 West End Avenue #28G, New York, NY 10023, (212) 724-6555, BA 52 Univ of MI - Ann Arbor; MA 68 Columbia Univ Teachers Coll; ED 73 (NS) Columbia Univ Teachers Coll; BOCES Southern Westchester, **SLP ACE**

Horwitz, Randi B 821 Timber Avenue, Dresher, PA 19025, (215) 728-2622, MS 87 Columbia Univ Teachers Coll; 87–Sp-Lang Path, Fox Chase Cancer Ctr/Moss Rehab Hosp, **SLP**

Horwitz, Susan B Worcester Speech & Lang Center, 111 Elm Street, Suite 101, Worcester, MA 01609, (617) 799-4626, BS 77 Northeastern Univ; MA 79 Northwestern Univ; Sp-Lang Path, Worcester Sp & Lang Cen, **SLP**

Horwitz-Danzinger, Mrs Helen 46 Pepper Creek Drive, Cleveland, OH 44124, (216) 382-7700, BA 75 Cleveland St Univ; MA 76 Cleveland St Univ; Sp/Lang Path, So Euclid/Lyndhurst Bd of Ed, **SLP**

Hosak, Mary Ann 25 East Fell Street, Summit Hill, PA 18250, (717) 645-5440, BA 72 Marywood Coll; MA 74 Univ of Pittsburgh - Pittsburgh; **SLP**

Hosbjor, Lila 1050 North Camino Seco #2003, Tucson, AZ 85710, (602) 290-1205, MS 87 Univ of AZ; Sp-Lang Path, Amphitheater Sch Dist, **SLP**

Hose, Mrs Marilyn K 80 Roanoke Street, Staten Island, NY 10314, (718) 494-8529, BA 68 CUNY - Brooklyn Coll; MS 80 CUNY - Brooklyn Coll; Sp-Lang Path, NYC Bd of Educ-Spec Educ Div, **SLP**

Hosek, Mrs Paula Ann 1181 Fieldgate Road, Lawrenceville, GA 30244, (404) 985-0557, BS 79 Univ of IL - Champaign; MS 80 Univ of IL - Champaign; **SLP**

Hosford, Joyce T 32 Lazarus Lovell Road, Centerville, MA 02632, (617) 362-4561, BS 61 Univ of MA - Amherst; MA 75 Univ of MA - Amherst; SLP, Cape Cod Collab, **SLP**

Hosford, Mrs Patti Miller 462 Carson Way, Paducah, KY 42003, (502) 898-6166, **SLP**

Hosford-Dunn, Dr Holly L Northwest Medical Plaza, 1980 Hospital Drive, Suite 109, Tucson, AZ 85704, BA 72 NM St Univ; MA 74 NM St Univ; PH 77 (NS) Stanford Univ; Asst Prof, Stanford U, **A**

Hoshiko, Dr Michael Comm Disorders Sciences, Southern Illinois Univ, Carbondale, IL 62901, (618) 453-2361, BA 48 Heidelberg Coll; MA 49 Bowling Green St Univ; PH 57 (Sp & Psych) Purdue Univ - West Lafayette; Prof, Southern IL Univ, **SLP LM**

Hosick, Heidi Ann Cary Medical Center, Department Of Audiology, Vanburen Road, Caribou, ME 04736, (207) 498-3111, BS 86 Bowling Green St Univ; MS 87 Bowling Green St Univ; 88–Aud, Otol Assoc, **A**

Hosier-Holt, Karen Leslie 3724 Spencer Street #114, Torrance, CA 90503-3236, (303) 399-0603, BA 84 Wichita St Univ; MA 85 Wichita St Univ; **SLP**

Hosken, Ann E 10480 East Op Avenue, Scotts, MI 49088, (616) 781-5141, BA 75 Western MI Univ; MA 77 Western MI Univ; SLP, Calhoun ISD, **SLP**

Hoskins, Dr Barbara B 285 West California Blvd, Pasadena, CA 91105, (818) 304-4774, BS 70 Syracuse Univ; MS 71 Southern IL Univ -Carbondale; PH 79 (NS) Northwestern Univ; Sp-Lang Path, Private Practice, **SLP**

Hoskins, Glee C 4440 Fairview Avenue, Downers Grove, IL 60515, (312) 960-1739, BS 75 Western IL Univ; MA 76 Western IL Univ; Sp-Lang Path, Naperville Sch Dist #203, **SLP**

Hoskins, Mrs Katherine Fleming 6840 Heathfield Drive, Atlanta, GA 30328, (404) 255-2033, BS 82 Auburn Univ - Auburn; MS 84 Vanderbilt Univ; Aud, Pediatric ENT of Atlanta, **A**

Hoskins, Dr Richard A 4402 Beulah Drive, La Canada, CA 91011, (818) 243-5566, BA 63 Augustana Coll; MS 70 Southern IL Univ -Carbondale; PH 73 (NS) Southern IL Univ -Carbondale; Teacher-Principal, Hoskins Sch & Educ Clinics, **SLP**

Hoskote, Vidya 4800 Chevy Chase Drive 404, Bethesda, MD 20815, (301) 762-0632, BS 75; MS 78; **SLP**

Hosmer, Mrs Teri Lynn Johnson 27670 U S Hwy 98, Apt 44, Daphne, AL 36526, (205) 626-8786, BS 83 Auburn Univ - Auburn; OM 85 Auburn Univ - Auburn; 87–Sp-Lang Path, Baldwin County Sch Bd, **SLP**

Hosner, Rochelle G 2805 Eagle Run Circle, Clearwater, FL 34620, (813) 535-0382, BA 75 OH St Univ; MA 78 Cleveland St Univ; Dir SLP, Rehab Assoc Inc, **SLP**

Hoss, Mrs Sarah Vance Route 2 Box 2560, Chuckey, TN 37641, (615) 639-2131, BS 79 East TN St Univ; MS 80 East TN St Univ; Sp-Lang Path, Greene Valley Dev Cen, **SLP**

Host, Leigh P O Box 972, Lake Geneva, WI 53147, (414) 248-1988, MS 82 Univ of WI - Whitewater; SLP, Delavan Darien Sch Dist, **SLP**

Hoste, Christine Marie Stratford General Hospital, 46 General Hospital Drive, Stratford, ON, Canada N5A 2Y6, (519) 271-2120, BS 80 Eastern MI Univ; MA 82 Eastern MI Univ; 86–Sp-Lang Path, Stratford Gen Hosp, **SLP**

Hosterman, Pamela Sue 206 Hickory Street, Rossville, GA 30741, (615) 472-4571, BS 83 PA St Univ - Univ Park; MS 84 Southern IL Univ-Edwardsvill; SLP, Bradley Co Schl Sys, **SLP ACE**

Hostetler, Sheila A 14 Cheverton Parade, Sandy Bay, Tasmania, Australia 7005, BA 75 Univ of IA; MA 76 Univ of IA; Sp-Lang Path, Douglas Parker Rehab Center, **SLP**

Hostetter, Melanie S 1517 Orange Grove Avenue, Orange, CA 92667, (714) 558-5766, BS 77 OH Univ - Athens; ME 81 Univ of GA; 87–Sp-Lang Path, Santa Ana USD, **SLP**

Hostetter, Patricia L 15 Springcreek Manor, Hershey, PA 17033, (717) 533-3688, BA 52 Goshen Coll; MA 53 Case Western Reserve Univ; **SLP**

Hostettler, Mrs Carmelita Ann P O Box 1066, Magalia, CA 95954, (916) 873-3170, BA 80 CA St Univ - Chico; MA 82 CA St Univ - Chico; **SLP**

Hosti, Bonnie S 707 Lovell Avenue, P O Box 1039, Tybee Island, GA 31328, (912) 786-5200, **SLP**

Hostler, Mrs Sandra Bradford 4214 North Locust, North Little Rock, AR 72116, (501) 758-0930, OB 77 Univ of Central AR; MS 81 Univ of AR - Little Rock; Sp-Lang Path, Little Rock Public Schools, **SLP**

Hosty, Kathleen A Metro Speech Path Group, 3223 Northampton Street N W, Washington, DC 20015, (202) 362-6337, BA 69 Catholic Univ of America; MA 72 Catholic Univ of America; Owner, Metro Sp Path Gr, **SLP ACE**

Hotard, Mark Drake 5176 Island Date Street, Sarasota, FL 34232, (813) 377-1231, BA 81 Nicholls St Univ; OM 87 LA St Univ - N O Medical Ctr

Hotchkiss, Dr John C 130 Circle Drive, Allegan, MI 49010, (616) 673-2167, BA 66 Albion Coll; MA 68 Western MI Univ; PH 73 (NS) Purdue Univ - West Lafayette; 86–Prin-Learning Ctr, Van Buren ISD, **SLP**

Hotchkiss, Karen Vail 32 James Drive, St Charles, MO 63301, (314) 839-3800, BA 78 Lindenwood Coll; MS 79 Fontbonne Coll; Sp-Lang Path, Christian Hospital NE-NW, **SLP**

Hotchkiss, Marcia Wheat 4544 Princeton, Memphis, TN 38117, (901) 685-2285, BS 82 LA St Univ - Baton Rouge; MA 83 LA St Univ - Baton Rouge; Sp-Lang Path, Memphis City Schools, **SLP**

Hotelling, Elaine Gracelyn 8903-D Harperpoint Drive, Cincinnati, OH 45249, (513) 423-9496, MA 84 Western MI Univ; **SLP**

Hotelling, Mrs Renee C 1520 South Norwood Drive, New Berlin, WI 53151, BS 73 Northeast MO St Univ; MA 74 Northeast MO St Univ; Sp-Lang Path, Milwaukee Pub Sch, **SLP**

Hotovy, Mrs Patricia E 303 East Weiler, West Point, NE 68788, (402) 372-5738, BS 76 Univ of NE - Lincoln; MA 79 Univ of NE - Lincoln; Sp-Lang Path, West Point Pub Sch, **SLP**

Hotson, Peggy Flach 323 Tower Drive, East Alton, IL 62024, (618) 377-7200, BA 74 Southern IL Univ-Edwardsvill; MS 77 Southern IL Univ-Edwardsvill; Sp-Lang Path, Bethalto Schs, **SLP**

Hotz, Gillian A 131 Bloor Street #1116, Toronto, ON, Canada M5S 1R1, (416) 927-7232, MS 85 Boston Univ; 86–Sp-Lang Path, St Michael's Hosp, **SLP**

Houchen, Ronald H 7700 West Pinehurst Drive, Fort Worth, TX 76134, **A**

Houchin, Dr Thomas D P O Box 621, Ansonia Station, New York, NY 10023, BA 46 Univ of IA; MA 50 Univ of IA; ED 63 Columbia Univ Teachers Coll; Professor, St Johns University, **SLP**

Houde, Dr Robert A 1895 Mt Hope Avenue, Rochester, NY 14620, (716) 271-3770, PH 65 (NS) Univ of MI - Ann Arbor; Pres, Cen for Commun Res

Houfek, Katherine Ann 5205-I Mereledge Court, Winston-Salem, NC 27106, (919) 744-1494, BS 82 Univ of KS; MA 85 Univ of KS; 87–Sp-Lang Path, Forsyth Memorial Hosp, **SLP**

Hougas, Wayne W Northland Medical Center, 1000 East 1st Street, Suite 403, Duluth, MN 55805, (218) 727-8581, BS 75 Univ of WI - Stevens Point; MS 76 Univ of WI - Stevens Point; Aud, Merrick Anderson Pa, **A**

Hough, Joanne McAleer 253 Atlanta Drive, Pittsburgh, PA 15228-1301, (412) 624-6571, MS 78 WV Univ; Clinical Super, U of Pgh, **SLP**

Hough, Judith M 908 Cardenas N E, Albuquerque, NM 87108, (505) 298-5009, BA 67 St Andrews Presbyterian Coll; MA 72 Univ of NM; Sp-Lang Path, Albuquerque Pub Sch, **SLP**

Hough, Mrs Karen S 1862 Castle Woods Drive, Clearwater, FL 33519, MS 75 Ithaca Coll; **SLP**

Hough, Dr Monica S School Of Allied Health Sciences, Speech/Language & Auditory Pathology, East Carolina University, Greenville, NC 27858, (919) 757-6961, BA 76 CUNY - Brooklyn Coll; MA 78 Univ of FL; PH 88 (Speech Pathology) Kent St Univ; Asst Prof, East Carolina Univ, **SLP**

Hough, Mrs Susan D 161 Lambeth Drive, Pittsburgh, PA 15241, (412) 521-9000, BS 76 PA St Univ - Univ Park; ME 79 Univ of Pittsburgh - Pittsburgh; Sp-Lang Path, Rehab I of Pittsburgh, **SLP**

Houghton, Marion F 3901 Franklin, Western Springs, IL 60558, (312) 883-9007, BS 79 Western IL Univ; MA 80 Western IL Univ; Sp-Lang Path, Dysfunctioning Child Center, **SLP**

Houghton, Martha H 40 School Street, Essex Junction, VT 05452, (802) 656-3861, BS 62 Univ of VT; ME 63 Boston Univ; Lect/Superv, U of VT, **A**

Houk, Mrs Melanie L 2205 South Pershing Drive, Muncie, IN 47302, (317) 288-8801, BS 79 Ball St Univ; MA 80 Ball St Univ; **SLP**

Houk, Ronald R 292 West Delevan Avenue, Buffalo, NY 14213, (716) 878-7371, BS 77 SUNY - Coll at Fredonia; MS 80 SUNY - Coll at Fredonia; Sp-Lang Path, Chldn Hosp of Buffalo NY, **SLP**

Houle, Dr Gail Ruppert PO Box 10103, Washington, DC 20018, (202) 667-3122, BA 73 SUNY - Center at Buffalo; MS 77 Univ of AL- Tuscaloosa; PH 88 (Administration) American Univ; 84–Sp-Lang Path, Dc Public Schools, **SLP**

Houle, Karen Rae 240 Dahlia Drive, North Kingstown, RI 02852, (401) 846-6400, BS 83 Univ of MA - Amherst; MS 85 Emerson Coll; 88–Sp-Lang Path, Vanderbilt Rehab Ctr Newport Hosp, **SLP ACE**

Houlihan, Mrs Jane Cooke 88 Hudson Road, Bellerose, NY 11001, (516) 328-9544, BA 71 Saint Joseph's Coll; MS 80 Adelphi Univ; Aud, Dr David Abraham, **A**

Houlihan, Patricia Ann 1606 Kraft Street, St Louis, MO 63139, (314) 595-2169, BA 81 Fontbonne Coll; MS 82 Fontbonne Coll; Sp-Lang Path, Spec Sch Dist, **SLP**

Hourigan, Mrs Rebecca B 8421 Ward Parkway, Kansas City, MO 64114, (913) 884-8711, BS 84 TX Christian Univ; MS 86 Univ of TX - Dallas; Sp-Lang Path, Meadowbrook Hosp, **SLP**

Hourihan, Dr John P 22 Mulberry Street, Newark, NJ 07102, (201) 623-0822, BA 45 Seton Hall Univ; OM 49 Catholic Univ of America; ED 74 (NS) Columbia Univ Teachers Coll; Consult, Private Practice, **A**

Hourlland, Mrs Sue Ann Elizabeth 324 Belford Court, Mars, PA 16046, (412) 772-1198, BS 86 Clarion Univ of PA; MS 87 Clarion Univ of PA; 88–Sp-Lang Path, S G Rehab Inc, **SLP**

House, Arthur S Institute For Defense Analyses, Thanet Road, Princeton, NJ 08540, (609) 924-4600, OB 42 CUNY - City College; MA 48 Univ of Denver; PH 51 (Experimental Phonetics) Univ of IL - Urbana; Inst for Defns Anal/Comm Res, **F LM**

House, Cynthia Schultz 6 Hazeltine Road, Upton, MA 01568, (508) 529-3950, BS 76 Boston Coll; MA 77 Central MI Univ; 87–Sp-Lang Path, BICO Collaborative, **SLP**

House, Donnita Ann 2205-H Champagne Drive, Albany, GA 31707, (912) 439-7061, BA 78 MI St Univ; MA 80 Case Western Reserve Univ; MA 81 Case Western Reserve Univ; 87–SLP, SW GA Easter Seal Rehab Ctr, **SLP A**

House, Jennifer A 808 Lakecrest Avenue #711, High Point, NC 27260, (919) 869-8487, BA 85 NC St Univ at Raleigh; MA 87 Univ of NC - Greensboro; 87–Sp-Lang Path, Davidson County Sch

House, Kathleen M 1304 Grand Avenue, St Paul, MN 55105, (612) 427-2200, BA 75 Univ of WI - Eau Claire; MS 79 Univ of WI - River Falls; SLP, Mercy Med Ctr, **SLP**

House, Len M 1317 Wiltshire Avenue, San Antonio, TX 78209, (512) 646-5060, BA 71 Univ of Northern IA; MA 73 Univ of Northern IA; Exec Dir, Rebound Inc, **SLP**

House, Dr Linda Infante 2159 Jones Bridge Road, Leicester, NY 14481, (716) 245-5331, BS 72 SUNY - Coll at Brockport; ME 73 SUNY - Coll at Geneseo; PH 79 Bowling Green St Univ; Asst Prof, SUNY at Geneseo, **SLP**

House, Mrs Mary R 20 Lambets Way, Alpharetta, GA 30201, (404) 887-9174, BA 66 Univ of NC - Greensboro; MA 68 Univ of NC - Greensboro; Retired, **SLP LM**

House, Thomas Duane 2159 Jones Bridge Road, Leicester, NY 14481, MS 85 Nazareth Coll of Rochester; Maryland State Sch for Blind

Householder, Julie A 2956 South Cherry Way, Denver, CO 80222, (303) 361-3888, BA 69 Univ of KY; MA 79 Univ of Northern CO; Sp-Lang Path, Fitzsimons Army Med Cen, **SLP**

Housel, Mrs Susan I 9375 Kemper Grove Lane, Loveland, OH 45140-8205, (513) 777-6128, BS 68; MS 72 IN St Univ - Terre Haute; Sp-Lang Path, Lakata Local Spec Serv, **SLP**

Houser, Jo M Texarkana Speech & Hearing, 4214 Texas Boulevard, Texarkana, TX 75503, (214) 794-0626, BS 71 Henderson St Univ; MS 74 Phillips Univ; Aud, Texarkana Sp-Hrng, **SLP A**

Houser, Michele M 2111 Lac Du Mont Drive, Apartment B-1, Haflett, MI 48840, (517) 339-2293, BA 84 MI St Univ; MA 86 Western MI Univ; **SLP**

Houser, Nancy E 1736 Humphrey, Birmingham, MI 48008-2406, BS 77 Western MI Univ; MA 82 MI St Univ; Sp/Lang Path, Southfield Rehab Hosp, **SLP**

Houston, Mrs Colleen Dibble 1-1A Consulate Drive, Tuckahoe, NY 10707, (914) 961-2499, BS 80 SUNY - Coll at Geneseo; MS 87 CUNY - Hunter Coll

Houston, Mrs Joan H 2251 Hunter Mill Road, Vienna, VA 22180, BS 62 Northwestern Univ; MA 68 Northwestern Univ; SLP, Fairfax Co Pub Sch, **SLP**

Houston, Mrs Ladonna 51 Yankee Folly Road, New Paltz, NY 12561, (914) 687-7631, BA 68 Fisk Univ; MA 76 Univ of AR - Fayetteville; Sp-Lang Path, Rondout Valley Central Schools, **SLP**

Houston, Mrs Mary Agnes HCR 69 Box 514, Sunrise Beach, MO 65079, (314) 374-6267, BA 32 Univ of KS; MA 57 Univ of MO - Columbia; Retired, **SLP LM**

Houston, Mrs Melaine Jayne 1071 Davie Street, Victoria, BC, Canada V8S 4E2, (604) 592-1923, **SLP**

Houston, Robin G 1009 East Mount Curve Avenue, Altadena, CA 91001, (818) 398-0934, BA 76 Univ of Denver; MA 78 George Washington Univ; Sp-Lang Path, Private Practice, **SLP**

Houth, Karen Kay 373 South Graham Street, Pittsburgh, PA 15232, (412) 394-5843, BS 80 9652; MA 83 Univ of Pittsburgh - Pittsburgh; 88–Aud, Allegheny Intermediate Unit, **A**

Hovden, Dawn L 3301 17th Avenue SW, Fargo, ND 58103, (701) 293-9996, MS 84 Moorhead St Univ; Sp-Lang Path, West Fargo PS, **SLP**

Hover-Parker, Teri Lynn 1907 Charles Street, Lafayette, IN 47904, (317) 742-1241, BS 85 Purdue Univ - West Lafayette; MS 87 Miami Univ - Oxford; 88–Sp-Lang Path, Woodlawn Ctr, **SLP**

Hoversten, Gloria H 1630 North Edgemont Street, Los Angeles, CA 90027, (213) 663-3022, BS 47 Univ of MN - Minneap-St Paul; MA 52 Univ of IA; 69–Aud, Los Angeles Co Ofc of Educ, **A F**

Hovey, Mrs Karen Kane 191 Park Avenue, Allendale, NJ 07401, (201) 967-4040, BS 80 West Chester Univ of PA; MS 83 William Paterson Coll; 86–Sp/Lang Path, Valley Home & Comm Health Care, **SLP**

Hovorka-White, Mrs Carolyn A 1833 Foxswallow Circle, Pleasanton, CA 94566, BA 74 San Francisco St Univ; MA 76 San Francisco St Univ; 86–Sp/Lang Path, American River Hosp, **SLP**

Howald, Mrs Carolyn Frances 5514 Rhone Drive, Wichita Falls, TX 76306, (815) 338-7411, BA 82 Univ of WI - Eau Claire; MS 83 Marquette Univ; Sp-Lang Path, Temporary Therapy Services, **SLP**

Howald, Mrs I Gayle 1018 Park Manor Terrace, Marietta, GA 30064, (404) 424-1416, BS 69 OH Univ - Athens; MA 72 Kent St Univ; Sp/Lang Path, Cobb County Pub Schs, **SLP**

Howard, Barbara H 6565 Taylor Mill, Independence, KY 41051-9293, (606) 331-0880, BS 72 Eastern KY Univ; MA 73 Univ of Cincinnati; Dir-Adult Svcs, Redwood Sch/Rehab Cen, **SLP**

Howard, Barbara Morrison P O Box 66, Barre, MA 01005, MS 85 UT St Univ; **SLP**

Howard, Craig L 27 Great Road, Bedford, MA 01730, (617) 275-9542, BS 78 SUNY - Coll at Geneseo; MS 80 CUNY - Brooklyn Coll; 87–Sp-Lang Path, Tewksbury Public Schools, **SLP**

Howard, Mrs Deborah Ann Route 1 Box 350, Prescott, WI 54021, (612) 388-6721, BS 73 Univ of WI - River Falls; MS 83 Univ of WI - River Falls; Sp-Lang Path, St Johns Hosp, **SLP**

Howard, Deborah K 1912 Regulus Court, Livermore, CA 94550, (415) 449-2611, MS 88 San Francisco St Univ; 88–Aud, Veterans Administration

Howard, Mrs Diane M 795 East 44th, Eugene, OR 97405, (503) 683-4627, BS 80 Univ of OR; MS 82 Univ of OR; SLP, Eugene District 4J, **SLP**

Howard, Eleanor W 2 Warren Street, Middletown, CT 06457, (203) 527-4155, BS 70 NY Univ; MS 73 Columbia Univ Teachers Coll; SLP, Hartford Bd of Ed, **SLP**

Howard, Elizabeth 14738 West 80th Street, Lenexa, KS 66215, **SLP**

Howard, Ellen Duncan c/o O H Duncan, 8708 Aragon Lane, Knoxville, TN 37923, (615) 693-3143, BS 79 Univ of AL-Birmingham; MS 84 Univ of OK - OK City; SLP, Speech Therapy Services, **SLP**

Howard, Mrs Jackie A 275 West Juniper Avenue #1113, Gilbert, AZ 85234, (602) 892-8624, BS 79 Univ of AZ; MA 82 IN Univ - Bloomington; 88–Sp-Lang Path, Gilbert PS, **SLP**

Howard, Janice Ann 105-B Fiddler Green, Stratford, CT 06497, (203) 787-0201, BA 83 Univ of CT; MA 85 Univ of CT; 86–Aud, Bernard Lipin Hrng Instruments, **A**

Howard, Mrs Jeni L 3015 Sothman Drive, Grand Island, NE 68801, (308) 381-1039, BA 77 Univ of NE - Lincoln; MA 78 Univ of NE - Lincoln; Sp-Lang Path, Educational Serv Unit 9, **SLP**

Howard, Joanne Catherine 896 Fellsway, Medford, MA 02155, (617) 565-9598, BA 79 Rutgers St Univ -N Brunswick; MA 81 Montclair St Coll; Aud, VA Outpatient Clin, **A**

Howard, Mrs Julie Marie 20343 S W Blaine, Aloha, OR 97006-2139, (503) 642-2340, MS 84 Western OR St Coll; Sp-Lang Path, Good Samaratin Hosp, **SLP**

Howard, Dr Karen J 6300 Humana Plaza, Suite 850, Abilene, TX 79606, (915) 698-9048, BA 67 Univ of TX - El Paso; MA 72 TX Tech Univ; ED 79 (NS) Univ of Houston - Univ Park; Owner, Assoc In Sp Lang & Hrng Svc, **SLP ACE**

Howard, Mrs Kay H 6049 Somerset Drive, Pensacola, FL 32506, BS 78 Baylor Univ; MS 79 Baylor Univ; **SLP**

Howard, Mrs Lauranne M 12950 Claymont Court, San Diego, CA 92130, (619) 259-5240, BA 80 CA St Univ - Northridge; MA 82 CA St Univ - Northridge; Sp-Lang Path, San Diequito Union HS Dist, **SLP**

Howard, Lisa Lynn 9600 Golf Lakes Trail, Apartment 1129, Dallas, TX 75231, (214) 826-7030, BA 83 TX Tech Univ; MS 85 Univ of TX - Dallas; 87–Sp-Lang Path, Baylor Rehab Hosp, **SLP**

Howard, Lori Ann S E 220 Water, Pullman, WA 99163, (817) 265-1466, BA 82 Univ of the Pacific; MA 85 Univ of Northern CO; Aud, Ritchey Hrng Lab, **A**

Howard, Marilyn R 21 Frothingham Road, Burlington, MA 01803-4021, (617) 666-5700, BA 70 Tufts Univ; ME 75 Univ of VA - Charlottesville; Sp-Lang Path, Somerville Pub Sch, **SLP**

Howard, Mrs Mary Ann 30411 Balewood, Southfield, MI 48076, (313) 757-5150, BS 51 Bowling Green St Univ; ME 57 Wayne St Univ; Retired, Fitzgerald PS, **SLP**

Howard, Mrs Mary Lynn 1116 Plateau Lane, Raleigh, NC 27615, (919) 847-7547, BS 62 MI St Univ; MA 70 Univ of MO - Columbia; Sp/Lang Path, Franklinton City Sch, **SLP**

Howard, Mrs Mary Tolton 3802 Charmouth Court, Marietta, GA 30062, (404) 578-9501, BA 75 Univ of MD - College Park; MA 76 Univ of MD - College Park; **A**

Howard, Dr Merle Ray Dept Speech Path & Audiology, Illinois State University, Normal, IL 61761, (309) 438-2654, BS 62 Southern IL Univ -Carbondale; MS 66 Southern IL Univ -Carbondale; PH 77 (Sp) Univ of Cincinnati; Asst Prof, Illinois State Univ, **SLP**

Howard, Mrs Myra N 52 Redding Ridge Drive, Gaithersburg, MD 20878, (301) 279-7206, BS 70 Univ of GA; MA 71 Univ of MD - College Park; **SLP**

Howard, Pamela 953 Locust Grove Road, Greenfield Center, NY 12833, (518) 382-4550, BS 77 SUNY - Coll at Geneseo; MS 80 Purdue Univ - West Lafayette; Sp-Lang Path, Sunnyview Rehabilitation Hosp, **SLP**

Howard, Phyllis 5800 Eubank Blvd N E #1524, Albuquerque, NM 87111, (505) 298-3174, **SLP**

Howard, R Ann 6890 West Archer Place, Denver, CO 80226, (303) 237-5707, BA Univ of Denver; MA 66 Western MI Univ; 68–Sp-Lang Path, Private Practice, **SLP**

Howard, Mrs Renee L P O Box 263, 639 11th Street, Fortuna, CA 95540, (707) 725-2987, BA 71 Humboldt St Univ; MA 73 Humboldt St Univ; Sp-Lang Path, Private Practice, **SLP**

Howard, Mrs Robin R 1511 East Emmaus Avenue, Allentown, PA 18103, (215) 759-3200, BS 78 Clarion Univ of PA; ME 79 Clarion Univ of PA; Sp-Lang Path, Northampton Co, **SLP**

Howard, Sharon J 752 Hartness Road, Statesville, NC 28677, (704) 872-1760, BS 79 East Carolina Univ; ME 81 Univ of NC - Greensboro; Aud, Private Practice, **A**

Howard, Sherril R 2665 North Indian Ridge Dr, Tucson, AZ 85715, (602) 721-1378, BS 80 Univ of AZ; MS 82 Univ of AZ; Sp-Lang Path, Univ Phys Inc, **SLP ACE**

Howard, Sherry H 7530 South Emerson Street, Littleton, CO 80122, (303) 797-8617, PH (NS); **SLP**

Howard, Mrs Sydney W 2411 Louisiana #G-84, Lawrence, KS 66046, (913) 843-8364, BA 66 George Washington Univ; MA 75 1606; Sp-Lang Path Consultant, Atwood USD #318, **SLP**

Howard, Tamaryn Means 3813 Haynsworth Place, Fairfax, VA 22031, BS 74 PA St Univ - Univ Park; MS 75 PA St Univ - Univ Park; Sp-Lang Path, Private Practice, **SLP**

Howard-Porter, Mrs Sara 8 Guide Place, Haskell, NJ 07420, (201) 977-6600, BS 79 SUNY - Coll at Fredonia; MA 80 Bowling Green St Univ; Sp-Lang Path, Passaic Co Elks Cerebral Palsy, **SLP**

Howatt, Kelly Ann 24 Sand Spurrey Road, Ballston Spa, NY 12020-9003, (518) 899-6935, SLP, UCP of Schnectady, **SLP**

Howatt, Sara L Clesson Brook Road, Charlemont, MA 01339, (413) 625-6135, MA 87 Univ of MA - Amherst; **SLP**

Howden, Dr Mary E P O Box 553, Burns, OR 97720, (503) 573-2122, BS 47 Univ of OR; MS 51 Univ of OR; PH 67 (NS) Univ of OR; Dir Spec Ed, Harney Co Educ Serv Dist, **SLP**

Howden, Shaune B 1160 Ring Street, Deltona, FL 32725, (407) 668-4315, BS 82 AL A & M Univ; MA 86 Univ of Central FL; 87–Sp-Lang Path, Volusia Co Schs, **SLP**

Howe, Mrs Camille 50 Clearwater Avenue, Massapequa, NY 11758, (516) 541-6681, MA 75 Hofstra Univ; Sp-Lang Path, Private Practice, **SLP**

Howe, Catherine Louise 22598 Veronica Drive, Salinas, CA 93908, (617) 661-1718, BA 82 Univ of the Pacific; MS 84 Boston Univ; Sp-Lang Path, New England Mem Hosp, **SLP ACE**

Howe, Elizabeth Boehme 152 Oak Street, Holliston, MA 01746, (617) 429-2916, MA 65 Middlebury Coll; ME 79 Northeastern Univ; PH 76 (Germanic Studies) Boston Coll; **SLP**

Howe, Mrs Janet Morse 1391 Heatherton Circle, Salt Lake City, UT 84121, (801) 565-6674, BS 82 Clarion St Coll; MA 84 Univ of Denver; 88–Sp-Lang Path, Western Rehab Inst, **SLP**

Howe, Katherine J Lakeland AEA 3, 401-1/2 Grand Avenue, Spencer, IA 51301, (712) 262-4020, BA 64 Univ of SD - Vermillion; MA 82 Univ of SD - Vermillion; SLP, Lakeland AEA 3, **SLP**

Howe, Linda B 25 Race Brook Road, West Hartford, CT 06107, (203) 521-8343, BS 75 Ithaca Coll; MS 77 Boston Univ; Sp-Lang Path, Private Practice, **SLP**

Howe, Mrs Marilyn K 687 North 350 West, Kaysville, UT 84037, (801) 399-5601, BA 74 Univ of Northern CO; MS 76 UT St Univ; Sp-Lang Path, Ogden Sp & Hrng Ctr, **SLP ACE**

Howe, Patricia Weston 8240 Ridge Road, Elsie, MI 48831, (517) 862-4887, BA 75 MI St Univ; MA 76 MI St Univ; Preprim Level Tchr Sp-Lang Imp, Clinton Co Inter Sch Dist, **SLP**

Howe, Mrs Pauline Elam 555 East Bledse, Gallatin, TN 37066-3046, (615) 860-0383, BA 42 Olivet Coll; MA 53; **LM**

Howe, Mrs Robin Lynne 5050 Garford Street, Apt 276, Long Beach, CA 90815, (213) 597-7616, BS 84 Purdue Univ - West Lafayette; MS 86 Purdue Univ - West Lafayette; 88–SLP, InSpeech Inc, **SLP**

Howe, Dr Susan W 3320 South 30th Street, Lincoln, NE 68502, (402) 464-8385, BA 65 Allegheny Coll; MA 80 Univ of NE - Lincoln; PH 83 (NS) Univ of NE - Lincoln; Aud, Dr J Fritsch & Assoc, **A**

Howell, Mrs Alison Shoulars 3 Four Seasons Lane, Charlotte, NC 28212, (704) 343-5533, BA 80 Univ of NC - Chapel Hill; MA 84 Univ of TX - Austin; Sp-Lang Path, Charlotte-Mecklenburg Schs, **SLP**

Howell, Ella M 311 Kossuth Street, Rome, NY 13440, (315) 336-2300, BS 80 Elmira Coll; MS 81 Ithaca Coll; SLP, Rome Developmental Center, **SLP**

Howell, Jenell L 11004 Leafwood Lane, Austin, TX 78750, (512) 258-6451, BS 77 Baylor Univ; MS 78 Baylor Univ; 79–Sp-Lang Path, Round Rock ISD, **SLP**

Howell, Mrs L J M 1704 Kingsbury Lane, Oklahoma City, OK 73116-6306, (405) 848-8129, **SLP**

Howell, Lynne M 8846 Pagoda Way, San Diego, CA 92126, (619) 260-7161, BS 76 Univ of WY; MS 78 Univ of WY; Sp-Lang Path, Mercy Hosp & Med Ctr, **SLP**

Howell, Marianne 1184 Hampden Street, Holyoke, MA 01040, (413) 533-1480, BA 78 Univ of MA - Amherst; MS 80 Univ of MA - Amherst; 84–Sp-Lang Path, Stewart Pediatric Clinic, **SLP**

Howell, Mrs Marsha Eidnier 705 Charles Avenue, Findlay, OH 45840, (419) 423-2592, BS 73 Bowling Green St Univ; MA 75 Bowling Green St Univ; Sp-Lang Path, Marsha Howell Speech/Lang Ther Svc, **SLP**

Howell, Mrs Nancy Hanks 9 Sunvalley, Jackson, TN 38305, (901) 422-4005, BS 77 Univ of AL- Tuscaloosa; MS 79 Univ of AL- Tuscaloosa; Aud, Wtn Hrng/Sp Cen, **A**

Howell, Mrs Nellie H 4695 Quince, Memphis, TN 38117-6548, (209) 634-1105, BA 68 Univ of AR - Fayetteville; MA 69 Univ of AR - Fayetteville; MA 81 CA St Univ - Stanislaus; **SLP**

Howell, Mrs Sara W C 14405 Haystack Court, Centreville, VA 22020, MS 81 Univ of HI - Manoa; SLP, Fairfax County Public Schools, **SLP**

Howell, Susan M 4404 Meadowbrook Drive, Fort Worth, TX 76103, (817) 534-4404, BS 70 OK St Univ; MS 72 Univ of OK Medical Center; Aud, Private Practice, **A**

Howell, Tina Marie 4621 Victoria Avenue, Los Angeles, CA 90043, (213) 673-4660, BA 81 CA St Univ - Los Angeles; MA 85 CA St Univ - Los Angeles; 88–Sp-Lang Path, Centrela Hosp Med Ctr, **SLP**

Howells, Mrs Cindy Wells P O Box 994225, Redding, CA 96099-4225, (916) 244-3260, MS 87 ID St Univ; **SLP**

Howells, Rod Carlyle P O Box 994225, Redding, CA 96099-4225, (916) 222-5629, BS 85 ID St Univ; MS 86 ID St Univ; **A**

Howerton, Mrs Jan DeMonde 2007 Woodlyn Drive #103, Fredericksburg, VA 22401, (919) 388-5592, BS 83 SUNY - Coll at Geneseo; MS 87 Nazareth Coll of Rochester; Sp-Lang Path, Healthcore Inc, **SLP**

Howey, Mrs Karla Buschle 2618 Edgemont, Trenton, MI 48183, (313) 671-1505, BS 82 Western MI Univ; MA 84 Bowling Green St Univ; Sp-Lang Path, Monroe PS, **SLP**

Howitz, Michael J Box M, Clear Lake, IA 50428, (515) 357-6125, BA 85 Univ of MN - Minneap-St Paul; MA 88 Univ of MN - Minneap-St Paul; 88–Aud, Northern Trails AEA

Howland, Denise Gayle 1005 E Jean Street, Tampa, FL 33604-6207, (813) 239-2422, BA 79 Univ of FL; MS 85 Univ of South FL; 88–Sp-Lang Path, Hillsborough Co Schs/Assoc Psych Svcs, **SLP**

Howland, Karole A 263 Farrwood Drive, Bradford, MA 01835, BA 81 Univ of MA - Amherst; MS 87 Emerson Coll; 88–Sp-Lang Path, North Shore Children's Hosp

Howle, Barbara K 30 Seabird Court, Newport Beach, CA 92663, (714) 848-1774, BS 64 Univ of MO - Columbia; MS 68 Univ of HI - Manoa; Sp-Lang Path, Huntington Bd Un Hs Dist, **SLP**

Howle, Mrs Nell T P O Box 1265, San Marcos, TX 78667, (512) 392-1224, BS 57 Southwest TX St Univ; ME 61 Rutgers St Univ -N Brunswick; Sp Ed Superv, San Marcos ISD, **SLP**

Howlett, Susan J S 19935 River Brook Drive, Humble, TX 77346, (713) 376-4180, BA 76 Jersey City St Coll; MA 78 OH Univ - Athens; Tchr, Klein ISD, **SLP**

Howse, Paula R 5394 Estate Office Drive, Suite 2, Memphis, TN 38119, (901) 682-1529, BS 78 Univ of TN - Knoxville; MA 79 Memphis St Univ; Sp/Lang Path, Mid-South Sp Path Group, **SLP**

Howse, Sandra F 455 Brookwood Drive, Mobile, AL 36606, (205) 431-3422, BS 80 Univ of South AL; MS 81 Univ of South AL; Sp-Lang Path, Rotary Rehab Hosp, **SLP**

Howton, Mrs Charlotte Powell Route 1 Box A-13, McCalla, AL 35111-9248, (205) 938-9266, BS 83 Univ of Montevallo; MS 85 Univ of Montevallo; **SLP**

Hoy, Carol Joan 531 Beechmont, Dearborn, MI 48124, BA 60 Univ of MI - Ann Arbor; MA 76 Eastern MI Univ; SLP, Clarenceville Public Schools, **SLP**

Hoy, Connie Lynn R R 1 Box 19, Onarga, IL 60955, (815) 939-8011, MS 86 Eastern IL Univ; **SLP**

Hoy, Rebecca B 31810 Bayview Drive, Avon Lake, OH 44012, (216) 459-6300, OB 78 Miami Univ - Oxford; MA 79 Bowling Green St Univ; SLP, Deaconess Hosp of Cleveland, **SLP**

Hoyes, Angela M 48 Hunter Road, Plymouth Meeting, PA 19462, (215) 825-4875, SLP, **SLP**

Hoyle, Marsha Audiology/Speech Path (126), VA Medical Center, 4951 Arroyo Road, Livermore, CA 94550, (415) 447-2560, BA 66 Univ of CA - Santa Barbara; MA 68 Univ of CA - Santa Barbara; **SLP**

Hoyman, Tami Lyn 245 Gridley, Platteville, WI 53818, (715) 835-4819, BA 85 Univ of WI - Eau Claire; MS 84 Univ of WI - Eau Claire; **SLP**

Hoynacke, Mrs Bonnie 17937 Rosecliff, Cleveland, OH 44119, (216) 481-7964, BA 75 Cleveland St Univ; MA 79 Cleveland St Univ; SLP, Shaker Hts Sch Sys, **SLP**

Hoyo, Elaine 95 Christopher Street #3-M, New York, NY 10014, (305) 447-1479, BA 79 CUNY - Hunter Coll; MA 86 San Diego St Univ; **A**

Hoyt, Mrs Dianna K E 1938 West 30th South, Wichita, KS 67217, (316) 326-8935, BA 77 Wichita St Univ; MA 78 Wichita St Univ; Sp-Lang Path, Sumner County Spec Ed Services, **SLP**

Hoyt, Katherine Marie 14-H Spindrift Circle, Baltimore, MD 21234, (301) 822-0397, BS 86 Towson St Univ; MS 87 Loyola Coll; **SLP**

Hoyt, Mrs Kathryn P 153 North 8th Avenue, Highland Park, NJ 08904, (609) 394-4177, BA 52 Wesleyan Coll; MS 56 Vanderbilt Univ; Dir Sp & Hrng, Mercer Med Cen, **A**

Hoyt, Mrs Linda P O Box 3, Buckeystown, MD 21717, (301) 791-4354, MA 72 OK St Univ; BS 71 Phillips Univ; SLP, Washington Co Bd of Ed, **SLP**

Hoyt, Margaret 1 Walnut Park Road, Natick, MA 01760, (617) 369-1400, BA 68 Univ of MI - Ann Arbor; MS 75 Univ of MI - Ann Arbor; Chief/Sp-Lang Path, Emerson Hospital, **SLP**

Hoyt, Michael B 30475 Birchway Drive, Franklin, MI 48025, (313) 773-6501, BA 70 MI St Univ; MA 78 Wayne St Univ - Sch of Med; 83–Aud, Hearing Lab Assoc, **A**

Hoza, Sherry T 4525 Lincoln Road, Louisville, KY 40220, (502) 452-1204, BS 76 PA St Univ - Univ Park; MA 77 George Washington Univ; Sp-Lang Path, Private Practice, **SLP**

Hoze, Brenda Joyce 21680 Stratford, Oak Park, MI 48237, (313) 967-1259, BS; MA; 78–Sp-Lang Path, Detroit PS, **SLP**

Hranichny, Kay Lynn 105 North George Street, Pottsville, PA 17901, (717) 622-5751, BS 82 Bloomsburg Univ of PA; MS 83 Bloomsburg Univ of PA; Aud, Schuylkill Otolaryngology Asoc, **A**

Hrdlicka, Jill 2930 S W Luradel Lane, Portland, OR 97219-6380, (503) 246-2820, BA 72 Univ of WI - Eau Claire; MS 73 Univ of WI - Eau Claire; SLP, N Clackmas Sch Dist #12, **SLP**

Hrinda, Mrs Mary L 1611 Peach Street, Suite 320, Erie, PA 16501, (814) 456-2031, BS 78 Edinboro Univ of PA; MA 79 Bowling Green St Univ; 79–Aud, ENT Assoc of Erie Inc, **A**

Hrivnak, Mrs Brenda Martin 572 Baysview Road, Kingsport, TN 37660, (615) 246-4600, BS 80 Univ Southern MS-Hattiesburg; MA 82 Memphis St Univ; Sp-Lang Path, Mt Reg Sp & Hrng Cen, **SLP**

Hrovat, Susan D 4000 Horizon Hill #1301, San Antonio, TX 78229, (512) 691-0737, BS 71 Phillips Univ; MA 72 Western MI Univ; 88–Sp-Lang Path, Rehab Inst of San Antonio, **SLP**

Hrubecky, Arlene E General Delivery, Eagle River, ON, Canada P0V 1S0, (807) 755-5541, BS 59 IL St Univ - Normal; MA 76 Governors St Univ; Sp-Lang Path, Private Practice, **SLP**

Hruby, Bernadette 624 Brooklyn Mountain Road, Hopatcong, NJ 07843, (201) 398-3171, MS 84 Bloomsburg Univ of PA; Aud, Roxbury Med Grp, **A ACE**

Hruschak, Jean M 5325-304 Portland Street, Columbus, OH 43220, (216) 743-1168, **SLP**

Hrycyna, Mrs Terry L 132 West Henry Clay, Whitefish Bay, WI 53217, (414) 962-3278, BS 75 Univ of WI - Milwaukee; MS 77 Univ of WI - Milwaukee; 88–Sp-Lang Path, Sch Dist of Shorewood, **SLP**

Hsu, Dr Jennifer R 434 Skyline Lake Drive, Ringwood, NJ 07456, (201) 595-2209, MA 69 Gallaudet Coll; MA 78 CUNY - Grad Sch & Univ Cntr; PH 81 (Linguistics) CUNY - Grad Sch & Univ Cntr; Assoc Prof, Wm Paterson Coll/Dept Comm Dis

Hu, Mrs Florence Sun 702 Camellia Drive, Salisbury, MD 21801, (301) 632-2582, MS 74 Southern IL Univ -Carbondale

Hu, Linda L 1071 Penn Circle #G311, King of Prussia, PA 19406, (215) 631-9300, BA 77 Univ of MD - College Park; MA 79 Trenton St Coll; Dir of Educ & Prog Dev, InSpeech Inc, **SLP ACE**

Hu, Mrs Lorna Kiyoko 537 Kealahou Street, Honolulu, HI 96825, (808) 735-4905, **SLP**

Huart, Steven A 2727 Plaza Drive, Wausau, WI 54401, (715) 847-3232, BS 83 Univ of WI - Stevens Point; MS 85 Univ of WI - Stevens Point; 86–Aud, Wausau Med Ctr, **A**

Hubatch, Dr Leona M West Surburban Speech Clinic, 1 South 224 Summit Avenue, Oakbrook Terrace, IL 60181, (312) 932-4599, BS 74 Western IL Univ; MA 75 Western IL Univ; PH 82 (NS) Northwestern Univ; Sp-Lang Path, West Suburban Speech Clinic, **SLP**

Hubbard, Carol P 858 N E 67th Street #102, Seattle, WA 98115, (206) 545-7400, BS 81 Univ of IL - Urbana; MS 82 Univ of IL - Urbana; Grad, Univ of WA, **SLP ACE**

Hubbard, Charlotte A 801 Gate Lane #706, Knoxville, TN 37909, (615) 974-5451, BS 75 Univ of KS; MA 76 Wichita St Univ; 88–Sp-Lang Path, Pro Health Svcs, **SLP**

Hubbard, Mrs Cynthia Hatley 2813 Paula Drive, West Plains, MO 65775, (417) 256-1938, BS 85 AR St Univ; OM 86 AR St Univ; **SLP**

Hubbard, Dr Dee Jay 1357 Haute Loire, St Louis, MO 63011, (314) 894-6675, BS 62 KS St Univ; MA 65 Univ of IA; PH 67 (Sp Path) Univ of IA; 77–Ch Aud & SLP, St Louis VA Med Cen, **SLP**

Hubbard, Mrs Frances L 420 Hollow Drive, Houston, TX 77024, BA 63 LA St Univ - Baton Rouge; MA 73 Univ of Houston - Univ Park; Sp-Lang Path, Houston ISD, **SLP**

Hubbard, Mrs Francine Bruster 10 Capewood Road #147, Simpsonville, SC 29681, (803) 967-2005, MA 83 SC St Coll; ME 85 SC St Coll; 86–Sp-Lang Path, Greenville County Sch Dist, **SLP**

Hubbard, Mrs Gail L 1073 Ross Avenue Suite C, El Centro, CA 92243, (619) 353-2525, BA 69 Univ of NM; MA 70 Univ of CA - Santa Barbara; Dir of Aud, Valley Hrng & Sp Consultants, **A**

Hubbard, Jenita Lynn 3314 South Verbena Court, Denver, CO 80231, (303) 773-1800, BS 81 Appalachian St Univ; MA 82 Memphis St Univ; Aud, Jewish Hosp at Wash U Sch Med, **A**

Hubbard, Mrs Karen D 10331 Esthner, Wichita, KS 67209, (316) 722-3943, BS 78 Baylor Univ; MA 79 Wichita St Univ; Sp-Lang Path, USD 259 Wichita Pub Sch, **SLP**

Hubbard, Dr Kenneth A 714 Dogwood Road, Boone, NC 28607, ED 79 (Administration and Supervision) Univ of NC - Greensboro; President, Alta Petens Inc, **SLP**

Hubbard, Kim Niemi 113 Carriage Hill Drive, Warner Robins, GA 31088, (912) 922-1320, BA 82 OH St Univ; MA 84 Univ of Cincinnati; Sp-Lang Path, Robins AFB Schs, **SLP**

Hubbard, Mrs Lynn R 714 Dogwood Road, Boone, NC 28607, (704) 264-0566, BA 74 Appalachian St Univ; MA 75 Appalachian St Univ; Sp-Lang Path, Alta Petens Inc, **SLP**

Hubbard, Nancy Ehle 14801 Zircon Circle, Anchorage, AK 99516, (907) 563-3175, BA 77; MA 85; Sp-Lang Path, Dynamic Communication Inc, **SLP**

Hubbard, Dr Patricia B 5102 Sansom Court, Columbus, OH 43220, (614) 221-7855, BS 63 OH St Univ; MA 66 OH St Univ; PH 71 (Sp and Hrng Science) OH St Univ; 74–Sp-Lang Path, Diocesan Chld Guid Cen, **SLP ACE**

Hubbard, Mrs Rebecca Johnson 523 Dearborn Street, Iowa City, IA 52240, (319) 337-4367, BS 82 CO St Univ; MA 84 Univ of IA; SLP, Grant Wood AEA, **SLP**

Hubbard, Mrs Sally A Suite 560 Dollar Fed Bldg, Third And High Streets, Hamilton, OH 45011, (513) 874-0990, BA 71 Univ of FL; MA 78 Univ of Cincinnati; Aud, Hamilton-Fairfield ENT Spec, **A**

Hubbard, Tana Witte P O Box 976, Crystal River, FL 32629, BA 78 Univ of Denver; MS 80 Univ of AZ; Coord Inpatient Rehabilitation, Nilliam Beaumont Hospital, **SLP**

Hubbard, William Conway 523 Dearborn Street, Iowa City, IA 52240, (319) 337-4367, BS 82 Western MI Univ; MA 84 Univ of IA; University of Iowa, **SLP**

Hubbard-Wiley, Pamela S 6619 Halm Avenue, Los Angeles, CA 90056-2225, (213) 290-1051, MA 75 CA St Univ - Los Angeles; Dir, Sp & Lang Ther Cen, **SLP**

Hubbell, Robert D Dept Speech Path & Audiology, California State Univ, Sacramento, CA 95819, PH (NS); **SLP**

Huber, Mrs Carol T 247 Keller Lane, Marion, VA 24354, (703) 783-2609, BS 74 Radford Univ; MA 75 Western MI Univ; Sp-Lang Path, Smyth Co Pub Sch, **SLP**

Huber, Connie M 1119 South Forest, Ann Arbor, MI 48104, (313) 662-0812, MA 86 Eastern MI Univ; Self Employed, **SLP**

Huber, Kimberly Ann 600 Country Club Drive #32, New Albany, IN 47150, BS 78 IN Univ - Bloomington; MS 80 Univ of Louisville; 83–Aud, The Rehabilitation Ctr, **SLP**

Huber, Mrs Linda K 1914 Brandon Avenue, Marion, IN 46952, (317) 674-3321, OB 72 Boston Univ; OM 74 IN Univ - Bloomington; Chief/Aud/Sp-Lang Path, Veterans Admini Medical Center, **SLP**

Huber, Mary Elizabeth 5431-A Gertrude Avenue, St Louis, MO 63116, (314) 752-3806, BS 83 Saint Louis Univ; MA 85 Saint Louis Univ; **SLP**

Huber, Dr Mary Wehe 1055 Olive Way, Palm Springs, CA 92262, (619) 323-3003, BS 39 Univ of WI - Madison; MA 40 Univ of WI - Madison; PH 45 (NS) Univ of WI - Madison; **SLP F LM**

Huber, Mrs Patricia Marie 27 Thorncliffe Drive, Rochester, NY 14617, (716) 359-3710, BA 79 SUNY - Coll at Potsdam; MA 81 SUNY - Coll at Geneseo; SLP, School of Holy Childhood, **SLP**

Huber, Thomas M 950 Marion Road, Indiana, PA 15701, (814) 472-7350, BS 67 Indiana Univ of PA; ME 77 Indiana Univ of PA; 79–Dir, Ebensburg Ctr, **SLP**

Hubert, Mrs Amy Bell 107 Strongwood Road, Owings Mills, MD 21117-2426, (404) 633-7105, BA 81 Emory Univ; OM 83 Emory Univ; **SLP**

Hubert, Mrs Donna A 403 High Street, Wilmington, OH 45177, (513) 382-0253, BS 53 Univ of IL - Urbana; MA 76 Univ of Cincinnati; SLP, Wilmington City Sch, **SLP**

Huberty, Marsha L 1645 Ridgeway Drive, Ellettsville, IN 47429, (812) 336-9484, OB 74 Central MO St Univ; MS 77 Central MO St Univ; Sp-Lang Path, Bloomington Hospital, **SLP**

Hubka, Beverly J 843 Hillview, Ashland, OR 97520, (503) 482-8383, BS 65 Univ of CO - Boulder; MS 75 FL St Univ; Providence Hosp, **SLP**

Hubner, Mary Ellen 3639 North Oakley, Chicago, IL 60618, (312) 283-6317, **SLP**

Hubschman, Dr Eva W 1817 West Claremont, Phoenix, AZ 85061, (602) 242-3484, BA 40 CUNY - Brooklyn Coll; MA 56 Columbia Univ Teachers Coll; PH 76 (Sp Path) CUNY - Grad Sch & Univ Cntr; **SLP LM**

Huck, Barbara 603 Whiting Road, Weiser, ID 83672, (208) 549-3131, BS 74 UT St Univ; MS 76 UT St Univ; SLP, Weiser School District #431, **SLP**

Huck, Jeanne E N 3433 West Capitol Drive, Peoria, IL 61614, (309) 672-6720, BA 67 Univ of IA; MA 69 Univ of IA; SLP, Peoria Pub Sch Dist #150, **SLP**

Huck, Mrs Nancy E Tawas Bay Hearing Instruments, 1395 Laidlaw Road, P O Box 267, Tawas City, MI 48764, (517) 362-4800, BA 68 MI St Univ; MA 69 MI St Univ; Dir/Aud, Tawas St Joseph Hospital, **A**

Huckabee, Mrs Kimberly Ann 2304 Forrest Park, Arkadelphia, AR 71923, (501) 246-4531, BA 83 Ouachita Baptist Univ; MS 85 Univ of AR - Little Rock; Supervisor, Ouachita Baptist Univ, **SLP**

Huckaby, Geraldine 3343 California Avenue, Signal Hill, CA 90807, **SLP**

Huckaby, Mrs Rose M Route 2 Box 303-B2, Jamestown, KY 42629, (502) 343-4621, BA 81 Western KY Univ; MS 82 Western KY Univ; Sp-Lang Path, Comm for Handicapped Children, **SLP**

Hucker, Mrs Patricia 4 N 595 Kildeer Lane, Elburn, IL 60119, (312) 365-6396, BS 73 Southern IL Univ -Carbondale; MS 74 Eastern IL Univ; Sp-Lang Path, Comm Unit Sch Dist #303, **SLP**

Huckleberry, Mrs Helen Carol B 57 Holiday Drive, Monroe, LA 71203, (318) 345-2533, BA 66 Southern Univ - Baton Rouge; MA 67 Western MI Univ; Sp-Lang Path, Ouachita Parish Sch Syst, **SLP**

Hudak, Mrs Deborah Wright 4882 Sawyer Pine Road, Sarasota, FL 33583, (813) 957-3890, BS 80 WV Univ; MS 81 WV Univ; **A**

Hudak, Mrs Diane C 280 Longview Lane, Kennett Square, PA 19348, (215) 444-1869, BA 73 Montclair St Coll; MA 78 West Chester Univ of PA; Sp-Lang Path, Private Practice, **SLP**

Huddart, M Susan F 508 East Polo Drive, Clayton, MO 63105, (314) 839-1515, BS 64 Coll of Saint Rose; MS 78 Coll of Saint Rose; 78–Sp-Lang Path, St Louis Co Spec Sch Dist, **SLP**

Huddleston, Delores Jeneal 373 Plantation N W, Orangeburg, SC 29115, (803) 531-2200, BA 74 SC St Coll; MA 86 SC St Coll; **SLP**

Huddleston, Lynne A 2915 North Texas Street, Apartment 140, Fairfield, CA 94533, (707) 437-4691, BA 78 Eastern WA Univ; MS 79 Eastern WA Univ; Sp-Lang Path, Offi Solano Co Supt of Sch, **SLP**

Huddleston, Ronald L MBAEA9, Audiological And Education Hearing Impared Services, 729 21st Street, Bettendorf, IA 52722, (319) 359-1371, BA 62 Univ of Northern CO; MA 63 Univ of Northern CO; ED 72 Central MO St Univ; Superv, Dept of Hrng Conserv Ed Serv, **SLP A**

Hudesman, Jill Aber 287 Cedarhurst Avenue #J2, Cedarhurst, NY 11516, (201) 992-0820, BA 82 George Washington Univ; MA 81 Kean Coll of NJ; Aud, Private Practice, **A**

Hudgins, Mrs Judith M 613 Mardon Avenue, Akron, OH 44303, (216) 836-7772, BA 76 Univ of Akron; MS 77 Univ of AL- Tuscaloosa; ED (Educational Administration) Univ of Akron; 88–Doctoral Research Asst, The Univ of Akron, **SLP**

Hudgins, Mrs Leslee E 11120 Swift Flight Lane, Glen Allen, VA 23060, (804) 266-2609, BA 79 Longwood Coll; ME 81 Univ of VA - Charlottesville; **SLP**

Hudock, John F 750 East Beau Street #101, Washington, PA 15301, (614) 264-7276, BA 73 Cleveland St Univ; MA 77 Cleveland St Univ; Aud, Private Practice, **A**

Hudock, Mrs Victoria Ann 12 Tracy Lane Rd #3, Shelburne, VT 05482, MS 86 Univ of VT; 87–Sp-Lang Path, North East Addison Supervisory Dist, **SLP**

Hudson, Mrs Alane B 2018 Brookwood Med Ctr Dr, Suite 214, Birmingham, AL 35209, (205) 871-4961, BS 76 Midwestern St Univ; MS 77 Univ of North TX; Aud, M Alan Goodson MD, **A**

Hudson, Dr Amelia I 5525 Valley Forge Avenue, Baton Rouge, LA 70808, (504) 388-5356, BS 65 Univ Southern MS-Hattiesburg; MS 66 Univ Southern MS-Hattiesburg; PH 77 (Sp Path) FL St Univ; Assoc Prof Sp/Lang Path, Louisiana St U, **SLP**

Hudson, Amy Jo Rte 8 Box 165, Harrison, AR 72601, (501) 741-3542, BS 83 Univ of AR - Fayetteville; MS 85 Univ of AR - Fayetteville; 87–Sp-Lang Path, Jasper PS, **SLP**

Hudson, Atwood 204 Sans Souci #1-D, Charleston, SC 29403, PH (NS); **SLP LM**

Hudson, Mrs Cheerie Gentry Route 1 Box 1405, Chula, GA 31733, (912) 468-7220, BS 83 Univ of GA; ME 84 Valdosta St Coll; 83–Sp-Lang Path, Irwin County Bd of Educ, **SLP**

Hudson, D Ann 233 173rd Street, Hammond, IN 46324, BS 51 Purdue Univ - West Lafayette; MA 56 Univ of AL- Tuscaloosa; Asst Dir SLP, Trade Winds Rehab Cen, **SLP**

Hudson, Delores Y 3257 Hester Drive, Tallahassee, FL 32308, **SLP**

Hudson, Diane Lorraine 2303 West Meadowview Road, Suite 49, Greensboro, NC 27407, (919) 292-7775, BS 82 East Carolina Univ; Director, Care-Pak Inc, **SLP**

Hudson, Gail C 3828 Silverstone, Plano, TX 75023, **SLP**

Hudson, Jan Elaine 7604 Fair Oaks Drive #2042, Dallas, TX 75231, (214) 348-4532, MS 85 Univ of TX - Dallas; SLP, Dallas ISD, **SLP**

Hudson, Mrs Judith T 3233-A Park Road, Charlotte, NC 28209, (704) 373-6977, BA 63 Pfeiffer Coll; ME 70 Univ of NC - Greensboro; **SLP**

Hudson, Karen Sue 235 South McLean #8, Memphis, TN 38104, (901) 528-6511, BA 82 Memphis St Univ; MA 84 Memphis St Univ; 87–Sp-Lang Path/Coord, Univ of TN Child Dev Ctr, **SLP**

Hudson, Mrs Laura Bachner North Park Street, Adams, NY 13605, (315) 232-4882, BA 85 SUNY - Coll at Cortland; MS 86 Ithaca Coll; 86–Sp-Lang Path, Watertown City Sch Dist, **SLP**

Hudson, Mrs Louise V 3765 Preakness Drive, Decatur, GA 30034, (404) 241-2742, BS 70 FL A & M Univ; MS 73 FL St Univ; **SLP**

Hudson, Martha Frances Special Children's Center, 355 West Green, Pasadena, CA 91105, (818) 795-9349, ME 86 Columbia Univ Teachers Coll; 88–Sp-Lang Path, Special Children's Ctr, **SLP**

Hudson, Mary S R R 2 Box 102-B, Freeport, ME 04032, (207) 865-1039, BS 80 Coll of Saint Rose; MS 81 Coll of Saint Rose; Sp-Lang Path, Rensselaer Co Assoc/Ret Chldn, **SLP**

Hudson, Nancy T P O Box 8, Harrison, AR 72602, (501) 741-7711, BS 75 Univ of TN - Knoxville; MA 76 Memphis St Univ; Sp-Lang Path, Private Practice, **SLP**

Hudson, Mrs Nellie H 103 Tomahawk Trail, Clinton, NC 28328, (919) 592-7487, BS 74 Univ of NC - Chapel Hill; MS 77 Univ of Montevallo; Sp-Lang Path, Clinton City Schs, **SLP**

Hudson, Mrs Susan B 253 Shade Drive, Fairborn, OH 45324, (512) 298-2089, OB 80 Univ of FL; ME 81 Univ of FL; **SLP**

Hudson, Mrs Tinamarie Petrillo University Of Miami, Mailman Center For Child Development, PO Box 016 820 (D-820), Miami, FL 33101, (305) 547-5937, BS 83 Towson St Univ; MS 87 Univ of South FL; 87–Aud, Mailman Ctr for Child Dev, **A**

Hudson, Tracy L 89 West Lane #5, Ridgefield, CT 06877, (203) 775-4700, BS 75 Univ of TN - Knoxville; MA 77 Univ of TN - Knoxville; 88–Sp-Lang Path, Datahr Inc A Comprehensive Rehab Agency, **SLP ACE**

Hudson, William E Audiologic Hearing Center, 2420 Professional Drive, P O Box 7309, Rocky Mount, NC 27804, (919) 937-4110, BA 75 Old Dominion Univ; MA 78 Univ of TN - Knoxville; Aud, Audiologic Hearing Center, **A**

Hudson-Edwards, Allison 906 Laurel Drive S E, Albuquerque, NM 87108, (505) 831-3301, OB 74 Univ of NM; MA 78 Univ of NM; MS 83 Univ of NM; Sp-Lang Path, Albuquerque Pub Schs, **SLP**

Hudson-Graham, Karen Marie 20514 Picadilly, Detroit, MI 48221, (313) 864-7803, MA 88 Eastern MI Univ

Hue, Mrs Eva M 618 Taraval Street, San Francisco, CA 94116, (415) 871-4898, OB 46 Univ of HI - Manoa; MA 64 San Francisco St Univ; 88–Tchr, San Mateo County Spec Schools, **SLP**

Huebner, Mrs Christie Elizabeth 77 Commonwealth Avenue, New Providence, NJ 07974, (201) 771-9453, BS 82 James Madison Univ; MS 84 Vanderbilt Univ; Aud, Manchester Hrng Cen, **A**

Huebner, Debbra K 3311 Lorton Avenue, Davenport, IA 52807, (319) 359-4574, BA 71 Univ of Northern IA; MA 75 Western IL Univ; **SLP**

Huebner, Mrs Debra S 2592 Hickory Lane, Arlington Heights, IL 60004, (312) 259-2592, BS 79 Northern IL Univ - De Kalb; MA 80 Northern IL Univ - De Kalb; **SLP**

Huebner, Sheila 37 Fairmount Avenue, Haverstraw, NY 10927, (914) 294-5431, BA 84 SUNY - Coll at Cortland; MA 88 Montclair St Coll

Huebsch-Lessmann, Noreen 167 Glenview Road, Wauwatosa, WI 53213, (815) 758-2082, OB 83 Governors St Univ; MA 86 Northern IL Univ - De Kalb; **SLP**

Hueffner, Debra Sue Arizona State University, Dept Of Sp & Hear Sciences, Tempe, AZ 85287, BS 83 Univ of IA; MS 85 Univ of AZ; Audiology Interne, University of Arizona, **A**

Huefner, Deborah Petro 4776 Debbie Drive, Medina, OH 44256, (216) 825-0863, BS 75 Kent St Univ; MA 79 Kent St Univ; Sp/Lang Path, Norton City Schools, **SLP**

Hue Gunawan, Marcia Denise Speech & Hearing, San Joaquin General Hospital, PO Box 1020, Stockton, CA 95201, (209) 468-6210, BA 82 CA St Univ - Chico; MA 86 CA St Univ - Chico; 88–Sp-Lang Path, San Joaquin General Hosp, **SLP**

Huelsberg, Susan R 2275 Willis Road, Saline, MI 48176, (517) 546-5550, BA 75 Univ of MI - Ann Arbor; MS 76 Univ of MI - Ann Arbor; 78–SLP, Livingston ISD, **SLP**

Huer, Dr Mary B University Of Wisconsin-Whitewater, Roseman 1020, Communicative Disorders, Whitewater, WI 53190, (414) 472-1485, BA 75 IN Univ - Bloomington; MA 76 IN Univ - Bloomington; PH 81 (Sp Science) IN Univ - Bloomington; 83–Asst Prof, U of WI-Whiterwater, **SLP**

Huerta, Dr Lynn Ellen ENT Associates, 171 Grandview Avenue, Waterbury, CT 06708, (203) 753-8833, BA 83 Univ of FL; MS 85 Vanderbilt Univ; PH 88 (Hrng Science) Vanderbilt Univ; Aud, ENT Assoc, **A**

Huet, Elizabeth M c/o A B Huet Iii, Box 23, Frankfurt Milcom, APO New York, NY 09710, **SLP ACE**

Huey-You, Dr Patricia 4826 South Dorchester, Chicago, IL 60615, PH 85 (NS) Southern IL Univ -Carbondale; Sp-Lang Path, Chicago Pub Schs, **SLP**

Hufana, Melinda Suyin 24 Willard Gardens, Toronto, ON, Canada M6S 1G1, (416) 890-1099, BS 78 Northern MI Univ; MA 85 Northern MI Univ

Huff, Mrs Brenda Kay 1 Lake Forest Drive, Roanoke, TX 76262, (817) 430-8998, BS 68 Southeast MO St Univ; MA 75 Saint Louis Univ; Richardson ISD, **SLP**

Huff, Mrs Carolyn Ditman 209 Raven Court, Modesto, CA 95350-4920, (209) 579-7046, BA 81 CA St Univ - Stanislaus; MA 84 CA St Univ - Stanislaus; 88–Sp-Lang Path, Ripon USD, **SLP**

Huff, Mrs Debra Sue 1310 Jefferson Drive, Boonville, MO 65233, (816) 882-7474, BS Central MO St Univ; MS 85 Central MO St Univ; **SLP**

Huff, Donna Todd 8120 Pagent, Downey, CA 90240, (213) 923-1797, BA 76 CA St Univ - Chico; MA 78 CA St Univ - Los Angeles; Sp-Lang Path, ABC USD, **SLP**

Huff, Elaine B 124 South Morgan Drive, Moore, OK 73160, (405) 691-4845, BA 74 Univ of OK - Norman; MS 75 Univ of OK Medical Center; Sp/Lang Path, Moore Pub Schs, **SLP**

Huff, Frances Ann 455 Rivergate Way #9, Sacramento, CA 95831, (916) 723-7050, MS 87 CA St Univ - Sacramento; **A**

Huff, Gary L 1682 NW 109th, Des Moines, IA 50322, (515) 225-7338, BS 67 SD St Univ; MA 69 Univ of NE - Omaha; Sp-Lang Path, Private Practice, **SLP**

Huff, Mrs Janet Lee 34 Pony Court, San Ramon, CA 94583, (415) 275-1571, BA 81 San Francisco St Univ; MS 83 San Francisco St Univ; 86–Sp/Lang Path, Private Practice, **SLP**

Huff, Lou Ann Gioannini Arkansas Department Of Health, Children's Hearing & Speech Clinic, 4815 West Markham Street, Little Rock, AR 72205-3867, (501) 661-2328, BS 74 Southern IL Univ -Carbondale; MS 76 Southern IL Univ -Carbondale; 88–Aud, AR Dept of Health, **A**

Huff, Mrs Marcia L 1741 Amherst Way, Woodland, CA 95695, (916) 666-3641, BA 77 Univ of the Pacific; MA 78 Univ of the Pacific; Sp-Lang Path, Yolo Co Offi of Ed, **SLP**

Huff, Mrs Marion Vonkolnitz 809 H Hideaway Drive, Mount Pleasant, SC 29464, (803) 881-3372, BA 84 Columbia Coll; OM 85 Univ of SC - Columbia; **SLP**

Huff, Ronna Lynn 508A Maple Avenue, Du Bois, PA 15801, (814) 371-7869, MA 88 Edinboro Univ of PA; 88–Sp-Lang Path

Huff, Mrs Sheryl Joy Serbin P O Box 493, Lakemore, OH 44250, (216) 784-7948, Sp-Lang Path, Lake Lical Schools, **SLP**

Huff, Dr Steven Jay 2020 Mercury Way, Sacramento, CA 95864, (916) 488-5729, BS 78 Northern AZ Univ; MS 81 ID St Univ; PH 88 (Aud) Univ of WA; 86–Aud, Alta Arden Hearing Ctr, **A**

Huffer, Mrs Frances C 4587 Terrace Drive, San Diego, CA 92116, (714) 463-9284, BA 71 Baylor Univ; MA 73 Northwestern Univ; **A**

Huffman, Dianna Lynne 25 Winter Street, Westerville, OH 43081, (614) 898-0605, BS 85 Miami Univ - Oxford; MS 86 Miami Univ - Oxford; **SLP**

Huffman, Dr Elna S 4300 Heather Road, Long Beach, CA 90808, (213) 425-2719, BA 36 Univ of IA; MS 38 Purdue Univ - West Lafayette; PH 71 (NS) Univ of Southern CA; **SLP LM**

Huffman, Frances H 2466 Green Canyon Road, Inkom, ID 83245, MS 77 4358; 85–Sp-Lang Path, Sch Dist #25, **SLP**

Huffman, James Raymond P O Box 852, Tillamook, OR 97141, (503) 842-9379, BA 72 Univ of Redlands; MS 76 Univ of Redlands; 81–Sp-Lang Path, Private Practice, **SLP**

Huffman, Mrs Jeanine Marie 802 West 2nd Street, Dixon, IL 61021, (815) 288-5572, BS 78 Central MI Univ; MA 79 Central MI Univ; Aud, Dixon Developmental Center, **A**

Huffman, Mrs Judith Bartels 6701 Airport Boulevard, Suite B-123, Mobile, AL 36608, (205) 633-2323, OB 84 Univ Southern MS-Hattiesburg; MS 86 Univ Southern MS-Hattiesburg; Aud, ENT Center PA, **A**

Huffman, Mrs Myra Jean 3416 Burrell Drive, Louisville, KY 40216-4371, (502) 636-7258, BS 78 Eastern KY Univ; MS 86 Nova Univ; SLP, Jo Lynn B Drury & Assoc, **SLP**

Huffman, Mrs Nancy P 590 Stearns Road, Churchville, NY 14428, (716) 377-4660, BS 64 SUNY - Coll at Buffalo; MS 65 SUNY - Coll at Geneseo; Chair Sp-Lang Path & Aud, Monroe Co BOCES #1, **SLP A F ACE**

Huffstetler, Mrs Donna Gail P O Box 25, Yadkinville, NC 27055, (919) 679-2297, BA 81 Univ of NC - Chapel Hill; MS 84 Univ of NC - Chapel Hill; **SLP**

Hufnagle, Dr Jon Dept Speech Path & Audiology, Illinois State University, Normal, IL 61761, (309) 438-8838, BS 66 Ball St Univ; ME 70 Wayne St Univ; PH 73 (NS) Wayne St Univ; Assoc Prof, Il St U, **SLP**

Hufnagle, Katy Kammer 2274 Ashley River Rd #116, Charleston, SC 29407, (803) 792-3004, BS 68 Ball St Univ; MS 73 Murray St Univ; Director, Med Univ of Sc, **SLP**

Hufstedler, Mrs Laurie C 2107 Dakota, Norman, OK 73069, (405) 360-0220, BS 67 Univ of OK - Norman; MA 73 Univ of OK - Norman; Sp-Lang Path, Norman Public Schools, **SLP**

Hug, Gerald August 1436-B Hidden Meadoews E, Walled Lake, MI 48088, (313) 661-4100, BS 81 Central MI Univ; MA 83 Central MI Univ; Aud, Ford Hosp, **A**

Hugar, Lily A Herbert J Dodd Md, 880 Cass, Suite 207, Monterey, CA 93940, BS 73 Univ of TN - Knoxville; MA 75 Univ of TN - Knoxville; Audiologist, Hj Dodd MD, **A**

Hugghins, Mrs Marcia L 479 Creighton Road, Orange Park, FL 32073, (904) 642-1611, BS 57 Univ of MD - College Park; MS 67 Catholic Univ of America; Sp-Lang Path, Duval County Schools, **SLP**

Huggins, Janice L 313 Swanee, Placentia, CA 92670, (714) 871-3280, BS 73 Univ of AZ; MS 75 Univ of AZ; 88–Dir Rehab Prog, St Jude Hosp & Rehab Cen, **SLP**

Huggins, Sharon DeNise 2013 Wilmich Drive, Akron, OH 44319, (216) 455-0022, BS 83 Univ of GA; MA 87 Kent St Univ; 88–Sp-Lang Path, Bes-Mont Sp & Lang Ctr, **SLP**

Huggins, Sherry A 41 Manhasset Trail, Medford Lakes, NJ 08055, (609) 726-1000, BA 78 Glassboro St Coll; MS 80 Rutgers St Univ - Newark; SLP, New Lisbon Develop, **SLP**

Huggins, Mrs Terri Sue 1405 Conti Lane, Kokomo, IN 46902, (317) 453-1901, SLP, Bona Vista Programs, **SLP**

Hughart, Jiovanne N 2100 Hilda Burns Place, Lithonia, GA 30058, (412) 831-2700, BS 79 CA Univ of PA; MA 81 OH Univ - Athens; Aud, American Audiology Associates, **A**

Hughes, Amy Jean 436 Hamburg Avenue, Egg Harbor, NJ 08215, (914) 883-5151, BA 83 SUNY - Coll at New Paltz; OM 84 SUNY - Coll at New Paltz; **SLP**

Hughes, Barbara E 59 Manchester Court, Wayne, NJ 07470, (201) 697-1700, BA 64 Paterson St Coll; MA 73 Northern MI Univ; Sp/Lang Path, W Milford Twp Bd of Ed, **SLP**

Hughes, Barbara S 12 Hilltop Terrace, Woburn, MA 01801, (617) 935-4486, BA 68 Suffolk Univ; ME 72 Northeastern Univ; **SLP**

Hughes, Christine M 1019 North McKinley Road, Arlington, VA 22205, (703) 522-2777, BS 79 Univ of VA - Charlottesville; MA 83 Univ of IA; Sp-Lang Path, Arlington Co Pub Sch, **SLP**

Hughes, David G 9822 Old Lincoln Trail, Fairview Heights, IL 62208, 68-398-1017, MA 87 Western IL Univ

Hughes, Deborah Dukes 2207 Biscayne Court, Sugar Land, TX 77478, (713) 342-4681, BS 79 FL St Univ; MS 80 FL St Univ; Dir/Sp-Lang-Hrng, Richmond State School, **SLP**

Hughes, Diana Fitz 11712 Lorene Avenue, Midwest City, OK 73130, (405) 769-3652, MS 85 Univ of OK Medical Center; Sp-Lang Path, Speech and Hearing Assoc, **SLP**

Hughes, Diana L Communication Disorders Prog, Central Michigan Univ, 417 Moore Hall, Mount Pleasant, MI 48859, (517) 774-3471, BS 69 Eastern IL Univ; MS 72 Southern IL Univ -Carbondale; PH 82 Univ of WA; Asst Prof, Cen Mi U, **SLP**

Hughes, Mrs Diane Hutchinson 7604 Thunder Mountain Dr, Boise, ID 83709, (208) 336-0712, MA 62 Case Western Reserve Univ; 79–Sp-Lang Path, Head Start, **SLP**

Hughes, Eileen Karen 14401 Buffalo Street, Anchorage, AK 99516-4201, (907) 753-8235, MS 82 Univ of WI - Madison; Tchr Presch Spec Ed, Anchorage Sch Dist, **SLP**

Hughes, Jacqueline Deets P O Box 325, Stockton, NJ 08559, (201) 234-0011, MA 83 2553; Sp-Lang Path, Matheny School/Hospital, **SLP**

Hughes, Mrs Jane S 6346 Argonne Boulevard, New Orleans, LA 70124, (504) 488-1815, BS 72 LA St Univ - Baton Rouge; OM 77 Tulane Univ; 83–Sp-Lang Path, Orleans Parish Sch Bd, **SLP**

Hughes, Joanne M 746 Los Palos Drive, Lafayette, CA 94549, (415) 654-3381, BA 77 Univ of CA - Santa Barbara; MS 80 San Francisco St Univ; SLP, Amy E Faltz, **SLP**

Hughes, Judy A G 5672 Singletree Drive, Frederick, MD 21701, **SLP**

Hughes, Kara L 454 East Taylor #2E, Barlett, IL 60103, (312) 213-3567, MA 87 Northern IL Univ - De Kalb; 88–Sp-Lang Path, School District U46

Hughes, Karen R 1221 Whitethorn Street, Bluefield, WV 24701, (304) 327-6189, BS 72 WV Univ; MS 73 WV Univ; Coordinator of Communication, Disorders & Audiology Programs, **SLP**

Hughes, Kathleen 2071 Penasquitas Drive, Aptos, CA 95003, (408) 758-1071, BA 71 Univ of AR - Fayetteville; MA 78 Univ of Tulsa; Sp-Lang Path, Speak E-Z Assoc, **SLP**

Hughes, Mrs Kathleen Gilbert 104 Elmwood Court, Hammond, LA 70403-9685, (504) 342-0018, BS 81 Univ Southern MS-Hattiesburg; OM 83 LA St Univ - N O Medical Ctr; Audiologist, Associates III, **A**

Hughes, Mrs Kathleen Homet 3615 Woodhaven Drive, Erie, PA 16506, (814) 453-5602, BS 76 Edinboro Univ of PA; MA 82 Edinboro Univ of PA; Sp-Lang Path, Dr Gertrude A Barber Center, **SLP**

Hughes, Mrs Kathy E H 2285 Tod Avenue N W, Warren, OH 44485-1917, (216) 632-0262, BS 76 Clarion Univ of PA; ME 77 Clarion Univ of PA; Sp-Lang Path, Cardinal Local School District, **SLP**

Hughes, Lela J Route 6 Box 48B, Manchester, KY 40962, (606) 598-2168, BS 73 Eastern KY Univ; MA 76 Univ of KY; Sp-Lang Path, Clay Co Bd of Ed, **SLP**

Hughes, Margaret E 603 East Glenside Avenue, Wyncote, PA 19095, (215) 545-3322, MS 84 Bloomsburg Univ of PA; 84–Aud, R T Sataloff MD, **A**

Hughes, Mary Catherine Gallaudet College, Dept Of Audiology, 800 Florida Avenue, Washington, DC 20002, (202) 651-5328, BS 78 Bloomsburg Univ of PA; MS 82 Syracuse Univ; Super Aural Rehab/Sp-Lang Path, Gallaudet College, **SLP**

Hughes, Mary H 3382 Fraserdale Drive, Lexington, KY 40503, (606) 255-9497, BA 70 Coe Coll; BA 76 Univ of KY; MA 77 Univ of KY; Fayette Co Pub Sch, **SLP**

Hughes, Nancy Lee 411 14th Street, Apartment N-10, Ramona, CA 92065, (619) 789-4600, SLP, Neurocare, **SLP**

Hughes, Mrs Nancy Marie 3204 West Germantown Pike, Norristown, PA 19403, (215) 539-3130, BA 81 Western WA Univ; MA 83 WA St Univ; SLP, **SLP**

Hughes, Pamela Jean 7160 Skillman #1624, Dallas, TX 75231, BS 82 Univ of WI - Milwaukee; MS 85 Univ of WI - Madison; **SLP**

Hughes, Patricia M 28 Ferry Street, Lawrence, MA 01841, BS 72 Northeastern Univ; MA 73 MI St Univ; Program Manager, MA UCP Assoc, **SLP**

Hughes, Mrs Patricia M 10 Spring Grove Street, Darien, CT 06820, (212) 379-4547, BS 77 Univ of MA - Amherst; MS 79 Columbia Univ Teachers Coll; 79–Sp-Lang Path, Citywide Speech Unit-NYC Bd of Educ, **SLP**

Hughes, Mrs Renee M 247 Louvett Street, Norfolk, VA 23503, BS 74 Old Dominion Univ; MS 78 Old Dominion Univ; Sp-Lang Path, VA Beach Cty Sch, **SLP**

Hughes, Mrs Sharon Kaye 1375 Metro Drive, Lebanon, PA 17042, (717) 274-3401, BS 84 Bloomsburg Univ of PA; MS 85 Bloomsburg Univ of PA; 86–Aud, Lebanon ENT Assoc, **A**

Hughes, Mrs Stacey B 241 West Main Street #205, Palatine, IL 60047-2351, (312) 395-0845, BS 81 Univ of IL - Urbana; MS 82 Univ of IL - Urbana; Sp-Lang Path, Antioch Sch Dist 34, **SLP**

Hughes, Mrs Suann 2612 Beaver Bend Drive, Plano, TX 75025, (214) 423-7440, BS 73 Northeast MO St Univ; MA 74 Northeast MO St Univ; Sp-Lang Path, Plano ISD, **SLP**

Hughes, Suzanne W 260 New Meadow Road, Barrington, RI 02806, (617) 675-7892, MS 80 Univ of RI; BA 76 Univ of RI; Sp-Lang Path, Plano ISD, **SLP**

Hughes, Vanessa 535 N Ridgeland Avenue, Oak Park, IL 60302, (312) 383-0700, BA 79 Mundelein Coll; MS 80 Bradley Univ

Hughes, Mrs Wendy L 4143 S Eloro Street, Las Vegas, NV 89121, (602) 978-6097, BS 68 Univ of CT; MS 71 Univ of OK Medical Center; Parent Adv, AZ at Sch for the Deaf & Blind, **SLP**

Hughes-Fenchel, Carolyn P 6120 Allan Drive, Woodridge, IL 60517, (312) 969-8607, MA 87 Northern IL Univ - De Kalb

Hughes-O'Sullivan, Jeanne M 19 Locust Avenue, Exeter, NH 03833, (603) 778-0934, BA 76; ME 79 Northeastern Univ; Sp-Lang Path, Portsmouth Pub School System, **SLP**

Hughey, Mrs Julianne C 5543 Ackerman Cove, Memphis, TN 38134, (901) 388-2152, BA 70 Western KY Univ; MA 71 OH St Univ; **SLP**

Hughley, Mrs Mary Michelle 107 Fourth Avenue, Columbia, MO 65203, (314) 442-3925, OB 85 Univ of MO - Columbia; OM 87 Univ of MO - Columbia; 88–Sp-Lang Path, Audrain City/Co Health Unit, **SLP**

Hugley-Priori, Martha Ann P O Box 682, Pittsburgh, PA 15230, (412) 232-7773, BA 75 Univ of Pittsburgh - Pittsburgh; MA 84 CA St Univ - Stanislaus

Huguet, Michelle 2205 Farrell Avenue #201, Redondo Beach, CA 90278, (213) 371-3830, BA 84 Univ of CA - Santa Barbara; MS 86 CA St Univ - Long Beach; 88–Sp-Lang Path, College Hosp, **SLP**

Huhman, Evelyn Nilges 405 Hutton Lane, Jefferson City, MO 65101, (314) 635-7141, BS 84 Univ of MO - Columbia; OM 86 Univ of MO - Columbia; **SLP**

Huhn, Mrs Kathleen L 4671 Katie Lee Way, Santa Rosa, CA 95403-1494, (707) 526-3160, BA 80 Univ of the Pacific; MA 81 Univ of the Pacific; Sp-Lang Path, Sonoma Co Dept of Ed, **SLP**

Huie, Mrs Nancy Eng 244 Senator Street, Brooklyn, NY 11220, (212) 732-0832, BS 81 Saint John's Univ - Jamaica; MA 83 CUNY - Queens Coll; 87–Sp-Lang Path, United Med Group, **SLP ACE**

Huisingh, Mrs Rosemary A 510 North 12th Street, Fulton, IL 61252-1912, (309) 762-5112, BS 70 Western IL Univ; MA 75 Western IL Univ; 85–Chief Operating Officer, LinguiSystems Inc, **SLP**

Hulbert-Wilson, Susan S 1640 Cascade Court, Jackson, MI 49203, (517) 787-8910, BS 72 Western MI Univ; MA 75 Eastern MI Univ; Sp/Lang Path, Jackson Inter Sch Dist, **SLP**

Hulett, Kelly Cavadel Route 1 Box 1180, Nicholson, GA 30565, (404) 757-2454, BS 85 Univ of GA; ME 86 Univ of GA; 88–Sp-Lang Path, Jackson Co Sch Sys, **SLP**

Hulit, Dr Lloyd M 1609 Barton Drive, Normal, IL 61761, (309) 438-5206, BS 67 Ashland Coll; MA 71 OH St Univ; PH 72 (NS) OH St Univ; 72–Prof of Sp-Lang Path & Aud, Il St U, **SLP**

Hull, Barbara B 24961 Calle Vecindad, El Toro, CA 92630, (714) 855-2043, BS 61 Washington Univ; MA 86 Wichita St Univ; 65–Sp-Lang Path, Private Practice, **SLP**

Hull, Mrs Christine Carter 412 Jerome, Marshalltown, IA 50158, (515) 752-1578, MA 84 Univ of IA; 85–Aud, AEA 6 Marshalltown IA, **A**

Hull, Mrs Corrine F 1500 Woods Road, Richmond, IN 47374, (317) 983-3000, BS 71 Miami Univ - Oxford; MA 72 Miami Univ - Oxford; 80–Sp-Lang Path, Reid Mem Hosp, **SLP**

Hull, Mrs Eileen M PO Box 144, 15 Colby Road, Danville, NH 03819, (603) 926-8788, BA 74 Salem St Coll; MA 75 Western MI Univ; 88–Sp-Lang Path, SAU #21, **SLP**

Hull, Mrs Johanna R 3 Canterbury Court, Toledo, OH 43606, (419) 536-6919, BS 74 Miami Univ - Oxford; MA 78 Eastern MI Univ; SLP, Private Practice, **SLP**

Hull, Mrs Joyce M 600 Abbey, Birmingham, MI 48008, (313) 494-9721, BA 59 Duke Univ; MA 78 Wayne St Univ; Sp/Lang Path, Rehab Inst, **SLP**

Hull, Karla M 23 Elmwood Road, Rutland, VT 05701-4639, (415) 436-0111, BS 74 4009; MS 76 4009; Dir Child Commun Ctr, Early Childhood Ed Ctr, **SLP**

Hull, Mrs La Donne Buck 505 Meadowcrest, Montgomery City, MO 63361, (314) 386-2214, BS 83 Central MO St Univ; MS 86 Central MO St Univ; 83–Sp-Lang Path, North Callaway R-I Sch Dist, **SLP**

Hull, Laura Kay 7340 Ethel Avenue #1E, St Louis, MO 63117, (314) 362-7489, BS 84 Univ of IL - Urbana; MA 86 Univ of IL - Urbana; **A**

Hull, Mary E 1937 Sheely Drive, Fort Collins, CO 80526, (303) 482-6795, BA 42 Wichita St Univ; MA 47 Wichita St Univ; **SLP LM**

Hull, Mrs Mary O'Shea 1600 Mill Creek Road #108, Jacksonville, FL 32211, (904) 744-4122, BS 80 Univ of VA - Charlottesville; MA 83 Univ of FL; SLP, Duval Co Pub Sch, **SLP**

Hull, Mrs Nancy D 22W147 McCarron Road, Glen Ellyn, IL 60137, (312) 858-8196, BS 73 Western IL Univ; MA 74 Northwestern Univ; 86–Sp-Lang Path, La Rabida Children's Hosp, **SLP**

Hull, Dr Raymond H Dept Of Communication Disorder, Univ Of Northern Colorado, Greeley, CO 80639, (303) 351-2734, BA 63 McPherson Coll; MA 64 Univ of SD - Vermillion; PH 71 (Aud/Neurophysiology) Univ of Denver; Prof -Dir of Aud, U of N Co/Dept Commun Dis, **SLP A F**

Hull, Robert A, Jr 2101 Gornto Road, Valdosta, GA 31602, (912) 333-5608, BS 69 Clarion Univ of PA; ME 75 Clarion Univ of PA; Asst Prof, Valdosta State College, **SLP**

Hull, Mrs Ruth Elmore 13941 Peach Grove Street, Sherman Oaks, CA 91423, (805) 251-2901, **SLP**

Hull, Virginia Anne 807 Jefferson Avenue, Memphis, TN 38105, (901) 525-2682, BS 80 Univ of Montevallo; MS 83 Univ of South AL; 86–Aud, Memphis Speech & Hearing Ctr, **A**

Hullen, Mrs Virginia B 232 West 42nd Street, Hialeah, FL 33012, (305) 822-0770, BA 64 Stanford Univ; MA 78 Univ of Miami; 78–Sp-Lang Path, Dade Co Pub Sch, **SLP ACE**

Hullihan, Mrs Michelle Martina 699 Norfleet Road, Atlanta, GA 30305, (404) 352-2962, BS 83 Southern IL Univ -Carbondale; MA 85 Saint Louis Univ; **SLP**

Hulme, Nancy A Slater 3096 Windrose Court, Chino Hills, CA 91709, (714) 624-9041, BA 76 CA St Univ - Fullerton; MA 79 CA St Univ - Fullerton; 88–Sp-Lang Path, Claremont USD, **SLP**

Hulse, Christine Jo 311 E Del Norte, Colorado Springs, CO 80904, (303) 471-9712, MS 86 CO St Univ; **SLP**

Hulsey, Carol J 114 Columbia Drive, Oak Ridge, TN 37830, **SLP**

Hulstine, Margaret M 824 South Santa Fe, Salina, KS 67401, (913) 827-5203, MA 75 Wichita St Univ; Sp-Lang Path, Kids Connection Dev Center, **SLP**

Hultz-Sheriff, Mrs Georgia Isdd, Indiana University, 2853 East 10th Street, Bloomington, IN 47405, (812) 335-0872, BS 76 Radford Univ; MA 78 Western IL Univ; Coordinator Program Prepare, Dev Training Ctr U of In, **SLP**

Hum, Mrs Carolyn C 3401 Bexhill Place, Kensington, MD 20895, (301) 942-4152, BS 72 Univ of MD - College Park; MA 74 Univ of MD - College Park; 86–Sp-Lang Path, Private Practice, **SLP**

Human, Mrs Carol A 3633 Saunders Settlement Rd, Sanborn, NY 14132, BS 67 SUNY - Coll at Geneseo; MS 70 SUNY - Coll at Geneseo; Sp-Lang Path, Orleans-Niagara BOCES, **SLP**

Hume, Dr Celia Bessel 6902 Haverhill Drive, Knoxville, TN 37909, (615) 588-3247, BS 71 OH St Univ; MS 73 Emory Univ; PH 84 (NS) Univ of TN - Knoxville; SLP, U of TN, **SLP**

Hume, Mrs Dayna Lisanne 23 Roosevelt Avenue, Leominster, MA 01453, (617) 792-8500, BS 83 Worcester St Coll; MS 85 Northeastern Univ; **A**

Hume, Dr William G 410 Wesley Road, Greenville, NC 27834-7132, BA 63 Trenton St Coll; MS 65 PA St Univ - Univ Park; PH 69 (NS) PA St Univ - Univ Park; Prof, E Carolina U, **A**

Humes, Dr Larry E 2003 Montclair Avenue, Bloomington, IN 47401, (812) 335-3507, BS 75 Purdue Univ - West Lafayette; MS 76 Central MI Univ; PH 79 (Audiology) Northwestern Univ; 86–Prof and Dir of Aud, Indiana Univ, **A**

Humlicek, Elizabeth Eledge 4561 Greene Avenue, Omaha, NE 68157, (402) 734-6040, BS 83 Univ of NE - Lincoln; MA 85 Univ of TX - Austin; Sp-Lang Path, **SLP**

Hummel, Karen S 331 Robin Way, Richardson, TX 75080, (214) 437-3119, **SLP**

Hummel, Lauren J 79B Pleasant Street, Plainville, MA 02762, (401) 434-3400, BA 76 Adelphi Univ; MA 78 Univ of CT; 85–Sp/Lang Path, Bradley Hosp, **SLP ACE**

Humphrey, Mrs Anita 1155 Old Monrovia Road, Apartment 5-D, Huntsville, AL 35806, BS 77 AL A & M Univ; MS 85 AL A & M Univ; 78–Head Start Dir, CAA of Huntsville

Humphrey, Brian D 432 Hamline Avenue South, St Paul, MN 55105-2943, (612) 293-8850, BA 72 Univ of Rochester; MA 75 Univ of MN - Minneap-St Paul; Sp-Lang Path, St Paul Schools, **SLP**

Humphrey, Cynthia T Ach Speech & Hearing Dept, 1820 Richmond Road S W, Calgary, AB, Canada T2T 5C7, (403) 229-7050, BS 67 Univ of MN - Minneap-St Paul; MA 68 Northwestern Univ; Sp-Lang Path Superv, Alberta Chldn's Hosp, **SLP**

Humphrey, Jane Ellen 2048 Lost Lake Place, Martinez, CA 94553, (415) 680-8891, MA; 83–Aud, CSG Hearing Services, **A**

Humphrey, Mary Lisa 4815 Mill Park Drive, Glen Allen, VA 23060, (804) 321-6666, BS 85 James Madison Univ; MS 87 James Madison Univ; **SLP**

Humphrey-Lahayne, Joan 14557 Mac Clintock Road, Glenwood, MD 21738-9626, (301) 854-6493, BA 80 Univ of MD - College Park; MS 81 Loyola Coll; Sp-Lang Path, Howard Co Pub Sch, **SLP**

Humphreys, Anita B HCR 64 Box 40, Thayer, MO 65791, (501) 625-7213, OM 86 AR St Univ; **SLP**

Humphreys, Paula Louise 2620 Meadowview Drive, Arlington, TX 76016, (817) 429-3573, BA 74 Roanoke Coll; MS 84 Univ of TX - Dallas; 87–Aud, Otology Consultants PA, **A**

Humphreys, Mrs Rita H 20 Silver Ridge Court N W, Calgary, AB, Canada T3B 4V5, (403) 270-3711, BS 68 Ithaca Coll; MA 69 Northwestern Univ; ME 78 Univ of Toronto - Ontario; 80–Sp-Lang Path, The Lrng Cen, **SLP**

Humphrey-Zika, Mrs Jean M 774 Trestle Glen Road, Oakland, CA 94610, BS 73 Southern IL Univ -Carbondale; MS 76 Southern IL Univ -Carbondale; **SLP**

Humphries, Mrs Patricia S 229 Ridgewood Court, Waconia, MN 55387, (612) 442-5321, BS 70 Univ of KS; MA 71 Univ of MO - Columbia; **SLP**

Hundley, Claire L Route 4 Box 257, Versailles, KY 40383, (606) 277-1949, BS 69 Vanderbilt Univ; MA 71 Univ of IA; Sp-Lang Path, Swigert & Associates Inc, **SLP ACE**

Hundley, Lucinda G 8 Campanero West, Irvine, CA 92720, BA 71 Univ of the Pacific; MA 72 Univ of the Pacific; Dir-Spec Educ, Santa Ana USD, **SLP**

Hund-Reid, Cecelia M 11427 42nd Avenue, Edmonton, AB, Canada T6J 0W2, (403) 437-7545, **SLP**

Hundt-Loss, Patricia A 1959 South 95th Street, West Allis, WI 53227, (414) 535-0300, BA 74 Univ of WI - Milwaukee; MS 80 Univ of WI - Milwaukee; SLP, Vna of Milwaukee, **SLP**

Huneke, Mary J 3040 Churchill Drive, Florissant, MO 63033, (314) 839-2099, BS 76 Southern IL Univ-Edwardsvill; MS 77 Southern IL Univ-Edwardsvill; Sp-Lang Path, Therapeutic Inter for Presch, **SLP**

Hunera, Darlene T P O Box 837, Oak Creek, CO 80467, BS 76 Bowling Green St Univ; MS 78 Miami Univ - Oxford; Sp-Lang Path, Horizons, **SLP**

Hungerford, Suzanne Mary 312 North 15th Street, Murphysboro, IL 62966, (618) 687-1638, BA 78 Southern IL Univ -Carbondale; MS 86 Southern IL Univ -Carbondale; Graduate Assistantship, Southern Illinois University, **SLP**

Hunker, Dr Chauncey Joseph 6612 Offshore Drive, Madison, WI 53705, (608) 263-2935, BS 72 Ball St Univ; MS 75 Bradley Univ; PH 84 (NS) Univ of WI - Madison; Sci, Dept of Rehab Med Univ of Wisc Med Sch, **SLP**

Hunnicutt, Darla Jo 991 River Drive #311, Kankakee, IL 60901-2274, **SLP**

Hunsberger, Deborah N 2436 Riverview Drive, Green Bay, WI 54303, (414) 497-3906, BS 77 Univ of WI - Stevens Point; MS 79 Univ of WI - Stevens Point; Sp/Lang Path, Green Bay Area Pub Sch, **SLP**

Hunsicker, Deborah Jane 55 Bargate Trail, Killingworth, CT 06417-1382, BA 83 Univ of CT; MS 86 Univ of NM; **SLP**

Hunsinger, Andrea S 401 37th Avenue N E, St Petersburg, FL 33704, (813) 823-6341, BS 74 WV Univ; MA 76 Univ of TN - Knoxville; 86–Sp-Lang Path, InSpeech Inc, **SLP ACE**

Hunsucker, Mrs Diann J RR 3 Box 1480, Cushing, OK 74023, (918) 225-3425, BS 76 OK St Univ; MA 79 OK St Univ; Sp-Lang Path, Cushing Pub Sch, **SLP**

Hunt, Mrs Aileen 2220 Densmore, Toledo, OH 43606, (419) 241-6219, BA 75 Ashland Coll; MA 77 Univ of Akron; Spec Proj Consultant, Toledo Hrng & Sp Cen, **SLP**

Hunt, Mrs Barbara Ann 810 Ninth Street Southwest, Rochester, MN 55902-6317, (507) 281-3424, BS 84 Univ of WI - Madison; MS 87 Mankato St Univ; 87–Sp-Lang Path, ISD #535

Hunt, Mrs Barbara S 921 Spanish Circle #332-E, Delray Beach, FL 33483, (407) 276-5212, BA 31 Univ of ME - Orono; ME 61 Univ of FL; **SLP LM**

Hunt, Deanna Johnson 17 Lateer Drive, Normal, IL 61761, (309) 454-3199, BS 64 Northern MI Univ; MS 65 Univ of MI - Ann Arbor; Sp-Lang Path, Private Practice, **SLP**

Hunt, Dr J Paul Northeast Missouri State Univ, Kirksville, MO 63501, (816) 665-8090, BS 65 Univ Southern MS-Hattiesburg; MA 69 Univ Southern MS-Hattiesburg; PH 70 (NS) Univ Southern MS-Hattiesburg; Aud, NE MO St U, **A**

Hunt, Mrs Jane Evelyn 11074 Manor Drive, Plymouth, IN 46563, (219) 935-5431, BS 83 Ball St Univ; MA 84 Ball St Univ; SLP, Joint Serv In Spec Ed, **SLP**

Hunt, Mrs Janeth Nash 707 I Street, Eureka, CA 95501, (707) 443-6638, BA 78 Univ of the Pacific; MA 84 Humboldt St Univ; 87–Sp-Lang Path, Private Practice, **SLP**

Hunt, Joanna Ruth 3816 Craighill Street, Lynchburg, VA 24502, (804) 528-6113, BA 82 Davidson Coll; MA 88 Univ of TN - Knoxville; 88–Sp-Lang Path, Central VA Training Ctr

Hunt, John Robert 79 Victoria Street, Revere, MA 02151, (617) 284-2251, MA 88 Univ of MA - Amherst

Hunt, Marline Elam 241 West Joseph Lane, Palmdale, CA 93551-2918, (805) 947-3627, BS 60 Northeast MO St Univ; MA 84 Northeast MO St Univ; 87–Sp-Lang Path, Los Angeles Co Office of Educ, **SLP**

Hunt, Mrs Mary Ida 4185 Wildwood Beach, Richland, MI 49083, BS 40 Western MI Univ; MA 65 Western MI Univ; Assoc Prof Emeritus, **SLP LM**

Hunt, Mrs Mary N 2616 Mesilla NE Suite 3, Albuquerque, NM 87110, (505) 881-1299, BA 70 Univ of Redlands; MA 72 CA St Univ - Los Angeles; Sp-Lang Path, Private Practice, **SLP ACE**

Hunt, Mrs Norma M 303 Bernard Drive, Warner Robins, GA 31093, BA 61 Wesleyan Coll; ME 62 Emory Univ; Sp-Lang Path, Houston County Board of Educ, **SLP**

Hunt, Mrs Sharon R Abingdon ENT Associates, 176 Valley Street, Abingdon, VA 24210, (703) 628-9547, BS 80 East TN St Univ; MS 81 East TN St Univ; Aud, Abingdon ENT Assoc, **A**

Hunt, Tracey L 52 Potawatomi, Urbana, IL 61801-2139, (217) 384-6089, BS 79 Central MI Univ; MA 80 Central MI Univ; Sp-Lang Path, U of IL Icbd, **SLP**

Hunt-Berg, Mary 1977 Hopkins Street, Berkeley, CA 94707, (415) 261-1343, BA 77 MI St Univ; MA 78 MI St Univ; Sp-Lang Path, Private Practice, **SLP**

Hunte, Frances 2400 South Fremont Avenue, Alhambra, CA 91803, BA 32 AZ St Univ; MS 43 Univ of Southern CA; **SLP LM**

Hunteman, Kathy L H 15 Daniel Street, Mooresville, IN 46158, (317) 831-8105, BS 77 IN Univ - Bloomington; MA 78 IN Univ - Bloomington; Sp-Lang Path, Mooresville Consol Sch Corp, **SLP**

Hunter, Mrs Ann E 55 Edgewood Drive, Mechanicsburg, PA 17055, (717) 766-4314, BS 77 Bloomsburg Univ of PA; MS 78 Bloomsburg Univ of PA; Sp-Lang Path, Polyclinic Medical Ctr, **SLP**

Hunter, Mrs Caroline J 308 Crestview, McPherson, KS 67460, (316) 241-1650, BS 75 Central MO St Univ; MS 76 Fort Hays St Univ; Sp-Lang Path, McPherson County Spec Ed Coop, **SLP**

Hunter, Carolyn Jean 15638 Southeast 90 Terrace, Summerfield, FL 32691, (904) 429-2533, BA 81 Univ of FL; MS 83 FL St Univ

Hunter, Deborah Chaney 1600 Race Track Road, New Bern, NC 28560, (919) 637-2329, **SLP**

Hunter, Mrs Donna J Speech/Language/Hearing Clinic, Western Washington University, Bellingham, WA 98225, (206) 676-3881, BA 71 Univ of Saskatchewan - Sask; MS 74 Minot St Univ; 86–Aud, Western Washington Univ, **A**

Hunter, Mrs Elaine J 119-16 103rd Avenue, New York, NY 11419, (718) 835-0711, BA 76 CUNY - Queens Coll; MA 77 NY Univ; 86–Sp-Lang Path, Bd of Educ City of NY, **SLP**

Hunter, Elizabeth Ann 72 Shore Road, Sydney Mines, Cape Breton, NS, Canada B1V 1B2, (902) 736-2831, BS 65 Purdue Univ - West Lafayette; MS 72 Syracuse Univ; MA 80 Bowling Green St Univ; Sp-Lang Path, Nova Scotia Hrng and Sp Clinic, **SLP**

Hunter, James L 11229 Walking Horse Lane, Charlotte, NC 28215, (704) 567-9916, MA 78 Univ of NC - Greensboro; Elb/Monitor Inc, **A**

Hunter, Mrs Janet L P O Box 236, Fairfax, MO 64446, (816) 686-3451, BS 74 Univ of MO - Columbia; MS 78 Bradley Univ; 88–Sp-Lang Path, Fairfax R-III Sch Dist, **SLP**

Hunter, Jenny Lynn 2149 E Sunshine #309-B, Springfield, MO 65804, BS 79 Southwest MO St Univ; MA 86 Southwest MO St Univ

Hunter, Mrs Joyce K 1774 Boulinwood Lane, Germantown, TN 38138, (901) 757-0595, BS 74 Univ of IL - Urbana; MS 75 Univ of IL - Urbana; Clinical Instructor, Memphis St Univ, **SLP**

Hunter, Mrs Judith P 4737 Bickford Avenue, Akron, OH 44319, (216) 644-7774, BA 66 Univ of Akron; MA 68 Univ of Akron; Sp-Lang Path, Timken Mery Med Ctr, **SLP**

Hunter, Margaret S 136 Flintfield Drive, Winston-Salem, NC 27103, (919) 788-8052, ME 79 Univ of NC - Greensboro; SLP, Winston-Salem/Forsyth Co Sch, **SLP**

Hunter, Marilyn B 1254 Armstrong Court, Derby, KS 67037, (316) 776-2142, BS 71 IN Univ - Bloomington; MS 72 IN Univ - Bloomington; Sp-Lang Path, Butler Co Sch Brd Council, **SLP**

Hunter, Mollie Annand 6471 N Tierra Catalinas, Apartment 72, Tucson, AZ 85718, (602) 299-7072, MA 76 Marshall Univ; 76–Sp-Lang Path, Tucson USD, **SLP**

Hunter, Patricia S 16312 Rambling Vine Drive, Tampa, FL 33624, (813) 968-1528, BA 74 5923; MS 79 Univ of South FL; Sp-Lang Path, Hillsborough Co Bd of Educ, **SLP**

Hunter, Mrs Sue Ann P O Box 823, Franklin, VA 23851, (804) 569-9425, BS 77 Bowling Green St Univ; MS 83 Old Dominion Univ; 87–Sp-Lang Path, Private Practice, **SLP**

Hunter-Morehead, Cindy L 1641 Southwest 37th Terr, #1028, Topeka, KS 66609, (913) 267-5468, BS 82 KS St Univ; MA 83 KS St Univ; Sp-Lang Path, Shawnee Heights Sch Dist, **SLP**

Huntington, Kathleen M P O Box 70, Oracle, AZ 85623, (602) 896-2403, Sp-Lang Path, **SLP**

Huntley, Jill Allison 326 West Walnut, Hastings, MI 49058, (616) 945-4412, BA 84 MI St Univ; MA 85 MI St Univ; 88–Sp-Lang Path, Grandville PS, **SLP**

Huntley, Jill E 8 Hillstar Court, Columbia, SC 29206, (803) 787-7547, BA 76 Columbia Coll; OM 77 Univ of SC - Columbia; Sp-Lang Path, Private Practice, **SLP**

Huntley, Ruth A Dept Of Communication Disorders, 6 Arnold House, Univ Of Massachusetts, Amherst, MA 01003, (413) 545-0131, BS 79 Univ of VA - Charlottesville; MA 81 Auburn Univ - Auburn; PH 87 (Experimental Phonetics) Univ of FL; Asst Prof, Univ of MA, **SLP ACE**

Huntley-Kraus, Nancy Ann McFarland Clinic, 1215 Duff Avenue, Ames, IA 50010, (515) 239-4480, MS 79 Univ of KS; Aud, McFarland Clinic, **A**

Huntress, Mrs Linda M 2350 Auburn Avenue, Suite 19, Cincinnati, OH 45219, (513) 784-0033, BA 64 IN Univ - Bloomington; MA 67 IN Univ - Bloomington; PH 87 (Sp-Lang Path) Univ of Cincinnati; 87–Sp-Lang Path, Private Practice, **SLP ACE**

Huntsinger, Marcy G 801 East Grant, Lebanon, OR 97355, (503) 451-5493, BS 51 Univ of MN - Duluth; MA 52 Northwestern Univ; OD 80 (NS) Drake Univ; Sp-Lang Path, Comm Home Health, **SLP**

Huntsman, Mrs Angela Abundis P O Box 69, Iona, ID 83427, (208) 525-4400, BS 73 ID St Univ; MS 86 ID St Univ

Hunt-Thompson, Jill Western Washington University, Parks Hall #25, Department SLP, Bellingham, WA 98225, (206) 676-3881, **SLP**

Huntzinger, Mrs Janet H 3265 Arroyo Road, Brookfield, WI 53005, (414) 679-1177, BA 56 IN Univ - Bloomington; MS 75 Univ of WI - Milwaukee; SLP, New Berlin Pub Schs, **SLP**

Hunyadi, Martha A 300 Battles Street, Brockton, MA 02401, (617) 587-2121, BS 75 SUNY - Coll at Fredonia; MA 76 Univ of TN - Knoxville; Rehabilitation Supvr, Brockton Visiting Nurse Assoc, **SLP**

Hunziker, Mrs Cheryl Copeland 221 Ringwood Avenue #22A, Pompton Lakes, NJ 07442, (201) 839-2332, BA 74 Montclair St Coll; MA 78 Montclair St Coll; 74–Sp-Lang Path, Wayne Board of Education, **SLP**

Huot, Germaine 4874 Cote Des Neiges #105, Montreal, PQ, Canada H3V 1H4, (514) 731-5252, MA 54 Northwestern Univ; 75–Consult, Cmsn Scolaire Ste Croix, **SLP LM**

Huotari, Mrs Janice Lynn 5440 West 98th Street, Los Angeles, CA 90045, (818) 986-1977, BS 81 Southern IL Univ-Edwardsvill; MA 84 CA St Univ - Los Angeles; Sp-Lang Path, South Pacific Rehab Services, **SLP**

Hupp, Randall 1435 Pacific Avenue, Laguna Beach, CA 92651-1928, (714) 494-2946, BA 74 CA St Univ - Chico; MA 76 CA St Univ - Chico; Sp-Lang Path, Private Practice, **SLP**

Huprich, Mrs Joann S S 270 Sterkel Boulevard, Mansfield, OH 44907, (419) 756-1133, BA 73 Univ of MI - Ann Arbor; MA 74 Western MI Univ; 81–Dir Phys Restoration Ser, Rehab Ser of N Cen Ohio, **SLP**

Hurd, Mrs Diane A 17 Andover Road, Hartsdale, NY 10530-2024, (914) 632-9000, MA 78 NY Univ; Sp/Lang Path, City Sch Dis of New Rochelle, **SLP**

Hurd, Joyce A E 5420 Pacifica Drive, La Jolla, CA 92037, (619) 273-1563, BS 62 Univ of Southern CA; SLP, San Diego City Sch, **SLP**

Hurd, Mrs Kathy Ann 7555 Timber Creek #4, Portage, MI 49002, (616) 329-4025, BA 81 Fort Hays St Univ; MS 82 Fort Hays St Univ; 87–Sp-Lang Path, Calhoun Intermediate Sch Dist, **SLP**

Hurd, Mrs Mary E 2550 Garland Street, Lakewood, CO 80215, BS 66 Univ of CO - Boulder; MA 71 Univ of CO - Boulder; **SLP LM**

Hurewitz, Mrs Karen Ellyce 2 Tedrence Drive, Englishtown, NJ 07726, (201) 446-1350, **SLP**

Hurlbert, Linda L 4728 East Oak, Phoenix, AZ 85008, (602) 838-6300, BS 75 AZ St Univ; MS 77 AZ St Univ; SLP, Mesa Pub Sch, **SLP**

Hurlburt, Skye 100 Grandview Avenue, Lincoln, RI 02865, (401) 728-0241, MS 88 Univ of RI

Hurley, Connie Lynn 16820 Pepper Lane, Brookfield, WI 53005, (414) 782-8791, BS 86 Univ of WI - Stevens Point; MS 87 Marquette Univ

Hurley, Mrs Holly Ann 3557 Collins Ferry Road, Apartment B33, Morgantown, WV 26505, (304) 293-4250, BS 82 Radford Univ; MS 83 Radford Univ; Aud, WV U Med Center, **A**

Hurley, Leah Ann 6308 Prospect #3, Dallas, TX 75214, (214) 827-9887, BA 75 Univ of MS; MA 76 Vanderbilt Univ; Law Clerk, Attorney General of Texas, **SLP**

Hurley, Margaret Rose 1659 South Riverstone Lane, Apartment 301, Boise, ID 83706-4062, (208) 345-3982, BA 85 Wichita St Univ; MA 87 Wichita St Univ; 87–Sp-Lang Path, Rehab Associates Inc, **SLP**

Hurley, Martin D 3549 Rutherford Road #159, Taylors, SC 29687, (803) 242-7713, BA 79 Marshall Univ; MA 80 Marshall Univ; Sp-Lang Path, Speech Hearing & Learning Center, **SLP**

Hurley, Mary M 4637 East Talmadge Drive, San Diego, CA 92116, (619) 281-4450, BA 69 Gonzaga Univ; MA 72 Univ of WA; **SLP**

Hurley, Michele 10928 Audelia Road #826, Dallas, TX 75243, (214) 270-0516, BS 85 Univ of OK - Norman; MS 87 Univ of North TX; 88–Aud, Ear Nose & Throat Med Ctr of TX

Hurley, Raymond Michael Dept Communicative Disorders, University Of Rhode Island, Kingston, RI 02881, (401) 792-5969, BS 66 Kent St Univ; MA 68 Kent St Univ; PH 75 (NS) Univ of MI - Ann Arbor; Assoc Prof, U of Rhode Island, **A**

Hurley, Robert Lee, Jr P O Box 169, Covina, CA 91724, (714) 599-8525, BA 60 Univ of LA Verne; MA 66 Univ of Redlands; Sp-Lang Path, Private Practice, **SLP**

Hurley, Mrs Wanda L 3032 Pascal Drive, Marrero, LA 70072, (504) 347-4741, BS 72 LA St Univ - Baton Rouge; MA 74 LA St Univ - Baton Rouge; Sp-Lang Path, Jefferson Parish Pub Sch, **SLP**

Hurley-Bularzik, Debra C 16 Golf Avenue, Clarendon Hills, IL 60514, (312) 354-5730, BA 77 Saint Xavier Coll; MA 78 Western MI Univ; 87–Sp-Lang Path, LaGrange Area Dept of Spec Educ, **SLP**

Hurley-Forget, Mrs Patricia Anne 15503 North Platte Drive, Bowie, MD 20716, (301) 986-8747, BA 83 Loyola Coll; MS 84 Loyola Coll; 88–Sp-Lang Path, Private Practice, **SLP**

Hurley-Sandell, Nancy Lee P O Box 28, Republic, KS 66964, (913) 361-2511, BA 80 KS St Univ; MA 82 Fort Hays St Univ; Sp-Lang Path, Private Practice, **SLP**

Hurley-Vangerud, Mrs Heather 3413 East Bermuda, Apartment 6, Tucson, AZ 85716, BS 76 Univ of AZ; MS 84 Univ of AZ; 88–Instr, Univ of Arizona, **SLP ACE**

Hurlock, Michael Thomas 71 Essex Park Drive, Hampton, VA 23669, (804) 727-7167, BA 78 Univ of VA - Charlottesville; ME 82 Old Dominion Univ; SLP, Hampton General Hospital, **SLP**

Hurni, Jill E 1929 Mary Street, Cadillac, MI 49601, (616) 775-8543, BA 71 MI St Univ; MA 76 Western MI Univ; Sp-Lang Path, Wexford Missaukee ISD, **SLP**

Hursala, Mrs Dafna 884 Surf Street, Lindenhurst, NY 11757, (516) 957-9274, MA 88 Long Island U - CW Post Ctr; 88–Sp-Lang Path, Variety Pre-School's Workshop

Hurst, Breta 21409 Greenbrier, Elkhorn, NE 68022, (402) 289-3090, BS 61 Ball St Univ; MA 63 Case Western Reserve Univ; **SLP**

Hurst, Dr Charles G, Jr 2322 Ladymeade Drive, Silver Spring, MD 20906, BS 53 Wayne St Univ; MS 59 Wayne St Univ; PH 61 (NS) Wayne St Univ; Prof, U of Lowell, **A F**

Hurst, Mrs June Manger 134 Queen Ann Road, Brick, NJ 08723, (201) 255-3125, MA 85 Trenton St Coll; Sp-Lang Path, Brick Twp Bd of Ed, **SLP**

Hurst, Karen Diane 2295 East Iliff #214, Denver, CO 80210, (303) 733-3780, BS 73 Ball St Univ; MA 78 Ball St Univ; **SLP**

Hurst, Kathleen M 6120 West Mississippi Pl, Lakewood, CO 80226, (303) 922-1404, BS 70 FL Atlantic Univ; MA 86 Univ of Denver; **SLP**

Hurst, Maria Antonietta 1507 Rugby Circle, Thousand Oaks, CA 91360, (805) 529-1149, BA 81 CA St Univ - Los Angeles; MA 84 CA St Univ - Los Angeles; **SLP**

Hurst, Nancy Ann Audiology Services, 404 University Avenue, Syracuse, NY 13210, (315) 428-0016, BS 82 Clarion Univ of PA; MS 84 Clarion Univ of PA; 87–Aud, Alan S Feldman PhD PC Aud Svcs, **A**

Hurstak, Jane M 30 Morrison Road, Braintree, MA 02184, (800) 922-8290, BA 83 Bridgewater St Coll; MS 85 Emerson Coll; **SLP**

Hurt, Jerri Johnson 6765 Yarrow Street, Arvada, CO 80004, (303) 556-4488, BS 75 Southwest TX St Univ; ME 76 Southwest TX St Univ; Sp-Lang Path, Univ of CO at Denver, **SLP**

Hurt, Mrs Linda Marie 1722 West Cape Rock Drive, Cape Girardeau, MO 63701, (314) 334-7173, BS 81 Southwest MO St Univ; MA 83 Southwest MO St Univ; Aud, SE Missouri ENT Consultants, **A**

Hurt, Mrs Rhonda K 2035 Emerald Crest Court, Chesterfield, MO 63017, BA 74 Fontbonne Coll; MA 76 Saint Louis Univ; Sp-Lang Path, Private Practice, **SLP**

Hurtig, Cynthia Ruth 10745 83rd Avenue, Apartment 207, Edmonton, AB, Canada T6E 2E5, (403) 422-0244, BS 80 Univ of Western Ontario; MA 84 Univ of Western Ontario; 82–Aud, Alberta Sch for the Deaf, **A**

Hurtubise, Gabrielle Marie 140-28 Quince Avenue, Flushing, NY 11355, (212) 430-0547, BA 85 SUNY - Coll at Oneonta; MS 87 Columbia Univ Teachers Coll; **SLP**

Hurtz, Mrs Kathryn S 34 North Hills Drive, Parkersburg, WV 26101, (304) 485-8679, BA 75 Univ of NE - Lincoln; MA 77 Univ of Houston - Univ Park; 88–Sp-Lang Path, Private Practice, **SLP ACE**

Hurvitz, Joel A Veterans Administration Medical Center, Audiology Department 126, 1611 Plummer Street, Sepulveda, CA 91343, (818) 891-7711, OB 62 CUNY - City College; MA 71 CA St Univ - Los Angeles; Aud, VA Medical Center, **A**

Hurvitz, Judith A 3705 George Mason Drive, Apartment 1404, Falls Church, VA 22041, (202) 675-7324, BA 66 Univ of MD - College Park; MA 67 OH St Univ; Sp-Lang Path, Hndcpd Chldn's Serv, **SLP**

Hurwitz, Mrs Diane Albert 9007 Avalon Drive, Richmond, VA 23229, (804) 741-8729, BA 74 0500; 87–Sp-Lang Path, Richmond City PS

Hurwitz, Mrs Jane S RFD 2 P O Box 295, Brookwood Road, Bedford, NY 10506, MA 71 Columbia Univ Teachers Coll; Sp-Lang Path, Private Practice, **SLP**

Hurwitz, Marcia Rogers 147 Henfield Avenue, Cherry Hill, NJ 08003, (609) 424-9428, BA 65 Temple Univ-Tyler Sch of Art; MA 81 Trenton St Coll; Sp-Lang Path, Private Practice, **SLP**

Hurwitz, Morton William 2691 N W 121st Drive, Coral Springs, FL 33065, (305) 344-5840, BS 64 SUNY - Coll at Fredonia; MS 68 Adelphi Univ; 88–Sp-Lang Path, Broward Co PS, **SLP**

Hurwitz, Mrs Renee Linda 571 Meadowland Avenue, Kingston, PA 18704, (717) 288-0727, BS 71 PA St Univ - Univ Park; MA 73 Temple Univ; Parent-Infant Prog Tchr, Scranton State Sch for Deaf, **SLP**

Huryn, Theodore F 621 Gordon Street, Allentown, PA 18102, (215) 776-3270, MA 75 Trenton St Coll; 85–Director, Good Shepherd Rehabil Hospital, **SLP**

Hus, Mrs Yvette 21 Crestwood Avenue, Montreal, PQ, Canada H4X 1N3, (514) 487-2763, BA 76 Concordia Univ - Quebec; MS 78 McGill Univ - Quebec; 88–Sp-Lang Path, Private Practice, **SLP**

Husa, Florence A Dept Communicative Disorders, Speech And Hearing Clinic, Northern Illinois Univ, De Kalb, IL 60115, (815) 753-1481, BS 52 Northern IL Univ - De Kalb; MA 71 Northern IL Univ - De Kalb; 74–Cl Assoc, Northern IL U, **SLP**

Husband, Susan 7 Oakwood Drive, London, ON, Canada N6K 2V5, (519) 657-9630, BS 74 Queens Univ - Ontario; OM 80 Univ of Western Ontario; **SLP**

Husby, Deborah Louise 1890 Newell Avenue, Walnut Creek, CA 94595, (415) 947-5859, BA 81 Univ of CA - Santa Barbara; MS 83 UT St Univ; Sp-Lang Path, Small Talk, **SLP**

Huschle, Mary Patricia Valley Childrens Hospital, 3151 North Millbrook, Fresno, CA 93703, (209) 225-3000, BA 81 Saint Cloud St Univ; MS 84 Univ of WI - Madison; Sp-Lang Path, Valley Childrens Hospital, **SLP**

Husemann, Mrs Diana A 324 Pinehurst, Sidney, OH 45365, (513) 492-3894, BS 73 OH St Univ; MA 74 OH Univ - Athens; Sp-Lang Path, Troy City Sch, **SLP**

Huseth, Nancy J 2457 Montgomery Avenue, Highland Park, IL 60035, (312) 234-5600, BA 61 Carthage Coll; MA 72 Northwestern Univ; 79–Sp-Lang Path, Lake Forest Hosp, **SLP**

Huskey, Marilyn R 20 Georgetown Green, Charlottesville, VA 22901, (804) 978-4031, BA 60 Univ of OK - Norman; ME 87 Univ of VA - Charlottesville; 87–Aud, Piedmont Reg Educ Prog

Huskey, Dr Robert L Special Sch Dist St Louis Cnty, 12110 Clayton Road, Town & Country, MO 63131, (314) 569-8222, BS 62 Southern IL Univ -Carbondale; ME 63 Southern IL Univ -Carbondale; PH 76 (NS) Saint Louis Univ; Assistant Superintendent, Spec Sch Dist of St Louis Co, **SLP**

Huskey, Mrs Sarah Farley 4270 Aloma Avenue #124, Suite 23A, Winter Park, FL 32792, (305) 677-5955, BS 78 Purdue Univ - West Lafayette; MA 82 Northwestern Univ; Aud, Private Practice, **A ACE**

Hussey, Deborah Heath 1809 20th Street N W #357, Washington, DC 20009, BA 85 George Washington Univ; MS 86 Univ of NC - Chapel Hill; **SLP**

Husted, Mrs Valerie Lynne 6788-1 Willowbrook Drive, Fayetteville, NC 28304, (919) 868-1347, OB 82 Univ of KS; MA 84 Univ of KS; Sp-Lang Path, **SLP**

Hustedde, Dr Carol G Department Of Audiology & Speech Pathology, Memphis State University, 807 Jefferson Avenue, Memphis, TN 38105, (901) 525-2682, BA 77 MI St Univ; MA 79 MI St Univ; PH 87 (Aud) Univ of WI - Madison; 87–Research Asst Prof, Memphis State Univ, **A**

Huston, Janet K 4207 Homestead Drive, Prairie Village, KS 66208, (913) 384-0059, BA 66 Univ of MO - KS City; MA 68 Univ of KS; SLP, St Lukes Hospital, **SLP**

Huston, Leona M 1011 Glen Avenue, Mount Pleasant, MI 48858, **SLP**

Hutaff, Mrs Susan East 523 Robin Drive, Monroe, NC 28110, (704) 527-5589, BA 78 Univ of NC - Chapel Hill; MS 83 Univ of NC - Chapel Hill; SLP, Charlotte Merklenburg Sch Syst, **SLP**

Hutcherson, Leslie Elaine 25 Proctor Court, Keene, NH 03431, (802) 885-5141, MA 81 CA St Univ - Fullerton; Sp-Lang Path, Springfield School District, **SLP**

Hutcheson, Deloris A 11245 84th Avenue #303, North Delta, BC, Canada V4C 2L9, (604) 638-0311, BA 78 Univ of Northern CO; MA 80 Univ of Northern CO; Sp-Lang Path, Min Hlth Div Sp/Hrng, **SLP**

Hutchings, Mrs Susan Lorraine RR2 P O Box 65 Site 208, St Albert, AB, Canada T8N 1M9, (403) 973-6477, BS 79 Univ of Alberta - Alberta; MA 81 Univ of MT; 81–Aud, Glenrose Rehab Hosp, **A**

Hutchings, Mrs Teresa C 7012 Escondido Drive, Arlington, TX 76016, ME 76 Southwest TX St Univ; 88–Sp-Lang Path, InSpeech Inc, **SLP**

Hutchins, Betty J Route 1, Geuda Springs, KS 67051, (316) 447-3242, BA 84 Wichita St Univ; MA 85 Wichita St Univ; **SLP**

Hutchins, Bradley Marianjoy Rehabilitation Center, Speech/Language Pathology & Audiology, PO Box 795, Wheaton, IL 60189-0795, (312) 462-4220, BS 79 Eastern MI Univ; MA 81 Eastern MI Univ; Dir Sp-Lang Path/Aud, Marianjoy Rehab Ctr, **SLP ACE**

Hutchins, Deborah D 16100 S W 87th Avenue, Miami, FL 33157, (305) 233-1266, OB 71 Univ of GA; MS 72 Univ of South FL; Sp-Lang Path, Private Practice, **SLP**

Hutchins, Jerilyn 3265 West Carefree Circle, Colorado Springs, CO 80917, (303) 596-7034, BA 81 Univ of CO - CO Springs; MA 82 Univ of CO - CO Springs; 88–Aud, Assoc in Otor, **A**

Hutchins, Mrs Kathryn J PO Box 215, Deer Harbor, WA 98243, (206) 376-5338, BA 70 Univ of WA; OM 71 Univ of WA; **SLP**

Hutchins, Lisa Anne 207 North Hills Drive, Apartment #4, McMinnville, TN 37110, (813) 275-9577, BA 85 Univ of TN - Knoxville; MA 86 Univ of TN - Knoxville; **A**

Hutchins, Mrs Mary M 2320 Braddock Road, Mount Airy, MD 21771, (301) 833-9300, BS 65 MT St Agnes Coll; MS 78 Loyola Coll; Sp-Lang Path, Bd of Ed of Balto Co, **SLP**

Hutchins, Mrs P Joan Route 2 Box 158-E, Gallatin, TN 37066, (615) 452-7009, BS 68 KS St Univ; MA 70 KS St Univ; Corporate Dir Rehab Therapies, Rebound Inc, **SLP**

Hutchins, Robin P 1425 Kensington Drive, Knoxville, TN 37922, BA 72 Univ of KY; MA 74 Memphis St Univ; **SLP**

Hutchins, Susan S 2763 South 1500 East, Salt Lake City, UT 84106, (801) 485-8713, BA 74 William Paterson Coll; MS 76 Univ of UT; Aud, Jordan Sch Dist, **A**

Hutchinson, Barbara J 3114 Terrace Linda Drive, Santa Rosa, CA 95404, BS 69 CA Univ of PA; MA 71 CA St Univ - Long Beach; Ch Program Specialist, Sonoma Co Offic of Ed, **SLP**

Hutchinson, Mrs Cheryl Schosek 13818 St Marys, Houston, TX 77079, (713) 493-6697, BS 74 Syracuse Univ; MS 80 Univ of NM

Hutchinson, Cynthia Baur 44 Bayview Avenue, Salem, MA 01970, (617) 745-9000, BS 75 UT St Univ; MS 76 UT St Univ; Sp-Lang Path, Lenox Hill Nursing Home, **SLP**

Hutchinson, Debra A 126 West Penn Street, Philadelphia, PA 19144, (215) 843-9450, BS 74 Ithaca Coll; MA 80 Temple Univ-Tyler Sch of Art; MA 80 Temple Univ-Tyler Sch of Art; 80–Sp-Lang Path, Camphill Special Schs Inc, **SLP**

Hutchinson, Dianna Ball 12 Rice Cove Road, Weaverville, NC 28787, BA 71 Univ of TN - Knoxville; MA 74 Univ of TN - Knoxville; **SLP**

Hutchinson, Mrs Dianne C 150 Hilltop Road, Oxford, OH 45056, (513) 529-2326, BS 66 SUNY - Coll at Geneseo; MS 67 SUNY - Coll at Geneseo; Instr/Cl Superv, Miami Univ, **SLP**

Hutchinson, Edward C Language Reading And, Exceptionalities, Appalachian State Univ, Boone, NC 28608, (704) 262-2185, BA 51 Hiram Coll; MA 55 Kent St Univ; PH 62 (Sp Science) OH St Univ; 77–Prof, Appalachian State University, **SLP F**

Hutchinson, Joan F 6672 Sims Drive, Oakland, CA 94611, (415) 351-7980, BA 76 Holy Names Coll; MS 80 Univ of San Francisco; SLP, San Lorenzo USD, **SLP**

Hutchinson, Dr John M Idaho State University, P O Box 8063, Pocatello, ID 83209, (208) 236-2362, BA 69 Univ of Redlands; MS 71 Purdue Univ - West Lafayette; PH 73 (Sp Path) Purdue Univ - West Lafayette; VP for Academic Aff, Idaho State U, **SLP**

Hutchinson, Julie Irene 603 Valerie Ruth Court, Santa Clara, CA 95050, (408) 246-4965, BS 84 Univ of CA - Santa Barbara; MS 87 San Francisco St Univ; **SLP**

Hutchinson, Lisa Katz 1232 Warwick Place, Allentown, PA 18104, (215) 395-0438, BS 77 CA Univ of PA; MS 80 Adelphi Univ; Sp-Lang Path, Cedarbrook County Home, **SLP**

Hutchinson, Pamela A 1701 June N E, Albuquerque, NM 87112, (505) 864-7799, BA 78 Loyola Coll; MS 79 Loyola Coll; Sp/Lang Path, Belen Consolidated Sch, **SLP ACE**

Hutchinson, Peggy Diane 5248 North Ridge West, Ashtabula, OH 44004, (216) 964-7111, OB 79 Cleveland St Univ; OM 85 Cleveland St Univ; 85–Sp-Lang Path, Ashtabula Soc Hndcpd Chldn Ad, **SLP**

Hutchinson, Mrs Tracy King Route 1 Box 1060, Silver Creek, MS 39663, (601) 886-7645, MS 87; 88–Sp-Lang Path, Monticello Elem Sch

Hutchinson, Mrs Valerie Jean 418 Hoover Street, Oceanside, CA 92054, (714) 559-0818, BA CA St Univ - Long Beach; MA 85 CA St Univ - Long Beach; **SLP**

Hutchinson-Clutter, Margaret L 1705 Potomac Place, Garland, TX 75042, (817) 267-1521, MS 83 Univ of TX - Dallas; 86–Research/Asst, Univ of TX SW Med Ctr-Dallas, **A**

Hutchison, Alice N 2702 South Compton Avenue, St Louis, MO 63118-1205, (314) 772-3477, BS 80 Fontbonne Coll; MS 81 Fontbonne Coll; President, Speech/Audi Services Corp, **SLP**

Hutchison, Donna M 803 North Fancher Avenue, Mount Pleasant, MI 48858-1521, (517) 773-7921, BS 77 Central MI Univ; MA 80 Central MI Univ; Clinical Supervisor, MI Dept of Ment Hlth, **SLP**

Hutchison, Kathleen 1242 Idylwild Drive, Lincoln, NE 68503, (402) 473-0278, BA 72 Univ of NE - Lincoln; MA 73 Univ of NE - Lincoln; Sp-Lang Path, Lincoln Pub Sch, **SLP**

Hutchison, Kathleen 2232 Belle Fontaine #11, Houston, TX 77030, (713) 790-5913, BS 80 PA St Univ - Univ Park; MA 82 OH St Univ; Aud, New Haven Hrng & Sp Cen, **A**

Hutchison, Mrs Leisa Smith Ohio County Board Of Education, 315 East Union Street, Hartford, KY 42347, (502) 298-3249, BA 84 Univ of KY; MS 86 Univ of KY; 88–Preschool Coord, Ohio Co Bd of Educ, **SLP**

Hutchison, Linda A 78 Creekport Drive, Columbia, KY 42728, (502) 384-6668, BA 62 KY Wesleyan Coll; ME 80 Univ of Louisville; 76–Sp/Lang Path, Adair Co Bd of Educ, **SLP ACE**

Hutchison, Lynne Michele 311 General Green Apts #C, Dover, DE 19901, (302) 674-3329, BS 85 Old Dominion Univ; MS 87 James Madison Univ; 88–Sp-Lang Path, InSpeech Inc, **F**

Hutchison, Mary Judith P O Box 344, Morrilton, AR 72110, (501) 354-3351, OM 83 Univ of Central AR; Sp-Lang Path, South Conway Co Pub Sch, **SLP**

Hutchison, Thomas L c/o Audiology Department, Naval Clinic Portsmouth, Portsmouth, NH 03801, BA 76 Kent St Univ; MS 77 Kent St Univ; Aud, US Dept of Defense, **A ACE**

Hutkoff, Mrs Emily I 8705 Hidden Hill Lane, Potomac, MD 20854, (301) 229-6111, BA 61 SUNY - Center at Buffalo; MS 65 CUNY - Brooklyn Coll; Sp-Lang Path, Montg Co Pub Schls, **SLP**

Hutson, Debra Kay 3300 South Tamarac Drive, Denver, CO 80231, (303) 879-0391, BS 80 Univ of ND; MA 81 Univ of MN - Duluth

Hutson, Grover Henry 27 Kingspark Drive, Maumelle, AR 72118, (501) 851-2215, BA 77 Univ of AR - Little Rock; MS 82 6901; 86–Dir of Aud, AR Ear Nose Throat Clinic, **A**

Hutson, Kathleen A Route 1 Box 94, Big Stone Gap, VA 24219, (703) 328-8017, BS 66 Saint Louis Univ; MS 72 Vanderbilt Univ; Sp-Lang Path, Wise Co Schs, **SLP**

Hutson, Mrs Patricia Fitzwillia 824 Seacrest Drive, Largo, FL 33540, (314) 962-8977, BS 67 Saint Louis Univ; MA 73 Saint Louis Univ; SLP, Spec Sch Dist St Louis County, **SLP**

Hutson-Nechkosh, Margaret Ruth 203 North Jones Street, Barneveld, WI 53507, (608) 935-3311, BS 81 Univ of WI - Madison; MS 82 Univ of WI - Eau Claire; 82–Sp-Lang Path, Dodgeville Sch Dist, **SLP**

Hutt, Donna Marie 3860 Davisville Road, Hatboro, PA 19040, (215) 295-1155, BA 77 Beaver Coll; MA 85 Temple Univ-Tyler Sch of Art; 85–Sp-Lang Path, Valley Day Sch, **SLP**

Hutt, Stephen Charles 9237 Dartford Road, Woodbury, MN 55125, (612) 738-2394

Hutterman, Lorraine G 625 Westridge, Idaho Falls, ID 83402, (208) 523-1967, BS 73 CO St Univ; MS 75 CO St Univ; Sp-Lang Path, Private Practice, **SLP**

Huttner, Mrs Sharon G Lang Sp & Myofunctional Thrpy, 65 River Road, North Haven, CT 06473, (203) 281-1098, BA 69 SUNY - Center at Buffalo; MA 72 SUNY - Center at Buffalo; Sp-Lang Path, Private Practice, **SLP**

Hutto, Brenda 3131 Homestead Road #5N, Santa Clara, CA 95051, (408) 272-7967, BA 71 Univ of AL- Tuscaloosa; MA 73 Univ of AL- Tuscaloosa; Sp-Lang Path, Cupertino Union Sch Dist, **SLP**

Hutto, Charles L 402 Hartman Drive, Severna Park, MD 21146, (301) 647-7795, BA 72; Pres, Chesapeake Hrng Cntrs Inc, **A**

Hutton, Dr Chas L, Jr Audiology & Speech Pathology, V A Medical Center (126), 1670 Clairmont Road, Decatur, GA 30033, (404) 321-6111, BA 49 Univ of Pittsburgh - Pittsburgh; MA 51 Univ of Pittsburgh - Pittsburgh; PH 54 (NS) Univ of IL - Urbana; Chief SLP & Aud Ser, VA Med Cen, **SLP A**

Hutton, Mary McCoy 277 East 15th, Eugene, OR 97701, (503) 687-2504, BS 77 Univ of OR; MS 86 Univ of OR; **SLP**

Hutton, Mrs Terri J 53 Coachlight, Little Rock, AR 72207, (501) 569-3155, BS 70 Marquette Univ; OM 71 Southern Methodist Univ; Instructor-Clinical Supervisor, Univ Arkansas Little Rock, **SLP**

Hutton-Johnson, Mrs Iona Irene 613 Benninghaus Road, Baltimore, MD 21212, (301) 789-6200, **SLP**

Hux, Karen Ann 1927-G Sherman, Evanston, IL 60201, (312) 869-5981, OB 81 MI St Univ; BA 81 MI St Univ; MA 83 MI St Univ; **SLP**

Huxel, Mrs Linda Noyes 3005 Corydon Road, Cleveland Heights, OH 44118, (216) 371-7230, BS 71 Kent St Univ; MA 76 Kent St Univ; 88–Sp-Lang Path, Cleveland Hts Univ, **SLP**

Huxtable, Susan J P O Box 229 R R 01, Old Stone House, West Winifield, NY 13491, (315) 822-6748, BS 66 Univ of VT; MA 74 Coll of Saint Rose; BS 66 Univ of VT; Sp-Lang Path, BOCES, **SLP**

Huzzard-Trombly, Deborah 2079 S Quintero Street, Aurora, CO 80013, (303) 320-2140, BA 80 Univ of MI - Ann Arbor; MS 82 Univ of MI - Ann Arbor; Sp-Lang Path, Rose Medical Center, **SLP ACE**

Hwang, Dora K P O Box 4344, Austin, TX 78765, (512) 926-2410, MA 73 Western MI Univ; Sp-Lang Path, Travis State School, **SLP**

Hyams, Mrs Sheila S 2324 Boston Road, Bronx, NY 10467, (212) 882-2035, BA 57 CUNY - City College; Sp-Lang Path, New York City Board of Educ, **SLP**

Hyatt, Bonnie D 1714 Woodmore Oaks, Manchester, MO 63011, **SLP**

Hyde, Caroline C Yarmouth Audiology, 18 Main Street, Yarmouth, ME 04096, (207) 846-3308, BA 73 Univ of PA; MS 75 McGill Univ - Quebec; Aud, Private Practice, **A**

Hyde, Mrs Eileen T 18625 West Cavendish Drive, Castro Valley, CA 94546, (415) 562-7788, BA 69 Univ of Redlands; MS 71 Univ of Redlands; Spec Day Class Commun Hndcpd, Amador Valley High Sch Dist, **SLP**

Hyde, Lawrence Dow P O Box 81, Charing Cross, ON, Canada N0P 1G0, (519) 352-0048, BS 78 Western MI Univ; MA 87 Univ of SD - Vermillion; **SLP**

Hyde Phd, Charlene J 10611 Wilkins Apts #3, Los Angeles, CA 90024, PH (NS); **SLP**

Hyder, Elizabeth 752 N Mission, Wichita, KS 67206, (316) 687-5239, BA 76 Wichita St Univ; MA 79 Wichita St Univ; SLP, **SLP**

Hyde-Smith, Mrs Jennifer 10007 Crestwood Road, Kensington, MD 20895, (301) 493-8395, BS 83 Brigham Young Univ; OM 85 Brigham Young Univ; **SLP**

Hye, Jane Linda 21-15 Fox Run Drive, Plainsboro, NJ 08536, (609) 734-4616, **SLP**

Hyink, Mrs Pamela J 271 South Cedarbrook, Boulder, CO 80302, (303) 443-6089, BA 71 Univ of CO - Boulder; MA 74 Univ of Northern CO; Sp-Lang Path, Private Practice, **SLP**

Hyland, Jennifer Denise 1218 Sweeney Drive #1, Middleton, WI 53562, (608) 267-6174, BS 84 Univ of WI - Madison; MS 86 Univ of WI - Madison; Sp-Lang Path, Meriter/Madison Gen Hosp, **SLP**

Hyland, Mrs Sandra Ann Colema U S Defense Attache Office, American Embassy Paris, APO New York, NY 09777, (703) 360-1997, BA 64 Univ of CT; MS 77 Univ of HI - Manoa; **SLP**

Hylander, Diana Jo 545 Elm Street, El Cerrito, CA 94530, (301) 270-1388, BA 75 MD Inst Coll of Art; OB 82 CA St Univ - Sacramento; MA 83 Univ of the Pacific; SLP, The Lab School of Washington, **SLP**

Hyman, AnnJoan 74 2nd Avenue, Apartment #4B, New York, NY 10003, (212) 505-6636, MA 82 New York Univ; 85–Sp-Lang Path, New York Sp Improvement Ctr, **SLP**

Hyman, Mrs Joy Anne K 5950 Airport Highway, Suite #17, Toledo, OH 43615, (419) 865-7500, BA 68 Parsons Coll; MA 75 Univ of Akron; Co-Director, Hyman Speech Lang Hearing Serv, **SLP**

Hyman, Dr Melvin 63 Back Bay Road, Bowling Green, OH 43402, (419) 865-7500, BA 49 CUNY - Brooklyn Coll; MA 50 OH St Univ; PH 53 (Sp Science) OH St Univ; Co-Director, Hyman Speech Lang Hearing Serv, **SLP F**

Hyman, Susan M 2020 Higgins Circle, Beaumont, TX 77706, (813) 366-9222, BA 78 MI St Univ; MA 78 MI St Univ; Aud, Dr George Swanson, **A**

Hymel, Susan Cassagne 245 Lakewood Drive, Luling, LA 70070, (504) 785-9031, OM 88 LA St Univ - N O Medical Ctr; Sp-Lang Path, Jefferson Parish Schl Bd

Hymes, Enid F U Of Rochester/Strong Mem Hosp, P O Box 629, 601 Elmwood Avenue, Rochester, NY 14642, (716) 275-4803, BA 71 Northern IL Univ - De Kalb; MA 77 Trenton St Coll; Sp/Lang Path, Strong Memorial Hospital, **SLP**

Hynes, Ann Maureen 7574 Buckingham #3, St Louis, MO 63105, (314) 391-5630, BS 74 Fontbonne Coll; MS 82 Fontbonne Coll; Sp-Lang Path, Sp Sch Dis of St Louis Co, **SLP**

Hynes, Ann P F 17 The Rise Mount Merrion, Co Dublin, Ireland, BS 76 Boston Univ; MS 79 Rutgers St Univ -N Brunswick; Sp-Lang Path, Central Remedial Clinic, **SLP**

Hynes, Patricia A 435 Dahlia, Denver, CO 80220, (303) 394-7691, BS 71 Saint Louis Univ; MA 73 Univ of Denver; **SLP**

Hyre, Mrs Noreen Marie 8783 Village Green Court, Alexandria, VA 22309, (703) 360-1539, BS 83 WV Univ; MA 84 George Washington Univ; SLP, Fairfax Cty Public Schools, **SLP**

Hyre, Rickey J 203 Lothrop Street, Pittsburgh, PA 15213, (412) 647-2030, BS 79 Indiana Univ of PA; MA 81 Univ of Pittsburgh - Pittsburgh; Aud, Eye & Ear Hosp, **A**

Hyter, Yvette Delaine 3511 Cambridge, Detroit, MI 48221, (313) 579-4400, BS 82 Western MI Univ; MA 84 Western MI Univ; Sp-Lang Path, Samaritan Health Ctr, **SLP**

I

Iacarino, Judith E 1010 Cecil Avenue, Millersville, MD 21108, (301) 321-4022, BA 68 CUNY - Queens Coll; MS 78 Towson St Univ; Cl Superv, Towson St U, **SLP**

Iacono, Mrs Jacqueline 40 Birchwood Drive, Narragansett, RI 02882, (401) 792-9652, BS 71 Saint Louis Univ; MA 72 Saint Louis Univ; Ed Diagn, S Kingstown Sch Dept, **SLP**

Iams, Judith L 5660 Bartlett, Klamath Falls, OR 97603, (503) 883-3621, BA 65 Univ of HI - Manoa; MA 69 Univ of TX - Austin; MA 84 Univ of MT; Sp-Lang Path, Klamath Falls City Schs, **SLP**

Iandoli, Dr Edward W Twin Lakes Apartment, 89-C Carriage Hill, Clifton Park, NY 12065, (518) 445-3713, BS 50 Univ of VA - Charlottesville; MA 52 Univ of VA - Charlottesville; PH 58 (NS) Syracuse Univ; Assoc Dir/Commun Dis, Albany Med Cen Hosp, **SLP A**

Ianni, Marilyn Annette 2326 East 31st Street, Davenport, IA 52807, (319) 359-1371, BS 75 Northern IL Univ De Kalb; MA 76 Northern IL Univ - De Kalb; Sp-Lang Path, MS Bend AEA, **SLP**

Ianuzzi, Mrs Gayle S 17 Meadowview Terrace, Fair Lawn, NJ 07410, (201) 791-3816, BA 77 SUNY - Center at Buffalo; MA 79 Hofstra Univ; Sp-Lang Path, Private Practice, **SLP**

Iarussi, Jane M R R 13 Box 240, Concord, NH 03301, (603) 783-9561, BS 78 Univ of NH; MS 80 Univ of NH; Program Coord, Laconia Develop Svcs, **SLP**

Ibarra, Claire Kimie 734 North 94th Street, Apt 1, Seattle, WA 98103, (206) 784-3761, BS 85 Univ of HI - Manoa; MS 87 Univ of WA; 87–Sp-Lang Path, Good Samaritan Hosp, **SLP**

Ibbotson, Candace Baumgart 508 End O Trail, Harker Heights, TX 76543, (817) 547-8282, MS 81 Baylor Univ; 87–Sp-Lang Path, Private Practice, **SLP**

Ice, Sonia G 100 1/2 Kendall Drive, Pauls Valley, OK 73075, (405) 238-2341, BS 85 Univ of OK - OK City; MS 87 Univ of OK - OK City; 87–Sp-Lang Path, Pauls Valley State Sch, **SLP**

Iceton, Mrs Mary Lou 7943 48th Avenue N W, Calgary, AB, Canada T3B 2A7, (403) 270-1611, BS 75 Western MI Univ; MS 84 Univ of MI - Ann Arbor; 84–Sp-Lang Path, Foothills Hospital, **SLP**

Ickes, Mrs Claire R 1404 Wakefield Road, Lynchburg, VA 24503, (919) 682-8970, BA 71 SUNY - Center at Albany; MA 80 Univ of NC - Greensboro; **SLP**

Ickes, Mrs Michelle Ann 1024 Cedar Terrace, Columbia, SC 29209, (803) 783-6726, Aud, VA Med Cntr, **A**

Ickes, Dr William K P O Box 4266 Tech Station, Lubbock, TX 79409, (806) 742-3908, BS 48 Univ of UT; MS 49 Univ of UT; PH 60 (NS) Southern IL Univ -Carbondale; 62–Prof Emeritus, TX Tech U, **SLP A F**

Ifft, Linda Marie 7007 23rd Avenue, Hyattsville, MD 20783, (703) 941-8903, BA 82 George Washington Univ; MS 84 George Washington Univ; 84–Sp-Lang Path, Annandale Fluency Cl, **SLP ACE**

Igel, Joyce Diane 3219 Mountview Road, Columbus, OH 43221, (614) 451-8437, BS 85 Miami Univ - Oxford; MS 86 Miami Univ - Oxford; 87–Sp-Lang Path, Columbus Speech & Hearing Ctr, **SLP**

Iglesias, Dr Aquiles Temple University, 118 Weiss Hall, Philadelphia, PA 19122, (215) 787-8537, BS 70 Southern IL Univ -Carbondale; MS 72 Southern IL Univ -Carbondale; PH 78 (NS) Univ of IA; Assoc Prof, Temple Univ, **SLP**

Iglesias-Golden, Mrs Olga 8827 S W 123 Court, Bldg 3 #101, Miami, FL 33186, **SLP**

Igrisan, Lori J 35136 Elmira, Livonia, MI 48150, **SLP ACE**

Ihara, Grace R 1380 Lusitana Street #209, Honolulu, HI 96813, (808) 524-1432, BA 65 Univ of HI - Manoa; MS 66 Univ of OR; Sp-Lang Path, Sp Path Consult & Serv, **SLP**

Ihnat, Ruthanne Melfi 8888 West 102nd Street, Palos Hills, IL 60465, (312) 798-1060, BS 80 Saint Xavier Coll; MS 82 Governors St Univ; SLP, Flossmoor II, **SLP**

Ihns, Mary J 323 Runaway Bay Circle, Apartment 1B, Mishawaka, IN 46545, (219) 258-0257, BS 85 Purdue Univ - West Lafayette; MS 87 Purdue Univ - West Lafayette; 87–Sp-Lang Path, St Joseph's Med Ctr, **SLP**

Ihrig, Karen R 9322 West Mount Vernon, Milwaukee, WI 53226, **SLP ACE**

Ihrig, Steve 612 Road 36, Pasco, WA 99301, (509) 545-6742, BS 74 Western OR St Coll; MS 75 Western OR St Coll; Sp-Lang Path, Pasco Sch Dist, **SLP**

Ihrke, Mrs Ann G R R 4 Box 91, Mokena, IL 60448, BA 64 Univ of IL - Urbana; 88–Sch Admin, Trinity Sch & Dev Ctr, **SLP**

Ike, Tami Lee Piedmont Hearing Aid Center, 518 N Hamilton, High Point, NC 27262, (919) 883-2815, BS 81 Radford Univ; MS 84 Radford Univ; 86–Aud/Mgr, Piedmont Hrng Aid Ctr Inc, **A**

Ikeda, Mrs Pamela F 130 Halenani Drive, Wailuku, HI 96793, (808) 244-9706, BA 74 Univ of Northern CO; MA 75 Univ of Northern CO; 78–Sp-Lang Path, St of HI Dept of Ed, **SLP**

Ikeuye, Colleen Teruko 617-F North Rural Drive, Monterey Park, CA 91754, MA 76 CA St Univ - Long Beach; BA 73 CA St Univ - Long Beach; SLP, Los Angeles Cty USD, **SLP**

Ikner, Cynthia Lewis Route 4 Box 48-C, Lewisburg, WV 24901, (304) 647-5235, 84–Aud, WV Sch of Osteopathic Med, **A**

Ikuta, Brenda Laurel 1570 Adelaide St North, Apartment 253, London, ON, Canada N5X 2L7, (519) 434-4219, 88 Univ of Western Ontario

Ikuta, Michele J 2080 Century Park East, Suite 108, Los Angeles, CA 90067, (213) 201-0731, BA 74 CA St Univ - Northridge; MA 75 CA St Univ - Northridge; Owner/Aud, Sn CA Hearing Services, **A**

Ilecki, Dr Henry J Royal Victoria Hospital, Speech & Hearing Division, 687 Pine Avenue West, Montreal, PQ, Canada H3A 1A1, (514) 842-1231, BS 66 SUNY - Coll at Buffalo; MA 67 Syracuse Univ; PH 74 (Aud) Univ of WA; Dir Sp & Hrng Div, Royal Victoria Hosp, **A**

Iler, Mrs Becky B 1082 South Ellen Circle, Orem, UT 84058, (801) 224-5812, BA 78 Brigham Young Univ; MA 81 Brigham Young Univ; Sp-Lang Path, Private Practice, **SLP**

Ill, Mrs Karen A 1098 Oceanic Drive, Encinitas, CA 92024-4005, (619) 944-0047, BS 79 San Diego St Univ, MS 81 San Francisco St Univ; Sp-Lang Path, Associated Speech Pathologists, **SLP**

Illerbrun, Dr David W 310-410 Main Street East, Saskatoon, SK, Canada S7N 0B8, (306) 665-8228, OM 65 Univ of Toronto - Ontario; MS 68 Minot St Univ; PH 74 Univ of IL - Urbana; Sp-Lang Path, Univ of Saskatchewan, **SLP**

Illich, David Michael Professional Hearing Assoc, 1045 East Valley Parkway, Escondido, CA 92025, (619) 489-6901, BS 77 Univ Southern MS-Hattiesburg; MS 79 Univ Southern MS-Hattiesburg; Owner/Dir, Prof Hrng Assoc, **A**

Illingworth, Barbara M 529 Middle Street, North Babylon, NY 11703, BS 69 IN Univ - Bloomington; MA 72 Hofstra Univ; OM 74 Long Island U - CW Post Ctr; SLP, Brentwood Pub Sch, **SLP**

Illsley, Sylvia Jasso P O Box 1178, Bodega Bay, CA 94923, (707) 664-6108, BA 75 Univ of CA - Los Angeles; OB 81 CA St Univ - Los Angeles; MA 85 Univ of San Francisco; Sp-Lang Path, Northcoast Rehab Ctr, **SLP**

Ilott, Dr Helen G University Of Alberta, 1-135 Education, Edmonton, AB, Canada T6G 2G5, (403) 432-5350, OB 62 Western WA Univ; ME 67 Western WA Univ; PH 87 (Educational Psychology) Univ of Alberta - Alberta; 80–Dir of Sp Ctr, Univ of Alberta, **SLP**

Ilseman, Mrs Carmen B 14635 Woodridge Circle, Brookfield, WI 53005, (414) 785-2188, BS 62 Northwestern Univ; MS 70 Univ of WI - Milwaukee; Sp-Lang Path, Elmbrook Mem Hosp, **SLP ACE**

Imada, Dr Dixie H 1555 Barnett Circle, Carmichael, CA 95608, (916) 486-9455, BS 75 Clarion Univ of PA; MA 76 Bowling Green St Univ; PH 79 (NS) Bowling Green St Univ; Cl Superv, CA St U Sacramento, **A**

Imes, Mary Ellen 313 Tulane Court, Grand Forks, ND 58201, (701) 772-2091, MS 84 Minot St Univ; **SLP**

Imhoff, Karen L 4201 Drew Avenue South, Minneapolis, MN 55410, (612) 457-7260, BA 74 Saint Cloud St Univ; MS 78 Univ of UT; Sp-Lang Path, Inver Grove Hgts Sch Dist 199, **SLP**

Imhoff, Susan H 1111 West Montana Avenue, St Paul, MN 55108, (612) 626-3369, BS 69 Univ of MN - Minneap-St Paul; MA 71 Univ of MN - Minneap-St Paul; Sp-Lang Path, Univ of Minn Hosp & Clin, **SLP**

Imhoff, Timothy E 11803 Bernardo Terrace, Apartment G-104, San Diego, CA 92128, (715) 836-4905, BS 78 Univ of WI - Madison; MA 79 Univ of IA; Inst/Cl Super-Dept of Comm Dis, U of WI, **SLP ACE**

Imhoff-Smith, Georgia Ellen 2801 Brandon Road, Madison, WI 53719, (608) 273-9594, MS 84 Western OR St Coll; **SLP**

Imizu-Iwanaga, Darlene 5072 Pine Circle, La Palma, CA 90623, (714) 739-0269, BA 73 Univ of CA - Los Angeles; MA 80 Whittier Coll; **SLP**

Immer, Valerie J 5823 Filbert, Orangevale, CA 95662, (916) 685-9549, BA 77 CA St Univ - Chico; MA 79 CA St Univ - Chico; Sp-Lang Path, Elk Grove USD, **SLP**

Impey, Gillian M 679 Prospect Avenue, Little Silver, NJ 07739, **SLP**

Inamasu, Laura T 6700 Warner Avenue #5-D, Huntington Beach, CA 92647, (818) 962-3311, BA 73 Univ of CA - Irvine; Sp-Lang Path, Baldwin Park USD, **SLP**

Inbar, Mrs Betsy L 4438 Meadowcreek Circle, Sarasota, FL 34233, (813) 923-2012, BS 74 Boston Univ; MA 77 Case Western Reserve Univ; Sp-Lang Path, Private Practice, **SLP**

Indresano, Susan L 114 Front Street, Marblehead, MA 01945, (617) 631-2202, BS 65 Boston Univ; ME 68 Boston Univ; Sp-Lang Path, Salem Visiting Nurse Assn, **SLP**

Indursky, Beatrice 25 Tudor City Place #707, New York, NY 10017, BS 63 Syracuse Univ; MA 65 Stanford Univ; **A ACE**

Infante, Alicia Anne 8 Mackenzie Court, Bowling Green, OH 43402, (419) 353-3148, BA 84 SUNY - Coll at Plattsburgh; MS 86 Bowling Green St Univ; 88–Instr, Henry Co Bd of Men Ret & Dev Dis, **SLP**

Ingalls, Patricia M Highlands Hearing Center, 1369 Harrison Avenue, Butte, MT 59701, (406) 723-4373, BA 69 WA St Univ; MS 76 Univ of NM; Aud/Owner, Private Practice, **A ACE**

Ingberman, Jeanne Ellen 436 Prospect Street #5, Lakewood, NJ 08701, (201) 370-1438, MA 88 Univ of MD - College Park; 88–Aud, The Hearing Laboratory Inc

Ingebo, Mrs Mildred H Box 85, Apartment C-3, Crosby, ND 58730, (701) 965-6792, BS 64 Mankato St Univ; MS 71 Minot St Univ; Sp-Lang Path, Divide Co Sch Dist 1, **SLP**

Ingels, Ginger L 2205 New Garden Road #1902, Greensboro, NC 27410, (919) 282-7693, BA 84 San Jose St Univ; MA 86 San Jose St Univ; 86–Grad Researcher Asst, Univ of North Carolina

Ingenito, Debra J 2 Sunrise Drive, Kingston, MA 02364, (617) 585-8479, MS 88 Northeastern Univ; 88, Northeastern Univ

Ingersoll, Mary J 55-6 Thompson Street #D, East Haven, CT 06513, (203) 783-3410, BA 75 Southern CT St Univ; MS 78 Southern CT St Univ; Sp/Lang Path, Milford Publ Schs, **SLP**

Ingersoll, Solveig H 10703 Meadowhill Road, Silver Spring, MD 20901, (301) 949-8070, BA 69 George Washington Univ; MA 67 George Washington Univ; Dir, The Hearing Center, **A**

Ingerson, Mrs Linda Leigh 14708 Northeast 40th St, Apt S-104, Bellevue, WA 98007, (206) 869-1542, BA 84 Minot St Univ; MS 86 Minot St Univ; 88–Sp-Lang Path, Shoreline PS, **SLP**

Ingham, Dr Janis Costello Speech And Hearing Center, University Of California, Santa Barbara, CA 93106, (805) 961-2249, BS 64 Northwestern Univ; MA 66 Univ of KS; PH 69 (NS) Univ of KS; Prof, U of CA-Santa Barbara, **SLP F**

Ingham, Dr Roger J 1947 Eucalyptus Hill Road, Santa Barbara, CA 93108, (805) 961-2776, BS 66 Univ New So Wales-Australia; PH 72 (Psychology) Univ New So Wales-Australia; Chairperson and Prof, U of CA Santa Barbara, **F**

Ingison, Mrs Dianna Scott P O Box 17, Manchester Village, VT 05254, (802) 362-1878, BS 85 Bradley Univ; MS 86 Univ of VT; Sp-Lang Path, **SLP**

Ingle, Mrs Bobbie H 1118 Trevino Drive N E, Roanoke, VA 24019, (703) 387-6520, BA 73 Marshall Univ; MS 81 Radford Univ; Aud, Roanoke County Schs, **A**

Ingle, Catherine D Route 9 Box 103, Apartment C, Morgantown, WV 26505, (304) 291-0863, BS 83 WV Univ; MS 86 WV Univ; 87–Aud, T F Hall MD Fairmont ENT Assoc Inc, **A ACE**

Inglebret, Ella R 305 East Fifth, Moscow, ID 83843, (208) 799-3460, BA 75 Univ of MN - Duluth; MA 85 Univ of MT; 83–Sp-Lang Path, Adlt/Chld Develop Cen, **SLP**

Inglis, Mrs Beverly Shank 6727 Glenkirk Road, Baltimore, MD 21239, (301) 821-1088, BS 75 East Stroudsburg Univ of PA; MA 81 Trenton St Coll; 88–Sp-Lang Path, The Hannah More Center, **SLP**

Inglis, Joanne M 242 Elm Street, Winnipeg, MB, Canada R3M 3P2, (204) 284-1159, BA 75; MS 77 UT St Univ; Sp/Lang Path, St Boniface Hosp, **SLP**

Inglis, Mrs Marjorie K 1338 Poplar Estates Pkwy, Germantown, TN 38138, (901) 767-8333, BS 67 Boston Univ; MA 68 Columbia Univ Teachers Coll; Sp-Lang Path, Private Practice, **SLP**

Inglis, Robert H, Jr 10874 Mogadore Avenue, Uniontown, OH 44685, (216) 535-1300, BS 67 Youngstown St Univ; MA 74 Univ of Akron; Ind Hygienist, American Analytical Lab Inc, **A**

Inglisa-Vernetti, Mrs Marylou Joan 13915 Turnmore Road, Silver Spring, MD 20906, (301) 460-0833, MA 88 George Washington Univ

Ingmire, Mrs Janet U 522 Tanglewood Lane, Frankfort, IL 60423, (815) 469-1055, BS 71 Univ of NE - Lincoln; MA 73 Univ of KS; Sp-Lang Path, Frankfort Sch Dist 157C, **SLP**

Ingmire, Susan M P O Box 1261, Columbus, IN 47202, (812) 379-9386, BS 73 IN Univ - Bloomington; MA 75 IN Univ - Bloomington; 84–Priv Practioner, Private Practice, **SLP**

Ingraham, Mrs Velda Chemise 13907 Citrus Pointe Dr, Tampa, FL 33625, (904) 588-2210, MS 85 Univ of South FL; **SLP**

Ingraldi, Cynthia Ann 66 Woodcrest Avenue, Bridgeton, NJ 08302, (201) 289-4877, BA 85 Kean Coll of NJ; MA 86 Kean Coll of NJ; **SLP**

Ingram, Dr Beth A 134 North Moon Avenue, Brandon, FL 33511, (813) 681-5958, BA 68 OK St Univ; MS 71 Univ of OK Medical Center; Instr, Univ of S FL, **SLP**

Ingram, Mrs Catherine 3128 Grandview Boulevard, Los Angeles, CA 90066, (213) 390-2330, BA 75 Humboldt St Univ; MS 76 Ithaca Coll; Sp-Lang Path, Private Practice, **SLP**

Ingram, Dr David B 855 Mimosa, Oviedo, FL 32765, (305) 365-8730, BA 62 Western MI Univ; MS 66 Western MI Univ; PH 73 (NS) SUNY - Coll at Buffalo; Associate Professor, University of Central Florida, **SLP**

Ingram, Mrs Glenda Christine 204 East Holden, St Louis, MO 63125, (314) 544-2420, BS 80 Fontbonne Coll; MS 85 Fontbonne Coll; **SLP**

Ingram, James E 910 Pine Tree, Lake Orion, MI 48035, (313) 644-9300, BS 58 Northwestern Univ; ME 61 Wayne St Univ; Sp-Lang Path, Birmingham Public Schools, **SLP**

Ingram, Judith L S 3927 Windsor, Youngstown, OH 44512, **SLP**

Ingram, June M 5336 Kennedy Street, Columbus, GA 31907, MS 71 Univ of NE - Lincoln; Assistant Professor, Grambling State University, **SLP**

Ingram, Mrs Linda Liggett P O Box E, Catlin, IL 61817, (217) 427-5275, BS 65 Univ of IL - Urbana; MA 87 Univ of IL - Urbana

Ingram, Maria M 900 Calle DE Los Amigos, Apartment N3, Santa Barbara, CA 93105, (805) 687-5486, BA 29 PA St Univ - Univ Park; MA 55 CA St Univ - Fresno; **SLP LM**

Ingram, Mrs Nancy Murrow 4607-C East 93rd Court S, Tulsa, OK 74137, (918) 496-9251, BS 77 Southern Methodist Univ; MS 79 Baylor Coll of Medicine; Aud, Cty of Faith Med & Res Cen, **A**

Ingram, Rebecca Vinson P O Box 942, Troy, AL 36089-0942, (205) 566-6343, **SLP**

Ingram, Mrs Renee Morris 4441 Bay Villa Avenue, Tampa, FL 33611, (813) 831-2667, MS 84 Univ of South FL; 87–Sp-Lang Path, Sch Bd of Hillsborough Co, **SLP**

Ingram-Colotti, Mrs Allison 19-F Ari Drive, Somerset, NJ 08873, (201) 297-8902, BA 81 Rutger's St Univ - Douglas Coll; MS 82 Rutgers St Univ -N Brunswick; Sp-Lang Path, NJ St Trng Sch for Boys, **SLP**

Ingrisano, Dr Dennis R S Dept Communication Disorders, Univ Of Northern Colorado, Greeley, CO 80639, (303) 351-2734, BS 69 De Paul Univ; ME 71 PA St Univ - Univ Park; PH 78 (NS) IN Univ - Bloomington; Faculty, Univ of Northern Colorado, **SLP**

Ingrosso, Diana Chedoke-McMaster Hospital, Speech Dept Evel 1 Box 2000 Station A, 1200 Main Street West, Hamilton, ON, Canada L8N 3Z5, (416) 522-4941, MA 87 SUNY - Center at Buffalo; Sp-Lang Path, Chedoke-McMaster Hosp, **SLP**

Ingve, Kathleen Jane 1666 South Laredo Street, Aurora, CO 80017, (303) 861-5881, BS 84 Univ of WY; MS 86 Univ of WY; **A**

Inkles, Mrs Sharon M 47 Eastwood Lane, Valley Stream, NY 11581-2427, (516) 791-5980, BA 80 Adelphi Univ; MS 81 Adelphi Univ; **SLP**

Inkmann, Mrs Constance Marie 1460 Edgehill Lane, Redlands, CA 92373, BA 66 Marquette Univ; MS 81 Univ of Redlands; Sp-Lang Path, San Bernardino Comm Hosp, **SLP**

Inman, Mrs Denise Elaine 10962 East Vassar Drive, Aurora, CO 80014, (303) 428-0637, BA 79 San Francisco St Univ; MS 81 4689; Sp-Lang Path, Cherry Creek School District, **SLP**

Inman, Dr Margaret A Providence Speech & Hrng Ctr, 1301 Providence Avenue, Orange, CA 92668, (714) 639-4990, BA 36 Saint Mary-of-the-Woods Coll; MS 65 Marquette Univ; PH 81 (Learning Disabilities) Univ of Beverly Hills; Executive Director, Providence Speech & Hrng Cen, **SLP**

Inman, Nancy L 1005 Leighsford Lane, Apartment 10305, Arlington, TX 76006, BA 78 Univ of NC - Chapel Hill; MA 80 IN Univ - Bloomington; Sp-Lang Path, Child Study Center, **SLP**

Inman-Ebel, Mrs Beverly 842 South Germantown Road, Chattanooga, TN 37412, (615) 622-8255, BS 75 Univ of TN - Knoxville; MA 77 Univ of TN - Knoxville; Sp-Lang Path, Communication Clinic, **SLP**

Innerst, Mrs Shari Lynn 650 Chronister Street, York, PA 17402, (717) 755-6035, BS 85 Bloomsburg Univ of PA; MS 86 Bloomsburg Univ of PA; SLP, Mechanicsburg Rehab Cntr, **SLP**

Innes, Mary R 19 Harvest Hill, West Simsbury, CT 06092, BA 71 Boston Coll; MS 74 Boston Univ; **SLP**

Inniss, Melissa Elvira 172-20 133rd Avenue #12B, Jamaica, NY 11434, (212) 899-8800, BA 81 CUNY - Queens Coll; MS 83 Columbia Univ Teachers Coll; Audiologist, Lexington Hearing/Speech Ctr, **A**

Inouye, Mrs Karen Gail T 4264 Pepper Avenue, Yorba Linda, CA 92686, (714) 591-3129, BA 74 Univ of CA - Santa Barbara; MA 80 CA St Univ - Los Angeles; SLP, Chino USD, **SLP**

Insalaco, Deborah Michelle 116 Homestead Avenue, Albany, NY 12203, (518) 458-2604, BS 77 SUNY - Center at Albany; MS 85 Coll of Saint Rose; **SLP**

Inseth, Bette J 417 South Rodney #4, Helena, MT 59601, (406) 449-2590, BS 73 Portland St Univ; MS 75 Portland St Univ; Aud, Montana Developmental Center, **A**

Insler-Gross, Mrs Marilyn A 79-24 260th Street, Floral Park, NY 11004, (718) 377-8845, BA 76 CUNY - Hunter Coll; MA 78 CUNY - Queens Coll; SLP, NYC Bd of Ed, **SLP**

Iola, Judith Elaine 7839 South Gary Place, Tulsa, OK 74136, (918) 496-3451, BS 83 OK St Univ; MA 84 Univ of Tulsa; **SLP**

Ionin, Mrs Joyce M 24 Marigold Lane, Marlboro, NJ 07746, (201) 780-1241, BA 74 CUNY - Brooklyn Coll; MS 77 CUNY - Brooklyn Coll; Sp-Lang Path, Monmouth County Educ Svc Comm, **SLP**

Ip, Lai-Fan Renee 2825 South King Street, Apartment 1802, Honolulu, HI 96826, (808) 949-6382, BA 84; MS 87 Univ of HI - Manoa; **SLP**

Ipsen, Mrs Peggy Loretta 15238 Stradbrook Drive, Houston, TX 77062, (713) 486-7547, OM 76 Brigham Young Univ; **SLP**

Irby, Mrs Rachel Ragsdale 1435 Holiday Place, New Orleans, LA 70131, (504) 366-5572, BS 76 Univ of TN - Knoxville; MA 78 Memphis St Univ; 88–Research Assoc, Kresge Hearing Research Lab, **A**

Ireland, Jerry V 823 Prentice Road N W, Warren, OH 44481, (216) 841-3700, BS 73 Kent St Univ; MA 76 Kent St Univ; 79–Sp-Lang Path, Hillside Hosp, **SLP**

Ireland, JoAnn Chirakos 189 Brookside, Akron, OH 44301, (216) 929-6634, MA 85 Univ of Akron; Aud, MEO/SERRC, **A**

Ireland, Nancy D 5722 Field Street, Arvada, CO 80002, **SLP**

Ireland, Nancy E 85 Valleyview Drive, Westfield, MA 01085, (413) 568-6978, BS 82 Northern IL Univ - De Kalb; MA 84 Northern IL Univ - De Kalb; 85–Sp-Lang Path, Douglas A Thom Clinic, **SLP**

Ireland, Mrs Peggy G 3535 Constitution Court, Cincinnati, OH 45248, (513) 574-3397, BS 77 Univ of Cincinnati; MS 79 Miami Univ - Oxford; Sp-Lang Path, Cincinnati Bd of Educ, **SLP**

Irey, Linda 355 Hartman Drive, Severna Park, MD 21146, (301) 766-3390, BA 73 Univ of MD - College Park; MS 76 Towson St Univ; SLP, Anne Arundel Co Pub Sch, **SLP**

Irion, Loretta Snyder 53 Harrow Road, Levittown, PA 19056, (215) 750-2224, St Marys Hospital, **SLP**

Irish, Mrs Patricia White Sunland Center, Audiology Department, P O Box 1150, Gainesville, FL 32602, (904) 395-1793, BA 82 Univ of FL; MA 84 Univ of FL; Audiologist, Sunland Center, **A**

Irla, Joni 29075 Spoon, Madison Heights, MI 48071, (313) 399-8753, BA 80 Wayne St Univ; MA 82 Wayne St Univ; Sp-Lang Path, Mt Carmel Hosp, **SLP**

Irmen, Antonia Sares 1833 S Holland-Sylvania Rd, Maumee, OH 43537, (419) 866-6633, OB 81 Univ of Toledo; BA 81 Univ of Toledo; MS 86 Bowling Green St Univ; 82–Sp-Lang Path, Whiteford Agricultural Sch, **SLP**

Irons, Mrs Patricia Lynn 1322 Dominion, Katy, TX 77450-4310, (713) 558-7270, **SLP**

Irons, Susan K 5412 Treebound Court, Garner, NC 27529, (919) 779-8876, BA 78 Dana Coll; MA 81 Univ of NE - Lincoln; 87–Sp-Lang Path, Wake Co PS, **SLP**

Irvin, E C 2411 Nicholson Road, Sewickley, PA 15143, **SLP**

Irvin, Mrs Elaine H P O Box 902, Cornelia, GA 30531, (404) 778-9608, BS 77 Univ of GA; ME 78 GA St Univ; 81–Admin, Sp&Lang Path Sers, **SLP**

Irvin, Howard Van P O Box 507, 404 E Wilson Street, Fountain, NC 27829, (919) 749-6001, BS 76 Univ of CA - Davis; MS 82 Brigham Young Univ; 85–Sp-Lang Path, MultiCom, **SLP**

Irvin, Merle J 7962 Camino Tranquilo, San Diego, CA 92122, (619) 483-2986, BS 68 Univ of WI - Madison; MS 69 Univ of WA; 88–Sp-Lang Path, West Coast Sp Lang & Cognitive Ctr, **SLP**

Irvin, Mrs Susan Hegel 10221 N E Mattey Lane, McMinnville, OR 97128, (303) 753-9339, MS 83 CO St Univ; Coordinator Childrens Programs, Salem Speech & Language Center, **SLP**

Irving, Deborah A 713 Arno S E, Albuquerque, NM 87102, (505) 877-1278, BA 75 MI St Univ; MS 82 Univ of NM; MA 80 Univ of NM; Sp-Lang Path, Albuquerque Pub Sch, **SLP**

Irving, Mary Manzione 4655 Country Vale Court, Annandale, VA 22003, (703) 451-3985, BS 84 James Madison Univ; MS 86 Univ of UT; 88–Sp-Lang Path, Fairfax County PS, **SLP**

Irving, Susan Elizabeth 20 Riverside Street Apartment 27, Watertown, MA 02172, (716) 283-9295, BS 85 SUNY - Coll at Geneseo; MA 87 SUNY - Center at Buffalo; 88–Sp-Lang Path, New England Rehab Hosp, **SLP**

Irwin, Dr David L Dept Of Communication Arts, Northeast Louisiana Univ, Monroe, LA 71209-0320, (318) 342-3052, BS 75 Central MO St Univ; MS 76 Central MO St Univ; PH 83 (Sp-Lang Path) Univ of OK Medical Center; Dir of SLP & Hrng, NE LA Univ, **SLP ACE**

Irwin, Mrs Dina Minish 875 Stevens Street, #2311, Solana Beach, CA 92075, (619) 481-9632, BA 86 San Diego St Univ; MA 87 Univ of the Pacific; 87–Sp-Lang Path, Vista USD, **SLP**

Irwin, James Ross Travis Park Plaza Bd, 711 Navarro, Suite 204, San Antonio, TX 78205-1710, BA 67 Univ of TX - Austin; MA 79 Univ of TX - El Paso; Aud-Managing Dir, Audiphone Co of S Tx, **A**

Irwin, Janet S 103 Hazelpath, White Hall Bldg, Hendersonville, TN 37075, (615) 822-9010, BA 73 Univ of IA; MA 77 Univ of IA; 87–Asst VP, Rebound Inc, **SLP**

Irwin, Dr John V P O Box 22314, Lexington, KY 40522, (606) 269-1301, BA 37 OH Wesleyan Univ; MA 40 OH St Univ; PH 47 (NS) Univ of WI - Madison; Lec/Consul, En KY U, **SLP F H LM**

Irwin, Dr Margaret Louise South Community Medical Tower, 1044 S W 44th Street, Suite 310, Oklahoma City, OK 73109, (405) 631-0137, BS 63 Univ of TN - Knoxville; ME 67 Emory Univ; PH 86 (Sp-Lang Path) Univ of OK - Norman; 80–Owner/CEO, Med Sp Path/Aud Assoc, **SLP**

Irwin, Nedra H 1167 Edward Avenue, Allentown, PA 18104, **A**

Irwin, Dr Ruth B 2685 Henthorne Road, Columbus, OH 43221, (614) 486-1050, BS 29 Emporia St Univ; MA 36 Univ of IA; PH 40 (Sp Path & Psych) Univ of Southern CA; **SLP F H LM**

Irwin, Sandra Sue 7000 Magda Drive #202, Maple Grove, MN 55369, **SLP**

Irwin, Trudy Lorain 4320 East Murdock, Wichita, KS 67208, (316) 686-4274, BS 65 Univ of MO - Columbia; MA 85 Wichita St Univ; 86–Eng as a Second Lang Tchr, Wichita Public School, **SLP**

Irwin, Mrs Vickie Hammer 101 Brandywine Lane, West Monroe, LA 71291, (318) 323-3604, BA 77 Univ of OK - Norman; MS 79 Univ of OK Medical Center; Sp-Lang Path, Ouachita Parish Schs, **SLP**

Irzyk, Barbara Kathleen 320 Sheetz Street, West Lafayette, IN 47906, (219) 583-8227, BS 79 Purdue Univ - West Lafayette; MS 81 Purdue Univ - West Lafayette; SLP, Logansport School Corporation, **SLP**

Isaacs, Elizabeth Ellen 6548 Harco Street, Long Beach, CA 90808, (714) 558-5807, **SLP**

Isaacs, Gale Joann 419 Frank Street, Raleigh, NC 27604, (919) 755-4841, BA 77 Univ of MD - College Park; ME 79 NC Central Univ; MA 81 Univ of MD - College Park; 84–Asst Professor, Shaw U Sp & Hrng Cl

Isaacs, Mrs Laura J P 5428 Harleston Drive, Lyndhurst, OH 44124, (216) 687-3804, BS 75 OH Univ - Athens; MA 77 Cleveland St Univ; 88–Aud, Cleveland State Univ, **A**

Isaacs, Linda D 5167 Carlson Dairy Road, Summerfield, NC 27358, (919) 854-6420, BA 75 Univ of AR - Fayetteville; MA 81 Auburn Univ - Auburn; Sp-Lang Path, Wesley Long Comm Hosp, **SLP**

Isaacs, Lois E 3811 Fox Run Drive #1122, Cincinnati, OH 45236, (513) 751-1716, BS 76 Northwestern Univ; MS 78 Washington Univ; Aud, ENT Assoc of Cincinnati, **A**

Isaacson, Frances 5604 Meridian Hill Place, Burke, VA 22015-2142, (804) 440-5647, MS 77 Univ of WA; **SLP**

Isaacson, Nancy Lynn 33 Lancaster Terrace #202, Brookline, MA 02146, (617) 731-8786, BA 74 Syracuse Univ; MS 87 Emerson Coll; **SLP**

Isaacson, Rosalie 6216 Norvo Road, Baltimore, MD 21207, (301) 396-0833, BA 65 American Univ; MS 75 Loyola Coll; 75–Sp-Lang Path, Baltimore City Pub Sch, **SLP ACE**

Isaacson, Mrs Susan B 92 West Street, Warwick, NY 10990, (914) 986-5191, BA 70 CUNY - Lehman Coll; MA 72 CUNY - City College; Dir/Sp-Lang Path, Horton Mem Hosp, **SLP**

Isabell, Mrs Terry Lynn 7255 Richmond, Memphis, TN 38125, (901) 755-4993, BS 81 Memphis St Univ; MA 85 Memphis St Univ; Sp-Lang Path, St Francis Hospital, **SLP**

Isack, Audrey Helen 2111 East Darby Road, Havertown, PA 19083, (215) 885-0611, BS 83 NY Univ; MA 85 Temple Univ-Tyler Sch of Art; 88–Reg Mgr, Universal Rehab Services, **SLP**

Isacke, Mrs Bonnie W 6601 Darlington Road, Pittsburgh, PA 15217, (412) 647-5575, BS 70 Carlow Coll; ME 76 Univ of Pittsburgh - Pittsburgh; MA 71 Univ of Pittsburgh - Pittsburgh; Sp/Lang Path, Chldns Hosp of Pgh, **SLP**

Isakson, Mrs Carolyn Weiner 212 Mohawk Drive, West Hartford, CT 06117, (203) 232-4756, BA 64 McGill Univ - Quebec; MA 66 Northwestern Univ; Sp-Lang Path, Commun Therapy Serv, **SLP ACE**

Isbell, Lisa Angelyn 3712 Spring Creek Lane, Dunwoody, GA 30350, (404) 255-2918, BS 84 Auburn Univ - Auburn; MS 86 Univ of South AL; 88–Aud, North Suburban ENT Assoc, **A**

Isbell, Marie M 5216 Shelborne Circle #5, Memphis, TN 38134, (901) 529-0233, BS 77 Univ of TN - Martin; MA 81 Memphis St Univ; 86–Sp/Lang Path, Les Passees Childrens Rehab Ctr, **SLP**

Isdaner, Mrs Ellen Kalodner 357 Wyndmoor Lane, Huntingdon Valley, PA 19006, (215) 938-1030, BS 74 Emerson Coll; MA 76 Temple Univ; Sp-Lang Path, Private Practice, **SLP**

Isele, Ronald Woodward Ohio University, 215 Lindley Hall, Athens, OH 45701, (614) 593-1418, BS 63 Kent St Univ; MA 65 Kent St Univ; 67–Assoc Prof, OH U, **SLP A**

Isenberg, Mrs Leslie Z 2220 Calle Tiara, La Jolla, CA 92037, (619) 456-9161, BS 69 Boston Univ; MS 71 Columbia Univ Teachers Coll; President, Marketing Insight Inc, **SLP**

Isenhath, Dr J O Rd 1 Box 879, Conneaut Lake, PA 16316, (814) 333-5100, BS 74 OH Univ - Athens; MA 76 OH St Univ; PH 88 (Aud/Comm Science & Dis) Union for Experi Coll & Univ; 76–Dir Aud/Sp Ctr, Meadville Med Ctr, **A**

Iserman, Blake F 14035 Yucca Street N W, Andover, MN 55304, (612) 339-7296, BA 73 Ripon Coll; MS 80 Univ of WI - Stevens Point; Aud, Minneapolis ENT Cl, **A**

Iserman, Mrs Joan K 10435 Yucca Street N W, Andover, MN 55304, (612) 825-0978, BA 80 Univ of WI - Eau Claire; MA 81 Univ of MN - Duluth; Sp-Lang Path, Anoka-Hennepin District #11, **SLP**

Isert, Mrs Deanna S 700 S W 18th Street, Boca Raton, FL 33432, (305) 368-5975, BA 62 Upsala Coll; MA 73 Montclair St Coll; Ed Spec, Deanna S Isert and Assoc

Iseyama, Dee Ann 1926 Broadway, Chico, CA 95928, (916) 538-7241, BA 80 CA St Univ - Chico; MA 84 CA St Univ - Chico; 84–Sp-Lang Path, Bulte County Ofc of Educ, **SLP**

Isham, Cynthia Rochelle 4849 Haverwood #306, Dallas, TX 75287, (214) 250-3846, BS 86 Baylor Univ; MS 87 Baylor Univ; 88–Sp-Lang Path, Callier Ctr for Comm Dis

Isham, Lorie 1625 North Troy-Sidney Road, Troy, OH 45373, (513) 339-8313, BS 78 Miami Univ - Oxford; MA 82 OH Univ - Athens; Sp-Lang Path, Miami Co Riverside Sch (169), **SLP**

Ishimoto, Sharon Kiku 1479 Ukiah Way, Upland, CA 91786, (714) 982-7220, 88–Sp-Lang Path, San Bernardino Co Supt of Schs, **SLP**

Ison, Mrs Pamela A Hearing Serv Of Kentucky Inc, 212 West 18th Street, Hopkinsville, KY 42240, (502) 885-0034, BS 77 Univ of GA; ME 78 Univ of GA; Aud/Bd Dir, Hearing Serv of Kentucky Inc, **A**

Isquith, Mrs Amy E 26 Summer Street #9, Marblehead, MA 01945, (617) 639-2388, BS 82 Univ of MA - Amherst; MS 84 Boston Univ; 88–Sp-Lang Path, Private Practice, **SLP**

Israel, Hollis B R 17 Thomas Road, Rockville Centre, NY 11570, (516) 678-6545, BA 71 Monmouth Coll; MA 74 Hofstra Univ; **SLP**

Israel, Mrs Jaclyn Sue 10 Devonshire Road, New Rochelle, NY 10804, (914) 633-3156, BS 74 Northwestern Univ; MA 75 Northwestern Univ; Dir, Sound Shore Speech, **SLP**

Israel, Dr Leonard 309 Knotty Wood Lane, West Palm Beach, FL 33414, (407) 798-1142, BA 70 CUNY - Queens Coll; MA 72 CUNY - Queens Coll; PH 79 (NS) CUNY - Grad Sch & Univ Cntr; Sp-Lang Path, Private Practice, **SLP**

Israel, Mrs Marian A 3320 North 37th Street, Hollywood, FL 33021, BS 60; MS 67 CUNY - Brooklyn Coll; Sp-Lang Path, Private Practice, **SLP**

Israel, Dr Richard H 9801 Georgia Avenue, Suite 2-27, Silver Spring, MD 20902, (301) 681-7077, BA 60 Univ of VA - Charlottesville; ME 61 Univ of VA - Charlottesville; PH 67 (Aud) Case Western Reserve Univ; 81–Pres, Private Practice, **SLP A**

Israel, Sherri M 4040 San Felipe #232, Houston, TX 77027, (713) 797-3277, BS 76 Univ of TX - Austin; MS 79 Baylor Coll of Medicine; 85–Aud, Hermann Hosp, **A**

Israelsky, Mrs Roberta Schwartz 20 Jacamar Drive, Voorhees, NJ 08043, (609) 424-8970, BA 76 Temple Univ-Tyler Sch of Art; MA 78 Trenton St Coll; Sp-Lang Path, Camden Co Ed Serv Commission, **SLP**

Isserow, Mrs Rachelle Rosenberg 41 Brentwood Avenue, Newton Center, MA 02159, BA 53 CUNY - Hunter Coll; ME 57 Boston Univ; Sp-Lang Path, Winchester MA Pub Schs, **SLP ACE**

Issokson, Roberta G 37 Pinecrest Lane, Durham, NH 03824, (603) 742-5252, BS 70 Northeastern Univ; MS 81 Univ of NH; Sp-Lang Path Dept Coord, Wentworth-Douglass Hosp, **SLP ACE**

Istre, Dr Clifton O, Jr 109 Country Club Drive, Covington, LA 70434, BS 52; MA 56; PH 65 (NS); Owner, Med Hrng Serv Inc, **SLP A**

Ito, Arlene Karen 83 Mission Plaza Drive, Ventura, CA 93001-2611, (805) 644-4779, BS 76 Univ of CA - Davis; MA 82 CA St Univ - Stanislaus; SLP, Ventura Unif Sch Dist, **SLP**

Itoh, Dr Motonobu 1770 Toriyama-Cho, Kohoku-Ku, Yokohama, Japan 222, 45-473-0666, BA 64; MA 72 CA St Univ - Chico; PH 75 (NS) Purdue Univ - West Lafayette; Researcher, Tokyo Metro Gvnmnt

Itsines, Mrs Christina HCR 1 Box 25-A, Swiftwater, PA 18370, (717) 839-6460, Kent St Univ; **SLP**

Ittleman, Mark A Ittleman Communications, 2212 New Jersey Road, Lakeland, FL 33803, (813) 688-8765, OB 71 Univ of Miami; MS 72 Univ of South FL; Sp/Lang Path, Ittleman Commun, **SLP ACE**

Iturralde, Mrs Joy Harvey 12416 South Harrells Ferry, Apartment 4-C, Baton Rouge, LA 70816, (504) 292-4379, BS 85 LA St Univ - Baton Rouge; MA 87 LA St Univ - Baton Rouge

Iuorio, Mrs Barbara Baldwin 1219 Evergreen Court, Palatine, IL 60067, (312) 934-2887, BS 83 Elmhurst Coll; OM 85 Governors St Univ

Ivanick, Mrs Jane E 484 Hillcrest Road, Elmira, NY 14903, BA 75 SUNY - Coll at Cortland; MS 78 Univ of RI; **SLP**

Ivankovic, Susan E L 737 Tuckahoe Road #34, Yonkers, NY 10710, (914) 268-4101, BA 73 Iona Coll; MA 76 CUNY - Lehman Coll; Sp-Path, Clarkstown Central Sch, **SLP**

Ivans, William 100 Knollwood Drive, Cherry Hill, NJ 08002, (609) 667-5430, BA 73 Rutgers St Univ - Newark; MA 77 Temple Univ; Sp-Lang Path, Comm Hlth & Nurs Serv, **SLP ACE**

Iven, Cari Joanne 31 Central Street #2, Randolph, VT 05060, BS 84 OR St Univ; MS 86 Univ of AR - Little Rock; 88–Sp-Lang Path, Orange-Windsor Sup Union, **SLP**

Iversen, Mrs Judith A Carle Hearing Services, 709 West University Avenue, Urbana, IL 61801, (217) 337-3197, BA 69 Univ of Manitoba - Winnipeg; MA 72 Univ of ND; Aud, Carle Cl Assn, **A**

Iversen, Thomas Richard 102 Church Street #4, Holliston, MA 01746, (508) 429-2783, MS 88 Northeastern Univ; 88–Sp-Lang Path, Sp & Lang Resources

Iverson, Jane Elizabeth 8616 S E Yamhill Street, Portland, OR 97216, (503) 760-7700, BS 71 OR St Univ; MS 72 Western OR St Coll; Sp-Lang Path, David Douglas Sch Dist, **SLP**

Iverson, Jeannine 2445 Lyttonsville Road, Apartment 1401, Silver Spring, MD 20910, (301) 565-1351, BA 71 Univ of MD - College Park; MS 76 Towson St Univ; Sp-Lang Path, Holy Cross Hosp, **SLP ACE**

Iverson, Mrs Mary W 18914 Jonathan Lane, Homewood, IL 60430, (312) 747-4000, BS 73 Southern IL Univ -Carbondale; OM 79 Governors St Univ; **SLP**

Iverson, Sharon A 19623 Ronald Avenue, Torrance, CA 90503, (213) 371-7976, BA 79 CA St Univ - Los Angeles; MA 81 NM St Univ; SLP, LA Co Supt of Schls, **SLP**

Ives-Kline, Kathleen Mary 107 Euclid Avenue, Troy, NY 12180, (518) 356-5032, BS 80 SUNY - Coll at Geneseo; MS 83 Coll of Saint Rose; 83–Sp-Lang Path, Rotterdam-Mohonasen Cen Sch Dist, **SLP**

Ivey, Kathryn Teresa 18 Levan Avenue, Lockport, NY 14094-3114, (716) 434-1763, BS 76 SUNY - Coll at Buffalo; MS 82 SUNY - Coll at Buffalo; 85–Sp-Lang Path, UCP, **SLP**

Ivey, Dr Lillian P 13610 Pin Oak, Edmond, OK 73034, (405) 478-0384, BA 37 Central St Univ; MA 62 Univ of Tulsa; ED 68 (NS) Univ of OK - Norman; **SLP LM**

Ivey, Dr Robert G L103-240 Wharncliffe Rd N, London, ON, Canada N6H 4P2, (519) 673-5551, BA 67 Univ of FL; MS 69 CO St Univ; PH 78 (Aud) Univ of WI - Madison; 86–Aud, Private Practice, **A**

Ivey, Dr Sara M 119 Ingham, St Simons Island, GA 31522, (912) 638-7777, PH 52 (NS) LA St Univ - Baton Rouge; Consult, Physical Ther Rehab Serv, **SLP LM**

Ivinskas, Ann E 5829 Pinecone Court, Columbus, OH 43229, (614) 899-7311, BS 79 Western MI Univ; MA 82 Western MI Univ; SLP, **SLP**

Ivory, Dr Peter J 5113 Academy Drive, Metairie, LA 70003, (504) 588-5661, BA 75 Univ of CA - Santa Barbara; MS 78 Univ of WI - Stevens Point; PH 83 (NS) Univ of KS; Aud, Tulane Med Ctr, **A**

Ivory, SarahAnn 1835 Kepler Road, Pottstown, PA 19464, (215) 873-4900, BS 75 West Chester Univ of PA; MA 81 Trenton St Coll; 87–Sp-Lang Path, The Devereux Foundation, **SLP**

Ivsan, Carol Falbo 41 Solmar Drive, Rochester, NY 14624, (716) 245-5328, BS 80 SUNY - Coll at Geneseo; MA 82 SUNY - Coll at Geneseo; 88–Aud Supvr, SUNY-Coll at Geneseo, **A**

Iwamoto, Karen Chizuko 1348 Fruitdale Avenue, Apartment 68, San Jose, CA 95126, (408) 294-2351, BA 80 San Jose St Univ; MS 85 Univ of WA; **SLP**

Iwamoto, Valerie Iyeko 1551 Ala Mahamoe Street, Honolulu, HI 96819, (808) 839-5768, BA 83 Western WA Univ; MS 85 Univ of HI - Manoa; SLP, Department of Education, **SLP**

Iwamoto, Vickie M 46-229 Kahuhipa Street, #D404, Kaneohe, HI 96744, (808) 456-6338, BA 73 Univ of HI - Manoa; BS 73 Univ of HI - Manoa; MS 75 Univ of HI - Manoa; Superv SLP & Aud, St of HI Dept of Hlth-Wtsh, **SLP A**

Iwan, Susan Kelly 918 West Transit Avenue, Roseville, MN 55113, (612) 633-8150, BA 78 Univ of MN - Minneap-St Paul; MA 76 Univ of MN - Minneap-St Paul; SLP, Roseville Area Sch ISD #623, **SLP**

Iwankovitsch, Mrs Janet Jefferson 120 Wildhaven Drive, Albertville, AL 35950, (205) 891-1649, BA 72 Univ of NC - Greensboro; MS 76 Old Dominion Univ; Sp-Lang Path, Guntersville Cty Schs, **SLP**

Izdebski, Dr Krzysztof 632 Sonoma Street, Richmond, CA 94805, (415) 228-6800, OM 70 Univ of Lund - Sweden; MA 71 Univ of CA - Los Angeles; PH 76 (NS) San Francisco St Univ; Chief SLP, VA Med Cen, **SLP**

Izen, Joan M 74 Jones Street, Manchester, NH 03103, (603) 625-2810, BS 77 Emerson Coll; MA 80 Univ of ME - Orono; Sp-Lang Path, Private Practice, **SLP**

Izumi, Mrs Marsha 5265 Via Adela, Yorba Linda, CA 92686, (714) 779-0754, BA 72 CA St Univ - Fresno; MA 74 CA St Univ - Fresno; Sp-Lang Path, **SLP**

Izumi, Mutsumi I 3041 11th Avenue, Los Angeles, CA 90018, BA 73 Univ of CA - Los Angeles; MA 77 CA St Univ - Los Angeles; SLP, Los Angeles Cnty Supt Schools, **SLP**

J

Jabaay, Julie 664 Willowby Run, Pasadena, MD 21122, (301) 522-5450, BS 84 Baylor Univ; MA 86 Northwestern Univ; 87–Sp-Lang Path, Kennedy Institute, **SLP**

Jablon, Dr Ann D 670 West End Avenue #1-F, New York, NY 10025, (212) 799-9525, MA 76 CUNY - Queens Coll; OM 79 CUNY - Grad Sch & Univ Cntr; PH 86 (Psycholinguistics) CUNY - Grad Sch & Univ Cntr; 86–Sp-Lang Path, Private Practice, **SLP**

Jablonovsky, Melanie S 6-1/2 Geneva Street, Bath, NY 14810, (607) 776-4110, BS 80 Clarion Univ of PA; MS 82 Indiana Univ of PA; Sp-Lang Path, Haverling Ctrl Sch, **SLP**

Jablonski, Gregory Michael Usmca Ansbach, P O Box 293, APO New York, NY 09177, (313) 381-9434, MA 81 Wayne St Univ; Chief of Sp-Lang Path, 121 Evacuation Hosp, **SLP**

Jablonski, Mrs Terry Anne 212 West North Street, Tampa, FL 33604, (813) 544-8859, MS 86 Univ of South FL; 87–Sp-Lang Path, N Harris Exceptional Student Ctr, **SLP**

Jabre, Mrs Angele Debbane 1231 South Trimble Road, Mansfield, OH 44907, BS 80 Marquette Univ; MA 83 Univ of Cincinnati; Sp-Lang Path, **SLP**

Jacaruso, Mrs Maryanne Chesko 140 Weekeepeemee Road, Bethlehem, CT 06751, (203) 754-5141, BS 77 Southern CT St Univ; MS 79 Rutger's St Univ - Douglas Coll; Sp-Lang Path, Er Sl Rehab Cen-Gtr Waterbury, **SLP**

Jacavage, Gene 258 Indiana Avenue, Shenandoah, PA 17976, (717) 544-4737, BS 75 PA St Univ - Univ Park; MS 79 Bloomsburg Univ of PA; 75–Aud, Schuylkill IU #29, **A**

Jachym, Mrs Jane A 163 Debbie Drive, South Windsor, CT 06074, (203) 644-5155, BA 77 Elms Coll; MS 84 Worcester St Coll; Sp/Lang Path, **SLP**

Jack, Mrs Mary D 2833 Alexandria Pike, Anderson, IN 46012, (317) 643-6405, BS 71 Ball St Univ; MA 76 Ball St Univ; Sp-Lang Path, Private Practice, **SLP**

Jacka, Mrs Janice Christine 6008 S W 23rd Terrace, Topeka, KS 66614, (913) 232-0551, BS 71 KS St Univ; MA 73 KS St Univ; 88–Sp-Lang Path, Topeka Pub Schs, **SLP**

Jacke, Patti Jean 218 Pells Meadow Drive, Fairfield, CT 06430, (212) 828-9000, BA 72 CUNY - Lehman Coll; MA 76 CUNY - Lehman Coll; 83–Aud, St Joseph's Sch for the Deaf, **A**

Jackel, Rebecca B 5 Ashley Drive, Maple Glen, PA 19002, (215) 540-0366, BS 78 SUNY - Center at Albany; MA 80 Univ of Pittsburgh - Pittsburgh; 88–Sp-Lang Path, Albert Einstein Med Ctr, **SLP**

Jackerson, Cathy Briggs 19341 N E 22nd Avenue, North Miami Beach, FL 33180, (305) 932-8080, BS 72 Central MI Univ; MA 80 Central MI Univ; **SLP**

Jack-Hannan, Allison R P O Box 325, Myrtle Creek, OR 97457, (503) 863-6460, BA 77 Univ of CA - Santa Barbara; MA 80 WA St Univ; Sp-Lang Path, Private Practice, **SLP**

Jacklen, Kathleen Ann Route 1 Box 2006, Britt, MN 55710, (218) 749-5312, BS 77 Univ of MN - Minneap-St Paul; MS 79 Univ of WI - Stevens Point; Audiologist, Univ of Minn-Audiology Clinic, **A**

Jackowski, Mrs Linda A 7 Conifer Drive, Burnt Hills, NY 12027, (518) 885-5321, BA 72 Coll of Saint Rose; MA 73 Coll of Saint Rose; 80–Sp-Lang Path, Ballston Spa Ctrl Schs, **SLP**

Jackson, Mrs Adrianne 403 North Vine, Hinsdale, IL 60521, (602) 299-8763, BS 70 Univ of GA; MA 71 Univ of TN - Knoxville; **SLP**

Jackson, Audrey A 8324 Burkhart Circle, Houston, TX 77055, (713) 932-7069, BS 69 MS Univ for Women; MS 70 MS Univ for Women; **SLP**

Jackson, Mrs Barbara J 129 Atchison Road, Harrisville, MI 48740, (517) 355-8078, BA 86 MI St Univ; MA 88 MI St Univ

Jackson, Bernard R 911 Vireo Drive, Barefoot Bay, FL 32958, (305) 589-9329, BA 49 Western MI Univ; MA 50 Univ of Denver; PH 61 (NS) OH St Univ; **SLP LM**

Jackson, Mrs Betty J J P O Box 803, Grambling, LA 71245, (318) 274-2344, BS 63 Grambling St Univ; MA 73 LA Tech Univ; Asst Prof/Dir, Grambling State University, **SLP**

Jackson, Mrs Bonnie Lee N 114 Emmons Street, Newark, NY 14513, (315) 331-1700, BS 79 SUNY - Coll at Geneseo; MS 81 Southern IL Univ -Carbondale; 81–Sp-Lang Path, New Arcadia Day Treatment Prog, **SLP**

Jackson, Mrs Bonnie M V 800 Brentwood, Pella, IA 50219, (515) 842-2719, BS 73 IA St Univ; MA 74 Northeast MO St Univ; Sp-Lang Path, Heartland AEA, **SLP**

Jackson, Caroline R 104 Mountain Road, Cheshire, CT 06410, **SLP**

Jackson, Catherine 3723 N E 150th Street, Seattle, WA 98155, (206) 771-1414, BA 74 Univ of WA; BA 74 Univ of WA; OM 76 Univ of WA; Cl Mgr - SLP, Northwest Sp & Hrng, **SLP ACE**

Jackson, Catherine A 1203 10th Street, Hermosa Beach, CA 90254, (213) 379-9557, BA 75 Univ of Redlands; MS 77 Univ of WI - Madison; MA 84 Univ of CA - Los Angeles; 81–Sp-Lang Path, Private Practice, **SLP**

Jackson, Charline B Route 1 Box 59, Dardanelle, AR 72834, BS; **SLP LM**

Jackson, Dr Colleen O 4202 4th Avenue #202, San Diego, CA 92103, (619) 571-3801, BS 72 Univ of Cincinnati; MA 74 Wayne St Univ; PH 78 (Aud) Wayne St Univ; 86–Aud, Nu-Ear Electronics, **A ACE**

Jackson, Mrs Cynthia G 54 Coronado Avenue, Kenner, LA 70065, (504) 443-2342, BS 72 Univ of North TX; MS 75 Univ of North TX; 88–Sp-Lang Path, Jefferson Parish Pub Sch Sys, **SLP**

Jackson, Eleanor J 19836 Van Aken #303, Shaker Heights, OH 44122, (216) 382-7700, BS 76 Hampton Univ; MA 79 Case Western Reserve Univ; 87–Sp-Lang Path, So Euclid-Lyndhurst City Schs, **SLP ACE**

Jackson, Mrs Faith L 222 Baldwin Avenue, Bowling Green, OH 43402, (419) 372-2515, BS 58 Bowling Green St Univ; MA 59 Bowling Green St Univ; Assoc Prof of Commun Dis, Bowling Green St U, **SLP**

Jackson, Frances H P O Box 190, Mansfield, LA 71052, (318) 872-1696, BA 64 Southern Univ - Baton Rouge; ME 69 Northwestern St Univ; MA 71 Northwestern St Univ; Sp/Lang Path, De Soto Parish Sch Bd, **SLP**

Jackson, Janancy S 2844 East 3rd #310, Long Beach, CA 90814, (213) 433-6017, BA 32 CA St Univ - Los Angeles; MS 64 Univ of Southern CA; Sp/Lang Path, Private Practice, **LM**

Jackson, Janet L 900 Henderson Avenue #919, Houston, TX 77058, (713) 333-9187, BS 86 Univ of TX - Austin; MS 88 Southwest TX St Univ; InSpeech Inc

Jackson, Mrs Janet Sue 612-B Rockcreek, Charlottesville, VA 22903, (804) 924-5781, MA 87 MI St Univ; Sp-Lang Path, Univ of VA Med Ctr, **SLP**

Jackson, Janette Rhodes 1264 Lakeshore Drive, Orangeburg, SC 29115, (803) 534-8609, BA 84 SC St Coll; MA 86 SC St Coll; **SLP**

Jackson, Janice E 1171 Phillips Road, Yuba City, CA 95991, (916) 633-2473, BA 75 CA St Univ - Chico; MS 78 Univ of WY; SLP, Yuba Co Supt of Sch, **SLP**

Jackson, Jean Marie 1410 Checola Court, Santa Cruz, CA 95065, (408) 924-3679, BA 79 San Jose St Univ; MA 81 San Jose St Univ; Coord of Clin Svcs, San Jose State Univ, **SLP**

Jackson, Jerry John 1108 North 8th Street, Independence, KS 67301, (316) 331-1154, ME 85 Northeastern OK St Univ; 82–Sp-Lang Path, Tri-County Spec Educ #607

Jackson, Joanne K 6700 Luella Anne Drive N E, Albuquerque, NM 87109-4039, (505) 836-4387, BS 67 Indiana Univ of PA; MA 73 Univ of MD - College Park; SLP, Albuquerque Public Schools, **SLP**

Jackson, Mrs Jody Mayo 1208 North 8th Avenue, Lanett, AL 36863, (404) 645-4862, BS 82 Auburn Univ - Auburn; MS 85 Univ of South AL; Aud, West Point Pepperell, **A**

Jackson, Juaquita E Cumberland Hall Hospital, 804 Youngs Lane, Nashville, TN 37207, (615) 228-4848, BS 70 Northwestern Univ; MS 71 Univ of MI - Ann Arbor; 88–Sp-Lang Path, Cumberland Hall Hosp, **SLP**

Jackson, Mrs Judith Ann 41536 Myrtle St, Palmdale, CA 93551, (805) 943-1949, MA 81 CA St Univ - Northridge; BA 79 CA St Univ - Northridge; SLP, Burbank USD, **SLP**

Jackson, Judith Lynn 2338 18th Street, Boulder, CO 80302, (303) 444-0515, BS 77 Stockton St Coll; MA 80 Univ of CA - Santa Barbara; SLP, Memorial Hosp of Santa Barbara, **SLP**

Jackson, Dr Judith M 1471 Comstock Avenue, Los Angeles, CA 90024, BA 58 Univ of Denver; MA 74 Univ of Southern CA; PH 79 (Education) Univ of Southern CA; 81–Assoc Prof, CA St Univ Dominguez Hills, **SLP**

Jackson, Mrs Karen Ehrlich 21 Phyllis Drive, Pomona, NY 10970, (914) 577-6290, BA 74 CUNY - Queens Coll; MS 77 AZ St Univ; Sp-Lang Path, East Ramapo School District, **SLP**

Jackson, Kenneth J 6742 Jardines Drive, Huntington Beach, CA 92647, (714) 847-2551, BA 73 CA St Univ - Long Beach; MA 75 CA St Univ - Long Beach; Sp/Lang Path, Ocean View Sch Dist, **SLP**

Jackson, Lauri Sleeth 10104-H Woodlake Drive, Cockeysville, MD 21030, (301) 321-3095, MS; 88–Aud, Hearing Assessment Ctr, **A**

Jackson, Mrs Laurie Lynn K 3614 Bobcat Trail, Temple, TX 76502, (817) 773-0779, BA 77 Univ of MI - Ann Arbor; MA 79 Wayne St Univ; **SLP**

Jackson, Mrs Lee Ann 24725 Calle El Toro Grande, El Toro, CA 92630, BS 82 Eastern MI Univ; MA 83 Eastern MI Univ; **SLP**

Jackson, Linda Lee 2045 Clinton Avenue #34, Alameda, CA 94501, (415) 865-3636, BS 83 CA St Univ - Hayward; MS 85 CA St Univ - Hayward; SLP, Oakland Public School District, **SLP**

Jackson, Linda S 1635 Alvarado Street, Oceanside, CA 92054, **SLP**

Jackson, Lisa Gibson 15642 Madison, Dolton, IL 60419, (219) 949-4000, BS 81 Northwestern Univ; MS 85 Northeastern Univ; Sp-Lang Path, Trade Winds Rehab Ctr, **SLP ACE**

Jackson, Mrs Lorraine Mae 3211 Applewood, Midland, MI 48640, (517) 835-1556, BA 71 Central MI Univ; MA 74 Central MI Univ

Jackson, Mrs Maland Bunton 5453 Onacrest Drive, Los Angeles, CA 90043, (213) 296-1143, BA 73 CA St Univ - Los Angeles; MA 77 CA St Univ - Los Angeles; **SLP**

Jackson, Margaret 1307 Silver SW1, Albuquerque, NM 87102, BS 85 Univ of AZ; MS 87 Univ of AZ; **SLP**

Jackson, Margaret Kathleen 543 Blazedwood Drive, Ballwin, MO 63021, (314) 569-8311, BA 72 Southern IL Univ-Edwardsvill; MS 87 Southern IL Univ-Edwardsvill; 88–Sp-Lang Path Impaired Tchr, Spec Schl Dstr, **SLP**

Jackson, Mrs Mari Ann Levandowsk 10316 Woodhaven Circle, Indianapolis, IN 46229, (317) 849-2474, BA 80 IN Univ - Bloomington; MS 82 Univ of WI - Madison; Sp/Lang Path, Speak Listen and Learn, **SLP**

Jackson, Mrs Martha F P O Box 344, Bainbridge, IN 46105, (317) 522-2828, BS 74 IN St Univ - Terre Haute; MS 75 IN St Univ - Terre Haute; Sp-Lang Path/Consult, Putnam Co Comprehensive Serv, **SLP**

Jackson, Mary Ann 1310 West Race, Searcy, AR 72143, (501) 268-2333, BA 75 Univ of AR - Fayetteville; MA 76 Univ of AR - Fayetteville; **SLP**

Jackson, Mary G P O Box 615, Oakdale, CA 95361-0615, (209) 847-5151, BA 76 CA St Univ - Stanislaus; MA 78 CA St Univ - Stanislaus; SLP, Modesto Cty Sch, **SLP**

Jackson, Mrs Mary Kathleen 7848 Crossover Boulevard, West Worthington, OH 43235, (614) 766-9564, MA 88 OH Univ - Athens; 88–Sp-Lang Path, Delaware Sp & Hearing Ctr

Jackson, Maureen Therese 725 North 4th Street, Fort Dodge, IA 50501, (515) 576-7434, BA 86 Univ of Northern IA; MA 87 Western IL Univ; 88–Aud, Arrowhead AEA

Jackson, Melissa Foens 807 Ridge Drive #1019, De Kalb, IL 60115, BA 84 Univ of Northern IA; MA 86 Univ of IA; 88–Sp-Lang Path, Mid-Valley Spec Educ Coop, **SLP**

Jackson, Mrs Nina Jim 1711 Grant, Wichita Falls, TX 76309, (817) 322-0771, BS 50 TX Woman's Univ; ME 73 Midwestern St Univ; Supervisor of Speech/Language, North TX Easter Seal Rehab Cen, **SLP**

Jackson, Dr Pamela L Dept Communicative Disorders, Northern Illinois Univ, De Kalb, IL 60115, (815) 753-6510, BS 70 Purdue Univ - West Lafayette; MS 71 Purdue Univ - West Lafayette; PH 74 (Aud) Purdue Univ - West Lafayette; 74–Assoc Prof, No Il U Dept Commun Dis, **A**

Jackson, Patricia A 890 Bell Street, East Palo Alto, CA 94303, (408) 998-6317, BS 73 Univ of CA - Davis; MA 80 San Jose St Univ; SLP, San Jose USD, **SLP**

Jackson, Patricia Carol 501 West Street, Ahoskie, NC 27910, (919) 332-8121, BS 81 Longwood Coll; ME 83 Univ of VA - Charlottesville; Sp-Lang Path, Roanoke Chowan Hosp, **SLP**

Jackson, Dr Patricia Daugherty Department Of Communicative Disorders, Speech And Hearing Center, University, MS 38677, (601) 232-7271, BA 59 Univ of AL-Tuscaloosa; MS 68 Univ of MI - Ann Arbor; PH 86 (Aud) Univ of MI - Ann Arbor; Asst Prof, Univ of Mississippi, **A**

Jackson, Mrs Patricia P Child Guidance Clinic, 700 Elgin Avenue, Winnipeg, MB, Canada R3E 1B2, (204) 786-7841, MS 73 Univ of South FL; Sp-Lang Path, Child Guid Cl, **SLP**

Jackson, Patricia W 175 High Point Circle, Tallmadge, OH 44278, BS 56 Kent St Univ; ME 71 Kent St Univ; Aud Sp-Lang Superv, Akron Pub Sch, **SLP**

Jackson, Rhonda L 7406 Glen Manor, Houston, TX 77028, (713) 633-3126, BA 80 Univ of Houston - Univ Park; MA 86 Univ of Houston - Univ Park; **SLP**

Jackson, Mrs Rita H 1793 East Homer Road, Cortland, NY 13045, (607) 753-6444, MS 84 Syracuse Univ; SLP, Special Childrens Ctr, **SLP**

Jackson, Roberta E University Of California, Dept Of Speech, Santa Barbara, CA 93106, (805) 961-2148, BA 66 Univ of CA - Santa Barbara; MA 68 Univ of CA - Santa Barbara; Lecturer, U of CA-Santa Barbara, **SLP**

Jackson, Dr Rosemary H 4817 Clairmont Avenue, Birmingham, AL 35222, (205) 591-1222, BA 69 Southern IL Univ-Edwardsvill; MA 70 Univ of IL - Urbana; PH 77 (NS) Univ of MD - College Park; Private Practice, **SLP**

Jackson, Mrs Ruth M 464 Selby Lane, Atherton, CA 94025, MS; **SLP LM**

Jackson, Sandra Michelle 3314 Hemsworth Street, Durham, NC 27707, (919) 732-9348, **SLP**

Jackson, Shelley L #228 1298 Som Center Road, Mayfield Heights, OH 44124, (216) 442-2409, BA 77 Temple Univ; MA 79 Temple Univ; SLP, Nicolet, **A**

Jackson, Mrs Shirley W 13-3 Woods View Lane, Ossining, NY 10562-0025, (914) 941-7300, BS 45 Univ of Pittsburgh - Pittsburgh; MA 61 Columbia Univ Teachers Coll; 86–Admin Coord Alternative Care, Bethel Homes, **SLP**

Jackson, Mrs Sue M 80 30th Street Northwest, Barberton, OH 44203, (216) 263-8276, OB 85 Bowling Green St Univ; OM 86 Bowling Green St Univ; 88–Aud, Wooster Comm Hosp, **A**

Jackson, Susan Theresa 5562 Hobart Street #305, Pittsburgh, PA 15217, (412) 624-6807, BA 84 Dalhousie Univ - Nova Scotia; MS 86 Dalhousie Univ - Nova Scotia

Jackson, Terri A 8913 Cobble Crest Lane, Sandy, UT 84092, **A**

Jackson, Terri Alexa 279 8th Street, Jersey City, NJ 07302, (201) 795-7156, MA 85 Montclair St Coll; **A**

Jackson, Theresa L 220 East Sola Street #8, Santa Barbara, CA 93101, (805) 964-0529, BA 77 Univ of CA - Irvine; MA 83 Univ of CA - Santa Barbara; Sp-Lang Path, Seton School, **SLP**

Jackson, Mrs Valerie P 2402 South Dundee Blvd, Tampa, FL 33629, (813) 832-3685, BA 73; MS 77 Rutgers St Univ -N Brunswick; 87–Sp-Lang Path, Hillsborough County Sch Sys, **SLP**

Jackson, Valerie White 4050 Morgan Road, Apt #306, College Park, GA 30349, (404) 964-2339, BA 79 SC St Coll; MA 80 Univ of IL - Urbana; 87–Sp-Lang Path, Fulton Co Sch Dist, **SLP**

Jackson-Bruyn, Mrs Sherryl A P O Box 184, Southampton, NY 11968, (516) 283-8087, BS 82 SUNY - Coll at Fredonia; MS 83 SUNY - Coll at Fredonia; 88–SLP, Riverhead Central Sch Dist, **SLP**

Jackson-Colando, Patricia 18721 Portofino Drive, Irvine, CA 92715, (714) 854-1926, MS 73 Purdue Univ - West Lafayette; Sp-Lang Path, Private Practice, **SLP ACE**

Jackson-Menaldi, Dr Maria Cristina 699 Lakeshore Drive, Grosse Pointe, MI 48236, (313) 882-1638

Jacob, Barbara 36 Hooper Avenue, West Orange, NJ 07052, **A**

Jacob, Fae Jean 27415 Detroit Road #G-41, Westlake, OH 44145, (216) 282-9121, BS 83 Bowling Green St Univ; MA 86 OH St Univ; 86–Sp-Lang Path, Lorain Comm Hosp, **SLP**

Jacob, Lisa Anne 723 Tribal Trail, Woodstock, GA 30188-3062, (404) 926-4993, BS 79 PA St Univ - Univ Park; ME 83 Northeastern Univ; 88–Aud, AHAS Hearing & Speech, **A**

Jacob, Loyal J Dept Communication Disorders, Youville Hospital, 1575 Cambridge Street, Cambridge, MA 02238, (617) 876-4344, BS 66 Univ of KS; MA 68 Univ of KS; Sp-Lang Path, Youville Hosp, **SLP**

Jacob, Sheryl R 14 Barnaby Lane, Hartsdale, NY 10530, (212) 594-8945, **SLP**

Jacobelli-Glass, Lucia Jo Pine Lake, Kingman, AZ 86401, (602) 757-3629, BS 76 CA St Univ - Fresno; MS 82 Northern AZ Univ; 82–Sp-Lang Path, Lucia J-Glass Sp & Lang Svcs, **SLP**

Jacobi, Mrs Mary Elizabeth 1452 D'Angelo Drive, North Tonawanda, NY 14120, (716) 693-1553, BS 82 SUNY - Coll at Geneseo; MA 84 SUNY - Center at Buffalo; Sp-Lang Path, UCP Assoc, **SLP**

Jacobitti, Carmela A One Thomas Place, Ogdensburg, NJ 07439, (201) 827-2164, BA 66 Montclair St Coll; MA 71 Seton Hall Univ; Sp-Lang Path, Private Practice, **SLP**

Jacobs, Dr Anita Isaacson 1306 Clayton Drive, South Bend, IN 46614, (219) 291-1993, MS 72 Univ of VT; ME 74 Univ of VT; PH 77 (NS) GA St Univ; **SLP**

Jacobs, Mrs Arleen G Fairwood Professional Bldg, Route 37 P O Box 8895, New Fairfield, CT 06812, (203) 746-2459, BA 72 SUNY - Center at Buffalo; MA 73 Cleveland St Univ; 81 Southern CT St Univ; Sp/Lang Path, Private Practice, **SLP**

Jacobs, Arthur H 8 Prescott Place, Old Bethpage, NY 11804, (212) 470-2556, BA 73 CUNY - Lehman Coll; MS 74 PA St Univ - Univ Park; Sp-Lang Path, Li Jewish-Hillside Hrng/Sp Cen, **SLP**

Jacobs, Beverly Jean 271 Broad Avenue S #203, Naples, FL 33940, (813) 262-3131, BS 77 Univ of SD - Vermillion; MA 78 Univ of SD - Vermillion; 85–Chief Sp-Lang Path, Naples Comm Hosp, **SLP ACE**

Jacobs, Mrs Carol Donnelly 7321 Tiki Avenue, Cincinnati, OH 45243, (513) 369-4730, MA 87 Univ of Cincinnati

Jacobs, Mrs Dale H 1648 Bay Point, Virginia Beach, VA 23454, (804) 496-0700, BS 69 Boston Univ; MS 72 Vanderbilt Univ; Sp-Lang Path, Private Practice, **SLP**

Jacobs, Donald W 7177 West Kimberly Way, Glendale, AZ 85308, (602) 561-1080, BS 76 Univ of Tulsa; MA 78 Central MI Univ; Sp-Lang Path, Deer Valley USD, **SLP**

Jacobs, Ellen L P O Box 1282, Flagstaff, AZ 86002, (602) 526-7683, BS 78 Univ of AZ; MS 81 Univ of AZ; Sp/Lang Path, Prescott USD, **SLP**

Jacobs, Frederick Paul Jacobs And Saline Clinical Aud, 2 West Fern, Redlands, CA 92373, (714) 792-0074, Aud, Private Practice, **A**

Jacobs, Gary Michael 1977 Ramona Avenue, Salt Lake City, UT 84108, (801) 467-3618, BS 79 Univ of UT; MS 86 Univ of UT; Audiologist, University of Utah Medical Cen, **A**

Jacobs, Mrs Janet S 3064 Mildred Drive, Roseville, MN 55113, (612) 298-8288, BA 67 Elmira Coll; MA 70 Univ of MN - Minneap-St Paul; Sp-Lang Path, Utd & Chldn Hosp, **SLP**

Jacobs, Mrs Karen Ann P O Box 1983, Grand Rapids, MI 49501, (616) 459-7749, BS 83 Central MI Univ; MA 85 Central MI Univ; Aud, Kent Otolaryngology, **A**

Jacobs, Linda A 7089 Ward Eagle, West Bloomfield, MI 48033, (313) 875-5250, BA 78 Western MI Univ; MA 80 Eastern MI Univ; Sp-Lang Path, Detroit Pub Schs Sp & Hrng Cl, **SLP**

Jacobs, Linda W 5629 Bellaire Drive, New Orleans, LA 70124, **SLP**

Jacobs, Mrs Lori c/o Boxer, 100-56 Baker Court, Island Park, NY 11558, (516) 435-9111, BA 79 SUNY - Center at Albany; MS 81 Adelphi Univ; Sp-Lang Path, Brentwood Sch Dist, **SLP**

Jacobs, Luann 16 South Lexington Street, Arlington, VA 23430, (703) 578-1616, BS 69 IN Univ - Bloomington; MA 71 IN Univ - Bloomington; Sp-Lang Path, **SLP**

Jacobs, Mrs Lucille Karas 501 Lincoln Avenue, Takoma Park, MD 20912, (301) 464-5770, BS 78 PA St Univ - Univ Park; MA 80 George Washington Univ; Sp-Lang Path, Prince Geo Co Proj Head Start, **SLP**

Jacobs, Margaret A 5701 East Glenn #82, Tucson, AZ 85712, (602) 795-7947, BA 71 Western WA Univ; MS 73 Univ of AZ; Aud, Moore Duncan & Huerta Pa, **A**

Jacobs, Mary Kane 1347 Carlotta Avenue, Berkeley, CA 94703, (415) 526-0490, BA 78 SUNY - Center at Buffalo; MA 80 Univ of CA - Santa Barbara; SLP, Fairfield-Suisun USD, **SLP**

Jacobs, Mrs Mary T 1977 Ascot Drive #1, Moraga, CA 94556, (415) 376-7422, BA 38 Univ of IA; MA 39 Univ of IA; Retired, **SLP LM**

Jacobs, Merle 6575 North Glenwood #3S, Chicago, IL 60626, (312) 633-8691, BS 80 Boston Univ; MA 83 Northwestern Univ; SLP, Cook Cty Hosp, **SLP**

Jacobs, Molly Ann 39 B Stonegate Court, Fairfield, OH 48014, (513) 948-2500, BS 84 OH Univ - Athens; MA 86 Univ of Cincinnati; 86–Sp-Lang Path, Daniel Drake Mem Hosp, **SLP**

Jacobs, Mrs Nancy 3581 Aquarius Drive, Huntington Beach, CA 92649, (213) 866-6195, BS 69 CA St Univ - Los Angeles; MA 71 Univ of Southern CA; Administrator, Wonderland Primary Sch, **SLP**

Jacobs, Mrs Sharon R 3211 Roods Lake Road, Lapeer, MI 48446, (313) 664-2951, BS 73 Western MI Univ; MA 74 Western MI Univ; Sp-Lang Path, Oakdale Regional Cen, **SLP**

Jacobs, Dr Teri G 2309 Ocean Park Boulevard, Santa Monica, CA 90405, (213) 558-8400, BS 68 NY Univ; MA 76 CA St Univ - Los Angeles; PH 81 (NS) Univ of Southern CA; Sp-Lang Path, Los Angeles Cnty Supt Schools, **SLP**

Jacobs, Virginia V 804 Woodley Drive, Rockville, MD 20850, (301) 321-2437, BA 59 Univ of MD - College Park; MA 63 Univ of MD - College Park; Asst Prof, Towson St U, **SLP**

Jacobs-Condit, Linda 106 East Oxford Avenue, Alexandria, VA 22301, (202) 994-7360, BA 76 Newcomb Coll Tulane Univ; MS 78 Tulane Univ; 87–Clin Instr of Aud, George Washington Univ, **A**

Jacobsen, Dr Cynthia H Childrens Mercy Hospital, Hearing Speech Dept, 24th At Gillham Road, Kansas City, MO 64108, MA 71 Univ of PA; MA 73 Memphis St Univ; PH 82 (NS) Univ of KS; Dir Hrng & Sp, The Chldn's Mercy Hosp, **SLP**

Jacobsen, Ellen D 7 Chestnut Lane, Clifton Park, NY 12065, **SLP**

Jacobsen, Lee Ann G 691 Windfield Lane, Machesney Park, IL 61111, (815) 654-4508, BS 71 Northern IL Univ - De Kalb; MA 72 Northern IL Univ - De Kalb; Sp-Lang Path, Harlem Consolidated Schools, **SLP**

Jacobsen, Roxann K Audio-Technica US Incorporated, Hearing & Instrument Division, 1221 Commerce Drive, Stow, OH 44224, (216) 686-2600, BA 77 MI St Univ; MA 78 Central MI Univ; 87–Aud, Audio-Technica US Inc, **A**

Jacobson, Bonny S 842-B South American St, Philadelphia, PA 19147, (215) 351-7036, BS 69 Rutger's St Univ - Douglas Coll; MS 72 Columbia Univ Teachers Coll; 79–Sp-Lang Path, Sch Dist of Philadelphia, **SLP**

Jacobson, Brenda Rae 317 East 8th Street South, Ladysmith, WI 54848, (715) 532-5559, BA 80 Univ of WI - Eau Claire; MS 87 Univ of WI - River Falls; 81–Sp-Lang Path, Flambeau Sch Dist

Jacobson, Cheryl F 455 Canyon Vista Drive, Los Angeles, CA 90065, (213) 222-4902, BA 74 Univ of CA - Santa Barbara; MA 82 CA St Univ - Northridge; SLP, Los Angeles USD, **SLP**

Jacobson, Claire Adrienne 34 Overlook Drive, Danville, PA 17821, (717) 271-6378, BS 78 Univ of UT; ME 82 Dalhousie Univ - Nova Scotia; MS 86 Univ of MS; 87–Aud, Geisinger Med Ctr, **A**

Jacobson, Mrs Dana B 14028 93rd Avenue N E, Bothell, WA 98011, (206) 328-3285, BA 72 Univ of WA; MA 74 Univ of WA; SLP, Lake Washington Sch Dist 414, **SLP**

Jacobson, Mrs Deborah A 14439 89th Place N E, Bothell, WA 98011, (206) 827-4649, BA 75 WA St Univ; MA 76 WA St Univ; Dir of Christian Ed, Rose Hill Presbyterian Church, **SLP**

Jacobson, Deborah K 1705 Shetland, Laramie, WY 82070, (307) 742-7237, MS 80 Univ of WY; Sp-Lang Path, Wee Folks Developmental Center, **SLP**

Jacobson, Dr Edward J 9141 Grant Street, Suite 135, Thornton, CO 80229, (303) 252-9959, BS 64 ID St Univ; MA 67 Univ of CO - Boulder; PH 71 (NS) Univ of CO - Boulder; Aud, Communicology Ltd, **SLP A**

Jacobson, Eileen Roberts 9020 New Britain Circle, Manassas, VA 22110, (703) 369-3232, BS James Madison Univ; ME 82 Old Dominion Univ; Sp/Lang Path, Manassas Cty Pub Schs, **SLP**

Jacobson, Dr Gary P Dir Div Of Aud Dept Of Oto, Henry Ford Hospital, 2799 West Grand Blvd, Detroit, MI 48202, (313) 876-3280, BA 74 CA St Univ - Fullerton; MS 75 Univ of WI - Stevens Point; PH 78 (NS) Kent St Univ; Director, Henry Ford Hosp, **A**

Jacobson, Mrs Ina B 913 Oregon Trail, Cincinnati, OH 45215, (513) 821-0110, BS 53 Univ of Cincinnati; MA 81 Univ of Cincinnati; 84, Private Practice, **SLP ACE**

Jacobson, Joan Department Of Comm Disorders, St Cloud State University, St Cloud, MN 56301, (612) 255-4172, BA 44; MA 48 Syracuse Univ; PH 58 (Lang of the Achieving and Non-Achieving Retarded) Syracuse Univ; Prof, St Cloud St U, **SLP A ACE**

Jacobson, Dr John T Department Of Audiology & Speech Pathology 42-43, Geisinger Medical Center, Danville, PA 17822, (717) 271-6378, MA 70 San Francisco St Univ; MS 72 Western OR St Coll; PH 77 (Aud) Univ of UT; Dir /Aud, Geisinger Med Ctr, **A**

Jacobson, Mrs Kathy Jean 835 1st Street, Menasha, WI 54952, (414) 722-0458, BS 82 Univ of WI - Stevens Point; MS 84 Univ of WI - Stevens Point; Sp-Lang Path, Greenbay Area Pub Schs, **SLP**

Jacobson, Mrs Laura L 9720 West Center Street, Milwaukee, WI 53222, BS 80 Marquette Univ; MS 81 Marquette Univ; Sp-Lang Path, Menomonee Falls Public Schools, **SLP**

Jacobson, Lucille S 911 Brighton Avenue, Reading, PA 19606, (215) 371-5919, BA 61 Syracuse Univ; MS 64 Temple Univ; 61–Sp-Lang Path, Berks Co Iu, **SLP**

Jacobson, Norma S 1617 Butterfield Road, Flossmoor, IL 60422, (312) 957-9390, BS 75 Univ of IL - Urbana; MA 77 Governors St Univ; **SLP**

Jacobson, Paul Alan 641 Detroit, Iron Mountain, MI 49801, (906) 774-6837, BA 83 Univ of Northern CO; MA 85 Univ of Northern CO; Sp-Lang Path, **SLP**

Jacobson, Peggy F 14 Acorn Drive, East Northport, NY 11731, (516) 757-9414, BA 75 Univ of NM; MA 82 NM St Univ; Sp-Path, St Charles Hospital, **SLP ACE**

Jacobson, Mrs Rebecca M 4799 Adrian Circle, Prior Lake, MN 55372, (612) 440-4428, BS 81 Minot St Univ; MS 82 Minot St Univ; 87–Sp-Lang Path, Achievement Rehab Corp, **SLP**

Jacobson, Mrs Robin Lynn 3401 Deming Court, Bakersfield, CA 93309, (805) 833-3531, **SLP**

Jacobson, Mrs Rose 2630 Cropsey Avenue, Brooklyn, NY 11214, (718) 439-7000, BA 82 CUNY - Brooklyn Coll; MS 85 CUNY - Brooklyn Coll; Sp-Lang Path Dir, ACRMD Bklyn Day Treatment Prog, **SLP**

Jacobson, Susan Gail 225 Park Place #2-H, Brooklyn, NY 11238, (718) 871-2980, BA 74 Univ of Denver; MA 75 Univ of Northern CO; 86–Supvr/Aud, NYC Dept of Health, **A**

Jacobson, Susan M 17 West 64th Street, New York, NY 10023, (212) 868-1121, BA 66 CUNY - Brooklyn Coll; MA 67 NY Univ; SLP, NYC Bd of Ed-Sp Serv Ut, **SLP**

Jacobson, Terry A Communication Concepts, 3000 Pearl Street, Suite 106, Boulder, CO 80301, (303) 442-7769, BS 68 Washington Univ; MS 69 Washington Univ; Dir/Sp-Lang Path, Commun Concepts, **SLP**

Jacobson, Tracy L 1203 Dover Lane, Elk Grove Village, IL 60007, (312) 437-0550, BS 86 Univ of IL - Urbana; MA 88 Univ of IL - Urbana

Jacobs-White, Leona M 1535 Parker Street, Berkeley, CA 94703, (415) 843-2189, BA 62 Holy Names Coll; MA 63 Columbia Univ Teachers Coll; SLP, Richmond USD, **SLP**

Jacobus, Mrs Heather J 5223 Pine Street, Bellaire, TX 77401, (713) 661-3913, BA 70 Univ of Houston - Univ Park; MA 76 Univ of Houston - Univ Park; **SLP**

Jacobvitz, Lynda O 7 Harding Street, New Bedford, MA 02740, (508) 997-1570, BA 83 Univ of Denver; MS 84 Boston Univ; Sp-Lang Path, Kennedy-Donovan Center, **SLP**

Jacoby, Dr Beatrice F Rural Delivery, Copake, NY 12516, (518) 329-7473, BA 33 CUNY - Hunter Coll; MA 34 Columbia Univ Teachers Coll; PH 46 (Sp Path & Aud) Columbia Univ Teachers Coll; Retired, Columbia Co Dept Hlth, **SLP A LM**

Jacoby, Dr David I Zalman Aran, Ashdod, Israel, PH (NS); **SLP**

Jacoby, Randi Faith 1623 Third Avenue #14G, New York, NY 10128, (212) 831-7655, BS 80 Boston Univ; MS 82 Columbia Univ Teachers Coll; Sp/Lang Path, Private Practice, **SLP**

Jacopetti, Mrs Theresa M 269 Mountain View Drive, Nanticoke, PA 18634, (717) 735-5812, BS 79 Bloomsburg Univ of PA; MS 80 Bloomsburg Univ of PA; Sp-Lang Path, John Heinz I of Rehab Med, **SLP**

Jacquart, John E 55 Main Street, P O Box 463, Rosendale, NY 12472, (914) 338-8686, BA 85 MI St Univ; MA 86 MI St Univ; Aud, Aquinas Hearing Service, **A**

Jacques, Jeanette Marie Beaumont Hospital, Speech Lang Path Dept, 3601 West Thirteen Mile Rd, Royal Oak, MI 48072, (313) 258-1090, BS 82 Eastern MI Univ; MA 84 Eastern MI Univ; Sp-Lang Path, William Beaumont Hosp, **SLP**

Jacques, Dr Richard D Eastern Illinois University, Dept Communication, Charleston, IL 61920, (419) 372-2515, BS 70 UT St Univ; MA 73 UT St Univ; PH 84 (NS) Bowling Green St Univ; 87–Asst Prof, Eastern Illinois Univ, **SLP**

Jacques-Twichell, Mrs Kathy Ann 34 2nd Street, Ledminster, MA 01453, (617) 534-0027, MS 87 Worcester St Coll; 86–Sp-Lang Path, Shirley Sch Sys

Jacquez, Teddy M Department Of Audiology, 801 West Maple, Farmington, NM 87401, (505) 325-5011, BA 80 Eastern NM Univ; MA 85 Grand Canyon Coll; **A**

Jacquin, Mrs Diane Rubinski 1765 Alder Drive, Orange Park, FL 32073, (904) 269-0253, MS 76 Univ of South FL; Sp-Lang Path, Clay Co Sch Bd, **SLP**

Jacquot, Dr Willard S 717 Linwood Street, Denton, TX 76201-1170, (817) 565-2262, BA 48 Univ of Northern CO; MA 49 Univ of Northern CO; PH 59 (NS) Univ of Denver; Prof, N TX St U, **SLP A**

Jadd, Mrs Ellen Barron 32 Bradenham Place, Eggertsville, NY 14226, (716) 837-8180, BA 74 Elmira Coll; MS 76 Emerson Coll; Sp-Path, UCP of Western NY, **SLP**

Jadd, Lisa-Gaye Marie 34 Wendy Crescent, London, ON, Canada N5X 3J8, (519) 668-6391, BS 82 Univ of Western Ontario; OM 85 Univ of Western Ontario; 87–Sp-Lang Path, Parkwood Hosp, **SLP**

Jaeger, Ellen Louise 1150 Galapago #320, Denver, CO 80204-3576, (303) 441-0437, BS 83 Univ of WI - Stevens Point; MS 85 Univ of WI - Stevens Point; 85–Sp-Lang Path, Memorial Hosp of Boulder, **SLP**

Jaeger, Joan M 3434 10th Avenue West, Seattle, WA 98119, (206) 368-1848, BA 74 Univ of WA; MS 76 Univ of WA; Manager, Northwest Hosp, **SLP**

Jaeger, Karen S 3514 Norfolk Way, Boise, ID 83706, BA 77 Univ of WI - Eau Claire; MS 79 AZ St Univ; Sp-Lang Path, Boise Pub Sch Dist, **SLP**

Jaeger, Sharon Elizabeth 7165 South Elm Court, Littleton, CO 80122, (303) 761-1496, BA 82 Univ of Denver; MA 85 Univ of MN - Minneap-St Paul; SLP, Englewood Public Schools, **SLP**

Jaegli, Mrs Luanne 5814 Capello, Houston, TX 77035, (713) 463-7265, BS 78 Univ of TX - Austin; ME 80 Southwest TX St Univ; **SLP**

Jaekel, Mrs Susan M 1233 Yorkshire, Barrington, IL 60010, (312) 223-8223, BA 82 Saint Xavier Coll; MS 83 Marquette Univ; **SLP**

Jaekels, Anne L 321 Tower View Drive, Green Bay, WI 54301, (414) 435-9358, BS 75 Marquette Univ; MS 76 Marquette Univ; Sp-Path, **SLP**

Jaffa, Mrs Helen S 1844 South Beverly, Mesa, AZ 85202, (602) 967-3703, BS 76 Syracuse Univ; MA 78 CUNY - Queens Coll; Sp-Lang Path, Arizona Sp Path Assoc, **SLP**

Jaffe, Mrs Amy Goldman 24-4 Horseshoe Circle, Ossining, NY 10562, (212) 598-1340, BA 80 CUNY - Queens Coll; MA 82 CUNY - Queens Coll; Audiologist, NY Eye and Ear Infirmary, **A**

Jaffe, Brenda S 300 East 57th Street, New York, NY 10022, (212) 319-5429, BA 82 OH Wesleyan Univ; MA 87 NY Univ

Jaffe, Denise A 16 Far Hill Lane, Pleasantville, NY 10570-2524, (914) 747-0721, BA 73 Hofstra Univ; MS 74 Univ of WI - Madison; MA 81 Pace U -NY City; SLP, Sn Westchester BOCES, **SLP ACE**

Jaffe, Emily G 1055 Suntan Lane, Palm Springs, CA 92264, (619) 322-4118, MA 84 CA St Univ - Northridge; Aud, Private Practice, **A**

Jaffe, Mrs Louise C 4942 Heatherglen, Houston, TX 77096, (713) 728-1163, MA 85 Univ of Houston - Univ Park; Sp-Lang Path, Memorial Hospital Southwest, **SLP**

Jaffe, Dr Mata B 6370 Via Tierra, Boca Raton, FL 33433, (407) 495-3075, BS 67 Univ of Pittsburgh - Pittsburgh; MS 70 Univ of Pittsburgh - Pittsburgh; PH 79 (Sp-Lang Path) Univ of Pittsburgh - Pittsburgh; 86–Dir-SLP/Aud Dept, Pinecrest Rehab Hosp, **SLP ACE**

Jaffe, Mrs Nancy E R 425 Ronnie Drive, Buffalo Grove, IL 60090, (312) 634-0233, BS 73 Northwestern Univ; MS 74 Univ of WI - Madison; **SLP**

Jaffe, Norma S 39-15 Allwood Place, Fair Lawn, NJ 07410, (201) 797-7355, **SLP**

Jaffe, Robert 15738 Plaza South Drive, Taylor, MI 48180, **SLP**

Jaffe, Mrs Sharon B 28 Deforest Lane, Wilton, CT 06897, (516) 239-1258, BA 67 Univ of MD - College Park; MA 69 Univ of MD - College Park; **SLP**

Jaffee, Mrs Susan Ann 1104 Cerrito Feliz Lane, El Paso, TX 79912-2046, (915) 584-1189, Sp-Lang Path, El Paso Indep Sch, **SLP**

Jaffe-Karp, Alison P O Box 2278, Running Springs, CA 92382, (818) 287-6197, BA 80 IN Univ - Bloomington; OM 82 IN Univ - Bloomington; Sp/Lang Path, Private Practice, **SLP**

Jager, Lori L 203 Grant Street, Bettendorf, IA 52722, (319) 359-1371, BA 83 Augustana Coll; MA 86 Western IL Univ; 86–Sp-Lang Path, Miss Bend AEA, **SLP**

Jager, Mrs Susan H 29 Wychwood Road, Livingston, NJ 07039, (201) 893-7369, BA 73 CUNY - Queens Coll; MA 75 CUNY - Queens Coll; Sp-Lang Path, Montclair College, **SLP ACE**

Jagla, Mrs Virginia Abraham 11320 North Meadowbrook Dr, Mequon, WI 53092, (414) 474-4531, BS 80 Northwestern Univ; MS 82 Univ of WI - Madison; Sp/Lang Path, **SLP**

Jagoda, David R 13 Florence Court, Valley Cottage, NY 10989, (203) 325-1544, BA 74 CUNY - Brooklyn Coll; MA 75 Long Island U - CW Post Ctr; **SLP**

Jagodzinski, Mrs Mary Carolyn Route 1 Box 295-D1, Suring, WI 54174, BA 64 Edinboro Univ of PA; MS 65 Syracuse Univ; Sp-Lang Path, CES 8, **SLP**

Jahneke, Anna Maria 4954 Botanical Avenue, St Louis, MO 63110, (314) 773-1846, BS 75 Saint Louis Univ; MA 77 Saint Louis Univ; Sp-Lang Path, Sp Sch Dist-St Louis Co, **SLP**

Jahnes, Mrs Kim H 1206 Madison Street, Charleston, WV 25382, (304) 766-4875, BA 86 Marshall Univ; MA 87 Marshall Univ; 88–Sp-Lang Path, W VA Rehab Ctr, **SLP**

Jahnke, Jeanette M 250 88th Avenue NE, Norman, OK 73071, (405) 360-0220, BA 79 Univ of OK - Norman; MS 81 Univ of OK Medical Center; 82–Sp-Lang Path, Norman Pub Sch, **SLP**

Jahnke, Katherine Anne 610 West State Street #2, Marshalltown, IA 50158, (515) 754-6200, BS 84 Univ of WI - Stevens Point; MS 86 Univ of WI - Stevens Point; **A**

Jahnke, Kathryn Ann 34209 Banbury, Farmington Hills, MI 48331, (313) 593-7725, BA 82 Univ of Denver; MA 84 Univ of CO - Boulder; 87–Sp-Lang Path, Oakwood Hosp, **SLP**

Jahr, Mrs Katherine Layton 1262 East Elm Street, Anaheim, CA 92805, (213) 670-2305, BA 68 Univ of the Pacific; MA 71 CA St Univ - Long Beach; Sp-Lang Path, La Habra Cty Sch Dist, **SLP**

Jakielski, Mrs Kathy Jo 300 Phillips Cove, Driftwood, TX 78619, (512) 858-4443, BS 81 Towson St Univ; MA 88 Univ of TX - Austin; **SLP**

Jakimetz, Dr John R 47 Birchwood Drive West, Valley Stream, NY 11580, (212) 794-4821, BA 74 Iona Coll; MA 77 CUNY - Hunter Coll; PH 84 (NS) NY Univ; Aud, Manhattan Audiological Service, **A**

Jakischa, Mrs Katherine Pauer 14132 Franklyn Boulevard, Brook Park, OH 44142, (216) 826-2278, BA 83 Baldwin-Wallace Coll; MA 85 Cleveland St Univ; **SLP**

Jakosh, Terri Lynn 2510 Spruce Lane, Lynwood, IL 60411, (312) 474-1714, BS 80 Purdue Univ - West Lafayette; MS 81 IN St Univ - Terre Haute; Sp-Lang Path, Lansing School District 158, **SLP**

Jakubec, Mrs Christine Smith 6603 Rhode Island Trail, Crystal Lake, IL 60012, (815) 338-7411, BS 73 Univ of Cincinnati; MA 75 Univ of Cincinnati; Aud, Lake McHenry Reg Prog, **A**

Jakubiak, Dawn Marie 3372 Coolidge Highway #72, Royal Oak, MI 48072, (313) 435-3101, BS 84 Central MI Univ; MA 86 Wayne St Univ; 87–Sp-Lang Path, Sinai Hosp of Detroit, **SLP**

Jakubik, Dennis M 6012 East Lovers Lane, Apartment 217, Dallas, TX 75206, (214) 750-7307, MA 87 Wayne St Univ; 87–Sp-Lang Path, TruCare Rehab Services Inc, **SLP**

Jakubosky, Mrs Ann Leblanc 41 Putnam Park, Fitchburg, MA 01420, (617) 345-2151, BA 78 Assumption Coll; MS 82 Worcester St Coll; Sp-Lang Path, Fitchburg Pub Sch, **SLP**

Jakubovics, Helena Alter 1421 East 4th Street, Brooklyn, NY 11230, (718) 339-4751, **SLP**

Jakubowitz, Melissa D 5913 Kipling Drive, El Sobrante, CA 94803, (415) 881-5243, BS 79 Univ of OR; MA 80 Univ of the Pacific; Sp-Lang Path, Private Practice, **SLP**

Jakubowski, Allan J 5356 North 25th Street, Glendale, WI 53209, (414) 542-9811, BS 73 Univ of WI - Milwaukee; MS 74 Univ of WI - Milwaukee; Sp-Lang Path, Curative Rehab Ctr, **SLP**

Jakubowski, Barbara 36 Brandy Brook Road, North Scituate, RI 02857, (203) 928-7995, BA 76 Montclair St Coll; MA 78 Seton Hall Univ; Sp-Lang Path, Putnam Bd of Ed, **SLP**

Jalonack, Mary Louise T 85 Irving Terrace, Bloomfield, NJ 07003, (201) 429-8910, BA 75 SUNY - Center at Buffalo; MA 81 Montclair St Coll; Sp-Lang Path, Private Practice, **SLP**

Jaloszynski, Jacqueline M 1051 Penn Circle #G-205, King of Prussia, PA 19406, (800) 526-3921, BS 80 Clarion Univ of PA; MS 81 Clarion Univ of PA; Territorial Marketing Manager, Oticon Corporation, **SLP A**

Jalovaara, Rosemary A Planning For Living, 2355 Delta Road, Bay City, MI 48706, (517) 684-6832, **SLP**

Jalowayski, Mrs Irene R 6864 Lipmann Street, San Diego, CA 92122, (619) 452-4367, BS 64 Univ of Miami; MA 80 San Diego St Univ; 88–Dir, Pacific Sp and Lang Ctr, **SLP**

James, Anna Maria R D 5 Box 26, Selinsgrove, PA 17870, (717) 523-1155, BS 76 Indiana Univ of PA; MS 83 Bloomsburg Univ of PA; **SLP**

James, Carol C Route 2 Box 411, Mount Crawford, VA 22841, (703) 568-6491, ME 80 James Madison Univ; Audiologist, James Madison University, **SLP A**

James, Cynthia A 115 North Franklin Tnpk, Apartment 5, Ramsey, NJ 07446, (201) 934-1141, BA 73 Univ of MA - Amherst; MA 75 Montclair St Coll; ME 87 William Paterson Coll; 87–Sp-Lang Path, Private Practice, **SLP ACE**

James, Mrs Cynthia Dwyer Rt 1 Box 367, Prosperity, SC 29127, (803) 445-8333, OB 81 Northeast MO St Univ; MA 82 Northeast MO St Univ; 84–Sp-Lang Path, Saluda County School District, **SLP**

James, Cynthia Rae 931 Belle Court, Tracy, CA 95376, (209) 835-8732, BS 82 Kent St Univ; MA 86 San Jose St Univ; 86–Sp-Lang Path, Tracy PS, **SLP**

James, Daniel H Fort Lauderdale Hearing Center, 1122 Bayview Drive, Fort Lauderdale, FL 33304, (305) 563-3355, BS 73 Indiana Univ of PA; MA 75 Univ of FL; Owner/Aud, Ft Laud Hrng Cen, **A**

James, Evelyn Louise 11002 Annapolis Road, Bowie, MD 20715, (301) 464-3705, MS 88 Howard Univ

James, Mrs Jacquelyn 8941 Footed Ridge, Columbia, MD 21045, (301) 596-3844, BA 74 Case Western Reserve Univ; MS 76 Univ of South FL; **SLP**

James, Jan Lynnette 5900 Timbercreek Lane #304, Raleigh, NC 27612, (919) 790-2500, BS 84 WV Univ; MS 86 Univ of SC - Columbia; **SLP**

James, Mrs Jane G 3010 Valley Brook Drive, Champaign, IL 61821, BS 58 OH St Univ; MS 64 Univ of IL - Urbana; SLP, Champaign Unit #4 Schs, **SLP**

James, Mrs Julie Koehn 404 Woodhaven Court, Sheboygan, WI 53081, (414) 458-3149, BS 84 Univ of WI - Milwaukee; MS 86 Marquette Univ; 88–Sp-Lang Path, Sheboygan Memorial Med Ctr, **SLP**

James, Mrs Kay Robbins 12206 Fair Oaks Boulevard, Apartment 24, Fair Oaks, CA 95628, (916) 929-2277, BS 83 Pacific Union Coll; MS 85 San Francisco St Univ; SLP, Rehabilitation Service N Calif, **SLP**

James, Kellye A Speech Pathology Services, Hot Springs Rehab Center, P O Box 1358, Hot Springs, AR 71902, (501) 624-4411, BS 85 Univ of AR - Little Rock; MS 87 Univ of AR - Medical Sci; 88–Sp-Lang Path, Hot Springs Rehab Ctr Hosp, **SLP**

James, Mrs La Reeca Meador P O Box 740, Cadiz, KY 42211, (502) 522-3929, BS 74 G Peabody Coll-Vanderbilt U; MS 75 Vanderbilt Univ; 87–Sp-Lang Path, Private Practice, **SLP**

James, Laura S 35-B2 Second Street, Christiansburg, VA 24073, (703) 343-2753, BS 79 Radford Univ; MS 84 Radford Univ; 86–Sp-Lang Path, Ctr for Rehab and Dev, **SLP**

James, Linda L 9 East Trenton Boulevard, Fayetteville, AR 72701, (501) 442-9846, OB 75 Univ of AR - Fayetteville; MA 76 Univ of AR - Fayetteville; Sp-Lang Path:Chrprsn, Fayetteville Public Sch, **SLP**

James, Marcy Ann 425 S Hubbards Lane #3, Louisville, KY 40207, (502) 636-5241, BS 85 Western KY Univ; MS 87 Western KY Univ; SLP, InSpeech Inc, **SLP**

James, Mary Catherine 5235 West 5150 South, Kearns, UT 84118, (208) 967-2656, BS 83 Univ of UT; MS 86 Univ of UT; 86–Sp-Lang Path, Jordan Valley CDC, **SLP**

James, Mrs Mary-Teresa C Lewis-Gale Clinic Inc, 4910 Valley View Boulevard NW, Roanoke, VA 24012, (703) 265-1605, BS 85 SUNY - Coll at New Paltz; MS 87 PA St Univ - Univ Park; 88–Aud, Lewis-Gale Clinic Inc, **A**

James, Mrs Rae K 4412 Oakton Road, Fort Worth, TX 76116, (817) 738-9586, BS 68 TX Woman's Univ; MA 73 TX Woman's Univ; Sp-Lang Path, Ft Worth ISD, **SLP**

James, Sally Lynn P O Box 291, Basye, VA 22810, (919) 816-1401, BS 84 Indiana Univ of PA; MS 86 James Madison Univ; Sp-Lang Path, Northwestern Community Svcs, **SLP**

James, Mrs Sarah H 191 Robins Road, Harvest, AL 35749-9577, (205) 536-5243, BS 71 Auburn Univ - Auburn; ME 73 Univ of VA - Charlottesville; Sp-Lang Path, Private Practice, **SLP**

James, Dr Sharon L University Of Wisconsin System, 1652 Van Hise Hall, Madison, WI 53706, (608) 263-3680, BA 67 Univ of HI - Manoa; MS 72 Univ of WI - Madison; PH 75 (NS) Univ of WI - Madison; Academic Planner, Univ of Wisc, **SLP**

James, Mrs Sheryl G Rt 1 Box 172, Bassett, VA 24055, (703) 629-7206, MS 70 SUNY - Coll at Geneseo; BS 69 SUNY - Coll at Geneseo; Sp/Lang Path, Henry Co Pub Sch, **SLP**

James, Susan Kathleen 420 West Country Hills Drive, La Habra, CA 90631, (714) 871-8510, BS 84 Northern AZ Univ; MS 86 Univ of Redlands; 88–Sp-Lang Path, Lowell Joint Sch Dist, **SLP**

James, Sylvia E 227 Circle Drive, Mattoon, IL 61938, (217) 234-2179, BS 69 Eastern IL Univ; MS 67 Eastern IL Univ; SLP/Educ Diagnostician, Educational Consulting Service, **SLP**

James, Vivian Kirkpatrick 3365 Ridgeline Drive, Las Cruces, NM 88005, (505) 525-0972, BS 75 East Carolina Univ; MA 77 Univ of TN - Knoxville; 88–Sp-Lang Path, Private Practice, **SLP**

Jameson, Dean G 2026 Belmont, Abilene, TX 79602, (915) 692-1633, BA 76 TX Tech Univ; BA 77 TX Tech Univ; MA 80 Univ of North TX; Sp-Lang Path, W Tx Rehab Cen, **SLP**

Jameson, Janet W 21 Glen Valley Drive, Penfield, NY 14526, (716) 671-9450, **SLP**

Jameson, Mrs Joyce Eileen 123 Birchwood Drive, Hendersonville, NC 28739, (704) 894-8240, BS 75 Miami Univ - Oxford; MA 84 Western Carolina Univ; SLP, Polk Co Schools, **SLP**

Jameson, Mrs Michele B 2420 Ridgelea Avenue, Culpeper, VA 22701, (703) 825-0713, BA 71 Fisk Univ; MA 73 Catholic Univ of America; Sp-Lang Path, Culpeper County Schools, **SLP**

Jameson, Scott G 21 Glen Valley Drive, Penfield, NY 14526, (716) 671-9450, MS; **A**

Jameson, Shelby Denise 6777 Rasberry Lane #1023, Shreveport, LA 71129, (318) 688-6488, BA 85 Univ of North TX; MA 87 Univ of North TX; 88–Aud, Highland Clinic

James-Trychel, Michele 727 Swaying Palm Drive, Apopka, FL 32712, (305) 841-5111, BA 77 Univ of FL; MA 78 Univ of FL; Coord Infant Hrng Imp Scrn, Orlando Reg Med Cen, **SLP A**

Jamieson, Mrs Frances Rayman 4457 Starling Court, Woodbridge, VA 22193, (703) 899-1656, MS 88 James Madison Univ; 88–Sp-Lang Path, Mary Washington Hosp

Jamieson, Mrs Janet Lorraine 6717 Coleman Cr Road, Medford, OR 97501, (503) 776-8552, BA 75 Coll of Great Falls; MA 83 Coll of Great Falls; **SLP**

Jamison, Gayle 954 Ohayo Mountain Road, Woodstock, NY 12498, (914) 679-6138, BA 69 Montclair St Coll; MS 74 Vanderbilt Univ; 79–Sp-Lang Path, Private Practice, **SLP**

Jamison, Mrs Robin J R Rural Delivery #1, Halpin Road, Middlebury, VT 05753-1305, (802) 388-3338, BS 80 Radford Univ; MA 82 Marshall Univ; SLP, Pamela Kampf, **SLP**

Jamison, William J 712 13th Street #4, Auburn, NE 68305, (402) 274-5147, BA 69 Univ of NE - Lincoln; MA 74 Univ of NE - Lincoln; Aud, Esu #4, **A**

Jamroga, Elizabeth 23 Hardin Lane, Glastonbury, CT 06033, (203) 633-5321, BA 64; MA 69 Univ of Hartford; MS 82 Southern CT St Univ; Sp-Lang Path, Bd of Ed Glastonbury, **SLP**

Jamron, Susan Carol 126 East Gate Lane, Hamden, CT 06514, (203) 281-4664, MA 88 Vanderbilt Univ; 88–Sp-Lang Path, Easter Seal Rehab Ctr of Central CT Inc

Janak, Judy A 19802 Rustlewood, Humble, TX 77338, (713) 540-5097, BS 77 Univ of Houston - Univ Park; MA 78 Univ of Houston - Univ Park; Sp-Lang Path, Humble ISD, **SLP ACE**

Janes, Mrs Judith E 894 Grove Street, Meadville, PA 16335, (814) 432-3171, BA 70 Indiana Univ of PA; ME 75 Clarion Univ of PA; Dir of Sp & Hrng, Polk Cen/Sp & Hrng Dept, **SLP**

Janik, Mrs Rosa Lee 3126 Bonney Briar, Missouri City, TX 77459, (713) 498-8110, **SLP**

Jankeloff, Lois 32 Allevard Street, Lido Beach, NY 11561, (516) 889-2713, BA 81 CUNY - Brooklyn Coll; MS 82 CUNY - Brooklyn Coll; Sp/Lang Path, N Shore U Hosp, **SLP**

Jankowski, Mrs Ann Ericsson P O Box 147, Adamsville, RI 02801, (401) 635-2151, BA 74 Univ of CT; MS 77 Southern CT St Univ; 88–Sp-Lang Path, East Providence PS, **SLP**

Jankowski, Mrs Catherine Jane 912 Smithbridge Road, Wilmington, DE 19807, (302) 323-2786, BA 79 Univ of DE; MS 82 PA St Univ - Univ Park; **SLP**

Jankowski, Janet Marie 34 Huntington Court, Bethel, CT 06801, (203) 356-1989, BA 71 Anna Maria Coll; MS 74 Emerson Coll; **SLP**

Janota, Mrs Deloris A 318 Seneca Street, Park Forest, IL 60466, (312) 748-3322, BS 45 Univ of IL - Urbana; MA 74 Governors St Univ; Sp-Lang Path, Dist 163-Park Forest Il, **SLP**

Janovcik, Marita Harsanyl 212 Ranchero Place N W, Calgary, AB, Canada T3G 1C7, (204) 267-2225, MS 86 Univ of ND; **SLP**

Janow, Mrs Ethel W 8510 Bay Parkway, Brooklyn, NY 11214, (718) 996-4600, BA 61 CUNY - Queens Coll; MS 74 CUNY - Brooklyn Coll; Sp/Lang Path, Private Practice, **SLP**

Janowicz, Pamela J 239-B White Horse Pike, Audubon, NJ 08106, (609) 546-8155, BA 85 SUNY - Coll at New Paltz; ME 87 Univ of VA - Charlottesville; 87–Sp-Lang Path, Kingsway Learning Ctr, **SLP**

Jans, Mrs Deborah L 11 Embassy Court, Inglis Road, London, England, BS 78 Syracuse Univ; MS 80 Columbia Univ Teachers Coll; Sp-Lang Path, Ealing Health Authority, **SLP**

Jansen, Cindy Larson 9927 Brunswick Court, San Ramon, CA 94583, (415) 828-5050, BA 81 CA St Univ - Chico; MA 87 San Jose St Univ; Sp-Lang Path, Mt Diablo Hosp, **SLP**

Jansen, John W 1055 Clermont, Denver, CO 80220, (303) 393-2871, BS 62 Northern IL Univ - De Kalb; MA 65 Univ of IL - Urbana; PH 69 (PD) Univ of OK Medical Center; 85–Aud, VA Medical Center, **A**

Jansen, Kathleen M 15-A Robin Road, Mount Holly, NJ 08060, (609) 265-0148, BS 85 Clarion Univ of PA; MS 87 Clarion Univ of PA; **A**

Jansen-Petersen, Jane E 6852-A Hyde Park Drive, San Diego, CA 92119-2232, BS 84 IA St Univ; MA 86 Univ of Northern IA; **A**

Jans-Kaplan, Mrs Gayle S 442 North California, Mundelein, IL 60060, (312) 949-8017, BS 74 Southern IL Univ -Carbondale; MS 75 Southern IL Univ -Carbondale; Sp-Lang Path, Laremont Sch (Sedol), **SLP**

Janso, Christine Maria 297 Berkshire Avenue, New Milford, NJ 07646, (201) 836-0470, BS 85 Stockton St Coll; MS 87 William Paterson Coll; **SLP**

Janson, Diane B 59 Sampson Road, Bolton, MA 01740, **SLP**

Janson, Laura Jean 424 Chestnut Lane, Wayne, PA 19087, (215) 688-1732, BA 85 Coll of Wooster; MA 87 OH Univ - Athens; **SLP**

Janssen, Lynda D Tulsa Ear Nose & Throat Inc, 6565 South Yale #408, Tulsa, OK 74136, (918) 492-5577, BA 70 Washington Univ; MA 73 Univ of MD - College Park; **SLP A**

Jansson, Mrs Eraine Arndt #4-4 Chinook Drive SW, Medicine Hat, AB, Canada T1A 4B3, MS 65 Western MI Univ; 88–Sp-Lang Path, Medicina Hat Reg Hosp

Janusko, Mrs Claudia Ripinski 170 Highland Street, Rocky Hill, CT 06067, (203) 224-2631, BA 82 Univ of Toledo; MA 83 Bowling Green St Univ; Aud, ENT & Facial Plastic Grp Pc, **A**

Jaques, Mrs Julie McGee 2571 Redding Road, Atlanta, GA 30319, (404) 261-0205, BS 77 Univ of GA; ME 78 Univ of GA; 88–Sp-Lang Path, Bailey Sp Lang Svcs, **SLP**

Jaquith, Mrs Barbara A 4151 43rd Avenue South, Minneapolis, MN 55406, (612) 544-1579, BA 75 Univ of MN - Duluth; MS 79 Univ of WI - Eau Claire; Sp-Lang Path, Robbinsdale Sch Dist #281, **SLP**

Jaramillo, Aura Elena 4847 Borchers Drive, Kirby, TX 78219, (512) 245-2157, BS 80 Southwest TX St Univ; ME 81 Southwest TX St Univ; Sp-Lang Path, Commun & Lrng Clinic, **SLP ACE**

Jardin, Mrs Irene M 1429 Trout Brook Drive, West Hartford, CT 06117, (201) 491-3290, BA 71 Elmira Coll; ME 72 Boston Univ; SLP, Shared Services, **SLP**

Jardini, Mrs Linda P 77 Owendale Avenue, Pittsburgh, PA 15227, (412) 648-8389, BA 60 Hiram Coll; MS 74 Univ of Pittsburgh - Pittsburgh; Cl & Aud, U Pitt/Cleft Palate Craniofacial Ctr, **A**

Jarecki, Janis Marie 124 Duncan Drive, Butler, PA 16001, (814) 226-2445, BS 78 Allegheny Coll; MS 81 Clarion Univ of PA; 87–Asst Prof, Clarion Univ of PA, **SLP ACE**

Jared, Carol Beth c/o Institute Of Logopedics, 2400 Jardine Drive, Wichita, KS 67219, (316) 262-8271, BS 81 OK St Univ; MS 83 Univ of OK - OK City; Aud, Institute of Logopedics, **A**

Jared, Mrs Laura Lee 1032 Avenue H, Redondo Beach, CA 90277, (303) 663-2977, BA 83 Univ of Northern CO; MA 84 Univ of Northern CO; SLP, Poudre Ri Sch Dist, **SLP**

Jarema-Mongeau, Ann Univ Of Rochester Medical Cen, Dept Aud & Sp Path Box 629, 601 Elmwood Avenue, Rochester, NY 14642, (716) 275-4803, BS 81 Ithaca Coll; MS 83 Univ of WI - Madison; 83–SLP, Univ of Rochester Medical Ctr, **SLP ACE**

Jarett, Mrs Irene G 2163 Meadowbrook Court, Thousand Oaks, CA 91362, (818) 885-5330, BA 79 Univ of CA - Santa Barbara; MA 81 CA St Univ - Northridge; Dir Comm Disorders, Northridge Hosp Med Ctr, **SLP**

Jargosch, Debra L 213 Hillsborough, Columbia, SC 29212, BS 76 Univ of KS; MA 78 Univ of KS; 88–Dir-Sp-Lang Path, Babcock Ctr, **SLP**

Jarman, Susan M Rd 2 Box 48, Birdsboro, PA 19508, (215) 582-5203, BA 79 SUNY - Coll at Cortland; MA 81 OK St Univ; **SLP**

Jarmel, Mrs Fredi M 199-07 19th Avenue, Whitestone, NY 11357, (516) 560-5100, BA 73 CUNY - Queens Coll; MA 76 Hofstra Univ; 80–Aud - Proj Coord, Pre-Sch Hrng Council of Li Inc, **A**

Jarmolowski, Patricia Ann 313 Lasalle Avenue, Buffalo, NY 14215, BA 85 Thiel Coll; MA 87 SUNY - Center at Buffalo; 87–Sp-Lang Path, Lang Dev Prog of W NY, **SLP**

Jarrell, Rita Coval 1315 South Maple Road #305, Ann Arbor, MI 48103, (313) 429-1596, Program Admin, Sp & Com Inc, **SLP**

Jarrett, Catherine DeClerk Rt 6 Box 204, Pocahontas, AR 72455, (501) 892-9623, BS 83 AR St Univ; OM 86 AR St Univ; 88–Sp-Lang Path, St Paul Parochial Sch, **SLP**

Jarrett, Marian H 200 Forest Drive, Falls Church, VA 22046, (202) 994-6170, BS 66 WV Univ; MA 67 Northwestern Univ; ED 85 (NS) George Washington Univ; 88–Sp-Lang Path, George Wash Univ, **SLP**

Jarrick, Nancy A 429 South 6th Avenue, La Grange, IL 60525, (312) 579-0948, BS 75 Western IL Univ; MA 76 Univ of IL - Urbana; SLP, Darien School Dstr 61, **SLP**

Jarrosak, Mrs Nancy R 50 Campbell Road, Rutland, VT 05701, (802) 773-9265, BA 78 Univ of VT; MS 79 Univ of VT; Sp-Lang Path, Rutland South Supervisory Un, **SLP**

Jarrow, Dr Jane E 3537 Sunset Drive, Columbus, OH 43221, (614) 457-5681, BS 70 Purdue Univ - West Lafayette; MS 71 Purdue Univ - West Lafayette; PH 76 Wichita St Univ; Exec Dir, Assoc Hndcpd Stud Serv Sec Ed, **SLP**

Jarusek, Mrs Sandra L 5081 Hamer Lane, Placentia, CA 92670, (818) 969-2467, BS 70 OH Univ - Athens; MS 77 Southern CT St Univ; Sp-Lang Path, Azusa USD, **SLP**

Jarvis, Barbara S 6288 Willowgate Lane, Dallas, TX 75230, **A**

Jarvis, Carol A 60 Magnolia Avenue #F, San Anselmo, CA 94960, (415) 472-4110, BA 60 WA St Univ; ME 69 Univ of FL; Sp-Lang Path, Marin County Office of Educ, **SLP**

Jarvis, Cynthia Nick P O Box 2, Tomahawk, WI 54487, BS 73 Univ of WI - Stevens Point; MS 74 Univ of WI - Stevens Point; 82–Aud, Ear Nose Throat Assn of Wausau, **A**

Jarvis, Doris S 1230 Parkside Avenue, Hampton, VA 23669, **SLP**

Jarvis, Mrs Elizabeth Wolz 5392 Kenilworth Drive, Huntington Beach, CA 92649, (714) 960-6909, BA 83 Univ of CA - Santa Barbara; MA 86 San Diego St Univ; **SLP**

Jarvis, Hilary 410 17th Street, Apartment 207B, Knoxville, TN 37916, BA 80 George Washington Univ; MA 83 Northwestern Univ; Aud, **A**

Jarvis, Mrs Julie Ann 1702 E Sunnymede Avenue, South Bend, IN 46615, (219) 232-2065, BS 80 Ball St Univ; MA 83 Ball St Univ; Sp/Lang Path, Speech Plus Inc, **SLP**

Jarvis, Mrs Kelly Michele 4138 East Patricia Jane Dr, Phoenix, AZ 85018, (602) 954-6527, **SLP**

Jarvis, Ruthann Reis 13532 Prospect, Santa Ana, CA 92705-2612, (213) 436-7787, BA 81 CA St Univ - Long Beach; MA 83 CA St Univ - Long Beach; Sp/Lang Path, Long Beach Scottish Rite Ins, **SLP**

Jarvis, Susan E 220 Sullivan Way #B-8, Trenton, NJ 08628, (609) 924-8120, BS 79 Trenton St Coll; MA 82 Trenton St Coll; SLP, Lewis Clinic for Educ Therapy, **SLP ACE**

Jarvis, Susan Marie 355 Voorhees, Buffalo, NY 14216, BA 76 SUNY - Center at Buffalo; MS 80 SUNY - Coll at Buffalo; SLP, Buffalo Bd of Ed, **SLP**

Jasinski, Andrew Joseph 10513 Mountain Road N E, Albuquerque, NM 87112, (505) 356-2343, BS 79 Northern MI Univ; MS 80 Univ of WI - Stevens Point; Supervisor, River Ridge Rehab, **SLP**

Jasinski, Mrs Mary E W 235 55121 Otter Tr, Waukesha, WI 53186, (414) 548-0319, BS 73 Marquette Univ; MS 75 Marquette Univ; SLP, Waukesha Pub Schools, **SLP**

Jask, Barbara Ann 201 Wilton Street, New Hyde Park, NY 11040, (516) 921-7171, BA 85 Adelphi Univ; MA 86 SUNY - Coll at Geneseo; 87–Sp-Lang Path, Variety Pre-Sch Workshop, **SLP**

Jaskierski, Sheila P 726 Brighton Lane, La Grange, Il 60525, (312) 352-5264, BS 76 Bradley Univ; MA 77 Northwestern Univ; SLP, La Grange Area Dept Spec Ed, **SLP**

Jasman, Daniel Robert 12092 Manley Street, Garden Grove, CA 92645, (213) 625-6792, BA 78 San Diego St Univ; OM 81 CA St Univ - Long Beach; **SLP**

Jasnoch-Fairchild, Debra 1008 West B Street, North Platte, NE 69101, (308) 532-8269, BA 76 Kearney St Coll; MS 82 Univ of NE - Lincoln; Aud, Private Practice, **A**

Jason, Henry C, Jr P O Box 15142, San Francisco, CA 94115, (415) 573-2027, BA 68 Boston Coll; MA 70 Harvard Univ; MS 73 Emerson Coll; 88–Sp-Lang Path, Chope Community Hosp, **SLP**

Jassal, Sat Pal Thomas Jefferson Hospital, Hearing Center Suite 8168, 111 South 11th Street, Philadelphia, PA 19107, (215) 928-8897, BA 65; MA 71 Temple Univ; Ch of Aud, Thomas Jefferson U Hosp, **A**

Jassem, Harriet Lois 53 West 70th Street #2-B, New York, NY 10023, (212) 724-9404, BS 74 Emerson Coll; MS 76 Columbia Univ Sch of Gen St; 88–Pres, Speech Transformation Systems, **SLP**

Jaster, Mary L 4105 Colgate, Dallas, TX 75225, **SLP**

Jastrzab, Joyce A 6715 Pershing Court, Woodridge, IL 60517, (312) 832-6122, MS 72 IL St Univ - Normal; Sp-Lang Path, Salt Creek School District 48, **SLP**

Jasuta, Stephanie 10705 Little Thicket Road, Austin, TX 78736, (512) 346-9988, BS 72 Univ of TX - Austin; MA 74 Univ of TX - Austin; Co-Director, Sp Lang & Hrng Serv, **SLP**

Jauernig, Mrs Joan R 6 Sunset Road West, North Branford, CT 06471, (203) 468-3218, BS 66 Southern CT St Univ; MS 74 Southern CT St Univ; Dept Head Sp-Lang-Hrng Serv, East Haven Public Schools, **SLP**

Javid, Claudia M 4750 Lafayette Drive, Madison, WI 53705, (217) 788-3767, **SLP**

Javier, Nancy T Childrens Hospital, Speech & Hearing Dept, 200 Henry Clay Avenue, New Orleans, LA 70118, (504) 899-9511, **SLP**

Javor, John M 570 Meadow Road, North Huntingdon, PA 15642, (412) 863-7071, BS 71 PA St Univ - Univ Park; MS 72 PA St Univ - Univ Park; Sp-Lang Path, Westmoreland Iu #7, **SLP**

Jaworek, Sherry Ann 5546 Scranton Road, Roanoke Apartment 2, Hamburg, NY 14075, (716) 532-5522, BS 82 SUNY - Coll at Fredonia; MS 83 Ithaca Coll; Sp-Lang Path, J N Adam DDSO, **SLP**

Jaworski, Sandra Ann 13L Lakeside Drive, Ledyard, CT 06339, (203) 572-7221, BS 84 SUNY - Coll at Fredonia; MS 85 SUNY - Coll at Fredonia; 85–Sp-Lang Path, DMR-Region 6-Mystic Ctr

Jaworski, Mrs Suzanne Marie 11 Irma Place, Oceanport, NJ 07757, (201) 229-4089, BA 69 Newark St Coll; MA 70 Newark St Coll; 87–Aud, West Long Branch Sp & Hrng Ctr, **A**

Jax, Dr Vicki A P O Box 2809, Seal Beach, CA 90740, (213) 596-0675, BA 69 Univ of CA - Santa Barbara; MA 73 CA St Univ - Long Beach; PH 88 (Special Education) CA St Univ - Los Angeles; 81–Sp-Lang Path, Private Practice, **SLP**

Jay, Anne Octavia 3913 A Flad, St Louis, MO 63110, (314) 772-1713, BA 83 Kenyon Coll; MA 86 Saint Louis Univ; 88–Sp-Lang Path, Good Shepherd Sch for Children, **SLP**

Jay, Mrs Ellen R R 1046 North Main Avenue, Sidney, OH 45365, (513) 492-9209, BS 75 Miami Univ - Oxford; MS 77 Miami Univ - Oxford; Sp-Lang Path, Private Practice, **SLP**

Jay, Dr Robert E 3903 Bandak Court, High Point, NC 27260-9633, (919) 886-3430, BA 69 Univ of CO - Boulder; MS 71 Eastern NM Univ; PH 77 (NS) Vanderbilt Univ; Audiology Program Coordinator, Univ N Carolina Chapel Hill, **SLP A**

Jaye, Robin Lynne P O Box 1854, St Matthews Station, San Mateo, CA 94401-3113, (415) 930-8186, BA 81 Univ of Redlands; MS 84 San Francisco St Univ; Sp/Lang Path, John Muir Med Ctr, **SLP**

Jaynes, Beverly Ann 154 Eileen, Bloomfield Hills, MI 48013, (313) 574-0900, BS 74 1890; MA 76 Wayne St Univ; Asst Dir/Rehabilitation Servcs, Home Health Care Service-Macon, **SLP**

Jazzar, Carol Barbara 280 DE Chateauguay Street, Longueuil, PQ, Canada J4H 2K7, (514) 482-0500, BA 79 McGill Univ - Quebec; MS 84 Boston Univ; 84–Sp-Lang Path, Mackay Ctr

Jean, Mrs Jacqueline Willever 3580 Westwood Drive, Easton, PA 18042, (201) 859-1001, BS 72 Ithaca Coll; MS 73 Ithaca Coll; Sp/Lang Path, Harmony Twp Bd of Ed, **SLP**

Jeanes, Barbara Cree 1905 Bromley Estates, Pine Hill, NJ 08021, (609) 342-3064, BS 76 Bloomsburg Univ of PA; MA 77 Bowling Green St Univ; Director Dept of SLP, Cooper Hospital, **SLP**

Jeanmard, Frances Lee 5101-D Maple Court, Alexandria, LA 71303, (504) 628-8237, **SLP**

Jeans, Karen K 1616 Burnside Lane, St Charles, MO 63303, (314) 928-5402, BS 65 IL St Univ - Normal; ME 73 Drury Coll; 87–Dir-Early Childhood Learning Ctr, St Louis Univ Dept of Comm Dis, **SLP**

Jeans, Mrs Rowena Marie 11 Top Rail Lane, Rancho Palos Verdes, CA 90274, (213) 544-0088, MA 74 Univ of Southern CA; Sp-Lang Path, Private Practice, **SLP**

Jebb, Jeanne Frances Route 7 Box 124KZ, Santa Fe, NM 87505, BA 74 Eastern WA Univ; MS 76 Eastern WA Univ; MS 83 Univ of NH; Sp-Lang Path, Ctr for P T & Rehab, **SLP**

Jeddah, Janet Z 31 Cambria Road, Syosset, NY 11791, (212) 735-2669, BS 73 SUNY - Center at Albany; MS 76 Adelphi Univ; Aud, Kings Co Hosp Cen/Hrng Sp Cl, **A**

Jeffers, Donna P 20881 Crestview Lane, Huntington Beach, CA 92646-5951, (714) 968-1797, BS 76 Brigham Young Univ; OM 77 Brigham Young Univ; 88–Sp Lang Path, Long Beach USD, **SLP**

Jeffers, Mrs Florence K 1655 Vicksburg N W, Bend, OR 97701, (503) 382-2979, BA 43 Univ of OK - Norman; ME 58 Univ of OR; **SLP LM**

Jeffers, Sarah Jane 13106 West 88th Court #25, Lenexa, KS 66215, (913) 621-5155, BA 82 Augustana Coll; MA 88 Univ of KS; 84–Sp-Lang Path, Wyandotte Co Spec Ed Coop USD, **SLP**

Jeffers, Stephanie 84 Allandale Avenue, Rochester, NY 14610, (716) 377-4660, BS 76 SUNY - Coll at Geneseo; MA 77 Univ of ME - Orono; SLP, BOCES, **SLP**

Jefferson, Mary Catherine 104 Dublin Road, Muskogee, OK 74403, (918) 683-0321, BA 83 Northeastern OK St Univ; MA 87 Univ of Tulsa; 88–Sp-Lang Path, Muskogee Guidance Ctr, **SLP**

Jeffery, Carol 93 Sterling Place, Brooklyn, NY 11217, (718) 638-2728, BA 72 Montclair St Coll; MA 78 CUNY - Hunter Coll

Jeffery, Jill Coleen 2408 East Broadway, Long Beach, CA 90803, (213) 434-1320, BS 74 Bowling Green St Univ; MS 78 Miami Univ - Oxford; Sp-Lang Path, Long Beach USD, **SLP**

Jeffery, Mrs Karin L 245 Flax Hill Road, Norwalk, CT 06854, (203) 855-0118, BA 84 Univ of CT; MA 87 Memphis St Univ; 87–Sp-Lang Path, The Foundation Sch, **SLP**

Jeffrey, Mrs Jennifer S 11 Nob Circle, Newburgh, NY 12550, BA 76 Southern CT St Univ; MS 78 Southern CT St Univ; Sp-Lang Path, **SLP**

Jeffrey, Mrs Judith Lynn 5H Yester Oaks Circle, Greensboro, NC 27408, (919) 765-0550, BA 84 Marshall Univ; MA 85 Marshall Univ; 86–Sp-Lang Path, InSpeech Inc, **SLP**

Jeffreys, Hanna Helane 10533 Green Mountain Circle, Columbia, MD 21044, (301) 730-3310, MA 67 Univ of MD - College Park; 84, Private Practice, **SLP**

Jeffreys, Maureen B 131 Mill Road #8, Rhinebeck, NY 12572, (914) 373-9618, BS 77 SUNY - Coll at Geneseo; MS 86 Syracuse Univ; 88–Sp-Lang Path, Card Hayes Sch/Special Chldn, **SLP**

Jeffries, Angela L 3900 Fir Tree Drive #4-B, Riverside, CA 92505, (714) 736-6333, BS 83 Loma Linda Univ - Riverside; MS 85 Loma Linda Univ - Riverside; 87–Sp-Lang Path, Corona Comm Hosp, **SLP**

Jeffries, Cheryl Anita 6687 Wild Ridge Circle, Memphis, TN 38119, (901) 525-2682, BA 81 NC St Univ at Raleigh; MS 85 Univ of the DC; 86–Clin Supvr, Memphis State Univ, **SLP ACE**

Jeffries, Judith Ann 1504 Marlwood Circle, Charlotte, NC 28212-4023, BA 80 Marshall Univ; MA 83 Marshall Univ; MA 85 Kent St Univ; Audiology Interne, Huntington Ear Clinic, **A**

Jeffries, Mrs Mary Joan P 2621 Mollimar, Plano, TX 75075, (214) 596-4839, BS 62 OK St Univ; OM 63 Univ of OK Medical Center; SLP, Dr Ron Perkins, **SLP**

Jeglum, Mrs Marilynn J 1468 West Foster Avenue, Chicago, IL 60640, (312) 492-7986, BA 71 Mundelein Coll; MA 73 Northwestern Univ; Comm Consol Sch Dis 65, **SLP**

Jeje, Saeeda S N 325 Ranchglen Place N W, Calgary, AB, Canada T3G 1G2, (403) 229-7055, BA 71; ME 74 Boston Univ; OD 82 (NS) Boston Univ; Sp/Lang Path, Alberta Chld Hosp

Jelinek, Dr Janis A 1066 Bonita Road, Laramie, WY 82070, (307) 766-5710, BA 55 Fort Hays St Univ; MA 64 Univ of WY; PH 79 (EDADM) Univ of WY; 65–Assoc Dean, U of WY-Dept Sp Path & Aud, **SLP F**

Jelinek, Mrs Judith E M 28831 Shady Lane, Laguna Beach, CA 92651, (714) 751-5992, OB 59 0162; BA 72 CA St Univ - Fullerton; MA 73 CA St Univ - Fullerton; **SLP**

Jelinsky, Barbara M 27 Andover Drive, Wayne, NJ 07470, (201) 694-0118, BS 64 Emerson Coll; Sp-Lang Path, Hamilton Plaza Oakridge Nursing Home, **SLP**

Jelm, Judith Michels Pediatric Sp & Lang Ther Serv, 3033 Ogden Avenue, Lisle, IL 60532, (312) 983-6104, BS 75 Univ of IL - Urbana; MS 76 Univ of IL - Urbana; Sp-Lang Path, Pedia Sp & Lang Ther Serv Ltd, **SLP**

Jelonek, Susan Jean 1380 Oak Creek Drive #420, Palo Alto, CA 94304, (415) 325-3416, BA 72 Univ of CA - Berkeley; OM 76 Univ of PA; 88–Pres, Micro Sound Products

Jemelka, Victor J 4906 18th Street West #B, Bradenton, FL 34207-4006, BS 48 Southwest TX St Univ; MA 52 Northwestern Univ; Sp/Lang Path, Private Practice, **SLP LM**

Jenison, Marcia M Associated Children's Therapies Speech Services, 1200 Mountain Creek Road Suite C-9, Chattanooga, TN 37405, (615) 877-5042, BA 56 Univ of RI; MS 73 Western CT St Univ; ME 75 Univ of NC - Greensboro; Sp-Lang Path, Assoc Children's Ther & Sp Svcs, **SLP ACE**

Jenison, Virginia Williams 221 Cherry Street, Metairie, LA 70005, (504) 568-6511, BS 72 Univ of TN - Knoxville; MA 78 Univ of TN - Knoxville; Asst Prof, LA St U Med Cen Sch/Alio Hlth, **A**

Jenison-Hemmye, Susan 35718 Ravine Circle #27205, Farmington Hills, MI 48331, (313) 489-8860, BS 83 Western MI Univ; MA 84 Western MI Univ; 88–Sp-Lang Path, Total Therapy Management, **SLP**

Jenkin, Mrs Cynthia Miranne 110 Hope Street, Rumford, RI 02916, (401) 438-8874, BS 80 Saint Mary's Dominican Coll; OM 81 LA St Univ - N O Medical Ctr; Sp-Lang Path, Sargent Rehab Center, **SLP**

Jenkin, Mrs Laura Snodgrass Box 130, Kybunga, South Australia, Australia 5463, BS 68 Southern IL Univ-Edwardsvill; MS 72 Southern IL Univ-Edwardsvill; SLP, Ed Dept of South Australia, **SLP**

Jenkins, Barbara Benda 222 North Valley Road, Amherst, MA 01002, (413) 253-2929, BA 64 Grinnell Coll; MA 66 Univ of WA; Sp-Lang Path, Private Practice, **SLP**

Jenkins, Mrs Beverly J Rd #1 Box 1694, Honesdale, PA 18431, (717) 253-5401, BS 71 Bloomsburg Univ of PA; ME 76 Bloomsburg Univ of PA; SLP, Northeastern Iu #19, **SLP**

Jenkins, Carol 6 Falcon Court, Castle Hayne, NC 28429, (919) 675-2039, BA 68 Univ of Akron; MA 76 Univ of Akron; 82–Sp-Lang Path, Brunswick Co Schs, **SLP**

Jenkins, David W Hearing Associates, 16053 Victory Boulevard, Van Nuys, CA 91406, (818) 780-2669, BS 66 Eastern NM Univ; MS 68 UT St Univ; Aud, Hearing Assoc, **A**

Jenkins, Debra Lynne 4602 Tieton Drive #B10, Yakima, WA 98908, (509) 575-0100, Aud, Dr Abbenhaus, **A**

Jenkins, Mrs Donna L Route 2 Box 65A, Lexington, MO 64067, (816) 259-4341, BS 70 Central MO St Univ; MS 76 Central MO St Univ; SLP, Lexington R-V Sch Dist, **SLP**

Jenkins, Edna Margaret 33 North Main Street #9B, Lombard, IL 60148, (312) 495-2653, BA 43 Univ of GA; MA 52 Columbia Univ Teachers Coll; Sp-Lang Path/Aud/Academic Ther, Private Practice, **SLP A LM**

Jenkins, Mrs Helen Michelle 898 Douglas Court, Hemet, CA 92343, (714) 925-0724, BS 83 Brigham Young Univ; MA 84 Brigham Young Univ; SLP, Menifee Union Schl Dstr, **SLP**

Jenkins, Mrs Leslie A 417 Dearborne Avenue, Blackwood, NJ 08012, (609) 931-5353, BA 79 Loyola Coll; MS 81 Loyola Coll; Sp-Lang Path, Runnemede Public School Dist, **SLP**

Jenkins, Linda Jean 4096 Klondike Road, Delaware, OH 43015, (614) 363-1333, BS 77 Kent St Univ; MS 78 Univ of MI - Ann Arbor; Sp-Lang Path, Delaware County Supt Schools, **SLP**

Jenkins, Mrs Lucille B 4410 16th Street N E, Washington, DC 20017, (202) 724-4752, BA 50 Miles Coll; MA 75 Gallaudet Coll; 69, D C Pub Sch-Spec Ed

Jenkins, Mrs Marija M 2508 Jackson Drive, Woodridge, IL 60517, (312) 963-3167, BA 73 Saint Xavier Coll; MA 74 Northern IL Univ - De Kalb; 86–Aud, Senior Hrng Svcs Inc, **A**

Jenkins, Mary A 5979 Devecchi Avenue #121', Citrus Heights, CA 95621, (916) 334-5753, BA 85 Eastern WA Univ; MA 87 Univ of the Pacific; **SLP**

Jenkins, Mrs Melissa Kaye 128 Stone Meadow Lane, Madison, AL 35758, (205) 830-9034, BS 84 Auburn Univ - Auburn; OM 86 Auburn Univ - Auburn; SLP, Lakeshore Hospital, **SLP**

Jenkins, Paula Kay 811 Almeria Avenue, Coral Gables, FL 33134, (305) 448-9313, BA 79 CA St Univ - Long Beach; MA 83 CA St Univ - Long Beach; **SLP**

Jenkins, Mrs Sarah 10304 Delray Drive, Richmond, VA 23060, (804) 261-5880, BS 64 Radford Univ; ME 74 Univ of NC - Greensboro; Sp-Lang Path, Medical coll of VA, **SLP**

Jenkins, Mrs Sharon E F 2472 Beech Drive N E, Orangeburg, SC 29115, (803) 536-8074, BA 75 SC St Coll; MA 77 SC St Coll; 77–Instr of Aud, S C State College, **A**

Jenkins, Mrs Shelley L F 212 University Village, Athens, GA 30605, (404) 354-3190, BS 83 Univ of GA; ME 84 Univ of GA; 85–Sp-Lang Path, St Mary's Hosp, **SLP**

Jenkins, Susan Leonard 213 McRoberts, Mather AFB, CA 95655-3315, (916) 366-3748, BA 82 IN Purdue Univ -Indianapolis; MS 85 Minot St Univ; 86–Sp-Lang Path, InSpeech Inc, **SLP**

Jenkins, Terrilynn Faye P O Box 632, Atmore, AL 36502-0632, (205) 368-9342, BS 85 Southern Univ - Baton Rouge; MA 87 Western MI Univ; SLP, InSpeech Inc, **SLP**

Jenkins, Tina Louise 1722 Hawthorn Drive, Plainfield, IN 46168, (317) 872-4210, BS 79 Purdue Univ - West Lafayette; MS 84 Univ of Louisville; Sp-Lang Path, St Vincent New Hope, **SLP**

Jenkinson, Phillip H 3412 Crestmoor Place, Des Moines, IA 50310, (515) 270-9030, BA 64 Univ of Northern IA; MA 72 Univ of Northern IA; Supervisor, Heartland AEA, **SLP**

Jenks, Dr Randall Julian P O Box 6255, Bend, OR 97708, (503) 382-5882, BS 73 Phillips Univ; MS 73 Phillips Univ; PH 76 (Sp Path & Aud) Wichita St Univ; 86–Admin/Sp-Lang Path, Cen OR Home Health Agency, **SLP**

Jennerjohn, Mrs Carolyn J 631 Colonial Avenue, York, PA 17403, (717) 843-9089, BS 64 Univ of WI - Madison; MS 81 Towson St Univ; Sp-Lang Path, York ENT Assoc/Cl Pal Cl, **SLP**

Jennewine-Mullins, Jewelyn L Route 1 Box 80, Center Point Road, Thurman, OH 45685, **SLP**

Jennings, Amy Leigh 337 George Street, Winchester, VA 22601, (703) 667-7909, BS 84 James Madison Univ; ME 85 James Madison Univ; SLP, Grafton School, **A**

Jennings, Mrs Carol M 108 Beechwood Lane, Irmo, SC 29063, BA 79 Columbia Coll; MS 80 Univ of SC - Columbia; Sp-Lang Path, Pineview Elementary School, **SLP**

Jennings, Mrs Carole S 525 Winnepoge Drive, Fairfield, CT 06430, (203) 255-8300, BA 62 Coll of New Rochelle; MA 74 Seton Hall Univ; 78–Sp-Lang Path, Fairfield Pub Schs, **SLP**

Jennings, Mrs Diana R 1579 Fairway Drive #102, Naperville, IL 60540, (312) 961-8357, BS 86 IL St Univ - Normal; MS 87 IL St Univ - Normal

Jennings, Mrs Evelyn W Route 5 Box 388, Payne Spring Road, Dickson, TN 37055, (615) 446-8565, BS 75 Purdue Univ - West Lafayette; MA 80 Univ of TN - Knoxville; Aud, Private Practice, **A**

Jennings, Mrs Joan Bormann 11 Bayou Teche, Conroe, TX 77302, (713) 367-4677, BA 79 SUNY - Coll at Plattsburgh; MS 82 Adelphi Univ; 87–Sp-Lang Path, Conroe ISD, **SLP**

Jennings, Joan M 235 West 22nd Street, New York, NY 10011, **SLP**

Jennings, Joan Mary 1960 East 28th Street, Brooklyn, NY 11229, (718) 441-5333, MS 87 CUNY - Brooklyn Coll; 87–Sp-Lang Path, First Step Early Childhood Ctr

Jennings, Mrs Karen Jean Lucas CS-2478, Pullman, WA 99165, (509) 332-6597, BA 78 Lewis & Clark Coll; MA 83 Portland St Univ; Sp/Lang Path, North Clackamas PS, **SLP**

Jennings, Karen Sue 4225 Harding Road, Apt 301, Nashville, TN 37205, (615) 269-5323, SLP, Baptist Hospital, **SLP**

Jennings, Sara Easter 2032 Island Home Boulevard, Knoxville, TN 37920, (615) 562-8377, BS 81 Univ of TN - Knoxville; MA 83 Univ of TN - Knoxville; Aud, Campbell Co Bd of Ed, **A**

Jennings, Susan M 8100 Mountain Road N E, Suite 102, Albuquerque, NM 87110, (505) 255-7571, BA 70 Creighton Univ; MS 72 TX Tech Univ; Sp-Lang Path, Private Practice, **SLP**

Jennings-Reimer, Terry D 13702 Walnut Street, Whittier, CA 90602, (213) 922-7688, BA 79 CA St Univ - Long Beach; MA 81 Whittier Coll; Sp/Lang Path, Rancho Los Amigos Hosp, **SLP**

Jennison, Pamela Faye Route 1 Box 123, Healy, KS 67850, (316) 398-2288, BA 73 Univ of Northern CO; MA 77 Univ of Northern CO; **SLP**

Jensen, Mrs Becky J L South 3620 Smith, Spokane, WA 99223, BA 74 WA St Univ; MS 76 Eastern WA Univ; 87–Sp-Lang Path, Holy Family Hosp, **SLP**

Jensen, Betty L Tri St Hrd Aid/Audiology Ctr, 308 Delaware Road, Frederick, MD 21701, (301) 663-0553, BS 74 Univ of IA; MA 76 Univ of IA; Pres/Aud, Tri-Stae Hrng Aid/Aud Ctr Inc, **A**

Jensen, Cynthia A 3040 West St Germain #105, St Cloud, MN 56301, (612) 274-8218, MA 83 Saint Cloud St Univ; Sp-Lang Path, School District 876, **SLP**

Jensen, Darrell L 256 East 400 North, Nephi, UT 84648, (801) 623-0328, MS 81 UT St Univ; BS 79 Brigham Young Univ; SLP, Juab Sch Dist, **SLP**

Jensen, Mrs Debra A R 1019 Farmer Street, Tomah, WI 54660, (608) 372-4226, BA 77 Univ of WI - Eau Claire; MS 78 Univ of WI - Eau Claire; **SLP**

Jensen, Mrs Debra Cyd 835 Fireside Drive, Apple Valley, MN 55124, (612) 473-4636, BA 80 Univ of ND; MA 83 Western MI Univ; Sp-Lang Path, Minnetonka Public Schools, **SLP A**

Jensen, Denise A 1210 E Jackson Street, Orlando, FL 32801, (407) 897-1766, BS 81 Southern IL Univ -Carbondale; MS 83 Moorhead St Univ; Sp-Lang Path, FL Hosp, **SLP**

Jensen, Dianna Leah 2235 Normandy Drive #3A, Michigan City, IN 46360, (800) 331-8840, BS 86 Univ of SD - Vermillion; MA 87 Western IL Univ; **SLP**

Jensen, Janet K 4800 A Street, Lincoln, NE 68510, (402) 489-7496, BS 51 Univ of NE - Lincoln; PH 87 (Interdisciplinary) IN Univ - Bloomington; 87–Adjunct Asst Prof, Univ of NE-Lincoln, **SLP**

Jensen, Mrs Janet Kay 789 North 150 West, Logan, UT 84321, (801) 753-5780, BS 73 UT St Univ; MA 73 Northwestern Univ; **SLP ACE**

Jensen, Dr Jay R Dept Comm Disorders Umc 10, Utah State University, Logan, UT 84322, (801) 750-1388, BS 51 Univ of UT; MS 57 Univ of UT; PH 60 (Sp Path) Univ of WI - Madison; Prof, Utah St U, **SLP F**

Jensen, Jeffery Paul Hutchinson Clinic Pa, 2101 North Waldron, Hutchinson, KS 67502, (316) 663-6121, BS 81 Brigham Young Univ; OM 84 Brigham Young Univ; **A**

Jensen, Mrs Joyce H 1238 Kupau Street, Kailua, HI 96734, (808) 547-6511, BS 79 Univ of HI - Manoa; MS 81 Univ of HI - Manoa; 87–Sp-Lang Path, St Francis Med Ctr, **SLP**

Jensen, Julie Lynn 235 Nathan Lane #341, Plymouth, MN 55441, (612) 520-5614, OM 84 Emory Univ; 86–Sp-Lang Path, North Memorial Med Ctr, **SLP**

Jensen, Mrs Karen Hick 1111 Kingbolt Circle Drive, Apartment G, St Louis, MO 63129, (314) 892-1762, OB 84 Univ of MO - Columbia; MA 87 Univ of IL - Urbana; **SLP**

Jensen, Kris Kay 106-1460 Pandosy Street, Kelowna, BC, Canada V1Y 1P3, (604) 785-8916, BA 79 Univ of Northern CO; MA 81 Univ of Northern CO; Sp-Lang Path, British Columbia Ministry Hlth, **SLP**

Jensen, Mrs Linda Jeanne 467 Harrison Avenue, Schenectady, NY 12306, (518) 664-5066, BS 84 Coll of Saint Rose; MS 85 Coll of Saint Rose; **SLP**

Jensen, Marian Mahfood 2422 East Dragoon Avenue, Mesa, AZ 85204, (602) 949-7277, BA 79 OH St Univ; MA 80 OH St Univ; 81–Aud, Scottsdale Ear Nose Throat, **A**

Jensen, Mrs Marilyn 5197 Seminole Drive, Flagstaff, AZ 86001, (602) 523-2522, BA 64 Univ of OK - Norman; MS 81 Northern AZ Univ; Dir, Northern Arizona U, **SLP ACE**

Jensen, Mary P 17012 Peterson Way N E, Poulsbo, WA 98370, (206) 779-3707, BA 75 Univ of ID; MS 79 ID St Univ; SLP, Bainbridge Island Sch Dist, **SLP**

Jensen, Dr Michelle W 1011 N W 21st Street, Gainesville, FL 32605, (904) 378-0104, BA 58 Pomona Coll; MA 60 IA St Univ; PH 72 (NS) Univ of Southern CA; Sp-Lang Path, Private Practice, **SLP ACE**

Jensen, Dr Myltreda L 1117 Perimeter Center West, Suite W-304, Atlanta, GA 30338, (404) 396-0441, BS 64 Edinboro Univ of PA; MS 76 Coll of Saint Rose; PH 84 (Human Behavior) United States Int'l Univ; 87–SLP, Natl Ctr for Mediated Lrng, **SLP**

Jensen, Mrs Nancy L 2843 East Norcroft Circle, Mesa, AZ 85213, (602) 924-2318, BS 75 Southern Methodist Univ; MS 76 CO St Univ; Aud, **A**

Jensen, Dr Paul J 1011 N W 21st Street, Gainesville, FL 32605, (904) 392-2113, BA 52 Univ of IA; MA 54 Univ of IA; PH 62 (NS) Univ of IA; Prof, U of FL, **SLP F**

Jensen, Robert J 2843 East Norcroft Circle, Mesa, AZ 85203, (602) 924-2318, BS 72 Southern IL Univ -Carbondale; MS 81 AZ St Univ; Audiologist, Maricopa ENT Pc, **A**

Jensen, Mrs Senta H Beaver Brook 19-0, 550 South Dupont Parkway, New Castle, DE 19720, (302) 322-8998, MS; Retired, **SLP LM**

Jensen, Sherry E Kensington School, 201 South Evanston, Arlington Heights, IL 60004, (312) 577-7749, BS 68 Northern IL Univ - De Kalb; MS 70 Univ of IL - Urbana; 88–Sp-Lang Path, Northwest Suburban Spec Educ Organ, **SLP**

Jensen, Susan K 37 Mt Foraker Drive, San Rafael, CA 94903, (415) 456-9680, BA 66 Univ of MT; MA 68 Univ of MT; Dir-Patient Svcs, Kentfield Rehab Hosp, **SLP**

Jensen, Dr Thomas Wendell Section Of Comm Disorders, Rush Pres St Lukes Med Ctr, 1753 West Congress Pkwy, Chicago, IL 60612, BS 63 Mankato St Univ; MS 68 Univ of WI - Madison; PH 74 (NS) Univ of Cincinnati; Dir Commun Dis Sect, Rush Prebyterian Med Cen, **SLP**

Jensen, Mrs Valerie Carda 11206 North Post Road, Omaha, NE 68112, BA 78 Univ of SD - Vermillion; MA 79 Univ of SD - Vermillion; SLP, Loess Hills AEA, **SLP**

Jenson, Mrs Barbara Jean Martin Luther Home, P O Box 607, Beatrice, NE 68310, (402) 223-5209, Sp-Lang Path, Liberty Pub Schs, **SLP**

Jenson, Gloria R 721 Via Otogic, San Clemente, CA 92672, (714) 492-9874, MS 78 FL St Univ; Dir Sp-Lang Ctr, Orange Coast Coll, **SLP**

Jenson, Dr Pauline M 5 Murray Place, Princeton, NJ 08540, (609) 771-2399, BS 48 Trenton St Coll; MA 50 Columbia Univ Teachers Coll; PH 69 (Special Ed (Deaf)) Columbia Univ Teachers Coll; 70–Prof, Trenton State College, **SLP A**

Jentges, Helen C 33046 22nd Place South, Federal Way, WA 98003, **SLP**

Jentoft, Richard C 1517 Euclid Avenue, Beloit, WI 53511, (414) 472-1301, BS 60 Univ of MN - Duluth; MS 66 Univ of WI - Madison; Asst Prof/Dir Commun Dis, U of WI-Whitewater, **SLP**

Jenuwine, Karen Jean 427C Tradewinds Drive, Fayetteville, NC 28304, (919) 486-1605, BA 84 MI St Univ; MA 85 MI St Univ; Sp-Lang Path, Dev Eval Center of NC, **SLP**

Jepsen, Debbie L 302 1st Avenue N E, Oelwein, IA 50662, (319) 637-2206, BA 79 Univ of Northern IA; MA 80 Univ of Northern IA; Sp-Lang Path, Keystone AEA #1, **SLP**

Jepsen, Liane Marie 3217 Wright, Des Moines, IA 50316, (515) 262-1122, BA 84 Univ of Northern IA; MA 85 Univ of Northern IA; **SLP**

Jepsen, Mrs Maureen McGowan 3630 Rockingham Road, Royal Oak, MI 48072, (313) 828-6003, BS 83 Univ of WI - Madison; MS 85 Univ of WI - Madison; 87–Sp-Lang Path, Wm Beaumont Hosp-Troy, **SLP ACE**

Jeremiah, Mrs Kimberly W 5910 Westone Road, Mechanicsville, VA 23111, (804) 321-7774, BA 77 Allegheny Coll; MA 79 Case Western Reserve Univ; Sp-Lang Path, Richmond ARC Infant Intervent Svcs, **SLP**

Jeremic, Elisa D 984 Memorial Village, Private Drive, Houston, TX 77024, (713) 780-5857, BS 76 Univ of TX - Austin; MA 79 Univ of Houston - Univ Park; 86–Dir Sp-Lang Path, Rosewood Med Ctr, **SLP ACE**

Jerger, Dr James F Baylor College Of Medicine, Neurosensory Center #NA200, 6501 Fannin Street, Houston, TX 77030, (713) 799-5917, BS 51 Northwestern Univ; MA 52 Northwestern Univ; PH 54 (NS) Northwestern Univ; Professor of Audiology, Baylor College of Medicine, **A F H**

Jerger, Margaret A 216 East Charles Road, Elmhurst, IL 60126, (312) 851-6161, BS 62 Northwestern Univ; MA 85 Northwestern Univ; **SLP**

Jerger, Dr Susan Wood Baylor College Of Medicine, Neurosensory Center NA200, 6501 Fannin Street, Houston, TX 77030, (713) 799-5917, BA 61 Univ of Houston - Univ Park; MS 63 Purdue Univ - West Lafayette; PH 86 (NS) Baylor Univ; Assistant Professor, Baylor College of Medicine, **A**

Jerke, Thomas A 504-E Mananai Place #14-E, Honolulu, HI 96818, (808) 433-6488, BA 65 Univ of Northern CO; MS 67 Univ of HI - Manoa; Ch-SLP Cl, Tripler Army Med Cen, **SLP**

Jern, Mrs Lori E 6672 North Thorne Avenue, Fresno, CA 93711-1448, (209) 436-0788, BA 79 CA St Univ - Fresno; MA 84 CA St Univ - Fresno; Sp-Lang Path, Fresno USD, **SLP**

Jernigan, Mrs Anne L 3690 Glendale Drive, Horseheads, NY 14845, (607) 796-2338, MS 81 Nazareth Coll of Rochester; Sp-Lang Path, Stueben BOCES, **SLP**

Jernigan, Gina Merle Route 3 Box 281, Mount Olive, NC 28365, (919) 689-2679, MS 85 East Carolina Univ; **SLP**

Jernigan, Lesley Ray 4729 Annunciation, New Orleans, LA 70115, (504) 897-2606, BS 71 Univ Southern MS-Hattiesburg; MS 73 Univ Southern MS-Hattiesburg; 85–Exec Dir, New Orleans Sp & Hrng Ct, **SLP**

Jerome, Dr Eldon K 8715 Manhattan Drive, Houston, TX 77096, PH (NS); **SLP LM**

Jerome, Maj James J USA MEDDAC-Nuernberg, Box 141, APO New York, NY 09105-5000, BS 71 Univ of WI - Milwaukee; MA 73 Western IL Univ; Aud, USA MEDDAC-Nuernberg, **A**

Jerrels, Mrs Elaine Glynn R R 2 Box 599, Harrisburg, IL 62946, (618) 252-5241, BA 79 OH St Univ; MA 81 OH St Univ; Sp-Lang Path, Private Practice, **SLP**

Jervay, Debra M 8110 17th Place, Adelphi, MD 20783, (301) 942-2088, **SLP**

Jeske, Agnes N Bremerhaven Elementary School, P O Box 356, APO New York, NY 09069, BA 78 Central WA Univ; MA 82 Central MI Univ; Sp-Lang Path, Dept of Defense Schs, **SLP**

Jespersen, Rhonda M 3721 Vinton Avenue #9, Los Angeles, CA 90034, (818) 766-1715, BS 85 Univ of IA; MA 87 CA St Univ - Fresno; 87–Aud, Hearing Care Associates

Jessamy, Linda E 27 Midwood Street, Brooklyn, NY 11225, (718) 462-2386, BA 71 CUNY - Brooklyn Coll; MS 73 CUNY - Brooklyn Coll; OM 85 CUNY - Brooklyn Coll; 88–Supervisor, Bd of Ed-City of NY, **SLP**

Jesse, Barbara Lynne 3816 N Sheffield #3-W, Chicago, IL 60613, (312) 328-5180, BS 84 Eastern IL Univ; MA 86 Northern IL Univ - De Kalb; Aud, Audio-Vestibular, **A**

Jessen, Joanne K 9 Schindler Court, Silver Spring, MD 20903, (301) 897-5700, BS 66 Univ of WI - Madison; MA 67 Northwestern Univ; Director Publications Div, ASHA, **SLP A**

Jessiman, Sherril Daun 8747 South Appletree Place, Highlands Ranch, CO 80126-2148, (303) 744-1961, BA 82 Brandon Univ - Manitoba; MA 86 Univ of Denver; 86–Dir-Audiological Svcs, Assoc of Otolaryngology PC, **A**

Jessup, Georgia L 2101 Marine Street, Santa Monica, CA 90405, **SLP**

Jessup, Rita Ann 1377 Chippewa Drive, Greenville, OH 45331, (513) 548-8323, BS 83 Ball St Univ; MA 85 Eastern KY Univ; **SLP**

Jesteadt, Dr Walt Boys Town Natl Institute, 555 North 30th Street, Omaha, NE 68131, (402) 498-6704, BA 66 Johns Hopkins Univ; PH 71 (Psychology) Univ of Pittsburgh - Pittsburgh; 84–Dir of Research, Boys Town Natl Institute

Jester, Mrs Deanna Kay 6125 Pennyrich Court, Florissant, MO 63033, (314) 921-1111, MS 73 Southern IL Univ-Edwardsvill; SLP, Spec Sch Dist, **SLP**

Jesudowich, Mrs Barbara W 810 East Johnson Avenue, Southington, CT 06489, (203) 628-0331, BS 73 Nazareth Coll of Rochester; MS 74 Ithaca Coll; Sp-Lang Path, Southington Bd of Ed, **SLP**

Jetchick, Jeannie Marie 317 North Mill, Plymouth, MI 48170-1445, (313) 481-0625, BA 82 Wayne St Univ; MA 84 Wayne St Univ; **SLP**

Jeter, Mrs Amy Lee 64 Gayle Court, Huntington, WV 25704, (304) 429-4358, BS 81 WV Univ; MA 82 Marshall Univ; 84–Sp/Lang Path, Developmental Therapy Center, **SLP**

Jeter, Mrs Christine M 27505 Old Colony, Farmington Hills, MI 48018, (313) 626-2740, BA 81 MI St Univ; MA 83 Wayne St Univ; Sp/Lang Path, Morton Plant Hospital, **SLP**

Jeter, Mrs Patti A 2534 East 10th, Fremont, NE 68025, (402) 721-6720, BS 78 Northwest MO St Univ; MS 80 Univ of NE - Omaha; 88–Sp-Lang Path, Scribner-Snyder Comm Sch, **SLP**

Jeter-Krasnikoff, Michelle 18113 57A Avenue, Surrey, BC, Canada V3S 1J7, (604) 534-9221, BA 76 Univ of MI - Ann Arbor; MA 77 Eastern MI Univ; Sp/Lang Path, Ministry of Hlth, **SLP**

Jett, Ellen E 11528 North Lone Mountain Place, Tucson, AZ 85737, (602) 797-2540, MS 80 Univ of AZ; Aud, Loma Linda Surgery Med Group, **A**

Jett, Madonna T 3621 Candlewood Way N E, Marietta, GA 30066, **SLP**

Jett, Mrs Susanna Tingle 831 Spring Valley Drive, Fredericksburg, VA 22405-1910, (703) 659-2106, BS 76 James Madison Univ; MS 81 James Madison Univ; Sp/Lang Path, Stafford County Public Schools, **SLP**

Jetty, Dr Albert J 7411 Watford Avenue, Baton Rouge, LA 70808, (504) 766-9464, BS 63 Northern MI Univ; MA 65 Western MI Univ; PH 68 (Aud & Sp Sciences) MI St Univ; Dir of Aud Svcs, Private Practice, **SLP A**

Jevne, Robert B P O Box 663, Everett, WA 98206, (206) 353-5866, BS 63 Western WA Univ; BA 64 Western WA Univ; **SLP**

Jewell, Mary Carole Route 2, Dodgeville, WI 53533, (608) 935-2005, BS 85 Univ of WI - Madison; MA 87 Univ of IA; 87–Sp-Lang Path, Dodgeville PS, **SLP**

Jewell, Mrs Mary Kay 2617 Lakeridge Circle, Oklahoma City, OK 73170, (405) 737-7025, BA 72 Univ of OK - Norman; MA 73 Univ of OK - Norman; **SLP**

Jewett, Janet M 729 Emerson, Evanston, IL 60201, (312) 688-3000, BA 56 NE Wesleyan Univ; OM 59 Roosevelt Univ; MA 78 Univ of SD - Vermillion; Sp-Lang Path, Victory Mem Hosp, **SLP**

Jewett, Judith E 2405 Queensberry Road, Pasadena, CA 91104, (818) 997-2357, BA 77 Univ of CA - Santa Barbara; MA 80 CA St Univ - Northridge

Jiang, Tao Ns Hearing And Speech Clinic, Fenwick Place, 559 Fenwick Street, Halifax, NS, Canada B3H 1R2, (902) 423-7354, BA 82; MS 88; 88–Aud, Dr George T Mencher NS Hrng & Sp Cl

Jicha, John James, III 352 Summit Avenue, Hagerstown, MD 21740, (301) 791-4643, BA 82 Loyola Coll; MS 84 Loyola Coll; **SLP**

Jicha, Sandra Lynn 265 North Ballston Avenue, Apartment #4, Scotia, NY 12302, (518) 382-1043, BS 86 SUNY - Coll at Geneseo; MA 87 SUNY - Coll at Geneseo; 87–Sp-Lang Path, Newmeadow Preschool Program, **SLP**

Jillette, Mrs Janet D W 13 Highland Street, Concord, NH 03301, (603) 753-6561, BS 60 Boston Univ; ME 81 Notre Dame Coll; Sp-Lang Path, Merrimack Sch Dist, **SLP**

Jillson, Mrs Sheila Rose 279 West Street, Amherst, MA 01002, (413) 253-5136, MS 87 Emerson Coll; 88–Sp-Lang Path, Belchertown PS

Jillson-Cook, Kathryn Dayle 4750 S Dudley Street #29, Littleton, CO 80123, BA 79 Kearney St Coll; MA 80 Univ of Northern CO; 87–Teacher, Horizon HS, **SLP**

Jimenez, Dr Beatrice C 4 Alameda Park Circle, Chico, CA 95928, BA 66 San Jose St Univ; MA 75 CA St Univ - Fresno; PH 77 (Sp & Hrng Science) OH St Univ; 80–Assoc Prof, Calif State U Chico, **SLP**

Jimenez, Mary Rutledge 3496 Cedarwood Trail, Tallahassee, FL 32312, (904) 656-4800, BS 83 Baylor Univ; MS 85 Baylor Univ; 88–Sp-Lang Path/Aud, Capital Rehab Hosp, **SLP A**

Jimenez, Patricia Gordon 902 East Missouri, Kirksville, MO 63501, (816) 665-0957, BA 85 Chapman Coll; MA 86 Whittier Coll; 87–Sp-Lang Path, Kirksville R-III Sch Dist

Jingst, Judith Ann 2239 Cannon Drive, Virginia Beach, VA 23454, (804) 463-6670, BS 83 Western IL Univ; MA 84 Western IL Univ; 88–Sp-Lang Path, Easter Seal Soc, **SLP**

Jinks, Andrew F 2509 Harwood Road, Baltimore, MD 21234, (301) 877-1440, BS 76 Bloomsburg Univ of PA; MA 77 Bowling Green St Univ; Sp-Lang Path, National Rehabilitation Hosp, **SLP**

Jiran, Marygrace 10 Michigan Avenue, Massapequa, NY 11758, (516) 798-2739, BS 84 SUNY - Coll at Geneseo; MA 86 SUNY - Coll at Geneseo; **SLP**

Jirecek, Amy Louise Cleveland Hearing & Speech Center, 11206 Euclid Avenue, Cleveland, OH 44106, (216) 231-8787, BS 85 Bowling Green St Univ; MA 87 Kent St Univ; 88–Sp-Lang Path, Cleveland Hearing & Sp Ctr, **SLP**

Jirsa, Dr Robert E Sp & Hrng Ctr Ferguson 300, University Of N Carolina, Greensboro, NC 27412, (919) 334-5184, BS 65 Western IL Univ; MA 67 OH Univ - Athens; PH 70 (Aud) Univ of KS; 87–Asst Prof of Comm, Univ of NC, **A**

Joachim, Mrs Amy M Rd 1 Box 1200, Hookstown, PA 15050, (412) 573-4644, BA 74 Thiel Coll; MA 77 Univ of Pittsburgh - Pittsburgh; **SLP**

Joachim, Marilyn Jean 116 South Miller Road #2, Akron, OH 44313, (216) 927-3115, BA 75 Hiram Coll; MA 84 Kent St Univ; 81–Sp-Lang Path, Rittman Exempted Village Schs, **SLP**

Joachim, Mrs Pamela Christlieb 485 Terrace Road, Santa Barbara, CA 93109, (805) 965-8699, BA 83 Univ of VT; BA 83 Univ of VT; MA 85 Univ of CA - Santa Barbara; 87–Sp-Lang Path, Sally Burleigh Sp Path Assoc, **SLP**

Jobe, Brenda 111 Antelope Drive, Sedona, AZ 86336, (602) 282-7290, BS 61 CA Poly St Univ-San Luis Obi; MA 67 Stanford Univ; Aud, AZ St Sch for Deaf & Blind, **A**

Jobe, Meredith A 1918 North Tejon Street #4, Colorado Springs, CO 80907, (719) 520-2157, BS 73 CO St Univ; MS 74 CO St Univ; 88–Supvr-Spec Educ, Colorado Spgs Sch Dist #11, **SLP**

Jobe, Mrs Ruth B H 4406 Williams Dairy Road, Greensboro, NC 27406, (919) 674-0107, BA 61 Greensboro Coll; ME 76 Univ of NC - Greensboro; SLP, Guilford Co Sch Syst, **SLP**

Jobin, Mrs Barbara Ann 5 Terrace Road, Concord, NH 03301, (603) 225-1031, BA 74 Univ of NH; MS 82 Univ of NH; Sp-Lang Path, Associated Consultants Team, **SLP**

Joblin, Meryl A Main Line Speech Consult, 112 Harrogate Road, Overbrook Hills, PA 19151, (215) 649-8255, BA 72; MA 74 Temple Univ-Tyler Sch of Art; Dir, Main Line Sp Consult, **SLP**

Jochem, Macie J 1119 Braemar Court, Cary, NC 27511, (919) 469-2259, BA 71 Randolph-Macon Woman's Coll; MS 78 Univ of NC - Chapel Hill; **SLP**

Jockel, Mrs Carol M 7 Moonshadow Court, Kinnelon, NJ 07405, (201) 438-7675, BS 70 William Paterson Coll; MS 76 William Paterson Coll; SLP, Rutherford Board of Education, **SLP**

Joens, Mrs Vicky De Witte 10028 Caenen, Lenexa, KS 66215, MA 79 Northeast MO St Univ; SLP, Deporah King & Associates, **SLP**

Joest, Mrs Kathleen Fleming 10764 Oyster Bay Court, Indianapolis, IN 46236, (317) 871-2270, BS 83 Ball St Univ; MA 85 Ball St Univ; Sp-Lang Path, St Vincent Hosp, **SLP**

Joffee-Meszaros, Mrs Janis A East Way, Bedford, NY 10506, (914) 937-1632, MS 73 Adelphi Univ; Sp-Lang Path, Bedford Central Sch Dist, **SLP**

Joga, Mrs Regina Vilkas 23807 South Fulmar Avenue, Torrance, CA 90501, (213) 237-1820, BA 82 CA St Univ - Northridge; MA 84 CA St Univ - Northridge; 88–Sp-Lang Path, InSpeech Inc, **SLP**

Johannes, Susan Underwood 15918 Douglas Circle, Omaha, NE 68118, (402) 333-8744, BS 85 Univ of NE - Omaha; MS 86 Univ of NE - Omaha; 86–Sp-Lang Path, Millard Pub Schs, **SLP**

Johannesen, Mrs Jane Lizette 1581 NW 101st Street, Clive, IA 50322, (515) 262-8372, MA 83 Univ of Northern IA; 85–Aud, Heartland AEA, **A**

Johanningmeier, Mrs Marcia Kemp 7337 Scenic Court, Cedar Hill, MO 63016, (314) 629-3637, BS 79 Fontbonne Coll; MS 85 Fontbonne Coll; **SLP**

Johannis, Mrs Joyce Ann 58 Wayland Trail, Narragansett, RI 02882, (401) 847-2100, BS 75 Emerson Coll; MS 85 Univ of RI; **SLP**

Johanns, Mrs Cindy J 7567 Tenbury Drive, Dublin, OH 43017, (614) 267-0570, BS 80 OH Univ - Athens; MA 86 OH St Univ; Aud, Riverside Hrngservices, **A**

Johanon, Rebecca R 600 Starkey Road #914, Largo, FL 33541, (813) 585-5873, BS 81 Baylor Univ; MS 84 Univ of South FL; Sp-Lang Path, UCP, **SLP**

Johansen, Alice Elizabeth 31608 3rd Place South, Federal Way, WA 98003, (206) 848-6661, BS 82 Univ of WA; MS 84 Univ of WA; Sp-Lang Path, Good Samaritan Hospital, **SLP**

Johansen, Anna Lee 509-21st Street, Bemidji, MN 56601, (218) 751-2160, BS 77 ND St Univ; MS 85 Moorhead St Univ; 78–Sp-Lang Path, Bemidji Pub Sch, **SLP**

Johansen, Catherine Louise 2826 Powhattan Parkway, Toledo, OH 43606, (419) 385-0231, MA 82 Bowling Green St Univ; Sp-Lang Path, NW Ohio Developmental Center, **SLP**

Johansen, Connie Marie 417 Indiana Avenue, New Port Richey, FL 34652, (813) 847-9237, BS 85 FL St Univ; MS 86 FL St Univ; **SLP**

Johansen, David Duke 756 West 1150 South, Provo, UT 84601, (801) 373-5880, BS 81 Brigham Young Univ; MA 82 Brigham Young Univ; SLP, Provo Sch Dist, **SLP**

Johansen, Mrs Floye V 5515 Jessamine Lane, Orlando, FL 32809, (407) 855-8737, MA 51 Univ of FL; Sp-Lang Path, Private Practice, **SLP**

Johansen, Mrs Nancy E 53 Highland Avenue, Bangor, ME 04401, (207) 942-3882, BS 77 Eastern IL Univ; MS 78 Eastern IL Univ; **SLP A ACE**

Johansen, Mrs Sharon H 3015 Constitution Drive, Stafford, VA 22554, BS 79 Univ of NE - Lincoln; MA 80 Univ of Northern CO; 88–Sp/Lang Path, Comm Svcs Bd/Parent Educ, **SLP**

Johansen, Mrs Sheila Rae 333 Dennison Avenue, St Paul, MN 55126, (612) 481-0039, MS 84 Univ of ND; 88–Sp-Lang Path, Custom Contracts & Svcs Inc, **SLP**

Johlfs, Connie T 142 James Drive, Macomb, IL 61455, (309) 298-2917, BS 73 Western IL Univ; MA 76 Western IL Univ; Instr, W Ill Univ, **SLP**

John, Anne Farquhar 37 South Lindsey Street, Castle Rock, CO 80104, (303) 688-1273, BS 81 Univ of WY; MS 83 Univ of WY; SLP, Ctr for Hrng Sp & L, **SLP**

John, Mrs Lynda Barker 4616 Cooke Street, Duluth, MN 55804, (218) 525-4545, BA 86 Univ of MN - Duluth; MA 87 Univ of MN - Duluth

John, Martin B Yakima Valley Hrng & Sp Ctr, 303 South 12th Avenue, Yakima, WA 98902, (509) 453-8248, BA 76 WA St Univ; MS 78 Univ of WA; Aud, Yakima Valley Hrng & Sp Ctr, **A**

John, Sunita 5412 North Plaza Drive, Peioria, IL 61614, (309) 692-3414, MS 88 IL St Univ - Normal

John, Mrs Valerie L 1010 Sullivan Road, Ogden, UT 84403, (801) 394-9557, BS 78 ID St Univ; MS 80 ID St Univ; 85–Sp-Lang Path, Stewart Rehab Ctr, **SLP**

Johns, Mrs Catherine Beatrice 6891 Telephone Road, Pavilion, NY 14525, (716) 584-3807, BS 78 SUNY - Coll at Geneseo; MA 83 SUNY - Coll at Geneseo; **SLP**

Johns, Dr Donnell F Division Of Plastic Surgery, Univ Of TX S W Medical Sch, 5323 Harry Hines, Dallas, TX 75235, (214) 688-3571, BS 62 OH Univ - Athens; MS 64 FL St Univ; PH 68 (NS) FL St Univ; Dir Clin Res Plastic Surg Div, Univ of Texas SW Medical Sch, **SLP F**

Johns, Dr Elizabeth 3708 Maryland Street, Alexandria, VA 22309, (703) 845-6214, BS 55 VA St Univ; MA 57 Case Western Reserve Univ; ED 77 (NS) VA Polytechnic Inst St Univ; Chmn Div of Social Sciences, N VA Comm Coll, **SLP F**

Johns, Mrs Julie O'Donovan 1631 Buttercup Road, Encinitas, CA 92024, (619) 436-5418, MA 83 San Diego St Univ; Aud, Private Practice, **A**

Johns, Leslie A 2009 Clayton Avenue, Artesia, NM 88210, (505) 746-2581, BS 78 Eastern NM Univ; MS 80 Eastern NM Univ; Sp-Lang Path, Carlsbad Municipal Schools, **SLP ACE**

Johns, Mary Bloomquist 7039 San Pedro #PH12, San Antonio, TX 78216, (512) 655-3621, BS 75 Univ of North TX; ME 82 Southwest TX St Univ; Sp-Lang Path, NE ISD, **SLP**

Johns, Patricia Lynn Audiology (126), VA Medical Center, Allen Park, MI 48101, (313) 562-6000, BS 80 Central MI Univ; MA 83 Wayne St Univ; 83–Aud, VA Med Cen, **A**

Johns, Valerie C P O Box 8059, Fredericksburg, VA 22404, (703) 786-8263, BA 71 MI St Univ; MS 74 Univ of Pittsburgh - Pittsburgh; Dir, Fredericksburg Speech Pathology, **SLP**

Johns-Elmy, Mrs Lisa Anne 111 New Haven Road, Seymour, CT 06483, (203) 734-1018, BA 83 Skidmore Coll; MS 87 Southern CT St Univ

Johnsen, Mrs Marijane 9305 31st N W, Seattle, WA 98117, (206) 526-2154, BA 69 Gonzaga Univ; MA 71 Univ of WA; 87–Rehab Oper Mgr, Chldn's Hosp & Med Cen, **SLP**

Johnsen, Mrs Sue H 1904 Lake Crest, Plano, TX 75023, (214) 423-8001, BA 65 Univ of TX - Austin; MS 78 Lamar Univ; Sp-Lang Path, Plano ISD, **SLP**

Johnson, Adele S R R 1 Box 16A, So Kent Road, South Kent, CT 06785, (203) 355-3713, BA 76 Southern CT St Univ; MS 78 Western OR St Coll; SLP, New Milford Bd of Ed, **SLP ACE**

Johnson, Alan L 50 Vernon Avenue, Atlantic Beach, NY 11509, (516) 239-2598, BS 71 Univ of WI - Stevens Point; MA 74 AZ St Univ; MA 81 Hofstra Univ; Sp-Lang Path, Private Practice, **SLP**

Johnson, Dr Albert F Berks County Intermediate Unit, 2900 St Lawrence Avenue, Reading, PA 19606-2233, (215) 779-7111, BA 50 Univ of MI - Ann Arbor; MS 51 Univ of MI - Ann Arbor; ED 77 (Ed Admin) Temple Univ; 67–Sp-Lang Path, Berks Co Inter Unit, **SLP A**

Johnson, Mrs Aleta Marie 509 Tulip Street, Summerville, SC 29483, (803) 722-8461, BS 80 Western IL Univ; MS 82 Southern IL Univ-Edwardsvill

Johnson, Dr Alex F, Jr 3883 Wallingford Road, South Euclid, OH 44121, (216) 231-8787, BS 73 Kent St Univ; MA 76 Kent St Univ; PH 83 (NS) Case Western Reserve Univ; Dir of Sp-Lang Path, Cleveland Hrng & Sp Cen, **SLP**

Johnson, Dr Alice L 4129 Mildred Avenue, Los Angeles, CA 90066, (213) 454-4796, BA Northern MI Univ; MA Columbia Univ Teachers Coll; ED 58 (NS) Columbia Univ Teachers Coll; **SLP LM**

Johnson, Alison A 239 Central Street, Rowley, MA 01969, (617) 935-5050, BS 85 IN St Univ - Terre Haute; MS 86 Syracuse Univ; 88–Sp-Lang Path, New England Rehab Hosp, **SLP**

Johnson, Mrs Anita Faye 5160 N Sabino Foothills Dr, Tucson, AZ 85715, (602) 749-4264, BA 64 Elmhurst Coll; MA 70 Univ of AZ; Sp-Lang Path, Tucson USD #1, **SLP**

Johnson, Anita Lee 1560 North 115th, Suite 109, Seattle, WA 98133, (206) 361-1736, BA 82 Univ of IL - Urbana; MS 85 Washington Univ; **A**

Johnson, Mrs Ann F 1700 Liveoak Valley Circle, Waco, TX 76710, (817) 772-2341, BA 69 Nicholls St Univ; MS 73 Tulane Univ; Sp-Lang Path, Waco Independent Sch Dist, **SLP**

Johnson, Annette Simmon 1123 Glenview Avenue, Wauwatosa, WI 53213, MS 82 Univ of IL - Urbana; BS 81 Univ of IL - Urbana; **SLP**

Johnson, Dr Barbara Ann 2975 Mount Read Boulevard, Rochester, NY 14616, (716) 475-6267, BS 75 Worcester St Coll; MA 77 Univ of MA - Amherst; PH 82 (Adult Neurogenic Disorders) Univ of FL; Assistant Professor, NTID, **SLP**

Johnson, Barbara F 10801 S W 109th Ct #D305, Miami, FL 33176, (305) 595-3175, BA 71 Howard Univ; MS 75 Univ of the DC; SLP, Self Employed, **SLP**

Johnson, Mrs Barbara Faye 515 East Hillside Road, Naperville, IL 60540, (312) 983-4586, BS 74 Central MO St Univ; MA 84 Northern IL Univ - De Kalb; 85–Sp-Lang Path, Lockport Area Spec Ed Coop, **SLP**

Johnson, Mrs Barbara Jo 10465 Caenen Lake Road, Lenexa, KS 66215, (816) 234-3392, BS 72 Univ of SD - Vermillion; MA 75 Univ of WI - Milwaukee; Sp-Lang Path, Crpld Chldn Nurs Sch, **SLP**

Johnson, Barbara Louise 379 Crine Road, Morganville, NJ 07751, (201) 591-1668, BA 85 Kean Coll of NJ; MA 86 Kean Coll of NJ; 88–Sp-Lang Path, J L Scores Associates, **SLP**

Johnson, Mrs Barbara Powell 13168 Cabinwood Drive, Silver Spring, MD 20904, (202) 576-6161, BS 63; MS 78 Univ of the DC; Sp-Lang Path, District of Columbia Pub Sch, **SLP**

Johnson, Mrs Barbara Zintz 204 Cedar Circle, Charles City, IA 50616, (515) 228-2536, BS 76 Univ of IA; MA 77 Univ of Northern IA; 78–Sp-Lang Path, Northern Trails AEA, **SLP**

Johnson, Beth Ellen 2050 Allen Boulevard Apartment 8, Middleton, WI 53562, (608) 742-7114, BA 86 Univ of WI - Eau Claire; MS 87 Univ of WI - Eau Claire; **SLP**

Johnson, Dr Bonnie Diedrich 627 Ferndale Road North, Wayzata, MN 55391, (612) 291-2848, BS 72 Northwestern Univ; MA 73 Northwestern Univ; PH 85 CUNY - Grad Sch & Univ Cntr; Sp-Lang Path, Gillette Chldrns Hosp, **SLP**

Johnson, Mrs Bonnie F 6995 Mariann Drive, Eden Prairie, MN 55344, (612) 243-7191, BS 78 Univ of MN - Duluth; MA 79 Univ of MN - Duluth; **SLP**

Johnson, Mrs Bonnie J S 4444 South Meadow Court, Ellicott City, MD 21043, (301) 750-7738, BA 73 Pomona Coll; MA 75 Univ of Denver; Sp-Lang Path, Private Practice, **SLP**

Johnson, Bonnie Marshall 12409 Shirley Street, Omaha, NE 68144, (402) 572-2274, MS 84 Univ of ND; 87–Sp-Lang Path, Immanuel Medical Center, **SLP**

Johnson, Carla J Department Of Psychology, University Of Western Ontario, London, ON, Canada N6A 5C2, (519) 679-2111, BS 72 Univ of WI - Madison; MS 73 Univ of WI - Madison; Asst Prof, U West Ontario, **SLP**

Johnson, Carla W 16051 N W 18th Court, Opa-Locka, FL 33054, (305) 624-9671, MS 85 Univ of Tampa; **SLP**

Johnson, Carole Elizabeth 3500 Sutherland Avenue, C-209, Knoxville, TN 37919, (615) 974-5019, BA 82 Univ of CA - Santa Barbara; MA 86 Univ of TN - Knoxville

Johnson, Mrs Carole Fornell Sierra Speech & Hearing, 2950 Moony Boulevard, Suite E, Visalia, CA 93277, (209) 733-3818, BA 82 Univ of WI - Eau Claire; MA 84 Univ of IA; Audiologist, Sierra Speech & Hearing, **A**

Johnson, Carolyn 18032 Fairfield, Detroit, MI 48221, (313) 863-8337, SLP, Rehab Ins, **SLP**

Johnson, Mrs Carolyn Russell Route 9 P O Box 186-Cale, Boat Club Road, Fort Worth, TX 76179, (713) 342-5521, BS 80 Univ of TX - Austin; ME 82 Southwest TX St Univ; Sp-Lang Path, Birdville ISD, **SLP**

Johnson, Mrs Catherine Carty 1061 Westmore, Apt #205, Lombard, IL 60148, (312) 780-2492, BA 85 Augustana Coll; MA 86 Western MI Univ; SLP, School District #103, **SLP**

Johnson, Mrs Cathy J 5304 Lake Highlands, Waco, TX 76710, (817) 666-0033, BS 77 Baylor Univ; MS 78 Baylor Univ; Sp/Lang Path, Midway ISD, **SLP**

Johnson, Charita B 608 Blue Jay Drive, Hayward, CA 94544-6729, (415) 834-1261, BA 74 San Jose St Univ; **SLP**

Johnson, Dr Charles 1016 West Dorothy Lane, Dayton, OH 45409, (513) 299-3845, BA 53 Univ of IA; MS 55 Bowling Green St Univ; PH 69 (NS) OH St Univ; **SLP**

Johnson, Charles S Route 5 Shady Lane, Canton, GA 30114, (404) 479-1871, BS 68 East TN St Univ; ME 71 Univ of GA; Sp-Lang Path, Cherokee Co Bd of Ed, **SLP**

Johnson, Dr Charlotte E 5421 Normlee Place, Pittsburgh, PA 15217, (412) 647-5575, OB 64 Coll of Spch Therapists Eng; MS 66 Univ of Pittsburgh - Pittsburgh; PH 76 (NS) Univ of Pittsburgh - Pittsburgh; 87–Sp-Lang Path, Chldn Hosp of Pittsburgh, **SLP**

Johnson, Cherrel 2228 S W 78th Street, Oklahoma City, OK 73159, (405) 681-2841, BA 76 Univ of OK - Norman; MS 78 Univ of OK - Norman; 78–Sp-Lang Path, OK City Pub Sch, **SLP**

Johnson, Mrs Cheryl Bennett 208 Ellery Avenue, Newark, NJ 07106, (201) 385-4857, BS 75 Trenton St Coll; MA 77 Trenton St Coll; Sp-Lang Path, Bergen Ctr for Child Dev

Johnson, Cheryl Mae 1707 Woodbury Lane, Duluth, MN 55803, (218) 723-4150, BA 72 Univ of MN - Duluth; MA 74 Univ of MN - Duluth; Sp-Lang Path, ISD 709, **SLP**

Johnson, Christine 68 Cypress Drive, East Windsor, NJ 08520, (609) 448-1580, MA 80 Ball St Univ; **A**

Johnson, Mrs Christine L W R R Box 7, Altona, IL 61414, (309) 484-4981, BS 76 Eastern IL Univ; MS 77 Eastern IL Univ; Sp-Lang Path, St Mary's Hosp, **SLP**

Johnson, Mrs Christine Richter 7691 Traphill Court, Worthington, OH 43235, (614) 792-8332, BS 84 Kent St Univ; MA 86 Cleveland St Univ; **SLP**

Johnson, Mrs Christine Smith 517 Dentro Drive, Santa Barbara, CA 93111, (805) 964-5177, 74 Univ of CA - Santa Barbara; 75 Univ of Denver; 88–Aud, Univ of CA-Santa Barbara, **A**

Johnson, Mrs Cindy Jan 864 Cooper Road, Jackson, MS 39212, (601) 373-0968, BS 83 MS Univ for Women; MS 85 Vanderbilt Univ; Aud, VA Med Ctr, **A**

Johnson, Cindy Marie Casa Colina Hospital, Transitional Living Center, 255 East Bonita Avenue, Pomona, CA 91767, (714) 593-7521, BA 84 CA St Univ - Fullerton; MA 86 CA St Univ - Fullerton; 88–Sp-Lang Path, Casa Colina Hosp, **SLP**

Johnson, Cindy Smith 1308 John Road, Ardmore, OK 73401, (405) 223-9554, BS 85 Univ of OK - OK City; MS 87 Univ of OK - OK City; **SLP**

Johnson, Clayton R 10336 Military Road, Dubuque, IA 52001, (319) 589-9750, BS 66 Moorhead St Univ; MS 69 Purdue Univ - West Lafayette; 73–Aud, Medical Associates, **A**

Johnson, Clint Daniel 5407 Bryan #B-208, Dallas, TX 75206, (214) 638-6346, BS 84 TX Christian Univ; MS 86 TX Christian Univ; SLP, Memorial SE Hosp, **SLP**

Johnson, Constance Cowing 320 Van Buren Street, Wilmington, IL 60481-1162, (815) 727-4302, BS 59 Northwestern Univ; OM 79 Governors St Univ; **SLP LM**

Johnson, Craig W 4115 Century Town Road, Randallstown, MD 21133, (301) 944-3100, BA 74 Univ of MD - College Park; MS 75 Towson St Univ; **A**

Johnson, Cynthia Ann 734 North Bruns Lane #H, Springfield, IL 62704, (217) 793-1028, **SLP**

Johnson, Cynthia Clark 115 Harlan Way, Fortuna, CA 95540, (707) 725-9073, BA 81 Humboldt St Univ; MA 83 Humboldt St Univ; 85–Sp-Lang Path, Eureka City Schs, **SLP**

Johnson, Dr Cynthia J Dept Of Speech And Hearing Sci, University Of Illinois, 901 South 6th Street, Champaign, IL 61820, (217) 244-2540, BA 73 Univ of IA; MA 75 Univ of IA; PH 79 (Communication Disorders) Univ of MN - Minneap-St Paul; Assoc Prof, U of IL/Dept of Sp-Hrng Serv, **SLP**

Johnson, Mrs Cynthia Kelley 26291 Via Madrigal, San Juan Capistrano, CA 92675, (714) 661-4031, BS 78 Northern AZ Univ; MA 85 CA St Univ - Fullerton; **SLP**

Johnson, Cynthia L 12 Morningside Drive, Conway, AR 72032, (501) 329-6851, OB 79 Univ of Central AR; MA 80 Memphis St Univ; 81–Sp-Lang Path Superv, Conway Human Dev Cen, **SLP**

Johnson, Cynthia P 332 Old Babcock Trail, Gibsonia, PA 15044, **SLP**

Johnson, Cynthia W 1598 Mesa Verde Drive, Vista, CA 92083, BS 73 Univ of Redlands; MS 74 Univ of Redlands; **A**

Johnson, David Warren Hennepin County Medical Center, 701 Park Avenue, Audiology 824, Minneapolis, MN 55415, (612) 347-2429, BA 66 Univ of MN - Duluth; MA 69 Univ of OR; MS 71 Portland St Univ; 71–Aud, Hennepin Co Med Cen, **A**

Johnson, Deanna E 3326 West Riviera Court, Mequon, WI 53092, BS 72 Univ of WI - Stevens Point; MS 73 Univ of WI - Stevens Point; Sp/Lang Path, Ebenezer Soc, **SLP**

Johnson, Mrs Deborah K B 6 Hill Court, Roanoke, TX 76262, (817) 283-1583, BA 68 Grinnell Coll; MA 77 Univ of IA; Sp-Lang Path, Hurst-Euless-Bedford ISD, **SLP**

Johnson, Deborah L Boys Town Institute, 555 North 30th Street, Omaha, NE 68131, (402) 498-6624, BS 78 AZ St Univ; MS 80 AZ St Univ; 81–Sp-Lang Path, Boys Town I for Commun Dis, **SLP**

Johnson, Mrs Debra Ann 906 Campbell Drive, Grand Forks, ND 58201, (701) 772-0555, BS 76 Univ of ND; MS 82 Univ of ND; SLP, Grand Forks Pub Sch Dist 1, **SLP**

Johnson, Mrs Debra Brosseau 126 Quailwood Drive, Winter Haven, FL 33880-8617, (813) 967-7844, BS 77 FL St Univ; MS 78 FL St Univ; Sp-Lang Path, Polk Co Sch Bd, **SLP**

Johnson, Debra Lois 1019 23rd Avenue, Moline, IL 61265, (309) 762-1575, BA 81 Augustana Coll; MA 83 Northeast MO St Univ; SLP, Blackhawk Area Education Cen, **SLP**

Johnson, Mrs Debra Sue 644 Swain Avenue, Elmhurst, IL 60126, (312) 361-2121, BS 84 Northern IL Univ - De Kalb; MA 86 Northern IL Univ - De Kalb; 88–Aud, Sertoma Ctr for Comm Dis, **A**

Johnson, Deloris Marie 3525 Attucks Street, Houston, TX 77004, (713) 623-5011, **SLP**

Johnson, Deloris R P O Box 5309, Macon, GA 31208, BA 75 SC St Coll; MA 76 Univ of IL - Urbana; Sp/Lang Path, Ctrl GA Sp Hrng Cen, **SLP**

Johnson, Mrs Denise H 105 Portis Street, Union, MS 39365, (601) 635-2956, BS 76 MS St Univ - MS State; MS 77 MS Univ for Women; Sp-Lang Path, Newton Co Schs, **SLP**

Johnson, Mrs Denise L 2910 S W 22nd Circle #21-E2, Delray Beach, FL 33445, (305) 278-6282, MS 79 Univ of South FL; Sp-Lang Path, Private Practice, **SLP**

Johnson, Mrs Denise Loy 1938 Love Circle, Simi Valley, CA 93063, (805) 527-2462, BS 80 Univ of CA - Santa Barbara; MS 82 UT St Univ; Sp-Lang Path, Simi Valley Adventist Hosp, **SLP**

Johnson, Diane F 1016 Liberty Street, Arlington, VA 22205, (703) 435-0488, BS 79 Univ of VA - Charlottesville; MS 81 Vanderbilt Univ; Sp-Lang Path, Childrens Sp-Lang Services, **SLP**

Johnson, Diane L 23 Colonial Court, Absecon, NJ 08201, (609) 652-7000, BS 86 East Stroudsburg Univ of PA; MS 88 PA St Univ - Univ Park; 88–Sp-Lang Path, Betty Bacharach Rehab Hosp

Johnson, Diane M 1317 Willmar Avenue S W, Willmar, MN 56201, (612) 235-4613, BS 70 Wayne St Univ; MA 71 Univ of Denver; Sp-Lang Path, W Central Community Serv Ctr, **SLP**

Johnson, Dr Donald D Rochester Inst Of Technology, Ntl Tech Inst For The Deaf, One Lomb Memorial Drive, Rochester, NY 14623, (716) 475-6434, BS 61 Univ of IL - Urbana; MA 62 Northwestern Univ; PH 70 (NS) Univ of IL - Urbana; Prof of Aud/Sr Research Assoc, NTID, **A F**

Johnson, Donald F 1017 Cedar Drive, Sulphur, OK 73086, (405) 622-3186, BA 67 Univ of OK - Norman; ME 70 East Central OK St Univ; MA 73 Univ of North TX; Aud Servs Super, OK Sch for the Deaf, **A**

Johnson, Mrs Doris E Route 1 Box 95, P O Box 324, Loon Lake, WA 99148, (509) 233-8333, OB 64 Eastern WA Univ; BA 64 Eastern WA Univ; ME 70 Central WA Univ; 85–University Supervisor, Eastern Washington University, **SLP**

Johnson, Mrs Doris Emiko 2223 Nantucket Road, Johnson City, TN 37601, (615) 929-0753, MS 87 East TN St Univ

Johnson, Doris Joan Learning Disabilities Center, Communication Disorder Bldg, Northwestern University, Evanston, IL 60201, (312) 492-3183, BA 53 Augustana Coll; MA 55 Northwestern Univ; PH 71 (NS) Northwestern Univ; Prof/Prog Head Lrng Dis, Northwestern U, **SLP F**

Johnson, Mrs Dorothy C 18630 Polvera Drive, San Diego, CA 92128, (619) 485-9505, BA 49 MacAlster Coll; MA 51 Stanford Univ; **SLP LM**

Johnson, Mrs Dorothy E 3140 Oregon Street, Bakersfield, CA 93306, BS 54 Bradley Univ; MS 52 Bradley Univ; 78–Sp-Lang Path, Kern County Supt of Schs, **SLP**

Johnson, Mrs Dovie Jean 321 East Loma Alta Drive, Altadena, CA 91001, (707) 459-5376, BA 61 San Francisco St Univ; MA 69 San Francisco St Univ; SLP, Los Angeles USD, **SLP**

Johnson, E Suzanne 2821 Augusta Lane, Billings, MT 59102, (406) 255-3626, BS 76 CO St Univ; MS 79 CO St Univ; Aud, Billings PS, **A**

Johnson, Dr E W 4151 Colbath Avenue, Sherman Oaks, CA 91423, (213) 483-9930, BA 39 Gustavus Adolphus Coll; MA 53 Univ of Southern CA; PH 56 (NS) Univ of Southern CA; Consultant Prof Relations, Siemens Hrng Instruments, **A LM**

Johnson, Mrs Elaine S 108 Campfire Road North, Henrietta, NY 14467, (716) 377-0880, BS 72 SUNY - Coll at Geneseo; MS 73 SUNY - Coll at Geneseo; 83–Sp-Lang Path, Penfield Ctrl Sch, **SLP**

Johnson, Mrs Elizabeth 5448 Trinidy Avenue, Lowville, NY 13367, (315) 376-7531, BA 65 Bloomsburg Univ of PA; MA 69 Univ of Denver; SLP, Lewis Co Headstart, **SLP**

Johnson, Mrs Elizabeth Ann 1014 Glynn Oaks, Arlington, TX 76010, (817) 261-9191, BS 80 Univ of North TX; MS 82 Univ of North TX; Aud, Dr William Briggs, **A**

Johnson, Mrs Elizabeth Jackson 729 11th Avenue, Helena, MT 59601, (406) 442-7034, MS 84 Univ of MT; Sp-Lang Path, Missoula Comm Rehab Ctr, **SLP**

Johnson, Ellen Harshey 409 West South Street, Bluffton, IN 46714, (219) 824-0182, BS 85 Ball St Univ; MA 86 Ball St Univ; 87–Sp-Lang Path, Parkview Memorial Hosp, **SLP**

Johnson, Mrs Emily C 199 Kent Court, Summerville, SC 29485, (803) 871-9669, BS 76 Western Carolina Univ; MA 78 Univ of TN - Knoxville; 88–Aud/Owner, Hrng Care of Summerville, **A**

Johnson, Mrs Erin Dawn 2740-A N E 103rd Street, Seattle, WA 98125, (206) 524-9124, BS 80 Univ of WA; OM 83 Univ of WA; 88–Sp-Lang Path, Northshore SD #417, **SLP**

Johnson, Erin Michelle 29845 Avenue Cima Del Sol, Temecula, CA 92390, (714) 788-6630, BA 82 Univ of Redlands; MA 84 San Diego St Univ; **SLP**

Johnson, Faye Guttormson 106 17th Avenue S E, Minot, ND 58701, (701) 857-4410, BS 72 Minot St Univ; MS 74 Minot St Univ; Sp/Lang Path, Souris Valley Special Serv, **SLP**

Johnson, Flora Renee 4420 McClain Lane, Huntsville, AL 35810, (205) 859-7368, 88 AL A & M Univ

Johnson, Frances L 1501 Delmont Court #3, Urbana, IL 61801, (217) 367-7804, BA 44 Augustana Coll; MS 49 Univ of IL - Urbana; **SLP**

Johnson, Mrs Frances Y 111 Forest Hillcourt, Shawano, WI 54166, (715) 758-2234, BA 63 Univ of IA; Sp-Lang Path, Bonduel Sch, **SLP**

Johnson, Gail A 136 Callender, Fort Worth, TX 76108, (817) 237-1599, BS 73 Univ of TX - Austin; MS 75 Univ of North TX; 88–Dir-Spec Educ, Lake Worth ISD, **SLP**

Johnson, Gayl E 1821 Jelinek Avenue, Schofield, WI 54476, **SLP**

Johnson, George William, III Route 1 Box 63, Greenville, NC 27834, (919) 756-1262, BS 80 East Carolina Univ; MS 85 East Carolina Univ; Aud/Sp-Lang Path, Pitt County Schools, **SLP A**

Johnson, Georgia S Box 134-B, Big Foot, TX 78005, **SLP**

Johnson, Georgiana 3764 Telluride Lane, Boulder, CO 80303, (303) 444-7400, BA 40; MS 70 Univ of CO - Boulder; Therapy Coord, Boulder Pain Cen, **SLP LM**

Johnson, Dr Gerald F 301 Greenbriar Park Ridge, Stevens Point, WI 54481, (715) 346-3496, BS 55 Western MI Univ; MS 59 Western MI Univ; PH 63 (NS) MI St Univ; Prof, U of WI-Stevens Pt, **SLP A**

Johnson, Geraldine 13236 North 7th Street #4-194, Phoenix, AZ 85022, (602) 482-6779, BS 74 Univ of HI - Manoa; MS 76 Univ of HI - Manoa; **SLP**

Johnson, Mrs Gertrude L 462 Macon Street, Brooklyn, NY 11233, (718) 326-8272, BA 60 CUNY - Hunter Coll; MA 62 CUNY - Brooklyn Coll; MS 83 Pace U -NY City; Sp-Lang Path, Sp Serv UT/NYC Bd of Ed, **SLP**

Johnson, Glen W 7 Laughlin Square on Main, Greeneville, TN 37743-5039, (615) 638-2721, BS 74 East TN St Univ; MA 76 East TN St Univ; Dir, Greenville Aud Serv, **A**

Johnson, Mrs Glenda L Route 2 Box 24-C, Ceresco, NE 68017, (402) 564-0815, MS 87 Univ of NE - Lincoln

Johnson, Glenn A 8039 14th Avenue NE, Seattle, WA 98115, (206) 545-7400, BA 76 Temple Univ; MA 85 Univ of MT; 88–Sp-Lang Path, Univ of Washington, **SLP**

Johnson, Gloria J 7224 Roberts Road, Apex, NC 27502, (919) 872-0572, BA 67 Central MI Univ; MA 74 MI St Univ; **SLP**

Johnson, Mrs Grace Kane 2032 Old Hillsboro Road, Franklin, TN 37064, (615) 377-3357, BS 82 Auburn Univ - Auburn; MS 83 FL St Univ; Sp-Lang Path, Private Practice, **SLP**

Johnson, Helen Gutmann 108 Graymoor Lane, Olympia Fields, IL 60461, **SLP ACE**

Johnson, Mrs Hettie P 6500 Sugar Creek Drive S, Mobile, AL 36695, (205) 633-3348, BA 70 Auburn Univ - Auburn; MA 72 Univ of Montevallo; Sp/Lang Path, Private Practice, **SLP**

Johnson, Iris E 4516 45th Avenue South, Minneapolis, MN 55406, (612) 729-7672, BS 78 ND St Univ; MA 80 Univ of IA; Aud, Columbia Park Med Gp, **A**

Johnson, Mrs J Louise 29543 Pheasant Avenue, Corvallis, OR 97333, (503) 967-6108, BA 68 Minot St Univ; MS 69 Minot St Univ; Instructional Asst, Linn Benton Comm Coll

Johnson, James W 8906 Mansfield, San Antonio, TX 78251, **A**

Johnson, Mrs Jan Marsden 8541 Fernald Avenue, Morton Grove, IL 60053-2820, (312) 966-3739, **SLP**

Johnson, Jana Lee 5611 Carlisle Court, New Orleans, LA 70114, (504) 523-6419, BA 83 LA St Univ - Baton Rouge; MA 85 LA St Univ - Baton Rouge; 88–Dir of Patient Care, Assoc Healthfocus, **SLP**

Johnson, Mrs Jane C 5054 Oak Trail Drive, Dunwoody, GA 30338, (404) 252-5325, BS 51 Purdue Univ - West Lafayette; MS 51 Purdue Univ - West Lafayette; Director, Atlanta Rehabilitation Inst, **SLP**

Johnson, Dr Jane I 8 Debary Place, Summit, NJ 07901, (201) 533-5786, BA 45 American Univ; MA 72 Kean Coll of NJ; ED 77 (Aud) Columbia Univ Teachers Coll; Director Speech-Hearing, Rehab Cen-Sp-Hrng St Barnabas, **A**

Johnson, Mrs Janet A 4731 North Lake Drive, Whitefish Bay, WI 53211, (414) 259-1414, BS 76 Marquette Univ; MS 77 Marquette Univ; SLP, Curative Rehab Cen, **SLP**

Johnson, Janet L 779 Eastowne Drive, #506, Ravenna, OH 44266, (216) 296-8188, MA 88 Kent St Univ

Johnson, Janet Mary 515 College Avenue, South Milwaukee, WI 53172, (414) 353-6400, BS 86 Marquette Univ; MS 87 Marquette Univ

Johnson, Janice A 2229 Monterey Lane, Eugene, OR 97401, (503) 344-3070, BS 70 OH Univ - Athens; MS 76 Univ of OR; Dir Sp Lang & Cog Therapies, Center for Neuroeduc Therapies, **SLP**

Johnson, Mrs Janice F 226 Rio Verde Drive, Salinas, CA 93901, (408) 424-3415, BA 61 San Jose St Univ; **SLP**

Johnson, Janice L Tucson Unified School District, Davidson Elementary School, 3915 East Fort Lowell Road, Tucson, AZ 85712, (602) 798-2527, BA 72 Univ of OR; MS 74 Univ of AZ; 88–Sp-Lang Path, Tucson USD, **SLP**

Johnson, Janice M 3684 East 151st Street, Cleveland, OH 44120, (202) 244-4420, MS 87 Gallaudet Coll; **A**

Johnson, Mrs Janice R 3071 South Josephine St, Denver, CO 80210, (303) 757-5912, BS 72 CO St Univ; MS 74 Univ of OK Medical Center; Sp-Lang Path, Private Practice, **SLP**

Johnson, Jean T 1600 Hobart Drive, Camarillo, CA 93010, (805) 482-9838, BS 56 UT St Univ; MA 81 CA St Univ - Northridge; SLP, Pleasant Valley School Dist, **SLP**

Johnson, Dr Jeanne M Department Of Speech, Washington State Univ, Pullman, WA 99164-2420, (509) 335-4525, BA 73 Edison Univ; MA 78 Western WA Univ; PH 86 (Commun Dis & Sci) Southern IL Univ -Carbondale; 88–Asst Prof, Washington State Univ, **SLP**

Johnson, Dr Jeannette Seloover 1671 Century Circle #216, Woodbury, MN 55125-2116, (612) 778-5421, BS 62 Univ of WI - Milwaukee; MA 63 Northwestern Univ; PH 66 (Aud) Northwestern Univ; 88–Aud Research, 3M Co, **A**

Johnson, Jennifer A 2600 East Central, Wichita, KS 67214, (316) 684-2424, BA 75 Wichita St Univ; MA 76 Wichita St Univ; Sp-Lang Path, Related Therapies Inc, **SLP**

Johnson, Jerry E Ohio Div Of Special Education, 933 High Street, Worthington, OH 43085, (614) 466-2650, BS 61 OH Univ - Athens; MA 64 OH Univ - Athens; Sp-Lang Path, Ohio Div of Spec Ed, **SLP**

Johnson, Jill M 923 Bank Street, Cincinnati, OH 45214, (513) 579-0619, BS 76 Kent St Univ; MA 77 Kent St Univ; Oral Comm Instr, Springer Sch, **SLP**

Johnson, Jilonda L 2912 Vaughn #2, Cincinnati, OH 45219, (513) 751-6806, MA 88 Univ of Cincinnati

Johnson, Mrs Joanne Phelps 6 Roswell Road, Box 264, West Simsbury, CT 06092, (203) 651-0765, BA 63 CO St Univ; MS 65 CO St Univ; **SLP**

Johnson, Mrs Jody A 4021 Aldrich Avenue South, Minneapolis, MN 55409, (612) 421-1420, BS 77 Univ of WI - River Falls; MS 78 Univ of WI - River Falls; SLP, Anoka Hennepin School Dist #11, **SLP**

Johnson, John D, III Ctrl Florida Ear & Hearing Clinic, 827 Deltona Boulevard, Suite D, Deltona, FL 32725, (407) 574-1492, BA 78 Southern IL Univ-Edwardsvill; MA 81 Univ of Central FL; Dir Aud, Cen FL Ear & Hrng Cl, **A**

Johnson, Dr John P Northern Kentucky University, 214 Bep, Highland Heights, KY 41076, (606) 572-5666, BA 67 FL St Univ; MS 69 FL St Univ; PH 75 (Sp-Lang Path) Kent St Univ; 87–Dean Coll of Pro Studies, Northern Kentucky Univ, **SLP**

Johnson, Joni Lynn 4917 101st Place S W, Everett, WA 98204-3313, (206) 361-4252, BA 81 Univ of WA; OM 83 Univ of WA; Aud, Shoreline Pub Sch, **A**

Johnson, Mrs Josephine W 2945 Kimi Court N E, Bremerton, WA 98310, (203) 443-5380, BA 78 Metropolitan St Coll; MA 81 Univ of Central FL; 88–Sp-Lang Path, Bremerton Sch Dist, **SLP**

Johnson, Joy Clark 8234 Calabar Avenue, Playa Del Rey, CA 90293, **SLP**

Johnson, Joyce E P O Box 124, Jefferson, WI 53549, (414) 563-2437, BS 70 Univ of WI - Whitewater; MS 81 Univ of WI - Whitewater; Sp/Lang Path, Somed Inc, **SLP**

Johnson, Judith A 43 Brook Road, Upper Saddle River, NJ 07458, (201) 342-6311, BS 62 Fairleigh Dickinson U-Teanec; MA 74 Montclair St Coll; 77–Sp-Lang Path, Hackensack Med Ctr, **SLP ACE**

Johnson, Judith Ann 126 East Alcott, Fergus Falls, MN 56537, (218) 736-6987, BS 68 Moorhead St Univ; MS 72 Univ of WI - Eau Claire; Sp-Lang Path, Lakeland Ment Hlth Cen, **SLP**

Johnson, Judith C 1760 South Corona, Denver, CO 80210, BS 70 CO St Univ; MS 72 Univ of WA; Sp-Lang Path, **SLP**

Johnson, Mrs Judith Callan 414 South Caldwell Street, Brevard, NC 28712, (704) 252-1853, BA 74 Univ of FL; MS 76 FL St Univ; Aud, Wnc ENT Surgeons, **A**

Johnson, Mrs Judy C 2908 South Edwards, Wichita, KS 67217, (316) 942-6368, BA 85 Wichita St Univ; MA 87 Wichita St Univ

Johnson, Judy Lynn 3810 J Street, Sacramento, CA 95816, (916) 736-3399, BS 84 TX Christian Univ; MS 86 Univ of TX - Dallas; **A**

Johnson, Julia 2860 Masseyville Road, Macon, GA 31201, (912) 742-4699, **A**

Johnson, Mrs Kara L 1119 Lafond, St Paul, MN 55104, BS 80 ND St Univ; MS 83 Univ of WI - River Falls; SLP, St Paul Pub Sch, **SLP**

Johnson, Karen A Rd 1 Box 90, East Otto, NY 14729, (716) 822-1806, MA 84 Bowling Green St Univ; 85–Sp-Lang Path, Language Dev Prog of W NY, **SLP**

Johnson, Karen Ann 216-1/2 Byron, Mankato, MN 56001, (507) 625-1811, BS 81 Central MI Univ; MA 83 Central MI Univ; Aud, Mankato Cl Ltd, **A**

Johnson, Karen Christine 2232 Bellefontanie, Apt #11, Houston, TX 77030, (713) 790-5913, BA 76 Rutger's St Univ - Douglas Coll; MA 82 Auburn Univ - Auburn; Research Assist, Baylor College of Med, **A**

Johnson, Karen H 9961 N Placita Papalote, Tucson, AZ 85704, (602) 297-9947, BA 74 Augustana Coll; MS 76 Univ of AZ; Sp-Lang Path, Private Practice, **SLP**

Johnson, Karen L 4911 Fremont Avenue N #303, Seattle, WA 98103, (206) 364-0300, BA 75 WA St Univ; MA 77 WA St Univ; SLP, Dshs Fircrest School, **SLP**

Johnson, Karen Lee 2056 Bayard #2, St Paul, MN 55116, (612) 293-8970, BA 75 Augsburg Coll; MA 82 Univ of WI - River Falls; Sp-Lang Path, St Paul Pub Schools, **SLP**

Johnson, Mrs Karin L L 2806 27th Avenue, Rock Island, IL 61201, (309) 794-7273, BA 63 Augustana Coll; MA 67 Univ of KS; Instr/Cl Superv, Agustana Coll, **SLP**

Johnson, Mrs Katherine Vaughn 3225 Victoria Drive #2013, Baton Rouge, LA 70805, (504) 355-1955, BA 78 Siena Heights Coll; MA 81 LA St Univ - Baton Rouge; Sp/Lang Path, Ascension Parish School System, **SLP**

Johnson, Kathleen R 1812 East Secretariat, Tempe, AZ 85284, (602) 839-5267, BS 80 AZ St Univ; OM 86 AZ St Univ; **SLP**

Johnson, Mrs Kathleen Rose Michigan State University, Dept Audiology/Speech Sci, 101 Wilson Road, East Lansing, MI 48824, (517) 353-8780, BS 76 Bowling Green St Univ; MA 77 Kent St Univ; Clinical Supervisor, Michigan State University, **SLP**

Johnson, Kathleen Therese 19402 Ridgeland Avenue, Cleveland, OH 44135, (216) 267-1527, **SLP**

Johnson, Kathryn A 1004 St Albans Place, Leucadia, CA 92024, (619) 942-7005, BA 70 San Diego St Univ; MA 71 San Diego St Univ; Sp-Lang Path, Private Practice, **SLP**

Johnson, Kathryn Ann-Hagen 1348 Mississippi Avenue, Duluth, MN 55811, (218) 727-5083, BS 79 Univ of MN - Minneap-St Paul; MA 80 Univ of MN - Duluth; Sp-Lang Path, Polinsky Med Rehab Ctr, **SLP**

Johnson, Kenneth A 812 121st Street East, Tacoma, WA 98445, (206) 537-0211, **SLP**

Johnson, Dr Kenneth O 18630 Polvera Drive, San Diego, CA 92128, (619) 485-9505, BA 46 MacAlster Coll; MA 48 Univ of MN - Minneap-St Paul; PH 52 (NS) Stanford Univ; **SLP A F H LM**

Johnson, Dr Kenneth R Audiology Professionals, 224 East Fulton, Grand Rapids, MI 49503, (616) 459-7122, BS 62 Kent St Univ; MA 65 MI St Univ; PH 70 (NS) MI St Univ; Aud, Aud Professionals, **A ACE**

Johnson, Kevin Charles 4638 Seahurst, Everett, WA 98203, (206) 775-4555, BS 82 Univ of WA; MS 84 Univ of WA; Sp-Lang Path, Group Health Coop, **SLP**

Johnson, Mrs Kimberly Ann 612 South Armstrong, Litchfield, MN 55355, (612) 235-1058, BA 82 Univ of Northern IA; MA 83 Univ of Northern IA; Sp-Lang Path, ISD #347, **SLP**

Johnson, Kristin Matheson 8152 Monrovia, Lenexa, KS 66215, (913) 492-2585, BS 80 IA St Univ; MA 83 Univ of KS; Sp-Lang Path, Wyandotte Co Spec Ed Coop, **SLP**

Johnson, Kyle C 8831 Ashworth North, Seattle, WA 98103, (206) 883-5350, BA 82 Stanford Univ; MS 85 Univ of WA; **A**

Johnson, Lamont S 2315 Scholl Road, University Heights, OH 44118, (216) 481-4823, BA 73 Cleveland St Univ; MA 79 Cleveland St Univ; SLP, Johanna Grasselli Rehab & Ed, **SLP ACE**

Johnson, Mrs Laurie W 1930 Borland Road, Pittsburgh, PA 15243-1528, (412) 462-2903, **SLP**

Johnson, Mrs Lee Ann 225 Graham Road, Fern Park, FL 32730, (713) 633-0796, BA 79 Creighton Univ; MA 83 Univ of Houston - Univ Park; Sp-Lang Path, FL I of Rehab, **SLP**

Johnson, Mrs Leeda G 8761 Sailport Drive, Huntington Beach, CA 92646, (714) 968-1826, BA 71 Univ of CA - Los Angeles; MA 77 CA St Univ - Long Beach; 87–Sp-Lang Path, Placentia USD, **SLP**

Johnson, Lennette Ruby P O Box 1161, Tupelo, MS 38802-1161, MS 87 Univ of MS

Johnson, Mrs Leslie M 6007 Whitehaven Road, Columbus, GA 31909, (404) 561-6428, BS 81 James Madison Univ; MS 83 Univ of Louisville; Aud, Aud Med Cen, **A**

Johnson, Mrs Letitia L 1480 Roxbury Road, Ann Arbor, MI 48104, (313) 996-9544, BS 63 Univ of IL - Urbana; MA 64 Stanford Univ; SLP, **SLP**

Johnson, Mrs Lila Kay 5245 Mill Branch Road, Lavalette, WV 25535, **SLP**

Johnson, Linda Grassel 13307 Ramroo, Manchaca, TX 78652, (512) 396-8500, BS 76 Southwest TX St Univ; ME 79 Southwest TX St Univ; Superv SLP Aud, Brown Schs, **SLP**

Johnson, Linda J 1873 Ashland Avenue, St Paul, MN 55104, (612) 373-4116, BA 70 Fordham Univ; MA 72 Univ of Southern CA; Research Assistant, 3M, **SLP**

Johnson, Linda W 135 Frederick Drive, Apalachin, NY 13732, (701) 361-2144, BS 74 CO St Univ; MA 76 Coll of Saint Rose; Sp-Lang Path, Manassas Cty Sch, **SLP**

Johnson, Lisa Ann 318 Belmont Street #2, Watertown, MA 02172, (617) 926-9433, MA 84 Univ of Pittsburgh - Pittsburgh; Sp-Lang Path, **SLP**

Johnson, Mrs Lori 5 Lent Court #3, Schenectady, NY 12306-1205, (518) 597-3524, MS 84 Coll of Saint Rose; BS 81 Coll of Saint Rose; Sp-Lang Path, BOCES Clinton Essex Warren, **SLP**

Johnson, Mrs Lorraine Deutsch Audiology Srvs Pekin Memorial, Court At 14th Street, Pekin, IL 61554, (309) 353-0200, BS 78 Northern IL Univ - De Kalb; MA 79 Northern IL Univ - De Kalb; Supvr of Aud Svcs, Aud Srvs Pekin Mem Hosp, **A**

Johnson, Louise C 110 East Walnut Lane, Philadelphia, PA 19144, BS; **SLP LM**

Johnson, Lucie M 248 Parkridge Place S E, Calgary, AB, Canada T2J 5B7, (403) 229-7061, BA 77 Univ of Alberta - Alberta; MA 79 Northwestern Univ; Aud, Alberta Children's Hosp, **A**

Johnson, Mrs Lucille Mary 481 Deer Park Avenue, Babylon, NY 11702, (516) 422-6915, BA 79 Adelphi Univ; MS 85 Adelphi Univ; **SLP**

Johnson, Mrs Lynn A 13817 East 30th Street, Tulsa, OK 74134, (918) 272-8021, BS 67 OK St Univ; MA 79 Univ of Tulsa; Dir of Sp Serv, Owasso Pub Sch, **SLP**

Johnson, M K Maddie 6956 North Starshine, Tucson, AZ 85741, (602) 297-5006, BA 78 Grand Valley St Coll; MS 87 Univ of AZ; 87–Sp-Lang Path, University Physicians Inc, **SLP**

Johnson, Margaret Anne 1014 Countryside Trace, Louisville, KY 40223, (502) 583-8303, BS 81 Northwestern Univ; MA 82 Northwestern Univ; 88–Aud Supvr, University Surgical Associates, **A**

Johnson, Margaret L 1115 Woodfield Drive, Jackson, MS 39211, (601) 981-2611, BA 85 Univ of MS; MS 87 Univ of MS; Sp-Lang Path, Miss Methodist Rehab Center, **SLP**

Johnson, Mrs Margaret Mary 208 Brookside Lane, Willowbrook, IL 60514, (312) 383-1203, BA 82 Augustana Coll; MA 83 Western MI Univ; Sp-Lang Path, Dist 89-Stevensn Sch, **SLP**

Johnson, Marie H 2301 Hammond Road, Stoughton, WI 53589, (608) 884-9402, BS 80 Univ of WI - Stevens Point; MS 82 Univ of WI - Madison; SLP, Edgerton Sch Dist, **SLP**

Johnson, Dr Marie Love P O Box 2026, Vernon, CT 06066, (203) 875-7628, BS 51 IN Univ - Bloomington; ME 53 Univ of Hartford; PH 78 (NS) Univ of CT; **SLP F**

Johnson, Marilyn Kaye 1611 North Quincy, Arlington, VA 22207, (313) 885-8660, BS 81 CO St Univ; MA 85 Univ of CO - Boulder; SLP, Foundation for Excep Chldrn, **SLP**

Johnson, Mrs Marilyn Spears 263 Sumba Court, San Jose, CA 95123, (408) 246-7117, BA 83 Univ of TX - El Paso; MS 86 Univ of TX - El Paso; 88–Sp-Lang Path, Franklin-McKinley Sch Dist, **SLP**

Johnson, Mrs Mary A 669 Honey Way, Sacramento, CA 95831, (916) 429-6602, MA 87 CA St Univ - Fresno; 88–Sp-Lang Path, InSpeech Inc

Johnson, Mrs Mary Ann 1740 Moundview Drive, Topeka, KS 66604, (913) 296-7711, BS 79 Univ of KS; MA 80 Univ of KS; 85–Sp-Lang Path, Youth Center at Topeka, **SLP**

Johnson, Mrs Mary B 53 Elder Drive, Marquette, MI 49855, (906) 226-7613, BS 76 Northern MI Univ; MA 78 Northern MI Univ; SLP, Marquette Pub Sch, **SLP**

Johnson, Mrs Mary Blaine 6335 Riverton, Troy, MI 48098, (313) 745-3535, BS 81 Wayne St Univ; MA 82 Wayne St Univ; Sp-Lang Path, Detroit Rec Hosp U Hlth Cen, **SLP**

Johnson, Mary Elizabeth 1870-10, Columbus, OH 43212, (614) 488-9529, BA 26 Muskingum Coll; MA 33 Univ of MI - Ann Arbor; **LM**

Johnson, Mrs Mary J 932 Hamilton Avenue, Latrobe, PA 15650, (412) 539-9777, BS 64 CA Univ of PA; ME 67 Indiana Univ of PA; SLP, Westmoreland Iu #7, **SLP**

Johnson, Mrs Mary Kay 125 West Everett, Fergus Falls, MN 56537-3418, (218) 739-3712, BS 82 ND St Univ; MS 86 Moorhead St Univ

Johnson, Mrs Mary L T 809 Oakwood Drive, Castle Rock, CO 80104, (303) 688-3856, BS 75 Saint Cloud St Univ; MA 78 Saint Cloud St Univ; **SLP**

Johnson, Mary Lou Brecht 10456 East Powers Place, Englewood, CO 80111, (303) 861-6800, BA 73 OH Wesleyan Univ; MS 75 Washington Univ; Sp-Lang Path, The Childrens Hospital, **SLP**

Johnson, Mary R P O Box 1394, Opelousas, LA 70570, (318) 948-6094, BS 71 Southern Univ - Baton Rouge; ME 87 Southern Univ - Baton Rouge

Johnson, Mrs Mary T Kremeyer 1615 Tanglewood Drive, Clinton, MS 39056, (601) 987-3555, BA 52 Rockford Coll; OM 78 Univ of MS; Sp-Lang Path, Jackson Public Schools, **SLP**

Johnson, Mrs Maryann Shields 1113 Woodbrook Way, Garner, NC 27529, (919) 772-9003, BS 85 East Carolina Univ; MS 86 East Carolina Univ; Sp-Lang Path, **SLP**

Johnson, Maurita G 3806 Torre, Amarillo, TX 79109, (806) 378-5321, BS 73 West TX St Univ; MA 76 West TX St Univ; Dir of Adult Commun Dis, High Plains Baptist Hosp, **SLP**

Johnson, Mrs Maxine M 301 Grenbriar Avenue, Stevens Point, WI 54481, (715) 345-5417, BS 58 Western MI Univ; MS 70 Univ of WI - Stevens Point; Sp-Lang Path, Stevens Point Area Bd of Ed, **SLP**

Johnson, Meredith A 9023 Lunar Avenue, Apt 203, Orland Park, IL 60462, (312) 333-2300, BS 80 IL St Univ - Normal; MS 81 IL St Univ - Normal; SLP, Ingalls Mem Hosp, **SLP**

Johnson, Michael Dewees Crotched Mountain Rehabilitation Center, Department Of Communication Disorders, Greenfield, NH 03047, (603) 547-3311, BA 78 Univ of MD - Baltimore CO; MA 86 Towson St Univ; 86–Sp-Lang Path, Crotched Mountain Rehab Ctr, **SLP**

Johnson, Michael G Speech Language Hearing Clinic, 4701 Chicago Avenue, Minneapolis, MN 55407, (612) 823-6660, BA 67 Northern MI Univ; MA 69 Univ of NM; Pres, Sp Lang Hrng Cl, **SLP**

Johnson, Michael H 623 Chatham Road, Columbus, OH 43214, (614) 459-9657, BS 85 Bowling Green St Univ; MS 86 Bowling Green St Univ; **SLP**

Johnson, Mrs Michele A Box 295, Palmer Gulch Lodge, Hill City, SD 57745, (605) 574-2525, BA 75 Univ of SD - Vermillion; MA 77 Univ of SD - Vermillion; Sp-Lang Path, Hill Cty Pub Sch, **SLP**

Johnson, Mrs Michele B 3409 Woodbranch Road, Columbia, SC 29206, (803) 787-2657, BA 71 Coll of Wooster; MA 73 MI St Univ; Sp-Lang Path, Richland Co Sch Dist Two, **SLP**

Johnson, Mrs Michele F 721 Crystal Street, Mundelein, IL 60060, (312) 566-9180, BS 73 Northern IL Univ - De Kalb; MA 74 Northern IL Univ - De Kalb; 79–Sp-Lang Path, Spec Ed Dist of Lake Co, **SLP**

Johnson, Mrs Michelle McDonald 38944 162nd Street East, Palmdale, CA 93550, (805) 264-4634, BA 82 CA St Univ - Fullerton; MA 85 CA St Univ - Fullerton; Sp-Lang Path, **SLP**

Johnson, Mindy O 2330 West State Street, Janesville, WI 53546, (608) 882-4606, BA 84 Univ of WI - Eau Claire; MS 85 Univ of WI - Stevens Point; 88–Sp-Lang Path, Evansville Comm Sch Dist, **SLP**

Johnson, Mrs Mony Coey 695 Lincoln Avenue, Fennimore, WI 53809, (608) 822-6398, BS 82 Univ of WI - River Falls; OM 87 Univ of WI - River Falls

Johnson, Nancy Ellen 9300 Collegeview Road, Apartment #229, Bloomington, MN 55437, (612) 831-6634, BA 83 Univ of MN - Duluth; MA 84 Univ of MN - Duluth; 87–Sp-Lang Path, Eden Prairie ISD #272, **SLP**

Johnson, Mrs Nancy J 2051 Country Club Drive, Tallahassee, FL 32301, (904) 656-9683, BA 50 Univ of WI - Madison; MA 63 OH Univ - Athens; 69–Sp-Lang Path, Leon Co Sch, **SLP**

Johnson, Mrs Nancy Jean 3233 Sheridan Avenue North, Minneapolis, MN 55412, (612) 293-7693, BA Univ of MN - Minneap-St Paul; MA Univ of WI - River Falls; **SLP**

Johnson, Mrs Nancy S 1421 Coraopolis Heights Rd, Coraopolis, PA 15108, (412) 281-7244, BS 60 Carlow Coll; MA 63 Univ of CT; Sp-Lang Path, Er Sl So Allegheng Co, **SLP**

Johnson, Nancy Y 158 Herkimer Street, Hamilton, ON, Canada L8P 2H4, (416) 521-2100, MA 86 MI St Univ; **SLP**

Johnson, Neal Blanchard 6109 Ramsgate Road, Bethesda, MD 20816, (301) 229-5858

Johnson, Mrs Norma O 5802 Fern Avenue, Shreveport, LA 71105, (318) 865-2540, BA 71 Northwestern St Univ; MA 72 Northwestern St Univ; Sp-Lang Path, Caddo Parish Schs, **SLP**

Johnson, Mrs Pamela A 2814 Highway 61 South, Red Wing, MN 55066, (612) 388-2843, BS 81 Univ of WI - River Falls; MS 83 Univ of WI - River Falls; Sp-Lang Path, Red Wing Health Center, **SLP**

Johnson, Pamela C 3196-B Ginger Drive, Tallahassee, FL 32308, (904) 878-6539, BS 73 FL St Univ; MS 74 FL St Univ; Res Serv Dir, Sunland Cen Gainesville, **SLP**

Johnson, Pamela L 316 Lakeview Drive, Collingswood, NJ 08108, (215) 587-3000, BA 85 Rutger's St Univ - Douglas Coll; OM 87 Hahnemann Univ Grad Sch; Sp-Lang Path, Magee Rehab Hosp, **SLP**

Johnson, Pamela Lynn 4527 West Austin, Fresno, CA 93722, (209) 275-3043, BA 79 CA St Univ - Fresno; MS 85 CA St Univ - Fresno; 85–Sp-Lang Path, Madera County Supt of Schools, **SLP**

Johnson, Mrs Patricia A 2108 Commodore Court, Virginia Beach, VA 23454, (804) 496-0420, BS 77 James Madison Univ; ME 78 Univ of VA - Charlottesville; Sp-Lang Path, VA Beach Pub Sch, **SLP**

Johnson, Patricia Gasiciel 220 Sherman Avenue, Grand Haven, MI 49417, (616) 777-2667, BA 72 Eastern MI Univ; MA 73 Eastern MI Univ; 73–Sp-Lang Path, Muskegon Public Schools, **SLP**

Johnson, Mrs Patricia Rhyne 190 Forest Ridge Drive, Hickory, NC 28602, (704) 464-4766, BA 76 Elizabeth City St Univ; MA 78 SC St Coll; 81–Sp-Lang Path, Catawba Co Bd of Educ

Johnson, Mrs Paula Tenpas 1133 North 16th Street, Manitowoc, WI 54220-2606, (414) 684-2442, BA 76 Univ of WI - Eau Claire; MS 77 Univ of WI - River Falls; Sp-Lang Path, Holy Family Medical Center, **SLP**

Johnson, Pearl E 6733 Hyacinth Circle, Carlsbad, CA 92008, (619) 438-3707, BA 69 CA St Univ - Los Angeles; MA 72 CA St Univ - Los Angeles; **SLP**

Johnson, Dr Peter Roy 116 Maple Avenue, Wheeling, WV 26003, (304) 242-7395, BS 64 Northern IL Univ - De Kalb; MA 66 Univ of Pittsburgh - Pittsburgh; PH 71 (NS) Univ of Pittsburgh - Pittsburgh; Program Director, New Medico Meadowlands H C C, **SLP**

Johnson, R C P O Box 7353, New Orleans, LA 70186, (504) 482-4515, **SLP**

Johnson, Randall Kent 225 Iris Street, Mahtomedi, MN 55115, (612) 482-9093, BA 72 Valparaiso Univ; MA 75 Univ of MN - Minneap-St Paul; SLP, Reuben Lindh Lrng Ctr, **SLP**

Johnson, Randolph Scott 7029 Knighthood Lane, Columbia, MD 21045, (301) 455-0892, BS 57 Northern IL Univ - De Kalb; MS 61 Northern IL Univ - De Kalb; 74–Sp-Lang Path, Bd of Educ Baltimore Co, **SLP**

Johnson, Raymonde Crennel Box 154 Elon Road, Madison Heights, VA 24572, (804) 528-6254, BS 79 James Madison Univ; MA 84 Hampton Univ; SLP, Ctrl VA Trng Cen, **SLP**

Johnson, Rebecca C 10808 Whitaker Woods Drive, Richmond, VA 23233, (804) 644-1201, BS 75 East Carolina Univ; MA 76 Univ of TN - Knoxville; Dept Chrprson/Sp-Lang Path, Henrico Co Pub Sch, **SLP**

Johnson, Mrs Rebecca Lynn 3217 Meadowbrook Drive, Fort Worth, TX 76103, (817) 336-8311, BS 86 Univ of North TX; MS 86 Univ of North TX; **A**

Johnson, Mrs Rebekah Jahna P O Box 811, Lake Vales, FL 33853, (813) 676-3379, BA 78 Univ of Central FL; BS 81 FL St Univ; MS 82 FL St Univ; Sp-Lang Path, Private Practice, **SLP**

Johnson, Reid C PO Box 1114, Ocean Shores, WA 98569, (206) 289-2614, BS 86 Clarion Univ of PA; MS 87 Clarion Univ of PA; 88–Sp-Lang Path, Aberdeen Sch Dist No 5, **SLP**

Johnson, Richard M 820 North 3rd Street, Wahpeton, ND 58075, (701) 642-6687, BA 66 San Diego St Univ; MA 69 Univ of ND; SLP, Wahpeton Sch Dist, **SLP**

Johnson, Richard M 1501 Chukka Drive #108, Arlington, TX 76012-2553, (817) 265-0257, BS 78 Southwest TX St Univ; ME 79 Southwest TX St Univ; Cl Supvr, InSpeech Inc, **SLP**

Johnson, Richard W 3105 Meadow Lane, West Des Moines, IA 50265, (515) 270-9030, BA 71 Univ of IA; MA 79 Northeast MO St Univ; Sp-Lang Path, Heartland AEA #11, **SLP**

Johnson, Robert James 909 South 700 East, Marion, IN 46953, (317) 674-3321, BA 80 Geneva Coll; MS 82 Purdue Univ - West Lafayette; Aud, VA, **A**

Johnson, Dr Robert M 18400 S W Indian Creek Dr, Lake Oswego, OR 97034, (503) 225-8032, BS 61 ND St Univ; MA 63 Northwestern Univ; PH 68 (NS) Northwestern Univ; Aud, Kresge Hearing Research Lab, **A F**

Johnson, Robin Christine 6908 Irving Avenue South, Richfield, MN 55423, (612) 888-9284, BS 78 Mankato St Univ; MS 83 Mankato St Univ; 87–Sp-Lang Path, Bloomington Schs, **SLP**

Johnson, Roma Lee Fort Dodge Speech & Hearing Ct, 720 North 15th Street, Fort Dodge, IA 50501, (515) 573-4701, BA 64 Univ of IA; MA 66 Univ of IA; Owner/Aud, Ft Dodge Hrng & Sp Cen, **A**

Johnson, Ronald D 117 24th Avenue North, Fargo, ND 58102, (701) 280-3417, BS 70 ND St Univ; MA 71 Ball St Univ; Aud, Dakota Clinic, **A**

Johnson, Rose Mary Davis Southwest 245 Wyant Lane, Hamilton, MT 59840, (406) 363-1164, BA 78 Univ of MT; MS 80 WV Univ; Sp/Lang Path, Corvallis Sch Dist, **SLP**

Johnson, Roxanna M PO Box 1579, Solana Beach, CA 92075, (619) 481-2489, BA 73 San Diego St Univ; MA 76 San Diego St Univ; Pres, Mayer - Johnson Co, **SLP**

Johnson, Mrs Ruby Stradford P O Box 782, 700 Hamar Street, Beaufort, SC 29901-0782, (803) 524-6208, BA 75 SC St Coll; MA 87 SC St Coll; 75–Sp-Lang Path, Beaufort Co Schs

Johnson, Sally Grace 4605 S 184 Plaza, Omaha, NE 68135, (402) 895-8052, BS 75 Northwest MO St Univ; MS 85 Univ of NE - Omaha; Sp-Lang Path, Omaha Public Schools, **SLP**

Johnson, Sandra 5164 Mississippi Bar Drive, Orangevale, CA 95662, (916) 989-6924, BA 76 CA St Univ - Chico; MA 80 CA St Univ - Sacramento; Sp-Lang Path, Easter Seal Rehab Cen, **SLP**

Johnson, Sandra Stringham 409 West 3300 South, Bountiful, UT 84010, BS 79 Brigham Young Univ; OM 80 Brigham Young Univ; 84–Sp-Lang Path, State Dept of Health, **SLP**

Johnson, Mrs Sara Ann 603 North Broad Street, Suffolk, VA 23434, (804) 934-0416, **SLP**

Johnson, Sara Jane Communication Sci & Disorders, University Of Montana, Missoula, MT 59812, (406) 243-4131, BA 78 Univ of MT; MA 81 Northwestern Univ; Lecturer & Audiologist, University of Montana, **A ACE**

Johnson, Mrs Sara M General Delivery, Pound Ridge, NY 10576-9999, (203) 853-1225, BS 70 Ithaca Coll; MS 72 Columbia Univ Teachers Coll; Sp-Lang Path, Sara R Johnson, **SLP**

Johnson, Sarah Jo 3317 East 13th Terrace, Kansas City, MO 64137, (314) 882-1571, OB 84 Univ of MO - Columbia; OM 85 Univ of MO - Columbia; **A**

Johnson, Sharon Ann 266-B Kathann Drive, Hampton, VA 23605, (804) 825-0926, BS 83 Univ Southern MS-Hattiesburg; MS 85 Univ Southern MS-Hattiesburg; **SLP**

Johnson, Mrs Sharon J 4520 Quail Hollow Court, Fort Worth, TX 76133, (713) 373-3180, BS 74 TX Christian Univ; MS 75 TX Christian Univ; Sp-Lang Path, Ft Worth ISD, **SLP**

Johnson, Sharon K 25 Frontenac, Godfrey, IL 62035, (618) 463-5670, BA 66 Southern IL Univ -Carbondale; MS 80 Southern IL Univ-Edwardsvill; Practical Communication, Private Practice, **SLP**

Johnson, Mrs Sheryl L 26 Spruce Street, Jamestown, NY 14701, (716) 484-7351, BS 75 SUNY - Coll at Fredonia; MS 77 SUNY - Coll at Fredonia; Sp-Lang Path, SUNY Coll at Fredonia, **SLP**

Johnson, Sheryl R 3643 West Grace, Floor 2, Chicago, IL 60618, (312) 478-4291, BS 78 Southern IL Univ -Carbondale; MA 81 Northern IL Univ - De Kalb; Sp-Lang Path, United Homecare Ltd, **SLP ACE**

Johnson, Sue Burns 2125 Glenhollow, Westlake Village, CA 91361, (805) 495-1689, BA 66 Univ of HI - Manoa; MA 67 MI St Univ; Sp-Lang Path, InSpeech Inc, **SLP ACE**

Johnson, Mrs Susan H 287 Dushane Drive, Buffalo, NY 14223, (716) 837-2115, BS 80 SUNY - Coll at Buffalo; MA 82 Hofstra Univ; 88–Sp/Lang Path, Mary R Harris Sp/Lang Clinic, **SLP**

Johnson, Mrs Susan Hilburn 721 Ridgewood Road, Duluth, MN 55804, (218) 724-3671, MS 87 Univ of NE - Omaha; 88–Sp-Lang Path, Duluth PS

Johnson, Susan Hurt 1418 Hickory Drive, West Point, MS 39773, (601) 494-1000, BA 80 Univ of MS; OM 82 Univ of MS; Sp-Lang Path, West Point Mun Sep School Dist, **SLP**

Johnson, Susan K Box 263, Glenwood, IA 51534, (712) 527-4811, BS 75 Univ of NE - Omaha; MS 76 Univ of NE - Omaha; Sp-Lang Path, Glenwood St Hosp Sch, **SLP**

Johnson, Mrs Susan King Arkansas Rehabilitation Ins, 9601 Interstate 630 Ext 7, Little Rock, AR 72205-7249, (501) 223-7558, BS 80 Univ of Central AR; MA 82 Memphis St Univ; Sp-Lang Path, AR Rehab I, **SLP**

Johnson, Susan L 2232 Argonne, Long Beach, CA 90815, (213) 597-3531, **SLP**

Johnson, Mrs Susan L W 4608 South Harrington Avenue, Sioux Falls, SD 57103, (605) 528-3215, BA 77 Univ of SD - Vermillion; MA 78 Univ of SD - Vermillion; Sp-Lang Path, West Central Sch Dist, **SLP**

Johnson, Mrs Susan N 935 Deena Drive, Columbus, MS 39702, (601) 328-2598, BS 82 MS Univ for Women; MS 87 Univ of AL- Tuscaloosa; 88–Sp-Lang Path, Columbus Municipal Sch

Johnson, Mrs Susan Payne Route 9 Box 382-H, Winston-Salem, NC 27107, (919) 472-7965, BS 80 Appalachian St Univ; MA 82 Appalachian St Univ; SLP, Davdson Co Schs, **SLP**

Johnson, Susan Straute 954 East Congress Park Dr, Dayton, OH 45459, (513) 223-6192, MA 87 Miami Univ - Oxford; **SLP**

Johnson, Mrs Suzanne 3413-A 134th Place S W, Lynnwood, WA 98037, (206) 745-8369, BS 75 Edinboro Univ of PA; MS 84 TX Christian Univ; **SLP**

Johnson, Dr T Earle 1 Bellview Drive, Tuscaloosa, AL 35405, (205) 752-9898, BA 26 LA St Univ - Baton Rouge; MA 31 Univ of WI - Madison; PH 45 (NS) Univ of WI - Madison; **A F LM**

Johnson, Terri K P O Box 506, Natalbany, LA 70451, (504) 549-2214, BA 78 Southeastern LA Univ; ME 83 Southeastern LA Univ; Sp-Lang Path Owner, Educ Assoc of the South East I, **SLP**

Johnson, Therese Ann P O Box 1725, Tuba City, AZ 86045, (602) 283-4211, BA 77 Briar Cliff Coll; MA 84 Univ of SD - Vermillion; **SLP**

Johnson, Thomas R 8260 Bennett Drive, Stockton, CA 95212, (209) 477-4564, BA 74 San Jose St Univ; MA 75 Humboldt St Univ; MA 78 CA Lutheran Coll; Dir Ed, Lincoln Christian Academy, **SLP**

Johnson, Dr Thomas Stoddard 642 East 1900 North, Logan, UT 84321, (801) 750-1375, BS 64 UT St Univ; MS 67 UT St Univ; PH 69 (Sp Path & Aud) Univ of KS; Prof & Hd Dept Commun Dis, Utah State U, **SLP**

Johnson, Mrs Toni D 4443 Braemar Drive, Indianapolis, IN 46254, (317) 291-0809, BS 74 Ball St Univ; MA 78 Ball St Univ; Prog Consult, Ofc of Voc Rehab, **SLP**

Johnson, Valerie J 537 Lowell Street, Lexington, MA 02173, (617) 862-4205, BS 79 Northeastern Univ; ME 81 Northeastern Univ; 81–Sp-Lang Path, Private Practice, **SLP**

Johnson, Vicki Lynette 3312 Fairfax Street, Eau Claire, WI 54701, (608) 372-5828, BA 84 Univ of WI - Eau Claire; MS 85 Univ of WI - Eau Claire; Sp-Lang Path, Tomah Rehab Cntr, **SLP**

Johnson, Victor Ross 650 North Ross Street #C-6, Auburn, AL 36830, (205) 826-5545, BS 79 Auburn Univ - Auburn; OM 83 Auburn Univ - Auburn; Adjunct Inst, Auburn U Sp & Hrng Cl, **A**

Johnson, Virginia Ann 314 Buena Vista, Altus, OK 73521, (405) 482-2209, BS 85 ND St Univ; MS 87 Moorhead St Univ; **SLP**

Johnson, Mrs Virginia C P O Box 628, Columbus, TX 78934-0628, (409) 732-6956, BA 70 Univ of Houston - Univ Park; MA 71 Univ of Houston - Univ Park; Sp-Lang Path, Colorado Co Educ Co-op, **SLP**

Johnson, Dr Warren Edward HCR-63 Box 656-B, Newport, OR 97365, (503) 265-2360, BA 49 Wabash Coll; MA 50 Northwestern Univ; PH 70 (Aud) Univ of OR; 87–Dir, Lincoln County Food Share, **A F**

Johnson, William B 2116 North 51st Street, Milwaukee, WI 53208, (414) 449-2422, BS 69 IL St Univ - Normal; MS 75 Univ of IL - Urbana; Sp-Lang Path, Milwaukee Pub Schs, **SLP**

Johnson, William M Henry H North School, 333 East Miller Road, Lansing, MI 48910, (517) 887-3238, BA 73 MI St Univ; MA 75 MI St Univ; Aud, Lansing School District, **A**

Johnson, William Paul 56 Conant Street, Acton, MA 01720, (617) 343-5005, BS 82 Univ of MA - Amherst; MA 85 Univ of CT; 85–Supvr, Burbank Hosp, **SLP**

Johnsonbaugh, Mrs Susan H 804 Chicago Avenue, Portland, IN 47371, (217) 726-7731, BS 74 Ball St Univ; MA 77 Ball St Univ; SLP, Jay Randolph Dev Serv, **SLP**

Johnson-Casteel, Linda L 1345 South 4th East, Salt Lake City, UT 84115, (801) 485-4086, BS 76 Univ of WY; MS 79 Univ of WY; Sp-Lang Path, Developmental Disabilities Inc, **SLP**

Johnson-Elmore, Fannie Mason 715 57th Street Southeast, Charleston, WV 25304, (304) 925-4391

Johnson-Glaser, Mary Ann 8259 Windsail Court, Maineville, OH 45039, (513) 529-2504, BS 69 Miami Univ - Oxford; MS 70 Univ of WI - Milwaukee; Asst Prof, Miami Univ, **SLP**

Johnson-Janes, Janet 4306 Hummingbird, Houston, TX 77035, (713) 728-9187, BA 74 Univ of Houston - Univ Park; MA 76 Univ of Houston - Univ Park; Sp-Lang Path, Private Practice, **SLP**

Johnson-Lawrence, Paula Faith 2120 31st Street S E, Washington, DC 20020, (301) 870-3814, **A**

Johnson-Liscio, Christine 15 Fox Hill Road, Nahant, MA 01908-1109, (617) 581-2400, BA 78 SUNY - Coll at Cortland; MS 80 Syracuse Univ; Clin Dir of Sp-Lang Path, Lenox Hill, **SLP**

Johnson-Olsonk, Jeanne 614 N W 3rd Street, Wadena, MN 56482, (218) 631-3530, BA 66 Moorhead St Univ; MA 70 Northern MI Univ; Sp-Lang Path/Coord, Wadena Pub Sch, **SLP**

Johnson-Powell, Valerie K Rt 5 Box 186, Lawrence, KS 66046-9865, (913) 841-8463, OB 80 Northeast MO St Univ; MA 81 Northeast MO St Univ; Sp/Lang Path, USD 497, **SLP**

Johnson-Russell, Vickie 259 East Harney Road, Esko, MN 55733, (218) 728-5722, BA 75 Univ of MN - Duluth; MA 76 Western MI Univ; Clinical Instructor, U of MN Duluth 85, **SLP**

Johnson-Sollenne, Jeanene 3741 Jardin, Houston, TX 77005, (409) 938-5405, BS 76 Carlow Coll; MA 78 OH St Univ; Dir Sp-Lang Path/Aud, Mainland Ctr Hosp, **SLP**

Johnson-Thomas, Patricia Speech & Language Pathologist, 15315 Dawn Meadows Drive, Houston, TX 77068-2034, (713) 772-8532, **SLP**

Johnson-Weatherall, Mrs Ruth 11618 Spriggs Way, Houston, TX 77024, (713) 464-7870, BA 61 Wichita St Univ; MA 78 Univ of Houston - Univ Park; Sp-Lang Path, Private Practice, **SLP**

Johnson-Welch, Mrs Judith S 525 Arlington Drive, Metairie, LA 70005-5515, (504) 834-0313, BS 74 LA St Univ - Baton Rouge; MA 76 LA St Univ - Baton Rouge; **SLP**

Johnston, Sr Anna Mae 3175 Lexington Road, Louisville, KY 40206

Johnston, Mrs Annette Plourde 621 Westwood Drive #2-S, Clayton, MO 63105, (314) 727-6295, BS 83 Univ of UT; MS 86 Univ of UT; 88–Aud, Washington Univ Sch of Med, **A**

Johnston, Mrs Arlene M 323 Green Meadows Circle, Columbia, MO 65203, (314) 882-8409, BA 61 Univ of MI - Ann Arbor; MS 64 Univ of MI - Ann Arbor; 77–Cl Instr, U of MO-Col Sp & Hrng Cl, **SLP**

Johnston, Charles E 439 Washington Avenue, Glencoe, IL 60022, (312) 948-4750, BA 70 IN Central Univ; OM 73 Butler Univ

Johnston, Cheryl Ann 53 Losse Way, Chico, CA 95926, (408) 484-1172, MA 83 CA St Univ - Chico; **SLP**

Johnston, Mrs Clarion E 4450 Lamar Court, Richmond Heights, OH 44143, (216) 261-2900, BS 51 OH Univ - Athens; MA 73 Cleveland St Univ; Sp-Lang Path, Euclid Bd of Ed, **SLP**

Johnston, Mrs Diane T G 19 Linden Drive, Cohasset, MA 02025, (617) 383-0291, ME 75 Northeastern Univ; President, Private Practice, **SLP**

Johnston, Donna Lynn 3943 Kerri Circle, Montgomery, AL 36109, (205) 270-8736, Montgomery Rehab Hosp, **SLP ACE**

Johnston, Elizabeth Rd 2 Box 355, Pottstown, PA 19464, (215) 469-6654, BS 50 Temple Univ; ME 53 Temple Univ; **SLP LM**

Johnston, Dr Elizabeth 6424 Contrearas Road, Oxford, OH 45056, (513) 529-2326, BA 52 MT St Univ; MS 58 Univ of OR; ME 78 Univ of Cincinnati; Asst Prof, Miami Univ of Oh, **SLP**

Johnston, Mrs Elizabeth 1080 Braeburn Drive, Baton Rouge, LA 70815-5302, (504) 388-2995, BA 70 Univ of Southwestern LA; MS 78 Univ of Southwestern LA; 88–Instr, LSU, **SLP**

Johnston, Eloise R Eloise R Johnston & Associates, Alvarado Medical Center, 6505 Alvarado Rd Suite 107, San Diego, CA 92120, (619) 583-0777, BA 50; MA 68; Private Practice, **SLP**

Johnston, Dr Frances J ASHA, 10801 Rockville Pike, Rockville, MD 20852, (301) 897-5700, BA 61 Coll of Wooster; MA 65 Univ of IA; PH 73 (Sp Path & Aud) Univ of IA; Dir Con & Meetings Div, ASHA, **SLP**

Johnston, Gennie S 1966 Brookside Drive, Wooster, OH 44691, (216) 264-3673, BS 71 Kent St Univ; MA 74 Northwestern Univ; Assoc Dir Sp/Hrng Cl, Coll of Wooster, **SLP**

Johnston, Gerry P 1290 Lincoln Road, Suite 3, Yuba City, CA 95991, (916) 673-6039, BA 77 CA St Univ - Sacramento; MA 79 CA St Univ - Sacramento; 87–Sp-Lang Path, Sacramento Scottish Rite, **SLP**

Johnston, Jennifer 22 Weitz Street, Allston, MA 02134, BA 78 Univ of Northern CO; MS 84 Emerson Coll; 85–Sp-Lang Path, Children's Hosp, **SLP**

Johnston, Joann Carol 1710 Frisch Road, Madison, WI 53711, (608) 424-3371, BS 81 Univ of WI - Madison; MS 83 Univ of WI - Whitewater; Sp-Lang Path, Belleville Sch Dist, **SLP**

Johnston, Dr Judith Rae School Of Audiology & Speech Sciences, University Of British Columbia, Vancouver, BC, Canada V6T 1W5, (604) 228-5591, BA 64 Stanford Univ; MA 66 Stanford Univ; PH 79 (Psychology) Univ of CA - Berkeley; Prof/Dir, Univ of British Columbia, **SLP F**

Johnston, Judy Franke 2140 Dead Hollow Rd South, Harpersville, AL 35078, (205) 672-7588, BA 72 Univ of AL- Tuscaloosa; MA 73 Univ of AL- Tuscaloosa; MS 85 Univ of Montevallo; 73–Sp-Lang Path, AL Inst for Deaf & Blind, **SLP**

Johnston, Kathleen A 501 West High Street, Bellefonte, PA 16823, (814) 359-3421, BS 68 Edinboro Univ of PA; MS 71 PA St Univ - Univ Park; Dir of Sp-Lang Path, Nittany Valley Rehab Hosp, **SLP**

Johnston, Kathleen Kennelly 26 Orchard Street, Delmar, NY 12054, (518) 272-0767, BA 80 SUNY - Coll at Plattsburgh; MS 82 Ithaca Coll; Sp-Lang Path, Beginnings: Prog for Yng Chldn, **SLP**

Johnston, Kathleen L 550 North Snelling Avenue, Apartment 606, St Paul, MN 55104, (612) 221-3700, BS 60 Saint Olaf Coll; 81–Rsearch Coordinator, St Paul Ramsey Medical Center

Johnston, Laura Assante 18346 Collins Street #3, Tarzana, CA 91356, (213) 483-4431, BA 86 CA St Univ - Northridge; MA 87 CA St Univ - Northridge

Johnston, Linda S 451 North Jackson, St Louis, MO 63130, **SLP**

Johnston, Maureen M Speech Pathology Services, 24050 Madison Street, Suite 111, Torrance, CA 90505, (213) 378-0036, BA 70 CA St Univ - Long Beach; MA 73 CA St Univ - Long Beach; Owner/Sp-Lang Path, Sp-Lang Serv, **SLP**

Johnston, Michael Mary/Tiema 1147 Calle Cordoniz, Los Osos, CA 93402, (408) 779-5278, BA 76 San Jose St Univ; MA 82 San Jose St Univ; SLP, Morgan Hill USD, **SLP**

Johnston, Mrs Nancy N 519 Millwood Drive, Fallston, MD 21047, (301) 676-2400, BS 71 Towson St Univ; MA 72 Univ of MD - College Park; Sp-Lang Path, Harford Ct Bd of Ed, **SLP**

Johnston, Patricia A 38 St Georges Crescent, Edmonton, AB, Canada T5N 3M7, BS 72 Univ of Alberta - Alberta; OM 76 Univ of Western Ontario; Research Consult, **SLP**

Johnston, Dr Robert G 647 Fisher Road, Grosse Pointe, MI 48230, (313) 577-3337, BA 66 Adams St Coll; MA 67 Adams St Coll; PH 70 (NS) Univ of IL - Urbana; Head Commun Dis & Sciences, Wayne St U, **SLP**

Johnston, Mrs Robin Lee Drawer D, Mount Olive, MS 39119, (601) 797-4267, BS 81 MS Coll; MS 83 Univ of SC - Columbia; Sp-Lang Path, Private Practice, **SLP**

Johnston, Sally L P O Box 1459, Breckenridge, CO 80424, **SLP**

Johnston, Mrs Susan Yates 26 Morton Street, Andover, MA 01810, (617) 475-3806, BA 60 Middlebury Coll; MS 81 Southern CT St Univ; Sp-Lang Path, Prof Ctr for Hndcpd Chldrn, **SLP**

Johnston, Suzanne Flockhart 969 Garson Avenue, Rochester, NY 14609, (716) 288-7155, BS 81 SUNY - Coll at Geneseo; MA 83 SUNY - Coll at Buffalo; 88–Sp-Lang Path, Univ of Rochester-Strong Memorial Hosp, **SLP**

Johnston, Mrs Tracy R 496 Sweat Street, Walterboro, SC 29488, (803) 549-2712, BA 68 Univ of SC - Columbia; ME 71 Univ of SC - Columbia; 88–Sp-Lang Path, Colleton County Sch Sys, **SLP**

Johnston, Valerie Leigh Overton Speech & Language Center, 4763 Barwick Drive Suite 103, Fort Worth, TX 76132, (817) 294-8408, BS 75 TX Christian Univ; MS 78 TX Christian Univ; 82–Owner/Dir, Overton Sp & Lang Cen Inc, **SLP ACE**

Johnston, Virginia J 390 North Winchester Blvd, Apt 5-3G, Santa Clara, CA 95050, (707) 248-2386, **SLP**

Johnstone, Mrs Carol M 3009 Finley Place, Charlotte, NC 28210, (704) 552-5091, BS 76 Boston Univ; MA 78 Univ of Pittsburgh - Pittsburgh; 88–Sp-Lang Path, Mercy Home Care, **SLP**

Johnstone, Diane B 1317 Hillsdale Drive, Richardson, TX 75081, (214) 234-8111, BS 80 Kent St Univ; MA 81 Kent St Univ; Sp-Lang Path, Cntr for Neuro Skills, **SLP**

Johnstone, Patti Michele 2025 Fixlini, San Luis Obispo, CA 93401, (805) 543-0277, **SLP**

Johnstone, Mrs Rhetta 1096 Bath Lane, Ventura, CA 93001, (805) 487-3918, BA 80 Univ of Southwestern LA; MA 83 Whittier Coll; 86–Sp-Lang Path, Oxnard Elem Sch Dist, **SLP**

Johnston-Rowland, Mary F P O Box 775044, Steamboat Springs, CO 80477, (303) 824-6042, BA 74 Humboldt St Univ; MA 75 Humboldt St Univ; 87–Sp-Lang Path, Moffat County Sch Dist RE 1, **SLP**

Jojo, Susanne Marie Fenimore Trace Apts, Apt 4E, Watervliet, NY 12189-1631, (518) 273-6307, BS 83 Coll of Saint Rose; MS 84 Coll of Saint Rose; **SLP**

Jolie, Kim R 267 River Road, Andover, MA 01810, (603) 226-2900, BS 78 Univ of NH; MA 79 Univ of FL; Coord, Educ Dev Assoc Inc, **SLP**

Jolitz, Julie Lynne 177 East Washington, West Bend, WI 53095, (414) 423-7046, BS 85 Univ of WI - Milwaukee; MS 87 Marquette Univ

Jolley, Elaine Braithwait 1454 W Meadows Connection, Park City, UT 84060, (801) 649-9211, BS 78 Brigham Young Univ; MS 83 Univ of UT; **A**

Jolley, Ray Garth 1536 West Kerry Lane, Phoenix, AZ 85027-5419, (602) 582-4772, BS 81 Brigham Young Univ; MA 86 Brigham Young Univ; Audiologist, Metro Hrng Aid and Audiology, **A**

Jolls, Gwen Marie 6609 Canyon Cove Way, Las Vegas, NV 89108, (702) 731-8644, BS 80 Northern AZ Univ; MS 82 Univ of WA; 84–Chief Sp-Lang Path, Humana Hospital Sunrise, **SLP**

Jolly, Mrs Faith 256 East Green Street, Claremont, CA 91711, (714) 625-6257, BA 39 San Diego St Univ; MA 61 Univ of HI - Manoa; SLP, Private Practice, **SLP A LM**

Jolly, Peggy R P O Box 2986, Tupelo, MS 38803, (601) 842-1891, BS 76 Northwest MO St Univ; MA 82 Univ of MS; 85–Dir/Aud, Regional Rehabilitation Center Inc, **A**

Jolly, Mrs Sharon C P O Box 387, Central Valley, NY 10917, (914) 928-2579, BA 65 3104; MA 66 OH St Univ; Aud/Sp-Lang Path, Private Practice, **SLP A**

Jolly, Sharon T G 3790 N Dumbarton Street, Arlington, VA 22207, (703) 241-7057, BS 71 East Carolina Univ; MA 72 Saint Louis Univ; **SLP**

Jonakin, Mrs Karen Benfield 510 Carolina Avenue, Signal Mountain, TN 37377, (615) 624-1533, BA 80 Univ of NC - Chapel Hill; MA 83 Univ of TN - Knoxville; 87–Sp-Lang Path, Professional Health Services, **SLP**

Jonas, Mrs Carol F 3731 Lancelot Pl, Garland, TX 75043, (214) 494-8581, BA 75 Winthrop Coll; MA 77 Univ of SC - Columbia; MA 81 Univ of SC - Columbia; 87–Aud, Garland ISD, **A**

Jonas, Mrs Jane M 450 North Pine Crest, Milwaukee, WI 53208, (414) 527-0325, BA 75 Univ of WI - Eau Claire; MS 78 Marquette Univ; SLP, Milwaukee Public Schools, **SLP**

Jonas, Jill G 10627 Van Alden, Northridge, CA 91326, (213) 625-4185, BA 64 CA St Univ - Northridge; BA 69 CA St Univ - Northridge; Sp-Lang Path, LA USD, **SLP**

Jonas, Linda F 107 Randall Avenue, Port Jefferson, NY 11777, (516) 473-3010, BA 63 Adelphi Univ; MA 66 NY Univ; Sp-Lang Path, BOCES, **SLP**

Jonas, Dr Renai K 206 N W 41st Avenue, Deerfield Beach, FL 33442, (305) 421-0814, BA 74 CUNY - Hunter Coll; MS 75 CUNY - Brooklyn Coll; ED 85 (NS) Nova Univ; Sp-Lang Path, Private Practice, **SLP**

Jonatzke, Mary Elizabeth 2620 Thayer Drive, St Joseph, MI 49085, (616) 983-7420, BS 78 Western MI Univ; MA 85 Western MI Univ

Jonay, Adrienne 75-03 196th Street, Flushing, NY 11366, (212) 631-6284, BA 63 Adelphi Univ; MS 68 Adelphi Univ; Adj Lect, Queensborough Commun Coll, **SLP**

Joncas, Nancy Martin 162 Sea Road, Kennebunk, ME 04043, (207) 967-2121, BA 80 Univ of ME - Orono; MA 82 Univ of ME - Orono; Sp/Lang Path, Maine Sch Admin Dist #71, **SLP**

Jones, Alice Ott P O Box 114, Louisville, KS 66450, (913) 296-5391, BA 68 CA St Univ - Los Angeles; MA 72 CA St Univ - Los Angeles; 86–Sp-Lang Path, Kansas Neurological Institute

Jones, Mrs Alix N 32 Mount Well Avenue, Haddonfield, NJ 08033, (609) 667-1350, BA 67 Univ of AL- Tuscaloosa; ME 68 PA St Univ - Univ Park; Sp-Lang Path, Cherry Hill Pub Sch, **SLP**

Jones, Alyce W P O Box 172, Rescue, CA 95672, BA; **SLP**

Jones, Mrs Amy J 7645 North 4th Avenue, Phoenix, AZ 85021, (602) 222-6412, BA 75 IN Univ - Bloomington; MA 76 IN Univ - Bloomington; Audiologist, Veterans Administration Hosp, **A**

Jones, Andrea Andrews Route 3 Box 220E, Benson, NC 27504, (919) 934-7579, BA 84 NC St Univ at Raleigh; MS 86 East Carolina Univ; 87–Aud, N Daniel Catz MD, **A**

Jones, Mrs Ann C 908 Devere Drive, Silver Spring, MD 20903, (301) 439-2072, BS 75 Goucher Coll; BS 77 Towson St Univ; MS 78 Towson St Univ; **SLP**

Jones, Ann Katherine 4637 North Edgebrooke Pl, Tucson, AZ 85705, (602) 292-0444, BS 83 CO St Univ; MS 85 CO St Univ; **SLP**

Jones, Anna L 1018 Pearl River Avenue, McComb, MS 39648, **SLP**

Jones, Anna M 756 18th Court, Vero Beach, FL 32962, (407) 778-4116, MA 87 IN Univ - Bloomington; SLP

Jones, Mrs Anne Evans 45 Hopper Hills Way, Mendon, NY 14506, (716) 582-2115, BA 78 MI St Univ; MS 79 PA St Univ - Univ Park; 87–Sp-Lang Path, Neuro Rehab Associates Inc, **SLP**

Jones, Mrs Anne G 350 Thunderbird Street #25, El Paso, TX 79912, (915) 859-9113, BA 58 Univ of AL-Tuscaloosa; MA 67 Univ of AL- Tuscaloosa; Resource Tchr Lrng Disabled, Ysleta ISD, **SLP**

Jones, Anne M 5155 N E 3rd Street, Ocala, FL 32670, (904) 694-7966, **SLP**

Jones, Mrs Anne Marie 14407 US 24 RR #1, Sherwood, OH 43556, (419) 592-6451, BS 82; MA 84; 88–Sp-Lang Path, Filling Memorial Home of Mercy, **SLP**

Jones, Mrs Barbara Plunkert 881 Alameda, Abilene, TX 79605, (915) 698-2295, BS 79 TX Christian Univ; MS 80 TX Christian Univ; Associate SLP, Associates Speech & Language, **SLP**

Jones, Dr Barry W Dept Communicative Disorders, San Diego State University, 5300 Campanile Drive, San Diego, CA 92182, (619) 594-6774, BS 68 Eastern NM Univ; MS 74 Canisius Coll; PH 77 (Linguistics) Univ of IL - Urbana; 88–Actg Charmn-Dept of Comm Dis, San Diego State University

Jones, Bettie Maxine 12338 S E Foster Road, Portland, OR 97236, (503) 760-7755, BS 50 Drexel Univ; ME 67 Univ of OR

Jones, Dr Betty M E 134 Kilbuck Drive, Monroeville, PA 15146, (412) 856-2680, BS 67 Clarion Univ of PA; MA 68 Wayne St Univ; PH 83 (Commun Dis & Sciences) Wayne St Univ; 87–Dir Sp-Lang Path, Greater Pittsburgh Rehab Hosp, **SLP**

Jones, Mrs Betty Reingold 2243 Goldsmith, Houston, TX 77030, (713) 664-6546, BS 76 Univ of CA - Santa Barbara; MS 78 Columbia Univ Teachers Coll; Sp-Lang Path, Private Practice, **SLP**

Jones, Beverly 3610 Flintpoint Way, Cincinnati, OH 45227-4307, (513) 793-9949, BA 58 Huron Coll; MA 60 Northwestern Univ; Owner-Director, Read Write & Talk, **SLP**

Jones, Beverly Katrina 528 Galloway Road, Brundidge, AL 36010, (205) 774-2355, BS 81 AL A & M Univ; MS 84 AL A & M Univ; **SLP**

Jones, Bobby D 4002 21st Street, Lubbock, TX 79410, (806) 792-6135, BS 67 Eastern NM Univ; MS 68 Eastern NM Univ; Dir/Owner, Sp-Lang-Hrng Cen of Lubbock, **SLP**

Jones, Bradley L 500 Zimalcrest Road #2109, Columbia, SC 29210, (803) 252-2538, **SLP**

Jones, Bronwen L 16 Morehouse Lane, Norwalk, CT 06850, (203) 866-6012, BA 67 Univ of HI - Manoa; MA 69 Univ of CA - Santa Barbara; Independent Contractor, **A**

Jones, Byron Lee Route 2, Reynolds Bridge Road, Kingston, GA 30145, (404) 382-3813, MS 82 Univ of Montevallo; Sp-Lang Path, Bartow County Schools, **SLP**

Jones, Carla A 1995 Pinto Drive, Moscow, ID 83843, (509) 335-5826, BA 74 WA St Univ; MA 75 WA St Univ; SLP, Wash St Univ CDC, **SLP**

Jones, Carmen Lynne 8509 Sunlit Lane, Orlando, FL 32810, **SLP**

Jones, Carol 610 Martin Pointe Court, Ballwin, MO 63011, BS 75 Univ of VA - Charlottesville; ME 76 Univ of VA - Charlottesville; Dir, Wilmington Aud Serv, **A**

Jones, Carol A 103 Berryman Drive, Snyder, NY 14226, (716) 837-2441, BA 74 SUNY - Center at Buffalo; MA 76 SUNY - Center at Buffalo; Sp-Lang Path, Lang Dev Prog of W NY, **SLP**

Jones, Carol Elise 209-57th Avenue South, St Petersburg, FL 33705, (813) 892-4141, BS 85 FL St Univ; MS 86 FL St Univ; 87–Sp-Lang Path, All Childrens Hosp, **SLP**

Jones, Mrs Carol Johnston 1539 Twisted Oak Drive, Reston, VA 22094, (703) 437-7346, BS 77 Edinboro Univ of PA; MS 82 Indiana Univ of PA; **SLP**

Jones, Dr Carolane 403 West Oak Street, Suite 303, El Dorado, AR 71730, (501) 863-2666, BS 70; MS 71; PH 81 (NS); Dir, Commun Dis Cen, **SLP ACE**

Jones, Mrs Caroline Selig 2151 Marion Drive, La Place, LA 70068, (504) 652-6536, **SLP**

Jones, Mrs Charlene A 500 Center Grange Road #57, Monaca, PA 15061, (216) 726-8855, BA 84 2627; 87–Aud, Youngstown Hrng & Sp Ctr, **A**

Jones, Mrs Cheri Benge 5305 Redfield Road, Dunwoody, GA 30338-3723, (404) 390-0380, MA 84 Univ of Houston - Univ Park; Sp-Lang Path Associate, Speech and Language Services, **SLP**

Jones, Cheryl Phillips-W 11901 Jefferson Avenue, #22-G, Newport News, VA 23606, (804) 623-8600, BS 77 CA Univ of PA; MS 86 CA Univ of PA; **SLP**

Jones, Christine Ann 2728 Barcelona Drive, Modesto, CA 95354-3209, (209) 578-5003, **SLP**

Jones, Cynthia D 715 1/2 12th Avenue, Huntington, WV 25701, (304) 525-9151, BA 78 Marshall Univ; MA 79 Marshall Univ; Sp-Lang Path, Cabell Co Pub Sch Syst, **SLP**

Jones, Mrs Cynthia Pinney 430 Silver Valley Blvd, Munroe Falls, OH 44262, (216) 375-3882, BA 63 Mount Union Coll; MA 65 Case Western Reserve Univ; Sp-Lang Path, Akron Cty Hosp, **SLP**

Jones, Mrs Cynthia Winham 1546 West Lewis, Phoenix, AZ 85007, (602) 279-0003, MS 84 Univ of TX - Dallas; Aud, Hearing Consultants Ltd, **A**

Jones, David Lowry 421 South Lucas Street, Iowa City, IA 52240, (319) 335-8117, BS 80 Westminster Coll; MA 83 Univ of IA; **SLP**

Jones, Deanna Suenette 8101 Brixton Road #6, Louisville, KY 40222, (502) 456-5831, BS 84 Univ Southern MS-Hattiesburg; MS 86 Univ Southern MS-Hattiesburg; Aud, Louisville Hrng Aid Ctr Inc, **A**

Jones, Debra Leigh 7313 Woodlawn N E, Seattle, WA 98115, (206) 822-9588, **SLP**

Jones, Dena M 20 Violet Street, Weymouth, MA 02188, (617) 337-9970, **SLP**

Jones, Mrs Dianne Delaney 71 Christian Avenue, Setauket, NY 11733, (516) 724-3626, BA 82 SUNY - Coll at Plattsburgh; MS 84 PA St Univ - Univ Park; 88–Sp-Lang Path, Volz & Amato, **SLP**

Jones, Mrs Dinah R 409 East Tierra Buena, Phoenix, AZ 85022-3034, (602) 864-1300, BS 71 Southeast MO St Univ; MA 78 Southeast MO St Univ; Sp-Lang Path, UCP, **SLP**

Jones, Donna L 30011 Ivy Glenn #108, Laguna Niguel, CA 92677, MA; **A**

Jones, Mrs E Sharon L 1829 Senate Street #3-C, Columbia, SC 29201, BS 69 East TN St Univ; MA 73 Univ of Houston - Univ Park; Sp-Lang Path, **SLP**

Jones, Edith T 536 Lodge Avenue, Evansville, IN 47714, (812) 424-8628, BA 74 Roger Williams Coll; MA 80 Trenton St Coll; Sp-Lang Path, Green River Comp Care Cen, **SLP**

Jones, Elisa Saccardo 16 Morgan Road, Holbrook, MA 02343, (617) 331-7514, BA 75 Univ of MA - Amherst; MS 76 Marquette Univ; Sp-Lang Path, Judith Wisnia & Associates, **SLP**

Jones, Mrs Elizabeth 106 Niagara Street, Winnipeg, MB, Canada R3N 0T9, (204) 787-2740, BS 76 Univ of Western Ontario; OM 80 Univ of Western Ontario; Sp/Lang Path, Health Sciences Cen Chldn Hosp, **SLP**

Jones, Elizabeth A 14435 South 87th Avenue, Orland Park, IL 60462, (312) 349-0186, BA 86 Augustana Coll; MA 88 Univ of KS; 88–Sp-Lang Path, Oak Forest Hosp

Jones, Mrs Elizabeth Dillin PO Box 827, Melbourne, AR, (501) 268-4467, BA 80 Harding Univ; MS 86 AR St Univ; 88–Sp-Lang Path, Northcentral AR Educ Svc Ctr, **SLP**

Jones, Ellen Laetitia 2015 Ivy Road Suite 114, Charlottesville, VA 22901, (804) 977-8389, BA 76 Knox Coll; BS 78 Northern IL Univ - De Kalb; MS 82 Univ of NC - Chapel Hill; Sp/Lang Path, Sp-Lang-Learning Svcs, **SLP**

Jones, Ernest I 706 South 3rd Street, La Crescent, MN 55947, (608) 782-9760, BA 60 Univ of IA; MA 65 Univ of IA; Aud, Skemp Clinic Ltd, **SLP A**

Jones, Mrs Fay Linda Schlimper 4320 N W 3 Court, Coconut Creek, FL 33066, (305) 943-1155, BA 71 Univ of FL; MA 73 Univ of FL; SLP, Broward Co Sch Bd, **SLP**

Jones, Fay M 1616 Hoaaina Place, Honolulu, HI 96821, (808) 947-8234, OB 58; MS 77 Univ of HI - Manoa; Sp-Lang Path, Kapiolani Med Ctr, **SLP**

Jones, Mrs Frances Marie 404 Society Place, Newtown, PA 18940, (609) 683-8414, BS 77 CA Univ of PA; MA 82 Univ of Pittsburgh - Pittsburgh; Director of Sp & Hrng Dept, Med Cen at Princeton, **SLP ACE**

Jones, Frederick M 3322-B Drive South, East Leroy, MI 49051, (616) 966-5600, MA 80 Wayne St Univ; Aud, VA Med Ctr, **A**

Jones, Gary Lee 8955 La Verne Drive, Alta Loma, CA 91701, (714) 982-0579, BA 80 CA St Univ - Long Beach; MA 83 CA St Univ - Long Beach; Aud, Pacific Hearing Svcs, **A**

Jones, Dr Gary W 73 Carriage Road, Clifton Park, NY 12065, (518) 454-5256, BS 67 East Stroudsburg Univ of PA; ME 72 Bloomsburg Univ of PA; PH 81 (Sp Science) SUNY - Center at Buffalo; Program Director, College of St Rose, **SLP**

Jones, Grant W Department Of Speech Pathology, Hillside Hospital, 8747 Squires Lane N E, Warren, OH 44484, (216) 841-3700, BA 69 Linfield Coll; MS 71 Western OR St Coll; Dir Sp-Lang Path & Audiology, Hillside Hosp, **SLP**

Jones, Howard C 23642 Via San Gil, Mission Viejo, CA 92691, (213) 494-5414, BA 66 Univ of AZ; MA 67 Univ of AZ; Aud, VA Med Cen, **A**

Jones, Mrs I Terry 817 Long Cove Road, Gales Ferry, CT 06335, (203) 889-3217, BS 58 Ithaca Coll; MA 62 Columbia Univ Teachers Coll; Sp-Lang Path, Norwich Pub Sch, **SLP**

Jones, Mrs Irene E Jack Jones Hearing Aid Clinic, 400 South Henderson, Fort Worth, TX 76104, (817) 335-2583, BA 67 Hardin-Simmons Univ; MA 68 TX Christian Univ; MS 79 Southern Methodist Univ; Aud, Jack Jones Hrng Aid Cents Inc, **A**

Jones, J Paula 2275 Scenic Highway #126, Pensacola, FL 32503, (904) 455-0111, BS 70 MS Univ for Women; MS 71 MS Univ for Women; Sp-Lang Path, Escambia Co Sch Dist, **SLP**

Jones, Dr Jacqueline Lehman College, Dept Of Spec Services In, Education, Bronx, NY 10468, (212) 960-8173, BA 69 CUNY - Lehman Coll; MA 70 Northwestern Univ; PH 84 (NS) Northwestern Univ; 85–Coord, Lehman College

Jones, James L P O Box 7043, Napa, CA 94558, (707) 253-5571, BS 72 Kent St Univ; MS 76 Univ of ND; OM 83 Univ of San Francisco; Tchr, Napa St Hosp, **SLP**

Jones, Mrs Janet Hyde 8031 52nd Avenue West, Mukilteo, WA 98275, (206) 258-7850, BA 66 WA St Univ; MA 67 MI St Univ; Dir Sp-Lang Path, Providence Hosp, **SLP**

Jones, Janet P 25 Back River Way, Duxbury, MA 02332, (617) 749-9612, BS 75 PA St Univ - Univ Park; MA 76 OH St Univ; Sp-Lang Path, Cardinal Cushing Sch/Trng Cen, **SLP**

Jones, Mrs Janice Lohman 1821 Pine Road, Heath, OH 43056, (614) 323-0277, BA 78 LA Tech Univ; MA 84 LA St Univ - Baton Rouge; **SLP**

Jones, Jean T 128-16 150th Street, South Ozone Park, NY 11436, **SLP**

Jones, Jeremy K 8216 South Madison Avenue, Indianapolis, IN 46227, (317) 888-4244, BS 71 IN Univ - Bloomington; MA 73 IN Univ - Bloomington; Gen Mgr, Hearing Center Inc, **A**

Jones, Jeri A 3040 N W 58, Seattle, WA 98107, **SLP**

Jones, Jo Ann P 1405 South Kittredge, Aurora, CO 80017, (303) 368-8129, BS 76 KS St Univ; MA 78 KS St Univ; 87–Sp-Lang Path, Arapahoe Co Sch Dist 6, **SLP**

Jones, Joan Harris 2416 Pesquera Drive, Los Angeles, CA 90049-1225, (213) 471-6788, BA 73 George Washington Univ; MA 74 George Washington Univ; SLP, Private Practice, **SLP**

Jones, John F 134 Kilbuck Drive, Monroeville, PA 15146, (614) 695-4931, BA 74 Wayne St Univ; MA 72 Eastern MI Univ; 87–Sp-Lang Path, Belmont Habilitation Ctr, **SLP**

Jones, Judith Burch 1330 Marion Street, Denver, CO 80218, (303) 794-9460, BA 81 MI St Univ; MA 84 Univ of CO - Boulder; 88–Sp-Lang Path, Littleton PS, **SLP**

Jones, Mrs Judith J 1731 Auburn Avenue, Dayton, OH 45406, MA 70 Univ of KY; Sp-Lang Path, Dayton Board of Education, **SLP**

Jones, Mrs Judith S 1714 Lopshire Lane, New Haven, IN 46774, (219) 493-3491, BS 72 FL St Univ; MS 73 FL St Univ; 88–Sp-Lang Path, Fort Wayne State Dev Ctr, **SLP**

Jones, Judy Davidson Box 14-D, Zamora Road, Tijeras, NM 87059, (505) 831-6993, MS 76 Univ of NM; Sp-Lang Path, Albuquerque Pub Sch, **SLP**

Jones, Judy K 10 La Veta Avenue, Alamosa, CO 81101, (719) 589-6791, BA 74 Adams St Coll; MA 74 Adams St Coll; 75–SLP, Alamosa Pub Sch, **SLP**

Jones, Julia Mary Assoc In Audiology & Sp Path, 2233 West Lindsey, Suite 105, Norman, OK 73069, (405) 329-0390, BA 79 Univ of OK - Norman; MS 81 Univ of OK Medical Center; Sp/Lang Path, Assoc Aud & Sp Path, **SLP**

Jones, Julie 366 North 1000 West, Provo, UT 84601, (801) 373-7850, BS 83 Brigham Young Univ; MA 84 Brigham Young Univ; Sp-Lang Path, Utah Valley Reg Med Ctr, **SLP**

Jones, Julie Gail 2645 Battle Creek Highway, Charlotte, MI 48813-9023, (517) 372-6725, **A**

Jones, Dr Julie Kay 9232 Arlington Blvd, Fairfax, VA 22031, (703) 385-1466, BA 69 Univ of South FL; MA 73 G Peabody Coll-Vanderbilt U; PH 78 (NS) Univ of Pittsburgh - Pittsburgh

Jones, Mrs Julie Lavezzoli 53 Stoneheights Drive, Waterford, CT 06385, (203) 442-0711, BS 81 CA St Univ - Fresno; MA 83 Univ of MA - Amherst; Sp-Lang Path, Lebanon Sch Sys, **SLP**

Jones, Karen E 3106 Stratford Drive, Greensboro, NC 27408, MS 79 Univ of NC - Greensboro; SLP, W S /for Co Schs, **SLP**

Jones, Mrs Karen P P O Box 3525, Fremont, CA 94539, BS 57 Univ of NE - Lincoln; Sp-Lang Path, Pleasanton Sch Dist, **SLP**

Jones, Karin A 4458 Sandner Drive, Sarasota, FL 34243, (813) 798-6220, BA 78 Univ of FL; MA 80 Univ of FL; 81–Sp-Lang Path, HCA L W Blake Hosp, **SLP**

Jones, Kathleen 19 Elm Street, Geneseo, NY 14454, (716) 243-5191, BA 65 Coll of Wooster; MA 67 Univ of IL - Urbana; Doctoral /Assistant, State University of New York, **SLP**

Jones, Kathleen 92 Jeffrey Drive, Depew, NY 14043-4620, (716) 685-4594, BA 73 SUNY - Center at Buffalo; MA 77 San Jose St Univ; Sp/Lang Path, UCP Assoc W NY, **SLP**

Jones, Kathleen H 731 1/2 30th Street, Hermosa Beach, CA 90254, (408) 384-7524, BA 75 CA St Univ - Fresno; MA 82 CA St Univ - Fresno; **SLP**

Jones, Kathryn S 1110 Travis Heights Blvd, Austin, TX 78704, (512) 454-0341, BA 71 Univ of TX - Austin; MA 76 Univ of TX - Austin; Aud, Private Practice, **A**

Jones, Mrs Kay H 2613 Shasta Court, Fort Worth, TX 76133, (817) 737-6646, BA 59 Univ of North TX; MA 70 TX Christian Univ; Dir of Spec Ed, Fort Worth ISD, **SLP**

Jones, Kenneth E 2405 North Warner, Tacoma, WA 98406, (206) 456-0550, BS 75 Univ of WA; OM 77 Univ of WA; Audiologist, Multicare Speech/Hrng Services, **A**

Jones, Kristina Marie 27 Bowdoin Street #21, Worcester, MA 01609, (617) 792-8500, BS 84 Boston Univ; MA 86 George Washington Univ

Jones, Lenora L 774 Duff Avenue, La Puente, CA 91744, (818) 918-6975, BA 61 Univ of WA; **SLP**

Jones, Leslie E 547 Davis Road #4, Cincinnati, OH 45255, (513) 752-8427, BS 77 Miami Univ - Oxford; MA 78 Bowling Green St Univ; Sp-Lang Path, Hamilton Co Offi of Ed, **SLP**

Jones, Linda G 136 North Brooks Street, Pontotoc, MS 38863, (601) 489-3493, BA 69 Univ of MS; ME 71 MS Coll; Sp-Lang Path, North Pontotoc Attend Cen, **SLP**

Jones, Linda H 625 Lawrence Circle, Haughton, LA 71037, (318) 797-5099, BA 68 LA Tech Univ; MA 70 LA Tech Univ; Instr, LA LSU, **SLP**

Jones, Mrs Linda J 3335 Ridgerock Way, Snellville, GA 30278, (404) 985-6012

Jones, Linda Swindell 414 Olive, Lindsay, OK 73052, (405) 238-6401, BS 84 OK St Univ; MA 87 OK St Univ; 88–Sp-Lang Path, Pauls Valley St Sch

Jones, Lisa Kaye 1602 Cherry Street #E 5, Conway, AR 72032, (501) 327-5315, BS 84 Univ of Central AR; MS 86 Univ of Central AR; 86–Sp-Lang Path, S Conway Co PS, **SLP**

Jones, Lisa Marie Williams State Service Center, Speech - Language - Hearing Services, Rt 13 & River Road, Dover, DE 19901, (302) 736-5376, BS 84 East Stroudsburg Univ of PA; MS 86 PA St Univ - Univ Park; 86–Aud, State of DE, **A**

Jones, Lisa Petersen 8955 La Verne Drive, Alta Loma, CA 91701, (714) 829-5950, BA 80 Univ of CA - Santa Barbara; MA 81 San Diego St Univ; 84–Aud, Kaiser Permanente, **A**

Jones, Lou Ann 3409-B Alpine Court, Lexington, KY 40502, (606) 272-7015, MS 83 Univ of Louisville; Aud, Kentucky School for the Deaf, **A**

Jones, Lucille W 233 Manor Drive, San Francisco, CA 94127, PH (NS); **SLP LM**

Jones, Mrs Lyda B Rural Route 4, 3195 Sunderland Road, Lima, OH 45806, (419) 657-2019, BS 63 Miami Univ - Oxford; Sp-Lang Path, Lima Vna/Wapakonta Cty Schs, **SLP**

Jones, Mrs Lynette 4210 South Nonchalant, Colorado Springs, CO 80917, (303) 597-6012, **SLP**

Jones, Lynette Susan New York School For The Deaf, 555 Knollwood Road, White Plains, NY 10603, (914) 949-7310, BS 85 Western MI Univ; MS 87 Gallaudet Coll; 87–Aud, New York Sch for the Deaf, **A**

Jones, Mrs Lynn A 9451 Ambleside Drive, Cincinnati, OH 45241, (513) 825-2012, BA 77 Wright St Univ; MA 79 Univ of Cincinnati; Sp-Lang Path, Mt Healthy Cty Sch, **SLP**

Jones, Lynn M Office Of Drs Sibbitt & White, 514 West 2nd Street, Bloomington, IN 47401, (812) 332-9634, BA 79 IN Univ - Bloomington; MA 81 IN Univ - Bloomington; Aud, Private Practice, **A**

Jones, Dr M Carolyn 332 Audubon Street, New Orleans, LA 70118, (504) 861-8913, BS 55 LA St Univ - Baton Rouge; MA 58 LA St Univ - Baton Rouge; PH 65 (NS) Northwestern Univ; Sp-Lang Path, Private Practice, **SLP**

Jones, Mamie J 3747 Ptree Road N E #1709, Atlanta, GA 30319, PH (NS); **SLP F LM**

Jones, Margaret E 641 North Hine Avenue, Waukesha, WI 53188, (414) 544-2445, BS 83 Univ of WI - Madison; MA 85 Univ of KS; Sp-Lang Path, Waukesha Mem Hosp, **SLP**

Jones, Mrs Marietta R 3607 Valle Vista Drive, Chino, CA 91710, (714) 597-6253, BA 74 Wichita St Univ; MA 76 Wichita St Univ; SLP/Aud, Riverside USD, **SLP**

Jones, Marilyn 560 West 43rd #11-K, New York, NY 10036, (517) 835-5408, BA 65 Univ of IA; MA 87 Central MI Univ

Jones, Marlene L 150 Sheriff Street, Elyria, OH 44035, (216) 329-3740, BS 78 Univ of Cincinnati; MA 79 OH St Univ; Sp-Lang Path, Lorain Co Bd/Men Ret&Dev Disab, **SLP**

Jones, Mrs Marny S 75 Longwood Drive, San Rafael, CA 94901, (415) 454-9057, BA 44 Stanford Univ; MA 69 San Francisco St Univ; **SLP**

Jones, Dr Martha E 29 Highland Street, West Hartford, CT 06119-0000, (203) 233-2502, BA 37 Central CT St Univ; MA 43 Univ of IA; OM 58 Univ of CT; **SLP LM**

Jones, Mrs Martha Leigh 203 E Spring Street, Fayetteville, AR 72701, (501) 521-7843, BS 84 AR St Univ; MA 87 Univ of AR - Fayetteville

Jones, Mary B 13509 Granite Walk Drive, Chantilly, VA 22021, (703) 378-5410, BA 70 Univ of SC - Columbia; ME 73 Univ of SC - Columbia; **SLP**

Jones, Mrs Mary B 1092 Cliff View Lane, Carol Stream, IL 60188, (312) 908-6134, BS 84 Northwestern Univ; MA 85 Northern IL Univ - De Kalb; 87–Sp-Lang Path, Rehab Inst of Chicago, **SLP**

Jones, Dr Mary E 5021 Euclid Lane, Richton Park, IL 60471, (312) 534-5000, BS 72 Memphis St Univ; MA 75 MI St Univ; PH 80 (NS) Univ of Pittsburgh - Pittsburgh; Professor, Governors State University, **SLP**

Jones, Mary Elizabeth P O Box 3832, Bryan, TX 77805, (409) 776-2872, BS 80 OK St Univ; MA 83 OK St Univ; Reg Therapist II, St Sch, **SLP ACE**

Jones, Mary Ellen Therese 2051 Jonathan Avenue, San Jose, CA 95125, (408) 559-5963, BA 71 Holy Names Coll; MA 77 San Jose St Univ; 80–Sp-Lang Path, Fremont USD, **SLP**

Jones, Mary Lou Herceg 23642 Via San Gil, Mission Viejo, CA 92691, MS; **A**

Jones, Mary Lynne 1840 Englewood Drive S E, Grand Rapids, MI 49506, (616) 530-7558, BA 68 MI St Univ; MA 72 Ball St Univ; SLP, Wyoming Pub Sch, **SLP**

Jones, Mrs Marybeth D 3003 Applegate Lane, Glenview, IL 60025, (312) 724-6293, MS 74 IN Univ - Bloomington; Sp-Lang Path, New Horizon Center, **SLP**

Jones, Merrily M The Vanderbilt Clinic, Speech Pathology Dept, Room 1702, Nashville, TN 37232, (615) 322-0100, BA 79 Univ of TN - Knoxville; MS 82 Vanderbilt Univ; Sp-Lang Path, Vanderbilt Univ Medical Center, **SLP**

Jones, Mrs Merry M 1853-A North Dupont Hwy, Dover, DE 19901, (302) 734-1228, BS 68 Indiana Univ of PA; MS 69 Univ of HI - Manoa; 83–Sp-Lang Path, Caesar Rodney Sch Dist, **SLP**

Jones, Morris Val Speech And Hearing Center, California State Univ, 6000 J Street, Sacramento, CA 95819, PH (NS); **SLP A LM**

Jones, Nadine J 3711 Leroy Stevens Road, Mobile, AL 36619, (205) 639-0965, MA 79 OH St Univ; Sp/Lang Path, Private Practice, **SLP**

Jones, Mrs Pamela R L c/o LTC Michael J Jones, HHC 3AD G-3, APO New York, NY 09039, BA 68 IN Univ - Bloomington; MA 73 IN Univ - Bloomington; 88–Sp-Lang Path, Frankfurt American HS, **SLP**

Jones, Mrs Patricia 129 Centre Street, Haddonfield, NJ 08033, (609) 456-7116, BS 75 Univ of AR - Little Rock; MA 76 Univ of AR - Little Rock; Sp-Lang Path, Gloucester Cty Pub Schs, **SLP**

Jones, Mrs Patricia A Route 1 Box 161-A, Waverly, AL 36879, (205) 271-9355, BA 74 Temple Univ; OM 81 Auburn Univ - Auburn; Aud, Auburn Univ at Montgomery, **A**

Jones, Patricia A 3720 Midvale Avenue #2, Los Angeles, CA 90034, (213) 202-9049, BA 75 CA St Univ - Long Beach; MA 77 CA St Univ - Long Beach; SLP, LA USD, **SLP**

Jones, Mrs Patricia Marie 2566 Lee Road, Cleveland Heights, OH 44118, (216) 283-3402, **SLP**

Jones, Mrs Patricia Presnall 7774 Lewis Street, Arvada, CO 80005, (303) 428-3511, BA 63 OK St Univ; MA 82 Univ of Denver; Sp-Lang Path, Adams Co Sch Dist #50, **SLP**

Jones, Paula L 1113 Gibbon, Laramie, WY 82070, (307) 721-4460, BA 75 Univ of OK - Norman; MS 76 Univ of OK Medical Center; Aud, Albany Co Sch Dist #1, **A**

Jones, Mrs Priscilla Henderson 107 West Karnes, Waco, TX 76706, (817) 662-2686, BA 83 Harding Univ; MA 85 Abilene Christian Univ; 88–Sp-Lang Path, McLennan Co Coop for Excep Chldn, **SLP**

Jones, Rhonda Duman 4 Travis Place, Portsmouth, VA 23702, (804) 539-1744, BS 81 Old Dominion Univ; MS 86 James Madison Univ; 81–Sp-Lang Path, Suffolk City Schs, **SLP**

Jones, Robin R Bon Vista Apartment #A3, Morgantown, WV 26505, (304) 293-4241, BS 72 WV Univ; MS 73 WV Univ; 75–Asst Prof of Aud/Hrng Cl Coord, WV U, **A**

Jones, Mrs Roma B 20034 Shrewsbury Road, Detroit, MI 48221, (313) 345-6164, BS 56 Hampton Univ; MA 61 Columbia Univ Teachers Coll; SLP, Detroit Cty Sch, **SLP**

Jones, Dr Ronald Count 10501 Duryea Drive, Richmond, VA 23235-2104, (804) 230-1388, BS 71 Northern IL Univ - De Kalb; MA 73 Northern IL Univ - De Kalb; PH 81 (NS) Univ of Cincinnati; Aud, VA Med Ctr, **A**

Jones, Ronda Diane 1803 Morgan Smith Road, Greensboro, NC 27405, (919) 375-0311, BS 85 Univ of NC - Greensboro; ME 86 Univ of NC - Greensboro

Jones, Mrs Roseann D 230 South Firestone Blvd, Akron, OH 44301, (216) 253-2113, BS 65 Univ of Akron; MA 69 Univ of Akron; Doctoral, Kent State U, **SLP**

Jones, Mrs Ruth E 1970 G Street, Carson City, NV 89701, (702) 883-7682, BA 54 Whittier Coll; MA 68 Univ of Southern CA; Sp-Lang Path, Rsvp, **SLP LM**

Jones, Ruth E M 11114 Burdine, Houston, TX 77096, (713) 729-2518, BS 74 Univ of AZ; MS 75 Univ of AZ; Sp-Lang Path, St Lukes/Texas Chldns Hosp, **SLP**

Jones, Sandra Tucker Northeast Regional Office, P O Box 6118, Monroe, LA 71211, (318) 362-5234, BA 80 Univ of MS; MA 81 Univ of MS; Aud Region Viii, Dept of Hlth & Human Resources, **A**

Jones, Mrs Sara J 9947 N W 46th Court, Sunrise, FL 33351, (305) 749-0689, BS 81 Northern IL Univ - De Kalb; MA 84 Univ of Houston - Univ Park; 85–Sp-Lang Path, Broward Co Sch Brd, **SLP**

Jones, Sharen 713 Shepard Court, Gurnee, IL 60031, **SLP**

Jones, Sheila L N 7520 Maywood, Ralston, NE 68127, (402) 331-0540, BA 66 Creighton Univ; MA 68 Univ of NE - Lincoln; SLP, Ralston Public Schools, **SLP**

Jones, Mrs Sheryl K 7120 Carlson Circle, Apartment 269, Canoga Park, CA 91303, (818) 348-4351, BA 79 Univ of MT; MA 83 Univ of CO - Boulder; SLP, Burnwall Clinic, **SLP**

Jones, Shirley A 12016 Hunterton Street, Upper Marlboro, MD 20772, (202) 732-1092, BS 56 Hampton Univ; MA 63 Temple Univ-Tyler Sch of Art; OD 79 (Law) Georgetown Univ; Acting Chief, US Dept of Ed, **SLP F**

Jones, Mrs Sondra Carson 816 East Jackson, Fayetteville, AR 72701, (501) 273-1810, BA 79 Univ of AR - Fayetteville; MA 80 Univ of AR - Fayetteville; Sp-Lang Path, Benton County Sunshine School, **SLP**

Jones, Stacey Dawn 1707 Bedingfield Drive, Tampa, FL 33603, (813) 876-2230, MS 87 Univ of South FL

Jones, Mrs Susan C Route 6 Box 125, Martinsville, VA 24112, (703) 632-8115, BA 75 Mary Washington Coll; MA 78 CA St Univ - Northridge; Sp/Lang Path, Private Practice, **SLP**

Jones, Susan Lynne 236 Cypress Street #1, Brookline, MA 02146, (216) 758-9402, BS 82 Kent St Univ; MA 86 Univ of Akron; **A**

Jones, Mrs Teresa Marie 1074-7 Lancaster Boulevard, Mechanicsburg, PA 17055, (717) 737-6728, BS 84 Indiana Univ of PA; MS 86 Bloomsburg Univ of PA; 86–Sp-Lang Path, Capital Area Intermed Unit, **SLP**

Jones, Terri Lee 125 Valhalla Road, Southern Pines, NC 28387, (919) 582-2878, BS 79 Miami Univ - Oxford; MS 80 Miami Univ - Oxford; Sp-Lang Path, Southeastern Sp & Hrng, **SLP**

Jones, Mrs Theresa T 800 North Colusa Drive, Walnut, CA 91789, (818) 964-0034, BA 76 CA St Univ - Los Angeles; MA 78 CA St Univ - Los Angeles; SLP, Los Angeles Co Supt Sch, **SLP**

Jones, Vern 906 E Hastings Road, Spokane, WA 99218-1741, (509) 838-4567, BA 71 Eastern WA Univ; MS 73 Eastern WA Univ; Sp-Lang Path, Spokane Speech Rehab Center, **SLP**

Jones, Mrs Vickie Kay Handley 310 Northlake Drive #39, Warner Robins, GA 31093, (912) 987-1929, BS 84 Univ of GA; ME 85 Univ of GA; 85–Sp-Lang Path, Houston Co Bd of Educ, **SLP**

Jones, Virginia Sue 307 South 21st, Blue Springs, MO 64015, (816) 228-4786, BA 50 Hendrix Coll; MA 71 Northeast MO St Univ; Sp-Lang Path, **SLP**

Jones, Vivian Booker 304A Nazareth Road, Spartanburg, SC 29301, (803) 439-1825, BA 66 SC St Coll; MA 73 Univ of CT; Sp-Lang Path, Spartanburg Sch Dist 6, **SLP**

Jones, W Harold P O Box 781, Hot Springs, SD 57747, (605) 745-4101, OM 64 Northeastern OK St Univ; Sp/Lang Path, Uamc Hot Springs, **SLP**

Jones, William B Box 872, APO New York, NY 09019-0005, BS 73 East Carolina Univ; MS 79 East Carolina Univ; SLP, Dod Depend Schs, **SLP**

Jones, William Dixon 717 Northridge Street, Greensboro, NC 27403-2108, (919) 294-8984, BA 80 Wake Forest Univ; ME 83 Univ of VA - Charlottesville; 87–SLP, Cadwell Laboratories Inc, **A**

Jones, Dr William O 5 West Colorado Avenue, Haven Beach, NJ 08008, (609) 652-7000, BA 54 Capital Univ; MA 55 Columbia Univ Teachers Coll; ED 68 (Sp Path) Columbia Univ Teachers Coll; 72–Prof Sp-Lang Path & Aud, Trenton State Coll, **SLP A**

Jones, Winifred Brandt Rt 1 Box 70, Valley Center, KS 67147, (316) 688-1888, BA 78 Wichita St Univ; MA 80 Wichita St Univ; Dir Comm Outreach Prog, Cp Res Foundation of Ks, **SLP**

Jones-Boon, Gael A 1 Ellalong Road, Turramurra, Sydney, New South Wales, Australia 2074, **SLP A**

Jones-Brown, Mrs Robin Elane 3301 South Bear St, Apartment 61A, Santa Ana, CA 92704, (714) 751-8562, BS 82 Univ of NV - Reno; MS 85 Univ of NV - Reno; **SLP**

Jones-Lewis, Beverly L Route 3 Box 287 A-1, Dover, TN 37058, (502) 825-7200, BS 79 Murray St Univ; MS 81 Murray St Univ; Aud, Trover Cl, **A**

Jones-McNamara, Mrs Sara 5501 Seminary Road, 106 South Skyline Square, Falls Church, VA 22041, (703) 845-8190, BS 71 OH Univ - Athens; ME 80 Columbus Coll; 88–Reg Dir Cl Prog, InSpeech Inc, **SLP ACE**

Jones-Oleson, Mrs Linda Doreen 402 North Market Street, Staunton, VA 24401, BS 76 Madison Coll; MS 80 James Madison Univ; 80–Sp-Lang Path, Virginia Sch for Deaf & Blind, **SLP**

Jones-Owens, J Lyndelle 6804 South Canton Suite 1000, Tulsa, OK 74136, (918) 492-6292, BA 65 Univ of OK - Norman; OM 66 Univ of OK Medical Center; Sp-Lang Path, Private Practice, **SLP**

Jones-Prus, Mrs Debora 71 Birch Hill Lane, Oakville, ON, Canada L6K 2P1, (416) 845-5965, BS 76 Univ of Western Ontario; MA 77 MI St Univ; 86–Sp-Lang Path, Memorial Hosp, **SLP**

Jong, Nancy Tomi Hamai 755 Mandana Blvd, Oakland, CA 94610, (415) 832-5732, BA 82 CA St Univ - Long Beach; MA 84 Univ of CA - Santa Barbara; 88–SLP, Rehabilitation Svcs of N CA, **SLP**

Jons, Catherine Riedel Walter Reed Army Medical Ctr, Army Audiology & Spch Ctr, Washington, DC 20307-5001, (202) 576-1649, BA 81 Univ of MN - Duluth; MS 84 Univ of WI - Madison; 86–Aud, Walter Reed Army Med Ctr, **A**

Jons, Mrs Sarah M 1916 18th Avenue South #11, Moorhead, MN 56560, (218) 236-6400, BA 72 Univ of WY; MS 76 Univ of MN - Minneap-St Paul; Sp/Lang Path, ISD #152, **SLP**

Jopling, Bobbie Jean 800 Mallery Street, Village Green #88, St Simons Island, GA 31522, (912) 264-3141, BS 72 GA Southern Coll; ME 84 Armstrong St Coll; Sp-Lang Path, Easter Seal Sp & Hrng, **SLP ACE**

Joram, Mary Fazzino 29 Coumbia Drive, New Fairfield, CT 06812, (203) 796-1830, BA 79 Southern CT St Univ; SLP, New Fairfield Bd of Ed, **SLP**

Jordahl, Nanette J Route 1, Wilson, WI 54027, **SLP**

Jordan, Mrs Angela Fox 19 Pinehurst Lane, Boca Raton, FL 33431, (305) 368-7972, BS 79 FL St Univ; MS 80 FL St Univ; Sp-Lang Path, Nova Univ, **SLP**

Jordan, Annemarie H 33-C Grandview Drive, Farmington, CT 06032, (203) 677-1353, BA 79 Univ of CT; MS 80 PA St Univ - Univ Park; Sp/Lang Path, Private Practice, **SLP**

Jordan, Barbara May 36 Medford Indian Mills Road, Indian Mills, NJ 08088, (609) 654-9624, BS 76 West Chester Univ of PA; MA 82 Trenton St Coll; Sp-Lang Path, Private Practice, **SLP**

Jordan, Connie L 215 Yerba Buena Avenue, Los Altos, CA 94022-2212, **A**

Jordan, Corinne M 6446 West 89th Street #56, Overland Park, KS 66212, (816) 756-2250, BS 77 IA St Univ; MA 78 Univ of Northern IA; 88–Sp-Lang Path, Rehab Inst, **SLP**

Jordan, Craig Eugene PSC 3 Box 15646, APO San Francisco, CA 96432-0006, BS 80 IL St Univ - Normal; MS 82 IL St Univ - Normal; Aud, 13th Air Force Med Ctr, **A ACE**

Jordan, Deborah P 1380 Apple Cross Court, Kernersville, NC 27284, (919) 993-4859, BA 75 Univ of NC - Chapel Hill; MS 77 East Carolina Univ; Sp-Lang Path, **SLP**

Jordan, Mrs Ethel S 517 Coston, Boise, ID 83702, BS; **SLP A LM**

Jordan, Eugenia 301-B Park Avenue, La Grange, GA 30240, (404) 884-6578, BA 76 Columbus Coll; OM 81 Auburn Univ - Auburn; Sp-Lang Path, Lagrange City Sch Sys, **SLP**

Jordan, Gretchen B 2 Lancefield Crescent, Brampton, ON, Canada L6S 2R2, (416) 451-2515, BA 67 Stanford Univ; MA 68 Stanford Univ; Prin, Peel Bd Ed/McHugh Pub Sch, **SLP**

Jordan, Dr Herbert N Rural Route 2 Box 14, Iowa City, IA 52240, (319) 338-0581, BA 54 IN Univ - Bloomington; MA 57 Syracuse Univ; PH 62 (NS) Syracuse Univ; Sp-Lang Path, VA Med Ctr, **A**

Jordan, Mrs Jacqueline 690 Oleander Cricle, Virginia Beach, VA 23464, (804) 473-5029, BS 71 NC St Univ at Raleigh; MS 84 Old Dominion Univ; Sp-Lang Path, VA Beach City PS, **SLP**

Jordan, Janet W 104 Timber Drive, Storrs, CT 06268, (203) 429-1260, BS 75 Univ of WI - Madison; MS 76 Univ of WI - Madison; 87–Sp-Lang Path, Eastconn Infant/Toddler Interv Prog, **SLP**

Jordan, Mrs Jean Whitlock 3600 Keith Street N W #1504, Cleveland, TN 37312, (615) 479-8246, BS 81 Auburn Univ - Auburn; MS 83 Auburn Univ - Auburn; Sp/Lang Path, Cleveland City Sch Sys, **SLP**

Jordan, Mrs Karen Donna 253-32 61st Avenue, Littleneck, NY 11362, (718) 225-7230, BA 78 SUNY - Center at Stony Brook; MA 79 Adelphi Univ; MS 84 Adelphi Univ; SLP, Sp Serv Unit NYC, **SLP**

Jordan, Kaye 403 Oakwood, Roswell, NM 88201, (505) 347-5491, BS 64 Eastern NM Univ; MS 78 Eastern NM Univ; Dir Sp-Lang Pathology, NM Rehab Cen, **SLP**

Jordan, Lillian H 1 Mountain Top Road/High Knob, Front Royal, VA 22630, (703) 635-9311, BS 54 East Carolina Univ; MS 76 East Carolina Univ; Sp-Lang Path, Warren County PS, **SLP**

Jordan, Dr Linda S Rural Route 2, Box 14, Iowa City, IA 52240, (319) 356-2571, BA 62 Univ of IA; MA 64 Univ of IA; PH 72 (NS) Univ of IA; Sp-Lang Path, University of Iowa, **SLP**

Jordan, Mrs Maria Poon 425 Columbia Center Boulevard, F206, Kennewick, WA 99336, (509) 735-6126, MA 83 Univ of OR; 88–Sp-Lang Path, Kennewick Sch Dist #17, **SLP**

Jordan, Marjorie J 1315 Wilson Street #B, Eau Claire, WI 54701, (309) 697-3932, MS 83 Bradley Univ; **A**

Jordan, Marya T 1141 North President, Wheaton, IL 60187, (312) 668-1337, MS 80 Marquette Univ; **SLP**

Jordan, Mrs Miriam 2394 Hulick Place, Rahway, NJ 07065, (201) 321-7766, BS 82 San Diego St Univ; MA 87 Kean Coll of NJ; 87–Sp-Lang Path, John F Kennedy Med Ctr, **SLP**

Jordan, Patrick David 2213 Rivermont Avenue, Lynchburg, VA 24503, (804) 522-4520, ME 86 Univ of GA; Sp-Lang Path, Central VA Sp & Hrng Ctr, **SLP ACE**

Jordan, Rebecca Semenak 1145 Brookdale Avenue, Bay Shore, NY 11706, (516) 444-2599, BS 74 G Peabody Coll-Vanderbilt U; MS 76 Vanderbilt Univ; Aud, Neur Assoc Univ Hosp/SUNY, **A**

Jordan, Richard O P O Box 296, Huntington, MA 01050-0296, (413) 323-6311, BS 71 Ithaca Coll; MA 79 Case Western Reserve Univ; Superv/Speech-Hrng, Belchertown State School, **A**

Jordan, Mrs Sheryl A 56 High Ridge Road, West Hartford, CT 06117, (203) 232-6747, SLP, **SLP**

Jordan, Star M 223 East 85th Street #26, New York, NY 10028, (718) 963-8319, BA 84 Univ of New Brunswick - Nb; MS 87 Columbia Univ Teachers Coll; Sp-Lang Path, PC Associates Woodhull Hosp, **SLP**

Jordan, Mrs Terri Jolene 209 Clark Street, Gardner, MA 01440, (203) 486-2629, BS 82 Univ of MA - Amherst; MA 84 Univ of CT; SLP, Acton Boxborough Reg Sch Dist, **SLP**

Jordan, Vesper Quarti 3420 Broderick Street, San Francisco, CA 94123, (415) 545-3828, BS 67 Univ of KS; MA 77 Temple Univ-Tyler Sch of Art; **SLP**

Jordan-Trestik, Jill Marie P O Box 4514, Missoula, MT 59806, (406) 728-6199, BA 82 Univ of MT; MS 85 Portland St Univ; Aud, **A**

Jorgensen, Carol A B 13404 Byrds Nest Circle, Austin, TX 78736, (512) 263-9701, BS 73 Univ of IA; MA 74 Univ of IA; **SLP**

Jorgensen, Debra Ann 403 East Main Street #B-2, Bay Shore, NY 11706, (516) 581-2560, BS 83 SUNY - Coll at Oneonta; MS 85 Adelphi Univ; 84–Sp-Lang Path, ISLIP Union Free Sch Dist, **SLP**

Josefiak, William R 874 Main Street, West Seneca, NY 14224, (716) 674-6300, ME 81 SUNY - Coll at Buffalo; MS 75 SUNY - Coll at Geneseo; SLP, West Seneca Develop Ctr, **SLP**

Joselson, Dr Maurice Louis 3124 US Highway 441 SE Unit B1, Okeechobee, FL 34974-6874, (813) 467-6030, BA 65 Adelphi Univ; MS 66 Adelphi Univ; PH 70 (NS) Univ of FL; 88–Sp-Lang Path, InSpeech Inc, **SLP**

Joseph, Cynthia Beth Cleveland Hearing/Speech Cntr, 11206 Euclid Avenue, Cleveland, OH 44106, (216) 231-8787, BS 81 Miami Univ - Oxford; MA 85 Case Western Reserve Univ; Aud, Cleveland Hearing and Sp Ctr, **A**

Joseph, Mrs Ida M G 17889 Santa Valera, Fountain Valley, CA 92708, (714) 541-5991, BS 61 Univ of PR - Rio Piedras; MS 73 Univ of PR - Rio Piedras; Sp-Lang Path, Orange Co Dept of Ed, **SLP**

Joseph, Janet M 27 Schooner Ridge, Marblehead, MA 01945, (617) 631-0713, BS 73 Nazareth Coll of Rochester; MS 74 Syracuse Univ; Aud, MA Eye & Ear Inf, **A**

Joseph, Karyn Marie 29 Hudson Bay, Kirkland Lake, ON, Canada P2N 2H8, (705) 567-9355, BS 83 Eastern MI Univ; MA 84 Eastern MI Univ; 87–Sp-Lang Path, Timiskaming Health Unit, **SLP**

Joseph, Laura Sue 1815 Dogwood Drive, Fairmont, WV 26554, (304) 623-5661, BS 84 WV Univ; MS 85 WV Univ; Sp-Lang Path, Summit Center No 6, **SLP**

Joseph, Linda Dorr 294 Tavistock, Haddonfield-Berlin Road, Cherry Hill, NJ 08034, (609) 342-3060, BS 61 Northwestern Univ; MS 85 Hahneman Medical Coll; 85–Sp-Lang Path, Cooper Hospital Medical Center, **SLP**

Joseph, Phyllis Harris 1283 Southport Drive, Sarasota, FL 34242, BA 56 Albion Coll; MA 58 Univ of MI - Ann Arbor; MS 86 Univ of South FL; **SLP**

Joseph, Rosanne Miller 17522 Port O' Call, Crosby, TX 77532, (713) 328-6521, MA 79 Edinboro Univ of PA; Sp-Lang Path, Crosby Indepedent School, **SLP**

Joseph, Mrs Sheryl S 12400 Olivewood Place, Silver Spring, MD 20904, (301) 345-8481, BS 69 Purdue Univ - West Lafayette; MS 70 Univ of MI - Ann Arbor; 74–Sp-Lang Path, Prince Georges Co Sch, **SLP**

Joseph, Thomas S 1206 Vaughn Road, Burlington, NC 27215, (919) 226-0660, BS 78 East Carolina Univ; MS 80 East Carolina Univ; Aud, Burlington ENT, **A**

Joseph, Mrs Vivian 636 East 192nd Street, Glenwood, IL 60425, BA 62 Oakwood Coll; MS 72 Vanderbilt Univ; SLP/Remedial Reading Teach, Lake Region Conf (Shiloh Ady), **SLP**

Josephson, Glenda M 510 North Bryan, Little Rock, AR 72205, (501) 661-2328, BA 60 Univ of Northern CO; MA 73 Univ of IA; Sp-Lang Path, Chldn Hrng Sp Cl Ark Dept Hlth, **SLP**

Josephson, Mrs Jane C 10915 Lakeview Drive, Carmel, IN 46032, (317) 844-9851, BA 68 IN Univ - Bloomington; OM 70 IN Univ - Bloomington; Sp-Lang Path, Indianapolis Head Start, **SLP**

Josephson, Mrs Judith A St Josephs Medical Center, 127 South Broadway, Yonkers, NY 10701, (914) 378-7501, BS 60 Univ of CT; MA 75 Montclair St Coll; Admin-Sp & Aud Dept, St Joseph's Medical Center, **SLP ACE**

Josey, Anne F 1811 State Street, Nashville, TN 37203, (615) 327-3040, BA 66 Vanderbilt Univ; MS 67 Vanderbilt Univ; Aud, The Otology Gp, **A**

Joshu, Dan R 136 Appletree Lane, Edwardsville, IL 62025, BS 78 Southern IL Univ-Edwardsvill; MS 80 Southern IL Univ-Edwardsvill; Aud, Ten Co Spec Ed Dist, **A**

Jositas, Mrs Susan M 180 Shelton Road, Trumbull, CT 06611, (203) 966-9575, BA 74 Univ of CT; MA 76 Univ of CT; SLP, New Canaan Bd of Ed, **SLP**

Josof, Mrs Wadia Bolus 52 Medical Park Drive East, Suite 108, Birmingham, AL 35235, (205) 838-3098, BS 79 Univ of Montevallo; MS 80 FL St Univ; Owner/Dir, Area Sp and Rehab PC, **SLP**

Josserand, Mrs Deedra Quay 2046 Coast Guard Dr, Stafford, VA 22554, (703) 659-7799, BA 77 Wichita St Univ; MS 80 East Carolina Univ; 88–Sp-Lang Path, Stafford County Schs, **SLP**

Joswiak, Laura Marie 1179 Sycamore, Rochester, MI 48063, (313) 755-1520, BA 80 Wayne St Univ; MA 84 Wayne St Univ; **SLP ACE**

Jouras, Nikki A 7813 Jefferson, Kansas City, MO 64114, (816) 525-2950, BS 77 Univ of MO - Columbia; MA 79 OK St Univ; Sp-Lang Path, Rebound Inc, **SLP**

Jove-D'Amato, Martha 400 Davis Street #210, San Leandro, CA 94577, (415) 357-3821, Audiologist, Marilyn Righetti MD, **A**

Joy, Mrs Pamela Colston 339 Chesham, San Carlos, CA 94070, (415) 592-4381, MA 76 San Jose St Univ; SLP Dir, Private Practice Assoc Lang Spec, **SLP**

Joy, Patricia E 48 Trillium Road, Fairfield, CT 06430, (203) 255-5568, BS 74 NY Univ; MA 79 NY Univ; 87–Sp-Lang Path, Private Practice, **SLP**

Joyce, Jeanne M 109 Sperbeck Street, La Crosse, WI 54603, (608) 788-5700, BA 75 Coll of Saint Teresa; MS 76 Univ of WI - Eau Claire; 84–Sp/Lang Path, Bethany-St Joseph Care Ctr, **SLP ACE**

Joyce, Jerri Kaplan 58 Partridge Run, Amherst, NY 14228, (516) 585-0100, BA 78 SUNY - Center at Buffalo; MA 80 SUNY - Center at Buffalo; Aud, Niagara Cnty Sp-Hring-Lang Ctr, **A**

Joyce, Julia Beatrice 4225 Beach Drive S W, Seattle, WA 98116, (206) 932-1803, BA 79 FL St Univ; MA 82 Northwestern Univ; Sp-Lang Path, Northwest Hospital, **SLP**

Joyce, Margaret M 5705 Indian Court #2-C, Alexandria, VA 22303, (301) 894-5089, BA 67 Bradley Univ; MA 68 Univ of IA; Sp-Lang Path, Pg Brd of Ed, **SLP**

Joyce, Mrs Natalie J 1527 Tina Marie Circle, Indianapolis, IN 46229, (317) 894-8846, BS 75 Ball St Univ; MA 76 Ball St Univ; Sp-Lang Path, Private Practice, **SLP**

Joyce, Patricia E V A Medical Center, 2215 Fuller Road, Ann Arbor, MI 48105, (313) 769-7100, BA 82 Univ of RI; MS 84 Univ of MI - Ann Arbor; Aud, VA Med Ctr, **A**

Joyce, Mrs Patricia Pamela 748 Loridans Drive N E, Atlanta, GA 30342, (404) 377-3836, OM 84 Emory Univ; 87–Comm Dept Head, UCP of Atlanta, **SLP**

Joyce, Mrs Peggy M 378 Walmar Drive, Bay Village, OH 44140, (216) 871-7943, BS 82 Ball St Univ; MS 84 Kent St Univ; 88–Sp-Lang Path, Private Practice, **SLP**

Joyce-O'Toole, Patricia Edna 398 Pinewoods Avenue, Brunswick, NY 12180, (518) 274-7919, BS 81 Coll of Saint Rose; MS 85 Coll of Saint Rose; Sp-Lang Path, BOCES, **SLP**

Joyner, Mrs Gayle Merrix 4012 Fulton Avenue, Dayton, OH 45439, **SLP**

Joyner, Jeanette P O Box 2742, Washington, DC 20013, **SLP**

Joyner, Rhonda H 1517 Hollybriar Lane, Greenville, NC 27834, (919) 757-4448, BS 79 East Carolina Univ; MS 83 East Carolina Univ; Aud, Pitt County Memorial Hosp, **A**

Jozwick-Joseph, Mrs Denise M 128 Hillcrest Drive, Pittsburgh, PA 15237, (412) 734-1800, BS 75 Duquesne Univ; MS 77 Syracuse Univ; PH 88 (Communication Disorders) Univ of Pittsburgh - Pittsburgh; Sp-Lang Path, Private Practice, **SLP**

Juarez, Irma Estella 2918 West Poplar, San Antonio, TX 78207, (512) 224-7321, BA 82 Our Lady Lake Univ-San Anton; MA 84 Our Lady Lake Univ-San Anton; 84–Sp-Lang Path, San Antonio ISD, **SLP**

Juarez, Dr Manuela 202 Arcadia Place #108, San Antonio, TX 78209, (512) 821-3759, PH 83 (Communication Disorders) Univ of TX - Austin; Sp-Lang Path, Private Practice, **SLP ACE**

Juba-Jelusic, Karen Louise 25 Holland Avenue, Chatham, ON, Canada N7M 5X8, (519) 354-3770, MA 86 Wayne St Univ; **SLP**

Jubelirer, Mrs Amy R 2011 Woodland Road, Abington, PA 19001, (215) 886-5562, BS 75 PA St Univ - Univ Park; MA 78 Temple Univ-Tyler Sch of Art; Sp-Lang Pathologist, Private Practice, **SLP**

Jubelirer, Mrs Mary-Jo Kann 222 Beaumont Drive, Altoona, PA 16602, (814) 946-8392, BS 67 Boston Univ; MA 68 OH St Univ; Prin, Altoona Area Sch Dist, **SLP**

Jubien, Ghislaine 46 High Point Drive, Amherst, MA 01002, (413) 256-6726, BS 69 Emerson Coll; MA 70 Columbia Univ Teachers Coll; 71–Sp-Lang Path, Amherst Pub Sch, **SLP**

Juckett, Mrs Lauri Woods 210 Creswell Avenue, Scott, LA 70583, (318) 981-2219, BA 76 LA St Univ - Shreveport; OM 83 LA St Univ - N O Medical Ctr; Aud, Dept Health & Human Resources, **A**

Judd, Mrs Catherine Whitehouse 1476 Black Spruce Court, Lilburn, GA 30247, (404) 381-5739, BS 67 Cornell Univ; MS 79 Southern CT St Univ; Sp-Lang Path, **SLP**

Judd, Mrs Diane F 39 Elliot Street, Holyoke, MA 01040, (413) 532-8621, BS 73 Northwestern Univ; MA 78 Northwestern Univ; Cl Superv, **SLP**

Judd, Rebecca Muhleka 762 Pearlwood Way, San Jose, CA 95123, MS 85 Univ of NE - Omaha; **SLP**

Jude, Susan M 17535 41st Avenue North, Plymouth, MN 55446, (612) 557-0185, BS 75 Saint Cloud St Univ; MS 81 Saint Cloud St Univ; Sp-Lang Path, ISD #879, **SLP**

Judge, Mrs Annette Foreman 4909 Yale Street #B, Metairie, LA 70006, (504) 455-4878, BA 84 Univ of Southwestern LA; MS 86 Univ of Southwestern LA; 88–Sp-Lang Path, Psy Cog Associates, **SLP**

Judge, Mrs Jean 3831 Bailey Avenue, New York, NY 10463, (914) 949-9300, BA 77 CUNY - Hunter Coll; MS 78 Columbia Univ Teachers Coll; ME 79 Columbia Univ Teachers Coll; Sp-Lang Path, Westchester Assoc/Ret Citizens, **SLP**

Judge, Mrs Pamela Monroe 832 Rill Drive, Altamonte Springs, FL 32714, BS 79 East Carolina Univ; MA 83 Univ of Central FL; Sp-Lang Path, Seminole County School Board, **SLP ACE**

Judge, Robert D P O Box 581, Estero, FL 33928, **SLP**

Judice, Donna Felecia 782 Magnolia Woods Drive, Baton Rouge, LA 70808, (504) 922-5400, **SLP**

Judice, Kathy Theriot 1087 Southwest 28th Avenue, Boynton Beach, FL 33426, (305) 272-5445, BS 81 Saint Mary's Dominican Coll; MS 83 Univ of Southwestern LA; Sp-Lang Path, Palm Beach Co Sch Bd, **SLP**

Judkins, Mary Gold 2695 Stephens Road, Boulder, CO 80303, (303) 427-8484, BA 75 Univ of CO - Boulder; MS 77 Univ of OR; Sp-Lang Path, Rivendell Sch, **SLP**

Judkowitz, Mrs Helen F 18 Canterbury Way, Morristown, NJ 07960-3606, (203) 938-2519, BA 74 CUNY - Queens Coll; MA 75 Hofstra Univ; 88–Sp-Lang Path, Bernards Township Pub Sch, **SLP**

Judkowitz, Mrs Joyce Palefsky 10900 Gaynor Avenue, Granada Hills, CA 91344, BS 78 SUNY - Center at Albany; ME 81 Coll of Saint Rose; Sp-Lang Path, LA Sch Dist, **SLP**

Judlo, Jodi 1040 Lake Shore Drive #6A, Chicago, IL 60611, **SLP**

Judson, Mrs Dee Anne Barker 4534 Lorenzo Lane #516, Stockton, CA 95207, (209) 474-2844, BA 86 San Diego St Univ; MA 86 Univ of the Pacific

Judy, Joanna Michele 152 West Rockrimmon Boulevard #201, Colorado Springs, CO 80919, (719) 260-8559, BS 81 WV Univ; MA 83 Univ of MD - College Park; 88–Sp-Lang Path, InSpeech Inc, **SLP**

Juedes, Mrs Elizabeth Route 1 Box 217, Unity, WI 54488, (715) 683-2414, BS 72 Univ of WI - Madison; MS 76 Univ of WI - Stevens Point; Sp-Lang Path, Sch Dist of Marshfield, **SLP**

Juelich, Margaret Fritsch Washington Univ Medical School, Division Of Audiology, 517 South Euclid, St Louis, MO 63110, (314) 362-7489, BS 77 Saint Louis Univ; MS 79 Southern IL Univ-Edwardsvill; Aud, WA U Med Sch, **A**

Juengerman, Paula J 610 Eastcliff Drive, Euless, TX 76039, (817) 268-2010, BA 50 East TX St Univ - Commerce; MS 64 East TX St Univ - Commerce; Lrng Dis / Tchr, Hurst-Euless-Bedford Sch Dist, **SLP**

Juenke, Dorothy Ebersole 7750 Pipers Lane #104, San Antonio, TX 78251, (512) 532-9610, BA 69 Capital Univ; MA 71 Univ of Cincinnati; Sp-Lang Path, Northside ISD, **SLP**

Juergens, Mrs Karen Joy 895 Lake Forest Drive, Lake Oswego, OR 97034, (619) 747-6933, **SLP**

Juffer, Mary Jane Rural Route 6, Decorah, IA 52101, (319) 382-2672, BA 65 Univ of MO - Columbia; MS 68 Univ of KS; SLP, Mary Jane Juffer, **SLP**

Julian, Mrs Betty R P O Box 321, Goose Creek, SC 29455, (803) 569-1037, BA 73 Univ of SC - Columbia; OM 76 Univ of SC - Columbia; 87–Dir-SLP Svcs, Manor Care Nursing Ctr, **SLP**

Julian, Mrs Cynthia C 775 Tannery Drive, Wayne, PA 19087, (215) 783-6010, **SLP**

Julian, Mrs R Marlene 4640 Venturi Lane, Fort Collins, CO 80525, (303) 669-3940, BS CO St Univ; MS 85 CO St Univ; 85–Sp-Lang Path, Thompson Sch Dist R-2J, **SLP**

Juliano, Mrs Ethel D 16056 Givliano Place, Fontana, CA 92335, (714) 875-3000, BS 56 SUNY - Coll at Fredonia; MA 64 Loma Linda Univ - Loma Linda; **SLP**

Juliano, Mrs Janice Jerris 376 West Delavan Avenue, Buffalo, NY 14213, (716) 881-2266, MS 81 Univ of South FL; Sp-Lang Path, West Seneca Dev Cen, **SLP**

Julien, Joan E 24-6 Woodlake Road, Albany, NY 12203, (716) 473-5150, BS 70 SUNY - Coll at Fredonia; MS 71 SUNY - Coll at Geneseo; **SLP**

Julien, Mrs Judith Rae 19832 North 47th Avenue, Glendale, AZ 85308, (602) 582-8454, BS 78 Northern AZ Univ; MS 84 Northern AZ Univ; 82–Sp-Lang Path, Alhambra Elem Sch Dist, **SLP**

Julis, Thelma R 12 Milford Lane, Suffern, NY 10901, (914) 357-8439, BA 51 CUNY - Brooklyn Coll; MA 53 CUNY - Hunter Coll; Sp-Lang Path, Private Practice, **SLP**

Jumonville, Lynn Chisholm 24 Walker Street, Somerville, MA 02144, (617) 745-2100, BA 80 Univ of Central FL; MS 87 Boston Univ; Sp-Lang Path, North Shore Childrens Hosp

Jump, Jill Ellen 7750 Spicewood Lane, Cincinnati, OH 45255, (513) 932-4293, BS 79 OH Univ - Athens; MA 85 Univ of Cincinnati; SLP, Redwood Sch&Rehabilitation Ctr, **SLP**

Jumper, Mrs Eleshia Geno 509 Washington Street, Bonneville, MS 38829, (601) 728-4632, BS 80 MS Univ for Women; MS 83 Univ of MS; Sp/Lang Path, Prentiss County Schs, **SLP**

Jumper, Mrs Martha Melinda Rte 8 Box 757U, Pine Bluff, AR 71602-9448, (501) 247-9313, BA 82 Univ of MS; MS 84 Univ of MS; Audiologist, Jenkins Memorial Ctr, **A**

Junak, Shelly Ann 4807 Morton Road, New Bern, NC 28562, (919) 559-5281, BS 83 Northern MI Univ; MA 84 Northern MI Univ; 88–Sp-Lang Path, East Carolina Univ, **SLP**

Juneau, Cynthia Cheek 75 Ragan Drive, Alexandria, LA 71303, (318) 473-8415, BA 83 LA Tech Univ; MA 85 LA St Univ - Baton Rouge; 88–Sp-Lang Path, Assoc Healthfocus of LA, **SLP**

Jung, Mrs Cynthia Farkas 2107 East 4th Street, Duluth, MN 55812, (218) 724-8124, BA 80 Cleveland St Univ; MS 82 Purdue Univ - West Lafayette; 88–Aud, Mariner Med Clinic Ltd, **A**

Jung, Marjorie D 13 Hampton Court, Bristol, CT 06010, (203) 582-6215, **A**

Jungemann, Susan Elaine 2005 16th Street #C, Rock Valley, IA 51247, (712) 476-2743, BS 84 Northern St Coll; MS 86 Murray St Univ; SLP, AEA #4

Junker, Mrs Carolyn W 218 Pennsylvania Blvd, Pittsburgh, PA 15228, (412) 343-3834, BA 52 Univ of Cincinnati; MS 57 Univ of Pittsburgh - Pittsburgh; Offi Admin, Ch Aud, Pittsburgh Otol Assn, **A**

Junkins,, Robert William, Jr P O Box 1243, Drexel, NC 28619, (704) 433-2754, BS 82 Northeastern Univ; MA 87 Appalachian St Univ; 87–Sp-Lang Path, Western Carolina Center, **SLP**

Juntunen, Janet K Memorial School, Salisbury, MA 01952, (508) 462-2562, MS 70 Univ of NC - Chapel Hill; Sp-Lang Path, Salisbury Mem Sch, **SLP**

Juntunen, Lynn 179 East Little Canada Rd, Apartment 321, St Paul, MN 55117, (612) 481-0535, BS 83 Univ of MN - Duluth; MS 84 Univ of WI - Eau Claire; Sp-Lang Path, Metro Med Cen, **SLP**

Jupiter, Dr Tina Z 20 West 86th Street, New York, NY 10024, (212) 724-7294, BA 68 CUNY - Brooklyn Coll; MA 72 CUNY - Hunter Coll; PH 82 (NS) Columbia Univ Teachers Coll; Dir of Clin Svcs, Lexington Hrng & Sp Cen, **A**

Jurado-Hilton, Antoinette 224 Pond Street, Hopkinton, MA 01748, (617) 435-5507, BA 75 Univ of CO - Boulder; MA 79 Univ of CO - Boulder; 88 Sp Lang Path, Holliston HS, **SLP**

Jurecka, Joanne W 150 Glendale Avenue, Toronto, ON, Canada M6R 2T2, (416) 530-1094, BA 67 Univ of TX - Austin; MA 79 Univ of OR; 79–Sp-Lang Path, Private Practice, **SLP**

Jurey, Ruth A Advance-ability, PO Box 12, Carnelian Bay, CA 95711, (916) 546-2702, BA 71 Univ of Redlands; MS 72 Univ of Redlands; 77–Sp-Lang Path, Advance-ability, **SLP**

Jurgens-Haberlack, Mrs Cheryl Ann 2426 20th Avenue South #308K, Fargo, ND 58103, (701) 237-6424, BA 85 Univ of ND; MS 87 Univ of ND

Jurgill, Carol A Route 42 P O Box 1393, Centralia, PA 17927, (717) 875-2331, BS 75 Bloomsburg Univ of PA; ME 76 Bloomsburg Univ of PA; Resource Rm Tchr, Mt Carmel Area Sch Dist, **SLP**

Jurikson-Hankin, Helene Beth P O Box 12, Erwinna, PA 18920-0012, (609) 586-1979, ME 84 Trenton St Coll

Jurkowitz, Mrs Chaya B 6841 East Fieldstone Lane, Tucson, AZ 85715, (602) 721-0735, BA 68 OH Univ - Athens; MA 70 Univ of AZ; Sp-Lang Path, Tucson USD, **SLP**

Jury, Mrs Vernice Liljenberg 3 Egypt Road, Ellington, CT 06029, (203) 875-5733, BA 64 Saint Cloud St Univ; MA 66 Univ of CT; 87–Sp-Lang Path, Ellington CT PS, **SLP**

Juskie, Mrs Dorothy Bartosh 1531 Solway Court, Apopka, FL 32712, (407) 880-0196, BS 75 Governors St Univ; MS 77 Governors St Univ; 86–Sp-Lang Path, Orange County PS, **SLP**

Juskowitz, Susan 42 San Benito Way, Novato, CA 94945, (415) 892-9326, BA 75 SUNY - Center at Buffalo; MA 77 Univ of CA - Santa Barbara; MA 84 San Francisco St Univ; Program Mgr, Marin Co Offi of Ed, **SLP**

Just, Lynn B 2404 Valley Vista, Louisville, KY 40205, (812) 282-4381, BS 72 Murray St Univ; MS 73 Murray St Univ; **SLP**

Justen, Mary Sandra P O Box 3286, State University, AR 72467, (501) 972-1036, BS AR St Univ; OM 85 AR St Univ; **SLP**

Juster, Mrs Suzanne F 6587 Racquet Club Drive, Lauderhill, FL 33319, (305) 485-0905, BA 48 Russell Sage Coll; MA 49 SUNY - Center at Albany; Dir, S FL Sp/Lang Cen, **SLP**

Justice, Ann L 105 Real Road #I, Bakersfield, CA 93309, (805) 845-3719, BS 77 Marquette Univ; MS 78 Marquette Univ; 78–Sp-Lang Path, Kern Co Supt of Sch, **SLP**

Justice, Mrs Brenda Sue P O Box 1255, Pineville, WV 24874, (304) 732-7689, BS 80 Edinboro Univ of PA; MS 85 Radford Univ; 80–Sp-Lang Path, WY Co Bd of Educ, **SLP**

Justice, Mrs Frances L 430 Cypress Creek, Collinsville, IL 62234, (314) 868-5330, BS 72 Southern IL Univ -Carbondale; MS 76 Southern IL Univ -Carbondale; Sp-Lang Path, Spec Dis of St Louis Co Mo, **SLP**

Justice, Kathryn P 6147 Lakota Drive, Cincinnati, OH 45243, (513) 369-2474, BS 75 OH Univ - Athens; MA 76 Univ of TN - Knoxville; Dir/SLP & Audiology, The Christ Hospital, **SLP**

Justice, Natalie R R #1 Box 119, Hennepin, IL 61327, (815) 882-2496, BS 84 Univ of IL - Urbana; MA 86 Univ of IL - Urbana; **A**

Justice, Mrs Suzanne M 2820 Huntington Drive, Peoria, IL 61614, (309) 346-6013, BS 68 Bradley Univ; MA 70 Bradley Univ; Sp-Lang Path, U of IL /Coll of Med at Peoria, **SLP**

Justice-Brown, Mrs Joan L 205 Fairoaks Drive, Modesto, CA 95351, (209) 572-2505, BA 76 CA St Univ - Stanislaus; MA 79 CA St Univ - Stanislaus; 88–Sp-Lang Path, Strand-Kelley Sp Path, **SLP**

Justinger, Judith A 750 South Fork Drive, River Falls, WI 54022, (715) 246-6991, BS 70 Univ of WI - LA Crosse; OM 80 Univ of WI - River Falls; Sp-Lang Path, St Croix Co Hlth Cen, **SLP**

Juston, Loretta Adele 8224 Burholme Avenue, Philadelphia, PA 19111-1842, (215) 886-9500, BA 74 Carnegie-Mellon Univ; ME 77 Beaver Coll; MA 88 Temple Univ; 85–Sp-Lang Path, Sch Dist of Cheltenham

Justus, Molly Ann Soifer Goldenberg & Associates, 111 West First Street Suite 1000, Dayton, OH 45402, (513) 223-1234, BS 73 Marquette Univ; MA 74 Bowling Green St Univ; Aud, Nathaniel Soifer MD & Assoc, **A**

Jylkka, Margaret 1720 Republic Road, Silver Spring, MD 20902, (202) 466-7747, BA 70 Catholic Univ of America; MS 73 Gallaudet Coll; Aud, Feldman-Hausfeld Otolaryn Ass, **A**

K

Kaatz, Kathryn J P O Box 420, Redondo Beach, CA 90277-0420, BS 79 Univ of WI - Madison; MS 81 Univ of WI - Milwaukee; SLP, Long Beach USD, **SLP**

Kabaker, Mrs Barbara S 2805 Lexington Lane, Highland Park, IL 60035, (312) 433-6631, BS 68 Miami Univ - Oxford; MS 69 Univ of MI - Ann Arbor; Sp-Lang Path, Private Practice, **SLP**

Kabat, Deborah G 10 Pearl Street, Oneonta, NY 13820, (518) 462-6222, BS 75 SUNY - Coll at Brockport; ME 77 Nazareth Coll of Rochester; **SLP**

Kabatchnick, Ruth Karen 8139 Crabapple Lane, Gaithersburg, MD 20879, (301) 977-8411, BS 80 Univ of MD - College Park; MA 86 Univ of MD - College Park; 86–Sp-Lang Path, Montgomery Co PS, **SLP**

Kabath, Mrs Ellen 115 Lake Shore Drive, Lake Parsippany, NJ 07054, (201) 335-6006, BA 78 CUNY - Queens Coll; MA 79 CUNY - Queens Coll; Aud, N Jersey ENT & Hrng Ctr, **A**

Kaber, Dinneen L 6860 East 10th Street, Long Beach, CA 90815, (213) 596-0231, BA 78 Univ of WA; MS 80 Univ of WA; Sp-Lang Path, Dept of Defense Depedents Sch, **SLP**

Kach, Stacey Rabin 35 Summit Avenue, Port Chester, NY 10573, BS 80 SUNY - Coll at Geneseo; MA 81 Ball St Univ; Sp-Lang Path, Hallen School, **SLP**

Kachel, Robin B 2 The Glenada, Roslyn Estates, NY 11576, (516) 621-1606, BA 74 CUNY - Queens Coll; MA 86 Long Island U - CW Post Ctr; 86–Sp-Lang Path, Lowell Sch, **SLP**

Kacmarynski, Mrs Judith A 10571 Highlawn Court, Cedarburg, WI 53012, (414) 377-6105, BS 67 Marquette Univ; MS 74 Univ of WI - Milwaukee; Sp-Lang Path, Grafton Public Schools, **SLP**

Kaczmarek, Monica Carin 53 East Rocks Road, Norwalk, CT 06851, (203) 846-0926, BS 85 Ithaca Coll; MS 87 Rutgers St Univ -N Brunswick; 87–Sp-Lang Path, The Norwalk Bd of Educ, **SLP**

Kaczor, Kathy E R R 3 Box 255A, Freeport, ME 04032, (207) 775-4000, BS 81 Southern CT St Univ; MA 82 MI St Univ; Sp/Lang Path, New England Rehab Hosp, **SLP**

Kaczor-Czech, Bonita Marie 17491 Loranger, Mount Clemens, MI 48044, (313) 286-0587, MA 79 Wayne St Univ; SLP, Detroit Pub Sch, **SLP**

Kaczuk, Mrs Priscilla A 6454 Woodbury Drive, Solon, OH 44139, BS 68 Bowling Green St Univ; MA 83 Bowling Green St Univ; 87–Sp-Lang Path, Cuyahoga Co Bd of Mental Ret, **SLP**

Kadas, Thelma E 6800 Wydown Boulevard, c/o Fontbonne College Lib, St Louis, MO 63105, (314) 544-4224, BS 76 Fontbonne Coll; MA 77 Saint Louis Univ; Asst Prof Superv, Fontbonne Coll, **SLP**

Kadavy, Julie Rice 9806 Belfair Road, Bellevue, WA 98004, (206) 455-9775, BA 79 Stanford Univ; MA 81 Univ of IA; **SLP**

Kaderavek, Joan N 234 West 7th Street, Perrysburg, OH 43551, (419) 241-6219, BA 75 Miami Univ - Oxford; MA 77 OH St Univ; Prog Dev Coord, Toledo Hearing & Speech Center, **SLP**

Kadijevic, Vojislav Hearing Center, 631 Blomfield Avenue, Montclair, NJ 07042, (201) 744-2495, MS 71 Seton Hall Univ; Aud, Hearing Center, **A**

Kadin, Mrs Shelly M 5 Kimberly Drive, East Northport, NY 11731, (516) 368-4813, BA 76 CUNY - Queens Coll; MA 77 Hofstra Univ; Sp-Lang Path, Bldg Blks Develop Pre-School, **SLP**

Kadison, Jerilyn G 72 East Maple Street, Teaneck, NJ 07666, (914) 354-8917, BS 69 NY Univ; MA 70 NY Univ; Sp/Lang Path, Jerilyn Kadison MacCc, **SLP**

Kadulski, Mrs Jane W 1250 Circle Drive, Green Bay, WI 54304, (414) 336-1421, BS 77 Univ of WI - Stevens Point; MS 78 Univ of WI - Stevens Point; Sp-Lang Path, Sch Dist of Depere, **SLP**

Kaelin, Charlotte 2407 Meadow Drive, Louisville, KY 40218, BS 70; ME 71; Sp-Lang Path, Jefferson Co Bd of Ed, **SLP**

Kaemmerle, Ann W Otolaryngology Clinic F4/214, University Of Wisconsin Hospital, 600 Highland Avenue, Madison, WI 53792, (608) 263-6197, BA 73 Wichita St Univ; MS 75 Univ of AZ; Aud, Univ of Wisconsin Hosp, **A**

Kaetzel, Esther B 980 Howard Street, Des Plaines, IL 60018, (312) 283-8805, BA 70 Augustana Coll; MS 75 Bradley Univ; Sp-Lang Path, Visiting Nurse Assoc of Chicago, **SLP**

Kafer, Joan Desrochers 16631 North 56th Street, Apartment 2050, Scottsdale, AZ 85254, (602) 263-7131, BA 84 WA St Univ; MS 86 Univ of AZ; 88–Aud, St Joseph's Hosp, **A**

Kaffee, Mrs Jacqueline 427 Faletti Circle, River Vale, NJ 07675, (201) 573-8853, BS 73 NY Univ; MA 75 CUNY - Lehman Coll; **SLP**

Kaffel, Joyce W 22 Silver Spring Road, Short Hills, NJ 07078, (201) 376-5246, **SLP**

Kafkafi, Ilana 7002 Boulevard East #219B, Guttenberg, NJ 07093, (201) 731-3600, MA 74 Univ of MD - College Park; Kessler Inst For Rehabilitation, **SLP**

Kafoure, Dory Rigopoulos 17941 Aguamiel Road, San Diego, CA 92127, **SLP**

Kafton-Minkel, Carol 3425 N E 18th, Portland, OR 97212, (503) 280-6244, BA 74 San Francisco St Univ; MS 83 Portland St Univ; Sp-Lang Path, Portland Pub Sch, **SLP**

Kagan, Laurie 1475 South Quebec Way, Apartment B-11, Denver, CO 80231, (303) 861-3359, BA 70 Univ of MI - Ann Arbor; MS 71 Univ of WI - Madison; OM 87 Univ of CO - Denver; Fin Analyst, Kaiser Permanente of Co, **SLP**

Kagan, Marcia 21722 SE 28th Street, Issaquah, WA 98027, (206) 391-8717, BA 72 Hofstra Univ; MS 86 Southern OR St Coll; **SLP**

Kagan, Sara B 5100 Highbridge Street, Apartment 52E, Fayetteville, NY 13066, (315) 637-0349, BS 78 Univ of Cincinnati; MA 80 Univ of Cincinnati; **A**

Kagel, Mrs Marion C 410 Clearview Avenue, Wilmington, DE 19809, (215) 447-2428, BS 70 Old Dominion Univ; MA 74 Temple Univ; Ch of Sp-Lang Path Serv, Crozer-Chester Med Cen, **SLP**

Kagy, Jane E 6450 Stoneham Place, Cincinnati, OH 45236, (513) 793-9309, BS 74 Bowling Green St Univ; MA 80 Bowling Green St Univ; Sp/Lang Path, Private Practice, **SLP**

Kahalley, Barbara Jean 200 Pensacola Beach Road, Apartment G-1, Gulf Breeze, FL 32561, (904) 434-4957, BS 84 Univ of South AL; MS 86 Univ of South AL; Sp-Lang Path, Baptist Hosp, **SLP**

Kahan, Mrs Candace R 120 White Oaks Drive, Longmeadow, MA 01106, (413) 567-3993, BA 68 SUNY - Center at Buffalo; ME 70 Northeastern Univ; **SLP**

Kahan, Candace Wice 4818 Park Boulevard #2, Oakland, CA 94602, (415) 748-4072, BS 73 Kent St Univ; MA 80 Humboldt St Univ; Sp-Lang Path, Alameda USD, **SLP**

Kahane, Denise H 1705 Avenue X, Brooklyn, NY 11235, (718) 851-3700, BA 75 SUNY - Coll at Plattsburgh; MA 76 MI St Univ; 86–Aud, Metro Jewish Geriatric Ctr, **A**

Kahane, Dr Joel C 5337 Laurie Lane, Memphis, TN 38119, (901) 525-2682, BA 69 CUNY - Brooklyn Coll; MS 72 CUNY - Brooklyn Coll; PH 75 (Biocommunication) Univ of Pittsburgh - Pittsburgh; Assoc Prof-Dept/Aud & Sp-Lang Path, Memphis St U, **SLP**

Kahansky, Karen 10 Pitfield Road, Agincourt, ON, Canada M1S 1X7, (416) 654-9616, BA 81 Univ of Toronto - Ontario; MA 82 SUNY - Center at Buffalo; Aud, Private Practice, **A**

Kahgan, Arnold 318 East 70th Street, New York, NY 10021, (212) 772-1117, Self Employed, **A**

Kahl, W Bailey 92 Billings Drive, Dover, DE 19901, (302) 736-5376, BS 62 OH Univ - Athens; MS 66 Washington Univ; MA 73 Northwestern Univ; Sp-Lang Path, Off Sp-Lang & Hrng Del Pub Hl, **SLP A**

Kahlenberg-Picciano, Trudi 9628 72nd Road, Forest Hills, NY 11375, (718) 793-3128, BS 82 Northwestern Univ; MA 84 Northwestern Univ; Sp-Lang Path, Stepping Stone Day Sch, **SLP**

Kahler, Linda B 485 North Wellwood Avenue, Lindenhurst, NY 11757, (516) 321-3136, BA 71 SUNY - Coll at New Paltz; MS 75 SUNY - Center at Albany; Sp-Lang Path, W Babylon Sch Dist, **SLP**

Kahler, Mrs Sally A 5749 Chancellor Boulevard, Vancouver, BC, Canada V6T 1E4, (604) 222-4929, BA 71 Allegheny Coll; MA 73 Catholic Univ of America; **SLP**

Kahn, Adrienne L 20515 East Country Club Dr, Apartment 1142 Tower 2, North Miami Beach, FL 33180, (305) 932-4805, **SLP**

Kahn, Dr Alice R 44 Providence Drive #77, Fairfield, OH 45014, (513) 529-2500, BA 68 LA Tech Univ; MA 69 Univ of Houston - Univ Park; PH 84 (NS) Memphis St Univ; Asst Professor of Sp-Lang Path, Miami University, **SLP**

Kahn, Mrs Alison P Scripps Clinic, 15025 Innovation Drive, San Diego, CA 92128, (619) 487-1800, BA 77 Washington Univ; MA 82 San Diego St Univ; Aud, Scripps Cl Rancho Bernardo, **A**

Kahn, Mrs Andrea Port 5580 S W 8th Street, Plantation, FL 33317, (305) 581-2268, BA 68 Adelphi Univ; MA 69 Case Western Reserve Univ; Sp-Lang Path, Private Practice, **SLP ACE**

Kahn, Ange 228 Frederick, Athens, GA 30607-1602, (404) 354-3025, BA 71 Univ of NC - Chapel Hill; MA 74 Univ of OK - Norman; Sp-Lang Path, St Mary's Hosp Home Hlth Care Svcs, **SLP**

Kahn, Barbara 5005 Newport Avenue, Bethesda, MD 20816, (301) 320-2084, BA 68 George Washington Univ; MA 70 3912; **SLP**

Kahn, Betti E 155 West Washington Lane, Apartment H-4, Jenkintown, PA 19046, (215) 884-5661, BS 72 Temple Univ; MS 79 Marywood Coll; ME 85 Trenton St Coll; 86–Sp-Lang Path, Phila Bd of Educ, **SLP**

Kahn, Mrs Deborah Ann 817 Cherry, Big Rapids, MI 49307, (616) 796-3543, BS 69 Univ of IL - Urbana; MA 71 Northern IL Univ - De Kalb; MA 84 Central MI Univ; Sp-Lang Path/Tchr of Pre-Primary Impaired, Mecosta-Osceola ISD, **SLP**

Kahn, Mrs Debra W 210 Winne Road, Delmar, NY 12054, (518) 456-3771, BA 70 SUNY - Center at Albany; MS 72 SUNY - Center at Albany; Sp-Lang Path, Guilderland Central Schools, **SLP**

Kahn, Mrs Denise J 755 West Bigbeaver, Suite 404, Troy, MI 48084, (313) 362-4299, BS 76 Wayne St Univ; MA 77 Wayne St Univ; Dir, Medi-Sp Svc Inc, **SLP**

Kahn, Dr Gerri Division Of Developmental Disabilities, University Of Iowa, Iowa City, IA 52242, (319) 356-1168, BA 66 Temple Univ; MA 68 Univ of IA; PH 74 (Psychoacoustics) Univ of IA; Aud, Univ Hosp Sch Univ of Iowa, **A**

Kahn, Helen J P O Box 1957, Fargo, ND 58107, (218) 299-4213, BA 76 San Francisco St Univ; MA 80 San Jose St Univ; PH 88 (Psychology) Univ of ND; 87–Lecturer-Psych, Concordia Coll, **SLP**

Kahn, Janet S 2720 Banquos Trl, Pensacola, FL 32503, (904) 433-4681, BS 76 PA St Univ - Univ Park; MS 79 FL St Univ; Aud, Dr Donald R Todd, **A**

Kahn, Joan Herman 88-21 69th Road, Forest Hills, NY 11375, (718) 263-2041, **SLP**

Kahn, Mary Kay 3556 Georgetown Road, Roanoke, VA 24018, (703) 362-1656, BA 83 Southeastern LA Univ; MS 85 Univ of TX - Dallas; Sp-Lang Path, Easter Seal Soc of VA, **SLP**

Kahn, Melanie Susan 3815 Eleanor Drive, Mohegan Lake, NY 10547, (914) 528-4608, BS 81 Ithaca Coll; MS 84 Northeastern Univ; Sp-Lang Path, Putnan/Northern BOCES, **SLP**

Kahn, Dr Nancy T 21382 Fleet Lane, Huntington Beach, CA 92646, (213) 625-4183, BS 53 Univ of IL - Urbana; MA 66 CA St Univ - Los Angeles; PH 78 Univ of CA - Los Angeles; Sp-Lang Path, Los Angeles USD, **SLP**

Kahn, Robin Sue 333 East 43rd Street #917, New York, NY 10017, (212) 360-3726, BS 82 Boston Univ; MS 85 Columbia Univ Teachers Coll; 87–Sp-Lang Path, Terence Cardinal Cooke Health Care Center, **SLP**

Kahne, Mrs Lenore B 17 Ellis Drive, Syosset, NY 11791, (516) 496-8573, BA 74 SUNY - Coll at Cortland; MS 77 Adelphi Univ; SLP, Rainbow Presch of Suffolk Co, **SLP**

Kahoud, Mrs Judith L 3 Lyman Road, West Hartford, CT 06117, (203) 282-3364, BA 69 Adelphi Univ; MS 71 Adelphi Univ; Sp-Lang Path, E Hartford Pu Sch, **SLP**

Kahre, Mrs Vina Maureen Route 1 Box 78AA, Lockwood, MO 65682, (417) 232-4914, BS 75 Southeast MO St Univ; MA 86 Southeast MO St Univ; Sp-Lang Path, Lockwood R-1, **SLP**

Kahrs, Catherine 107 Bronwen Court, Goose Creek, SC 29445, BA 70 Winthrop Coll; MA 75 Univ of NC - Chapel Hill; **SLP**

Kahrs, Sharon Girardey R R 1 Box 95-A, Kent, CT 06757-9709, (203) 927-3023, BA 75 East Carolina Univ; MA 76 Univ of TN - Knoxville; Consult, Private Practice, **SLP**

Kail, Sandra L 3915 Paseo Del Prado, Boulder, CO 80301, (303) 441-1020, BA 67 CA St Univ - Northridge; BA 74 CA St Univ - Long Beach; MA 76 CA St Univ - Long Beach; Sp-Lang Path, Developmental Disabilities Cen, **SLP**

Kainrath, Marilyn Joyce 115 Cool Creek Boulevard, Apartment 8, Carmel, IN 46032, (317) 456-5635, BS 85 Purdue Univ - West Lafayette; MS 87 IN St Univ - Terre Haute; **SLP**

Kaires, Patti Lee 16677 IDA Center Road, Petersburg, MI 49270, (313) 341-1353, BA 83 Univ of Toledo; MA 85 Wayne St Univ - Sch of Med; **A**

Kaiser, Holle Aungst Ottawa Hearing Center, 417 West Madison Suite 101B, Ottawa, IL 61350, (815) 434-2244, BS 79 Ashland Coll; MA 81 Univ of Akron; Audiologist, Private Practice, **A**

Kaiser, Holly W 2415 Oregon Street, Berkeley, CA 94705, (415) 548-5660, BA 76 MI St Univ; MA 77 Central MI Univ; Sp-Lang Path, Private Practice, **SLP**

Kaiser, Paula Lynn Route 1 Box 54, Linville, VA 22834, (703) 943-6604, BS 62 Case Western Reserve Univ; MS 70 SUNY - Coll at Buffalo; 81–Dir of Lift Prog for Infants, Valley Comm Sers Bd, **SLP**

Kaji, Mrs Agnes O 7230 Woodrow Drive, Oakland, CA 94611-1435, (415) 339-1696, MS; **SLP A**

Kakuska, Mrs Frances W 2914 North Bay Shore Dr, La Crosse, WI 54603, (608) 782-7300, BS 67 Marquette Univ; MS 79 Univ of WI - Eau Claire; SLP-Dept of Neur, Lacrosse Luth Hosp/Gundersen Clin, **SLP ACE**

Kalas, Beth Hoffman 421 North Merrill Street, Park Ridge, IL 60068, (312) 318-0873, BA 79 Valparaiso Univ; MS 80 IN St Univ - Terre Haute; Aud, Gordon J Siegel MD, **A ACE**

Kalash, Mrs Sharon U 315 Crescent Drive, Thompson, ND 58278, (701) 780-2447, BA 69 Univ of ND; MA 70 Univ of ND; Sp-Lang Path, Med Center Rehab Hosp, **SLP**

Kalashian, Verjene Eileen 1016 Ripple, Pacific Grove, CA 93950, (408) 424-0654, BA 77 Univ of the Pacific; MA 80 Whittier Coll

Kalb, Mrs Madelyn G 11 Danemar Drive, Middletown, NJ 07748, (201) 530-9270, MS 74 Southern CT St Univ; Sp-Lang Path, Private Practice, **SLP**

Kalb, Marti B 1457 Old Tale Road, Boulder, CO 80303-1323, (303) 444-0119, BA 65 Baker Univ; MA 77 Univ of KS; Sp/Lang Path, Adams County District #12, **SLP**

Kalberer, Ann Elizabeth 555 North 30th Street, Omaha, NE 68131, (402) 449-6650, BS 80 Purdue Univ - West Lafayette; MS 82 Purdue Univ - West Lafayette; Aud, Boys Town Natl I for Commun Di, **A**

Kalbfleisch, Kathleen E P O Box 15612, San Francisco, CA 94115, (415) 397-2835, BA 51 Denison Univ, MA 53 Univ of IA; 59–Aud, Private Practice, **A**

Kaldor, Mrs Cindy O 7281 Pineview Lane, Maple Grove, MN 55369, (612) 574-0397, BS 80 IA St Univ; MA 82 Univ of KS; SLP, Anoka-Hennipin Schls, **SLP**

Kalec, Ann Elizabeth 7506 Westview Lane, Woodridge, IL 60517, (312) 910-3389, BA 85 MI St Univ; MA 87 Northwestern Univ; 88–Sp-Lang Path, Rehab Inst of Chicago, **SLP**

Kaleita, Dr Annette M 244 7th Street, California, PA 15419, (412) 938-4387, ME 60 Duquesne Univ; MA 62 Northwestern Univ; ED 71 (Education) Univ of MD - College Park; Prof, CA U of Pa, **A**

Kalfuss, Dr Helene A 1506 Chico Circle, Palm Springs, CA 92264, (619) 327-8595, BS 63 Wayne St Univ - Sch of Med; ME 63 Wayne St Univ - Sch of Med; PH 68 (Sp Path) Wayne St Univ - Sch of Med; 72–Sp-Lang Path, Private Practice, **SLP**

Kalhan, Mrs Behroze E 2807 Thatcher Court, Bloomington, IN 47401-8467, (812) 339-8190, BS 68 T.N. Medical Coll - Bombay, India; MS 71 Univ of OK Medical Center; 88–Sp-Lang Path, InSpeech Inc, **SLP**

Kalik, Barbara G 100 East Hartsdale Avenue, Apartment 6AW, Hartsdale, NY 10530, BA 72 CUNY - Lehman Coll; MS 74 Columbia Univ Teachers Coll; Spec Ed Tchr, NYC Bd of Ed, **SLP**

Kalin, George Audiology Service Inc, 363 South Cleveland Avenue, Hagerstown, MD 21740, (301) 790-3300, BS 68 Ball St Univ; MS 73 Univ of WI - Stevens Point; President, Aud Serv, Inc, **A**

Kalina, Andrea F 97 Cedarhurst Avenue #Qq, Cedarhurst, NY 11516, **SLP**

Kalina, Mrs Christine 16 Bedford Lane, North Kingstown, RI 02852, (401) 295-7921, BS 74 Southern IL Univ -Carbondale; MA 76 Northern IL Univ - De Kalb; Sp-Lang Path, Private Practice, **SLP**

Kalinka, Mrs Marian Quinn 105 North Busey #304, Urbana, IL 61801, (217) 337-6013, BS 86 Univ of IL - Urbana; MA 88 Univ of IL - Urbana; 88–Sp-Lang Path, United Samaritans Med Ctr

Kalinoski, Laurie A 1 Haven Court, Apt N-3D, Nyack, NY 10960, (914) 245-6023, **SLP**

Kalinosky, Mrs Sharon Marie 105 Edgevale Circle, Beaver Dam, WI 53916, (414) 887-7692, BS 83 Univ of WI - Madison; MS 85 Univ of WI - Madison; Sp-Lang Path, Private Practice, **SLP**

Kalinowski, Mrs Linda C 1602 Laurel Oaks, Richmond, TX 77469, (713) 342-8066, BA 74 Sam Houston St Univ; MA 81 Univ of Houston - Univ Park; Sp-Lang Path, Lamar Consolidated ISD, **SLP**

Kalish, Phylis L 89-11 63rd Drive #603, Rego Park, NY 11374, BA 77 CUNY - Queens Coll; MA 79 CUNY - Queens Coll; SLP, Bd of Ed NYC, **SLP**

Kaliski, Myra S 410 Lafayette Road, Harrington Park, NJ 07640, **SLP**

Kalix, Joan Smyrl 6220 North 5th Street, Philadelphia, PA 19120, (215) 548-5426, BS 75 PA St Univ - Univ Park; MA 79 Univ of CT; Priv Conslt, Communication Skills Inc, **SLP**

Kall, Mrs Maralyn Bettina 5620 Magda Court, Palmdale, CA 93550, (805) 944-3011, MA 83 CA St Univ - Los Angeles; SLP, Lancaster School District, **SLP**

Kalla, Mrs Barbara 5454 Guarino Road, Pittsburgh, PA 15217, (412) 441-1111, BS 82 Kent St Univ; MA 82 Kent St Univ; 83–Sp-Lang Path, Pace Sch, **SLP**

Kallail, Dr Ken James 807 Honeybrook, Derby, KS 67037, (316) 261-2607, BA 75 Wichita St Univ; MA 76 Wichita St Univ; PH 81 (NS) Univ of OK - OK City; Director of Research, Univ of Kansas-Sch of Med, **SLP**

Kallaus, Dan M P O Box 111, St Peter, MN 56082, (507) 931-3067, BA 78; MA 79; Aud Consult, S Cen Ecsu, **A**

Kallaus-Gay, Anne M Wendell Johnson Sp & Hrng Cntr, Hawkins Drive, University Of Iowa, Iowa City, IA 52242, (319) 353-5081, BA 78 Univ of IA; MA 79 Univ of IA; Clinical Supervisor, University of Iowa, **SLP**

Kallem, Ellen 11 Saul Place, Plainview, NY 11803, (516) 681-0289, BA 75 CUNY - Brooklyn Coll; MA 77 CUNY - Queens Coll; **SLP**

Kallen, Deborah 1610 Nme Tillamook Unit 2, Portland, OR 97212, (503) 282-1536, BA 72 CT Coll; MS 80 Portland St Univ; Dept Mgr-Sp-Lang Path, Holladay Park Hosp, **SLP**

Kallet, Mrs Adele M 803 Winding Way, Riverdale, NJ 07675-6140, MS 76 SUNY - Center at Albany; Sp-Lang Path, Ramsey Public Schools, **SLP**

Kallio, Pamela DeBoer 5308 South Lee Court, South Bend, IN 46614, (219) 237-6849, BA 70 Ball St Univ; MA 74 IN Univ - Bloomington; Sp-Lang Path, St Joseph's Med Ctr, **SLP**

Kallstrom, Rolfe D Box 11535, 8325 Maywood, Raytown, MO 64138, **SLP**

Kalman, Janet 1701 Rock Springs Drive, Apartment 1083, Las Vegas, NV 89128, (702) 739-7771, BS 72 Univ of TX - Austin; MA 74 Univ of TX - Austin; SLP, NV Easter Seals, **SLP**

Kalodoukas, Debra Economos 4712 Seminole Trail, Holiday, FL 34690, (813) 531-0457, BA 76 Univ of FL; OM 77 Auburn Univ - Auburn; SLP, Pinellas Co Sch Bd, **SLP**

Kalotkin, Madoline 18 Lake Shore Court, Brighton, MA 02135, **SLP**

Kaloustian, Houri Khatcher Children's Seashore House, 4100 Atlantic Avenue, Atlantic City, NJ 08401, (609) 347-6150, MA 85 Temple Univ-Tyler Sch of Art; 85–Sp-Lang Path, Children's Seashore House, **SLP**

Kalowsky, Leora B Box 821, Conyngham, PA 18219, (717) 788-3502, BA 69 MI St Univ; ME 75 Wayne St Univ; **SLP**

Kaltenborn, Arthur L, Jr 1370 Athena Drive, Kent, OH 44240, (216) 673-7642, BA 37 Coll of Wooster; MA 48 Northwestern Univ; **SLP LM**

Kaltenborn, J Dean 8 Rambo Road, Red Lion, PA 17356, (717) 244-1232, BS 63 Indiana Univ of PA; ME 69 PA St Univ - Univ Park; Sp-Lang Path, Easter Seal Soc York Co, **SLP**

Kalter, Mrs Carol Cepler 755 Westover Road, Stamford, CT 06902, (203) 357-1139, BA 67 Hofstra Univ; MS 68 Adelphi Univ; Sp-Lang Path, Private Practice, **SLP**

Kalter, Eleanor R 3440 Lebon Drive #4213, San Diego, CA 92122, (619) 452-0313, BS 79 Boston Univ; MA 83 Univ of MN - Minneap-St Paul; 88–Sp-Lang Path, NeuroCare, **SLP**

Kalweit, Linda M 22 Greenbrier Drive, Athens, OH 45701-3202, (618) 594-6455, BS 79 Central MI Univ; MA 81 Central MI Univ; Aud, Mankato Clinic LTD, **A**

Kam, Elizabeth Y F NE 1425 Valley Road #4, Pullman, WA 99163, (509) 332-4403, OB 84 Gonzaga Univ; MA 88 WA St Univ; 88–Sp-Lang Path, Lewiston-Clarkston Early Child Development Prog

Kam, Ernie K 500 Clark, Scott City, MO 63780, (314) 785-0131, BA 71; MA 74 Southeast MO St Univ; SLP, Butler Co Hlth Cen, **SLP**

Kam, Kellie W J 2755 Peter Street, Honolulu, HI 96816, (808) 737-3585, BS 83 Univ of HI - Manoa; MS 84 ID St Univ; Sp-Lang Path, Dept of Educ/Central, **SLP**

Kamaka, Mrs Anita Riebeling 1618 Burrows Street, San Francisco, CA 94134, (415) 239-1703, BA 56 San Francisco St Univ; MA 65 San Francisco St Univ; Sp-Lang Path, San Francisco USD, **SLP**

Kamalic, Linda J S 2939 Brighton 5th Street, Brooklyn, NY 11235, BS 67 Boston Univ; MS 68 Univ of WI - Madison; Sp-Lang/Educational Evaluator, New York City Bd Educ D22 Coh, **SLP**

Kamara, Dr Carol Anne 7314 Oskaloosa Drive, Derwood, MD 20855, (301) 990-0859, BS 63 OH Univ - Athens; MS 69 Univ of WI - Milwaukee; PH 74 OH Univ - Athens; **SLP A**

Kamber, Mrs Beverly F 16426 Septo Street, Sepulveda, CA 91343, (818) 997-2357, BA 60 Univ of CA - Los Angeles; SLP, LA USD, **SLP**

Kambic, Laura Esler 16829 South 93rd Avenue, Orland Hills, IL 60477, BS 85 IL St Univ - Normal; MA 86 Northern IL Univ - De Kalb; 86–Sp-Lang Path, UCP of Will Co, **SLP**

Kamdar, Aditi Vijay 20530 Anza Avenue #263, Torrance, CA 90503, (213) 370-4755, **SLP**

Kamen, Ruth Saletsky 5705 Brookstown Drive, Dallas, TX 75230, **SLP**

Kamer, Mrs Arlene R 116 Gail Drive, New Rochelle, NY 10805, (914) 235-7772, BA 57 CUNY - Hunter Coll; 88–Sp-Lang Path, Vol Amer Bronx Erly Lrng Ctr, **SLP**

Kamerman, Joan D 14737 Charter Road, Jamaica, NY 11435, (516) 338-4204, BA 72 CUNY - Queens Coll; MA 74 CUNY - Queens Coll; Sp/Lang Path, N Shore U Hosp Pre-Sch Dev Prg, **SLP**

Kamhi, Dr Alan G Dept Audiology & Speech Path, Memphis State University, 807 Jefferson Avenue, Memphis, TN 38105, (901) 525-2682, BA 72 Univ of WI - Madison; MA 76 IN Univ - Bloomington; PH 79 (Lang Development and Disorders) IN Univ - Bloomington; Assoc Prof, Memphis St U, **SLP**

Kamholz, Pamela Kay 2908 Panama, Carmichael, CA 95608, (916) 485-8706, BS 81 Northern AZ Univ; MS 83 Northern AZ Univ; Sp-Lang Path, Scottish Rite Clinic, **SLP**

Kamhoot, Judi Kaye 518-B Street, Salt Lake City, UT 84103, (801) 363-4104, BS 74 4556; MS 79 ID St Univ; PH 84 (NS) Univ of UT; Dir/Commun Dis, Holy Cross Hosp, **A**

Kamian, Colette Alice 3522 Gross Road, Santa Cruz, CA 95062, (408) 475-5382, BA 81 CA St Univ - Chico; MA 83 CA St Univ - Chico; SLP/Aud, Santa Cruz City Schools, **SLP**

Kamil, Mrs Eileen B 14 Brandywine Drive, Setauket, NY 11733, (516) 751-6122, BA 66 CUNY - Brooklyn Coll; MS 67 Univ of WI - Madison; 87–Sp-Lang Path, Shoreham-Wading River Sch Dist, **SLP**

Kamin, Alice M R 1655 Oakwood Drive #N-323, Penn Valley, PA 19072-1023, (215) 664-0224, MS 72 PA St Univ - Univ Park; BS 70 PA St Univ - Univ Park; Sp-Lang Path, Private Practice, **SLP**

Kaminaga, Gail Naomi 1154 Puu Poni Street, Pearl City, HI 96782, (808) 622-4123, BA 64 Univ of HI - Manoa; ME 82 Univ of HI - Manoa; Special Education Teacher, St of HI-Dept of Ed, **SLP**

Kaminetzky, Aviva L 328 Benner Street, Highland Park, NJ 08904, **SLP**

Kamino, Mrs Maureen Kay 5623 Fieldcrest Drive, Camarillo, CA 93010, (805) 654-2743, BA 78 Univ of CA - Santa Barbara; MA 83 CA St Univ - Fullerton; **SLP**

Kaminski, Mrs Sherri A 6593 Royal Parkway South, Lockport, NY 14094, (716) 434-4558, BA 78 SUNY - Center at Buffalo; MA 80 SUNY - Center at Buffalo; 80–Sp/Lang Path, Niagra Chld Educ of Trent Ctr, **SLP**

Kaminski, Mrs Susan Gold 4498 South Buffalo Road, Orchard Park, NY 14127, (716) 662-1334, BA 85 SUNY - Coll at Buffalo; MA 87 SUNY - Coll at Buffalo; 88–Sp-Lang Path, Erie 2 BOCES

Kaminski-Thorpe, Carol Ann 1519 Judith Drive, Yardley, PA 19067, (215) 321-0104, BS 79; MA 83; Sp-Lang Path, Sch Dist of Phila, **SLP**

Kaminsky, Barbara M 3470 Clare Cottage Trace, Marietta, GA 30060, (404) 439-1222, BS 71 Univ of GA; ME 74 Univ of GA; 74–Sp-Lang Path, Atlanta Cty Sch Syst, **SLP**

Kaminsky, Mrs Maryann P 9521 Heather Spring Drive, Richmond, VA 23233-4461, (804) 270-9462, BA 77 Longwood Coll; ME 78 Univ of VA - Charlottesville; **SLP**

Kamish, Stacey Jean 10 Piney Run Road, Rd 21, Medford, NJ 08055-9752, (609) 596-0060, BS 85 Univ of WI - River Falls; MA 87 Trenton St Coll

Kamitomo, Gail A 5503-108 Street, Edmonton, AB, Canada T6H 2Y8, (403) 432-6630, BS 74 Univ of Alberta - Alberta; MA 75 Univ of KS; Sp/Lang Path, U of Ab Hosp, **SLP**

Kamitses, Kim L 1373 Labella Avenue, Sunnyvale, CA 94087, (408) 736-3624, MA 85 San Jose St Univ; SLP, San Jose Hospital, **SLP**

Kamiyama, Dr Goro No 24 Isogodai 3-chome, Isogo-ku, Yokohama, Japan 235, 03-305-4976, DD 49 8142; MD 56 Univ of Tokyo - Japan; PH 63 (Stuttering) Wichita St Univ; 86–Dir, Karasuyama Medical Clinic

Kamke, Mrs Jo K N17W5191 Garfield Circle, Cedarburg, WI 53012, (414) 375-4176, BS 79 Marquette Univ; MS 81 Marquette Univ; 81–Sp-Lang Path, Therapy Assoc, **SLP**

Kamm, Dr Candace A Bell Communications Research, MRE 2E-256 Box 1910, 445 South Street, Morristown, NJ 07960-1910, (201) 829-4519, MA 74 CA St Univ - Los Angeles; MA 78 Univ of CA - Los Angeles; PH 80 (Psychology) Univ of CA - Los Angeles; Bell Commun Res Inc, **A**

Kammermeier, Dr Martin A 1226 14th Street North, St Cloud, MN 56301, (612) 255-4145, BS 59 Saint Cloud St Univ; MS 62 Saint Cloud St Univ; PH 69 (NS) Univ of MN - Minneap-St Paul; Prof, St Cloud State University, **SLP**

Kammersell, Mrs Nancy M 325 Ridgewood Avenue, Pittsburgh, PA 15229, (412) 741-9500, OB 78 Univ of Pittsburgh - Pittsburgh; BA 78 Univ of Pittsburgh - Pittsburgh; MA 81 Univ of IA; 87–Sp-Lang Path, D T Watson Rehab Hosp, **SLP**

Kammlade, Mrs Helen S 703 Taylor Drive, Carbondale, IL 62901, BA 48 Univ of IL - Urbana; MS 72 Southern IL Univ -Carbondale; Retired, Carbondale District 95, **SLP**

Kampe, Mary Angela 1914 47th Street, Galveston, TX 77551, (409) 765-4303, BS 77 Univ of North TX; MA 83 Univ of Houston - Univ Park; 87–Sp-Lang Path, Univ of Tex Med Branch, **SLP**

Kampen, Karen Lynn 12011 East 186th Street, Artesia, CA 90701, (714) 973-0307, BA 82 CA St Univ - Fullerton; MA 85 CA St Univ - Fullerton; **SLP**

Kampf, Pamela D 2109 Berkley Avenue S W, Roanoke, VA 24015, (703) 772-3124, BS 74 Univ of KS; ME 75 Univ of VA - Charlottesville; Owner, The Sp & Comm Ctr, **SLP A**

Kamrad, Joseph F 397 Cummings Avenue, Trenton, NJ 08611, **A**

Kamrath, Mrs Gail C 7449 Columbia Court, Woodbury, MN 55125, (612) 731-2896, BS 78 Univ of WI - Madison; MS 79 Purdue Univ - West Lafayette; SLP, ISD 832, **SLP**

Kanagy, David N 12417 Evergreen, Delta, OH 43515, (419) 782-2921, BA 62 Goshen Coll; MA 71 Bowling Green St Univ; 88–Sp-Lang Path, Defiance Co Bd of Educ, **SLP**

Kanar, Fay Carol 21470 Winchester, Southfield, MI 48076, (313) 353-8549, MA 86 Wayne St Univ; 88–Sp-Lang Path, William Beaumont Hosp Barnum Health Ctr, **SLP**

Kanar, Mrs Robin Rochelle 1 Laurel Drive, Hollidaysburg, PA 16648, (703) 963-5765, BS 77 CA Univ of PA; MS 81 CA Univ of PA; Sp/Lang Path, Keystone Rehab Systems, **SLP**

Kandel, Mrs Bonnie Daduk 3172 Drexel Road, Bensalem, PA 19020, (215) 757-0605, BA 71 CUNY - Queens Coll; MA 72 George Washington Univ; Coord Ther Serv, UCP Asso, **SLP**

Kandel, Ellen B Childrens Specialized Hospital, New Providence Road, Westfield, NJ 07091, (201) 233-3720, BA 71 Univ of VT; MA 72 Univ of IL - Urbana; 78–Dir Sp & Hrng, Chldns Specialized Hosp, **SLP ACE**

Kandel, Mrs Jodi Murayama 3522 Hillcrest Drive, Los Angeles, CA 90016, (714) 623-5251, BA 81 CA St Univ - Long Beach; MA 84 CA St Univ - Long Beach; **SLP**

Kandle, Virjean Camp 3 Poplar Circle, Londonderry, NH 03053, (603) 437-0601, BS 83 SUNY - Coll at Fredonia; MS 84 SUNY - Coll at Fredonia; 85–Sp-Lang Path, Nashua Memorial Hospital, **SLP**

Kane, Mrs Angela Marie 8 Tallwood Road, Farmington, CT 06032, (203) 747-2112, **SLP**

Kane, Bridget R 3934 Linden Avenue, Western Springs, IL 60558, (312) 333-2300, BA 78 SUNY - Center at Buffalo; MA 80 SUNY - Center at Buffalo; Aud, Ingalls Mem Hosp, **A**

Kane, Christina Marie 4635 Coronet Avenue, Virginia Beach, VA 23455, (804) 497-3289, BS 84 Old Dominion Univ; ME 86 Univ of FL; **SLP**

Kane, Deborah A 61-15 97th Street #9R, Rego Park, NY 11374, (212) 473-8152, BA 72 CUNY - Queens Coll; MA 78 CUNY - Hunter Coll; Sp-Lang Path, NYC Bd of Ed-Sp Servs Ut, **SLP**

Kane, Debra S 1988 Peterson Road, Muskegon, MI 49445, (616) 773-3297, BS 74 Eastern MI Univ; MA 75 Eastern MI Univ; Sp/Lang Path, Muskegon Pub Sch, **SLP**

Kane, Ellen M 765 Keith Lane, West Islip, NY 11795, (516) 348-5079, BS 78 Ithaca Coll; MA 80 Montclair St Coll; 83–Sp-Lang Path, Central Islip Public Schools, **SLP**

Kane, Dr James K Keystone Audiological Assoc, 121 Main Street, Johnstown, PA 15901, (814) 536-0745, BS 70 CA Univ of PA; MS 73 Univ of Pittsburgh - Pittsburgh; PH 76 (NS) Univ of Pittsburgh - Pittsburgh; Pres, Keystone Aud Assoc Inc, **A**

Kane, Jane F 316 16th Avenue Southeast, Minot, ND 58701, (512) 680-7789, BS 75 Univ of ND; MS 76 Univ of ND; Instructor, Ctl U of Nd, **SLP**

Kane, Jane Lois 26 Horton Street, Gloucester, MA 01930, (617) 283-0912, BS

Kane, Janet T 2527 Parkside Drive, Fremont, CA 94536, (415) 347-8968, BS 77 CA St Univ - Hayward; MS 79 San Francisco St Univ; 86–Sp-Lang Path, San Mateo Co Sch Dist, **SLP**

Kane, Joan G Univ Of Southwestern Louisiana, Box 43532, Lafayette, LA 70504, (318) 261-1455, BA 62 Stephen F Austin St Univ; MA 63 Stephen F Austin St Univ; Asst Prof, U of Swn LA, **SLP**

Kane, Joann S 3528 Woody Lane, Minnetonka, MN 55343, (612) 421-9172, BS 77 Mankato St Univ; MA 79 Northeast MO St Univ; SLP, Anoka-Hennysin Sch Dist 22, **SLP**

Kane, Karen Hilary 9900 Spain N E, #X1132, Albuquerque, NM 87111, (505) 883-9116, BA 83 MI St Univ; MA 85 MI St Univ; Sp-Lang Path, Albuquerque Public Schools, **SLP**

Kane, Linda A 14 Andover Court, Brookfield, CT 06804, (203) 744-2170, BA 78 CUNY - Lehman Coll; MA 80 CUNY - Lehman Coll; Sp-Lang Path, Danbury Hospital, **SLP**

Kane, M Eileen 204 Spencer Road, Webster Groves, MO 63119, (801) 943-7731, BA 74 Saint Louis Univ; MA 76 Saint Louis Univ; Sp-Lang Path, **SLP**

Kane, Margaret Mary 12802 South Greenwood, Blue Island, IL 60406, (312) 389-1235, BS 81 Southern IL Univ -Carbondale; MS 84 Univ of WI - Stevens Point; 87–Sp-Lang Path, Sch Dist 132-Calumet Park IL, **SLP**

Kane, Michele G 607 West Mt Vernon Street, Lansdale, PA 19446, (215) 278-8680, BA 79 Univ of MI - Ann Arbor; MA 82 Univ of CA - Santa Barbara; 85–Sp-Lang Path, Sacred Heart Hosp & Rehab Ctr, **SLP**

Kane, Sandra Bordner 17411 Irvine Boulevard, Suite D, Tustin, CA 92680, (714) 544-2730, MS 79 Univ of SC - Columbia; Pres, Rehab Connection Ltd, **SLP**

Kane, Mrs Susan B 98 Algonquin Trail, Oakland, NJ 07436, (201) 337-4161, BA 68 CUNY - Hunter Coll; MA 70 Montclair St Coll; Sp-Lang Path, Mahwah Bd of Educ, **SLP ACE**

Kane, Susan Beverly P O Box 531025, Miami Shores, FL 33153, (305) 835-6148, BS 82 FL St Univ; MS 84 FL St Univ; 87–Dir of Sp-Lang Path, N Shore Med Ctr, **SLP**

Kane, Mrs Wendy Louise 6143 Craig Avenue, Bensalem, PA 19020, (215) 671-7535, BA 80 Univ of Pittsburgh - Pittsburgh; MA 82 Memphis St Univ; Sp-Lang Path, Memorial Hosp of Burlington Co, **SLP**

Kanelos, Frank T 612 22nd Avenue South, Birmingham, AL 35205, (205) 868-2245, BA 71 Univ of AL- Tuscaloosa; MS 75 Southern Methodist Univ; 86–Admin Dir-Sp & Hrng, Lakeshore Hosp, **SLP**

Kane-Markowitz, Rochelle 102-55 67th Drive, Forest Hills, NY 11375, (212) 454-3636, BA 68 CUNY - Queens Coll; MA 74 CUNY - Queens Coll; Sp-Lang Path, Sp Serv Unit NYC Bd of Ed, **SLP**

Kaner, Mrs Debra 4153 Woodcrest Road, Las Vegas, NV 89121, BA 71; ME 73 Boston Univ; **SLP**

Kaner, Richard P Brooklyn Audiology Associates, 8502 4th Avenue, Brooklyn, NY 11209, (718) 745-6363, BA 77 CUNY - Queens Coll; MA 79 CUNY - Queens Coll; Brooklyn Aud Assoc, **A**

Kanfer, Ruthe T 561 Hunter Avenue, Scotch Plains, NJ 07076-1603, (201) 464-9006, BS 66 Univ of Pittsburgh - Pittsburgh; MA 69 OH St Univ; SLP, Union Co Ed Serv Comm, **SLP ACE**

Kang, Poh-Sim 114-I Bukit Serindit, 75400 Melaka, Melaka, Malaysia, BS 84 IL St Univ - Normal; MS 86 IL St Univ - Normal; **SLP**

Kangas, Kathleen A 118 Rockland Drive, West Lafayette, IN 47906, (317) 494-7341, BS 74 Northern MI Univ; OM 77 Univ of WA; 86–Grad Asst, Purdue Univ, **SLP**

Kania, Mrs Cathy S 5044 Cumberland Lane, Spring Hill, FL 33526, (904) 683-3636, BS 78 SUNY - Coll at Buffalo; MS 81 SUNY - Center at Buffalo; Sp-Lang Path, Hernando Co Sch, **SLP**

Kania, Deborah A 839 Chalmers Place, Pittsburgh, PA 15243, (412) 624-6571, BS 73 CA Univ of PA; MS 74 WV Univ; Asst Cl Dir, U of Pitt Sp/Hrng Cen, **SLP**

Kania, Mrs Eileen S 506 West Center Street Ext, Southington, CT 06489, (203) 249-0665, BA 76 Univ of CT; MS 79 Southern CT St Univ; SLP, Hartford Board of Education, **SLP**

Kanis, Mrs Karen Lee Rd 3 Box 323-B, Barry Road, Monroe, NY 10950, (914) 782-5731, BS 69 CUNY - Brooklyn Coll; MS 71 CUNY - Brooklyn Coll; SLP, NYC Bd of Ed Sp Serv, **SLP**

Kankelborg, Carol G 1516 South 44th Street, Tacoma, WA 98408, (206) 596-2325, BA 70 Holy Names Coll; MA 73 Univ of WA; Sp-Lang Path, Tacoma Pub Sch, Dist #10, **SLP**

Kann, Cheryl M 418 East 77th Street, New York, NY 10021, (212) 772-6636, BA 70 Long Island U - Brooklyn Ctr; MA 72 CUNY - Lehman Coll; **SLP**

Kanna, Rhoda Mae 927 Clover, Kalamazoo, MI 49008, (616) 344-5707, BS 83 Pacific Union Coll; MS 86 Loma Linda Univ - Loma Linda; 87–Sp-Lang Path, Kalamazoo Valley ISD, **SLP**

Kannenberg, Patricia C 2580 Robb Street, Lakewood, CO 80215, (303) 232-0877, BA 83 Univ of CO - Boulder; MA 86 Univ of TX - Austin; 86–Sp-Lang Path, Wheat Ridge Regional Center, **SLP**

Kanno, Dr Leila Okino 523 West Lanikaula Street, Hilo, HI 96720-4091, (808) 933-3542, PH 71 (Sp Path) Univ of MO - Columbia

Kanofsky, Dorrie Lynne 201B 7th Street, St Augustine, FL 32084, (904) 471-8357, BA 72 Univ of MD - College Park; OM 74 Emory Univ; Aud, Private Practice, **A**

Kansas-Zahn, Mrs Kathleen Marie 25605 Paseo La Cresta, Laguna Niguel, CA 92677, (714) 495-2242, BA 82 Chapman Coll; MS 84 Chapman Coll; Sp-Lang Path, Capistrano USD, **SLP**

Kanski, Mrs Cynthia R 310 Elk Avenue, Johnsonburg, PA 15845, (814) 965-3170, BS 80 PA St Univ - Univ Park; MS 81 PA St Univ - Univ Park; SLP, Seneca Highlands I U #9, **SLP**

Kanter, Mrs Ann B 1131 Laurel Avenue, Deerfield, IL 60015, (312) 564-9230, BA 75 Elmhurst Coll; MA 76 Northwestern Univ; Dir Ped Serv Nonsp Commun, Gottfred Speech Associates, **SLP**

Kanter, Mrs Carol S 70 Fawn Drive, Stamford, CT 06905, (203) 854-4000, BS 76 Ithaca Coll; MA 77 Hofstra Univ; Sp-Lang Path, Norwalk Board of Education, **SLP**

Kanter, Mrs Karen 501 Concord Avenue, Lexington, MA 02173, BA 76 Wheaton Coll; ME 81 Northeastern Univ; 88–Sp-Lang Path, Concord Area Spec Educ Collab, **SLP**

Kanter, Mrs Nancy E 3550 Beauclerc Circle No, Jacksonville, FL 32217, (904) 733-4768, BA 69 Case Western Reserve Univ; MA 72 CUNY - Queens Coll; Aud, I Stanton Hudmon MD Pa, **A**

Kantner, Elizabeth 5303 Brandy Lane, Sylvania, OH 43560, (419) 882-0923, BA 69 Univ of Toledo; MA 73 Bowling Green St Univ; **SLP**

Kantor, Elaine B 67 Gottlieb Drive, Chestnut Ridge, NY 10965, (914) 735-4326, BS 80 Mercy Coll; MA 85 Seton Hall Univ; Sp-Lang Path, Greenburgh 11 Usfd Chldrns Vil, **SLP**

Kantor, Mrs Rita H 15 Honeyman Drive, Succasunna, NJ 07876, (201) 539-9631, BA 64 William Paterson Coll; MA 69 Montclair St Coll; Sp/Lang Path, NJ Dir Servcs, **SLP**

Kapassakis, Georgea 230 81st Street, Brooklyn, NY 11209, (212) 750-6788, BS 78 CUNY - Hunter Coll; MS 79 Columbia Univ Teachers Coll; Asst Chief, NYU Med Cen/Goldwtr Hosp, **SLP**

Kapilow, Carin P 2 Bruce Street, Newburgh, NY 12550, (914) 561-7643, 62 CUNY - City College; MS 63 Univ of WI - Eau Claire; MA 65 Northwestern Univ; Sp-Lang Path/Aud, Private Practice, **SLP A**

Kapke, Christine Ruth 452 Brookshire Drive, Apt 6, Valparaiso, IN 46383, (219) 464-9580, BA 86 IN Univ - Bloomington; MA 87 IN Univ - Bloomington; Aud, Professional Hearing Managemen

Kaplan, Barbara F 4 Ocean Avenue, Rockport, MA 01966, (201) 249-9097, BA 68 CUNY - Queens Coll; MA 69 Montclair St Coll; 87–Sp-Lang Path, Private Practice, **SLP**

Kaplan, Beth 905 Woodhollow Drive, Marlton, NJ 08053, (609) 342-2187, BA 71 SUNY - Coll at Cortland; MA 73 Case Western Reserve Univ; Admin, Cooper Hosp/U Med Cen, **SLP**

Kaplan, Betty Marsha 1548 East 14th Street, Brooklyn, NY 11230, (718) 376-0406, MS 86 0500; SLP, Broioklyn Childhood Cntr, **SLP**

Kaplan, Beverly L 315 Fawn Hill Road, Narberth, PA 19072, BA 69 American Univ; MA 71 Temple Univ-Tyler Sch of Art; **A**

Kaplan, Mrs Carol Beth 1722 Dove Field Place, Brandon, FL 33511, (813) 689-8076, MS 84 Univ of South FL; 86–Sp-Lang Path, Hillsborough Co PS Sys, **SLP**

Kaplan, Carol M 2492 Lenola Road, Cinnaminson, NJ 08077, (609) 428-0830, BS 67 Temple Univ; MA 68 MI St Univ; 88–Sp-Lang Path, Lumberton PS, **SLP**

Kaplan, Mrs Carrie Levine 625 Alice Drive, Northbrook, IL 60062, BS 74 Northwestern Univ; MA 75 Northwestern Univ; **A**

Kaplan, Mrs Claire G 32-20 92nd Street, Jackson Heights, New York, NY 11369, (212) 520-7074, BA 47 CUNY - Queens Coll; MS 50 CUNY - City College; Adjunct Lecturer, Queens College, **SLP**

Kaplan, David B 9200 Bustleton Avenue, 1408 Earle Bldg, Scotch Lane, Philadelphia, PA 19115, (215) 671-0608, BA 71 Towson St Univ; MS 73 PA St Univ - Univ Park; **SLP**

Kaplan, Donald E 8485 Mariners Cove, Huntington Beach, CA 92646, (714) 773-3617, BA 51 Univ of CA - Los Angeles; MA 54 CA St Univ - Long Beach; Prof Emeritus, CA St U Fullerton, **SLP A LM**

Kaplan, Mrs Ellen D 93 Somerset Drive, Suffern, NY 10901, (914) 357-6104, BA 74 SUNY - Coll at New Paltz; MS 76 William Paterson Coll; Dir, Rockland Co Sp/Hrng Cen, **SLP**

Kaplan, Mrs Ellen W 630 Perth Avenue, Flossmoor, IL 60422, (312) 957-3781, BA 68 Kean Coll of NJ; MS 84 Governors St Univ; Sp-Lang Path, Sch Dist 128, **SLP**

Kaplan, Dr Harriet F 12812 Middlevale Lane, Silver Spring, MD 20906, (202) 651-5317, BA 55 CUNY - Brooklyn Coll; MS 57 PA St Univ - Univ Park; PH 74 (NS) Univ of MD - College Park; Assoc Prof, Gallaudet Univ, **A**

Kaplan, Mrs Helene E One Sutton Place, Easton, PA 18042, (201) 859-6758, BA 56 CUNY - Brooklyn Coll; MS 57 PA St Univ - Univ Park; Dir Sp-Lang Path, Warren Hosp, **SLP**

Kaplan, Holly Sue 28 North Main Street #1, Muncy, PA 17756, BS 82 Bradley Univ; MS 84 Gallaudet Coll; Aud, Geisinger Med Ctr, **A**

Kaplan, Mrs Ilene L 289 Chicory Lane, Buffalo Grove, IL 60089, (312) 689-0070, BA 82 IN Univ - Bloomington; MA 83 Northwestern Univ; Sp/Lang Path, N Chi Sch Dist 64, **SLP**

Kaplan, Jacqueline L 322 Marston Avenue, Madison, WI 53703, MS 74 Univ of IL - Urbana; Sp-Lang Path, Madison Metro Sch Dist, **SLP**

Kaplan, Jerome H 60 Trapelo Road, Belmont, MA 02178, (617) 720-6734, BA 70 SUNY - Center at Albany; MA 74 NY Univ; Sp-Lang Path, Spaulding Rehab Hosp, **SLP ACE**

Kaplan, Mrs Joan R 973 East End, Woodmere, NY 11598, (718) 454-8855, BS 59 Boston Univ; MA 61 CUNY - Brooklyn Coll; Sp-Lang Path, Bd of Ed-NY Cty, **SLP**

Kaplan, Joel J P O Box 42632, San Francisco, CA 94142, (415) 431-4585, BA 68 CUNY - Hunter Coll; MA 72 OH Univ - Athens; Sp-Lang Path/Aud, Private Practice, **SLP**

Kaplan, Judith G 1205 South Ogden Drive, Los Angeles, CA 90019, (213) 931-4860, BA 63 Univ of CA - Los Angeles; MA 68 Univ of CA - Los Angeles; SLP, LA USD, **SLP**

Kaplan, Mrs Judith L 22 Waughaw Road, Towaco, NJ 07082, (201) 777-4600, BS 61 Boston Univ; MA 71 2571; SLP, Clifton Nj Bd Ed, **SLP**

Kaplan, Karen E 2014 Christie Lane, Carrollton, TX 75007, MA 72 Case Western Reserve Univ; Practicum Supervisor, University of Texas - Dallas, **SLP**

Kaplan, Mrs Kathleen L Pachappa Elementary School, 6200 Riverside Avenue, Riverside, CA 92506, (714) 788-7355, BA 86 CA St Univ - Fullerton; MA 88 CA St Univ - Fullerton; 88–Sp-Lang Path, Riverside USD

Kaplan, Mrs Lynda 6224 Ballsford Drive, Fairfax Station, VA 22039, BA 69 MI St Univ; MA 70 MI St Univ; **A**

Kaplan, Mrs Marsha Helene 20 Jules Drive, Staten Island, NY 10314, (718) 761-9028, MS 83 Adelphi Univ; Sp-Lang Path, Private Practice, **SLP**

Kaplan, Mrs Marsye W 8 Mission Wood Way, Reisterstown, MD 21136, (301) 848-7022, BS 74 Towson St Univ; MS 76 Loyola Coll; Sp-Lang Path, Baltimore County Board of Educ, **SLP**

Kaplan, Max 19 Carlton Lane, Monsey, NY 10952, (914) 356-4100, BS 51 Bloomsburg Univ of PA; ME 52 PA St Univ - Univ Park; **SLP**

Kaplan, Dr Michael A P O Box 9530, Santa Fe, NM 87504, (505) 827-6541, BS 70 Saint John's Univ - Jamaica; MA 72 CUNY - Queens Coll; PH 85 (NS) Univ of NM; Sp-Lang Path, NM Dept of Ed, **SLP**

Kaplan, Dr Netta R 185 Randolph, Windsor, ON, Canada N8B 2J2, BA 51 Antioch Coll; MA 67 Univ of Cincinnati; PH 72 (NS) Wayne St Univ; **SLP**

Kaplan, Robin Jacobs 11724 S W 115th Terrace, Miami, FL 33186, (305) 221-0284, OB 75 Univ of Miami; MA 76 Univ of Miami; 75–Sp-Lang Path, Dade County Public Schools, **SLP**

Kaplan, Ronald Marc 2135 Woodbox Lane #A, Baltimore, MD 21209, (301) 653-0112, BS 79 Towson St Univ; MS 81 Towson St Univ; Sales Rep, Audiology Associates Inc, **A**

Kaplan, Mrs Sharon R 542 Putnam Road, Merion, PA 19066, (215) 668-8128, BA 79 Temple Univ; MA 81 Temple Univ; Sp-Lang Path, Private Practice, **SLP**

Kaplan, Shelley A 136 Peachtree Memorial Drive, Rhode Island #5, Atlanta, GA 30309, (404) 352-1279, BA 74 Case Western Reserve Univ; MS 77 Univ of WI - Madison; Southeast Reg Proj Dir, UCP, **SLP**

Kaplan, Susan K 3757 Lewis Avenue, Long Beach, CA 90807, BA 80 CA St Univ - Long Beach; MA 82 CA St Univ - Long Beach; Chief Audiologist, Harbor/UCLA Medical Center, **A**

Kaplan, Mrs Tola E P O Box 708, 241 Highway 33, Freehold, NJ 07728, (201) 462-8440, BA 66 Long Island U - Brooklyn Ctr; MS 69 Emerson Coll; Sp/Lang Path, Vna, **SLP ACE**

Kaplan-Greenberg, Mrs Vicki 55 Buckingham Court, Pomona, NY 10970-2524, (914) 362-0964, BA 78 Montclair St Coll; MA 80 Montclair St Coll; Aud, Metro Aud Assoc, **A**

Kapleau-Lebov, Mrs Nancy B 43 Fox Hill Road, Woodbridge, CT 06525, (203) 387-6992, BA 73 Univ of CT; MA 75 Univ of CT; Clinical Supervisor, Southern Connecticut St Univ, **SLP**

Kaplon, Mrs Marsha J 2438 Sylvale Road, Baltimore, MD 21209, (301) 484-6955, BS 63 Towson St Univ; MS 77 Towson St Univ; Sp/Lang Path, Balto Cty Pub Sch, **SLP**

Kaplowitz, Mrs Lotte T 39 Brower Avenue, Woodmere, NY 11598, (516) 374-0797, BS 55 Syracuse Univ; MA 60 Northwestern Univ; Hrng Res Tchr, Hrng Ed Serv NYC Bd of Ed, **A**

Kapner, Mary 1002 Williams, League City, TX 77573, (713) 554-7352, BS 72 Baylor Univ; MA 73 Baylor Univ; Sp-Lang Path, Private Practice, **SLP**

Kapp, Mrs Helen H Veterans Administration Hosp, 109 Bee Street, Charleston, SC 29405, (803) 577-5011, OB 75 Univ of SC - Columbia; MS 77 Univ of SC - Columbia; Aud, VA Medical Center, **SLP A**

Kapp, Sharon W 23 Shirley Road, Wellesley, MA 02181, **SLP**

Kappe, Mrs Terry Highstreet 708 Abbot Avenue, San Gabriel, CA 91776, (818) 575-2336, MA 80 CA St Univ - Los Angeles; SLP, LA Co Supt of Sch, **SLP**

Kappelman, Mrs Joan G 2124 Western Run Drive, Baltimore, MD 21209, MS 75 Towson St Univ; Sp-Lang Path, Baltimore City Public Schools, **SLP**

Kapper, Mrs Carol Sisler 1729 Prather Lane, De Kalb, IL 60115, (312) 365-5116, **SLP**

Kapur, Mrs Revati D 8 North Drive, East Brunswick, NJ 08816, (201) 549-5580, BA 59; MS 66 Univ of Pittsburgh - Pittsburgh; Supervisor Early Intervention, Cerebral Palsy Association, **SLP**

Kapur, Dr Y P Audiology And Speech Sciences, Michigan State University, East Lansing, MI 48823, MD (NS); **A**

Kapura, Mrs Diane Kaczka 19 Lawrence Road, Wayne, NJ 07470, BA 70 Kean Coll of NJ; MS 83 William Paterson Coll; 73–Sp-Lang Path, BOCES/City of Garfield, **SLP**

Kapusta, Mrs Carol-Lynn 5725 Lockwood Avenue, Cote St Luc, Montreal, PQ, Canada H4W 1Z1, (514) 487-3534, MS 88 Columbia Univ Teachers Coll

Kapusta, Mrs Lauri Walting 1031 Rill Road, Reading, PA 19606, (215) 376-9728, BA 81 Univ of Pittsburgh - Pittsburgh; MA 83 Univ of Pittsburgh - Pittsburgh; Aud, Berks ENT Surgical Assoc Inc, **A**

Karabacz, Mrs Nancy C 7267 Pheasant Run, Gaylord, MI 49735, (517) 939-8544, BA 69 San Jose St Univ; MA 71 MI St Univ; Sp/Lang Path, Northern Speech Services, **SLP**

Karam, Mrs Laurie Montgomery 123 Tilney Avenue, Griffin, GA 30223, (404) 227-9478, BS 82 Valdosta St Coll; ME 87 GA St Univ

Karam, Marilyn R 2620 Chancer Drive, Richmond, VA 23233, (804) 780-7809, BA 75 Univ of NC - Greensboro; MA 76 Univ of NC - Greensboro; Supvr, Richmond Public Schools, **SLP**

Karamourtopoulos, Donna Hollander 46 Mount Vernon Street, Lawrence, MA 01843, (617) 774-5000, Supervisor of Speech N Hearing, Hogan Regional Center, **SLP**

Karas, Irene D 10 Emerson Place #11-D, Boston, MA 02114-2227, ME 73 Northeastern Univ; Sp-Lang Path, Boston Pub Sch, **SLP**

Karas, Karen Joy 264 Kelton Street #8, Brighton, MA 02134, (617) 232-9500, OB 85 Univ of MA - Amherst; MS 87 Northeastern Univ; **A**

Karasik, Mrs Rozalyn Z 388 St Clements Avenue, Toronto, ON, Canada M5N 1M1, (416) 881-8423, BA 77; OM 79 McGill Univ - Quebec; 82–Sp-Lang Path, Scarborough Bd of Ed, **SLP**

Karastathas, Mrs Susan E C 660 Rambler Road, Merced, CA 95340, (209) 385-6629, BA 72 CA St Univ - Fresno; MA 75 CA St Univ - Fresno; SLP, Merced Cty Sch, **SLP**

Karbelnig, Amy Bade 238 6th Avenue, Venice, CA 90291, (213) 824-3100, BA 80 CA St Univ - Fullerton; **SLP**

Karbowski, Laurie L 9385 S W 77th Avenue #2035, Miami, FL 33156, (305) 547-6350, MA 83 Central MI Univ; Aud, U of Miami Mailman Ctr, **A**

Karcher-Hewitt, Mrs Sherry Lynne 38 North Pine Avenue #4, Albany, NY 12203, (518) 783-1644, BS 85 Coll of Saint Rose; MS 86 Coll of Saint Rose; SLP, NY Assoc for the Learning Dis, **SLP**

Kareff, Gary R Hearing Consultants, 8888 N W 3rd Court, Coral Springs, FL 33071, (305) 973-6200, BS 79 SUNY - Coll at Buffalo; MA 80 SUNY - Center at Buffalo; Audiologist, Hearing Consultants, **A**

Karenz, Mrs Sandra M W125 Oosty Avenue, Oconomowoc, WI 53066, (414) 261-3050, BS 75 Univ of WI - Milwaukee; MS 76 Univ of WI - Milwaukee; Sp-Lang Path, Bethesda Lutheran Home, **SLP**

Karger, Vera V 301 Park Street, New Canaan, CT 06840, (203) 966-3416, BA 74 Southern CT St Univ; MS 77 Southern CT St Univ; 84–Sp-Lang Path, Stamford Bd of Ed, **SLP**

Karibian, Dana 600 North Pantano #719, Tucson, AZ 85710, (602) 795-0553, **A**

Kariyasu, Makoto Elegant Haruyama #103, 1-7-12 Haruyama, Tukui City, Japan 910, MA 86 Univ of KS; 86–Instr Sp-Lang Path, Fukui Inst of Tech for Med

Karkowsky, Faith G 925 Mayfield Road, Woodmere, NY 11598, (516) 569-1962, BA 73 CUNY - Hunter Coll; MS 76 CUNY - Brooklyn Coll; Audiologist, St Vincents Hospital, **SLP A**

Karl, Mrs Belinda Louise 3504 Wakefield Drive, Columbia, MO 65203, (314) 449-7309, BS 79 Univ of MO - Columbia; MA 80 Univ of MO - Columbia; Area Admin, Assoc Rehab Serv, **SLP**

Karl, Mrs Edith L 11820 Smoke Tree Road, Potomac, MD 20854, (301) 983-0033, BA 59 CUNY - Brooklyn Coll; Sp/Lang Path, Private Practice, **SLP**

Karlan, Mrs Andrea 976 Cherrywood Drive, Baldwin Harbor, NY 11510, (516) 868-5601, BS 71 Emerson Coll; MS 75 Adelphi Univ; 79–Sp/Lang Path, Bay Shore Un Free Sch Dist, **SLP**

Karlberg, Janice M T 8 Oaks Drive, Tonasket, WA 98855, BA 73 Western WA Univ; MA 74 Western WA Univ; Sp-Lang Path, Omak Sch Dist 19, **SLP**

Karlberg, Philip L Crumbacher Estates, 8 Oakes Drive, Tonasket, WA 98855, (509) 486-4933, BA 72 Western WA Univ; MA 74 Western WA Univ; Sp-Lang Path, Tonasket School District, **SLP**

Karle, Mrs Linda J 200 East 72nd Street #20-K, New York, NY 10021, (212) 734-7541, BA 62 Marygove Coll; MA 77 Wayne St Univ; 87–Sp-Lang Path, Kennedy Child Study Ctr, **SLP**

Karlin, Andrea S 9607 North Kostner, Skokie, IL 60076, (312) 679-7170, BS 81 Univ of IL - Urbana; OM 82 Univ of IL - Urbana; **A**

Karlin, Torrey S 2757 Santa Ana Drive, Reno, NV 89502, (702) 825-7628, BA 71 CA St Univ - Chico; MS 82 Western OR St Coll; **SLP**

Karlovich, Dr Raymond S Dept Communicative Disorders, University Of WI/Madison, 1975 Willow Drive, Madison, WI 53706, (608) 262-3951, BS 61 Bloomsburg Univ of PA; MS 65 Purdue Univ - West Lafayette; PH 67 (Aud) Purdue Univ - West Lafayette; Prof, U of WI-Madison, **SLP A**

Karlow, Carol Marie 805 Pine Valley Court, Rockledge, FL 32955, (305) 452-1234, BA 79 Univ of NE - Lincoln; MA 82 Univ of KS; SLP, Sch Brd of Brevard Co Sch, **SLP**

Karlquist, Mrs Suzanne Winslow 15330 W Street, Omaha, NE 68137, (402) 896-1701, BS 82 Abilene Christian Univ; MA 84 TX Woman's Univ; 87–Sp-Lang Path, Omaha PS, **SLP**

Karlsen, Dr Elizabeth Kansas University Medical Center, Otolaryngolgy Head & Neck Surgery Foundation, 39th & Cambridge, Kansas City, KS 66103, (913) 588-6706, BS 72 SUNY - Coll at Geneseo; MA 74 Univ of KS; PH 78 (NS) Univ of KS; Asst Prof, Ks U Med Cen, **A ACE**

Karlsen, Else 5576 Winsome Way, Oregon, WI 53575, (608) 246-5030, BS 80 Univ of WI - Madison; MS 82 Univ of WI - Madison; Sp-Lang Path, Madison Metro Sch Dist, **SLP**

Karmelek, Eugene Joseph Suite 505, 1655 Main Street, Springfield, MA 01103, (413) 731-9615, BS 74 SUNY - Coll at Fredonia; MS 77 SUNY - Coll at Fredonia; 87–Sp-Lang Path, Private Practice, **SLP**

Karn, Mrs Regina-Jo 15 Autumn Drive, East Northport, NY 11731, (516) 754-2256, BA 80 Hofstra Univ; MA 81 Hofstra Univ; Sp-Lnag Path, Suffolk Chld Dev Cen Day Treat, **SLP**

Karnack, Mrs Romaine S 103 Hazel Street, Bentleyville, PA 15314, (412) 239-3518, BS 60 CA Univ of PA; BS 60 CA Univ of PA; Sp-Lang Path, Intermediate Unit 1, **SLP**

Karneboge, Mrs Monica D Speech And Language Services, 430 West Francis Road, New Lenox, IL 60451, (815) 485-0111, BA 71 Coll of Saint Francis; MA 72 Northwestern Univ; Sp-Lang Path/Comm Dev, Private Practice, **SLP**

Karnell, Dr Michael Peter 2246 Willow Road, Homewood, IL 60430, (312) 962-6695, BS 78 Western MI Univ; MA 79 Western MI Univ; PH 83 (NS) Univ of IA; Asst Prof, U of Chicago, **SLP**

Karner, Mrs Karen Kay 1617 Pennsylvania Street, El Dorado, KS 67042-4221, (913) 483-5577, BA 84 Fort Hays St Univ; MS 84 Fort Hays St Univ; Sp-Lang Path, USD 465, **SLP**

Karnes, Mrs Dianne E 3600 Eldorado Drive, Rocky River, OH 44116, (216) 231-0400, BA 69 Saint Xavier Coll; MA 73 Cleveland St Univ; SLP, Positive Education Program, **SLP**

Karnuta, Maryann L 618 Millard Drive, Bay Village, OH 44140, (216) 331-4822, BA 77 Cleveland St Univ; MA 79 Cleveland St Univ; 87–Aud, Clev Met Gen Hosp, **A**

Karolak, Mrs Donna Lucia 252 Steeplechase Circle, Weddington, NC 28713, (704) 846-8672, BA 79 Saint John's Univ - Jamaica; MA 80 Hofstra Univ; Prog Dir, Assn Advancmnt Blind & Retard, **SLP**

Karow, Mrs Colleen Marie 2087 Hunters Glen Drive, Apartment #104, Dunedin, FL 34698, **SLP**

Karp, Mrs Adrienne 71 Davis Road, Port Washington, NY 11050, (212) 355-2200, BA 56 CUNY - Queens Coll; MA 63 CUNY - Brooklyn Coll; Aud, NY Assoc for Blind, **A**

Karp, Elaine Barbara 229 Meadowbrook Drive, Syracuse, NY 13210, (315) 473-6931, **SLP**

Karp, Mrs Roxanne L 7440 S W 18th Street, Plantation, FL 33317, (305) 792-5542, BA 79 Univ of Miami; MA 81 Univ of Miami; Sp-Lang Path, Dade County Public Schools, **SLP**

Karpati, Janet M Knutson 24953 Paseo DE Valentia, Suite 14-C, Laguna Hills, CA 92653, (714) 581-2800, BS 83 Univ of WI - Stevens Point; MS 84 Univ of WI - Stevens Point; Sp-Lang Path, Newport Lang Speech Audiology, **SLP**

Karpe, Mrs Donna N 8 Dove Circle, Little Rock, AR 72205, (501) 227-6974, MS 78 Univ of South FL; **SLP**

Karpe, Larry M 8 Dove Circle, Little Rock, AR 72205, (501) 370-6651, MS 78 Univ of South FL; Aud, VA Med Cen, **SLP A**

Karpel-Freilich, Anne R 88 Bleecker Street #1D, New York, NY 10012, (212) 475-1385, BS 73 Emerson Coll; MS 75 Columbia Univ Teachers Coll; Sp-Lang Pathology Consultant, Private Practice, **SLP**

Karpinski, Lauren Barbara 44 Newport Place, Fairfield, CT 06430, (203) 374-5124, **SLP**

Karpoff, Marilyn A 201 East 21st Street, New York, NY 10010, (212) 777-2307, BA 71 CUNY - City College; MA 74 NY Univ; Sp-Lang Path & Aud, Bur for Sp Improvement, **SLP**

Karr, David R 2207 North Maryland Avenue, Peoria, IL 61603, (309) 672-6515, MA 70 Bradley Univ; BS 65 Bradley Univ; Sp-Lang Path, Peoria Pub Sch Dist 150, **SLP**

Karr, Lawana R P O Box 369, Fort Myers, FL 33902, **SLP**

Karr, Linda A RD 2 Box 423, Red Hook, NY 12571, (914) 758-6537, BA 75 SUNY - Coll at New Paltz; MA 76 Coll of Saint Rose; 88–Sp-Lang Path, Astor Day Treatment Center, **SLP**

Karr, Mrs Susan T 9 Enid Court, Potomac, MD 20854, (301) 897-5700, BA 76 SUNY - Center at Buffalo; MS 78 Ithaca Coll; Consult, American Sp-Lang Hearing Assoc, **SLP**

Karsh, Abbie Jean 3411 Hennepin Avenue South, Apartment 7, Minneapolis, MN 55408, (612) 627-2402, BA 77 Univ of MN - Minneap-St Paul; MA 85 Univ of MN - Minneap-St Paul; Sp-Lang Path, Minneapolis PS, **SLP**

Karsh, Mrs Diane M 700 South Flower Street, Apartment 2300, Los Angeles, CA 90017-4210, (213) 275-4574, BA 73 Univ of OR; MA 74 Case Western Reserve Univ; Sp-Lang Path, Private Practice, **SLP**

Karson-Bach, Mrs Lisa Ann 217 Foxmoor, Fox River Grove, IL 60021, (312) 639-7549, BS 82 Marquette Univ; MS 83 Marquette Univ; SLP, School District 54, **SLP**

Karson Gries, Allyson Sue 675 Portsmouth Drive, Island Lake, IL 60042, (815) 338-7411, BS 83 Marquette Univ; MS 84 Marquette Univ; **SLP**

Karstaedt, Marcelle M 220 Harmon Court, Winston-Salem, NC 27106, (919) 748-3103, BA 75; MS 79 Washington Univ; Aud, N C Baptist Hosp, **A**

Karwandy, Elizabeth R 391 London Street #3, Peterborough, ON, Canada K9H 3A1, (705) 748-2221, OB 86 Minot St Univ; MS 87 Minot St Univ

Karwowski, Mrs Lucianne Pitard 10437 Grovedale Drive, Knoxville, TN 37922, (615) 522-7714, BS 71 Univ of TN - Knoxville; MS 73 Memphis St Univ; 88–Sp-Lang Path, Daniel Arthur Rehab Ctr, **SLP**

Karz, Mrs Lynn Anita 1301 Ozone Avenue, Santa Monica, CA 90405, (213) 392-7591, BA 70 Univ of CA - Los Angeles; MA 74 CA St Univ - Long Beach; 88–Dir, Emanuel Streisand Sch, **SLP**

Karzon, Dr Roanne K 217 Spencer, Webster Groves, MO 63119, (314) 454-6171, BA 74 Univ of CT; ME 76 Univ of VA - Charlottesville; PH 82 (Communication Sciences) Washington Univ; 84–Aud, ENT Wash Univ, **SLP A**

Kasa, Felicia Marie 9028 S Baltimore Avenue, Chicago, IL 60617, (312) 375-9660, BA 79 Univ of IL - Chicago; OM 86 Governors St Univ; **SLP**

Kasan, E A Lee Department Of Communication Sciences & Disorders, Univ Of South Florida, BHA 255, Tampa, FL 33620, (813) 974-2006, BA 54 Univ of FL; MA 56 Univ of FL; Lecturer Coord, Univ of South Florida, **SLP ACE**

Kasan, Mrs Marilyn F 10302 Cliff Circle, Tampa, FL 33612, BA 52 FL St Univ; Sp-Lang Path, Hillsborough Co Pub Sch Syst, **SLP**

Kasanoff, Julie Lynn Speech Hearing & Neurosensory Center, 8001 Frost Street, San Diego, CA 92123, (619) 576-5838, BA 80 Univ of CA - Santa Barbara; MS 82 UT St Univ; Coord, Children's Hosp, **A**

Kasden, Stephen Douglas 333 School Street, Suite 306, Pawtucket, RI 02860, (401) 723-5110, BS 64 Emerson Coll; MS 67 Emerson Coll; Sp-Lang Path/Aud, Private Practice, **SLP A**

Kasdorf, Susan Cohen 4336 Bedford Avenue, Brooklyn, NY 11229, (718) 963-8319, BS 80 SUNY - Coll at Buffalo; MS 84 Columbia Univ Teachers Coll; Sp-Lang Path, Woodhill Med & Mental Health Ctr, **SLP**

Kase, Lynn C 100 Prospect Avenue, Hackensack, NJ 07601, (201) 343-1068, **A**

Kasewurm, Mrs Gyl Ann 3301 Lakeshore Drive, St Joseph, MI 49085, (616) 471-9080, BS 80 Andrews Univ; MA 83 Western MI Univ; Owner, Professional Hearing Services, **A**

Kashani, Joanne S 486 Amhurst Road, Valparaiso, IN 46383, (219) 886-6585, BA 74 Worcester St Coll; MA 76 Ball St Univ; Sp/Lang Path, Gary Sch Corp, **SLP**

Kashinsky, Mrs Eileen D 1340 Miette Way, Sunnyvale, CA 94087, (408) 730-1771, BA 68 Rutger's St Univ - Douglas Coll; MA 70 Univ of Southern CA; Sp-Lang Path, Sunnyvale Sch Dist, **SLP**

Kasica, Antoinette P 125 South Central, Somerset, KY 42501, (606) 679-8450, BS 69 WV Univ; MA 72 SUNY - Coll at Geneseo; Sp-Lang Path, Lifeline Home Health, **SLP**

Kaslon, Karen W 9 Hickory Road, West Orange, NJ 07052, (201) 325-1754, BA 70 CUNY - Brooklyn Coll; MS 75 Univ of Pittsburgh - Pittsburgh; Sp-Lang Path, Priv Practice, **SLP**

Kasmer, Mrs Shelia H 52 Country Lane, Bristol, CT 06010, (203) 747-2466, BS 56 Univ of KS; MS 78 Southern CT St Univ; SLP, Plainville Board of Education, **SLP**

Kasner, Mrs Lois J P O Box 84, Washougal, WA 98671, (714) 788-7468, **SLP**

Kaspar, Mrs Susan M 3 Sherwood Lane, Setauket, NY 11733, (516) 689-8873, BA 69 Hofstra Univ; MA 73 Hofstra Univ; Sp-Lang Path, Three Vill Pub Sch, **SLP**

Kasper, Mrs Andrea G 2203 Sand Castle Lane, Grand Junction, CO 81501, (702) 482-5617, BS 69 Fort Hays St Univ; MS 72 Univ of WY; SLP, Carbon County School District, **SLP**

Kasper, Helen Hall 113 E 37th Street, New York, NY 10016, (212) 523-6280, BA 78 Depauw Univ; MS 80 Univ of IL - Urbana; 86–Sp-Lang Path, St Luke's-Roosevelt Hosp, **SLP**

Kasper-Marrello, Marie Yvonne 20 Tall Pines Trail, Holland Lndg, ON, Canada L0G 1H0, (416) 853-0405, BS 81 Univ of WI - Stevens Point; MA 82 Central MI Univ; Sp-Lang Path, Private Practice, **SLP**

Kasprisin, Dr Arlene 165 Port Royal Avenue, Foster City, CA 94404, (415) 493-5000, BA 67 Indiana Univ of PA; MA 69 Northwestern Univ; PH 76 (NS) Univ of Pittsburgh - Pittsburgh; Chief Audiology & SLP, VA Medical Center, **SLP**

Kasprzak, Carolyne Mary 73 Murdock Road, Baltimore, MD 21212, (301) 377-6020, MS 84 Loyola Coll; BA 82 Loyola Coll; 85–Sp-Lang Path, Baltimore Co Bd of Educ, **SLP**

Kasprzyk, Mrs Sarah J 4528 Deerfield Drive, Hamburg, NY 14075, (716) 649-3212, BS 83 Univ of NV - Reno; MS 84 Univ of NV - Reno; 88–Sp-Lang Path, West Seneca Central Sch Dist, **SLP**

Kasriel, Mrs Ernestine 926 Northcliffe Drive N W, Atlanta, GA 30318, (404) 351-8441, BS 45 Coll of William & Mary; ME 61 Emory Univ; Retired, **SLP**

Kass, Mrs Carole L 3 Frost Court, Morganville, NJ 07751, BA 74 Kean Coll of NJ; BA 74 Kean Coll of NJ; MA 76 Montclair St Coll; **SLP**

Kassees, Kenneth Salim 7206 W Plainfield Avenue, Greenfield, WI 53220, (414) 544-8970, BS 81 Univ of WI - Madison; MS 83 Univ of WI - Madison; 83–Sp-Lang Path, Waukesha PS, **SLP**

Kassel, Karen Hochstein 43-60 Douglaston Parkway, Apartment 121, Douglaston, NY 11363, (718) 423-1534, BS 70 Ithaca Coll; ME 71 Boston Univ; Sp-Lang Path, NYC Bd of Ed, **SLP**

Kasselmann, Mrs Amanda Bennett PO Box 8321, Camp Lejeune, NC 28542, (919) 328-1518, BS 85 Miami Univ - Oxford; MS 87 OH St Univ; 88–Sp-Lang Path, Onslow Co Sch Sys, **SLP**

Kassel- Petrocco, Mrs Janice 20 Hill Street, Morristown, NJ 07960, (201) 539-5636, MA 85 Montclair St Coll; Sp-Lang Path, The Morris County Society, **SLP ACE**

Kassi, John Rd 4 Box 766, Belmar Road, Franklin, PA 16323, (814) 432-8353, BS 70 Edinboro Univ of PA; ME 73 Clarion Univ of PA; Unit Manager, Commonwealth of PA Polk Center, **SLP**

Kassing, Jane M 405 Carryback Drive, Marietta, GA 30068, (404) 233-5332, BS 67 Northwestern Univ; ME 68 Univ of VA - Charlottesville; Aud, Atlanta Sp Sch Inc, **A**

Kass-Levy, Maxanne 94 Knollwood Road, West Hartford, CT 06110, (203) 521-7830, BA 72 Sarah Lawrence Coll; MA 76 Univ of CT; 80–Sp-Lang Path, Newington Bd of Ed, **SLP**

Kastagir, Penelope A 3605 Long Beach Boulevard Suite 210, Long Beach, CA 90807, (213) 595-4878, BA 78 CA St Univ - Long Beach; MA 81 CA St Univ - Long Beach; 82–Sp-Lang Path, Bernard A Landes PhD & Assoc, **SLP**

Kastel, Joan H 1847 N Sedgwick Street, Chicago, IL 60614, (312) 446-6060, BS 64 Northwestern Univ; Sp-Lang Path, Winnetka Pub Sch, **SLP**

Kasten, Dr Roger N Communicative Disorders & Sci, Wichita State University, Wichita, KS 67208, (316) 689-3240, BS 55 Bowling Green St Univ; MA 56 Bowling Green St Univ; PH 64 (NS) Northwestern Univ; Prof of Aud, Wichita St U, **A F**

Kasten-Feintuch, Dr Frances 140 Cooper Drive, Great Neck, NY 11023, (516) 829-8908, BA 75 CUNY - Queens Coll; MA 77 CUNY - Queens Coll; PH 85 (NS) CUNY - Grad Sch & Univ Cntr; Clinical Supervisor, Queens College, **SLP**

Kastenholz, Maribeth Ann 3146 South Harlem Avenue, Apartment 2E, Riverside, IL 60546, (312) 531-3771, BS 82 Marquette Univ; MS 83 Marquette Univ; 87–Sp-Lang Path, Loyola University Medical Ctr, **SLP**

Kastner, Deborah Butler 17003 Ainsworth, Torrance, CA 90504, **SLP**

Kaswinkel, Mrs Patricia T 584 William Ellery Street, Orange Park, FL 32073, (904) 725-8972, BA 79 Univ of FL; MA 81 Univ of FL; Sp-Lang Path, S Allen Smith Clinic, **SLP**

Katagi, Dr Roland K 8520 Cruickshank Drive, Richmond, BC, Canada V6Y 2X6, (604) 270-9300, BA 65 Biola Univ; MS 67 Univ of OR; PH 73 (Sp Path) Univ of OR; 82, Ministry of Health, **SLP**

Katauskas, Linda Marie 502 Bell Court #7, Alamosa, CO 81101, (719) 589-5851, BA 83 Coll of Saint Teresa; MA 84 Univ of MN - Duluth; 88–Sp-Lang Path, San Luis Vall Bd of Coop Svcs

Katayama, Kerri Misao 1422 Cooper Street, Selma, CA 93662, (209) 896-6348, BA 79 CA St Univ - Fresno; MA 83 CA St Univ - Fresno; Sp-Lang Path, Kings Co Supt of Sch, **SLP**

Katerberg, Jane E 849 Brownwood N W, Grand Rapids, MI 49504, (616) 453-5370, BA 70 Western MI Univ; MS 71 Western MI Univ; 88–Sp-Lang Path, Christian Learning Center, **SLP**

Kates, Mrs Adele Dalinsky Adele Kates Med & Assoc Pa, 1 N E 168th Street, North Miami Beach, FL 33162, (305) 651-6442, BA 64 CUNY - Brooklyn Coll; ME 65 PA St Univ - Univ Park; 75–Sp-Lang Path, Humana Hospital-Biscayne, **SLP ACE**

Kates, Alison Dale 79 Cheshire Drive, Absecon, NJ 08201, (609) 652-7000, BA 83 Univ of MD - College Park; MA 85 Temple Univ-Tyler Sch of Art; Aud, Betty Bacharach Rehab Hosp, **A**

Kates, Leslie V 47 Penniman Road, Brookline, MA 02146, BS 63 Emerson Coll; Sp-Lang Path, Malden Pub Sch, **SLP**

Kathrein, Paula C 6242 North Greenview, Chicago, IL 60660, (312) 743-1152, BS 77 Northwestern Univ; MA 79 Univ of IA; **SLP**

Katko, Mrs Suzanne M 133 Eureka Street, Syracuse, NY 13204, (315) 479-5719, BS SUNY - Coll at Geneseo; MA 85 SUNY - Coll at Geneseo; 88–Aud, Veterans Administration

Katkov, George W 918 Aaron Drive, Redlands, CA 92374, (213) 452-6155, SLP, Bell Speech Pathology, **SLP**

Kato, Wendy Yuriko 2381 Ahakapu Street, Pearl City, HI 96782, (808) 455-3215, MS 84 Univ of HI - Manoa; Sp-Lang Path, Hawaii State Gov, **SLP**

Katsantonis, Joann V 1104 Harvard Place, Fort Lee, NJ 07024, (201) 224-8834, Columbia Univ Teachers Coll; **A**

Katsuki-Nakamura, Dr Jun 2-26 Yokogawa-Cho, Kanazawa-Shi, Japan 921, 76-286-2211, BA 80 Radcliffe Coll; MA 82 Univ of MN - Minneap-St Paul; PH 85 (Sp-Lang Path) Univ of MN - Minneap-St Paul; 88–Sp-Lang Path, Kaga Yahata Onsen Rehab Hosp

Katsuyama, Laurel H 25322 DE Salle, Laguna Hills, CA 92653, (714) 730-7398, BA 71 San Jose St Univ; MA 72 Univ of the Pacific; Sp-Lang Path, Tustin USD, **SLP**

Katt, David F 2228 Fairfax Road, Lansing, MI 48910, BS 63 Rockford Coll; MA 64 Univ of MI - Ann Arbor; Audiology/Sp-Lang Path Consultant, Michigan Dept of Public Health, **SLP A**

Katten, Mrs Laurie 58 Egan Road, Middletown, CT 06457, (203) 346-2481, BA 78 MI St Univ; MA 79 MI St Univ; SLP, Middletown Bd of Ed, **SLP**

Kattermann, Debora Ann 3 King Philip Road, Mattapoisett, MA 02739, (508) 824-6911, BS 81 Ithaca Coll; MS 83 PA St Univ - Univ Park; Sp-Lang Path, Morton Hospital, **SLP ACE**

Katz, Mrs Barbara Ruth 7 Lake Street #4R, White Plains, NY 10603, (914) 948-6746, MA 84 Northwestern Univ; Sp-Lang Path, Dennis Hampton PhD & Assoc, **SLP**

Katz, Mrs Betsy H 2130 Penn Avenue, West Lawn, PA 19609, (215) 678-0858, BS 71 Boston Univ; ME 72 Boston Univ; Sp-Lang Path, Private Practice, **SLP**

Katz, Carolyn 18802 64th Avenue #8J, Flushing, NY 11365, (516) 678-1200, BA 74 Hofstra Univ; MA 76 Hofstra Univ; **SLP**

Katz, Cindy Miller 6 Whittier Place #12C, Boston, MA 02114, (617) 596-8837, BA 77 Univ of MI - Ann Arbor; MS 80 Univ of WI - Madison; Sp/Lang Path, Swampscott Pub Schs, **SLP**

Katz, Debra Friedland 3209 Dungarvin Drive, Tallahassee, FL 32308, (904) 656-4800, BA 77 Univ of MD - College Park; MA 79 OH St Univ; 87–Clin Coord, Capital Rehab Hosp, **SLP**

Katz, Mrs Debra R 603 Ridge Road, Highland Park, IL 60035, (312) 635-6763, BS 75 Northwestern Univ; MA 76 Northwestern Univ; SLP, Private Practice, **SLP**

Katz, Mrs Erica J 8 Hazamir Street, Ramat Gan, Israel 52596, BA 43 Witwatersrand Univ S Africa; **SLP LM**

Katz, Francine H 2250 Montecito Drive, San Marino, CA 91108, (213) 796-2124, BS 55 Northwestern Univ; MA 61 CA St Univ - Los Angeles; Lip Reading Spec & Asst Prof, Pasadena City College, **SLP**

Katz, Mrs Gloria B 38 Central Avenue, East Brunswick, NJ 08816, (201) 613-6833, BA 63 CUNY - Brooklyn Coll; MA 65 Columbia Univ Teachers Coll; Sp-Lang Path, East Brunswick Bd of Educ, **SLP**

Katz, Mrs Heidi Rathe 48 Tenby Chase Drive, Voorhees, NJ 08043, (609) 768-1753, BA 81 Montclair St Coll; MA 82 Montclair St Coll; Sp-Lang Path, Self Employed-Sturbridge Sp & Lang Ctr, **SLP**

Katz, Herman G 54-09 253rd Street, Little Neck, NY 11362, (212) 470-2271, BA 52 NY Univ; MA 56 CUNY - Brooklyn Coll; Chairman/Sp & Hrng Dept, Sewanhaka Cen Hs Dist, **SLP**

Katz, Mrs Iris L 3158 Cardinal Drive, Westminster, MD 21157, (301) 356-0710, BS 71 Towson St Univ; MA 72 Univ of MD - College Park; Sp/Lang Path, Bd of Ed of Balto Co, **SLP**

Katz, Dr Jack Communicative Disorders & Sci, Univ At Buffalo - SUNY, 109 Park Hall, Buffalo, NY 14260, (716) 636-3400, BA 56 CUNY - Brooklyn Coll; MS 57 Syracuse Univ; PH 61 (NS) Univ of Pittsburgh - Pittsburgh; Prof, Univ at Buffalo - SUNY, **SLP A F ACE**

Katz, James B P O Box 4880, Louisville, KY 40204, (502) 458-5445, Territory Mgr, Phonic Ear, **A**

Katz, Jean Becker 410 North Lincoln, Moscow, ID 83843, **SLP**

Katz, Mrs Jean Yager 10383 Rochester Avenue, Los Angeles, CA 90024, (213) 922-6326, BS 54 Univ of WI - Madison; MA 70 Univ of Chicago; Consult, LA Co Supt of Schs, **SLP**

Katz, Jeffrey A 908 Bowman Road, Elmira, NY 14905, (607) 733-6541, BA 74 CUNY - Lehman Coll; MA 76 CUNY - Lehman Coll; OM 81 Alfred Univ; Admin Dir Rehab, Twin Tiers Rehab Cen St Jos H, **A**

Katz, Jodi Robin Barrow Neurological Institute, St Joseph's Hospital, 350 West Thomas Road, Phoenix, AZ 85013, (602) 285-3284, BS 79 Univ of AZ; MS 82 Univ of AZ; 88–Sp-Lang Path, Barrow Neurological Institute, **SLP**

Katz, Dr Karyn Bobkoff Dept Communicative Disorders, University Of Akron, Akron, OH 44325, (216) 375-7883, BS 73 Univ of TX - Austin; MA 74 Case Western Reserve Univ; PH 82 (Sp Path) Kent St Univ; 79–Assoc Prof, U of Akron, **SLP**

Katz, Lisa Beth 179 Maplewood Street, Watertown, MA 02172, (608) 263-6190, BS 82 Univ of WI - Madison; MS 85 Univ of WI - Madison; Aud, Harvard Comm Hlth Plan, **A**

Katz, Lori E 49 Winthrop Road, Plainview, NY 11803, (516) 938-7810, BA 84 Hofstra Univ; MA 86 Hofstra Univ; **SLP**

Katz, Melanie W 255 Bronx River Road, Apartment 8-P, Yonkers, NY 10704, (212) 360-6148, BA 76 Adelphi Univ; MA 77 Hofstra Univ; Audiologist, New York Medical College, **A**

Katz, Nancy Suslick 8 South Michigan Avenue, Suite 2120, Chicago, IL 60603, (312) 236-3518, BS 80 Univ of IL - Urbana; MA 82 Univ of IL - Urbana; 83–Aud, Irwin D Horwitz MD SC, **A**

Katz, Nina 2327 Columbia, Eugene, OR 97403, **SLP**

Katz, Dr Richard C 11750 Sunset Boulevard, Suite 414, Los Angeles, CA 90049, (213) 894-3850, BA 71 Univ of MA - Amherst; MA 73 Univ of MA - Amherst; PH 77 (NS) Univ of FL; 77–Asst Chief Aud, VA, **SLP**

Katz, Roberta Ann 178 Burlington Avenue, Deer Park, NY 11793, (516) 243-3812, BS 85 SUNY - Coll at Buffalo; MS 86 SUNY - Coll at Buffalo; 86–Sp-Lang Path, Suffolk Child Devel Ctr, **SLP**

Katz, Robin Beth 10810 Carrollwood Drive, Tampa, FL 33618, (813) 933-5630, BA 84 Univ of FL; MA 86 Univ of TN - Knoxville; SLP, Sulphur Springs Elem School, **SLP**

Katz, Mrs Sally L 1621 Old Trenton Road, Rural Delivery 4, Trenton, NJ 08691, (609) 443-3184, BA 64 William Paterson Coll; MA 68 Columbia Univ Teachers Coll; **SLP**

Katz, Mrs Sally M 811 Pointer Ridge Drive, Gaithersburg, MD 20878, (301) 330-3443, BA 73 Univ of MD - College Park; MS 75 Univ of WI - Madison; Sp/Lang Path, Mont Co Pub Sch, **SLP**

Katz, Mrs Sarabeth B 3533 Chaparral Drive SW, Roanoke, VA 24018, (703) 981-2867, BA 70 Univ of NC - Greensboro; MA 72 Univ of MD - College Park; 85–Sp-Lang Path, Roanoke City PS, **SLP**

Katz, Mrs Sheila E 908 Bowman Road, Elmira, NY 14905, (607) 739-5601, BA 73 CUNY - Lehman Coll; MS 75 Columbia Univ Teachers Coll; Tchr, BOCES, **SLP**

Katz, Susan J 537 Sheridan Road, Evanston, IL 60202, (312) 864-8122, MA 74 Our Lady Lake Univ-San Anton; 83–Sp/Lang Path, Northern Suburban Spec Ed Dist, **SLP**

Katz, Susan L 60 Pattison Street E-28, North Abington, MA 02351, (617) 871-8048, BS 76 Boston Univ; MS 77 Columbia Univ Teachers Coll; Sp-Lang Path, Weymouth Public Schools, **SLP**

Katz-Brown, Mrs Barbara D 110 Eastwood Avenue, Ithaca, NY 14850, (607) 274-2241, BS 74 Ithaca Coll; MS 75 Ithaca Coll; Sp-Lang Path, Ithaca Cty Sch Dist, **SLP ACE**

Katzen, Sheri H 1623 Avenue R, Brooklyn, NY 11229, (718) 990-5026, BA 81 CUNY - Brooklyn Coll; MS 83 CUNY - Brooklyn Coll; Sp-Lang Path, Private Practice, **SLP**

Katzenberger, Kathleen Anne 5216 Cromarty Road, Baltimore, MD 21229, (301) 355-0100, BS 85 Towson St Univ; MS 87 Towson St Univ; 87–Sp-Lang Path, The Easter Seal Soc of MD Inc, **SLP**

Katzin, Betsy Sue 51 Chestnut Way, Manalapan Township, NJ 07726, (718) 332-5829, BA 83 CUNY - Brooklyn Coll; MS 85 CUNY - Brooklyn Coll; 86–Aud, Kingsbrook Jewish Med Ctr, **A**

Katzman, Dr Elizabeth A 1412 Willow Avenue, Louisville, KY 40204, BA 72 Univ of Louisville; MS 74 Univ of Louisville; ED 87 (Supervision) Univ of Louisville; 85–Tchr, Jefferson Co Pub Sch, **SLP**

Katzman, Mrs Jeanne 2811 Wilshire Boulevard, Suite 800, Santa Monica, CA 90403, (213) 829-5968, BA 68 Univ of Southern CA; MA 70 Catholic Univ of America; Sp-Lang Path, Private Practice, **SLP**

Katzman, Mrs Karen B 459 Rose Lane, Rockville, NY 11570, (516) 663-1084, BA 68 Queens Coll; MS 69 Adelphi Univ

Katzman, Mrs Sherry Hecht 34 Powder Creek Drive, Belleville, IL 62223, (618) 537-4553, BA 76 Newcomb Coll Tulane Univ; MS 83 Southern IL Univ-Edwardsvill; Sp-Lang Path, Lebanon District 9, **SLP**

Katzman, Mrs Shirley Rose 7255 S W 140th Terrace, Miami, FL 33158, (305) 238-8113, BA 63 IN Univ - Bloomington; MS 79 FL Int'l Univ; Sp-Lang Path, Joy E Felton/Assoc, **SLP ACE**

Katz-Weintraub, Sharon Elaine 11131 Leisure Lane, St Louis, MO 63146, (314) 567-3598, BS 72 Univ of IL - Urbana; MA 76 Univ of MN - Minneap-St Paul; 85–Clinical Supervisor, St Louis University, **SLP**

Kau, Darlene M 3610 Pahoa Avenue, Honolulu, HI 96816, (808) 521-2992, BA 64 Univ of HI - Manoa; OM 82 Univ of HI - Manoa; MA 66 Univ of HI - Manoa; Owner, Darlene MI Kau, **SLP A**

Kaucher, Gail Louise 1007 North 8th Street, Wyomissing, PA 19610, (215) 374-0048, BS 84 Bloomsburg Univ of PA; MS 85 Bloomsburg Univ of PA; 85–Aud, Penta & Shelby ENT Assoc Ltd, **A**

Kaucic, Cheryl Ann 2969 North 54th Street, Milwaukee, WI 53210, (414) 442-0172, BS 85 Marquette Univ; MS 86 Marquette Univ; **SLP**

Kauffman, Carol L 7263 Rising Way, Columbus, OH 43235, (614) 852-1372, BA 73 Baldwin-Wallace Coll; MA 77 OH St Univ; Sp-Lang Path, Madison County Hosp, **SLP**

Kauffman, Catherine The Winston L Prouty Ctr, 2 Oak St, Brattleboro, VT 05301, **SLP**

Kauffman, Mrs Cynthia A 17555 144th Avenue #B, Spring Lake, MI 49456-9522, (616) 674-8091, BS 80 Western MI Univ; MA 82 Western MI Univ; SLP, Van Buren Intermed School Dist, **SLP**

Kauffman, Dorothy Carlson 17364 Fielding, Detroit, MI 48219, (313) 538-4586, BS 84 Eastern MI Univ; MA 86 Eastern MI Univ

Kauffman, Ellen K 160 Gordonhurst Avenue, Apartment G32, Upper Montclair, NJ 07043, (201) 744-0567, BA 30 9660; MA 45 Columbia Univ Teachers Coll; **SLP LM**

Kauffman, Mrs Laura Lee 76 Pearl Street, Bangor, ME 04401, (207) 942-3871, BS 80 Radford Univ; MS 82 James Madison Univ; **SLP**

Kauffman, Mary Jane 1134 Lakeview Crescent, Birmingham, AL 35205, (205) 939-3183, BA 67 LA St Univ - Baton Rouge; MA 80 Univ of TN - Knoxville; **SLP**

Kauffman-Mally, Mrs Helene 25576 Wareham, Huntington Woods, MI 48070-1663, (313) 542-4786, BS 79 Wayne St Univ; MA 80 Wayne St Univ; Tchr, Detroit Pub Sch, **SLP**

Kaufman, Carol C 1 Green Briar Lane, Dix Hills, NY 11746, (516) 269-6000, MA 85 Long Island U - CW Post Ctr, 80–Sp-Lang Path, Kings Park Central Sch Dist, **SLP**

Kaufman, Mrs Carol M 152 Cornflower Drive, Milford, CT 06460, (203) 783-3533, BS 61 Boston Univ; MS 73 Southern CT St Univ; Sp-Lang Path, Milford Bd of Ed, **SLP**

Kaufman, Debra Watson 1108 Sioux Terrace, Madison, TN 37115, (615) 322-7995, BS 82 Western KY Univ; MS 83 Western KY Univ; Sp-Lang Path, Vanderbilt Univ Med Ctr, **SLP**

Kaufman, Diana Kay 7949 Montgomery Avenue, Elkins Park, PA 19117, (215) 635-6445, BA 61 Temple Univ; MA 63 Temple Univ; **SLP**

Kaufman, Mrs Diane Boehler 3239 Southwest 18th Street, Okeechobee, FL 34974, (813) 923-2686, BS 75 Nazareth Coll of Rochester; MS 81 Nazareth Coll of Rochester; Sp-Lang Path, Private Practice, **SLP**

Kaufman, Mrs Eleanor G 1 Laurel Hill Place, Armonk, NY 10504, (914) 273-8231, BA 50 Adelphi Univ; **SLP**

Kaufman, Elise S 233 Taber Avenue, Providence, RI 02906, (401) 353-4010, BS 72 Southern Methodist Univ; MS 74 Vanderbilt Univ; **SLP**

Kaufman, Dr Gale A 316 West 79th Street #6W, New York, NY 10024, (212) 787-0527, BA 66 CUNY - City College; MA 72 CUNY - City College; PH 82 (NS) CUNY - Grad Sch & Univ Cntr; **SLP**

Kaufman, Glenda F 5674 South Fulton Way, Englewood, CO 80111, (303) 694-2237, BA 64 Univ of Denver; MA 65 Univ of Denver; **SLP**

Kaufman, Janis Mae 1335 Tamera Drive, Klamath Falls, OR 97601, (503) 882-0259, BS 82 Portland St Univ; 86–Sp-Lang Path, Klamath Co Sch Dist, **SLP**

Kaufman, Mrs Jennifer R 4000 Cordova Drive, Austin, TX 78759, (512) 452-6471, BS 74 Univ of TX - Austin; MS 76 Baylor Coll of Medicine; Aud, Children's Otolaryngology Assoc, **A**

Kaufman, Mrs Joyce E 3510 Brook Drive, Muncie, IN 47304, (317) 747-5416, BS 50 Ball St Univ; MA 64 Ball St Univ; SLP, Muncie Comm Sch, **SLP**

Kaufman, Kathy E 34 Heritage Drive, Reading, PA 19607, (215) 775-8287, BS 79 Bloomsburg Univ of PA; MS 80 Bloomsburg Univ of PA; Sp-Lang Path, Reading Rehabilitation Hosp, **SLP**

Kaufman, Mrs Marilyn J 520 Murray Canyon Drive, Apartment 511, Palm Springs, CA 92264, (619) 322-7864, BS 53 Univ of MN - Duluth; MA 70 Univ of MN - Duluth; Resource Spec, Palm Springs, **SLP**

Kaufman, Mrs Marjorie J Rd 1 Box 202, 35 Leslie Avenue, Conklin, NY 13748, (607) 775-1838, BA 68 CUNY - Brooklyn Coll; MS 71 CUNY - Brooklyn Coll; 79–Sp/Lang Path, Private Practice, **SLP**

Kaufman, Mary E 1619 North Normandy, Chicago, IL 60635, **SLP**

Kaufman, Mary F 414 Fifth Street, Oakmont, PA 15139, (412) 795-1052, BS 73 Duquesne Univ; MS 75 Univ of Pittsburgh - Pittsburgh; 76–Sp-Lang Path, Pittsburgh-Mt Oliver IU, **SLP**

Kaufman, Nancy Hope 7127 Northampton Way, Houston, TX 77055, BA 50 MI St Univ; ME 56 Univ of FL; MA 74 Univ of Houston - Univ Park; Instructor, Houston Comm Coll, **SLP**

Kaufman, Nancy R William Beaumont Hospital, Speech Pathology Dept, 3601 West 13 Mile Road, Royal Oak, MI 48072, (313) 288-2370, BA 78 MI St Univ; MA 79 Wayne St Univ; SLP, William Beaumont Hospital, **SLP ACE**

Kaufman, Mrs Nancy W 380 South Coldbrook Avenue, Chambersburg, PA 17201, (717) 264-7578, BS 74 Clarion Univ of PA; ME 75 Clarion Univ of PA; Exec Dir, Easter Seal Society, **SLP**

Kaufman, Paula W 5577 Naiche Road, Columbus, OH 43213, MS

Kaufman, Randi E 119 Clark Street, Hillside, NJ 07205, (201) 926-7645, BS 74 NY Univ; MA 76 NY Univ; Sp-Lang Path, Newark Beth Israel Med Cen, **SLP**

Kaufman, Renee C 136-A Tierney Drive, Cedar Grove, NJ 07009, (201) 676-1000, BS 71 Syracuse Univ; MS 72 Columbia Univ Teachers Coll; Sp-Lang Path, VA Medical Center, **SLP ACE**

Kaufman, Rosalind E 49 La Salle Avenue, Rye, NY 10580, (212) 519-4000, BA 69 George Washington Univ; MA 70 Columbia Univ Teachers Coll; Sp-Lang Path, Montefiore Med Cen, **SLP**

Kaufman, Sharon F 364 Lloyd Avenue, Providence, RI 02906, **SLP**

Kaufman, Mrs Tobie Nan 89 Green Way, Allendale, NJ 07401, (201) 265-9653, BA 68 William Paterson Coll; MS 85 William Paterson Coll; 85–Sp-Lang Path, Spec Svcs of Bergen Co, **SLP**

Kaufman-Katz, Valerie F 3109 Abington Drive, Beverly Hills, CA 90210-1101, (818) 706-2370, BA 74 CA St Univ - Northridge; MA 75 CA St Univ - Northridge; Private Practice, **SLP**

Kaufman-Lennon, Andrea 1192 Cumberland Road, Atlanta, GA 30306, (404) 634-2321, BS 78 Univ of IL - Urbana; MS 79 Univ of IL - Urbana; Sp-Lang Path, Fulton Co Bd of Ed, **SLP**

Kaufman-Mamon, Mrs Lauren Jan 100 Rosemary Way #119, Needham, MA 02194, (617) 444-8363, MS 85 Columbia Univ Teachers Coll; **SLP**

Kaufmann, Mrs Arlene J 8824 Stage Ford Road, Raleigh, NC 27615, (919) 848-1427, BS 57 Bradley Univ; MA 59 Univ of KS; Sp-Lang Path, InSpeech Inc, **SLP**

Kaufmann, Evelyn M 14246 Cedar Road #210, University Heights, OH 44121, (216) 835-8888, BA 76 Cleveland St Univ; MA 77 Cleveland St Univ; Sp/Lang Path, Cuyahoga Co Bb of Ment Retard, **SLP**

Kaufmann, Linda B 3465 South Columbine Circle, Englewood, CO 80110, (303) 753-0491, BA 75 Univ of Northern CO; MA 76 Univ of Northern CO; OM 81 Univ of Denver; SLP, Private Practice, **SLP**

Kaufmann, Tiphanie J 3046 Jackson, Apt B, San Francisco, CA 94115, (415) 563-6541, BA 85 Univ of CA - Santa Barbara; MS 87 UT St Univ; 88–Sp-Lang Path, Spectrum, **SLP**

Kaufman-Plenn, Beth 1628 Mayflower Lane, Cherry Hill, NJ 08003, (609) 795-7570, BA 70 Oglethorpe Univ; MA 82 Trenton St Coll; President - Sp-Lang Path, BKP Rehabilitation Assoc, **SLP**

Kauhane, Mrs Jere A 332 Puamamane Street, Honolulu, HI 96821, (808) 423-2477, BA 69 Elmhurst Coll; MS 76 Univ of HI - Manoa; Sp/Lang Path, Dept Ed, **SLP**

Kaul, Joan W 42 Rutherford Avenue, San Anselmo, CA 94960, (415) 472-4110, BA 73 San Francisco St Univ; MA 74 San Francisco St Univ; SLP, Marin Co Offi of Ed, **SLP**

Kautsch, Mrs Elaine M 3015 West 9th Street, Lawrence, KS 66044, (913) 841-4652, BS 67 Mankato St Univ; ME 77 GA St Univ; **SLP**

Kautzman, Laura Katherine 7003 Terry Place, Anchorage, AK 99502, (907) 248-3759, **SLP**

Kavanagh, Mrs Heddy Lee 2303 Hewitt Drive, Houston, TX 77018, MS 54 Univ of Houston - Univ Park; **SLP LM**

Kavanagh, Dr James F 909 Winhall Way, Silver Spring, MD 20904, (301) 496-5097, BA 49 George Washington Univ; MS 50 Univ of WI - Madison; PH 60 (Sp Path & Aud) Univ of WI - Madison; Assoc Dir Cen Res Mothers/Chldn, NIH, **SLP F**

Kavanaugh, D Jane 3809 Birch Street, Windsor, ON, Canada N9C 1Z4, (519) 977-5637, BA 78 Univ of Windsor - Ontario; MA 83 Wayne St Univ; 85–Sp-Lang Path, Grace Hosp, **SLP**

Kavanaugh, Diane E Rural Delivery 8, 6 Cindy Lane, Ballston Spa, NY 12020, **SLP**

Kavanaugh, Mrs Kirsten P 808 6th Avenue, Dixon, IL 61021, (815) 857-3619, BS 74 Western IL Univ; MA 75 Western IL Univ; Sp-Lang Path, Amboy Sch Dist #272, **SLP**

Kavanaugh, Mrs Michelle M 61 Havenwood Lane, Grand Island, NY 14072, (716) 694-8040, BS 76 SUNY - Coll at Buffalo; MS 78 SUNY - Coll at Buffalo; Asst Prin, North Tonawanda City Schs, **SLP**

Kavarsky, Mrs Joan M 80 Anderson Avenue, Scarsdale, NY 10583, (914) 592-7555, BA 74 CUNY - City College; MA 76 CUNY - City College; 88–Dir of Sp-Lang Path & Aud, Blythedale Chldn Hosp, **SLP**

Kavouriaris, Kathleen Waldron 7601 South Roberts Road, Bridgeview, IL 60455, (312) 598-5711, BA 77 Mundelein Coll; MS 79 Emerson Coll; Sp-Lang Path, SW Coop Assoc for Special Ed, **SLP**

Kavulla, Patrick S 4113 Forrest Heights, Stow, OH 44224, (216) 253-5290, BS 69 Kent St Univ; MA 72 Kent St Univ; Super of Sp & Lang Serv, Summit Co Bd of Ed, **SLP**

Kawaguchi, Jean Noriko 625 North Marvista #4, Pasadena, CA 91106, (213) 263-9818, BA 75 CA St Univ - Los Angeles; MA 78 CA St Univ - Los Angeles; Sp-Lang Path, LA USD, **SLP**

Kawell-Meskan, Mary E Illinois Eye And Ear Infirmary, 1855 West Taylor Street, Chicago, IL 60612, (312) 996-6520, BS 82 Univ of IL - Urbana; MA 84 Univ of IL - Urbana; 87–Audiologist, Univ of Ill-Chicago, **A**

Kay, Aimee 21321 N E 23th Avenue, Miami, FL 33180, (305) 666-6511, BA 79 Univ of FL; MA 80 FL St Univ; Aud, Miami Childrens Hosp, **A**

Kay, Mrs Janice Terry 28890 Nottoway, Farmington Hills, MI 48331, (313) 594-6110, BA 78 MI St Univ; MA 79 Central MI Univ; 85–Sp-Lang Path, Outer Drive Hosp, **SLP**

Kay, Mrs Lois F 3870 Bethany Road, Cleveland, OH 44118, BA 52 OH Univ - Athens; MA 84 John Carroll Univ; Sp-Lang Path, Cleveland Bd of Ed, **SLP**

Kay, Melinda Harrison 603 14th Avenue Southwest, Rochester, MN 55902-2016, (507) 281-1180, BS 75 Marquette Univ; MA 76 Kent St Univ; **SLP**

Kay, Mrs Nancy S 2112 Campus Drive, South Euclid, OH 44121, (216) 382-7123, BS 59; MA 62; **SLP**

Kay, Mrs Pamela M Route 2 Box 221B, Sparta, TN 38583, (615) 738-3052, BA 77 Univ of Northern CO; MA 80 Univ of TN - Knoxville; Sp-Lang Path, Putnam Cty Schs, **SLP**

Kay, Vicki D 9365 Silverleaf Way, Alta Loma, CA 91701, (714) 967-2841, BS 68 Southwest TX St Univ; ME 69 Southwest TX St Univ; SLP, Offi of LA Co Supt Sch, **SLP**

Kayata, Mary Ellen 301 Wood Have Road, Pawtucket, RI 02861, BA 84 Univ of VT; MS 86 James Madison Univ; **SLP**

Kaye, Mrs Arlene D 17 Hunters Trail, Bethany, CT 06525, (203) 393-0006, BA 75 Elmira Coll; MS 78 Southern CT St Univ; Sp-Lang Path, Shelton Pub Sch, **SLP**

Kaye, Debra Naiztat 2020 East 67th Street, Brooklyn, NY 11234-6008, (212) 436-7600, BA 79 CUNY - Brooklyn Coll; MS 81 CUNY - Brooklyn Coll; Sp-Lang Path, UCP, **SLP**

Kaye, Helen Donaldson 421 Warren Avenue, Cary, NC 27511, (919) 467-1180, BA 67 Rutger's St Univ - Douglas Coll; ME 68 PA St Univ - Univ Park; 87–Admin, Cary Counseling Ctr, **SLP**

Kaye, Jennifer E 10066 Foxboro Circle, San Ramon, CA 94583, (415) 577-1435, BA 77 Wesleyan Univ; MA 79 San Diego St Univ; Project Leader Comp Install, Fairmont Hosp, **SLP**

Kaye, Roberta Loren 6209 Resesa Boulevard #210, Reseda, CA 91335, (213) 824-3100, **SLP**

Kayfes, Mareve Box 513, Buhl, MN 55713, BS 74 Marquette Univ; MA 75 Univ of Denver; **SLP**

Kayl, Susan N 20748 Exhibit Place, Woodland Hills, CA 91367, (818) 884-5606, BA 72 CA St Univ - Northridge; MA 75 CA St Univ - Northridge; MA 77 CA St Univ - Northridge; SLP, Los Angeles USD, **SLP A**

Kaylor, Carol L 497 East California Blvd, Apartment 113, Pasadena, CA 91106, **SLP**

Kaylor, Kristen A 945 Oakcrest #C-22, Iowa City, IA 52246, (319) 369-7491, BS 73 Bowling Green St Univ; MA 75 Bowling Green St Univ; Sp-Lang Path, St Lukes Hosp, **SLP**

Kaynatma, Martha Janecky 8414 West 100th Street, Bloomington, MN 55438, (612) 642-4030, BS 75 Univ of WI - Madison; MS 76 Univ of WI - Madison; Sp-Lang Path, St Paul Sch Dist #625, **SLP**

Kayner, Mrs Janet G 19W 083 Avenue Chateaux North, Oak Brook, IL 60521, (312) 852-1607, BS 64 Northwestern Univ; **SLP**

Kay-Newman, Mrs Susan 74 Hawthorne Avenue, Floral Park, NY 11001, (212) 423-7323, BA 79 CUNY - Queens Coll; MA 81 CUNY - Queens Coll; Sp-Lang Path, Visiting Therapy Assoc, **SLP**

Kay-Rainingbird, Elizabeth 2924 Harvey Street #3D, Madison, WI 53705, (406) 395-4474, BA 78 Queens Univ - Ontario; MS 80 Columbia Univ Teachers Coll; **SLP**

Kays, Linda A 2302 S W 114th Street, Seattle, WA 98146, (206) 433-2149, BA 67 Univ of WA; MA 74 Univ of WA, Early Chldhd Spec Ed Tchr, Highline Pub Sch, **SLP**

Kayser, Dean J 613 Polk Boulevard, Des Moines, IA 50312, (515) 255-2300, BS 77 Purdue Univ - West Lafayette; MA 79 Central MI Univ; 88–Aud, Woodard Hearing Aid Centers, **A**

Kayser, Dr Hortense Garcia Texas Christian University, Box 30793, Fort Worth, TX 76129, (817) 921-7620, BS 73 Univ of AZ; MS 75 Univ of AZ; PH 85 (Bilingual Language Development) NM St Univ; 85–Assistant Professor, Texas Christian University, **SLP**

Kayser, Kathy Ann 80 East Irvin Avenue, Hagerstown, MD 21740, (301) 791-5157, **A**

Kayser, Marianne Catherine 2964 Hatherly Drive, St Louis, MO 63121, (314) 355-2300, SLP, Christian Hosp NE, **SLP**

Kayser, Mrs Virginia C 2 Grouse Terrace, Lake Oswego, OR 97035, (503) 288-6036, BS 60 Portland St Univ; MS 72 Portland St Univ; 68–Sp-Lang Path, Portland Public Sch, **SLP**

Kazandjian, Marta S 119 South Bay Avenue, Islip, NY 11751, (516) 581-1774, BA 85 SUNY - Center at Binghamton; MA 87 CUNY - Hunter Coll; **SLP**

Kazdan, Mrs Phyllis Parks 4507 South Fortuna Way, Salt Lake City, UT 84124, (801) 278-7602, BS 70 IN St Univ - Terre Haute; MS 71 IN St Univ - Terre Haute; SLP, **SLP**

Kazek, Mrs Ruth Elizabethk 860 Lake Catherine Drive, Maitland, FL 32751, (305) 331-4770, MS; **A**

Kazer, Mrs Joan G Two Grove Street, Mount Kisco, NY 10549, (914) 241-0139, BA 74 Case Western Reserve Univ; MS 75 Columbia Univ Teachers Coll; Sp-Lang Path, Bedford Hills Elem Sch, **SLP**

Kea, Mrs Christa Langston 1766 Colony Road, Rock Hill, SC 29730, (803) 285-8439, MS 84 Univ of AR - Little Rock; Sp-Lang Path, Winthrop College, **SLP**

Keahon, Sonia M V P O Box 821, Setauket, NY 11733, **SLP**

Keally, Mrs Maryann Wilson 1213 Misty Hollow Way, Virginia Beach, VA 23454, (804) 481-3468, BS 73 PA St Univ - Univ Park; MS 74 PA St Univ - Univ Park; **SLP**

Kean, Mrs Sally Ann 106 Hickory Drive, Pataskala, OH 43062, MS 66 PA St Univ - Univ Park; SLP, The Columbus Academy, **SLP**

Keane, Mrs G Marie c/o Hawley School, 29 Church Hill Road, Newtown, CT 06470, (203) 426-7666, BA 70 Univ of Bridgeport; ME 74 SUNY - Coll at Geneseo; Sp/Lang Path, Newtown Public Schools, **SLP**

Keane, Marta M 3474 Caledonia Circle, Woodbridge, VA 22192, (703) 497-0799, BA 76 Univ of VA - Charlottesville; ME 78 Univ of VA - Charlottesville; Sp-Lang Path, InSpeech Inc, **SLP ACE**

Keane, Mrs Sandra O'Neill 506 Brightwaters, Cocoa Beach, FL 32931, (305) 268-6181, MA 80 Trenton St Coll; SLP, North Brevard Rehab Cen, **SLP**

Keane, Dr Vincent E P O Box 953, Belmar, NJ 07719, (201) 681-0512, BA 54 Seton Hall Univ; MA 61 Univ of IA; PH 70 (NS) Univ of OR; SLP, St Rose Hgh & Gram Schs, **SLP**

Kearney, Anne Ferguson 21 Roslyn Park East, Sea Cliff, NY 11579, (516) 671-9057, BS 76 PA St Univ - Univ Park; MS 79 Adelphi Univ; 80–Sp-Lang Path, Private Practice, **SLP**

Kearney, Kathleen M 296 Randolph Street, Abington, MA 02351, (508) 676-3411, BA 86 Bridgewater St Coll; MA 88 Univ of MA - Amherst; 88–Aud, R H Fitton Jr MD Inc

Kearney, Margaret Mary 96 Kim Louise Drive #3, Campbell, CA 95008, (408) 259-2396

Kearney, Ruth S 71 Sawmill Road, Bricktown, NJ 08724, (201) 458-5363, BA 73 Geneva Coll; ME 75 Clarion Univ of PA; Sp/Lang Path, Ocean Co Health Dept, **SLP**

Kearns, Barbara A 10 West Parsons Court, East Setauket, NY 11733, (516) 348-2729, BA 71 CUNY - Queens Coll; MA 73 CUNY - Queens Coll; Aud, Suffolk Co Dept of Hlth Servs, **A**

Kearns, Mrs Dacia L 13919 Adamson Road, Huntley, IL 60142, (312) 365-5116, BS 84 IL St Univ - Normal; MS 86 IL St Univ - Normal; **SLP**

Kearns, Mrs Felicia J 137 North Main Street, Manchester, PA 17345, (717) 767-6941, BS 80 Indiana Univ of PA; MS 82 Univ of AZ; Head Injury Prog Dir, Rehab Hosp of York, **SLP**

Kearns, Geralyn Harvey 1806 Colfax Street, Evanston, IL 60201, (312) 880-3430, BA 74 Univ of VT; MA 76 IN Univ - Bloomington; Sp-Lang Path, Children's Memorial Hosp, **SLP**

Kearns, Kevin P VA Medical Center, Audiology/Speech (126), 3001 Greenbay Road, North Chicago, IL 60064, (312) 578-3759, BS 74 SUNY - Center at Buffalo; MA 75 Saint Louis Univ; PH 79 (Sp Path) Univ of KS; 86–Chief-Aud/Sp-Lang Path, VA Med Ctr, **SLP**

Kearns, Thomas J 18810 Springdale Avenue, Cleveland, OH 44135, (216) 267-4378, MA 87 Cleveland St Univ; 87–Sp-Lang Path, PSI Affiliates Inc, **SLP**

Kearns, Timothy M 8739 Falls Road, West Falls, NY 14170, (716) 674-6300, **SLP**

Kearns-Crockett, Patricia M 3304 Shoreline Drive, Las Vegas, NV 89117, (702) 254-1363, BS 79 CA St Univ - Hayward; MS 81 Univ of AZ; 87–Sp-Lang Path, Univ Med Ctr of Southern NV, **SLP**

Kearsley, Nancy Conlin 78 Stony Brook Lane, Norwell, MA 02061, (617) 749-3435, BS 50 Simmons Coll; ME 70 Boston Univ; Sp-Lang Path, Hingham Pub Sch, **SLP**

Keaster, Jacqueline 4192 Palmer Drive, Los Angeles, CA 90065, MS; **A F LM**

Keating, Mrs Carol Ann 2549 Hillridge Lane, Spring Valley, CA 92078, MA 84 Univ of CA - San Diego; Sp-Lang Path, Scottsdale Schools, **SLP**

Keating, Mrs Linda Susan 2 Baldwin Court, Hamilton, OH 45013, (513) 894-6351, BS 81 Univ of Cincinnati; MA 82 MI St Univ; Sp-Lang Path, Hamilton Cty Schs, **SLP**

Keating, Lisa Beekman 5521 Eagles Nest Drive, Wilmington, NC 28403, (919) 763-1308, BS 81 Miami Univ - Oxford; MA 83 Kent St Univ; Sp-Lang Path, Hearing and Speech Services, **SLP**

Keating, Maryann Pozycki 13 Corinth Drive, Madison, CT 06443, (203) 245-4029, BA 74 Southern CT St Univ; MS 76 Southern CT St Univ; 78–Sp-Lang Path, Private Practice, **SLP**

Keating, Shirley M 14774 Pioneer Blvd, Norwalk, CA 90650, (213) 868-1441, BA 75 CA St Univ - Long Beach; MA 78 CA St Univ - Long Beach; Sp/Lang Path, Private Practice, **SLP**

Keatinge, Connie Laguna Honda Hosp-Sp/H Clinic, 375 Laguna Honda Blvd, San Francisco, CA 94116, (415) 664-1580, Univ of OR; Director Speech-Hearing Clinic, Laguna Honda Hospital, **SLP**

Keatley, Dr Mary A W 2310 Juniper, Boulder, CO 80302, (303) 440-0056, BA 72 Univ of CO - Boulder; MA 75 Univ of CO - Boulder; PH 80 (NS) Univ of CO - Boulder; 88–Sp-Lang Path, Private Practice, **SLP**

Keaton, Mrs Larue M 4700 Lake Park Drive, Arlington, TX 76016, (817) 478-7504, BS 75 Baylor Univ; MA 76 Baylor Univ; **SLP**

Keats-Rigby, Mrs Caren S 1877 El Rancho #179, Sparks, NV 89431, (702) 329-5108, BA 82 CUNY - Brooklyn Coll; MS 85 CUNY - Brooklyn Coll; 88–Sp-Lang Path, Nevada Communication Services, **SLP**

Keblusek, Sue J 35 Ronada Avenue, Oakland, CA 94611, (415) 633-5248, BA 70 Mary Washington Coll; MA 71 Univ of FL; 83–Sp/Lang Path, Oakland Naval Hosp, **SLP ACE**

Keck, Deborah Ann 5866 59th Street, Sacramento, CA 95824, (916) 457-1004, MS 87 CA St Univ - Sacramento; Audiologist, Dr Balfour, **A**

Keck, Mrs Patricia Joan 2402 Lucille Drive, Omaha, NE 68147, (402) 572-5952, BS 83 Miami Univ - Oxford; MS 84 Miami Univ - Oxford; Sp-Lang Path, Omaha Public Schools, **SLP**

Kee, Donna Katherine P O Box 561, Franklin, WV 26807, (304) 358-7093

Kee, Linda M 9235 Butte Mtn Lane West, Jackson, CA 95642, (209) 736-4662, BA 77 CA St Univ - Sacramento; MA 80 CA St Univ - Sacramento; SLP, Calaveras Co Off of Ed, **SLP**

Keefe, Karen R 337 East Bodley, Kirkwood, MO 63122, **SLP**

Keefe, Kristen Ann 5733 Phillips Avenue 1st Fl, Pittsburgh, PA 15217, (412) 647-8094, BA 84 Case Western Reserve Univ; MA 86 Univ of Pittsburgh - Pittsburgh; Phd, Univ of Pittsburgh, **SLP**

Keefe, Mrs Linda Marie 1982 Alta Court, Oakdale, CA 95361, (209) 571-6600, **SLP**

Keefe, Mary Jo 30894 Morlock, Livonia, MI 48152, (313) 771-3305, BA 74 Loyola Coll; MS 75 Loyola Coll; 88–Sp-Lang Path, Lakeshore ENT Clin, **SLP**

Keefer, Mrs Barbara L 200 Bershire Circle West, Longwood, FL 32779, (703) 361-3444, BS 74 Middle TN St Univ; MA 75 Univ of TN - Knoxville; C O R E Instructor, Seminole Comm College, **SLP**

Keefer, C Helen Box 541, Cave Spring, GA 30124-0451, (404) 777-8878, BS 68 GA Southern Coll; ME 71 GA St Univ; ES 87 GA St Univ; 71–Assoc Sch Psych, State Dept of Educ Sch for the Deaf

Keegan, Frances P 4 Country Court, East Greenwich, RI 02818, (401) 885-1236, BA 84 Univ of RI; MS 86 Univ of RI; 88–Sp-Lang Path, Cranston PS, **SLP**

Keegan, Mrs Melody Ann 121 Melbourne Street, Vestal, NY 13850, (607) 748-6455, BS 82 Clarion Univ of PA; MS 83 Clarion Univ of PA; 84–Sp-Lang Path, Lourdes Hosp, **SLP**

Keel, Franklin D 10449 Dover, Yukon, OK 73099, (405) 231-5581, BS 78 Univ of Science & Arts of OK; MS 80 TX Tech Univ; Chief/Commun Dis Branch, OK Area Indian Hlth Ser, **A**

Keel, Mrs Jennifer Lynn W 10449 Dover Drive, Yukon, OK 73099, (405) 324-0350, MS 80 Southern IL Univ-Edwardsvill; Private Practice, **SLP**

Keele, Judy Smith 1512 Wildrose Avenue, Box 1154, Gardnerville, NV 89410, (702) 782-5232, BS 75 Univ of NV - Reno; MA 76 Univ of UT; 83–Sp-Lang Path, Totland Presch, **SLP**

Keele, Susan Laraine 521-A West Main, Fairfield, IL 62837, (618) 842-2529, BS 86 Eastern IL Univ; MS 87 Eastern IL Univ; Sp-Lang Path, Fairfield Comm HS, **SLP**

Keelen-D'Amore, Mrs Karen Ann 157 Spring Street, Red Bank, NJ 07701, (201) 747-9399, BA 78 Trenton St Coll; MS 87 Rutgers St Univ -N Brunswick; 88–Sp-Lang Path, CP Assn

Keeler, Andrew S 823 Lay Boulevard, Kalamazoo, MI 49001, (616) 385-3493, MA 87 Western MI Univ

Keeler, Dr Christine Siss 45 Shadyside Drive, Wyckoff, NJ 07481, (201) 977-2435, BA 71 Muhlenberg Coll; MS 73 Columbia Univ Teachers Coll; PH 83 (Sp-Lang Path) 2162; 88–Sp-Lang Path, St Josephs Hosp & Med Ctr, **SLP**

Keeler, Darlene D 938 East Porter Avenue, Naperville, IL 60540, MS; **LM**

Keeler, Janice W 217 Carolwood Drive, San Antonio, TX 78213, (512) 690-1276, BA 73 SUNY - Center at Albany; MA 74 Our Lady Lake Univ-San Anton; Administrator, Northside ISD, **SLP**

Keeler, Mrs Linda W 504 S 15th Street, Norfolk, NE 68701, (402) 379-0478, BS 65 Phillips Univ; MS 66 Southern IL Univ -Carbondale; Sp-Lang Path, Educational Service Unit #1, **SLP**

Keeler, Patricia Sue 5128 Calvin Road, Sylvania, OH 43560, (419) 243-5191, BS 83 Western MI Univ; MS 85 Univ of MI - Ann Arbor; **SLP**

Keeley, Jane Lee Box 190-A R R #4, Viroqua, WI 54665, (608) 675-3308, BA 81 Humboldt St Univ; MA 85 Humboldt St Univ; Sp-Lang Path, CES 4, **SLP**

Keeley, Mrs Susanne Phillips 9 Salem Lane, Evanston, IL 60203, (312) 883-8527, BA 82 Univ of CO - Boulder; MA 84 Northwestern Univ; Sp-Lang Path, Chicago Neurosurgical Ctr, **SLP**

Keeling, James D 1383 Ginger, Poplar Bluff, MO 63901, (913) 877-3301, BA 74 Univ of AR - Fayetteville; MA 76 Univ of AR - Fayetteville; Asst Dir for Habilitation, Poplar Bluffs Regional Ctr, **SLP**

Keeling, Leslie Thompson 1383 Ginger, Poplar Bluff, MO 63901-2107, (314) 785-6809, BA 74 Univ of AR - Fayetteville; MA 75 Univ of AR - Fayetteville; 85–Sp-Lang Path, Private Practice, **SLP**

Keeling, Sandra D Audiology Services, 2310 Belmont Drive, Reidsville, NC 27320, (919) 342-5250, BS 73 Radford Univ; MA 75 Univ of VA - Charlottesville; Aud, Aud Serv, **A**

Keels, Edward W 1522 Forrestal Street, Philadelphia, PA 19145, **A**

Keels-Miller, Mrs Rita Ann 8520 Delmar Lane, Prairie Village, KS 66207, (816) 276-4023, **SLP**

Keely, Cynthia Meier 601 Greenbriar Drive, Williamstown, NJ 08094, (609) 342-7600, BA 71 Seton Hall Univ; MA 83 Temple Univ-Tyler Sch of Art; Sp/Lang Path, Mediplex Rehab-Camden, **SLP**

Keen, Gerald Lawrence 455 Barbara Lane, West Hempstead, NY 11552, (516) 265-3001, BA 75 CUNY - Queens Coll; MA 79 Hofstra Univ; Sp/Lang Path, Suffolk Chld Dev Cen, **SLP**

Keen, Mrs Janis Dyar 2114 Crestwood Drive, Picayune, MS 39466, (601) 798-4555, BS 74 Univ Southern MS-Hattiesburg; MS 78 Univ Southern MS-Hattiesburg; Sp-Lang Path, Communication Ltd, **SLP**

Keen, Mrs Jeanmarie 910 Surrey Lane, Algonquin, IL 60102, (312) 658-0795, BA 78 Northern IL Univ - De Kalb; MA 79 Northern IL Univ - De Kalb; Aud, Illinois Dept of Health, **A**

Keen, Mrs Joyce M 40 Florida Place, Durango, CO 81301, (303) 259-2452, BA 70 CA St Univ - Fullerton; MA 72 CA St Univ - Fullerton; Sp-Lang Path, Mercy Med Ctr, **SLP**

Keen, Mrs Lynn E 1411 Wheaton Way, Bremerton, WA 98310, (206) 479-4065, BS 75 Purdue Univ - West Lafayette; OM 78 Univ of WA; Owner/Aud, Private Practice, **A**

Keen, Mrs Peggy A 3913 Burning Bush Road, Louisville, KY 40222, (502) 425-8755, BS 74 Eastern KY Univ; MA 75 Univ of KY; Sp/Lang Path, Home Hlth Care, **SLP**

Keenan, Allison Faye St Vincent Professional Bldg, ORL Associates Of Northwestern PA PC, 311 West 24th Street Suite 500, Erie, PA 16502, (814) 452-2405, BA 80 Allegheny Coll; MS 83 Clarion Univ of PA; Audiologist, ORL Assoc of Northwestern PA PC, **A**

Keenan, Dr Joseph S 4142 Betty Ford Road, Murfreesboro, TN 37130, (615) 893-4464, BA 50 Univ of ID; MA 57 Univ of VA - Charlottesville; PH 60 (Sp Path) Univ of FL; 88–Sp-Lang Path, Private Practice, **SLP**

Keenan, Mrs Judy E 18792 Via Verona, Irvine, CA 92715, (714) 832-9200, BA 63 CA St Univ - Long Beach; MA 84 CA St Univ - Fullerton; Dir of SLP, Western Neuro Care Cen, **SLP**

Keenan, Kathleen L Spring Creek Rehabilitation Hospital, 8383 Meadow Road, Dallas, TX 75231, (214) 891-0880, BA 79 William Paterson Coll; MS 83 Vanderbilt Univ; Dir of SLP, Spring Creek Rehab Hosp, **SLP**

Keenan, Laura Jean 101 Granlee Road, San Rafael, CA 94903, (707) 938-5581, BA 77 Univ of CA - Santa Barbara; MA 84 CA St Univ - Los Angeles; **SLP**

Keenan, Mary Colleen 34 Willow Avenue, Somerville, MA 02144, (617) 666-4944, MS 88 Northeastern Univ

Keenan, Nancy C 148 Academy Street, Poughkeepsie, NY 12601, (914) 883-5151, BA 69 CUNY - Lehman Coll; MS 72 Eastern IL Univ; Sp-Lang Path, Early Educ Ctr, **SLP**

Keenan, Mrs Patricia M 275 Bryn Mawr Avenue #H-11, Bryn Mawr, PA 19010, (215) 565-4585, BA 52 Univ of CO - Boulder; MA 53 Univ of Denver; MA 57 Northwestern Univ; 80–Sp-Lang Path, Delaware Co Inter Ut, **SLP A**

Keenan, Robert A 766 Chestnut Street, Meadville, PA 16335, MS

Keene, Mrs Lisa C 5038 East Mulberry, Phoenix, AZ 85018, (602) 952-9772, BS 77 Northern AZ Univ; MS 79 Univ of OK - Norman; Sp-Lang Path, Scottsdale PS, **SLP**

Keene, Risa G 11 Maple Street, Keene, NH 03431, (603) 352-4111, BS 76 Syracuse Univ; MS 78 Syracuse Univ; Sp-Lang Path, Cheshire Med Ctr, **SLP**

Keener, Christine Bebee 628 Placer Street, Grand Junction, CO 81504, (303) 464-5614, BS 69 CO St Univ; MA 73 Kent St Univ; Newspaper Publisher, Palisade Tribune, **SLP**

Keener, Lynn Diane 167 South Allen Street, Albany, NY 12208, (518) 438-4565, BS 81 SUNY - Coll at Geneseo; ME 84 Coll of Saint Rose; Sp-Lang Path, Parsons Child & Family Ctr, **SLP**

Keener, Sandy K 39th & Rainbow Boulevard, 33CRU, Kansas City, KS 66103, (913) 588-5730, BA 84 Univ of KS; MA 87 Univ of KS; **A**

Keeney, Janice Marie 680 Jamestown Boulevard, Apartment 2350, Altamonte Springs, FL 32714, (407) 897-1766, Sp-Lang Path, Rebound, **SLP**

Keeney, Linda E 866 Kellogg Avenue, Santa Barbara, CA 93111, (805) 964-7557, BA 66 CA St Univ - Los Angeles; MA 67 CA St Univ - Los Angeles; **SLP**

Keeney, Mrs Sandra D Route 1 Box 12, Pomona, MO 65789-9701, (417) 256-3113, BS 72 Southeast MO St Univ; MA 73 Southeast MO St Univ; Sp-Lang Path, Private Practice, **SLP**

Keepnews, Susan B 144 Hawk's Hill Road, New Canaan, CT 06840, **SLP**

Keer, Mrs Barbara D 2601 Marian Lane, Wilmette, IL 60091, (312) 622-3626, BA 75 Northwestern Univ; MA 77 Northwestern Univ; Sp-Lang Path, Chicago Pub Sch, **SLP**

Keer, Mrs Francine E 4136 Benedict Canyon Avenue, Sherman Oaks, CA 91604, (213) 984-3870, BS 72 Ithaca Coll; MA 76 CA St Univ - Northridge; Sp/Lang Path, New Sch for Chld Dev, **SLP**

Kees, Mrs Mary A HC 33 Box 73, Alliance, NE 69301, (308) 762-4331, BS 77 West Chester Univ of PA; MA 79 Trenton St Coll; SLP, Alliance City Sch, **SLP**

Kees, Maxwell G 2150 Pericles, Baton Rouge, LA 70808, **SLP A**

Keesee, Mrs Denise Renee 5558 93rd St, Lubbock, TX 79424, (806) 794-7122, BS 81 Univ of North TX; MS 87 TX Tech Univ; **SLP**

Keesee, Mrs Linda Lee 4308 Harcourt, Austin, TX 78727, (512) 834-9420, BA 72 Augustana Coll; MA 78 Western IL Univ; Sp-Lang Path, Linda L Keesee Sp Path, **SLP**

Keesee, Patricia D 600 Westgate, Iowa City, IA 52246, (319) 356-1415, BS OH Univ - Athens; MS Purdue Univ - West Lafayette; U of Iowa, **SLP**

Keesling, Julie Tate 270 International Circle, ENT Department, San Jose, CA 95119, (408) 448-5533, BA 80 San Jose St Univ; MA 82 San Jose St Univ; **A**

Keetay, Victoria Department Of Audiology & Speech Sciences, Purdue University, West Lafayette, IN 47907, (317) 494-7743, BS 80 Ball St Univ; MA 83 Ball St Univ; 88–Aud, Purdue Univ, **A**

Keeter, Dr Larry G 100 Hewlett, Bakersfield, CA 93309, MA 76 CA St Coll - Bakersfield; MA 72 CA St Univ - Chico; ED 81 (NS) Brigham Young Univ; Coord Sp & Lang Serv, Kern Co Supt of Sch Offi, **SLP**

Keeton, Mary F 2720 Westbrook N W, Grand Rapids, MI 49504, **SLP**

Keever, Mrs Aelise H 647 Kenesaw Avenue, Knoxville, TN 37919, (615) 522-1673, BA 71 Univ of TN - Knoxville; BA 74 Univ of TN - Knoxville; MA 75 Univ of TN - Knoxville; 88–Sp-Lang Path, Ft Sanders Hosp Home Hlth & Hospice, **SLP**

Keever, Lyn G 615 Price, Calumet City, IL 60409, (312) 868-6408, BA 63 Coll of Saint Francis; MA 70 Northwestern Univ; 81–Admin, Most Holy Redeemer, **SLP**

Kefauver, Leslie F 4831 Park Avenue, Bethesda, MD 20816, (301) 229-8576, MA 87 Univ of MD - College Park; 88–Sp-Lang Path, Montgomery Co PS

Kegg, Stephen Earl 111 Windsor Circle, Chapel Hill, NC 27514, (919) 732-6138, MS 83 Univ of NC - Chapel Hill; SLP, Orange Co Schs, **SLP**

Kehl, Cynthia Ann 34366 WCR 37, Eaton, CO 80615, (303) 454-2301, MA 88 Univ of Northern CO

Kehn-Nichols, Judith Lynn 109 Potter Drive, Belleville, MI 48111, (313) 782-2716, MA 85 MI St Univ; Riverside Elementary School, **SLP**

Kehoe, Katherine M 977 Golf Course Road #8, Crystal Lake, IL 60014, (312) 381-4340, BA 73 Univ of MI - Ann Arbor; MS 74 Univ of MI - Ann Arbor; 74–Sp-Lang Path, Comm Ut Sch Dist 220, **SLP**

Kehoe-Murray, Karen L 215 Pine Road, Wallingford, PA 19086, (215) 565-4585, BA 77 Rutger's St Univ - Douglas Coll; MS 79 Boston Univ; Aud, Delaware City Intermed Unit, **A**

Kehrli, Karen S Rd 3 Box 343, Pleasant Valley, NY 12569, **SLP**

Keidar, Anat 701 Limit Avenue #2-N, St Louis, MO 63130, (314) 454-7875, MA 78 Univ of IA; MA 81 Univ of IA; PH (NS) Univ of IA; **SLP**

Keidel, Susan M 1116 Cleveland Road, Blue Bell, PA 19422, (215) 444-1601, BS 82 West Chester Univ of PA; MA 87 West Chester Univ of PA; 87–Sp-Lang Path, Team Rehabilitation Inc, **SLP**

Keighley, Patricia 63-A Highland Avenue, Montague, MA 01351, BA 79 Univ of VT; MA 83 Univ of MA - Amherst; Sp-Lang Path, Franklin Med Cen, **SLP ACE**

Keil, Mrs Sharon G 8637 Jefferson Avenue, Munster, IN 46321, (219) 836-4397, BS 76 Ball St Univ; MS 84 Governors St Univ; Sp-Lang Path, Lincoln Sch Dist 156, **SLP**

Kein, Joni Suzanne 3201 14th Street North, Apartment 125, St Cloud, MN 56303, (612) 252-0415, MS 84 Univ of WI - Eau Claire; 88–Tchr, Dist 742 Comm Schs, **SLP**

Keirn, Susan Green 3249 Colby Avenue, Los Angeles, CA 90066, (213) 595-2411, BA 64 Univ of HI - Manoa; MS 69 SUNY - Center at Albany; 88–Prog Dir-Brain Injury Svcs, Memorial Med Ctr of Long Beach, **SLP**

Keisch, Christine C 10 Apple Avenue, Apartment B, Gettysburg, PA 17325, (717) 334-0745, BS 86 Bloomsburg Univ of PA; MS 87 Bloomsburg Univ of PA; 87–Sp-Lang Path, Easter Seal Soc of Franklin, **SLP**

Keiser, Mrs Diane 230 West Kendall Street, Vacaville, CA 95688, BA 79 Univ of WI - Eau Claire; MS 80 Univ of WI - Eau Claire; SLP, Solano Co Offi Ed, **SLP**

Keiser, Mrs Gay K 4101 Wimbledon Drive, Harrisburg, PA 17112, (717) 652-7371, BA 76 Allegheny Coll; MA 79 Temple Univ-Tyler Sch of Art; **SLP**

Keiser, Dr Janet Hope 510 North Bryan Street, Little Rock, AR 72205, (501) 569-3155, BS 62 IN Univ - Bloomington; MA 65 Northwestern Univ; PH 80 (Aud) Univ of IA; Assoc Prof, U of Ark for Med Sci, **A**

Keiser, Nancy Jo 1704 Edgebrook Drive, Apartment 6, Marshalltown, IA 50158, (515) 752-1578, BA 85 Univ of Northern IA; MA 87 Univ of Northern IA; 87–Sp-Lang Path, AEA 6, **SLP**

Keitel, Stephanie P O Box 1555, Montpelier, VT 05602, (802) 223-1034, BA 74 CA St Univ - Fullerton; MA 76 CA St Univ - Fullerton; Sp-Lang Path & Aud, **SLP A**

Keith, Mary Russell 979 East 3rd Street, Suite 508, Chattanooga, TN 37403-4227, (615) 756-2773, MA 83 Univ of TN - Knoxville; Aud, Head & Neck Spec, **A**

Keith, Mrs Melanie P 10005 Springlake Terrace, Fairfax, VA 22030, (703) 691-0115, BS 74 James Madison Univ; MA 78 George Washington Univ; Sp-Lang Path, Arlington County School Board, **SLP**

Keith, Odilia F 803 Terryhollow, Channelview, TX 77530, (713) 462-7708, BS 77 Lamar Univ; MS 79 Lamar Univ; Sp-Lang Path, Region IV Educ Svc Ctr, **SLP**

Keith, Robert Lee 1901 65th Street N E, Rochester, MN 55904, (507) 284-3112, BS 57 Minot St Univ; MS 62 Univ of ND; Sp-Lang Path/Asst Prof, Mayo Cl, **SLP F**

Keith, Dr Robert W Speech And Hearing Division, Univ Of Cincinnati Med Ctr, Mail Loc 528, Cincinnati, OH 45267, (513) 872-4893, BA 62 Univ of IA; MA 64 Univ of IA; PH 67 (NS) Univ of IA; Dir-Div of Aud & SLP, U of Cincinnati, **A F ACE**

Keizer, Kathleen B R R 1 Box 77, Sutton, VT 05867, (802) 525-4012, BA 75 William Paterson Coll; MS 79 Univ of VT; Sp-Lang Path, Orleans Cen Superv Un, **SLP**

Kelchner, Lisa K N 3049 Beech Hill Drive, Spring Valley, OH 45370, (513) 229-6081, BA 76 Baldwin-Wallace Coll; MS 77 Miami Univ - Oxford; Chief SLP, St Elizabeth, **SLP**

Keleher, Elizabeth Lee 85 Scotland #B-4, Royal Plaza, Pueblo, CO 81001, (303) 543-8321, MA 87 George Washington Univ

Kelke, Dr Carl A 21831 Highview, Mount Clemens, MI 48043, PH (NS); **A**

Kelke, Sandra A 210 West Park, Harrison, MI 48625, (517) 386-3851, BS 63 Central MI Univ; MA 68 Central MI Univ; Sp-Lang Path, Clare-Gladwin 1SD, **SLP**

Kelleher, Candice J 25 Blackstone Street, West Peabody, MA 01960, (508) 535-4056, BS 78 Salem St Coll; ME 81 Northeastern Univ; 82–Sp-Lang Path/Tchr, Cambridge Pub Schs, **SLP**

Kelleher, Loleati A 312 Dochan Circle, Montebello, CA 90640, BA 43 Univ of Northern IA; **SLP LM**

Kelleher, Sheila H 7 Longmeadow Drive, Staatsburg, NY 12580, (914) 229-2668, BA 72 Univ of NH; MA 76 Coll of Saint Rose; Sp-Lang Path, **SLP**

Kelleher, Mrs Tamara Jo 3830 North Greenview Avenue, Apartment 8, Chicago, IL 60613-2763, (312) 929-6527, **SLP**

Kelleher, Thomas Peter 424 East 238th Street, Bronx, NY 10470, (212) 324-0645, BA 80 Pace U -NY City; MA 82 NY Univ; Sp-Lang Path Consult, Private Practice, **SLP**

Kelleher-Assael, Kathleen Rd 3 Box 63, Fox Street, Selkirk, NY 12158, (518) 756-6998, BA 76 SUNY - Coll at Cortland; MS 80 Coll of Saint Rose; Sp-Lang Path, Early Childhood Lrng Ctr, **SLP**

Kellenberger, Mrs Paula Hansen 204 South 4th, Sabetha, KS 66534, (913) 284-2175, BS 82 Northwest MO St Univ; MS 83 Northwest MO St Univ; Sp-Lang Path, Holton Spec Ed Coop, **SLP**

Keller, Barbara R 439 Manhattan Road S E, Grand Rapids, MI 49506, (616) 949-7633, BS 59 Miami Univ - Oxford; Sp-Lang Path, Hearing & Speech Center of Gr, **SLP**

Keller, Cindy Melanie 47 Nimbus Road, Holbrook, NY 11741, (516) 472-3985, MA 88 SUNY - Coll at Fredonia

Keller, Mrs Claire B 2951 Stanley Place, Oceanside, NY 11572, (516) 473-2800, BA 55 Adelphi Univ; MS 72 Adelphi Univ; Super Sp & Hrng Ctr, St Charles Hosp, **SLP**

Keller, Dana Renee 1504 North Broadway, Blytheville, AR 72315, (501) 763-1637, OM 87 AR St Univ

Keller, Gary A 18 Xyris Road, P O Box 362, Rocky Point, NY 11778, BA 76 Queens Coll; MA 78 Hofstra Univ; 81–Sp-Lang Path, Long Island Dev Ctr, **SLP**

Keller, Dr Geraldine Bermay Department Of Preventive Medicine, Ohio State University, 320 West 10th Avenue, Columbus, OH 43210, (614) 293-3908, BA 51 CUNY - Hunter Coll; MA 52 NY Univ; PH 78 (Communication) OH St Univ; 70–Res Assoc, OH St U, **SLP A**

Keller, Karen Leone P O Box 248, Centerville, UT 84014-0248, (801) 399-5601, BS 84 Brigham Young Univ; OM 86 Brigham Young Univ; Aud, Ogden Speech & Hearing, **A**

Keller, Mrs Kathleen 510 Pennsylvania Avenue East, Warren, PA 16365, (814) 726-1427, BS 70 Indiana Univ of PA; ME 74 Indiana Univ of PA; Sp-Lang Path, NW Tri-County Indepen Unit 5, **SLP**

Keller, Mrs Linda Takahata 2243 Norman, Stow, OH 44224, BS 79 Kent St Univ; MA 81 Kent St Univ; SLP, Akron Pub Sch, **SLP**

Keller, Margo I 7614 S E 19th Street, Portland, OR 97202, (503) 266-5878, BS 74 Portland St Univ; MS 75 Portland St Univ; Sp-Lang Path, Canby Elem Sch Dist 86, **SLP**

Keller, Dr Mildred G 805 Hillendale Drive, Hattiesburg, MS 39401, (601) 477-9384, BS 63 Univ Southern MS-Hattiesburg; MS 64 Univ Southern MS-Hattiesburg; PH 68 (NS) Univ Southern MS-Hattiesburg; 87–Dir QA Dept, Ellisville State School, **SLP A**

Keller, Mrs Pamela A 3231 Betsy Lane, Herndon, VA 22070, (703) 476-9272, BA 72 MI St Univ; ME 73 Univ of VA - Charlottesville; 73–Sp-Lang Path, Loudoun Co PS, **SLP**

Keller, Sarah E 60 Whitney Ridge Road #F-1, Fairport, NY 14450-1612, (716) 377-4660, BA 65 SUNY - Center at Albany; MA 81 SUNY - Coll at Geneseo; Sp-Lang Path, Monroe BOCES I, **SLP**

Keller, Sharon Pillsbury 24414 Bernard Drive, P O Box 1745, Crestline, CA 92325, (714) 336-2035, BA 78 Univ of LA Verne; MS 83 Univ of LA Verne; 86–Sp-Lang Path, Rim of the World USD, **SLP**

Keller, Sheri Glass 332 Plymouth Street, West Hempstead, NY 11552, (516) 483-3003, BA 81 Long Island U - CW Post Ctr; MA 85 Hofstra Univ; **SLP**

Keller, Mrs Sherry C 2003 Dragonfly, El Dorado, KS 67042, (316) 321-4310, BS 72 Fort Hays St Univ; MA 74 Fort Hays St Univ; SLP, USD 490, **SLP**

Keller, Mrs Susan B 3224 Sherwood Drive, Walworth, NY 14568, (716) 232-2310, BS 81 SUNY - Coll at Brockport; MS 87 Nazareth Coll of Rochester; 87–Sp-Lang Path, Rochester City Sch Dist, **SLP**

Keller, Mrs Susan L F 12515 Larkwood Drive, Creve Coeur, MO 63146, (314) 432-3597, BS 71 LA St Univ - Baton Rouge; MA 72 OH Univ - Athens; Sp/Lang Path, Spec Sch Dist of St Louis Co, **SLP**

Keller, Winifred Jean 8730 North Himes Avenue, Apartment 104, Tampa, FL 33614-8301, (813) 251-7762, BA 81 Univ of FL; MS 85 Univ of South FL; Aud, Univ Med Clinics, **A**

Kellerhouse, Sylvia Pittman 5820 Amaro Drive, San Diego, CA 92124, (619) 560-1391, BS 70 East Carolina Univ; MS 75 East Carolina Univ; SLP, Poway USD, **SLP**

Kellerman, Mrs Sandra Volusher 1018 Dell Drive, Cherry Hill, NJ 08003, (609) 966-8840, BA 71 Univ of CT; MS 74 Southern CT St Univ; 87–SLP, Camden Bd of Educ, **SLP**

Kelley, Mrs Anita Jaime 577 West Magdalena Drive, Tempe, AZ 85283, (602) 730-6126, BS 79 Univ of Southern CO; MS 83 Northern AZ Univ; 88–Sp-Lang Path, Tempe Elem Sch Dist, **SLP**

Kelley, Arthur L 740 Cordell Court, St Louis, MO 63132, **SLP**

Kelley, Carolyn A 2225 Wallis Avenue, Overland, MO 63114, (314) 427-0623, BS 73 Univ of MO - Saint Louis; ME 74 Univ of MO - Saint Louis; MS 87 Fontbonne Coll; **SLP**

Kelley, Mrs Donna P 1110 Sugarloaf Lane, Anniston, AL 36201, (205) 835-0091, BA 76 Univ of AL- Tuscaloosa; MS 79 Univ of AL- Tuscaloosa; Sp/Lang Path, UCP Ctr, **SLP**

Kelley, Edward L 605 1st Street East, Lyndon, IL 61261, (815) 537-2345, BA 59 Fort Hays St Univ; MA 68 Univ of Northern IA; Sp-Lang Path, Prophetstown/Lyndon Schools, **SLP**

Kelley, Elisa Meredith 130 Northway Road, Greenbelt, MD 20770, (301) 345-8975, BA 84 Univ of MD - College Park; MS 87 Univ of AZ; 88–Sp-Lang Path, Mount Vernon Hosp, **SLP**

Kelley, Elizabeth Anne 2 Colonial Village Drive, Apartment B-10, Arlington, MA 02174, (617) 641-4417, BS 82 Northeastern Univ; MS 83 Rutgers St Univ -N Brunswick; 83–Sp-Lang Path, Shore Educ Collaborative, **SLP**

Kelley, Kara Beth 28 Manemet Road, Newton, MA 02159, (617) 244-1121, MS 87 Emerson Coll

Kelley, Mrs Karin Wolverton 18 Center Court, Walnut Creek, CA 94595, (415) 256-4406, BA 76 Occidental Coll; MA 78 Vanderbilt Univ; Sp/Lang Path, **SLP**

Kelley, Mrs Kathleen Janice 720 Flicker Court, Anaheim, CA 92807, (714) 983-0042, OB 68 Plymouth St Coll; MA 87 CA St Univ - Fullerton; 87–Sp-Lang Path, San Bernardino Schs, **SLP**

Kelley, Kathy A 2814 South Steele Street, Denver, CO 80210, (303) 773-2858, BS 73 CO St Univ; MS 75 CO St Univ; 77–Sp-Lang Path, Cherry Creek Pub Sch, **SLP**

Kelley, Laura N 6627 East Hummingbird Lane, Paradise Valley, AZ 85253, (602) 998-7979, BA 73 OH St Univ; MA 74 OH St Univ; **A**

Kelley, Mrs Leanne Brittany 62 Country Club Drive, Danville, IL 61832, (217) 446-5610, OB 84 Univ of MO - Columbia; MS 87 Southern IL Univ -Carbondale; 87–Aud, RJ Hearing LTD, **A**

Kelley, Leslie L 1701 Ellis Lake Drive #74, Marysville, CA 95901, (916) 743-3225, BA 85 CA St Univ - Chico; MA 87 CA St Univ - Chico; 87–Sp-Lang Path, Yuba Co Supt of Schs

Kelley, Pamela J 11570 Panay Street, Cypress, CA 90630, (714) 432-5505, BA 75 CA St Univ - Fresno; MA 77 CA St Univ - Fresno; 87–Spec Day Class Tchr, Fullerton Sch Dist, **SLP**

Kelley, Patrick R 35 Doctors Park, Cape Girardeau, MO 63701, (314) 339-0135, MS 88 Lamar Univ; 88–Aud, Cape Co Otol

Kelley, Rhonda 1 Cedar Hills Drive, Cabot, AR 72023, (501) 490-2000, BS 76 Univ of AR - Fayetteville; MS 84 Univ of Central AR; Sp-Lang Path, Pulaski County Spec Sch Dist, **SLP**

Kelley, Dr Rhonda H 4143 Seminary Place, New Orleans, LA 70126, (504) 838-3900, BA 74 Baylor Univ; MS 75 Baylor Univ; PH 83 (NS) Univ of New Orleans; Dir, Ochsner Cl, **SLP ACE**

Kelley, Roberta Ann Harbor Speech & Hearing Center, P O Box 693, Aberdeen, WA 98520, (206) 533-8300, BA 70 Coll of New Rochelle; MS 72 Univ of WI - Madison; Sp-Lang Path, Harbor Speech & Language Ctr, **SLP**

Kelley, Ronald W 2916 Hillanbrook Drive, Kalamazoo, MI 49008, (616) 966-5600, BS 67 IN St Univ - Terre Haute; MA 71 Western MI Univ; 74–Chief Aud/Sp-Lang Path, VA Med Cen, **SLP**

Kelley, Susan Deanne 4925 Yorkshire Drive, Enid, OK 73703, (405) 237-1027, BA 82 Univ of Tulsa; MA 83 Univ of Tulsa; Sp-Lang Path, Enid State Sch, **SLP**

Kelley, Susan P 2755 Kapiolani Boulevard, Apartment 32, Honolulu, HI 96826, (808) 455-2885, BS 81 Worcester St Coll; MS 83 CO St Univ; Sp & Hrng Path, Dept/Ed-Spec Serv-Leeward Dist, **SLP**

Kelley-Manzella, Mary Ann 517 McKinley Avenue, Dunkirk, NY 14048, (716) 366-6700, BS 72 PA St Univ - Univ Park; MS 78 SUNY - Coll at Fredonia; 85–Sp-Lang Path, Dunkirk PS, **SLP**

Kelley-McCarthy, Leigh Anne 7904 Schuyler Court, Annandale, VA 22003, (703) 750-1189, BA 86 George Washington Univ; MA 86 George Washington Univ; 88–Sp-Lang Path, Cheryl Person & Assoc, **SLP**

Kelley-Smith, Mrs Susan 8 Vine Way, Bordentown, NJ 08505, (609) 298-4366, BS 77 PA St Univ - Univ Park; MS 82 Indiana Univ of PA; Sp-Lang Path, Abington Sch Dist, **SLP**

Kellinger, Denise Litrenta 3808 Font Hill Drive, Ellicott City, MD 21043, BA 76 Catholic Univ of America; MA 78 Catholic Univ of America; **SLP**

Kellison, Carol Sue 168 West Zaun, Blue Springs, MO 64015, (816) 584-2142, OB 84 Univ of KS; MS 86 Central MO St Univ; Sp-Lang Path, Higginsville Hab Ctr, **SLP**

Kellman, Mrs Marianne J 2411 Norwood Place, Madison, WI 53705, (608) 233-4637, BS 52 Univ of WI - Madison; MS 76 Univ of WI - Madison; Sp-Lang Path, Madison Metro Sch Dist, **SLP**

Kellner, Judith Roach 230 Randolph Drive #208, Madison, WI 53717, (608) 833-3028, BS 75 Univ of WI - Madison; MS 76 Univ of WI - Madison; 86–Sp-Lang Path, Wisconsin Heights PS, **SLP**

Kellogg, Mrs Debra J HCO 1 Box 11-A, Arnegard, ND 58835, BS 78 Northern St Coll; MS 81 Minot St Univ; SLP, Makenzie County Schools, **SLP**

Kells, Mrs Lynn D 1520 Peth Road, Manlius, NY 13104, (315) 655-9408, BA 81 SUNY - Coll at Cortland; OM 82 Univ of SC - Columbia; 88–Sp/Lang Path, Syracuse Cty Sch Dist, **SLP**

Kellum, Dr Gloria Dodwell Box 556, University, MS 38677, (601) 232-7271, BA 65 LA St Univ - Baton Rouge; MS 67 LA St Univ - Baton Rouge; PH 81 (Sp-Lang Path) LA St Univ - Baton Rouge; Assoc Prof & Dir of Clin Serv, U of MS, **SLP F**

Kellum, Jane M G 600 South Graves #305, Mc Kinney, TX 75069, (214) 542-3158, BS 77 Univ of IL - Urbana; MS 78 Univ of IL - Urbana; Sp-Lang Path, Med Temporaries, **SLP**

Kelly, Ann Marie 51 Thorndike Avenue, Arlington, MA 02174, (617) 648-5427, SLP, Mass Gen Hosp, **SLP**

Kelly, Mrs Bea B 514 Miller Road, Coral Gables, FL 33146, BA 64 Univ of AL- Tuscaloosa; MA 78 Univ of Miami; Sp-Lang Path, Dade Co Pub Sch, **SLP**

Kelly, Dr Ben R Dept Of Communicative Disorder, California State Univ, Fresno, CA 93740, (209) 294-4220, BA 64 Univ of FL; MS 68 FL St Univ; PH 71 (NS) Case Western Reserve Univ; Prof of Aud, CA St U-Fresno, **A**

Kelly, Mrs Carole R Southern Arizona Speech Path, 6840 North Casas Adobes Dr, Tucson, AZ 85704, (602) 742-7958, BA 70 Univ of ND; MA 72 Univ of ND; Sp-Lang Path, So Arizona Sp Path Assoc, **SLP**

Kelly, Catherine P O Box 493, 35 Park Street, Republic, PA 15475, (412) 246-8828, BS 70 CA Univ of PA; ME 71 CA Univ of PA; SLP, Intermediate Unit One, **SLP**

Kelly, Charleen A 8228 30th Avenue N E, Seattle, WA 98115, **SLP**

Kelly, Cheryl Mills 1253 38th Street S E, Cedar Rapids, IA 52403, (319) 399-6700, BS 77 Univ of IA; MS 80 Southern IL Univ -Carbondale; SLP, Grant Wood AEA, **SLP**

Kelly, Mrs Chris-Anne PO Box 221, Northville, MI 48167, (313) 347-3418, BA 83 MI St Univ; MA 84 MI St Univ; 88–Sp-Lang Path, Northville PS, **SLP**

Kelly, Mrs Christine 5235 101st Avenue North, Pinellas Park, FL 34666, (813) 546-9897, MS 72 Univ of South FL; Sp-Lang Path, Pinellas Co Sch Bd, **SLP ACE**

Kelly, Christine Delort R R 1 Box 558, Kittery, ME 03904, (207) 439-1386, BA 72 Loyola Univ of Chicago; MA 76 Univ of Cincinnati; Aud, **A**

Kelly, Mrs Claudia M 10 Brianwood Lane, Granby, CT 06035, (203) 653-4873, BS 76 Wayne St Univ; MA 77 Wayne St Univ; Sp-Lang Path, Cranby PS, **SLP**

Kelly, Dr Dan H 300 Chillicothe Avenue, Hillsboro, OH 45133, (513) 393-1740, BA 65 OH Univ - Athens; MA 66 Western MI Univ; PH 73 (Sp Path Sp Science) OH Univ - Athens; 88–Sp-Lang Path, Speech Language & Hearing Associates, **SLP**

Kelly, Mrs Dawn M 2003 Tremont Street, Cedar Falls, IA 50613, (319) 273-8250, BA 80 Univ of Northern IA; MA 81 Univ of Northern IA; Sp/Lang Path, AEA 7, **SLP**

Kelly, Deborah A 200 Yorkshire Drive, New Market, ON, Canada L3Y 6J7, (416) 853-1484, BA 75 Southern CT St Univ; MS 78 SUNY - Coll at Buffalo; 80–Sp-Lang Path, York Region Separate Sch Bd, **SLP**

Kelly, Mrs Deborah R 1001 Redbud, Crockett, TX 75835, (713) 370-1096, BA 72 Baylor Univ; MS 73 Baylor Univ; **SLP**

Kelly, Debra Parr 4821 S E Tattershall Way, Lawton, OK 73501, (405) 248-5909, BA 82 Univ of OK - Norman; MS 84 Univ of OK - OK City; Sp-Lang Path, Lawton Pub Schs, **SLP**

Kelly, Delores L 300 South Haywood #203, Waynesville, NC 28786, (704) 456-9858, BA 33 Coll of Saint Francis; MS 60 Univ of IL - Urbana; **SLP LM**

Kelly, Donna J 839 New York Street, Lawrence, KS 66044, (913) 588-5952, BA 77 IN Univ - Bloomington; MA 79 IN Univ - Bloomington; Sp-Lang Path/ Instuctor, Chldn Rehab Ut/ Ku Med Ctr, **SLP**

Kelly, Dorothy Ann Regional Educ Serv Agency, 615 West King Street, Martinsburg, WV 25401, (304) 263-8948, BA 75 Univ of VA - Charlottesville; ME 82 James Madison Univ; Aud, Reg Ed Ser Agency Viii, **A**

Kelly, Edward Joseph 2406 Avon Road, Ardmore, PA 19003, (215) 543-1418, BS 69 Villanova Univ; MS 80 Hahneman Medical Coll; SLP, Don Guanella Sch, **SLP**

Kelly, Ellen M 410 Deerfield Road #5, East Syracuse, NY 13057-1325, (315) 423-2370, BA 81 Saint Bonaventure Univ; MS 84 Syracuse Univ; **SLP**

Kelly, Ellen Maderski Center For Speech & Hearing Sciences Inc, 5 Brunswick Woods Drive, East Brunswick, NJ 08816, (201) 238-1664, BA 78 Rutgers St Univ -N Brunswick; MS 79 PA St Univ - Univ Park; Aud/Dir, Cen for Sp & Hrng, **A ACE**

Kelly, Mrs Eloise Kathleen 709 West Oak, Independence, KS 67301, (316) 331-6303, BA 79 Murray St Univ; MA 85 Wichita St Univ; **SLP**

Kelly, Erma F 917 Pleasant Street, Richmond, VA 23223, (804) 737-6071, BS 75 Hampton Univ; ME 76 Univ of VA - Charlottesville; Sp/Lang Path, Sheltering Arms Rehab Hosp, **SLP**

Kelly, George J 504 Winding Way, Warminster, PA 18974, (215) 539-8550, BS 69 Georgetown Univ; OM 73 Northwestern Univ; Sp-Lang Path, Mont Co Inter Ut, **SLP**

Kelly, Mrs Geralyn Helen 6674 Breckenridge Road, Lisle, IL 60532, (312) 961 0736, BA 73 Coll of Saint Francis; MS 77 Fontbonne Coll; 88–Sp-Lang Path, Naperville Sch Dist #203, **SLP**

Kelly, Mrs Gloria J R 343 Hampshire Street, Buffalo, NY 14213, (716) 834-1419, BA 74 SUNY - Center at Buffalo; MA 76 SUNY - Center at Buffalo; Sp/Lang Path, Buffalo Bd of Educ, **SLP**

Kelly, Mrs Jackie Miller 4931 So Melrose Avenue, Tampa, FL 33629, (817) 699-9556

Kelly, Jacqueline Lou 162 Linde Circle, Marina, CA 93933-2205, (408) 649-1455, BA 78 CA St Univ - Sacramento; MA 85 CA St Univ - Sacramento; SLP, Monterey Peninsula USD, **SLP**

Kelly, Jacquelyn F Ntl Technical Inst For Deaf, 1 Lomb Memorial Drive, Rochester, NY 14623, (716) 475-6865, BA 64 Nazareth Coll of Rochester; MS 69 SUNY - Coll at Geneseo; Sp-Lang Path, NTID, **SLP**

Kelly, Janet Anne 399 Old Main Street, Rocky Hill, CT 06067, (203) 721-8192, BA 80 Univ of CT; MA 83 Univ of CT; Sp-Lang Path, **SLP**

Kelly, Mrs Jean A 12687 C Street, Omaha, NE 68144, BA 74 Creighton Univ; MS 75 Univ of NE - Omaha; Sp-Lang Path, Omaha Public Schools, **SLP**

Kelly, Joann Linda Box 37, Eaton, NH 03832, (603) 383-6863, BS 80 Univ of NH; MS 85 Univ of NH; **SLP**

Kelly, Jody Goggins 91 Shepard Street, New Haven, CT 06511, (203) 787-8994, BA 79 Southern CT St Univ; MA 81 SUNY - Coll at Geneseo; Sp-Lang Path, New Haven Pub Sch Syst, **SLP**

Kelly, Mrs Judith Cox P O Box 514, Greencastle, IN 46135, (317) 658-4496, BS 56 Purdue Univ - West Lafayette; MS 59 Purdue Univ - West Lafayette; 67–Instr-Dept Comm Arts & Sci, DePauw Univ, **SLP**

Kelly, Kathleen A 123 Maple Terrace, Pittsburgh, PA 15211, (412) 745-8000, BA 85 Duquesne Univ; MA 87 Univ of Pittsburgh - Pittsburgh

Kelly, Kerry A 375 34th Street, Sacramento, CA 95816, (916) 921-3660, BA 78 CA St Univ - Sacramento; MA 82 CA St Univ - Sacramento; SLP, Grant Joint Union H Sch Dist, **SLP**

Kelly, Mrs Kristina Larsen Rehab Center For Chld & Adults, 300 Royal Palm Way, Palm Beach, FL 33480, (305) 655-7268, MS 84 FL St Univ; Sp-Lang Path, Rehab Center for Chld & Adults, **SLP**

Kelly, Laura J 2 Bachelor Hall, Miami University, Oxford, OH 45056, (513) 529-2500, BS 75 Bradley Univ; MA 76 MI St Univ; PH 88 (NS) MI St Univ; 88–Aud, Miami Univ, **A**

Kelly, Lela M PO Box 8448 SVL, Victorville, CA 92392, (619) 243-2825, BA 74 Univ of Redlands; MS 77 Univ of Redlands; 87–SLP, Apple Valley USD, **SLP**

Kelly, Mrs Linda A Challenge Center Inc, 39 North 25th Street East, Superior, WI 54880, (715) 394-2771, MA 84 Univ of MN - Duluth; SLP, Challenge Cen Inc, **SLP**

Kelly, Linda Lee 2996 Louise Avenue, Grove City, OH 43123, (614) 263-2448, BS 74 OH St Univ; MA 78 OH St Univ; SLP, Columbus Pub Sch, **SLP**

Kelly, Mrs Louise Ellen 2500 Eastway Dr #32A, Charlotte, NC 28205, (704) 338-4430, BS 82 Univ of WI - Stevens Point; MS 85 James Madison Univ; Sp-Lang Path, Charlotte Rehab Hosp, **SLP**

Kelly, Mrs Martha K 1745 Fawnvalley Drive, St Louis, MO 63131, (314) 966-5700, BS 55 Purdue Univ - West Lafayette; Sp-Lang Path, Spec Sch Dist of St Louis Co, **SLP**

Kelly, Maureen Theresa 28-26 200 Street, Bayside, NY 11360, (212) 863-4925, SLP, These Our Treasures Inc, **SLP**

Kelly, Michael A 266 Melbourne Street, North Adelaide, South Australia, Australia 5006, (08) 267-1001, BA 78 Worcester St Coll; MS 81 Univ of Redlands; 88–Sp-Lang Path, Private Practice, **SLP**

Kelly, Michele Yvonne 8621 Rook Road, Indianapolis, IN 46234, (317) 872-3131, BA 84 Univ of Northern IA; MS 85 CO St Univ; 88–Sp-Lang Path, Communicology Inc, **SLP**

Kelly, Mrs Nancy G D 3190 Green Corners Road, Lapeer, MI 48446, (313) 678-3300, BS 75 Central MI Univ; MA 77 Wayne St Univ; Sp-Lang Path, Lapeer Comm Sch, **SLP**

Kelly, Mrs Nancy Sue 207 North 4th Street, Patterson, CA 95363, (209) 892-8937, BA 80 Westmont Coll; MA 86 CA St Univ - Stanislaus

Kelly, Paula E P O Box 304, Soquel, CA 95073, (408) 476-0525, BA 76 Univ of RI; MS 78 Columbia Univ Teachers Coll; Spec Day Class Tchr, Soquel Elem Sch Dist, **SLP**

Kelly, Richard James 58 Elizabeth Street, Kingston, NY 12401, (914) 895-3301, BS 78 SUNY - Coll at Geneseo; MA 81 SUNY - Coll at Geneseo; Sp/Lang Path, Wallkill Sch Dist, **SLP**

Kelly, Robert 6735 Ridge Boulevard, Brooklyn, NY 11220, (914) 877-6821, BA 67 CUNY - Brooklyn Coll; MS 68 SUNY - Coll at Geneseo; Sp-Lang Path, Wassaic Dev Ctr, **SLP**

Kelly, Sarah T 212 West 30th Street, Farmington, NM 87401, **SLP**

Kelly, Sheila D 6529 43rd Avenue NE, Seattle, WA 98115, (206) 527-9020, BA 70 Queens Univ - Ontario; OM 72 Univ of Toronto - Ontario; Case Mgr, Greenery Rehabilitation Ctr, **SLP**

Kelly, Mrs Sondra I Box 244 Mountain Road, Stanfordville, NY 12581, (914) 485-9813, BS 73 SUNY - Center at Albany; MS 77 SUNY - Center at Albany; 78–Sp-Lang Path, Rehab Prog Inc Day Treat Prog, **SLP**

Kelly, Susan White Box 1624, Edgartown, MA 02539, (617) 627-1033, BA 63 Univ of Akron; MA 68 Northwestern Univ; Sp-Lang Path/Teacher, Martha's Vineyard Regnl H Sch, **SLP**

Kelly, Vanessa McIntosh Rt 2 Box 8-P, Wimberley, TX 78676, (512) 847-5134, BS 84 Western KY Univ; MS 86 Southwest TX St Univ; 87–Sp-Lang Path, New Braunfels ISD, **SLP**

Kelly-Ballweber, Denise Multicare Speech & Hearing Ser, 1220 Division Avenue, Tacoma, WA 98403, (206) 572-5252, BS 77 Northern IL Univ - De Kalb; MA 79 Northern IL Univ - De Kalb; Aud, Multicare Sp & Hrng Ser, **A**

Kelman-Maziuk, Margot E 701 Woburn Drive, Spring Hill, Camillus, NY 13031, (315) 425-4386, BS 78 SUNY - Coll at Fredonia; MS 81 Syracuse Univ; Sp-Lang Path, Syracuse City School Distr, **SLP**

Kelmenson, Florence 4000 North Charles Street, Apartment 903, Baltimore, MD 21218, (301) 235-9753, BA 44 Goucher Coll; MA 68 Univ of MD - College Park; Sp-Lang Path, Baltimore Cty Pub Schs, **SLP LM**

Kelner, Mrs Gail Siegel 8 Greenbrier Lane, Scotch Plains, NJ 07076, (201) 756-5397, BA 69 SUNY - Center at Buffalo; MA 80 Kean Coll of NJ; 84–Sp-Lang Path, Winfield Township Sch Sys, **SLP**

Kelner, Morgan Martha Rural Route 2, #1 Lewis Lane, New Paltz, NY 12561, (914) 255-4392, BA 69 Rutgers St Univ - Newark; MS 87 SUNY - Coll at New Paltz; **SLP**

Kelnhofer, Cheryl D 904 West Browning Street, Appleton, WI 54914, BA 80 Univ of WI - Eau Claire; MS 81 Univ of WI - Eau Claire; Sp-Lang Path, Freedom Area School District, **SLP**

Kelsay, Mrs Danielle Rubino 442 Holiday Road, Coralville, IA 52241, (319) 354-2328, BS 84 Univ of IA; MA 87 Univ of IA; 88–Aud, Univ of Iowa Hosp and Clin, **A**

Kelsch, Carol 830 North 700 West, Provo, UT 84604, (801) 375-9986, BS 67 Brigham Young Univ; MS 68 Brigham Young Univ; Sp-Lang Path, Commun Cl, **SLP**

Kelsey, Nancy Dorothy 40-H Adirondack Lane, Plattsburgh, NY 12901, (518) 298-4031, BA 80 SUNY - Coll at Plattsburgh; MA 83 SUNY - Coll at Plattsburgh; Tchr, N E Clinton Cen Sch, **SLP**

Kelsey, Susan G 5863 Winslow Road, Whitehouse, OH 43571, (419) 877-0207, BS 72 Cornell Univ; MS 75 Univ of NC - Chapel Hill; 82–Sp-Lang Path, St Vincent Medical Center, **SLP**

Kelsey, Valerie B Rd 1 Box 200A, Verona, NY 13478, (315) 338-3229, BS 73 Bloomsburg Univ of PA; MS 74 Syracuse Univ; MS 75 SUNY - Coll at Oswego; Dir/Spec Ed, Rome City Sch Dist, **SLP**

Kelso, Mrs Joanne P 3N714 Ferson Creek Road, St Charles, IL 60174, (312) 742-1106, BS 71 Central MI Univ; MA 72 Central MI Univ; Aud, Elgin ENT & Allergy Assoc, **A**

Kelso, Peggy D 12017 Tall Oaks, Houston, TX 77024, BS 66 Univ of TX - Austin; ME 68 Boston Univ; Sp-Lang Path, Baylor Coll of Medicine, **SLP**

Keltner, Jerry L 710 1st Avenue, Aberdeen, WA 98520, (206) 533-2911, BA 63 Western WA Univ; MA 80 Western WA Univ; Aberdeen Sch Dist 5, **SLP**

Kelton, Debra D 8022 South La Fayette, Chicago, IL 60620, (312) 881-1005, BA 74 Mundelein Coll; MS 76 Howard Univ; 86–Sp-Lang Path, Beacon Therapeutic Sch, **SLP**

Kelty, Mrs Kimberly Renee 806 Circle Drive, Bellaire, TX 77401, (713) 432-1217, BS 85 Univ of Houston - Univ Park; MA 87 Univ of Houston - Univ Park; 88–Sp-Lang Path, HCA-Med Ctr Hosp Del Oro Inst for Rehab, **SLP**

Kelty, Mrs Pauline Cotaya 3717 Pecan Drive, Chalmette, LA 70043, (504) 271-0780, BA 73 Univ of New Orleans; OM 82 LA St Univ - N O Medical Ctr; Sp-Lang Path, Private Practice, **SLP**

Kemble, Sr Carita Sisters Of Charity, Mount St Joseph, OH 45051, (513) 244-4692, BA 42 Coll of Mount Saint Joseph; MA 52 Xavier Univ; MA 74 Univ of Cincinnati; Sp-Lang Path, Mothr Margaret Hall Nursng Hom, **SLP LM**

Kemerling, Julie Ann 244 Wickford Court #7, Fayetteville, NC 28314, (919) 323-6079, BS 83 Phillips Univ; MS 85 Univ of MS; 88–Sp-Lang Path, Southeastern Reg Rehab Ctr, **SLP**

Kemker, Dr Francis Joseph 1019 N W 94th Street, Gainesville, FL 32606, (904) 395-0174, BS 63 Univ of TN - Knoxville; MA 64 Univ of TN - Knoxville; PH 71 (NS) Univ of Denver; Chief Aud/Prof, U of Florida Dept/Commun Dis, **A F**

Kemmerer, Eileen Ann 9451 Lee Highway #3-804, Fairfax, VA 22031, (617) 969-7880, BS 82 Elmira Coll; MS 83 Boston Univ; Sp-Lang Path, Community Center School, **SLP**

Kemp, Dr James Charles Rehabilitative Services, Miami Children's Hospital, 6125 SW 31st Street, Miami, FL 33155, (305) 666-6511, BS 63 Syracuse Univ; MS 65 Univ of FL; PH 72 (Sp-Lang Path) Univ of WA; Admin Coord, Miami Chldn Hosp, **SLP F ACE**

Kemp, John Patrick 606 Rhodes Street, Clarksville, AR 72830, (501) 442-3090, BS 77 Univ of Central AR; MS 82 Univ of LA Verne; **SLP**

Kemp, Martha Jane 908 Wyoming Avenue, Erie, PA 16505, (814) 868-4609, BS 75 Edinboro Univ of PA; MA 79 Edinboro Univ of PA; SLP, Com Rehab Spec, Inc, **SLP**

Kemp, Pamela J 4 Elderkin Street, Potsdam, NY 13676, BS 78 SUNY - Coll at Geneseo; MA 82 SUNY - Coll at Plattsburgh; Sp-Lang Path, St Lawrnce Co Bd-Coop Ed Serv, **SLP**

Kemper, Mrs Marilyn Ruth 640 E McArthur Dr, Springfield, MO 65810, (417) 882-6976, BA 76 Evangel Coll; MA 84 Southeast MO St Univ; 85–Sp-Lang Path, St John's Regional Health Ctr, **SLP**

Kemper, Dr Robert L 11 Felt Street, Salem, MA 01970, (617) 745-2100, BA 69 MI St Univ; MS 74 Purdue Univ - West Lafayette; PH 85 (Dev Psycholinguistics) Kent St Univ; Director Lang-Sp-Hearing Dept, North Shore Childrens Hospital, **SLP**

Kempf, Mrs Connie Lynn Route 2 Box 1-C, Harrisburg, AR 72432, (501) 578-5391, OB 83 AR St Univ; OM 84 AR St Univ; SLP, Truman Public Schools, **SLP**

Kempler, Dr Daniel 6338 West 6th Street, Los Angeles, CA 90048, (213) 824-3100, MA 84 CA St Univ - Los Angeles; PH 84 (Linguistics) Univ of CA - Los Angeles; 88–Sp-Lang Path/Asst Prof, Univ of Southern CA Med Ctr, **SLP**

Kempner, Heidi N 14527 Darkwood Drive, Rockville, MD 20853, **SLP ACE**

Kempster, Dr Gail B 328 North Scoville Avenue, Oak Park, IL 60302, (312) 534-5000, BA 75 Valparaiso Univ; MS 76 Purdue Univ - West Lafayette; PH 84 (Sp-Lang Path) Northwestern Univ; Prof, Governors State Univ, **SLP**

Kempster, Marjory I 6803 North 68th Plaza #107, Omaha, NE 68152, BA 37 Univ of IA; MA 38 Univ of IA; **SLP LM**

Kenaston, Alicia Ann Avenida Italia 1465, Comuna DE Providence, Santiago, Chile, BA 75 Eckerd Coll; MS 78 Georgetown Univ; MS 82 Univ of the DC; Sp-Lang Path, Private Practice, **SLP**

Kendall, Deborah Anne 4719 North Tenth Street, Phoenix, AZ 85014, (602) 279-2299, BA 68 MI St Univ; MA 78 AZ St Univ; MS 87 Northern AZ Univ; 74–Sp-Lang Path, Phoenix Elem Dist #1, **SLP**

Kendall, Geralyn M 2358 North Sheffield #212, Chicago, IL 60614, (312) 472-1858, MS 87 Rush Univ

Kendall, Melody Walsh 9208 South 93rd E Avenue, Tulsa, OK 74133, (918) 299-4411, BS 80 OK St Univ; MA 82 OK St Univ; Sp/Lang Path, Jenks Publ Schs, **SLP**

Kendrick, Mrs Clara A Yourman 900 Alturas Way, Mill Valley, CA 94941, (415) 383-8852, BA 79 Univ of Redlands; MS 82 Univ of Redlands; Tchr, Marin County Office of Educ, **SLP**

Kendrick, Mrs Julie E 3241 Running Cedar Drive, Marietta, GA 30062, (404) 578-9104, BS 80 Brigham Young Univ; OM 81 Brigham Young Univ; 88–Sp-Lang Path, Sp Path Services Inc, **SLP**

Kendrick, Kathryn Ann 112 Estonia Drive, Richmond, KY 40475, (606) 723-2181, BS 80 Eastern KY Univ; MA 82 Eastern KY Univ; Sp-Lang Path, Estill Co Bd of Ed, **SLP**

Kendrick, Mrs Marian M 1434 Greenmont Court, Reston, VA 22090, (703) 437-8611, BS 76 Purdue Univ - West Lafayette; MA 78 George Washington Univ; **SLP**

Kendrick, Nancy B 1605 Heard Drive, Maple Glen, PA 19002, (215) 663-1121, Aud, Wilf-Silberman MD Assoc, **A**

Kendrick, Norma L 4006 Homestead Drive, Prairie Village, KS 66208, (913) 432-1912, BS 74 Central MO St Univ; BA 58 Univ of MO - KS City; Sp-Lang Path, Shawnee Mission School Dist, **SLP**

Kendrick, Teresa Louise 15705 Ambiance Drive, Gaithersburg, MD 20878, (301) 951-7144, BA 78 Univ of MD - College Park; BS 78 Univ of MD - College Park; MA 80 Univ of MD - College Park; Aud, Private Practice, **A**

Kendzior, Laurel R 33 Boretz Road, Colchester, CT 06415-1026, (203) 537-3714, BA 84 Univ of CT; MA 86 Univ of CT; **SLP**

Kenefick, Kimberly Lindell 655 East 145th Street, Burnsville, MN 55337, (612) 431-4944, BA 85 Univ of ND; MS 86 Univ of ND; **SLP**

Kenfield, Ann E 8395 S E 53rd Place, Mercer Island, WA 98040-4653, (206) 236-9741, BA 77 Univ of the Pacific; MA 79 Univ of the Pacific; **SLP**

Kengersky, Mrs Donna Ann Rd #7 Box 24, Punxsutawney, PA 15767, (814) 938-3406, BS 73 Indiana Univ of PA; MS 77 Indiana Univ of PA; 86–SLP, Private Practice, **SLP**

Kenig, Mrs Janet A 569 Tate Creek Court, Acworth, GA 30101, (404) 751-2500, BS 84 Northwestern Univ; MA 85 Northwestern Univ; 87–Sp-Lang Path, N Fulton Regional Hosp, **SLP**

Kenna, Ellen Therese 1517 Balltown Road #2, Schenectady, NY 12309, (518) 393-5205, MA 87 SUNY - Center at Buffalo; 87–Sp-Lang Path, Helping Hands Preschool, **SLP**

Kenna, Mrs Marcia Jo 4886 East Costilla Place, Littleton, CO 80122, (303) 778-1955

Kenna, Peggy T 723 West Curry Street, Chandler, AZ 85224, (602) 839-7530, BA 58 Univ of MT; MA 60 Univ of MT; 88–Sp-Lang Path, Kenna & Posner Inc, **SLP**

Kennalley, Mrs Teresa L 4440 East English, Wichita, KS 67218, (316) 686-6608, BA 78 Wichita St Univ; MA 79 Wichita St Univ; Aud, Wichita Ear Cl Pa, **A**

Kennard, Carol Ann 641 N W 79th Street, Seattle, WA 98117, (206) 784-0333, BA 82 Univ of WA; MS 84 Univ of WA; **SLP**

Kennard-MacKenzie, Kathy 33 Tower Hill Drive, Port Chester, NY 10573, (212) 750-6785, OB 77; OB 78; MA 84 NY Univ; Sp-Lang Path, Private Practice, **SLP**

Kennedy, Alexanne 159 Pringle Street, Kingston, PA 18704, (717) 826-3768, MS 87 PA St Univ - Univ Park; 87–Sp-Lang Path, John Heinz Institute of Rehab Med Allied Svcs, **SLP**

Kennedy, Alicia Quinn 5 Placer Lane, Hot Springs, AR 71909, (516) 587-0663, BA 42 Coll of New Rochelle; MS 70 Adelphi Univ; **SLP LM**

Kennedy, Anne Aileen 1762 Euclid, Lincoln, NE 68502, (402) 470-2244, BA 75 Montclair St Coll; MS 82 Univ of NE - Lincoln; Sp-Lang Path, Lincoln Pub Sch, **SLP**

Kennedy, Mrs Anne Louise 686 Glen Road, Warminster, PA 18974, (215) 757-7620, BA 78 West Chester Univ of PA; MA 81 Temple Univ; Aud, ENT & Facial Plastic Surg Asso, **A**

Kennedy, Catherine 636 Crandall Street, Madison, WI 53711-1837, (608) 271-7711, BA 72 Portland St Univ; MA 75 Western WA Univ; SLP, Madison School District, **SLP**

Kennedy, Darlene A Greasewood School, Ganado, AZ 86505, (602) 729-5041, BA 72 Univ of CO - Boulder; MA 79 Univ of CO - Denver; Sp/Lang Path, Bureau of Indian Affairs, **SLP**

Kennedy, Elizabeth 118 Woodland Avenue, Barrington, NJ 08007, (215) 581-6082, BA 77 Univ of MA - Amherst; MA 79 Temple Univ-Tyler Sch of Art; Instr, Temple Univ, **A**

Kennedy, Glenda Lynette Route #2 Box 89, McCool, MS 39108, (601) 924-5664, BS 84 Jackson St Univ; MS 86 Mankato St Univ; 87–Sp-Lang Path, Clinton PS

Kennedy, Grace M 48 Edward Road, Watertown, MA 02172, MS; **SLP LM**

Kennedy, Mrs Jacqueline 5512 91st, Lubbock, TX 79424, (806) 792-6135, BS 73 West TX St Univ; MS 78 TX Tech Univ; Sp-Lang Path, Sp-Lang & Hrng Cen, **SLP**

Kennedy, Mrs Janice D 2728 State Route 132, New Richmond, OH 45157, (513) 481-6894, BS 80 Univ of Cincinnati; MA 84 Univ of Cincinnati; Sp-Lang Path, St Elizabeth Med Center North, **SLP**

Kennedy, Jera J 17902 Cypress Springs, Spring, TX 77373, (713) 469-2152, BS 65 Sam Houston St Univ; MA 71 Univ of Houston - Univ Park; 88–Sp-Lang Path, Northwest Harris County Deaf Co-op, **SLP**

Kennedy, Josephine 2648 Baker Street, San Francisco, CA 94123, (415) 239-3000, BA 64 Stanford Univ; MA 66 Stanford Univ; Instructor, Cty College of San Francisco, **SLP**

Kennedy, Judith L 344 Berkeley Street, Rochester, NY 14607, **SLP**

Kennedy, Dr June Ford 95 West Columbia, Orlando, FL 32806, (407) 422-2200, BA 58 MI St Univ; MA 65 Wayne St Univ; PH 72 (NS) Wayne St Univ; Aud Owner, June F Kennedy Ph & Assoc Pa, **SLP A ACE**

Kennedy, Mrs Karen Darlene 1601 Tobie Layne, Fort Worth, TX 76126, (817) 882-2045, BS 85 Univ of North TX; MS 87 Univ of North TX; 87–Sp-Lang Path, Harris Methodist Hosp-Ft Worth, **SLP**

Kennedy, Kathleen A Good Samaritan Hospital, 407 14th Avenue S E, Puyallup, WA 98372, (206) 848-6661, BA 74 Univ of CA - Santa Barbara; MS 76 Univ of NM; 82–Dir Sp-Lang Path Dept, Good Samaritan Hosp, **SLP**

Kennedy, Dr Kathleen B 135 George, New Brunswick, NJ 08903, (201) 932-9335, OB 64 Southwest TX St Univ; ME 72 Southwest TX St Univ; PH 81 (Clinical Supervision) Univ of OR; 88–Asst Prof, Rutgers Univ, **SLP**

Kennedy, Mrs Kathleen D 46-17 193rd Street, Flushing, NY 11358, (212) 683-6970, MA 74 CUNY - Queens Coll; MS 78 CUNY - Queens Coll; OM 81 CUNY - Queens Coll; Superv, Citywide Sp Svc NYC Bd of Educ, **SLP LM**

Kennedy, Mrs Kathryn Ann/Isaac 444 Northeast Donald Terr, Myrtle Creek, OR 97457, (503) 673-6306, BA 78 CA St Univ - Sacramento; MA 81 CA St Univ - Sacramento; **SLP**

Kennedy, Kathy S Route One Box 269, Coolidge, GA 31738, (912) 985-3143, BS 86 Valdosta St Coll; ME 87 Valdosta St Coll; 88–Sp-Lang Path, Mitcheh County PS Sys

Kennedy, Kim B 5265 SE Nowata Road #104, Bartlesville, OK 74006, (918) 335-1513, BA 79 OK St Univ; MA 82 OK St Univ; 88–Sp/Lang Path, Private Practice, **SLP**

Kennedy, Linda E 5590 Leesway Boulevard, Pensacola, FL 32504, (904) 478-4976, BA 67 Saint Mary's Dominican Coll; MS 71 FL St Univ; 86–Sp-Lang Path, Escumbia Co Sch Sys, **SLP ACE**

Kennedy, Louise A 5714 Kenmore Road, Baltimore, MD 21210, BA 78 WV Univ; MS 81 Loyola Coll; Sp-Lang Path, Baltimore City Pub Sch, **SLP**

Kennedy, Mrs Lynn G 5247 St Genevieve Place, Alexandria, VA 22310, (703) 768-3237, BS 74 Ithaca Coll; MA 75 Montclair St Coll; SLP, Charles Co Bd of Ed, **SLP**

Kennedy, Margaret F 3425 Tulane Court, Iowa City, IA 52245, (319) 354-2421, BA 38 Univ of IA; MA 66 Univ of IA; **SLP LM**

Kennedy, Margaret M 830 West Roscoe #3, Chicago, IL 60657, (312) 774-6945, BA 84 Baldwin-Wallace Coll; MA 86 Northwestern Univ; 86–Sp-Lang Path, Chicago Bd of Educ, **SLP**

Kennedy, Mrs Marianne D 36 Gardner Lake Heights, Salem, CT 06415, (203) 447-7545, BA 71 Trinity Coll; MA 77 Univ of CT; Sp-Lang Path, CT Coll, **SLP**

Kennedy, Mrs Marilyn A 201 Ridge Road, Bel Air, MD 21014, (301) 833-0129, BA 52 Univ of IA; Sp-Lang Path, Harford Co Pub Sch, **SLP**

Kennedy, Mary K W 2506 Hillcrest, Greenville, TX 75401, (214) 455-2112, BS 79 East TX St Univ - Commerce; MS 81 Univ of North TX; 88–Sp-Lang Path, Greenville ISD, **SLP**

Kennedy, Mary M 1988 Commonwealth Avenue, Apartment 3, Brighton, MA 02135, (617) 265-6060, MS 72 Catholic Univ of America; Sp-Lang Path, Boston Public Schools, **SLP**

Kennedy, Mrs Mary Zimmerman 250 Phelps Road, Ridgewood, NJ 07450, (201) 447-1471, BS 64 WV Univ; MS 84 William Paterson Coll; Sp-Lang Path, Private Practice, **SLP**

Kennedy, Patricia A 4949 Donalson Road, Panama City, FL 32401, (904) 769-1431, 74 Univ of Tampa; BS 76 FL St Univ; MS 77 FL St Univ; Sp-Lang Path, Bay Co Sch Bd, **SLP**

Kennedy, Mrs Patricia P 4238 Morriswood Drive, Nashville, TN 37204, (615) 322-6117, BA 75 Univ of AL-Tuscaloosa; MA 76 Memphis St Univ; SLP-Rehab Unit, Vanderbilt University Hospital, **SLP**

Kennedy, Regina M Z 710 Washington Street, Sewickley, PA 15143, BS 72 Clarion Univ of PA; ME 76 Clarion Univ of PA; Sp-Lang Path, Hardin Co Bd of Ed, **SLP**

Kennedy, Mrs Robin G R Box 168, Elk Mountain, WY 82324, (307) 348-7374, BA 77 Univ of Northern IA; MS 79 Univ of WY; Sp-Lang Path, Carbon County School Dist 2, **SLP**

Kennedy, Susan Liff P O Box 83057, Fairbanks, AK 99708-3057, (907) 353-5280, BA 71 Rutger's St Univ - Douglas Coll; MA 73 Vanderbilt Univ; Aud, US Army, **A**

Kennedy, Mrs Suzanne N 941 Bryans Place Road, Winston-Salem, NC 27104, (919) 768-6271, BA 69 Univ of TX - Austin; MS 73 CO St Univ; **SLP**

Kennedy, Timothy J Park Falls Elementary School, 380 North 9th Street, Park Falls, WI 54552, (715) 762-3393, BS 77 Univ of WI - River Falls; MS 79 Univ of WI - River Falls; Sp-Lang Path, Park Falls Public Schools, **SLP**

Kennedy, William W, II Rd 2 Box 377, Old Kennedy Road, Troy, PA 16947, (717) 297-2379, BS 46 Syracuse Univ; MA 63 Syracuse Univ; Retired, Blast I U #17, **SLP LM**

Kenner, Patricia 2726 Cupid Street, New Orleans, LA 70114, **SLP**

Kenney, Arthur Joseph 4 Edgewood Drive, Baldwinsville, NY 13027, (315) 475-4276, BS 82 Syracuse Univ; MS 86 Syracuse Univ; **SLP**

Kenney, Karen Jean 12 Holland Avenue, Westfield, MA 01085, (413) 562-1037, BA 83 Elms Coll; MA 85 OH Univ - Athens; 87–Sp-Lang Path, Westfield PS, **SLP**

Kenney, Katherine Mary 2264 Woodview #379, Ypsilanti, MI 48198, (517) 423-2141, MA 83 Eastern MI Univ; Sp-Lang Path, Herrick Memorial Hlth Care Ctr, **SLP**

Kenney, Kathryn W P O Box 1203, Gilbert, AZ 85234, (602) 965-2373, BS 77 AZ St Univ; MS 79 AZ St Univ; Sp-Lang Path, Arizona State University, **SLP**

Kenney, Mrs Kerry Ann 232 Oak Avenue, Harahan, LA 70123, (504) 738-0641, BS 76 Saint Mary's Dominican Coll; OM 77 LA St Univ - N O Medical Ctr; Sp-Lang Path, Jefferson Parish Public Schs, **SLP**

Kenney, Mary E 31 Forest Valley Road, Pleasant Valley, NY 12569, (914) 635-8840, BA 69 SUNY - Coll at New Paltz; MA 71 Coll of Saint Rose; Sp-Lang Path, Wappingers Central Schools, **SLP**

Kenney, Mary Kathryn 84 North Walkup, Crystal Lake, IL 60014, (815) 965-6745, BA 82 Temple Univ; MA 84 Temple Univ; 85–Sp-Lang Path, Chldn Dev Ctr, **SLP**

Kenney, Michael J 515 Fitzgerald N W, Albuquerque, NM 87107, (505) 754-2020, MA 73 NM Highlands Univ; MS 82 4815; Sp-Lang Path, Albuquerque Pub Sch, **SLP**

Kenney, Rosita L 66 Town Square Drive, Newport News, VA 23607, (804) 838-5551, BS 72 Hampton Univ; MA 79 Hampton Univ; Sp-Lang Path, Hampton City Schs, **SLP**

Kenney, Susan P Eye & Ear Associates, 923 Eliza Street, Green Bay, WI 54301, (414) 432-9261, BS 77 Univ of WI - Stevens Point; MS 78 Univ of WI - Stevens Point; Audiologist, Eye and Ear Associates, **A**

Kenney, Mrs Teresa Plevyak 7134 Dogwood Road, Baltimore, MD 21207, (301) 391-1000, BS 80 Towson St Univ; MA 82 Univ of MD - College Park; Sp-Lang Path, Baltimore Co Board of Educ, **SLP**

Kenney, Yvonne C 167 Woodgate Lane, Paoli, PA 19301, (215) 640-0420, MA 86 West Chester Univ of PA; 88–Sp-Lang Path, Chester County Inter Unit #24, **SLP**

Kenngott, Carolyn L 1112 Hamilton Heights Road, Corvallis, MT 59828, (406) 363-2287, BA 73 Univ of Akron; MA 74 Univ of Akron; Sp Lang Cl, Hamilton Publ Sch, **SLP ACE**

Kennington, Mrs Sabra Grant 1311 St Paul's Way, Crownsville, MD 21032, (301) 849-3766, BA 57 Cl Coll; MS 82 Univ of HI - Manoa; Sp-Lang Path, Innovative Learning Ctr, **SLP**

Kenny, Mrs Elena F 108 Nottingham Road, Ramsey, NJ 07446, (201) 790-7909, BA 74 Jersey City St Coll; MS 82 William Paterson Coll; Sp-Lang Path, Prospect Pk Bd of Ed, **SLP**

Kenny, Maureen Elizabeth RD2 Box 745 Chateaugay Lake, Chateaugay, NY 12920, (518) 425-6150, BS 75 SUNY - Coll at Geneseo; MS 80 Coll of Saint Rose; Sp/Lang Path, Malone School District, **SLP**

Kent, Mrs Ann Kaiser 2804 Dublin, Austin, TX 78745, (512) 442-1402, BA 77 Our Lady Lake Univ-San Anton; MA 79 Our Lady Lake Univ-San Anton; Sp-Lang Path, Plaguemines Parish Sch Bd, **SLP**

Kent, Mrs Carrie E Route 3 Box 90, Lexington Park, MD 20653, (301) 862-1557, BS 61 Tuskegee Inst; ME 62 Tuskegee Inst; ME 69 Univ of VA - Charlottesville; Sp/Lang Path, Consumer Health Services Inc, **SLP**

Kent, Mrs Connie L 2751 27th Avenue, Marion, IA 52302, (319) 373-2084, BA 75 Augustana Coll; MA 77 Northwestern Univ; **SLP**

Kent, Daphne H 2688 Hibbert Avenue, Columbus, OH 43202, (614) 263-0023, BS 72 Univ Southern MS-Hattiesburg; MS 76 Univ Southern MS-Hattiesburg; **A**

Kent, Debora D 83 Newburg Street, Roslindale, MA 02131, **SLP**

Kent, Edythe K 153 Sierra View Road, Pasadena, CA 91105, **SLP**

Kent, Helen 18820 Lenross Court, Castro Valley, CA 94546, (415) 538-8993

Kent, Margaret S 1001 Carroll Parkway #207, Frederick, MD 21701, (301) 695-1669, BS 42 Columbia Univ Teachers Coll; MA 49 Columbia Univ Teachers Coll; **LM**

Kent, Marilyn Louise 10047 Westpark Drive #H-89, Houston, TX 77042, (713) 462-5351, BS 70 Univ of ND; MS 71 Univ of ND; Aud, Cypress-Fairbanks ISD, **SLP A**

Kent, Dr Raymond D Dept Communicative Disorders, University Of Wisconsin, 1975 Willow Drive, Madison, WI 53706, (608) 262-3951, BA 65 Univ of MT; MA 69 Univ of IA; PH 70 (NS) Univ of IA; Prof, Dept of Commun Dis U of WI, **F**

Kent, Mrs Sandra Ferguson 1411 Bentwood Drive, Missouri City, TX 77489, (713) 499-9244, BS 80 Univ of VA - Charlottesville; ME 82 Univ of VA - Charlottesville; Sp-Lang Path, AMI Twelve Oaks Hosp, **SLP**

Kent, Thomas P, Jr 4642 Wooddale Lane, Pelham, AL 35124, (215) 691-4431, BA 72 Glassboro St Coll; MA 79 Temple Univ-Tyler Sch of Art; Dir of Rehab Serv, St Lukes Hosp, **A**

Kent, Mrs Wanda Z 1600 Plantation, Mountain Home, AR 72653, (501) 425-9333, BS 62 Univ of AR - Fayetteville; MA 68 Univ of AR - Fayetteville; **SLP**

Kent, William C 377 Calle Lupita, San Luis Obispo, CA 93401, (805) 543-7732, BA 66 Wichita St Univ; MA 68 Wichita St Univ; Sp-Lang Path, San Luis Obispo Co Supt of Sch, **SLP**

Kenton, Mrs Hedda S 103 Emily Drive, Rockville, MD 20850, (301) 279-9040, BA 62 Temple Univ-Tyler Sch of Art; MA 64 Univ of CT; SLP, Mont County Proj Head Start, **SLP**

Kent-Udolf, Dr Louise 715 South Broadway, Suite 701, Corpus Christi, TX 78401, (512) 883-8273, MA 83 Corpus Christi St Univ; MA 57 IN Univ - Bloomington; PH 66 (NS) Univ of IA; Spec Educ Prog Mgr, Ed Serv Cen Reg II, **SLP**

Kenvin, Kathy Elyse 338 East 83rd Street, New York, NY 10028-4251, (212) 420-2760, BS 81 Boston Univ; MS 83 Univ of MI - Ann Arbor; 87–Aud, Beth Israel Med Ctr, **A**

Kenworthy, Diane VA Medical Center West LA, (691/126), Wilshire & Sawtelle Boulevard, Los Angeles, CA 90073, (213) 824-3100, BA 79 Univ of NH; MA 85 CA St Univ - Los Angeles; 87–Aud, VA Med Ctr West LA, **A**

Kenworthy, Dr O T 1426 North Freeman, Santa Ana, CA 92706, (714) 673-8701, BA 74 Univ of WA; MA 76 Univ of WA; PH 84 (NS) Univ of WI - Madison; Dir of Aud, Providence Speech & Hearing Ctr, **A ACE**

Kenyherz, Mrs Janet Z 936 Elizabeth Street, Pittsburgh, PA 15221, (412) 648-6025, BS 64 CA Univ of PA; ME 71 CA Univ of PA; Sp-Lang Path, Mary Jo Truschel, **SLP**

Kenyon, Mrs Diana Lynn 200 N E 19th Ct, Apt M209, Wilton Manors, FL 33305, (305) 565-4518, BS 81 Univ of IL - Urbana; MS 83 Univ of IL - Urbana; Sp/Lang Path, Lauderhill Pt Elem, **SLP**

Kenyon, Mrs Julie Hudson 8289 Stub Highway, Eaton Rapids, MI 48827, (517) 646-0558, BS 81 Western MI Univ; MA 83 MI St Univ; 83–Sp-Lang Path, Lansing PS, **SLP**

Kenyon, Karen K Speech Pathology Services, Saint Francis Memorial Health Center, 2116 West Faidley PO Box 2046, Grand Island, NE 68802, (308) 382-3890, BS 68 Kearney St Coll; MS 80 Kearney St Coll; Sp-Lang Path, Private Practice, **SLP ACE**

Kenyon, Kirsten M 575 Hacienda Avenue #203, Campbell, CA 95008, (408) 295-6115, BA 78 San Diego St Univ; MA 82 San Jose St Univ; SLP, L J Francia Ma, **SLP**

Kenyon, V Talley P O Box 412, Milford, NJ 08848, (803) 420-2455, BA 70 FL St Univ; MA 77 San Francisco St Univ; Sp-Lang Path, Hunterdon Med Cen, **SLP**

Kenzel, Sherri Lynn 360 Whisper Way, Dacula, GA 30211, (404) 822-5945, BS 85 Valdosta St Coll; MS 86 Valdosta St Coll; Sp-Lang Path, Gwinnett Co Ps, **SLP**

Kenzik, Mark Anthony 512 Park Hill Court, Hendersonville, NC 28739, (704) 693-0706, BA 74 Univ of Central FL; MA 76 Univ of Central FL; 77–Audiologist, Hendersonville ENT Pa, **A**

Kenzy, Karol 238 SW Gage Boulevard 501, Topeka, KS 66606, (913) 582-4081, BS 73 Northern St Coll; MA 78 KS St Univ; Sp-Lang Path, USD #372, **SLP**

Keough, Kristine Marie 8047 38th N E, Seattle, WA 98115, (206) 326-3482, BA 78 Univ of WA; MS 82 Univ of WA; 82–Sp-Lang Path, Puget Sound-Central Hosp, **SLP**

Keough, Mrs Sharon Alexander 3675 Schooner Ridge, Alpharetta, GA 30201, (404) 664-3602, BA 80 Univ of KY; MS 84 Univ of South FL; **SLP**

Keough, Susan Ann 248-B Elm Street, Schenectady, NY 12304, (518) 842-3100, BS 85 FL St Univ; ME 87 Univ of VA - Charlottesville; 87–Aud, Amsterdam Mem Hosp, **A**

Keown, Therese Marie 713 Oak, Spooner, WI 54801, (715) 635-2238, BS 79 IN St Univ - Terre Haute; MA 85 Univ of MN - Duluth; SLP, Spooner School District, **SLP**

Keperling, Marcia Lynn 11641 Cedarview Drive, Cincinnati, OH 45249, (513) 489-3231, BS 73 Northern IL Univ - De Kalb; MA 85 Western IL Univ; Cincinnati Pub Schools, **SLP**

Kephart, Beth Casey 156 Crest Drive, Mount Olive, NC 28365, (919) 735-1480, BA 76 Univ of NC - Greensboro; MS 85 East Carolina Univ; 86–Sp-Lang Path, Wayne County Schs, **SLP**

Kephart, Lucy Rosauer 1316 Forest Street, Brookings, SD 57006, (605) 334-4220, BS 85 IA St Univ; MA 86 Northwestern Univ; 88–Sp-Lang Path, Brookings Hosp, **SLP**

Kephart, Maggie B 1818 Douglass Avenue, Minneapolis, MN 55403, MS 77 Univ of WI - Madison; 81–Sp-Lang Path, Private Practice, **SLP**

Kephart, Mary Lisa 5527 Sierra Ridge Drive, Columbus, OH 43231, (614) 228-5523, BA 81 OH St Univ; MA 82 OH St Univ; Sp-Lang Path, Easter Seal Society, **SLP**

Kepler, Laura Jennings 17857 West Lunnonhaus Drive, Apartment 11, Golden, CO 80401, (317) 743-0365, BS 85 Purdue Univ - West Lafayette; MS 87 Purdue Univ - West Lafayette; 87–Instr, Dept of Comm Dis & Sp Sci Univ of CO at Boulder, **A**

Kepper, Mrs Jo Nelle S 6528 Canal Boulevard, New Orleans, LA 70124, (504) 488-0586, BS 72 Univ Southern MS-Hattiesburg; BS 74 Univ Southern MS-Hattiesburg; MS 76 Univ Southern MS-Hattiesburg; **SLP**

Keramedjian, Lisa 4490 Strathdale, West Bloomfield, MI 48033, BA 78 Univ of MI - Ann Arbor; ME 79 Univ of MI - Ann Arbor; **SLP**

Kerbow, Kendra L 9409 South Fresno, Fort Smith, AR 72903, (501) 785-3300, MS 82 Univ of AR - Fayetteville; 86–Dir, Ft Smith Rehabilitation Hosp, **SLP**

Kerby, Mary Ellen 290 North Iowa, East Wenatchee, WA 98801, (509) 884-4365, BA 63 Central WA Univ; ME 85 Heritage Univ; SLP, Wenatchee Sch Dist #246, **SLP**

Kercher, Robyn K 2817 Urwiler #1, Cincinnati, OH 45211, (513) 324-2081, BS 77 Bowling Green St Univ; MA 79 Univ of Cincinnati; Sp-Lang Path, Good Samaritan Hosp, **SLP**

Kerensky, Nancy A 35 Berle Road, South Windsor, CT 06074, (203) 644-8697, BS 65 Univ of MN - Minneap-St Paul; MS 66 CO St Univ; **SLP**

Kerg, Mrs Gail B 233 Park Drive, Mansfield, OH 44906, (419) 526-1141, BA 78 Baldwin-Wallace Coll; MA 80 Univ of Akron; Aud, William H Kaye MD Inc, **A**

Kerin, Alberta Rugh 1838 Gulf Stream Way, West Palm, FL 33411, ME 61; President, Kanga Rugh Enterprise, **SLP**

Kerins, Mrs Elynore P 82 Briarwood Drive, Terre Haute, IN 47803, (812) 877-1264, BS 49 IN St Univ - Terre Haute; 62–Retired, Vigo Co Sch Corp, **SLP**

Kerins, Marie R 6260 Gilston Park Road, Baltimore, MD 21228, (301) 526-5000, BS 79 Marquette Univ; MS 81 Loyola Coll; Sp-Lang Path, Hannah More Cen, **SLP**

Kerins, Marilyn A 565 West 26th Street, Eugene, OR 97405, (503) 686-3575, BA 70 Western MI Univ; OM 75 IN Univ - Bloomington; Res Assoc, Crpld Chldn Div, OR Hlth Sci U, **SLP**

Kerksiek, Charlotte Psc Box 1384, APO Miami, FL 34002, BS 63 CO St Univ; ME 87 Univ of OK - Norman; 68–Sp-Lang Path, Dodds Panama Reg, **SLP**

Kerley, Mrs Paula Wall 7842 Holiday Road So, Jacksonville, FL 32216, (904) 725-3824, BA 64 FL St Univ; MS 65 FL St Univ; 67–Sp-Lang Path, Sp & Hrng Ctr Inc, **SLP**

Kerman-Lerner, Patricia 501 East 79th Street #5-A, New York, NY 10021, (212) 750-6790, BA George Washington Univ; MA 65 Columbia Univ Teachers Coll; Director SLP Aud Services, Goldwater Memorial Hospital, **SLP A**

Kern, Carolyn A 124 Mary Way, Los Gatos, CA 95032, (408) 356-4771, BA 72 Case Western Reserve Univ; OM 74 Univ of WA; SLP, Private Practice, **SLP**

Kern, Diane P 106 South Madison Street, Harrisburg, PA 17109, **SLP**

Kern, Nelda Jean 911 North Easton Road, Willow Grove, PA 19090, BS 66 Bob Jones Univ; MA 69 Temple Univ-Tyler Sch of Art; **SLP**

Kern, Mrs Sandra Paulson Century Village #A6-11, 1451 Pineville Road, Neosho, MO 64850, (417) 451-7457, BS 85 Southwest MO St Univ, MS 88 Central MO St Univ; 88–Sp-Lang Path, St John's Reg Med Ctr

Kern, Susan Wilson 54 Brookline Avenue, Haverhill, MA 01830, (617) 396-5800, MS 86 Northeastern Univ; 86–Sp-Lang Path, Medford PS, **SLP**

Kernaghan, Mrs Jean F 811 Aumond Place East, Augusta, GA 30909, (404) 790-2123, BS 59 GA Southern Coll; ME 61 Univ of GA; ES 84 Univ of GA; SLP/Aud, Gracewood St Sch & Hosp, **SLP**

Kerner, Debra Hanovich Southwest Speech, 10103 Fondren #160, Houston, TX 77096, (713) 771-2461, BS 71 Syracuse Univ; MS 73 Columbia Univ Teachers Coll; Co-Dir, Southwest Speech, **SLP**

Kernoschak, Jeanne Opeil 201 Mockingbird Lane, Swedesboro, NJ 08085, (614) 353-7774, BS 80 Marywood Coll; MA 82 OH Univ - Athens; Sp-Lang Path, Crozer-Chester Med Ctr, **SLP**

Kerns, Barbara J 430 Biggs Highway, Rising Sun, MD 21911, (301) 642-2144, BS 68 Towson St Univ; MS 72 Towson St Univ; Sp-Lang Path, Cecil County Board of Educ, **SLP**

Kerns, Mrs Cynthia Newton 3158 University Avenue, Morgantown, WV 26505, (301) 337-0759, BA 79 Univ of MD - College Park; MS 81 Towson St Univ; Aud, **A**

Kerns, Pamela A 1114 22nd St Apartment 4, Santa Monica, CA 90403, (213) 453-3839, **SLP**

Kerr, Allison Joan B3-255 Kingsmere Blvd, Saskatoon, SK, Canada S7J 4J6, (306) 569-0826, **SLP**

Kerr, Mrs Barbara Benson 1039 Cheyenne Meadows, Katy, TX 77450, (713) 392-7149, BS 82 Miami Univ - Oxford; MS 86 Univ of TX - Austin; 88–Sp-Lang Path, Private Practice, **SLP**

Kerr, Mrs Carol M 336 Chandler Street, Duxbury, MA 02332, (617) 878-1367, BS 73 Northeastern Univ; ME 76 Northeastern Univ; Sp-Lang Path, Rockland Pub Sch, **SLP**

Kerr, Mrs Caroline J 1004 North 6000 West, Rexburg, ID 83440, (208) 356-9340, BS 79 Northern IL Univ - De Kalb; MA 80 Northern IL Univ - De Kalb; Aud, Hearing Clinic, **A**

Kerr, Mrs Cynthia Canipe 4300 Crystal Lake Dr, Apartment F-8, Pompano Beach, FL 33064, (305) 946-2503, BS 76 Univ of TN - Knoxville; MA 78 Univ of TN - Knoxville; Sp-Lang Path, **SLP**

Kerr, Debra L 3914 Delmont Avenue, Oakland, CA 94605, (415) 521-5600, BS 77 CA St Univ - Hayward; MS 79 San Francisco St Univ; Sp-Lang Path Supervisor, Hillhaven, **SLP**

Kerr, Mrs Dee Schaefer Rural Route 4, Warrensburg, MO 64093, (816) 429-1462, BA 66 AZ St Univ; MA 68 AZ St Univ; Sp-Lang Path, Lafayette C-1 Schs, **SLP**

Kerr, Kathie Reid RR 1 Box 111, Tripoli, IA 50676, (319) 882-3097, BS 72 Univ of UT; MS 73 Univ of UT; Sp-Lang Path, **SLP**

Kerr, Linda G T 14409 Manor Road, Phoenix, MD 21131, **A**

Kerr, Linda M 625 31st Avenue North, Apartment B-11, Columbus, MS 39701, (213) 491-9788, BA 83 CA St Univ - Chico; MA 85 CA St Univ - Chico; **SLP**

Kerr, Mrs Linda Susan 78 Netherwood Drive, Jackson, TN 38305, (901) 427-8269, **SLP**

Kerr, Mrs Marlys Mae 805 Augusta Road, Wilmington, DE 19807, (302) 651-2750, BS 58 TX Tech Univ; Sp-Lang Path, Red Clay Consolidated Sch Dist, **SLP**

Kerr, Mrs Miriam G 1810 Carmel Road, Greensboro, NC 27401, ME 75 IN Univ - Bloomington; SLP, Margie Cheshire & Associates, **SLP**

Kerr, Mrs Robin R 12816 Valleyhill Street, Woodbridge, VA 22192, (703) 494-6677, BS 78 Indiana Univ of PA; ME 81 Indiana Univ of PA; 85–Sp-Lang Path, Prince William County Schools, **SLP**

Kerr, Rosellen PO Box 3247, Wichita Falls, TX 76309, (817) 767-5041, BS 65 Univ of North TX; MS 71 Univ of North TX; Sp-Lang Path, Private Practice, **SLP**

Kerr, Victoria A 3801 Willow Lake Drive, Apartment 313, Kalamazoo, MI 49008, (616) 375-7370, BA 79 Western MI Univ; MA 80 Western MI Univ; Sp-Lang Path, Private Practice, **SLP**

Kerrigan, Ann H 11270 30 Mile Road, Romeo, MI 48065, (313) 628-5440, BA 76 MI St Univ; MS 77 MI St Univ; Teacher Ppi, Oxford Area Community Schools, **SLP**

Kerrigan, Mrs Janet B 19 Clifdon Drive, Simsbury, CT 06070, (203) 658-0845, BA 71 Univ of CT; MS 72 Purdue Univ - West Lafayette; Sp-Lang Path, Avon Speech Associates, **SLP**

Kerrigan, Patricia Leann 9408 W 88 Terrace #101, Overland Park, KS 66212, (816) 861-4700, BS 86 Univ of NE - Omaha; 87–Sp-Lang Path, VA Med Ctr

Kerrin, Rosemary G 11 Gortgranagh Drive, Coleraine, County Derby, Northern Ireland, BA 75 LA St Univ - Baton Rouge; MA 77 George Washington Univ; Lecturer, University of Ulster, **SLP**

Kerschen, Kim Elizabeth 14309 Marquette N E, Albuquerque, NM 87123, (505) 292-8001, BA 82 NM St Univ; MA 84 NM St Univ; 84–Sp-Lang Path, Albuquerque PS, **SLP**

Kershlis, Kimberley Ingrid 31 Alvord Street, South Hadley, MA 01075, (413) 533-4635, BS 86 Univ of MA - Amherst; MA 88 Univ of MA - Amherst

Kerst, Kathryn A 3617 Davission Road, Des Moines, IA 50310, (515) 283-1548, BS 72 Univ of NE - Lincoln; MA 74 Univ of NE - Lincoln; Aud, Private Practice, **A**

Kersting, Frank M 668 Windmill Way, Bowling Green, KY 42101-3833, (502) 745-4541, ED 83 (NS) Vanderbilt Univ; Cl Coord/Assoc Prof, Wn KY U, **SLP**

Kertesz, Laurie Ann 154 Mount Kemble Avenue, Morristown, NJ 07960-2773, (201) 533-5786, BS 85 James Madison Univ; MA 87 Univ of TN - Knoxville; 87–Sp-Lang Path, St Barnabas Med Ctr, **SLP**

Kertoy, Marilyn K 15-A Park Street, Orono, ME 04473-1525, (608) 263-6940, BA 70 OH St Univ; MA 75 Western MI Univ; Res Asst, U of WI-Waisman Cen, **SLP**

Kervick, Mrs Janice H A 29 Westwood Drive, Worcester, MA 01609, (617) 756-6104, BA 73 Univ of RI; MS 75 Univ of RI; **SLP**

Keshgegian, Mrs Patrice Anne 45 Sugar Maple Drive, Newtown Square, PA 19073, (215) 356-6484, **SLP**

Kesler, Mrs Lucy C Route 6, Watergate Addn, Olney, IL 62450, (618) 393-2191, BS 72 Eastern IL Univ; MS 80 Eastern IL Univ; Sp-Lang Path, E Richland Sch Dist, **SLP ACE**

Kesler, Sharon S 9920 Cove View Drive East, Jacksonville, FL 32217, (904) 725-8972, BS 61 Univ of WI - Madison; BS 61 Univ of WI - Madison; Sp/Lang Path, S Allen Smith Cl, **SLP**

Kesling, Randy Ann Marshall 4344 Mac Ronald Drive, La Mesa, CA 92041, (619) 464-3204, BA 70 Univ of Redlands; MS 71 Univ of Redlands; Sp-Lang Path, La Mesa/Spring Valley Sch Dist, **SLP**

Keslinger, Annette S 53 Hawley Avenue, Port Chester, NY 10573, (212) 430-0479, BA 76 CUNY - Queens Coll; MA 78 Hofstra Univ; OM 83 New Sch for Social Research; Sp-Lang Path, OMRDD, **SLP**

Kesner, Mrs Betsy Bannen 6021 Rosslyn, Indianapolis, IN 46220, (317) 251-6812, BS 82 Purdue Univ - West Lafayette; MA 84 Univ of IL - Urbana; **SLP**

Kesner, Mrs Catherine I P O Box 446, Fort Ashby, WV 26719, (301) 724-6632, BS 73 WV Univ; MS 74 WV Univ; Sp-Lang Path, Allghy Cy Bd Ed, **SLP**

Kespohl, Beverly J 4412 Arden View Court, Arden Hills, MN 55112, (612) 781-2681, BS 64 Univ of MN - Minneap-St Paul; MA 78 Univ of MN - Minneap-St Paul; Sp/Lang Path, St Anthony Vill-ISD #282, **SLP**

Kessaris, Mrs Claire Connolly 28 Bow Street, Woburn, MA 01801, (617) 933-6429, BA 75 Univ of MA - Amherst; ME 80 Northeastern Univ; **SLP**

Kessel, Marjorie Wasserman 560 Compton Road, Cincinnati, OH 45231, (513) 521-3378, BA 74 IN Univ - Bloomington; MA 76 Univ of Cincinnati; Sp/Lang Path, Private Practice, **SLP**

Kesselman, Toby 396 West 18th Street, Deer Park, NY 11729, (718) 793-2431, BA 86 CUNY - Queens Coll; MA 88 CUNY - Queens Coll; 88–Sp-Lang Path, Peninsula Hosp Ctr

Kesselring, Christina Leigh 2101 No Parish Place #G, Burbank, CA 91504, (818) 843-5231, BA 76 San Diego St Univ; MA 81 CA St Univ - Los Angeles; SLP, Los Angeles Co Schools, **SLP**

Kessing, Elizabeth Ann 1927 Hidden Circle, Tallahassee, FL 32308-4507, (904) 877-8195, MS 72 Univ of South FL; Sp-Lang Path, InSpeech Inc, **SLP**

Kessinger, Jacque L 4820 Cherryvale Avenue, Soquel, CA 95073, (408) 476-3119, BS 71 Univ of MO - Columbia; MA 73 San Jose St Univ; **SLP**

Kessler, Dorcas 2330 Roosevelt Street, Berkeley, CA 94703, (415) 666-2464, BA 64 Univ of CA - Berkeley; OM 65 Univ of CA - Berkeley; MA 77 San Francisco St Univ; Coord Cochlear Implant Proj, U CA/San Francisco, **A**

Kessler, Geraldine 145 Lowell Court, Langhorne, PA 19047, (215) 322-6555, BA 55 Temple Univ-Tyler Sch of Art; ME 73 Trenton St Coll; ME 78 Trenton St Coll; SLP, Bucks Co Schools IU22, **SLP**

Kessler, Joan 58 Apache Ridge Road, Santa Fe, NM 87505, (505) 982-2604, BS 70 Syracuse Univ; MA 72 Long Island U - CW Post Ctr; Sp-Lang Path, Santa Fe Pub Sch, **SLP**

Kessler, Jodell Peterson Box 5123, St Cloud, MN 56302, (612) 253-1455, BS 83 Saint Cloud St Univ; MS 85 Saint Cloud St Univ; SLP, Rehab Therapy Ctr, **SLP**

Kessler, Kathy Sharon 1814 Friendship Drive, Indianapolis, IN 46217, (317) 274-8868, BA 80 MI St Univ; MS 83 Purdue Univ - West Lafayette; Sp-Lang Path/Aud, Indiana Univ Med Ctr, **SLP A**

Kessler, Lue Ann 700 Shoshone #11, Green River, WY 82935, (307) 382-2474, BS Univ of SD - Vermillion; MA 85 Univ of SD - Vermillion; **SLP**

Kessler, Maurine E 22 Hamlin Drive, West Hartford, CT 06117, (203) 397-4573, BS 47 Univ of NE - Lincoln; MA 69 Univ of CT; PH 78 (Aud) Univ of CT; Prof-Commun Dis, Sn CT St U, **A**

Kessler, Mitchell Ray 16 Caledonia Street, St Johnsbury, VT 05819, (802) 748-8761, MA 84 Univ of CO - Boulder; Sp-Lang Path, St Johnsbury Pub Sch, **SLP**

Kessler, Mrs Monica Balsano 960 War Eagle Drive, Colorado Springs, CO 80919, (303) 635-6560, BA 74 Univ of Northern CO; MA 75 Univ of Northern CO; SLP, Private Practice, **SLP**

Kessler, Myles A 242 Talcottville Road #305, Vernon, CT 06066, (203) 932-5711, BA 83 SUNY - Center at Buffalo; MA 85 Univ of Cincinnati; Aud, VA Med Ctr West Haven Ct, **A**

Kessler, Robin Ann 241 South West 87th Terr, Plantation, FL 33324, (305) 472-5800, BA 83 Univ of FL; MA 85 Univ of FL; Aud, Hearing Ctrs of America, **A**

Kessler, Stewart C 61-15 98th Street, Rego Park, NY 11374, (718) 830-1457, BA 75 Yeshiva Univ; MA 79 CUNY - City College; 86–Sp/Lang Path, Mt Sinai Svcs-Elmhurst Hosp Ctr, **SLP**

Kessler-Heiberg, Mrs Heike A 9630 Benavente Street, San Diego, CA 92129, (619) 541-4415, BA 80 Georgetown Univ; MS 82 George Washington Univ; Sp/Lang Path, Sp-Hrng & Neurosensory Ctr, **SLP**

Kessman, Barbara A 1692 Tarleton Way, Crofton, MD 21114, (301) 262-3013, BS 74 Trenton St Coll; MA 77 Montclair St Coll; Sp-Lang Path, Prince George's Co Bd of Ed, **SLP**

Kestel, Lisa Marie 2284 Highland Parkway #305, St Paul, MN 55116, (612) 347-8550, MS 84 Mankato St Univ; 87–SLP, Hennepin County Med Ctr, **SLP**

Kester, Mrs Sandra Isaacman 4172 South 36th Street, Arlington, VA 22206, (703) 820-7630, MS 83 WV Univ; **A**

Kesterson, Randall K 639 College Avenue, Pittsburgh, PA 15232, (412) 647-2030, MA 72 Univ of IA; Aud, Eye & Ear Hosp of Pittsburgh, **A**

Kesterson, Suzanne B 241 St Andrews Drive, Aptos, CA 95003, (408) 688-3803, BS 53 Northwestern Univ; MA 71 San Jose St Univ; Sp-Lang Path, Cabrillo Coll Stroke Cen, **SLP ACE**

Kesting, Mrs Lisa Mortimer 1755 Bighorn Trail, Colorado Springs, CO 80919, (719) 598-2566, BS 80 CO St Univ; MA 83 Univ of Denver; 86–Sp-Lang Path, Academy Sch Dist #20, **SLP**

Kestler, Carla J 12315 Brink Avenue, Norwalk, CA 90650, (213) 434-8421, BA 77 Univ of IA; MA 79 Univ of TN - Knoxville; 88–Sp-Lang Path, Alamitos-Belmont Rehab Hosp, **SLP**

Kestner, Joanne B Forge Gate Apts #G-16, Snyder Road, Lansdale, PA 19446, **SLP**

Ketaineck, Mrs Francie E 229 Sage Hollow Road, Guilford, CT 06437, (203) 457-0691, BA 73 Adelphi Univ; MS 75 Southern CT St Univ; Sp/Lang Path, Project Learn, **SLP**

Ketay, Barbara Biggin 487 Jefferson Road, Princeton, NJ 08540-3418, (516) 825-8800, BA 72 SUNY - Coll at New Paltz; MS 78 Univ of MI - Ann Arbor; SLP, Franklin Gen Hosp, **SLP**

Ketcham, Julie F 8442 Cerco Court, Fort Wayne, IN 46815, (219) 485-7554, BA 65 IN Univ - Bloomington; OM 66 IN Univ - Bloomington; Dir of Sp & Hrng Dept, Ft Wayne St Hosp & Trng Cen, **SLP**

Ketcherside, Jane 401 South 2nd Street, St Charles, MO 63301, (314) 946-6546, BS 77 Southeast MO St Univ; ME 78 Southeast MO St Univ; Coord Sp-Lang Dept, Utd Serv for Hndcpd Inc, **SLP**

Ketchum, Mrs Linda Harrison 1236 To-Lani Drive, Stone Mountain, GA 30083, (404) 482-6700, BS 81 Auburn Univ - Auburn; MA 83 Auburn Univ - Auburn; Sp-Lang Path, Dekalb County School System, **SLP**

Ketelsen, Mrs Mary J P O Box 1767, Parksville, BC, Canada V0R 2S0, (604) 754-5521, BS 76 SD St Univ; MA 77 Univ of SD - Vermillion; 87–Sp-Lang Path, Sch Dist #68-Nanaimo, **SLP**

Ketkar, Dr Indira S 1752 Burrstone Road, New Hartford, NY 13413, (315) 733-6264, ME 58 Poona Univ - India; MS 68 Syracuse Univ; PH 71 (Aud) Syracuse Univ; Hearing and Speech Consultant, Private Practice, **SLP A**

Ketner, Mrs Holly C 63 Waters Edge, Salisbury, NC 28144, (704) 636-6750, BS 77 East Carolina Univ; ME 80 Western Carolina Univ; Sp-Lang Path, Rowan County Schs, **SLP**

Ketter, Mrs Nancy R 1900 West 31st Street #L-4, Lawrence, KS 66046, (913) 842-5122, BS 77 Fort Hays St Univ; MS 78 Fort Hays St Univ; Sp-Lang Path, USD 501, **SLP**

Ketterer, Connie 1141 Williams Boulevard, Springfield, IL 62704, (217) 544-6464, BA 67 IN Univ - Bloomington; MA 69 IN Univ - Bloomington; Sp-Lang Path, St Johns Hosp, **SLP**

Ketterman, Mrs Mary T 10115 West Cold Spring Rd, Apartment 201, Greenfield, WI 53228, (414) 529-9380, OB 84 Univ of WI - Whitewater; MS 85 Univ of WI - Whitewater; 88–Sp-Lang Path, Kenosha USD, **SLP**

Kettler, Mrs Sandra D Box 545, Needville, TX 77461, (409) 793-6886, BS 70 Southwest TX St Univ; ME 71 Southwest TX St Univ; SLP, Needville ISD, **SLP**

Kevech, John James 40 Baytree Drive, Wheeling, WV 26003, **SLP**

Kevelson, Margery Gale 1511 East Sandpiper Circle, Pembroke Lakes, FL 33026-0005, (305) 431-4720, BA 81 Univ of FL; MS 82 FL St Univ; SLP, Dept of Defense Overseas Schs, **SLP**

Kevitt, Christine 505 Volland Drive, Columbus, IN 47203, (812) 376-9404, BA 71 IN Univ - Bloomington; MS 74 IN Univ - Bloomington; 84–Sp-Lang Path, Developmental Services Inc, **SLP**

Kew, Joyce Margaret 44203 North Fine Circle, Lancaster, CA 93536-6164, (805) 949-0627, BA 78 WA St Univ; MA 81 WA St Univ; SLP, Kern Co Supt of Sch, **SLP**

Kewak, Debra Lynn 14010 15 Mile Road #209, Sterling Heights, MI 48077, (313) 343-2029, BS 86 Central MI Univ; MA 87 Central MI Univ

Kewley-Port, Dr Diane 2619 Poplar Drive, Bloomington, IN 47401, (812) 335-6622, BS 64 Univ of MI - Ann Arbor; MS 68 Univ of MI - Ann Arbor; PH 81 (NS) CUNY - Grad Sch & Univ Cntr; Research Scientist, IN U Dept Sp & Hrng

Key, Jan C 155 Cabro Court, Novato, CA 94947, (415) 898-9836, BA 74 Univ of IA; MA 76 Univ of MT; Sp/Lang Path, Novato USD, **SLP**

Keyes, Mrs Alison M 1901 York, Napa, CA 94559, (707) 252-7116, BS 71 Univ of ND; MS 76 Univ of ND; Sp-Lang Path, Napa County Supt of Schools, **SLP**

Keyes, Carynne A 15009 Dunn Drive, Traverse City, MI 49684, (616) 223-7571, BS 77 Eastern MI Univ; MA 78 Eastern MI Univ; **SLP**

Keylon, Mrs Judy G 1101 Windsong Trails, Richardson, TX 75081, (214) 644-3317, BS 72 OK St Univ; MS 78 Univ of North TX; Sp-Lang Path, Richardson ISD, **SLP**

Keys, Mrs Tracy L 806 1/2 South Bayfront, Balboa Island, CA 92662, (714) 675-0675, BS 79 CA St Univ - Fullerton; MA 81 CA St Univ - Fullerton; SLP, Anaheim Union High School Dist, **SLP**

Keys, Wade Tyrone 503 North Hickory, Apartment 3, De Soto, IL 62924, (618) 453-4301, BA 79 LA Tech Univ; MA 83 Northwestern St Univ; Sp-Lang Path, **SLP**

Keyser, Beverly Ann 105 Seabreeze Avenue, Delray Beach, FL 33483, (703) 955-2400, BS 75 Univ of VA - Charlottesville; MS 78 Univ of South FL; 88–Sp-Lang Path, Palm Beach County Schs

Keyser, MaryAnn C 109 North Main Street, P O Box 116, Cassadaga, NY 14718-0116, (716) 672-4371, OB 77 SUNY - Coll at Fredonia; OM 79 SUNY - Coll at Fredonia; SLP, Chautauqua Co Bd of Coop Ed S, **SLP**

Keyser, Mrs Nancy S 120 Newell Lane, Oak Ridge, TN 37830, (615) 482-6370, BA 59 Denison Univ; MA 75 Univ of TN - Knoxville; SLP, Oak Ridge Sch, **SLP**

Keystone, Lori B 2 Quimper Court #3A, Baltimore, MD 21208, (301) 578-5601, BA 86 Univ of MD - College Park; MA 87 George Washington Univ; 88–Sp-Lang Path, Sinai Hosp

Khan, Linda M L P O Box 340295, San Antonio, TX 78234, (512) 434-6711, BA 71 Valparaiso Univ; MS 76 Syracuse Univ; 87–Cl Superv, Harry Jersig Center-OLLU, **SLP ACE**

Khan, Susan Antaki 402 Berry Hill Drive, Carrboro, NC 27510, BA 74 CUNY - Queens Coll; MA 78 Hofstra Univ; SLP, Home Health Services, **SLP**

Khoo, Mrs Keiko I 26061 Hinckley Street, Loma Linda, CA 92354-3945, (714) 824-4998, BA 68; MA 87 Univ of CA - Los Angeles; Asst Prof of Aud, Loma Linda Univ, **A**

Kian, Mrs Martie A 604 Silverthorn Road, Gulf Breeze, FL 32561, (904) 932-6444, BS 64 Troy St Univ - Troy; ME 69 Vorhees Coll; Regional Dir, InSpeech Inc, **SLP ACE**

Kibbe, Kathleen McGrann 1385 Amsterdam Court, Colorado Springs, CO 80907, (303) 473-5866, BS 72 PA St Univ - Univ Park; MS 73 Univ of WI - Madison; Sp-Lang Path, Harrison Sch Dist, **SLP**

Kibby, Carol M 5 August Avenue, Baltimore, MD 21228, BA 79 Univ of MD - College Park; MA 81 Univ of FL; Aud, Balto Co Health Dept, **A**

Kibler, Janice Marie 4102 Providence Road #A, Charlotte, NC 28211, (704) 338-4430, BA 83 Univ of Pittsburgh - Pittsburgh; ME 85 Univ of VA - Charlottesville; Sp-Lang Path, Charlotte Rehab Hosp Inc, **SLP**

Kibler, Lucy Maud Box 43 Stonehaven, Valdese, NC 28690, (704) 437-4663, BA 48 Shorter Coll; MA 51 Northwestern Univ; **SLP**

Kibler, Melinda A 1022 West 31st Street, Erie, PA 16508, (814) 456-2031, BS 84 Clarion Univ of PA; MS 85 Clarion Univ of PA; 88–Aud, Ear Nose & Throat Assoc, **A**

Kidd, Cynthia Louise 5363 Mississippi Bar Drive, Orangevale, CA 95662, (714) 581-2800, BA 81 CA St Univ - Sacramento; MA 83 CA St Univ - Sacramento; SLP, Olga Ramirez Assoc, **SLP**

Kidd, Danielle O 3343 Windsor Drive, Charlotte, NC 28209, (704) 283-3566, BA 60 Univ of NC - Greensboro; MA 76 Univ of NC - Greensboro; 86–Aud, Mecklenburg Ctr Human Dev, **A**

Kidd, Gerald D, Jr 128 Taylor Avenue, Dedham, MA 02026, (617) 495-3859, BA 75 Univ of OK - Norman; MS 77 Univ of OK Medical Center; PH 81 (NS) Purdue Univ - West Lafayette; Assistant Prof, Boston U, **A**

Kidd, Joyce E 370 Wisconsin #304, Long Beach, CA 90814, (213) 421-8424, BS 69 Bradley Univ; MS 70 Bradley Univ; Sp-Lang Path, Bernard A Landes PhD and Assoc, **SLP**

Kidd, Margaret L 1012 7th Street #18, Santa Monica, CA 90403, (213) 208-5380, BS 76 Univ of KS; MS 78 Tulane Univ; SLP, LA City Sch, **SLP**

Kidd, Mrs Margaret R 3028 South Holly Place, Denver, CO 80222, (303) 758-4565, BA 78 Univ of Denver; MA 80 CA St Univ - Long Beach; **SLP**

Kidder, Claude K 11653 Lally Drive, Lowell, MI 49331, Central MI Univ; Sp-Lang Path, Grand Rapids Public Schools, **SLP**

Kidder, Dr Herman C U S Naval Hospital, P O Box 98, FPO Seattle, WA 98778, (804) 444-7599, BS 68 Central MI Univ; MA 71 SUNY - Center at Buffalo; PH 77 (NS) Wichita St Univ; Head Operational Audiology, US Navy, **A**

Kidder, Mrs Roselyn J 120 North Jefferson, Lowell, MI 49331, BS; **SLP**

Kido, Patricia F 99-931A Lalawai Drive, Aiea, HI 96701, (808) 841-8304, BA 75 Univ of HI - Manoa; OB 75 Univ of HI - Manoa; MS 79 Univ of HI - Manoa; 79–Sp-Lang Path, Hi St Dept/Ed Ctrl Oahu Dist, **SLP ACE**

Kidron, Charles A 520 Arrowhead Trail, Sinking Spring, PA 19608, BS 59 Bloomsburg Univ of PA; ME 69 Bloomsburg Univ of PA; Sp-Lang Path, Berks County Intermed Unit 14, **SLP**

Kidwell, Marcella Elizabeth 2414 Kevsway Court, Baltimore, MD 21207, **SLP**

Kidwell, Mrs Susan Marie 4383 Wilmarth Road, Stockton, CA 95205, (209) 931-4926, BA 84 CA St Univ - Sacramento; MA 85 Univ of the Pacific; SLP, Escalon USD, **SLP**

Kieber, Mrs Carol Ann 14810 Palmerston Square, Centreville, VA 22020, (703) 830-5815, BA 82 SUNY - Center at Buffalo; MA 84 SUNY - Center at Buffalo; **SLP**

Kieburtz, Mrs Nancy Jean c/o Marsha Eidlin, 20 S W 97th Avenue, Portland, OR 97229, (503) 668-8011, BA 59 Univ of WA; MA 63 CUNY - Hunter Coll; Sp-Lang Path, Sandy Un Hgh Sch, **SLP**

Kiec-Lehmier, Cheryl 412 Rome Road, Lititz, PA 17543, (215) 631-9300, BS 78 Old Dominion Univ; MS 83 SUNY - Coll at Buffalo; **SLP**

Kiefaber, Mrs Victoria L 5084 Far Hills, Kettering, OH 45429, (513) 434-8827, BS 72 Northern MI Univ; MA 74 Northern MI Univ; 74–Sp-Lang Path, Hrng & Sp Cen for Chldn&Adults, **SLP**

Kiefer, Julie A 4817 Briarwood, Royal Oak, MI 48073, (313) 288-2734, BS 80 Western MI Univ; MA 82 Wayne St Univ; Coord-Rehab Unit Svcs, William Beaumont Hosp, **SLP**

Kiefer, Mrs Marlene 671 Tobulynn Drive, Nashville, TN 37211, (615) 832-8310, BA 73 Saint Olaf Coll; MA 77 Vanderbilt Univ; SLP, Bd of Ed Nashville/Davidson Co, **SLP**

Kiefer, Patricia J 2825-C Sherwood Road, Columbus, OH 43209, (614) 252-0731, BA 76 OH St Univ; MA 80 OH St Univ; Sp-Lang Path, St Vincent Chldn's Cen, **SLP**

Kiefer, Mrs Susan Deborah 520 Cedar Crest Court, Lafayette, LA 70501, (318) 662-5421, BA 82 Southeastern LA Univ; ME 85 Southeastern LA Univ; Sp-Lang Path, St Landry Parish Sch Bd, **SLP**

Kieft, Susan D 1707 Hillshire Drive, Kalamazoo, MI 49008, (616) 387-8045, BA 74 MI St Univ; MA 75 MI St Univ; 81–Asst Prof, Wn MI U/Dept of Sp Path & Aud, **A**

Kiel, Carol Ann 1690 Vintner Way, San Jose, CA 95124, (408) 269-0401, **SLP**

Kiel, Mrs Julia J 201 Fourth Street #224, Del Mar, CA 92014, (619) 792-1548, BS 81 Univ of TX - Austin; MA 84 Abilene Christian Univ; Sp-Lang Path, West Texas Rehabilitation Ctr, **SLP**

Kielbasa, Mrs Maureen Greichen 141 Rhode Island Boulevard, Portsmouth, RI 02871, (401) 683-9743, BA 77 Univ of RI; MS 79 Univ of RI; Sp/Lang Path, Warwick Sch Dept, **SLP**

Kielhold, Mrs Nancy Louise 505 East 17th Street, Interstate Apartment #24, South Sioux City, NE 68776, (402) 494-5382, BS 84 Northern St Coll; MA 85 Univ of SD - Vermillion; **SLP**

Kielmeyer, Mrs Kristine Marie Route 1, Wilson, WI 54027, (715) 772-4203, OM 85 Univ of WI - River Falls; 88–Sp-Lang Path, CES #11, **SLP**

Kielp, Therese Anne 57 Malden, La Grange, IL 60525-5843, (312) 346-1136, BS Southern IL Univ -Carbondale; MS 84 Southern IL Univ -Carbondale; **A**

Kielty, Pamela J 813 Villa Court, Bowling Green, KY 42101, (502) 842-0387, BS 69 Clarion Univ of PA; MS 71 Vanderbilt Univ; ES 83 Univ of KY; 77–Sp-Lang Path, Bowling Green Indep Sch, **SLP A**

Kiely, Michael A 1938 Farrel Drive, Coralville, IA 52240, (319) 351-2510, BA 72 Univ of MT; MA 73 Univ of MT; Coordinator Special Education, Grant Wood AEA, **SLP**

Kiem, Tami Sue 14559 Tramore Drive, Chesterfield, MO 63017, (314) 946-3557, BS 84 Fontbonne Coll; MS 85 Fontbonne Coll; **SLP**

Kienapple, Jean Ann Box 11033, 87 Carlheath Drive, Windsor Junction, NS, Canada B0N 2V0, (902) 429-4180, BA 78 Univ of Waterloo - Ontario; MS 83 Purdue Univ - West Lafayette; 85–Aud, Audiometric Consultants, **A**

Kienle, Marjorie L 536 East New York Street, Indianapolis, IN 46202, (317) 632-9391, BS 71 OH St Univ; ME 73 Bloomsburg Univ of PA; Coord Cochlear Implant Project, Methodist Hospital of Indiana, **SLP**

Kienlen-Trujillo, Mrs Kyle 660 Bonnie Brae, Lander, WY 82520, (307) 332-6967, BS 78 Univ of WY; MS 79 Eastern WA Univ; Sp-Lang Path, Fremont Co Sch Dist, **SLP**

Kienow, Mrs Barbara McGilvray 8780 SW Parkview Loop, Beaverton, OR 97005, (503) 645-4242, MS 80 Portland St Univ; Sp-Lang Path, Washington Cnty Educ Serv Dist, **SLP**

Kienzle, Mrs Nancy L 710 22nd Avenue N W, Minot, ND 58701, (701) 857-4680, BS 77 Univ of ND; MS 78 Univ of ND; Sp-Lang Path, Minot Pub Sch, **SLP**

Kiernan, Kim L 9013 Satyr Hill Road, Baltimore, MD 21234, MS 78 Loyola Coll; Sp-Lang Path, Baltimore Co Bd of Ed, **SLP**

Kiernan, Robert Leddy, Jr 231 Burgundy Hill Lane, Middletown, CT 06457, (203) 679-8365, BA 81 RI Coll; MS 83 Univ of MI - Ann Arbor; SLP, St of CT Dept of Mr, **SLP**

Kiernan, Susan C 1355 Woodmoor Drive, Monument, CO 80132, (719) 630-5200, BA 71 Univ of SD - Vermillion; MA 72 Univ of SD - Vermillion; Sp/Lang Path, Penrose Hosp, **SLP**

Kiersh, Nancy E 25 Monroe Place #8-F, Brooklyn, NY 11201, (718) 237-2218, BA 76 Duke Univ; MS 79 Columbia Univ Teachers Coll; 85–Sp-Lang Path Super, Long Island Coll Hosp, **SLP**

Kierstead, James M 607 North Platte Street, Fremont, NE 68025, (402) 721-0743, BS 60 Univ of NE - Lincoln; MS 65 Univ of NE - Lincoln; **SLP LM**

Kiesel, Lucinda J 161 Clinton Avenue, Tiffin, OH 44883, (419) 447-7521, BS 75 Bowling Green St Univ; MA 76 Bowling Green St Univ; 84–Sp-Lang Path, Seneca Co Opportunity Ctr, **SLP**

Kiesling, Elizabeth Heath 556 Vista Avenue, Palo Alto, CA 94306, (415) 573-4021, BA 73 Univ of the Pacific; MA 74 Univ of the Pacific; Sp-Lang Path, San Mateo Co Sch, **SLP**

Kiesow, James R Route 3 Box 243, Colfax, WI 54730-9167, BS 69 Univ of WI - River Falls; MS 76 Univ of WI - Eau Claire; Aud, Private Practice, **A**

Kiesow, Marion Sabrina 19924 Sweetgun Circle, #31, Germantown, MD 20874, (301) 540-6721, BA 83 Univ of MD - College Park; MA 86 Univ of MD - College Park; **SLP**

Kiester, Mrs Jeanette L 18269 Greenbay Avenue, Lansing, IL 60438, MS 77 Univ of IL - Urbana; BS 76 Univ of IL - Urbana; Sp-Lang Path, Private Practice, **SLP**

Kiester, Jerry D 5001 Bel Aire Road, Des Moines, IA 50310, (515) 276-6834, BS 73 Univ of NE - Lincoln; MA 74 Univ of NE - Lincoln; Audiologist, Private Practice, **A**

Kiester, Vicki A 2648 Rio Bravo Circle, Sacramento, CA 95826-2212, (916) 929-2277, BA 73 Univ of San Diego; MA 77 Univ of San Diego; Aud, Sutter Hrng & Sp Cen, **A**

Kieta, Mrs Mary Julie 3702 Warner Avenue, Louisville, KY 40207, BS 84 Western KY Univ; MS 85 Western KY Univ; 87–SLP, Dept of Defense Dependent Schs, **SLP**

Kievman-Young, Mrs Lisa M 19 Fairview Place, Hauppauge, NY 11788, (516) 582-8431, BS 77 Northeastern Univ; MS 78 Adelphi Univ; Sp-Lang Path, Private Practice, **SLP**

Kiewel, Mrs Linda Lou 2142 Park Avenue, St Paul, MN 55110-2321, (612) 721-1631, **SLP**

Kight, Mrs Carolyn Rizer 21 Courtney Court, Sumter, SC 29154, (803) 481-4517, BA 83 Columbia Coll; MS 84 Univ of SC - Columbia; Sp-Lang Path, Home Health Services, **SLP**

Kight, Jana Brown 102 I Windy Cove, Hampton, VA 23666, (804) 865-8253, BS 81 WV Univ; MS 82 WV Univ; Audiologist, Newport News Shipbldg & Drydoc, **A**

Kihara, Jane J 508 W Imperial Avenue, Apartment 3, El Segundo, CA 90245, (213) 640-6831, MS 86 Portland St Univ; **SLP**

Kiihnl, Linda L 2208 Chasefield, Shreveport, LA 71118, **SLP**

Kilar, Carolyn Yandura 3271 Bloomfield Lane #613, Auburn Hills, MI 48057, (313) 689-2043, BS 85 Central MI Univ; MA 86 Central MI Univ; **SLP**

Kilbey, Gretchen Carla Rural Route 2 Box 237, Praire Du Chien, WI 53821, (454) 426-1582, BS 84 Univ of WI - Oshkosh; MS 86 Univ of WI - Oshkosh; SLP, Cesa #6

Kilburg, Dr Gail Donahue 5 Barrow Court, Towson, MD 21204, (301) 321-3099, BA 69 Skidmore Coll; MS 71 Univ of Pittsburgh - Pittsburgh; PH 80 (Sp-Lang Path) Univ of Pittsburgh - Pittsburgh; Assoc Prof, Towson St U, **SLP**

Kilcher, Mary Frances Hillcrest Village #11, Route 3, Pittsburg, KS 66762, (316) 231-4527, BA 73 Marygove Coll; MS 81 Central MO St Univ; Sp-Lang Path, Webb City R-7, **SLP**

Kilcoyne, Claire N 701 Sidney Baker, Kerrville, TX 78028, (512) 896-8700, BS 72 Saint Louis Univ; MA 74 Saint Louis Univ; 88–Aud, R F Montgomery MD, **A ACE**

Kilday, Theresa Claire 12421 S Dairy Ashford, Houston, TX 77099, (713) 498-8110, 88–Resource Tchr, Alief ISD, **SLP**

Kile, Dr Jack E 1430 Valley Road, Oshkosh, WI 54901, (414) 424-4416, BS 61 Ashland Coll; MA 64 OH St Univ; PH 66 (NS) OH St Univ; Prof & Audiologist, University of Wisconsin, **A**

Kileny, Dr Paul R 2344 Dundee, Ann Arbor, MI 48103, (313) 936-8013, BA 73; MA 75; PH 78 (NS) Univ of IA; 85–Aud, Univ Michigan Med Ctr, **A**

Kiley, Kathy 6907 Ponderosa Drive, North Little Rock, AR 72116, **SLP**

Kilgo, Deborah Cherie D 207 Willow Way, Vicksburg, MS 39180, (601) 638-2771, BA 74 LA Tech Univ; BA 74 LA Tech Univ; MA 78 LA Tech Univ; 88–Sp-Lang Path, Vicksburg Warren Schs, **SLP**

Kilgren, Lori Ann 6143 Knoll Wood Road #105, Willowbrook, IL 60514, BS 80 Purdue Univ - West Lafayette; MA 81 Univ of TN - Knoxville; Sp-Lang Path, Rehabilitatn Services/Chicago, **SLP**

Kilhoffer, Royce L 32 Algonquin Forest, Millstadt, IL 62260, (618) 476-7963, BS 76 Western IL Univ; MA 77 Western IL Univ; SLP, Christian Hosp NE, **SLP**

Kilian, Mrs Marianne M 6048 Leafwood, Carmichael, CA 95608, (916) 481-1272, BA 66 Southwest TX St Univ; MA 73 Our Lady Lake Univ-San Anton; **SLP**

Killam, Alma Ellis 814 Arbor Road, Winston-Salem, NC 27104, (919) 725-8035, BA 32 Carson-Newman Coll; MA 57 Univ of MI - Ann Arbor; **SLP LM**

Killam, Mrs Doris 1632 Shafter Street, San Angelo, TX 76901, (915) 653-8329, BS 50 Southwest TX St Univ; ME 65 Univ of Houston - Univ Park; **SLP**

Kille, Judi C Westman Regional Hearing Ctr, 340 9th Street, Brandon, MB, Canada R7A 6C2, (204) 726-6171, BA 80 Minot St Univ; MS 80 Minot St Univ; 81–Aud, Westman Reg Hrng Cen, **A**

Killeen, Alicia M 132 North Berger Parkway, Apartment B-6, Fond Du Lac, WI 54935, (319) 351-4986, BS 85 Marquette Univ; MA 87 Univ of IA; 88–Sp-Lang Path, St Agnes Hosp, **SLP**

Killeen, Denise M 556 Tudor Road, San Leandro, CA 94577, (415) 783-1357, BS 75 CA St Univ - Hayward; MS 86 CA St Univ - Hayward; 87–Sp-Lang Path, Hayward USD, **SLP**

Killian, Bobbye N M 364 Vista Baya, Newport Beach, CA 92660, (714) 751-9776, BA 75 CA St Univ - Fullerton; MA 79 CA St Univ - Fullerton; Instr/Coastline Comm Coll, Private Practice, **SLP**

Killian, Dr Patricia 7220 West Jefferson, Suite 219, Denver, CO 80235, (303) 986-1133, BA 66 Univ of NE - Omaha; MS 67 Univ of NE - Omaha; PH 74 (NS) Univ of IA; 81–Proprietor, Killian PhD & Assoc, **SLP**

Killinger, Pamela J 475 North Green Bay Road, Apartment 10, Grafton, WI 53024, (414) 673-2100, BA 80 Univ of WI - Eau Claire; MS 81 Univ of WI - Stevens Point; Sp-Lang Path, Hartford Jt Sch Dist #1, **SLP**

Killingsworth, Carol A 2560 152nd N E Ste A, Redmond, WA 98052, (206) 883-5110, BA 72 WA St Univ; MA 74 Univ of WA; Manager, The Hear Cntr, **A**

Killion, Duree Gail 1407 West Stassney Lane, Austin, TX 78745, (512) 444-9561, BS 84 Baylor Univ; MS 85 Baylor Univ; 85–Sp-Lang Path, Oaks Treatment Ctr, **SLP**

Killion, M'Lizabeth 10102 Inwood Shadows, Houston, TX 77088, (713) 820-1723, BS 72 Univ of TX - Austin; MA 75 Univ of Houston - Univ Park; Private Practice, **SLP**

Killion, Mead C Etymotic Research, 61 Martin Lane, Elk Grove Village, IL 60007, (312) 228-0006, BA 61 Wabash Coll; MS 70 IL Inst of Tech; PH 79 (Aud) Northwestern Univ; President, Etymotic Research

Killius, Kristin Ann 8600 East Alameda Avenue, Apartment 17-207, Denver, CO 80231, (303) 321-3063, BS 84 Miami Univ - Oxford; MA 86 Cleveland St Univ; 86–Sp-Lang Path, Developmental Pathways Inc, **SLP**

Killoren, Mary Jo P O Box 683, Festus, MO 63028-0683, (314) 937-5407, BS 82 Northwest MO St Univ; MA 84 Univ of Northern IA; Sp-Lang Path, Private Practice, **SLP**

Killorin, Victoria Stewart 2044 South Clack, Apartment #638, Abilene, TX 79606, (915) 692-1633, BA 85 Univ of KY; MA 87 Univ of Northern CO; Sp-Lang Path, West Texas Rehab Center, **SLP**

Killough, Mrs Candace L 12 East Voorhees, Danville, IL 61832, (217) 443-2900, BA 76 IL St Univ - Normal; MA 77 IL St Univ - Normal; Sp-Lang Path/Interpreter, Danville Sch Dist #118, **SLP**

Killyon, Mrs Jeanine L 3105 Wildwood Drive, Nashville, TN 37217, (615) 329-2837, BS 74 Univ of NE - Lincoln; MS 75 Adelphi Univ; Sp-Lang Path, Metro Nashville Pu Sch Syst, **SLP**

Kilmer, Mark T 2731 West Elm Road, Franklin, WI 53132-9170, (414) 684-2011, BS 84 Univ of WI - Whitewater; MS 85 Univ of WI - Whitewater; **SLP**

Kilpatrick, Janet I c/o R Hilton Kilpatrick, Box 319, Nelliston, NY 13410, (315) 376-7394, BS 34 Columbia Univ Teachers Coll; MA 38 Columbia Univ Teachers Coll; **SLP LM**

Kilpatrick, Kathryn M 2404 Tyre Drive, Hudson, OH 44236, (216) 650-1958, BA 67 Univ of MA - Amherst; MA 68 Univ of MA - Amherst; Sp-Lang Path, Private Practice, **SLP**

Kilpatrick-Staubus, Jean M 1301 Willowood Lane, Virginia Beach, VA 23454, (804) 481-5635, BA 76 NC St Univ at Raleigh; MS 79 Univ of NC - Chapel Hill; 83–Sp-Lang Path, VA Beach Cty PS, **SLP**

Kilzer, Jeanne Marie 327 Clark Avenue, Billings, MT 59102, (406) 248-4778, BA 86 Univ of ND; MS 87 Univ of ND; 88–Sp-Lang Path, St Vincent Hosp

Kim, Dr Byoung W 7831 North Rockledge Avenue, Glendale, WI 53209, (414) 229-4290, DD 62 Seoul Nat'l Univ; OM 65 Seoul Nat'l Univ; PH 71 (NS) Univ of WI - Madison; 78–Assoc Prof, Univ of Wisconsin Milwaukee

Kim, Erin Jamie 2245 River Run Drive #4201, San Diego, CA 92108-1678, (408) 243-6792, MA 87 San Diego St Univ; **A**

Kim, Munah 156 Miles Avenue, Syracuse, NY 13210, (315) 479-9165, BA 85; MS 87 Clarion Univ of PA

Kim, Young Tae 303-11 Diamond Village, Gainesville, FL 32603, MA 86 Univ of FL

Kimata, Cheryl Lynn 1968 Nehoa Place, Honolulu, HI 96822, **SLP**

Kimball, Dr B D P O Box 306, Vernal, UT 84078, (801) 789-4479, BA 57 Brigham Young Univ; MA 58 Northwestern Univ; PH 62 (NS) Southern IL Univ -Carbondale; 84–Aud, State Department of Health, **A**

Kimball, Mrs Carol 5810 S W Nevada Court, Portland, OR 97219, (503) 777-4505, BA 70 Western MI Univ; MS 75 Portland St Univ; Classroom Teacher, Hollady Cen-Phys Hndcpd-Portl, **SLP**

Kimball, Roberta R 3207 22nd Avenue South, Minneapolis, MN 55407, (612) 721-6605, MA 86 Univ of MN - Minneap-St Paul; **SLP**

Kimbarow, Dr Michael L Cleveland Hearing & Speech Cen, 11206 Euclid Avenue, Cleveland, OH 44106, (216) 231-8787, BA 75 CUNY - Lehman Coll; MS 76 Univ of MI - Ann Arbor; PH 82 (Communication Disorders) Univ of MN - Minneap-St Paul; 88–Dir Sp-Lang Path & Hosp Svcs, Cleveland Hearing & Speech Cen, **SLP ACE**

Kimberlin, Karen T 30 Columbia Drive, Tinton Falls, NJ 07724, (201) 826-3360, BS 74 Trenton St Coll; MS 78 Rutgers St Univ -N Brunswick; Sp-Lang Path, Perth Amboy Pub Sch, **SLP**

Kimberly, Pamela Silva 24 Plymouth Court, Milford, CT 06460, (203) 783-3410, BA 76 Bridgewater St Coll; MS 78 Southern CT St Univ; Sp/Lang Path, Milford Pub Sch, **SLP**

Kimble, Carline S 4 Hamilton Avenue, Princeton, NJ 08542, (609) 924-6057, BS 68 Indiana Univ of PA; MS 71 WV Univ; Sp/Lang Path, Mercer Co Spec Serv Sch Dist, **SLP**

Kimble-Smith, Carlotta 314 Flora, Clinton, MO 64735-1932, **SLP**

Kimbrell, Steve Morris, Jr P O Box 315, Greenwood, MS 38930, (601) 453-1888, BS 82 Delta St Univ; MS 85 Univ Southern MS-Hattiesburg

Kimbrough, Channing Michelle 3900 Hamilton Street, Apartment K-304, Hyattsville, MD 20781, (301) 779-5922, MS 88 Howard Univ

Kimbrough, Mrs Deborah A 1501 1/2 Ester Street, Vancouver, WA 98660, (206) 256-7951, BA 81 WA St Univ; MA 82 WA St Univ; SLP, N W Theropy Services, **SLP**

Kimbrough, Graham F P O Box 51, Varnell, GA 30756, (404) 259-8421, BS 73 SUNY - Coll at Geneseo; MS 75 SUNY - Coll at Buffalo; Sp/Lang Path, Whitfield County, **SLP**

Kimelman, Dr Mikael D Z Dept Of Communication Disorder, LSU Medical Center, 1900 Gravier Street, New Orleans, LA 70112, (504) 568-4348, BS 78 CA St Univ - Hayward; MA 80 Univ of FL; PH 86 (Communication Disorders) Univ of WI - Madison; 86–Asst Prof, LSU Med Ctr, **SLP**

Kimes, Cheryl Jane 86 Maegan Place #1, Thousand Oaks, CA 91362, (805) 496-6683, BA 74 Pepperdine Univ - Los Angeles; MA 83 CA St Univ - Northridge; SLP, Conejo Valley USD, **SLP**

Kimes, Mrs Patricia Klesel 416 Flock Street, Georgetown, SC 29440, (803) 546-1056, BS 76 Southwest TX St Univ; ME 77 Southwest TX St Univ; Sp-Lang Path, La Porte ISD, **SLP**

Kimm, Gayle A 611 South Street #B-1, Marshalltown, IA 50158, (515) 753-4248, BA 78 Univ of Northern IA; MA 79 Univ of Northern IA; Sp/Lang Path, Iowa Veterans Home, **SLP**

Kimmel, Barry L Hearing Healthcare Center Inc, 3525 Ensign Road N E, Olympia, WA 98506, (206) 491-9733, BA 69 Portland St Univ; MS 72 Portland St Univ; Aud-Dir, Hearing Healthcare Ctr Inc, **A**

Kimmel, Mrs Theresa Marie 1918 Gustavus, Laredo, TX 78040, (512) 723-2926, BS 80 Univ of TX - Austin; ME 85 Southwest TX St Univ; **SLP**

Kimmerly, Susan L Rural Delivery 3 Box 1450, Montpelier, VT 05602, (802) 828-3141, BA 77 McGill Univ - Quebec; MS 83 Univ of VT; Consultant Speech/Lang/Hearing, Coord of Sch Dist Svcs, **SLP**

Kimoto, Kathleen Y 2734 Nakookoo Street #9, Honolulu, HI 96826, (808) 941-8495, BS 69 Western OR St Coll; MS 70 Univ of OR; 76–Sp-Lang Path, HI Dept of Educ, **SLP**

Kimpel, Mrs Linda Sue 508 Maona Avenue, Fond Du Lac, WI 54935, (414) 922-6670, BS 70 Univ of WI - Oshkosh; MS 84 Univ of WI - Oshkosh; 88–Sp-Lang Path, Sp Path Svc of Fond Du Lac, **SLP**

Kimpel, M Anne c/o Meyer Center, 8080 North Stadium Drive Suite 2300, Houston, TX 77054, (713) 794-2526, BS 79 Southern Methodist Univ; MS 81 Univ of OK Medical Center; Sp-Lang Path, Baylor College of Medicine, **SLP**

Kimura, Mrs Kathleen C 335-A Olomana Street, Kailua, HI 96734, (808) 544-3310, BS 81 Univ of HI - Manoa; MS 83 Univ of AZ; Sp-Lang Path, Rehab Hosp of Pacific, **SLP**

Kimzey, Mary Whitfield 2697 Golden Fawn Trail, Shingle Springs, CA 95682, (916) 985-0112, BA 74 Univ of CA - Davis; MS 82 San Francisco St Univ; Sp-Lang Path, El Dorado Co Ofc of Educ, **SLP**

Kinarti, Ruth Kibbutz Kineret, Mobile Post, Emek Hayarden, Israel, MS

Kinas, Christophe N 552 East Broadway, South Boston, MA 02127, (617) 268-1424, BS 58 Boston Univ; MS 62 Boston Univ; Sp-Lang Path, Framingham Pub Sch, **SLP**

Kincaid, Kathy K 1120 Nebraska Court N E, Salem, OR 97301, (503) 378-3447, BA 75 Western OR St Coll; BA 75 Western OR St Coll; MS 76 Western OR St Coll; Sp/Lang Path, Fairview Trng Cen, **SLP**

Kincaid, Laura Leanne 5608-4 Woodshire Drive, Fort Wayne, IN 46815, (219) 485-7554, BS 83 Ball St Univ; MA 85 Ball St Univ; **SLP**

Kincaid, Vicki S Y 8592 Bayonne Drive, Huntington Beach, CA 92646, **SLP**

Kincheloe, Dr John W Minot State University, Minot State University, Minot, ND 58701, (701) 857-3150, BA 52 Wichita St Univ; MA 58 Wichita St Univ; ED 72 (Special Education) Univ of Northern CO; Dean Sch of Educ & Human Serv, Minot State Coll, **SLP**

Kinde, Dr Stewart 285 Salem Avenue, Palm Harbor, FL 33563, (813) 974-2006, BS 60 Central MI Univ; MS 62 Central MI Univ; PH 72 (NS) MI St Univ; Retired, U of S FL, **SLP A**

Kinder, Deborah L Health Sciences Center U Of C, Box B210, 4200 East Ninth Avenue, Denver, CO 80262, (303) 394-7856, BS 79 Boston Univ; MA 81 Univ of Northern CO; Aud, U of CO Hlth Sci Cen, **A**

Kinder, Kathy Meyer 522 Chapparal Drive, O'Fallon, MO 63366, (314) 272-2850, MS 86 Fontbonne Coll; **SLP**

Kinder, Mrs Mary Beth P O Box 444, Flemingsburg, KY 41041, (606) 845-5111, BS 81 Eastern KY Univ; MA 83 Eastern KY Univ; Sp-Lang Path, Fleming County, **SLP**

Kindler, Mrs Barbara Hickey 3051 Hickory Woods, Greenfield, IN 46140, (317) 529-0900, BS 81 Ball St Univ; MA 82 Ball St Univ; Dir Sp & Hrng, New Castle State Dev Ctr, **SLP**

Kindred, Mrs Sheryl A PO Box 483, Northome, MN 56661, (218) 897-5275, BS 70 Northeast MO St Univ; MA 70 Northeast MO St Univ; 88–Sp-Lang Path, S Koochiching Rainy River Sch, **SLP**

Kindt, Jacqueline L 26837 Lake Vue #4, Perrysburg, OH 43551, (419) 874-5959, BS 86 Bowling Green St Univ; MS 87 Bowling Green St Univ; 87–Sp-Lang Path, InSpeech Inc, **SLP**

King, Annabelle Joyce 6750 El Colegio Road #76, Goleta, CA 93117, (805) 685-2849, MA 88 Univ of CA - Santa Barbara

King, Barbara S 2311 12th Street S W, Calgary, AB, Canada T2T 3N7, (403) 245-1642, BS 64 Bloomsburg Univ of PA; ME 68 PA St Univ - Univ Park; **SLP**

King, Betty A M 8147 South Downing, Littleton, CO 80122, (303) 795-6342, MA 74 Univ of Northern CO; SLP, Littleton Pub Schs, **SLP**

King, Bonnie L 505 Circle Drive, Oroville, CA 95965, MA 72 San Jose St Univ; **SLP**

King, Brian G ENT Surgical Associates, 201 North Lakemont Avenue, Suite 100, Winter Park, FL 32792, (407) 644-4883, BA 76 FL St Univ; MA 80 Univ of TN - Knoxville; 84–Dir of Aud, Central FL Hearing Ctr, **A**

King, Burton B Duke Univ Medical Center, P O Box 3887, Durham, NC 27710, (919) 684-3859, BS 54 Southwest TX St Univ; MA 55 Northwestern Univ; 65–Aud, Duke U Med Cen, **A**

King, Carol Leigh 505 Lookout #202, Richardson, TX 75080, (214) 238-8111, OB 77 TX A & M Univ; MS 87 Univ of TX - Dallas; **SLP**

King, Carolyn V 560 Gaylord Mountain Road, Hamden, CT 06518, **SLP**

King, Mrs Catherine Arthur 2630 Washington Street, Columbus, IN 47201, (812) 372-9044, BS 77 Purdue Univ - West Lafayette; MS 78 Vanderbilt Univ; Sp-Lang Path, Brown County Sch Corp, **SLP**

King, Catherine H 338 1st Avenue E #33, Dickinson, ND 58601, (701) 225-1968, BS 78 Minot St Univ; MA 81 Western MI Univ; 81–Sp-Lang Path, Dickinson Pub Schs, **SLP**

King, Mrs Cheryl Ann 37840 State Route 124, Pomeroy, OH 45769, (614) 992-6895, **SLP**

King, Mrs Cheryl L Rd #2 Box 135A, Waymart, PA 18472, (717) 348-2141, BS 79 Marywood Coll; MS 80 Loyola Coll; 87–Sp-Lang Path, PA Home Health, **SLP**

King, Christi Lee 6605 Beck Drive Northeast, Albuquerque, NM 87109, (505) 298-7486, BA 81 Univ of NM; MS 84 Univ of NM; **SLP**

King, Danielle Coppes 45 Grant Avenue, Norwood, MA 02062, (617) 769-6579, BS 84 Elmira Coll; MS 87 Emerson Coll; **SLP**

King, Deborah A 10000 West 75th Street, Suite 121, Shawnee Mission, KS 66204, (913) 362-7518, MA 75 Wichita St Univ; Sp-Lang Path, Private Practice, **SLP**

King, Deborah A 4832 Martin Mill Pike, Knoxville, TN 37920, (615) 974-5451, BS 74 Auburn Univ - Auburn; MA 77 Univ of TN - Knoxville; Sp-Lang Path, U of TN, **SLP ACE**

King, Mrs Deborah Crow Affiliated Audiology & Sp Path, 4900 Reed Road, Suite 105, Columbus, OH 43220, (614) 457-1548, BA 79 Heidelberg Coll; MA 82 OH St Univ; Regional Dir, Affiliated Aud & Sp Path, **SLP**

King, Debra Arslain 125 Lamplighter Drive, Morgantown, WV 26505, (304) 594-1151, BS 80 WV Univ; MS 81 WV Univ; Sp-Lang Path, Monongalia County Board of Ed, **SLP**

King, Mrs Dona D 2207 Seneca Drive, Charleston, IL 61920, (217) 235-5446, BS 72 Eastern IL Univ; BS 72 Eastern IL Univ; MS 74 Eastern IL Univ; Sp-Lang Path, Cusd #2 Mattoon Il, **SLP**

King, Emily M 1145-D North 11th Street, Beaumont, TX 77702, **SLP**

King, Mrs Fannie E 3806 Dryades Street, New Orleans, LA 70115, (504) 899-6874, BS 30 Dillard Univ; MA 70 Univ of MN - Minneap-St Paul; **SLP LM**

King, Franklin T 108 East Belmont, Milo, IA 50166, MA 74 Univ of Northern IA; Sp-Lang Path, Heartland AEA, **SLP**

King, Glynis Dawn 8112 Saint Lawrence Avenue, Chicago, IL 60619, (312) 487-0316, BS 80 Univ of IL - Urbana; MA 82 Memphis St Univ; Sp-Lang Path, Chicago Bd of Ed, **SLP**

King, Gregory P 2704 Costello Road, Sioux Falls, SD 57105, (605) 331-7948, BA 72 Kearney St Coll; MA 75; Coord, Sioux Falls School Dist 49-5, **SLP A**

King, Gwen Sparkman 224 Bienville Road, Folsom, LA 70437, (504) 796-9825, BS 80 LA St Univ - Baton Rouge; ME 86 Southeastern LA Univ; **SLP**

King, Dr Henry L 204 South Avenue D, Portales, NM 88130, (402) 472-2081, BS 65 Eastern NM Univ; MS 67 Eastern NM Univ; PH 84 (NS) Wichita St Univ; Aud, High Plains Reg Ctr, **A**

King, Mrs Iva L 175 Rockspray Ridge, Peachtree City, GA 30269, (404) 487-3491, BA 69 FL St Univ; MS 70 FL St Univ; Sp-Lang Path, Coweta Co Sch Sys, **SLP**

King, Janet Little P O Box 1244, Oxford, MS 38655, (601) 234-1091, BA 83 Univ of MS; MS 86 Univ of MS; **SLP**

King, Mrs Jillian Suzanne 2135 31st Avenue, San Francisco, CA 94116, (415) 342-7364, BS 81 Pacific Union Coll; MA 83 Univ of MD - College Park; Sp-Lang Path, The Bridge Sch, **SLP**

King, Joan 1213 Forest Street, Inglewood, CA 90302, **SLP**

King, Jody Lynette 1284 East Fallbrook, Fresno, CA 93710, (209) 292-5840, BA 79 CA St Univ - Fresno; MA 83 CA St Univ - Fresno; Sp-Lang Path, Madera Co Dept of Ed, **SLP**

King, Judy Bell 900 34th Street, Boulder, CO 80303, (303) 492-6445, MS 75 Humboldt St Univ; Graduate Instructor, University of Colorado, **SLP**

King, Karen Lynn W179 N8652 Village Court #8, Menomonee Falls, WI 53051, BA 85 Univ of CT; MS 87 Southern CT St Univ; 87–Sp-Lang Path, Campbellsport Sch, **SLP**

King, Karolyn Louise 1266 8th Avenue, San Francisco, CA 94122, (415) 334-5000, BA 68 Univ of OR; MA 71 San Francisco St Univ; 71–Sp-Lang Path, San Francisco USD, **SLP**

King, Kathleen 3010 Montrose Avenue #32, La Crescenta, CA 91214, (818) 248-4515, MA 85 CA St Univ - Los Angeles; Aud, **A**

King, Kathleen Anne 1027 Cherry Lane, Lombard, IL 60148, (312) 620-4433, BS 82 Univ of WI - Stevens Point; MS 84 Univ of WI - Stevens Point; Sp-Lang Path, Dupage Easter Seal Trtmtn Cen, **SLP**

King, Kayla Rochelle 501 Houston, Apartment 103-C, Waxahachie, TX 75165, (214) 937-5904, MS 88 Baylor Univ; 88–Sp-Lang Path, Waxahachie ISD

King, Kerry B P O Box 6, Prosperity, PA 15329, (304) 686-3305, BS 76 Clarion Univ of PA; MS 78 WV Univ; Sp/Lang Path, Marshall Co Sch, **SLP**

King, Mrs Laurie R 2682 Dalto Court, Oceanside, NY 11572, (516) 763-1366, BS 77 SUNY - Coll at New Paltz; MA 78 Hofstra Univ; Sp-Lang Path, NY Cty Bd of Ed, **SLP**

King, Linda Johnston 2844 Embassy Circle N W, Roanoke, VA 24019, (703) 387-6517, BS 74 Radford Univ; MS 81 Radford Univ; Sp/Lang Path, Roanoke Co Sch, **SLP**

King, Linda Marian 3306 Highbrook Drive, Dallas, TX 75234, (214) 358-8339, BS 79 OK St Univ; MA 82 OK St Univ; SLP, Dallas Rehab Center, **SLP**

King, Mrs Margaret F 10 Offut Court, Woodstock, MD 21163, (301) 461-5365, BS 73 Towson St Univ; MS 76 Johns Hopkins Univ; Sp-Lang Path, Chatsworth Sch, **SLP**

King, Marie L 1104 Aspen Circle, Birmingham, AL 35215, BS 79 Univ of Montevallo; MS 80 Univ of Montevallo; Sp-Lang Path, Blout Co Bd of Ed, **SLP**

King, Marilyn O 2214 Fruitland, Kennewick, WA 99336, (509) 582-2072, BS 65; Sp-Lang Path, Children's Sp & Lang Ctr, **SLP**

King, Mrs Marjorie C 127 Hillside Drive, Delaware, OH 43015, (513) 644-6115, MS 71 Univ of South FL; Dir/Sp & Hrng, Mem Hosp of Union Co, **SLP**

King, Mary Ella P O Box 8, Seagrove, NC 27341, (919) 873-7897, BS 83 Appalachian St Univ; MA 86 Appalachian St Univ; 88–Sp-Lang Path, Mary E King & Assoc, **SLP**

King, Mary L A 13923 Castle Blvd #13, Silver Spring, MD 20904, (601) 355-4818, BS 72 Jackson St Univ; MS 79 Univ Southern MS-Hattiesburg; SLP, Jackson Pub Sch, **SLP**

King, Mary T 423 South Scoville, Oak Park, IL 60302, (312) 450-2725, BS 79 Eastern IL Univ; MS 80 Eastern IL Univ; 84–Sp-Lang Path, Westchester School Dist 92 5, **SLP**

King, Dr Michael D McV Station Box 55, Richmond, VA 23298, (804) 786-0240, 79–Assoc Prof, Medical Coll of VA, **SLP**

King, Michelle F Commission Handicapped Childre, 982 Eastern Parkway, Louisville, KY 40217, (502) 588-4459, BA 79 Bellarmine Coll; MS 81 Univ of Louisville; Audiologist, Commission Handicapped Childrn, **A**

King, Mrs Nelda K 5524 76th Street, Lubbock, TX 79424, (806) 794-6096, BA 79 TX Tech Univ; MS 81 TX Tech Univ; Director, Communication Disorders Ctr, **SLP ACE**

King, Mrs Patricia S 206 Magnolia, Republic, MO 65738, (417) 463-2514, BS 76 Central MO St Univ; MS 79 Central MO St Univ; 88–Sp-Lang Path, Marionville Sch Dist, **SLP**

King, Mrs Patricia Schovanec 1101 Sequoyah Drive, Enid, OK 73703, (405) 242-6413, BS 76 Phillips Univ; MA 78 Wichita St Univ; 84–Sp-Lang Path, Hedges Comm Sp & Hrng Ctr, **SLP**

King, Mrs Peggy A Rd 2 Box 195A, Staver Road, Reinholds, PA 17569, (215) 378-0481, BS 76 Bloomsburg Univ of PA; MS 77 Bloomsburg Univ of PA; Sp-Lang Path, Berks Vstng Nurse Home Hlth Ag, **SLP**

King, Penney Reissis 1486 Quaker Street, Northbridge, MA 01534, (617) 234-6196, SLP, Newton P S, **SLP**

King, Richard N 33 Huntington Avenue, Hamilton, ON, Canada L8T 1X5, (416) 440-0641, BA 72 Brock Univ - Ontario; MA 75 SUNY - Center at Buffalo; Exec Dir, Canadian Assoc of Sp-Lang Path, **SLP**

King, Robert S Route 11 Box 551, Jonesboro, TN 37659, (615) 926-1171, BA 67 AR St Univ; MA 72 Univ of MO - Columbia; Sp-Lang Path, VA, **SLP**

King, Roger D 5546 Monica Drive, Fairfield, OH 45014, (513) 829-0281, MA 76 Miami Univ - Oxford; SLP, Community Multicare Center, **SLP**

King, Sally 2553 2nd Avenue East, La Crosse, WI 54603, (608) 783-5644, BS 76 Univ of WI - Stevens Point; MS 78 Univ of WI - Eau Claire; Sp-Lang Path, Onalaska Pub Sch, **SLP**

King, Shelley L 1128 Cordell, Excelsior Springs, MO 64024, (816) 637-6044, BA 78 William Jewell Coll; MS 81 Central MO St Univ; Sp-Lang Path, Excelsior Springs Sch Dist, **SLP**

King, Sheri-Lyn R 627 South Estelle, Wichita, KS 67211, (316) 662-8566, BA 80 Wichita St Univ; MA 82 Wichita St Univ; Sp-Lang Path, USD 260, **SLP**

King, Dr Susan H 445 Arenas Street, La Jolla, CA 92037, (619) 454-9947, BA 62 Saint Mary's Coll; MA 64 Univ of WI - Madison; PH 70 (NS) LA St Univ - Baton Rouge; **SLP**

King, Susan J 2307 Claridge Circle, South Charleston, WV 25303, **SLP**

King, Dr Thomas W 108 Shorewood Drive, Menomonie, WI 54751, (715) 235-4747, MS 72 Univ of WI - Eau Claire; OM 78 Univ of WI - Superior; ED 78 (Adapted PE/Spec Ed Adm) Clayton Univ; 87–Lecturer/Supvr, Private Practice, **SLP**

King, Mrs Wilma G 20 Gulf Manor Drive, Venice, FL 34285, (813) 484-2469, BS 48 PA St Univ - Univ Park; ME 49 PA St Univ - Univ Park; **SLP**

King-Debaun, Patricia P O Box 440051, Kennesaw, GA 30144, BS 83 CO St Univ; MS 85 CO St Univ; Sp-Lang Path, Bartow Public Schools, **SLP**

King-Grant, Mrs Caryl 3928 Blackburn Lane #24, Burtonsville, MD 20866, (301) 421-9422, BA 81 Saint John's Univ - Jamaica; MA 83 NY Univ; SLP, City of New York Board of Educ, **SLP**

Kingkade, Sandra Kirchmann 4607 North View Drive, Omaha, NE 68134-2938, (402) 330-2770, SLP, Esu #3, **SLP**

Kingma, Lora Leigh 160 Wooden Shoe Court, Christiansburg, VA 24073, (703) 356-2833, BS 84 Radford Univ; MS 85 Radford Univ; **SLP**

Kingman, Mrs Janice L 320 Hudson Avenue, Clarendon Hills, IL 60514, (312) 887-2740, BS 61 Purdue Univ - West Lafayette; MA 65 Univ of Southern CA; Sp-Lang Path, Mercy Health Care & Rehab Ctr, **SLP**

Kingman, Mrs Wendy S 5 Sanford Lane, Box 841, Monument Beach, MA 02553, (508) 759-4120, BA 75 Bridgewater St Coll; MA 82 Univ of MA - Amherst; Sp-Lang Path, Bourne PS, **SLP**

King-Reeves, Mrs L Carole 1805 34th Street, Parkersburg, WV 26104, (304) 863-3321, BA 83 Marshall Univ; MA 84 Marshall Univ; MA 88 WV Univ; Sp-Lang Path, Wood County Board of Education, **SLP**

Kingsbury, Karen Basting W177 N9032 St Stevens Court, Menomonee Falls, WI 53051, (414) 461-8850, BS 84 Univ of WI - Madison; MS 86 Univ of WI - Madison; 87–Sp-Lang Path, Marian Franciscan Home, **SLP**

Kingsbury, Nancy 7542 West Harrison, Forest Park, IL 60130, (312) 996-3714, MS 84 Rush Univ; Sp-Lang Path, Univ of IL Hospital, **SLP**

Kingsley, Mrs Georgia F 2900 Charolais Drive, Greensboro, NC 27406, (919) 584-5571, BA 68 Lamar Univ; ME 81 Univ of NC - Greensboro; 87–Cl Supvr, Univ of NC, **SLP**

Kingsley-Douglas, Susan 4917 Morris Avenue, Fort Worth, TX 76103, (817) 336-9371, BS 74 TX Tech Univ; MS 76 TX Tech Univ; 88–Chief-Lang Path, St Joseph Hosp, **SLP**

Kingston, Mary E 180 Osborne, St Lambert, PQ, Canada J4R 1B2, (514) 671-6970, BS 73 Univ of MN - Minneap-St Paul; MA 75 Mankato St Univ; **SLP**

King-Streit, Mrs Suzanne 8904 Weatherby Court, Granite Bay, CA 95661, (916) 966-8722, BA 76 CA St Univ - Sacramento; MA 78 CA St Univ - Sacramento; 81–Resource Specialist, San Juan USD, **SLP**

King-Webb, Robin 527 University Place, Redlands, CA 92373-4392, (714) 781-1725, BS 76 Pacific Union Coll; MS 82 Loma Linda Univ - Riverside; SLP, Rubidoux Hs/Jurapa USD, **SLP**

Kinigopoulos, Mrs Helen Galinis 9757 Michaels Way, Ellicott City, MD 21043, (301) 461-3650, BS 73 Towson St Univ; MS 87 Towson St Univ

Kinion, Renee Louise 7520 Potranco Road #2510, San Antonio, TX 78251, (512) 622-3436, BS 85 Southwest TX St Univ; MS 86 Southwest TX St Univ; 88–Sp-Lang Path, S/W ISD

Kinkead, Rebecca J 91 South 5th Avenue, Clarion, PA 16214, BS 78 Clarion Univ of PA; ME 79 Clarion Univ of PA; **SLP**

Kinkead, Steven Dale 206 West Hardy Street, St James, MO 65559-1309, (314) 265-8949, BA 77 Univ of MO - Columbia; MA 78 Univ of MO - Columbia; Sp-Lang Path, InSpeech Inc, **SLP**

Kinker, Joyce R 2743 West Central Avenue, Toledo, OH 43606, (419) 473-9949, BA 71 Bowling Green St Univ; MA 72 Bowling Green St Univ; Dir of Aud, Toledo Otolaryngology, **A**

Kinlaw, Sarah H B 1429 Lincoln Avenue, St Paul, MN 55105, (612) 698-4644, BA 73 Skidmore Coll; MS 76 Boston Univ; SLP, St Paul Pub Sch, **SLP**

Kinloch, Dr Diane L 5706 South Kimbrough, Springfield, MO 65807, (417) 883-4993, BA 72 Wichita St Univ; MA 73 Wichita St Univ; PH 85 (NS) Univ of MO - Columbia; Ment Retard Classroom Teacher, Univ of Missouri, **SLP**

Kinnard, Kristi K 93 Signal Hill Court, Holland, PA 18966, (609) 394-4177, BA 77 OH Univ - Athens; MA 84 OH Univ - Athens; Sp-Lang Path, Mercer Med Ctr, **SLP**

Kinne, Mrs L Kay Lakeland Area Education #3, 1-1/2 State Street, Algona, IA 50511, (515) 295-7784, BS 61 OH Univ - Athens; MA 80 Univ of Northern CO; Aud, Lakeland AEA, **A**

Kinney, Brenda L 533 West Guadalupe Road, Apartment 2052, Mesa, AZ 85210, (602) 994-1996, BS 78 Miami Univ - Oxford; MS 79 Miami Univ - Oxford; Sp-Lang Path, Scottsdale Public Schools, **SLP**

Kinney, Kimberley Ann 550 Pearl Street #205, Reading, PA 19602, (215) 775-8334, BS 84 Bloomsburg Univ of PA; MS 85 Bloomsburg Univ of PA; 85–Sp-Lang Path, Reading Rehab Hosp, **SLP**

Kinney-White, Dr Barbara A Live Oak Mobile Home Park, 1225 17th Avenue #29, Santa Cruz, CA 95062, (408) 462-2903, BA 48 San Jose St Univ; MA 52 San Jose St Univ; PH 83 (Education) American National Inst; **SLP LM**

Kinnish, Kathleen Monica 10095 Avondale Lane, Traverse City, MI 49684, (616) 922-9537, BS 72 IL St Univ - Normal; MS 84 IL St Univ - Normal; Sp-Lang Path, Munson Med Cntr, **SLP**

Kinoshita, Mrs Sheryl M HC 81 Box 64, Chappell, NE 69129, (308) 874-3406, MS 78 Univ of WY; Sp-Lang Path, Rehab Therapy Inc, **SLP**

Kinsberg, Helene K 2971 Voorheis Avenue, Brooklyn, NY 11235, BA 71 CUNY - Hunter Coll; MA 73 NY Univ; SLP, New York City Bd of Ed

Kinsella, Colleen Therese 908 South Briggs, Joliet, IL 60433, (815) 740-3196, BS 84 Northern IL Univ - De Kalb; MS 87 Governors St Univ; Sp-Lang Path, Joliet PS Dist 86

Kinsella, Debra A 6920 Lake Park Circle, St Louis, MO 63123-1600, (314) 645-6961, MS 80 Southern IL Univ-Edwardsvill; SLP, St Louis Spec Sch Dist, **SLP**

Kinsella-Meier, MaryAnn 13100 Wilton Oaks Drive, Silver Spring, MD 20906, (202) 651-5377, BA 79 Univ of MD - College Park; MS 82 Gallaudet Coll; 85–Aural Rehab, Gallaudet Univ, **A**

Kinsey, Charles R 4154 Bennetts Corners Road, Holley, NY 14470, (716) 461-2800, BA 74 SUNY - Coll at Brockport; MA 79 SUNY - Coll at Geneseo; Sp/Lang Path, Monroe Dev Cen, **SLP**

Kinsey, Joanmarie Therese 1435 Malibu Circle #105, Palm Bay, FL 32905, (305) 984-4600, BS 85 FL St Univ; MS 86 FL St Univ; **SLP**

Kinsinger, Susan I 26660 Players Circle, Lutz, FL 33549, BS 71 Murray St Univ; ME 74 Univ of Louisville; 87–Sp-Lang Path, District Sch Bd of Pasco Co, **SLP**

Kinsman, Mrs Georgene J Fairview School, 28500 Oakcrest, Farmington Hills, MI 48050, (313) 626-8335, BS 69 Eastern MI Univ; MA 69 Eastern MI Univ; 69–Sp-Lang Path, Farmington PS, **SLP**

Kinsora-Joseph, Mrs Peggy 15298 S W 104th Str #9-11, 1, Miami, FL 33196, (305) 382-9534, BS 74 Univ of San Diego; MS 78 Univ of PR - Rio Piedras; Teacher, Paul Davis School, **SLP**

Kinstle, Frances Lillian 917 Brookfield Drive #8, Mansfield, OH 44907, (419) 522-1214, **SLP**

Kinstler, Dr Donald B 3488 Kingmont Drive, Loomis, CA 95650, (916) 652-4000, BA 38 Lafayette Coll; MA 54 CA St Univ - Los Angeles; PH 59 (Sp Aud) Univ of Southern CA; **SLP A LM**

Kintigh, Marcella Louise Bridge Street, Rd #1 Box 142, Hunker, PA 15639, (412) 925-7828, MS 86 CA Univ of PA; **SLP**

Kintz, Julia Aileen R R 2 Box 829, Woodstock, VT 05091, (802) 457-1213, BS 83 Northern MI Univ; MA 85 MI St Univ; **SLP**

Kinzie, Coralene Box 193, Ainsworth, NE 69210, (402) 387-2083, BA 74 Kearney St Coll; MS 77 Kearney St Coll; Sp-Lang Path, Ainsworth City Sch, **SLP**

Kipfmueller, Dr Leo J 420 South Franklin Street, Mount Pleasant, MI 48858, (517) 774-3471, BA 55 Central MI Univ; MA 59 Central MI Univ; PH 69 (NS) Univ of MI - Ann Arbor; Professor, Central Michigan University, **SLP**

Kipnis, Mrs Joan E K 146 North Mansfield Blvd, Cherry Hill, NJ 08034, BA 72 PA St Univ - Univ Park; MA 76 Temple Univ; Audiologist, Private Practice, **A**

Kipper-Hall, Mechele 20800 Starshine Road, Walnut, CA 91789, (213) 861-4357, BA 73 CA St Univ - Northridge; MA 81 CA St Univ - Los Angeles; Sp-Lang Path, Los Angeles Co Supt of Sch, **SLP**

Kipps, Helen A 1301 Fox Run N W, Bremerton, WA 98310, (206) 692-8363, BS 79 Marywood Coll; MA 81 Univ of ME - Orono; SLP, **SLP**

Kippur, Mrs Mary Scharpf 949A Heritage Village, Southbury, CT 06488, (203) 575-1224, BA 73 Alverno Coll; MS 84 Southern CT St Univ; SLP, Waterbury Brd of Educ, **SLP**

Kirby, Sr Alice M Special Education Department, Bridgewater State College, Bridgewater, MA 02324, (617) 697-1200, BA 55 Regis Coll; ME 60 Boston Univ; Asst Prof, Bridgewater State Coll, **SLP**

Kirby, D'Lyla A Abilene Christian University, Box 8160, Abilene, TX 79699, (915) 674-2074, BS 73 Abilene Christian Univ; MS 78 TX Tech Univ; Cl Dir, Abilene Christian V, **SLP**

Kirby, Mrs Karen Berg 3683 Riedham Road, Shaker Heights, OH 44120, (216) 268-6648, BA 63 LA St Univ - Baton Rouge; MA 69 Univ of WA; Sp/Lang Path, East Cleveland Bd of Ed, **SLP**

Kirby, Kathleen F 82 Elm Street, Worcester, MA 01609, MS; **A LM**

Kirby, Kristy A 7327 Creekwood Quorum Dr, Apartment 203, Charlotte, NC 28212, (704) 536-0787, BA 84 Marshall Univ; MA 85 Marshall Univ; 87–Sp-Lang Path, Charlotte-Mecklenburg PS, **SLP**

Kirby, Mrs Sherry Maddox 3139 Suffolk Drive, Shelby, NC 28150, (704) 553-2826, MA 83 Western Carolina Univ; Sp-Lang Path, Cleveland Home Health Agcy, **SLP**

Kirby, Virginia M Biosciences Laboratory, Life Sciences Sector/3M, Bldg 270-4S-11/3M Center, St Paul, MN 55144, (612) 733-4951, BS 77 Univ of MN - Minneap-St Paul; MS 81 Purdue Univ - West Lafayette; Biosciences Laboratory 3M Co, **A**

Kirby, Wayne H P O Box 72, Knoxville, TN 37901, (615) 522-7121, BA 73 Univ of TN - Knoxville; MA 74 Univ of TN - Knoxville; 87–Aud, Hearing Aid Spec, **A**

Kirchdoerfer, Diana G 370 Pine Way, Oregon, WI 53575, (608) 221-7679, BS 77 Univ of MO - Columbia; MA 79 Univ of IA; Sp-Lang Path, Monona Grove Schools, **SLP**

Kirchenbauer, Susan H Potomac Center, 1380 Marshall Street, Hagerstown, MD 21740, (301) 791-4643, MS 76 Loyola Coll; Sp-Lang Path, Potomac Center, **SLP**

Kirchgasler, Claudia Roberts 1012 East 21st Street, Idaho Falls, ID 83401, (208) 524-3740, BA 76 Northern St Coll; MA 77 Univ of SD - Vermillion; Sp-Lang Path, Private Practice, **SLP**

Kirchgessner, Janice A P 6479 Almond Lane, Clarkston, MI 48016, (313) 625-5773, BS 69 Bowling Green St Univ; MA 71 Eastern MI Univ; 86–Sp-Lang Path, Clarkston Comm Schs, **SLP**

Kirchmann, Olivia Augustina P O Box 1026, Joshua Tree, CA 92252, (619) 366-8064, BA 74 CA St Univ - Fresno; MA 80 San Diego St Univ; Sp-Lang Path, Morongo USD, **SLP**

Kirchner, Dr Diane M 2550 9th Street, Suite #115, Berkeley, CA 94710, (415) 644-1266, BA 73 Univ of MT; MA 75 Univ of Denver; PH 84 (Sp & Hrng Science/Lang Emphasis) Univ of CA - Santa Barbara; 82–Dir/Owner, Private Practice, **SLP**

Kirchner, Maryanne 3406 Pebble Beach Drive, Wilmington, DE 19808, BA 76 Kean Coll of NJ; MA 78 OH St Univ; SLP, **SLP**

Kirchner, Mrs Patricia Johnson 12301 Rivers Edge Drive, Potomac, MD 20854, (301) 963-5847, BS 84 WV Univ; MA 85 George Washington Univ; **SLP**

Kirchner, Mrs Therese Ear Nose And Throat Treat Ctr, 2300 North Mayfair Rd #630, Wauwatosa, WI 53226, (414) 259-1211, MS 83 Univ of WI - Stevens Point; Audiologist, Ear Nose Throat Treatment Cen, **A**

Kirchner-Smudde, Mrs Patricia Lynn 221 East Plainfield Avenue, Milwaukee, WI 53207, (414) 769-1781, BS 80 Univ of WI - Milwaukee; MS 84 Univ of WI - Milwaukee; 84–Sp-Lang Path, Milwaukee PS, **SLP**

Kirdzik, Constance B 37 Washington Street, Naugatuck, CT 06770, (203) 729-7890, BA 84 Central CT St Univ; MS 86 Southern CT St Univ; 86–Sp-Lang Path, New Britain Bd of Educ, **SLP**

Kiriluk, Ellaine A 1812 South Ashland Avenue, Park Ridge, IL 60068, (312) 823-5868, BS 74 Bradley Univ; MS 76 IN Univ - Bloomington; Sp-Lang Path, Chldrns Mem Hosp, **SLP**

Kirk, Barbara C 69 Allen Street, Suite 2, Rutland, VT 05701, (802) 773-8469, BS 70 SUNY - Coll at Fredonia; MA 72 Univ of CT; Dir Aud, Vermont Achiev Cen, **A**

Kirk, Bonnie Jo University Of Bristol, Junior Year Abroad Program, 12 Priory Road, Bristol, England BS8 ITU, BA 76 CA St Univ - Northridge; MA 79 CA St Univ - Northridge; Sp-Lang Path, Porterville Developmental Center, **SLP**

Kirk, Mrs Carolyn S 11734 Sela Lane, Houston, TX 77072, (713) 498-8110, **SLP**

Kirk, Joni Rogers Speech & Hearing Clinic, Dept Of Speech Communication, CMA 2 200, Austin, TX 78712, (512) 471-3841, BS 82 Southwest TX St Univ; ME 83 Southwest TX St Univ; Sp-Lang Path, Univ of Texas, **SLP**

Kirk, Mrs Karen Iler 326 Hutchinson Avenue, Iowa City, IA 52240, (213) 483-4431, BA 78 Univ of CA - Santa Barbara; MA 80 Univ of CA - Santa Barbara; MS 87 Univ of Southern CA; Research Asst, Univ of IA, **SLP**

Kirk, Mrs Karen Lee 411 E 9th Avenue, Collegeville, PA 19426, (215) 489-2105, BS 72 Kent St Univ; MA 74 Kent St Univ; Prog Support Spec/SLP, Montgy Co Interm Unit, **SLP**

Kirk, Mary L 7902 Calhoun, Dearborn, MI 48126, **SLP**

Kirk, Nancy C 9763 East Elizabeth Street, Parker, CO 80134, (303) 841-9615, **SLP**

Kirk, Rita A A-8 Whitegate Drive, Nashua, NH 03060, MS 75 Univ of South FL; Sp-Lang Path, Nashua Sch Dist, **SLP**

Kirkes, Mrs Bette L 2251 Cowper Street, Palo Alto, CA 94301, (415) 877-5677, BA 68 San Jose St Univ; MA 71 San Jose St Univ; Sp-Lang Path, County of San Mateo, **SLP**

Kirkey, Karen P 249 Chili Avenue, Rochester, NY 14611, BS 76 Rochester Inst of Tech; MS 87 Gallaudet Coll; **A**

Kirkham, Cherie Cooper 286 Hedstrom Drive, Buffalo, NY 14226-2528, (217) 328-2462, BS 85 Miami Univ - Oxford; MS 86 Miami Univ - Oxford; **SLP**

Kirkland, Erin E Box 626, Meade, KS 67864, (316) 873-2049, BS 80 KS St Univ; MA 82 KS St Univ; Sp-Lang Path, Swn Area Sp Ed Coop #613, **SLP ACE**

Kirkland, James Wade 1118 Scaleybark #317-C, Charlotte, NC 28209, (704) 525-1951, BA 83 Univ of FL; MA 87 Univ of FL; 88–Aud, Charlotte EENT Associates, **A**

Kirkland, Jean Clennon 3839 Los Feliz Blvd #303, Los Angeles, CA 90027, (213) 669-2809, BA 73 Lawrence Univ; MS 80 Univ of NC - Chapel Hill; 87–Sp-Lang Path, Cucamonga Sch Dist, **SLP**

Kirkland, Mrs Julie Ann 29 Wagonwheel Court, Little Rock, AR 72211-4160, (501) 666-8686, SLP, Eliz Mitchell Chldrns Ctr, **SLP**

Kirkland, Mrs Sheila Laney 1006 Anne Street, Chipley, FL 32428, (904) 638-4550, MS 84 FL St Univ; Sp-Lang Path, Washington Co Schs, **SLP**

Kirkland, Mrs Susan Rice 1111 Dorris Road, Douglasville, GA 30339, BS 81 Auburn Univ - Auburn; OM 83 Auburn Univ - Auburn; Sp-Lang Path, Carroll Co Sch, **SLP**

Kirkland, Wendy Rita 5050 Wilder Drive, Apt C, Soquel, CA 95073, (408) 462-3691, BA 74 CA St Univ - Sacramento; MA 75 CA St Univ - Sacramento; Sp-Lang Path, San Benito County Off Ed, **SLP**

Kirkman, Judith A 3765 Lakeshore Drive, Marietta, GA 30067, (404) 257-2075, BA 72; MA 74 Montclair St Coll; Sp-Lnag Path, Med Cen at Princeton, **SLP**

Kirkmeyer, Reva D M 3218 Aspen Drive, Casper, WY 82601, (307) 237-9571, BS 74 Univ of WY; MS 75 Univ of WY; **SLP**

Kirkpatrick, Anita G 2538 Wilma, Wichita, KS 67211, (316) 686-3388, BA 81 Wichita St Univ; MA 82 Wichita St Univ; SLP, St Josephs Med Ctr Hhc, **SLP**

Kirkpatrick, Mrs Bonita Smith 558 South Queen Street, Lancaster, PA 17603, (717) 898-2451, BA 75 Univ of MD - College Park; MS 77 PA St Univ - Univ Park; Audiologist, Lancaster Intermediate Unit 13, **A**

Kirkpatrick, Mrs Diane Yvonne 415 North Turnpike Road, Santa Barbara, CA 93111, (805) 964-4711, BS 70 Univ of CA - Santa Barbara; MA 73 Univ of CA - Santa Barbara; Sp-Lang Path, Santa Barbara Co Sch, **SLP**

Kirkpatrick, Mrs Julie M Lasalle Co Spec Ed Co-Op, Easter Seal Center, 1013 Adams Street, Ottawa, IL 61350, (815) 434-0857, BS 81 Univ of WI - Stevens Point; MA 84 Northern IL Univ - De Kalb; 84–Aud, LEASE/Easter Seal Ctr, **A**

Kirkpatrick, Lorie Lyn 473 Laswell Avenue, San Jose, CA 95128-2234, (408) 277-2646, BA 24 San Jose St Univ; MA 86 San Jose St Univ; **SLP**

Kirkpatrick, Mrs Mary Jill 109 S E 101st Avenue, Vancouver, WA 98664, (206) 256-7951, BS 72 Purdue Univ - West Lafayette; MS 73 Purdue Univ - West Lafayette; 83–Sp/Lang Path/Dir, NW Thrpy Serv, **SLP**

Kirkpatrick, Nancy Shay 110 Imperial Avenue, Bennington, VT 05201, (802) 362-4104, MS; 88–Sp-Lang Path, Bennington-Rutland Supvy Union, **SLP**

Kirkpatrick, Mrs Sandra Lee 5531 Vaden, The Colony, TX 75056, (214) 370-7635, MS 77 TX Christian Univ; 87–Sp-Lang Path, Lewisville ISD, **SLP**

Kirkpatrick, Tara L 9807 Covered Wagon, Converse, TX 78109, (512) 659-4824, BS 78 Southwest TX St Univ; ME 79 Southwest TX St Univ; Sp-Lang Path, Schertz-Cibolo-Univrsl Cty ISD, **SLP**

Kirkwood, Mrs Catherine Faust 709 Pere Marquette Bldg, New Orleans, LA 70112, BA 76 LA St Univ - Baton Rouge; OM 77 LA St Univ - N O Medical Ctr; Aud, Audiphone Hrng Inst, **A**

Kirkwood-Hodge, Alledi J 7262 Pinedale Drive, Columbia, SC 29223, (803) 452-5454, BS 74 UT St Univ; MA 75 Univ of Houston - Univ Park; 88–Sp-Lang Path, Sumter Sch Dist II, **SLP**

Kirkwood-Johnson, Mrs Karla 5604 32nd Avenue Court, Moline, IL 61265, BA 76 Augustana Coll; MA 77 Western IL Univ; 88–Sp-Lang Path, CARES of Rock Island, **SLP**

Kirley, Mrs Mary S 319 West 6th Avenue, Shakopee, MN 55379, (612) 445-6482, BS 77 Univ of WI - Stevens Point; MA 78 OH Univ - Athens; Sp/Lang Path, Sch Dist 110 Waconia, **SLP**

Kirn, June H 145 Ridge Avenue, Idaho Falls, ID 83402, (208) 525-7236, BA 46 North Central Coll; BS 48 Univ of IL - Urbana; MS 76 ID St Univ; SLP, Adlt/Chld Dev Cen, **SLP**

Kirn, Tamara Sue 2842 Whitener #B-4, Cape Girardeau, MO 63701, (314) 334-5817, BS 85 Southeast MO St Univ; MA 87 Southeast MO St Univ; **SLP**

Kirpalani, Mrs Pamela Tadlock 9801 Tamarack Lane, Escondido, CA 92025, (619) 746-7381, BS 72 Bowling Green St Univ; MA 74 Bowling Green St Univ; 80–Sp-Lang Path, Poway USD, **SLP**

Kirsch, Christine Lynn 3074 Dwight Street, San Diego, CA 92104-4260, (619) 281-1949, MA 82 San Diego St Univ; Audiologist, Sp-Hrng Neurosensory Center, **A**

Kirsch, Ida 1 Garden Street, Great Neck, NY 11021, (718) 464-7500, BA 75 CUNY - Queens Coll; MA 76 Hofstra Univ; Sp-Lang Path, Creedmoor Psychi Ctr, **SLP**

Kirsch, Jane 3109 Goose Creek Road, Louisville, KY 40222, BS 71 Purdue Univ - West Lafayette; MA 72 CA St Univ - Los Angeles; Sp/Lang Path, Jeff Co Pub Sch, **SLP**

Kirsch, Laurie Jean 2010 E Santa Clara Avenue #46, Santa Ana, CA 92701, (714) 832-9200, OB 85 Univ of MN - Duluth; MA 86 Univ of MN - Duluth; SLP, Western Neuro Care Ctr, **SLP**

Kirsch, Mrs Martha Rose 13 Webster Avenue, Exeter, NH 03833, (603) 926-8708, BA 72 Univ of NH; MA 83 SUNY - Coll at Plattsburgh; Sp-Lang Path, Sau #21 Hampton Sch District, **SLP**

Kirsch, Theresa Ann 709 Mojave Court, Sidney, OH 45365, (513) 498-4565, BS 75 Miami Univ - Oxford; MA 86 Univ of Cincinnati; SLP, Shelby Co Bd of Mental Retard, **SLP**

Kirschbaum, Mrs Laurel L 326 Lake Bay Court, Lake Oswego, OR 97034-3046, (503) 232-2458, BA 76 WA St Univ; MS 81 Portland St Univ; Sp-Lang Path, Portland Pub Schs, **SLP**

Kirschblum, Mrs Elyse K 51 Schuyler Avenue #6G, Stamford, CT 06902, (203) 327-7406, MA 87 Univ of CT; **A**

Kirschenbaum, Mrs Bonnie L 13 Soundview Lane, Sands Point, NY 11050, (516) 767-1576, MS 72 CUNY - Hunter Coll; SLP, New York City Board of Educ, **SLP**

Kirschner, Doris Ann 1413 East 54th Place, Chicago, IL 60615, (312) 241-7641, BS 57 Northwestern Univ; MA 61 Northwestern Univ; Michael Reese Hosp & Med Ctr, **SLP**

Kirschner, Mrs Ellyn Goodman 1725 Chatham Avenue, Charlotte, NC 28205, (704) 537-9238, MA 71 Western MI Univ; ME 83 Univ of NC - Charlotte; Sp/Lang Path, Char-Meck Sch Sys, **SLP**

Kirschner, Neil L 1725 Chatham Avenue, Charlotte, NC 28205, (704) 343-3625, BA 66 American Univ; MA 71 Western MI Univ; Sp-Lang Path, Charlotte-Mecklenburg Schools, **SLP**

Kirschner, Mrs Randi 140-08 Jewel Avenue, Flushing, NY 11367, (718) 793-6546, MA 87 CUNY - Queens Coll; 87–Aud, Lexington Hrng & Sp Ctr, **A**

Kirschner, Sandra A 136 Berger Parkway #A-4, Fond Du Lac, WI 54935, (414) 921-5865, BA 78 Univ of WI - Eau Claire; MS 79 Univ of WI - Stevens Point; SLP, Cambridge Comm Schools, **SLP**

Kirschner, Susan B 801 Twisted Oak, Buffalo Grove, IL 60090, BS 64 Syracuse Univ; MA 67 De Paul Univ; Sp/Lang Path, Oak Park River Forest H Sch, **SLP**

Kirsh, Isidore M 3303 Janellen Drive, Baltimore, MD 21208, (301) 484-2373, BA 83 Univ of MD - Baltimore CO; ME 87 Univ of VA - Charlottesville

Kirsh, Risa 254-03 58 Avenue, Little Neck, NY 11362, (212) 920-5445, BS 81 Boston Univ; MS 83 Univ of MI - Ann Arbor; SLP, N Shore U Hosp, **SLP**

Kirshenbaum, Rachelle P 366 Divot Road, Oceanside, NY 11572-5607, (516) 766-1364, BA 75 CUNY - Brooklyn Coll; MS 77 Columbia Univ Teachers Coll; Private Practitioner, Private Practice, **SLP**

Kirshner, Mrs Sheri Weiner 2120 Crestmoor Road, Nashville, TN 37215, (615) 297-3939, Aud, Hearing Serv of TN, **A**

Kirszbraun, Mrs Arlene F 1960 Eva Drive, Lansdale, PA 19446, (215) 539-8550, BA 66 CUNY - Brooklyn Coll; ME 67 PA St Univ - Univ Park; SLP, Mont Co Inter Ut #23, **SLP**

Kirtland, Mrs Margaret T 3416 Hyman Place, New Orleans, LA 70114, (504) 367-3120, BA 77 Univ of NC - Greensboro; OM 78 LA St Univ - N O Medical Ctr; Sp-Lang Path, Jefferson Parish Sch Syst, **SLP**

Kirton, Mrs Susan J 4205 South Grant, Englewood, CO 80110, (303) 789-3102, BS 76 CO St Univ; **SLP**

Kirts, Mrs Celine F 827 North Chestnut Street, Lansdale, PA 19446, (215) 362-2196, BS 77 West Chester Univ of PA; MA 81 West Chester Univ of PA; **SLP**

Kirven, Laura Ann P O Box 2006, Massillon, OH 44646-0006, BS Kent St Univ; MA 85 Kent St Univ; **SLP**

Kisatsky, Thomas J 315 Williamson Circle, Oakville, CT 06779, (203) 754-5141, BS 59 Bloomsburg Univ of PA; ME 66 Bloomsburg Univ of PA; Superv of Aud, Es Rehab Cen, **SLP A**

Kiselewich, Mrs Anne S 577 Rosa Linda Way, Santa Barbara, CA 93111, (805) 964-2894, BS 69 Northwestern Univ; MS 70 Univ of MI - Ann Arbor; Sp-Lang Path, Private Practice, **SLP**

Kiser, Patricia M 510 Carnation Drive, Clarks Summit, PA 18411, (717) 348-1424, BS 69 Ball St Univ; MS 71 Purdue Univ - West Lafayette; Sp-Lang Path, InSpeech Inc, **SLP**

Kish, Edward L 5254 Edenshire Avenue, Memphis, TN 38117, (901) 522-5651, BS 74 Northern IL Univ - De Kalb; MA 75 Northern IL Univ - De Kalb; Chief of Audiology, Baptist Mem Hosp, **A**

Kish, Karen L 107 Woakley Drive North, Apartment 111, Westmont, IL 60559, (312) 620-3700, BA 75 Western IL Univ; MS 76 Western IL Univ; Sp-Lang Path, Lombard School District 44, **SLP**

Kishon-Rabin, Mrs Liat 2365 Matthews Avenue, Bronx, NY 10467, (212) 642-2174, BA 85 Tel Aviv Univ - Israel; MA 87 CUNY - City College

Kishter, Mrs Helen H M 21500 Johnson Street, Box 61, Pembroke Pines, FL 33029, (305) 431-8280, BA 38 James Madison Univ; ME 57 Univ of VA - Charlottesville; **SLP LM**

Kisich, Esther S Ocean Speech & Language Serv, 5321 Appian Way, Long Beach, CA 90803, (213) 434-5941, BA 55 Univ of CA - Los Angeles; MA 80 CA St Univ - Long Beach; Sp-Lang Path, Ocean Sp & Lang Svcs, **SLP**

Kisiday, Cynthia T Audiological And Speech Asso, 736 Church Street, Indiana, PA 15759, (412) 349-5070, BS 77 Indiana Univ of PA; MS 81 Indiana Univ of PA; Dir of Serv, Sp-Lang Path, Audiological & Sp Assoc, **SLP ACE**

Kisiel, Dr Dennis L 126 Waverly Place #3-B, New York, NY 10011, (718) 780-1755, BA 73 Case Western Reserve Univ; MA 74 Cleveland St Univ; PH 79 (NS) Memphis St Univ; Dir/Aud Div, Long Island Coll Hosp, **A**

Kisler, Nancy C Robert D Craig MD Inc, 3400 S E Frank Phillips, Suite 601, Bartlesville, OK 74006, (918) 333-8910, BS 77 Univ of Tulsa; MA 79 Univ of Tulsa; Aud, Robert D Criag MD Inc, **A**

Kisner, Carol Helen 180 Beatrice Drive, West Haven, CT 06516, (203) 937-0449, MS 84 Southern IL Univ -Carbondale; 87–Aud, Med Ctr Pharmacy, **A**

Kisner, Rita P 818-B Jennifer Lane, Costa Mesa, CA 92626, (714) 751-2024, BA 76 CA St Univ - Fullerton; MA 78 CA St Univ - Fullerton; SLP, Huntington Beach Union Hs Dis, **SLP**

Kissel, Ellen Elizabeth 201 Confederate Drive, Spanish Fort, AL 36527, (205) 626-7136, BA 74 Univ of Central FL; MA 76 Univ of Central FL; Dir of SLP, Med Serv Corp, **SLP**

Kissel, Mrs Joan S 1140 South Orlando #D-14, Maitland, FL 32751, (305) 423-9293, BA 56 Univ of MI - Ann Arbor; MA 88 Univ of Central FL

Kissel, Sr Judith Ann 3450 Bucks Branch Road, Martin, KY 41649, (606) 886-9624, BS 73 IN St Univ - Evansville; MS 81 Murray St Univ; 86–Sp-Lang Path, Private Practice, **SLP**

Kissel, Robert J 18350 Hatteras Street #166, Tarzana, CA 91356, (818) 609-1931, **SLP**

Kissell-Ariel, Veronica C 20 Railroad Street, Northbridge, MA 01534, (617) 234-4556, MS 83 Worcester St Coll; BS 78 CA Univ of PA; **SLP**

Kissh, H Laura 4575 Kensington Drive #1, San Diego, CA 92116, (619) 284-1015, BS 68 Brigham Young Univ; OM 72 Brigham Young Univ; 76–Sp-Lang Path, La Mesa-Spring Valley Sch Dist, **SLP**

Kissick, Mrs Donann Hoopingarn Route 1 Box 208, Springport, IN 47386, (317) 755-3618, MA 84 Ball St Univ; SLP, South Henry School Corp, **SLP**

Kissick, Mrs Kara Miller 1821 Cheryl, Wichita, KS 67212, (316) 283-5011, BS 81 Fort Hays St Univ; MS 82 Fort Hays St Univ; 82–SLP, Harvey Co Spec Ed Coop, **SLP**

Kistenberg, Lisa B 90 Lexington Avenue, Apt 9-G, New York, NY 10016, (212) 779-9270, BA 79 CUNY - Brooklyn Coll; MS 82 CUNY - Brooklyn Coll; 79–Sp-Lang Path, NYC Bd of Ed-Comm-Spec Educ, **SLP**

Kistenbroker, Mrs Valerie Spera 1935 Smith Road, Northbrook, IL 60062-5829, (312) 480-0306, BS 77 Marquette Univ; MS 78 Marquette Univ; Supvr of Sp-Lang Path, InSpeech Inc, **SLP**

Kistler, Blaze W Covina Valley Unified, School District, 519 East Badillo Street, Covina, CA 91723, (818) 331-3371, BA 76 CA St Univ - Northridge; MA 79 CA St Univ - Los Angeles; Aud, Covina-Valley USD, **A**

Kita, Mrs Virginia E 1401 Prairie Heights, Bartlesville, OK 74006, (918) 333-5225, BS 76 Univ of Tulsa; MA 78 Univ of Tulsa; Sp/Lang Path, Tri-Quad Special Services, **SLP**

Kitagawa, Yoko c/o National Defense Medical College, Rehabilitation Section, 3-2 Namiki Tokorozawa-Shi, Saitama-Ken, Japan 359, MS 85 Univ of HI - Manoa; 88–Sp-Lang Path, National Defense Med Coll

Kitain, Mrs Sonia S 5511 Greenbriar Drive, West Bloomfield, MI 48033, (313) 661-5554, BS 72 OH St Univ; MS 73 Northeast MO St Univ; MS 79 Univ of Dayton; Sp/Lang Path, Private Practice, **SLP**

Kitaoka, Jennifer Yoshiko 219 East Ashland, Visalia, CA 93277, (209) 625-6500, MA 83 CA St Univ - Fresno; **SLP**

Kitch, Mrs Connie Joan S 6838 Shelbyville Road, Indianapolis, IN 46237, (317) 882-4288, BS 79 Ball St Univ; MA 80 Ball St Univ; Aud, Indy Otol Assoc, **A**

Kitchell, Dr Pat S 3736 El Campo Court, Concord, CA 94519, (425) 686-3398, MS 78 Univ of WA; Dir, S Bay Comm Re-Entry Ser, **SLP**

Kitchen, Dr Dale Western 311 Parson Street, Alpena, MI 49707, (517) 356-4834, BA 63 MI St Univ; MA 65 MI St Univ; PH 68 (NS) MI St Univ; Sp-Lang Path, Iosco ISD, **SLP A**

Kitchen, Mrs Linda L R 6556 South Graham Road, St Charles, MI 48655, (517) 776-0289, BS 70 Bowling Green St Univ; MA 71 Bowling Green St Univ; Sp-Lang Path, Saginaw Bd of Ed, **SLP**

Kitchen, Mrs Mary C 7519 Wilderness Way, Fairfax Station, VA 22039, BS 69 Auburn Univ - Auburn; MA 74 Univ of AL- Tuscaloosa; 88–Sp-Lang Path, Fairfax County PS

Kitchings, Mrs Anne H 17415 Thunder Road, Jupiter, FL 33478-5301, (407) 694-7359, OB 62 Univ of FL; ME 63 Univ of FL; 66–Sp-Lang Path, Palm Beach Co Sch Bd, **SLP**

Kitchings, Donald A 17415 Thunder Road, Jupiter, FL 33478-5301, (407) 744-7979, OB 62 Univ of FL; ME 63 Univ of FL; 66–Sp-Lang Path, Palm Beach Co School Board, **SLP**

Kite, LeAnn 710 Rilla Drive, Garland, TX 75041, (214) 494-8581, BS 78 Baylor Univ; MS 79 Baylor Univ; 79–Sp-Lang Path, Garlnad ISD, **SLP**

Kite, Robert H P O Box 3626, Boone, NC 28607, (704) 295-4521, BA 85 Univ of SC - Columbia; MA 88 Univ of SC - Columbia; 88–Coord, Alta Petens Inc

Kitley, Mrs Deborah Sweeney 211-5 Echelon Road, Voorhees, NJ 08043, (609) 767-2600, BA 81 Univ of Scranton; MA 84 Temple Univ; 86–Sp-Lang Path, Children's Seashore House, **SLP ACE**

Kitselman, Dr Kurt Dept Of Speech Communications, California State Univ, 800 N State College Blvd, Fullerton, CA 92634, (714) 773-3617, BS 72 Univ of CA - Irvine; MA 74 CA St Univ - Fullerton; PH 78 (NS) Univ of CA - Santa Barbara; Assoc Prof, CA St U-Dept of Sp Commun, **SLP**

Kitson, Mrs Laura G J 1539 Woody Hills Drive, El Cajon, CA 92020, (619) 579-0684, BA 70 Univ of the Pacific; MA 71 San Diego St Univ; Resource Specialist, Cajon Valley Sch Dist, **SLP**

Kitson, Nancy Carolan 4501 Glen Street, La Mesa, CA 92041, (619) 421-1611, BA 74 San Diego St Univ; MA 77 San Diego St Univ; SLP, Chula Vista Cty Sch, **SLP**

Kittay, Mrs Judith L 209 Kuyper Drive, Upper Nyack, NY 10960, (914) 358-4979, BA 66 CUNY - City College; MS 68 Adelphi Univ; **SLP**

Kittredge, Deborah Luff 52018 Helena Beach Drive, Three Rivers, MI 49093, (616) 496-4795, BS 78 Western MI Univ; MS 86 Western MI Univ; 87–Sp-Lang Path, Portage PS, **SLP**

Kittson, Susan A 622 Brooks Place, Wausau, WI 54401, (715) 257-7571, BA 78 Univ of WI - Eau Claire; MS 79 Univ of WI - Eau Claire; Sp-Lang Path, Marathon Co Spec Ed, **SLP**

Kitz, Janice H 100 Cold Spring Road, Barrington, IL 60010, (312) 381-2841, BA 70 Univ of IL - Chicago; MA 72 Northern IL Univ - De Kalb; **A**

Kitz, Margaret D 804 John Glen Boulevard, Webster, NY 14580, (716) 473-1533, BS 66 SUNY - Coll at Geneseo; MS 71 SUNY - Coll at Geneseo; SLP, City Sch Dist - Rochester, **SLP**

Kitzman, George H 3308-B East Grant Road, Tucson, AZ 85716, (602) 326-4425, BS 59 Univ of WI - Oshkosh; MA 65 Univ of Northern CO; Owner-Mgr/Aud, Aamsco Hearing Aid Center, **A**

Kiyan, Beverly Ng 1311 Drakeridge Crest, Redlands, CA 92373, BA 75 San Francisco St Univ; MA 77 CA St Univ - Los Angeles; **A**

Kiyota, Linda K 1470 South Quebec Way #196, Denver, CO 80231, (303) 351-2012, BA 80 Univ of Northern CO; MA 81 Univ of Northern CO; Aud, Univ of Northern Colorado, **A**

Kizer, Mrs Julia Bante 1726-B East Florida, Urbana, IL 61801, (217) 892-2131, BS 83 Northeast MO St Univ; MA 84 Northeast MO St Univ; Sp-Lang Path, Rantoul City Schs, **SLP**

Kizewski-Hill, Cynthia Maria 8412 Louwanda, Little Rock, AR 72205-1629, (501) 223-3722, BS 76 Univ of WI - Oshkosh; MA 77 Univ of TN - Knoxville; Aud, **A**

Kjellson, Mrs Sylvia Yeaton 70 Riverview Drive, Fishkill, NY 12524, (914) 285-8187, BS 83 Univ of NH; MA 85 Univ of CT; Audiologist, Westchester Co Med Ctr, **A**

Klacan, Ann Marie 812 Whittier Placet N W, Washington, DC 20012, (202) 291-1711, BS 85 Univ of WI - Stevens Point; MS 87 Gallaudet Coll; **A**

Kladde, Annette G 5944 North 108th Court, Omaha, NE 68164, (402) 493-3230, BA 59 Univ of IA; MA 63 Univ of IA; Sp-Lang Path, Omaha Pub Schls, **SLP**

Klafter, Carmem E 5100 North Marine Drive, Chicago, IL 60640, (312) 769-3439, BA 54 Univ of MI - Ann Arbor; MA 68 De Paul Univ; Sp-Lang Path Consult, Private Practice, **SLP**

Klages, Mrs Catherine 28 Ball Pond Road East, New Fairfield, CT 06812, BA 74 Southern CT St Univ; MS 76 Univ of WI - Stevens Point; Private Practice, **SLP**

Klahr, Lynn R 659 Reads Lane, Far Rockaway, NY 11691, (718) 851-3700, MA 86 CUNY - Hunter Coll; 88–Sp-Lang Path, Metro Jewish Geriatric Ctr, **SLP**

Klaiman, Mrs Paula Gayle 1111 Beacon Street, Brookline, MA 02146, (617) 232-1213, BS 83 Univ of Western Ontario; MS 85 Univ of Western Ontario; **SLP**

Klamut, Mrs Kathryn L 6046 Hawthorne Drive, Sylvania, OH 43560-5010, (419) 882-0509, BS 79 Miami Univ - Oxford; BA 79 Miami Univ - Oxford; MS 80 Miami Univ - Oxford; Sp-Lang Path, Med Coll of OH Hosp, **SLP**

Klane, Bonnie E 66 Crawford Road, Middletown, NJ 07748, (201) 671-3742, BA 70 Rutgers St Univ - Newark; MA 73 Newark St Coll; 88–Sp-Lang Path, Union Beach-Bd of Educ, **SLP**

Klapholz, Renee 68-36 108th Street #B-54, Flushing, NY 11375, (718) 793-3566, BA 83 CUNY - Brooklyn Coll; MS 85 CUNY - Brooklyn Coll; 88–Sp-Lang Path, New York Childhood Ctr, **SLP**

Klapman, Mrs Phyllis L 2045 Gulf Of Mexico Drive, Apartment 416, Longboat Key, FL 34228, (813) 383-6346, BA 64 Northwestern Univ; MA 68 Northeastern IL Univ; **SLP**

Klapper, Mrs Deborah 15 Oak Spring Road, West Nyack, NY 10994, (914) 358-9667, BA 61 Adelphi Univ; MS 64 Adelphi Univ; 79–Sp-Lang Path, Tuckahoe Sch Dist, **SLP**

Klaras, Mrs Denise Demaret 3625 Fort, Waco, TX 76710, (817) 752-8839, MS 81 Baylor Univ; Aud, Private Practice, **A**

Klas, Lisa Marie 82 Leaside Drive, West Seneca, NY 14224, (716) 674-0818, BS 85 SUNY - Coll at Buffalo; MS 86 SUNY - Coll at Buffalo; **SLP**

Klash, Donna Marie 214 Barthel Avenue, Gardner, MA 01440, (508) 630-1180, BS 77 Worcester St Coll; MS 82 Worcester St Coll; Sp-Lang Path, Gardner Sch Dept, **SLP**

Klasner, Estelle R 65 Ellerslie Avenue #359, Willowdale, ON, Canada M2N 1Y1, (416) 762-7316, BS 80 Southern IL Univ -Carbondale; MA 84 CUNY - Hunter Coll; Sp-Lang Path, Runnymede Hosp, **SLP**

Klatsky, Mrs Iris Ann 45 Kerry Lane, Chappaqua, NY 10514, (212) 605-3740, BA 70 Case Western Reserve Univ; MA 71 George Washington Univ; 85–Asst Dir Commun Dis, Manhattan Eye Ear Throat Hosp, **SLP**

Klatt, Carolyn A 826 Winford Avenue, Green Bay, WI 54303, (414) 497-6041, BA 70 Univ of WI - Eau Claire; MS 77 Univ of WI - Eau Claire; 70–Sp-Lang Path, Green Bay Area Pub Sch, **SLP**

Klatt, Mrs Sallyanne Eichler 262 Aristocrat, Billings, MT 59105, (406) 255-3624, BA 83 MT St Univ; MS 85 Univ of WY; 85–Sp-Lang Path, Billings Sch Dist #2, **SLP**

Klauk, Susan W 707 Avenue Chaumont, Delray Beach, FL 33445, (407) 498-0406, BA 75 Univ of FL; ME 76 Univ of FL; 80–Sp-Lang Path, Bethesda Mem Hosp, **SLP**

Klaus, S Elizabeth 532 Howell Lane #A, Indianapolis, IN 46224, (317) 241-7035, BS 74 Northern IL Univ - De Kalb; MA 76 Northern IL Univ - De Kalb; Coordinator of Audiology Serv, Communicology Inc, **A**

Klaver, Mary Melissa 5415 North Sheridan #2910, Chicago, IL 60640, (312) 263-7171, BA 74 MI St Univ; MA 85 Northwestern Univ; 86–Aud, Hearing Health Center Inc, **A**

Klawinski, Donna Marie 9609 Grayce Drive, Sturtevant, WI 53177, (414) 442-9000, BS 82 Univ of WI - Whitewater; MS 84 Univ of WI - Stevens Point; **A**

Klawiter, Mrs Pamela Sue 1081 New Haven Road, Unit 12-B, Naugatuck, CT 06770, (203) 723-1203, MA 82 MI St Univ; Sp-Lang Path, Southbury Training School, **SLP**

Kleber, Patricia E 8405 Ridgemont Drive, Urbandale, IA 50322, (515) 672-2546, BS 85 IA St Univ; MA 88 Northeast MO St Univ; 88–Sp-Lang Path, Southern Prairie AEA #15

Klebes, Martha S 1175 Meadowbrook Road, Southampton, PA 18966, **SLP**

Klecak, Lucinda B 491 Massapoag Avenue, Sharon, MA 02067, (617) 848-5353, BS 77 SUNY - Coll at Geneseo; MS 80 Boston Univ; 80–SLP, Braintree Hospital, **SLP**

Klecan-Aker, Joan S Dept Communication Disorders, University Of Houston, Central Campus, Houston, TX 77004, (904) 644-2238, BS 68 Middle TN St Univ; MA 71 Memphis St Univ; PH 81 (NS) FL St Univ; **SLP**

Kleckner, Ann Marie 216 North Franklin Street, Stoughton, WI 53589, (608) 263-7334, BS 74 Univ of WI - Milwaukee; MS 84 Univ of WI - Madison; Sp-Lang Path, University of WI-Madison, **SLP**

Kleckner, Glen T 3625 Congress Street, Allentown, PA 18104, (215) 395-7895, BS 74 Brescia Coll; ME 76 Bloomsburg Univ of PA; Aud, Allen Aud/Hrng Instruments, **A**

Kleczewska, Maria K 36214 Salisbury, Newark, CA 94560, (415) 493-5000, BS 79 Univ of WI - Milwaukee; MS 81 Univ of WI - Madison; SLP, Palo Alto VA, **SLP**

Klee, Margaret A 500 Stuart Circle, Norfolk, VA 23502, BS 72 Univ of MO - Columbia; MS 73 Univ of WY; 88–Comm Ofcr, US Govt, **SLP**

Klee, Dr Thomas M Vanderbilt University, School Of Medicine, Nashville, TN 37232-8700, (615) 320-5353, BS 75 IN Univ - Bloomington; MA 76 IN Univ - Bloomington; PH 81 (NS) Univ of WI - Madison; Asst Prof, Vanderbilt U Sch of Med

Kleehammer, Kimberly Smith 1606 Melody Lane, Chattanooga, TN 37412, (615) 629-1451, BS 84 IN St Univ - Terre Haute; MA 86 IN Univ - Bloomington; 88–Sp-Lang Path, Orange Grove Center, **SLP**

Kleffner, Frank R Director, Institute Of Logopedics, 2400 Jardine Drive, Wichita, KS 67219, (316) 262-8271, BS 49 Univ of WI - Madison; MS 51 Univ of WI - Madison; PH 52 (Sp Path) Univ of WI - Madison; Pres, I of Logopedics, **SLP F H**

Klegon, Ilene Z 30952 Perry Crossing, Farmington Hills, MI 48331, (313) 661-2672, MS 73 Univ of WI - Madison; BA 71 MI St Univ; **SLP**

Kleid, Terry Lynne 2404 Bush Street, San Francisco, CA 94115, (415) 922-1714, BA 72 Antioch Coll; OM 84 San Jose St Univ; Tchr, San Francisco USD, **SLP**

Kleidon, Mrs Brenda K 11380 South Horseshoe Dr, Three Rivers, MI 49093, (616) 244-8525, BA 76 Valparaiso Univ; MA 77 Our Lady Lake Univ-San Anton; Sp-Lang Path, Three Rivers Community School, **SLP**

Kleifges, Mrs Elena Munero 2430 Edgeview Lane, Midlothian, VA 23113, (804) 230-0297, BS 84 James Madison Univ; MA 86 Univ of MD - College Park; 88–Aud/Mgr, AARP, **A**

Kleiman, Mrs Kay Seaton 1136 Chickasawba, Blytheville, AR 72315, (501) 762-1036, BS 85 Southwest MO St Univ; MS 87 Central MO St Univ; 88–Sp-Lang Path, Osceola PS Dist #1

Kleiman, Larry I 11231 Weatherby Road, Los Alamitos, CA 90720, (714) 638-0801, MA 80 CA St Univ - Northridge; Sp-Lang Path, Private Practice, **SLP**

Klein, Dr Alan J Dept Of Oto & Comm Sciences, Medical Univ Of S Carolina, Charleston, SC 29425, (803) 792-3004, OB 72 Univ of NM; MA 76 Univ of FL; PH 79 (NS) Univ of FL; 84–Asst Prof, Med Univ of S Carolina, **A**

Klein, Barbara Greenstein P O Box 127, Cross River, NY 10518, BA 73 Montclair St Coll; MA 79 Trenton St Coll; **SLP**

Klein, Mrs Barbara Jones 5640 Baines Holding, Milford, OH 45150, (513) 221-4243, BS 83 Univ of Cincinnati; MA 87 Univ of Cincinnati; 88–Sp-Lang Path, Butler Co Bd of MR/DD

Klein, Mrs Camille S 9459 Shouse Drive, Vienna, VA 22180, (202) 745-5600, BA 67 George Washington Univ; MA 70 George Washington Univ; **A**

Klein, Carla L 17110 N E 11th Court, North Miami Beach, FL 33162, (305) 549-6397, MA 69 Case Western Reserve Univ; Sp/Lang Path, Jackson Mem Hosp, **SLP**

Klein, Mrs Carol A Rd 4 Box 156-A, Milford, NJ 08848, (201) 788-6424, BA 71 Adelphi Univ; MA 72 Seton Hall Univ; Dir Sp & Hrng, Hunterdon Med Cen, **SLP ACE**

Klein, Mrs Carolyn G 8659A South Market Place, Oak Creek, WI 53154, (414) 694-8300, BS 82 Univ of WI - Milwaukee; MS 84 Univ of WI - Milwaukee; Sp-Lang Path, InSpeech Inc, **SLP**

Klein, Cynthia F 6785 Andiron Court, West Bloomfield, MI 48322, (313) 649-6505, BA 75 Univ of MI - Ann Arbor; MA 76 Eastern MI Univ; 88–Sp-Lang Path, Rehab Placement Associates, **SLP**

Klein, Dale Ginny 55C Friars Gate, Clifton Park, NY 12065, BS 77 SUNY - Coll at Geneseo; MA 81 CA St Univ - Long Beach; **SLP**

Klein, Mrs Deanna Lynne 172 North Washington, Apartment 3, Ypsilanti, MI 48197, (313) 487-1887, BS 86 Eastern MI Univ; MA 87 Eastern MI Univ; 87–Sp-Lang Path, Oakwood Hosp, **SLP**

Klein, Edward D 25 Cobb Avenue, White Plains, NY 10606, (914) 668-6580, BS 57 NY Univ; MA 59 NY Univ; 57–Sp-Lang Path, Mt Vernon Bd of Ed, **SLP**

Klein, Dr Edward S 6532 Bright Avenue, Whittier, CA 90601, (213) 693-0771, BA 73 George Washington Univ; MA 75 George Washington Univ; PH 81 (Special Education) PA St Univ - Univ Park; Chrmn, Whittier Coll, **SLP**

Klein, Mrs Ellen R 2147 Oakawana Road, Atlanta, GA 30345, (404) 524-5614, BA 75 SUNY - Coll at New Paltz; MA 77 NY Univ; Sp-Lang Path, Private Practice, **SLP**

Klein, Ellen S 134 7th Street #9, Seal Beach, CA 90740, BS 84 Univ of MA - Amherst; MS 86 Emerson Coll; SLP, **SLP**

Klein, Dr Estelle E 16040 East Loyola Drive, Aurora, CO 80013, (303) 693-7658, BA 70 CUNY - Brooklyn Coll; MS 72 CUNY - Brooklyn Coll; PH 77 (NS) CUNY - Grad Sch & Univ Cntr; Sp-Lang Path, Aurora Pub Sch, **SLP**

Klein, Mrs Estelle R 225 Albemarle Road, White Plains, NY 10605, BA 43 CUNY - Queens Coll; MA 44 Columbia Univ Teachers Coll; SLP, Pub Sch of the Tarrytowns, **SLP**

Klein, Dr Harriet B 110 Bleecker Street #11B, New York, NY 10012-2103, (212) 998-5267, BA 58 CUNY - Brooklyn Coll; MA 60 CUNY - Brooklyn Coll; PH 78 (NS) Columbia Univ Teachers Coll; Assoc Prof, NYU, **SLP**

Klein, Helen P G 910 Riverside Drive East, Bradenton, FL 33508, **SLP A**

Klein, Mrs Jill W 24 Carriage Road, Great Neck, NY 11024, BS 76 NY Univ; MA 77 NY Univ; **SLP**

Klein, Mrs Judy B 65 Prescott Place, Freehold Township, NJ 07728, (201) 780-9559, BS 68 SUNY - Coll at Geneseo; MA 69 CUNY - City College; Sp-Lang Path, MCOSS Nursing Svcs Inc, **SLP**

Klein, Leah Abigail 23598 Civic Center Drive, Apartment 235, Southfield, MI 48034, (313) 357-2032, BA 79 Univ of MI - Ann Arbor; MS 84 Univ of VT; Aud, Harper Hospital, **A**

Klein, Lorraine E Medical Col VA Commonwealth Univ, Ambulatory Care Center, Box 150 McV Station, Richmond, VA 23298, (804) 786-0431, BS 76 Univ of VA - Charlottesville; MA 77 Univ of TN - Knoxville; Aud/Super, Med Coll of VA Hosp, **A**

Klein, Dr M Diane 6633 Wheeler, La Verne, CA 91750, (714) 593-9325, BA 67 Central MI Univ; MA 69 Western MI Univ; PH 80 (Developmental Psychology) MI St Univ; Associate Professor, Cal St University Los Angeles, **SLP**

Klein, Marc I 1727 Crystal Lane, Mount Prospect, IL 60056, (312) 896-2181, BS 69 IL St Univ - Normal; MS 77 IL St Univ - Normal; Aud, Sound Resources, **A**

Klein, Marie 39 Irving Street Apartment 2, Boston, MA 02114, (617) 723-5283, BA 83 SUNY - Coll at Cortland; MA 86 Hofstra Univ; Sp-Lang Path, Cambridge PS, **SLP**

Klein, Marilyn 7000 Boulevard East, Guttenberg, NJ 07093, BA 66 Caldwell Coll; MA 68 Columbia Univ Teachers Coll; Director/Dept Commun Disorders, Mental Retardation Ins Uafucmc, **SLP**

Klein, Mrs Mary Ann 1020 Polk Street, Franklin Square, NY 11010, (516) 997-9700, BS 83 Long Island U - CW Post Ctr; MS 85 Adelphi Univ; **SLP**

Klein, Michelle Gloria 100 Bennett Avenue, New York, NY 10033, **SLP**

Klein, Patricia K 2394-I Pleasant Way, Thousand Oaks, CA 91362, (805) 497-9511, BA 63 Univ of AZ; MA 64 Univ of AZ; 82–Sp-Lang Path, Conejo Valley USD, **SLP**

Klein, Mrs Patricia L 2659 Parkview Boulevard, Robbinsdale, MN 55422, (612) 574-6570, BS 83 Mankato St Univ; MA 85 Univ of MN - Duluth; SLP, ISD 13, **SLP**

Klein, Patty A 449 Orange Grove Avenue, San Fernando, CA 91340, (818) 365-1544, BA 78 CA St Univ - Northridge; MA 79 CA St Univ - Los Angeles; Aud, ENT Head & Neck Associates, **A**

Klein, Phyllis 657 East 80th Street, Brooklyn, NY 11236, (718) 763-4245, BA 74 CUNY - Brooklyn Coll; MS 75 Columbia Univ Teachers Coll; Sp-Lang Path & Audiologist, Private Practice, **SLP A**

Klein, Selma Alperen El Camion Medical Center, 8100 Constitution Place NE, Suite 1100, Albuquerque, NM 87110, (505) 294-9556, Private Practice, **SLP**

Klein, Shelia 65 Minna Street, Brooklyn, NY 11218, **A**

Klein, Susan Shadyside Hospital-East Wing, 510 South Aiken Avenue Suite 210, Pittsburgh, PA 15232, (412) 621-0123, BA 78 Univ of Pittsburgh - Pittsburgh; MA 80 Univ of Pittsburgh - Pittsburgh; 81–Aud, Facial Paralysis Testing Lab, **A**

Kleinert, Jane E O'Regan 637 Severn Way, Lexington, KY 40503, (606) 276-1352, BA 72 Bellarmine Coll; OM 75 Univ of WA; Sp-Lang Path, Horn Richardson & Assoc, **SLP**

Kleinert, Sheila B 854 Cross Hill, Danville, KY 40422, (606) 238-7386, BS 74 Bellarmine Coll; MA 80 Univ of KY; Sp-Lang Path, Burgin Indep Schs, **SLP**

Kleingartner, Michelle Stock 1726 3rd Avenue N E, Jamestown, ND 58401, (701) 252-4100, Supervisor of Audiology, Speech & Hearing Services Inc, **A**

Klein-Hall, Karen J 57 Florida Avenue, Commack, NY 11725, (516) 543-2031, MS 73 PA St Univ - Univ Park; Sp-Lang Path, Private Practice, **SLP**

Klein-Koonin, Mrs June E 13 Fabish Drive, Buffalo Grove, IL 60089, (312) 459-7029, BS 76 Univ of IL - Urbana; MA 78 Northwestern Univ; Sp-Lang Path, St Joseph Hosp, **SLP**

Kleinline, Lisa Jane 6233 Harrisbrg-Georgesvile, Grove City, OH 43123, (614) 461-2420, BA 81 OH St Univ; MA 83 OH St Univ; Aud, Columbus Childrens Hosp, **A**

Kleinman, Mrs Frances R 2839 Arthur Lane, Wantagh, NY 11793, (516) 679-8584, BA 75 SUNY - Center at Buffalo; MA 77 NY Univ; Sp-Lang Path, NY Cty Bd of Ed, **SLP**

Kleinman, Madeline Karter 34 Forest Park Avenue, Larchmont, NY 10538, (914) 738-4610, BS 65 Univ of Cincinnati; MA 70 NY Univ; 84–Sp-Lang Path, Pelham Bd of Educ, **SLP**

Kleinman, Marvin A 11 Broad Street, Elizabeth, NJ 07201, (201) 353-8866, BA 72 CUNY - Brooklyn Coll; MS 74 CUNY - Brooklyn Coll; Aud-Owner, Prof Hrng Serv, **A**

Kleinman, Sandra Nan 95 Prescott Street #32, Cambridge, MA 02138, (617) 576-2256, BA 71 SUNY - Center at Albany; ME 72 Northeastern Univ; ME 78 Harvard Univ; 78–Sp-Lang Path, The Children's Hosp, **SLP**

Kleinmeyer, Mrs Kathleen Joanne 3601 South Bend Road, New Milford, IL 61109, (815) 874-9063, BS 79 Univ of IA; MS 81 Bradley Univ; **SLP**

Kleinschmidt, Mary Jo 1467 South 13th East, Salt Lake City, UT 84105, BA 54 Univ of IA; MS 72 Univ of UT; Sp-Lang Path, Salt Lake Head Start, **SLP**

Kleinworth, Roxie Cummings 14910 Aldine-Westfield Rd, Houston, TX 77039, (713) 449-1011, BA 61 Baylor Univ; MA 73 Univ of Houston - Univ Park; **SLP**

Klemens, James A 2217 Woodbine Drive, Decatur, IL 62526, (217) 877-0730, BS 72 SUNY - Coll at Geneseo; MA 73 Univ of IL - Urbana, Aud, Dr Griffith/Pettit/Chadwick, **A**

Klemens, Mrs Miriam P 2217 Woodbine Drive, Decatur, IL 62526, (217) 424-3073, BS 67 SUNY - Coll at Geneseo; MS 70 SUNY - Coll at Geneseo; Sp-Lang Path, Macon/Platt Spec Ed Dist, **SLP**

Klemin, Mrs Lisa Maria 3726 East 14th Street, Long Beach, CA 90804-2904, (213) 868-6603, BA 81 CA St Univ - Long Beach; MA 84 CA St Univ - Fullerton; **SLP**

Klemka, Lisa Michelle 550 Pearl Street #305, Reading, PA 19602, (215) 374-1026, BS 84 Bloomsburg Univ of PA; MS 86 Hahnemann Univ Grad Sch; 86–Sp-Lang Path/Aud, Reading Rehab Hosp, **SLP A**

Kleppe, Kamela Joy Department Speech-Language Pathology, Mercy Health Center, Mercy Drive, Dubuque, IA 52001, (319) 589-9026, BS 85 Univ of IA; MS 87 Univ of AZ; 87–Sp-Lang Path, Mercy Health Ctr, **SLP**

Klescewski, Sue 342 Cheviot Chase #24, Waukesha, WI 53186, (414) 548-0734, BA 72 Univ of WI - Eau Claire; MS 73 Univ of WI - Stevens Point; Sp-Lang Path, Waukesha School District, **SLP**

Klevans, Dr Deborah R 103 West Marylyn Avenue, State College, PA 16801, (814) 865-7679, BA 60 Univ of MI - Ann Arbor; MA 65 Univ of Southern CA; PH 75 (Human Development & Family Studies) PA St Univ - Univ Park; 86–Research Proj Assoc, Penn St Univ, **SLP ACE**

Klibert, Mrs Elizabeth W 4713 Janice Avenue, Kenner, LA 70065, (504) 455-0918, BA 77 LA St Univ - Baton Rouge; OM 81 Tulane Univ; **SLP**

Klich, Dr Richard John Sch Of Speech Path & Audiology, Kent State University, Kent, OH 44240, (216) 672-2672, BS 66 Univ of IL - Urbana; MA 67 Univ of IL - Urbana; PH 73 (NS) Univ of IA; Assoc Prof, Kent St U

Klick, Mrs Pamela 9609 South Mayfield, Oak Lawn, IL 60453, (312) 425-7036, BS 71 Loyola Univ of Chicago; MA 74 Northwestern Univ; Sp-Lang Path, Aero Special Education Dist, **SLP**

Klick, Susan Lee 106 Cherry Street, Statesboro, GA 30458, (912) 764-5810, Speech Language Pathologist, Screven County School District, **SLP**

Klien, Karen Ann Box 400 Rd #3, Clarks Summit, PA 18411, (607) 847-6554, BS 83 Marywood Coll; MA 85 OH Univ - Athens; **SLP**

Klien, Mrs Mary Hewson Route 1 Box 972, 592 Congers Lane, Mc Gaheysville, VA 22840, (602) 239-4755, **SLP**

Kligerman, Dr Anne Barbara 64 Rutgers Street, Closter, NJ 07624, (201) 767-3625, BS 61 Syracuse Univ; MS 62 Syracuse Univ; ED 78 (Aud) Columbia Univ Teachers Coll; 87–Consult, Private Practice, **A**

Kligman, Mrs Audrey 20165 North Greenway, Southfield, MI 48076, (313) 355-1506, BA 60 Univ of MI - Ann Arbor; MS 65 Univ of MI - Ann Arbor; Sp-Lang Path, Lamphere Schools, **SLP**

Kligman, Mrs Roberta A 810 Cortijo, El Paso, TX 79912-2502, (915) 581-8858, BA 74 Univ of OK - Norman; MA 77 Univ of TX - El Paso; **SLP**

Klim, Dr Charles J 52 Fairmont Street, Malden, MA 02148, (617) 536-7255, BA 50 Emerson Coll; MA 53 Emerson Coll; PH 59 (Sp & Hrng Disorders) Univ of Pittsburgh - Pittsburgh; Chmn Commun Dis, Emerson Coll, **SLP**

Klim, Mrs Helen S 52 Fairmont Street, Malden, MA 02148, (617) 893-8050, BA 51 Emerson Coll; MA 54 Syracuse Univ; Sp/Lang Path, Waltham Pub Schs, **SLP**

Klimcheck, Mary Ann 5358 Overland Trail, Pittsburgh, PA 15236, (412) 653-7335, BA 86 Univ of Pittsburgh - Pittsburgh; MA 87 Univ of Pittsburgh - Pittsburgh

Klimovitch, Mrs Michele O 162 Harvest Lane, Lincoln Park, NJ 07035, (201) 299-0166, BA 76 Montclair St Coll; MS 77 Loyola Coll; Sp/Lang Path, Lake Drive Sch/Hrng Imp Chldn, **SLP**

Klimowicz, Mrs Donna Hug 405 Arbour Drive, Newark, DE 19713, (301) 885-5003, BS 75 WV Univ; MS 80 Towson St Univ; Sp-Lang Path, Cecil Co Pub Schs, **SLP**

Klinar, Charles A Texas Childrens Hospital, 6621 Fannin #O-174, Dept Of Otolaryngology, Houston, TX 77030, (713) 791-4440, MA 85 Univ of TX - Austin; TX Childrens Hosp, **A**

Kline, Catherine 4720 Circle Lazy J Road, Riverside, CA 92501, (714) 684-0818, BA 67 CA St Univ - Fullerton; MA 72 CA St Univ - Fullerton; 73–SLP, Moreno Valley USD, **SLP**

Kline, Mrs Cindi M 109 Westgate Drive, Edison, NJ 08820-1161, (201) 757-3811, BA 78 Rutger's St Univ - Douglas Coll; MS 79 PA St Univ - Univ Park; Sp-Lang Path, Private Practice, **SLP**

Kline, Constance Church 11215 North Street, Port Richey, FL 34668, (813) 868-6508, BS 80 Univ of North TX; MA 83 Univ of Northern IA; Sp-Lang Path, Comm Disorders Clinic, **SLP**

Kline, Mrs Jamie Kay 1702 Bright Well Court, Waldorf, MD 20601, (301) 373-8100, BS 79 Indiana Univ of PA; MS 81 Bradley Univ; Prog Coord/SLP, St Marys Co Dev Cen, **SLP**

Kline, Joann I 890 McClure Road, Aurora, IL 60504, **SLP**

Kline, Karen K 1325 Whippoorwill Trail, Stow, OH 44224, (216) 678-3106, BA 79 OH St Univ; MA 82 Kent St Univ; Aud, Dr A A Kuri, **A**

Kline, Kathy Kay 1610 North Broom Street, Wilmington, DE 19806, (302) 651-6052, **SLP**

Kline, Lorrie L S 156 Valleyview Drive, Pocatello, ID 83204, (208) 232-0735, BS 77 ID St Univ; MS 78 ID St Univ; **SLP**

Kline, Marcia S Usis, Suva Dos, Washington, DC 20521-4290, **SLP**

Kline, Margaret L 834 Chestnut Street #1526, Philadelphia, PA 19107, (215) 448-7698, BS 74 Indiana Univ of PA; MA 79 Temple Univ-Tyler Sch of Art; 87–Sp-Lang Path, Hahnemann Univ, **SLP**

Kline, Margaret S 1339 Wauchope Drive, Elgin, IL 60123, (312) 888-1339, BA 66 Elmhurst Coll; MA 71 Northern IL Univ - De Kalb; Sp-Lang Path, Sp-Lang Assoc Inc, **SLP**

Kline, Mary Barbara Nmsu, Speech And Hearing Clinic, Violette Hall #146, Kirksville, MO 63501, (816) 785-4345, BS 69 Marquette Univ; MA 73 Northeast MO St Univ; Superv, Northeast Mo St U, **SLP**

Kline, Nancy Lee 4002 Adrienne Drive, Alexandria, VA 22309, (703) 664-7190, MS 84 Bloomsburg Univ of PA; SLP, Mt Vernon Hosp, **SLP ACE**

Kline, Paula Jo 3584 Lieb Street, Columbus, OH 43214, (614) 387-1035, BA 84 OH St Univ; MA 86 OH St Univ; **SLP**

Kling, Irene Frances 140 Riverside Drive #2-A, New York, NY 10024, (212) 340-6027, BS 63 NY Univ; MA 88 NY Univ; 88–Sp-Lang Path, Rusk Inst of Rehab Med

Kling, Mrs Sandra Tiffany 1304 Edinburgh Drive, Friendswood, TX 77546, (713) 481-4262, BS 81 Univ of Houston - Univ Park; MA 83 Univ of Houston - Univ Park; Sp/Lang Path, Clear Creek ISD, **SLP**

Klinge, Donald J 71 Columbia Avenue, Vineland, NJ 08360, MS

Klingelhoefer, Paula H 9 Fawn Place, Smithtown, NY 11787, (516) 549-4900, BS 78 SUNY - Coll at New Paltz; MA 80 CUNY - Queens Coll; 85–Educ Planner, Suffolk BOCES III, **SLP**

Klingensmith, Judith Kay 405 Penn Circle, Apt A, Allentown, PA 18102, (215) 776-0586, BS 82 PA St Univ - Univ Park; MS 84 Boston Univ; Sp-Lang Path, **SLP**

Klingensmith, Ruth E 163 West Kenworth Road, Columbus, OH 43214, (216) 267-4900, BS 74 Kent St Univ; MA 76 OH Univ - Athens; **SLP**

Klinger, Mrs Deborah S P O Box 5324, San Mateo, CA 94402, (415) 784-2820, BA 78 CA St Univ - Los Angeles; MA 82 CA St Univ - Los Angeles; Sp-Lang Path, Hayward USD, **SLP**

Klinger, Dr Herbert N 90-60 Union Turnpike, Flushing, NY 11385, (212) 690-5377, BS 49 CUNY - Brooklyn Coll; MS 54 PA St Univ - Univ Park; PH 59 (Sp Path) NY Univ; 68–Assoc Prof Speech, City Clg of NY, **SLP F**

Klinger, Mrs Susan Ames P O Box 631, Cardiff By Sea, CA 92007, (619) 436-1857, **SLP**

Klingler, Laura Rae 8869 Thomas Lea Terrace, Gaithersburg, MD 20879, (301) 869-6749, 1983; MA 83 Univ of MD - College Park; Aud, Treatment & Learning Centers, **A**

Klingler, Mrs Mona L 1757 16th Street, Cuyahoga Falls, OH 44221, (216) 253-1161, BA 79 Univ of Akron; MA 81 Univ of Akron; Assistant Professor, University of Akron, **A ACE**

Klingman, Kathy C 15119 Naturewalk Drive, Tampa, FL 33624, (813) 963-3599, BA 78 SUNY - Coll at Plattsburgh; MA 81 Univ of TX - Austin; 88–Sp-Lang Path, Private Practice, **SLP**

Klingman-Palk, Paula C 2506 Nancy Lane, Atlanta, GA 30345, (404) 634-3862, OB 74 Univ of GA; ME 75 Univ of GA; 87–Mgr/Owner, Metro Rehab Svcs, **SLP**

Klink, Dr Marcia L 768 Goffle Road, Hawthorne, NJ 07506, (201) 427-3542, BA 70 Montclair St Coll; MA 71 CUNY - City College; PH 83 (NS) CUNY - Grad Sch & Univ Cntr; Sp-Lang Path, Fair Lawn Bd of Ed, **SLP**

Klinkert, Mrs Laurie Jackson 262 North Goldenspur Way, Orange, CA 92669, BA 72 Univ of Redlands; MS 73 Univ of Redlands; **SLP**

Klinkhamer, Luci H 430 Lake Avenue, Northville, MI 48167, (313) 348-9693, BA 73 MI St Univ; MS 75 Univ of MI - Ann Arbor; Sp-Lang Path, Willow Run Comm Schs, **SLP**

Klinski, Lee N 8507 N E 71 Street, Vancouver, WA 98662, (503) 280-5730, BA 76 WA St Univ; MA 77 WA St Univ; Sp-Lang Path, Holladay Cen/Phys Hndcpd Chldn, **SLP**

Klinsky, Shirley Dombrow 3517 Avenue L, Brooklyn, NY 11210, (718) 258-1441, BA 71 2067; MS 81 CUNY - Brooklyn Coll; Sp-Lang Path, NYC Bd of Ed, **SLP**

Klipp, Abbie J 140 Hamden Avenue Unit E, Waterbury, CT 06704, (203) 754-9648, BA 81 Southern CT St Univ; MA 83 OH Univ - Athens; Sp-Lang Path, Sp Lang Path Assoc of NW CT, **SLP**

Klipper, Rhonda D 1 Bay Club Drive #W-6-G, Bayside, NY 11360, (516) 681-0212, BA 80 Univ of MD - College Park; MA 81 Hofstra Univ; Sp-Lang Path, Long Is Jewish-Hillside Hosp, **SLP**

Klipsch, Marcia S 5301 Brickson Park Road, Madison, WI 53704, **SLP**

Klisanin, Mrs Joan 1020 Catalina Avenue, Seal Beach, CA 90740, (213) 598-2722, BA 67 CA St Univ - Fullerton; MA 71 CA St Univ - Long Beach; Coord Sp & Lang Serv, Anaheim Un Hs Dist, **SLP**

Kliszczuk-Gilbert, Mrs Mary Ann 4440 Monticello Boulevard, South Euclid, OH 44143, (216) 826-8010, BA 77 Case Western Reserve Univ; MA 79 Case Western Reserve Univ; Sp-Lang Path, Southwest Gen Hosp, **SLP**

Klitzke, Carol Ann 11270 East French Lake Rd, Osseo, MN 55369, (612) 337-4302, BS 70 Univ of WI - Oshkosh; MS 71 Univ of WI - Madison; Chief of Sp-Lang Path, Riverside Med Ctr, **SLP**

Kloberdanz, Mrs Brenda K 1021 Chestnut Street, Osage, IA 50461, (515) 732-4856, BA 78 Univ of Northern IA; MA 79 Univ of Northern IA; Sp-Lang Path, NM Trails AEA, **SLP**

Kloberdanz, Jennie A 304 Fourth Avenue #6, Coralville, IA 52241, (319) 369-7491, MA 88 Univ of IA; 88–Sp-Lang Path, St Luke's Hosp

Klobucar, Mrs Cheryl L 22615 Colgate, Farmington Hills, MI 48024, (313) 425-5660, BS 68 Wayne St Univ; MA 75 Oakland Univ; MA 79 Eastern MI Univ; **SLP**

Klock, Mrs Lila 509 Cumberland Road, De Land, FL 32724, (904) 734-2647, MS 73 Univ of South FL; 88–Sp/Lang Path, Private Practice, **SLP**

Klockenkemper, Barbara Anne 3951-5 Cornerwood Lane, Charlotte, NC 28212, (704) 364-0746, BS 82 Univ of IL - Urbana; MS 84 Univ of IL - Urbana; Sp-Lang Path, Community Re-Entry Services, **SLP**

Klodd, Dr David 6723 Lockwood Avenue, Lincolnwood, IL 60646, (312) 942-5332, BS 73 Univ of WI - Whitewater; MS 75 Univ of WI - Stevens Point; PH 77 (NS) Bowling Green St Univ; Aud, Rush-Presby St Lukes Med Cen, **A**

Kloep, Karen Langenfeld Cook Co Hospital, 657 Kensington Way, Bolingbrook, IL 60439, (312) 633-7168, **A**

Kloer, Cheryl N St Cloud ENT Clinic, 1225 West St Germain St, St Cloud, MN 56301, (612) 252-0233, BA 67 Elmhurst Coll; MA 70 Northern IL Univ - De Kalb; Aud, St Cloud ENT Clinic, **A**

Kloet, Marilyn Jean 2915 North 50th Street, Milwaukee, WI 53210, **SLP**

Kloiber, Margaret A 269 Secret Way, Casselberry, FL 32707, (305) 695-1014, BS 86 FL St Univ; MS 87 FL St Univ; 87–Sp-Lang Path, Orange Co Sch Bd, **SLP**

Kloosterboer, Linda Jean 5885 Schumann Drive, Madison, WI 53711, (608) 271-4909, BS 80 Univ of WI - Madison; MS 82 Univ of WI - Madison; **SLP**

Klor, Dr Barry 1677 Henry, Des Plaines, IL 60016, (312) 343-7200, BS 71 Northwestern Univ; MA 72 Northwestern Univ; PH 77 (NS) Northwestern Univ; Sp-Lang Path, VA Hospital-Hines, **SLP**

Klor, Laura A 1677 Henry, Des Plaines, IL 60016, (312) 620-4433, BS 74 Northern IL Univ - De Kalb; MS 75 Eastern IL Univ; Sp-Lang Path, Du Page Easter Seal Society, **SLP**

Kloske, Mrs Margaret L 3907 Brookridge Drive, Mechanicsburg, PA 17055, (717) 732-5721, BA 68 Allegheny Coll; MS 70 Washington Univ; 82–Sp/Lang Path, Vstng Nrs Assoc of Harrisburg Inc, **SLP**

Klossman, Mrs Patricia N Rd #1 Box 181B, Spring City, PA 19475, BS 82 West Chester Univ of PA; ME 83 Smith Coll; 86–Dir of Sp-Lang Svcs, Leader Nursing & Rehab Ctr, **SLP**

Kloster-Doohan, Kristine Kay 15 West Winthrope Road, Kansas City, MO 64113-1707, (816) 444-4274, BA 78 Univ of KS; MS 84 Central MO St Univ; 86–Sp-Lang Path, Spelman Memorial Hosp, **SLP**

Klosterman, Julie A Minneapolis ENT Clinic, 801 Phys & Surg Bldg, 63 South 9th Street, Minneapolis, MN 55402, (612) 339-7296, OB 75 Univ of ND; MS 76 CO St Univ; Dir Aud, Minneapolis ENT Cl, **A**

Klotz, Marianne R Ski Lane, Mill Neck, NY 11765, (516) 626-1000, 69; BA 72 Hofstra Univ; MA 74 Hofstra Univ; Coord of Cl Serv, Assoc Ret Chldn, **SLP**

Klotz, Susan Lisa 6200 Meadowood #1106, Reno, NV 89502, (702) 329-5108, BS 83 Univ of NV - Reno; MS 85 Univ of NV - Reno; **SLP**

Kluck, Jana Benge 4829 N W 62nd Terrace, Oklahoma City, OK 73122, (405) 722-7021, BA 75 OK St Univ; MA 77 Wichita St Univ; Sp-Lang Path, Private Practice, **SLP**

Klueger, Mrs Ruth Elizabeth 25264 Branchaster, Farmington Hills, MI 48018, (313) 493-6315, BS 78 Wayne St Univ; MA 85 Wayne St Univ; Sp-Lang Path, St Joseph Mercy Hosp, **SLP**

Kluesing, Mrs Marsha A 80 Torchwood Avenue, Plantation, FL 33324, (305) 487-2130, BS 73 FL St Univ; MS 74 FL St Univ; Aud, Private Practice, **A**

Klug, Pamela Sue 109 3rd Street, Oak Hill, WV 25901-2205, (304) 252-0790, BA 80 OH St Univ; MA 82 OH St Univ; Aud/Dir, Beckley Hrng Cen, **A**

Kluge, Mrs Mary Beth 2000 Kingsdale, Stow, OH 44224, (216) 434-1661, BS 57 Univ of IL - Urbana; MA 60 Univ of IL - Urbana; PH 74 (NS) Univ of IL - Urbana; Interim Coord Spec Educ, Akron Pub Sch, **A**

Kluin, Karen J University Of Michigan Medical Center, Speech Pathology/Department PMR, 1500 Medical Center Drive, Ann Arbor, MI 48109-0050, (313) 936-7080, BA 77 Univ of MI - Ann Arbor; MS 78 Univ of MI - Ann Arbor; 80–Sp-Lang Path, Univ of MI Med Ctr, **SLP**

Klukan, Katherine Ann 16975 Spanghurst Drive, Walton Hills, OH 44146, (216) 232-1680, MA 87 Univ of Akron; **SLP**

Klump, Margaret A 8717 George F Bunker, Sterling Heights, MI 48077, (313) 739-4854, BS 85 Northeast MO St Univ; MA 87 Memphis St Univ; 88–Aud, Dr Davis & Dr Dickson, **A**

Klumpp, Mrs Jean Ann 3825 East 36th Street, Sioux Falls, SD 57103, (515) 424-7611, BS 84 IA St Univ; MS 85 Central MO St Univ; **SLP**

Klungtvedt, Steven L 3812 Washington Avenue, Des Moines, IA 50310, (515) 247-3061, BA 77 Minot St Univ; MS 78 Minot St Univ; Aud, Iowa Head and Neck Associates, **A**

Klute, Mrs Jacqueline Monk 280 Redmond Way, Gahanna, OH 43230, (614) 471-3705, BS 77 Purdue Univ - West Lafayette; MS 78 Purdue Univ - West Lafayette; Sp-Lang Path, Columbus City Sch, **SLP**

Kluz, Ellen L 2008 Portland, St Paul, MN 55104-5856, (612) 644-7966, BA 75 MacAlster Coll; MS 80 Saint Cloud St Univ; **SLP**

Kmetz, John W 806 Furman Drive, Monroeville, PA 15146-1912, (412) 678-8671, BS 72 CA Univ of PA; ME 74 CA Univ of PA; Sp-Lang Path, Vna of Allegheny Co, **SLP**

Kmetz, Julianne 1115 Campbell Street, Wheaton, IL 60187, (312) 682-2000, BA 64 Coll of Saint Francis; MS 65 Univ of MI - Ann Arbor; Sp-Lang Path, Comm Sch Dist #200, **SLP**

Knaack, Patricia Schweinfurt American School, APO New York, NY 09033-0005, (206) 455-6077, BA 73 Univ of WA; MA 75 Univ of WA; SLP, Bellevue Sch Dist, **SLP**

Knabe, Mrs Judith Milisen 1101 Weeber Circle, Iowa City, IA 52240, (319) 338-9208, BA 63 IN Univ - Bloomington; MS 64 Univ of WI - Madison; Sp-Lang Path, Grant Wood AEA, **SLP**

Knackendoffel, Mrs Becky S 240 Columbus Canyon Road, Grand Junction, CO 81503, (303) 241-4014, BS 74 KS St Univ; MA 75 KS St Univ; **SLP**

Knafelc, Valerie 5616 Osage Way, Larkspur, CO 80118, (303) 681-3303, BS 79 CO St Univ; MA 84 Univ of Northern CO; SLP, School Dist 20, **SLP**

Knapp, Brenda Kelly Birmingham Sp & Hrng Assoc, 4 Office Park Circle, Suite 301, Birmingham, AL 35223, (205) 871-3878, BA 78 Univ of AL- Tuscaloosa; MS 80 Univ of AL- Tuscaloosa; Coord Sp-Lang Serv, Birmingham Sp & Hrng Assoc, **SLP**

Knapp, Cynthia 4 Dalton Road, Newton, MA 02178, MA 75 Kent St Univ; Comm Dept Head, The Carroll Sch, **SLP**

Knapp, Gerald A Prof Hearing Services, 315 South Main, Suite 316, Minot, ND 58701, (701) 852-6565, BS 67 Western MI Univ; MA 68 Western MI Univ; Owner, Prof Hrng Serv, **A**

Knapstein, Mary K 412 West Main Street #4, Merrill, WI 54452, (414) 826-5819, BA 78 Univ of WI - Eau Claire; MS 79 Univ of WI - Eau Claire; Sp-Lang Path, Antigo Public Sch, **SLP**

Knarr, Stacey Collins 203 South Railroad Street, Hummelstown, PA 17036, (717) 273-5382, BS 81 West Chester Univ of PA; MS 84 Syracuse Univ; SLP, Lancaster Independent Unit 13, **SLP**

Knauf, Mrs Loren W 3370 Lookout Place, Reno, NV 89503, (702) 323-6917, BS 62 Univ of NV - Reno; ME 66 Univ of NV - Reno; **SLP LM**

Knauf, Mrs Marguerite 2161 North Fort Thomas Avenue, Fort Thomas, KY 41075, BS 46 Miami Univ - Oxford; MA 71 Univ of Cincinnati; Sp-Lang Path, Private Practice, **SLP**

Knauf, Mrs Marilyn G 5709 Texas Drive, Vancouver, WA 98661, (503) 284-2157, BA 58 Pacific Univ; MS 77 Portland St Univ; Sp-Lang Path, Portland Pub Sch, **SLP**

Knauf, Dr Vincent H 3370 Lookout Place, Reno, NV 89503, (702) 329-7017, BS 42 Univ of WI - Madison; MS 48 Univ of WI - Madison; PH 52 (NS) Univ of WI - Madison; Aud-Owner, Sierra Aud Cen, **SLP A LM**

Knauss, Mrs Genevieve M 7626 North 79th Plaza, Omaha, NE 68122, (402) 554-6044, BA 79 Creighton Univ; MS 81 Univ of NE - Omaha; 80–Sp-Lang Path, Omaha Pub Sch, **SLP**

Knauss, Judith D S 103 Briarwood Drive, Versailles, KY 40383, (606) 299-1020, BS 67 Univ of ND; MS 70 Univ of ND; SLP, Fayette County Schools, **SLP**

Kneale, Mrs Patricia Susan 2220 East Peak Court, Martinez, CA 94553, (415) 687-0202, BA 83 Univ of the Pacific; MA 84 Univ of the Pacific; 84–Sp-Lang Path, Mt Diablo USD, **SLP**

Knebel, Karlene 212 West University Drive, Chapel Hill, NC 27514, **SLP**

Knecht, Mrs Gail B 12748 Goodwood Blvd, Baton Rouge, LA 70815, (504) 655-5534, BS 69 LA St Univ - Baton Rouge; MA 71 LA St Univ - Baton Rouge; Sp-Lang Path, Livingston Parish Sch Bd, **SLP**

Kneeter, Judith 1645 Merritt, Novato, CA 94949-3059, (415) 654-9906, BA 56 Univ of IA; MA 76 Univ of IA; 88–Admin Dir, Transitions-Bay Area Recovery Center, **SLP**

Kneier, Barbara Louise 32 West Vine, Oxford, OH 45056, (513) 548-2509, BS 85 Miami Univ - Oxford; MS 86 Miami Univ - Oxford; 86–Sp-Lang Path, Greenville City Schs, **SLP**

Kneil, Dr Thomas R Communicative Disorders & Sci, Wichita State Univ Box 75, Wichita, KS 67208, (316) 689-3240, BA 55 Bowdoin Coll; MS 60 Syracuse Univ; PH 72 (NS) Univ of IA; Assistant Professor, Wichita State University

Knell-Berg, Caron Anne 3582 Silverwood, Redding, CA 96002, (916) 222-5537, BA 77 Western WA Univ; MA 80 Western WA Univ; SLP, Shasta County School, **SLP**

Knepflar, Dr Kenneth J Communication Services Center, 1156 East Green Street, Suite 102, Pasadena, CA 91106, (818) 449-1843, BA 52 SUNY - Center at Buffalo; MS 55 Univ of UT; PH 64 Univ of CA - Los Angeles; Dir, Commun Serv Cen, **SLP F**

Knepka, Mrs Cynthia W 15 Cresthill Drive, Whitesboro, NY 13492, (315) 736-1195, BS 78 Nazareth Coll of Rochester; MA 80 SUNY - Center at Buffalo; Sp/Lang Path, New Hartford Cen Sch, **SLP**

Knepp, Cynthia Susanne 2809 February Court, Modesto, CA 95351, BA 78 CA St Univ - Fresno; MA 80 CA St Univ - Fresno; SLP, Modesto Cty Sch, **SLP**

Knerl, Mary K 2045 Lyans Drive, La Canada, CA 91011, (213) 997-2395, BA 48 Stanford Univ; MA 68 Univ of Southern CA; SLP, Los Angeles USD, **SLP**

Knicely, Dena Marie 1666 7th Avenue, Huntington, WV 25703-1428, (304) 522-0307, BA 84 Marshall Univ; MA 85 Marshall Univ; 86–Sp-Lang Path, Kentucky Easter Seal, **SLP**

Knigge-Dartt, Ann E 122 Woodbine Avenue, East Rochester, NY 14445, (716) 381-0964, MS 80 SUNY - Coll at Geneseo; SLP, Monroe Development Center, **SLP**

Knight, Carolyn L P O Box 3502, Chico, CA 95927, (916) 345-6525, MA 77 CA St Univ - Chico; Sp-Lang Path, Chico Comm Hosp, **SLP**

Knight, Colleen W 1133 Sleepy Hollow Drive, Olathe, KS 66062, (913) 764-6955, BS 75 Univ of NE - Omaha; MS 76 Univ of NE - Omaha; Sp-Lang Path, Olathe USD #233, **SLP**

Knight, Dan P, Jr 214 Fairfield Drive, Thibodaux, LA 70301, (504) 446-8111, BS 64 Univ of Montevallo; MA 66 LA St Univ - Baton Rouge; Assoc Prof-Sp/Cl Superv, Nicholls St U, **SLP**

Knight, Doris Lee 5958 Jared Court, Satsuma, AL 36572, (205) 452-0421, BA 66 Univ of OK - Norman; MS 70 Phillips Univ; 78–Sp-Lang Path, Mobile Co Pub Sch, **SLP**

Knight, Dr Elmo L Siesta Sands Apartment #211, 1001 Point Of Rocks Road, Sarasota, FL 34242, (813) 349-3568, BA 48 Syracuse Univ; MS 51 Syracuse Univ; PH 65 Syracuse Univ; Retired, Childrens Hosp of Buffalo, **SLP A F LM**

Knight, Mrs Georgianne 14017 Painted Desert Road, Poway, CA 92064, (916) 972-0665, MS 80 4807; MA 71 (NS) Western OR St Coll; **SLP**

Knight, Mrs Helen Sullivan 717 Hunter Road, Glenview, IL 60025, (312) 724-3632, BA 31 AR Coll; MA 36 Northwestern Univ; Retired, **SLP F H LM**

Knight, Jane Kiser 3900 Fallen Timber Drive, Louisville, KY 40241, (502) 426-5337, BA 63 Univ of AL- Tuscaloosa; **SLP**

Knight, Jane Sanders 110 Bellevue Road #31, Nashville, TN 37221, (615) 327-5529, MS 84 Saint Louis Univ; Sp-Lang Path, Home Health Services, **SLP ACE**

Knight, Mrs Janice Knapp 4410CHAPMAN Road, Millbrook, AL 36054-2513, (205) 285-3746, BS 75 Univ of South AL; MS 87 Univ of Montevallo; 87–Sp-Lang Path, Elmore Co Bd of Educ, **SLP**

Knight, Jody L 281 Marna Drive, Vacaville, CA 95688, (707) 446-6939, BS 77 Univ of IA; MA 78 Univ of IA; SLP, Solano County Office of Educ, **SLP**

Knight, Mrs Judy W 5227 Old Stage Road, Morristown, TN 37814, (615) 586-7744, BS 70 East TN St Univ; MA 71 Vanderbilt Univ; Aud, Hamblen Co Schs, **A**

Knight, Karen F 5961 Brynthrop, Utica, MI 48087, (313) 651-6210, BS 78 Wayne St Univ; MA 79 Western MI Univ; Sp-Lang Path, Rochester Comm Sch, **SLP**

Knight, Mrs Karen Jean/Bell 5 Bradley Court, Rochester, NH 03867, (207) 384-2210, BS 79 Univ of ME - Farmington; MS 84 Univ of NH; Sp-Lang Path, School Administrative Dist 35, **SLP**

Knight, Kathryn Elaine 8451 Thousand Oaks #8-H, North Richland Hills, TX 76180, (817) 581-8370, BS 84 TX Woman's Univ; MA 87 TX Woman's Univ; **SLP**

Knight, Kimberly K 126 Long Lane, Bristol, CT 06010, (203) 753-2124, BA 80 Auburn Univ - Auburn; MS 82 Syracuse Univ; 87–Aud, Prof Hearing Services Inc, **A**

Knight, Linda L 416 Market Street, Spencer, WV 25276, **SLP**

Knight, Mrs Marion H R R 1 Box 256, Brookfield, VT 05036, (802) 276-3418, BA 33 Plymouth St Coll; MA 49 Univ of MI - Ann Arbor; **SLP LM**

Knight, Mrs Nancy F 49 Norwood Avenue, Summit, NJ 07901, (201) 273-0793, BS 51 Northwestern Univ; MA 53 Washington Univ; 79–Sp/Lang Path, Mendham Boro Pub Sch, **SLP**

Knight, Mrs Patricia D 4542 East Bluebird Avenue, Orange, CA 92669, (714) 525-3584, BA 56 Univ of the Pacific; MA 67 CA St Univ - Long Beach; Resource Spec, Fullerton Elem Sch Dist, **SLP**

Knight, Paul D 717 Hunter Road, Glenview, IL 60025, (312) 724-3632, BS 26 Univ of IL - Urbana; MA 40 Northwestern Univ; **SLP F H LM**

Knight, Mrs Regina C 2410 North Maryland, Peoria, IL 61603, (309) 682-1433, BS 46 Northern IL Univ - De Kalb; MS 66 Bradley Univ; Retired, Peoria Public Schools, **SLP**

Knight, Mrs Shelly Kay 321 East 50th Street, Indianapolis, IN 46205, (317) 226-4128, BS 83 Ball St Univ; MA 84 Ball St Univ; Aud, Indianapolis Pub Schs, **A**

Knight, Terryl M 636 Galaxie Drive, Lexington, KY 40502, **SLP**

Knightly, Carol Ann 4410 Township Line Avenue, Apartment A-1B, Drexel Hill, PA 19026, (215) 449-0890, BA 83 Thiel Coll; MA 85 OH Univ - Athens; **A**

Knight-McKenna, Mary T 47 Winfield Street, East Freetown, MA 02717, (617) 823-9860, BS 77 Nazareth Coll of Rochester; ME 79 Northeastern Univ; Sp-Lang Path, Reg Ed Assessment & Diag Serv, **SLP**

Knighton, Robert D 730 Lavina Drive, Ogden, UT 84403, (801) 476-1113, BS 69 ID St Univ; MA 71 Univ of WA; Sp-Lang Path, Intermountain Health Care, **SLP**

Knip-Ness, Rebecca L 3 Rock Bluff, Pomona, CA 91766, (714) 990-7820, BA 81 CA St Univ - Fullerton; MA 84 CA St Univ - Fullerton; **SLP**

Knipp, Anne 2027 Red River Road, Sykesville, MD 21784, (201) 788-9298, **SLP**

Knipprath, Mrs Cathleen H 17685 Beech Street, Fountain Valley, CA 92708, (502) 267-4321, MS 75 Univ of Houston - Univ Park; **SLP**

Knisley, Marianne Murray Rt 1 Box 658, Magnolia Avenue, East Palatka, FL 32031, (904) 824-0428, OB 84 Brigham Young Univ; OM 85 Brigham Young Univ; **SLP**

Knittel, June M 2705 Vine, Hays, KS 67601, (913) 628-2514, BS 82 Univ of SD - Vermillion; MS 84 Univ of WY; 87–Aud, Private Practice, **A**

Knittel, Mary Ann Lyon Oakland Schools, 2100 Pontiac Lake Road, Pontiac, MI 48054, (313) 858-1922, BA 76 Univ of IA; MA 77 Univ of IA; 86–Aud, Oakland Schs Sp & Hearing Clinic, **A**

Knize, Mrs Evelyn B 128 Brannan Drive, Ennis, TX 75119, (214) 875-3664, BS 71 TX Christian Univ; MS 72 TX Christian Univ; Self-Employed, **SLP**

Knobeloch, Dr F X Calvin 121 Larkspur Circle, Durham, NC 27713, (919) 966-5171, BS 49 IN Univ - Bloomington; PH 59 (Sp Path/Aud) Univ of FL; 88–Dir of Clin Svcs, Ctr for Dev & Learing-UNC, **SLP A F**

Knoblauch, Elizabeth Renee 3201 32nd Avenue South, Minneapolis, MN 55406, (612) 884-8550, MA 84 Univ of MN - Minneap-St Paul; Sp-Lang Path, Bloomington Pub Sch/Dist 271, **SLP**

Knoch, Mrs Joni K Rd 2 Box 300, Tarentum, PA 15084, (412) 224-2163, BS 77 Indiana Univ of PA; MS 81 Indiana Univ of PA; Sp-Lang Path, Private Practice, **SLP ACE**

Knockel, Mrs Brenda Renee 6942 Dupre Road, Centerville, MN 55038, (612) 938-5511, BS 83 Winona St Univ; BS 83 Coll of Saint Teresa; OM 85 Univ of WI - River Falls; Sp-Lang Path, Achievement Rehab Corp, **SLP**

Knodle, Mrs Lauren M 4324 Lori Drive Apt 2, Rockford, IL 61111, (815) 968-6861, BS 82 Bowling Green St Univ; MS 84 Univ of WI - Stevens Point; 88–Sp-Lang Path, Rockford Memorial Hosp, **SLP**

Knoebel, Mrs Constance 120 6th Avenue, Nyack, NY 10960, (914) 634-4941, BA 60 Coll of New Rochelle; MS 76 Columbia Univ Teachers Coll; Teacher of the Deaf, Clarkstown Ctrl Sch Dist, **SLP**

Knoegel, Mrs Roberta G 197 Glendale Drive, Bristol, CT 06010, (203) 628-0331, BA 76 Univ of CT; MS 80 Southern CT St Univ; SLP, Southington Co Bd of Ed, **SLP**

Knoerl, Annmarie 68 Niagara Street, Oswego, NY 13126, (315) 342-2818, MS 88 Nazareth Coll of Rochester; 84–Sp-Lang Path, Oswego County BOCES

Knoff, Mrs Shari Rohloff 314 Elm Avenue, Burlington, NJ 08016, (609) 877-1430, BS 75 Trenton St Coll; MA 80 Trenton St Coll; Sp-Lang Path, Edgewater Park Township Sch, **SLP**

Knoll, Cheryl L Willmar Medical Center, 101 Willmar Avenue S W, Willmar, MN 56201, (612) 231-5019, BA 70 Saint Cloud St Univ; MA 79 Wichita St Univ; 85–Aud, Willmar Med Cen, **A ACE**

Knolle, Janie H 5314 Musket Ridge, Austin, TX 78759, (512) 483-3115, BA 70 Baylor Univ; MS 71 Baylor Univ; Sp-Lang Path, Austin ISD, **SLP**

Knorr, Geralynn Snyder 8859 Alcott Street, Los Angeles, CA 90035, (213) 273-4375, BA 75 Univ of MI - Ann Arbor; MS 77 Univ of MI - Ann Arbor; Sp-Lang Path, Cognitive Rehab Service, **SLP**

Knott, Margaret R 11020 Running Ridge Road, Charlotte, NC 28226, (704) 541-5053, BS 77 WV Univ; MA 79 Univ of NC - Greensboro; Sp-Lang Path, Private Practice, **SLP ACE**

Knott, Mary Carolyn Speech Pathology Clinic-Annex, WM Beaumont Army Med Ctr, El Paso, TX 79920, (915) 569-2065, BA 63 Univ of Northern CO; MA 70 NM St Univ; Sp-Lang Path, Wm Beaumont Army Med Cen, **SLP**

Knott, Monica Cathrine 200 Wentworth Street North, Hamilton, ON, Canada L8L 5V7, BA 80 Univ of Winnipeg - Manitoba; MS 83 Minot St Univ; 87–Sp-Lang Path, Bd of Educ for Hamilton City, **SLP**

Knotts, Jennifer L 5364 Primrose Avenue, Indianapolis, IN 46220-3317, (317) 266-4283, **SLP**

Knourek, Marge Ann 209 East River Parkway #32, Champlin, MN 55316, (612) 422-9119, BS 65 Univ of MN - Duluth; MA 81 Univ of MN - Minneap-St Paul; 88–Sp-Lang Path, St Francis PS, **SLP**

Knowles, Brooke O 266 St Joseph Avenue, Long Beach, CA 90803, (714) 848-0656, BA 75 Univ of Southern CA; MA 78 CA St Univ - Long Beach; Sp-Lang Path, Huntington Beach Union Hsd, **SLP**

Knowles, Cynthia Dixon 5147 Jackwood, Houston, TX 77096, (713) 771-9966, BA 78 Univ of FL; MS 79 FL St Univ; Sp-Lang Path, Sp & Lang Remed Cen, **SLP A**

Knowles, Gillian E 3836 13th Street S W, Calgary, AB, Canada T2T 3R3, (403) 268-9590, BA 63 Dalhousie Univ - Nova Scotia; OM 65 Univ of Toronto - Ontario; Div Dir SLP, Calgary Gen Hosp, **SLP**

Knowles, Mary Susan 628 Ponte Vedra Boulevard, Apartment #A-10, Ponte Vedra Beach, FL 32082, (904) 285-1324, BS 77 Saint John's Univ - Jamaica; ME 84 Columbus Coll; Sp-Lang Path, Duval County Sch Board, **SLP**

Knowles, Mrs Patti Rose 16623 74th Place West, Edmonds, WA 98020, (206) 485-0497, BA 79 Univ of WA; OM 83 Univ of WA; SLP, Northshore Sch Dist, **SLP**

Knowles, Russell D Route 5 Box 284, Lebanon, MO 65536-9336, **SLP**

Knowles-McCall, Mrs Amy S 9425 244th Street SW E-208, Edmonds, WA 98020, (206) 546-5798, BS 84 Univ of IA; MS 87 Univ of WA; Pacific ENT CLinic, **A**

Knowlton, Mrs Janice Lynne Route 1 Box 216, North Vernon, IN 47265, (217) 735-2361, BS 81 Southern IL Univ -Carbondale; MS 83 Southern IL Univ -Carbondale; Sp-Lang Path, Muscatatuck Developmental Ctr, **SLP**

Knowlton, Linda M M Rd 1 Box 253, Accord, NY 12404, (914) 338-8686, BA 76 SUNY - Coll at New Paltz; MA 78 Kent St Univ; 87–Aud, St Francis Hosp, **A**

Knox, Dr Albert W 6300 Granada, Prairie Village, KS 66208, (913) 722-2173, BA 50 Univ of CA - Los Angeles; MA 52 UT St Univ; PH 59 (Sp Path & Aud) Univ of Southern CA; 88–Consult, Private Practice, **SLP A F LM**

Knox, Alexandra Brittain 304 Southern Boulevard, Chatham, NJ 07928, (201) 966-0318, OB 63 Wellesley Coll; MA 85 NY Univ; 87–Sp-Lang Path, Saint Barnabas Med Ctr, **SLP**

Knox, Ann Elizabeth 100 Hickory, Box 195, Villa Grove, IL 61956, BS 84 IL St Univ - Normal; MA 86 Univ of IL - Urbana; **SLP**

Knox, Barbara D 55 Fulton Street #6-M, Middletown, NY 10940, BS 51 Ithaca Coll; MS 55 Syracuse Univ; **SLP A LM**

Knox, Brenda Bonuccelli 6 Breeze Branch Court #G, Timonium, MD 21093, (301) 683-7478, BA 83 Loyola Coll; MS 85 Loyola Coll; Sp-Lang Path, Balto Co Bd of Educ, **SLP**

Knox, Mrs Jane Hastings 4100 Wallahatchie Road, Pike Road, AL 36064, (205) 272-7230, BA 78 Univ of FL; OM 81 Emory Univ; Sp-Lang Path, **SLP**

Knox, Dr Jeffrey A 1012 Tower Court, Iowa City, IA 52240, (319) 351-2464, BA 63 Lawrence Univ; MA 68 Univ of IA; PH 75 Univ of IA; SLP, Grant Wood AEA, **SLP**

Knox, Joanne Elles Route 2, 21A Carriage Lane, Contoocook, NH 03229, (603) 746-5868, BA 66 MI St Univ; MA 81 Western MI Univ; Sp-Lang Path, Private Practice, **SLP**

Knox, John Gerard 826 South Main #112, Racine, WI 53403, (414) 886-9733, MS 86 Univ of WI - Stevens Point; **A**

Knox, Mrs Leona L 6273 Stonewood Lane, Solon, OH 44139, (216) 248-7023, BA 78 Cleveland St Univ; MA 79 Cleveland St Univ; **SLP**

Knox, Nancy Shapiro 4841 Swinton Avenue, Encino, CA 91436-1317, (213) 761-2801, BA 74 CUNY - Queens Coll; MA 75 Hofstra Univ; SLP, Los Angeles USD, **SLP**

Knox, Susan C 1627 Camino Uva, Los Alamos, NM 87544, (505) 662-4141, BA 71 TX Tech Univ; MS 75 TX Tech Univ; Sp/Lang Path, Los Alamos Sch, **SLP**

Knox, Dr Thomas E 2611 Babcock Road, Vienna, VA 22180, (713) 938-8171, DD 33 Washington Univ; **LM**

Knudsen, Mrs Jana L 1303 Marbee Drive #5, Omaha, NE 68124, OB 65 Univ of NE - Omaha; MS 70 Univ of NE - Omaha; **SLP**

Knudsen, Karen E 55 Wellington Drive, Farmington, CT 06032, (203) 242-2274, BA 73; MS 75 Univ of NE - Omaha; Sp-Lang Path, Oak Hill Sch, **SLP**

Knudsen, Lisa Anne P O Box 1124, Fraser, CO 80442, (303) 726-9541, BS 86 Baylor Univ; MS 87 Baylor Univ; 87–Sp-Lang Path, NW Co BOCES

Knudsen, Nancy Willard 920 Hoyt Avenue, Everett, WA 98201, (206) 326-3485, BA 74 Univ of Rochester; MA 77 Northwestern Univ; Sp-Lang Path, Sp Lang & Hrng Svcs, **SLP**

Knudson, Cherylanne 142 Quincy Shore Dr #150, North Quincy, MA 02171-2924, (617) 727-5608, BA 76 SUNY - Coll at Plattsburgh; MA 80 Univ of KS; 88–Superv SLP, Dept of Mental Retard of MA, **SLP**

Knudson, Mrs Wendy K P O Box 894, Estes Park, CO 80517, (303) 586-4439, BS 77 CO St Univ; MS 78 CO St Univ; Aud, Wendy's Hearing Svc, **A**

Knudten, Lisa A 2105 Glen Cove Lane, Brookfield, WI 53005, (414) 351-0450, BA 84 Univ of WI - Madison; MS 86 Univ of WI - Madison; **SLP**

Knuff, Mrs La Vonne 27 Lakeview Drive, Marquette, MI 49855, (906) 226-6067, BS 67 Marquette Univ; OM 69 Marquette Univ; **SLP**

Knupp, Diane T 4225 Amanda Lane, Schenectady, NY 12303, (518) 374-4551, MS 75 SUNY - Center at Albany; Sp/Lang Path, Mohawk Reg Cen, **SLP**

Knupp, Laura L 15 Mulberry Street, Rhinebeck, NY 12572, (518) 325-4471, BA 69 Carthage Coll; ME 71 Univ of VA - Charlottesville; 84–Sp-Lang Path, Taconic Hills Central Schs, **SLP**

Knuter, Lynnette M 1401 East Girard Avenue, #13-289, Englewood, CO 80110, (303) 399-0603, BS 79 CO St Univ; MA 81 Univ of Northern CO; 84–Special Needs Coord, Chld Opportunity Prog Inc, **SLP**

Knuteson, Mrs Christine Owen 1511 25th Avenue, Monroe, WI 53566, (608) 325-4879, BA 66 Baylor Univ; MA 68 Univ of TN - Knoxville; **A**

Knuth, Renee Marie 3305 S 100th Street, Greenfield, WI 53227, (414) 241-5530, BS 85 Univ of WI - Stevens Point; MS 87 Univ of WI - Stevens Point; **SLP**

Knutilla, Cynthia Cooper 430 8th Street, Lincoln, IL 62656, (217) 735-2361, MA; Sp-Lang Path, Lincoln Dev Ctr, **SLP**

Knutson, Andrea J 5712 Morgan Avenue South, Minneapolis, MN 55419, (612) 926-8610, BA 77 Carleton Coll; MS 83 Saint Cloud St Univ; Sp-Lang Path, Minneapolis Public Schools, **SLP**

Knutson, Mrs Diane K 909 North Madison Street, Stoughton, WI 53589, (608) 873-7257, BS 73 Univ of WI - Madison; MS 74 Univ of WI - Madison; Sp-Lang Path, Stoughton PS, **SLP**

Knutson, Mrs Leah Joy 43502 Gadsden Avenue, Apartment 220, Lancaster, CA 93534, (805) 945-7062, BS 83 FL St Univ; MS 84 FL St Univ; Sp-Lang Path, Snowline Uni Schl Dstr, **SLP**

Knutzen, Mrs Robin H 19035 68th Street East, Bonney Lake, WA 98390, (206) 863-3267, BS 76 SUNY - Coll at Geneseo; MS 81 Southern CT St Univ; Sp-Lang Path, Old Saybrook Pub Schs, **SLP**

Koan, Margaret A Box 454, Tyndall, SD 57066, (605) 589-3388, BS 83 Univ of SD - Vermillion; MA 85 Univ of SD - Vermillion; **SLP**

Koan, Phyllis A 1881 Johnson Drive, Concord, CA 94520, (415) 254-0521, BA 79 MI St Univ; MA 80 Central MI Univ; Sp-Lang Path, Orinda Sch Dist, **SLP**

Kobara-Mates, Mrs Mindy S 2227 Lincolnwood Drive, Evanston, IL 60201, (312) 866-9502, BS 81 Univ of WA; MA 84 Northwestern Univ; **SLP**

Kobayashi, Lynn M 745 Paani Street #B, Honolulu, HI 96826, (808) 941-0410, MS 88 Univ of HI - Manoa; 88–Sp-Lang Path, Dept of Educ

Kobernick, Deena Bornstein 922 Edwina Way, Cardiff, CA 92007, **SLP**

Kobiernicki, Mrs Brenda Bwel 3234 Grand Route Street, New Orleans, LA 70119, (504) 488-5395, **SLP**

Koblas, Linda Tutewohl 5201 Frost Point Circle, Prior Lake, MN 55372, BS 80 Univ of MN - Minneap-St Paul; MA 82 Univ of MN - Minneap-St Paul; Aud, Audiometrics Inc, **A**

Koble, Carolyn A 1509 Bison Drive #514, Williston, ND 58801, (701) 572-4519, MS 88 Minot St Univ; 88–Sp-Lang Path, Wilmac Multidistrict Spec Educ Unit

Koblenz, Mrs Marta B R 149 Colonial Avenue, Albany, NY 12208-1408, (518) 438-4387, BS 77 SUNY - Center at Albany; MS 81 Coll of Saint Rose; Sp-Lang Path, Albany Med Cen, **SLP**

Koblenz, Mrs Maxine 3175 Falmouth Road, Shaker Heights, OH 44122, (216) 561-6070, BS 56 Syracuse Univ; ME 80 John Carroll Univ; **SLP ACE**

Kobrin, Mrs Marjorie S 133 Commander Shea Blvd, Apartment 802, North Quincy, MA 02171, BS 77 Univ of MA - Amherst; MA 79 NY Univ; Sales Representative, Welch Allyn, **A**

Kobrin, Meryl Audiology Department, Northwestern University, Frances Searle Bldg, 2299 Sheridan Road, Evanston, IL 60208, (312) 491-3164, BA 84, MA 87 Northwestern Univ

Kobritz, Lauren Susan 529 West Fullerton #22, Chicago, IL 60614, BS 75 Univ of IL - Urbana; MS 76 Univ of IL - Urbana; 88–Chief of Sp-Lang Path, La Rabida Children's Hosp, **SLP**

Kobus, Mrs Anna H 15 Holly Springs Court, Baltimore, MD 21236, (301) 882-5163, BS 77 Towson St Univ; MS 78 Towson St Univ; Sp-Lang Path, Baltimore City Public Schools, **SLP**

Koch, Carol Anne 4819 Boonsboro Road #B, Lynchburg, VA 24503, (505) 397-2828, BS 80 OK St Univ; MS 83 Univ of OK Medical Center; Sp-Lang Path, Hobbs Mun Sch, **SLP**

Koch, Catherine Marie 595 Berkley, Elmhurst, IL 60126, MA 83 Univ of Northern CO; BA 82 Augustana Coll; 88–Sp-Lang Path, LaGrange Area Dept of Spec Educ, **SLP**

Koch, Mrs Deborah Georgian 7165 Peace Chimes Court, Columbia, MD 21045, (301) 955-6240, BA 76 Geneva Coll; MA 78 Northwestern Univ; 87–Sp-Lang Path, Johns Hopkins Med Inst, **SLP**

Koch, Elaina Sunas 8337 Twin Pointe Circle, Indianapolis, IN 46236-8901, (803) 758-4632, MA 82 Univ of TN - Knoxville; Sp-Lang Path, Scdmr Midlands Ctr, **SLP**

Koch, Evanne N S 339 Ridge Road, Cedar Grove, NJ 07009, **SLP ACE**

Koch, Gerald C 1207 West River Road #D-3, Elyria, OH 44035, (419) 447-2927, BS 70 Bowling Green St Univ; MA 77 Bowling Green St Univ; Elem Superv, Seneca Cty Bd of Ed, **SLP**

Koch, Larry John 1814 Weldon Boulevard, Ann Arbor, MI 48103, (313) 665-0550, BS 64 Univ of WI - Madison; MS 67 Univ of WI - Madison; Aud, Saline Community Hosp, **A**

Koch, Mrs Lisa McHugh 312 Sanders Drive, Gallipolis, OH 45631, (614) 446-7619, BS 77 Clarion Univ of PA; MS 79 Gallaudet Coll; Owner, Inhearing, **A**

Koch, Lynnette J 2830 Santa Barbara Drive, Brookfield, WI 53005, (414) 782-6407, MS 87 Univ of WI - Whitewater; 88–Sp-Lang Path, New Medico Rehab Ctr of WI, **SLP**

Koch, Sarah Cooper 1600 N E Dixie Highway, Apartment 10-206, Jensen Beach, FL 33457, (305) 287-5200, BS 85 Miami Univ - Oxford; MS 86 Miami Univ - Oxford; **SLP**

Koch, Mrs Victoria W 104 North Marilyn Avenue, Northlake, IL 60164, (312) 825-0144, BS 81 Eastern IL Univ; MS 82 Eastern IL Univ; Sp-Lang Path, Rosemont Elem Sch #78, **SLP**

Kochans, Joyce B 21325 Woodhill, Northville, MI 48167, BS 80 Northern MI Univ; MA 82 Western MI Univ; SLP, Detroit Receiving Hospital, **SLP ACE**

Kochenash, Mrs Susan D 812 Stoughton Avenue, Chaska, MN 55318, (612) 448-2890, BS 75 Bloomsburg Univ of PA; ME 76 Bloomsburg Univ of PA; SLP, Shakopee School District, **SLP**

Kocher, Beth Karen 61 Par Court, Pennsauken, NJ 08109, (609) 261-7030, BS 66 Bob Jones Univ; MA 68 Temple Univ; Mgr Sp-Hrng/Pedia Rehab, Memorial Hosp/Burlington Co, **SLP**

Kocher, Judith L 2948 Strathaven Lane, Abingdon, MD 21009-1823, (301) 676-7890, BS 72 WV Univ; MA 74 Cleveland St Univ; **SLP**

Koches, Mrs Lisa C 1402 Southwind Court, Vienna, VA 22180, (703) 691-4063, BA 77 Univ of CT; ME 78 Univ of VA - Charlottesville; Sp-Lang Path, Comm Rehab Services PC, **SLP**

Kocipak, Susan P O Box 53686, Albuquerque, NM 87153, (505) 298-5009, BA 81 CA St Univ - Sacramento; MA 84 CA St Univ - Sacramento; Sp-Lang Path, Albuquerque Pub Sch, **SLP**

Kocs, Diane S 12165 Wensley Road, Florissant, MO 63033, (314) 831-8798, BS 64 Marquette Univ; MA 78 Saint Louis Univ; Sp-Lang Path, Ferguson-Florissant Early Educ Prog, **SLP**

Kodama, Mrs Mildred Riley 1113 Applegrove Road N W, North Canton, OH 44720, MS; **SLP LM**

Kodama, Sakie 145 Montreal Road #2, Cornwall, ON, Canada K6H 1B2, (613) 932-3300, OM 88 Univ of Western Ontario; 88–Dir of Sp-Lang Path, Cornwall Gen Hosp

Kodman, Dr Frank, Jr 1503 Glendale Road, Murray, KY 42071, (502) 762-2851, BA 48 2727; MA 51 Univ of Pittsburgh - Pittsburgh; PH 54 Univ of IL - Urbana; **SLP A**

Koebli, Mrs Judith Rose 185 Valley Rd, Clark, NJ 07066, (201) 351-1665, BA 84 Kean Coll of NJ; MA 87 CUNY - Hunter Coll; **SLP**

Koebsell, Katherine Allison 2105 Graham Avenue, Redondo Beach, CA 90278, (213) 226-5073, BA 78 Univ of the Pacific; MS 84 Syracuse Univ; Aud, Lac/Usc Medical Center, **A**

Koegel, Lynn Kern 2335 Foothill Lane, Santa Barbara, CA 93105, (805) 684-7657, BA 80 Univ of CA - Santa Barbara; MA 82 Univ of CA - Santa Barbara; SLP, Carpinteria USD, **SLP**

Koegel, Mrs Marian T Rural Delivery 2, 52 Lay Road, Delta, PA 17314, (717) 456-5734, BS 78 Bloomsburg Univ of PA; MS 79 Bloomsburg Univ of PA; Sp-Lang Path, Harford Co Pub Sch, **SLP**

Koehl, Dolores I 201 West Creighton, Fort Wayne, IN 46807, (219) 449-1433, BA 75 IN Univ - Bloomington; OM 77 IN Univ - Bloomington; SLP, Rehab Hlth Serv, **SLP**

Koehler, Mrs Ann Malcolm c/o Dr Richard Koehler, A L Lee Memorial Hospital, 510 South 4th Street, Fulton, NY 13069-0607, (318) 377-7605, Coord SLP, Claiborne Parish Sch Bd, **SLP**

Koehler, Mrs Dorothy M W230 S9085 Clark Street, Big Bend, WI 53103, (414) 662-4401, BA 78 Univ of WI - Eau Claire; MS 79 Univ of WI - Eau Claire; Mukwonga Area Schools, **SLP**

Koehler, Gwen Ensley 3023 Stratford Drive, Greensboro, NC 27408, (919) 282-0052, BA 78 Univ of NC - Greensboro; MA 79 Univ of NC - Greensboro; Private Practice, **SLP**

Koehler, Lisa Claire 1306 Wayland Street, Beaver Dam, WI 53916, (414) 885-6081, BS 83 Univ of WI - Whitewater; MS 84 Marquette Univ; 88–Sp-Lang Path, Beaver Dam USD, **SLP**

Koehler, Mrs Mary P 4944 Golden Arrow Drive, Rancho Palos Verdes, CA 90274, (213) 533-4481, BS 57 Univ of Southern CA; MA 77 CA St Univ - Long Beach; SLP, Los Angeles County Sup Schools, **SLP**

Koehler, Sheree Lynn 9260 190th Street North, Forest Lake, MN 55025, (612) 464-3313, BS 82 Univ of WI - River Falls; MA 84 MI St Univ; Sp-Lang Path, Forest Lake Sch Dist #831, **SLP**

Koehn, Beth 9715 East 75th #917, Tulsa, OK 74133, (918) 366-4421, BS 79 Univ of MO - Columbia; MA 81 Univ of KS; SLP, Bixby Public Schools, **SLP**

Koehnemann, Donald F 811 Bristol Avenue, Westchester, IL 60153, (312) 344-1373, BA 54 Ball St Univ; MA 58 Northwestern Univ; 55–Sp-Lang Path, Private Practice, **SLP**

Koehnke, Dr Janet D Boston University, Department Of Communication Disorders, 48 Cummington Street, Boston, MA 02155, (617) 353-5640, BS 76 Univ of MA - Amherst; MA 77 SUNY - Coll at Geneseo; PH 83 (NS) Univ of CT; Research Asst Prof, Boston Univ, **A**

Koelemay, Mrs Fon W 4012 Andover Drive, Plano, TX 75023, (214) 422-5389, BS 74 Fairleigh Dickinson U-Madisn; MS 76 Old Dominion Univ; Sp-Lang Path, Private Practice, **SLP**

Koelliker, Deborah Lee Route 3 Box 376, Mount Pleasant, TX 75455, (214) 572-9194, BS 82 Ball St Univ; MA 83 Ball St Univ; **SLP**

Koeneke-Varley, Meridith Ann 7518 Brava Street, Carlsbad, CA 92009, (619) 746-3223, BS 75 CO St Univ; MS 77 AZ St Univ; Prog Dir, Lrng Svcs-Escondido Comm Re-Entry Prog, **SLP**

Koenen, Susan Kathryn 2840 North Murray Avenue, Milwaukee, WI 53211, (414) 964-9527, MS 88 Univ of WI - Milwaukee

Koenig, Mrs Brenda P 116 Kirkside Drive, Starkville, MS 39759, (601) 324-1511, BS 81 MS Univ for Women; MS 82 MS Univ for Women; Sp-Lang Path, Starkville Mun Separate Sch, **SLP**

Koenig, Mrs Ellen Gitter 25 Alhambra Drive, Oceanside, NY 11572, (718) 738-1800, BA 81 Univ of MD - College Park; MA 83 CUNY - Queens Coll; Sp-Lang Path, Spec Kids Intervention Prog, **SLP ACE**

Koenig, Linda A 4455 Cushing Lane, Richmond Heights, OH 44143, (216) 371-7230, OB 71 OH Univ - Athens; MA 72 OH Univ - Athens; Coord/Language Services, Cleveland Heights City Schools, **SLP**

Koenig, Mrs Marcia L 1714 Kenwick Place, Pasadena, TX 77504, (713) 487-2712, BS 79 Lamar Univ; MS 80 Lamar Univ; **SLP**

Koenig, Dr Mareile A 3858 Florence Drive #4, Alexandria, VA 22305, (703) 836-5315, BS 70 Southern IL Univ -Carbondale; MS 75 Southern IL Univ -Carbondale; PH 82 (NS) Univ of IL - Urbana; Assistant Professor, Childrens Hosp Natl Med Ctr, **SLP**

Koenig, Mary A 4520 25th, Columbus, NE 68601, (402) 563-1019, BS 82 Kearney St Coll; MS 83 Kearney St Coll; Sp-Lang Path, Esu #7 Special Ed Cooperative, **SLP**

Koenig, Vera Lee C 1905 9th Avenue, Kearney, NE 68847, (308) 237-3542, BA 71 Kearney St Coll; MS 77 Kearney St Coll; Sp-Lang Path, Kearney Pub Sch, **SLP**

Koenigsberg, Linda R 235 North Long Street, Williamsville, NY 14221, (716) 837-2441, BS 76 SUNY - Coll at Geneseo; MA 79 SUNY - Center at Buffalo; Sp-Lang Path, Lang Dev Prog of W NY, **SLP**

Koenigsberger, Mrs Bobbie Ariz 927 Skeel Drive, Camarillo, CA 93010, (805) 482-8861, BA 70 Central WA Univ; MA 83 CA St Univ - Los Angeles; SLP, Pleasant Valley Sch Dist, **SLP**

Koenigsknecht, Dr Roy A 720 Gatehouse Lane, Worthington, OH 43085, (614) 888-8339, BA 64 Central MI Univ; MA 65 Northwestern Univ; PH 68 (NS) Northwestern Univ; 85–Dean of Grad Sch, Ohio St Univ, **SLP F**

Koepke, Sandra Hann 1902 Dial Court, Springfield, IL 62704, (217) 793-8619, BS 82 IL St Univ - Normal; MS 84 IL St Univ - Normal; 88–Sp-Lang Path, Springfield Sch Dist #186, **SLP**

Koepp-Baker, Dr Herbert Route 1 Box 308, Highlands, NC 28741, (704) 526-2244, BS 26 Univ of MI - Ann Arbor; MS 33 PA St Univ - Univ Park; PH 38 (NS) Univ of IA; Retired, So IL Univ, **SLP F H LM**

Koerbel, Jane McCann 6963 Newbury Circle, Wichita, KS 67226, (316) 686-8861, BA 80 Univ of Northern IA; MA 82 Univ of WI - Madison; Sp-Lang Path, Private Practice, **SLP**

Koerner, Sr Janet E 111 East 2nd Street, Fond Du Lac, WI 54935-4341, (414) 898-4208, OB 76 Southeast MO St Univ; MS 79 Univ of WI - Madison; Sp-Lang Path, New Holstein Public Schools, **SLP**

Koerner, Mrs Susanne L 105 High Pine Court, Cary, NC 27513, (919) 469-5265, BA 83 Univ of NC - Chapel Hill; MS 84 Univ of NC - Chapel Hill; 88–Sp-Lang Path, Chldn Spec Hlth Svc, **SLP**

Koerth, Rosemarie 950 Willow Glen Drive, Bethel Park, PA 15102, (412) 488-5673, BS 58 Univ of Pittsburgh - Pittsburgh; MA 61 NY Univ; Sp/Lang Path, South Side Hosp, **SLP**

Koessler, Mrs Susan Grace 2236 Old Colony Drive, York, PA 17402, (717) 741-4399, MA 82 OH Univ - Athens; 87–Sp-Lang Path, Community Progress Council Inc, **SLP**

Koester, Mrs Margaret M 1465 Dorthen, Grosse Pointe Woods, MI 48236, (313) 884-5314, BS 70 Marquette Univ; MS 74 MI St Univ; 87–Sp-Lang Path, Detroit Bd of Educ, **SLP**

Koffler, Lori H Sunshine School, 231-10 Hillside Avenue, Queens Village, NY 11437, (718) 468-9000, **SLP**

Kogen-Scharf, Mrs Kim 2801 North University Dr, Suite 101, Coral Springs, FL 33065, (305) 752-7760, BA 76 Emory Univ; MA 78 Univ of Miami; Sp-Lang Path, Private Practice, **SLP**

Kogler, Clare 1092 St Vincent Place, Santa Ana, CA 92705, (714) 832-8529, MA 74 CA St Univ - Fullerton; **SLP**

Koglin, Diane Campoli Audiological Health Services, 209 Glenwood Avenue, Port Huron, MI 48060, BA 76 MI St Univ; MA 78 MI St Univ; Aud, Audiological Hlth Serv, **A**

Kohama, Mrs Kathleen Albertoni 339 South Pomelo Apt F, Monterey Park, CA 91754, (818) 280-9021, BA 79 CA St Univ - Long Beach; MA 82 CA St Univ - Los Angeles; Sp-Lang Path, LA USD, **SLP**

Kohen, Francine P 5316 Ellsworth Avenue, Pittsburgh, PA 15232, (412) 681-4101, BA 76 Univ of Pittsburgh - Pittsburgh; MS 78 PA St Univ - Univ Park; Rehab Inst of Pittsburgh, **SLP**

Kohl, Mrs Cecilia M 624 Marine Avenue, Manhattan Beach, CA 90266, (213) 543-1223, BA 75 Univ of Redlands; MA 82 CA Lutheran Coll; Sp-Lang Path, L A Co Supt of Sch, **SLP**

Kohl, Mrs Cynthia Ann 26609 Julia Street, Wind Lake, WI 53185, (414) 895-7780, BS 74 Univ of WI - Whitewater; MS 81 Marquette Univ; **SLP**

Kohl, Mrs Evelyn P 3429 West Golden Lane, Phoenix, AZ 85051, BA 63 Minot St Univ; MS 65 Minot St Univ; **SLP LM**

Kohlbus, Mrs Carin Marie 19 Ann Pl, Quarryville, PA 17566, (301) 272-1470, MS 84 James Madison Univ; Sp-Lang Path, Harford County Pub Schs, **SLP**

Kohlenberger, Lisa Karen 3805 Forest Avenue, Yorba Linda, CA 92686, (714) 634-5168, BA 81 Univ of CA - Santa Barbara; MA 83 Northwestern Univ; Sp-Lang Path, Univ of CA Irvine Med Ctr, **SLP ACE**

Kohler, Polly Wagner 116-4 Deerhurst Lane, Webster, NY 14580, (716) 671-0710, BS 84 Nazareth Coll of Rochester; MS 85 Nazareth Coll of Rochester; **SLP**

Kohler, Dr R Ramon Box 3311 University Sta, Laramie, WY 82071, (307) 766-6426, BS 58 Brigham Young Univ; MS 61 Brigham Young Univ; PH 67 (Sp Path) Univ of UT; 79–Prof, U of Wyoming, **SLP**

Kohler, Susan 11744 Darlington Avenue, Apartment 102, Los Angeles, CA 90049, (602) 990-0037, BS 77 AZ St Univ; MS 79 AZ St Univ; Sp-Lang Path, Private Practice, **SLP**

Kohlin, Carol Marie 4420 North New England, Harwood Heights, IL 60656, (312) 425-6972, BS 85 Northern IL Univ - De Kalb; MA 87 Northern IL Univ - De Kalb; 88–Aud, Sound Resources Inc, **A**

Kohlman, Sandra N 140 Dodge Street, Helper, UT 84526, (801) 472-5405, BS 61 Univ of UT; MS 76 Univ of UT; Sp-Lang Path, **SLP**

Kohlmeyer, Anne M 1656 Bowling Green Drive, Lake Forest, IL 60045, (312) 295-1842, BS 86 Northwestern Univ; MA 87 Northwestern Univ

Kohn, Connie Rae 4901 Chalet Gardens Road, Apartment 211, Madison, WI 53711, (414) 241-5530, BS 85 Univ of WI - Stevens Point; MS 87 Univ of WI - Stevens Point; **SLP**

Kohn, Mrs Debra Glass 2202 East 28th Street, Brooklyn, NY 11229, (212) 743-0220, BS 73 SUNY - Center at Albany; MS 74 Adelphi Univ; SLP, NYC Bd of Ed, **SLP**

Kohn, Lawrence L 2605 Gregory Street, Madison, WI 53711, **SLP**

Kohn, Mrs Sybil W 19614 Gifford Street, Reseda, CA 91335, BA 65 Univ of CA - Berkeley; MA 77 CA St Univ - Northridge; SLP, Los Angeles USD, **SLP**

Kohner, Pamela K R R 3 Box 204, Elizabeth, WV 26143, (304) 275-4263, BA 67 Central MI Univ; MA 68 Northwestern Univ; MA 88 WV Univ; 81–Sp-Lang Path, Wirt Co Bd of Ed, **SLP**

Kohn-Lau, Annette M 1822 Kiest, Northbrook, IL 60062, (312) 696-6274, BA 74 Washington Univ; MA 76 Northwestern Univ; Sp/Lang Path, Lutheran Gen Hosp, **SLP**

Kohring, Mrs Sandra K 95 Bayard, Providence, RI 02906, (401) 272-6323, BS 68 Northwestern Univ; MA 70 Univ of MO - Columbia; Sp-Lang Path, Ctrl Falls Pub Sch, **SLP**

Kohrs, Charlotte 3876 Belmont Avenue, San Diego, CA 92116, (619) 281-0691, BA 30 Univ of WI - Madison; MA 38 Univ of CA - Berkeley; Owner/Mgr/Author, Creative Chldn Press, **SLP LM**

Kohtz, Mrs Jane K 2906 Hancock Place, Grand Island, NE 68803, (308) 384-5590, BA 75 Fort Hays St Univ; MA 77 Univ of KS; Sp-Lang Path, Grand Island Pub Sc, **SLP**

Kohut, Carrie Ann 16941 Green Street #8, Huntington Beach, CA 92649, (714) 241-6545, BA 82 CA St Univ - Long Beach; MA 84 CA St Univ - Los Angeles; Aud, Taft Hrng Impaired Sch, **A**

Kohut, Ellen Allen 3918 Modlin Avenue, Fort Worth, TX 76107, (904) 862-9199, ME 84 Southwest TX St Univ; SLP, Okaloosa County School System, **SLP**

Koike, Dr Kazunari J Speech-Lang Path & Audiology, University Of Utah, 1201 Behavioral Science, Salt Lake City, UT 84112, (801) 581-6725, BA 74 Sophia Univ - Japan; MA 77 Univ of TN - Knoxville; PH 81 (NS) Univ of TN - Knoxville; Asst Prof, U of UT, **A**

Koike, Mary A 3835 South 2780 East, Salt Lake City, UT 84109, (801) 272-1063, BS 72 Univ of TN - Knoxville; MA 80 Univ of TN - Knoxville; Audiologist, Utah School for the Deaf, **A**

Kojak, Mrs Dolores J 37 Carol Drive, Succasunna, NJ 07876, (201) 398-4400, BA 71 Newark St Coll; ME 78 William Paterson Coll; MA 72 Newark St Coll; 72–Sp-Lang Path, Mount Arlington Bd of Ed, **SLP ACE**

Kok, Mrs Jean H 10028 Alice Court, Oak Lawn, IL 60453, (312) 389-0555, BA 68 Chicago St Univ; MA 77 Governors St Univ; 71–Sp-Lang Path, Elim Christian Sch for Hndcpd, **SLP**

Kokot, Mrs Nadyne T Franklin School, 4215 Alder, East Chicago, IN 46312, (219) 391-4156, BA 61 IN Univ - Bloomington; MS 67 IN Univ - Bloomington; Dir-Finance, Sch Cty of E Chi, **SLP**

Kolano, S Kay Wiseman 1874 Deer Park Circle, Grand Junction, CO 81503, BS 70 WV Univ; MA 75 Marshall Univ; 88–Sp-Lang Path, Private Practice, **SLP**

Kolarov, Margaret 93 Seward Apartment 405, Detroit, MI 48202, (313) 927-7000, BA 76 Eastern MI Univ; MA 77 Eastern MI Univ; Doctoral /Admin, Wayne State Univ, **SLP**

Kolas, Christy 21090 Eaton Road, Fairview Park, OH 44126, (216) 251-3714, BS 53 Kent St Univ; MA 56 Kent St Univ; Sp-Lang Path/Audiologist, West Park Sp-Hrng Clinic, **SLP A**

Kolatch, Mrs Francine R 141-13 68th Drive, Flushing, NY 11367, (212) 920-5838, BA 51 CUNY - Hunter Coll; MA 82 CUNY - Queens Coll; SLP, Beth Abraham Hosp, **SLP**

Kolb, Jacqueline S 3312 West Amherst Road, Muncie, IN 47304, (317) 747-3772, BS 81 Ball St Univ; MA 82 Western IL Univ; 88–Sp-Lang Path, Ball Memorial Hosp, **SLP**

Kolb, Karen C 7600 West Military Drive, Lot 94, San Antonio, TX 78227, (512) 921-4750, BS 78 Southwest TX St Univ; ME 79 Southwest TX St Univ; 88–Sp-Lang Path, Harlandale ISD, **SLP**

Kolb, Maxine Angel 908 Ireland Avenue, Muskegon, MI 49445, (616) 759-8142, BS 73 1093; MS 78 Univ of MI - Ann Arbor; **SLP**

Kolbe, Joyce B P O Box 518, La Grange, TX 78945-0518, (512) 863-6048, BS 78 Univ of TX - Austin; ME 80 Southwest TX St Univ; **SLP**

Kolbeck, Mrs Cathleen M 4225 S W 314th Place, Federal Way, WA 98023, (619) 434-0219, BA 78 WA St Univ; MA 79 WA St Univ; **SLP**

Kolberg, Mrs Carolyn K 1086 Dyer Place, Laguna Beach, CA 92651, (714) 838-5440, BA 78 CA St Univ - Long Beach; MA 80 CA St Univ - Long Beach; SLP, Irvine USD, **SLP**

Kolbrenner, Mrs Susan G 66 Fawn Drive, Stamford, CT 06905, (203) 329-2517, BS 69 Southern CT St Univ; MA 71; MA 76 Southern CT St Univ; Sp-Lang Path, Norwalk Bd of Ed, **SLP**

Kolda, Sr Felice Marie 725 California Avenue, Santa Monica, CA 90403, (213) 395-1689, BA 57 Holy Names Coll; MA 64 Stanford Univ; 83–Aud, Hope for Hearing Foundation, **A**

Koleda, Carolyn M 7629 West Pearson, Washington, MI 48094, (313) 781-2673, BS 84 Central MI Univ; MA 85 Central MI Univ; 86–Sp-Lang Path, Hurley Med Ctr, **SLP**

Kolenovsky, Mrs Gladys W Texas Scottish Rite Hospital, 2222 Welborn, Dallas, TX 75219, (214) 559-7525, BA 73 Baylor Univ; MA 74 Univ of Denver; 76–Sp/Lang Path, TX Scottish Rite Hosp, **SLP**

Kolff, Andrew J Rt 2 Box 668, N9523 18th Avenue, Necedah, WI 54646, (608) 565-2659, BS 86 Univ of WI - Stevens Point; MS 88 Univ of WI - Stevens Point; 88–Sp-Lang Path, CESA #5

Kolker, Maura F 626 Harrison Avenue, East Meadow, NY 11554-3627, (516) 538-6720, BA 75 CUNY - Queens Coll; MA 77 Univ of MA - Amherst; Sp-Lang Path, Stepping Stone Day Sch Inc, **SLP**

Kollender, Mrs Rona P 1786 North Beverly Glen, Los Angeles, CA 90024, (213) 475-0376, BA 74 SUNY - Coll at Cortland; MA 77 CA St Univ - Fullerton; Owner/Dir, Private Practice, **SLP**

Koller, Donald E 5017 Hopewood Lane, Peoria, IL 61607, (309) 676-7611, BS 50 Bradley Univ; MA 53 Bradley Univ; Assoc Prof-Asst Dir, Bradley U, **SLP**

Koller, Jerry J 1038 East 3rd Street, Brooklyn, NY 11230, (718) 780-5186, BA 72 Yeshiva Univ; MA 74 CUNY - Lehman Coll; 87–Supvr of Clin Svcs, Brooklyn Coll, **SLP**

Kollia, Haralambia 304 Mulberry Street, Apartment 5H, New York, NY 10012, (212) 431-6334, BS 85 Univ of MN - Minneap-St Paul; MA 87 CUNY - Hunter Coll

Kollinger, Mrs Dorothy P 82 Tamenend Avenue, New Britain, PA 18901, (215) 348-2940, MA 84 Trenton St Coll; SLP, Bucks Co Intermediate Unit 22, **SLP**

Kollofski, Cindy 3515 S W Veterans Hosp Rd, Portland, OR 97201, (503) 228-6479, BA 78 Univ of MT; MA 80 Univ of MT; Aud, Portland Ctr for Hrng & Sp, **A**

Kolman, Dr Ira H 5712 Oakshire Road, Baltimore, MD 21209, (301) 664-0533, OM 74 Johns Hopkins Univ; MA 66 Univ of MD - College Park; OD 70 (NS) Johns Hopkins Univ; Dir, Hearing Resources, **SLP A**

Kolmodin, Sally J 1181 Termino #7105, Long Beach, CA 90815, (213) 483-9930, BS 84 Bradley Univ; MS 86 Rush Univ; **A**

Kolo, Mrs Lori E Solberg 10906 West Michigan Street, Milwaukee, WI 53226, (414) 463-4161, BS 82 Univ of WI - Milwaukee; MS 83 Univ of WI - Milwaukee; Sp-Lang Path, Mequon-Thiensville School Dist, **SLP**

Kolodny, Dr Marvin R 5 Sleepy Hollow Lane, Carmel, IN 46032-2051, (317) 925-7077, BA 67 CUNY - Queens Coll; MA 69 IN Univ - Bloomington; PH 74 (Aud) IN Univ - Bloomington; 88–Dir of Aud, Meridian Otology Lab, **A**

Kolpon, Mrs Suzanne W 1600 Grand Avenue #P1, Baldwin, NY 11510, (516) 546-9633, BS 78 SUNY - Center at Albany; MA 79 Hofstra Univ; 79–Sp-Lang Path, Island Trees Sch Dist, **SLP**

Kolsch, Angela M 8703 Banyan Way, Cape Canaveral, FL 32920, (305) 784-2572, MS 76 FL St Univ; Sp-Lang Path, Brevard Homecare, **SLP ACE**

Kolts, Mary Hoover P O Box 182, Ochelata, OK 74051, (918) 535-2501, BS 70 KS St Univ; MA 86 Univ of Tulsa; 86–Sp-Lang Path, Tri-Quad Spec Svcs Coop, **SLP**

Komarek, Rachel Ann 125 East Buffalo Street, Duluth, MN 55811, (218) 727-5083, BA 83 Univ of WI - Eau Claire; MA 85 Univ of MN - Duluth; **SLP**

Komarow, Patricia W 1210 North Farragut, Colorado Springs, CO 80909, (719) 578-9418, MS 72 Wichita St Univ; 88–Sp-Lang Path, Colorado Springs Dist 11 Schs, **SLP**

Komendat, Karen Ann 2612 Elmore Drive, Springfield, OH 45505, (513) 324-2081, BA 81 Univ of MI - Ann Arbor; MS 83 Univ of MI - Ann Arbor; Sp-Lang Path, W Ctrl Oh Hrng & Sp Cen, **SLP**

Komerous, Sharon Sahrmann 9133 Pennant Lane, St Louis, MO 63126, (314) 726-2460, BA 75 Saint Louis Univ; MA 77 Saint Louis Univ; Sp-Lang Path, Spec Sch Dist of St Louis Co, **SLP**

Komes, Linda W 945 Greensboro Court, Naperville, IL 60540, (312) 629-7272, BS 74 Eastern IL Univ; MS 74 Eastern IL Univ; Communication Development Cons, Dupage/W Cook Spec Educ Assoc, **SLP**

Kominsky, Mrs Perrie M Speech Pathology & Audiology, Illinois Masonic Med Ctr, 836 West Wellington, Chicago, IL 60657, (312) 975-1600, BS 69 Univ of IL - Urbana; MA 70 Northwestern Univ; Sp-Lang Path, Il Masonic Med Cen, **SLP**

Komisarof, Miriam S 16 Rolling Road, Overbrook Hills, Philadelphia, PA 19151, (215) 642-2396, BA 59 George Washington Univ; MA 63 Temple Univ; SLP, Sch Dist of Phila, **SLP**

Kommers, Mary S 519 Fairman Lane, Langhorne, PA 19047, (215) 757-4038, BA 73 Univ of NE - Lincoln; MA 74 Univ of IA; **SLP**

Komros-Hachenburg, Mrs Gail 16 Waterview Drive, Medway, MA 02053, (617) 429-6787, BS 76 Syracuse Univ; MA 78 SUNY - Coll at Buffalo; Sp-Lang Path, Private Practice, **SLP**

Konarska, Keith P 5961 Robin Hill Northeast, Belmont, MI 49306-9664, (616) 246-5173, BA 79 Central MI Univ; MA 80 Central MI Univ; ME 87 Grand Valley St Coll; 88–Dir/Ken-O-Sho Ctr, Grand Rapids Pub Sch, **SLP**

Konarska, Kevin A 3378 Keswick N E, Belmont, MI 49306, (616) 866-9665, BS 79 Central MI Univ; MA 80 Central MI Univ; Sp-Lang Path, Grand Rapids Public Schools, **SLP**

Konarska, Laurie Hughes 3378 Keswick N E, Belmont, MI 49306, (616) 866-9665, BS 80 Central MI Univ; MA 81 Central MI Univ; Sp-Lang Path, Greenville Public Schools, **SLP**

Koncen, Ruth Kay 1156 Kram Road, Creve Coeur, MO 63141, (314) 776-4320, BA 63 Fontbonne Coll; MA 71 Saint Louis Univ; Outreach Dir, Mo Sch for Blind, **SLP**

Konchan, Teresa Briguglio 110 Fisher Avenue #6A, Eastchester, NY 10709-2622, (212) 828-9000, BA 80 CUNY - Queens Coll; MA 83 CUNY - Queens Coll; SLP, NY League for Early Learning, **SLP**

Kondas, Lois Flavin Route 4 Box 4049, La Plata, MD 20646, (301) 645-6540, **SLP**

Kondis, Marilyn D 152 E Main Street 2nd Fl, Kutztown, PA 19530, (215) 562-6244, BS 73 Clarion Univ of PA; ME 80 Clarion Univ of PA; SLP, Hamburg Cen, **SLP**

Kondra, Jeanne Smith 150 Ocean Park Blvd #519, Santa Monica, CA 90405-3573, (213) 396-3974, BA 75 Jersey City St Coll; MA 81 Montclair St Coll; Sp-Lang Path, Private Practice, **SLP**

Kone, Chris Jay 4 Hoills Road, South Easton, MA 02375, **SLP**

Konefal, Dr Joanne 3417 Lincoln Road, Hattiesburg, MS 39401, (504) 986-2661, BA 67 Paterson St Coll; MA 72 OH St Univ; PH 81 (NS) OH Univ - Athens; SLP, Washington Parish Sch, **SLP**

Kongable, Trisha Marie 1021 N Fifth #2, Burlington, IA 52601, (319) 753-3384, BS 86 Northeast MO St Univ; MA 87 Northeast MO St Univ; 87–Sp-Lang Path, Burlington Med Ctr, **SLP**

Koniditsiotis, Dr Cornelia Y 1055 Homestead Avenue, Metairie, LA 70005, (504) 885-7929, BA 66 Univ of AL- Tuscaloosa; MA 68 Univ of AL- Tuscaloosa; PH 79 (NS) Univ of New Orleans; Sp-Lang Path/Counsellor, Private Practice, **SLP**

Konig, Diana G 900 Lydig Avenue, Bronx, NY 10462, (212) 870-6372, OB 84 SUNY - Center at Buffalo; MS 86 Columbia Univ Teachers Coll; **SLP**

Konikoff, Mrs Anita C 2312 Parklands Road, St Louis Park, MN 55416, (612) 871-8144, BA 75 MI St Univ; MA 76 MI St Univ; Aud, Park Nicollet Medcenters, **A**

Konitzer, Nancy McCue 251 Old Haymaker Road, Monroeville, PA 15146, (412) 664-2468, MS 82 IL St Univ - Normal; Sp-Lang Path, McKeesport Hosp, **SLP**

Konkle, Dr Dan F Dir Communication Disorder Ctr, Childrens Hosp Philadelphi, One Civic Center Boulevard, Philadelphia, PA 19104, (215) 596-9829, BS 65 Central MI Univ; MA 70 Central MI Univ; PH 75 (NS) MI St Univ; Dir/Commun Dis Cen, The Chldns Hosp of Phila, **A**

Konnerth, Lynn A 20 Chestnut Street #202, Malden, MA 02148-3631, (617) 979-7013, BA 73 Case Western Reserve Univ; MA 76 Univ of CT; 85–Sp-Lang Path, New England Memorial Hospital, **SLP**

Kononen, Mrs Patricia T 786 Highway 5 North, Woodstock, GA 30188, (404) 928-2910, BA 71 Kennesaw Coll; BS 73 Univ of GA; ME 74 Univ of GA; Sp-Lang Path, Cherokee Co Bd of Ed, **SLP**

Konopisos, Mrs Melinda J 25682 Nugget, El Toro, CA 92630, (714) 380-8781, BS 75 Marquette Univ; MS 76 Marquette Univ; **SLP**

Konopka, Mrs Glenda B 565 Covered Bridge Road, Greenwood, IN 46142, (317) 929-3311, BS 73 Northwestern Univ; MA 74 Northwestern Univ; 86–Sp-Lang Path, Methodist Hosp of Indiana, **SLP**

Konrad-Wood, Patricia 716 Kathy Court, Naperville, IL 60540-6369, (312) 355-9833, BS 75 Purdue Univ - West Lafayette; MS 77 Purdue Univ - West Lafayette; Owner, S/L Services, **SLP**

Konrath, Mrs Eileen Finucane 12097 West Jewell Drive, Lakewood, CO 80228, (303) 288-6881, BS 81 Nazareth Coll of Rochester; MA 84 Univ of CO - Boulder; 84–Sp-Lang Path, Mapleton Pub Schs, **SLP**

Kons, Jane Marie 202 West Main Street, Little Chute, WI 54140, (414) 433-8263, **SLP**

Konstam, Mrs Marilyn Leah 3 Olympia Lane, Monsey, NY 10952, (914) 423-9800, BA 73 CUNY - Brooklyn Coll; MA 82 NY Univ; **SLP**

Konz, Ruth A 7200 Leighton Avenue, Lincoln, NE 68507, (402) 464-8246, BS 63 Univ of NE - Lincoln; MA 65 Univ of NE - Lincoln; SLP, Lincoln Pub Sch, **SLP**

Konzen, Dolores Anne Marie 2107-D Sidneywood Road, West Carrollton, OH 45449, (513) 859-1934, BS 86 Miami Univ - Oxford; MS 87 Miami Univ - Oxford; 88–Sp-Lang Path, Dayton PS, **SLP**

Koocher, Aida Louise 32 Matthew Drive, Salem, NH 03079, (603) 893-9329, BA 77 Rutgers St Univ -N Brunswick; MA 79 Montclair St Coll; Sp-Lang Path, Salem Sch Dist, **SLP ACE**

Kools, Dr Joseph A 530 Holman Avenue #1, Athens, GA 30606, (404) 542-1685, BS 53 Marquette Univ; MA 56 Univ of IA; PH 66 (NS) Univ of IA; Assoc Prof-Sp-Lang Path, U of Georgia, **SLP**

Koonmen, Karin Elizabeth 1403 West Cuyler #2, Chicago, IL 60613, (312) 848-9750, BS 83 Bradley Univ; MA 85 Univ of IL - Urbana; **SLP**

Koonter, Martha M 3225 Alco, Pontiac, MI 48055, (313) 746-7350, BS 73 MI St Univ; MA 74 Northwestern Univ; Sp-Lang Path, Southfield Pub Schs, **SLP**

Kooper, Rebecca F 55 Monroe Boulevard #4-S, Long Beach, NY 11561, (516) 432-6085, BA 71 SUNY - Center at Buffalo; MA 73 SUNY - Center at Buffalo; OD 81 (NS) Pace U -Coll of White Plains; Aud, Nassau Co BOCES Hrng Imp Prog, **A**

Koopmans, Sherri Lynn 140 Park Place #2, Fort Thomas, KY 41075, (513) 948-2735, BS 84 IL St Univ - Normal; MA 86 Univ of IL - Urbana; 88–Sp-Lang Path, Daniel Drake Memorial Hosp, **SLP**

Kooy, Dr Linda Klesker 20084 Crescent Avenue, Lynwood, IL 60411, **SLP**

Kopay, Kathleen Naval Medical Clinic, San Francisco, CA 94130-5030, (415) 675-5975, MA 84 OH Univ - Athens; **A**

Kopecky, Adele 427 Hazel Drive, Corona Del Mar, CA 92625, (714) 261-0102, BA 73 CA St Univ - Fullerton; MA 74 CA St Univ - Fullerton; Sp-Lang Path, Sp Commun Assoc, **SLP**

Kopel, Lydia Ann 4575-L Northside Parkway, Atlanta, GA 30339, (404) 961-2151, BS 80 Indiana Univ of PA; ME 84 GA St Univ; 80–Sp-Lang Path, Clayton Co Bd of Educ, **SLP**

Kopelow, Nancie Lynn 246 Rennie Avenue, Venice, CA 90291, (213) 825-0118, BA 82 CA St Univ - Northridge; MA 84 CA St Univ - Northridge; **SLP**

Koperski, Ben Joseph Audiological Services, 721 Sheridan, Suite 100, Cody, WY 82414, (307) 527-6472, BS 72 Univ of NE - Lincoln; MA 73 Univ of NE - Lincoln; Aud, Coe Med Cen, **A**

Kopetsky, Marilyn Blick 116 East Glendale Avenue, Appleton, WI 54911, (414) 735-0232, BS 73 Univ of WI - Madison; MS 74 Univ of WI - Madison; Sp-Lang Path, Private Practice, **SLP**

Kopf, Karen P 44 Paumanake Road, Blue Point, NY 11715, (516) 363-5154, BS 77 SUNY - Coll at Geneseo; MS 79 Adelphi Univ; Sp-Lang Path, Little Village Sch, **SLP**

Kopff-Schaefer, Helen L 72 Russell Street, Hamden, CT 06517, (203) 789-8991, BA 81 Univ of VT; MA 82 Western MI Univ; Sp/Lang Path, Prospect Regional Sch Dist, **SLP**

Kopilow, Ellen D 1259 Capitol Drive #123, San Pedro, CA 90732, (213) 514-8363, BA 72 Univ of CO - Boulder; MA 74 Univ of Denver; Sp-Lang Path, LA Co Office of Education, **SLP**

Kopin, Sr Marie Central Michigan University, 448 Moore Hall, Mount Pleasant, MI 48859, (517) 774-3471, BS 59 Central MI Univ; MS 68 Univ of MI - Ann Arbor; Cl Superv-Sp-Lang Path, Central Mich Univ, **SLP ACE**

Kopmeier, Mrs Mary K 8395 North Pelican Lane, Milwaukee, WI 53209, (414) 355-3636, BS 69 Univ of WI - Stevens Point; MA 70 Univ of WI - Milwaukee; **SLP**

Kopp, Mrs Christine 6309 Swan Landing Court, Burke, VA 22015, (703) 451-1057, BA 75 Case Western Reserve Univ; MA 76 George Washington Univ; Sp-Lang Path, Pg Co Pub Sch, **SLP**

Kopp, Dr Harriet G 6711 Golfcrest Drive, San Diego, CA 92119, (619) 265-6775, BA 37 CUNY - Brooklyn Coll; MA 39 CUNY - Brooklyn Coll; PH 62 (NS) Columbia Univ Teachers Coll; 70–Prof, San Diego St U, **A F LM**

Kopp, Irene Rudzinski 83 Nevin Road, South Weymouth, MA 02190, (617) 749-2180, **SLP**

Kopp, Mrs Margaret B 6921 N W 15th Street, Fort Lauderdale, FL 33313, (305) 792-1285, BA 75 Montclair St Coll; MS 76 Rutgers St Univ -N Brunswick; Clinical Supervisor, InSpeech Inc, **SLP ACE**

Koppel, Mrs Tina R 149 Hampton Road, Sharon, MA 02067, (617) 784-2129, BS 70 Univ of MI - Ann Arbor; MS 71 Emerson Coll; 88–Sp-Lang Path, Judith Wisnia & Assoc, **SLP**

Koppelman, Mark Lee Dept Of Otolaryngology-Aud Ser, TX Chldrns St Lukes Hosp, P O Box 20269 6621 Fannin, Houston, TX 77225, (713) 791-4440, BS 71 Univ of ND; MS 72 Univ of ND; Aud, Texas Chldn St Lukes Hosp, **A**

Kopra, Dr Lennart L Department Of Speech, University Of Texas, Austin, TX 78712, (512) 471-3841, BA 51 Wittenberg Univ; MA 52 Northwestern Univ; PH 54 (Aud) Northwestern Univ; Professor Emeritus, U of TX/Austi, **A F**

Kopra, Leonard F 40 Honorine, Depew, NY 14043, **SLP**

Koprowski, Pamela A N 7562 Buckingham Drive, St Louis, MO 63105, **A**

Kopsch, Janet H 10319 William Penn Lane, Matthews, NC 28105, BA 67 Univ of MI - Ann Arbor; MA 69 Univ of Northern IA; **SLP**

Kopun, Mrs Judy G 555 North 30th Street, Omaha, NE 68132, (402) 498-6536, BS 82 Univ of MN - Minneap-St Paul; MA 85 Univ of MN - Minneap-St Paul; 85–Aud, Boys Town Natl Inst, **A**

Korabic, Dr Edward W Marquette University, Speech Pathology-Audiology, College Of Speech, Milwaukee, WI 53233, (414) 224-5190, BS 72 Siena Coll; MA 74 Coll of Saint Rose; PH 81 (Aud) Syracuse Univ; Asst Prof, Marquette U, **A**

Korany, Mrs Dielynda Sue 3620 Rookshire Drive, Trenton, MI 48183, (313) 671-6116, MA 88 Eastern MI Univ; 88–Sp-Lang Path, Beyer Memorial Hosp

Korb, Mrs Loree Vivatson 13304 Cardinal Creek Road, Eden Prairie, MN 55344-5223, (612) 937-5913, BS 74 Univ of ND; MS 77 Univ of WI - Eau Claire; **SLP**

Korczynski, Mrs Beth Ann 1300 Rusnak Trail, Broadview Heights, OH 44147, (216) 526-2276, BS 80 PA St Univ - Univ Park; MA 84 Cleveland St Univ; Sp-Lang Path, Parma City School District, **SLP**

Kordek, Dolores A Audiology Associates Of Az, 1901 East Thomas, Suite 100, Phoenix, AZ 85016, (602) 279-9030, BA 68 TX Tech Univ; MS 69 Univ of HI - Manoa; Exec Dir, Aud Assoc of AZ, **A**

Kordell, Karen Ann 14816 Rocking Spring Drive, Rockville, MD 20853, (301) 972-3327, BA Univ of MD - College Park; MA 85 Univ of MD - College Park; **A**

Korek, Pamela Jean 870 Buttercup Road, Carlsbad, CA 92009, (619) 431-9277, BS 83 Univ of WI - Milwaukee; MS 85 Univ of WI - Milwaukee; Sp-Lang Path, Carlsbad USD, **SLP**

Korenvaes, Cynthia B 9000 S W 51th Street, Miami, FL 33165, **SLP**

Korf, Mrs Patricia C 95 Huntington Place, Colorado Springs, CO 80906, (719) 520-2285, BS 67 Northeast MO St Univ; MA 74 Univ of MO - Columbia; Sp-Lang Path, Colorado Sprgs Sch Dist #11, **SLP**

Korkes, Nancy L 1790 East 22nd Street, Brooklyn, NY 11229, (212) 741-7698, BS 84 NY Univ; ME 86 Univ of VA - Charlottesville; 86–Sp-Lang Path, NY League for the Hard of Hearing, **SLP**

Korman, Arlene C 4106 West Touhy, Lincolnwood, IL 60646, (312) 677-4957, MA 76 Univ of IL - Urbana; Sp-Lang Path, Stratford Sch, **SLP**

Korman, Darlene Marie 22410 Champaign, Taylor, MI 48180, (312) 450-2139, BS Eastern MI Univ; MA 85 Eastern MI Univ; **SLP**

Korman, Rebecca B 20 West Bridlewood Trail, Durham, NC 27713, **SLP**

Korn, Jeffrey Michael 141-D La Bonne Vie Dr West, East Patchogue, NY 11772, (516) 654-5249, BA 80 CUNY - Queens Coll; MS 82 SUNY - Coll at Buffalo; Sp-Lang Path, South Country PS, **SLP**

Kornberg, Michelle Caren 304 East 65th Street, Apartment 12B, New York, NY 10021, (516) 921-7650, BA 82 Syracuse Univ; MA 86 Hofstra Univ; 87–Dir-Sp-Lang Path, Nassau Ctr for Dev Disabled, **SLP**

Kornberg, Stanley Saul 20 Doone Drive, Syosset, NY 11791, (212) 683-6970, BA 67 CUNY - Queens Coll; OM 72 Saint John's Univ - Jamaica; MA 87 Long Island U - CW Post Ctr; 85–Sp-Lang Path, NY Bd of Educ

Kornblatt, Mrs Debra Fink 42 Witherspoon Court, Wayne, PA 19087, (215) 925-2717, BS 81 PA St Univ - Univ Park; MA 83 George Washington Univ; Sp-Lang Path, Ai Dupont I, **SLP**

Kornbluth, Joanne Z 161 Evergreen Place, Teaneck, NJ 07666, (201) 833-1239, BS 76 SUNY - Center at Albany; MS 78 Columbia Univ Teachers Coll; Sp-Lang Path, Private Practice, **SLP**

Kornburg, Mrs Caroline Semler 5250 Southwest Landing Dr, Apartment 205-B1, Portland, OR 97201, (503) 279-8356, BA 84 Univ of Southern CA; MS 87 Portland St Univ; 88–Sp-Lang Path, Emanuel Hosp, **SLP**

Kornegay, Mrs Lisa Felterman P O Box 177, 1519 Main Street, Patterson, LA 70392, (504) 384-8355, BA 80 Nicholls St Univ; OM 82 LA St Univ - N O Medical Ctr; 83–Sp/Lang Path, St Mary Parish Sch Bd, **SLP**

Korneliussen, Barbara Ann Hatleberg Studenthjem, 5035 Bergen, Sandviken, Norway, MS 83 ID St Univ; **SLP**

Kornell, Mrs Tamara Ann 8028 Glenoak Parkway, Fort Wayne, IN 46815, (219) 485-1231, BS 83 Ball St Univ; MA 85 Ball St Univ; 87–Aud, Beltone Hearing Aid Ctr, **A**

Kornet, Renee H 29 Delaware Avenue, Jericho, NY 11753, (212) 520-7358, BA 76 CUNY - Queens Coll; MA 78 CUNY - Queens Coll; Adjunct Lecturer, Queens Coll Sp & Hrng Cen, **SLP**

Kornfield, Mrs Roberta T 5989 Meadow Lark Lane, East Petersburg, PA 17520, (717) 560-0441, BS 75 Indiana Univ of PA; MS 76 PA St Univ - Univ Park; Priv Pract, **SLP**

Korngold, Mrs Debra L 101 Dalton Terrace, Cherry Hill, NJ 08003, MS 77 Rutgers St Univ -N Brunswick; SLP, Cherry Hill Board of Education, **SLP**

Kornhaber, Arlene Cohen 44 Gentry Drive, Englewood, NJ 07631, (212) 379-5020, BA 76 CUNY - Queens Coll; MS 77 Columbia Univ Teachers Coll; Dir-Sp&Hrng, Hebrew Hosp for Chronic Sick, **A**

Kornhauser, Debora S 15735-A 26th Avenue North, Plymouth, MN 55447, (612) 472-1600, BS 75 Miami Univ - Oxford; MA 76 MI St Univ; SLP, Westonka Sch Dist #277, **SLP**

Kornkven, Colleen 403 West 10th Street, Bottineau, ND 58318, (701) 228-3114, BS 70 Minot St Univ; MS 71 Minot St Univ; Sp/Lang Path, Belcourt Sch Dist, **SLP**

Kornov, James J 4621 South Cedar Lake Road, Minneapolis, MN 55416, (612) 755-8220, BA 61 Saint Cloud St Univ; MA 68 Saint Cloud St Univ; Consultant, Anoka-Hennepin Dist #11, **SLP**

Kornsweig, Mrs Carole Linda 35 Cloverfield Road South, Valley Stream, NY 11581, (516) 791-7904, BA 72 SUNY - Center at Albany; MA 74 Queens Coll; Sp-Lang Path, Private Practice, **SLP**

Korona, Karen Joyce 3560 East Orchard Road, Littleton, CO 80121, (303) 850-0689, Sp-Lang Path, Private Practice, **SLP**

Korosa, Mrs Luan Davidson 4548 Rex Lake Drive, Akron, OH 44319, (216) 896-2341, BA 75 Kent St Univ; MA 77 Univ of Akron; Sp-Lang Path, Green Local Sch, **SLP**

Korpela, Mrs Shirley M 5163 Bobs Court South, Salem, OR 97306, (503) 399-3173, BS 52 Univ of OR; Sp-Lang Path, Salem Pub Sch, **SLP**

Korsgard, Mrs Susan Victoria 1837 Prentiss Drive, Downers Grove, IL 60516, (312) 852-6288, **A**

Korte, Carol Lynn 7594 Watson Road Apartment 301, St Louis, MO 63119, (314) 962-4678, BS 86 Central MI Univ; MA 87 Central MI Univ; 88–Sp-Lang Path, Deaconess Hosp, **SLP**

Korte, Solveig Sperati 2130 Grant, Blair, NE 68008, (402) 426-2145, BA 74 Luther Coll; MA 79 OH Univ - Athens; 88–Sp-Lang Path, Blair Comm Schs, **SLP**

Kortekamp, Mrs Carol W 6997 Queensway Lane, Cincinnati, OH 45230, BS 60 Miami Univ - Oxford; ME 84 Univ of Cincinnati; SLP, Sycamore Comm Schools, **SLP**

Korth, Gail Dennison 259 Sherwood Place, Stratford, CT 06497, (203) 377-4874, BA 74 Gettysburg Coll; MS 86 Southern CT St Univ; Dir of Sp-Lang, UCP Special Needs Center, **SLP**

Kortyka, Mrs Alice Ann 5253 Bear Lake Drive, East Lansing, MI 48823, (517) 332-0149, MS 81 MI St Univ; 83–Aud, Edward Berg, **A**

Korwatch, Yvonne N P O Box 695, Boothbay Harbor, ME 04538, (207) 633-6622, BS 74 Univ of KY; ME 75 Union Coll; MS 76 Univ of Cincinnati; 88–Sp-Lang Path, Private Practice, **SLP**

Korza, Laurie Jane 30 Grant Avenue, Northampton, MA 01060, (413) 584-8271, BS 80 Univ of MA - Amherst; MA 84 Univ of MA - Amherst; 86–Sp-Lang Path, Pioneer Valley Head Injury Ctr, **SLP**

Korzeniowski, Mrs Roxanne F 11912 Weatherby Road, Los Alamitos, CA 90720, (213) 538-8414, BA 61 Univ of CA - Los Angeles; MA 64 Univ of CA - Los Angeles; VP-Oper, Pace Therapy Inc, **SLP**

Kos, Sue Dusenbery Grant Wood Area Education Agency #10, 200 Holiday Road, Coralville, IA 52241, (319) 656-2621, BS 81 IA St Univ; MA 83 Univ of IA; Sp-Lang Path, Grant Wood AEA #10, **SLP**

Kos, Susanne 1000 North Davis Suite D, Arlington, TX 76012, (817) 261-7484, MA 75 Univ of North TX; Aud, Private Practice, **A**

Kosary, Therese Ann 320 Mary Street, San Marcos, TX 78666, (512) 392-9904, MS 87 Southwest TX St Univ; 88–Sp-Lang Path, Sequin ISD, **SLP**

Kosater, Leigh Bowen 5155 Holly Springs Drive, Douglasville, GA 30135, (404) 942-2427, BS 81 Univ of GA; ME 84 Univ of GA; Sp-Lang Path, Douglas Co Bd of Ed, **SLP**

Koschkee, Danna L Dept Communicative Disorders, University Of Wisconsin, 1975 Willow Drive, Madison, WI 53706, BS 73 Northern IL Univ - De Kalb; MA 74 Northern IL Univ - De Kalb; Cl Instr, U of WI - Madison, **SLP**

Koschmann, Dawn Arleen Dept Of Aus Heavilon Hall, Purdue University, West Lafayette, IN 47907, (317) 494-3789, BS 83 Univ of South AL; MS 85 Univ of WI - Stevens Point; Aud, Purdue, **A**

Koschnitzke, Carol D 8550 Roosevelt, Taylor, MI 48180, (313) 295-5801, BS 74 Wayne St Univ; MA 75 Wayne St Univ; Sp-Lang Path, Taylor Pub Sch, **SLP**

Kosek, Steven Sister Kenny Institute, Dept Of Speech Pathology, Chicago At 27th, Minneapolis, MN 55407, (612) 863-4407, BA 73 Saint Cloud St Univ; MS 74 Saint Cloud St Univ; Sp-Lang Path, Sister Kenny Inst, **SLP**

Kosel, Denise A PO Box 425, Placentia, CA 92670, (714) 524-7804, BA 80 CA St Univ - Fresno; MA 82 CA St Univ - Fresno; Sp-Lang Path, Private Practice, **SLP**

Koser, Larry A 16702 Castle Fraser Drive, Houston, TX 77084, (713) 463-8919, BA 78 Univ of Houston - Univ Park; MA 82 Univ of Houston - Univ Park; SLP, Memorial Hospital System, **SLP**

Kos-Flanagan, Mrs Stephanie Jo 204 Parsonage Hill, Northford, CT 06472, (203) 669-5723, BS 85 Univ of RI; MS 87 Southern CT St Univ; 87–Sp-Lang Path, Clinton PS Sys

Kosh, Mrs Zelda H 4041 North 41st Street, Arlington, VA 22207, (703) 538-4032, BA 33 Adelphi Univ; MA 34 Columbia Univ Teachers Coll; Sp-Lang Path, Private Practice, **SLP LM**

Koshak, Karen K P O Box 177, Cascade, CO 80809, (719) 684-2506, BA 77 Univ of CO - Boulder; MA 79 Univ of Northern CO; Sp-Lang Path, El Paso County School Dist 11, **SLP**

Koshnick, Tami Rose 2823 Case Avenue, Bradenton, FL 34207, (813) 753-8941, OB 83 Governors St Univ; OM 85 Governors St Univ; Sp-Lang Path, Mediplex Rehab-Bradenton, **SLP**

Kosinski, Mrs Diane T 23 Columbia, Park Ridge, IL 60068, (312) 647-9752, BA 75 Northeastern IL Univ; MA 77 Northern IL Univ - De Kalb; SLP, Niles Pub Elem Sch, **SLP**

Kosinski, Patricia Jean 108 Stonecliff Court, Stone Mountain, GA 30083, (404) 498-2743, BA 73 Marshall Univ; MA 74 Marshall Univ; Sp-Lang Path, Speech and Language Services, **SLP**

Koski, Kathleen M 503 Rosemere Lane #1, Maquoketa, IA 52060, (319) 652-5621, BA 81 Augustana Coll; MS 82 Eastern IL Univ; 85–Sp-Lang Path, Mississippi Bend AEA, **SLP**

Koski, Ruby Vitalis 9363 Wentlock Road, Woodbury, MN 55125, (612) 731-8665, BS 70 Univ of WI - River Falls; OM 86 Univ of WI - River Falls; **SLP**

Koski, Mrs Sandra Jennings 2125 Golfside #B-107, Ypsilanti, MI 48197-1355, (313) 434-1411, BS 84 Eastern MI Univ; MA 85 Eastern MI Univ; 87–Sp-Lang Path, Rainbow Tree Ctr Inc, **SLP**

Koskus, Dr Michael W Burns Clinic Medical Center, 560 West Mitchell, Petoskey, MI 49770, (616) 347-7000, BA 64 MI St Univ; ME 68 Wayne St Univ; PH 79 (NS) Wayne St Univ - Sch of Med; Dir of Aud, Burns Cl Med Cen Pc, **A**

Kosmo, Helen L P O Box 32, Lincolnville, ME 04849, **SLP**

Kosoff, Tess O 209 Berkeley Drive, Syracuse, NY 13210, (315) 472-3711, BS 54 Syracuse Univ; MA 62 Syracuse Univ; OM 74 Syracuse Univ; Adj Instr, Onondaga Co Comm Coll, **SLP**

Kososki, Carrie Lee Saint Joseph's General Hospital, 70 Spine Road, Elliot Lake, ON, Canada P5A 1X2, (705) 848-8140, MA 87 Northern MI Univ; 87–Dir Sp-Lang Path, St Joseph's General Hosp, **SLP**

Kosowsky, Alice Puchalsky 35 Barrett Street, Hamden, CT 06517, (203) 287-1390, BA 76 Univ of CT; MA 79 Univ of CT; MS 82 Purdue Univ - West Lafayette; **SLP**

Koss, Mrs Anita Diamond 46 Yarmouth Bluffs, Yarmouth, ME 04096, (207) 282-7504, BS 83 Ithaca Coll; MS 84 Boston Univ; Sp-Lang Path, York Co Counseling Services, **SLP ACE**

Koss, Lynn C R 219 Locksley Road, Syracuse, NY 13224, (315) 446-0227, BS 73 SUNY - Center at Binghamton; MS 78 Syracuse Univ; Sp-Lang Path, Private Practice, **SLP**

Koss, Penny Sue 2111 Michie Drive #32, Charlottesville, VA 22901, (804) 977-2076, BS 85 Univ of VA - Charlottesville; ME 87 Univ of VA - Charlottesville; 87–Sp-Lang Path, Charlottesville City Schs, **SLP**

Kossel, Mrs Sylvia K 5175 Monches Road, Colgate, WI 53017, (418) 628-4529, BS 73 Marquette Univ; MS 76 Marquette Univ; Sp-Lang Path, Germantown Pub Sch, **SLP**

Kossick, Laurie Ann 1911 Hualalai #302, Hilo, HI 96720, (808) 935-4760, BA 77 Grand Valley St Coll; MA 85 Eastern MI Univ; **SLP**

Kossover-Wechter, Denise 2244 Southwest Vermont St, Portland, OR 97219, BA 77 SUNY - Center at Buffalo; ME 88 Lewis & Clark Coll; Aud, **A**

Kosta, Dr Joan C 297 Engle Street, Tenafly, NJ 07670, (201) 967-4040, OB 62 Ithaca Coll; MA 65 Columbia Univ Teachers Coll; ED 72 (Sp Path) Columbia Univ Teachers Coll; Dir Sp & Hrng Cen, Bergen Pines Co Hosp, **SLP ACE**

Kostakis, Cynthia 12045 East Bay Drive #321, Largo, FL 34641, (813) 585-0975, BA 84 Rutger's St Univ - Douglas Coll; MA 86 Univ of FL; **SLP**

Koste, Marilyn B 1347 Gasparilia Drive, Fort Myers, FL 33901, **SLP**

Kostecki, Cami Alayne 3736 West 45th Street, Casper, WY 82604, (307) 577-6730, BS 83 CO St Univ; MS 85 CO St Univ; 87–Aud, Natrona Co Sch Dist #1, **A**

Kostek, Mary J 7 Evergreen Circle, Wilbraham, MA 01095, BA; MA 72 Univ of MA - Amherst; Sp-Lang Path, Springfield PS, **SLP**

Koster, Marilyn H 2030 Norway, Ann Arbor, MI 48104-6204, (313) 429-1596, BA 71 Eastern MI Univ; MS 72 Eastern MI Univ; 74–Dir-Sp & Lang Prog, Speech & Communication Services, **SLP**

Kostes-Fiorella, Ellen H 11 Arbor Lane, Merrick, NY 11566, (516) 581-1600, BA 75 CUNY - Hunter Coll; MA 78 CUNY - Hunter Coll; Sp-Lang Path, E Islip Sch Dist, **SLP**

Kostis, Sandy Hughes 19628 Back Nine Drive, Boca Raton, FL 33498, (305) 487-2311, MS 84 Univ of AL-Tuscaloosa; Sp-Lang Path, Tuscaloosa Co Boe, **SLP**

Kostka, Mrs Candice E 9 Towantic Hill Road, Oxford, CT 06483, (203) 888-4752, BS 79 Long Island U - CW Post Ctr; MS 80 Southern CT St Univ; Sp-Lang Path, Waterbury Bd of Ed, **SLP**

Kostrzeba, Susan Marie 2008 N Sturdy Road, Valparaiso, IN 46383, (219) 465-7808, MS 82 Purdue Univ - West Lafayette; Cl Coord Instr, Valparaiso U, **SLP**

Kostura, Michelle Marie 3517 East 46th Street, Cleveland, OH 44105, (216) 441-2932, MA 88 Cleveland St Univ

Kostyshock, Linda Marie R R #3 Box 75, Edwardsville, IL 62025, (618) 656-1182, BS 85 Southern IL Univ-Edwardsvill; MS 86 Southern IL Univ-Edwardsvill; **SLP**

Kosuda, Mrs Maria A Charlotte Rehabilitation Hosp, 1100 Blythe Boulevard, Charlotte, NC 28203, (704) 338-4430, BS 75 FL St Univ; MS 76 FL St Univ; Sp-Lang Path, Charlotte Rehab Hosp, **SLP**

Koszczuk, Georgette 1469 Ashland Avenue #3-N, Des Plaines, IL 60016, (312) 696-6274, BS 79 IL St Univ - Normal; MS 80 IL St Univ - Normal; Aud, Lutheran Gen Hosp, **A**

Koszykowski, Mrs Karen Elizabeth Brumley Apartment D2-8, Stillwater, OK 74074, (405) 258-0850, BS 83 OK St Univ; MA 85 OK St Univ; **SLP**

Kotacska, Rosina M G 42 Davenport Road, Big Flats, NY 14814, (607) 562-7549, BA 73 Newark St Coll; MA 80 SUNY - Coll at Geneseo; Sp/Lang Path, Steuben Allegany BOCES, **SLP**

Kotek, Mrs Beth Schuldiner 15-15 Alden Terrace, Fair Lawn, NJ 07410, (212) 920-5445, BA 79 Rutgers St Univ -N Brunswick; MS 81 Columbia Univ Teachers Coll; Sp-Lang Path, Montefiore Med Cen-Sp&Hrng Cen, **SLP ACE**

Kotelnicki-Martin, Deborah Joann 3520 Washington Pike #404, Bridgeville, PA 15017-1065, (412) 941-4434, BS 82 Indiana Univ of PA; MS 83 Indiana Univ of PA; Sp-Lang Path/Reg Coord, Crossroads Speech and Hearing, **SLP**

Koth, Margaret A 220 Lowell Hall, 610 Langdon Street, Madison, WI 53703, (608) 836-1045, BS 75 Univ of WI - Stevens Point; MA 78 Univ of FL; 85–Prog Coord, UW-Madison

Kothe, James Donald 2000 Friendship Lane, Burnsville, MN 55337, (612) 892-3499, BA 79 Univ of WI - Eau Claire; MS 81 Univ of WI - River Falls; Reg Mktg Dir, Oticon Corp, **A**

Kothe, Sylvia Lynn 2000 Friendship Lane, Burnsville, MN 55337, (612) 892-1150, **A**

Kotis, Christine Kelly 5213 South Maudelayne Drive, Mobile, AL 36693, (205) 661-6975, BS 83 Univ of South AL; MS 85 Univ of South AL; Sp-Lang Path, Knollwood Long Term Care Hosp, **SLP**

Kotkas, Karen P 63 Gray Road N Yarmouth, Cumberland Center, ME 04021, **SLP**

Kotler, Ava-Lee 115 Eglinton Avenue West, Apartment 26, Toronto, ON, Canada M4R 1A4, (416) 493-8693, BA 84 Univ of Western Ontario; MS 86 Purdue Univ - West Lafayette; 86–Sp-Lang Path, Hugh MacMillan Med Ctr, **SLP**

Kotler, Mrs Sheila B 16 Salisbury Court, Holmdel, NJ 07733, (201) 264-5578, BA 63 Montclair St Coll; MA 81 Monmouth Coll; Sp-Lang Path, Marlboro Bd of Educ, **SLP**

Kotorac, Rita Erlbaum 471 Sierra Vista Lane, Valley Cottage, NY 10989, (914) 358-0509, BS 77 SUNY - Center at Albany; MA 80 NY Univ; 83–Sp-Lang Path, First Step Early Childhood Cen, **SLP**

Kottenstette, Claire M 2736 South Pennsylvania St, Englewood, CO 80110, (303) 690-7972, BA 77 Univ of Denver; MA 78 Univ of Denver; Sp/Lang Path, Cherry Creek Sch Dist #5, **SLP**

Kottman, Yvette Fischbach 515 Buckeye Lane, Napoleon, OH 43545, (419) 278-3050, BS 82 Bowling Green St Univ; MA 83 Bowling Green St Univ; Sp-Lang Path, Henry Co Bd Ment Ret/Dev Disab, **SLP**

Kotula, Carol A 4 Townridge Court #E, Baltimore, MD 21236, (301) 668-0291, BS 76 Towson St Univ; MS 77 Loyola Coll; Sp-Lang Path, Baltimore Co Bd of Ed, **SLP**

Kotula, Mrs Heather Bloecher 4625 Saratoga Avenue, Downers Grove, IL 60515, (312) 532-1771, BS 78 IN Univ - Bloomington; MA 79 IN Univ - Bloomington; Sp-Lang Path, District 146 Tinley Park II, **SLP**

Kotula, Mrs Nora R 235 Gaywood Road, Baltimore, MD 21212, (301) 396-9381, BA 75 Loyola Coll; MS 76 Loyola Coll; Sp-Lang Path, Baltimore Cty Pub Sch, **SLP**

Kotula, Ona C 1092 Lane Avenue, Phoenixville, PA 19460, (215) 363-2532, BS 81 West Chester St Coll; OM 86 Hahnemann Univ Grad Sch; SLP, Dr Alfred Mauriello, **A**

Kouba-Monda, Mrs Virginia A 1680 N W 14th Drive, Gresham, OR 97030, (503) 666-3019, BS 75 Portland St Univ; MS 77 Western OR St Coll; Sp-Lang Path, Portland Public Schools, **SLP**

Koudelka, Garry Anthony 2826 North Main #3, Flagstaff, AZ 86002, (602) 289-3107, MS 83 Northern AZ Univ; SLP, Winslow Uni Schls #1, **SLP**

Koudelka, Teri 426 Springboro Lane, Worthington, OH 43085, (614) 431-5443, BA 84 OH St Univ; MA 86 OH St Univ; **A**

Koupal, Mrs Margaret Thomson 181 Fairway Circle, Norwalk, OH 44857, (419) 668-8101, BS 70 Univ of WI - Whitewater; MS 76 Univ of WI - Whitewater

Kouri, Theresa A 607 North Water Street, Kent, OH 44240-2446, (216) 672-2672, MS; PH 88 (Sp-Lang Path) Kent St Univ; 88–Postdoctoral Fellow, Akron Children's Hosp, **SLP**

Koury, Laurie Nash 860 Murfreesboro Road #J-5, Nashville, TN 37217-1105, (615) 865-3489, BS 79 Syracuse Univ; MS 80 SUNY - Center at Albany; MA 86 SUNY - Center at Buffalo; 87–Sp-Lang Path, Nashville Memorial Hosp, **SLP**

Koury-Parker, Dr Danielle I 630 Bittersweet Road, Center Valley, PA 18034, (215) 791-5020, BS 66 Bloomsburg Univ of PA; MS 71 SUNY - Coll at Geneseo; PH 83 (Comm Disorders) Northwestern Univ; Dir of QA, InSpeech Inc, **SLP**

Koussa, Mrs Therese 22 Sylvan Avenue, Cranston, RI 02905, (416) 785-0976, BA 81 Southern CT St Univ; MA 83 SUNY - Center at Buffalo; 88–Aud, Cranston Aud & Lab Svcs, **A**

Koutstaal, Dr Cornelis W 21736 Cheswold Lane, Saugus, CA 91350, MS 63 Springfield Coll; PH 66 (NS) Case Western Reserve Univ; Exec Dir, Delano Med Corp, **SLP A**

Kovac, Lisa Barone 30 Fawn Ridge, Millwood, NY 10546, (914) 941-3435, BA 81 SUNY - Coll at Cortland; MA 83 Hofstra Univ; Sp-Lang Path, Mamaroneck Sch Dist, **SLP**

Kovacevic, Mrs Jan D 12559 Cross Ridge Way, Germantown, MD 20874, (301) 694-1620, BA 83 PA St Univ - Univ Park; MS 86 Loyola Coll; 86–Sp-Lang Path, Frederick Co Bd of Educ, **SLP**

Kovach, Pamela Gay 131 Auburn Avenue, Colombus AFB, MS 39701, (601) 434-9352, BS 85 Valdosta St Coll; ME 86 Valdosta St Coll; Sp-Lang Path, W Phoenix Sp/Lang Rehab Agency Inc, **SLP**

Kovach, Therese M 1759 South Lee Street #C, Lakewood, CO 80226, (303) 861-6800, BA 72 Univ of CO - Boulder; MA 74 Univ of CO - Boulder; Sp-Lang Path, The Children's Hosp, **SLP**

Kovacic, James 315 W 8th Street #3, Erie, PA 16502, (814) 453-5602, BS 82 Indiana Univ of PA; MS 84 CA Univ of PA; **SLP**

Kovacik, Mrs Dawn R 216 Poppy Lane, Plainfield, IL 60544, (815) 744-3550, BS 79 Ball St Univ; MA 80 Ball St Univ; Aud, Joliet Audio Vestibular Lab In, **A**

Kovacs, Colleen Braden 115 Milton Circle, Lititz, PA 17543, (717) 569-8262, BS 73 OH St Univ; MA 82 OH St Univ; 83–Sp-Lang Path, Lancaster-Lebanon Iu 13, **SLP**

Kovacs, Mrs Kathleen Ann 5377 Burning Tree, Kalamazoo, MI 49002, (616) 385-0785, BS 69 Eastern MI Univ; MA 80 Western MI Univ; Sp-Lang Path, Kalamazoo Pub Sch, **SLP**

Kovalovich, Andrew RD #2 Box 289, Johnstown, NY 12095, (315) 724-5101, BS 83 SUNY - Coll at Geneseo; MA 87 SUNY - Center at Buffalo; 88–Aud, Chldrn Hosp & Rehab Ctr-Utica, **A**

Kovar, Nancy Christine 5607 Palatine Place N, Seattle, WA 98103, (206) 591-6763, BA 81 Univ of MI - Ann Arbor; MS 83 Univ of MI - Ann Arbor; Sp-Lang Path, St Joseph Hosp, **SLP**

Kovarik, Anne M P O Box 4933, San Jose, CA 95125, (408) 268-5105, BA 81 Univ of Northern CO; MA 82 Univ of Northern CO; Sp-Lang Path, Santa Clara Office of Educ, **SLP**

Kovars, Mrs Louise J 3528 Lynn Hill Road, Nekoosa, WI 54457, (715) 886-3771, BS 69 Univ of WI - Stevens Point; MS 75 Univ of WI - Stevens Point; Sp-Lang Path, Nekoosa Pub Sch, **SLP**

Kove, Mrs Rose 75 East End Avenue 11C, New York, NY 10028, (914) 632-9000, BA 69 CUNY - Hunter Coll; MA 71 CUNY - Lehman Coll; Sp/Lang Path, New Rochelle Cty Sch Dist, **SLP**

Koven, Marvin V 1100 Glendon Avenue, Suite 1119, Los Angeles, CA 90024, PH (NS); **SLP**

Kovian, Theresa Maria R R #1 Keller Drive, Box 224B, Fonda, NY 12068, (518) 853-3856, BA 82 SUNY - Coll at Plattsburgh; MA 83 SUNY - Coll at Plattsburgh; 88–Sp-Lang Path, BOCES Hamilton-Fulton Mont Co, **SLP**

Kowalczyk, Deborah Jean 145 Chestnut Lane, Bldg G #226, Richmond Heights, OH 44143, (216) 729-1919, BA 75 Cleveland St Univ; MA 81 Cleveland St Univ; Sp-Lang Path, Cleveland Hearing & Speech Center, **SLP ACE**

Kowalik, Mrs Norene Davitt Rd 1 Box 197, New Hampton, NY 10958, (914) 355-1598, BA 72 SUNY - Coll at New Paltz; MS 81 Montclair St Coll; Sp/Lang Path, Warwick Valley Cen Sch, **SLP**

Kowalka, Linda H 203 Winding Way, San Carlos, CA 94070, (408) 998-6255, BA 71 Univ of Redlands; MS 72 Univ of Redlands; SLP, San Jose USD, **SLP**

Kowalkowski, Katharine 92 Beacon Street Apt #11, South Lawrence, MA 01843, (508) 682-0877, BS 79 SUNY - Coll at New Paltz; MS 81 Univ of WI - Milwaukee; **SLP**

Kowalski, Gwen Laura 455 Douglas Avenue Suite 2655, Altamonte Springs, FL 32714, (407) 774-8049, BS 77 Eastern KY Univ; MA 79 Northern MI Univ; Vice President, Professional Communication Ser, **SLP ACE**

Kowalski, Mrs Joanne D 243 Sagewood Terrace, Williamsville, NY 14221, BA 79 SUNY - Center at Buffalo; MA 81 SUNY - Center at Buffalo; 81–Sp-Lang Path, Erie #1 BOCES, **SLP**

Kowalski, Mrs Joanne M 19 Tallowood Drive, Mount Holly, NJ 08060, (609) 267-4367, MA 88 Trenton St Coll

Kowalski, Kathryn R 1 Dartmouth Street, Beverly, MA 01915, (508) 927-9623, BA 75 Univ of WI - Madison; ME 82 Northeastern Univ; 82–Sp-Lang Path, Middlesex Co Hosp, **SLP**

Kowalski, Mrs Susan Swartz 1411 M W Edgerton, Milwaukee, WI 53221-3563, BS 79 Univ of WI - Milwaukee; MS 81 Univ of WI - Milwaukee; SLP, School District of Waukesha, **SLP**

Kowalski, Timothy P Prof Communication Services Inc, 455 Douglas Avenue Suite 2655, Altamonte Springs, FL 32714, (407) 774-8049, BA 76 Southern CT St Univ; MA 78 Case Western Reserve Univ; Pres, Prof Commun Serv, **SLP**

Kowba, Mrs Joyce B 150 Thronton Road, Rochester, NY 14617, (716) 467-3306, BS 80 SUNY - Coll at Buffalo; MA 82 SUNY - Center at Buffalo; 80–Sp/Lang Path, Rochester Cty Sch Dist, **SLP**

Kowker, Mrs Kathleen Ann 31 Mohican Drive, Schnecksville, PA 18078, (215) 778-2544, OB 83 Bloomsburg Univ of PA; MS 84 Bloomsburg Univ of PA; 88–Sp-Lang Path, The Allentown Hosp, **SLP**

Kozan, Anita L 3305 2nd Avenue South, Minneapolis, MN 55408, (612) 298-8288, BS 69 Univ of MN - Minneap-St Paul; MA 72 Univ of MN - Minneap-St Paul; 88–Tchg Asst, Dept of Communication Disorders Univ of MN, **SLP ACE**

Kozar, Nadia E 329 Center Street #3, Huron, OH 44839, (419) 433-6343, BA 77 Baldwin-Wallace Coll; MA 84 Central MI Univ; **SLP**

Kozel, Monica Marie 400 Beech Street, Park Hill, PA 15945, (814) 539-9447, BS 79 Indiana Univ of PA; MS 85 Indiana Univ of PA; **SLP**

Kozelsky, Joseph D 1000 Elmond Avenue, Rochester, NY 14620, (716) 271-0680, BS 64 Le Moyne Coll; MS 68 Syracuse Univ; Dir/Aud, Hrng & Sp Cen of Rochstr Inc, **A**

Kozicki, Michelle M 958 Alpine Drive, Green Bay, WI 54311, (414) 494-5231, BA 86 Univ of WI - Eau Claire; MS 87 Univ of WI - Milwaukee; 88–Sp-Lang Path, San Luis Manor

Kozikowski, Mary A 301 West Minnesota Street, Spring Valley, IL 61362, (815) 223-2567, BS 73 Western IL Univ; MS 76 Bradley Univ; Sp/Lang Path, Peru Publ Schs, **SLP**

Kozin, Linda P 8736 Glenwick Lane, La Jolla, CA 92037, (619) 457-2317, BA 66 Univ of IL - Urbana; MA 69 Univ of IL - Urbana; **SLP**

Koziol, L Steve Aud & Speech Path Serv (126), VA Medical Center, Fort Howard, MD 21052, (301) 687-8853, BA 70 IN Univ - Bloomington; OM 74 Univ of WI - Madison; MA 80 Univ of NE - Lincoln; 80–Sp-Lang Path, United States Vets Admin, **SLP**

Kozlik, Ethel Weimer R R 1 Box 267-G, Route 516, Matawan, NJ 07747, (201) 566-1800, BA 73 Montclair St Coll; MA 81 Trenton St Coll; SLP, Matawan Board of Education, **SLP**

Kozlosky, Michaline 490 Philmont Drive, Lancaster, PA 17601, (717) 898-2231, BS 70 Clarion Univ of PA; ME 72 Clarion Univ of PA; Sp-Lang Path, Lancaster-Lebanon Iu #13, **SLP**

Kozlov, Enid M 1820 Ticonderoga Lane, Cherry Hill, NJ 08003, **SLP**

Kozlovsky, Eva B Rt 2 Box 29, Rockwall, TX 75087, (214) 373-3988, BA 79 Sam Houston St Univ; MS 80 Southern Methodist Univ; Sp/Lang Path, Private Practice, **SLP ACE**

Kozlowski, Barbara A 211 Niagara Street, Lockport, NY 14094, (716) 837-2441, BA 82 SUNY - Center at Buffalo; MA 84 SUNY - Center at Buffalo; Sp-Lang Path, Wny Lang Dev Prog, **SLP**

Kozlowski, Mrs Colleen Cook R R 3 Box 268, St Johnsbury, VT 05819, (802) 748-9246, OB 81 Univ of Pittsburgh - Pittsburgh; OM 83 Temple Univ; 86–Sp-Lang Path, St Johnsbury Sch Dist, **SLP**

Kozlowski-Willmarth, Jean M 74 Colgate Street, Rochester, NY 14619, (716) 328-1836, **SLP**

Kozubal, Judith A 1026 Girard Avenue, Swarthmore, PA 19081, (215) 543-4142, BS 72 Bloomsburg Univ of PA; MA 80 Temple Univ; Director, St Christophers Hosp for Chld, **A**

Kraai, Mrs Rhonda V 3808 Penbrook, Marion, IN 46952, (317) 285-8160, BS 79 Western MI Univ; MS 81 Marquette Univ; 88–Prof, Ball State Univ, **SLP**

Kraak, Christie L 2609 Charlesgate, Wyoming, MI 49509, (616) 459-8277, BS 72 Western MI Univ; MS 73 Vanderbilt Univ; Sp/Lang Path, Hrng & Sp Cen- Grand Rapids, **SLP**

Kraat, Arlene 19-10 Parsons Boulevard, Whitestone, NY 11357, (718) 520-7358, MS 70 IN Univ - Bloomington; Asst Prof, CUNY-Queens Coll, **SLP**

Kraayeveld, Sandra Jean Route 1 Box 8, Delavan, WI 53115, (414) 741-4118, OB 84 Univ of WI - Whitewater; MS 86 Univ of WI - Whitewater; 87–Sp-Lang Path, Lakeland Sch of Walworth Co

Krabbenhoeft, Cathy A 403 13th Avenue, Rock Falls, IL 61071, (815) 625-4715, MA 87 Northern IL Univ - De Kalb

Krabbenschmidt, Mrs Katie J 1401 Alamo, P O Box 371267, Montara, CA 94037, (415) 573-2235, BA 68 San Jose St Univ; MA 73 San Francisco St Univ; Sp-Lang Path, San Mateo Co Bd Ed, **SLP**

Kracht, Colleen H 335 Morningside Drive, Battle Creek, MI 49015, (616) 965-3206, BS 75 IN Univ - Bloomington; MS 77 Univ of Denver; 86–Aud, Private Practice, **A**

Krackenfels, Doreen 38 Hughes Street, Wilkes-Barre, PA 18702, (717) 823-5555, BS 85 Marywood Coll; MA 87 OH Univ - Athens; **SLP**

Kracov, Mrs Marion 1121 University Blvd West, Wheaton, MD 20902, (301) 942-4847, BA 55 CUNY - Brooklyn Coll; Sp-Lang Path, Montgomery County Pub Schools, **SLP**

Krady, Kimberly Ann 401 North Main Street #223-B, Williamstown, NJ 08094, BS 80 Mansfield Univ of PA; ME 85 James Madison Univ; 85–Aud, Vineland Dev Ctr, **A**

Kraemer, Iris T 4539 Trails Drive, Sarasota, FL 34232, (813) 377-1232, BA 79 Univ of FL; MA 81 Univ of FL; Sp-Lang Path, **SLP**

Kraemer, Maxine G 675 7th Avenue, San Francisco, CA 94118, (415) 668-5919, BS 65 PA St Univ - Univ Park; MS 80 San Francisco St Univ; **SLP**

Kraemer, Mrs Nancy B 452 Richmond Avenue, Maplewood, NJ 07040, (201) 763-5195, BS 62 Adelphi Univ; MS 68 CUNY - Queens Coll; Sp-Lang Path, Nancy Kraemer Priv Pract, **SLP**

Kraemer, Stacey Fordham 2214 Round Lake, Houston, TX 77077, (713) 497-5179, BS 81 Univ of TX - Austin; MA 84 Univ of Houston - Univ Park; 87–Sp-Lang Path, Memorial City Rehab Hosp, **SLP**

Krafcheck, Mrs Debbie J 1500 Croston, Plano, TX 75075, BS 77 Western MI Univ; MS 80 Marquette Univ; **SLP**

Krafft, Karen Marie 7 West Main Street, Canton, NY 13617, (315) 386-3830, BS 83 SUNY - Coll at Buffalo; MS 87 SUNY - Coll at Buffalo; **SLP**

Kraft, Dr Anita R 46 Walnut Place, Briarcliff Manor, NY 10510, (914) 762-1348, MS 59 PA St Univ - Univ Park; MA 77 Columbia Univ Teachers Coll; PH 85 (Lang & Learning Disabilities) Fordham Univ; Sp-Lang Path, Briarcliff Manor School Dist, **SLP**

Kraft, Arlene F 6 Phyllis Court, Wayne, NJ 07470, BA 73 Montclair St Coll; MS 74 Columbia Univ Teachers Coll; Sp-Lang Path, Morris Sch Dist, **SLP**

Kraft, Mrs Frances L 105 Pearl Street, Lumberton, MS 39455, (601) 266-5216, BA 74 Univ of MS; MS 75 Univ of MS; 81–SLP, U of Southern Mississippi, **SLP**

Kraft, Kathryn Irene 1107 Ruhlman Avenue, Portsmouth, OH 45662, (614) 353-7774, SLP, Scioto Mem Hosp S & H Ctr, **SLP**

Kraft, Stephanie A 6795 Hunters Oak Drive, Apartment 203, Memphis, TN 38119-4473, (901) 757-2476, BS 86 Univ of GA; MA 87 Memphis St Univ; 88–Sp-Lang Path, Les Passees Childrens Rehab Ct

Kraft, Mrs Susan E 12 Brookside Road, Succasunna, NJ 07876, (412) 561-8664, BS 69 PA St Univ - Univ Park; ME 70 Northeastern Univ; 87–Sp-Lang Path, Madison Sch Dist, **SLP**

Kragt, Cynthia A 3699 David Lane, Lansing, MI 48910, BA 69 MI St Univ; MA 70 MI St Univ; **SLP**

Krah, Mrs Kerrie Mc Manus 111 Plymouth Drive #2-D, Norwood, MA 02062, (617) 848-5353, MA 85 Hofstra Univ; Sp-Lang Path, Braintree Hosp, **SLP**

Krainen, Gordon 5994 Kingsfield, West Bloomfield, MI 48033, (314) 895-4148, BA 77 Univ of MI - Ann Arbor; MA 79 Wayne St Univ; 88–Sp-Lang Path, Rehab Institute of Detroit, **SLP**

Krais, Janelle Graveline 3325 East Hayes Road, Norristown, PA 19403, (215) 584-6095, BS 84 West Chester Univ of PA; MA 86 Trenton St Coll; 86–Dir-SLP, Leader Nursing/Healthcare Ctr, **SLP**

Krajewski, Mrs Christine 90 Schlemmer Road, Lancaster, NY 14086-9727, BS 74 SUNY - Coll at Buffalo; MS 77 SUNY - Coll at Buffalo; Tchr, BOCES Dist 1, **SLP**

Krakower, Barbara J 218 Hendricks Isle, Fort Lauderdale, FL 33301-3705, (305) 985-3157, **SLP**

Krakowiak, Mrs Marianne V 3501 Nassau Drive, Augusta, GA 30909, (404) 733-9859, BA 52 Univ of MI - Ann Arbor; MA 56 Univ of MI - Ann Arbor; Sp-Lang Path, Richmond Co PS, **SLP**

Kral, Rhonda S 9424 Henrietta, Brookfield, IL 60513, (312) 387-0356, BA 76 Elmhurst Coll; MA 78 Northern IL Univ - De Kalb; Sp-Lang Path, Dist 48 Villa Park Sch, **SLP**

Krall, Mrs Cindy Martin 1 North Harmon Drive, Mitchell, SD 57301, (605) 996-3113, BS 85 SD St Univ; MA 86 Northern IL Univ - De Kalb; **SLP**

Kralovic, Mrs Susan Dora Rd #1 Route 159 Box 239-C, Pattersonville, NY 12137, MS 80 Coll of Saint Rose; **SLP**

Kramer, Mrs Bonnie S 18100 Darnell Drive, Olney, MD 20832, (301) 570-4208, BA 68 Univ of FL; ME 69 Univ of FL; 87–Sp-Lang Path, Ctrs for the Hndcpd Inc, **SLP ACE**

Kramer, Mrs Carol Anne 50 3rd Avenue, Berea, OH 44017, (216) 243-6317, BS 69 OH Univ - Athens; MA 85 Cleveland St Univ; **SLP**

Kramer, Mrs Carol W 3707 Gardenview Road, Baltimore, MD 21208, SLP, Fallstaff Middle School, **SLP**

Kramer, Mrs Catharine Milligan 2725 Modaff, Naperville, IL 60565, MS 81 Univ of WA; **SLP**

Kramer, Charles G 561 Scott Circle, Decatur, GA 30033, (404) 894-5798, BS 69 SUNY - Coll at Geneseo; ME 79 GA St Univ; Sp-Lang Path, Learning Svcs Co, **SLP**

Kramer, Heidi A 7121 Brecken Ridge Avenue, Raleigh, NC 27615, (919) 847-3600, BS 75 SUNY - Center at Albany; MS 76 SUNY - Center at Albany; Sp-Lang Path, Wake Co PS Sys, **SLP**

Kramer, Mrs J Beverly 401 W Linden Street, Abbotsford, WI 54405, (715) 229-2172, BA 69 Univ of WI - Eau Claire; MA 70 Univ of IA; 88–Sp-Lang Path, Midwest Rehab Svcs, **SLP**

Kramer, Mrs Judith A 2920 S W Wembley Park Road, Lake Oswego, OR 97034, (503) 636-5366, BS 57 Univ of WI - Madison; Sp-Lang Path, Tigard Public Schools, **SLP**

Kramer, Mrs Julie Miller 208 Henderson Circle, Harrisburg, NC 28075, (704) 455-3034, BS 83 Bloomsburg Univ of PA; MS 84 Bloomsburg Univ of PA; Sp-Lang Path, Cabarrus Cnty Schs, **SLP**

Kramer, Kathleen Laura 3607 Jamieson #1 South, St Louis, MO 63109, (314) 644-8400, BS 84 Fontbonne Coll; MS 85 Fontbonne Coll; **SLP**

Kramer, Laura K 2711 Rochester Road, Shaker Heights, OH 44122, **SLP**

Kramer, Lisa 408 Central Avenue #D, Alameda, CA 94501, (415) 769-8828, 88–Sp-Lang Path, NeuroCare, **SLP**

Kramer, Lynne C 2740 Brettwood Drive, Henderson, KY 42420, (812) 479-1666, BA 67 Univ of KY; MA 74 NY Univ; Asst Exec Dir, The Rehab Cen, **A**

Kramer, Dr Marc B 159 East 69th Street, New York, NY 10021, (212) 734-8900, BA 65 Temple Univ; MA 67 Temple Univ; PH 72 (NS) CUNY - Grad Sch & Univ Cntr; Aud, Private Practice, **A F**

Kramer, Mrs Marilyn L 163 San Juan Avenue, Albertson, NY 11507, (212) 263-2940, BA 72 CUNY - Queens Coll; MA 74 Hofstra Univ; Spec Educ Tchr, Forest Hills Hs, **SLP**

Kramer, Dr Mitchell B Mid-Vermont ENT, 69 Allen Street Suite 4, Rutland, VT 05701, (802) 775-3314, BA 71 CUNY - Brooklyn Coll; MS 73 CUNY - Brooklyn Coll; PH 77 (Aud) Northwestern Univ; 86–Aud, Mid-Vermont ENT, **A ACE**

Kramer, Mrs Pamela M 1234 South Feather Street, Anaheim, CA 92802, (714) 774-4307, BA 79 CA St Univ - Fullerton; MA 82 CA St Univ - Fullerton; Sp-Lang Path, Santa Ana USD, **SLP**

Kramer, Mrs Patricia R 216 North 27th Street, Allentown, PA 18104, (215) 435-8798, BA 75 Baldwin-Wallace Coll; MS 76 PA St Univ - Univ Park; **SLP**

Kramer, Mrs Patricia Roberts 6040 Comfort Court, Carmichael, CA 95608, (916) 485-6711, BS 74 Miami Univ - Oxford; MS 83 Whittier Coll; Dir Sp-Lang Path, Easter Seal Soc, **SLP**

Kramer, Mrs Roberta J 104 Taymil Road, New Rochelle, NY 10804, (914) 576-3982, BA 68 CUNY - Queens Coll; BA 72 CUNY - Hunter Coll; MA 84 Pace U -NY City; **SLP**

Kramer, Sallie Phyliss 11957 Villa Dorado, St Louis, MO 63146, (314) 441-0996, BS 83 Univ of MO - Saint Louis; MA 87 Saint Louis Univ; 87–Sp-Lang Path, St Louis Dev Disab Treatment Ctr, **SLP**

Kramer, Mrs Sharon Parker 4089 Woodland Court, Mims, FL 32754, (407) 269-1023, MA 84 Univ of Central FL; Sp-Lang Path, South Lake Elem Sch, **SLP**

Kramer, Dr Steven J San Diego State University, Dept Communicative Disord, San Diego, CA 92182, BA 76 Univ of CA - Santa Barbara; MA 78 Univ of FL; PH 81 (NS) Univ of FL; Associate Professor, San Diego State University, **A**

Kramer, Mrs Susan Elizabeth 3279 Owasso Heights Road, St Paul, MN 55126-3015, (612) 546-6437, BA 81 Univ of WI - Eau Claire; MS 82 Univ of WI - Eau Claire; Sp-Lang Path, United Rehab Inc, **SLP**

Kramer, Mrs Tamar Feder 69-82B 136th Street, Flushing, NY 11367, (718) 793-1912, BA 79 CUNY - Queens Coll; MA 81 CUNY - Queens Coll; Aud, Intl Ctr for Disabled, **A**

Kramer, Dr William L 1906 White River Boulevard, Muncie, IN 47303, (317) 285-8135, BA 64 SUNY - Center at Buffalo; MA 65 Ball St Univ; PH 72 (NS) OH Univ - Athens; Assoc Prof, Ball State U, **SLP**

Kramer-Kohlbrenner, Mrs Claudia 1314 Crane Boulevard, Libertyville, IL 60048, (312) 367-4555, BS 72 Clarion Univ of PA; ME 73 Clarion Univ of PA; Sp-Lang Path, Sp Ed Dist of Lake Co, **SLP**

Kramerson, Mrs Sherri F 8 Alva Street, East Greenbush, NY 12061, (518) 434-4103, BA 75 SUNY - Coll at New Paltz; MS 77 Ithaca Coll; Sp-Lang Path, Er Sl Sp & Hrng Cen, **SLP**

Krammer, Katherine 3138 Waialae Avenue #230, Honolulu, HI 96816, (808) 834-9472, BS 77 Univ of HI - Manoa; MS 80 Univ of HI - Manoa; Sp-Lang Path, Kaiser Permanente, **SLP**

Krammes, Mrs Lynn H Route 4, 73 Shady View Drive, Floyds Knobs, IN 47119, (812) 923-7283, BS 85 Brescia Coll; MS 86 Univ of Louisville; 87–Sp-Lang Path, Rauch Rehab & Dev Svcs, **SLP**

Kramp, H Ned P O Box 253, Bena, VA 23018, (804) 642-9617, ME Bloomsburg Univ of PA; 87–Hearing Conservation Coord, Dept of the Navy, **A**

Kramp, Mrs Lynn M 1801 SW Cloverleaf Road, Lake Oswego, OR 97034, (503) 636-3968, BS 77 Baylor Univ; MA 79 Wichita St Univ; **SLP**

Kranefuss, Mrs Ellen Norton 24 Castano Court, Needham, MA 02192, (617) 720-6728, BS 82 PA St Univ - Univ Park; MA 84 Northwestern Univ; 86–Sp-Lang Path, Spaulding Rehab Hosp, **SLP ACE**

Kranich, Jane G 2119 Watertown Place, Clarksville, TN 37043, (615) 645-8163, BA 75 CUNY - Queens Coll; MA 76 Hofstra Univ; Sp-Lang Path, Private Practice, **SLP**

Krantz, Mrs Henrietta C P O Box 1087, Sequim, WA 98382, (206) 683-6878, BA 37 Univ of HI - Manoa; MA 43 Univ of HI - Manoa; **SLP A LM**

Krantz, Mrs Joan Berkowitz 220 Passaic Avenue, Pompton Lakes, NJ 07442, (201) 492-2079, BS 58 Boston Univ; MS 81 Paterson St Coll; Sp/Lang Path, Butler New Jersey Bd of Ed, **SLP**

Krantz, Mrs Joan H 11315 N W 10th Place, Coral Springs, FL 33071, (301) 755-3589, BA 68 CUNY - Brooklyn Coll; MA 71 NY Univ; 88–Sp-Lang Path, **SLP**

Krantz, Mrs Miriam L 4010 West 97th, Overland Park, KS 66207, (913) 642-6953, BA 46 Univ of IA; MA 47 Univ of IA; Retired, Hrng/Sp Dept U KS Med Cen, **A LM**

Krantz, Mrs Susan Eileen 3055 Roxburgh Drive, Roswell, GA 30076, (404) 475-0325, OB 72 Univ of FL; MS 73 Univ of South FL; Sp-Lang Path, Counseling and Assessment Ctr, **SLP**

Krantz, Susan Sanders 628 Lebanon, Aurora, IL 60505, (312) 896-8518, BS 79 Eastern IL Univ; MS 80 Eastern IL Univ; Sp-Lang Path, Aurora E Dist #131, **SLP**

Kranz, Karen A 1993 Lowell Lane, Merrick, NY 11566, **SLP**

Krapp, Dr Dwight E Audio Serv Of Cincinnati Inc, 199 William Howard Taft Rd, Cincinnati, OH 45219, (513) 861-2888, BS 71 Univ of ND; MS 72 Univ of ND; PH 76 (NS) Univ of Cincinnati; 77–Aud, Aud Svcs of Cincinnati Inc, **A**

Krappes, Mrs Teresa Kathleen 4212 Golden Ridge Way, Fort Collins, CO 80526-4108, (303) 669-3940, BS 82 CO St Univ; MS 85 CO St Univ; **SLP**

Krasner, Mrs Gladys R 10 Magnolia Lane, Jericho, NY 11753, (516) 487-0690, BA 48 Univ of MI - Ann Arbor; MA 70 Hofstra Univ; Sp-Lang Path, Private Practice, **SLP**

Krasner, Sherri L 94 Rumford Street, #4, Concord, NH 03301, (603) 228-3822, BS 84 Ithaca Coll; MS 87 NY Univ; 87–Sp-Lang Path, Lakes Region Gen Hosp, **SLP**

Krasniewski, Christine 4437 Bromley, Toledo, OH 43623, (419) 472-7707, BS 77 Univ of Toledo; MA 81 Eastern MI Univ; Sp/Lang Path, Lucas County Office of Ed, **SLP**

Krasny, Lori Ellen 1128 Broadway E #302, Seattle, WA 98102, (206) 543-4011, BA 82 San Francisco St Univ; MS 85 Univ of WA; 85–Sp-Lang Path, University of Washington, **SLP**

Krasow, Mrs Dyane Schrager 2176 Bunkerhill Drive, San Mateo, CA 94402, (415) 593-1647, BA 78 San Francisco St Univ; MA 80 CA St Univ - Sacramento; **SLP**

Krass, Jay J 11 Kristy Drive, Beacon, NY 12508, (914) 669-5414, BA 73 CUNY - Hunter Coll; MA 77 CUNY - City College; OM 85 CUNY - City College; Sp-Lang Path, N Salem Cen Sch Dist, **SLP**

Krassowski, Mrs Elaine Burke 4726 Huntley Lane, Sarasota, FL 34232, (813) 377-6476, MS 77 Rutgers St Univ - Newark; Sp-Lang Path, Sarasota Co Sch Dist, **SLP**

Krasuski, Mrs Mary J A 11 Johnson Road, Mechanicville, NY 12118, (518) 664-3572, BS 77 SUNY - Coll at Geneseo; MS 79 Coll of Saint Rose; SLP, Albany Medical Center Hospital, **SLP**

Kratchman, Robynne F 5 Vine Street, Waldwick, NJ 07463, (212) 240-5141, BA 75 SUNY - Center at Stony Brook; MS 78 Columbia Univ Teachers Coll; Sp-Lang Path, Private Practice, **SLP**

Krater, Mary K 13 Copley Place, Laguna Niguel, CA 92677, (714) 240-0803, BA 71 CA St Univ - Fresno; MA 73 Univ of Southern CA; **SLP**

Kratville, Mrs Carol A D Richardson Development Center, P O Box 835066, Richardson, TX 75083, (214) 490-9055, BS 74 Southern Methodist Univ; MS 75 Southern Methodist Univ; 76–Exec Dir, Richardson Dev Cen, **SLP**

Kratze, Alexa Romain 2554 Luciernaga Street, Carlsbad, CA 92008, (619) 576-5837, BA 72 Univ of CA - Santa Barbara; MA 74 San Diego St Univ; Cl Superv, Sp-Hrng & Neurosensory Cen, **SLP**

Krauklis, Mrs Rita H 468 Tittabawassee Road, Sanford, MI 48657, (517) 790-1234, BS 75 Purdue Univ - West Lafayette; MA 77 MI St Univ; Dept Head/Sp-Lang Path, Saginaw Comm Hosp, **SLP**

Kraus, Mrs Kirsten Lacy 421 Ben Oaks Drive West, Severna Park, MD 21146, (301) 578-5601, BS 79 Towson St Univ; MS 81 Towson St Univ; 86–Chief Sp-Lang Path, Sinai Hospital of Baltimore, **SLP**

Kraus, Dr Nina J Michael Reese Hosp & Med Ctr, Siegel Institute, 3033 South Cottage, Chicago, IL 60613, (312) 791-5487, BA 74 Swarthmore Coll; PH 80 (Auditory Physiology) Northwestern Univ; Assistant Professor, Siegel Institute/Univ of Chicago, **SLP**

Krause, Eloise M 2915 N Avenue Del Conquistado, Tucson, AZ 85749, **SLP**

Krause, Karlene Ann Soegel Elementary School, APO New York, NY 09069-0005, (414) 887-2938, BS 84 Univ of WI - Madison; MS 85 Marquette Univ; **SLP**

Krause, Linda S 28578 Tonnor Drive, Highland, CA 92346, BS 69 Polytechnic Inst of Brooklyn; MA 71 Saint Louis Univ; Sp-Lang Path, San Bernardino City Sch Dist, **SLP**

Krause, Dr SueEllen 333 East Ontario Street, #2908-B, Chicago, IL 60611, (312) 942-7240, BA 71 MI St Univ; MA 73 Northwestern Univ; PH 78 (NS) Northwestern Univ; Dir, Krause Comm Assoc, **SLP**

Kraushar, Saundra Ann 4554 Peck Circle, La Verne, CA 91750, (714) 599-6787, BA 82 CA St Univ - Fullerton; MS 84 Univ of LA Verne; **SLP**

Krauss, Jeffrey D 356 Rockway Parkway, Valley Stream, NY 11580, (516) 561-7415, BA 77 CUNY - Brooklyn Coll; MS 79 CUNY - Brooklyn Coll; Aud, NY City Board of Educ, **A**

Krauss, Mrs Zehava 6034 North St Louis, Chicago, IL 60659, (312) 463-6611, BA 77 CUNY - Brooklyn Coll; MS 80 CUNY - Brooklyn Coll; **SLP**

Krauss-Lehrman, Patricia L 3353 Norcross Lane, Dallas, TX 75229, (214) 905-3136, BA 78 Washington Univ; OM 80 Emory Univ; Sp/Lang Path, Callier Cen for Commun Dis, **SLP**

Kraut, Mrs Beverly H 1007 Russell Lane, West Chester, PA 19382, (215) 399-0922, BA 73 Temple Univ; MA 75 Temple Univ; Sp-Lang Path, Private Practice, **SLP**

Krautter, Mary E 7311 Halbert, Austin, TX 78750, ME 76 Southwest TX St Univ; **SLP**

Kravit, Mrs Deborah S 9290 North Broadmoor Road, Milwaukee, WI 53217, (414) 351-4435, BS 76 Univ of WI - Madison; MS 77 Univ of WI - Milwaukee; Sp-Lang Path, Milwaukee Hearing Society, **SLP**

Kravitz, Dena S 1626 North Prospect, Apartment 705, Milwaukee, WI 53202, (414) 273-2321, BS 78 SUNY - Coll at Buffalo; MS 81 Univ of WI - Milwaukee; Sp/Lang Path, Milwaukee Pub Schs, **SLP**

Kravitz, Ellen M 27 Fuller Road, Watertown, MA 02172, (617) 894-3600, BA 74 Hamilton Coll; MS 76 Purdue Univ - West Lafayette; Sp-Lang Path, W E Fernald St Sch, **SLP**

Krawczyk, Rita A 4972 Armor Drive, Hamburg, NY 14075, (716) 648-6211, BS 67 SUNY - Coll at Buffalo; OM 85 SUNY - Coll at Buffalo; **SLP**

Krawitz, Beverly G 5166 Candlewood Drive, Fayetteville, NY 13066, BA 63 Univ of Toronto - Ontario; OM 65 Univ of Toronto - Ontario; **SLP**

Kraynick, Linda I 326-D Oak Road, Gibsonia, PA 15044, (412) 665-4985, BS 79 Clarion Univ of PA; ME 74 Clarion Univ of PA

Krchnavek, Elizabeth Pfeiffer Center For Head Injuries-Cog Rehab, 2048 Oaktree Road, Edison, NJ 08820, BA 82 Rutgers St Univ -N Brunswick; MS 84 Columbia Univ Teachers Coll; 85–Sp-Lang Path, The Ctr For Head Injuries, **SLP**

Krcmar, Jean Gebhart 24 Elmwood Drive, Indian Head Park, IL 60525, (312) 246-0068, BA 75 Coll of Saint Teresa; MS 76 Univ of WI - Eau Claire; 86–Sp-Lang Path, Dist 95, **SLP**

Krebs, Mrs Ann Winn 1424 Leo Avenue, Fruita, CO 81521-9006, BS 67 Purdue Univ - West Lafayette; MS 73 MI St Univ

Krebs, Mrs Barbara Ballard 41 Solana Drive, Los Altos, CA 94022, (408) 274-9500, BS 68 Purdue Univ - West Lafayette; MA 73 Northwestern Univ; Spec Ed Principal, Santa Clara Co Schs, **SLP**

Krebs, Dr Donald F Speech Hrng & Neurosensory Ctr, 8001 Frost Street, San Diego, CA 92123, (619) 576-5842, BS 53 CA St Univ - Los Angeles; MA 57 CA St Univ - Los Angeles; PH 72 (Leadership and Human Behavior) United States Int'l Univ; Vice Pres Ambul Serv/Res, Chldns Hosp & Hlth Cen, **A F**

Krebs, Janet Misita 391 South Maple Avenue, Ridgewood, NJ 07450, (201) 670-0707, BA 75 CUNY - Brooklyn Coll; MS 77 CUNY - Brooklyn Coll; Dir/Sp-Lang Path, Communication Therapy Ctr, **SLP**

Krebs, Mrs Kay D 2724 Walker Street, South Bellmore, NY 11710, (516) 781-8154, BA 63 CUNY - Brooklyn Coll; MS 76 Adelphi Univ; Audiologist, Private Practice, **A**

Krebs, Mrs Leslie B 1208 Glyndon Drive, Plano, TX 75023, (214) 526-8901, BS 78 Univ of GA; MS 80 Tulane Univ; **SLP**

Krebs, Mary Ann P 518 Sunlight Drive, Rochester, MI 48309-1329, (313) 375-2628, BS 62 Saint Louis Univ; MA 79 Wayne St Univ; 87–Sp-Lang Path, The Childs Place, **SLP ACE**

Krebs, Mrs Mary B V 3602 Lexington Road, Louisville, KY 40207, (502) 451-6200, BA 71; ME 76 Univ of Louisville; Sp-Lang Path, Jefferson Co Bd of Ed, **SLP**

Kreeger, Deborah 229 West 105th Street #35, New York, NY 10025, (718) 946-9700, OB 83 IN Univ - Bloomington; MS 85 Columbia Univ Teachers Coll

Kreeger, Sandra F 6318 St James Drive, Carmichael, CA 95608, (916) 736-3399, BA 57 Univ of CA - Los Angeles; MA 76 CA St Univ - Sacramento; Aud, Sacramento ENT, **A**

Kreeger, Virginia Flechtner 4360 Colony Hills Drive, Akron, OH 44313, (216) 762-9491, BS 67 Kent St Univ; MA 85 Univ of Akron; 88–Sp-Lang Path, PSI Affiliates, **SLP**

Krehbiel, Mary B 5547 Old Highway 410, Olympia, WA 98502, (206) 456-7637, BA 76 MI St Univ; MA 77 Central MI Univ; 88–Sp-Lang Path, North Thurston Sch Dist, **SLP**

Krei, Mrs Barbara Nall 5708 N W 110th Street, Oklahoma City, OK 73132, (405) 721-5108, BA 73 Univ of MS; ME 77 Tulane Univ; SLP, Western Hts Sch Dist, **SLP**

Kreider, Mrs Gloria A 9 Gull Drive, Hauppauge, NY 11788, (516) 265-2612, BA 51 CUNY - Hunter Coll; MA 53 CUNY - Hunter Coll; 88–Sp-Lang Path, Private Practice, **SLP**

Kreider, Thomas N Dept Of Hearing And Speech, Bethesda Hospital, 2951 Maple Avenue, Zanesville, OH 43701, (614) 452-2915, BA 67 Univ of Cincinnati; MA 69 Univ of Cincinnati; Dept Head/Aud, Bethesda Hosp, **A**

Kreier, Kathi Sue 1406 Little Main Street, Streator, IL 61364, (815) 249-6225, MS 84 IL St Univ - Normal; MS 86 IL St Univ - Normal

Kreifels, Mary Margaret 3126 South 69th Avenue #16, Omaha, NE 68106, (402) 978-7078, BS 82 Univ of NE - Lincoln; MS 83 Univ of NE - Lincoln; Sp-Lang Path, Omaha Pub Schs, **SLP**

Kreinbihl, Mrs Beth A 136 Creston Road, Mansfield, OH 44906, (419) 756-1133, BA 77 OH Wesleyan Univ; MA 79 Univ of Cincinnati; Superv Sp-Lang Serv, Rehab Serv of N Cen Oh Inc, **SLP**

Kreinik, Mrs Andrea Dorice 240-58 66th Avenue, Douglaston, NY 11362, (212) 683-6970, BA 68 CUNY - Queens Coll; MA 70 Long Island U - CW Post Ctr; MA 85 Long Island U - CW Post Ctr; 85–Teacher, NYC Bd of Ed/Dist 28 Queens, **SLP**

Kreis, Mrs Mary Katherine 4521 North 96th Street, Omaha, NE 68134, (402) 572-6747, BS 81 Univ of NE - Lincoln; MS 82 Univ of NE - Lincoln; Sp-Lang Path, Millard Public Schools, **SLP**

Kreisle, Alice E 10430 Londonderry Court, Montgomery, OH 45242, (513) 724-2022, BS 75 IN Univ - Bloomington; MA 76 IN Univ - Bloomington; 86–Aud, Cincinnati Sp Lang & Hrng Ctr, **A**

Kreitzman, Jackie L 5955 Jamieson, Encino, CA 91316, (818) 708-2288, BA 76 CA St Univ - Northridge; MA 78 CA St Univ - Northridge; SLP, Los Angeles USD, **SLP**

Kreitzman, Natalie Rae Middlesex Day Training Center, 1377 Rahway Avenue, Avenel, NJ 07001, (201) 488-5035, MA 82 Seton Hall Univ; Sp-Lang Path, State of NJ, **SLP**

Krejci, Evelyn C 2071 Parasol Drive, Chesterfield, MO 63017, BS 75 Univ of KS; MA 77 Saint Louis Univ; SLP, Spec Sch Dist, **SLP**

Krejmas, Mrs Jodee 3427 Meadow Court, Maineville, OH 45039, BA 78 Clarion Univ of PA; ME 80 Clarion Univ of PA; Sp-Lang Path, Hamilton Co Office of Educ, **SLP**

Kremer, Linda Susan 4693 Pettit Avenue, Niagara Falls, ON, Canada L2E6L4, (416) 356-0137, BS 67 SUNY - Coll at Buffalo; MS 85 SUNY - Coll at Buffalo; 72–Sp-Lang Path, Niagara South Bd of Educ, **SLP**

Kremer, Mrs Susan Elaine 6932 Violet Court, Rancho Cucamonga, CA 91739, (714) 899-3362, BA 81 CA St Univ - Fullerton; MA 84 CA St Univ - Fullerton; Sp-Lang Path, Rowland USD, **SLP**

Kremer-Stern, Mrs Sharon L 629 Leafydale Terrace, Baltimore, MD 21208, (301) 396-9165, BS 77 Towson St Univ; MS 79 Loyola Coll; Sp-Lang Path, Baltimore City PS, **SLP**

Krengulec, Kathleen 221 Virgil Avenue, Buffalo, NY 14216, (716) 883-1366, MA 85 SUNY - Center at Buffalo; **A**

Krenkel, Paula S 21 Hillside Road, Larchmont, NY 10538, (914) 833-0203, BA 72 CUNY - Queens Coll; MA 74 CUNY - Queens Coll; Private Practice, **SLP**

Krentcil, Bonnie 98 Elm Street, Andover, MA 01810, **SLP**

Krenzke, Lorre 704 Schuller #314, Lufkin, TX 75901, (409) 634-3353, **SLP**

Krepps, Mrs Cathleen Stowe 6415 Fawnwood, Spring, TX 77389-3624, MA 80 Univ of CO - Denver; SLP, Conroe ISD, **SLP**

Krepsky, Dr Judith C 1251 Guns Road, Green Bay, WI 54311-6003, (414) 497-3886, PH 81 (NS) Southern IL Univ -Carbondale; Sp-Lang Path, Green Bay Schl, **SLP**

Kresheck, Dr Janet Dept Communicative Disorders, Northern Illinois Univ, De Kalb, IL 60115, (815) 753-1484, BS 60 FL St Univ; MA 61 OH St Univ; PH 69 (NS) Northwestern Univ; Prof, Nn IL U, **SLP**

Kress, Linda Elizabeth R R #1 Box 454, New Ipswich, NH 03071, (603) 547-3311, BS 77 Ithaca Coll; MS 83 Univ of NH

Kress, Mary F 4302 Westover Place N W, Washington, DC 20016, **SLP**

Kressner, Mrs Debra F 9 Marbourne Drive, Mamaroneck, NY 10543, (914) 381-2595, BA 73 George Washington Univ; MS 75 SUNY - Coll at Buffalo; Sp-Lang Path, Private Practice, **SLP**

Kressner, Kathrine 425 Hawthorne Street, Neenah, WI 54956, (414) 722-2371, BS 71 SUNY - Center at Albany; MA 75 Coll of Saint Rose; 86–Sp-Lang Path, Infant Preschool Program, **SLP**

Kretschmer, Dr Laura W University Of Cincinnati, Mail Station 379, Cincinnati, OH 45221, (513) 556-4490, MA 61 Northwestern Univ; MA 66 Columbia Univ Teachers Coll; ED 72 (NS) Columbia Univ Teachers Coll; Prof, U of Cincinnati, **A**

Kretschmer, Dr Robert E 70 Lasalle Street #3-B, New York, NY 10027, (212) 678-3864, BS 66 Northwestern Univ; MA 67 Northwestern Univ; PH 76 (NS) Univ of KS; Assoc Prof, Tchrs Coll Columbia U

Kreuk, Lydia M Department Of Audiology, The Mississauga Hospital, 100 Queensway West, Mississauga, ON, Canada L5B 1B8, (416) 848-7281, BS 77 Univ of Western Ontario; MA 79 Univ of KS; Dir of Aud, The Mississauga Hosp, **A**

Kreul, Dr E James California State University, Speech Pathology & Aud, Chico, CA 95929, (916) 895-5949, BS 50 Univ of WI - Madison; MS 52 Univ of WI - Madison; PH 66 (NS) Stanford Univ; Prof-Dir of Res, CA State U, **SLP A**

Kreutzer, Mrs Robin Jeanine 7090 Homewood Drive, Oakland, CA 94611, (213) 813-1971, BA 82 CA St Univ - Long Beach; MA 84 Univ of the Pacific; 88–Sp-Lang Path, Private Practice, **SLP**

Krevolin, Mrs Evelyn S 11 Grove Hill Road, Woodbridge, CT 06525, (203) 397-1223, BS 57 Syracuse Univ; Sp-Lang Path, Orange Bd of Educ, **SLP**

Krezmien-Grasso, Susan M 115 Rauch Drive, Springville, NY 14141, BS 74 SUNY - Coll at Brockport; ME 78 SUNY - Coll at Fredonia; Coordinator Sp-Lang Path Serv, Livingston County BOCES, **SLP**

Kricheff, Adele M 293 Hooker Avenue, Poughkeepsie, NY 12603, MS 73 SUNY - Coll at Geneseo; 85–Sp-Lang Path, Dover Union Free Schs, **SLP**

Kricheff, Barry 293 Hooker Avenue, Poughkeepsie, NY 12603, **A**

Kricheff, Mrs Marjorie G 946 Red Road, Teaneck, NJ 07666, (201) 836-7667, BS 53 Syracuse Univ; Sp-Lang Path, Saddle River Bd of Ed, **SLP A**

Kricos, Dr Patricia Department Of Speech, University Of Florida, 337 Dauer Hall, Gainesville, FL 32611, (904) 392-2113, BA 70 Univ of TX - El Paso; MA 71 OH St Univ; PH 73 (Aud) OH St Univ; Assoc Prof, U of Florida, **A**

Krider, Jane A 7 Adams Court, Hopewell Junction, NY 12533, (914) 221-0795, BS 76 Saint John's Univ - Jamaica; MS 78 PA St Univ - Univ Park; 88–Sp-Lang Path, Danbury Hosp, **SLP**

Kriege, Mari S 25678 Clover Road, Hayward, CA 94542, (415) 577-1579, BS 80 CA St Univ - Hayward; MA 81 Univ of the Pacific; Sp-Lang Path Asst Chief, Fairmont Hosp, **SLP**

Kriegel, Ellen S 9 Glenwood Road, New York, NY 10956, BA 73 CUNY - Queens Coll; MA 75 CUNY - Queens Coll; Sp-Lang Path, Palisades Early Childhood Prog, **SLP**

Kriegel, Janice Manolopoul 272 Bellehurst Drive, Rochester, NY 14617, MA 78 SUNY - Center at Buffalo; Sp-Lang Path, Rochester Cty Sch, **SLP**

Krieger, Mrs Dorothy H 4015 West 44th Street, Minneapolis, MN 55424, (612) 627-2494, BS 43 Univ of MN - Minneap-St Paul; MA 76 Coll of St Thomas; Sp-Lang Path, Minneapolis Pub Sch, **SLP**

Krieger, Mrs Janet Carmichael 303 South 12th Avenue, Yakima, WA 98902, (509) 453-8248, BA 77 Eastern WA Univ; MS 78 Eastern WA Univ; Sp/Lang Path, Yakima Valley Hrng & Sp Cen, **SLP**

Krieger, Mrs Judith 134 Miles, Santa Cruz, CA 95060, (408) 427-3684, BA 63 Our Lady Lake Univ-San Anton; MA 64 Northwestern Univ; Sp-Lang Path, Santa Cruz City Schs, **SLP**

Krieger, Kim M 9205 O Street, Omaha, NE 68127, BA 77 Univ of NE - Omaha; MS 78 Univ of NE - Omaha; Sp-Lang Path, Department of Defense, **SLP**

Krieger, Dr Miriam R 326 Rutgers Avenue, Swarthmore, PA 19081, (215) 328-3035, BA 44 Univ of PA; MA 46 Univ of PA; ED 67 (NS) Univ of PA; Psychologist, Swarthmore Academy, **LM**

Krieger, Richard C 2412 Melbourne Drive, Harrisburg, PA 17112-1083, (717) 782-4350, BS 70 SUNY - Coll at Geneseo; MS 71 SUNY - Coll at Geneseo; Dir, Polyclinic Med Cen, **A**

Kriegisch, Patricia Smiddy Hall, Ithaca College, Ithaca, NY 14850, (607) 274-3714, BS 75 Indiana Univ of PA; MA 78 OH St Univ; 87–Clinic Coord, Ithaca Coll, **SLP**

Kriegman, Mrs Lois S 26 Malvern Avenue, Richmond, VA 23221, (804) 358-2161, BA 40 Univ of IL - Chicago; MA 41 IA St Univ; Cl Psychol, The Kriegman Cl Ltd

Kriegsmann, Elinor L 2350 McGilvra Blvd East, Seattle, WA 98112, (206) 455-4042, MA 63 San Francisco St Univ; Assoc Dir, Sp/Lang Hrng Serv Gp Hlth Coop, **SLP**

Kriendler, John C 3251 North Six Bar Spur, Tucson, AZ 85745-9776, (602) 622-5833, MA 73 Univ of AZ; MS 80 Univ of AZ; Sp-Lang Path, Sp-Lang Cl St Marys Hosp, **SLP**

Kriendler, Mrs Sandra L 8740 Westheimer #42, Houston, TX 77063, (713) 784-3455, BA 63 Univ of FL; MA 67 CUNY - Hunter Coll; OM 80 Univ of NM; 81–Sp/Lang Path, Houston ISD, **SLP**

Krier, Marcia Ann 860 6th Street #2, New Richmond, WI 54017, (715) 268-9771, BA 85 Univ of WI - Eau Claire; MS 86 Univ of WI - Eau Claire; **SLP**

Kriesel, Mrs Leslie J 2616 Prindle Road, Belmont, CA 94002, (415) 595-1447, BA 70 Univ of WA; MA 71 Northwestern Univ; SLP, San Mateo Co Bd of Ed, **SLP**

Krieski, Sandra Nan 2807 East Sunnyside Drive, Phoenix, AZ 85028, (602) 264-1157, BS 79 Univ of AZ; MS 81 Univ of AZ; Sp/Lang Path, Sunnyside Sch Dist, **SLP**

Krieter, Mrs Mary Kathleen 1687 Cumberland, Aurora, IL 60504, (312) 820-8340, BS 76 Purdue Univ - West Lafayette; MA 82 Ball St Univ; Sp-Lang Path, NW In Spec Ed Coop, **SLP**

Krikelas, Mrs Alma Laurila 49 South Erie Street, Aurora, MN 55705, (218) 229-3321, BA 74 Univ of MN - Duluth; SLP, Aurora-Hoyt Lakes Sch ISD 691, **SLP**

Krikorian, Carol Ann 5705 Spanish Oak Drive, Greensboro, NC 27409-2727, (919) 294-7350, BS 79 James Madison Univ; MS 81 James Madison Univ; Sp-Lang Path, Greensboro City Pub Sch, **SLP**

Krikorian, Mrs Lynn A 6211 North Tamera, Fresno, CA 93711, (209) 442-3967, BA 76 CA St Univ - Fresno; MA 79 CA St Univ - Fresno; Aud, Central CA ENT Medical Group, **A**

Krikorian, Marvel J 1434 West Monte Vista Avenue, Visalia, CA 93277, (209) 733-9102, BA 75 CA St Univ - Sacramento; OM 78 CA St Univ - Chico; 88–Admin/Prog Dir, Home Stretch Inc, **SLP**

Krill, Mrs Mary Louise 2226 Pemberton, Toledo, OH 43606, (419) 537-2244, BS 63 Saint Louis Univ; ME 77 Univ of Toledo; OM 81 Univ of Toledo; Cl Superv, U of Toledo, **SLP**

Krimmel, Mrs Margaret W P O Box 545, 26540 Fairfield Road, Wauconda, IL 60084, (312) 395-1105, BS 46 Northwestern Univ; MS 72 Central WA Univ; Sp-Lang Path, Emmons Sch Dist 033, **SLP**

Kriney, Valerie Pinto 50 Euclid Avenue Unit 1-H, Hackensack, NJ 07601, (201) 967-4040, BS 74 Ithaca Coll; MA 75 NY Univ; Aud, Bergen Pines County Hosp, **A ACE**

Krinkin, Mrs Naomi K 44 Shderot Eshkol, Jerusalem, Israel, MS 72 Bradley Univ; Sp-Lang Path, Board of Education, **SLP**

Krino, Mrs Susan F 1840 South Williamston Rd, Williamston, MI 48895, (517) 339-8208, OB 68 OH Univ - Athens; MA 69 OH Univ - Athens; 86–Tchr, Haslett PS, **SLP**

Krinock, Mrs Pamela S Speech & Language Therapy Serv, 929 Harmony Lane, South Charleston, WV 25303, (304) 744-3212, BA 79 Marshall Univ; MA 80 Marshall Univ; Sp-Lang Path, Sp-Lang Ther Serv, **SLP**

Krinsky, Martin S 22 Eisenhower Road, West Peabody, MA 01960, (508) 535-4923, BS 70 Boston Univ; MS 71 Univ of VT; OM 78 Boston Univ; 78–Sp-Lang Path, Greater Lynn Visiting Nurse Assoc, **SLP**

Krinsky, Ruth Tammi 65 Devon Road, Bethpage, NY 11714, (516) 261-9000

Kripal, Joni Peters Bio-Logic Systems, 1 Bio-Logic Plaza, Mundelein, IL 60060, (800) 323-8326, MS 84 UT St Univ; Aud, Bio-Logic Systems, **A**

Krische, Karen L 750 1/2 South Marengo, Pasadena, CA 91106, BA 76 Univ of CA - Santa Barbara; MA 80 CA St Univ - Northridge; SLP, Los Angeles USD, **SLP**

Krish, Geneva A Office Of Dr Michael C Reese, 1110 West Elm, Rogers, AR 72756, (501) 636-0110, BS 71 Univ of TX - Austin; MS 79 Univ of NM; Aud, Dr Michael C Reese, **A**

Krishna, Suzanne 330 Longwood Road, Kennett Square, PA 19348, (215) 869-8737, **SLP**

Krishnan, Dr Ananthanarayan 509 South Highland Avenue #14, Pittsburgh, PA 15206, (412) 624-7790, BS 73 Univ of Mysore - India; MA 80 Memphis St Univ; PH 83 (Hrng Science) Univ of TX - Dallas; 87–Asst Prof, Univ of Pitt, **A**

Krishnan, Ranjani 55 Reservoir Road #3, Chestnut Hill, MA 02167, (401) 331-5511, BS 84 Topiwala Nat'l Med Coll Bombay Univ - India; MS 87 Northeastern Univ; 88–Aud, Dudley Audiology Services

Krishnaswamy, Latha 16 Prospect Avenue, Douglaston, New York, NY 11362, (718) 279-3465, MS 87 CUNY - Brooklyn Coll; BS 85; **SLP**

Kriske, Mrs Lydia Lucio 12240 Ridge Crown, San Antonio, TX 78247, (512) 396-8500, BS 84 Southwest TX St Univ; MA 86 Southwest TX St Univ; **SLP**

Kriss, Charles Anthony, Jr 400 Timber Creek Drive, Apartment 405, Richwood, TX 77531, (409) 297-2477, BS 80 Univ Southern MS-Hattiesburg; MS 82 Univ Southern MS-Hattiesburg; 86–Aud, Dr Meyer & Dr Lunsford, **A**

Krissman, Mrs Rosalynn 250 South Bedford Drive, Beverly Hills, CA 90212, (213) 557-3618, MA 74 CA St Univ - Northridge; Sp-Lang Path, Private Practice, **SLP**

Kristal-Bryant, Linda Gail 1530 N W 40th Drive, Gainesville, FL 32605, (904) 376-5656, BA 71 Univ of Miami; MA 85 Univ of FL; SLP, Sunland Center, **SLP**

Kristall-Sclar, Anita Joy 5010 Lakeview Drive, Fayetteville, NY 13066, (716) 473-8417, BA 76 SUNY - Center at Buffalo; MS 78 SUNY - Coll at Buffalo; Sp-Lang Path, Private Practice, **SLP**

Kristiansen, Mrs Mary Ann 5755 East River Road Apartment 412, Tucson, AZ 85715, (602) 577-9542, MA 74 Governors St Univ; Sp-Lang Path, Tucson USD, **SLP**

Kristoff, Mrs Barbara L 9 Miriam Drive, Matawan, NJ 07747, (201) 932-9137, BA 76 Montclair St Coll; MS 79 Rutgers Coll; 78–Sp-Lang Path, Douglas Dev Disabl Cen, **SLP**

Kritz, Kenneth W Maryland School For The Deaf, P O Box 250, Frederick, MD 21701, (301) 662-4159, BA 55 Univ of WI - Stevens Point; MS 60 Gallaudet Coll; MA 67 Northwestern Univ; Prin, MD Sch for the Deaf

Krivacek, Paul Louis 210 Linda Drive, Greensburg, PA 15601, (412) 836-2460, BS 64 CA Univ of PA; MA 66 WV Univ; Super/Spec Progs, Westmoreland Inter Ut, **SLP**

Krivak, Brenda Marie 212 N W 32nd Street, Corvallis, OR 97330, (503) 485-8521

Krival, Catherine R c/o Mediplex Rehab-Bradenton, 5627 Ninth Street East, Bradenton, FL 34203, (813) 753-8941, BA 83 Univ of WI - Madison; MS 85 Univ of WI - Whitewater; 87–SLP, Mediplex Rehab-Bradenton, **SLP**

Krival, Dr Molly P 736 Durion Court, Sanibel, FL 33957, (414) 472-5203, BA 47 Univ of MO - Columbia; MA 49 Univ of MO - Columbia; PH 65 (NS) Univ of WI - Madison; 88–Retired, U of WI-Whitewater, **SLP**

Krivarchka, Mrs Cheryl M 781 Oakridge Drive, Lisbon, ND 58054, (701) 683-5761, BS 75 Univ of ND; MA 76 Univ of ND; Sp-Lang Path, Sheyene Valley Spec Ed Unit, **SLP**

Kriynovich, Linda G 5163 Joseph Street, Maple Heights, OH 44137, (216) 663-1694, BA 74 Cleveland St Univ; MA 75 Cleveland St Univ; Sp-Lang-Hrng Spec, Euclid Pub Schs, **SLP**

Krizic, Lynn Soprych 106 Cornwall Drive, Crete, IL 60417, (815) 740-3196, BS 77 Univ of IL - Urbana; MS 78 Univ of IL - Urbana; Coord, Joliet Sch Dist #86, **SLP**

Krizman, Mrs Debora Johnson 1950 Littlecreek Road, Auburn, CA 95603-9604, (716) 823-7532, MA 82 San Jose St Univ; Sp-Lang Path, Placer Sp & Hrng Serv, **SLP**

Kroc, Robin RFD 1 Box 1474, Brunswick, ME 04011, (207) 729-1669, BA 68 Univ of Denver; MA 69 Univ of Denver; Sp-Lang Path, Brunswick Sch Dept, **SLP**

Kroell, Mrs Anne Carroll 135 Harlan Drive, Bloomfield Hills, MI 48013, (313) 644-9300, OM 66 Wayne St Univ; BA 62 Marygove Coll; Sp-Lang Path, Birmingham Schools, **SLP**

Kroese, Judith M G 3059 Sleepy Hollow Drive, Stockton, CA 95209, (209) 952-7546, BA 67 Univ of IA; MA 69 Univ of IA; SLP, Stockton USD, **SLP**

Krogh, Stanley O 2609 9th Street, North Fargo, ND 58102, (701) 237-2441, BA 66 ND St Univ; BA 66 ND St Univ; MS 69 ND St Univ; Dir of Aud, Fargo Cl, **A**

Krogul, Mrs Valerie A PO Box 359, 18 Walker Drive, Quinebaug, CT 06262, (203) 923-9581, BS 80 Univ of MA - Amherst; MS 82 Worcester St Coll; Sp-Lang Path, Thompson Mem Sch, **SLP**

Krogulski, Priscilla Mary Reading Rehabilitation Hosp, Route 1 Box 250, Reading, PA 19607, (215) 777-7615, **SLP**

Krohel, Mary Beth K The Village Preschool, P O Box 269, West Sand Lake, NY 12196, (518) 674-2881, BA 75; MA 76 Coll of Saint Rose; 81–Dir, Village Preschool & Comm Ctr, **SLP**

Krohn, Mrs Myrna L 1427 South 85th Avenue, Omaha, NE 68124, **SLP A**

Krol, Mrs Mary Chambers P O Box 1201, Sterling Heights, MI 48311-1201, (313) 463-1115, BS 82 Central MI Univ; MA 84 Central MI Univ; Sp-Lang Path, Grosse Pointe Sch Sys, **SLP**

Krol, Mrs Sheree Sarko 2309 Foliage Lane, Dyer, IN 46311, (219) 865-3406, BS 82 Purdue Univ - West Lafayette; MS 85 Purdue Univ - West Lafayette; Aud, **A**

Krolikowski, David Milker 9 Gregg Lane, Coram, NY 11727, (516) 474-1647, BS 81 Nazareth Coll of Rochester; MA 85 Hofstra Univ; Sp-Lang Path, BOCES II, **SLP**

Kroll, Dr Allan P O Box 924, 547 Glenridge Avenue, St Catharines, ON, Canada L2R 6Z4, (416) 688-2980, BS 64 McGill Univ - Quebec; MS 68 CUNY - Brooklyn Coll; PH 70 (Speech Pathology) Purdue Univ - West Lafayette; Dir/Sp-Lang Path-Aud, Niagra Peninsula Rehab Cen, **SLP**

Kroll, Linda J 6732 N E McKinstry, Suquamish, WA 98392, (206) 598-3510, BA 65 Elmhurst Coll; MS 75 Eastern WA Univ; Sp-Lang Path, Private Practice, **SLP**

Kroll, Mrs Mercedes San Patricio Plaza, PMC Suite #334, San Juan, PR 00920, BS 53 Northwestern Univ; MA 59 Northwestern Univ; PH 69 (NS) Univ of MI - Ann Arbor; Retired, **SLP**

Kroll, Paulette 315 Goldenrod, Corona Del Mar, CA 92625, (213) 985-4594, BS 75 Marquette Univ; MA 77 CA St Univ - Long Beach; Lect, CA St U-Long Beach, **SLP**

Kroll, Susan Faye Language Clinic, Hawthorn Center, 18471 Haggerty, Northville, MI 48167, (313) 928-0144, MA 85 Eastern MI Univ; **SLP**

Kroll, William J 906 Jones Street, Berkeley, CA 94710, (415) 524-9210, BA 71; MA 76; 84–Sp-Lang Path, Oakland USD, **SLP**

Kronberg, Linda Ann 6214 South 43rd Street, Phoenix, AZ 85040, BS 72 AZ St Univ; MS 80 AZ St Univ; 84–Sp-Lang Path, Kyrene School District #28, **SLP**

Kronman, Mrs Joan Safier 9 Estate Road, P O Box 916, Center Moriches, NY 11934, (516) 878-1683, MA 84 Long Island U - CW Post Ctr; Adj Prof, St Joseph's Coll, **SLP**

Kronman, Mrs Sharon M 485 Longview Road, South Orange, NJ 07079, (201) 762-8784, BS 72 Univ of GA; MS 73 Rutger's St Univ - Douglas Coll; 87–Sp-Lang Path, Suburban Sp & Lrng Ctr, **SLP**

Kropa, Jean J 1006 Viscount Court, Avondale Estates, GA 30002, (404) 299-1738, ME 85 GA St Univ; **SLP**

Kropf, Anne N 8 Meadowbrook Lane, Old Westbury, NY 11568, (516) 626-0077, BA 66 Hofstra Univ; MA 69 Hofstra Univ; SLP, Nassau BOCES, **SLP**

Kropf, Mrs T Janet 21913 Grant Avenue, Torrance, CA 90503, (213) 546-3488, BA 76 CA St Univ - Long Beach; MA 78 CA St Univ - Long Beach; Sp-Lang Path, Manhattan Beach City Sch, **SLP**

Krostich, Mrs Linda Gordon 28 Oakwood Lane, Plainview, NY 11803, (516) 822-9240, BS 77 SUNY - Center at Albany; MS 79 Hahneman Medical Coll; 84–Sp-Lang Path, Private Practice, **SLP**

Krotick, Mindy Gayle 33-53 82nd Avenue #A-1, Jackson Heights, NY 11372, (212) 565-1024, BS 80 Syracuse Univ; MA 82 NY Univ; SLP, NYC Bd of Ed, **SLP**

Kroupa, Molly J 1135 South Pine Avenue, Arlington Heights, IL 60005, (312) 228-1985, BA 73 Univ of CA - Santa Barbara; MS 75 Marquette Univ; Sp-Lang Path, Pro Rehab Assoc, **SLP**

Krouse, Dr Carl W 3924 Bishop, Detroit, MI 48224, PH 76 (Aud) Wayne St Univ; 75–Aud, Wayne County Intermed Sch Dist, **SLP A**

Krouse, Maureen Casey 14 Laurel Lane, Princeton, MA 01541, (508) 799-4171, BS 74 Salem St Coll; MA 79 Univ of MA - Amherst; 85–Dir & Sp-Lang Path, Sp Path Assoc PC, **SLP ACE**

Krowchenko, Laura L 602-4105 Maywood Street, Burnaby, BC, Canada V5H 4A3, (604) 534-7891, BA 71; MA 73 Univ of ND; Sp-Lang Path, Sch Dist #35, **SLP**

Krowiorz, Pamela Jeanne 516 Saratoga Street, Green Bay, WI 54303, BS 76 Univ of WI - Madison; MS 78 Univ of WI - Madison; 78–Sp-Lang Path, Green Bay Area Pub Sch, **SLP**

Krueger, Mrs Barbara A 976 Antelope N E, Albuquerque, NM 87122, (505) 296-6660, BA 85 Univ of NM; MA 88 Univ of NM

Krueger, Beverly M 2136 South Central Avenue, Burlington, IA 52601, (319) 752-2255, BA 73 MacAlster Coll; BA 77 Univ of MN - Minneap-St Paul; MA 79 Univ of IA; Sp-Lang Path, Private Practice, **SLP**

Krueger, Charles Kent 3675 Pecos-McLeod, Las Vegas, NV 89121, (702) 733-4066, BS 74 ID St Univ; MS 76 ID St Univ; 88–Sp-Lang Path, Paradise Valley Speech & Hearing, **SLP**

Krueger, Kathleen M 2300 Crestwood Road, North Little Rock, AR 72116, (501) 660-2008, BS 66 Univ of MN - Minneap-St Paul; MS 68 Univ of OK Medical Center; 78–Sp-Lang Path, VA Med Ctr, **SLP ACE**

Krueger, Kathy Ann 719 Edgestone Place #351, Arlington, TX 76006, (214) 277-1674, BS 78 Southwest TX St Univ; ME 80 Southwest TX St Univ; Sp-Lang Path, Trinity Easter Seals Soc for Child, **SLP**

Krueger, Michele Sabol 238 Anne Drive, Newport News, VA 23601, (804) 596-1203, BS 86 OH Univ - Athens; MA 87 OH Univ - Athens; 88–Sp-Lang Path, VA Sch for the Deaf & Blind

Krueger, Sharon Lee 15511 Stefan Circle S E, Prior Lake, MN 55372, (612) 469-4461, BS 81 Mankato St Univ; MS 83 Saint Cloud St Univ; 84–Sp-Lang Path, ISD 194 Lakeville PS, **SLP**

Krug, Karen A 61 Crystal Forest, Heber Springs, AR 72543, (501) 362-7700, BA 80 IA St Univ; MA 81 Northeast MO St Univ; **SLP**

Krug, Karen E 2928 Lydia, Topeka, KS 66614, BS 79 KS St Univ; MA 81 KS St Univ; 88–Sp-Lang Path, St Francis Hosp & Med Ctr, **SLP**

Krug, Dr Richard F 2765 Juilliard Street, Boulder, CO 80303, (303) 494-0766, BS 49 IL St Univ - Normal; MA 51 Northwestern Univ; PH 60 (NS) Univ of OK Medical Center; Prof Emeritus, U of CO-Boulder, **SLP A LM**

Krug, Terri L 2950 Broadway #7, Boulder, CO 80302-0020, (303) 938-8810, MS 79 IL St Univ - Normal; Sp-Lang Path, InSpeech Inc, **SLP**

Kruger, Anita L 3401 Skycroft Circle N E, St Anthony, MN 55418, (612) 487-1445, BA 73 Univ of MN - Duluth; MA 79 Mankato St Univ; SLP, Spec Interm Dist #916, **SLP**

Kruger, Dr Barbara 37 Somerset Drive, Commack, NY 11725, (212) 430-8386, BA 67 CUNY - Queens Coll; MA 70 CUNY - Queens Coll; PH 75 (NS) CUNY - Grad Sch & Univ Cntr; Dir, Aud & Comm Svcs, **SLP A F**

Kruger, Dr Frederick M 37 Somerset Drive, Commack, NY 11725, (516) 543-5392, BA 61 Washington Square Coll - NYU; PH 69 (NS) CUNY - Grad Sch & Univ Cntr; Consult/Pres, Scitronix Inc

Kruhm, Carolyn M 321 Imperial Blvd #99-J, Lakeland, FL 33803, (813) 647-3213, BS 84 FL St Univ; MS 86 FL St Univ; **SLP**

Kruh-Meyer, Nancy L 17 Alfred Road West, Merrick, NY 11566, (516) 378-0263, Aud, Larry Deutsch PhD, **A**

Krull, Mrs Alice M 945 157th Avenue N E, Anoka, MN 55304, (612) 444-5506, BA 52 Capital Univ; MA 53 Case Western Reserve Univ; Sp-Lang Path, Cambridge-Isanti Sch Dist #911, **SLP**

Krum, Susan Elizabeth 11881A Academy Road, Philadelphia, PA 19154, (215) 829-5182, BS 82 East Stroudsburg Univ of PA; MA 85 Temple Univ; Aud, Atkins-Keane Otol Associates, **A**

Krumm, John B 4028 France Avenue North, Robbinsdale, MN 55422, (612) 535-9399, BA 67 Univ of WI - River Falls; MA 72 Univ of MN - Minneap-St Paul; Superv/Itinerant&Shared Servcs, ISD 281, **SLP**

Krumm, Kent M P O Box 1418, Hazard, KY 41701, (606) 439-2900, BA 69 TX Tech Univ; MA 72 Univ of KY; Dir, Sp Cl Inc, **SLP**

Krumm, Laurence Charles 3270 Hebron Court #3, San Jose, CA 95121, (908) 270-5046, BA 73 OH Northern Univ; MA 75 Kent St Univ; **SLP**

Krumm, Mark Paul 2924 East 33rd St North, Wichita, KS 67219, BS 80; MS 82 Univ of WY; Aud, Wichita St U-Sp &Hrng Dept, **A**

Krupat, Barbara R 151 Elgin Street, Newton Center, MA 02159, BA 68 CUNY - Hunter Coll; MS 69 Univ of MI - Ann Arbor; 87–Sp-Lang Path, Newton PS, **SLP**

Krupic, Kathryn Lynn 22236 Innsbrook Drive, Northville, MI 48167, (616) 343-2601, **SLP**

Krupit, Mrs Felicia Mindy 846 Paseo Estero Drive, San Jose, CA 95122, (408) 286-8729, MA 88 San Jose St Univ

Krupke, David L 729 21st Street, Bettendorf, IA 52722, (319) 359-1371, BS 70 Western IL Univ; MA 73 Western IL Univ; Sp-Lang Path, MS Bend AEA, **SLP**

Krupp, Rita S 11326 Olympia Fields Row, San Diego, CA 92128, (619) 451-0336, BA 77 Univ of MN - Duluth; MA 78 Univ of MN - Duluth; SLP, Grossmont High Sch Dist, **SLP**

Kruppa, John R 34 Hurst Avenue, Clair Manor, Belle Vernon, PA 15012, (412) 929-5141, BS 67 CA Univ of PA; ME 75 CA Univ of PA; Dir Commun Dev, S W Habilitation Cen, **SLP**

Kruppert-Hayes, Ursula c/o F W Kruppert, Rural Route 1, Goulais River, ON, Canada P0S 1E0, (313) 971-7610, BA 78 Lake Superior St Coll; MA 81 Northern MI Univ; 88–Sp-Lang Path, Sault Ste Marie Bd of Educ, **SLP**

Kruse, Caroline Gann 4405 Canal Street, New Orleans, LA 70119, (504) 482-8351, OM 82 LA St Univ - N O Medical Ctr; Aud, Orleans Parish Schs, **A**

Kruse, Mrs Lisa Polino 2328 Archwood Lane #67, Simi Valley, CA 93063, (805) 527-3109, BA 83 CA St Univ - Northridge; MA 86 CA St Univ - Northridge; **SLP**

Kruse, Dr R J Main At Maple, Lightstreet, PA 17839, (717) 389-4436, BA 60 Temple Univ; MA 64 Temple Univ; PH 72 (Sp-Lang Path) Temple Univ; Professor, Bloomsburg University, **SLP**

Kruse, Prof Richard W 9 Maple Circle, Westborough, MA 01581, (617) 345-2151, BA 57 Denison Univ; ME 65 Boston Univ; Asst Prof Sp, Fitchburg State Coll, **SLP**

Kruse, Mrs Sydney Lynne B General Delivery, Walthill, NE 68067, (402) 846-5488, BS 61 Univ of NE - Lincoln; MS 82 Univ of NE - Lincoln; Sp-Lang Path, Educational Service Unit I, **SLP**

Krush, Mrs Gail Owan 1326-14th Avenue South, Fargo, ND 58103, (701) 232-4641, BS 81 ND St Univ; MS 86 Univ of ND

Kruszewski, Christine 783 Quince Orchard Blvd, Apartment #22, Gaithersburg, MD 20878, (512) 451-6539, BS 78 Trenton St Coll; MA 79 Trenton St Coll; Sp/Lang Path, Dev Cen Aisd, **SLP**

Krutt, Susan Sidranksy 813 Cypress Road, Newington, CT 06111, (203) 237-7835, MS 84 Gallaudet Coll; Aud, Easter Seal Rehab Ctr, **A**

Kruzer, Mrs A Tammy 2076 Hillcrest Avenue, Cleveland, OH 44109, (216) 459-3178, MA 84 Case Western Reserve Univ; 87–Sp-Lang Path, Cleveland Metro Gen Hosp, **SLP**

Kruzshak, Lauren L 930 Old Town Road, Trumbull, CT 06611, (203) 261-3691, BS 75 Ithaca Coll; MA 76 OH St Univ; **SLP**

Krych, David K Centre For Neuro Skills, 2658 Mount Vernon, Bakersfield, CA 93306, (805) 324-9565, BS 77 Southern IL Univ -Carbondale; MS 79 Southern IL Univ -Carbondale; Exec Dir, Centre for Neuro Skills, **SLP**

Kryder, Mrs Cynthia Landis 984 Fox Chase Drive, West Chester, PA 19380, (215) 251-5434, BS 76 Bloomsburg Univ of PA; MS 77 Bloomsburg Univ of PA; 88–Dir of Comm Disorders, Bryn Mawr Rehab Hosp, **SLP**

Kryzer, Mrs Katherine 805 Kerwin Road, Silver Spring, MD 20901, (301) 593-6334, BA 80 Univ of MT; MA 82 George Washington Univ; **SLP**

Krzywicki, Joanne K Rd 1 Lot 11, 1500 Zion Road, Middletown, PA 17057, BS 71 Bloomsburg Univ of PA; MS 72 Bradley Univ; 78–Sp/Lang Path, Pro Home Hlth Care Agcy, **SLP**

Kuba, Janis M 1707 N Outagamie Street, Appleton, WI 54914, (414) 424-0053, BS 78 Univ of WI - Stevens Point; MA 79 MI St Univ; 87–Sp-Lang Path, Univ of WI-Oshkosh, **SLP**

Kubala, Virginia 5408 Royal Drive N E, Albuquerque, NM 87111, (505) 822-9622, BA 72 Univ of OK - Norman; MA 73 Univ of OK - Norman; **SLP**

Kuberry, Gjoa 34 Spotted Deer, The Woodlands, TX 77381, **SLP**

Kubiak, Mrs Margaret Kristen 6034 North 21st Street, Arlington, VA 22205-3406, (303) 733-5181, MS 80 Northwestern Univ; **A**

Kubiak-Cherkaski, Lisa D 70 McLaughlin Street, Staten Island, NY 10305, (718) 720-0054, BA 85 Long Island U - Brooklyn Ctr; MA 87 Kean Coll of NJ; **SLP**

Kubik, Dr Alexander W 1704 Landrake Road, Ruxton, MD 21204, BS 53 Bloomsburg Univ of PA; MA 59 Univ of MD - College Park; PH 78 (NS) Univ of MD - College Park; Sp-Lang Path & Audiologist, Univ of MD-Inst of Emerg Med, **SLP A**

Kubin, Mrs Leigh Ann 5901 West 84th Terrace, Overland Park, KS 66207-1643, (913) 341-4827, BS 80 Univ of KS; MA 82 Univ of KS; Sp-Lang Path, Shawnee Mission Sch Dist, **SLP**

Kubler, Mrs Paula S 209 Tremont Avenue, Greensburg, PA 15601, (412) 836-2792, BS 74 Carlow Coll; MS 75 Univ of HI - Manoa; Sp-Lang Path, Easter Seals/L Doerfler Aud As, **SLP**

Kucera, Stephen Alan 4911 Berryhill Circle, Perry Hall, MD 21128, (301) 256-6520, BA 69 Towson St Univ; MS 72 Loyola Coll; Sp-Lang Path, Baltimore Co Bd of Ed, **SLP**

Kucharski, Mrs Kimberlea Panuce 918 Thames Court, Schaumburg, IL 60172, (312) 980-1849, BA 79 Northern IL Univ - De Kalb; MA 81 Northern IL Univ - De Kalb; Sp/Lang Path, NW Sub Spec Ed Organization, **SLP**

Kucherawy, David A P O Box 94, Polk, PA 16342, (814) 432-3171, BS 74 CA Univ of PA; MA 78 West Chester Univ of PA; Facility Director, Polk Center, **SLP**

Kuchmaner, Mrs Lauri Dahman 266 Bradford Drive, Canfield, OH 44406, (216) 533-7495, BS 80 Bowling Green St Univ; MA 81 Bowling Green St Univ; Eap Proj Coord, Neo/Serrc, **SLP**

Kuchon, Dr Patricia P 24 Martindale Road, Short Hills, NJ 07078, (201) 761-9075, BA 66 Montclair St Coll; MS 68 Adelphi Univ; PH 76 (NS) CUNY - Grad Sch & Univ Cntr; Vice-Chancellor, Seton Hall U, **SLP F**

Kudritz, Joann Monica 8 Coldwater Street East #4, Orillia, ON, Canada L3V 6L2, (705) 326-7361, BA 80 SUNY - Coll at Potsdam; MA 82 SUNY - Center at Buffalo; 84–Aud, Huronia Regional Centre, **A**

Kudszus, Ursula R 1557 Newburg Drive, Fairfield, CA 94533, (707) 425-0281, OB 64; MA 78 CA St Univ - Sacramento; Coord/SLP, Fairfield-Suisun USD, **SLP**

Kuebler, Mrs Linda K 1324 Sunnyvale Drive, Jefferson City, MO 65109, (314) 893-5021, BS 78 Central MO St Univ; MS 80 Central MO St Univ; 87–Sp-Lang Path, The "Special" Lrng Ctr, **SLP**

Kuehn, Dr David P University Of Illinois, Dept Sp & H Science, 901 S 6th Street, Champaign, IL 61820, (217) 244-2539, BA 67 Northern IL Univ - De Kalb; MA 70 Univ of IA; PH 73 (NS) Univ of IA; 86–Assoc Prof, U of IL, **F**

Kuehn, Marilyn K 770 Anderson Avenue #20-K, Cliffside Park, NJ 07010, (201) 833-5490, BA 54 CUNY - Brooklyn Coll; MA 72 CUNY - Brooklyn Coll; 68–Sp-Lang Path, Teaneck Bd of Ed, **SLP**

Kuehner, Suzanne June 115 Chicora Road, Butler, PA 16001, (412) 283-8602, BS 85 Clarion Univ of PA; MS 86 Clarion Univ of PA; Sp-Lang Path, Easter Seal Soc of Butler Co, **SLP**

Kuehnle, Lisa G 66168 48th Avenue, Hartford, MI 49057, 84–Sp-Lang Path, Watervliet PS, **SLP**

Kueht, James D 6413 West Clarke Street, Milwaukee, WI 53213, (414) 646-3319, BS 79 Univ of WI - Milwaukee; MS 81 Univ of WI - Milwaukee; Sp-Lang Path, Sch Dist Kettle Moraine, **SLP**

Kueht, Margaret Lynn 209 Wright Street Upper, Waukesha, WI 53186-5531, (414) 542-8036, BS 85 Univ of WI - Whitewater; MS 86 Univ of WI - Whitewater; 87–Sp-Lang Path, Lutheran Social Svcs, **SLP**

Kuemmel, Robbie E 3715 Green Trails South, Austin, TX 78731, (512) 483-3120, BS 69 Univ of TX - Austin; MA 76 Univ of Houston - Univ Park; Sp-Lang Path, Austin ISD, **SLP**

Kuenzli, Timothy R 1463 Deanforest Road, Savannah, GA 31405, (912) 925-4402, BS 82 Northern MI Univ; MA 86 Central MI Univ; **SLP**

Kuerbis, Tracy L 2464 Tunlaw Road N W, Washington, DC 20007, (202) 651-5045, BA 84 San Diego St Univ; MS 86 Gallaudet Coll; **A**

Kuergeleis, Bonita Jean 55 North Bompart, Apartment G-2-D, St Louis, MO 63119, (314) 968-1081, MS 81 Univ of OR; Sp-Lang Path, PFT-Webster Groves Sch Dist, **SLP**

Kufahl, Mrs Susanne Suther R R 2 Box 39, Wheaton, KS 66551, MA 81 KS St Univ; **SLP A**

Kuffel, Constance F 4150 Northmeadow Circle, Tampa, FL 33624, (813) 974-2006, BA 64 MI St Univ; MA 68 Univ of South FL; Coor Clin Services/Trng In Aud, University of South Florida, **SLP A ACE**

Kugelman, Sandra Marli 2963 West Tower Avenue, Cincinnati, OH 45238, (513) 451-5299, BS 84 Univ of Cincinnati; MA 86 Univ of Cincinnati; **SLP**

Kugler, Karen J 1109 Otero, San Clemente, CA 92672, **SLP**

Kuhl, Kathryn Trcka 1923 East Highview Drive, Sauk Rapids, MN 56379, (612) 255-5678, BS 85 Saint Cloud St Univ; MS 87 Saint Cloud St Univ; 87–Sp-Lang Path, Saint Cloud Hosp, **SLP**

Kuhl, Susan Lisa 325 West 77th Street, New York, NY 10024, (212) 420-2760, BA 84 Queens Coll; MA 86 CUNY - Queens Coll; 87–Sp-Lang Path, Beth Israel Med Ctr, **SLP**

Kuhles, Nancy Lillian 1190 Manor Drive, Reno, NV 89509, (702) 348-0272, BA 80 CA St Univ - Sacramento; MS 82 Univ of NV - Reno; **SLP**

Kuhlmann, Marcia D P O Box 484, Rankin, TX 79778, (915) 693-2445, BS 77 Southwest TX St Univ; ME 78 Southwest TX St Univ; Spec Ed, Rankin ISD, **SLP**

Kuhn, Beth Ann 10875-6 Scripps Ranch Boulevard, San Diego, CA 92131, (619) 586-7168, BS 81 Coll of Saint Rose; MS 82 Coll of Saint Rose; Sp/Lang Path, Sp Hrng & Neuro Ctr, **SLP**

Kuhn, Mrs Charleene L 204 Dayton Avenue, Huron, OH 44839, (419) 433-6098, MS 85 Howard Univ

Kuhn, Mrs Cheryl Thomas 119 Rochester Drive, Sheboygan Falls, WI 53085, (414) 459-3886, BS 78 Univ of WI - Stevens Point; MS 80 Univ of WI - Eau Claire; Sp-Lang Path, Sheboygan Co Hndcpd Chld Ed Bd, **SLP**

Kuhn, Deborah Jean 12231 Clifton #3, Lakewood, OH 44107, (216) 362-6450, BS 76 Old Dominion Univ; MA 82 Cleveland St Univ; Sp/Lang Path, Cuyahuga Co Bd of Mr/Dd, **SLP**

Kuhn, Mrs Elizabeth Ellen 8702 Matchlock Court, Indianapolis, IN 46256, (317) 462-9219, BS 79 Purdue Univ - West Lafayette; MA 83 Ball St Univ; Sp-Lang Path, Hancock/S Madison Joint Serv, **SLP**

Kuhn, Janeen G 323 Mill Street, Williamston, MI 48895, (517) 655-5142, BA 77 MI St Univ; MS 79 Rutgers St Univ - Newark; SLP, **SLP**

Kuhn, Joan C Box 199, 8700 West Wisconsin Avenue, Milwaukee, WI 53226, (414) 257-7344, MS 68 Marquette Univ; BS 67 Univ of IL - Urbana; Sp-Lang Path, Medical College of Wisconsin, **SLP ACE**

Kuhn, Joan Smith 6500 Monroe, Evansville, IN 47715-6022, (812) 429-0700, BS 74 Purdue Univ - West Lafayette; MS 76 Purdue Univ - West Lafayette; Chief/SLP, Tallahassee Mem Reg Med Cen, **SLP**

Kuhn, Mrs Kathleen Beskid 105 North Liberty Street, Apartment C-5, Centerville, MD 21617, (215) 783-6010, BA 81 Loyola Coll; MS 82 Loyola Coll; Sp-Lang Path, Anne Arundel County Pub School, **SLP**

Kuhn, Lynn Erica 2585 South Lansing Way, Aurora, CO 80014, (303) 368-8504, BA 73 SUNY - Center at Buffalo; MA 79 Univ of Denver; SLP, Cherry Creek School District, **SLP**

Kuhn, Mrs Margaret E 3105 Mill Springs Road, Belleville, IL 62221, BS 80 Southern IL Univ-Edwardsvill; MS 81 Southern IL Univ-Edwardsvill; SLP, Spec Sch Dist of St Louis Co, **SLP**

Kuhn, Marilynn Harvit 8208 Tinkerton Court, Charlotte, NC 28212-5376, BS 79 Univ of Cincinnati; MA 82 Univ of Cincinnati; SLP, Charlotte Rehabilitation Hosp, **SLP**

Kuhn, Michael Robert 4421 Avenida Manana NE, Albuquerque, NM 87108, (505) 873-0710, BA 82 Univ of NM; MS 87 Univ of NM; 88–Sp-Lang Path, Educ Assess Systems Inc, **SLP**

Kuhn, Ruby M 579 Coventry Lane, West Chester, PA 19380, (215) 237-4388, BS 75 Radford Univ; OM 78 Hahneman Medical Coll; Director Speech & Hearing Serv, Fitzgerald Mercy Hospital, **SLP**

Kuhne, Sylvia Marie 129 Bishop Street, Watertown, NY 13601, BS 59 Syracuse Univ; MA 86 CA St Univ - Northridge; 88–Sp-Lang Path, BOCES, **SLP**

Kuhns, Evelyn Mae 9 Woloski Park, Middleboro, MA 02346, (508) 947-8394, BA 80 Goshen Coll; MS 83 James Madison Univ; 85–Sp-Lang Path, READS Inc Hrng Impaired Prog, **SLP**

Kuhns, Mrs Linda Lister 302 East Chatham Street, Fredericksburg, VA 22405, (304) 636-4120, BS 81 CA Univ of PA; MS 85 CA Univ of PA; **SLP**

Kuhnsman, Liane M 2299 Sheridan Road, Frances Searle Bldg, Northwestern University, Evanston, IL 60208, (312) 491-4171, BA 78 Univ of MD - College Park; MS 79 James Madison Univ; 88–Sp-Lang Path, Chicago NeuroSurgical Ctr, **SLP**

Kuipers, Kenneth E 709 Williams Street, Hamburg, PA 19526, (215) 562-6312, BS 76 Edinboro Univ of PA; MA 80 Edinboro Univ of PA; Sp-Lang Path, Hamburg Center, **SLP**

Kujawa, Sharon Guilds University Medical Center, 1501 North Campbell, Tucson, AZ 85724, (602) 626-7222, BA 75 MI St Univ; MS 82 ID St Univ; Aud, U of AZ, **A**

Kujawski, Mrs Cindy D 511-80 Pheasant Run Drive, Granger, IN 46530, (219) 289-7765, BS 74 Purdue Univ - West Lafayette; MA 75 MI St Univ; ES 83 IN Univ - Bloomington; Sp-Lang Path, So Bend Comm Sch Corp, **SLP**

Kujawski, Claudia Ezman 26635 Huntington Road, Huntington Woods, MI 48070, (313) 547-6380, BA 80 Wayne St Univ; MA 82 Wayne St Univ; Sp-Lang Path, Hamtramck Public Schools, **SLP**

Kujolic, Carolyn Ann 4006 Balwynne Park Road, Philadelphia, PA 19131, (609) 424-9084, MA 87 Gallaudet Coll

Kuk, Dr Francis Kok-Ming Department Of Otolaryngology, University Of Iowa, Hospital And Clinic, Iowa City, IA 52242, (319) 356-3970, BS 80 Miami Univ - Oxford; MA 83 Univ of IA; PH 86 (Aud/Hrng Science) Univ of IA; 86–Asst Research Sci, Univ of Iowa Hosp, **A**

Kukelka, Mrs Tina R 63 Winthrop Road, Plainview, NY 11803, (516) 931-1949, BA 73 CUNY - Queens Coll; MS 74 Univ of WI - Madison; Sp-Lang Path, Arlene Falk, **SLP**

Kukich, Boyana 1237 Avenue Road Apartment 2, Toronto, ON, Canada M5N 2G5, (416) 471-4782, BS 76 Univ of Toronto - Ontario; MS 79 Emerson Coll; 87–Sp/Lang Path, York Reg RCSS Bd, **SLP**

Kukla, Janis Ann 1014 4th Avenue, Sacramento, CA 95818, (916) 366-8434, MS 85 CA St Univ - Sacramento; Sp-Lang Path, Folsom USD, **SLP**

Kukler, Linda B 2556 West Coyle, Chicago, IL 60645-3213, (312) 769-6997, **SLP**

Kuklewski, Karen Marie 2830 Crosby Avenue, Pittsburgh, PA 15216, (412) 341-3913, BS 84 Clarion Univ of PA; MA 85 OH Univ - Athens; SLP, Sewickley Valley Hosp, **SLP**

Kukol, Dr Robert J Speech Pathology (117H), VA Medical Center, Canandaigua, NY 14424, (716) 394-2000, BA 68 Univ of OK - Norman; MA 70 Univ of NM; PH 79 (Sp-Lang Path) Wichita St Univ; Sp-Lang Path, VA Med Cen, **SLP**

Kukula, Jane M Marymount Hearing-Bal Center, 12000 McCracken Road, Garfield Heights, OH 44125, (216) 662-3373, BA 77 Cleveland St Univ; MA 79 Cleveland St Univ; Aud, Marymount Hearing-Bal Center, **A**

Kukurudz, Kim Marie MSU, Head Res Dakota Hall, Minot, ND 58701, (701) 857-3500, 88 Minot St Univ

Kulcak-Studer, Mrs Bridget # 30 Sandy Creek Est, Brenham, TX 77833, (409) 836-7116, BS 75 Lamar Univ; MS 76 Southern Methodist Univ; Sp-Lang Path, Brenham Sp Lang Lrng Cen, **SLP**

Kuliberda, Theresa A 3112 Sherwood Avenue #244, Modesto, CA 95350-1381, **SLP**

Kulick, Kathleen Callan 27555 Middlebelt, Farmington Hills, MI 48018, (313) 476-4622, BS 74 Wayne St Univ; MA 76 Wayne St Univ - Sch of Med; Assoc Dir of Aud, Michigan Ear Institute, **A**

Kulig, Dr Sharon G 2109 Beverly Court, San Angelo, TX 76901, (915) 942-1294, BA 66 Univ of TX - Austin; ME 67 Univ of NC - Chapel Hill; PH 69 (NS) Univ of FL; Sp-Lang Path, Private Practice, **SLP**

Kulik, Mrs Linda 5745 Hempstead Drive, Agoura Hills, CA 91301, BA 72 CA St Univ - Northridge; MA 73 Univ of Denver; **SLP**

Kulkarni, Shridhar Govind 105-1588 Juniper Street, Prince George, BC, Canada V2L 1N5, (604) 563-1754, BS 82 0500; MA 85 Trenton St Coll; **A**

Kulla, Karen Kirsten 615 1/2 South 9th Street, Moorhead, MN 56560, (218) 233-8012, MS 88 Moorhead St Univ

Kuller, Mary Ehrlich 5 Berrien Avenue, Princeton Junction, NJ 08550, (212) 605-3740, BA 72 Case Western Reserve Univ; MS 74 Univ of MI - Ann Arbor; Aud, Manhattan ENT Hosp, **A**

Kully-Martens, Deborah A 401 8540 109 Street, Edmonton, AB, Canada T6G 1E6, (403) 432-2619, BS 80 Univ of Alberta - Alberta; MS 85 Univ of WA; 85–Clin Dir, Inst for Stuttering Treat & Res, **SLP**

Kulpa, Judith I 2938 North 61st Street, Milwaukee, WI 53210, (414) 937-2203, BS 68 Marquette Univ; MS 70 Marquette Univ; 88–Asst VP-Specialty Svcs, St Anthony's Family Med Ctr, **SLP ACE**

Kuluris, Mrs Joan J M 4715 East Bluebird Avenue, Orange, CA 92669, (714) 538-0912, BA 75 CA St Univ - Fullerton; MA 80 CA St Univ - Fullerton; Clinical Services, Orange USD, **SLP**

Kulway, Joann M E B Brown Hearing Aid Centers, 1549 East 30th Street, Cleveland, OH 44114, (216) 241-0474, BA 78 Cleveland St Univ; MA 79 Cleveland St Univ; 84–Aud/Dir, E B Brown Opticians/Hrg Ctrs, **A**

Kulzick, Mary Lynn 2946 South 80th Street, West Allis, WI 53219, (414) 321-0756, BS 84 Marquette Univ; MA 86 Kent St Univ; **SLP**

Kumiega, Santina Mantione 6411 Versailles Road, Lake View, NY 14085, (716) 649-6850, BS 75 SUNY - Coll at Buffalo; MS 77 SUNY - Coll at Buffalo; Sp-Lang Path, Hamburg Ctrl Sch, **SLP**

Kumin, Dr Libby B 5438 Thunder Hill Road, Columbia, MD 21045, (301) 323-1010, BA 65 Long Island U - Brooklyn Ctr; MA 66 NY Univ; PH 69 (NS) NY Univ; Sp-Lang Path, Loyola College, **SLP**

Kummer, Ann W Children's Hosp Medical Center, Dept Of Sp Path/Room 3-22, Elland And Bethesda Avenue, Cincinnati, OH 45229-2899, (513) 559-4341, BA 72 IN Univ - Bloomington; MA 73 IN Univ - Bloomington; PH 86 (Sp Path) Univ of Cincinnati; Dir of SLP Dept, Chldn's Hosp Med Cen, **SLP**

Kumnick, Mrs Laurie C 55 Hampshire Road, Meriden, CT 06450, (203) 238-9756, BS 76 Ithaca Coll; MA 79 OH Univ - Athens; 85–Sp-Lang Path, Meriden Health Dept, **SLP**

Kumpf, Donna M 580 Pleasant View Road, Lewisberry, PA 17339, (717) 737-6728, BS 80 Bloomsburg Univ of PA; MS 81 Bloomsburg Univ of PA; SLP, Capital Area Inter Ut, **SLP**

Kundel, Dr Karl J 4505 West 44th Street, Edina, MN 55424, (612) 922-3026, BS 72 Univ of IA; MA 75 Univ of IA; PH 79 (NS) Univ of IA; Asst Prof, U of OK, **A**

Kundel, Mrs Margaret N 1204 Northwood Lane, Muscatine, IA 52761, (319) 263-2412, BA 63 Univ of IA; MA 64 Stanford Univ; **SLP**

Kundin, Mrs K R 1 East Aster Drive, Phoenix, AZ 85022, (602) 978-1100, BS 70 AZ St Univ; MS 72 AZ St Univ; School Administrator, Peoria USD, **SLP**

Kundo, Mrs Peggy Diane P O Box 76, Capeville, VA 23313, (804) 331-3160, BA 83 Univ of West FL; BS 84 FL St Univ; MS 86 Vanderbilt Univ; 88–Sp-Lang Path, Northampton Co Schs, **SLP**

Kundrat, Donna M 3 Buttrick Court #304, Timonium, MD 21093, (301) 554-5372, BS 81 PA St Univ - Univ Park; MS 84 WV Univ; 86–Sp-Lang Path, MD Inst Emergency Med Services, **SLP**

Kundrot, Mrs Theresa Marie MRC Lab Of Molecular Biology, c/o Dr Craig Kundrot, Holl Road, Cambridge, England CB2 2QH, (203) 468-3261, BA 84 Northwestern Univ; MA 85 Northwestern Univ; Sp-Lang Path, East Haven Bd of Ed, **SLP**

Kunes, Ellen Blair 7342 Ventura Canyon #2, Van Nuys, CA 91405, (818) 908-8738, BS 76 Syracuse Univ; MA 78 2856; 88–Aud, Valley Hosp Med Ctr, **A**

Kunicki, Mrs Elizabeth 1816 Settlers Reserve Oval, Westlake, OH 44145, (216) 871-8909, BA 71 Cleveland St Univ; MA 71 Cleveland St Univ; Cl Superv, Cleveland St U, **SLP**

Kunin-Phillips, Cathy 183 Bear Hill Road, North Andover, MA 01845, BS 75 Northwestern Univ; MS 77 Boston Univ; SLP, Walpole Pub Sch, **SLP**

Kunkel, Mrs Amy Elizabeth 42-F Hudson View Drive, Beacon, NY 12508, (914) 737-6021, MS 83 Univ of MI - Ann Arbor; 85–Sp-Lang Path, Yorktown Bd Coop Educ Services, **SLP**

Kunken, Mrs Naomi S 156 Greystone Lane #4, Rochester, NY 14618, (716) 244-9091, BS 39 Columbia Univ Teachers Coll; MA 38 Columbia Univ Teachers Coll; **A LM**

Kunreuther, Mrs Gene R 141-34 71st Avenue, Kew Gardens, NY 11367, (718) 544-7492, BA 66 CUNY - Hunter Coll; MS 72 CUNY - Brooklyn Coll; Sp-Lang Path, Residential Health Care Facility, **SLP**

Kunstman, Mrs Mary J Bahr 1280 Wayne Road #201, West Bend, WI 53095, (414) 626-2160, **SLP**

Kuntz, Mrs Marlene B 6615 Chelwood Road, Baltimore, MD 21209, (301) 484-6228, MS 75 Towson St Univ; **SLP**

Kuntz, Patricia A 2027 Acero #49, Pueblo, CO 81004, (303) 547-3950, BS 78 Univ of Southern CO; MS 81 Phillips Univ; Sp-Lang Path, Pueblo Sch Dist #60, **SLP**

Kunz, Audrey J 853 Tifft Street, Buffalo, NY 14220, (716) 883-9880, BS 74 SUNY - Coll at Buffalo; ME 77 SUNY - Coll at Buffalo; Sp-Lang Path, Buffalo Bd of Ed, **SLP ACE**

Kunze, Mrs Barbara Lou 1131 Indian Springs Drive, Glendora, CA 91740, (818) 969-8636, BA 76 Univ of Redlands; MS 78 Univ of Redlands; Sp-Lang Path, LA Co Supt of Schs, **SLP**

Kunze, Dr Luvern H Ctr For Speech & Hearing Dis, Duke Univ Medical Center, P O Box 3887, Durham, NC 27710, (919) 684-6271, BA 50 Dakota Wesleyan Univ; MA 54 Univ of Northern CO; PH 62 (NS) Univ of IA; Sp-Lang Path, Duke U Med Cen, **SLP F**

Kupchak, Linda S 6311 Creek Bend, Houston, TX 77096, (713) 771-3353, BA 75 Montclair St Coll; MA 77 SUNY - Center at Buffalo; Sp-Lang Path, Private Practice, **SLP**

Kupensky, Sandra S 8318 Portsmouth Drive, Darien, IL 60559, **SLP**

Kuper, Mrs Eolin C 1221 Boyce Avenue, Ruxton 4, Baltimore, MD 21204, BS 49 Johns Hopkins Univ; MA 51 Johns Hopkins Univ; **SLP A LM**

Kupets-Mannon, Deborah L PO Box 640, Glen Gardner, NJ 08826, (201) 730-8045, BS 78 Radford Univ; MA 80 Univ of Pittsburgh - Pittsburgh; Sp-Lang Path, Sp Path Assoc, **SLP**

Kupferer, Albert F 25 McKinley Avenue, West Orange, NJ 07052, (201) 736-7900, BA 53 Montclair St Coll; MA 57 Columbia Univ Teachers Coll; Instr, **SLP**

Kuphall, Susan S Box 187, Plainfield, WI 54966, (414) 787-3405, BA 77 Univ of WI - Stevens Point; MS 78 Univ of WI - Stevens Point; **SLP**

Kupiec, Karen Jean 101 North Caroline Place, Suite #103, Dover, DE 19901, (302) 674-3752, BS 74 Nazareth Coll of Rochester; MA 75 SUNY - Coll at Geneseo; Aud, ENT Assoc of Dover, **A ACE**

Kupperman, Dr Gerard L 1078 Timberline Court East, Oconomowoc, WI 53066, (414) 567-7639, BA 66 CUNY - Brooklyn Coll; MS 68 Univ of WI - Madison; PH 70 (Aud) Univ of WI - Madison; Pres, Hrng Serv Ltd, **A**

Kupperman, Phyllis P 1132 North Ridgeland, Oak Park, IL 60302, (312) 530-8551, BS 63 Univ of IL - Urbana; MA 64 Univ of IL - Urbana; 79–Co Dir, Cen for Sp & Lang Dis, **SLP**

Kupperman, Susan J 1115 North East Avenue, Oak Park, IL 60302, (312) 848-9629, BS 74 Syracuse Univ; OM 76 San Jose St Univ; Sp-Lang Path, Private Practice, **SLP**

Kupperman, Mrs Suzan L 1078 Timberline Court, Oconomowoc, WI 53066, (414) 567-1727, BS 67 Carlow Coll; MS 68 Univ of WI - Madison; Sp-Lang Path, Arrowhead AEA, **SLP**

Kuprenas, Sandra V The Mason Clinic, 1100 9th Avenue, Seattle, WA 98111, (206) 223-6392, BA 72 Univ of IL - Chicago; MA 75 Univ of IL - Urbana; Aud, The Virginia Mason Clinic, **A**

Kupris, Joseph J 1681 Mells Lane, Anaheim, CA 92802, (714) 772-7525, BS 78 Univ of MN - Minneap-St Paul; MS 80 Mankato St Univ; Sp/Lang Path, Garden Grove USD, **SLP**

Kupsky, Barbara L 1125 St Christopher St, Apartment 57, Russell, KY 41169, (606) 324-0465, BS 84 Bradley Univ; MA 85 Northern IL Univ - De Kalb; **SLP**

Kuratko, Charles Patrick 4321 Brownfield Highway, Lubbock, TX 79407, (806) 792-0546, MS 77 TX Tech Univ; Aud, Audio Acoustics, **A**

Kuratomi, Christine 4262 Warren Avenue, Sacramento, CA 95822, (916) 442-3114, BA 71 CA St Univ - Sacramento; MA 73 CA St Univ - Sacramento

Kurbanick, Gloria 193 Woodland Way, Pass Christian, MS 39571, (601) 865-3030, BS 64 TX Woman's Univ; 88–Sp-Lang Path, Sun Coast Ctr for Rehab, **SLP**

Kurcz, Mrs Karen Brasie 333 Buttonwood, Bowling Green, OH 43402, (419) 865-1738, BA 82 MI St Univ; MA 83 Western MI Univ; 88–Doctoral Fellow, Bowling Green State Univ, **SLP**

Kurek, Mrs Patricia A 3526 Young Road, Millersville, MD 21107, (301) 744-3151, BA 81 Loyola Coll; MS 82 Loyola Coll; 82–Sp-Lang Path, UCP Cent MD, **SLP**

Kurick-McAnally, Mrs Linda 8215 North Venus Court, Tucson, AZ 85704-2130, (602) 575-8524, BA 74 OH St Univ; MS 77 Univ of AZ; Sp-Lang Path, Sunnyside Sch Dist, **SLP**

Kurjack, Mrs Paula Reed 1975 Sarno Access Road, Melbourne, FL 32935, (407) 242-0079, BS 73 FL St Univ; MS 77 FL St Univ; Sp/Lang Path, Brevard County School System, **SLP**

Kurjan, Mrs Randy M 9917 Durango Drive, Damascus, MD 20872, (301) 253-5568, MS 74 Rutgers St Univ -N Brunswick; Sp-Lang Path, Mont Co Pub Sch, **SLP**

Kurland, Mrs Carol L 354 Salisbury Street, Worcester, MA 01609, (617) 799-7855, BA Hofstra Univ; MA NY Univ; **SLP**

Kurland, Mrs Cecelia J 11 Neal Drive, East Brunswick, NJ 08816, (201) 739-5955, BA 64 Rutger's St Univ - Douglas Coll; MA 65 Columbia Univ Teachers Coll; Sp-Lang Path, Bayshore Comm Hosp, **SLP**

Kurland, Mrs Linda Roberts Route 1 Box 41-R, Purdon, TX 76679, (817) 562-2821, BS 75 East TX St Univ Commerce; MS 76 East TX St Univ - Commerce; Sp-Lang Path, Navarro Freestone Coop, **SLP**

Kurland, Linda Sue 580 Bucknell Avenue #L, Claremont, CA 91711, BA 82 Univ of CA - Los Angeles; MA 85 CA St Univ - Los Angeles; Sp-Lang Path, Casa Colina Hospital, **SLP**

Kurland, Miriam B R R 2 Box 81, Maria Drive, Holmes, NY 12531, MS 78 Univ of MO - Columbia; Sp-Lang Path, Private Practice, **SLP**

Kurland, Paul F Bay Hearing Conservation, 1600 Shawano Avenue, Suite 110W, Green Bay, WI 54303, (414) 499-6366, BS 71 East TN St Univ; MA 76 East TN St Univ; Owner, Bay Hrng Conservation, **A**

Kurman, Barbara L c/o Guinta Associates, 67 Leuning Street, South Hackensack, NJ 07606, (201) 488-4425, BA 73 CUNY - Brooklyn Coll; MS 78 Syracuse Univ; Dir of Aud Serv, Guinta Assoc, **A**

Kurmin, Kathi E 82 Robbins Court, Bricktown, NJ 08723, BS 75 Ithaca Coll; MA 78 Univ of Pittsburgh - Pittsburgh; Aud, Chldns Hosp of Pittsburgh, **A**

Kurn, Mrs Barbara A 7151 North 15th Street, Phoenix, AZ 85020, **SLP**

Kurowski, Karen Susan 2566 Woodmeadow S E, Grand Rapids, MI 49506, (616) 942-1660, BS 82 Western MI Univ; MA 83 Western MI Univ; Aud, Comprehensive Aud Services, **A**

Kurpita, Barbara J 4195 North Mill Grove Road, Alden, NY 14004, (416) 688-2980, MA 85 SUNY - Center at Buffalo; MA 87 SUNY - Center at Buffalo; 88–Aud, Niagara Rehab Ctr, **A**

Kurtenbach, Mrs Janet Ruth 4912 South 63rd Street, Lincoln, NE 68516, (402) 464-1289, BS 82 Kearney St Coll; MS 83 Kearney St Coll; Sp-Lang Path, Malcolm PS, **SLP**

Kurth, Cathy E Audiology & Hearing Aid Center, 3271 N Civic Center Plaza, Suite 4, Scottsdale, AZ 85251, (602) 941-0519, BS 73 Loyola Univ of Chicago; MA 75 Univ of IL - Urbana; Dir Aud, Aud & Hrng Aid Cen, **A**

Kurth, Donald D 4513 96th Street, Urbandale, IA 50322, (515) 276-1143, BA 62 Univ of Northern CO; MA 62 Univ of Northern CO; Aud, Indust Hrng Conserv Serv Pc, **A**

Kurtz, Mrs Carla Ann 925 Tracy Place, Mason, OH 45040, (513) 825-5454, BA 79 OH St Univ; MA 81 Univ of Cincinnati; 81–Aud, Tri County ENT Head & Neck Assoc, **A**

Kurtz, Mrs Connie JoAnn 325 Randall, Troy, MI 48098, (313) 528-2459, MA 86 MI St Univ; Sp-Lang Path, Lakeshore Ear Nose Throat, **SLP**

Kurtz, Deborah Ann 422 63rd Street, Holmes Beach, FL 34209, (813) 778-2575, BS 82 Univ of NH; MS 85 Univ of NH; 87–Sp-Lang Path, Mediplex Rehab-Brandenton, **SLP**

Kurtz, Debra J Shawler Brook Road, Rd#2 Box 89A, Sherburne, NY 13460, (607) 334-2771, BA 83 SUNY - Center at Buffalo; MA 85 SUNY - Center at Buffalo; 87–Sp-Lang Path, Delaware-Chenango BOCES, **SLP**

Kurtz, Janet Leigh 8533 Tiwn Pointe Circle, Indianapolis, IN 46236, (202) 651-5960, BS 74 Towson St Univ; MS 82 Loyola Coll; Sp-Lang Path, Model Sec Sch for Deaf, **SLP**

Kurtz, Joellen 2395 South Cook Street, Denver, CO 80210-5526, (303) 733-7054, MA 77 Our Lady Lake Univ-San Anton; Sp-Lang Path, Private Practice, **SLP**

Kurtz, Paula Marie Zanker 1358-J Lincoln Avenue, San Rafael, CA 94901, (415) 457-3908, BS 83 Edinboro Univ of PA; MA 84 Edinboro Univ of PA; 87–Sp-Lang Path, Oakland USD, **SLP**

Kurtz-Califf, Mrs Rebecca A 2740 Lake Way, Hollywood, FL 33026, (305) 432-1841, OB 77 Univ of FL; MA 79 Memphis St Univ; Sp-Lang Path, Private Practice, **SLP**

Kurtzer, Denise Wynne 1239 23rd Street #1, Santa Monica, CA 90404, (213) 515-3084, SLP, La High School District, **SLP**

Kurtzer, Ellen A 369 Old Post Road, North Attleboro, MA 02760, (401) 277-3525, BA 75 Univ of RI; MS 78 Vanderbilt Univ; Aud, Ri Sch Deaf, **A**

Kurtzer-Metter, Mrs Karen 7821 East Briarwood Road, Orange, CA 92669, (714) 529-4538, BA 77 CA St Univ - Fullerton; MA 80 CA St Univ - Northridge; Sp-Lang Path, Placentia USD, **SLP**

Kurtz-Myers, Mrs Lisa 800 S Arlington Mill Drive, Apartment #202, Alexandria, VA 22204, (703) 931-4067, BS 85 Kent St Univ; MA 85 Kent St Univ; SLP, Annandale Fluency Clinic, **SLP**

Kurtzrock, Dr George H 4807 Cypress Ridge Place, Tampa, FL 33624, (813) 961-5146, BA 49 Univ of MO - Columbia; MA 51 Univ of IL - Urbana; PH 56 (NS) Univ of IL - Urbana; Professor Emeritus, Sn IL U, **SLP A**

Kurz, Christine Shaver 149 West 600 North, Salt Lake City, UT 84103, (801) 467-0332, BA 78 Western WA Univ; MA 80 Univ of Northern CO; Aud, Mt Aud/Mt Hd & Nk Surg, **A**

Kurz, Mary Ann 30 Breezy Acres, Wheeling, WV 26003, (304) 243-0375, BS 74 OH Univ - Athens; MS 80 WV Univ; Sp-Lang Path, Ohio Co Pub Sch, **SLP**

Kurz, Olivia Dee 601 Delaine Drive, Corpus Christi, TX 78411, (512) 888-7911, BA 80 East TX St Univ - Commerce; MA 82 East TX St Univ - Commerce; Elem Spec Ed Consultant, Corpus Christi ISD, **SLP**

Kurz, Mrs Sue E 9 Harav Bar Shaul, Rechovot, Israel 76251, BA 67 CUNY - Queens Coll; MS 70 Adelphi Univ; Sp-Lang Path, **SLP**

Kurzawski, Bernadette Ann 3146 Bieler Road, Orchard Park, NY 14127-1116, BA 77 SUNY - Center at Buffalo; MA 79 SUNY - Center at Buffalo; Sp-Lang Path, West Seneca Development Center, **SLP**

Kurzeja, Barbara A 643 North 9th Avenue, Kankakee, IL 60901, MS 77 Eastern IL Univ; Sp-Lang Path, Riverside Medical Center, **SLP**

Kurzius, Colette E 99 Lamarck Drive, Snyder, NY 14226, (716) 839-1774, BA 75 Elmira Coll; MA 79 LA St Univ - Baton Rouge; Sp/Lang Path, Sch Adm Dist #4, **SLP**

Kurzman, Esther Rachel 182-27 80 Drive, Jamaica Estates, NY 11432, (718) 591-5176, MS 82 CUNY - Brooklyn Coll; 83–Sp-Lang Path, Prospect Pk Nursing Home, **SLP**

Kusamura, Yoshimi 701-155 Wellington Crescent, Winnipeg, MB, Canada R3M 0A3, (204) 786-7841, BA North-Kyushu Univ; MS 77 Univ of WI - Stevens Point; Sp-Lang Path, Child Guidance Clinic, **SLP**

Kush, Christine Rd #3 Box 2812, Aliquippa, PA 15001, (412) 374-5010, BS 82 Indiana Univ of PA; MS 86 Indiana Univ of PA; **SLP**

Kusher-Smith, Ilyse Beth 1 Horizon Road, Fort Lee, NJ 07024, (212) 496-8400, BA 82 CUNY - Brooklyn Coll; MS 84 CUNY - Brooklyn Coll; **SLP**

Kushinsky, Sharon L 44 Dinsmore Avenue #606, Framingham, MA 01701, (617) 542-5900, BS 79 Ithaca Coll; MS 80 Univ of NC - Chapel Hill; Aud, Thomas W Fell Co Inc, **A**

Kushmeider, Susan Lynn 10307 Montrose Avenue #101, Bethesda, MD 20814, (301) 424-5200, BA 83 Mary Washington Coll; MA 85 George Washington Univ; 86–Sp-Lang Path, Treatment & Learning Centers, **SLP**

Kushner, Laura 90 Lincoln Street, Apt 2, Winthrop, MA 02152, (617) 539-0635, BS 74 PA St Univ - Univ Park; MS 78 PA St Univ - Univ Park; SLP, New Medico, **SLP**

Kushner, Mrs Linda Ross 11380 Prosperity Farms Road, Suite 203B, Palm Beach Gardens, FL 33410, (407) 627-7207, BS 63 Boston Univ; MA 80 Univ of Miami; Sp-Lang Path, Private Practice, **SLP**

Kushner, Marcia R 3501 South 35th Street, Lincoln, NE 68506, (402) 473-0374, BS 50 Univ of NE - Lincoln; MA 72 Univ of NE - Lincoln; Aud, Lincoln Pub Sch, **A**

Kushner, Mrs Roslyn Schachter 2946 Lee Place, Bellmore, NY 11710, (516) 781-1005, BA 72 CUNY - Brooklyn Coll; MS 83 CUNY - Brooklyn Coll; Sp-Lang Path, Private Practice, **SLP A**

Kushner, Mrs Sandra Gerson 16 Medoc Court, Marlton, NJ 08053, (609) 983-4308, BS 78 PA St Univ - Univ Park; MA 83 Trenton St Coll; Sp-Lang Path, Robin Muller & Associates, **SLP**

Kushner-Johnson, Mrs Miriam Leslie 1314 Maxwell, Ames, IA 50010-5657, (913) 682-5932, OB 76 Univ of MO - Columbia; OM 85 Univ of MO - Columbia; **SLP**

Kushner-Rulnick, Mrs Rhonda L 1406 Autumn Lane, Cherry Hill, NJ 08003, MS 77 George Washington Univ; Sp-Lang Path, Private Practice, **SLP**

Kusik, Mrs Lanita J 519 North Oak, Hennessey, OK 73742, **SLP**

Kuske, Trudy Kay Box 28-A Route 1, Dickinson, ND 58601, (701) 227-4301, BS 84 Northern St Coll; MS 86 Univ of WY; **SLP**

Kusko, Mrs Cheryl W 142 North Broad Street, Allentown, PA 18104, (215) 759-7600, BS 76 Kutztown Univ of PA; MA 81 Temple Univ; Sp-Lang Path, Colonial Northampton Iu # 20, **SLP**

Kuster, Judith Maginnis 1018 South Payne Street, New Ulm, MN 56073, (507) 389-5840, BS 65 Univ of WI - Madison; MS 67 Univ of WI - Madison; OM 87 Mankato St Univ; 87–Instr/Clinic Dir, Mankato St Univ-Mankato MN, **SLP**

Kustron, Mrs Janice M 104 Marble Drive, Bridgeville, PA 15017-1726, (412) 225-2226, BS 74 WV Univ; MS 75 WV Univ; Dir of Sp & Lang Dept, Swn Pennsylvania Easter Sl Soc, **SLP**

Kuta, Joan E 6901 Agave Cove, Austin, TX 78750, (512) 345-6830, BS 77 Coll of Saint Rose; MS 78 Coll of Saint Rose; Sp-Lang Path, Private Practice, **SLP ACE**

Kuta, Mary D 57 Louise Street, Delmar, NY 12054, **SLP**

Kutcher, Evelyn Gong 5719 Eveward Road, Culver City, CA 90230, (213) 393-0511, BA 80 Univ of CA - Santa Barbara; MA 82 Univ of CA - Santa Barbara; Aud, Hearing Care Associates, **A**

Kutler, Debra 441 South 153rd Circle, Omaha, NE 68154, **SLP**

Kutlik, Mrs Roberta Emilie 12511 South 73rd Court, Palos Heights, IL 60463, (312) 687-0500, BS 58 Northern IL Univ - De Kalb; MS 82 Governors St Univ; Sp-Lang Path, SW Cook Co Coop Assoc, **SLP**

Kuttesch, Cynthia Rose 214 Ashland Avenue, Buffalo, NY 14222, (716) 883-5347, BS 79 SUNY - Coll at Buffalo; MS 85 SUNY - Coll at Buffalo; **SLP**

Kutz, Mrs Jane Ann Talmage 1386 Green Mist Drive, Fenton, MO 63026, (913) 384-1789, BS 77 Univ of IL - Urbana; MS 78 Univ of IL - Urbana; Sp-Lang Path, Special School District, **SLP**

Kutz, Sheila L 106 N Windmill, Box 344, Marine, IL 62061, (618) 887-4406, BS 81 Southern IL Univ-Edwardsvill; MS 82 Southern IL Univ-Edwardsvill; Aud, St Elizabeth Med Ctr, **A**

Kuusisto, Rita Paal 4012 Cavalry, Plano, TX 75023, (713) 460-3985, BA 81 Univ of Houston - Univ Park; MA 84 Wichita St Univ; Sp-Lang Path, Richardson ISD, **SLP**

Kuvshinoff, Mrs Barbara Elizabeth 804 Ashcroft Court, Springdale, OH 45240, (513) 742-9037, MS 84 Loyola Coll; Sp-Lang Path, Cincinnati City Public Schools, **SLP ACE**

Kuzan, Mrs Kathleen Massotto 1365 Oakland Avenue, Union, NJ 07083, (201) 688-1200, BA 77 Montclair St Coll; MA 83 Montclair St Coll; 80–Sp-Lang Path, Union Township Bd of Educ, **SLP**

Kuzel, Christina M 14 Alonzo Street, Rochester, NY 14612, (716) 325-4560, BA 84 SUNY - Coll at Buffalo; MA 86 SUNY - Coll at Geneseo; **SLP**

Kuzio, Beverlee M 524 Fairview Road, Medford, NJ 08055, (609) 596-9670, BS 85 Trenton St Coll; MA 87 Montclair St Coll; 88–Aud, Family Hrng Ctr

Kuzmik, Susan D 3 Rustic Drive, Monsey, NY 10952, **SLP**

Kvaal, Jolene Teresa 739 Ensenada Court, San Diego, CA 92109, (619) 488-4258, MA 84 Southeastern Coll; SLP, Sandiego City Schools, **SLP**

Kvietok, Camilla Maria 4 Ridge Drive, Glen Cove, NY 11542, (212) 860-7800, BS 77 SUNY - Coll at Fredonia; MS 81 Columbia Univ Teachers Coll; 88–Sp-Lang Path, Shore View Nursing Home, **SLP**

Kviklys, Karen Anne 4384 Ivywood Drive, Marietta, GA 30062-6431, (404) 257-2077, SLP, Scottish Rite Hosp, **SLP**

Kvols, Martha 6630 Buckthorn Road N W, Rochester, MN 55901, (507) 288-0064, BA 65 Baylor Univ; MA 69 Univ of Houston - Univ Park; Sp-Lang Path, Stanley Jones & Assoc, **SLP**

Kwait-Cohen, Mrs Darcee 2471 Warrensville Center Road, University Heights, OH 44118, (216) 397-0004, BA 87 OH St Univ; MA 88 Cleveland St Univ; 88, Cleveland Hrng & Sp Ctr

Kwarta, Keri L 4010 North Brandywine, #1113, Peoria, IL 61614, (312) 381-4060, MS 88 Southern IL Univ -Carbondale

Kwasniewski, Kenneth James 3328 Piedmont Avenue, Pittsburgh, PA 15216, (412) 561-0242, BS 71 PA St Univ - Univ Park; MA 74 Univ of Pittsburgh - Pittsburgh; SLP, Pittsburgh Board of Pub Educ, **SLP**

Kwass, Susan M Lake Shore Tower Apartment #802, 6260 South Lake Drive, Cudahy, WI 53110, (414) 529-2932, BA 79 Marquette Univ; BS 83 Marquette Univ; MS 86 Marquette Univ; 87–Sp-Lang Path, Sacred Heart Rehab Hosp, **SLP**

Kwiatkoski, Mrs Janet E 391 Forest Avenue, Glen Ridge, NJ 07028, (201) 744-4441, BS 77 East Stroudsburg Univ of PA; MS 78 Ithaca Coll; 87–Aud, Private Practice, **A**

Kwiatkowski, Mrs Ellen B R D 2 Box 307-C, Mertztown, PA 19539, (215) 682-9892, BS 81 West Chester Univ of PA; MS 83 WV Univ; 87–Sp-Lang Path, Carbon-Lehigh Intermed Unit, **SLP ACE**

Kwiatkowski, Joan Dept Communicative Disorders, University Of Wisconsin, 1975 Willow Drive, Madison, WI 53706, (608) 262-3951, BA 58 Univ of IL - Urbana; MA 64 Univ of CT; Cl Instructor, U of Wisconsin-Mad, **SLP**

Kwiatkowski, Mrs Susan Mack 30 Ridge Meadows Drive, Spencerport, NY 14559, (716) 352-2440, BA 82 Allegheny Coll; MS 87 Nazareth Coll of Rochester

Kwiecinski, Bruce Gerard 22960 Apple Hill Lane #204, Prairie View, IL 60069, (312) 567-8661, BA 80 IL Coll; MS 83 Washington Univ; 86–Aud, Chic Ps, **A**

Kwit, Paula D Don Johnston Developmental Equipment Incorporated, PO Box 639, Wauconda, IL 60084, (312) 526-2682, BS 76 Eastern IL Univ; MS 77 Univ of WI - Milwaukee; 87–Mktg Dir, Don Johnston Dev Equip Inc, **SLP**

Kwitowski, Mrs Clare N 2150 Stonebrook Road, Winchester, VA 22601-6612, (703) 635-3125, BS 76 Univ of KY; MS 77 Univ of KY; 86–Sp-Lang Path, Warren County Sch Sys, **SLP**

Kwock, Dana S Y 382 - 7 S W 62nd Blvd, Gainesville, FL 32607, (904) 335-0534, MS 87 Univ of UT; **A**

Kyea, Mrs Gail G 7 Siwanoy Lane, Plattsburgh, NY 12901, (518) 561-0100, BS 62 SUNY - Coll at Geneseo; MS 67 SUNY - Coll at Geneseo; Sp-Lang Path, BOCES, **SLP**

Kyker, Mrs Judy Catherine 1228 North Heidelberg Avenue, Walnut, CA 91789, (714) 594-5064, BA 82 CA St Univ - Los Angeles; MA 84 CA St Univ - Los Angeles; Sp-Lang Path, South Pacific Rehab Services, **SLP**

Kyle, Amy Louise 9340 D Kungsholm Drive, Indianapolis, IN 46250, (317) 841-9450, BA 84 IN Univ - Bloomington; OM 85 IN Univ - Bloomington; 88–Sp-Lang Path, Hancock-So Madison Jt Svcs, **SLP**

Kyle, Mildred W 204 Timberlane Drive, Carthage, TX 75633, (214) 693-6567, BA 58 Univ of North TX; MA 86 Univ of TX - Tyler; 83–Classroom Teacher, Carthage ISD, **SLP**

Kyllo, Mrs Teresa Marie 1510 9th Avenue N W #712, Williston, ND 58801, (701) 572-6609, MS 87 Univ of ND; **SLP**

Kynett, Deanna 132 April Waters North, Montgomery, TX 77356, (409) 760-7764, BS 74 Northwest MO St Univ; MS 78 Central MO St Univ; ME 81 Central MO St Univ; 88–Spec Educ Supvr, Conroe ISD, **SLP**

Kyriakides, Laura 9945 Ivy Lane, Munster, IN 46321, (219) 924-2933, BS Marquette Univ; MS 87 Marquette Univ

Kyrk, Rochelle Racanelli 28 Steven Place, Smithtown, NY 11787, (516) 979-7714, BA 78 Boston Coll; MS 80 Univ of IL - Urbana; Superv Speech & Lang Dept, Cleary School for the Deaf, **SLP**

Kyros, Mrs Victoria H 9930 O Circle, Omaha, NE 68127, (402) 339-6499, BS 76 Univ of NE - Lincoln; MS 77 Univ of NE - Omaha; **SLP**

Kysar, Carol B 4076 Meadowlark Drive, Calabasas, CA 91302, (818) 594-7609, BA 79 Rutger's St Univ - Douglas Coll; MS 81 Rutgers Coll; 83–Sp-Lang Path, Private Practice, **SLP**

L

Laakman, Mrs Mary J 2248 Semmes Drive, Montgomery, AL 36106, (205) 271-1232, BS 71 Univ of NE - Omaha; MA 74 Univ of NE - Lincoln; Sp/Lang Path, Private Practice, **SLP**

Labarge, Joann Mareen 6643 Dana Drive, Macon, GA 31210, (912) 477-8128, BS 83 Auburn Univ - Montgomery; OM 85 Auburn Univ - Auburn; **SLP**

La Barge-King, Karen Elaine 5619 N E 204th Street, Seattle, WA 98155, (206) 326-3485, BA 81 Univ of CA - Santa Barbara; MS 83 Univ of WA; 85–Sp/Lang Path, Group Hlth Coop, **SLP ACE**

Labatt, Mrs Laura M 135 West Elsmere, San Antonio, TX 78212, (512) 732-2493, BA 65 Our Lady Lake Univ-San Anton; MA 67 Our Lady Lake Univ-San Anton; **SLP**

La Bauve, Sonya M 200 Henry Clay Avenue, New Orleans, LA 70118, (504) 899-9511, BS 83 Univ of Southwestern LA; MA 84 LA St Univ - N O Medical Ctr; Aud, Childrens Hosp, **A**

La Bella, Georgianna Teresa 1760 E 52nd Street, Brooklyn, NY 11234, (212) 258-5143, BA 74 CUNY - Brooklyn Coll; MA 79 NY Univ

La Bella, Renee 214 North Prospect Street, Rockford, IL 61107, (815) 964-4130, BS 84 Northern IL Univ - De Kalb; MA 86 Northern IL Univ - De Kalb; **SLP**

Labelle, Dr Joseph L 606 East Bryn Mawr, Roselle, IL 60172, (312) 794-3965, BS 62 Univ of MN - Minneap-St Paul; MA 66 Univ of MN - Minneap-St Paul; PH 71 (NS) Univ of WI - Madison; Hd/Sp-Lang-Hrng Serv, Il Dept of Mental Hlth, **SLP**

Laberge, Mrs Patricia Christine 16304-100 Street #407, Edmonton, AB, Canada T5X 5J6, (403) 457-0974, MA 87 Western WA Univ

Labiak, James M Dept Of Speech & Hearing Sci, University Of Washington, 4131 15th Avenue N E, Seattle, WA 98195, (206) 545-2187, BS 69 Central MI Univ; MA 71 Univ of WA; Lecturer, U of WA Sp-Hrng Cl, **A**

Labick, John M Rd 2 Box 312, Latrobe, PA 15650-9411, (412) 539-2540, BS 73 Indiana Univ of PA; MS 76 Indiana Univ of PA; Sp-Lang Path, Family Home Health Services, **SLP**

Labier, Francesca M 25 D-8 Pine Lane, Albany, NY 12203, (518) 432-2590, BS 77 Nazareth Coll of Rochester; MS 79 Coll of Saint Rose; Sp-Lang Path, Eleanor Roosevelt Dev Serv, **SLP**

Lablance, Dr Gary R 7516 Terri Lynn, St Louis, MO 63123, (314) 658-2939, BS 76 Saint Louis Univ; MA 77 Saint Louis Univ; PH 83 (Sp-Lang Path) Northwestern Univ; Asst Prof, St Louis U Dept of Comm Disorders, **SLP**

Laborde, Mrs Karen Dorsey 205 Presence Drive, Lafayette, LA 70506, (318) 984-4160, BA 83 Univ of Southwestern LA; MA 85 LA St Univ - Baton Rouge; SLP, Our Lady of Lord Hospital, **SLP**

Laborde, Mrs Suzanne Mayer 2410 State Street, New Orleans, LA 70118, (504) 897-8563, BS 82 LA St Univ - Baton Rouge; OM 83 LA St Univ - N O Medical Ctr; 85–Sp-Lang Path, Touro Infirmary, **SLP ACE**

La Borwit, Dr Louis J 12809 Babcock Lane, Bowie, MD 20715, (301) 262-2578, BA 54 Univ of VA - Charlottesville; ME 57 Univ of VA - Charlottesville; PH 77 (Counseling) Catholic Univ of America; 87–Sp-Lang Path, Private Practice, **SLP ACE**

Labourdette, Janet Marie 96 Kim Louise Drive, Apartment #3, Campbell, CA 95008, (408) 370-3348, BA 84 San Jose St Univ; MA 87 San Jose St Univ; **SLP**

Labrake, Mrs Barbara A 5115 Branch Avenue, Tampa, FL 33603, (813) 237-4232, BA 74 SUNY - Coll at Plattsburgh; MS 78 Coll of Saint Rose; **SLP**

Labrecque, Janet 84 School Street, Central Falls, RI 02863, (401) 568-2551, BS 75 Univ of RI; MS 77 Univ of RI; Sp-Lang Path, Dr Ue Zambarano Mem Hosp, **SLP**

Labriola, Mrs Cheryl Hicklen 2606 Cropsey Avenue, Brooklyn, NY 11214, (718) 373-5900, BA 81 CUNY - Brooklyn Coll; MS 84 CUNY - Brooklyn Coll; SLP, New York City Board of Educ, **SLP**

Labrot, Mrs Marquerite Wilford 23 West Charlton Street, Savannah, GA 31401, (803) 757-2618, BS 71 Ithaca Coll; MS 73 Univ of WI - Madison; **A**

Labrozzi, Karen M 6134 West Corrine Drive, Glendale, AZ 85304, (602) 878-8355, BS 72 PA St Univ - Univ Park; MS 76 AZ St Univ; 87–Sp-Lang Path, Peoria USD, **SLP**

Labrutto-Wilson, Janis D 5040 Society Place E #3C, West Palm Beach, FL 33415, (305) 585-6494, BS 72 FL St Univ; MS 73 FL St Univ; Sp/Lang Path, Palm Beach County Sch, **SLP**

Labudde, Mrs Dorothy E 5755 Summit Drive, Rocklin, CA 95677, (415) 564-0357, BS 45 Univ of WI - Oshkosh; MS 49 Univ of WI - Madison; 88–Retired, San Francisco USD, **SLP F**

Labuskes, Debra Hettinger 205 South Broad Street, Mechanicsburg, PA 17055-4102, (412) 787-2350, BS 79 James Madison Univ; MS 81 James Madison Univ; Sp/Lang Path, Robinson Dev Cen, **SLP**

Lacalle, Mrs Evelyn S 410 South 5th Street, Eunice, LA 70535, (318) 457-2215, BA 74 Univ of Southwestern LA; MS 75 Univ of Southwestern LA; Sp-Lang Path, St Landry Parish School Board, **SLP**

Laccinole, Dr Michael D 3425 Wayne, Amarillo, TX 79109, (806) 359-7681, BA 71; MS 78 Univ of OR; PH 82 (Adult Communication Disorders) Univ of OR; Sp-Lang Path, Amarillo Speech Lang Hrng Cen, **SLP**

Lacelle, Dr Barbara D 175 Albert Street East, Sault Ste Marie, ON, Canada P6A 2J2, (705) 759-1234, BS 66 AZ St Univ; MS 68 AZ St Univ; PH 71 (Sp Path & Aud) Univ of KS; Sp-Lang Path, Group Health Center, **SLP**

Lacey, Christine 380 Carmelita Place, Fremont, CA 94538, **SLP**

Lacey, Cynthia A Saint Christopher's Hospital For Children, Speech And Hearing Department, 5th Street And Lehigh Avenue, Philadelphia, PA 19133, (215) 427-5518, BS 79 PA St Univ - Univ Park; MA 83 Temple Univ; 87–Dir-Sp & Hrng Dept, St Christophers Hospital, **A**

Lacey, Elaine Marie 14008 Edmore Drive, Detroit, MI 48205, (313) 527-8747, BS 84 Eastern MI Univ; MA 85 Eastern MI Univ

Lacey, Mrs Francis Karen 1450 Encina Road, Santa Fe, NM 87501, (505) 256-1423, BA 80 Univ of MT; MS 87 Univ of NM; **SLP**

Lacey, Susan F L Rd 1 Box 75, Swan Lake, NY 12783, **SLP**

Lacey-Scholze, Brenda A West 906 Falcon Avenue, Spokane, WA 99218, (509) 467-6189, BA 80 Univ of CA - Santa Barbara; MS 82 UT St Univ; 87–Sp-Lang Path, Mead Sch Dist, **SLP**

Lach, Edythe T 58 Summertree Court, Nicholasville, KY 40356, (606) 223-1526, BS 73 Northeastern Univ; MA 74 Univ of VA - Charlottesville; Sp-Lang Path, Humana Inc, **SLP**

La Chance, Patti A 97 Kenson Drive, East Greenwich, RI 02818, BS 82 Northeastern Univ; MS 84 Boston Univ; Sp-Lang Path, Sargent Rehab Ctr, **SLP**

La Chance, Susan Carol ENT & FPS, 5125 Beacon Hill Road #103, Columbus, OH 43228, (614) 299-1111, Aud, ENT & Facial Plastic Surg Inc, **A**

Lacher, Linda Lea 1429 Como Avenue #3, St Paul, MN 55108, (612) 645-1427, BA 85 Univ of MN - Duluth; MA 86 Univ of MN - Duluth; Sp-Lang Path, Dakota County Intermed Sch Dist 917, **SLP**

Lachmann, Teresa D 6101 Warwick Court, New Orleans, LA 70131, **SLP**

Lachowsky, Mrs Pamela Smith 2500 Fairway Drive, Apartment 803, Alvin, TX 77511, (713) 585-5318, BA 83 MI St Univ; MS 85 Univ of Central AR; **SLP**

Lack, Mrs Barbara S 5888 N W 66th Way, Parkland, FL 33067, (305) 943-2130, BS 59 OH St Univ; MS 77 FL Inst of Tech; SLP, Broward Co Sch Bd, **SLP A**

Lacken, Vivienne E R R 4 Box 337, Blairstown, NJ 07825, (201) 362-9384, BA 69 Rutger's St Univ - Douglas Coll; MS 71 Rutgers St Univ -N Brunswick; 82–Sp-Lang Path, Frelinghuysen Bd of Ed, **SLP**

Lackey, Mrs Cathy Lynn 1316 Clifton Lane, Nashville, TN 37215, (615) 298-3579, BA 78 Middle TN St Univ; MS 80 Vanderbilt Univ; Sp-Lang Path, Vanderbilt University Med Ctr, **SLP**

Lackner, Susan L 3620 East Floyd Drive, Denver, CO 80210, **SLP**

Lacko-Pries, Mrs Diane 1154 Granville Road, Newark, OH 43055, (614) 763-3525, BS 76 Purdue Univ - West Lafayette; MA 78 Northern IL Univ - De Kalb; Sp/Lang Path, Licking Valley Local Sch Dist, **SLP**

Lacombe, Mrs Idell H 103 Cindy, Lafayette, LA 70508, MS 76 Univ Southern MS-Hattiesburg; SLP, Lafayette Parish School Board, **SLP**

Lacon, Mrs Donna Lynn 8711 Castlecreek Drive, Contorville, OH 45459, (513) 426-5787, BS 76 Miami Univ - Oxford; MA 81 Montclair St Coll; Sp-Lang Path, Greene Co Bd of Ed, **SLP**

LaCoss, Mrs Joan Harkin Childrens Hearing & Speech Ctr, Childrens Hosp Ntl Med Ctr, 111 Michigan Avenue N W, Washington, DC 20010, (202) 745-5600, BS 76 Univ of MA - Amherst; MA 77 George Washington Univ; Aud, Chldn Hosp Natl Med Ctr, **A**

Lacosse, Mrs Brenda J S 35501 Purcell Place, Fremont, CA 94536, (415) 794-3666, BA 71 Univ of CA - Santa Barbara; ME 75 Western MD Coll; MA 73 Univ of CA - Santa Barbara; Aud, Calif School for Deaf-Fremont, **A**

La Coste, Patricia A 110 Bonita Drive, Birmingham, AL 35209, **A**

Lacroix, Dr Paul G 11 Jana Lane, Stratham, NH 03885, (203) 449-3870, BA 74 Univ of CT; MA 76 Univ of CT; PH 80 (Communication Science) Univ of CT; Aud, Naval Medical Command NE, **A ACE**

La Croix, Zane E Oklahoma Dept Of Human Service, Speech & Hearing Services, P O Box 25352, Oklahoma City, OK 73125, (405) 521-3765, BA 61 Northeastern OK St Univ; MS 71 Phillips Univ; Superv Sp & Hrng Serv, OK Dept of Human Serv, **SLP**

LaCross, Kimberly A 203 Eagle Drive, Alpena, MI 49707-2563, (517) 354-4289, MA 87 Central MI Univ; 86–Aud, Northern Hearing Services, **A**

Lacy, Mrs Aleyce Bluestein 102 Tallowood Drive, Lafayette, LA 70508, (318) 856-6798, BA 79 Univ of Southwestern LA; MS 82 Univ of Southwestern LA; SLP, Sp Dis Ctr Inc, **SLP**

Lacy, Mrs Brigitte Gil 502 Cardinal Court, South Boston, VA 24592, (804) 575-3339, BS 85 James Madison Univ; MS 87 James Madison Univ; 86–Sp-Lang Path, InSpeech Inc, **SLP**

Lacy, Debra D 6400 N W Expressway #928, Oklahoma City, OK 73132, (405) 787-4801, BS 78 Phillips Univ; MS 80 Phillips Univ; Sp-Lang Path, Bethany Guidance Clinic, **SLP**

Lacy, Donna F 3845 Everett Street, Lincoln, NE 68506, (402) 473-0322, BS 54 Univ of NE - Lincoln; MA 57 Univ of NE - Lincoln; Sp-Lang Path, Lincoln Pub Sch, **SLP**

Lacy, Susan D 141 Brookway, Ithaca, NY 14850, (607) 257-0379, BA 70 Univ of CA - Berkeley; OB 72 Sonoma St Univ; MS 76 Univ of VT; **SLP**

Laczay, Mary Koltay 4 Lisa Court, Dobbs Ferry, NY 10522, (914) 693-1511, BS 79 Mercy Coll; MA 80 Hofstra Univ; SLP, Pelham Pub Schools, **SLP**

Lada-Butterworth, Joan E 3 Loring Street, Auburn, MA 01501, (617) 832-5331, BS 76 Northeastern Univ; MS 77 Purdue Univ - West Lafayette; Sp-Lang Path, Burbank Hosp, **SLP ACE**

Ladd, Mrs Ruth A P O Box 324, 135 North Humboldt Street, Marine, IL 62061, (618) 637-2131, BA 75 Southern IL Univ-Edwardsvill; MS 76 Southern IL Univ-Edwardsvill; SLP, Livingston & Worden Pub Sch, **SLP**

Ladd, Mrs Sandra Jane 55 North Street, Marcellus, NY 13108, (315) 425-4444, MS 83 Syracuse Univ; Sp-Lang Path, Syracuse City Schs, **SLP**

Laddbush-Lecompte, Mrs Diane M 1726 Laurel Highway, Seaford, DE 19973, (302) 398-8197, BA 79 Univ of MD - College Park; MS 81 Loyola Coll; Sp-Lang Path, Lake Forest Sch Dist, **SLP**

Lade, Mrs Debra Moseley 3104 Mary Ann Lane, San Bernardino, CA 92404, (714) 886-1755, BA 83 Univ of Redlands; MS 84 Univ of Redlands; Sp-Lang Path, Bonita USD, **SLP**

Ladefoged, Dr Peter N Linguistics Department, University Of California, Los Angeles, CA 90024, (213) 825-0829, MA 51 0110; PH 59 (NS); Prof, UCLA, **F**

Laden, Mrs Joan 627 Maple Street, River Vale, NJ 07675, (201) 391-5491, BA 71 Univ of Miami; MA 72 NY Univ; Sp-Lang Path, River Vale Bd of Ed, **SLP**

Laderberg, Mrs Cathy M 6063 Newport Point, Norfolk, VA 23505, (804) 489-7933, BA 74 Univ of Miami; MS 77 Old Dominion Univ; Sp-Lang Path, Private Practice, **SLP**

Laderta, Paul P 720 Gordon Terrace, Chicago, IL 60613-2262, (312) 570-4171, **SLP**

La Dew, Lisa A Center For Communication Dis, 250 Pond Street, Braintree, MA 02184, (617) 848-5353, BA 77 Univ of WI - Eau Claire; MS 78 Univ of WI - Eau Claire; 86–Asst Dir Ctr for Comm Dis, Braintree Hosp, **SLP**

Ladmer, Linda A K-6 Jordan Drive, Whitehall, PA 18052, (215) 391-1111, BS 76 Kutztown Univ of PA; MS 78 Rutger's St Univ - Douglas Coll; Sp-Lang Path, Carbon-Lehigh Iu, **SLP**

Ladnier, Carol A D 1045 Wicker Lane, Wichita, KS 67207, **SLP**

La Due, Mrs Cecilia M 6716 158th Avenue N W, Anoka, MN 55303, (612) 429-4704, BA 66 Moorhead St Univ; MS 78 Saint Cloud St Univ; SLP, Centennial Schs Dist 12, **SLP**

Ladzik, Mrs Kathleen M 119 Farrier Drive, Kitchener, ON, Canada N2P 1K1, (519) 578-3660, BS 69 Northern MI Univ; MS 72 CO St Univ; Sp-Lang Path, Waterloo Reg Roman Cath Sch Bd, **SLP**

Laeder, Ronald L 1558 Maplewood Drive, Caro, MI 48723, (517) 673-2144, BS 60 Central MI Univ; MA 64 Central MI Univ; Chair-Dept SLP, Tuscola Inter Sch Dist, **SLP F**

Laemmle, Jane M 10002 Tuppence Trace, Louisville, KY 40223, (502) 245-7622, BA 75 Bellarmine Coll; MS 79 Univ of Louisville; Sp-Lang Path, Bullitt Co Bd of Ed, **SLP**

Laesch, Kelley Bowers 312 Lorraine Road, Wheaton, IL 60187, (312) 682-1600, BS 81 Univ of WI - Eau Claire; MA 83 Univ of TX - Austin; 88–Sp-Lang Path, Edward Hosp, **SLP**

Lafaver, Joan B 227-1/2 East Elgin Street, Broken Arrow, OK 74012, **SLP**

Lafayette, Carol Jean 4675 Mink Livsey Road, Lithonia, GA 30058, (404) 483-4713, BS 82 Towson St Univ; OM 85 Emory Univ; 85–Sp-Lang Path, Rockdale Co Bd of Educ, **SLP**

Laferle, Kenneth R 630 West Berkley Lane, Hoffman Estates, IL 60194, (312) 463-9173, BA 80 Univ of MI - Ann Arbor; MS 82 Univ of Montevallo; Aud Services Admin, Oto-Sonic Inc, **A**

Laferriere, Darlene Margaret St Joseph's Hospital, 720 McLaren Street, North Bay, ON, Canada P1B 3L9, (705) 472-6100, BS 78 Univ of Western Ontario; MS 83 ID St Univ; 83–Sp-Lang Path, St Josephs Hosp, **SLP**

Lafevers, Nancy E 5115-C Del Monte, Houston, TX 77056, (713) 794-2526, BA 66 OK St Univ; MA 71 Univ of MO - Columbia; 75–Coord Sp/Lang Path, Baylor Coll of Med/Meyer Ctr, **SLP**

Lafevor, Mrs Julia S 120 West Meade Drive, Lebanon, TN 37087, (615) 444-0823, BA 56 Vanderbilt Univ; ME 73 Middle TN St Univ; Sp/Lang Path, Private Practice, **SLP**

Lafferty, Mrs Deborah Ann 2504 Leticoe Street, Pittsburgh, PA 15203, (412) 761-6062, BS 77 Carlow Coll; ME 85 Indiana Univ of PA; 84–Sp-Lang Path, Rehab Specialists, **SLP**

Lafferty, Roxane Kreger 16 Shenandoah Lane, Vincentown, NJ 08088, (609) 859-2942, BS 79 PA St Univ - Univ Park; MS 85 Indiana Univ of PA; 86–Sp-Lang Path, Medford Township Schs, **SLP**

Laffey, Mrs Bonnie Jean 1009 North Cambridge Court, Waunakee, WI 53597, (608) 643-2343, MS 83 Univ of WI - Whitewater; Dir-Rehab & Educ Svcs, Rural Wisconsin Hospital Coop, **SLP**

Laffy, Glenn Joseph 35 Simmons Avenue, Whitman, MA 02382, (617) 331-0686, BS 80 Salem St Coll; MS 82 Boston Univ; 85–Sp-Lang Path, Sp-Lang-Hrng Assoc, **SLP**

Laflamme, Joanne R R #2 Dukeland Drive, Woodstock, CT 06281, (203) 928-7751, Senior Communications Therapis, Johndempsey Regional Center, **SLP**

Laflamme, Karen A 414-A Main Street, Sanford, ME 04073, (207) 324-6117, BS 83 Univ of ME - Farmington; MS 86 Syracuse Univ; SLP, York County Counceling Service, **SLP**

Laflamme, Mrs Laurel L 20 Oak Knoll Drive, Hampden, MA 01036, (413) 566-8037, BA 73 Univ of MA - Amherst; MA 78 Univ of CT; Sp-Lang Path, Town of Stafford, **SLP**

La Fleur, Mrs Kathryn E 253 E Blenkner, Columbus, OH 43206, (614) 457-1548, BS 82 Bowling Green St Univ; MA 84 OH Univ - Athens; Sp-Lang Path, Affiliated A & Sp, **SLP**

La Fleur, Mrs Michele B Svcbtry 2/75 Fa Box 452, APO New York, NY 09165, (609) 234-5121, BS 86 Univ of NE - Lincoln; MA 87 Trenton St Coll

Laflure, Mrs Dorothy Drobny 1515 Earl Of Dunmore, Katy, TX 77449, (713) 347-4377, BS 75 Univ of Pittsburgh - Pittsburgh; OM 83 LA St Univ - N O Medical Ctr; **SLP**

Lafollette, Lisa Marie 1114 Pauline, Madison, WI 53705, (608) 233-6958, MS 88 Univ of WI - Madison

Lafond, James Rolland R R 3 Box 251A, Manchester, IA 52057, (319) 927-2143, BS 68 Saint Louis Univ; MA 73 Northeast MO St Univ; SLP, Keystone AEA #1, **SLP**

Lafontaine, Linda M 40 Norwood Terrace, Holyoke, MA 01040, (413) 532-0925, BA 79 Elms Coll; MA 81 Univ of MD - College Park; 88–Instr, Coll of Our Lady of the Elms, **SLP**

Lafontaine, Sandra D Calkins Road, Plattsburgh, NY 12901, (518) 561-5826, BA 73 SUNY - Coll at Plattsburgh; MA 85 SUNY - Coll at Plattsburgh; **SLP**

Lafoon, Cynthia Lynn Route 1 Box 120, Rawlings, VA 23876, (804) 848-3209, BS 78 Longwood Coll; MS 82 James Madison Univ; SLP, Brunswick Co Pub Schs

Laforest, Mary Pat 1725 Arlington Drive, Missoula, MT 59801, (406) 728-2402, BA 71 Univ of MT; MA 73 Univ of MT; SLP, Missoula Co High Schs, **SLP A ACE**

Lafortune, Mrs Cheryl Collins 1136 East 26th Street, Tulsa, OK 74114, BS 77 Univ of Tulsa; MA 79 Univ of Tulsa; 87–Sp-Lang Path, Private Practice, **SLP**

LaFosse, Maryann Hillcrest Hearing Aids, 111 West First Street, Suite 1000, Dayton, OH 45402, (513) 223-1513, BS 78 Univ of MA - Amherst; ME 80 Northeastern Univ; Aud, Hillcrest Hearing Aids, **A**

Lage, Ray V 5768 Mendocino Avenue, Oakland, CA 94618, (415) 255-0293, 86–Aud, Castro Hearing Center, **SLP A**

Lager, Mrs Mary Jo 3204 Random, Kalamazoo, MI 49004, (616) 345-9602, BS 83 Western MI Univ; MA 84; **SLP**

Lagler, Mrs Claudia A 7174 East 13th Street, Indianapolis, IN 46219, (317) 356-1856, BA 74 Purdue Univ - West Lafayette; MA 79 Ball St Univ; **SLP**

Lagno, Joan A 80 Highmeadow Road, Watertown, CT 06795, (203) 945-0147, BS 74 Northeastern Univ; ME 75 Northeastern Univ; 88–Coord/Sp-Lang Path, Watertown Bd of Educ, **SLP**

Lagourgue, Helen F 32172 Sea Island Drive, Laguna Niguel, CA 92677, MS; **SLP**

Lagourgue, John R 32172 Sea Island Drive, Laguna Niguel, CA 92677, MD (NS) 0101

Lagrant, Margaret A 264 Stonetree Circle, Rochester Hills, MI 48309-1143, (313) 373-9645, **SLP**

Laguaite, Dr Jeannette Tulane University Medical Sch, 1430 Tulane Avenue, New Orleans, LA 70112, (504) 588-5493, BA 37 6839; MA 40 6839; PH 52 (NS) LA St Univ - Baton Rouge; Prof Emeritus, Tulane U, **SLP A F LM**

Lahaie, Dr Ralph V 19285 Cedarcrest N W, North Fort Myers, FL 33903, BS 41 Central MI Univ; MA 49 Univ of FL; PH 58 (NS) Univ of Denver; Prof Emeritus, Old Dominion U, **SLP LM**

Lahey, Dr Margaret M P O Box B, Oxford, NH 03777, (212) 481-4464, BS 52 SUNY - Coll at Geneseo; MA 53 OH St Univ; ED 72 (Lang Development & Disorders) Columbia Univ Teachers Coll; Prof, Hunter Coll, **SLP A F**

Lahm, Mary Elizabeth 1696 Green Bay Road, Highland Park, IL 60035, (608) 784-8660, BS 76 Univ of WI - Oshkosh; MA 77 Univ of WI - Oshkosh; Sp-Lang Path, Edgerton School District, **SLP**

Lahrmer, Mrs Jackie S 1365 Firethorne Drive, Mason, OH 45040, (513) 398-9638, MA 88 Univ of Akron; 88–Sp-Lang Path, Kings Local Sch Dist

Lahti, Dr Ganea P 3234 Ellenda Avenue, Los Angeles, CA 90034, (213) 477-5033, BA 65 San Diego St Univ; ME 67 Boston Univ; PH 79 (Special Education) Univ of CA - Los Angeles; 86–Sp-Lang Path, Private Practice, **SLP**

Laiche, Grace Marie 248 Papworth Avenue, Metairie, LA 70005, (504) 443-1603, BS 84 Nicholls St Univ; MS 88 Southeastern LA Univ

Laidig, Margaret Anne 185 Pine Street #302, Manchester, CT 06040, (203) 334-2118, BS 80 Univ of WI - Madison; MS 83 FL St Univ; Sp-Lang Path, Easter Seals Rehabilitatn Ctr, **SLP**

Laikko, Paul E 15260 Cuming St, Omaha, NE 68154, (402) 559-5755, BA 76 WA St Univ; MA 78 WA St Univ; Sp-Lang Path, Meyers Children Rehab Inst, **SLP**

Laikko, Terry McGrath 14233 North 21st Street, Phoenix, AZ 85022, (602) 971-4007, BS 81 Northern AZ Univ; MS 84 AZ St Univ; SLP, Cartwright Sch Dist, **SLP**

Lail, Mrs Lorie Fox 123 Pennsylvania Place, El Paso, TX 79903, (915) 562-7611, BA 78 Univ of TX - El Paso; MA 80 Univ of TX - El Paso; Sp-Lang Path, El Paso Ind Sch Dis Reg Pro Df, **SLP**

Lainer, Harriet 21 Fairview Terrace, Maplewood, NJ 07040, (201) 753-5014, MA 67 Kean Coll of NJ; Pub Relations-Superv, Hrng & Sp Consult, **SLP**

Laing, Pamela J 737 Admiralty Way, Fort Worth, TX 76108, ME 79 Southwest TX St Univ; Sp-Lang Path, Ft Worth ISD, **SLP**

Lainoff, Janice S 9843 South 262nd Place, Kent, WA 98031, (206) 854-1885, BA 68 Our Lady Lake Univ-San Anton; MA 69 Our Lady Lake Univ-San Anton; SLP, Kent Sch Dist, **SLP**

Laird, Mrs Beverly K 1151 4th Avenue #609, Chula Vista, CA 92011, (501) 236-3653, BS 80 AR St Univ; MS 81 AR St Univ; Sp-Lang Path, Paragould Pub Sch, **SLP**

Laird, Mrs Emily W G 530 Woodland Avenue, Bowling Green, KY 42101, (502) 842-3477, BS 75 Western KY Univ; MA 78 Western KY Univ; 84–Sp-Lang Path, Barren River MH/MR Bd Inc, **SLP**

Laird, James Bryan Rd 1 Box 68-A, Hartstown, PA 16131, (412) 588-2500, **SLP A**

Laird, Mrs Jane Ellen 802 Holly Street, St Marys, OH 45885, (419) 394-2116, BS 79 Purdue Univ - West Lafayette; MA 82 Ball St Univ; **SLP**

Laird, Mrs Kathryn A 2303 Barberry Drive, Champaign, IL 61821, (217) 893-4141, BS 77 Eastern IL Univ; MS 78 Eastern IL Univ; Sp-Lang Path, Rantoul Cty Schs, **SLP**

Laird, Ralph F 854 Avenue E, Traverse City, MI 49684, (616) 947-3874, BA 51 Univ of Northern IA; MA 57 Univ of MI - Ann Arbor; Retired, Traverse Bay Intermed Sch Dist, **SLP**

Lajoie, Claudette S P O Box 377, Waquoit, MA 02536, (508) 477-9190, BA 62 Assumption Coll; MA 66 Assumption Coll; MS 76 Emerson Coll; Sp-Lang Path, Sp Path Assoc of Cape Cod, **SLP**

Lakatos, Mrs Catherine 12 Hearthstone Drive, Bethel, CT 06801, (203) 743-6628, BS 77 Bloomsburg Univ of PA; MS 78 Bloomsburg Univ of PA; Sp-Lang Path, Private Practice, **SLP**

Lakawicz, Judith Anne 112-B Marchand Drive, Westover, WV 26505, (304) 292-5836, BS 83 Clarion Univ of PA; MS 84 WV Univ; **SLP**

Lake, Albert E 44 Weber Avenue, Warwick, RI 02886, BA 74 Nasson Coll; MS 76 Univ of RI; Aud, Hearing Speech Language Assoc, **A**

Lake, Constance Ann 5134 Woodstock Drive, Swartz Creek, MI 48473, (313) 732-9131, BA 79 MI St Univ; MA 80 MI St Univ; Indep Contr, Bay Valley Corp, **SLP**

Lake, Mrs Donna Bland P O Box 496, Jane Lew, WV 26378, (304) 269-4585, BS 81 Indiana Univ of PA; MS 82 Indiana Univ of PA; Sp/Lang Path, Lewis County Board of Educ, **SLP**

Lake, Mrs Ethel P 3028 Castle Street, Los Angeles, CA 90039, (213) 664-0052, BA 42 Univ of IL - Urbana; MA 75 CA St Univ - Los Angeles; SLP, El Rancho Un Sch Dist, **SLP**

Lake, Hope G 10921 Bloomingdale Drive, Rockville, MD 20852, (301) 770-7220, MS 88 Emerson Coll; 88–Sp-Lang Path, National Rehab Hosp

Lake, Janet E 5316 Paso Del Rio Way, Concord, CA 94521, BS 73 Univ of FL; MA 82 CA St Univ - Sacramento; SLP, Pittsburg USD, **SLP**

Lake, Kathleen T 44 Weber Avenue, Warwick, RI 02886, (401) 438-9500, BA 74 Iona Coll; MS 76 Univ of RI; Sp-Lang Path, Meeting St Sch, **SLP**

Lake, Nancy A 934 South 21st Street, South Bend, IN 46615, (219) 288-2391, BS 77 Ball St Univ; MA 78 Ball St Univ; Sp-Lang Path, United Health Services, **SLP**

Lake, Patricia 6690 East Eastman Avenue, Denver, CO 80224, **SLP**

Lake, Mrs Sandra J 1530 Hamilton Avenue, Palo Alto, CA 94303, (415) 327-4663, BS 62 Case Western Reserve Univ; MA 67 Kent St Univ; 86–Sp-Lang Path, Private Practice, **SLP**

Lake, Shirley K 1038 Brown, Junction City, KS 66441, (913) 238-6184, BA 63 Wichita St Univ; Sp-Lang Path, Geary Co USD, **SLP**

Lake, Mrs Susan E 830 Hover Road, Longmont, CO 80501, BS 75 Southwest TX St Univ; ME 76 Southwest TX St Univ; Sp-Lang Path, Poudre Valley Hosp Rehab Dept, **SLP**

Lake, Teresa Manlove 1224 Temple City Blvd #E, Arcadia, CA 91006, (213) 595-9521, BA 85 CA St Univ - Long Beach; MA 86 CA St Univ - Los Angeles; **A**

Laker, Etta-Jo 35 Jacaruso Drive, Spring Valley, NY 10977, (914) 425-8618, BA 78 Yeshiva Univ; MA 81 NY Univ; Research Asst, IBM-T J Watson Research Ctr, **SLP**

Lakes, Mrs Dana L 1724 Jackson Street, Anderson, IN 46016, (317) 646-8412, BS 80 Ball St Univ; MA 81 Ball St Univ; Sp-Lang Path, St Johns Med Cen, **SLP**

Lakis, Mrs Karen Terhune 909 Brookfield Lane, Perrysburg, OH 43551, (419) 874-5400, BS 79 SUNY - Coll at Geneseo; MA 80 SUNY - Coll at Geneseo; 88–Sp-Lang Path, Private Practice, **SLP**

Laky, Mrs Mildred H 572 Jefferson Street, Lehighton, PA 18235, (215) 377-0417, BS 40 East Stroudsburg Univ of PA; ME 61 PA St Univ - Univ Park; Sp-Lang Path, Palmerton Hosp, **SLP LM**

La Lance, Linda L 1506 Ashlawn Drive, Murfreesboro, TN 37129, (615) 896-5795, BS 63 WV Univ; ME 67 Univ of FL; **SLP**

Laliberte, Mrs Jeannie S 210 McClellan St, Suite 405, Wausau, WI 54401, (715) 848-1313, BA 70 Univ of MN - Minneap-St Paul; MA 73 Univ of MN - Minneap-St Paul; Sp-Lang Path, Private Practice, **SLP ACE**

Lalich, Margaret Myrtle 2047 Coronado Avenue, Napa, CA 94558, (707) 253-5674, BS 83 CA St Univ - Hayward; Sp-Lang Path, Napa State Hospital, **SLP ACE**

Lally, Eleanore Coomes Rt 1 Box 8, Mount Olivet, KY 41064, (606) 724-5950, MS 84 Univ of KY; 75–Sp-Lang Path, Robertson Co Bd of Educ, **SLP**

Lally-Barton, Judy Ann 9405 Holtwood, Overland, MO 63114, BS 77 Fontbonne Coll; MS 78 Fontbonne Coll; Sp-Lang Path, Associated Rehab Services, **SLP**

La Loggia, Mary Messina 2000 Laura Lane, Waukesha, WI 53186, (414) 228-9440, **SLP**

Lalone, Dale T Maxwell & Roediger MDPA, 43 Baxter Boulevard, Portland, ME 04101, (207) 775-6381, BA 78 SUNY - Coll at Potsdam; MS 79 Ithaca Coll; Audiologist, Maxwell & Roediger Mdpa, **A**

Lalone, Mrs Faye Bonnie c/o Maxwell & Roediger, MDPA 43 Baxter Blvd, Portland, ME 04101, (207) 775-6381, BA 81 Univ of Denver; MA 83 Univ of Denver; Aud, Maxwell & Roediger MD Pa, **A**

La Luzerne, Dawn Marie 3412 Colfax Avenue S #106, Minneapolis, MN 55408, (612) 823-6660, BA 86 Univ of WI - Eau Claire; MS 87 Univ of WI - Eau Claire; **SLP**

Lam, Mrs Barbara B 1209 Amsterdam, Madison, WI 53716, (608) 222-7564, BA 68 Univ of WI - Whitewater; MA 69 Temple Univ; Sp-Lang Path, Madison Metro Sch Dist, **SLP**

Lam, Vivian Wai Wan 9215-93A Street #402, Fort St John, BC, Canada V1J 5V4, (604) 787-3360, BS 83 Univ of HI - Manoa; MS 85 Univ of HI - Manoa; 87–Sp-Lang Path, British Columbia/Ministry-Hlth, **SLP**

Lam, Mrs Winona Lau 99-370 Paint Street A9, Aiea, HI 96701, (808) 487-5882, BS 83 OR St Univ; MS 85 Univ of WA; 85–Sp-Lang Path, Dept of Educ, **SLP**

Lamanna, Mary Lyon 266-A Lake Kitchawan Drive, South Salem, NY 10590, (914) 628-3415, **SLP**

Lamaster, Craig A 2828 Valley Drive, Sioux City, IA 51104, **SLP**

Lamaster, Sandra K 2828 Valley Drive, Sioux City, IA 51104, MS; **SLP**

Lamay, Mrs Linda P 421 Benton, El Paso, TX 79927, (915) 852-4373, BA 64 FL St Univ; 87–Sp-Lang Path, Ysleta ISD, **SLP**

Lamb, Donald P 1925 Ridgefield, Naperville, IL 60565-2251, (312) 888-0663, MA 86 Northern IL Univ - De Kalb; **A**

Lamb, Mrs Kathryn Marie 112 Columbus Road, Bedford, OH 44146, (216) 274-2598, BS 82 Kent St Univ; MA 84 Kent St Univ; 84–Sp-Lang Path, Crestwood Local School Dist, **SLP**

Lamb, Leigh A Rt 4 Box 37, Loudon, TN 37774, (615) 376-5592, BA 76 Univ of TN - Knoxville; MA 78 Univ of TN - Knoxville; Aud, Roane County Schools, **A**

Lamb, Mrs Lisa Guy 37 Napa Valley Circle, Madison, MS 39110-9546, (901) 454-1333, MA 84 Memphis St Univ; Sp-Lang Path, Baptist Memorial Hospital, **SLP**

Lamb, Dr Lloyd E 1004 Morina Court N E, Albuquerque, NM 87112, (505) 277-2948, BA 60 Univ of North TX; MS 62 Purdue Univ - West Lafayette; PH 64 (NS) Purdue Univ - West Lafayette; Prof, U of New Mexico, **A**

Lamb, Mrs Mary Londergan Rt 5 Box 217, Detroit Lakes, MN 56501, (216) 847-3917, BS 62 Univ of ND; **SLP LM**

Lamb, Nancy L 7415 El Monte, Shawnee Mission, KS 66208, (913) 362-8386, BA 50 Ottawa Univ; MA 64 Univ of KS; SLP, Shawnee Missim USD #512, **SLP**

Lamb, Noelle L School Of Audiology And Speech Science, University Of British Columbia, 5804 Fairview Avenue, Vancouver, BC, Canada V6T 1W5, (604) 228-5953, MS 66 Purdue Univ - West Lafayette; 81–Sen Instrctr, U of BC, **A**

Lamb, Mrs Patricia A 4713 North Shore, Wichita Falls, TX 76310-3514, (817) 322-0771, MA 84 TX Woman's Univ; Sp-Lang Path, North TX Easter Seal Rehab, **SLP**

Lamb, Stanford H 6 Hermosa Place, Menlo Park, CA 94025, PH (NS); **SLP A**

Lamb, Wendy Meredith 702 West Cherry #A, Flagstaff, AZ 86001, (602) 779-3366, BS 82 Northern AZ Univ; MS 83 Northern AZ Univ; Consult Sp/Lang Path, Sp/Hrng Consult Serv, **SLP**

Lambden, Kristi Ann 625 Country Club Drive #621, Simi Valley, CA 93065, (805) 582-0237, BS 88 Univ of SC - Columbia; 88–Sp-Lang Path, Camarillo State Hosp

Lambdin, Janis Elaine 509 West 33rd Street, Sand Springs, OK 74063-2934, BA 83 Wichita St Univ; MA 86 Wichita St Univ; **SLP**

Lambert, Mrs Alice M 408 Old Mill Creek Drive, Waco, TX 76712, (817) 772-9181, BA OH Wesleyan Univ; MA 53 Univ of AL-Birmingham; Sp-Lang Path, Midway Schs, **SLP LM ACE**

Lambert, Mrs Beatrice Baker 12825 Short Avenue, Los Angeles, CA 90066, (213) 391-3626, BA 76 Radcliffe Coll; MA 79 Northwestern Univ; 88–Sp-Lang Path, New Pathways Ctr for Brain Inj Rehab (DFMH/Inglewood CA), **SLP ACE**

Lambert, Carol A 6355 East Skelly Dr, Tulsa, OK 74135, (918) 622-7064, BA 72 Univ of Tulsa; MA 77 Univ of Tulsa; Aud, Private Practice, **A**

Lambert, Mrs Carolyn 752 Bay Road, Belchertown, MA 01007, (413) 586-8692, BS 84 Univ of MA - Amherst; MA 85 OH Univ - Athens; 86–Sp-Lang Path, Franklin/Hampshire Comm Health Ctr, **SLP**

Lambert, David Armstrong P O Box 1472, St George, UT 84770, (801) 628-1646, BS 83 Univ of UT; MS 86 Univ of UT; Sp-Lang Path, Washington Co School Dstr, **SLP**

Lambert, Dennis E 423 12th Avenue East #3, Seattle, WA 98102, BS 71 Northern MI Univ; MA 72 Western MI Univ; Aud, **A**

Lambert, Evalyn Feller 2 Aberdeen Place, Fair Lawn, NJ 07410, (201) 796-4389, BA 77 Univ of RI; MA 78 NY Univ; Sp-Lang Path, Private Practice, **SLP**

Lambert, Gerald T 621 Checker Drive, Buffalo Grove, IL 60089

Lambert, Dr James David Mexia State School, Dept Of Habilitative SVC, P O Box 1132, Mexia, TX 76667, (817) 562-2821, PH 54 (NS) Purdue Univ - West Lafayette; 86–Aud, Mexia State Sch, **SLP A ACE**

Lambert, Judith C 11 Hearth Lane, Westbury, NY 11590, BA 65 Hofstra Univ; MA 66 NY Univ; Aud, Adelphi U, **A**

Lambert, Karen Marie 2724 Jennings Road, Kensington, MD 20895, (301) 984-4444, BA 81 Emmanuel Coll; MS 85 Univ of NH; **SLP**

Lambert, Laura J 152 Henry Drive, Orion, IL 61273, (309) 752-1669, BS 78 IL St Univ - Normal; MA 81 Univ of IL - Urbana; SLP/Lrng Dis Instr, United Township High Sch, **SLP**

Lambert, Lorna J 330 West Gray #315, Norman, OK 73069, (405) 366-0123, BA 77 Univ of OK - Norman; MS 79 Univ of OK Medical Center; Sp-Lang Path, Private Practice, **SLP**

Lambert, Mrs Lynn O 3326 Creekbend Drive, Garland, TX 75042, (214) 234-8866, BA 68 Univ of AL- Tuscaloosa; MS 74 Southern Methodist Univ; Sp/Lang Path, Richardson ISD, **SLP**

Lambert, Mrs Nancy B 8439 Holly Leaf Drive, Mc Lean, VA 22102, (703) 448-9877, BA 71 Univ of NC - Greensboro; MA 74 George Washington Univ; **SLP**

Lambert, Mrs Nancy N Route 5 Box 234A, Canton, TX 75103, (214) 896-1761, BS 73 East TX St Univ - Commerce; MS 75 East TX St Univ - Commerce; Spec Educ Supvr, Van Zandt/Rains Bi-Co Coop, **SLP**

Lambert, Mrs Susan Therese 1504 East Glen, Peoria Heights, IL 61614, (309) 686-1898, **SLP**

Lambert-Galtman, Mrs Pennie 1550 Worcester Road #501-W, Framingham, MA 01701, (617) 793-8055, BA 65 CUNY - Hunter Coll; MA 70 CUNY - Hunter Coll; **A**

Lamberth, Mrs Ellen McGuirk 2148 Camino La Vista, Fullerton, CA 92633, (213) 926-5566, BA 81 CA St Univ - Fullerton; MA 84 CA St Univ - Fullerton; 88–Sp-Lang Path, ABC USD, **SLP**

Lambeth, Robert Scott 3162-107 Berry Lane SW, Roanoke, VA 24018, (804) 239-2657, MS 87 Univ of Montevallo; Sp-Lang Path, Communicare of VA, **SLP**

Lambiase, Barbara A 56 12th Street, Somerset, NJ 08873, (201) 247-9266, BA 77 SUNY - Coll at Geneseo; BS 77 SUNY - Coll at Geneseo; MA 80 CUNY - Queens Coll; Sp-Lang Path, JFK Med Ctr, **SLP**

Lambie, Charlene L 1303 Walnut Street, Pittsburgh, PA 15221, (608) 249-2151, BA 78 Univ of Pittsburgh - Pittsburgh; MA 80 Univ of Pittsburgh - Pittsburgh; Sp-Lang Path, Rehab Institute of Pittsburgh, **SLP**

Lambrecht, Karen J 5115 S W Grayson Street, Seattle, WA 98116, (206) 368-1848, BS 77 Portland St Univ; MS 83 Portland St Univ; Sp-Lang Path, Northwest Hospital, **SLP**

Lambright, Barbara L 15112 Barnwall, La Mirada, CA 90638, BA 75 CA St Univ - Fullerton; MA 77 CA St Univ - Fullerton; Aud, Centralia School District, **A**

Lambright, Laura G 5600 Green Court, Durham, NC 27713, (919) 544-4963, BA 79 Univ of MD - College Park; OM 80 LA St Univ - N O Medical Ctr; Aud, State of North Carolina, **A**

Lambros, Georgette Koskovolis 1956 Central Drive N, East Meadow, NY 11554, (718) 523-1874, BA 83 Saint John's Univ - Jamaica; MA 85 CUNY - Queens Coll; **SLP**

Lamden, Mrs Frances F 3240 North Riverbend Circle W, Tucson, AZ 85715, (602) 885-7150, BA 68 Univ of NC - Greensboro; MA 70 Univ of CA - Santa Barbara; SLP, Sunnyside USD, **SLP**

Lamendola, Paula Fueller Syosset Speech And Hearing, 175 Jericho Turnpike, Syosset, NY 11791, (516) 364-1234, BS 84 Bloomsburg Univ of PA; MS 85 Bloomsburg Univ of PA; Aud, Albert M Nalevanko MD, **A**

Lamendola, Rita Gandelman 3 Springhill Drive, Lawrenceville, NJ 08648, BA 77 Temple Univ; MA 80 Trenton St Coll

Lamich, Mrs Kathleen Horan 1526 Bristol Avenue, Westchester, IL 60153, (312) 865-1586, BS 83 Marquette Univ; MS 84 Marquette Univ; **SLP**

Lamkey, Mrs Becky Marie Rural Route 1, Ames, IA 50010, BS 80 Eastern IL Univ; MS 81 Eastern IL Univ; Sp-Lang Path, Heartland AEA 11, **SLP**

Lamm, Joanne Schwartz 2423 Tunlaw Road N W, Washington, DC 20007, (202) 373-7374, BA 69 Univ of MD - College Park; MA 71 Univ of IA; Sp-Lang Path, St Elizabeth Hosp, **SLP**

Lamm, Tina Senders 144 West 86th Street #5C, New York, NY 10024, (212) 340-6027, BA 83 Yeshiva Univ; MA 86 CUNY - Queens Coll; **SLP**

Lammel, Julie K 510 Countrywood Drive, Franklin, TN 37064, (615) 360-2912, BS 70 Univ Southern MS-Hattiesburg; MS 73 TN St Univ; Sp-Lang Path, Metro - Nashville Pub Sch, **SLP**

Lammon, Mrs Kay L 1843 Heatherton Drive, Montgomery, AL 36106-3034, BS 74 Univ of AL-Tuscaloosa; MS 80 Univ of South AL; Sp/Lang Path, Montgomery Co Board of Educ, **SLP**

La Mora, Christine M 17 Lamoille River Road, Milton, VT 05468, (802) 658-9060, BS 73 SUNY - Coll at Fredonia; MS 76 SUNY - Coll at Fredonia; Sp-Lang Path, S Burlington Sch Dist, **SLP**

Lamorey, Suzanne Grace 520 West Wilson Apt #211, Glendale, CA 91203, (213) 465-4231, BA 75 Univ of CA - Berkeley; MS 83 AZ St Univ; Aud, Cedar Sinai Med Ctr, **A**

Lamorte, Mrs Frances B 609 Forest Hill Circle, Elizabeth City, NC 27909, (919) 426-5741, BS 75 West Chester Univ of PA; MS 76 Loyola Coll; Sp-Lang Path, Perquimans Co PS, **SLP**

La Motte, Carolyn 543 Sun Ridge #201, Altamonte Springs, FL 32714, BA 82 SUNY - Coll at Cortland; MA 86 Univ of Central FL; **SLP**

La Moy, Juli R Box 14-A, Bernhart Road, Wallkill, NY 12589, **SLP**

Lamp, Mrs Gayle 2532 20th Street Road, Greeley, CO 80631, (303) 330-3889, BA 67 Univ of Southern CA; MA 69 Univ of Southern CA; Sp-Lang Path, Northern Colorado Medical Cen, **SLP**

Lampard, Lucille Brinz 1008 Martin Behrman, Metairie, LA 70005, (504) 482-7110, BS 80 Tulane Univ; OM 82 Tulane Univ; Sp-Lang Path, Jefferson Par Pub Sch, **SLP**

Lampe, Henrica C 48 Avery Heights, Hartford, CT 06106, (203) 524-1880, **SLP LM**

Lampert, Jeffrey J San Mateo Hearing Center, 149 South B Street, San Mateo, CA 94401, (415) 342-8841, BA 79 San Diego St Univ; MA 82 San Diego St Univ; Dir of Aud, San Mateo Hearing Ctr, **A**

Lamphear, Judith M 804 Forest Hill Court, Columbia, MO 65203, (314) 874-7977, BA 67 Univ of GA; OB 67 Univ of GA; MS 69 Univ of GA; Dir, Columbia Sp,Lang,Hrng Serv, **SLP**

Lampros, Nancy P 2339 Winstead Circle, Wichita, KS 67226, BA 85 Wichita St Univ; MA 86 Wichita St Univ; 86–SLP, USD #259 Wichita Ps System, **SLP**

Lampson, Joyce M 1715 Third Street, Brookings, SD 57006, (605) 688-6131, BA 71 SD St Univ; MA 72; Asst Prof, Sd St U, **SLP**

Lamson-Uhelski, Karen Dianne 2428 Sebastian, Grand Blanc, MI 48439, (313) 257-3900, BS 85 Western MI Univ; MA 86 Western MI Univ

Lamy, Mrs Lori Kay 5636 M-32 West, Gaylord, MI 49735, (616) 546-3291, BS 85 Northern MI Univ; MA 86 Central MI Univ; **SLP**

Lamzik, Mrs Jean Marie 5 Gold Run Drive, St Peters, MO 63376, (314) 447-4463, OB 81 Northeast MO St Univ; MA 82 Northeast MO St Univ; Sp-Lang Path, Howell Sch Dist, **SLP**

Lancaster, Ernest Arthur, Jr 6724 18th Avenue N W, Seattle, WA 98117, (206) 453-0233, BA 83 Western WA Univ; **SLP**

Lancaster, Leslie Ann 6917 Yorktowne Drive, Charlotte, NC 28226-7659, (502) 781-2490, MA 84 Univ of TN - Knoxville; Aud, Comm for Handicapped Children, **A**

Lance, Mrs Beverly Ann 777 Walter Reed Boulevard, Suite 305, Garland, TX 75042, (214) 494-5691, BS 75 Southwest TX St Univ; ME 76 Southwest TX St Univ; Sp-Lang Path, Private Practice, **SLP**

Lance, Karen Lloyd 5117 Secor Road #2, Toledo, OH 43623, (419) 531-4465, BA 85 Univ of Toledo; MS 86 Bowling Green St Univ; Sp-Lang Path, InSpeech Inc, **SLP**

Lanctot, Virginia L 8719 Hillswick Terr, Brooklyn Park, MN 55443, (612) 533-2246, BA 73 Univ of MN - Duluth; MA 75 CA St Univ - Sacramento; Sp-Lang Path, Robbinsdale Area Schools, **SLP**

Land, Mrs Carol R 17210 South Mill Creek Rd, Noblesville, IN 46060, (317) 776-0370, BS 74 Ball St Univ; MA 78 Ball St Univ; Sp-Lang Path, Noblesville Schools, **SLP**

Landa, Dr Rebecca 21012 Middletown Road, Freeland, MD 21053, (301) 955-7018, BS 77 Towson St Univ; MS 78 PA St Univ - Univ Park; PH 85 (Language Science) Univ of WA; 86–Asst Prof, Johns Hopkins Univ Sch of Med, **SLP**

Landau, Cecelia Charest 2101 Country Club Road, Ann Arbor, MI 48105, (313) 769-8725, BA 75 Univ of MI - Ann Arbor; MS 86 Univ of MI - Ann Arbor; **SLP**

Landau, Claudia 1182 Glenwood Trails, De Land, FL 32720, (904) 736-9856, BA 75 SUNY - Coll at Cortland; MS 76 Univ of South FL; Sp-Lang Path, Private Practice/Clinic, **SLP ACE**

Landau, Ellen Jill 300 Mercer Street #321, New York, NY 10003-6744, (212) 254-4284, MA 85 NY Univ; **SLP**

Landau, Mrs Sharon 70-14 141 Street, Flushing, NY 11367, (718) 520-0693, **A**

Landay, Sheila D H 204 Tudor Road, Needham, MA 02192, (617) 444-4100, BA 63 Boston Univ; ME 71 Northeastern Univ; Sp-Lang Path, Needham Pub Sch, **SLP**

Lande, Anita 325 Central Park West, New York, NY 10025, (212) 220-6246, BA 40 CUNY - Hunter Coll; MA 58 Columbia Univ Teachers Coll; **SLP LM**

Lande, Mrs Briana L N 600 North Brookdale Drive, Schaumburg, IL 60194, (312) 843-8117, BS 75 Bradley Univ; MS 77 Bradley Univ; **SLP**

Lander, Mrs Joyce I P P O Box 11, Accident, MD 21520, (301) 826-8165, BS 77 Clarion Univ of PA; ME 78 Clarion Univ of PA; Sp/Lang Path, Garrett Co Bd of Ed, **SLP**

Landers, Mrs Kristine S 1585 Seawind Drive, Charleston, SC 29407-9658, (803) 571-4708, BS 71 Central MO St Univ; MA 73 Univ of MO - Columbia; **SLP**

Landers, Mrs Madie L 38 El Jer Drive, Cedar Hill, MO 63016, (314) 285-4569, BS 44 Southeast MO St Univ; MA 50 Univ of Denver; 88–Retired, **SLP LM**

Landers, Millard T 38 El Jer Drive, Cedar Hill, MO 63016, (314) 285-4569, BS 53 Northwestern Univ; MS 57 Southern IL Univ -Carbondale; MS 59 Syracuse Univ; 88–Retired, **LM**

Landes, Dr Bernard A 3605 Long Beach Boulevard, Suite 210, Long Beach, CA 90807, (213) 595-4878, BS 51 Purdue Univ - West Lafayette; MS 53 Purdue Univ - West Lafayette; PH 58 (Sp Path & Aud) Univ of MI - Ann Arbor; 61–Sp-Lang Path & Aud, Private Practice, **SLP A F ACE**

Landes, Mrs Eileen Schaefer 26587 Simmons Way, Hemet, CA 92344, (714) 654-7349, BA 76 Univ of Redlands; MS 77 Univ of Redlands; Sp-Lang Path, San Jacinto USD, **SLP**

Landesberg, Ann Simpson 311 Elysian Street, Pittsburgh, PA 15206, MA 81 Univ of Pittsburgh - Pittsburgh; Sp-Lang Path, Private Practice, **SLP**

Landess-Towne, Susan Carol Route 20 Box 2108, Springfield, MO 65803, (617) 885-3282, BA 78 Southern CT St Univ; MS 81 Southern IL Univ -Carbondale; 84–Director Sp-Lang Path, St Johns Regio Health Ctr, **SLP**

Landin-Bohbot, Deborah Pears University Of Minnesota, Communication Disorders, 5 Montague Hall, Duluth, MN 55812, (218) 726-6135, BS 74 FL St Univ; MS 75 FL St Univ; Aud, Duluth Pub Sch, **A**

Landino, Daniel 215 Quinnipiac Avenue, North Haven, CT 06473, (203) 734-9209, BA 79 Southern CT St Univ; MS 82 Southern CT St Univ; Sp-Lang Path, Derby Board of Ed, **SLP**

Landis, Keith Duane 600 East Harding, La Grange, IL 60525, (312) 438-6319, BA 83 Elmhurst Coll; OM 86 Governors St Univ; **SLP**

Landis, Lydia J 196 Harrison Road, Cheshire, CT 06410, BA 57 Rockford Coll; MA 62 Univ of IL - Urbana; OM 88 Yale Univ; 73–Sp-Lang Path, St of CT, **SLP**

Landis, Marcia H 2370 Valencia Court, San Jose, CA 95125, (415) 794-2033, BA 76 Univ of CA - Santa Barbara; MA 80 San Jose St Univ; 79–Sp-Lang Path, Newark USD, **SLP**

Landis, Marjorie A Box 4347, Aspen, CO 81612, (303) 925-8057, BS 70 Univ of PA; MA 75 Univ of CO - Boulder; Sp-Lang Path, Aspen Sch Dist, **SLP**

Landis, Patricia Ann 1745-F Champlain Drive, Baltimore, MD 21207, (301) 225-5581, BA 55 Heidelberg Coll; MA 56 Case Western Reserve Univ; Sp-Lang Path, MD St Dept of Health Ment Hyg, **SLP**

Landman, Chana 896 East 8th Street, Brooklyn, NY 11230, **SLP**

Lando, Mrs Leah F 3602 Clarks Lane, Baltimore, MD 21215, (301) 396-6380, BS 72 CUNY - Brooklyn Coll; MS 81 Towson St Univ; Sp-Lang Path, Baltimore Cty Publ Schs, **SLP**

Landoe, Jurine 4627 Beach Boulevard, Buena Park, CA 90621, (213) 864-2593, MS 81 Chapman Coll; SLP, Norwalk-La Mirada Sch Dist, **SLP**

Landon, Connie L 345 Kinsmen Way, Hampton, VA 23666-2448, (804) 825-4642, BA 79; ME 82 Trenton St Coll; Sp-Lang Path, Hampton City Schools, **SLP**

Landrey, Mrs Lynne Herring 2450 Montchanin Road, Greenville, DE 19807, (302) 654-2161, BA 77 Gettysburg Coll; MA 83 Temple Univ; 87–Sp-Lang Path, Al DuPont Inst, **SLP**

Landrock, Rose-Marie 285 East Shore Trail, Sparta, NJ 07871, **SLP**

Landrum, Mrs Anne T Route 70, P O Box 380, Mount View, AR 72560, (501) 363-4568, ME 87 Univ of Central AR; 88–Sp-Lang Path, Shirley Sch Dist, **SLP**

Landry, Mrs Anne Ligocki 24 Carey Lane, Norwich, CT 06360, (203) 887-1654, BA 75 Emory Univ; OM 77 Emory Univ; 85–Sp-Lang Path, SE CT Hrng & Sp Ctr, **SLP**

Landry, Beth M 2950 N Broadway #10, Redarrow Apartment, Boulder, CO 80302, (303) 938-9271, MA 87 Univ of CO - Boulder; 87–Sp-Lang Path, Boulder Mem Hosp, **SLP**

Landry, David D 20 Kimberly Drive, South Hadley, MA 01075, (508) 781-9100, BA 74 Univ of MA - Amherst; MS 79 Emerson Coll; 86–Sp-Lang Path, Mercy Hosp Reg Rehab Ctr, **SLP**

Landry, Katherine Denise 2444 Dogwood Drive Circle, Alexandria, LA 71301, BS 73 AZ St Univ; MS 81 MS Univ for Women; **SLP**

Landry, Mrs Laura Christman 102 Chickasaw, Lafayette, LA 70501, (318) 234-5053, BS 77 Saint Mary's Dominican Coll; MS 85 Univ of Southwestern LA; 88–Sp-Lang Path, Lafayette Parish Sch Bd, **SLP**

Landry, Mrs Lisa D North Brookfield Road, Barre Plains, MA 01005, (617) 885-3319, **SLP**

Landsman, Carol D 1480 Mill Plain Road, Fairfield, CT 06430, (203) 384-8681, BA 68 CUNY - Queens Coll; MA 71 Univ of CT; Dir, Rehab Assoc, **SLP**

Landsverk, Carolyn J 6120 S E 32nd, Portland, OR 97202, (503) 222-9221, BS 68 1859; MS 71 1859; Aud, Portland-VA Med Cen, **SLP A**

Landy, Mrs Barbara Jo 404 Clear Ridge Road, Linwood, MD 21764, (301) 775-7138, BA 71 Towson St Univ; MS 75 Towson St Univ; Sp-Lang Path, Howard Co Dept of Ed, **SLP**

Lane, Allison Wilhite 3892 Bald Eagle Drive #220, Memphis, TN 38115, (901) 366-7168, BA 83 Univ of AR - Fayetteville; MS 85 Univ of AR - Little Rock; 88–Aud, VA, **A**

Lane, Angela Bollich 4120 N W 19th Terrace, Gainesville, FL 32605, (904) 373-9168, BS 83 LA St Univ - Baton Rouge; MA 86 Univ of FL; **SLP**

Lane, Audrey Lynn 6596 Rocky Park Drive, Memphis, TN 38115-7256, (901) 523-8990, BS 83 Purdue Univ - West Lafayette; MA 85 Memphis St Univ; **SLP**

Lane, Barbara D 5609 Whitman Avenue, Fort Worth, TX 76133, **SLP**

Lane, Bette 600 N E 36th Street, Miami, FL 33137, (305) 576-6606, BA 59 CUNY - Brooklyn Coll; MS 73 CUNY - Brooklyn Coll; Sp-Lang Path, Private Practice, **SLP**

Lane, Mrs Carol Ann 2003 Elysian Fields Drive, Austin, TX 78727, (512) 454-4869, **SLP**

Lane, Mrs Cathy Walker P O Box 2646, Oroville, CA 95965, BA 72 Univ of Northern CO; MA 74 Univ of Northern CO; **SLP**

Lane, David M 45 Liberty Street, Warsaw, NY 14569, (716) 493-2581, BS 64 Emerson Coll; MA 69 SUNY - Coll at Geneseo; Sp/Lang Path, Letchworth Ctrl Sch, **SLP**

Lane, Dr Helen S 7290 Greenway, St Louis, MO 63130, (314) 652-3200, BA 26 OH St Univ; MA 28 OH St Univ; PH 30 (NS) OH St Univ; **F LM**

Lane, Mrs Jerrie N 2905 Bransford Road, Augusta, GA 30909, (404) 736-0183, BA 67 Univ of GA; ME 68 Univ of GA; Sp-Lang Path, Richmond Co Bd of Ed, **SLP**

Lane, Mrs Joanne W Box 124, Hickory Lane, Glenford, NY 12433, BA 76 CUNY - Hunter Coll; MS 77 SUNY - Coll at Buffalo; Sp-Lang Path, Onteora Central Sch Dist, **SLP**

Lane, Kathleen Ann 112 B Water Gate Drive, Lynchburg, VA 24502, (804) 522-2124, BS 81 CA Univ of PA; MA 84 Univ of Akron; 85–Sp-Lang Path, Central Virginia Training Cen, **SLP**

Lane, Linda Carolyn 207 Naples Road, Fort Ord, CA 93941, (408) 394-6037, BA 79 MI St Univ; MS 86 Columbia Univ Teachers Coll; **SLP**

Lane, Mrs Lynne S 50 Elizabeth Avenue, Stamford, CT 06907, BS 66 Northwestern Univ; MA 68 Case Western Reserve Univ; Sp-Lang Path, Stamford Bd of Ed, **SLP**

Lane, Mara H 140 Greenbriar East Drive, Deerfield, IL 60015, (312) 945-8977, BA 75 CUNY - Brooklyn Coll; MS 78 CUNY - Brooklyn Coll; Sp-Lang-Path, Private Practice, **SLP**

Lane, Marilyn J 10416 Conser #1-H-2, Overland Park, KS 66212, (913) 648-8422, BS 59 Fort Hays St Univ; MS 65 Emporia St Univ; MS 76 Kearney St Coll; Sp-Lang Path, Shawnee Mission Sch Dist, **SLP**

Lane, Pamela Pruitt 6310 Gander Road East, Dayton, OH 45424, (513) 222-5597, BS 80 Southern IL Univ-Edwardsvill; MS 86 Howard Univ

Lane, Mrs Rhonda Smith 22 Fawnwood East, Aiken, SC 29801, (803) 649-0060, BS 76 Appalachian St Univ; MA 78 Appalachian St Univ; Sp-Lang Path, Private Practice, **SLP ACE**

Lane, Scott Robert General Delivery, Angoon, AK 99820, (907) 788-3460, BS 74 Portland St Univ; MS 78 Portland St Univ; 87–Prin, Chatham Sch Dist, **SLP**

Lane, Susan 403 Furnace Dock Road, Peekskill, NY 10566, (914) 347-4677, BA 70 CUNY - Brooklyn Coll; MA 72 Univ of CT; Supervisor/Audiology Services, Westchester County Med Center, **A**

Lane, Susan A Rural Route 5, 15712 Mountainview, Surrey, BC, Canada V4B 4Z5, (604) 584-7404, BA 73 Western WA Univ; MA 76 Univ of MT; 86–Sp-Lang Path, Bc Elks Aud Rehab Cen, **SLP**

Lane, Susan Melinda 3 Chimney Rock Road, Rutherfordton, NC 28139, (704) 287-5090, BS 83 Univ of NC - Greensboro; MA 86 Univ of NC - Greensboro; 88–Sp-Lang Path, Rutherford Co Sch Sys, **SLP**

Lane, Mrs Tracie L 829 Royal Lane, West Dundee, IL 60118, (312) 428-8721, MS 87 Eastern IL Univ; 87–Sp-Lang Path, Comm Consolidated Dist #15, **SLP**

Lane, Dr Vera Wall 544 Miller Avenue, Pacifica, CA 94044, (415) 469-1001, BA 63 PA St Univ - Univ Park; MS 65 PA St Univ - Univ Park; PH 74 (Special Education) San Francisco St Univ; Professor, San Francisco State U, **SLP**

Lane-Hill, Carol A R R 2 Box 215A, Adel, IA 50003, (515) 283-6344, BS 73 Univ of IA; MA 76 Univ of IA; Sp-Lang Path, IA Meth Med Cen, **SLP**

Lane-Johnson, Mrs Catherine Ann Rt 1 Box 58C, Constable, NY 12926, (518) 483-6149, BS 83 Eastern NM Univ; MA 86 SUNY - Coll at Plattsburgh; 86–Sp-Lang Path, Franklin County ARC, **SLP**

Lane-Marko, Joanne Hq 7th Medcom, Box 211, APO New York, NY 09102-3304, BS 79 Coll of Saint Rose; MS 81 Columbia Univ Teachers Coll; 85–Sp-Lang Path, Exceptional Family Member Serv, **SLP**

Laneve, Mrs Cathy Kash 4022 West 38th Street, Erie, PA 16506, (814) 838-6823, BS 82 Edinboro Univ of PA; MA 83 Edinboro Univ of PA; **SLP**

LaNeve, Marion Yavener 10607 Muirfield Drive, Potomac, MD 20854, (301) 230-2840, BA 65 Rutger's St Univ - Douglas Coll; MA 66 Temple Univ; Sp-Lang Path, Montgomery Co Pub Sch, **SLP**

Laneve, Natalie Rose 538 Rossmore Road, Richmond, VA 23225, (804) 230-1388, BS 83 Univ of VA - Charlottesville; ME 85 Univ of VA - Charlottesville; **A**

Lanford, Elizabeth Davis 211 Wilderness Lane, Fredericksburg, VA 22401, (804) 321-7474, BS 85 Univ of VA - Charlottesville; ME 87 Univ of VA - Charlottesville; Sp-Lang Path, Ricmond Childrens Hosp, **SLP**

Lang, Dr Adrianne Escondido Union School Dist, 980 North Ash, Escondido, CA 92025, BA 64 Univ of TX - Austin; MA 79 San Diego St Univ; PH 72 (NS) Australian Nat'l Univ; SLP, Escondido USD, **SLP**

Lang, Mrs Anne A 6178 Clarks Road, Winneconne, WI 54986, (414) 729-6980, MS 83 Univ of WI - Oshkosh; Sp-Lang Path, Neenah Joint Sch Dist, **SLP**

Lang, Mrs Carol E 180 Southvue Drive, Pittsburgh, PA 15236, (412) 647-2030, BA 59 Oberlin Coll; MS 62 Univ of Pittsburgh - Pittsburgh; Sp-Lang Path, Eye & Ear Hosp Ctr Sp-Lang Path, **SLP**

Lang, Edmonia L 702 Brown Street, Washington, NC 27889, (919) 537-5617, MS 87 Univ of NC - Chapel Hill

Lang, Mrs Elizabeth 1888 Temblethurst Drive, South Euclid, OH 44121, (216) 382-2240, OD 50 Northwestern Univ; MA 42 Northwestern Univ; **LM**

Lang, Georgie Lee P O Box 8263, Paducah, KY 42002-8263, (502) 442-2947, **SLP**

Lang, Mrs Grace L 51 Paolino Street, Johnston, RI 02919, (401) 272-4075, BA 84 Bridgewater St Coll; MS 86 Southern CT St Univ; 87–Sp-Lang Path, Woonsocket Education Dept, **SLP**

Lang, Mrs Jane D 4924 Burke Drive, Metairie, LA 70003, (504) 282-5151, BS 76 Baylor Univ; MS 78 Univ of Southwestern LA; Sp-Lang Path, St Charles Parish Sch Bd, **SLP**

Lang, Dr Janna Smith 2-2790 East Cliff Drive, Santa Cruz, CA 95062, (408) 288-7777, BS 61 Univ of IL - Urbana; MA 62 Univ of IL - Urbana; PH 69 (NS) Stanford Univ; 70–Aud, Private Practice, **A ACE**

Lang, Mrs Judith Ann 12247 South Oak Park Avenue, Palos Heights, IL 60463, (312) 371-0378, BS 60 MI St Univ; MS 84 Governors St Univ; Sp-Lang Path, CHSD 218

Lang, Mrs Kathryn Samway 24 Joanie Lane, North Tonawanda, NY 14120, (716) 689-9730, BS 72 Nazareth Coll of Rochester; MS 82 SUNY - Coll at Buffalo; Sp-Lang Path, Kenmore School District, **SLP**

Lang, Mrs Linda J 4001 Pepperwood Court, Sonoma, CA 95476, (209) 478-3911, BA 71 CA St Univ - Northridge; MA 87 Univ of the Pacific; 88–Sp-Lang Path, Sonoma Developmental Ctr, **SLP**

Lang, Mrs Lori Jean 2460 Riveredge Drive S E, Grand Rapids, MI 49506, (616) 772-1844, **A**

Lang, Micheal D 104 East 13th, Hutchinson, KS 67501, (316) 663-7178, BA 78 Fort Hays St Univ; MS 79 Fort Hays St Univ; Sp-Lang Path, Reno Co Ed Coop, **SLP**

Lang, Roxanne M Route 1 Box 357, Nipton, CA 92364, (213) 457-1112, BS 73 Univ of KS; MA 74 KS St Univ; **SLP**

Lang, Dr Stanley R 4720 South Harvard, Suite 202, Tulsa, OK 74135, (918) 745-9052, BS 77 Univ of Tulsa; MA 79 Univ of Tulsa; PH 82 (Aud) Wichita St Univ; 83–Owner, Aud of Tulsa Inc, **A**

Lang, Susan K 1922F Hohnson Ferry Road, Atlanta, GA 30319, (404) 475-4559, SLP, Fulton Co Schools, **SLP**

Lang, Mrs Tammy T 37 Sharmont Drive, Hattiesburg, MS 39401, (601) 582-0251, OB 79 LA St Univ - Shreveport; MS 80 LA St Univ - N O Medical Ctr; 85–Sp-Lang Path, Hattiesburg Public Schools, **SLP**

Langdon, Frances P P O Box 221198, Charlotte, NC 28222, (704) 365-3246, BA CA St Univ - Long Beach; MA CA St Univ - Long Beach; SLP, Charlotte Mecklenburg Sch Dist, **SLP**

Langdon, Dr Henriette W 21354 Dexter Drive, Cupertino, CA 95014, (408) 257-4183, BS 68 Universidad Del Museo Social Argentino; ME 70 Tufts Univ; ED 77 (Psycholinguistics) Boston Univ; Sp-Lang Path, Private Practice, **SLP ACE**

Langdon, Jo Ann Mills Route 2 Box 264, Limekiln Road, Malone, NY 12953, (518) 483-7370, BA 81 SUNY - Coll at Plattsburgh; MA 86 SUNY - Coll at Plattsburgh

Langdon, S Fruzan P O Box 5978, Nassau, Bahamas, (809) 325-5396, OB 65 Oldrey Fleming Sch of Speech Therapy - London, England; MS 78 Purdue Univ - West Lafayette; 85–Sp-Lang Path, Ministry of Educ, **SLP**

Lange, Barbara L 17085 San Bruno #D, Fountain Valley, CA 92708, (714) 581-2800, BA 73 Univ of Redlands; MS 75 Univ of Redlands; Sp-Lang Path, Sp & Lang Path Servs, **SLP**

Lange, Diana Louise 629 7th Avenue, New Hyde Park, NY 11040, (516) 352-3089, BA 84 SUNY - Center at Buffalo; MA 86 SUNY - Center at Buffalo; 87–Sp-Lang Path, Agency VTA Mgmt Svcs, **SLP**

Lange, Gail Larson Rt 4 Box 72, Pine City, MN 55063, (612) 679-3731, BA 72 Southwest St Univ; MA 78 Mankato St Univ; Sp/Lang Path, ISD 332 Mora Pub Schs, **SLP**

Lange, Gail T Psc Box 1476, APO New York, NY 09292, **SLP**

Lange, Geraldine A 40 Princess Avenue East, Brandon, MB, Canada R7A 1R9, (204) 727-1066

Lange, Michael W 4524 14th Avenue, Rock Island, IL 61201, (309) 793-0330, BA 73 Augustana Coll; MA 79 Univ of IL - Urbana; **SLP**

Lange, Mrs Nancy Slate 265 Roman Avenue Northeast, Palm Bay, FL 32907, (305) 724-6129, BS 79 West Chester St Coll; MS 83 Univ of NM; 88–Sp-Lang Path, InSpeech Inc, **SLP**

Lange, Ruth Anne 505 McKay Avenue North #2, Alexandria, MN 56308, (612) 762-2141, BS 83 Marquette Univ; MA 86 Univ of IA; 86–Sp-Lang Path, ISD #206, **SLP**

Lange, Terry Ann 18525 Millar Road, Mount Clemens, MI 48043, (519) 542-3471, BA 84 MI St Univ; MA 85 MI St Univ; 87–Sp-Lang Path Coord, Sarnia Children's Treat Ctr, **SLP**

Langella-Pristera, Mrs Lori Lynn 6 Riverview Avenue, Oakdale, NY 11769, (516) 758-0886, BS 82 SUNY - Coll at Geneseo; MA 83 Hofstra Univ; 83–Sp-Lang Path, Sachem Central Schl Dstr, **SLP**

Langenfeld, Kelene Kelly 13708 Edna St, Omaha, NE 68138, (402) 895-5007, BA 78 Univ of NE - Omaha; MS 79 Univ of NE - Omaha; Sp-Lang Path, Omaha Public Schools, **SLP**

Langer, Mrs Deana K 10133 Amigo Avenue, Northridge, CA 91324, (818) 993-8939, BA 66 Univ of MD - College Park; MA 69 Univ of MD - College Park; Aud, Micahel Reder MD, **A**

Langer, Dr Roy M 14540 S W 80th Avenue, Miami, FL 33158, (305) 666-5983, BA 60 CUNY - Brooklyn Coll; MA 64 CUNY - Brooklyn Coll; PH 68 (NS) Northwestern Univ; 85–Pres, Ctr for Effective Comm, **SLP**

Langford, Mrs Ann L 3927 West Schafer Road, Pinckney, MI 48169, (517) 546-5550, BS 78 Eastern MI Univ; MA 79 Eastern MI Univ; 79–Sp-Lang Path, Livingston Inter Sch Dist, **SLP**

Langford, Marietta M 311 Pebble Beach, Portland, TX 78374-4005, (512) 884-5131, BA 60 Marshall Univ; 88–Sp-Lang Path, Corpus Christi ISD, **SLP**

Langford, Dr Ted L 1703 Westgate Parkway, Dothan, AL 36303, (205) 255-6820, BA 54 Univ of TX - Austin; PH 64 (Experimental Psychology) Univ of TX - Austin; Proj Supv, Univ of TX at Dallas

Langham, Diane Elizabeth 112 1/2 Park Drive, Fayetteville, WV 25840, (304) 574-0311, BA 85 Univ of Pittsburgh - Pittsburgh; MA 87 Univ of Pittsburgh - Pittsburgh; 87–Sp-Lang Path, Fayette Co Bd of Educ, **SLP**

Langhans, Dr Joseph J 14077 80th Avenue North, Seminole, FL 34646-3312, (813) 398-6661, BA 73 Univ of CT; MS 75 Univ of AZ; PH 85 (Sp-Lang Hrng Sciences) Univ of AZ; Sp-Lang Path, VAMC, **SLP**

Langhauser, Karen A 724 N E 113th Street, Biscayne Park, FL 33161, (305) 651-1100, BS 75 Nazareth Coll of Rochester; MA 80 Univ of Miami; Sp-Lang Path, Parkway Regional Medical Ctr, **SLP**

Langhaus-Herrmann, Terry 8517 Ordinary Way, Annandale, VA 22003, (703) 425-5159, BA 73 IN Univ - Bloomington; MA 75 Univ of FL; Sp-Lang Path, Private Practice, **SLP**

Langhenry, Mrs Debra Dlouhy 31509 Bexley Drive, Bay Village, OH 44140, (216) 871-7300, BS 74 OH St Univ; MA 79 Cleveland St Univ; SLP, Westlake City Sch, **SLP**

Langhorn, Mary C 25 Hillview Avenue, Providence, RI 02908, BA 61 Salve Regina - Newport Coll; MA 67 Univ of RI; MS 71 Emerson Coll; 85–Sp-Lang Path, Sargent Rehabilitation Center, **SLP ACE**

Langkabel, Terry Lynn 4530 54th Street #6, San Diego, CA 92115, (619) 470-4226, BS 83 Univ of WI - Milwaukee; MA 87 San Diego St Univ; 88–Sp-Lang Path, Paradise Valley Hosp, **SLP**

Langkopt, Linda Kay Route 5 Number 45, Washington Park Townhouse, Twin Falls, ID 83301, (208) 733-9498, BS 82 Southeast MO St Univ; MS 87 Central MO St Univ; **SLP**

Langland, Julia Ann 1331 South Maple #C-38, Sioux City, IA 51106, (712) 279-2144, BS 85 SD St Univ; MA 87 Univ of Northern IA; 87–Sp-Lang Path, Marian Health Ctr, **SLP**

Langland, Mrs Martha F 502 Washington Avenue, Red Oak, IA 51566, (712) 623-9617, BS 75 IL St Univ - Normal; MA 77 Northwestern Univ; **SLP**

Langley, Elizabeth McCoy 3717 Forest Green Drive, Lexington, KY 40503, (606) 272-0567, BA 84 1873; MS 86 1873; **SLP**

Langley, Sharon B 4200 Colonial Drive, Columbia, SC 29203, (803) 796-8060, BA 77 Columbia Coll; MS 80 Univ of NC - Chapel Hill; 86–Aud, Carolina Ear Nose & Throat Assoc, **A**

Langlois, Dr Aimee Dept Speech & Hearing Sciences, Humbolt State University, Arcata, CA 95521, (707) 826-3476, BA 65 Univ of Montreal - Quebec; MA 67 Univ of Montreal - Quebec; ED 75 (Sp Science and Sp-Lang Path) Columbia Univ Teachers Coll; 80–Assoc Prof, Humboldt St U, **SLP A**

Langlois, Jean Ann 3120 St Paul Street #317-H, Baltimore, MD 21218, (301) 522-5450, MS 82 Purdue Univ - West Lafayette; Sp-Lang Path, The Kennedy Institute, **SLP**

Langlois, Mary Ane #1 Hanging Tree Court, St Peters, MO 63376, (219) 949-4000, MA 86 Saint Louis Univ; **SLP**

Langman, Iris 1472 12th Avenue, San Francisco, CA 94122, (415) 452-0243, BA 77 Univ of MD - College Park; OM 80 Hahneman Medical Coll; Coord of Hrng Outreach Prog, Hrng Soc for the Bay Area, **A**

Langmore, Dr Susan L 233 Crest Avenue, Ann Arbor, MI 48103, (313) 769-7100, BA 66 Univ of CA - Los Angeles; MA 68 Stanford Univ; PH 80 Northwestern Univ; Sp-Lang Path, VA, **SLP**

Langnau-Morris, Candace J 3405 Westridge Court, Lawrence, KS 66044, (913) 749-0619, BA 77 MI St Univ; MA 78 MI St Univ; **SLP**

Langot, Helene 9069 55th Avenue, Elmhurst, NY 11373, (718) 699-9079, BS 81; OM 86 LA St Univ - N O Medical Ctr

Langridge, Mrs Diane R 3906 Jose Court, Chino, CA 91710, (714) 627-3286, BA 74 CA St Univ - Fullerton; MA 78 CA St Univ - Fullerton; 87–SLP, Upland USD, **SLP**

Langsam, Susan Klaif 4222 Levelside Avenue, Lakewood, CA 90712, BA 62 CUNY - Brooklyn Coll; MS 66 CUNY - Brooklyn Coll; Sp-Lang Path, Private Practice, **SLP**

Langsdorf, Anne M Speech - Language - Hearing, Hudson State Service Center, 501 Ogletown Road, Newark, DE 19711, (302) 368-6925, BA 71 Coll of Wooster; MA 00 West Chester Univ of PA; 88–Sp-Lang Path, St Dept of Pub Health

Langston, Mrs Patricia S 2113 Crestline Drive, Nashville, TN 37214, (615) 885-8918, BS 67 Auburn Univ - Auburn; MA 68 Auburn Univ - Auburn; Sp/Lang Path, Metro Nashville Pub Sch Syst, **SLP**

Langtry, Donna Martin 25 Mansion Street, West Harwich, MA 02671, (617) 432-3132, BS 80 Kutztown Univ of PA; MA 82 Univ of ME - Orono; Sp-Lang Path, Hd Injury Cntr at Lewis Bay, **SLP**

Langue, Mrs Jill Silverman 127 Crofton Drive, Pittsburgh, PA 15238, (412) 963-0608, BS 78 PA St Univ - Univ Park; MA 80 Univ of Pittsburgh - Pittsburgh; SLP, Allegheny Inter Un/Pgh Pa, **SLP**

Langworthy, Jack Allen 6401 Ninth Street North, St Petersburg, FL 33702, (813) 526-6966, MS 74 Univ of South FL; Dir, Hearing Labs Inc, **A**

Lanham, Mrs Tammy Kay 1721 Live Oak Court, Lewisville, TX 75067, (817) 481-6342, BS 82 Univ of TX - Austin; MS 85 Univ of North TX; **A**

Lanier, Delores Spaid 305 East Willow Lake Drive, Metter, GA 30439, (912) 685-5052, OB 84 Univ of GA; ME 85 Univ of GA; 85–Sp-Lang Path, Candler County Bd of Educ, **SLP**

Lanier, Janet Crismore 14125 S E Bryn Mawr Court, Milwaukie, OR 97267, (503) 653-5113, OB 84 Northern IL Univ - De Kalb; OM 85 IL St Univ - Normal; **SLP**

Lanius, Julia K 12311 Inletridge, Maryland Heights, MO 63043, BS 80 Southern IL Univ-Edwardsvill; MS 81 Southern IL Univ-Edwardsvill; Sp-Lang Path, Spec Sch Dist of St Louis Co, **SLP**

Lankford, Holly M 12 Granada, Briarcrest Gardens, Hershey, PA 17033, (717) 533-7397, BS 80 Towson St Univ; MS 82 Towson St Univ; **A**

Lankford, Mrs Isabelle S 614 South 9th Street, Vincennes, IN 47591, (618) 943-2326, BA 78 Univ of Miami; MS 81 IN St Univ - Terre Haute; Sp/Lang Path, Comm Ut Sch Dist #20, **SLP**

Lankford, James E 325 Joanne Lane, De Kalb, IL 60115, BS 64 OK Christian Coll; MS 68 Univ of OK - Norman; PH 69 (NS) Univ of OK - Norman; Professor, Northern Illinois University, **A**

Lankford, Nila Kay 1000 Pine Gate Drive #B-34, Spartanburg, SC 29303, (803) 472-8403, BS 78 Western Carolina Univ; MA 85 Western Carolina Univ; Sp-Lang Path, Spartanburg Co Sch Dist I, **SLP**

Lanna-Farris, Karyn M 24438 Park Street, Torrance, CA 90505, (213) 378-4823, BS 77 Rutgers St Univ - Newark; MA 80 Montclair St Coll; SLP, L A City Unified, **SLP**

Lannig, Mrs Joanne Wiegand 22 Greenway Circle, Syosset, NY 11791, (516) 921-1453, BS 81 Saint John's Univ - Jamaica; MS 82 Adelphi Univ; SLP, Patchogue-Medford Un Sch Dist, **SLP**

Lanning, Jackie Christine 920 Four Mile Road #3-B, Grand Rapids, MI 49504, (313) 995-1317, MA 88 Eastern MI Univ

Lannon, Mary Beth 50 Chester Street #4, Brighton, MA 02135, (603) 883-5521, BS 80 Northeastern Univ; MA 81 MI St Univ; Aud, MA Eye & Ear Infirmary-Boston, **A**

Lanphere, Teresa 1003 East Pine Avenue Apt#8, El Segundo, CA 90245, (213) 322-5935, BA 83 CA St Univ - Long Beach; MA 86 CA St Univ - Northridge; 86–Sp-Lang Path, Manhattan Beach City Sch Dist, **SLP**

Lanphier, Melanie Ledyard 200 East Burgess Rd, Apartment 51B, Pensacola, FL 32503, BA 82 Univ of AL-Tuscaloosa; MS 86 Univ of AL- Tuscaloosa; SLP, **SLP**

Lansberry, Carole Miller 5418 Bondy Drive, Erie, PA 16509, (814) 453-6784, BS 78 SUNY - Coll at Plattsburgh; MA 82 Edinboro Univ of PA; 86–Sp-Lang Path, NW Tri-County Intermed Unit, **SLP**

Lansing, Dr Charissa R 730 Kekokuk Court, Iowa City, IA 52240, (319) 356-2222, MS 73 Univ of IL - Urbana; PH 84 (NS) Univ of IA; Assistant Research Scientist, University of Iowa, **SLP A**

Lansing, Jeanne Georgia 4856 Crockett Court, Raleigh, NC 27606, (919) 851-9032, BS 84 Univ of IA; ME 86 Univ of VA - Charlottesville; 88–Aud, Raleigh Ear Nose & Throat Inc, **A**

Lansky, Pamela Stewart 644 Kingman Avenue, Santa Monica, CA 90402, (213) 459-8424, BS 79 Univ of Alberta - Alberta; MA 84 Univ of CO - Boulder; Sp-Lang Path, Blind Chdrn Cen, **SLP**

Lantello, Debra 14874 Highway 66, Ashland, OR 97520, **SLP**

Lantz, Eleanor Piazza 405 Port Penn Road, Middletown, DE 19709, (302) 684-8522, BS 79 PA St Univ - Univ Park; ME 82 Univ of VA - Charlottesville; Sp-Lang Path, Cape Henlopen School District, **SLP**

Lantz, Mrs Karen G 2904 Cross Bend, Plano, TX 75023, (214) 867-0010, BA 72 Univ of Redlands; MA 74 Univ of Houston - Univ Park; Consultant, Private Practice, **SLP**

Lantz-Dey, Susan Ann P O Box 201, North Hero, VT 05474, (518) 562-1614, OB 76 Western WA Univ; BA 79 Univ of WA; MA 82 WA St Univ; 84–Sp/Lang Path, NY Assoc for Ret Chldn, **SLP**

Lanza, Carol K 1219 Davidson Drive, Bldg R #8, Fort Collins, CO 80526-2484, (715) 357-3771, MS 88 CO St Univ

Lanza, Mrs Elaine Rehgio 2510 Consaul Road, Schenectady, NY 12304, (518) 393-7867, MS 79 Coll of Saint Rose; 79–Sp-Lang Path, Albany PS Sys, **SLP**

Lanza, Elizabeth Hope 141 Horizon Terrace, Hawthorne, NJ 07506, (212) 523-3127, BS 82 Boston St Coll; MS 83 Columbia Univ Teachers Coll; 85–Aud, St Luke's/Roosevelt Hosp, **A**

Lanza, Mrs Janet Royer 4308 Winding Way, Fort Worth, TX 76126, (817) 731-4149, BS 75 TX Christian Univ; MS 76 TX Christian Univ; Sp/Lang Path, Private Practice, **SLP**

Lapas, Annette Kuzdenyi 807 West Road, Kinston, NC 28501, (919) 638-6519, BA 76 Univ of Pittsburgh - Pittsburgh; MA 78 Marshall Univ; Executive Director, Our Homes Inc, **SLP**

Lapenna, Aimee M 508 Everdell Avenue, West Islip, NY 11795, (516) 661-5620, BA 83 Boston Coll; MS 87 Adelphi Univ; **SLP**

Lapidge, Barbara L 31 Carriage Drive, Naugatuck, CT 06770, (203) 264-8231, BS 74 SUNY - Center at Albany; MS 78 Southern CT St Univ; Sp/Lang Path, St of CT, **SLP**

Lapidus, Deborah Cohen 39 Cherry Drive East, Plainview, NY 11803, (516) 349-9878, BA 73 CUNY - Queens Coll; MA 75 CUNY - Hunter Coll; **SLP**

Lapidus, Ghita A 1843 North Dayton, Chicago, IL 60614, (312) 266-7948, BA 72; MA 74 Northwestern Univ; Sp-Lang Path/LD Spec, Private Practice & Psychol Assoc, **SLP**

Lapierre, Rhonda Irion P O Box 551, Milldale, CT 06467, (203) 584-7815, BA 79 Trenton St Coll; MS 80 Syracuse Univ; 85–Sp-Lang Path, Bristol Public Schools, **SLP**

Lapin, Mrs Monica Ann M 26478 N E Lake Shore Drive, Wauconda, IL 60084, (309) 475-2061, BS 76 IL St Univ - Normal; MS 78 IL St Univ - Normal; 85–Sp-Lang Path, Prospect Heights Dist #23, **SLP**

LaPine, Dr Peter R 634 Butterfield Drive, East Lansing, MI 48823, (517) 353-8780, BA 73 MI St Univ; MA 76 Northern MI Univ; PH 83 (Aud & Sp Sciences) MI St Univ; Asst Prof / Clin Dir, MI St U, **SLP**

Lapin-Pastorella, Robin 39 Grad Avenue, Lawrenceville, NJ 08648, (609) 683-8414, BA 78 Temple Univ; MS 80 Columbia Univ Teachers Coll; 81–Sp/Lang Path, Med Ctr at Princeton, **SLP**

Lapish, Marisa Joy Stony Glen Camp, Ford Road, Madison, OH 44057, (216) 298-3264, **SLP**

Laplaca, Mary Grace 225 East Eight Avenue, Conshohocken, PA 19428, (215) 828-3314, BS 79 Northern IL Univ - De Kalb; MA 81 Northern IL Univ - De Kalb; 87–Sp-Lang Path, Albert Einstein Med Ctr, **SLP**

Laplante, Elaine N 460 Lombardi Road, Le Mars, IA 51031, (515) 432-6345, BA 79 Univ of Northern IA; MA 80 Univ of Northern IA; SLP, Western Hills AEA, **SLP**

Lapointe, Constance 37 Tumelty Road, Peabody, MA 01960, **SLP**

LaPointe, Dr Leonard Lyell Dept Of Speech & Hrg Science, Arizona State University, Tempe, AZ 85287-0102, (602) 965-2905, BA 61 MI St Univ; MA 66 Univ of CO - Boulder; PH 69 (Sp-Lang Path) Univ of CO - Boulder; 84–Chmn-Dept Sp & Hrng, AZ St U, **SLP F**

Lapon, Mrs Donna M 44 Boylston Street, Randolph, MA 02368, (617) 963-6426, BA 75 Adelphi Univ; MA 76 Wayne St Univ; **SLP**

LaPorta, Rosemary A 102 Oviedo Street, Gulf Breeze, FL 32561, (904) 243-8741, BS 67 Loyola Univ of Chicago; MA 69 Northern IL Univ - De Kalb; 82–Asst Dir Sp-Lang Path, Sp & Hrng Cir of Ft Walton Beach, **SLP ACE**

Laporte, Lynn M 1684 Saint David Drive, Danville, CA 94526, (415) 831-3426, BS 76 LA St Univ - Baton Rouge; OM 79 LA St Univ - N O Medical Ctr; **SLP**

Laporte, Patricia Lynn 134 East Mosholu Parkway, Apartment 2H, Bronx, NY 10458, (212) 584-7679, BA 79 Univ of FL; MA 82 Univ of FL; Sp-Lang Path, Mount Saint Ursula Sp Cen, **SLP**

La Posta Donohue, Mrs Constance A 12 Gaslight Drive, Albany, NY 12205, (518) 382-4550, BS 80 Coll of Saint Rose; MA 82 Northwestern Univ; Aud, Sunnyview Hosp & Rehab Ctr, **A**

Lapping, Leslye 404 Barton, Evanston, IL 60202, (312) 869-7164, BS 75 Univ of WI - Madison; MA 77 Northwestern Univ; SLP, Cook County Hosp, **SLP**

Laprad, Debra C 549 Spokane, Lansing, MI 48910, (517) 393-5319, BA 79 Northern MI Univ; MA 80 Western MI Univ; 88–Sp-Lang Path, St Mary's Med Ctr, **SLP**

Laquer, Mrs Mary Jane W 207 South 5th Street, North Wales, PA 19454, (215) 647-3150, BS 78 PA St Univ - Univ Park; ME 80 Univ of VA - Charlottesville; Sp-Lang Path, Doylestown Hosp, **SLP**

Lara, Anastasia M 6036½ Friends Avenue, Whittier, CA 90601, (213) 693-9682, BA 82 Univ of the Pacific; MA 87 Whittier Coll; 88–Sp-Lang Path, InSpeech Inc

Lara, Cynthia 2324 Caballero Lane, Santa Maria, CA 93454, **SLP**

Laragione, Mrs Evelyn Keeler 36 Cole Avenue, Pittsfield, MA 01201, (413) 442-8592, BS 80 Ithaca Coll; MA 82 Univ of MA - Amherst; Sp-Lang Path, Lenox Public Schools, **SLP**

Laraia, Karen Marie 30132 Blancke, Warren, MI 48093, (517) 773-0619, BS 85 Central MI Univ; MA 86 Central MI Univ; **SLP**

Laraway, Mrs Ginette Marie 4027 Brewster Drive, Westlake, OH 44145, BA 82 Univ of Toledo; MA 84 Case Western Reserve Univ; SLP, InSpeech Inc, **SLP**

Laraway, Lee Ann 3488 Manda Drive, San Jose, CA 95124, (408) 723-9057, BA 80 San Jose St Univ; MA 83 San Jose St Univ; SLP, Oak Grove Sch Dist, **SLP**

Larcher, Elaine W 107 Macon Lane, Oak Ridge, TN 37830, (615) 376-3416, BS 77 Univ of TN - Knoxville; MA 78 Univ of TN - Knoxville; Sp-Lang Path, Dunn Cen, **SLP**

Lardent, Jeanne P 440 South Victor Way, Aurora, CO 80012, (303) 758-3415, BA 68 Univ of Northern CO; MA 71 Univ of Northern CO; Business Consultant, Private Practice, **SLP**

Lardner, Mrs Mary L 5403 Redfield Circle, Atlanta, GA 30338, (404) 396-1902, BS 65 Emerson Coll; MA 66 Syracuse Univ; **SLP**

Large, Julie Gwynne 2711 Oakland Avenue, Nashville, TN 37212, (615) 297-1483, BS 84 West Chester Univ of PA; MA 86 West Chester Univ of PA; **SLP**

Largura, Marjorie Jo Box 611 Ogden Dunes, Portage, IN 46368, (219) 762-2326, **SLP**

Larimore, Dr Howard W 5235 Apple Drive, Fort Collins, CO 80526, (303) 491-6981, BA 57 Univ of NE - Omaha; MA 58 Univ of Denver; PH 70 (Sp-Lang Path) Univ of Denver; 69–Associate Professor, Colorado State University, **SLP**

Larimore, Mrs Jody Kelly 4509 Hildring Drive East, Fort Worth, TX 76109, (817) 926-5984, BS 83 Radford Univ; ME 85 Univ of GA; 85–Aud, General Dynamics

Laris, Emily Joan 13356 Cumpston Street, Van Nuys, CA 91401, (818) 241-3111, BA 76 Occidental Coll; MA 82 CA St Univ - Los Angeles; Sp-Lang Path, Glendale USD, **SLP**

La Riviere, Dr Conrad Louis P O Box 49, Costigan, ME 04423, (207) 581-2006, BA 64 Providence Coll; MA 67 Univ of AZ; PH 71 Univ of FL; **A**

Lariviere, Mrs Lisa Ann 120 Willow Lane, Scotia, NY 12302, (518) 489-7429, BS 84 Univ of MA - Amherst; MS 86 Syracuse Univ; Aud, Benway-Haworth-Lawlor E Aid Co, **A**

Larke, Lynn Marie 4644 7th Street S W, Canton, OH 44710, (216) 492-8136, BS 81 Univ of Akron; MA 87 Univ of Akron; Sp-Lang Path, Stark Co Bd of Educ, **SLP**

Larkin, Mrs Alecia Stafford 900 Thorney Lea Terrace, Schaumburg, IL 60193, (312) 351-3032, MA 84 Memphis St Univ; 88–Sp-Lang Path, Private Practice, **SLP**

Larkin, Mrs Ann A 109 Lynnfield Road, Memphis, TN 38119, (901) 761-5211, OB 69 Southern Methodist Univ; OM 70 Southern Methodist Univ; Aud, Drs Turley and Turley, **A**

Larkin, Carol D B 1897 Malden Street, San Diego, CA 92109, (617) 466-4137, Sp-Lang Path, Lemesa Spring Valley Schl Dstr, **SLP**

Larkin, Elizabeth Anne 214 Cynthia Drive, Raynham, MA 02767, (508) 823-4604, BA 64 Boston Univ; ME 70 Northeastern Univ; OM 84 Boston Coll; **A ACE**

Larkin, Mrs Marilyn K East End Hearing & Speech, 619 Roanoke Avenue, Riverhead, NY 11901, (516) 369-1917, BA 73 OH St Univ; MS 74 Adelphi Univ; Dir, E End Hrng & Sp, **A**

Larkin, Mrs Mary Ann Amplimed Corporated, 315 Calhoun Street, Suite 300, Charleston, SC 29401, (803) 722-8387, BS 81 Purdue Univ - West Lafayette; MS 83 Purdue Univ - West Lafayette; Aud, Amplimed Corporated, **A ACE**

Larkin, Patricia G 16711 Greenview Lane, Huntington Beach, CA 92649, (714) 847-2516, **SLP**

Larkin, Mrs Patricia Jo 1739 Harrow Court #D, Wheaton, IL 60187-8346, (312) 682-1232, BS 81 Univ of WI - Eau Claire; MS 86 Univ of WI - Stevens Point; 86–Sp-Lang Path, Marianjoy Rehab Ctr, **SLP**

Larkins, Deborah A Kapiolani/Childrens Med Center, Communication Disorders Clin, 1319 Punahou Street, Honolulu, HI 96826, (808) 947-8235, BA 72 Case Western Reserve Univ; MA 73 Case Western Reserve Univ; 80–Aud, Kapiolani/Chldn's Med Cen, **A**

Larkins, Dr Patricia Gail 2101 Briggs Road, Silver Spring, MD 20906, (301) 897-5700, BS 71 Hampton Univ; MA 72 MI St Univ; PH 80 (NS) Memphis St Univ; Dir Sp-Lang Path Liason Branch, Amer Speech-Lang-Hearing Soc, **SLP**

Larks, Mrs Sheri Moeckler 100 E Detroit #301, Indianola, IA 50125, (515) 961-8191, BS 85 Univ of IL - Urbana; MA 87 Univ of IL - Urbana; Aud, Heartland AEA, **A**

L'Armee, Claudette 5111 Glen Ridge #J25, San Antonio, TX 78229, (512) 690-0345, BA 75 Our Lady Lake Univ-San Anton; MA 76 Our Lady Lake Univ-San Anton; Sp-Lang Path, Sp-Lang-Hrng Assoc, **SLP**

Larner, Mrs Carolynn 1645 Oakhaven Drive, Arcadia, CA 91006, (818) 355-3644, MS 82 San Francisco St Univ; SLP, Los Angeles Co Supt of Schools, **SLP**

Larner, Mrs Deborah Ann 5965 Murdock Avenue, Bethel Park, PA 15102, (412) 262-3500, BS 83 Bloomsburg Univ of PA; MS 85 CA Univ of PA; 87–Sp-Lang Path, Allegheny Valley Sch, **SLP**

Larock, Mrs Beatrice B 16558 Zuni Street N W, Anoka, MN 55303, MS 66 OH Univ - Athens; Consult, Anoka Hennepin Dist 11, **SLP**

Laroque, Mrs Roseann T 3004 Fronklin Drive, Morehead City, NC 28557, (919) 726-0186, BS 82 East Carolina Univ; MS 83 East Carolina Univ; Sp-Lang Path, New Bern Craven Co Schools, **SLP**

LaRosa, Janell B 3630 46th SW, Seattle, WA 98116, (206) 223-6393, BS 78 Univ of UT; MA 79 Univ of WA; 88–Aud, Virginia Mason Cl, **A**

LaRosa, Mrs Marianne Kuhar 981 Bricker Boulevard, Columbus, OH 43221, (614) 459-3328, BS 84 Miami Univ - Oxford; MA 86 Univ of FL; 86–Sp-Lang Path, Columbus Speech & Hearing Ctr, **SLP**

Larose, Giselle Mary 2208 Country Club Drive#12, Woodridge, IL 60517, (312) 325-6133, BS 83 Univ of IA; MA 85 Northern IL Univ - De Kalb; **A**

Larose, Roger Walter 201 East Ogden Avenue, Hinsdale, IL 60521, (312) 323-7970, BS 74 Univ of IL - Urbana; MA 76 Univ of IL - Urbana; President, Sound Resource Inc

Larowe, Mrs Barbara 25W659 Coventry Court, Wheaton, IL 60187, (312) 510-0713, BA 76 Univ of MI - Ann Arbor; MS 77 Univ of MI - Ann Arbor; Sp-Lang Path, Winfield PS Dist 34, **SLP**

Larrabee, Holly A H 72 Newland Avenue, Augusta, ME 04330, **SLP**

Larranaga, Catherine A 144 Redwood Avenue, Wayne, NJ 07470, (201) 835-0907, BA 85 Rutgers St Univ -N Brunswick; ME 87 Univ of VA - Charlottesville; 87–Sp-Lang Path, Kessler Institute for Rehab, **SLP**

Larrick, Susan Marie 59 Deer Lane, Hicksville, NY 11801, (516) 931-4385, BA 84 SUNY - Coll at Cortland; MA 87 Hofstra Univ; **SLP**

Larrick, William Raymond 12202 Fairpoint, Houston, TX 77099, (713) 795-0891, MA 78 Univ of TX - Austin; OM 83 LA St Univ - Baton Rouge; 88–Sp-Lang Path, Associated Healthfocus, **SLP**

Larrigan, Lynn B East 2121 Upriver Dr #28, Spokane, WA 99207, (509) 456-3275, BA 64 Eastern WA Univ; MS 74 Eastern WA Univ; Coord/Intern Prog, W A St U, **SLP**

Larrimore, Elizabeth F 9 Pelican Cove, Savannah, GA 31410, **SLP**

Larsen, Mrs Connie S 2700 Country Club Lane, Kearney, NE 68847, (308) 236-5236, BA 72 Kearney St Coll; MA 73 Univ of KS; ES 88 Kearney St Coll; Sp/Lang Path Superv, Ed Serv Ut #10, **SLP**

Larsen, Mrs Debra Penzi 43 Jefferson Avenue, Northport, NY 11768, (516) 931-6622, SLP, Private Practice, **SLP**

Larsen, Mrs Donna A 764 Cielo Lane, Evergreen, CO 80439, (303) 674-4303, BA 65 Pepperdine Univ - Los Angele; MA 66 Pepperdine Univ - Los Angele; Sp/Lang Path, Private Practice, **SLP**

Larsen, Dr George Lars VA Hospital, 4435 Beacon Avenue South, Seattle, WA 98108, (206) 764-2404, BS 57 Univ of UT; MS 58 Univ of UT; PH 62 (Sp Path) Univ of WA; Sp-Lang Path, VA Med Cen, **SLP**

Larsen, Janell Marie 1220 1/2 Hennepin Avenue, Glencoe, MN 55336, (612) 587-2860, OM 84 Univ of WI - River Falls; SLP, Crow River Special Educ Coop, **SLP**

Larsen, Joan Ellen 4407 Harpoon Court, Fort Collins, CO 80525, (303) 491-6981, BA 66 Univ of KS; MS 67 CO St Univ; Cl Instr, Co St U, **SLP**

Larsen, Joni K 1116 North 154 Avenue Circle, Omaha, NE 68154, (402) 291-4088, MS 86 Univ of NE - Omaha; **SLP**

Larsen, Mrs Joyce F 1369 Laurel Avenue, Ukiah, CA 95482, (707) 462-7447, BA 68 Univ of WY; MA 69 CA St Univ - Los Angeles; Aud, Private Practice, **A**

Larsen, Judith Persoon 2505 Clearwater Road #305, St Cloud, MN 56301, (612) 252-2594, BA 84 Coll of Saint Teresa; MA 86 Univ of MN - Minneap-St Paul; 88–SLP, ISD 882, **SLP**

Larsen, Jule Anne 439 Ash Street N E, Albuquerque, NM 87106, (602) 247-2950, BA 85 Univ of ND; MS 87 Univ of ND; **SLP**

Larsen, Mrs Kay 9146 Glocca Morra Circle, Lakeville, MN 55044, (612) 445-1194, Purdue Univ - West Lafayette; Coord Mh and Pohi Services, Minnesota Rv Valley Sp Ed Coop, **SLP**

Larsen, Kristine Marie North Okanagan Health Unit, 1277-15 Street, Vernon, BC, Canada V1T 8S7, (604) 549-5700, MS 88 Univ of Alberta - Alberta; 83–Sp-Lang Path, BC Ministry of Health

Larsen, Leanne Shaff R R 1 Box 59, Camanche, IA 52730, (319) 242-6454, BA 79 Augustana Coll; MA 80 Univ of Northern IA; SLP, Mississippi Bend AEA, **SLP**

Larsen, Lori Jean 11502 Northpark Avenue North, Seattle, WA 98133, (206) 367-6061, BA 84 Western WA Univ; MA 87 Western WA Univ; 86–Sp-Lang Path, Children's Hosp & Med Ctr, **SLP**

Larsen, Maren Lynn 904 Sibley Road, Towson, MD 21204, (301) 296-3495, BS 86 Towson St Univ; MS 87 Loyola Coll; 88–Sp-Lang Path, Care Rehab Inc, **SLP**

Larsen, Robert E 15 Howard Street, Patchogue, NY 11772, (516) 475-9490, BS 50 NY Univ; MS 68 Adelphi Univ; 67–Sp-Lang Path, Private Practice, **SLP**

Larsen, Mrs Sandra M P O Box 99, 251 South 100th West, Mendon, UT 84325, BS 72 UT St Univ; MS 74 UT St Univ; SLP, Logan City Schools, **SLP**

Larsen, Sveinar Y 2505 Clearwater Road #305, St Cloud, MN 56301, (612) 255-6370, BS 84 Univ of MN - Minneap-St Paul; MA 86 Univ of MN - Minneap-St Paul; Aud, VA Med Ctr, **A**

Larsen, Ulla Tang Navarro Villoslada 1-8° 01012, Vitoria-Gasteiz, Spain, MA 83 WA St Univ; Sp-Lang Path, Private Practice, **SLP**

Larsen, William G 441 East Union Street, River Falls, WI 54022, (715) 425-3801, BS 60 Univ of AZ; MA 61 Univ of AZ; Assoc Prof, U of Wisconsin - Riv Falls, **SLP**

Larson, Arthur Francis 68 Goethals Street, Fort Leonard Wood, MO 65473, (314) 368 9591, MS 82 IL St Univ - Normal; BS 79 IL St Univ - Normal; **A**

Larson, Beth Ann 3322 Tropic Lane Apartment 7, Waterloo, IA 50702, (319) 273-8250, MA 88 Univ of Northern IA; 88–Aud, AEA #7

Larson, Christine 7720 190th Avenue East, Bonney Lake, WA 98390, (206) 829-1111, BA 76 Western WA Univ; MA 78 Western WA Univ; Sp-Lang Path, Rainier Sch, **SLP**

Larson, D Jayne 809 Rio Grande Suite 102, Austin, TX 78701, (512) 478-9131, BS 78 Southwest TX St Univ; MS 80 Univ of TX - Dallas; 88–Sp-Lang Path, Live Oak Ctr for Comm Disorders, **SLP**

Larson, Debra A 425 East Hill, Box 265, Lehigh, IA 50557, (515) 576-7434, BA 74 Univ of Northern IA; MA 75 Univ of Northern IA; 75–Sp-Lang Path, Arrowhead AEA, **SLP**

Larson, Doreen A 1708 West Murdock, Oshkosh, WI 54901, (414) 426-3151, BS 83 Univ of WI - Oshkosh; MS 85 Univ of WI - Oshkosh; **SLP**

Larson, Fonda Rae 1511 West Kamps, Appleton, WI 54914, (414) 734-1675, BA 84 Univ of WI - Eau Claire; MS 86 Univ of WI - Stevens Point; 86–Sp-Lang Path, Freedom Sch Dist, **SLP**

Larson, Dr George W Div Of Communication Disorders, North Texas State Univ, P O Box 5008, Denton, TX 76203, BA 66 Baylor Univ; MA 67 Baylor Univ; PH 70 (NS) Northwestern Univ; Assoc Prof, North Texas State U, **SLP**

Larson, Mrs Gladys Jacobson Rt 1 CPR Box 39, Buffalo, WY 82834, (307) 684-5521, BA 55 William Jewell Coll; MS 59 Univ of KS; MS 77 Univ of WY; Sp-Lang Path/Aud, Johnson Co Mem Hosp, **SLP A**

Larson, Glen A 1285 Westwood Drive N W, Salem, OR 97304-3749, (503) 280-6524, BS 76 Western OR St Coll; MS 78 Western OR St Coll; 87–Sp-Lang Path, Portland PS, **SLP**

Larson, Jamie A 200 South Chrisalta Way, Anaheim, CA 92807, (714) 998-6921, BA 84 CA St Univ - Fullerton; MA 87 CA St Univ - Fullerton; **SLP**

Larson, Janet Inga 7777 East Main Street, Apartment 319, Scottsdale, AZ 85251, (602) 990-9231, 85–Sp-Lang Path, Good Samaritan Med Ctr, **SLP ACE**

Larson, Joy Elspeth 5156 Santa Clara Avenue, Victoria, BC, Canada V8Y 1W4, (604) 263-4486, BA 74 Univ of Victoria - Bc; MA 78 Western WA Univ; **SLP**

Larson, Katherine O'Neil 44 East 7th Street, Springfield, CO 81073, MA 77 Kean Coll of NJ; Audiologist, **A**

Larson, Mrs Kendra Sue 3931 Storm Circle, Rapid City, SD 57702, (605) 394-4036, MA 84 Univ of SD - Vermillion; SLP, Rapid City Area Schools, **SLP**

Larson, Mrs Kristen Hansen 4220 Fox Meadow Dr S E, Cedar Rapids, IA 52403, (319) 363-3967, BA 74 Univ of WI - Stevens Point; MS 75 Univ of WI - Stevens Point; SLP, Grant Wood AEA, **SLP**

Larson, Kristin 505 Ogden Street, Denver, CO 80218, (303) 778-6542, MA 88 Univ of CO - Boulder

Larson, Leslie A 4610 Natick Avenue #110, Sherman Oaks, CA 91403, (213) 240-8000, BS 77 Univ of WI - Stevens Point; MA 79 CA St Univ - Long Beach; Sp-Lang Path, Glendale Adven Med Cen, **SLP**

Larson, Lillian C Dept Of Sp Ed And Com Disorder, West Center, Kearney State College, Kearney, NE 68849, (308) 234-8300, BA 68 Augustana Coll; MA 71 Western MI Univ; PH 81 (Sp Path) IN Univ - Bloomington; 87–Assistant Professor, Kearney State Coll, **SLP**

Larson, Linda Elizabeth 33 Richmond Avenue, Worcester, MA 01602, (617) 791-2793, BS 84 Univ of MA - Amherst; MA 86 Univ of MA - Amherst; 88–Sp-Lang Path, Fairlawn Rehab Hosp, **SLP**

Larson, Linda J 11803 Plum Point, Houston, TX 77099, (713) 776-5225, BA 68 Univ of AR - Fayetteville; MA 70 TX Christian Univ; Director of Speech Pathology, Memorial Hosp Syst, **SLP**

Larson, Lori Beth 3810 South 13th Street #29, Omaha, NE 68107, (402) 734-2777, BS 81 IA St Univ; MA 83 Northeast MO St Univ; 86–Sp-Lang Path, Omaha PS, **SLP**

Larson, Mrs Mardell R Route 1 Box 6, Funk, NE 68940, (308) 995-4269, BA 75 Kearney St Coll; MS 78 Kearney St Coll; Sp-Lang Path, Holdrege City Sch, **SLP**

Larson, Mark H 3451 Apollo Street, San Diego, CA 92111, (619) 230-2072, BS 39 UT St Univ; MA 49 Univ of Denver; PH 55 (NS) Univ of Denver; Retired, **SLP LM**

Larson, Mrs Mary K 2172 Center Street, Marquette, MI 49855, (906) 228-8419, BS 70 Northern MI Univ; MA 75 Univ of WI - Stevens Point; **SLP**

Larson, Mary Lynn 837 East Apple Tree Lane, Appleton, WI 54911-1503, (414) 749-1174, MA 88 Northern MI Univ; 88–Sp-Lang Path, Cent Wisconsin Rehab Assoc Inc

Larson, Mrs Micki McGuire 6421 Barrett, Downers Grove, IL 60516, (312) 654-2188, BS 80 Western IL Univ; MA 81 Western IL Univ; Sp-Lang Path, Commun Sch Unit #201, **SLP**

Larson, Nancy M 10726 South St Louis, Chicago, IL 60655, (312) 567-5557, BS 86 Northern IL Univ - De Kalb; MA 87 Northern IL Univ - De Kalb; 88–Sp-Lang Path, Mercy Hosp & Med Ctr

Larson, Mrs Nancy S 1005 Holly Springs Drive, Louisville, KY 40242, (502) 423-8224, BA 73 Mary Washington Coll; ME 74 Univ of VA - Charlottesville; Sp/Lang Path, Nancy S Larson M Ed Ccc, **SLP**

Larson, Patricia 128 Crawford Drive, Martinez, GA 30907, (404) 737-7681, BA 82 Univ of MD - College Park; MA 84 Univ of MD - College Park; 87–Sp-Lang Path, St Joseph's Hosp, **SLP**

Larson, Penny S 3605 Gene Field #A-27, St Joseph, MO 64506, (816) 271-7577, BS 85 Northwest MO St Univ; MA 87 Univ of Northern IA; Sp-Lang Path, Heartland Hosp W, **SLP**

Larson, Mrs Rita F 738 Winchester Drive, Burlingame, CA 94010, (415) 589-5900, BA 67 San Francisco St Univ; MA 70 San Francisco St Univ; Sp-Lang-Hrng Spec, San Bruno Park Sch Dist, **SLP**

Larson, Rose Mary Route 2 Box 23, Galva, KS 67443, (316) 241-1650, BS 77 Carlow Coll; MS 81 PA St Univ - Univ Park; Sp-Lang Path, McPherson Spec Ed Coop, **SLP**

Larson, Mrs Sharon Kay 2083 Arrowhead Trail, Marietta, GA 30062, (404) 980-9373, BS 80 Central MI Univ; MA 82 Wayne St Univ; 85–Sp-Lang Path, Chldrns Therapy Serv Inc, **SLP**

Larson, Sherri C 1835 Northbrook, Ann Arbor, MI 48103-6035, (313) 668-6610, BS 72 Eastern MI Univ; MA 73 Eastern MI Univ; Sp-Lang Path, Milan Area Schools, **SLP**

Larson, Mrs Stephanie Brock 507 North Vermont, Iola, KS 66749, (316) 365-3925, BA 81 Wichita St Univ; MA 82 Wichita St Univ; Sp-Lang Path, ANW Coop, **SLP**

Larson, Steven Kenneth 4520 East Base Line #1102, Phoenix, AZ 85044, (602) 438-0205, BS 85 Univ of WI - Stevens Point; MS 87 Univ of WI - Madison

Larson, Mrs Susan J 6833 North Chance, Fresno, CA 93710, (209) 488-3250, BA 68 Univ of the Pacific; MA 74 CA St Univ - Fresno; SLP, Diag Sch for Neurohndcpd Chldn, **SLP**

Larson, Mrs Thalia W 2318-B Via Puerta, Laguna Hills, CA 92653, (714) 830-4588, BA 32 Univ of Southern CA; MA 57 CA St Univ - Long Beach; **SLP LM**

Larson, Dr Vernon Dale VA Medical Center-126, 2460 Wrightboro Road, Augusta, GA 30910, (404) 823-2228, BA 65 Augustana Coll; MS 66 CO St Univ; PH 73 (Aud) Univ of OK Medical Center; 80–Ch Aud/Sp-Lang Path, VA Med Cen, **A**

Larson, Dr Vicki Lord School Of Graduate Studies & Office Of University Research, Schoolfield 201, University Of Wisconsin, Eau Claire, WI 54702, (715) 836-2721, BS 66 Univ of WI - Madison; MS 68 Univ of WI - Madison; PH 74 (CDIS Sp-Lang Path) Univ of WI - Madison; Asst Dean, U WI-Eau Claire, **SLP ACE**

Larson-Fagre, Mrs Kristen M 1105 9th Street NW, Waverly, IA 50677, (319) 352-2741, BS 83 OH Univ - Athens; MA 85 Univ of IA; 88–Sp-Lang Path, Bremer Co Care Facility, **SLP**

Larson-Schofield, Mrs September 8 Fowlers Lane, Ipswich, MA 01938-1338, (617) 475-3806, BS Miami Univ - Oxford; MA Emerson Coll; Sp-Lang Path, Pro Ctr for Early Intervention, **SLP**

Larson-Tuttle, Claudine Sandra 1139 7th Place, Hermosa Beach, CA 90254, (213) 372-7658, BA 84 CA St Univ - Long Beach; MA 86 CA St Univ - Long Beach; 87–Aud, Newport Lang Sp and Aud Ctr Inc, **A**

Larssen, Karen 134 Luz Place, Davis, CA 95616, (916) 661-2710, BA 67 CA St Univ - Northridge; MA 74 CA St Univ - Northridge; 88–Sp-Lang Path, Yolo Co Ofc of Educ, **SLP**

La Rue, Janet Ruth P O Box 369, Cobb, CA 95426, (707) 263-3595, BS 77 Univ of WI - Oshkosh; MS 84 San Francisco St Univ; 87–Sp-Lang Path, Lakeport USD, **SLP**

La Russa, Mrs Karen M 11 Vanderbilt Road, West Hartford, CT 06119, (203) 236-5732, BA 74 CUNY - Hunter Coll; MA 76 CUNY - Queens Coll; 88–Sp-Lang Path, Private Practice, **SLP**

Larvadain, Janice M 319 Wynwood Apartment, Pineville, LA 71360, (318) 640-0754, BS 75 Southern Univ - Baton Rouge; MA 76 Western MI Univ; Asst Dir SLP IV, Pinecrest State School, **SLP**

Larvick, Jenny C 792 Wildcat Canyon, Berkeley, CA 94708, (415) 222-2161, BA 68 Univ of CA - Santa Barbara; MA 73 Univ of CA - Santa Barbara; MS 81 San Francisco St Univ; 81–Sp-Lang Path, Richmond USD, **SLP**

Lasalle, Lisa Renee 807 Mortimer Avenue, Fredericksburg, VA 22401, (703) 373-0162, MA 88 Univ of VA - Charlottesville

La Salle, Lori Jo 22 Quailbush Drive, Fairport, NY 14450, (716) 223-9124, BS 83 Nazareth Coll of Rochester; MS 86 Nazareth Coll of Rochester; Private Practice, **SLP**

Laschkewitsch, John M 5401 N W 83rd Terrace, Kansas City, MO 64151, **SLP A**

Lasensky-Curtin, Judith A 7401 Rhoads Street, Philadelphia, PA 19151, (302) 656-6510, BS 73 Marquette Univ; MS 75 Marquette Univ; Aud/Sp-Lang Path, Del Val Cd Speech Assoc, **SLP A**

Laseter, Carrell 1740 Meadowdale Avenue N E, Atlanta, GA 30306, (404) 925-9543, BS 80 TX Christian Univ; MA 82 Univ of MD - College Park; Sp-Lang Path, Gwinnett Co Ps, **SLP**

Lash, Mrs Susan Bour 22450 Ethel, Strongsville, OH 44136-1030, (216) 678-0388, **A**

Lashley, Clare Oliveri 1893 Northview Road, Largo, FL 34640, (813) 546-2106, BA 82 Univ of FL; MA 84 Univ of FL; 85–Sp-Lang Path, Lashley & Associates Inc, **SLP**

Lashley, Luann L Route 5 Box 163A, Portsmouth, OH 45662, (614) 353-7774, BS 75 OH Univ - Athens; MA 76 OH Univ - Athens; Director Speech and Hearing, Scioto Memorial Hospital, **SLP**

Lashley, Mrs Rebecca E 8318 Ridgemoor Drive, Riverdale, GA 30296, (404) 477-2894, BS 45 Northern IL Univ - De Kalb; MA 62 G Peabody Coll-Vanderbilt U; Sp-Lang Path, Clayton Co Schs, **SLP**

Lashway, Mrs Carolanne Polizzi 57A Jackman Drive, Poughkeepsie, NY 12603, (914) 279-2905, BA 75 Saint John's Univ - Jamaica; MA 76 SUNY - Coll at Geneseo; MS 85 Western CT St Univ; Treatment Team Leader, Wassaic Dev Ctr, **SLP**

Laskey, Ann Lynn 6115 North Boston Avenue, Portland, OR 97217, (503) 635-0347, BS 73 Portland St Univ; MS 75 Portland St Univ; Sp-Lang Path, Lake Oswego Sch Dist #7, **SLP**

Laskey-Kemnitz, Alisa J 1216B Gilmore Drive, Key West, FL 33040, (305) 294-9985, BA 77 Univ of FL; MA 79 Univ of Miami; Sp-Lang Path, Monroe County PS, **SLP**

Laskin, Mrs Rebecca D 5953 Lake Trace Circle, Jackson, MS 39211, (601) 981-3711, BS 71 Northern IL Univ - De Kalb; OM 76 Univ of MS; Sp-Lang Path, Private Practice, **SLP**

Lasko, Teresa Helen 151-B Louise Drive, Newport News, VA 23601, (919) 767-9435, BA 83 OH St Univ; MS 86 Clarion Univ of PA; **SLP**

Laskowski, Margaret M 19 Winters Street, City Island, NY 10464, (212) 885-0136, BS 77 Trenton St Coll; ME 86 Columbia Univ Teachers Coll; 88–Sp-Lang Path, Tchrs Coll Sp & H Clinic, **SLP**

Laskowski, Randy Paul Mult-District HI Program, Hansel Lowe School, 16th & Vesper, Blue Springs, MO 64015, (913) 588-5937, BS 78 Univ of KS; MA 82 Univ of KS; Aud, Multi-Dist Hlp R-IV Sch, **A**

Lasky, Mrs Helene 66 Bayview Avenue, Great Neck, NY 11021, (516) 482-8762, BA 63 CUNY - Brooklyn Coll; MA 78 CUNY - Queens Coll; Sp-Lang Path, Variety Preschoolers Workshop, **SLP**

Lasky-Broecker, Brenda 1705 Colonial Drive, Avenel, NJ 07001, (201) 396-8039, BA 84 SUNY - Center at Buffalo; MA 86 CUNY - Hunter Coll; 87–Research Asst, City Univ Grad Ctr, **A**

Lasky-Case, Mrs Lynnemarie 59 Oakland Avenue, Amsterdam, NY 12010, (518) 843-3180, BS 80 SUNY - Coll at Geneseo; MS 81 Ithaca Coll; SLP, Amsterdam Sch Dist Tecler Cen, **SLP**

Laspisa, Lisa A 415 Huntington Avenue, Buffalo, NY 14214, (716) 895-2334, BS 79 SUNY - Coll at Buffalo; MA 81 SUNY - Center at Buffalo; Aud, Buffalo Bd of Ed, **A**

Lasris, Mrs Manette E 231 Banburn Court, Longwood, FL 32750, (305) 862-7848, BS 68 Memphis St Univ; MA 69 Univ of TN - Knoxville; Sp-Lang Path, Seminole County Schools, **SLP**

Lass, Dr Norman J 1374 Braewick Drive, Morgantown, WV 26505, (304) 293-4242, BA 65 CUNY - Brooklyn Coll; MS 66 Purdue Univ - West Lafayette; PH 68 (Sp Path/Sp Science) Purdue Univ - West Lafayette; 69–Prof, W V Univ, **F**

Lasser, Amy B 412 Morris Avenue #29, Summit, NJ 07901, (201) 234-0011, BS 85 Ithaca Coll; MA 87 George Washington Univ; 88–Sp-Lang Path, Matheny Sch/Hosp, **SLP**

Lasseter, Mrs Susanne Wilkinson 941 North Caribe Avenue, Tucson, AZ 85710, (602) 296-8247, BS 80 Univ of AZ; MS 82 Univ of AZ; 88–Sp-Lang Path, Tucson USD, **SLP**

Lassin, Mrs Bonnie Sue 125 Beechwood Avenue, Langhorne, PA 19047, (215) 225-5385, BS 77 Trenton St Coll; MA 81 Trenton St Coll; **SLP**

Lassiter, Josephine J P O Box 17141, Huntsville, AL 35810, BS 62 Univ of the DC; MA 69 CA St Univ - Los Angeles; 85–Sp-Lang Path, Lassiter Sp Path Assoc, **SLP**

Lassman, Dr Frank M Department Of Otolaryngology, University Of Minnesota, Box 283, University Hospital, Minneapolis, MN 55455, (612) 626-5775, BA 41 CUNY - Brooklyn Coll; MA 42 Univ of IA; PH 50 (Sp-Lang Path) Univ of Southern CA; 62–Prof, U of MN, **SLP A F**

Lasson, Sheryl R 14801 Lincoln Drive #104, Oak Park, MI 48237, (313) 968-5958, MS 88 CUNY - Brooklyn Coll

Lassonde, Mrs Christena L RR1 Box 1252, Route 149, Weare, NH 03281, (603) 624-6338, BS 79 Northwestern Univ; MA 80 Northwestern Univ; Sp/Lang Path, Manchester Publ Schs, **SLP**

Lasswell, Mrs Carolyn Jean 1338 Calle Colnett, San Marcos, CA 92069, (619) 741-1642, BA 75 San Diego St Univ; MA 82 San Diego St Univ; 87–Sp-Lang Path, Children's Hosp & Health Ctr, **SLP ACE**

Last, Stephanie 3740 Riviera Drive #F, San Diego, CA 92109, (619) 270-2276, BS 76 SUNY - Coll at Fredonia; MA 81 CA St Univ - Los Angeles; SLP, San Diego USD, **SLP**

Laster, Mrs Cheryl Elizabeth 2620 Farmington Drive, Marietta, GA 30060, (404) 432-0431, BA 78 Univ of OK Medical Center; OM 81 Auburn Univ - Auburn; **SLP**

Laster, Mrs Jan Colwick 938 North Cumberland Circle, Riverdale, GA 30296, (404) 477-5300, BA 82 Univ of TN - Knoxville; ME 84 GA St Univ; Sp-Lang Path, Clayton Co Brd of Ed, **SLP**

Lastrapes, Carolyn Hall 820 Burgin, Baton Rouge, LA 70808, (504) 927-9050, BS 77 Univ of Southwestern LA; MS 81 Univ of WI - River Falls; Sp-Lang Path, Med Therapy Rehab Svcs Inc, **SLP**

Lasure, Mrs Laurie Lou 1341 Dodge Street, Lake Geneva, WI 53147, (414) 248-6609, BS 83 Univ of WI - Madison; MS 84 Univ of WI - Eau Claire; **SLP**

Laszewski, Carol Lynn 644 North Ashbury, Bolingbrook, IL 60439-1164, (312) 848-9750, BS 82 Univ of NH; MA 85 IN Univ - Bloomington; Oak Park Sp & L Cntr, **SLP**

Lataille, Charlene Frances 19 Methyl Street, Providence, RI 02906, (401) 944-4760, BA 82 Univ of RI; MS 84 PA St Univ - Univ Park; Sp-Lang Path, Ocean State Rehab Services Inc, **SLP**

Latham, Mrs Elizabeth 387 St George Street, London, ON, Canada N6A 3A9, (519) 438-6185, BA 62 Univ of KY; MS 64 Univ of Pittsburgh - Pittsburgh; Sp-Lang Path, **SLP**

Latham, Mrs Nancy J P O Box 2101, Idyllwild, CA 92349, (714) 659-2068, BA 70 Univ of Redlands; MS 72 Univ of Redlands; Sp-Lang Path, Vip Tots, **SLP**

Latham, Mrs Sandra 4501 Indian School Road NE, Albuquerque, NM 87110, (505) 266-5934, BS 67 Univ of DE; MS 74 Radford Univ; MA 75 Central MI Univ; Aud, DNM, **A**

Lathen, Jill E 1002 Kim Street, Halstead, KS 67056, (316) 835-2055, BA 84 Wichita St Univ; MA 85 Wichita St Univ; **SLP**

Lather, James E Box 161, Brenham, TX 77833, (409) 836-4511, BS 71 Univ of North TX; MS 72 Univ of North TX; Admissions Coord, Tdmhmr Brenham State Sch, **SLP**

Lathrop, Mrs Debra C 142 Fogarty Avenue, Jewett City, CT 06351, (203) 376-4342, BA 77 SUNY - Coll at Plattsburgh; MA 79 CUNY - Lehman Coll; Sp/Lang Path, Franklin Bd of Ed, **SLP**

Lathrop, Mrs Debra Lantz 310 Abbey Lane, Franklin, TN 37064, (919) 851-8560, BS 79 IA St Univ; MA 80 Univ of NE - Lincoln; Sp-Lang Path, Duke U Med Ctr, **SLP**

Lathrop, Jennifer Fargo Pacific Hearing Service, 960 North San Antonio Road, Suite 101, Los Altos, CA 94022, (415) 941-0664, BA 72 Univ of Redlands; MA 73 Kent St Univ; Owner, Pacific Hrng Serv, **A**

Latino, Susan B 68 Sorghum Road, Huntington, CT 06484, (203) 926-0077, BS 77 Univ of MA - Amherst; MS 80 Columbia Univ Teachers Coll; Sp-Lang Path, Bridgeport Pub Sch, **SLP**

Latocha, Mrs Diane C 1 Longspur Drive, Limestone Hills, Wilmington, DE 19808, (302) 992-5574, BS 74 Trenton St Coll; MA 81 West Chester Univ of PA; 82–Sp-Lang Path, Red Clay Consol Sch Dist, **SLP**

Latona, Madelaine J 156 Bell Street, Belleville, NJ 07109, (201) 751-9537, BA 82 Rutgers St Univ -N Brunswick; MS 84 PA St Univ - Univ Park; Sp-Lnag Path, New York Univ Medical Center/RIRM, **SLP**

Latona, Patricia C 10000 Oakland Street, Dalton, NY 14836, (607) 776-9800, BS 63 SUNY - Coll at Geneseo; MS 66 SUNY - Coll at Geneseo; Treatment Team Leader (MR), Craig Dev Cen, **SLP ACE**

Latta, Angela Trautman Outpatient Rehabil Inst Inc, 999 Northwest Circle Blvd, Corvallis, OR 97330, (503) 753-2273, BA 70 CUNY - Queens Coll; MA 75 CA St Univ - Los Angeles; President, Outpatient Rehabil Inst Inc, **SLP**

Latta, Mrs Diane C West 613 14th Avenue #1, Spokane, WA 99204, (509) 624-7120, BS 74 OR St Univ; MS 76 Portland St Univ; 88–Sp-Lang Path, Spokane PS, **SLP**

Latta, Mary 315 Richards Road, Melbourne Beach, FL 32951, (305) 723-4474, BS 65 Southern IL Univ -Carbondale; MS 68 Southern IL Univ -Carbondale; Sp-Lang Path, Easter Seal Center Inc, **SLP**

Lattig, Marcia Jo 104 Strickland, Mather AFB, CA 95655, BA 73 CA St Univ - Northridge; MS 81 Univ of Redlands; **SLP**

Lattof, Mrs Marian T 6401 Cedar Bend Court-Unit 4, Mobile, AL 36608, (205) 343-3402, BA 67 Univ of AL-Tuscaloosa; MA 69 Univ of AL- Tuscaloosa; **SLP**

Lattz, Audrey L Route 1 Box 243, New Sharon, ME 04955-9761, (207) 778-9173, BA 80 Augustana Coll; MS 84 Southern IL Univ -Carbondale; Sp-Lang Path, Private Practice, **SLP**

Latzo, Mrs Michele Marie 1058 West 4th Street, Erie, PA 16507, (814) 452-5100, BS 84 Clarion Univ of PA; MS 85 Clarion Univ of PA; **SLP**

Lau, Dr Aileen C 19 Barony Lane, Hilton Head, SC 29928, (803) 525-7404, BS 46 Northwestern Univ; MA 49 Univ of MI - Ann Arbor; ED 84 (NS) Univ of SC - Columbia; Adjunct Assistant Professor, U of S Carolina, **SLP F**

Laub, Billie 603 North Howard Street, Apartment 401, Alexandria, VA 22304, (301) 274-3182, MS 76 George Washington Univ; SLP, Charles County Public Schools, **SLP**

Laub, Mrs Clarice C 1700 Rexford Drive, Las Vegas, NV 89104, (702) 735-1279, BA 42 Southwestern OK St Univ; MA 57 Western St Coll of CO; **SLP LM**

Laubach, Mrs Connie L 1035 Archer Lane, Lansdale, PA 19446, (215) 539-8550, BS 72 Bloomsburg Univ of PA; ME 73 Bloomsburg Univ of PA; Sp-Lang Path, Montgomery Cty Indepen Unit 23, **SLP**

Laubach, Mrs Victoria H Route 2 Box 709AC, New Braunfels, TX 78130, (512) 625-8575, BS 71 Southwest TX St Univ; ME 73 Southwest TX St Univ; Sp-Lang Path, Private Practice, **SLP ACE**

Laubacher, Marci P 836 Manitowish Place, Depere, WI 54115-3667, (414) 336-0203, BS 83 Univ of Cincinnati; MS Univ of Cincinnati; **SLP**

Lauber, Mrs Vicky Sue N P O Box 254, Sunman, IN 47041, (812) 623-2836, BS 75 Purdue Univ - West Lafayette; MA 80 Ball St Univ; Sp-Lang Path, Private Practice, **SLP**

Laucius, Gail 1025 Arboretum Road, Wyncote, PA 19095, (215) 288-2102, BA 68 Temple Univ-Tyler Sch of Art; MA 70 Temple Univ-Tyler Sch of Art; Aud, Ear Nose & Throat Consult, **A**

Laudenslager, Mrs Wanda Lee 37733 Logan Drive, Fremont, CA 94536, (415) 793-4064, BA 62 San Jose St Univ; MA 65 San Jose St Univ; SLP, Newark USD, **SLP**

Lauder, Edmund 11115 Whisper Hollow, San Antonio, TX 78230, (512) 492-1984, MA 59 George Washington Univ; BS 56 Univ of MD - College Park; Sp-Lang Path, Amer Cancer Soc, **SLP LM**

Lauderdale, Linda F Route 2 Box 57, Archer Grove School Road, Athens, GA 30607, (404) 353-2903, BS 71 Univ of GA; ME 76 Univ of GA; Clin Superv, U of GA, **SLP**

Lauer, Marianne 1020 Tiverton Court, Schaumburg, IL 60193, (312) 934-2853, BS 73 Northern IL Univ - De Kalb; MA 74 Northern IL Univ - De Kalb; 74–Com Cons Sch Dist 15, Ccsd #15, **SLP**

Lauer, Therese P 60 Tecumseth, Orillia, ON, Canada L3V 1X9, (705) 737-1991, BS 73 SUNY - Coll at Geneseo; MS 74 Univ of OK Medical Center; Owner/Aud, Barrie Aud Clinic, **A**

Laufer, Debora 1815 Beacon Street, Brookline, MA 02146, (617) 731-0848, OB 76 Hebrew Coll; BS 77 Boston Univ; MS 79 Boston Univ; Sp-Lang Path, Private Practice, **SLP**

Laufer, Dr M Barbara 3819 Grosvenor Drive, Ellicott City, MD 21043-4910, (301) 321-2436, BS 72 Towson St Univ; MS 73 PA St Univ - Univ Park; PH 85 (Human Development-Gerontology) Univ of MD - College Park; 75–Asst Professor, Towson St U, **A**

Laufer, Dr Marsha Z 3 Jackson Drive, Setauket, NY 11733, (516) 751-8311, BA 64 Univ of MD - College Park; MA 65 Columbia Univ Teachers Coll; PH 72 (NS) Northwestern Univ; Res Assoc Prof, St U of NY Stony Brook, **SLP**

Laufer-Turk, Mrs Stella Claire 2375 Ocean Avenue #1-B, Brooklyn, NY 11229, (718) 769-4239, BA 84 CUNY - Brooklyn Coll; MS 86 CUNY - Brooklyn Coll; **A**

Lauffenburger, Angela T 1943 Cheyenne Drive, Carrollton, TX 75010, (214) 394-1720, BS 81 OK St Univ; MS 87 Univ of North TX

Laughery, Virginia M P O Box 964, Astoria, OR 97103, (503) 325-4843, MS 76 Eastern WA Univ; Sp-Lang Path, Private Practice, **SLP**

Laughlin, John Bohan, Jr 4520 Cascade Place, Vernon, BC, Canada V1T 8M8, (604) 545-8962, **SLP**

Laughlin, Veronica 6501 Paces Arbor Circle, Apartment 618, Raleigh, NC 27609, (919) 560-6470, BS 80 NC St Univ at Raleigh; MA 82 LA St Univ - Baton Rouge; 88–Supvr, North Carolina Central Univ, **SLP**

Laughlin, Mrs Yvonne O Mountain School, North Road, Los Alamos, NM 87544, (505) 662-4367, BS 74 Kent St Univ; MS 78 Univ of NM; 78–Sp-Lang Path, Los Alamos Sch, **SLP**

Laughton, Dr Joan University Of Georgia, Department Of Communication Sciences/Disorders, 570 Aderhold Hall, Athens, GA 30602, (404) 542-1685, BS 60 Kent St Univ; ME 68 Kent St Univ; PH 76 (NS) Kent St Univ; 85–Coord Hrng Impairmnt, U of GA, **SLP**

Laukka, Suzanne Mary 4513 Browndale Avenue, Edina, MN 55424, (612) 920-5360, BA 85 Univ of CO - Boulder; MA 87 IN Univ - Bloomington; **SLP**

Laul, Alfred Christopher 70-33 68th Place, Glendale, NY 11385, (516) 385-2700, BA 70 Saint John's Univ - Jamaica; MS 76 CUNY - Brooklyn Coll; 70–Treat Team Leader, Long Island Dev Ctr, **SLP**

Lauless, Sandra L 1335 Appleton #8, Long Beach, CA 90802, (213) 865-2064, BS 78 Univ of IL - Urbana; MS 79 Univ of IL - Urbana; 80–Sp-Lang Path, ABC USD, **SLP**

Launer, Dr Patricia B 4627 Ocean Boulevard #206, San Diego, CA 92109, (619) 594-2684, MA 71 SUNY - Center at Buffalo; OM 81 CUNY - Grad Sch & Univ Cntr; PH 82 (Sp & Hrng Sciences) CUNY - Grad Sch & Univ Cntr; 80–Lecturer, Dept Commun Dis-San Diego St U, **SLP**

Laurel, Marci K Albuquerque Therapy Services, 2412 Monroe Street N E, Suite C, Albuquerque, NM 87110, (505) 883-9791, BA 80 Univ of FL; MA 81 Univ of FL; Sp-Lang Path, Albuquerque Therapy Services, **SLP**

Lauren, Maureen A 3825 South 25th Street, Omaha, NE 68107, (402) 734-7046, PH (NS); **SLP**

Laurence, Deanna Glaser 28331 Osborn Road, Bay Village, OH 44140, (216) 231-8787, BS 69 Cleveland St Univ; MA 85 Cleveland St Univ; 85–Sp-Lang Path, Cleveland Hearing & Speech Ctr, **SLP**

Laurence, Mrs Elizabeth Wilkey 2111 Savanna Court South, League City, TX 77573, (713) 332-8281, BS 85 Baylor Univ; MS 87 Baylor Univ; 87–Sp-Lang Path, Goose Creek Consolidated ISD, **SLP**

Laurence, Marianna Louise 3262 Thompson Avenue, Alameda, CA 94501, (415) 428-3344, **SLP**

Laurent, Deborah 686 Black Rock Turnpike, Fairfield, CT 06430, (203) 846-9531, BS 86 WV Univ; MA 88 Univ of Pittsburgh - Pittsburgh; 88–Sp-Lang Path

Laurent, Jan Claire 6595 Wilder Drive, Beaumont, TX 77706, (713) 428-2553, BS 85 Lamar Univ; MS 87 Lamar Univ; **SLP**

Lauria, Joanne 342 North Claremont, Fresno, CA 93727, (209) 255-7809, BA 77 CA St Univ - Fresno; MA 79 CA St Univ - Fresno; SLP, Fresno Co Offi of Ed, **SLP**

Lauria, Toni Ann M 876 Park Avenue, Huntington, NY 11743, (516) 673-2115, BA 84 Hofstra Univ; MA 87 Hofstra Univ

Laursen, Mrs Charlene Ann St Mary's Hospital, 1044 Kabel Avenue, Rhinelander, WI 54501, (715) 369-6605, BS 83 Univ of WI - Madison; MS 84 Marquette Univ; Sp-Lang Path, Sacred Heart St Marys Hosp, **SLP ACE**

Lauten, Kathleen W c/o Aramco, P O Box 10844, Dhahran, Saudi Arabia, BS 67 Univ of TX - Austin; MA 70 Univ of TX - Austin; 86–Sp-Lang Path, Rehab Unit-Dhahran Health Ctr, **SLP**

Lauter, Karen 1911 Darlee Court, Lakewood, CO 80215, BS 72 Stephen F Austin St Univ; MS 75 Univ of North TX; **SLP**

Lautz, John R, II 345 San Marcos Street #5, San Gabriel, CA 91776-1012, (818) 284-1000, MA 79 CA St Univ - Los Angeles; Aud, Hearing Specialists, **A**

Lauve, Jane F The Speech Pathology Center, 431 Colonial Drive, Baton Rouge, LA 70806, (504) 923-1140, BS 66 LA St Univ - Baton Rouge; MA 69 LA St Univ - Baton Rouge; Sp-Lang Path, The Sp-Path Center, **SLP**

Lauze, Susan Flanders 62 Dunklee Street, Concord, NH 03301, (603) 225-0858, BA 75 Univ of NH; ME 82 Northeastern Univ; Sp-Lang Path/Asst Prin, Concord School District, **SLP**

Lavallee, Mrs Donna Marlin 3396 Greenway Road, Grand Island, NY 14072, (716) 883-6800, BA 83 SUNY - Center at Buffalo; MA 85 SUNY - Center at Buffalo; Aud, Buffalo Otological Group, **A**

LaVallee-Kennedy, Mrs Janet Mary 41 Ball Road, Walnut Creek, CA 94596, (415) 757-7110, BS 79 CA St Univ - Hayward; MA 82 Western WA Univ; 82–Sp-Lang Path, Antioch USD, **SLP**

Lavallie, Patrick Dennis Palm Garden Of West Palm Beach, 300 Executive Center Drive, West Palm Beach, FL 33401, (407) 471-5566, BS 85 Univ of WI - River Falls; OM 86 Univ of WI - River Falls; 86–Sp-Lang Path, Pro Health Svcs, **SLP**

Lavan, Mrs Leah D A 30530 Camino Porvenir, Palos Verdes Peninsula, CA 90274-4537, BA 60 MI St Univ; MA 78 Whittier Coll; Sp-Lang Path, Off of LA Co Supt of Sch, **SLP**

La Velle, Connie Marie 2204 Lynch, Granite City, IL 62040, (618) 451-7209, BS 82 Southern IL Univ-Edwardsvill; MS 83 Southern IL Univ-Edwardsvill; Sp-Lang Path, Special School Dist St Louis, **SLP**

Lavelle, Renee Marie 534 Stephenson #C, Shreveport, LA 71104, (318) 222-5935, BS 82 Baylor Univ; MS 83 Baylor Univ; **SLP**

Lavely-Planisek, Debra Sue 469 Topaz Lane, Brunswick Hills, OH 44212, (216) 920-1516, **SLP**

Laven, Frances J 2810 Aquila Avenue South, Minneapolis, MN 55426, (612) 935-5057, BA 67 Washington Univ; MA 74 Univ of WI - Milwaukee; Executive Secretary, MN Sp-Lang-Hrng Assn, **SLP**

Lavender, Mrs Barbara Comstock 3253 Valley Park Place, Birmingham, AL 35243, (205) 967-9245, BS 76 Bowling Green St Univ; MS 85 Univ of Montevallo; Sp-Lang Path, Jefferson County Board of Educ, **SLP**

Lavender, Mrs Celia Curcio 741 Maple, Clarksdale, MS 38614, (601) 627-3231, BS 81 Delta St Univ; MS 87 Univ of MS; 81–Sp-Lang Path, Clarksdale Sch Dist, **SLP**

Lavene, Mrs Phyllis L 4025 Gull Hills, Richland, MI 49083, BS 53 Western MI Univ; MA 60 Western MI Univ; **SLP**

Laverdure, Mrs Edythe S Rural Delivery 1, 1113 Steelmanville, Linwood, NJ 08221, (609) 641-5044, BA 68 Trenton St Coll; MA 81 Trenton St Coll; Sp/Lang Path, Northfield Bd of Ed, **SLP**

Lavergne, Mrs Angela Marie 8215 Killian Street, Beaumont, TX 77706, (409) 985-9303, BS 84 Bowling Green St Univ; MS 87 Lamar Univ; **SLP**

Laverick, Mrs Charlotte Lorraine 10945 Fox Mill Lane, Matthews, NC 28105, (704) 846-8280, BS 83 Univ of NC - Greensboro; ME 85 Univ of NC - Greensboro; **SLP**

La Verne, Mrs Dianne A 142 Thomas Street, South Plainfield, NJ 07080, (201) 757-6610, BA 81 Rutger's St Univ - Douglas Coll; MS 83 Rutgers St Univ -N Brunswick; Sp-Lang Path, Laurie Neurodev Inst, **SLP**

Laverty, Barbara Ann 604 Cocheco Court, Dover, NH 03820, (603) 749-2446, BS 84 Univ of NH; MA 85 George Washington Univ; 88–Sp-Lang Path, New England Sp Svcs, **SLP**

Laverty-Reves, Robin M 9764 Treetop Drive, Stockton, CA 95209, (209) 953-8370, BA 76 CA St Univ - Sacramento; MA 81 CA St Univ - Sacramento; 86–Sp-Lang Path, Lodi USD, **SLP**

Lavigne, Mrs Benjie Panesh 23 Applewood Lane, Morris Township, NJ 07960, (201) 263-7200, BS 79 Immaculata Coll; MA 82 Montclair St Coll; **SLP**

Lavigne, Cheryl Ann 6540 Kirkville Road #173, East Syracuse, NY 13057, (315) 437-6010, BS 83 Coll of Saint Rose; MS 84 Ithaca Coll; E Syracuse Minoa Central Schls

Laville, Lisa J 1504 63rd Street, Des Moines, IA 50311, (815) 942-8598, BA 83 Univ of NE - Lincoln; MA 85 Univ of TX - Austin; 87–Sp-Lang Path, Des Moines Hrng & Sp Ctr, **SLP**

Lavin, Mrs Ellen 532 Clavery Court, Highland Park, IL 60035, (312) 432-1941, BS 67 Northwestern Univ; MA 68 Northwestern Univ; SLP, Madison School, **SLP**

Lavin, Kathryn D 1729 Beachway Lane, Odessa, FL 33556, (813) 996-3600, BA 73 SUNY - Center at Buffalo; MA 74 Memphis St Univ; Sp-Lang Path, Florida Diag&Learning Res Sys, **SLP**

Lavin, Marian 22812 9th Street, Newhall, CA 91312, (805) 252-9580, BA 78 CA St Univ - Northridge; MA 81 CA St Univ - Northridge; SLP, Los Angeles Co, **SLP**

Lavin, Nancy J 306 Mulhern Court #2, Yorkville, IL 60560, (815) 467-2900, BA 85 Augustana Coll; MA 87 Western IL Univ; **SLP**

Lavin-Arcand, Maureen 137 Lawson Road, Scituate, MA 02066, (617) 471-3263, BA 71 Coll of New Rochelle; ME 75 Northeastern Univ; Bus Mgr, Quincy Surgical Associates, **SLP**

La Vine, Mrs Arlene K 5410 Forest Brook Parkway, Marietta, GA 30067, (404) 977-1247, BS 72 Univ of IL - Urbana; MA 74 Saint Louis Univ; Sp/Lang Path, Cobb Co Bd of Ed, **SLP**

Lavine, Mrs Janice Helene 12250 Castlegate Drive, Los Angeles, CA 90049, (818) 795-0679, BA 81 Univ of CA - Los Angeles; MA 85 CA St Univ - Northridge; **A**

Lavine, Laura Beth 303 Dewitt Road, Syracuse, NY 13214, (315) 469-6926, BS 77 Ithaca Coll; MS 82 Ithaca Coll; Supvr of Spec Educ, Onondaga Central Schools, **SLP**

LaVoi, Dr Gerald W Department Of Communication Disorders, St Cloud State University, A216 Education Bldg, St Cloud, MN 56301, (612) 255-2092, BS 63 Univ of MN - Minneap-St Paul; MS 69 Univ of ND; PH 84 (NS) Univ of MO - Columbia; 88–Asst Prof, St Cloud St U, **SLP**

Lavoie, Mrs Evelyn Fairchild 13401 S W 100th Court, Miami, FL 33176, (305) 238-6110, BS 74 Southern CT St Univ; MS 77 Southern CT St Univ; Sp-Lang Path, Dade Co PS, **SLP**

Lavoie, Mary E 2680 Shanley Road, Auburn, CA 95603, (916) 624-0995, MA 86 San Jose St Univ; **A**

Lavorato, Dr Alfred S 820 Falmouth, Thousand Oaks, CA 91362, (213) 854-5702, BS 69 Portland St Univ; MS 70 Portland St Univ; PH 76 (Sp Path) Univ of Pittsburgh - Pittsburgh; 82–Sp-Lang Path, Private Practice, **SLP**

LaVoy, Mrs Anita Kay R R 1 Box 216, Waubun, MN 56589, (218) 327-2261, BS 84 Moorhead St Univ; MS 86 Moorhead St Univ; 88–Sp-Lang Path, Bemidji Regional Interdis Council, **SLP**

Lavriha, Nancy Anne Ntid At Rit 1 Lomb Mem Dr, P O Box 9887, Lbj-2241, Rochester, NY 14623-0887, (716) 475-6413, BS 82 SUNY - Coll at Geneseo; MA 86 SUNY - Coll at Geneseo; SLP, NTID, **SLP**

Law, Deborah A Hearing Dynamics, 728 Robinson Avenue, San Diego, CA 92103, (619) 294-2506, BA 76 San Diego St Univ; MA 77 San Diego St Univ; Aud, Hearing Dynamics, **A**

Law, Debra L T 7148 Amberwood Lane, Highland, CA 92346, (714) 881-3427, BA 76 Univ of Redlands; MS 77 Univ of Redlands; SLP, San Bernardino City USD, **SLP**

Law, Elaine M 32 Grove Street, Branford, CT 06405, (203) 789-8055, BA 75 Southern CT St Univ; MS 78 Southern CT St Univ; Aud, Hearing Balance & Sp Ctr, **SLP**

Law, Gail E 1531 Dell Dale, Channelview, TX 77530-2141, (713) 527-5499, BS 73 Univ of North TX; MS 75 Univ of North TX; Aud, Park Plaza Hearing Services, **A**

Law, Mrs Kathleen L 445 Blanchard Lake Road, Whitefish, MT 59937, BS 72 Univ of MT; MS 80 Eastern WA Univ; Sp-Lang Path, Sch Dist #44 Whitefish, **SLP**

Law, Mrs Lyana L S 3024 Burnt Mill Road, Charlotte, NC 28210, (704) 366-3282, BA 59 OH St Univ; MA 61 Case Western Reserve Univ; SLP/Aud, Charlotte Mecklenberg Sch, **SLP A**

Law, Mrs Marilyn Ayers 1902 Angels Hollow, Tallahassee, FL 32308, MS 76 FL St Univ; Sp-Lang Path, John S Rose and Associates, **SLP**

Law, Patricia L 4001 West Eva, Phoenix, AZ 85021, **SLP**

Law, Mrs Sibylla M 5537 Cajon, Buena Park, CA 90621, (714) 522-6131, BS 66 Univ of MN - Minneap-St Paul; MS 74 Vanderbilt Univ; Resource Spec/Admin, Centralia Schl Dist, **SLP**

Lawhead, Douglas R 5325 Dole Road, Myrtle Creek, OR 97457, (503) 440-4031, BA 73 Humboldt St Univ; MA 77 Humboldt St Univ; SLP, Roseburg PS, **SLP**

Lawler, Mrs Marcia Putzel 2505 Cockrell, Fort Worth, TX 76109, (817) 923-1098, BA 70 Univ of North TX; MA 73 Univ of North TX; **SLP**

Lawler, Terri Ann 131 Cherry Hill Avenue, Goose Creek, SC 29445, (803) 572-1738, BS 81 Coll of Saint Rose; MS 83 Univ of SC - Columbia; 88–Sp-Lang Path, Berkeley Co Schs, **SLP**

Lawless, Kimberly H 325 Transylvania Park, Lexington, KY 40508, (606) 255-6841, BA 78 Univ of KY; MA 81 Univ of Cincinnati; Aud, Lexington Cl, **A**

Lawless-Lane, Charlene Ann 14 Decatur, Gloucester, MA 01930, (617) 281-0452, MS 86 Northeastern Univ; **SLP**

Lawlor, Mrs Josephine Losito 1206 Doris Avenue, Wanamassa, NJ 07712, (201) 946-1811, BA 71 Adelphi Univ; MS 72 Adelphi Univ; Sp-Lang Path, Holmdel Bd of Ed, **SLP**

Lawrence, Mrs Barbara Cullen 320 High Meadow Drive, Marietta, GA 30067, (404) 993-6947, BS 75 Univ of FL; MS 77 Univ of MN - Minneap-St Paul; 77–Sp-Lang Path, Fulton County Board of Educ, **SLP**

Lawrence, Dr Carol W 945 Mull Avenue, Apartment PH2, Akron, OH 44313, (216) 375-6803, BS 70 OH St Univ; MA 72 Kent St Univ; PH 80 (Sp Path) Kent St Univ; 85–Associate Professor, University of Akron, **SLP**

Lawrence, Clara Jane 2637 R Suffolk Avenue, High Point, NC 27260, (919) 885-5161, BS 84 Appalachian St Univ; MA 86 Appalachian St Univ; 86–Sp-Lang Path, High Point PS, **SLP**

Lawrence, Mrs Cynthia Louise 7554 Iron Horse Lane, Indianapolis, IN 46256, (317) 924-4374, BS 81 Ball St Univ; MA 82 Ball St Univ; 85–Audiologist, Indiana School for the Deaf, **A**

Lawrence, Dr Donald L 10713 West 70th Terrace, Shawnee, KS 66203, (816) 561-4423, BA 59 Univ of WY; MS 60 Univ of WI - Madison; PH 67 (NS) LA St Univ - Baton Rouge; Aud, **SLP A**

Lawrence, Mrs Francine M 3652 Anderson Parkway, Toledo, OH 43613, (419) 243-9311, BS 68 Bowling Green St Univ; MA 69 Bowling Green St Univ; Sp-Lang Path, Toledo Pub Sch, **SLP**

Lawrence, Dr Frank R 2536 Ramsay Way, Fairfield, CA 94533, (707) 422-8330, BS 51 Univ of OR; MA 61 San Francisco St Univ; ED 75 (Educ Admin) Nova Univ; 60–Sp-Lang Path, Offi of Solano Co Supt of Sch, **SLP**

Lawrence, Jacqueline Deirdre 45 Ridout Street S Upper, London, ON, Canada N6C 3W8, (519) 336-1500, OM 83 Univ of Western Ontario; **SLP**

Lawrence, Jan J 12091 Sky Lane, Santa Ana, CA 92705, (714) 997-3023, BA 71 UT St Univ; MA 72 UT St Univ; **SLP**

Lawrence, Kimberly Ann Route 7 Box 183, Dothan, AL 36301, (205) 665-3259, BS 85 Univ of Montevallo; MS 86 Univ of Montevallo; **SLP**

Lawrence, Lois K 3583 Herschel Street, Jacksonville, FL 32205, (904) 272-0557, BA 76 George Washington Univ; MS 78 FL St Univ; SLP, Clay Co Sch Bd, **SLP**

Lawrence, Suzanne M 708 Elkmont Road, Knoxville, TN 37922-3650, (615) 624-1533, BS 77 Boston Univ; MA 79 Univ of TN - Knoxville; Sp-Lang Path, Forrt Sanders Regional Med Ctr, **SLP**

Lawrence, Mrs Telete Z 3860 South Hills Circle, Fort Worth, TX 76109, (817) 927-2339, BA 32 Univ of CA - Berkeley; MA 63 TX Christian Univ; **SLP LM**

Lawrence, Teresa Gail 1066 South Line Street, Grenada, MS 38901, (601) 226-8900, BS 82 Univ Southern MS-Hattiesburg; MS 84 Univ Southern MS-Hattiesburg

Lawrence, Thomas George 505 Euclid Street, Grandview, WA 98930-1522, BA 74 Western OR St Coll; ME 77 Western OR St Coll; SLP, Grandview School Dstr, **SLP**

Lawrence, Mrs Wanda Sue 3518 Stanton Drive, Lee's Summitt, MO 64063, (816) 331-2131, BA 73 Evangel Coll; MS 86 Central MO St Univ; **SLP**

Lawrence-Dederich, Susan Michele 305 Westgate Road, Kenmore, NY 14217, (716) 873-1578, MA 87 SUNY - Center at Buffalo; 87–Sp-Lang Path, Erie #1 BOCES, **SLP**

Lawrie, Patricia Marie S 1168 North Del Sol Lane, Diamond Bar, CA 91765, (714) 988-8511, BA 76 CA St Univ - Fullerton; MA 79 CA St Univ - Fullerton; Sp-Lang-Hrng Spec, Chaffey Joint Uhs Dist, **SLP**

Laws, Dr Douglas W University Of Wyoming, Box 3311 University Sta, Laramie, WY 82071, (307) 766-6426, BS 67 Brigham Young Univ; MS 68 Brigham Young Univ; PH 76 (Diagnostic Aud) Univ of NE - Lincoln; Dir of Aud, U of WY, **A**

Lawson, Audrey C 3717 East 2nd Street #5, Long Beach, CA 90803, BA 83 CA St Univ - Chico; MA 86 Univ of CA - Santa Barbara; **SLP**

Lawson, Mrs Cathy S 4316 Ponce, McHenry, IL 60050, (815) 338-7411, BS 75 AR St Univ; OM 76 AR St Univ; Coord Sp-Lang Serv, Sp Ed Dist of McHenry Co, **SLP**

Lawson, Mrs Cynthia King 4345 Cider Mill Drive, Cincinnati, OH 45245, (513) 553-3181, BS 82 Univ of Cincinnati; MA 84 Univ of Cincinnati; Sp-Lang Path, New Richmond Schs, **SLP**

Lawson, Mrs Donna H 6004-A Westcreek Drive, Austin, TX 78749, (512) 892-4702, BS 67 Univ of Houston - Univ Park; MA 69 Univ of Houston - Univ Park; Sp-Lang Path, Austin ISD, **SLP**

Lawson, Mrs Dorothy M 11201 Country Place, Oakton, VA 22124, (703) 620-2407, BA 59 Sweet Briar Coll; ME 61 Emory Univ; Sp-Lang Path, Sp & Lang Ctr of N VA, **SLP**

Lawson, Mrs Elisabeth M 4610 West Clifford Street, Tampa, FL 33611, BA 71 WV Univ; ME 75 Univ of NC - Greensboro; **SLP**

Lawson, Mrs Gail Marie Cook 531 Somerville, Tonawanda, NY 14150, (716) 833-7598, BS 75 SUNY - Coll at Buffalo; MS 77 SUNY - Coll at Buffalo; Sp-Lang Path, St Mary's Sch for Deaf, **SLP**

Lawson, Gary D 2608 Strathmore, Kalamazoo, MI 49009, (616) 383-0963, BA 64 Univ of TN - Knoxville; MA 69 Univ of TN - Knoxville; PH 80 (NS) MI St Univ; Assoc Prof, Western MI Univ, **SLP A**

Lawson, Mrs Jane Withers 1571 Beacon Hill Road, Lexington, KY 40504, (606) 233-3789, BA 63 Univ of KY; MA 69 Univ of KY; Sp-Lang Path, Private Practice, **SLP**

Lawson, Janet Lee 29 Crooks, Loma Linda, CA 92354, (714) 796-8929, BS 75 Pacific Union Coll; MA 78 Loma Linda Univ - Riverside; SLP, Fontana USD, **SLP**

Lawson, Jeanne Marie 3160 Linwood Avenue, Apartment 203, Cincinnati, OH 45208, (513) 321-4631, BS 83 OH Univ - Athens; MS 86 Miami Univ - Oxford; **SLP**

Lawson, Kathryn Chaffin 435 East Nelson Avenue, Alexandria, VA 22301, (703) 549-2573, BA 85 Mary Washington Coll; MS 87 James Madison Univ; InSpeech Inc, **SLP**

Lawson, Kris A 490 Golf Club Road, Pleasant Hill, CA 94523-5856, (415) 682-9000, Sp-Lang Path, California Ctr Rehabiltn Servs, **SLP**

Law-Till, Cindy B Daniel Freeman Memorial Hosp, Dept Of Communication Dis, 333 North Prairie Avenue, Inglewood, CA 90301, (213) 674-7050, BA 80 Univ of CA - Santa Barbara; MA 82 Northwestern Univ; Sp/Lang Path, Daniel Freeman Mem Hosp, **SLP**

Lawton, Ellen Lynn 778 Old Brook Road, Charlottesville, VA 22901, (804) 924-8245, BS 81 FL St Univ; MS 83 FL St Univ; SLP, Southeastern Sp Hrng Serv, **SLP**

Lawton, Joan S 200 Winston Drive #1916, Cliffside Park, NJ 07010, (201) 894-3287, BS 77 NY Univ; MS 78 Columbia Univ Teachers Coll; SLP, Private Practice, **SLP**

Lawton, Kathleen W Baptist Medical Center, Speech Pathology Service, 3300 N W Expressway, Oklahoma City, OK 73112, (405) 949-3280, BS 67 Duke Univ; MS 75 Univ of OK Medical Center; Dir-SLP Serv, Baptist Med Cen, **SLP**

Lawton, Suzan Pflug 333 Arnold Street, Reese AFB, Lubbock, TX 79416, (806) 885-2680, BS 74 Emerson Coll; ME 79 Northeastern Univ; 88–Sp-Lang Path, Lubbock State Sch, **SLP**

Lawyer, Mrs Sharon Harmes Rd #1, East Fairfield, VT 05448, (802) 868-4457, BA 82 Univ of VT; MS 84 Univ of VT; Sp-Lang Path, Franklin NW/NE Ess Early Ed, **SLP**

Lax, Linda Sue 4583 Fairway Ridge, West Bloomfield, MI 48033, (313) 855-1888, BA 69 Univ of MI - Ann Arbor; MS 70 Univ of MI - Ann Arbor; Sp-Lang Path, Private Practice, **SLP**

Lay, Christine L 308-180 Cherryhill Circle, London, ON, Canada, (519) 432-8858, OM 88 Univ of Western Ontario

Lay, Deborah Anne 3222-5 Selwyn Farms Lane, Charlotte, NC 28209, (704) 333-6634, BA 80 Univ of NC - Chapel Hill; MA 82 Univ of TN - Knoxville; SLP, Charlotte Rehab Hosp, **SLP**

Lay, Jacqueline 9417 Jane Court, Lake Elmo, MN 55042, (612) 293-8745, BS 70 Univ of WI - River Falls; MS 79 Univ of WI - River Falls; **SLP**

Lay, Karen Susan 3215 E 98th Avenue, Thornton, CO 80229, (303) 289-2208, BA 86 Univ of Northern CO; BA 86 Univ of Northern CO; MA 87 Univ of Northern CO; 88–Spec Educ Tchr, Mapleton PS Dist #1

Lay, Mary Francis 192 Safe Harbor, Goodlettsville, TN 37072, (615) 451-1662, MA 85 Eastern MI Univ; BS 83 Eastern MI Univ; **SLP**

Lay, Ruth Ann 1500 East 10th #7-B, Winfield, KS 67156, (316) 221-7519, BA 76 Wichita St Univ; MA 77 Wichita St Univ; 86–Sp-Lang Path, Serendipity Spec Purpose Sch, **SLP**

Lay, Dr Thomas N 3601 Lindell Boulevard, St Louis, MO 63103, (314) 658-2588, PH 64 (Communication Disorders) North Park Coll; 88–Prof, St Louis Univ, **SLP**

Laycob, Carol L 4 Greenridge Road, Englewood, CO 80111, (303) 773-6861, BA 83 Univ of Denver; MA 85 Univ of Denver; 88–Sp-Lang Path, Janet Haglund

Layden, Doris L 1071 Farmington Avenue, West Hartford, CT 06107, BA 51; MA 74; SLP, Hartford Pub Schs, **SLP**

Layes, Mrs Holly R Davis Route 2 Box 1780, Paris, AR 72855, OM 88 Univ of Central AR; 88–Sp-Lang Path, Mansfield PS

Layne, Martha A Industrial Audiology, 1 Portland Pier, Portland, ME 04101, (207) 775-1364, BS 70 OH Univ - Athens; MA 71 OH Univ - Athens; Owner, Indust Aud, **A**

Layte, Donna L 16 West Chardon Road, Winchester, MA 01890, (617) 720-6730, BS 75 Emerson Coll; MS 76 Columbia Univ Teachers Coll; Asst Dir/Sp-Lang Path Dept, Spaulding Rehab Hosp, **SLP**

Layton, Mrs Carolyn D 115 Kencrest Drive, Gulfport, MS 39503, (601) 832-2701, BS 64 Univ Southern MS-Hattiesburg; MS 76 Univ Southern MS-Hattiesburg; Sp-Lang Path, Harrison Co Sch Syst, **SLP**

Layton, Mrs Donna K William Monroe Elem School, Monroe Drive, Stanardsville, VA 22973, (804) 985-2580, BS 76 Univ of VA - Charlottesville; MS 84 James Madison Univ; Sp-Lang Path, Greene Co Sch Sys, **SLP**

Layton, Dr Thomas L 5727 Williamsburg Way, Durham, NC 27713, (919) 966-1006, BS 66 Univ of NE - Lincoln; MA 68 Univ of NE - Lincoln; PH 76 (NS) Univ of NE - Lincoln; Assoc Prof, U Div Sp & Hrng Sci, **SLP**

Lazar, Gloria Schertz 3 School Street Suite 206, Glen Cove, NY 11542, (516) 674-3900, MA 87 Columbia Univ Teachers Coll; 88–Sp-Lang Path, Private Practice, **SLP**

Lazar, Mrs Sandra E 9856 Middle Meadow Road, Ellicott City, MD 21043, (301) 674-2241, BA 67 SUNY - Center at Buffalo; MS 73 Towson St Univ; Sp-Lang Path, Anne Arundel County Pub Sch, **SLP**

Lazaros, Mrs Sandra L 18409 Sandringham Court, Northridge, CA 91326, (805) 251-2901, BA 76 CA St Univ - Northridge; MA 79 CA St Univ - Northridge; SLP, Los Angeles, **SLP**

Lazarov, Debbie Sue 155 N Rembert, Memphis, TN 38104, (901) 454-1333, BS 83 Boston Univ; MA 85 Memphis St Univ; **SLP**

Lazar-Reskakis, Julie 80 Oak Street, Teaneck, NJ 07666, (212) 360-3716, BA 79 Alfred Univ; MS 83 Adelphi Univ; 86–Aud, Terence Cardinal Cooke Hlth Care Ctr, **A**

Lazarus, Mrs Barbara A 38 Gordon Avenue, Shelton, CT 06484-4411, (203) 735-7048, BA 76 Southern CT St Univ; MS 79 Southern CT St Univ; Sp-Lang Path, Monroe Ct Bd of Ed, **SLP**

Lazarus, Cathy L Northwestern University Medical School, 303 East Chicago Avenue, Ward 3-140, Chicago, IL 60611, (312) 908-8035, BS 79 Northwestern Univ; MA 80 Northwestern Univ; 80–Sp-Lang Path, Northwestern U, **SLP ACE**

Lazarus, Gloria J 3333 N W 54th Avenue, Gainesville, FL 32606, (904) 336-2710, BA 73 Univ of FL; ME 75 Univ of FL; Sp-Lang Path, Alachua Co Sch Bd, **SLP**

Lazarus, Susan B 250 West 103rd Street #5A, New York, NY 10025, (212) 678-3409, BS 75 Syracuse Univ; MS 79 Columbia Univ Teachers Coll; Aud, Teachers Coll Columbia Univ, **A**

Lazarus, Susan Beth 12 Olympia Lane, Stony Brook, NY 11790, (516) 751-5638, BA 85 SUNY - Coll at Plattsburgh; MS 86 Ithaca Coll; **SLP**

Lazenby, Mrs Blake B 3910 Wayland Drive, Nashville, TN 37215, (615) 320-5353, BS 65 Univ of TN - Knoxville; MS 69 Vanderbilt Univ; 69–Aud/Coor, Bill Wilkerson Hrng & Sp Ctr, **A**

Lazer, Dianne Ellen 4540-B Lakeside North, Columbus, OH 43232, (614) 252-5200, BA 79 OH St Univ; MA 82 Hofstra Univ; Sp-Lang Path, Ctrl Islip Psychi Cen, **SLP**

Lazere, Mrs Jane P 1220 S W Morrison, Suite 805, Portland, OR 97205, (503) 223-3238, BS 65 Emerson Coll; MS 69 Portland St Univ; **SLP**

Lazerov, Florence Elise 1312 Mc Dowell, Naperville, IL 60540, (312) 717-9167, BA 85 IN Univ - Bloomington; MA 87 Northern IL Univ - De Kalb

Lazerson-Ross, Mrs Susan Gail 2573 Piccadilly Circle, Thousand Oaks, CA 91362, (805) 498-3686, MA 84 CA St Univ - Northridge; SLP, Conejo Valley USD, **SLP**

Lazich, Richard W c/o Drs Cohen/Silk Psc, 225 Abraham Flexner Way, Apartment 401, Louisville, KY 40202-1817, (502) 583-9425, BA 77 IN Univ - Bloomington; MA 79 IN Univ - Bloomington; Aud, Cohen and Silk, **A**

Lazik, Michael Jerome 8740 Boyce Road, Corfu, NY 14036, (716) 674-6300, **SLP**

Lazor, Mrs Judy L 333 Olenview Circle East, Powell, OH 43065, (614) 293-8065, BA 79 OH St Univ; MA 81 OH St Univ; Aud, Ohio St U, **A**

Lazowski, Laura Elizabeth 5114 North Wolcott #2-N, Chicago, IL 60640, (312) 334-1739, MS 83 Univ of WI - Madison, **A**

Le, Tuyet Mai Thi 49 Howard Street, Pompton Lakes, NJ 07442, (914) 358-6200, MS 84 William Paterson Coll; BA 79 Univ of DE; 86–Sp-Lang Path, Nyack Hosp, **SLP**

Lea, Joan Pickens 208 Patti Drive, Westerville, OH 43081, (614) 263-2448, OB 64 OH Univ - Athens; MA 85 OH St Univ; **SLP**

Lea, Leeanne Joy 1404 Timberidge Drive, Bethel Park, PA 15102, (412) 831-7042, BA 83 Muhlenberg Coll; MS 85 Columbia Univ Teachers Coll; **SLP**

Lea, Mrs Sue Ellen 138 Keifer Street, Owosso, MI 48867, (517) 723-2375, BS 77 Central MI Univ; MA 87 Central MI Univ; 85–Sp-Lang Path, Shiawassee Inter Schs, **SLP**

Leach, Mrs Carol N 221 Riverdale Drive, Durham, NC 27712, (919) 383-8854, BA 75 Univ of NC - Greensboro; ME 76 Univ of NC - Greensboro; 88–Sp-Lang Path, Durham City Schs, **SLP**

Leach, Clifford J Dogwood Drive Box 1, Centerbrook, CT 06409, **SLP**

Leach, Dr Edwin A Dept Communications, Pan American University, Edinburg, TX 78539-2999, (512) 381-3587, BA 56 Millikin Univ; MA 58 Southern IL Univ -Carbondale; PH 65 (NS) Univ of KS; Dir-Sp & Hrng Prog, Pan American Univ, **SLP F**

Leach, Helen M 5537 Dumfries Court E, Dublin, OH 43017, (614) 761-0164, BS 70 James Madison Univ; MA 72 OH Univ - Athens; Sp-Lang Path, Hudson Local Sch, **SLP**

Leach, Mrs Judy S 1603 Pecan Street, Nokomis, FL 34275, (813) 484-3908, MS 72 Univ of South FL; **SLP**

Leach, Mrs Linda R 32288 Avenue 12, Madera, CA 93638, BA 73 Univ of the Pacific; MA 74 Univ of the Pacific; Sp-Lang Path, Madera Co Supt of Schs, **SLP**

Leach, Marilyn M Univ Of N E Ctr For Faculty Development, A & S #217, 60th & Dodge, Omaha, NE 68182-0050, (402) 554-2427, BA 57 Southern IL Univ -Carbondale; MA 62 Univ of KS; Dir-Cen for Faculty Dev, U NE-Omaha, **SLP**

Leach, Mary S 801 Wilson Drive, New Orleans, LA 70119, (504) 443-1604, BA 70 Southeastern LA Univ; OM 77 LA St Univ - N O Medical Ctr; Sp-Lang Path, Jefferson Parish Sch Bd, **SLP**

Leach, Mrs Susan M 7235 M 119, Harbor Springs, MI 49740, (616) 526-6673, BS 65 Univ of MN - Duluth; MA 68 Western MI Univ; **SLP**

Leacy, Mrs Lorelle Barrett 1108 North Cedar Street, Tacoma, WA 98406, **SLP**

Leadbitter, Elizabeth 6116 Kemberly Street, Columbia, SC 29209, (803) 776-4000, MS; **A ACE**

Leaden, Lynn Wagner 55 Woodridge Road, Hampton Bays, NY 11946, (516) 728-0368, BS 84 SUNY - Coll at Geneseo; MA 86 CUNY - Lehman Coll; **SLP**

Leader, Barbara J 6 West 77th Street #15B, New York, NY 10024, (718) 780-1281, BA 71 CUNY - Queens Coll; MA 74 CUNY - Hunter Coll; 86–Dir of Sp-Lang Path, Long Island Coll Hosp, **SLP ACE**

Leaders, Mrs Linda 137 Heather Ridge Road, Battle Creek, MI 49017, (616) 965-9446, BS 72 IN St Univ - Terre Haute; MS 74 IN St Univ - Terre Haute; 85–Spec Educ Supvr, Battle Creek Pub Sch, **SLP**

Leadford, Mrs Julia Hensley 1412 Denson Drive, Pauls Valley, OK 73075, (405) 238-6760, BA 82 OK St Univ; MA 84 OK St Univ; Sp-Lang Path, Pauls Valley PS, **SLP**

Leadon, Margaret Rose 412 N E 13th Avenue, Gainesville, FL 32601, (904) 372-7672, BA 80 Coll of Saint Catherine; MA 86 Univ of FL; **SLP**

Leaf, Antony 1801 Chaparral Road, Santa Rosa, CA 95404, (707) 527-5585, BS 74 OR St Univ; MS 78 Western OR St Coll; Real Estate Broker, Own Office, **SLP**

Leaf, Mrs Kim D 6914 Floyd, Overland Park, KS 66204, (816) 932-3262, OB 84 Univ of KS; MA 87 Univ of KS; 87–Sp-Lang Path, St Lukes Hosp of KS City, **SLP**

Leaf, S Michael William F Herholtz Inc, 708 North Tejon Street, Suite C, Colorado Springs, CO 80903, (303) 635-9966, BA 74 Fort Hays St Univ; MA 75 Wichita St Univ; Aud, Private Practice, **A**

Leafstedt, Carla Hagemeyer 809 Blue Ridge Drive, Edmond, OK 73034, (405) 271-8046, BS 84 Univ of SD - Vermillion; MA 86 Univ of SD - Vermillion; 87–Sp-Lang Path, Unif of OK Coll of Med ENT Dept, **SLP**

League, Roslynn P 230 Arlington Road North, Jacksonville, FL 32211, (904) 725-8972, MS 65 Univ of MI - Ann Arbor; 76–Sp-Lang Path, S Allen Smith Clinic, **SLP**

Leahy, Mrs Deborah 8 Lincoln Street, Stoneham, MA 02180, (617) 623-3480, BA 77 Suffolk Univ; ME 80 Northeastern Univ; Sp-Lang Path, **SLP**

Leahy, Mrs Jane Dennis 512 Crescent Drive, Midland, MI 48640, (517) 774-3471, MA 83 Central MI Univ; 87–Clin Supvr, Cen Mich Univ, **SLP ACE**

Leahy, Mrs Patricia M 844 South 76th Street, West Allis, WI 53214, (414) 259-0606, BS 76 Univ of WI - Milwaukee; MS 77 Univ of WI - Milwaukee; Sp-Lang Path, Private Practice, **SLP**

Leake, Guy Dudley, Jr Department Of Speech, Louisiana Tech University, P O Box 3165, Ruston, LA 71272, (318) 257-4764, BA 60 LA Tech Univ; MA 62 Univ of AL- Tuscaloosa; Head of Sp-Lang Path, LA Tech U, **SLP A**

Leake, Mrs Harriet B 201 East Arizona Avenue #1, Ruston, LA 71270, (318) 247-3721, MA 54 LA St Univ - Baton Rouge; MA 66 LA Tech Univ; MA 75 LA Tech Univ; Sp-Lang Path, Ruston St Sch, **SLP**

Leake, Linda S 4407 Sunscape Lane, Raleigh, NC 27612, (919) 876-1401, BS 68 Western MI Univ; MA 74 Wayne St Univ; Dir/Owner, Private Practice, **SLP**

Leaks, Denise 1332 North Lockwood, Chicago, IL 60671, BS 77 IL St Univ - Normal; OM 86 Governors St Univ; **SLP**

Leal, Sr Lourdes 1622 East Jackson, Harlingen, TX 78550, (512) 428-6111, BA 60 Our Lady Lake Univ-San Anton; MA 64 Our Lady Lake Univ-San Anton; PH 69 (Communication Disorders) Univ of OK Medical Center; 87–Pastoral Asst, St Anthony Harlingen, **SLP**

Leamy, Donald P Ventura Hearing & Speech Cen, 2674 East Main Street, Suite 1, Ventura, CA 93003, BA 68 Univ of MO - Columbia; MA 73 CA St Univ - Long Beach; Director, Ventura Hearing & Speech Cen, **A**

Leaney, A Pearl 2125 Topaz Street, Clearbrook, BC, Canada V2T 3W7, (604) 853-1293, BS 84 Univ of Alberta - Alberta; MS 86 Univ of Western Ontario; **SLP**

Lear, Dorothy Ann 1860 West Navarro, Mesa, AZ 85202, BS 71 UT St Univ; MS 73 UT St Univ; Sp-Lang Path, Mesa Pub Schls, **SLP**

Learman, Lindsay McIntyre 515 South Linwood Beach, Linwood, MI 48634, (517) 697-3369, BA 82 MI St Univ; MS 85 Marquette Univ; 85–Sp-Lang Path, St Mary's Med Ctr, **SLP**

Learned, Mrs Helen S 1065 Gulf Of Mexico Drive, Apartment 505, Longboat Key, FL 34228, (813) 383-2295, BS 68 AZ St Univ; MS 72 Univ of South FL; Sp/Lang Path, Florida Commun Cen, **SLP**

Leary, Judith E Box 1595, APO New York, NY 09179, (203) 442-6179, **SLP**

Leary, Kimberly Anne 4634 South Frasier Court, Apartment B, Aurora, CO 80015, (303) 320-2140, MS 84 CO St Univ; **SLP**

Leary, Martha H 54 Mackenzie Crescent, Toronto, ON, Canada M6J 1T1, (416) 968-7877, BS 70 SUNY - Coll at Brockport; MA 74 SUNY - Coll at Geneseo; Sp-Lang Path, Private Practice, **SLP**

Leath, Laurie Jones 70 Country Club Drive, Danville, IL 61832, (217) 443-5275, BS 84 Univ of IL - Urbana; MA 86 Univ of IL - Urbana; Chief of Aud, United Samaritans Med Ctr, **A**

Leatherwood, Elaine M 3705 Medical Parkway #320, Austin, TX 78705, (512) 454-0392, BS 79 Univ of TX - Austin; MA 83 Univ of TX - Austin; Aud, Austin Ear Nose Throat Clinic, **A**

Leavell, Suanne M 546 Atkins Street, Shreveport, LA 71104, (318) 227-5156, BS 68 LA St Univ - Baton Rouge; MA 70 Univ of TN - Knoxville; Instructor, Lousiana State Univ Med Center, **SLP**

Leaver, Mrs Kathleen Ann 1226 Talcott Street, Fort Atkinson, WI 53538-2725, (414) 563-7115, BS 84 Univ of WI - Stevens Point; MS 85 Univ of WI - Stevens Point; **SLP**

Leavitt, Jane Freiberg Beachwood City Schools, 24601 Fairmount Blvd, Beachwood, OH 44122, (216) 464-2600, BA 75 MI St Univ; MA 77 Case Western Reserve Univ; 78–Aud, Beachwood Bd of Ed, **A**

Leavitt, Mrs Nancy J R 195 Steamboat Road, Great Neck, NY 11024, (516) 783-9515, BA 65 KS Wesleyan; MS 78 Adelphi Univ; SLP, Wantagh Pub Sch, **SLP**

Leavitt, Phillip A 2240 Denevi Drive, Sparks, NV 89431, (702) 359-3643, BS 71 Weber St Coll; MS 87 Univ of NV - Reno

Leavitt, Ron J University Of Texas Austin, Dept Of Sp Commun & Disord, Austin, TX 78712-1089, (512) 471-3841, MS 78; Aud, Tacoma Ps, **A**

Lebel, Mrs Debra Karen 176 Little East Neck Rd S, Babylon, NY 11702, (516) 567-8518, BA 79 Adelphi Univ; MS 80 Adelphi Univ; Sp-Lang Path, BOCES #2/Suffolk, **SLP**

Lebel Curran, Mrs Jana M 95 Starboard Drive, Cape Elizabeth, ME 04107, (207) 799-1871, BS 82 Boston Univ; MS 83 Univ of VT; 88–Sp-Lang Path, Cape Elizabeth Sch Sys, **SLP**

Leberknight, Jean C 4401 Old Farm Road, Baldwin, MD 21013, (301) 592-2058, BS 64 Bloomsburg Univ of PA; ME 67 PA St Univ - Univ Park; **SLP**

Le Blanc, Mrs Barbara M 12503 Jim Babin Road, St Amant, LA 70774, (504) 647-7949, BS 72 LA St Univ - Baton Rouge; MA 85 LA St Univ - Baton Rouge; Coord Sp-Lang Path, Ascension Parish School Board, **SLP**

Leblanc, Denise Pendergast 41 Conant Street, Danvers, MA 01923, (617) 774-3386, BA 70 Salem St Coll; ME 83 Northeastern Univ; **A**

Leblanc, Jane H 1305 South Main Street, Jonesboro, AR 72401, (501) 932-6799, OM 82 AR St Univ; MS 68 Vanderbilt Univ; Aud, Wm C Young MD, **SLP A ACE**

Leblanc, Marcelle Catherine 99 Keasler Road, Asheville, NC 28805, (704) 252-2255, BA 78 Nicholls St Univ; MA 85 Western Carolina Univ; 88–Sp-Lang Path, Visiting Health Professionals, **SLP**

Leblanc, Mrs Marie K 538 South Market, Opelousas, LA 70570, (318) 948-8940, BA 73 Univ of Southwestern LA; MS 75 Univ of Southwestern LA; **SLP**

Le Blanc, Sherry A 14641 Stoneberg Avenue, Baton Rouge, LA 70816, (504) 272-6242, BS 64 LA St Univ - Baton Rouge; MA 65 LA St Univ - Baton Rouge; Dir, Assoc III Hrng Sp & Lrng Ctr, **SLP**

LeBlanc, Valerie Foster 38 Lakeside Trail, Kinnelon, NJ 07405, (201) 881-6184, BA 64 Catholic Univ of America; MA 66 Univ of CO - Boulder; 85–Coord of Special Services, Paterson Nj Bd of Ed, **SLP ACE**

LeBlanc-Ward, Mrs Linda Fay 2401 Lazy Hollow #129-A, Houston, TX 77063, (713) 783-4564, MS 83 Univ of Southwestern LA; BA 77 Nicholls St Univ; Sp-Lang Path, HealthSouth Rehab Hosp, **SLP**

Le Blon, Deirdre H 34 Hollander Street, South River, NJ 08882, (201) 257-8300, BA 76 Rutger's St Univ - Douglas Coll; MS 77 Columbia Univ Teachers Coll; **SLP**

Lebo, Christina Ann F Fairfax County Public Schools, Camelot Center, 8100 Guinevere Drive, Annandale, VA 22003, (703) 560-5880, BS 73 PA St Univ - Univ Park; MS 75 PA St Univ - Univ Park; 79–Aud, Fairfax Co PS, **A**

Leboeuf, Mrs Julie D Psc Box 4388, APO New York, NY 09057-5374, (501) 661-2328, BS 78 LA St Univ - Baton Rouge; MS 80 Univ of AR - Little Rock; Sp-Lang Path, Private Practice, **SLP**

Lebold, Christine Laurie 1835 Franklin St, Denver, CO 80220, (303) 837-7021, MA 86 Univ of Northern CO; 88–Aud, St Joseph Hosp, **A**

Lebold-Ruska, Mrs Suzanne 1018 Thomas Fox Drive East, North Tonawanda, NY 14120, (716) 282-1836, BS 76 Nazareth Coll of Rochester; MS 78 SUNY - Coll at Buffalo; **SLP**

Leboutillier, Mrs Merrianne L 103 Mariners Cove, Hilton Head, SC 29928, (803) 681-3623, BA 79 Clemson Univ; ME 81 Univ of GA; SLP, Beaufort Co Sch Dist, **SLP**

Lebow, Catherine 3712 Southwest Kelly #3, Portland, OR 97201, (503) 229-7071, BA 75 Univ of CA - Riverside; MA 85 Humboldt St Univ; 88–Sp-Lang Path, Good Samaritan Hosp & Med Ctr, **SLP**

Lebow, Mrs Katherine 808 North Tyrol Trail, Golden Valley, MN 55416, (612) 377-5539, BA 72 Univ of MN - Minneap-St Paul; MA 79 Univ of MN - Minneap-St Paul; **SLP**

Lebowitz, Mrs Sandra S 5 English Ivy Court, Rockville, MD 20854, (301) 279-4955, BA 55 Univ of MD - College Park; MA 67 Univ of MD - College Park; 86–Supvr, Montgy Co PS Sp-Lang Prog, **SLP**

Lebowitz, Mrs Trudy Eilbaum 2624 Lake Shore Boulevard, Apartment 2171, Euclid, OH 44132, (216) 289-5290, **SLP**

Lebron-Ortiz, Maria G 6905 Taylor Street, Landover Hills, Landover, MD 20784, (202) 576-8608, BA 78 Jersey City St Coll; MS 88 Univ of the DC; 85–Sp-Lang Path, Dist of Columbia PS, **SLP**

Lebrun, Jackie D 826 Foots Creek Road, Gold Hill, OR 97525, (319) 652-5621, BA 78 Univ of CA - Santa Barbara; MA 81 Univ of Northern CO; Audiologist, Klamath Speech & Hearing Cen, **A**

Le Brun, Mrs Karen Lee Colorado Ear Nose & Throat Grp, 2020 Wadsworth Boulevard, Denver, CO 80215, (303) 234-1366, BA 80 Univ of CO - Boulder; MA 81 Univ of Northern CO; Aud, Co ENT, **A**

Leccese, Linda R 110-26 65th Avenue, Forest Hills, NY 11375, (718) 997-0328, BA 74 CUNY - Hunter Coll; MS 76 Southern CT St Univ; 85–Sp-Lang Path, Private Practice, **SLP**

Leccia, Jocelyn M A 471 Nantucket, Naperville, IL 60565, (312) 462-4220, BS 80 Univ of WI - Stevens Point; MS 81 Univ of WI - Stevens Point; Sp-Lnag Path, Marianjoy Rehab Ctr, **SLP**

Lechner, Barbara K 1520 Welsh Hills Road, Granville, OH 43023, (614) 522-2162, BA 60 Marietta Coll; MA 71 OH St Univ; PH 76 (NS) OH St Univ; 80–Administrator, Lang Experience Center, **SLP**

Lechner, Roberta E 544 Galen Drive, State College, PA 16803, (814) 364-1481, BS 58 OH St Univ; MS 71 PA St Univ - Univ Park; Sp Lang Cl, Penns Valley Area Sch Dist, **SLP**

Lecholop, Carol R 13850 Crested Rise, San Antonio, TX 78217, (512) 590-4437, BA 75 Columbia Coll; ME 76 Univ of GA; SLP, **SLP**

Lechtenberg, Mrs Cheryl Lynn 4050 N E 12th Terrace #38, Oakland Park, FL 33334, (305) 566-7565, BS 85 Univ of IA; MS 86 FL St Univ; 88–Aud, Hear X Ltd, **A**

Lechthaler, Denise Ann 1103 Doe Court, Roseville, CA 95678, (916) 782-7532, BS 79 Brigham Young Univ; OM 82 Brigham Young Univ; Sp/Lang Path, Alpine Sch Dist, **SLP**

Leciejewski, Ruth Klonowski 206 North Marvine Avenue, Auburn, NY 13021, (315) 473-4806, BS 82 Marquette Univ; MA 84 Cleveland St Univ; Sp-Lang Path, SUNY Health Science Ctr, **SLP**

Lecks-Chernett, Nancy 2274 Shuford Drive, Dublin, OH 43017, (614) 792-2049, BA 73 Case Western Reserve Univ; MA 75 Case Western Reserve Univ; Aud Super, Toledo Hrng & Sp Ctr, **A**

Leclercq, Mrs Julie P 1625 Westbury Drive, Hoffman Estates, IL 60195, (312) 359-7852, BS 78 IL St Univ - Normal; MS 79 IL St Univ - Normal; **SLP**

Lecomte, Dr Barbara V 159 Briarwood Drive East, Berkeley Heights, NJ 07922, (201) 527-2218, BA 66 Newark St Coll; MA 68 Newark St Coll; PH 83 (Lang Disorders) NY Univ; Asst Prof SLP & Aud, Kean Coll of Nj, **SLP**

Lecrone, Susan Kay 7335 Holly Court, 2nd Floor, River Forest, IL 60305, (312) 366-7664, BS 77 Southern IL Univ -Carbondale; MA 86 Univ of IL - Urbana; **SLP**

L'Ecuyer, Mrs Rebecca Lee 5501 Medow Heights Drive, Shawnee, KS 66226, (913) 441-0037, BS 80 Northeast MO St Univ; MA 82 Univ of KS; Sp-Lang Path, Ks Cty Ks Dist #500, **SLP**

Ledbetter, Dixie Acton 5801 N W 31st Terrace, Oklahoma City, OK 73122, **SLP**

Ledbetter, Mrs Jane Frances Route 2 Box 66, Linneus, MO 64653, (816) 895-5442, BS 76 Northeast MO St Univ; MA 80 Northeast MO St Univ; Sp-Lang Path, Meadville R-IV Pub Sch, **SLP**

Ledbetter, Patricia 2232 Commonwealth Drive, Apartment F, Charlottesville, VA 22901-1537, MS; **SLP**

Ledbetter, Tamra Sue 12609 Whispering Hollow Dr, Oklahoma City, OK 73142, (405) 728-7529, BS 85 Univ of OK - OK City; MS 87 Univ of OK - OK City

Leddo, John J 226 Mill Hill Avenue, Bridgeport, CT 06610, (203) 366-7551, BA 56 CUNY - Brooklyn Coll; MA 58 Wayne St Univ; 74–Dir Dept of Aud, Rehab Cen of En Fairfield Co, **SLP A**

Leddy, Karen A 59 Boston Avenue #2, Worcester, MA 01604, (617) 792-2864, BS 83 Univ of MA - Amherst; MS 87 Emerson Coll; 86–Sp-Lang Path, Harrington Memorial Hosp, **SLP**

Leddy, Mark Hodge 99 Joralemon St #1-A, Brooklyn Heights, NY 11201, (212) 750-6737, BS 84 Trenton St Coll; MS 86 Columbia Univ Teachers Coll; Sp-Lang Path, Goldwater Mem Hosp, **SLP**

Leddy, Mrs Sharon F Wright 529 Olympic Drive, Brandon, MS 39042, (601) 939-8640, BS 83 Delta St Univ; MS 84 Univ Southern MS-Hattiesburg; 88–Sp-Lang Path, Husdpeth Ctr, **SLP**

Leder, Arthur Lawrence 101 Ray Street, Schenectady, NY 12309, (518) 374-9515, BS 76 SUNY - Center at Albany; MS 77 SUNY - Center at Albany; Sp-Lang Path, Bethlehem Central Schs, **SLP**

Leder, Dr Steven B 19 Fairway Drive, Cheshire, CT 06410, (203) 785-2467, BS 74 Ithaca Coll; MA 76 Univ of MD - College Park; PH 83 (Sp-Lang Path) Univ of CT; 88–Sp-Lang Path, Yale-New Haven Hosp, **SLP**

Lederer, Barbara Anne 1431 Park Avenue, Baltimore, MD 21217, (301) 383-9021, BS 85 Towson St Univ; MS 86 Towson St Univ; **SLP**

Lederer, Mrs Barbara Freedman 37 Constantine Place #6, Summit, NJ 07901, (201) 277-1475, BA 60 Kean Coll of NJ; MA 67 Kean Coll of NJ; Sp-Lang Path, Morris Sch Dist, **SLP**

Lederer, Barbra 14 Buckingham Road, Rockville Centre, NY 11570, (516) 536-1007, BS 78 Ithaca Coll; MS 81 Columbia Univ Teachers Coll; Self Employed, **SLP**

Lederman, Mrs Donna G 110 Glenway, Syosset, NY 11791, (516) 935-8322, BA 72 Adelphi Univ; MA 74 Hofstra Univ; Sp-Lang Path, Nassau BOCES, **SLP**

Ledinsky, Judith A 9769 East River Rd North, Olmsted Falls, OH 44138, (216) 235-3401, BA 75 Ursuline Coll; MA 78 Cleveland St Univ; Sp-Lang Path, Cuyahoga Co Bd Ment Retard, **SLP**

Lednicky, Mrs Ann Blaize 4011 Heather Court, Knoxville, TN 37919, (615) 588-6607, BA 84 Southeastern LA Univ; OM 86 LA St Univ - N O Medical Ctr; 87–Sp-Lang Path, Blount Hearing & Sp Svcs Inc, **SLP**

Le Donne, Diana Frances 307 Academy Avenue, Reisterstown, MD 21136, (301) 740-2105, BS 69 Univ of UT; MS 78 Johns Hopkins Univ; MS 83 Loyola Coll; Private Practice, **SLP**

Le Donne, Marianne 702 10th Street #A, St Albans, WV 25177, (304) 727-4517, BS 79 Indiana Univ of PA; ME 85 CA Univ of PA; 86–Sp-Lang Path, Kanawha County Schs, **SLP**

LeDoux, Leonelle M 805 East Tremont Avenue, Charlotte, NC 28203, (704) 375-3894, BA 71 Univ of Southwestern LA; ME 72 Univ of VA - Charlottesville; Sp-Lang Path, Charlotte-Mecklenburg Schs, **SLP**

Le Duc, Judith A 2120 North Fremont #1109, Chicago, IL 60614, (312) 363-6700, MA 71 Univ of IL - Urbana; Sp/Lang Path, Siegal Inst/Reese Hosp/Med Cen, **SLP**

Leduc, Mrs Sandra S 9317 Viento Fuerte Way, La Mesa, CA 92041, (619) 463-7721, BA 72 Univ of Redlands; MA 77 San Diego St Univ; Sp-Lang-Hrng Spec, Lamesa Sprng Valley Sch Dist, **SLP**

Ledvina, Mrs Catherine Anne 823 North Chestnut Avenue, Green Bay, WI 54303, (414) 242-4260, BS 79 Univ of WI - Green Bay; MS 81 Univ of WI - Eau Claire; Sp-Lang Path, Mequon-Thiensville PS, **SLP**

Ledwon-Robinson, Elaine 2100 Independence, Ann Arbor, MI 48104, (313) 936-7080, BA 73 Univ of MI - Ann Arbor; MS 74 Univ of MI - Ann Arbor; Dir Sp-Lang Path, University of Michigan Med Cen, **SLP**

Lee, Ann S 1801 West Church, Mena, AR 71953, (501) 394-6091, BA 76 Univ of KY; MA 81 OH St Univ; **SLP**

Lee, Mrs Barbara B 12351 Buckingham, Baton Rouge, LA 70815, (504) 644-8683, BS 61 Southwest MO St Univ; MA 76 LA St Univ - Baton Rouge; ME 83 LA St Univ - Baton Rouge; Aud/Deaf Ed Coord, Ascension Parish Pub Sch, **A**

Lee, Barbara Dean 22 Rachel Drive #1, Jackson, TN, (615) 885-2178, BS 71 East TN St Univ; MS 83 East TN St Univ; Sp-Lang Path, Rebound Inc, **SLP**

Lee, Dr Bonnie Engel 1800 Centennial Lane, Racine, WI 53406, (602) 942-8125, BA 71 Univ of FL; MS 72 PA St Univ - Univ Park; PH 79 (NS) Temple Univ; 87–VP-SLP Svcs, M J Therapy Svcs, **SLP**

Lee, Carol E 308 Bolner Lane, Delrio, TX 78840, BS 67 Southwest TX St Univ; ME 73 Southwest TX St Univ; San Felipe Del Rio Consol ISD, **SLP**

Lee, Carol T 2500 Duncan Street, Columbia, SC 29205, (803) 256-3328, BA 72 Furman Univ; OM 78 Univ of SC - Columbia; Sp-Lang Path, Reach, **SLP**

Lee, Caroline M 50 Laurel Creek, Laguna Hills, CA 92653, (714) 458-0544, MA 88 CA St Univ - Fullerton

Lee, Corinne C 2032 North Clybourn, Chicago, IL 60614, (312) 929-8200, BS 51 Northwestern Univ; MA 57 Northwestern Univ; 58–Dir, Commun Dis, Ctr-Rehab of Persons with Dis, **SLP F ACE**

Lee, Mrs Deborah Ann 1675 Helmsley Way, Arnold, MD 21012, (301) 224-5000, BS 81 Worcester St Coll; MS 85 Loyola Coll; **SLP**

Lee, Mrs Dee Ann H 3045 Ala Napuaa Place, Apartment 1705, Honolulu, HI 96818, (808) 836-7724, BS 85 Univ of HI - Manoa; MA 87 Univ of Northern CO; 86–Sp-Lang Path, Dept of Educ, **SLP**

Lee, Diane M 514 Rue DE La Parc, Slidell, LA 70461, (504) 641-7065, BS 78 Univ of TN - Knoxville; MS 80 Vanderbilt Univ; Sp/Lang Path, Private Practice, **SLP**

Lee, Eileen J 23 Highland Street East, Massapequa, NY 11758, (516) 293-0060, BS 59 Fordham Univ; MS 74 Adelphi Univ; **SLP**

Lee, Geralyn Marie 17 Washburn Street, Centereach, NY 11720, (516) 737-5012, BA 84 Adelphi Univ; MS 85 Adelphi Univ; Sp-Lang Path, St Charles Hosp, **SLP**

Lee, Mrs Heidi Marie 3428 Cove View Blvd #212, Galveston, TX 77551, (409) 761-7383, MA 83 Central MI Univ; 85–Aud, U of TX-Medical Branch, **A**

Lee, Jane 6 Cortez Court, Oakland, CA 94611, (415) 682-6330, **SLP**

Lee, Karen 2089 North Michelle, Sanger, CA 93657, (209) 638-6976, BA 80 CA St Univ - Fresno; MA 82 CA St Univ - Fresno; Sp-Lang Path, Kings Canyon USD, **SLP**

Lee, Mrs Karen M Ogden City Schools, 2444 Adams Bldg 2, Ogden, UT 84401, (801) 625-8742, BA 63 ID St Univ; 88–Dir of Comm Dis, Ogden City Sch, **SLP**

Lee, Mrs Kathleen Collier 461 Calle Poctilla, Camarillo, CA 93010, (805) 987-8621, BS 74 Univ of CA - Davis; MA 76 Univ of the Pacific; Sp-Lang Path, Christian Chruch Sch, **SLP**

Lee, Kathleen D 6736 Walnut Avenue, Pennsauken, NJ 08109, (609) 342-3064, BA 79 Temple Univ; MA 82 Temple Univ; 88–Supvr of Sp-Lang Path, Cooper Hosp/Univ Med Ctr, **SLP**

Lee, Kathleen Kehoe 4514 Loftwood Drive, Owensboro, KY 42303, (812) 426-3353, BS 80 Brescia Coll; MS 84 Western KY Univ; 87–Sp-Lang Path, Deaconess Hosp, **SLP**

Lee, Mrs Kathryn Lyness 1404 Washington Street, Michigan City, IN 46360, (219) 769-8957, BS 80 IN Univ - Bloomington; MS 87 Purdue Univ - West Lafayette

Lee, Lana K 1920 Estelle Drive, Durant, OK 74701, (405) 924-1117, BS 73 Univ of KS; MA 74 Univ of KS; Sp-Lang Path, Durant Public Schools, **SLP**

Lee, Laurie 35 Berlin Street #17, Clinton, MA 01510, (508) 365-2728, MA 88 Univ of MA - Amherst; 88–Aud, Boston Guild for the Hard of Hearing

Lee, Dr Linda University Of Cincinnati, Speech Pathology, Mail Location 379, Cincinnati, OH 45221, (513) 556-4491, BS 74 Univ of WI - Whitewater; MS 76 Univ of WI - Madison; PH 79 (NS) Univ of WI - Madison; Sp-Lang Path, Univ of Cincinnati, **SLP**

Lee, Linda L 3315 Highland, Joplin, MO 64804, (417) 624-7286, BA 73 Univ of OK - Norman; MA 74 Univ of MO - Columbia; SLP, Joplin R-8 School District, **SLP**

Lee, Mrs Loretta B MSHLC, 2300 West Michigan, Suite 8, Midland, TX 79701, (915) 684-4345, BS 72 Abilene Christian Univ; MS 74 Univ of OK Medical Center; Dir, Midland Sp/Hrng/Lang Cen, **SLP**

Lee, Lynne M 6917 Lake Kenilworth Drive, Apartment 102, New Orleans, LA 70126, (504) 483-7690, BA 75 Tulane Univ; OM 76 LA St Univ - N O Medical Ctr; Asst Prof & Cl Superv, Xavier U of La, **SLP**

Lee, May L 2925 East 148th Avenue, Lutz, FL 33549, (813) 977-1846, MS 87 Univ of South FL; Aud, Speech Hearing & Stress Clinic, **A**

Lee, Myra Amy 1716 1st Street, Jacksonville, FL 32225, (904) 575-6198, BS 82 Valdosta St Coll; MS 86 FL St Univ; **SLP**

Lee, Mrs Nancy B 1 Mill River Road, Setauket, NY 11733, (516) 689-9453, BS 73 Ithaca Coll; MS 74 Columbia Univ Teachers Coll; **A**

Lee, Mrs Patricia B 23 Amherst Road, Port Washington, NY 11050, (516) 944-6633, BA 43 Univ of NC - Chapel Hill; MA 67 CUNY - Queens Coll; Sp-Lang Path, Visiting Nurse Assn of LI, **SLP**

Lee, Patricia Clark P O Box 184, Garfield, AR 72732, (501) 451-8827, BS 84 Univ of AR - Fayetteville; MS 85 Univ of AR - Fayetteville; SLP, Ozark Guidance Center, **SLP**

Lee, Patricia Spears 9 Penasco Court, Sacramento, CA 95833, (916) 924-9338, BA 76 Univ of CA - Davis; Specialist Teacher, Public Education, **SLP**

Lee, Rebecca Mance 425 11th Street West, Owen Sound, ON, Canada N4K 3T1, (807) 597-6941, OM 85 Univ of Western Ontario; **SLP**

Lee, Dr Rene Friemoth 1479 Carr Avenue, Memphis, TN 38104, (901) 324-1702, BS 75 Univ of Cincinnati; MA 78 Univ of TX - Austin; PH 85 (NS) Memphis St Univ; Sp-Lang Path, Lee, Stimbert & Associates, **SLP**

Lee, Robert E 2974 Federal Avenue, Alliance, OH 44601, **A**

Lee, Robyn Ladean 646 East 1700 South #10, Salt Lake City, UT 84105, (801) 467-8977, BS 76 UT St Univ; MS 78 UT St Univ; SLP, Davis Co P S, **SLP**

Lee, Sarah Britt 1204 Harrington Drive, Champaign, IL 61821, (217) 351-3866, BS 73 Southern Methodist Univ; MA 74 Univ of IL - Urbana; 88–Sp-Lang Path, Champaign Unit #4 Sch Dist, **SLP**

Lee, Sharon J 436 Redford Lane, Modesto, CA 95350-1025, (213) 273-8480, MA 85 Humboldt St Univ; **SLP**

Lee, Sheila R 7902 South Grove, Wichita, KS 67233, BS 71 MS Univ for Women; MS 72 MS Univ for Women; Ed Coord, I of Logopedics, **SLP**

Lee, Soon-Hee Park Kung Gee DO, Kwachun City, Jugong Apartment 407, Dong, Korea 1102, (904) 375-6759

Lee, Stephanie M 1112 Arlington Place #1, Blue Springs, MO 64015, (417) 866-4849, MA 88 Southwest MO St Univ

Lee, Mrs Susan D 2735 Whitewood Road, Bethlehem, PA 18017, (215) 776-3270, BS 78 WV Univ; MS 79 WV Univ; 87–Asst Dir, Good Shepherd Rehab Hosp, **SLP**

Lee, Mrs Susan E 8940 North Main Street #2, Mc Kean, PA 16426, (814) 453-7661, BS 85 Edinboro Univ of PA; MA 86 Edinboro Univ of PA; SLP, Dr Gertrude A Barber Ctr, **SLP**

Lee, Mrs Susan K T 5810 131st Place S E, Snohomish, WA 98290, (206) 355-4338, BS 77 Univ of WA; MA 79 Western WA Univ; SLP, Seattle Sch Dist, **SLP**

Lee, Teresa Dawn S RR 3 Box 216, Mitchell, IN 47446, (812) 275-3331, BS 75; MS 80; 85–SLP, Dunn Memorial Hosp, **SLP**

Lee, Terry L 506 4th Street S E, Hillsboro, ND 58045, (701) 436-5860, BS 77 Univ of ND; MS 78 Univ of ND; Spec Ed Coord, Gst Ed Svcs, **SLP**

Lee, Virginia G 132 Maple Grove, Springfield, IL 62707, (217) 529-5689, BS 67 Univ of Houston - Univ Park; MA 71; Aud/SLP, Dept of Mental Hlth, **SLP A**

Lee, Wanda W 148 Floral Parkway, Floral Park, NY 11001, **SLP A**

Leeb, Mrs Sherry Samson 9526 Kedvale Avenue, Skokie, IL 60076, (312) 982-1484, BA 77 Yeshiva Univ; MA 84 NY Univ; Self Employed, **SLP**

Leech, Melissa Frances 3523 Greystone Drive #102, Austin, TX 78731, (512) 346-2213, MA 84 Univ of TX - Austin; SLP, Austin ISD, **SLP**

Leeds, Linda Nadelman 1217 Avocado Isle, Fort Lauderdale, FL 33315, (305) 581-3730, BS 67 Boston Univ; MA 72 Univ of MA - Amherst; Sp/Lang Path, Broward Co Pub Sch-FL, **SLP**

Leeds, Sherry Ann 137 Woodridge Road, Kirkwood, MO 63122, (314) 569-8311, BS 55 Washington Univ; OM 79 Webster Univ; Teacher, Special Sch Dist St Louis Co, **SLP A**

Leeds-Horwitz, Susan B 21330 Kingsbury Street, Chatsworth, CA 91311, (805) 257-3550, BA 72 CA St Univ - Northridge; ME 73 Univ of SC - Columbia; OM 84 Univ of LA Verne; 88–Dir of Spec Proj, Castaic Union Sch Dist, **SLP**

Leedy, Mrs Susan C 1314 Byron Street, Huntington, IN 46750, (219) 356-6210, BS 81 Ball St Univ; MA 84 Ball St Univ; Sp-Lang Path, Huntington Co Comm Sch System, **SLP**

Leek, Dr Marjorie R Army Audiology & Speech Center, Walter Reed Army Medical Center, Washington, DC 20307-5001, (202) 576-1685, BA 69 Univ of KS; MA 77 Univ of KS; PH 80 (NS) Univ of KS; 88–Aud, Walter Reed Army Med Ctr, **A**

Leeker, Mrs Linda 880 St Paul Road, St Louis, MO 63021, (314) 569-6640, BA 78 Fontbonne Coll; MA 80 Memphis St Univ; Clin Coord, St John's Mercy Med Ctr, **SLP**

Leelman, Maryellen Alicia 67 Lowell Street, Lexington, MA 02173, **SLP**

Leeman, Mrs Martha Wahl 65 South Milton Avenue, Campbell, CA 95008, (408) 379-4185, BS 61 Univ of VT; ME 65 Boston Univ; Tchr-Deaf/HOH, Santa Clara USD, **SLP**

Leemans, Mrs Christine Marie 220 North 12th Street, Le Claire, IA 52753, (319) 242-6554, BA 81 Augustana Coll; MA 83 Northeast MO St Univ; SLP, Mississippi Bend AEA, **SLP**

Leemhuis, Jane E 135 Chatham Road, Columbus, OH 43214, (614) 272-2000, BA 78 OH St Univ; MA 80 OH St Univ; 87–Dir-Lang Dev, Heinzerling Development Ctr, **SLP**

Leenheers, Mrs Karen Woerner 4240 Clausen Avenue, Western Springs, IL 60558, (312) 246-9025, BS 82 Purdue Univ - West Lafayette; MS 86 Rush Univ; 86–Sp-Lang Path, Saint Margaret Hosp, **SLP**

Leeper, Dr Herbert Andrew, Jr Department Of Communicative Disorders, London, ON, Canada N6G 1H1, (519) 661-2001, BS 63 Bloomsburg Univ of PA; MS 66 Purdue Univ - West Lafayette; PH 69 (Sp Path) Purdue Univ - West Lafayette; Assoc Prof, U of Wn Ontario, **SLP F**

Leeper, Dr Linda H Route 3 Box 169, Versailles, KY 40383, (606) 257-1332, MS 72 Univ of South FL; PH 81 (NS) Univ of FL; Asst Prof, Univ of Kentucky, **SLP**

Leeper, Nancy S 4614 Dundee Drive, Tyler, TX 75703, BA 69 Mary Washington Coll; MS 72 Univ of OK Medical Center; Pre-Schl Tchr, Pollard Method Church, **SLP**

Lees, Andrew B 62 Meander Lane, Southington, CT 06489, (203) 282-3115, BA 68 Montclair St Coll; MA 72 Univ of CT; SLP, E Hartford PS, **SLP**

Lees, Cheryl K Rd 2 Box 182-E, Pleasantville, NJ 08232, (609) 465-2721, BA 74 Rutgers St Univ - Camdem; ME 76 Trenton St Coll; Sp/Lang Path, Cape May Co Spec Ser Sch Dist, **SLP**

Lee-Sheridan, Sharon M 312 Highland Avenue, Morgantown, WV 26505, (304) 292-4780, BS 74 IA St Univ; MS 79 Saint Cloud St Univ; Sp/Lang Path, Minneapolis Publ Schs, **SLP**

Leeson-Forner, Linda P O Box 1116, Chico, CA 95927, (916) 345-2411, MA 84 CA St Univ - Chico; SLP, Stephen Forner MD, **SLP**

Leet, Mrs Sandra P 4066 Phoenix Way, Lilburn, GA 30247-2674, (404) 921-6694, BS 82 James Madison Univ; MS 80 James Madison Univ; Speech Language Pathologist, Davison School, **SLP**

Leever, Karen N 5510 Willow Circle, Fort Worth, TX 76112, (817) 870-1393, BS 75 TX Tech Univ; MS 76 TX Tech Univ; Sp-Lang Path, Speech Pathology Inc, **SLP**

Leever, Lynn C 419 West 4th Suite 700, Odessa, TX 79761, (915) 337-2611, BS 74 TX Tech Univ; MS 75 TX Tech Univ; 88–Sp-Lang Path, Private Practice, **SLP**

Lefebvre, Richard H 201 West Montgomery Street, Johnstown, NY 12095, (518) 725-2117, BS 61 Emerson Coll; MA 67 Coll of Saint Rose; Dept Chmn, Gloversville Enlarged Sch Dist, **SLP**

Lefevre, Mrs Cecily S Dept Comm/Studies CSUS, 801 West Monte Vista, Turlock, CA 95380, (209) 667-3371, BA 71 CA St Univ - Chico; MA 80 Central MI Univ; Asst Professor & Audiologist, California St Univ Stanislaus, **A**

Lefevre, Margaret C 7401 Central Avenue #206, St Petersburg, FL 33710, (813) 347-4250, BA 32 Western MI Univ; MA 46 Univ of MN - Minneap-St Paul; PH 57 (NS) Case Western Reserve Univ; **SLP F LM**

Leff, Mrs Ruth B 6589 North Crestwood Drive, Milwaukee, WI 53209, (414) 351-0311, BS 67 Univ of WI - Milwaukee; MS 68 Univ of WI - Milwaukee; Sp-Lang Path, Private Practice, **SLP**

Leffel, Myra P 225 West 12th Street #2-E, New York, NY 10011, (212) 691-6683, BA 75 SUNY - Coll at Buffalo; MA 76 New York Univ; 86–Sp-Lang Path, Private Practice, **SLP**

Leffke, Gary S Virginia Audiology Associates, 1821 Old Donation Parkway, Suite 7, Virginia Beach, VA 23454, (804) 481-4003, BS 73 SUNY - Coll at Geneseo; MS 75 Univ of WY; Owner, VA Aud Assoc, **A**

Leffler, Mrs Donna Marie 11740 Ivy Lane, Moreno Valley, CA 92387, (714) 242-9262, **SLP**

Leffler, Pamela 4242 Stansbury #105, Sherman Oaks, CA 91423, (818) 788-3762, BA 84 Univ of CA - Santa Barbara; MS 87 Univ of WA; 88–Sp-Lang Path, LA Ctr for Therapy Educ, **SLP**

Lefker, Madeleine Sherwood c/o Sojourner Inn, 605 Gold Star Highway, Groton, CT 06340, (313) 662-9552, BA 81 Univ of MI - Ann Arbor; MA 83 Western MI Univ; Sp-Lang Path, **SLP**

Lefkov, Carol S 4314 Lakeway Drive, Orlando, FL 32809, (305) 422-3200, BA 70 Univ of MD - College Park; MA 74 IN Univ - Bloomington; Sp-Lang Path, Orange County Public Schools, **SLP**

Lefkowitz, Mrs Beverly B 33 Melbury Road, Babylon, NY 11702, (516) 266-5250, BS 60 Boston Univ; MA 67 Temple Univ; Sp-Lang Path, Commack Pub Sch, **SLP**

Lefkowitz, Freya 444 Neptune Avenue, Brooklyn, NY 11224, (718) 859-8850, **SLP**

Lefkowitz, Laurie E 2951 Ocean Avenue #5-C, Brooklyn, NY 11235-3280, **SLP**

Lefkowitz, Nancy G 13 Michael's Green Quail Run, Woburn, MA 01801, (617) 720-6727, BA 70 CUNY - Brooklyn Coll; MS 72 Univ of MI - Ann Arbor; Dir-Sp-Lang Path, Spaulding Rehab Hosp, **SLP ACE**

Lefler, Cynthia Ann 537 Lefler Street, Mountain City, TN 37683, (615) 727-8118, **SLP**

Lefler, Mary Anne 2627 Eagle Avenue, Alameda, CA 94501-1501, **SLP**

Lefort, Claudia A 15 Gate Hill Drive, The Woodlands, TX 77381-3291, (713) 751-4471, **A**

Lefton-Greif, Maureen A 1917 Old Court Road, Baltimore, MD 21204, (301) 821-7484, BA 72 CUNY - Brooklyn Coll; MA 73 Case Western Reserve Univ; PH 88 (Sp Path) Temple Univ; **SLP**

Leftwich, Emily G 101 Lynnbrook Court, Nashville, TN 37215, (615) 832-8955, BA 74 Emory Univ; MS 76 Vanderbilt Univ; Sp/Lang Path, M E Lynch Ms, **SLP**

Lefty, Dianne K 9011 Westmoreland Lane, St Louis Park, MN 55426, (612) 544-2615, BS 64 Univ of AZ; MA 70 San Jose St Univ; Sp-Lang Path, Private Practice, **SLP**

Lege, Mrs Niki Smith 1203 Canal Avenue, Nederland, TX 77627, (409) 832-8326, BS 79 Lamar Univ; MS 81 Lamar Univ; Sp/Lang Path, Beaumont ISD, **SLP**

Legg, Mrs Bonnie Kay 26 Winston Road, East Lyme, CT 06333, (203) 739-4579, BS 67 Univ of KS; MA 68 Univ of KS; Sp-Lang Path, Private Practice, **SLP**

Legg, Mrs Hettie F 1329 University Drive, Nacogdoches, TX 75961, (409) 564-6907, BA 69 Auburn Univ - Auburn; MS 70 MI St Univ; Sp-Lang Path, Private Practice, **SLP**

Legler, Mrs Danielle Michaelene 328 Little John Drive, Schererville, IN 46375, (219) 464-9607, **SLP**

Legler, Mrs Lannie T 25392 Avenida Cappela, Valencia, CA 91355, (805) 259-8833, BA 76 CA St Univ - Northridge; MA 78 CA St Univ - Northridge; MA 82 CA St Univ - Los Angeles; 77–Sp-Lang Path, Los Angeles County Office of Educ, **SLP**

Le Grand, Carol Devine 6 Hagers Mill Court, Manchester, MO 63021, (314) 768-3222, OM 84 Univ of MO - Columbia; 87–Aud, Park Central Institute, **A**

Legrand, Roseanne 172 Carlyle Green, Staten Island, NY 10312, (718) 948-7508, BS 67 CUNY - City College; MA 70 CUNY - City College; Sp-Lang Path, Sp Serv UT-NYC Bd of Ed, **SLP**

Legresley, Mrs Kelly G 4901 Fairwood Boulevard NE #106, Tacoma, WA 98422, (206) 952-6289, BA 81 WA St Univ; MA 82 WA St Univ; 88–Sp-Lang Path, Tacoma Sch Dist #10, **SLP**

Legrow, Lori Novek Callier Ctr For Comm Disorders, University Of Texas, 1966 Inwood Road, Dallas, TX 75235, (214) 783-3060, BS 78 Kent St Univ; MA 78 Kent St Univ; Practicum Super, U of TX/Dallas, **SLP**

Lehenbauer, B Ellen 246 Evelyn Avenue #6, Loves Park, IL 61111, (815) 654-4506, BS 71 Concordia Coll; MA 73 Univ of IL - Urbana; Sp-Lang Path, Harlem Sch Dist #122, **SLP**

Leher, Mrs Phyllis M 3518 Montclair Road, Springfield, OH 45503, (513) 328-2082, BS 72 Miami Univ - Oxford; MA 73 Univ of IL - Urbana; Sp-Lang Path, Springfield City Schs, **SLP**

Lehman, Mrs Annie Laurie H 16511 28th Avenue North, Plymouth, MN 55447, BA 75 Univ of NC - Greensboro; MA 76 Memphis St Univ; SLP, All Speech and Language, **SLP**

Lehman, Mrs Donna Brooks 1805 Mountain Brook Drive, Huntsville, AL 35801, (205) 536-3364, BA 81 Univ of NC - Chapel Hill; MS 82 Univ of NC - Chapel Hill; Sp/Lang Path, Mahone-Cen for Sp & Lang Path, **SLP**

Lehman, Maj Jay W 131 Shenandoah Trail, Robins AFB, Warner Robins, GA 31088, (912) 926-4411, BA 70 FL Southern Coll; ME 72 Seton Hall Univ; 88–Dir, Robins AFB, **A**

Lehman, Jean S 16195 Mt Lowe Circle, Fountain Valley, CA 92708, BS 55 Univ of TX - Austin; MA 73 CA St Univ - Fullerton; Retired, Whittier Cty Sch Dist

Lehman, Karen Jane 4070 S W 173rd Avenue, Beaverton, OR 97007, (503) 251-7433, BA 75 Pacific Univ; MA 76 Pacific Univ; OM 84 Portland St Univ; 87–Aud, Multhomah Co ESD, **A**

Lehman, Kimberly Ann 438 Steele Avenue, Lincoln, NE 68510, (402) 476-2482, BS 79 Univ of NE - Lincoln; MA 81 Univ of NE - Lincoln; Sp-Lang Path, Lincoln Pub Sch, **SLP**

Lehman, Linda Maurer 227 Peel Road, Langhorne, PA 19047, (215) 752-8819, BS 79 West Chester Univ of PA; MA 82 Trenton St Coll; Sp-Lang Path, Bciu #22, **SLP**

Lehman, Mark Edward 3179 Braeburn Circle, Ann Arbor, MI 48108, (313) 973-6541, BA 79 Univ of MI - Ann Arbor; MA 81 Univ of MI - Ann Arbor; PH 87 (Sp-Lang Path) Univ of MI - Ann Arbor; 88–Lecturer, Wayne State Univ, **SLP**

Lehman, Tamra Lea 458 South Spring Road, Westerville, OH 43081, (513) 644-6115, BA 82 OH St Univ; MA 85 OH St Univ; **SLP**

Lehmann, Mrs Billie Kay 3303 N Elmcroft Terrace, Peoria, IL 61604, (309) 686-1724, OB 67 Univ of KY; MS 77 IL St Univ - Normal; MS 86 IL St Univ - Normal; **SLP**

Lehmann, Mrs Joanne Laatsch 110 Hillcrest, Box 123 Ogden Dunes, Portage, IN 46368, (219) 763-4688, Sp-Lang Path, Community School District 303, **SLP**

Lehmann, M Drue 680 Overland #1, Cincinnati, OH 45226, (513) 558-7461, BS 71 Bowling Green St Univ; MA 73 OH St Univ; Phys Med & Rehab, U of Cinti Med Cen, **SLP ACE**

Lehmann, Martha G R 1200 Stonehurst Drive, Huntsville, AL 35801, **SLP**

Lehmann-Epstein, Mrs Carolyn 4040 East 129th Way, Denver, CO 80241, (303) 650-6070, BA 75 Univ of WA; OM 76 Univ of WA; 86–Sp-Lang Path, SD #12 Adams Co, **SLP**

Lehmkuhler, Mrs Elaine R 2206 Howell Street, Dodge City, KS 67801, (316) 227-8002, BS 79 Univ of NE - Lincoln; MA 80 Univ of NE - Lincoln; 84–Sp/Lang Path, SW Kansas Coop, **SLP**

Lehn, Mrs Ann Marie 130 South Ninth Avenue, P O Box 1993, Page, AZ 86040, (602) 645-8801, BS 83 Northern AZ Univ; MS 84 Northern AZ Univ; 85–Sp-Lang Path, Page Uni Sch Dist, **SLP**

Lehne, Mrs Kathryn Audette 100 Arrow Mound, San Antonio, TX 78231, (512) 691-0737, BS 86 Southwest TX St Univ; MS 88 Southwest TX St Univ; 88–Sp-Lang Path, Rehab Inst of San Antonio

Lehner, Leslie H 2323 Lincolnwood Drive, Evanston, IL 60201, BA 70 George Washington Univ; MS 72 Washington Univ; **SLP**

Lehr, Janet S 34 Cranwell Avenue, South Burlington, VT 05401, (802) 862-8789, MS 84 Univ of VT; **SLP**

Lehrer, Mrs Carol M 1229 North Dutton Avenue Suite D, Santa Rosa, CA 95401, (707) 578-1988, BS 79 Wayne St Univ; MA 80 Wayne St Univ; Sp-Lang Path, Speech-Language Pathways Group, **SLP**

Lehrer, Stuart 124 Sycamore Avenue, Freehold, NJ 07728, (201) 431-3313, BA 66 Long Island U - Brooklyn Ctr; MA 68 NY Univ; Dir, Commun Cl, **SLP**

Lehrhaupt, Judith R 1515 Esther Lane, Yardley, PA 19067, (215) 736-0713, BS 67 NY Univ; MA 69 Columbia Univ Teachers Coll; 88–Sp/Lang Path, Trenton St Coll, **SLP**

Lehrhoff, Dr Irwin Wilshire Landmark, 11755 Wilshire Boulevard, Suite 1830, Los Angeles, CA 90025, (213) 477-2497, BA 49 Univ of Southern CA; MA 51 Univ of Southern CA; PH 54 (NS) Univ of Southern CA; Director, Private Practice, **SLP ACE**

Lehrhoff, Terri L 6001 Oakdale Avenue, Woodland Hills, CA 91367, (213) 997-2357, BA 75 Univ of CA - Los Angeles; MA 79 CA St Univ - Northridge; Sp-Lang Path, LA USD, **SLP**

Lehrman, Mrs Aliza 2414 Avenue T, Brooklyn, NY 11229, (718) 763-8300, BA 81 CUNY - Brooklyn Coll; MS 86 CUNY - Brooklyn Coll; **SLP**

Lehrman, Karen E 21313 San Miguel, Woodland Hills, CA 91364, (818) 346-1562, BA 77 SUNY - Coll at Cortland; MA 81 CA St Univ - Northridge; Sp-Lang Path, Los Angeles USD, **SLP**

Lei, Linnea 2430 West Winchcomb Drive, Phoenix, AZ 85023, **SLP**

Leibach, Ronna B 661 Wyngate, Buffalo Grove, IL 60089, BS 74 Univ of IL - Urbana; MS 75 Univ of IL - Urbana; Sp-Lang Path, Northwest Speech Path Assoc, **SLP**

Leibensberger, Gail Ruth 1707 West 8th Street, Irving, TX 75060, (213) 253-7791, MS 88 Univ of North TX

Leibman, Joyce A 6052 Olinger Circle, Edina, MN 55436, **SLP**

Leibner, Aimee Kyle 37243 28th Street East, NBU 93, Palmdale, CA 93550, (805) 273-7335, BA 84 SUNY - Coll at Cortland; MA 86 SUNY - Coll at Plattsburgh; **SLP**

Leibner, Fran Reiner 60 Edwina Court, Dayton, NJ 08810, (201) 329-3006, BS 75 SUNY - Center at Albany; MA 77 Univ of Pittsburgh - Pittsburgh; Sp-Lang Path, **SLP**

Leiboff, Francine R 35 Lionel Avenue #E, Waltham, MA 02154, (617) 264-4700, BA 70 SUNY - Coll at New Paltz; ME 73 Northeastern Univ; SLP-Dept Chrperson, Acton Pub Sch, **SLP**

Leiboff, Mrs Jean A 50 Mann Street, Mansfield, PA 16933, (717) 827-2171, BA 66 Creighton Univ; MA 68 Univ of NE - Lincoln; Sp-Lang Path, North Penn Home Health Agency, **SLP**

Leibowitz, Hope 15 Cranford Road, Plainview, NY 11803, (212) 899-8800, BA 75 Hofstra Univ; MA 76 Hofstra Univ; Sp-Lang Path, Lexington Sch for the Deaf, **SLP**

Leibowitz, Mrs Jane S 1401 Ocean Avenue, Brooklyn, NY 11230, (718) 258-8517, BA 69 CUNY - Brooklyn Coll; MA 71 NY Univ; 85–Sp-Lang Path, William O'Connor Sch, **SLP**

Leibowitz, Mrs Martha Sue 357 Brittany Farms Road, Apt #136, New Britain, CT 06053, (203) 229-3551, BA 81 Univ of Rochester; MA 83 Univ of MD - College Park; Sp-Lang Path, Charles County Board of Educ, **SLP**

Leicht-LeBron, Rachelle 160 Princeton Road, Rockville Centre, NY 11570, (516) 561-8686, BA 64 Adelphi Univ; MS 68 CUNY - Queens Coll; 65–Sp-Lang Path, Bd of Ed Valley Str Hs Dist, **SLP**

Leidecker, Catherine Beardsley 1313 Calder Road, Mc Lean, VA 22101, (703) 556-8769, BS 61 Univ of the DC; MA 68 Catholic Univ of America; **SLP LM**

Leidenheimer, Cathy L 636 Beverly Garden Drive, Metairie, LA 70002, (504) 834-4623, BS 76 Univ of TX - Austin; MS 79 Tulane Univ; Sp-Lang Path, Eye-Ear-Nose-Throat Hospital, **SLP**

Leidholt, Kathleen W 1012 Driftwood Drive #3, Fort Collins, CO 80525, (303) 226-5979, BA 72 Univ of Denver; MA 73 Univ of Denver; Sp-Lang Path, Poudre Valley Hosp-Rehab Serv, **SLP**

Leidwinger, Lewis E 1415 Esplanade, Klamath Falls, OR 97601, (503) 883-3621, BS 69 Allegheny Coll; MS 77 Syracuse Univ; Aud, Klamath Speech & Hearing Ctr, **A**

Leidy, Dr Gerald A 608 Woodland Avenue, Mount Holly Springs, PA 17065, (717) 532-1731, BS 55 Indiana Univ of PA; ME 58 Univ of Pittsburgh - Pittsburgh; PH 71 (Special Education) Univ of MD - College Park; 88–Prof Emeritus, Shippensburg U of Pa, **SLP**

Leidy, Dr Gordon Alan 276 Lucky Hill, West Chester, PA 19382, (302) 994-2511, BA 63 Temple Univ; MA 65 Temple Univ; PH 73 (NS) Case Western Reserve Univ; 87–Aud, VA, **A**

Leidy, Susan W 37 Del Ord Lagoon, Novato, CA 94947, **SLP**

Leight, Gilbert 3004 Malibu Place, Plano, TX 75023, (214) 867-2152, PH 60 (Sp Path) Columbia Univ Teachers Coll; 88, Private Practice, **SLP**

Leighton, Gregory Scott Route 4 Box 276, Viroqua, WI 54665, (608) 637-3934, BA 76 Univ of WI - Eau Claire; MS 81 Univ of WI - Milwaukee; Sp/Lang Path, Private Practice, **SLP**

Leighton, Kellie Ann 3833 Harriet Avenue South, Minneapolis, MN 55409, (612) 422-5180, BA 81 Univ of MN - Minneap-St Paul; MA 86 Univ of MN - Minneap-St Paul; 86–Sp-Lang Path, Anoka-Hennepin Sch Dist #11, **SLP ACE**

Leighton, Terry True 13002 Monroe Avenue, Fort Washington, MD 20744, (301) 292-0834, BA 83 Allegheny Coll; MA 86 Univ of MD - College Park; **SLP**

Leighty, Elizabeth G Murdale Homes #3, Route 9, Carbondale, IL 62901, MS; **SLP**

Leiman, Lori I 1240-A Hampton Hill Court, Harrisburg, PA 17111, (717) 540-1024, BA 84 Univ of MD - College Park; ME 86 James Madison Univ; 88–Aud, Polyclinic Med Ctr Sp & Hrng Ctr, **A**

Leiman, Mrs Sheilla Irene 24105 Albers Street, Woodland Hills, CA 91367, (818) 347-6339, BA 81 CA St Univ - Northridge; MA 83 CA St Univ - Northridge; SLP, Los Angeles USD, **SLP**

Leinaar, Mrs Anne Rhodes Route 4 Box 764, Havana, FL 32333, (904) 488-7526, BA 78 FL St Univ; MS 80 FL St Univ; Sp/Lang Path, Leon Co Sch Bd, **SLP**

Leinbach, Cs Martha A Y 1302 Kenwood Lane, Charlottesville, VA 22901, (804) 973-5031, BA 74 Univ of TN - Knoxville; MA 75 Univ of TN - Knoxville; Sp-Lang Path, Blue Ridge Rehab Assoc, **SLP**

Leininger, Gail Lynn 4 Commodore #229, Emeryville, CA 94608, (415) 494-1000, BA 85 OH St Univ; ME 87 Univ of VA - Charlottesville; 88–Aud, Calif Ear Institute, **A**

Leiper, Mrs Norah Mary 345 Hoyt Street, Buffalo, NY 14213, (716) 892-9210, BS 63 SUNY - Coll at Buffalo; MS 67 SUNY - Coll at Buffalo; **SLP LM**

Leipert, Mrs Nancy J 43 Hawthorne Road, Sicklerville, NJ 08081, (609) 468-2015, BA 80 Glassboro St Coll; MA 85 Trenton St Coll; 81–Sp-Lang Path, Gloucester Co Educ Svcs Comm, **SLP**

Leiphart, Janet R 267 Vendome Court, Grosse Pointe Farms, MI 48236, (313) 884-5564, BA 67 MI St Univ; MS 72 Eastern MI Univ; **SLP**

Leiser, Mrs Ann Gail 3098 Greenlake Drive, Decatur, IL 62521, (217) 428-8507, BS 54 1399; Sp-Lang Path, Private Practice/Foreign Accents, **SLP**

Leiser, Mrs Jane Bronstien 10956 E Crestline Place, Englewood, CO 80111, (303) 740-0300, BA 76 Univ of CO - Boulder; MA 78 Univ of Denver; Sp-Lang Path, St Lukes Hospital, **SLP**

Leiser, Rosalind P 27365 Red Leaf Lane, Southfield, MI 48076, (313) 779-7610, MA 78 Wayne St Univ; Aud, Lakeshore Ear Nose Throat Cen, **A**

Leishman, Kim B P O Box 875, Centerville, UT 84014, (801) 533-3830, MS 70 UT St Univ; Dir Sp/Lang/Hrng Svcs, Intermountain Health Care, **SLP**

Leising, Mrs Kathleen P 3300 South 91st Street, Lincoln, NE 68520, (402) 483-0628, BA 75 Univ of NE - Lincoln; MA 76 Univ of NE - Lincoln; PH 88 (NS) Univ of NE - Lincoln; Sp-Lang Path, Wadonna Professional Care Cen, **SLP**

Leis-Rossio, Dr Beverly c/o Veteran Admin Medical Ctr, Veteran's Road, Bldg 5, Tomah, WI 54660, (608) 372-2624, BA 76 Wichita St Univ; MA 77 Wichita St Univ; PH 86 (Sp & Hrng Science) Univ of IA; **SLP A**

Leiss, Dr Robert H Box 642, Lansdale, PA 19446, (215) 539-8550, BS 60 Bloomsburg Univ of PA; ME 68 Temple Univ; ED 74 (NS) Temple Univ; Asst Dir-Spec Ed, Montgomery Co Inter Ut, **SLP**

Leister, Mrs Catherine M 6401 Carmel Road Suite 101, Charlotte, NC 28226, (704) 541-3737, BA 76 Depauw Univ; ME 81 Univ of NC - Greensboro; 84–Sp-Lang Path, Private Practice, **SLP**

Leister, Cheryl M 107 Millard Avenue, West Babylon, NY 11704, (201) 688-2750, BA 78 CUNY - Brooklyn Coll; MS 81 CUNY - Brooklyn Coll; 87–Dist Supvr, Hearing Laboratory, **A**

Leisz, Jacquelin 7241 Encelia Drive, La Jolla, CA 92037, (619) 456-0739, BA 68 CA St Univ - Fullerton; MA 77 CA St Univ - Long Beach; Sp-Lang Path, Grossmont Dist Hosp-Rehab Ut, **SLP**

Leite, Jane M 808 South Thompson, Sioux Falls, SD 57103, (605) 335-0732, BA 76 SD St Univ; MS 79 Saint Cloud St Univ; Sp-Lang Path, Crippled Children's Hosp & Sch, **SLP ACE**

Leiter, Mrs Ann Cheryl 4125 Indian Runn Drive, Dayton, OH 45415, (513) 275-1208, BA 79 Univ of Toledo; MS 81 Miami Univ - Oxford; Sp-Lang Path, Western County Mental Retard, **SLP**

Leiter, Everett R 201 West 16th Street #3-F, New York, NY 10011, (212) 929-0384, BA 74 Brown Univ; MA 78 CUNY - Hunter Coll; OM 81 CUNY - Grad Sch & Univ Cntr; Sp-Lang Path, Advanced Commun Serv, **SLP**

Leitgeb, Mrs Diane D 1341 Turner Drive, Victor, NY 14564, (716) 924-7207, MS 75 Nazareth Coll of Rochester; BS 72 Ithaca Coll, Sp-Lang Path, Fingerlakes Dev Serv, **SLP**

Leith, Dr William R Communication Disorders & Sci, Wayne State University, 555 Manoogian Hall, Detroit, MI 48202, (313) 577-3337, BS 51 Western MI Univ; MS 52 Purdue Univ - West Lafayette; PH 54 (NS) Purdue Univ - West Lafayette; Prof, Wayne St U, **SLP F**

Leitner, Lisa Helen 640 Fort Washington Avenue, Apartment 3-F, New York, NY 10040-3965, (212) 927-3784, BA 85 Barnard Coll; MS 87 Columbia Univ Teachers Coll; 87–Sp-Lang Path, Beth Abraham Hosp, **SLP**

Leitner-Lockwood, Judith C State Tower Bldg, Suite 929, 109 South Warren Street, Syracuse, NY 13202, (315) 479-9171, BS 67 Roosevelt Univ; MS 76 Syracuse Univ; Sp-Path, Private Practice, **SLP**

Lejeune, Joseph B 3943 A Utah, St Louis, MO 63116-3504, BA 77 Univ of Southwestern LA; MA 82 Memphis St Univ; Sp-Lang Path, Joplin Reg Cen, **SLP**

Lejeune, Sarah C 4821 Pike Drive, Metairie, LA 70003, (504) 897-8563, BA 71 LA St Univ - Baton Rouge; MA 73 George Washington Univ; Sp-Lang Path, Touro Infirmary, **SLP ACE**

Lekberg, Mrs Rebecca Stetson 29 Powder Hill Road, East Longmeadow, MA 01028, (413) 567-0374, BS 68 Tufts Univ; MA 81 Univ of MA - Amherst; Sp-Lang Path, Willie Ross Sch for the Deaf, **SLP**

Leland, Leslie Culbertson 4650 Lake Jeanette Road, Greensboro, NC 27408, (919) 342-1611, BA 79 Univ of NC - Greensboro; ME 82 Univ of NC - Greensboro; 87–Sp-Lang Path, Rockingham Co Enrichment Ctr, **SLP ACE**

Leland-Philbrook, Mrs Marilyn 10 Deepwood Drive, Portland, ME 04103-3777, (207) 797-2021, BA 76 IN Univ - Bloomington; MS 78 Univ of VT; 88–Sp-Lang Path, Gorham PS, **SLP**

Lelchook, Alex K 13 Notre Dame Road, Acton, MA 01720, (508) 635-0139, MS 76 Univ of OK Medical Center; 88–Sp-Lang Path, Newton PS Sys, **SLP**

Le Levier, Suzanne Marie P O Box 562, Girdwood, AK 99587, (907) 274-4582, BA 76 Univ of CA - Santa Barbara; MA 78 Univ of Denver; 88–Aud, Anchorage Sch Dist, **A**

Lelli, Janet S 16767 Quail Court, Portland, OR 97229, (404) 963-6713, BS 77 Univ of PA; MA 79 Wayne St Univ; **SLP**

Lemahieu, Thomas William 920 First Avenue NW, Grand Rapids, MN 55744, (218) 326-1538, BA 80 Univ of MN - Duluth; MA 82 Univ of MN - Duluth; 82–Sp-Lang Path, Sch Dist #318, **SLP**

Leman, Mrs Lori Berry 48 Ledgeview Drive, Rochester, NH 03867, (603) 749-2446, BS 82 Univ of ME - Farmington; MS 84 Northeastern Univ; Sp-Lang Path, New England Sp Services, **SLP**

Le Mark, Mary Elizabeth 59 Elm Street, Albany, NY 12202, (518) 436-3949, BS 83 Elmira Coll; MA 85 SUNY - Coll at Geneseo; 86–Sp-Lang Path, NYS Easter Seal Society, **SLP**

Lemaster, Mrs Beverly Joan Norton Sound Health Corp, Audiology Department, P O Box 966, Nome, AK 99762, (907) 443-3311, BS 79 Northern AZ Univ; MS 82 ID St Univ; Audiologist, Norton Sound Health Corp, **A**

LeMaster, Sharon Lyn 1522 East Felming Drive North, Arlington Heights, IL 60004, (312) 593-4359, BS 85 IL St Univ - Normal; MS 86 IL St Univ - Normal; 87–Sp-Lang Path, Reg Hrng Imp Prog

Lemay, Laurie Keefe 515 North 81st, Seattle, WA 98103, (206) 859-7491, BA 80 Western WA Univ; MA 82 Western WA Univ; 87–SLP, Kent Sch Dist, **SLP**

Lemieux, Janice M 2601 Ashe Road #45, Bakersfield, CA 93309, (805) 835-2272, BS 76 Edinboro Univ of PA; MA 81 Edinboro Univ of PA; Sp/Lang Path Group, Bakersfield Assoc Ret Cit, **SLP**

Lemke, Alison Easley 1415 44th Street, Des Moines, IA 50311, (515) 277-0672, BA 83 Valparaiso Univ; MA 85 Univ of IA; 86–Sp-Lang Path, Central Rehab, **SLP**

Lemley, Colleen Belle 824 Lakeview Drive, Apartment 102-C, Parkersburg, WV 26101, (304) 485-0610, MS 87 WV Univ; 87–Spec Educ Tchr, Wood County Bd of Educ

Lemli, Jayne Abrams 53 June Avenue, Northport, NY 11768, (516) 271-6263, **SLP**

Lemma, James Dominic 6473 Benfield Road, Macungie, PA 18062, (215) 327-7539, BS 82 SUNY - Coll at New Paltz; MS 84 OH Univ - Athens; Sp-Lang Path, InSpeech Inc, **SLP**

Lemme, Dr Margaret L 7321 South Columbine Way, Littleton, CO 80122, (303) 871-2385, BS 65 Univ of OK - Norman; MS 67 Univ of OK Medical Center; PH 74 (NS) Univ of CO - Boulder; Associate Professor, University of Denver, **SLP F**

Lemoine, Noma R Los Angeles Unified Sch Dist, 6505 Zelzah Avenue, Reseda, CA 91335, (818) 997-2357, BA 72 Pepperdine Univ - Los Angele; MA 77 CA St Univ - Los Angeles; OM 81 CA Lutheran Coll; Administration, Los Angeles USD, **SLP**

Lemon, Pamela G 1519 22nd Avenue, Rock Island, IL 61201, (309) 793-2009, BA 73 Augustana Coll; MS 76 Univ of WI - Madison; SLP, Franciscan Med Cen, **SLP**

Lemon, Phyllis D 4710 Manposa Way, Englewood, CO 80110, **SLP**

Lemon-Updike, Dr Claudia D 2304 West Cambridge Drive, Muncie, IN 47304, (317) 285-8166, BA 72; MA 74 SUNY - Center at Buffalo; PH 77 (NS) IN Univ - Bloomington; Prof of Aud, Ball State U, **A**

Lemp, Janice Wright 620 West Stetson Street, Orlando, FL 32804, (407) 293-6252, BS 79 FL St Univ; MS 80 FL St Univ; 86–Sp/Lang Path, Orange County Sch Sys, **SLP**

Lenahan, Joan Frances 13 North Dorado Circle, Apartment 1-J, Hauppauge, NY 11788, (516) 234-7268, BA 81 CUNY - Queens Coll; MA 83 Hofstra Univ; 83–Sp-Lang Path, Northport VA, **SLP**

Lenertz, Ann Schweitzer 15618 W 146th Terrace, Olathe, KS 66062, (913) 782-8221, BA 81 Minot St Univ; MA 86 Univ of KS; SLP, **SLP**

Lengefeld, Joyce Mary 178 Greystone Lane #12, Rochester, NY 14618, (716) 243-0245, BS 83 SUNY - Coll at Geneseo; MA 85 SUNY - Coll at Geneseo; Sp-Lang Path, Geneseo Cen Sch, **SLP**

Lenhardt, Dr Martin Louis Route 3 Box 1339, Hayes, VA 23072, (804) 786-9687, BS 66 Seton Hall Univ; MA 68 Seton Hall Univ; PH 70 (NS) FL St Univ; Assoc Prof, VA Commonwealth U, **SLP A**

Lenhart, Mrs Brenda Craig 256 Iroquois Road, Virginia Beach, VA 23462, (804) 473-5007, BS 75 Clarion Univ of PA; ME 83 Clarion Univ of PA; Sp-Lang Path, Virginia Beach City Schs, **SLP**

Lenich, Jennifer Komnick 11502 Autumn Ridge Road, Austin, TX 78759, (512) 458-4276, BS 83 Purdue Univ - West Lafayette; MA 86 Univ of TX - Austin; 86–Aud, Associates in Otolaryngology, **A**

Lenke, Nancy E 1107 East Center Street, Warsaw, IN 46580, MA 80 Ball St Univ; Audiologist, Dr Steven B Ashton, **A**

Lenkey, Laura E 7710 Anterier Rd, Dixon, IL 61021, (815) 284-4440, BS 81; MA 82; Sp-Lang Path, Private Practice, **SLP**

Lenkner, Lucretia A 407 Vine Street, Munhall, PA 15120, (412) 572-6166, BS 78 Clarion Univ of PA; MS 79 Indiana Univ of PA; 86–Sp-Lang Path/Aud, Dr Edward Elmer & Hrng Svc, **SLP A**

Lenkner, Melody A Route 2 Box 5249, Twin Falls, ID 83301, (208) 734-8324, BA 68 WA St Univ; MA 72 WA St Univ; Owner/Sp-Lang Path, Lenkner Michener & Assoc Inc, **SLP ACE**

Lenk-Roberts, Susan Colleen 821 Stockbridge Drive, Hockessin, DE 19707, (609) 757-3973, BA 80 Rutger's St Univ - Douglas Coll; MS 83 Hahneman Medical Coll; Sp-Lang Path/Aud, Middlesex General Hospital, **SLP A**

Lenling, Camille M 5298 Candy Cove Trail S E, Prior Lake, MN 55372, (612) 895-7313, BS 70 Saint Cloud St Univ; ME 77 Univ of WI - River Falls; SLP, Burnsville Pub Sch, **SLP**

Lennes, Mrs Karna 16720 Norell Avenue North, Marine St Croix, MN 55047, (612) 433-3063, BA 66 Augustana Coll; MA 70 Univ of MN - Minneap-St Paul; 71–Sp-Lang Path, Dist 281 Robbinsdale Schs, **SLP**

Lennon, Dr E James 1302 George Street, Brunswick, GA 31520, BA 49 Anderson Coll; MS 50 Univ of WI - Madison; PH 52 (Sp) Univ of WI - Madison; 74–Sp/Lang Path, E James Lennon, **SLP LM**

Lennon, Kim 28318 Bayberry, Farmington Hills, MI 48018, BA 78 MI St Univ; MA 79 Eastern MI Univ; **SLP**

Lennox, Barbara E 1205 Taylor Avenue, Richmond, VA 23225, (804) 737-2060, BS 71 OH Univ - Athens; MA 72 OH Univ - Athens; Sp/Lang Path, Henrico Co Schs, **SLP**

Lent, Alexandra 457 Old Farm Road, Wyncote, PA 19095, (215) 221-3661, BA 73 Clark Univ; MA 81 Temple Univ-Tyler Sch of Art; Aud, Temple Univ Hosp/Dept of Aud, **A**

Lent, Barbara Claire 2422 New Berne Road, Richmond, VA 23228, (804) 786-0207, BS 80 Univ of VA - Charlottesville; ME 82 Univ of VA - Charlottesville; Supervisor Sp-Lang Path, Medical College of Virginia, **SLP**

Lenters-Hansen, Marjorie S 6038 Marsh Place, North Ridgeville, OH 44039, (216) 327-0637, BA 65 Univ of SD - Vermillion; MA 66 Univ of SD - Vermillion; Sp-Lang Path, No Ridgeville Cty Schs, **SLP**

Lentz, Mrs Barbara S 26565 Mazur Drive, Rancho Palos Verdes, CA 90274, (503) 620-1147, BA 77 Univ of Denver; MA 79 Univ of Denver; Aud, Kresge Hearing Research Lab, **A**

Lentz, Mrs Terri Colleen 10643 West 84th Place, Arvada, CO 80005-4710, (303) 797-7394, **SLP**

Lentz, Dr William Edwin 2001 South Shields #J, Fort Collins, CO 80526, (303) 221-5249, BS 62 CO St Univ; MS 65 CO St Univ; PH 70 (NS) Univ of UT; Owner, Private Practice, **A**

Lenz, Carol F 1120 5th Avenue, New York, NY 10028, (212) 430-2200, BS 61 Univ of IL - Urbana; MA 70 NY Univ; **SLP**

Lenz, Judith A 1131 Palmertown Road, Blairsville, PA 15717, (412) 459-5954, BS 82 OH St Univ; MS 87 Indiana Univ of PA

Lenz, Mrs Susan Roberta Rt 1 Box 368, Boonville, MO 65233, BS 83 Univ of MO - Columbia; MA 85 Univ of KS; Sp-Lang Path, Associated Rehab Services, **SLP**

Lenza, Mrs Aurora B 5724 Hidden Stone, St Louis, MO 63129, (314) 966-1557, BA 69 Fontbonne Coll; MA 71 Saint Louis Univ; **SLP ACE**

Lenzen, Mrs Polly Metzger 12808 Pointe Drive, St Louis, MO 63127-1742, (314) 889-1407, BS 78 Fontbonne Coll; MS 77 Fontbonne Coll; 85–Instr/Cl Supvr, Fontbonne College, **SLP**

Leo, Mrs Ellen Deborah P O Box 32, 865 Cherry Lane, Penns Park, PA 18943, (201) 782-6464, BS 80 PA St Univ - Univ Park; MS 83 Rutgers St Univ - Newark; SLP, East Amwell Township Sch, **SLP**

Leo, Victoria Ireland 4929 Tiffany Park Circle, Santa Maria, CA 93455, (805) 922-7171, BS 72 CA Poly St Univ-San Luis Obi; MA 75 CA St Univ - Long Beach; Sp-Lang Path, Santa Monica Elem School Dist, **SLP**

Leombruno, Joseph A 236 Yorktown Court, Voorheesville, NY 12186, (518) 237-9100, MS 73 SUNY - Center at Albany; MS 82 SUNY - Center at Albany; Prin, Berne-Knox-Westerlo CSD, **SLP**

Leon, Julian P 2956 Washington Boulevard, Cleveland, OH 44118, **SLP**

Leonard, Barbara A McCleaf 347 South Main Street, Marysville, PA 17053, (717) 732-0771, BS 78 Univ of WA; MA 80 Western WA Univ; SLP, Capital Area Iu #15, **SLP**

Leonard, Mrs Bernita Elin Z 208 Manor Circle, Takoma Park, MD 20912, BA 79 George Washington Univ; MA 81 George Washington Univ; Sp-Lang Path, Pw Co Pub Sch, **SLP**

Leonard, Carol Jane 1521 Longview Drive, Latrobe, PA 15650, (412) 537-6177, BS 75 Clarion Univ of PA; MS 85 Indiana Univ of PA; **SLP**

Leonard, Cathy Marie 7743B Oxford Avenue, Philadelphia, PA 19111, (215) 221-7042, BS 79 PA St Univ - Univ Park; MA 81 Temple Univ; Dir of SLP, Temple Univ Hosp, **SLP**

Leonard, Mrs Cheryl M 2134 Eve Circle, Charleston, SC 29414, (803) 763-1555, BS 74 Coll of Charleston; OM 75; Sp-Lang Path, Charleston Co Sch, **SLP**

Leonard, Colleen C 30½ George Street, Kittery, ME 03904, (207) 324-1550, BA 83 Bridgewater St Coll; MS 85 Univ of WI - Madison; 87–Aud, York Co Counseling Svcs, **A**

Leonard, Jacqueline F 5 Trillium Place, Huntington, NY 11743, (516) 223-8100, BA 75 Hofstra Univ; MA 76 Hofstra Univ; Sp/Lang Path, Baldwin Pub Sch, **SLP**

Leonard, Jeanette S Dept Of Audiology & Speech Sci, Purdue University, West Lafayette, IN 47907, (317) 494-3789, MA 70 Univ of South FL; Superv Sp-Lang Path, Purdue Univ, **SLP A**

Leonard, Mrs Kathleen M 2800 N Lake Shore Drive, Apartment 2014, Chicago, IL 60657, (312) 477-2115, BS 57 Marquette Univ; MS 66 Marquette Univ; Sp-Lang Path, Chicago Bd of Educ, **SLP**

Leonard, Kimberly Sue Rt 5 Box 464-K, Salisbury, NC 28144, (704) 636-8213, BA 79 Univ of NC - Charlotte; MA 85 Appalachian St Univ; **SLP**

Leonard, Dr Laurence B Dept Of Audiology & Speech Sci, Purdue University, West Lafayette, IN 47907, (317) 494-3794, BA 69 Univ of South FL; MS 70 Univ of South FL; PH 73 (NS) Univ of Pittsburgh - Pittsburgh; Prof, Prudue Univ, **SLP F**

Leonard, Laurie A 7157 Crittenden Street, Philadelphia, PA 19119, (215) 242-3412, BS 76 PA St Univ - Univ Park; OM 80 Hahneman Medical Coll; Sp-Lang Path, Children's Hosp of Philadelphia, **SLP**

Leonard, Lisa Jean 2529 Camelot Court, Colorado Springs, CO 80904, (303) 578-1367, BA 81 Univ of Northern CO; MA 83 Univ of Northern CO; 86–Sp/Lang Path, Falcon School Dstr, **SLP**

Leonard, Lois L 6 Willow Lane, Scotia, NY 12302, BS 72 Univ of WI - Stevens Point; MS 75 Univ of WI - Stevens Point; SLP, Grantwood AEA, **SLP**

Leonard, Lois M Avenue Winston Churchill 119 1180, Brussels, Belgium, BA 64 Adelphi Univ; MS 69 Adelphi Univ; 83–Coord, St John's Intl Sch, **SLP**

Leonard, Loretta Ann 8838 Birch Street, New Orleans, LA 70118, (504) 821-7622, **SLP**

Leonard, Mrs Marilyn Greene Route 10 Box 149, Columbus, MS 39702, (601) 328-2598, **SLP**

Leonard, Mrs Melodie Kincaid Brescia College Speech And Hearing Clinic, Brescia College, 718 Allen Street, Owensboro, KY 42301, (502) 684-8622, BS 80 Brescia Coll; MS 85 Western KY Univ; 87–Sp-Lang Path, Brescia Sp & Hrng Cl

Leonard, Muriel J 22 Meadowbank Avenue, Mattapan, MA 02126, (617) 726-6200, BS 72 Boston Univ; MS 74 Emerson Coll; Special Education Dept Head, City Boston-Public Schools, **SLP**

Leonard, Perry C PO Box 276603, Sacramento, CA 95827-6603, (916) 685-9525, BS 73 Southern IL Univ -Carbondale; MS 77 Southern IL Univ -Carbondale; Sp-Lang Path, Private Practice, **SLP**

Leonard, Dr Ralph Northern Hearing Service Inc, P O Box S, Woodruff, WI 54568, (715) 356-3292, BA 58 Central MI Univ; MA 62 MI St Univ; PH 68 (NS) MI St Univ; Aud, Northern Hearing Serv Inc, **A**

Leonard, Dr Rebecca J 2500 Stockton Boulevard, Sacramento, CA 95817, (916) 453-3729, BA 67 IN Univ - Bloomington; MS 72 Purdue Univ - West Lafayette; PH 76 (NS) Purdue Univ - West Lafayette; Assoc Adj Prof, U Cal/Davis Med Sch, **SLP**

Leonard, Mrs Roberta Millrod 11 Hilltop Road, Stony Brook, NY 11790, (516) 751-0287, BA 75 SUNY - Center at Buffalo; MS 76 Adelphi Univ; SLP, BOCES II, **SLP**

Leonard, Sarah L M 469 Ponderosa Drive, Thomaston, GA 30286, (404) 647-9621, BA 64 Auburn Univ - Auburn; OM 71 Auburn Univ - Auburn; Asst Supt, Upson Co Sch Syst, **SLP**

Leonard Allen, Patricia Ann 1324 Middlebury Drive, Aurora, IL 60504-6802, (312) 267-0722, BS 80 Marquette Univ; MS 81 Southern IL Univ-Edwardsvill; Sp/Lang Path, Kankakee Sch Dist #111, **SLP**

Leonard-Fleckman, Star C 5041 Ivanhoe Place N E, Seattle, WA 98105, (206) 525-7256, BA 71 OR St Univ; MA 73 Washington Univ; MS 81 Univ of CT; Aud, Private Practice, **A**

Leonard-Harper, Gayle S 135 Demers Drive, Fort McMurray, AB, Canada T9H 2B3, MA 74 KS St Univ; Sp-Lang Path, Private Practice, **SLP**

Leonard-Pitts, Lori A 1307 South Chestnut, Arlington Height, IL 60005, (312) 593-6976, SLP, Community Therapy Services, **SLP**

Leone, Mrs Susan L 96 Kerry Lane, Whitinsville, MA 01588, (617) 234-8509, **SLP**

Leong, Kathleen Jayne 75-12 195th Street, Flushing, NY 11366, (212) 924-2912, BA 82 Saint John's Univ - Jamaica; MS 84 Adelphi Univ; **SLP**

Leong, Marci Kim 3212 Beacon Avenue South, Apartment 301, Seattle, WA 98144, (206) 725-4662, BS 84 Univ of WA; MS 87 Univ of WA; 88–Aud, Valley ENT Clinic, **A**

Leon-Rodriguez, Mrs Maria E 9710 S W 15th Street, Miami, FL 33174-2925, (305) 554-1517, BA 74 Univ of FL; ME 76 Univ of FL; Sp-Lang Path, Dade Co Pub Sch, **SLP**

Leonti, Mrs Susan L 10715 S W 63rd Place, Portland, OR 97219, (503) 232-2458, BS 66 Portland St Univ; MS 73 Portland St Univ; Sp-Lang Path, Portland Pub Sch, **SLP**

Leopold, Mrs Leslie Peterson 3623 Chadwick Court, Pasadena, MD 21122, (301) 255-4477, BA 76 Univ of Northern CO; MS 80 Univ of AZ; **SLP**

Leorza, Mrs Susan C 11 Sycamore Circle, Ormond Beach, FL 32074-3411, (904) 677-2737, BS 70 FL St Univ; ME 73 Univ of GA; SLP, Volusia Co Sch, **SLP**

Le Page, Mrs Linda Theresa 412 Penrod Place, Cape Girardeau, MO 63701, (314) 334-1969, Physcian's Office, **SLP**

Lepczyk, Mrs Susan Guess 206 Marion-Quimby Way, Stevensville, MD 21666, (301) 643-2942, BA 79 MI St Univ; MA 81 Wayne St Univ; **SLP**

Le Peau, Nancy S 114 South Mt Vernon Drive, Iowa City, IA 52240, (319) 353-5140, BS 65; MA 71 IN Univ - Bloomington; Assoc Prof: Dental Hygiene, U of IA, **SLP**

Lepelstat, Anita R 937 Franklin Avenue, South Plainfield, NJ 07080, (201) 231-8541, BA 59 CUNY - Queens Coll; MA 65 CUNY - Brooklyn Coll; Sp-Lang Path, Manville Public Schools, **SLP**

Lepi, Mrs Carol L 3339 Tyler Drive, Brunswick, OH 44212, (216) 775-2786, BS 74 OH Univ - Athens; MA 76 Kent St Univ; Aud, N OH Spec Educ Reg Resource Ctr, **A**

Lepkowski, Mary Ellen Burns 4903 Augusta Circle, Glendale, AZ 85308, (602) 978-6268, BS 78 Marquette Univ; MS 79 Marquette Univ; MA 84 Cardinal Stritch Coll; Sp-Lang Path, Peoria Sch Dist, **SLP**

Lepoire, Mrs Deborah J 2119 White Owl, Okemos, MI 48864, (517) 334-6982, BA 73 MI St Univ; MA 74 MI St Univ; Sp-Lang Path, MI Sch for the Blind, **SLP**

Lepold, Mrs Lori Richter 614 Parkside Avenue, Elmhurst, IL 60126, (312) 260-6159, **SLP**

Lepore, Nancy P RR #1 Box 347 L, Stanfordville, NY 12581, (914) 877-6821, BS 77 SUNY - Coll at Geneseo; MA 78 Bowling Green St Univ; Sp-Lang Path, Wassaic Dev Cen, **SLP**

Lepp, Daniel S 2610 University, Dubuque, IA 52001, (319) 588-0538, BA 74 McKendree Coll; MA 76 Western IL Univ; SLP, Keystone AEA, **SLP**

Leppla, Mrs Patricia Lindenmuth 130 Farmersville Pk, Germantown, OH 45327, (513) 855-7401, BS 77 Eastern KY Univ; MA 85 Univ of Cincinnati; 88–Sp-Lang Path, Private Practice, **SLP**

Lepre-Clark, Mrs Camille 2455 Bernice Boulevard, Binghamton, NY 13903, (607) 770-0424, BA 80 SUNY - Center at Binghamton; MS 82 PA St Univ - Univ Park; Sp-Lang Path, Broome Dev Serv, **SLP ACE**

Lerea, Dr Louis 45 Beecher Road, Woodbridge, CT 06525, (203) 389-6117, BA 49 CUNY - Brooklyn Coll; MA 51 Univ of IA; PH 54 (NS) Univ of Pittsburgh - Pittsburgh; Prof, Sn CT St U, **SLP A F**

Lerer, Pamela Batson 1251 Nilles Road, #7 Clock Tower Place, Hamilton, OH 45014, BA 65 Central MI Univ; MA 66 Univ of MA - Amherst; 87–Sp-Lang Path, Associates in Sp Aud & Psych, **SLP**

Le Resche, Mrs Marilyn M 1057 Brockton Street, El Cajon, CA 92020, MS 72 Univ of IL - Urbana; Asst Dir, Grossmont Union HS Dist, **SLP**

Leri, Mrs Susan M 785 Highmeyer Road, Harborcreek, PA 16421, (814) 452-5510, BA 70 Allegheny Coll; MS 71 Univ of MI - Ann Arbor; Sp-Lang Path, St Vincent Reg Rehab Cen, **SLP**

Lerman, Dr Jay William 35 Thomas Drive, Storrs, CT 06268, (203) 486-2817, BA 55 Temple Univ-Tyler Sch of Art; MA 57 Temple Univ-Tyler Sch of Art; PH 61 (NS) Univ of Pittsburgh - Pittsburgh; Prof & Dept Head, U of CT, **SLP F**

Lerman, Joanne Linda 42 North Main Street #54, West Hartford, CT 06107, (203) 521-9667, BA 81 Clark Univ; MS 83 Columbia Univ Teachers Coll; SLP, Crec

Lerner, Dr Brenda J 2709-B Rue St Martin, Hammond, LA 70402, (504) 542-2214, PH 77 (Sp Path) Univ of IL - Urbana; 87–Asst Prof, Southeastern LA Univ, **SLP**

Lerner, Mrs Carol J 9306 Chelsea Drive North, Plantation, FL 33324, (305) 731-0767, BA 66 Adelphi Univ; MS 71 CUNY - Queens Coll; Sp-Lang Path/Pres, Communispeech Intl Inc, **SLP**

Lerner, Mrs Janet 8 Pipestem Court, Potomac, MD 20854, (301) 424-9014, BA 80 Univ of MD - College Park; MS 81 Columbia Univ Teachers Coll; Sp-Lang Path, InSpeech Inc, **SLP ACE**

Lerner, Judith L S 420 Santa Ynez Way, Sacramento, CA 95816, (916) 456-8261, BA 72 LA St Univ - Baton Rouge; MS 75 LA St Univ - Baton Rouge; **SLP**

Lernihan, Andrea Joyce 370 High Street #214, New Britain, CT 06051, (802) 775-3264, BS 82 Indiana Univ of PA; MS 83 Indiana Univ of PA; Sp-Lang Path, Rutland S Superv Un, **SLP**

Leroi, Mrs Ellen S 4431 Elmwood Drive, Okemos, MI 48864, (517) 349-1027, MA 69 MI St Univ; **A**

Le Roy-Rojek, Mrs Patricia Marie 7001 Brandywine Drive, Derby, NY 14047-9610, (716) 947-5981, BS 77 Daemen Coll; MA 84 Edinboro Univ of PA; 86–Sp-Lang Path, Eden Central School, **SLP**

Lescher, Mrs Ellen B 17 Old Barge Road, Simsbury, CT 06070, (203) 658-1795, BS 74 Boston Univ; MA 75 Case Western Reserve Univ; Sp-Lang Path, W Hartford Pub Sch, **SLP**

Lesczynski-Weber, Mrs Dorene Lisbeth 20 Pamela Court, Spotswood, NJ 08884, (201) 251-9106, MS; **SLP**

Lesesne, Mrs Jean P 607 Long Leaf Drive, Chapel Hill, NC 27514, (919) 929-2578, BA 63 Vanderbilt Univ; MA 64 Univ of FL; **SLP**

Lesher, Judith L 803 Monroe Drive, Elizabethtown, KY 42701, (502) 765-7703, BS 72 Spalding Coll; OM 73 Brigham Young Univ; Director, Regional Hearing/Speech Center, **SLP**

Leshin, Mrs Phyllis 555 Muskingum Avenue, Pacific Palisades, CA 90272, (213) 454-9427, BA 57 Univ of MI - Ann Arbor; MA 61 Univ of CA - Los Angeles; **SLP**

Leshyn, Mrs Carolyn B 9645 South Harding Avenue, Evergreen Park, IL 60642, (312) 838-5120, BS 63 Eastern IL Univ; MS 86 Governors St Univ; Sp-Lang Path, Chicago Bd of Ed, **SLP ACE**

Lesiecki, William 1585 Clemson Drive #B, Eagan, MN 55122, (612) 681-0249, MA 84 Univ of IL - Urbana; Aud, Nicolet Aud, **A**

Lesinski, Mrs Kathleen Niven 50 Wentworth Street, Dedham, MA 02026, (617) 326-6237, BA 83 Boston Coll; MA 87 Wayne St Univ; Sp-Lang Path, MA Easter Seal Soc, **SLP**

Lesinski, Mrs Marilyn Feicht 1601 Shannon Road, Girard, OH 44420, (216) 539-4665, **SLP**

Lesiuk, Lorraine 31 Blundell Bay, Winnipeg, MB, Canada R2P 1Z2, (204) 334-7484, BA 84 Univ of Winnipeg - Manitoba; MS 86 Minot St Univ; 87–Sp-Lang Path, Child Guidance Clinic, **SLP**

Lesley, Marie G 6274 Marbut Farms Road, Lithonia, GA 30058-2861, (404) 985-1933, BA 79 Saint Xavier Coll; MS 81 Governors St Univ; 86–Sp-Lang Path, Gwinnett Co PS, **SLP**

Leslie, Dr Carol Prahl 3021 Vernon Place, Cincinnati, OH 45219, (513) 221-0527, BA 68 Valparaiso Univ; MA 70 Univ of IA; PH 80 (NS) Univ of Cincinnati; Exec Dir, Cincinnati Sp and Hrng Cen, **SLP F**

Leslie, Mrs Christina 15853 Marmac, Ramona, CA 92065, BA 74 San Diego St Univ; MA 79 San Diego St Univ; SLP, Poway USD, **SLP**

Leslie, Mrs Cynthia M 9628 Kingsford Drive, Raleigh, NC 27606, (919) 755-6626, BA 79 Univ of Houston - Univ Park; MS 81 Univ of NC - Chapel Hill; SLP, Wake County Public Schools, **SLP**

Leslie, Gail W 662 Cheshire Avenue, Eugene, OR 97402, (503) 485-8521, BS 65 Carlow Coll; MS 70 Tulane Univ; Aud, Eugene Hrng & Sp Cen, **A**

Leslie, Mrs Susan P 2757 Wendell Lane, Yorktown Heights, NY 10598, (914) 245-7444, BA 71 Univ of CT; MS 77 Columbia Univ Teachers Coll; Sp-Lang Path, Lakeland Ctrl Sch Dist, **SLP**

Leslie, T Anne Harris Tri Valley Speech & Language, 2040 Emory Avenue, Simi Valley, CA 93063, (805) 522-4471, BA 72 CA St Univ - Fresno; MA 74 CA St Univ - Fresno; SLP, LA Co Supt of Schls, **SLP**

Lesmez, Rebecca Mohn 939 G Cherry Lane, East Lansing, MI 48823, (517) 787-1343, BA 85 MI St Univ; MA 87 MI St Univ; 87–Aud, S H Ancerewicz MD PC, **A**

Lesner, Dr Sharon A Speech And Hearing Center, University Of Akron, Akron, OH 44325, (216) 375-7884, MA 75 Kent St Univ; MA 76 Wayne St Univ - Sch of Med; PH 79 (Aud) OH St Univ; Prof, U of Akron, **A**

Lesniak, Dennis P Kaiser-Permanente Medical Offices, 50 Severance Circle, Cleveland Heights, OH 44118, (216) 291-1100, BA 77 Cleveland St Univ; MA 80 Cleveland St Univ; Aud, Ohio Permanente Medical Group, **A**

Lesniak, Mrs Donna Lynn 13 Ascot Circle, Schaumburg, IL 60194, (312) 884-0592, **SLP**

Lesniak, Peggy S 1216 North Pine, Tacoma, WA 98406, (206) 473-8732, **SLP**

Leson, Mary A 4010 Brandywine Drive, Apartment In, Peoria, IL 61614, (309) 685-6129, **SLP**

Lesowski, Kristin Ann 53 Gough Avenue, West Warwick, RI 02893, (401) 828-3459, BS 83 Syracuse Univ; MS 85 Southern CT St Univ; **SLP**

L'Esperance, Mrs Merry L 2051 Ladera Court, Carlsbad, CA 92008, (714) 722-1641, BS 75 Univ of Redlands; MS 76 Univ of Redlands; **SLP**

Lessac, Prof Arthur 826 2nd Street #306, Santa Monica, CA 90403, (213) 395-7055, BS 41 NY Univ; MA 48 NY Univ; Emeritus Professor, **SLP LM**

Lesselyong, Mrs Lisa Marie 905 Jacobsen Road, Unit F, Neenah, WI 54956, (414) 735-9977, BS 84 Univ of WI - Stevens Point; MS 86 Univ of WI - Stevens Point; 86–Sp-Lang Path, Gmeiner Clinic for Commun Dis and Lrng Disabilities, **SLP**

Lessem, Margot L 74 Beals St, Brookline, MA 02146, (617) 277-6674, BA 85 Rutgers St Univ -N Brunswick; MS 87 Boston Univ

Lesser, Karen Anne 223 Terrace Drive, Vista, CA 92083, (619) 743-0034, BS 81 Stephen F Austin St Univ; MS 83 Univ of TX - Dallas; **SLP**

Lessley, Elizabeth J 607 Garden Ridge Circle, Birmingham, AL 35244, (205) 991-9679, MA 87 Auburn Univ - Auburn

Lestage, Rosemary B P O Box 151, De Ridder, LA 70634, BS 69 LA St Univ - Baton Rouge; MA 71 LA St Univ - Baton Rouge; Sp-Lang Path, Beauregard Parish School Board, **SLP**

Lester, Karen Sue 2315 Irving Avenue S #3, Minneapolis, MN 55403, (612) 338-2156, BA 85 Univ of WI - Madison; MA 86 Northwestern Univ; **SLP**

Lester, Leatrice Burgess 900 North Avalon Street, Memphis, TN 38107, (901) 722-2092, BS 74 Univ of TN - Knoxville; MA 84 Memphis St Univ; **SLP**

Lester, Leigh Ann 222 Rochester Road, Mobile, AL 36608, (205) 342-4452, MA 88 Vanderbilt Univ; 88–Aud, Mobile County PS Sys

Lester, Mrs Patricia A 907 Woodbrook Drive, Purcell, OK 73080, (405) 527-5059, BA 74 Univ of OK - Norman; MS 76 Univ of OK Medical Center; **SLP**

Lester, Rhonda A 3037 3rd Avenue #6, Huntington, WV 25702, (304) 429-1328, BS 79 WV Univ; MS 81 WV Univ; Aud, Res A ll, **A**

Lester, Mrs Rochelle Monica 1956 Georgian Road, Philadelphia, PA 19138, (215) 549-2053, BA 80 Duquesne Univ; MA 85 Temple Univ-Tyler Sch of Art; **SLP**

Lestz, Mrs Nancy Morris 3001 125th Avenue S E, Apartment 3-B, Bellevue, WA 98005, (805) 962-7661, BA 78 Univ of WA; MA 80 Northwestern Univ; Sp-Lang Path, Sally Burleigh Sp/P Assoc, **SLP ACE**

Letcavage, Noryn Ann 9278-B Jamison Avenue #B, Philadelphia, PA 19115-4281, (215) 677-7069, BS 82 Univ of AZ; MA 85 Temple Univ-Tyler Sch of Art; **SLP A**

Letcher-Glembo, Dr Lisa 3050 Old Highway 8, Apartment 319, Roseville, MN 55113, (612) 631-9577, MS 85 Univ of South FL; PH (Sp-Lang Path) Univ of MN - Minneap-St Paul; 88–Sp-Lang Path, U Minnesota Cleft Palate Clin, **SLP**

Letey, Abbie J San Juan Regional Medical Ctr, 801 West Maple, Farmington, NM 87401, (505) 325-5011, BS 74 TX Tech Univ; MS 76 TX Tech Univ; Dir of Aud Electro, San Juan Reg Med Cen, **A**

Lethlean, B Sue 5709 Cedar Ridge Road, Middleton, WI 53562, (608) 833-2877, BS 72 Univ of WI - Madison; MS 79 Univ of WI - Whitewater; 88–Reg VP, Rehab Associates, **SLP ACE**

Letien, W Cary Hearing Healthcare Associates, North Shore Acoustic Aids, 266 Cabot Street Lindsey Bldg Box 207, Beverly, MA 01915, (508) 922-1888, BA 73 Old Dominion Univ; MA 74 Central MI Univ; Owner, North Shore Acoustic Aids, **A**

Letizia, Mrs Marina Roberta 58 Oak Street, Lynbrook, NY 11563-1832, (516) 334-3100, SLP, The East Meadow School Dis, **SLP**

Leto, Mrs Deborah Leonard 24 Leto Road, Albany, NY 12203, (518) 482-3331, **SLP**

Letostak, Jody Terry 2162 Maple Street, Costa Mesa, CA 92627, (714) 650-3113, BA 71 OH Wesleyan Univ; MA 73 OH Univ - Athens; Sp/Lang Path, Newport Mesa USD, **SLP**

Letowski, Dr Tomasz R 1611 Laurel Avenue #502, Knoxville, TN 37916, (615) 974-1807, MS 65 Warsaw Tech Univ - Poland; PH 73 (Acoustics) Wroclaw Tech Univ - Poland; 81–Research Assoc Prof, Univ of Tennessee

Lettieri, Mrs Mary M 185 Alta Drive, Munroe Falls, OH 44262, (216) 678-2400, BS 77 Kent St Univ; MA 78 Kent St Univ; 78–Sp-Lang Path, Portage Co Bd of Ment Ret, **SLP**

Lettieri, Teresa Jo 3428 Cove View Boulevard, Apartment 611, Galveston, TX 77554-8047, (409) 761-6365, MS 82 Univ of North TX; Sp-Lang Path, U of TX Medical Branch, **SLP**

Lettko, Mrs Carol Shearer Westview Lane, Norwalk, CT 06854, (203) 797-7504, BS 80 Coll of Saint Rose; MA 81 SUNY - Coll at Geneseo; Sp-Lang Path, Kent County Hospital, **SLP**

Letto, Claire 12772 Newhope, Garden Grove, CA 92640, (818) 338-4013, BA 69 9154; MA 74 9154; Sch Prin, Baldwin Pk USD, **SLP**

Letzter, Carol B 162-16 85th Street, Howard Beach, NY 11414, (718) 745-5191, BA 81 CUNY - Queens Coll; MA 82 Hofstra Univ; Aud, American Hearing Ctr Inc, **A**

Leue, Debra Ann P O Box 937, Evergreen, CO 80439, (303) 674-3329, BS Univ of Cincinnati; MA Univ of Cincinnati; SLP, Jefferson Co Pub Sch, **SLP**

Leutholt, Mrs Barbara Dugger Rd 1 Box 549-A, Pleasant Run Road, Flemington, NJ 08822, (201) 356-5196, BS 64 East TN St Univ; Coord Sp-Lang Path Dept, Center Sch, **SLP**

Levan, Dee A 10643 Bragg Avenue, Grass Valley, CA 95945, (916) 888-7053, Special Education Teacher, Placer County Office of Educ, **SLP**

Levan, Mrs Kathleen 327 East Benton Avenue, Stockton, IL 61085, (815) 947-2596, BS 73 Univ of IL - Urbana; MS 74 Univ of IL - Urbana; Sp-Lang Path, Community Unit Dist 206, **SLP**

Levander, Jane M 3550 South Kendall #5-203, Denver, CO 80235, BA 85 Univ of SD - Vermillion; MS 87 Univ of NE - Lincoln; 88–Aud, Denver Ear Nose Throat PC, **A**

Levandowski, Mary Kaye 32400 Glen Cove #6, Farmington Hills, MI 48018, (313) 592-3332, BA 85 Western MI Univ; MA 87 Western MI Univ; 87–Aud, Redford Union Ord Prog for HI

Levar, Lavonne 3145 Dana Road, Duluth, MN 55811, (612) 781-6571, **SLP**

Levary, Mrs Esther Feldman 13173 Royal Pines Drive, Unit 7, St Louis, MO 63146, (314) 469-7843, BA 70 Univ of WI - Madison; MS 72 Univ of WI - Madison; Sp-Lang Path, Spc Sch Dist St Louis Co, **SLP**

Levasseur, Mrs Mary T 9 Channel View Road, Cape Elizabeth, ME 04107, (518) 785-9529, BA 73 Univ of ME - Orono; MS 75 Univ of VT; Sp-Lang Path, Portland Pub Sch, **SLP**

Levatter, Theodore D 12957 Moorpark Street, Studio City, CA 91604, BA 71 Univ of CA - Santa Barbara; MA 83 CA St Univ - Los Angeles; 85–Instr, Glendale Comm Coll, **SLP**

Leveen, Mrs Nancy C 14807 S W 139th Place, Miami, FL 33186, BS 78 FL St Univ; MS 80 FL St Univ; SLP, Dade Co Publ Schls, **SLP**

Levell, Mrs Marilyn M 305 Concord Circle, Papillion, NE 68046, (712) 527-5261, BA 73 Univ of SD - Vermillion; MA 74 Univ of SD - Vermillion; Sp-Lang Path, Loess Hills AEA 13, **SLP**

Leven, Kathy Breese 1721 47th Street, Pennsauken, NJ 08110, (609) 342-3060, BA 79 Rutger's St Univ - Douglas Coll; OM 81 Hahneman Medical Coll; Sp-Path/Aud, Coorer Hosp/U, **SLP A**

Levenhagen, Tracy Ann 1182 Kavanaugh Place, Wauwatosa, WI 53213, (414) 259-1414, **SLP**

Levenson, Jodi Lynn P 37 Pine Terrace, Demarest, NJ 07627-1214, (212) 356-1719, BS 77 Boston Univ; MS 80 Adelphi Univ; SLP, Richmond Mem Hosp Cl, **SLP**

Levenson, Mrs Roberta M 2359 Edgerton Road, University Heights, OH 44118, (216) 371-2445, BS 65 OH St Univ; MA 67 Case Western Reserve Univ; Sp-Lang Path, Private Practice, **SLP**

Levenson, Mrs Sally Kanner 6452 Monitor Street, Pittsburgh, PA 15217, (412) 521-8896, BS 86 OH Univ - Athens; MA 87 OH Univ - Athens; 87–Sp-Lang Path, Allegheny Valley Sch

Levenson, Mrs Sondra H 40 Princeton Road, Chestnut Hill, MA 02167, (617) 232-5987, Sp-Lang Path, Malden Hosp, **SLP**

Leventer, Dr Susan L 810 Medical Arts Bldg, 277 Alexander Street, Rochester, NY 14607, (716) 232-5620, BA 69 Barnard Coll; MA 72 SUNY - Coll at Geneseo; PH 85 (Psychology) Univ of Rochester; 77–Dir, Private Practice, **SLP**

Leventhal, Mark L 26 Darewood Lane, Valley Stream, NY 11581, (212) 642-6096, BS 72 Ithaca Coll; MS 76 CUNY - Brooklyn Coll; Sp-Lang Path, Brooklyn Dev Cen, **SLP**

Leveque, Mrs Grace 10956 El Chino Avenue, Fountain Valley, CA 92708, (714) 963-7257, BA 85 CA St Univ - Fullerton; MA 87 CA St Univ - Fullerton; 88–SLP, Anaheim Cty Elem Sch Dist

Lever, Mrs Katharine Rando 14 Bayberry Lane, Scarborough, ME 04074, (207) 839-4484, BA 79 Boston Coll; MS 81 Boston Univ; Sp-Lang Path, Gorham Sch Dept, **SLP**

Leverenz, A Florence 2000 Vale Road, San Pablo, CA 94806, (415) 235-7000, BA 68 San Jose St Univ; MA 71 San Jose St Univ; Sp/Lang Path, Private Practice, **SLP**

Leverett, Dr Ralph G Missouri Southern State College, Newman & Duquesne Roads, Joplin, MO 64801-1595, (417) 625-9623, MA 69 G Peabody Coll-Vanderbilt U; MS 74 Vanderbilt Univ; PH 83 (Prog Devt/Hrng & Sp Sci) G Peabody Coll-Vanderbilt U; Prof of Spec Ed, MO Southern St Coll, **SLP**

Levernier, Mrs Christine Marie South 3615 Mercy Court, Spokane, WA 99206, (509) 455-3287, BA 83 WA St Univ; MS 85 Eastern WA Univ; 86–Sp-Lang Path, Sacred Heart Med Ctr, **SLP**

Levert, Stephanie M 7511 Sunbury Circle, Baton Rouge, LA 70808, (504) 767-1846, BA 71 Univ of AL- Tuscaloosa; MA 74 Tulane Univ; Sp-Lang Path, Our Lady of the Lake Reg Med Ctr, **SLP A**

Levesque, Caren Ann 6 Leech Street, Beverly, MA 01915, (617) 774-5000, BS 84 Univ of NH; MS 86 Boston Univ; 86–Sp-Lang Path, Hogan/Berry Rehab Ctr, **SLP**

Levesque, Mrs Cynthia Hyatt 600 Canyon Drive, Auburn, CA 95603, (916) 888-1321, BA 80 CA St Univ - Sacramento; MA 83 CA St Univ - Chico; Sp/Lang Path, Private Practice, **SLP**

Levesque, Ute D 6740 Baxter Terrace Circle, Anchorage, AK 99504, (907) 338-6279, BA 79 CA St Univ - Fresno; MS 85 Univ of WA; **A**

Levett, Mrs Colleen Ann 4519 McDonald Road, Syracuse, NY 13215, (315) 492-2577, BS 76 Marywood Coll; MS 77 Ithaca Coll

Levey, Mary Jean 1339 Shoecraft Road, Webster, NY 14580, (716) 671-4205, BS 74 Nazareth Coll of Rochester; MS 79 Nazareth Coll of Rochester

Levey, Sandra K 235-A Christopher Street, Upper Montclair, NJ 07043-1702, (415) 493-2156, BA 78 Wayne St Univ; MA 81 Wayne St Univ; Private Practice, **SLP**

Levi, Ellen Carol University Of Washington, Sp & Hrng Sciences Jg-15, 1417 N E 42nd Street, Seattle, WA 98105, (206) 545-2212, BS 78 Univ of TX - Austin; MA 81 Univ of TN - Knoxville; Research Assistant, University of Washington, **A**

Levin, Mrs Angela Fuoco 10046 South Homan Avenue, Evergreen Park, IL 60642, (312) 425-9473, BA 83 Augustana Coll; MA 84 Western MI Univ; Sp-Language Pathologist, Evergreen Park School District, **SLP**

Levin, Betsy 330 West Diversey, Chicago, IL 60657, (312) 666-6500, BS 63 Univ of IL - Urbana; MA 66 De Paul Univ; 82–Sp-Lang Path Admin Ofcr/Ambulatory Care, VA W Side Med Cen, **SLP**

Levin, C Lynn 4724 Sherman, Galveston, TX 77550, BS 68 Univ of TX - Austin; MA 74 Univ of Houston - Univ Park; **SLP**

Levin, Julie Anne 6923 North Kedvale, Lincolnwood, IL 60646, BA 82 Mundelein Coll; MS 84 Rush Univ; SLP, Hinsdale Hospital, **SLP**

Levin, Lynne S 11 Windsor Drive, Voorhees, NJ 08043, **SLP**

Levin, Molly 164 Stratford Road, Painesville, OH 44077, BA 63 OH St Univ; **SLP**

Levin, Patricia Ann 5452 Munila Avenue, Oakland, CA 94618, (415) 527-7411, BA 70 Univ of CA - Berkeley; MS 84 CA St Univ - Hayward; SLP, Herrick Hospital, **SLP**

Levin, Stephanie Lynn 1030 West 72nd Street, Indianapolis, IN 46260, (317) 255-7291, BS 73 IN Univ - Bloomington; MA 75 Univ of MA - Amherst; **A**

Levin, Mrs Susan Schwartz 35 Park Drive, Mount Kisco, NY 10549, (914) 285-8172, BS 81 Ithaca Coll; MS 83 Boston Univ; 84–Sp-Lang Path, Westchester Co Medical Cntr, **SLP ACE**

Levin, Wendy Gail 22 Adams Street, Arlington, MA 02174, (617) 782-5552, **SLP**

Levin-Charns, Dr Judy 29 Braeburn Road, Newton, MA 02166, (617) 969-9219, BA 73 SUNY - Center at Stony Brook; MS 75 Boston Univ; ED 86 (Psycholinguistics) Boston Univ; 83–Sp/Lang Path/Core Team Ldr, Wellesley Publ Schs, **SLP**

Levine, Mrs Arlene Greneman 116 Main Street, Farmington, CT 06032, (203) 677-4475, **SLP**

Levine, Mrs Beth Shapiro ENT Specialists Inc, 825 Washington Street Suite 310, Norwood, MA 02062, (617) 769-8910, BS 80 Univ of GA; MS 82 Boston Univ; Aud, ENT Specialists Inc, **A**

Levine, Carol A 227 Storm Drive, Holtsville, NY 11742, (516) 289-9262, BA 80 SUNY - Coll at Cortland; MA 82 CUNY - Queens Coll; Sp-Lang Path, Unit Cereb Palsy Assn Suffolk, **SLP**

Levine, Mrs Cynthia S 400 Ponderosa Court, Lafayette, CA 94549, (415) 939-1720, BS 66 Univ of MO - Columbia; MA 67 Univ of MO - Columbia; **SLP**

Levine, David S St Louis Hearing & Speech Ctr, 9526 Manchester, St Louis, MO 63119, (314) 968-4710, BS 54 Washington Univ; MA 58 Washington Univ; Chief of Clinical Staff, St Louis Hearing & Sp-Center, **SLP A**

Levine, Deborah Biskin 151 Colonial Avenue, Albany, NY 12208, (518) 489-5018, BS 78 CUNY - Brooklyn Coll; ME 82 Coll of Saint Rose; 86–Sp-Lang Path, Kids' Samples Ltd, **SLP**

Levine, Elizabeth 55-1501 River Drive South, Jersey City, NJ 07310-1501, (201) 626-1216, BA 84 SUNY - Coll at Cortland; MA 85 Bowling Green St Univ; 86–Aud, New York Eye and Ear Infirmary, **A**

Levine, Elizabeth Fernandez 4301 East English, Wichita, KS 67218, (316) 689-8146, BS 82 Valdosta St Coll; MA 84 Univ of Central FL; **SLP**

Levine, Esther S 12202 Drakemill, Houston, TX 77077, (713) 558-8200, BS 70 Univ of TX - Austin; MA 76 Univ of Houston - Univ Park; Sp-Lang Path, Private Practice, **SLP ACE**

Levine, Mrs Helene B 24 Stonegate Road, Ossining, NY 10562, (914) 941-2636, BS 63 Univ of IL - Urbana; MA 65 Univ of IL - Urbana; Sp-Lang Path, Ossining Public Schools, **SLP**

Levine, Irma L 1200-18 Warburton Avenue, Yonkers, NY 10701, (914) 967-8948, BA 53 NY Univ; MA 63 Seton Hall Univ; 88–Sp-Lang Path, Private Practice, **SLP**

Levine, Mrs Jan W 291 Orchard Drive, Pittsburgh, PA 15228, (412) 394-5815, BS 65 Northwestern Univ; MS 68 Univ of WI - Madison; Sp-Lang Path, Allegheny Intermediate Unit, **SLP**

Levine, Jodie L 3747 Tallsman Place #C, Boulder, CO 80301, BS 82 West Chester Univ of PA; MA 86 Univ of MD - College Park; **SLP**

Levine, Judith 15 Cygnet Drive, Smithtown, NY 11787, (516) 265-2065, BA 58 CUNY - Queens Coll; MA 71 Hofstra Univ; SLP, Smithtown Cen Sch Dist, **SLP**

Levine, Mrs Judith D 7902 Ivy Mount Terrace, Potomac, MD 20854, (301) 983-8176, BA 65 Univ of MD - College Park; MA 67 Univ of MD - College Park; SLP, Montg Co Pub Sch, **SLP**

Levine, Judith G 5 Deepwood Lane, Westport, CT 06880, (203) 227-8451, BS 68 Boston Univ; MS 70 George Washington Univ; Sp-Lang Path, Westport Board of Education, **SLP**

Levine, Mrs Linda K 5023 Sentinel Dr, Apt 123, Bethesda, MD 20816, (301) 229-0694, BA 77 Brandeis Univ; MA 79 George Washington Univ; Sp-Lang Path, Private Practice, **SLP**

Levine, Marion 304 Sea Isle Key, Secaucus, NJ 07094, **SLP A**

Levine, Nancy 16846 Royal Crest Drive, Houston, TX 77058, (713) 488-8949, BS 62 Univ of Houston - Univ Park; MA 66 Univ of Houston - Univ Park; Owner/Dir, Bay Area Sp-Lang-Learning Cen, **SLP**

Levine, Mrs Nioma K 316 Curtis Drive, Wyncote, PA 19095, (215) 887-2681, BA 62 Temple Univ; MA 67 Temple Univ; SLP, Montgomery Co Intermediate Ut, **SLP LM**

Levine, Phylis Cedar Swamp Road, Jericho, NY 11753, (516) 932-1462, BS 77 SUNY - Center at Albany; MS 78 Syracuse Univ; SLP, Onodaga-Madison BOCES, **SLP**

LeVine, Mrs Ricki 1609 Thayer Avenue, Los Angeles, CA 90024, (213) 855-2109, BA 66 Long Island U - Brooklyn Ctr; MA 81 Whittier Coll; 82–Sp-Lnag Path, Cedars-Sinai Med Cen, **SLP**

Levine, Mrs Risa F 1602 Hearthglow Lane, Richmond, VA 23233, (804) 740-3635, BA 70 CUNY - Queens Coll; MS 72 Columbia Univ Teachers Coll; Sp-Lang Path, Restreat Hospital, **SLP**

Levine, Rochelle 52 Chester Court, Peekskill, NY 10566, (212) 430-8386, MA 73 Univ of IL - Urbana; Aud, Albert Einstein College of Med, **A**

Levine, Mrs Ronnie Elaine Freedman 1 Ivy Way, Dayton, NJ 08810, (201) 274-2509, BA 74 Hofstra Univ; MA 76 Hofstra Univ; Sp-Lang Path, **SLP**

Levine, Mrs Rose Beverly 4 Woodstone Road, Morris Plains, NJ 07950, (201) 267-3343, BA 66 Montclair St Coll; ME 80 Paterson St Coll; **SLP**

Levine, Mrs Ruth 7 Woodford Lane, Manalapan Township, NJ 07726, (201) 246-4255, BA 60 CUNY - Brooklyn Coll; MA 62 CUNY - Brooklyn Coll; Sp-Lang Path, Univ of Medicine & Dentistry-NJ, **SLP ACE**

Levine, Mrs Sandra Young 59 Verbena Drive, Commack, NY 11725, (516) 542-0339, OB 68 OH Univ - Athens; OM 88 New Sch for Social Research; 86–Family Svcs Coord, NY State Head Injury Assoc, **SLP**

Levine, Sharon W 4984 Northwest 82 Terrace, Coral Springs, FL 33067, (201) 763-6801, BS 74 Northeastern Univ; MA 75 Case Western Reserve Univ; Sp-Lang Path, Private Practice, **SLP ACE**

Levine, Susan 5835 Conway Road, Bethesda, MD 20817, (202) 363-6261, BA 75 Case Western Reserve Univ; MA 75 Case Western Reserve Univ; Sp-Lang Path, Private Practice, **SLP**

Levine, Susan B 111 Goldenrod, Irvine, CA 92714, (714) 786-2757, BA 73 Hofstra Univ; MA 74 Hofstra Univ; SLP, Susan Levine, **SLP**

Levine, Terri 21 Poppy Court, Brick, NJ 08723, (201) 920-4815, BA 78 Univ of Pittsburgh - Pittsburgh; MS 79 Ithaca Coll; **SLP**

Levine Esq, Mrs Barbara Pearlman 5520 15th Avenue #6C, Brooklyn, NY 11219, (212) 270-2960, BA 53 CUNY - Brooklyn Coll; MA 55 CUNY - Brooklyn Coll; OD 83 (NS) Brooklyn Law Sch; Attorney Law Assistant, Civil Court Kings Co NYC, **SLP**

Levine-Stern, Ilene Easter Seal, 555 Auburn Street, Manchester, NH 03103, (603) 623-8863, BS 72 Boston Univ; MS 73 Univ of WI - Madison; Aud, Easter Seal of NH, **A**

Levinger, Bonnie Kwasman 22676 Shadow Pine Way, Novi, MI 48050, (313) 348-9542, BS 83 Univ of AZ; MS 85 Univ of MI - Ann Arbor; **SLP**

Levinn, Mrs Karen A Rural Delivery 4, 49-B Fairmount Avenue, Chester, NJ 07930, BS 79 SUNY - Coll at Geneseo; MS 80 Syracuse Univ; Sp-Lang Path, Rehab Ctr for the Handicapped, **SLP**

Levinson, Dianne Mihic 7200 S E 34th Avenue, Portland, OR 97202, MS; **SLP**

Levinson, Elizabeth Arla 165-20 Jewel Avenue, Flushing, NY 11365, (718) 821-6880, MS 84 CUNY - Queens Coll; 86–Tchr, NY City Bd of Educ, **SLP**

Levinson, Janice Sue 66-10 Thornton Place Lh, Forest Hills, NY 11375, (212) 852-3220, BA 82 CUNY - Queens Coll; MS 83 Adelphi Univ; Sp-Lang Path, Lowell School, **SLP**

Levinson, Karen Beth 12000 Old Georgetown Road, Apartment S-705, Rockville, MD 20852, (301) 881-1974, BS 81 Syracuse Univ; MS 83 Towson St Univ; Sp-Lang Path, Speech Pathology Associates, **SLP**

Levinson, Dr Philip J Scottish Rite Clinics, 1507 S W Morrison Street, Suite A, Portland, OR 97205, (503) 226-1048, BA 63 Univ of CA - Los Angeles; MA 70 CA St Univ - Los Angeles; PH 73 (Sp Path) Univ of WA; Dir, Scottish Rite Clinic/Chldhd Lang Di, **SLP ACE**

Levinson, Renee Presbyterian University Hosp, Dept Of Otoneurology #591, 230 Lothrop Street, Pittsburgh, PA 15213, (412) 647-3130, MA 74 Case Western Reserve Univ; Aud, Presbyterian University Hosp, **A**

Levinson, Shelly K 4105 Centralea, Lakewood, CA 90712, (213) 925-2285, BA 75 CA St Univ - Northridge; MA 80 Whittier Coll; **SLP**

Levinson, Steven M 346 Sequine Avenue, Staten Island, NY 10309, (212) 356-1719, BA 70 CUNY - Queens Coll; MS 73 Univ of RI; Sp-Lang Path, Private Practice, **SLP**

Levinson, Susan Kings Highway Towers #D310, Maple Shade, NJ 08052, (609) 722-1088, MA 87 West Chester Univ of PA

Levinson, Mrs Teri Solomon 2 Bartlett Court, Matawan, NJ 07747, (201) 679-3981, BA 79 Rutgers St Univ -N Brunswick; MA 81 Montclair St Coll; SLP, Passaic Cerebral Palsy Center, **SLP**

Levinston, Mrs Donna H Adler 457 Brookside Lane, Somerville, NJ 08876, (201) 297-7800, BS 65 Wayne St Univ; ME 66 Wayne St Univ; 68–Sp-Lang Path, South Brunswick Twp Bd of Educ, **SLP**

Levis, Mrs Gayle Ann Route 3, Audubon, IA 50025, (712) 563-4459, BA 69 Grinnell Coll; MA 71 Univ of IA; Sp-Lang Path, Private Practice, **SLP**

Levi-Shandler, Karen L 5358 Pooks Hill Road, Bethesda, MD 20814, (301) 649-3162, BA 73 Univ of CA - Santa Barbara; MS 76 Emerson Coll; Sp-Lang Path, Montgy Co Pub Sch, **SLP**

Levisohn, Ruth L 5290 East Yale Circle, Suite 207, Denver, CO 80222, (303) 777-5015, **SLP**

Levitan, Mrs Peggy 71 Warner Lane, Syosset, NY 11791, (516) 921-4125, BS 73 SUNY - Center at Albany; MA 76 Hofstra Univ; **SLP**

Levitan, Tamar K 5-D Ashmore 630 Mix Avenue, Hamden, CT 06514, (203) 932-5711, BA 77 SUNY - Center at Buffalo; MS 79 Columbia Univ Teachers Coll; Sp-Lang Path, VA West Haven, **SLP**

Levithan, Lisa 5450 Carversville Road, Doylestown, PA 18901, BS 83 Trenton St Coll; MA 87 Trenton St Coll; 84–Sp-Lang Path, Bucks County Intermediate Unit, **SLP**

Levitin, Mrs Rochelle 39 Carlton Road, Monsey, NY 10952, (914) 352-6925, BA 77 CUNY - Brooklyn Coll; MA 79 NY Univ; Sp-Lang Path, Private Practice, **SLP**

Levitt, Ellen 105 Colonial Village, Route 9, Amherst, MA 01002, (203) 423-8401, MA 82 CUNY - Lehman Coll; Sp-Lang Path, Willimantic Public Schools, **SLP**

Levitt, Dr Harry 46 Tanglewood Drive, Livingston, NJ 07039, (212) 790-4366, BS 58; PH 64 (NS); Professor, City University of New York, **F**

Levitt, Joyce Barbara P O Box 38 Sles, FPO Seattle, WA 98767-0005, (619) 291-2506, BS 76 Univ of CO - Boulder; MA 82 CA St Univ - Sacramento; Sp/Lang Path, Scottish Rite Cl, **SLP**

Levitt, Mrs Linda Ruth 4230 Christy Way, Reno, NV 89509, (702) 747-5795, BA 73 Univ of the Pacific; MA 74 Univ of the Pacific; 79–Sp-Lang Path, Washoe Co Sch Dist, **SLP**

Levitt, Nina 7 Fairmount Avenue, Morristown, NJ 07960, (201) 455-1435, BA 70 CUNY - Hunter Coll; MS 71 Columbia Univ Teachers Coll; Sp-Lang Path, Nina Levitt, **SLP**

Levitt, Mrs Patricia Joseph 287 Wayne Avenue, Haddonfield, NJ 08033, BS 80 Ithaca Coll; MA 81 Trenton St Coll; Sp-Lang Path, Private Practice, **SLP**

Levitt, Robert Olin 492 4th Avenue, Salt Lake City, UT 84103, (801) 521-1680, BS 80 Western MI Univ; MS 84 Univ of UT; **SLP**

Levitz, Mrs Ingrid 31 Chinook Crescent, Nepean, ON, Canada K2H 7C9, (613) 226-5367, BS 69 Emerson Coll; MS 70 Adelphi Univ; **SLP**

Le Vos, Mrs Sandra Clawson Route 1 Box 131-A, Pennsboro, WV 26415, (304) 659-3915, BA 68 Pacific Union Coll; MA 70 Univ of Redlands; **SLP**

Levy, Alice Marie 2006 Maury #3N, St Louis, MO 63110, (314) 569-8100, **SLP**

Levy, Mrs Barbara G 12 Nome Drive, Woodbury, NY 11797, (516) 692-4085, BS 71 Long Island U - CW Post Ctr; MS 74 Hofstra Univ; Aud, Jewish Inst for Geriatric Care, **A**

Levy, Mrs Cara S 24 Carling Drive, New Hyde Park, NY 11040, (516) 294-0275, BS 74 SUNY - Center at Albany; MS 78 CUNY - Brooklyn Coll; 87–Dir of Sp Svcs, Inst of Applied Human Dynamics, **SLP**

Levy, Carol B 648 Washington Street, Brookline, MA 02146, (617) 720-6818, MA 68 IN Univ - Bloomington; ME 73 Harvard Univ; ED 77 (Applied Psycholinguistics) Boston Univ; 88–Mgr of Consulting Svc, Spaulding Rehab Hosp, **SLP**

Levy, Dr Constance Andrea 200 East 71st Street #76, Apartment 5-H, New York, NY 10021, (212) 737-3502, BA 73 CUNY - Hunter Coll; MA 86 NY Univ; PH 81 (Comparative Literature-Spanish Russian French & English) NY Univ; 88–Sp-Lang Path, Card Cooke Med Ctr, **SLP**

Levy, Mrs Cynthia 144 Irving Place, Basking Ridge, NJ 07920, (201) 674-6934, BA 80 Rutger's St Univ - Douglas Coll; MA 83 NY Univ; Sp-Lang Path, Kessler Inst, **SLP**

Levy, David H 7019 Kingston Pike, Knoxville, TN 37919-5760, (615) 588-3277, BS 72 Univ of TN - Knoxville; MA 76 Univ of TN - Knoxville; Pres, Bal Enterprises Inc, **A**

Levy, Debra Renee 2 Crawford Drive, Dix Hills, NY 11746, (516) 499-3420, MS 88 SUNY - Coll at Buffalo

Levy, Diane D 3703 Blue Heron Drive, Fort Myers, FL 33908, (813) 337-8367, OB 69 Univ of FL; ME 73 Univ of FL; Sp-Lang Path, Lee County School Board, **SLP ACE**

Levy, Mrs Ellyn B 54-44 Little Neck Parkway, Little Neck, NY 11362-2285, (718) 224-8246, BS 78 SUNY - Coll at New Paltz; MS 80 Columbia Univ Teachers Coll; Sp-Lang Path, Private Practice, **SLP**

Levy, Mrs Hillary Brook 2323 Sharon Road #211, Menlo Park, CA 94025, (415) 854-3123, **SLP**

Levy, Mrs Inez B 8841 North Laramie, Skokie, IL 60076, **SLP**

Levy, Mrs Joan R 227 East 57th Street #11C, New York, NY 10022, (212) 470-8910, BA 51 CUNY - Brooklyn Coll; MA 68 CUNY - Queens Coll; Chief Sp-Lang Path, L Isl Jewish-Hillside Med Cen, **SLP ACE**

Levy, Joanne Schnee Dept Communication Disorders, Daniel Freeman Hospital, 333 North Prarie Avenue, Inglewood, CA 90301, (213) 674-7050, BA 77 Univ of CA - Santa Barbara; MA 80 Univ of WA; SLP, Daniel Freeman Mem Hosp, **SLP**

Levy, Mrs Karen Brannigan 1860 Jefferson Street, Concord, CA 94521, (415) 825-5254, BS 82 LA St Univ - Baton Rouge; MS 85 Univ of Southwestern LA; Sp-Lang Path, **SLP**

Levy, Laura Robin 3270 N Lake Shore Drive, Apartment 10C, Chicago, IL 60657, (312) 327-0595, BS 76 MI St Univ; MS 78 Univ of WI - Madison; Sp-Lang Path, Private Practice, **SLP**

Levy, Lisa Jan 4156-A Cove Lane, Glenview, IL 60025, (312) 275-8822, **SLP**

Levy, Louise 301 Lincoln Plaza #16V, New York, NY 10023, (212) 420-2760, BS 79 Boston Univ; MS 81 Columbia Univ Teachers Coll; Aud/Chief, Beth Israel Med Cen, **A**

Levy, Mrs Marcia K 5 Patton Boulevard, New Hyde Park, NY 11040, BS 75 SUNY - Center at Albany; MA 76 Hofstra Univ; **SLP**

Levy, Mrs Mary A R 15208 Court Road, Minnetonka, MN 55345, (612) 520-5614, BA 76 Univ of OR; MA 77 Univ of ND; 87–Sp-Lang Path, North Memorial Med Ctr, **SLP ACE**

Levy, Mrs Miriam S 18 Walnut Parkway, Montclair, NJ 07042, (305) 475-2020, BA 74 Adelphi Univ; MS 75 FL St Univ; **SLP**

Levy, Regina H 9980 Central Park Blvd N, Suite 104, Boca Raton, FL 33428, (407) 483-6000, BA 75 Univ of Miami; MA 78 Univ of Miami; 84–Sp-Lang Path, Private Practice, **SLP**

Levy, Robin C W 3716 Sixth Street, P O Box 699, North Beach, MD 20714, (301) 535-2212, BS 75 WV Univ; MA 77 Catholic Univ of America; Sp-Lang Path, Calvert Co Pub Sch, **SLP**

Levy, Mrs Robyn K 9403 E Lake Avenue, Englewood, CO 80111, (303) 694-6378, **SLP**

Levy, Mrs Rosalind R 301 East 21st Street, New York, NY 10010, (212) 561-3564, BA 52 CUNY - Hunter Coll; 55–Sp-Lang Path, Bellevue Hosp, **SLP**

Levy, Sharon H 7431 Baltimore Avenue, Takoma Park, MD 20912, (301) 589-0155, MA 72 Case Western Reserve Univ; Sp-Lang Path, Montgomery Co School System, **SLP**

Levy, Sheila Z 5901 Donlyn Drive, Huntington Beach, CA 92649, (714) 558-5591, BA 72 Univ of CA - Los Angeles; MA 77 CA St Univ - Long Beach; Coord Comm Handicapped, Santa Ana USD, **SLP**

Levy, Stephanie 7 Leeward Lane, Commack, NY 11725, (516) 289-2200, BA 80 SUNY - Coll at New Paltz; MS 82 Adelphi Univ; Tchr, BOCES-Secondary Dist, **SLP**

Levy, Mrs Susan F Sacred Heart Hospital & Rehabilitation Center, Speech-Language Pathology, 1430 DeKalb Street, Norristown, PA 19401, (215) 278-8620, BA 80 Univ of Pittsburgh - Pittsburgh; MA 82 Univ of Cincinnati; Chief Sp-Lang Path, Sacred Heart Hosp & Rehab Cntr, **SLP**

Levy-Millen, Mrs Meta J 176 Hartman Road, Newton, MA 02159, (617) 552-7673, BA 74 Northeastern Univ; ME 76 Northeastern Univ; 87–Chmn-Sp-Lang Dept, Newton Pub Sch, **SLP**

Lew, Beverly 5745 Chicopee, Encino, CA 91316, (818) 996-6395, BA 85 CA St Univ - Northridge; MA 87 CA St Univ - Northridge; **A**

Lew, Linda 12549 Cuesta Drive, Cerritos, CA 90701, (213) 926-7727, BA 81 Univ of CA - Santa Barbara; MA 85 CA St Univ - Los Angeles; Assoc Clin Dir, Head Injury Rehab Svcs Inc, **SLP**

Lew, Mrs Rhoda M B 225 Lyncroft Road, New Rochelle, NY 10804, (914) 632-9000, BA 67 CUNY - Brooklyn Coll; MA 72 NY Univ; Sp-Lang Path, New Rochelle Bd of Ed, **SLP**

Lewallen, Barbara Hewitt Professional Hearing Services, 2354 Hassell Road, Hoffman Estates, IL 60195, (312) 490-1670, BS 83 Northern IL Univ - De Kalb; MA 85 Northern IL Univ - De Kalb; 86–Aud, Pro Hrng Svcs Ltd, **A**

Lewandowski, Mrs Carole C 1767 East 60th Place, Tulsa, OK 74105, (918) 495-6869, BA 59 MI St Univ; MA 72 Univ of Tulsa; Assistant Professor, Oral Roberts U, **SLP**

Lewandowski, Deborah Lynne 1-B Stadler Place, Greensboro, NC 27410-2744, (304) 325-2471, MA 84 Univ of NC - Greensboro; **A**

Lewandowski, Elaine Cecilia 21-36 Himrod Street, Ridgewood, NY 11385, (212) 904-2677, BA 83 CUNY - Queens Coll; MA 85 CUNY - Queens Coll; 85–Aud, Hosp Albert Einstein Coll Med, **A**

Lewark, Mrs Nancy Marie 1808 South State Road, Apartment 135, Greenwood, IN 46143, (317) 535-9792, BA 74 Ball St Univ; MA 79 Ball St Univ; Admin, Southside Rehab Cen, **SLP**

Lewellen, Sherri Ann 1550 North Verdugo Road, Apartment 31, Glendale, CA 91208, (213) 660-2430, BA 84 CA St Univ - Northridge; MA 86 CA St Univ - Northridge; **A**

Lewin, Jan S University Of Michigan Hospital, Department Of Otolaryngology Speech Pathology Division, TC-1904-0312 1500 East Medical Center Drive, Ann Arbor, MI 48109-0312, (313) 936-7507, BA 77 Univ of MI - Ann Arbor; MS 78 Univ of MI - Ann Arbor; Dir-SLP Div, U of MI Hosp-Dept of Otor, **SLP**

Lewis, Andrea Jill 185 Lakeshore Road #2, Brighton, MA 02135-3819, (617) 782-2463, BS 81 Ithaca Coll; ME 84 Northeastern Univ; **SLP**

Lewis, Angela Utena 2810 Oakley Avenue, Baltimore, MD 21215, (301) 396-1357, **SLP**

Lewis, Mrs Arlene 300 Windsor Lane, Marlton, NJ 08053, (609) 596-0319, BA 75 CUNY - Brooklyn Coll; MA 78 Temple Univ; Sp-Lang Path, Private Practice, **SLP**

Lewis, Barbara Jean 5950 Southwest 74th Street, Apt 207, South Miami, FL 33143, (305) 662-8050, BS 81 Miami Univ - Oxford; MA 83 Univ of IL - Urbana; Sp-Lang Path, University of Miami, **SLP**

Lewis, Mrs Barbara M 7451 Briar Hill, Kirtland, OH 44094, (216) 844-3669, BS 76 Saint Mary's Coll; MA 79 Case Western Reserve Univ; PH 87 (Sp Path) Case Western Reserve Univ; Sp-Lang Path, Case Western Reserve Univ, **SLP**

Lewis, Brenda S 1419 Surrey Lane, Philadelphia, PA 19151, (215) 642-7197, BA 71 CUNY - Queens Coll; MA 72 NY Univ; SLP, Sch Dist of Phila, **SLP**

Lewis, Carolyn Jean 7901 Nolen Drive, Little Rock, AR 72209, (501) 568-6970, BS 78 Univ of Central AR; MS 85 Univ of Central AR; **SLP**

Lewis, Dawna E Boystown Institute, 555 North 30th Street, Omaha, NE 68131, (402) 498-6607, BS 80 Univ of VA - Charlottesville; MA 82 Univ of TN - Knoxville; 82–Aud, Boys Town Natl I, **A**

Lewis, Debra A 3823 South Campbell, Springfield, MO 65807, (417) 882-7284, BS 78 Southwest MO St Univ; MA 79 Univ of MO - Columbia; Sp-Lang Path, Sp-Lang Serv of SW MO, **SLP**

Lewis, Debra Karen 19-A Surrey Hills, Hannibal, MO 63401, (314) 221-0414, MA 80 Univ of Denver; Dir of SLP, Hannibal Reg Healthcare Sys, **SLP**

Lewis, Debra Lyn 3918 Penbrook Lane, Lafayette, IN 47905-4140, (317) 659-1339, BS 82 Eastern IL Univ; MS 83 Eastern IL Univ; SLP, Clinton Prairie Sch Corp, **SLP**

Lewis, Debra Marie 1263 Devonshire Drive, Vacaville, CA 95688, (215) 631-9300, BS 85 CA St Univ - Sacramento; MS 88 San Francisco St Univ

Lewis, Delinda 646 East 1700 South #5, Salt Lake City, UT 84105, (801) 451-1158, BS 77 UT St Univ; MS 78 UT St Univ; Sp-Lang Path, Davis Co Schl Dist, **SLP**

Lewis, Diane 2035 Lyttonsville Road, Silver Spring, MD 20910, (703) 548-0209, MA 71 MI St Univ; Sp/Lang Path, Private Practice, **SLP**

Lewis, Mrs Diane H 2710 China Lake Drive, St Louis, MO 63129, BS 72 Southeast MO St Univ; MA 74 Saint Louis Univ; Sp-Lang Path, **SLP**

Lewis, Donna Lee 7300 Gran Vida, El Paso, TX 79912, (915) 569-2071, BA 77 Univ of TX - El Paso; MA 82 Univ of TX - El Paso; 87–Sp-Lang Path, William Beaumont Army Med Ctr, **SLP ACE**

Lewis, Douglas Augustus 1246-R Sheridan Drive, Lancaster, OH 43130, (614) 687-8150, MA 83 OH Univ - Athens; OM 85 Wright St Univ; Aud, Lancaster Fairfield Comm Hosp, **A**

Lewis, Frederick, Jr 1238 Maplewood Avenue, Portsmouth, NH 03801, (603) 862-2110, BS 63 Southern CT St Univ; MS 67 Southern CT St Univ; PH 70 (Sp Path) OH Univ - Athens; Assoc Prof, U of NH, **SLP**

Lewis, Dr Harold Donell 225 Bracken Court, Raleigh, NC 27615, (919) 560-6470, BS 72 Shaw Univ; MA 73 Central MI Univ; PH 79 (Aud) Univ of IL - Urbana; 84–Assoc Prof/Dir, North Carolina Central Univ, **A**

Lewis, Mrs Helga Lauretta 1850 Linden Street, East Lansing, MI 48823, (517) 676-1051, BS 83 Central MI Univ; MA 85 Central MI Univ; 88–Aud, Ingham Intermediate Sch Dist, **A**

Lewis, Mrs Jacquelyn B 1719 Prince George Court, Katy, TX 77449, (713) 347-1580, BA 74 Univ of Houston - Univ Park; MA 78 Univ of Houston - Univ Park; 82–Sp/Lang Path, Sp & Comm Consult Inc, **SLP**

Lewis, James A 5250 Saber Drive, Merrill, WI 54452, (715) 536-5011, BA 54 Univ of MN - Minneap-St Paul; MS 59 Univ of WI - Madison; 88–Retired, **SLP**

Lewis, Jan Summers 9429 Freedom Way N E, Albuquerque, NM 87109, (505) 843-2336, BA 74 Univ of NM; MA 77 Univ of KS; Instr/Cl Super, U of NM-Dept Commun Dis, **A**

Lewis, Janet E 1135 20th Street, Hermosa Beach, CA 90254-3315, **SLP**

Lewis, Mrs Janet S 21 Staples Place, West Hartford, CT 06107, (203) 521-7635, BA 75 Univ of CT; MA 77 Univ of CT; 86–Sp-Lang Path, Private Practice, **SLP**

Lewis, Mrs Janice Rechnitz 14 Alton Place #3, Brookline, MA 02146, (617) 254-3800, BA 76 Univ of CA - Santa Barbara; MS 79 Univ of NM; Sp-Lang Path, Kennedy Mem Hosp, **SLP**

Lewis, Mrs Jean S 1516 4th Avenue North, Great Falls, MT 59401, (406) 727-6303, BA 75 MI St Univ; MS 76 Purdue Univ - West Lafayette; Sp-Lang Path, N Central Learning Resource Ctr, **SLP ACE**

Lewis, Dr Jeffrey Ian 1504 SW 8th Street, Topeka, KS 66604, (913) 235-6600, BA 70 CUNY - Brooklyn Coll; MS 72 CUNY - Brooklyn Coll; PH 75 (NS) Purdue Univ - West Lafayette; Dir Commun Dis Serv, The Kansas Rehab Hosp, **SLP**

Lewis, Jennifer 5827 Corley Street, Columbia, SC 29210, (803) 786-3745, BS 71 Univ Southern MS-Hattiesburg; MS 72 Univ Southern MS-Hattiesburg; Asst Prof/Cl Dir, Columbia Coll, **SLP**

Lewis, Mrs Johanna L 20313 30th Street N E, Seattle, WA 98155, (206) 339-4595, BS 71 Bowling Green St Univ; MA 76 Univ of WA; Sp-Lang Path, Everett Sch Dist #2, **SLP**

Lewis, Mrs Judith Kay 825 South Miller Street, Litchfield, MN 55355, (612) 693-2436, BS 84 Winona St Univ; MS 85 Univ of WI - Eau Claire; 85–SLP, Lichfield Pub Sch ISD 465, **SLP**

Lewis, Judy L 8534 131st Avenue N E, Kirkland, WA 98033, (206) 828-3201, BA 77 San Diego St Univ; MA 83 Univ of MT; 87–Sp-Lang Path, Lake Washington School District, **SLP**

Lewis, Mrs Judy L 7060 Westview Drive, Worthington, OH 43085, (614) 369-3650, BA 79 Marshall Univ; MA 80 Marshall Univ; SLP, Delaware Sp & Hear Center, **SLP**

Lewis, Karla Clair Broome Developmental Center, Upper Glenwood Road, Binghamton, NY 13905, (607) 770-0441, **A**

Lewis, Kathryn Carroll P O Box 245, Worcester, NY 12197-0245, (607) 397-8990, BA 82 SUNY - Coll at Plattsburgh; MS 86 Coll of Saint Rose; **SLP**

Lewis, Mrs Kathy E Rural Delivery 1, Woodbury Road, Highland Mills, NY 10930, (914) 534-7553, BA 73 Mercy Coll; MS 79 Southern CT St Univ; Sp-Lang Path, Private Practice, **SLP**

Lewis, Kerry E 1526 S E Knight Street, Portland, OR 97202, BS 75 Portland St Univ; MS 77 Portland St Univ; Sp/Lang Path, **SLP**

Lewis, Kristy A 6788 Rolling Hills Drive, Riverside, CA 92505, (714) 785-8175, BA 83 CA St Univ - Long Beach; MA 85 CA St Univ - Long Beach; Sp-Lang Path, Corona-Norco USD, **SLP**

Lewis, Mrs Lesley L 25 Borochov Street, Givatayim, Israel 53204, (213) 337-1820, BA 80 Tel Aviv Univ - Israel; MA 84 Univ of SC - Columbia; Sp-Lang Path, InSpeech Inc, **SLP**

Lewis, Lisa Beth 183 Saybrook Lane, Wallingford, PA 19086, (302) 654-1011, BS 83 PA St Univ - Univ Park; MA 86 Temple Univ-Tyler Sch of Art; **A**

Lewis, Mrs Louise Y 1205 Briar Creek Road, Enid, OK 73703, (405) 237-9221, BS 71 Phillips Univ; MS 74 Univ of OK Medical Center; Sp/Lang Path, Private Practice, **SLP**

Lewis, Lynda Patricia 56 Arlington Avenue, Toronto, ON, Canada M6G 3K8, (416) 651-1973, BA 80 Ryerson Polytech Inst - On; MA 84 SUNY - Center at Buffalo; 88–Sp-Lang Path, City of York Bd Educ Adven Pl, **SLP**

Lewis, Mrs Margaret Kyle 208 Oak Street, Timberville, VA 22853, (703) 896-8956, BS 53 Univ of WI - Madison; SLP, Rockingham Co Pub Sch, **SLP**

Lewis, Marlene M 863 Cuaulta Crescent, Victoria, BC, Canada V9C 3H2, (604) 387-2663, BA 77 Univ of Winnipeg - Manitoba; MA 80 Univ of ND; Sp-Lang Path, Ministry of Hlth, **SLP**

Lewis, Mrs Marti C 433 Delaware Avenue, Oak Ridge, TN 37830, BS 75 East TN St Univ; MA 81 Univ of TN - Knoxville; SLP, Knox County Schools, **SLP**

Lewis, Mary Anne 2539 Puesta Del Sol, Santa Barbara, CA 93105, (805) 687-0402, 84–Sp-Lang Path, Rehab Inst at Santa Barbara, **SLP**

Lewis, Mary C 247 Washington Avenue, Winthrop, MA 02152, MS; **SLP LM**

Lewis, Mary F 516 Coolidge Court, Davis, CA 95616, (619) 267-9139, MS; **SLP**

Lewis, Mary Frances 6745 Parkside Avenue, San Diego, CA 92139, (619) 267-9139, **SLP**

Lewis, Mary Grady 211 Mt View Boulevard, Maryville, TN 37801, MS; **SLP LM**

Lewis, Mrs Mary Jane Star Route 194-A, Lonsdale, AR 72087, (501) 939-2635, BS 82 Univ of AR - Little Rock; MS 86 Univ of Central AR; 88–Sp-Lang Path, NM Head Injury Sys-AR, **SLP**

Lewis, Michael A St Dept Ed Prog For Handicapped, Koger Executive Center, Santee Bldg Suite 210, Columbia, SC 29210, (803) 737-8710, BA 70 Univ of Akron; MA 71 Kent St Univ; Consult/Hrng Hndcpd, S Carolina Dept of Ed, **A**

Lewis, Nancy Delaney 3800 Ridgeway Drive, Birmingham, AL 35259, (205) 868-2245, BS 80 Auburn Univ - Auburn; MA 84 Univ of Montevallo; **SLP**

Lewis, Nancy E 7730 S W 56th Avenue #3, Miami, FL 33143, (305) 665-7595, BA 75 Mary Washington Coll; ME 76 Univ of VA - Charlottesville; Aud, Insight, **A**

Lewis, Mrs Nancy J H 4949 Rockne Circle, Carmel, IN 46032, (317) 848-6928, BA 69 Univ of OK - Norman; MA 76 Univ of Tulsa; **SLP**

Lewis, Nancy P 3900 San Isidro Northwest, Albuquerque, NM 87107, (505) 266-8811, BA 78 Univ of FL; MS 80 Univ of AZ; Sp-Lang Path, Albuquerque Special Preschool, **SLP**

Lewis, Mrs Nancy S 6618 Belle Isle Place, Fort Wayne, IN 46835, (219) 485-4404, BS 77 Purdue Univ - West Lafayette; MA 78 Ball St Univ; **A**

Lewis, Mrs Nancy Shackman 2159 Nites, St Paul, MN 55116, (312) 848-9845, BS 77 Univ of WI - Madison; MS 79 Univ of WI - Madison; **A**

Lewis, Peta Janice ICS Medical Corporation, 2227 Hammond Drive, Schaumburg, IL 60173, (312) 397-2150, MA 84 Northwestern Univ; 88–Customer Svc Rep, ICS Medical Corp, **A**

Lewis, Mrs Roberta A 362 Angola Road, Cornwall, NY 12518, (914) 534-9864, BA 73 Mercy Coll; MA 75 SUNY - Coll at Geneseo; 86–Sp-Lang Path, Newburgh Dev Learning Ctr, **SLP**

Lewis, Rosemary Brown 1056 High Point Drive N E, Atlanta, GA 30306, (404) 851-7586, BS 78 FL St Univ; MS 79 FL St Univ; Sp-Lang Path, St Joseph's Hosp, **SLP ACE**

Lewis, Rosemary M 212 Hibiscus Lane, San Antonio, TX 78213, (512) 658-5373, OB 44 Baylor Univ; MA 68 Our Lady Lake Univ-San Anton; Dir of Spec Ed, Judson Sch Dist, **SLP**

Lewis, Sally M 25 Sugarbush Lane, Chagrin Falls, OH 44022, (813) 797-9931, BS 69 Kent St Univ; MA 75 Kent St Univ; PH 88 (Aud) Kent St Univ; **A**

Lewis, Sharon Klich 1929 Featherwood Street, Silver Spring, MD 20904, (202) 722-2323, BS 78 PA St Univ - Univ Park; MA 80 Univ of MD - College Park; Sp-Lang Path, Ntnl Chdns Cen Inc, **SLP**

Lewis, Sheila Renee 3441 North 13th Street, Milwaukee, WI 53206, (414) 263-1149, BA 83 Univ of WI - Eau Claire; OM 86 Univ of WI - River Falls; **SLP**

Lewis, Mrs Shirley M 1167 Loma Portal Drive, El Cajon, CA 92020, (619) 448-1865, BS 59 SD St Univ; MA 69 CA St Univ - Los Angeles; Tchr, Cajon Val Union Sch Dist, **SLP**

Lewis, Stephen W 1847 Barclay Street #108, Vancouver, BC, Canada V6G 1K7, (604) 687-7900, BS 70 Univ of NE - Lincoln; MS 72 Univ of WY; Sp-Lang Path, Cty of Vancouver Hlth Dept, **SLP**

Lewis, Steven Edward Norfolk Naval Shipyard, Code 720 7 Bldg 277, Portsmouth, VA 23709, (804) 396-7791, BS 71 OH Univ - Athens; MS 72 Univ of WY; Aud, Norfolk Naval Shipyard, **A**

Lewis, Susan K 20 Woodcrest Avenue, Wolcott, CT 06716, (317) 845-8128, BS 82 IN St Univ - Terre Haute; MA 83 IN Univ - Bloomington; Sp-Lang Path/Cognitive Rehab, Cen for Neuropsych Rehab, **SLP**

Lewis, Susan Myra 11310 Brill Drive, Studio City, CA 91604, (213) 894-3850, BA 85 CA St Univ - Long Beach; MA 88 CA St Univ - Northridge; 88–Sp-Lang Path, VA Outpatient Clinic

Lewis, Susan R S 510 Washington Street, Glendale, WV 26038, (304) 845-7650, BA 76 West Liberty St Coll; MS 78 WV Univ; **SLP**

Lewis, Terry K 303 Main Street West, Hamilton, ON, Canada L8P 1J7, (416) 529-5373, BA 70 OH St Univ; MA 72 OH St Univ; President/ Aud, Private Practice, **A**

Lewis, Valerie Tenney 6019 Creekstone Lane, Centreville, VA 22020, (703) 263-0636, MA 80 Central MI Univ; Sp-Lang Path, Washington Adventist Hospital, **SLP**

Lewis, Mrs Virginia Morgan 8358 Greenvale Drive, Nashville, TN 37221, (615) 298-8085, BS 63 Auburn Univ - Auburn; MS 66 Vanderbilt Univ; Sp-Lang Path, Nashville-Davidson Co Bd of Ed, **A**

Lewis, Yvonne J 3904 South Plaza Trail, Virginia Beach, VA 23452, (804) 463-7370, BA 71 Howard Univ; MA 73 Howard Univ; Sp-Lang Path, Chesapeake Pub Sch, **SLP**

Lewis-Barnette, Helen Candice 6819 Concord Road, Savannah, GA 31410, (912) 352-1230, BA 72 Univ of AL- Tuscaloosa; MA 73 Univ of AL- Tuscaloosa; Sp-Lang Path, InSpeech Inc, **SLP**

Lewis-Hyde, Mrs Mary Lee 305 Walnut, Batavia, IL 60510, (312) 520-9850, BS 84 Univ of IA; MA 87 Northern IL Univ - De Kalb

Lewison, Mrs Nancy M 300 East Lancaster Avenue, Apartment 1004, Wynnewood, PA 19096-2139, (201) 567-7875, BA 64 CUNY - City College; MA 65 Columbia Univ Teachers Coll; Director, Commun Cen Inc, **SLP**

Lewis-Strong, Cheryl M 230 West Nicolet Boulevard, Marquette, MI 49855, (715) 623-5822, BA 80 Univ of WI - Green Bay; MA 83 Northern MI Univ; Sp-Lang Path, Marquette Gen Hosp, **SLP**

Lewman, Mrs Linda A Route 1 Box 293, Eddyville, IA 52553, (515) 682-8591, BS 72 Northeast MO St Univ; MA 73 Northeast MO St Univ; Sp-Lang Path, S Prairie Area Ed Agen 15, **SLP**

Lewman, Mrs Lucie E 13743 Ridge Road, Whittier, CA 90601, (818) 960-3802, BA 62 Whittier Coll; MA 71 Whittier Coll; Program Administrator, Los Angeles County Supt of Sch, **SLP**

Lewsley, Mrs Sandra J 30231 Wicklow Court, Farmington Hills, MI 48018, (313) 476-8277, BA 77 MI St Univ; MA 79 Wayne St Univ; SLP, Garden City Public Schools, **SLP**

Lew-Stolzoff, Angela A 1614 18th Avenue, Sterling, IL 61081, (815) 625-7931, BA 74 SUNY - Center at Buffalo; MA 75 Univ of IA; Aud, Northwestern Illinois Assn, **A**

Lex, Mrs Sandra B 280 Argonne Avenue, Long Beach, CA 90803, (213) 868-0871, BS 64 Univ of WI - Madison; MA 68 CA St Univ - Long Beach; SLP, LA Co Supt Sch, **SLP**

Ley, Mrs Kathleen Ann 18495 East Progress Avenue, Aurora, CO 80015, (303) 696-0944, BS 76 CO St Univ; MS 78 CO St Univ; **SLP**

Leyba, Naomi E 1861 West Richland Circle, West Jordan, UT 84084, (801) 566-2984, BA 76 Univ of UT; MS 78 Univ of UT; Sp-Lang Path, Granite Sch Dist, **SLP**

Leyrer, Gina Raie 1416 Marigny Street, Mandeville, LA 70448, (504) 897-8563, BS 85 Univ of Houston - Univ Park; MA 86 Univ of Houston - Univ Park; Sp-Lang Path, Touro Inf, **SLP ACE**

Lezak, Mrs Mary H W 3693 Latimore, Shaker Heights, OH 44122, (216) 421-3212, BS 65 Northwestern Univ; MS 67 Gallaudet Coll; Aud, Cleveland Bd of Ed, **A**

Lezak, Dr Raymond J 3693 Latimore Drive, Shaker Heights, OH 44122, (216) 475-8689, BA 51 Univ of MI - Ann Arbor; MA 52 Univ of MI - Ann Arbor; OD 61 (NS) PA St Univ - Univ Park; Private Practice, **SLP A**

Lezynski, Jeffrey Mark 1265 Ontario Street, Apartment 801, Burlington, ON, Canada L7S 1X8, (416) 681-0224, BA 84 SUNY - Center at Buffalo; MA 86 SUNY - Center at Buffalo; 88–Dir of Aud, Dr William Love Sr, **A**

Li, Dr Edith C 2206 Camino Del Sol, Fullerton, CA 92633, (714) 773-3617, BA 73 Univ of Southern CA; MA 75 Northwestern Univ; PH 81 (NS) Northwestern Univ; Asst Prof, CA State U Fullerton, **SLP**

Libbey, Stephen R P O Box 358, Enosburg Falls, VT 05450, (802) 933-2171, BS 67; MS 69 Univ of VT; Sp-Lang Path, Franklin NE Superv Un, **SLP**

Libby, Mrs Christina Aldea 322 Muldoon Road #C, Anchorage, AK 99504, (907) 337-9434, BS 72 Loma Linda Univ - Riverside; MS 75 Loma Linda Univ - Loma Linda; **SLP**

Liber, Teena J 3313 Darlington Road, Toledo, OH 43606, (419) 535-1473, **SLP**

Libera, Mrs Jan A 1529 East Hedrick Drive, Tucson, AZ 85719, (602) 323-2279, BA 83 IL St Univ - Normal; MS 85 IL St Univ - Normal; Sp-Lang Path, Tucson USD, **SLP**

Liberman, George A 23 Brookfield Lane, Centereach, NY 11720, (516) 544-2525, BA 71 Adelphi Univ; MS 76 CUNY - Brooklyn Coll; Treatment Team Leader, Kings Park Psychiatric Center, **SLP**

Liberman, Jane R B 17 Diana Lane, Lexington, MA 02173, MS; 84–Aud, MA Eye & Ear Infirmary, **A**

Liberman, Robin L L 1623 Third Avenue 20-J West, New York, NY 10128, (212) 534-0036, MA 74; 74–Sp-Lang Path, Yonkers Pub Sch, **SLP**

Liberman, Thelma Wattenberg 3014 Lightfoot Drive, Baltimore, MD 21208, (301) 484-6616, BA 58 Montclair St Coll; MS 79 Towson St Univ; 79–Sp-Lang Path, Baltimore City Schs, **SLP**

Libertini, Mrs Kim E 19 Hilltop Drive, R D #1, New Freedom, PA 17349, (301) 396-0670, BA 79 Towson St Univ; MS 81 Towson St Univ; Sp-Lang Path, Baltimore Cty Pub Sch, **SLP**

Libertini, Nancy S 3780 Hollyberry Drive, Huntingtown, MD 20639, (203) 651-8853, BS 73 Towson St Univ; MS 74 Towson St Univ; Sp-Lang Path, Private Practice, **SLP ACE**

Liberto, Samuel 37 Parliament Court, Baltimore, MD 21212, (301) 532-3740, BS 72 Towson St Univ; MS 74 PA St Univ - Univ Park; Sp-Lang Path, Good Samaritan Hosp, **SLP**

Liberty, Dr Timothy D Med Visit Incorporated, 411 Andrews Road, Suite 240, Durham, NC 27705, (919) 383-4444, BS 69 Western MI Univ; MA 70 Western MI Univ; PH 78 (Sp-Lang Path) Wayne St Univ; 88–Admin, Med Visit Inc, **SLP**

Licausi, Josephine 6824 Rockhill Road, Kansas City, MO 64113, (913) 897-2381, BS 73 Univ of KS; MS 75 Central MO St Univ; SLP, Blue Vy Sch Dist, **SLP**

Lichlyter, Cynthia A R R 1 Box 194, Jasper, IN 47546, (812) 482-2563, OM 87 IN Univ - Bloomington; 88–Sp-Lang Path, Daviess-Martin Spec Educ Coop

Lichman, Mrs Jeanne M 2110 Wildflower Circle, Brea, CA 92621, BA 68 Univ of AZ; MA 71 Univ of AZ; **SLP**

Lichtenberg, Dr Eva F 3920 Lake Shore Drive, Chicago, IL 60613, (312) 332-2787, BA 52 Univ of Chicago; MA 55 Univ of Chicago; PH 60 (NS) Univ of Chicago; Cl Psychol, Private Practice

Lichtenstadter, Anne Elizabeth 8007 5th Avenue N E, Seattle, WA 98115-4112, (206) 524-7327, BS 79 Western WA Univ; MS 84 Univ of OR; Sp-Lang Path, Kent Sch Dist, **SLP**

Lichtenstein, Sandra 200 West 16th Street #3G, New York, NY 10011, (212) 262-3370, BS 78 Northwestern Univ; MA 80 Northwestern Univ; SLP, VA Med Cen E Orange Nj, **SLP**

Lichter, Kathryn M 8008 Rodgers Avenue, Wauwatosa, WI 53213, MS 76 Marquette Univ; **SLP**

Lichtig, Christine 1241 Charles Street, State College, PA 16801, (814) 234-4261, BS 73 PA St Univ - Univ Park; MS 75 PA St Univ - Univ Park; **SLP**

Lichtman, Andrea R 1717 El Rito Avenue, Glendale, CA 91208, (818) 956-5878, BS 68 Northern IL Univ - De Kalb; MA 69 Univ of IL - Urbana; SLP, Los Angeles USD, **SLP**

Lichtman, Mrs Heather Novy 63 Springbrook Road, Livingston, NJ 07039, (201) 992-3988, BA 70 George Washington Univ; MS 72 Columbia Univ Teachers Coll; Sp-Lang Path, S Orange/Maplewood Nj Sch Dist, **SLP**

Lichty, Jill K 37 Victoria Way, Camp Hill, PA 17011-1727, BS 73 Bloomsburg Univ of PA; MS 78 Bloomsburg Univ of PA; Sp/Lang Path, Carbon Lehigh Iu 21-Proj Conec, **SLP**

Lickhart, Candy Ann 1612 Santa Fe, Atchison, KS 66002, MS 84 Northwest MO St Univ; SLP, Boe USD #409, **SLP**

Liddell, Richard A 4460 South Lone Lake Road, Langley, WA 98260, (206) 221-7538, BS 70 Brigham Young Univ; MS 72 Brigham Young Univ; Director, Whidbey Speech Clinic, **SLP**

Liddle, Mrs Brenda H Chestnut Hill Rehabilitation Hospital, 8601 Stenton Avenue, Wyndmoor, PA 19118, (215) 233-6253, BS 83 Clarion Univ of PA; MS 85 Hahneman Medical Coll; 86–Sp-Lang Path, Communication Skills Inc, **SLP**

Liddle, Mrs Lorene Swanson 2316 Lafayette, Columbus, IN 47201, (812) 376-5319, BS 66; MA 67 Univ of IA; Sp-Lang Path, Bartholomew Co Hosp, **SLP**

Lidell, Stacy C 7331 Brentwood Rd, Apt A, Philadelphia, PA 19151, (215) 477-5233, BA 78 SUNY - Center at Binghamton; MA 86 Temple Univ-Tyler Sch of Art; **SLP**

Lider, Barbara R 10351 Hummingbird Street, Coon Rapids, MN 55433, (612) 786-5570, BS 72 Moorhead St Univ; MS 78 Saint Cloud St Univ; Sp-Lang Path, Springlake Park Sch Dist #16, **SLP**

Lieber, Mrs Starr Ehmke 2171 Ackerman Drive, Pittsburg, CA 94565, (415) 427-4582, MS 87 San Francisco St Univ

Lieberburg, Ellen H 1165 East 54th Street, Brooklyn, NY 11234, (718) 763-3420, BA 82 CUNY - Brooklyn Coll; MS 85 CUNY - Brooklyn Coll; Sp-Lang Path, UCP-New York, **SLP**

Liebergott, Dr Jacqueline 33 Beaumont Street, Newton, MA 02160, PH 73 (NS); Dean of Graduate Studies, Emerson College, **SLP**

Lieberman, Beth Susan 260 Northern Boulevard, St James, NY 11780, (516) 679-1822, BA 84 SUNY - Coll at Cortland; MS 85 Adelphi Univ; 85–Sp-Lang Path, Sch for Lang & Comm Dev, **SLP**

Lieberman, Mrs Bobbi M 13 Filmont Drive, New City, NY 10956, (914) 638-2928, BA 69 CUNY - Queens Coll; MA 74 Hofstra Univ; Sp-Lang Path, Private Practice, **SLP**

Lieberman, Mrs Elaine F 3 President Avenue, Providence, RI 02906, (401) 751-4499, BA 39 Brown Univ; ME 62 Boston Univ; SLP, Meeting St School, **SLP LM**

Lieberman, Gayle 1301 West Fletcher #410, Chicago, IL 60657, (312) 327-1550, BS 73 Bradley Univ; MS 74 Bradley Univ; Sp-Lang Path, Private Practice, **SLP**

Lieberman, Jody 925 Huntingdon Pike #112, Huntingdon Valley, PA 19006, (215) 663-8829, BS 80 PA St Univ - Univ Park; MA 82 Temple Univ; Sp-Lang Path, Private Practice, **SLP**

Lieberman, Mrs Maura Elizabeth 3425 New Heritage Drive, Alpharetta, GA 30201, (404) 292-9220, BS 76 Edinboro Univ of PA; MS 80 Towson St Univ; 88–Aud, Dr Willis Paul Callins, **A**

Lieberman, Mrs Nancy K Hearing/Visually Impaired Prog, Exceptional Student Educ, 1400 N E 6th Street, Pompano Beach, FL 33060, (305) 765-6661, BA 68 CUNY - Brooklyn Coll; MS 72 CUNY - Brooklyn Coll; ED 82 (NS) Nova Univ; Curr Superv Hrng & Visual Imp, Schl Bd Broward Co Sch, **SLP ACE**

Lieberman, Dr R Jane Communication Disorders Program, Appalachian State Univ, Boone, NC 28608, (704) 262-2185, BS 68 OH St Univ; MS 70 Univ of MI - Ann Arbor; PH 81 (NS) Univ of FL; Assoc Prof, Appalachian St U, **SLP**

Lieberman, Mrs Rochelle Rotblatt 35305 Valley Forge Drive, Farmington Hills, MI 48018, (313) 493-6315, BA 73 Univ of MI - Ann Arbor; MA 75 Wayne St Univ; Sp/Lang Path, Sinai Hosp of Detroit, **SLP**

Lieberman, Mrs Shelley M 2443 Fair Avenue, Bexley, OH 43209, (614) 252-8789, BA 74 OH St Univ; MA 75 OH St Univ; **SLP**

Lieberman, Susan B 259 Bellington Lane, St Louis, MO 63141, **SLP**

Lieberman, Mrs Susan G H 39085 Lancaster, Farmington Hills, MI 48331, (313) 857-8520, BA 82 MI St Univ; MA 84 Wayne St Univ; 85–Sp-Lang Path, Pontiac Sch Dist, **SLP**

Lieberman-Altman, Denise Elayne 450 Island Road #118, Ramsey, NJ 07446, (201) 934-1640, BA 79 SUNY - Center at Buffalo; MS 81 Adelphi Univ; **SLP**

Lieberth, Dr Ann K 7332 Kingswood Circle, Fort Worth, TX 76133, (817) 921-7620, BA 67 Marygove Coll; MA 70 Bowling Green St Univ; PH 84 (NS) NY Univ; Assistant Professor, Texas Christian University, **SLP A**

Lieblich, Dr Malcolm 424 Shady Lane, Edwardsville, IL 62025, (618) 656-5604, BA 48 Univ of WI - Madison; MS 50 NY Univ; PH 60 (NS) NY Univ; Prof, Sn IL at Edwardsville, **SLP**

Liebman, Aaron H 902 Washington Avenue, Albany, NY 12203, (518) 458-8811, BS 78 SUNY - Center at Albany; MS 82 CUNY - Brooklyn Coll; Aud, Aud Consult, **A**

Liebman, Anita H 14 Tall Oaks Drive, Summit, NJ 07901, (201) 635-9455, BA 72 Univ of CA - Los Angeles; MA 76 San Diego St Univ; 88–Sp-Lang Path, Chatham Sch Dist, **SLP**

Liebman, Eve 13000 S E Almond Court, Clackamas, OR 97015, (503) 280-6528, BA 79 CA St Univ - Northridge; MS 82 Portland St Univ; Sp-Lang Path, Portland Public Schools, **SLP**

Liebman, Dr Jerome 979 Balltown Road, Schenectady, NY 12309, (518) 370-0407, BA 54 CUNY - Brooklyn Coll; MA 57 CUNY - Brooklyn Coll; PH 66 (NS) Purdue Univ - West Lafayette; Aud, Private Practice, **SLP A**

Liebman, Joyce Kay 1602 Abell Circle, Crestwood, KY 40014, (502) 845-2761, BA 73 Univ of KY; MA 75 Univ of KY; 88–Sp-Lang Path, No Cen Dist Home Health Agency, **SLP ACE**

Liebman, Mrs Roberta N 3407 Thornapple Street, Chevy Chase, MD 20815, (202) 651-5658, BA 55 Radcliffe Coll; MA 71 Catholic Univ of America; 88–Clin Supvr, Gallaudet Univ, **SLP**

Liebner, Mrs Catherine 35 Summit Avenue, Chadds Ford, PA 19317, (215) 284-8570, BA 73 George Washington Univ; MA 75 Northwestern Univ; 88–Aud, Del Co Mem Hosp, **A**

Liebowitz, Barbara Joan 4626 S W 35th Place, Portland, OR 97221, (503) 222-9221, **SLP**

Liebowitz, Mrs Linda J 52 Littlewood Court, Wayne, NJ 07470, (201) 441-2161, BA 77 CUNY - Queens Coll; MS 79 PA St Univ - Univ Park; 86–Aud, Hackensack Med Ctr, **A**

Liebowitz, Mrs Maxine A 44 Glen Way, Cold Spring Harbor, NY 11724, (516) 385-2787

Liebowitz, Mrs Roni S 78 Stratton Road, Scarsdale, NY 10583, (914) 698-9000, BS 65 Boston Univ; MA 66 Columbia Univ Teachers Coll; Sp-Lang Path, Mamaroneck Bd of Ed, **SLP**

Liedman, James 4225 Hawksley Drive, Chesapeake, VA 23321-5427, (804) 398-5363, BS 73 Western IL Univ; MA 74 Univ of IL - Urbana; 78–Coord Sp-Lang Path, Oto-H&Ns Serv Naval Hosp, **SLP ACE**

Lief, Rebecca L P O Box 616, Moose Lake, MN 55767, (218) 485-8443, BA 77 Univ of MN - Minneap-St Paul; MA 82 Univ of MN - Duluth; 82–Sp-Lang Path, Moose Lake Reg Treatment Ctr, **SLP**

Liemberger, Kathleen A 8262 Old Post Road East, East Amherst, NY 14051-1514, (716) 741-9790, BS 71 SUNY - Coll at Buffalo; ME 74 SUNY - Coll at Buffalo; Sp-Lang Path, Kenmore Un Free School Dist, **SLP**

Liening, Maryellen Gleason 632 Barrington, Grosse Pointe Park, MI 48230, (313) 745-8903, BA 83 MI St Univ; MA 85 Wayne St Univ; 85–Sp-Lang Path, Children's Hosp of MI, **SLP ACE**

Liensch, Lynne W 1910 S W 112th, Seattle, WA 98146, BA 72 Univ of WA; OM 76 Univ of WA; SLP, Federal Way School District, **SLP**

Lierman, Mrs Cynthia L 6247 Chattanooga Drive, Baton Rouge, LA 70817, (504) 292-6232, BS 78 Univ of Southwestern LA; MS 80 Univ of WY; **SLP**

Lies, Mrs Leigh A 1752 South Market, Wichita, KS 67211, (316) 262-8271, BA 78 Wichita St Univ; MA 79 Wichita St Univ; Sp/Lang Path, Inst of Logopedics, **SLP**

Ligas, Michael J 150 W Woodstock Circle Dr, The Woodlands, TX 77381-2716, (713) 292-6360, BA 76 Cleveland St Univ; MA 79 Cleveland St Univ; SLP, Tri County M Hlth & M Ret Serv, **SLP**

Light, Mrs Giselle Hope 7 Casino Court, Silver Spring, MD 20906, (301) 933-9385, **SLP**

Light, Mrs Leah Karen 611 North 32nd Court, Hollywood, FL 33021, (305) 446-5597, BS 82 Univ of FL; MS 86 Univ of South FL; Audiologist, Hrng & Sp Ctr of FL Inc, **A**

Light, Malcolm H, II Kendall Professional Bldg, 9150 S W 87th Avenue, Suite 103, Miami, FL 33176, (305) 595-1530, BS 73 Univ of TN - Knoxville; MA 75 Univ of TN - Knoxville; Aud, Aud and Vestibular Cen Inc, **A**

Lighter, Mrs Audrey Gail PO Box 120512, Peoria, IL 61614, (309) 692-6252, BS 82 IL St Univ - Normal; MS 84 IL St Univ - Normal; Aud, Dr Adel El-Deiry, **A**

Lightfoot, Adrienne R 3000 Majestic Ridge #69, Las Cruces, NM 88001, (505) 522-6766, BA 76 Univ of IL - Chicago; MA 81 Western MI Univ; Sp-Lang Path, Las Cruces PS, **SLP**

Lightfoot, Jean E 211 Donnelly Drive, Anderson, IN 46011, (317) 646-5171, BS 64; MA 66 Ball St Univ; Sp & Hrng Path-Dept Head, Community Hosp, **SLP**

Lightfoot, Mrs Pamela S E 1551 South Chase Street, Lakewood, CO 80226, BA 77 Metropolitan St Coll; MA 79 Univ of Denver; **SLP**

Lightle, Mrs Susan Hall 9480 Princeton Sq Blvd S, Apartment 2509, Jacksonville, FL 32216, (904) 733-4808, OB 82 Valdosta St Coll; ME 84 GA St Univ; SLP, St Johns Co School Bd, **SLP**

Lightman, Mrs Karen Mandelkehr 1620 Plymouth Rock Drive, Cherry Hill, NJ 08003, (609) 354-1028, MA 84 Temple Univ; Sp-Lang Path, State of New Jersey, **SLP**

Ligon, Judith Carol 2500 Quartermill Road, Richmond, VA 23229, (804) 786-0207, BS 80 Eastern KY Univ; MA 81 Univ of IL - Urbana; Sp-Lang Path, Medical College of Virginia, **SLP**

Likavec, Judith Marie 1910 Rockefeller Lane, Redondo Beach, CA 90278, (213) 940-7680, BS 80 Wayne St Univ; MS 82 Univ of MI - Ann Arbor; Sp/Lang Path, Rancho Los Amigos Med Ctr, **SLP**

Likens, Barbara A 1130 Idaho Avenue, Santa Monica, CA 90403, (213) 394-1899, BS 55; ME 61 Univ of WA; PH 86 (Counseling Psychology) International Univ; Sp-Lang Path, Los Angeles PS

Likman, Edward A 53 Mountain Ridge Drive, Wayne, NJ 07470, (201) 694-2028, BA 62 Paterson St Coll; MA 66 Montclair St Coll; Pres/Owner, Sp/Hrng Assoc Inc, **SLP**

Liles, Barbara H 21913 Linda Drive, Torrance, CA 90503, (213) 868-0431, BA 55 Univ of CA - Los Angeles; MA 79 CA St Univ - Long Beach; SLP, Norwalk - La Miranda USD, **SLP**

Liles, Dr Betty Zoe Dept Of Communication Science, University Of Connecticut, Storrs, CT 06268, (203) 486-2628, BA 65 Our Lady Lake Univ-San Anton; MA 66 Our Lady Lake Univ-San Anton; PH 73 (NS) Univ of MN - Minneap-St Paul; Prof, U of CT, **SLP**

Liles, Patricia A 56 Tamalpias Road, Berkeley, CA 94708, (415) 843-4288, BA 70 San Francisco St Univ; MA 72 San Francisco St Univ; Sp-Lang Path, Albany USD, **SLP**

Liles, Sara J 3507 Holly, Denison, TX 75020, **SLP**

Lilienfeld, Mrs Riselle S 1283 Yale Drive, Yardley, PA 19067, (215) 493-5811, BA 67 Temple Univ; MA 69 Temple Univ; Sp-Lang Path, E J Constance & Associates, **SLP ACE**

Lilienthal, Andrea Elsita 1901 12th Avenue, Watervliet, NY 12189, (518) 465-5201, BA 84 SUNY - Coll at Cortland; MS 85 Coll of Saint Rose; 87–Sp-Lang Path, NYS Easter Seal Society, **SLP**

Lilienthal, Jeanette Roberta Route 10 Box 146, Puesta Del Sol, Santa Fe, NM 87501, (505) 471-4158, MS 83 Univ of NM; **SLP**

Liljeblad, Mrs Astrid University Station, P O Box 8463, Reno, NV 89507, BA 56 ID St Univ; MA 62 Stanford Univ; **SLP LM**

Liljefors, Janet Lee 3204-5 Selwyn Farms Lane, Charlotte, NC 28209, (704) 338-4430, BA 80 CUNY - Queens Coll; MA 85 CUNY - Hunter Coll; 87–Sp-Lang Path, Charlotte Rehab Hosp, **SLP**

Liljegren, Mrs Susanne F 6312 150th Avenue, Redmond, WA 98052, (206) 455-5855, BA 67 Univ of AZ; MA 69 Univ of AZ; SLP, Private Practice, **SLP**

Liljeqvist, Christine 7 Assissi Way, Norwalk, CT 06851, (203) 847-5131, BA 75 Univ of the Pacific; MA 76 Univ of Denver; Sp/Lang Path, Greenwich Bd of Ed, **SLP**

Lillegard, Linda R 5119 Burt, Omaha, NE 68132, (717) 322-7354, BS 64 Univ of MN - Minneap-St Paul; MS 74 Univ of NE - Omaha; SLP, Loess Hills AEA 13, **SLP**

Lillevig, Mrs Diana W 3383 Whipple Court, Annandale, VA 22003, (703) 532-3697, BA 55 Univ of MD - College Park; MA 65 Univ of MD - College Park; Sp-Lang Path, Fairfax Co Sch Bd, **SLP**

Lilley, Georgetta Sue Box 747, Everson, WA 98247, (305) 382-1944, ME 69 CA Univ of PA; **SLP**

Lilley, Lois Anne 1045-B Moore Street, Harrisonburg, VA 22801, (703) 434-8352, BS 72 James Madison Univ; MS 78 James Madison Univ; Sp-Lang Path, Harrisonburg City Sch, **SLP**

Lilley, Pat Krchmar 307 Dolores N W, Albuquerque, NM 87105, (505) 836-3386, BA 75 Montclair St Coll; MS 81 Univ of NM; 87–Sp-Lang Path, U of NM/Sch of Med Ped, **SLP**

Lilley, Mrs Patricia Reed 7074 South Elm Street, Littleton, CO 80122, (303) 779-9016, BA 70 Wichita St Univ; MS 78 Univ of North TX; 88–Sp-Lang Path, Denver PS

Lilley, Mrs Terri A C Route 2 Box 1, 1104 West Grant, Dexter, MO 63841, (314) 624-7500, BS 75 AR St Univ; MS 76 AR St Univ; Sp-Lang Path, Semo Reg Home Hlth Agcy, **SLP**

Lillich, Mrs Maureen Cronan 5 Bourg Court, Harahan, LA 70123, (504) 738-5851, BA 75 Tulane Univ; MS 79 Tulane Univ; **SLP**

Lillie, Sue M 5032 Marc Drive, Nashville, TN 37211-6724, (615) 790-2249, BA 59 Vanderbilt Univ; MS 61 Vanderbilt Univ; Sp/Lang Path, Ashland Indep Sch, **A**

Lillo, Mrs Margaret A 7600 Nutwood Court, Derwood, MD 20855, (301) 251-6942, BA 72 Valparaiso Univ; BS 78 Univ of MA - Amherst; MA 80 Univ of MA - Amherst; Aud, Reg I/Chldn & Adolescents, **A**

Lilly, Dr David J Good Samaritan Hosp & Med Ctr, Director Of Audiology, 1040 N W 22nd Avenue, Portland, OR 97210, (503) 229-7860, BA 54 Univ of Redlands; MA 57 Univ of Redlands; PH 61 (NS) Univ of Pittsburgh - Pittsburgh; Director of Audiology, Good Samaritan Hosp & Med Cen, **A F**

Lilly, Mrs Karen Bates 13112 Price Distillery Rd, Clarksburg, MD 20871, (301) 253-2905, BS 82 WV Univ; MS 83 WV Univ; Sp-Lang Path, Montgomery Co Pub Schs, **SLP**

Lilly, Mrs Karen C B Rd 3 Box 3805, East Stroudsburg, PA 18301, (717) 629-4931, BA 74 Univ of Pittsburgh - Pittsburgh; MA 76 Univ of Pittsburgh - Pittsburgh; Sp-Lang Path, InSpeech Inc, **SLP ACE**

Lilly, Mrs Linda P 1110 Valewood Road, Towson, MD 21204, (301) 687-6500, BS 69 Univ of IA; MA 70 Univ of IA; 87–Chief of Div of Sp-Lang-Hearing, Baltimore Co Dept of Hlth, **SLP**

Lillywhite, Beth Ann 595 So Dunas Road, Orange, CA 92669, (714) 532-5842, BS 83 Brigham Young Univ; MA 86 San Diego St Univ; **A**

Lillywhite, Dr Herold 570 N 10th Avenue #30, Cornelius, OR 97113, (503) 548-5458, PH 43 (NS) NY Univ; **SLP F H LM**

Lim, Kerk Chan 487 North Highland #5, Memphis, TN 38122, (901) 867-2921, BS 80 Univ of AL- Tuscaloosa; MS 82 Univ of AL- Tuscaloosa; Aud, Arlington Developmental Center, **A**

Limb, Terence Alford c/o Evergreen Sp & Hear Clinic, 8301 161st Avenue N E, Suite 304, Redmond, WA 98052, (206) 882-4347, BS 83 Univ of WA; MS 86 Univ of WA; **A**

Limbacher, Maureen Allegheny General Hospital, 320 East North Avenue, Pittsburgh, PA 15221, (412) 359-3782, BA 82 Univ of Pittsburgh - Pittsburgh; MA 84 Univ of TN - Knoxville; Aud, Allehgeny Gen Hosp, **A**

Limbacher, Rosemarie Barbara 60-44 Catalpa Avenue, Ridgewood, NY 11385, (718) 386-1023, BA 83 CUNY - Hunter Coll; MS 86 Columbia Univ Teachers Coll; 88–Sp-Lang Path, Private Practice, **SLP**

Limbert-Lerch, Carol Sue 5350 Barton Road, North Ridgeville, OH 44039, (216) 327-2681, MA 87 Univ of Cincinnati; 87–Sp-Lang Path, PSI Affiliates Inc

Limburg, Mrs Laura Anne 404 Thurber Drive West, Apartment #2, Columbus, OH 43215, (614) 476-0530, BS 84 Miami Univ - Oxford; MA 86 OH St Univ; 88–Sp-Lang Path, Franklin Co Bd of Mentl Ret, **SLP**

Limmer, Kathleen 708 Tefft Avenue, Jackson, MI 49203, (517) 788-8706, BS 74 Central MI Univ; MA 75 MI St Univ; Aud, Stahl Jackson Sp & Hrng Cl, **A**

Limoges, Mrs Suzanne D 1602 Westminster Place, Ann Arbor, MI 48104, (313) 429-5429, BA 69 Alma Coll; MS 72 Univ of MI - Ann Arbor; 87–Sp-Lang Path, Saline Area Schs, **SLP ACE**

Limtiaco, Theresa M G 62 Bay State Road #6, Boston, MA 02215, (617) 479-7980, BA 81 Univ of Southern CA; MS 87 Boston Univ; **SLP**

Linam, Ruth 1239 Deane Street, Fayetteville, AR 72703, (501) 751-4659, BS 76 Univ of AR - Fayetteville; MA 77 Univ of AR - Fayetteville; Sp-Lang Path, Springdale Pub Sch, **SLP**

Linam, Virginia L 2536 E Vogel- Dreamy Draw, Phoenix, AZ 85028, (602) 482-5908, BA 56 Univ of CO - Boulder; BS 57 Univ of CO - Boulder; MA 71 Univ of Denver; Aud, Private Practice, **A ACE**

Linander, Mrs Esther S 564 West Greendale, Detroit, MI 48203, (313) 883-1680, BA 38 Univ of Western Ontario; ME 54 Wayne St Univ; **SLP LM**

Linane, Mrs Valerie Ann 3528 Encinal Avenue, La Crescenta, CA 91214-3219, (818) 243-5176, BA 81 Univ of NM; MA 85 CA St Univ - Fullerton; **SLP**

Linares-Orama, Dr Nicolas G-101 Quintas DE Cupey, Rio Piedras, PR 00926, (809) 764-6035, **SLP**

Lincoln, Joyce Marie 1243 Marlon Street, Owosso, MI 48867, (517) 725-6966, BS 69 Western MI Univ; MA 86 MI St Univ; 87–Sp-Lang Path, Ingham Inter Sch Dist, **SLP**

Lincoln, Karen Lee 2 Chapman Street, Arlington, MA 02174, (617) 735-6471, BS 80 Univ of NH; MS 82 Univ of NM; Aud, Chldn Hosp Med Cen, **A**

Lincoln, Laura 965 East 38th Avenue, Vancouver, BC, Canada V5W 1J2, (604) 324-7308, MA 79 Northern IL Univ - De Kalb; Sp-Lang Path, **SLP**

Lind, Mrs Cheryl G 4 Wagon Wheel Drive, Spearfish, SD 57783, (605) 642-2570, BS 76 SD St Univ; MA 78 Univ of SD - Vermillion; 86–Sp-Lang Path, Spearfish P S System, **SLP**

Lind, Mary N 2104 13th Street, Moline, IL 61265, (309) 757-3505, BA 72 Augustana Coll; MS 76 Univ of WI - Madison; Sp-Lang Path, Moline Pub Sch, **SLP**

Lind, Richard C Marysville Medical Group, 800 3rd Street, Marysville, CA 95901, (916) 741-1300, BA 69 San Francisco St Univ; MA 77 CA St Univ - Sacramento; Aud, Marysville Medical Group, **A**

Lind, Terrie Lee 866 Apricot Avenue #D, Campbell, CA 95008-3251, (408) 559-2700, BA 70 WA St Univ; MA 71 WA St Univ; Prgm Coor, Health Dimmensions Inc, **SLP**

Lindahl, Raymond F Deaf Hearing & Speech Center, 19185 Wyoming Street, Detroit, MI 48221, (313) 341-1353, BS 59 Wayne St Univ; ME 64 Wayne St Univ; Pres/CEO, Deaf Hearing & Speech Center, **SLP**

Lindaman, Sandra L 1225 West Lunt #2-B, Chicago, IL 60626, (312) 328-1900, BA 72 Augustana Coll; MA 76 Northwestern Univ; 88–Comm Rel Coord, Visiting Nurse Assoc, **SLP**

Lindamood, Linda Phelps 11311 Stormy Ridge Road, Austin, TX 78739, (612) 715-8220, MA 85 Univ of MN - Minneap-St Paul; SLP, Anoka School District 11, **SLP**

Lindamood, Lori Hope 310 Washington Street #7, Lynchburg, VA 24504, (804) 239-7711, MS 83 Radford Univ; BS 81 Radford Univ; Sp-Lang Path, Lynchburg City Schools, **SLP**

Lindamood, Patricia Conway Lindamood-Bell Learning Processes, 416 Higuera Street, San Luis Obispo, CA 93401, (805) 541-3836, BS 49 Univ of MN - Minneap-St Paul; MS 67 Univ of OR; 67–Director, Private Practice, **SLP**

Lindberg, Mrs Jodie Ann 3640 Lynx Drive, San Jose, CA 95136, (408) 448-4357, BA 84 CA St Univ - Sacramento; MA 87 San Jose St Univ; 87–Sp-Lang Path, Leonette J Francia & Assoc, **SLP**

Lindberg, Karen W 835 Lee Avenue, Harrisonburg, VA 22801, (703) 433-0662, BS 81 Indiana Univ of PA; MS 86 James Madison Univ; 88–Sp-Lang Path, Shenandoah Val Prog Op Educ

Lindberg, Mrs Patricia B 1020 Kensington, Peoria, IL 61614, (309) 692-0404, BS 68 Bradley Univ; MA 69 Bradley Univ; Sp-Lang Path, Tazewell-Mason Co Spec Educ Assoc, **SLP ACE**

Lindberg, Paul William 2959 Bright Star N W, Albuquerque, NM 87120, (505) 831-9371, OB 76 Univ of MN - Duluth; MS 82 Univ of NM; Sp-Lang Path, Developmental Disabilities Ov, **SLP**

Lindberg, Dr Robert F 6010 North Keenland, Peoria, IL 61614, (309) 676-3131, BA 62 Marietta Coll; MA 64 OH Univ - Athens; PH 71 (Aud) MI St Univ; 86–Pres, Cn Il Hrng Aid Centers Inc, **A**

Linde, Diane Marie 5325 Chicago Avenue South, Minneapolis, MN 55417, (612) 824-8350, BS 79 Univ of WI - River Falls; MS 86 Univ of WI - River Falls; 86–Sp-Lang Path, Hennepin Tech Inst ISD #287, **SLP**

Linde, Lisa M 183 S Main Street, Yardley, PA 19067, (814) 226-3020, MS 86 Clarion Univ of PA; **SLP**

Lindeen, Ruth N RR #5, Mount Pleasant, IA 52641, (319) 385-4130, MA 79 Univ of Northern IA; 86–Sp-Lang Path, AEA #16, **SLP**

Lindell, Dr Gary A Speech Language & Hearing Clinic, Ball State University, Muncie, IN 47306, (317) 285-8174, BA 66 Carthage Coll; ME 68 Univ of VA - Charlottesville; ED 75 (Sp-Lang Path) Univ of VA - Charlottesville; 70–Assoc Prof, Ball St U, **SLP**

Lindell, Gloria Jean Rd 3 Box 3182, Russell, PA 16345, (814) 723-5500, MS 84 Clarion Univ of PA; Sp-Lang Path, PA Dept of Welfare, **SLP**

Lindell, Helen Alma Long Park Route, Estes Park, CO 80517, MS; **LM**

Lindell, Mrs Melinda J 1508 West Yale, Muncie, IN 47304, (317) 284-6749, BS 75 Univ of Cincinnati; MA 76 Ball St Univ; Sp-Lang Path, Private Practice, **SLP**

Lindelof, Laura 1412 Columbine, Mount Prospect, IL 60056, (312) 296-8716, BS 86 Eastern IL Univ; MS 87 Eastern IL Univ; **SLP**

Lindeman, Janet M 1703 Pulaski Road, Buffalo, MN 55313, (612) 682-5597, BS 75 Univ of IA; MA 76 Northern IL Univ - De Kalb; Aud, Minnesota Ear Head & Neck, **A**

Lindeman, Mrs Mary Ann 311 Pleasant Drive, Hudson, IA 50643, (319) 472-5221, BA 65 Univ of Northern IA; MA 81 Univ of Northern IA; Sp/Lang Path, IA Braille & Sight Sau Sch, **SLP**

Lindemann, Larisa 9433 244th Street S W, Apartment A-203, Edmonds, WA 98020, (206) 546-4994, BS 69 CO St Univ; MA 74 Western WA Univ; Sp-Lang Path, Home Call of Edmonds Inc, **SLP**

Lindemann, Norma M V 19655 Green Mountain Drive, Newhall, CA 91321, **SLP**

Lindemann, Patricia Ann 304-A 67th Street, Holmes Beach, FL 34217, (813) 778-9235, BA 73 Skidmore Coll; MS 83 Univ of TX - Dallas; Sp-Lang Path, Sch Bd Manatee Co FL, **SLP**

Linden, Neil J 243 West 70th #5B, New York, NY 10023, **SLP**

Linden, Patricia L The Good Samaritan Hospital, 5601 Loch Raven Blvd, Baltimore, MD 21239, (301) 532-3740, BS 74 Univ of MD - College Park; MA 76 Univ of MD - College Park; Sp-Lang Path, The Good Samaritan Hosp of MD, **SLP ACE**

Linden, Sharon 5801 Lowell N E #20B, Albuquerque, NM 87111, (505) 291-0705, MS 85 Univ of NM; Slp, InSpeech Inc, **SLP**

Lindenman, Dr Michael Dept Communication Sci & Dis, Montclair State College, Upper Montclair, NJ 07043, (201) 894-5279, BA 68 Trenton St Coll; MA 70 Columbia Univ Teachers Coll; PH 80 (NS) NY Univ; Prof, Montclair St Coll, **A**

Lindenstein, Margaret G 214 Highland Avenue, Piedmont, CA 94611, (415) 654-9973, BA 65 Univ of CA - Los Angeles; MA 74 Univ of CA - Berkeley; Sp-Lang Path, Berkeley USD, **SLP**

Linder, Mrs Barbara C 226 Gladstone Road, Pittsburgh, PA 15217, **SLP**

Linder, Lori Renee 606 Ravens Crest Drive, Plainsboro, NJ 08536-2448, (305) 684-5107, BA 84 IN Univ - Bloomington; MA 85 Saint Louis Univ; **SLP**

Linderman, Timothy D 3 South 154th Burr Oak Dr, Glen Ellyn, IL 60137-7382, (312) 462-4220, **SLP**

Lindevig, Kathy Ann 309 Ulland Avenue, Westby, WI 54667, (608) 634-3918, BS 82 Univ of WI - River Falls; MS 87 Univ of WI - River Falls; 82–Sp-Lang Path, Norwalk-Ontario Sch Dist

Lindgren, John H 10657 Queen Avenue South, Bloomington, MN 55431, (612) 887-9165, BS 61 Univ of MN - Duluth; MS 67 Univ of WI - Madison; Coor of Spec Ed, Bloomington Pub Sch, **SLP**

Lindholm, Sylvia B 1425 4th Street S W #A-703, Washington, DC 20024, MS; **SLP**

Lindhorst, Suzanne L S 470 Maymont, Ballwin, MO 63011, (314) 391-9504, BS 73 Univ of MO - Columbia; MA 79 Univ of MO - Columbia; Sp-Lang Path, Speech Lang Serv Inc, **SLP**

Lindley, Mrs Connie Lou 8441 Filmore Lane, Wheelersburg, OH 45694-1847, (614) 574-4520, BA 73 Marshall Univ; MS 84 Univ of KY; **SLP**

Lindley, Katherine E 333 East 5th Street #B1, New York, NY 10003, (212) 947-5770, BS 78 Central MI Univ; MA 80 Central MI Univ; Sp-Lang Path, VTA Mgmt Svcs, **SLP**

Lindmark, Janice Clare 14 Dogwood, Park Forest, IL 60466, (312) 747-3535, BA 79 Augustana Coll; MA 80 Univ of IL - Urbana; 80–Sp-Lang Path, Matteson School District 162, **SLP**

Lindner, Dr Laurie Gilden 48 Birch Hill Road, Stow, MA 01775, (617) 638-7370, BA 68 CUNY - City College; MS 72 CUNY - Brooklyn Coll; PH 81 (NS) CUNY - Grad Sch & Univ Cntr; Dir/SLP, Boston U Med Cen, **SLP**

Lindner, Ruth Jean 7021 W Wellauer Drive, Wauwatosa, WI 53213, (612) 546-5411, BS 84 Marquette Univ; MS 87 Univ of WI - Whitewater

Lindorff, Mrs Vicki M 21 Pleasant Place, Kearny, NJ 07032, (201) 991-4011, BA 76 Montclair St Coll; MA 78 Montclair St Coll; 82–Sp Ed Admin-Prin, Early Childhood Learning Ctr, **SLP**

Lindsay, Ann M 1922 Delaware Avenue, Apartment 2-R, Wilmington, DE 19806, (302) 654-1011, ME 88 Univ of VA - Charlottesville; 88–Aud, Wilmington Aud Svcs

Lindsay, Charles Hunter 44 West Lancaster Avenue, Downingtown, PA 19335, (215) 269-3223, BS 64 Univ Southern MS-Hattiesburg; MA 66 MI St Univ; 75–Aud, Assoc in Aud Inc

Lindsay, Mrs Elissa G 104 Michigan Avenue, Beckley, WV 25801, (304) 252-1925, BS 73 WV Univ; MS 74 WV Univ; 80–Owner/Sp-Lang Path, Beckley Sp Ther Serv, **SLP**

Lindsay, Mrs Jean Horton 17 Farmington Drive, Charlottesville, VA 22901, (804) 924-7107, **SLP**

Lindsay, Kathleen 1106 North Josephine, Madison, SD 57042, (605) 256-4235, BA 73 Univ of SD - Vermillion; MA 74 Univ of SD - Vermillion; Sp-Lang Path, Private Practice, **SLP**

Lindsay, Mrs Nadean F Route 4 Box 206, Long Street, Fuquay-Varina, NC 27526, (919) 893-8151, BS 78 Meredith Coll; MS 81 Univ of NC - Chapel Hill; Sp-Lang Path, Harnett Co Sch Syst, **SLP**

Lindsay, Ted J 8821 Knoll Court, Franklin, WI 53132, (414) 534-2301, BA 75 Univ of MI - Ann Arbor; MA 75 Western MI Univ; 88–Mktg Assoc, New Medico Head Injury System, **SLP**

Lindsay, Thomas N P O Box 938, Deming, NM 88031, (505) 546-6568, BA 71 NM St Univ; MA 72 NM St Univ; Sp-Lang Path, Deming Public Schools, **SLP**

Lindsey, Deanne Michelle 5715 Baltimore #113, La Mesa, CA 92041, (619) 463-4515, MA 87 San Diego St Univ; 87–Sp-Lang Path, Children's Hosp, **SLP**

Lindsey, Deborah A 45 327 Makalani Street, Kaneohe, HI 96744, (808) 247-8994, BS 75 Univ of HI - Manoa; MS 80 Univ of HI - Manoa; Aud, Roland Fs Tam MD, **A**

Lindsey, Mrs Pamela Sloan Route 4 Box 4841, Palestine, TX 75801, (214) 729-6120, BS 80 Stephen F Austin St Univ; MS 83 Univ of AR - Little Rock; SLP, Good Shepherd Med Cen, **SLP**

Lindsey, Patricia B 2354 Gavinley Lane, Columbus, OH 43220, (614) 875-0116, BS 77 Kent St Univ; MA 78 Kent St Univ; Sp-Lang Path, Private Practice, **SLP**

Lindstedt, D Elise 1003 Mitchell Street, Laramie, WY 82070, (307) 721-8001, BA 71 CA St Univ - Los Angeles; MS 74 Univ of AZ; Doctoral, Univ of Denver, **SLP**

Lindstrom, Mrs Karen I 211 East Lake, Silver Lake, KS 66539, (913) 582-4209, BA 73 Wichita St Univ; MA 74 Wichita St Univ; 84–Sp-Lang Path, Seaman Spec Services USD #345, **SLP**

Lindstrom, Mrs Kathryn S 1725 Danbury Lane, Rochester Hills, MI 48063, (313) 626-3652, BS 77 Purdue Univ - West Lafayette; MS 80 Purdue Univ - West Lafayette; Aud, **A**

Lindstrom, Mrs Sandra Harris 273 Prospect Avenue, East Aurora, NY 14052, (716) 549-2300, BS 81 SUNY - Coll at Buffalo; MS 85 SUNY - Coll at Buffalo; 84–Sp-Lang Path, Lake Shore Central School Dist, **SLP**

Lindstrom, Mrs Sue A 6276 Station Mill Drive, Norcross, GA 30092, (404) 441-7578, BA 72 IN Univ - Bloomington; MA 73 IN Univ - Bloomington; **SLP**

Linebaugh, Dr Craig W George Washington University, Speech & Hearing Center, 2201 G Street N W, Washington, DC 20052, (202) 994-7364, BA 70 Lebanon Valley Coll; MA 74 Temple Univ; PH 76 (Sp & Hrng Science) Temple Univ; Prof Sp & Hrng Res Prof of Med, George Wash U, **SLP**

Lineberger, Robert D 354 Terrace Drive, Springfield, OH 45503, (513) 324-2081, BA 73 Marshall Univ; MA 74 Marshall Univ; Exec Dir, W Ctrl Oh Hrng & Sp Cen, **SLP**

Lineberger, Susan Todd 308 Hemlock Drive, Chapel Hill, NC 27514, (919) 942-1434, BA 85 Univ of NC - Chapel Hill; MS 87 Univ of NC - Chapel Hill; 87–Sp-Lang Path, Durham Co Schs, **SLP**

Lineberry, Mrs Nancy Caplitcka 77 Ebony Drive, East Greenwich, RI 02818, (401) 846-6400, **SLP**

Linehan, Mrs Cynthia Konow 22857 Hilton Head Drive #192, Diamond Bar, CA 91765, (714) 860-4024, BA 84 CA St Univ - Northridge; MA 87 CA St Univ - Northridge; Sp-Lang Path, Bassett Uni Schl Dstr, **SLP**

Lines, David L 644 Ashbourne Lane, Greenwood, IN 46142-2036, (317) 882-1523, BS 63 Ball St Univ; MA 68 Ball St Univ; Sp-Lang Path, Central State Hospital, **SLP**

Ling, Dr Daniel Dean Faculty Of Applied, Health Sciences, Univ Of Western Ontario, London, ON, Canada N6G 1H1, OB 51; MS 66 McGill Univ - Quebec; PH 68 (NS) McGill Univ - Quebec; Dean Faclty Applied Hlth Sci, U of Western Ontario, **F**

Lingard, William E Lethbridge School District #51, 433 15th Street South, Lethbridge, AB, Canada T1J 2Z5, (405) 327-4521, BA 61 Univ of MT; Sp-Lang Path, Lethbridge Sch Dist #51, **SLP**

Lingenfelter, D C 3933 Tonquin Street, Erie, PA 16506, **SLP A**

Lingenfelter-Proper, Lisa Marie 12141 Cheyenne Trail, Jacksonville, FL 32223, (904) 739-3711, BS 82 SUNY - Coll at Fredonia; MS 84 Univ of Louisville; 85–Sp-Lang Path, InSpeech Inc, **SLP ACE**

Lingerfelt, Gwendolynn F 355 Mooreland Road, Richmond, VA 23229, (804) 321-7474, BA 74 Mary Washington Coll; ME 75 Univ of VA - Charlottesville; Sp-Lang Path, Children's Hosp, **SLP**

Lingo, Mrs Maryann S 62 Oak Meadow, Evansville, IN 47711, (812) 867-6054, BS 74 Murray St Univ; MA 77 Saint Louis Univ; **SLP**

Lingo, Mida Evans 8103 Seminary Ridge, Austin, TX 78745, (817) 292-9723, BS 76 Univ of North TX; MS 78 Univ of North TX; Sp-Lang Path, Fort Worht St Sch, **SLP**

Lingor, Mrs Gail J 10074 Delano Drive East, Jacksonville, FL 32217, (904) 268-1399, BA 76 Northern St Coll; MS 77 Phillips Univ; Associate Director, New Medico Rehabilitation Serv, **SLP**

Lingras, Robyn Levine 497 Lionville Road, Downingtown, PA 19335, (215) 777-0255, BA 72 CUNY - Queens Coll; MS 73 PA St Univ - Univ Park; Sp-Lang Path, Berks Co Inter Ut Spec Ed Sers, **SLP**

Lingwall, Dr James Bernard 12034 Devilwood Drive, Potomac, MD 20854, (301) 762-6051, BS 57 Univ of MN - Minneap-St Paul; MA 61 Univ of MN - Minneap-St Paul; PH 67 (Sp-Lang Path) Univ of MN - Minneap-St Paul; **SLP ACE**

Lingwall, Maxine Campbell 12034 Devilwood Drive, Potomac, MD 20854, (703) 430-4350, MA 74 Univ of KS; Sp-Lang Path, Fairfax Co Pub Sch Dist, **SLP**

Linhart, Julie G 317 Mahaley Avenue, Salisbury, NC 28144, **SLP**

Liniger, Harriet W 820 Weaver Lane, Concord, CA 94518, (415) 682-1078, BA 65 Blue Mountain Coll; OM 67 IN Univ - Bloomington; Sp/Lang Path, Mt Diablo USD, **SLP**

Linik, Frank Joseph P O Box 1023, Exeter, CA 93221, (209) 592-4236, BA 67 The Citadel; MA 74 CA St Univ - Fresno; **A**

Link, Karen E Route 1 Box 198-A, Mohrsville, PA 19541, (215) 371-5632, BS 74 Bloomsburg Univ of PA; MS 80 Bloomsburg Univ of PA; Sp-Lang Path, Berks Co Inter Unit, **SLP**

Link, Mrs Linda R 66 Parkway Drive, Syosset, NY 11791, (516) 938-6578, BA 71 CUNY - Queens Coll; MS 74 CUNY - Brooklyn Coll; Sp-Lang Path, Private Practice, **SLP**

Link, Mrs Miriam Ruth 4815 Todd #73, Ames, IA 50010, (515) 296-2299, BS 85 Northeast MO St Univ; MS 87 CO St Univ; SLP, Childrens Rehab Ctr

Linke, Charles E Route 1 Box 376, Santa Rosa Beach, FL 32459, (504) 524-5611, BA 49 Univ of IA; MA 52 Univ of IA; PH 53 (NS) Univ of IA; **SLP A F LM**

Linkenheld, Debbie A 607 West Fullerton #3, Chicago, IL 60614-2613, (312) 935-0685, BS 79 IL St Univ - Normal; MS 80 IL St Univ - Normal; Sp-Lang Path, Rush-Pres St Lukes Medical Ctr, **SLP**

Linker, Mrs Barbara Jean 100 Krimminger Road, Concord, NC 28025, (704) 788-8354, BS 77 Western Carolina Univ; ME 82 Univ of NC - Greensboro; 86–Sp-Lang Path, Cabarrus County Sch System, **SLP**

Linker, Mrs Elizabeth L 8605 Rockdale Court, North Richland Hills, TX 76180, (817) 281-0031, MS 87 Univ of TX - Dallas

Linklater, Diane K 10902 Montverde Lane, Houston, TX 77099, (713) 933-9069, BS 67 Univ of Houston - Univ Park; MA 68 Univ of Houston - Univ Park; Sp-Lang Path, Upjohn Hlthcr-Rehab Conroe, **SLP**

Linko-Bellavia, Mrs Susan Claire 476 Village Oaks Lane, Babylon, NY 11702-3123, (516) 661-5015, BA 81 Boston Coll; MA 83 Univ of MA - Amherst; Sp/Lang Path, East Islip Cen Sch Dist, **SLP**

Linkous, Mrs Pamela Thornton P O Box 145, Elliston, VA 24087, (703) 343-2753, MS 87 Radford Univ; **SLP**

Linn, Debra R 318 East 5th Street, Albert Lea, MN 56007, (507) 373-1766, MS 88 Mankato St Univ

Linn, Dr George B 1229 Woodland Drive, Santa Paula, CA 93060, (805) 525-5641, BA 36 Univ of WY; MA 41 Univ of WY; ED 65 (Exceptional Children) Univ of Southern CA; **SLP LM**

Linnan, Mrs Kathy B Speech Pathology Services, 34 North 8th Avenue, Clarion, PA 16214, (814) 226-9541, BS 73 Clarion Univ of PA; MA 74 Kent St Univ; Sp/Lang Path, Sp Path Serv, **SLP**

Linnell, Dr Craig O Shekeda Hearing Conservation, 4528 North Highway 61, P O Box 10747, White Bear Lake, MN 55110, (612) 429-8333, BS 61 Univ of MN - Duluth; MA 63 Univ of Southern CA; PH 67 (NS) Northwestern Univ; Pres, Shekeda Hrng Conserv Inc, **A**

Linnelli, Mrs Donna C 1433 Greystone Drive, Pittsburgh, PA 15206, BS 74 Carlow Coll; MS 78 Indiana Univ of PA; Sp-Lang Path, Pittsburgh-Mt Oliver IU #2, **SLP**

Linovitz, Maeva P 8525 East Rovey, Scottsdale, AZ 85253, BA 62 Kean Coll of NJ; Sp-Lang Path, Cartwright Sch Dist, **SLP**

Linrud, Mrs Carlotta Jean R R 2 - Box 36A, Velva, ND 58790, (701) 624-5414, MS 87 Minot St Univ; 88–Sp-Lang Path, Souris Valley Spec Svcs

Linsky, Sharon E 20 Hammond Pond Parkway, Apartment 15, Chestnut Hill, MA 02167, (617) 965-4623, MS 74; Sp-Lang Path, Private Practice, **SLP**

Linson, Mrs Linda Carol 411 Forest Avenue, Jackson, MS 39206, (601) 981-9397, **SLP**

Lintner, Mary Emily 76 Linda Avenue #1, Oakland, CA 94611, (415) 836-8229, BA 35 Univ of San Francisco; MA 50 Stanford Univ; Aud, Oakland USD, **A LM**

Linton, Anita L 6351 Burnett Court, Ventura, CA 93003, **SLP**

Linton, Mrs Regina Dreher 308A Scales Street, Starkville, MS 39759, (601) 323-4795, BS 85 Univ Southern MS-Hattiesburg; MA 86 Univ Southern MS-Hattiesburg; 87–Sp-Lang Path, West Point Sch Dist, **SLP**

Linville, Mrs Debra Devore 2710 Strong Oak, San Antonio, TX 78247, (512) 490-6063, **SLP**

Linville, Dr Raymond N Dept Of Speech & Hrng Sciences, Box 4266 TX Tech Univ, Lubbock, TX 79409, (806) 742-1575, BA 74 East Carolina Univ; MS 78 East Carolina Univ; PH 82 (NS) Univ of IA; 88–Asst Prof, Texas Tech Univ, **SLP**

Linville, Dr Sharon S 3603 Roundtree Court, Boulder, CO 80302, (303) 444-7544, BS 73 Univ of Western Ontario; MA 79 Univ of KS; PH 87 (Hrng & Sp Science) Univ of KS; **A**

Linville, Dr Sue Ellen Speech Pathology & Audiology, Marquette University, 619 North 16th Street, Milwaukee, WI 53233, (414) 224-7349, BS 71 Boston Univ; MA 72 Univ of TX - Austin; PH 81 (Sp-Lang Path) Northwestern Univ; Assoc Prof, Marquette U, **SLP**

Linz, Joseph R 6139 Lakota Drive, Cincinnati, OH 45243, (513) 278-2612, BS 73 Univ of Cincinnati; MA 77 Univ of Cincinnati; Superv, Good Samaritan Hosp, **SLP**

Linzer, Deborah R 3640 Floral Drive, Santa Cruz, CA 95062, (408) 476-7140, BS 73 Boston Univ; MS 74 Univ of WI - Madison; Sp-Lang-Hrng Spec, Santa Cruz Co Office of Ed, **SLP**

Linzie, William Robert 2035 7th Avenue, Las Vegas, NM 87701, BA 82 Univ of NM; MS 86 Univ of NM; 86–Sp-Lang Path, Northern New Mexico Rehab Ctr, **SLP**

Lipchak, Andrea M 2936 Baywood Drive, Gretna, LA 70056, (504) 367-3120, BS 72 Clarion Univ of PA; ME 79 CA Univ of PA; Sp-Lang Path, Jefferson Parish School System, **SLP**

Lipe, Barbara C 10936 South Richmond, Tulsa, OK 74136, **SLP**

Lipe, Lisa Ann 4972 Berton Circle, La Palma, CA 90623, (213) 860-5435, BA 85 CA St Univ - Long Beach; MA 87 CA St Univ - Long Beach; **A**

Lipin, Bernard Hearing Services, Temple Medical Center, 60 Temple Street, New Haven, CT 06510, (203) 787-0201, BA 56 Long Island U - Brooklyn Ctr; MA 58 Columbia Univ Teachers Coll; Dir, B Lipin Hrg Serv, **A ACE**

Lipkind, Vicki L 18-70 211th Street, Bayside, NY 11360, **SLP**

Lipman, Mrs Heidi Rappaport 220 Lakeland Court, Roswell, GA 30076, (404) 594-1179, BA 83 Univ of GA; ME 85 GA St Univ; 87–Sp-Lang Path, Fulton County Schs, **SLP**

Lipman, Joan Michelle 805 N Howard Street #340, Alexandria, VA 22304, (703) 823-1279, MA 86 Northwestern Univ, **SLP**

Lipman, Mrs LeAnn Carol 8325 La Prada East #2047, Dallas, TX 75228, (214) 328-4409, BS 77 IL St Univ - Normal; MS 79 IL St Univ - Normal; 86–Aud, Chung-Sen HSU MD, **A**

Lipman, Lori H 127 Voorhis Avenue, River Edge, NJ 07661, (914) 636-4367, BA 80 2935; MA 82 SUNY - Center at Buffalo; 83–Sp-Lang Path, BOCES of Southern Westchester, **SLP**

Lipman, Roberta B 317 Berry Drive, Naperville, IL 60540, (312) 355-1833, BA 68 Adams St Coll; MS 74 SUNY - Center at Albany; 83–Sp-Lang Path, Sch Dist 204, **SLP**

Lipman, Sharon H 315 Hampton Lane, Key Biscayne, FL 33149, (305) 361-6598, BA 77 CA St Univ - Northridge; MA 80 CA St Univ - Northridge; Sp-Lang Path, Dade Co Pub Sch, **SLP**

Lipnack, Robin Lori 6301 Boca Colony Dr #1422, Boca Raton, FL 33433, (305) 325-1050, BA 84 Hofstra Univ; MA 84 Univ of FL; Prof Assoc, InSpeech Inc, **SLP**

Lipner, Hildy S 99 32nd 66th Road, Rego Park, NY 11374, (212) 860-7800, BS 77 SUNY - Center at Albany; MA 80 Kent St Univ; Sp-Lang Path, Cardinal Cooke Healthcare Cen, **SLP**

Lipp, Linda A 2101 Waterford Road #B, New Waterford, OH 44445, BS 73 OH St Univ; MA 81 Kent St Univ; Sp-Lang Path, Columbiana Co Bd of Ed, **SLP**

Lipp, Lori S 2660 Losantiville Avenue, Cincinnati, OH 45237, (606) 261-3605, BS 79 Miami Univ - Oxford; MS 81 IL St Univ - Normal; 81–Aud, Dr R C Kratz, **A ACE**

Lipp, Rhandee Gail 6950 Commerce Boulevard, Suite 4, Rohnert Park, CA 94928, **SLP**

Lippe, Mrs Shirel W Hackensack High School, 1st & Beech Streets, Hackensack, NJ 07601, (201) 488-4100, BA 49 Montclair St Coll; MA 62 Montclair St Coll; OM 69 Columbia Univ Teachers Coll; Sp-Lang Path, Hackensack Bd of Ed, **SLP**

Lippe, Sylvia P 69 Spenser Drive, Short Hills, NJ 07078, (201) 376-6758, BA 57 CUNY - Brooklyn Coll; MA 74 Montclair St Coll; Sp/Lang Path, Private Practice, **SLP**

Lippert, Emily Anne 939 East End Avenue, Pittsburgh, PA 15221, (412) 751-0267, BA 74 Beloit Coll; MA 81 Univ of Pittsburgh - Pittsburgh; Sp-Lang Path, Rehab Inst of Pgh, **SLP**

Lippert, Mrs Janet C 1309 Farwell Drive, Madison, WI 53704, (608) 249-2151, BS 64 Univ of WI - Madison; MS 73 Univ of WI - Madison; SLP, State of WI Dept of Health, **SLP**

Lippes, Beth C 1026 Palm Lane, Redondo Beach, CA 90278, **SLP**

Lippincott, Charles V Holiday Station #8100, Anaheim, CA 92802, (714) 772-3121, BA 58 Univ of Redlands; SLP, Anaheim Union H J District, **SLP**

Lippke, Mrs Barbara A 4560 East Mercer Way, Mercer Island, WA 98040, (206) 232-3288, BS 56 Purdue Univ - West Lafayette; MS 71 Univ of WA; Sp-Lang Path, **SLP**

Lippman, Mrs Leslie Gaye 150 Burnt Plains Road, Milford, CT 06460, (203) 877-6374, BA 82 Boston Coll; MA 83 MI St Univ; 86–Sp-Lang Path, InSpeech Inc, **SLP**

Lippmeier, Linda Lee 5 Lane Avenue, Greenland, NH 03840, (603) 436-0442, BS 83 Syracuse Univ; MS 85 Columbia Univ Teachers Coll; Sp-Lang Path, Whittier Rehabilitation Hosp, **SLP**

Lippold, Timothy Alan 1230 10th Street South, Wisconsin Rapids, WI 54494, (715) 423-7224, BS 74 Univ of WI - Eau Claire; MS 76 Univ of WI - Stevens Point; Aud, Private Practice, **A**

Lipschultz, Rochelle W 205 Davis Avenue, Brookline, MA 02146, (617) 536-7255, BS 75 Univ of MD - College Park; MS 77 Univ of WI - Madison; Sp-Lang Path, Emerson Coll, **SLP**

Lipscomb, Dr David M 30531 15th Avenue NE, Stanwood, WA 98292, (206) 629-4865, BA 57 Univ of Redlands; MA 59 Univ of Redlands; PH 66 (NS) Univ of WA; Pres, Correct Service Inc, **A F**

Lipscomb, Mrs Gwendolyn 16400 N W 39th Court, Miami, FL 33054, (305) 921-8103, BS 75 FL St Univ; MS 76 FL St Univ; SLP, Broward Co Sch Bd, **SLP**

Lipscomb, Marsha Ann 163 Parker Drive, Marietta, GA 30060, (404) 522-7272, OB 78 Kennesaw Coll; BS 81 Univ of GA; ME 82 Univ of GA; Aud, Atlanta Public Schools, **A**

Lipscomb, Mary Winders 1018 Pope Circle, McComb, MS 39648, (601) 684-6220, BS 67 MS Univ for Women; ME 86 Southeastern LA Univ; 88–Sp-Lang Path, McComb PS, **SLP**

Lipsett, Robert K 3 Avalon Cove, Laguna Niguel, CA 92677, (714) 496-1215, BS 77 Boston Univ; MA 78 Ball St Univ; Sp-Lang Path, Capistrano USD, **SLP**

Lipsey, Mrs Judy M 144 Green Road, Kersey, PA 15846, (814) 885-6152, BS 81 Gannon Univ; MS 84 Clarion Univ of PA; Sp-Lang Path, Bradford Hosp, **SLP**

Lipshaw, Mrs Lori Robin 32466 Chesterbrook, Farmington Hills, MI 48018, (313) 489-4172, BA 85 MI St Univ; MA 87 Wayne St Univ - Sch of Med

Lipsi, Kathy Ann 6269 Gentle Lane, Alexandria, VA 22310, (202) 745-3223, BS 82 Elmira Coll; MA 83 OH St Univ; Dev Spec, Children's Hosp, **SLP**

Lipsitz, Mrs Margaret A 92 Alexandra Drive, Stamford, CT 06903, (203) 322-8464, BS 77 Boston Univ; MA 78 Hofstra Univ; Sp-Lang Path, **SLP**

Lipsky, Adrianne 17 Laura Drive, Monsey, NY 10952, (914) 357-2161, BA 68 Adelphi Univ; MA 69 NY Univ; Sp-Lang Path, NYC Bd of Ed/Commit On Hndcpd, **SLP**

Lipsky, Mrs Sharon Braver 2423 Young Avenue, Bronx, NY 10469, (212) 549-4753, MA 86 CUNY - Queens Coll; 86–Sp-Lang Path, Herbert G Birch Early Child Ctr, **SLP**

Lipsky, Walter 495 West End Avenue, New York, NY 10024, (212) 650-6153, BA 71 CUNY - Brooklyn Coll; MA 78 CUNY - Hunter Coll; Audiologist, Mount Sinai Medical Center, **SLP A**

Lipsmeyer, Gregory Anderson 85 Lincolnshire, Mineralwells, WV 26150-9603, (304) 684-2441, BS 76 AR St Univ; MS 82 AR St Univ; 86–Sp-Lang Path, Colin Anderson Ctr Dept of Educ, **SLP**

Lipson, David Mintz 35/11 Ramot 04, Jerusalem, Israel, **SLP**

Lipson, Mrs Joni Freed 6085 Pickwood Drive, West Bloomfield, MI 48322, (313) 280-8403, BA 77 MI St Univ; MA 78 Wayne St Univ; Sp-Lang Path, Wm Beaumont Hosp, **SLP**

Lipson, Mrs Marilyn E 12109 Heathertree Court, Cincinnati, OH 45242, (513) 489-8565, BA 70 Rutger's St Univ - Douglas Coll; MA 71 Univ of Cincinnati; Sp-Lang Path, Ind Contractor Home Health Ag, **SLP**

Lipson-Ticker, Mrs Denise 3809 West 15th #700, Plano, TX 75075, (214) 596-4005, BS 75; MS 77 Southern Methodist Univ; MS 77 Southern Methodist Univ; Aud, Wm B Cobb MD, **A**

Lipuma, Cynthia L 943 Olive Road #1-B, Homewood, IL 60430, (312) 799-1067, BS 74 Eastern IL Univ; MS 75 Eastern IL Univ; **SLP**

Lisabeth, Mrs Susan Fern 1 Daniel Drive, Plainview, NY 11803, (516) 932-7365, BS 82 Univ of MD - College Park; MA 83 Hofstra Univ; Sp/Lang Path, BOCES Fern Place, **SLP**

Lisak, Mrs Myriam Tobon 17256 Rinaldi Street, Granada Hills, CA 91344, (805) 252-9580

Lisbona, Bonnie Zients 3304 Wildwood Court, Monmouth Junction, NJ 08852, (201) 297-5691, SLP, Self Employed, **SLP**

Liscic, Debra Schumann 825 Oakland Avenue, Joliet, IL 60435, (312) 361-2121, BS 85 Northern IL Univ - De Kalb; MA 87 Northern IL Univ - De Kalb

Lisemby, Doris M 1 Holly Oak Drive, Arkadelphia, AR 71923, MS; **SLP LM**

Lisenbee, Catherine 9100 Loveless Drive, Rockford, MI 49341, (616) 874-8401, MA 80 MI St Univ; 87–Aud, Hearing & Speech Ctr, **A**

Liseski, LuAnn Davis Rd #1 Box 287-A, Wallkill Avenue, Wallkill, NY 12589, (914) 744-5266, BA 85 SUNY - Coll at New Paltz; MS 86 SUNY - Coll at New Paltz

Lish, Mrs Jane Gesler 1439 Ripchak Road, Corona, CA 91719, (714) 735-5568, MA 86 CA St Univ - Fullerton; 86–Sp-Lang Path, Lake Elsinore Sch Dist, **SLP**

Lisicia, Katherine Ann 2213 Druid Oaks, Atlanta, GA 30329, (404) 296-5440, BS 85 Armstrong St Coll; ME 87 Univ of GA; 87–Sp-Lang Path, Americana Hlth Care Ctr, **SLP**

Liska, Jill M 5643 South Hately Avenue, Cuaahy, WI 53110, (414) 769-6176, BS 86 Univ of WI - Whitewater; MS 87 Univ of WI - Whitewater; 88–Sp-Lang Path, Round Lake Comm Sch Dist #116

Liska, Mrs Robin Susan 35 Putter Drive, Wallingford, CT 06492, (203) 265-9379, BS 85 Northeastern Univ; MS 87 Southern CT St Univ; **SLP**

Liss, Mrs Bonnie S 7325 Imperial Drive, Franklin, WI 53132, (414) 931-4065, BS 68 Univ of WI - Milwaukee; MS 69 Univ of WI - Milwaukee; Sp-Lang Path, Milwaukee Chldn Hosp, **SLP**

Liss, Julie Marie 5810 Russett Road #2, Madison, WI 53711, (608) 274-6753, BA 84 Univ of WI - Madison; MA 86 Univ of Denver; SLP, VA Hosp, **SLP**

Liss, Lorri P 2500 Johnson Avenue #3S, Riverdale, NY 10463, (212) 601-3679, BA 80 CUNY - Queens Coll; MS 82 Columbia Univ Teachers Coll; Sp-Lang Path, Private Practice, **SLP**

Liss-Bronstein, Linda 5 Sage Road, Rocky Hill, CT 06067, (203) 635-5507, BS 77 SUNY - Center at Albany; MS 78 Syracuse Univ; Sp-Lang Path, Hartford Public Schools, **SLP**

Lisson, Mrs Jennifer Kaye 12714 Willowyck, St Louis, MO 63146, (314) 434-4112, BS 78 Univ of Southwestern LA; MS 83 Univ of Southwestern LA; **SLP**

List, Catherine Oas 1202 134th Avenue N E, Bellevue, WA 98005, (206) 562-1589, BA 78 Univ of MI - Ann Arbor; MS 79 Univ of MI - Ann Arbor; Sp-Lang Path, Issaquah Sch Dist 411, **SLP**

Lister, Jocelyn 4 David Drive, Raymond, NH 03077, (605) 895-4346, BS 75; MA 77 Western MI Univ; Sp-Lang Path, Raymond Jr-Sen High School, **SLP**

Lister, Paul B P O Box 508, Birchwood Hills, Bethlehem, NH 03574, (603) 869-2408, BA 72 Long Island U - Brooklyn Ctr; MA 75 Central MI Univ; Owner/Dir, Private Practice, **SLP**

Listoe, Kim M 319 South 2nd West, Riverton, WY 82501, (307) 856-5250, BS 80 Univ of WY; MS 82 Univ of WY; 82–Aud, Fremont Co Sch Dist #25, **A**

Listokin, Sandra Arlene 6865 Bridlewood Court, Boca Raton, FL 33433, (305) 394-8265, MA 79 Trenton St Coll

Liston, Mrs Joan F 9 Valley Lane, Toms River, NJ 08753, (201) 244-6829, BA 66 Kean Coll of NJ; MA 68 Kean Coll of NJ; Sp-Lang Path, Private Practice, **SLP**

Liston, Lynn R 325 Fairview, Belvidere, IL 61008, (815) 962-5252, BS 72 Univ of MI - Ann Arbor; MA 75 Northern IL Univ - De Kalb; Aud, Midwest Sp and Hrng Assoc, **A**

Liston, William J 1923 Wilson Avenue, Salt Lake City, UT 84108, (801) 974-8307, MS 62 Univ of UT; 69–Dir Sp & Hrng, Salt Lake City Schs, **SLP A**

Listwa, Mrs Sharon P 1425 Lincoln Parkway West, Allentown, PA 18104, (215) 395-4433, BA 69 Temple Univ; MA 72 Temple Univ; Sp/Lang Path, Carbon-Lehigh IU #21, **SLP**

Litchfield, Mrs Marilyn K 23 Covered Bridge Lane, Newark, DE 19711, BS 72 Univ of IL - Urbana; MA 74 MI St Univ; Sp-Lang Path, Cristina School District, **SLP**

Litecky, Mrs Rene Dubois 12085 Ilex Street N W, Coon Rapids, MN 55433, (612) 421-9190, BS 74 Saint Cloud St Univ; MS 81 Saint Cloud St Univ; SLP, Anoka-Hennepin Dist #11, **SLP**

Lithgow, Joan Ann 208 Mount Shasta Drive, San Rafael, CA 94903, (415) 223-2595, BA 59 IN Univ - Bloomington; MA 86 Univ of San Francisco; 86–Sp-Lang Path, San Francisco USD, **SLP**

Litinas, Nikos 30 Mihael Nomikov, Patisia, Athens, Greece GR 112, (01) 862-0988, BA 83 Univ of IL - Chicago; MS 85 Governors St Univ

Litke, Robert E Speech & Hearing Center, University Of South Dakota, Vermillion, SD 57069, (605) 677-5474, BA 55 San Jose St Univ; MS 60 SD St Univ; PH 75 (NS) Univ of NE - Lincoln; Prof, U S Dak, **SLP A**

Litsey, Mrs Lisa Everhard 4205 South Eastern Parkway, Owensboro, KY 42303, (502) 686-7333, **SLP**

Litsky, Jay 200 West 79th Street #5C, New York, NY 10024, (212) 683-6970, BA 60 CUNY - Brooklyn Coll; MA 61 Univ of WI - Madison; 80–Sp-Lang Path, NY City Bd of Ed, **A**

Litt, Bonnie 436 East Cross Street, Baltimore, MD 21230, (301) 685-8240, BS 58; MS 72 Loyola Coll; **SLP**

Litten, Mrs Janet R 13560 Crestmoor, Dallas, TX 75234, (214) 243-6326, BS 69 Purdue Univ - West Lafayette; MS 70 Purdue Univ - West Lafayette; **SLP**

Littke, Jean M 417 40th Avenue, Greeley, CO 80634, BS 73 ND St Univ; MA 81 Univ of IA; Sp-Lang Path, Rehab / Visiting Nurse Assoc, **SLP**

Little, Cassandra A 556 Willow Place, La Verne, CA 91750, (714) 599-7162, BA 70 Howard Univ; MS 71 PA St Univ - Univ Park; PH 85 (Curriculum & Supervision) Univ of Pittsburgh - Pittsburgh; Sp-Lang Path, Azusa USD, **SLP**

Little, Charlotte P O Box 816, Winnsboro, LA 71295, **SLP**

Little, Mrs Cheryl D S 10207 Greenwillow Street, Houston, TX 77035, (713) 728-8947, BS 77 IN St Univ - Terre Haute; MS 78 IN St Univ - Terre Haute; Self Contained Teacher, Fort Bend ISD, **SLP**

Little, Mrs Deborah Joy 2773 Yuma Circle, Salt Lake City, UT 84109, (801) 565-7100, BA 83 CA St Univ - Fresno; MA 86 CA St Univ - Fresno; 86–Sp-Lang Path, Jordan Sch Dist, **SLP**

Little, Jane K Department Of Communication Disorders, 3560 Bathurst Street, North York, ON, Canada M6A 2E1, (416) 785-2377, BA 73 Univ of Toronto - Ontario; MA 76 Univ of ME - Orono; Sp/Lang Path, Baycrest Centre for Geriatrics, **SLP**

Little, Mrs Janet M 657 Ridgecrest Road, Akron, OH 44303, (216) 864-8359, BS 75 Kent St Univ; ME 87 Univ of Akron; 88–Supvr, Medina Co Achievement Ctr, **SLP**

Little, Jimmie L 9170 Forest Lane #132, Dallas, TX 75243, (214) 699-3311, BS 73 West TX St Univ; MA 76 West TX St Univ; Sp/Lang Path, Richardson ISD, **SLP**

Little, Mrs Joyce E 4035 47th Avenue N E, Salem, OR 97305, (503) 588-5124, BS 73 OR St Univ; MA 75 Northern MI Univ; Sp-Lang Path, Marion Co Educ Serv Dist, **SLP**

Little, Julie Arlen 544 Pine Ridge Road, Raleigh, NC 27609-4634, (919) 934-6031, BS 83 Appalachian St Univ; MA 84 Appalachian St Univ; SLP, Johnston Co Schs, **SLP**

Little, Kathy L 1376 Hibiscus Court, Banning, CA 92220-2049, (714) 849-4786, BA 76 CA St Univ - Fresno; MA 78 CA St Univ - Fresno; Sp-Lang Path, Riverside Co Schs, **SLP**

Little, Marilyn D 1910 Devlin Drive, Fayetteville, NC 28303, (919) 323-4411, BA 80 Wake Forest Univ; MS 82 Univ of NC - Chapel Hill; 87–Sp-Lang Path, Home Health Care of Cumberland County, **SLP**

Little, Mrs Mary E 1405 Meadow Glen, Valparaiso, IN 46383, (219) 464-9621, BS 70 Western MI Univ; MS 72 Purdue Univ - West Lafayette; 86–Sp-Lang Path, Porter Co Assoc Retarded Cit, **SLP**

Little, Noreen Hughes 31 Sylvan Lane, Feeding Hills, MA 01030, (413) 534-4563, BA 82 Univ of MA - Amherst; MS 83 WV Univ; Sp-Lang Path, Hampshire Educ Collaborative, **SLP**

Little, Odette Kay 543 North Orchard, Pittsfield, IL 62363, (217) 285-2147, BS 84 Western IL Univ; MA 85 Western IL Univ; **SLP**

Little, Mrs Patricia S 2729 Main, Vernon, TX 76384, (817) 552-9901, BS 74 TX Woman's Univ; MA 77 TX Woman's Univ; Sp-Lang Path, Texas Dept Men Health/Men Retd, **SLP**

Little, Patricia Wright 2040 Shady Branch Trail, Richmond, VA 23233-3262, (804) 786-0207, BS 82 Radford Univ; OM 83 Univ of SC - Columbia; 85–Sp-Lang Path, Medical College Virginia Hosp, **SLP**

Little, Sharon F 9351 East Calle Kuehn, Tucson, AZ 85756, (602) 327-1541, BS 83 Andrews Univ; MS 86 Univ of AZ; SLP/Aud, Tucson Med Cntr, **SLP A**

Little, Tom Anthony, III 920 West Main, Blytheville, AR 72315, (501) 763-2778, BA 77 Hendrix Coll; MS 81 AR St Univ; **SLP**

Littledike, Lila Jaclyn 450 East 800 South, Lewiston, UT 84320, (801) 750-1375, BA 65 UT St Univ; MS 67 UT St Univ; Asst Prof, Utah St U, **SLP**

Littlefield, Mrs Catherine M 9411 Shore Road, Brooklyn, NY 11209, (212) 855-6789, BS 80 CUNY - Brooklyn Coll; MS 82 Columbia Univ Teachers Coll; Dir Sp-Lang Path & Aud, Cobble Hill Nurs Home, **SLP**

Littleton, Mrs Katherine 104 Lamplighter Way, O'Fallon, MO 63366, (314) 474-9562, BS 79 Southeast MO St Univ; MA 80 Southeast MO St Univ; Sp-Lang Path, Occupational Resource Cen, **SLP**

Littman, Thomas A 1919 Boulevard DE Province, Apartment 28, Baton Rouge, LA 70816-8703, (504) 388-2545, MS; **A**

Litton, Mrs Alene L 4522 Cervato Street, Long Beach, CA 90815, (213) 679-9705, BA 73 CA St Univ - Chico; MA 75 CA St Univ - Chico; Sp-Lang Path, LA Co Ofc of Educ, **SLP**

Litton, Mrs Ellen Freeman 50 Knollridge Drive, Asheville, NC 28804, (704) 658-2680, **SLP**

Litvinas, Carol J Fao Detachment, Usdho Box 50, APO San Francisco, CA 96346-0001, (408) 394-7835, BA 76 Univ of Northern CO; MA 78 Univ of Northern CO; **A**

Litwack, Ellen P 517 South Roberts Road, Bryn Mawr, PA 19010, **SLP**

Litwin, Zelda 56 Whitman Drive, Brooklyn, NY 11234, (718) 375-1231, BA 59 CUNY - Brooklyn Coll; MA 61 CUNY - Brooklyn Coll; Sp-Lang Path, NYC Bd Ed, **SLP**

Litz, Mrs Laurie Donelan 12918 Cady Street, Omaha, NE 68164, (402) 493-5430, MA 83 Univ of SD - Vermillion; Sp-Lang Path, **SLP**

Litz, Nancy F 7-C Ashwood Court, Maple Shade, NJ 08052, (609) 482-2538, BA 85 Loyola Coll; MS 86 Loyola Coll; Lourdes Rehab Services, **SLP**

Litz, Paulette J 3490 Twin Oaks Court, Napa, CA 94558, (707) 253-6865, BS 72 Northwestern Univ; ME 74 Boston Univ; Sp-Lang Path, Napa County Ofc of Educ, **SLP**

Litz, Stacy L 21622 Marguerite Pkwy, #155, Mission Viejo, CA 92692, (714) 837-3061, BA 83 IN Univ - Bloomington; MA 85 Case Western Reserve Univ; Sp-Lang Path, Orange Speech and Language Ctr, **SLP**

Litzelman-Scoles, Janne 90 Monmouth Street, Suite 201, Red Bank, NJ 07701, (201) 747-7481, BA 70 Univ of NC - Greensboro; MA 72 Univ of NC - Greensboro; Sp-Lang Path, Private Practice, **SLP ACE**

Liu, Margaret Eichel 401 East 34th Street, Apartment N-11H, New York, NY 10016, (212) 988-4800, BA 76 SUNY - Center at Buffalo; MA 81 Univ of Miami; Sp/Lang Path, Private Practice, **SLP**

Liuzza, Nancy Merlotti 5717 Itaska, St Louis, MO 63109, (314) 771-0010, MA 85 Saint Louis Univ; 86–Sp-Lang Path, Spec Sch Dist of St Louis Co, **SLP**

Liuzza, Rosalie 301-B Live Oak Boulevard, Mandeville, LA 70448, (504) 796-9611, BA 76 Southeastern LA Univ; OM 78 LA St Univ - N O Medical Ctr; Sp-Lang Path, New Medico Rehab Center of LA, **SLP**

Livecchi, Patricia Rosato 22 Rydal Drive, Lawrenceville, NJ 08648, (609) 771-3630, BA 83 Boston Coll; MA 85 George Washington Univ; SLP, Mercer Cty Spec Svc/Private Pr, **SLP**

Livesay, Alesia Good Rt 1 Box 420B, Maurertown, VA 22644, (703) 459-8023, BS 84 Radford Univ; MS 85 James Madison Univ; 87–Sp-Lang Path, Shenandoah Co Sch Sys, **SLP**

Livesay, Laurel Y 24035 Windward Drive, Laguna Niguel, CA 92677, MS; **SLP LM**

Livesay, Luanne L 10 Cleveland Street #1, Somerville, MA 02143, (617) 625-0390, BS 82 Boston Univ; MA 84 George Washington Univ; Sp-Lang Path, KLK Assoc Inc, **SLP**

Livingston, Andrea Dawn Hearing Consultants Inc, 3838 U S 27 South, Sebring, FL 33870, (813) 382-4800, BS 80 Russell Sage Coll; OB 82 Coll of Saint Rose; MS 84 Syracuse Univ; Aud, Private Practice, **A**

Livingston, Cheryl 1459 Pine Row Court, Creve Coeur, MO 63146, (314) 993-2956, BS 83 Fontbonne Coll; MS 85 Fontbonne Coll; **SLP**

Livingston, Dana Lou Usmca-Kitz, Box 427, APO New York, NY 09031, (205) 739-0486, BS 76 Univ of Montevallo; MS 81 Univ of Montevallo; Sp-Lang Path, Cullman Co Bd of Ed, **SLP**

Livingston, Gregory Merrill 3100 Ashe Road #2, Bakersfield, CA 93309, (805) 397-5444, BA 75 CO St Univ; BS 82 CO St Univ; MS 85 CO St Univ; 87–Sp-Lang Path, Kern County Supt of Schs, **SLP**

Livingston, Mrs Janetta P 1328 23rd Avenue, Bradenton, FL 33508, ME 81 Nova Univ; Ese Program Coordinator, Exceptional Student Ed Dept, **SLP**

Livingston, Laura A 73 North Main Street, Uxbridge, MA 01569, (508) 278-6947, MS 88 Worcester St Coll; 79–Sp-Lang Path, Woonsocket PS, **SLP**

Livingston, Mary Brace 15015 Foothill Road, Golden, CO 80401, (303) 278-2161, BA 85 Univ of Northern CO; MA 86 Univ of Northern CO; 86–Sp-Lang Path, Jefferson Co Sch Dist, **SLP**

Livingston, Mary Lou Route 1, Box 168, Captain Cook, HI 96804, (808) 328-2303, BS 77 Northwest MO St Univ; MS 81 Central MO St Univ; SLP, Speech-Language Services, **SLP**

Livingstone, Deborah Kay 5502 29th Avenue N E, Apt #1, Seattle, WA 98105, (206) 525-2104, BA 76 San Jose St Univ; BA 81 San Jose St Univ; MS 84 Univ of WA; Sp-Lang Path, VA Med Cen, **SLP**

Livingston-Keller, Rachael Route 1 Box 144-V, Coweta, OK 74429, (918) 486-6331, BA 77 KS St Univ; MA 79 KS St Univ; Sp/Lang Path, Owasso Pub Schs, **SLP**

Livoni, Mrs Linda E 1145 West Highland Avenue, Redlands, CA 92373, (714) 793-3557, BA 74 Univ of Redlands; MS 75 Univ of Redlands; Sp-Lang Path, Alta Loma Sch Dist, **SLP**

Lix, Jean D 31606 126th Avenue S E, Auburn, WA 98002, (206) 941-0100, BS 69 SUNY - Coll at Geneseo; MS 73 SUNY - Coll at Geneseo; Sp-Lang Path, Fed Way Pub Sch Dist, **SLP**

Lizzul, Lee Ann 3660 Knoll Lane #90, Colorado Springs, CO 80917, (719) 597-3390, BS 82 CO St Univ; MS 84 CO St Univ; 85–Aud, Center for Hrng Speech & Lang, **A**

Llewellyn, Deborah Daniels 1727 Red Barn Road, Encinitas, CA 92024, (619) 576-5837, BA 80 Our Lady Lake Univ-San Anton; MA 81 Our Lady Lake Univ-San Anton; 86–Sp-Lang Path, Sp Hrng & Neurosensory Ctr, **SLP**

Llorente, Renee Ann 7094 Paoli Road, Verona, WI 53593, (608) 267-6174, OB 84 Boston Coll; MA 86 OH Univ - Athens; Aud, Madison General Hospital, **A**

Lloyd, Janet M 10935 S E 23rd Street, Bellevue, WA 98004, (206) 848-6661, BA 55 Univ of WA; OM 76 Univ of WA; Sp-Lang Path, Good Samaritan Hosp Rehab Cen, **SLP**

Lloyd, Jay C Route 3 Box 6410, Twin Falls, ID 83301, (208) 734-4555, BA 66 ID St Univ; MS 70 ID St Univ; Aud, Majic Valley ENT Assoc, **A**

Lloyd, Dr Lyle L 1717 Sheridan Road, West Lafayette, IN 47906, (317) 494-7333, BS 56 Eastern IL Univ; MA 59 Univ of IL - Urbana; PH 64 (NS) Univ of IA; Prof & Chair/Spec Ed, Prudue Univ, **SLP A F**

Lloyd, Peggy Allen 88 Rice Drive, Whitby, ON, Canada L1N 7N2, (416) 668-8220, BA 75 McGill Univ - Quebec; MS 76 Syracuse Univ; Sp/Lang Path, Durham Bd of Ed, **SLP**

Lloyd, Rachel U S A Meddac, Box 463, APO New York, NY 09221-3544, **SLP**

Lloyd, Mrs Rose M 241 Avenida Santa Elena, La Habra, CA 90631, (714) 525-2272, BA 75 CA St Univ - Fullerton; MA 80 CA St Univ - Fullerton; SLP, Fullerton Sch Dist, **SLP**

Lloyd, Shelley Hornik 321 Oxbow Drive, Torrington, CT 06790-4225, (203) 693-8164, BS 73 OH Univ - Athens; MA 76 Western IL Univ; Sp-Lang Path, Canton Pub Sch, **SLP**

Lloyd, Susan 3290 Professional Drive, Suite C, Auburn, CA 95603, (916) 823-7532, BS 72 CA St Univ - Hayward; OM 82 CA St Univ - Sacramento; MA 73 Univ of the Pacific; Aud/SLP, Placer Sp & Hrng Ser, **SLP A**

Lloyd, Mrs Susan R 3450 South Maryland Parkway, Las Vegas, NV 89109, (702) 733-6811, BA 78 Univ of FL; MA 81 Univ of FL; Aud, International Hrng Aids, **A**

Lloyd, Mrs Therese H Rural Delivery 5, 1276 Hemlock Street, Bloomsburg, PA 17815, (717) 784-5051, SLP, **SLP**

Lloyd-Jones, Mrs Rebecca Jo 7130 Fairway Bend Lane, Unit 292, Sarasota, FL 34243, (813) 798-6220, Coor of Dysphasic Prog, Hca Blake Hosp, **SLP ACE**

Lo, Dawn R 1704 SHA Court, Longview, TX 75605, (214) 236-2791, BS 79 Clarion Univ of PA; MA 81 Kent St Univ; 85–Sp-Lang Path, Good Shepherd Medical Center, **SLP**

Loafman, Mrs Debra Gwaltney Route 1 Box 398, Bartlesville, OK 74003, (918) 337-0035, BS 80 OK St Univ; MA 82 OK St Univ; Sp/Lang Path, Bartlesville PS, **SLP**

Loaiza-Suarez, Rosario Maria 61-45 98th Street #11M, Rego Park, NY 11374, (201) 596-3766, BS 78 Syracuse Univ; MA 81 NY Univ; 84–Sp-Lang Path, Mt Carmel Guild Cath Comm Serv, **SLP**

Loavenbruck, Dr Angela M Loavenbruck Lynn & Cohen PC, 500 New Hempstead Road, New City, NY 10956, (914) 362-1350, BA 65 SUNY - Center at Buffalo; MA 68 Columbia Univ Teachers Coll; ED 73 (NS) Columbia Univ Teachers Coll; Pres, Loavenbruck Lynn & Cohen PC, **SLP A F**

Lobaina, Elizabeth Sarah 15 Drexel Hill Drive, Kendall Park, NJ 08824, (201) 821-4124, BA 77 Rutgers St Univ -N Brunswick; MA 83 NY Univ; 84–Sp-Lang Path, Private Practice, **SLP**

Lobato, Mrs Cecelia B 2340 Jowett Place, Rahway, NJ 07065, (201) 862-3004, BA 60 Univ of Miami; SLP, Linden Board of Education, **SLP**

Lobb, Barbara Routley 2640 Killarney Road, Victoria, BC, Canada V8P 3G8, (604) 721-0565, Sp-Lang Path, Sch District #61, **SLP**

Lobdell, Mary Moseley 612 Girard Park Drive, Lafayette, LA 70503, (318) 236-6800, BA 77 Univ of Southwestern LA; MS 86 Univ of Southwestern LA; **SLP**

Lobelle, Donald E 7140 Camelot Drive, Canton, MI 48187, **A**

Loch, Lucinda 5111 Skillman #125, Dallas, TX 75206, (214) 905-3000, BA 86 Univ of Northern CO; MS 88 Univ of TX - Dallas; 88–SLP, Univ of TX

Loch, Michael C 3130 Lamar Avenue, Paris, TX 75460, (214) 784-8100, MA 72 San Francisco St Univ; Aud, Loch Hearing Center, **A**

Lochansky, Sydney Beth 92-44 213th Street, Queens Village, NY 11428, (212) 947-5770, BA 81 Queens Coll; MA 83 Queens Coll; Sp-Lang Path, NY State Ucp Assoc, **SLP**

Locher, Tracy Christine Rd 2 Box 130, Johnstown, PA 15904, (814) 539-2010, MS 87 Indiana Univ of PA

Lochman, Mrs Linda K Bauwens 9 Dobbs Place, Durham, NC 27707, (919) 968-3473, BS 71 Purdue Univ - West Lafayette; MS 81 Univ of North TX; Sp-Lang Path, Chap H-Carrboro Cnty Sch Sys, **SLP**

Lochner, Mrs Nancy Kaufman 37 Putnam Street, Quincy, MA 02169, (617) 749-7518, BS 84 Western OR St Coll; MS 87 Western OR St Coll; **SLP**

Lochow, Carol A 513 18th Street S W #2, Jamestown, ND 58401, (701) 252-2795, BS 83 ND St Univ; MS 86 Moorhead St Univ; 83–Dept Head-Sp-Lang Path, Anne Carlsen Sch for Multi-Hndcpd Stu, **SLP**

Locicero, Jeanne Marie 60 Raintree Island #9, Tonawanda, NY 14150, (716) 877-6800, BS 82 SUNY - Coll at Buffalo; MS 83 SUNY - Coll at Buffalo

Lock, Patricia Swinburne 332 Gerald Drive, Lafayette, LA 70503, (318) 824-6250, MS 84 Univ of Southwestern LA; **SLP**

Lock, Robin B 43W519 Main Street Road, Elburn, IL 60119, (312) 365-2952, BS 78 Northern IL Univ - De Kalb; MA 80 Northern IL Univ - De Kalb; 88–Sp/Lang Path, Horizons Speech Path Consultants, **SLP**

Lock, Mrs Sally A R R 1 Box 128, Avon, IL 61415, (309) 465-3863, BA 78 Miami Univ - Oxford; MA 80 Univ of IA; **SLP**

Lockamyeir, Mrs Judith Ann 43 Hermitage Road, Rochester, NY 14617, (716) 352-2440, BS 64 Nazareth Coll of Rochester; MA 67 SUNY - Center at Buffalo; Sp/Lang Path, BOCES #2, **SLP**

Lockard, Mrs Cheryl Smith 236 Hardy Avenue, Eugene, OR 97404, MA 68 Univ of OR; 88–Sp-Lang Path, Springfield Sch Dist #19, **SLP**

Lockart-Neilon, Ina Jeane Route 1 Box 1389, Boerne, TX 78006, (512) 755-8948, BS 76 0500; MS 82 Lamar Univ; **A**

Locke, Dr John L Massachusetts General Hospital, Neurolinguistics Lab, 15 River Street, Boston, MA 02108, (617) 726-8017, BA 63 Ripon Coll; MA 65 OH Univ - Athens; PH 68 OH Univ - Athens; Director Neurolinguistics Lab, Massachusetts General Hospital, **SLP F**

Locke, Mrs Miriam G P O Box 285, Triangle, VA 22172, BS 51 Bob Jones Univ; MS 55 FL St Univ; Sp-Lang Path, Quantico Dependents Sch Sys, **SLP**

Locke, Patricia 589 Northpark Court, Bossier City, LA 71111-2263, (318) 746-6890, BA 72 LA Tech Univ; MA 75 LA Tech Univ; SLP/Aud, Bossier Parish Sch Syst, **SLP**

Locke, Sandy R Route 1 Box 391, Muskogee, OK 74401, (918) 682-0490, BA 67 Northeastern OK St Univ; MA 71 Univ of Tulsa; **SLP**

Locke, Shirley Walker 1973 Sever Drive, Clearwater, FL 34624, (813) 585-1156, BA 79 Univ of MI - Ann Arbor; MS 81 Univ of MI - Ann Arbor; 86–Sp-Lang Path, Sun Coast Hosp, **SLP ACE**

Locke, William L 55 Keith Drive, Battle Creek, MI 49017-2705, (616) 963-0234, **SLP**

Locker, Mrs Christine 118 Washington Avenue North, Hopkins, MN 55343, (612) 479-1530, BS 80 Western MI Univ; MA 81 Western MI Univ; Sp-Lang Path, Orono PS, **SLP**

Lockett, Ann Victoria 5223 Columbine Court, Gahanna, OH 43230, (614) 461-2420, BS 83 OH Univ - Athens; MS 85 PA St Univ - Univ Park; **SLP**

Lockhart, Charles R 702 1st Avenue, Chula Vista, CA 92011, BA 67; MS 73 Southern CT St Univ; SLP, San Diego USD, **SLP**

Lockhart, Janet Lee 1265 Waller Street SE, Salem, OR 97302, (503) 371-6486, BS 83 OR St Univ; MS 86 ID St Univ; 85–Coord of Children's Prog, Salem Sp & Lang Ctr, **SLP**

Lockhart, Maureen Flannery 9103 Woodchat Way, Louisville, KY 40272, (502) 454-8322, BS 84 Brescia Coll; MA 85 Bowling Green St Univ; 87–Sp-Lang Path, Jefferson County PS, **A**

Lockhart, Sarah K 1932 Park Road, Charlotte, NC 28203, BA 70 Univ of MS; MS 74 Univ of NC - Chapel Hill; Sp/Lang Path, Childevelopment, **SLP**

Lockrem, Mrs Tracey MaryEllen PO Box 193, 305 First Avenue SW, Dilworth, MN 56529, (218) 287-2554, MS 87 Minot St Univ; Sp-Lang Path, Private Practice

Locks, Francis M 2529 Corning Avenue #203, Fort Washington, MD 20744, (301) 725-3600, BA 69 Howard Univ; MS 71 Gallaudet Coll; Aud, Dc Govt, **A**

Lockwood, Belva 7102 Lantana Terrace, Carlsbad, CA 92009, MS 70 AZ St Univ; Spec Reading Tchr, Harold W Smith Sch, **SLP**

Lockwood, Dr Dean D Speech And Hearing Center, University Of South Dakota, Vermillion, SD 57069, (605) 677-5474, BA 59 Augustana Coll; MA 61 Stanford Univ; PH 72 (NS) Univ of OK Medical Center; 70–Dir & Prof - Commun Dis Prog, U of SD, **SLP A F**

Lockwood, Elizabeth Loring 201 North Rogers, Northville, MI 48167, (313) 467-1362, BS 53 Western MI Univ; MA 59 Western MI Univ; Coord of Monitoring, Wayne County Indepen Sch Dist

Lockwood, Mette Norma 30 Roslyn Crescent, Winnipeg, MB, Canada R3L 0H7, (204) 452-7591, BA 85 Univ of Winnipeg - Manitoba; MA 87 SUNY - Coll at Plattsburgh; 87–Sp-Lang Path, Child Guidance Clinic

Lockwood, Sally 4601 Watergap, Manlius, NY 13104-9321, (315) 425-4404, BA 76 Univ of MI - Ann Arbor; MS 78 Syracuse Univ; Sp-Lang Path, Syracuse Cty Sch, **SLP**

Lockwood, Mrs Susan Alta 2647 Skyline Drive, Salt Lake City, UT 84108, (801) 583-2718, BA 82 Univ of UT; MS 84 Univ of NM; **SLP**

Lococo, Jomar K 22 Skylark Drive #222, Larkspur, CA 94939, (415) 499-5807, BA 70 Dominican Coll of San Rafael; MS 74 Univ of OR; Sp-Lang Path, Marin Co Ofc of Educ, **SLP ACE**

Loda, Robert A 9 Marshall Lane, Ansonia, CT 06401, (203) 261-6411, MS 65 Southern CT St Univ; Sp-Lang Path, Trumbull Pub Sch, **SLP**

Lodewick, Mrs Christine Lobeck 201 Spring Valley Road, Ridgefield, CT 06877, (203) 431-0147, BS 65 Univ of WI - Madison; MA 66 Univ of CT; **SLP**

Lodholz, Mrs Colleen A 5025 Stonehaven Drive, Madison, WI 53716, (608) 222-9670, BS 78 Univ of WI - Stevens Point; MS 80 Univ of WI - Stevens Point; SLP, Madison Metro School District, **SLP**

Lodholz, Mrs Dorleta Oetting 584 Andrews, St Louis, MO 63122, (314) 842-4674, BS 80 Univ of MO - Columbia; MS 81 Central MO St Univ; Sp/Lang Path, Private Practice, **SLP**

Lodholz-Horton, Rita M 100 Lakeaires, Peachtree City, GA 30269, (404) 599-6621, BS 75 Southwest MO St Univ; MS 83 Sonoma St Univ; MS 76 Central MO St Univ; Sp/Lang Path, Homehlth, **SLP**

Lodwick, Mrs Helen c/o Pat Carroll, 3200 East Renner Road, Richardson, TX 75081, BA 52 Univ of IA; MA 71 Southern Methodist Univ; President, Lodwick Sp & Lang Serv Inc, **SLP**

Loeb, Mrs Diane Frome 515 Dexter Lane, West Lafayette, IN 47906, (702) 972-0443, BS 82 Univ of NV - Reno; MS 84 Univ of NV - Reno; 85–Grad Asst, Purdue University, **SLP**

Loeb, Elise 20023 Tuba Street, Chatsworth, CA 91311-3445, **SLP**

Loeb, Mrs Marlene L 9300 N Broadmoor, Bayside, WI 53217, (414) 352-5632, BS 69 PA St Univ - Univ Park; ME 71 Boston Univ; Sp-Lang Path, **SLP**

Loeb, Randi Chudnow 1409 Commonwealth Avenue #201, Brighton, MA 02135, (617) 783-9633, BA 82 CT Coll; MS 87 Emerson Coll; 88–Sp-Lang Path, Kennedy Mem Hosp Chldr

Loechel, June E 55 Rock Crest, Hicksville, NY 11801, (212) 376-8780, BA 70 Hofstra Univ; MA 77 Hofstra Univ; SLP, NY Cty Bd of Ed-Sp Serv Ut, **SLP**

Loeding, Barbara L 219-10 Nimitz Drive, West Lafayette, IN 47906, (317) 743-1015, BA 75 Univ of MN - Minneap-St Paul; BA 75 Univ of MN - Minneap-St Paul; MS 79 Mankato St Univ; 84–Research Fellow, Prudue Univ, **SLP**

Loeffelhardt, Jean 421 Martin Grove Road, Islington, ON, Canada M9B 4M1, (416) 848-1711, BA 75 Univ of Northern IA; MA 76 Univ of Northern IA; Sp-Lang Path, Private Practice, **SLP**

Loeffert, Richard H 427 Gilfillan Street, Franklin, PA 16323, (814) 437-5885, BS 72 Bowling Green St Univ; ME 75 Clarion Univ of PA; **SLP**

Loeffler, Dr Donald Lee Western Carolina University, Dept STA, P O Box 473, Cullowhee, NC 28723, (704) 227-7491, OB 52 Univ of Dayton; MA 53 Columbia Univ Teachers Coll; PH 69 (NS) Bowling Green St Univ; Prof Dept Sp & Theatre Arts, Western Carolina University, **SLP**

Loeffler, Kathryn E 13003 Oak Creek Court, Midlothian, VA 23113, (804) 379-3698, BA 78 Univ of MD - College Park; MS 80 James Madison Univ; Sp-Lang Path, Chesterfield Co Public Schools, **SLP**

Loeffler, Susanne Ellen 7481 South Forest Court, Littleton, CO 80122, BS 79 Northern AZ Univ; MA 82 Univ of Denver; Sp-Lang Path, Porter Memorial Speech & Hrng, **SLP**

Loeffler, Susanne M 1686 Ebbets Drive, Campbell, CA 95008, (408) 379-4244, BA 84 Univ of CA - Santa Barbara; MA 85 Univ of the Pacific; **SLP**

Loehr, Lynda K B 4537 Snowdrift, St Louis, MO 63128, **SLP**

Loeper, Sr Donna Jo 209 East Price Street, Philadelphia, PA 19144, (215) 525-8800, BS 75 Clarion Univ of PA; ME 77 Clarion Univ of PA; 87–Sp-Lang Path, St Edmond's Home, **SLP**

Loera, Barbara G 606 W 17th #411, Austin, TX 78701, (512) 471-3841, BA 75 TX A & I Univ; MA 76 Our Lady Lake Univ-San Anton; Coord Bilingual Sp-Path Proj, Univ of TX of Austin, **SLP**

Loeser, Gregory J 10402 Nall Avenue, Overland Park, KS 66207-3835, (816) 444-0077, BA 71 Univ of WI - Milwaukee; MA 72 Western MI Univ; 85–Sp-Lang Path, Kansas City (Mo) School Dist, **SLP**

Loeser, Mrs Nancy A 133 Lighthouse Drive, Jupiter, FL 33469, (407) 746-0424, BS 54 OH St Univ; MA 76 Seton Hall Univ; Sp-Lang Path, Private Practice, **SLP ACE**

Loest, Deborag Gaye 2680 Curtis Way, Sacramento, CA 95818, (916) 452-0844, BA 82 CA St Univ - Sacramento

Loest, Patricia L 416 South German Street, Mayville, WI 53050, BS 83 Univ of WI - Milwaukee; MS 85 Univ of WI - Milwaukee; **SLP**

Loetzbeier, Mrs Anne H 2830 Derhammer Road, Bath, PA 18014, (215) 837-1234, BA 50 Ursinus Coll; ME 57 PA St Univ - Univ Park; **SLP**

Loewe, Elaine H 83-26 Lefferts Boulevard #6F, Kew Gardens, NY 11415, (212) 904-4264, BA 76 SUNY - Center at Buffalo; MS 78 Columbia Univ Teachers Coll; OM 86 Adelphi Univ; 88–Aud, NYC Dept of Health, **A**

Loewenthal, Terri 432 Ward Street, Newton, MA 02159, (617) 735-6475, BS 73 Ithaca Coll; MS 75 Washington Univ; Aud, Chldn Hosp Med Cen, **A**

Loewy, Eva Susanna 2225 College Drive #29, Baton Rouge, LA 70808, (318) 235-7216, OB 80 Beaver Coll; MA 86 Temple Univ

Lof, Gregory L 2525 University Avenue #C, Madison, WI 53705, BS 79 Moorhead St Univ; MS 81 Moorhead St Univ; **SLP**

Loffler, Mrs Tanya Lambert 1507 Taylor, Denver City, TX 79323, (806) 592-2277, BA 81 TX Tech Univ; MS 84 TX Tech Univ; 83–Sp-Lang Path, Denver City Independ Sch Dist, **SLP**

Loffredo, Lisa Catherine 147 New Broadway, North Tarrytown, NY 10591, (914) 631-0892, BS 85 Elmira Coll; MS 87 Columbia Univ Teachers Coll; 87–Sp-Lang Path, Bronx VA Med Ctr, **SLP**

Lofink, Joanne L T 5003 East Lakeside, Orange, CA 92667, (714) 997-6275, BA 71 CA St Univ - Fullerton; MS 78; Sp-Lang Path, Private Practice, **SLP**

Lofland, Kristie Brown Ap & S Clinic, 221 South 6th Street, Terre Haute, IN 47807, (812) 232-0564, BS 72 IN St Univ - Terre Haute; MS 78 IN St Univ - Terre Haute; Aud, Assocd Physn & Surg Cl, **A**

Lofquist, Beverly Henke PO Box 993, Wilmington, DE 19899, (302) 654-4327, BS 84 Indiana Univ of PA; MS 87 Univ of TX - Dallas; Sp-Lang Path, New Castle Hring Spech Vest Ct, **SLP**

Loftesnes, Mrs Lucille M Route 1 Box 120, Granville, ND 58741, BS 71 Minot St Univ; MS 75 Minot St Univ; Sp-Lang Path, Minot Pub Schs Spec Ser, **SLP**

Loftin, Mrs Joni Grey Route 1 Box 457-B, Blowing Rock, NC 28605, (704) 264-1280, BS 84 Appalachian St Univ; OM 86 Univ of SC - Columbia; 86–Sp-Lang Path, Dev Eval Ctr, **SLP**

Loftin, Rosemary B 4204 Bloomington Avenue, Apartment 102, Arlington Heights, IL 60004, (312) 520-9850, BS 76 IL St Univ - Normal; MS 78 IL St Univ - Normal; 87–Sp-Lang Path, Excellcare Rehab Inc, **SLP**

Loftiss, Eugene W 2018 Fletcher, Urbana, IL 61801, (217) 337-5977, PH (NS); **A**

Loftus, Mrs Paula Megan 22 Joaquin Avenue, Assonet, MA 02702, (617) 823-8181, BA 75 Bridgewater St Coll; MS 85 Northeastern Univ; 75–Sp-Lang Path, Taunton PS, **SLP**

Logan, Carol Lynn 1289 East Ridge Meadow Ln, Apt 8-U, Midvale, UT 84047, (801) 571-1223, BA 84 Univ of CA - Santa Barbara; MS 86 UT St Univ; **A**

Logan, Kenneth J 510 Fremont Street, Laramie, WY 82070, (307) 745-3014, BS 79 CO St Univ; MS 81 CO St Univ; Clinical Supervisor, Univ of Wy, **SLP**

Logan, Kimberly Denise 1933 West Street, Annapolis, MD 21401, (301) 224-4560, BA 84 Univ of NC - Chapel Hill; MS 86 Univ of NC - Chapel Hill; 88–Aud, Hearing Lab, **A**

Logan, Lorri Backer 15 Hillcrest Avenue, Ellenville, NY 12428, (914) 339-1416, BS 80 SUNY - Coll at Geneseo; MS 85 SUNY - Coll at New Paltz; 87–Sp-Lang Path, Ulster Co BOCES, **SLP**

Logan, Patricia Mary 2611 North University Dr, Apt 1, Waukesha, WI 53188, (414) 521-0544, BS 85 Univ of WI - Whitewater; MS 86 Univ of WI - Whitewater; Sp-Lang Path, Oconomowoc Public Schools, **SLP**

Logan, Dr Richard Lanham 179 Hines Terrace, Macon, GA 31204, (912) 746-0090, BA 59 Univ of AL- Tuscaloosa; MA 62 Univ of AL- Tuscaloosa; PH 77 (Learning Disabilities-Early Childhood Spec Ed) GA St Univ; 84–Sp-Lang Path, Sp Lang Lrng Serv, **SLP**

Logan, Dr Robert 30 Tucker Creek Road, Conway, AR 72032, (501) 450-3176, MS 76 FL St Univ; MS 76 FL St Univ; PH 85 (NS) FL St Univ; Asst Prof, Univ of Central Ar, **SLP A**

Logan, Robert A 4541 Chuckwood Drive, Charlotte, NC 28212, (704) 545-3164, BS 62 Wayne St Univ; ME 64 Wayne St Univ; 87–Sp-Lang Path, St Joseph of the Pines Hosp, **SLP**

Logan, Susan A 4710 Belmont Park Terrace, Nashville, TN 37215, **A**

Logan, Mrs Susan Anderson Drawer G, Vail, CO 81658, (303) 949-5675, BA 77 Univ of Denver; MA 79 Univ of Denver; **SLP**

Loganbill, Dr G Bruce California State University, McIntosh 701, 1250 Bellflower Boulevard, Long Beach, CA 90840, (213) 498-4305, BA 56 Bethel Coll; MA 58 Univ of KS; PH 61 (NS) MI St Univ; Prof-Logoped Path, CA St U-Long Beach

Logeman, Mrs Deborah J 3215 Everglade, Woodridge, IL 60517, (312) 985-6269, BS 78 Univ of IL - Urbana; MS 79 Univ of IL - Urbana; Sp-Lang Path, Commun Dis Cen, **SLP**

Logemann, Jerilyn Ann 1002 Greenleaf, Wilmette, IL 60091, (312) 491-3066, BS 63 Northwestern Univ; MA 64 Northwestern Univ; PH 68 (Sp Path) Northwestern Univ; 70–Prof, Northwestern U, **SLP F**

Logerfo, Catherine 6653 San Benito Avenue, Alta Loma, CA 91701, (714) 944-8448, BA 76 CA St Univ - Los Angeles; MA 80 CA St Univ - Los Angeles; Sp-Lang Path, Ontario-Montclair School Dist, **SLP**

Loggie, Bonnie Lee 656 West Gordon Terrace #2E, Chicago, IL 60613, (312) 323-5656, BS 82 Purdue Univ - West Lafayette; MA 84 Univ of IL - Urbana; Sp-Lang Path, Paulson Ctr for Rehab Med, **SLP**

Loggins, Janice Ellen 2318 S Cuatro Drive, Rowland Heights, CA 91748, (714) 639-4990, BA 84 4359; MA 86 CA St Univ - Los Angeles; **A**

Logsdon, Mrs Celia W 15 Francis Drive, Reading, MA 01867, (617) 944-3618, BA 74 MI St Univ; MA 75 MI St Univ; Aud, John G Hernandez & Assoc, **A**

Logsdon, John Paul 2255 Josh Court #427, Melbourne, FL 32904-8934, (305) 724-5489, MS 87 Western KY Univ; InSpeech Inc, **SLP**

Logston, Sharee Lu 11737 Jefferson Avenue #26B, Newport News, VA 23606, (804) 878-5412, BS 81 Univ of UT; MS 84 Univ of OK - OK City; Chief Audiologist, Mc Donald Army Hospital, **A**

Logue, Anne L 2213 North Spruce, Santa Ana, CA 92706, **SLP**

Logue, Mrs Barbara H 2919 Colony Road, Durham, NC 27705, BA 72 Univ of NC - Chapel Hill; ME 74 Univ of NC - Chapel Hill; Sp/Lang Path, Barbara H Carr & Assoc, **SLP**

Lohman, Mrs Tricia M 37474 Fountain Park Circlr, Apartment 477, Westland, MI 48185, (313) 459-5925, MA 87 Wayne St Univ

Lohman-Ruiz, Patricia S 5631 Palm Avenue, Sacramento, CA 95841, (916) 334-4853, BS 86 CA St Univ - Sacramento; MA 87 Univ of the Pacific; 88–Sp-Lang Path, Burger Rehab, **SLP**

Lohmeier, Jean A 202 11th Avenue N W, Altoona, IA 50009, (515) 967-3771, BS 72 Univ of NE - Lincoln; MA 73 Univ of NE - Lincoln; SLP, Heartland AEA, **SLP**

Lohner, Mrs Denise M 22 Summertree Run, Sparta, NJ 07871, (201) 729-8447, BA 78 Loyola Coll; MS 79 Loyola Coll; **SLP**

Lohr, Dr Frances E 2430 Glenwood Drive, Kalamazoo, MI 49008, (616) 383-0963, BA 51 MI St Univ; MA 55 Northwestern Univ; PH 68 (NS) Univ of MI - Ann Arbor; Prof SLP/Clinic Coord, Western Michigan University, **SLP**

Lohse, Katherine A 4876 Goethe, St Louis, MO 63116, (314) 942-2565, BS 84 Saint Louis Univ; MA 85 Saint Louis Univ; **SLP**

Lohsen, Brenda W 6932 Cameron Glen Drive, Charlotte, NC 28210, (704) 552-8193, BA 70 Univ of NC - Greensboro; MA 72 Univ of MD - College Park; **SLP**

Loigman, Mrs Sonia Spielberg 631 Colebrook Road, Philadelphia, PA 19115, (215) 698-0980, **SLP**

Loiry, Mrs Carol J 7812 Deerfield Lane, Panama City, FL 32404-8610, (904) 871-6488, **SLP A**

Loiselle, Louise Hathaway 6501 Fannin NA200, Houston, TX 77030, (713) 529-9146, BA 75 Trinity Univ; MS 83 UT St Univ; 83–Aud, Methodist Hosp, **A**

Lojacono, Marie S 392 Dalewood Drive, Orinda, CA 94563, (415) 254-8197, BA 55 MI St Univ; **SLP**

Lolan, Thomas C Audiology & Hear Aid Services, 704 East Stroop Road, Kettering, OH 45429, (513) 299-5613, BS 71 Univ of Cincinnati; MA 75 Univ of Cincinnati; Aud Consultant, Private Practice, **A ACE**

Lollos, Mrs Virginia Farese 86 Beach Street, Bloomfield, NJ 07003, (201) 748-6023, Sp-Lang Path, Bd of Ed, **SLP**

Loman, Mrs Renee Coleen 11008 17 Mile Road, Sterling Heights, MI 48078, (207) 873-7186, BS 83 Northern MI Univ; MS Northern MI Univ; **SLP**

Lomax, Brenda S P O Box 1774, Laurel, MS 39440, (601) 477-9384, BS 71 Univ Southern MS-Hattiesburg; MS 73 Univ Southern MS-Hattiesburg; Sp/Lang Path, Jaycee Eval Cen, **SLP**

Lomax, Mrs Teresa Ann 601 Joe Farris Drive, Hammond, LA 70403, (504) 345-8494, BS 77 Univ Southern MS-Hattiesburg; ME 87 Southeastern LA Univ; 82–Sp-Lang Path, Tangipahoa Parish Sch Bd, **SLP**

Lombard-Brundage, Eileen 4065 Lorrea Road, Las Cruces, NM 88001, (505) 546-6546, **SLP**

Lombardino, Linda Jean Department Of Speech, University Of Florida, Arts And Science Bldg, Gainesville, FL 32611, (904) 376-3682, BA 72 OH Univ - Athens; MA 74 Seton Hall Univ; PH 78 (NS) OH Univ - Athens; Assoc Prof, U of FL, **SLP**

Lombardo, Frank C 113 Brian Way, Middletown, NJ 07748, (201) 477-0833, BA 79 Temple Univ-Tyler Sch of Art; MA 80 Kean Coll of NJ; Aud, Alhac Inc, **A**

Lombardo, James C Wausau Medical Center, 2727 Plaza Drive, Wausau, WI 54401, (715) 847-3232, BS 70 Univ of WI - Stevens Point; MS 71 Univ of WI - Stevens Point; Aud, Wausau Med Cen, **A**

Lombardo, Maureen F 1080 Sun Valley Drive, Annapolis, MD 21401, (301) 757-2600, BA 69 Univ of MD - College Park; MA 71 Univ of MD - College Park; Sp-Lang Path, Anne Arundel Co PS, **SLP**

Lombardo, Mrs Rose Ann Schirripa 48-B Mine Road, Monroe, NY 10950, (917) 782-7466, BA 81 CUNY - Hunter Coll; MA 87 Long Island U - CW Post Ctr

Lomonaco, Mrs Beatrice Joros 855 10th Street #204, Santa Monica, CA 90403, (818) 905-0243, BA 81 CA St Univ - Los Angeles; MA 86 CA St Univ - Los Angeles; **SLP**

Loncarich, Patricia A 1260 Camelot Drive, Las Cruces, NM 88005, (505) 522-0909, BS 77 Univ of IA; MA 79 Univ of IA; Sp-Lang Path, Las Cruces Pub Schs, **SLP**

Loncke, Jane Marie 200 Bay Street South #201, Hamilton, ON, Canada L8P 4S4, (416) 522-4941, BS 82 Univ of Western Ontario; MS 86 Univ of WI - Madison; 86–Sp-Lang Path, St Joseph's Hosp, **SLP**

London, Cynthia J 87 E Padonia Road, Timonium, MD 21093, (301) 252-0904, **SLP**

London, Mrs Denise Marie 509 Towson Avenue, Lutherville, MD 21093, (301) 561-8468, BS 82 Towson St Univ; MA 86 George Washington Univ; 87–Sp-Lang Path, The Hrng & Sp Agency, **SLP**

London, Janet S 1430 Kew Avenue, Hewlett, NY 11557, (718) 322-1210, BS 67 CUNY - Queens Coll; MS 73 CUNY - Queens Coll; 88–Sp-Lang Path, NYC Bd of Educ-Dist 27, **SLP**

London, Louise A 37 Magnolia Street, Malden, MA 02148, (617) 324-8000, BS 74 Emerson Coll; MS 76 Emerson Coll; Sp-Lang Path, Malden PS, **SLP**

London, Mrs Sylvia Claire 7023 Waldheim Court, San Jose, CA 95120, **SLP**

London-Samuels, Mrs Shelley D 170-5 Dreiser Loop #5-E, Bronx, NY 10475, (212) 379-5960, BA 77 CUNY - Lehman Coll; MA 79 NY Univ; Sp-Lang Path, Bd of Ed Sp Serv Unit, **SLP**

Lonegan, Dr Charles PO Box 24204, Fort Lauderdale, FL 33307, (305) 568-9196, BS 64 Montclair St Coll; MS 66 PA St Univ - Univ Park; PH 72 (NS) MI St Univ; Sp-Lang Path, Private Practice, **SLP ACE**

Lonergan, Mary Ann 5349 Amesbury #604, Dallas, TX 75206-3488, (214) 348-5180, BS 78 Univ of TX - Austin; MS 80 Southern Methodist Univ; Sp-Lang Path, Richardson ISD, **SLP**

Loney, Helen E P O Box 442, East Millinocket, ME 04430, (207) 746-3633, BA 79 Univ of ME - Orono; MA 76 Univ of ME - Orono; Sp-Lang Path, Sp Path Serv, **SLP**

Long, Mrs Alice Jo 3108 Temple, Springfield, IL 62704, **SLP**

Long, Mrs Beverly E 6452 North Fourth Street, Fresno, CA 93710-4107, (209) 431-9700, BA 71; MA 72; **SLP**

Long, Carla L 200 26th Street #U-203, Atlanta, GA 30309, (404) 875-5018, BA 84 Spelman Coll; ME 87 GA St Univ

Long, Mrs Cathy Brown 2413 Meadow Creek, Bedford, TX 76021, (817) 267-9456, BS 79 Stephen F Austin St Univ; MS 87 Univ of TX - Dallas

Long, Charles L 1724 Virginia Street N E, Albuquerque, NM 87110, (505) 299-1212, BS 38 Pittsburg St Univ; MA 52 Univ of NM; Sp-Lang Path, Albuquerque Bd of Ed, **SLP**

Long, Mrs Cynthia Lynne 6143 Belle Meade Drive, Villa Rica, GA 30180, ME 85 West GA Coll; **SLP**

Long, Debra Northup P O Box 22, Henderson, WV 25106, (304) 675-4540, BA 78 Marshall Univ; MA 87 Marshall Univ

Long, Dr Edgarita E 1523 North Jardot, Stillwater, OK 74075, (405) 377-8264, BS 71 Univ of OK - Norman; MA 73 Univ of OK - Norman; PH 81 (NS) Southern IL Univ -Carbondale; 88–Owner SLP, Private Practice, **SLP**

Long, Elaine K 1813 Armory Road, Barstow, CA 92311, (714) 256-0611, BS 62 Ball St Univ; Barstow USD, **SLP**

Long, Dr Glenis Raewyn Department Of Audiology & Speech Sciences, Purdue University, West Lafayette, IN 47907, (317) 494-3815, BA 65; MA 68; PH 71 (Psychology) Princeton Univ; 84–Asst Prof, Purdue Univ

Long, Gloria K 3321 South 400 East Road, Kokomo, IN 46902, (317) 455-0206, BS 77 Purdue Univ - West Lafayette; MA 80 Ball St Univ; Sp-Lang Path, Private Practice, **SLP**

Long, Helen J 25052 West 8 Mile #407, Southfield, MI 48034, (313) 283-9200, BA 75 MI St Univ; MA 76 MI St Univ; **A**

Long, Janice M 33 Duden Hills Road North, Marthasville, MO 63357, (314) 433-2889, BS 75 Univ of MO - Columbia; MS 76 Central MO St Univ; **SLP**

Long, Joann Verville 3478 Hazelwood #2, Cincinnati, OH 45211, (513) 661-1856, BA 80 Univ of KY; MS 85 Southern IL Univ-Edwardsvill; 88–Sp-Lang Path, Cincinnati PS, **SLP**

Long, Dr John B Box 365, Cape Girardeau, MO 63702-0365, (314) 334-1422, BS 50 Southeast MO St Univ; MA 62 Univ of MO - Columbia; PH 65 (Sp Path & Aud) Univ of MO - Columbia; Retired, Southeast Missouri State Univ, **SLP A**

Long, Kai M 605 22nd Street, North Beach, St Augustine, FL 32084, (904) 824-8174, BA 69 Univ of MS; MA 72 Univ of Northern IA; Sp-Lang Prgm Coord, St Johns Co Sch Dist, **SLP**

Long, Karen Dene 100 East Lake Drive, Greensboro, NC 27403, (919) 272-5117, **SLP**

Long, Karen Madison 3700BUSH River Road #M-1, Columbia, SC 29210, (803) 772-8147, BS 79 East Carolina Univ; MA 82 Auburn Univ - Auburn; Sp-Lang Path, Univ of SC, **SLP**

Long, Mrs Karen V 292 Ramble Ridge Drive, Thousand Oaks, CA 91360, (213) 225-6187, BA 73 CA St Univ - Northridge; MA 75 CA St Univ - Northridge; Dis Sp-Lang Path, CA State Dept of Ed, **SLP**

Long, Mrs Kari Sue 5402 Pembrook, Wichita, KS 67220, (716) 688-0748, BS 80 OK St Univ; MS 82 Univ of OK Medical Center; SLP, Buffalo Pub Sch, **SLP**

Long, Kathleen E 11142 Campbell, Chicago, IL 60655, (312) 233-8419, BA 79 Saint Xavier Coll; MS 81 IL St Univ - Normal; Sp-Lang Path, Private Practice, **SLP ACE**

Long, Mrs Laurie Constance 7414 East Grand Avenue, Apartment 431, Dallas, TX 75214, (214) 841-2645, BA 84 Kean Coll of NJ; ME 86 Univ of VA - Charlottesville; SLP, Callier Center -Baylor Rehab, **SLP**

Long, Leland L 1829 West Luther Road, Janesville, WI 53545, (608) 756-8324, BS 53 Univ of WI - Platteville; MS 61 Univ of WI - Madison; Sp-Lang Path, Janesville Bd of Ed, **SLP A**

Long, Lisa Dawn 214 Crescent Road, Beckley, WV 25801, (304) 256-4555, BS 86 WV Univ; MS 87 WV Univ

Long, Mrs Marsha M Y 520 South Shore Boulevard, Land O'Lakes, FL 33539, (813) 996-6403, MS 76 Univ of South FL; SLP, Dist Sch Bd of Pasco County, **SLP**

Long, Mrs Martha S 6410 Kreil Street, Baltimore, MD 21207, (301) 661-2800, MA 71 Univ of Northern CO; ME 72 CO St Univ; OM 77 Johns Hopkins Univ; Aud, Baltimore Co Bd of Ed, **SLP A**

Long, Nancy Michelle 631 Franklin Square, Michigan City, IN 46360, (219) 879-6221, BA 84 Valparaiso Univ; MS 86 Purdue Univ - West Lafayette; 86–Clin Supvr, Argabright Comm, **SLP**

Long, Dr Nancy V 2120 Laguna Vista Drive, Novato, CA 94945, (415) 897-7109, BA 70 Queens Coll; MA 73 Marshall Univ; PH 79 (NS) Northwestern Univ; Sp-Lang Path, Private Practice, **SLP**

Long, Patricia B 1 Old Wilderness Road, Summersville, WV 26651, (304) 872-3481, BS 75 TX Christian Univ; MS 76 TX Christian Univ; Sp-Lang Path, Sp & Lang Serv, **SLP**

Long, Dr Steven H P O Box 740, Arcata, CA 95521, (707) 826-3476, BA 74 Haverford Coll; MA 78 San Diego St Univ; PH 82 (Sp-Lang Path) Northwestern Univ; Asst Prof, Humboldt St Univ, **SLP**

Long, Susan D Dept Of Communication Skills, Lufkin State School, PO Drawer 1648, Lufkin, TX 75902, (409) 634-3353, OB 73 Stephen F Austin St Univ; ME 77 Southwest TX St Univ; 79–Dir of Comm Skills, Lufkin State Sch, **SLP ACE**

Long, Susan Michele P O Box 791, Tuba City, AZ 86045, (602) 283-4878, BS 76 East Carolina Univ; MS 81 East Carolina Univ; Sp/Lang Path, Tuba City USD, **SLP**

Long, Suzanne C 2518 East 54th Street, Tulsa, OK 74105, (918) 749-0919, BS 69 Univ of Tulsa; MS 71 Washington Univ; Aud, Springer Clinic, **A**

Long, Suzanne L 23304 Grant Avenue, Torrance, CA 90505, (213) 375-8761, BS 74 Univ of KS; MA 76 Univ of KS; SLP, Villa Serena, **SLP**

Long, Wanda Baltes 1516 Bradshire Drive, Columbus, OH 43220, (614) 261-5364, BA 78 OH St Univ; MA 82 OH St Univ; Sp-Lang Path, Riverside Methodist Hosp, **SLP**

Longa, Robin L 43 Overlook Road, Poughkeepsie, NY 12603, (914) 431-8800, St Francis Hospital, **A**

Longacre, Mrs Kathleen D 1738 Forest Hills Drive, Vienna, WV 26105, (304) 295-5025, BS 78 Bloomsburg Univ of PA; MS 79 Bloomsburg Univ of PA; Sp/Lang Path, Wood County Bd of Educ, **SLP**

Longerich, Dr Mary C 1930 Wilshire Boulevard, Suite 1416, Los Angeles, CA 90057, (213) 484-9749, BA 31 Univ of Akron; MA 35 Univ of WI - Madison; PH 42 (Sp Path) LA St Univ - Baton Rouge; 44–Sp-Lang Path, Private Practice, **SLP F LM**

Longhurst, Lynn D 608 Irwin Avenue, Albion, MI 49224, (517) 629-4228, **SLP**

Longhurst, Dr Thomas M Speech Pathology & Audiology, Idaho State University, Box 8116, Pocatello, ID 83209, (208) 236-3495, BS 66 Brigham Young Univ; MS 67 UT St Univ; PH 70 (N/S) Univ of MN - Minneap-St Paul; Prof, ID St U, **SLP**

Longinotti, Cheryl S 3624 North Greenview, Chicago, IL 60613, BA 74 Univ of CA - Berkeley; MA 77 Northwestern Univ; PH 85 (Aud) Northwestern Univ; 87–Aud, VA, **A**

Longnecker, Beth Anne 734 Mesa Hills #184, El Paso, TX 79912, (915) 779-5866, BA 78 WA St Univ; OM 80 Univ of WA; 85–Aud, El Paso ENT Associates, **A ACE**

Longo, Mrs Barbara L 15 Scott Drive, Smithtown, NY 11787, (516) 736-4679, BS 64 Ithaca Coll; MS 68 Adelphi Univ; Sp-Lang Path, Middle Country Csd #11, **SLP**

Longo, Elizabeth A Wilcox Street, Bristol, RI 02809, (401) 254-0426, BA 85 Bridgewater St Coll; MA 87 Univ of MA - Amherst; 87–Sp-Lang Path, Charlton Memorial Hosp, **SLP**

Longo, Mrs Janine Marie 6041 La Chateau Court, St Louis, MO 63129, (314) 577-5671, BS 82 Southeast MO St Univ; MS 84 Southern IL Univ-Edwardsvill; **SLP**

Longo, Karen Brode 6419 Bricktown Circle, Glen Burnie, MD 21061, (202) 675-5225, BA 85 Univ of MD - College Park; MA 87 Univ of MD - College Park; **A**

Longoria, Margarita L P O Box 66098, Houston, TX 77266-6098, (713) 271-8456, BS 80 Univ of Houston - Univ Park; MA 82 Univ of Houston - Univ Park; Sp/Lang Path, St Anthony Center, **SLP**

Longo-Silvestri, Joann 70 Manchester Road, Eastchester, NY 10709, (914) 337-7971, BA 80 CUNY - Lehman Coll; MA 82 CUNY - Lehman Coll; Sp/Lang Path, Private Practice, **SLP**

Longstreet, Eric J 717 South Pitt Street, Alexandria, VA 22314, (703) 683-0730, MS

Longstreth, Dana G 5001 North Elkhart Avenue, Whitefish Bay, WI 53217, (414) 649-6252, BA 78 IN Univ - Bloomington; MS 80 Univ of WI - Madison; Sp-Lang Path, St Lukes Hospital, **SLP**

Longtin, Dr Susan E 110-07 73rd Road #5F, Forest Hills, NY 11375, (212) 544-4176, BA 70 CUNY - Hunter Coll; MA 74 CUNY - Hunter Coll; PH 84 (Lang Development & Lang Disorders) CUNY - Grad Sch & Univ Cntr; Asst Prof, Hunter Coll, **SLP**

Lonsway, John Alan G 2076 West Reid Road, Flint, MI 48507, (313) 235-8971, BA 66 MI St Univ; MA 70 Wayne St Coll; 85–Aud, Private Practice, **A**

Lontos, Nancy Bywaters 7617 Larchview, Dallas, TX 75240, (214) 387-0041, BS 79 Univ of TX - Dallas; MS 81 Univ of TX - Dallas; Sp/Lang Path, Richardson ISD, **SLP**

Look, Lois Neff 3000 Masters Point, Castle Rock, CO 80104, (303) 744-7205, BA 83 Univ of CO - Boulder; MA 85 Univ of CO - Boulder; 86–Aud, Roy Jones MD, **A**

Looker, Susan N Dover Public Schools, 3 Autumn Street, Dover, NH 03820, (603) 742-1202, BA 76 Univ of VT; MS 78 Univ of VT; **SLP**

Loomer, Delores M 8095 Gandy Court, Grosse Ile, MI 48138, **SLP**

Loomis, Janet Paider 6146 West 65th South, Idaho Falls, ID 83402, (208) 524-5067, BA 78 OH St Univ; MS 81 UT St Univ; Sp-Lang Path, Sch Dist #91-Idaho Falls, **SLP**

Loomis, Robert A Jewish Hospital Of St Louis, Dept Of Otolaryngology, 4910 Forest Park Suite 212, St Louis, MO 63108, (314) 454-7875, BA 77 Univ of Rochester; MS 79 Washington Univ; Aud, Washington Univ Med Sch, **A**

Loomis, Mrs Selene G 9816 Stukey Lane, Chardon, OH 44024, (216) 439-4363, BS 58 Case Western Reserve Univ; ME 68 Kent St Univ; Sp-Lang Path, Bedford Board of Education, **SLP**

Loomis, Susan Roberta 3515 Cheffield Manor Terrace, Apartment 202, Silver Spring, MD 20904, (202) 745-5600, BS 82 Ithaca Coll; MS 85 Univ of MI - Ann Arbor; **SLP**

Loomis, Wilda Brown Route 3 Box 418, Waynesville, NC 28786, (704) 649-2217, MA 81 Western Carolina Univ; SLP, Madison Co Sch, **SLP**

Loomos, Dimitra J 300 Capricorn, Oakland, CA 94611, (415) 654-2067, BS 74 Univ of CA - Berkeley; MS 78 Univ of AZ; Aud, Fresno Community Hospital, **A**

Loonan, Diane Bourhis 225 Bedford Avenue, Buffalo, NY 14216, BS 77 SUNY - Coll at Buffalo; MS 81 SUNY - Coll at Buffalo; SLP, Buffalo Bd of Ed, **SLP**

Looney, Carol Ruch Rt 1 Box 126-H, Gridley, IL 61744, BS 78 IL St Univ - Normal; MS 81 IL St Univ - Normal; SLP, Il Univ-Lab School, **SLP**

Looney, Nancy A 1135 Ridgemont Drive, Aiken, SC 29801, (803) 649-6264, BS 78 TX Christian Univ; MS 79 TX Christian Univ; Sp-Lang Path, Natl Hlth Corp, **SLP**

Looney, Shawn Spangle 2525 N E Knott, Portland, OR 97212, (503) 287-3320, MS 88 Portland St Univ

Looney-Burman, Patricia L 1349 Ulupuni Street, Kailua, HI 96734, (808) 261-7647, BA 64 Grinnell Coll; MA 68 Emerson Coll; OM 85 Univ of HI - Hilo; 83–Sp-Lang Path, CA-Hi Elks Major Proj Inc, **SLP ACE**

Looper, Callie A 103 Avenida Espana, San Jose, CA 95139, **SLP**

Loos-Cosgrove, Margaret Myriah 23 Compton St, New Haven, CT 06511-3509, (203) 562-8964, BA 79 Univ of CT; MS 85 Southern CT St Univ; 86–Sp-Lang Path, The Gaylord Hosp, **SLP**

Loose, Dr Frances F 4950 Chipping Camden, Okemos, MI 48864, (517) 332-2545, BS 69 Univ of MI - Ann Arbor; MA 71 Univ of MI - Ann Arbor; PH 84 (Special Education) MI St Univ; 74–Tchr Consult, East Lansing PS

Loosveldt, Sylvia L 1911 West 40th Avenue, Kennewick, WA 99337-3903, (509) 582-1250, BA 81 Eastern WA Univ; MS 82 Eastern WA Univ; Sp-Lang Path, Kennewick Sch Dist, **SLP**

Loovis, Dr Carl F 97th General Hospital, Box 60, APO New York, NY 09757-3398, BS 63 Seton Hall Univ; MS 66 Univ of WI - Madison; PH 72 (NS) LA St Univ - Baton Rouge; Aud, US Army, **A**

Lopacki, Sandra R 106 Athelstane Road, Newton Center, MA 02159, (617) 735-8394, BS 74 SUNY - Coll at Buffalo; MA 76 Northwestern Univ; **SLP**

Lopata, Leslie Faden 15749 Hesby Street, Encino, CA 91436, (818) 789-5967, BA 66 CUNY - Brooklyn Coll; ME 68 PA St Univ - Univ Park; Sp-Lang Path, Dubnoff Cen, **SLP**

Lopatin, Nina S 5540 Poppleton Court, West Bloomfield, MI 48033, (313) 858-3111, BA 82 MI St Univ; MA 84 Case Western Reserve Univ; Aud, St Joseph Mercy Hosp, **A**

Lopatin, Rickey N 15 Wheeler Road, Westborough, MA 01581, (508) 481-5046, BS 69 Boston Univ; MS 82 Worcester St Coll; Sp-Lang Path, Assabet Valley Presch Prog, **SLP**

Lopes, Charlotte Marie 6665 Golfcrest Drive, San Diego, CA 92119, (619) 453-7500, BA 81 San Diego St Univ; MA 85 San Diego St Univ; **SLP**

Lopez, Alina 1700 Benjamin Franklin Pkw, Apartment 2008, Philadelphia, PA 19103, (215) 988-9670, BA 83 George Washington Univ; MA 88 Temple Univ

Lopez, Mrs Amye Humphreys 6011 Appletree, Apartment 3, Memphis, TN 38115, (901) 726-7684, BS 81 Univ Southern MS-Hattiesburg; MA 85 LA St Univ - Baton Rouge; Sp-Lang Path, Methodist Hosp, **SLP**

Lopez, Arlys N 5890 Bandolero, Apartment 3003, El Paso, TX 79912, (915) 833-2852, BA 82 TX Tech Univ; MA 85 Univ of TX - Austin; **SLP**

Lopez, Beth B 5034 Park Plaza, Houston, TX 77018, **SLP**

Lopez, Mrs Carolyn Calhoun 5688 Swan Creek, Toledo, OH 43614, (419) 729-8219, BA 66 Univ of NM; MA 67 Univ of NM; SLP, Toledo Pub Schs, **SLP**

Lopez, Elizabeth Swanson 233 Glenmere Way, Toledo, OH 43615, (419) 531-2463, BA 83 1485; MS 87 Miami Univ - Oxford

Lopez, Gilda Irene 3148 West Rockcreek Road, Apartment 902, Norman, OK 73072, (405) 236-3131, BA 74 Univ of PR - Rio Piedras; MS 85 Univ of OK Medical Center; 86–Sp-Lang Path, Health South Rehab Ctr, **SLP**

Lopez, Mrs Jeanette B 1905 Septiembre, El Paso, TX 79935, (915) 593-0747, BA 76 Our Lady Lake Univ-San Anton; MA 77 Our Lady Lake Univ-San Anton; **SLP**

Lopez, M B Alaska Comm Disorders Program, P O Box 1048, Bethel, AK 99559, (907) 543-3711, BA 75 CUNY - Queens Coll; MA 77 Northwestern Univ; Aud, AK Dept Hlth & Soc Serv, **A**

Lopez, Sandra 52 Moriarity Drive, Wilton, CT 06897, (212) 520-7358, BS 73 IN Univ - Bloomington; MS 75 IN Univ - Bloomington; **A**

Lopez, Sharon Rosen 16 Brevoort Road, Chappaqua, NY 10514, (914) 238-8093, BA 71 Univ of WI - Madison; MA 81 Univ of WA; **SLP**

Lopez, Susanne R 325 West Barnard Street, 3rd Floor, West Chester, PA 19382, (215) 351-7036, BS 78 West Chester Univ of PA; MA 81 West Chester Univ of PA; Sp-Lang Path, Sch Dist of Phila, **SLP**

Lopez-Chaney, Anna Marie 12848 Blossom, Alsip, IL 60658, (312) 597-1624, BS 82 Northern IL Univ - De Kalb; MA 83 Northern IL Univ - De Kalb; Sp/Lang Path, Southwest Cooperative, **SLP**

Lopez-Valladares, Jose A Calle 5 #1112, Villa Nevarez, Rio Piedras, PR 00927, (809) 758-2525, BA 71 Catholic Univ Puerto Rico; MS 73 Univ of PR - Rio Piedras; Assoc Prof, Dept of Commun Dis-UPR, **SLP**

Lopopolo, Mrs Theresa J 2695 Coit Drive, San Jose, CA 95124, (408) 249-5200, BA 79 Temple Univ; MA 81 Temple Univ; 87–Sp-Lang Path, Meadowbrook Neuro Care Ctr, **SLP ACE**

Lopushinsky, Mrs Anne Martha 3221-112-A Street, Edmonton, AB, Canada T6J 3X1, (403) 471-7934, OB 79 Univ of Alberta - Alberta; OM 80 Univ of WA; Sp-Lang Path, Glenrose Rehab Hosp, **SLP**

Lorah, April D 600 Alison Avenue, Mechanicsburg, PA 17055, (717) 766-4490, BS 86 Bloomsburg Univ of PA; MS 87 Bloomsburg Univ of PA; 87–Sp-Lang Path, Capital Area Intermediate Unit, **SLP**

Lorand, Mrs Marjorie J 1434 Corey Way South, South Pasadena, FL 33707, (813) 343-0855, BS 76 Eastern IL Univ; MS 77 Eastern IL Univ; Sp-Lang Path, Pinellas County Schools, **SLP**

Lorang-Schmirler, Mrs Karen Marie 1928 S W 6th Avenue, Camas, WA 98607, (206) 256-6022, BA 73 Eastern WA Univ; MS 74 Eastern WA Univ; Dept Hd/Sp-Lang Path, Evergreen Sch Dist #114, **SLP**

Lorber, Douglas Radman 1906 Old Dominion Road, Albany, GA 31707, (912) 435-7161, BA 79 Mary Washington Coll; ME 81 Univ of VA - Charlottesville; Aud, Albany ENT, **SLP A**

Lorber, Nina P 13245 Bavarian Drive, San Diego, CA 92129, **SLP**

Lorber, Pamela Ann 770 West Ferry #32-B, Buffalo, NY 14222, (716) 885-5572, BS 81 SUNY - Coll at Buffalo; MS 84 SUNY - Coll at Buffalo; Sp-Lang Path, Buffalo Bd of Educ, **SLP**

Lorber, Sharyn S 60 Scudder Avenue, Northport, NY 11768, (516) 757-0440, MA 88 CUNY - Hunter Coll

Lord, Cheryl C Route 5 Box 229, Charlottesville, VA 22901, (804) 645-8149, **SLP**

Lord, Mrs Joan Cashin 815 Louisa Drive, Santa Rosa, CA 95404, (707) 544-9487, MA 81 Saint Louis Univ; Sp-Lang Path, N Coast Rehab Ctr, **SLP**

Lord, Karen Sampson 2290 South 1st Street, Lake City, FL 32055, (904) 752-1652, BA 84 Univ of FL; MA 86 Univ of FL; 88–Sp-Lang Path, Private Practice, **SLP**

Lord, Mrs Katharine Berry 1935 Copenhaffer Road, Dover, PA 17315, (717) 266-7169, BS 80 Emerson Coll; OM 82 Hahneman Medical Coll; Aud/Sp-Lang Path, Alfred J Mauriello II MD, **SLP A**

Lord, Kathleen M Heritage Village, 337-A Condo 10, Southbury, CT 06488, (914) 277-3661, BS 76 SUNY - Coll at Geneseo; MS 81 Columbia Univ Teachers Coll; 85–Sp-Lang Path, Datahr Inc, **SLP**

Lord, Sherman G 8110 Commandant Way, Manlius, NY 13104, (315) 682-4840, BS 75 Bloomsburg Univ of PA; MS 77 Bloomsburg Univ of PA; 87–Reg Mgr, Instrumentation Assoc, **A**

Lorden, Jill B 1420 Wildwood Drive, Midland, MI 48640, (517) 631-7500, BS 75 IN Univ - Bloomington; MA 77 IN Univ - Bloomington; 82–Aud, Herbert L Camp MD, **A**

Lore, Dr James I 5103 S Tenth Street, Apartment 1, Arlington, VA 22204, (703) 931-7844, **SLP A LM**

Lorell, Daryl M 4110 Elmwood Road, South Euclid, OH 44121, (216) 444-5142, BS 75 Boston Univ; MS 79 Univ of WI - Madison; Sp/Lang Path, Cleveland Clinic Found, **SLP ACE**

Loren, Blanche M 4555 Henry Hudson Parkway, New York, NY 10471, BA 71 CUNY - Lehman Coll; MS 73 Columbia Univ Teachers Coll; SLP, NYC Bd of Ed-Sp Serv Unit, **SLP**

Loren, Dr Catherine Ann 5401 Chimney Rock #616, Houston, TX 77081, (713) 660-9719, BS 83 Bowling Green St Univ; MA 84 Bowling Green St Univ; Doctoral Candidate, Bowling Green State University, **SLP**

Lorence, Karen Carr 2075 Legion Avenue, Lake Elmo, MN 55042, (612) 777-7788, BS 62 IA St Univ; MA 68 Univ of IA; **SLP**

Lorendo, Leah C Northeastern University, Department Of Speech-Language Pathology & Audiology, 360 Huntington Avenue, 133 Forsyth Bldg, Boston, MA 02115, (617) 437-3117, BA 76 Auburn Univ - Auburn; MA 78 Auburn Univ - Auburn; PH 88 (Health Care Administration) Univ of MS; 88–Lecturer/Clin Supvr, Northeastern Univ, **SLP**

Lorenz, Deborah G 2102 Winchester Street, Temple, TX 76502, (817) 774-9404, SLP, Temple loc, **SLP**

Lorenz, Mrs Delores Rustad 1809 East 54th Avenue, Spokane, WA 99203, (509) 458-3836, BA 73 Chapman Coll; MS 76 Eastern WA Univ; Sp-Lang Path, Spokane Sch Dist #81, **SLP**

Lorenz, Mrs Lori J 6021 N 107 Street, Omaha, NE 68134, (402) 496-4151, BS 84 ND St Univ; MS 87 Univ of NE - Omaha

Lorenz, Lynn U 6700 Evergreen Canyon, Oklahoma City, OK 73162, (405) 524-4885, BA 82 Univ of OK - Norman; MS 84 Univ of OK Medical Center; 85–Sp-Lang Path, Oklahoma Cty PS, **SLP**

Lorenz, Mary Grace 2 Belknap Place, Cincinnati, OH 45218, (513) 825-5788, MA 84 Univ of Cincinnati; Sp-Lang Path, Hamilton Co Office of Educ, **SLP**

Lorenzen, Mrs Anna L 71 Glen Lake Drive, Pacific Grove, CA 93950, (408) 375-1876, BA 51 Univ of IA; MA 70 Auburn Univ - Auburn; Aud, Private Practice, **SLP A**

Lorenzen, Mrs Geraldine 143 North James Street, Woodbridge, NJ 07095, (201) 636-8709, BA 77 Univ of RI; MS 79 Columbia Univ Teachers Coll; Sp-Lang Path, Franklin Twp Bd of Educ, **SLP**

Lorenzen, Susan R 1038 Sanford 2N, St Louis, MO 63139, (314) 647-1586, BS 83 Northern IL Univ - De Kalb; MS 86 Fontbonne Coll; **SLP**

Lorenzo, Adrienne M 17 Gulls Cove, Manhasset, NY 11030, (212) 735-2667, BS 57 East Stroudsburg Univ of PA; MS 75 Adelphi Univ; Audiologist, Kings Cty Hosp, **A**

Lorenzo, Jackie C 37 Bradford Drive, Little Rock, AR 72207, (501) 371-1919, BA 68 Univ of AR - Fayetteville; MS 78 Univ of AR - Little Rock; Sp-Lang Path, AR Sch for the Deaf, **SLP**

Lorenzut, Mrs Geraldine 5 Brown House Road, Old Greenwich, CT 06870, (203) 863-3240, BA 65 CUNY - Hunter Coll; MA 68 Northwestern Univ; Dir Hrng & Sp, Greenwich Hosp, **A**

Lorig, Linda R 375 North 22nd, Springfield, OR 97477, (503) 485-8521, BS 72 Southern IL Univ -Carbondale; MS 74 Univ of OK Medical Center; Sp-Lang Path, Eugene Hearing & Speech Center, **SLP**

Loring, Mrs Arlene G 70 Shenandoah Road, Deerfield, IL 60015, (312) 945-3550, BS 71 Univ of WI - Madison; MS 72 Univ of WI - Madison; **SLP**

Loring, Diane 533 Redwood Avenue, Corte Madera, CA 94925-1331, (415) 388-5999, BS 82 CA St Univ - Hayward; MA 86 Univ of San Francisco; 83–Sp-Lang Path, Lucie Alexander Mill Valley Developmental Preschool, **SLP**

Loring, Mrs Julie K 160 East Myrna Lane, Tempe, AZ 85284, (602) 839-5682, BS 77 Univ of NM; MS 79 CO St Univ; **SLP**

Lorman, Janis S 1738 Gorge Park Boulevard, Stow, OH 44224, (216) 375-3882, BS 66 Kent St Univ; MA 69 Kent St Univ; Superv Communication Disorders, Akron City Hosp, **SLP A**

Lorowitz, Lori Michele 930 East 81st Street, Brooklyn, NY 11236, (718) 241-0652, BA 85 SUNY - Center at Buffalo; MA 87 SUNY - Center at Buffalo; 88–Sp-Lang Path, UCP of NYC Inc, **SLP**

Lorson, Ann W 145 Oakridge, Iowa City, IA 52240, (319) 351-2449, BA 64 CO Coll; MA 69 Univ of IA; **SLP**

Los, Mrs Donna Weaver Metropolitan ENT Associates, 3107 Passavant Prof Bldg, 9104 Babcock Boulevard, Pittsburgh, PA 15237, (412) 366-3471, MS 83 PA St Univ - Univ Park; Aud, Metropolitan ENT Associates, **A**

Losasso, Sharon A 436 East Chester Lane, Boise, ID 83706, (208) 378-2397, BS 74 CO St Univ; MS 76 CO St Univ; Sp-Lang Path, St Luke's Reg Med Ctr, **SLP**

Loscheider, Mary Jo 350 East Forestwood, Morton, IL 61550, (309) 925-4841, BS 79 Eastern IL Univ; MS 81 Eastern IL Univ; Sp/Lang Path, Tremont Comm Unit Schl, **SLP**

Losching, Mrs Susan Ruth 626 Sunset, Janesville, WI 53545, (608) 756-1865, BS 78 Univ of WI - Madison; MS 80 Univ of WI - Madison; 88–Sp-Lang Path, Sch Dist of Beloit, **SLP**

LoSciuto, Mrs Ruth Ann 74 Rice Avenue, Rockland, MA 02370, (617) 878-8593, BS 82 Worcester St Coll; MS 84 Emerson Coll; 85–Sp-Lang Path, Plymouth PS, **SLP**

Loser, Cindy P Butler University, Speech Department, 4600 Sunset Avenue, Indianapolis, IN 46208, **A**

Losey, Jana P 900 Kings Mountain Drive, Little Rock, AR 72211, BA 74 Univ of AR - Fayetteville; MS 76 Univ of OK Medical Center; PH 86 (Speech Pathology) Univ of OK Medical Center; 84–Sp-Lang Path, Private Practice, **SLP**

Losey, Sue Ann S 7721 Tremayne Place #110, Mc Lean, VA 22102, BS 68 Univ of KY; MA 73 Univ of KY; Office Mgr - Leg Asst, House of Representatives, **SLP**

Losinski, Mrs Jayne F 8362 Meadowdale, Grand Blanc, MI 48439, **SLP**

Lothers, Dr William T Department Of Communications, Wheaton College, Wheaton, IL 60187, (312) 260-5095, MA 59 Univ of OK - Norman; MS 81 Governors St Univ; PH 66 (NS) MI St Univ; Associate Professor Speech, Wheaton College, **SLP**

Lothrop, Sondra Swartz 204 East 11th St #4, Crete, NE 68333, (402) 759-3143, BS 84 Univ of NE - Lincoln; MS 85 Univ of NE - Lincoln; 85–Sp-Lang Path, Geneva Support Svcs Coop, **SLP**

Lotierzo, Mrs Christine 136 Fawn Hill Road, Upper Saddle River, NJ 07458, (201) 934-1788, BS 73 SUNY - Coll at Geneseo; MA 75 Univ of ME - Orono; SLP, Allendale Sch Sys, **SLP**

Lotito, Heather Tobias RR 1 111 Pine Street, West Hurley, NY 12491, (914) 679-5761, BS 77 SUNY - Coll at New Paltz; MS 78 Adelphi Univ; Sp-Lang Path, Private Practice, **SLP**

Lotlikar, Swati M 645 Western Avenue, Grafton, ND 58237, (701) 352-2140, BS 85; MS 87 Syracuse Univ; **A**

Lotowycz, Mrs Nancy Carol 12361 Teal Run Court, Jacksonville, FL 32223, (904) 390-2079, BS 72 MS Univ for Women; MS 84 East Carolina Univ; MA 84 East Carolina Univ; 88–Sp-Lang Path, Duval Co Sch Bd, **SLP**

Lotspeich, Nancy Ruonavaara 930 Olive Drive #7, Bakersfield, CA 93308-4166, (805) 398-3799, BA 70 CA St Univ - Chico; MA 86 CA St Univ - Chico; 86–Sp-Lang Path, Kern Co Supt of Schs

Lott, Carol Lusco 1524 2nd Place N W, Birmingham, AL 35215, (205) 665-6720, BS 81 Univ of Montevallo; MS 82 Univ of Montevallo; ES 88 Univ of Montevallo; Sp-Lang Path, Chilton County Sch Sys, **SLP**

Lott, Kay Ritchie Foothill Speech & Language Services, 226 West Foothill Boulevard Suite F, Claremont, CA 91711, (714) 621-1520, BS 64 CO St Univ; MS 65 CO St Univ; Sp-Lang Path, Foothill Sp and Lang Servs, **SLP**

Lott, Mrs Linda M 2605 Sunset Drive, Hattiesburg, MS 39401, (601) 582-7454, BS 72 Univ Southern MS-Hattiesburg; MS 75 Univ Southern MS-Hattiesburg; 88–Sp-Lang Path, Petal PS Sys, **SLP**

Lott, Rosalie 7735 Millicent Circle, Shreveport, LA 71105, (318) 631-5110, BA 64 Northwestern St Univ; MS 70 Northwestern St Univ; Director of Special Education, Caddo Parish Sch Bd, **SLP**

Lotterman, Dr Stephen H Gallaudet College, Department Of Audiology, 7th & Florida Avenue N E, Washington, DC 20002, BA 60 Univ of CA - Los Angeles; MA 61 Univ of Southern CA; PH 64 (NS) Northwestern Univ; Associate Professor, Gallaudet College, **A**

Lotz, Wendy Kay Boys Town National Institute, 555 North 30th Street, Omaha, NE 68131, (402) 498-6666, BS 72 Univ of WI - Madison; MS 73 Univ of WI - Madison; Sp-Lang Path, Boys Town National Institute, **SLP**

Loucks, Mrs Natalie Frappolli 16 Mumford Street, Seneca Falls, NY 13148, (315) 789-4222, BA 75 Elmira Coll; MS 76 SUNY - Coll at Buffalo; **SLP**

Loucks, Sr Yvonne Mary 63 Crane Hollow Road, Bethlehem, CT 06751, (301) 486-2629, BA 72 Mercy Coll of Detroit; MA 77 Central MI Univ; PH 87 (Sp-Lang Path); 87–Sp-Lang Path, Univ of Connecticut, **SLP**

Loudamy, Mrs Shelly Renea 2427 Palo Alto, Arlington, TX 76015, (817) 860-1248, BS 82 Baylor Univ; MS 83 Baylor Univ; SLP, Arlington Indep School Dist, **SLP**

Loudenslagel, Jean F 7543 North 16th Drive, Phoenix, AZ 85021, (602) 848-5886, BS 75 Northeastern Univ; MS 77 Phillips Univ; SLP, Maryvale Sam Hospital, **SLP ACE**

Loudenslagel, Mark W 7543 North 16th Drive, Phoenix, AZ 85021, (602) 943-4521, BS 75 Bowling Green St Univ; MA 76 Kent St Univ; OM 83 AZ St Univ; 87–Bus Svcs Admin, Maricopa Co Long Term Care, **SLP**

Louderback, Frances Mae 704 Valencia Avenue, Davis, CA 95616, (916) 666-8710, BA 73 CA St Univ - Chico; Sp-Lang Path, Yolo Co Schs, **SLP**

Louderback, Mrs Kristen Wakelin 5204 Mockingbird Lane, St Joseph, MO 64506, (816) 364-6543, BS 82 Northwest MO St Univ; MS 83 Northwest MO St Univ; 88–Sp-Lang Path, Heartland Health System Inc, **SLP ACE**

Lougeay-Mottinger, Janice W 2105 Nob Hill, Carrollton, TX 75006, (214) 905-3114, BS 69 Southern IL Univ -Carbondale; MA 70 Bowling Green St Univ; Practicium Coord, U of TX-Dallas, **SLP**

Lough, Mrs Charlotte Benefield 4904 Larchmont N E, Albuquerque, NM 87111, (505) 294-7932, BA 61 Mercer Univ - Macon; MS 82 Univ of OK - Norman; 88–Sp-Lang Path, St Jos Rehab Ctr, **SLP**

Loughery, James H Pittsford Garden Apts #47, 3660 Monroe Avenue, Pittsford, NY 14534, PH (NS); **SLP LM**

Loughery, Jean M 3660 Monroe Avenue #47, Pittsford, NY 14534, (716) 381-3661, BA 39 Nazareth Coll of Rochester; MA 43 Cornell Univ; PH 54 (NS) Univ of MI - Ann Arbor; **SLP LM**

Loughran, Colleen 1816 Red Queen Court, Richmond, VA 23235, (804) 323-7429, BS 81 WV Univ; MS 82 WV Univ; Aud, Fairmont ENT Assoc Inc, **A**

Loughran, Mrs Judith Tanner 542-H Shady Pine Way, West Palm Beach, FL 33415, (407) 439-3150, BS 74 FL St Univ; MS 75 FL St Univ; **SLP**

Loughrey, Susan Elizabeth 406 Court Street, Keene, NH 03431, (603) 547-3311, BA Univ of FL; MA 85 Univ of MA - Amherst; **SLP**

Loughridge, Anne H 3830 Central Avenue, Apartment 112, Fort Myers, FL 33901, (813) 939-0974, BS 77 OK St Univ; MA 79 Univ of Tulsa; 87–Sp-Lang Path, Lee County Schools, **SLP**

Loui, Calvin M 2626 South Gaucho, Mesa, AZ 85202, (602) 996-2115, BA 71 Univ of CO - Boulder; MS 73 CO St Univ; Aud, Valley Aud Serv, **A**

Louick, Mrs Bettye A 2326 Malraux Drive, Vienna, VA 22180, (703) 574-2044, BA 64 Univ of TX - Austin; MS 66 Vanderbilt Univ; **SLP ACE**

Louick, Mrs Karen Kronheim 17 7th Avenue, Brooklyn, NY 11217, (718) 768-5995, BA 73 CUNY - Queens Coll; MA 74 CUNY - Queens Coll; SLP, Private Practice, **SLP**

Louis, Timothy C 427 West 20th Street, Suite 703, Houston, TX 77008, (713) 868-4451, BS 86 Northwestern Univ; MA 87 Northwestern Univ; 88–Dir of Aud, Dr Eduardo M Diaz, **A**

Louis-Dodson, Dr Patricia Jo 926 Willowleaf Drive #204, San Jose, CA 95128, (408) 258-4923, BS 84 Univ of WI - Madison; MA 86 San Jose St Univ; 87–Sp-Lang Path, Alum Rock Union Elem Schs, **SLP**

Louiselle, Theresa Lahood 1517 J Oak Forest Spur Dr, St Louis, MO 63146, (314) 432-1661, OB 84 Univ of NE - Omaha; OM 86 Saint Louis Univ; **SLP**

Louisos-Kramer, Elaina 23-D Marion Road, Salem, MA 01970-4460, (508) 741-2111, BS 77 Univ of MA - Amherst; MA 81 Univ of MA - Amherst; 88–Sp-Lang Path, The Children's Hosp-Dept of Neur, **SLP**

Louko, Linda J Dept Of Sp Path & Audiology, McDonald Bldg, SUNY College At Cortland, Cortland, NY 13045, (607) 756-5423, BS 72 SUNY - Coll at Brockport; MA 77 Univ of NE - Lincoln; Sp/Lang Path, Ithaca Hearing & Speech Assoc, **SLP**

Loumbas, Dean George P O Box 14642, San Francisco, CA 94114, **SLP**

Lounsbury, Kathrin Ilona Comp A-7 Site 29, R R 12, Fredericton, NB, Canada E3B 6H7, (506) 452-5931, BA 83 Univ of New Brunswick - Nb; MS 85 McGill Univ - Quebec; 85–Sp-Lang Path, Dr Everett Chalmers Hosp, **SLP**

Loup, C Lorioux 540 28th Avenue, Seattle, WA 98112, (206) 324-3886, SLP, Auburn School District 408, **SLP**

Lourie, Bonita F L 6706 Old Stage Road, Rockville, MD 20852, (301) 984-5657, BA 67 Univ of MD - College Park; MA 80 George Washington Univ; Aud, Treat Cen for Dis Chldn, **A**

Louro, Gina P 1837 Sherwood Street, Allentown, PA 18103, (215) 691-7342, **A**

Loushine, Patricia L Box 123 Route 2, Lawrence, KS 66044, (913) 764-1993, BA 76 William Paterson Coll; MA 79 Univ of KS; Aud, Ks St Sch for Deaf, **A**

Loutas, Mrs Shirla S 431 South Pennsylvania, Casper, WY 82609, (307) 237-9571, BA 68 Phillips Univ; MS 72 Phillips Univ; 86–Sp-Lang Path, Natrona Co Sch Dist #1, **SLP ACE**

Loutrel, Barbara H 8410 East 32nd Street #A, Anchorage, AK 99504, (907) 333-7527, BS 71 TX Tech Univ; MS 72 TX Tech Univ; SLP, Anchorage School District, **SLP**

Lovall, Susan Marie 530 Reynolds Drive Lot 90, Charleston, IL 61920, (217) 268-4961, BS 82 Eastern IL Univ; MS 84 Eastern IL Univ; Sp-Lang Path, Arcola Comm Unit 306, **SLP**

Lovdahl, Ann S 2875 Jordan Avenue, Minnetonka, MN 55343, (612) 566-4780, OB 81 Univ of MN - Duluth; MA 82 Univ of MN - Duluth; Clinical Supervisor, InSpeech Inc, **SLP**

Love, James M 318 South Prairie, Miles City, MT 59301, (406) 232-3812, BA 71 Central WA Univ; MS 72 Central WA Univ; Sp-Lang Path, Miles Cty Sch Dist #1, **SLP**

Love, Mrs Joni Emm 1843 Wythe Street, Worthington, OH 43085, (614) 687-6666, MA 87 OH St Univ; 87–Sp-Lang Path, Pro Rehab Assoc Inc

Love, Kathleen Mary 1405 Jackson, Missoula, MT 59802-3832, (406) 338-2715, BA Univ of Northern IA; MA 84 Univ of Northern IA; **SLP**

Love, Mrs Patricia Lehner 3120 Gretchen Drive N E, Warren, OH 44483, (216) 847-0455, BA 71 OH Univ - Athens; 83–Sp-Lang Path, Champion Local Schs

Love, Dr Russell J Hearing And Speech Sciences, Vanderbilt University, School Of Medicine, Nashville, TN 37232-8700, (615) 320-5353, BS 53 Northwestern Univ; MA 54 Northwestern Univ; PH 62 (Sp-Lang Path) Northwestern Univ; 67–Prof of Sp and Lang Path, Vanderbilt Med Sch, **SLP F**

Love, Mrs Susan Odegaard 7542 Ivystone Avenue South, Cottage Grove, MN 55016, (612) 772-2451, BS 85 Moorhead St Univ; MS 87 Saint Cloud St Univ; 88–Sp-Lang Path, ELR Systems Inc

Love, Teresa Carnese 7900 South West 66th St, Portland, OR 97223, (503) 244-6536, BS 75 Portland St Univ; MS 77 Portland St Univ; Sp-Lang Path, Providence Hospital, **SLP**

Lovecky, Drusilla Dulcy P O Box 452, Tarrytown, NY 10591, (914) 428-9258, **SLP**

Lovegreen, Mrs Valerie Ann 352 Canoe Trail Lane, Orlando, FL 32825, (305) 275-5635, BS 80 RI Coll; MA 88 Univ of Central FL

Lovejoy, Donna Akers 5507 Knights Court, Lake Dallas, TX 75065, (817) 497-4801, BS 81 Baylor Univ; MS 82 Baylor Univ; Sp-Lang Path, Private Practice, **SLP**

Lovelace, Lynne C 563 31st Street, Manhattan Beach, CA 90266, (213) 545-8363, BA 61 Univ of Louisville; MA 81 CA St Univ - Long Beach; SLP, Lennox Sch Dist, **SLP**

Lovelady, Jane 2954 Wembley Park Road, Lake Oswego, OR 97034, (503) 280-6282, OB 67 Southern Methodist Univ; OM 80 Univ of MT; Sp-Lang Path, Portland Public Sch, **SLP**

Loveland, Mrs Christine Kina 10754 Peach Street, Waterford, PA 16441, (814) 453-5602, MS 83 WV Univ; 84–Sp-Lang Path, Lake Erie Institute of Rehab, **SLP**

Loveless, Mrs Barbara Louise 4072 South Atchison Way, Apartment 302, Aurora, CO 80014, BA 74 MI St Univ; MA 75 MI St Univ; SLP, Denver Pub Sch, **SLP**

Lovell, Mrs Debra Mase 8454 Timber Belt, San Antonio, TX 78250-4476, (512) 299-6809, BS 81 Baylor Univ; MA 84 Univ of Houston - Univ Park; Sp-Lang Path, Irwin Lehroff and Associates, **SLP**

Lovell, Mary E 324 Altamira, Las Vegas, NV 89128, (702) 363-3791, BS 76 AZ St Univ; MA 77 Univ of MO - Columbia; **SLP**

Lovell, Sheryl Dee 1000 Illinois Street, Des Moines, IA 50314, (515) 244-5225, BS 82 Ball St Univ; MA 83 Ball St Univ; 84–Aud, Phillip A Linquist Do Pc, **A**

Lovely, Leslee Susan 7481 Beagle Street, San Diego, CA 92111, (619) 281-5511, Sp-Lang Path, Vista Hill Found, **SLP**

Lovely, Nancy J 2899 Fagleysville Road, Gilbertsville, PA 19525, (215) 323-2696, **A**

Loven, Dr Faith C University Of Minnesota-Duluth, Department Of Allied Clinical Health, 246 Montgue Hall, Duluth, MN 55812, (218) 726-8204, BS 79 Univ of IA; MA 81 Univ of IA; PH 85 (NS) Univ of IA; Asst Prof, U of MN-Duluth, **A**

Lovendahl, Crisler Magor 1145 Russellwood Court, Buffalo Grove, IL 60089-6859, (312) 634-2467, MA 83 Northwestern Univ; SLP, Waukegan Pub Sch, **SLP**

Lovering, Dr Larry J Professional Hearing Healthcare Centers, 13200 North 103rd Avenue Suite 17, Sun City, AZ 85351, (602) 933-0000, BS 58 Univ of MT; MA 60 Univ of AZ; PH 70 (NS) MI St Univ; Aud, Private Practice, **A**

Loverso, Dr Felice L Ctr Communication Disorders, Braintree Hospital, 250 Tond Street, Braintree, MA 02184, (617) 848-5353, BA 74; MA 76 Univ of CO - Boulder; PH 80 (NS) Univ of CO - Boulder; Dir-Sp-Lang Path, Braintree Hosp, **SLP**

Lovestedt, Lucille K 105 Betty Way, Grass Valley, CA 95949, (916) 272-7454, BA 70 CA St Univ - Los Angeles; MA 72 CA St Univ - Los Angeles; Sp-Lang Path, Vna, **SLP LM**

Lovett, Mrs Janet A 59438 Downey Avenue, Mishawaka, IN 46544, (219) 237-7246, BA 79 Univ of MI - Ann Arbor; MS 81 Univ of MI - Ann Arbor; Sp-Lang Path, St Josephs Med Cen, **SLP**

Loving, Susan H 444 Country Club, Stansbury Park, UT 84074, (801) 882-1293, BS 69 SUNY - Coll at Geneseo; MS 70 Univ of HI - Manoa; Sp-Lang Path, Tooele Co Sch Dist, **SLP**

Lovins, Mrs Julia Feola 118 Locust Street, Huntington, WV 25705, (304) 525-7639, BS 77 WV Univ; MA 78 Marshall Univ; Sp-Lang Path, Cabell County Board of Educ, **SLP**

Lovis, Mrs Emmy A 2030 North 76th Court, Elmwood Park, IL 60635, (312) 794-3966, BS 54; MS 62 Southern IL Univ -Carbondale; Sp-Lang Path, Il Dept of Ment Hlth & Dev, **SLP**

Lovorn, Sallie Beraud Box 17 ENT Clinic, 97th General Hospital, APO New York, NY 09757, (318) 233-9779, **A**

Lovorn, Mrs Vickey G 3818 Alandale, Pascagoula, MS 39567, (601) 938-6559, BS 81 Univ Southern MS-Hattiesburg; MS 82 Univ Southern MS-Hattiesburg; Sp-Lang Path, Pascagoula Schools, **SLP**

Lovrinic, Dr Jean Hahn P O Box 24, Westtown, PA 19395, (215) 787-1870, BS 62 Univ of NE - Lincoln; MA 62 Univ of NE - Lincoln; PH 65 (NS) Univ of Pittsburgh - Pittsburgh; Prof, Temple Univ, **A F**

Lovrinic, Dr William S P O Box 24, Westtown, PA 19395, (215) 692-7559, BS 59 PA St Univ - Univ Park; MD 63 (Medicine) Thomas Jefferson Coll; 70–Phys & Owner, Chester County ENT Ltd

Lovsin, Carol 28626 Karam Drive, Madison Heights, MI 48071, (313) 548-0294, BA 82 Eastern MI Univ; MA 83 Eastern MI Univ; 84–Sp-Lang Path, Lakeshore ENT Cen, **SLP ACE**

Lovus, Dr Yvonne A 880 North Hilldale Avenue, Apartment 5, Los Angeles, CA 90069, (213) 659-5773, BA 73 Univ of CA - Los Angeles; MA 77 CA St Univ - Northridge; Sp-Lang Path, Los Angeles City USD, **SLP**

Low, Mrs Annie Chui 740 North Myers Street, Burbank, CA 91506, (213) 625-4183, BA 81 Univ of CA - Los Angeles; MA 85 CA St Univ - Northridge; SLP, Lausd, **SLP**

Low, Cynthia H R R #3 Site 310 C-8, Port Alberni, BC, Canada V9Y 7L7, (604) 724-3839, BA 79 Carleton Univ - Ontario; MA 84 Western WA Univ; Sp-Lang Path, Private Practice, **SLP**

Low, Elaine Yee Ling 110 North Chapel Avenue, Unit 11, Alhambra, CA 91801, (818) 282-2616, BA 76 CA St Univ - Los Angeles; MA 78 CA St Univ - Los Angeles; Pres, Speech Image Inc, **SLP**

Low, Dr Gordon M 525 East 3950 North, Provo, UT 84604, (801) 225-2269, BS 49 Univ of UT; MS 50 Univ of UT; PH 55 (NS) Univ of MN - Minneap-St Paul; **SLP LM**

Low, Mrs Linda K M 13111 Marcy Circle, Omaha, NE 68154, (402) 498-1820, BA 68 Univ of Northern CO; MS 76 Univ of NE - Omaha; SLP, Boys Town, **SLP**

Low, Patricia 840 Viewridge Drive, San Mateo, CA 94403, (415) 572-0145, BA 75 San Francisco St Univ; MA 79 San Francisco St Univ; SLP, San Mateo City Sch Dist, **SLP**

Lowary, Susann M 13303 Barrett Road, Yakima, WA 98908, (509) 575-3284, BA 71 Kearney St Coll; MS 76 Kearney St Coll; SLP, Yakima Sch Dist #7, **SLP**

Lowder, Kenneth L Hearing Aid Services Inc, 415 10th Avenue, Coralville, IA 52241, (319) 338-6043, BS 64 Eastern IL Univ; MA 68 De Paul Univ; Aud, Hrng Aid Serv Inc, **SLP A**

Lowder, Mary W Department Of Otolaryngology, Univ Of Iowa Hospital, Iowa City, IA 52242, (319) 356-2222, BA 69 Univ of IA; MA 70 Univ of IA; Aud, U of IA Hosp, **A**

Lowe, Albert G, III P O Box 852, Marianna, FL 32446, (904) 482-9352, BS 70 Auburn Univ - Auburn; MS 72 FL St Univ; 83–QA Dir, State of Florida, **SLP**

Lowe, Mrs Audrey D VA Medical Center, 1670 Clairmont Road, Atlanta, GA 30033, (404) 321-6111, BA 57 Univ of FL; ME 64 Emory Univ; Aud, VA Med Cen, **A**

Lowe, Mrs Fonda 409 Bostwick Lane, Gaithersburg, MD 20878, (301) 963-2465, BA 75 Univ of MD - College Park; MA 77 Univ of MD - College Park; Sp-Lang Path, Ivymount Sch, **SLP**

Lowe, Dr John, III Dean College Of Health Prof, Governors State University, University Park, IL 60466, BS 64 Eastern IL Univ; MA 66 Univ of IL - Urbana; PH 69 (NS) Univ of IL - Urbana; 82–Dean Coll of Hlth Prof, Governors State U, **SLP**

Lowe, Mrs Linnea Katherine 295 East Niles, Fresno, CA 93710, (209) 441-3000, **SLP**

Lowe, M Kathleen 7644 Yarmouth Drive, Richmond, VA 23225, (804) 254-0330, BA 76 Baldwin-Wallace Coll; MS 78 Miami Univ - Oxford; SLP, Private Practice, **SLP**

Lowe, Mrs Marsha S 144 Fairway, Missoula, MT 59803, (406) 728-2520, BA 72 Univ of MT; MA 74 Univ of MT; **SLP**

Lowe, Mary Elizabeth 1000 West Forest, Jackson, TN 38301, (901) 668-1317, BA 81 Southern IL Univ -Carbondale; MA 83 Southern IL Univ -Carbondale; Sp-Lang Path, Jackson-Madison Co Gen Hosp, **SLP**

Lowe, Dr R Gregory State & Beacon Medical Bldg, 2730 East State Boulevard, Fort Wayne, IN 46808, (219) 484-4175, BA 73 IN Univ - Bloomington; MA 75 Ball St Univ; PH 79 (NS) Purdue Univ - West Lafayette; Pres, Hrng Rehab Lab, **A**

Lowe, Raymond L 301 Brockmont Drive, Glendale, CA 91202, (818) 243-4405, BA 49 Univ of Southern CA; MA 55 Univ of Southern CA; **SLP LM**

Lowe, Mrs Rebecca J 1797 Camellia Street, Greenville, MS 38701-7521, (601) 335-3731, BS 69 MS Coll; MS 70 MS Univ for Women; **SLP**

Lowe, Dr Robert Joel P O Box 322, Mifflinville, PA 18631, (717) 752-2166, BA 73 Slippery Rock Univ of PA; ME 77 Clarion Univ of PA; PH 86 (Sp Path) OH Univ - Athens; 86–Asst Prof, Bloomsburg Univ, **SLP**

Lowe, Sandra Rae 55 Lafayette Street, Hopewell, NJ 08525, (609) 466-4679, MS 87 Ithaca Coll; 87–Sp-Lang Path, Eden Institute Inc, **SLP**

Lowe-Bell, Dr Sena E S 686 Oahu Street, Bay St Louis, MS 39520, (504) 646-4920, BA 53 Univ of Southwestern LA; MA 62 CA St Univ - Long Beach; PH 70 (Sp Path/Aud) LA St Univ - Baton Rouge; Sp-Lang Path, St Tammany Parish Schs, **SLP**

Lowe-Heistad, Mrs Mardi E 15759 95th Avenue, Surrey, BC, Canada V3R 9G3, (604) 589-3236, BS 78 Univ of Western Ontario; MS 82 Western WA Univ; Dir Sp-Lang Path, Surrey Mem Hosp, **SLP**

Lowell, Edgar Lafayette 3165 Motor Avenue, Los Angeles, CA 90064, (213) 748-5481, BA 49 Reed Coll; MA 51 Wesleyan Univ; PH 52 (NS) Harvard Univ; 88–Consult, John Tracy Clinic, **F LM**

Lowell, Mrs Elizabeth L 6814 Burke Court, Chino, CA 91710, (213) 257-3006, BA 69 Saint Xavier Coll; MA 75 Northern IL Univ - De Kalb; 86–Sp-Lang Path, The Almansor Ctr, **SLP ACE**

Lowell, Judy Z Box 17648, Plantation, FL 33318-7648, SLP, Broward Co Schl District, **SLP**

Lowell, Mrs Marilyn Olsen 3165 Motor Avenue, Los Angeles, CA 90064, (213) 836-6142, BA 58 Univ of WA; MA 63 Univ of WA; 88–Sp-Lang Path/Aud, Private Practice, **SLP A**

Lowell, Sarah L 620 2nd Street, Ann Arbor, MI 48103, (313) 663-9294, MS 88 Eastern MI Univ

Lowenfels, Barbara B 30 Paddington Road, Scarsdale, NY 10583, (914) 723-8697, BS 70 Skidmore Coll; MA 75 Columbia Univ Teachers Coll; SLP, Private Practice, **SLP**

Lowenthal, Mrs Laura Lee 2854 Erie Avenue, Cincinnati, OH 45208, BA 53 Duke Univ; MA 82 Univ of Cincinnati; Aud, Cincinnati Sp & Hrng Cen, **A**

Lowenthal, Phyllis 6 Glenside Terrace, Upper Montclair, NJ 07043, (201) 783-6096, BA 73 SUNY - Center at Buffalo; MS 76 Columbia Univ Teachers Coll; 88–Sp-Lang Path, Newark Beth Israel Hosp, **SLP**

Lowery, Deborah Hodges 3616 Peartree Court, Apartment #44, Silver Spring, MD 20906, (703) 670-8126, BS 84 East Carolina Univ; MS 85 East Carolina Univ; 88–Aud, Prince William Sp & Hrng Ctr, **A**

Lowery, Jeffery 2511 North Lexington St, Arlington, VA 22207, (919) 739-8286, BS 80 East Carolina Univ; MS 82 East Carolina Univ; Sp-Lang Path, Comprehensive Home Health, **SLP**

Lowery, Rita L 775 Pershing #2A, Glen Ellyn, IL 60137, (312) 790-3567, BS 77 IL St Univ - Normal; MA 78 Univ of IL - Urbana; Sp-Lang Path, Dupage Easter Seal, **SLP**

Lowery, Dr Scott D 12111 Stoney Crown, San Antonio, TX 78247, (512) 490-7144, BS 74 Western IL Univ; MA 75 Western IL Univ; PH 82 (Aphasia) Univ of IL - Urbana; 87–Sp-Lang Path, Private Practice, **SLP**

Lowes, Mrs Victoria Sue 7 Marvin Place, Westport, CT 06880, (203) 227-1544, BA 68 MI St Univ; MA 77 Univ of Pittsburgh - Pittsburgh; Sp-Lang Path, **SLP**

Lowry, James Keith 436 Tenth Court, Pleasant Grove, AL 35127, (205) 251-7169, BA 81 Univ of AL- Tuscaloosa; MS 83 Univ of AL- Tuscaloosa; 85–Aud, Pappas Ear Clinic PC, **A**

Lowry, Dr Jean 11700 Valiant, Riverside, CA 92505, (714) 785-2157, BA 66 Loma Linda Univ - Riverside; MA 68 Univ of Redlands; PH 73 (NS) Kent St Univ; Assoc Prof, Loma Linda U La Sierra, **SLP**

Lowry, Kathleen Mary 26243 Newport Avenue, Loma Linda, CA 92354, (213) 273-8480, **SLP**

Lowry, Mrs Laura D G 1119 Vine Street, Denver, CO 80206, (303) 355-4101, BS 79 Univ of Tulsa; MA 80 Our Lady Lake Univ-San Anton; 87–Sp-Lang Path, Craig Hosp, **SLP**

Lowry-Romero, Mary Frances Speech-Language Rehab Section, Fitzsimons Army Med Center, Bldg 600, Aurora, CO 80045, (303) 361-8120, BS 64 Southern IL Univ -Carbondale; MS 65 Southern IL Univ -Carbondale; Sp-Lang Path, Fitzsimons Army Med Cen, **SLP**

Lowsky, Debra C 6907 Townbridge Road, Fayetteville, NC 28306, BS 75 Trenton St Coll; MS 76 Rutgers St Univ - Newark; SLP, **SLP**

Lowther, Maria Anne 848 Park Avenue, Syracuse, NY 13204, (315) 488-2951, BA 84 SUNY - Coll at Plattsburgh; MS 86 Syracuse Univ; Sp-Lang Path, St Camillus, **SLP**

Loy, Betty Ann 5808 N Pennsylvania Avenue, Apartment 205A, Oklahoma City, OK 73112, (405) 636-7434, BA 73 OK City Univ; MS 82 Univ of OK Medical Center; Aud, Self Employed, **A**

Loy, Mrs Carla Fogleman 2628 Cambridge Road, Burlington, NC 27215, (919) 226-4085, BS 81 Appalachian St Univ; ME 83 Univ of NC - Greensboro; Sp/Lang Path, Alamance County Schs, **SLP**

Loy, Kent Matthews 8 Heaton Orchard Road, West Kingston, RI 02892, (401) 789-1256, BA 67 Wilson Coll; MS 79 Univ of RI; 88–Aud, So County Hearing Svcs, **A**

Loyborg, Troels V 2264 Loma Heights Road, Napa, CA 94558, (707) 646-2424, BS 68 Univ of UT; MS 69 Univ of UT; Hrng Cons Prog Mgr, Mare Island Naval Shipyard, **A**

Loyd, Rebecca R 1362 South 143rd Street, Omaha, NE 68144, (402) 334-5798, BS 74 Southwest MO St Univ; MA 76 Univ of NE - Lincoln; **SLP**

Loyd, Sharon K 7509 Vista Del Arroyo N E, Albuquerque, NM 87109, (505) 294-3713, BA 66 Univ of Science & Arts of OK; MA 71 Univ of NM; Sp-Lang Path, Albuquerque Pub Schs, **SLP**

Loyer, Mrs Barbara C 90 State Street, Windsor, VT 05089, (603) 643-6050, BA 68 Univ of VT; MS 78 Univ of VT; Sp-Lang Path, Sch Admin Unit 22, **SLP**

Loy-Every, Marilyn J 3120 25th Avene Court S E, Puyallup, WA 98374, (206) 841-0255, BS 84 Kearney St Coll; MS 87 Univ of WY; **A**

Lozano-Rodriguez, Jose Rafael 2651 West End Road, West Palm Beach, FL 33406-7739, (305) 433-3500, BA 77 Univ of FL; MA 80 FL St Univ; Sp-Lang Path, Palm Beach School Board, **SLP**

Lozeau, Mrs Colleen Doody P O Box 122, Michigan, ND 58259, (701) 259-2261, BS 78 Minot St Univ; MS 79 Minot St Univ; Sp-Lang Path, Private Practice, **SLP**

Lozier, Barbara L 17 East Colfax, Logansport, IN 46947, (219) 722-5288, BS 69 Purdue Univ - West Lafayette; MS 70 Purdue Univ - West Lafayette; Aud/Sp-Lang Path, Logansport Comm Schs, **SLP A**

Lozier, Dr Carol Whitcomb 3471 Summit Boulevard, Pensacola, FL 32503, (904) 474-6148, PH 84 (NS) OH St Univ; Dir Hrng & Spch, Sacred Heart Hosp, **A**

Lozo, Deborah A 4629 Sammy Drive, Powder Springs, GA 30073, (404) 943-9611, BS 76 SUNY - Coll at Fredonia; ME 81 GA St Univ; 88–Sp-Lang Path, Cobb Co Bd Educ, **SLP**

Lozow, Mrs Karen Simmons 7794 East Hampden Circle, Denver, CO 80237, (303) 741-1559, BA 80 Univ of CO - Boulder; MS 82 Purdue Univ - West Lafayette; Sp-Lang Path, Laradon Early Ed Prog, **SLP**

Lozoya, Mrs Maria Uribe 11250 Campbell Avenue, Riverside, CA 92505, (714) 627-9638, BA 82 CA St Univ - Long Beach; MA 85 CA St Univ - Fullerton; SLP, R Gird Elementary School, **SLP**

Lu, Fang-Ling P O Box 754, Clinton, MS 39056, OM 85 Univ of SC - Columbia

Lubach, Karly S 9401 244th Street SW #W106, Edmonds, WA 98020, (206) 542-7523, MS 87 Univ of WA; 88–Sp-Lang Path, InSpeech Inc, **SLP**

Lubanski, Mrs Cathy Michele 37601 Lancaster, Farmington Hills, MI 48018, (313) 646-1150, SLP, Professional Therapy Staffing, **SLP**

Lubar, Phyllis 371 Russett Road, Brookline, MA 02167, (617) 965-0764, BS 69 Syracuse Univ; ME 71 Boston Univ; Sp-Lang Path, Needham Pub Sch, **SLP**

Lubbers, Dr Donald E 1521 Kessler, Keego Harbor, MI 48320, (313) 682-9647, BS 61 Minot St Univ; ME 63 Wayne St Univ; PH 68 (NS) Wayne St Univ; Dir of Aud, Oakland ENT Cen Pc, **A**

Lubbert, Larry L 901 Maple Avenue, Decorah, IA 52101-2119, (319) 382-8053, BS 64 Univ of KS; MA 68 Univ of KS; 68–Sp/Lang Path, Keystone AEA #1, **SLP**

Lubell, Patricia A 1813 Geiberger Drive, Fayetteville, NC 28303, (919) 822-5287, BS 67 Univ of WI - Madison; MA 71 George Washington Univ; OM 77 Saint John's Univ - Jamaica; 87–Sp-Lang Path, Cumberland Co Bd of Educ, **SLP**

Luber, Lucille M 204 Gremer Street, Edwardsville, IL 62025, (314) 741-0055, BS 80 Southern IL Univ-Edwardsvill; MS 81 Southern IL Univ-Edwardsvill; Sp-Lang Path, Spec Sch Dist of St Louis Co, **SLP**

Lubert, Mrs Barbara D 16808 Rolling Rock Drive, Tampa, FL 33618-1115, (813) 962-2629, BS 71 Purdue Univ - West Lafayette; MA 74 Cleveland St Univ; Sp-Lang Path, Hillsborough County Schs, **SLP**

Lubin, Joyce R 7 Deer Lodge Court, Owings Mills, MD 21117, (301) 363-6325, BS 74 Towson St Univ; MS 76 Johns Hopkins Univ; Sp-Lang Path, Balt City Pub Schs, **SLP**

Lubinski, Dr Rosemary B 115 Park Hall Department Of CDS, SUNY At Buffalo, Amherst, NY 14260, (716) 836-3400, BS 68 Bloomsburg Univ of PA; MA 69 Columbia Univ Teachers Coll; ED 76 (Sp Path) Columbia Univ Teachers Coll; Assoc Prof, SUNY-Buffalo, **SLP F ACE**

Lubinsky, Dr Jay 13823 Timber Trails Road, Orland Park, IL 60462, (312) 534-5000, BA 67 CUNY - Brooklyn Coll; MS 72 CUNY - Brooklyn Coll; PH 77 (Aud) Case Western Reserve Univ; Chmn Div of Commun Dis, Governors St U, **SLP A ACE**

Lubinsky, Natalie B 1169 Fairfield Road, Bridgewater, NJ 08807, (201) 722-6465, BA 75 Rutger's St Univ - Douglas Coll; MS 76 Columbia Univ Teachers Coll; Sp-Lang Path, Natalie B Lubinsky Children's Spec Hosp, **SLP**

Lubinsky-Zubrycky, Mary-Anne 28 Sioux Crescent, Nepean, ON, Canada K2H 7E5, (613) 828-9950, BA 79 Univ of Western Ontario; MA 81 Wichita St Univ; SLP, St Vincent Hosp, **SLP**

Lubin-Sulzman, Mrs Karen 30 Fox Hunt Court, Staten Island, NY 10301, (718) 448-1246, MS 84 Saint Johns Univ - Staten Is; Sp-Lang Path, NYC Bd of Ed, **SLP**

Lubker, Dr Bobbie B University Of North Carolina, Cb 3500 014 Peabody Hall, Chapel Hill, NC 27599, (919) 962-5579, BA 53 Troy St Univ - Troy; MA 56 Univ of KY; PH 82 (NS) Univ of NC - Chapel Hill; Asst Professor/Sp-Lang Path, Univ of N Carolina-Chapel Hill, **SLP**

Lubker, Dr James Fredrick University Of Vermont, Comm Science And Disorders, Allen House, Burlington, VT 05405, (802) 656-3861, PH 67 (Sp Science) Univ of IA; Professor and Chairman, University of Vermont, **F**

Lubnau, Kathryn Lee PO Box 1028, Gillette, WY 82717, (307) 682-5171, BS 83 Univ of WY; MS 85 Univ of WY; Sp-Lang Path, Campbell County School Dist, **SLP**

Lubowicz, Patricia Barniak 3395 Scranton Road, Cleveland, OH 44109, (216) 459-3165, MA 84 Cleveland St Univ; Aud, Cleveland Metro Gen Hosp, **A**

Lucas, Annie Hall 1011 Ironbound Avenue, Plainfield, NJ 07060, (201) 754-4980, BA 72 SUNY - Coll at Buffalo; MA 81 Kean Coll of NJ

Lucas, Elizabeth Creech 1814 Broadmoor Road, Johnson City, TN 37604, (615) 461-6981, BS East TN St Univ; MS Vanderbilt Univ; 86–Sp-Lang Path Dir, Johnson City Med Cntr Hosp, **SLP ACE**

Lucas, Gary Allen P O Box 1164, Claremont, CA 91711, (714) 593-7521, BS 73 Phillips Univ; MS 74 Vanderbilt Univ; Sp-Lang Path, Casa Coliva Hosp/Rehab Med, **SLP**

Lucas, Jeanne Rossmiller 1014 14th Street, Boone, IA 50036, (515) 432-6345, BA 83 Augustana Coll; MA 85 Univ of IA; 85–Sp-Lang Path, Heartland AEA, **SLP**

Lucas, Dr Karen Hawver Northeast Rehabilitation Hospital, 70 Butler Street, Salem, NH 03079, (603) 893-2900, PH 78 (Sp Path) Univ of Cincinnati; 88–Sp-Lang Path, Northeast Rehab Hosp, **SLP**

Lucas, Linda J 11 West Alhambra Avenue, Lindenhurst, NY 11757, (516) 225-2047, BS 79 SUNY - Coll at Geneseo; MS 80 Indiana Univ of PA; Sp-Lang Path, Smithtown Ctrl Sch Dist, **SLP**

Lucas, Mary Anne General Delivery, Hornby, ON, Canada L0P 1E0, (416) 522-0466, MS 87 Univ of NC - Chapel Hill; 87–Sp-Lang Path, C Hess & Associates

Lucas, Mary Anne L 4612 G Colony Road, Charlotte, NC 28226, BA 80 Univ of NC - Chapel Hill; ME 83 Univ of NC - Greensboro; 87–Sp-Lang Path, VCP of North Carolina, **SLP**

Lucas, Minnie B 305 Wayne Circle, Durham, NC 27707, MS; **SLP**

Lucas, Mrs Patricia J 1309 Lincolnshire Blvd, Marion, IN 46952, (317) 662-6592, BS 71 Bowling Green St Univ; MA 77 MI St Univ; Sp-Lang Path, **SLP**

Lucas, Tana Roush 211 South High Street, Hillsboro, OH 45133, (513) 393-4234, BS 69 Miami Univ - Oxford; MA 71 Univ of TN - Knoxville; Sp-Lang Path, Private Practice, **SLP**

Lucas-Alexander, Mrs Nancy 12321 Marlowe Place, Ocean Springs, MS 39564, (601) 872-2472, BS 75 Northwestern Univ; MA 77 George Washington Univ; 88–Sp-Lang Path, Jackson County Sch Dist, **SLP**

Lucas-Cooley, Mrs Ann Marie 3 Annawon Avenue, West Haven, CT 06516, (203) 783-3553, BA 74 Univ of CT; MS 78 Southern CT St Univ; Sp-Lang Path, Milford Public Schools, **SLP**

Lucci, Mrs Bonnie D 4 Parton Court, Lincolnshire, IL 60045, (312) 295-7137, BS 72 Univ of CT; MS 74 Ithaca Coll; Sp-Lang Path, Barrington PS, **SLP ACE**

Luce, Michael S 720 West Conn, Council Grove, KS 66846, (316) 767-5192, MA 78 IN Univ - Bloomington; Sp-Lang Path, Flint Hills Spec Ed Coop, **SLP**

Luce, Roberta E 862 West Chicago, Detroit, MI 48202, MA 78 Wayne St Univ; Tchr, Detroit Board of Education, **SLP**

Lucente, Mrs Laura Dykes 2573 Shenandoah Drive S, Orange Park, FL 32073, (904) 355-3403, **SLP**

Lucente, Maria Frances 4102 Greenpoint Drive, Greensboro, NC 27407, (919) 294-6534, BS 84 Univ of NC - Greensboro; ME 85 Univ of NC - Greensboro; SLP, Winston-Salem Forsyth Co, **SLP**

Lucente, Warren R 2573 Shenandoah Dr South, Orange Park, FL 32073, BA 72 Hofstra Univ; MA 74 Hofstra Univ; Aud, VA, **A**

Lucey-Sparacio, Patricia 4 Stockton Drive, Marlboro, NJ 07746, BS 78 SUNY - Coll at Brockport; MA 79 Hofstra Univ; SLP, State of New York (Sidc), **SLP**

Luchini, Ann 52 School Street, Milford, MA 01757, (617) 478-0723, BA 69 Fontbonne Coll; MS 76 Southern IL Univ-Edwardsvill; **A**

Luchini, Mrs Lizabeth Torres P O Box 117, Hatch, NM 87937, (505) 524-3522, **SLP**

Luchko, Christine D'Altilio 2349 South Howard Street, Allentown, PA 18103, (215) 866-8092, BS 80 Marywood Coll; MS 82 PA St Univ - Univ Park; 84–Coordinator of Speech Services, Lehigh Valley Easter Seals, **SLP**

Luchs, Mrs Deana M 29 Brookside Road, Succasunna, NJ 07876, (201) 584-4331, BA 69 Trenton St Coll; MS 80 William Paterson Coll; 87–Sp-Lang Path, Roxbury Twp Bd of Educ, **SLP**

Lucht, James L 1066 Oxford Court, Neenah, WI 54956, (414) 734-7181, BS 76 Univ of WI - Oshkosh; MS 77 Univ of WI - Oshkosh; 77–Aud, ENT Surg Assoc SC, **A ACE**

Luciani, Ann Kristen 829 North Irving Avenue, Scranton, PA 18510, (717) 342-5630, BS 85 Marywood Coll; MS 87 Columbia Univ Teachers Coll; 87–Aud, St Luke's Hosp

Lucido, Mrs Bonnie R Brigham Young University, 133 Tlrb, Provo, UT 84602, (801) 378-6461, BS 64 Brigham Young Univ; MS 66 Brigham Young Univ; Instr, Brigham Young U, **SLP**

Lucie, Mrs Riel 12135 Paul Contant, Montreal, PQ, Canada H4K 1S3, (514) 337-2994, BA 67 Univ of Montreal - Quebec; OM 69 Univ of Montreal - Quebec; Aud, Sacre-Coeur Hosp, **A**

Lucier, Penny J 829 South Main Street, Fall River, MA 02724, (508) 678-8336, BS 79 Boston Univ; ME 82 Northeastern Univ; Aud, Azhar Q Mustafa MD Inc, **A**

Luck, Mrs Georgia H Route 3 Box 930, Ashland, VA 23005, (804) 798-4809, BS 67 Univ of GA; ME 68 Univ of VA - Charlottesville; Dir/Owner, Private Practice, **SLP**

Luck, Mrs Sheryl F R 3754 Bobbitt, Shreveport, LA 71107, (318) 227-8363, BA 74 LA Tech Univ; MA 75 LA Tech Univ; **SLP**

Luckenbaugh, Mrs Sharon Hughes 16B Dix Avenue, Glens Falls, NY 12801, (518) 761-5333, BS 81 Coll of Saint Rose; MS 82 Coll of Saint Rose; Sp-Lang Path, Glens Falls Hosp, **SLP**

Lucker, Dr Jay R 95 Croton Avenue, P O Box 1048, Ossining, NY 10562, (914) 762-7712, BA 69 CUNY - Lehman Coll; MA 72 CUNY - Hunter Coll; ED 79 (NS) Columbia Univ Teachers Coll; 80–Aud, Private Practice, **SLP A**

Lucker, Nancy J 7515 North Damen Avenue, Chicago, IL 60645, (312) 465-0563, BS 83 Univ of Hartford; MA 85 Northwestern Univ; 88–Sp-Lang Path, Northbrook PS Dist 27, **SLP**

Luckern, Marie P 731 Chenango Street, Binghamton, NY 13901, (607) 724-2693, BA 43 Coll of New Rochelle; MS 56 SUNY - Coll at Cortland; MS 65 Syracuse Univ; **SLP LM**

Luckett, Catherine 1720 DE Anza Court, San Luis Obispo, CA 93401, MA 71 CA St Univ - Sacramento; SLP, San Luis Coastal USD, **SLP**

Luckett, Joan L 805 Weatherwood Drive, Manchester, MO 63021, (314) 256-2647, BA 77 Bellarmine Coll; MA 82 Univ of Cincinnati; Aud, **A**

Luckey, Richard S, Sr 10938 Belmar Avenue, Northridge, CA 91326, (818) 709-9854, BA 50 Univ of Denver; MS 67 Univ of Southern CA; MA 74 CA St Univ - Northridge; Co-Owner, Santa Susana School, **A**

Luckhurst, Mrs Joan A 465 East Main Street, Owego, NY 13827, BS 74 SUNY - Coll at Geneseo; MS 75 SUNY - Center at Albany; Sp/Lang Path, Owego Apalachin Ctrl Sch Dist, **SLP**

Luckhurst, John M 465 East Main Street, Owego, NY 13827, BA 74 SUNY - Coll at Geneseo; MS 84 Ithaca Coll; 86–Aud, Rehab Svcs Inc, **A**

Lucking, Victoria Bradley 26 Ridge Road, Greenville, SC 29611, (803) 294-0261, BS 76 Western Carolina Univ; ME 80 Univ of GA; Sp-Lang Path, Greenville Co Sch Dist-NW Area, **SLP ACE**

Lucks, Dr Lisa Ellen 102 Moore Bldg, State College, PA 16802, (814) 863-2013, BS 83 Univ of GA; ME 84 Univ of GA; PH 88 (Sp & Hrng) Univ of CA - Santa Barbara; Asst Prof, Penn St Univ

Lucky, Joan Route 1, 207 River Oaks, Luling, LA 70070, (504) 785-6289, ME 78 6839; BA 57 Northwestern St Univ; Head Ther, St Charles Parish Sch Bd, **SLP**

Lucov-Lenox, Mrs Jerilyn 660 Harrell Avenue, Woodbridge, NJ 07095, (201) 549-5580, BA 85 2565; MS 87 2565; 87–Sp-Lang Path, Cerebral Palsy Assoc of Middlesex Co, **SLP**

Ludden, Sr Mary A 3700 West 103rd Street, Chicago, IL 60655, (312) 779-3300, BA 34 CUNY - Hunter Coll; MA 35; Cl Supvr, St Xavier College, **SLP LM**

Ludden, Sarah Margaret 2341 Acton Street, Berkeley, CA 94702, (415) 548-6354, BA 75 Northwestern Univ; MA 77 Northwestern Univ; 88–Aud, Alta Bates-Herrick Hosp, **A**

Ludington, Harriet Jane R 2 Buttons Road, Chapel Hill, NC 27514, (919) 966-1006, BA 57 Middlebury Coll; MS 81 Univ of NC - Chapel Hill; Clin Instr, Univ of NC, **SLP**

Ludington, Mrs Noreen Malone 34 King Street, Morristown, NJ 07960, (914) 986-1181, BS 80 SUNY - Coll at Brockport; MA 84 Seton Hall Univ; **SLP**

Ludke, Judy Lavon 11906 Beltsville Road #24, Beltsville, MD 20705, (301) 772-0990, BA 80 Univ of MD - College Park; MA 83 Univ of MD - College Park; Aud, Prince Georges Co Hlth Dept, **A**

Ludlow, Dr Christy L Speech Pathology Unit NINCDS, NIH Bldg 10 Room 5N226, 9000 Rockville Pike, Bethesda, MD 20892, (301) 496-9365, BS 65 McGill Univ - Quebec; MS 67 McGill Univ - Quebec; PH 73 (NS) NY Univ; Sp-Lang Path, Natl I Neur & Commun Dis Stror, **SLP F**

Ludlow, Ellen D 584 First Avenue South, Apartment B-6, Naples, FL 33940, (215) 368-6464, **SLP**

Ludlow, Patricia A 1244 Clairmont Road, Suite 208-209, Decatur, GA 30033, (404) 321-9107, ME 81 Univ of NC - Greensboro; BA 73 Saint Xavier Coll; 84–Director /Sp-Lang Services, Emory-Clairmont Diag Ctr, **SLP ACE**

Ludolph, Leslie Baker 124 Walford Drive, Moraga, CA 94556, (415) 783-4880, BA 78 OH St Univ; MS 84 CA St Univ - Hayward; Sp-Lang Path, Hayward USD, **SLP**

Ludtke, Beverly M 4526 Cheltenham Drive, Bethesda, MD 20814, (202) 576-1676, BA 74 Humboldt St Univ; MA 77 Humboldt St Univ; Sp-Lang Path, Walter Reed Army Med Cen, **SLP ACE**

Luduena, Linda G 6711 Country View, San Antonio, TX 78240, (512) 691-1882, BS 76 Baylor Univ; MA 78 Kent St Univ; Sp-Lang Path, Private Practice, **SLP**

Ludwick, Dianne Marie 800 Thompson Street, Turtle Creek, PA 15145, (412) 261-3950, BA 84 Univ of Pittsburgh - Pittsburgh; MA 86 Univ of Pittsburgh - Pittsburgh; Aud, Allegheny ENT Assoc Inc, **A**

Ludwig, Mrs Alisa L 25 Hickory Lane, Long Valley, NJ 07853, (201) 876-4986, BA 69 Temple Univ; MA 71 CUNY - Hunter Coll; Sp-Lang Path, Private Practice, **SLP**

Ludwig, Dr Carol S K Route 1 Box 18-A, Jackson, MO 63755, (314) 335-7279, BS 70 Southeast MO St Univ; MA 74 Southeast MO St Univ; PH 84 (Communication Disorders & Sci) Southern IL Univ -Carbondale; 84–Sp-Lang Path, Sp-Lang Path Assoc, **SLP**

Ludwig, Cheryl L C 529 Latona Avenue, Trenton, NJ 08618, (609) 393-8228, BS 75 Trenton St Coll; MA 79 Trenton St Coll; Sp/Lang Path, Ej Constance and Assoc, **SLP**

Ludwig, Denise A 4099 South Norway SE, Grand Rapids, MI 49506, (616) 957-4057, BS 80 Western MI Univ; MS 81 Univ of MI - Ann Arbor; Exec Dir, Residential Resources, **SLP**

Ludwig, Gail Ann 5048 Merrimac Court, San Diego, CA 92117, (619) 465-0711, BA 80 Univ of MD - College Park; MA 82 Univ of Northern IA; SLP, Grossmont Dist Hosp-La Mesa, **SLP**

Ludwig, Janelle Lynne 1815 Evergreen Street, San Diego, CA 92106, (619) 276-2832, BA 83 San Diego St Univ; MS 86 Univ of Redlands

Ludwig, Jeanne Law 3621 East Van Norman, Cudahy, WI 53110, (414) 481-8428, BS 79 Univ of WI - Milwaukee; MS 82 Univ of WI - Stevens Point; **SLP**

Ludwig, Karen Lanice 1541 S E 27th Street #F, Ocala, FL 32671, (904) 351-7225, BS 83 Southern IL Univ -Carbondale; MS 86 Southern IL Univ -Carbondale; 87–Sp-Lang Path, Munroe Regional Med Ctr, **SLP**

Ludwig, Lynne Marie 5914 Baymeadows Lane #1716, Arlington, TX 76017, (817) 468-7402, MS 88 6401; 88–Sp-Lang Path, Arlington ISD

Ludwig, Mrs Marsha S P O Box 728, Loyalton, CA 96118, (916) 993-4611, BS 81 Univ of NV - Reno; MS 82 Univ of NV - Reno; 88–Tchr, Sierra Co Ofc of Educ, **SLP**

Ludwig-Macaulay, Anita M 55 Walnut Lane, Morrisville, PA 19067, (215) 736-2349, BS 77 Trenton St Coll; MA 81 Trenton St Coll; Sp-Lang Path, Private Practice, **SLP**

Ludwikoski, Steven P 918 Hilly Haven Court, Green Bay, WI 54301, (414) 433-8263, BA 69 Univ of WI - Eau Claire; MS 74 Univ of WI - Eau Claire; **SLP ACE**

Luebbe, Judith M 1907 Ashbrook Drive, Cincinnati, OH 45238, (513) 921-1750, BS 76 Univ of Cincinnati; MA 78 Univ of Cincinnati; Sp-Lang Path, Cincinnati Pub Sch, **SLP**

Luebbe-Gearhart, Mrs Mary Lou Luebbe Hearing Services, 3327 North High Street, Columbus, OH 43202, (614) 267-9249, BS 73 OH St Univ; MA 79 OH St Univ; Luebbe Hrng Serv Inc, **A ACE**

Luebkert, Mrs Frances R 1712 Waldorf Court, Crofton, MD 21114, (301) 225-5605, BS 57 Univ of MD - College Park; MA 60 Univ of MD - College Park; Dir-Offi Prog Sup-Chldns Serv, MD Dept of Hlth & Men Hygiene, **SLP A**

Luecht, Kim L 8325 North Menard Avenue, Morton Grove, IL 60053, (312) 965-1426, BS 77 Northwestern Univ; MA 78 Northwestern Univ; 85–Sp/Lang Path, C C Sch Dist 96, **SLP**

Lueck, Dr Anne Gillespie Scott And White Clinic, 2401 South 31st Street, Temple, TX 76508, (817) 774-3950, BA 64 TX Tech Univ; MA 68 Baylor Univ; PH 87 (Sp) Univ of TX - Austin; Ch Sect of Sp-Lang Path, Scott & White Cl, **SLP ACE**

Lueck, Mrs Margaret F 32844 Co Rd 58, Iliff, CO 80736, (303) 522-8330, BS 73 CO St Univ; MA 74 Univ of Northern CO; SLP, Re-1 Valley Sch Dist, **SLP**

Luellen, Betty Ruth 2054 Locust, Denver, CO 80207, (316) 832-7506, BA 68 Univ of Denver; ME 69 Boston Univ; Manager, At & T Info Syst, **SLP**

Luensman, Karen Butler 248 West Russell Street, Barrington, IL 60010-4233, (312) 662-1877, BS 79 Northwestern Univ; MA 80 Northwestern Univ; Parent-Infant Ed/Sp-Lang Path, Lake McHenry Reg Prog, **SLP**

Luers, Ann E R R 51 Box 50, Terre Haute, IN 47805, (812) 877-3575, BA 79 Univ of NE - Lincoln; MA 81 Univ of KS; Sp-Lang Path, Union Hosp, **SLP**

Luessenhop, Stephanie K 237 Washington Avenue, Providence, RI 02905, (401) 828-3020, BA 74 Univ of CO - Boulder; MA 78 Univ of Denver; 87–Sp/Lang Path, In Motion PT Svcs Inc, **SLP**

Lufrano, Nancy 232 Elm Place, Mineola, NY 11501, BA 81 SUNY - Center at Buffalo; MA 83 Hofstra Univ; 88–Sp-Lang Path, Hofstra Univ Sp & Hearing Ctr, **SLP**

Luft, Cynthia Burt 3204 Lubbock, Fort Worth, TX 76109, (817) 927-5307, OB 85 Baylor Univ; OM 86 Baylor Univ; **SLP**

Luger, Linda Suzanne 2500 North 6th Street, Burbank, CA 91504, (213) 838-6110, SLP, Los Angeles School District, **SLP**

Lugo, Mabeline 27 Nebraska Street, Long Beach, NY 11561, (718) 451-1800, BA 84 Hofstra Univ; MA 87 Temple Univ; **SLP**

Luhman, Annalee D 9816 Vineyard Crest, Bellevue, WA 98004, (206) 454-6878, MS; **SLP**

Luhn, Kathleen Krabacher 641 Conina Drive, Cincinnati, OH 45233, (513) 451-3685, **A**

Luhr, Mrs Vernae Ivone R R 1 Box 181, Wakefield, NE 68784, (402) 287-2061, BS 82 Univ of SD - Vermillion; MA 84 Univ of SD - Vermillion; Aud, Educational Service Unit One, **A**

Luis, Deborah N 357 1/2 North Spaulding, Los Angeles, CA 90036, (213) 471-6768, BS 79 Univ of AZ; MS 82 Univ of AZ; SLP, The Parish School, **SLP**

Luis, Maureen Elizabeth 6416 Oakland #207, St Louis, MO 63139, (314) 362-2362, BS 82 Univ of WA; MS 85 Univ of WI - Madison; **SLP**

Lujan, Beverly Ann 2955 East 3900th South, Salt Lake City, UT 84124, (801) 272-3109, **SLP**

Lujan, Erin Hayes 113 Mateo Circle N, Santa Fe, NM 87501, (505) 988-3124, BS 61 Washington Univ; MA 78 Marshall Univ; Educational Diagnostician, Albuquerque Public Schools, **SLP**

Lujan, Kathleen Wheeler 9105 Locura Place S W, Albuquerque, NM 87105, (505) 831-3716, BA 84 Univ of NM; MS 86 Univ of NM; **A**

Lukach, Lynne M 605 Clifton Boulevard, Mansfield, OH 44907, **SLP**

Lukach, Sharon D 3610 Montridge Court, Arlington, TX 76016, (817) 478-2719, BA 73 Univ of NM; MS 71 Univ of NM; 87–Aud, Fort Worth ISD, **A**

Lukanic, Bill A 2352 S Gray Drive, Denver, CO 80227-3956, MS

Lukas, Elaine K 4204 West Mequon, Mequon, WI 53092, MS 77 Univ of WI - Milwaukee; Nursing Home Administrator, Beverly Enterprises, **SLP**

Lukas, Julie S 2327 East Mountain View Rd, Phoenix, AZ 85028-3632, (602) 867-4142, MS 79 San Francisco St Univ; Consultant Aud, Comprehensive Audio Eval Inc, **A**

Lukas, Margaret Kay 13 Peach Tree Road, Glastonbury, CT 06033, (203) 659-1778, MA Univ of CT; BS Univ of CT; 85–Sp-Lang Path, Colchester Bd of Educ, **SLP**

Lukas, Patricia A 89 Pond Point Avenue, Milford, CT 06460, (203) 874-7143, BA 77 Southern CT St Univ; MA 86 Univ of TX - Austin

Lukas, Robert Alan 350 Route 210, Stony Point, NY 10980, (914) 947-3000, BA 75 SUNY - Center at Buffalo; MA 78 SUNY - Center at Buffalo; 79–Dir-SLP & Aud, Helen Hayes Hosp/Sp & Hrng, **A**

Lukaskiewicz, Janet 1 Lower Windbrook Drive, Auburn, MA 01501, (413) 289-1241, MA 87 Univ of MA - Amherst; Aud, Kirtikant P Kantesaria MD PC, **A**

Lukaszewski, Carolyn A 555 St Mary Avenue #1125, Winnipeg, MB, Canada R3C 3X4, (204) 787-2740, BA 78 MI St Univ; MA 81 MI St Univ; 87–Sp-Lang Path, Health Sciences Ctr, **SLP**

Lukat, R Michael Route 1 Box 427-D, Fayetteville, NC 28301, (502) 769-5561, BS 72 Murray St Univ; ME 76 Univ of Louisville; Aud, Owner, Private Practice, **A**

Lukat, Rita K 3920 South Dixie Highway, Elizabethtown, KY 42701, **SLP**

Lukavich, Susan E 8-40 Chester Street, Fair Lawn, NJ 07410, (201) 441-2158, BA 72 Rutger's St Univ - Douglas Coll; MA 79 Montclair St Coll; Ch/Sect Commun Dis, I for Chld Dev Hackensack Med, **SLP**

Luke, Charlene M 8208 Kingslee Road, Bloomington, MN 55438, (612) 370-8361, BA 75 Adams St Coll; MA 75 Adams St Coll; 87–Sys Analyst, Pillsbury World Headquarters

Luke-Gysin, Patricia A 17 Corona Street #1, Denver, CO 80218-3803, (303) 296-2400, SLP, Laradon Hall, **SLP**

Lukenda, Mrs Karen Bornheimer 24 Lehigh Boulevard, Jackson, NJ 08527, (201) 244-3100, BS 81 West Chester Univ of PA; MS 83 Univ of NM; 88–Dir-Outpatient Head Inj Prog, Garden State Rehab Hosp, **SLP**

Lukens, Mrs Ann M 1205 Virginia Avenue, Libertyville, IL 60048, (312) 367-9189, BS 73 Univ of KY; MA 75 Xavier Univ; MS 78 Marquette Univ; **SLP**

Luker, Edward E Ear Nose & Throat Clinic, 2003 Kentucky Avenue, Paducah, KY 42001, (502) 444-9936, BA 77 Univ of AR - Little Rock; MS 79 Univ of AR - Little Rock; 79–Aud, Hawkins-McCracken-Zellmer PSC, **A**

Luker, Janice K Courage Center, 3915 Golden Valley Rd, Golden Valley, MN 55422, (612) 520-0409, BS 76 Univ of WI - Oshkosh; OM 79 Univ of WI - Oshkosh; Prog Dir Sp-Lang-Hrng, Courage Center, **SLP ACE**

Lukes-Miller, Mrs Barbara E 7760 Cedarville Court, Cincinnati, OH 45255, (513) 742-2200, BS 79 Miami Univ - Oxford; MS 80 Miami Univ - Oxford; Sp/Lang Path, Hamilton Co Off Ed, **SLP**

Lukin, Susan S 30-11 Parsons Boulevard, Flushing, NY 11354, (718) 762-3321, BA 62 SUNY - Coll at Buffalo; MA 69 CUNY - Hunter Coll; Sp-Lang Path, Private Practice, **SLP**

Lukins, Margaret Roblee 311 Santo Tomas, Costa Mesa, CA 92627, (714) 631-8360, BS 81 Marquette Univ; MS 83 Purdue Univ - West Lafayette; 88–Sp-Lang Path, Irvine USD, **SLP**

Lukmire, Nan K 4266 South 35th Street, Arlington, VA 22206, (703) 578-4844, BA 70 Mary Washington Coll; ME 71 Univ of VA - Charlottesville; 88–Aud, WRAMC-Aud & Sp Ctr, **A**

Lukoff, Mrs Linda G 22872 Via Genoa, South Laguna, CA 92677, (714) 499-5075, BA 77 Univ of CA - Santa Barbara; MA 79 Univ of WA; Sp-Lang Path, Private Practice, **SLP**

Lukomski, Mrs Joy Ellen 4141 16th St Bldg 15 #10, Vero Beach, FL 32960, (407) 562-7752, BS 84 Purdue Univ - West Lafayette; MA 86 Memphis St Univ; Sp-Lang Path, Donna S Brown & Assoc Inc, **SLP**

Lukomski, Thomas Stephen 4141 16th St Bldg 15 #10, Vero Beach, FL 32960, (215) 631-9300, BS 83 Univ of WI - Milwaukee; MA 86 Memphis St Univ; InSpeech Inc, **SLP**

Lukos, Lizz 602 Alsmeyer Drive, O'Fallon, MO 63366, (314) 272-6620, BA 82 CA St Univ - Los Angeles; MA 85 CA St Univ - Los Angeles; **SLP**

Luks, Susan Beall UAB Audiology Service, Surgery Outpatient Clinic, 1813 6th Avenue South, Birmingham, AL 35294, (205) 934-9783, MS 84 CO St Univ; Aud, U of AL-Birmingham, **A**

Luloff, Arlyne K 1 Foley Drive, Southborough, MA 01772, (508) 481-5328, BA 69 George Washington Univ; MS 86 Emerson Coll; 86–Sp-Lang Path, Learning Ctr for Deaf Children, **SLP**

Lum, Mrs Eydie Emi 45-552 Poliahu Place, Kaneohe, HI 96744, (808) 247-4809, BS 80 Univ of HI - Manoa; MS 82 Univ of HI - Manoa; SLP, Dept of Ed/Spec Serv Hi, **SLP**

Lum, Laura S F 630 Janet Avenue, Lancaster, PA 17601, (717) 397-4741, BA 51 Univ of HI - Manoa; MA 53 Northwestern Univ; Aud, Hrng Conserv/Deaf Serv Cen, **A**

Lumadue, Carol E J 5643 Carvesville Road, Doylestown, PA 18901, BA 74 Bloomsburg Univ of PA; MA 77 Trenton St Coll; Sp-Lang Path, Bucks County I U #22, **SLP**

Lumaghi, Nancy Dowd 19 Ellsworth Lane, Ladue, MO 63124, Sp-Lang Path, Spec Sch Dist St Louis County, **SLP**

Lumm, Mrs Crystal Wells 1130 Howard Avenue, Nashville, TN 37216, (615) 227-3332, BS 84 PA St Univ - Univ Park; MS 86 Vanderbilt Univ; 86–Sp-Lang Path, PS, **SLP**

Lumpkin, Sindy Stickler 102-55 67th Drive #La, Forest Hills, NY 11375, (718) 830-0353, BS 64 FL St Univ; MS 72 CUNY - Queens Coll; Sp-Lang Path, Private Practice, **SLP**

Lumsden-Boehling, Nancy C 4606 Ordinary Court, Annandale, VA 22003, (703) 664-7190, BS 76 Longwood Coll; ME 77 Univ of VA - Charlottesville; Sp-Lang Path, Mount Vernon Hospital, **SLP**

Lumsden-Owen, Patricia A 126 Charbonneau Crescent, Winnipeg, MB, Canada R3X 1C1, (204) 257-0202, BA 76; MA 78 Univ of IA; Sp-Lang Path, Chld Guid Cl of Gtr Winnipeg, **SLP**

Luna, Ann L W 435 Green Acres Circle, Howard, OH 43028, (614) 397-2854, BA 73 Capital Univ; MA 81 OH St Univ; Sp/Lang Path, Affi Aud & Sp-Path, **SLP**

Luna, Denise E Lee Memorial Hospital, PO Drawer 2218, Fort Myers, FL 33902, (813) 334-5284, BS 68 FL St Univ; MS 73 FL St Univ; Sp-Lang Path, Lee Mem Hosp, **SLP ACE**

Lunak, Bridget F 1639 Meadowbrook Lane, Paradise, CA 95969, (916) 896-5342, BA 72 Fontbonne Coll; MA 81 CA St Univ - Chico; 86–Dir of Rehab Svcs, Chico Community Hospital, **SLP**

Lund, Mrs Carrol G 69 Talcott Road, Guilford, CT 06437, (203) 457-0301, BS 66 Carlow Coll; ME 67 Boston Univ; Sp-Lang Path, Guilford Public Schools, **SLP**

Lund, Josette V 2407 El Brio Court, Henderson, NV 89014, (702) 451-2307, BS 71 AZ St Univ; MS 74 AZ St Univ; Sp-Lang Path, Univ Med Ctr-S NV, **SLP**

Lund, Lori Ellen 15165 Danbury Avenue, Rosemount, MN 55068, (612) 423-6795, BA 85 Augustana Coll; MS 86 Eastern IL Univ; 88–Sp-Lang Path, Sp Lang Hrng Clinic, **SLP**

Lund, Mrs Marion 1600 Ponder Point Loop, Sandpoint, ID 83864, (208) 263-2914, BA 71 Univ of MT; MA 73 Univ of MT; Bonner Co Schl Dist, **SLP**

Lund, Mary Melissa 30965 Tamarack #32211, Wixom, MI 48096, (313) 624-0364, BA 83 Univ of ND; MS 84 Minot St Univ; **SLP**

Lund, Dr Nancy J 58 Lincoln Road, Snyder, NY 14226, (716) 878-5306, BS 63 Univ of ND; MS 68 Rutgers St Univ -N Brunswick; PH 72 (Sp Path) Univ of MD - College Park; 73–Prof, St U Coll, **SLP**

Lund, Mrs Shanna J E 13662 Park Street, Whittier, CA 90601-3852, MS 76 CA St Univ - Fullerton; SLP, Los Angeles Office of Educ, **SLP**

Lunda, Todd A 3440 Girard Avenue South, Apartment 1, Minneapolis, MN 55408-3853, (612) 339-0304, **A**

Lunday, Dr Audrey Mostoller Dept Communication Disorders, Minot State University, Minot, ND 58701, (701) 857-3030, BS 58 Saint Cloud St Univ; MA 59 OH St Univ; PH 67 (NS) OH St Univ; Professor, Minot State College, **SLP**

Lundblad, Anne Marie 4689 Greentree #A, Columbus, OH 43220, (614) 451-9409, **SLP**

Lunde, Mrs Florence K 2112 Starling Avenue, Bronx, NY 10462, (212) 491-1538, BS 62 NY Univ; MA 63 NY Univ; SLP Rehab Med, Columbia U Med Cen/Harlem Hosp, **SLP**

Lunde, Laura Katherine 782 South Vine Street, Denver, CO 80209, (303) 321-0651, BA 80 Univ of CA - Santa Barbara; MA 83 Univ of Denver; Aud-Neuro Spec, Denver Ear Inst, **A**

Lundeen, Dr Conrad Dept Speech Path & Audiology, West Virginia University, 805 Allen Hall P O Box 6122, Morgantown, WV 26506, (304) 293-4241, BA 72 SUNY - Center at Albany; MA 74 Northwestern Univ; PH 79 (Aud) Univ of IA; Assistant Professor, West Virginia University, **A**

Lundeen, Dr Dale J 1925 15th Avenue, Greeley, CO 80631, (303) 353-6843, BS 47 Western MI Univ; MA 49 IN Univ - Bloomington; PH 55 (NS) Univ of MN - Minneap-St Paul; Retired, U N Col, **SLP LM**

Lundeen, Mrs Deedra Jane West Virginia University, Box 6122, 805 Allen Hall, Morgantown, WV 26506-6122, (405) 232-6262, **A**

Lundergan, Mrs Mia Houk 711 Sperry Drive, Las Vegas, NM 87701-4939, (505) 425-6784, OB 74 Univ of NM; MS 84 Univ of NM; **SLP**

Lundgren, Gerry H Route 1 Box 43, Stanton, IA 51573, (712) 623-3488, BA 76 MS Univ for Women; MS 78 Memphis St Univ; SLP, Green Valley AEA #14, **SLP**

Lundgren, Kristine M P O Box 115, Cohasset, MA 02025, (617) 545-3417, BA 79 Univ of CT; MS 81 Boston Univ; Sp-Lang Path, Private Practice, **SLP ACE**

Lundstrom, Sheila L 575 Sunnywood Lane, Woodland Park, CO 80863, (719) 687-0771, MS 73 Univ of South FL; Sp-Lang Path, Penrose Hosp, **SLP**

Lundwall, Cherilyn J 3331 Jackson Avenue, Ogden, UT 84403, (801) 392-3658, BS 72 Brigham Young Univ; MS 74 Brigham Young Univ; **SLP**

Lundy, Donna S Department Of Otolaryngology, University Of Miami, P O Box 016960 (D-48), Miami, FL 33101, (305) 549-6101, BA 76 Univ of FL; MA 78 Univ of Miami; Sp-Lang Path, Jackson Mem Hosp, **SLP ACE**

Lundy, Mrs Marcia Cohn 2286 Autumn Lane, Lafayette Hill, PA 19444, (215) 828-8134, BA 76 Rutger's St Univ - Douglas Coll; OM 78 Hahnemann Univ Grad Sch; Sp-Lang Path, Private Practice, **SLP A**

Lundy, Mrs Nancy Lynn Heatherbank Rehab Center, 745 Chiques Hill Road, Columbia, PA 17512, (717) 684-7555, BS 82 CA Univ of PA; MS 83 CA Univ of PA; **SLP**

Luneckas, Mrs Ina Kristina 8431 Forest Drive, Hickory Hills, IL 60457, (312) 420-6540, BA 82 Saint Xavier Coll; MS 84 Governors St Univ; Sp-Lang Path, Assn Special Ed Dupage County, **SLP**

Lunger, Judith Gloria 1671 Woodland Avenue, Palo Alto, CA 94303, (408) 258-4923, **SLP**

Lunn, Mrs Joan Morgan 3 Boardman Lane, Topsfield, MA 01983, (508) 887-8297, BS 63 Emerson Coll; MS 68 Emerson Coll; SLP, Vna of N Shore, **SLP**

Lunn, Ronald A 43 Highview Road South, Denville, NJ 07834, (201) 977-2435, BA 70 KY Wesleyan Coll; MA 73 Newark St Coll; Aud, St Josephs Hosp & Med Cen, **SLP**

Lunsford, Mrs Deanna Roberts 1200 Arapahoe #A-1, Lincoln, NE 68502, (402) 223-2302, BA 86 LA Tech Univ; MA 88 LA Tech Univ; 88–Sp-Lang Path, Lincoln PS

Lunsford, Deborah B 10332 Lee Manor Drive, Manassas, VA 22110, (703) 369-1811, BA 75 Radford Univ; MA 77 George Washington Univ; Sp-Lang Path, Manassas City Public Schools, **SLP**

Lunsford, Marla Dee Route 1, Metropolis, IL 62960, (618) 524-4975, BS 84 1294; MS 87 Murray St Univ; 87–Sp-Lang Path, Dr Laurie Ballew Inc, **SLP**

Lunstad, Mrs Penny E 627 10th Street N E, Minot, ND 58701, (701) 838-8581, MS 87 Minot St Univ

Lunsted, Carol Lappin 6419 East Reynolds Road, Haslett, MI 48840, (517) 339-2820, MA 70 MI St Univ; MA 71 MI St Univ; MA 77 MI St Univ; **SLP**

Lunz, Ellen D 808 Leyden Lane, Wilmette, IL 60091, (312) 508-4050, BA 72 Univ of WI - Madison; MS 73 Univ of MI - Ann Arbor; 79–Sp-Lang Path, Chicago Board of Educ, **SLP**

Luongo, Patricia Marie 17 Turner Street, Salem, MA 01970, (508) 741-2748, MS 86 Boston Univ; 88–Sp-Lang Path, Perkins Sch for the Blind, **SLP**

Luongo, Rhonda Ruth 1080 Parrott Drive, Hillsborough, CA 94010, (415) 344-8865, BA 70 Univ of IA; ME 72 Univ of NC - Chapel Hill; SLP, Palo Atlo USD, **SLP**

Lupatkin, Robin Mara 14 Washington Avenue, Cobleskill, NY 12043, (607) 547-3291, BS 85 SUNY - Coll at Geneseo; MA 87 George Washington Univ; 88–Aud, The Mary Imogene Bassett Hosp, **A**

Lupella, Dr Robert O Cincinnati Ctr For Devel Dis, Speech And Hearing, 3300 Elland Avenue, Cincinnati, OH 45229, (513) 559-4628, OB 52 Southern IL Univ -Carbondale; MA 53 Southern IL Univ -Carbondale; PH 66 (NS) Northwestern Univ; 71–Dir Aud/Sp-Lang Path, Cincinnati Cen for Dev Dis, **SLP**

Luper, Dr Harold L Dept Audiology & Speech Path, University Of Tennessee, Knoxville, TN 37996-0740, (615) 974-5019, BA 49 Western MI Univ; MA 50 OH St Univ; PH 54 (Sp Science) OH St Univ; 63–Prof, U of TN, **SLP A F**

Lupinski, Michael Felix 743 North Van Dyke, Bad Axe, MI 48413, (517) 269-2251, BS 77; MA 78 1216; SLP, Hearing & Speech Clinic, **SLP**

Luplow, Catherine Ann 345 Fox Run, Libertyville, IL 60048, (312) 367-0242, BS 85 Northern IL Univ - De Kalb; MA 87 Northern IL Univ - De Kalb; 88–Sp-Lang Path, Darien SD #61, **SLP**

Lupo, Judith L 614 Langwood Drive, Houston, TX 77079, (713) 497-6947, BA 62 Emory Univ; ME 63 Emory Univ; SLP, Private Practice, **SLP**

Lupoletti, Nina L 17 Sparrow Lane, Huntington, NY 11743, (516) 367-3629, BA 84 NC St Univ at Raleigh; MS 86 Southern CT St Univ; **SLP**

Luppino, Marilyn A 400 Taunton Place, Buffalo, NY 14216-2019, BS 79 SUNY - Coll at Buffalo; MS 82 5533; SLP, Buffalo Bd of Ed, **SLP**

Lupton, Mrs Linda K 8485 N Pennsylvania Street, Indianapolis, IN 46240, (317) 646-8172, BS 72 Purdue Univ - West Lafayette; MS 74 Purdue Univ - West Lafayette; Aud, St Johns Med Cen, **A ACE**

Lupu, Susan Picker 982 Wenwood Drive, North Bellmore, NY 11710, (516) 679-0054, MA 84 Hofstra Univ; Audiologist, **A**

Lurie, Bonnie American Hearing Center Inc, 533 86th Street, Brooklyn, NY 11209, (212) 748-2630, BA 70 SUNY - Center at Buffalo; MA 73 IN Univ - Bloomington; Vp Dir Aud, Amer Hrng Cen Inc, **A**

Lusaitis, John Robert 6577 Hollow Drive, East Petersburg, PA 17520, (717) 397-9483, BS 81 PA St Univ - Univ Park; MS 83 PA St Univ - Univ Park; Aud, Audio Mobile Hearing Service, **A**

Lusby, Mrs Barbara Peterson 711 Beauregard Road, Summerville, SC 29483, (802) 745-5141, BS 75 Western MI Univ; MA 77 Temple Univ-Tyler Sch of Art; Sp-Lang Path, Healthcare Rehab Ctr, **SLP ACE**

Lusco, Alene M S 644 Helen Avenue, Terre Haute, IN 47802, (812) 234-8918, OB 43 Southern IL Univ -Carbondale; MS 51 IN St Univ - Terre Haute

Luse, Dr Eleanor M 325 Kempton Street #256, Spring Valley, CA 92077, (619) 267-7017, BS 28 Northwestern Univ; MS 34 Northwestern Univ; PH 48 (Voice Problems) Northwestern Univ; **SLP F LM**

Lusk, Elise Bernadette Laguna Honda Hospital Ward K-4, 375 Laguna Honda Hospital, San Francisco, CA 94116, (415) 664-1580, BS 81 CA St Univ - Hayward; MA 82 Univ of the Pacific; Sp-Lang Path, County of San Francisco, **SLP**

Lusk, Susan Lay 11033 Ferncliff Drive, Seneca, SC 29678, (803) 882-3237, BS 80 Winthrop Coll; MS 83 Univ of SC - Columbia; Sp-Lang Path, Center for Dev Pediatrics, **SLP**

Luskin, Wendy Marie 318 Avenue A, Doylestown, PA 18901, (215) 345-0554, BS 81 West Chester Univ of PA; MA 85 Trenton St Coll; **SLP**

Luss, Sandra L 5802 Lincoln Road, Newark, NY 14513, (315) 331-1700, BS 80 SUNY - Coll at Geneseo; MA 81 SUNY - Coll at Geneseo; Aud, Newark Dev Cen, **A**

Lustbader, Wendy 25-22 120th Street, Flushing, NY 11354, (718) 358-3704, BS 83 Boston Univ; MS 84 Boston Univ; Sp-Lang Path, The Herbert Birch Early Child, **SLP**

Luster, Mrs Thelma B 1300 Lafayette East #301, Detroit, MI 48207, (313) 393-2439, BS 59 Wayne St Univ; ME 64 Wayne St Univ; Tchr-Coord Hrng Conserv Prog, Detroit Pub Sch, **SLP**

Luster-Carpenter, Mary J 620 South Euclid, Pasadena, CA 91106, (818) 962-3311, BA 73 Coll of Saint Teresa; MS 75 Univ of WI - Madison; Sp-Lang Path, Baldwin Park USD, **SLP ACE**

Lustiber, Mrs Laurie A 619 Bennettwood Court, Cincinnati, OH 45230, (513) 231-7995, BA 78 Harvard Univ; MS 80 Boston Univ; 86–Mgr of Sp-Lang Path, Providence Hosp, **SLP**

Lustig, Beth E 15 O'Neill Court, Lawrenceville, NJ 08648, (609) 584-1359, BA 84 Univ of MD - College Park; MA 85 George Washington Univ; **SLP**

Lustig, Dr Vincent Frank P O Box 2229, Charleston, WV 25328, (304) 345-8522, BS 64 OH St Univ; MA 66 OH St Univ; PH 70 (NS) OH St Univ; Aud, Aud & Hrng Aid Sers, **SLP A**

Lustri, Jessye J J 309 El Rio, Modesto, CA 95351, **SLP**

Lute, Virginia M 166 Spruce Street #5, North Tonawanda, NY 14120, (716) 693-4254, BS 86 SUNY - Coll at Geneseo; MA 87 SUNY - Coll at Geneseo; 87–Sp-Lang Path, Niagara Co Sp Hrng and Lang Ctr, **SLP**

Luter, Dr James G, Jr 13117 Balboa Boulevard, Granada Hills, CA 91344, (213) 669-4355, BA 56 Univ of CA - Los Angeles; MA 63 Univ of CA - Los Angeles; PH 77 (NS) Univ of Southern CA; Sp/Dept Chair, Los Angeles City College, **SLP**

Luterman, Dr Barry F VA Medical Center, Asps (126), University & Woodland Avenue, Philadelphia, PA 19104, (215) 382-2400, BA 67 CUNY - Brooklyn Coll; MS 69 Univ of WI - Madison; PH 82 (Aud) Univ of MO - Columbia; 87–Aud, VA, **A**

Luterman, David M 5 Manning Street, Lexington, MA 02173, (617) 862-8658, BA 56 CUNY - Brooklyn Coll; MS 58 PA St Univ - Univ Park; ME 60 PA St Univ - Univ Park; Prof Commun Dis, Emerson Coll, **A F**

Luterman, Mrs Lillian B 65 Old Hill Road, Westport, CT 06880, (203) 227-6255, BA 67 McGill Univ - Quebec; MA 69 Emerson Coll; 85–Sp-Lang Path, Trumbull Bd of Educ, **SLP**

Lutey, James Christophe 4405 Concord, Saginaw, MI 48603, (517) 792-8771, BS 70 Central MI Univ; MA 83 Central MI Univ; 70–Sp-Lang Path, Saginaw Township Comm Schs, **SLP**

Lutgen, Mrs Kathleen Duerinck 6115 Spring Creek Oaks Dr, Spring, TX 77379, BS 77 Bradley Univ; MS 78 Bradley Univ; Sp-Lang Path, **SLP**

Luth, Mrs Tracy R 17902 San Leandro Lane, Huntington Beach, CA 92647, (213) 538-8414, BA 80 CA St Univ - Long Beach; MA 83 CA St Univ - Long Beach; Sp-Lang Path, Pace Therapy Inc, **SLP**

Luthanen, Mrs Carol Jokisch 505 North Walsh, Joliet, IL 60435, (815) 838-8080, BS 77 IL St Univ - Normal; MS 79 IL St Univ - Normal; 79–Sp-Lang Path, Lockport Area Spec Ed Coop, **SLP**

Luthas, Pamela J The Hear Center, 304 15th Avenue East, Seattle, WA 98112, (206) 562-9441, BS 78 Andrews Univ; MA 81 Western MI Univ; 84–Dir, The Hear Ctr, **A**

Luther, Mrs Laurie Lynn 15 Fisher Avenue, Nanuet, NY 10954, (914) 362-1350, BS 86 Bloomsburg Univ of PA; MS 87 Bloomsburg Univ of PA; 87–Sp-Lang Path, Loavenbruck Lynn & Cohen PC, **SLP**

Luther, Mary C 2857 Lasalle Avenue, Bronx, NY 10461, (212) 792-8750, BA 81 CA St Univ - Chico; MA 83 CA St Univ - Chico; Sp-Lang Path, Private Practice, **SLP**

Luthy, Sheila Snell 7226 Blanco Road #2504, San Antonio, TX 78216, (512) 532-9610, BA 79 Our Lady Lake Univ-San Anton; MA 86 Our Lady Lake Univ-San Anton; SLP, San Antonio State School, **SLP**

Lutolf, John J 27 Chatham Street, Chatham, NJ 07928, (201) 676-1000, BA 61 Seton Hall Univ; MA 69 Seton Hall Univ; Aud, VA Med Cen-E Orange, **A**

Luttrell, Mrs Sherri Robin 3708 15th Street West, Lehigh Acres, FL 33971, (605) 996-4932, BS 82 Northern St Coll; MS 84 Moorhead St Univ; SLP, Lee County School District, **SLP**

Lutz, Arlene Mae 7300 Beverly Street N E #16, North Canton, OH 44721, BA 74 Univ of Akron; MA 85 Kent St Univ; **SLP**

Lutz, Mrs Carol M 719 East Main, Mexia, TX 76667, (817) 562-6045, BA 75 Northeastern OK St Univ; MA 76 Univ of Tulsa; Sp-Lang Path, Private Practice, **SLP**

Lutz, Mrs Carolyn Louise 723 South Meridian Road, Mount Pleasant, MI 48858, BS 73 Central MI Univ; MA 79 Central MI Univ; SLP, Mount Pleasant Pub Sch, **SLP**

Lutz, Dennis R 1907 Loire Valley Road, Johnson City, TN 37601, (615) 926-1171, BS 72 WV Univ; MS 74 WV Univ; Sp-Lang Path, VA Med Cen, **SLP**

Lutz, Ellen Ruth Rd #1 Box 4, Tuthills Lane, Riverhead, NY 11901, (516) 289-2200, BA 75 SUNY - Coll at Geneseo; MA 82 SUNY - Coll at Geneseo; SLP, BOCES Supervisory District 2, **SLP**

Lutz, Mrs Judith G 25161 Burning Trail, Wheaton, IL 60187-5023, MS 73 Saint Louis Univ; Sp-Lang Path, Sch Dist of Clayton, **SLP**

Lutz, Konnie Clarke 506 East Osage, Paola, KS 66071, (913) 294-3190, BS 82 East TX St Univ - Commerce; MA 85 Southwest TX St Univ; **SLP**

Lutz, Margaret Mary 5781 Rayburn Avenue, Apartment A, Alexandria, VA 22311, (703) 379-0746, BS 77 Georgetown Univ; MA 82 George Washington Univ; Sp Lang Path, Private Practice, **SLP**

Lux, Cecelia Marie 4312 Crystal Circle, Cypress, CA 90630, (714) 826-4019, BA 72 CA St Univ - Long Beach; MA 84 CA St Univ - Long Beach; 87–Sp-Lang Path Dir, Private Practice, **SLP**

Lux, Mrs Elizabeth Pluim 205 Floyd Avenue #18, Modesto, CA 95350, (209) 522-8888, BA 37 Univ of CA - Berkeley; **SLP LM**

Lux, Lynn Louise 1105 North Depot, Apt #9, Knoxville, IA 50138, (515) 842-2719, BA 84 Univ of Northern IA; MA 85 Univ of Northern IA; 86–Sp-Lang Path, Heartland AEA, **SLP**

Luxenberg, Jan 26 Manor Road, Greenbrae, CA 94904, (415) 461-0336, MS 86 Gallaudet Coll; Aud, **A**

Lyall, Lisa Ann 25897 Butternut Ridge, North Olmsted, OH 44070, (216) 779-1520, BA 85 Baldwin-Wallace Coll; MA 86 Cleveland St Univ; **SLP**

Lybarger, Mrs Marceda W 7847 Park North Circle, Indianapolis, IN 46260, (317) 875-0898, BS 68 Purdue Univ - West Lafayette; MS 69 Purdue Univ - West Lafayette; **SLP**

Lybolt, Dr John T 2317 Oak, Northbrook, IL 60062, (312) 564-9230, BS 69; MS 70; PH 77 (NS) Northwestern Univ; SLP, Gottfred Speech Assoc, **SLP**

Lybrand, Roberta H 3501 Cotillion Avenue, Charlotte, NC 28210, (704) 861-1156, 80–Sp-Lang Path, Private Practice, **SLP**

Lybyer, Mrs Mary J HCR 9 Box 200, Huggins, MO 65484, (417) 967-3395, BS 75 Southwest MO St Univ; MA 78 Univ of MO - Columbia; Sp/Lang Path, Houston Missouri Sch Dist, **SLP**

Lydon, Kathleen Ann 5 Latania Lane, Chico, CA 95926, (916) 824-4891, BA 74 CA St Univ - Chico; MA 79 CA St Univ - Chico; Teacher, Tehama County Schools, **SLP**

Lydon, Mary D 4125 Lusk Drive, Sacramento, CA 95864, (916) 485-6711, BA 65 CA St Univ - Sacramento; MA 71 CA St Univ - Sacramento; 86–Dir of Prog, Easter Seal Soc of Sacra, **SLP ACE**

Lye, Mrs C Kathryn 115 Louisa Street, St Catharines, ON, Canada L2R 2K2, (416) 682-8608, BA 67 Univ of TX - Austin; MA 82 SUNY - Center at Buffalo; 87–Sp-Lang Path, Hotel Dieu Hosp, **SLP**

Lykes, Aloma Reed 1216 Riviera Avenue, New Orleans, LA 70122, (504) 483-7690, BS 74 Xavier Univ of LA; OM 76 LA St Univ - N O Medical Ctr; 88–Instr, Xavier Univ, **SLP**

Lyle, Mrs Barbara A 3433 Court Street, Sioux City, IA 51104, (712) 274-6040, BS 76 TX Christian Univ; MA 78 Univ of SD - Vermillion; SLP, Western Hills AEA 12, **SLP**

Lyle, Mrs Cheryl W 690 Carollo Drive, Slidell, LA 70458, (504) 641-2370, OM 84 LA St Univ - N O Medical Ctr; SLP, St Tammany Parish Sch Bd, **SLP**

Lyle, Dr Martha B 3158 Greenwood Street, Winter Park, FL 32792-1718, (305) 679-8274, BA 66 Montclair St Coll; ME 68 Univ of VA - Charlottesville; PH 72 (NS) Univ of FL; Sp-Lang Path, Seminole Co Schls, **SLP A**

Lyles, Melanie Kay 122 Lazy Lane, Sumter, SC 29150-4652, (803) 224-2173, BA 81 Univ of SC - Columbia; MA 85 Univ of SC - Columbia; **SLP**

Lyles, Mrs Sarah B J 7215 Smithfield Road, Columbia, SC 29223, (803) 786-1638, BA 72 SC St Coll; MA 77 SC St Coll; Sp-Lang Path, Lexington Sch Dist #5, **SLP**

Lyman, Charlotte Kay 1125 St Christopher Drive, Apartment 57, Russell, KY 41169, (606) 324-0465, BS 83 OH Univ - Athens; MA 86 Kent St Univ; Aud, Geiger Eastr Sls Sp & Hrng Cen, **A**

Lyman-McCann, Mrs Janet M 768 Long Hill Road, Middletown, CT 06457, (203) 633-5231, BA 76 Southern CT St Univ; MS 78 Emerson Coll; Sp/Lang Path, Town of Glastonbury, **SLP**

Lynaugh, Mae A 1425 Shoreline Drive, Santa Barbara, CA 93109, (805) 963-4331, BA 46 Coll of New Rochelle; ME 53 Boston Univ; Ch Sp-Lang Path, Santa Barbara Sch Dist, **SLP**

Lynch, Amy R P O Box 207, Waveland, MS 39576, BS 73 LA St Univ - Baton Rouge; MA 76 Memphis St Univ; Sp/Lang Path, St Tammany Parish Schs, **SLP**

Lynch, Anna M 5700 Ming Avenue #58, Bakersfield, CA 93309-0101, (805) 845-2946, BS 79 Northern AZ Univ; MA 86 Pacific Univ; Sp-Lang Path, Kern Co Supt of Schs, **SLP**

Lynch, Beverly Jean P O Box 125, Anderson, IN 46015, (317) 644-3617, BS 82 Purdue Univ - West Lafayette; MA 85 Ball St Univ; **A**

Lynch, Mrs Carol L 227 Beach Street, Northwood, OH 43619, (419) 698-2631, BS 78 Bowling Green St Univ; MA 87 Eastern MI Univ; **SLP**

Lynch, Mrs Carol Queen 56 Burkleigh Road, Towson, MD 21204, (301) 337-8668, BS 74 Towson St Univ; MS 75 Loyola Coll; SLP, **SLP**

Lynch, Constance E 13300 Ewood Lane, Silver Spring, MD 20906, (301) 897-5700, BS 68 Miami Univ - Oxford; MA 72 Univ of MD - College Park; Asst Dir State& Regulatory Pol, ASHA, **SLP**

Lynch, Dr Constance J P O Box 2384, APO New York, NY 09130-5368, BA 74 Univ of Northern IA; MA 75 Univ of Northern IA; PH 81 Univ of MN - Minneap-St Paul; **SLP**

Lynch, Eileen Marie 44 Atkins Street #3, Brighton, MA 02135, (617) 254-6892, BS 86 James Madison Univ; MS 88 Boston Univ; 88–Sp-Lang Path, Northeast Rehab Hosp

Lynch, Mrs Elizabeth J 1310 Parliament Drive, South Bend, IN 46637, (219) 282-4130, BA 46 Univ of the Pacific; MA 48 Univ of IA; Director of Spec Educ, South Bend Community Schools, **SLP**

Lynch, Mrs Gere C 5901 Searl Terrace, Bethesda, MD 20816, (301) 320-4365, BA 49 Catholic Univ of America; MA 63 Catholic Univ of America; Sp-Lang Path, Montgomery County Public Schs, **SLP**

Lynch, Mrs Gwendolyn 3628 Forest Garden Avenue, Baltimore, MD 21207, (301) 944-8171, MA 66 Temple Univ; BA 60 Morgan St Univ; **SLP**

Lynch, Dr Joan I Speech And Hearing Institute, University Of Texas, 1343 Moursund, Houston, TX 77030, (713) 792-4511, BA 53 IN Univ - Bloomington; MA 55 Northwestern Univ; ED 69 (Sp Path) Columbia Univ Teachers Coll; Assoc Prof, U of TX Hlth Sci Cen-Houston, **SLP F ACE**

Lynch, Mrs Joann L V 20 Niles Avenue, Middletown, NJ 07748, BS 49 Adelphi Univ; MA 67 Newark St Coll; Dir Sp-Hrng Dept, Riverview Med Ctr, **A ACE**

Lynch, Kathleen E 516 Andover Street, Lawrence, MA 01843, **SLP**

Lynch, Kelly J 701 North 2nd Street #8, Blytheville, AR 72315, (501) 762-1400, MA 88 Central MI Univ; 87–Aud, James L Canale MD FACS

Lynch, Laurel Rebecca 1105 West Inwood, Arlington, TX 76013, (817) 275-0452, MS 84 TX Christian Univ; BS 83 Baylor Univ; **SLP**

Lynch, Lauren L 307 South Oakland Avenue, Villa Park, IL 60181, (312) 345-9870, BA 74 Elmhurst Coll; MS 79 Governors St Univ; Sp-Lang Path, Madden Mental Health Center, **SLP**

Lynch, Linda Lee P O Box 463, Ellensburg, WA 98926, (509) 925-9921, BA 66 Univ of MT; MA 68 Univ of MT; Consultant, Private Practice, **SLP**

Lynch, Mrs Margaret Mary D 6733 Errick Road, North Tonawanda, NY 14120, (716) 694-3200, BS 75 SUNY - Coll at Buffalo; MS 81 SUNY - Coll at Buffalo; SLP, N Tonawanda Pub Sch

Lynch, Martha E 4712 Trousdale Drive, Nashville, TN 37220, (615) 832-8955, BS 58 Middle TN St Univ; MS 64 Vanderbilt Univ; Sp-Lang Path, Private Practice, **SLP**

Lynch, Mrs Mary P 215 Stanley Avenue, Hasbrouck Heights, NJ 07604, (201) 393-7179, BA 84 Iona Coll; MA 87 CUNY - Lehman Coll; 86–Sp-Lang Path, NY City Bd of Educ, **SLP**

Lynch, Onita C PO Box 843, Storrs, CT 06268, (203) 486-2629, BS 68 OK St Univ; MA 69 Univ of KS; MA 75 Gallaudet Coll; Aud, University of Connecticut, **A**

Lynch, Mrs Sharon A 76 Elmwood Drive, Clifton, NJ 07013, (201) 523-4037, BA 74 Montclair St Coll; MA 75 Montclair St Coll; Sp-Lang Path, Private Practice, **SLP**

Lynch, Susan L T 5406 South Kimbrough, Springfield, MO 65810-6742, (417) 864-3813, BA 73 Western KY Univ; ME 76 Univ of Louisville; 86–Sp-Lang Path, Speech & Language Clinic, **SLP**

Lynch, Teresa Ryan 4356 Nokomis Avenue South, Minneapolis, MN 55406, (612) 895-7240, Sp-Lang Path, Burnsville PS, **SLP**

Lynch-Bennett, Maureen E 86 Sunset Trail West, Fairport, NY 14450, (716) 377-4189, BA 71 Loyola Coll; MS 72 Syracuse Univ; 84–SLP, Rochester City Sch Dist, **SLP**

Lynch-Kenyon, Mrs Terri 9880 Bustleton Avenue, Centre One Bldg Suite 305, Philadelphia, PA 19115, (215) 673-6800, BS 84 PA St Univ - Univ Park; MA 87 Temple Univ; 88–Aud, Leonard Berenholz MD, **A**

Lyndes, Dr Kellogg O 2611 Arcadia Drive, Missoula, MT 59803, (406) 251-2653, BS 52 Univ of Denver; MA 70 Univ of Denver; PH 72 (NS) Univ of Denver; Associate Prof, U of Mt, **SLP LM**

Lyness, Elizabeth Susanne 7910 Wellesley Court, Pasadena, MD 21122, (301) 437-2400, BA 75 Loyola Coll; MA 76 Saint Louis Univ; 76–Sp-Lang Path, Anne Arundel County Pub Sch, **SLP**

Lynn, Anne H 18 Jenny Lane, Oxford, CT 06483, (203) 366-7551, MS 84 3019; Aud, Rehabilitation Center, **A**

Lynn, Cheryl 7642 Harbour Isle, Indianapolis, IN 46240, BA 62 IN Univ - Bloomington; MA 66 IN Univ - Bloomington; 75–Sp-Lang Path, Indiana School for the Blind, **SLP**

Lynn, Cindy F 122 Druid Oaks NE, Atlanta, GA 30329, (404) 237-6141, BA 86 Univ of FL; MA 88 Univ of FL; 88–Aud, Auditory Educ Ctr

Lynn, Mrs Corinne W 373 Hickory Grove, Thousand Oaks, CA 91320, (805) 583-6157, BA 76 CA St Univ - Northridge; MA 78 CA St Univ - Northridge; 88–Sp-Lang Path, Private Practice, **SLP**

Lynn, Mrs Cornelia Conrad 207 Pine Avenue, Severna Park, MD 21146, (301) 766-5511, BA 80 George Washington Univ; MA 82 George Washington Univ; Sp-Lang Path, Anne Arundel County Bd of Educ, **SLP**

Lynn, Deborah J 3240 Cambridge Avenue, Riverdale, NY 10463, (914) 362-1350, BS 75 SUNY - Coll at New Paltz; MS 77 Columbia Univ Teachers Coll; Audiologist, Loavenbruck Associates Pc, **A**

Lynn, Diana 221 Drakes Bay Avenue, Los Gatos, CA 95030-2769, (408) 227-8300, BS 69 West TX St Univ; ME 75 Southwest TX St Univ; Sp-Lang Path, Oak Grove School District, **SLP**

Lynn, Doyle L 527 Sharpless Street, West Chester, PA 19382, (215) 383-3850, BS 56 Bloomsburg Univ of PA; Asst Director/Special Educ, Chester County Indepen Unit 24, **SLP**

Lynn, Mrs Elizabeth A Route 254 Box 53, Northfield, CT 06778, (203) 567-9459, BS 78 Eastern MI Univ; MA 79 Eastern MI Univ; Sp-Lang Path, Litchfield PS, **SLP**

Lynn, Mrs Gail G 3804 Niami Street, Seaford, NY 11783, (516) 221-4025, BA 74 CUNY - Brooklyn Coll; MA 78 Hofstra Univ; Sp-Lang Path, Private Practice, **SLP**

Lynn, Mrs Gerene Rd 1, 165 Glenridge Road, Scotia, NY 12302, (518) 465-9060, BS 73 SUNY - Coll at Fredonia; MA 76 Coll of Saint Rose; Sp/Lang Path, Albny-Schoharie-Schen Co-BOCES, **SLP**

Lynn, Dr James M Dept Communicative Disorders, University Of Akron, Akron, OH 44325, (216) 375-7884, BS 67 Univ of IA; MA 69 Univ of IA; PH 75 (Aud) Univ of IA; Assoc Professor & Audiologist, U of Akron, **A**

Lynn, Jeannine 2213 Rogers Circle, Norman, OK 73071, (405) 321-4830, BA 74 Univ of OK - Norman; MS 75 Univ of OK Medical Center; 82–Sp-Lang Path, McCarty Cen Hndcpd Children, **SLP**

Lynn, Karen Lee 24565 Ashland Drive, Laguna Hills, CA 92653, (714) 839-3730, BA 73 Univ of LA Verne; MS 77 Univ of LA Verne; 85–Tchr-SDC-CH, Capistrano USD, **SLP**

Lynn, Mrs Karen Sue 145 Hunt Club Drive, #1-D, Akron, OH 44321, (216) 379-8645, BA 82 Univ of Akron; MA 84 Univ of Akron; 88–Aud, Childn's Hosp Med Ctr of Akron, **A**

Lynn, Mrs Margaret H 527 Sharpless Street, West Chester, PA 19382, (215) 692-6778, BS 55 West Chester Univ of PA; ME 60 PA St Univ - Univ Park; Superv/Sp-Lang-Hrng Services, Chester County Head Start Inc, **SLP**

Lynn, Mrs Mary Martha 383 Oradell Avenue, Oradell, NJ 07649, OB 70 Univ of VA - Charlottesville; MA 72 Univ of MD - College Park; **SLP**

Lynn, Michelle 7777 Southwest Freeway, Suite 812, Houston, TX 77074, (713) 995-0119, OB 65 TX Christian Univ; MS 68 Univ of WI - Madison; Owner, Private Practice, **SLP**

Lynn, Mrs Phyllis A 7900 N W 18th Court, Margate, FL 33063, (305) 979-3940, BA 75 Univ of Miami; MS 78 Univ of Miami; ME 86 Nova Univ; 88–Sp-Lang Path, Broward Co Sch Sys, **SLP**

Lynn, Susan G Rural Route 2, Cedar Rapids, IA 52404, (319) 369-7491, BS 74 Univ of IA; MA 76 Univ of IA; 85–Aud, St Luke's Hosp, **A**

Lynn, William M Route 254 Box 53, Northfield, CT 06778, (203) 482-0196, BS 78 Eastern MI Univ; MA 80 Eastern MI Univ; 81–Sp-Lang Path, Dmr Northwest Cen, **SLP**

Lynott, Mrs Cheryl Ann P O Box 353, Cresco, PA 18326, (717) 595-3756, BS 81 Marywood Coll; MS 84 Rutgers St Univ -N Brunswick; Slp, Intermed Unit 20, **SLP**

Lyon, Barbara J Coronet #803, 1314 Victoria Street, Honolulu, HI 96814, (808) 735-9003, BA 54 Univ of Cincinnati; MS 77 Univ of HI - Manoa; 83–Prog Craniofacial Coord, St of HI Dept of Health Svc, **SLP**

Lyon, Carolyn Kassel 308 N Canton Club Circle, Jackson, MS 39211, (601) 859-1440, BA 80 Univ of MS; MA 82 LA St Univ - Baton Rouge; Sp-Lang Path, Methodist Rehab Cen, **SLP ACE**

Lyon, Deborah Lee P O Box 3128, South Attleboro, MA 02703, (401) 277-5485, MS 80 Univ of RI; 88–Aud, Rhode Island Hosp, **A ACE**

Lyon, Dr Jon G Speech Pathology, VA Medical Center, 1000 Locust Street, Reno, NV 89502, (702) 786-7200, BA 67 Univ of CO - Boulder; MA 70 Univ of CO - Boulder; PH 74 (NS) Univ of CO - Boulder; Sp-Lang Path, VA Medical Center, **SLP**

Lyon, Jonathan Victor 1808 Sacramento Street, Berkeley, CA 94702, **SLP**

Lyon, Karen F 4714 South 30th Street, Arlington, VA 22206, (703) 671-9758, BS 82 Univ of WI - Stevens Point; MS 83 Ithaca Coll; SLP, The Lab School of Washington, **SLP**

Lyon, Katherine 5 Crystal Street, Melrose, MA 02176, **SLP**

Lyon, Mrs Maureen C 800 Prospect Street, Plantsville, CT 06479, (203) 574-8056, BA 76 Southern CT St Univ; MS 79 Southern CT St Univ; Sp-Lang Path, Bd of Ed Waterbury Ct, **SLP**

Lyons, Mrs Charisse Diane 14006 Princeton Avenue South, Savage, MN 55378-2037, (612) 451-1331, BA 83 Univ of MN - Duluth; MA 84 Univ of MN - Duluth; **SLP**

Lyons, Mrs Denise E 2326 Cripple Creek, Arlington, TX 76014, (817) 467-0568, BS 79 Baylor Univ; MS 80 Baylor Univ; 84–Sp-Lang Path, Arlington ISD, **SLP**

Lyons, Joy I 9608 Quail Run, Des Moines, IA 50322, (515) 993-4596, BA 77 Univ of Northern IA; MA 78 Univ of Northern IA; Sp-Lang Path, Heartland AEA, **SLP**

Lyons, Joy Lynn PO Box 34, Maddison, AL 35758, (205) 232-1379, MS 84 Univ Southern MS-Hattiesburg; SLP, **SLP**

Lyons, Leslie Ann 711 West Mount Drive, Apt 104, Los Angeles, CA 90069-5132, (213) 659-9365, MS 78 San Francisco St Univ; Administrator, Meadowbrook Head Inj Ctr of La, **SLP**

Lyons, Sr M Justine 4212 Karl Road, Columbus, OH 43224, (614) 267-5563, BA 57 Daemen Coll; MA 68 Catholic Univ of America; 85–Sp-Lang Path, Private Practice, **SLP ACE**

Lyons, Patricia Rose 769 Watertown Street, West Newton, MA 02165-2143, (215) 562-6312, **SLP**

Lyons, Mrs Shelley Byas Route 20 Box 316, Gray, TN 37615, (615) 477-2947, BS 84 East TN St Univ; MS 86 East TN St Univ; 88–Sp-Lang Path, Greene Valley Developmental Ctr, **SLP**

Lyons, Susan Blake 703 Pond Street, Syracuse, NY 13208-2801, (315) 422-6713, BA 80 SUNY - Center at Buffalo; MA 82 NY Univ; Sp-Lang Path, Seguin Community Svcs, **SLP**

Lyons, Teresa S 12831 North 42nd Street, Los Senderos #147, Phoenix, AZ 85032, (602) 953-0263, BA 69 Miami Univ - Oxford; MS 75 AZ St Univ; **SLP**

Lyons, Theresa M 1969 S W Park Avenue #907, Portland, OR 97201, (503) 280-6171, BS 55 Northern IL Univ - De Kalb; MA 62 Northern IL Univ - De Kalb; Sp-Lang Path, Sch Dist #1, **SLP**

Lysaght, Mrs Mary Conn 570 Hawthorne Drive, Adrian, MI 49221, BA 63 Univ of Tulsa; MS 65 Univ of OK Medical Center; **SLP**

Lystrup, Laura D 3077 Sand Dollar Way, Sacramento, CA 95821, (916) 991-1006, BS 76 IA St Univ; MA 77 Wichita St Univ; Sp-Lang Path, Private Practice, **SLP**

Lytle, Mrs Mary E A 322 Fowles Street, Oceanside, CA 92054, (619) 721-6511, BA 77 UT St Univ; OM 79 Univ of WA; Aud, **A**

Lytle, Pauline 738 Benicia Road, Vallejo, CA 94591, (707) 642-0942, BA 72 Coll of New Rochelle; MA 74 Northwestern Univ; MA 87; 76, **SLP**

Lytton, Beverly J 1800 7th Street, East Moline, IL 61244, (309) 755-1118, BA 61 Augustana Coll; MA 75 Western IL Univ; **SLP LM**

Lytton, Richard E 77 Blackstone Boulevard, Providence, RI 02906, (401) 438-9500, BA 72 George Washington Univ; MA 74 George Washington Univ; 79–Sp-Lang Path, Easter Seal Soc-RI, **SLP**

M

Maag, Gregory J 2 St Anthony's Way, Suite 109, Alton, IL 62002, (618) 465-0124, BS 79 Southern IL Univ-Edwardsvill; MA 80 Univ of IL - Urbana; Dir of Aud, Oto-Metrics Inc, **A**

Maag, O Eugene Speech And Hearing Center, Southern Illinois Univ, Edwardsville, IL 62026, (618) 465-0124, BA 49 Univ of Northern CO; MA 52 Univ of Northern CO; PH 66 (NS) Southern IL Univ -Carbondale; Prof of SLP & Aud, Southern Illinois University, **SLP A**

Maahs, Anne Marie 6655 Jackson Road, Lot 110, Ann Arbor, MI 48103, (517) 263-8931, BS 81 Central MI Univ; MA 82 Central MI Univ; 84–Sp-Lang Path, Lenewee Intermediate Sch Dist, **SLP**

Maas, Anne D 1321 Washington, Evanston, IL 60202, BA 73 Cornell Univ; MA 86 Northwestern Univ; **SLP**

Maas, Mrs Lynne Bradbury 184 Holiday Mobile Home Ct, North Liberty, IA 52317, BS 81 Worcester St Coll; MA 83 Univ of IA; SLP, Grant Wood AEA, **SLP**

Maatta, M'Elizabeth Ritchie 614 Fairchild Terrace, Manhattan, KS 66502-3718, (913) 233-5033, BS 79 Ithaca Coll; MA 83 Northwestern Univ; Aud, The Menninger Foundation, **A**

Mabbs, Linda Lu 1641 Dayton, St Paul, MN 55104, (612) 823-6660, BA 74 Univ of SD - Vermillion; MA 86 Univ of SD - Vermillion; **SLP**

Mabe, Denise M 2539 Porter, Wichita, KS 67204, (316) 838-1819, BA 80 Wichita St Univ; MA 81 Wichita St Univ; 87–Sp-Lang Path, Wesley Med Ctr, **SLP**

Mabe, Joan Loeffler Easter Seal Hr/Sp Center, 233 East Broadway, Louisville, KY 40202, (502) 584-9781, MS 84 Univ of Louisville; Audiologist, Easter Seal, **A**

Mabee, Mrs Ila Pirtle 1321 Pierce, Oregon City, OR 97045, (503) 653-3691, BS 61 Univ of OR; 73–SLP, N Clackamas Sch Dist, **SLP**

Mabee, Susan 9900 West Murdock, Wichita, KS 67212, (316) 833-3555, BA 77 Humboldt St Univ; MA 82 Humboldt St Univ; Sp-Lang Path, USD 259, **SLP**

Mabel, Suzanne S 11909 Paso Robles Avenue, Granada Hills, CA 91344, BS 58 Univ of CA - Los Angeles; MA 76 CA St Univ - Northridge; Aud, Los Angeles USD, **A**

Maben, Nancy E 1720 Camino DE La Costa #1, Redondo Beach, CA 90277, (213) 373-2946, BA 76 CA St Univ - Northridge; MA 78 CA St Univ - Northridge; SLP, Los Angeles Cnty Supt Schools, **SLP**

Mabie, Denise Ann 8241 Courtland Drive N E, Rockford, MI 49341-9401, (616) 961-7404, MA 85 Western MI Univ; **SLP**

Mabie-DeRuyter, Ann Moninne 3201 Mount Curve Avenue, Altadena, CA 91001, (213) 669-4593, MA 81 Univ of WA; Clinical Supervisor, Childrens Hospital Los Angeles, **A**

Mabis, Janet H R R 3 Box 180, Heim Road, Chandler, IN 47610, (812) 925-7258, BS 71 Univ of Cincinnati; MS 72 Vanderbilt Univ; Sp-Lang Path, Private Practice, **SLP**

Mabry, Lisa Rai 3820 Nicolasvillle Road, Apartment 1209, Lexington, KY 40503-4485, (606) 271-3916, BA 85 Univ of KY; MS 87 Univ of KY; **SLP**

MacAllister, Lance J P O Box 2571, Salisbury, MD 21801, (301) 742-4977, BA 70 Univ of AZ; ME 74 Bloomsburg Univ of PA; Dir Sp & Hrng, Holly Cen, **SLP ACE**

Macaluso, James T 301 East Avenue, Lockport, NY 14094, (716) 433-7090, BS 72 Syracuse Univ; MA 75 SUNY - Center at Buffalo; Owner, Lockport Hrng Consults, **A**

MacAngus, Shona Jane 82 Thatcher Drive, Winnipeg, MB, Canada R3T 2L5, (204) 945-7912, BA 86 Univ of ND; MA 87 SUNY - Coll at Plattsburgh; 87–Sp-Lang Path, Manitoba Educ

Macari, Marylou 80 Fallwood Parkway, Farmingdale, NY 11735, (516) 454-0026, BA 84 Hofstra Univ; MA 86 Hofstra Univ; 87–Aud, Wilks Hearing Ctr, **A**

MacArthur, Karen 43 Edgemere Road, Mount Arlington, NJ 07856, (201) 770-3760, Sussex County Educ Commission, **SLP**

MacAuley, Kelly Ann 227 South Oak Park Avenue, Oak Park, IL 60302, (312) 848-1641, BS 80 Univ of WI - Madison; MA 83 Univ of IA; 86–Lecturer/Aud, Northwestern Univ, **A**

MacCalous, Jean 454 Norfolk Road, Torrington, CT 06790, (203) 482-7183, BA 80 Kean Coll of NJ; MA 85 Univ of MA - Amherst; Sp-Lang Path, State of CT/Dept of Mental Ret, **SLP**

MacCammond, Mrs Mickie S, III Mid-Cities Sp & Hrng Clinic, 1701 W Euless Boulevard, Suite 210, Euless, TX 76040, (817) 283-3191, BA 75 LA Tech Univ; MA 76 LA Tech Univ; Owner, Mid Cities Sp/Hrng Cl, **SLP**

MacChello, Ronda M 3614 McNulty Way, Redwood City, CA 94061, BA 72 Stanford Univ; MS 74 Univ of WI - Madison; **SLP**

MacChio, Elaine A 95 Elwyn Street, Cranston, RI 02920, (401) 942-8826, **SLP**

MacCracken, Ellen Louise 22130 Millard Avenue, Richton Park, IL 60471, (312) 702-1923, BS 83 Bradley Univ; MS 85 Rush Univ; 86–Sp-Lang Path, Univ of Chicago Med Ctr, **SLP**

MacDonald, Carol A 505 Fishermans Road, Norfolk, VA 23503, (804) 587-5092, BS 73 Bradley Univ; MS 75 Bradley Univ; Sp-Lang Path, **SLP**

MacDonald, Catherine 5321 Irving Avenue South, Minneapolis, MN 55419, **SLP**

Macdonald, Charlene Alexandra Cratt Apartment 203, 1 Clark Street, St Catharines, ON, Canada L2R 7L5, (416) 688-3550, BA 82; MA 86 SUNY - Center at Buffalo; 86–Sp-Lang Path, Niagara Peninsula Children's Ctr, **SLP**

MacDonald, Mrs D Hannah 1106 Navaho Trail, Richardson, TX 75080, (214) 235-4825, BA 59 Univ of CO - Boulder; MS 75 Southern Methodist Univ; Sp-Lang Path, Richardson ISD, **SLP**

MacDonald, Deborah Crabbs 426 South Street, Bennington, VT 05201, (802) 442-6361, BS 79 Ithaca Coll; MS 82 Purdue Univ - West Lafayette; Sp-Lang Path, Vermont Med Center, **SLP**

MacDonald, Mrs Diane Newell R R 4 Box 330, Minot, ND 58701, (701) 857-4410, MA 84 Minot St Univ; Aud, Souris Valley Spec Serv, **A**

MacDonald, Elizabeth Anne 2722 Inverloch Circle, Duluth, GA 30136, (404) 623-0153, BS 83 Western MI Univ; ME 86 Univ of GA; 86–Aud, VA Med Ctr, **A**

MacDonald, Dr James D The Nisonger Center, 1580 Cannon Drive, Columbus, OH 43210, PH (NS); **SLP**

MacDonald, Shirley R 25202 Rouge River Drive, Dearborn Heights, MI 48127, (313) 493-6315, BA 59 Wayne St Univ; MA 70 Wayne St Univ; Sp-Lang Path, Sinai Hosp of Detroit, **SLP**

MacDonald, Mrs Theresa D 3210 Danville Road, Brandywine, MD 20613, (202) 877-6717, BS 80 Univ of MD - College Park; MA 81 George Washington Univ; Aud, Washington Hosp Cen, **A**

MacDonell, Mrs Ellen Mindy 1435 Landis Circle, Bel Air, MD 21014, (301) 893-2397, BA 83 Univ of MD - College Park; ME 86 Trenton St Coll; 88–Sp-Lang Path, Harford Co Sch Sys, **SLP**

MacDougall, Mrs Mary Donnelly P O Box 198, HHC Setaf, APO New York, NY 09168, BA 75 Univ of MA - Amherst; MS 83 Univ of NC - Chapel Hill; Sp-Lang Path, Dept of the Army, **SLP**

MacDougall, Maryann Izzo 7 Purvis Street, Watertown, MA 02172, (617) 926-9863, BA 78 Northeastern Univ; ME 80 Northeastern Univ; Sp-Lang Path, Choate Symmes Health Svcs, **SLP**

Mace, Mrs Linda S St Josephs Hospital, Speech Therapy Department, 19th And Murdoch Avenue, Parkersburg, WV 26101, (304) 424-4277, BS 70 Kent St Univ; MA 72 Kent St Univ; Dept Hd/SLP, St Joseph's Hosp, **SLP**

Mace, Mrs Shirley C Route 3 Box 249, Marion, SC 29571, (803) 423-3927, BS 74 Longwood Coll; ME 75 Univ of VA - Charlottesville; **SLP**

MacElrevey, Mary Denise 8878 Rising Sun Avenue, Philadelphia, PA 19115, (215) 671-9084, MS 83 Hahneman Medical Coll; MA 83 Hahneman Medical Coll; Aud/Sp-Lang Path, Private Practice, **SLP A**

Macey, Mrs Esther B 515 East Poplar Avenue, San Mateo, CA 94401, (415) 342-3558, BA 40 Stanford Univ; Assoc Dir/SLP, Poplar Center, **SLP**

MacGill, Debra Anne Deer Lodge Centre, 2109 Portage Avenue, Winnipeg, MB, Canada R3J 0L3, (204) 831-2147, MS 85 Minot St Univ; 86–Sp-Lang Path, Deer Lodge Centre, **SLP**

MacGregor, Mrs Charlene J 10532 South Oak Avenue, Chicago Ridge, IL 60415, (312) 636-9088, BS 64 IL St Univ - Normal; 88–Sp-Lang Path, SW Cook Co Coop for Spec Educ, **SLP**

MacH, Mary Ann L PO Drawer B, Gulfport, MS 39502, (601) 863-0583, BS 56 Univ Southern MS-Hattiesburg; MS 65 Univ Southern MS-Hattiesburg; 76–Sp-Lang Path, Harrison Co Trng Cen Excep Chd, **SLP**

MacHado, Elisa Celeste P O Box 784513, Sandton 2146, Transvall, South Africa, BS 86 Univ of NH; MS 88 Univ of NH

Machart, Victor Eugene Box 44, Underwood, ND 58576, (701) 442-3201, MS 82 Minot St Univ; 80–Sp-Lang Path, Souris Valley Spec Svcs, **SLP**

MacHefsky, Kathryn A 725 Swarthmore Lane, University City, MO 63130, (314) 361-4565, **SLP**

Machella, Mary W 2021 Sunshine Avenue, Johnstown, PA 15905, (800) 722-0097, BS 75 Indiana Univ of PA; MS 80 Indiana Univ of PA; 83–Sp-Lang Path, Lee Hosp, **SLP**

MacHen, Mrs Nancy Knapp 423 Croydon Road, Baltimore, MD 21212, (301) 368-6078, BS 81 Towson St Univ; MS 83 Loyola Coll; Sp-Lang Path, Audiology Associates Inc, **SLP**

MacHin, Mrs Karen Louise 428 A Street, Encinitas, CA 92024-3222, (619) 943-1279, BA 80 CA St Univ - Chico; MA 83 CA St Univ - Long Beach; Sp-Lang Path, Private Practice, **SLP**

MacHinske, Kevin Arthur 3659 W 11th Street, Indianapolis, IN 46222, (317) 635-7401, MS 86 Purdue Univ - West Lafayette; 88–Aud, VA, **A**

MacHiorlatti, Mrs Carol Oddo 2335 Brighton Drive S E, East Grand Rapids, MI 49506, (616) 243-2840, ME 71 Wayne St Univ; **SLP**

Machon, Marsha W 4 Sunnyside Drive, Durham, NH 03824, (603) 868-5527, BA 68 Univ of MD - College Park; MA 69 Univ of MD - College Park; **SLP**

MacHtolff, Kim M 355 South Bayly Avenue, Louisville, KY 40206, BS 78 Eastern KY Univ; ME 82 Eastern KY Univ; 87–Sp-Lang Path, UCP Kids Ctr, **SLP ACE**

Maclas, Lori Anne 5412 Bret Court, Jefferson City, MO 65101, (314) 893-7786, MA 86 Univ of MO - Columbia; **SLP**

Maclejewski, Theresa Marie 11630 Blackhawk #6, Mokena, IL 60448, (312) 479-5583, BS 85 Northern IL Univ - De Kalb; MS 87 IL St Univ - Normal

Maclel, Karen J 13751 DE Vries Road, Lodi, CA 95240, (209) 948-8762, BA 75 CA St Univ - Stanislaus; MA 75 CA St Univ - Stanislaus; Sp-Lang Path, Private Practice, **SLP**

Maclel, Sabrina Dunham 729 Pawnee, Hewitt, TX 76643, (817) 666-3957, OB 85 Hardin-Simmons Univ; MS 87 Baylor Univ; 88–Sp-Lang Path, Hillcrest Baptist Med Ctr, **SLP**

MacIntosh, Karen M 900 Minnesota Avenue, Owatonna, MN 55060-3647, **SLP**

MacIntosh, Rita G 744 Carpenter Lane, Philadelphia, PA 19119, MS; **SLP LM**

MacIntyre, Patricia G 3108 Huntington Road, Shaker Heights, OH 44120, (216) 231-8787, BA 45 Case Western Reserve Univ; MA 68 Case Western Reserve Univ; 86–Dir Infant/Toddler Proj, Cleveland Hearing & Sp Ctr, **SLP ACE**

Maclone, Michael John 12 Water Street #111, Mystic, CT 06355, (203) 447-0301, BA 84 Univ of CT; MA 85 SUNY - Coll at Plattsburgh; Aud, CT St Dept of Mr, **A**

Maclone, Mrs Nancy E L 215 Glenwood Avenue, New London, CT 06320, (203) 536-4957, BA 75 Southern CT St Univ; MS 78 Southern CT St Univ; Sp/Lang Path, Groton Bd of Ed, **SLP**

Maclosek, Rae Ann 1776 Freemont Avenue South, Minneapolis, MN 55403, (612) 489-8035, BS 76 Univ of MN - Duluth; MA 77 Univ of MN - Duluth; SLP, St Paul Pub Sch, **SLP**

MacIsaac, Diane M 754 Golfview Terrace, Buffalo Grove, IL 60089, (312) 537-8055, BS 82 OK St Univ; OM 83 LA St Univ - N O Medical Ctr; 86–SLP-Parent Infant Educ Prog, Nsseo, **SLP**

MacIsaac, Mrs Lorri W 2815 Broadlawn Drive, Erie, PA 16506, (814) 459-2755, BS 69 Edinboro Univ of PA; MA 74 SUNY - Coll at Fredonia; Sp/Lang Path, Erie Co Crpld Chldn Cen, **SLP ACE**

MacIver, Mrs Margaret L 10111 Colesville Road, Silver Spring, MD 20901, (301) 434-4854, BA 35 OH Univ - Athens; OB 38 Univ of Cincinnati; MA 64 George Washington Univ; **SLP LM**

MacIver, Nora L 133 Saratoga Road, Apt #J16, Scotia, NY 12302, (518) 842-2100, BS 83 Central MI Univ; MA 86 Western MI Univ; Aud, Amsterdam Memorial Hospital

Mack, Mrs Constance P Fearn P O Box 539, Lanham, MD 20706, (301) 336-1262, BS 63 Univ of the DC; 70–Sp-Lang Path, Prince George's Co Pub Sch, **SLP**

Mack, Erminia D 481 Grove Street, Glencoe, IL 60022, (312) 835-0064, BS 72 Marquette Univ; MS 75 Marquette Univ; Sp-Lang Path, Cove Sch, **SLP**

Mack, Janne Himes Randolph ENT Associates, 3535 Randolph Road, Randolph Bldg Suite 100, Charlotte, NC 28211, (704) 365-0711, BS 70 Miami Univ - Oxford; ME 75 Univ of VA - Charlottesville; Aud, Private Practice, **A**

Mack, Karolyn J CSHS Speech & Hearing Clinic, Lenox Baker Children's Hosp, 3000 Erwin Road, Durham, NC 27705, (919) 684-6669, BA 63 San Jose St Univ; MS 64 Purdue Univ - West Lafayette; 86–Dir CS Cl, St of NC-Dept of Human Res, **SLP**

Mack, Linda 1247 SE 11th Avenue, Gainesville, FL 32601, (904) 371-4153, BA 82 SC St Coll; MA 84 Univ of FL; **SLP**

Mack, Ronald Andrew 6209 Reseda Blvd, Apartment 227, Reseda, CA 91335, (818) 705-7903, BS 85 Northwestern Univ; MS 87 Univ of AZ; Sp-Lang Path, Kaiser Permanente, **SLP**

Mackall, Jane M 6404 Charles Avenue, Parma, OH 44129, (216) 888-0924, BS 83 John Carroll Univ; MA 87 Cleveland St Univ; **A**

Mackay, Ann Catherine 7650 Courtney Campbell CSY, Suite 300, Tampa, FL 33607, (813) 888-7700, BS 77 Univ of VA - Charlottesville; MA 80 Univ of FL; Training Supervisor, NY Life Ins Co, **SLP**

Mack-Balitz, Mrs Aileen 115 Emann Drive, Camillus, NY 13031, (315) 488-2951, BA 71 Saint Bonaventure Univ; MS 72 Syracuse Univ; OM 85 Syracuse Univ; Dir-Prof Serv, St Camillus Resident Care Fac, **SLP**

MacKenzie, Barbara B 10210 Hadley Avenue N, White Bear Lake, MN 55110, BA 69 Univ of MN - Minneap-St Paul; MS 83 Univ of WI - River Falls; **A**

MacKenzie, Charla Bodimer 61 Halliday Heights, Gallipolis, OH 45631, (614) 446-0318, BS 69 OH St Univ; MA 71 OH Univ - Athens; Tag Prog Coord, Gallia County Local Schools, **SLP**

MacKenzie, Douglas Joseph Audiology Department, NTID, One Lomb Memorial Drive, Rochester, NY 14623, (716) 475-6384, BA 80 SUNY - Coll at Oswego; MA 82 SUNY - Coll at Geneseo; Aud, NTID, **A ACE**

MacKenzie, Dr Elizabeth H 1200 Sixth Street SW #802, Calgary, AB, Canada T2R 1H3, (403) 233-2283, BA 70 Univ of Manitoba - Winnipeg; MA 74 Univ of ND; PH 82 (NS) Univ of WI - Madison; Sp-Lang Path, E H MacKenzie & Associates Inc, **SLP**

MacKenzie, Janet Hanbery 19 Victoria Drive, Atherton, CA 94025, (415) 854-4433, BA 81 San Jose St Univ; MA 83 San Jose St Univ; Sp-Lang Path, Menlo Park City School Dist, **SLP**

MacKenzie, Shirley R 254 Taylor Street, Granby, MA 01033, (413) 323-6311, BS 74 Univ of MA - Amherst; MS 76 Univ of RI; Superv Speech/Hearing Services, Belchertown State School, **SLP**

MacKenzie, Vicki 26 Strawberry Patch Lane, Stamford, CT 06902, (203) 359-1185, BA 73 CUNY - Queens Coll; MA 76 Hofstra Univ; Sp-Lang Path, Private Practice, **SLP**

MacKenzie-Laxague, Judy L 821 North Rios Avenue, Solana Beach, CA 92075, (619) 259-7678, BA 79 San Diego St Univ; MA 82 San Diego St Univ; Sp-Lang Path, Private Practice, **SLP**

MacKenzie-Stepner, Mary Karen 348 Mapleleaf Drive, Toronto, ON, Canada M6L 1P6, (416) 598-6105, MS 82 Univ of Toronto - Ontario; 85–Sp-Lang Path, Hospital for Sick Children, **SLP ACE**

MacKersie, Carol L 320 West 96th Street 3F, New York, NY 10025, (212) 308-5855, BA 77 Univ of MI - Ann Arbor; MA 80 San Diego St Univ; 88–Aud, Columbia-Presbyterian Eastside Assoc, **A**

Mackey, April F 340 Oak P O Box 427, Presho, SD 57568, (605) 895-2662, BA 76; MA 79 Univ of SD - Vermillion; Sp-Lang Path, Lyman District Schools, **SLP**

Mackey, Barbara Raymond 2892 Fischer Place, Cincinnati, OH 45211, (606) 344-2221, BS 80 Univ of Cincinnati; MA 81 Western MI Univ; Aud, St Elizabeth Medical Center, **A**

Mackey, Catherine Hadley 3906 Council Crest, Madison, WI 53711, (608) 231-2186, BS 78 Univ of WI - Madison; MS 80 Univ of WI - Madison; Sp-Lang Path, New Glarus Schs, **SLP**

Mackey, Maureen Jane 38255 Fairway Court #81C, Mount Clemens, MI 48044, (313) 939-2290, BA 82 MI St Univ; MA 83 SUNY - Coll at Geneseo; Sp-Lang Path, MacOmb ISD, **SLP**

Mackey, Mrs Sandra M O 2 Lisa Lane, Spring Valley, NY 10977, (914) 735-0361, MS 78 Montclair St Coll; Sp-Lang Path, Private Practice, **SLP**

Mackey, Mrs Teresa Ann 1866 Muchacha Drive, Henderson, NV 89015, (702) 329-1075, BS 81 Univ of NV - Reno; MS 83 Univ of NV - Reno; Sp-Lang Path, Private Practice, **SLP**

Mackey, Mrs Thada W P O Box 994, League City, TX 77573, (713) 332-9575, BS 69 Univ of Houston - Univ Park; MA 70 Univ of Houston - Univ Park; Sp-Lang Path, Clear Creek ISD, **SLP**

Mackey, Mrs Virginia R 126 White Oak Drive, Lancaster, PA 17601, (717) 295-8327, BA 75 Univ of OK - Norman; MA 76 George Washington Univ; Administrative Director P M R, Lancaster Gen Hosp, **SLP**

Mack-Hess, Mrs Joalyn Dawn 1170 Yank Street, Golden, CO 80401, BA 79 Univ of Northern CO; MA 80 Univ of Northern CO; **SLP**

MacKie, Mrs Elizabeth Ann 6207 Hibbling Avenue, Springfield, VA 22150, (703) 943-3101, BA 83 Boston Coll; ME 85 Univ of VA - Charlottesville; **SLP**

MacKin, Mrs Anita Marion Box 275, 603 Hatherly Road, Minot, MA 02055, (617) 545-6700, BA 65 San Diego St Univ; MA 69 Boston Univ; Sp-Lang Path, Scituate Pub Sch, **SLP ACE**

MacKin, Christine Lynn 832 Rose Boulevard, Highland Heights, OH 44143, (216) 449-0152, BA 85 Cleveland St Univ; MA 87 Cleveland St Univ; 87–Sp-Lang Path, So Euclid-Lyndhurst City Schs, **SLP**

MacKin, Karen Marie 189-04 64th Avenue #9I, Fresh Meadows, NY 11365, (212) 454-7866, BA 82 CUNY - Queens Coll; MA 85 Long Island U - CW Post Ctr; **SLP**

MacKin, Susan C 641 212th Street, Dyer, IN 46311, (219) 931-8420, BA 77 Ball St Univ; MA 79 Ball St Univ; Mgr, Buchele Hrng Aid Cen, **A**

MacKinnon, Elizabeth 26 Guildford Court, London, ON, Canada N6J 3Y1, (519) 472-3095, **SLP**

MacKins, Cynthia Campos 1255 5th Avenue #5-E, New York, NY 10029, (212) 598-4327, BA 82 Saint John's Univ - Jamaica; MS 87 CUNY - Brooklyn Coll

MacKisack-Morin, Eleanor Louise 837 Botetourt Gardens, Norfolk, VA 23507, (804) 928-8250, BS 82 Univ of HI - Manoa; MA 84 George Washington Univ; 87–Dir Sp-Lang Path, Riverside Rehab Institute, **SLP**

MacKlem, Mrs Janet Sixel 21768 Poppleton Avenue, Elkhorn, NE 68022, (402) 289-2298, BS 63 Univ of NE - Lincoln; MS 87 Univ of NE - Omaha; 87–Sp-Lang Path, Westside Comm Schs Dist 66, **SLP**

Mack Nair, Mrs Anne Elizabeth 15 Wellesley Court, Londonville, NY 12211, (518) 462-6222, BS 83 Coll of Saint Rose; MS 82 Coll of Saint Rose; 88–Sp-Lang Path, Britton Kill Central Sch, **SLP**

Mackowiak, Diane Stec 8936 South 83rd Court, Hickory Hills, IL 60457, (312) 687-0900, BS 79 IL St Univ - Normal; MS 82 Governors St Univ; Sp/Lang Path, SW Cook Co Coop Assoc/Sp Ed, **SLP**

MacLachlan, Dr Barbara Gayle 75-66 199th Street, Fresh Meadows, NY 11366, (212) 947-5770, BA 74 Univ of Redlands; MS 76 Univ of Redlands; PH 87 (Communicative Disorders) Univ of WI - Madison; 88–Sp-Lang Path, Brooklyn Coll-CUNY, **SLP**

MacLaren, Jeanne E 121 South Navarra, Scotts Valley, CA 95066, (408) 462-7735, BA 71 CA St Univ - Long Beach; MA 73 CA St Univ - Long Beach; Coordinator Communication Dis, Dominican Santa Cruz Hospital, **SLP**

MacLaren, Suzanne Carol 5301-6651 Ranchview Dr N W, Calgary, AB, Canada T3G 1P3, (403) 270-1358, BA 81 Univ of British Columbia; MA 85 Western WA Univ; **A**

MacLean, Mrs Carol Pavlick 526 West Sedgwick Street, Philadelphia, PA 19119, (215) 848-1620, BS 78 PA St Univ - Univ Park; MA 83 West Chester Univ of PA; SLP, Sch Dist of Phil, **SLP**

MacLean, Christina Marie 169 Washington Street #5, Newton, MA 02158, (617) 965-3366, BA 84 Boston Coll; MA 85 George Washington Univ; **SLP**

MacLean, Sandra C Washington Audiology Services, 7001 Perimeter Road South, Seattle, WA 98108, (206) 764-3330, BS 77 Univ of WA; MA 78 Western WA Univ; Audiologist/President, Washington Audiology Services, **A**

MacLearie, Elizabeth 1742 Diamond Street #8, San Diego, CA 92109, (619) 270-0134, MS; **SLP F LM**

MacLellan, Maryanne 3675 Barnard Drive #206, Oceanside, CA 92056, (619) 471-1198, BA 76 San Diego St Univ; MA 84 San Diego St Univ; Sp-Lang Path, Associated Speech Pathologists, **SLP**

MacLeod, Mrs Cynthia Soforenko 105 Harvest Drive, Lafayette, LA 70508, (318) 232-7604, OB 81 Univ of Southwestern LA; MS 84 Univ of OK - OK City; **SLP**

MacLeod, Mrs Kimberly S Route 1 Box 360, Orrington, ME 04474, BS 78 Bloomsburg Univ of PA; MS 79 Bloomsburg Univ of PA; Sp-Lang Path, Griffiths-Larrabee, Inc, **SLP**

MacLeod, Mrs Nancy J N2503 Ullom Road, Monroe, WI 53566, (608) 328-0130, BS 63 Univ of WI - Madison; MS 64 Univ of WI - Madison; Tchr, Sch Dist of Monroe, **SLP**

MacMillan, Claudia J 605-5750 Larch Street, Vancouver, BC, Canada V6M 4E2, (604) 266-8496, BA 72 Simon Fraser Univ - Bc; MA 74 WA St Univ; 84–Coord of Spec Educ, BC Ministry of Educ, **SLP**

MacMillan, Dana Lillian Rt 2 Box 134, Aberdeen, NC 28315, (919) 295-0243, BS 83 Univ of GA; ME 86 Univ of GA; Aud, Pinehurst Surg Clnc, **A**

MacMillan, Kathleen W 213 Seville Place, Starkville, MS 39759, (601) 323-7486, BA 74 Univ of WA; MS 76 Univ of WA; 88–Sp-Lang Path, Private Practice, **SLP**

MacMullin, Keith A 184 City View Drive, Rochester, NY 14625, (716) 271-0680, BS 75 SUNY - Coll at Geneseo; MA 78 Univ of CT; Sp-Lang Path, Rochester City School District, **SLP**

MacNeil, Donna M Waltr Reed Army Medical Ctr, Army Aud & Speech Center, Washington, DC 20307-5001, (202) 576-1650, BS 74 Towson St Univ; MA 76 Univ of MD - College Park; Audiologist, Army Aud & Sp Cen, **A**

MacNeil-Brint, Kathleen M 919 Nardo #4, Encinitas, CA 92024, (619) 944-7573, BA 82 San Diego St Univ; MA San Diego St Univ

MacOmb, Mrs Carol Krause 1759 Salem Drive, Emmaus, PA 18049, (215) 965-5349, BA 80 Univ of CT; MS 82 Southern CT St Univ; Sp-Lang Path, Private Practice, **SLP**

Macon, Cynthia Rutherford 4111 Lone Oak Road, Nashville, TN 37215, (615) 327-4658, BS 78 TN Tech Univ; MS 81 Vanderbilt Univ; Sp-Lang Path, Baptist Hospital, **SLP**

MacPeek, June Marie R R 1 Box 110A, Millbrook, NY 12545, (914) 677-5471, BS 85 SUNY - Coll at Buffalo; MS 86 SUNY - Coll at Fredonia; **SLP**

MacPhail, Mrs Josephine Ruth R R 2 Box 88, c/o Ned Macphail, Greencastle, IN 46135, (317) 653-9771, BS 73 IN St Univ - Terre Haute; MS 85 IN St Univ - Terre Haute; **SLP**

MacPherson, Colin A 1964 Woodmont Court, Canton, MI 48188, (313) 764-8442, BS 77 Central MI Univ; MA 79 Central MI Univ; Asst Director/Speech Camp, University of Michigan, **SLP**

MacPherson, Helen Margaret 118 Village Green North, Riverside, RI 02915, (401) 438-0806, BS 27 Boston Univ; MA 52 Case Western Reserve Univ; PH 70 (NS) RI Coll; **A LM**

MacPherson, Mary A 2840 Washington Street, Alameda, CA 94501, (816) 521-5908, BA 72 Holy Names Coll; MA 83 Univ of San Francisco; Sp-Lang Path, Private Practice, **SLP**

MacPherson, Mrs Mary E 1611 North Pontiac Drive, Janesville, WI 53545, (608) 755-0306, BS 75 Univ of WI - Whitewater; MS 80 Univ of WI - Whitewater; Sp-Lang Path, Private Practice, **SLP**

MacPherson, Dr Robert H P O Box 9573, Asheville, NC 28815, (704) 298-7911, BA 47 Tufts Univ; MA 65 Syracuse Univ; PH 68 (NS) Syracuse Univ; Chief Aud of Sp-Lang Path, VA Medical Center, **SLP A ACE**

MacQuilken, Christine Marie 1435 First Avenue #3FS, New York, NY 10021, (212) 220-8014, BS 75 PA St Univ - Univ Park; MS 77 Rutgers St Univ - Newark; **SLP**

Macri, Constance Leigh 8610-6 Beacontree Lane, Richmond, VA 23229, (804) 747-8122, BS 86 Bowling Green St Univ; ME 88 Univ of VA - Charlottesville; 88–Aud, Maico Hearing Aid Service Inc

Mactague, Mrs Janet Mary 3214 West Sierra Drive, Westlake Village, CA 91362, (805) 496-4542, BA 83 CA St Univ - Northridge; MA 84 CA St Univ - Northridge; Sp-Lang Path, Las Virgenes USD, **SLP**

MacWhirter-Holbrook, Carol A 1110 North Harvey, Oak Park, IL 60302, (312) 880-3430, BS 73 Univ of MN - Minneap-St Paul; MA 78 Northern IL Univ - De Kalb; 88–Sp-Lang Path, Childrens Memorial Hosp, **SLP**

MacWilliam, Dalene D 2966 Bay Oaks Drive, Dallas, TX 75229, (214) 357-7378, BA 69 Emporia St Univ; MS 75 Southern Methodist Univ; 77–Sp-Lang Path, Dallas ISD, **SLP**

Madak, Terri Wilson 9 Buckeye, St Peters, MO 63376, (314) 724-5560, BS 75 KS St Univ; MA 77 KS St Univ; **SLP**

Madar, Mrs Glenda Falovitch 205 DE La Roche, Dollard Des Ormeaux, PQ, Canada H9A 9Z7, (514) 626-8314, BA 78 McGill Univ - Quebec; MS 80 McGill Univ - Quebec; SLP, Sir M B Davis-Jewish Gen Hosp, **SLP**

Madden, Barbara Jane 158 Bishops Drive, Aston, PA 19014, (215) 891-3370, BS 82 PA St Univ - Univ Park; MS 85 PA St Univ - Univ Park; 88–Dir of Sp & Hrng Svcs, Riddle Memorial Hosp, **A**

Madden, Dr Deirdre Peters Baldwin-Wallace College, Berea, OH 44017, (919) 270-3209, OB 58 OH Univ - Athens; MA 67 Case Western Reserve Univ; PH 82 (Spec Ed Administration) Kent St Univ; 67–Prof, Baldwin Wallace Coll, **SLP**

Madden, Mrs Shirley 3315 South Avenue, Springfield, MO 65807, (417) 864-3719, BA 72 Augustana Coll; MA 75 Western IL Univ; Sp-Lang Path, Springfield Pub Sch R-12, **SLP**

Madding, Carolyn 5372 Rockledge Drive, Buena Park, CA 90621, (714) 544-6043, BS 59 OH St Univ; MA 82 CA St Univ - Fullerton; 82–Sp-Lang Path, Newport Lang/Sp/Aud Inc, **SLP**

Maddock, Mrs Janet Lyle 1625 North Dayton, Chicago, IL 60614, **SLP**

Maddock, Mary Laird 5201 Lord Tennyson, Wilmington, NC 28405, (919) 791-3845, BS 78 Univ of Tulsa; MA 83 Univ of TX - Austin; 87–Aud, Wilmington Ear Nose & Throat, **A**

Maddox, Carol M 2901 North Seminary #103, Chicago, IL 60657-4323, (312) 996-6520, BS 79 Vanderbilt Univ; MS 81 Purdue Univ - West Lafayette; Sp-Lang Path, U of IL-Coll of Med, **SLP**

Maddox, Carol Maria 3225 Gwynns Falls Parkway, Baltimore, MD 21216, (301) 947-1823, BS 82 Elmira Coll; MS 85 Towson St Univ; **SLP**

Maddox, Chere 1734 New Hampshire Avenue N W, Washington, DC 20009, (202) 232-0211, MA 88 Howard Univ

Maddox, Mrs Gail G Route 9 Box 301, Sour Lake, TX 77659, (409) 838-5261, BA 59 Univ of Southwestern LA; ME 72 Lamar Univ; Dir, Hardin Jefferson ISD, **SLP**

Maddox, Sarah Payne 38 1/2 King Street, Charleston, SC 29401, (803) 577-5011, SLP, VA Hosp, **SLP**

Maddry, Ellen Ann 503 Lawndale Street, Garner, NC 27529-4220, (919) 752-2029, **SLP**

Maddy, Mrs Julie Kay 413 West 5th, Hays, KS 67601, (913) 625-8499, MS 88 Fort Hays St Univ

Madeira, Mrs Shelley S 803 Arbor Avenue, Wheaton, IL 60187, (312) 668-0748, BA 72 Wheaton Coll; MA 75 IN Univ - Bloomington; Sp-Lang Path, Private Practice, **SLP**

Madell, Dr Jane Reger 450 West 23rd Street #D, New York, NY 10011, (212) 741-7674, BS 64 Emerson Coll; MS 65 Univ of WI - Madison; PH 69 (Comm Dis) Univ of WI - Madison; 70–Aud, NY League for Hard of Hearing, **SLP A F ACE**

Madell-Charles, Mrs Nancy Lake Magdalene Manor, 14038 Shady Shores Drive, Tampa, FL 33612, (813) 969-2848, **SLP**

Mader, Mrs Marjorie A 72 Bellerive Acres, St Louis, MO 63121, (314) 569-1503, BS 73 Southeast MO St Univ; MA 78 Saint Louis Univ; Sp-Lang Path, Spec Sch Dist/St Louis Co, **SLP**

Madianos, Lorette D 1081 Fox Chase Road, Jenkintown, PA 19046, (215) 886-8913, BA 84 Univ of DE; MA 86 Temple Univ; 88–Sp-Lang Path, Northwest Child Develop Ctr, **SLP**

Madigan, Mrs Anne McClave 119 Adams Road, Londonderry, NH 03053, (603) 622-3623, BA 81 Univ of CT; MA 83 Univ of CT; Aud, So Nh Ear Nose & Throat Assoc, **A**

Madison, Dr Charles L Communication Disorders Clinic, Daggy Hall, Pullman, WA 99164, (509) 335-4222, BS 66 9533; MA 67 OH Univ - Athens; PH 70 (NS) OH Univ - Athens; Assoc Prof Coor Cl Serv, WA St U, **SLP**

Madison, Kathy W 211 East 29th Street, Tulsa, OK 74114, (918) 664-9464, BS 69 OK St Univ; MA 71 Univ of Tulsa; Sp-Lang Path, Union Public Schools, **SLP**

Madison, Lawanda D 3401 Orange Drive, Yuma, AZ 85365, (602) 726-7385, BA 50 Wichita St Univ; 79–Retired

Madison, Nancy K N W 905 Bryant, Pullman, WA 99163, (509) 334-7387, BS 65 SUNY - Coll at Buffalo; MA 67 Case Western Reserve Univ; Aud, Early Hearing Svcs, **A**

Madison, Mrs Patricia Trippe 7A Statesboro Circle, Belle Fourche, SD 57717, (605) 892-2112, BA 82 Univ of Central FL; MA 83 Univ of Central FL; 88–Sp-Lang Path, Belle Fourche Health Care Ctr, **SLP**

Madison, Ted Keith 5432 Harvard, Raytown, MO 64133, (816) 765-7772, BS 82 Univ of IA; MA 84 Univ of IA; 86–Asst Dir, Timbre Hearing & Sp Ctr, **A**

Madison Isaac, Sherryl Luane Elwyn Institute, 111 Elwyn Road, Dept Of Audiology, Elwyn, PA 19063, (215) 891-2189, Elwyn Inst, **A**

Madison-Land, Mrs Sharron R 1498-G Edwards Place, Bolling Afb, Washington, DC 20336, (703) 360-4260, BA 80 MI St Univ; MA 82 MI St Univ; Sp-Lang Path, **SLP**

Madkin, Mrs Mary E A 1681 Glenwood Avenue, Upland, CA 91786, (714) 987-0755, BA 68 CA St Univ - Los Angeles; MA 76 CA St Univ - Los Angeles; SLP, San Bernardino Co Supt of Sch, **SLP**

Madlock, Mrs Rosalind Dewitt 2201 Cambridge Drive, Memphis, TN 38116, (901) 396-8973, MA 78 Memphis St Univ; Sp-Lang Path, U of Louisville, **SLP**

Madoff, Gretchen G Dept Of Communication, SUNY New Paltz, New Paltz, NY 12561, (914) 257-2030, BA 66 MI St Univ; MS 72 SUNY - Coll at Buffalo; Dir/Cl Ser, New Paltz, **SLP**

Madonia, Julie Anne 141 East 89th Street #2-L, New York, NY 10028, (212) 996-5830, **SLP**

Madore, Donna P RFD 1 Box 1742, Dresden, ME 04342, (207) 737-8193, MA 87 0587

Madory, Robert David San Francisco Hrng & Sp Ctr, 1234 Divisadero, San Francisco, CA 94115, (415) 921-7658, BS 75 Univ of IA; MA 78 Central MI Univ; Audiologist, San Francisco Hrng/Speech Ctr, **A**

Madrid, Joe 1106 Rancho Road, Roswell, NM 88201, (505) 324-0987, MS 70 Western MI Univ; Executive Director, Idtc Inc, **SLP**

Madsen, Betsy P O Box 7566, 68 Hatton Avenue, Spreckels, CA 93962, (408) 455-1757, BA 72 Univ of CA - Santa Barbara; MA 74 Seton Hall Univ; MA 74 Seton Hall Univ; Sp/Lang Path, Private Practice, **SLP**

Madsen, Sitka Ann 2129 Belle Vue Way, Tallahassee, FL 32304, (904) 575-6069, BS 81 FL St Univ; MS 82 FL St Univ; 83–Sp-Lang Path, Thomas Co Sch Syst, **SLP**

Madura-Carroll, Karin 3320 Serpentine Drive, Antioch, CA 94509, (415) 778-8863, BS 74 Univ of IL - Urbana; MS 77 IL St Univ - Normal; **SLP**

Maegli, Mary 8505 West Hawthorne Avenue, Wauwatosa, WI 53226, (414) 541-8080, BS 57 Univ of WI - Madison; Sp-Lang Path, West Allis-West Milw PS, **SLP**

Maehl, Mrs Cheri P 1320 13th Avenue North, Fort Dodge, IA 50501, (515) 955-3119, BA 71 Univ of Northern IA; MA 72 Univ of Northern IA; Sp-Lang Path, AEA #5, **SLP**

Maemori, Kathy Sadanaga 1252 Kinau Street #4, Honolulu, HI 96814, (808) 841-8304, BS 81 Univ of HI - Manoa; MS 82 Univ of HI - Manoa; Sp/Lang Path, State of HI-Dept of Ed, **SLP**

Maenaga, Linda A 1228 Deerpark Drive #49, Fullerton, CA 92631, (714) 996-9928, MA 88 CA St Univ - Northridge

Maeno, Alice H 632 Nandina Circle, Oxnard, CA 93030, (213) 397-8555, BA 73 Univ of CA - Santa Barbara; MA 74 Univ of the Pacific; Sp-Lang Path, Los Angeles Co Supt of Schools, **SLP**

Maertens, Mrs Maria Hidalgo 1250 Eudora Street, Denver, CO 80220, (801) 350-4723, BA 82 CA St Univ - Fullerton; **SLP**

Maes, Daniel R Pl Box 162, Dixon, NM 87527, (505) 753-2256, BA 72 NM St Univ; MA 74 NM St Univ; SLP, Espanola Municipal School, **SLP**

Maesaka, Michele Lynn 1750 Kyllo Lane, Eagan, MN 55122, (612) 927-3736, BS 85 Univ of MN - Minneap-St Paul; MS 86 Boston Univ; 88–Sp-Lang Path, Park Nicollet Med Ctr, **SLP**

Maes-Serazio, Audrey Susan 6626 West Mercer Lane, Glendale, AZ 85304, (602) 285-3605, BS 82 Univ of Southern CO; MS 84 Eastern NM Univ; SLP, Aspra, **SLP**

Maffeo, Angela Marie 35 Bell Waver Way, Oakland, CA 94619, (415) 531-0960, MA 88 Univ of CA - Santa Barbara

Magdinec, Melanie 11900 Edgewater Drive #406, Lakewood, OH 44107, (216) 531-9000, BS 74 Bowling Green St Univ; ME 76 Univ of Louisville; MA 83 Cleveland St Univ; Dept Mgr-Sp & Aud, Meridia Euclid Hosp, **SLP A**

Magee, Dorothy Lynn 6060 Oak Bay #1225, Houston, TX 77091, (713) 695-2772, OB 77 Stephen F Austin St Univ; MA 84 Univ of Houston - Univ Park; Sp-Lang Path, Houston ISD, **SLP**

Magee, Helmtrud Maria 30357 Camino Porvenir, Palos Verdes Peninsula, CA 90274, (213) 757-1226, **SLP**

Magee, Janet Clark P O Box 1631, Shepherdstown, WV 25443, (304) 876-6240, BS 74 WV Univ; MS 76 WV Univ; 88–Sp-Lang Path, **SLP**

Magee, Mrs Linda B Univ S Mississippi, Box 5092, Speech & Hearing Dept, Hattiesburg, MS 39406, (601) 266-5232, MS 75 Univ Southern MS-Hattiesburg; Clinic Coordinator, Univ S Mississippi Sp&Hrng Cln, **SLP**

Magee, Mrs Rebecca D 278 Kings College Court, Arnold, MD 21012, (301) 544-5020, BS 73 Univ Southern MS-Hattiesburg; MS 75 Univ Southern MS-Hattiesburg; **SLP**

Magee, Sheryl Kinsey 2712 Windy Crossing, Winston-Salem, NC 27107, BA 80 Univ of Northern IA; MA 81 Univ of Northern IA; SLP, Winston-Salem Forsyth Co Schs, **SLP**

Magelky, Mrs Phyllis J 1314 N 10th St, Moorhead, MN 56560, (218) 233-2597, BA 78 Coll of Saint Teresa; MS 84 Moorhead St Univ; Sp-Lang Path, Gst Educ Serv, **SLP**

Magelssen, Liane 9876 Adams Street, Fort Lewis, WA 96433, (206) 964-3378, BS 76 UT St Univ; MS 77 UT St Univ; Audiologist, **A**

Mager, Mrs Lisa Z 9308 Augusta N E, Albuquerque, NM 87111, MS 82 Univ of NM

Magers, Mrs Claudia A 132 South Crescent, Independence, MO 64053-1232, (816) 234-3677, BA 74 Cedarville Coll; MS 78 Central MO St Univ; 79–Sp-Lang Path, Children's Mercy Hosp, **SLP**

Magers, J L, Jr 1517 Adams, Great Bend, KS 67530, (316) 793-3862, BA 69 Kearney St Coll; MS 74 Univ of AZ; Audiologist, Private Practice, **A**

Magers, Mrs K Diane 1517 Adams, Great Bend, KS 67530, (316) 793-3862, BS 64 Fort Hays St Univ; ME 73 Univ of AZ; SLP, Private Practice, **SLP**

Magers, Mary Alberta 1300 N E 16th Avenue #821, Portland, OR 97232, (503) 280-2488, BS 41 Univ of OR; MA 65 Univ of WA; **LM**

Maggio, Mrs Laura Lynn Fort Dodge Hearing & Speech C, 1099 Kenyon Road, Fort Dodge, IA 50501, (515) 573-4701, BA 79 IA St Univ; MA 85 Univ of IA; 85–Sp-Lang Path, Fort Dodge Hearing/Sp Ctr, **SLP**

Maggio, Mrs Michele W 17 Community Road, Bay Shore, NY 11706, (516) 666-7282, BS 80 SUNY - Coll at Geneseo; MA 81 Hofstra Univ; 87–Sp-Lang Path, Private Practice, **SLP**

Maggi-Thomas, Debra Jane 6539 Moonshell Court, Orlando, FL 32819-0144, (305) 290-0071, BS 77 WV Univ; ME 80 GA St Univ; Sp-Lang Path, Cobb County School System, **SLP**

Magid, Lee T 1645 Branch Valley Drive, Roswell, GA 30076, (404) 894-3226, BS 71 Univ of VA - Charlottesville; MA 73 Univ of Cincinnati; OM 84 Univ of HI - Manoa; 87–Sp-Lang Path, Georgia Dept/Human Resources, **SLP**

Magiera, Beverly D 505 Lochmoor Place, Eugene, OR 97405, (503) 686-6442, BS 75 Carlow Coll; MA 77 Univ of Pittsburgh - Pittsburgh; Sp-Lang Path, Sacred Heart Home Health, **SLP**

Magiera, Nancy Snidow 4006 Keywest, Corpus Christi, TX 78411-5009, (512) 881-4757, BS 74 East TN St Univ; MA 76 Univ of TN - Knoxville; Dir/Aud, Mem Med Cen, **A**

Magill, Mrs Kathleen O'Grady 6264 Hallen Avenue, Belvidere, IL 61008, (815) 544-9851, BS 73 Northern IL Univ - De Kalb; MA 74 Northern IL Univ - De Kalb; 74–Sp-Lang Path, Boone Co Spec Educ, **SLP**

Magill, Shanda Barger 733 S W Hibiscus Street, Port St Lucie, FL 34983-8764, (305) 879-4163, MA 84 Wichita St Univ; 86–Sp-Lang Path, InSpeech Inc, **SLP**

Maginn, Mary Margaret 1424 East Goldspur Drive, Fort Wayne, IN 46804, (219) 456-1469, BA 73 Univ of Miami; ME 75 Univ of Miami; Pres, Ft Wayne Commun Dis Cen Inc, **SLP**

Magley, Gail Susan 6832 Merwood Street, Worthington, OH 43235, (614) 263-5151, BS 74 OH St Univ; MA 76 Univ of Houston - Univ Park; **SLP**

Magnan, Elaine A R Rd 2 Route 7, St Albans, VT 05478, **SLP**

Magnani, Mrs Bernadette 435 Carol Place, Pelham Manor, NY 10803, (914) 738-1220, BS 67 Fordham Univ; MA 72 CUNY - Hunter Coll; **SLP**

Magnani, Nancy M 346 Sunset Street, Plymouth, MI 48170, (313) 453-0441, BA 78 CUNY - Queens Coll; MS 79 PA St Univ - Univ Park; 87–Sp-Lang Path, Communication Disorders Inc, **SLP ACE**

Magnera, Dr Georgia Elizabeth 3611 Winfield Cove, Austin, TX 78704, (512) 441-2230, PH 82 (NS) Univ of Alberta - Alberta; Sp/Lang Path, **SLP**

Magness, Lana Jaton 626 Green Oak Drive, Longview, TX 75604, (214) 759-4404, BA 80 TX Tech Univ; MS 82 Univ of Dallas; 88–Sp-Lang Path, Spring Hill ISD, **SLP A**

Magnotta, Olive Hughes 129 Le Grande Drive, Pittsburgh, PA 15221, BS 72 Carlow Coll; MA 76 Univ of WA; Sp-Lang Path, Allegheny Inter Unit, **SLP**

Magnusdottir, Mrs Sigridur Hjardarlandi #1 270, Varma, Iceland, OB 67; MS 77 Boston Univ; Sp-Lang Path, Reykjalundur Rehab Cen, **SLP**

Magnuson-Jongsma, Mrs Cleo Grace 416 South 975 East, Layton, UT 84041, BA 74 Univ of Saskatchewan - Sask; MS 83 Minot St Univ; Sp-Lang Path, Mc Kay-Dee Hosp, **SLP**

Magnusson, Dr Deanne L 3742 West Sunrise Drive, Minnetonka, MN 55345, (612) 935-9274, BS 84 Univ of MN - Minneap-St Paul; MA 59 Univ of MN - Minneap-St Paul; PH 68 (NS) Univ of MN - Minneap-St Paul; Administrator SLP Programs, Minneapolis Public Schools, **SLP**

Magnusson, Ronald L 3418 Loma Vista Road #2A, Ventura, CA 93003, (805) 654-8551, BA 76; MA 79 CA St Univ - Los Angeles; Aud, Hrng Aid Aud & Sp Assoc, **A**

Magsam, Loren A 10432 102nd Place, Maple Grove, MN 55369, Instructor, St Cloud State U, **SLP**

Maguire, Jeanette Porter 272 West Waterloo Street, Canal Winchester, OH 43110, (614) 860-9434, BS 84 OH Univ - Athens; MA 86 OH Univ - Athens; Sp-Lang Path, Jeanette P Maguire MA CCC, **SLP**

Maguire, Mrs Katherine Cypher 23 Gulf Road, Peterborough, NH 03458, (603) 924-7503, BS 71 MT St Agnes Coll; MS 72 Loyola Coll; 88–Sp-Lang Path, Contoocook Valley Sch Dist, **SLP**

Maguire, Mrs Lisa Carlson 350 Illinois Boulevard, Hoffman Estates, IL 60194, (312) 884-6957, BA 82 TX Tech Univ; MS 84 TX Tech Univ; 87–Sp-Lang Path, Proviso Area for Excep Chldn, **SLP**

Maguire, Mabel C 25-A-3 Pine Lane, Albany, NY 12203, (518) 452-0384, BS 78 Coll of Saint Rose; MS 80 Coll of Saint Rose; Sp-Lang Path, UCP of Schenectady, **SLP**

Maguire-Bradley, Sheila Ann 7464 N Ellison Drive, Tucson, AZ 85704, (602) 293-0737, BS 80 Univ of AZ; MS 82 Univ of AZ; Sp-Lang Path, Amphitheater Sch Dist, **SLP**

Magyar, Karla J W 305 Manor Drive, Warrensburg, MO 64093, (612) 831-5345, BS 75 Univ of WI - Madison; MS 76 Univ of WI - Stevens Point; **SLP**

Mahaffey, Mrs Joy A 4011 Chester Street, Tyler, TX 75701, (214) 581-1671, BS 71 Stephen F Austin St Univ; MS 75 Univ of North TX; 88–Sp-Lang Path, Tyler ISD, **SLP**

Mahaffey, Kevin Brooks 93 North Main Street, West Hartford, CT 06107, (203) 521-9492, BA 82 Drew Univ; MA 87 Univ of CT; Mercy Hosp

Mahaffey, Dr Robert B Division Speech & Hearing Sci, Univ Of North Carolina, School Of Medicine, Chapel Hill, NC 27514, (919) 966-1006, BA 62 OH St Univ; MA 63 OH St Univ; PH 66 (NS) OH St Univ; Dir Div of Sp & Hrng Sci, U of NC, **SLP**

Mahaffie, Mrs Catherine Jean 911 Hazel Avenue, Campbell, CA 95008, (408) 773-0204, BA 82 San Jose St Univ; MA 84 San Jose St Univ; Aud, Golden State Aud Assoc, **A**

Mahan, Mrs Anne Marie 11 Westview Drive, Mansfield, MA 02048, (617) 593-2727, BA 79 Manhattanville Coll; MS 82 Southern CT St Univ; Sp/Lang Path, Mansfield Public Schools, **SLP**

Mahan, Mrs Carla S 2619 24th Street, Lubbock, TX 79410, (806) 763-5401, OB 79 Sam Houston St Univ; MS 87 TX Tech Univ

Mahan, Dr Guy H 4557 Howard, Western Springs, IL 60558, (312) 246-3501, PH 68 (NS) Loyola Univ of Chicago; SLP, Private Practice, **SLP**

Mahanna, Mary Christine R R 2 Box 5, Barneveld, NY 13304, (518) 449-8829, BS 82 Nazareth Coll of Rochester; OM 85 Coll of Saint Rose; **SLP**

Mahanna-Boden, Susan Vickers Village #932, Richmond, KY 40475, (606) 622-4442, BS 75 Univ of KS; MS 77 Phillips Univ; PH 87 (Sp Path Child Lang) Wichita St Univ; 86–Assistant Professor, Eastern Kentucky University, **SLP**

Mahecha, Mrs Nancy R 715 9th Avenue #2R, New York, NY 10019, (212) 581-3593, BS 72; MA 81 CUNY - Hunter Coll; Sp-Path, Private Practice, **SLP**

Maher, Mrs Angela Maria 613 North Lincoln, Pittsfield, IL 62363-1213, (217) 285-2147, BS 84 Western IL Univ; MA 85 Western IL Univ; **SLP**

Maher, Barbara Anne 9503 S Plaza #5-201, Omaha, NE 68127, (402) 593-9358, BS 83 Univ of NE - Lincoln; MS 86 Univ of NE - Lincoln; 88–Sp-Lang Path, Bellevue PS, **SLP**

Maher, Betty Jane Claridge House 1 #505, Verona, NJ 07044, (201) 733-8401, BS 45 Fordham Univ; MA 49 NY Univ; 46–Sp-Lang Path, Newark Bd of Ed, **SLP**

Maher, Catherine A 1100 North Ferncreek Avenue, Orlando, FL 32803, MS 74 FL St Univ; Regional Director, Florida Easter Seal Society, **SLP**

Maher, Mrs Elaine Dubois 13800 83rd Way, Maple Grove, MN 55369, (612) 753-2554, BA 74 Univ of MD - College Park; MS 76 Univ of MD - College Park; **SLP**

Maher, John J, III 10740 Meridian Avenue North, Suite 108, Seattle, WA 98133, (206) 367-9030, OM 80 Univ of Puget Sound; MA 71 CA St Univ - Sacramento; Dir, Hrng Healthcare Ctr Inc, **A**

Maher, Lynn M 4336 N W 69th Street, Gainesville, FL 32606, (904) 338-1938, BA 78 Catholic Univ of America; MA 79 George Washington Univ; 88–Sp-Lang Path, Univ of FL Dept of Neurology, **SLP ACE**

Maher, Mrs Lynne Meyer 3842 Basilone Street #4, San Diego, CA 92110, (619) 274-9871, BA 73 San Diego St Univ; MA 83 CA St Univ - Fresno; Sp-Lang Path, San Diego Cty Sch, **SLP**

Maher, Mary E 707 Montezuma Drive, Pacifica, CA 94044-4030, (415) 355-1913, BA 73 Univ of Southern CA; MA 78 CA St Univ - Long Beach; Sp-Lang Path, Private Practice, **SLP**

Maher, Patricia L 319 Browning Avenue, Altoona, PA 16602, (814) 946-5411, BS 72 Carlow Coll; ME 78 CA Univ of PA; Sp/Lang Path, Hme/Nur Agy Blair Hunt Fult Co, **SLP**

Maher, Roger Lee Box 257 Mink Road, Cotton, MN 55724, (218) 482-5589, BS 73 Univ of MN - Duluth; MA 74 Univ of MN - Duluth; Sp-Lang Path, Communication Disorder Spec, **SLP**

Maher, Mrs Sherri Rae 171 Village Drive, Taylor, PA 18517, (717) 562-2746, BS 83 PA St Univ - Univ Park; MS 87 Bloomsburg Univ of PA; 88–Sp-Lang Path, NEIU #19, **SLP**

Maher, Suzanne Rachael 133 Walnut Street, East Providence, RI 02914, (401) 434-3400, BS 82 Worcester St Coll; MS 86 CO St Univ; 86–Sp-Lang Path, Comm Disord Dept Bradley Hosp, **SLP**

Mahle, Mrs Carla Brooks 9803 Roark Road #2149, Houston, TX 77099, (713) 668-1438, MA 88 Univ of Houston - Univ Park; 88–Sp-Lang Path, Alief ISD

Mahler, Mrs Linda Marie 47 Presidential Circle, Hampton, NH 03842, (603) 926-4695, MA 88 Univ of NH; 88–Sp-Lang Path, Exeter Hosp

Mahler, Marla Cooper 1320 York Avenue, Apartment 31-M, New York, NY 10021, (212) 628-4191, SLP, Kennedy Child Study Center, **SLP**

Mahlmann, Dr Jeanne E 117 Arch Avenue, Pittsburgh, PA 15202, (412) 683-3000, BS 69 Boston Univ; ME 70 PA St Univ - Univ Park; PH 88 (Sp Path) Univ of Pittsburgh - Pittsburgh; 72–Sp-Lang Path, VA Med Cen, **SLP**

Mahn, Kathleen E 3700 Hobbs Road, Nashville, TN 37215-2331, (615) 322-2709, BS 77 Middle TN St Univ; MS 79 Vanderbilt Univ; Sp/Lang Path, Child Dev Ctr of Vanderbilt, **SLP**

Mahnke, Nancy C 1274 Corberosa, Arroyo Grande, CA 93420, (805) 489-1351, BA 75 CA St Univ - Fresno; MA 77 CA St Univ - Fresno; Sp-Lang Path, Lucia Mav USD, **SLP**

Mahometa, Mrs Maryann Retkwa 110 Beverly Road, Hawthorne, NJ 07506, (201) 427-1300, BA 71 William Paterson Coll; MA 72 Seton Hall Univ; Sp-Lang Path, Hawthorne Board of Education, **SLP**

Mahon, Christine Shannon 41 Abington Lane, Alamo, CA 94507, (415) 938-8686, MA 85 San Jose St Univ; **A**

Mahon, Mrs Donna Weckerle 22 Coolbrook Court #C, East Amherst, NY 14051-1205, (716) 834-9200, **A**

Mahon, Mrs Florence L 196 Reed Street, New Bedford, MA 02740, (617) 992-5331, BS 56 Boston Univ; ME 58 Boston Univ; ED 62 Boston Univ; Licensed Psychologist, Private Practice, **SLP LM**

Mahon, Julia Weiss 70 Wampanog Lane, Tiverton, RI 02878, (401) 624-6167, BA 70 Temple Univ; MS 80 Univ of RI; Sp-Lang Path, Salve Regina College, **SLP**

Mahone, Mrs Melissa McDonald Center For Speech & Lang Path, 719 Franklin Street S E, Huntsville, AL 35801, (205) 536-3364, BA 66 FL St Univ; MS 67 FL St Univ; Dir, Cen for Sp-Lang Path, **SLP ACE**

Mahoney, Mrs Barbara Katherine 22995 Caminito Brisa, Laguna Hills, CA 92653, (213) 861-2891, BA 75 Univ of Redlands; MS 77 Univ of Redlands; 75–Prog Admin-Sp Prog, Los Angeles Cnty Ofc of Educ, **SLP**

Mahoney, Mrs C Michelle 12234 Arbor Trail, Palos Heights, IL 60463, (312) 908-3637, OB 85 Univ of Western Ontario; MS 87 IN St Univ - Terre Haute; Sp-Lang Path, Rehab Institute of Chicago

Mahoney, Carol Ann 20 Hutchinson Boulevard, Scarsdale, NY 10583, (914) 737-3300, **SLP**

Mahoney, Dennis G 4 Cogswell Avenue #41, Cambridge, MA 02140, (617) 661-1829, BA 69 Fordham Univ; MA 78 Emerson Coll; **SLP**

Mahoney, Elaine Marie 1135 North Vista Street, West Hollywood, CA 90046, (607) 277-0316, BS 84 Ithaca Coll; MA 85 Bowling Green St Univ; **SLP**

Mahoney, M Elaine 4208 Lea Court, Bakersfield, CA 93306, (805) 325-1137, BA 72 Univ of Redlands; MS 73 Univ of Redlands; Dir-SLP Servs, E M Speech Path, **SLP**

Mahoney, Mary H 91 Academy Hill Road, Brighton, MA 02135, (617) 478-3400, BS 77 Nazareth Coll of Rochester; MS 79 Boston Univ; SLP, Visiting Nurse Assoc of Boston, **SLP**

Mahoney, Melanie 556 Bald Mountain Drive, Livermore, CO 80536, (303) 221-2782, MS; **A LM**

Mahoney, Patricia 6 Dexter Park Boulevard, Cincinnati, OH 45241, (513) 683-6818, BS 76 Kent St Univ; MA 79 Kent St Univ; Sp/Lang Path, Loveland Bd of Ed, **SLP**

Mahoney, Ruth Elizabeth 48 Cary Avenue, Milton, MA 02186, (617) 447-4408, BA 73 Mount Saint Mary Coll; MS 84 Boston Univ; **SLP**

Mahoney, Mrs Susan Ann 8526 West Grand Avenue, River Grove, IL 60171, (312) 452-7414, BS 82 Northern IL Univ - De Kalb; MA 86 Northern IL Univ - De Kalb; 88–Sp-Lang Path, NW Suburban Spec Educ Organ, **SLP**

Mahoney, Susan Mary 5771 South 121 Street, Hales Corners, WI 53130, (414) 649-6400, BS 86 Marquette Univ; MS 87 Marquette Univ; 87–Sp-Lang Path, St Luke's Med Ctr

Mahoney, Theresa Ann 375 Mt Sinai-Coram Road, Miller Place, NY 11764, (516) 689-9850, BS 77 Univ of WI - Madison; MS 83 Univ of NH; Sp-Lang Path, Suffolk Child Dev Dtr, **SLP**

Mahoney, Dr Thomas M Utah State Dept Of Health, Bureau Of Communicative Disorders, 44 Medical Drive, Salt Lake City, UT 84113, (801) 533-6175, OB 63 Univ of ND; MA 68 Univ of ND; PH 73 (NS) Univ of OR; Dir Bur of Commun Dis, State Dept of Hlth, **SLP A**

Mahood, Mrs Gina Marie 1255 Lakeview Drive, Butler, PA 16001, (412) 282-6806, MS 84 Indiana Univ of PA; Sp-Lang Path, Visiting Nurses Assoc/Butler, **SLP**

Mahood, Mrs Lynne Temple 186 Rollin Irish Road, Milton, VT 05468, (802) 893-4921, BS 77 PA St Univ - Univ Park; MA 78 OH Univ - Athens; Sp-Lang Path, Grand Isle Superv Un Dist, **SLP**

Mahorney, Mrs Lori Jean 4410 Grove Avenue, Cincinnati, OH 45227, (513) 471-5792, BS 76 2833; MA 79 Univ of South FL; 81–Sp-Lang Path, Hamilton County Ofc of Educ, **SLP**

Mahosky, Katherine Passmore 3501 West Lois Lane, Flagstaff, AZ 86001, (602) 774-4791, BS 77 East Stroudsburg Univ of PA; MS 82 Northern AZ Univ; 83–Sp-Lang Path, Inst for Human Dev Northern AZ Univ, **SLP**

Mahrt, Vickie Krause 1316 Vernon Street, Normal, IL 61761, (309) 452-6926, BA 76 William Jewell Coll; MA 78 Univ of NE - Lincoln; Sp-Lang Path, Octavia Sch Dist, **SLP**

Mahshie, Dr James J Department Of Audiology, Gallaudet College, Washington, DC 20002, (202) 651-5328, BS 70 Le Moyne Coll; MS 73 Syracuse Univ; PH 80 (NS) Syracuse Univ; Associate Professor Audiology, Gallaudet Univ, **SLP**

Mai, Mrs Deborah L 9135 Delano, Wichita, KS 67212, (316) 722-6166, BA 76 Baylor Univ; MA 81 OK St Univ; Sp-Lang Path, Rainbows United Inc, **SLP**

Maiani, Mrs Rhonda Jeannette 1754 Santa Clara Street, Santa Clara, CA 95050, (408) 554-8845, BA 81 San Jose St Univ; MA 85 San Jose St Univ; **SLP**

Maibor, Debra K 52 Briarwood Circle, Needham, MA 02194, (617) 449-6554, BS 73 OH Univ - Athens; MS 74 Univ of MI - Ann Arbor; Sp-Lang Path, Private Practice, **SLP**

Maida, Lorraine Ann 33715 North Royaloak Lane, Apartment 204, Gages Lake, IL 60030, (312) 566-2420, BA 76 Elmhurst Coll; MA 78 Northern IL Univ - De Kalb; Sp-Lang Path, Special Ed Dist of Lake Co, **SLP**

Maida, Michele S 83 Abingdon Avenue, Staten Island, NY 10308, (718) 356-5286, BA 75 Jersey City St Coll; MA 79 Kean Coll of NJ; Sp-Lang Path, Sp Serv UT/NY Cty Bd of Ed, **SLP**

Maida-Cantone, Kathleen 8820 Butterfield, Orland Park, IL 60462, (312) 448-9350, BA 74 Saint Xavier Coll; MS 76 Bradley Univ; Sp-Lang Path, Private Practice, **SLP**

Maida-Schmieder, Debora 8020 4th Avenue #E8, Brooklyn, NY 11209, (212) 683-0736, BS 77 Saint Joseph's Coll; MA 79 NY Univ; Sp-Lang Path, NY Cty Bd of Ed, **SLP**

Maidlow, Gail Marie P O Box 801, Gleneden Beach, OR 97388, (503) 994-5296, BA 72 Univ of FL; MA 81 Western WA Univ; 82–Sp-Lang Path, Lincoln Co School District, **SLP**

Maier, Mrs Deborah M 10212 Eden Court N E, Albuquerque, NM 87112, (505) 293-3175, BA 80 Univ of NM; MS 81 Univ of NM; SLP, St Maries Sch Dist, **SLP**

Maier, Kathleen M 5840 West 104th Street, Apartment 211, Oak Lawn, IL 60453, (312) 838-4909, BA 69 Saint Xavier Coll; MA 70 Northwestern Univ; Sp-Lang Path, Chicago Bd of Ed, **SLP ACE**

Maier, Linda Carol 7402 Six Mile Lane #10, Louisville, KY 40220, (502) 584-9781, BS 83 Purdue Univ - West Lafayette; MS 85 Purdue Univ - West Lafayette; 85–Sp-Lang Path, Easter Seal Hearing & Sp Ctr, **SLP**

Maier, Valerie Judith 2251 Middletown Drive, Campbell, CA 95008, (415) 794-2141, MA 86 San Jose St Univ

Maierle, Victoria M 422 East Bradley Avenue, Milwaukee, WI 53207, (414) 482-0535, BS 78 Univ of WI - Milwaukee; MS 80 Univ of WI - Milwaukee; Sp-Lang Path, Milwaukee Pub Sch, **SLP**

Maiers, Mary A 4525 Appletree Circle, Racine, WI 53405, (414) 886-3431, BS 65 Marquette Univ; MS 73 Univ of WI - Stevens Point; Pres, Medical Support Services Inc, **SLP**

Maietta, Dr Donald Francis 22 Banister Road, Andover, MA 01810, (617) 353-3215, BS 50 Bloomsburg Univ of PA; MS 51 Univ of Pittsburgh - Pittsburgh; PH 55 (NS) Univ of Pittsburgh - Pittsburgh; **SLP A**

Maile-Freese, Jill R 3222 North 49th Street, Milwaukee, WI 53216, (414) 442-3645, BA 80 Valparaiso Univ; MS 82 Univ of WI - Milwaukee; Sp-Lang Path, **SLP**

Maillet, Cassandra Joan 3588 Woodfront Court, Indianapolis, IN 46222, (317) 848-3620, MA 87 Ball St Univ; 88–Aud, Hrng Lab/Hrng Ctr, **A**

Mailloux, Sally S 69 East Street, Bristol, VT 05443, (802) 388-4421, MS 76 Univ of VT; Sp/Lang Path, Middlebury ISD #4, **SLP**

Maimbourg, Mrs Odette M 3362 Glencairn Road, Shaker Heights, OH 44122, (216) 561-2344, BS 82 Southern Methodist Univ; MS 83 Univ of North TX; **SLP**

Main, Kimberly L 902-B 16th Street, Port Royal, SC 29935, (803) 525-7404, BS 78 Northern IL Univ - De Kalb; MA 80 Univ of IL - Urbana; Sp-Lang Path, Coastal Sp & Hrng Clinic, **SLP**

Main, Mary Ann 22 Hillside Avenue, Marblehead, MA 01945, **SLP**

Maine, Mrs Candy R 2798 Britwell Court, Miamisburg, OH 45342, (513) 434-9191, BS 79 Miami Univ - Oxford; MS 80 Miami Univ - Oxford; Kindergarten Tchr, Miamisburg Cty Sch, **SLP**

Mainess, Karen Joanne 15767 Tuscola Road #6, Apple Valley, CA 92307, (619) 244-9323, BS 79 Loma Linda Univ - Riverside; MS 86 Loma Linda Univ - Riverside; **SLP**

Mainguy, Susan E 1209 Morgans Landing Drive, Dunwoody, GA 30350, (404) 396-6971, BA 78 Univ of FL; MA 80 Univ of TN - Knoxville; Sp-Lang Path, Scottish Rite Childrens Hosp, **SLP**

Mains, Sheryl Southwest Therapy Services, 626 North Main Street, Greensburg, PA 15601, (412) 837-2070, BS 79 Indiana Univ of PA; MS 80 WV Univ; Chief Sp-Lang Path, Southwest Therapy Services, **SLP**

Maio, Carmela A 159-23 85th Street, Howard Beach, NY 11414, (718) 843-2767, BS 73 CUNY - York Coll; MS 76 Columbia Univ Teachers Coll; Sp-Lang Path, Private Practice, **SLP**

Maio, Mrs Debra Dawkins 1528 Shenta Oak Drive, Norcross, GA 30093, (404) 921-2000, OM 83 Emory Univ; Sp-Lang Path, Gwinnett Co Pub Sch, **SLP**

Maio-Duffy, Maureen E 244 Martin Road, Hebron, CT 06248, (203) 688-4971, BA 79 Univ of CT; MA 81 Univ of CT; SLP, Windsor Publ Schs, **SLP**

Maisel, Clare G 205 Montvue Road, Knoxville, TN 37919, (615) 693-9241, BA 52 Univ of TX - Austin; ME 56 Univ of TX - Austin; Retired, **SLP F**

Maisel, Vivian T Ambi-Lingual Associates, 1140 West 50th Street, Suite 402, Hialeah, FL 33012, (305) 556-0121, BS 74 Univ of GA; ME 78 Univ of Miami; Dir, Ambi-Lingual Assoc, **SLP ACE**

Maisenhalder, Laurie Evelyn 7061 N W 49th Place, Lauderhill, FL 33319, (305) 739-7720, MS 84 CUNY - Brooklyn Coll; Sp-Lang Path, Ctr for Pediatric Therapy, **SLP**

Maitland, Mrs Holly McKinley 1441 Laurel SE, Grand Rapids, MI 49506, (616) 242-0424, MS 87 Miami Univ - Oxford; 87–Sp-Lang Path, Mary Free Bed Hosp/Rehab Ctr, **SLP**

Maitland, Mrs Merryl G 710 East Fishers Creek Rd, Smithville, NJ 08201, (609) 645-3138, BA 75 Univ of MN - Minneap-St Paul; MA 77 SUNY - Center at Buffalo; SLP, Shirley Eves Center, **SLP**

Maj, Barbara J 2825 North Sunrock Lane, Tucson, AZ 85745, (602) 622-7241, BA 75 Univ of CO - Boulder; MS 77 Univ of AZ; Owner-Sp-Lang Path, Speech & Language Associates, **SLP ACE**

Maj, Mrs Elizabeth 12 Trina Court, Walnut Creek, CA 94596, (415) 825-5398, BA 64 Mills Coll; MA 70 San Francisco St Univ; Sp-Lang Path, Mt Diablo USD, **SLP**

Maj, Jennifer Rea 7544 Tempo Terrace, Minneapolis, MN 55432, (612) 781-6571, BA 83 MI St Univ; MA 85 MI St Univ; **SLP**

Maj, Mary B 66 Russell Road, Garden City, NY 11530, MS

Majdic, Lynn Napkori 649 S Henderson Road, King of Prussia, PA 19406, (215) 251-5602, BS 82 PA St Univ - Univ Park; MA 86 West Chester St Coll; 82–Sp-Lang Path, Bryn Mawr Rehab Hosp, **SLP**

Majernik, Mrs Sylvia R 1403 South Galemont Avenue, Hacienda Heights, CA 91745, (818) 997-2434, BA 73 Univ of Redlands; MA 77 CA St Univ - Los Angeles; Audiologist, Los Angeles USD, **A**

Majerus, Anita 1503 Rochester #4, Iowa City, IA 52240, (319) 356-2485, BS 85 IA Wesleyan Coll; MA 88 Univ of Northern CO; 88–Aud, Univ of Iowa Hosp

Majeska, Jo Anne W 1373 Epping Forrest Dr N E, Atlanta, GA 30319, **SLP**

Majlinger, Kathleen A 43 Waterview Avenue, Massapequa, NY 11758, (516) 799-6813, BA 79 CUNY - Queens Coll; MA 81 CUNY - Queens Coll; Sp-Lang Path, Developmental Therapy Cons, **SLP**

Maki, Mrs Francyne A 1035 Redwood Place, Owatonna, MN 55060, (507) 451-9513, BA 67 Saint Cloud St Univ; MS 70 Saint Cloud St Univ; Sp-Lang Path, Owatonna Pub Sch, **SLP**

Maki, Dr Jean E Department Speech-Language Pathology And Audiology, Andrews University, Berrien Springs, MI 49104, (616) 471-3468, BS 72 Northeastern Univ; MA 73 MI St Univ; PH 75 (NS) MI St Univ; 87–Assoc Prof, Andrews Univ, **SLP**

Maki, Jerilyn Satomi 2830 Waialae Avenue, Honolulu, HI 96826, (808) 949-7948, BS 84 Univ of HI - Manoa; MS 87 Univ of HI - Manoa

Maki, Mrs Linda G 4429 North Maryland Avenue, Milwaukee, WI 53211, (414) 354-7733, BS 65 Univ of MN - Duluth; MS 68 Univ of WI - Milwaukee; Sp-Lang Path, Brown Deer Bd of Ed, **SLP**

Maki, Mrs Paula D R R 1 Box 726, Newberry, MI 49868, (906) 293-5022, BS 70 Ball St Univ; MA 74 MI St Univ; Sp-Lang Path, Tahqamenon Area Sch, **SLP**

Maki, Ruanna Kuykendall 218 War Highway, Lubbock, TX 79416, (806) 885-2767, BS 83 Univ of IL - Urbana; MS 85 Univ of IL - Urbana; 88–Sp-Lang Path, Sp-Lang Hrng Ctr of Lubbock, **SLP**

Makie, Patricia A 17 Rose Circle, Peabody, MA 01960, (617) 531-6338, BS 75 Salem St Coll; ME 77 Northeastern Univ; SLP, Lowell Pub Sch, **SLP**

Makman, Judith M 316 E 84th St Apartment 2E, New York, NY 10028, (212) 517-4107, BA 84 Univ of MI - Ann Arbor; MS 87 Columbia Univ Teachers Coll

Makovec, Julie A 15350 Cascade Drive, Elm Grove, WI 53122, (414) 576-1133, BA 86 Univ of WI - Eau Claire; MS 87 Univ of WI - Eau Claire; **SLP**

Makres-Polites, Olga D 25 Lovett Court, Timonium, MD 21093, (301) 243-3800, BA 80 Loyola Coll; MS 81 Loyola Coll; 83–Sp-Lang Path, The Hrng & Sp Agcy Metro Balt, **SLP**

Makrynioti, Athina 119 Himittou Street, Athens, Greece 116, **SLP**

Maks, Wendy W 59 Hampton Drive, Langhorne, PA 19047, (215) 757-6716, BS 78 Trenton St Coll; MA 80 Trenton St Coll; 87–Sp-Lang Path, Private Practice, **SLP**

Maksail, Tricia C 86 Baldwin Road, Scotia, NY 12302, (518) 872-1117, BA 62 Russell Sage Coll; MS 80 Coll of Saint Rose; 88–Jr-Sr HS Prin, Berne-Knox Westerlo Sch Dist, **SLP**

Makuch, Mrs Denise Regina 7739 30th Street S E, Ada, MI 49301, BS Western MI Univ; MA Western MI Univ; SLP, Mary Free Bed Hosp & Rehab Cen, **SLP**

Malach, Randi S 6444 Admiral Rickover N E, Albuquerque, NM 87111, (505) 867-3396, BA 71 Univ of CO - Boulder; MS 76 Univ of Western Ontario; 81–Sp-Lang Path, S W Communication Resources, **SLP ACE**

Malacrida, Mrs Joan K 429 Farview Avenue, Paramus, NJ 07652, (201) 261-6537, BA 74 Rutger's St Univ - Douglas Coll; MA 75 Univ of IL - Urbana; **SLP**

Malakoff, Iris Mae 1022 Prospect Avenue, San Gabriel, CA 91776, (818) 966-8331, BA 56 CA St Univ - Los Angeles; MA 87 4703; 79–Sp-Lang Path, Charter Oak USD, **SLP**

Malamud, Mrs Gloria S 3290 Woodward Street, Oceanside, NY 11572, (516) 766-0588, BA 77 CUNY - Brooklyn Coll; MA 79 NY Univ; Sp-Lang Path, Temple Israel-Lawrence, **SLP**

Malanaphy, Kathleen A 157 East 18th Street #5G, New York, NY 10003, (212) 605-3796, BA 78 SUNY - Coll at Cortland; MA 81 CUNY - Hunter Coll; 87–Supvr of Sp Lang Path, Manhattan Eye Ear & Throat Hosp, **SLP**

Malavenda, Anthony 79 Couture Drive, Bristol, CT 06010, (203) 722-8635, BA 73 Southern CT St Univ; MS 74 Univ of VT; OM 81 Southern CT St Univ; Coor Lang Sp & Hrng, Hartford Bd of Ed, **SLP**

Malavey, Mohan Rao 1463 Sunbeam Circle, Sunshadow MHC, San Jose, CA 95122, (408) 432-8500, MA 72 Temple Univ-Tyler Sch of Art; Aud, Agnews Developmental Center, **A**

Malazdrewicz, Edward John #1-390 Riverview Road, Yorkton, SK, Canada S3N 2L8, (306) 786-1360, BA 84 Brandon Univ - Manitoba; MS 86 Minot St Univ; 86–Aud, Saskatchewan Hrng Aid Plan

Malbon, Pamela 1895 Somerset Drive #1-D, Glendale Heights, IL 60139, (312) 858-3554, BS 85 Univ of IL - Urbana; MS 87 Univ of IL - Urbana; 87–Sp-Lang Path, Schaumburg Sch Dist #54, **SLP**

Malchow, Mary K Route 1 Box 193, Yankton, SD 57078, (605) 665-2073, BS 76 Univ of SD - Vermillion; MA 78 Univ of SD - Vermillion; 78–Sp/Lang Path, Yankton Sch Dist 63-3, **SLP**

Malchow-McCarty, Deborah Lee 1780 Chalcedony, San Diego, CA 92109, (619) 576-5838, BA 76 San Diego St Univ; MA 79 San Diego St Univ; Superv/Aural Rehab-Aud, Chldn's Hosp & Hlth Cen, **A**

Malcomson, David L 101 East 6th Street, Room 211, East Liverpool, OH 43920, (216) 385-7200, BA 69 Slippery Rock Univ of PA; MS 75 Univ of Pittsburgh - Pittsburgh; Dir-Comm Dis, E Liverpool City Hosp, **SLP**

Maldonado, Miguel E Jardines DE Cuenca 201-2A, Avenue Arterial Hostos, Hato Rey, PR 00918, (809) 852-6415, BA 75 Univ of PR - Rio Piedras; MS 80 Univ of PR - Rio Piedras; Aud, Audio Logos Asociados, **A**

Maldonado, Monica 4521 North Delta Avenue, Rosemead, CA 91770, (213) 824-3100, **SLP**

Malecky, Susan M 438 Main Street, Portland, CT 06480, BS 74 Emerson Coll; MA 76 Cleveland St Univ; Sp-Lang Path, Middleton Pub Sch, **SLP**

Malekos, Karen Marie 439 Greenhills Drive, Millbrae, CA 94030, (415) 696-4886, BA 82 Univ of the Pacific; MA 83 Univ of the Pacific; Sp-Lang Path, Mills-Peninsula Hosp, **SLP**

Malepeai, Brenda Bertsch Idaho State University, P O Box 8116, Pocatello, ID 83209, (208) 236-2852, BS 76 ID St Univ; MS 77 ID St Univ; 86–Clin Coord, Idaho State University, **SLP**

Malerba, Louis 256 Artist Lake Drive, Middle Island, NY 11953, (516) 345-3847, BA 80 Adelphi Univ; MA 84 Hofstra Univ; Sp-Lang Path, BOCES II, **SLP**

Maleski, Mrs Diane P 330 Broad Street, Kingsport, TN 37660, (615) 246-4600, BS 67 Purdue Univ - West Lafayette; MS 69 Purdue Univ - West Lafayette; 86–Exec Dir, Mt Reg Sp & Hrng Cen, **SLP**

Maletto, Mrs Patricia M 31 Garfield Avenue, Linwood, NJ 08221, (609) 399-1290, BS 74 Trenton St Coll; MA 78 Trenton St Coll; Sp-Lang Path, Ocean City Public Schools, **SLP**

Maletzke, Ann M 28607 Burma Lane, Waterford, WI 53185, **SLP**

Maley, Susan P H 380 Church Street, Marshfield, MA 02050, (617) 837-8234, BS 75 Univ of RI; MS 78 Boston Univ; Sp-Lang Path, Pilgrim Area Collaborataive, **SLP**

Malfer, Nancy Rose Old Bedford Road, Goldens Bridge, NY 10526, (203) 863-3240, BA 73 Univ of AR - Fayetteville; MA 76 CUNY - Hunter Coll; SLP, Greenwich Hosp Hrng Sp Cen, **SLP**

Malfitano, Amanda A 161 77th Street, Brooklyn, NY 11209, (718) 238-7847, BS 86 Saint John's Univ - Jamaica; MS 88 Columbia Univ Teachers Coll; 88–Sp-Lang Path, LICH-LAMM Institute

Malgeri, Roberta 110 North Bluff, Alpharetta, GA 30201, (404) 751-3851, **SLP**

Malgeri, Mrs Suzanne Elizabeth 20 Cheshire Avenue, Syosset, NY 11791, (516) 921-2909, BS 78 SUNY - Center at Albany; MS 82 Adelphi Univ; Sp-Lang Path, Comm-Sults, **SLP**

Malik, Joan M 18 Bridgeport Lane, Geneva, IL 60134, (312) 426-1261, BA 75 Adelphi Univ; MA 76 Univ of IL - Urbana; 76–Sp-Lang Path, Commun Unit Sch Dist 300, **SLP**

Malilay, Marirose Martha 3109 Lakehurst Avenue, Forestville, MD 20747, (301) 420-8255, BA 84 Univ of MD - College Park; MA 87 Univ of MD - College Park; 86–Sp-Lang Path, Prince George's Co PS, **SLP**

Malin, Jerald A 8918 Allenswood Road, Randallstown, MD 21133, PH (NS); **SLP A**

Malin, Susan S 1128 Laurel Drive, Lafayette, CA 94549, (415) 820-2911, BA 73 Univ of the Pacific; MA 75 Univ of the Pacific; SLP, Sonoma Co Office of Ed, **SLP**

Malina, Mrs Sheila 3512 Lawson Road, Glenview, IL 60025, (312) 453-6813, BS 74 Southern IL Univ -Carbondale; MS 75 Marquette Univ; Sp/Lang Path, Rhodes Elem Sch, **SLP**

Malinak, Betty S 14723 Armin Avenue, Lakewood, OH 44107, (216) 521-4266, BA 69 Case Western Reserve Univ; MA 70 Case Western Reserve Univ; Sp-Lang Path, Private Practice, **SLP**

Malinoff, Dr Rochelle L 131 Perry Street, New York, NY 10014, (212) 598-1343, PH 85 (NS) CUNY - Grad Sch & Univ Cntr; Dir Sp & Hrng, NY Eye & Ear Infirmary, **A**

Malinowski, Marylou 270 Paterson Avenue, Little Falls, NJ 07424, (201) 233-3720, BA 73 William Paterson Coll; MA 77 Montclair St Coll; Sp-Lang Path, Private Practice, **SLP**

Malinowski, Pamela Ann 253 Old Haymaker Road, Monroeville, PA 15146, (412) 622-3865, MA 84 Univ of Pittsburgh - Pittsburgh; BA 82 Univ of Pittsburgh - Pittsburgh; Sp-Lang Path, Pittsburgh Public Schools, **SLP**

Malinsky, Ann Elizabeth 2480 Krumroy Road, Akron, OH 44312-4313, (813) 792-6611, BS 76 Southern IL Univ -Carbondale; MS 85 Southern IL Univ -Carbondale; **SLP**

Malis, Mrs Alexis Pervanis 910 Lakepointe Avenue, Grosse Pointe Pk, MI 48230, (313) 548-1950, BA 79 Wayne St Univ; MA 80 Wayne St Univ; Sp-Lang Path, Sch Dist of Ferndale, **SLP**

Maliszewksi, Michelle Barbara 14 Casey Lane, Wethersfield, CT 06109-3801, (413) 786-8000, Sp-Lang Path, Woodmere Health Care Ctr, **SLP**

Malitz-Katz, Mrs Karen L 49 Lovell Road, Watertown, MA 02172, (617) 924-0783, BA 72 Northwestern Univ; MS 74 Boston Univ; Sp-Lang Path, Private Practice, **SLP**

Malke, Mrs Tracy L 991 Box Elder, St Louis, MO 63122, (314) 569-8100, BS 79 Univ of MO - Columbia; MA 80 Univ of MO - Columbia; Sp-Lang Path, Spec Sch Dist of St Louis Co, **SLP**

Malkiewicz, Jane M 147 Reed Avenue, Trenton, NJ 08610, (609) 599-5220, BA 72 Rosemont Coll; MA 74 Seton Hall Univ; Superv Sp & Hrng Dept, St Francis Med Cen, **A**

Malkin, Cheryl Felmus 24 Burlwood Drive, Burlington, CT 06013, (203) 667-5320, BA 84 Univ of CA - Santa Barbara; MS 86 Univ of WI - Madison; 87–Sp-Lang Path, Newington Children's Hosp, **SLP**

Malkin, Darcie Ellen 4 Countryside Drive, Basking Ridge, NJ 07920, (201) 232-3711, BS 75 Emerson Coll; MS 77 Emerson Coll; 83–Sp-Lang Path, Mountainside Sch Dist, **SLP**

Malkin, Edward S 463 Millburn Avenue #4A, Millburn, NJ 07041, (201) 937-8655, BA 73 Fairleigh Dickinson U-Ruther; MA 78 Montclair St Coll; 88–Dir of Rehab Svcs, Robert Wood Johnson Univ Hosp, **SLP**

Mallahan, Michael Stephen Pacific ENT Clinic, 1515 Pacific Avenue, Everett, WA 98201, (206) 259-5166, Director of Audiology, Pacific ENT Clinic, **A**

Mallar, Mrs Mary M 5010 State Road, Hillsdale, MI 49242, (517) 287-4651, BS 72 OH Univ - Athens; MA 75 Marshall Univ; 87–Sp-Lang Path, Head Injury Therapy Services Inc, **SLP**

Mallard, Dr A Dick 7 Timbercrest, San Marcos, TX 78666, (512) 245-2344, BA 64 Univ of North TX; MA 66 Univ of North TX; PH 74 (Sp-Lang Path) Purdue Univ - West Lafayette; 79–Prof, SW TX St U, **SLP**

Malle, Mrs Joyce Marie 5375 College Avenue, Riverside, CA 92505-3122, BA 82 CA St Univ - Fullerton; MA 84 CA St Univ - Fullerton; 87–Sp-Lang Path, Children's Ctr of Riverside, **SLP**

Malles, Dr Irwin Hal 1163 Highway 37 West, Bldg A1, Toms River, NJ 08753, (201) 505-9090, BA 56 Long Island U - CW Post Ctr; MA 59 CUNY - Brooklyn Coll; PH 81 (Public Health) Univ of Santa Monica; 63–Aud, Private Practice, **A**

Mallette, Julie Lynn 500 East Orchard Street, Odessa, MO 64076, (816) 633-5334, MA 85 Southeast MO St Univ; SLP, Odessa R7 School District, **SLP**

Mallette-Tschaepe, Judi S-4451 Windsor Terrace, Hamburg, NY 14075, (716) 827-9760, BS 77 Eastern KY Univ; MA 83 SUNY - Center at Buffalo; Sp-Lang Path, Olv Infant Home Nursery Sch, **SLP**

Mallon, Christine Box 261, Ardenvoir, WA 98811, (509) 663-7117, BA 72 Univ of MI - Ann Arbor; MS 74 Univ of WI - Madison; 79–Sp-Lang Path, Wenatchee Sch Dist #246, **SLP ACE**

Mallory, Donna M P O Box 7218, Redlands, CA 92375, (714) 782-3830, BS 82 Eastern NM Univ; MS 84 Univ of Redlands; Aud, Clinical ENT Practices, **A**

Mallory, Jocelyn Elaine 3742 Fenley Drive, Los Alamitos, CA 90720, (714) 663-6384, BA 69 CA Poly St Univ-San Luis Obi; MA 71 CA Poly St Univ-San Luis Obi; MA 84 CA St Univ - Long Beach; Sp-Lang Path, Garden Grove Sch Dist, **SLP**

Mallory, Kathleen E The Children's Hospital, 1056 East 19th Avenue, Denver, CO 80218, (303) 861-6800, BS 76 CO St Univ; MA 79 Univ of Denver; 88–Sp-Lang Path, Chldn Hosp Denver, **SLP ACE**

Mallow, Pamela Ann 13400 Beacon Hill Drive, Plymouth, MI 48170, (517) 351-6808, **SLP**

Malloy, Brenda Lane 2816 Ellis Avenue, P O Box 933, Eaton Park, FL 33840-9999, (813) 665-3629, BS 73 Eastern KY Univ; MA 82 Univ of Central FL; SLP, Polk Co Sch Bd, **SLP**

Malloy, Mrs Deborah Marlitt 919 Arizona Street #B, La Grange, GA 30240, (404) 672-1368, **SLP**

Malloy, Mrs Jacquelynn A 3315 Beacon Hill Avenue, Pittsburgh, PA 15216-2203, (412) 675-8716, BA 79 Duquesne Univ; MS 80 WV Univ; Sp-Lang Path, South Hills Health System, **SLP ACE**

Malloy, Mrs Mylene Tamayo 2514 Sunset Drive, Tampa, FL 33629, (813) 239-1179, BS 85 FL St Univ; ME 87 Univ of FL; 88–Sp-Lang Path, UCP of Tampa, **SLP**

Malmad, Susan J P O Box 306, Chestnut Hill, MA 02167, (617) 323-3265, BS 72 Emerson Coll; ME 75 Northeastern Univ; Sp-Lang Path, Sp Ther Assoc, Inc, **SLP**

Malmgren, Virginia A 3533 Pueblo Way, Las Vegas, NV 89109, (608) 655-3345, BS 74 AZ St Univ; MA 76 Univ of Denver; Sp-Lang Path, Marshall Pub Sch, **SLP**

Malnar, Debra D 2506 Clarke Street, River Grove, IL 60171, (312) 455-4818, BA 80 Augustana Coll; MA 81 Univ of IL - Urbana, Sp/Lang Path, Mannheim Sch Dist 83, **SLP**

Malnati, Cheryl P O Box 1168, Fort Bragg, CA 95437, (707) 964-4044, BS 85 CA St Univ - Sacramento; MS 87 San Francisco St Univ; 88–Resource Spec, Mendocino USD

Malof, Leah Berkowitz 10750 Westbrae Parkway, #1808, Houston, TX 77031, (713) 792-4500, BA 85 Emory Univ; MA 88 IN Univ - Bloomington; 88, Sp & Hrng Inst Univ of TX

Malone, Mrs Charleen Campbell 2936 Thunderbird Drive, Poland, OH 44514, (216) 757-9058, BA 64 Carlow Coll; SLP, Poland Bd of Ed, **SLP**

Malone, Christina 133 Grand Avenue, Rockville Centre, NY 11570, (516) 766-8036, BA 75 CUNY - Queens Coll; MS 76 Adelphi Univ; Infant Spec, Suffolk Child Dev Ctr, **SLP**

Malone, Dr James Charles Route 2 Box 797, Beaufort, NC 28516, (919) 247-5570, BA 62 Vanderbilt Univ; MS 63 Vanderbilt Univ; PH 70 (Aud) Univ of OK Medical Center; Private Practice, **A**

Malone, Mrs Jane Grace 19 Draeger Place, South River, NJ 08882, (201) 238-5783, MA 84 Seton Hall Univ; 88–Sp-Lang Path, Milltown PS, **SLP**

Malone, Margueritte S 4801 Bel Pre Road, Rockville, MD 20853, BS 59 Central MO St Univ; MS 61 PA St Univ - Univ Park; 78–Sp-Lang Path, Montgomery County PS, **SLP**

Malone, Martha L 3758 Fremantle Drive, Palm Harbor, FL 34684, (813) 787-5508, MS 80 FL St Univ; SLP, Dunedin High School, **SLP**

Malone, Michael J 1138 Glendale, Saginaw, MI 48603, (517) 776-0545, BA 75 MI St Univ; MA 76 MI St Univ; Aud, Saginaw Pub Sch, **A**

Malone, Sr Patricia 51 Medford Street, Arlington, MA 02174, (617) 893-1820, MA 64 9160; OM 70 Boston Univ; ED 80 (NS) Boston Univ; **SLP**

Malone, Patricia A 9715 Darien Road, West Falls, NY 14170, (716) 592-3260, BS 76 SUNY - Coll at Buffalo; MS 78 SUNY - Coll at Buffalo; 77–Sp-Lang Path, Springville Griffith Institute, **SLP**

Malone, Dr Russell L 10801 Rockville Pike, Rockville, MD 20852, (301) 897-5700, BA 54 Univ of AL- Tuscaloosa; MS 60 Univ of UT; PH 66 (Sp-Lang Path & Aud) Case Western Reserve Univ; 78–Dir Pub Info, ASHA, **SLP F**

Malone, Susan M 3675 Misty Meadows Drive, Colorado Springs, CO 80920, (719) 531-5782, BS 76 Clarion Univ of PA; ME 77 Clarion Univ of PA; Sp-Lang Path, Rocky Mt Rehab Ctr, **SLP**

Malone, Terry P Box 205, Woodson, IL 62695-0205, (217) 673-4721, BS 75 Western IL Univ; MA 76 Western IL Univ; Sp-Lang Path, Jacksonville School Dist 117, **SLP**

Maloney, Anita Louise 161 Atlantic Street, North Quincy, MA 02171-1608, BS 83 Worcester St Coll; MS 85 Emerson Coll; Sp-Lang Path, Morton Hosp, **SLP ACE**

Maloney, Ann P O Box 434, Wheatland, WY 82201, (307) 322-5480, **SLP**

Maloney, Mrs Beth Ann 1796 West Lake Avenue, Littleton, CO 80120, (303) 794-6806, BS 83 CO St Univ; MS 85 CO St Univ; **SLP**

Maloney, John B 16100 Cogan Drive, Independence, MO 64055, (816) 461-0930, BS 64 Central MO St Univ; MS 74 Central MO St Univ; SLP, Independence Bd of Ed, **SLP**

Maloney, John Stevens P O Box 1573, Pawleys Island, SC 29585, (803) 546-2561, BS 71 Appalachian St Univ; MA 73 Appalachian St Univ

Maloney, Nina Belle c/o Jan Marsh, Route 1 Box 165-A, Kirksville, MO 64601, MS; **SLP LM**

Malott, Mrs Celeste Marie 801 South Thomas, Saginaw, MI 48603, (517) 792-8771, BA 82 MI St Univ; MA 83 MI St Univ; **SLP**

Malott, Paul James Speech And Hearing Clinic, Miami University, Oxford, OH 45056, (513) 529-2549, BS 62 Miami Univ - Oxford; MA 63 Bowling Green St Univ; PH 70 (NS) Bowling Green St Univ; Dir/Sp-Lang Path, Miami U, **SLP**

Maloy, Mrs Janet Y 1120 6th Street, Huntington, WV 25701, (304) 523-0461, BA 56 MI St Univ; MA 72 Marshall Univ; Sp/Lang Path, Cabell Cty Bd of Ed, **SLP**

Maloy, Marianne C 16 Phillips Road, Rensselaer, NY 12144, (215) 645-2210, BS 76 SUNY - Coll at Geneseo; MA 79 Temple Univ; Sp-Lang Path, VA Hosp, **SLP**

Malphurs, Dr Ojus, Jr 5605 Warwick Drive, Jackson, MS 39211, (601) 956-3364, BA 59 Univ of VA - Charlottesville; ME 64 Univ of VA - Charlottesville; PH 70 (NS) Univ of VA - Charlottesville; Asst Prof & Dir, U of MS Med Cen, **SLP A**

Malpica, Frida L 209 Garth Road #2-A, Scarsdale, NY 10583-3965, (914) 723-8252, BA 74 CUNY - Lehman Coll; MS 76 PA St Univ - Univ Park; Aud, Private Practice, **A**

Malsin, Janie 11706 Southwest 108 Lane, Miami, FL 33186-3921, (305) 649-2811, **SLP**

Malstrom, Linda K 2215 Birchwood, Wilmette, IL 60091, (312) 251-1069, BS 68 Northern IL Univ - De Kalb; MA 69 Univ of IL - Urbana; **SLP**

Maltby, Robert L 4160 Ross Road, Nanaimo, BC, Canada V9T 493, (604) 756-7885, OB 78 Univ of Western Ontario; OM 82 Univ of WA; Sp/Lang Path, Min of Hlth, **SLP**

Malte, Patricia L 2434 130th Avenue N E, Bellevue, WA 98005, (206) 885-2460, BS 62 Saint Cloud St Univ; MS 68 Univ of MI - Ann Arbor; OM 84 Univ of WA; **SLP**

Maly, Mrs Debra Rhein 18251 Cummings Street, Fontana, CA 92336, BS 82 Univ of Cincinnati; MA 84 Univ of Cincinnati; Sp-Lang Path, Redwood School, **SLP**

Mamey, Joan F 929 Chudleigh Lane, Glendale, CA 91207, **SLP**

Mammoser, Lisa Marie 26106 Lamuera, Farmington Hills, MI 48018, (313) 288-8085, MA 85 Wayne St Univ; **SLP**

Mamolen, Eleanor G 1201 Alta Vista Road #106, Santa Barbara, CA 93103, (805) 962-8284, BA 36 CUNY - Hunter Coll; MA 37 Columbia Univ Teachers Coll; **SLP LM**

Mamrila, Mrs Suzanne 8613 Cline Avenue, Crown Point, IN 46307, (219) 365-8577, BA 80 Purdue Univ - West Lafayette; MA 81 Univ of IL - Urbana; SLP, West Lake Special Ed Coop, **SLP ACE**

Man, Hilda 996 Springview Circle, San Ramon, CA 94583, (415) 938-4722, BA 80 Humboldt St Univ; MS 83 San Francisco St Univ; 88–Sp-Lang Path, Diablo Valley Rehab Clinic, **SLP**

Manasco, Mrs Betty Jo P 1016 Ramsgate Lane, Chesapeake, VA 23320-1963, BA 75 Mary Washington Coll; ME 76 Univ of VA - Charlottesville; **SLP**

Manassero, Robynn 2505 4th Street #211, Santa Monica, CA 90405, (213) 399-5213, BA 77 CA St Univ - Northridge; MA 79 CA St Univ - Northridge; SLP, LA USD, **SLP**

Mancano, Bridget Barnard 706 Argyle Road, Wynnewood, PA 19096-2503, (215) 642-5972, MA 84 Temple Univ; Audiologist, Washington Univ Sch Medicine, **A**

Mancha, Ellen Padget 672 Abington, El Paso, TX 79912, (915) 598-8121, BS 77 Univ of TX - Austin; MA 79 CA St Univ - Northridge; Sp/Lang Path, Edgewood ISD, **SLP**

Manchester, Ellen Morris 67 Lane Drive, Norwood, MA 02062, MS 79 Hofstra Univ; Sp-Lang Path, Walthamweston Hospital Eip, **SLP**

Manchester, Karen Z 15 Rectory Lane, Scarsdale, NY 10583, (212) 988-5556, BS 70 NY Univ; MS 71 Univ of MI - Ann Arbor; Sp-Lang Path, Private Practice, **SLP**

Manchester, Mary Elizabeth 1118 Montclaire N E, Albuquerque, NM 87110, (505) 884-5275, BS 78 Univ of NM; MS 82 Univ of NM; Sp-Lang Path, Albuqquerque Pub Schs, **SLP**

Mancina, Mary Rose 1714 Henderson Avenue, Clarksburg, WV 26301, (304) 623-2931, BS 84 WV Univ; MS 85 WV Univ; **SLP**

Mancinelli, James Mark 141 Fitzwater Street, Philadelphia, PA 19147, (215) 448-7698, BA 72 Rutgers St Univ - Camdem; MS 84 Rutgers St Univ -N Brunswick; Sp-Lang Path, Hahnemann Univ, **SLP**

Mancini, Frederic J P O Box 1268, Ellicott City, MD 21043, (800) 521-5400, BA 81 MI St Univ; MA 83 MI St Univ; Aud, Hrng & Sp Cen/Grand Rapids, **A**

Mancini, Mrs Susan B 12418 Mossycup, Houston, TX 77024, (713) 932-9601, BS 71 Univ of MN - Minneap-St Paul; MA 75 Univ of MN - Minneap-St Paul; **SLP**

Mancino, Diane Marie 14 Park Place #4, New Britain, CT 06051, (203) 666-1434, BA 79 Central CT St Univ; MS 84 Southern CT St Univ; Sp-Lang Path, Private Practice, **SLP**

Mancusco, Catherine 4219 1st Avenue East, Bradenton, FL 34208, (414) 259-1414, BS 80 Univ of WI - Eau Claire; MS 82 Univ of WI - Milwaukee; **SLP**

Mancuso, Robert A 126 Culler Road, Weirton, WV 26062, (304) 723-1615, OB 73 West Liberty St Coll; MS 75 WV Univ; Sp-Lang Path, Brooke Co Sch, **SLP**

Mandel, Mrs Ellen W 9 Hamden Heights Court, New City, NY 10956, (914) 362-1350, MS 70 CUNY - Brooklyn Coll; OM 84 Columbia Univ Teachers Coll; PH 84 (NS) Columbia Univ Teachers Coll; Assistant Professor, Pace University, **SLP**

Mandel, Jeri Lynn 68 Welsh Tract Road #208, Newark, DE 19713, (302) 656-2521, BA 76 Univ of MD - College Park; OM 78 Hahneman Medical Coll; Sp-Lang Path, De Curative Workshop Inc, **SLP**

Mandel, Mrs Jill New York School For The Deaf, 555 Knollwood Road, White Plains, NY 10603, (914) 949-7310, BA 76 SUNY - Center at Buffalo; MA 78 Univ of CT; 80–Aud, NY Sch for the Deaf, **A**

Mandel, Rae L K 1475 Wellesley, Mount Clemens, MI 48043, (313) 286-8800, BS 74 Miami Univ - Oxford; MA 75 MI St Univ; 76–Sp/Lang Path, MacOmb ISD, **SLP**

Mandel, Mrs Susan Y 51 Raymond Terrace, Elizabeth, NJ 07208, (201) 527-6361, BS 78 Southern CT St Univ; MS 85 Saint Joseph Coll; MA 84 Boston Univ; **SLP**

Mandelbaum, Mrs Nancy J 920 Manhattan Beach Boulevard, Suite 4, Manhattan Beach, CA 90266, (213) 546-6468, BA 76 CUNY - Queens Coll; MA 78 NY Univ; Sp-Lang Path/Dir of Serv, South Bay Sp & Lang Svcs, **SLP**

Mandelbaum, Tricia Ann 5417 Dexter Falls Road, Hilliard, OH 43206, (614) 263-5151, BA 80 IN Univ - Bloomington; MA 82 IN Univ - Bloomington; Audiologist, Columbus Speech Hearing Center, **A**

Mandel-Herbert, Mrs Jody 2255 West Club View Drive, Glendale, WI 53209, (414) 352-9036, BS 75 Univ of WI - Madison; MA 76 George Washington Univ; Sp-Lang Path, Fox Point-Bayside Schs, **SLP**

Mandelker, Mrs Cheryl Z 33 Winthrope Road, Manhasset, NY 11030, (516) 365-7516, BA 72 Univ of AZ; MS 73 Univ of AZ; 79–Sp-Lang Path, Private Practice, **SLP**

Mandell, Elizabeth Ann 1636 North Wells Street, Apartment 611, Chicago, IL 60614, (312) 943-9283, BA 73 Univ of MI - Ann Arbor; MA 75 Wayne St Univ - Sch of Med; Aud, Private Practice, **A**

Mandell, Jacqueline Kramer 9053 S W 78th Place, Miami, FL 33156, (305) 596-5929, BS 66 Univ of Cincinnati; MS 87 Nova Univ; 88–Sp-Lang Path, Baptist Hosp of Miami, **SLP**

Mandell, Mrs Roni K 14 Millbury Lane, Centereach, NY 11720, (516) 732-2444, BS 72 Long Island U - CW Post Ctr; MS 73 Long Island U - CW Post Ctr; Dir, Pedia Cen for Sp Path, **SLP**

Mandell, Mrs Sue-Ellen 430 Littleton Road North, New City, NY 10956, (914) 358-8830, BA 65 CUNY - Hunter Coll; MA 80 CUNY - Lehman Coll; Sp-Lang Path, Clarkstown Central Sch Dist, **SLP**

Mandell, Dr Theodore 21460 Constitution Drive, Southfield, MI 48076, (313) 494-1643, BA 40 Univ of MI - Ann Arbor; MA 41 Univ of MI - Ann Arbor; ED 56 (NS) Wayne St Univ; Retired, Detroit Pub Sch, **SLP F LM**

Mandeltort, Susan G 1229 Trinity Place, Libertyville, IL 60048, (312) 623-0021, BA 80 MacAlster Coll; MA 84 Northwestern Univ; 85–Sp-Lang Path, Spec Educ Dis, **SLP**

Manding, Mrs Glorilynn O 94-1109 Kahuanui Street, Waipahu, HI 96797, (808) 671-0587, BS 87 Univ of HI - Manoa; MS 87 Univ of HI - Manoa

Mandiola, Mrs Claudine Allamand 1372 Smokewood Drive, Santa Ana, CA 92705, (714) 835-3314, BA 81 CA St Univ - Fullerton; MA 84 CA St Univ - Fullerton; 88–Consult/Sp-Lang Patn, Private Practice, **SLP**

Mandke, Kalyani Narsinha 964 Sadashive Peth, Pune, India 411030, (617) 478-0723, BS 75 Bombay Univ - India; ME 82 Northeastern Univ; 84–Aud, Private Practice, **A**

Mandor, Sandra A 36 Oxford Road, Old Bethpage, NY 11804, (516) 231-8000, BA 75 CUNY - Queens Coll; MA 77 CUNY - Queens Coll; **SLP**

Manek, Mrs Doris J Route 1 Box 24, Libertyville, IL 60048, MS 71 Northwestern Univ; SLP, Special Educ Dist of Lake Cnty, **SLP**

Manela, Mrs Temmy L 1752 45th Street, Brooklyn, NY 11204, BA 72 CUNY - Brooklyn Coll; MS 80 CUNY - Brooklyn Coll; Sp-Lang Path, NYC Bd of Ed, **SLP**

Manelli, Leslie Thedford 81 Martinique Avenue, Tampa, FL 33606, (813) 254-9419, **SLP**

Manello, Mrs Ephros 265 Warren Avenue, Rochester, NY 14618, (716) 244-4738, BS 63 Syracuse Univ; MA 64 Columbia Univ Teachers Coll; 83–Sp-Lang Path, Rochester Gen Hos/Private Practice, **SLP**

Maneri, Mrs Dina A 712 Blue Ridge Drive, Medford, NY 11763, (516) 724-3626, BS 82 Univ of IA; MS 86 Hofstra Univ; 86–Consult, LI Ctr for Comm Disorders, **SLP**

Maneri, Mrs Marilyn S 17 Brookside Road, Ridgefield, CT 06877, (203) 797-4797, BS 57 Syracuse Univ; MS 74 Southern CT St Univ; OM 79 Southern CT St Univ; SLP, Danbury Pub Schs, **SLP**

Maness, Lisa Diana 31717 Edgeworth, Madison Heights, MI 48071, (313) 589-0123, BA 84 Harding Univ; MS 86 Univ of AR - Little Rock; 86–Sp-Lang Path, Rehab Inst, **SLP**

Manetta-Lawson, Margaret A 2675 Stonebury Drive, Rochester, MI 48063-6127, **SLP**

Mangan, Debra Hashimoto 264 North Whisman #20, Mountain View, CA 94043, (408) 730-4220, **A**

Mangan, Dr James 931 Rue Crozat, Baton Rouge, LA 70818, (504) 766-6113, BA 66 Carroll Coll; MA 72 Univ of MT; PH 77 (NS) Univ of IA; SLP/Aud, Prof Sp & Hrng Serv Inc, **SLP A**

Mangels, Barbara J 3553 Emerald Street #315, Torrance, CA 90503, (213) 530-0401, BA 69 Mary Washington Coll; ME 70 Univ of VA - Charlottesville; Sp-Lang Path, The Speech Cen, **SLP**

Mangiapane, Patricia Ann 6449 Aspinwall Road, Oakland, CA 94611, (415) 339-1259, BS 81 CA St Univ - Hayward; MA 83 Univ of the Pacific; **SLP**

Mangin, Nancy L 15516 Riverdale Avenue East, Baton Rouge, LA 70816, (504) 272-6242, BA 74 Univ of South AL; MA 76 LA St Univ - Baton Rouge; SLP, Assoc II Sp-Lang Cl, **SLP**

Mangino, Patrick N 1180 Smoke Burr Drive, Westerville, OH 43081, (614) 267-5128, BA 72 Kent St Univ; MA 73 Kent St Univ; Pres, Aud & Hrng Aid Serv Inc, **A**

Mangipudi, Latha D 210 Church Street, Waltham, MA 02154, (617) 893-4112, OB 82; OM 84; 88–Sp-Lang Path, Lang & Cognative Dev Ctr, **A**

Mango, Frances 53 Heritage Drive, Tewksbury, MA 01876, (617) 273-1870, BS 73 Edinboro Univ of PA; MA 81 Edinboro Univ of PA; Sp-Lang Path, LABB-Preschool Lang Delayed Class, **SLP**

Mango, Howard T 500 North Newport, Suite 101, Newport, CA 92660, (714) 642-7935, BA 73 Univ of Southern CA; ME 75 Univ of VA - Charlottesville; Dir of Aud & Vestibular Lab, Newport Mesa Aud Inc, **A**

Mangold, Lorraine S 1435 Funderburg Street, Keyser, WV 26726, (304) 298-3632, BS 81 PA St Univ - Univ Park; MA 83 Univ of Pittsburgh - Pittsburgh; Sp-Lang Path, Mineral County Board of Educ, **SLP**

Mangrum, Mrs Julia Gayle P O Box 954, Hugo, OK 74743, (405) 326-7645, BS 84 Southeastern OK St Univ; MS 85 Univ of North TX; 86–Sp-Lang Path, Bryan Co Child Guidance Clinic, **SLP**

Mangum, Mrs Connie West 4483 Kinkead Ct, Fayetteville, NC 28304, (919) 867-4227, BA 83 Univ of NC - Chapel Hill; MS 85 Univ of NC - Chapel Hill; **SLP**

Mangum, Mrs Susan B 5115 McCormick, Durham, NC 27713-2339, (919) 544-6896, BA 73 Univ of NC - Chapel Hill; MS 79 Univ of NC - Chapel Hill; 88–Aud, Cary Ear Nose/Throat Clinic, **A**

Mangurten, Mrs Brucene B 602 Warwick Road, Deerfield, IL 60015, (312) 945-1844, BS 66 Univ of IL - Urbana; MA 67 Northwestern Univ; Sp-Lang Path, Deerfield Pub Sch, **SLP**

Mangus, Robin Elizabeth 2023 North 104th Street, Omaha, NE 68134, (303) 574-8300, **SLP**

Manheimer, Mrs Sandra 26 Hemlock Terrace, Springfield, NJ 07081, (201) 233-3720, BA 51 Rutgers St Univ - Newark; MA 66 Kean Coll of NJ; Sp-Lang Path, Chldn Specialized Hosp, **SLP**

Manidok, Renee Ann 7107 Ming Avenue #42, Bakersfield, CA 93309, (805) 397-4734, OB 84 IL St Univ - Normal; OM 85 IL St Univ - Normal; **A**

Manigold, Mrs Jo Ann W 7749 Wenda Way, El Paso, TX 79915, (915) 598-0861, BA 71 Univ of TX - El Paso; MA 81 Univ of TX - El Paso; Sp-Lang Path, Ysleta ISD, **SLP ACE**

Manigold, Mrs Rebecca D 435 McKee Street, Batavia, IL 60510, (312) 393-9413, BS 80 IL St Univ - Normal; MS 81 IL St Univ - Normal; Sp-Lang Path, Wheaton-Warrenville Dist 200, **SLP**

Manion, Kathleen H 1150 Alviria Drive, Ojai, CA 93023, BA 72 Univ of CA - Santa Barbara; MA 83 CA St Univ - Northridge; Sp-Lang Path, Ventura USD, **SLP**

Manion, Mary Beth 1708 Jeanette, Wichita, KS 67203, (316) 263-3004, BA 72 Wichita St Univ; MA 73 Wichita St Univ; Sp-Lang Path, Wichita Pub Sch USD #259, **SLP**

Manji, Shelina T 15 Torrance Road #1801, Scarborough, ON, Canada M1J 3K2, (416) 439-7640, MS 85 Univ of South FL; **SLP**

Manley, Anita Odell 1616 Smith Road, Columbus, OH 43207, (614) 274-7123, BS 76 NC A & T St Univ; MA 78 OH St Univ; SLP, State of Ohio, **SLP**

Manley, Rita O 1501 Forest Street, Columbus, OH 43206, (614) 443-9425, BS 76 NC A & T St Univ; MA 78 OH St Univ; Sp-Lang Path, The Childhood League Center, **SLP**

Manlove, Sr Christine 3725 Ellerslie Avenue, Baltimore, MD 21218, (301) 235-3378, BA 74 Loyola Coll; MS 75 Loyola Coll; MS 81 Johns Hopkins Univ; Doctoral /Instructor, St Francis Sch for Spec Ed, **SLP**

Manly, Dr Carol Ann 360 East 65th Street, Suite 21-D, New York, NY 10021, (212) 691-3434, BS 69 Kent St Univ; MA 70 Univ of Cincinnati; 88 (Sp-Lang Path) New York Univ; Sp-Lang Path, Private Practice, **SLP**

Mann, Andrea L 27 Pineneedle Road, Boulder, CO 80302-0436, (303) 441-0493, BS 75 SUNY - Coll at Geneseo; MA 77 SUNY - Coll at Geneseo; Sp-Lang Path, Boulder Memorial Hosp, **SLP**

Mann, Brenda Pakier 2505 Loring Street, San Diego, CA 92109, (619) 260-7161, BS 75 Univ of IL - Urbana; MS 76 Univ of MI - Ann Arbor; Superv Sp-Lang Path, Mercy Hosp, **SLP**

Mann, Mrs Donna J 645 Central Avenue, Buellton, CA 93427, (805) 683-3788, BA 78 Univ of NM; MS 83 Eastern NM Univ; Sp-Lang Path, Fort Stanton Hospital, **SLP ACE**

Mann, Mrs Ellen K 8551 North Point Drive, Fox Point, WI 53217, OM 73 Southern IL Univ -Carbondale; MA 75 Southern IL Univ -Carbondale; **SLP**

Mann, Mrs Jeri Lynn 519 Nottingham Oaks Trail, Houston, TX 77079, (713) 589-7123, BS 80 Miami Univ - Oxford; MA 82 OH St Univ; SLP, Robbin Parish Sp/P Assoc, **SLP**

Mann, Mrs Judith G 2313 Woodcreek Drive, Birmingham, AL 35226, (205) 939-9253, OB 71 Auburn Univ - Auburn; OM 72 Auburn Univ - Auburn; Sp-Lang Path, The Childrens Hosp, **SLP**

Mann, Karen Eileen 1007 Forest Oak Drive #502, Charlotte, NC 28209, (704) 522-8535, BS 83 East Carolina Univ; MS 84 East Carolina Univ; Sp-Lang Path, Assoc Healthfocus, **SLP**

Mann, Marcia P 603 East 23rd Street, Brooklyn, NY 11210, BS 59 New York Univ; MA 63 Stanford Univ; 72–Sp-Lang Path, NYC Bd of Educ, **SLP**

Mann, Mrs Mary Ann 318 East Oklahoma Avenue, Milwaukee, WI 53207, (414) 483-4820, BS 79 Marquette Univ; MS 85 Univ of WI - Milwaukee; **SLP**

Mann, Dr Mary B 24 Columbine Drive, Williamsville, NY 14221, (716) 831-3395, BA 36; MA 37 Univ of IA; PH 41 (Clinical Psychology) Univ of IA; Assoc Prof Emeritus, State University of New York, **SLP F LM**

Mann, Neal E 11422 East Lake Road, North East, PA 16428, (814) 833-9533, BA 67 Univ of MA - Amherst; MA 68 Univ of MA - Amherst; 86–Aud, Erie Aud & Hrng Aid Ctr, **A**

Mann, Richard Clarke 19 Stephanie Drive, Bear, DE 19701, (302) 328-7758, BA 83 SUNY - Coll at Plattsburgh; MA 85 SUNY - Coll at Plattsburgh; **A**

Manna-Levin, Karen Lee 9630 Vanalden Avenue, Northridge, CA 91324, (818) 772-2668, BA 86 CA St Univ - Northridge; MA 88 CA St Univ - Northridge

Mannarelli, Julie A 7169 Sugar Spring Court, St Louis, MO 63129, **SLP**

Mannello, Deborah C 231 Clifton Avenue, Kingston, NY 12401, (914) 331-2568, BS 70 SUNY - Coll at Geneseo; MS 76 SUNY - Center at Albany; 85–Sp-Lang Path, Private Practice, **SLP**

Manners, Lori Sue 8235 Southwest 151 Street, Miami, FL 33158, (305) 253-7253, BA 79 Univ of FL; MA 81 Univ of FL; Sp/Lang Path, Broward Co Sch, **SLP**

Manney, Anne M R R 2 Box 123, Ashby, MA 01431, (508) 386-5579, BA 69 Univ of MA - Amherst; MA 70 Univ of MA - Amherst; Audiologist, Cheong H Kim MD, **A**

Mannigel, Mrs Pamela A Box 91, Pulaski, WI 54162, (414) 822-3191, BA 69 Univ of WI - Eau Claire; MS 70 Univ of WI - Stevens Point; Sp-Lang Path, Pulaski Comm Schs, **SLP**

Manninen, Mrs Debra Lynn 4312 Renas Road, Gladwin, MI 48624, (517) 275-5137, MA 80 Central MI Univ; Sp-Lang Path, Coor ISD, **SLP**

Manninen, Jean L M 168 Parkview, Golden, CO 80401, (303) 571-1003, BS 61; MA 79; SLP, Jefferson Co Pub Sch, **SLP**

Manning, Annette Louise 2867 Norma Street, Cuyahoga Falls, OH 44223, (216) 923-6162, BA 85 Univ of Akron; MA 87 Univ of Akron; Sp-Lang Path, Kent St Univ, **SLP**

Manning, Mrs Bonnie Krawczyk 4477 St Michaels Drive, Lilburn, GA 30247, (404) 292-7272, BA 72 Univ of KY; ME 78 GA St Univ; Sp/Lang Path, De Kalb County Board of Educ, **SLP**

Manning, Carol Ann Middlesex Hearing Aids Inc, West Meeting House, 86 Pleasant Street, Marlboro, MA 01752, BS 78 Worcester St Coll; MS 79 Ithaca Coll; Owner & Operator, Middlesex Hearing Aids Inc, **A**

Manning, Dr Charlie C C C Manning Phd And Assoc, 33515 10th Place South, Suite 12-A, Federal Way, WA 98003, (206) 874-2599, BA 52 WA St Univ; MA 57 Univ of WA; PH 64 (NS) Univ of WA; Owner, C C Manning & Assoc, **SLP A**

Manning, Mrs Colleen M 138 Branch Street, Scituate, MA 02066, BA 74 Univ of MA - Amherst; ME 75 Northeastern Univ; SLP, Quincy Public Schools, **SLP**

Manning, Cynthia Wheeler 18 Cortez Drive, Nashua, NH 03062, (603) 432-6937, BS 84 Univ of NH; MS 85 Syracuse Univ; 87–Sp-Lang Path, Londonderry Sch Dist, **SLP**

Manning, Mrs Joan B 1738 The 12th Fairway, West Palm Beach, FL 33414, (305) 433-1907, BS 66 PA St Univ - Univ Park; MS 69 Purdue Univ - West Lafayette; SLP, Palm Beach County School Board, **SLP**

Manning, Judy Ellen 1309 5th Avenue #6B, New York, NY 10029, (212) 596-5725, BA 80 Pace U -NY City; MS 82 Adelphi Univ; SLP, Speech Services Unit Bd of Ed, **SLP**

Manning, Kathy Lynn Tau Valley Estates #S3, 237 Winstead Avenue, Rocky Mount, NC 27804, (919) 443-8858, BS 80 Purdue Univ - West Lafayette; MS 82 Vanderbilt Univ; 83–Sp-Lang Path, Dev Eval Cen, **SLP**

Manning, Mrs Marlynn C 4237 Selkirk Drive West, Fort Worth, TX 76109, (713) 350-0332, BA 73 IN Univ - Bloomington; MA 76 Ball St Univ; **SLP**

Manning, Mrs Mary C 55 Rogers Court, Pleasant Hill, CA 94523, (415) 682-8000, BS 67 Northern MI Univ; MS 68 CO St Univ; Admin, Mt Diablo USD, **SLP**

Manning, Mary E 348 Collingswood Street, San Francisco, CA 94114, (415) 921-7658, BS 59 Univ of MN - Minneap-St Paul; MA 64 Case Western Reserve Univ; Dir-Sp Servs, San Francisco Hrng & Sp Cen, **SLP**

Manning, Robert Dean Eastern Kentucky Sp & Hrng Clinic, 2101 Nicholasville Road, Suite 104, Lexington, KY 40503, (606) 277-0491, BA 76 IL St Univ - Normal; MS 77 IL St Univ - Normal; Aud/Owner, En KY Sp&Hrng Cl, **A**

Manning, Mrs Susan Slack 2026 Gurney Court, Burlington, NC 27215, (919) 584-1149, BA 76 Marshall Univ; MA 77 Univ of TN - Knoxville; Sp-Lang Path, Private Practice, **SLP**

Manning, Dr Walter Harne Dept Audiology & Speech Path, Memphis State University, 807 Jefferson Avenue, Memphis, TN 38105, (901) 525-2682, BA 64 Lycoming Coll; ME 67 PA St Univ - Univ Park; PH 72 (Speech Science and Path) MI St Univ; 77–Prof, Memphis State University, **SLP**

Mannion, Marianne Theresa 1222 South 18th Street, St Louis, MO 63104, BS 78 Univ of MO - Columbia; MA 80 Univ of CO - Boulder; Sp-Lang Path, Cardinal Glennon Mem Hosp, **SLP**

Mannisto, Marilisa 542 Lake Avenue, Apartment 10, Hancock, MI 49930, **SLP**

Mannix, Mrs Maureen McMahon South 4412 Sheri Court, Spokane, WA 99223, (509) 455-3024, BA 82 Carroll Coll; OM 85 Univ of MT; 86–Sp-Lang Path, Sacred Heart Med Center, **SLP**

Manno, Mrs Carol Eve 3708 Pinewood Street, Redford, TX 76021, (817) 354-5584, BS 76 FL St Univ; MS 82 Univ of HI - Manoa; **SLP**

Manno, Cecilia J 1060 Churchville Road, Southampton, PA 18966, BS 76 Indiana Univ of PA; MS 80 Indiana Univ of PA; Sp-Lang Path, Appalachia Intermediate Unit 8, **SLP**

Manno, Lorane 727 Bronx River Road, Bronxville, NY 10708, (914) 237-4239, BA 72 CUNY - Lehman Coll; MA 74 CUNY - Lehman Coll; Superv-Sp/Lang Path, **SLP**

Mannon, Janice Evelyn 1045 Via Tranquila, Santa Barbara, CA 93110, (805) 682-3642, **SLP**

Mannos, Mrs Ronnie S 236 Delphi Circle, Los Altos, CA 94022, (415) 948-1869, BS 68 Emerson Coll; MA 70 San Francisco St Univ; **SLP**

Mannschreck, Brenda S R R 1 Box 163, Fairbury, NE 68352, (402) 729-5956, BA 71 Kearney St Coll; MA 76 Univ of NE - Lincoln; Head of Dept SLP, Beatrice Comm Hosp, **SLP**

Manolson, Ayala A 252 Bloor Street West, Suite 4-126, Toronto, ON, Canada M5S 1V6, (416) 967-0417, BA 52 1859; MS 72 McGill Univ - Quebec; Dir, Hanen Early Lang Prog, **SLP**

Manoogian, Mrs Judy L 47 Vine Street, North Attleboro, MA 02760, (617) 226-0630, BA 77 Bridgewater St Coll; MS 78 Rutgers St Univ -N Brunswick; **SLP**

Manscuk, Mrs Theresa C 1324 Shoecraft Road, Webster, NY 14580, (716) 383-2244, BA 79 SUNY - Center at Buffalo; MA 81 SUNY - Center at Buffalo; Sp-Lang Path, Monroe BOCES #1, **SLP ACE**

Mansell, Bruce Edmonton Audiological Center, 215-10113 104th Street, Edmonton, AB, Canada T5J 1A1, (403) 422-6734, MS 72 Southern IL Univ -Carbondale; BS 70 Emerson Coll; Aud, Edmonton Aud Cen, **A**

Mansell, Mrs Teresa M Rd 4 Box 4105, Pottsville, PA 17901, (717) 622-3350, BS 77 Marywood Coll; MS 79 Bloomsburg Univ of PA; **SLP**

Manser, Joseph Stephen, III 4373 Stoneybrook Drive S E, Warren, OH 44484, BS 72 Kent St Univ; MA 76 Kent St Univ; **A**

Mansfield, Mrs Carol S 73 Muskoka, Grosse Pointe Farms, MI 48236, (313) 882-7866, BA 72 Gonzaga Univ; MA 76 Wayne St Univ; Sp-Lang Path, Private Practice, **SLP**

Mansfield, Kelly Lyn 418 East Belmar Street, Lakeland, FL 33803, (813) 682-7149, BS 84 0880; MS 86 Western KY Univ; 88–Sp-Lang Path, InSpeech Inc, **SLP**

Mansfield, Lynn A 232 Leighway Drive, Westerville, OH 43081, (614) 888-3221, BS 73 Miami Univ - Oxford; MS 74 Miami Univ - Oxford; Sp/Lang Path, Ohio Sch Deaf, **SLP**

Mansfield, Mrs Lynne N 1174 Northwood Lake, Northport, AL 35476, (205) 339-9678, BS 67 TX Woman's Univ; MA 73 TX Woman's Univ; SLP, Neurology Cl, **SLP**

Mansfield, Mrs Mary Lee 1370 Ridgewood, Salem, OH 44460, (216) 332-0316, BS 73 Kent St Univ; MA 84 Kent St Univ; 73–Sp-Lang Path, Salem City Schs, **SLP**

Mansfield, Miriam C 5607 Spring Lodge Drive, Kingwood, TX 77345, **A**

Mans-Leary, Linda L Route 1 Box 168, Kearney, MO 64060, (816) 792-1437, BS 76 Fort Hays St Univ; MA 80 Univ of KS; **SLP**

Mansolillo, Angela 92 Carver Street, Springfield, MA 01108, (413) 739-6874, BA 83 RI Coll; MA 85 Univ of CT; 86–Sp-Lang Path, Mercy Rehab Ctr, **SLP**

Mansourian, Anne Louise Myrtle Avenue, RFD 11 Box 268, Mahopac, NY 10541, (914) 621-2250, BA 79 Iona Coll; MS 82 CUNY - Brooklyn Coll; SLP, NYC Bd of Ed, **SLP**

Mansour-Shousher, Mrs Randa 3050 Hopewell Place, Toledo, OH 43606-3104, (419) 381-4012, BS 79 Univ of Toledo; MS 81 Univ of MI - Ann Arbor; 84–Aud, Randa Mansour-Shousher MD Inc, **A**

Mansur, Cs Wade A 180 Olinda Drive, Brea, CA 92621, (213) 726-1225, BA 55 San Diego St Univ; MA 59 CA St Univ - Los Angeles; Sp-Lang Path, Private Practice, **SLP**

Mantel, Heather P 1970 Cabriolet Court, Naperville, IL 60565, (312) 983-9712, BS 80 Northern IL Univ - De Kalb; MA 81 Northern IL Univ - De Kalb; 88–Sp-Lang Path, Naperville CUSD #203, **SLP**

Mantel, Pamela Marie 7124 St Edmands Drive, Cincinnati, OH 45230, (513) 232-9053, **SLP**

Mantenfel, Ellen McDonald 28 Triangle Circle, Sandwich, MA 02563, (617) 888-6620, MA 84 Case Western Reserve Univ; 86–Sp-Lang Path, Carver PS Sys, **SLP**

Manthie, Mrs Martha A 5209 16th Avenue South, Minneapolis, MN 55417, (612) 724-8912, BA 70 Univ of MN - Minneap-St Paul; MA 72 Univ of AZ; MA 75 Univ of MN - Minneap-St Paul; **SLP**

Mantilla, Mary W 1201 North Mitchel, Arlington Heights, IL 60004, (312) 259-2679, BS 76 Univ of WI - Madison; MS 77 Univ of WI - Madison; Sp-Lang Path, Private Practice, **SLP**

Mantione, Denise Ann 892 N Landing Rd, Rochester, NY 14625, (716) 458-5982, BS 81 SUNY - Coll at Fredonia; MS 84 Nazareth Coll of Rochester; 83–Sp-Lang Path, Rochester City Schs, **SLP**

Manton, Judee Anne 145 North Auburndale, Memphis, TN 38104, (901) 278-7205, MA 88 Memphis St Univ

Manucia, Dr Charles F 1508 Circa Del Lago #B-111, Lake San Marcos, CA 92069, (619) 744-1196, BS 40 NY Univ; MA 42 NY Univ; PH 68 (Clinical Psychology) United States Int'l Univ; Retired, **SLP LM**

Manuel, Bettina R 3091 Lincoln Boulevard, Cleveland Heights, OH 44118, (216) 464-0950, BA 73 Univ of CA - Santa Barbara; MS 75 Boston Univ; Sp-Lang Path, Cuyahoga County Bd Mental Retn, **SLP**

Manuell, Karen E Hassmer 6 Quail Court, Woodridge, IL 60517, (312) 985-3603, BS 77 Marquette Univ; MS 78 Marquette Univ; Sp-Lang Path, PS Dist 68-Woodridge, **SLP**

Manus, Louis J, Jr 1019 North Huron, Pierre, SD 57501, (605) 773-3678, BA 66 WA St Univ; MA 71 WA St Univ; Sp-Lang Path, Sd Sect for Spec Ed, **SLP**

Many, Mrs Marina Teglia 6713 Charleston Drive, Darien, IL 60559-3805, (312) 963-0620, BA 79 Northern IL Univ - De Kalb; MA 81 Northern IL Univ - De Kalb; Sp/Lang Path, Dist 98 North Berwyn, **SLP**

Manz, Mrs Laura 1004 Vanier House, Michener Park, 69 7604-29 Avenue, Edmonton, AB, Canada, (403) 432-2619, BS 85 Univ of Alberta - Alberta; MS 88 Univ of Alberta - Alberta; 86–Cl Coord, Inst-Stuttering Treat & Res

Manz, Michael J 734 Hillary Street, Sarnia, ON, Canada N7T 7T8, (519) 332-6386, BS 75 Western IL Univ; MA 76 Western IL Univ; Instr, Wn Il U, **A**

Manzek, Mrs Noralee B 3176 Margate Road, Bethlehem, PA 18017, (215) 759-7600, BS 64 Indiana Univ of PA; MA 68 Temple Univ; Sp-Lang Path, Colonial Northampton Iu #20, **SLP**

Manzella, Dr Diane S Gardner Manzella & Associates, 15301 Ventura Boulevard, Suite 300, Sherman Oaks, CA 91403, (818) 789-0662, BA 65 Montclair St Coll; MA 72 CA St Univ - Northridge; ED 82 (NS) Univ of CA - Los Angeles; Co-Owner, Gardner Manzella & Assoc, **SLP A**

Manzella, Dr Robert A 517 McKinley Avenue, Dunkirk, NY 14048, (716) 673-3203, BS 64 SUNY - Coll at Fredonia; ME 67 SUNY - Coll at Fredonia; PH 75 (NS) SUNY - Center at Buffalo; Dept Chmn, State Univ of New York, **SLP ACE**

Manzo, Barbara J 313 Wheeler Place, First Floor, Endicott, NY 13760, (607) 770-0544, BS 77 Marywood Coll; MS 81 Ithaca Coll; Sp-Lang Path, Broome Developmental Services, **SLP**

Manzo, Frances Marie 640 East 2nd Street #B-3, Brooklyn, NY 11208, (718) 965-4800, BA 78 SUNY - Center at Stony Brook; **SLP**

Manzy, Y'Shua School Of Allied Health Professionals, LSU Medical Center, 1900 Gravier Street, New Orleans, LA 70112, (504) 568-4348, BA 74 Univ of AR - Little Rock; MS 76 Purdue Univ - West Lafayette; Assistant Professor, Louisiana St Univ Medical Cen, **A**

Mapes, Mrs Lonna K 3721 Ray Hardy Drive, Clovis, NM 88101, (505) 762-3781, BS 67 Eastern NM Univ; MS 79 Eastern NM Univ; Sp-Lang Path, Clovis Mun Sch, **SLP**

Maples, Barbara Milillo 49 Flint Road, Langhorne, PA 19047, (215) 750-7442, BA 80 Temple Univ; MA 82 Temple Univ; Sp-Lang Path, Private Practice, **SLP ACE**

Mar, Margaret A 5200 Greenwood Circle, Excelsior, MN 55331, (612) 474-3566, BA 72 Univ of MN - Minneap-St Paul; MS 76 Saint Cloud St Univ; Sp-Lang Path, **SLP**

Marable, Denise L 223 Banyan Drive, Lake Jackson, TX 77566, (409) 297-5270, BS 74 Southwest TX St Univ; ME 75 Southwest TX St Univ; Sp-Lang Path, Private Practice, **SLP**

Maramaldi, Mrs Carolyn Roger 278 Homestead Road, Paramus, NJ 07652, (201) 261-1496, BA 65 Montclair St Coll; MS 83 William Paterson Coll; **SLP**

Maranga, Gina 141 Bay 20th Street #2, Brooklyn, NY 11214, (718) 780-1986, BS 83 Boston Univ; MS 84 Boston Univ; 87–Sp-Lang Path, Lamm Institute Long Island Coll Hosp, **SLP**

Marano, Mrs Deborah F 2 Poplar Woods, Wedgewood Addition, Morgantown, WV 26505, (304) 233-4343, BS 70 WV Univ; MS 72 WV Univ; **SLP**

Marano, Karen A 28 Mariner Drive, Washington Township, Sewell, NJ 08080, (609) 582-1748, BA 75 Rutger's St Univ - Douglas Coll; MS 76 PA St Univ - Univ Park; **SLP**

Marans, Wendy Dalton 143 Vista Terrace, New Haven, CT 06515, (203) 387-6823, BS 77 Nat'l Hosp Coll of Speech Sci - London, England; MS 84 Inst of Neurology - London, England; 85–Assoc Research Scientist, Yale Chld Study Ctr, **SLP**

Maranzano, Nanci A 3019-K Ordway Drive N W, Roanoke, VA 24017, (703) 343-9113, BA 75 SUNY - Coll at Oswego; ME 76 Univ of VA - Charlottesville; 86–Sp-Lang Path, City of Salem Schs, **SLP**

Marascalchi, Carole Anne 236 Caroline Avenue, Solvay, NY 13209, (315) 433-2631, BS 82 SUNY - Coll at Geneseo; MS 85 Nazareth Coll of Rochester; 85–Sp-Lang Path, Onondaga-Cortland-Madison BOCES, **SLP**

Marasco, Kendra L 18 Bridgewood Drive, Fairport, NY 14450, (716) 475-6251, BS 68 Northern IL Univ - De Kalb; MA 72 Kent St Univ; 88–Sp-Lang Path, NTID, **SLP A**

Marashi, Mrs Melinda O 3286 Lakebrook Boulevard, Knoxville, TN 37909-1141, (615) 588-7319, MA 85 Univ of TN - Knoxville; 85–Sp-Lang Path, Fort Sanders Reg Med Center, **SLP**

Marasovich, Mary Louise 1380 Lusitana Street, Suite 615, Honolulu, HI 96813, (808) 537-4030, BA CA St Univ - Stanislaus; MA CA St Univ - Stanislaus; 88–Sp-Lang Path, Oahu Sp & Lang Path Consult, **SLP**

Marber, Mrs Marilyn Seltzer 30 Halley Drive, Pomona, NY 10970, (914) 354-4644, BA 64 OH St Univ; MA 65 Columbia Univ Teachers Coll; Sp-Lang Path, Summit Sch at Nyack, **SLP**

Marble, Elaine Mary 359 7th Avenue, Troy, NY 12182, (518) 658-3895, BS 85 Nazareth Coll of Rochester; MS 88 Coll of Saint Rose; 87–Sp-Lang Path, Capl Dist Beginnings, **SLP**

Marburger, Mrs Marianne Rebholz 1204 South Derby, Denison, TX 75020, (214) 893-7457, BS 67 Univ of IA; MA 69 Univ of IA; Sp-Lang Path, Grayson Co Cen Crpld Chld/Adul, **SLP**

Marbury, Mrs Sharon Jeffcoat 3612 Park Lane, Birmingham, AL 35213, (205) 838-3098, BA 84 Univ of AL-Tuscaloosa; MS 85 FL St Univ; Clin Supvr, Area Sp and Rehab PC, **SLP**

Marcano, Maria Amelia 25 Street SE 942, Reparto Metropolitan, Rio Piedras, PR 00921, (809) 783-2387, BA 83 Univ of PR - Rio Piedras; MS 85 Univ of PR - San Juan; 88–Sp-Lang Path, Hartford Bd of Educ

Marcantel, Kathleen Doherty P O Box 1094, Jennings, LA 70546, (318) 824-4327, **SLP**

Marcarelli, Karen H 306 Union Street, Braintree, MA 02184, (617) 735-3171, BA 77 Southern CT St Univ; MA 79 Univ of CT; 81–Aud Coor, Beth Israel Hosp, **A**

Marceau, Mrs Frances Kaldenbach P O Box 180, Lower Plains Road, East Middlebury, VT 05740, (802) 247-5757, BA 82 Wichita St Univ; MA 83 Wichita St Univ; Sp/Lang Path, Rutland N E Superv Union, **SLP**

Marcel, Mrs Beth Marie 4511 Majestic Oaks Drive, New Orleans, LA 70126, (504) 652-8927, BA 80 Western WA Univ; MA 83 Western WA Univ; Sp-Lang Path, St Charles Parish Sch Bd, **SLP**

March, Harold H 01510 S W Carey Lane, Portland, OR 97219, (503) 636-4295, BA 33 WA St Univ; ME 59 Univ of OR; **SLP LM**

Marchant, Calvin R 5066 South 4460 West, Kearns, UT 84118, (801) 533-6165, BS 54 Univ of UT; MS 61 Univ of UT; Aud/Sp/Lang Path, UT St Dept Hlth, **SLP A**

Marchese, Dr Judith 505 East 79th Street, New York, NY 10021, (212) 472-0083, BA 67 Syracuse Univ; MA 68 Columbia Univ Teachers Coll; ED 85 (NS) Columbia Univ Teachers Coll; Sp-Lang Path, Private Practice, **SLP**

Marchesseault, Marie Ann 1 Oak Street, Plainfield, CT 06374, (203) 564-4086, BA 80 Univ of CT; MA 82 Univ of CT; Sp-Lang Path, Plainfield Bd of Educ, **SLP**

Marchette, Mrs Susan Nealon 11097 Pegasus Avenue, San Diego, CA 92126-4415, (619) 566-3162, BA 80 Univ of CA - San Diego; MA 82 CA St Univ - Northridge; 85–Palomar Pomerado Hosp Dist, I Lehrhoff PhD & Assoc, **SLP**

Marchetti, Patricia 2709 Woosdale Avenue, Baltimore, MD 21214, (301) 323-1010, BS 73 Towson St Univ; MS 76 Towson St Univ; SLP Cl Superv, Baltimore City Pub Sch, **SLP**

Marchewka, Carol C 1769 Crane Street, Schenectady, NY 12303, (518) 456-6010, BS 65 SUNY - Coll at Geneseo; MS 79 SUNY - Center at Albany; MS 69 SUNY - Center at Albany; Sp/Lang Path, Guilderland Central Schs, **SLP**

Marchildon, Claudia E 16001 West Nine Mile Road, PO Box 2043, Southfield, MI 48037, (313) 424-3907, BA 72 Wayne St Univ; MA 79 Central MI Univ; 81–Sp-Lang Path, Providence Hosp, **SLP**

Marchionda, Mrs Jeannie Anne 1130 Blueberry Hill, Brunswick, OH 44212, BS 85 Kent St Univ; MA 87 Univ of Akron; 88–Aud, Adnan Mourany MD, **A**

Marchitelli-Martin, Mrs Karen A 730 Champagne Avenue, Bowling Green, OH 43402, (419) 381-4012, BA 77 SUNY - Coll at Cortland; MA 78 Bowling Green St Univ; Sp-Lang Path, Med Coll of Ohio, **SLP**

Marcin, Mrs Kathy Elaine 21411 Highland Knolls, Katy, TX 77450, (713) 578-6473, BS 80 Univ of GA; MA 82 OK St Univ; **SLP**

Marcinkevich, Mrs Paula Ruth 122 E Summerfield Avenue, Collingswood, NJ 08108, (215) 465-8800, BS 80 IL St Univ - Normal

Marcinko, Mrs Michele Brady 319 East Highland Avenue, Ebensburg, PA 15931, (814) 472-7350, BS 84 Indiana Univ of PA; MS 88 Indiana Univ of PA; 84–Sp-Lang Path, DPW-Ebensburg Ctr, **F**

Marcks, Erin Alley Rt 1 Box 1669, Hager City, WI 54014, (715) 792-2777, BS 84 Univ of WI - River Falls; MS 86 Univ of WI - River Falls; 86–Sp-Lang Path, Ellsworth Comm Sch Dist

Marco, Catherine Mary Meadowview Apt #3-C, Augusta Road, Topsham, ME 04086, (207) 725-8587, **SLP**

Marcon, Doris Louise 22 Chicora Avenue, Toronto, ON, Canada M5R 1T6, (416) 848-7286, **SLP**

Marcopulos, E Gail 4725 Hoen Avenue #B, Santa Rosa, CA 95405, (707) 542-1154, BA 76 San Francisco St Univ; MA 77 San Francisco St Univ; Aud, Santa Rosa Speech & Hearing Ctr, **A**

Marcot, Mrs Maryanne A 10319 Parkman Road, Silver Spring, MD 20903, (301) 445-4912, BA 73 Loyola Coll; MA 74 Univ of MD - College Park; Acct/CPA, Private Practice, **SLP**

Marcotte, Beth Anne 1066 Smithfield Avenue, Lincoln, RI 02865, (401) 884-5999, BA 83 Univ of RI; MA 86 Worcester St Coll; **SLP**

Marcotte, Mrs Sally B 25000 West 10 Mile Road, Southfield, MI 48075, **A**

Marcovici, Mrs Selma Goldstein 98-09 64th Road #4G, Rego Park, NY 11374, (718) 459-5314, BA 72 CUNY - Queens Coll; MA 74 Univ of IL - Urbana; 74–Sp/Lang Path, Long Island Jewish Hosp, **SLP**

Marcucci, Carol Ann 911 Teaneck Road, Teaneck, NJ 07666, **SLP**

Marcum, Debra L Lifeline Home Health, Cundiff Square, Somerset, KY 42501, BA 75 Western KY Univ; MA 76 Western KY Univ; Sp-Lang Path, Lifeline Home Health, **SLP ACE**

Marcum, Gladys Charlene 9 Fairview Avenue, Holtsville, NY 11742, (516) 727-0733, BA 69 Eastern KY Univ; MA 85 Long Island U - CW Post Ctr; 86–Sp-Lang Path, Private Practice, **SLP**

Marcum, Mrs Terry D 6111 Boulder Creek Lane, Harrisburg, NC 28075, (704) 343-5835, BA 78 Univ of NC - Chapel Hill; MA 79 Univ of NC - Greensboro; 80–Sp-Lang Path, Charlotte-Mecklenburg Sch, **SLP**

Marcus, Mrs April Came 30160 Westbrook Pkwy, Southfield, MI 48076, (313) 258-6226, BA 75 MI St Univ; MA 76 Wayne St Univ; SLP, Detroit Bd of Ed, **SLP**

Marcus, Mrs Beth Kraus 1440 Sherwood, Highland Park, IL 60035, (312) 831-0343, BS 69 Univ of IL - Urbana; MA 71 Western MI Univ; 78–Ch Sp-Lang Path, M Reese Hosp & Med Cen, **SLP**

Marcus, Debbie Beth 3457 Turf Road, Oceanside, NY 11572, (718) 498-2500, BA 80 CUNY - Queens Coll; MA 86 CUNY - Hunter Coll; Sp-Lang Path, League School, **SLP**

Marcus, Mrs Geraldine Suite 1406, 1 Datran Center, 9100 South Dadeland Boulevard, Miami, FL 33156, (305) 665-0333, BS 66 Cornell Univ; MA 69 Newark St Coll; 77–Sp-Lang Path, Geraldine Marcus MA, **SLP ACE**

Marcus, Ivy April 106 Brite Avenue, Scarsdale, NY 10583, (914) 472-9116, BS 78 Dickinson Coll; MA 82 NY Univ; **SLP**

Marcus, Mrs Rovena S 233 East Shore Road, Great Neck, NY 11023, (516) 482-7505, BA 69 CUNY - Brooklyn Coll; MA 70 NY Univ; Sp-Lang Path, Rovena Marcus Ma, **SLP**

Marcus, Mrs Sandra S 12 Iron Gate, Metuchen, NJ 08840, (201) 826-3360, BS 64 Boston Univ; Sp-Lang Path, Perth Amboy Bd of Ed, **SLP**

Marcus, Sharon Lee 299 Rosemary Street, Needham, MA 02194, (617) 444-8895, BS 83 Univ of MA - Amherst; MS 85 Boston Univ; 88–Sp-Lang Path, MA Easter Seal Society, **SLP**

Marcus, Sheryl 40 Roseland Avenue #A-3, Caldwell, NJ 07006, (201) 464-7616, BA 81 Kean Coll of NJ; MA 82 Kean Coll of NJ; Sp-Lang Path, Morris Union Jointure Commission, **SLP**

Marder, Linda J Post Office Box 230, Copeville, TX 75018, (214) 853-2531

Mardis, Mrs Emily J 6 South State Street, Apartment 22, Dover, DE 19901, (302) 736-5376, BS 84 James Madison Univ; MS 86 James Madison Univ; **SLP**

Marean, Prof Charles E P O Box 416, Geneseo, NY 14454, (716) 243-3766, BS 50; MS; PH (NS); Professor, State Univ College at Geneseo, **SLP A ACE**

Mareing, Robert J 506 Coachlight Lane, Hazelwood, MO 63042, (314) 863-9161, BS 70 IL St Univ - Normal; MS 74 IL St Univ - Normal; 84–Aud/Owner, Private Practice, **A**

Marencin, Gary Joseph Medical Center Of Delaware, Speech And Hearing Center, 4755 Ogletown-Stanton Rd, Newark, DE 19718, (302) 428-2286, BS 83 PA St Univ - Univ Park; MS 86 PA St Univ - Univ Park; Aud, Med Ctr of DE, **A**

Maresco, Kathy D 2124 Eldred Avenue, Lakewood, OH 44107, (216) 382-9979, BA 78 Cleveland St Univ; MA 79 Cleveland St Univ; 87–Sp-Lang Path/Consult, DIVA Assoc, **SLP**

Maresh-Ericksen, Bernadette M 610 Jefferson, Oregon City, OR 97045, BA 79 Portland St Univ; MS 81 Portland St Univ; 85–Sp-Lang Path, Willamete Valley Family Ctr, **SLP**

Marfurt, Malinda Kay 568 Meadoway Park, Worthington, OH 43085, (614) 263-5151, BA 83 Miami Univ - Oxford; MA 85 IN Univ - Bloomington; **SLP**

Margagliotti-Money, Sandra 6 Troy Place, Schenectady, NY 12309, (518) 370-7574, BA 77 CUNY - Queens Coll; MS 81 Coll of Saint Rose; Sp-Lang Path, Mys-Od Heck Dev Cen, **SLP**

Marge, Dorothy K 111 Clarmar Road, Fayetteville, NY 13066, (315) 425-2987, BA 60 Montclair St Coll; MA 64 Seton Hall Univ; OM 78 Syracuse Univ; Deputy Cmsnr, Onondaga Co Dept of Social Ser, **SLP**

Marge, Dr Michael 111 Clarmar Road, Fayetteville, NY 13066, (315) 443-9643, BA 52 Emerson Coll; MA 53 Harvard Univ; ED 59 (Child Development) Harvard Univ; 74–Prof of Commun Sciences & Dis, Syracuse U, **SLP F**

Margolies, Mrs Judy K 2628 Mimi Circle, Philadelphia, PA 19131, (215) 477-0127, BA 74 CUNY - Queens Coll; MS 75 Ithaca Coll; Sp-Lang Path, Sch Dist of Phila, **SLP**

Margolis, Janet C 1355 Arden View Drive, Arden Hills, MN 55112, (612) 639-1985, BS 71 Marquette Univ; MS 75 Univ of WI - Madison; **SLP**

Margolis, Leonard H Bergen Co Vocational/Technical, High School District, 200 Hackensack Avenue, Hackensack, NJ 07601, (201) 343-6000, BA 66 Curry Coll; MA 69 Montclair St Coll; 87–Dir, Bergen County Vocational/Tech SD, **SLP**

Margolis, Lynn A 23 Lanark Road #6, Brookline, MA 02146-1837, (617) 329-1400, BS 80 Syracuse Univ; MA 82 Univ of Pittsburgh - Pittsburgh; Aud, Dedham Med Ctr, **A**

Margolis, Natalie M 61 Livingston Lane, Manalapan, NJ 07726, (718) 987-9400, BA 64 CUNY - Brooklyn Coll; MS 67 CUNY - Brooklyn Coll; Dir/Pres, Our PLACE Sch Inc, **SLP**

Margolis, Norma C 9009 North Kenton, Skokie, IL 60076, (312) 676-0876, BS 73 Univ of IL - Urbana; MS 74 Univ of IL - Urbana; Sp-Lang Path, Chicago Board of Education, **SLP**

Margolis, Dr Robert H University Of Minnesota, Department Of Otolaryngology, Box 283 UMHC, Minneapolis, MN 55455, (612) 626-3872, BS 68 Kent St Univ; MA 69 Kent St Univ; PH 74 (NS) Univ of IA; Aud, Univ of Minnesota, **A**

Margolis, Wendy M 1311 North 49th Street #2, Seattle, WA 98103, (206) 547-1621, BA 83 Univ of CA - Santa Barbara; MS 85 Univ of WA; **A**

Marguglio, Gloriann 2211 Reagan Boulevard, Carrollton, TX 75006, (214) 706-1364, BS 68 Loyola Univ; MS 70 Marquette Univ; 88–Consult, American Heart Assn, **SLP**

Margulies, Cecele 120 West 86th Street, New York, NY 10024, **SLP**

Margulies, M Lee 1070 Sussex Road, Teaneck, NJ 07666, (212) 481-4339, BS 53 Julliard School; MA 59 Columbia Univ Teachers Coll; Lect, Hunter Coll Cuny, **A**

Margulies, Dr Maris K 1070 Sussex Road, Teaneck, NJ 07666, (212) 445-1400, MA 68 CUNY - Hunter Coll; OM 78 CUNY - Grad Sch & Univ Cntr; PH 80 (NS) CUNY - Grad Sch & Univ Cntr; Aud, L J Deutsch & Assoc, **SLP A**

Margulies, Mrs Selma K 949 West End Avenue, New York, NY 10025, (212) 666-2635, BA 53 CUNY - Hunter Coll; MA 56 CUNY - Brooklyn Coll; Ch Sp-Lang Path, St Johns Queens Hosp, **SLP**

Margulies, Vivian 729 New Scotland Avenue, Albany, NY 12208, (518) 473-4666, BA 57 Emerson Coll; MA 59 Emerson Coll; Prin Med Facilities Auditor, Nys Dept of Hlth, **SLP A**

Mariani, Felix Joseph 81 Clover Drive, Hollidaysburg, PA 16648, (814) 944-3535, BS 73 PA St Univ - Univ Park; MS 74 PA St Univ - Univ Park; Asst Admin, Rehab Hosp of Altoona, **SLP**

Maricle, Carlton A 117 Church Street, Little Falls, NY 13365, (315) 823-1400, BS 74 SUNY - Coll at Geneseo; MA 75 SUNY - Coll at Geneseo; Audioligist, Self Employed, **A**

Marie, Mrs Georgia Breaux 210 Kathryn Street, New Iberia, LA 70560, (318) 364-6180, BS 79 Univ of Southwestern LA; OM 80 LA St Univ - N O Medical Ctr; Aud, Ideria Hrng Cen, **A**

Marienthal, Pamela P 8728 Nielson Road #12, Oak Hills, CA 92371-9611, (714) 558-5766, BA 74 Univ of Redlands; MS 76 Univ of NE - Omaha; Sp-Lang Path, Santa Ana USD, **SLP**

Marietti-Benito, Mrs Valerie Ann 430 Sumner Avenue, Rio del Mar, CA 95003, (408) 728-6337, BA 84 Univ of the Pacific; MA 85 Univ of the Pacific; 86–Sp-Lang Path, Pajaro Valley USD, **SLP**

Marillo, Mrs Marie J 2214 Willow Lane, Niagara Falls, NY 14304, **SLP**

Marin, Mrs Beatriz Gumucio 1604 Sunrise Lakes Drive, #8, Erie, PA 16509, (814) 453-4309, BS 86 UT St Univ; MS 87 UT St Univ; **SLP**

Marinak, Joseph M 1157 Wintertide Drive, Harrisburg, PA 17111, (717) 782-4350, BA 77 Temple Univ; MA 79 Temple Univ; Aud, Poly Cl Med Cen-Sp&Hrng Cen, **A**

Marincov, Mrs Elizabeth Ellen 506 White River Drive, Orlando, FL 32828, (305) 275-9275, BA 83 Univ of Pittsburgh - Pittsburgh; MS 84 CA Univ of PA; Sp-Lang Path, Orange County PS, **SLP**

Marincovich, Dr Peter J Audiology Associates, 4000 Montgomery Dr, Suite A, Santa Rosa, CA 95405, (707) 545-7348, BA 76 Univ of CA - Santa Barbara; OM 78 LA St Univ - N O Medical Ctr; PH 86 (Aud) Memphis St Univ; 84–Owner, Audiology Associates, **A**

Marineau, Robyn Lee Ridgeview At Lewiston Apartment 123, 4877 Eddy Drive West, Lewiston, NY 14092, (416) 521-5003, BA 86 SUNY - Center at Buffalo; MA 88 SUNY - Center at Buffalo; 88–Aud, Chedoke-McMaster's Hosp

Marinelli, Karen Cook 28 Belmar Road, Hatboro, PA 19040, (215) 671-5143, BS 85 Bloomsburg Univ of PA; MS 86 Bloomsburg Univ of PA; SLP, Temple University, **SLP**

Marinelli, Mrs Kathleen A 3 Hepburn Court, Stony Brook, NY 11790, (516) 266-5420, BA 78 SUNY - Coll at Plattsburgh; MS 79 Adelphi Univ; SLP, Elwood Ufsd, **SLP A**

Marinello, Robert P 126 Oswego Street, Staten Island, NY 10301, (718) 448-2172, BA 70 Fordham Univ; MS 72 Columbia Univ Teachers Coll; Sp-Lang Path, Spec Educ Dist 27, **SLP**

Maring, Lana J 2310 East Bradford Avenue, Apartment 1, Milwaukee, WI 53211, (414) 276-4897, BA 75 Univ of IA; MA 76 Northeast MO St Univ; 78–Sp-Lang Path, Milwaukee Public Schools, **SLP**

Marinkovich, Gayle E 2416 Dresden Place, La Jolla, CA 92037, (619) 270-7658, BA 79 San Diego St Univ; MA 81 San Diego St Univ; Sp-Lang Path, La Mesa-Spring Valley Sch Dist, **SLP**

Marino, Anne Jean 11823 Bernardo Terrace, C203, San Diego, CA 92128, (619) 451-1343, BS 84 TX Christian Univ; MA 86 TX Woman's Univ; **SLP**

Marino, Mrs Catherine 1811 Brabham Street, El Cajon, CA 92019, (619) 588-3053, BS 64 Marquette Univ; MA 68 Case Western Reserve Univ; Spec Educ Coord, Cajon Valley USD, **SLP**

Marino, Mrs Corinne A 1133 Rhinelander Avenue Apartment 3C, New York, NY 10461, (212) 822-2171, BA 79 CUNY - Lehman Coll; MA 80 CUNY - Lehman Coll; SLP, Citywide Sp Unit, **SLP**

Marino, Gina Patricia 1215-F Court DE Ville, Birmingham, AL 35209, (205) 945-0767, MS 86 Univ of Montevallo; 88–Sp-Lang Path, Medtherapy Inc, **SLP**

Marino, Marcia L 3293A S Springfield Avenue, Milwaukee, WI 53207, BS 75 Marquette Univ; MS 77 Univ of WI - Milwaukee; Sp-Lang Path, St Josephs Hosp, **SLP**

Marino-Tomey, Mrs Denise T 12 Merryweather Drive, Cambridge, MD 21613, (301) 228-4747, BS 74 Univ of MD - College Park; MS 75 Towson St Univ; Sp/Lang Path, Dorchester Co Bd of Ed, **SLP**

Marion, Mrs Laurel J 5800 Santa Rosa Road, Suite 123, Camarillo, CA 93010, (805) 482-9821, BA 75 Univ of Redlands; MS 76 Univ of Redlands; Owner/Aud, The Hearing Ctr, **A**

Marion, Lori Marie 233 Hallam Avenue, Mahtomedi, MN 55115, (612) 426-8503, BA 83 Univ of MN - Duluth; MA 84 Memphis St Univ; Aud, Columbia Park Medical Group, **A**

Marion, Michael W 5800 Santa Rosa Road, Suite 123, Camarillo, CA 93010, (805) 482-9821, BS 68 Univ of UT; MS 71 Univ of UT; Owner/Aud, The Hearing Ctr, **A**

Marion, Michelle Renee 306 Raymond Drive, O'Fallon, MO 63366, (314) 239-7711, BS 85 Southwest MO St Univ; OM 87 Univ of MO - Columbia; 88–Sp-Lang Path, St John's Mercy Hosp, **SLP**

Mariotti, Mrs Margaret Q 1630 Wyoming Avenue, Scranton, PA 18509, (716) 424-3034, BA 75 Marywood Coll; MA 77 Temple Univ-Tyler Sch of Art; Aud, Marywood College, **A**

Mark, Carol 57 Falkland Street, Brighton, MA 02135, (617) 683-4000, BA 76 Univ of CT; MA 80 Univ of CT; Sp/Lang Path, Lawerence Gen Hosp, **SLP ACE**

Mark, Kathy Jane 41135 Via Puerta, Temecula, CA 92390, (714) 674-7731, BA 78 Univ of CA - Santa Barbara; OM 82 San Jose St Univ; SLP, Lake Elsinore School District, **SLP**

Markel, Edith G 94 Cresent Beach Drive, Huntington, NY 11743, (516) 294-8700, BA 52; MA 70; Instr/Super, Adelphi University, **SLP**

Markell, Debra L 2 Firwood Drive, Bricktown, NJ 08723, **A**

Markello, Mrs Carol G 5415 Rawlings, Flower Mound, TX 75028, (214) 539-8844, BS 76 SUNY - Coll at Geneseo; MA 81 LA St Univ - Baton Rouge; **SLP**

Marker, Margaret M 7039 East State Road 45, Bloomington, IN 47401, (317) 342-0528, BS 75 Bowling Green St Univ; MA 76 Bowling Green St Univ; Sp-Lang Path, Metro Sch Dist of Martinsville, **SLP**

Marker, Sheila R 9661 Haney Street, Pico Rivera, CA 90660, (213) 865-1257, BA 77 Whittier Coll; MA 78 Whittier Coll; Tchr, ABC Sch Dist, **SLP**

Markeson, Judith M Box 943, FPO Seattle, WA 98774, MA 80 CA St Univ - Fullerton; Preschool Handicapped Teacher, Department of Defense, **SLP**

Markey, Mrs Shari Kligman 15440 Huntridge Road, Davie, FL 33331, (305) 557-4016, BS 83 Univ of TX - Austin; MS 85 Univ of TX - Dallas; 87–Aud, Dr Julio D Torres MD FACS PA, **A**

Markey, Susan Anne 92 Woodlake Villas, Hilton Head Island, SC 29928, (803) 681-3496, BS 84 SUNY - Coll at Fredonia; OM 86 Univ of SC - Columbia; **A**

Markham, Amy Joyce 3914 Taylor Road #46, Fort Wayne, IN 46804, (219) 426-8117, BA 84 MI St Univ; MA 86 MI St Univ; Aud, ENT Assoc, **A**

Markiewicz, Lori Ann 107 Winding Way #F, Covington, KY 41011, (513) 221-4243, BS 83 Purdue Univ - West Lafayette; MA 85 Memphis St Univ; Sp-Lang Path, Hrng Sp & Language Service, **SLP**

Markin, Lori Ann 9707 E Colorado Avenue, Apartment 107, Denver, CO 80231-3014, (303) 797-8453, BS 81 Univ of North TX; MS 82 Univ of North TX; SLP, Littleton Pub Schs, **SLP**

Markland, Sandra Hill Route 3 Box 547C, Cherryville, NC 28021, (704) 482-4416, BA 81 Univ of NC - Greensboro; ME 82 Univ of NC - Greensboro; Sp/Lang Path, Dev Eval Ctr, **SLP**

Markley, Mary F 4159 Steck #R197, Austin, TX 78759, (512) 346-2856, BS 77 OH Univ - Athens; MS 79 Baylor Univ; Sp-Lang Path, Austin ISD, **SLP ACE**

Markoe, Ruth 7 Holly Lane, Lawrenceville, NJ 08648, (609) 895-9660, BA 69 CUNY - City College; MS 70 Univ of WI - Madison; Sp-Lang Path, Private Practice, **SLP**

Markoff, Maxine N 157 Falmouth Road, Scarsdale, NY 10583, (212) 605-3740, BA 73 CUNY - Lehman Coll; MA 74 CUNY - Queens Coll; Aud, Manhattan ENT Hosp, **A**

Markotic, Klare K 9648 Larchmede Court, Ellicott City, MD 21043, **SLP**

Markowitz, Meryl Lynn 8 Waterford Drive, Wheatley Heighs, NY 11798, (516) 643-4899, MS 87 Adelphi Univ

Markowitz, Michelle 108 Stature Drive, Newark, DE 19713, (301) 356-7667, BS 83 Towson St Univ; MS 85 Towson St Univ; **SLP**

Markowski, Mrs Ruth Ann 24 Kimball Ridge Court, Baltimore, MD 21228, (301) 788-1231, BA 82 Univ of DE; MS 85 Loyola Coll; **SLP**

Marks, Adrienne L 333 East 34th Street #7-G, New York, NY 10016-4947, (212) 689-5538, BA 63 OH St Univ; MA 73 CUNY - Hunter Coll; OM 86 Yale Univ; Audiologist, State Dept of Health, **A**

Marks, Dr Colleen J Dept Of Comm Dis & Special Ed, Bloomsburg University, Navy Hall, Bloomsburg, PA 17815, (717) 389-4119, BS 62 Edinboro Univ of PA; MA 64 Univ of IL - Urbana; ED 78 (NS) Lehigh Univ; Prof, U of PA/Bloomsburg, **SLP**

Marks, Mrs Elizabeth 42 Middlefield Drive, West Hartford, CT 06107, (203) 233-6652, BS 71 Boston Univ; MS 72 Univ of WI - Madison; Sp-Lang Path, Division of Health Services, **SLP**

Marks, Janet A 1611 Davinbrook Lane, Stillwater, OK 74074, (405) 744-6021, BS 70 Emporia St Univ; MA 75 OK St Univ; Instr, Oklahoma St Univ, **SLP**

Marks, Joan Marie 1 Lee Court, Rockville, MD 20850, (206) 622-6987, BS 80 Univ of WA; OM 82 Univ of WA; Aud, Depot of the Army, **A**

Marks, Mrs Julie F 900 East Woodchase Lane, Marietta, GA 30067, (516) 378-2000, BS 83 Boston Univ; MS 84 Boston Univ; Sp-Lang Path, Marshall Rehab Ctrs of GA, **SLP**

Marks, Mary B 3964 Brendan Lane #407F, North Olmsted, OH 44070, (216) 687-3807, BA 72 Cleveland St Univ; MA 74 Cleveland St Univ; 86–Sp-Lang Path, Cleveland VA Med Ctr, **SLP**

Marks, Mary Jane 5850 Riverside Drive, Greendale, WI 53129, (414) 327-6670, BS 67 Univ of WI - Madison; MS 68 Univ of WI - Madison; Sp/Lang Path, Physical Therapy Svcs, **SLP**

Marks, Dr Maura G 459 Fruit Street, Mansfield, MA 02048, (508) 339-0855, BA 73 CUNY - Queens Coll; MA 75 CUNY - Queens Coll; PH 81 (Aud) Univ of MA - Amherst; Aud Consult, Private Practice, **A**

Marks, Mrs Nancy R F 325 Richey Avenue, West Collingswood, NJ 08107, (609) 858-6568, BS 75 Millersville Univ of PA; ME 81 Trenton St Coll; Sp-Lang Path, Bd of Ed Borough of Audubon, **SLP**

Marks, Mrs Robin D 116 Forest Avenue, Elsmere, DE 19805, (302) 429-4118, BS 82 Miami Univ - Oxford; MA 83 Wichita St Univ; 87–Sp-Lang Path, Christina Sch Dist, **SLP**

Marks, Sharyn E 10220 S W 141st Street, Miami, FL 33176, BA 75 Univ of FL; ME 76 Univ of Miami; MA 80 Univ of Miami; Sp/Lang Path & Deaf Educator, Private Practice, **SLP**

Marks, Sheila Gay 5012-B Cana Cove, Austin, TX 78749, (512) 483-3115, BA 73 Univ of TX - El Paso; MA 78 Univ of TX - El Paso; SLP, Austin ISD, **SLP**

Marks, Dr Sidney 67-05 167th Street, Flushing, NY 11365, (212) 479-5280, BA 54 CUNY - Brooklyn Coll; MA 56 CUNY - Brooklyn Coll; PH 68 (NS) NY Univ; Special Education Supervisor, New York City Board of Educ, **SLP**

Marks, Susan F 14226 Greenspan Lane, Rockville, MD 20853, (301) 933-0020, BS 70 Kent St Univ; MS 72 Univ of CT; Prin, Montgy Co Pub Sch, **SLP**

Marks, Susan L N 4790 S W 189th Place, Aloha, OR 97007, (503) 645-4242, MS; **SLP**

Marks, Susan M Children Hospital Of Wisconsin, 1700 West Wisconsin Avenue, P O Box 1997, Milwaukee, WI 53201, (414) 931-4065, BS 65 Univ of WI - Madison; MS 66 Univ of WI - Madison; Sp-Lang Path, Chldrns Hosp of WI, **SLP**

Marks-Hershey, Leslie A 140-8 Asch Loop, Apt 8-G, Bronx, NY 10475, (212) 320-2126, BA 74 Univ of RI; MS 76 Univ of RI; Sp/Lang Path, **SLP**

Markt, Maureen F 257 Franklin Street, Holyoke, MA 01040, (413) 532-3692, BA 70 Univ of MA - Amherst; ME 76 Amer Int'l Coll; Sp-Lang Path, Holyoke Pub Sch, **SLP ACE**

Markum, Mrs Patricia L 804 Hardin Drive, Norman, OK 73072, (405) 272-5545, BA 63 Univ of OK - Norman; ME 79 Central St Univ; **SLP**

Markus, Theodore 319 Faneuil Street #3, Brighton, MA 02135, (617) 969-7336, BA 73 SUNY - Coll at Plattsburgh; MA 76 OH Univ - Athens; **SLP**

Markwiese, Beth Mary 12151 W Godsell Avenue, Hales Corners, WI 53130, (414) 961-4174, BS 84 Marquette Univ; MS 85 Marquette Univ; 87–Sp-Lang Path, Columbia Hosp, **SLP**

Markwitz, Adele 890 Park Avenue, New York, NY 10021, (212) 988-4718, BA 50 CUNY - Brooklyn Coll; MA 52 CUNY - Brooklyn Coll; Aud-Sp-Lang Path, Private Practice, **SLP A**

Marler, Sharon Ellen G 2489 Senate Way, Medford, OR 97504-8538, (503) 772-8337, BA 60; MA 82 OR St Univ; SLP, Jackson Cty Chld Dev Cen, **SLP**

Marlette, Amy 1417 Elizabeth Circle #2, Idaho Falls, ID 83404, (208) 524-1031, BS 81 ID St Univ; MS 87 ID St Univ; 87–Sp-Lang Path, Adult/Child Dev Ctr, **SLP**

Marley, Melinda M 9 Hillside Place, Ilion, NY 13357, (315) 724-5101, BS 71 Nazareth Coll of Rochester; MS 73 Syracuse Univ; Sp-Lang Path, Chldn Hosp & Rehab Cen, **SLP**

Marley-Leedom, Suzanne Marie 4609 Silverhill Drive, Knoxville, TN 37921, (615) 558-8554, BS 84 Univ of TN - Knoxville; MA 86 Univ of TN - Knoxville; 86–Sp-Lang Path, Anderson County Schs

Marlin, Mrs Elaine A 9310 S W 83rd Street, Miami, FL 33173, (305) 279-0734, BA 75 Univ of FL; ME 76 Univ of FL; **SLP**

Marlis, Jane A L 1959 Thayer Avenue, Los Angeles, CA 90025, (213) 757-1226, BS 70 Western MI Univ; MA 77 CA St Univ - Northridge; SLP, Los Angeles USD, **SLP**

Marlow, Mrs Lisa Burnett 27405 Greenfield #8, Southfield, MI 48076, (313) 286-8500, BA 85 MI St Univ; MA 86 Western MI Univ; **A**

Marlow, Mrs Mollie Zaffos 23 Pittsford Way, Nanuet, NY 10954, (914) 623-6264, BA 64 CUNY - Hunter Coll; MA 71 CUNY - Brooklyn Coll; 86–Sp-Lang Path, Clarkstown Sch Dist, **SLP**

Marlow, Patricia A 47 South Main Street, Pittsford, NY 14534, (716) 247-1480, MS 84 Nazareth Coll of Rochester; SLP, BOCES #2 Monroe-Orleans

Marlowe, Cynthia L 519 North Kentucky Street, Corbin, KY 40701, **SLP**

Marlowe, Judith A 2081 Dundee Drive, Winter Park, FL 32792, (305) 629-5073, BA 69 Thomas More Coll; MA 71 Univ of Cincinnati; PH 86 (Behavioral Sci/Hlth Pro) Walden Univ; 85–Director/Owner, Judith A Marlowe Audiology, **A ACE**

Marmo, Deborah Marie F 130 Stewart Street, Old Forge, PA 18518, (717) 457-6898, BS 78 Marywood Coll; MS 80 Bloomsburg Univ of PA; Sp/Lang Path, Private Practice, **SLP**

Marmonti, Mrs Mary Kathleen 4741 Langtree, St Louis, MO 63128, (314) 938-5513, BS 81 Southeast MO St Univ; MS 83 Fontbonne Coll; SLP, Sp Sch Dist of St Louis Co, **SLP**

Marmor, Mrs Francine Levy 9496 N W 39th Street, Sunrise, FL 33351, (305) 748-8367, BA 80 Hofstra Univ; MA 82 NY Univ; Sp-Lang Path, **SLP**

Marohn, Mrs Judith Riley 6700 Kingsview Lane, Maple Grove, MN 55369, (619) 557-1015, BA 76 Univ of MN - Minneap-St Paul; OM 79 Univ of WI - River Falls; 87–Sp-Lang Path, Hennepin Tech Ctrs Dist #287, **SLP**

Marois, Denis A 95 North St Andrews Drive, Ormond Beach, FL 32074, (904) 677-6095, MS 73 Univ of South FL; **SLP**

Marold, Jacqueline 4237 Wilson Street, Minnetonka, MN 55345, (612) 561-9077, BS 77 Univ of MN - Minneap-St Paul; MA 79 Mankato St Univ; SLP, Osseo Sch Dist #279, **SLP**

Maron, Linda R 103B Eagle Heights Apts, Madison, WI 53705, (608) 238-9989, BA 78 Univ of ND; MA 79 Univ of ND; 84–Lecturer/Supervisor, Univ of WI-Oshkosh, **SLP**

Marotta, Mrs Beth Karol 16 Maple Street, Latham, NY 12110, (518) 785-3336, MS Coll of Saint Rose; 84–Sp-Lang Path, Private Practice, **SLP**

Marotta, Louis Jude 10214 Barwood, Houston, TX 77043, (713) 847-7302, BS 80 Stephen F Austin St Univ; MS 82 Univ of North TX; SLP, InSpeech Inc, **SLP**

Marousek, Diane R 376 Telegraph Road, Rising Sun, MD 21911, (301) 658-2495, BS 73 Towson St Univ; MS 77 Towson St Univ; Sp-Lang Path, Baltimore City Pub Sch, **SLP**

Marple, Mrs Christine Anne 2125 Niagara Street, Buffalo, NY 14207, (716) 873-3574, BS 78 SUNY - Coll at Buffalo; MS 81 SUNY - Coll at Buffalo; Sp/Lang Path, Buffalo Bd of Ed, **SLP**

Marquard, Mrs Virginia K 1104 Ironwood Court #176, Bellevue, NE 68005, (712) 366-0505, BA 73 Creighton Univ; MA 75 Univ of IA; Sp-Lang Path, Loess Hills AEA, **SLP**

Marquardt, Mrs Lillian A 17517 Shirley Drive, Lansing, IL 60438, (312) 895-1186, BA 69 CA St Univ - Fullerton; MA 72 CA St Univ - Fullerton; **SLP LM**

Marquardt, Dr Thomas P Department Of Speech Communication, University Of Texas, CMA7 246, Austin, TX 78712, (512) 471-7596, BS 68 Univ of WI - Madison; MS 70 Univ of WI - Madison; PH 73 (NS) Univ of WA; 76–Prof, U of TX-Austin, **SLP**

Marquardt, Valerie Anne Mercy Medical Center, Speech Pathology Dept, 4050 Coon Rapids Boulevard, Coon Rapids, MN 55433, (612) 427-2200, BS 83 Univ of WI - Stevens Point; MS 85 Univ of WI - Stevens Point; Sp-Lang Path, Mercy Medical Center, **SLP**

Marques, Corinne L 16511 31st Street S E, Bellevue, WA 98008, BS 77 SUNY - Coll at Brockport; MA 80 WA St Univ; **SLP**

Marquez, Mrs Frima K 3030 Majestic Ridge, Las Cruces, NM 88001, BA 80 NM St Univ; MA 82 NM St Univ; 86–Sp-Lang Path, R L Marquez MD PA, **SLP**

Marquez, Tamara Elizabeth 17 Lincoln Avenue, N Bay Shore, Long Island, NY 11706, (212) 491-8037, BS 84 Andrews Univ; MA 86 Hofstra Univ; 87–Aud, Columbia Univ Harlem Hosp Ctr, **A**

Marquis, Brenda Sue 5438-B Bishops Circle, Norcross, GA 30093, (404) 325-3011, BS 63 Univ of KY; ME 74 Univ of GA; ED 88 (Sp Path) Univ of GA; Coord/Sp-Lang Dis Prog, Dekalb Co Sch Syst, **SLP ACE**

Marquis, Mrs Catherine Toney 3265 Hembree Court, Marietta, GA 30062, BS 80 LA St Univ - Baton Rouge; MA 82 LA St Univ - Baton Rouge; Aud, La Otol Assoc, **A**

Marquis, Marjorie A 1714 Solano Drive N E, Albuquerque, NM 87110, (505) 294-5061, BA 73 FL Int'l Univ; MS 78 Univ of NM; Sp-Lang Path/Cl Supvr, Albuquerque Pub Sch, **SLP**

Marquis-Canham, Mrs Celeste 100 Bleachery Court, Apartment C, Warwick, RI 02886, (401) 737-8919, BS 79 Coll of Saint Rose; MA 81 Northwestern Univ; 88–Sp-Lang Path, J Arthur Trudeau Memorial Ctr, **SLP**

Marr, Molly Kay 1436-1/2 Avon Park Terrace, Los Angeles, CA 90026, (213) 922-6205, BA 71 Univ of Southern CA; MA 73 Univ of Southern CA; Teacher On Spec Assighnment, Los Angeles Co Office of Ed, **SLP**

Marra, Cynthia Keller 82 Alpine Drive, Latham, NY 12110, (518) 434-4104, MS 84 Coll of Saint Rose; MS 84 Coll of Saint Rose; Sp-Lang Path, Private Practice, **SLP**

Marra, Mrs Pamela S 5410 Crescent Beach Road, Vaughn, WA 98394, (206) 884-2551, BS 70 Univ of WY; OM 76 Univ of WA; SLP, Peninsula Sch Dist, **SLP**

Marrah, Sr Marita Anne Cardinal Glennon Children's Hospital, 1465 South Grand, St Louis, MO 63104, (314) 577-5671, BS 66; MA 68; Chief Sp-Lang Path, Cardinal Glennon Chldn Hosp, **SLP**

Marrero, Francenia 10309 Calle Hidalgo N W, Albuquerque, NM 87114, **SLP**

Marrin, Joan P O Box 121, Georges Mills, NH 03751, (603) 763-9207, BA 76 SUNY - Center at Stony Brook; MS 80 Columbia Univ Teachers Coll; Sp-Lang Path, Newport Sch Dist, **SLP**

Marrinan, Diane Margaret MN Ear Head & Neck Clinic, 701 25th Avenue South, Minneapolis, MN 55454, (612) 339-2836, BA 85 Coll of Saint Teresa; MS 87 Univ of WI - Stevens Point; Aud, MN Ear Head & Neck Clinic, **A**

Marrinan, Eileen 38 Bracebridge Road, Newton Center, MA 02159, (617) 735-6165, BS 78 CO St Univ; MS 86 Univ of WI - Madison; 86–Sp-Lang Path, Childrens Hosp Boston, **SLP**

Marriott, Mrs Kay Joyce 13342 Huntsman Road, San Antonio, TX 78249, (512) 647-2100, BA 67 KS St Univ; MS 83 Western KY Univ

Marron, Kathleen Hutchinson Miami University, 2 Bchelor Hall, Oxford, OH 45056, (814) 863-3118, BA 76 Univ of NE - Lincoln; MS 78 Univ of NE - Lincoln; PH 86 (Geriatric Aud) PA St Univ - Univ Park; Asst Prof, Miami Univ of Ohio, **A**

Marrs, Mrs Elizabeth Gage 1409 Westover Gardens Blvd, Richmond, VA 23225, (804) 272-5652, BS 82 Univ of VA - Charlottesville; ME 84 Univ of VA - Charlottesville; 86–Aud, Otolaryngology Assoc, **A**

Marrs, Mrs Sandra Lorentz 4315 143rd Northeast, Bellevue, WA 98007, (206) 828-3201, BA 73 Univ of WA; OM 74 Univ of WA; Sp-Lang Path, Lake Washington Sch Dist, **SLP**

Mars, Mrs Julie Burkholder 251 Andover Drive, Glenmoore, PA 19343, (215) 524-5059, BS 75 West Chester Univ of PA; MA 81 West Chester Univ of PA; 75–Sp-Lang Path, Chester County IU #24, **SLP**

Marsala, Penelope D 4229 30th Avenue South, Minneapolis, MN 55406, (612) 435-8121, BS 78 Bradley Univ; MA 82 Univ of MN - Minneap-St Paul; Audiologist, Park Nicollet Medical Center, **A**

Marschall, Ellen J F 131 West Lincoln Avenue, Gettysburg, PA 17325, (717) 337-1865, BA 69 Univ of WI - Madison; MS 71 Univ of WI - Madison; MS 79 Towson St Univ; **SLP**

Marseille, Patricia A 29W064 Batavia Road, Warrenville, IL 60555-9506, (312) 393-2072, BA 72 Elmhurst Coll; MA 74 Northern IL Univ - De Kalb; Sp-Lang Path, Dupage Easter Seal Treatmt Cen, **SLP**

Marsh, Mrs Carolynn K R R 1 Box 937, Kittery, ME 03904, (207) 439-2016, BA 73 Pomona Coll; MA 76 Univ of CT; 88–Sp-Lang Path, Private Practice, **SLP**

Marsh, Debra Rose 3560 S W 110th Avenue, Beaverton, OR 97005, (503) 649-5566, BA 77 OR St Univ; MS 83 Western OR St Coll; **SLP**

Marsh, Diana M Box 3183, Soldotna, AK 99669, (907) 262-9006, BA 74 Univ of VT; MS 76 CO St Univ; Special Preschool Teacher, Kenai Peninsula Boro Sch Dist, **SLP**

Marsh, Mrs Janet H 8626 Northport Drive, Cincinnati, OH 45255, (513) 559-4341, BS 73 Univ of Cincinnati; MA 75 Univ of Cincinnati; Sp/Lang Path, Children's Hosp Med Ctr, **SLP**

Marsh, Janice Ruth 6460 229th Avenue N W, Elk River, MN 55330, (612) 255-5678, BS 84 Ball St Univ; MA 85 Ball St Univ; 88–Sp-Lang Path, St Cloud Hosp, **SLP**

Marsh, Lucille T Rural Free Delivery, Steele City, NE 68440, MS; **LM**

Marsh, Mary Beth 133 Garden Road, Columbus, OH 43214, (614) 261-4940, MA 73 OH St Univ; BA 72 Otterbein Coll; Manager Neuro Rehab Ctr, Riverside Methodist Hosp, **SLP**

Marsh, Mary G 2810 Kingfisher, Humble, TX 77338, (713) 441-2321, BA 74 Univ of OK - Norman; MS 77 Phillips Univ; **SLP**

Marsh, Mrs Michele Poynton 422-M Barreda Boulevard, Lusby, MD 20657, (301) 326-2453, MA 87 George Washington Univ; **SLP**

Marsh, Nancy C 261 10th Avenue, Bethlehem, PA 18018, BS 56 PA St Univ - Univ Park; ME 63 PA St Univ - Univ Park; Sp/Lang Path, Bethlehem Area Sch Dist, **SLP**

Marsh, Niki Pappas 37 Lambeth Bridge Court, Lutherville, MD 21093, (301) 683-3243, BS 76 CA Univ of PA; MS 79 PA St Univ - Univ Park; Sp-Lang Path, Baltimore Co Bd of Educ, **SLP**

Marsh, Rochelle I 1100 South Barton Street Apartment 287, Arlington, VA 22204, (703) 979-3633, BS 71 Saint Mary's Coll; MS 77 Howard Univ; 75–Sp-Lang Path, Fairfax County PS, **SLP**

Marsh, Sandra Evers 16039 Partnership Road, Poolesville, MD 20837, (301) 972-7410, BA 78 OH Wesleyan Univ; MS 80 Towson St Univ; 87–Sp/Lang Path, Montgomery Co PS, **SLP**

Marsh, Susan A G 1264 Wesley #302, Memphis, TN 38116, (901) 332-3782, BA 73 Memphis St Univ; MA 78 Memphis St Univ; 87–Aud, Robert M Fisher MD, **A**

Marshak, Mrs Elizabeth 20 William Street, Needham, MA 02194, (617) 668-5400, BS 67 Emerson Coll; ME 78 Wheelock Coll; MS 81 Emerson Coll; Sp-Lang Path, Walpole Public Schools, **SLP**

Marshall, Mrs Bonnie B P O Box 769, Sonoma, CA 95476, (707) 938-2525, BA 76 PA St Univ - Univ Park; OM 79 LA St Univ - N O Medical Ctr; Sp/Lang Path, Sonoma Valley USD, **SLP**

Marshall, David Paul Route 1 Box 170A, Stillwell, OK 74960, (907) 279-6661, MS 83 Univ of AZ; Aud, WW Hastings Hosp, **A**

Marshall, Deborah Durst 116 Deerfield Lane North, Pleasantville, NY 10570, BS 73 SUNY - Center at Albany; MS 75 Columbia Univ Teachers Coll; Sp-Lang Path, Private Practice, **SLP**

Marshall, Edwina Catherine 101 East Montezuma Avenue, Cortez, CO 81321, (303) 565-3080, BS 71 CO St Univ; MA 87 Univ of Northern CO; 74–Sp-Lang Path, Montezuma RE-1 Sch Dist

Marshall, Eileen Frances 20 Walnut Avenue, North Hampton, NH 03862, (603) 964-9303, BA 75 Univ of MA - Amherst; ME 79 Northeastern Univ; **A**

Marshall, Elizabeth 1220 Jackson S E, Albuquerque, NM 87108, **SLP**

Marshall, Elizabeth T Route 3 Box 1782, Danville, VA 24540, (804) 793-TALK, BA 72 Univ of NC - Greensboro; MA 77 Univ of NC - Greensboro; Dir-Sp-Lang Path, Danville Sp & Hrng Cen, **SLP**

Marshall, Ellen Frances GCMP Box 139, Pryor, OK 74361, (918) 256-5529, BS 77 OK St Univ; MA 84 Univ of Tulsa; **SLP**

Marshall, Ethel C 2074 Lorne Terrace, Victoria, BC, Canada V8S 2H8, (604) 386-2464, BS 74 Univ of Alberta - Alberta; OM 78 Univ of WA; Dir Therapy Svcs LTC, Greater Victoria Hosp Society, **SLP**

Marshall, Dr George Matthews, Jr 940 Stanford Avenue #120, Baton Rouge, LA 70808, (504) 642-3306, BA 59 Univ of MS; MS 64 Vanderbilt Univ; PH 72 (NS) LA St Univ - Baton Rouge; SLP/Aud, LA Spec Sch Dist #1, **SLP**

Marshall, Mrs Jean M 4812 Wayside Drive, Old Hickory, TN 37138, (615) 244-6900, BS 73 TN St Univ; MS 74 Vanderbilt Univ; Sp-Lang Path, Trevecca Health Care Center, **SLP**

Marshall, Mrs Linda 2215 Tyler Place, Charlottesville, VA 22901-9571, (804) 295-9250, BS 75 James Madison Univ; MS 76 James Madison Univ; SLP, Thomas Jeff Hlth Dept, **SLP**

Marshall, Linda 1211 Brunswick Lane, Ventura, CA 93001, (805) 648-3411, BA 82 CA St Univ - Northridge; MA 85 CA St Univ - Northridge; **SLP**

Marshall, Mrs Lori J 220 Shady Lea Road #2, North Kingstown, RI 02852, (401) 295-2385, BA 81 RI Coll; MS 83 Univ of RI; Sp/Lang Path, Cumberland Sch Dept, **SLP**

Marshall, Luan F 915 West Michigan Street, New Buffalo, MI 49117, (616) 469-0640, BS 77 Ball St Univ; MA 82 Western MI Univ; Sp-Lang Path, Speech Plus Inc, **SLP**

Marshall, Dr Lynne Naval Sub Medical Research Lab, Naval Sub Base New London, Groton, CT 06349, (203) 449-2550, MA 73 Univ of KS; MA 76 Univ of KS; PH 77 (NS) Univ of KS; Aud, US Government, **A**

Marshall, Dr Mary H Management And Planning Serv, 3821 Paces Ferry West, Atlanta, GA 30339, (404) 436-6277, BA 62 Columbia Coll; ME 70 Univ of SC - Columbia; PH 74 (Sp & Hrng Sciences) Univ Southern MS-Hattiesburg; 82–Pres, Management & Planning Services, **SLP**

Marshall, Merri Lea 809 N E Holliman Lane, Lee's Summit, MO 64063, (816) 524-9112, OB 85 Univ of MO - Columbia; MS 86 Central MO St Univ; 87–Sp-Lang Path, Lee's Summit R-7 Sch Dist, **SLP**

Marshall, Nancy B 2800 Vestavia Forest Drive, Birmingham, AL 35216, (615) 528-7531, BA 68 Univ of Louisville; MS 71 Washington Univ; ED 87 (NS) Univ of AL-Birmingham; 87–Dir Hosp & Spec Progs, MedTherapy Inc, **SLP A**

Marshall, Paulette A 2713 Craig Circle, Fullerton, CA 92635, **SLP**

Marshall, Pauline D 7516 Vanessa Drive, Fort Worth, TX 76112, BS 59 TX Woman's Univ; MA 65 Western MI Univ; 88–Dir Sp-Lang Path, Fort Worth State School 85, **SLP**

Marshall, Mrs Phyllis 1700 Syracuse Drive, Richardson, TX 75081, (214) 238-0683, BA 59 Our Lady Lake Univ-San Anton; MA 68 TX Woman's Univ; Sp-Lang Path, Richardson ISD, **SLP**

Marshall, Dr Rita K 3410 South Calumet, Chicago, IL 60616-3936, MA 77 Governors St Univ; MA 78 Governors St Univ; PH 85 (NS) Southern IL Univ -Carbondale; Sp-Lang Path, **SLP**

Marshall, Dr Robert C 6425 SW Burlingame Avenue, Portland, OR 97201, (503) 220-8262, BA 61 Univ of CA - Santa Barbara; MS 65 Univ of OR; PH 69 (NS) Univ of OK Medical Center; Chief Aud & Sp-Lang Path, VA Med Center, **SLP F**

Marshall, Mrs Robin A H 2514 Northumberland Avenue, Richmond, VA 23220, (804) 727-5432, MA; Asst Prof, Hampton Univ, **A**

Marshall, Sheri Caplan 2143 Country Club Drive, Lawrenceville, GA 30243, (404) 962-8282, BA 77 Univ of MD - College Park; MS 79 Towson St Univ; Aud, Gwinnett Otolaryngology, **A**

Marshall, Stephanie Scott 835 Crittenden Street N E, Washington, DC 20017, (202) 636-6990, BS 77 Hampton Univ; MS 79 Gallaudet Coll; Cl Superv, Howard U, **A**

Marshall, Sue J 3118 East 84th Street, Tulsa, OK 74137-1429, (918) 481-3118, **SLP**

Marshall, Susan A V 4244 Shenandoah, St Louis, MO 63110, (314) 991-5986, MA 78 Northern IL Univ - De Kalb; BS 75 Northern IL Univ - De Kalb; Aud, Spec Sch Dist of St Louis Co, **A**

Marshall, Mrs Susan L 4473 Falcon Avenue, Long Beach, CA 90807, (213) 926-5566, BA 72 Whittier Coll; MA 75 CA St Univ - Fullerton; 74–Sp-Lang Path, ABC USD, **SLP**

Marshall, Dr Thomas D Audiology & Speech Path Serv, VA Hospital, Pittsburgh, PA 15240, (412) 683-3000, BA 63 Colgate Univ; MA 65 Western MI Univ; PH 75 (NS) Univ of WI - Madison; Sp-Lang Path, VA Med Cen, **SLP**

Marshalla, Pamela R 131 N W Bowdoin, Seattle, WA 98107, (206) 633-0780, BS 75 Univ of IL - Urbana; MA 76 Univ of IL - Urbana; Writer/Consult, Innovative Concepts, **SLP**

Marshall-Siegel, Mrs Susan 2609 South Quebec #6, Denver, CO 80231, (303) 753-1564, BS 61 Miami Univ - Oxford; MA 77 Univ of CO - Denver; Sp-Lang Path, Private Practice, **SLP**

Marshall-Thoreen, Janet S 4012 44th Avenue South, Minneapolis, MN 55406, (612) 722-4479, OB 81 Univ of MN - Minneap-St Paul; MA 83 Univ of MN - Minneap-St Paul; **SLP**

Marsicek, Jeanne Marie 13305 Arden Way #22, Laurel, MD 20708, (703) 824-8056, BS 84 FL St Univ; MS 86 Univ of NE - Omaha; SLP, Easter Seal Society of VA, **SLP**

Marsrow-Jablonski, D'Orcie 225 East State Line Road, Toledo, OH 43612, BA 81 Univ of Toledo; MA 82 Bowling Green St Univ; SLP, Lucas Co Bd of Men Ret, **SLP**

Marston, Dr Larry E 109 Providence Road, Lawrence, KS 66044-1110, (913) 843-8479, BA 64 KS St Univ; MA 68 Univ of KS; PH 71 (Aud) Univ of KS; Assoc Prof, U of KS, **A**

Marston, Mrs Linda J 1022 Indiana Avenue, Wisconsin Dells, WI 53965, (608) 742-4131, BS 78 Univ of WI - Stevens Point; MS 82 Univ of WI - Madison; **SLP**

Marston, Mark Dewayne Woodward State Hospital, c/o Speech & Hearing, Woodward, IA 50276, (515) 438-2600, BS 83 Northern IL Univ - De Kalb; MA 85 Northern IL Univ - De Kalb; **A**

Mart, Mrs Margaret J 2957 Panama Avenue, Carmichael, CA 95608, (916) 965-3398, BA 60 Univ of IA; MA 62 Univ of IA; Sp/Lang Path, Private Practice, **SLP**

Martel, Susan Lynne 904 C Ridgefield Circle, Clinton, MA 01510, (508) 345-5250, BA 82 Univ of VT; MA 87 San Diego St Univ; 87–Sp-Lang Path, FLLAC Educ Collaborative, **SLP**

Martelli, Lisa 34 Acorn Drive, Bridgeton, NJ 08302, (609) 696-6843, SLP, Vineland Dev Cntr, **SLP**

Martello-Shepard, Nadine J 4865 Mannboro Drive, Upper Arlington, OH 43220, BS 79 Purdue Univ - West Lafayette; MA 80 Univ of IL - Urbana; Aud, Univ of Chicago Medical Center, **A**

Marten, Mrs Treasure A 3422 50th Street, Moline, IL 61265, (309) 764-6211, BA 78 Augustana Coll; MS 79 Eastern IL Univ; 86–Sp-Lang Path, Sherrard Dist #200, **SLP**

Martenis, Mrs Barbara Jeanne 41-B Doorstone Drive, Latham, NY 12110, (518) 271-8637, BS 82 Coll of Saint Rose; MS 84 Coll of Saint Rose; 84–Sp-Lang Path, Enlarged City Sch Dist of Troy, **SLP**

Martens, Colleen Finnen Chedoke Hospital, Evel 1 Speech Department, Box 2000 Station A, Hamilton, ON, Canada L8N 3Z5, (416) 521-7951, BA 84 Univ of ND; MS 85 Univ of ND; 88–Sp-Lang Path, Chedoke-McMaster Hosp, **SLP**

Martens, Dale M 9826 Corella, Whittier, CA 90603, **SLP**

Martens-Pitts, Lucinda A 2891 Bronson Hill Road, Avon, NY 14414, (315) 462-3216, BA 76 SUNY - Coll at Geneseo; MA 77 SUNY - Coll at Geneseo; Sp-Lang Path, Monroe BOCES, **SLP**

Marth, Julie E 8 Cleveland Lane, Petaluma, CA 94952, (707) 938-6472, BA 75 San Diego St Univ; MA 77 San Francisco St Univ; Aud, Sonoma Dev Cen, **A**

Marth, Mrs Suzanne S 11282 Burr Ridge Lane, Eden Prairie, MN 55344, (612) 941-7814, BA 67 Univ of MI - Ann Arbor; MA 69 Univ of CT; 88–Aud, ISD 287, **A**

Martien, Brenda M Route 3 Box 444, Ozark, MO 65721, (417) 334-5112, BS 73 Southwest MO St Univ; MS 78 Central MO St Univ; SLP, Hollister R-5 Sch, **SLP**

Martin, Amy Jane 4225 Village Lane #62, West Des Moines, IA 50265, (515) 266-5079, BA 85 Univ of Northern IA; MA 87 Univ of Northern IA; 87–Sp-Lang Path, Des Moines PS Hrng Imp, **SLP**

Martin, Amy Rose 3862 Isabella #1, Cincinnati, OH 45209-2127, (513) 420-5233, OB 83 Miami Univ - Oxford; MA 85 Miami Univ - Oxford; Sp-Lang Path, Middletown Regional Hosp, **SLP**

Martin, Anita C 2307 N Congress Avenue #11, Boynton Beach, FL 33426, (407) 737-4203, BS 82 Edinboro Univ of PA; MS 86 Univ of SC - Columbia; Sp-Lang Path, Communitherapy Inc, **SLP**

Martin, Mrs Anita P 3841 Campbell, Kansas City, MO 64109, (816) 453-5050, BS 73 Univ of IA; MS 74 Central MO St Univ; Sp-Lang Path, N KS Cty Sch Dist, **SLP**

Martin, Mrs Ann O'Neill 1585 Poes Lane, Charlottesville, VA 22901, (804) 296-5885, BA 72; ME 74 Univ of VA - Charlottesville; Sp-Lang Path, Albemarle Co Pub Schs, **SLP**

Martin, Ann W 3650 Windemere Drive, Ann Arbor, MI 48105, (313) 665-2168, BS 69 Northwestern Univ; MS 70 Univ of MI - Ann Arbor; 84–Sp-Lang Path, Chelsea Community Hosp, **SLP**

Martin, Mrs Anne H 1950 S E 23rd Avenue, Fort Lauderdale, FL 33316, (305) 523-8516, BA 73 Univ of FL; MS 77 Univ of South FL; Sp-Lang Path, Private Practice, **SLP**

Martin, Barbara H 17 Lancaster Road, Burlington, NJ 08016, (609) 386-3520, BS 56 Hampton Univ; MS 79 Rutgers St Univ -N Brunswick; Sp-Lang Path, Burlington Township Bd of Ed, **SLP**

Martin, Mrs Barbara Jeanne Rdi Box D-10 Cora Lane, Chester, NJ 07930, (201) 879-6380, BA 64 William Paterson Coll; MS 86 William Paterson Coll; **A**

Martin, Mrs Barbara K 32447 Woodyard Road, Albany, OH 45710, (614) 698-2106, BA 67 Univ of MO - KS City; MA 69 Univ of KS; 87–Sp-Lang Path, Echoing Meadows Res Fac, **SLP**

Martin, Barbara Lynn 2276-B Winterberry Drive, Lexington, KY 40504, (606) 234-1001, MA 84 Eastern KY Univ; Sp-Lang Path, Excepticon, **SLP**

Martin, Mrs Beth Miller 22 Fairview Lane, Shawnee, OK 74801, (405) 275-8277, MA 83 Univ of Tulsa; Sp-Lang Path, Pottawatomie Co Guidance Cen, **SLP**

Martin, Mrs Bette J S 176 Stoke Drive, Kitchener, ON, Canada N2N 2C1, (519) 749-4201, BA 74 Elmhurst Coll; MA 75 Univ of IL - Urbana; 75–Aud, Kitchener-Waterloo Hosp, **A**

Martin, Mrs Bobette Susanne White Mountain Hearing Serv, P O Box 2707, Pinetop, AZ 85935, (602) 367-5659, **A**

Martin, Mrs Bonita L 300 Chessington Circle, Summerville, SC 29483, (803) 899-4308, BA 77 SC St Coll; MA 78 SC St Coll; Sp-Lang Path, Berkeley Co Sch Syst, **SLP**

Martin, Bonnie Marie 2518 Somerset Drive, New Orleans, LA 70114, (504) 392-7292, BS 84 Saint Mary's Dominican Coll; OM 86 LA St Univ - N O Medical Ctr; **SLP**

Martin, Mrs Bonnie S 126 Shore Drive, Nashua, NH 03062, (603) 883-4437, BS 76 Coll of Saint Rose; ME 77 Coll of Saint Rose; **SLP**

Martin, Mrs Brenda K 7956 Thunder Mountain Road, Boise, ID 83709, (208) 384-1465, BS 76 ID St Univ; MS 77 ID St Univ; Sp-Lang Path, Private Practice, **SLP**

Martin, Brett A 379 Henry Street #3, Brooklyn, NY 11201, (718) 797-1316, BS 85 Northwestern Univ; MA 85 Northwestern Univ; 86–Aud, Columbia Presbyterian Med Ctr, **A**

Martin, Carol F 1426 North Riata, Gilbert, AZ 85234, (602) 892-6963, BA 66 Univ of AR - Fayetteville; MA 68 Univ of AR - Fayetteville; **SLP**

Martin, Mrs Carolyn C 817 Corbett Road, Monkton, MD 21111, (301) 293-4607, BS 69 Old Dominion Univ; MS 73 Loyola Coll; SLP, Private Practice, **SLP**

Martin, Carolyn F 2426 Inglewood Court, Falls Church, VA 22043, **SLP**

Martin, Mrs Cathryn P 261 Hiddenlake Road, Hendersonville, TN 37075, (615) 822-5890, BS 72 Univ of TN - Knoxville; MA 75 Memphis St Univ; Sp-Lang Path, The Learning Lab, **SLP**

Martin, Dr Charles W 5000 Cardinal Drive, Muncie, IN 47304, **SLP**

Martin, Charyleen 4530 Harlem Road, Amherst, NY 14226, (716) 686-2017, BS 79 SUNY - Coll at Buffalo; MS 80 SUNY - Coll at Buffalo; Sp-Lang Path, Erie BOCES I, **SLP**

Martin, Mrs Cheryl Ann 1905 Corbitt Street, Shreveport, LA 71108, (318) 636-0210, BA 78 LA St Univ - Shreveport; OM 84 LA St Univ - N O Medical Ctr; **SLP**

Martin, Cheryl L 351 Orchard Street, East Lansing, MI 48823, **SLP**

Martin, Mrs Cheryl Sprout 891 King Street, Lewisberry, PA 17339, (717) 737-6728, BS 78 PA St Univ - Univ Park; MS 81 Bloomsburg Univ of PA; Aud, Capital Area Intermed Unit, **A**

Martin, Colleen Marie 717 Cape Cod Drive, South Lyon, MI 48178, (313) 581-2600, BS 83 Central MI Univ; MA 84 Western MI Univ; Aud, Midwest Health Center, **A**

Martin, Mrs Cynthia J 4443 South Roxborough Park, West Valley City, UT 84119, (801) 481-7110, BA 76 Univ of UT; MS 78 Univ of UT; 78–Sp-Lang Path, Granite Sch Dist, **SLP**

Martin, Dr Daniel E 1080 Greenhills, Ann Arbor, MI 48105-2722, (313) 833-0710, BS 64 Kent St Univ; MS 66 Purdue Univ - West Lafayette; PH 70 (NS) Univ of MI - Ann Arbor; Director Sp-Lang Pathology, Lake Shore Ear Nose Thr Center, **SLP**

Martin, Deborah J 402 North Sheridan Road, Apartment 304-A, Lawton, OK 73501, (405) 357-6117, BA 86 Wichita St Univ; MA 87 Wichita St Univ

Martin, Mrs Deborah S 317 Avon Street, New London, WI 54961, (715) 258-5140, BS 76 Marquette Univ; MS 77 Univ of WI - Eau Claire; Sp-Lang Path, Waupaca Sch Dist, **SLP**

Martin, Debra Lynn 1630 S W Allen Street, Corvallis, OR 97333, (812) 825-7224, BA 80 IN Univ - Bloomington; MA 84 Ball St Univ; Sp-Lang Path, Union Hospital, **SLP**

Martin, Denise A 163-14 Booth Memorial Avenue, Flushing, NY 11365, (212) 240-5809, BA 74 CUNY - Queens Coll; MS 76 Columbia Univ Teachers Coll; Director of Clinical Services, Center for Child Development, **SLP**

Martin, Denise Louise 2106 West Park Avenue, Napa, CA 94558, (707) 255-1115, BA 84 CA St Univ - Sacramento; MS 86 CA St Univ - Sacramento; **A**

Martin, Denise Marie 1504 North Robertshaw, Greenville, MS 38701, (601) 335-5678, Ms St Supervisor, National Speech & Hearing Ser, **SLP**

Martin, Diane C 1001 Douglas, Alton, IL 62002, (618) 465-3594, BA 75 Eastern IL Univ; MS 82 Southern IL Univ-Edwardsvill; 82–Sp/Lang Path, Alton Catholic Children's Home, **SLP**

Martin, Douglas R 3248 Cranberry, Wichita, KS 67226, (316) 689-3289, BA 81 Wichita St Univ; MA 83 CA St Univ - Fresno; Aud, Valley Chldn Hosp, **A**

Martin, Dr Edwin W Human Resources Center, I-U Willets Road, Albertson, NY 11507, (516) 747-5400, BA 53 Muhlenberg Coll; MA 55 Univ of AL- Tuscaloosa; PH 61 (NS) Univ of Pittsburgh - Pittsburgh; Pres & Ch Exec Off, Human Resources Center, **SLP F**

Martin, Elaine G 408 Bridle Path, Marietta, GA 30068, (404) 325-3011, BA 69 Vanderbilt Univ; MS 71 Vanderbilt Univ; Sp/Lang Path, De Kalb Co Bd of Ed, **SLP**

Martin, Mrs Elizabeth 5306 Outrigger, Oxnard, CA 93035, (805) 388-4438, BA 73 Univ of WA; MS 73 Univ of WA; 74–Aud, Jentura Co Supt of Schs, **A**

Martin, Elizabeth L Baptist Medical Center, Cochlear Implant Clinic, 3300 N W Expressway, Oklahoma City, OK 73112, (405) 949-3398, BA 81 Memphis St Univ; MA 78 Memphis St Univ; Sp/Lang Path, Baptist Med Cen, **SLP**

Martin, Elizabeth Pleune 4468 Harbor Circle, Hoffman Estates, IL 60195, (312) 893-7995, BS 83 Univ of IA; MA 85 Northern IL Univ - De Kalb; SLP, Community Therapy Services, **SLP**

Martin, Faith Suzanne 6123 Ellsworth, Dallas, TX 75214, (817) 460-4611, BS 81 Baylor Univ; MA 85 TX Woman's Univ; 87–Sp-Lang Path, Private Practice, **SLP**

Martin, Dr Frederick N Dept Of Speech Communication, University Of Texas, Austin, TX 78712, (512) 471-3841, BA 57 CUNY - Brooklyn Coll; MA 58 CUNY - Brooklyn Coll; PH 68 (Aud) CUNY - Grad Sch & Univ Cntr; 68–Prof, U of TX, **SLP A F**

Martin, Glenn Thomas 2156 Anita Drive, Point Coquitlam, BC, Canada V3C 1H3, (403) 532-4441, OM 83 Univ of Philippines; **A**

Martin, Gloria Rodriguez 512 Brookwood Drive, Waco, TX 76710, (817) 776-3830, **SLP**

Martin, Hubert 1120 Greenlawn Drive, Pittsburgh, PA 15220, (412) 622-4485, BA 76 Univ of Pittsburgh - Pittsburgh; MA 79 Univ of Pittsburgh - Pittsburgh; Sp/Lang Path, St Francis Gen Hosp, **SLP**

Martin, James P 1705 Blossom Lane, Redondo Beach, CA 90278, (213) 824-3100, BA 79 CA St Univ - Los Angeles; MA 82 CA St Univ - Los Angeles; Aud, VA Medical Cen West LA, **A**

Martin, Mrs Janet B 9 Tulip Drive, Gaithersburg, MD 20877, (301) 963-0227, BA 69 PA St Univ - Middletown; ME 70 PA St Univ - Middletown; 78–Sp-Lang Path, Montgomery Co Pub Schs, **SLP**

Martin, Janice L 889 Woodtick Road #11, Waterbury, CT 06705, (203) 754-5141, BA 85 SUNY - Center at Binghamton; MS 87 Syracuse Univ; 87–SLP, Easter Seal Rehab Ctr, **SLP**

Martin, Jannette J 13471 West Dakota Avenue, Lakewood, CO 80228, (303) 987-1285, MA 81 Univ of CO - Boulder; Sp-Lang Path, **SLP**

Martin, Joanne C 11444 North 88th Place, Scottsdale, AZ 85260, (602) 581-7730, BA 75 Hofstra Univ; MA 76 Hofstra Univ; Admin, Deer Valley USD #97, **SLP**

Martin, Mrs Joanne Wilbur 11590 Mohican Road, Woodbridge, VA 22192, (518) 377-8519, BA 78 SUNY - Coll at Cortland; MS 79 Ithaca Coll; Sp/Lang Path, Fairfax Co Pub Sch, **SLP**

Martin, Karen Maria 1921 Carnot Street, New Orleans, LA 70122, **A**

Martin, Mrs Karen Marie Sr 2 Box 860, Clam Gulch, AK 99568, (907) 567-3306, BA 74 Univ of MT; MS 75 Western OR St Coll; 88–Aud, **A**

Martin, Karin Kligfield 9 Cheyenne Way, Corte Madera, CA 94925, BA 69 Univ of WA; MA 74 San Francisco St Univ; Sp/Lang Path, San Fran USD, **SLP**

Martin, Katherine 912 Jamieson Road, Lutherville, MD 21093, MS; **SLP LM**

Martin, Katherine Louise Star Route Box 23, Placitas, NM 87043, (505) 867-3133, BS 82 CO St Univ; MA 87 Univ of Northern CO; **SLP**

Martin, Kathleen Anne 1024 West Scott, Springfield, MO 65802, (417) 831-4523, **SLP**

Martin, Mrs Kathleen Sheehan 37 Tamarack Lane, Peabody, MA 01960, (617) 531-0065, OB 85 Salem St Coll; MS 87 Boston Univ; **SLP**

Martin, Kellie Sue 1835 Winding Hills Road, Apartment 1418, Davenport, IA 52807, (319) 355-2012, BS 83 IA St Univ; MA 84 Univ of Northern IA; SLP, MS Bend AEA 9, **SLP**

Martin, Mrs Kristen Kosisko 1445 East 36th Street, Erie, PA 16504-3008, (814) 453-5602, BA 84 Thiel Coll; ME 86 Univ of VA - Charlottesville; 86–Sp-Lang Path, Lake Erie Inst of Rehab, **SLP**

Martin, Mrs Kristi Jean 502 Glenview Heights Drive, New Albany, IN 47150, (812) 944-3646, BS 82 Purdue Univ - West Lafayette; MS 84 Purdue Univ - West Lafayette; 88–Aud, Jefferson Co PS, **A**

Martin, Laurel Campbell 1527 Farragut Street N W, Washington, DC 20011, (202) 723-4096, BA 80 Univ of MD - College Park; MA 86 Univ of MD - College Park; 88–Sp-Lang Path, Mont County PS

Martin, Le'Ann L P O Box 5833, Asheville, NC 28813, (704) 254-6478, BA 69 Marshall Univ; MA 71 Marshall Univ; Dir/Owner, Mountain Area Sp Assoc Inc, **SLP**

Martin, Leona Dee Rd 1 Box 312-E, Conklin Hill Road, Chenango Fork, NY 13746-9730, BS 83 SUNY - Coll at Geneseo; MA 85 SUNY - Coll at Geneseo; 86–Sp-Lang Path, Sheila R Gitlitz Sp and Hrng Assoc, **SLP**

Martin, Lesa A 6825 East Iliff #414, Denver, CO 80224-2545, (303) 753-6643, BS 81 Univ of Tulsa; MA 84 Univ of CO - Boulder; Aud, Private Practice, **A**

Martin, Leslie Schroeder 3140 Frances Avenue, La Crescenta, CA 91214, (818) 249-6012, BA 84 CA St Univ - Northridge; MA 86 CA St Univ - Northridge; 86–Sp-Lang Path, Los Angeles Co Ofc of Spec Educ

Martin, Linda D Marquez 4310 Avenue B Apt 214, Austin, TX 78751, (512) 453-5671, MA 78 Northwestern St Univ; SLP, Austin State Hospital, **SLP**

Martin, Linda J 101 Arthur Street, Hartwell, GA 30643, **SLP**

Martin, Mrs Lisa King 2008 Village Wood Road, Encinitas, CA 92024, (619) 632-1362, BS 82 Univ of Cincinnati; MS 84 OH Univ - Athens; 87–Sp-Lang Path, San Dieguito Union HS Dist, **SLP**

Martin, Lynda M 3 Sibley Street, Grafton, MA 01519, (617) 839-4873, BS 69 SUNY - Coll at Geneseo; MS 71 Ithaca Coll; Terr Markt Man, Oticon Corp, **A**

Martin, Margaret 2922 East Claire Drive, Phoenix, AZ 85032, (602) 949-7823, BS 72 AZ St Univ; MS 76 AZ St Univ; Consult, Private Practice, **SLP**

Martin, Margaret Allison 3766 Freemont Road, South Euclid, OH 44121, (216) 291-3592, BA 85 Cleveland St Univ; MA 87 Cleveland St Univ; 87–Sp-Lang Path, Meredia Euclid Hosp, **SLP**

Martin, Margaret H 4443 Palisades Park, Billings, MT 59106, (406) 657-7945, BS 69 CO St Univ; MS 71 CO St Univ; Dir-Rehab Therapies, St Vincent Hosp & Rehab Ctr, **SLP**

Martin, Mrs Marilyn Morse 363 East Linn Street, Bellefonte, PA 16823, (717) 748-3928, BA 67 Muskingum Coll; MS 81 PA St Univ - Univ Park; 85–Sp-Lang Path, Infant Dev Program, **SLP**

Martin, Marlene M 718 Welty Street, Greensburg, PA 15601-4114, (412) 537-1000, BS 74 OH Univ - Athens; MA 75 OH Univ - Athens; 80–Sp-Lang Path, Private Practice, **SLP**

Martin, Martha A 1125 Batey Drive, Nashville, TN 37204, (615) 259-8702, BA 49 David Lipscomb Coll; MA 51 G Peabody Coll-Vanderbilt U; Sp/Lang Path, Metro Pub Sch, **SLP**

Martin, Mary Arney 503 West 10th, Sterling, IL 61081, (815) 625-0400, BS 81 Bradley Univ; MS 83 Bradley Univ; Aud, Commun Gen Hosp, **A**

Martin, Mrs Mary Kay C 139 Olive Street, Huntington, WV 25705, (216) 923-7534, BS 80 WV Univ; MA 81 Marshall Univ; **SLP**

Martin, Maryann Leathem 4230 Camden, Dallas, TX 75206-5402, (214) 340-6256, BS 83 Western MI Univ; MA 84 Central MI Univ; 86–Sp-Lang Path, Dallas Rehabilitation Institute, **SLP**

Martin, Maureen K 105 Commanche Drive, Hattiesburg, MS 39401, (601) 266-5223, BS 75 Univ Southern MS-Hattiesburg; MS 76 Univ Southern MS-Hattiesburg; PH 85 (NS) Nat'l Univ of Ireland; Sp-Lang Path & Asst Director, Usm Sch/Chldn Lang Dis, **SLP**

Martin, Maureen McHugh 28686 Roanoke Street, Hayward, CA 94544, (415) 783-0471, MS 88 CA St Univ - Hayward; 88–Sp-Lang Path, Castro Valley USD

Martin, Michael E 2415 18th Avenue No, Nashville, TN 37208, (615) 889-8802, BA 70 Fisk Univ; MS 74 Emerson Coll; Aud, C K Hiranya Gowda, M D P C, **A**

Martin, Michele Hurst 2561 West Bovino Way, Tucson, AZ 85741, (602) 622-5833, BA 80 Columbia Coll; MS 81 Univ of AL- Tuscaloosa; Sp-Lang Path, St Marys Hosp, **SLP**

Martin, Molly A Box 338, Red Creek, NY 13143, (315) 594-8051, BS 77 SUNY - Coll at Oswego; MA 80 SUNY - Coll at Geneseo; SLP, North Rose-Wolcott Cent Sch Dist, **SLP**

Martin, Dr Nadine Villagebridge, 98 Oak Avenue #1305, Lindenwold, NJ 08021, (609) 435-0191, BA 74 Hofstra Univ; ME 75 Northeastern Univ; Res Asst, Temple Univ Med Sch, **SLP**

Martin, Nancy Jane 8057 West Dianne Court, Michigan City, IN 46360, **SLP**

Martin, Nancy S 2 Marilyn Drive, Belleville, IL 62221, (618) 235-0931, **SLP**

Martin, Nancy Schoenhut 22 Hirth Drive, Yardville, NJ 08620, (609) 588-8515, BA 81 Marshall Univ; MA 83 Univ of TN - Knoxville; Sp-Lang Path, Mercer Co Project Chld, **SLP**

Martin, Nancy Stuart 3517 49th Street, Lubbock, TX 79413, (806) 763-7041, MA 72; Sp-Lang Path, Lubbock St Sch, **SLP**

Martin, Orville W 8199 Priestley Drive, Reynoldsburg, OH 43068, (614) 466-2235, BS 59 OH St Univ; MA 68 OH St Univ; SLP, Ohio Dept Hlth, **A**

Martin, Mrs Patricia Arnold 408 South Greene Street, Wadesboro, NC 28170, (704) 694-9397, BS 78 Saint John's Univ - Jamaica; MA 80 Univ of Miami; Sp/Lang Path, Wadesboro Dev Center, **SLP**

Martin, Patti F Arkansas Childrens Hospital, Audiology Clinic, 804 Wolfe Street, Little Rock, AR 72203, (501) 370-1225, BA 81 Univ of AR - Fayetteville; MS 83 Univ of AR - Little Rock; Aud, Arkansas Childrens Hospital, **A**

Martin, Paul G P O Box 1284, Bluefield, WV 24701, (304) 325-3007, MS 76 5094; Owner, Aud Consult & Hrng Instruments, **A**

Martin, Dr Richard R Department Comm Dis, University Minnesota, 110 Shevlin Hall, Minneapolis, MN 55455, (612) 373-4116, BA 55; MA 58 Univ of IA; PH 63 (NS) Univ of MN - Minneap-St Paul; Prof, Univ Minnesota Dept Comm Dis, **SLP F**

Martin, Mrs Rosalind Shope 38 Oakleaf Drive, Mansfield, MA 02048, (508) 339-0990, BA 79 Lesley Coll; ME 83 Northeastern Univ; Aud, Martin Audiology Associates, **A**

Martin, Sandra Beth 17 Washburn Avenue, Auburndale, MA 02166, (617) 726-2763, BA 82 Univ of MD - College Park; MS 84 Univ of WI - Madison; 86–Sp-Lang Path, Mass Gen Hosp, **SLP**

Martin, Sandra H 1521 Isleview Drive, Ballwin, MO 63011, (314) 532-1681, BA 66 CUNY - Brooklyn Coll; MS 71 Eastern MI Univ; MA 67 Univ of MI - Ann Arbor; 88–Sp-Lang Path, Spec Sch Dist St Louis Co, **SLP**

Martin, Sandra Kay 2915 Forest Rim Court South, Puyallup, WA 98374, (206) 841-1331, BS 84 Brigham Young Univ; OM 86 Brigham Young Univ; 86–Aud, ENT Head & Neck Surgery Clinic, **A**

Martin, Mrs Sara Lee M 17910 Jashua Drive, Yorba Linda, CA 92686, (714) 524-8583, BA 68 Univ of the Pacific; MA 70 CA St Univ - Long Beach; Tchr, La Habra City Sch Dist, **SLP**

Martin, Sharil 19814 Kinzie Street, Chatsworth, CA 91311, (213) 997-2357, BA 66; MA 74; SLP, Los Angeles USD, **SLP**

Martin, Sharon Robinson Route 1, West Salem, WI 54669, BA 76 Univ of CO - Boulder; MA 79 Univ of Denver; Aud, Gundersen Cl, **A**

Martin, Shena Wileman 1187 East Herndon, Suite 101, Fresno, CA 93710, (209) 432-3303, BA 74 San Diego St Univ; MA 75 San Diego St Univ; Audiologist, Central California ENT Med Gp, **A**

Martin, Sherrie 5719 Fisherman's Landing, Bradenton, FL 34209, (813) 794-2223, BA 86 Ouachita Baptist Univ; MS 86 FL St Univ; 88–Sp-Lang Path, L W Blake Hosp, **SLP**

Martin, Sherry Ann 315 North Daniels, Carthage, TX 75633, (214) 693-8380, BS 83 Stephen F Austin St Univ; ME 85 Stephen F Austin St Univ; SLP, **SLP**

Martin, Mrs Sheryl Branan 331 Elder Road, Griffin, GA 30223, (404) 228-4555, BS 83 Tift Coll; ME 86 Univ of GA; 86–Sp-Lang Path, Griffin-Spalding Sch Sys, **SLP**

Martin, Stephanie Tarrant 4638 Briars, Eugene, OR 97404, (503) 686-3591, BS 77 OR St Univ; MA 80 Univ of KS; PH 88 (Central Auditory Processing) Univ of OR; 88–Dir of Aud/Sp-Lang Path, Eugene Clinic, **SLP A**

Martin, Steven Leroy 127 Palani Street, Hilo, HI 96720, (808) 935-3285, BA 83 Humboldt St Univ; MA 85 Humboldt St Univ; **SLP**

Martin, Mrs Susan C 3300 West Cooper Drive, Flagstaff, AZ 86001, (406) 259-6901, BA 75 Univ of Northern IA; MA 76 Univ of Northern IA; 85–Sp-Lang Path, Northern Arizona University, **SLP**

Martin, Mrs Susan J 8199 Priestley Drive, Reynoldsburg, OH 43068, (614) 864-1472, BS 69 OH Univ - Athens; MA 71 OH Univ - Athens; Aud, Bethesda Hosp, **A**

Martin, Susan K Madison Elementary School, 4120 Constitution Avenue, Colorado Springs, CO 80909, (719) 520-2300, BA 76 Adams St Coll; MA 77 Adams St Coll; Sp-Lang Path, Colorado Spr Sch Dist II, **SLP**

Martin, Terry M P O Box 3664, Evansville, IN 47735, (812) 425-2646, BS 72 IN St Univ - Terre Haute; MS 73 IN St Univ - Terre Haute; Dir/Aud, Hearing & Speech Assoc Inc, **A**

Martin, Vicky Cecile 421 Church Street, St Martinville, LA 70582, (318) 394-9119, BA 79 Univ of Southwestern LA; MS 82 Univ of Southwestern LA; **SLP**

Martin, Mrs Virginia Bruce 3214 Paces Station Ridge, Atlanta, GA 30339, (404) 252-5325, BS 81 Appalachian St Univ; ME 82 Univ of NC - Greensboro; 87–SLP, Atlanta Rehab Inst, **SLP**

Martin, Mrs Virginia E 149 Oxford Street, Winnipeg, MB, Canada R3M 3H7, (204) 786-7841, BS 53 Purdue Univ - West Lafayette; MA 56 Univ of SD - Vermillion; SLP, Child Guidance Clinic, **SLP**

Martina, Mark Charles 11450 Capistrano Court, Fort Myers, FL 33908-4034, (813) 466-0526, BA 83 SUNY - Center at Buffalo; MA 85 SUNY - Center at Buffalo; **A**

Martinat, Mrs Martha G P O Box 556, Rutherford College, NC 28671, (704) 322-4453, BS 77 Univ of TN - Knoxville; MA 78 Univ of TN - Knoxville; 85–Sp-Lang Path, Private Practice, **SLP**

Martinazzi, Vicci L 1752 S W Bonnie Brae Drive, Lake Oswego, OR 97034, (503) 280-6527, BS 66 Univ of OR; MS 68 Southern IL Univ -Carbondale; Sp-Lang Path, Portland PS, **SLP**

Martin-Boehs, Mrs Sally Sue 1518 Gatehouse Circle, South B-2, Colorado Springs, CO 80904, (719) 574-8300, MS 83 CO St Univ; 86–Sp-Lang Path, Child Development Ctr, **SLP**

Martindale, Mrs Eleanor N 731 Berry Avenue, Los Altos, CA 94022, MA 73 San Francisco St Univ; Tchr, Co of San Mateo, Spec Ed, **SLP**

Martindale-Whipple, Dr Kathy 120 Brenda, Hewitt, TX 76643, BS 72 Ouachita Baptist Univ; MS 73 Southern Methodist Univ; PH 82 (NS) Memphis St Univ; Asst Prof, Baylor U, **SLP**

Martine, Catherine Jane 2766-8 Jobee Drive, Charleston, SC 29414, (803) 792-3004, BS 75 Bloomsburg Univ of PA; OM 84 Univ of SC - Columbia; 85–Instructor of Aud, Med U of Sc, **A**

Martineau, Deborah R 500 Kane Street, Mount Pleasant, MI 48858, (517) 774-3471, BA 69 Univ of MI - Ann Arbor; MA 74 Central MI Univ; Temporary Instruct, Central Michigan U, **SLP**

Martinelli, Mrs Ann U 107 Circle Drive, St Clairsville, OH 43950-1001, (614) 695-5786, BS 77 WV Univ; MS 78 WV Univ; Aud, M Merrick & Associates, **A**

Martinelli, Mrs Laureen J 19 Brewerton Drive, Rochester, NY 14624, (716) 271-2520, BS 82 Med Coll of GA; MS 88 Nazareth Coll of Rochester; 85–Sp-Lang Path, Rochester Rehab Ctr, **SLP**

Martinet, Lenore A 10754 East La Jara, Cerritos, CA 90701, (213) 644-9728, BA 72 4873; MA 73 4873; SLP, LA County Supt of Sch, **SLP**

Martinetti, Mrs Helen Catherine 29 Crane Neck Drive, Sound Beach, NY 11789, MA 81 Hofstra Univ; Sp-Lang Path, Longwood Ctrl Sch, **SLP**

Martinetti, John Alan 5225-10 Nesconset Hwy, Port Jefferson Station, NY 11776, (516) 331-1888, MA 78 Hofstra Univ; Aud, Port Jefferson Sp-Hrng Ctr, **SLP A**

Martinez, Mrs Catherine Chreitzber 4691 North Avenida Ronca, Tucson, AZ 85715, (602) 294-1411, BS 80 Indiana Univ of PA; MS 82 Univ of AZ; Sp/Lang Path, Sunnyside U S D #12, **SLP**

Martinez, Catherine Rose 11262 East By Ways Street, South El Monte, CA 91733, (714) 383-7373, BA 83 CA St Univ - Los Angeles; MA 86 CA St Univ - Los Angeles; **SLP**

Martinez, Cecilia A 302 Cleveland, Pueblo, CO 81004, **SLP**

Martinez, Cecilia Monica Audiology Department, Lovelace Medical Center, 5400 Gibson S E, Albuquerque, NM 87108, (505) 262-7261, BS 79 Northern AZ Univ; MS 83 CO St Univ; 85–Aud, Lovelace Med Ctr, **A**

Martinez, Charles D West Los Angeles VA Med Ctr, (691/126), Wilshire & Sawtelle Blvd, Los Angeles, CA 90073, (213) 824-3100, BA 77 IN Univ - Bloomington; MA 79 Northwestern Univ; 86–Asst Chief-Aud, West Los Angeles VA Med Ctr, **A**

Martinez, Mrs Cynthia Rose 1113 Winecup Circle, College Station, TX 77840, (409) 361-5399, BS 79 Southwest TX St Univ; ME 81 Southwest TX St Univ; Sp-Lang Path, Bryan Independent School Dist, **SLP**

Martinez, Frieda Bleeck 120 Sunnyland Drive, San Antonio, TX 78228, (512) 433-8035, BA 66 Merrimack Coll; MA 73 Our Lady Lake Univ-San Anton; Sp-Lang Path, Edgewood ISD, **SLP**

Martinez, Mrs Janet R 3605 Paul Harris Court, Ellicott City, MD 21043, (301) 938-3000, BA 72 Univ of MD - College Park; MS 78 Towson St Univ; 88–Sp-Lang Path, Sheppard Pratt Hosp, **SLP**

Martinez, Martha R 3010 Valentine Avenue Apt 3G, Bronx, NY 10458, (601) 656-7950, BA 82 Univ of MS; MS 83 TX Christian Univ; **SLP**

Martinez, Mrs Regina Ann 7706 Buckboard, San Antonio, TX 78227, (512) 534-6851, BA 82 Our Lady Lake Univ-San Anton; MA 85 Our Lady Lake Univ-San Anton; 84–Sp-Lang Path, San Antonio ISD, **SLP**

Martinez, Rita Teran 4201 6th Avenue #307, San Diego, CA 92103, (619) 297-5208, BA 83 CA St Univ - Northridge; MA 86 San Diego St Univ

Martinez, Shannon Kay 2017 Algodones N E, Albuquerque, NM 87112, BS 85 Univ of WY; MS 86 Univ of HI - Manoa; 86–Sp-Lang Path, Educ Assesment Systems Inc, **SLP**

Martinez, Shari L 24 Knob Hill, Laguna Niguel, CA 92677-5903, BA 77 San Diego St Univ; MA 80 CA St Univ - Long Beach; Sp-Lang Path, Irvine USD, **SLP**

Martinez-Pita, Mrs Rowena Lee 20 East 9th Street 5F, New York, NY 10003, (212) 790-8678, BA 60 CUNY - Brooklyn Coll; MA 65 Univ of MN - Minneap-St Paul; Ch Sp-Lang Path, St Vincent's Hosp & Med Cen-NY, **SLP**

Marting, Ann McCay 15 Perthshire Drive, Peachtree City, GA 30269, (404) 487-7800, ME 85 GA St Univ; **SLP**

Marting, Debra Abplanalp 112 Fairview Street, Irwin, PA 15642, (412) 321-6995, BS 82 Indiana Univ of PA; MS 83 Univ of NC - Chapel Hill; Sp-Lang Path, Pressley Ridge Sch, **SLP**

Martin-Hantas, Ann E Gorgiou 14, Athens, Greece 11636, (914) 922-3359, BS 77 Auburn Univ - Auburn; MA 83 SUNY - Center at Buffalo; Sp-Lang Path, Private Practice, **SLP**

Martini, Jerry B 74 Woodland Terrace, Dunancsville, PA 16635-9295, (814) 946-6929, BS 71 CA Univ of PA; ME 76 Indiana Univ of PA; Dir of SLP & Aud, Dept of Pub Welfare-Altoona, **SLP**

Martini, Regina M 482 Chestnut Road, Severna Park, MD 21146, (301) 747-3940, BS 67 Towson St Univ; MS 74 OH St Univ; Sp/Lang Path, Balto Co Bd Ed, **SLP**

Martini, Mrs Valerie Fitch 1280 Inverness Drive, Elgin, IL 60120, (312) 742-7458, MA 86 Northern IL Univ - De Kalb; **A**

Martinkosky, Dr Stanley J 132 Hunters Ridge Road, Chapel Hill, NC 27514, (919) 966-3325, BS 66 OH Univ - Athens; MA 67 Western MI Univ; PH 75 (NS) OH St Univ; Dir Hearing & Sp Ctr, Nc Mem Hosp, **SLP**

Martin-Nadeau, Kimberly P O Box 672, North Hampton, NH 03862, (603) 964-5779, BS 79 Univ of NH; MS 80 Ithaca Coll; 80–Sp-Lang Path, Hampton Sch Dist, **SLP**

Martino, Jane H Box 126, Jefferson, IA 50129, (515) 386-8264, BS 73 Clarke Coll; MA 75 Univ of IA; PH 88 (Child Development) IA St Univ; Sp-Lang Path, Iowa State University, **SLP**

Martino, Nancy L 3404 Park Avenue #4, Richmond, VA 23221, (804) 264-9185, BS 78 PA St Univ - Univ Park; MA 85 Univ of TN - Knoxville; Sp-Lang Path, Communi-Care Inc, **SLP**

Martin Ochsner, Deborah Ann 2020 North 8th Street, Grand Junction, CO 81501-2934, (303) 241-1262, BS 75 CO St Univ; MA 82 Univ of Northern CO; 86–Sp-Lang Path, Hilltop Rehab Hosp & Private Practice, **SLP ACE**

Martinoff, Rosemary V 3417 Palos Verdes Drive N, Palos Verdes Estates, CA 90274, (213) 674-7050, SLP, Daniel Freeman Mem Hosp, **SLP ACE**

Martinson, Mrs Elizabeth 9141 Grant Street, Suite 135, Thornton, CO 80229, BA 70 Univ of CO - Boulder; MA 72 Univ of CO - Boulder; Sp-Lang Path, Private Practice, **SLP**

Martis, Janet A The Medical Plaza, 1300 Andrea Suite 101, Bowling Green, KY 42102-3380, (502) 782-7768, BS 73 PA St Univ - Univ Park; MA 75 Vanderbilt Univ; Aud, W G Begley MD PSC, **A**

Marto, Robert J Communispeech International, 4850 W Oakland Park Blvd, Fort Lauderdale, FL 33313, (305) 731-0767, BA 78 Temple Univ; MA 81 Univ of Pittsburgh - Pittsburgh; 85–Vice President, Communispeech International, **SLP**

Marton, Karen D 5336 North 45th Place, Phoenix, AZ 85018, (602) 279-0003, BS 79 AZ St Univ; MS 81 AZ St Univ; Aud, ENT Assoc, **A**

Marttila, Joan D 4660 Lindbergh Drive, Bettendorf, IA 52722, (319) 386-7662, BS 72 Univ of SD - Vermillion; MA 74 Univ of IA; Aud, MS Bend AEA 9, **A**

Martucci, Mrs Julie S 6825 Cherry, Kansas City, MO 64131, (816) 444-7334, BA 78 Univ of AR - Fayetteville; MA 79 Univ of TN - Knoxville; **SLP**

Martucci, Phyllis Joy 244-24 57th Drive Upper, Douglaston, NY 11362, (218) 224-8769, BA 78 CUNY - City College; MA 86 CUNY - Queens Coll; 87–Sp-Lang Path, Visiting Nurse Assoc, **SLP**

Marty, Mrs Mary J Pershing School, 9010 Pershing Avenue, Orangevale, CA 95662, (916) 966-8747, BA 72 CA St Univ - Sacramento; MA 75 CA St Univ - Sacramento; Sp-Lang Path, San Juan USD, **SLP**

Martz, Mrs Cynthia S 828 Pine, Los Alamos, NM 87544, (505) 662-4790, BS 80 Baylor Univ; MS 81 Baylor Univ; Sp-Lang Path, Los Alamos Pub Schs, **SLP**

Marven, Elaine Maria 70 Farmington Avenue, New London, CT 06320, (518) 434-2141, **SLP**

Marvin, Dr Christine A Department Of Special Education, 202 Barkley Memorial Center, University Of Nebraska, Lincoln, NE 68583-0732, (402) 472-5483, BS 72 Eastern MI Univ; MA 74 Eastern MI Univ; PH 85 (NS) Univ of OR; 88–Assist Prof, Univ of Neb-Dept of Spec Educ, **SLP**

Marvin, Joanne 9 Brigade Court, Bedminster, NJ 07921, (201) 430-5947, BA 78 William Paterson Coll; MS 79 William Paterson Coll; Audiologist, Pub Ser Electric & Gas, **A**

Marvin, Lynda 162 Lake Avenue, Tuckahoe, NY 10707, (212) 860-8400, OB 62 Cornell Univ; MS 85 Columbia Univ Teachers Coll; **SLP**

Marvis, Elenny Michelle 2232 West Eleventh Street, Cleveland, OH 44113, (216) 781-0462, **SLP**

Marwit, Dr Karen L 8000 Maryland Avenue, Suite 420, Clayton, MO 63105, (314) 721-6500, BA 68 SUNY - Center at Buffalo; ME 68 SUNY - Coll at Buffalo; PH 78 (NS) Saint Louis Univ; Sole Proprieter, Private Practice, **SLP**

Marx, Barbara Ruth S 13627 Sunset Boulevard, Pacific Palisades, CA 90272, (213) 454-2184, BS 59 Univ of IL - Urbana; MA 80 CA St Univ - Los Angeles; Sp-Lang Path, Private Practice, **SLP**

Marx, Mrs Brenda Vest 6800 Peachtree Industrial, Blvd Apt L-16, Doraville, GA 30360, BS 79 Ball St Univ; MA 81 Ball St Univ; Sp-Lang Path, InSpeech Inc, **SLP ACE**

Marx, Charles Gordon 504 Lamar Avenue, Hattiesburg, MS 39401, (601) 268-8490, BA 75 MS St Univ - MS State; MS 83 Univ Southern MS-Hattiesburg; Aud, Methodist Hospital, **A**

Marx, Francis N 358 South Gramercy Place, Apartment 305, Los Angeles, CA 90020, (213) 382-0738, BA 58 CA St Univ - Los Angeles; MA 62 CA St Univ - Los Angeles; **SLP LM**

Marx, Joann K 209 Rolling Fork Court, Nashville, TN 37205, (615) 352-4835, **SLP**

Marx, Linda Carol 2211 S W 92nd Terrace, Apt 1802, Fort Lauderdale, FL 33324, (305) 473-5417, MA 83 Hofstra Univ; 85–Sp-Lang Path, Broward County Schs, **SLP**

Marx, Mrs Maureen G 215 East Yeiser Street, Macomb, IL 61455, (309) 837-3660, BA 72 Univ of Philippines; MA 79 Western IL Univ; Clinic Coordinator, **SLP**

Marxheimer, Mrs Suzette 15201 75th Avenue, Edmonton, AB, Canada T5R 2Y9, (403) 489-1301, BS 53 Univ of IL - Urbana; MA 54 Univ of MI - Ann Arbor; Sp/Lang Path, Edmonton Pub Sch Bd, **SLP**

Marzano, Lisa Ann 706 N Forest, St Louis, MO 63119, (314) 768-5338, BS 85 Fontbonne Coll; MS 86 Fontbonne Coll; 86–Sp-Lang Path, SSM Rehabilitation Inst, **SLP**

Marzell, Miriam S 22 Old Short Hills Road, Livingston, NJ 07039, (201) 994-4468, BA 69 Hofstra Univ; MA 70 Seton Hall Univ; Sp-Lang Path, Private Practice, **SLP ACE**

Marzitelli, Mrs Gail Russin 113 Krakow Street, Garfield, NJ 07026, (201) 772-9213, BA 77 Montclair St Coll; MA 87 Montclair St Coll; **SLP**

Marzonie-Devine, Monica Star Route Box 1710, Eagle River, AK 99577, (907) 694-3402, BA 76 Central MI Univ; MA 78 Northern MI Univ; Sp-Lang Path, Eagle River Sp Path Ser, **SLP**

Marzouk, Mrs Sheila Warren 3 Shorehaven Lane, Manhasset, NY 11030, (516) 365-2383, BA 80 SUNY - Center at Buffalo; MS 82 Columbia Univ Teachers Coll; Aud, Audionics Corp, **A**

Masarsky, Iris Abbe 9450 Poinciana Place, Apartment 111, Fort Lauderdale, FL 33324, (305) 765-6000, BA 81 Long Island U - CW Post Ctr; MA 82 Long Island U - CW Post Ctr

Masayda, Barbara Lynn 96 Franklin Avenue, Oakville, CT 06779, (203) 272-0341, BS 78 Univ of CT; MS 83 Southern CT St Univ; MS 85 Southern CT St Univ; **SLP**

Mascara, Mrs Eleanor S 914 Hippocket Road, Peachtree City, GA 30269-0092, (404) 460-3560, BA 59 CUNY - Queens Coll; MA 78 GA St Univ; ES 88 Univ of GA; Sp/Lang Path, Fayette Co Bd of Ed, **SLP**

Mascaro, Mrs Janet M 1745 Outlook Drive, Verona, PA 15147, BS 73 Indiana Univ of PA; MA 75 Univ of Pittsburgh - Pittsburgh; Sp-Lang Path, Allegheny Inter Ut, **SLP**

Masche, Patricia A 42 Browns River Road, Sayville, NY 11782, (516) 581-3020, BA 76 Adelphi Univ; MA 79 Hofstra Univ; SLP, Wm Floyd School Distr, **SLP**

Maschgan, Marilyn G 670 Inglenook Drive, Las Vegas, NV 89123, (702) 382-4327, BS 75 PA St Univ - Univ Park; MA 79 San Diego St Univ; Aud, Sp & Hrn Ctr, **A**

Maschmann, Carolyn R Rural Route 1, Hartwick, IA 52232, (319) 525-3355, BA 76 Univ of Northern IA; MA 77 Univ of Northern IA; SLP, AEA #6, **SLP**

Mascia, John 107 15th Street, Apartment 2B, Garden City, NY 11530, (212) 360-3724, BA 83 Hofstra Univ; MA 85 Hofstra Univ; **A**

Mascitelli, Anna Marie Speech Lang Diag & Treat Services, 83 Pine Street North, Thorold, ON, Canada L2V 2P3, (416) 227-9209, BA 76 Brock Univ - Ontario; MA 79 SUNY - Center at Buffalo; Sp-Lang Path, Greater Niagara Gen Hosp, **SLP**

Mascow, Susan Zievers 10575 Silver Lake Road, Brighton, MI 48116, (313) 231-1335, BS 77 Marquette Univ; MS 78 Marquette Univ; **SLP**

Masden, Susan L 1723 Payne Street, Louisville, KY 40206-1940, (502) 454-8285, BS 79 Spalding Coll; MS 81 Univ of Louisville; Sp-Lang Path, Jefferson Co Board of Ed, **SLP**

Mase, Dr Darrel J 3944 NW 25th Circle, Gainesville, FL 32606, (904) 376-6384, BS 28 Emporia St Univ; MA 32 Univ of MI - Ann Arbor; PH 45 (NS) 9905; Sp-Lang Path, **SLP F LM**

Masek, Mrs Carol M P O Box 121, Valparaiso, NE 68065, (402) 665-3651, BS 77 Univ of NE - Lincoln; MA 78 Univ of NE - Lincoln; Sp-Lang Path, Raymond Cen Pub Sch, **SLP**

Masella, Alice Karen Box 342, 24 Oak Leaf Drive, Stuyvesant, NY 12173, (518) 799-3471, BS 83 Coll of Saint Rose; MS 87 Coll of Saint Rose; 84–Sp-Lang Path, Hudson City Sch Dist, **SLP**

Mashaw, Susan L Salem Speech & Language Center, 1265 Waller Street, Salem, OR 97302, (503) 371-6486, BS 72 Univ of IA; MA 73 Univ of IA; Salem Speech & Language Center, **SLP ACE**

Mashima, Pauline Matsumoto 1492 Ala Hahanui, Honolulu, HI 96818, (808) 948-8279, OB 75 Univ of HI - Manoa; BA 75 Univ of HI - Manoa; MS 78 Univ of HI - Manoa; 81–Instr, U of HI-Manoa, **SLP ACE**

Mashiyama, Dee K 2499 Kapiolani Blvd #2300, Honolulu, HI 96826, (802) 944-3678, BA 83 Univ of HI - Manoa; MS 87 Univ of AZ

Mashunkashey, Vickie A 801 Pueblo, Ardmore, OK 73401, **SLP**

Masica, Martha Denise 4180 Crest Road, Pebble Beach, CA 93953, (408) 899-7015, ME 82 Old Dominion Univ; Sp-Lang Path, Monterey Peninsula USD, **SLP**

Maskevich, Judith S 524 Olive Terrace, Union, NJ 07083, BA 69 Rutger's St Univ - Douglas Coll; MS 73 Columbia Univ Teachers Coll; 73–Sp-Lang Path, Sp & Hrng Assoc, **SLP ACE**

Maskin, Mrs Lynn N 30595 Country Club Drive, Redlands, CA 92373, (714) 884-6836, BA 72 CUNY - Queens Coll; MS 73 Univ of MI - Ann Arbor; SLP, San Bernardino USD, **SLP**

Masland, Mary W 118 East Hamilton Avenue, Englewood, NJ 07631, MS; **SLP LM**

Maslin, Mrs Joyce L 7943 Holmes, Kansas City, MO 64131, (816) 331-2131, BA 70 William Jewell Coll; MA 77 Univ of KS; SLP, Con Sch Dist No 4, **SLP**

Maslow, Lisa Abell 3610 Peartree Court #32, Silver Spring, MD 20906, (703) 979-8544, MA 87 George Washington Univ

Maslow, Shari Debra 816 Hurley Court, Far Rockaway, NY 11691, BA 84 CUNY - Queens Coll; MA 86 Temple Univ; **SLP**

Maslyn, Mary Lisa 3683 Arcadia-Zurich Road, Lyons, NY 14489, (315) 331-2429, MS 80 SUNY - Coll at Buffalo; 80–Sp-Lang Path, Newark Dev Ctr, **SLP**

Mason, Carolyn G Route 1 Box 97A, Martinsburg, Pekin, IN 47165, (812) 949-4250, BA 69 Elmhurst Coll; MS 72 IN Univ - Bloomington; ME 74 Univ of Louisville; 70–Sp-Lang Path, New Albany-Floyd Co Sch Corp, **SLP**

Mason, Christine 128 Taylor Avenue, Dedham, MA 02026, (617) 353-3252, BA 75 Boston Coll; MS 79 Purdue Univ - West Lafayette; Research Associate, Boston University, **A**

Mason, Clarice Jaynes 2230 Shady Creek, Richardson, TX 75080, (214) 231-0341, BA 63 Southern Methodist Univ; MS 74 Southern Methodist Univ; Sp-Lang Path, Richardson ISD, **SLP**

Mason, Dr David I 320 Annondale, Ballwin, MO 63011, (314) 652-3200, **A**

Mason, Deborah B 320 Annondale, Ballwin, MO 63011, **SLP**

Mason, Jane Marie 34 Neponset Avenue, Apartment #3, Hyde Park, MA 02136, (617) 566-1408, BA 74 Univ of MA - Amherst; MS 86 Boston Univ; 86–Sp-Lang Path, The Therapeutic Ctr/Vinfen Corp, **SLP**

Mason, Mrs Judith Asbury 2039 Puna Street, Honolulu, HI 96817, (808) 834-9218, BA 70 Univ of HI - Manoa; MS 76 Univ of HI - Manoa; Aud, Kaiser Med Ctr, **A**

Mason, Mrs Kathleen Marie P O Box 422, 65 Lake Street, Stillwater, NY 12170, (518) 237-0800, BA 78 SUNY - Coll at Plattsburgh; MS 82 Coll of Saint Rose; 79–Sp-Lang Path, Waterford-Halfmoon Sch Dist, **SLP**

Mason, Mrs Kelly Ann 31364 San Andreas Drive, Union City, CA 94587, (415) 487-0474, BA 85 San Francisco St Univ; MS 87 San Francisco St Univ; 87–Sp-Lang Path, Easter Seal Society, **SLP**

Mason, Kristen Elizabeth P O Box 706, Culbertson, MT 59218, (406) 787-6392, BA 84 Univ of ND; MS 86 Minot St Univ; Sp-Lang Path, Roosevelt Co Coop, **SLP**

Mason, LaRita 2223 South Ong, Amarillo, TX 79109, (806) 376-6200, BA 69 Phillips Univ; MS 70 Vanderbilt Univ; 72–SLP, Private Practice, **SLP ACE**

Mason, Mrs Luane C 6285 Tanglewood Drive N E, St Petersburg, FL 33702, (813) 527-7304, BA 74 Univ of FL; MA 75 Univ of FL; Sp-Lang Path, Pinellas Co Sch, **SLP**

Mason, Mrs Lynn M P O Box 1686, Laurinburg, NC 28352, (919) 276-2121, BS 77 East Carolina Univ; MA 82 Appalachian St Univ; Sp-Lang Path, Scotland County Schools, **SLP**

Mason, Marcia L DODDS-P/DSO-KOREA, APO San Francisco, CA 96301, BS 68 OK St Univ; MA 70 OK St Univ; 86–Spec Educ Coord, Dept of Defense Dept Sch-Korea, **SLP**

Mason, Mrs Mary Golsen 3914 Kincaid Terrace, Kensington, MD 20895, (301) 949-3851, BS 85 WV Univ; MS 86 Univ of SC - Columbia; Sp-Lang Path, Pro Rehab Network Inc, **SLP**

Mason, Mrs Mickie Flora 121 Cedar, Mulvane, KS 67110, (316) 777-4321, BA 83 Wichita St Univ; MS 85 Northwest MO St Univ; 86–Sp-Lang Path, USD #263, **SLP**

Mason, Molly Ann 21320 Woodland #202, Northville, MI 48167, (313) 348-6442, BA 85 Univ of MI - Ann Arbor; MS 86 Univ of MI - Ann Arbor; **SLP**

Mason, Nancie C 1822 McDonal Avenue, Lexington, KY 40503, (606) 223-5680, BA 68 Univ of KY; MA 72 Our Lady Lake Univ-San Anton; Sp/Lang Path, Fayette Co Sch, **SLP**

Mason, Mrs Nancy Kite 1914 Franconia Drive, Fairmont, WV 26554, (304) 367-0318, BS 85 WV Univ; MA 87 WV Univ; **SLP**

Mason, Pamela Ann 5513 Brite Drive, Bethesda, MD 20817, (202) 994-3632, MA 74 Mary Washington Coll; ME 75 Univ of VA - Charlottesville; 86–Aud, George Wash Univ, **A**

Mason, Pamela Jean 4417 Harbor Country Drive, Apartment D-7, Gig Harbor, WA 98335, (206) 851-2063, BA 80 WA St Univ; MA 82 WA St Univ; Sp-Lang Path, Dept of Social & Health Svcs, **SLP**

Mason, Pamela K 649 Montebello Circle, Chesapeake, VA 23320, (804) 487-4644, MS 79 Northern IL Univ - De Kalb; SLP, Chesapeake Public Schools, **SLP**

Mason, Mrs Pamela M 899 Hill Drive, Zephyrhills, FL 34248, (813) 788-0411, BA 68 IN Univ - Bloomington; MA 69 IN Univ - Bloomington; Sp-Lang Path, East Pasco Med Ctr, **SLP**

Mason, Mrs Rachel J Route 1 Box 530-Xx, Mullins, SC 29574, (803) 423-2891, BA 72 SC St Coll; MS 75 Phillips Univ; 86–Coord of Spec Svcs, Marion Sch Dist III, **SLP**

Mason, Richard D 3615 Tilden Avenue, Los Angeles, CA 90034-6909, (213) 559-7078, BA 76 CA St Univ - Northridge; MA 78 CA St Univ - Northridge; **SLP**

Mason, Dr Robert M 110 Ironwood Place, Chapel Hill, NC 27514, (919) 684-5113, MS 61 Univ of IL - Urbana; DD 77 Univ of KY; PH 65 (Sp Path) Univ of IL - Urbana; 79–Prof of Orthodontics, Duke U Med Cen, **SLP F**

Mason, Ruth SLP, Carney Hospital, 2100 Dorchester Avenue, Boston, MA 02124, (617) 296-4000, BS 73 Syracuse Univ; MS 74 Purdue Univ - West Lafayette; Director Sp-L Path Dept, Carney Hos, **SLP**

Mason, Mrs Sharon Lee 9333 Everett Court, Westminster, CO 80020, (303) 422-3490, BS 69 Western IL Univ; MA 82 Univ of CO - Boulder; Sp/Lang Path, Adams Co Sch Dist #12, **SLP**

Mason, Susan Reddan 7429 Baltimore Avenue, Takoma Park, MD 20912, (301) 495-3337, BA 73 Catholic Univ of America; MA 76 Catholic Univ of America; 88–Prog Dir, Job Discovery Inc, **SLP**

Mason, Susan S 71 West 12th Street #2D, New York, NY 10011, (212) 430-5595, BA 71 SUNY - Center at Buffalo; MS 74 Columbia Univ Teachers Coll; Sp/Lang Path, Albert Einstein Coll of Med, **SLP ACE**

Mason, Susan Shaw 2523 Stanley Avenue, Roanoke, VA 24014, BS 69 Pacific Union Coll; MS 82 Radford Univ; Sp-Lang Path, Roanoke City Schools, **SLP**

Mason, Mrs Sydney Brooks 4501 Old Greenwood Road, Apartment #9, Fort Smith, AR 72903, (501) 646-0093, BS 85 Univ of Central AR; MS 86 Univ of Central AR; **SLP**

Mason-Clendaniel, Charlene Magaki Uab Speech & Language Clinic, 1717 6th Avenue South, Birmingham, AL 35294, (205) 934-4467, BS 81 Univ of NC - Chapel Hill; MS 83 Univ of NC - Chapel Hill; Med SLP, Uab Sp & Lang Cl, **SLP**

Masone, Patrick Great Neck Audiology Assoc, 525 Northern Boulevard, Great Neck, Long Island, NY 11021, (516) 482-0660, BS 67 SUNY - Coll at Plattsburgh; MS 69 Adelphi Univ; Great Neck Audiology Associate, **A**

Masoner, Judith Collins 46 Hillcrest, Carbondale, IL 62901, (618) 457-6762, BA 69 Univ of OK - Norman; MS 86 Southern IL Univ -Carbondale; Aud

Mass, Mrs Hagit Pur 595 Mohawk Court, Suffern, NY 10901, (914) 634-4648, BA 79 Hebrew Univ-Jerusalem Israel; MS 86 Columbia Univ Teachers Coll; **SLP**

Massa, Mrs Georgiann K 322 Eagleston, Elmhurst, IL 60126, (312) 833-8614, BS 83 IL St Univ - Normal; MS 86 IL St Univ - Normal; **SLP**

Massa, Michael V 5037 Backlick Road #A, Annandale, VA 22003, (703) 941-4594, BS 74 OH Univ - Athens; ME 79 Univ of VA - Charlottesville; Owner-Aud, Audiology Cen, **A**

Massaro, Mrs Donna M 64 Chaucer Drive Rd 2, Hackettstown, NJ 07840, (201) 637-6810, BA 81 Rutgers St Univ -N Brunswick; MA 85 NY Univ; Sp-Lang Path, Barnert Mem Hosp Ctr, **SLP**

Massarotto, Caroline E 1170 Varsity Estates Dr N W, Calgary, AB, Canada T3B 5E8, MA 74 Univ of MT; 88–Sp-Lang Path, Alberta Children's Hosp, **SLP**

Masse-Arikian, Jody Lynne 339 Broad Street, Nashua, NH 03063, (617) 772-0935, BA 79 Bridgewater St Coll; ME 82 Northeastern Univ; Sp-Lang Path, Ayer Sch Sys, **SLP**

Massenberg, Angela Renee 22531 West McNichols, Detroit, MI 48219, (313) 487-4410, BS 81 Wayne St Univ; MA 82 Eastern MI Univ; 88–Asst Prof, Eastern Michigan Univ, **SLP**

Massengill, Dr Raymond, Jr 61 Kingsbridge, Bristol, TN 37620, (615) 968-1821, BS 59 Univ of TN - Knoxville; MS 59 Univ of TN - Knoxville; ED 68 (NS) Univ of VA - Charlottesville; **SLP F**

Massett, Mrs Kathryn H 5900 Goshen Road, Goshen, OH 45122, (513) 722-2223, BS 79 Univ of Cincinnati; MA 81 Univ of Cincinnati; Sp-Lang Path, Clermont Co Bd of Ed, **SLP**

Massey, Mrs Amy Reichard 2577 Ridgewood Terrace NW, Atlanta, GA 30318, (404) 653-4775, BS 84 Southwest MO St Univ; MS 86 IN Univ - Bloomington; 86–Sp-Lang Path, Georgia Baptist Med Ctr, **SLP**

Massey, April 1424 Decatur Street N W, Washington, DC 20011, (202) 726-3536, BA 80 OH St Univ; MA 82 Univ of Cincinnati; Sp-Lang Path, Howard University, **SLP**

Massey, Cathey L A 6076 Donnybrook Drive, Clay, NY 13041, **SLP**

Massey, Claire A 3411 Massengale Road, Chattanooga, TN 37419, (615) 837-7875, BS 74 Univ of TN - Knoxville; MA 75 Univ of TN - Knoxville; 86–Sp-Lang Path/Dir, Marion Co Sp & Hrng Clinic, **SLP**

Massey, Mrs E Jeannette Route 1 Lot 5, Midway Mobile Home Park, Stroud, OK 74079, (918) 352-9519, BS 77 OK St Univ; MS 86 Univ of OK Medical Center; Sp-Lang Path, Drumright Schools, **SLP**

Massey, Elizabeth 9348 Rocky Valley Cove, Cordova, TN 38018, (901) 346-7906, BA 70 Univ of MS; MA 71 Univ of AL- Tuscaloosa; Sp-Lang Path, Chatterbox Sp-Lang Cen, **SLP**

Massey, Holly Joyce 1285 Bordeaux Street, Livermore, CA 94550, (415) 447-9500, MA 87 San Jose St Univ; 80–Sp-Lang Path, Livermore Unif Sch Dist, **SLP**

Massey, Mrs Joan Benanzer 7870 Fort Loramie Swanders, Rural Route 2, Anna, OH 45302-9802, (419) 628-4023, BS 84 Ball St Univ; MA 77 Purdue Univ - West Lafayette; 86–Sp-Lang Path, Private Practice, **SLP**

Massey, Mrs Michele Miller 2128 Falcon Ridge, Carrollton, TX 75010, (214) 370-5552, BS 85 Univ of North TX; MS 86 Univ of North TX; 88–Sp-Lang Path, Lewisville ISD, **SLP**

Massie, Sherin L T 6570 North Backer Avenue, Fresno, CA 93710, (209) 299-8957, BA 71 CA St Univ - Fresno; MA 75 CA St Univ - Fresno; Inst/Supv, CA St U Fresno, **SLP**

Massimi, Mrs Theresa Shanley Box 130, Bloomington, NY 12411, (914) 331-1774, BS 73 SUNY - Coll at Geneseo; MS 76 Hofstra Univ; Sp-Lang Path, Private Practice, **SLP**

Massine, Donna White 825 East Dry Creek Road, Sandy, UT 84070, (801) 565-7100, BS 80 ND St Univ; MA 81 Minot St Univ; MS 83 Minot St Univ; 88–Sp-Lang Path, Jordan Sch Dist, **SLP A ACE**

Massingill, Joyce L Lyle 1109 College Street, Port Gibson, MS 39150, (601) 437-5620, BS 69 Univ Southern MS-Hattiesburg; MS 75 Univ Southern MS-Hattiesburg; Sp/Lang Path, Vicksburg Warren Sch Dist, **SLP**

Massini, Paula A 90 Morgan Avenue, East Haven, CT 06512, (203) 467-7122, BA 84 Univ of CT; MS 87 Southern CT St Univ; 87–Sp-Lang Path, North Branford PS

Massoglia, Ann Tomasin Rural Route 3, 4426 Townline Road, Milton, WI 53563-9406, **SLP**

Masson, Mrs Ella Marie 4810 Whitechapel Boulevard, Alexandria, LA 71303, (318) 445-8395, BA 61 Northwestern St Univ; ME 72 Northwestern St Univ; Dir Sp-Lang Svcs, Rehab Ctr of Rapides Parish, **SLP**

Massucci, Ellen Marie 257 Old Turnpike Road, Southington, CT 06489, (203) 628-7920, BA 83 Boston Coll; MA 86 Univ of CT; **SLP**

Mast, Barbara D 4741 El Rancho Verde Drive, La Palma, CA 90623, (213) 698-9531, BA 74 Whittier Coll; MA 76 Whittier Coll; 76–Sp-Lang Path, Whittier City Sch Dist, **SLP**

Mastalerz, Vickie R 191 Hoff Road, Union Bridge, MD 21791, (301) 775-7638, BS 72 Juniata Coll; MS 77 WV Univ; Aud, Western Maryland College, **A**

Masten, Irving 104 Lincoln Drive, Oakdale, NY 11769, (516) 435-2215, BA 54 Long Island U - Brooklyn Ctr; MA 62 CUNY - Brooklyn Coll; Dept Head/Sp & Hrng, Brentwood Sch, **SLP**

Masterman, Mrs Sandra J 539 Berry Avenue, Hayward, CA 94544, (415) 582-9194, BA 79 Harding Univ; MS 87 Old Dominion Univ

Masters, Eileen T 20 Redwood Road, Newton Center, MA 02159, (617) 969-8374, BS 67 Boston Univ; MA 68 NY Univ; Sp-Lang Path, Needham Pub Sch, **SLP**

Masters, Mrs Janis M 80 Prospect Trail, North Little Rock, AR 72118, (501) 758-8269, MS 88 Univ of AR - Little Rock; 88–Sp-Lang Path, Little Rock Sch Dist

Masters, Dr Joseph J 5723 Arcturus Drive S W, Roanoke, VA 24018, (703) 982-2463, BA 64 SUNY - Center at Buffalo; MA 67 SUNY - Center at Buffalo; PH 70 (Sp Path) SUNY - Center at Buffalo; 73–Chief Audiol&SLP Service, VA Medical Center, **SLP**

Masters, M Gay 310 Taunton Place, Buffalo, NY 14216, (716) 636-3401, BA 76 OH Wesleyan Univ; MA 78 Univ of Cincinnati; 86–Clin Asst Prof, State U NY at Buffalo, **SLP**

Masters, Nancy E 76 Colonial Terrace, Bridgeton, NJ 08302, (609) 451-0345, BS 72 FL St Univ; ME 73 Univ of FL; 83–SLP, Vineland Bd of Educ, **A**

Masters, Susan Roberta Alden Place, P O Box 1051, Millbrook, NY 12545, (914) 431-8800, BS 81 TX Christian Univ; MS 83 Gallaudet Coll; Audiologist, St Francis Hospital, **A**

Masters, Vera E 11809 Goshen Avenue #11, Los Angeles, CA 90049, (213) 474-7216, BA 63 Univ of CA - Los Angeles; MA 61 Univ of CA - Los Angeles; Sp-Path Assoc, Mj D'Asaro & Assoc, **SLP**

Masters-Moore, Christine Aileen 24039 Preakness Drive, Damascus, MD 20872, (301) 490-3359, **SLP**

Masterson, Dr Julie J Dept Of Comm Disorders, Sp & Hrng Center, University, MS 38677, (601) 232-7271, BA 77 Ouachita Baptist Univ; MS 79 Baylor Univ; PH 85 (Sp-Lang Path) Memphis St Univ; 88–Asst Prof, Univ of MS, **SLP ACE**

Mastin, Bonnie Yegge 142 Parkridge Drive, Mason City, IA 50401, (515) 357-6125, BS 80 IA St Univ; MA 83 Univ of Northern IA; SLP, Northern Trais AEA, **SLP**

Mastman, Mrs Ellen Sue 18951 Saratoga Glen Place, Saratoga, CA 95070, (408) 973-1352, BA 71 Univ of Rochester; MA 74 SUNY - Center at Buffalo; Aud, **A**

Mastrandreas, Margaret 125 Peterborough Street, Apartment 25, Boston, MA 02215, (617) 935-5050, BS 84 Boston Univ; MS 85 Boston Univ; **SLP**

Mastri, Stephanie Mirchel 13140 Thornapple Place, Herndon, VA 22071, (301) 593-3797, BS 80 Marywood Coll; MA 82 MI St Univ; Sp-Lang Path, Montgomery Primary Achiev Cen, **SLP**

Mastriano, Barbara P 205 Park Lane, Haddonfield, NJ 08033, (215) 787-7593, BA 66 Temple Univ; MA 68 Temple Univ; Asst Prof, Temple Univ Sp Dept, **SLP**

Mastrocinque, Mrs Meryl 171 Birch Road, Kings Park, NY 11754, (516) 543-5100, BA 80 SUNY - Coll at Cortland; MA 81 Hofstra Univ; Sp-Lang Path, South Huntington OFSD, **SLP**

Mastrocola, Mrs Phyllis A 815 Salem Avenue, Burlington, NJ 08016, (609) 386-0178, BA 61 Adelphi Univ; MS 68 Adelphi Univ; Sp-Lang Path, **SLP**

Mastrogiacomo, Sharon Jean 303 Boston Post Road, Box G-5, Marlboro, MA 01752, (617) 745-9000, BS 83 Univ of NH; MS 85 Emerson Coll; Sp-Lang Path, Shaughnessy-Kaplan Rehab Hosp, **SLP**

Mastroianni, Mary Ann P 1420 Chilton Drive, Silver Spring, MD 20904, **A**

Mastronardi, Mrs Debra Longawa 67 Coe Hill Drive #2, Toronto, ON, Canada M6S 3E2, (416) 769-1929, BS 78 Purdue Univ - West Lafayette; MS 80 Purdue Univ - West Lafayette; 88–Sp-Lang Path, Humber Mem Hosp, **SLP**

Masuda, Ann House Ear Institute, 256 South Lake Street, Los Angeles, CA 90057, (213) 483-4431, BA 85 Univ of CA - Santa Barbara; MS 87 Univ of AZ; 87–Aud, House Ear Institute, **A**

Masuda, Mrs Irene S 1077 Lunalilo Home Road, Honolulu, HI 96825, (808) 737-2321, BS 70 Univ of HI - Manoa; MS 71 Univ of HI - Manoa; Sp-Lang Path, Hi St Dept of Ed, **SLP**

Mata-Pistokache, Mrs Teri 502 Elmwood #205, Austin, TX 78705, (512) 478-2137, MS 83 TX Christian Univ; Assistant Professor/Clin Supv, **SLP**

Matas, Judy A 3040 W Laurelhurst Dr N E, Seattle, WA 98105, (206) 527-3314, BS 78 Univ of WA; MS 79 Univ of WA; Sp/Lang Path, Private Practice, **SLP**

Mate, Cynthia A 389 Old Bedford Road, Concord, MA 01742, (617) 264-4700, BA 74 Rutger's St Univ - Douglas Coll, MA 75 Temple Univ; SLP, Acton Sch Dist, **SLP**

Matejka, Karen A 4970 Galen Court, Lake Oswego, OR 97034, (503) 692-1190, BA 68 Lewis & Clark Coll; MS 76 Portland St Univ; Aud, Private Practice, **A**

Materna, Mary E P O Box 603, Romeo, MI 48065-0603, **SLP**

Mates, Dr Barbara 390 West End Avenue, New York, NY 10024, (212) 873-8866, MA 54 CUNY - Brooklyn Coll; MA 63 Columbia Univ Sch of Gen St; PH 65 (Neuropsychology) Columbia Univ Sch of Gen St; 77–Dir, Amer Diag Lrng & Rdng Cen, **SLP**

Matesich, Charlene 611 North Beatty Street, Pittsburgh, PA 15206, (412) 648-6000, BS 72 Univ of Pittsburgh - Pittsburgh; MS 74 Univ of Pittsburgh - Pittsburgh; Audiologist, Montefiore Hospital, **A**

Matesich, Martha Anne 1565 North 21st Street, Newark, OH 43055, (614) 454-5862, BS 78 Marquette Univ; MS 83 Univ of WI - Milwaukee; Sp-Lang Path, Good Samaritan Med Cen, **SLP**

Matheny, Mrs Mary Palmer 61-A Street, Hillcrest Apartment, Salt Lake City, UT 84103, (801) 322-2324, BS 84 Brigham Young Univ; MA 85 Brigham Young Univ; SLP, Jordons School Dstr, **SLP**

Matheny, Nancy 25 Fullerton Road, New Castle, PA 16102, (412) 458-6700, BS 70 Kent St Univ; MA 75 Kent St Univ; SLP, Midwn Intermediate Unit 4, **SLP**

Matheny, Dr Patricia A 11260 Chalon Road, Los Angeles, CA 90049, (213) 476-1317, BS 52 Univ of Tulsa; MA 54 Univ of Tulsa; PH 71 Univ of Southern CA; Research Consult, Private Practice, **SLP A**

Mather, Diann P O Box 14965, Lenexa, KS 66215, (913) 780-2811, BS 79 Univ of KS; MS 80 Central MO St Univ; Sp-Lang Path, Private Contractor, **SLP**

Mather, Jennifer Leigh 3 Schilke Drive, Westerly, RI 02891, (203) 449-2568, MA 86 Univ of MD - College Park; **A**

Mather, Ronnie K 2841 North Forgeus, Tucson, AZ 85716, (602) 881-8740, BA 73 OH St Univ; MS 74 Columbia Univ Teachers Coll; Aud, Self Employed, **A**

Mather, Mrs Susan O 832 East Georgiana, Port Angeles, WA 98362, MS 66 Vanderbilt Univ; MA 74 Pacific Univ; **A**

Matherne, Roberta T 105 Lawnes Circle, Williamsburg, VA 23185, (804) 966-2775, BA 72 Mary Washington Coll; ME 73 Univ of VA - Charlottesville; Sp-Lang Path, New Kent County Public Schools, **SLP**

Mathers, Jolayne R RFD1 Box 1450, Farmington, ME 04938, (207) 685-3336, Maranacook School District, **SLP**

Mathers, Marilyn Sue 39 W 441 Homeward Hill Dr, St Charles, IL 60175, (312) 888-5285, BS 68 IL St Univ - Normal; MA 83 Northern IL Univ - De Kalb; Sp-Lang Path, School District U-46, **SLP**

Mathers, Dr Pamela L 2160 Fairway Drive, Birmingham, MI 48009, (313) 689-6000, BA 72 MI St Univ; MA 73 MI St Univ; PH 82 (NS) Wayne St Univ; SLP, Troy Sch Dist, **SLP**

Mathers-Schmidt, Barbara A 7003 54th Avenue N E, Seattle, WA 98115, (206) 223-6618, BA 72 Lewis & Clark Coll; MS 78 Portland St Univ; PH 87 (Sp Path) Univ of WA; 88–Sp-Lang Path, Virginia Mason Med Ctr, **SLP**

Matheson, Barbara Gail 9427 Longlake, Wichita, KS 67207, (316) 684-2838, BS 78 East Stroudsburg Univ of PA; MA 82 Wichita St Univ; MA 86 Wichita St Univ; Aud, Institute of Logopedics, **SLP A**

Matheson, Mrs Joan 44-016 Aina Moi Place, Kaneohe, HI 96744, (808) 254-3834, BA 71 Auburn Univ - Auburn; MS 73 Southern Methodist Univ; **A**

Matheson, Linda A 4322 North Parkway Avenue, Scottsdale, AZ 85251, **SLP**

Mathew, Karen F 2743 N E 16th Avenue, Portland, OR 97212, (503) 280-5240, BS 77 Portland St Univ; MS 81 Portland St Univ; Sp-Lang Path, Portland Public Schools, **SLP**

Mathews, Barbara Lucy Route 3 Lot 14 Betty Drive, Arnaudville, LA 70512, (318) 394-6162, BA 80 LA Tech Univ; MS 84 Univ of Southwestern LA; **SLP**

Mathews, Mrs Bertha B 2007 Greenland Drive, Murfreesboro, TN 37130, (615) 893-1151, OB 34 Univ of IA; BS 54 Wayne St Univ; ME 59 Wayne St Univ; **SLP LM**

Mathews, Burma J 1470 South 7th, Kankakee, IL 60901, (815) 933-0720, BA 74 Mundelein Coll; MS 75 Marquette Univ; Coord of Sp-Lang Path, Kankakee Sch Dist #111, **SLP**

Mathews, Mrs Cheri Rene 9375 Pagoda Way, Reno, NV 89506, BA 80 Northwest Nazarene Coll; MS 82 ID St Univ; SLP, Washoe County School District, **SLP**

Mathews, Gwendolyn Shereese 2413 Townhouse Lane, Kalamazoo, MI 49001, (616) 349-8925, MA 85 Western MI Univ

Mathews, Lynne L 18873 Warwick Drive, Birmingham, MI 48009, **SLP**

Mathews, Pamela J M 21 Turkey Lane, Cold Spring Harbor, NY 11724, (516) 367-3718, BA 64 Univ of London - England; MA 79 Hofstra Univ; Sp/Lang Path, Private Practice, **SLP ACE**

Mathews-Ayres, Carol 323 Stadium Drive South, Monmouth, OR 97361, BS 74 Western OR St Coll; MS 76 Western OR St Coll; Sp-Lang Path, Salem Hosp, **SLP**

Mathewson, David Richard 2405 Rogers Street, Milwaukee, WI 53215, (414) 567-1133, MS 81 Univ of WI - Madison; Sp-Lang Path, Somed Inc, **SLP**

Mathewson, Peggy A 777 Monterey Street, Santa Cruz, CA 95060, (408) 426-6911, BA 73 Univ of AZ; MS 82 Univ of AZ; Sp-Lang Path, Speech Plus, **SLP**

Mathianas, Mrs Karen Obringer B-9 Market Square, 1001 Market Street, Beaver, PA 15009, (412) 774-5632, BS 80 CA Univ of PA; ME 81 CA Univ of PA; Sp-Lang Path, Crossroads Speech Hrng Inc, **SLP**

Mathias, Mrs Daisy E 19 Fomer Road, South Hampton, MA 01073, (413) 527-9485, BA 62 Wells Coll; MS 73 McGill Univ - Quebec; Sp-Lang Path, Massachusetts Dept of Pub Hlth, **SLP**

Mathias, Mrs Dana 2735 Black Diamond Terrace, Colorado Springs, CO 80918, (303) 636-5186, BS 74 CO St Univ; MS 75 CO St Univ; Sch Aud, Co Sch for the Deaf & Blind, **A**

Mathias, Mrs Deborah Ann 316 Bishop Court, Westminster, MD 21157, BA 82 Loyola Coll; MS 83 Loyola Coll; 88–Sp-Lang Path, MCDS, **SLP**

Mathias, Gerald A Route 1 Box 86K, Sunrise Summit, Romney, WV 26757, (304) 822-3050, BS 61 WV Univ; MS 65 WV Univ; OM 78 WV Univ; Dir/Spec Ed, Hampshire Co Bd of Ed, **SLP**

Mathias, Mrs Karen Peterson P O Box 387, Wardensville, WV 26851, (304) 874-3551, BS 77 Indiana Univ of PA; MS 83 Indiana Univ of PA; Sp-Lang Path, Hardy Co Bd of Educ, **SLP**

Mathiasen, Antoinette Tucker 10614 East Maplewood Drive, Englewood, CO 80111, (303) 694-6835, MS 84 Rutgers St Univ -N Brunswick; 88, Private Practice, **SLP**

Mathieu, Ardie E 6811 North Bryant, Brooklyn Center, MN 55430, (612) 427-2200, BA 80 Univ of MN - Minneap-St Paul; MA 81 Univ of MN - Minneap-St Paul; Sp-Lang Path, Methodist Hosp, **SLP**

Mathieu, Lawrence H Lawrence Mathieu Associates, 408 West Church Street, Elmira, NY 14901, (607) 734-3329, BA 58 West Liberty St Coll; MA 69 WV Univ; 76–Aud, Lawrence Mathieu Assoc, **A**

Mathieu, Lori Elizabeth 3 Eagle Court, Goshen, NY 10924, (201) 688-0100, BA 82 SUNY - Coll at Plattsburgh; MS 84 Syracuse Univ; **A**

Mathis, Brian Roger 4111 2nd Street, Riverside, CA 92501-2311, (714) 788-7135, MS 86 Univ of Redlands; **SLP**

Mathis, Carla L 452 East 35th Street, Paterson, NJ 07504, (212) 523-3127, BA 86 SC St Coll; MS 88 Columbia Univ Teachers Coll

Mathis, Mrs Kathy Chandler Mathis Therapy Associates, 317 8th Street, Henderson, KY 42420, (502) 827-4857, BA 75 Brescia Coll; MS 81 Western KY Univ; Sp-Lang Path, Private Practice, **SLP**

Mathrani, Jolanda W 8704 Liberty Lane, Potomac, MD 20854, BS 75 Univ of WI - Milwaukee; MA 79 Wayne St Univ; **SLP**

Mathy-Laikko, Pamela 15260 Cuming St, Omaha, NE 68154, (402) 559-5557, BA 75 Univ of MA - Amherst; MA 78 WA St Univ; Sp-Lang Path, Meyers Child Rehab Inst, **SLP**

Matis, Dr Edward Eugene Route 1 Box 228, Natchitoches, LA 71457, (318) 352-8930, BS 51 Lock Haven St Coll; OM 52 Univ of AL- Tuscaloosa; PH 68 (Educational Psychology) Univ of AL- Tuscaloosa; Retired, **SLP A LM**

Matis, Mary J Route 1 Box 228, Natchitoches, LA 71457, (318) 352-1270, OB 43; MS 49 Univ of MI - Ann Arbor; Sp-Lang Path, Private Practice, **SLP LM**

Matkin, Dr Noel D University Of Arizona, Speech Bldg, Room 103, Tucson, AZ 85721, (602) 621-5599, BA 54 Wichita St Univ; MA 59 Northwestern Univ; PH 65 (NS) Northwestern Univ; Prof Aud, U of AZ, **A F ACE**

Matkin, Mrs Susan Stewart 3608 Jason Avenue, Pocatello, ID 83204, (208) 226-2391, BS 80 Northern AZ Univ; MS 82 ID St Univ; SLP, American Falls School District, **SLP**

Matlock, Dr Mildred P 1941 Orleans #611, Detroit, MI 48207, (313) 745-9753, BS 68 Wayne St Univ; ME 72 Wayne St Univ; PH 76 (Sp-Lang Path) Wayne St Univ; Asst Admin Clin Svcs, Rahab I-Detroit, **SLP**

Matlock, Renee H 20916 Corinth Road, Olympia Fields, IL 60461, (312) 799-7520, BS 73 Southern IL Univ -Carbondale; MA 75 Northern IL Univ - De Kalb; 80-Dir/Owner, Cen for Commun Dis Ltd, **SLP ACE**

Matolyak, Joye E 308 Sherwood Drive, Johnstown, PA 15905, (814) 472-9821, BS 76 Indiana Univ of PA; MS 81 Indiana Univ of PA; Sp-Lang Path, Intermediate Unit 08, **SLP**

Matonak, Kathy Elaine 3550 California Street #3, San Francisco, CA 94118, (415) 922-6985, BS 77 PA St Univ - Univ Park; MS 82 San Francisco St Univ; 82–Aud, Agnews Developmental Ctr, **A ACE**

Matos, Karen Ann 5 Lacava Lane, Wethersfield, CT 06109, (203) 524-5732, BA 85 Elms Coll; MS 86 Adelphi Univ; 87–Sp-Lang Path, Glastonbury PS, **SLP**

Matricardi, Mrs Natalie L 168 Southwood Drive, Buffalo, NY 14223, BS 73 SUNY - Coll at Geneseo; MS 77 SUNY - Coll at Buffalo; Sp-Lang Path, Kenmore-Town of Tonawanda Sch, **SLP**

Matrow, Mrs Elizabeth 146 Munn Road, Monson, MA 01057, (413) 967-6236, BA 78 Elms Coll; MS 82 Worcester St Coll; 86–Sp-Lang Path, Ware PS, **SLP**

Matrozzo, Mrs April Joy 3547 Dunedin Drive, Apartment #202, Chesapeake, VA 23321, (804) 487-2559, BS 85 James Madison Univ; MS 87 James Madison Univ; 87–Sp-Lang Path, Chesapeake PS, **SLP**

Matsko, Thomas A Moss Rehabilitation Hospital, 12th Street & Tabor Road, Philadelphia, PA 19141, (215) 456-9292, BS 64 CA Univ of PA; MS 66 PA St Univ - Univ Park; 70–Dir/Cen for Commun Dis, Moss Rehab Hosp, **SLP**

Matson, Denise Kay P O Box 773321, Steamboat Springs, CO 80477, (303) 879-7550, BS 80 Portland St Univ; MA 83 OH Univ - Athens; Sp-Lang Path, Steamboat Springs Schl Dstr, **SLP**

Matson, Mrs Shari S Rural Route 1 Box 92, Gideon, MO 63848, (314) 448-5326, MS 79 Eastern IL Univ; Sp-Lang Path, Portageville School District, **SLP**

Matsuda, Dr Maryon M 5151 State University Dr, Los Angeles, CA 90032, PH 81 (NS) PA St Univ - Univ Park; Assoc Prof, **SLP**

Matsui, Lisa 15410 S E 9th Street, Bellevue, WA 98007, MS; 86–Sp-Lang Path, Highline Sch Dist, **SLP**

Matsumoto, Ann S T 388 Kailva Road, Kailua, HI 96734, (808) 735-1796, BS 76 Univ of HI - Manoa; MS 78 Univ of HI - Manoa; SLP, Dept of Ed, **SLP**

Matsumoto, Dale T 94-428 Hokulewa Place, Mililani Town, HI 96789, (808) 623-8213, BS 83 Univ of HI - Manoa; MS 86 Univ of HI - Manoa

Matsumoto, Mrs Haunani K P O Box 17082, Honolulu, HI 96817, (808) 623-4005, MS 86 Univ of HI - Manoa; **SLP**

Matsumoto, Judy Ann 6484 Brevard Street, St Augustine, FL 32084, (904) 471-8484, MS 83 Washington Univ; 86–Aud, Flagler Coll, **A**

Matsumoto, Mrs Lillian S 8347 Elsmore Drive, South San Gabriel, CA 91770, (818) 288-9784, BA 78 CA St Univ - Los Angeles; MA 81 CA St Univ - Los Angeles; Sp/Lang Path, Private Practice, **SLP**

Matsunaga, Faye A T 45-310 Puali Street, Kaneohe, HI 96744, **A**

Matsusaka, Eileen Kiyomi 6801 Par Lane #811, Wichita, KS 67212-3333, (816) 234-3677, MA 83 Univ of KS; Aud, Chldns Mercy Hosp, **A**

Matsuwaki, Mrs Beverly A 95-199 Kaopua Loop, Mililani Town, HI 96789, (808) 622-2269, BA 66 Univ of HI - Manoa; MS 69 Univ of HI - Manoa; Sp-Lang Path, Hi Dept of Ed, **SLP**

Matt, David W 338 Key West Drive, Charlottesville, VA 22901-8426, (804) 295-3720, BS 74 SUNY - Coll at Brockport; ME 78 Univ of VA - Charlottesville; Sp-Lang Path, Charlottesville VA Pub Sch, **SLP**

Matt, Mrs Doris E 5445 Jackson Drive #327, Mounds View, MN 55112, (612) 780-1556, **SLP**

Mattai, Susan Lentz 3107 Lawn Avenue, Tampa, FL 33611, (813) 839-5144, MS 83 Univ of WI - Madison; Sp-Lang Path, InSpeech Inc, **SLP**

Mattas, Maureen C 4852 Lowell Avenue, Lincoln, NE 68506, (402) 474-4311, BA 76 Univ of NE - Lincoln; MA 78 Univ of NE - Lincoln; SLP/Classroom Teach, Lincoln Public Schools, **SLP**

Matteo, Jo-Anne B 365 Mather Street, Unit 34, Hamden, CT 06514, (203) 966-9575, BA 79 Southern CT St Univ; MS 80 Adelphi Univ; OM 83 Southern CT St Univ; 84–Sp-Lang Path, New Canaan Bd of Ed, **SLP**

Matter, Dr Linda S RR 1 Box 61 Birchwood, Fergus Falls, MN 56537, (218) 739-2807, BA 65 Univ of IA; MA 66 Univ of IA; PH 80 (Sp-Lang Path) Univ of IA; SLP, Fergus Falls Area Spec Ed Coop, **SLP**

Mattern, Ann Louise 582 Graymont Drive, Santa Rosa, CA 95405, (707) 542-2771, BA 80 San Francisco St Univ; MS 82 San Francisco St Univ; Sp-Lang Path, Brookwood Hospital, **SLP**

Mattern, Patricia C EFMD AUDIO LARMC, Box 61, APO New York, NY 09180-3460, MS 81 Univ of AL- Tuscaloosa; Aud, 2nd Gen Army Med Hosp, **A ACE**

Mattes, Dr Lawrence J 3917 Marvin Street, P O Box 6044, Oceanside, CA 92056, (619) 758-9593, BA 73 Univ of CA - Santa Barbara; MA 76 Univ of CA - Santa Barbara; ED 82 (NS) Univ of San Diego; Sp/Lang Path, Oceanside USD, **SLP**

Mattes, Nancy Ann 6840 Edgewood Road, Palos Heights, IL 60463, (312) 361-3984, BA 80 Saint Xavier Coll; MA 81 Northern IL Univ - De Kalb; Sp-Lang Path, Little Co of Mary Hosp, **SLP**

Matteson, Susan Lori 14321 Northeast 30th St, Apartment B, Vancouver, WA 98682-8179, (206) 254-4485, BA 82 Eastern WA Univ; MS 83 Eastern WA Univ; 84–Sp-Lang Path, Evergreen Sch Dist, **SLP**

Mattheis, Mrs Susan A 92 East Lynn Street #102, Seattle, WA 98102, (206) 324-5703, BA 86 Univ of CA - Santa Barbara; MA 87 Univ of the Pacific; 87–Sp-Lang Path, InSpeech Inc

Matthes, Dr Elisa Fuchs 11 Charred Oak Lane, East Windsor, NJ 08520, (609) 924-2809, BS 66 Cornell Univ; MA 71 Columbia Univ Teachers Coll; PH 81 (NS) Columbia Univ Teachers Coll; Sp-Lang Path, Private Practice, **SLP**

Matthes, Mrs Paula K 19 Crystal Springs #14, San Mateo, CA 94401, (415) 348-0739, BS 73 Southwest TX St Univ; ME 75 Southwest TX St Univ; Sp-Lang Path, San Mateo City Schs, **SLP**

Matthes, Dr Richard W VA Administration Med Center, 800 Poly Place, Aud & Sp Service (126), Brooklyn, NY 11209, (718) 836-6600, BA 66 Rutgers St Univ -N Brunswick; MA 70 Montclair St Coll; ED 80 (NS) Columbia Univ Teachers Coll; Aud/SLP, VA Med Cen Brooklyn NY, **A**

Matthews, Mrs Ann 3508 Arden Circle, Raleigh, NC 27612, (214) 542-9306, BS 68 Univ of TN - Knoxville; MS 74 Southern Methodist Univ; Sp/Lang Path, **SLP**

Matthews, Mrs Bonnie G 300 Winter Street, Walpole, MA 02081, (617) 668-6209, BS 66 Indiana Univ of PA; MA 68 Western MI Univ; **SLP**

Matthews, Cheryl L T 2503 Nature Bend Lane, Carrollton, TX 75006, (214) 688-0666, **SLP**

Matthews, Dr Claire 478 Clemens, St Louis, MO 63122, (314) 894-4672, BA 69 Univ of KS; MA 78 Univ of KS; PH 80 (NS) Univ of KS; Asst Prof, St Louis U, **SLP ACE**

Matthews, Cynthia A 6725 Whaley Drive, Boulder, CO 80303, (303) 492-5375, BS 75 Univ of NE - Lincoln; MA 76 Univ of NE - Lincoln; Cl Superv In Aud, U of CO-Dept Commun Dis, **A**

Matthews, Cynthia B 5501 Greenbrier, Dallas, TX 75209, (214) 826-9852, BS 77 Southern Methodist Univ; MS 78 Southern Methodist Univ; OM 83 Univ of Dallas; Sp/Lang Path, Baylor Inst for Rehab, **SLP**

Matthews, Debbie S Star Route Box 50-D, South Pittsburg, TN 37380, (615) 942-3434, BS 78 Middle TN St Univ; OM 80 Auburn Univ - Auburn; Sp/Lang Path, Warren Co Sch Syst, **SLP**

Matthews, Hannah 825 Old Mill Road, Pittsburgh, PA 15238, (412) 963-8046, BA 39 OH St Univ; MA 42 OH St Univ; U of Pittsburgh, **SLP LM**

Matthews, Jack 825 Old Mill Road, Pittsburgh, PA 15238, (412) 624-6570, BA 38 Heidelberg Coll; MA 40 OH Univ - Athens; PH 46 (NS) OH St Univ; Prof of Commun, U of Pitts, **SLP F H LM**

Matthews, Mrs Judith L 13322 Malena Drive, Santa Ana, CA 92705, (714) 731-2844, BA 71 CA St Univ - Long Beach; MA 74 CA St Univ - Long Beach; Aud, Dr Wilbur Suesberry, **A**

Matthews, Karen Bettina P O Box 5372, Cary, NC 27511, (919) 467-7380, BA 80 Univ of NC - Chapel Hill; ME 82 Univ of NC - Greensboro; Aud, Wake Co Pub Sch/Cary ENT Cl, **A**

Matthews, Kathleen Marie 319 East Madison Suite 2C, Springfield, IL 62701, (217) 522-6462, BS 84 IL St Univ - Normal; MS 85 IL St Univ - Normal; 85–Aud, Richard Bass MD SC, **A**

Matthews, Kathleen McGinnis 1542-B Maple Drive, Blytheville AFB, AR 72315, (501) 532-8122, BA 79 Ouachita Baptist Univ; MS 84 Univ of AR - Fayetteville; **SLP**

Matthews, Leslie Kandee 2628 Eagle Avenue, Alameda, CA 94501, BS 76 Univ of MA - Amherst; MA 78 Univ of CO - Boulder; Sp-Lang Path, Faltz Associates Inc, **SLP**

Matthews, Linda Jenkins Rd Box 38 Howe Road, Lake Lucerne, NY 12846, (518) 696-5203, BS 82 CO St Univ; MS 84 Ithaca Coll; 86–Sp-Lang Path, Queensburg Sch Dist, **SLP**

Matthews, Lois Jean 21 Rivers Point Row #8-F, Charleston, SC 29412, (803) 792-3004, BA 81 Univ of Miami; MS 84 Purdue Univ - West Lafayette; Instuctor of Aud, Medical U of Sc, **A**

Matthews, Lynn Hale 2814-B Partridge Drive, Albany, GA 31707, (912) 759-6806, BS 76 Ball St Univ; ME 81 GA St Univ; OM 83 GA St Univ; Sp/Lang Path, Lee Co Bd of Ed, **SLP**

Matthews, Mary J K 7022 Copperwood Way, Columbia, MD 21046, (301) 381-5659, BS 77 James Madison Univ; MA 80 George Washington Univ; Sp-Lang Path, Delaware Dept of Public Health, **SLP**

Matthews, Mrs Nancy Shubella P O Box 88, Calhan, CO 80808, (719) 347-2392, BA 70 Coll of Saint Francis; MA 71 Univ of IL - Urbana; Sp-Lang Path, Sch Dist, **SLP ACE**

Matthews, Mrs Shellie B 113 Tower Drive, Vicksburg, MS 39180, (601) 636-4371, BA 73 Univ of MS; MA 80 Univ of MS; Sp-Lang Path, Vicksburg Warren Schs, **SLP**

Matthey, Mrs Doris S 120 West Ridgewood Avenue, Ridgewood, NJ 07450, (201) 445-9381, BA 67 Paterson St Coll; MA 69 Paterson St Coll; Sp-Lang Path, Bergen Co Spec Serv Sch Dist, **SLP ACE**

Matthias, Karen Killian 54 Weaver Avenue, Harrisonburg, VA 22801, (703) 337-2535, BS 77 James Madison Univ; MS 81 James Madison Univ; Sp-Lang Path, The Augusta County Schools, **SLP**

Matthies, Dr Melanie L 901 South 6th Street, Champaign, IL 61820, (217) 244-2558, BA 76 SUNY - Center at Buffalo; MS 78 Purdue Univ - West Lafayette; PH 84 (Hrng Science) Univ of IL - Urbana; Visiting Research Asst Prof, Univ of Illinois, **A**

Matthiesen, Mrs Linda L 1840 South 138th Street, Omaha, NE 68144, (402) 895-8320, BA 69 Univ of MI - Ann Arbor; MA 72 Eastern MI Univ; SLP, Millard Pub Sch, **SLP**

Mattie, Mrs Linda Larosa 78 East Mountain Drive, Southington, CT 06489, Sp-Lang Path, Town of West Hartford, **SLP**

Mattimoe, Mrs Susan Gleespen 8539 Alderwood Court, Jacksonville, FL 32244, (904) 772-0879, BS 82 Bowling Green St Univ; MA 83 Bowling Green St Univ; Sp-Lang Path, **SLP**

Mattingly, Marilyn T 12809 Dulaney Valley Road, Glen Arm, MD 21057, (301) 465-0110, BA 69 Univ of WI - Madison; MS 75 Loyola Coll; Sp-Lang Path, Howard Co Pub Sch, **SLP**

Mattingly, Dr Susan C 160 Timber Ridge Drive, Nashville, TN 37217, (615) 832-8955, BA 68 Towson St Univ; MA 69 OH St Univ; PH 71 (Speech & Hearing Science) OH St Univ; 84–Sp-Lang Path, Private Practice, **SLP A**

Mattise, Mary Ellen 1038 JFK Blvd #3, Endwell, NY 13760, (607) 798-7117, BS 82 PA St Univ - Univ Park; MS 86 Ithaca Coll; SLP, Hndcpd Childrens Assoc, **SLP**

Mattison, Kelly Mack Route 1 Box 39-A, Ridgeland, WI 54763, (715) 234-1515, MS 84 Univ of WI - Eau Claire; BS 83 Univ of WI - Stevens Point; 84–Sp-Lang Path, Lakeview Med Ctr, **SLP**

Mattison, Mindy Susan 4965 Maynard Street, San Diego, CA 92122, (619) 457-3588, 84–Sp-Lang Path, Private Practice, **SLP**

Mattison, Roger W 3770 Janes Road, Arcata, CA 95521, BA 70 Humboldt St Univ; MA 75 Humboldt St Univ; MS 76 Phillips Univ; Aud, Private Practice, **A**

Mattock, Regis A Box 355, Mars, PA 16046, (412) 283-1010, BS 75 Edinboro Univ of PA; ME 78 Clarion Univ of PA; 87–Supvr Sp-Lang Path, Easter Seal Society of Butler, **SLP ACE**

Mattox, Helen M 4144 Tall Tree Drive, Orlando, FL 32810, BS; **LM**

Mattox, Katrina Ann Route 2 Box 103-C, Boone, NC 28607, (704) 264-7190, **SLP**

Mattson, Laurinda R 2205 Bridlewood Drive, Rancho Cordova, CA 95670, (916) 638-8244, MA 84 CA St Univ - Sacramento; Audiologist, Placer Speech & Hearing Serv

Mattson, Mrs Mary Mueller East 15106 26th, Veradale, WA 99037, (509) 245-3211, BA 84 WA St Univ; MS 85 Eastern WA Univ; **SLP**

Mattson, Mrs Patty J 15750 West 137th Street, Olathe, KS 66062, (913) 780-4127, BS 74 AZ St Univ; MS 80 AZ St Univ; Sp-Lang Path, Tempe Elem Dist #3, **SLP**

Matty, Betty Jean 2400 Robbins Station Road, North Huntingdon, PA 15642, (412) 379-4183, OB 82 CA Univ of PA; BS 61 CA Univ of PA; MS 87 Duquesne Univ; Sp-Lang Path, Allegheny Inter Ut, **SLP**

Matuga, Patricia 115 Warwick Drive, Monaca, PA 15061, (412) 775-6602, BA 86 Duquesne Univ; MA 88 OH Univ - Athens; Aud, Bell Froman Orsini & Associates

Matulle, Terry V 115 South Franklin Street, Janesville, WI 53545, (608) 752-3529, BS 79 Univ of WI - Oshkosh; MS 81 Univ of WI - Oshkosh; Pres, Hrng Care Assoc Inc, **A**

Matuszewski, Mrs Domencia 219 Grace Street, Old Forge, PA 18518, BS 77 Marywood Coll; MS 81 Bloomsburg Univ of PA; Sp-Lang Path, Luzerne Inter Unit #18, **SLP**

Matyk, Mrs Karen A 3879 South Biscay Street, Aurora, CO 80013, (303) 693-4242, BS 65 CO St Univ; MA 77 CA St Univ - Northridge; Special Education Teacher, Cherry Creek Schools, **SLP**

Matz, Dr Rita B 82-34 Grenfell Street, Kew Gardens, NY 11415, (212) 846-6033, BA 65 CUNY - Queens Coll; MS 69 CUNY - Queens Coll; ED 82 (NS) Columbia Univ Teachers Coll; Sp/Lang Path, Private Practice, **SLP**

Matz, Susan C 2128 Georgetown Boulevard, Ann Arbor, MI 48105, (313) 439-1525, OB 76 Univ of Toledo; MA 78 Eastern MI Univ; SLP, Milan Area Schs, **SLP**

Matzinger, Darcy 441-G Tradewinds Drive, Fayetteville, NC 28304, (919) 485-5145, BS 84 Univ of Cincinnati; MA 85 Northeast MO St Univ; **SLP**

Mauceri, Patricia Murphy 50 Harrison Avenue, Swampscott, MA 01907, (617) 979-7126, BA 74 Univ of MA - Amherst; MS 77 Boston Univ; 87–Sp-Lang Path/Aud, New England Mem Hosp, **A**

Mauch, Mrs Janice 7805 Kugler Mill, Cincinnati, OH 45243, (513) 791-0016, BS 68 CO St Univ; MS 73 CO St Univ; Sp-Lang Path, Madeira City Schools, **SLP**

Mauer, Joanna Marie 2710 Hemlock Avenue, Alexandria, VA 22305, (703) 836-8508, BA 78 Washington & Jefferson Coll; MS 85 Univ of VT; **SLP**

Mauk, Mrs Cornelia L 715 East Boundary, Perrysburg, OH 43551, (419) 352-7588, BS 51 Northwestern Univ; MA 71 Bowling Green St Univ; Superv Sp/Lang/Hrng Serv, Bowling Gr St U Chldrn Cen, **SLP**

Maul, Mrs Rosalie W 142 Melrose Court, Vacaville, CA 95687, (707) 446-1526, BS 72 IL St Univ - Normal; MS 82 Southern IL Univ-Edwardsvill; Sp-Lang Path, Yolo Co Schools, **SLP**

Maule, Bettyjo 13627 N E 14th Street #18-1, Bellevue, WA 98005, (206) 746-6207, BS 84 PA St Univ - Univ Park; MS 86 Univ of WA

Maulsby, Emily Potts 7508 La Madera Road N E, Albuquerque, NM 87109, (505) 821-7337, BS 72 Univ of TN - Knoxville; MS 74 Memphis St Univ; **A**

Maultra, Alisa L 7053 Hampstead Lane, Indianapolis, IN 46256, (317) 849-3913, BA 82 IN Univ - Bloomington; MA 84 IN Univ - Bloomington; 87–Aud, Comm Hosp Indianapolis, **A**

Maulucci, Fred V Mountain View Drive, Pleasant Valley, NY 12569, (914) 257-2600, BS 53 SUNY - Coll at Oswego; ME 57 PA St Univ - Univ Park; Assoc Dean La & S, SUNY-New Paltz, **SLP**

Maund, Mrs Christie Young 3035 Pine Needle Road, Augusta, GA 30909-3047, (404) 737-7310, BS 78 Univ of GA; MA 79 Univ of TN - Knoxville; **SLP**

Maund, Gay 1601 Camino DE Villas, Burbank, CA 91501, (213) 894-7135, BA 67 Loyola Marymount Univ; MA 69 Univ of Southern CA; Aud, Veterans Administration, **A**

Mauner, Gail Ann 3212 Sawtelle Boulevard, Apartment 2, Los Angeles, CA 90066, (213) 397-3264, BA 77 Pomona Coll; MA 86 CA St Univ - Los Angeles; **SLP**

Mauney, Mrs Mardi J 24 Northview Avenue, Upper Montclair, NJ 07043, (201) 783-1365, BA 66 Duke Univ; MA 77 Univ of RI; Aud, Private Practice, **A**

Maupin, Dianne C 100-28th Street S W, Minot, ND 58701, (701) 857-3030, BS 71 Minot St Univ; MS 72 Minot St Univ; 85–Asst Prof, Minot State Univ, **SLP**

Maurer, Anne Berg P O Box 1084, Joshua Tree, CA 92252, (619) 365-3223, MA 68 MI St Univ; Sp-Lang Path, Morongo USD, **SLP**

Maurer, Charlo Jean 18 Laurel Street, Cambridge, MA 02139, (617) 267-7050, BA 75 Univ of WI - Madison; ME 79 Boston Univ; MS 87 Emerson Coll; 87–Sp-Lang Path, Boston PS

Maurer, Dr James F Speech & Hearing Sciences, Portland State University, Box 751, Portland, OR 97207, (503) 229-3527, MA 61; PH 68 (NS) Univ of OR; 68–Prof, Portland State Univ, **SLP A F**

Maurer, Joan E 42 Williams Avenue, Hillcrest, NY 10977, (914) 634-4648, BS 74 Nazareth Coll of Rochester; MS 78 Coll of Saint Rose; Sp/Lang Path, Rockland Co Cen/Phys Hndcpd, **SLP**

Mauro, Darla M Route 1 Box 114-2, Swanton, MD 21561, (304) 446-5141, BS 76 Clarion Univ of PA; ME 77 Clarion Univ of PA; Sp-Lang Path, Mineral Co Bd of Ed, **SLP**

Maury, Cynthia Ann 107 Harlan Street, Manchester, CT 06040, (203) 236-1919, BA 80 Univ of CA - Santa Barbara; MS 82 Boston Univ; Sp/Lang Path, Es Cen Conn, **SLP**

Maust, Mrs H Madelein 2312 South Valley Road, Berwyn, PA 19312, (215) 647-6140, BS 73 PA St Univ - Univ Park; MA 78 West Chester Univ of PA; Sp/Lang Path/Cen Lead, De Co Iu, **SLP**

Mautner, Mrs Diane S 23330 Gonzales Drive, Woodland Hills, CA 91367, (818) 997-2357, BA 62 Univ of CA - Los Angeles; MA 80 CA St Univ - Northridge; Diagnostic Examiner, Los Angeles USD, **SLP**

Mauzy, Mrs Anne 5000 Crestway Drive, Austin, TX 78731, (512) 459-1617, BA 48 Univ of TX - Austin; ME 54 Univ of Houston - Univ Park; **A**

Mawdsley, Brenda 2819 Oriole, Wichita, KS 67204-5342, (316) 689-3240, BA 71 Wichita St Univ; MA 72 Wichita St Univ; Inst Commun Dis & Sciences, Wichita St U, **SLP**

Mawhiney, Allan L Medfield State Hospital, 45 Hospital Road, Rehab Department D-1, Medfield, MA 02052, (617) 359-7312, BA 76 Hofstra Univ; MA 78 Hofstra Univ; 88–Dir-Speech & Hearing Dept, Medfield State Hosp, **SLP**

Mawhinney, Dr Clara K 2724 West Reservoir Blvd, Peoria, IL 61614, (309) 682-0936, BA 19 Univ of MN - Minneap-St Paul; MA 30 Univ of WI - Madison; PH 37 (NS); **SLP LM**

Mawhinney, Mrs Linda M 612 Dewsbury Court, Bel Air, MD 21014, (301) 836-9123, BS 73 Edinboro Univ of PA; MS 77 Loyola Coll; Sp/Lang Path, Harford Co Bd of Educ, **SLP**

Max, Mrs Becky Sue P O Box 297, Wilber, NE 68465, (402) 821-3164, BA 80 Univ of NE - Lincoln; MA 82 Univ of KS; 88–Sp/Lang Path, Milford PS, **SLP**

Max, Mrs Phyllis R 14 Neylon Court, Rockville Centre, NY 11570, (516) 766-8984, BA 55 Bryn Mawr Coll; MS 69 Adelphi Univ; Sp-Lang Path, **SLP**

Maxam, Patricia D 6254 East Owens Avenue, Las Vegas, NV 89110-1844, (904) 678-3615, **SLP**

Maxfield, Kathrine M 2409 Cypress Drive, Lewisville, TX 75067-6523, (214) 393-0576, BS 77 Southwest TX St Univ; ME 78 Southwest TX St Univ; Doc Stud/Tchng Asst, U of TX at Dallas/Callier Cen, **SLP**

Maxon, Dr Antonia Brancia 131 Chaffeeville Road, Mansfield Center, CT 06250, (203) 486-2628, BA 69 CUNY - Queens Coll; MA 71 CUNY - Queens Coll; PH 77 (Hrng Science) CUNY - Grad Sch & Univ Cntr; Assoc Prof, Univ of Conn, **A**

Maxon, Carleen O P O Box 455, North Chatham, MA 02650, (617) 945-1797, BA 72 Univ of NM; MS 73 Univ of NM; **SLP**

Maxsimic, Mrs Katherine 161 Clinton Street, Portland, ME 04103, (207) 774-3626, BA 73 Univ of ME - Orono; MA 79 Univ of OR; SLP, S Portland Sch Dept, **SLP**

Maxwell, Mrs Barbara Hafner 13305-A Saddlebrook Trace, Austin, TX 78729-5701, (512) 335-1071, BS 82 Southwest TX St Univ; ME 83 Southwest TX St Univ; Sp-Lang Path, Brenham State School, **SLP**

Maxwell, Mrs Bess Sirmon 1704 Thomasville Road #164, Tallahassee, FL 32303, (904) 656-4800, BS 84 FL St Univ; MS 87 FL St Univ; 87–Sp-Lang Path, Cap Rehab Hosp, **SLP**

Maxwell, Camille M 37 Lawrencia Drive, Lawrenceville, NJ 08648, **SLP**

Maxwell, Mrs Catherine T 232 Lagoon Drive, Fort Myers, FL 33905, (813) 336-6913, MS 80 Univ of South FL; Sp-Lang Path, Lee Memorial Hosp Rehab Ctr, **SLP ACE**

Maxwell, Dr David L 320 Farmlane, Westwood, MA 02090, (617) 578-8525, BS 62 Southern IL Univ -Carbondale; MS 65 Southern IL Univ -Carbondale; PH 70 (NS) Southern IL Univ -Carbondale; Professor, Emerson College, **SLP**

Maxwell, Mrs Donna Hesslau 20 North Roslyn, Westmont, IL 60559, (312) 246-7590, BS 84 Western IL Univ; MA 85 Western IL Univ; 87–Sp-Lang Path, Western Springs Dist 101, **SLP**

Maxwell, Mrs Elizabeth D 124 Ridge Road, Perry, FL 32347, (904) 584-6635, BS 74 FL St Univ; MS 75 FL St Univ; Sp-Lang Path, Taylor Co Sch Bd, **SLP LM ACE**

Maxwell, Jean A 3610 Waterside Court #H, Richmond, VA 23229, (804) 270-5242, BA 75 Denison Univ; MA 79 OH St Univ; Sp/Lang Path, Med Coll of VA, **SLP**

Maxwell, Jeannene 872 South 1100 East, Eden, ID 83325, (208) 734-8324, MS 84 Univ of UT; SLP, Preston School District 201, **SLP**

Maxwell, Joellen 4101 West Lake Echo Road, Tucson, AZ 85741, (602) 744-9277, MS 83 Northeast MO St Univ; Sp-Lang Path Preschool, Kendall County Special Ed Coop, **SLP**

Maxwell, Lesley Anne 12 Stearns Road #2, Brookline, MA 02146, (617) 734-0631, BA 84 Univ of CA - Santa Barbara; MS 85 Boston Univ; **SLP**

Maxwell, Martha Lynn 3707 Southway Drive #96, Roanoke, VA 24014, (703) 982-7023, MS 84 Radford Univ; Sp-Lang Path, Roanoke City PS, **SLP H**

Maxwell, Pamela A 2604 Creekside Drive, Newark, DE 19711, (302) 368-6790, Sp-Lang Path, Speech-Lang-Hearing Services, **SLP**

Maxwell, Mrs Patricia 810 Astro, Rocky Ford, CO 81067, (719) 384-6825, BA 72 Boston Coll; MA 73 Central MI Univ; 83–Coord Hndcp Serv/Sp-Lang Path, Child Develop Serv, **SLP**

Maxwell, Mrs Rosalou S 2821 Burleson Street, Florence, AL 35630, (205) 764-8940, BS 72 TX Tech Univ; MA 74 Univ of OK Medical Center; Sp-Lang Path, UCP Center, **SLP**

Maxwell, Sandra Rose Rural Route 4 Box 103-C, Maryville, MO 64468, (816) 562-3233, BS 83 Northwest MO St Univ; MS 85 Northwest MO St Univ; 88–Sp-Lang Path, Maryville RII Sch Dist, **SLP**

Maxwell, Sara Elizabeth 320 Farm Lane, Westwood, MA 02090, (617) 326-7500, BS 63 Southern IL Univ -Carbondale; ME 82 Boston Coll; MS 64 Southern IL Univ -Carbondale; 69–Dir, Sp-Lang Path Prog, Westwood Pub Sch, **SLP**

Maxwell, Stephen Allen 37 Saturn Drive, Lr Sackville, NS, Canada B4C 1V6, (902) 865-9459, BA 74 Brigham Young Univ; MS 81 IA St Univ; 81–Aud, NS Hrng & Sp Cl, **A**

Maxwell, Susan 191 Chandler Drive, West Chester, PA 19380, **SLP**

May, Ann R 2415 Edwards Street, Berkeley, CA 94702, (415) 372-4348, BA 77 Holy Names Coll; MS 79 Columbia Univ Teachers Coll; Sp-Lang Path, Contra Costa Co Hosp, **SLP**

May, Dr Annette Anisman 807 Alisal Court, Santa Monica, CA 90402, (213) 454-5353, BA 47 Univ of WI - Madison; MA 60 Univ of CA - Los Angeles; PH 68 (Sp-Lang Path) Univ of CA - Los Angeles; 79–Dir, Lincoln Cen for Sp Path Inc, **SLP ACE**

May, Mrs Betty Ann 2720 Cherry Street, Montgomery, AL 36107-2806, (205) 284-5470, BS 73 Univ of AL-Tuscaloosa; MS 77 Auburn Univ - Auburn; Audiologist, Drs Kitchens & Chapman PA, **A**

May, Charlene M 8444 Seabridge Way, Indianapolis, IN 46240, (317) 896-2016, SLP, Carmel Clay & Westfield Schls, **SLP**

May, Diana P 900 Sturbridge Drive, Richmond, VA 23236, (804) 320-1895, BS 76 James Madison Univ; MS 78 James Madison Univ; Sp/Lang Path, Private Practice, **SLP**

May, Mrs Elizabeth 83 Ostego Street, Ilion, NY 13357, (315) 894-4912, BS 80 Elmira Coll; MA 81 Western MI Univ; Sp-Lang Path, Private Practice, **SLP**

May, Mrs Gaylene M 21 Wilson Avenue, Morgantown, WV 26505, (913) 843-5821, BS 73 Kent St Univ; MA 80 Kent St Univ; Sp-Lang Path, Communication Disorders Center, **SLP**

May, Mrs Helen C P 306 Joor Street, Rolling Fork, MS 39159, (601) 873-6540, BA 62 Univ of MD - College Park; MA 73 Univ of MS; SLP, Sharkey-Issaquena Consol Sch, **SLP**

May, Helen M 8609 Northwest Plaza Drive, Suite 330, Dallas, TX 75225, (214) 521-7355, BS 79 Univ of TX - Dallas; MS 81 Univ of TX - Dallas; Owner, Private Practice, **SLP**

May, Dr Jane V 76 Crossgates Drive, Brandon, MS 39042, (601) 987-3925, BS 52 Univ Southern MS-Hattiesburg; MS 66 Univ Southern MS-Hattiesburg; PH 68 (Audiology) Univ Southern MS-Hattiesburg; 85–Teacher Supervisor, Mississippi Sch for the Deaf, **A**

May, Janet E 414-C Clearview Court, Greenwood, IN 46143, (317) 882-6635, BA 84 IN Univ - Bloomington; OM 87 IN Univ - Bloomington; **SLP**

May, Dr Jo Whitten P O Box 958, Bermuda Run, Advance, NC 27006, (919) 750-2693, BA 59 Univ of VA - Charlottesville; MA 69 Univ of NC - Greensboro; PH 77 (NS) Univ of NC - Greensboro; Dir Stu Tchg, Winston-Salem St U, **SLP ACE**

May, Mrs Joan P 2910 Woodside Drive, Tallahassee, FL 32312, (904) 681-5446, OB 78 Univ of FL; OM 80 Auburn Univ - Auburn; Sp-Lang Path, Tallahassee Mem Hosp, **SLP**

May, Dr John M 525 N W 17th Street, Oklahoma City, OK 73103, (405) 272-9876, BA 66 Univ Southern MS-Hattiesburg; OM 67 Univ of OK Medical Center; PH 82 (NS) Univ Southern MS-Hattiesburg; Aud, VA Medical Center, **A**

May, John P 5295 South Moorland Road, New Berlin, WI 53151, (414) 384-2000, BA 70 SD St Univ; MA 76 Univ of Denver; Aud, VA Hosp, **A**

May, Judith S 320 West 90th Street #1F, New York, NY 10024, (212) 799-0471, BS 57 Univ of NE - Lincoln; MS 74 Columbia Univ Teachers Coll; Aud, Private Practice, **A**

May, June E 813 S E 95th Avenue, Vancouver, WA 98664, (206) 696-7256, BS 71 Portland St Univ; MS 73 Portland St Univ; SLP, Vancouver School District 37, **SLP**

May, Mrs Marilyn P 5008 Farming Ridge Blvd, Reading, PA 19606, (215) 779-5511, BS 75 Bloomsburg Univ of PA; ME 76 Bloomsburg Univ of PA; Sp-Lang Path, Berks County Intermediate Unit, **SLP**

May, Mrs Mary Rural Delivery 2, 40 Lackawanna Road, Stanhope, NJ 07874, (201) 533-5786, BS 75 William Paterson Coll; MS 79 William Paterson Coll; Sp-Lang Path, St Barnabas Medical Center, **SLP**

May, Mary E 1403 Willowview Court, Encinitas, CA 92024, (619) 758-1620, BA 85 CA St Univ - Chico; MA 86 CA St Univ - Chico; 88–Sp-Lang Path, Children's Hosp

May, Mona M 8001 Havenwood, Austin, TX 78759, **SLP**

May, Patricia 2900 20th Street, Bakersfield, CA 93301, (805) 589-4242, BA 69 Univ of CA - Santa Barbara; MS 71 Univ of OK Medical Center; Hd Tchr/Prog Spec, Kern Co Supt of Sch, **SLP**

May, Regina Margaret 4203 Martyridge Drive, Oakville, MO 63129, (314) 638-6358, BS 80 Southwest MO St Univ; MS 82 Southern IL Univ-Edwardsvill; Sp-Lang Path, Irwin Lehrhoff, **SLP**

May, Sally L 200 Lowood Lane, Greenville, SC 29605, (803) 235-8176, BS 70 Nazareth Coll of Rochester; MS 71 SUNY - Coll at Geneseo; **SLP**

May, Samye Louise 2015 Cervin Boulevard, Austin, TX 78727, (512) 451-2931, MA 84 Univ of TX - Austin; Audiologist, Austin Regnl Day Sch Prog-Deaf, **A**

May, Mrs Sarah Jane 2398 Kellogg Road, Hinckley, OH 44233, **SLP**

May, Susan J 6106 C Alexandria Drive, Evansville, IN 47715, (812) 479-1411, BS 86 Western KY Univ; MS 88 Vanderbilt Univ; 88–Sp-Lang Path, Rehabilitation Ctr

May, Suzanne 4730 Oyes Street #313, San Diego, CA 92109, (619) 426-2448, MA 86 San Diego St Univ; **SLP**

May, Suzanne J 211 Georgetown Drive, Glastonbury, CT 06033, (203) 667-5320, BS 84 Bowling Green St Univ; MA 87 Kent St Univ; 87–Sp-Lang Path, Newington Children's Hosp, **SLP**

May, Mrs Thomasena Glover 6521 Idle Brook Drive, Charlotte, NC 28212, (704) 568-7008, BA 72 SC St Coll; MA 79 Montclair St Coll; 84–Sp-Lang Path, Charlotte Mecklenburg Sch, **SLP**

Mayberry, Jill Marian 16 Chapin Avenue, Reading, MA 01867, (617) 942-1444, MA 86 Humboldt St Univ; **SLP**

Mayberry, Dr Rachel I Department Of Education, University Of Chicago, 5835 South Kimbark, Chicago, IL 60637, (312) 702-3645, BA 70 Drake Univ; MS 73 Washington Univ; PH 79 (Communication Disorders) McGill Univ - Quebec; 83–Research Prof, U of Chicago, **SLP**

Mayberry-Langston, Claudia L 7839 Parallel, Kansas City, KS 66112, (913) 788-7740, BS 73 Univ of IA; MA 79 Case Western Reserve Univ; Aud, Family Hearing Ctr, **A**

Maybruck, Dr Iris L 1920 South Pandora Avenue, Los Angeles, CA 90025, (213) 474-0819, BS 61 OH St Univ; MA 64 OH St Univ; ED 86 (NS) Pepperdine Univ - Los Angele; Sp/Lang Path, Private Practice, **SLP**

Maydew, Linda S 709 Lexington, Chicago Heights, IL 60411, (312) 996-9058, BA 81 Univ of Northern CO; MA 82 Univ of Northern CO; 86–Aud, Univ of Illinois-Div of Svc for Crippled Children, **A**

Mayeda, M Melinda Gaminde 8606 N Third Street, Fresno, CA 93710, (209) 439-1054, BA 79 CA St Univ - Long Beach; MA 83 Whittier Coll; 86–Sp-Lang Path, Abell Sp & Lang Ctr, **SLP**

Mayer, Carol A M 4148 Forest Avenue, Western Springs, IL 60558, (312) 469-5505, BS 63 Univ of IL - Urbana; MS 77 Southern CT St Univ; Sp-Lang Path, Glen Ellyn #89, **SLP**

Mayer, Dr Carole L 104 Elmhurst Circle, Sacramento, CA 95825, (916) 278-6601, BA 57 CUNY - Hunter Coll; MA 67 Seton Hall Univ; PH 80 (Hrng Science) CUNY - Grad Sch & Univ Cntr; 77–Prof, CSU-Sacramento, **A**

Mayer, Mrs Carolyn M 504 Holly Hill Drive, Evansville, IN 47710, (812) 254-1530, BA Bellarmine Coll; MS IN St Univ - Terre Haute; SLP, Daviess-Martin Spec Ed Coop, **SLP**

Mayer, Mrs Judith H 11752 Parish, Bridgeton, MO 63044, (314) 291-4090, BA 65 Fontbonne Coll; MS 68 Marquette Univ; Sp-Lang Path, St Louis Hearing & Speech Cen, **SLP**

Mayer, Katherine K 7963 West Rue Du Chateau, Dixon, IL 61021, (815) 288-5531, BS 79 Univ of WI - Madison; MA 80 Western MI Univ; Sp/Lang Path, Midwest Sp/Hrng Assoc Inc, **SLP**

Mayer, Margaret Jean 3634 Douglas Avenue #719, Racine, WI 53402, (414) 681-2369, BS 86 Marquette Univ; MS 87 Marquette Univ; 87–Sp-Lang Path, Racine USD, **SLP**

Mayer, Mrs Mavis E P O Box 7984, Metairie, LA 70010, (504) 641-1061, BS 64 Univ of WI - River Falls; MA 66 Stanford Univ; Cl Coord, New Orlean Sp & Hrng Cen, **SLP**

Mayer, Mrs Melanie H Route 3 Box 303-Hb, Wilmington, NC 28403, (919) 799-7749, MS 78 Appalachian St Univ; 79–Sp-Lang Path, New Hanover County Bd of Educ, **SLP**

Mayer, Nancy E 609 Northwood Avenue, Charlottesville, VA 22901, **SLP**

Mayer, Mrs Sharon Peach 8132 Pawtucket Drive, Huntington Beach, CA 92646, (714) 556-3482, MA 84 1389; 85–Sp-Lang Path, Newport-Mesa USD, **SLP**

Mayer, Mrs Shelli Susan 18181 N E 31st Court #1607, North Miami Beach, FL 33160, (305) 581-7662, Adjunct Prof / Cl Superv, Nova U Grad Sch, **SLP**

Mayer, Mrs Theresa K 5708 Old Leeds Road, Birmingham, AL 35210, (205) 871-8191, BA 73 Univ of AL- Tuscaloosa; MA 75 Univ of AL- Tuscaloosa; Sp-Lang Path, Mountain Brook Board of Educ, **SLP**

Mayerak, Dawn A 703 East 144th Street, Dolton, IL 60419, (312) 841-1299, OB 81 Governors St Univ; OM 86 Governors St Univ; **SLP**

Mayerhoff, Caryn Sue 401 Marlborough Road, Cedarhurst, NY 11516, (516) 569-6025, BA 85 CUNY - Queens Coll; MA 87 CUNY - Queens Coll; **A**

Mayerik, Mrs Christine Annette 6453 Bella Vista Drive, Rockford, MI 49341, (616) 874-8728, BA 82 Wayne St Univ; MS 85 IL St Univ - Normal; 88–Sp-Lang Path, Mary Free Bed Rehab Ctr, **SLP**

Mayerovitch, Julie R 140 Elm Ridge Drive #811, Toronto, ON, Canada M6B 1B1, (416) 826-4000, BS 72 McGill Univ - Quebec; MA 74 Case Western Reserve Univ; Sp-Lang Path, Peel Bd of Educ, **SLP**

Mayer-Weinstock, Daniela 1211 5th Avenue, New Hyde Park, NY 11040, (516) 775-5244, BA 75 CUNY - Queens Coll; MA 82 CUNY - Hunter Coll; Sp-Lang Path, Private Practice, **SLP**

Mayette, Mrs Sue Anne Rd 3 Box 3778, Montpelier, VT 05602, (802) 229-9909, BS 77 Coll of Saint Rose; MS 85 Worcester St Coll; Sp-Lang Path, Washington Cent Super Union, **SLP**

Mayeux, Deborah Anne M 5707 North Drive, Alexandria, LA 71301, (318) 487-5472, BA 77 Northwestern St Univ; MA 80 Northwestern St Univ; Sp/Lang Path, LA Spec Ed Cen, **SLP**

Mayfield, Bonnie L 1337 East Coronado, Phoenix, AZ 85006, (602) 253-0385, BS 75 Univ of WY; MS 77 Phillips Univ; Sp-Lang Path, Mesa Publ Schs, **SLP**

Mayfield, Mrs Francine A 6180 East Owens, Las Vegas, NV 89110, BA 74 Univ of CA - Los Angeles; ME 79 Southwest TX St Univ; SLP, Clark Co Sch Dist, **SLP**

Mayfield, Mrs Margaret Topian 20 Tobin Avenue, Chelmsford, MA 01824, (617) 595-1840, BS 77 SUNY - Coll at Oneonta; MS 79 Purdue Univ - West Lafayette; Program Case Mgr/Head Injuries, Community Reentry Services, **SLP**

Mayfield, Norman K Allied Hearing & Audiology, 323 North Lincoln, PO Box 554, Santa Maria, CA 93456, (805) 925-7323, BS 74 UT St Univ; MA 74 UT St Univ; Aud, Allied Hearing & Audiology, **A**

Mayfield, Mrs Rhonda Moore 1-A Kamakani Place, Honolulu, HI 96818, (808) 423-1541, BS 71 Old Dominion Univ; ME 81 Old Dominion Univ; 88–Sp-Lang Path, St Francis Med Ctr, **SLP**

Mayfield, Dr Sandra A 2605 South Indiana #1602, Chicago, IL 60616, (312) 791-0109, BS 71 CO St Univ; MA 72 Case Western Reserve Univ; PH 80 (Comm Disorders-Child Lang) Univ of WI - Madison; **SLP**

Mayfield, Sheryl Melinda 500 Circulo Gallegos N W, Albuquerque, NM 87107, (505) 345-1432, BA 67 Miami Univ - Oxford; MS 71 Univ of NM; Sp/Lang Path, Albuquerque Pub Sch, **SLP**

Mayger-Gwyn, Tara 905 Sampson Street, Taylor, PA 18517, (607) 539-7155, BA 79 Ithaca Coll; MS 81 Ithaca Coll; Sp-Lang Path, Visiting Nurse Assoc, **SLP**

Mayhew, Nancy Craig 1456 Stanley Boulevard, Birmingham, MI 48009, (313) 646-1452, BA 79 MI St Univ; MS 81 Univ of MI - Ann Arbor; **SLP**

Mayhew, Preston W, II CHAR-EM ISD, Mercer Boulevard, Charlevoix, MI 49720, (616) 547-9947, BS 69 Central MI Univ; MA 73 Central MI Univ; 80–Early Childhood Development, Charlevoix-Emmet ISD, **SLP**

Maykulsky, Vicki W 3506 West 25th St Terrace, Lawrence, KS 66044, (913) 841-0054, BA 73 Wichita St Univ; MA 76 Wichita St Univ; Sp-Lang Path, Lawrence USD 497, **SLP**

May-Landes, Annette Lynn 1206 Sorrento Drive, Colorado Springs, CO 80910, (719) 636-5186, BS 80 Northern IL Univ - De Kalb; MA 82 Northern IL Univ - De Kalb; Sp-Lang Path, Co School of Deaf & Blind, **SLP**

Maylath, Mrs Pamela J 156 Virginia Avenue, Reading, PA 19606, (215) 775-8334, BS 80 Bloomsburg Univ of PA; MS 81 Bloomsburg Univ of PA; Sp/Lang Path, Reading Rehab Hosp, **SLP**

Maynard, Mrs Conita S RR 1 Box 159A, Tipton, IN 46072, (317) 675-8500, BS 63 IN Univ - Bloomington; OM 67 IN Univ - Bloomington; Sp-Lang Path, Tipton Co Mem Hosp, **SLP**

Maynard, Margaret E Ochoa 9455 Viscount #160, El Paso, TX 79925, (915) 851-2714, BA 81 Univ of TX - El Paso; MA 84 Univ of TX - El Paso; SLP, Clint ISD, **SLP**

Mayne, Mrs Pat L 9 Country Lane, Wimberley, TX 78676, (512) 847-5126, BA 80 Southwest TX St Univ; ME 82 Southwest TX St Univ; **SLP**

Maynor, Joyce Lynn 10444 North 69th Street, #225, Scottsdale, AZ 85253, (602) 483-8126, BS 80 AZ St Univ; OM 84 AZ St Univ; Sp-Lang Path, John C Lincoln Hosp & Hlth Ctr, **SLP**

Mayo, Dr Carolyn M P O Box 63215, 800 Madison, Memphis, TN 38163, MA 73 OH St Univ; PH 78 (Sp-Lang Path) MI St Univ; 87–Exec Dir, W Tenn Area Hlth Educ Ctr, **SLP ACE**

Mayo, Kathleen Tina P O Box 6191, Hayward, CA 94540, (415) 948-3383, BA 85 CA St Univ - Stanislaus; MA 86 Univ of the Pacific; SLP, Altos Sp Lang & Learn Ctr, **SLP**

Mayo, Mrs Lizabethe Route 3 Box 539, Proctorville, OH 45669, (614) 354-4526, BA 76 Marshall Univ; MA 77 Marshall Univ; Sp/Lang Path, Pilasco Ross Spec Ed Resrc Cen, **SLP**

Mayo, Mrs Patricia Jean 620 South 44th Avenue, Wausau, WI 54401, (715) 359-0511, MS 83 Univ of WI - Stevens Point; BA 81 Univ of WI - Eau Claire; SLP, Dc Everest Jr Hgh Sch, **SLP**

Mayo, Robert P O Box 63215, 800 Madison, Memphis, TN 38163, (901) 525-2682, BA 75 George Washington Univ; MA 77 OH St Univ; Doctoral Asst, Memphis St Univ, **SLP**

Mayo, Robert A 4436 West Melvina, Milwaukee, WI 53216, (414) 461-5810, BA 69 Saint Francis Seminary; MA 72 Univ of WI - Milwaukee; 73–Sp-Lang Path, Milwaukee Publ Sch, **SLP**

Mays, Carla Marie 250 Moonglow #D-6, Alamogordo, NM 88310, (505) 437-3040, BA 83 San Francisco St Univ; MS 85 Univ of AR - Little Rock; 86–Sp-Lang Path, Zia Therapy Ctr Inc, **SLP**

Mays, Cheryl Ann 4001 Anderson Road, Unit I-56, Nashville, TN 37217, (615) 366-0214, MA 73 Western MI Univ; Audiologist, Dr Downey, **A**

Mays, Nancy Miller Route 1 Box 548, South Point, OH 45680, (614) 532-6698, BS 78 OH Univ - Athens; MA 82 Marshall Univ; **SLP**

Mayster, Lynda W 1440 West State Parkway, Chicago, IL 60610, (312) 751-2140, BA 64 CUNY - Hunter Coll; MA 67 CUNY - Hunter Coll; Sp-Lang Path, Private Practice, **SLP**

Mayton, Mrs Linda Mary 2473 Phillips Road, Stanley, NY 14561, (716) 526-6351, **SLP**

Mayton, Mrs Pamela Sue 124 Cottonwood Cove, Marion, AR 72364, (501) 633-9188, BS 79 AR St Univ; MA 81 AR St Univ; Sp-Lang Path, Forrest City Public Schools, **SLP**

Mayworm, Sylvia L 337 East Elm Street, Villa Park, IL 60181, (312) 345-9870, BA 72 Univ of IL - Chicago; MA 74 Northwestern Univ; Sp-Lang Path, Madden Mental Health Ctr, **SLP**

Mazar, Linda Nylen 800 8th Avenue South, South St Paul, MN 55075-2909, (612) 780-7666, OM 87 Univ of WI - River Falls; 88–Sp-Lang Path, Centennial Schs

Mazeau, Zoe Ann 7626 South Biscay Street, Aurora, CO 80016, (516) 757-4615, **SLP**

Maziarz, Jennifer Lynn 30905 Tamarack #31310, Wixom, MI 48096, (517) 684-3845, MA 87 Central MI Univ

Mazor, Marvin Mallios, 788 Columbus Avenue, Apartment 6A, New York, NY 10025, (212) 520-7358, BA 62 CUNY - Brooklyn Coll; MA 65 CUNY - Brooklyn Coll; PH 71 (NS) NY Univ; Asst Prof of Commun Arts, Queens Coll of Cty U of NY, **SLP A**

Mazor, Rosemarie 1117 West Park Avenue, Long Beach, NY 11561, MS; **A**

Mazow, Mrs Maxine S 12 Robert Road, Marblehead, MA 01945, BA 63 Univ of CT; MS 82 Boston Univ; SLP, Winthrop Pub Sch, **SLP**

Mazur, Mrs Barbara P 179 Blue Ridge Drive, Manchester, CT 06040, (203) 649-6590, MA 71 SUNY - Center at Buffalo; SLP, E Hartford Bd of Ed, **SLP**

Mazur, Carol L 33 Kenneth Street #7-B, West Haven, CT 06516, (203) 933-8516, BS 86 WV Univ; MA 88 Univ of Northern CO; 88–Aud, New Haven Ear Nose Throat

Mazur, Carolyn 7974 Versailles Road, Angola, NY 14006, (716) 532-4942, BS 77 SUNY - Coll at Fredonia; ME 81 SUNY - Coll at Fredonia; SLP, J N Adam Ddso, **SLP**

Mazur, Jill Gleason 606 4th Street, Niagara Falls, NY 14301, (716) 282-4130, BS 82 WV Univ; MA 84 Temple Univ; 88–Aud/Owner, The Hearing Aid Ctr, **A**

Mazurek, Mrs Susan McHugh 5314 Tramore Road, Baltimore, MD 21214, (301) 665-0820, BA 71 MT St Agnes Coll; MS 73 Loyola Coll; MS 84 Loyola Coll; SLP, Baltimore Co Bd of Ed, **SLP**

Mazurski, Phyllis A 170 Main Street, Hatfield, MA 01038, (413) 247-5506, BS 78 Emerson Coll; MS 81 Boston Univ; Sp-Lang Path, **SLP**

Mazursky, Mrs Marcie Alpert 6868 East Kings Avenue, Scottsdale, AZ 85254, (602) 839-7100, **SLP**

Mazuzan, Marsinah Anne 2900 S 13th Street #201, Arlington, VA 22204, (703) 323-4058, MS 84 Vanderbilt Univ; Sp-Lang Path, Washington Hrng & Sp Soc, **SLP**

Mazza, Michael A 1226 Strieff Lane, Flossmoor, IL 60422, (312) 453-5265, Sp-Lang Path, South Metropolitan Assoc, **SLP**

Mazzaro, Mrs Patricia E 392 Doane Avenue, Staten Island, NY 10308, BA 71 CUNY - Brooklyn Coll; MS 73 CUNY - Brooklyn Coll; **SLP**

Mazzella-Gordon, Mrs Carmella 1591 Green Valley Road, Danville, CA 94526, (209) 223-1416, BA 76 San Francisco St Univ; MS 78 San Francisco St Univ; Dept Head Sp-Lang Path, Amador Hosp, **SLP**

Mazzeo, Larry Paul 755 Pineview Drive, San Jose, CA 95117, (408) 243-5008, MA 86 San Jose St Univ

Mazzetta, Kay Box 7, White House Station, NJ 08889, MA 76 CUNY - Lehman Coll; **SLP**

Mazzocco, Diane M 4249 Virginia Road, Long Beach, CA 90807, **SLP**

Mazzola, Lynda J RFD 1 Box 2800, Leeds, ME 04263, (207) 582-2571, BS 65 Univ of Southern CA; MS 75 Univ of Southern ME; MS 83 Univ of OR; Sp-Lang Path, Private Practice, **SLP**

Mazzucco, Mrs Sandra B 692 Pelton Avenue, Staten Island, NY 10310, (718) 442-6006, BA 76 CUNY - Brooklyn Coll; MA 78 NY Univ; 78–Sp-Lang Path, UCP NYC, **SLP**

McAdam, Carol C 15901 Longmeadow, Dearborn, MI 48120, BS 65 SUNY - Coll at Geneseo; MS 68 SUNY - Coll at Geneseo; Sp-Lang Path, Dearborn Public Schools, **SLP**

McAdam, Daniel L 157 Gentle Avenue, Monmouth, OR 97361, (503) 378-5286, BS 80 Western OR St Coll; MS 82 Western OR St Coll; Aud, St of or/Fairview Trng Cen, **A**

McAdam, Malcolm A 15901 Longmeadow, Dearborn, MI 48120, (313) 867-6000, BS 68 SUNY - Coll at Geneseo; MS 70 Purdue Univ - West Lafayette; 73–Aud, ENT Center of Detroit, **A**

McAdams, Mrs Lisa Rasenti 23260 Road 148, Tulare, CA 93274, (415) 493-8111, BA 86 Univ of the Pacific; MS 87 Univ of Redlands

McAfee, Dena P 235 Roosevelt Avenue, Eau Claire, WI 54701, BS 72 CO St Univ; MA 74 Case Western Reserve Univ; **SLP**

McAfee, Jacqulea S Sandybrook Center, 1005 Limit Avenue, Mount Dora, FL 32757, (904) 383-6007, BS 67 Sul Ross St Univ; MA 74 Our Lady Lake Univ-San Anton; 88–Coord of Sp-Lang Path, Rebound Inc, **SLP**

McAfee, Mrs Mary Cincotta 760 Sugar Creek Trail, Webster, NY 14580, (716) 475-6863, BS 82 Nazareth Coll of Rochester; MS 83 Nazareth Coll of Rochester; Instructor, NTID, **SLP**

McAfee, Mrs Patricia H 2611 Laporte Avenue, Valparaiso, IN 46383, (219) 464-3860, BS 71 Purdue Univ - West Lafayette; MS 73 Purdue Univ - West Lafayette; 88–Clin Supvr, Valparaiso Univ, **SLP ACE**

McAleer, Dr Colleen A 38 Frampton Street, Clarion, PA 16214, (814) 226-2326, BS 73 PA St Univ - Univ Park; ME 75 Clarion Univ of PA; PH 79 (Aud) Kent St Univ; 82–Assoc Prof, Clarion U of Pa, **SLP A ACE**

McAleer, Patricia Kathleen 71 Stony Hill Village, Brookfield, CT 06804, (203) 775-9519, BA 81 Glassboro St Coll; MA 86 Trenton St Coll; 87–Sp-Lang Path, Region 14 Schs, **SLP**

McAleese, Patricia Marie 5764 Thornhill Drive, Oakland, CA 94611, (415) 947-5300, BA 78 Syracuse Univ; MS 84 Univ of WI - Madison; 88–Sp-Lang Path, John Muir Med Ctr, **SLP**

McAlerney, Colleen Ann 6518 Cleopatra Place N W, Seattle, WA 98117, (206) 783-8227, BS 83 Univ of WA; MS 86 Univ of WA; **SLP**

McAlexander, Mary Lee 100 Briar Meade Drive, Clinton, MS 39056, (502) 782-7720, BA 83 MS Coll; MS 85 Univ Southern MS-Hattiesburg; Aud, William T Moore MD, **A**

McAlister, Mrs Sarah Long P O Box 912, Laurens, SC 29360, (803) 682-5415, BA 79 Clemson Univ; MS 81 Univ of SC - Columbia; Sp-Lang Path, Private Practice, **SLP**

McAlister, Shirley W 13112 Ireland Lane, San Diego, CA 92129, (619) 484-6170, BS 73 Pacific Union Coll; MS 75 Loma Linda Univ - Riverside; Sp-Lang Path, Communication Health Services, **SLP**

McAllister, Judith Boyden 18125 Kingsport Drive, Malibu, CA 90265, (213) 454-6977, BA 61 MI St Univ; MA 65 Western MI Univ; **SLP**

McAllister, Mrs Linda Ruth 322 River Road, Maumee, OH 43537, (419) 893-4656, **SLP**

McAllister, Mary Elizabeth 2609 Taylorsville Road #3, Louisville, KY 40205, (502) 451-0110, BS 35 Eastern KY Univ; MA 51 Univ of KY; **SLP LM**

McAllister-Strong, Mrs Laurie Anne 1148 Ontario Street Apt 1, Oak Park, IL 60302, MA 84 Edinboro Univ of PA; BS 83 Clarion Univ of PA; **SLP**

McAloose, Jennifer Mary 19 S Norrison Street, Mc Adoo, PA 18237, (717) 826-3800, BS 85 Bloomsburg Univ of PA; MS 88 Bloomsburg Univ of PA

McAlpine, Mrs Catherine A 1902 East Red River, Victoria, TX 77901, (512) 573-9774, BS 58 Southwest TX St Univ; 77–Sp-Lang Path, Victoria Home Hlth Agcy, **SLP LM**

McAndrew, Joyce Kathryn 18 Newcastle Road, Rochester, NY 14610, (716) 377-4660, BS 74 Nazareth Coll of Rochester; MS 79 Nazareth Coll of Rochester; Sp-Lang Path, BOCES 1 Monroe, **SLP**

McAndrew, Patricia Burke 2074 Arthur Avenue, Lakewood, OH 44107, (216) 521-2702, BS 65 Bowling Green St Univ; MA 86 Cleveland St Univ; **SLP**

McArdle, Mrs Mary 236 Paterson Avenue, Paterson, NJ 07502, (201) 256-1700, BA 86 Kean Coll of NJ; MA 87 Kean Coll of NJ; 87–Sp-Lang Path, North Jersey Developmental Ctr, **SLP**

McArthur, Mrs Barbara Mattson 4 Forest Street, Lake Ronkonkoma, NY 11779, (516) 585-1235, BS 81 Northeastern Univ; MA 87 Hofstra Univ; Aud, Dr Chase, **A**

McArthur, Cindy Biss 766 Granite Hills Circle, El Cajon, CA 92019-3157, (619) 440-1540, BA 83 San Diego St Univ; MA 85 Univ of MN - Duluth; **SLP**

McArthur, Eileen Birchett 2 Chadwick Rd, White Plains, NY 10604, (914) 949-7310, BS 75 Saint Lawrence Univ; MA 77 Seton Hall Univ; Sp-Lang Path, NY Sch for the Deaf, **SLP**

McArthur, Madelyn 124 North 300 West, Apt #1, Cedar City, UT 84720, (801) 586-7802, BS 73 Brigham Young Univ; MS 85 UT St Univ; Sp-Lang Path, Southern Utah State College, **SLP ACE**

McAsey, Danila B 1213 E Forrest Hill Avenue, Peoria, IL 61603, (309) 672-6308, BS 72 Marquette Univ; MA 74 Univ of IA; 79–Sp/Lang Path, Peoria Assoc/Retarded Citizens, **SLP**

McAtee, Mrs Linda Jo 1829 Tony, Wichita, KS 67212, (316) 721-1579, MS 81 Fort Hays St Univ; BA 80 Fort Hays St Univ; Sp-Lang Path, Haysville PS, **SLP**

McAughan, Margaret Ann 11626 Sagecanyon, Houston, TX 77089, (713) 481-0454, MA 86 Univ of Houston - Univ Park; 78–Sp-Lang Path, Pasadena ISD, **SLP**

McAuley, Mrs Nancy C Rd 1 Box 240B, Scenery Hill, PA 15360, (412) 267-3192, BS 78 Clarion Univ of PA; MS 79 Indiana Univ of PA; 85–Sp-Lang Path, S G Rehabilitation Agency, **SLP**

McAuliffe, Christine Matrice 718 West Algonquin #8, Des Plaines, IL 60016, (217) 337-7034, MA 87 Univ of IL - Urbana; **SLP**

McAuliffe, Mrs Shelley A 4625 Smokey Wreath Way, Ellicott City, MD 21043, (301) 253-2333, BS 80 Towson St Univ; MS 81 Towson St Univ; Sp/Lang Path, Montg Co Pub Schs, **SLP**

McAvoy, Kathleen Anne 114 Wellington Place #5, Cincinnati, OH 45219, (513) 241-6369, MA 88 Univ of Cincinnati

McBeath, Karen Haymond 98-F Escondido Village, Stanford, CA 94305, **SLP**

McBeath-Benner, Susan 361 4th Court East, Carmel, IN 46032, (317) 844-2281, BS 61 Univ of WI - Madison; MS 62 Univ of WI - Madison; MA 87 Butler Univ; **SLP**

McBee, Gala S Childrens Medical Center, 5300 East Skelly Drive, Tulsa, OK 74135, (918) 664-6600, BA 77 Univ of AR - Fayetteville; MA 78 Univ of AR - Fayetteville; Sp-Lang Path, Chldn's Med Cen, **SLP**

McBee, Mrs Lucy Rush 560 Lees Trace, Marietta, GA 30064, (404) 479-1871, **SLP**

McBeth, Mrs Gloria J P O Box 92, Spring Lake, MI 49456, (616) 846-6925, BA 64 Univ of CA - Santa Barbara; MA 66 Univ of WA; Sp-Lang Path, Private Practice, **SLP**

McBratnie, Barbara P 1521 Gull Road, Kalamazoo, MI 49001, (616) 343-2601, BS 63 SUNY - Center at Buffalo; MA 67 Western MI Univ; Coord-Adult Sp-Lang Svcs, Constance Brown Hrng & Sp Cen, **SLP**

McBride, David Lawrence 730 East McKellips, Suite C-722, Tempe, AZ 85281, (602) 481-9462, MS 86 AZ St Univ; 86–Aud, Drs' Hrng Aid Svcs Inc, **A**

McBride, Debra L 12312-B Furrow Cove, Austin, TX 78753, (512) 836-4939, **SLP**

McBride, Gilda Chauvin 2035 Brandylin, Anchorage, AK 99516-1965, (318) 235-7812, BS 77 Univ of Southwestern LA; MA 81 Univ of Southwestern LA; Spec Educ Teacher of Autism, Lafayette Parish School Board, **SLP**

McBride, Glen Dale, Jr 924 North Demint Avenue, Dixon, IL 61021, (815) 288-4830, BA 80 Northern IL Univ - De Kalb; MA 83 Univ of SD - Vermillion; SLP, AEA 4, **SLP**

McBride, Mrs Janet E Blue Bell Woods, 234 Tulip Tree Court, Blue Bell, PA 19422, (215) 539-8550, BA 68 Mundelein Coll; MA 70 Northwestern Univ; 75–Supvr Sp-Lang Path, Montgomery Co Intermed Unit, **SLP**

McBride, Karen L 506 C Street, Antioch, CA 94509, (415) 439-7516, BA 78 CA St Univ - Long Beach; MA 81 CA St Univ - Long Beach; Sp-Lang Path, Lynn Center, **SLP**

McBride, Laura A 208 Lafayette NE, Grand Rapids, MI 49503, (616) 527-1820, BS 85 Central MI Univ; MA 86 MI St Univ; 86–SLP, Ionia PS, **SLP**

McBride, Lloyd A 315 Glassmere Avenue, Interlaken, NJ 07712, (201) 761-9000, BA 53 Seton Hall Univ; Instr In Commun, Seton Hall U

McBride, Mrs Lois A 1150 Hillcrest Avenue, Tulare, CA 93274, (209) 686-4576, BA 49 Fort Hays St Univ; MA 55 Univ of Denver; Sp-Lang Path, **SLP**

McBride, Marie Francesca 25 Daniel Street, Rensselaer, NY 12144, (518) 479-7622, BA 84 Bridgewater St Coll; MS 86 Coll of Saint Rose; Sp-Lang Path, Unity House, **SLP**

McBride, Martha Louise 3549 Curry Lane, Apt #2808, Abilene, TX 79606, (915) 691-7300, BA 83 Wichita St Univ; MA 82 Wichita St Univ; 84–Sp-Lang Path, W Texas Rehab Cen, **SLP**

McBride, Teresa Lyn 77 South Ogden Street #403, Denver, CO 80209, (303) 788-0533, BS 80 IL St Univ - Normal; MS 85 Southern IL Univ -Carbondale; Sp-Lang Path, Private Practice, **SLP**

McBride, Mrs Vivian D 509 Forest Drive, South Boston, VA 24592, (804) 572-1335, BA 72 Wake Forest Univ; ME 73 Univ of VA - Charlottesville; **SLP**

McBroom, Gail B 2402 Gateshead Circle, Austin, TX 78745, (512) 447-9729, BS 79 Eastern NM Univ; MS 80 Eastern NM Univ; Sp-Lang Path, Austin ISD, **SLP**

McBryde, Mrs Terri Moore 2611 James, San Marcos, TX 78666, (512) 396-8500, BS 78 Baylor Univ; MA 82 Baylor Univ; Prog Coord, Hlth Care Intl - Brown Sch, **SLP**

McBurnett, William M, Jr 3674 S E Roanoke Court, Hillsboro, OR 97123, (503) 649-0461, BS 73 Walla Walla Coll; ME 81 Western OR St Coll; Sp-Lang Path, Beaverton Sch Dist #48, **SLP**

McCabe, Barbara Ann 959 Independence Hill, Morgantown, WV 26505, (304) 291-4500, BS 77 WV Univ; MS 79 WV Univ; **A**

McCabe, Mrs Barbara Michalak 11035 West Bobolink Avenue, Milwaukee, WI 53225, (414) 353-2395, OB 76 Univ of WI - Oshkosh; MS 77 Western MI Univ; SLP, Waukesha Public Schools, **SLP**

McCabe, Carol Lee 7100 East Mississippi #13-308, Denver, CO 80224, (303) 753-1421, BA 82 WA St Univ; MS 84 CO St Univ; 87–Sp-Lang Path, Denver PS, **SLP**

McCabe, Deborah Ann 106 Camino Pablo, Orinda, CA 94563, (415) 254-2651, BA 58 Univ of CA - Berkeley; ME 77 Holy Names Coll; Sp-Lang Path, Private Practice

McCabe, Mrs Janice L 119 Campbell Drive, Lowell, MA 01851, (617) 334-4500, BS 72 Kent St Univ; MS 74 Univ of Pittsburgh - Pittsburgh; Sp-Lang Path, Town of Tewksbury, **SLP**

McCabe, Margaret K 1818 Glade Court, Annapolis, MD 21403, (301) 454-6924, BS 74 Univ of WI - Madison; MS 76 Univ of WI - Madison; Dir of Aud Serv, U of MD, **A**

McCabe, Margaret R 19 Bacon Street, Winchester, MA 01890, (617) 237-4521, BS 75 Northeastern Univ; ME 77 Northeastern Univ; **SLP**

McCabe, Marianne Michele 205 West Fern Avenue #7, Redlands, CA 92373, BA 84 Univ of Redlands; MS 87 Univ of Redlands

McCabe, Mary Ann 712 Doctors Drive #E, Kinston, NC 28501, (919) 522-1261, BS 76 Marquette Univ; MA 81 Marshall Univ; Sp/Lang Path, Caswell Cen, **SLP**

McCabe, Mrs Mary Ann Jenkins 6 Cavan Way, Pittsford, NY 14534, (716) 248-5481, BS 58 Univ of MN - Minneap-St Paul; MS 75 Nazareth Coll of Rochester; Sp-Lang Path, BOCES #1-Monroe, **SLP**

McCabe, Mrs Melanie S 5661 Clark Avenue, Bethel Park, PA 15102, (412) 665-5000, BS 76 Edinboro Univ of PA; MA 80 Univ of Pittsburgh - Pittsburgh; Sp-Lang Path, Pittsburgh Pub Sch, **SLP**

McCabe, Robert B Dept Speech Lang & Aud Path, East Carolina University, Greenville, NC 27834, (919) 757-6961, BS 67 Univ of OR; MS 69 Univ of OR; Assoc Prof, E Carolina U, **SLP ACE**

McCabe, Ronald L 5505 West Pershing, Visalia, CA 93291, (209) 625-6761, BA 72 Wichita St Univ; MA 73 Wichita St Univ; Supervisor/Special Education, Visalia USD, **SLP**

McCafferty, Mrs Mary A M 225 Dover Street, Jefferson City, MO 65109, (314) 893-5502, BA 58 Univ of AR - Fayetteville; MS 64 Purdue Univ - West Lafayette; 88–Sp-Lang Path, St Mary's Health Ctr, **SLP**

McCaffrey, Mrs Anne Randler 737 Whittier Street, Idaho Falls, ID 83401, (208) 524-5376, BA 77 SUNY - Center at Buffalo; MA 79 Univ of CT; Sp/Lang Path, Joint Jefferson Co Sch Dist, **SLP**

McCaffrey, Helen A 3901 Ridgelea Drive, Austin, TX 78731, (512) 471-3841, BA 74 Trinity Univ; MS 76 Univ of OK Medical Center; Faculty, SW Texas St Univ Sp & Hrng Ctr, **A**

McCaffrey, Dr Patrick K 2219 Santa Clarta Avenue, Chico, CA 95928, (916) 895-6421, BA 69 Curry Coll; ME 71 Montclair St Coll; PH 75 (NS) OH Univ - Athens; Coord/SLP-Aud Prog, California State University, **SLP**

McCain, Mrs Kathleen C 725 3rd Street, Helena, MT 59601, (406) 443-7527, BA 69 Northern St Coll; MA 74 Univ of MT; Sp-Lang Path, Wmt Commun Care Inc, **SLP**

McCain, Mrs Permelia A 150 Indian Trail, North Haledon, NJ 07508, (201) 875-8820, BS 69 MS Coll; MA 71 Univ of AL- Tuscaloosa; ES 73 Univ of AL- Tuscaloosa; 88–Sp-Lang Path, Sussex Wantage Sch Dist, **SLP**

McCairns, Mrs Lillian O'Leary 20 Weatherby Avenue, Clarksboro, NJ 08020, (609) 423-7489, **SLP**

McCaleb, Mrs Mary L P O Box 237, Yellowstone Park, WY 82190, (307) 344-7772, ME 81 Western OR St Coll; 87–Sp-Lang Path, Livingston Sch Dist, **SLP**

McCaleb, Peggy Ann 18 Moorland, Cranston, RI 02905-3513, (401) 461-5945, BA 72 North Park Coll; MS 81 Southern IL Univ -Carbondale; Sp-Lang Path, New Eng Comm Svcs, **SLP**

McCall, Mrs Carolyn M 111 East Sierra Circle, San Marcos, TX 78666, (512) 245-2157, BS 71 Southwest TX St Univ; ME 73 Southwest TX St Univ; Dir Academic Learning Clinic, Southwest Texas State Univ, **SLP**

McCall, Colleen K 24 King Street, Danbury, CT 06811, (914) 528-8092, BS 77 SUNY - Coll at New Paltz; MS 82 Southern CT St Univ; SLP, Putnam Valley Sch Dist, **SLP**

McCall, Eleanor T 7350 57th Avenue, Seattle, WA 98115, (206) 281-6943, BA 63 Univ of WA; OM 73 Univ of WA; Sp-Lang Path, Seattle Pub Sch, **SLP**

McCall, Dr Gerald N Dept Of Hearing And Speech, Samar College Park, University Of Maryland, College Park, MD 20742, (301) 454-5832, BS 59 FL St Univ; MA 62 Northwestern Univ; PH 64 (Communication Disorders) Northwestern Univ; Professor, University of Maryland, **SLP F**

McCall, Gerard A 301 Cedar Road, Goldsboro, NC 27530, (919) 735-9146, BA 66 Univ of Notre Dame; OB 66 Univ of Notre Dame; MA 75 Univ of NC - Greensboro; Aud/Sp-Lang Path, Goldsboro ENT Associates P A, **SLP A**

McCall, J Louise Box 202, Adair, IL 61411, (309) 837-3911, MA 85 Western IL Univ; 85–Sch Aud, West Cen Illinois Spec Educ Coop, **A**

McCall, Judith Ann 492-2 Silver Oaks Drive, Kent, OH 44240, (216) 297-2771, BA 77 Youngstown St Univ; MA 82 Kent St Univ; Dir-Rehab Svcs-Aud/Neur, Robinson Mem Hosp, **A**

McCall, Kathryn J 2037 South Main, Moultrie, GA 31768, (912) 985-7408, BS 77 MS Univ for Women; MS 78 MS Univ for Women; Sp-Lang Path, Visiting Nurses Assoc, **SLP**

McCall, Mrs Laurie Elizabeth P O Box 834, Summerland, CA 93067, (805) 969-4026, BA 82 Univ of CA - Santa Barbara; MS 84 San Francisco St Univ; **SLP**

McCall, Margaret Ann 331 Elmora Avenue #5F, Elizabeth, NJ 07208, (201) 233-3720, BS 80 Western MI Univ; MA 82 Western MI Univ; Sp-Lang Path, UCP/Nassau Co, **SLP**

McCall, Mrs Nancy Demeter 301 Cedar Road, Goldsboro, NC 27530, (919) 731-2234, BS 76 East Carolina Univ; MS 79 East Carolina Univ; Sp-Lang Path, Home Health & Hospice Care Inc, **SLP**

McCall, Patricia Lynn 2800 N E 14th Street #241, Pompano Beach, FL 33062, (305) 395-8655, BS 83 East Carolina Univ; MS 84 East Carolina Univ; **A**

McCall, Rosanne Bennion 7800 Greenway Drive, Louisville, KY 40222, (502) 429-5407, BS 79 Brigham Young Univ; OM 80 Brigham Young Univ; SLP, **SLP**

McCallister, Mrs Kimberly Sue 7103 Fieldshire Court, Mechanicsville, VA 23111, (804) 746-2547, MS 84 James Madison Univ; Sp-Lang Path, Private Practice, **SLP**

McCallister, Robin R P O Box 793, Shady Spring, WV 25918, BA 77 Marshall Univ; MA 78 Marshall Univ; **SLP**

McCallum, James T, Jr P O Box 2182, Chapel Hill, NC 27515, (919) 966-1006, BA 67 Mercer Univ - Macon; ME 72 Univ of GA; 88–Asst Prof, Univ of North Carolina at Chapel Hill, **A**

McCaman, Gary E 409 North Columbia, Warsaw, IN 46580, (219) 269-2059, BS 77 Univ of IA; MA 79 Univ of IA; Aud, Hearing Shop, **A**

McCammond, Mrs Shirley Pease 410 West 33rd Street, Kearney, NE 68847, (308) 234-7183, BA 81 Kearney St Coll; MS 82 Kearney St Coll; Consul SLP, Good Samaritan Hosp, **SLP**

McCampbell, Pamela M Box 225, Westside, IA 51467, (712) 263-4625, BS 75 Northwest MO St Univ; MS 78 Univ of North TX; SLP, Wn Hills AEA 12, **SLP**

McCandless, Phillip Todd 2985 East Brookburn Road, Salt Lake City, UT 84109, (801) 272-8738, BS 85 Univ of UT; MS 87 Univ of UT; 88, Wasatch Aud Assoc

McCanless, Mrs Carol S P O Box 459, Oxford, GA 30267, (404) 786-4674, BA 59 Converse Coll; ME 79 Univ of GA; Sp-Lang Path, Newton Co Sch Syst, **SLP**

McCann, Mrs Ann H 21530 Via La Naranja, Yorba Linda, CA 92686, (714) 779-0631, BS 71 Univ of North TX; MS 73 Univ of North TX; Sp-Lang Path, Santa Ana USD, **SLP**

McCann, Beth 12 Woodside Villas, 7200 S W 8th Avenue, Gainesville, FL 32607, (904) 392-2041, BA 69; MA 73 Univ of ME - Orono; **SLP**

McCann, Carole J 6 Vermont Avenue, Worcester, MA 01603, (617) 765-9771, BS 76 Worcester St Coll; MA 77 Kean Coll of NJ; Sp-Lang Path, Harrington Mem Hosp, **SLP**

McCann, Donna S 7722 19th Avenue N E, Seattle, WA 98115, (206) 361-4259, ME 75 Univ of FL; Sp-Lang Path, Shoreline Sch Dist Seattle WA, **SLP**

McCann, James Edward, Jr 35 Arnold Street, New Bedford, MA 02740, (617) 994-1680, BA 82 Univ of RI; MS 84 Univ of RI; **A**

McCann, Janet S 8 Quailways, Creve Coeur, MO 63141, **SLP**

McCann, Kim L Box 124, Ulm, MT 59485, (406) 761-0471, BA 78 Univ of MT; MA 80 Univ of MT; 82–Sp-Lang Path, Joe Luckman PT Physical Ther & Sp Path, **SLP**

McCann, Mrs Lawrette Jane 3432 Southern Road, Richfield, OH 44286, (216) 375-3882, BS 68 Kent St Univ; MA 69 Univ of Denver; Sp-Lang Path, Akron Cty Hosp, **SLP**

McCanna, Donald Ashland College, Speech & Hearing Clinic, Ashland, OH 44805, (419) 289-5037, BA 57 Bowling Green St Univ; MA 60 Univ of MI - Ann Arbor; Assoc Prof Aud & SLP, Ashland Coll, **SLP A**

McCants, Diana J 17115 Red Oak Drive, Suite 101-A, Houston, TX 77090, (713) 537-0107, BS 75 Southern Methodist Univ; MS 76 Southern Methodist Univ; 78–Sp/Lang Path, Dj McCants Ms Ccc Pc, **SLP**

McCardle, Dr Peggy D Dept Pediatrics EFMP, Walter Reed Arm Med Ctr, Washington, DC 20307-5001, (202) 576-4185, BA 69 Juniata Coll; MA 74 PA St Univ - Univ Park; PH 80 (NS) PA St Univ - Univ Park; Sp-Lang Path, D Peds Wramc, **SLP ACE**

McCarney, Teresa D 3768 Hawkins N E, Albuquerque, NM 87109, (505) 345-2568, BS 70 FL St Univ; MA 74 Univ of FL; ED 76 (NS) Univ of FL; Asst Dir, Albuquerque Rehab Ctr, **SLP**

McCarron, Jeanne Marie 189-15 39th Avenue, Apt#114, Flushing, NY 11358, (718) 468-9000, BA 82 CUNY - Queens Coll; MS 83 Adelphi Univ; 86–Sp-Lang Path, Sunshine Developmental School, **SLP**

McCarron, Maureen P 76 Lozier Street, Rochester, NY 14611, (716) 546-2540, BS 75 SUNY - Coll at Geneseo; MA 78 SUNY - Center at Buffalo; Sp-Lang Path, Craig Dev Ctr, **SLP**

McCartan, Daniel Edward 1408 East Dayton Street, Madison, WI 53703, (608) 221-6620, BA 77 Univ of WA; MA 79 Univ of WA; Sp/Lang Path, Madison Metro Sd, **SLP**

McCartan, Dr Kathleen Child Development Department, Iowa State University, Ames, IA 50010, (515) 294-8957, BA 72 WA St Univ; MA 74 Univ of WA; PH 81 (NS) Univ of ID; Assoc Prof, IA St U, **SLP**

McCarthy, Mrs Bridget S Westchester Association For, Retarded Citizens, 567 Yonkers Avenue, Yonkers, NY 10704, (914) 963-1600, BA 74 CUNY - Lehman Coll; MS 76 Columbia Univ Teachers Coll; Sp-Lang Path, Westchester Assn Ret Citz, **SLP**

McCarthy, Christine M 4245 Pechin Street, Philadelphia, PA 19128, (215) 335-6120, BA 78 Temple Univ; MA 81 Temple Univ; Radiologic Tech, Nazareth Hosp, **A**

McCarthy, Mrs Constance 4560 West Larkspur Drive, Glendale, AZ 85304, (602) 995-1801, BS 53 Syracuse Univ; MS 56 Syracuse Univ; Sp-Lang Path, Washington Elementary Sch Dist, **SLP**

McCarthy, David Max Hearing Systems Co, 10802 Lazy Meadow, Houston, TX 77064, (713) 466-5351, BA 78 SUNY - Center at Buffalo; MA 81 SUNY - Center at Buffalo; Aud/Parent-Infant Adv, NW Harris Co Coop/Ed Hrng Imp, **A**

McCarthy, Mrs Debra Porco 43 Waddell Court, Wyckoff, NJ 07481, **SLP**

McCarthy, Diane Elizabeth HHD 95th MP BN, APO New York, NY 09086-3813, 011 49 621 738251, BS 85 SUNY - Coll at Fredonia; MS 86 SUNY - Coll at Fredonia; **A**

McCarthy, Diane L 2179 43rd Street S E, Grand Rapids, MI 49508, (313) 455-7143, BA 83 MI St Univ; MA 85 Eastern MI Univ; **SLP**

McCarthy, Eileen M 46 Ivy Lane West, East Windsor, NJ 08520, (609) 426-4042, BS 80 Trenton St Coll; MS 81 Rutgers St Univ - Newark; Sp-Lang Path, Private Practice, **SLP**

McCarthy, Dr Geraldine MacAvoy 6829 McLean Province Circle, Falls Church, VA 22043-1666, (301) 899-9490, BA 57 CUNY - Queens Coll; MA 75 Catholic Univ of America; ED 81 (Educational Admin) Vanderbilt Univ; 86–Prin, Prince George's Co PS, **SLP**

McCarthy, Mrs Jean D 535 Heritage Drive, Rochester, NY 14615, (716) 392-9471, BS 61 SUNY - Coll at Geneseo; MS 65 SUNY - Coll at Geneseo; Sp-Lang Path, Hilton Ctrl Sch, **SLP**

McCarthy, Mrs Jean Marie 204 Church Street #3-B, Boonton, NJ 07005, (201) 989-3118, BA 84 Univ of RI; MS 87 Univ of RI; SLP, Dover Gen Hosp, **SLP**

McCarthy, Mrs Kathleen Byrnes 2920 Davis Street, Oceanside, NY 11572-2028, (516) 536-9395, BA 78 Loyola Coll; MS 79 Loyola Coll; 88–Sp-Lang Path, Assoc Children Down's Syndrome, **SLP**

McCarthy, Mrs Linda Palin 101 Old Saratoga Road, Gansevoort, NY 12831, (518) 587-5048, BS 72 SUNY - Coll at Buffalo; MA 87 SUNY - Coll at Plattsburgh; 87–Sp-Lang Path, UCP Ctr of Tri Counties Inc, **SLP**

McCarthy, Mrs Mary 717 Bolivar Drive, San Jose, CA 95123, (408) 779-5220, BA 57 Univ of CA - Santa Barbara; Sp-Lang Path, Morgan Hill USD, **SLP ACE**

McCarthy, Mrs Mary C 506 Main Street, Childs, PA 18407, (717) 282-3135, BS 77 Marywood Coll; MS 78 Ithaca Coll; **SLP**

McCarthy, Mrs Mary E Payne 249 South Hoopes Avenue, Auburn, NY 13021, (315) 253-0301, BS 71 Nazareth Coll of Rochester; MS 72 SUNY - Coll at Geneseo, Sp-Lang Path, Auburn Enl Rgd Cty Sch Dist, **SLP**

McCarthy, Mary Melissa 28-L Brandywine Drive, Shrewsbury, MA 01545, (215) 631-9300, BS 83 Univ of NH; ME 86 Univ of VA - Charlottesville; **SLP**

McCarthy, Mary Pat 62 Ski Run Trail, Carroll Valley, PA 17320-3516, BS 85 Clarion Univ of PA; MS 86 Clarion Univ of PA; **SLP**

McCarthy, Mrs Monica Van Vleet 681 Ryan Lane #1-W, West Dundee, IL 60118, (815) 648-2606, BS 83 Marquette Univ; MS 84 Marquette Univ; Sp-Lang Path, Woodstock School District 200, **SLP**

McCarthy, Dr Patricia A University Of Georgia, 565 Aderhold Hall, Athens, GA 30602, (404) 542-1685, BS 72 Univ of IL - Urbana; MA 74 Univ of MD - College Park; PH 79 (Aud) Univ of Denver; Associate Professor, University of Georgia, **A**

McCarthy, Valerie Baldwin 3326 Hazelwood Drive, Fallston, MD 21047, (301) 356-0775, BA 68 MT St Agnes Coll; MS 71 Loyola Coll; 85–Sp-Lang Path, Baltimore County PS

McCarthy-O'Donnell, Mrs Lyn Ann 700 Norway Avenue, Trenton, NJ 08629, (609) 987-0099, BS 84 Trenton St Coll; MA 87 Trenton St Coll; **SLP**

McCartin-Clark, Marguerite 12 Eastwood Road, Miller Place, NY 11764, BA 76 CUNY - Queens Coll; MA 77 Hofstra Univ; Sp/Lang Path, Pilgrim Psychiatric Cen, **SLP**

McCartney, Mrs Jacqueline M 506-F Sarah Lane, Creve Coeur, MO 63141, (314) 532-1762, OB 86 Univ of MO - Columbia; OM 87 Univ of MO - Columbia; **SLP**

McCartney, Dr James H Dept Speech Path & Audiology, California State Univ, Sacramento, CA 95819, (916) 454-6601, BS 66 Geneva Coll; MA 68 Case Western Reserve Univ; PH 74 (NS) Univ of WA; Prof & Chmn of Dept, CA St U-Sacramento, **A**

McCartney, Mary Eileen 3904 Teacher's Lane #3, Orchard Park, NY 14127, (716) 662-9211, BS 83 CA Univ of PA; MS 87 CA Univ of PA; 87–Sp-Lang Path, People Inc, **SLP**

McCarty, Cynthia Ann Route 3 Box 106, Guthrie Center, IA 50115, (515) 747-2201, BS 74 Northwest MO St Univ; MA 75 Univ of SD - Vermillion; Sp-Lang Path, InSpeech Inc, **SLP**

McCarty, Janet Platt 6443 Old Chesterbrook Road, Mc Lean, VA 22101, (703) 448-7797, BS 77 Univ of VA - Charlottesville; ME 78 Univ of VA - Charlottesville; Sp-Lang Path Dir, Blue Ridge Sp & Hrng Cen, **SLP**

McCarty, Mary Margaret 11626 Maple Glen Court, Creve Coeur, MO 63146, (314) 926-2020, BS 74 Univ of IL - Urbana; MA 75 Wichita St Univ; Aud, Lawrence Levine MD, **SLP A**

McCarty, Patricia A P O Box 25051, Main Minneapolis Post Off, Minneapolis, MN 55440, BS 68 Univ of ND; MA 72 Univ of WA; ME 83 Univ of MN - Minneap-St Paul; Head Tchr, U of MN, **SLP**

McCarty, Thomas A 3208 Latouche B-5, Anchorage, AK 99508, (907) 276-5354, BA 75 Univ of MD - College Park; MA 77 Univ of MD - College Park; Aud, St of AK Commun Dis, **A**

McCarty-Leet, Patricia A 1320 Fitch Way, Sacramento, CA 95864, (916) 481-4441, BS 75 Saint Louis Univ; MA 76 Univ of IL - Urbana; **SLP**

McCarus, Carol H 254 Westwood, Birmingham, MI 48009, (313) 333-3983, BA 58 Univ of MI - Ann Arbor; MA 76 Wayne St Univ; Sp-Lang Path, Pontiac Mi Sch Dist, **SLP**

McCarver, Melodie Carol 011188, 2002 Belle Terrace #D, Knoxville, TN 37923, (615) 693-4063, BS 82 Univ of TN - Knoxville; MA 83 Univ of TN - Knoxville; Sp-Lang Path, Pro Health Svcs, **SLP**

McCaskey, Monica E F 6173 South Wasatch Drive, Ogden, UT 84403, (801) 627-4283, MS 88 Univ of UT; 88–Sp-Lang Path, Ped Rehab Ctr of Northern UT, **SLP**

McCaughey, Mrs Vicki Rowe 510 Westshore Drive, Madison, WI 53715, (608) 257-1464, MS 88 Marquette Univ; 88–Sp-Lang Path, Rehab Associates

McCaughrin, Dr Wendy B 36 Hillside Lane, Briarcliff, Mahomet, IL 61853, (217) 586-4356, MA 77 Wayne St Univ; MS 81 Univ of IL - Urbana; PH 88 (Educational Research) Univ of IL - Urbana; 88–Asst Prof, Univ of Illinois-Urbana, **SLP**

McCauley, Mrs Linda Hall 3405 25th Street #32, Parkersburg, WV 26101, (304) 428-6198, BA 84 Marshall Univ; MA 85 Marshall Univ; **SLP**

McCauley, Dr Rebecca Joan University Of Vermont, Dept Comm Science/Disorder, Allen House, Burlington, VT 05405, (802) 656-3861, BS 73 LA St Univ - Baton Rouge; MA 74 Univ of Chicago; PH 81 (Behavioral Sciences) Univ of Chicago; 86–Asst Prof, The Univ of Vermont, **SLP**

McCauley, Susanne Mary 1379 Randolph Avenue, St Paul, MN 55105, (612) 699-4014, BS 82 Saint Cloud St Univ; MS 84 Univ of WI - River Falls; 84–Sp-Lang Path, Midwest Rehabilitation Specialists, **SLP**

McCauley-Fisher, Mrs Heather R 1940 Pometacom Drive, Hanover, MD 21076, (301) 551-3258, BS 78 Univ of AZ; MS 80 Univ of AZ; SLP, Tucson USD, **SLP**

McCauliff, Mrs Claire A 21 Shawmont Lane, Stony Brook, NY 11790, (516) 689-8980, BA 71 CUNY - Queens Coll; MS 81 Adelphi Univ; **SLP**

McCharen, Martha Sanger 5209 Long Branch Lane, Edmond, OK 73034, (405) 799-5551, BA 67 Univ of OK - Norman; ME 86 Central St Univ

McChesney, Kathleen Ann 323 Ridge Point Circle, Bridgeville, PA 15017, (412) 221-0635, BS 80 Indiana Univ of PA; ME 86 Valdosta St Coll

McCladdie, Michelle R 6150,Buckingham Parkway, #107, Culver City, CA 90230, **A**

McClafferty, Kathleen M 3450 Wharton, Butte, MT 59701, (406) 494-4223, BS 74 Gonzaga Univ; MS 76 Eastern WA Univ; Sp-Lang Path, Butte School District #1, **SLP**

McClain, Linda S 622 Bunting Drive, Delray Beach, FL 33444, (305) 278-8395, BA 66 Univ of Science & Arts of OK; MA 67 Univ of MI - Ann Arbor; Sp-Lang Path, Private Practice, **SLP**

McClain, Sandra D 2047 Mac Arthur, Houston, TX 77030, (612) 823-6760, BS 61 Southern IL Univ-Edwardsvill; MA 65 Univ of IL - Urbana; Parish Assistant, St James Church, **SLP**

McClain, Sara C Glenrose Hospital, 10230 111th Avenue, Edmonton, AB, Canada T5G 0B7, (403) 471-2262, BA 46 IN Univ - Bloomington; MA 59 IN Univ - Bloomington; 79–Superv, Glenrose Rehab Hosp, **A**

McClain, Thora H 328 Sunfield West #4, Sun Prairie, WI 53590, (608) 249-2151, BS 74 Univ of WI - Eau Claire; MS 80 Univ of WI - Eau Claire; Sp-Lang Path, Ctrl WI Ctr Dev Dis, **SLP**

McClain, Wendy L 113 Bayberry Lane, Bedford, OH 44146, (216) 241-5643, BA 78 Cleveland St Univ; MA 79 Cleveland St Univ; Aud, Union Eye Care Ctr, **A**

McClamroch, Linda A Speech Pathology Dept, Magnolia Hospital, Alcorn Drive, Corinth, MS 38834, (601) 286-6961, BA 73 SUNY - Center at Stony Brook; OM 76 Univ of MS; Sp/Lang Path, Magnolia Hosp, **SLP**

McClanahan, Mrs Anne R 1665 Labrador, Costa Mesa, CA 92626, (714) 546-1500, MA 88 CA St Univ - Fullerton

McClanahan, Mrs Barbara A 341 Barberry, Cape Girardeau, MO 63701, (314) 335-5797, BS 76 Southeast MO St Univ; ME 82 Southeast MO St Univ; Sp-Lang Path, Cape Giradeau Pub Sch, **SLP**

McClanahan, Mrs Carolyn A Rural Route 5, Kirksville, MO 63501, (816) 665-7854, BS 70 Northeast MO St Univ; MA 71 Northeast MO St Univ; Sp-Lang Path, Private Practice, **SLP ACE**

McClanahan, Deana Sue 4715 N Black Canyon Hwy, #2055, Phoenix, AZ 85015, (602) 994-9667, BS 84 AZ St Univ; MS 87 AZ St Univ; 87–Aud, Drs Cohen & Weiss ENT's

McClanahan, Mrs Sharolyn A 7939 Village Drive, Cincinnati, OH 45242, (513) 489-5253, MS 88 Univ of TX - Dallas; 88–Sp-Lang Path, SpeechPath

McClanahan, Mrs Sharon Lynn Star Route 13-P, Poca, WV 25159, (301) 768-1982, BS 77 Marshall Univ; MA 80 Marshall Univ; SLP, Kanawha County Board of Educ, **SLP**

McClannahan, Sharon K 1111 Windsor Park Lane, Hendersonville, TN 37075, (615) 451-9810, BS 79 Middle TN St Univ; MS 87 Univ of TX - Dallas

McClary, Annette Edmonds 2273 Primrose Lane #2507, Clearwater, FL 34623, (813) 786-6697, BS 81 Middle TN St Univ; OM 83 Auburn Univ - Auburn; 83–Sp/Lang Path, Professional Health Services, **SLP ACE**

McClary, Barbara A 3410 South Ravenwood Drive, Augusta, GA 30907, (404) 863-2232, BA 77 SC St Coll; MA 79 SC St Coll; Sp-Lang Path, Gracewood State School & Hosp, **SLP**

McClatchie, Mrs Adeline D 5 Donald Drive, Orinda, CA 94563, (415) 428-3344, OB 62; OM 66; Coord Audiological Services, Childrens Hospital Medical Cen, **A**

McClatchy, Mrs Callie R 216 Station Avenue, Coopersburg, PA 18036, (215) 778-2240, BS 77 Bloomsburg Univ of PA; MS 78 Bloomsburg Univ of PA; Sp-Lang Path, Graduate Hosp, **SLP ACE**

McClean, Marsha D 3200 Willing, Fort Worth, TX 76110, (817) 336-8611, BS 68 East TX St Univ - Commerce; MA 72 IN Univ - Bloomington; Dept Head Communications, Easter Seal Society, **A**

McClean, Dr Michael D Graduate Dept Of Speech Path, University Of Toronto, 88 College Street, Toronto, ON, Canada M5G 1L4, BA 66 CA St Univ - Fresno; MA 69 Univ of WA; PH 71 (NS) Univ of WA; Assoc Professor, Univ of Toronto

McCleary, Diana S 1460 Camelot, Corona, CA 91720, (714) 558-5591, OB 64 Oberlin Coll; OM 65 Univ of WI - Madison; MA 80 CA St Univ - Fullerton; Sp-Lang Path, Santa Ana USD, **SLP**

McCleary, Mrs Gail Vontobel 545 Echo Lake Road, Watertown, CT 06795, (203) 584-7740, BS 82 Southern CT St Univ; MA 84 Southern CT St Univ; Regional School District 15, **SLP**

McClellan, Gary E 1515 7th Street, Oregon City, OR 97045, (503) 656-0601, BS 72 Brigham Young Univ; MA 77 Brigham Young Univ; Aud, ENT Cl of or Cty, **A**

McClellan, Mrs Lucile E 4304 Woodstone, Temple, TX 76502-3132, (806) 659-3761, BA 76 Southwest TX St Univ; MS 78 Southwest TX St Univ; **SLP**

McClellan, Max E VA Medical Center 126, 2100 Ridgecrest Drive S E, Albuquerque, NM 87108, (505) 265-1711, BS 60 SUNY - Coll at Buffalo; MA 64 Univ of IA; PH 65 (NS) Univ of IA; Chief Aud Sec, VA, **A**

McClellan, Sara Greer Box 116 County Road 550, Marquette, MI 49855, (906) 226-3206, BA 56 MI St Univ; MA 68 MI St Univ; Dir-Commun Rehab Dept, Marquette Gen Hosp, **SLP**

McClellan, Sherry Jaynes 59 Weatheridge Drive, Jackson, TN 38305, (615) 528-9205, BS 78 Murray St Univ; MS 79 Murray St Univ; Sp-Lang Path, Cumberland Mt Home Hlth Care, **SLP**

McClelland, Mrs Alison P 876 Old England Avenue, Winter Park, FL 32789, (407) 629-5925, BA 74 Univ of Central FL; MA 76 Univ of TN - Knoxville; **SLP**

McClelland, Mrs Brenda Kelly Route 1 Box 43-V, Portage Dessioux, MO 63373, (314) 899-1618, BS 76 Southern IL Univ-Edwardsvill; MS 87 Southern IL Univ-Edwardsvill; 87–Sp-Lang Path, Southern IL Sp & Hrng Assoc

McClelland, Dr Keener D 110 Southampton Road, Hattiesburg, MS 39401, (601) 583-4327, BA 61 Univ of TN - Knoxville; MA 64 Univ of TN - Knoxville; PH 68 (Psychoacoustics) Univ of FL; Owner, Audiology & Speech Associates, **A**

McClelland, Linda G 1065 Zang Street, Golden, CO 80401, (303) 273-6698, BS 64 Univ of WI - Madison; MA 74 Univ of Denver; 82–Cord of Related Service, Jefferson Co Sch Dist R-1, **SLP**

McClelland, Dr William D 905 Poplar Lane, Kirksville, MO 63501, (816) 785-4671, BS 51 Univ of KS; MS 53 Univ of KS; PH 69 (Sp Path and Aud) Univ of KS; Program Dir, NE MO St Univ, **SLP**

McClendon, Mrs Carol S North East Independent School, Office Of Student Resource, 10333 Broadway, San Antonio, TX 78217, (512) 657-8715, ME 72 Southwest TX St Univ; Sup of Sp-Path & Early Ch Ed, North East ISD, **SLP**

McClendon, Marian E 3315 Sacramento Street, Apartment 246, San Francisco, CA 94118-1911, BA 55 Univ of TX - Austin; MS 74 Columbia Univ Teachers Coll; **SLP**

McClendon, Mary Kay 12991 Middlebrook Square, San Diego, CA 92128, (619) 475-1666, BA 79 San Diego St Univ; MA 81 San Diego St Univ; Sp-Lang Path, Natl Sch Dist, **SLP**

McCleskey, Mrs Katrina Sanders 350 North Festival #1415, El Paso, TX 79912, (915) 833-7348, MA 88 Univ of TX - El Paso

McCleskey, Mrs Marla G 6220 Lakeview Drive, Paris, TX 75460, (214) 785-8686, BA 72 Wichita St Univ; MA 74 Wichita St Univ; 87–Sp-Lang Path, North Lamar ISD, **SLP**

McClintock, Mrs Ferne E ECHO Foundation, 2937 7th Avenue South, Birmingham, AL 35233, (205) 251-2193, MS 83 Univ of South FL; 88–Sp-Lang Path, ECHO Foundation, **SLP**

McClorin, Cynthia V P O Box 228, Lane, SC 29564, (803) 435-8195, MA 83 SC St Coll; SLP, Clarendon County District III, **SLP**

McCloskey, Deborah Burns 77 Shelley Drive, Mill Valley, CA 94941-1520, (415) 587-7529, BA 80 CA St Univ - Chico; MA 82 Univ of San Francisco; Sp-Lang Path, Private Practice, **SLP**

McCloskey, Mrs Debra Vitello 1 Tryon Avenue, Bldg 7 #8, Scotia, NY 12302, (518) 370-0872, ME 88 Coll of Saint Rose; Sp-Lang Path, Amsterdam Preschool Prog

McCloud, Elizabeth 6782 South Las Olas, Malibu, CA 90265, (805) 983-0444, BA 48 Univ of MI - Ann Arbor; MA 63 Univ of CA - Los Angeles; Dir, CA Hrng & Sp Cen, **SLP A**

McCloud, Mark Allen 11 Merrill Way, Newnan, GA 30263, (404) 882-1411, BA 82 West GA Coll; ME 84 GA St Univ; Chief of Dept of SLP, West GA Med Cntr, **SLP**

McClow-Kinsey, Sheila 2060 Cather Drive, Colorado Springs, CO 80915, (303) 473-3475, BA 73 Whittier Coll; MA 76 CA St Univ - Los Angeles; Sp-Lang Path, Rocky Mountain Rehab Center, **SLP**

McClowry, Dr Danny P 4013 Empedrado, Tampa, FL 33629, (813) 985-7711, BS 70 OH St Univ; ME 74 Southwest TX St Univ; PH 78 (NS) OH St Univ; Sp-Lang Path, Private Practice, **SLP**

McCluggage, Mrs Vicki Sue 5141 W 127th Terrace, Leawood, KS 66209, (913) 681-3631, BA 74 Harding Univ; MA 83 Whittier Coll; Clinic Supervisor, **SLP**

McClung, Dr Betty Beranek 3356 Harding, Dearborn, MI 48124, (313) 562-6000, BS 56 Univ of UT; MA 62 Univ of NE - Lincoln; PH 81 (NS) Wayne St Univ; Cooridnator SLP, VA Medical Ctr, **SLP**

McClung, Emily Weiss 81 Buffam Road, Pelham, MA 01002, (413) 549-1378, BS 77 Ithaca Coll; MA 82 Univ of MA - Amherst; Sp/Lang Path, Swift River Elem Sch, **SLP**

McClung, Mrs Janice Wester 733 HI Lo Way, Tallahassee, FL 32308, (904) 893-1265, MS 80 FL St Univ; Sp-Lang Path, Leon County School System, **SLP**

McClung, Linda N 4716 Waterwich Point Road, Orlando, FL 32806, (305) 857-1136, BS 71 FL St Univ; MS 72 FL St Univ; **SLP**

McClure, Mrs Bernadette A Ross 404 Lexington Drive, Aliquippa, PA 15001-9551, (412) 378-9935, BS 76 Edinboro Univ of PA; MA 77 Edinboro Univ of PA; 77–Sp-Lang Path, Beaver Valley Inter Unit, **SLP**

McClure, Mrs Elisa Markle 816 Oakland Park Avenue, Columbus, OH 43224, (614) 447-8547, BA 85 OH St Univ; MA 87 OH St Univ

McClure, Mrs Janice K 3303 Tiley Drive N E, Albuquerque, NM 87110-1743, (505) 275-2451, **SLP**

McClure, Lavonne K 4 East White Oak, Arlington Heights, IL 60005, (312) 593-1977, BA 70 Univ of WI - Madison; MS 74 Univ of IL - Urbana; SLP, Spec Ed Dist of Lake Co, **SLP**

McClure, Mrs Lisa Marie 109 North Warren Street, Orwigsburg, PA 17961, (717) 366-8898, BS 85 Marywood Coll; MS 86 Bloomsburg Univ of PA; 87–Sp-Lang Path, Pottsville Hosp & Warne Cl, **SLP**

McClure, Mrs Mona W 7826 La Manga, Dallas, TX 75248, (214) 233-5326, BS 61 Abilene Christian Univ; MA 63 Univ of Houston - Univ Park; **SLP**

McClure, Pamela Sue 300 Clark Street #8, Saline, MI 48176, (313) 429-1524, BA 83 Eastern MI Univ; MA 84 Eastern MI Univ; **SLP**

McClure, Ramona Anne 2922 Cascade Drive, Ann Arbor, MI 48104, (313) 572-5121, BA 78 IN Univ - Bloomington; MA 80 IN Univ - Bloomington; 88–Sp-Lang Path, Cath McAuley Health Ctr, **SLP ACE**

McClure, Mrs Susan D 108 Robins Drive, Roswell, NM 88201, (505) 623-8180, BA 72 Univ of NM; MS 74 Univ of NM; SLP, Roswell ISD, **SLP**

McClure-Beck, Jane A 529 Miles, Centralia, MO 65240, (314) 682-3506, BS 78 Southwest MO St Univ; MA 80 Univ of MO - Columbia; Sp-Lang Path, Boone Co Rvi Sch, **SLP**

McClurg, Lisa B 410 Pleasant Hill Lane, Sierra Madre, CA 91024, (818) 355-1714, BA 83 CA St Univ - Los Angeles; MA 85 CA St Univ - Los Angeles; Aud, Cigna Healthplans of Sn Ca, **A**

McClurken, Rita W 250 Wenner Way, Fort Washington, PA 19034, (215) 643-6207, BA 72 Univ of Northern CO; MA 73 Univ of Northern CO; **A**

McClurkin, Robert H Kay Elemetrics Corp, 12 Maple Avenue, Pine Brook, NJ 07058, (201) 227-2000, BA 76 Univ of NC - Chapel Hill; MS 80 Univ of NC - Chapel Hill; Product Specialist, Kay Elemetrics Corp, **SLP**

McCluskey, Mrs Kathryn Marie 3610 S W 90th Avenue, Portland, OR 97225, (503) 228-6479, MS 84 Portland St Univ; Sp-Lang Path, North Clackamas School Dist, **SLP**

McColgin, Leslie S R R 1 Box 146, Cunningham, KY 42035, (502) 674-5654, BS 75 IL St Univ - Normal; MS 77 IL St Univ - Normal; 88–Sp-Lang Path, Lourdes Home Care, **SLP**

McCollister, Mrs Faye Perry Box 313 University Station, 1720 7th Avenue South, Birmingham, AL 35294, (205) 934-5448, BA 65 Univ of AL- Tuscaloosa; MA 67 Univ of AL- Tuscaloosa; ED 87 (Education); Coord of Aud Serv, Cen for Dev & Lrng Dis, **A**

McCollom, Herbert F, Jr Hearing Services Of Lancaster, 202 Butler Avenue, Lancaster, PA 17601, (717) 393-5761, BA 53 PA St Univ - Univ Park; ME 59 Franklin & Marshall Coll; 77–Owner, Hrng Ser of Lancaster, **SLP A ACE**

McCollough, Yvonne D 600 Edgewater Bldg, Apartment 204-C, Foster City, CA 94404, **SLP**

McCollum, Mrs Carolyn W 1431 Millington Road, Columbus, GA 31904, (404) 324-3320, ME 84; SLP, Fort Benning Dependents School, **SLP**

McCollum, Diane Elaine 510 Hale Court, Burlington, NC 27215, (919) 227-3343, MA 87 Univ of NC - Greensboro

McComas, Anne W 15935 Raven Rock Road, Brookfield, WI 53005, (703) 931-6071, BS 74 Northwestern Univ; MS 75 Univ of WI - Madison; Sp/Lang Path, Ridley and Fill Sp Lang Assoc, **SLP**

McComas, Mrs Karen Leigh 4 Louie Court, Barboursville, WV 25504, (304) 696-3640, BA 77 Marshall Univ; MA 78 Marshall Univ; 86–Asst Prof, Marshall Univ, **SLP**

McComas, Mrs Robin Lynn 14 Washington Court, Barboursville, WV 25504, (304) 736-4737, BA 79 Marshall Univ; MA 83 Marshall Univ; **SLP**

McComb, Kathryn F 1107 Taurus Drive, Edmond, OK 73034, **SLP**

McCombs, Dr Richard P Roosevelt Hear & Speech Center, 6300 9th Avenue N E, Seattle, WA 98115, (206) 523-3400, PH 85 (Aud) Univ of WA; 85–Dir, Roosevelt Hearing & Speech Ctr, **A**

McConaghy, Mrs Kathleen D 962 Merrimac Circle, Naperville, IL 60540, (312) 420-7013, BS 70 Marquette Univ; MA 71 Univ of IL - Urbana; **A**

McConahy, Regina Ellen 2370 Ansley, Alliance, OH 44601, (216) 489-0800, BS 83 Miami Univ - Oxford; MS 85 Miami Univ - Oxford; **SLP**

McConahy, Mrs Renee L 4629 Vorhies Road, Ann Arbor, MI 48105, (313) 697-6385, BS 78 Eastern MI Univ; MA 79 Eastern MI Univ; Teacher Speech-Lang Impaired, Van Buren Public Schools, **SLP**

McConaughey, Lori A 777 South Federal Highway, Jasmine 203, Pompano Beach, FL 33062, (305) 941-1452, BA 77 West Liberty St Coll; MS 78 WV Univ; Sp/Lang Path, Broward Co Schs, **SLP**

McConkie, Mrs Karen E 1021 Vassar, Alma, MI 48801, (517) 463-5911, BA 81 MI St Univ; MA 84 Central MI Univ; **A**

McConnell, Betty D 104 Surrey Hill Point, Hendersonville, TN 37075, (615) 822-0622, BA 66 Univ of TN - Knoxville; MS 67 Vanderbilt Univ; Sp-Path, At Home Hlth Care, **SLP**

McConnell, Diane 325 East Meadow Lane, Monrovia, CA 91016, (818) 918-3131, MA 87 CA St Univ - Los Angeles; **SLP**

McConnell, Prof Freeman E 3828 Richland Avenue, Nashville, TN 37205, (615) 383-8264, BS 39 Univ of IL - Urbana; MA 46 Univ of IL - Urbana; PH 50 (Aud) Northwestern Univ; Prof Emeritus, Vanderbilt U, **A F H LM**

McConnell, Mrs Jill B Box 68, Firth, NE 68358, (402) 791-5344, BA 65 Lebanon Valley Coll; MA 75 Cleveland St Univ; Consult, St of NE, **SLP**

McConnell, Mrs Leisa Kay 3618 Avenue M, Kearney, NE 68847-3256, (308) 743-2401, **SLP**

McConnell, Nancy L 1459 Woodberry Avenue, San Mateo, CA 94403, (415) 345-3948, BA 80 San Francisco St Univ; MS 82 San Francisco St Univ; Sp-Lang Path, San Mateo City Sch District, **SLP**

McConnell, Patricia 964 Woodlyn Drive North, Cincinnati, OH 45230, (513) 742-2200, MS 77 Univ of South FL; Sp-Lang Path, Hamilton Co Offi of Ed, **SLP**

McConnell-Stephen, Patricia Lynn 2956 Ridgewood Avenue, Cincinnati, OH 45213-1060, (513) 531-5999, BS 84 Univ of Cincinnati; MA 86 Univ of Cincinnati; 86–Sp-Lang Path, Kenton Co PS, **SLP**

McCool, Mrs Kathryn B 104 Halstead Road, Ocean Springs, MS 39564, (601) 875-5847, BS 77 Univ Southern MS-Hattiesburg; MS 78 Univ Southern MS-Hattiesburg; Sp-Lang Path, Ocean Springs Sch Dist, **SLP**

McCool, Mrs Linda Jean 33852 Del Obispo Street, Apartment 28, Dana Point, CA 92629-2111, (714) 661-4913, BA 75 Montclair St Coll; MA 82 Univ of Central FL; Clinical Supervisor, InSpeech Inc, **SLP ACE**

McCool, Mrs Patti J 1540 Thomas Lake Pointe Rd, Apartment 101, Eagan, MN 55122, (612) 681-0025, BS 78 Univ of WI - Stevens Point; MS 80 Univ of WI - Madison; Sp-Lang Path, **SLP**

McCord, Christine Jo 902 Williamsburg Drive, Hendersonville, TN 37075, (615) 824-5615, BS 81 Ball St Univ; MA 83 Ball St Univ; 87–Sp-Lang Path, Rebound Inc, **SLP**

McCord, Jill Stewart Route 1 Box 495, Woodland, AL 36280, (205) 449-6491, BS 84 Auburn Univ - Auburn; MS 86 Auburn Univ - Auburn; Sp-Lang Path, Chambers Co Bd of Ed, **SLP**

McCorkel, Mrs Stephanie Lynn 8115 Tifton Road, Charlotte, NC 28226, (704) 541-8664, BS 78 Southern IL Univ -Carbondale; MS 81 Southern IL Univ-Edwardsvill; Sp-Lang Path, Jamaica Consol School Dist 12, **SLP**

McCormack, Jane Ellen 562 South Main Street, Manchester, NH 03102, (603) 641-6336, BS 83 Univ of NH; MS 85 Ithaca Coll; **SLP**

McCormack, Joan E New England Rehab Hospital, Comm Disorders Dept, Rehabilitation Way, Woburn, MA 01801, (617) 935-5050, BS 78 Northeastern Univ; MA 80 Univ of CT; Dir Commun Dis, New Eng Rehab Hosp, **A**

McCormack, Judy J 5321 Hollow Bend, Garland, TX 75043, **SLP**

McCormack, Julie Ellen Singapore Association For The Deaf, 227 Mountbatten Road, Singapore, Singapore 1439, BA 82 Univ of CO - Boulder; MS 87 Univ of WA; 88–Aud, S'pore Assn f/t Deaf

McCormack, Susan M 22-14 Williamsburg Court, Shrewsbury, MA 01545, (508) 856-2398, BS 80 Marywood Coll; MA 82 MI St Univ; Sp-Lang Path, Univ of MA Med Ctr, **SLP**

McCormick, Mrs Candace A 8929 Larchwood Court, St Louis, MO 63126, (314) 851-0094, BS 77 Fontbonne Coll; MS 78 Fontbonne Coll; Sp-Lang Path, Spec Sch Dist of St Louis Co, **SLP**

McCormick, Cecilia M 1408 East Dayton Street, Madison, WI 53703, (608) 263-5824, BA 76 Catholic Univ of America; MS 79 Univ of WA; PH 87 (Early Childhood Special Education) Univ of WI - Madison; Lecturer, U of WI, **SLP**

McCormick, Eileen P 19 Skycrest Avenue, East Providence, RI 02914, (508) 679-7026, BA 80 Univ of RI; MA 82 Univ of MA - Amherst; Sp-Lang Path, Charlton Mem Hosp, **SLP**

McCormick, Mrs Frances H 2894 Carrousel Court, Stone Mountain, GA 30087, (404) 284-0600, BS 74 Univ Southern MS-Hattiesburg; MS 76 Univ of MS; Sp-Lang Path, DeKalb Schs, **SLP**

McCormick, Dr Glen P Chief Aud & Speech Path Serv, VA Medical Service, P O Box 92, Butler, PA 16001, (412) 287-4781, BA 59 WV Univ; MA 60 WV Univ; PH 65 (NS) Purdue Univ - West Lafayette; Ch Aud & SLP Serv, VA Med Cen, **SLP A**

McCormick, Jean Tedford 2310 Bengal Lane, Plano, TX 75023, (214) 867-0010, BS 79 Miami Univ - Oxford; MS 80 Miami Univ - Oxford; 88–Sp-Lang Path, Plano ISD, **SLP**

McCormick, Kathleen Ann 59-A Mount Vernon Street, Boston, MA 02108, (617) 720-6735, BS 82 Boston Univ; MS 84 Emerson Coll; Sp-Lang Path, Spaulding Rehab Hosp, **SLP**

McCormick, Mrs Mary Helen 1901 Nipper Road, Raleigh, NC 27614, (919) 876-2418, BS 76 Marquette Univ; MS 77 Marquette Univ; 87–Sp-Lang Path, Wake Cnty Pub Schools, **SLP**

McCormick, Michael John 11121 Normandy Place #1, Tampa, FL 33617-2919, (813) 870-1931, BA 80 Univ of Central FL; MA 82 Univ of Central FL; Sp/Lang Path, Bay Area Rehab Inc, **SLP**

McCormick, Mrs Suzanne 205 Hilltop Lane, Brea, CA 92621, (714) 731-7331, BA 78 Humboldt St Univ; MA 80 Humboldt St Univ; 87–Sp-Lang Path/Asst Dir, Riler's Sp & Lang I, **SLP ACE**

McCormick, Mrs Wendy Lu 1810 N W Broadway, Albany, OR 97321, (503) 928-1712, BS 73 Univ of WI - Milwaukee; MS 75 Univ of WI - Milwaukee; SLP, First Christian Sch Dist, **SLP**

McCormick-Dunsmore, Virginia 825 South Harvey, Oak Park, IL 60304, (312) 567-5650, BS 83 Western MI Univ; MA 85 Memphis St Univ; 88–Aud, Mercy Hosp, **A**

McCornack, Mrs Mariann W 26011 Fairfield, Warren, MI 48089, (313) 582-6232, BS 57 OH St Univ; ME 63 Boston Univ; 74–Sp-Lang Path, Dearborn Pub Sch, **SLP**

McCorry, Mrs Lori Eisenberg 200 Scottsdale Drive, Coraopolis, PA 15108, (412) 728-6410, BA 78 SUNY - Coll at Brockport; MA 81 Univ of Denver; Aud, Kenneth S Skolnick MD, **A**

McCorry, Mrs Suzanne B 111 9th Avenue, Belmar, NJ 07719, (201) 240-2400, BS 84 Ithaca Coll; MA 85 Northwestern Univ; Audiologist, Ellen B Gerner, **A**

McCort, Tricia Anne P O Box 1081, Shepherdstown, WV 25443, (304) 263-0811, BA 75 Univ of MD - College Park; MS 81 Loyola Coll; Sp-Lang Path, VA Med Ctr, **SLP**

McCoskey, Anita M Box 223, Altamont, KS 67330, (316) 784-5726, MA 86 Wichita St Univ; 88–Sp-Lang Path, Tri-Co Special Educ Cooperative No 607, **SLP**

McCowan, Leslie S 4 Hemlock Drive, Hopkinton, MA 01748, (508) 435-5881, BS 78 Univ of NH; MS 79 PA St Univ - Univ Park; **A**

McCowen, Mrs Judith E 8908 Moye, El Paso, TX 79925, (915) 778-4209, BA 78 Univ of TX - El Paso; MA 81 Univ of TX - El Paso; Sp-Lang Path, El Paso ISD, **SLP**

McCown, Mrs Barbara Lorraine 7143 Parkside Place, Rancho Cucamonga, CA 91701, (213) 965-2331, MA 84 Whittier Coll; SLP, Charter Oak USD, **SLP**

McCown, Mrs Donna E 5615 Waterview, Arlington, TX 76016, (817) 277-0100, BA 75 Baylor Univ; MA 76 Baylor Univ; Sp-Lang Path, Private Practice, **SLP**

McCown, Mrs Jacqueline 1183 Dover Center Road, Westlake, OH 44145, (216) 574-8514, BA 70 Cleveland St Univ; MA 71 Cleveland St Univ; Sp/Lang Path, Cleveland Pub Sch, **SLP**

McCown, Marilyn C 4236 Paces Ferry Road, Atlanta, GA 30339, (404) 434-7193, BS 73 Univ of TN - Knoxville; ME 78 GA St Univ; Sp-Lang Path, Vinings Sp-Lang Cl, **SLP**

McCoy, Barbara Isabel 17 N 665 Hidden Hills Trl, West Dundee, IL 60118, (312) 428-7408, MA 86 Northern IL Univ - De Kalb; 86–Sp-Lang Path, Comm Consolidated Sch Dist #54, **SLP**

McCoy, Dr Carolyn Hearing & Speech Services, Dr Carolyn McCoy, 1001 Windsor Drive PO Box 1504, Lodi, CA 95241-1504, (209) 946-2381, BS 67 Univ of OR; MS 68 CO St Univ; PH 77 (Aud) Univ of OR; Aud/Sp-Lang Path, Private Practice, **SLP A**

McCoy, Catherine Gordon 9859 Siegen Lane, Baton Rouge, LA 70810, (504) 767-2057, BS 84 LA St Univ - Baton Rouge; MA 86 LA St Univ - Baton Rouge

McCoy, Christine 5209 Barton Road, Madison, WI 53711, **SLP**

McCoy, Mrs Ellen D 7239 Steamerbell Row, Columbia, MD 21045, (301) 381-4489, OB 79 Muhlenberg Coll; MS 85 Syracuse Univ; **SLP**

McCoy, Lois T R Route #2 Box 268, South Royalton, VT 05068, BA 73 Mount Union Coll; MS 82 Southern CT St Univ; 88–Sp-Lang Path, Hartford Sch Dist, **SLP**

McCoy, Lou Ann 2904 S E Yamhill, Portland, OR 97214, (503) 266-2744, BS 75 Northern IL Univ - De Kalb; MS 77 Portland St Univ; Sp-Lang Path, Canby Elem Sch Dist 86, **SLP**

McCoy, Dr Malcolm B 270 Cedar Creek Drive, Athens, GA 30605, (404) 549-4801, BA 49 Univ of VA - Charlottesville; MA 51 Univ of VA - Charlottesville; PH 54 (NS) Case Western Reserve Univ; Aud, Private Practice, **A**

McCoy, Margaret Jane 9734 Bevlyn, Houston, TX 77025, (713) 666-2625, **A**

McCoy, Mary K 21410 9th Street S E, Bothell, WA 98021, (206) 361-4238, BA 66 Western WA Univ; MS 74 Univ of WA; Dir, Scottish Rite Ctr for Sp Dis, **SLP**

McCoy, Michael J 22404 Charlotte Drive, Torrance, CA 90505-2170, (213) 644-4478, BA 76 CA St Univ - Long Beach; MA 78 CA St Univ - Long Beach; SLP, Los Angeles Co Supt Sch, **SLP**

McCoy, Nancy Ellen 2250 Lake View Avenue, Los Angeles, CA 90039, (213) 693-0771, BA 81 CA St Univ - Northridge; MA 83 CA St Univ - Northridge; Aud, Whittier Coll, **A**

McCoy, Noreen Lynn 15 Michigan Road, Bellerose, NY 11001, (516) 488-2815, BS 85 Saint John's Univ - Jamaica; MS 86 Adelphi Univ; 86–Sp-Lang Path, Sch for Lang & Comm Dev, **SLP**

McCoy, Mrs Patricia Helen 303 Evergreen, Kosciusko, MS 39090, (601) 289-7193, BS 73 Bowling Green St Univ; MA 82 Bowling Green St Univ; 86–Sp-Lang Path, Kosciusko Mun Separate Sch, **SLP**

McCracken, Mrs Patrice Marie 5201 Marcel Drive, Fairfield, OH 45014, (513) 829-6300, BS 73 Eastern IL Univ; MA 77 Univ of IL - Urbana; Sp-Lang Path, Fairfield School District, **SLP**

McCracken, Mrs Rosanne D 10523 Des Moines Avenue, Northridge, CA 91326, (818) 360-8643, BS 57 Northwestern Univ; Sp-Lang Path, Los Angeles USD, **SLP**

McCracken, Wendy Margaret 918 20th Avenue Place #9, Coralville, IA 52241-5098, (319) 338-2288, BA 80 McGill Univ - Quebec; MS 86 Purdue Univ - West Lafayette; 86, Univ of Iowa

McCrarey, Mrs Rebecca Ann 314 Shetland Lane, Lexington, SC 29072-8232, (803) 252-2538, **SLP**

McCrary, Debra S 471 Woodland Hills, Tuscaloosa, AL 35405, (205) 348-7131, BA 74 Univ of AL- Tuscaloosa; MA 75 Univ of AL- Tuscaloosa; Coord-Preschool Ut-U of Al, Tuscaloose Co Schs, **SLP**

McCrary, Judith Anne 717 North Midvale Blvd #4, Madison, WI 53705, (608) 238-8514, MS 88 Univ of WI - Madison

McCraven, Patricia Leslie 9219 South Euclid, Chicago, IL 60617, (312) 754-1644, BS 83 Northwestern Univ; MA 85 Univ of IL - Urbana; Early Childhood Sp-Lang Path, School District #161, **SLP**

McCraw, Virginia L Kendall Center, 4015 W Wendover Avenue, Greensboro, NC 27407, (919) 373-7563, BS 79 Atlantic Christian Coll; MS 81 Univ of NC - Chapel Hill; Sp-Lang Path, Guilford County, **SLP**

McCray, Jeri L 10150 East Virginia Avenue, Bldg 2 #303, Denver, CO 80231, **SLP**

McCray, Mrs Phyllis E 2039 Challeux Drive West, Jacksonville, FL 32225, (904) 261-0556, BA 52 LA St Univ - Baton Rouge; MA 53 LA St Univ - Baton Rouge; 88–Exec Dir, Sp-Lang & Hrng Svcs, **SLP**

McCrea, Dr Elizabeth S 700 South Jordan Avenue, Bloomington, IN 47401, (812) 335-6251, BA 66 IN Univ - Bloomington; ME 69 Univ of VA - Charlottesville; PH 80 (Supervisory Process) IN Univ - Bloomington; 87–Clin Asst Prof, Indiana Univ, **SLP**

McCready, Carolyn V 4942 Harvest Road, McLeansville, NC 27301, (919) 334-5184, BA 65 Univ of AL- Tuscaloosa; MA 67 Case Western Reserve Univ; Cl Superv, U O Nc Greensboro, **SLP**

McCready, Lynn R 20-D Shore Drive, Peabody, MA 01960, (401) 277-5485, BA 75 Univ of RI; MA 77 Catholic Univ of America; SLP, North Shore Spec Ed Consortium, **SLP**

McCreary, Dawn Evans 6810 25th Avenue, Hyattsville, MD 20782, (202) 576-6161, BA 74 Marshall Univ; MS 77 Howard Univ; Sp/Lang Path, Sharpe Hlth Sch, **SLP**

McCrory, Ana Moran 4719 110th Avenue N E, Kirkland, WA 98033, (206) 822-5887, BA 84 Univ of OR; MA 85 Univ of OR; Sp-Lang Path, **SLP**

McCrory, Mrs Barbara G 408 Ark Lane, Petal, MS 39465, (601) 764-2033, BS 73 Univ Southern MS-Hattiesburg; MS 79 Univ Southern MS-Hattiesburg; Sp-Lang Path, Petal Mun Separate Sch Dist, **SLP**

McCrory, Mrs Elizabeth Flynn 196 Brenton Drive, Newark, OH 43055, (614) 653-5501, BS 81 OH St Univ; MA 83 OH St Univ; Sp-Lang Path, Newark Speech Services, **SLP**

McCroskey, Dr Robert L 7413 Pagent Lane, Wichita, KS 67206, (316) 689-3240, BS 48 OH St Univ; MA 52 OH St Univ; PH 56 (NS) OH St Univ; Prof Commun Dis, Wichita St U, **SLP A F**

McCrossen, Karen B 36 Long Park Drive, Rochester, NY 14612, **SLP**

McCue, Susan Kay 23 Block 6 Enue S E, 742 Kingsmore Cres S W, Calgary, AB, Canada T2V 2H8, (403) 255-6165, BS 83 Brigham Young Univ; MA 84 Brigham Young Univ; **SLP**

McCuiston, Patricia Robinson 1660 Ryan Avenue, Murray, KY 42071-9804, (502) 753-9983, BS 83 Murray St Univ; MS 86 Murray St Univ; 88–Sp-Lang Path, Marshall County Bd of Educ, **SLP**

McCullagh, Mrs Bette C 5914 Wild Plum Road, Crystal Lake, IL 60014, (815) 459-5280, MS 81 IL St Univ - Normal; Sp/Lang Path, Easter Seals for McHenry Co, **SLP**

McCulley, Mrs Marilyn Joy 4586 Stauffer Avenue S E, Kentwood, MI 49508, (616) 281-1963, **SLP**

McCulloch, Barbara J 2435 Scott Avenue, Lincoln, NE 68506, (402) 464-8385, BA 67 Univ of NE - Lincoln; MA 68 Univ of NE - Lincoln; Aud, Great Plains ENT/HNS Inst, **A**

McCulloch, Frances Harriet 835 23rd Avenue North, St Petersburg, FL 33704, (813) 894-6903, MS 86 Univ of South FL; 86 Sp-Lang Path, Pinellas Co Sch Bd, **SLP**

McCulloch, Mrs Joan Helene 22524 Jameson Drive, Woodland Hills, CA 91364, (213) 840-7900, BA 76 Occidental Coll; MS 78 Vanderbilt Univ; Sp-Lang Path, Inaba Foto Consultants, **SLP**

McCullough, Brenda Carol 8972 Allenbrook Way, San Diego, CA 92103, (619) 484-6369, BS 85 FL St Univ; MS 87 FL St Univ; **SLP**

McCullough, Cheryl Ann 3221 Apt #C, Zuider Zee Drive, Winston-Salem, NC 27127, (919) 785-9630, MA 87 OH St Univ; SLP, InSpeech Inc, **SLP**

McCullough, Mrs Eleanor B Route 1 Box 137, Winfield, AL 35594, (205) 487-2305, BS 75 Univ of Montevallo; MS 77 Univ of Montevallo; Sp-Lang Path, Winfield City Bd of Ed, **SLP**

McCullough, Dr June Antablin 6168 Springer Way, San Jose, CA 95123-5129, (408) 578-7423, BA 78 CA St Univ - Fullerton; MA 79 CA St Univ - Fullerton; PH 86 (Hrng Science) Univ of IA; 88–Aud, California Ear Inst, **A**

McCullough, Maryann Desch 434 Norristown Road, Horsham, PA 19044, (215) 247-4404, BA 84 Univ of Pittsburgh - Pittsburgh; MA 86 Temple Univ-Tyler Sch of Art; 86–Aud, Otolaryngology Associates Inc, **A**

McCullough, Mrs Pamela S 2883 Carrousel Court, Stone Mountain, GA 30087, (404) 292-7272, BS 70 Univ of GA; ME 74 Univ of GA; 71–Sp/Lang Path, Dekalb Co Bd of Ed, **SLP**

McCullough, Patricia J 1025 Wonderview Drive, Dunlap, IL 61525, (309) 243-7128, **SLP**

McCullough, Mrs Peggy Crooks 5425 Martis Court, El Sobrante, CA 94803, (415) 222-2161, BS 80 Univ of IA; MA 81 Univ of IA; SLP, Richmond USD, **SLP**

McCune, Ellen Carol 3-C Kingcrest Court, Baltimore, MD 21207, (703) 434-6585, BS 79 Towson St Univ; MS 84 James Madison Univ; Sp-Lang Path, Baltimore Co Board of Ed, **SLP**

McCurdy, Joanne Lee 136 Cynthia Drive, Hackettstown, NJ 07040, (201) 234-3803, BS 79 Bloomsburg Univ of PA; MS 80 Syracuse Univ; **SLP**

McCurry, Jeanne K 1421 West Norwood, Chicago, IL 60660, **SLP**

McCusker, Ann 2636 Enterprise Road E, Apartment C-13, Clearwater, FL 34619, (813) 799-6858, BA 80 Loyola Coll; MS 81 Loyola Coll; Sp-Lang Path, Pinnellas Co Sch, **SLP ACE**

McCutcheon, Gloria K 1201 W McGaffey #12, Roswell, NM 88201, (505) 625-1525, BA 57 Univ of North TX; MA 63 Univ of Denver; Sp-Lang Path, Roswell ISD, **SLP**

McDade, Dr Hiram L Dept Communicative Disorders, Univ Of South Carolina, Columbia, SC 29208, (803) 777-4813, BA 70 Baldwin-Wallace Coll; MA 74 Univ of TN - Knoxville; PH 76 (Sp Science) Univ of TN - Knoxville; Assoc Prof, U of SC, **SLP**

McDaniel, Adalyn R 50 East Main Street, Uniontown, PA 15401, (412) 437-3887, BS 74 WV Univ; MS 75 WV Univ; Sp-Lang Path, Sewickley Valley Hosp, **SLP**

McDaniel, Mrs Ann S R R 2 Box 287, Shelbyville, IN 46176, (317) 392-4429, BS 70 IN Univ - Bloomington; MA 71 IN Univ - Bloomington; Sp/Lang Path, Self Employed, **SLP**

McDaniel, Barbara C 1401 Timberwood Drive, Columbia, TN 38401, (615) 381-1111, BA 71 Memphis St Univ; MA 72 Memphis St Univ; 84–Sp-Lang Path, Maury Reg Hosp, **SLP**

McDaniel, David Michael 1222 Trotwood Avenue #411, Columbia, TN 38401, (615) 381-0843, BS 70 AR St Univ; MA 72 Memphis St Univ; Aud, Robert Stewart MD, **A**

McDaniel, Mrs Diane F Route 7 Box 126, Haleyville, AL 35565, (205) 486-3405, BS 70 Auburn Univ - Auburn; MS 75 Univ of Montevallo; 88–Sp-Lang Path, Haleyville Cty Bd of Ed, **SLP**

McDaniel, Jane R G 3220 Anchor Drive, Plano, TX 75023, (214) 867-4719, BA 77 CA St Univ - Sacramento; MA 79 CA St Univ - Sacramento; Sp-Lang Path, Private Practice, **SLP**

McDaniel, Kathy Johnson 1920 Jefferson Street, Conway, AR 72032, (501) 968-3967, BA 80 Hendrix Coll; MS 84 Univ of Central AR; Sp-Lang Path, Russellville Pub Sch, **SLP**

McDaniel, Mary M 5810 6th Avenue N W, Seattle, WA 98107, (206) 764-3330, BS 75 ND St Univ; MS 77 Minot St Univ; Coordinator Audiology Services, Washington Audiology Services, **A**

McDaniel, Mrs Mary Therese 126 W Calle La Guerra Ct, Camarillo, CA 93010, (805) 482-4606, BA 79 CA St Univ - Northridge; MA 81 CA St Univ - Northridge; Sp-Lang Path, Pleasant Valley School Dist, **SLP**

McDaniel, Mrs Ruth H 12314 Walker Drive, Omaha, NE 68123, (402) 292-5853, BS 84 LA St Univ - Baton Rouge; MS 87 Univ of NE - Omaha; 87–Sp-Lang Path, Bellevue PS, **SLP**

McDaniels, Janis M 659 Lake Pine Drive, Shoreview, MN 55126, (612) 490-1109, BA 81 Univ of MN - Duluth; MA 82 Univ of MN - Duluth; 86–Sp-Lang Path, White Bear Lake Sch Dist 624, **SLP**

McDaniels, Karen E 701 Calle Vallarta, San Clemente, CA 92672, (213) 978-4606, **SLP**

McDanniels, Nora Lee 3005 19th Street, Columbus, NE 68601, (402) 563-4500, BS 83 Clarion Univ of PA; MS 85 Clarion Univ of PA; Aud, Columbus Otolaryngology, **A**

McDannold, Steven Bernard Route 5 Box 251, Mexico, MO 65265, (314) 581-5268, BA 76 Northeast MO St Univ; MA 83 Northeast MO St Univ; Sp-Lang Path, Mexico Pub Schls, **SLP**

McDavid, Dorothy S 11580 Calle Corvo, Colorado Springs, CO 80926, (719) 579-9267, BS 67 IL St Univ - Normal; MS 70 IL St Univ - Normal; 86–Sp-Lang Path, Coloada Sch/Deaf & Blind, **SLP**

McDavid, Mary E F 2033 Stratford Road, South Charleston, WV 25303, (304) 343-5200, BS 75 WV Univ; MS 77 WV Univ; Sp-Lang Path, Kanawha Co Bd of Ed, **SLP**

McDearman, Mrs Terri Turner 7332 Hernando Road, Jacksonville, FL 32217, (904) 389-2230, BS 79 Auburn Univ - Auburn; MS 82 Auburn Univ - Auburn; Sp-Lang Path, Fishweir Elem Sch, **SLP**

McDearmon, Dr James R 2160 Julie, Turlock, CA 95380, BA 40 Univ of CA - Berkeley; MA 50 Univ of the Pacific; PH 60 (NS) Univ of Denver; **SLP LM**

McDermid, Mrs Susan Renee 6259 Sager Way, Blossom Hill Road, San Jose, CA 95123-4644, (408) 629-9190, BA 80 Univ of CO - Boulder; MA 82 Univ of Northern CO; Sp-Lang Path, Private Practice, **SLP**

McDermott, Barbara B 1716 N E 52nd Avenue, Portland, OR 97213, (503) 255-1841, BS 70 Univ of NE - Omaha; MS 75 Univ of NE - Omaha; Sp/Lang Path, Multnomah Ed Serv Dist, **SLP**

McDermott, Catherine Ann 2712 North 112th Street, Omaha, NE 68164, (402) 496-0661, **SLP**

McDermott, Glenn W 502 1st National Bank Bldg, Richmond, IN 47374, (317) 966-4915, BS 59 IN St Univ - Terre Haute; MA 66 IN Univ - Bloomington; SLP, Private Practice, **SLP**

McDermott, Dr John C 2013 N E Fremont Street, Portland, OR 97212, (503) 220-8262, BA 73 Univ of Akron; MA 75 Kent St Univ; PH 80 (Sp & Hrng Sciences) Univ of AZ; 85–Aud, VA Med Ctr, **A**

McDermott, Patricia Lynn 7 North Goodman Street Apartment #602, Rochester, NY 14607, (716) 473-2858, BS 82 SUNY - Coll at Buffalo; MS 84 SUNY - Coll at Buffalo; Sp-Lang Path, Hearing & Sp Ctr of Rochester, **SLP**

McDermott, Patrick J 4733 La Villa Marina #A, Marina Del Rey, CA 90292-7016, (805) 496-7511, OB 66; MA 67 Univ of Redlands; Private Practice, **SLP**

McDermott, Dr Richard P University Of Minnesota, 110 Shevlin Hall, 164 Pillsbury Drive, Minneapolis, MN 55455, (612) 624-3322, BS 53 Western MI Univ; MA 55 OH St Univ; PH 62 (Sp Lang Path) Univ of IA; Prof, U of MN, **SLP F**

McDermott, Mrs Rita P 732 Atkins Street, Middletown, CT 06457, (203) 344-2337, BS 73 Ithaca Coll; MS 75 Southern CT St Univ; Sp-Lang Path, Riverview Hosp for Chldn, **SLP**

McDermott, Sandra 27 Zemek Street, Valley Stream, NY 11580, (718) 520-7358, BA 80 Saint John's Univ - Jamaica; MA 82 CUNY - Queens Coll; 86–Instr, Queens Coll, **A**

McDermott, Susan 12216 Izard, Omaha, NE 68154, **SLP**

McDermott, Therese M 361 South Nelson, Kankakee, IL 60901, (815) 933-0720, BS 78 IL St Univ - Normal; OM 82 Governors St Univ; Sp-Lang Path, Kankake School District 111, **SLP**

McDevitt, Amy Michelle 2461 Cunningham Road, Salem, OH 44460, (216) 743-1168, BS 84 Miami Univ - Oxford; MA 87 Kent St Univ

McDevitt, Marcella Gertrude 3941 Largo Lane, Beaver Creek, OH 45430, (513) 426-8257, BS 77 Cornell Univ; MA 82 Univ of IA; Aud, Robert A Tennant MD Inc, **A**

McDevitt, Marcie E 10811 88th Street, Kenosha, WI 53142, (312) 336-3100, BA 69 Univ of ND; MA 76 Univ of WI - Milwaukee; Sp-Lang Path, Waukegan Pub Schs, **SLP**

McDevitt, Mary A 828 Chippewa Avenue, St Paul, MN 55107-3553, (612) 224-2305, BS 75 SUNY - Coll at Geneseo; MS 77 Southern IL Univ -Carbondale; 87–Sp-Lang Path, Minnesota Dept of Educ, **SLP**

McDilda, Dalzell G 3705 S W 20th Street, Gainesville, FL 32608, (904) 378-4608, BA 66 Univ of FL; ME 75 Univ of FL; **SLP**

McDill, Dr Jim D Mobile Eye Ear Nose, 2880 Dauphin Street, Mobile, AL 36606-2457, (205) 433-8421, BS 66 William Carey Coll; MS 67 Univ Southern MS-Hattiesburg; PH 69 (NS) Univ Southern MS-Hattiesburg; Aud, Mobile Eent Cen, **A**

McDonald, Mrs A Joan Ronan 8580 Hendrie Boulevard, Huntington Woods, MI 48070, (313) 832-6400, BA 55 CUNY - Hunter Coll; MA 56 OH Univ - Athens; Aud, Detroit Day Sch for the Deaf, **A**

McDonald, Alexis C 1700 S E 15th Street #104, Fort Lauderdale, FL 33316, (305) 523-9035, MS 87 Nova Univ; **SLP**

McDonald, Amelia A 27585 West 83rd, Shawnee Mission, KS 66227, (913) 441-2136, BS 85 Marquette Univ; MA 87 Wichita St Univ; **SLP**

McDonald, Mrs Ann M 5127 Timber Gale, San Antonio, TX 78250, (512) 680-2824, BA 77 Our Lady Lake Univ-San Anton; MA 76 Our Lady Lake Univ-San Anton; Sp/Lang Path, Northside ISD, **SLP**

McDonald, Mrs Barbara A 20610 Camino DE Los Cantos, Yorba Linda, CA 92686, MS 70 IL St Univ - Normal; **SLP**

McDonald, Barbara Jean 3675 Desert Rose Drive, Lake Havasu City, AZ 86403, (714) 855-4697, BA 50 Grinnell Coll; MA 57 Univ of Southern CA; **SLP**

McDonald, Betty Y 3000 Weslayan Suite 255, Houston, TX 77027, (713) 871-8007, MA 71 Univ of Houston - Univ Park; Sp-Lang Path, Private Practice, **SLP**

McDonald, Crystal Lynne 427 East 71st Street, Los Angeles, CA 90003, (818) 893-7562, MA 86 CA St Univ - Northridge; **SLP**

McDonald, Mrs Dawn Daganhardt 642 Hudson Avenue, Main Post Office, Tampa, FL 33606, (813) 251-3686, MS 80 Univ of South FL; 88–Sp-Lang Path, James A Haley VA Hosp, **SLP**

McDonald, Denise Marie 206 1/2 Adams Street, Philipsburg, PA 16866, (814) 944-5014, BS 83 1660; MS 86 Indiana Univ of PA; Sp-Lang Path, Blair County Easter Seal Soc, **SLP**

McDonald, Edward J 2569 Kennedy, Laramie, WY 82070, (307) 766-5711, BS 75 Univ of WY; MS 79 Univ of WY; Supvr of Clin Svcs, U of WY, **A ACE**

McDonald, Elaine Ketner 2681 Lafayette Avenue, Columbus, IN 47201, (317) 637-1303, BA 82 IN Univ - Bloomington; MA 85 IN Univ - Bloomington; 86–Aud, John Payne Assoc, **A**

McDonald, Elizabeth 8112 Weblank Way, Clay, NY 13041-8935, (315) 470-3276, BS 76 SUNY - Coll at Geneseo; MA 78 OH St Univ; Sp-Lang Path, N Syracuse Early Ed Prog, **SLP**

McDonald, Elizabeth Jean 1903 East Highland Drive, Seattle, WA 98112, (206) 575-4718, BA 79 Gonzaga Univ; MS 81 Eastern WA Univ; 87–Dir-Sp Lang Dept, Valley Med Ctr, **SLP**

McDonald, Erin E 1843 Acuba Lane, Atlanta, GA 30345, **SLP**

McDonald, Eugene T 510 Glenn Road, State College, PA 16801, PH (NS); **SLP F H LM**

McDonald, Dr F Douglas 300 Black Friars Road, Columbia, SC 29209, (803) 776-4000, BS 54 Middle TN St Univ; MS 60 Vanderbilt Univ; PH 69 (NS) Univ of OK Medical Center; Ch Aud SLP Serv, Dorn Veterans Hosp, **A F**

McDonald, Mrs Gertrude R 700 Eveningtide Avenue, Altoona, PA 16602, (814) 695-5643, BS 41 CA Univ of PA; ME 50 PA St Univ - Univ Park; **SLP LM**

McDonald, Dr James M 1407 York Road, Suite 201, Lutherville, MD 21093, (301) 583-7021, BS 49 CA Univ of PA; ME 50 PA St Univ - Univ Park; ED 72 (NS) PA St Univ - Univ Park; Dir Diag & Consult Serv, Appalachia Int Unit 8, **A**

McDonald, Dr James M 1407 York Road, Suite 201, Lutherville, MD 21093, (301) 583-7021, BA 75 Towson St Univ; MA 76 Univ of MD - College Park; OD 79 (NS) Johns Hopkins Univ; Director of Clinical Services, The Hearing Assessment Ctr, **A**

McDonald, Jane E 2171 Hamble, Eugene, OR 97403, (503) 485-8521, BA 68 Univ of MO - Columbia; MA 66 Univ of MO - Columbia; Dir Sp & Lang, Eugene Hrng & Sp Cen, **SLP ACE**

McDonald, Janet M 105B3 Charles Drive, Bryn Mawr, PA 19010, (215) 527-8257, BS 78 Marywood Coll; MS 79 Ithaca Coll; Sp/Lang Path, Fairfax County Public Schools, **SLP**

McDonald, Joan K 248 Dewhurst Boulevard North, Toronto, ON, Canada M4J 3K6, (416) 622-8833, BS 76; MA 78 Wichita St Univ; Sp/Lang Path, George Hull Ctr for Children & Fam, **SLP**

McDonald, Joan K 48 Mesa Road, Springfield, IL 62702, (217) 793-2796, BS 84 Eastern IL Univ; MS 85 Eastern IL Univ; 88–Sp-Lang Path, Springfield PS Dist #186, **SLP**

McDonald, Judith B 4529 Bagley Avenue North, Seattle, WA 98103, (206) 633-2610, BS 69 Saint Louis Univ; MS 70 Univ of WI - Madison; VP, Adaptive Peripherals Inc, **SLP**

McDonald, Kathleen A 108 Hawthorne Avenue, Utica, NY 13502, (315) 733-5083, BA 73 SUNY - Coll at Brockport; MA 78 Montclair St Coll; Sp-Lang Path, Rome Dev Disabl Serv Offi, **SLP**

McDonald, Mrs L Christine 6290 Greenwood Parkway, Apartment 102, Sagamore Hills, OH 44067, (216) 888-1800, BA 78 Coll of Wooster; MA 81 Univ of Akron; Sp-Lang Path, Parma Commun Gen Hosp, **SLP**

McDonald, Lynn Price Route 1 Box 410 C, Espanola, NM 87532, (505) 455-2892, BA 76 CA St Univ - Fresno; MA 78 9312; 78–Aud, Northern NM Rehab Ctr, **A**

McDonald, Sr Margaret M 800 North Main Street, Randolph, MA 02368, (617) 963-8150, BS 49 Regis Coll; MA 53 Case Western Reserve Univ; **A LM**

McDonald, Marie G 204 Nelson Road, Ithaca, NY 14850, (607) 687-3360, BS 73 Ithaca Coll; MS 81 Ithaca Coll; Sp-Lang Path/Prog Coord, Spec Chldns Cen, **SLP**

McDonald, Mrs Mary Ann Lefavour P O Box 114, 505 Laura Lane, Sweetser, IN 46987, (317) 662-2546, BA 60 IN Univ - Bloomington; MA 64 Northwestern Univ; Sp-Lang Path, Marion Comm Sch, **SLP**

McDonald, Mary O'Farrell 9733 Westview, Houston, TX 77055, (713) 464-9393, BS 76 WV Univ; MS 77 WV Univ; Aud, Private Practice, **A**

McDonald, Mrs Maryalyce 1961 Knox Road, Vancouver, BC, Canada V6T 1S5, (604) 261-8272, MA 77 0500; MS 84 Univ of British Columbia; **A**

McDonald, Maureen 219 Grand Avenue, Rochester, NY 14609, (716) 275-4852, BS 83 Nazareth Coll of Rochester; MS 86 Gallaudet Coll; 87–Aud, Univ of Rochester-Med Ctr, **A**

McDonald, Mrs Melanie Dalrymple 2404 Northcrest, Plano, TX 75075, (214) 423-3346, BA 80 SUNY - Coll at Cortland; MS 82 Univ of TX - Dallas; Sp-Lang Path, Plano ISD, **SLP**

McDonald, Nancy 2 Cimino Lane #14, Schenectady, NY 12306, BS 83 Winona St Univ; OM 85 Coll of Saint Rose; SLP, Earle Childhood Ed Cntr, **SLP**

McDonald, Mrs Nancy Chamberlain 87 Celia Terrace, Belleville, NJ 07109, (201) 759-1851, BA 80 William Paterson Coll; MS 84 William Paterson Coll; 83–Sp-Lang Path, Paterson Bd of Educ, **SLP**

McDonald, Mrs Pamela Bonnette 3608 Castle Road, Alexandria, LA 71301, (318) 445-8395, BS 80 LA St Univ - Shreveport; MA 84 Northwestern St Univ; **SLP**

McDonald, Patricia Marie 39 Aspen Ledges Road, Ridgefield, CT 06877, (203) 438-8953, BA 85 Univ of CT; MA 87 Univ of CT

McDonald, R Hilton 215 North 5th, Arkadelphia, AR 71923, (501) 246-4531, BS 78 Ouachita Baptist Univ; MA 82 Univ of Northern CO; Sp-Lang Path, Quachita Baptist U, **SLP**

McDonald, Ryta E 754 S E Englewood Drive, Hillsboro, OR 97123, MS; **SLP LM**

McDonald, Sharon L 476 West 40th Avenue, Vancouver, BC, Canada V5Y 2R4, (604) 327-0161, BA 78 Univ of British Columbia; MS 83 Univ of OR; **SLP**

McDonald, Mrs Vesta Betonte 18701 Lamson Road, Castro Valley, CA 94546, (415) 886-7549, BS 76 CA St Univ - Hayward; MS 78 San Francisco St Univ; Audiologist, Fairmont Hosp, **A**

McDonald-Bell, Connie R 211 Forbush Mt Drive, Chapel Hill, NC 27514, (919) 966-3325, BS 77 East Carolina Univ; MA 79 OH Univ - Athens; 83–Sp-Lang Path, NC Memorial Hosp, **SLP**

McDonald-Judd, Margaret J 27 Evelyn Avenue, Toronto, ON, Canada M6P 2Z2, (416) 424-3855, BS 78 Univ of Western Ontario; OM 83 Univ of Western Ontario; Sp/Lang Path, On Crpld Chldns Cen, **SLP**

McDoniel, Margaret Burke 923 26th Street, Moline, IL 61265, (309) 797-4879, BS 76 SUNY - Coll at Geneseo; MA 79 Northern IL Univ - De Kalb; 86–Aud, Mississippi Bend AEA, **A**

McDonnel, Annette 1561 Sinks Canyon Rd, Lander, WY 82520, (307) 332-3430, MA 87 Univ of Northern CO; 87–Sp-Lang Path, Wyoming State Training Sch, **SLP**

McDonnell, Eileen 139 Surrey Lane, Harleysville, PA 19438, **SLP A**

McDonnell, John J 13718 Starlite Drive, Brook Park, OH 44142, (216) 676-8355, MA 88 Cleveland St Univ

McDonnell, Patricia Kim 615 Westwood Drive #7, St Louis, MO 63105, (314) 569-8100, BS 76 Southern IL Univ -Carbondale; MA 80 Saint Louis Univ; SLP, Spec Sch Dist of St Louis Co, **SLP**

McDonough, Mrs Alanna May 4843 Nordegg Cres N W, Calgary, AB, Canada T2K 2M3, (403) 270-1256, BA 83 Univ of Manitoba - Winnipeg; MS 85 Univ of ND; 85–Sp-Lang Path, Foothills Hosp, **SLP**

McDonough, Dr Dayle Davis 401 Crescentwood Loop, Slidell, LA 70458, (504) 643-7248, BS 72 Univ of Southwestern LA; MS 73 Univ Southern MS-Hattiesburg; PH 86 (Comparison of Lang Abilities in Autistic Aphasic & Learning Disabled Children) Univ of New Orleans; Sp-Lang Path, St Tommany Parish Sch Bd, **SLP**

McDonough, Mrs Diane T 73 Yawpo Avenue, Oakland, NJ 07436, MS 78 Southern CT St Univ; Sp-Lang Path, Ho-Hokus Board of Education, **SLP**

McDonough, Donna M 8641 Golfview Drive, Orland Park, IL 60462-1417, (312) 403-2122, OM 86 Governors St Univ; Sp-Lang Path, SW Cook Co Coop, **SLP**

McDonough, Mrs Mary C 2805 Jutland Road, Kensington, MD 20895, (301) 946-5166, BA 77 Univ of MD - College Park; MA 80 Univ of MD - College Park; Sp-Lang Path, InSpeech Inc, **SLP ACE**

McDonough, Mrs Mary Young 2015 South Finley Road, #611, Lombard, IL 60148, (312) 852-8914, BS 85 Northern IL Univ - De Kalb; MA 86 Northern IL Univ - De Kalb; 87–Aud, The Hammond Clinic, **A**

McDonough, MaryEllen 35 Hector Road, Morris Plains, NJ 07950, (201) 539-4618, BA 57 Coll of New Rochelle; MA 62 NY Univ; **SLP**

McDonough, Paula Sharkey 387 Pleasant Street, Tewksbury, MA 01876-2746, (617) 894-3600, BA 79 Univ of CT; ME 82 Northeastern Univ; 86, Private Practice, **SLP**

McDonough, Roberta F 14041 Preston Road #2313-E, Dallas, TX 75240-3498, BS 73 Marquette Univ; MA 74 Univ of Denver; Aud, Auditory-Verbal Consult, Private Practice, **A**

McDonough, Mrs Ruth Ann Stergar 5575 El Dorado Court, Helena, MT 59601, **SLP**

Mc Dougal, Carol Langreck 230 East North Avenue, Antigo, WI 54409, (715) 623-2394, BS 81 Univ of WI - Stevens Point; MS 83 Univ of WI - Stevens Point; Sp-Lang Path, Langlade Health Care Ctr, **SLP**

McDougal, Cheryl M 5609 Oldtowne Road, Raleigh, NC 27612, (919) 783-7476, BS 76 Appalachian St Univ; MA 77 Appalachian St Univ; Sp/Lang Path, Dev Eval Cen, **SLP**

McDougal, Kathleen A 210 South Franklin, Shawano, WI 54166, (715) 524-4616, BA 76 Univ of WI - Eau Claire; MS 77 Univ of WI - Eau Claire; 77–Sp-Lang Path, Shawano-Gresham Sch Dist, **SLP**

McDougald, Mrs Claire Conrad 3604 Junior Place, Shreveport, LA 71109, (318) 667-6700, BS 79 LA St Univ - Baton Rouge; MA 76 LA St Univ - Baton Rouge; SLP, St Martin Par Sch Bd, **SLP**

McDougall-Gibbs, Betsy E Putnam Heights Elementary School, 635 West MacArthur Avenue, Eau Claire, WI 54701, (715) 836-5520, OM 80 Univ of WI - Whitewater; BA 74 Univ of MN - Duluth; MA 75 Western MI Univ; Instructor Early Chld Hndcpd, Eau Claire Sch Dist, **SLP**

McDougall-Thompson, Mrs Martha 1283 Lakevue Drive, Butler, PA 16001, (412) 287-4781, BS 73 Southwest TX St Univ; ME 74 Southwest TX St Univ; Sp-Lang Path, VA Med Ctr, **SLP**

McDowall, Dr Mark T Condominium Ponciana 7C, Box 7515, Ponce, PR 00732, (809) 844-8595, BA 65 Univ of SD - Vermillion; MA 67 Univ of IA; PH 76 (Aud) Univ of OK Medical Center; Director, Dr Mark T McDowall, **A**

McDowell, Mrs Angela P 28925 Geronimo Drive, Rancho Palos Verdes, CA 90274, (213) 377-1087, BA 62 OH Univ - Athens; **SLP**

McDowell, Betty M 3210 Clinton Avenue, Richmond, CA 94804, BS

McDowell, Cheryl L 5121 West 12th Street, Los Angeles, CA 90019, (213) 931-8618, MA 87 CA St Univ - Los Angeles; **SLP**

McDowell, Elizabeth Parkway Nursing Home, 1201 Parkway Avenue, Trenton, NJ 08628, PH; **SLP F LM**

McDowell, Kathleen Ana 426 Ridge Street #1, Honesdale, PA 18431-1627, (717) 253-6846, BS 75 Union Coll; ME 80 Northeastern Univ; Sp/Lang Path, St Josephs Med Cen, **SLP**

McDowell, Mary Louise 113-1/2 Dantzler Court, Lexington, KY 40503, (606) 278-3807, BA 31 Univ of KY; MS 51 Univ of AL- Tuscaloosa; Retired, **SLP LM**

McDowell, Thomas J 616 North Longview Place, Longwood, FL 32779, (305) 322-1252, BS 69 Ball St Univ; MA 76 Ball St Univ; 87–Asst Prin, Seminole Co Sch Bd, **SLP ACE**

McDowell-Fleming, Martha M 30901 Vodie Watts Road, Spanish Fort, AL 32527, (904) 434-4957, BA 70 Duke Univ; MS 77 Univ of NC - Chapel Hill; 87–Sp-Lang Path, Baptist Hosp, **SLP ACE**

McDuffee, Mrs Cynthia Delores 27 Hopyard Road, Stafford Springs, CT 06076, (203) 646-4316, BS 84 Univ of NH; MA 86 Univ of CT; Aud, Manchester Hearing Ctr, **A**

McDuffie, Mrs Andrea S 4209 Hiawatha Drive, Knoxville, TN 37919, (615) 523-3014, BA 72 Emory Univ; MA 75 Univ of TN - Knoxville; Sp-Lang Path, U of TN/Dept of Aud, **SLP**

McElduff, Mary Kathleen 501 Napa Valley Road #1022, Little Rock, AR 72211, (501) 370-1830, BA 84 Ouachita Baptist Univ; MS 86 Univ of AR - Little Rock; 88–Sp-Lang Path, Arkansas Children's Hosp, **SLP**

McElhaney, Paula R S 7159 South Clay Street, Littleton, CO 80120, (303) 837-1000, MA 77 Adams St Coll; Sp-Lang Path, Denver Public Schools J8, **SLP**

McElhinney, Dana 752 Islay, San Luis Obispo, CA 93401, (805) 541-3433, MA 87 Univ of CA - Santa Barbara; 88–Sp-Lang Path, San Luis Obispo Co Schs, **SLP**

McElhinney, Gwynne 209 North 4th Street, Boise, ID 83702, (208) 338-3655, BA 73 Univ of San Francisco; MS 75 Univ of OR; Sp-Lang Path, Boise Pub Sch, **SLP**

McElmurry, John David 9372 West 176th Street, Lakeville, MN 55044, (612) 892-5403, **A**

McElmurry, Mrs Susan P 265 Bluff View, Batesville, AR 72501, (501) 793-7372, BA 63 Univ of AR - Fayetteville; Sp-Lang Path, Newark Public Sch, **SLP**

McElrath, Mrs Lesli Overbey 12621 Timber Bend, Little Rock, AR 72211, (501) 224-4031, BA 81 Univ of AR - Fayetteville; MA 82 Univ of Tulsa; **SLP**

McElroy, Mrs Anne-Marie C 21 W009 Mayfair, Lombard, IL 60148, (312) 953-1904, BS 79 Bradley Univ; MA 80 Univ of IL - Urbana; Sp-Lang Path, **SLP**

McElroy, Mrs Jo 183 Harlow Street #118, Bangor, ME 04401, (207) 945-7365, BS 84 Univ of ME - Farmington; MA 86 Univ of ME - Orono; **SLP**

McElroy, Margaret D 2315 Glenn Court, Charlottesville, VA 22901, (804) 924-4613, BA 63 Saint Mary-of-the-Woods Coll; ME 65 Univ of VA - Charlottesville; MS 70 Vanderbilt Univ; Clin Instr-Aud, Uva, **SLP A F ACE**

McElroy, Nancy T 144 Placer Mine Road, Folsom, CA 95630, (916) 351-0956, BA 76 CA St Univ - Chico; MA 78 CA St Univ - Chico; 88–Sp-Lang Path, Folsom Cordova USD, **SLP**

McElroy, Trecia Lewis 2011 South Olympia, Tulsa, OK 74107, BA 84 Univ of Tulsa; MA 86 Univ of Tulsa; 86–Sp-Lang Path, Collinsville PS, **SLP**

McElwain, Judy Ann M 275 Hickory Drive, Greenville, OH 45331, **SLP**

McElwee, Amy Salitsky 101 Stacey Court, Downingtown, PA 19335, (215) 873-8783, BA 79 George Washington Univ; MA 81 Hahneman Medical Coll; 87–Sp/Lang Path, Bryn Mawr Rehab Hosp, **SLP A**

McEneaney, Joseph Peter 2112 North Seminary #16, Chicago, IL 60614-4141, (312) 567-5559, BS 80 Univ of MA - Amherst; MS 82 Columbia Univ Teachers Coll; 88–Sp-Lang Path, Mercy Hosp & Med Ctr, **SLP**

McEnroe, Catherine Voice 271 Spadina Road, Toronto, ON, Canada M5R 2V3, (416) 928-1006, BA 71 MI St Univ; OM 81 IN Univ - Bloomington; 86–Aud, Voice for Hrng Impaired Child, **A**

McEntee, Maureen K 101 Van Zandt Avenue, Warwick, RI 02889, (401) 861-2080, BA 80 RI Coll; MA 82 Univ of Northern IA; TDD Prog Coord, Vocational Resources Inc, **SLP**

McEntire, Beverly Lynn P O Box 7272, Canyon Lake, CA 92380, (714) 674-7731, BA 80 CA St Univ - Long Beach; MA 82 CA St Univ - Long Beach; 83–Sp-Lang Path, Lake Elsinore Sch Dist, **SLP**

McEntyre, Carol Mitchell 1935 Waybridge Lane, Fenton, MO 63026, (314) 343-1659, BS 78 Miami Univ - Oxford; MS 79 Miami Univ - Oxford; 87–Sp-Lang Path, Rehab Network, **SLP**

McEntyre, Karen 3007 36th Street, Meridian, MS 39305, BA 74 Univ of AL- Tuscaloosa; MA 76 Memphis St Univ; Sp-Lang Path, Meridian City Schools, **SLP**

McErlain, Eileen Margaret 1419 5th Street West, Palmetto, FL 33561, (813) 729-7000, ES 86 3828; 88, Private Practice, **SLP**

McEuen, Gayle Appling Orange Grove Center, 615 Derby Street, P O Box 3249, Chattanooga, TN 37404, (615) 629-1451, BA 76 Western KY Univ; MA 78 Univ of TN - Knoxville; Sp/Lang Path, Orange Grove Cen Inc, **SLP**

McEver, Mrs Janease Graham 1801 N W 35th, Oklahoma City, OK 73118, (913) 863-2919, **SLP**

McEvoy, Jane P 33 Evelyn Place, Staten Island, NY 10305, (718) 447-0200, BS 73 Saint John's Univ - Jamaica; MA 75 Long Island U - CW Post Ctr; 88–Aud, UCP, **SLP A**

McEwen, Beth Ann 1732-25 A Street S W, Calgary, AB, Canada T3C 1J9, (403) 291-0894, OB 81 Carleton Univ - Ontario; OM 84 Univ of Western Ontario; **SLP**

McEwen, Mrs Judy Laura 60 School Street, Arlington, MA 02174, MS; 82–Sp-Lang Path, City of Boston, **SLP**

McEwen, Susan K 1254 Coronado #5, Sunnyvale, CA 94086, (415) 797-1111, BA 78 MI St Univ; MA 79 Univ of IL - Urbana; Sp-Lang Path, Wash Hosp Rehab Ser Dept, **SLP**

McEwen-Sosnovich, Dr Kathleen 112 Church Street, Woodbridge, NJ 07095, (201) 634-5980, BS 78 Bloomsburg Univ of PA; MS 79 Bloomsburg Univ of PA; Sp-Lang Path, Overlook Hospital Jfk Med Cen, **SLP ACE**

McFadden, Dr Dennis Department Of Psychology, Mezes Hall 330, University Of Texas, Austin, TX 78712, (512) 471-4324, BA 62 CA St Univ - Sacramento; PH 67 (Experimental Psychology) IN Univ - Bloomington; 67–Professor of Psychology, University of Texas

McFadden, Mrs Janice E 4490 Clearwater Harbor Dr, Largo, FL 34640, (813) 581-5774, BA 73 Univ of FL; MA 75 Univ of FL; **A**

McFadden, Maureen Ann 331 Weymouth Road, Norristown, PA 19401, (215) 539-8550, BS 83 Indiana Univ of PA; MA 85 Temple Univ; 85–Sp-Lang Path, Montgomery Co Intermediate Unit, **SLP**

McFadden-Wittrock, Mrs Margaret C P O Box 1085, Pacific Grove, CA 93950, (408) 624-4815, BS 60 Miami Univ - Oxford; MS 71 Purdue Univ - West Lafayette; Learning Specialist, Briarcliff Academy, **SLP**

McFall, Mrs Bonnie Lois 301 Baytree Drive, Greenville, NC 27834, (919) 522-1261, BA 80 VA Intermont Coll; MS 83 East Carolina Univ; Sp-Lang Path, Caswell Center, **SLP**

McFall, Bonnie U 402 West Main Street, Elmwood, IL 61529, **SLP**

McFarland, Mrs Alice Anne P O Box 354, Lutesville, MO 63762, (314) 238-2333, BS 79 Midwestern St Univ; MA 86 Southeast MO St Univ; 88–Sp-Lang Path, Woodland R-4 Schs

McFarland, Mrs Ann D 91 Yale Street, Medford, MA 02155, (617) 395-2508, BS 74 Emerson Coll; ME 76 Northeastern Univ; Sp/Lang Path, Arlington Pub Sch, **SLP**

McFarland, Brenda Kay 7325 S W 33rd, Topeka, KS 66614, (913) 267-3961, BA 83 Wichita St Univ; MA 85 Wichita St Univ; Sp-Lang Path, Auburn/Washburn USD 437, **SLP**

McFarland, David Harmon, II Dept Of Aud & Sp Science, Heav Hall, Purdue University, West Lafayette, IN 47907

McFarland, Robert Taylor 515 Warder Avenue, St Louis, MO 63130, (314) 889-6591, MA 85 Univ of KS; Dis Aud, Lawrence USD, **A**

McFarland, Dr William H Otologic Medical Groups Inc, 2122 West Third Street, Los Angeles, CA 90057, (202) 651-5328, BA 65 San Francisco St Univ; MA 66 San Francisco St Univ; PH 69 (Aud) Univ of WA; 85–Dir of Aud, Otologic Med Group, **A**

McFarlane, Christine Mazurk 5180 Saratoga, Dubuque, IA 52001, (319) 588-0538, BA 75 Univ of Northern IA; MA 77 Univ of Northern IA; Sp-Lang Path, Keystone AEA, **SLP**

McFarlane, Jean L 36 Ridgewood Avenue, Kitchener, ON, Canada N2H 4L2, (519) 578-7228, BA 72 Queens Univ - Ontario; MA 75 Northern MI Univ; Sp-Lang Path, Kitchener-Waterloo Hosp, **SLP**

McFarlane, Dr Stephen C 10180 Deadwood Drive, Reno, NV 89506, (702) 784-4887, BS 67 Portland St Univ; MS 68 Portland St Univ; PH 75 (NS) Univ of WA; Prof & Ch Sp-Lang Path Dept, U of NV Sch of Med, **SLP F ACE**

McFarling, Mrs Faith Ann 420 Tungsten Place, Longmont, CO 80501-3938, (303) 772-2779, BS 78 West Chester Univ of PA; MA 81 Univ of SD - Vermillion; Sp-Lang Path, St Brain Valley Schools, **SLP**

McFeely, Susan P 513-B Center Street, Chambersburg, PA 17201, (717) 264-7578, BS 81 Clarion Univ of PA; MS 82 FL St Univ; Sp-Lang Path, Easter Seal Soc of Franklin & Adams Co, **SLP**

McFeeters, Donna S 14 Cottage Circle, Pelham, AL 35080, (205) 987-7267, BS 83 Univ of Montevallo; MS 85 Univ of Montevallo; Aud, Jefferson Co Bd of Educ, **A**

McFerren, Druscilla Kaye 305 South 9th Street #A-15, Lafayette, IN 47901, (317) 884-0850, BS 64 Purdue Univ - West Lafayette; MS 68 Purdue Univ - West Lafayette; Sp-Lang Path, Benton Comm Sch, **SLP**

McGaan, Mary Ellen P O Box 882, Elkader, IA 52043-0882, (319) 245-1480, BS 83 Northwest MO St Univ; MA 85 Univ of Northern IA

McGann, David 37180 Oak View Road, Yucaipa, CA 92399, (714) 796-4824, BS 71 Pacific Union Coll; MS 73 CO St Univ; Chief Aud, Loma Linda Surg Medical Group, **A**

McGann, William Morris 427 Camino Del Remedio, Santa Barbara, CA 93110, (805) 683-3788, BA 74 Univ of CA - Davis; MA 85 Univ of CA - Santa Barbara; 88–Sp-Lang Path, Rehab Inst of Santa Barbara, **SLP**

McGargill, Dr Roger L, Jr 3611 South 114th Street, Omaha, NE 68144, (402) 558-0440, BS 68 Creighton Univ; MS 69 Univ of NE - Omaha; PH 74 (NS) Univ of NE - Lincoln; Owner, Professional Audiol & Hrng Ctr, **SLP A**

McGarr, Dr Nancy S Speech And Hearing Sciences, Graduate Center Room 901, 33 West 42nd Street, New York, NY 10036, (212) 790-4385, BA 70 Adelphi Univ; MS 72 Adelphi Univ; PH 78 (Sp & Hrng Sciences) CUNY - Grad Sch & Univ Cntr; 78–Res Assoc, Haskins Labs-Cuny, **SLP A**

McGarrell, Mrs Stephanie L 41 Straw Hat Road #3-C, Owings Mills, MD 21117, (301) 356-5519, MS 88 Towson St Univ

McGarry, Mrs Amy H 325 Clearspring Road, Lansdale, PA 19446, (215) 539-8550, BS 81 Bloomsburg Univ of PA; MS 82 Bloomsburg Univ of PA; SLP, Mont Co Inter Un #23, **SLP**

McGarry, Jane Elizabeth 4040 Crow Road #1406, Beaumont, TX 77706-7058, (409) 899-4099, MA 87 LA St Univ - Baton Rouge; 87–Sp-Lang Path, Speech Language Assoc Inc, **SLP**

McGarry, Marian M 1969 Richmond Road, Staten Island, NY 10306, (212) 349-5701, BA 76; MA 77 NY Univ; Aud, Hrng Ed Serv NYC Bd of Ed, **A**

McGarry, Maureen Elizabeth 3711 North Cedar, Davenport, IA 52806, (319) 383-1499, MA 84 Univ of IA; BS 83 Univ of IA; Sp-Lang Path, Mercy Hosp, **SLP**

McGartland, Marilyn A 4355 Laclede, St Louis, MO 63108, (314) 535-4303, BS 75 Fontbonne Coll; MA 76 Saint Louis Univ; 88–Sp-Lang Path, Private Practice, **SLP**

McGarvey, Judith Lombardo 1668 St Albans Court, Columbus, OH 43220, (614) 459-1986, SLP, **SLP**

McGarvey, Margaret Zeis 706 Prospect Boulevard, Waterloo, IA 50701, (319) 235-7423, BA 64 Univ of Denver; MA 66 Univ of IA; **SLP**

McGarvey, Susan Denise 1481 West 10th Street, Indianapolis, IN 46202, (317) 635-7401, BS 80 Purdue Univ - West Lafayette; MS 83 Purdue Univ - West Lafayette; Sp-Lang Path, VA Admin Med Ctr, **SLP**

McGary, Robin Jo 14915 Havenridge, Houston, TX 77083, (713) 890-0100, BS 81 Northern IL Univ - De Kalb; MA 82 Northern IL Univ - De Kalb; Aud, Northwest ENT Assoc, **A**

McGary-Fynmore, Susan 3418 East Roma, Phoenix, AZ 85018, (602) 285-3284, BA 73 Univ of IL - Urbana; MS 74 Univ of IL - Urbana; Barrow Neur I St Joseph's Hosp, **SLP**

McGaughey, Derrick L 10520 Maple Ridge Road, Medina, NY 14103, (716) 778-7101, BS 74 SUNY - Coll at Geneseo; MS 75 SUNY - Coll at Geneseo; OM 87 SUNY - Coll at Brockport; Sp-Lang Path, Private Practice, **SLP**

McGaughy, Sandra L Box C 50 G, New Windsor, IL 61465, (309) 596-2114, BS 74 Western IL Univ; MA 75 Western IL Univ; SLP, Winola School Dist, **SLP**

McGee, Dr Annell 57 Antigua Drive Unit B, Kenner, LA 70065, (504) 443-5021, BS 52 Northwestern Univ; MS 64 Tulane Univ; PH 74 (NS) Univ of Denver; SLP, Jefferson Parish Sch Bd, **SLP**

McGee, Dr Donald I 332 M Street S W, Washington, DC 20024, (703) 691-2395, BS 57 Univ of IL - Urbana; MA 59 Univ of IL - Urbana; PH 75 (NS) Univ of MD - College Park; Sp-Lang Path, Fairfax Co Pub Sch, **SLP**

McGee, Mrs Laura Ferreira 3950 Mahaila Avenue, Apartment B-27, San Diego, CA 92122, (619) 587-8244, BA 82 Univ of NC - Chapel Hill; MS 83 Univ of NC - Chapel Hill; **SLP**

McGee, Marylee N R R 2 Box 78, Newman, IL 61942, (217) 837-2685, BS 74 Eastern IL Univ; MS 75 Eastern IL Univ; Sp-Lang Path, Newman Grade Sch Dist #303, **SLP**

McGee, Sandra R 778 Raymond Drive, Idaho Falls, ID 83401, **SLP**

McGeehan, Mrs Maryellen Gallagher 253 Prince Rd, Rocky Point, NY 11778, (516) 360-7891, BA 81 SUNY - Coll at Cortland; ME 84 Univ of NC - Greensboro; 87–Sp-Lang Path, The Opportunity Preschool, **SLP**

McGettrick, Peggy 2 Sandra Circle, Chico, CA 95926, (916) 534-4241, BA 75 CA St Univ - Chico; MA 77 CA St Univ - Chico; SLP, Butte Co Supt of Sch, **SLP**

McGhee, Connie D Route 3 Box 203-1, Leesburg, GA 31763, (912) 439-8078, BA 79 Columbus Coll; ME 83 Columbus Coll; Sp-Lang Path, Healthmaster Home Health, **SLP**

McGhee, Judith L 3255 Ferry St, Eugene, OR 97405, (503) 687-3373, BA 65 Univ of OR; OM 70 Simmons Coll; MA 87 Univ of OR

McGhee, Wendy Gale 14101 Michoud Boulevard #353, New Orleans, LA 70129, (504) 254-2907, BA 81 Grambling St Univ; MS 83 Univ of IL - Urbana; Sp-Lang Path, NM Rehab & Skilled Nursing Ctr, **SLP**

McGiffert, Mrs Maura Robinson 9323 Pawnee, Leawood, KS 66206, (913) 383-9014, BS 70 Univ of KS; MA 71 Saint Louis Univ; 83–Sp-Lang Path, Children's Therapy Group, **SLP**

McGill, Barbara A 2717 Urbana Drive, Silver Spring, MD 20906, (301) 949-7767, BA 80 Loyola Coll; MS 81 Loyola Coll; **SLP**

McGill, Mrs Haley P 4412 Trenton Road, Chapel Hill, NC 27514, (919) 286-0411, BA 49 Oberlin Coll; MA 72 Univ of NC - Greensboro; Aud, Durham VA Med Ctr, **A**

McGill, Mrs Pamela C W 3262 East Tusc Avenue Ext, Barberton, OH 44203, (216) 745-5850, BS 74 Univ of Akron; MA 78 Univ of Akron; Sp-Lang Path, Springfield Local Sch, **SLP**

McGillick, Maureen C 1 Raylon Drive, Apartment K, Baltimore, MD 21236, (301) 363-2758, BA 79 Loyola Coll; MS 80 Loyola Coll; Sp/Lang Path, Rosewood Ctr-State of MD, **SLP**

McGillicuddy, Marjorie 26 Hillcrest Road, Medfield, MA 02052, (617) 444-4100, BS 77 Univ of MA - Amherst; ME 80 Northeastern Univ; Sp-Lang Path, Needham Pub Sch, **SLP**

McGillivray, Larae A 413 37th Avenue South, Moorhead, MN 56560, (218) 236-2286, BS 71 Minot St Univ; MS 76 Minot St Univ; Sp-Lang Path, Moorhead State U, **SLP**

McGillivray, Mrs Vickie 2030 Coventry Way, Eugene, OR 97405, (503) 342-6240, BA 79 WA St Univ; MA 80 WA St Univ; Sp-Lang Path, Creswell Sch Dist, **SLP**

McGinity, Lori Jean 48 Kristee Circle, West Warwick, RI 02893, (401) 821-3518, MS 88 Univ of RI

McGinley, Heather L 2327 West Tremont Court, Richmond, VA 23225, (804) 524-7561, BS 86 Radford Univ; MS 87 Radford Univ; **A**

McGinley, Joan Marie 104 Washington Terrace, Audubon, NJ 08106, (609) 547-0071, BS 85 Bloomsburg Univ of PA; MS 86 Bloomsburg Univ of PA; 87–Sp-Lang Path, Washington Township BOE, **SLP**

McGinley, Mrs Mary R 2665 Summer Lane, Salina, KS 67401, (913) 827-9963, BS 72 Fort Hays St Univ; MS 73 Fort Hays St Univ; Sp-Lang Path, McGinley Sp/Lang Serv, **SLP**

McGinn, Carey Elizabeth 245 Pleasant Street #4, Worcester, MA 01609, (617) 753-2564, BS 77 Worcester St Coll; MS 86 Worcester St Coll; **SLP**

McGinn, Joan M 32 Fairlawn Drive, Worcester, MA 01602, (617) 756-9752, BA 71 SUNY - Coll at Plattsburgh; MA 73 Univ of Denver; Consulting Sp-Lang Path, League Sch of Boston, **SLP**

McGinn, Nancy 1633 North Prospect 10 E, Milwaukee, WI 53202-0622, (414) 272-3407, BS 52 Marquette Univ; MS 76 Marquette Univ; Sp-Lang Path, Private Practice, **SLP**

McGinness, Mrs Joanne P 2406 Single Tree Lane, Norristown, PA 19403, (215) 539-3071, BS 76 West Chester Univ of PA; MA 79 Trenton St Coll; Sp-Lang Path, Chester Co Intermediate Unit, **SLP**

McGinnis, Amy R 1453 Brockton Avenue #5, Los Angeles, CA 90025, (213) 473-7851, BA 79 Brown Univ; MS 81 Vanderbilt Univ; MA 86 Univ of CA - Los Angeles; SLP, LA USD, **SLP**

McGinnis, Mrs Carol Boyle 800 Greenwich Green Lane, Manchester, MO 63011, (203) 775-6348, BS 61 Carlow Coll; MA 63 Case Western Reserve Univ; SLP, Brookfield Sch Syst, **SLP**

McGinnis, Carolyn S 1528 Luzerne Street, Bethlehem, PA 18017, (215) 821-1168, BA 79 Univ of Pittsburgh - Pittsburgh; MS 81 Bloomsburg Univ of PA; Aud, Allen ENT Assoc, **A**

McGinnis, Diane S 312 Kirkman Avenue, Elmont, NY 11003, (516) 354-5424, BS 80 WV Univ; MS 82 WV Coll of Graduate Studies; 87–Aud, A Holly Patterson Geriatric Ctr, **A**

McGinnis, Mrs Landa J Soifer Goldenberg & Assoc Inc, 111 West 1st Street, Dayton, OH 45402, (513) 223-1234, BA 74 Ball St Univ; MA 76 Ball St Univ; 78–Aud, Soifer Goldenberg & Assoc Inc, **A**

McGinnis, Linda Rieser 916 Berkshire Road, Dayton, OH 45419-3737, (513) 276-5285, BA 80 OH St Univ; MA 82 OH St Univ; Audiologist, Soifer Goldenberg and Assoc, **A**

McGinnis, Lisa M 3125 Medford Court, Aurora, IL 60505, (312) 420-6477, BS 80 IL St Univ - Normal; MS 81 IL St Univ - Normal; Sp-Lang Path, Naperville Sch Dist 203, **SLP**

McGinnis, Maxine S 130 Mt Lassen Drive, San Rafael, CA 94903, (415) 239-1192, BS 67 Univ of IL - Urbana; MA 69 Univ of CT; Sp-Lang Path, San Francisco USD, **A**

McGinnis, Mrs Wanda M 15500 Lakeshore Blvd #509, Cleveland, OH 44110, (216) 481-7457, MS 88 Cleveland St Univ

McGinty, Mrs Barbara Peloquin P O Box 887, Lotus Beach, CA 95651-0887, (415) 664-4646, MS 85 San Francisco St Univ; **SLP**

McGinty, Patricia Josephine 8430 Germone Lane, Sebastopol, CA 95472, (707) 527-2271, BA 68 Univ of IL - Urbana; MS 70 Univ of IL - Urbana; **SLP**

McGinty-Pace, Patricia L 1908 Hunts Neck Court, Virginia Beach, VA 23456, (804) 461-5001, BS 64 Univ of MI - Ann Arbor; MS 69 Washington Univ; Dir of Sp-Lang Path, Lake Taylor Hosp, **SLP**

McGlasson, Julie A 6000 Hollister #2416, Houston, TX 77040, (817) 537-0700, BS 81 Baylor Univ; MS 82 Baylor Univ; Sp-Lang Path, MedTherapy Inc, **SLP**

McGlasson, Mrs Peggy Adele 4553 Clayborne Drive, Kalamazoo, MI 49009, (616) 372-4482, **SLP**

McGlinchey, Kathleen S 103 Old Toll Road, Madison, CT 06443, (203) 669-5768, BA 83 Southern CT St Univ; MS 86 Southern CT St Univ; 85–Sp-Lang Path, Clinton CT Bd of Educ, **SLP**

McGlothlin, Beth A 5269 Batavia Road, South Gate, CA 90280, (213) 862-9269, BA 85 CA St Univ - Long Beach; MA 88 CA St Univ - Long Beach

McGlothlin, Martha 8414 Stillwood Lane, Austin, TX 78758, (512) 450-1177, BS 69 Univ of TX - Austin; MA 71 Univ of TX - Austin; Sp-Lang Path/Dir, Austin Ctr for Sp-Lang-Lrng, **SLP**

McGlynn, Becky A 711 North Weber Street, Suite 2, Colorado Springs, CO 80903, (303) 633-1494, BA 74 Univ of Akron; MA 76 Univ of Akron; Aud, Private Practice, **A**

McGoldrick, Catherine 340B Saybrook Lane, Wallingford, PA 19086, (215) 358-6612, BS 75 West Chester Univ of PA; MA 78 West Chester Univ of PA; Sp-Lang Path, Elwyn Inst, **SLP**

McGonigle, Mrs Patricia 702 Fairview, Elmhurst, IL 60126, (312) 279-4963, BA 74 Augustana Coll; MA 75 Univ of IL - Urbana; **SLP**

McGorman, Margot Maureen 301-20 Gore Street, Kingston, ON, Canada K7L 2L1, (613) 544-3310, BS 80 Univ of Western Ontario; MA 82 Wayne St Univ; Sp-Lang Path, Hotel Dieu Hosp, **SLP**

McGough, Mrs Donna Woods 564 Lynn Valley Way, Stone Mountain, GA 30087, (404) 938-6855, **A**

McGough, Mrs Sandra C 115 Will Scarlet Drive, Mc Murray, PA 15317, BS 68 WV Univ; MA 70 Temple Univ-Tyler Sch of Art; 88–Sp-Lang Path, Crossroads Sp-Hearing Inc, **SLP**

McGovern, Dona M 40 Central Street, Beverly, MA 01915, (508) 922-3000, BA 78 MI St Univ; MA 80 Western MI Univ; Aud, Beverly Hosp, **A**

McGovern, Mrs Ella Jo C 4803 Villa Vera Drive, Arlington, TX 76017, (817) 467-2707, BS 70 SUNY - Center at Buffalo; MS 77 TX Christian Univ; Early Childhood Teacher, Arlington ISD, **SLP**

McGovern, Mrs Tara Diehl 24 Cumberland Avenue, Shippensburg, PA 17257, (717) 530-1682, BS 85 Bloomsburg Univ of PA; MS 86 Bloomsburg Univ of PA; 86–Sp-Lang Path, Easter Seal Soc of Franklin Co, **SLP**

McGovern, Theresa L 824 Marvin Parkway, Park Ridge, IL 60068, (312) 885-6700, BS 84 IL St Univ - Normal; MS 86 IL St Univ - Normal; **SLP**

McGovern-Lawler, Janine M 34 Maple Place, Nutley, NJ 07110, (201) 893-4357, BA 83 Rutger's St Univ - Douglas Coll; MA 86 Montclair St Coll; **SLP**

McGowan, Charlene Green 2020 Diamond Street, San Diego, CA 92109, (619) 483-3472, BA 73 Univ of the Pacific; MS 83 Univ of LA Verne; SLP, San Diego USD, **SLP**

McGowan, Deborah Mirra 13 Rufus Jones Lane, Easton, MA 02356, (315) 470-3322, BS 79 Nazareth Coll of Rochester; MS 81 Syracuse Univ; Program Director, R E A D S Collaborative, **SLP**

McGowan, Jean Marie 84 Old Stage Road, Chelmsford, MA 01824, (617) 459-6363, BS 83 Worcester St Coll; MA 85 Univ of CT; **A**

McGowan, Joy Silverman 1207 Wharton Street, Philadelphia, PA 19147, (215) 222-1300, BS 77 Emerson Coll; MS 78 Columbia Univ Teachers Coll; 85–Sp-Lang Path, Childrens Seashore House, **SLP**

McGowan, Judith D 94 White Avenue, West Hartford, CT 06119, (203) 284-2880, BA 76 Univ of CT; MA 77 Western MI Univ; Sp/Lang Path, Gaylord Hosp, **SLP**

McGowan, Mrs Laurie Hendricks 447 Alameda Drive, Livermore, CA 94550, (415) 447-9500, BA San Jose St Univ; MA 84 San Jose St Univ; SLP, Livermore USD, **SLP**

McGowan, Margaret M 85 Grannis Road, Orange, CT 06477, (203) 264-8283, BS 54 Diocesan Teachers Coll; MA 63 Catholic Univ of America; Sp-Lang Path, Reg Sch Dist #15, **SLP ACE**

McGowan, Marie E 40 Herman Avenue, Wellsville, NY 14895, BS 73 SUNY - Coll at New Paltz; MS 74 Central MI Univ; 86–Sp-Lang Path, Allegany BOCES, **SLP**

McGowan, Mrs Neita B 8210 Blemont, Lubbock, TX 79424, (806) 794-9833, BS 79 Univ of North TX; MS 78 Univ of North TX; 83–Sp-Lang Path, Sp-Lang Hrng Ctr of Lubbock, **SLP**

McGowin, Katherine Brown 1598 Gilmer Avenue, Montgomery, AL 36104, (205) 288-5999, BA 72 Univ of South AL; MA 74 Auburn Univ - Auburn; Cl Dir, Sp Ther Serv, **SLP**

McGown, Christine L R R 3 Box 802, Fairland, IN 46126, (317) 862-5290, BS 79 Purdue Univ - West Lafayette; MS 81 Purdue Univ - West Lafayette; Sp-Lang Path, Prather & Assoc, **SLP**

McGrady, Dr Harold J, Jr 4600 South Four Mile Run Drive #641, Arlington, VA 22204, (703) 358-6040, BS 54 Bowling Green St Univ; MA 55 OH St Univ; PH 64 (Lang Path-Learning Disabilities) Northwestern Univ; Dir of Special Educ, Arlington PS, **SLP**

McGrail, Louis J 1006 Oriole Avenue, Rogers, AR 72756, (501) 273-3271, BS 70 Southwest MO St Univ; MA 78 Univ of AR - Fayetteville; Aud, Private Practice, **A**

McGranahan-Eiring, Sarah 130 Midvale Road, Mountain Lakes, NJ 07046, (516) 588-0530, **SLP**

McGrane, Rhonda L 3640 Smuggler Way, Boulder, CO 80303, MA 86 Univ of CO - Boulder; **SLP**

McGrane, Mrs Susan Driver 3260 West Fox Run Way, San Diego, CA 92111, BS 73 AZ St Univ; MA 76 Univ of TX - Austin; Sp-Lang Path, San Diego Cty Sch, **SLP**

McGrath, Dr Carl O 503 North 203rd Court, Seattle, WA 98133, (206) 524-0712, BA 65 CA St Univ - Long Beach; MA 66 CA St Univ - Long Beach; PH 70 (Sp Lang Path) Univ of WA; Sp-Lang Path, Assoc In Behav & Child Develop, **SLP**

McGrath, Mrs Christine P O Box 251, New Milford, CT 06776, **SLP**

McGrath, Mrs Cynthia Lundgren 4133 Coolidge Avenue, Oakland, CA 94602, (415) 531-8257, BA 76 Augustana Coll; MA 77 Ball St Univ; Sp-Lang Path, Private Practice, **SLP**

McGrath, Mrs Jeanne Z 16 Quailways Drive, Creve Coeur, MO 63141, (314) 872-7133, BA 58 Univ of MI - Ann Arbor; MA 81 Saint Louis Univ; Sp/Lang Path, St Johns Mercy Hosp, **SLP**

McGrath, Mrs Julia B R R 1 Box 694, Paulding, OH 45879, (419) 258-5421, BS 73 Brigham Young Univ; MS 76 ID St Univ; Sp-Lang Path, Paulding Co Sch Dist, **SLP**

McGrath, Karen Marie 21 Norseman Avenue, Watertown, MA 02172-1527, (617) 254-3800, BA 78 Westfield St Coll; MS 83 Emerson Coll; Speech Language Pathologist, Kennedy Memorial Hospital, **SLP**

McGrath, Mrs Kathe E K 7447 North Artesiano, Tucson, AZ 85743, (602) 744-4525, MS 87 Univ of AZ; 88–Sp-Lang Path, Tucson Med Ctr Cerebral Palsy Fnd, **SLP**

McGrath, Kim Irene 509 Lockwood Road, Fairfield, CT 06430, (203) 374-6868, BA 80 Boston Coll; MS 82 Purdue Univ - West Lafayette; SLP, Fairfield Pub Schools, **A**

McGrath, Mrs Maryann Cooney 19 Middle Road, South Hampton, MA 01073, (203) 741-3567, BA 77 Elms Coll; MS 84 Worcester St Coll; **SLP**

McGrath, Mrs Muiriel Jean 503 North 203 Court, Seattle, WA 98133, (206) 542-2339, MS 78 Univ of WA; Sp-Lang Path, Highline Comm Hosp, **SLP**

McGrath, Patricia L 807 Nottingham Road, Syracuse, NY 13224, (315) 476-7461, BS 70 Syracuse Univ; MS 71 Syracuse Univ; Aud, VA Med Cen, **A**

McGrath, Patricia M 36 Fayette Street, #2, Cambridge, MA 02139, (617) 876-2652, BS 77 Emerson Coll; MA 79 Univ of Pittsburgh - Pittsburgh; Sp-Lang Path, Youville Hospital, **SLP**

McGrath, Susan R 224 Windy Drive, Waterbury, CT 06705, (203) 754-1794, BA 78 Southern CT St Univ; MS 81 Southern CT St Univ; Sp/Lang Path, Bd of Ed-Waterbury Ct, **SLP**

McGraw, Charlene S 98-500 Koauka Loop #9-G, Aiea, HI 96701, **SLP**

McGraw, Mrs Paula Louise 2707 Anderson Road, White Hall, MD 21161, (301) 838-2120, BS 71 Towson St Univ; MS 78 Towson St Univ; Sp-Lang Path, Harford County Public Schools, **SLP**

McGraw, Mrs Sandra A 2439 Hermitage, Montgomery, AL 36111, (205) 263-7274, BS 70 Auburn Univ - Auburn; MA 71 Our Lady Lake Univ-San Anton; Sp-Lang Path, Montgomery PS, **SLP**

McGraw, Wilmer Tracy 1802 South Grand, Stuttgart, AR 72160, (501) 673-1770, MS 87 Univ of AR - Little Rock

McGraw-House, Mrs Deborah 5322 Leatherwood Drive, West Chester, OH 45069, (513) 522-0071, BS 79 Miami Univ - Oxford; MS 80 Miami Univ - Oxford; Sp-Lang Path, Hamilton Co Off of Ed, **SLP**

McGreevy, Patricia 5127 Sheila Drive, Toledo, OH 43613, (419) 241-6191, BA 73 Univ of VT; MA 74 Western MI Univ; Coord of Screening Serv, Cummings Zucker Cen, **SLP**

McGregor, Mrs Crystal Higgins 1272 Devonshire Place, Greenville, MS 38701, (601) 335-5678, BA 79 Univ of AR - Fayetteville; MA 81 Univ of TN - Knoxville; Sp-Lang Path, National Sp and Hrg Services, **SLP**

McGregor, Joyce E Hansen 2830 Beltline Road #220, Garland, TX 75044-1606, (214) 298-7323, BA 76 Jersey City St Coll; MS 81 Rutgers St Univ -N Brunswick; 88–Sp-Lang Path, PsyCog Associates Inc, **SLP**

McGregor, Karla Kay Purdue University, Aus Heavilon Hall, West Lafayette, IN 47907, (317) 494-3789, BS 84 Univ of NC - Chapel Hill; MS 87 Purdue Univ - West Lafayette

McGregor, Kathleen J 5108 Tree Mountain Pkwy, Stone Mountain, GA 30083, (404) 469-2864, BS 78 Univ of TN - Knoxville; MA 79 Univ of TN - Knoxville; Dir/SLP, Central Health Serv, **SLP**

McGregor, Sarah S 22 Stallion Drive, Newark, DE 19713, (302) 429-4046, MS 83 Univ of IL - Urbana; Sp-Lang Path, Colonial Sch Dist, **SLP**

McGregor, Mrs Theodora F 3109 Hillside Drive, West Covina, CA 91791, (213) 919-4237, BA 54 Univ of CA - Santa Barbara; **SLP**

McGrew, Mrs Winifred C West 4624 34th Avenue, Spokane, WA 99204, (509) 624-7997, BA 67 Eastern WA Univ; ME 68 Eastern WA Univ; Retired, **SLP**

McGroarty, Jane L 94 Cherokee Drive, New Britain, PA 18901, (215) 348-5424, BS 68 Clarion Univ of PA; ME 70 Clarion Univ of PA; Private Practice, **SLP**

McGuckin, Cynthia Jean 5801 Eubank N E #21, Albuquerque, NM 87111-6187, (505) 884-8282, BS 76 SUNY - Coll at Geneseo; MA 85 Western WA Univ; **SLP**

McGuckin, Mrs Virginia Bader 1266 Romayne Drive, Akron, OH 44313, (216) 836-4491, BA 70 Univ of Akron; MA 71 Univ of Akron; 80–Asst Dir of SLP Svcs, PSI Affiliates, **SLP**

McGuffey, Mrs Annice Houston 5457 Mimosa Drive, Jackson, MS 39206, **SLP**

McGuffie, Mrs Alyce Lynne Rt 4 Box 203, Hollywood, MD 20636, (301) 862-2194, BS 61 WV Univ; MS 84 Towson St Univ; Sp/Lang Path, St Mary's Co Pub Sch, **SLP**

McGuffin, Mrs Barbara D Speech And Language Services, Park Ridge Professional Ctr, 1303 S W Park Ridge Blvd, Lawton, OK 73505, (405) 248-5300, BS 63 Univ of OK - Norman; MS 77 Univ of OK Medical Center; Sp-Lang Path/Owner, Speech and Language Services, **SLP**

McGuffin, Donaldine E 315 Wooddard, Kent, OH 44240, (216) 326-2511, BA 57 Grinnell Coll; MA 88 Kent St Univ; 85–Sp-Lang Path, Windham Exempted Village Sch, **SLP**

McGuine, Mrs Jane Barden 2518 East Hamilton, Eau Claire, WI 54701, (608) 348-2648, MS 82 Univ of WI - Eau Claire; SLP, Deforest Public Schools, **SLP**

McGuinness, Gretchen M Rd 2 Box 141-E, Slippery Rock, PA 16057, (412) 654-8608, BS 72 Edinboro Univ of PA; MA 73 Western IL Univ; Sp-Lang Path, SPEAC-AID Ltd, **SLP**

McGuinness, Kevin Rd 1 Box 357-C, Slippery Rock, PA 16057-9119, (412) 794-2330, BS 72 Edinboro Univ of PA; MA 73 Western IL Univ; Aud, VA Med Cen, **A**

McGuinness, Rosemarie Contini 6512 Dryden Drive, Mc Lean, VA 22101, (703) 698-1600, BA 67 Catholic Univ of America; ME 69 Kent St Univ; SLP, Fairfax Co Pub Sch, **SLP**

McGuire, Mrs Ann C 407 Est 3rd Avenue, Rome, GA 30161, (404) 234-3907, BS 68 Univ of TN - Knoxville; MA 69 Univ of TN - Knoxville; Sp-Lang Path, Hoople Hearing & Speech Center, **SLP**

McGuire, Carol A 196-53 69th Avenue #2, Fresh Meadows, NY 11365, (212) 539-4343, BS 69 Saint John's Univ - Jamaica; MS 72 Adelphi Univ; Aud, NYC & NYS DOH, **A**

McGuire, Mrs Carole L K Box 156 Amy Road, Falls Village, CT 06031, (203) 824-5639, BS 66 Miami Univ - Oxford; MA 73 Montclair St Coll; District SLP, Regional School District #1, **SLP**

McGuire, Cynthia L 5-B Lee Terrace, Easton, MD 21601, (301) 822-8805, MS 87 Loyola Coll; 81–SLP, Caroline Co Bd of Educ, **SLP**

McGuire, Eileen J 96 Westville Avenue, Caldwell, NJ 07006, (201) 256-1700, BA 80 Montclair St Coll; MS 82 Columbia Univ Teachers Coll; SLP, North Jersey Developmental Cen, **SLP**

McGuire, Jane Ann 415 East 80th Terrace, Kansas City, MO 64131, (816) 523-5940, BS 64 Univ of MO - Columbia; Sp-Lang Path, Kansas City Mo Bd of Ed, **SLP**

McGuire, Jane E 8787 E Mountain View Road #1008, Scottsdale, AZ 85258, (602) 266-5976, BS 78 Eastern IL Univ; MS 79 Eastern IL Univ; 84–Sp-Lang Path, Southwest Human Dev, **SLP**

McGuire, Jesse B 1934 S W Wembley Place, Lake Oswego, OR 97034, (503) 684-1583, BA 57 Univ of WA; MA 60 Univ of WA; Pres, Metro Hrng & Sp Cl, **A**

McGuire, Karen A 2021 Downsville Pike #22, Hagerstown, MD 21740, (301) 694-8527, BS 85 WV Univ; MS 87 WV Univ; **A**

McGuire, Dr Kenneth Martin Northeast Missouri State Univ, 166 Violette Hall, Kirksville, MO 63501, (816) 785-4672, BS 50 Southeast MO St Univ; MA 56 Univ of MO - Columbia; PH 67 (NS) Univ of MO - Columbia; Prof of SLP, Northeast Missouri State U, **SLP**

McGuire, Laurie D P O Box 32173, Tucson, AZ 85751, (602) 327-5461, BA 77 Univ of AZ; MS 82 Univ of Redlands; Sp-Lang Path, Tucson Med Ctr, **SLP**

McGuire, Mrs Madelyn T 188 Knotty Oak Drive, Mount Laurel, NJ 08054-2115, (609) 273-0237, BA 74 Iona Coll; MA 76 CUNY - Lehman Coll; Sp-Lang Path, Private Practice, **SLP**

McGuire, Marion 1212-1/2 South 2nd Street, Alhambra, CA 91801, (818) 281-2147, BA 26 Western MI Univ; MA 36 Univ of Southern CA; **LM**

McGuire, Marjorie S 2842 Lilac Lane, Fargo, ND 58102, BS 71 Univ of KS; MA 72 Univ of KS; **SLP**

McGuire, Maureen A Bi State Mental Health Fdnt, P O Box 951, Ponca City, OK 74602, (405) 762-0470, BA 62 Univ of CA - Berkeley; MA 79 OK St Univ; Sp-Lang Path, Bistate Mental Health Found, **SLP**

McGuire, Dr Richard A 2902 Raintree Circle, Norman, OK 73072, (405) 271-3345, BS 78 Northern MI Univ; MA 82 Northern MI Univ; Asst Prof, Univ of Ok Hlth Sci Ctr, **SLP**

McGuire, Tamara Jane 1055 Heather Drive, Salinas, CA 93906, (408) 758-9825, BA 71 CA St Univ - Chico; MA 82 CA St Univ - Chico; Sp-Lang Path, Salinas City Schools, **SLP**

McGuire, Mrs Wendy Lynn 11727 Arguello Drive, Mira Loma, CA 91752, (714) 685-9100, **SLP**

McGuirt, Mrs Janice Spakes 2225 Ashley River Road, #175, Charleston, SC 29414, (803) 766-8386, SLP, Charleston School District, **SLP**

McGurk, Mary Pat 736 Cumberland Drive, Waukesha, WI 53188, (414) 548-0090, BS 74 Univ of WI - Stevens Point; MS 75 Univ of WI - Stevens Point; SLP, Waukesha Pub Sch, **SLP**

McHale, Jane Elizabeth 156 Keets Road, Deerfield, MA 01342, (413) 586-8692, MA 84 Univ of MA - Amherst; Early Intervention Specialist, Reach Program, **SLP**

McHale, Kathleen Patricia 1198 Ragley Hall Road N E, Atlanta, GA 30319, (404) 233-5332, BS 85 Univ of GA; ME 86 Univ of GA; **SLP**

McHan, Kathryn Carson 3605 58th Street, Camrose, AB, Canada T4V 4A4, (403) 672-3161, BS 72 Univ of IA; MA 72 Univ of IA; Sp-Lang Path, Alberta East Central Hlth Unit, **SLP**

McHatton, Mrs Laurene Hanlon 393 Addison Road, Riverside, IL 60546, (312) 890-8000, BA 71 Coll of Saint Francis; MA 73 Univ of IL - Urbana; Sp-Lang Path, Chicago Bd of Ed, **SLP**

McHenry, Eileen M 609 Burns Street #206, Carol Stream, IL 60188-2514, (312) 653-7157, BS 85 Purdue Univ - West Lafayette; MS 87 Purdue Univ - West Lafayette

McHenry, Dr Monica A Dept Of Speech & Hrng Sciences, J-G15 Univ Of Washington, Seattle, WA 98195, (206) 545-2212, BS 77 Bloomsburg Univ of PA; MS 78 PA St Univ - Univ Park; PH 83 (Voice Disorders) Univ of WA; 86–Sp-Lang Path, Univ of WA, **SLP**

McHone, Mrs Molly Miller 726 Fisk Street, Piqua, OH 45356, (513) 773-5545, OB 78 Bowling Green St Univ; MS 86 Univ of Cincinnati; Sp-Lang Path, Shelby Co Brd of Mr/Dd, **SLP**

McHugh, Dr Eugene Rice McHugh Center For Hearing, North Weber Professional Bldg Suite 280, Colorado Springs, CO 80907, (719) 520-1155, BA 75 Univ of Northern CO; MA 76 Univ of Northern CO; ED 85 (Spec Educ/Aud) Univ of Northern CO; Aud, Private Practice, **A**

McHugh, Joan E M 322 East Gill Avenue, Kirkwood, MO 63122, (314) 822-0761, BS 75 Marquette Univ; MS 76 Marquette Univ; Sp-Lang Path, **SLP**

McHugh, Lea M 135 Shaw Street, Manchester, NH 03104, **SLP**

McHugh, Mrs Maria Stella P O Box 1891, North Conway, NH 03860, (603) 224-3346, BS 85 Univ of RI; MS 87 Univ of RI; Aud, Aud & Hrng Instrments of Nh

McHugh, Mary Susan 1075-M Court Drive, Duluth, GA 30136, (305) 977-2180, BS 85 Univ of GA; ME 86 GA St Univ

McIlrath, Mrs Pauline R Box 801, Bloomfield Hills, MI 48013, (313) 645-6003, OB 68 Oberlin Coll; BA 68 Oberlin Coll; MA 81 Western IL Univ; Sp-Lang Path, Wm Beaumont Hospital, **SLP ACE**

McIlwain, Cheri McDaniel 1522 Mt Vernon Road, Charleston, WV 25314, (304) 342-3261, BA 72 Univ of Northern CO; MA 76 Univ of IL - Urbana; 87–Sp-Lang Path, Kanawha Co Schs

McIlwain, Mrs Judith W 9628 Robin Meadow, Dallas, TX 75243, (214) 348-5180, BA 68 Saint Mary's Dominican Coll; MS 70 Minot St Univ; Sp-Lang Path, Richardson ISD, **SLP**

McInally, Mrs Lynn Torigoe 5534 East Del Amo Blvd, Lakewood, CA 90713, (213) 496-1250, BA 80 Univ of Southern CA; MA 82 WA St Univ; 88–Sp-Lang Path, Lynn McInally & Assoc, **SLP ACE**

McInerney, Judy Peplowski 1-S 312 Windsor Lane, Villa Park, IL 60181, (312) 255-6350, BA 79 Mundelein Coll; MS 80 Marquette Univ; Sp Lang Path, NW Sub Spec Ed Org, **SLP**

McInerney, Mrs Laurie Stehwien 1628 West 19th Avenue, Covington, LA 70433, (504) 796-3820, BS 80 Univ of NM; MS 82 Lamar Univ; SLP, St Tammany Sch Bd, **SLP**

McInerney, Louise M 14 Grandview Boulevard, Derby, CT 06418, (203) 735-8870, BA 72; MS 77 Southern CT St Univ; Sp-Lang Path, Derby Bd of Ed, **SLP**

McInerney, Maryrose Hannon 246 Meadowbrook Road, Wyckoff, NJ 07481, (201) 441-2161, BA 78 Catholic Univ of America; MA 79 Western MI Univ; Aud, Hackensack Med Ctr, **A**

McIngvale, Gayelene K P O Box 682313, Houston, TX 77268, (713) 583-8455, BS 79 LA St Univ - Baton Rouge; MA 87 Univ of Houston - Univ Park; **SLP**

McInnes, Alison Jean Grey Bruce Regional Health Centre, 1400 8th Street East Box 1400, Owen Sound, ON, Canada N4K 6M9, (204) 787-2326, BA 75; OM 78 Univ of Western Ontario; Sp-Lang Path, Grey Bruce Reg Hlth Ctr, **SLP**

McInnes, Mrs Vera K 5945 Porto Alegre Drive, San Jose, CA 95120, (408) 268-0607, BS 70 Bloomsburg Univ of PA; MS 71 PA St Univ - Univ Park

McInnis, Ellen M 23 Borelle Square, Parlin, NJ 08859, (718) 636-7500, BA 65 Saint Joseph's Coll; MA 66 NY Univ; Coord of Rehab Services, Private Practice, **SLP**

McInroy, Mrs Cynthia Kay 7222 Lyndale Avenue S, Richfield, MN 55423, (612) 866-3573, BA 83 Univ of IA; MA 85 Univ of Northern IA; **SLP**

McInroy, Mrs Judy W 907 West Ridge Drive, Ravenna, NE 68869, (308) 452-3202, BA 76 Kearney St Coll; MS 77 Kearney St Coll; Sp-Lang Path, Esu #10 Kearney NE, **SLP ACE**

McIntosh, Bonnie J 42 Rockview Street #4, Jamaica Plain, MA 02130, (617) 491-0600, BA 80 Castleton St Coll; MA 84 Univ of OR; Early Interven Sp-Lang Path, Preschool Unit Camb-Somerville, **SLP**

McIntosh, Mrs Evelyn Jean 436 North Church Street, 2nd Floor Rear, West Chester, PA 19380, (215) 436-6688, BS 82 Indiana Univ of PA; MS 84 Clarion Univ of PA; **A**

McIntosh, Mrs Jennifer Baur 808 NW 20th Terrace, Gainesville, FL 32603, (904) 335-7231, BA 85 Emory Univ; MS 87 Vanderbilt Univ; 88–Sp-Lang Path, Upreach Rehab Hosp, **SLP**

McIntosh, Margaret Swanson 4052 East Aster, Phoenix, AZ 85032, (602) 943-2481, MA 82 CA St Univ - Stanislaus; Sp-Lang Path, John C Lincoln Hosp, **SLP**

McIntosh-Skupen, Mrs Nancy Linden 2121 W Magnolia Blvd, Burbank, CA 91506, (818) 848-6933, SLP, CA Sp & L Ctr, **SLP**

McIntyre, Annagail M 11623 Briar Rose, Houston, TX 77077, (713) 462-7708, BA 70 LA St Univ - Baton Rouge; MA 72 LA St Univ - Baton Rouge; 82–Consul, Region IV Ed Serv Cen, **SLP**

McIntyre, Christine 1144 Maple Street, Carlisle, PA 17013, (717) 243-2633, BS 39 CA Univ of PA; ME 54 PA St Univ - Univ Park; Retired, **SLP LM**

McIntyre, Claire Galloway 18859 West Louise Drive, Lansing, IL 60438, **SLP**

McIntyre, Donna Kudzy 56 Williams Street, North Easton, MA 02356-1533, (617) 369-8798, **SLP**

McIntyre, Judith R 22692 Jubilo Place, El Toro, CA 92630, (714) 855-8775, BA 66 Univ of MI - Ann Arbor; MS 68 Univ of WI - Madison; 87–Sp-Lang Path, Saddleback Valley USD, **SLP**

McIntyre, Mrs Mary Ann 1824-3 Cherokee Drive, Salinas, CA 93906, (408) 443-6549, BA 78 Auburn Univ - Auburn; MA 79 Memphis St Univ; High Risk Infant Couns, San Andreas Reg Ctr, **SLP**

McIntyre, Mary Elizabeth 814 East Kensington Blvd, Apartment 4, Milwaukee, WI 53211, (313) 963-1684, MS 74 Marquette Univ; Freelance Instructor, McIntyre & Assoc, **SLP**

McIntyre, Mrs Patricia A 5929 5th Street North, Arlington, VA 22203, BS 53 Northwestern Univ; MA 60 American Univ; **SLP**

McIntyre, Patricia M Speech & Language Services, P O Box 945, Ponchatoula, LA 70454, (504) 294-3112, BS 73 LA St Univ - Baton Rouge; ME 78 Southeastern LA Univ; SLP, Private Practice, **SLP**

McIntyre, Rebecca J 17 Town Colony Drive #923, Middletown, CT 06457-1618, (203) 484-0400, BA 83 Southern CT St Univ; MS 85 Southern CT St Univ; 85–Sp-Lang Path, North Branford Sch Sys, **SLP**

McIntyre, Regina A 637 Banks Road, Margate, FL 33063, (305) 979-3511, MA 77 Trenton St Coll; Sp-Lang Path, InSpeech Inc, **SLP**

McIntyre, Sue Ellen Glenda P O Box 16214, Las Cruces, NM 88004, (505) 524-8581, BA 81 Western WA Univ; MA 85 Western WA Univ; 86–Sp-Lang Path, Las Cruces Pub Schs, **SLP**

McIsaac, Mrs Pamela Dianne 15130 Brookhurst #214, Westminster, CA 92683, (714) 973-0307, BA 83 CA St Univ - Fullerton

McIvers, Janice P O Box 675, Santa Cruz, CA 95060, (408) 429-3879, **SLP**

McJenkin, Mrs Dorothy F 25502 Ponce Court, Laguna Hills, CA 92653, (714) 667-3397, BA 51 Univ of CA - Berkeley; MA 76 Chapman Coll; Coord Commun Dis Prog, Rancho Santiago Coll, **SLP**

McJunkin, Leslie D 540 Fox Hunt Circle, Highlands Ranch, CO 80126, **A**

McJunkin, Suzanne R 902 Marticville Rd, Pequea, PA 17565-9998, (717) 569-7331, MA 60; MS 62; SLP, IV 13, **SLP**

McKaig, Michael Dean 2321 Westchester, Oklahoma City, OK 73120, **SLP**

McKain, Virginia Kraft 1318 Jackson, Boise, ID 83705-2913, (208) 385-0962, MA 79 Univ of WA; 86–Sp-Lang Path, Rehab Assoc, **SLP**

McKamey, Mrs Laura Jo Rt 1 Box 138, Warden, WA 98857, (509) 349-8036, BS 79 Brigham Young Univ; MS 84 UT St Univ; **SLP**

McKamy, Mrs Vicky L W 897 East 132nd Drive, Thornton, CO 80241, (303) 457-1097, BA 77 OH St Univ; MA 79 OH St Univ; Sp-Lang Path, **SLP**

McKann, Mrs Sallie M 11644 Cline Drive, Baker, LA 70714, (504) 929-5334, BA 72 LA Tech Univ; MA 75 LA St Univ - Baton Rouge; Instructional Specialist, E Baton Rouge Parish Sch Bd, **SLP**

McKanna, Mrs Susan I P O Box 4598, Virginia Beach, VA 23454, (804) 340-1592, BA 78 San Diego St Univ; MA 82 San Diego St Univ; 88–Sp-Lang Path, De Paul Hosp, **SLP**

McKay, Mrs Janet Lea 50104 Flintrock, Georgetown, TX 78626, (512) 837-1102, BS 83 Univ of TX - Austin; ME 85 Southwest TX St Univ; **SLP**

McKee, Bruce L 398 B Rose Lane, Zanesville, OH 43701, (614) 453-2823, BS 84 WV Univ; MS 85 WV Univ; **SLP**

McKee, Mrs Dianne Kay 1020 East 5th Street, Lee's Summitt, MO 64063, (816) 363-1411, **SLP**

McKee, Dorothy L Rural Route 1, Decorah, IA 52101, (319) 382-2870, BS 69 Western OR St Coll; ME 70 Western OR St Coll; **SLP**

McKee, Mrs Gail 776 10th Street, Charleston, IL 61920, (217) 346-2166, BS 55 Eastern IL Univ; 62–Sp-Lang Path, Ks & Oakland Ut Sch, **SLP**

McKee, Gill Grimsley 19001 Huron Drive, Twain Harte, CA 95383, (209) 533-5866, BA 71 Univ of Redlands; MS 72 Univ of Redlands; Coord/Lang-Sp-Hrng, Calaveras Co Office of Bd, **SLP**

McKee, Mrs Joan Tolley 4029 East Whitton, Phoenix, AZ 85018-5939, (602) 956-0541, Infincom, **SLP**

McKee, Loralee 3942 Josh Street, Eugene, OR 97402, (503) 686-7085, BA 75 9345; MA 76 Humboldt St Univ; OD 85 (Law Doctor of Jurisprudence) Univ of OR - Sch of Law; 85–Sp-Lang Path, Eugene Hrng Sp Ctr, **SLP**

McKee, Mrs Lynda C PO 701, Gonzales, TX 78629, (512) 672-6441, BS 77 Southwest TX St Univ; OB 81 Trinity Univ; ME 78 Southwest TX St Univ; SLP, Gonzales ISD, **SLP**

McKee, Maribeth Caya 136 43rd Avenue, Vero Beach, FL 32962, (509) 747-4899, BA 85 Eastern WA Univ; MS 86 Eastern WA Univ; **SLP**

McKee, Sally Bradshaw Speech Pathology Services, 2027 Elmen, Houston, TX 77019, (713) 526-8181, BS 72 Univ of Houston - Univ Park; MA 74 Univ of Houston - Univ Park; Dir, Sp Path Serv, **SLP**

McKee, Sonna Cherie 221 Cresent Drive, Rupert, ID 83350, (208) 436-1152, OB 69 OK St Univ; OM 86 CA St Univ - Stanislaus; 87–Sp-Lang Path, Idaho Health and Welfare, **SLP**

McKee, Suzanne Wagnon 2117 Breconridge Drive, Marietta, GA 30064, (404) 843-1893, BA 75 LA Tech Univ; MA 78 Auburn Univ - Auburn; Sp-Lang Path, Adaptive Learning Center, **SLP**

McKee, Teresa J 424 Haldeman Boulevard #B, New Cumberland, PA 17070-1232, BA 83 Univ of Pittsburgh - Pittsburgh; MS 86 Bloomsburg Univ of PA; **SLP**

McKee, Thomas L 418 Webster, Clay Center, KS 67432, (913) 632-3178, BS 71 KS St Univ; MA 73 KS St Univ; Sp-Lang Path, Twin Lakes Educational Coop, **SLP**

McKeehan, Ann Lee 563 Foxridge Drive, Providence, UT 84332, (801) 750-1377, BS 69 UT St Univ; MS 70 Univ of UT; Cl Superv, Utah Sta Univ, **SLP ACE**

McKeirnan, Mrs Karla K 3003 Brentmoor Drive, Arnold, MO 63010-3770, BS 79 Southern IL Univ-Edwardsvill; MS 80 Southern IL Univ-Edwardsvill; Sp-Lang Path, InSpeech Inc, **SLP**

McKelvey, Mrs Judy F 1605 Elmwood, Harlingen, TX 78550, (512) 428-1795, BA 68 Univ of TX - Austin; MA 76 Univ of TX - Austin; Director & SLP, Private Practice, **SLP**

McKelvey-Burbage, June 10 Luau Drive, North Little Rock, AR 72116-3262, (501) 327-2715, **SLP**

McKendall, Maureen D 19 Mt Vernon Road, Upper Montclair, NJ 07043, (212) 688-9400, **SLP**

McKenna, Mrs Beth Wheelock 15 Maple Avenue, Fredonia, NY 14063, (716) 672-8852, BS 80 Boston Univ; MS 82 Boston Univ; **SLP**

McKenna, Ellen Mary P O Box 36, Baptistown, NJ 08803, (201) 256-3337, MS 49 Fordham Univ; Sp-Lang Path, Passaic Co Day Training, **SLP ACE**

McKenna, James C 102 Pratt Street, Lunenburg, MA 01462, MS 79 Univ of MA - Amherst; Clinical Superv/Sp-Lang Path, Burbank Hospital, **SLP**

McKenna, Lori Kay 1328 Boynton Drive, Lansing, MI 48917, (517) 543-0661, MA 84 Central MI Univ; Sp-Lang Path, Eaton Intermed School Dist, **SLP**

McKenna, Mrs Marla 3101 Allendale Drive, Kettering, OH 45409, (513) 299-8948, BS 82 Bowling Green St Univ; MA 84 Bowling Green St Univ; Sp-Lang Path, **SLP**

McKenna, Patricia S 14 Fairholm Drive, Rochester, NY 14624, (716) 546-5554, BS 62 Nazareth Coll of Rochester; ME 69 SUNY - Coll at Geneseo; Sp-Lang Path, Monroe Dev Serv, **SLP**

McKenna, Sue M 8370 Estes Court, Arvada, CO 80005, (303) 424-1660, BS 68 Marquette Univ; MS 78 Univ of WI - Milwaukee; Sp/Lang Path, Adama Co Dist 14, **SLP**

McKenna, Teresa E 1710 Meadowgate, Richardson, TX 75081, (214) 231-4521, BA 74 TX Tech Univ; MS 78 Univ of TX - Dallas; 84–Sp-Lang Path, Plano Therapeutic Svcs, **SLP**

McKenney, Mrs Ann Therese 3913 Stoneybrook, Zachary, LA 70791, (617) 747-6065, MS; **SLP**

McKenny, Mrs Irene F 511 Forest View Road, Linthicum, MD 21090, (301) 766-4222, BS 73 Towson St Univ; MS 74 Towson St Univ; Sp-Lang Path, Anne Arundel County Bd of Ed, **SLP**

McKenny, M Joseph, Jr 511 Forest View Road, Linthicum, MD 21090, (301) 768-2321, BS 73 Towson St Univ; MS 75 Towson St Univ; Sp-Lang Path, Anne Arundel Co Bd of Ed, **SLP**

McKenzie, Bonnie Sue 2831 Accomac, St Louis, MO 63104, (314) 968-4710, MS 82 Univ of AZ; Sp-Lang Path, St Louis Hearing & Speech Cen, **SLP**

McKenzie, Earl V 148th Street, Michael's Cres, Lorette, MB, Canada R0A 0Y0, (204) 942-3715, BS 68 Univ of ND; MA 70 Univ of WA; 88–Aud, Winnipeg Hearing Aid Ctr, **A**

McKenzie, Mrs Emma R 109 Aspen Lane, Columbia, SC 29212, (803) 781-2730, BA 72 Columbia Coll; ME 73 Univ of SC - Columbia; Hd/Sp-Lang Path, Lexington Co Sch Dist V, **SLP**

McKenzie, Kimberly Rhodes 4318 Kiser Lane, Ashland, KY 41101, **SLP**

McKenzie, Mrs Margaret 2411 Gentle Oaks Lane, Fayetteville, AR 72703, (501) 443-5642, BA 69 Southern AR Univ; MA 74 LA Tech Univ

McKenzie, Terri A 2 Lyndhurst Place, Champaign, IL 61820, (217) 359-0442, BS 71 Eastern IL Univ; MS 80 Univ of IL - Urbana; Sp-Lang Path, UT 4 Sch Champaign II, **SLP**

McKenzie, Thelma M P O Box 440, 4000 Lafayette Road, Hopkinsville, KY 42240, (502) 885-0034, BS 58 Austin Peay St Univ; MA 73 Murray St Univ; 82–Sp-Lang Path, Sp Hrng & Counseling Inc, **SLP ACE**

McKenzie-Goodwin, Phyllis D Route 3 Box 327E, Water Valley, MS 38965, (601) 473-3388, BS 74 MS Univ for Women; MS 76 MS Univ for Women; Sp-Lang Path, Water Valley Consolidated Sch, **SLP**

McKeon, Barbara J Mari-Castle, 41 South Main Street, Randolph, VT 05060, (802) 728-4400, BA 79 Rutgers St Univ -N Brunswick; MS 81 Univ of VT; Sp/Lang Path, Interdisciplinary Educ Assoc, **SLP**

McKeon, Gerald Joseph 2351 Warwick Avenue, Apartment 32, Los Angeles, CA 90032, (213) 225-2085, BA 80 Univ of WI - Eau Claire; MS 84 Univ of WI - River Falls; SLP, Self Employed, **SLP**

McKeown, Carol Petito 376-W West Lake Road, Geneseo, NY 14454, (315) 462-3216, BS 76 Ithaca Coll; MA 77 SUNY - Coll at Geneseo; Instr Sp Lang Hrng Impaired, Wayne-Finger Lakes BOCES, **SLP**

McKeown, Maureen 166 Highland Avenue, San Francisco, CA 94110, (415) 696-4885, BA 73 Boston Coll; MA 76 Univ of TN - Knoxville; Dir Sp-Lang Path/Aud, Mills-Peninsula Hosp, **SLP**

McKeown, Mrs Milfred R 13220 Nassau Drive #209-A, Seal Beach, CA 90740, (213) 596-4217, MA 40 Northern AZ Univ; **SLP LM**

McKerns, Dorothy M , Blue Hills Falls, ME 04615, PH (NS); **SLP**

McKey, Frances D 4336 South Maiden Drive, Baton Rouge, LA 70809, (504) 925-9988, BA 79 LA St Univ - Baton Rouge; MS 80 Univ Southern MS-Hattiesburg; Sp-Lang Path, Private Practice, **SLP**

McKibben, Dr Margaret Anne 1925 Mount Royal Blvd, Glenshaw, PA 15116, (412) 486-4911, MA 73 Univ of Pittsburgh - Pittsburgh; PH 83 (Counseling) Univ of Pittsburgh - Pittsburgh; Sp-Lang Path, Pgh Bd of Public Ed, **SLP**

McKillop, Mrs Marcia Ann 8675 113th Street North, Seminole, FL 34642, MA 70 Univ of South FL; Sp-Lang Path, Pinellas Co Sch Bd, **SLP**

McKinley, Anne C 11407 Woodcrest Drive S E, Huntsville, AL 35803, (205) 536-3364, BS 82 Univ of Montevallo; ME 86 AL A & M Univ; 88–Sp-Lang Path, Ctr for Sp & Lang Path, **SLP**

McKinley, Nancy L 7021 West Lowes Creek Road, Eau Claire, WI 54701, (715) 836-4186, BS 73 Moorhead St Univ; MS 74 Univ of WI - Eau Claire; Inst, University of Wisconsin, **SLP**

McKinley, Mrs Sheila Ison Route 2, Box 555, Russell Springs, KY 42642, (502) 866-6248, BS 76 Eastern KY Univ; MA 78 Western KY Univ; **SLP**

McKinley, Mrs Susan H 1123 Purdue Drive, Longmont, CO 80501, (303) 776-8861, BA 73 Univ of CO - Boulder; MA 74 Univ of Denver; SLP, St Vrain Vlly Pub Sch, **SLP A**

McKinley, Susanna C 702 South 26th Street, South Bend, IN 46615, (405) 271-4214, BA 82 IN Univ - Bloomington; MS 84 Univ of OK - OK City; Professional Associate, InSpeech Inc, **SLP**

McKinney, Beverly M 585 East Parkway South #4, Memphis, TN 38104, (901) 726-7684, BS 59 Middle TN St Univ; MA 75 Memphis St Univ; Chief SLP, Methodist Hosp of Memphis, **SLP**

McKinney, Mrs Beverly Sue 1009 Rutledge Place, Modesto, CA 95355, (209) 526-9007, MA 85 CA St Univ - Stanislaus; **SLP**

McKinney, Mrs Christine Lee East 26010 Olympic Avenue, Newman Lake, WA 99025, (509) 922-6865, BA 82 Univ of CA - Santa Barbara; MS 84 Eastern WA Univ; **SLP**

McKinney, Elizabeth Ann 5622 Silkwood Lane, Orange Park, FL 32073, (904) 399-6713, BS 79 OH Univ - Athens; MA 80 Kent St Univ; Sp-Lang Path, Memorial Regional Rehab Cen, **SLP ACE**

McKinney, Mrs Lee Ann Scharbach 4174 Oakledge Drive, Liverpool, NY 13090, (315) 470-3196, OB 78 SUNY - Coll at Buffalo; ME 79 SUNY - Coll at Buffalo; Sp-Lang Path, N Syracuse Cen Sch, **SLP**

McKinney, Marcia Ann 6734 Bowie Drive, Springfield, VA 22150, **SLP**

McKinney, Marnette P P O Box 215, North, SC 29112, (803) 247-2366, BS 74 Hampton Univ; MA 75 Case Western Reserve Univ; Instr, South Carolina State Coll, **SLP**

McKinney, Stephen Kent P O Box 567, New Liskeard, ON, Canada P0J 1P0, (705) 647-4305, BS 82 Howard Payne Univ; MS 84 Univ of TX - Dallas; Sp-Lang Path, Timiskaming Health Unit, **SLP**

McKinney, Susan Aiken 7824 El Dorado Drive, Austin, TX 78737, (512) 288-4655, BS 76 Univ of TX - Austin; MA 79 Univ of TX - Austin; SLP, St Davids Comm Hosp, **SLP**

McKinney, Dr Virginia 420 North Louise Street, Apartment 22, Glendale, CA 91206, (213) 483-0943, BA 68 CA St Univ - Los Angeles; MA 69 CA St Univ - Northridge; PH 83 (NS) Claremont Graduate Sch; Dir, Cen Commun Dev Inc

McKinnis, Mrs Sandra K 1955 Rosemary, Anchorage, AK 99508, (907) 272-0586, BS 72 Purdue Univ - West Lafayette; MA 75 Memphis St Univ; 85–Prog Mgr-Pediatrics, Alaska Treatment Ctr, **SLP**

McKinnon, Frances Louise 518 Forest Point Drive, Macon, GA 31210, (912) 474-9440, BS 86 Valdosta St Coll; ME 87 Valdosta St Coll; 88–Sp-Lang Path, Bibb Co PS

McKinster, Mrs Katherine RFD 4 Box 440, Valley Drive, Gilford, NH 03246, (603) 279-6442, BA 77 Dalhousie Univ - Nova Scotia; MA 79 Ball St Univ; SLP, Wolfboro Childrens Center, **SLP**

McKirdy, Dr Laura Spielvogel Rd 1 Box 202-A, Far Hills, NJ 07931, (201) 299-0166, BS 62 PA St Univ - Univ Park; MA 63 Northwestern Univ; PH 78 (Developmental Psychology) Rutgers St Univ -N Brunswick; Principal, Lake Drive Sch for Hrng Imp Ch, **SLP**

McKissick, Mrs Karen E Bernardo 758 River Road, Binghamton, NY 13901, BS 82 SUNY - Coll at Cortland; MS 83 Coll of Saint Rose; Sp-Lang Path, Broome Dev Ctr, **SLP**

McKissick, Kelly A 1381 Grove Way, Concord, CA 94518, **SLP**

McKitish, Mrs Dianne M 2220 South Ellsworth St, Allentown, PA 18103, (215) 252-3461, BS 81 Bloomsburg Univ of PA; MS 82 Bloomsburg Univ of PA; SLP, Helen Beebe Sp Hrng Center, **SLP**

McKitrick, Edward F 13530 Moorpark Street #2, Sherman Oaks, CA 91423, (805) 251-4010, BA 70 Univ of Akron; MA 78 Ball St Univ; SLP, LA Co Pub Sch, **SLP**

McKittrick, Julie Linn 3637 North 20th Place, Sheboygan, WI 53083, (414) 457-0915, MS 83 Univ of WI - Madison; BS 81 Univ of WI - Stevens Point; SLP, Sheboygan County, **SLP**

McKnerney, Lorraine 91 Murielle Drive, South Windsor, CT 06074, (203) 647-3346, BA 73 CUNY - Hunter Coll; MA 74 Univ of CT; SLP, Bd of Ed, **SLP**

McKnight, Mrs Anne Elmore 11036 North Oak Hills Pkwy, Baton Rouge, LA 70810, BA 62 Univ of MS; MA 65 LA St Univ - Baton Rouge; Aud, Drs Braud & Breaux, **SLP A**

McKnight, Mrs Catherine Margaret 110 Ocean Drive, Richardson, TX 75081, (214) 669-9225, BA 81 SUNY - Coll at Buffalo; MS 83 Univ of TX - Dallas; Sp-Lang Path, Richardson ISD, **SLP**

McKnight, Deborah E 861 Via Colinas, Westlake Village, CA 91362-5046, (805) 373-8619, MA 87 CA St Univ - Northridge

McKnight, Donna Rountree 4027 Barton Street, Niagara Falls, NY 14305-1515, (716) 278-5665, BS 73 Nazareth Coll of Rochester; MS 74 SUNY - Coll at Geneseo; SLP, Board of Education, **SLP**

McKnight, Evelyn Vinduska 410 East 22nd, Fremont, NE 68025, (402) 721-7077, BA 77 Univ of NE - Lincoln; MA 79 Univ of IA; Aud, Private Practice, **A ACE**

McKnight, Mrs Kathleen N 4625 Pine Ridge, Baton Rouge, LA 70809, (504) 928-3081, BS 71 LA St Univ - Baton Rouge; OM 76 LA St Univ - N O Medical Ctr; Sp-Lang Path, Gables Academy, **SLP**

McKnight, Laura W 520 N Street S W, Washington, DC 20024, MS; **SLP LM**

McKnight, Mrs Roxanne Crum 3120 N W 61st Terrace, Oklahoma City, OK 73112, **SLP**

McKone, Ann M 6 Florence Street, Dover, NH 03820-3403, (603) 749-1519, BA 74 Univ of NH; MS 79 Syracuse Univ; 86–Sp-Lang Path, Dover Sch Sys, **SLP ACE**

McKown, Mary Frances 2263 Jefferson, Lower, Memphis, TN 38104, (901) 726-6134, BS 83 East TN St Univ; MA 84 Memphis St Univ; **A**

McKown, Mrs Patricia D P O Box 2199, 1600 Breckenridge, Owensboro, KY 42302, (502) 686-1335, BA 75 Southern IL Univ -Carbondale; MS 76 Kent St Univ; 84–Aud, Commision for Handicap Childrn, **A**

McLachlan, Catherine Dunn 803 Jefferson Circle, Martinsville, VA 24112, (919) 658-5083, BS 84 Radford Univ; MS 85 Radford Univ; **SLP**

McLain, Mrs Judy Lynne 2435 Glenridge, Cape Girardeau, MO 63701, (314) 471-3511, BS 77 Southeast MO St Univ; ME 83 Southeast MO St Univ; Sp-Lang Path, Scott Co R-V Sch Dist, **SLP**

McLain, Julie Ann 7767 England, Overland Park, KS 66204, (816) 756-2250, BS 82 KS St Univ; MS 84 Univ of OK - OK City; Sp-Lang Path, Rehab Institute, **SLP**

McLauchlin, Dr Robert M Interim Dean, School Of Education Health & Human Services, Ronan Hall 307, Mount Pleasant, MI 48859, (517) 774-6995, BS 62 Western MI Univ; MA 63 Northwestern Univ; PH 70 (NS) Wayne St Univ; Prof & Interim Dean, Ctrl Michigan U, **SLP A F**

McLaughlin, Barbara Ann 328 Huntington Avenue #1, Hyde Park, MA 02136, (617) 364-5908, BS 82 Univ of MA - Amherst; MS 84 Boston Univ; **SLP**

McLaughlin, Colette M 3918 Stone Avenue, Sioux City, IA 51106, (712) 276-0252, BA 86 Univ of Northern IA; MA 88 Univ of SD - Vermillion; Siouxland Easter Seals

McLaughlin, Colleen Marie 4321 Beard Avenue S, Minneapolis, MN 55410, (612) 920-6306, BS 83 Univ of MN - Minneap-St Paul; MA 86 Univ of MN - Minneap-St Paul; 86–Sp-Lang Path, Bloomington Ps, **SLP**

McLaughlin, Diane Jean P O Box 2066, Greensboro, NC 27402-2066, (919) 755-1708, MS 87 Univ of NC - Chapel Hill; 87–Sp-Lang Path, Chatham County Schs

McLaughlin, Donna C Mansfield Training School, Speech & Hearing Dept, P O Box 51, Mansfield Depot, CT 06251, (203) 429-6451, BS 73 Univ of CT; MA 76 Univ of CT; Dept Supvr, Mansfield Training School, **A**

McLaughlin, Donna Marie 1452 Glenbrook Lane, West Chester, PA 19380, (302) 454-2202, BS 77 West Chester Univ of PA; MA 81 West Chester Univ of PA; **SLP**

McLaughlin, Florence E Rural Route 2, Salem, IL 62881, (618) 548-0163, BA 33 Cedarville Coll; BS 37 Univ of IL - Urbana; MA 45 Univ of IL - Urbana; **SLP LM**

McLaughlin, Jean Marie 32 Meadowbrook Road, North Wales, PA 19454, (215) 643-1386, BS 81 Univ of RI; MS 82 SUNY - Coll at Buffalo; Sp/Lang Path, Private Practice, **SLP**

McLaughlin, Joann Nancy 3341 Euclid Heights Blvd, Cleveland Heights, OH 44118, (216) 321-9098, BS 75 West Chester St Coll; MS 76 Syracuse Univ; 88, Univ of Akron, **SLP**

McLaughlin, John F 14 Darnell Road, Worcester, MA 01606, (508) 853-3849, BS 56 Coll of the Holy Cross; ME 62 Worcester St Coll; Assoc Prof, Worcester St Coll, **SLP ACE**

McLaughlin, Joseph G 141 Lorraine Drive, Storrs, CT 06268, (203) 429-4895, BA 73 Stonehill Coll; MA 76 Univ of CT; Dir Resource Svcs, Mansfield Trng Sch, **SLP**

McLaughlin, Karen Neilan 41 Fanning Road, Ledyard, CT 06339, (203) 464-8941, BA 75 Univ of CT; MS 76 Adelphi Univ; Sp-Lang Path, New London Pub Sch, **SLP**

McLaughlin, Kathy S 3616 Glenmanor Circle, Midwest City, OK 73110, (405) 737-4461, BA 76 Univ of OK - Norman; MS 78 Univ of OK Medical Center; 78–Sp-Lang Path, Midwest Cty Sch, **SLP**

McLaughlin, Mrs Nancy Cookle 404 Siegert Street, Marion, WI 54950, (715) 754-2821, MS 83 Univ of WI - Stevens Point; Sp-Lang Path, Sch Dist of Marion, **SLP**

McLaughlin, Noreen A 5800 Arlington Avenue, New York, NY 10471, **A**

McLaughlin, Patricia 110 Dean Street #51, Taunton, MA 02780, (617) 787-3390, BS 84 Northeastern Univ; MS 86 Northeastern Univ; SLP, The Greenery Rehab, **SLP**

McLaughlin, Patricia A 10205 Reavie Gardens Drive, St Louis, MO 63123-1965, (314) 638-2612, BS 79 Bloomsburg Univ of PA; MS 80 Bloomsburg Univ of PA; **A**

McLaughlin, Dr Scott F 3616 Glenmanor Circle, Midwest City, OK 73110, (405) 321-2980, BS 76 Winona St Univ; MS 78 Univ of OK Medical Center; PH 83 (Sp-Lang Path) Univ of OK Medical Center; 83–Assoc Prof, Central St U, **SLP**

McLaughlin, Susan M 1621 Berkley Lane, Belleville, IL 62233, (305) 274-8428, MS 84 Univ of NM; BS 81 Bradley Univ; Sp-Lang Path/Aud, Easter Seals Society Dade Co, **SLP A**

McLaughlin, Wendy Irene 416 1/2 North 3rd Avenue, Newton, IA 50208, (515) 792-4870, BS 84 Univ of WI - Stevens Point; MS 86 Univ of WI - Oshkosh; 86–Aud, Heartland AEA #11, **A**

McLaughlin-Wheat, Mrs Darlene L 7348 North Ridge Boulevard, Unit 12-A, Chicago, IL 60645, (312) 869-6610, BA 64 Mundelein Coll; MA 65 Northwestern Univ; 87–Dir, Shore Comm Svc for Retarded Cit, **SLP**

McLaurin, Paul Andrew Amos Cottage Rehab Hospital, Bowman Gray School Of Med, 3325 Silas Creek Parkway, Winston-Salem, NC 27103, (919) 765-9916, BS 76 Univ of NC - Chapel Hill; MS 78 Univ of NC - Chapel Hill; OM 87 Univ of NC - Greensboro; Superv of Sp-Lang Path, Bowman Gray Sch of Med, **SLP**

McLaurine, Mary A Quarters E-5 McDec, Quantico, VA 22134, BS 75 Hampton Univ; OM 79 Univ of SC - Columbia; Sp-Lang Path, Fairfax Co Hlth Dept, **SLP ACE**

McLean, Darlene 3431 West Glen Holly Drive, Anaheim, CA 92804, (213) 698-8121, MA 87 Whittier Coll; **SLP**

McLean, Mrs Elizabeth Ann 3051 Branford Court, Marietta, GA 30062, (404) 565-8658, BS 77 Nazareth Coll of Rochester; MS 80 Ithaca Coll

McLean, Dr James E Parsons Research Center, Bureau Of Child Research, P O Box 738, Parsons, KS 67357, (316) 421-6550, BS 51 IN Univ - Bloomington; MA 59 Univ of KS; PH 65 (Sp Path and Aud) Univ of KS; 76–Sp-Lang Path, Bur/Chld Res U Ks, **SLP F**

McLean, John M 1008 Almaden, Eugene, OR 97402, (503) 687-2505, BA 70 CA St Univ - Stanislaus; MA 71 Univ of KS; MS 78 Univ of OR; Sp-Lang Path, Eugene Sch Dist 4J, **SLP**

McLean, Kathleen Ann 2765 Via Seville, Fullerton, CA 92635, (714) 255-1015, BA 80 CA St Univ - Long Beach; MA 83 CA St Univ - Fullerton; Sp-Lang Path, Anaheim Union High Sch Dist, **SLP**

McLean, Linda B 1301 Wendover Road, Charlotte, NC 28211, BS 70 Univ of TN - Knoxville; ME 73 Univ of NC - Greensboro; 74–Sp-Lang Path, Charlotte-Mecklenburg Schs, **SLP**

McLean, Mrs Nancy J 191 Claremont Avenue, Tonawanda, NY 14223, (716) 937-9116, BS 78 SUNY - Coll at Buffalo; MS 81 SUNY - Coll at Buffalo; Sp/Lang Path, Alden Cen Sch Dist, **SLP**

McLean, Robin Rae 3102 Futura Drive, Roswell, NM 88201, (505) 623-7000, BA 68 KS St Univ; MA 84 Wichita St Univ; Sp-Lang Path, Roswell ISD, **SLP**

McLean, Sharon Nellis 17 Benjamin Road, Belmont, MA 02178, (617) 720-6732, **SLP**

McLean, Shelle Donn 138 Education Bldg, Fort Collins, CO 80523, (303) 491-1949, BA 77 Univ of Northern CO; MA 78 Univ of Northern CO; Clin Supvr Instr, Colorado State Univ, **A**

McLean-Muse, Dr Ann 125 Longfellow Road, Worcester, MA 01602, (617) 755-1692, BA 75 Univ of AL- Tuscaloosa; MS 77 Univ of AL- Tuscaloosa; PH 85 (Sp-Lang Path) Northwestern Univ; Sp-Lang Path, Worcester State Coll, **SLP**

McLean-Stead, Constance 7 Nottingham Drive, Yarmouth Port, MA 02675, **SLP**

McLeer, Mrs Una Lee 23 Hillside Lane North, Syosset, NY 11791, BA Univ of Miami; MS 64 Adelphi Univ; SLP, Syosset Public Schools, **SLP**

McLellan, Elaine A 1011 Smithfield Avenue, Lincoln, RI 02865, (401) 353-7000, MS 71 Univ of RI; Sp-Lang Path, J E Fogarty Center, **SLP**

McLelland, Mrs Rosann Elizabeth 2045 Hall Street S E, Grand Rapids, MI 49506-4071, (616) 247-0210, BA 83 MI St Univ; MA 84 MI St Univ

McLemore, Brenda Davis 434 Tanglewood Drive, Slidell, LA 70458, (601) 798-4555, **SLP**

McLemore, Mrs Sarah Lee 4721 Olde Village Lane, Dunwoody, GA 30338, BS 69 Univ of GA; MS 85 GA St Univ; **SLP**

McLennan, Roderick O, Jr 9905 Perry Drive, Overland Park, KS 66212, PH (NS); **A**

McLeod, Mrs Dara B 57295 Buckhorn Road, Three Rivers, MI 49093, (616) 273-8809, BA 80 Univ of Northern IA; MA 81 Univ of Northern IA; **SLP**

McLeod, Dr H Lee Casas Adobes Hearing Center, 6812 North Oracle Road, Suite 144, Tucson, AZ 85704, (602) 297-4571, BS 71 Brigham Young Univ; MS 73 Brigham Young Univ; PH 77 (NS) Bowling Green St Univ; Owner/Corp Pres, Southern AZ Aud Assoc, **A**

McLeod, Joye L 16402 South 111th Street, Omaha, NE 68138, (402) 339-3411, BA 71 Univ of NE - Omaha; MS 75 Univ of NE - Omaha; 75–Sp-Lang Path, Papillion-LaVista PS, **SLP**

McLeod, Mrs Susan Seagroves General Delivery, Aberdeen, NC 28315-9999, (919) 485-5145, **SLP**

McLeroy, Mrs Carol M 2106 East Dolphin Circle, Portland, TX 78374, (512) 643-7767, BA 79 Univ of AR - Fayetteville; MA 80 Univ of AR - Fayetteville; Sp/Lang Path, Corpus Cristi State School, **SLP**

McLeroy, Kathleen Plano Hearing Aid Dispensary, 926 15th Street, Suite 102, Plano, TX 75074, (214) 423-8500, BS 77 Univ of TX - Austin; MS 78 Univ of North TX; 82–Aud/Owner, Plano Hrng Aid Dispensary, **A**

McLoughlin, Judy L Rd 5 3 Denmark Lane, Jackson, NJ 08527, (201) 370-5438, BA 71 William Paterson Coll; MA 72 Montclair St Coll; SLP, Jackson Sch Jackson Nj, **SLP**

McLoughlin, Mrs Patricia J 7702 Diagonal Road, Kent, OH 44240, (216) 678-6470, MA 83 Kent St Univ; Sp-Lang Path, Private Practice, **SLP**

McMahan, Mrs Maxine Marilyn 3817 Merriman Drive, Plano, TX 75074, (214) 423-8330, BS 69 PA St Univ - Univ Park; MS 85 Univ of TX - Dallas; Sp-Lang Path, ISD, **SLP**

McMahon, Mrs Ann Carney 22 Hemlock Court, Cromwell, CT 06416, (203) 342-4046, BA 83 Univ of CT; MA 85 Univ of CT; Aud, Prof Hrng Services, **A**

McMahon, Ann Fleming 152 Sylvan Way, Bremerton, WA 98310, (206) 373-2536, BA 84 Univ of NM; MS 85 Univ of NM; 86–Sp-Lang Path, Holly Ridge Ctr, **SLP**

McMahon, Constance 5 Fair Oaks Circle, Ormond Beach, FL 32074, MA 77 1933; SLP, Volusia County School District, **SLP**

McMahon, Cynthia Marie P O Box 984, Wautoma, WI 54982, (414) 787-4696, BS 79 Marquette Univ; MS 81 Marquette Univ; Sp-Lang Path, Rehabilitation Associates, **SLP**

McMahon, Mrs Helen M 1007 South Stone Avenue, La Grange, IL 60525, (312) 579-5913, BA 68 Saint Xavier Coll; MA 70 Univ of IL - Urbana; Sp-Lang Path, Private Practice, **SLP**

McMahon, Joan 1516 S E Knight, Portland, OR 97202, (503) 229-3533, BS 69 Portland St Univ; MS 70 Portland St Univ; Assoc Prof, Portland St U, **SLP**

McMahon, Judith A 30 Knowles Drive, Warwick, RI 02888, (401) 463-7740, MS 87 Univ of RI; 88–Sp-Lang Path, Warwick PS, **SLP**

McMahon, Mrs Judith A 18 Sunnyfield Drive, Cortland, NY 13045, (607) 753-9301, MS 87 Ithaca Coll

McMahon, Kathleen Mary 64 Quincy Drive, Levittown, PA 19057, (215) 946-5016, BS 77 Trenton St Coll; MA 82 Trenton St Coll; 87–Sp-Lang Path, Mercer Co Spec Svcs, **SLP**

McMahon, Kelley Kay 644 Prescott Avenue, El Cajon, CA 92020, (619) 588-3146, BA 80 San Diego St Univ; MA 83 San Diego St Univ; Tchr, Cajon Valley School District, **SLP**

McMahon, Mrs Kelly Ann 2690 Greenwich, San Francisco, CA 94123, (707) 644-8388, BA 84 San Francisco St Univ; MS 86 San Francisco St Univ; **SLP**

McMahon, Margaret A 670 Lake Pine Drive, Shoreview, MN 55126, (612) 457-7245, BA 75 Univ of MN - Duluth; MS 76 Univ of WI - Eau Claire; SLP, ISD, **SLP**

McMahon, Nancy B 1700 Indian Plaza NE #49, Albuquerque, NM 87106, (505) 843-2336, BA 85 Univ of CA - Santa Barbara; MS 87 Univ of NM; 87–Aud, Univ of NM-Dept of Surgery, **A**

McMahon-Llaurado, Kathleen D 6624 West Lloyd Street, Wauwatosa, WI 53213, BS 80 Univ of WI - Madison; MS 81 Univ of WI - Stevens Point; SLP, Waukesha Publ Schs, **SLP**

McMain, Deanna G 1265 East Escalon, Fresno, CA 93710, (209) 432-2728, BS 67 Univ of NM; MS 78 Univ of NM; MA 88 The Fielding Inst; 88–Psychology Intern, Allan G Hedberg PhD & Assoc, **A**

McMains, Lynn A 1218 West 2nd, Pella, IA 50219, (515) 628-1162, BS 77 Northeast MO St Univ; MA 78 Northeast MO St Univ; Sp-Lang Path Icfmr Supervisor, Christian Opportunity Center, **SLP**

McManamon, Donna W 2421 Fairbanks Avenue, Clearwater, FL 34624, (813) 443-3511, **SLP**

McManaway, Emily Paula 593 East Shelldrake Circle, Fresno, CA 93710-1232, BS 75 OH Univ - Athens; MA 86 Memphis St Univ; **SLP**

McManus, Deborah M P O Box 656, Daleville, IN 47334, BA 77 IN Univ - Bloomington; MA 78 IN Univ - Bloomington; **SLP**

McManus, Edna L 919 Terry Lane, Oakdale, LA 71463, (504) 342-3631, BA 64 Southeastern LA Univ; ME 70 LA St Univ - Baton Rouge; Academic Supervisor, State Department of Education, **SLP**

McManus, Margaret Theresa 853 Chalcedony, San Diego, CA 92109, (619) 283-5953, BS 82 SUNY - Coll at Fredonia; **SLP**

McManus, Mrs Nancy L Route 2, 530 Lakewood Circle, Washington, WV 26181, (304) 422-8411, BA 68 CA Univ of PA; ME 72 CA Univ of PA; Ch Sp/Lang Path, Wood Co Sch, **SLP**

McManus, Natalie Gutow 9139 Everett Court, Springfield, VA 22152, (703) 451-6032, BA 81 PA St Univ - Univ Park; MA 83 Univ of IA; 88–Sp-Lang Path, Speech-Language Services of McLean, **SLP**

McManus, Penny E 4655 Sullivan Way, Santa Rosa, CA 95405, (707) 527-2271, BA 79 CA St Univ - Chico; MA 81 CA St Univ - Chico

McManus, Sharon G 1243 Upton Circle, West Chester, PA 19380, (215) 696-4919, BA 70 Mary Washington Coll; MA 77 Univ of Miami; Sp-Lang Path, Chester Co Intermed Unit, **SLP**

McMartin, Colleen M 21 Hoosick Street, Hoosick Falls, NY 12090-1727, (518) 686-9492, BS 78 Coll of Saint Rose; ME 79 Coll of Saint Rose; **SLP**

McMartin, Heidi Therese 2995 Redwood, Ann Arbor, MI 48104, (313) 764-8442, BA 77 Univ of MI - Ann Arbor; MS 82 Univ of MI - Ann Arbor; Sp-Lang Path, Rainbow Tree Center, **SLP**

McMaster, Nancy R 935 Stagecoach, Wichita, KS 67230, (318) 322-1255, BA 74 Wichita St Univ; MA 75 Wichita St Univ; Sp/Lang Path, **SLP**

McMellor, Gladys M 22 Birch Court, North Liberty, IA 52317, (319) 399-6835, BA 60 Univ of IA; MA 76 Univ of TN - Knoxville; Sp-Lang Path, Grant Wood AEA, **SLP**

McMenamin, Cathy Elizabeth 680 Mason Drive, Warminster, PA 18974, (215) 675-8042, BS 85 Bloomsburg Univ of PA; MS 86 Bloomsburg Univ of PA; **SLP**

McMenamin, Sr Therese Resurrection Convent, 2035 Vista Street, Philadelphia, PA 19152, BS 63 Trinity Coll; MA 74 Temple Univ; 77–Sp-Lang Path, Sch Dist of Phil, **SLP**

McMenimen, Annemary M 97 Leonardine Avenue, South River, NJ 08882, (201) 238-1968, MS; 87–Sp-Lang Path, Sayreville PS, **SLP**

McMichael, Mrs Shirley O Route 2 Box 724, Reidsville, NC 27320, (919) 342-4671, BA 72 Univ of NC - Greensboro; ME 77 Univ of NC - Greensboro; SLP, Private Practice, **SLP**

McMicken, Dr Betty Lou Dir Westmed Speech & Hrng Ctr, 1001 North Tustin Avenue, Santa Ana, CA 92705, (714) 953-3328, BA 64 Univ of Southern CA; MA 67 Univ of Southern CA; PH 87 (Sp Science) Univ of Southern CA; Director Speech & Hearing, Western Medical Center, **SLP**

McMillan, Aundria R 19 Cambridge Place, Brooklyn, NY 11238, (212) 678-3410, BA 71 CUNY - City College; MS 72 Columbia Univ Teachers Coll; Ch Superv/Lang Path, Columbia U Tch Coll, **SLP**

McMillan, Deborah Mosely 3128 McAdams Drive, Raleigh, NC 27604, (919) 438-4027, MA 76 Univ of IL - Urbana; 87–Sp-Lang Path, Wake County PS, **SLP**

McMillan, Don Fraizer 1720 W Coolidge Street, Phoenix, AZ 85015, (602) 255-1181, BS 81 Univ of AZ; MS 84 ID St Univ; Aud, Arizona Dept Health Svcs, **A**

McMillan, Jeanette Lum 44904 18th Street West, Lancaster, CA 93534, (805) 948-8749, BA 84 CA St Univ - Northridge; MA 86 Univ of the Pacific

McMillan, Mrs Jeanne Kay R R 3 Box 253A, Portland, IN 47371, (219) 726-7240, BS 83 Ball St Univ; MA 84 Ball St Univ; Sp-Lang Path, Celina City Schools, **SLP**

McMillan, Mrs Olga Christina President 8th District GaFWC, 962 North Beachview Drive, Jekyll Island, GA 31520, (912) 635-2273, BS 34 Univ of MD - College Park; MA 35 Univ of MD - College Park; Retired, Washington DC PS, **SLP LM**

McMillan, Mrs Pamella M 594 South 7th Street, Ann Arbor, MI 48103, (313) 936-7507, BA 75 Case Western Reserve Univ; MA 75 Case Western Reserve Univ; Aud, Univ of MI Hosp, **A**

McMillan, Susan B 2139 N E 56th Place, Fort Lauderdale, FL 33308, (813) 343-2180, MS 84 Univ of South FL; Sp-Lang Path, North Broward Hosp Dist, **SLP**

McMillen, Anne Purdy 11 Van Buren Street, Massapequa Park, NY 11762, BS 41 Columbia Univ Teachers Coll; **SLP A LM**

McMillen, Joanne Lynn 2727 Camino Del Rio South, Suite 228, San Diego, CA 92108, (619) 296-5360, BS 83 Kutztown Univ of PA; MA 85 Univ of Northern CO; 87–Sp-Lang Path, Counselling & Sp Ther Ctr

McMillen, Malcolm E Newington Childrens Hospital, Newington, CT 06111, (203) 667-5320, BS 63 Western MI Univ; MA 70 Eastern MI Univ; MA 82 Hartford Grad Cen; Asst Dir SLP, Newington Chldn Hosp, **SLP**

McMillen, Dr Margaret H University Of Wisconsin, Dept Commun Disorders, Eau Claire, WI 54701, (715) 836-4185, PH 77 (NS); Assistant Professor, University of Wisconsin, **SLP**

McMillian, Jennifer H c/o Center Spch/Lng/Lrng, 14740 Barryknoll, Houston, TX 77079-2802, (713) 496-1636, BA 76 Univ of Houston - Univ Park; MA 77 Univ of Houston - Univ Park; Sp-Lang Path, Center for Spch/Lang/Learning, **SLP**

McMillian, Susan McPherson 106 Holly Trail, Cumming, GA 30130, (404) 536-6681, **SLP**

McMillin, Lois C 908 Maplewood Lane, Iowa City, IA 52245, (319) 351-2510, BS 74 Univ of IA; MA 75 Univ of IA; Grantwood AEA, **SLP**

McMillion, Mrs Leslie Ann 1713 Brenda, Bellevue, NE 68005, (402) 291-7708, BA 80 CA St Univ - Chico; MS 87 Univ of NE - Omaha; **SLP**

McMonigal, Lizabeth J 11210 52nd Avenue #N, Minneapolis, MN 55442, BS 78 Univ of WI - River Falls; MS 79 Univ of WI - River Falls; SLP, St Paul School District 625, **SLP**

McMorrow, Mrs Dorothy Murray P O Box 228, Monument Beach, MA 02553, (617) 548-0151, BA 74 Bridgewater St Coll; MS 78 Emerson Coll; SLP, Falmouth Pub Sch, **SLP**

McMullen, Catherine Therese 21 South Lasalle Street, Apartment 21-C, Durham, NC 27705-3017, (617) 787-3390, MS 84 Northeastern Univ; **SLP**

McMullen, Mrs Gayle Mohorcich Lovelace Medical Center, Audiology Section, 5400 Gibson Boulevard S E, Albuquerque, NM 87108, (505) 262-7261, BS 78 CO St Univ; MS 80 CO St Univ; 84–Aud, Lovelace Med Ctr, **A**

McMullen, Mary Chattin 23 Preston Avenue, Trenton, NJ 08618, (609) 695-4485, BS 83 Trenton St Coll; MA 86 Trenton St Coll; **SLP**

McMullen, Mrs Maureen 95 Summit Avenue, West Warwick, RI 02893, (401) 821-2917, MS 88 Univ of RI

McMullin, Brent R 1505 Columbia Avenue, Gladstone, OR 97027, (503) 643-5454, BS 73 ID St Univ; MS 74 ID St Univ; Aud, Consult, **A**

McMullin, Mrs Carolyn R 35 Parsonage Lane, Topsfield, MA 01983, (508) 535-6197, BA 66 Albion Coll; MA 68 Western MI Univ; Sp-Lang Path, North Shore Spec Ed Consortium, **SLP ACE**

McMullin, Jane A 645 Niagara Street, Victoria, BC, Canada V8V 1J1, (604) 652-1151, BA 76 Univ of Lethbridge - Alberta; MA 80 WA St Univ; 80–Sp/Lang Path, Sch Dist #63 (Saanich), **SLP**

McMullin, Kelly Kristine 178 Greystone Lane #12, Rochester, NY 14618, (716) 243-5470, BS 83 SUNY - Coll at Geneseo; MA 85 SUNY - Coll at Geneseo; Sp-Lang Path, Livingston County BOCES, **SLP**

McMurray, Christine Ann 4517 62nd Street, Des Moines, IA 50322, (515) 276-5690, BA 74 Univ of Northern IA; MA 75 Univ of Northern IA; SLP, Des Moines Indep Comm Sch Dist, **SLP**

McMurray, Mrs Mary Erdani 24049 Glenbrook, Euclid, OH 44117, (216) 241-8230, BA 81 Cleveland St Univ; MA 83 Cleveland St Univ; Sp-Lang Path, Cuyahoga Co Bd of Ment Ret, **SLP**

McMurry, Mrs Claudia 2620 Mockingbird Lane, Amarillo, TX 79109, (806) 353-7650, BA 74 Wichita St Univ; MA 75 Wichita St Univ; Sp-Lang Path, Private Practice, **SLP**

McMurtrey, Mrs Lisa G 2317 Hickory Nut Court, Little Rock, AR 72211, (501) 834-0217, BS 84 Univ of Central AR; MS 87 Univ of Central AR; 87–Sp-Lang Path, N Hills Services for Hndcpd

McMurtry, Mrs Carol A W 679 Riverlake Way, Sacramento, CA 95831, (916) 453-2666, BA 64 San Francisco St Univ; MA 66 Stanford Univ; Chief Aud, Ucd Med Cen, **A**

McMurtry, Mrs Janice Marshall 5744 Monticello, Chino, CA 91710, (714) 628-9527, BA 61 Univ of MA - Amherst; MA 65 Univ of MA - Amherst; **SLP**

McMurtry, Marilyn Holt 224 South Paul, Pauls Valley, OK 73075, (405) 238-6401, BS 82 Univ of AR - Fayetteville; MS 83 Univ of AR - Fayetteville; 86–Sp-Lang Path, OK Dept of Human Svcs, **SLP**

McNab, Teresa Marie 708 Remington #4, Fort Collins, CO 80524, (303) 778-5645, BS 86 Moorhead St Univ; MS 88 CO St Univ

McNabb, Mrs Kathy O 740 Crab Orchard Court, Roswell, GA 30076, (404) 296-5440, BS 75 East TN St Univ; MA 78 Univ of TN - Knoxville; 88–Dir of Mktg, ManorCare The Reach Program, **SLP**

McNair, Mrs Kay M Route 5 Box 42-Aa, Liberty, MO 64068, (816) 781-2474, BA 73 Univ of MO - KS City; MS 74 Central MO St Univ; Sp/Lang Path, School Distr 500, **SLP**

McNairn, Mrs Peggi H 215 Spanish Moss, Arlington, TX 76018, (817) 460-7211, BS 77 TX Christian Univ; MS 78 TX Christian Univ; Sp-Lang Path, Arlington ISD, **SLP**

McNally, Geralyn M 1310 Rose Hill Drive, Charlottesville, VA 22903-1412, (804) 924-5781, BA 80 Univ of DE; MA 81 George Washington Univ; 84–Sp-Lang Path, Univ of Virginia Med Ctr, **SLP**

McNally, Mrs Helen Strobel 28 Carol Street, Lynbrook, NY 11563, (516) 378-8220, BA 80 Molloy Coll; MS 82 Adelphi Univ; Sp-Lang Path, Roosevelt Un Free Sch Dist, **SLP**

McNally, Mrs Lorraine P O Box 119, Niagara Falls, NY 14304, (716) 885-8318, BS 72 SUNY - Coll at Buffalo; MS 73 SUNY - Coll at Buffalo; Sp/Lang Path & Superv Deaf, Buffalo Hrng & Sp Cen, **SLP**

McNally, Mrs Michele Gauthier 14 Annawamscutt Road, Barrington, RI 02806, (401) 294-4581, **SLP**

McNamara, Christine T 1100 West Chester Pike, Apartment M-26, West Chester, PA 19382, (215) 692-6946, BS 86 Bloomsburg Univ of PA; MS 87 Bloomsburg Univ of PA; Sp-Lang Path, Elwyn Inc, **SLP**

McNamara, Mrs Gail Marie 24220 Shaker Blvd, Shaker Heights, OH 44122, (216) 751-9053, BA 68 CUNY - Queens Coll; MS 71 CUNY - Queens Coll; 86–Sp-Lang Path, PSI Affiliates, **SLP ACE**

McNamara, James Patrick Child Study Center, Old Dominion University, Norfolk, VA 23529-0136, (804) 683-4117, MS 85 Old Dominion Univ; 88–Sp-Lang Path, Old Dominion Univ, **SLP**

McNamara, Jean 6616 Chauncey Drive, Memphis, TN 38115-6153, (901) 367-1933, **SLP**

McNamara, John Joseph 519 Lakeview Park, Rochester, NY 14613, (716) 647-2802, MA SUNY - Coll at Geneseo; 88–Aud, Ontario Hearing Instru Corp, **A**

McNamara, Mrs June Bilotta 918 Floral Drive, Orlando, FL 32803, (305) 894-7843, **SLP**

McNamara, Kevin Michael 149 Harkness Drive, Milford, CT 06460, (203) 579-6906, BA 77 Montclair St Coll; MA 81 Univ of CT; Sp-Lang Path, CT Dept Mental Retardation Region 4, **SLP**

McNamara, Sheila Marie 9651 Springfield, Evergreen Park, IL 60642, (312) 423-9746, MS 88 Eastern IL Univ; 88–Sp-Lang Path, Easter Seal Soc of Metro Chicago

McNamara, Stephen D P O Box 61, Hollidaysburg, PA 16648, (814) 696-9574, BS 65 Villanova Univ; OM 70 Villanova Univ; MA 76 Temple Univ-Tyler Sch of Art; President, Management System Consultants, **SLP ACE**

McNamara, Mrs Tena Workman 5317 N Diane Court, Peoria, IL 61615, (309) 692-6252, BS 80 Bradley Univ; MS 83 Bradley Univ; Aud, Adel El-Deiry MD, **A**

McNamee, Melissa St George 210 Linder Lane, Rochelle, IL 61068, (815) 758-0651, BS 78 IL St Univ - Normal; MS 80 IL St Univ - Normal; Sp/Lang Path, Bangor Area Sch, **SLP**

McNary, Doris 13372-B Huston Street, Sherman Oaks, CA 91423, (818) 767-8014, OB 72 Univ of MS; OM 83 Univ of MS; 86–Tchr, Los Angles USD

McNay, Valerie J P O Box 533, Parsons, KS 67357, (316) 421-6550, BA 73 MI St Univ; MA 74 Wayne St Univ; MA 78 Western MI Univ; Proj Coor, Parsons Resear Cen, **SLP**

McNeal, Mrs Julia Ann Verhey 4674 S W Stoddard Drive, Aloha, OR 97007, (503) 591-7573, BA 78 Gonzaga Univ; MS 80 Eastern WA Univ; 88–Sp-Lang Path, Washington Co Educ Svc Dist, **SLP**

McNeal, Kathryn Marie 20055 Westhaven Lane, Rocky River, OH 44116, (216) 231-8787, BS 84 Purdue Univ - West Lafayette; MS 86 Purdue Univ - West Lafayette; **SLP**

McNealy, Karen K 1 Aspen Road, Huntington, WV 25705, (606) 324-0465, BA 74 Marshall Univ; MA 75 Univ of TN - Knoxville; Aud, Geiger Er Sl So Sp & Hrng Cen, **A**

McNear, Claire Tyrrell 34499 Weld County Road #31, Greeley, CO 80631, BA 80 Univ of Northern CO; MA 81 Univ of Northern CO; Sp-Lang Path, Weld County BOCES, **SLP**

McNee, Mrs Margaret D 2880 N W Circle A Drive, Portland, OR 97229, BA 70 San Francisco St Univ; **SLP**

McNeese-Elliott, Linda S R 5125, Wasilla, AK 99687, (907) 376-5683, BS 84 ID St Univ; MS 85 ID St Univ; **SLP**

McNeil, Dr Ellen E 950 S W 29th Street, Albany, OR 97321, (503) 926-8092, **A**

McNeil, Mrs Lystra E 8822-10 East Lemon Creek, Berrien Springs, MI 49103, (616) 471-3468, BS 79 Andrews Univ; MA 84 SUNY - Coll at Buffalo; 84–Prof/Aud, Andrews Univ, **A**

McNeil, Dr Malcolm R Dept Of Communicative Disorders, U Of Wisconsin - Madison, 1975 Willow Drive, Madison, WI 53706, (608) 262-6468, BS 69 Northern MI Univ; MA 71 Northern MI Univ; PH 77 (Sp-Lang Path) Univ of Denver; Prof, U of WI-Madison, **SLP**

McNeill, Mrs Donna M D 2710 Friar Tuck Lane, Austin, TX 78704, (512) 445-0681, BA 78 Univ of MS; MA 79 Univ of MS; Sp/Lang Path, Brown Sch-Ranch Treat Cen, **SLP**

McNeill, Linda D 4404 North Thornwood Avenue, Davenport, IA 52806, (319) 383-1499, BS 81 IL St Univ - Normal; MS 82 IL St Univ - Normal; Sp-Lang Path, Mercy Hospital, **SLP**

McNeill, Linda E 7339 Eastwick Lane, Indianapolis, IN 46256, **SLP**

McNeill, Mrs Mannon B 18368 Colville Street, Fountain Valley, CA 92708, (714) 828-8660, MA 70 CA St Univ - Long Beach; Sp-Lang Path, Cypress ISD, **SLP**

McNeill, Marguerite 1332 Audubon Road, Maitland, FL 32751, (409) 856-6895, **A**

McNeillie, Mrs Lynn K 105 New Deer Lane, Cary, NC 27511, (919) 851-6196, BS 72 Edinboro Univ of PA; MS 76 PA St Univ - Univ Park; Sp-Lang Path, Wake County Schs, **SLP**

McNeilly, Mrs Lemmietta Jones 1531 Northgate Square, 11-B, Reston, VA 22090, (202) 636-6990, BS 77 Hampton Univ; MA 79 SC St Coll; 88–Sp-Lang Path, Howard Univ, **SLP**

McNelis, Mrs Linda Marie 28311 Blum, Roseville, MI 48066, (313) 573-5123, MA 83 Wayne St Univ; SLP, Mike Evans & Assoc, **SLP**

McNiece, Dr Elaine M 1410 Prince, Conway, AR 72032, (501) 450-3175, OB 70 Univ of Central AR; MA 71 Memphis St Univ; ED 82 (NS) Univ of AR - Fayetteville; 87–Asst Dean, Un Cent Ark, **SLP ACE**

McNiece, Mrs Judith Ann 401 Sandy Lane, Deltona, FL 32738, (407) 574-6783, BA 82 Cleveland St Univ; MA 84 Cleveland St Univ; Sp-Lang Path, Volusia Co Pub Schools, **SLP**

McNiel, Mrs Bernadine Ledwig 2222 North Florence, El Paso, TX 79902, (915) 533-2387, BS 45 TX Woman's Univ; MA 78 Univ of TX - El Paso; Retired, El Paso Public Schools, **SLP**

McNish, Mrs Lynn M 4143 Meadow Lane, Eau Claire, WI 54701, (715) 834-8104, BA 77 Univ of WI - Eau Claire; MS 78 Univ of WI - Eau Claire; Sp-Lang Path, Eau Claire Public Schools, **SLP**

McNown, Vicki P 1900 Anderson Place S E, Albuquerque, NM 87108, (913) 296-5451, BS 68 Southwest MO St Univ; MA 74 Univ of KS; Sp-Lang Path, Ks Neur I, **SLP**

McNutt, Eileen Sharon 595 Sunnyside Drive, Eugene, OR 97404, (503) 689-6326, BA 80 Univ of OR; MS 85 Portland St Univ; 88–Sp-Lang Path, Triangle Lake Sch Dist, **SLP**

McNutt, Dr James C 1266 Pine Avenue West, Montreal, PQ, Canada H3G 1A8, (514) 392-5957, BS 56 Edinboro Univ of PA; ME 68 PA St Univ - Univ Park; PH 73 (NS) Kent St Univ; 76–Assoc Prof, McGill Univ Sch of Hum Comm Dis, **SLP**

McOsker, Cynthia Crandall 995 Sawyer Street, South Portland, ME 04106, (207) 775-3491, BA 78 Allegheny Coll; ME 80 Allegheny Coll; MA 81 Case Western Reserve Univ; Sp-Lang Path, Cape Elizabeth Sch Sys, **SLP**

McOsker, Thomas Gerard 995 Sawyer Street, South Portland, ME 04106, (207) 795-2482, BA 79 Coll of the Holy Cross; MA 81 Case Western Reserve Univ; Sp-Lang Path, Private Practice, **SLP**

McPartland, Mrs Tracy Stoecker 7305 Summit Street, Kansas City, MO 64114, (816) 523-3066, BA 81 Univ of IA; MA 83 Univ of IA; Sp-Lang Path, Center School Dist, **SLP**

McPhail, Mrs Barbara E 2005 Brockman McClimon Rd, Greer, SC 29651, (803) 288-7618, BS 74 Auburn Univ - Auburn; MA 75 Memphis St Univ; **SLP**

McPhail, Fay Lois 412 Alpha Avenue #204, Grand Forks, ND 58201, **SLP**

McPhail, Paula A 4771 Pennswood Drive, Huber Heights, OH 45424, (513) 257-8756, BA 76 Univ of NC - Greensboro; ME 79 Univ of NC - Greensboro; 87–Chief-Audiology Svcs, USAF Med Ctr Wright-Patterson AFB, **A**

McPheeters, Deborah H Star Rt 2-A Box 3498-L, Tehachapi, CA 93561, (805) 945-8553, BA 80 Univ of CA - Santa Barbara; MA 83 Univ of CA - Santa Barbara; 85–Sp-Lang Path, High Desert Hosp, **SLP**

McPhee-Van Hevel, Judith A 11018 Peninsula Drive, Traverse City, MI 49684, (616) 922-6259, BA 76 Western MI Univ; MA 77 Western MI Univ; SLP, Traverse Bay Area ISD, **SLP**

McPherson, Betsy Nan 1837 Longcress Drive, Knoxville, TN 37918-2297, (615) 544-1277, BS 80 Auburn Univ - Auburn; MA 82 Univ of TN - Knoxville; 88–Sp-Lang Path, Knox Co Bd of Educ, **SLP**

McPherson, Cynthia Keddy 8 Acorn Acres, Rye, NH 03870, (603) 431-6871, BS 78 0500; MS 86 Univ of NH; **SLP**

McPherson, David L Univ Of Calif Medical Center, Department Of Neurology, DSC 2223 Rt 13, 101 City Drive South, Orange, CA 92668, (714) 634-5776, BS 67 Brigham Young Univ; MA 69 George Washington Univ; PH 71 (NS) Univ of WA; Assoc Prof of Neur & Pedia, U of CA-Irvine, **SLP A**

McPherson, Hal C 436 Diana Place, Marina, CA 93933, (408) 757-0374, BA 78 CA St Univ - Fresno; MA 80 Univ of WA; Aud, Natividad Med Cen, **A**

McPherson, James H 2908 South Phillips Avenue, Sioux Falls, SD 57105, (605) 336-3503, BS 68 East TN St Univ; MS 73 Univ of WY; Aud, Private Practice, **A**

McPherson, Larry T Lancaster Audiology Services, 44241 North 15th St West, Suite 204, Lancaster, CA 93534, (805) 948-7377, BA 73 CA St Univ - Northridge; MA 75 CA St Univ - Northridge; Aud/Owner, Lancaster Aud Serv, **A**

McPherson, Mrs Lillian Lother P O Box 129, Lowdesboro, AL 36752, (205) 288-5999, BS 60 Auburn Univ - Auburn; MA 61 Univ of AL- Tuscaloosa; Sp/Lang Path, Sp Therapy Servs, **SLP**

McPherson, Lorrane Marie 209 Alamosa Avenue, Alamosa, CO 81101, (602) 386-4471, BS 77 Univ of WY; MS 82 Chadron St Coll; 88–Sp-Lang Path, Maricopa Spec Svcs Consortium, **SLP**

McPherson, Neal I 21518 Green Hill Road #239, Farmington Hills, MI 48024, (313) 494-1643, BS 79 Wayne St Univ; MA 81 Eastern MI Univ; 88–Sp-Lang Path, Walled Lake Schs

McPherson, Mrs Shirley Smith P O Box 310, Euless, TX 76039, (817) 571-2821, BS 78 Southwest TX St Univ; ME 79 Southwest TX St Univ; SLP, Floresville Int School Dist, **SLP**

McPherson, Mrs Wendy B Rd 2 Box 325, Brookville, PA 15825, (814) 849-5384, BA 77 Clarion Univ of PA; ME 82 Clarion Univ of PA; SLP, Clarion Manor Iu #6, **SLP**

McPhillips, M Regina P O Box 326, Centerville, MA 02632-0326, MS; **A LM**

McQuade, MaryAlice 370-C Montaque Road, Sunderland, MA 01375, (413) 772-0211, BA 70 Coll of New Rochelle; MS 72 Columbia Univ Teachers Coll; 77–Dept Mgr, Franklin Med Cen, **SLP**

McQuade, Rosalyn F 2404 Augusta Street, San Luis Obispo, CA 93401, (805) 543-0441, BA 71 Univ of CA - Berkeley; MA 75 CA St Univ - Northridge; SLP, San Luis Coastal USD, **SLP**

McQuade, Mrs Veronica Balicki South 5111 Orchard Avenue, Hamburg, NY 14075, (716) 823-1324, BS 77 SUNY - Coll at Buffalo; MS 81 SUNY - Coll at Buffalo; 77–Sp-Lang Path, Buffalo Board of Educ, **SLP**

McQuaid, Mrs Patricia W 4441 Mendenhall Drive, Dallas, TX 75244, (214) 960-6810, BA 68 Marietta Coll; MS 70 Univ of North TX; **SLP**

McQuaide, Karen Lynn Aud Dept Temple Univ Hospital, West Bldg 3440 No Broad St, Philadelphia, PA 19140, (215) 221-3661, BA 83 Montclair St Coll; MA 84 Northwestern Univ; Aud, Temple University Hospital, **A ACE**

McQuaide, Marilyn H 66 Lake View Drive, Gettysburg, PA 17325-7413, (717) 334-8331, BS 74 PA St Univ - Univ Park; MS 79 PA St Univ - Univ Park; Sp-Lang Path, Easter Seals, **SLP**

McQuaig, Jean S 101 Lenora Street, Pineville, LA 71360, **SLP**

McQuain, Johnny D 2606 Barton Avenue, Nashville, TN 37212, (615) 320-5353, BA 81 Harding Univ; MS 83 Vanderbilt Univ; Sp-Lang Path, Bill Wilkerson Hrng/Sp Cen, **SLP**

McQuay, Sue M Route 4 Box 278-B, Jonesboro, AR 72401, (501) 932-4043, BS 84 AR St Univ; MS 85 AR St Univ

McQueen, Ann B 7015 Shamrock Drive, Little Rock, AR 72205, (501) 227-2118, BA 75 Univ of AR - Little Rock; MS 78 Univ of AR - Little Rock; Super-SLP Servs, Baptist Med Syst, **SLP**

McQueen, Mrs Carol B 15643 Yellowbrook Lane, La Mirada, CA 90638, (213) 943-9461, BA 67 Columbia Coll; MS 75 Univ of SC - Columbia; **SLP**

McQueen, Jo Ella 1342 Leegate Street N W, Washington, DC 20012, MS; **SLP**

McQueen, Karen Connor 3301 Loop Road #1803, Tuscaloosa, AL 35404, (205) 553-4550, BS 78 Towson St Univ; MS 79 Univ of AL- Tuscaloosa; Sp/Lang Path, Dept of Ment Hlth St of Al, **SLP**

McQuilkin, Jean S 261 Stanton Avenue, Columbiana, OH 44408, (216) 424-9561, BS 64 Kent St Univ; MA 74 Kent St Univ; Sp-Lang Path, Columbiana Co Bd of Ed, **SLP ACE**

McQuirk, Susan Jean 3448 Las Palmas Avenue, Glendale, CA 91208, (818) 409-8023, BA 84 CA St Univ - Northridge; MA 87 CA St Univ - Northridge; Sp-Lang Path, Glendale Adventist Med Ctr

McQuown, Maureen E 1410 West 11th, Apt #9, Erie, PA 16502, (814) 453-7661, BS 84 2641; MA 86 2641; SLP, Dr Gertrude A Barber Ctr, **SLP**

McRae, Mrs Carol 4408 Somerset Blvd S E, Bellevue, WA 98006, (206) 455-6077, BS 62 Univ of KS; MA 65 Univ of WA; SLP, Bellevue Public Schools, **SLP**

McRae, Catherine L 1520 Viscount, Tallahassee, FL 32304, (904) 627-9651, BS 75 Central MI Univ; MS 81 FL St Univ; Coordinating Specialist, Gadsen County, **SLP**

McRae, Mrs Martha Polk 2404 Syon, Memphis, TN 38119, (901) 767-5354, BS 69 Univ of TN - Knoxville; MA 72 Univ of IA; SLP, Private Practice, **SLP**

McRandle, Dr Carol C 905 Racine, Bellingham, WA 98226, (206) 676-3885, BS 58 Univ of MN - Duluth; MS 61 Purdue Univ - West Lafayette; PH 64 (NS) Purdue Univ - West Lafayette; Aud, Wn WA U, **SLP A**

McReynolds, Barbara L 409 South A Street, Lompoc, CA 93436, **SLP**

McReynolds, Dr Leija V 10745 Oakmont, Shawnee Mission, KS 66210, (913) 469-9187, BS 46 IL St Univ - Normal; MA 59 Univ of IL - Urbana; PH 64 (NS) Stanford Univ; Prof Sp-Lang Path, U of KS Med Cen, **SLP F LM**

McRight, K Renee H 2797 Marico Place, Greenville, MS 38701, **SLP**

McShane, William Thomas 806 West Fifth Street, Marshfield, WI 54449, (715) 387-1896, MS 87 Univ of WI - Stevens Point; **SLP**

McSharry, Edward J Rural Free Delivery 8, Bartlett Road, Plymouth, MA 02360, (617) 293-5411, BS 66 Emerson Coll; MS 69 CUNY - Brooklyn Coll; Sp-Lang Path, Pembroke-Pub Sch, **SLP**

McSharry, Mrs Margaret Tassinari Rural Free Delivery 8, Barlett Road, Plymouth, MA 02360, (617) 548-0411, BS 66 Emerson Coll; ME 67 PA St Univ - Univ Park; 88–Dir Rehab Dept, Barnstable Co Hosp, **SLP**

McSorley, Mrs Mary Kim Rd 3 Box 77, Chestertown, MD 21620, BS 76 Radford Univ; MS 78 Towson St Univ; Sp-Lang Path, Bewedictine Sch, **SLP**

McSpaden, Corlene H Lebanon Med Ctr Bldg, 33171 North Santiam Hgwy, Lebanon, OR 97355, (503) 451-1631, BA 68 Univ of KS; OM 68 Western OR St Coll; Sp/Lang Path/Aud, Corlene H McSpaden, **SLP A**

McSpaden, Dana Kirsten 3141 Northshore Drive S E, Apartment 10, Albany, OR 97321-4527, (503) 327-2742, BS 84 Willamette Univ; MS 86 Western OR St Coll

McSpaden, Dr Jay B Lebanon Medical Center Bldg, 33171 North Santiam Highway, Lebanon, OR 97355, (503) 451-1631, BA 67; MS 68 Western OR St Coll; PH 71 (NS) Univ of WA; Aud, Private Practice, **A**

McSween, Mrs Nena Etheridge 382 Valley Brook Drive, Atlanta, GA 30342, (404) 451-1756, OB 76 Univ of GA; MS 78 Univ of AL- Tuscaloosa; Sp-Lang Path, Dekalb County Board of Educ, **SLP**

McSweeney, Aileen Marie 13828 Edgewater, Lakewood, OH 44107, (216) 856-2107, BS 83 Eastern MI Univ; MA 84 Eastern MI Univ

McTeer, Vidalia G Speech Services Inc, P O Box 1131, 514 West Liberty Street, Sumter, SC 29150, (803).775-5965, BS 68 SC St Coll; MS 73 Vanderbilt Univ; Sp-Lang Path, Sp Ser Inc, **SLP**

McTernan, Mrs Carolyn L 5215 Wissioming Road, Bethesda, MD 20816, (301) 770-8437, BA 61 Our Lady Lake Univ-San Anton; MA 71 George Washington Univ; Sp-Lang Path, Hebrew Home/Greater Washington, **SLP**

McTighe, Audrey R 130 East 94th Street, Apartment #7-E, New York, NY 10128, (907) 474-8663, BS 75 NY Univ; MA 78 NY Univ; Sp-Lang Path, **SLP**

McVann, Owen J 3702 South Whitnall Avenue, Milwaukee, WI 53207, (414) 384-2000, BA 79 Univ of MN - Duluth; MS 86 Univ of WI - Milwaukee; Sp-Lang Path, VA Hosp, **SLP**

McVay, Mary 2026 Saint Charles Avenue, Suite 806, New Orleans, LA 70130, BA 69 CA St Univ - Los Angeles; MA 76 CA St Univ - Los Angeles; Sp-Lang Path, Private Practice, **SLP**

McVay, Maureen Elizabeth 1330 5th Street N E #43, Hickory, NC 28601, (804) 792-0650, BS 82 Nazareth Coll of Rochester; MS 83 Radford Univ; Sp/Lang Path, Frye Regional Medical Center, **SLP**

McVay, Robyn 109 Hawley Avenue, Milford, CT 06460, (203) 734-3355, BA 84 Univ of RI; MS 87 Southern CT St Univ; **SLP**

McVeigh, Patricia Sutley 211 Concord Drive, River Edge, NJ 07661, **SLP**

McVey, Diane E Diles Hearing Center, 326 West Union, Athens, OH 45701, (614) 594-3571, BS 75 OH Univ - Athens; MA 76 OH Univ - Athens; Aud, Private Practice, **A**

McVey, Kerry Lea 15532 Signall Hill Ct, Granger, IN 46530, (219) 277-0705, BS 86 Purdue Univ - West Lafayette; BA 86 Purdue Univ - West Lafayette; MA 88 OH St Univ; 88–Sp-Lang Path, Therapeutic Sys

McVey, Lola C Box 315, Kismet, KS 67859, (316) 563-7650, BA 64 Wichita St Univ; Sp-Lang Path, Private Practice, **SLP**

McVey, Richard K 45 Ridge Lane Drive, Decatur, IL 62521, (217) 424-3423, BS 70 Northern IL Univ - De Kalb; MA 74 Northern IL Univ - De Kalb; Aud, St Marys Hospital, **A**

McVey, Mrs Theresa A 10219 Fairway Drive, Ellicott City, MD 21043, (301) 661-2400, BA 77 Loyola Coll; MS 78 Loyola Coll; Sp-Lang Path, Baltimore County Pub Schools, **SLP**

McVicar, Mrs Denise Yvonne 9 Whitehill Avenue, Nepean, ON, Canada K2G 3A9, (613) 737-2372, BA 76 Univ of CA - Berkeley; MS 79 San Francisco St Univ; 84–Sp/Lang Path, Chldns Hosp of E Ont, **SLP**

McVoy, Esther Marie 6409 N W 192nd Terrace, Miami, FL 33015, (305) 836-2820, BS 78 WV Univ; MA 79 Univ of Miami; Sp-Lang Path, Dade County Schools, **SLP**

McWeeney, Leeann Di Salvia 25 Phillips Road, East Greenwich, RI 02818, (401) 739-2700, BA 78 Univ of FL; MS 81 Univ of RI; Sp/Lang Path, J Arthur Trudeau Mem Cen, **SLP**

McWhorter, Mrs Sue Jordan 769 Canyon Road, Logan, UT 84321-4316, (304) 525-8586, BA 76 Marshall Univ; MA 77 Marshall Univ; Sp-Lang Path, Region III Child Dev Services, **SLP**

McWhorter, Susan Jane 4003 Wynbrook Way, Monroe, NC 28110, (704) 764-7086, MA 87 Appalachian St Univ

McWhorter, Tina D 415 North Rock Hill Road, Webster Groves, MO 63119, (314) 968-0143, BS 77 Saint Louis Univ; MA 79 Univ of KS; Ch Aud, Jewish Hosp at Wash U, **A**

McWilliams, Dr Betty J 512 Bigham Road, Pittsburgh, PA 15211, (412) 624-3198, BS OH St Univ; MS Univ of Pittsburgh - Pittsburgh; PH (Sp Path/Psych) Univ of Pittsburgh - Pittsburgh; Director Cleft Palate Center, University of Pittsburgh, **SLP F**

McWilliams, Bonnie L 5940 Sawmill Road, Paradise, CA 95969, BA 74 Univ of CA - Santa Barbara; MA 86 CA St Univ - Chico; 88–Sp-Lang Path, Yuba County Schs

McWilliams, Carol S 3295 Norwood Road, Shaker Heights, OH 44122, (216) 561-1023, BS 61 Univ of KS; MA 65 Northwestern Univ; Sp-Lang Path, Private Practice, **SLP**

McWilliams, Linda Leverenz 10000 Pandora Drive, La Mesa, CA 92041, (619) 691-5455, BA 77 Univ of the Pacific; MA 85 San Diego St Univ; 84–Tchr, Sweetwater Union HS Dist

McWilliams, Mrs Maren L 3310 Morning Dew Road, Greensboro, NC 27407, (919) 272-5117, BA 67 Univ of WA; MA 69 Univ of WA; Sp-Lang Path, Karen Long & Assoc, **SLP**

Meach, Mrs Barbara S 2372 N Pine Center Drive, West Bloomfield, MI 48033, (313) 681-9211, BA 59 Univ of MI - Ann Arbor; MA 66 Univ of MI - Ann Arbor; SLP, Private Practice, **SLP**

Mead, Brenda Cammon 320 Manhattan Avenue #29, New York, NY 10026, (212) 491-8029, BA 75 Case Western Reserve Univ; MS 76 Columbia Univ Teachers Coll; SLP, Private Practice, **SLP**

Mead, Mrs Denise M Route 1 Box 359, Thornton, WV 26440, (304) 265-4090, MS 75 WV Univ; BS 73 WV Univ; Special Services Coordinator, Taylor County Board of Educ, **SLP**

Meade, Edwina P O Box 60, Cape May Court House, NJ 08210, (609) 465-1557, MA 81 Temple Univ; 86–Sp-Lang Path, Cape May Co Spec Sch Dist, **SLP**

Meade, Kathleen N 11994 Carrington Court, Cincinnati, OH 45249-1765, (513) 677-1537, BS 76 Univ of VA - Charlottesville; MA 78 Vanderbilt Univ; Sp-Lang Path, Children's Hosp Outpatient N, **SLP**

Meade, Mrs Lynn T 140 Rosewood Drive, Metairie, LA 70005, (504) 835-5958, BS 74 Saint Mary's Dominican Coll; OM 79 LA St Univ - N O Medical Ctr; Sp-Lang Path, Private Practice, **SLP**

Meade, Mrs Margaret B 239 Emmans Road, Flanders, NJ 07836, (201) 540-5202, BA 72 George Washington Univ; MS 73 Rutgers St Univ -N Brunswick; Dir, Morristown Mem Hosp, **SLP ACE**

Meade, William F 135 Ashland Place #12-A, Brooklyn, NY 11201, (212) 875-2084, BA 54 CUNY - Brooklyn Coll; MA 56 CUNY - Brooklyn Coll; Assoc Prof, Long Island U Bklyn Cen, **SLP**

Meader, Diane D P O Box 563, Bermuda Run, Advance, NC 27006, (919) 768-9090, BA 77; ME 78 Univ of NC - Greensboro; Director, Speech Pathology Associates, **SLP**

Meader, Nancy Kay 504 Eastview S W, Albuquerque, NM 87105, (505) 883-9116, OB Univ of NM; MS 83 Univ of NM; 87–Sp-Lang Path/Evaluator, Albuquerque PS, **SLP**

Meador, Dr Helen Elisa P O Box 7488, Ann Arbor, MI 48107, (313) 747-2504, BA 77 CUNY - Hunter Coll; MA 79 NY Univ; PH 87 (Sign Lang Use of Hrng Imp'd Childr) Univ of MI - Ann Arbor

Meador, Mrs Jeanette D 2524 North Central Drive, Chandler, AZ 85224, (602) 899-2445, BS 80 Northern AZ Univ; MS 81 Northern AZ Univ; SLP, Mesa Pub Sch Dist, **SLP**

Meador, Joan Route 5 Box 591-B, Boone, NC 28607, (704) 264-9659, MS; **SLP**

Meador, Kathryn A 17 Salter Place, Maplewood, NJ 07040, (201) 937-8758, BS 82 Nazareth Coll of Rochester; MS 84 Nazareth Coll of Rochester; **SLP**

Meador, Dr Millard M Route 5 Box 591-B, Boone, NC 28607, (704) 262-2184, BS 53 Wayne St Univ; MA 57 1998; PH 62 (NS) Wayne St Univ - Sch of Med; Prof, Appalachian St U, **A**

Meadors, Deborah Lynn 717 Ramsdell, Tacoma, WA 98466, (206) 565-1570, BA 81 Western WA Univ; MA 83 WA St Univ; Sp-Lang Path, Tacoma Public Schools, **SLP**

Meadows, Amanda L 3427-I S W 30th Terrace, Gainesville, FL 32608, (904) 375-4159, MA 88 Univ of FL

Meadows, Cynthia Kay 285 Boulevard, Suite 210, Atlanta, GA 30312, (404) 524-2438, BA 82 Univ of TN - Knoxville; MA 83 Univ of TN - Knoxville; 85–Aud, Metropolitan Aud Ctr, **A**

Meadows, Cynthia Lynn 7905 Piper Lane, Lake Worth, FL 33436, (407) 736-8599, BS 79 WV Univ; MS 80 WV Univ; Aud, Hearx Ltd, **A**

Meadows, Mrs Jan H Route 2 Box 170, Elgin, TX 78621, (512) 285-4143, BA 72 LA St Univ - Baton Rouge; MA 75 Univ of TX - Austin; Instr/Prin, Meadows Country Sch, **SLP**

Meadows, Joseph D P O Box 6682, Houston, TX 77265-6682, (713) 529-9804, BA 84 Eastern MI Univ; MA 85 Eastern MI Univ; SLP, Ind Contractor, **SLP**

Meadows, Mary Beth M 1233 Center Point Road, Carrollton, GA 30117, (404) 832-0181, BA 78 Univ of FL; OM 80 Auburn Univ - Auburn; Sp-Lang Path, Private Practice, **SLP**

Meadows, Mrs Polly E Office Of Speech - Language - Hearing, Hudson State Service Center, 501 Ogletown Road, Newark, DE 19711, (302) 368-6790, BA 74 Univ of FL; ME 75 Univ of FL; 77–Aud, St Dept of Pub Hlth, **A**

Meadows, Sally B Sweet Briar College, Box AJ, Sweet Briar, VA 24595, (804) 381-5624, BS 66 East TN St Univ; MS 68 Vanderbilt Univ; **SLP**

Meagher, Mary Kane 23462 Crestwood Drive, Elkhart, IN 46514, (219) 293-7506, BS 64 Nazareth Coll of Rochester; MS 69 SUNY - Coll at Geneseo; Sp-Lang Path, Assn for the Dis of Elkhart Co

Mealins, Amy P O Box 1165, Glendale Heights, IL 60139, (714) 658-5595, BA 77 Augustana Coll; MA 79 Northern IL Univ - De Kalb; Warner Lambert, **SLP**

Mealler, Mrs Jo-An Murch 483 Fruitwood Drive, Grand Junction, CO 81504-5841, (303) 245-2100, BS 76 CO St Univ; MS 80 CO St Univ; Aud, Grand Junction Regional Center, **A**

Means, Mrs D Yvonne N 5 Brookspring Circle, Columbia, SC 29223, (803) 777-2614, BA 75 Columbia Coll; MA 77 Univ of TN - Knoxville; Aud, U Sc Sp/Hrng Cl, **A**

Means, Mrs Pamela Ingram PO Box E, Corsicana, TX 75110, (214) 874-4423, BS 82 Univ of AR - Fayetteville; MS 84 Univ of AR - Fayetteville; 88–Sp-Lang Path, Freestone-Navarro Co Educ Coop, **SLP**

Means, Paulette G 16805 Sunderland, Detroit, MI 48219, (313) 467-2664, BA 71 Univ of MI - Ann Arbor; MS 72 Univ of MI - Ann Arbor; SLP, Wayne Co General Hosp, **SLP ACE**

Means, Sharon H 1435 Bedford Street #7-G, Stamford, CT 06905, (203) 348-4686, BS 63 Purdue Univ - West Lafayette; MA 74; OM 79; 63–Sp/Lang Path, Private Practice, **SLP**

Means, Teresa Elizabeth 425 Oak Hills Parkway, Baton Rouge, LA 70810, (301) 948-8230, **SLP**

Means, Wanda R 30330 Suzanne Circle, Springfield, MO 65807, **SLP**

Mearan, Judith U 1464 Fahlander Drive North, Columbus, OH 43229, **SLP**

Mearns-Brown, Mrs Marily Ann 1791 Allison Road, Vancouver, BC, Canada V6T 1S7, (604) 261-4943, BA 69 Univ of the Pacific; MA 71 Univ of Southern CA; Sp-Lang Path, Private Practice, **SLP**

Mears, Kathleen Lazgin 503 Hill Avenue, Langhorne, PA 19047, BS 78 DE Valley Coll of Sci & Agr; ME 83 Trenton St Coll; SLP, Davidson School, **SLP**

Mears, Mrs Treva J 2512 Rolling Green Drive, Independence, KS 67301, (316) 331-6303, BA 57 Wichita St Univ; ME 65 Wichita St Univ; 76–Sp-Lang Path, Tri Co Spec Ed Coop, **SLP**

Mease, Mrs Deborah Kay Box 702 Susan Road, Coopersburg, PA 18036, (215) 776-3270, BS 84 Bloomsburg Univ of PA; MS 85 Bloomsburg Univ of PA; 85–Sp-Lang Path, Good Shepherd Rehab Hosp, **SLP**

Mease, Richard P 1790 Lisa Drive #9, Indiana, PA 15701, PH (NS); **SLP**

Measeles-Allen, Larwin Michele 3201 Carriage Lane, Chandler, AZ 85224, (602) 279-5801, BA 73 Scripps Coll; MA 76 Northern AZ Univ; OM 84 AZ St Univ; **SLP**

Mecca, Annamaria 918 East University Avenue, Bloomington, IN 47401, (812) 855-6508, BA 75 SUNY - Center at Buffalo; MA 78 IN Univ - Bloomington; 85–Sp-Lang Path, Indiana University, **SLP**

Meccia, Nancy 51 Curie Rd #B-7, Cornwall, NY 12520, (914) 534-9290, BA 83 Hofstra Univ; MS 84 Adelphi Univ; 85–Sp-Lang Path, Monroe Woodbury Sch Dist, **SLP**

Mecham, Dr Merlin J 1785 South 400 East, Bountiful, UT 84010, (801) 581-6725, BA 48 Brigham Young Univ; MS 49 UT St Univ; PH 54 (NS) OH St Univ; Prof, U of UT, **SLP F**

Mecham, Richard W 61 North 200 West, American Fork, UT 84003, Director Special Education, Alpine School District, **SLP**

Mecham, Steven G 3710 North Diana Street, Fresno, CA 93726, (209) 224-9696, BS 81 UT St Univ; OM 82 Brigham Young Univ; Aud, MacK E Patterson MD, Inc, **A**

Mechanic, Janis B 2228 West Appletree Road, Milwaukee, WI 53209, (414) 354-0900, BS 70 Univ of WI - Milwaukee; MS 72 Univ of WI - Milwaukee; 88–Sp-Lang Path, Franciscan Home Health, **SLP**

Meche, Peggy A 407 Sonny Street, Lafayette, LA 70501, (318) 231-2166, BS 76 Univ of Southwestern LA; MA 78 Univ of Southwestern LA; Sp-Lang Path, Our Lady/Lourdes Reg Med Cen, **SLP**

Mechelis, Mrs Koula S K 312 Penwood Road, Silver Spring, MD 20901, (301) 345-7612, BA 76 Univ of MD - College Park; MS 78 Loyola Coll; Sp/Lang Path, Pr Georges Co Proj-Hd Start, **SLP**

Meck-Eisenberg, Diane Marie 1924 Curtiss, Downers Grove, IL 60515-4324, (312) 276-4000, BS 81 Northern IL Univ - De Kalb; MS 83 Univ of IL - Chicago; SLP, Easter Seal of Metro Chicago, **SLP**

Mecklenborg, Mrs Janis Pohlman 4175 Janward Drive, Cincinnati, OH 45211, (513) 481-9386, BS 78 Bowling Green St Univ; MS 82 Miami Univ - Oxford; Sp-Lang Path, Cincinnati Pub Sch, **SLP**

Mecklenburg, Mrs Deborah V 1315 St Andrews Drive East, Schererville, IN 46375, (219) 865-8901, BS 58 Northwestern Univ; MA 76 OH St Univ; Sp-Lang Path, City of Hammond, **SLP**

Mecklenburg, Dr Dianne Jorgi Cavale Consulting, 975 8th Street, Boulder, CO 80302, (303) 772-4471, BA 70 CA St Univ - Los Angeles; MA 71 CA St Univ - Los Angeles; PH 78 (NS) Bowling Green St Univ; North Amer Cl Coord, Cochlear Corp, **SLP A**

Mecklenburger, Jill E 411 West Fullerton Parkway #702W, Chicago, IL 60614, (312) 787-0199, BS 85 Univ of IL - Urbana; MA 87 Univ of IL - Urbana; 88–Aud, Neurotology inc, **A**

Meckler, Mrs Deanna L Route 7 Deacon Hills, Lake Shore Drive, Richmond, KY 40475, (606) 622-4442, BA 67; MS 68; **A**

Meckler, Marlys 17525 Ventura Boulevard, Suite 307, Encino, CA 91316, (818) 907-7499, BA 60 Univ of MI - Ann Arbor; MA 70 CA St Univ - Northridge; Dir, Tarzana Sp-Lang Cen, **SLP**

Meckley, Mrs Stacy Lynn 518 Greeves Street, Kane, PA 16735, (814) 837-8475, BA 84 Thiel Coll; MA 86 SUNY - Center at Buffalo; **SLP**

Medall, Lisa Zee 4210 Raintree Circle, Culver City, CA 90230, (714) 581-2800, BA 83 CA St Univ - Long Beach; MA 85 CA St Univ - Long Beach; 85–Sp-Lang Path, Newport Lang Sp Aud Ctr Inc, **SLP**

Medanich, Melanie 112 Woodmont Boulevard, Nashville, TN 37205-2212, (615) 292-8384, MS 77 TX Christian Univ; 87–Sp-Lang Path, Bill Wilkerson Sp & Hrng Cl, **SLP**

Meday-Rozwod, Mrs Susan 4073 Kidron Lane, Liverpool, NY 13090, (315) 487-4631, BA 84 SUNY - Coll at Cortland; MS 85 Syracuse Univ; **SLP**

Medders, Emily A 7342 Northwest 116th, Oklahoma City, OK 73162, (405) 720-0839, BS 80 Phillips Univ; MS 82 Phillips Univ; Sp-Lang Path, OK Cty Pub Sch, **SLP**

Medeiros, Myra Ann 218 Plantation Court, St Marys, GA 31558, (912) 882-2241, BS 73 Bridgewater St Coll; MA 78 Bowling Green St Univ; **SLP**

Medeles, Sandra Silva 1641 Labrador, Costa Mesa, CA 92626, (714) 957-5147, BA 76; MA 79 Univ of TX - El Paso; 88–Sp-Lang Path, Fairview Developmental Center, **SLP**

Medford, Cydney M 424 Brady Lane, Austin, TX 78746, (512) 444-4835, BS 79 Baylor Univ; MS 80 Baylor Univ; 85–Sp-Lang Path, Healthcare Rehab Ctr, **SLP**

Medina, Mrs Alma Lizette Calle Las Mesas Q-8 Colina, Metropolitan Ii, Guaynabo, PR 00657, (809) 790-2416, MS 86 Univ of PR - Rio Piedras; **SLP**

Medina, Mrs Sherri Larson 27800 Medical Center Road, Bldg 1 Suite 206, Mission Viejo, CA 92691, (714) 364-4778, BA 82 Univ of Redlands; MS 84 Univ of Redlands; 88–Sp-Lang Path/Owner, South Coast Rehab Svcs, **SLP**

Medinger, Sue Ellen Rd 3 Box 105, Ten Mile Road, Allegany, NY 14706, (716) 375-4453, BA 75 Univ of Pittsburgh - Pittsburgh; MA 83 Univ of FL; Sp-Lang Path, Allegany-Cattaraugus BOCES, **SLP**

Medland, Julie Community Rehabilitation Ctr, 1009 Maitland Ctr Commons, Suite 200A, Maitland, FL 32751, (407) 660-2936, BA 76 Univ of Central FL; MA 78 Univ of Central FL; Admin/Vp/Treas, Communty Rehab Cen, **SLP**

Medler, Diane 52 Kenview, Tonawanda, NY 14217, (716) 884-1937, BS 80 SUNY - Coll at Buffalo; MS 87 SUNY - Coll at Buffalo; 88–Sp-Lang Path, Lang Dev Prog of W NY, **SLP**

Medley, Kennard E 3736 Blue Grouse, Pocatello, ID 83201, (208) 236-2852, BS 86 ID St Univ; MS 87 ID St Univ; 88–Aud, Sp & Hearing Ctr

Medlock, Sophia Anderton 2003 Wildflower Drive, Hoover, AL 35244, (205) 424-1450, MS 83 Univ of AL-Tuscaloosa; Aud, ENT Clinic, **A**

Medsker, Susan A 5350 Olive Drive, Concord, CA 94521, MS

Meduna, Marian Kay 6100 Vine #D-23, Lincoln, NE 68505, (402) 464-5511, BS 85 Univ of NE - Lincoln; MS 86 Univ of NE - Lincoln; **A**

Medved-Diangelo, Mrs Karen 1243 Whitlock Ridge Drive, Marietta, GA 30064, (404) 427-5666, BS 78 Univ of GA; MS 80 Univ of GA; Sp-Lang Path, Cobb Co Pub Schs, **SLP**

Medvidovich, Patricia A 222 Connecticut Avenue, Clairton, PA 15025, (412) 233-9762, BS 71 CA Univ of PA; ME 75 CA Univ of PA; Sp-Lang Path, Allegheny Intermediate Unit, **SLP**

Medwetsky, Leslie Weigel 56 Heling Boulevard, Lindenhurst, NY 11757, (516) 226-7931, BA 81 SUNY - Center at Stony Brook; MA 84 Long Island U - CW Post Ctr; Sp-Lang Path, Nassau BOCES, **SLP**

Meech, Mrs Sandy Swank 612 40th Street North, Great Falls, MT 59401, (406) 727-3430, BA 63 Univ of MT; MA 74 Univ of MT; Sp-Lang Path, Great Falls Pub Sch, **SLP**

Meehan, Mrs Carolyn Schindler 136 Quail Springs Road, Martinez, GA 30907, (404) 790-2123, BS 68 Lamar Univ; ME 87 Univ of North FL; 88–Sp-Lang Path, Columbia Co Schs

Meehan, Mrs Maria Gonzalez 1 Knightsbridge Court, Baltimore, MD 21236, (301) 574-4950, BA 81 Loyola Coll; MS 82 Loyola Coll; SLP, Balto County Pub Sch, **SLP**

Meehan, Mary H 2712 Middletown Road, Pittsburgh, PA 15205, (412) 394-5815, BS 71 Indiana Univ of PA; MS 72 PA St Univ - Univ Park; SLP, Allegheny Inter Ut, **SLP**

Meek, Mrs Denise Patricia R 940 Linda Lane, Barstow, CA 92311, (619) 256-0611, MS 81 Univ of Redlands; 88–Sp-Lang Path, Barstow USD, **SLP**

Meek, Kathleen Stauffer 408 Ridgewood Drive, Richardson, TX 75080, (214) 495-8250, MA 77 IN Univ - Bloomington; Sp-Lang Path, Richardson ISD, **SLP**

Meek, Merry Mina 6217 S E 41st, Portland, OR 97202, (503) 279-8356, BS 64 WA St Univ; MS 66 Purdue Univ - West Lafayette; Sp-Lang Path, Oregon Health Sciences Univ, **SLP F**

Meek, Stephanie 1035 11th #5, Eureka, CA 95501, (707) 445-5111, BA 81 CA St Univ - Fresno; MA 83 CA St Univ - Sacramento; Sp-Lang Path, General Hosp, **SLP**

Meek, Mrs Sylvia D 6576 Devonwood Drive, Cincinnati, OH 45224, (513) 521-3407, BS 64 Univ of IL - Urbana; ME 65 Southern IL Univ -Carbondale; 86–Sp-Lang Path, Univ of Cinti Med Ctr, **SLP**

Meeker, Joan B 2700 Dexter, Terre Haute, IN 47805, (812) 466-2998, BS 78 IN St Univ - Terre Haute; MS 79 IN St Univ - Terre Haute; **SLP**

Meeker, Sidney A R R 1 Box 190-A, Mulvane, KS 67110, (316) 689-3240, BS 76 KS St Univ; MA 77 KS St Univ; 86–Instr/Clin Supvr, Wichita State Univ, **SLP**

Meeker, Susan Scott 29550 Bolingbrook, Pepper Pike, OH 44124, (216) 444-4961, BS 80 Miami Univ - Oxford; MA 81 OH St Univ; 86–Sp-Lang Path, Cleveland Clinic Foundation, **SLP**

Meeks, Mrs Constance Dove 405 Pitman Avenue, Pitman, NJ 08071, MS 81 Univ of South FL; Sp-Lang Path, Cerebral Palsy Ctr, **SLP**

Meeks, Mrs Kathryn R 10 Carriage Drive, Country Club Estates, Greer, SC 29651, (803) 585-0322, BS 72 Eastern KY Univ; MA 74 Univ of TN - Knoxville; Coord Sp-Lang Path, Spartanburg Co Pub Sch, **SLP**

Meeks, Linda 214-B East Gaston Street, Savannah, GA 31401, (912) 232-8551, BA 68 Univ of AL- Tuscaloosa; MA 71 Univ of AL- Tuscaloosa; Sp-Lang Path, Savannah Pub Sch, **SLP**

Meeks, Lisa Rene 9600 Meandering Way, Apartment 6, Fort Smith, AR 72903, (501) 452-0656, BS 82 Henderson St Univ; MS 84 Univ of AR - Little Rock; 88–Sp-Lang Path, West AR Guidance Cnsl Ctr, **SLP**

Meeks, Peggy N 114 North 4th Street, Alvin, TX 77511, (713) 776-9432, BS 72 TX Tech Univ; MA 73 Univ of Houston - Univ Park; Ed Diagn, Houston ISD, **SLP**

Meengs, Della K 11211 Takilma Road, Cave Junction, OR 97523, **SLP**

Meester, Cindy Lee Dickinson 12710 50th Avenue North, Plymouth, MN 55442, (612) 533-2297, BS 77 Saint Cloud St Univ; MS 85 Univ of WI - River Falls; 77–Sp-Lang Path, Osseo Area Schs Dist 279, **SLP**

Megargee, Mary Eigler 40 Wauwinet Court, Guilford, CT 06437, (203) 669-5701, BA 81 0500; MS 85 Southern CT St Univ; SLP, Clinton Bd of Ed, **SLP**

Megel, Mary J 15250 Brandy Lane, Utica, MI 48087, (313) 247-1228, BS 75 Western MI Univ; MA 80 Wayne St Univ; Sp-Lang Path, Macomb ISD, **SLP**

Meglasson, Katherine 418 Iven Avenue, St Davids, PA 19087, (215) 251-5434, BA 77 Univ of Houston - Univ Park; MA 79 Univ of Houston - Univ Park; Director Dept Commun Disorders, Bryn Mawr Rehabilitation Hosp, **SLP**

Mehlbrech, Mrs Debra A G 1009 2nd Street N E, Sibley, IA 51249, (712) 754-2320, BS 75 Univ of SD - Vermillion; MA 76 Univ of SD - Vermillion; 88–Sp-Lang Path, AEA #4 Sioux Ctr IA, **SLP**

Mehler, Mrs Beth M 7 Clark Court, Kendall Park, NJ 08824, (201) 688-0100, BA 73 Rider Coll; MA 85 Kean Coll of NJ; **A**

Mehler, Mrs Esther 5120 9th Avenue, Brooklyn, NY 11220, (203) 468-0312, BA 82 CUNY - Queens Coll; MA 86 CUNY - Hunter Coll; **SLP**

Mehlhorn, Mrs Noelle R 9433 Thornton N E, Albuquerque, NM 87109, (505) 242-3425, BA 75 Univ of MI - Ann Arbor; MS 76 Univ of MI - Ann Arbor; Aud, Private Practice, **A ACE**

Mehlmann, Mrs Marybeth Ames 7017 East Fair Avenue, Englewood, CO 80111, (303) 693-1500, BS 72 CO St Univ; MA 76 Univ of Northern CO; SLP, Cherry Creek Schls, **SLP**

Mehmel, Mrs Norma J 815 East 4th Street, Willmar, MN 56201, (612) 231-1100, BA 51 Univ of MI - Ann Arbor; MA 57 Case Western Reserve Univ; Sp-Lang Path, Little Crow Spec Educ Coop, **SLP**

Mehner, Robert O 5225 South 100th Street, Hales Corners, WI 53130, **SLP**

Mehr, Dr Allan S 939 Oak Street SE, Salem, OR 97301, (503) 364-2828, BA 76 CUNY - Queens Coll; MS 77 Western OR St Coll; OD 83 (NS) Adelphi Univ; Aud, Private Practice, **A**

Mehring, Martha Jane 1821 Mt Zion Drive, Golden, CO 80401, (303) 837-7021, BS 81 CO St Univ; MS 86 CO St Univ; 87–Sp-Lang Path, St Joseph Hosp, **SLP**

Mehring, Mrs Sheila Osman 607 East 33rd Street, Baltimore, MD 21218, (301) 355-0100, BS 76 Towson St Univ; MS 78 Towson St Univ; 87–Dir, Easter Seal Society of MD, **SLP**

Mehrman, Mrs Normajean 3210 Wells Road, Peconic, NY 11958, (516) 728-0420, BA 77 SUNY - Coll at Plattsburgh; MA 81 Long Island U - CW Post Ctr; Sp-Lang Path, Hampton Bay Sch Dist, **SLP**

Mehta, Annette M P O Box 1311, Murfreesboro, TN 37133, (615) 890-0935, BS 70 Middle TN St Univ; ME 74 Middle TN St Univ; MA 82 Memphis St Univ; 83–Sp-Lang Path, Private Practice, **SLP**

Meiburg, Mrs Diane Sanderson 1004 Blackoak Court, Apex, NC 27502, (919) 362-4496, BS 82 Appalachian St Univ; MA 87 Appalachian St Univ; **SLP**

Meier, Mrs Ann Lynn 6035 Miakonda Trail, Sylvania, OH 43560, (419) 882-1579, BA 69 OH Wesleyan Univ; MA 70 Bowling Green St Univ; Sp-Lang Path, Private Practice, **SLP**

Meier, Gary A 1120 East 8th Street, Port Angeles, WA 98362, (206) 772-1224, BA 74 Northwest Nazarene Coll; MS 76 ID St Univ; 87–Sp-Lang Path, Port Angeles Sch Dist #121, **SLP**

Meier, Irene Marie 2970-I Walnut Forest Court, Apartment 5-I, Winston-Salem, NC 27103, (919) 760-0352, MA 77 Univ of South FL; ME 84 Univ of NC - Greensboro; Sp-Lang Path, Frye Regional Medical Center, **SLP**

Meier, Mrs Susan M R R 4 Box 94, Clay Center, KS 67432-8941, (913) 643-3178, BS 75 KS St Univ; MA 76 KS St Univ; Sp-Lang Path, Twin Lakes Ed Coop, **SLP**

Meigs-Haislop, Mrs Amy Jo 1710 Market Street, Parkersburg, WV 26101, (304) 424-4277, BS 83 Clarion Univ of PA; MA 85 OH Univ - Athens; Sp-Lang Path, St Josephs Hospital, **SLP**

Meikle-Neelley, Louise D 9207 79th Street, Edmonton, AB, Canada T6C 2R6, (403) 468-7268, OB 50 Sch of the Art Inst -Chicago; MS 61 Southern IL Univ -Carbondale; Sp-Lang Path, Univ of Alberta Hospital, **SLP**

Meilahn, Kristine 19903 164th N E, Woodinville, WA 98072, (206) 258-7311, MS 79 Univ of OR; SLP, Providence Hosp, **SLP**

Meilinger, Cynthia Smith 1414 Beaufort Drive, Lexington, KY 40502, (606) 236-5132, BS 82 Univ of KY; MS 84 Univ of KY; Sp-Lang Path, Kentucky Sch for the Deaf/Outreach Prog, **SLP**

Meine, Cathy L 628 North Cliff Street, Carrollton, GA 30117, (404) 834-5373, BS 81 Central MO St Univ; MA 83 Univ of TN - Knoxville; 88–Sp/Lang Path, Fulton Co PS, **SLP ACE**

Meinert, Mrs Lisa Pieger 2508 Merrick Court, Abingdon, MD 21009, (301) 676-2838, BS 80 Edinboro Univ of PA; MS 81 Columbia Univ Teachers Coll; 86–Sp-Lang Path, Maryland Gen Hosp, **SLP**

Meinke, Mrs Deanna Kay 1900 16th Street, Greeley, CO 80631, (303) 350-2411, BA 79 CO St Univ; MS 80 Northern IL Univ - De Kalb; Aud, Greeley Medical Clinic, **A**

Meintel, Mary Kay 845 Navarre Avenue, New Orleans, LA 70124, (504) 486-4833, OB 71 Northwest MO St Univ; ME 74 Southwest TX St Univ; SLP, **SLP**

Meiring, Peggy L 65 St Francis Avenue, Betty Jane Mem Reba Ctr, Tiffin, OH 44883, (419) 447-9811, BA 83 Wright St Univ; MA 86 OH St Univ; **A**

Meis, Mrs Marcia D 1228 Idlewilde Heath Drive, Winston-Salem, NC 27106, (919) 765-2403, BA 55 Univ of IA; MA 57 Univ of IA; Aud, Ann Q Bogard-Prac of Otol, **A**

Meisel, Diane Leslie 569 Pontiac Road, East Meadow, NY 11554, (516) 221-1706, MS 82 CUNY - Brooklyn Coll; **SLP**

Meisel, Edith Schneider 37 Continental Avenue, Newark, DE 19711, (914) 292-9082, BA 74 OK St Univ; MA 76 OK St Univ; Sp-Lang Path, UCP of Sullivan Co, **SLP**

Meisel, Janice B 1248 Dubonnet Court, Agoura, CA 91301, SLP, **SLP**

Meisel, Ruth M 69 Parker Street #3, Watertown, MA 02172-3913, (617) 926-4621, BS 82 Ithaca Coll; ME 84 Northeastern Univ; Sp-Lang Path, Lynn PS, **SLP**

Meisel, Mrs Sara M 107-19 70th Avenue, Forest Hills, NY 11375, (212) 836-6600, BA 74 CUNY - Queens Coll; MS 75 Univ of MI - Ann Arbor; Sp-Lang Path, Brooklyn VA Med Cen, **SLP**

Meiser, Amy Maria 4201 236th Street SW H-304, Mountlake Terrace, WA 98043, (206) 364-6500, MA 88 Western WA Univ; 88–Aud, Sound Assoc, **A**

Meisler, Mrs Barbara Altman HDI Wing, 11710 Hunters Lane, Rockville, MD 20852, (301) 649-5333, BA 65 George Washington Univ; MA 67 George Washington Univ; Sp-Lang Path, Private Practice, **SLP**

Meisler, Beatrice R 6328 Longboat Lane W, Box 304B, Boca Raton, FL 33433-5234, MS; **SLP A LM**

Meisner, John R 149 Bridge Street, Northampton, MA 01060, (413) 781-9100, BA 82 Adelphi Univ; MS 84 Gallaudet Coll; 84–Aud, Mercy Hospital, **A**

Meissner, Mrs Alice N 735 Fir, St Charles, MO 63301, (314) 946-2765, BA 61 IN Univ - Bloomington; 86–SLP, Lincoln Co RIV Sch Dist, **SLP**

Meissner, Mrs Deborah E 115 68th Street N W, Bradenton, FL 34209, (813) 794-8001, BA 80 Univ of FL; MS 81 FL St Univ; Sp-Lang Path, Manatee Co Sch, **SLP**

Meissner, James H 12 Chesler Square, Succasunna, NJ 07876, (201) 584-8311, BA 41 Dartmouth Coll; MA 44 Univ of IA; SLP, Meissner's Consult Servs, **SLP LM**

Meissner, Mrs Nancy Fay 1005 Hacienda Drive, Sun City Center, FL 33570, (813) 634-9612, BS 55 Miami Univ - Oxford; Sp-Lang Path, Professional Health Services, **SLP**

Meissner, Dr William August Peoria ENT Group Sc, 2627 North Knoxville Avenue, Peoria, IL 61604, (309) 686-5900, BA 65 Valparaiso Univ; MA 67 Northern IL Univ - De Kalb; PH 70 (Aud) Univ of OK Medical Center; Dir of Aud, Peoria,Ear,Nose, Throat Group, **A**

Meister, Mrs Beth A 10685 Mitchell Road, Columbia Station, OH 44028, (216) 933-5108, BA 82 Baldwin-Wallace Coll; MA 84 Cleveland St Univ; 85–Sp-Lang Path, Avon Lake Schs, **SLP**

Meister, Mrs Martha J 542 Ballas Trails Drive, St Louis, MO 63122, (314) 965-3073, BA 83 CA St Univ - Long Beach; MS 85 Washington Univ; Aud, Barnes Hospital, **A**

Meitl, Mrs Pamela A 1217 North 1st, Mulvane, KS 67110, (316) 777-4402, BS 74 Univ of Montevallo; MS 75 Univ of Montevallo; 88–Sp-Lang Path, Unif Sch Dis #263, **SLP**

Meitus, Vicki L 114 Pinecrest Lane, King of Prussia, PA 19406, (215) 265-0402, BS 77 CO St Univ; MA 79 Memphis St Univ; Sp-Lang Path, InSpeech Inc, **SLP ACE**

Meizel, Ellen Stacey 3695 Coral Tree Circle, Forest Pointe At The Township, Coconut Creek, FL 33073, (305) 749-0300, BA 82 Kean Coll of NJ; MA 87 NY Univ; 88–Sp-Lang Path, Sunrise Rehab Hosp

Mejeur, Mrs Judy L 5464 Overhill Drive, Saginaw, MI 48603, (517) 781-4911, BA 71 Millikin Univ; MS 75 IL St Univ - Normal; Sp-Lang Path, Bridgeport-Spaulding Comm Sch, **SLP**

Mejia-Hershberger, Mrs Yvonne M 103 West Rutherford Drive, Newark, DE 19713, (302) 737-4682, BA 79 Mary Washington Coll; MS 81 Univ of AL- Tuscaloosa; Sp-Lang Path, Christina Sch Dist, **SLP**

Mekrut-Suzio, Mrs Joy M Oak Terrace, Durham, CT 06422, (203) 267-2585, BA 76 Boston Coll; MS 79 Southern CT St Univ; Sp-Lang Path, E Hampton Pub Sch, **SLP**

Mekus, Mrs Deborah Drake 7004 Carmen Boulevard, Las Vegas, NV 89128, (702) 799-4223, BA 79 San Diego St Univ; MA 83 CA St Univ - Sacramento; Sp-Lang Path, Clark Co Sch Dist, **SLP**

Melamid, Juliet A 355 West Olive Street, Suite 208, Sunnyvale, CA 94086-3137, (408) 733-0345, **SLP**

Melander, Laura B 2505 Ensign Street, Duluth, MN 55811, (218) 722-3935, BA 73 Univ of MN - Duluth; MA 74 Univ of MN - Duluth; SLP, ISD #709, **SLP**

Melarkey, Barbara Alexina 966 Piedmont Drive, Sacramento, CA 95822, (916) 447-1716, MA 84 Univ of the Pacific; Sp-Lang Path, Yolo Co Office of Education, **SLP**

Melby, Mrs Carol Rhoades 2020 North 8th Street, Bismarck, ND 58501, (701) 255-3285, BS 66 Minot St Univ; MS 69 Minot St Univ; 78–Sp-Lang Path, Utd Tribes Tech Coll, **SLP**

Melcer, Martin P 59-15 47th Avenue #17-E, Woodside, NY 11377, (212) 489-5700, BA 71 CUNY - Queens Coll; MA 72 Univ of MA - Amherst; OM 79 Columbia Univ Teachers Coll; SLP, Vns of NY, **SLP**

Melcher, Dr Joe A 815 Desire, New Orleans, LA 70117, (504) 483-7690, BA 65 TX Tech Univ; MA 66 TX Tech Univ; PH 73 (NS) LA St Univ - Baton Rouge; Prof, Xavier U of La, **A ACE**

Melcher, Mrs Keli L W1764 Circle Drive, Sullivan, WI 53178, (414) 261-3050, BS 86 Univ of WI - Oshkosh; MS 87 Univ of WI - Milwaukee; 88–Sp-Path, Bethesda Lutheran Home

Melcon, Melinda A 14208 Greenleaf, Sherman Oaks, CA 91423, (818) 997-2357, BA 77 Univ of CA - Los Angeles; MA 82 CA St Univ - Northridge; SLP, LA USD, **SLP**

Melda, Keith A 4330 Hickory Road #2-C, Mishawaka, IN 46545, (219) 232-4040, BS 85 Purdue Univ - West Lafayette; MS 87 Washington Univ; Aud, Hrng Clinic Inc, **A**

Mele, Maryteresa Colette 2261-B Washington Street, Newton Lower Falls, MA 02162, (617) 665-1740, BS 82 Univ of NH; MS 84 Boston Univ; Sp-Lang Path, Lang & Cognitive Develpmnt Cen, **SLP**

Mele-McCarthy, Joan A 12102 Northwood Drive, Upper Marlboro, MD 20772, (301) 952-0778, BA 76 Adelphi Univ; MS 77 Adelphi Univ; Sp-Lang Path Dir, Commun Therapies, **SLP ACE**

Melendy, Lorna K 413 4th Street S E, Washington, DC 20003, (202) 546-6317, BA 70 George Washington Univ; MS 72 Emerson Coll; **SLP**

Melgares, Nancy 3057 Murray Lane, Costa Mesa, CA 92626, (714) 552-4211, BS 74 Univ of CA - Irvine; MA 81 CA St Univ - Long Beach; Tchr, Irvine USD, **SLP**

Melhus, Marina L 10151 Prado Vista Drive, Cupertino, CA 95014, (408) 253-4495, BA 73 San Jose St Univ; MA 75 San Jose St Univ; Sp/Lang Path, Private Practice, **SLP**

Meline, Nannette C 449 Crestview Drive East, Montevallo, AL 35115, (205) 665-4128, BS 77 Northwest MO St Univ; MS 80 IL St Univ - Normal; Assist Prof, Univ of Montevallo, **A**

Meline, Dr Timothy J PO Box 523, Montevallo, AL 35115, (205) 665-6730, BS 72 Western IL Univ; MA 73 Western IL Univ; PH 76 (NS) Univ of IL - Urbana; Sp-Lang Path, Univ of Montevallo, **SLP ACE**

Melizzi, Mary A 1 Baldwin Court #B, Catonsville, MD 21228-6006, (312) 397-6979, **SLP**

Mellblom, Caron 6820 Evers Boulevard, Cheyenne, WY 82009, (307) 634-5853, BA 79 CA St Univ - Fullerton; MS 81 Univ of WY; Instr, Laramie Co Commun Coll, **SLP**

Mellen, Mrs Mary Ellen 276 Parum Road, Colchester, CT 06415, BS 68 Kent St Univ; MA 70 Univ of CT; Sp-Lang Path, Colchester Board of Education, **SLP**

Mellencamp, Sheila F Route 3 Box 54, Clarinda, IA 51632, (712) 246-1716, BS 73 Northwest MO St Univ; MS 75 Univ of NE - Omaha; SLP, Loess Hills AEA 13, **SLP ACE**

Mellencamp, Virginia L 529 Juniper Drive, Santa Fe, NM 87501, (505) 983-9948, MS 53; Retired, **SLP A LM**

Melley, Clare 137 East 36th Street #6H, New York, NY 10016, (212) 870-5000, BA 66 Tufts Univ; MA 68 Catholic Univ of America; MA 77 NY Univ; Dir of Sp/Lang Path Svc, Jewish Home & Hosp for Aged, **SLP**

Mellis, Eugenia 35709 Indigo Drive, Sterling Heights, MI 48310, (313) 979-2361, BS 74 Wayne St Univ; MA 76 Wayne St Univ; Sp-Lang Path, Wm Beaumont Hosp, **SLP**

Mellisy, Carolyn R 65 Williams Road, Oakdale, CT 06370, (203) 859-1800, BS 76 Southern CT St Univ; MS 78 Southern CT St Univ; Sp-Lang Path, Montville Bd Ed, **SLP**

Mello, Mrs Mary L 18 Crescent Lane, Putnam Valley, NY 10579, (914) 526-3845, BS 84 Mercy Coll; MA 87 CUNY - Lehman Coll; 84–Sp-Lang Path, BOCES Putnam/N Westchester, **SLP**

Mello, Mrs Maureen Murphy 246 Green Street, Fairhaven, MA 02719, (617) 997-4511, BA 81 Bridgewater St Coll; MS 82 Univ of VT; Sp/Lang Path, New Bedford PS, **SLP**

Melloh, Mrs Crispin Mary 52 South 20th Street, Terre Haute, IN 47803, (812) 238-7537, BS 84 IN St Univ - Terre Haute; MA 86 Ball St Univ; **SLP**

Mellon, Mrs Karen M Percy 4035 49th Avenue South, St Petersburg, FL 33711, (813) 867-4380, BS 82 Stockton St Coll; ME 84 Trenton St Coll; Sp-Lang Path, Mediplex Rehab, **SLP**

Mello-Smither, Susan A 3801 Rexford Drive, Modesto, CA 95356, (209) 524-2406, BA 69 CA St Univ - Fresno; MA 71 CA St Univ - Fresno; Resource Specialist, Modesto City Schools, **SLP**

Mellott, Kathleen Eccard 11402 Howard Court, Beltsville, MD 20705, (202) 687-8186, BA 76 Univ of MD - College Park; MS 77 Towson St Univ; Aud, Georgetown University Hospital, **A ACE**

Mellott, Mrs Patricia Klimas 6011 Creekstone Lane, Centreville, VA 22020, (301) 423-4595, MS 84 WV Univ; **SLP**

Melmed, Dr Paul J 957 Dewing Avenue, Lafayette, CA 94549, (415) 283-6777, BA 64 Univ of Northern CO; MA 66 Stanford Univ; PH 69 (NS) Univ of CA - Berkeley; Director, Melmed Reading Cl Inc, **SLP**

Melnick, Beth K 164 Whitney Street, Hartford, CT 06105, (203) 232-8781, MS 79 Southern CT St Univ; SLP, Meriden Board of Education, **SLP**

Melnick, Carol R 711 Gordon Terrace #307, Chicago, IL 60613, (312) 996-7202, BS 70 Boston Univ; MA 71 Northwestern Univ; Sp-Lang Path/Instr, U of IL Med Cen, **SLP**

Melnick, Robyn H Rolling Hill Apartment, 26 Township Line Road, Apartment C-32, Elkins Park, PA 19117, (215) 539-8550, BS 76 PA St Univ - Univ Park; MA 79 Temple Univ-Tyler Sch of Art; SLP, Moorestown Public Schools, **SLP**

Melnick, Dr William Ohio State University, University Hosp Clinic #4024, 456 Clinic Drive, Columbus, OH 43210, (614) 293-8065, BA 53 Univ of Pittsburgh - Pittsburgh; MS 57 Univ of Pittsburgh - Pittsburgh; PH 61 (NS) Univ of Pittsburgh - Pittsburgh; Prof, Dept/Otol Ohio St U, **A F**

Melnychuk, Mrs Kathleen 140 Andrien Road, Glen Mills, PA 19342, BS 68 Northern MI Univ; MA 69 Northern MI Univ; Sp-Lang Path, Delaware Co Intermed Unit, **SLP**

Melnyk, Lesia Anna 812 Center Drive, Ann Arbor, MI 48103, (313) 761-8274, MA 88 Eastern MI Univ

Melough, Mrs Nancy S 1 Park Lane, Darien, CT 06820, (203) 348-8024, BA 77 Univ of CT; MS 79 Southern CT St Univ; Sp-Lang Path, **SLP**

Meloy, Melette L 6346 Del Monte, Houston, TX 77057, (713) 520-0066, BS 75 Southern Methodist Univ; MS 76 Southern Methodist Univ; Aud, Health Testing Inc, **A**

Melrose, Dr Jay 61 Cottage Street, Amherst, MA 01002, (413) 545-0551, BA 48 CUNY - Queens Coll; MA 53 Univ of IL - Urbana; PH 54 (NS) Univ of IL - Urbana; Prof of Commun Dis, Univ of MA, **SLP A F**

Melton, Barbara Ann North 1525 Marguerite Road, Spokane, WA 99212, (509) 928-7272, BA 79 Eastern WA Univ; MA 83 Western WA Univ; Aud, Drs McClelland & Rutter, **A**

Melton, Donna Hicks 266 North Star Road, Newark, DE 19711, (302) 994-7086, **SLP**

Melton, Mrs Mary E 11 Buckskin Circle, Rogers, AR 72756, (501) 636-5204, BS 77 Henderson St Univ; MS 78 AR St Univ; 83–Sp-Lang Path, Private Practice, **SLP**

Melton, Ray E 324 West Bower, Harrison, AR 72601, (501) 741-7684, BS 71 Univ of Central AR; MA 73 Memphis St Univ; 77–Aud, Chambers Cl, Ltd, **A**

Melton, Mrs Sally A 46 Rotary Way #P, Vallejo, CA 94591, (707) 554-8113, MA 87 Univ of the Pacific

Melton, Suzanne Spears 8012 Field Court, Arvada, CO 80005, (303) 420-6663, BS 72 Univ of TX - Austin; MS 74 Univ of North TX

Meltsner, Sheryl Eve 1619 Third Avenue #12-B, New York, NY 10028, (212) 831-9489, BA 78 Long Island U - CW Post Ctr; MA 85 NY Univ; 88–Sp-Lang Path, New York City Bd of Educ, **SLP**

Meltzer, Mrs Bonnie Rosett 2510 Cobblewood Dr, Northbrook, IL 60062, (312) 564-4062, BS 72 Univ of IL - Urbana; MA 72 Univ of IL - Urbana; **SLP**

Meltzer, Mrs Elaine F Gantman 4100 N W 7th Lane, Delray Beach, FL 33445, (407) 495-1725, BA 80 CUNY - Queens Coll; MA 83 CUNY - Queens Coll; 86–Sp-Lang Path, Palm Beach Co Sch Bd, **SLP**

Meltzer, Mrs Evelyn S 8335 North Karlov Avenue, Skokie, IL 60076, (312) 492-7965, BS 60 Washington Univ; Elementary School Teacher, Evanston School District 65, **SLP**

Meltzer, Mrs Jill B H 3026 Margo Lane, Northbrook, IL 60062, (504) 588-5451, BA 74 Univ of Denver; OM 77 Tulane Univ; Aud, N Shore Aud Vestibular Lab, **A**

Meltzer-Weller, Cynthia R 3062 Shepard Road, Bensalem, PA 19020, (215) 331-6878, BA 73 Univ of Pittsburgh - Pittsburgh; MA 75 Temple Univ-Tyler Sch of Art; Aud, Arnold K Brenman, M D P C, **A**

Melum, Arla J 9045 N W Sherry Court, Portland, OR 97229, (503) 229-7526, MS 82 Portland St Univ; Aud, Infant Hrng Res, **A**

Melvey, Mary K 8246 4th Avenue N E, Seattle, WA 98115, (206) 525-6117, BS 79 Ithaca Coll; MA 80 Western MI Univ; 84–Sp/Lang Path, Sp Lang & Hrng Svcs, **SLP**

Melvin, Mrs Julie Terese 20 Pleasant Street, Hopkinton, MA 01748, **SLP**

Melvin, Mrs Patricia W 7535 East Edison, Tucson, AZ 85715, (602) 887-5500, BS 63 Bradley Univ; MA 64 Univ of Northern CO; Sp/Lang Path, Amphitheater Pub Schs, **SLP**

Melvin-Hines, Mrs Darshell Devore P O Box 1683, Front Royal, VA 22630, (703) 635-4870, BS 83 Longwood Coll; MS 85 James Madison Univ; 85–Sp-Lang Path, Warren Cty Public Sch, **SLP**

Membrino, Mrs Irene F 107 Oakwood Drive, Hendersonville, TN 37075, (615) 320-5353, MS 88 Vanderbilt Univ

Memminger, Anna Belle 5638 Swamp Fox Road, Jacksonville, FL 32210-7312, **SLP**

Menard, Mrs Donna M 10600 South Sacramento, Chicago, IL 60655, (312) 496-3330, BA 71 Saint Xavier Coll; OM 81 Governors St Univ; Sp-Lang Path, Aero Spec Ed Center, **SLP**

Menard, Mrs Karen Lynne 389 Fenno Street #2, Revere, MA 02151, (617) 289-0883, BS 79 Boston Univ; MS 84 Northeastern Univ; 80–Sp-Lang Path, City of Revere PS, **SLP**

Mencel, Mrs Elizabeth 784 Springbank Drive, London, ON, Canada N6K 1A4, BA 78 Univ of Windsor - Ontario; OM 81 Univ of Western Ontario; Sp-Lang Path, Ministry of Comm & Soc Serv, **SLP**

Mencher, Dr George T 15 Birchview Drive, Halifax, NS, Canada B3P 1G5, (902) 423-7354, BA 58 Pepperdine Univ - Los Angele; MA 64 CA St Univ - Long Beach; PH 68 (Sp-Lang Path and Aud) Univ of MI - Ann Arbor; 73–Dir, NS Hrng & Sp Clin, **SLP A F**

Mencke, Dr Eugene O Dept Of Communication Disorders, Univ Of Ok Health Sci Ctr, P O Box 26901, Oklahoma City, OK 73190, (405) 271-4214, BS 52 Concordia Coll; MA 55 Columbia Univ Teachers Coll; PH 63 (NS) Univ of OK - Norman; Prof of Aud & Ed of Deaf, U of OK Hlth Sci Cen, **A F**

Mendel, Dr Maurice I Memphis Speech & Hearing Ctr, Memphis State University, 807 Jefferson Avenue, Memphis, TN 38105, (901) 525-2682, BA 65 Univ of CO - Boulder; MS 67 Washington Univ; PH 70 (Aud) Univ of WI - Madison; 88–Chr & Dir, Memphis State University, **A F**

Mendelewicz, Mrs Dianne S 5400 S W 148th Avenue, Fort Lauderdale, FL 33330, MS 78 Univ of South FL; SLP, Dade Co Pub Sch, **SLP**

Mendelsohn, Mrs Bernice L 6 Thurlow Road, Hampstead, PQ, Canada H3X 3G5, (514) 342-3111, BA 70 McGill Univ - Quebec; OM 75 Univ of WA; Dir-Aud & SLP, Sir M B Davis Jewish Gen Hosp, **SLP**

Mendelsohn, Mrs Priscilla 103 Cypress Drive, Woodbury, NY 11797, (516) 367-4527, BA 71 Hofstra Univ; MA 72 Hofstra Univ; Sp-Lang Path, **SLP**

Mendelson, Gary L 11604 Bunnell Court South, Potomac, MD 20854, (301) 299-6714, BA 70 Univ of MD - College Park; MA 72 Univ of MD - College Park; Aud, Private Practice, **A**

Mendenhall, Mrs Janella Annette 1405 Hollyhead Terrace, Yukon, OK 73099, (307) 789-2128, BA 82 Wichita St Univ; MA 83 Wichita St Univ; Sp-Lang Path, Moore School District, **SLP**

Mendenhall, Kay 1710 Alpha Street, North Platte, NE 69101, (308) 534-5979, BA 81 Kearney St Coll; ME 82 Kearney St Coll; 88–Sp-Lang Path, Sidney PS, **SLP**

Mendenhall, Marcia Ann 3503 101st Street, Lubbock, TX 79423-5120, (806) 745-3226, BS 82 KS St Univ; MS 84 TX Tech Univ; **SLP**

Mendenhall, Patricia Ann 18700 Cordata Street, Fountain Valley, CA 92708, (714) 968-5473, BA 79 CA St Univ - Long Beach; MA 82 CA St Univ - Long Beach; Sp-Lang Path, Sp-Lang Dev Cen, **SLP**

Mendes, Diane G 547 Highland Avenue, Malden, MA 02148, (617) 256-6531, BS 82 Univ of MA - Amherst; MA 84 Univ of MA - Amherst; SLP, Chelmsfor Ps, **SLP**

Mendez-Kurtz, Lucy P 2245 Ryder Street, Brooklyn, NY 11234, (718) 780-5186, BA 82 CUNY - Brooklyn Coll; MS 84 CUNY - Brooklyn Coll; Aud, Aud Diagnostics, **A**

Mendicino, Michael 36 N Tenney Drive, Buckhannon, WV 26201, (304) 472-5480, MS 85 CA Univ of PA

Mendlik, David F 37 Kentucky Street, Long Beach, NY 11561, (516) 889-7245, BS 85 Univ of NE - Lincoln; MA 87 Temple Univ; 88–Aud, Hrng & Sp Assoc Inc/Plainview, **A**

Mendola, Noreen G 67 Lovering Avenue, Buffalo, NY 14216, (716) 837-2441, BA 78 SUNY - Center at Buffalo; MA 80 SUNY - Center at Buffalo; Diag Sp-Lang Path/Cfy Aud, Lang Dev Prog of W NY, **SLP**

Mendoza, Sylvia Ann 5503 Eglise Avenue, Pico Rivera, CA 90660, (213) 855-6265, BA 80 Univ of Southern CA; MA 82 Whittier Coll; Sp-Lang Path, Cedars-Sinai Medical Center, **SLP**

Menefee, John Thomas, II 105 Yorktown Drive, Franklin, TN 37064, (615) 794-0912, BA 85 Univ of TN - Knoxville; MA 86 Univ of TN - Knoxville

Meneghel, Susan L 1155 Ingerson Road, Arden Hills, MN 55112, **SLP**

Menges, Joanna L 106 North Gow, Wichita, KS 67203, (316) 263-9949, BA 79 Wichita St Univ; MA 81 Wichita St Univ; 84–Sp-Lang Path, Wesley Med Ctr, **SLP**

Menicucci, Andrea Lynn 2601 West Seventh Street, Reno, NV 89503, (702) 747-3940, BS 85 Univ of NV - Reno; MS 87 Univ of NV - Reno

Menist, Mrs Cynthia R 6 Laurie Lane, Little Silver, NJ 07739, (201) 842-7326, MA 64 NY Univ; BA 63 CUNY - City College; 70–Sp-Lang Path, Private Practice, **SLP ACE**

Menken, Dr Gregory E 18900 Pacific Drive, Fort Bragg, CA 95437, (707) 964-1444, BA 73 Univ of OR; MA 74 Northwestern Univ; PH 81 (Spec Ed/Instruct Tech) Univ of Southern CA; Pres, Winning Images, **SLP**

Menking, Mrs Elizabeth Polizos 6030 Netherton Street, Centreville, VA 22020, (703) 378-9528, BS 85 Old Dominion Univ; MA 87 George Washington Univ; 88–Sp-Lang Path, Fairfax Hosp, **SLP**

Menks, Alice H General Delivery, Graves Mill, VA 22721, (703) 948-4516, BS 72 Univ of UT; MS 73 Univ of UT; **SLP**

Menlo, Louise P O Box 160843, Austin, TX 78716, (512) 440-7140, PH (NS); Management Consultant, Private Practice, **SLP**

Mennis, Mrs Selma Tres 721 Paseo Del Mar, Palos Verdes Estates, CA 90274, (213) 373-3270, BA 41 CUNY - Hunter Coll; MA 65 Temple Univ-Tyler Sch of Art; Teacher, Torrance Adult School System, **SLP**

Menno, Kathleen Ann 43 Strathmore Road #3, Brookline, MA 02146, (617) 277-0261, BS 83 SUNY - Coll at Geneseo; MS 85 Boston Univ; 86–Sp-Lang Path, North Suffolk Mental Hlth Assoc, **SLP**

Mentch, Mace W 624 Oberlin Avenue, Lorain, OH 44052, (216) 721-5400, BS 73 PA St Univ - Univ Park; MS 76 Indiana Univ of PA; 86–Dir/Comm Dis, Health Hill Hosp, **SLP**

Mentges, Carol J 4150 Pembrook Road #103, Youngstown, OH 44515-4634, (216) 799-5911, **SLP**

Mentis, Michelle 485 Terrace Road, Santa Barbara, CA 93109, (805) 564-3157, MA 85 Univ of CA - Santa Barbara; **SLP**

Mentzer-Dice, Mrs Joan L 120 Longmeadow Lane, State College, PA 16803, BS 78 PA St Univ - Univ Park; MA 82 Univ of Pittsburgh - Pittsburgh; Sp-Lang Path, **SLP**

Menyuk, Prof Paula 162 Mason Terrace, Brookline, MA 02146, (617) 353-3194, BS 51 NY Univ; ME 55 Boston Univ; ED 62 (NS) Boston Univ; 72–Professor, Boston University, **F**

Menza, Marie A 3016 Hall Avenue, Marinette, WI 54143, (414) 567-1133, **SLP**

Menzel, Otto J Rt 4 Box 144, Bristol, TN 37620, BA 49 WV Univ; MA 50 Northwestern Univ; PH 58 (Aud) Univ of IA; Retired, **A LM**

Menzel, Mrs Rita H 461 North Wilson, La Habra, CA 90631, (213) 602-6912, BA 68 CA St Univ - Los Angeles; MA 72 CA St Univ - Los Angeles; SLP, Paramount USD, **SLP**

Menzies-O'Leary, Pamela Jeanne 334 Croaton Street, Ronkonkoma, NY 11779, (516) 474-3400, BS 83 SUNY - Coll at Geneseo; MS 85 SUNY - Coll at Buffalo; Sp-Lang Path, Maryhaven Therapeutic Presch, **SLP**

Menzin, Roberta Szalavetz 10839 Whiterim Drive, Potomac, MD 20854, (301) 365-9012, MS 83 Boston Univ; Sp/Lang Path, **SLP**

Mercadante, Anthony J 6122 Donegal East, Lakeland, FL 33813, (813) 533-7879, BS 73 Seton Hall Univ; MA 78 Kean Coll of NJ; Aud, Polk Co Sch, **A**

Mercaitis, Dr Patricia A 81 Bay Road, Belchertown, MA 01007, (413) 545-2565, BA 71 Boston Coll; MA 79 Univ of MA - Amherst; PH 83 (NS) Univ of MA - Amherst; Asst Prof Sp-Lang Path, U Mass Dept Commun Disorders, **SLP**

Mercer, Anne L 1017 South 17th Street, Grand Forks, ND 58201, (701) 775-7513, BA 70 IL St Univ - Normal; MA 74 Univ of ND; **SLP**

Mercer, Deena L 2301 Albert Street, Alexandria, LA 71301, (318) 443-7352, BA 82 LA Tech Univ; MA 86 LA Tech Univ; **SLP**

Mercer, Mrs Elizabeth Lawson 1936 3rd Street S E, Moultrie, GA 31768, (912) 769-3612, BA 67 Univ of GA; MS 73 Univ of OK Medical Center; 86–Sp-Lang Path, Colquitt Co Bd of Educ, **SLP**

Mercer, Ellen F 112 Sycamore Court, Sanford, FL 32773, (305) 322-7933, BA 75 Temple Univ; MA 77 Univ of FL; Prog Coord/Sp-Lang Path, Seminole Co Sch Bd, **A**

Mercer, Mrs Linda Marie 1400 Wildhorse Creek Road, Glencoe, MO 63038, (314) 968-4710, BS 80 Univ of MO - Columbia; MS 82 Fontbonne Coll; Sp-Lang Path, St Louis Hearing & Speech Ctr, **SLP**

Mercer, Linda R 227 Crescent Road, Wanaque, NJ 07465, (201) 831-1953, BS 66 Univ of WI - River Falls; ME 76 Univ of FL; SLP, East Orange Pub Sch, **SLP**

Mercer, Louise B 4861 East Missouri Avenue, Denver, CO 80222, (303) 861-0504, BA 73 CO St Univ; MS 75 CO St Univ; Sp-Lang Path, Swedish Hosp/Spalding Hosp, **SLP**

Mercer, Mrs Lynn Weismiller 16102 West 125th Street, Olathe, KS 66062, (316) 681-1344, BA 79 Univ of Waterloo - Ontario; MA 84 Wichita St Univ; SLP, USD 259, **SLP**

Merchant, Mrs Cheryl Terese 519 S Rantoul Street, Lena, IL 61048, (815) 369-5383, BA 80 Augustana Coll; MA 84 Northeastern IL Univ; **SLP**

Merchant, Penelope Watson 44 Auchmar Road, Hamilton, ON, Canada L9C 1C5, (519) 966-2211, BA 73 Univ of Western Ontario; MA 75 Western MI Univ; 84–Mgr, The Child's Place, **SLP**

Mercure, Roland 15 Diane Avenue, Plymouth, MA 02360, PH (NS); **SLP**

Mercurio, Mary Ann R 509 Clifton Avenue, Newark, NJ 07104, (201) 265-9653, BA 60 Kean Coll of NJ; MA 61 Columbia Univ Teachers Coll; MA 72 Seton Hall Univ; 73–Dir, Bergen Co Spec Serv Sch Dist, **SLP A**

Meredith, Grace 5212 Cote Brilliante, St Louis, MO 63113, (314) 569-8509, BA 80 Univ of MS; OM 82 Trinity Coll; Sp-Lang Path, Irwin Lehroff PhD and Associates, **SLP**

Meredith, James E P O Box 1301, Bluefield, WV 24701, (304) 325-2471, BA 65 Concord Coll; MS 67 WV Univ; Dir Sp&Hrng, Mem Gen Hosp, **SLP A**

Meredith, Mrs Marti A County Diagnostic Center, 5451 Beaver Kill Road, Columbia, MD 21046, (301) 964-8483, BA 76 Univ of MD - College Park; MS 77 Towson St Univ; Sp-Lang Path, Co Diag Cen Howard Co Pub Sch, **SLP**

Meredith, Rebecca Lynn 7085 Via Pacifica, San Jose, CA 95139, (408) 773-9933, BA 84 San Jose St Univ; MA 86 San Jose St Univ; 86–Aud, Golden State Aud Assoc, **A**

Meredith, Mrs Renita R Box 536, Panora, IA 50216, (515) 747-2212, BA 73 Univ of Northern IA; MA 74 Univ of Northern IA; Sp-Lang Path, Heartland AEA II, **SLP**

Meredith, Mrs Theresa P O Box 145 Services, Binghamton, NY 13903, (607) 798-7117, BA 80 SUNY - Coll at Cortland; MS 81 James Madison Univ; Sp/Lang Path, Handicapped Childrens Assoc, **SLP**

Merenda, Irene B Delaware County Intermediate Unit, Indian Lane School, 309 South Middletown Road, Media, PA 19063, (215) 565-4585, BA 77 Rutgers St Univ - Newark; MA 83 Trenton St Coll; 88–Aud, Delaware Co Inter Unit, **A**

Merenstein-Brooks, Mrs Debra Karen 185 West Park Avenue #321, Long Beach, NY 11561, (516) 678-1200, **SLP**

Merin, Diane S 2937 Cape Sebastian Place, Cardiff, CA 92007, (619) 695-8469, BS 79 FL St Univ; BS 80 FL St Univ; MS 81 FL St Univ; Sp-Lang Path, Childrens Hosp & Health Center, **SLP**

Merkel, Amanda Schneider 6865 Brandon Mill Road, Atlanta, GA 30328, (404) 255-2517, BA 78; MS 81 Emory Univ; Sp-Lang Path, Private Practice, **SLP**

Merker, Mrs Corina E 5088 Chapin Street, Dayton, OH 45429, (513) 233-8080, BA 81 Wright St Univ; MA 83 Univ of Akron; Aud, Apple Creek Hearing Aids & Aud, **A**

Merklein, Richard A 4857 North Woodruff Avenue, Whitefish Bay, WI 53217, (414) 647-2767, BS 57 Univ of WI - Milwaukee; MA 59 Northwestern Univ; Aud, Milwaukee Pub Sch, **A**

Merkley, Dr Frances A Giannino 165 Fairway Lane, Ojai, CA 93023-3001, (805) 485-0068, BS 54; ME 59; PH 77 (NS); Exec Dir, Asst Lgue Sch

Merkley, Mary J P O Box 1025, Alamosa, CO 81101, (303) 589-5434, BA 78 Univ of Northern CO; MA 79 Univ of Northern CO; Audiologist, Intermountain Audiology Assoc, **A**

Merle, Kathleen S University Of Rochester, 601 Elmwood Avenue, Box 629, Rochester, NY 14642, (716) 275-2501, BS 65 Nazareth Coll of Rochester; MS 75 Nazareth Coll of Rochester; Aud, Univ of Rochester Med Ctr, **A**

Merlini, Mary Elizabeth 92 Main Street Unit 412, Deep River, CT 06417, (203) 526-5708, BA 80 Boston Coll; MS 83 Columbia Univ Teachers Coll; **SLP**

Mermelstein, Pamela B 137-36 70 Road, Flushing, NY 11367, (718) 544-2002, MA 88 Saint John's Univ - Jamaica

Mermelstein-Epner, Lillie E 1557 East 66th Street, Brooklyn, NY 11234, (212) 968-7454, BA 74 CUNY - Brooklyn Coll; MS 79 CUNY - Brooklyn Coll; SLP, Cty of NY Bd of Ed, **SLP**

Mero, Mrs Janette Lee Route 365 R R 4, Stewarts Mobile Home Park, Rome, NY 13440, (315) 336-2300, BS 79 SUNY - Coll at Fredonia; MS 80 SUNY - Coll at Fredonia; Sp-Lang Path, Rome Develop Cen, **SLP**

Merrefield, Gayle Emery 80 Sherman Avenue, Staten Island, NY 10301, (718) 727-1515, BA 72 Fairmont St Coll; ME 78 Univ of GA; Sp-Lang Path, Toddler/Infant Prog for Sp Ed, **SLP**

Merrell, Dr Hal B 6727 67th East Avenue S, Tulsa, OK 74133, (918) 592-6000, BS 54 Univ of UT; MS 57 Univ of UT; PH 63 (NS) Southern IL Univ -Carbondale; Dir/Cl Servs, U of Tulsa, **A**

Merrell, Mrs Laquita Southall 2915 South Osage, Fort Smith, AR 72901, (501) 646-6854, BA 79 Univ of AR - Little Rock; MS 83 Univ of AR - Fayetteville; 79–Sp-Lang Path, Van Buren Sch Dist, **SLP**

Merrell, Mrs Mary Bishop Route 1 Box 370-A, Fletcher, NC 28732, (704) 274-7955, MA 81 Western Carolina Univ; BS 73 Western Carolina Univ; 73–Sp-Lang Path, Buncombe Co PS, **SLP**

Merrer, Mrs Christine M 12 High View Circle, Danbury, CT 06811, (203) 748-6834, BA 66 Loyola Coll; OM 68 Univ of CT; 75–Sp/Lang Path, Danbury Bd of Ed, **SLP**

Merrick, Kathleen 2745 North Hampden Court, Apartment #3E, Chicago, IL 60614, (312) 791-2900, **SLP**

Merrick, Niki P 1017 North Lombard Avenue, Oak Park, IL 60302, (312) 848-2286, BS 74 Univ of IL - Urbana; MS 75 Univ of IL - Urbana; **SLP**

Merrick, Mrs Paula Lenocker 4480 Ocean Valley Lane, San Diego, CA 92130, (619) 792-1147, BA 76 Univ of Redlands; MS 77 Univ of Redlands; SLP, San Diego USD, **SLP**

Merrick, Roy L 4480 Ocean Valley Lane, San Diego, CA 92130, (619) 792-1147, BA 73 CA St Univ - Fullerton; MA 74 OH Univ - Athens; SLP, San Diego USD, **SLP**

Merrick, Mrs Theadora Smith 12839 War Horse Street, San Diego, CA 92129, (619) 484-0099, BA 64 CA St Univ - Long Beach; MA 66 CA St Univ - Long Beach; Sp-Lang Path, Poway USD, **SLP**

Merrifield, Elizabeth 1601 East Knoll Drive, Marion, IA 52302, (319) 356-2154, BS 62 Univ of WI - Madison; MS 64 Univ of WI - Madison; PH 78 (NS) Univ of IA; SLP, Dept of Pedia U of IA, **SLP**

Merrill, Elizabeth Warner 26 Abbott Street Apartment 1, Beverly, MA 01915, (508) 774-5000, BS 79 Elmira Coll; MA 82 SUNY - Center at Buffalo; 88–Sp-Lang Path, Hogan Reg Ctr, **SLP**

Merrill, Gloria S 2403 Sandy Lane, Omaha, NE 68123-9444, (402) 293-1890, BA 54 Univ of NE - Lincoln; **SLP**

Merrill, Judith L 14 Linden Road, Melrose, MA 02176, BS 77 Worcester St Coll; MA 80 Univ of Miami; 88–Sp-Lang Path, MA Easter Seal Soc, **SLP**

Merrill, Laurel J P 7509 Penn Lane N E #D, Albuquerque, NM 87110, (505) 345-8531, OB 72 Univ of NM; MS 75 Univ of NM; SLP, Albuquerque Public Schools, **SLP**

Merrill, Patricia N 506 Grants Trail, Centerville, OH 45459, (513) 222-5597, BA 79 Univ of MI - Ann Arbor; MS 81 Univ of MI - Ann Arbor; SLP, Dayton Hrng/Sp Cen, **SLP**

Merrill, Pauline Reid 739 Bennett Place, Severna Park, MD 21146, (301) 647-8958, MS 84 Towson St Univ; Sp-Lang Path, Anne Arundel Co Bd of Ed, **SLP**

Merrill, Mrs Sharon Mares 6461 N E Mantova Street, Long Beach, CA 90815, (213) 598-9261, BA 70 CA St Univ - Fresno; MA 76 CA St Univ - Los Angeles; Sp-Lang Path, Private Practice, **SLP**

Merriman, Mrs Elizabeth 1387 Willshire Road, Lyndhurst, OH 44124, (216) 442-4656, BA 78 Catholic Univ of America; MA 79 Case Western Reserve Univ; Aud, Consultant Part Time, **A**

Merriman, Ronda Gaita 10 Panthorn Trail, Southington, CT 06489, (203) 521-0110, BA 75 Univ of MA - Amherst; MA 76 CUNY - Queens Coll; Sp-Lang Path, West Hartford Board of Educ, **SLP**

Merriman, Mrs Ruth Alice 6258 North Colfax, Coeur d'Alene, ID 83814, (208) 687-0551, BA 64 ID St Univ; MA 67 ID St Univ; Retired, Lakeland Dist 272, **SLP**

Merriman-Sorensen, Christine Ainsworth P O Box 2371, Polson, MT 59860, (406) 883-4459, BA 77 Univ of MT; MA 79 Univ of MT; SLP, Polson Pub Sch Dist #23, **SLP**

Merris, Mrs Margaret 2324 Scyene Way, Boise, ID 83712, (208) 338-3655, BA 67 Our Lady Lake Univ-San Anton; MA 68 Our Lady Lake Univ-San Anton; Sp-Lang Path, Boise Pub Sch, **SLP**

Merritt, Audree Huhn 8220 Vincetta Drive #21, La Mesa, CA 92042, (619) 460-5736, BS 83 Brigham Young Univ; OM 85 Brigham Young Univ; Private Contractor SLP, Eloise Johnson & Associates, **SLP**

Merritt, Cynthia Smith 9029 Lismore Drive, Elk Grove, CA 95624, (916) 685-8711, BA 82 San Jose St Univ; MS 88 Sacramento St Univ; 86–Aud, Stuart Gherini MD, **A**

Merritt, Mrs Dana M 10197 Classic Oaks Road N, Jacksonville, FL 32225, (904) 641-8389, MS 80 Univ of South FL; Sp-Lang Path, Private Practice, **SLP**

Merritt, Debra Reynolds Box 7 Site 7 R R 1, Tantallon, NS, Canada B0J 3J0, (902) 823-3208, BS 75 PA St Univ - Univ Park; MA 76 Western MI Univ; 84–Asst Supervisor SLP, Nova Scotia Hrng/Sp Cl, **SLP**

Merritt, Dr Donna D 21 Robin Road, Willimantic, CT 06226, (203) 423-4972, BA 73 RI Coll; MS 74 Univ of MI - Ann Arbor; PH 85 (NS) Univ of CT; Dir of Sp-Lang, Delta Consultants, **SLP**

Merritt, Joanna Z 1949 Evergreen Avenue, Fullerton, CA 92635, (714) 990-4577, BS 74 SUNY - Center at Albany; MS 75 SUNY - Center at Albany; Tchr, Fullerton Union High School, **SLP**

Merritt, Judith A 25088 West 8 Mile Apartment 708, Southfield, MI 48034, (517) 373-0668, BA 77 Wayne St Univ; BS 78 Wayne St Univ; MA 80 Wayne St Univ; Dept Analyst, Michigan Dept of Mental Health, **SLP**

Merritt, Mrs Sarah Luanne Abbey Lane, Hagerstown, MD 21740, (301) 797-2170, BS 85 WV Univ; MS 87 WV Univ; **A**

Merritt, Mrs Sharon Route 25 Box 112, Conroe, TX 77385, (713) 367-4414, BA 62 East TX St Univ - Commerce; ME 63 East TX St Univ - Commerce; Sp-Lang Path, Conroe ISD, **SLP**

Merritt, Mrs Susan J 1109 West Madero Avenue, Mesa, AZ 85210, (602) 838-8624, BS 77 Univ of Cincinnati; MS 78 Miami Univ - Oxford; Sp-Lang Path, Gilbert Pub Sch, **SLP**

Merry, Carol D 604 7th Avenue, Coralville, IA 52241, (319) 399-6889, BS 75 Univ of IL - Urbana; MA 80 NM St Univ; **SLP**

Merry-Aranyos, Mrs Elizabeth Jane 621 Athletic Street, Vassar, MI 48768, (517) 673-2144, BS 85 Central MI Univ; MA 87 Central MI Univ; 87–Sp-Lang Path, Tusola Inter School Dstr

Mershon, Dr Patricia M Pm Sp-Lang-Educational Serv, 7812 Sugarland Drive, Fort Worth, TX 76179, (817) 236-1265, BS 60 Univ of NM; MA 65 Univ of NM; PH 68 (NS) Univ of NM; Director Speech/Special Educ, Kennedale Independent Sch Dist, **SLP**

Mershon, Virginia R 1403 Schoolhouse Road, Montecito, CA 93108, (805) 969-0972, **SLP**

Mersinger, Sue Ann RR1 Box 97A, Troy, IL 62294, (618) 667-3393, BS 85 Southern IL Univ-Edwardsvill; MS 86 Southern IL Univ-Edwardsvill

Merson, Dr Richard M Communicative Disorders, 220 East Mermaid Lane #206, Philadelphia, PA 19118-3217, (215) 248-5018, BS 64 Wayne St Univ; MS 67 Wichita St Univ; PH 70 (NS) Univ of WI - Madison; Pres-Admin, Commun Dis Consult, **SLP**

Merten, Mrs Joyce G 1838 South Gunderson, Berwyn, IL 60402, (312) 484-5828, BS 85 Univ of IL - Urbana; MA 87 Univ of IL - Urbana; 87–Sp-Lang Path, Cicero Elem Sch Dist #99, **SLP**

Merten, Dr Karol Kay 1751 Glen Garry Drive, Lakewood, CO 80215, (303) 871-4328, BS 56 Univ of KS; MA 63 Univ of KS; PH 76 (NS) Univ of Denver; 88–Assoc Prof, Dept of Sp Comm-U of Denver, **SLP F**

Mertens, Debra Sue Route 3 12474 Road 27, Sterling, CO 80751, (303) 522-3361, MA 81 Univ of Northern CO; SLP, Re-1 Valley Sch Dist, **SLP**

Mertens, Patricia Lynne 462 Annie Place, Cheney, WA 99004, (509) 235-4807, BA 79 Univ of Northern CO; MA 80 Univ of Northern CO; Sp-Lang Path, Deer Lodge Sch Dist I, **SLP**

Mertesdorf, Donna H 408 Normandy Court, North Mankato, MN 56001, (507) 388-4826, BS 67 Mankato St Univ; MA 74 Univ of MN - Minneap-St Paul; Sp-Lang Path, Dist #77 Mankato MN, **SLP**

Mertz-Garcia, Sara J 5464 Quail Run West, Theodore, AL 36582, (205) 653-5314, BS 78 KS St Univ; MS 81 Univ of NE - Lincoln; **SLP**

Merwin, Alice K 21 Elm Street, Great Neck, NY 11021, (516) 487-9209, BA 59 CUNY - Queens Coll; MS 60 Univ of MI - Ann Arbor; Sp-Lang Path, Private Practice, **SLP**

Mery, Dr Barbara D 11 Novato Street #11, San Rafael, CA 94901, (415) 897-4269, BS 59 Northwestern Univ; MS 67 Syracuse Univ; PH 75 (NS) Syracuse Univ; Sp-Lang Path, Private Consultant, **SLP A**

Mery-Rutledge, Mrs Renee Louise 105 Calvert Court, Ukiah, CA 95482, (707) 462-1476, BA 70 Our Lady Lake Univ-San Anton; MA 71 Our Lady Lake Univ-San Anton; Sp-Lang Path, **SLP**

Mesa, Mrs Linda S 15403 Forest Land, San Antonio, TX 78232-1803, (512) 735-5461, BS 70 Sul Ross St Univ; MA 75 Our Lady Lake Univ-San Anton; SLP, San Antonio ISD, **SLP**

Mesa-Ariss, Mrs Maria E 84-01 Main Street, #105, Briarwood, NY 11435, (718) 846-7998, MS 86 Adelphi Univ; 86–Sp-Lang Path, Herbert G Birch Sch for Excep Chldn, **SLP**

Mesalam, Linda M 9542 Falkirk Drive, Indianapolis, IN 46256, (317) 871-2270, BS 77 Purdue Univ - West Lafayette; MS 79 Purdue Univ - West Lafayette; 79–Sp-Lang Path, St Vincent Hosp, **SLP**

Meschnark, Nancy Newell 16223 North 40th Place, Phoenix, AZ 85032, (602) 493-6070, BS 77 AZ St Univ; MS 84 AZ St Univ; Sp-Lang Path, Paradise Valley Schools, **SLP**

Meska, Mrs Susan Boldon Route 4 Box 99A, Winona, MN 55987, (507) 643-6627, BA 76 Univ of WI - Eau Claire; MS 77 Univ of WI - Eau Claire; **SLP**

Meske, Mrs Pauline L 3232 Interlaken Drive, Oconomowoc, WI 53066, (414) 567-5642, BS 54 Univ of WI - Madison; MS 75 Univ of WI - Milwaukee; 75–Sp-Lang Path, Oconomowoc Area Sch Dist, **SLP**

Mesmer, Lisa H 1347 East 26th Place, Tulsa, OK 74114, (918) 749-6973, BS 78 Univ of Tulsa; MA 80 Univ of Tulsa; **A**

Messano, Mrs Risa Lamia 61 Deppe Place, Staten Island, NY 10314, (212) 596-5742, BA 79 Saint Johns Univ - Staten Is; MS 83 CUNY - Brooklyn Coll; SLP, NYC Board of Ed Speech Service, **SLP**

Messerly, Dr Carol L 1307 Hereford Road, Cleveland Heights, OH 44118, (216) 442-2200, BS 60 OH St Univ; ME 69 Kent St Univ; PH 83 (NS) Kent St Univ; Coord Sec Hrng Impaired Prog, Mayfield Board of Education, **SLP**

Messerschmidt, Anita Borsdorf 2541 Prospect Avenue, Evanston, IL 60201, BS 77 Univ of IL - Urbana; MA 84 Northwestern Univ; Sp-Lang Path, **SLP**

Messer-Smith, Mrs Patricia D 1216 Valley Forge Drive, Dothan, AL 36301, (205) 794-0802, BS 77 Univ of Montevallo; MS 79 Univ of Montevallo; Sp/Lang Path, Private Practice, **SLP ACE**

Messick, Anna M N 3107 Grand, Parsons, KS 67357, MS; **SLP LM**

Messick, Mrs Carolyn M 11608 Bevenshire Road, Oklahoma City, OK 73162, (405) 728-1001, BS 85 OK St Univ; MS 87 Univ of OK Medical Center; 87–Sp-Lang Path, Oklahoma City PS, **SLP**

Messick, Cheri Fox Lakeview Medical Center, 1100 North Main Street, Rice Lake, WI 54868, (715) 234-1515, BS 77 Northwest MO St Univ; MS 82 Univ of NE - Lincoln; Director Sp-Lang Path, Lakeview Medical Center, **SLP**

Messick, Dr Cheryl K 90 West Overdale Drive, Tallmadge, OH 44278, (216) 633-2055, BA 76 Univ of CA - Santa Barbara; MA 80 San Diego St Univ; PH 84 (NS) Purdue Univ - West Lafayette; Program Director, Akron Childrens Hospital, **SLP**

Messier, Mrs Susan Gail 11 Scenic Avenue, Webster, MA 01570, (508) 791-6351, BS 83 Worcester St Coll; MA 85 Univ of CT; 87–Sp-Lang Path, Fairlawn Rehab Hosp, **SLP**

Messier-Grilli, Mrs Nancy Ann RD 1 Box 67AA, Croll Road, Valley Falls, NY 12185, (518) 753-6948, BS 82 Coll of Saint Rose; MS 86 Coll of Saint Rose; Sp-Lang Path, Cohoes City Sch Dist, **SLP**

Messineo, Marc Joseph 2654 Sheridan Dive, Apartment 3, Tonawanda, NY 14150, (716) 834-2712, MA 88 SUNY - Center at Buffalo

Messineo, Maryanne D 1007 Central Avenue, New Providence, NJ 07974, (201) 755-1707, BA 75 Kean Coll of NJ; MA 77 Temple Univ; 77–Aud, Floyd B Gusack MD, **A**

Messineo-Cowles, Jacqueline 1178 Earl's Dirve, Victor, NY 14564, (716) 924-7846, BS 83 Nazareth Coll of Rochester; MS 86 Nazareth Coll of Rochester; 85–Sp-Lang Path, West Irondequoit Sch Dist, **SLP**

Messing, Barbara Pisano 636 Portland Street, Baltimore, MD 21230, (301) 730-1118, BS 82 Appalachian St Univ; MA 85 Appalachian St Univ; **SLP**

Messinger, Laura Grabell 468 Wingate Road, Huntingdon Valley, PA 19006, (215) 947-4681, BA 81 Rutger's St Univ - Douglas Coll; MS 83 Boston Univ; Sp-Lang Path, Rolling Hill Hosp, **SLP**

Messinger, Maris S 257 Bronson Road, Southport, CT 06490, (203) 259-5590, BA 71 George Washington Univ; ME 72 Northeastern Univ; Sp/Lang Path, Private Practice, **SLP**

Messinger, Sue A 829 East 10th Street #1-J, Brooklyn, NY 11230, (212) 598-1340, BA 83 SUNY - Coll at Cortland; MS 87 CUNY - Brooklyn Coll; 87–Aud, NY Eye & Ear Infirm, **A**

Messner, Karen Courtney 8510 Joseph Avenue, Brentwood, MO 63144, (314) 961-7793, BS 82 Univ of KS; MS 85 Univ of WA; **SLP**

Messonnier, Mrs Pamela G 106 Maurice Street, Lafayette, LA 70506, (318) 235-3725, BS 84 LA St Univ - Baton Rouge; MS 88 Univ of Southwestern LA; 88–Sp-Lang Path, Acadiana Speech Svcs Inc

Mester, Leslie J 6403 Mariana Drive, Parma Heights, OH 44130, (216) 886-4200, BA 70 Cleveland St Univ; BA 73 Cleveland St Univ; MA 74 Cleveland St Univ; Aud, Tj Stefanik, **A**

Mester, Lori Marie 767 West 17th Street, Marshfield, WI 54449, (715) 389-2326, MS 87 Univ of WI - River Falls; 87–Sp-Lang Path, Midwest Rehab Specialists Inc, **SLP**

Mesulam, Mrs Audrey S 126 Drake Road, Somerset, NJ 08873, (201) 874-4600, BA 59 CUNY - Queens Coll; MS 76 Rutgers St Univ -N Brunswick; Sp/Lang Path, Montgomery Tnsp Bd of Ed, **SLP**

Metarelis, Mrs Sharon Eilzabeth 828 Hope Place N E, Albuquerque, NM 87123, **SLP**

Metcalf, Mrs Kathleen Highland 704 Breen Drive, Champaign, IL 61820, (217) 384-3572, BS 79 IL St Univ - Normal; MA 80 Univ of IL - Urbana; Sp-Lang Path, Univ of Illinois, **SLP**

Metcalf, Mikealiene Gail 7307 Major Avenue, Norfolk, VA 23505, (804) 423-2789, BS 73 Old Dominion Univ; MS 86 Old Dominion Univ; 86–Sp-Lang Path, City of VA Beach PS, **SLP**

Metcalfe, Dr Jean V 29 Willow Road, Menlo Park, CA 94025, PH (NS); **SLP LM**

Meth, Mrs Margaret Ann 28 Peter Bush Drive, Monroe, NY 10950, (914) 294-8544, MA 83 Montclair St Coll; Sp-Lang Path, Lovenbruck Assoc, **SLP ACE**

Meth, Phyllis R 92 Blamey Circle, Stratford, CT 06497, (203) 385-4225, BA 51 Mount Holyoke Coll; MA 77 Fairfield Univ; 68–Sp-Lang Path, Stratford PS, **SLP**

Methling, Mrs Catherine Camasto 262 Michigan Street, Elmhurst, IL 60126, (312) 833-2352, BA 76 Augustana Coll; MA 78 Northwestern Univ; **SLP**

Methven, Dr Margaret P 3931 South Uinta Street, Denver, CO 80237, (303) 770-1593, BA 40 Washburn Univ; MA 60 Univ of Denver; ED 76 (NS) Univ of Denver; Retired, Sch Dist No 1 Denver Co, **SLP**

Metilly, Mrs Doris G 10138 Turkey Oak Drive, New Port Richey, FL 34654, (813) 841-8848, BS 58 Boston Univ; Sp-Lang Path, Pawtucket Ri Sch Sys, **SLP**

Metke, Debra L 967 Pletcher Road, Youngstown, NY 14174, (716) 754-8178, BS 86 SUNY - Coll at Fredonia; MS 87 SUNY - Coll at Fredonia; 88–Sp-Lang Path, Niagra Children's ETC, **SLP**

Metraux, Ruth W 35 Rte DE Taillepied 1095, Lutry, Switzerland, BA 34 Marshall Univ; MA 41 Univ of MI - Ann Arbor; **SLP LM**

Metrik, Lynn R 36-40 Bowne #4Q, Flushing, NY 11354, (718) 353-0983, BA 73 Univ of Houston - Univ Park; MA 74 Univ of Houston - Univ Park; Instr/Consult-Voice-Sp, Amer Acad-Dramatic Arts, **SLP**

Metrione, Mrs Mary Ann L 341 Longwood Drive, Haddonfield, NJ 08033, (609) 933-3725, BS 57 Syracuse Univ; MA 80 Temple Univ; Sp-Lang Path, LARC Sch, **SLP**

Metrogen-Prieto, Karen Lea 15th Med Dept Box 3596, APO New York, NY 09114, BA 74 CA St Univ - Sacramento; MA 80 CA St Univ - Sacramento

Metropoulos, Theresa S 823 8th Avenue, Helena, MT 59601, (406) 443-0971, BA 79 Univ of MT; OM 81 Univ of MT; Sp-Lang Path, St Peter's Comm Hosp, **SLP ACE**

Metsch, Susan Ellen Winding Road Farm, Ardsley, NY 10502, (914) 378-7501, BA 79 Smith Coll; MA 88 CUNY - Lehman Coll; 88–SLP, St Joseph's Med Ctr Dept Sp & Aud

Metting, Mrs Pamela Jean 103 West Gibson Street, Canandaigua, NY 14424, (315) 789-3595, BS 70 Bowling Green St Univ; MA 72 Bowling Green St Univ; 84–Aud, Finger Lakes Hearing Ctr Inc, **A**

Mettler, Mrs Laura Lynn 402 Adare Road, Norfolk, NE 68701, (402) 379-2915, BA 82 Univ of SD - Vermillion; MA 84 Univ of SD - Vermillion; Sp-Lang Path, Ed Serv Unit #8, **SLP**

Mettler-Stephenson, Jean Marie 300 North 39th Avenue, Hattiesburg, MS 39401, BS 83 Univ of SD - Vermillion; MA 84 Univ of SD - Vermillion; Sp-Lang Path, Hattiesburg PS, **SLP**

Metts, Mrs Cheri Cobb 102 Dogwood Court, Cayce, SC 29033, (803) 739-4648, BA 86 Univ of AL- Tuscaloosa; MS 87 Univ of AL- Tuscaloosa; 88–Sp-Lang Path, Lexington County Sch Dist 2, **SLP**

Metts, Marlene 941 Dougherty Road, Aiken, SC 29801, (803) 648-3268, **SLP**

Metty, Debra I 60 Pinney Street #86, Ellington, CT 06029, (203) 528-2136, BS 78 WV Univ; MA 80 Univ of CT; 81–Sp/Lang Path, S Windsor Bd of Ed, **SLP**

Metz, Mrs Carol Neuner 709 Froome Avenue, Cincinnati, OH 45232, (513) 541-5213, BS 78 Univ of MO - Columbia; MA 79 Univ of MO - Columbia; **SLP**

Metz, Mrs Cheryl Lynn 4513 Cupid Drive, El Paso, TX 79924, (915) 598-8121, BA 73 Univ of TX - El Paso; MA 81 Univ of TX - El Paso; Sp-Lang Path, Ysleta ISD, **SLP**

Metz, Dr Dale E Ntid-Rit, 1 Lomb Memorial Drive, Rochester, NY 14623, (716) 475-6802, BS 70 SUNY - Coll at Geneseo; MS 72 Purdue Univ - West Lafayette; PH 76 (NS) Syracuse Univ; Res Assoc, Rochester I of Tech, **SLP**

Metz, Dr David Abraham 3680 Berkeley Road, Cleveland Heights, OH 44118, (216) 687-3803, BA 60 Case Western Reserve Univ; MA 65 Case Western Reserve Univ; PH 67 (NS) Case Western Reserve Univ; Prof/Assoc Dean, Cleveland St U, **A**

Metz, Mary A 3619 Mapleway Drive, Toledo, OH 43614, BS 72 Bowling Green St Univ; MA 74 Bowling Green St Univ; **SLP LM**

Metz, Dr Michael J 12665 Garden Grove Blvd, Suite 606, Garden Grove, CA 92643, (714) 638-8122, BS 66 Univ of IA; MS 67 CO St Univ; PH 72 (NS) Univ of Denver; Pres, Aud Assoc Inc, **A**

Metz, Mrs Pandora Frank 184 Pyramid Pines Estates, Saratoga Springs, NY 12866, (518) 584-0762, BA 82 Univ of NC - Greensboro; ME 83 Univ of NC - Greensboro; Sp-Lang Path, Private Practice, **SLP**

Metz, Mrs Stephanie S 978 Lincoln Way East, Chambersburg, PA 17201, (717) 737-6728, BS 83 Bloomsburg Univ of PA; MS 84 Bloomsburg Univ of PA; 84–Sp-Lang Path, Capital Area Intermed Unit #15, **SLP**

Metz, Mrs Wendy Susan 215 Scholfield Road, Rochester, NY 14617-4214, (716) 663-7070, BS 79 Nazareth Coll of Rochester; ME 82 Nazareth Coll of Rochester; Sp-Lang Path, Rocheser City, **SLP**

Metzendorf, Diane E 16 Taylor Street, Port Jefferson Station, NY 11776, (516) 474-4684, BA 83 Adelphi Univ; MS 84 Adelphi Univ; Sp-Lang Path, Sch for Lang & Comm Dev, **SLP**

Metzgar, Mrs Kim Marie 226 E 4th Avenue, Redfield, SD 57469, (605) 472-2400, BS 83 Univ of SD - Vermillion; MA 84 Univ of SD - Vermillion; 85–Sp-Lang Path, Redfield State Hospital/School, **SLP**

Metzger, Barbara Ann 505 West Point Drive, Akron, OH 44313, (216) 434-1661, BA 83 Duquesne Univ; MA 86 Kent St Univ

Metzger, Dr Hope H 7670 Blome Road, Cincinnati, OH 45243, (513) 825-5393, BA 59 OH St Univ; MA 62 Univ of MD - College Park; PH 85 (Aud) Univ of Cincinnati; Tchr for Hrng Imp/Aud, Greenhills-Forrest Park Sch, **A**

Metzger, Janet Marie 248 Lark Street #1, Albany, NY 12210, (518) 432-9193, BA 84 SUNY - Coll at Plattsburgh; MA 86 SUNY - Coll at Plattsburgh; 88–Sp-Lang Path, Early Childhood Learning Ctr, **SLP**

Metzger, Jayne W 824 West 28th Street, Richmond, VA 23225, (804) 230-4806, OB 84 Univ of KY; OM 86 Univ of SC - Columbia; Sales Representative, Elb Monitor, **A**

Metzger, Jean Frances 1340-1 South 9th Street, Park Terrace Apartment, Allentown, PA 18103, (215) 776-3270, **SLP**

Metzger, Mrs Judy A 13 Christy Street, Silver Creek, NY 14136, (716) 934-4274, BS 74 SUNY - Coll at Buffalo; MS 77 SUNY - Coll at Buffalo; Sp-Lang Path, Silver Crk Montessori Presch, **SLP**

Metzger, Kathleen Marie 6106 East 82nd Place #7, Tulsa, OK 74137, (918) 245-5911, **SLP**

Metzger, Maria Jusko 2637 Amhurst Road #2, Middleton, WI 53562, (608) 836-6605, **SLP**

Metzger, Mrs Mary E 1509 Lincoln Court, Arlington Heights, IL 60004, (312) 259-2338, BA 78 IN Univ - Bloomington; MA 79 Ball St Univ; **SLP**

Metzger, Mrs Mary Jean B Rural Delivery 4, 7 Monroe Court, Princeton, NJ 08540, (201) 329-2459, BA 50 Emerson Coll; MA 51 Univ of Southern CA; Sp-Lang Path, Private Practice, **SLP**

Metzger, Mrs Mary L 10500 Bond, Overland Park, KS 66214, (316) 263-9557, MA 81 Wichita St Univ; BA 71 Univ of KS; SLP, USD 233, **SLP**

Metzger, Patricia R 4550 S E 8th Street, Ocala, FL 32671, (904) 694-5621, **SLP**

Metzger, Rolland 832 North Brinton Avenue, Dixon, IL 61021, (815) 284-2956, BS 46 Univ of Chicago; MA 55 Northwestern Univ; PH 57 (Psychology) Northwestern Univ

Metzger, Thomas G 2025 Belvedere, Toledo, OH 43614, (419) 385-5236, OB 78 Univ of Toledo; MS 80 Boston Univ; 87–Pres, T G Metzger & Associates Inc, **SLP**

Metzker, Mrs Peggy L P O Box 642, Minden, LA 71058-0642, (318) 371-2426, BA 73 Univ of AR - Fayetteville; MA 80 Univ of AR - Fayetteville; 88–Sp-Lang Path, Webster Parish Sch Bd, **SLP**

Metzl, Dr Marilyn N Psychological-Educ Assoc Inc, 1000 West 59th Street, Kansas City, MO 64113, (816) 361-3633, BA 59 CUNY - Queens Coll; MA 68 CUNY - Hunter Coll; PH 78 (NS) Univ of KS; Dir, Psychological Ed Assoc Inc, **SLP**

Metzler, Robin Sedor 3461 Forest Road, Bethel Park, PA 15102, BS 79 Northwestern Univ; MA 82 Northwestern Univ; **SLP**

Meuel, Ann S 69 El Molino Drive, Clayton, CA 94517, (415) 672-6118, BA 76 San Francisco St Univ; MS 78 San Francisco St Univ; **SLP**

Meunier, Kathy C 8 Richmond Place, New Orleans, LA 70115, (504) 899-4950, BA 70 LA St Univ - Baton Rouge; MA 71 George Washington Univ; Sp/Lang Path, Jefferson Sp/Lang Cen, **SLP**

Meuse, Dr Sheila A 1219 Greenbriar Loop, Round Rock, TX 78664, (304) 293-4241, BA 77 Univ of CT; MA 80 Univ of TX - Austin; PH 84 (NS) Univ of TX - Austin; Sp-Lang Path, Private Practice, **SLP**

Meves, Mrs Julia Renee 12761 Dunas Road, Santa Ana, CA 92705, (714) 559-0100, BA 81 CA St Univ - Long Beach; MA 84 CA St Univ - Long Beach; SLP, Irvine USD, **SLP**

Meydag, Mrs Vana L 15925 Stanmont Street, Whittier, CA 90603, (714) 730-7546, BA 76 CA St Univ - Fullerton; MA 81 CA St Univ - Fullerton; SLP, Tustin USD, **SLP**

Meyer, Mrs Amalie 433 Sylvan Avenue #48, Mountain View, CA 94041, (415) 964-7262, BA 63 CUNY - Queens Coll; MA 64 Stanford Univ; 88–Retired, Los Gatos USD, **SLP**

Meyer, Mrs Andrea M 518 West Van Buren Street, Ottawa, IL 61350, (815) 434-0857, BS 77 IL St Univ - Normal; MA 79 Northwestern Univ; Sp-Lang Path, Lasalle Co Easter S Rehab Cen, **SLP**

Meyer, Annalisa K Rte 2 Box 38, Ogallala, NE 69153, (308) 284-8220, BS 79 Univ of NE - Lincoln; MA 83 Western WA Univ; Audiologist & Sp Pathologist, Pikes Peak Center for Sp & Hrg, **SLP A**

Meyer, Mrs Barbara S 2043 Sunflower Court, Chesterfield, MO 63017, (314) 889-1407, BS 73 Univ of MO - Columbia; MA 74 Saint Louis Univ; Asst Prof, Fontabonne Coll, **SLP**

Meyer, Becky Blodgett Speech And Hearing Department, McLaren General Hospital, 401 South Ballenger Hwy, Flint, MI 48502, (313) 762-2362, BA 79 MI St Univ; MS 81 Univ of MI - Ann Arbor; Audiologist, McLaren Genl Hosp, **A**

Meyer, Beth D 108 Woodridge Lane, Oak Ridge, TN 37830, (615) 482-1145, BS 73 Univ of MI - Ann Arbor; MS 75 Univ of WI - Madison; Sp-Lang Path, Private Practice, **SLP**

Meyer, Mrs Courtland Gunn 201 Spring Street, Culpeper, VA 22701, (703) 825-9153, BS 79 Univ of VA - Charlottesville; ME 83 Univ of VA - Charlottesville; 86–Sp-Lang Path, Easter Seal Society, **SLP**

Meyer, Mrs Deborah Scully 4760 Shadylawn Terrace, Cincinnati, OH 45238, (513) 471-9622, BS 78 Miami Univ - Oxford; MS 81 Miami Univ - Oxford; **SLP**

Meyer, Denise K 8132 Sanborn Drive, Lincoln, NE 68505, (402) 464-5940, BS 77 Univ of NE - Lincoln; MA 79 Univ of NE - Lincoln; **SLP**

Meyer, Mrs Diane Lynn 11722 Ruggles Circle, Omaha, NE 68164, (402) 496-1419, BS 84 Univ of NE - Omaha; MS 86 Univ of NE - Omaha; 86–Sp-Lang Path, Omaha PS, **SLP**

Meyer, Dr Dianne 434 East Hickory, Hinsdale, IL 60521, (312) 996-6520, BS OH Univ - Athens; MA Univ of IL - Urbana; Director Audiology Section, U of IL at Chicago, **A ACE**

Meyer, Mrs Donna L 604 Claymont Drive, Ballwin, MO 63021, (314) 569-8100, BA 76 Fontbonne Coll; MS 77 Fontbonne Coll; SLP, Spec Sch Dist of St Louis Co, **SLP**

Meyer, Dr Edward L 910 8th Street, Brookings, SD 57006, (605) 688-6131, BA 51; MA 53 Univ of SD - Vermillion; PH 75 (NS) Univ of MN - Minneap-St Paul; Professor of Speech, South Dakota State University, **SLP**

Meyer, Eileen R 2708 M Street, Belleville, KS 66935, (913) 527-2330, BS 71 KS St Univ; MA 73 KS St Univ; **SLP**

Meyer, Mrs Eileen R 228 Radcliff, Bolingbrook, IL 60439, (312) 759-7623, BS 82 Eastern IL Univ; MS 83 Eastern IL Univ; Sp/Lang Path, LaGrange Dept of Spec Educ, **SLP**

Meyer, Mrs Hope Bonnie 702 Kildare Court, Seaford, NY 11783, (516) 735-5514, MA 87 Hofstra Univ; 88–Tchr, Nassau BOCES

Meyer, Mrs Jacqueline 17 Horseshoe Lane Road #1, Chittenango, NY 13037, (315) 455-7571, BA 68 KS St Univ; OM 81 Univ of MO - Columbia; Sp/Lang Path, Lyncourt Sch, **SLP**

Meyer, Mrs Jeanne D 10202 Desert Willow, Dallas, TX 75243, (214) 680-3537, BS 72 KS St Univ; MA 73 KS St Univ; Sp-Lang Path, Richardson Sp & Lang Cl, **SLP**

Meyer, Joanne L 76 Ross Avenue, #7, San Anselmo, CA 94960, (415) 461-5304, BA 68 Southern Methodist Univ; MA 70 Univ of Denver; Sp/Lang Serv of Marin/Sonoma, **SLP**

Meyer, Judith A Goodhouse Road, Litchfield, CT 06759, (203) 567-0256, BA 61 CUNY - Queens Coll; MS 82 Southern CT St Univ; Sp/Lang Path, Priv Pract, **SLP**

Meyer, Judith Pollack 3411 North 5th Avenue, Suite 203, Phoenix, AZ 85013, (602) 266-9315, BA 66 Rutger's St Univ - Douglas Coll; MA 74 CUNY - City College; 77–Owner/Dir, Certified Sp Path Inc, **SLP**

Meyer, Mrs Karen A G 506 Village Drive, Brewster, NY 10509, (914) 279-9575, BA 69 CUNY - Lehman Coll; MA 71 Northwestern Univ; Sp-Lang Path, Westch Exceptional Chldrns Sch, **SLP**

Meyer, Kathy Sue Dean Box 162, Orchard, NE 68764, BA 80 SD St Univ; MA 81 SD St Univ; Sp-Lang Path, Educational Service Unit 8, **SLP**

Meyer, Mrs Kay B 445 North Pinecrest Road, Bolingbrook, IL 60439, (312) 739-7735, BA 76 Univ of IA; MA 78 Northwestern Univ; Sp-Lang Path, Downers Grove South HS, **SLP**

Meyer, Mrs Lauren Rene 60 North Beretania Street, Apartment 2306, Honolulu, HI 96817, (808) 524-7985, BA 80 Univ of CA - Santa Barbara; MA 83 Univ of CT; Sp-Lang Path, State of Hawaii Dept of Educ, **SLP**

Meyer, Dr Linda Anne Dir Communication Disorders, Woodrow Wilson Rehab Ctr, Fishersville, VA 22939, (703) 332-7086, BS 71 Old Dominion Univ; MS 74 Old Dominion Univ; PH 82 (NS) Vanderbilt Univ; 83–Dir/Comm Serv, Woodrow Wilson Rehab Cen, **SLP**

Meyer, Mrs Madeline D 5800 Kirkside Drive #A', Bakersfield, CA 93309-3670, (805) 398-3600, BA 64 Univ of CT; MA 65 Univ of CT; Sp-Lang Path, Kern Co Supt of Sch, **SLP**

Meyer, Marcia Ann 8123 Starview Drive, El Cajon, CA 92021, (619) 272-9023, **SLP**

Meyer, Mary F 801 Evans Road, Fieldbrook, CA 95521, (707) 826-3476, BA 78 Humboldt St Univ; MA 81 Humboldt St Univ; Sp-Lang Path, **SLP**

Meyer, Nancy E M Route 2 Box 78, Valley View Road, Roberts, WI 54023, (612) 426-3214, BS 71 Saint Cloud St Univ; MS 76 Univ of WI - Eau Claire; SLP, ISD 832, **SLP**

Meyer, Neil N P O Box 246, Idyllwild, CA 92349, (714) 925-1265, BA 69 CA St Univ - Long Beach; MA 74 CA St Univ - Long Beach; 88–Sp-Lang Path, Riverside County Ofc of Educ, **SLP**

Meyer, Phyllis R 5133 Troy Road, Delaware, OH 43015, (614) 421-3818, BA 77 OH St Univ; MA 80 Bowling Green St Univ; SLP, OH State U Hosp, **SLP**

Meyer, Robert C Louisiana Tech University, P O Box 3165, Ruston, LA 71270, PH (NS); **A**

Meyer, Robert G Dept Communicative Disorders, Northern Illinois Univ, De Kalb, IL 60115, (815) 753-6513, BS 50 Univ of IL - Urbana; MS 61 Univ of IL - Urbana; Coord Undergraduate Advisement, Northern Illinois University, **SLP**

Meyer, Robert R Medically Approved Hrng Ctr, 578 First Avenue North, St Petersburg, FL 33701, (813) 894-2775, MS 73 Univ of South FL; Aud Coor & Sect-Treasurer, Medically Approved Hearing Cen, **A**

Meyer, Sandra Jilek 2595 Saybrook Road, University Heights, OH 44118, (216) 231-8787, BS 75 Univ of IL - Urbana; MS 76 Univ of IL - Urbana; Coord of Continuing Educ, Case Western Reserve Univ, **SLP**

Meyer, Mrs Sheila Rose 196 Eastland Drive, Ottawa, OH 45875, (419) 226-9019, BS 85 Bowling Green St Univ; MS 86 Bowling Green St Univ; 86–Aud, St Ritas Med Ctr, **A**

Meyer, Susan Marie 1166 Killarney, Livermore, CA 94550, (415) 651-1190, BS 73 Northern St Coll; MA 76 Univ of MT; Sp-Lang Path, Fremont USD, **SLP**

Meyer, Dr Toby 1320 Chicago Avenue #6A, Evanston, IL 60201, (312) 492-5076, BA 79 CUNY - Lehman Coll; MA 80 CUNY - Lehman Coll; PH 85 (NS) Northwestern Univ; Res Asst, Nwn U, **SLP**

Meyer, Vicki L 1611 Grand Avenue, Davenport, IA 52803, (319) 242-6454, BS 80 Univ of MN - Duluth; MS 82 Univ of WI - Madison; SLP, **SLP**

Meyer, Mrs Victoria 12452 Glengate, Maryland Heights, MO 63043, (314) 727-8340, BS 71 Southeast MO St Univ; MA 73 Univ of KS; 87–Consult, Managed Health Care Svcs Inc, **SLP**

Meyer, Dr William H Sch Of Communicative Disorders, University Of Wisconsin, Stevens Point, WI 54481, (715) 346-3667, BS 67 Defiance Coll; MA 68 Kent St Univ; PH 73 (Sp-Lang Path) Southern IL Univ -Carbondale; 87–Assoc Vice Chancellor, U of Wis-Stevens Point, **SLP**

Meyer-Boldon, Carol A P O Box 537, 804 Williams Street, Sparta, WI 54656, (608) 269-3687, BS 81 Univ of WI - Stevens Point; MS 82 Univ of WI - Eau Claire; SLP, Private Practice, **SLP**

Meyerer, Mrs Margaret Lloyd 5515 Roosevelt Street, Bethesda, MD 20817, (301) 897-8260, BA 68 Univ of MD - College Park; MA 72 Catholic Univ of America; Sp-Lang Path, Private Practice, **SLP**

Meyerhoff, Mrs Linda M T 4351 S 50 W, Greenfield, IN 46140, (317) 861-4451, BS 73 Univ of CA - Davis; ME 75 Western OR St Coll; **SLP**

Meyerowitz, Elizabeth Ann 18404 West 114th Terrace, Olathe, KS 66061, (913) 383-9014, **SLP**

Meyers, Annette L 12345 Upper Preston Rd S E, Issaquah, WA 98027, (206) 222-5820, BA 76 Univ of WA; BS 76 Univ of WA; OM 78 Univ of WA; SLP, Lake Washington Sch Dist, **SLP**

Meyers, Mrs Barbara J 4617 Kingston Court, Midland, MI 48640, (517) 631-6467, **SLP**

Meyers, Carol A 3512 Johnson Street, High Point, NC 27260, (704) 246-2726, BA 73 Stetson Univ; ME 75 Univ of FL; Sp-Lang Path, Lexington Cty Sch, **SLP ACE**

Meyers, Mrs Carol A 711 North Weber Suite 2, Colorado Springs, CO 80903, (719) 633-1494, BS 79 Univ of NE - Lincoln; MA 80 Univ of NE - Lincoln; Aud, Hearing Cons of Col Springs, **A**

Meyers, Carolyn Ann 3834 Oaklake Circle South, Indianapolis, IN 46268, (812) 853-2993, BS 85 Univ of MO - Columbia; MS 86 Univ of SC - Columbia; Prof Assoc, InSpeech Inc, **SLP**

Meyers, Edward Frederick 2328 Cedar, Bakersfield, CA 93301, (805) 872-3408, BS 74 Eastern IL Univ; MS 80 Southern IL Univ -Carbondale; 88–Sp-Lang Path, Kern Co Supt of Schs, **SLP**

Meyers, Esther K 9536 Texhoma Avenue, Northridge, CA 91325, BA 67 CA St Univ - Northridge; MA 69 CA St Univ - Northridge; MA 80 CA St Univ - Northridge; Sp-Lang Path, LA USD, **SLP**

Meyers, Francine G 1960 Lincoln Park West, Apartment 603, Chicago, IL 60614, (312) 281-3396, BS 79 Eastern MI Univ; MA 80 Eastern MI Univ; Sp-Lang Path, Private Practice, **SLP**

Meyers, Dr Harold W, Jr Southwest Missouri State Univ, Communications Disorders, 901 South National, Springfield, MO 65804, (417) 836-5275, BA 65 Albion Coll; MS 70 Univ of OK Medical Center; PH 76 (NS) Wayne St Univ; Aud, SW Mo St U, **A**

Meyers, Jeanne C 3858 Joslin Lane, Vacaville, CA 95688, (707) 429-3798, BS 68 Univ of WI - Oshkosh; MA 71 Univ of IA; Sp-Lang Path, Solano Co Supt of Sch, **SLP**

Meyers, Judith A 3306 Delicious Drive, Clifton, CO 81520, (303) 434-7546, BA 74 Univ of CO - Boulder; MA 85 Univ of Northern CO; Sp-Lang Path, Mesa County Valley Sch Dist 51, **SLP**

Meyers, Karen L 329 Ronnie Drive, Buffalo Grove, IL 60090, (312) 975-3390, **SLP**

Meyers, Laura I 2134 Homecrest Avenue, Brooklyn, NY 11229, (718) 998-3284, BA 75 CUNY - Brooklyn Coll; MA 77 Hofstra Univ; Sp-Lang Path, HCHC Inc at Kingsbrook Hosp, **SLP**

Meyers, Linda Suzanne 2423 Espanola Northeast #C, Albuquerque, NM 87110, (505) 298-3766, MS 79 Auburn Univ - Auburn; Sp/Lang Path, Albuquerque Public Schools, **SLP**

Meyers, Lynn Denise 94239 27th Street, Marcellus, MI 49067, (616) 685-8543, BA 83 MI St Univ; MA 86 Central MI Univ; **SLP**

Meyers, Margaret Mae 56 Leonard Road, Boxborough, MA 01719, (508) 635-0002, BS 83 Northern IL Univ - De Kalb; MA 85 Northern IL Univ - De Kalb; 88–Sp-Lang Path, Bedford PS, **SLP**

Meyers, Martha M 949 Golfview Road, Glenview, IL 60025, (312) 729-3629, **SLP**

Meyers, Dr Susan C 101 Blithe Court, Charlottesville, VA 22901, (804) 924-4622, BA 73 Univ of Denver; MA 74 Univ of Denver; PH 83 (NS) Univ of TX - Dallas; Assistant Prof, U of Virginia, **SLP**

Meyers-Hafner, Ellen Joan R R 1 Box 87, Monee, IL 60449, (312) 371-0720, BS 79 IL St Univ - Normal; MS 80 IL St Univ - Normal; Sp/Lang Path, Sch Dist #126, **SLP**

Meyerson, Dr Marion D 225 Bay Street #203, San Francisco, CA 94133, (415) 433-1382, BA 55 CUNY - Hunter Coll; MA 64 CUNY - Brooklyn Coll; PH 71 (Sp Path) Univ of IL - Urbana; Lecturer, San Jose State University, **SLP A**

Meyrowitz, Gail S 140 Riverside Drive #1-0, New York, NY 10024, BS 79 Univ of MD - College Park; MA 81 NY Univ; Sp-Lang Path, Private Practice, **SLP**

Meythaler, Mrs Gwendolyn J 1301 J Street, Salida, CO 81201, (303) 539-2593, BA 75 Univ of Denver; MA 77 Univ of Denver; Sp-Lang Path, Salida Pub Sch Sys, **SLP**

Miccio, Adele Whiting 1923 14th Street Road, Greeley, CO 80631, (303) 352-0488, MA 86 Univ of Northern CO; 88–Sp-Lang Path, Univ of Northern Colorado, **SLP**

Miceli, Bernard Vincent 10 Aspinwood Way #C, Baltimore, MD 21237, (301) 687-1789, BS 82 Towson St Univ; MS 84 Towson St Univ; 85–Sp-Lang Path, MIEMSS/Montebello Rehab Hosp, **SLP**

Michael, Ann 261 Pinnacle Drive, Boone, NC 28607, **SLP**

Michael, Liane E 1983 Kobara Lane, San Jose, CA 95124, (408) 299-5617, BA 65 Univ of the Pacific; MA 66 Univ of the Pacific; Dir SLP Dept, Santa Clara Valley Med Cen, **SLP ACE**

Michael, Mrs Mary W 2278 Komo Mai Drive, Honolulu, HI 96782, BA 50 ID St Univ; ME 64 Univ of HI - Hilo; Instructor of English, Univ of HI

Michael, Dr Paul L 667 Franklin Street, State College, PA 16803, (814) 238-8533, BS 48 Fairmont St Coll; MS 49 WV Univ; PH 55 (Occupational Health) Univ of Pittsburgh - Pittsburgh; Environmental Acous, Paul L Michael & Associates Inc, **F**

Michaelides, Mrs Jackie K 940 Highview Drive, Worthington, OH 43085, (614) 885-0330, BS 76 Univ of MD - College Park; MA 79 Cleveland St Univ

Michaelis, Lucinda Jane 3775 E Denton #85, St Francis, WI 53207, (414) 482-4490, BS 82 Augustana Coll; MS 84 IL St Univ - Normal; Sp-Lang Path, Waukesha PS Dist, **SLP**

Michaels, Kathleen Cichocki W223 N2828 Pinewood Court, Waukesha, WI 53186, (414) 423-0593, BS 77 Univ of WI - Milwaukee; MS 79 Univ of WI - Milwaukee; SLP, Greendale School System, **SLP**

Michaels, Mrs Lisa R 23 Cranford Terrace, Cranford, NJ 07016, (201) 272-0842, BA 73 Long Island U - Brooklyn Ctr; MA 75 NY Univ; Program Manager, St Ils Boro Dev Serv Off, **SLP**

Michaels, Meredith G 3972 19th Street, San Francisco, CA 94114, (415) 981-6405, BA 73 Hofstra Univ; MA 74 CA St Univ - Long Beach; MA 80 Claremont Graduate Sch; **SLP**

Michaels, Susan Liz E 826 South Gammon Road #3, Madison, WI 53719, (608) 273-1637, BS 80 Univ of WI - Whitewater; MS 81 Univ of WI - Whitewater; 87–Sp-Lang Path, InSpeech Inc, **SLP ACE**

Michaelson, Mrs Melanie C 3164 Gilbert Drive, Baton Rouge, LA 70809, (504) 388-2545, BA 71 LA St Univ - Baton Rouge; MA 72 LA St Univ - Baton Rouge; 88–Clin Fac, LA State Univ, **SLP**

Michaletz, Mary Patricia 12244 Caminito Del Mar San, San Diego, CA 92130, BA 80 San Diego St Univ; MA 82 San Diego St Univ; 86–Sp/Lang Path, Private Practice, **SLP**

Michalowski, Mrs Alice J 2701 Cherry Street, Park Ridge, IL 60068, (312) 462-3180, BA 74 Mundelein Coll; MS 75 Marquette Univ; Co-Director, United Sp & Aud Consultants, **SLP**

Michalski, John A Ear Nose & Throat Assoc, 347 West Berry Street, Fort Wayne, IN 46802, (219) 426-8117, BS 72 Bowling Green St Univ; MA 76 Bowling Green St Univ; Aud, ENT Assoc, **A**

Michalski, Mrs Mary J Marshfield Clinic, Speech Pathology, 1000 North Oak Avenue, Marshfield, WI 54449, (714) 387-5128, BS 71 Marquette Univ; MS 72 Univ of WI - Milwaukee; Sp-Lang Path, Marshfield Cl, **SLP**

Michalson, Mrs Cheryl Kay Burt 4118 Mercier, Kansas City, MO 64111, (816) 221-7565, BA 81 Univ of MO - KS City; MS 85 Central MO St Univ; 85–Sp-Lang Path, Kansas City Sch Dist, **SLP**

Michaud, Mrs Janet Sullivan P O Box 2101, West Scarborough, ME 04074, (207) 284-7427, BA 82 Boston Coll; MA 84 OH Univ - Athens; 84–Sp-Lang Path, York Co Counseling Svcs Inc, **SLP**

Michaud-Patterson, Mrs M 4 Hege Drive, Lexington, NC 27292, (602) 835-8925, BS 71 LA St Univ - Baton Rouge; MS 73 Vanderbilt Univ; SLP, Private Practice, **SLP**

Michel, Dr John Frederich Dept Of Sp-Lang-Hrng, University Of Kansas, 290 Haworth Hall, Lawrence, KS 66045, (913) 843-0627, BA 59 OH St Univ; MA 60 OH St Univ; PH 64 (NS) Univ of FL

Michel, Mrs Karen Elaine 4 Page Street, Rochester, NH 03867, (603) 778-7311, MS 84 Univ of NH; Sp-Lang Path, Exeter Hospital, **SLP ACE**

Michel, Linda Beth 1731 Pacific Avenue, Glendale, CA 91202, (213) 245-5338, MA 72 Univ of Southern CA; BA 69 San Francisco St Univ; Prog Spec, Los Angeles USD, **SLP**

Michel, Dr Lorraine I 230 Concord Drive, Lawrence, KS 66044, (913) 296-6136, BA 59 Adelphi Univ; MA 60 OH St Univ; PH 65 (Sp-Lang Path) Univ of FL; 88–Coord of Sp-Lang Path, Kansas Dept of Health & Environment, **SLP**

Michele, Judith Louise 828 St James Drive, Virginia Beach, VA 23455, (804) 499-2306, ME 84 Old Dominion Univ; Sp-Lang Path, Commonwealth Healthcare Inc, **SLP**

Michelman, Margot 21542 Juego Circle #27C, Boca Raton, FL 33433, (305) 483-1166, BS 74 Boston Univ; MA 75 George Washington Univ; Sp-Lang Path, Private Practice, **SLP**

Michelow, Diane 63 Saco Street, Newton Upper Falls, MA 02164, (617) 824-6911, BA 78 Witwatersrand Univ S Africa; ME 80 Harvard Univ; Clin Superv, Morton Hosp, **SLP ACE**

Michels, Catherine Jean 218 North Wilson, Jefferson, IA 50129, (515) 386-8180, BA 84 Univ of Northern IA; MA 85 Univ of Northern IA; 86–Sp-Lang Path, Arrowhead AEA, **SLP**

Michels, Ida Ann 621 Belle Isle Avenue, Belleair Beach, FL 34635, (813) 596-2579, BA 55 OH St Univ; MS 82 Nova Univ; Sp-Lang Path, Aetna Ins Co, **SLP**

Michels, Linda V 2555 Fairmount Boulevard, Eugene, OR 97403, (503) 485-5915, MA 72 CA St Univ - Northridge; **SLP**

Michels, Mrs Marsha M 11126 East 37th, Spokane, WA 99206, (509) 326-1651, BA 76 Eastern WA Univ; MS 77 Eastern WA Univ; 88–Sp-Lang Path, Spokane Guilds Sch, **SLP**

Michels, Mrs Sonia L H Psc 1 Box 28009, San Francisco, CA 96230, (919) 477-0456, BS 77 Northwest MO St Univ; MS 80 Univ of NE - Omaha; Sp-Lang Path, Alamogordo Pub Sch, **SLP**

Michels, Mrs Suzanne Goenner St Mary's Hospital, Speech Language Path, 35 Grosvenor Street, London, ON, Canada N6A 1Y6, (519) 438-6185, BS 77 Univ of Western Ontario; OM 81 Univ of Western Ontario; 86–Sp-Lang Path, St Joseph's Health Centre, **SLP**

Michener, Mary C J Route 1, Eden, ID 83325, (208) 734-8324, BS 72 UT St Univ; MS 73 UT St Univ; Sp-Lang Path, Lenkner Michener & Assoc Inc, **SLP ACE**

Michie, Laura Audia 234 South Virginia Avenue, Falls Church, VA 22046, (703) 664-7190, ME 84 Univ of VA - Charlottesville; 87–Sp-Lang Path, Mt Vernon Hosp, **SLP**

Miciotto, Deanna P 4149 Bordeaux Drive, Kenner, LA 70065, (504) 830-4424, BA 76 Northeast LA Univ; OM 82 Tulane Univ; 82–Sp-Lang Path, Jefferson Parish PS Sys, **SLP**

Mickan, Mrs Penny Pierce 1606 Williams Drive, Georgetown, TX 78628, (512) 863-5486, BS 84 Baylor Univ; MS 85 Baylor Univ; Sp-Lang Path, Georgetown ISD, **SLP**

Mickelson, Mrs Carol Mohan 2516 22nd Avenue N E, Minneapolis, MN 55418, (612) 788-1940, BA 86 Univ of WI - Eau Claire; MS 87 Univ of WI - Eau Claire; **SLP**

Mickelson, Mrs Faye E Programs And Services Wheatley, 1200 Ritchie Road, Capitol Heights, MD 20743, (301) 336-7615, BA 68 George Washington Univ; MA 72 OH Univ - Athens; Aud, Prince Georges County Pub Sch, **SLP A**

Mickelson, William D 731 Alamo Drive, Vacaville, CA 95688, (707) 429-6691, BS 68 UT St Univ; MS 70 UT St Univ; SLP, Solano County Supt of Schools, **SLP**

Micken, Darrell J 366 Coulee Drive, Bozeman, MT 59715, (406) 586-0914, BS 62 MT St Univ; MA 69 Univ of MT; Aud, Medical Arts Hearing Center, **A**

Micken, Lee E 366 Coulee Drive, Bozeman, MT 59715, (406) 586-0914, BA 69 Univ of MT; MA 71 Univ of MT; Aud, Med Arts Hrng Cen, **A**

Mickey, Robin Reid 486 Cherry Court, Pittsburgh, PA 15237, (412) 323-4160, SLP, Pittsburgh Bd of Ed, **SLP**

Mickleberry, Darlene Marie 829 Libra Lane, Kenner, LA 70065, (504) 464-0973, BS 78 LA St Univ - Baton Rouge; OM 80 LA St Univ - N O Medical Ctr; Sp-Lang Path, Jefferson Parish School System, **SLP**

Mickowski, Jois Ann 4794 Arizona Street #109, San Diego, CA 92116, (619) 291-9506, **SLP**

Micucci, Betsy C 91 Acorn Street, Millis, MA 02054, (617) 642-0221, BA 74 George Washington Univ; MS 76 Emerson Coll; 84–Dir, Sp-Lang Path, E K Shriver Center UAP, **SLP**

Micucci, Debbie E 100 Lindsey Place, North Wales, PA 19454, (215) 368-5058, BS 79 West Chester Univ of PA; MA 85 West Chester Univ of PA; Communication Services Coord, Ken-Crest Services, **SLP**

Middaugh, Mrs Linda Welch 736 Alice Avenue, Rural Route 14, Thunder Bay, ON, Canada P7B 5E5, (807) 767-4842, BA 70 Univ of CO - Boulder; MS 77 Southern IL Univ-Edwardsvill; Sp-Lang Path, George Jeffrey Child Treat Ctr

Middel, Mrs Lori Ann 67 Flyers Drive, Norwich, CT 06360, (203) 887-7242, BS 82 SUNY - Coll at Geneseo; MS 88 Southern CT St Univ; 88–Sp-Lang Path, Connecticut/Dept Mental Retard, **SLP**

Middendorf, Kathi Ann 5301 Collinswood Drive, Raleigh, NC 27609, MS; **SLP**

Middleby, Maria Theresa 204 Pleasant Avenue, Rome, NY 13440, (315) 724-5101, **A**

Middleswarth, Mrs Karen L P O Box 116, Bellevue, OH 44811, (419) 483-5171, BS 74 Bowling Green St Univ; MA 77 Kent St Univ; Sp-Lang Path, Bellevue Bd of Ed, **SLP**

Middleton, Mrs Barbara M 324 Tremont Drive, Hopkinsville, KY 42240, (502) 887-1170, BA 81 Univ of KY; MS 84 Univ of KY; Sp-Lang Path, Christian Cty Sch Sys, **SLP**

Middleton, Mrs Carol L K 535 S E 68th, Portland, OR 97215, (503) 252-6534, BS 78 Portland St Univ; MS 82 Portland St Univ; Sp-Lang Path, N Clackamas Sch Dist, **SLP**

Middleton, Dr Grace Frederick 4804 Caseta, El Paso, TX 79922, (915) 747-5255, BS 63 OK St Univ; OM 64 Univ of OK Medical Center; ED 80 (Higher Education) TX Tech Univ; 70–Assoc Prof, U of TX-El Paso, **SLP**

Middleton, Janet B 68 Centre Street, Danvers, MA 01923-1427, **SLP**

Middleton, Mrs Janet M 155 Eagen Mountain Drive, Hope, ID 83836-9724, (208) 263-1128, BA 56 CO Coll; MS 83 San Francisco St Univ; Sp-Lang Path, Bonner County Sch Dist, **SLP**

Middleton, Lisa Annise 1304-D Nakomis N E, Albuquerque, NM 87112, (505) 275-3685, BA 82 TX Tech Univ; MS 85 Univ of TX - Dallas; **SLP**

Middleton, Lorraine D 17625 Ludlow Street, Granada Hills, CA 91344, (818) 368-1540, BA 85 CA St Univ - Northridge; MA 87 CA St Univ - Northridge; 88–Health Care Coord, Therapeutic Living Ctr for Blind

Middleton, Renee Annette 3501 Birmingham Highway, Ski Lodge Apartment #804, Opelika, AL 36801, (404) 834-1332, MA 83 Univ of TN - Knoxville; Instructor In Audiology, West Georgia College, **A**

Middleton, Rita Danneker 103 Roberts Road, Brookhaven, PA 19015, (215) 358-0536, BS 84 Bloomsburg Univ of PA; MS 86 Bloomsburg Univ of PA

Middleton, Mrs Susan H 3238 Park Place, Evanston, IL 60201, (312) 869-3619, BS 73 Northwestern Univ; MA 74 Northwestern Univ; SLP, Sch Dist 73, **SLP**

Middleton, Mrs Suzanne S 113 Sparrow Way, Beaumont, TX 77707, (409) 832-4588, BS 75 Lamar Univ; MS 78 Lamar Univ; **SLP**

Middleton, Tammy Louise 1061 Marcia S W, Wyoming, MI 49509, (616) 530-1608, BS 84 Central MI Univ; MA 85 Central MI Univ; **SLP**

Midgette, Laurie L 337 Windsor Park Lane, Havertown, PA 19083, (215) 247-9700, BS 73 Univ of MD - College Park; MA 74 Univ of MD - College Park; Aud, PA Sch for the Deaf, **A**

Midkiff-Borunda, Shelley S 19 Agassiz Street #24, Cambridge, MA 02140, **SLP**

Miech, Mrs Maureen Rose 217 Erbes Road #210, Thousand Oaks, CA 91362, (805) 494-0929, MA 88 Univ of CA - Santa Barbara

Mieczkowski, Susan Lynn 1025 Reynolds Road #R-1, Johnson City, NY 13790, (607) 798-7117, BS 85 SUNY - Coll at Geneseo; MA 87 SUNY - Center at Buffalo; **SLP**

Miehl, Frances Margaret Rd #1 Box 116, Springboro, PA 16435, BS 70 Villa Maria Coll; MA 86 Edinboro Univ of PA; 86–Sp-Lang Path, S G Rehab Agency Inc

Miele, Ellen Bronson 60 Creekview Drive, Rochester, NY 14624, (716) 244-3510, BS 82 SUNY - Coll at Geneseo; MS 83 Syracuse Univ; Aud, Rochester Otol Group, **A**

Mielke, Mrs Debra Nault 119 Northbreeze, Appleton, WI 54911, (414) 233-2372, BA 81 Univ of WI - Eau Claire; MS 83 UT St Univ; 87–Aud, CESA #6, **A**

Mielke, Mrs Martha Mary 128 Northview Avenue, Findlay, OH 45840, (419) 423-5732, BS 80 Northern MI Univ; MA 84 Northern MI Univ; Sp-Lang Path, **SLP**

Mielnik, Mrs Lynn K P O Box 712, Pataskala, OH 43062, (614) 461-2420, BS 80 Miami Univ - Oxford; MS 81 Miami Univ - Oxford; 88–Sp-Lang Path, Children's Hosp, **SLP**

Mient, Mrs Mary G Allegheny Intermediate Unit, 200 Commerce Court, Pittsburgh, PA 15219, (412) 394-5823, BS 69 Indiana Univ of PA; MA 73 Univ of Pittsburgh - Pittsburgh; Instruct Adv-Sp/Lang, Allegheny Intermediate Unit, **SLP**

Miers, Deanne Kaye Village Of Pine Run, 56-E, Blackwood, NJ 08012, (215) 237-4388, BA 85 Wichita St Univ; MA 87 Wichita St Univ; 88–Aud, Mercy Catholic Med Ctr-Fitzgerald

Miers-Lazas, Mrs Debby Rae 136 West Silver Street, Westfield, MA 01085, (312) 392-2250, BS 83 0681; MS 85 0681; Aud, NW Sp & Hrng Ctr, **A**

Mieszkowski, Mrs Gail B 220 Emerson Avenue, Pittsburgh, PA 15215, (412) 782-3361, BA 67 Univ of OR; MS 70 CO St Univ; Personal Care Home Manager, Outlook Menegement Co, **SLP**

Migaki, Karen Jo 1836 North Stapley #183, Mesa, AZ 85203, (602) 263-7140, BS 79 Bradley Univ; MA 81 Univ of IL - Urbana; 87–Aud, St Joseph's Med Ctr, **A**

Migdel, Mrs Meryl Marla Placid Pond Lane, Monroe, NY 10950, (914) 782-6557, BA 76 CUNY - Brooklyn Coll; MS 80 CUNY - Brooklyn Coll; Sp-Lang Path, Private Practice, **SLP ACE**

Migliore, Lawrence Edward 71-A North Street, Madison, NJ 07940-1104, (201) 765-9458, BA 84 Montclair St Coll; MA 87 Montclair St Coll

Miguel, Dr Shirley A 3353 Rolling Hills, Flower Mound, TX 75028, (214) 221-9570, BA 72 CA St Univ - Fresno; MA 73 CA St Univ - Fresno; PH 88 (Special Education Early Childhood) Univ of TX - Austin; Sp-Lang Path, Comprehensive Testing/Therapy Ctr, **SLP**

Mihalker-Scrudato, Mrs Diane 622 Cumberland Street, Westfield, NJ 07090, (201) 232-8423, BS 77 Syracuse Univ; MS 78 Columbia Univ Teachers Coll; Sp-Lang Path, Overlook Hosp, **SLP**

Mihalo, Mrs Deborah A 1421 Lake Avenue, Whiting, IN 46394, (219) 659-8066, BS 75 Purdue Univ - West Lafayette; MA 78 Ball St Univ; Sp/Lang Path, Hammond Pub Sch, **SLP**

Mihaly-Waldman, Janet Sue 1514 Laguna Court, Wheeling, IL 60090, (312) 577-9265, BS 81 IL St Univ - Normal; MS 83 IL St Univ - Normal; Sp-Lang Path, Woodland Dist So, **SLP**

Mika, Mrs Ann Marie 1272 Claire Court, Carol Stream, IL 60188, (312) 420-1610, BS 85 Univ of IL - Urbana; MA 87 Northwestern Univ; 87–Sp-Lang Path, Lombard Sch Dist #44, **SLP**

Mikaelian, Dr Diran O Jefferson Hospital, 1025 Walnut, Philadelphia, PA 19107, BS 50; MD 54 (NS); Otolaryngologist & Prof, Thomas Jefferson U Hosp

Mikami, Charlene Mieko Audiology 126, Veterans Administration Medical Center, 5901 East Seventh Street, Long Beach, CA 90822, (213) 494-5414, BA 82 CA St Univ - Los Angeles; MA 83 CA St Univ - Los Angeles; 87–Research Asst, VA Med Ctr/Univ of Cal-Irvine, **A**

Mikami, Judith Hinds 33 Smith Garrison Road, Newmarket, NH 03857, (603) 883-5521, BS 81 Northeastern Univ; MA 83 Univ of Denver; Sp-Lang Path, Nashua Memorial Hosp, **SLP**

Mikami, Karen Akemi 4369 South Quebec #6310, Denver, CO 80237, (303) 790-9010, BS 80 Univ of HI - Manoa; MA 83 Univ of KS; Aud, Cochlear Corp, **A**

Mikesell, Stephanie L 1825 Van Hise Avenue, Madison, WI 53705, (608) 233-2079, BA 75 Univ of FL; MS 81 East TN St Univ; 87–Rehab Svcs Mgr, MARC-Dev Ctrs Corp, **SLP**

Mikiewicz, Patricia Treacy 41 Broad Avenue, Paramus, NJ 07652, (201) 262-7311, MS 85 William Paterson Coll; 87–Sp-Lang Path, Communication Disorders Center, **SLP**

Mikita, Stephen F Riverside Regional Medical Center, Speech Pathology & Audiology, 500 J Clyde Morris Boulevard, Newport News, VA 23601, (804) 599-2094, BS 69 Southern IL Univ -Carbondale; MS 70 Southern IL Univ -Carbondale; Dir-Sp & Hrng, Riverside Hosp, **SLP**

Mikkelsen, Debra Kay 4520 East Baseline #1032, Phoenix, AZ 85044, (602) 431-0467, BS 83 ND St Univ; MS 86 Minot St Univ; 88–Sp-Lang Path, Tempe Elem Sch Dist #3, **SLP**

Mikkelsen, Marie E Psc Box 2159, APO New York, NY 09179-5367, MA 76 San Diego St Univ; Ch/Aud Sect, USAF, **A ACE**

Miklas, Mary Kathleen 2827 South 32nd Street, Omaha, NE 68105, (402) 291-3595, MS 85 Univ of NE - Omaha; 85–Sp-Lang Path, Bellevue Public Schools, **SLP**

Mikol, Mrs Page Norris 318 Grove Park Avenue, Winston-Salem, NC 27103, (919) 723-2360, BS 84 Western Carolina Univ; MA 85 Western Carolina Univ

Mikola, Judy Marie 1517 West 14th Street #5, Wilmington, DE 19806, (302) 888-1534, BS 82 MI St Univ; MS 84 MI St Univ; Sp-Lang Path, Med Ctr of DE, **SLP**

Mikolaski, Martha Ann 125 North Bond, Saginaw, MI 48602, (517) 790-0130, BA 85 Univ of MI - Ann Arbor; MS 87 Gallaudet Coll; 87–Aud, Dr Nicholas P Redfield MD, **A**

Mikon, Deena 25409 Sherwood, Huntington Woods, MI 48020, **SLP**

Mikrot, Dee Ann Lynn 2380 Mikrot Road, Willow River, MN 55795-9719, (715) 394-2771, BS 85 Saint Cloud St Univ; MA 86 Univ of MN - Duluth

Mikrut, Terry Agnes 14305 Palmer Avenue, Posen, IL 60469, (312) 519-0666, BS 81 Northern IL Univ - De Kalb; MA 84 Northern IL Univ - De Kalb; **A**

Miks, Mrs Marilyn G 2909 Morning Dew Street, Las Vegas, NV 89117, (702) 364-8321, BS 63 Marquette Univ; MS 84 George Washington Univ; Tchr, Clark Co Sch Dist, **SLP**

Miksak, Joseph A 10 Graystone Terrace, San Francisco, CA 94114, (415) 626-0790, BA 38 Univ of IL - Urbana; MA 50 Columbia Univ Teachers Coll; PH 59 (NS) Stanford Univ; **SLP LM**

Mikulich, Danielle M 335 Via Rosario, Fremont, CA 94539, (415) 428-3344, BA 76 Holy Names Coll; MA 78 CA St Univ - Sacramento; Aud, Chldn's Hosp of Oakland, **A**

Mikus, Mrs Linda D 110 Larose Drive, St Albert, AB, Canada T8N 2R5, (403) 471-7934, BA 69 Univ of MT; MA 71 Univ of MT; Superv SLP, Glenrose Rehab Hosp, **SLP**

Milane, Lynne A 1009 So Miller Street #203, Lakewood, CO 80226, (303) 986-1555, BA 74 Univ of IA; MA 75 Univ of Northern IA; Sp-Lang Path, Jefferson Co PS, **SLP**

Milbrandt, Mrs Mariette 5121 Pleasant View, Chubbuck, ID 83202, (208) 237-2503, BA 72 UT St Univ; MS 74 UT St Univ; SLP, Pocatello Sch Dist #25, **SLP**

Milburn, Dr Braxton 1929 Plymouth Road #2025, Ann Arbor, MI 48105, (313) 769-7100, BS 54 Univ of TX - Austin; MA 56 Univ of TX - Austin; PH 63 (NS) Univ of OK Medical Center; Ch Aud & Sp-Lang Path Services, VA Med Cen, **A**

Milburn, Mrs Lana Jo 230 Aspen Way, Noblesville, IN 46060, (317) 457-8273, BS 77 Purdue Univ - West Lafayette; MA 78 Ball St Univ; Coordinator of Speech & Audio, Bona Vista Prog Inc, **SLP**

Milburn, Mrs Rosemary L 28152 Bluebell Drive, Laguna Niguel, CA 92677, (714) 831-9035, BA 73 Univ of UT; MS 74 Univ of UT; **SLP**

Milch, Karole K 182 East 95th Street, New York, NY 10128, (212) 682-7500, BA 64 George Washington Univ; MA 72 NY Univ; **SLP**

Milchen, Mrs Selma B 13 Hewitt Drive, RR 1 Box 331, North Bennington, VT 05257, (802) 442-4373, BS 52 Boston Univ; ME 64 Framingham St Coll; MS 81 Worcester St Coll; 81–Sp-Lang Path, Swn VT Superv Un, **SLP**

Milenki, Kathy Helen 1-F Bluebonnet Hills, Brenham, TX 77833, (409) 836-8130, BS 84 Lamar Univ; MS 86 Lamar Univ; **SLP**

Mileris, Ramona 152 Kensington Avenue South, Hamilton, ON, Canada L8M 3H5, (416) 522-4941, MA Western MI Univ; Head Sp-Lang Path, St Joseph's Hospital, **SLP**

Miles, Amy Fulton 12821 East Shelby Lane, Brandywine, MD 20613, (813) 343-2180, BS 83 Northeast MO St Univ; MA 84 Northeast MO St Univ; **SLP**

Miles, Elizabeth 32 Catherine Road, Reading, MA 01867, (617) 391-1686, BS Salem St Coll; ME 51 Boston Univ; Dir of Chap I, Medford School Department, **SLP**

Miles, Mrs Janet A 28442 El SHR, Laguna Niguel, CA 92677-4407, (707) 448-1253, BA 73 CA St Univ - Long Beach; MA 75 CA St Univ - Long Beach; **SLP**

Miles, John C 155 Kipling, Ben Lomond, CA 95005, (408) 354-1316, BA 77 Humboldt St Univ; MS 80 San Francisco St Univ; Audiologist, Center for Hearing Health Inc, **A**

Miles, Linda F B 816 Watt Drive, Tallahassee, FL 32303-4627, (904) 878-3743, MS; **SLP**

Miles, Marcia C 208 Park Place, Fort Collins, CO 80525, BS 65 SUNY - Coll at Geneseo; MA 69 Univ of NM; 86–Proj Coord, Univ of Northern Colo, **SLP**

Miles, Mrs Mary Suzanne 3402 South 121st Street, Omaha, NE 68144, (712) 366-0571, BS 79 Univ of NE - Omaha; MS 82 Univ of NE - Lincoln; Sp-Lang Path, Iowa School for the Deaf, **SLP**

Miles-Fahs, Margaret Ellen 183 Treadwell Road, Tonawanda, NY 14150, (716) 837-2441, BS 83 SUNY - Coll at Fredonia; MA 84 Kent St Univ; 88–Sp-Lang Path, Lang Dev Prog of W NY, **SLP**

Mileur, Mari C 1007 West Stokes Street, Ahoskie, NC 27910, (919) 332-8224, BS 82 East Carolina Univ; ME 85 Univ of NC - Greensboro; Sp-Lang Path, Gates Co PS Sys, **SLP**

Milewski, Diane Marie 20 Washington Street #77, Methuen, MA 01844-0001, (617) 975-5476, MA 85 Univ of MA - Amherst; Sp-Lang Path, Hogan Regional Ctr, **SLP**

Milgrom, Patricia Mondro 2309 27th Street, Santa Monica, CA 90405, (213) 450-5491, BS 80 Eastern MI Univ; MA 81 Eastern MI Univ; Sp-Lang Path, **SLP**

Milhauser, Lynn 15 North Clover Drive, Great Neck, NY 11021, (516) 829-8611, BA 71 Univ of MD - College Park; MA 72 Univ of MD - College Park; SLP, Great Neck Pub Sch, **SLP**

Milianti, Dr Franklin J 3 North 445 Crown Road, Elmhurst, IL 60126, (312) 343-7200, PH 71 (Sp Path) Univ of OK - OK City; 71–Chief Sp-Lang Path/Aud, Hines VA Hosp, **SLP**

Miliman, Susan 8207 Bendon Road, Baltimore, MD 21208, **SLP**

Milisen, Dr Robert L 4180 Old State Road #37-N, Bloomington, IN 47401, (812) 336-6092, MA 33 Univ of IA; PH 37 (NS) Univ of IA; **SLP F H LM**

Militana, Mrs Norma K S 430 C Dodson Lane, Russellville, KY 42276, (502) 726-8482, BA 72 Univ of FL; ME 74 Univ of FL; **SLP**

Mill, Dr Gerald P Audiology & Hrng Aid Serv Inc, 1646 South Woodruff, Idaho Falls, ID 83404, (208) 529-1514, BA 64 Univ of OR; MS 69 Univ of OR; PH 72 (Aud) Univ of UT; Aud, Aud & Hrng Aid Servs Inc, **A**

Millar, Stewart Wilson 16357 Redington Drive, Redington Beach, FL 33708, (813) 253-5829, BA 53 Case Western Reserve Univ; MA 54 Case Western Reserve Univ; Sp-Lang Path, Hillsborough Co Hosp Tampa Gen, **SLP A**

Millard, Robert T 1420 Hollywood Drive, Lancaster, PA 17601, (717) 394-3334, BS 49 Bloomsburg Univ of PA; MA 50 Univ of IA; 50–Sp-Lang Path, Hk Cooper Cl, **SLP LM**

Millard, Mrs Rosemarie Lynn 4505 Live Oak Boulevard, Fort Wayne, IN 46804, (219) 425-3053, BS 81 Purdue Univ - West Lafayette; MA 83 Univ of Northern CO; 83–Sp-Lang Path, St Joseph Med Ctr, **SLP**

Millard, Sidney Ann 14118 Berwyn, Redford, MI 48239, (313) 341-1353, BS 78 Wayne St Univ; MA 79 Western MI Univ; Sp-Lang Path, Detroit Hrng & Sp Cen, **SLP**

Millay, Karyl Sue 7760 Boteler Road, Philpot, KY 42366, (502) 686-1100, **SLP**

Millay, Kathleen K 318 North Rosemont, Dallas, TX 75208, (214) 942-7654, BA 68 Wittenberg Univ; MA 69 MI St Univ; PH 84 (NS) Univ of TX - Dallas; Asst Instr, Callier Cen U Tx-Dallas, **SLP A**

Milledge, Ruth A The Methodist Hospital, 6501 Sannin Street, Suite #Na 200, Houston, TX 77030, (713) 790-5916, BA 68 TX Christian Univ; MA 71 Western MI Univ; SLP, The Methodist Hosp, **SLP**

Milleman, Mrs Vicky B 5924 Northern Dancer Drive, Macon, GA 31210, (912) 474-7441, BS 75 FL St Univ; MS 76 FL St Univ; Sp-Lang Path, Private Practice, **SLP**

Miller, A Elizabeth 4071 Glenwood Avenue #412, Youngstown, OH 44512, (216) 782-1813, BA 28; MA 37 Columbia Univ Teachers Coll; **SLP LM**

Miller, Dr Alfred L 5801 West Cascade Drive, Franklin, WI 53132, PH 61 (NS) Univ of WI - Madison; Audiologist, Kenosa Memorial Hospital, **A**

Miller, Mrs Andrea Jeanne 38 Coolidge Lane, East Quogue, NY 11942, (516) 653-4359, MA 81 Hofstra Univ; Sp-Lang Path, BOCES 1 Suffolk, **SLP**

Miller, Andrea Sue 322 East Rangely Avenue, P O Box 292, Rangely, CO 81648, (303) 675-2267, BS 82 Univ of IL - Urbana; MS 83 Univ of IL - Urbana; Sp-Lang Path, Rio Blanco Co Bocs, **SLP**

Miller, Mrs Ann Rochelle 1723 Country Club Drive, Cherry Hill, NJ 08003, (609) 429-0010, **SLP**

Miller, Anne H 641 Avondale Road, Philadelphia, PA 19118, **SLP**

Miller, Sr Annette Marie OLL Mission, Box 7, Porcupine, SD 57772, (605) 867-5568, BS 83 Univ of NE - Omaha; MS 84 Univ of NE - Omaha; Sp-Lang Path, Holy Rosary Mission, **SLP**

Miller, Mrs Antoinette Marie 1716 #A Front Street, Alhambra, CA 91803, (213) 681-4641, BA 83 CA St Univ - Long Beach; MA 84 CA St Univ - Los Angeles; Aud, Glendale Adventist Med Ctr, **A**

Miller, Barbara B 1871 Maude, Chicago, IL 60614, (312) 248-1676, BS 76 Miami Univ - Oxford; MS 77 Univ of MI - Ann Arbor; Owner, Allied Hlth Professionals, **SLP**

Miller, Mrs Barbara Kamm 7 Glenwood Circle, East Windsor, NJ 08520, (609) 448-3440, BA 74 CUNY - City College; MA 81 Trenton St Coll; Sp-Lang Path, Private Practice, **SLP**

Miller, Mrs Barbara R 20116 Valley Mill Road, Freeland, MD 21053, BA 72 Towson St Univ; MS 73 OH Univ - Athens; 88–Sp-Lang Path, Private Practice, **SLP**

Miller, Mrs Bethany Wilson 9220-Q Traders Crossing, Laurel, MD 20707, (301) 725-2873, MA 88 Univ of MD - College Park; 88–Sp-Lang Path, MIEMSS

Miller, Mrs Beverly L 1 Breton Drive, Pine Brook, NJ 07058, (201) 575-9240, BA 68 Montclair St Coll; MA 69 Columbia Univ Teachers Coll; Sp/Lang Path, Kinnelon Bd of Ed, **SLP**

Miller, Beverly Rycz Rd 3, Emlenton, PA 16373, BS 79 Clarion Univ of PA; ME 80 Clarion Univ of PA; SLP, Clarion Manor Intermediate #6, **SLP**

Miller, Bonnie G 1060 Middle Road, East Greenwich, RI 02818, **SLP**

Miller, Burnice D 3218 Tate Road, Augusta, GA 30906, **SLP**

Miller, Candace Johnson 1704 S Owasso Avenue, Tulsa, OK 74120, (918) 587-1978

Miller, MS3C Carole Ann 6700 Northwest 25 Terrace, Fort Lauderdale, FL 33309, (305) 973-3733, MS 86 Nova Univ; **SLP**

Miller, Carole S 220 East Walton Place, Chicago, IL 60611, **SLP**

Miller, Catherine Ann 755 West Big Beaver, Suite 404, Troy, MI 48084, (313) 362-4299, BS 86 IN St Univ - Terre Haute; MA 87 MI St Univ; 88–Sp-Lang Path, Medi-Sp Svc

Miller, Mrs Catherine S 1209 East Wausau Avenue, Wausau, WI 54401, BS 84 Univ of WI - Milwaukee; MS 86 Univ of WI - Milwaukee; 88–Sp-Lang Path, Merrill PS, **SLP**

Miller, Cecilia C 200 North 45th Street, Belleville, IL 62223, (618) 234-1553, BS 71 Saint Louis Univ; MA 72 Saint Louis Univ; SLP, Belleville Area Spec Ed Dist, **SLP**

Miller, Charlene W 825 Richard Street #E, Aurora, IL 60506, (312) 844-5550, BA 67 Univ of Northern IA; SLP, East Aurora School Dist 131, **SLP**

Miller, Dr Charles James 2121 Bonsallo Avenue, Los Angeles, CA 90007, (213) 749-0588, BA 51 Univ of Southern CA; MA 52 Univ of Southern CA; PH 57 (Sp) Univ of Southern CA; Sp-Lang Path, Private Practice, **SLP LM**

Miller, Mrs Cheryl Harding 147 Laurelwood Drive, Hopedale, MA 01747, (508) 856-2398, BA 81 Univ of Akron; MA 83 OH Univ - Athens; 87–Sp-Lang Path, Univ of Massachusetts Med Ctr, **SLP**

Miller, Cheryl J 13301 Waterside Circle, Germantown, MD 20874-3734, (301) 972-4674, BS 76 Univ of MD - College Park; MS 79 WV Univ; Sp-Lang Path, Montgomery Co Pub Sch, **SLP**

Miller, Cheryl U 1073 Karen Way, Mountain View, CA 94040, (408) 867-2200, BA 75 Univ of VT; MA 77 Northwestern Univ; Sp-Lang Path, Miller Sp Path Mission Coll, **SLP**

Miller, Mrs Cindy B 1 Meadowview Terrace, Fair Lawn, NJ 07410, (201) 797-4849, BA 79 Rutgers St Univ -N Brunswick; MS 81 Emory Univ; Sp-Lang Path, **SLP**

Miller, Claire Kane 3317 Lambert Place, Cincinnati, OH 45208, (513) 559-4341, BS 80 Miami Univ - Oxford; MS 81 Miami Univ - Oxford; Sp-Lang Path, Childrens Hospital Medical Ctr, **SLP**

Miller, Claudia F 18325 Gulf Boulevard #502, Redington Shores, FL 33708, (813) 323-4100, MS 77 Univ of South FL; Sp-Lang Path, Pinellas Co Sch Bd, **SLP**

Miller, Connie Jean 8604 East Long Place, Englewood, CO 80112-2714, (303) 796-7881, BA 78 SD St Univ; MS 83 Univ of NE - Omaha; 86–Sp-Lang Path, Cherry Creek Sch Dist, **SLP**

Miller, Mrs Cynthia Cox 9508 Fenwin Drive, Grand Blanc, MI 48439, (517) 337-2042, BA 81 MI St Univ; MA 82 Central MI Univ; Sp-Lang Path, Genesee Inter Sch Dist, **SLP**

Miller, Cynthia Lee 1544 Bentley Circle, Bel Air, MD 21014, (301) 642-2144, **SLP**

Miller, Cynthia Stewart 48 Apache Lane, Huntley, IL 60142, (312) 438-6319, **SLP**

Miller, Deborah Ann 2402 17th Street South, Apartment 305, Fargo, ND 58103, (701) 280-4493, BS 83 Univ of MN - Minneap-St Paul; MA 80 Univ of MN - Minneap-St Paul; 85–Coord Sp-Lang Path Svcs, Dakota Med Ctr, **SLP ACE**

Miller, Deborah S 926 Parcher Street, Wausau, WI 54401, (715) 842-1636, BS 71 Eastern NM Univ; MS 72 Univ of WI - Stevens Point; Superv Commun Dis Dept, N Central Hlth Care Facilities, **SLP**

Miller, Mrs Deborah W Akron ENT Assoc Inc, 452 East Market Street, Akron, OH 44304, (216) 762-8959, BA 75 Univ of Akron; MA 77 Univ of Akron; Aud, Private Practice, **A**

Miller, Debra L 722 Cherry, Missoula, MT 59802, (406) 777-5679, BA 77 Univ of MT; MA 83 Univ of MT; Clinician, Stevensville Schools, **SLP**

Miller, Denise Renee 942 East Park Avenue #2, Ottumwa, IA 52501, (515) 682-5098, BA 85 Univ of Northern CO; MA 86 Univ of Northern CO; Aud, Easter Seals, **A**

Miller, Diana L Dept Of Speech Pathology, Erlanger Hospital, 975 East 3rd Street, Chattanooga, TN 37403, (615) 778-7916, BS 78 Univ of TN - Knoxville; MA 79 Univ of TN - Knoxville; 87–Sp-Lang Path, Erlanger Hosp, **SLP**

Miller, Mrs Diane O 38 South Henry Street, Franklin, IN 46131, MS 68 IN Univ - Bloomington; SLP, Bartholomew County School Corp, **SLP**

Miller, Donna P O Box 1118, Buena Vista, CO 81211, (719) 395-6517, BA 75 Univ of Northern CO; MA 77 Univ of Northern CO; 84–Sp-Lang Path, Canon City Co, **SLP**

Miller, Doris Jane 1692 Franquette Drive, Yuba City, CA 95991, (916) 741-6112, BA 83 CA St Univ - Chico; MA 85 CA St Univ - Chico; 85–Sp-Lang Path, Yuba County Ofc of Educ, **SLP**

Miller, Mrs Dorothy S Route 3 Box 56, Oklawaha, FL 32679, (914) 471-9226, BA 63 SUNY - Center at Albany; MA 69 SUNY - Center at Albany; Sp/Lang Path, Wassaic Dev Cen, **SLP**

Miller, Earl Lewis P O Box 2142, Concord, CA 94521, (415) 432-3584, BA 47 San Jose St Univ; MA 48 Northwestern Univ; Sp-Lang Path, Pittsburg USD, **SLP A LM**

Miller, Eddie Jack 2310 44th Street N W, Washington, DC 20007, (202) 337-8202, BA 62 East TN St Univ; BA 62 East TN St Univ; MA 63 Univ of TN - Knoxville; **A**

Miller, Mrs Elizabeth G 2311 Brisbane Street, Apt 51, Clearwater, FL 34623, (813) 791-4066, BA 53 Univ of IL - Urbana; MS 66 Univ of IL - Urbana; 88–Sp-Lang Path, Pinellas County Sch Bd, **SLP ACE**

Miller, Elizabeth Lonam 714 Owens Street, Rockville, MD 20850, (301) 424-5722, BA 80 Loyola Coll; MS 81 Loyola Coll; Sp/Lang Path, Private Practice, **SLP**

Miller, Ellen R 137 Herbert Road, Arlington, MA 02174, (617) 641-1028, MS; **SLP**

Miller, Ellen S 15340 Falconbridge Terrace, Gaithersburg, MD 20878, (301) 977-6915, **SLP**

Miller, Eric G 3806 Johns Street, Madison, WI 53714, (608) 271-3333, BS 76 SUNY - Coll at Buffalo; MA 78 Univ of WA; Technical Liason, Nicolet Dionostics, **A**

Miller, Erik G 1451 West Water Street, Elmira, NY 14905, **SLP**

Miller, Erin Louise 7477 Huntington Dr #3, Youngstown, OH 44512, (216) 726-8155, BS 83 Clarion Univ of PA; MA 86 Kent St Univ; Aud, Neuro Com Services, **A**

Miller, Esther F Maryland Rehabilitation Center, 2301 Argonne Drive, Baltimore, MD 21218, (301) 554-3170, BA 69 Montclair St Coll; MS 71 Gallaudet Coll; 73–Chief Hrng/Sp Dept, Maryland Rehab Cen, **A**

Miller, Mrs Gabriella 116 Cedar Ridge Drive #26, Monroeville, PA 15146, (412) 372-3599, MA 87 Univ of Pittsburgh - Pittsburgh; 88–Sp-Lang Path, Allegheny Inter Unit, **SLP**

Miller, Gabrielle Judith 33 Kimlo Road, Wellesley, MA 02181, (508) 588-0230, BA 76 Case Western Reserve Univ; OB 82 Boston Conservatory of Music; MS 85 Boston Univ; 88–Sp-Lang Path, Avon PS, **SLP**

Miller, Mrs Gail Kingfisher County Guidance Center, 124 East Sheridan, Kingfisher, OK 73750, (405) 375-5763, BA 75 Univ of OK - Norman; MS 78 Univ of OK Medical Center; 78–Sp-Lang Path, Oklahoma State Dept of Health, **SLP**

Miller, Dr George H 3909 North Murray Avenue, Shorewood, WI 53211, (414) 962-3557, BS 49 Syracuse Univ; MA 51 Syracuse Univ; PH 62 (NS) Univ of WI - Madison; College Super, College of St Rose, **SLP**

Miller, Geraldine 327 Oak Meadow Drive, Los Gatos, CA 95030, BA 74 San Jose St Univ; MA 76 San Jose St Univ; Dispensing Aud, Private Practice, **A**

Miller, Gerard A 1705 Lombard Street, Philadelphia, PA 19146, BS 74 Univ of VA - Charlottesville; ME 76 Univ of VA - Charlottesville; Aud Consult, Private Practice, **A**

Miller, Dr Glenn D, Jr Dept Communication Disorders, Bloomsburg University, Bloomsburg, PA 17815, (717) 389-4436, BS 65 Indiana Univ of PA; MA 70 Temple Univ; PH 81 (NS) Temple Univ; 70–Prof of Aud, Bloomsburg U, **A**

Miller, Harriet R Rd 3 Box 398, Kingston, NY 12401, (914) 687-7631, BA 70 CUNY - Queens Coll; MS 75 SUNY - Center at Albany; Sp/Lang Path, Rondout Vy Cn Sch, **SLP**

Miller, Harriett Leggett 1710 West 9th Street, Anderson, IN 46016-2613, (317) 643-9987, MA 79 Ball St Univ; BS 64 Ball St Univ; SLP, New Castle St Dev Cen, **SLP**

Miller, Heather Neary 406 Riverdale Street, Mancelona, MI 49659, BA 71 Alma Coll; MA 86 Univ of WI - Oshkosh; 86–Sp-Lang Path, Traverse Bay Area Intermed Sch Dist, **SLP**

Miller, Mrs Irene W 1060 Sylvan Point Drive, Mount Dora, FL 32757, (904) 383-2904, BA 72 Univ of FL; ME 73 Univ of FL; Sp-Lang Path, Sch Bd of Lake Co, **SLP ACE**

Miller, J Michael 3317 Lambert Place, Cincinnati, OH 45208, (513) 853-5071, BS 81 Univ of Cincinnati; MA 83 Univ of Cincinnati; Sp-Lang Path, Providence Hospital, **SLP**

Miller, James R Route 1, 215 Vine Arbor Drive, Hickory, NC 28601, (704) 254-0754, OB 66 Memphis St Univ; MA 74 Memphis St Univ; Audiologist, Blue Ridge Hearing Aid Service, **A**

Miller, Jamie A 1430 Hood Avenue, Baton Rouge, LA 70808, (504) 338-9032, MA 87 LA St Univ - Baton Rouge; 88–Sp-Lang Path, Ochsner Clinic of Baton Rouge

Miller, Mrs Jan K Hearing & Speech Assoc Inc, 120 West Park Avenue, Long Beach, NY 11561, (516) 432-1800, BA 69 Brandeis Univ; MA 71 Columbia Univ Teachers Coll; Exec Dir, Hearing & Speech Assoc Inc, **A**

Miller, Jane E 936 Hamilton Street #2, Lockport, IL 60441-3424, BS 85 Northern IL Univ - De Kalb; MA 86 Northern IL Univ - De Kalb; 88–Sp-Lang Path, SPEED Dev Ctr, **SLP**

Miller, Jane P 7799 Owens Drive, Newburgh, IN 47630, (812) 649-2626, BA 66 Baker Univ; BS 78 Brescia Coll; MA 79 Western KY Univ; Sp-Lang Path, S Spencer Schs, **SLP**

Miller, Janet E 3208 Haywood Avenue, Chattanooga, TN 37415, (615) 698-8528, BS 76 James Madison Univ; MA 79 OH Univ - Athens; 87–Sp-Lang Path, Signal Center, **SLP**

Miller, Mrs Janice E 10441 Waterfowl Terrace, Columbia, MD 21044, (301) 997-2137, BA 74 WV Univ; BS 77 WV Univ; MS 80 WV Univ; Sp-Lang Path, Private Practice, **SLP**

Miller, Dr Janice Gritti 5526 145th Place S W, Edmonds, WA 98020, (206) 364-0500, BS 73 Univ of MN - Minneap-St Paul; MS 75 Saint Cloud St Univ; PH 78 (NS) Univ of OR; Clinical Manager, NW Hospital Sp-Hrng Center, **SLP**

Miller, Jean Ellen 7920 San Felipe Blvd #1707, Austin, TX 78729-7903, (512) 335-5304, BS 85 Southwest TX St Univ; MS 87 Southwest TX St Univ; 87–Sp-Lang Path, InSpeech Inc, **SLP**

Miller, Mrs Jean M A 3433 Fleetwood Drive, Lexington, KY 40502, (606) 281-0194, BS 66 Nazareth Coll of Rochester; MS 68 SUNY - Coll at Geneseo; 86–Sp-Lang Path, Fayette County Schs, **SLP ACE**

Miller, Mrs Jeannine Antoinnett 402 East Suffolk Drive, Tucson, AZ 85704, (602) 297-7416, BS 79 Univ of AZ; SLP, Southwest Human Dev, **SLP**

Miller, Jennie L 5140 N E 34th, Portland, OR 97211, (503) 281-1496, BS 79 Portland St Univ; MS 81 Portland St Univ; **SLP**

Miller, Mrs Jennifer Stump 1140 Wasena Avenue, Roanoke, VA 24015, (703) 982-3691, BS 84 James Madison Univ; MS 85 James Madison Univ; Sp-Lang Path, Rehab Services of Roanoke Inc, **SLP**

Miller, Jill M E Box 461, Atlantic, IA 50022, (712) 243-1480, BS 72 Univ of NE - Lincoln; MA 73 Univ of NE - Lincoln; Sp-Lang Path, Loess Hills AEA #13, **SLP**

Miller, Joan 555 North Avenue #22-N, Fort Lee, NJ 07024, (201) 944-7595, **SLP**

Miller, Joan 4504 Cannes Lane, Olney, MD 20832

Miller, Mrs Joan Mostoller Route 1 Box 154, Lake City, IA 51449, (712) 792-3102, BS 66 Saint Cloud St Univ; MS 87 Saint Cloud St Univ; 88–Sp-Lang Path, Heartland AEA, **SLP**

Miller, Joan P 73-63 Bell Boulevard, Apartment 4-M Bayside, New York, NY 11364, (718) 776-8910, MA 88 NY Univ

Miller, Mrs Joan S 1314 Brighton, Urbana, IL 61801, (217) 359-7347, BA 53 Radcliffe Coll; MS 75 Univ of IL - Urbana; SLP, Champaign Commun Sch UT4, **SLP**

Miller, Dr Joanne L Department Of Psychology, 125 Nightingale Hall, Northeastern University, Boston, MA 02115, (617) 437-3076, PH 74 (NS) Univ of MN - Minneap-St Paul; Professor of Psychology, Northeastern University

Miller, John P 1327 5th Avenue North, Denison, IA 51442, (712) 263-4625, BA 72 Univ of SD - Vermillion; MA 73 Univ of SD - Vermillion; Sp/Lang Path, W Hills AEA, **SLP**

Miller, John W 17 East 34 #21-C, Kansas City, MO 64111, (816) 531-4777, BS 70 Southwest MO St Univ; MS 73 Murray St Univ; Aud, Old Westport Medical Assn, **A**

Miller, Jon F 4414 Keating Terrace, Madison, WI 53711, (608) 265-5807, BA 64 San Diego St Univ; MS 66 Univ of Redlands; PH 69 (NS) Univ of WI - Madison; Professor, U of WI Madison Dep Com Dis, **SLP**

Miller, Jonathan P 9917 N E Harrison Drive, Kansas City, MO 64155, (913) 649-4400, BA 73 Univ of TX - Arlington; MS 80 Univ of TX - Dallas; Off Mgr, Hrng Aid Disp, **A**

Miller, Joseph William 6951 Warner Avenue #171, Huntington Beach, CA 92647, (714) 848-4375, MA 79 KS St Univ; Sp-Lang Path, Private Practice, **SLP**

Miller, Mrs Josephine Schulze Box 1363 26 Trw, APO New York, NY 09860-5362, 06332-43107, BS 85 MS Univ for Women; MS 87 Southwest TX St Univ; **SLP**

Miller, Judith A 811-B Bong Boulevard, Duluth, MN 55811, (218) 727-5083, BS 73 Miami Univ - Oxford; MA 75 Ball St Univ; OM 83 Univ of Notre Dame; Dir of Physical Med, Polinsky Med Rehab Cen, **SLP**

Miller, Judith Ann 5650 Rosemary Place, New Orleans, LA 70124, (504) 486-3091, BS 81 Saint Mary's Dominican Coll; ME 85 Southeastern LA Univ; **SLP**

Miller, Judith C 3209 Burning Tree Drive, Hoover, AL 35226, (205) 665-6720, BS 59 CA Univ of PA; MA 61 Univ of IA; Asst Prof, U of Montevallo, **SLP**

Miller, Mrs Judy Lynne P O Box 31, Jennerstown, PA 15547, (215) 631-9300, BS 83 Indiana Univ of PA; MS 84 WV Univ; Sp-Lang Path, InSpeech Inc, **SLP A**

Miller, Julia Ann 303 South Prairie Street, Chippewa Falls, WI 54729, (715) 237-2202, BA 81 Univ of WI - Eau Claire; MS 82 Univ of WI - Eau Claire; Sp-Lang Path, New Auburn Pub Sch, **SLP**

Miller, Mrs Julie L 11529 Springhill Drive, Austin, TX 78753, (512) 834-1885, BS 78 Southwest TX St Univ; ME 79 Southwest TX St Univ; 88–Sp-Lang Path, Private Practice, **SLP**

Miller, Dr June B 6401 Ensley Lane, Shawnee Mission, KS 66208, (913) 362-2474, BS 40 Washington Univ; MA 48 Columbia Univ Teachers Coll; ED 58 (NS) Columbia Univ Teachers Coll; Prof Emerita, **A F LM**

Miller, Karan K 2590 Yarrow Court, Boulder, CO 80303, **SLP**

Miller, Karen Teresa 312-3999 Enemark Cres, Prince George, BC, Canada V2N 2X8, (306) 682-2482, OB 85 Minot St Univ; MS 86 Minot St Univ; **A**

Miller, Kathleen Grace 4171 Bloomington Avenue, Apartment 103, Arlington Height, IL 60004, (312) 392-6573, BS 83 IL St Univ - Normal; MS 86 IL St Univ - Normal; **SLP**

Miller, Kathryn A 3915 East Larkspur Drive, Phoenix, AZ 85032, BS 63 Univ of IA; MS 76 Univ of WI - Madison; Sp/Lang Path, Stoughton Pub Schools, **SLP**

Miller, Mrs Kathryn A 3915 East Larkspur Drive, Phoenix, AZ 85032, (602) 285-3605, BS 74 Marquette Univ; MS 75 Marquette Univ; 88–Sp-Lang Path, St Joseph Hosp, **SLP**

Miller, Mrs Kelly McFann 1110 South Cowen, Garrett, IN 46738, (219) 357-3237, MA 87 Univ of Houston - Univ Park; 88–Sp-Lang Path, Northeast Ind Spec Educ Coop, **SLP**

Miller, Keri Ann 4040 Orleans Lane North, Plymouth, MN 55441, (612) 879-2896, OB 82 Univ of MN - Duluth; MA 85 Univ of KS; 88–Sp-Lang Path, ELR Systems Inc, **SLP**

Miller, Mrs Kimberly Inez 303 N Grant, Fort Collins, CO 80521, (303) 221-0743, BS 81 CO St Univ; MS 84 CO St Univ; **A**

Miller, Mrs Kimberly Marie 10424 South Mayfield, Oak Lawn, IL 60453, (312) 423-3078, BA 82 Saint Xavier Coll; MS 84 Governors St Univ; Sp-Lang Path, Atwood Hieghts Sch Dist 125, **SLP**

Miller, Laura Blanco C-4 McIntosh Manor, Pocatello, ID 83209, (208) 236-3857, OB 83 Univ of IA; MA 86 Univ of IA; 87–Sp-Lang Path, Pocatello Regional Med Ctr, **SLP**

Miller, Laura Dean 5110 East Vernon Street, Long Beach, CA 90815-1950, (213) 861-1218, BA 68 Loyola Marymount Univ; OM 72 CA St Univ - Los Angeles; MA 82 (NS) CA St Univ - Los Angeles; Asst Prin, LA Co Office of Education, **A**

Miller, Mrs Laurie W 1731 Eagle Meadow, San Antonio, TX 78248, (512) 696-2211, BS 71 Saint Cloud St Univ; MA 75 Our Lady Lake Univ-San Anton; SLP, Northside ISD, **SLP**

Miller, Leigh Ann 1004 North Main Street, Apartment 3, Rockford, IL 61103, (815) 965-2848, BA 85 MI St Univ; MA 87 MI St Univ; **A**

Miller, Leonard G 911 Downey Lane, Monroe, LA 71201, (318) 323-4406, BA 72 Northeast LA Univ; MS 73 Minot St Univ; Sp-Lang Path, LA Trng I-Monroe, **SLP**

Miller, Mrs Lillie C F Rd 1, Box 1091, Mercer, PA 16137, (412) 662-4176, BS 76 Clarion Univ of PA; MA 79 Kent St Univ; Sp-Lang Path, Reynolds Sch Dist, **SLP**

Miller, Mrs Linda Boczany Rd #2 Box 4270, Bristol, VT 05443, (802) 879-7173, BA 69 Rutger's St Univ - Douglas Coll; MS 77 Univ of VT; 87–Sp-Lang Path, Essex Town Sch Dist

Miller, Mrs Linda O 8 Franklin Valley Circle, Reisterstown, MD 21136, (301) 833-4221, BS 70 Bloomsburg Univ of PA; MS 75 Loyola Coll; Supervising Sp-Lang Path, The Chimes Inc, **SLP**

Miller, Linda R 7 Woodland Road, Roslyn, NY 11576, (516) 365-7182, BA 70 CUNY - Queens Coll; MA 73 CUNY - Queens Coll; **SLP**

Miller, Linda S 1247 Clearview Drive, Ringgold, GA 30736, (404) 935-2240, ME 83 GA St Univ; Sp-Lang Path, Dalton Public Schools, **SLP**

Miller, Linda S 13317 Nokoni Drive, Poway, CA 92064, **SLP**

Miller, Lindsay N 105 Toll Drive, Southampton, PA 18966, (215) 322-8943, BA 72 CUNY - Lehman Coll; MA 74 Trenton St Coll; Sp-Lang Path, Bucks Assoc for Retarded Cit, **SLP**

Miller, Mrs Lisa C 15 Springwalk Court, Lancaster, PA 17601, (717) 898-9315, BA 79 Longwood Coll; MA 83 Montclair St Coll; Sp-Lang Path, Home Hlth Care Agen Lancaster, **SLP**

Miller, Lisa Marie 200 Lodge Drive #610, Lafayette, LA 70506, (318) 332-3388, BA 78 Univ of Southwestern LA; MS 83 Univ of Southwestern LA; **SLP**

Miller, Lisa Wigington 111 Blake Drive, Summerville, SC 29485, (803) 873-8460, BA 79 Univ of KS; MA 80 Univ of KS; **A**

Miller, Lloyd 5048 Winfield Court, Bensalem, PA 19020, (215) 757-0227, BA 70 Glassboro St Coll; MA 71 Temple Univ-Tyler Sch of Art; ME 74 Trenton St Coll; SLP, Bucks County Intermediate Unit, **SLP**

Miller, Lori G 5708 Greenbush, Van Nuys, CA 91401, (818) 997-6466, BA 73 CA St Univ - Northridge; MA 74 CA St Univ - Northridge; Private Practice, **SLP**

Miller, Lori Lynn 105 Main Street B, Orono, ME 04473, (207) 873-7186, BS 81 Northern MI Univ; MA 84 Northern MI Univ; **SLP**

Miller, Mrs Louise Gervais 515 Deerwood Street, Columbia, SC 29205, (903) 787-5979, BA 78 Columbia Coll; MS 81 Univ of SC - Columbia; 81–Sp-Lang Path, Richland School District #1, **SLP**

Miller, Mrs Louise H 2332 San Paula, Dallas, TX 75228, (214) 327-3826, BA 38 Baylor Univ; MA 40 Baylor Univ; Retired, Private Practice, **SLP A LM**

Miller, Mrs Lynn Ann 1905 South Early Dawn, Veradale, WA 99037, (208) 664-7435, BS 61 Univ of ID; ME 63 Eastern WA Univ; Sp-Lang Path, Kootenai Med Ctr, **SLP**

Miller, Lynn M P O Box 536321, Orlando, FL 32853, BA 79 Univ of Central FL; MS 80 FL St Univ; Sp-Lang Path, Private Practice, **SLP**

Miller, Mrs M Annette 392 Man O War, Cantonment, FL 32533, (904) 474-5358, BS 64 TX Woman's Univ; 87–Sp-Lang Path, Rehab Inst of West FL, **SLP**

Miller, M Katherine 11586 Holmes #102, Kansas City, MO 64131, (816) 231-2432, Sp-Lang Path, Kansas City School District, **SLP**

Miller, Dr M Lynda 4304 Shoalwood Avenue, Austin, TX 78756, BA 64 Univ of CO - Boulder; MA 69 Univ of CO - Boulder; PH 76 (NS) Univ of CO - Boulder; 88–Dir, Language & Learning Institute, **SLP**

Miller, Madge B 290 Brady Court, Sacramento, CA 95820, MS; **SLP LM**

Miller, Marcia Lynne Route 3 Box 236, Rupert, ID 83350, (208) 934-4457, BS 72 ID St Univ; MS 80 ID St Univ; SLP, ID St Sch for the Deaf & Blind, **SLP**

Miller, Margaret A 6230 S Kinney Creek Road, Evergreen, CO 80439, (303) 674-4267, BA 66 Baylor Univ; MA 70 TX Christian Univ; **SLP**

Miller, Mrs Margaret Bumgardner 7 Oak Meadow, Evansville, IN 47711, (812) 867-5454, OB 63 OH Univ - Athens; MS 64 Univ of WI - Madison; **SLP**

Miller, Mrs Margaret T Ancortes Speech, 1258 Marine Drive, Anacortes, WA 98221-9719, (206) 293-8622, BS 69 OR St Univ; BA 69 OR St Univ; MA 71 Northwestern Univ; SLP, Anacortes Sp, **SLP**

Miller, Mrs Margery S 12316 Triple Crown Road, Gaithersburg, MD 20878, (301) 460-9393, BA 71 Elmira Coll; MA 72 NY Univ; MS 75 SUNY - Center at Albany; 88–Interim Dir-Natl Academy, Gallaudet Univ, **SLP**

Miller, Mrs Marianne Flowers 6823 Corintia Street, Carlsbad, CA 92009-5911, (619) 431-1418, BS 74 Bowling Green St Univ; MA 85 CA St Univ - Long Beach; **SLP**

Miller, Marilyn W 611 Cedar Hill Road NE, Albuquerque, NM 87122, (505) 296-1525, BA 61 Univ of MD - College Park; MS 75 Univ of NE - Omaha; 88–Sp-Lang Path, Albuquerque PS, **SLP**

Miller, Marita Murphy 904 Shilo Road, West Chester, PA 19382, (215) 692-9668, BS 75 East Stroudsburg Univ of PA; MA 81 West Chester Univ of PA; **SLP**

Miller, Marta G 27W088 Evelyn Street, Winfield, IL 60190, (312) 623-0021, BS 84 Western IL Univ; MA 85 Western IL Univ; Sp-Lang Path, Sedol, **SLP**

Miller, Martha Louise 222 Washington Avenue, Savannah, GA 31405, (912) 927-5479, Chief Aud, St Josephs Hosp, **A**

Miller, Mary Alice 10202 Hickory Ridge Road, Apartment 302, Columbia, MD 21044, BA 79 Eastern IL Univ; MA 85 Univ of IL - Urbana; **A**

Miller, Mary Frances Coniglio 1191 Hedgewood Lane, Niskayuna, NY 12309, (518) 346-4187, BS 85 SUNY - Coll at Fredonia; MS 86 SUNY - Coll at Fredonia; 86–Sp-Lang Path, St Peter's Hosp, **SLP**

Miller, Mrs Mary Kay 109 Elizabeth Circle, Kingwood, WV 26537, (304) 296-5962, BS 75 WV Univ; MS 77 WV Univ; **SLP**

Miller, Mary M 2480 East Broadway, Helena, MT 59601, (406) 449-6002, OB 85 Univ of KS; MS 87 Wichita St Univ; 87–Sp-Lang Path, State of Montana, **SLP**

Miller, Mary Margaret 1002 North 5th Street, Boise, ID 83702, (208) 343-2583, BS 79 ID St Univ; MA 81 WA St Univ; Sp-Lang Path, ID Elks Rehab Hosp, **SLP**

Miller, Mrs Maureen A 141 Cornfield Road, Milford, CT 06460, (203) 735-4327, BS 79 Southern CT St Univ; MS 81 Southern CT St Univ; Aud, The Hearing Center, **A**

Miller, Maureen L 36 Janet Drive, Plainview, NY 11803, (516) 935-4560, MA 74 CUNY - Queens Coll; Sp-Lang Path, Valley Stream Sch Dist #24, **SLP**

Miller, Maureen Marie 82 Green Street, Slatersville, RI 02876, (401) 769-0209, MA 87 Univ of CT; **A**

Miller, Dr Maurice H 7 Regent Drive, Lawrence, NY 11559, (212) 439-3385, BA 50 CUNY - Brooklyn Coll; MA 52 CUNY - Brooklyn Coll; PH 56 (Aud) Columbia Univ Teachers Coll; 72–Chief of Aud, Lenox Hill Hosp, **SLP A F**

Miller, Mrs Maxine Christa 321 Skyline Drive, Lewiston, ID 83501, (208) 743-8930, BS 69 Univ of AZ; MA 86 WA St Univ; Aud, Valley ENT Group, **A**

Miller, Dr Melvin D Dept Of Comm Dis, Univ Of OK Health Sciences Center, PO Box 26901, Oklahoma City, OK 73190, (405) 271-4214, BA 78 Brigham Young Univ; OM 79 Brigham Young Univ; PH 88 (Aud) Univ of OK - OK City; 88–Asst Prof, Univ of Oklahoma Health Sciences Ctr, **A**

Miller, Meredith Lee 142 Missouri Street, San Francisco, CA 94107-2425, (415) 861-2750, MA 82 CA St Univ - Northridge; SLP, Hastings On Hudson USD, **SLP**

Miller, Michele T 1278 Kashandra Drive, Marietta, GA 30067, (404) 427-4631, BS 80 Ball St Univ; MA 81 Ball St Univ; Sp-Lang Path, Marietta Cty Sch, **SLP**

Miller, Mrs Naida F Box 432, Wakita, OK 73771, (316) 842-5332, BS 63 Northeastern OK St Univ; MS 68 Phillips Univ; Sp-Lang Path, S Ctrl Ks Spec Ed Coop, **SLP**

Miller, Mrs Nancy E 1799 Estates Way, Chico, CA 95928, (916) 343-6416, BA 47 CA St Univ - Chico; MA 67 CA St Univ - Chico; **SLP**

Miller, Mrs Nancy J 59 Williams Road, Sharon, MA 02067, (617) 784-8114, BS 61 IL St Univ - Normal; MA 67 Northwestern Univ; 86–Aud, Private Practice, **A**

Miller, Nancy Joan 2414 Polk Drive, Huntsville, AL 35801, BA 74 Univ of RI; MS 76 Univ of RI; Sp-Lang Path, Huntsville Achi Sch, **SLP**

Miller, Dr Nancy K 5928 Glenway Avenue, Cincinnati, OH 45238, (513) 922-3333, BA 76 IN Univ - Bloomington; MA 78 Univ of Cincinnati; PH 86 (Sp Path) Univ of Cincinnati; 82–Sp-Lang Path, Private Practice, **SLP ACE**

Miller, Dr Nancy L 236 Francis Street, Longmont, CO 80501, (303) 499-2237, BS 72 SUNY - Coll at Geneseo; MS 74 Univ of CO - Boulder; PH 85 (NS) Univ of Denver; Director of Patient Education, Centennial Peaks Hosp, **SLP**

Miller, Nancy R 1133 Mayfair Lane, Glencoe, IL 60022, **SLP**

Miller, Nancy White 2841-B Phantom Street, Tyndall AFB, FL 32403-5000, (803) 722-8387, BA 80 Univ of FL; MA 82 Univ of FL; Aud, ENT Assoc/Amplimed, Inc, **A**

Miller, Mrs Nanette Malicki 19114 Orangepath, Glendora, CA 91740, (818) 963-8328, MA 84 Univ of GA; SLP, Los Angeles Cnty Off Education, **SLP**

Miller, Mrs Nola Moore N5748 Coffee Road, Johnson Creek, WI 53038, (414) 257-7344, BS 83 Univ of WI - Madison; MS 85 Univ of WI - Madison; Sp-Lang Path, Med Coll of WI, **SLP**

Miller, Mrs Nora Kathleen 246 2nd Avenue, Ripley, WV 25271-1522, (304) 273-3511, BA 85 Marshall Univ; MA 86 Marshall Univ; 88–Sp-Lang Path, Jackson Co Sch Sys, **SLP**

Miller, Mrs Pamela Crowe 6324 Odessa, West Bloomfield, MI 48033, (313) 360-1356, BS 78 Central MI Univ; MA 80 Eastern MI Univ; Sp-Lang Path/Case Manager, New Medico Rehabilitation Ser, **SLP**

Miller, Pamela Elizabeth 2490 Dearborn Street, Salt Lake City, UT 84106, (801) 487-3409, BA 76 Univ Southern MS-Hattiesburg; MS 80 Univ Southern MS-Hattiesburg; Sp-Lang Path, Primary Chldn Med Ctr, **SLP**

Miller, Pamela Moore 10013 118th Way North, Seminole, FL 34642, (813) 398-4540, BS 83 Auburn Univ - Auburn; MS 84 Auburn Univ - Auburn; **SLP**

Miller, Patricia D 2 Sappington Spur, St Louis, MO 63122, (314) 658-2939, BA 70 Univ of AL- Tuscaloosa; MS 72 Washington Univ; Instructor, St Louis U, **SLP**

Miller, Patricia J 4222 Beverly Road, Madison, WI 53711, (608) 274-6788, BS 73 Univ of WI - Madison; MS 79 Univ of WI - Whitewater; 85–Field U/w, New York Life, **SLP**

Miller, Patricia Kay 1703 14th Street #1, Boulder, CO 80302-6348, BS 77 Univ of MO - Columbia; MA 78 Univ of MO - Columbia; 86–Sp-Lang Path, Spalding Rehab Hosp, **SLP ACE**

Miller, Patricia M 3800 Inverary, Lansing, MI 48911, (517) 394-5100, BA 73 MI St Univ; MA 74 MI St Univ; Sp-Lang Path, Commun & Men Health Csdd, **SLP**

Miller, Patricia Wheeler 1389 Mackenzie Court, Tucker, GA 30084, (404) 843-3684, BS 74 GA St Univ; ME 78 GA St Univ; Sp/Lang Path, Northside Hospital, **SLP**

Miller, Paul S 511 Esplanade, Apartment M, New Orleans, LA 70116-2035, (504) 386-6014, OB 71 Wichita St Univ; MA 73 Marshall Univ; Consult, Interactive Comm Svcs, **SLP F**

Miller, Phyllis Jane 9 Susquehanna Road, Ossining, NY 10562, BA 78 MI St Univ; MA 81 Univ of Cincinnati; Sp-Lang Path, Chappaqua Ctr Sch Dist, **SLP**

Miller, Randi 2357 Bush Street Apt 9, San Francisco, CA 94115, (415) 931-4047, BA 85 San Francisco St Univ; MS 87 San Francisco St Univ; 87–Sp-Lang Path, San Francisco USD

Miller, Mrs Randi J 9990 South Florence Way, South Jordan, UT 84065, (801) 254-4458, BA 74 Univ of TX - El Paso; MS 80 Univ of UT; Sp/Lang Path, Salt Lake City Sch Dist, **SLP ACE**

Miller, Ravenna P 1505 Beechwood Boulevard, Pittsburgh, PA 15217, (412) 963-0334, BA 56 Univ of Pittsburgh - Pittsburgh; ME 60 Univ of Pittsburgh - Pittsburgh; Sp-Lang Path, Allegheny Intermed Unit, **SLP**

Miller, Rebecca Ballard 163 Jefferson Park Drive, Huntington, WV 25705, **SLP**

Miller, Rebecca Ward 1104 East Main Street, Clairton, PA 16214, (814) 226-7827, BA 68 Brenau Coll; MS 84 Clarion Univ of PA

Miller, Mrs Renee S 1422 Forres Avenue, St Joseph, MI 49085, (616) 983-8172, MA 77 Kent St Univ; Sp-Lang Path, Mercy Memorial Med Ctr, **SLP**

Miller, Mrs Rhonda Rene 2106 Gemini Drive, Bastrop, LA 71220, (318) 325-0601, BA 82 Northeast LA Univ; MS 85 Univ of North TX; 87–Sp-Lang Path, Monroe City Sch Sys, **SLP**

Miller, Dr Robert M VA Medical Center, 1660 South Columbian Way, Seattle, WA 98108, (206) 764-2829, BA 68 Univ of Redlands; MA 69 Univ of Redlands; PH 76 (NS) Univ of WA; 86–Chief Aud & SLP, Seattle VA Med Ctr, **SLP**

Miller, Robin P 1833 11th Street #101, Santa Monica, CA 90404, (213) 273-4952, BS 74 Emerson Coll; MS 75 Loma Linda Univ - Loma Linda; Sp-Lang Path, Bravos-Miller/Sp-Lang Path, **SLP**

Miller, Mrs Robin Schelzi 12 Blackberry Lane, Andover, MA 01801-4861, (617) 682-1938, **SLP**

Miller, Ronald W 1635 Jefferson Circle, Webb City, MO 64870, (417) 781-2311, BS 85 Brigham Young Univ; MA 87 Brigham Young Univ; Aud, Area Hrng & Sp Clinic Inc, **A**

Miller, Mrs Rosamond L 332 Windbrook Drive, Norman, OK 73072, (918) 335-1840, BA 51 OK Coll for Women; MA 71 Univ of Tulsa; Dir, Sp-Lang Path Dis Cen, **SLP**

Miller, Ruth A Star Route Box 26, Rosendale, NY 12472, (914) 339-3024, BS 71 Emerson Coll; MS 72 PA St Univ - Univ Park; Sp-Lang Path, Ruth A Miller, **SLP**

Miller, Sallie Annette 402 Huntington, Mount Clemens, MI 48043, (313) 784-9195, BS 76 Western MI Univ; MA 82 Eastern MI Univ; Sp-Lang Path, Armada Area Schools, **SLP**

Miller, Sally L 1225 Lyndale Drive, Charleston, WV 25314, (304) 348-1920, BS 78 WV Univ; MA 78 Marshall Univ; SLP, Kanawha Co Bd of Ed, **SLP**

Miller, Mrs Sandra E 453 Arbor Circle, Youngstown, OH 45505, (216) 792-1822, BS 57 OH Univ - Athens; MA 78 Kent St Univ; Teacher Multiple Handicapped, Youngstown County Schools, **SLP**

Miller, Mrs Sandra Lynne 845 Dawn Avenue #204, Ephrata, PA 17522, (717) 295-8327, BS 84 Bloomsburg Univ of PA; MS 85 Bloomsburg Univ of PA; Sp-Lang Path, Lancaster General Hosp, **SLP**

Miller, Mrs Sandra Malyn P O Box 9533, Midland, TX 79708, (512) 775-9328, BS 85 Baylor Univ; MS 85 Baylor Univ; **SLP**

Miller, Sandra Petersen 147 East 100 North, Providence, UT 84332, (801) 752-2050, BA 80 Univ of CA - Santa Barbara; MS 86 UT St Univ; Supervisor SLP, Logan Regional Hospital, **SLP ACE**

Miller, Sara F 9859 Caminitio Pudregal, San Diego, CA 92131, (619) 566-8163, BS 75 Northwestern Univ; MA 77 Temple Univ; Sp/Lang Path, Mercy Hosp, **SLP**

Miller, Mrs Sara M 4770 N W 177th Pl, Portland, OR 97229-2172, (503) 648-1162, BS 73 Univ of OR; MS 75 Portland St Univ; Sp-Lang Path, Hillsboro Elem Sch Dist #7, **SLP**

Miller, Sarah Ann 211 E 18th Street, New York, NY 10003, (212) 420-2760, MS 84 Columbia Univ Teachers Coll; **A**

Miller, Seth Bruce 782 Orange Street #1 Rear, New Haven, CT 06511, (203) 795-6075, **SLP**

Miller, Sheila Marie 725 South 6th West, Missoula, MT 59801-3834, (406) 728-2633, BA 84 Carroll Coll; MA 87 Univ of MT; **A**

Miller, Mrs Shelby Victoire 8631 Eagle Glen Terrace, Fairfax, VA 22039-2679, (703) 920-1489, MS 88 George Washington Univ

Miller, Sherri F 25 Wilmont Road, Framingham, MA 01701, (508) 620-9094, BS 76 Northeastern Univ; ME 80 Northeastern Univ; Sp-Lang Path, Self Employed, **SLP**

Miller, Mrs Stacey Anderson 16852 Passage #7, Paramount, CA 90723, (213) 630-2243, MA 88 CA St Univ - Fullerton; Sp-Lang Path, Cox & Associates

Miller, Stacy Lee Route 2 Box 110, Thompson Station, TN 37179, (615) 327-9313, BS 80 Northwestern Univ; MS 82 San Francisco St Univ; 88–Sp-Lang Path, Therapeutic Consultants Inc, **SLP**

Miller, Stephanie Mcllwain 616 Wellington Court, Lafayette, IN 47904-2770, (317) 448-6791, BS 84 OH Univ - Athens, MA 85 OH Univ - Athens; School Readiness Teacher, Grace United Methodist Church, **SLP**

Miller, Stephen E 10300 North Central Expressway, Bldg II #275, Dallas, TX 75231, (214) 696-9955, BS 74 FL St Univ; MS 75 FL St Univ; 85–Aud, Private Practice, **A**

Miller, Mrs Sue F 577 Greencraig Road, Los Angeles, CA 90049, (213) 857-2815, BA 56 Univ of CA - Los Angeles; MA 79 CA St Univ - Northridge; Sp-Lang Path, Private Practice, **SLP**

Miller, Suellen 52 Little Sewickley Creek, Sewickley, PA 15143, **SLP**

Miller, Susan D 311 East 75th Street #2-C, New York, NY 10021, (212) 794-5856, BS 73 Indiana Univ of PA; MS 75 Univ of OK Medical Center; Dir of Sp-Lang Path, Memorial Sloan Kettering, **SLP ACE**

Miller, Susan L 3934 Brennan Drive, Memphis, TN 38122, (901) 324-3765, BS 70 Northwestern Univ; MS 72 Emerson Coll; 86–Sp-Lang Path, Memphis City Schs, **SLP**

Miller, Susan Lynn 4616 Nagle Avenue, Sherman Oaks, CA 91423, Los Angeles Cnty Supt Schools, **SLP**

Miller, Mrs Susan Lynn 2613 Huntleigh Drive, Oklahoma City, OK 73120, (405) 751-3098, BS 83 Central St Univ; ME 86 Central St Univ; **SLP**

Miller, Mrs Susan Matteson 86 Buckthorn Drive, Littleton, CO 80127, (303) 973-7651, BS 83 CO St Univ; MA 85 Univ of CO - Boulder; 85–Aud, Cherry Creek Schs, **A**

Miller, Suzanne D 4243 W Bethany Home Road, Phoenix, AZ 85019, (602) 841-9151, BS 82 Univ of KS; MA 83 Wichita St Univ; Sp-Lang Path, Glendale Sp & L Ctr, **SLP**

Miller, Suzanne Marie 5110 N 32nd Street #111, Phoenix, AZ 85018, (602) 239-4755, BS 81 AZ St Univ; MS 86 AZ St Univ; 86–Sp-Lang Path, Good Samaritan Med Ctr, **SLP**

Miller, Mrs Suzanne Slayback 905 Lima Court N E, Albuquerque, NM 87123, (505) 294-0321, BS 79 WV Univ; MS 80 WV Univ; Audiologist, Albuquerque Hearing & Spch Cen, **A**

Miller, Syndee F W 359 Hazelwood Terrace, Buffalo Grove, IL 60090, **SLP**

Miller, Tammi Lynn 2002 Westlake Way, Houston, TX 77084, (713) 579-9457, BS 83 Univ of Tulsa; MA 85 Univ of Tulsa; **SLP**

Miller, Mrs Teresa C 5209 Lanton Drive, Gainesville, GA 30501, (404) 534-1080, BS 81 Univ of GA; ME 82 Univ of GA; ES 86 Univ of GA; 82–Sp/Lang Path, Hall County School System, **SLP**

Miller, Teresa Mary 4023 Heathersage Drive, Houston, TX 77084, (713) 855-1869, BA 83 Univ of FL; MA 88 Univ of FL; **SLP**

Miller, Terri Lynn Rural Route 3, Novinger, MO 63559, (816) 488-6785, BS 86 Northeast MO St Univ; MA 87 Northeast MO St Univ; 87–Sp-Lang Path, Milan C-II Sch, **SLP**

Miller, Terri Lynne 6599 East Thomas, #2154, Scottsdale, AZ 85251, (602) 946-0820, BA 86 Central MI Univ; MA 87 MI St Univ; 88–Sp-Lang Path, Camelback Communication Ctr, **SLP**

Miller, Dr Thomas D 88 Squirrels Heath Road, Fairport, NY 14450-9720, (716) 586-2525, BA 69 SUNY - Center at Buffalo; MS 72 SUNY - Coll at Buffalo; PH 83 (Sp-Lang Path & Aud) SUNY - Center at Buffalo; 76–Assoc Prof, Nazareth Coll of Rochester, **SLP**

Miller, Thomas W 2264 South Jefferson, Lorain, OH 44052, (216) 984-2416, BA 74 Univ of Akron; MA 76 Univ of Akron; Asst Dir, Rehab Cen of Lorain County Inc, **SLP**

Miller, Mrs Tracey Anne 1516 Courtship Drive, Lancaster, OH 43130, (614) 653-4154, BS 83 Miami Univ - Oxford; MS 84 Miami Univ - Oxford; 84–Sp-Lang Path, Amanda-Clearcreek Local Schs, **SLP**

Miller, Trudy K 2970 Lake Shore Drive 4F, Chicago, IL 60657, (312) 908-6138, BA 72 OH Univ - Athens; MA 73 OH Univ - Athens; Clinical Supervisor, Rehabilitation Inst of Chicago, **SLP**

Miller, Vaughn P 1182 Shallows Court, Port Orange, FL 32019, (904) 767-4935, MS 74 Kent St Univ; Sp-Lang Path, Volusia Co Sch, **SLP**

Miller, Mrs Vickie Barnes 1218 Oak Park, Maryville, TN 37801, (615) 546-9221, **A**

Miller, Victoria H Nalle Clinic, 1350 South Kings Drive, Charlotte, NC 28207, (704) 372-8750, BS 74 East Carolina Univ; MS 77 Univ of NC - Chapel Hill; 83–Aud, Nalle Cl, **A**

Miller, Dr Viola P Murray State University, Center For Continuing Education And Academic Outreach, Murray, KY 42071, (502) 436-2595, BS 64 Northwestern St Univ; MA 66 Tulane Univ; ED 78 (NS) Univ of AL- Tuscaloosa; Dean Ctr for Cont Educ, Murray St U, **SLP**

Miller, Virginia Carol 1435 Williams Grove Road, Mechanicsburg, PA 17055, (717) 737-6728, BS 83 Indiana Univ of PA; MS 86 Towson St Univ; 87–Sp-Lang Path, Capital Area Interm Unit, **SLP**

Miller, Wanda Louise 6308 Westbrook Drive, New Carrollton, MD 20784, (301) 373-3118, BA 82 Univ of MD - College Park; MA 85 Univ of MD - College Park; **SLP**

Miller, Warren M 12334 North Fairwood Drive, Apartment 58, Spokane, WA 99218, (509) 276-6881, BA 68 Kearney St Coll; MS 75 Eastern WA Univ; Sp-Lang Path, Deer Park Sch Dist #414, **SLP**

Miller, Wayne D Speech Pathologist-Audiologist, 76 Short Street, South Easton, MA 02375, (508) 238-7634, BA 58 Staley Coll; ME 71 Suffolk Univ; 65–Sp-Lang Path/Aud, Private Practice, **SLP A ACE**

Miller, Yolanda E 11 Hillendale Road, Asheville, NC 28805, (704) 669-3159, BS 77 Shaw Univ; MA 78 OH St Univ; Sp-Lang Path, Black Mountain Cen, **SLP**

Miller-Arnst, Charlene 212 East Weldon Avenue, Fresno, CA 93704, (209) 237-0883, BA 79 CA St Univ - Fresno; MS 81 San Francisco St Univ; Sp-Lang Path, Fresno Community Hospital, **SLP ACE**

Miller-Cook, Mrs Stephanie 443 Hollis Street, Framingham, MA 01701, (617) 879-3931, BA 83 Univ of MD - College Park; MS 84 Boston Univ; 87–Sp-Lang Path, Private Practice, **SLP**

Miller-Fritz, Mrs Jayne Ellen Abingdon ENT, P O Box 1328, Abingdon, VA 24210, (703) 628-9547, BS 84 East TN St Univ; MS 87 East TN St Univ; 86–Aud, Abingdon ENT Associates PC, **A**

Miller-Gordon, Deborah 405 Rancho Arroyo Parkway #311, Fremont, CA 94536, (415) 745-0312, MS 88 CA St Univ - Hayward

Miller-Linville, Beth Ann 8214 Clinton Avenue, Lubbock, TX 79424, (806) 793-4125, BA 85 MI St Univ; MA 87 Univ of Pittsburgh - Pittsburgh; 88–Sp-Lang Path, Methodist Hospital, **SLP**

Miller-Requarth, Marilyn Ann P O Box 221, Montpelier, VT 05602, (505) 455-3208, **SLP**

Miller-Van Veghel, Mrs Jeri L 200 Bay Street #1011, Hamilton, ON, Canada L8P 4S4, (416) 523-4175, BS 82 Univ of WI - Milwaukee; MS 84 Purdue Univ - West Lafayette; Sp-Lang Path, Chedoke-Mc Master Hosp, **SLP**

Miller Wilson, Grace Christine 16215 Clay Road #1502, Houston, TX 77084, (713) 550-1903, BS 84 Univ of TX - Austin; MS 86 Univ of TX - Dallas; 88–Sp-Lang Path, ISD, **SLP**

Miller-Wood, Deborah J 303 Green Street, Auburn, AL 36830-6122, (205) 826-7515, MS; **SLP**

Miller-Zuidema, Mrs Valerie Jean 12 Sutton Avenue, Oxford, MA 01540, (617) 869-2406, BS 85 Worcester St Coll; MS 88 Worcester St Coll; 87–Sp-Lang Path, Berlin-Boylston Reg Sch Sys

Millett, Mrs Ann Fantauzzi 565 Vera Circle, Bethlehem, PA 18017, (717) 424-3247, BS 79 Coll of Saint Rose; MS 80 Coll of Saint Rose; 88–Instr, E Stroudsburg Univ, **SLP**

Millett, Karen J 701-1/2 West Court Street, Rome, NY 13440, BS 80 Ithaca Coll; MA 82 Edinboro Univ of PA; Sp/Lang Path/Supervisor, BOCES, **SLP**

Millhiser, Mrs Rochelle D 8703 Berwickshire Drive, Richmond, VA 23229, (804) 285-0338, BS 71 Georgetown Univ; MA 73 George Washington Univ; **SLP**

Millhollen, Marjory M 38744 Flowerdale Drive, Springfield, OR 97478, (503) 687-3373, BA 65 Univ of OR; MS 67 Univ of OR; SLP, Eugene Sch Dist 45, **SLP**

Millhouse-Smith, Mrs Susan A 34063 Nebraska Lane, Yucuipa, CA 92399, (714) 983-0042, BA 64 CA St Univ - Fresno; MS 82 Univ of Redlands; Sp-Lang Path, San Bernardino Co Sch, **SLP**

Milligan, Mrs Mary Louise 1089 Oneida Trail, Hartville, OH 44632, (216) 438-2554, BS 60 Bowling Green St Univ; MA 82 Kent St Univ; Sp-Lang Path, Canton City Schools, **SLP**

Milligan, Terri P P O Box L-164, Langhorne, PA 19047, (215) 741-1651, BS 78 Southwest TX St Univ; ME 79 Southwest TX St Univ; Sp/Lang Path, The Woods Schs, **SLP**

Millikan, Mrs Cynthia Diane 8017 Moss Rock Drive, Fort Worth, TX 76123-1393, (806) 355-6501, BS 79 Yankton Coll; ME 83 West TX St Univ; Sp/Lang Path, Canyon ISD, **SLP**

Milliken, Deborah Lynne 4206 Arborwood, Lindenwold, NJ 08021, (609) 451-9000, BS 75 Trenton St Coll; MA 83 West Chester Univ of PA; **SLP**

Milliken, Joy J 666 6th Street South, St Petersburg, FL 33701, (813) 821-5435, BS 77 WV Univ; MS 79 WV Univ; Aud, Michael H Diamond MD, **A**

Millikin, Cynthia C 11621 Rivershore Drive, Dunkirk, MD 20754, (301) 297-5815, BA 75 Univ of MD - College Park; MS 77 Loyola Coll; Sp-Lang Path, P G Co Sch, **SLP**

Millikin, Paula A 1012 Kings Road, Erin Meadows, Hartford, WI 53027, **SLP**

Millin, Jennybel M 238 Dunbar Road, Tallmadge, OH 44278, MS; **SLP**

Millin, Dr Joseph P 238 Dunbar Road, Tallmadge, OH 44278, (216) 633-0039, BA 50 Case Western Reserve Univ; MA 65 Case Western Reserve Univ; PH 68 (Aud) Case Western Reserve Univ; 66–Prof of Aud, Kent State U, **A F**

Millington, Mrs Kelly Ann 20 Greensboro Boulevard, Clifton Park, NY 12065, (518) 382-1201, BA 80 SUNY - Coll at Plattsburgh; MS 82 Ithaca Coll; Sp-Lang Path, Scotia-Glenville PS, **SLP**

Million, Dr Phillip C 1114 McCann Drive, Winchester, KY 40391, (606) 744-7513, BS 75 Phillips Univ; MS 77 Univ of OK Medical Center; PH 83 (Aud) Univ of OK Medical Center; Aud, Private Practice, **A**

Milliren, Brenda F R R 15 Box 440, West Terre Haute, IN 47885, (812) 238-4425, BS 67 IN St Univ - Terre Haute; MS 72 IN St Univ - Terre Haute; 82–Sp/Lang Path, Vigo Cty Sch Corp, **SLP**

Millis, Robert Guy Clarksdale Speech & Hearing Ct, P O Box 182, Clarksdale, MS 38614, (601) 627-5247, BS 57 Univ Southern MS-Hattiesburg; MS 64 Univ Southern MS-Hattiesburg; Director, Clarksdale Speech & Hrng Cen, **SLP**

Millman, Mrs Arlene 21031 Winchester, Southfield, MI 48076, (313) 355-2527, BS 78 Eastern MI Univ; MA 79 Eastern MI Univ; Sp-Lang Path, Detroit Pub Schools, **SLP ACE**

Millman, Gladys 24 Cricket Club Drive, Roslyn, NY 11576-2910, (516) 365-7448, BA 79 CUNY - Queens Coll; MA 81 CUNY - Queens Coll; Asst Dir, Sch for Lang & Comm Dev, **SLP**

Millman, Ilene K 4 Fern Way, Belle Mead, NJ 08502, **SLP**

Millns, Jennifer 7 Hammock Place, Safety Harbor, FL 34695, BA 72 OH St Univ; MA 75 Univ of MO - Columbia; **SLP**

Millott, Mrs Marian Schlicht 1316 Columbus Avenue, Sandusky, OH 44870, (419) 626-3328, BS 63 Bowling Green St Univ; MA 65 Bowling Green St Univ; Sp-Lang Path, Betty Rinderle Sch, **SLP**

Mills, Mrs Anne E P O Box 55, Commerce, TX 75428, (214) 886-6792, BS 70 East TX St Univ - Commerce; MS 80 East TX St Univ - Commerce; Sp-Lang Path, Commerce ISD, **SLP**

Mills, Carlon Scott 1420 Plaza Drive, Winston-Salem, NC 27103, (919) 765-4922, BA 84 Harding Univ; MA 86 Univ of TN - Knoxville; 88–Dir of Hrng Ctr, Forsyth Head & Neck Assoc, **A**

Mills, Mrs Charlotte 1407 North Vassar, Wichita, KS 67208, (316) 262-3891, BA 62 Wichita St Univ; MA 67 Wichita St Univ; Sp-Lang Path, Private Practice, **SLP LM**

Mills, Mrs Cheryl Renee 4197 Stilmore Road, South Euclid, OH 44121, (216) 464-1000, BA 81 OH St Univ; MS 83 Univ of WI - Madison; 85–Sp-Lang Path, Beach Haven Health Care Ctr, **SLP**

Mills, Dawna Mitchell 4543 Hackett Avenue, Lakewood, CA 90712, (213) 483-9930, BS 84 Worcester St Coll; MA 86 CA St Univ - Long Beach; Aud, Otologic Med Gp, **A**

Mills, Debra Q 7137 Chelsea Drive N E, Cedar Rapids, IA 52402, (319) 399-6821, BA 74 Univ of CA - Davis; MA 78 San Jose St Univ; SLP, Grant Wood AEA, **SLP**

Mills, Denise Marie 345 Telegraph Road, Stafford, VA 22554, (703) 371-1263, BS 81 Bowling Green St Univ; MA 82 Bowling Green St Univ; 84–Aud, Hearing Resources Inc, **A**

Mills, Donna S 16804 Bridgeport Street, Fountain Valley, CA 92708, (714) 558-5501, BA 85 CA St Univ - Fullerton; MA 87 CA St Univ - Fullerton; **SLP**

Mills, Dr Jack R Communication Diagnostic Ctr, Nova University, 3301 College Avenue, Fort Lauderdale, FL 33303, (305) 475-7329, BA 57 Univ of TX - Austin; MA 59 Univ of TX - Austin; OD 69 (NS) Johns Hopkins Univ; Prog Dir, Nova Univ, **SLP A**

Mills, Jane Burrington 301 Village Run East, Encinitas, CA 92024, **SLP**

Mills, Janice Adele Woodrow Wilson Rehab Ctr, Dept Of Comm SVC, Box 499, Fishersville, VA 22939, (703) 332-7086, ME 83 Univ of VA - Charlottesville; Aud, Woodrow Wilson Rehab Ctr, **A**

Mills, Janice F 1170 Chersonese Round, Mount Pleasant, SC 29464, MS; **SLP**

Mills, Mrs Janis Ellyn 42 Wilshire Drive, Chestnut Ridge, NY 10977, (914) 425-4370, BS 69 SUNY - Coll at Buffalo; MS 71 Syracuse Univ; Sp-Lang Path, BOCES Serv, **SLP ACE**

Mills, Jeri Munger 529 N W 141st, Edmond, OK 73013, (405) 751-2166, BS 78 CO St Univ; MS 80 Univ of OK Medical Center; Asst Prof, U of OK Hlth Sci Cen, **A**

Mills, John H Department Otolaryngology, Medical Univ Of S Carolina, Charleston, SC 29425, (803) 792-7976, BA 63; MA 64; PH 68 (Aud) Univ of IA; 80–Prof, Med Univ S Carolina, **A**

Mills, Joyce S P O Box 2762, Ocala, FL 32678, (904) 732-8041, BS 63 SUNY - Coll at Geneseo; MS 65 SUNY - Coll at Geneseo; ED 83 (NS) Stetson Univ; Sp-Lang Path, Marion Co Bd of Pub Instr, **SLP**

Mills, Leigh Ear Medical Group, 2037 N W Lovejoy, Portland, OR 97209, (503) 227-3666, BA 75 Univ of CO - Boulder; OM 80 Univ of WA; Aud, Ear Med Group, **A**

Mills, Marion 303-255 Wellington Cres, Winnipeg, MB, Canada R3M 3V4, (204) 284-0156, BA 46; MA 59 Northwestern Univ; 85–Retired, Winniped Sch Div #1 Chld G Cl, **SLP**

Mills, Mrs Mary A 3711 High Bank Place, West Lafayette, IN 47906, (317) 463-7696, BS 72 Auburn Univ - Auburn; MS 76 Purdue Univ - West Lafayette; **SLP**

Mills, Mary Cathleen 1344 Minter, Plano, TX 75023, (214) 231-5303, BS 82 Univ of North TX; MS 84 Univ of North TX; 85–Sp-Lang Path, Richardson ISD, **SLP**

Mills, Mary E 442 Brentwood Drive, Benicia, CA 94510, (707) 643-0341, BS 73 CA St Univ - Hayward; MA 76 CA St Univ - Sacramento; Sp-Lang Path, Vallejo USD, **SLP**

Mills, Mrs Mary L 1901 Hammann Avenue, Muscatine, IA 52761, (319) 263-8476, MA 69 Univ of IA; Audiologist, Miss Bend AEA, **A**

Mills, Mrs Norma B 4268 Woodside Circle, Lake Oswego, OR 97035, (503) 620-1620, BS 53 Univ of IL - Urbana; ME 73 Western OR St Coll; Sp-Lang Path, Tigard Sch Dist 23J, **SLP**

Mills, Dr Russell H Audiology & Sp Path Serv (126), VA Medical Center, 2215 Fuller Road, Ann Arbor, MI 48105, (313) 769-7100, BA Univ of SD - Vermillion; MA 70 Univ of SD - Vermillion; PH 75 (NS) Univ of KS; Asst Chief & Sr SLP, VA Medical Center, **SLP**

Mills, Sharyn Sapp 11300 North Robinhood Lane, Kansas City, MO 64154, (816) 276-7123, MS 73 FL St Univ; Dir Sp-Lang Path/Aud, Baptist Med Ctr, **SLP**

Mills, Sherry Lisa 350 Park Place, Porterville, CA 93257, (209) 782-7099, BA 78 Univ of CA - Davis; MA 85 CA St Univ - Stanislaus; SLP, Porterville Schools, **SLP**

Mills, Susan J P O Box 8567, Scottsdale, AZ 85252, (602) 894-2080, BS 68 Marquette Univ; MS 74 AZ St Univ; **SLP**

Mills, Thelma B 645 North 3rd Street, Danville, KY 40422, (606) 236-5132, BS 70 Univ of TX - Austin; MA 72 Univ of TX - Austin; Tchr, Kentucky School for the Deaf, **A**

Mills, William David Div For Excep Chldrn St Dept, Raleigh, NC 27603, BS 65 Auburn Univ - Auburn; MA 69 Auburn Univ - Auburn; Asst Dir, Nc Dept Pub Instr, **SLP**

Mills, Dr Yvonne L 11 Tivoli Lake Court, Silver Spring, MD 20906, (202) 832-4400, BA 68 Howard Univ; MA 73 George Washington Univ; PH 85 (Bilingualism-Child Language) Howard Univ; Dir of Rehab Svcs/Chief of Sp & Hrng, Hosp for Sick Children, **SLP**

Millsap, Mrs Lynn N 116 Elmdale, Ottumwa, IA 52501, (515) 682-7397, BA 73 Univ of Northern IA; MA 74 Univ of Northern IA; SLP, Sn Prairie AEA, **SLP**

Millsaps, Mrs Deborah M Route 1 Box 152, Louisville, TN 37777, (615) 971-3911, BS 74 East TN St Univ; MA 77 Univ of TN - Knoxville; Sp-Lang Path, UT Hosp/Birh Dfcts&Humn Dev Ce, **SLP**

Millstone, Eileen M 27415 Aberdeen, Southfield, MI 48076, (313) 544-5890, BS 59 Wayne St Univ; MA 80 Wayne St Univ; Sp/Lang Path, Sch Dist Cty of Berkley, **SLP**

Millward, Dorothy D 610 Stone Street, Osceola Mills, PA 16666, (814) 339-6282, BS 45 Lock Haven St Coll; ME 50 PA St Univ - Univ Park; **SLP LM**

Millwood, Mrs Dessa Hampton Route 6 Box 235, Lincolnton, NC 28092-9017, (704) 922-5259, BS 81 Univ of TX - Dallas; MS 83 Univ of TX - Dallas; Sp-Lang Path, Gaston-Lincoln Ment Hlth Prog, **SLP**

Millwood, Rebecca R 2 Anchorage Court, Savannah, GA 31410, (912) 897-7863, BA 73 Univ of GA; ME 77 GA St Univ; 86–Sp-Lang Path, Savannah/Chatham Co PS, **SLP**

Milne, Charlynn J 22316 Dolorosa Street, Woodland Hills, CA 91367, (213) 997-2357, BS 57 Univ of UT; MA 74 CA St Univ - Northridge; Sp-Lang Path, Los Angeles USD, **SLP**

Milne, Ruth I 375 Armadale Avenue, Toronto, ON, Canada M6S 3X7, (416) 922-8820, BA 71; MS 85; 88–Asst Exec Dir, Metro Toronto Dist Hlth Council, **SLP**

Milner, Anna Mae 3015 North Aberndroth, Appleton, WI 54914, (414) 731-0619, BS 70 Univ of WI - Oshkosh; MS 77 Univ of WI - Stevens Point; Sp/Lang Path, Private Practice, **SLP**

Milner, Floyd Eugene 1380 West 48th Street #77, San Bernardino, CA 92407, (714) 787-4900, **A**

Milner, Mrs Joyce Browning 11035 Culver Blvd, Culver City, CA 90230, (213) 559-2410, MA 83; 88–Sp-Lang Path, **SLP**

Milner, Mrs Lynnette Kay 1615 Westgate Lane, Mattoon, IL 61938, (217) 253-2712, BS 82 Eastern IL Univ; MS 83 Eastern IL Univ; **SLP**

Milner, Dr Paul 403 Massapoag Avenue, Sharon, MA 02067, (617) 784-5058, BS 63 MA Inst of Tech; MS 70 Polytechnic Inst of Brooklyn; PH 82 (Sp & Hrng Sciences) CUNY - Grad Sch & Univ Cntr; 88–Dir of Pro Svcs, Wilner-Greene Associates, **A**

Milner, Ruth K 1215 Glen Burnie Lane, Dresher, PA 19025, (215) 331-6878, BS 74 Northeastern Univ; MA 79 Temple Univ; Aud, Arnold K Brenman, **A**

Milone, Kate 1671 New Windsor Court, Crofton, MD 21114, (301) 261-3174, BA 82 Univ of MD - College Park; MS 83 Memphis St Univ; Sp-Lang Path, Kate Milone & Assoc, **SLP**

Milone, Marjorie 13 Croyden Place, Kankakee, IL 60901, **SLP**

Milone, Mrs Sheri Sullivan Rd 5 Box 630, Honesdale, PA 18431, (717) 253-1300, MS 77 Univ of AZ; Rehab Services Director, Wayne County Memorial Hospital, **SLP A**

Milosch, Lizabeth Lynn 3030 West Southland Drive, Franklin, WI 53132, (414) 251-6714, **SLP**

Milosky, Linda M Communication Sci & Disorders, Syracuse University, 805 S Crouse Avenue, Syracuse, NY 13244-2280, (315) 423-4121, BS 74 Northwestern Univ; MS 75 Univ of MI - Ann Arbor; PH 86 (Lang Develop/Disorders in a Comm Dis Dept) Univ of WI - Madison; 88–Asst Prof, Syracuse Univ, **SLP**

Milstead, Kim F 923 Terrace Mountain Drive, Austin, TX 78746, (512) 327-1066, BS 74 Univ of North TX; ME 77 Southwest TX St Univ; 88–Sp-Lang Path, Austin State Sch, **SLP**

Milstein, Leslie J 15930 S E 43rd Street, Bellevue, WA 98006, (206) 747-4004, BS 63 Univ of MN - Minneap-St Paul; MS 68 Univ of MN - Minneap-St Paul; Sp-Lang Path, Merrywood Sch, **SLP**

Milstein, Rochelle Fern 29970 Fox Club Drive, Farmington Hills, MI 48018, (313) 280-8416, BA 80 Wayne St Univ; MA 82 Wayne St Univ; MA 84 Wayne St Univ; Sp-Lang Path, William Beaumont Hospital, **SLP**

Miltenberger, Damaris S PO Box 325, Dongola, IL 62926, (618) 827-3524, BS 65 Bethel Coll; MA 70 Univ of AL- Tuscaloosa; Sp-Lang Path, Dongola Unit Schs, **SLP**

Miltenberger, Gerald E Route 2, Dongola, IL 62926, (618) 827-4298, BS 57 Southern IL Univ -Carbondale; MA 63 CO St Univ; Sp-Lang Path, Choate Mental Health Dev Ctr, **SLP A**

Miltich, Dr Suzanne Hogan 2934 Shady Lane, Ann Arbor, MI 48104, (313) 973-9281, BA 63 Central St Univ; MA 66 Univ of MO - Columbia; PH 76 (NS) IN Univ - Bloomington; Sp-Lang Path, Private Practice, **SLP**

Milton, Mrs Janice Leah 1038 East 35th, Tulsa, OK 74105, (918) 560-5798, BS 85 Midwestern St Univ; MA 88 Univ of Tulsa; 88–Sp-Lang Path, Kaiser Rehab Ctr

Milton, Mary P 533 Crofton Avenue #4, Oakland, CA 94610, BA 61 Temple Univ; MA 63 Univ of PA; MA 65 Univ of WI - Madison; Sp-Lang Path, Richmond USD, **SLP**

Milton, Octavia W Atlanta Public Schools, 2730 Forrest Hills Dr SW, Atlanta, GA 30315, (404) 761-5411, BS 54 Hampton Univ; MA 68 Atlanta Univ; ED 86 (NS) Atlanta Univ; Director Prog for Except Chldn, Atlanta Public Schools

Milton, Sandra B 1044 20th Street Unit I, Santa Monica, CA 90403, (213) 653-7067, BS 78 Univ of MA - Amherst; MA 80 Univ of CA - Santa Barbara; Cl Dir, Head Inj Rehab Services, **SLP**

Mims, Dr Howard A 15608 Glynn Road, East Cleveland, OH 44112, (216) 687-6986, MA 54 Wayne St Univ; MA 63 Case Western Reserve Univ; PH 71 (NS) Case Western Reserve Univ; Assoc Prof Sp & Hrng, Cleveland State University, **SLP**

Mims, Mrs Lisa N 9116 West 90, Overland Park, KS 66212-3803, (913) 642-9343, MS 87 Univ of AR - Fayetteville

Mims, Sarah S Route 1 Box 369, Chapel Hill, NC 27514, (919) 942-8241, BA 72 Coker Coll; ME 77 Univ of GA; Sp-Lang Path, Durham Cty Schools, **SLP**

Mims, Sondra F K 1850 Blackwater Drive, Marietta, GA 30066-6712, MS 74 Univ of AL- Tuscaloosa; SLP, Neva King Cooper Educ Center, **SLP**

Mina, Mrs Sheila D 170 Sherry Lane, Chicago Heights, IL 60411, (312) 754-3766, BS 75 Northern IL Univ - De Kalb; MA 77 Northern IL Univ - De Kalb; Sp-Lang Path, Cen for Comm Dis, **SLP**

Minard, B Gail 248 Bluejay Drive, Worthington, OH 43085, (614) 263-2448, BS 74 Univ of MO - Columbia; MA 75 Univ of MO - Columbia; SLP, Columbus Pub Sch, **SLP**

Minard, Mrs Charlotte 14857 High Valley Road, Poway, CA 92064, (619) 486-1382, BA 52 Stanford Univ; MA 53 Stanford Univ; MA 82 CA St Univ - Los Angeles; Sp-Lang Path, Oceanside USD, **SLP**

Minard, Edwin E, II R R 5 Box 431, Burlington, IA 52601, (319) 753-6561, BA 73 Western KY Univ; MA 74 Western KY Univ; MA 75 Western IL Univ; Superv Hrng Conserv/Ed Ser, Gr River AEA 16, **A**

Minard, Nora Ann 539 Quinlan Drive, Williamston, MI 48895, (517) 655-3872, MA 88 MI St Univ

Minard, Mrs Pamela Dickinson St Joseph's Hospital Professional Bldg, 3070 North 51st Street Suite 407A, Milwaukee, WI 53210, (414) 442-9000, BS 86 Kent St Univ; MA 87 Kent St Univ; 86–Aud, Physicians' Hrng Svcs, **A**

Minardi, Mrs Lisa M S 44 D Civic Drive, Walnut Creek, CA 94596-2412, (605) 622-2558, OB 83 Northern St Coll; OM 84 Moorhead St Univ; **SLP**

Minarovic, Kathryn A 3003 Ritchie Avenue, Baltimore, MD 21219, (301) 391-3916, BS 76 Towson St Univ; MS 77 Towson St Univ; SLP, Balto Co Pub Sch, **SLP**

Mincer, Shelia Rae 0031 Sunlight Road, Glenwood Springs, CO 81601, (303) 945-8989, BA 68 Univ of CO - Boulder; MA 72 Univ of CO - Boulder; SLP, Mountain Valley Develomntl Ser, **SLP**

Mindel, Maxine C 5215 South Orchard #D, Tacoma, WA 98467, (206) 591-6763, BA 77 Univ of CT; MS 79 Univ of AZ; 85–Sp-Lang Path, St Joseph Hospital, **SLP**

Mindell, Audrey Robin 9983 Nob Hill Lane, Sunrise, FL 33351, (305) 485-5928, BA 84 Univ of FL; MA 86 Univ of FL; Aud, United Hearing & Deaf Svcs, **A**

Mindes, Miriam Joane 839 Larrabee Street, West Hollywood, CA 90069, MA 80 CA St Univ - Northridge; Sp-Lang Path, Los Angeles USD, **SLP**

Minear, Dr David J 79-35 210th Street, Hollis Hills, NY 11364, (212) 830-1015, BA 62 Loma Linda Univ - Riverside; MA 64 Univ of Denver; PH 69 (NS) Univ of CO - Boulder; Dir Sp Hrng Clinic, Elmhurst Hosp, **SLP**

Minear, Kenneth Edward 8095 S W 71th Avenue, Portland, OR 97223, (503) 245-4386, SLP, Beaverton Schl Dstr #48, **SLP**

Minekime, Karen Johnstone 3708 Monahan Lane, Dublin, OH 43017, (614) 761-3032, BS 71 Purdue Univ - West Lafayette; MA 72 Univ of NM; Aud, US Dept of Labor-OWCP, **A**

Minell, Jane F Northwest ENT Clinic, 1035 North Main Street, Rice Lake, WI 54868, (715) 234-6965, BS 80 Univ of WI - Stevens Point; MS 82 Univ of WI - Stevens Point; Aud, Northwest ENT Cl, **A**

Minella, Trina C 7100 Stella Lane #6, Carmichael, CA 95608, (916) 944-0260, **SLP**

Mineo, Dr Beth Ann 819 Stockbridge Drive, Hockessin, DE 19707, (302) 651-6836, BS 79 PA St Univ - Univ Park; MA 81 Univ of Pittsburgh - Pittsburgh; PH 85 (NS) Univ of Pittsburgh - Pittsburgh; Dir Info Lab, Univ of DE, **SLP**

Miner, Dr Adah L 350 North 190th Street, Cristwood 403-A, Seattle, WA 98133, (206) 363-9753, BA 43 Univ of WA; MA 48 Univ of WA; PH 62 (NS) Univ of WI - Madison; **SLP F LM**

Miner, Kathleen 1578 E Street, Anchorage, AK 99501, (907) 279-7755, BA 72 Marquette Univ; MS 74 Marquette Univ; SLP, Private Practice, **SLP**

Miner, Mrs Lista G R 554 Princeton Park, Madisonville, KY 42431, (502) 821-8234, BS 61 Northwestern Univ; BS 61 Northwestern Univ; **SLP**

Mines, Arthur B Route 1 Box 150, Hillsborough, NC 27278, (919) 286-9797, BA 72 SUNY - Coll at New Paltz; MA 73 Bowling Green St Univ; Exec Dir, Beginnings for Parents of HI Child, **SLP A**

Mines, Ethel S BA 31 CUNY - Hunter Coll; MA 33 Columbia Univ Teachers Coll; **LM**

Mines, Sondra 1401 Randall Court, Los Angeles, CA 90065, MA 67 Millersville Univ of PA; **SLP**

Minges, Geraldine S University Of South Carolina, Speech And Hearing Clinic, 1601 St Julian Place, Columbia, SC 29204, (807) 777-2614, BS 54 Wayne St Univ; ME 73 Univ of SC - Columbia; Cl Instr, U of SC, **SLP**

Minghetti, Nancy J 723 South Charles Street, Apartment 301, Baltimore, MD 21230, (301) 897-5700, BS 74 Kent St Univ; MA 75 Kent St Univ; 86–Prog Dir, American Sp-Lang-Hrng Found, **SLP**

Mingledorff, Tracy L 2506 Houser Road, Knoxville, TN 37919, (615) 585-5381, MA 88 Univ of TN - Knoxville

Mingo, Carla SJ Route 1, Eden, ID 83325, **SLP**

Miniaci, Karen J 725 Coronado Avenue #202, Long Beach, CA 90804, (213) 436-9931, BS 76 CA St Univ - Hayward; MA 79 CA St Univ - Stanislaus; Sp-Lang Path, Long Beach USD, **SLP**

Miniard, Holly P 222 Michigan Avenue, Monticello, KY 42633, (606) 348-5313, BA 80 Univ of KY; MA 82 Eastern KY Univ; 86–Sp/Lang Path, Lifeline Home Health Agency, **SLP**

Minick, Ellen G Gottfred Speech Associates, 1535 Lake Cook Road, Suite 100, Northbrook, IL 60645, (312) 564-9230, BS 75 Northwestern Univ; MS 76 Univ of WI - Madison; Dir, Gottfred Speech Associates, **SLP**

Minick Starke, Heidi 7725 Woodlands Trail, Chesterland, OH 44026, BA 77 Allegheny Coll; MA 78 Case Western Reserve Univ; Sp-Lang Path, Cuyahoga Co Bd for Ment Ret, **SLP**

Minifie, Mrs Ferne 1800 Adams Street, St Helena, CA 94574, (707) 963-7477, BA 36 Pacific Union Coll; MA 60 Univ of CA - Los Angeles; Sp-Lang Path, Primetime-Adult Day Hlth Care, **SLP LM**

Minifie, Dr Fred D Dept Of Speech & Hearing Sci #JG-15, University Of Washington, 1417 N E 42nd Street, Seattle, WA 98195, (206) 543-7974, BA 58 Linfield Coll; MS 62 Univ of IA; PH 63 (NS) Univ of IA; Prof/Chairman Dept Sp-Hrng Sci, University of Washington, **F**

Minix, Paula Vanlaanen 3021 W Wanda Street #1, Milwaukee, WI 53221, (414) 632-9790, BS 82 Univ of WI - Madison; MS 84 Univ of WI - Madison; **SLP**

Mink, Amy Sipes 31 West Coleman Avenue, Chatham, NJ 07928, (201) 906-2649, BA 76 Jersey City St Coll; MA 78 OH Univ - Athens; 83–Prog Coord, Robt W Johnson Jr Lifestyles I, **SLP ACE**

Minkler, Donna Beth 2932 Partridge Avenue, Oakland, CA 94605, (213) 885-8500, MA 77 Case Western Reserve Univ; BA 71 Univ of CA - Berkeley; 86–SLP, Childrens Hosp Med Ctr, **SLP**

Minkler, Pearllynne 2789 South Ivan Way, Denver, CO 80227, (303) 989-9972, BA 71 Univ of FL; ME 72 Univ of FL; 87–Sp-Lang Path, Craig Hosp, **SLP**

Minnich, Julie Anne 3607 West Biddison, Fort Worth, TX 76109, (817) 921-2247, BA 82 TX Christian Univ; MS 84 Univ of TX - Dallas; **SLP**

Minogue-Byrne, Mrs Maureen 61 Exeter Drive, Berkeley Heights, NJ 07922, (201) 988-3347, BS 73 Seton Hall Univ; MA 78 Montclair St Coll; **SLP**

Minor, Birdie J Communication Services, Woodrow Wilson Rehab Ctr, Fishersville, VA 22939, (703) 885-9718, BA 65 FL St Univ; MA 69 Univ of MO - Columbia; Superv Sp-Path, Woodrow Wilson Rehab Cen, **SLP**

Minor, Mrs Carla McNeely 1306 Pinon, Mansfield, TX 76063, (817) 473-1178, BA 71 Univ of TX - Arlington; MS 74 TX Tech Univ

Minor, Mrs Judy Kelley 110 Lakeview Drive #B-4, Morgantown, WV 26505, (304) 291-9217, BA 67 Salem Coll; MS 69 WV Univ; Coord Spec Educ, Monongalia Co Bd of Ed, **SLP**

Minor, Mrs Wendy Mary P O Box 406, Connell, WA 99326, (509) 234-2021, BA 82 Eastern WA Univ; MS 83 Eastern WA Univ; 85–Sp-Lang Path, North Franklin Sch Dist

Minot-Seabrook, Jill Michele 285 Richards Avenue, Portsmouth, NH 03801, (617) 498-9206, BS 75 Emerson Coll; MS 86 Univ of the DC; **SLP**

Minshew, Susan Ricks 4630 Kensington Avenue, Richmond, VA 23226, (804) 786-0431, BS 84 Univ of VA - Charlottesville; ME 86 Univ of VA - Charlottesville; **A**

Minsker, Marilyn c/o Back House, 4588 Elm Wood Court, Riverside, CA 92506-1011, (714) 781-8127, BS SUNY - Coll at Fredonia; MS SUNY - Coll at Fredonia; SLP, Palm Springs USD, **SLP**

Minsky, Mrs Shelley W 28 Lambert Common, Wilton, CT 06897, (914) 285-7294, BA 73 CUNY - Brooklyn Coll; MS 74 Columbia Univ Teachers Coll; 85–Aud, Westchester County Medical Cen, **A**

Minson, Adrienne Ann 15336 Faysmith Avenue, Gardena, CA 90249, (213) 978-0443, MA 88 Univ of Northern CO; 88–Sp-Lang Path/Asst, Rancho Los Amigos Med Ctr

Minson, Mrs Joyce E M 3740 South 96th East Avenue, Tulsa, OK 74145, (918) 252-3561, BS 55 Eastern IL Univ; MA 74 Univ of Tulsa; Sp-Lang Path, Un Pub Sch, **SLP**

Minton, Denise Casimir 12409 Blossomwood, Austin, TX 78759, (512) 926-2410, BS 81 Southwest TX St Univ; ME 82 Southwest TX St Univ; Sp-Lang Path, Travis State School, **SLP**

Minton, Sheila Cohen 1080 Victoria Avenue, Windsor, ON, Canada N9A 4N6, (519) 255-3300, BA 61 PA St Univ - Univ Park; MS 64 PA St Univ - Univ Park; ME 82 Univ of Windsor - Ontario; Consultant Spec Ed Services, Windsor Bd of Ed, **SLP**

Mintz, Mrs Barbara W 29 Pleasant Street, Houlton, ME 04730, (207) 532-6523, BA 73 Rutger's St Univ - Douglas Coll; MS 74 PA St Univ - Univ Park; Coord Sp & Hrng Serv, Aroostook Men Hlth Cen, **SLP**

Mintz, Mrs Laura Brill 24 Edgemount Road, Edison, NJ 08817, (201) 985-8355, BA 72 CUNY - Brooklyn Coll; MA 74 Saint Louis Univ

Mintz, Sandra Lee Arizona State University, Speech & Hearing Science, Tempe, AZ 85287, (602) 965-2373, BA 82 IN Univ - Bloomington; MS 84 Univ of AZ; 86–Aud Supervisor, AZ St U, **A**

Mintz, Susan M 12 Henmar Drive, Closter, NJ 07624, (201) 768-5185, BA 78 Hofstra Univ; MA 79 Univ of Rochester; Sp-Lang Path, Private Practice, **SLP ACE**

Mintz-Bitman, Sari 37 Sumac Court, Mount Laurel, NJ 08504, (609) 342-7600, BS 80 Ithaca Coll; MA 81 George Washington Univ; 88–Sp-Lang Path, Mediplex Rehab-Camden, **SLP**

Mintzes, Dr Susan S 429 Camway Drive, Wilmington, NC 28403, (919) 763-6254, BS 69 Northwestern Univ; MA 70 Northwestern Univ; ED 85 (Educational Administration) Univ of NC - Chapel Hill; 86–Asst Prin, Wrightsboro Elem Sch, **SLP**

Minus, Mrs Bertha D 5905 Southgate Drive, Temple Hills, MD 20748, (202) 727-2639, BA 73 George Washington Univ; MA 74 Univ of the Pacific; Asst Prof, Udc, **SLP**

Minutilli, James Benjamin 1034 Cambridge Station Rd, Apartment A, Centerville, OH 45458, (513) 220-2066, MA 84 OH St Univ; Sp-Lang Path, Miami Valley Hosp, **SLP**

Minyard, Lisa A 2914 Aftonshire Way, Apartment 18201, Austin, TX 78748, BS 85 Southwest TX St Univ; MS 86 Southwest TX St Univ; **SLP**

Mira, Mrs Janet C 1312 Bosler Place, Carlisle, PA 17013, (717) 243-6904, BS 71 Univ of NE - Lincoln; MS 74 Univ of NE - Omaha; **SLP**

Mirabella, Joann 314 Liston Road, Buffalo, NY 14223, (716) 439-6169, BA 81 SUNY - Center at Buffalo; MA 82 SUNY - Center at Buffalo; SLP, Niagara County Speech/Hearing, **SLP**

Mirabella, Mrs Susan M 15435 Sunset Ridge Drive, Orland Park, IL 60462, (312) 349-5335, BS 69 De Paul Univ; MA 76 Governors St Univ; Sp-Lang Path, SW Cook Co Coop Assn Spec Ed, **SLP**

Mirafuentes, Noreen Nenita 1412 St Louis Drive, Honolulu, HI 96816-2036, (808) 735-1359, OB 80 Univ of HI - Manoa; MS 83 Univ of HI - Manoa; SLP, Dept Ed/Leonard Oahu Sch Dist, **SLP**

Miraglia, Jean Ann M 1431 Hendrix Avenue, Thousand Oaks, CA 91360, (805) 495-8370, BA 73 CA St Univ - Northridge; MA 77 CA St Univ - Northridge; Los Angeles USD, **SLP**

Mirakian, Barbara Y 172 Notch Hill Rd, North Branford, CT 06471, **SLP**

Miranda, Carla Yvette 7 Hickory Lane, Cabot, AR 72023, (501) 676-2786, BS 83 Henderson St Univ; MS 85 Univ of Central AR; 86–Sp-Lang Path, Lonoke Exceptional Sch, **SLP**

Miranda, Mrs Judith T 1428 Sunnyvale Court N W, Olympia, WA 98502, (206) 866-8847, BA 72 Mary Washington Coll; ME 73 Univ of VA - Charlottesville; SLP, Shelton Sch Dist #309, **SLP**

Mirandona, Mrs Kathleen B 73-14 220th Street, Bayside, NY 11364, (212) 998-3951, BA 78 SUNY - Coll at New Paltz; MS 79 Adelphi Univ; SLP, NYC Bd of Ed, **SLP**

Mirau, Mrs Maureen M 700 Alvarado Street, Redlands, CA 92373, (714) 792-0098, BA 75 Univ of Redlands; MS 76 Univ of Redlands; Sp-Lang Path, Beaumont USD, **SLP**

Mirch, Marie Brown 1365 Canyon Creek Road, Reno, NV 89523, (702) 747-3495, BS 79 Univ of NV - Reno; MS 80 Univ of NV - Reno; 87–Contr, Gold Club Casino, **SLP**

Mire, Steve P 412 Louis Drive, Houma, LA 70364, (504) 876-4465, BA 79 Nicholls St Univ; OM 80 LA St Univ - N O Medical Ctr; Sp-Lang Path, Terrebonne Parish Sch Bd, **SLP ACE**

Mireles, Mrs Laura Ann 443 North Orange Grove, Los Angeles, CA 90036, (213) 625-4183, BA 81 CA St Univ - Northridge; MA 85 CA St Univ - Northridge; **SLP**

Mirenda, Dr Pat Univ Of Nebraska-Lincoln, 204 F Barkley Memorial Ctr, Lincoln, NE 68583, (402) 472-5479, BA 71 Univ of South FL; MS 83 Univ of WI - Madison; PH 84 (NS) Univ of WI - Madison; Asst Prof, U of NE- Lincoln

Mires, Joann M 4617 North Arna Way, Atwater, CA 95301, (209) 394-7456, BA 63 San Jose St Univ; **SLP**

Miric, Leigh Anne 4503 Atlantic Boulevard, Apartment 1424, Coconut Creek, FL 33066, (305) 786-3515, MA 85 Kent St Univ; **SLP**

Mirman, Anne M 6283 Rutherford Place, Columbus, OH 43213, (614) 263-5151, BS 63 OH St Univ; MA 76 OH St Univ; 88–Prog Dir, Columbus Sp & Hearing Ctr, **SLP**

Mirmelstein, Mrs Marcy R 6020 Timber Creek Lane, Dallas, TX 75248, (214) 248-1570, BS 77 Bradley Univ; MS 78 Univ of WI - Milwaukee; Sp-Lang Path, **SLP**

Miron, Mrs Helen K 612 West Nevada Street, Urbana, IL 61801, (217) 431-5400, BS 53 Northwestern Univ; ME 83 Univ of IL - Urbana; Sp-Lang Path, Danville Comm Sch Dist 118, **SLP**

Mirrett, Penny L 217 Lochridge, Durham, NC 27713, (919) 684-5417, BS 69 CO St Univ; MA 70 Univ of Northern CO; Coord Child Lang Svcs, Duke Univ Med Ctr, **SLP**

Mirro, Janice F 1804 Forrest Avenue, Memphis, TN 38112, (901) 522-6606, BS 74 Temple Univ; MA 76 Temple Univ; 82–Sp-Lang Path, Baptist Mem Hosp, **SLP**

Misback, Mrs Peggy S 4505 Amherst Road, College Park, MD 20740, **SLP**

Misch, Mrs Diane L P O Box 3239, Napa, CA 94558, (707) 255-0143, BA 68 Univ of OK - Norman; MA 69 Univ of OK - Norman; Sp-Lang Path, Napa County Supt of Schools, **SLP**

Mischell-Schnitzer, Alane Myra 196-15C 65 Crescent #1-B, Fresh Meadows, NY 11365, (718) 263-1587, MA 88 CUNY - Queens Coll; 88–Sp-Lang Path, Inter Ctr for Child Develop

Mischke, Renetta M 10 Timm Place, Sheridan, WY 82801, (307) 672-6610, BS 77 Univ of NE - Omaha; MS 78 Univ of NE - Omaha; 85–Sp-Lang Path, Children's Ctr Region II, **SLP**

Miscioscia, Mrs Elizabeth S 21 Maple Avenue, Tarrytown, NY 10591, (914) 332-1580, BS 80 Southeast MO St Univ; ME 81 Southeast MO St Univ; Sp-Lang Path, BOCES Southern Westchester, **SLP**

Misenhelder, Mrs Faye Cagle 3530 Tyrone Boulevard N, Lot 68, St Petersburg, FL 33710, (813) 381-2729, MA; **SLP**

Mishcon, Victoria Louise Elbow Pond Road, RFD 1 P O Box 2202, Andover, NH 03216-9801, (603) 934-4449, Sp-Lang Path, Kearsarge Reg Sch District, **SLP**

Mishkin, Mrs Lois W 1579 Rising Way, Mountainside, NJ 07092, (201) 937-7952, BS 67 NY Univ; MA 70 NY Univ; OM 80 Montclair St Coll; Prog Coord, Ctr for Cognitive Rehab, **SLP ACE**

Mishler, Pamela J 29 Rue Royale #K, Kettering, OH 45429, (513) 268-6511, BS 73 Univ of Akron; MS 76 Univ of South FL; PH 87 (Aud) Univ of Cincinnati; Aud, Dayton VA Hospital, **A**

Mishler, Mrs Shelley Steel Audiological Laboratory Ltd, 8780 Golf Road, Suite 200, Des Plaines, IL 60016, (312) 824-8789, BA 80 MI St Univ; MA 82 George Washington Univ; Aud, Audiological Laboratory Ltd, **A**

Mishler, Mrs Tracy Mehan Washington University, Dept Of Otolaryngology, 517 South Euclid, St Louis, MO 63144, (314) 362-7489, BS 80 Northwestern Univ; MA 81 Northwestern Univ; 84–Aud, Washington Univ Sch of Med, **A**

Miskell, John J P O Box 292, Jersey City, NJ 07303, (212) 369-0500, BA 67 Univ of MO - Columbia; MA 69 Univ of MO - Columbia; MA 72 Northeast MO St Univ; SLP, Manhattan Psychiatric Cen, **SLP**

Miskin, Kathryn Ann 12 126 Thompkins Drive #B, Austin, TX 78753, (512) 451-2931, BA 84 Univ of Pittsburgh - Pittsburgh; MA 86 Univ of TX - Austin; 86–Sp-Lang Path, Austin Reg Day Sch for the Deaf, **SLP**

Miskinis, Mrs Angela Lalla 5 Chestnut Street, Amsterdam, NY 12010, (518) 842-4809, BA 83 SUNY - Coll at Plattsburgh; MA 85 SUNY - Coll at Geneseo

Misler, Mrs Donna T 2202 Caves Road, Owings Mills, MD 21117, (301) 655-9070, BA 76 Univ of MD - College Park; MS 78 Towson St Univ; Sp-Lang Path, Anne Arundel County Public Sch, **SLP**

Mis-Palley, Cindy 35 Harkness Rd, Pelham, MA 01002-9704, (413) 536-3900, BA 77 Univ of MA - Amherst; MA 79 Univ of MA - Amherst; Sp-Lang Path, Presch Enrichment Team Inc, **SLP**

Missal, Mrs Donna M 4289 South Atlantic Avenue, Daytona Beach, FL 32019, BS 67 De Paul Univ; MA 75 Governors St Univ; Sp-Lang Path, Volusia County Schools, **SLP**

Misso, Mrs Anita S 815 N Forest Road, Williamsville, NY 14221, (716) 626-9336, MS 67 SUNY - Coll at Buffalo; BS 60 SUNY - Coll at Buffalo; Sp-Lang Path, Buffalo Bd of Ed, **SLP**

Mistal, Gregory Joseph P O Box 91, Arva, ON, Canada N0M 1C0, (519) 453-4400, BA 70 Northern MI Univ; MA 71 Western MI Univ; Coord Cl Serv, Ministry of Ed, **A**

Mistretta, Anna 2359 Cambridge Street, East Meadow, NY 11554, (516) 542-3455, BS 71 Columbia Univ Teachers Coll; MS 73 Columbia Univ Teachers Coll; SLP, Dewitt Nurs Home, **SLP**

Mistric, Mrs Catherine 2609 Price, Nederland, TX 77627, (409) 838-8170, BS 78 Lamar Univ; MS 80 Lamar Univ; Cl Superv, Lamar Univ, **SLP**

Mitaly, Mrs Barbara J 68 Jennifer Lane, Milford, CT 06460, (203) 878-9653, BA 71 Univ of CT; MS 73 Southern CT St Univ; **SLP**

Mitch, James L 822D Cabell Avenue, Charlottesville, VA 22903, (804) 924-3562, OB 80 Clarion Univ of PA; MA 82 Univ of IA; Asst Prof, Univ of VA, **SLP**

Mitchell, Mrs Amy Burns 2790 Hamilton Creek Drive, Mobile, AL 36695, (205) 431-3425, BS 81 Univ of South AL; MS 83 Univ of South AL; 87–Sp-Lang Path, Univ of South Alabama, **SLP**

Mitchell, Mrs Ann B 8903 Meadowknoll Drive, Dallas, TX 75243, (214) 788-0491, BS 76 Southern Methodist Univ; MS 77 Southern Methodist Univ; Sp-Lang Path, Associated Health Focus, **SLP**

Mitchell, Cecile A 927 South Westmoreland Avenue, #207, Los Angeles, CA 90006, (213) 387-6546, BA 73 Adelphi Univ; MS 75 Columbia Univ Teachers Coll; **A**

Mitchell, Mrs Christine D 6138 Tamilynn Street, San Diego, CA 92122, (619) 452-6207, BA 71 Paine Coll; MS 74 Univ of IL - Urbana; Sp-Lang Path, Chicago Board of Education

Mitchell, Clydie K 9419 Shartel Drive, Shreveport, LA 71118, (318) 226-5106, BA 59 Northwestern St Univ; ME 64 Northwestern St Univ; Dir Chldn Cen, LA St U Med Cen, **SLP**

Mitchell, Edgar D 408 Brookside Avenue, Redlands, CA 92373, (714) 792-3223, BA 60 Univ of WA; MA 67 Univ of Redlands; Sp-Lang Path, Private Practice, **SLP**

Mitchell, Mrs Gail H Rd N 2 Box 10, Addison, NY 14801, (607) 776-7631, BS 70 SUNY - Coll at Geneseo; MS 73 SUNY - Coll at Geneseo; 88–Sp-Lang Path, Steuben-Allegany BOCES, **SLP**

Mitchell, Harold R 519 Weeping Elm Road, Mount Juliet, TN 37122, (615) 320-3229, PH (NS); **SLP**

Mitchell, Jacqueline 519 Weeping Elm Road, Mount Juliet, TN 37122, PH (NS); **SLP**

Mitchell, Mrs Jane O'Connor 27 Patrick Road, Tewksbury, MA 01876, (617) 851-4693, BA 83 Univ of Miami; MS 85 Univ of TX - Dallas; **SLP**

Mitchell, John C, Jr 32969 Lyndon, Livonia, MI 48154, **SLP**

Mitchell, Judy M 1426 Wayside Drive, Tyler, TX 75701, (214) 593-8313, **SLP**

Mitchell, Mrs Karen K 7631 Ashworth Street, Worthington, OH 43085, (614) 294-6403, BS 78 WV Univ; MS 79 WV Univ; Audiologist, Columbus Sp & Hrng Cen, **A**

Mitchell, Karyn S 5858 Beacon Street, Pittsburgh, PA 15217, (412) 421-6607, BA 67 Columbia Union Coll; MS 76 Univ of the DC; Sp-Lang Path, Private Practice, **SLP**

Mitchell, Mrs Lillian R 1619 Washington Avenue, Findlay, OH 45840, (419) 423-1693, BA 66 Bowling Green St Univ; MA 68 Bowling Green St Univ; Aud, Roy E Hutchison MD, **A ACE**

Mitchell, Linda Sue 100 Walnut Street, Bordentown, NJ 08505, (215) 757-0227, BS 77 Trenton St Coll; MS 80 Trenton St Coll; 77–Sp-Lang Path, Bucks Co Intermed Unit #22, **SLP**

Mitchell, Mrs Lisa A Rd 1 Box 123-B, Beavertown, PA 17813, (717) 658-3405, BS 82 Bloomsburg Univ of PA; MS 83 Bloomsburg Univ of PA; SLP, Private Practice, **SLP**

Mitchell, Mrs Lisa Ann 26 Harris Road, Salem, NH 03079, BA 82 Boston Coll; MS 84 Emerson Coll; 88–Sp-Lang Path, Pentucket Reg Schs, **SLP**

Mitchell, Lora Porter 673 Exmoor Court, Crystal Lake, IL 60014, (815) 455-5513, BS 72 OR St Univ; MA 87 Northern IL Univ - De Kalb; 87–Sp-Lang Path, Comm Unit Sch Dist 220, **SLP**

Mitchell, Mrs Louann S 1003 Forrest Drive, Tullahoma, TN 37388, (615) 455-1506, BS 54 Auburn Univ - Auburn; MA 70 G Peabody Coll-Vanderbilt U; Sp-Lang Path, Tullahoma City Sch Sys, **SLP**

Mitchell, Mrs Lynn Farrell 1481 Hodges Mill Rd, Bogart, GA 30622, (404) 769-6002, BS 77 Univ of GA; ME 85 Univ of GA; **SLP**

Mitchell, Mrs Marilyn P 31 Earle Avenue, Bangor, ME 04401, (207) 848-3370, BS 71 SUNY - Coll at Buffalo; MS 73 SUNY - Coll at Buffalo; 80–Sp-Lang Path, School Union 34, **SLP**

Mitchell, Mary Wagner 5407 Fairway Road, Fairway, KS 66205, (913) 621-6610, OB 84 Univ of MO - Columbia; MA 87 Univ of KS; **SLP**

Mitchell, Megan Anne 5456 Dallas Street, P O Box 167, Lexington, MI 48450, (313) 987-5000, BA 86 MI St Univ; MA 87 Central MI Univ; 87–Sp-Lang Path, C & C Health Care Assoc, **SLP**

Mitchell, Mrs Michelle Cullerton P O Box 804, 700 Main Street, Boylston, MA 01505, (617) 824-6911, BS 84 Univ of MA - Amherst; ME 86 Univ of VA - Charlottesville; SLP, Morton Hosp & Med Ctr, **SLP**

Mitchell, Nancy A Route 4, 304 Brandys Place, Columbus, MS 39702, (601) 328-3365, **SLP**

Mitchell, Norma C 923 Lillooet Street West, Moose Jaw, SK, Canada S6H 4Z7, (306) 693-4631, BA 73 Univ of Regina -Saskatchewan; MS 83 Minot St Univ; Sp-Lang Path, Moose Jaw Shared Services, **SLP**

Mitchell, Dr Oscar, Jr Southern University, Box 9888, Baton Rouge, LA 70813, (504) 771-3950, BS Univ of Pittsburgh - Pittsburgh; MS Univ of Pittsburgh - Pittsburgh; PH 69 (NS) Univ of Pittsburgh - Pittsburgh; Prof & Chmn, Sn U A M Coll, **SLP A LM**

Mitchell, Dr Pamela R 805 Allen Hall, Assistive Technology Center/ACCESS, West Virginia University, Morgantown, WV 26506-6122, (304) 293-4242, BA 76 OH St Univ; MA 78 OH St Univ; PH 88 (Commun Disord) Univ of WA; 84–Asst Prof, West VA U, **SLP**

Mitchell, Mrs Patricia D 1049-8 Chena Road, Fort Wainwright, AK 99703, (914) 356-1219, BS 73 IN Univ - Bloomington; MA 74 IN Univ - Bloomington; 87–Sp-Lang Path, Fairbanks North Star Sch Dist, **SLP**

Mitchell, Robin S 10 Kallista Avenue, St Ives, New South Wales, Australia 2075, BS 78 Ithaca Coll; MA 83 CUNY - Hunter Coll; Sp-Lang Path, Lady Davidson Hosp, **SLP**

Mitchell, Sarah F 3000 Yorktown, Mesquite, TX 75149, (214) 288-7394, OB 70 Southern Methodist Univ; OM 69 Southern Methodist Univ; **SLP**

Mitchell, Terry P O Box 5538, Berkeley, CA 94705, (415) 461-9770, BA 72 Univ of CA - Los Angeles; MS 78 San Francisco St Univ; Aud, Aud Svcs, **A**

Mitchell, Thomas R 675 West Lake Street #339, Oak Park, IL 60302, (312) 383-2233, BS 81 Univ of North TX; MS 84 Univ of North TX; Reg Rep

Mitchell, Willa May 14819 East 46th Street, Independence, MO 64055, (816) 478-1677, BS 73 Central MO St Univ; MS 86 Central MO St Univ; **SLP**

Mitchener, Karl K R R 1 Box 524, Carbondale, IL 62901, (618) 833-5161, BS 74 Southern IL Univ -Carbondale; MS 78 Southern IL Univ -Carbondale; Sp-Lang Path, Choate Mental Hlth & Dev Ctr, **SLP**

Mitchener, Mrs Marilyn H R R 1 Box 524, Carbondale, IL 62901, (618) 724-2631, BS 74 Southern IL Univ -Carbondale; MS 77 Southern IL Univ -Carbondale; Sp/Lang Path, Christopher Grade Sch Unit 34, **SLP**

Mitchener-Colston, Mrs Wanda K 4312 13th Place Northeast, Washington, DC 20017, (202) 635-3160, MS 73 Univ of the DC; BA 72 Shaw Univ; Sp-Lang Path, Howard U Chld Dev Cen, **SLP**

Miterman, Gail Pamela 559 Joralemon Street, Belleville, NJ 07109, (201) 233-3720, BS 82 PA St Univ - Univ Park; MS 84 Boston Univ; Clin Coord, Childrens Spec Hosp, **SLP**

Mito, Marion J 2616 Wilshire Lane, Arlington Heights, IL 60004, BA 75 Univ of PA; MA 77 Northwestern Univ; Cl Super, Rehab I of Chicago, **SLP**

Mitrani, Mrs Laurie Cohen 2333 Brickell Avenue #1816, Miami, FL 33129, (305) 856-1096, BS 83 Univ of VA - Charlottesville; ME 85 Univ of VA - Charlottesville; 86–Aud, Miami Mailman Ctr Child Dev, **A**

Mitson, Linda A 34106 Avenue J, Yucaipa, CA 92399, BA 71 Univ of Western Ontario; MA 74 Univ of Western Ontario; SLP, **SLP**

Mitsuda, Patricia M 5525 28th N E, Seattle, WA 98105, (206) 223-3166, BS 72 Portland St Univ; OM 74 Univ of WA; SLP Cl Superv, VW Hosp/Harborview Med Cen, **SLP**

Mitsunaga, Faye F 6626 Picasso Road #34, Isla Vista, CA 93117, (805) 968-6858, MA 88 Univ of CA - Santa Barbara

Mittag, Lori Anderson 514 5th Street Ct, West Fargo, ND 58078, (701) 237-6424, BS 80 Moorhead St Univ; MS 87 Moorhead St Univ; **SLP**

Mittleman, Penny S 10 East Cedar Lane, Maplewood, NJ 07040, (201) 763-1980, BA 75 Adelphi Univ; MS 77 Gallaudet Coll; Aud, Haskill Hearing Aid Center, **A**

Mittler, Amy 527 Thrid Avenue, #216, New York, NY 10016, (212) 340-6027, MA 85 CUNY - Queens Coll; 88–Sp-Lang Path, NYU Med Ctr Rusk Inst, **SLP**

Mittler, Thomas F 14407 South Tripp, Midlothian, IL 60445, (312) 747-8100, BA 76 Coll of Saint Francis; MS 79 Governors St Univ; 88–Dir of Training, E Ludeman Dev Ctr, **SLP**

Mittman, Mrs Ellen K 14 Longmeadow Road, Newton, MA 02159, (617) 965-6280, BA 70 George Washington Univ; MS 74 Rutgers St Univ - Newark; 88–Sp-Lang Path, Walker Sch, **SLP**

Mittnight, Helen Hill 72 Morris Avenue, Haworth, NJ 07641, (201) 385-5162, BS 53 Univ of IL - Urbana; MA 83 Montclair St Coll; 87–Sp-Lang Path, UCP New York State, **SLP**

Mitton, Rosemary P S70 W23425 Millbrook Circle, Big Bend, WI 53103, **SLP**

Mitz, Mrs Lynda R 9265 North Regent Road, Bayside, WI 53217, (414) 351-6623, BS 73 Univ of WI - Milwaukee; MS 74 Univ of WI - Milwaukee; Sp-Lang Path, Brown Deer Sch Dist, **SLP**

Mitz, Mary E P O Box 69, Joshua Tree, CA 92252, **SLP**

Mixdorf, Mrs Carol F T 2500 South Carpenter, Appleton, WI 54915, MA 71 Univ of Northern IA; Sp-Lang Path, Appleton Area School District, **SLP**

Mixon, Mrs Carolyn Johnson 4616 Chiappero, Austin, TX 78731, (512) 451-9564, BS 77 Midwestern St Univ; MA 82 Univ of TX - Austin; Sp-Lang Path, ISD, **SLP**

Miyamoto, Kay D 4261 North 5th, Fresno, CA 93726, (209) 431-2231, BA 78 CA St Univ - Fresno; Sp-Lang Path, Fresno Co Dept of Ed, **SLP**

Miyamoto, Naomi H 507 Melemele Street, Wailuku, HI 96793, (808) 871-6881, **SLP**

Miyamura, Kelly Hisae 273 Casuda Canyon #B, Monterey Park, CA 91754, (818) 282-0824, MA 86 CA St Univ - Los Angeles

Mizar-Ortiz, Kathryn A P O Box 2083, Las Cruces, NM 88004, (505) 233-3236, BA 68 Univ of TX - El Paso; MA 83 NM St Univ; Sp-Lang Path, Gadsden ISD, **SLP**

Mize, Carole G 5307 West 14th, Topeka, KS 66604, (913) 272-1600, BA 64 KS St Univ; MA 77 KS St Univ; Sp-Lang Path, Topeka USD #501, **SLP**

Mize, Cathleen S 710 Seventh Street Apartment 7, Bowling Green, OH 43402, (419) 353-3109, BS 81 Ball St Univ; MA 82 Western IL Univ; **SLP**

Mize, Christina Joyce 1015 Narciso Court, San Jose, CA 95129, (415) 349-9922, BA 83 San Jose St Univ; MA 85 San Jose St Univ; **SLP**

Mize, David Lee Speech And Hearing Services, Nash General Hospital, Rocky Mount, NC 27801, (919) 443-8730, BA 78 Univ of MS; MA 79 Univ of MS; Aud, Nash Gen Hosp, **A**

Mize, Dr Jean C Route 1 Box 135D, Union, SC 29379, (803) 427-9040, ME 73 Winthrop Coll; MS 76 Winthrop Coll; ED 84 (Sp Ed Adm) Univ of SC - Columbia; Sp-Lang Path, Cherokee Co Sch Dist #1, **SLP**

Mize, Mrs Maura C Acadian Hearing & Speech Services, 555 South Ryan, Lake Charles, LA 70601, (318) 436-3277, BA 74 LA St Univ - Baton Rouge; ME 83 Tulane Univ; MA 76 Univ of TN - Knoxville; Sp-Lang Path, Private Practice, **SLP**

Mize, Pamala Dawn 1470 West Main Street, Wytheville, VA 24382, (703) 326-2635, BS 81 Radford Univ; MS 82 Radford Univ; Aud, Dr David M Harris, **A**

Mizell, Dr Diann 739 Boyd Avenue, Richmond, CA 94805-1719, (415) 232-1355, BS 61 Henderson St Univ; MA 66 Univ of Houston - Univ Park; PH 83 (Sp & Hrng Sciences) Univ of CA - San Francisco; 80–Sp-Lang Path, San Francisco USD, **SLP**

Mizell, Marilyn Purvis 740 West Gibson Street, Arcadia, FL 33821, (813) 494-4222, BA 52 Stetson Univ; ME 58 Univ of FL; Director Exceptional Stud Educ, Desoto County School Board, **SLP**

Mizerak, Deborah Jean 377 Fellsway West, Medford, MA 02155, (617) 391-8184, BA; MS; **SLP**

Mizuko, Dr Mark I Allied Clinical Health, Univ Of Minnesota-Duluth, 242 Montague Hall, Duluth, MN 55812, (218) 726-8203, BS 72 Univ of HI - Manoa; MS 74 Univ of HI - Manoa; PH 85 (NS) Univ of WI - Madison; Asst Prof, U of MN, **SLP A**

Mizushima, Margaret 2550 East Co Road #62E, Wellington, CO 80549, (303) 482-4111, BA 74 Univ of Northern CO; MS 75 CO St Univ; Dept Hd/SLP, Poudre Valley Hosp, **SLP**

Mlacnik, Mrs Victoria Sowinski 1529 W Cook, Springfield, IL 62704, (217) 788-3767, MS 83 Univ of IL - Urbana; Sp-Lang Path, Memorial Medical Center, **SLP**

Mlcoch, Dr Anthony G Dept Speech Path & Audiology, Hines VA Hospital, Hines, IL 60141, (312) 343-7200, MA 72 SUNY - Coll at Geneseo; PH 80 (NS) Purdue Univ - West Lafayette; Sp-Lang Path, Hines VA Hospital, **SLP**

Mlinar, Theresa Patricia 11517 Ivywood Street N W, Coon Rapids, MN 55433, (612) 753-2557, BA 81 Univ of ND; MS 83 Univ of ND; **SLP**

Mlotek, Mrs Janet Ritter 2918 South 116th Avenue, Omaha, NE 68144, (402) 978-7069, BA 80 Univ of SD - Vermillion; MA 81 Univ of SD - Vermillion; Sp-Lang Path, Omaha Pub Schs, **SLP**

Moake, Mary E 4222 Swarthmore, Houston, TX 77005, **SLP**

Moat, Mrs Dorothy J Bridges & Hardy, Medical Plaza 901, 601 East Dixie Avenue, Leesburg, FL 32748, (904) 728-2404, BS 82 FL St Univ; MS 85 FL St Univ; 85–Aud, Bridges & Hardy MD PA, **A**

Moats, Barbara H 4780 North Delno, Fresno, CA 93705, (209) 485-8560, BA 79 CA St Univ - Fresno; MA 80 CA St Univ - Fresno; Sp-Lang Path, Fresno County Headstart, **SLP**

Mobeck, Mrs Jeanette G 25 Elizabeth Street, Branford, CT 06405-5528, (203) 481-4187, BS 71 Southern CT St Univ; MS 73 Southern CT St Univ; Sp/Lang Path, Bd of Ed-Cty of New Haven, **SLP**

Mobley, Cynthia L 4900 Pear Ridge Drive, Apartment 2402, Dallas, TX 75287, (214) 248-4373, BS 78 Univ of North TX; MS 79 Univ of North TX; 87–Sp-Lang Path, Richardson Spo & L Clinic, **SLP**

Mobley, Mrs Mary Morgan 308 Ash, Amite, LA 70422, (504) 748-5412, **SLP**

Mobley, Mrs Patricia A 19860 Dorset, Southfield, MI 48075, (313) 355-2735, BA 68 Univ of MI - Ann Arbor; MA 69 Eastern MI Univ; Sp-Lang Path, Hawthorn Cen, **SLP ACE**

Moccia, Diane T 2134 Beechcreek Lane, Cincinnati, OH 45238, **SLP**

Moch, Mrs Corinne Sylvia 6007 North Sheridan Road, Apartment 21C, Chicago, IL 60660, (312) 275-2543, OB 50; MA 65 De Paul Univ

Moch, Ozzie Ree 1612 Glen Avenue, Shreveport, LA 71109, BS 73 0500; OM 83 LA St Univ - N O Medical Ctr; **SLP**

Mochel, Anne Louise North 12229 Ruby Road, Spokane, WA 99218, (509) 466-2938, MS 88 Eastern WA Univ

Mockbee, Mrs Jo Anne Valcho 130 Waldorf Drive, Akron, OH 44313, (216) 867-0057, BS 84 Univ of Cincinnati; MA 86 Univ of Akron; 88–Sp-Lang Path, Allied Health Rehab Center, **SLP**

Mockridge, Candace A 224 Ridgeview Drive, Venetia, PA 15367, **SLP**

Modahl, Mrs Jackie P 10907 Kewanee Drive, Temple Terrace, FL 33617, (813) 985-6047, BS 77 Saint Louis Univ; MA 79 Saint Louis Univ; Sp-Lang Path, Hillsborough Co Bd of Educ, **SLP**

Modde, Mrs Karen A 9766 Purcell Road, Richmond, VA 23228, (804) 261-7669, BS 85 Southeast MO St Univ; MA 87 Southeast MO St Univ; SLP, Hanover County Schools

Modell, Lisa Fern 3133 Rochambeau Avenue, Bronx, NY 10467, (212) 645-3773, MS 86 Columbia Univ Teachers Coll; **SLP**

Modin, Mrs Nancy G Box 782, Salina, KS 67401, (913) 827-0301, BS 72 Fort Hays St Univ; MA 73 KS St Univ; Sp/Lang Path, Central KS Coop In Ed, **SLP**

Modlin, Diane M 578 West Armitage, Elmhurst, IL 60126, (312) 832-3151, BA 80 Augustana Coll; MA 81 Western MI Univ; Sp-Lang Path, Leyden Hs-Dist 212, **SLP**

Modlin, Mrs Marika G 4301-B Myrtlewood Drive, Huntsville, AL 35816, (205) 837-4430, MS 87 Univ of Montevallo; **SLP**

Modreck, George A 102 Hawthorne Road, Pittsburgh, PA 15221, (412) 242-1834, BA OH St Univ; MA OH St Univ; Aud, Chldns Hosp of Pittsburgh, **A**

Modugno Okin, Paula 90 Schenck Avenue #1E, Great Neck, NY 11021, (516) 466-3451, BA 79 CUNY - Queens Coll; MA 81 CUNY - Queens Coll; Dir, North Shore Sp-Lang Assoc, **SLP ACE**

Moe, Eunice W 16705 Briardale Road, Rockville, MD 20855, Aud Tchr/Spec, Montgomery Co Pub Sch, **SLP**

Moe, Janet M S 1310 Childs Road West, Omaha, NE 68147, (402) 291-4976, BS 61 ND St Univ; MS 79 Towson St Univ; 88–Sp/Lang Path, Omaha PS, **SLP**

Moellenbeck, Karen Ann Box 205A Rt 24, Lewes, DE 19958, (302) 856-5213, BS 82 Southwest MO St Univ; MA 85 Southwest MO St Univ; 87–Sp-Lang Path, Div of Public Health, **SLP**

Moeller, Mrs Debra Ann 1301 East 48th Street, Savannah, GA 31404, (912) 355-2148, SLP, ABC Health Services, **SLP**

Moeller, Mrs Leslie A 117 Cedar Road, Severna Park, MD 21146, BS 70 OH Univ - Athens; MA 71 OH Univ - Athens; Sp-Lang Path, Baltimore Cty Pub Sch, **SLP**

Moeller, Mrs Mary P Boys Town National Institute, 555 North 30th Street, Omaha, NE 68181, (402) 449-6521, BS 72 Purdue Univ - West Lafayette; MS 73 Purdue Univ - West Lafayette; Aud, Boys Town National Institute, **A F**

Moeller, Sharon A 3726 West Augusta Avenue, Phoenix, AZ 85051, (602) 965-6796, BS 66 AZ St Univ; OM 80 LA St Univ - N O Medical Ctr; 88–Sp/Lang Path, US West/Arizona State Univ, **SLP ACE**

Moeller, Susan Jeannette 1626 Williams Street, Boise, ID 83706, (208) 746-2337, **SLP**

Moelter, Mary Kathryn R R 3 Box 182, River Falls, WI 54022, (612) 388-2843, BS 86 Univ of WI - River Falls; MS 88 Univ of WI - River Falls; 88–SLP, Red Wing Health Ctr

Moen, Christine Spece Rt 1 Box 225, Fergus Falls, MN 56537, (218) 739-3824, BS 81 Saint Cloud St Univ; MS 83 Saint Cloud St Univ; **SLP**

Moen, Gayl L 5017 Galano Drive, Camarillo, CA 93010-5234, (805) 482-9838, BA 78 CA St Univ - Northridge; MA 80 CA St Univ - Northridge; **SLP**

Moen, Mrs Lucille A 516 River Oak, Ames, IA 50010, (515) 232-7583, BS 62 Univ of ND; BS 67 Mankato St Univ; MA 74 Univ of Northern IA; Sp-Lang Path, Heartland AEA, **SLP**

Moering, Betty C 6022 Vassar Avenue N E, Seattle, WA 98115, (206) 543-8799, BA 73 San Diego St Univ; MS 75 Univ of WA; Lecturer, U of WA, **SLP**

Moerman, Jane Francis 404 West Northpoint Court, Peoria, IL 61614, (309) 692-8607, **SLP**

Moestue, Mrs Mary Jean P O Box 194, Eureka, IL 61530, (309) 444-3943, BS 56 Northern IL Univ - De Kalb; MS 75 IL St Univ - Normal; Sp-Lang Path, Central Grade Sch Dist 51, **SLP**

Moffa, Mrs Barbara C 119 Duncannon Road, Bel Air, MD 21014, (301) 879-6188, BA 74 Univ of MD - College Park; MS 75 Ithaca Coll; Sp-Lang Path, Private Practice, **SLP**

Moffa, Carol Ludwig 259 Kings Grant Road, Marborough, MA 01752, (617) 852-1626, **SLP**

Moffatt, Mrs Bridgett G Box 979, George West, TX 78022, **SLP ACE**

Moffatt, Mrs Karen Baird Rt 8 Box 101, Maryville, TN 37801, (615) 977-8890, BS 85 Univ of TN - Knoxville; MA 86 Univ of TN - Knoxville; 87–Sp-Lang Path, Blount County Schs, **SLP**

Moffatt, Rose Ann 116 McLeod, Missoula, MT 59801, (406) 777-2494, BS 77 Univ of MT; MA 85 Univ of MT; **SLP A**

Moffet, Bethann 7806 Shadow Bend Drive, Huntsville, AL 35802, (615) 433-7026, BS 86 Auburn Univ - Auburn; MS 87 Auburn Univ - Auburn; 87–Sp-Lang Path, Elk Valley Prof Affiliates

Moffitt, Mrs Peggie Collins 116 Bernhurst Road, New Bern, NC 28560, (919) 633-8892, BS 77 East Carolina Univ; MS 81 East Carolina Univ; 86–Sp-Lang Path, Craven Reg Med Ctr, **SLP**

Mogensen, Mrs Mary Beringer 57 Basket Shop Road, Hebron, CT 06248, (203) 228-9458, BS 69 Southern CT St Univ; MS 71 Southern CT St Univ; 70–Sp-Lang Path, Hebron Bd of Ed, **SLP**

Mogi, Mrs Jonet Ahuna P O Box 4162, Kaneohe, HI 96744, (808) 239-7727, BS 83 Univ of HI - Manoa; MS 85 Univ of HI - Manoa; Sp-Lang Path, Department of Education, **SLP**

Mogil, Shelley I Rehab Institute Of Chicago, 345 East Superior Street, Chicago, IL 60611, (312) 908-6020, BA 72 Ithaca Coll; MS 73 Columbia Univ Teachers Coll; 86–Asst Dir Allied Hlth & Nursing, Rehab Insti of Chicago, **SLP**

Mohardt, Karen Diane 3857 Coraltree Circle #303, Coconut Creek, FL 33073, (407) 487-6443, BS 86 East Carolina Univ; ME 88 Univ of FL; 88–Sp-Lang Path, Palm Beach Co Schs

Moheet, Denise M K 12011 Laneview Drive, Houston, TX 77070, (713) 462-6192, BA 76 Bloomsburg Univ of PA; MA 81 Univ of Houston - Univ Park; Sp-Lang Path, Cypress Fairbanks ISD, **SLP**

Mohler, Sally A 1716 Creasy Lane North, Lafayette, IN 47905, (317) 494-3792, BA 73 Purdue Univ - West Lafayette; MS 74 Purdue Univ - West Lafayette; 88–Supvr, Purdue Univ, **SLP**

Mohn, Mrs Nichole Aline 5135 Redwood Drive, Indiana, PA 15701, (412) 349-5070, **SLP**

Mohr, Ann H O 7215 8th Avenue, Regina, SK, Canada S4T 0X1, (306) 545-2635, BS 72 Southern IL Univ -Carbondale; MS 75 Univ of WI - Milwaukee; **SLP**

Mohr, Mrs Barbara A 1535 Foster Court, Longmont, CO 80501, (303) 772-7700, BA 63 Univ of IA; MA 78 Univ of Northern CO; Sp-Lang Path, St Vrain Valley Sch Dist, **SLP**

Mohr, Cheryl Kay 333 Cinnamon Drive #76, Lemoore, CA 93245, (209) 584-1441, BS 79 Univ of IA; MA 80 Univ of IA; SLP, Kings Co Supt of Sch, **SLP**

Mohr, Waynette F 52 Tfw-Psc Box 3135, APO New York, NY 09123, BS 77 MS Univ for Women; MS 76 MS Univ for Women; **SLP**

Mohs, Mrs Margaret Jo K 1621 Cedarberry Road, North Platte, NE 69101, (308) 532-3300, BS 72 Moorhead St Univ; MA 79 Univ of NE - Lincoln; Sp-Lang Path, N Platte Pub Sch Sys, **SLP**

Moidel, Barbara 5317 Randolph Road #6, Rockville, MD 20852, (202) 295-2307, BS 72 OH Univ - Athens; MA 73 Western MI Univ; 86–Sp-Lang Path, Naval Hosp Naval Med Command, **SLP**

Moir, Jane Magennis 26844 Grayslake Road, Rancho Palos Verdes, CA 90274, (213) 543-1223, BA 62 Westminster Coll; MA 65 Univ of Southern CA; Prog Admin, Los Angeles Co Ofc of Educ, **SLP**

Moisan, Patricia Lee Audiology/ENT Clinic, Ft Carson U S Army Hospital, Fort Carson, CO 80913, (719) 579-7450, BA 76 Univ of CO - Boulder; MS 81 Southern CT St Univ; Aud, Dept of Defense, **A**

Mokotoff, Mrs Barbara C 9049 Bywood Park Drive, Seminole, FL 34647, (813) 392-9292, BA 70 Case Western Reserve Univ; MA 72 Case Western Reserve Univ; **A**

Mokry, Deborah L 503 North Washington Street, Apartment 12, Rome, NY 13440, (315) 738-1366, BA 80 SUNY - Coll at Plattsburgh; MA 82 SUNY - Coll at Plattsburgh; 87–Sp/Lang Path, Oneida County Assoc for Retarded Citizens, **SLP**

Molacek, Mrs Vicki Louise 5805 Nicholas, Omaha, NE 68132, (402) 572-2279, BS 72 Univ of IA; MS 84 Univ of NE - Omaha; Sp-Lang Path, Immanuel Medical Center, **SLP**

Molchan, Ann Marie Sherry Lake Apartment, 150 Greenwich House, Conshohocken, PA 19428, (215) 233-9559, BS 78 Bloomsburg Univ of PA; MS 79 Bloomsburg Univ of PA; Sp-Lang Path, Montgomery Co Intermediate Ut, **SLP**

Molck-Ude, Roberta 4142 Burton Lane, Minneapolis, MN 55406, **SLP**

Molden, Ivy Tutein P O Box 14122, Gainesville, FL 32604, BA 82 Univ of FL; MA 86 Univ of FL; **A**

Mole, Arlene F 1227 East 172nd Street, Cleveland, OH 44119, (216) 687-3804, BA 70 John Carroll Univ; MA 76 Saint Louis Univ; Sp/Lang Path, Cleveland St U, **SLP**

Molecke, Constance 12100 St Marys Street N E, Albuquerque, NM 87111, **SLP**

Molek, Christine 625 North Court, Attumwa, IA 52501, (515) 683-1861, BS 84 De Paul Univ; MA 86 Northwestern Univ; **A**

Molek, Mrs Christine Marie 2908 83rd Street, Woodridge, IL 60517-4138, (312) 971-0840, BA 83 Saint Xavier Coll; MS 87 Governors St Univ; 87–Sp-Lang Path, Rehab Services of Chicago, **SLP**

Moler, Robin Seltzer 5 Mapleview Court, Cincinnati, OH 45236, (513) 281-6700, **SLP**

Moler, Sandra T 1205 Juniper Street, Longmont, CO 80501, (303) 772-7700, BS 68 OH St Univ; MA 83 Univ of Northern CO; Sp-Lang Path, St Urain Valley Schools, **SLP**

Molestatore, Mrs Patricia Ann Rd #2 Box 521 #21, Homer City, PA 15748, (412) 479-3341, BS 84 Indiana Univ of PA; MS 85 Indiana Univ of PA; 85–Sp-Lang Path, Indiana Sp Path and Aud Svcs, **SLP**

Molidor, Mrs Rebecca A 9099 Hillside, Frisco, TX 75034, (214) 377-9443, BS 79 Univ of North TX; MS 81 Univ of North TX; Sp-Lang Path, Private Practice, **SLP**

Molinari-Defusco, Mrs Elizabeth Plaza Hill Bldg, 646 Route 18, East Brunswick, NJ 08816, (201) 238-0744, BA 74 Kean Coll of NJ; MS 75 Columbia Univ Teachers Coll; Sp-Lang Path, Private Practice, **SLP**

Molinaro, Michelle T 1446 Cheshire Lane, Houston, TX 77018, (713) 522-1051, BS 77 Marywood Coll; MS 78 Ithaca Coll; Dir/Dept Commun Dis, Childrdens Ctr Develpmntl Ther, **SLP**

Molinary, Dolores H 687 Hill Road, Winnetka, IL 60093, BA 65 Univ of FL; MA 67 Univ of OK Medical Center; **SLP**

Molinelli, Clifford J, Jr 101 Washington Street, South Farmingdale, NY 11735, (516) 826-6200, BA 74 Hofstra Univ; MA 76 Hofstra Univ; Sp-Lang Path, Bellmore USD, **SLP**

Molinelli-Spatz, Mrs Roseann Judy 535 Willow Street, South Hempstead, NY 11550, (718) 236-0010, BA 81 SUNY - Coll at Cortland; MA 83 Hofstra Univ; Aud, Center for Hearing Services, **A**

Molineux, Barry R 2925 S W Maupin Lane #205, Topeka, KS 66614, (913) 272-4060, BS 66 Univ of KS; MA 68 KS St Univ; Dir Sp-Lang Path, The Capper Found, **SLP**

Molineux, Mrs Mary F 910 University, Helena, MT 59601, (406) 225-3311, BA 70 Univ of MT; MA 73 Univ of MT; Sp-Lang Path, Speech and Language Clinic, **SLP**

Molinski, Mrs Kathleen A 10174 St Paul Drive, Thornton, CO 80229-2832, (303) 252-9522, BA 76 Saint Joseph's Coll; MA 79 NY Univ; Sp-Lang Path, Denver Public Schools, **SLP**

Molitor, Guy Thomas 519 Chelsea Avenue, Rockford, IL 61107, (815) 398-8465, BS 81 Northern IL Univ - De Kalb; MA 83 Northern IL Univ - De Kalb; 84–Aud, Health Evaluation Prog Inc, **A**

Molitores, Jan Marie 1598 Deer Hollow Drive, Toms River, NJ 08753, (201) 270-5096, BS 85 Trenton St Coll; MS 87 PA St Univ - Univ Park; **SLP**

Moll, Mrs Delores M 206 Thomas, Sikeston, MO 63801, (314) 472-0707, BS 70 Southeast MO St Univ; ME 75 Southeast MO St Univ; Sp-Lang Path, Sikeston Pub Sch, **SLP**

Moll, Denise Zapach 201 South 15th Street, Emmaus, PA 18049, (215) 439-1501, BS 83 Kutztown Univ of PA; MA 85 Temple Univ-Tyler Sch of Art; Aud, Private Practice, **A**

Moll, Dr Dianne-Lynn L 12 Messmate Street, Aspley, Brisbane, Queensland, Australia 4034, (07) 263-1220, OB 62 8139; MS Univ of Pittsburgh - Pittsburgh; PH 78 (Linguistics) Univ of Pittsburgh - Pittsburgh; 88–Sp-Lang Path, Dept of Education Queensland, **SLP**

Moll, Judith Northeastern University, Stearns Hall, 360 Huntington Avenue, Boston, MA 02115, (617) 437-3453, BA 68 Univ of MN - Minneap-St Paul; MS 72 Mankato St Univ; Asso Prof Coord of Coop Ed, Northeastern University

Moll, Karla K W-7051 North 2nd Street Rd, Watertown, WI 53094, (414) 563-2437, BS 78 Univ of WI - Madison; MS 79 Univ of WI - Stevens Point; Sp-Lang Path, Rehabilitation Assoc, **SLP**

Moll, Dr Kenneth L 111 Jessup Hall, University Of Iowa, Iowa City, IA 52242, (319) 335-3565, BS 54 Southeast MO St Univ; MA 59 Univ of IA; PH 60 (Sp Science) Univ of IA; Prof/Assoc Vice Pres Acad Aff, University of Iowa, **SLP F H**

Moll, Mrs Mollie A M 8452 Greenleaf Drive, Cincinnati, OH 45255, (513) 553-3181, BS 75 Univ of Cincinnati; MA 77 Univ of KY; 77–Sp-Lang Path, New Richmond Sch, **SLP**

Moller, Dr Karlind Theodore 686 Arbogast Street, Shoreview, MN 55126, (612) 373-7966, BS 64 Univ of MN - Minneap-St Paul; MA 67 Univ of MN - Minneap-St Paul; PH 70 (NS) Univ of MN - Minneap-St Paul; Prof & Dir, U of MN, **SLP F**

Moller, Mary Scott 510 Kingswood Avenue, Eugene, OR 97405, (406) 752-0101, **SLP**

Moller, Mrs Miriam 4215 North 100th Street, Apartment 326, Milwaukee, WI 53222, (414) 224-1407, OB 47 Marquette Univ; MA 49 Marquette Univ; Prof, Marquette U, **SLP**

Mollerud, Theodore 714 West Hamilton, Eau Claire, WI 54701, (715) 834-3448, 69 ND St Univ; 69 ND St Univ; 69–Aud, Ear Nose Throat Cl, **A**

Mollica-Butfilowski, Diane P O Box 572, Greenwood Lake, NY 10925, (201) 429-6011, BA 79 CUNY - Brooklyn Coll; MS 80 CUNY - Brooklyn Coll; Dir-Dept of Aud & SLP, The Mountainside Hosp, **A**

Mollison, Karen Kelly 4602 East Sunset Drive, Phoenix, AZ 85028, (602) 991-6140, BS 77 Univ of AZ; MS 80 Univ of AZ; Sp-Lang Path, Private Practice, **SLP**

Molloy, Debra A 1032 Tyler, Gainesville, TX 76240-5735, (817) 665-3867, BS 73 OK St Univ; MA 74 OK St Univ; Sp-Lang Path, Private Practice, **SLP ACE**

Molloy, Janet Lynn 27306 Parkview Boulevard, Apartment 7309, Warren, MI 48092, (313) 745-9721, BS 85 Central MI Univ; MA 86 Central MI Univ; 88–Sp-Lang Path, Rehab Inst of Detroit, **SLP**

Molloy, Jill Marie 311 Spencer Road, Devon, PA 19333, (215) 596-9171, BS Ithaca Coll; MA 83 Univ of IL - Champaign; 88–Aud, Children's Seashore House at Children's Hosp of Philadelphia, **A**

Molloy, Julia Sale 230 Crest Road, Atco, NJ 08004, MS; **LM**

Molloy, Sr R 1483 82nd Boulevard, University City, MO 63132, MS; **LM**

Moll-Richmond, Mrs Deborah 423 Walton Drive, Cheektowaga, NY 14225, (711) 625-8795, BS 74 SUNY - Coll at Buffalo; MS 75 SUNY - Coll at Buffalo; Sp-Lang Path, Orleans-Niagara BOCES, **SLP**

Molly, Leda S 622 Greenwich Street #1A, New York, NY 10014, (718) 338-1729, BA 80 CUNY - Brooklyn Coll; MS 82 CUNY - Brooklyn Coll; Sp-Lang Path/Aud, Private Practice, **SLP A**

Molnar, Suzanne 16 Marlow Court, Hamilton, NJ 08610, (609) 581-3828, BS 85 Trenton St Coll; MA 87 Trenton St Coll; **SLP**

Molner, Janet Ann 155 Sheppler Street, Rochester, NY 14612, (716) 663-3307, BS 82 Nazareth Coll of Rochester; MS 84 Nazareth Coll of Rochester; Sp-Lang Path, Rochester City School, **SLP**

Molrine, Charlotte J 10 Parkway, Cambridge Springs, PA 16403, BA 78 Stephens Coll; MA 82 Edinboro Univ of PA; 88–Asst Prof/Sp-Lang Path, Edinboro University of Pa, **SLP**

Molstad, Mary Anne 116 Keeney, Evanston, IL 60202, (312) 578-3759, BS 83 IL St Univ - Normal; MS 85 Rush Univ; SLP, Chicago VA Hosp, **SLP**

Molt, Alexandra Rowland 22167 Serenata Circle East, Boca Raton, FL 33433-5336, (407) 394-8392, BA 75 Auburn Univ - Auburn; MS 76 Univ of South FL; 86–Sp-Lang Path, Palm Beach Co Sch Bd, **SLP**

Molt, Dr Lawrence F Department Of Exceptional Student Education, Florida Atlantic University, Boca Raton, FL 33431-0991, (407) 393-3280, MS 77 Univ of South FL; PH 86 (Sp & Hearing Science) Univ of TN - Knoxville; 86–Prog Dir, Florida Atlantic Univ, **SLP A**

Molter, Mrs Sandra Schneider 2568 North 71 Street, Milwaukee, WI 53213, (414) 259-1414, BS 78 Univ of WI - Milwaukee; MS 79 Univ of WI - Milwaukee; Sp-Lang Path, Curative Rehabilitation Center, **SLP**

Moltz, Mrs Candace C 200 Clearview Drive, Midlothian, TX 76065, (214) 905-3110, BA 72 Baylor Univ; MS 76 Univ of TX - Dallas; Clinical Supervisor, University of Texas at Dallas, **SLP ACE**

Molyneaux, Dr Dorothy Munz 27 Rosewood Drive, San Francisco, CA 94127, (415) 333-7637, BA 44 Univ of IL - Urbana; MS 45 Northwestern Univ; PH 49 (Sp-Lang Path) Stanford Univ; 87–Prof Emeritus, San Francisco State U, **SLP A**

Molyneux, Mrs Carol Snapp Route 2 Box 35, Alachua, FL 32615, (904) 454-1958, BS 71 FL St Univ; MS 72 FL St Univ; Sp-Lang Path, Alachun Co Sch Bd, **SLP ACE**

Momper, Anita F 1041 East 38th Place, Tulsa, OK 74105, (918) 749-7508, BS 77 OK St Univ; MA 79 Univ of Tulsa; Sp-Lang Path, St John Medical Center, **SLP**

Momsen, Mrs Joy J 15 Gilman Terrace, Sioux City, IA 51104, (712) 274-6040, BA 50 Morningside Coll; MA 66 Univ of SD - Vermillion; SLP, Western Hills AEA 12, **SLP**

Momtaz, Mrs Anita Ruth 155-56 North Singingwood, Orange, CA 92669, (714) 771-2845, BA 79 CA St Univ - Long Beach; MA 82 CA St Univ - Long Beach; Sp/Lang Path, Bernard A Landes PhD & Assoc, **SLP**

Monacelli, Mrs Melanie Lynn Box 146 Route 20, Sheridan, NY 14135, (716) 934-4274, BS 76 SUNY - Coll at Fredonia; MS 82 SUNY - Coll at Fredonia; Sp-Lang Path, Silver Creek Elem Sch, **SLP**

Monachese, Teresa 377-C Barker Circle, West Chester, PA 19380, (215) 647-3150, BS 76 West Chester Univ of PA; MA 79 West Chester Univ of PA; 82–Asst Dir & Brain Inj Coord, Bryn Mawr Rehab Hosp, **SLP**

Monachino, Mrs Julie Kay 2481 Delavan Drive, Dayton, OH 45459, (513) 434-5780, BS 81 Western KY Univ; MS 83 Bloomsburg Univ of PA; Audiologist, Miami Valley Regional Center, **A**

Monachino, Sandra Bullock 8 El Dorado Drive, Allegany, NY 14706, (716) 372-8293, BS 71 SUNY - Coll at Brockport; ME 82 SUNY - Coll at Fredonia; Sp-Lang Path, Cattaraugus-Allegany Co BOCES, **SLP**

Monaco, Christine 1729 South 139th Street, Omaha, NE 68144, (402) 978-7074, BS 74 Univ of NE - Omaha; MS 75 Univ of NE - Omaha; Sp/Lang Path, Omaha Pub Sch, **SLP**

Monaco, H Cynthia 6025 South Major Avenue, Chicago, IL 60638, (312) 343-7200, **A**

Monaghan-Maxson, Mrs Cindy M 3454 Voyager Circle, San Diego, CA 92130, (619) 792-1134, BA 80 San Diego St Univ; MA 84 San Diego St Univ; Sp/Lang Path, Naval Hosp, **SLP**

Monagle, Cathy Moira 821 Auburn, Buffalo, NY 14222, (716) 826-7000, BA 84 NM St Univ; MS 86 Univ of MI - Ann Arbor; 88–Sp-Lang Path, Mercy Hosp, **SLP**

Monahan, Mrs Dana O 1712 Shenandoah Drive, Lexington, KY 40504, (606) 885-5351, BA 72 Univ of KY; MS 81 Univ of KY; Sp-Lang Path, Jessamine Cosch, **SLP**

Monahan, Gail P 382 E California Blvd #201, Pasadena, CA 91106, (213) 824-3100, BS 68 Saint Lawrence Univ; MS 70 SUNY - Center at Albany; Chief Sp-Lang Path Serv, VA, **SLP**

Monahan, Judith A 11531 South Sacramento Dr, Merrionette Park, IL 60655, (312) 385-6800, BA 70 Coll of Saint Francis; MA 72 Central MI Univ; Sp-Lang Path, Sch Dist 130, **SLP**

Monahan, Mrs Sarah McGinnis Cinn Speech & Hearing Center, 3021 Vernon Place, Cincinnati, OH 45219, (513) 221-0527, OB 78 Morehead St Univ; MA 84 Univ of Cincinnati; Aud, Cin Sp & Hearing Ctr, **A**

Monahan-Tomasino, Christine 314 Reedwood, Joliet, IL 60436, (815) 725-2194, BA 76 Coll of Saint Francis; MA 78 Northern IL Univ - De Kalb; Dir-Clin Rehab, Er Sl Rehab Cen Will Grundy Co, **SLP**

Monaloy, Gail E 414 Passaic Avenue, Passaic, NJ 07055, (201) 777-8604, BS 64 PA St Univ - Univ Park; MA 66 Stanford Univ; Sp-Lang Path, Private Practice, **SLP**

Monane, Ellen 150-43 72nd Drive #2-G, Flushing, NY 11367, (718) 261-8505, MA 88 CUNY - Hunter Coll

Monast, Shelia A 1024 Quincy S E, Albuquerque, NM 87108, (505) 268-0313, BA 79 MI St Univ; MA 80 Eastern MI Univ; MA 81 Wayne St Univ; Sp-Lang Path, Educational Assessment Systems, **SLP**

Monat-Haller, Mrs Rosalyn K 104 Martin Lane, Summerville, SC 29485, (803) 873-5750, BS 66 Emerson Coll; ME 67 Boston Univ; Director Therapeutic Services, Coastal Cen Sc Dept Ment Retd, **SLP**

Moncarz-Attinson, Freda Deborah 235 East 22nd Street #14L, New York, NY 10010, (212) 689-4898, BS 78 SUNY - Coll at Buffalo; MS 83 CUNY - Brooklyn Coll; Sp-Lang Path, NY Assn for the Blind, **SLP**

Moncur, Dr John P 9873 East Sabrena Lane, Tucson, AZ 85748, BA 46 Univ of CA - Los Angeles; MA 47 Univ of WA; PH 50 (NS) Stanford Univ; **SLP A F LM**

Mondello, Mrs Debra Ford 26 Hume Road, Bedford, MA 01730, (617) 787-3390, BS 78 Univ of MA - Amherst; MS 80 Emerson Coll; Sp-Lang Path, Greenery Rehab/Skl Nursing Cen, **SLP**

Mondello, Linda Jean 1223 Newcastle Lane, Fullerton, CA 92633, (714) 821-3620, BA 68 Notre Dame Coll; MA 71 Case Western Reserve Univ; Sp/Lang Path, Sp & Lang Dev Cen, **SLP**

Mondor, Mrs Blair Gauthier 409 Main Street, Danielson, CT 06239, (203) 546-9026, BA 78 Univ of CT; MS 84 Worcester St Coll; 84–Sp-Lang Path, Dr Helen Baldwin Sch, **SLP**

Moneghan, Pamela Annette Audiology Department, Massachusetts Eye & Ear Infirmary, 243 Charles Street, Boston, MA 02114, (617) 573-3266, BS 84 Univ of MA - Amherst; MS 86 Northeastern Univ; Aud, MA Eye & Ear Inf, **A**

Moneka, Mrs Wynnette J 5536 Virginia, Clarendon Hills, IL 60514, (312) 647-8107, BS 67 Western IL Univ; MA 68 Northern IL Univ - De Kalb; Audiologist, Christ Hospital, **A**

Monet, Mrs Natalie S 1132 Templeton Place, St Louis, MO 63011, BA 64 Univ of CA - Los Angeles; MA 80 CA St Univ - Long Beach; 82–Sp-Lang Path, Spec Sch Dist of St Louis Co, **SLP**

Moneta, Deborah K 100 Grove Circle, Chalfont, PA 18914, (215) 345-2230, BS 78 PA St Univ - Univ Park; MS 79 Indiana Univ of PA; Sp/Lang Path, Doylestown Hosp/Rehab Cen, **SLP**

Money, Merrie R P O Box 293, Advance, NC 27006, BS 74 FL St Univ; ME 76 Univ of GA; **SLP**

Mong, Tracy Irene 3800 East Gibbon Mt Place, Apartment 12205, Tucson, AZ 85718, (602) 886-5074, BS 83 Northern AZ Univ; MS 84 Northern AZ Univ; **SLP**

Monger, Mrs Marilyn M 2615 West 2nd Avenue, Durango, CO 81301, (303) 247-3261, BS 72 PA St Univ - Univ Park; MS 74 PA St Univ - Univ Park; Sp-Lang Path, San Juan BOCES, **SLP**

Monger-Massie, Mrs Tamara Jo 3611 Niblick Drive, San Diego, CA 92041, (619) 463-9181, **SLP**

Mongiello, Mrs Ann 96 Golden Beach Drive, Golden Beach, FL 33160, (305) 932-1253, BA 55 CUNY - Hunter Coll; MA 57 NY Univ; Sp-Lang Path, **SLP**

Mongoven, Mary Elizabeth 3500 North Hayden Road, Apt 706, Scottsdale, AZ 85251, (602) 945-3530, BS 82 Marywood Coll; MS 84 Univ of WI - Madison; Assoc Dir, Camelback Communication Ctr, **SLP ACE**

Monhart, Charlotte Knaus 1415 North Dearborn #26-D, Chicago, IL 60610, (312) 787-4353, BA 81 Univ of MI - Ann Arbor; MS 83 Univ of MI - Ann Arbor; 85–Sp-Lang Path, Schwab Rehab Ctr, **SLP ACE**

Monicken-Johnson, Mrs Teresa Marie 110 East Wynoka Street, Pierre, SD 57501-2134, (605) 224-8848, MS 84 Minot St Univ; Aud, Mt Plains Aud Assoc, **A**

Monin, Stacey Schlaff 893 Princeton Road, Woodmere, NY 11598, (516) 569-6563, BA 77 CUNY - Brooklyn Coll; MS 81 CUNY - Brooklyn Coll; Sp-Lang Path, Private Practice, **SLP**

Monjure, Joann 1138 North Foster Drive, Apt #111, Baton Rouge, LA 70806, (504) 926-3086, BS 75 LA St Univ - Baton Rouge; OM 79 LA St Univ - Shreveport; **SLP**

Monk, Barbara P 6033 Citrus Avenue, Los Angeles, CA 90043, **SLP**

Monk, Dr Janice Walls Instructional Service Center, 2930 Forrest Hill Drive S W, Atlanta, GA 30315, (404) 827-8703, BS 74 Univ of GA; ME 75 Univ of GA; PH 87 (Mental Retardation) GA St Univ; Coord Sp-Lang Hrng Imp Serv, Atlanta Pub Sch, **SLP**

Monk, Janis Smith 8654 Jackson Square Place, Shreveport, LA 71115, (318) 222-9558, BA 53 Northwestern St Univ; MA 67 Northwestern St Univ; OM 70 LA Tech Univ; 88–Sp-Lang Path, Marshall ISD, **SLP**

Monk, Mrs Sharon P 132 Dogwood Drive, Winnfield, LA 71483, (318) 628-3595, BA 71 Northwestern St Univ; MA 81 Northwestern St Univ; SLP, Winn Parish School Board, **SLP**

Monk, Vicki R B 1413 South 7th Street, La Crosse, WI 54601, (608) 782-0740, MS 76 Univ of WI - Eau Claire; Sp-Lang Path, Private Practice, **SLP**

Monk, William H 317 Linwood Avenue, Bel Air, MD 21014, (301) 671-3829, BA 77 SUNY - Coll at Cortland; MA 80 CUNY - Hunter Coll; Chief Aud Sect, US Army USA Meddac Ft Lenrd Wd, **A**

Monkhouse, Dr Kay M 57 Elliot Road, East Greenbush, NY 12061, (609) 924-3487, BA 68 Univ of IA; MA 70 Univ of IA; PH 72 (NS) Univ of IA; Sp/Lang Path, Private Practice, **SLP ACE**

Monnier, Wilnette E 2005 Arthur Drive, Waukegan, IL 60085, MS 71 TX Tech Univ; SLP, Waukegan Public School Dist 60, **SLP**

Monnin, Mrs Jean A 6865 Ridgeway Court, Pickerington, OH 43147, (614) 837-4044, BS 77 Kent St Univ; MA 78 Kent St Univ; Sp/Lang Path, Bloom-Carroll Local Schs, **SLP**

Monnin, Dr Lorraine M 944 Country Road, Monterey Park, CA 91754, (213) 343-4690, BA 50 Saint Mary-of-the-Woods Coll; MA 59 CA St Univ - Los Angeles; PH 70 (Sp-Lang Path) Stanford Univ; Prof/Sp-Lang Path, CA St U/Los Angeles, **SLP**

Monofo, Mary Ellen 59 Princeton Place, Orchard Park, NY 14127, (716) 674-5300, **SLP**

Monoson, Dr Patricia Komiss Dept Speech Path & Audiology, Illinois State University, 204 Fairchild Hall, Normal, IL 61761, (309) 438-8934, BS 64 Univ of IL - Urbana; MA 65 Univ of IL - Urbana; PH 76 (NS) Univ of IL - Urbana; Sp-Lang Path, Illinois State University, **SLP**

Monroe, Alice D 9810 Kingsbridge Drive, Fairfax, VA 22031, BA 43 Univ of NH; ME 51 Boston Univ; Retired, Fairfax Hosp, **SLP LM**

Monroe, Mrs Cindy M F 548 Terrace Drive, Traverse City, MI 49684, (616) 922-9455, BA 74 Central MI Univ; MS 75 Univ of MI - Ann Arbor; 76–Sp-Lang Path, Munson Medical Center, **SLP**

Monroe, Mrs Cora M 3923 Elmer Lane, Shreveport, LA 71109, (318) 221-6782, BA 71 LA St Univ - Baton Rouge; MS 72 Miami Univ - Oxford; SLP, Caddo Parish School Board, **SLP**

Monroe, Cynthia E 6411 Harrison Road, Charlotte, NC 28226, (704) 365-5145, BS 80 Univ of South AL; MS 82 Univ of South AL; Sp/Lang Path, Private Practice, **SLP**

Monroe, Jeanne Cotters 110 Roslyn Drive, Youngstown, OH 44505, (216) 545-5777, BS 74 Clarion Univ of PA; ME 75 Clarion Univ of PA; Sp-Lang Path, Trumbull County Bd of Educ, **SLP**

Monroe, Dr Nancy J E 2805 West 27th Street, Stillwater, OK 74074, (405) 624-6020, BA 65 Univ of IA; MA 67 Univ of IA; PH 71 (NS) Univ of KS; Assoc Prof, Oklahoma State Univ, **SLP**

Monroe, Patricia A Southeast Communication Services, 7581 South Xanthia Court, Englewood, CO 80012, (303) 369-1096, BA 64 Creighton Univ; MA 68 Univ of CO - Boulder; Sp-Lang Path, Southeast Communication Svcs, **SLP**

Monroe, William M 15516 Detroit Avenue, Lakewood, OH 44107, BS 58 Kent St Univ; Aud, E-N-T Head & Neck Surgery Assc, **SLP**

Monsees, Mrs Harriet Kidwell 11116 Lakeridge Run, Oklahoma City, OK 73170, (405) 681-4833, BS 73 Univ of HI - Manoa; MS 81 Univ of NM; Sp-Lang Path, Moore Pub Sch, **SLP**

Monsen, Dr Randall B Dept Communication Arts & Sci, Howard University, Washington, DC 20059, (202) 636-6990, BA 66 Univ of Southern CA; MA 68 Columbia Univ Sch of Gen St; PH 72 (NS) Columbia Univ Sch of Gen St; Assoc Prof, Howard University

Monsey-Kavanaugh, JoAnn 7630 Washington Blvd, Indianapolis, IN 46240, BS 79 Purdue Univ - West Lafayette; MA 82 Univ of Cincinnati; Sp-Lang Path, Private Practice, **SLP**

Monsky, Ann Lebowitz 410 Wheeler Avenue, Scranton, PA 18510, (717) 342-8933, BS 75 Emerson Coll; MS 82 Bloomsburg Univ of PA; Sp-Lang Path, Scranton School District, **SLP**

Monson, Deborah Jean 1112 Moraine Way #202, Green Bay, WI 54303, (414) 434-4002, BS 81 Univ of WI - Stevens Point; MA 83 Univ of MN - Duluth; Sp-Lang Path, Sch Dist of Howard-Suamico, **SLP**

Monson, Donna L 1742 S Madaline Terrace, Springfield, MO 65804, (417) 885-6862, BS 79 KS St Univ; MA 81 Wichita St Univ; Sp-Lang Path, Cox Med Ctr, **SLP**

Monson, Kay E 2747 Royal Court, Lincoln, NE 68502, (402) 421-1235, BA 77 Univ of NE - Lincoln; MA 79 Univ of NE - Lincoln; Sp-Lang Path, Lincoln Pub Sch, **SLP**

Monson, Mrs Loretta J 5616 North Pascal Street, Shoreview, MN 55126, (919) 447-5146, BA 74 Univ of MN - Duluth; MA 75 Western MI Univ; **SLP**

Monson, Mark A Western Hills Area Educ Agency, 1520 Morningside Avenue, Sioux City, IA 51106, (712) 274-6040, BA 67 Wayne St Coll; MA 71 Univ of SD - Vermillion; Superv-Cl Sp-Lang Path, Wn Hills AEA 12, **SLP**

Monson, Mrs Susan K 4 Turin Way, Springfield, MA 01119, (413) 783-5999, BA 77 Elms Coll; MS 86 Worcester St Coll; 87–Sp-Lang Path, Mass Easter Seal Society, **SLP**

Monsoor, Mary R 115 South 11th Street, La Crosse, WI 54601, (608) 784-1697, BA 76 Univ of WI - Eau Claire; MS 77 Univ of WI - Eau Claire; Sp-Lang Path, La Crosse Sch Dist, **SLP**

Monsour, Rosemary J 1800 Hampton Road, Grosse Pointe Woods, MI 48236, MA 70 Western MI Univ; SLP, East Detroit Public Schools, **SLP**

Montag, Mary M 315 North Forest Street, Bellingham, WA 98225, **SLP**

Montag, Mrs Maxine S 1333 East 80th Street, Brooklyn, NY 11236, (718) 723-3427, BA 79 CUNY - Queens Coll; MS 81 CUNY - Brooklyn Coll; 88–Sp-Lang Path, N Westchester Ctr for Sp Dis, **SLP**

Montague, Barbara P Rd 2 Box 213, Five Mile Road, Allegany, NY 14706, (716) 372-8909, BS 67 Carlow Coll; MS 69 SUNY - Coll at Buffalo; Sp-Lang Path, BOCES, **SLP**

Montague, Dr James C, Jr Speech Language & Hearing Clinic-UALR, 2801 South University, Little Rock, AR 72204, (501) 569-3155, BS 59 FL Southern Coll; MA 67 Univ of FL; PH 71 (Sp-Lang Path) Univ of FL; Prof & Chair, U of Arkansas at Little Rock, **SLP F**

Montague, Jean L 233 Newport #4, Long Beach, CA 90803, (714) 826-0443, BA 74 Univ of MA - Amherst; MS 78 IL St Univ - Normal; 88–Human Resources Rep, InSpeech Inc, **SLP**

Montague, Mrs Karen Alm 6708 E Pleasant Valley Rd, Independence, OH 44131, (216) 531-9000, BA 81 IN Univ - Bloomington; MA 83 IN Univ - Bloomington; Sp/Lang Path, Euclid General Hosp, **SLP**

Montague, Kathryn Marie 31 Periwinkle Road, Narragansett, RI 02882, (203) 599-5832, BA 78 Univ of RI; MS 82 Southern CT St Univ; Sp-Lang Path, Stonington Bd of Ed, **SLP**

Montague, Melanie F 1809 Paseo Del Sol, Palos Verdes Estates, CA 90274, (213) 377-7854, BA 71 Univ of Southern CA; MA 73 Univ of Southern CA

Montali, Phyllis M 1367 Weymouth Lane, Charlotte, NC 28226, (704) 846-4507, BA 75 Cleveland St Univ; MA 76 Cleveland St Univ; Sp-Lang Path, Private Practice, **SLP**

Montalvo, Cathryn F 3278 Wynndale Circle, Woodbridge, VA 22192, (804) 254-7261, BS 75 Hampton Univ; ME 76 Univ of VA - Charlottesville; SLP, Springwood Elem, **SLP**

Montana, Amy L 2107 Napoleon Boulevard, Louisville, KY 40205, (502) 452-6204, BS 73 Ithaca Coll; MS 87 Univ of Louisville; 88–Sp-Lang Path, Floyd Memorial Hosp

Montanari, Mrs Therese Marie 432 36th Avenue N E, St Petersburg, FL 33703, (813) 892-4141, BS 84 FL St Univ; MS 85 FL St Univ; Sp-Lang Path, All Childrens Hosp, **SLP**

Montanaro, Mrs Janet J 14 Bavarian Lane, Wilmington, DE 19810, (215) 645-2723, Columbia Univ Teachers Coll; Sp-Lang Path, Lankenau Hosp, **SLP**

Montanez, Mrs Virginia F 1123 Presidio Boulevard, Pacific Grove, CA 93950, (408) 372-7930, BA 77 Humboldt St Univ; Sp-Lang Path, Alisal District

Montano, Joseph J 47-12 190th Street, Flushing, NY 11358, (212) 605-3739, BA 76 CUNY - Queens Coll; MA 77 NY Univ; Dir-Comm Dis, Manhattan Eye Ear Throat Hosp, **A**

Montano, Mrs Marleen Graf 47 Bentwood Road, West Hartford, CT 06107, (203) 548-5443, BS 74 Marquette Univ; ME 75 Bloomsburg Univ of PA; SLP, St Francis Hosp & Med Cen, **SLP**

Montanti, Dr John C 4300 Bayview Drive, Fort Lauderdale, FL 33308, (305) 525-2700, BA 74 Jersey City St Coll; MA 75 Kean Coll of NJ; ED 81 (NS) Nova Univ; **SLP A**

Montaug-Martin, Linda J 515 Fermoore Street, San Fernando, CA 91340, (818) 241-3111, BA 76 CA St Univ - Northridge; MA 78 CA St Univ - Northridge; Sp-Lang Path, Glendale USD, **SLP**

Monte, Denise Anne 68 Byron Drive, Avon, CT 06001, (203) 727-1315, BS 84 Univ of TN - Knoxville; MS 86 Syracuse Univ; 88–Aud, American Sch for the Deaf, **A**

Monte, Karen L 213 Commonwealth Avenue #7, Boston, MA 02116, (617) 424-1608, BA 77 Univ of FL; MA 80 Memphis St Univ; Sp-Lang Path, Don Orione Nursing Home, **SLP**

Montefusco, Mrs Marta Baucom 604 Montrose Drive, Greensboro, NC 27410, (919) 299-3911, BA 75 Wake Forest Univ; ME 79 Univ of NC - Greensboro; Sp-Lang Path/Aud, Marta Baucom Montefusco, **SLP A**

Monteith, Mrs Martha 6505 Main Street, Columbia, SC 29203, BA Allen Univ; MA Case Western Reserve Univ; Coordinator of SLP, Richland County School Dist #1, **SLP LM**

Monteleone, Ila K 4659 Wright Road, New Orleans, LA 70128, (504) 822-6590, BA 56 Northwestern St Univ; MA 71 Tulane Univ; Coord, New Orleans Pub Sch, **SLP**

Montelibano, Michelle Burg 4905 36th Avenue South, Minneapolis, MN 55417, (612) 298-8288, BS 84 Univ of WI - River Falls; MS 86 Mankato St Univ; Sp-Lang Path, United and Childrens Hospital, **SLP**

Montero, Mrs Gloria B 9 Erin Place, Kincheloe, MI 49788, (906) 478-7931, BS 85 Central MI Univ; MA 86 Central MI Univ; SLP, Eastern Upper Peninsul Schl, **SLP**

Montes, Michelle L Box 607 Jacobsen Hall, 175 Elizabeth Blackwell St, Syracuse, NY 13210, (315) 473-5937, BS 84 Purdue Univ - West Lafayette; MS 87 Purdue Univ - West Lafayette; 88–Aud, SUNY Health Sci Ctr, **A**

Montes, Michelle Marie 1900 Dufour Avenue #31, Redondo Beach, CA 90278, (213) 379-6694, BS 85 CA St Univ - Sacramento; MS 87 CA St Univ - Sacramento; 88–Sp-Lang Path, The ECHO Center, **SLP**

Montet, Thomas Herman 406 1st N E, Waukon, IA 52172, (319) 568-3411, **SLP**

Montgomery, Dr Allen A Dept Of Communicative Disorders, Univ Of South Carolina, Columbia, SC 29208, (803) 777-4813, BS 60 Miami Univ - Oxford; MA 61 Western MI Univ; PH 67 (Speech Science) Purdue Univ - West Lafayette; 88–Research Prof/NIH Fellow, Univ of South Carolina, **SLP**

Montgomery, Barbara S 237 South Holmes, Memphis, TN 38111, (901) 529-0233, BS 73 Univ of TN - Knoxville; MA 79 Memphis St Univ; Ch SLP, Les Passees Rehab Cen, **SLP**

Montgomery, Mrs Brenda Lynette 616 W Skyline Drive, Mobile, AL 36609, (205) 431-3424, BS 84 Talladega Coll; MS 85 Talladega Coll; **SLP**

Montgomery, Dianne Dickey P O Box 443, Chatom, AL 36518, (205) 847-2503, BA 78 Univ of AL- Tuscaloosa; MS 79 Univ of AL- Tuscaloosa; 88–Sp-Lang Path, Washington Co Bd of Educ, **SLP**

Montgomery, Gay Ann 14234 Woodmont, Detroit, MI 48227, BS 79 Wayne St Univ; MA 82 Wayne St Univ; Sp-Lang Path, Ferndale Pub Sch, **SLP**

Montgomery, Mrs Helena Cefalu 3151 The Pines, Opelousas, LA 70570, (318) 948-7472, **SLP**

Montgomery, James Wasson Audiology And Speech Sciences, West Lafayette, IN 47907, (317) 494-7738, BA 79 Depauw Univ; MA 82 IN Univ - Bloomington; PH 88 (Comm Disorders & Sciences) Wichita St Univ; 88–Postdoctoral Research Assoc, Purdue Univ, **SLP**

Montgomery, Mrs Janet K 1212 Graceland, Newport, AR 72112, (501) 523-6468, BS 69 Univ of Central AR; MA 75 Univ of AR - Fayetteville; 87–Sp-Lang Path, Private Practice, **SLP**

Montgomery, Dr Judith K Fountain Valley School, 17210 Oak Street, Fountain Valley, CA 92708, (714) 843-3280, BS 69 Univ of WI - Milwaukee; MA 73 CA St Univ - Long Beach; PH 85 (NS) Claremont Graduate Sch; 84–Sp-Lang Path, Fountain Valley Sch Dist, **SLP F ACE**

Montgomery, Karen Lynn Sixpenny Thatch, The Street, North Salisbury, Wiltshire, England, BS 78 TX Christian Univ, MA 80 Northwestern Univ; SLP, Salisbury Health District, **SLP**

Montgomery, Mrs Kathryn D 2389 White Wing Drive, Jamulpur, CA 92035, (303) 841-3000, BA 72 Univ of NE - Lincoln; MA 81 Univ of Denver; Owner/Sp-Lang Path, Douglas Co Cen for Commun Dis, **SLP**

Montgomery, Lillian L 6202 Turtle Point, Austin, TX 78746, MS; **SLP**

Montgomery, Marcia M 6732 Cary Lane, Columbia, SC 29206, (803) 788-1875, BS 64 Northern IL Univ - De Kalb; MS 74 Purdue Univ - West Lafayette; **SLP**

Montgomery, Mrs Maureen Maguire 3135 Roxanne Avenue, Long Beach, CA 90808, (213) 378-0036, BA 74 William Paterson Coll; MS 82 Univ of LA Verne; Sp-Lang-Hrng Spec, La Office of Ed, **SLP**

Montgomery, Patricia B 1711 Phantom Avenue, San Jose, CA 95125, (415) 493-5000, BS 70 Univ of TN - Knoxville; MA 72 Memphis St Univ; Aud, Palo Alto VA Med Cen, **A**

Montgomery, Mrs Rose B 4708 Hannett N E, Albuquerque, NM 87110, (505) 242-4995, BA 74 Univ of NM; MS 80 Univ of NM; Sp-Lang Path, Albuquerque Aphasia & Sp Cnslt, **SLP**

Montgomery, Mrs Suzanne V 735 Eagle Creek Court, Zionsville, IN 46077, (317) 873-6102, **SLP**

Montgomery-Loy, Mrs Nancy L 8503 Lucerne Road, Randallstown, MD 21133, (301) 922-1630, BA 74 Augustana Coll; MS 75 PA St Univ - Univ Park; 88–Sp-Lang Path, Carroll County Bd of Educ, **SLP**

Monthey, Joanne C 102 East 21st Street #15, Goldendale, WA 98620, (509) 773-3814, MS 88 Western OR St Coll

Montilla, Florence Mary G 4352 Hampshire Place, San Jose, CA 95136, BA 75 San Jose St Univ; MA 79 San Jose St Univ; Sp/Lang Path, Oak Grove Sch Dist, **SLP**

Montini, Mrs Maria 22 Portico Drive, Scarborough, ON, Canada M1G 3R3, (416) 839-1541, **SLP**

Montoya-Maestas, Mrs Mary K PO Box 424, Espanola, NM 87532-0424, (505) 753-4464, BA 82 NM St Univ; MA 84 NM St Univ; 84–Sp-Lang Path, Private Practice-Sole Proprietor, **SLP**

Montpetit, Isabelle 8 Hewlett Road, Red Hook, NY 12571, (914) 758-8730, MS 83 McGill Univ - Quebec; **SLP**

Montserrat-Hopple, Mrs Maria 6765 S W 179th Avenue, Aloha, OR 97007, (503) 642-7928, BA 81 Univ of WA; BS 82 Univ of IA; MS 85 Portland St Univ; 88–Aud, Portland St Univ, **A**

Monzon, Robert 60 East 42nd Street, New York, NY 10165, BA 58 CUNY - Hunter Coll; MA 72 Columbia Univ Teachers Coll; Aud, Audionics Corporation, **A**

Moock, Mrs Judy N 6331 Celestial Drive, Baton Rouge, LA 70816, (504) 622-4011, BS 77 LA St Univ - Baton Rouge; MA 79 LA St Univ - Baton Rouge; SLP, Ascension Parish School Board, **SLP**

Moody, Mrs Candice A'Lora 1572 Locust Street, Pasadena, CA 91106, (213) 681-1160, MA 86 CA St Univ - Los Angeles; **SLP**

Moody, Carla Susann 254-A South Berkeley St, Pasadena, CA 91107, BA 82 Univ of Chicago; MA 86 Univ of CA - Santa Barbara; Huntington Mem Hosp, **SLP**

Moody, Donna K Stuttgart Elementary & Jr High, Robinson Barracks, APO New York, NY 09154, OB 75 AR St Univ; MS 78 Univ of AR - Little Rock; Sp-Lang Path, Dept Defense Dep Sch, **SLP**

Moody, Donna Michelle 4894 Kilauea Avenue #4, Honolulu, HI 96816, (808) 521-4531, OB 80 Univ of HI - Manoa; BS 83 Univ of HI - Manoa; Sp/Lang Path, Honolulu Comm Act Prog, **SLP**

Moody, Mrs Laurie J 340 Chatham Drive, Aurora, OH 44202, (216) 562-8835, BS 78 Bloomsburg Univ of PA; MS 81 PA St Univ - Univ Park; Sp-Lang Path, Private Practice, **SLP**

Moody, Mary E 14905 Dufief Drive, Gaithersburg, MD 20878, (301) 340-3040, BA 68 Coll of New Rochelle; MA 70 Catholic Univ of America; 70, Private Practice, **SLP**

Moody, Mrs Mary H 600 So College Avenue, Univ Of Tulsa, Tulsa, OK 74104-3189, (918) 631-2914, BS 63 West TX St Univ; MS 75 Univ of North TX; 86–Clin Supvr, The Univ of Tulsa, **SLP**

Moody, Pauline F P O Box 1351, Chadron, NE 69337-1351, MS; **SLP LM**

Moody, Rosemary 2018 Atascadero Drive, Columbia, SC 29206, (803) 781-1523, BA 65 Univ of SC - Columbia; ME 72 Univ of SC - Columbia; Sp-Lang Path, Lexington School District 5, **SLP**

Mooers, Janet E 11012 Red Rock Drive, San Diego, CA 92131, (619) 465-3131, BA 71 Univ of CA - Santa Barbara; MA 74 San Diego St Univ; SLP, Grossmont Un Hs Dist Spec Ed, **SLP**

Moog, Ellen Reiter 425 Allentown Road, Parsippany, NJ 07054, (201) 386-1420, BS 69 Ball St Univ; MA 72 Univ of TN - Knoxville; 88–Sp-Lang Path, Mountain Lakes Pub Schs, **SLP**

Moog, Mrs Jean S Central Institute For Deaf, 818 South Euclid Avenue, St Louis, MO 63110, (314) 652-3200, BA 55 Smith Coll; MS 64 Washington Univ; Prin, Cen Inst for the Deaf

Moomaw, Douglas Edward Wenatchee Valley Clinic, 820 North Chelan Street, Wenatchee, WA 98801-5000, (509) 663-8711, Aud, Wenatchee Valley Clin, **A**

Moomaw, Mrs Edna L 2812 Wadsworth Road, Barberton, OH 44203, (216) 336-3571, BA 49 Lagrange Coll; MA 63 Univ of Akron; Sp-Lang Path, Wadsworth Cty Sch, **SLP**

Moon, Mrs Caryl 11144 Archer Avenue, Mishawaka, IN 46544, (219) 875-6565, BS 70 Purdue Univ - West Lafayette; MS 71 Purdue Univ - West Lafayette; Sp-Lang Path, Concord Comm Sch, **SLP**

Moon, Dr Jerald B Wendell Johnson Sp & Hearing, University Of Iowa, Iowa City, IA 52242, (319) 335-8722, BS 78 Univ of Western Ontario; OM 80 Univ of Western Ontario; PH 85 (NS) Purdue Univ - West Lafayette; Assistant Research Scientist, U of IA

Moon, Marjorie M Dept Speech & Lang Devel, 11234 Anderson Street, Loma Linda, CA 92354, (714) 824-4401, BS 81 Andrews Univ; MS 83 Univ of Redlands; Sp/Lang Path, Loma Linda U Med Cen, **SLP**

Moon, Sharon E P O Box 133, Orion, IL 61273, (309) 526-3587, **SLP**

Moon, Dr Susan L Rd 2 Box 298-G, Mertztown, PA 19539, (215) 683-4293, BS 71 PA St Univ - Univ Park; MS 72 PA St Univ - Univ Park; PH 83 (Clinical Sp) Temple Univ; Prof, Kutztown U, **SLP ACE**

Moonay, Ruth J 183 Londonderry Lane, Getzville, NY 14068, (716) 689-3191, MA 88 SUNY - Center at Buffalo

Moone, Marianne F 336 Acre Lane, Hicksville, NY 11801, **SLP**

Moonen, Diane E 7801 Colony Circle South, Apartment 210, Tamarac, FL 33321, (305) 720-8237, BA 78 MI St Univ; MA 80 MI St Univ; 87–Aud, Easter Seal Soc of Broward Co, **A**

Mooney, Darlene Rose 3 Brookview Court, Westerly, RI 02891, (401) 596-6136, MS 86 Southern CT St Univ; 87–Sp-Lang Path, New London PS, **SLP**

Mooney, Mrs Diane K 160 Emerald Hills Lane, Newnan, GA 30263, (404) 631-3250, ME 87 GA St Univ; SLP, Fayette Co Bd of Ed

Mooney, Dorothy D 620 Gaudet Drive, Marrero, LA 70072, (504) 366-7000, BS 69 Univ Southern MS-Hattiesburg; MS 70 Univ Southern MS-Hattiesburg; SLP, Jefferson Parish Pub Schools, **SLP**

Mooney, Mrs Janice Griffin 6768 East Leafwood Drive, Anaheim Hills, CA 92807, (714) 282-0682, BA 79 San Francisco St Univ; MA 80 Univ of the Pacific; **SLP**

Mooney, Marilyn Decker 25 Dresden Court, Albany, NY 12203, (518) 382-4550, BS 83 SUNY - Coll at Buffalo; MS 84 SUNY - Coll at Buffalo; 88–Sp-Lang Path, Sunnyview Hosp, **SLP**

Mooney, Mary L 1717 Jerry Abbott, El Paso, TX 79936, (915) 594-2432, BA 75 Univ of TX - El Paso; MA 76 Univ of TX - El Paso; Instr, El Paso Commun Coll, **SLP**

Mooney, Patricia V 912 West Beach Avenue #4, Inglewood, CA 90302, (213) 595-2411, BA 64 Univ of CA - Los Angeles; MA 82 CA St Univ - Northridge; Sp-Lang Path, Daniel Freeman Marina Hospital, **SLP**

Mooney, Thomas G 6205 Pheasant Run, McFarland, WI 53558-9123, (608) 241-5006, BS 75 Univ of WI - Whitewater; MS 76 Univ of WI - Whitewater; MA 80 Univ of WI - Madison; Sp-Lang Path, Janesville Pub Sch, **SLP**

Mooney Majeski, Mrs Sandra L 2902 Darlington Road, Unit 503, Beaver Falls, PA 15010, (412) 843-8702, MA 84 Edinboro Univ of PA; 87–Sp-Lang Path, Columbiana Co Bd Educ, **SLP**

Moon-Luethke, Mrs Alison 305 Dumbarton Road, Baltimore, MD 21212, (301) 377-5707, BA 83 Univ of FL; MS 85 Vanderbilt Univ; 88–Sp-Lang Path, Sinai Hosp, **SLP**

Mooradd, Mrs Theresa H 4 Greenhurst Road, West Hartford, CT 06107, (203) 521-2709, **SLP**

Moore, Alan Gregg 308 Mary Avenue, Castle Hayne, NC 28429, (919) 675-2858, MS 88 Univ of NC - Chapel Hill

Moore, Ann S 8637 Beacon Avenue South, Seattle, WA 98118, (206) 825-6393, BS 79 Univ of OR; MS 81 Univ of WA; SLP, Enumclaw Sch Dist, **SLP ACE**

Moore, Mrs Ann Siman 2416 Peterson Rd, Lakeland, FL 33813, (813) 682-5101, BA 73 Univ of Miami; ME 74 Univ of Miami; 84–Sp-Lang Path, Polk Co PS, **SLP**

Moore, Anna Cornell 181 Shamrock Lane, Ronceverte, WV 24970, (304) 647-4239, **SLP**

Moore, Anne White Abilene State School, Audiology, Box 451, Abilene, TX 79604, (915) 692-4053, MA 83 Univ of Denver; Supervisor of Aud Services, Abilene State School, **A**

Moore, Mrs B Jane M 519 Sutherland Drive, Toronto, ON, Canada M4G 1K9, (416) 425-0426, BA 67 0222; MA 69 Case Western Reserve Univ; SLP, Riverdale Hospital, **SLP**

Moore, Mrs Betty E 11292 Betlen Drive, Dublin, CA 94568, (415) 828-8780, BS 76 Northwestern Univ; MA 77 Northwestern Univ; Sp-Lang Path, Santa Clara Co Spec Schs, **SLP**

Moore, Betty Jean 745 South 19th Street, Pocatello, ID 83201, (208) 232-3563, BS 66 ID St Univ; MS 68 ID St Univ; SLP, Sch Dist #25, **SLP**

Moore, Dr Brian Cecil University Of Cambridge, Dept Of Experimental Psy, Downing Street, Cambridge, England CB2 3EB, BA 68 Univ of Cambridge - England; MA 71 Univ of Cambridge - England; PH 71 (Psycho-Acoustics) Univ of Cambridge - England; Lecturer, University of Cambridge

Moore, Dr Carmen E 8496 Grenache Court, San Jose, CA 95135, (408) 923-1842, BA 70 San Jose St Univ; MA 71 San Jose St Univ; ED 82 (NS) Univ of San Francisco; Dir of Pupil Serv, Berryessa Un Sch Dist, **SLP**

Moore, Carol Linda 820 Casanova Avenue #46, Monterey, CA 93940, (408) 755-6450, BA 80 0500; MS 86 Purdue Univ - West Lafayette; 87–Sp-Lang Path, Monterey County Ofc of Educ, **SLP**

Moore, Charles Glenn 20275 Johnson Road, South Bend, IN 46614, (219) 282-4128, BS 64 Purdue Univ - West Lafayette; MA 69 Ball St Univ; Superv Commun Hndcpd Prog, S Bend Comm Sch Corp, **SLP**

Moore, Charlotte Marie 1534 Hayes Street, San Francisco, CA 94117, (415) 885-0331, BS 83 Purdue Univ - West Lafayette; MS 85 ID St Univ; Aud, Audiology Associates, **A**

Moore, Mrs Charlotte W 509 Primm Circle, Thomasville, NC 27360, (919) 476-9783, BS 73 Eastern KY Univ; ME 78 Univ of Louisville; Sp-Lang Path, Lexington City Schools, **SLP**

Moore, Mrs Christine E 5035 Silica Drive, Sylvania, OH 43560, (419) 729-8219, BS 76 Bowling Green St Univ; MA 83 Bowling Green St Univ; 77–Sp-Lang Path, Toledo Bd of Ed, **SLP**

Moore, Dr Christopher Alden CDS Department Box 75, Wichita State University, Wichita, KS 67208, (316) 689-3240, BA 78 Univ of CA - San Diego; MS 82 Purdue Univ - West Lafayette; PH 85 (Sp Science) Purdue Univ - West Lafayette; 85–Asst Prof, Wichita St Univ

Moore, Mrs Cindy S 2777 Buckingham #204, Lisle, IL 60532, (312) 357-9260, BS 82 FL St Univ; MS 83 FL St Univ; Sp-Lang Path, Speech-Language Hearing Clinic, **SLP**

Moore, Claudia Contess 102 Woodlawn Avenue, Albany, NY 12208, (518) 459-5422, BS 77 SUNY - Center at Albany; MA 82 Gallaudet Coll; MS 87 Coll of Saint Rose; **SLP**

Moore, Dana 900 Mountain Creek Road, Apartment Q-265, Chattanooga, TN 37405, (615) 756-2609, BS 78 Eastern KY Univ; MS 81 Univ of Louisville; 88–Sp-Lang Path, Hamilton Co Schs, **SLP**

Moore, Darlene Yvonne 11501 February Circle #304, Silver Spring, MD 20904, (202) 651-5031, BA 83 Wichita St Univ; MA 84 Wichita St Univ; 87–Sp-Lang Path, Gaulladet Univ-Kendall, **SLP**

Moore, Mrs Dawn Marie 4505 Harding Road #119, Nashville, TN 37205, (615) 322-0100, BS 83 Univ of TN - Knoxville; MA 84 Univ of TN - Knoxville; Sp-Lang Path, Vanderbilt Univ Med Ctr, **SLP**

Moore, Mrs Debra E 38 Walnut Street, Tanglewood Hills, NY 11727, (516) 928-7740, BA 76 CUNY - Queens Coll; MA 78 Hofstra Univ; Sp-Lang Path, Ann E Gordon Associates, **SLP**

Moore, Denis G 3649 West 84th Street, Chicago, IL 60652, (312) 633-2169, BS 83 Northern IL Univ - De Kalb; MA 85 Northern IL Univ - De Kalb; 85–Aud, VA West Side Med Ctr, **A**

Moore, Denise Knisel 3421 Remington, Indianapolis, IN 46227, (317) 252-9132, BA 77 MI St Univ; MA 78 MI St Univ; Sp-Lang Path, National Therapy Svc, **SLP**

Moore, Denise P 6337 Sun High Place, Columbia, MD 21045, (301) 498-6280, BA 74 Univ of MD - College Park; MA 76 Univ of MD - College Park; Sp-Lang Path, Anne Arundel Co Pub Sch, **SLP**

Moore, Donna K 631 Holmes Street, Bettendorf, IA 52722, (319) 355-8130, BA 64 Univ of IA; MA 76 Univ of IA; 82–Sp-Lang Path, MS Bend AEA, **SLP**

Moore, Mrs Edith Young 5158 Garry Owen Road, El Paso, TX 79903, (915) 566-7304, BA 53 Univ of TX - El Paso; MA 56 Univ of TX - El Paso; **SLP LM**

Moore, Mrs Edra Lurae 4447 Cowell Boulevard #64, Davis, CA 95616, (916) 756-3450, **SLP**

Moore, Elizabeth 36 Ingraham Road, Wellesley, MA 02181, **A**

Moore, Ellen H 1919 Chestnut Street #2324, Philadelphia, PA 19103, BS 40 Univ of PA; MA 46 Univ of PA; **SLP LM**

Moore, Emily Katharine S11309 Highway C, Spring Green, WI 53588, (608) 546-4104, BA 84 Bowdoin Coll; MS 87 Univ of WI - Madison; 87–Sp-Lang Path, Richland Sch Dist, **SLP**

Moore, Dr Ernest J Michigan State University, Dept Aud & Speech Sci, 378 Comm Arts Bldg, East Lansing, MI 48824-1212, (517) 353-8788, BS 64 TN St Univ; MA 67 Northern IL Univ - De Kalb; PH 71 (NS) Univ of WI - Madison; 83–Professor/Chmn Dept Aud&Speech, Michigan State University

Moore, Evette Renee 11428 Red Jade Court, Upper Marlboro, MD 20772, (301) 350-9015, BS 81 Quinnipiac Coll; MS 85 Southern CT St Univ; 85–Sp-Lang Path, Private Practice, **SLP**

Moore, Dr G Paul 2234 N W 6th Place, Gainesville, FL 32603, (904) 376-1314, BA 29 WV Univ; MA 30 Northwestern Univ; PH 36 (NS) Northwestern Univ; **SLP F H LM**

Moore, George Wayne 3338 Woodland Drive, Roanoke, VA 24015, (703) 343-0165, BS 78 Radford Univ; MS 80 Radford Univ; Aud, Roanoke Valley Sp-Hrng Cen Inc, **A**

Moore, Mrs Gladys B 110 Calvin Avenue, Ruston, LA 71270, (318) 255-1336, MA 66 LA Tech Univ; Assoc Prof Sp, LA Tech U, **SLP**

Moore, Gregory K Moore Hearing Clinic, 1313 North Court Street, Ottumwa, IA 52501, (515) 683-3458, BS 74 Univ of IA; MA 76 Univ of IA; Owner/Aud, Moore Hearing Clinic, **A**

Moore, Gregory Robert 921 West University Drive, #1115, Mesa, AZ 85201, (602) 898-8165, BS 85 CO St Univ; MS 86 CO St Univ; 88–Dir of Lab, US Hearing Centers, **A**

Moore, Mrs Ilene S 18561 Misty Lake Drive, Jupiter, FL 33458-3702, (407) 575-0250, BS 76 Univ of MA - Amherst; MS 78 Boston Univ; 86–Sp/Lang Path, Palm Beach Co School Dist, **SLP**

Moore, Jacklyn Minnick 7008 Corsica Drive, Germantown, TN 38138, (901) 522-3051, BS Univ of Tulsa; MS Univ of OK Medical Center; VP-Spec Projs, American Medical Resources, **SLP**

Moore, Jacquelyn Custer State Hospital, Route 1 Box 98, Custer, SD 57730, (605) 673-4960, **SLP**

Moore, James E 780 Thornton Way, San Jose, CA 95118, (408) 298-2009, BA 63 San Jose St Univ; MA 69 San Jose St Univ; SLP, Santa Clara County Supt Sch, **SLP**

Moore, Jan Allison Northern United Clinic, P O Box 10, Yellowknife, NT, Canada X1A 2N1, (403) 229-7054, **SLP A**

Moore, Janaan Schmuhl 620 South 9th Avenue, La Grange, IL 60525, (312) 482-9091, MA 85 Northern IL Univ - De Kalb; Aud, Arthur Katz MD, **A**

Moore, Mrs Janet 11043 Longwood, Chicago, IL 60643, (312) 481-3450, BS 76 Governors St Univ; MS 81 Governors St Univ; SLP, School Dist #163 Park Forest, **SLP**

Moore, Mrs Janet Marie 1050 Chokecherry Drive, Winter Springs, FL 32708, (305) 423-9293, BA 83 Univ of Pittsburgh - Pittsburgh; MA 85 Univ of Central FL; **SLP**

Moore, Mrs Janice L H Route 3 Box 33-D, Hardinsburg, KY 40143, (502) 756-2959, BA 76 Auburn Univ - Auburn; MS 75 Auburn Univ - Auburn; Sp-Lang Path, Private Practice, **SLP ACE**

Moore, Janie Lee 910 NW Front I20, Portland, OR 97209, (503) 357-6171, BS 56 Univ of OR; MS 69 Western OR St Coll; Sp-Lang Path, Forest Grove Sch Dist, **SLP**

Moore, Jean P 3633 Bangor Street S E, Washington, DC 20020, (202) 651-5286, MA 67 Catholic Univ of America; Asst to Dean, Kendall Sch/Gallaudet Coll, **A**

Moore, Mrs Jeneen Graves 304 Westview Court, Vienna, VA 22180, (703) 938-8088, BS 85 James Madison Univ; MS 87 James Madison Univ; **SLP**

Moore, Jill D 4233 N W 56th Terrace, Oklahoma City, OK 73112, (405) 947-3449, BS 74 OK St Univ; MS 76 Univ of OK Medical Center; Sp-Lang Path, Private Practice, **SLP**

Moore, Joanna M 6073 Willowbrook Drive, Morrison, CO 80465, (303) 697-1765, **SLP**

Moore, Johanna Lee 2207 Clark Lane #3, Redondo Beach, CA 90278, (213) 372-7980, BS 83 Univ of CA - Davis; MA 87 CA St Univ - Northridge; 88–Sp-Lang Path, Los Angeles USD, **SLP**

Moore, John Mick 1919 East Blaine, Seattle, WA 98112, (206) 242-9400, BA 69 CA St Univ - Fullerton; MA 73 Univ of WA; State Coord, WA St Progs-Deaf/Blind Chldn, **A**

Moore, Joseph H 12616 Westport Lane, Woodbridge, VA 22192, (703) 339-5418, BS 75 James Madison Univ; MS 77 Purdue Univ - West Lafayette; SLP, Fairfax Co Pub Sch, **SLP**

Moore, Mrs Joy Reed 1711 Shades Park Drive, Birmingham, AL 35209, (205) 870-1704, BA 83 Univ of AL-Tuscaloosa; MS 84 Univ of AL- Tuscaloosa; Sp-Lang Path, Jefferson Co Bd of Educ, **SLP**

Moore, Joyce Ann Route 1, Afton, TN 37616, (615) 639-2131, BS 64 East TN St Univ; MA 68 East TN St Univ; Sp-Lang Path, Greene Valley Dev Cen, **SLP**

Moore, Mrs Judith A 6080 North Robin Avenue, Livingston, CA 95334, (209) 357-6140, MA 81 CA St Univ - Stanislaus; Sp-Lang Path, Atwater Elem Sch Dist, **SLP**

Moore, Kate C 11 Dwight Street, Watertown, MA 02172, (617) 484-6015, MS 87 Boston Univ; 88–Sp-Lang Path, Cotting Sch Inc, **SLP**

Moore, Mrs Kathanne Kelly 3018 20th Street, Lubbock, TX 79410, (313) 797-6778, BS 74 Baylor Univ; MS 75 Baylor Univ; Associate SLP, **SLP**

Moore, Katherine Knox 5024 King David Boulevard, Annandale, VA 22003, (703) 920-0952, BA 73 CT Coll; MA 77 Catholic Univ of America; Sp-Lang Path, Private Practice, **SLP**

Moore, Kathleen A 1218 East Carter, Tempe, AZ 85282, **SLP**

Moore, Kathleen Claire 1004 Magnolia, Bowling Green, KY 42101, (502) 745-4541, BS 78 Murray St Univ; MS 86 Western KY Univ; 88–Clin Supvr and Instr, Western Kentucky Univ, **SLP**

Moore, Kem E 211 North Eddy, PO Box 1755, South Bend, IN 46634, (219) 237-9200, BA 80 Ball St Univ; MA 82 Ball St Univ; Aud, S Bend Cl, **A**

Moore, Mrs Kerry L 1513 25th, Woodward, OK 73801, (405) 254-3235, BS 79 OK St Univ; MA 81 OK St Univ; 80–Sp-Lang Path, Coop Ed Prog, **SLP**

Moore, Leslie Virginia 2880 North Wickham Road, Apartment 1517, Melbourne, FL 32935, **SLP**

Moore, Linda L Box 145, Paragould, AR 72450, (501) 239-7151, OB 70 AR St Univ; MA 71 Southeast MO St Univ; Sp-Lang Path, Private Practice, **SLP ACE**

Moore, Mrs Linda R 7706 Ashley View Drive, Cincinnati, OH 45227-3948, (513) 561-5502, BS 69 Miami Univ - Oxford; MS 70 Univ of MI - Ann Arbor; 71–Sp-Lang Path, Cint Pub Sch, **SLP**

Moore, Lois Ann 2011 West Flormann Street, Rapid City, SD 57702, (605) 343-0576, BA 68 Univ of SD - Vermillion; MA 70 Univ of SD - Vermillion; **SLP**

Moore, Lori J 7 Meadow Lane, Mount Holly, NJ 08060, (609) 267-0814, BA 81 Rutger's St Univ - Douglas Coll; MA 87 Trenton St Coll

Moore, Mrs Lynda S 138 Deepwood Dr, Manchester, CT 06040, (203) 684-4211, BA 78 Univ of CT; MS 80 Southern CT St Univ; Sp/Lang Path, Stafford Springs Bd of Ed, **SLP**

Moore, Mrs Lynn Savasta 2-20 30th Street, Fair Lawn, NJ 07410, (201) 429-6011, BS 79 SUNY - Center at Albany; MA 81 Univ of CT; 88–Aud, Mountainside Hosp, **A**

Moore, M Patricia 846 Upper Glencoe Road, Glen Echo, MD 21152, (301) 472-4331, BA 74 Loyola Coll; MS 75 Loyola Coll; 85–Sp-Lang Path, Bd of Educ-Harford Co, **SLP**

Moore, Malinda K 1070 Scenic Drive N W, Albany, OR 97321, (503) 926-2244, BA 69 OH Wesleyan Univ; MS 70 Univ of MI - Ann Arbor; Sp-Lang Path, Albany Gen Hosp, **SLP**

Moore, Mrs Mania F K Route 1 Box 162, Emerald, WI 54012, (715) 246-2116, BS 70 Univ of WI - River Falls; MS 79 Univ of WI - River Falls; SLP, New Richmond Sch Dist, **SLP**

Moore, Mrs Marcia Czyewski 107 West Van Buren Street, Oswego, NY 13126, (315) 341-3521, BS 63 SUNY - Coll at Geneseo; MA 69 Univ of CT; Assoc Prof, SUNY at Oswego, **SLP**

Moore, Margaret Holland 57 Green Street, Watertown, MA 02172, (617) 769-9810, BA 85 SUNY - Center at Buffalo; MA 87 SUNY - Center at Buffalo; **A**

Moore, Marguerite 11815 Eton Drive, Colton, CA 92324, (714) 825-9312, BA 57 Univ of Redlands; MS 61 Loma Linda Univ - Loma Linda; **SLP LM**

Moore, Marlyn D 655 Nelson Drive, Baton Rouge, LA 70808, (504) 346-8342, BA 55 Univ of Southwestern LA; MA 57 LA St Univ - Baton Rouge; Superv of Related Serv, E Baton Rouge Parish Sch Bd, **SLP A**

Moore, Marti 1024 Las Lomas Drive #D, La Habra, CA 90631, (714) 553-9226, BS 79 OR St Univ; MA 81 CA St Univ - Fullerton; Sp-Lang Path, Craig & Ford Inc, **SLP**

Moore, Mary Ann 11455 Fallbrook #201-B, Houston, TX 77065, (713) 894-6009, BA 80 Univ of Houston - Univ Park; MA 83 Univ of Houston - Univ Park; Sp-Lang Path, Private Practice, **SLP**

Moore, Mrs Mary C 601 East 74th Terrace, Kansas City, MO 64131, (816) 276-4023, BS 79 Western KY Univ; MS 81 Vanderbilt Univ; Sp-Lang Path Supvr, Research Med Cen, **SLP**

Moore, Mary Virginia M 510 South Dean Road, Auburn, AL 36830, (205) 727-0550, BA 53 Valdosta St Coll; MS 56 Purdue Univ - West Lafayette; PH 82 (Neuropsychology) Auburn Univ - Auburn; Sp-Lang Path, VA Medical Center, **SLP F**

Moore, Maryevelyn R 14 Briarwood Avenue, Bloomington, IL 61701, (309) 438-5762, BS 65 Hardin-Simmons Univ; MS 71 FL St Univ; MS 80 IL St Univ - Normal; Instr/SLP Dept, Il St U, **SLP**

Moore, Melissa M 726 West Clay #2, Collinsville, IL 62234-3215, (618) 624-8805, BS 82 Southern IL Univ-Edwardsvill; MA 85 Univ of IL - Urbana; Aud, Dahlberg Inc at Sears, **A**

Moore, Mrs Myrna Fladeland 109 Polk Avenue S W, Fertile, MN 56540, (218) 945-6931, BS 72 Univ of ND; MS 76 Univ of ND; SLP, Fertile-Beltrami Pub Sch, **SLP**

Moore, Mrs Pamela Ann Route 3 Box 190, Ripley, WV 25271, (304) 372-6552, BS 85 WV Univ; MS 86 WV Univ; **SLP**

Moore, Pamela Gale 1904 Westridge Drive #A, Austin, TX 78704-3223, (512) 327-7285, **SLP**

Moore, Patti E 3301 Old Field Road, Route 3, Columbia, MO 65202, (314) 445-8594, BS 73 Univ of MO - Columbia; ME 74 Univ of MO - Columbia; 87–Sp-Lang Path, Columbia PS, **SLP**

Moore, Mrs Paula E 9328 Ewers, St Louis, MO 63126, (314) 849-3544, BA 71 Univ of MO - Columbia; MA 72 Univ of MO - Columbia; Sp-Lang Path, St Louis County Spec Sch Dist, **SLP**

Moore, Mrs Penny Louise W 26145 Windsor Drive, Loma Linda, CA 92354, BA 77 CA St Univ - Long Beach; MA 81 CA St Univ - Long Beach; Tchr, Colton Joint USD, **SLP**

Moore, Phyllis C Martin Memorial Hospital, Box 9010, Stuart, FL 34995, (407) 746-1907, BS 68 Saint Louis Univ; MA 69 Saint Louis Univ; 83–Dir Sp-Lang Path & Aud, Martin Memorial Hosp, **SLP ACE**

Moore, Mrs Rebecca N 585 Monroe Mill Drive, Ballwin, MO 63011, (314) 256-3606, BS 75 Appalachian St Univ; MS 80 Vanderbilt Univ; 85–Sp-Lang Path, St Anthony's Med Ctr, **SLP**

Moore, Robert E Route 1 Box 2074, Elmbrook, Rockford, TN 37853, (615) 632-5899, BA 75 Univ of TN - Knoxville; MA 76 Univ of TN - Knoxville; 88–Asst Dir/Sp Lang & Hrng Svcs, East Tennessee Baptist Hosp, **A**

Moore, Rosalie Marie 5120 Berkley Court, Fort Wayne, IN 46815, (219) 485-7554, BS 60 Bowling Green St Univ; Sp-Lang Path, Ft Wayne State Dev Cev, **SLP**

Moore, Roslyn H 116-39 167th Street, Jamaica, NY 11434, (212) 276-1819, BA 75 CUNY - Queens Coll; MS 77 Columbia Univ Teachers Coll; Sp-Lang Path, Queens Chldn's Psychiatric Hosp, **SLP**

Moore, Rowene Caley Route 9, 209 Springlake Drive, Pine Bluff, AR 71603, (501) 879-0220, BS 78 Univ of AR - Pine Bluff; MS 84 6901; Sp-Lang Path, Watson Chapel Sch Dist, **SLP**

Moore, Sandra Lynne 1720 Geranium Avenue, Carlsbad, CA 92008, (405) 273-2157, BA 78 San Diego St Univ; MS 84 Univ of OK - OK City; Sp-Lang Path, Sp & Hrng Neurosensory Ctr, **SLP**

Moore, Sharon L 2610 Mulberry Lane, Greenville, NC 27858, (919) 355-5334, **SLP**

Moore, Mrs Sherri A 119 Bramber Drive, Lafayette, LA 70508, (318) 264-5322, BS 80 LA St Univ - Baton Rouge; MA 81 LA St Univ - Baton Rouge; SLP, LA Dept Hlth/Commun Dis, **SLP**

Moore, Sherye Leigh Sherye M Hall, 2015 Stonewood Drive, Winston-Salem, NC 27103, (919) 760-5770, BA 84 Univ of NC - Chapel Hill; ME 86 Univ of NC - Greensboro; **SLP**

Moore, Stacy Jane 5507 Barker Ten Mile Road, Apartment 3, Lumberton, NC 28358, (919) 738-6071, BA 85 Univ of TN - Knoxville; MA 86 Univ of TN - Knoxville; 87–Sp-Lang Path, Linda A Smith & Associates, **SLP**

Moore, Dr Sulyn E 1626 Hollywood Drive, Columbia, SC 29205, BA 73 Univ of SC - Columbia; OM 75 Univ of SC - Columbia; PH 87 (Communication Arts & Science) Univ of San Francisco; 86–Sp-Lang Path, Sumter Sch District 2, **SLP**

Moore, Mrs Susan B 7801 Stewart Avenue, Los Angeles, CA 90045, (213) 649-6854, BA 70 Univ of CA - Santa Barbara; MA 75 Univ of CA - Santa Barbara; Sp-Lang Path, San Mon-Malibu Unif Sch Dist, **SLP**

Moore, Susan Beth 43 Olde Stage Stop Village, Marshfield, MA 02050, (617) 746-2001, BS 66 Univ of MN - Minneap-St Paul; MS 68 Univ of OK Medical Center; 81–Dir Sp-Lang Path Dept, The Jordan Hosp, **SLP ACE**

Moore, Susan M University Of Colorado, Box 409 COSS, Boulder, CO 80309, (303) 492-5284, BA 70 Coll of New Rochelle; MA 72 Univ of Denver; 88–Clin Dir, Univ of Colorado, **SLP**

Moore, Mrs Susan Rowe 146 Winnfield Road, West Monroe, LA 71291, (318) 396-4521, BS 74 Southern Methodist Univ; MA 76 Memphis St Univ; Instructor/Audiologist, Northeast Louisiana University, **A**

Moore, Mrs Susan Williams 5573 Afton Drive, Birmingham, AL 35242, (205) 871-3878, BA 83 Univ of AL-Tuscaloosa; MS 84 Univ of AL- Tuscaloosa; 85–Sp-Lang Path, Birmingham Speech & Hrng Assoc, **SLP**

Moore, Mrs Sylvia Pope 310 Travis Lane, Salisbury, NC 28144, (704) 869-2126, BS 77 East Carolina Univ; MA 83 Appalachian St Univ; Sp-Lang Path, Davidson Co Sch, **SLP**

Moore, Mrs Terri 1350 North Lake Shore Dr, Apt 618, Chicago, IL 60611, (312) 831-3028, BA 84 IN Univ - Bloomington; MA 86 IN Univ - Bloomington; Aud, Oak Forest Hospital, **A**

Moore, Thomas 906 8th Avenue S W, Suite 205, Calgary, AB, Canada T2P 1H9, (403) 261-0687, BS 71 ID St Univ; MS 72 ID St Univ; Aud, Private Practice, **SLP**

Moore, Dr Walter H, Jr 2422 North Hathaway Street, Santa Ana, CA 92701, (213) 498-4583, BA 69 Univ of South FL; MS 70 Univ of South FL; PH 73 (NS) Kent St Univ; Prof, CA State U Long B, **SLP**

Moore, Wendy Ann 2137 Surrey Lane, Rock Hill, SC 29730, (803) 327-1062, BA 84 Winthrop Coll; MS 86 Univ of NC - Chapel Hill; 88–Sp-Lang Path, InSpeech Inc, **SLP**

Moore-Brown, Barbara Joann 140 Calle Diaz, Anaheim Hills, CA 92807, (714) 964-3339, BA 80 CA St Univ - Fullerton; MA 82 Whittier Coll; **SLP**

Moorer, Mrs Laura Poteet Lakewood Estates #60, Denton, TX 76205, (817) 382-1018, BS 82 TX Woman's Univ; MA 85 TX Woman's Univ; Sp-Lang Path, Denton State School, **SLP**

Moorhead, Mary Katherine 3125 Autumnwood Avenue, Apartment 95, Memphis, TN 38115, (901) 522-6593, BS 86 Auburn Univ - Auburn; MS 88 Univ of South AL; 87–Sp-Lang Path, Baptist Mem Hosp Rehab Ctr

Moorman, Mrs Marilyn S 30710 Ivywood Trail, Stacy, MN 55079, BA 70 Univ of North TX; MA 71 Univ of North TX; SLP, N Branch Pub Sch, **SLP**

Moorse, Mrs Deborah L 1415 Minnesota Avenue, Benson, MN 56215, (612) 843-4246, BS 75 Saint Cloud St Univ; MS 80 Saint Cloud St Univ; Sp-Lang Path, Appleton Pub Sch & SW/Wc Ecsu, **SLP**

Moosmann, Anne F 1086 Everwild View, Webster, NY 14580, (716) 271-0680, BA 80 SUNY - Coll at Plattsburgh; MA 81 SUNY - Coll at Geneseo; Sp-Lang Path, Hearing & Speech Ctr-Rochester, **SLP**

Mopper, Marjorie Ann 7991 Playmor Terrace, San Diego, CA 92122, (619) 744-6730, BA 73 Univ of MI - Ann Arbor; MA 76 Eastern MI Univ; 81–SLP, San Marcos USD, **SLP**

Morabito, Cindy Palatka 103 Windsor Court, Summerville, SC 29483, (803) 873-2945, **SLP**

Morales, Amparo Elsa 66 Madison Avenue, New York, NY 10016, (212) 689-5878, BS 80 Ithaca Coll; MA 82 NY Univ; Sp-Lang Path, Private Practice, **SLP**

Morales, Diana Carol 1300 Valparaiso Drive, Apartment P-24, Florence, SC 29501, (803) 669-7732, BA 86 Univ of Northern CO; MA 88 Univ of Northern CO; 88–Sp-Lang Path, Pee Dee Sp & Hrng Ctr

Morales, Joanne Lynn 73-8 Woodlands Condo, Mays Landing, NJ 08330, (201) 458-8575, BS 86 Stockton St Coll; MS 86 Bloomsburg Univ of PA

Morales, Laura Rufina 4036 Bellefontaine #3, Houston, TX 77025, (713) 664-0511, BA 81 Our Lady Lake Univ-San Anton; MA 83 Our Lady Lake Univ-San Anton; Sp-Lang Path, Houston ISD, **SLP**

Morales, Mrs Susan M P O Box 12, Delhi, NY 13753, (607) 746-2105, BS 73 SUNY - Coll at Geneseo; MS 79 Ithaca Coll; Sp-Lang Path, De Acad & Cen Sch, **SLP**

Morales-Pena, Blanca M 2008 Stanford, Las Cruces, NM 88005, (505) 523-7519, MA 83 NM St Univ; Sp-Lang Path, Providence Memorial Hospital, **SLP**

Moran, Alison Jane 435-D Willow Circle, Allentown, PA 18012, (215) 437-1489, BS 82 PA St Univ - Univ Park; MA 84 Kent St Univ; **SLP**

Moran, Carolann 29 Raymond Street, Nashua, NH 03060, (603) 881-4404, BA 68 Rivier Coll; ME 76 Northeastern Univ; 88–Preschool Coord, Nashua Sch Dist, **SLP**

Moran, Catherine Ann 28 Crescent Street, Middletown, CT 06457, (203) 344-6012, BA 83 Univ of RI; MS 85 PA St Univ - Univ Park; 88–Sp-Lang Path, Middlesex Memorial Hosp, **SLP**

Moran, Cynthia Ann P O Box 318, Warren, RI 02885, (401) 245-6464, BS 79 Elmira Coll; MA 81 Montclair St Coll; SLP, Private Practice, **SLP**

Moran, Mrs Cynthia J P O Box 118, Plainfield, VT 05667, (802) 454-8022, MS 83 Univ of VT; Sp-Lang Path, Washington Ctrl Spvr Union, **SLP**

Moran, Joyce A 34953 Persimmon Avenue, Yucaipa, CA 92399, (714) 887-6333, BA Loma Linda Univ - Riverside; MA 70 Univ of Redlands; Sp-Lang Path, San Bernardino Comm Hosp, **SLP**

Moran, Laurette 1008 Woodbury Road, Edmond, OK 73034, (703) 552-7733, BS 73 Univ of MD - College Park; MS 75 Univ of OK Medical Center; Sp-Lang Path, Private Practice, **SLP**

Moran, Lynn Ryan 1137 Wilhelm Drive, Hellertown, PA 18055, (215) 838-7969, BS 63 Saint Louis Univ; ME 66 Boston Univ; 86–Dir/Sp-Lang Path, Good Sheperd Home, **SLP**

Moran, Marion C 123 Highland Avenue, Somerville, MA 02143, (617) 625-2863, BS 39 Salem St Coll; MS 52 Boston Univ; **A LM**

Moran, Mrs Mary Ann Route 1 Box 48B, Westernport, MD 21562, (301) 359-3567, BS 70 WV Univ; MS 71 WV Univ; **SLP**

Moran, Dr Michael J 1610 Millbranch Drive, Auburn, AL 36830, (205) 826-5545, BS 71 East Stroudsburg Univ of PA; MA 72 Wichita St Univ; PH 80 (Communication Disord) PA St Univ - Univ Park; 83–Prof, Auburn U Dept Comm Dis, **SLP**

Moran, Patricia Ann Cussen 806 West Kentucky, Anadarko, OK 73005, (405) 247-6688, BA 56 Univ of Science & Arts of OK; ME 72 Central St Univ; Admin, Anadarko Reg Ed Serv Cen, **SLP**

Moran, Patricia Elizabeth 25 Milton Avenue, West Seneca, NY 14224, (716) 672-4992, OB 80 SUNY - Coll at Fredonia; OM 81 SUNY - Coll at Fredonia; SLP, Erie 2-Chautauqua-Cattaraugus, **SLP**

Moran, Rosalyn Soares 2416 Payne Avenue, Modesto, CA 95351, (415) 784-2745, BA 59 CA St Univ - Fresno; Sp-Lang Path, Hayward USD, **SLP**

Moran, Susan Schutz 3305 King Richard Court, Seffner, FL 33584, (813) 236-5589, MS 84 Univ of South FL; Sp-Lang Path, Easter Seal Rehab Cen, **SLP**

Moran, Veronica Carreras C D Consultants, 1615B Don Rosery Drive, Las Cruces, NM 88001, (505) 522-8092, BS 79 NM St Univ; MA 81 NM St Univ; Sp-Lang Path, Private Practice, **SLP ACE**

Moran-Burton, Mrs Judith A 15 Birch Street, Binghamton, NY 13903, (607) 723-0262, BS 72 SUNY - Center at Albany; MA 74 SUNY - Coll at Geneseo; Supervisory Sp-Lang Path, Rehabilitation Service, **SLP**

Morand, Kate W220 N7454 Cherry Hill Rd, Sussex, WI 53089, (414) 644-6669, BS 78 Marquette Univ; MS 80 Marquette Univ; Sp-Lang Path, Sch Dist of Slinger, **SLP**

Moran-Grap, Mrs Lynn Marie 14 West End Court, Relay, MD 21227, (301) 242-0862, BS 82 Towson St Univ; MS 84 Towson St Univ; Sp-Lang Path, Prince Georges Board of Educ, **SLP**

Morasch, Candace M Saddletime Farm, 345 Sheraton Drive, Williams, OR 97544, (503) 474-5700, BA 68 Eastern WA Univ; BA 69 Eastern WA Univ; MA 81 Univ of Cincinnati; Sp-Lang Path, Sch Dist #7-Grants Pass, or, **SLP**

Moravek, Mrs Peggy Mulcrone 523 Callery Road, Evans City, PA 16033, (412) 538-4233, BA 72 Marygove Coll; MS 73 Southern CT St Univ; 75–Sp-Lang Path, Allegheny Intermediate Unit 3, **SLP**

Morawetz, Mary Jean 331 Overbrook Road, Birmingham, AL 35213, (205) 870-7243, BA 68 FL St Univ; MS 71 Univ of UT; Sp/Lang/Rdng Cen, **SLP**

Mordecai, Dr Dennis R 14 West Brooke Drive, Novato, CA 94947, (415) 892-4746, BA 72 Univ of CA - Santa Barbara; MS 73 Univ of IL - Urbana; PH 79 Northwestern Univ; 79–Exec Dir, Team Rehab, **SLP**

Mordue, Mrs Lavella Y 513 Byron, Mankato, MN 56001, (507) 388-5971, BS 76 Mankato St Univ; MS 81 Mankato St Univ; Sp-Lang Path, **SLP**

Moreau, Leonard J 115 Hanover Avenue, Pawtucket, RI 02861, (401) 725-4530, BS 48 Univ of RI; ME 52 Boston Univ; Sp-Lang Path, Pawtucket Sched Dept, **SLP**

Moreau, Mrs Maryellen Rooney 10 Coed Drive, Easthampton, MA 01027, (413) 527-6836, BA 68 Univ of MA - Amherst; ME 69 PA St Univ - Univ Park; Sp-Lang Path, American International Coll, **SLP**

Moreau, Vaughn K 40 Eichelberger Drive, Coraopolis, PA 15108, (412) 394-5826, BS 69 CA Univ of PA; MS 73 WV Univ; Sp-Lang Path, Allegheny Inter Ut, **SLP**

Morehouse, Charles Robin Kresge Hearing Research Laboratory, LSUMC 2020 Gravier Street Suite A, New Orleans, LA 70112-2234, (504) 568-4785, BS 72 Dalhousie Univ - Nova Scotia; MA 75 Univ of FL; MS 78 Dalhousie Univ - Nova Scotia; 87–Aud, Hearing Resch, **A**

Morehouse, Mrs Julie J P O Box 68, Mass City, MI 49948, MA 72 Western MI Univ; BS 71 Western MI Univ; SLP, Gogebic-Ontonagon Ind Sch Dist, **SLP**

Morehouse, Katherine Route 1 Box 58, Dayton, VA 22821, (703) 332-9048, **A**

Morehouse, Margaret P 26 May Apple Way, Ballston Spa, NY 12020, (518) 434-4103, BA 81 SUNY - Coll at Plattsburgh; MS 85 Coll of Saint Rose; **SLP**

Morehouse, Toni B 2740 Jane Lane, Lincoln, NE 68516, (402) 472-5471, BS 73 Univ of NE - Lincoln; MA 74 Univ of NE - Lincoln; 87–Instr, Univ of Nebraska, **SLP**

Morejohn, Linda Celeste 3336 Rocky Mountain Drive, San Jose, CA 95127, (408) 923-1940, BA 76 San Jose St Univ; MA 84 San Jose St Univ; Special Day Class Tchr, Beryessa Union School District, **SLP**

Morejohn, Nikki Lynn 1240 Forest Creek Drive, Hollister, CA 95023, (408) 637-3805, **SLP**

Moreken, Mrs Betty C 1328 Myrtle Street, Scranton, PA 18510, (717) 348-3455, BA 69 East Stroudsburg Univ of PA; ME 72 Bloomsburg Univ of PA; Sp-Lang Path, Scranton School District, **SLP**

Moreland, Mrs Elizabeth Bondurant 537 Harrow Road, Knoxville, TN 37922-4741, (912) 997-7809, BA 77 Emory & Henry Coll; MA 80 Univ of TN - Knoxville; Sp-Lang Path, Houston County Board of Educ, **SLP**

Moreland, Judith Pickett Box 543, Guilderland, NY 12084, (518) 370-7593, BS 75 SUNY - Center at Albany; MS 80 Univ of South FL; Sp-Lang Path, Od Heck Developmental Center, **SLP**

Morell, Susan A W 10825 N E 64th Street, Kirkland, WA 98033, (206) 827-4262, **SLP**

Morelli-Neddy, Mrs Aimee Beth 1211 Holland, Birmingham, MI 48009, (313) 524-2650, BS 82 Bowling Green St Univ; MA 86 Kent St Univ; 88–Sp-Lang Path, Neurorehab Day Trtmt Hlth S, **SLP**

Morelock-Maddamma, Cynthia Elizabeth 272 Lynn Drive, Pittsburgh, PA 15236, (412) 882-4321, BS 82 Southwest MO St Univ; MS 84 Central MO St Univ; Sp-Lang Path, Meadowlands Nerou Center, **SLP**

Morency, Claire D 3106 Chateau Knoll, Bettendorf, IA 52722, (319) 332-5012, BS 78 Augustana Coll; MS 79 Eastern IL Univ; Sp/Lang Path, MS Bend AEA, **SLP**

Morency, Janet M Unitron Industries Ltd, 20 Beasley Drive, P O Box 9017, Kitchener, ON, Canada N2G 4J3, (519) 893-6800, MA 77 Wayne St Univ - Sch of Med; Manager of Prof Relations, Unitron Indus, **A**

Morency-Hnat, Mrs Rachelle Anne 145 Oakwood Road, Mc Murray, PA 15317, (412) 521-9000, MA 84 Univ of Pittsburgh - Pittsburgh; SLP, Neurological Center Meadowland, **SLP**

Moreno, Cynthia E 715 Gayley, Apartment 202, Los Angeles, CA 90024, (213) 824-5142, BS 78 Boston Univ; MS 80 Columbia Univ Teachers Coll; 88–Sp-Lang Path, LA Co USC Med Ctr, **SLP**

Moreno, Melinda V 140 El Dorado Road, Walnut Creek, CA 94595-1503, (415) 935-6639, BS; **SLP**

Moreno, Mrs Yolanda Flores 2220 Sea Side, El Paso, TX 79936, (915) 595-5500, BA 83 Univ of TX - El Paso; MS 85 Univ of TX - El Paso

Morenz, Kim Renee 10514 Garnett #21, Overland Park, KS 66214-2742, (913) 829-0891, BA 83 Univ of Northern IA; MA 85 Memphis St Univ; 88–Sp-Lang Path, Assoc Audiologists Inc, **SLP**

Morenzi, Mrs Andria R 112 East Shore Road, Jamestown, RI 02835, (401) 456-9330, BA 77 Univ of Central FL; MS 79 Univ of RI; Sp-Lang Path, Providence Public Schools, **SLP**

Morere, Karen L Univ Of Ms Medical Center CDL, 2500 North State Street, Jackson, MS 39216, (601) 984-4550, BA 72 Southeastern LA Univ; OM 73 Univ of MS; Instr/Sp-Lang Path, Commun Dis Lab, **SLP**

Moretti, Margaret E 25001 Oak, Lomita, CA 90717, (714) 581-2800, BA 80 CA St Univ - Long Beach; MA 83 CA St Univ - Long Beach; Aud, Newport Lang Sp & Aud Cen, **A**

Moretz, Mrs Linda P 57 Carrington Avenue, Milford, CT 06460, (203) 878-1812, BA 64 Augustana Coll; Sp-Lang Path, Trinity Day Sch, **SLP**

Morey, Mrs Ann Patrice P O Box 71, Cambridge, IL 61238, (309) 342-0155, BA 82 Augustana Coll; **SLP**

Morey, Mrs Kathryn Downs 5100 North 1st Street, Arlington, VA 22203-1208, (703) 698-1600, BA 77 SUNY - Coll at Plattsburgh; MS 85 Coll of Saint Rose; SLP, Fairfax County Public Schools, **SLP**

Morey, Kathryn R 4136 West 157th Street, Cleveland, OH 44135, (216) 749-0356, 84–Sp-Lang Path, Cuyahoga Co Bd of Men Retard, **SLP**

Morgan, Alice A 1502 South Washington, Marshall, TX 75670, (318) 227-5158, BS 59 East TX Baptist Coll; MS 64 East TN St Univ; PH 79 (Sp-Lang Path) Univ of MO - Columbia; 81–Assoc Prof, LA St Unive Med Ctr Allied Hlt, **SLP**

Morgan, Dr Alisa L R 2 Pleasant Street, Concord, MA 01742, (617) 232-9500, 84 Univ of WI - Madison; MS 79 Univ of KS; PH (NS); Sp-Lang Path, Boston VA Medical Center, **SLP**

Morgan, Ann F P O Box 895, Winter Garden, FL 32787, (305) 293-1421, MS 78 Univ of WI - Eau Claire; BA 76 Univ of WI - Eau Claire; SLP/Aud, Sunland Cen-St of FL, **SLP**

Morgan, Ann M Grossmont Union High Sch Dist, Special Education, P O Box 1043, La Mesa, CA 92041, (619) 442-3463, BA 73 Univ of MN - Minneap-St Paul; MA 75 Univ of MN - Minneap-St Paul; Sp-Lang Path, Grossmont Un Hs Dist, **SLP**

Morgan, Barbara M 4020 Dunster Way, Sacramento, CA 95825, (916) 488-8172, BS 67 Northern IL Univ - De Kalb; MS 73 Phillips Univ; **SLP**

Morgan, Mrs Carol Wasson 630 Nolia Street, El Dorado, AR 71730-6740, (501) 863-3541, BA 81 Univ of AR - Fayetteville; MS 82 Univ of AR - Fayetteville; SLP, El Dorado Pub Schs, **SLP**

Morgan, Mrs Deborah Jones 107 Clark Hill Drive, Inman, SC 29349, (803) 592-9257, BS 77 WV Univ; MS 82 WV Univ; Sp-Lang Path, Spartanburg Co Schs Dist 2, **SLP**

Morgan, Debra Lynn 606 Foxcroft Avenue #3-B, Martinsburg, WV 25401, BS 82 Univ of Cincinnati; MA 84 OH St Univ; **A**

Morgan, Mrs Denise L 2226 Kings Avenue South, Brandon, FL 33511, (813) 974-2006, BA 79 Univ of FL; MS 82 Univ of South FL; Asst In Res Cl Superv, U of So FL, **SLP**

Morgan, Mrs Diane B 863 Timber Lane, Dresher, PA 19025, (215) 884-8333, BA 69 Temple Univ; MA 73 Temple Univ; Owner/Admin, Diane Morgan & Assoc, **SLP ACE**

Morgan, Dr Donald E Director Audiology Clinic, UCLA Medical Center, Chs 62-202, Los Angeles, CA 90024, (213) 825-5721, MA 65 San Diego St Univ; PH 68 (NS) Northwestern Univ; Assoc Prof/Dir Aud Cl, UCLA Sch of Med, **A**

Morgan, Mrs Donna Lynn R 1912 Westwood Drive, Cape Girardeau, MO 63701, (314) 334-0674, OB 75 AR St Univ; OM 76 AR St Univ; 87–SLP, Cape Girardeau Sch Dist, **SLP**

Morgan, Elizabeth Ash 517 West Tenth Street, Taylor, TX 76574, (512) 440-5427, BS 84 Southwest TX St Univ; ME 86 Southwest TX St Univ; **SLP**

Morgan, Gary L 518 North Owen Drive, Madison, WI 53705, (608) 238-6664, **A**

Morgan, Mrs Gerry Gardner 132 Old Post Drive, Hauppauge, NY 11788, (516) 360-3771, BA 69 Adelphi Univ; MS 87 Adelphi Univ; Sp-Lang Path, Assoc for Children with Down Syndrome, **SLP**

Morgan, Gilda Fay 2434 Gore Road, Baton Rouge, LA 70807, (504) 775-0725, ME 88 Southern Univ - Baton Rouge

Morgan, Jane Kirschbaum 510 Piper Drive, Madison, WI 53711-1319, (608) 822-3276, BS 83 Univ of WI - Madison; MS 85 Univ of WI - Madison; **SLP**

Morgan, Mrs Janet 1410 Club Parkway, Nashville, TN 37221, (615) 662-1758, BA 80 Univ of AL- Tuscaloosa; MS 85 Univ of KY; 88–Sp-Lang Path, Vanderbilt Univ Med Ctr, **SLP**

Morgan, Janet L 11108 Country River Drive, Parrish, FL 34219, (813) 758-2350, BS 70 Kent St Univ; MA 71 Kent St Univ; PH 88 (Special Education) Univ of South FL; 88–Sp-Lang Path, Manatee Co Sch, **SLP**

Morgan, Jeanne Boose 302 Orleans Avenue, Bossier City, LA 71112, (916) 741-8091, BS 73 LA St Univ - Baton Rouge; MA 75 LA Tech Univ; Sp-Lang Path, Bossier Parish Sch Bd, **SLP**

Morgan, Jeffrey Lynn 816 Shady Lake Drive, Bedford, TX 76021, (817) 735-8505, BS 82 IN Univ - Bloomington; MS 83 Univ of North TX; 86–Owner, Bowie Speech and Hearing, **A**

Morgan, Mrs Karen Gough 2802 Quanah, Round Rock, TX 78681, (512) 863-3030, BS 74 Southern Methodist Univ; MS 80 TX Tech Univ; SLP, Georgetown Indep School Dist, **SLP**

Morgan, Mrs Karen S 23-824 Del Cerro Circle, West Hills, CA 91304, (818) 716-1626, BS 69 Univ of UT; MA 72 CA St Univ - Los Angeles; Sp/Lang Path, LA Ctr for Therapy & Educ, **SLP**

Morgan, Kathleen Elizabeth 2418 A Spencer Avenue, St Louis, MO 63114, (314) 426-4077, BS 85 Fontbonne Coll; MA 87 Saint Louis Univ; **SLP**

Morgan, Mrs Kathleen I Box 209, Commerce, TX 75428, (214) 454-3805, BS 64 Univ of OK - Norman; MS 76 East TX St Univ - Commerce; 85–Sp-Lang Path, Rehab Assoc of Northeast Texas, **SLP ACE**

Morgan, Mrs Kay Hutchinson 2524 Plank Road, Keokuk, IA 52632, (319) 524-5032, BS 63 Univ of MO - Columbia; MA 80 Northeast MO St Univ; SLP, Great River AEA, **SLP**

Morgan, Mrs Linda M Rd 2, Sugarloaf, PA 18249, (717) 459-3154, BS 69 Bloomsburg Univ of PA; MS 71 Bloomsburg Univ of PA; SLP, Hazleton Area Sch Dist, **SLP**

Morgan, Mrs Lori Jean 5016 Frontier Lane, Plano, TX 75023, (214) 424-5602, BS 82 Southern IL Univ -Carbondale; MS 83 Southern IL Univ -Carbondale; SLP, Plano ISD, **SLP**

Morgan, Lynne Clark 13226 Memory Lane, Fairfax, VA 22033-3505, (704) 541-1309, BS 78 East Carolina Univ; MS 81 East Carolina Univ; Clinical Supervisor, InSpeech Inc, **SLP**

Morgan, Maria L 4725 Kynnelworth Drive Unit 6, Bettendorf, IA 52722, (309) 762-5112, BA 78 Wichita St Univ; MA 80 Wichita St Univ; 88–Editor, LinguiSystems Inc, **SLP**

Morgan, Marian T Trover Clinic, Clinic Drive, Madisonville, KY 42431, (502) 825-7363, BA 60 Univ of KY; MA 64 Univ of KY; Aud, Trover Cl, **A**

Morgan, Marianne Marie 1733 Cambridge Circle, Redlands, CA 92374, (714) 794-1976, MS 86 Univ of Redlands; 88–Sp-Lang Path, Palm Springs USD, **SLP**

Morgan, Marlene S 40 Rocky Pond Road, Brookline, NH 03033, (603) 673-6520, Self Employed, **SLP**

Morgan, Mrs Mary L 6528 117th Place Southeast, Renton, WA 98056, (206) 455-6260, BS 77 Univ of WA; MA 79 Univ of WA; SLP, Bellevue School District, **SLP**

Morgan, Mrs Michele Cole Route 4 Box 408-14, Clarkesville, GA 30523, (404) 754-8469, BS 86 Univ of GA; ME 87 Univ of GA

Morgan, Michele M 351 Maple Ridge Road, Twining, MI 48766, (517) 894-3144, BS 80 Northern MI Univ; MA 81 MI St Univ; Sp-Lang Path, **SLP**

Morgan, Mike David 2004 North Wilson, Hutchinson, KS 67502, (405) 234-4198, BS 83 Phillips Univ; MA 85 Wichita St Univ; **SLP**

Morgan, Nancy Patton 8400 Rockwood Lane, Austin, TX 78758, (512) 452-6360, **SLP**

Morgan, Mrs Noel Garvin 1921 Floyd Street, Sarasota, FL 34239, (813) 365-0367, BS 83 FL St Univ; MS 85 FL St Univ; 85–Aud, Ear Research Foundation, **A**

Morgan, Pamela Lynne 3449 So 2770 East, Salt Lake City, UT 84109, (801) 466-3846, BS 82 Brigham Young Univ; MS 86 Univ of UT; 84–Sp-Lang Path, Granite Sch Dist, **SLP**

Morgan, Mrs Patsy Hardin 925 North Tropical Trail, Merritt Island, FL 32953, (305) 452-0064, **SLP**

Morgan, Mrs Patti A 9453 Heatherdale, Dallas, TX 75243, BA 62; MA 80 Univ of North TX; 88–Sp/Lang Path, Private Practice, **SLP**

Morgan, Mrs Ruth Howells Route 4 Box 262, Warrenton, VA 22186, (606) 268-8356, **SLP**

Morgan, Sherrill Davis 6560 Saroni Drive, Oakland, CA 94611, (415) 339-8143, BA 64 Stanford Univ; MS 81 San Francisco St Univ; **SLP**

Morgan, Susan 354 Pilgrim Road, West Palm Beach, FL 33405, (407) 848-4371, BS 86 Western IL Univ; MA 87 Western IL Univ; 87–Sp-Lang Path, Palm Beach County School Dist, **SLP**

Morgan, Suzanne E 6605 Cypress Drive, Omaha, NE 68137, (402) 391-7948, BA 61 Purdue Univ - West Lafayette; MA 66 IN Univ - Bloomington; Sp-Lang Path, Westside Comm Sch, **SLP**

Morgan, Sylvia 42 Lafayette Avenue, Dumont, NJ 07628, (201) 387-0614, BS 47 OH St Univ; MA 54 Columbia Univ Teachers Coll; Aud, Columbia-Presbyterian Med Cen, **A**

Morgan, Mrs Tamara Snyder 504 Murdoch Road, Philadelphia, PA 19119, (215) 482-3100, BS 80 PA St Univ - Univ Park; MS 82 PA St Univ - Univ Park; Aud, Alan Berger MD, **A**

Morgan, Teresa Gail 3207 Lincoln Boulevard, Marion, IN 46953, (219) 293-7506, BS 83 Ball St Univ; MA 84 Ball St Univ; 88–Sp-Lang Path, Assoc for the Disabled of Elkhart County, **SLP**

Morgan, Terri Ann 1101 Lindsay Road, Carnegie, PA 15106, (412) 276-3655, BS 84 Clarion Univ of PA; MS 85 Clarion Univ of PA; 86–Sp-Lang Path, Easter Seal Soc of Allegheny Co, **SLP**

Morgan, Terry A 2217 Plymouth Street, Midland, MI 48640, **SLP**

Morgan, Yvonne 8060 Calico Street, San Diego, CA 92126, (619) 274-9842, BA 76 Univ of CA - Santa Barbara; MS 79 UT St Univ; Sp-Lang Path, San Diego USD, **SLP**

Morgan-Landing, Kathleen Anne 304 Timberlane Road, Tallahassee, FL 32312, (904) 386-8364, BA 75 Univ of MI - Ann Arbor; MS 78 Univ of WA; **A**

Morganstein, Shirley 145 East 15th Street, Apartment 5M, New York, NY 10003, (212) 241-6335, BA 68 NY Univ; MA 72 Univ of MN - Minneap-St Paul; 86–Coord Sp-Lang Path, Dept of Rehab Med-Mt Sinai Hosp, **SLP**

Morganti, Mrs Denise Ann Borek 11 Pleasant Drive, Rome, NY 13440, (315) 338-3268, BS 76 Ithaca Coll; MS 79 Ithaca Coll; 77–Sp-Lang Path, Rome Cty Sch, **SLP**

Morgan-Wasserman, Leslie L 223 Woodview Drive, Decatur, GA 30030, (404) 427-1314, BA 79 Univ of NC - Chapel Hill; ME 81 Univ of GA; 86–Aud, Byron Perry MD, **A**

Morgenroth, Nancy L 123-35 82nd Road, Kew Gardens, NY 11415, (212) 794-4821, BS 75 Boston Univ; MS 76 Univ of MI - Ann Arbor; SLP, The Summit Sch, **SLP**

Morgenstern, Carol S 60 Juniper Lane, Muttontown, NY 11791, **SLP**

Morgenstern, Doris A 59 Vernon Street, Waltham, MA 02154, (617) 899-4709, BA 55 Brown Univ; MS 70 Emerson Coll; Dir, Commun Hlth Care Assoc, **SLP ACE**

Morgenstern, Nancy 46 Mountain View Drive, West Hartford, CT 06117, (203) 233-7304, BA 72 SUNY - Center at Buffalo; MA 73 MI St Univ; SLP Consult, Nancy Morgenstern Ma Ccc-Spech, **SLP**

Morgese, Zoe L 506 N W 30th Street, Gainesville, FL 32607, (904) 376-4896, BA 74 Univ of Denver; MA 76 Univ of Denver; Sp-Lang Path, Special Communications, **SLP**

Moriarty, Daniel Gerard Easter Seal Hrng & Sp Ctr, 233 East Broadway, Louisville, KY 40202, (502) 584-9781, MS 84 Univ of Louisville; Coor of Ind Aud, Easter Seal, **A**

Moriarty, Michele Rae 1616 South Street, Whitehall, WI 54773, (715) 538-4013, BA 84 Univ of WI - Eau Claire; MS 86 Univ of WI - Stevens Point; **SLP**

Moriarty, Patricia L 1424 Fallsmead Way, Rockville, MD 20854, (301) 424-6282, BS 68 Marquette Univ; MA 70 Columbia Univ Teachers Coll; 88–Sp-Lang Path, Montgomery County PS, **SLP ACE**

Morico, Patricia Helen 597 Whispering Hills Drive, Chester, NY 10918, (914) 947-1000, BS 75 Bowling Green St Univ; OM 82 Tulane Univ; Sp-Lang Path, Letchworth Village Devel Cen, **SLP**

Morilak, Deborah Jeanne 504 Florida Street, Orlando, FL 32806, BS 85 Bowling Green St Univ; MA 86 Memphis St Univ; **SLP**

Morin-Connolly, Gisele 6975 Bendbough Court, Columbia, MD 21045-4607, (301) 992-7094, BA 76 Providence Coll; MA 79 Case Western Reserve Univ; SLP, McOss, **SLP**

Morisato, Teale Misae 3228 Esther Street, Honolulu, HI 96815, BS 84 Univ of HI - Manoa; MS 85 Univ of HI - Manoa; **SLP**

Morisco, Jacqueline 310 Riverside Drive #1121, New York, NY 10025, (212) 549-4753, BS 76 SUNY - Coll at Fredonia; MS 78 Columbia Univ Teachers Coll; Sp-Lang Path, H G Birch Early Chldhd Ctr, **SLP**

Morissette, Charmaine Lynne 2-325 3rd Street, Estevan, SK, Canada S4A 0N8, (306) 634-4741, BA 82 Univ of ND; MS 83 Univ of ND; 83–Sp-Lang Path, Moose Mountain Shared Services, **SLP**

Moritz, Susan Ann 10 North Main Street #401, Beacon Falls, CT 06403, (203) 729-9224, BA 86 George Washington Univ; MA 88 Univ of Pittsburgh - Pittsburgh; 88–Sp-Lang Path, New Britain Memorial Hosp

Mork-Adix, Delores Arlene R R 2 Box 198, Clearwater, MN 55320-9568, (612) 253-5857, MS 84 Univ of WI - Eau Claire; Sp-Lang Path, District 742, **SLP**

Morley, Dr Alonzo John 387 East 300 North, Provo, UT 84601, (801) 373-8987, BA 25 Brigham Young Univ; MA 31 Brigham Young Univ; PH 35 (Sp-Lang Path) IA St Univ; 71–Prof Emeritus SLP & Aud, Brigham Young Univ, **SLP A F LM**

Morley, D E 701 Barton Drive, Ann Arbor, MI 48105, (313) 663-2884, PH 49 (NS) Univ of MI - Ann Arbor; **SLP F LM**

Morley, Elizabeth Hird 114 Col Christopher Green, Road, Portsmouth, RI 02871, (617) 993-7374, BA 80 Univ of RI; MS 81 Syracuse Univ; Sp-Lang Path, Taunton Erly Intervent Prog, **SLP**

Morley, Lisa J 3004 Waterway Blvd, Isle of Palms, SC 29451, (803) 766-9455, BA 75 Memphis St Univ; MA 78 Memphis St Univ; Sp-Lang Path, Self Employed, **SLP**

Morley, Russell D Montgomery County I U #23, 1605-B West Main Street, Norristown, PA 19403, (215) 539-8550, BS 62 Indiana Univ of PA; ME 67 PA St Univ - Univ Park; Superv Sp & Lang, Montgy Co Inter Ut, **SLP F**

Morlier, Mrs Robin Eiserloh 2600 Aquaduct Court, Bedford, TX 76022, (817) 882-2045, BS 82 Baylor Univ; MS 83 Baylor Univ; Sp-Lang Path, Harris Meth Hosp, **SLP**

Morlock, Julianne M 383 Coventrey Court, Clarendon Hills, IL 60514, (312) 857-1325, BS 75 Saint Louis Univ; MS 76 Southern IL Univ-Edwardsvill; Sp/Lang Path, Christ Hosp, **SLP**

Morman, Mrs Patricia C 5161 Swift Street, Oswego, NY 13126-1717, (315) 343-3864, BS 68 Bowling Green St Univ; MS 76 Ithaca Coll; **SLP**

Mormer, Elaine A 1522 Denniston Street, Pittsburgh, PA 15217, (412) 521-6404, BS 79 Univ of MA - Amherst; MA 81 Univ of MA - Amherst; Aud, St Francis Med Ctr, **A**

Morningstar, Janet C 7133 Maple Avenue, Cincinnati, OH 45243, **SLP**

Mornout, Mrs Claudia W 2965 Mission Blvd #2C, San Diego, CA 92109-1732, (619) 488-1540, BS 70 Purdue Univ - West Lafayette; MS 71 Purdue Univ - West Lafayette; 88–Sp-Lang Path, Private Practice, **SLP ACE**

Morocco, Katherine Creen 158 Beechwood Road, Holden, MA 01520, (617) 829-2813, BA 67 Emmanuel Coll; MS 82 Worcester St Coll; Sp-Lang Path, Worcester Public Schools, **SLP**

Moroge, Mrs Phyllis A 2812 Morton Road, Raleigh, NC 27604, BS SUNY - Center at Buffalo; MS 80 Univ of NM; SLP/Superv, Duke U Med Cen, **SLP**

Morone, Mrs Rebecca S 2745 Chestnut Court, Columbus, IN 47201, (812) 376-6329, BS 78 Purdue Univ - West Lafayette; MA 79 Univ of IL - Urbana; Sp-Lang Path, Jackson County Schneck Memorial Hosp, **SLP**

Moroney, Donna Patrice 7402-91 Mission Trails Dr, Santee, CA 92071-3397, (619) 562-7206, BA 78 San Diego St Univ; MA 83 San Diego St Univ; Aud, Southern CA Permanente Med Grp, **A**

Moroney, Patricia Ann 149 N E 62nd Street, Seattle, WA 98115, (206) 526-2104, BA 79 San Diego St Univ; MA 82 Western WA Univ; 87–Sp-Lang Path, Childrens Hosp, **SLP**

Moroni, Mrs Susan M H 230 Belmeade Road, Rochester, NY 14617, (716) 467-3131, BS 79 Nazareth Coll of Rochester; MS 80 SUNY - Coll at Buffalo; Sp/Lang Path, Rochester Cty Sch Dist, **SLP**

Moroux, Danielle M P O Box 4926, Winter Park, FL 32793, (305) 647-2921, MA 79 Univ of TN - Knoxville; SLP, Valencia Comm College, **SLP**

Morphis, Gayle Thompson 1441 North Rock Road #2202, Wichita, KS 67206, (316) 833-4550, BA 73 Wichita St Univ; MA 75 Univ of TN - Knoxville; Sp-Lang Path, Wichita Pub Sch, **SLP**

Morreale, Carol Clifford 1903 Kiowa Lane, Mount Prospect, IL 60056, (312) 942-5332, BS 83 CO St Univ; MA 84 Northwestern Univ; Aud, Rush Presbyterian-St Luke's Med Ctr, **A**

Morrell, Mrs Ruth Ann 12373 Sunrise Drive, Indianapolis, IN 46229, (317) 894-5952, BS 74 Purdue Univ - West Lafayette; MS 78 Purdue Univ - West Lafayette; 75–Sp-Lang Path, Indianapolis Pub Sch, **SLP**

Morrell-Trussell, Carol Anne 2672 Stonecreek Drive #184, Sacramento, CA 95833, (916) 966-5055, BA 84 CA St Univ - Sacramento; MS 86 CA St Univ - Sacramento; **A**

Morren, Mrs Jeanette A 1206 South Seaman, Eastland, TX 76448, (817) 734-2020, OB 82 Hardin-Simmons Univ; Sp-Lang Path, East End Ed Co-Op, **LM**

Morriconi, Alfonso 45 King Road, Telford, PA 18969, (215) 234-4694, ME 57 Temple Univ; **SLP LM**

Morrin, Mrs Catherine Anne 333 Dixie Highway, Chicago Heights, IL 60411, (312) 756-0100, 79–Aud, Suburban Hts Med Ctr, **A**

Morris, Alison Lee 35 Fairview Avenue, Watertown, MA 02172, (617) 848-5353, MS 82 Univ of WI - Madison; 87–Sp-Lang Path, Braintree Hospital, **SLP**

Morris, Mrs Amy Catherine 3878 Shady Wood Drive #4, Jefferson, MD 21755, (301) 473-8613, BS 86 Towson St Univ; MA 88 Univ of Pittsburgh - Pittsburgh; 88–Sp-Lang Path, Frederick Co Bd of Educ

Morris, Barbara B 732 Schmitz Street #1, Denton, TX 76201, (817) 382-2397, BS 85 East TX St Univ - Commerce; MS 86 East TX St Univ - Commerce; 88–Sp-Lang Path, Private Practice, **SLP**

Morris, Mrs Barbara K 401 Pinoak Way, Easton, MD 21601, (301) 758-1320, BS 73 IN Univ - Bloomington; OM 74 IN Univ - Bloomington; Sp-Lang Path, Queens Anne County Board of Ed, **SLP**

Morris, Belinda Denise 6260 Greenwood Road, Apartment 1002, Shreveport, LA 71119, (318) 631-5110, BA 83 LA Tech Univ; MS 85 LA Tech Univ; 85–Sp-Lang Path, Caddo Parish Sch Bd, **SLP**

Morris, Mrs Cheryl A 1901 Lazy Branch, Independence, MO 64058, (816) 453-0353, BS 75 Southwest MO St Univ; MS 82 Central MO St Univ; Sp-Lang Path, N Kansas City Sch Dist, **SLP**

Morris, Colleen L 1611 St Paul Street, Apartment 3, Baltimore, MD 21202, (301) 955-6151, BA 86 Univ of FL; MA 88 George Washington Univ; 88–Aud, Johns Hopkins Hospital

Morris, Mrs Cynthia G 13357 Sherwood, Huntington Woods, MI 48070, (313) 697-9123, BS 78 MI St Univ; MA 80 Wayne St Univ; Sp-Lang Path, Van Buren Public Schools, **SLP**

Morris, Diane M 114 Edson Street, Buffalo, NY 14210, (716) 674-6300, BS 40 SUNY - Coll at Buffalo; MS 76 SUNY - Coll at Buffalo; SLP, Wn NY Chldn Psychi Con, **SLP**

Morris, Mrs Elizabeth 414 Chesney Street, Kenton, OH 43326, (419) 675-2700, BS 70 FL St Univ; MS 71 FL St Univ; 88–Sp-Lang Path, Hardin Co Spec Educ, **SLP**

Morris, Mrs Gail Marie 1600 Tanbark Circle, Jackson, MI 49203, (517) 787-2800, BS 74 Western MI Univ; MA 84 Eastern MI Univ; Sp-Lang Path, Jackson ISD, **SLP**

Morris, Harry A 3141 East Jackson Avenue, Orange, CA 92667, (714) 821-3620, BA 66 CA St Univ - Fullerton; MA 71 CA St Univ - Fullerton; Cl Administrator, Sp & Lang Dev Cen, **SLP**

Morris, Mrs Helen Anderson 809 Bray Avenue, Rolla, MO 65401, (314) 341-2638, BS 54 Minot St Univ; MS 57 Purdue Univ - West Lafayette; Sp-Lang Path, Univ of Missouri-Rolla, **SLP**

Morris, Dr Hughlett L Department Of Otolaryngology, University Hospital, Iowa City, IA 52242, (319) 356-2292, BA 52 Univ of IA; MA 57 Univ of IA; PH 60 (NS) Univ of IA; Sp-Lang Path, The U of IA, **SLP F**

Morris, Jacqueline P O Box 44011, Tucson, AZ 85733, (602) 325-2108, BA 68 Univ of OR; MS 76 Univ of AZ; Sp-Lang Path, Private Practice, **SLP**

Morris, Joyce M 13541 Point Pleasant Drive, Chantilly, VA 22021, **SLP**

Morris, Mrs Julie P 118 Cowell Avenue, Oil City, PA 16301, (814) 677-5443, BS 74 Indiana Univ of PA; MS 76 Indiana Univ of PA; Sp-Lang Path, Private Practice, **SLP**

Morris, Karen Elaine 8700 Basil, El Paso, TX 79925, (915) 533-2266, BA 81 TX Tech Univ; MA 85 Univ of KS; **A**

Morris, Mrs Karen Pawlowski 35396 North Adelphi, Waukegan, IL 60085-2210, (312) 662-2825, BS 81 Univ of IL - Urbana; MS 83 Purdue Univ - West Lafayette; Audiologist, VA Medical Center, **A ACE**

Morris, Mrs Kathleen Elizabeth 6371 Mercedes, Dallas, TX 75214, (214) 821-9083, BS 75 Univ of North TX; MS 79 Univ of TX - Dallas; Sp-Lang Path-Owner, Lakewood Sp & Lang Serv, **SLP**

Morris, Mrs Linda Beth 469 South Elm Street, Maywood, NJ 07607, (201) 843-2636, BA 82 Adelphi Univ; MA 86 Montclair St Coll; 82–Sp-Lang Path, Private Practice, **SLP**

Morris, Lizbeth T 1405 W Country Club Court, Spokane, WA 99218, (509) 458-6203, BA 80 Gonzaga Univ; MS 81 Eastern WA Univ; Coord/Off-Campus Clinic, Eastern Washington University, **SLP**

Morris, Mrs Lynn Mae 5544 W Sunwood Court, Rocklin, CA 95677, (916) 624-9260, BS 75 CA St Univ - Hayward; MA 78 CA St Univ - Sacramento; 87–Sp-Lang Path, Lynn Morris CCC, **SLP**

Morris, Margaret Fraser 36A Brainerd Road, Branford, CT 06405, (203) 483-1798, BA 81 Univ of IA; MA 83 Northeast MO St Univ; 87–Sp-Lang Path, Foundation Sch, **SLP**

Morris, Mrs Marion G 122 Highland, Ripley, TN 38063, (901) 635-2224, BS 52 Memphis St Univ; MS 58 Univ of TN - Knoxville; **SLP LM**

Morris, Mary Ann P O Box 2154, Covina, CA 91722, (818) 960-3802, BA 73 VA Polytechnic Inst St Univ; ME 76 Univ of VA - Charlottesville; SLP, LA Co Supt of Sch, **SLP**

Morris, Mary Clare 3036 Bennett Street North, St Petersburg, FL 33713, (813) 522-2938, BA 84 Univ of FL; MS 86 Univ of South FL; 86–Sp-Lang Path, Pinellas Co Sch Bd, **SLP**

Morris, Dr Mary Jane 5200 Framton Court, Lincoln, NE 68516-4939, (402) 472-5469, BS 72 Univ of NE - Lincoln; MA 73 Univ of KS; PH 85 (Lang and Ed Administration) Univ of NE - Lincoln; Asst Prof, Univ of Nebraska, **SLP**

Morris, Mary W 510 Randall Street #2, Waukesha, WI 53188, (414) 549-6960, SLP, Rehab Associates, **SLP**

Morris, Mrs Michele Diane 163-B Berkley Avenue, Lansdowne, PA 19050, (215) 662-2784, BA 82 Wake Forest Univ; MS 85 Syracuse Univ; 87–Aud, Hosp of the Univ of PA Sp & Hearing Ctr, **A**

Morris, Norman W 79 Meadow Lane, Greenfield, MA 01301-9703, **A**

Morris, Oranell D 3345 West Highland Blvd, Apartment 206, Milwaukee, WI 53208

Morris, Patricia A 183 Cobalt Ridge Dr South, Levittown, PA 19057, (609) 848-4700, BS 79 Trenton St Coll; MA 81 Trenton St Coll; **SLP**

Morris, Mrs Paula F 2720 North Woodhaven Drive, Peoria, IL 61604, (309) 685-7889, BS 72 IL St Univ - Normal; MS 73 Bradley Univ; Sp-Lang Path, I of Physical Medicine, **SLP**

Morris, Mrs Renee Warshaw 152 Terrace Avenue, Albany, NY 12203, (518) 459-3155, BS 80 Coll of Saint Rose; MS 81 Coll of Saint Rose; Sp-Lang Path, Albany City Sch Dist, **SLP**

Morris, Dr Richard J Dept Of Communication Disorder, 113 R R C, Florida State University, Tallahassee, FL 32306-2007, (904) 644-2238, BA 78 MI St Univ; MA 82 Memphis St Univ; PH 86 (Speech Science/Voice) Univ of FL; 88–Asst Prof, FL St Univ, **SLP**

Morris, Robert C Speech And Hearing Center, James Madison University, Harrisonburg, VA 22807, (703) 433-6491, BS 57 Univ of VA - Charlottesville; ME 59 Univ of VA - Charlottesville; Asst Prof/Aud, James Madison U, **SLP A**

Morris, Sandra Ann 1510 Normandy, Ann Arbor, MI 48103, (313) 665-2168, **SLP**

Morris, Mrs Sandra R 320 Arrowhead Drive, Montgomery, AL 36117, (205) 272-4993, BA 80 Auburn Univ - Montgomery; OM 82 Auburn Univ - Auburn; Aud, **A**

Morris, Mrs Shelia D 6021 Spring Glen Drive, Dallas, TX 75232, (214) 375-0306, BS 72 Hampton Univ; MS 74 Columbia Univ Teachers Coll; Sp-Lang Path, Dallas ISD, **SLP ACE**

Morris, Steven W 555 South Ryan Street, Colonnade Place, Lake Charles, LA 70601, (318) 436-3277, BS 74 ND St Univ; MS 75 Minot St Univ; Aud, Acadian Hearing Serv, **A**

Morris, Mrs Susan Edberg 1657 46th Street, Brooklyn, NY 11218, (718) 972-4210, BA 71 Univ of CA - Los Angeles; MA 76 CA St Univ - Los Angeles; SLP, UCP, **SLP**

Morris, Susan L 9514 Trojan Court, Richmond, VA 23229, BS 79 Univ of VA - Charlottesville; MA 80 Univ of TN - Knoxville; Sp/Lang Path, Johnston-Willis Hosp, **SLP ACE**

Morris, Dr Suzanne E Route 1 Box 175-S, Faber, VA 22938, (608) 238-8985, BA 60 Wichita St Univ; MA 62 Northwestern Univ; PH 72 (NS) Northwestern Univ; Sp-Lang Path, Private Practice, **SLP**

Morris, Mrs Terry L 11818 Robindale Road, Louisville, KY 40243, (502) 239-5338, BS 73 Murray St Univ; ME 76 Univ of Louisville; **SLP**

Morris, Mrs Thelma L 920 Clarissa Street, Pittsburgh, PA 15219, (412) 622-5900, BS 70 Carlow Coll; MA 76 Univ of Pittsburgh - Pittsburgh; Sp-Lang Path, Pittsburgh Pub Sch, **SLP**

Morris, Thomas W Nevada Hearing Service, 1701 Lakeside Drive, Reno, NV 89509, (702) 322-3264, BS 76 Univ of NV - Reno; MS 79 Univ of NV - Reno; Aud, Nevada Hearing Serv, **A**

Morris, Tom M 1950 Wall, Butte, MT 59701, (406) 782-8351, BA 66 Carroll Coll; MA 74 Univ of MT; Sp-Lang Path, Sch Dist #1, **SLP**

Morris, Valerie Ann 6830 Northwest Beaver Dr, Johnston, IA 50131-1244, (515) 270-6736, BA 83 Univ of Northern IA; MA 84 Univ of Northern IA; 88–Sp-Lang Path, Heartland AEA II, **SLP**

Morris-Gonzales, Ellen Kathryn 51 Springs Drive, Doylestown, PA 18901, (302) 734-7277, BA 81 Loyola Coll; MS 83 Loyola Coll; Sp/Lang Path, Private Practice, **SLP**

Morris-Lent, Mrs Valerie Sue 6005 Corliss Avenue North, Seattle, WA 98103, (206) 523-0167, BA 79 WA St Univ; MA 86 WA St Univ; **SLP**

Morris-Neufeld, Vonnie V 37 Treadwell Lane, Weston, CT 06883, (203) 226-1930, BS 66 Miami Univ - Oxford; MA 79 Southern CT St Univ; **SLP**

Morrison, Annette Yvonne 614 Bremer Drive, Lawrence, KS 66044, (913) 296-5452, BS 80 Univ of KS; MA 86 Univ of KS; **SLP**

Morrison, Mrs Carol Roberts 2806 Rebecca Drive, Tallahassee, FL 32312, (904) 488-7110, BS 79 FL St Univ; MS 80 FL St Univ; 82–Sp-Lang Path, Leon County School System, **SLP**

Morrison, Mrs Carolyn 11 Green Knoll Court, Northport, NY 11768, Aud, Kings Park Psyc Cen, **A**

Morrison, Claire V 3313 Mission Drive, Santa Cruz, CA 95065, (408) 476-1333, BA 71 Converse Coll; MS 73 Vanderbilt Univ; Aud, Santa Cruz ENT Med, **A**

Morrison, Dr Eleanor B 106 Morningside Drive, New York, NY 10027, (212) 678-3889, BA 57 CUNY - City College; MA 59 Columbia Univ Teachers Coll; PH 67 (NS) Columbia Univ Teachers Coll; Assoc Prof/Sp-Lang Path, Tchrs Coll-Columbia U, **SLP**

Morrison, George S, Jr 1211 10th Street #3, Alamogordo, NM 88310, (505) 437-3708, BA 69 Univ of NM; MA 74 NM St Univ; Aud/Owner, SW Hrng Serv, **SLP A**

Morrison, Glenda G P O Box 143, Monmouth, OR 97361, BS 79 Western OR St Coll; MS 82 Western OR St Coll; Sp-Lang Path, Salem Hosp, **SLP**

Morrison, Mrs Helen M 3410 Christmas Tree Lane, Bakersfield, CA 93306, (805) 392-2106, BA 50 Hiram Coll; ME 79 CA Lutheran Coll; MA 52 OH St Univ; Sp-Lang Path, Kern Co Supt of Sch, **SLP A**

Morrison, Judith A University Of Redlands, Dept Of Comm Disorders, P O Box 3080, Redlands, CA 92373-0999, (714) 793-2121, BA 71 WA St Univ; MS 78 Univ of WA; Assoc Prof, U of Redlands/Dept Comm Dis, **SLP**

Morrison, Mrs Judith G H 1439 43rd Street, Sacramento, CA 95819, (916) 381-5496, BA 59 Elmhurst Coll; MA 78 CA St Univ - Sacramento; Sp-Lang Path, Elk Grove USD, **SLP ACE**

Morrison, Kathleen A 15654 South 82nd Avenue, Orland Park, IL 60462, OB 82 Governors St Univ; OM 85 Governors St Univ; **SLP**

Morrison, Mrs Linda A 431 Rockingham Lane, Woodstock, GA 30188, **SLP**

Morrison, M Elizabeth 129 Otter Crescent, Oakville, ON, Canada L6H 1E7, (416) 842-6765, BA 78 Univ of Western Ontario; OM 81 Univ of Western Ontario; 84–Sp/Lang Path, Private Practice, **SLP**

Morrison, Margaret 314 17th Street, Seal Beach, CA 90740, (213) 598-0944, BA 72 CA St Univ - Northridge; MA 78 CA St Univ - Northridge; SLP, LA City U S D, **SLP**

Morrison, Mary M 6727 Larmanda #259, Dallas, TX 75231, (214) 591-3217, OB 71 Southern Methodist Univ; MS 75 Univ of North TX; **A**

Morrison, Michelle Kaleen 207 East 13th Street, Lockport, IL 60441, (815) 838-1568, BS 84 Western IL Univ; MA 86 Western IL Univ; 86–Sp-Lang Path, Cook Cty Dist #89, **SLP**

Morrison, Mrs Patricia Walters 209 Whispering Oaks, Bethalto, IL 62010, (618) 259-7150, BA 67 Southern IL Univ-Edwardsvill; MS 77 Southern IL Univ -Carbondale; SLP, East Alton, Il Sch Dist #13, **SLP**

Morrison, Mrs Priscilla 663 Pheasant Hill, Nagog Woods, MA 01718, (508) 667-8300, BS 61 Bridgewater St Coll; ME 75 Northeastern Univ; **SLP**

Morrison, Regina Z 1304 Biltmore Street, Dormont, PA 15216, BS 69 CA Univ of PA; MA 70 Emerson Coll; SLP, Pittsburgh Board of Education, **SLP**

Morrison, Rhoda K Massachusetts Eye & Ear Infirm, Audiology Department, 243 Charles Street, Boston, MA 02114, (617) 523-7900, BS 53 Univ of MN - Minneap-St Paul; MA 65 Univ of MN - Minneap-St Paul; Dir Aud Dept, MA Eye/Ear Infm, **A**

Morrison, Rick Alan 614 Miami, Hiawatha, KS 66434, (913) 742-2464, BS 76 Univ of KS; MA 77 Wichita St Univ; 86–Sp-Lang Path, Comm Therapeutics Inc, **SLP ACE**

Morrison, Mrs Roberta Jane 5133 Bison Drive, Lincoln, NE 68516, (402) 488-2165, BS 78 Univ of NE - Lincoln; MA 79 Univ of NE - Lincoln; Sp-Lang Path, Lincoln Public Schools, **SLP**

Morrison, Sally 4 Linwood Avenue, Wareham, MA 02571, MS 77 Univ of ME - Orono; Superv, Paul A Dever St Sch, **SLP**

Morrison, Sandra H 126 Folly Road, Charleston, SC 29407, (803) 766-2050, BA 69 Clemson Univ; ME 72 Univ of SC - Columbia; 88–Sp/Lang Path, James B Edwards Elem Sch, **SLP**

Morrison, Mrs Sheila Kies 5881 Marengo, Jackson, MI 49201, (517) 787-2800, MA 83 Eastern MI Univ; **SLP**

Morrison, Susan Tinker 2611 Princeton, Alamogordo, NM 88310, (505) 437-3200, BA 72 NM St Univ; MA 74 NM St Univ; 87–Sp-Lang Path, Alamogordo PS, **SLP**

Morrison, Mrs Vida R 9601 Tanoan Drive N E, Albuquerque, NM 87111, (505) 344-9478, BA 65 CUNY - City College; MA 68 CUNY - Hunter Coll; 88–Sp-Lang Path, Healthsouth Rehab Ctr, **SLP**

Morriss, Mrs Debra M 9807 Louisville, Lubbock, TX 79423, (806) 293-4475, BS 86 TX Tech Univ; MS 88 TX Tech Univ; 88–Sp-Lang Path, Children's Development Ctr

Morriss, Mrs Judy M 3 Salem Place, Valhalla, NY 10595, (914) 238-3911, BA 59 Coll of New Rochelle; MA 72 CUNY - Lehman Coll; Sp/Lang Path, Chappaqua Pub Sch, **SLP**

Morris-Scharl, Barbara 15 Bruuer Avenue, Wilbraham, MA 01095, (203) 741-3551, BS 77 Purdue Univ - West Lafayette; MS 79 Purdue Univ - West Lafayette; 85–Sp-Lang Path, Enfield Pub Sch, **SLP**

Morrisseau, Mrs Charlene R 2850 Claremont, Clovis, CA 93612, (209) 294-1255, BS 73 Moorhead St Univ; MS 74 Univ of WI - Stevens Point; Sp-Lang Path, CA-Hi Elks Major Proj, **SLP**

Morrissey, Elizabeth 82 Woodstock Lane, Cranston, RI 02920, **SLP**

Morrissey, Mrs Elizabeth C Rd 2 Box 2311-8, Anne Road, Windsor, NY 13865, (607) 775-3893, BS 84 2571; MS 86 SUNY - Coll at Buffalo; **SLP**

Morrissey, Mrs Emily Rollins 1912 Francis Street, Orangeburg, SC 29115-1932, (803) 534-8742, MA 85 SC St Coll; **SLP**

Morrissey, Kathleen M 410 N E 36th Street, Boca Raton, FL 33431, (407) 392-0218, BS 73 Trenton St Coll; MA 77 Trenton St Coll; OM 81 Rider Coll; 88–Nursing Home Admin, Natl Heritage Inc, **SLP ACE**

Morros, Joy S 1808 Park Drive, Raleigh, NC 27605, BS 68 Washington Univ; MA 71 Northwestern Univ; **A**

Morrow, Mrs Deanna R 3332 L Street, Lincoln, NE 68510, (402) 559-5557, MS 88 Univ of NE - Lincoln; 88–Sp-Lang Path, Meyer Children's Rehab Inst

Morrow, Elise Wilbanks 4001 Pelham Road #374, Greer, SC 29651-5973, (803) 297-7942, BS 77 OH Univ - Athens; MA 87 Univ of TN - Knoxville; Sp-Lang Path, Greenville Co School District, **SLP**

Morrow, Mrs Jean Levan 12 Melken Court, Baltimore, MD 21236, BA 54 Bloomsburg Univ of PA; MA 58 Univ of MD - College Park; Sp-Lang Path, Baltimore County Bd of Educ, **SLP**

Morrow, Mrs Jeanne Shuster Rd 3 Box 181, Newport, PA 17074, (717) 761-2181, BS 74 Indiana Univ of PA; MA 75 Temple Univ-Tyler Sch of Art; Sp-Lang Path, Prof Home Hlth Agcy, **SLP**

Morrow, Julia T 11092 Thrush Ridge Road, Reston, VA 22091, (703) 860-3932, BA 74 Univ of Pittsburgh - Pittsburgh; MA 75 Univ of Pittsburgh - Pittsburgh; Sp-Lang Path, Fairfax Co PS, **SLP**

Morrow, Mrs Mary Jo McCune 1507 West 36th Street, Kearney, NE 68847, (308) 234-8300, BS 58 Univ of NE - Lincoln; MA 63 Northwestern Univ; Instr Superv, Kearney St Coll, **SLP**

Morrow, Michelle Renee 7285 Greylock Avenue, Riverside, CA 92507, BA 84 Univ of Redlands; MS 86 Univ of Redlands; **SLP**

Morrow, Patricia Ellen 203 North 48th Street, Omaha, NE 68132-3116, (402) 559-4069, BA 80 Univ of NE - Lincoln; MS 85 Univ of NE - Lincoln; Aud, Univ of NE Med Ctr, **A**

Morrow, Rose A 146 Springside Avenue #B14, New Haven, CT 06515, (203) 239-5656, BA 78 Univ of RI; MS 81 Southern CT St Univ; Sp-Lang Path, Aces-Village School, **SLP**

Morse, Anita Wooten 623 West Peralta, Mesa, AZ 85210, (602) 926-0648, MS 84 AZ St Univ; BS 82 AZ St Univ; Sp-Lang Path, Mesa Pub Sch, **SLP**

Morse, Mrs Carol J 580 Pinon Drive, Billings, MT 59105, (406) 259-9047, BS 72 Minot St Univ; MS 79 Minot St Univ; Sp-Lang Path, Billings Public Schools, **SLP**

Morse, Diane M 1543 North Lake Circle, Jackson, MS 39211, (601) 956-7084, BS 69 Univ Southern MS-Hattiesburg; MS 70 Univ Southern MS-Hattiesburg; Sp-Lang Path, Private Practice, **SLP**

Morse, Diantha 36 Tulip Drive, Meriden, CT 06450, (203) 524-2735, BA 60 Univ of CT; MA 62 Univ of CT; Asst Prof, Uni of CT, **SLP A**

Morse, Elizabeth Desomery 46 Washington Avenue, Waltham, MA 02154, (617) 899-4709, BA 80 Univ of the Pacific; MA 81 Univ of the Pacific; Sp-Lang Path, Commun Hlth Care Assoc, **SLP**

Morse, Elizabeth Goss Box 141, St Germaine, MB, Canada R0G 2A0, (204) 837-1301, BS 73 SUNY - Center at Albany; MA 81 George Washington Univ; 84–Dir Sp-Lang Path, Deer Lodge Ctr, **SLP ACE**

Morse, Mrs Julie A A 5219 South Joliet Way, Englewood, CO 80111, BA 78 Univ of OK - Norman; MS 79 Southern Methodist Univ; Aud, **A**

Morse, Mrs Lynn Allison 3336 Kordes Way, Sacramento, CA 95826, (916) 921-3660, BA 79 CA St Univ - Sacramento; MA 83 CA St Univ - Sacramento; 82–Sp-Lang Path, Grant Joint Union HS, **SLP**

Morse, Mrs Nancy Elizabeth Route 4, Box 324, Poplar Bluff, MO 63901, (314) 785-0101, BS 83 Southwest MO St Univ; MA 86 Southeast MO St Univ; **SLP**

Morse, Mrs Rachel Cates 8901 Leatrice, Little Rock, AR 72207, (501) 225-1342, BS 80 Stephen F Austin St Univ; MS 82 Univ of AR - Medical Sci; 84–Sp-Lang Path, Private Practice, **SLP**

Morse, Stephen D Star Route 4314 HP R, Sitka, AK 99835, (907) 966-2417, BS Southeast MO St Univ; ME 74 Southeast MO St Univ; Sp-Lang Path, Sitka Pub Sch, **SLP**

Morse, Wendy Lynn 150-15 79th Avenue, Flushing, NY 11367, (718) 591-8971, BA 67 Long Island U - CW Post Ctr; MA 83 Long Island U - CW Post Ctr; 82–Sp-Lang Path, NYC Bd of Educ, **SLP**

Morseon, Mrs Marlene Volpe 15 Blue Spruce Lane, Commack, NY 11725, (516) 543-7698, BA 78 SUNY - Center at Stony Brook; MA 80 Long Island U - CW Post Ctr; Sp-Lang Path, Li Dev Cen, **SLP**

Mortensen, Mrs Camille Heward 440 South 5th East, Rexburg, ID 83440, (208) 356-8650, BA 75 Brigham Young Univ; OM 77 Brigham Young Univ; 81–Sp-Lang Path, Madison Mem Hosp, **SLP**

Mortensen, Sydnee Jean B 2141 South Rice Road, Ojai, CA 93023, (805) 488-4441, MA 76 Humboldt St Univ; SLP, Ocean View School District, **SLP**

Mortensen-Mascia, Nancy Ann 107 15th Street #2B, Garden City, NY 11530, (516) 294-5997, BS 83 Nazareth Coll of Rochester; MA 85 Hofstra Univ; Aud, Creedmoor Psy Ctr, **A**

Mortenson, Erin Kathleen 22 Nashawannuck #10-B, Easthampton, MA 01027, (413) 586-7145, BA 79 Mount Holyoke Coll; MA 85 Univ of OR; 86–Sp-Lang Path, Valley Rehab Inc, **SLP**

Mortimer, Mrs Emily Church 2011 Highland Drive, State College, PA 16803, (513) 751-1716, BS 73 PA St Univ - Univ Park; MA 79 Univ of Cincinnati; **A**

Mortimer, Mrs Jean A W 302 Salmon Falls Road, Rochester, NH 03867, (603) 652-4539, BS 76 Boston Univ; ME 78 Northeastern Univ; Sp-Lang Path, Milton Sch Dist, **SLP**

Morton, Mrs Ann N 635 Spartan Road, York, PA 17403, (717) 763-9501, BS 76 Bloomsburg Univ of PA; MS 77 Bloomsburg Univ of PA; Sp-Lang Path, Capital Area Inter Unit, **SLP ACE**

Morton, Mrs Betty Jean 6 Towne House Road, Hamden, CT 06514, (203) 272-0341, MS; 85–Qualified Mental Retardation Pro, State of CT, **SLP**

Morton, Mrs Cheryl Myers 4141 W Glendale Avenue, #3104, Phoenix, AZ 85051, (602) 973-3314, BS 86 Southern IL Univ -Carbondale; MS 88 Southern IL Univ -Carbondale; 88–Sp-Lang Path, Phoenix Cen Sp Lang Ctr, **F**

Morton, Deanna R 50 Brompton Road #2P, Great Neck, NY 11021, (212) 947-8150, BA 64 CUNY - Queens Coll; MS 71 CUNY - Queens Coll; Director, Private Practice, **SLP**

Morton, Mrs Karen D 200 Pitman, Nacogdoches, TX 75961, (409) 560-2688, BA 74 TX Tech Univ; MA 77 Univ of TX - Austin; Sp-Lang Path, Lufkin Indepen Sch Dist, **SLP**

Morton, Mrs Karen Deann 7020 Ces Box 754, APO New York, NY 09125, MS 87 Univ of South FL; **SLP**

Morton, Kathleen Susan 59 Tudor Village, Seneca Falls, NY 13148, (315) 255-2271, BS 86 SUNY - Coll at Geneseo; MS 87 Bowling Green St Univ; 87–Sp-Lang Path, Comprehensive Training Ctr, **SLP**

Morton, Larry H 6000 Lubbock Avenue, Fort Worth, TX 76133, (817) 346-8111, BS 72 TX Christian Univ; MS 73 TX Christian Univ; Private Contract Therapist, Private Practice, **SLP**

Morton, Natalie L 800 Hunt Road #812, Baytown, TX 77521, (713) 421-4839, MS 87 Lamar Univ; Sp-Lang Path, InSpeech Inc

Morton-Anderson, K Anne 6724 Francis, Lincoln, NE 68505, (402) 489-7102, OB 83 Univ of KS; MA 85 Univ of KS; Sp-Lang Path, Madonna Care Centers, **SLP**

Morvay, Christine Marie 1938 Rockville Drive, Baldwin, NY 11510, (516) 378-3900, BA 88 Adelphi Univ; MS 88 Adelphi Univ; 88–Sp-Lang Path, Merrick Union Free Sch Dist

Morvay, Ruth McConnell P O Box 3746, Mammoth Lakes, CA 93546-3746, OB 57 CA St Univ - Los Angeles; MA 68 CA St Univ - Long Beach; 88–Sp-Lang Path, Centinela Mammoth Hosp, **SLP**

Morvay, Torrey Lee 17387 Rodeo Drive, Madera, CA 93638, (209) 673-3466, BA 81 San Diego St Univ; MA 85 San Diego St Univ; **SLP**

Morvitz, Mrs Sandra Alperin 34 Lillian Lane, Plainview, NY 11803, (516) 822-6954, BA 78 Pace U -NY City; MA 81 Hofstra Univ; Sp-Lang Path, **SLP**

Mory, Mrs Kimberly Dews 10806 Hillcrest Court, Rancho Cucamonga, CA 91730-9704, (714) 593-7521, BA 80 CA St Univ - Fullerton; MA 83 CA St Univ - Fullerton; 84–Sp-Lang Path, Casa Colina Hosp for Rehab Med, **SLP**

Mos, Mrs Martha A 1215 Stratford Road, Kansas City, MO 64113, (816) 333-0233, MA 71 Univ of San Francisco; BA 66 Univ of MO - Columbia; Sp-Lang Path, Private Practice, **SLP**

Mosallem, Lynn C 4726 Aspen Street, West Mifflin, PA 15122, (412) 462-8544, BA 80 Univ of Pittsburgh - Pittsburgh; MA 82 Memphis St Univ; Reg Coord, Crossroads Sp-Lang-Hearing Inc, **SLP**

Mosca, Susan Roy 33 Witch Hazel Drive, Deep River, CT 06417, (203) 526-3111, BA 84 Univ of RI; MS 86 Southern CT St Univ; 87–Sp-Lang Path, Old Saybrook Bd of Educ, **SLP**

Mosca-Heisig, Dawn 267 Clark Boulevard, Massapequa Park, NY 11762, (516) 541-7368, BS 83 SUNY - Coll at Geneseo; MA 85 OH St Univ; 87–Sp-Lang Path, Brunswick Hosp Ctr Inc, **SLP**

Moscarello, Mrs Kathleen C 1560 Arroyo View Drive, Pasadena, CA 91103, (818) 793-4390, MA 85 CA St Univ - Northridge; Sp-Lang Path, Huntington Memorial Hospital, **SLP**

Moscato-Biondino, Mrs Paula 866 Wolf Hill Road, Cheshire, CT 06410, (203) 272-3549, BA 72 Long Island U - CW Post Ctr; MS 75 Southern CT St Univ; Sp-Lang Path, Chesire Board of Education, **SLP**

Mose, Mrs Janyce K 2019 Centerwood Drive, Olympia, WA 98501, BA 73 WV Wesleyan Coll; MA 80 Univ of IA; Aud, Private Practice, **A**

Mosehauer, Anne Lally 58 Erie Avenue, Newton, MA 02161, (617) 963-7703, BS 86 SUNY - Coll at Fredonia; MS 87 SUNY - Coll at Fredonia; **SLP**

Mosele, Mardelle B 2722 La Costa Avenue, Carlsbad, CA 92008, (619) 271-8050, BA 72 Roosevelt Univ; MA 76 Ball St Univ; SLP, San Diego USD, **SLP**

Moseley, Cathy 2910 West 66th Terrace, Shawnee Mission, KS 66208, **SLP**

Moseley, Mrs Donna J 131 Parkview Drive, Amarillo, TX 79106, (806) 354-4488, BS 61 Miami Univ - Oxford; MA 69 Southern Methodist Univ; Sp/Lang Path, Amarillo ISD, **SLP**

Moseley, Mrs Faye 2809 South Robertson, Tyler, TX 75701, MS; **LM**

Moseley, Jacqueline 3730 Quail Meadow, Missouri City, TX 77459, (713) 437-3849, BA 74 Northwestern St Univ; MA 75 Univ of Houston - Univ Park; Sp-Lang Path, Richmond State Sch, **SLP**

Moseley, Juanita 9553 South Winchester, Chicago, IL 60643, PH (NS); **SLP**

Moseley, Dr Mac R Sch Of Education & Psychology, University Of Texas, 3900 University Boulevard, Tyler, TX 75701, (214) 566-7052, BA 52 Baylor Univ; MA 59 San Francisco St Univ; ED 73 (Spec Educ/Sp Path) Univ of Houston - Univ Park; 76–Prof & Chairman & Grad Coord, Univ of Texas at Tyler, **SLP**

Moseley, Dr Mary June 2911 Hickory Leaf Way, Silver Spring, MD 20904, (202) 651-5336, BS 60 Phillips Univ; MA 77 Kent St Univ; PH 83 (Sp Path) Kent St Univ; Assoc Prof, Gallaudet College, **SLP**

Moseley, Mrs Susan M 1569 Dauphin Street, Mobile, AL 36604, (205) 344-8468, BA 71 Univ of AL- Tuscaloosa; MA 72 Univ of AL- Tuscaloosa; Sp-Lang Path, Private Practice, **SLP**

Mosely, Marcella M 276 Chimney Top Drive, Antioch, TN 37013, (615) 320-3227, BS 72 Vanderbilt Univ; MS 73 Vanderbilt Univ; Instr, TN St U, **SLP**

Moser, Ann Allen 2338 Ravenwood, Grand Prairie, TX 75050, (214) 264-6141, BA 73 Baylor Univ; MS 74 Baylor Univ; **SLP**

Moser, Mrs Claire Blackwell 415 2nd Street, Seymour, TN 37865, (615) 453-1036, BS 83 Appalachian St Univ; MA 85 Univ of TN - Knoxville; 85–Sp-Lang Path, Sevier Co Sch

Moser, Mrs Elizabeth Mills 1960 Leighton Court, Clarksville, TN 37043, (615) 648-5685, BA 83 Univ of KY; MS 84 Univ of KY; 85–Sp-Lang Path, Clarksville-Montgomery Schs, **SLP**

Moser, Georgia Jean 25844 Willowbend Road, Perrysburg, OH 43551, (419) 885-1444, MA 84 Bowling Green St Univ; Sp-Lang Path, Flower Mem Hosp, **SLP**

Moser, Mrs Hannah S 415 Audubon Road, Riverside, IL 60546, (312) 641-8234, BA 54 CUNY - Hunter Coll; MA 56 Northwestern Univ; 88–Aud, Private Practice, **A**

Moser, Mrs Miriam T 539 35th Avenue South, Seattle, WA 98144, BS; **SLP LM**

Moses, Mrs Andra A 4 Shannon Place, Newark, DE 19711, (302) 738-9756, BA 74 Univ of TN - Knoxville; MA 75 Univ of TN - Knoxville; 84–Coord Rehab Svcs, Prof Home Health Care, **SLP**

Moses, Mrs Christine Cefalu 5026 Regent Street, Madison, WI 53705, (608) 233-9327, BS 74 Univ of WI - Madison; MS 75 Univ of WI - Madison; 78–Sp-Lang Path, McFarland Comm Schs, **SLP**

Moses, Dr Elbert R, Jr 2001 Rocky Dells Drive, Prescott, AZ 86303, (602) 778-7804, BA 32 Univ of Pittsburgh - Pittsburgh; MS 34 Univ of MI - Ann Arbor; PH 36 (NS) Univ of MI - Ann Arbor; **SLP LM**

Moses, Frances R 6656 Locust, Kansas City, MO 64131, (816) 921-9600, BS 70 Central MO St Univ; MA 74 Univ of MO - Columbia; Sp-Lang-Hrng Spec, Mc Mo Sch Dist, **SLP**

Moses, Dr Gerald R 16518 Fox Den, San Antonio, TX 78247-1139, (512) 221-2595, BS 61 Loyola Univ of Chicago; MA 65 Western MI Univ; PH 69 (Sp Science) OH St Univ; 88–Sr Army Advisor, Health Svcs Command, **SLP**

Moses, Mrs Maryann C 16518 Fox Den, San Antonio, TX 78247, (512) 532-9610, BA 71 Eastern MI Univ; MA 76 Eastern MI Univ; 86–Sp-Lang Path, San Antonio St Sch, **SLP**

Moses, Mrs Nancy Johnson Rt 1 Box 277, O'Brien, FL 32071, (904) 364-5307, BA 80 Saint John's Univ - Jamaica; MA 82 NY Univ; 88–Sp-Lang Path, InSpeech Inc, **SLP ACE**

Moses, Dr Nelson 7243 Elm Court, Monmouth Junction, NJ 08852, (201) 932-9335, BA 71 CUNY - City College; MA 79 CUNY - City College; PH 82 (NS) NY Univ; Asst Prof, Rutgers U, **SLP**

Moseson, Susan Shedd 19 Linden Avenue, Bloomfield, NJ 07003, (201) 680-8017, BA 78 Montclair St Coll; MS 80 Columbia Univ Teachers Coll; 88–Pvt Consult, St Vincent's Nursing Home, **SLP**

Mosey, Mrs Gail Patricia 570 West Southmoor, Morris, IL 60450, (815) 695-5143, BS 81 Univ of WI - Stevens Point; MS 85 Univ of WI - Whitewater; Sp-Lang Path, Newark Pub Schs, **SLP**

Mosher, Mrs Beth 402 Senter, Farney, TX 75126, (214) 661-7221, BS 80 Univ of KS; MA 81 Univ of MO - Columbia; SLP, Dallas Rehabilitatn Institute, **SLP**

Mosher, Robert A 5678 New Meadow Drive, Ypsilanti, MI 48197, **A**

Mosier, Karen L P O Box 3444, Farmington Hills, MI 48433-3444, (313) 553-3641, BS 72 Central MI Univ; MA 77 Eastern MI Univ; Sp/Lang Path, Genesee ISD, **SLP**

Mosier, Laura F 4731 North Warner Terrace, Tucson, AZ 85705, (602) 385-2335, BS 79 Univ of AZ; MS 81 Univ of AZ; Sp/Lang Path, Mammoth San Manuel USD #8, **SLP**

Mosig, Mrs Edna Alice Ramsey 3715 Avenue F, Kearney, NE 68847, (308) 872-6441, BS 66 Eastern NM Univ; MS 78 Kearney St Coll; Sp/Lang Path, Sandhills Ed Coop, **SLP**

Moskal, Nancy 200 West Stadium, West Lafayette, IN 47906, (217) 235-5471, BS 80 Purdue Univ - West Lafayette; MA 82 Univ of IL - Urbana; Research Assistant, Purdue University, **A**

Moskovitz, Laurie Jane 1135 North Patterson Avenue, Santa Barbara, CA 93111, (805) 683-1995, BA 81 Univ of CA - Santa Barbara; MS 84 Univ of AZ; Sp-Lang Path, The Devereux Foundation, **SLP**

Moskowitz, Mrs Sheila I F 15057-B Sherman Way, Van Nuys, CA 91405, (818) 909-9988, BA 77 Univ of CA - Santa Barbara; MA 80 CA St Univ - Northridge; 85–Sp-Lang Path, Private Practice, **SLP**

Moskowitz, Susan Baer 3205 Lakeridge Drive, Marietta, GA 30067, (404) 634-2098, BS 77 Vanderbilt Univ; MA 79 Memphis St Univ; SLP, Private Practice, **SLP**

Moskowitz, Vickie L A 1822 Avocado Road, Oceanside, CA 92054, **A**

Mosley, Mrs Adrian Tureaud 1121 30th Street, Meridian, MS 39305, (601) 482-5438, MS 78 Univ Southern MS - Natchez; **SLP**

Mosley, Carol Ann 100 Bellegrove Circle, Brandon, MS 39042, (601) 981-4270, BS 81 Univ Southern MS-Hattiesburg; MS 82 Univ Southern MS-Hattiesburg; Exec Dir, Dogwood Sch, **SLP**

Mosley, Mrs Eleanor R 113 Whitefield Road, Springfield, IL 62704, BS 53 IN St Univ - Terre Haute; MS 60 Univ of IL - Urbana; Sp/Lang Path, Spfld Pub Sch Dist #186, **SLP**

Mosnik, Mrs Susan M 1293 Skylark Lane, Green Bay, WI 54303, BS 76 Univ of WI - Oshkosh; MS 77 Univ of WI - Oshkosh; **SLP**

Moss, Mrs Amy F 1004 West Main Street, Brownsville, TN 38012, (901) 772-2519, OB 68 Southern Methodist Univ; MA 69 Auburn Univ - Auburn; Sp-Lang Path, Trenton Sp Sch Dist, **SLP**

Moss, Mrs Amy Lee 4327 Windergate Drive, Jacksonville, FL 32217, (904) 630-4149, BS 81 Auburn Univ - Auburn; MS 83 Auburn Univ - Auburn; Sp/Lang Path, St Vincents Hosp, **SLP**

Moss, Mrs Arlene S 619 Skyline Drive, Jackson, TN 38301, (901) 424-3682, BA 73 Memphis St Univ; MA 74 Memphis St Univ; 74–Aud, West Tennessee ENT Clinic Pa, **A**

Moss, Barbara Ann 2650 Canada Drive, Dallas, TX 75212, (214) 630-1547, BS 65 Univ of North TX; MS 67 Univ of North TX; Early Chldn Intervention Coord, Dallas Co Ment Hlth/Ret Cen, **SLP A**

Moss, Mrs Barbara Castiglion 68 Maple Avenue, Cortland, NY 13045, BA 70 SUNY - Center at Albany; MS 76 SUNY - Center at Albany; **SLP**

Moss, Mrs Beverly A 9307 125th Avenue North, Largo, FL 34643-2532, (813) 462-7600, BA 71 Univ of KY; MA 72 Univ of KY; Rehab Coord, Morton Plt Hosp Rehab & Nsg Ctr, **SLP**

Moss, Catherine Route 2 Box 2146, Grayling, MI 49738, (517) 773-4356, BS 78 Northern MI Univ; MA 80 Northern MI Univ; 88–Sp-Lang Path/Asst Admin, STRIDE Inc, **SLP**

Moss, Mrs Cheryl Ann 5 Forest Meadow Trail, Rochester, NY 14624, (716) 594-0103, BA 80 SUNY - Coll at Plattsburgh; MA 85 Nazareth Coll of Rochester; **SLP**

Moss, Mrs Deborah C 452 Fort Pickens Road, Pensacola Beach, FL 32561, (904) 455-0111, BS 76 FL St Univ; MS 77 FL St Univ; Sp-Lang Path, Escambia Co Sch Bd, **SLP**

Moss, Mrs Donna J 719 Turner, Hastings, NE 68901, (402) 463-5611, BS 76 Creighton Univ; MA 77 Univ of NE - Omaha; Sp-Lang Path, Educational Service Unit #9, **SLP**

Moss, Ellen N 7616 38th Avenue North, St Petersburg, FL 33710, (813) 345-4859, BS 71 Boston Univ; MS 72 Univ of WI - Madison; Dir, Sp and Lang Ctr, **SLP**

Moss, Lynne R 36 Shore Road, Waterford, CT 06385, (203) 447-0301, BA 74 SUNY - Coll at New Paltz; MA 76 CUNY - Brooklyn Coll; OM 83 Southern CT St Univ; Supervisor of Speech Services, Seaside Center, **SLP**

Moss, Margaret Lynn 8954 Hollywood Hills Road, Hollywood, CA 90046, (213) 654-1912, MA 65 CA St Univ - Los Angeles; Sp-Lang Path, **SLP LM**

Moss, Mary M 30399 East Lee Road, Escalon, CA 95320, **SLP**

Moss, Pamela G 6640 Crosstimber Ct, Las Vegas, NV 89108, BS 68 Bloomsburg Univ of PA; ME 70 Univ of Pittsburgh - Pittsburgh; 88–Tchr, Clark Co PS, **SLP**

Moss, Sharon Elizabeth Department Of Comm Arts & Sciences, Howard University, Washington, DC 20059, (202) 636-6711, BS 81 SC St Coll; MA 85 Univ of FL; PH 88 (Sp-Lang Path) Univ of FL; 88–Asst Prof, Howard Univ, **SLP**

Moss, Stephanie Ecker 870 Shasta Avenue, Morro Bay, CA 93442, (805) 772-3277, MA 76 CA St Univ - Northridge; 82–Aud/Owner, Morro Bay Hrng Aid Ctr, **A**

Moss, Susan A 5 Pin Oak Drive, Conway, AR 72032-3412, (501) 450-3172, BS 73 Western IL Univ; MA 74 Western IL Univ; Grad Asst-Instructor/Superv, U of IL Urbana, **SLP**

Mosser, Mrs Sharon U 4229 Cedar Creek, Garland, TX 75043, (214) 240-2235, BA 73 Univ of AR - Fayetteville; MS 78 Southern Methodist Univ; Sp-Lang Path, Garland ISD, **SLP**

Mosshammer, Mrs Deborah E 2217 Foxboro Drive, Fort Wayne, IN 46818, (219) 484-4175, BS 86 Ball St Univ; MA 87 Ball St Univ; **A**

Mossman, Mary M 25380 Water Street, Olmsted Falls, OH 44138, BA 73 Cleveland St Univ; MA 74 Cleveland St Univ; Sp/Lang Path Consult, Cuyahoga Co Bd of Ment Ret, **SLP**

Mostel, Rebecca 98 Fairview Avenue, Great Neck, NY 11023, (516) 487-0039, BA 73 SUNY - Center at Stony Brook; MS 75 Columbia Univ Teachers Coll; Assoc Ch Sp-Lang Path, Private Practice, **SLP**

Moster, Mrs Jean Ann MacGregor 10820 West 115th Terrace, Overland Park, KS 66210, (913) 642-2646, BS 77 Univ of TX - Austin; MS 79 Southern Methodist Univ; 88–Sp/Lang Path, Shawnee Mission Sch Dist, **SLP**

Mostoller, Theresa Keating 50 Concord Street, New Britain, CT 06053, (203) 229-8323, BA 85 IN Univ - Bloomington; MA 87 Univ of MA - Amherst

Mote, Mrs Nina S 333 North 91st Street, Omaha, NE 68114, (713) 366-0503, BA 67 Wichita St Univ; MA 69 Wichita St Univ; SLP, Council Bluffs AEA, **SLP**

Motiwala, Tina S 11 Bretton Woods Drive, Rochester, NY 14618, (716) 385-1635, BA 74 SUNY - Center at Buffalo; MA 77 SUNY - Center at Buffalo; 86–Sp/Lang Path, Rochester City Schs, **SLP**

Motley, Mrs Carla H 8901 Kiowa, Boise, ID 83709, (208) 334-5475, BS 75 Phillips Univ; MS 77 Univ of NM; 85–Sp-Lang Path, Dept Health & Welfare Acdc, **SLP**

Moto, Eric Hiroshi 2847 Waialae Avenue #308, Honolulu, HI 96826, (808) 735-3744, BS 82 Univ of HI - Manoa; MS 84 Univ of HI - Manoa; Sp-Lang Path, Dept of Ed / Pohukaina School, **SLP**

Motola, Mrs Natalie G 15 Cobblers Lane, Dix Hills, NY 11746, (914) 963-4567, BS 58 NY Univ; MS 60 NY Univ; Sp-Lang Path, Yonkers Board of Education, **SLP**

Motteler, Elizabeth P O Box 7363, Wilmington, NC 28403-7363, (919) 672-2339, BS 76 East Carolina Univ; ME 77 Univ of NC - Greensboro; Sp/Lang Path, Randolph Co Hlth Dept, **SLP**

Mottershead, Janet Lee 17159 Los Padres Drive, Tracy, CA 95376, (415) 471-1039, BS 83 CA St Univ - Hayward; MS 86 CA St Univ - Hayward; 86–Sp-Lang Path, New Haven USD, **SLP**

Motto, Mrs Jane R 9 Rye Court, Gaithersburg, MD 20878, OB 61 Glenville St Coll; MS 66 WV Univ; **SLP**

Mouk, Betty Jean 48 Creekwood Drive, Cincinnati, OH 45246, (513) 761-8420, BS 45 OH St Univ; MS 65 Univ of WI - Madison; Sp-Lang Path/Reading Spec, Private Practice, **SLP**

Moul, Laura L 904 Florida Street, Milton, WV 25541, (304) 562-3610, BA 74 Marshall Univ; MA 80 Marshall Univ; MA 77 Marshall Univ; Lrng Disabl Tchr, Putnam Co Bd of Ed, **SLP**

Moul, Maj Michael J 8431 Kings Meade Way, Columbia, MD 21046, (202) 576-2414, BA 71 CO St Univ; MS 73 CO St Univ; PH 85 (NS) Univ of FL; Aud, U S Army, **A**

Moules, Mrs Pamela Susan 2688 Hunters Point Drive, Wexford, PA 15090-7991, (412) 935-8116, BS 81 PA St Univ - Univ Park; MS 83 Bloomsburg Univ of PA; Sp-Lang Path, D T Watson Rehab Hosp, **SLP**

Moulin, Dr Linda K 3750 Loch Highland Parkway, Roswell, GA 30075, (404) 475-2055, BS 59 Kent St Univ; MA 62 Kent St Univ; PH 68 (Law Aud) Case Western Reserve Univ; Dir Aud/Atty, Enviro Tech Corp, **SLP A**

Moulos, Tammy Jean 336 Basin Street, Navarre, OH 44662, (216) 879-5228, BS 84 Bowling Green St Univ; MS 86 Clarion Univ of PA; **SLP**

Moulton, Byron Jess Surgical Consultants Professional Corporation, 2928 Hamilton Boulevard, Sioux City, IA 51104, (712) 252-5203, BS 79 Brigham Young Univ; MA 80 Brigham Young Univ; Aud, Surgical Consult, **A**

Moulton, Mrs Christine J 5930 Sladen Avenue, Gladstone, OR 97027, (503) 655-7423, BA 74 CA St Univ - Fullerton; MS 83 Portland St Univ; Aud-Owner, Hollywood Aud Cl, **A**

Moulton, Mrs Janet Elizabeth 9-1 Nicole Circle, Ossining, NY 10562, (914) 285-8175, BS 80 Ithaca Coll; MA 82 NY Univ; Sp/Lang Path, Westchester County Med Ctr-MRI/UAP, **SLP**

Moulton, Dr Robert D Office Of Graduate Studies & Research, Lamar University, PO Box 10078, Beaumont, TX 77710, (409) 880-8230, BS 67 Univ of UT; MS 69 Univ of UT; PH 74 (NS) MI St Univ; 88–Assoc VP for Research, Lamar U, **SLP**

Moultrie, Mary Ann Taylor 1659 Glenwood Avenue, Dublin, CA 91786, (714) 949-8733, BA 76 MI St Univ; MA 78 MI St Univ; SLP, Los Angeles Co-Ofc of Ed, **SLP**

Mounce, Deborah Downing 4251-D Mapleleaf Drive, New Orleans, LA 70114, (504) 394-0117, BA 83 LA Tech Univ; MA 86 LA Tech Univ; **SLP**

Mounger, Dorothy C General Delivery, Glynn, LA 70736, (504) 694-2130, BA 64 LA Tech Univ; ME 71 LA St Univ - Baton Rouge; SLP, Pointe Coupee Parish Sch Bd, **SLP**

Mount, Mrs Amelia Willis 6333 Porcupine Court, Waldorf, MD 20603, (703) 280-5239, BS 82 WV Univ; MS 83 WV Univ; Aud, Fairfax Co Schools, **A**

Mount, Kathy Requarth 7843 Heatherglen Drive, Cincinnati, OH 45255, (513) 231-8067, BS 75 Miami Univ - Oxford; MS 77 Miami Univ - Oxford; Sp-Lang Path, Cincinnati PS, **SLP**

Mount, Dr Kay Hand P O Box 206, Okmulgee, OK 74447, (918) 267-3636, BS 67 OK St Univ; MA 68 OK St Univ; PH 81 (Sp-Lang Path) Univ of MO - Columbia; 88–VP & Mgr, Beggs Telephone Co, **SLP**

Mount, Marianne Route 7 Box 653-C, Chapel Hill, NC 27514, (919) 933-0882, BA 78 SUNY - Coll at New Paltz; MS 79 Univ of NC - Chapel Hill; SLP, Private Practice, **SLP**

Mountain, Catherine Angele 2950 N E 25th, Portland, OR 97212-3459, (213) 413-6005, BA 80 Univ of OR; MA 83 Univ of OR; **SLP**

Mountain, Mary C 3820 S E Alder, Portland, OR 97214, (503) 232-2458, BS 74 Portland St Univ; MS 80 Portland St Univ; Sp/Lang Path, Portland Pub Schs, **SLP**

Mountjoy, Marjorie P 4040 Greenleaf Circle #409, Kalamazoo, MI 49008, (616) 375-6463, BA 47 Lawrence Univ; MA 51 IN Univ - Bloomington

Mountsier, Mrs Deborah R 3912 Melanie Court, Des Moines, IA 50322, (515) 262-4881, BS 77 Univ of KS; MS 78 FL St Univ; Aud, Heartland AEA, **A**

Mountzouris, Christine Farakos 29 Revere Place, Milford, CT 06460, (203) 385-4212, MS 84 Southern CT St Univ; Sp-Lang Path, Stratford Board of Education, **SLP**

Moura, Rosangela 2750 Holly Hall #1404, Houston, TX 77054, (713) 795-5343, **A**

Moura-Durkin, Yvonne 21 West Holly Street, Cranford, NJ 07016, (201) 548-7610, MA; 88–Sp-Lang Path, JFK Med Ctr-Pediatric Rehab, **SLP**

Mourtada, Mrs Patricia R 23505 Lakeview Drive C304, Mountlake Terrace, WA 98043, (206) 339-4575, BA 66 Western WA Univ; ME 67 Western WA Univ; Sp-Lang Path, Everett Sch Dist, **SLP**

Movitz, Linda 4519 East Marconi Avenue, Phoenix, AZ 85032, BA 75 Univ of MD - College Park; MA 76 Univ of MD - College Park; 87–Aud, Hearing Consultants Ltd, **A**

Mow, Mrs Sally Mulder 2541 East Manoa Road, Honolulu, HI 96822, (808) 988-6668, BS 75 IA St Univ; MA 76 Central MI Univ; 88–Sp-Lang Path, Rehab Hosp of the Pacific, **SLP**

Mowbray, Mary L 716 Thorncrest Court, Janesville, WI 53545, (608) 752-6080, BS 80 Univ of WI - Whitewater; MS 82 Univ of WI - Whitewater; Sp-Lang Path, Wausau Hosp Cen, **SLP**

Mower, Laura D 722 Bounty Drive #2216, Foster City, CA 94404, (415) 574-1374, BS 81 Miami Univ - Oxford; MA 83 Univ of TN - Knoxville; 87–Asst Area Mgr, InSpeech Inc, **SLP**

Mower, Mrs Paula T 3945 Spoonwood, Fort Worth, TX 76137, (817) 924-2385, BS 77 Baylor Univ; MS 78 Baylor Univ; Sp-Lang Path, Fort Worth ISD, **SLP**

Mowers, Mrs Karen Chesser 9240 New Orleans Drive, Orlando, FL 32818, (305) 299-0934, 88–Sp-Lang Path, Comm Systems Evaluation Ctr, **SLP**

Mowery, Charlane W 3705 West Clover, McHenry, IL 60050, (815) 344-2411, BS 69 Northwestern Univ; MA 73 Northwestern Univ; Sp-Lang Path, Private Practice, **SLP**

Mowrer, Dr Donald Dept Of Speech & Hrng Science, Arizona State Univ, Tempe, AZ 85287-0201, (602) 965-3960, BA 51 FL St Univ; MA 53 FL St Univ; PH 64 (Elem Educ) AZ St Univ; 64–Prof, AR St U, **SLP F**

Mowrey, Marinnette 627 Rue Des Ursulines, New Orleans, LA 70116, (504) 340-4941, BS 80 Univ of Houston - Univ Park; MA 81 Univ of Houston - Univ Park; 82–Sp-Lang Path, Metairie Language & Learning Inc, **SLP**

Mowry, Lisa Jeannine 680 Mix Avenue 2E, Hamden, CT 06514, (203) 366-7551, BS 84 Ithaca Coll; MA 86 Univ of CT; Sp-Lang Path, The Rehab Ctr of Fairfield Co, **SLP**

Mowry, Richmond Bruce 328 Eardley Avenue, Pacific Grove, CA 93950, (408) 375-3806, BS 74 Univ of South FL; MS 77 Univ of South FL; 88–Aud, Pro Hearing Aid Ctr, **A**

Moy, Marcia E H 575 Dellbrook Avenue, San Francisco, CA 94131, **SLP**

Moy, Susan 1301 South Saltair Avenue, Apartment 3, Los Angeles, CA 90025, (213) 478-6234, BA 73 Univ of CA - Los Angeles; MA 77 CA St Univ - Los Angeles; SLP, Los Angeles USD, **SLP**

Moya, Mrs Manuela Helen 1424 La Mora Lane S W, Albuquerque, NM 87105, (915) 566-2929, BA 79 Univ of NM; MS 82 Univ of NM; Sp-Lang Path, El Paso Indep Sch, **SLP**

Moyano, Mrs Anne M 1814 10th Avenue North, Moorhead, MN 56560, (218) 236-6400, BS 71 Univ of MN - Minneap-St Paul; MA 72 Northwestern Univ; 76–Sp-Lang Path, ISD #152, **SLP**

Moyer, Deborah L 1614-C Helena Avenue, Norfolk, VA 23505, (804) 451-8697, MS 84 Old Dominion Univ; Sp-Lang Path, Virginia Speech and Lang Assoc, **SLP ACE**

Moyer, Donna J 372 Union Street, South Weymouth, MA 02190, (617) 573-3266, BA 72 Univ of MA - Amherst; MA 75 Northwestern Univ; Sp-Lang Path, Massachusetts Eye & Ear Infirmary, **A**

Moyer, Mrs Joyle Wiederspan 3612 Holiday Court N E, Albuquerque, NM 87111, (505) 247-8283, BS 58 Univ of NE - Lincoln; MS 82 Univ of NM; Sp/Lang Path, Albuquerque Pub Schs, **SLP**

Moynihan, Donna B 225 West Summit Avenue, Lakewood, NY 14750, (716) 483-4407, BS 78 SUNY - Coll at Fredonia; MS 82 SUNY - Coll at Fredonia; Sp-Lang Path, Jamestown Pub Sch, **SLP**

Moynihan, E A 3082 South Laredo Circle, Aurora, CO 80013, (303) 751-8862, BS 68 Univ of CO - Denver; MA 79 Univ of CO - Denver; SLP, Aurora Pub Sch, **SLP**

Moynihan, Judith B 27 Rockland Street, Swampscott, MA 01907, (617) 598-8981, BA 64 Univ of CT; MA 67 Temple Univ; Sp-Lang Path, Wakefield Public Schools, **SLP**

Moysan, Beth Ann 30 Oak Street, Gilbertsville, PA 19525-9411, (215) 367-9127, BS 84 East Stroudsburg Univ of PA; MA 87 Temple Univ; 88–Aud, Richard C Laucks, **A**

Mozena-Fetty, Mrs Jane Nile 408 1/2 University, Pella, IA 50219, (515) 628-3551, BA 85 Univ of IA; MA 87 Univ of IA; 87–Sp-Lang Path, Heartland AEA, **SLP**

Mozley, Audrey Marie 25 Dorest Court, Edwardsville, IL 62025, (314) 869-2505, BA 74; MS 81 Southern IL Univ-Edwardsvill; SLP, Spec Sch Dist of St Louis Cty, **SLP ACE**

Mraz, Norma Rivera 449 Talbrook Road, North Port, FL 34287, (813) 426-6047, BA 85 Univ of FL; MA 87 Univ of FL; **A**

Mroczek, Michael R 1278 Willa Drive, Clearwater, ON, Canada N7S 1T7, (519) 336-6139, BS 76 Eastern MI Univ; MA 78 Eastern MI Univ; Sp-Lang Path, Lambton Co Catholic Sch Bd, **SLP**

Mroczkowski, Marcia M 2109 Cedar Run Drive #106, Camp Hill, PA 17011, (717) 737-6728, BS 63 Emerson Coll; MS 67 Emerson Coll; Instr Advisor, Capital Area Intermediate Unit, **SLP**

Mrowca, Mrs Susan Ann 18919 N E 146th Way, Woodinville, WA 98072, (206) 524-7145, BA 73 Western MI Univ; MA 78 Western MI Univ; 88–Sp/Lang Path, Bellevue PS, **SLP**

Mrozek, Nancy J 217 South Webster Street, New Buffalo, MI 49117, (616) 469-3410, **SLP**

Mrozowski-Starr, Mrs Marianne 5902 Madison Street, Bethesda, MD 20817, (301) 762-2211, BA 73 Adelphi Univ; MA 80 Univ of MD - College Park; SLP, Montg Co Pub Schs, **SLP**

Mryglot, Kimberly Smith 1533 Belaire Drive, Horseheads, NY 14845, (804) 239-5523, **SLP**

Mucci, Mrs Kathleen A 40471 Olympia Drive, Sterling Heights, MI 48078, BS 71 Wayne St Univ; ME 75 Wayne St Univ; Sp-Lang Path, Detroit Bd Ed, **SLP**

Mucci, Mrs Vicki Lee 1338 Ottawa Avenue #2-S, Ottawa, IL 61350, (815) 434-5342, BS 82 IL St Univ - Normal; MS 83 IL St Univ - Normal; SLP, Lasalle Co Easter Seal Cen, **SLP**

Muccio, Maria A E 2281 Antigua Drive, Apt 1-D, Columbus, OH 43235, (614) 459-5860, BS 85 Miami Univ - Oxford; BS 86 Miami Univ - Oxford; MS 87 Miami Univ - Oxford; SLP, St Anthony Hospital

Muchmore, Teresa Ann 1313 Potomac #2-N, Bourbonnais, IL 60914, (815) 939-0356, BS 83 Eastern IL Univ; MS 84 Eastern IL Univ; SLP, Kankakee School District 111, **SLP**

Muchow, Mary Katherine Route 2 Box 164, Lorena, TX 76655, BS 85 Baylor Univ; MS 86 Baylor Univ; 86–Sp-Lang Path, NcClennan County Dept of Educ, **SLP**

Muck, Jane E 17 North Street, Geneseo, NY 14454, (716) 243-5480, BA 69 SUNY - Center at Albany; MA 78 SUNY - Coll at Geneseo; 78–Sp-Lang Path, Craig DDSO Doty Day Treatment, **SLP**

Muckerman, Cynthia Bell 109 Third Avenue, Columbia, MO 65203, (314) 875-3502, BA 81 Univ of CO - Boulder; MA 83 Univ of CO - Boulder; Sp-Lang Path, Boone Hosp Ctr, **SLP**

Muckian, Mrs Cathy A 384 Luella, Calumet City, IL 60409, (312) 868-2243, BS 77 IL St Univ - Normal; MS 78 IL St Univ - Normal; Sp-Lang Path, Sch Dist 140 John A Bannes Sch, **SLP**

Muckle-Davis, Lori K 111 West 1st Street #1, West Mifflin, PA 15122, (412) 856-2696, BS 83 Edinboro Univ of PA; MS 85 PA St Univ - Univ Park; 88–Sp-Lang Path, Greater Pittsburgh Rehab Hosp, **SLP**

Mudd, Mrs Mary Ann 104 Bellemeade Road, Louisville, KY 40222, (502) 429-6109, BA 78 Bellarmine Coll; MS 82 Univ of Louisville; **SLP**

Mudd, Sherri G 5125 Briggs Avenue, La Crescenta, CA 91214, (818) 957-0957, BA 73 Univ of CA - Los Angeles; MA 80 CA St Univ - Northridge; Sp-Lang Path, Los Angeles Co Sch, **SLP**

Mueh, Mrs Ferne H 651 Sinex Avenue, Pacific Grove, CA 93950, MS; **A LM**

Muehling, Linda Schutz 5806 South 96th Street, #127, Omaha, NE 68127, MA 88 LA St Univ - Baton Rouge; 88–Sp-Lang Path, Methodist Midtown Hosp

Mueller, Alison M 1858 Guernsey Avenue, Abington, PA 19001, (215) 885-1517

Mueller, Cathy Lynn 2149 Michelle Court #F, Appleton, WI 54914, (414) 733-3560, **SLP**

Mueller, Evelyn K 250 Harrogate Road, Lower Merion, PA 19151, **SLP**

Mueller, Grace A 644 Morris Street, Albany, NY 12208, (518) 584-3239, BA 57 SUNY - Center at Albany; MA 66 Coll of Saint Rose; Sp-Lang Path, Saratoga-Warren County BOCES, **SLP**

Mueller, Dr H Gustav Division Of Audiology, Letterman Army Medical Ctr, San Francisco, CA 94129, (415) 561-5267, BS 69 ND St Univ; MA 71 NM St Univ; PH 76 (NS) Univ of Denver; Supervisor of Audiology, Walter Reed Army Medical Cen, **A**

Mueller, James Charles 1919 13th Street, Moline, IL 61265, (309) 764-8161, BS 81 IL St Univ - Normal; MS 83 IL St Univ - Normal; 87–SLP, Moline PS, **SLP**

Mueller, Jill Elizabeth 6810 High Road, Darien, IL 60559, (312) 655-3818, BS 84 Elmhurst Coll; MA 86 Univ of IL - Urbana; Sp-Lang Path, Lyons Sch Dist #103, **SLP**

Mueller, Kathleen J 3527 Somerset Way, Carlsbad, CA 92008, (619) 720-0897, BS 80 Eastern MI Univ; MA 82 Eastern MI Univ; Sp-Lang Path, Oceanside USD, **SLP**

Mueller, Mrs L Jeannie 4706 McIlroy, St Louis, MO 63128, (314) 487-7569, MA 75 Saint Louis Univ; Sp-Lang Path, Special Sch Dist, **SLP**

Mueller, Laura J 2351 North 59th Street, Milwaukee, WI 53210, (414) 259-1977, **SLP**

Mueller, Mrs Linda L F 307 South Ash, North Platte, NE 69101, (308) 636-2252, BA 74 Kearney St Coll; MS 80 Kearney St Coll; SLP, Ed Serv Ut #16, **SLP**

Mueller, Lois Goetsch St Elizabeth Hospital, 1506 South Oneida Street, Appleton, WI 54911, (414) 738-2587, BS 63 Univ of WI - Madison; MS 68 Univ of WI - Eau Claire; Dir Rehab, St Elizabeth Hosp, **SLP**

Mueller, Mrs Michele Marie 516 West Cedar Street, Vermillion, SD 57069, (605) 624-4902, BA 83 Univ of SD - Vermillion; MA 85 Univ of SD - Vermillion; **SLP**

Mueller, Nancy Bitto 8210 Lanyard, Parma, OH 44129, (216) 888-7394, BA 75 Cleveland St Univ; MA 77 Cleveland St Univ; Sp-Lang Path, **SLP**

Mueller, Pam Brescia College Speech & Hearing Clinic, Brescia College, 718 Allen Street, Owensboro, KY 42301, (502) 685-3131, BS 74 Brescia Coll; MS 81 Univ of Louisville; Cl Superv, Brescia Coll Sp & Hrng Cl, **SLP**

Mueller, Dr Peter B Dept Of Communication Disorder, University Of North Texas, P O Box 5008, Denton, TX 76203, (817) 565-2262, BA 63 Univ of ND; MS 64 Purdue Univ - West Lafayette; PH 69 (Communication Disorders) Univ of WI - Madison; 88–Prof, Univ of N Texas, **SLP**

Mueller, Phoebe S 12 Berry Hill, Fort Smith, AR 72903, (501) 785-0202, BA 57 Univ of OK - Norman; ME 76 Univ of OK - Norman; **SLP**

Mueller, Rita J Park Nicollet Medical Center, 5000 West 39th Street, Minneapolis, MN 55416, (612) 927-3250, BA 76 Univ of IA; MA 77 Univ of IA; 83–Coord of Aud, Park Nicollet Med Cen, **A**

Mueller, Susan Jane 54 Congress Street, Williams Bay, WI 53191-9744, (414) 723-6811, MS 84 Univ of WI - Madison; Aud, Dr Robert Wolter, **A**

Mueller, Theresa Pinsky 206 East 25th Street, New York, NY 10010, MS; **SLP**

Mueller-Alms, Mrs Elizabeth A 604 Irvine, Champaign, IL 61821, BS 80 IL St Univ - Normal; MA 82 Univ of IL - Urbana; 88–Sp-Lang Path, Champaign Comm Sch Dist #4, **SLP**

Muellerleile, Steve Dystech Inc, 63 Deer Hills Court, North Oaks, MN 55110, (612) 484-3528, BA 73 Saint Cloud St Univ; MS 74 Saint Cloud St Univ; OM 84 Univ of MN - Minneap-St Paul; Executive Vice President, Dystech Inc, **SLP**

Muenster, Ann Powers 2025 West Harvest Drive, Appleton, WI 54914, (414) 735-6253, **SLP**

Muenzenberger, Mrs Elizabeth 309 Old Hunt Road, Fox River Grove, IL 60021, BS 78 Purdue Univ - West Lafayette; MS 80 Univ of TX - Dallas; Aud, Lake-Mc Henry Reg Prog, **A**

Mues, Catlin 10 Mirabella, Rancho Santa Margarita, CA 92688, (714) 858-3958, BA 73 CA St Univ - Long Beach; MA 74 CA St Univ - Long Beach; **SLP**

Mues, Dwana Urbom 33 Lakeside Drive, Kearney, NE 68847, (308) 237-5927, BS 71 Univ of NE - Lincoln; MS 86 Kearney St Coll; Sp-Lang Path, Educational Service Unit #10, **SLP**

Mueth, Mrs Patricia F 9336 Cherry Brook, St Louis, MO 63126, (314) 849-5547, BS 76 IL St Univ - Normal; MA 77 Univ of IL - Urbana; 81–Sp-Lang Path, Private Practice, **SLP**

Mueting, Mrs Karen H Box 111, Alton, IA 51003, (712) 756-8865, BA 77 Univ of SD - Vermillion; MA 78 Univ of SD - Vermillion; SLP, AEA #4, **SLP**

Muffley, Mrs Charlotte 7 Wagon Road, Asheville, NC 28805, (704) 254-9526, BS 64 TX Woman's Univ; MA 68 Univ of NE - Lincoln; 73–Sp-Lang Path, Asheville Pedia Assoc, **SLP**

Muffly, Debra Lowe RD 5 Box 11A, Muncy, PA 17756, (717) 546-7121, BS 78 Bloomsburg Univ of PA; MS 79 Bloomsburg Univ of PA; **SLP**

Muhleisen, Mrs Deborah G 327 South Fulton Street, Allentown, PA 18102, (215) 866-5555, BS 76 Indiana Univ of PA; MS 77 WV Univ; Aud, Rc Hunsicker MD Prof Hrng Assn, **A**

Muhr, Diane I 1408 Spear Street, South Burlington, VT 05403, (802) 656-3970, BS 75 OH Univ - Athens; MS 76 Univ of NM; Aud, Cen for Dis of Comm, **A**

Muilenburg, Diane D Wells Ridge Condos, 85 Debarry Road #3044, Orange Park, FL 32073, (904) 272-8332, BS 84 Univ of GA; MA 85 Memphis St Univ; 86–Aud, Audiology & Hearing Center, **A**

Muir, Katherine C Jones 22558 Greer Avenue, Port Charlotte, FL 33952, (904) 392-2041, BA 81 Wheaton Coll; MA 87 Univ of FL; **A**

Muir, Mrs Sue S 437 East Broadway, Bel Air, MD 21014, (301) 836-7905, BS 76 Towson St Univ; MA 78 Univ of MD - College Park; Sp-Lang Path, Harford Co Pub Sch, **SLP**

Mukherjee, Constance S 6-A Cornell Avenue, Taunton, MA 02780, (508) 880-2423, BS 75 IN Univ - Bloomington; OM 76 IN Univ - Bloomington; Sp-Lang Path, Taunton PS, **SLP**

Mukherjee, Mrs Sarah W 4500 East Sunrise Drive, Apartment Q-16, Tucson, AZ 85718, (513) 429-1623, BS 64 Syracuse Univ; ME 69 Boston Univ; **SLP**

Mulcahy, Juli Panepinto 600 Fulton Street #K-2, Farmingdale, NY 11735, (516) 352-2580, BA 83 SUNY - Coll at Cortland; MA 85 Hofstra Univ; SLP, School for Language & Comm Dev, **SLP**

Mulcahy, Mrs Kathryn Salo 16040 Siesta Lane, Brookfield, WI 53005-5170, (414) 937-2660, BS 75 Marquette Univ; MS 76 Univ of WI - Milwaukee; **SLP**

Muldoon-Donohue, Mrs Maureen 2607 Hawkshead Court, Silver Spring, MD 20904, (301) 890-2554, BS 77 Univ of MD - College Park; MA 80 Loyola Coll; Sp-Lang Path, Howard Co Pub Sch, **SLP**

Muldrow, Beverly Jo 4822 Eden Court, Indianapolis, IN 46254-2108, (317) 266-4721, BS 70 Ball St Univ; MA 76 Ball St Univ; Sp/Lang Path, Indianapolis Pub Sch, **SLP**

Mule, Lisa Nystrom 9 East View Drive, Simsbury, CT 06070, (203) 667-5320, BA 79 Univ of VT; MS 81 Boston Univ; 81–Sp-Lang Path, Newington Childrens Hospital, **SLP**

Mulford, Julie J 3272 Thorncrest S E, Grand Rapids, MI 49506, (616) 791 9757, BA 70 MI St Univ; MA 71 MI St Univ; Teacher, Region 1 Preschool, **SLP**

Mulford, Nicki M 124 Haymac Drive, Parchment, MI 49004, **A**

Mulford, Mrs Terri R 5432 Fossil Court North, Fort Collins, CO 80525, (303) 223-5649, MS 79 Univ of ND; BS 76 Northern St Coll; Sp-Lang Path, Poudre School District R-1, **SLP**

Mulhall, Alice Marie 2120 Queens Drive #B-2, Harrisburg, PA 17110, (717) 737-6728, **SLP**

Mulhaney, Mrs Laurie Elizabeth 650 North Terrace Drive, Elm Grove, WI 53122-2325, (414) 567-1133, BS 82 Marquette Univ; MS 84 Marquette Univ; Sp-Lang Path, Somed Inc, **SLP**

Mulhaupt, Mrs Dorothy Ellen 591 Old Farm Road, Lafayette, IN 47905, (317) 447-4102, BS 56 Purdue Univ - West Lafayette; MS 72 Purdue Univ - West Lafayette; Sp-Lang Path, Americana Healthcare, **SLP**

Mulhern, Margaret Dianne 8067 South Trenton Court, Englewood, CO 80112, (303) 771-8836, **SLP**

Mulhern, Mrs Susan Taber 1090 Beverly Place, Lake Forest, IL 60045, (312) 492-5012, BA 66 Catholic Univ of America; MA 67 Northwestern Univ; Clinic Director, Northwestern University, **SLP**

Mulhern, Mrs Vickie 14436 Kings Grant Street, Gaithersburg, MD 20878, (301) 279-3463, BS 75 Towson St Univ; MS 76 Towson St Univ; Sp-Lang Path, Montgomery Co Publ Schs, **SLP**

Mulholland, Dr Ann M 560 Riverside Drive, New York, NY 10027, (212) 749-4758, ME 36 Boston St Coll; MA 56 Northwestern Univ; PH 71 (NS) Fordham Univ; **A LM**

Mulholland, Elizabeth Lucille 320 South Lincoln, Springfield, IL 62704, (217) 525-0398, BS 85 IL St Univ - Normal; MS 87 IL St Univ - Normal

Mulholland, Mrs Julie B 530 South Hamilton, Georgetown, KY 40324-1542, (502) 863-1170, BA 82 Univ of KY; MS 84 Univ of KY; Sp-Lang Path, Scott County Schs, **SLP**

Mulick-Altuna, Dianne Jean 5245 Canoga Avenue, Woodland Hills, CA 91364, (818) 953-4449, BA 80 Univ of CA - Santa Barbara; MS 84 UT St Univ; Sp-Lang Path, St Joseph Med Ctr, **SLP**

Mulkern, Marie T 6430 Sun Eagle Lane, Bradenton, FL 34210, BS 54 Boston Univ; MA 55 Univ of FL; **SLP**

Mulkey, Katherine Ann 14066 West 88th Street, Lenexa, KS 66215, (913) 642-0415, BA 82 Wichita St Univ; MA 85 Wichita St Univ; 84–Sp-Lang Path, Wyandotte Spec Educ Coop USD 500, **SLP**

Mull, Rebecca J 41 North Park Drive, Rochester, NY 14612, (716) 872-1320, BS 74 SUNY - Coll at Brockport; MS 78 Nazareth Coll of Rochester; Sp-Lang Path, Webster Ctrl Sch Dist, **SLP**

Mullee, Cynthia Ann 1250 Shelly, Maumee, OH 43537, (313) 973-7465, BS 83 Northwestern Univ; MA 84 Miami Univ - Oxford; SLP, Ann Arbor Pub Sch, **SLP**

Mullen, Ann Marie 44 Apache Court, San Ramon, CA 94583, (619) 233-2241, BS 78 Brigham Young Univ; OM 79 Brigham Young Univ; Aud, Naval Hosp San Diego Ca, **A**

Mullen, Mrs Charlotte Houck 23 Lambert Street, Medford, MA 02155, (617) 735-6469, BS 82 Univ of MA - Amherst; MA 84 Western MI Univ; Aud, The Children's Hosp-Boston, **A**

Mullen, Mrs Elisa Celeste 1507 Stag Point, San Antonio, TX 78248-1345, (512) 344-4341, MA 72 Greensboro Coll; BS 61 Incarnate Word Coll; Sp/Lang Path, NE ISD, **SLP**

Mullen, Georgine Frank 250 Elgin Avenue, Forest Park, IL 60130, (312) 795-2454, BS 84 Northern IL Univ - De Kalb; MS 86 IL St Univ - Normal; **SLP**

Mullen, Jennifer Olson 1190 Rushbrooke Drive, Oakville, ON, Canada L6M 1H7, (402) 847-1646, BS 80 Univ of NE - Lincoln; MS 81 Univ of NE - Lincoln; **SLP**

Mullen, Joan M Dodds-P/Korea, Box 87 Seoul, American Elementary School, APO San Francisco, CA 96301-0005, BA 78 Univ of RI; MA 80 Univ of Denver; Sp/Lang Path, Department of Defense, **SLP ACE**

Mullen, Linda Lee 15121 Doug Road, Canyon Country, CA 91351-1958, (818) 982-9030, BS 82 Univ of CA - Los Angeles; MA 85 CA St Univ - Northridge; 85–Sp-Lang Path, Miller & Standel Sp Path Svcs Inc, **SLP**

Mullen, Sharon Fries 101 Lexington Square, Columbia, MO 65201, (314) 642-3301, BA 62 Wichita St Univ; MS 81 Univ of MO - Columbia; Dir Sp-Lang Path Dept, Fulton State Hosp, **SLP**

Mullendore, Dr James M 203 West Northgate Road, Peoria, IL 61614, (309) 691-2181, BS 41 Northwestern Univ; MA 42 Northwestern Univ; PH 48 (Sp Path & Aud) Northwestern Univ; **SLP A F LM**

Mullenix, Mrs Betty G 1332 Center Lane Drive, Ashland, OH 44805, (419) 524-4178, BA 61 OH Univ - Athens; Sp-Lang Path, Mansfield Mem Homes Inc, **SLP**

Mullen-Lynn, Patricia A 27428 Lathrup Boulevard, Lathrup Village, MI 48076, (313) 557-5070, BS 74 Univ of WY; MS 75 Univ of WY; Community Serv Dir, UCP, **SLP**

Muller, Barbara W RFD 1 Box 102, Belleville, WI 53508, **SLP**

Muller, Beth L F 28 Walnut Hill Road, Bethel, CT 06801, (203) 794-8677, BS 60 SUNY - Coll at Buffalo; MS 74 Southern CT St Univ; OM 79 Southern CT St Univ; 67–Sp-Lang Path, Bethel Bd of Ed, **SLP ACE**

Muller, Mrs Carolyn Wheeler Christiana Hospital, 4755 Ogletown-Stanton Road, PO Box 6001, Newark, DE 19718, (302) 733-1010, BS 77 Bloomsburg Univ of PA; MS 78 Bloomsburg Univ of PA; Sp-Lang Path, Med Ctr of DE, **SLP ACE**

Muller, George Childrens Hospital, 4480 Oak Street, Vancouver, BC, Canada V6H 3V4, (604) 875-2112, BA 62; OB 63; MA 69 Univ of WA; 74–Dir Aud & Sp-Lang Path Dept, Children's Hosp, **A**

Muller, Julie Anne 9941 Broadmoor, Omaha, NE 68114, (402) 393-0907, BA 81 Creighton Univ; MS 84 Univ of NE - Omaha; **SLP**

Muller, Mrs Robin W 1216 Washington Lane, Rydal, PA 19046, (215) 884-1736, BS 78 Stockton St Coll; MA 80 Temple Univ; Sp-Lang Path, Private Practice, **SLP**

Muller, Mrs Windie Karen 4504 Rebecca Boulevard, Metairie, LA 70003, (504) 467-1947, BA 81; MS 83 LA St Univ - N O Medical Ctr; Sp-Lang Path, Rutin Sp/Lang Ctr, **SLP**

Mullett, Carolyn M 1330 Morningside Drive, Charleston, WV 25314, **SLP**

Mullica, Karyn L 708 West Solano Drive, Phoenix, AZ 85013, (602) 246-4163, BS 65 IA St Univ; MA 70 CA St Univ - Northridge; President, Ecl Publications, **SLP**

Mullican, Megan McDaniel 731 Longstreet Drive, Hattiesburg, MS 39401, (601) 544-5057, BA 72 Univ of CO - Boulder; MS 79 Univ Southern MS-Hattiesburg; OM 87 Univ Southern MS-Hattiesburg

Mullican, Willis L 201 Stubbs, Monroe, LA 71201, (318) 387-7611, **SLP**

Mullies, Ronna McClanahan 18907 Manor Court, Independence, MO 64058, (816) 836-8100, OB 81 Northeast MO St Univ; MA 82 Northeast MO St Univ; 85–Sp-Lang Path, Independence Reg Health Ctr, **SLP**

Mulligan, Dr Kathleen 595 East Third Street, Bloomsburg, PA 17815, (717) 784-5000, BS 67 Bloomsburg St Coll; ME 69 Bloomsburg St Coll; PH 84 (Curriculum & Instruction) PA St Univ - Univ Park; 85–Coord, Bloomsburg Area Sch Dist, **SLP**

Mulligan, Laurie S 7741 West 154th Terrace, Overland Park, KS 66223, (913) 362-7518, BA 78 Univ of MO - KS City; MS 80 Central MO St Univ; 83–Sp-Lang Path, Deborah King and Assoc, **SLP**

Mulligan, Margo McKay 234 Lynn Cove Road, Asheville, NC 28804-1913, (704) 252-2255, BA 67 Chatham Coll; MS 82 East Carolina Univ; Sp-Lang Path, Visiting Health Professionals, **SLP**

Mulligan, Marilyn G 1288 Southfield Place, Virginia Beach, VA 23452, (804) 486-5194, BS 71 Purdue Univ - West Lafayette; MS 74 Rutgers St Univ - Newark; **SLP**

Mulligan, Moira Center Disorders Of Communication, CDC-MCHV, 1 South Prospect Street, Burlington, VT 05401, (802) 656-3970, BS 80 Univ of NH; MS 86 Univ of WI - Madison; 88–Sp-Lang Path, MCHV-CDC, **SLP**

Mullin, Cynthia M 521 Wall Street, Joplin, MO 64801, (417) 623-4944, BS 78 Indiana Univ of PA; MA 80 Memphis St Univ; 83–Owner/Sp-Lang Path, Cynthia M Mullin & Associates, **SLP**

Mullin, Mrs Sandra C 10 Forestedge Road, Amherst, MA 01002, (413) 467-9237, BS 58 Saint Louis Univ; MA 73 Univ of MA - Amherst; Sp-Lang Path, Granby Sch Dist, **SLP ACE**

Mullin, Dr Thomas A Dept Of Com Dis, Univ Of Central Florida, Orlando, FL 32816, (305) 275-2172, BS 61 SUNY - Coll at Geneseo; MS 67 Long Island U - CW Post Ctr; PH 72 (Aud & Sp Path) Syracuse Univ; Assoc Prof, U Cen FL, **SLP A**

Mullin, Vivian L S 6210 Mountain Brook Lane, Atlanta, GA 30328, **SLP**

Mulling, Mrs Sherry Lynne 51 Pop Runnels Road, Petal, MS 39465, (601) 545-2103, BS 83 Univ Southern MS-Hattiesburg; MS 86 Univ Southern MS-Hattiesburg; **SLP**

Mullins, Mrs Lynn D 556 Elm Street, Paintsville, KY 41240, (606) 789-1732, BA 72 Univ of KY; MA 73 Univ of KY; Sp-Lang Path, Private Practice, **SLP**

Mullins, Mrs Marion M Allied Center Speech, 1930 Fall Meadow, Missouri City, TX 77459-3446, (713) 438-2019, MS 69 Vanderbilt Univ; Dir, Allied Cen for Sp Lang Lrng, **SLP**

Mullins, Paul Leroy Rd #2 Box 56A, Hallstead, PA 18822, (607) 722-0028, BS 71 East Stroudsburg Univ of PA; MS 85 Bloomsburg Univ of PA; 88–Aud, Private Practice, **A**

Mullins, Mrs Tina Ruth 2909 Parklawn Court, Herndon, VA 22071, (202) 373-7367, BS 74 Univ of MD - College Park; MA 76 Univ of MD - College Park; Aud, Saint Elizabeths Hosp, **A**

Mullins, Vernon N Logan Audio & Hearing Aid Ctr, 417 White And Brownig Bldg, Logan, WV 25601, (304) 052-6018, BS 76 Marshall Univ; MA 78 Univ of TN - Knoxville; Aud, Logan Aud & Hrng Aid Cen Inc, **A**

Mulpeter, Virginia A 4 Greenwoods Lane, Farmington, CT 06085, BS 80 Coll of Saint Rose; MS 81 Emerson Coll; Superv-Communication Disorders, Danbury Hosp, **SLP**

Mulreany, Sue 22 Cove Lane, Levittown, NY 11756, (516) 581-2560, MA 75 Hofstra Univ; Sp-Lang Path, Islip Public Schools, **SLP**

Mulroy, Mrs Esther D 95 Bellevue Avenue, Swampscott, MA 01907, (617) 595-7049, BS 74 Simmons Coll; MS 79 Univ of VT; Sp-Lang Path, Private Practice, **SLP**

Mulson, Terri Lee Old Stage Road, East Berne, NY 12059, (518) 582-4550, BA 80 SUNY - Coll at Plattsburgh; MS 82 Univ of AZ; Sp-Lang Path, Sunnyview Rehabilitation Hosp, **SLP**

Multari, Bruno D 445 Eastern Boulevard, Bayville, NJ 08721, (201) 244-3100, BA 72 CUNY - Brooklyn Coll; MS 76 CUNY - Brooklyn Coll; Sp-Lang Path, Private Practice, **SLP**

Multer, Mrs Patricia C 41 Church Lane, West Islip, NY 11795, BA 45 Emerson Coll; MA 51 Columbia Univ Teachers Coll; **SLP LM**

Multer, Mrs Regina Hedberg 13 Adams Court, Oyster Bay, NY 11771, (516) 922-7487, BS 82 2008; MS 79 Ball St Univ

Muma, Diane B 3811 62nd Drive, Lubbock, TX 79413, (806) 797-8739, BS 67 Auburn Univ - Auburn; MA 71 Univ of Montevallo; Pres/Owner, Natural Child Publishing Co, **SLP**

Muma, John Ronald Speech And Hearing Sciences, Texas Tech Unversity, Lubbock, TX 79409, (806) 742-3908, BS 60 Central MI Univ; MA 63 Central MI Univ; PH 67 (NS) PA St Univ - Univ Park; Prof, Texas Tech Univ, **SLP F**

Mumford, Albert 101 Williams Drive, Battle Creek, MI 49015, (616) 965-3085, BA 63 Western MI Univ; MA 67 Western MI Univ; 63–Tchr, Lakeview Sch Dist, **SLP**

Mumm, Myrna N 64 South Gould Road, Columbus, OH 43209, (614) 263-2448, BS 52 OH St Univ; MA 68 OH St Univ; PH 73 (NS) OH St Univ; Diagnostic Clinic Coord, **SLP**

Mun, Coralee K 98-1944 Hoala Street, Aiea, HI 96701, BS 70 Univ of HI - Manoa; MA 72 San Jose St Univ; SLP, Dept of Ed, **SLP**

Muncy, Mrs Denise B 1717 Twinbrook Drive, Sellersburg, IN 47172, (502) 454-8209, BS 74 Bowling Green St Univ; MA 75 Western MI Univ; SLP, Jefferson Cty Publ Sch, **SLP**

Muncy, Mrs Julie Kehl 1408 Teasley #1313, Denton, TX 76205, (817) 565-9612, BS 81 Eastern IL Univ; MS 82 Eastern IL Univ; Sp-Lang Path, Tarrant County MHMR Services, **SLP**

Muncy, Dr M Jean 10532 La Morada Drive, San Diego, CA 92124, (619) 277-3325, BS 64 Univ of NE - Lincoln; MA 67 Univ of NE - Lincoln; ED 76 (NS) Univ of Northern CO; 88–Resource Spec, San Diego USD, **SLP**

Munday, Mrs Becky Sue 3002 Indian Drive, Enid, OK 73703, (405) 237-8341, MS 80 Phillips Univ; BA 78 Univ of OK - Norman; Sp-Lang Path, Enid State School, **SLP**

Munden, Mrs Anne D 111 Covebrook Lane, Mechanicsville, VA 23111, MS 75 Univ of VA - Charlottesville; SLP, Hanover County Schools, **SLP**

Mundil, Donna B 3150 South Tamarac Drive, Apartment C-203, Denver, CO 80231, (303) 752-4065, MA 87 Univ of Northern CO; **A**

Mundy, Mrs Alice Ann Edwards 1340 Dixon Circle, Gainesville, GA 30501, (404) 532-4383, BA 63 Greensboro Coll; Sp-Lang Path, Lakeview Acad, **SLP**

Mundy, Martha R 104 Pompano Avenue, Galveston, TX 77550-3130, (409) 762-2365, BA 74 Univ of AR - Fayetteville; MA 75 Vanderbilt Univ; Aud, Univ of TX Dept of Sp & Hearing, **A**

Mundy, Rosanna McGraw 83 Log Barn Road, Salisbury, NC 28144, (704) 279-8562, BA 75 WV Univ; MS 79 WV Univ; Sp-Lang Path, Rowan Co Schs, **SLP**

Mungall, Teresa Kelly 619 Maryland Avenue, St Cloud, FL 32769, (305) 348-7000, MA 84 Univ of Central FL; BA 81 Univ of Central FL; Sp-Lang Path, Osceola Co Sch Bd, **SLP**

Munger, Mrs Carol P 34 Sylvan Lake Road, Hopewell Junction, NY 12533, (914) 223-3641, BA 75 SUNY - Coll at New Paltz; MA 76 CUNY - Lehman Coll; 85–Sp-Lang Path, Private Practice, **SLP**

Muni-Thompson, Lynnette A Star Route Box 52, Gilbert, PA 18331, MS 81 Bloomsburg Univ of PA; Sp-Lang Path, Private Practice, **SLP**

Munk, Mrs Marilyn W 16 Pine Street, Walton, NY 13856, (607) 865-6551, BA 77 Univ of WA; MA 79 Univ of WA; Sp/Lang Path, Delaware Regional Center, **SLP**

Munkers, Mrs Linda Sue 3705 North Walrond, Kansas City, MO 64117, (816) 453-5050, BS 66 Central MO St Univ; MS 86 Central MO St Univ; **SLP**

Munn, Cynthia Ann 4504 Cherrywood Lane, Sioux City, IA 51106-3610, (712) 374-1408, BS 82 OK St Univ; MA 83 OK St Univ; Sp/Lang Path, Amarillo Sp Hrng Lang Cen, **SLP**

Munn, Janice C 5945 South New Haven, Tulsa, OK 74135, (918) 749-9068, BA 68; MS 70 Univ of Tulsa; Sp-Lang Path, Private Practice, **SLP**

Munn, Kimberly Stump 4906 Melbeth Drive, Greenville, OH 45331, (513) 548-3299, BS 80 Miami Univ - Oxford; MS 81 Miami Univ - Oxford; 88–Sp/Lang Path, Private Practice, **SLP**

Munneke, Mrs Margaret F 114 East Harvey, Mc Allen, TX 78501, (512) 682-9156, BA 42 Coe Coll; ME 60 Univ of Houston - Univ Park; Pvt Practice, **SLP LM**

Munoa, Marissa Hunt 5445 Castleton Drive, San Diego, CA 92117, (619) 292-1701, BA 84 Brigham Young Univ; OM 85 Brigham Young Univ; **SLP**

Munoz, Dr Orlando 6912 Oveja Avenue, El Paso, TX 79912, (915) 581-9677, MS 87 Univ of TX - El Paso; DD 56 (Doctor of Dental Science) Loyola Univ; **SLP**

Munro, Betsy Craig 3638 Covert Road, Pontiac, MI 48054, (313) 252-0440, BS 61 Western MI Univ; MA 76 Oakland Univ; Sp/Lang Path, Sch Dist of Pontiac J85, **SLP**

Munro, Carolyn B 18626 132nd Avenue N E, Woodinville, WA 98072, (206) 281-6855, BA 70 Univ of WA; MA 72 Univ of WA; SLP, Seattle Sch Dist 1, **SLP**

Munroe, Kathleen A 8001 Castle Cove Road, Indianapolis, IN 46256, (317) 353-5429, BS 78 Purdue Univ - West Lafayette; MS 80 Boston Univ; Dir, Castleton Sp-Lang Serv, **SLP**

Munroe, Susan Bessette 14 Old Meadow Plain Road, Simsbury, CT 06070, (203) 674-2831, BA 80 Univ of CT; MA 79 Univ of CT; Cl Superv, U Ct, **SLP**

Munsey, Mrs Bernice Wilson 4801 Massachusetts Avenue, Suite 400, Washington, DC 20016, (703) 524-4682

Munson, Deborah 6160 Melshore Drive, Mentor, OH 44060, (216) 257-0478, BS 77 SUNY - Coll at Oneonta; MS 80 Syracuse Univ; Sp-Path, Private Practice, **SLP**

Munson, Doris M 332 North Farragut, Colorado Springs, CO 80909, (719) 520-2595, BS 74 Western IL Univ; MA 75 Univ of Northern CO; 75–Sp-Lang Path, Sch Dist #11, **SLP**

Munson, Joan Mary 20 Claredon Terrace, Dover, NJ 07801, (201) 366-6831, BS 55 Newark St Coll; MA 56 Columbia Univ Teachers Coll; **A**

Munson, Mrs Joy E 23 Charles Street, Northampton, MA 01060, (413) 586-3762, BS 71 OH St Univ; MA 72 Western MI Univ; 86–Sp-Lang Path, Univ of Massachusetts, **SLP**

Munson, Karen Slavens 100 Am Windham Drive #205, Dadeville, AL 36322, BA 79 Univ of Akron; MA 85 Kent St Univ; **SLP**

Munson, Leslie Jean 1001 8th Avenue S E, St Cloud, MN 56304, (612) 259-4204, BA 70 Univ of NC - Chapel Hill; MS 73 Univ of NC - Chapel Hill; Sp-Lang Path, St Cloud Hosp, **SLP ACE**

Munson, Patricia Ann 4301 Lizshire Avenue C212, Orlando, FL 32822, (407) 422-7873, BS 82 Univ of Central AR; MS 85 Univ of AR - Little Rock; 87–Sp-Lang Path, Orange County Pub Schs, **SLP**

Munson, Mrs Theresa J 524 Avenue A Circle, Odessa, TX 79763, (915) 337-6793, BA 78 TX Tech Univ; MA 80 Univ of North TX; Sp-Lang Path, Ector Co ISD, **SLP**

Munson-Davis, Dr Joyce A 3538 South East Harold Ct, Portland, OR 97202, (503) 279-8356, BA 63 Yankton Coll; MA 72 Univ of IA; PH 88 (Sp Path) Univ of IA; 88–Dir-Environmental Access Prog, Oregon Health Sciences Univ, **SLP**

Munsterteiger, Kay D 2008 Gregg, Worland, WY 82401, (307) 347-2435, BS 78 Univ of WY; MS 80 Univ of NV - Reno; Sp/Lang Path, Washakie Co Sch Dist, **SLP**

Munzer, Mrs Susan W 531 Mesa Way, Long Beach, CA 90807, (504) 589-5266, BS 75 East Stroudsburg Univ of PA; MS 76 Rutger's St Univ - Douglas Coll; Sp-Lang Path, Private Practice, **SLP**

Murabito, Lucia 525 Grove Street, Morgantown, WV 26505, (304) 329-0580, MS 84 WV Univ; MS 84 WV Univ; **SLP**

Murakami, Karen Ayako 530 Shannon Way, Apartment 4202, Redwood City, CA 94065, BS 85 San Francisco St Univ; 88, Ellen Gilbert

Muramaru, Mrs Ruth Y 625 Iolani Avenue #1023, Honolulu, HI 96813-1867, (808) 531-2565, OB 69 Univ of HI - Manoa; MS 70 Univ of HI - Manoa; SLP, Hawaii Department of Education, **SLP**

Muraoka, Mrs Eileen Kikue 46-472 Kuneki Way, Kaneohe, HI 96744-3537, (808) 262-7737, MS 84 Univ of HI - Manoa; Sp-Lang Path, Dept of Ed Hawaii State, **SLP**

Murata, Hiroko 8014 Flower Avenue #2, Takoma Park, MD 20912, (301) 531-6686, MS 87 Miami Univ - Oxford; **SLP**

Murawski, Mrs Donna L 53 Oxford Road, Colonia, NJ 07067, (201) 549-5580, BA 75 Case Western Reserve Univ; MS 77 CO St Univ; Sp-Lang Path, Cpa-Middlesex County, **SLP**

Murbarger, Susan D M 520 Whispering Oaks Drive, Bethalto, IL 62010, (618) 259-3657, BS 78 Southern IL Univ-Edwardsvill; MS 79 Southern IL Univ-Edwardsvill; Sp/Lang Path, Region 3 Special Ed District, **SLP**

Murch, Mrs Donna Nicole 11 Arlene Street, Farmingville, NY 11738, (516) 736-4978, BA 82 Hofstra Univ; MA 84 Hofstra Univ; 88–Sp-Lang Path, Port Jefferson Sp-Lang-Hrng Center, **SLP**

Murdoch, Mrs Cynthia Watjen 295 Pebble Creek Court, Morgan Hill, CA 95037, (408) 779-4603, BS 83 Syracuse Univ; MS 84 Columbia Univ Teachers Coll; 86–Sp-Lang Path, InSpeech Inc, **SLP**

Murdock, Dr Betty Jane 68 Carnegie Drive, Milpitas, CA 95035, (408) 262-1958, BS 47 Pittsburg St Univ; MA 53 WA St Univ; PH 69 Univ of MO - Columbia; **SLP LM**

Murdock, Michael Joseph P O Box 202, West Central Speech Services, Lander, WY 82520, (307) 332-4420, MS 74 Univ of WY; Sp-Lang Path, Private Practice, **SLP**

Murdock, Mrs Susan A 1590 Hill Street, Suffield, CT 06078, BA 75 Univ of MA - Amherst; MA 78 Univ of MA - Amherst; Sp-Lang Path, Springfield Ma Pub Sch, **SLP**

Murdock-Abell, Roberta Ann 66 Tuttle Court, Bethany, CT 06525, (203) 393-1410, MA 82 CUNY - City College; OM 86 Southern CT St Univ; Sp-Lang Path, Waterbury Board of Education, **SLP**

Murley, Judith Lynn 10445 South Hale Avenue #3D, Chicago, IL 60643, (312) 333-7812, BA 79 Western MI Univ; MS 82 PA St Univ - Univ Park; Sp/Lang Path, South Metro Assoc, **SLP**

Murley, Mrs Laura Lynne 920 Riverstone Way, Woodstock, GA 30188-2970, (404) 928-5658, BS 83 0583; OM 87 Southern IL Univ -Carbondale; **SLP**

Murnen, Kathleen Sackman 1640 Cedarwood #132, Westlake, OH 44145, BA 84 Bowling Green St Univ; MA 85 Bowling Green St Univ; **SLP**

Murph, Jane Vallery 1936 Westminster, Carrollton, TX 75007, (214) 239-1413, MS 83 Univ of TX - Dallas; **SLP**

Murph, Jennifer Tallulah Route 1 Box 510, St Matthews, SC 29135, (803) 274-8288, BA 85 SC St Coll; MA 87 SC St Coll; 88–Sp-Lang Path, Branchville Elem Sch

Murph, Laura B 1042 Roberts Street, Reno, NV 89502, (702) 885-9591, BA 73 Univ of NV - Reno; MS 83 Univ of NV - Reno; **SLP**

Murphree, George D, Jr 205 St Clair Avenue, Huntsville, AL 35801, (205) 536-7405, BS 73 Univ of Montevallo; MA 76 Univ of AL- Tuscaloosa; Aud, Hrng Sp Cl, **A**

Murphree-Holden, Crystal 17 Kathleen Court, Columbia, SC 29210, (803) 252-0303, BS 78 Univ of TN - Knoxville; MA 80 Univ of TN - Knoxville; Sp-Lang Path, Richland School District One, **SLP**

Murphy, Mrs Alicia Ranon 3222 Palmira Avenue, Tampa, FL 33629, MS; **SLP**

Murphy, Mrs Amy Waters 3540 Southwest Archer Road, Apartment 277, Gainesville, FL 32608, (904) 371-1287, BS 85 Brigham Young Univ; MA 87 Univ of FL; **A**

Murphy, Mrs Angela M 34 Weir Crescent, Saskatoon, SK, Canada S7H 3A9, (306) 343-0323, BA 51 Univ of Manitoba - Winnipeg; ME 74 Univ of Saskatchewan - Sask; SLP, Saskatoon Cath Sch Bd, **SLP**

Murphy, Ann E PO Box 178, Ashburnham, MA 01430, (617) 827-5750, BA 74 Worcester St Coll; MA 84 Case Western Reserve Univ; 84–Sp-Lang Path, Reg Sch Dist Ashburnham/Westminster, **SLP**

Murphy, Anne Marie 110 Jefferson Avenue, Endicott, NY 13760, (607) 722-5308, BS 76 Coll of Saint Rose; MS 81 Ithaca Coll; Supervisor Speech & Hrng Dept, Rehab Services Inc, **SLP ACE**

Murphy, Mrs Barbara R 2 North Evanston, Arlington Heights, IL 60004, (312) 367-4300, BA 64 Northwestern Univ; MA 67 Northwestern Univ; 83–Coord-Aud Serv, Lake McHenry Regional Prog, **A ACE**

Murphy, Beverly S 12150 Saraglen Drive, Saratoga, CA 95070, BA 85 San Jose St Univ; MA 86 San Jose St Univ; 87–Aud, Donald A Belt PhD, **A**

Murphy, Blanche M 279 East Effin Green, Port Hueneme, CA 93041, BA 56 CA St Univ - Los Angeles; MA 70 Saint Thomas Univ - Phillipines; MA 75 Ball St Univ; 88–Sp/Lang Path, Dept of Def Dep Sch, **SLP LM**

Murphy, Carol A 1101 Wellington Street, Oakland, CA 94602, (415) 568-3112, BS 70 Northwestern Univ; MA 73 Northwestern Univ; Spec Day Cl Tchr, Oakland USD, **SLP**

Murphy, Mrs Carol L 410 Semple Avenue, Aptos, CA 95003, (408) 427-2753, MA 76 San Jose St Univ; BA 70 San Jose St Univ; Sp-Lang Path, Sp & Learning Services, **SLP**

Murphy, Catherine 634 Oakdale #2, Chicago, IL 60657, (312) 528-9503, BS 83 Marquette Univ; MS 86 Vanderbilt Univ; **SLP**

Murphy, Catherine R 913 Greenway Court #12, Norfolk, VA 23507, (804) 623-0526, MS 87 Univ of South FL; 87–Aud, Ear Nose & Throat Ltd, **A**

Murphy, Mrs Connie J 9214 Picture Ridge Road, Peoria, IL 61615, (309) 691-5225, BS 79 Bradley Univ; MS 80 Bradley Univ; **SLP**

Murphy, Conrad V 818 Wilkie Street, Dunedin, FL 33528, MS 77 Univ of South FL; SLP, Pinellas Co Sch, **SLP**

Murphy, Mrs Cynthia R 69 Pleasant Place, Kearny, NJ 07032, (201) 997-8624, BA 63 Chestnut Hill Coll; MA 79 Montclair St Coll

Murphy, Debora Sandquist 1211 Roberts Street, Lafayette, IN 47904, (317) 494-3785, BS 84 IA St Univ; MS 86 Purdue Univ - West Lafayette; 88–Sp-Lang Path, Purdue Univ, **SLP**

Murphy, Dolores Marie 57 Days Park, Buffalo, NY 14201, (716) 877-6800, MA 85 SUNY - Coll at Buffalo; Sp-Lang Path, Kenmore Schools, **SLP**

Murphy, Mrs Donna Caswell 200 Sugarpine, Gretna, LA 70056, (504) 367-3120, **SLP**

Murphy, Mrs Donna K 4804 Edinburgh Drive, Tyler, TX 75703, (214) 581-0913, BS 79 Univ Southern MS-Hattiesburg; MS 80 Univ Southern MS-Hattiesburg; Sp-Lang Path, Vaughn Speech & Hearing Ctr, **SLP**

Murphy, Eileen M 412 5th Street N W, Jamestown, ND 58401-3037, (701) 251-2840, MS 87 TX Christian Univ; 88–Sp-Lang Path, Speech & Hearing Svc Inc, **SLP**

Murphy, Frieda M 3026 S W 89th #F, Oklahoma City, OK 73159, (405) 794-1591, BA 72 Univ of OK - Norman; MA 74 Univ of OK - Norman; Sp-Lang Path, Clev Co Hlth Dept-Moore, **SLP**

Murphy, Gail E San Angelo Ind School Dist, 4717 South Jackson #247, San Angelo, TX 76903-9447, (915) 658-5187, MS 85 Univ of VT; 86–Sp-Lang Path, San Angelo ISD, **SLP**

Murphy, Mrs Glynis Barbosa 7945 Falmouth, Prairie Village, KS 66208-4043, (913) 341-1078, MA 86 Univ of KS; Aud, Children's Mercy Hosp, **A**

Murphy, Mrs Jan Hughes 563 Dirlam Lane, Mansfield, OH 44904, (419) 756-5588, **SLP**

Murphy, Jan Marie 179 Ridgewood Drive, Daphne, AL 36526, (719) 473-6852, BS 84 Auburn Univ - Auburn; OM 86 Auburn Univ - Auburn; **SLP**

Murphy, Jane W 4504 H Street, Sacramento, CA 95819, (916) 924-0280, BS 76 Univ of OR; MS 80 CO St Univ; 83–Manager of Client Serv, CA St U Sacramento, **SLP**

Murphy, Mrs Janice Cox 1516 Everhart Drive N W, Cleveland, TN 37311, (615) 479-7274, BS 77 Univ of TN - Knoxville; MA 81 Univ of TN - Knoxville; **SLP**

Murphy, Mrs Janice E 3311 North Parker Street, Columbia, MO 65202, BA 61 Augustana Coll; MA 75 Univ of MO - Columbia; Sp-Lang Path, Columbia Public Schools, **SLP**

Murphy, Janice E 2407 Sonora Drive, Carlsbad, CA 92008, (619) 720-9457, BS 71 Portland St Univ; MS 74 Portland St Univ; 87–Sp-Lang Path, Private Practice, **SLP**

Murphy, Janice S 226A Behrends Avenue, Juneau, AK 99801, (907) 463-3577, BA 70 Univ of Denver; MA 71 Univ of Denver; SLP, Private Practice, **SLP**

Murphy, Jerome E Department Of Audiology, Janeway Child Health Ctr, 15 Newfoundland Drive, St Johns, NF, Canada A1A 1R8, (709) 778-4541, BS 59 Gordon Coll; MS 65 Emerson Coll; MA 71 Univ of Rochester; Dir Aud, Janeway Chld Hlth Cen, **A**

Murphy, Jerry B Hearing And Speech Clinic, Alton State Hospital, Alton, IL 62002, (618) 465-5593, MA 60 Univ of OK - Norman; Superv Hrng & Sp Dept, Alton Ment Alth Cen, **A**

Murphy, Joan F 211 West Dogwood Drive, Gulfport, MS 39503, (601) 832-5639, BA 75 Tulane Univ; MS 77 CO St Univ; **SLP**

Murphy, John F 4 Camelot Drive, Hingham, MA 02043, (617) 749-2097, BA 55; ME 61 Emerson Coll; ME 63 Salem St Coll; Dir-Sp Ed, Hingham Pub Sch, **SLP**

Murphy, Mrs Jolyn Luna 250 Eaton Road, Rio Rancho, NM 87124, (505) 881-5124, MS 85 Univ of NM; **SLP**

Murphy, Julie A 23 Valley View Drive, St Peters, MO 63376, (314) 278-5271, BA 85 Univ of Northern IA; MA 87 Saint Louis Univ; **SLP**

Murphy, Karla B A 2413 Sunset Hills Terrace, Richmond, VA 23236, (804) 320-7711, MS 85 James Madison Univ; 86–Sp-Lang Path, Sheltering Arms Day Rehab Prog, **SLP**

Murphy, Kathleen Radnor Place, 1 Radnor Drive #F-4, Newtown Square, PA 19073, BA 78 Emerson Coll; MA 80 Emerson Coll; Sp-Lang Path, Devereaux Foundation, **SLP**

Murphy, Mrs Kathleen K 945 Old Metairie Drive, Metairie, LA 70001, (504) 361-4469, BS 81 LA St Univ - Baton Rouge; OM 83 LA St Univ - N O Medical Ctr; Sp-Lang Path, Jefferson Parish Sch Sys, **SLP**

Murphy, Kathleen M 5 Elmwood Road, Deer Park, NY 11729, **SLP**

Murphy, Kathy S 6707 North Sheridan, Chicago, IL 60626, (312) 908-8107, BS 74 Bradley Univ; MA 76 Northwestern Univ; 85–Lecturer/Clin Supvr, Northwestern Univ, **A**

Murphy, Kinzie S 809 Cobble Cove Lane, Sacramento, CA 95831, BA 64; MS 86 CA St Univ - Sacramento; 87–Sp-Lang Path, Rehab Svcs Sutler Comm Hosp, **SLP**

Murphy, Mrs Laura McNavage 405 Suffolk Road, Flourtown, PA 19031, (215) 233-3348, BA 80 Temple Univ-Tyler Sch of Art; MA 82 Temple Univ-Tyler Sch of Art; SLP, Private Practice, **SLP**

Murphy, Mrs Letitia Wicker Psc 1 Box 1075, APO New York, NY 09292, BS 84 Univ of North TX; MS 85 Univ of North TX; **SLP**

Murphy, Mrs Linda F 846 Waveland Road, Lake Forest, IL 60045, (312) 234-5656, MA 80 Elmhurst Coll; MS 82 Rush Univ; Sp-Lang Path, **SLP**

Murphy, Mrs Linda J T 808 South Michigan, PO Box 322, South Bend, IN 46624, (219) 287-7221, BS 76 IN Univ - Bloomington; MA 79 Ball St Univ; Aud, Acoustic-Aud Servs, Inc, **A**

Murphy, Mrs Lisa A 6083 Suellen Court, Goleta, CA 93117-1025, (805) 967-8774, MS; Program Cordinator, Solutions, **SLP ACE**

Murphy, Lori Lillian 851 Grix Court, Lake Orion, MI 48035, (313) 648-3770, BA 82 MI St Univ; MA 83 MI St Univ; Sp-Lang Path, Oakdale Regional Ctr, **SLP**

Murphy, Lynn B 411 Deer River Way, Sacramento, CA 95831-2456, (817) 387-8525, BS 82 Univ of MN - Duluth; MA 86 TX Woman's Univ; **SLP**

Murphy, Lynne Brackett 32 Carlisle Street, Worcester, MA 01602, (617) 365-4531, BS 79 Univ of MA - Amherst; MS 86 Worcester St Coll; Sp-Lang Path, The Clinton Hospital, **SLP**

Murphy, Margaret A 7205 Patton Drive, Woodbine, MD 21797, (301) 489-7400, BS 73 Towson St Univ; MS 77 Towson St Univ; Sp/Lang Path, Howard Co Bd of Ed, **SLP ACE**

Murphy, Margaret E 7438 Meridian Hills Court, Apartment A, Indianapolis, IN 46260, (317) 251-6713, BA 75 Saint Mary-of-the-Woods Coll; MA 77 Ball St Univ; Sp-Lang Path, Msd of Washington Twsp, **SLP**

Murphy, Margaret Kelley 5926 Langdon Avenue S W, Cedar Rapids, IA 52404, (319) 399-6700, BA 76 Benedictine Coll; MA 81 Univ of Northern IA; SLP, Grant Wood AEA, **SLP**

Murphy, Mrs Marie B 314 West 17th, Spokane, WA 99203, (509) 922-6810, BS 72 Eastern WA Univ; MS 78 Eastern WA Univ; SLP, Central Valley Sch Dist 356, **SLP**

Murphy, Marilyn Holm 1550 Daytonia, Miami Beach, FL 33141, (305) 865-7300, BA 66 OH Wesleyan Univ; MA 67 Columbia Univ Teachers Coll; Sp-Lang Path, Speech Institute, **SLP**

Murphy, Mrs Mary Ann P O Box 20452, Waco, TX 76702, (817) 753-5709, BS 67 Indiana Univ of PA; ME 71 Indiana Univ of PA; 85–Professional Associate, InSpeech Inc, **SLP**

Murphy, Mary J 311 North Eton #D, Birmingham, MI 48008, (313) 649-6149, BS 74 Wayne St Univ; MA 77 Wayne St Univ; **SLP**

Murphy, Maureen A 3616 South Depew #203, Denver, CO 80235, (303) 794-3160, BA 78 Univ of Northern CO; MA 79 Univ of Northern CO; Sp-Lang Path, Littleton Pub Sch, **SLP**

Murphy, Michele L 149 West Park Lane, Waterloo, IA 50701, BS 70 Saint Louis Univ; MA 72 Univ of IA; SLP, AEA 7, **SLP**

Murphy, Mrs Nancy 27 Forest Club Drive, Chesterfield, MO 63017, (201) 635-1627, BS 68 Saint Louis Univ; MS 70 Purdue Univ - West Lafayette; **SLP**

Murphy, Mrs Nancy R 1408 Lincoln Terrace, Peekskill, NY 10566, (914) 997-2295, BA 78 Univ of CT; MS 80 Southern CT St Univ; SLP, White Plains NY Pub Sch, **SLP**

Murphy, Patricia 4298 Farm Meadows Court, Okemos, MI 48864, (517) 349-3740, BS 73 MI St Univ; MA 75 MI St Univ; Sp-Lang Path, Durand Area Schools, **SLP**

Murphy, Patricia A 103 Chelsea Way, Bridgewater, NJ 08807, (201) 937-8655, BS 80 FL St Univ; MS 81 FL St Univ; Sp-Lang Path, Robert Wood Johnson Hospital, **SLP ACE**

Murphy, Patricia Ann 1619 Third Avenue #3CE, New York, NY 10128, (212) 230-7169, BA 68 CUNY - Hunter Coll; MA 70 CUNY - Hunter Coll; OM 77 NY Univ; Sp-Lang Path & Lrng Spec, Metropolitan Hosp & Mary Manning Walsh Nursing Home, **SLP**

Murphy, Patricia Daniels 4044 Kurt Drive, Macon, GA 31204, (912) 477-4434, BS 77 Univ of GA; MS 80 GA St Univ; Sp-Lang Path, Bibb Co Bd of Ed, **SLP**

Murphy, Mrs Patricia Mary Paolino 677 Plumtree Road, Springfield, MA 01118, (413) 782-3507, BA 82 Elms Coll; MA 84 Univ of MA - Amherst; Sp-Lang Path, Somers Pub Sch, **SLP**

Murphy, Patrick Maxwell 600 Valley Road E-57, Warrington, PA 18976-2251, (201) 688-2750, BS 80 Frostburg St Coll; ME 87 Univ of VA - Charlottesville; **A**

Murphy, Dr Pollie Saunders 3005 Kecoughtan Road, Hampton, VA 23661-3047, BS 73 Hampton Univ; MA 74 Univ of MA - Amherst; PH 82 (Sp Path/Aud) Memphis St Univ; Assistant Professor, Hampton University, **SLP**

Murphy, Mrs Rita Ann 95 Athens Avenue, South Amboy, NJ 08879, (212) 836-5773, **SLP**

Murphy, Sharon Rae 1604 Big Tree Drive, Fairmont, WV 26554, (304) 363-4579, BS 82 Marshall Univ; MA 83 Marshall Univ; Sp-Lang Path, Harrison County Schools, **SLP**

Murphy, Shawn A 314 1/2 35th Avenue, Newport Beach, CA 92663, (714) 639-4990, BA 85 Univ of Redlands; MS 87 Univ of WA; 87–Sp-Lang Path, Providence Sp & Hrng Ctr, **SLP**

Murphy, Mrs Susan Granger 764 Corbett Place, Florence, SC 29501-9198, (803) 669-4141, **SLP**

Murphy, Mrs Susan Lee 16130 Ozark, Tinley Park, IL 60477, (815) 469-2415, BS 81 Northern IL Univ - De Kalb; OM 84 Governors St Univ; Sp-Lang Path, Lincoln Way Area Spec Educ, **SLP**

Murphy, Mrs Susan Phillips 1001 McCarty, Route 1 Box 455-C, Brookland, AR 72417, (501) 933-0525, BS 83 AR St Univ; MS 84 AR St Univ; 84–Sp-Lang Path, Bay PS, **SLP**

Murphy, Mrs Suzanne McKeever 1400 Cedar Crossing Trail, Midlothian, VA 23113, (804) 794-7652, BS 79 Longwood Coll; ME 81 Univ of VA - Charlottesville; Sp-Lang Path, Richmond Intervention Servies, **SLP ACE**

Murphy, Mrs Tempe L C 1183 Emerson, Sheridan, WY 82801, (307) 672-7346, BS 71 Univ of WY; MS 76 Univ of WY; 78–Sp-Lang Path, Sheridan County Sch Dist #2, **SLP ACE**

Murphy, Tracey Dawn 3207 Hardisty Avenue, Cincinnati, OH 45208, (513) 223-6192, MS 84 Miami Univ - Oxford; Sp-Lang Path, Miami Valley Hosp, **SLP**

Murphy, Mrs Tracy Agne 6747 Blackwater Drive, St Louis, MO 63129, (314) 487-3601, BS 82 Southeast MO St Univ; MA 83 Saint Louis Univ; Sp-Lang Path, Washington Univ Medical School, **SLP**

Murphy, Valerie H 121 South Yellowstone, Madison, WI 53705, (608) 233-1776, BA 76 Northern IL Univ - De Kalb; MA 78 Northern IL Univ - De Kalb; **SLP ACE**

Murphy, William P Dept Of Audiology & Speech Sci, Purdue University, Heavilon Hall, West Lafayette, IN 47905, (317) 494-3810, BA 69 Univ of Northern IA; MA 71 Univ of Northern IA; Supvr-Sp-Lang Path, Purdue Univ, **SLP**

Murrans, Linda E 61 Deer Hills Court, North Oaks, MN 55127, (612) 780-9155, BS 74 Western IL Univ; MA 76 Northwestern Univ; Aud, Coon Rapids Med Ctr, **A**

Murray, Allison Slaughter 2153 West McLean Avenue #2, Chicago, IL 60647-4557, (312) 486-6540, BA 82 Mount Holyoke Coll; MA 86 Northwestern Univ; **SLP**

Murray, Mrs Anne M 3875 Prairie Lane, Bettendorf, IA 52722-2248, (319) 359-1371, BA 66 Univ of Northern IA; MA 76 Univ of Northern IA; 77–Sp-Lang Path, MS Bend AEA 9, **SLP**

Murray, Carol A 44 Pomeroy Terrace #2, North Hampton, MA 01060, (413) 772-0211, BS 85 Coll of Saint Rose; MA 87 Univ of MA - Amherst; SLP, Franklin Medical Center, **SLP**

Murray, Catherine A 1111 Delafield Street, Waukesha, WI 53188, (414) 549-5150, BS 78 Univ of WI - Stevens Point; MA 79 Western MI Univ; Aud, Prof Hrng Serv, **A**

Murray, Mrs Cheryl A 4424 West 63rd Street, Prairie Village, KS 66208, (913) 831-1567, BS 81 Univ of KS; MA 82 Wichita St Univ; Sp/Lang Path, Shawnee Mission Pub Schs, **SLP**

Murray, Cheryl Anne 5 Grecian Street, Parsippany, NJ 07054, (201) 487-6860, BA 63 Montclair St Coll; MA 67 Stanford Univ; Aud, Audiological Associates, **A**

Murray, Cynthia Lee Eent Phy & Surg Of Charleston, 1306 Kanawha Boulevard E, P O Box 3107, Charleston, WV 25331, (304) 343-4371, BS 78 WV Univ; MS 79 WV Univ; Dept Head/Aud, ENT Physn & Surg of Charleston, **A**

Murray, Dennis Paul 3011 Cedar Lane, Eureka, CA 95501, (707) 443-6055, BA 77 Humboldt St Univ; MA 81 Humboldt St Univ; Special Day Class Teacher, Eureka City Schools, **SLP**

Murray, Donna E P O Box 286, Pearsall, TX 78061, (512) 334-2440, **SLP**

Murray, Donna Smith 9250 Deercross Parkway #2D, Blue Ash, OH 45236-4533, (513) 351-7878, BS 84 Eastern KY Univ; MS 85 Univ of Louisville; 88–Sp-Lang Path, SpeechPath, **SLP**

Murray, Dr Elaine C 123 Crest View Lane, Martin, TN 38237, (901) 587-4231, BA 64 Univ of TN - Knoxville; MA 74 Univ of AL- Tuscaloosa; PH 81 (NS) Vanderbilt Univ; SLP/Asst Team Coord, Cane Creek Rehab Ctr, **SLP**

Murray, Mrs Eloise P 345 Riva Avenue, Milltown, NJ 08850, (201) 613-6753, BA 64 Rutger's St Univ - Douglas Coll; MS 70 Rutgers St Univ -N Brunswick; SLP, E Brunswick Pub Sch, **SLP ACE**

Murray, Elsaree D P O Box 4484, Modesto, CA 95352, **SLP**

Murray, Mrs Elvira Lalli 3401 West Marlene Street, Tucson, AZ 85741, (602) 744-2495, BA 68 CUNY - Brooklyn Coll; MS 72 Columbia Univ Teachers Coll; Sp-Lang Path, Sunnyside Sch Dist, **SLP**

Murray, Elwood 3455 South Corona, Englewood, CO 80110-2876, PH (NS); **SLP F LM**

Murray, Eugene Raymond 46-31 Bowne Street, Flushing, NY 11355, (212) 436-7600, **SLP**

Murray, Dr Frederick P 12 Old Landing Road, Durham, NH 03824, (603) 868-7376, BA 48 Stanford Univ; MA 50 Univ of Southern CA; PH 66 (Sp Path) Univ of Denver; Retired, **SLP F**

Murray, Dr Gail S Berkshire Road, Gates Mills, OH 44040, (216) 844-3668, BA 75 Mary Washington Coll; ME 76 Univ of VA - Charlottesville; PH 87 (Aud) Case Western Reserve Univ; 88–Asst Prof, Case Wn Res U/Rainbow Chld Hos, **A**

Murray, Mrs Gina Whatley 2201 Cahaba Road, Birmingham, AL 35223, (205) 669-3135, MS Auburn Univ - Auburn; 74–Supvr Sp-Lang Path, Shelby County Bd of Educ, **SLP**

Murray, Mrs Herbye Micheale 230 East Thornton, Houston, TX 77022-2820, **SLP**

Murray, Mrs Jane E 3307 Goldenrod Court, Walworth, NY 14568, (315) 986-2825, BS 79 Nazareth Coll of Rochester; MS 80 SUNY - Coll at Buffalo; Sp-Lang Path Supvr, UCPA, **SLP**

Murray, Jeanette E 10711 North Siderman Road, Roscommon, MI 48653, (517) 275-4177, BA 80 MI St Univ; MA 81 MI St Univ; **SLP**

Murray, Mrs Jeanne McAmis 112 Spruce Street, Washington, NC 27889-5251, (919) 975-3024, **SLP**

Murray, Mrs Judy Ann 408 North Henney Road, Choctaw, OK 73020, BA 69 Univ of OK - Norman; MA 70 Univ of OK - Norman; Sp-Lang Path, Crooked Oak School, **SLP ACE**

Murray, Mrs Kathleen A 14999 Ridge Lake Drive, Chesterfield, MO 63017, (314) 532-5605, BS 75 Fontbonne Coll; MS 77 Southern IL Univ-Edwardsvill; SLP, Special School District, **SLP**

Murray, Mrs Leslie Tishler 35 Platt Street, Milford, CT 06460, (203) 877-0371, BA 83 George Washington Univ; MA 85 George Washington Univ; **SLP**

Murray, Mrs Leslie Wright 2723 Quail Ridge St, Stillwater, OK 74074, (405) 624-1315, BS 79 OK St Univ; MA 80 OK St Univ; **SLP**

Murray, Lisa Elizabeth 3934 Bonnett Drive, Stow, OH 44224, (216) 922-0991, BA 73 OH Univ - Athens; MA 77 Case Western Reserve Univ; MA 81 Kent St Univ; **SLP**

Murray, Margaret A 122 Manor Street, Delmont, PA 15621, **SLP**

Murray, Marie Elsie P O Box 144, Tilton, NH 03276, (603) 286-8901, BA 80 Univ of ME - Orono; MA 84 Univ of ME - Orono; 84–Sp-Lang Path, Spaulding Youth Center, **SLP**

Murray, Mary E 2 Windsor Terrace #3-F, White Plains, NY 10601, **SLP**

Murray, Mrs Mary Scanlon 51 School House Road, Wallingford, CT 06492, (203) 265-4843, BA 80 Southern CT St Univ; MS 82 Southern CT St Univ; SLP, Hamden Board of Education, **SLP**

Murray, Matthew Richard 1933 Maple Avenue, Palmyra, NY 14522, (315) 331-1700, BA 84 SUNY - Coll at Plattsburgh; MS 85 Nazareth Coll of Rochester; 86–Sp-Lang Path, Newark Dev Disabilities Svc, **SLP**

Murray, Maurice E 2407 Palamar, Ventura, CA 93003, (805) 648-5391, BA 54 Univ of Denver; MA 55 Univ of Denver; SLP, Ventura USD, **SLP**

Murray, Murraileen P O Box 28241, Cleveland, OH 44128, **SLP**

Murray, Nancy Ann 810 East Oakland Avenue, Apt 204, Urbana, IL 61801, (217) 337-3100, BA 82 Univ of MT; OM 86 Univ of MT; Aud/Sp-Lang Path, Carle Clinic, **SLP A**

Murray, Mrs Ninevah W 2210 Coley Forest Place, Raleigh, NC 27607, (919) 790-2500, BA 74 Univ of NC - Greensboro; MS 79 Univ of NC - Chapel Hill; 88–Sp-Lang Path, Wake Co PS, **SLP**

Murray, Nuala Ann 608 Richmond Drive, Norman, OK 73071, (405) 321-4830, BA 79 Univ of OK - Norman; MA 81 OK St Univ; Sp-Lang Path, **SLP**

Murray, Patricia Snow 5582 Hamstead Crossing, Raleigh, NC 27611, (919) 493-7575, BA 75 Univ of NC - Charlotte; MS 82 Winthrop Coll; Sp-Lang Path, Med Personnel Pool, **SLP**

Murray, Mrs Patti Z 1058 Deepwood Drive, Westlake Village, CA 91362-4215, (805) 526-0200, BS 71 Purdue Univ - West Lafayette; MS 72 Purdue Univ - West Lafayette; SLP, Simi Valley USD, **SLP**

Murray, Rosemary M 1522 Vine, Lansing, MI 48912, (517) 485-6116, BA 68 MI St Univ; MA 70 MI St Univ; 88–Sp-Lang Path, Private Practice, **SLP**

Murray, Sandra R Narh, Hospital Avenue, North Adams, MA 01247, (413) 663-3701, BS 58 Montclair St Coll; MA 65 Montclair St Coll; Sp-Lang Path, Private Practice, **SLP**

Murray, Dr Sharon L Childrens Hear & Speech Center, Childrens Hosp Nat Med Cen, 111 Michigan Avenue N W, Washington, DC 20010, (202) 745-5600, BA 63 Univ of OR; MA 69 Univ of KY; PH 72 (NS) Univ of KS; 77–Dir Sp-Lang Path, Chld Hrng Sp Cen, **SLP**

Murray, Sharon S 219 East 26th Street #14, New York, NY 10010, (516) 338-4204, BA 63 Marymount Coll; MA 71 NY Univ; Sp/Lang Path, Private Practice, **SLP**

Murray, Shelly Arthur 8356 Garden Gate Place, Boca Raton, FL 33433, (305) 338-1468, MS 85 Univ of South FL; 85–Sp-Lang Path, Palm Beach Co Sch Sys, **SLP**

Murray, Susan E Mountain View Apartment, Vosburg Road Bldg 1, Apartment 3, Averill Park, NY 12018, (518) 674-8813, BS 84 Ithaca Coll; MS 85 Bloomsburg Univ of PA; **SLP**

Murray-Branch, Jamie 457 Agnes Drive, Madison, WI 53711, (303) 546-0356, BS 79 Univ of Southern CO; MA 81 Univ of TX - Austin; Clinic Instructor, University of Wisconsin, **SLP**

Murray-Hoff, Kelly Ann Box 464, Quakertown, NJ 08868, (201) 788-6396, BS 80 Stockton St Coll; ME 82 Trenton St Coll; Sp-Lang Path, Hunterdon Medical Center, **SLP**

Murray-Johnson, Gwendolyn 4319 Deep Springs Court, Kennesaw, GA 30144, (404) 926-5920, BS 78 Jackson St Univ; MA 80 Memphis St Univ; Independent Contractor, Private Practice, **SLP**

Murray-Peterson, Mrs Marilyn Ann #6 Willow Run, Salisbury, NC 28144, (704) 279-7342, BA 74 Univ of the Pacific; MA 76 Univ of KS; Sp-Lang Path, Private Practice, **SLP**

Murrell, Darlene Y 5518 Beaver Lodge, Kingwood, TX 77345, (713) 540-5097, BA 69 Univ of MT; MA 75 IN Univ - Bloomington; Sp-Lang Path/Aud, Humble ISD, **SLP A**

Murrell, Mrs Karen T 143 Terrace Road, Sanger, TX 76266, (817) 458-4985, BS 78 Baylor Univ; MS 80 TX Christian Univ; 88–Sp-Lang Path, Krum ISD, **SLP**

Murrin, Mary Ruth 8813 Maple Street, Allison Park, PA 15101, (412) 856-9250, Sp-Lang Path, Transact Health Systems Inc, **SLP**

Murry, Laura Silverberg 2770 Ocean Avenue #1-M, Brooklyn, NY 11229, (718) 646-2475, MS 86 CUNY - Brooklyn Coll; **SLP**

Murry, Dr Thomas 3737 Moraga Suite 105, San Diego, CA 92117, (619) 483-2986, BS 64 Indiana Univ of PA; MA 65 OH St Univ; PH 69 (NS) Univ of FL; Pres, West Coast Sp Lang Cog Ctr, **SLP F ACE**

Murskyj, Chrystyne L 98 Florence, Mokena, IL 60448, (815) 485-6969, OM 85 Governors St Univ; Sp-Lang Path, Lincolnway Area Spec Ed Coop, **SLP**

Murtagh, Mrs Patricia J 18 Greenfield Street, Cranston, RI 02920, (914) 668-6580, BA 81 SUNY - Center at Buffalo; BA 82 SUNY - Coll at Cortland; MA 85 CUNY - Lehman Coll; **SLP**

Murtha, Susan C 122 Elderwood Drive, Ebensburg, PA 15931, (814) 944-3535, BS 86 WV Univ; MS 87 Indiana Univ of PA; SLP, Rehab Hosp of Altoona

Murthy, Vasudha K 2021 Downing Street, Lombard, IL 60148, BS 69; MS 72; Aud, Mercy Hosp & Med Cen, **A**

Murvay, Terri Elizabeth 1283 N Thorne Avenue, Fresno, CA 93728, (209) 268-0343, BS 82 Western IL Univ; MA 86 CA St Univ - Fresno; 86–Sp-Lang Path, Fresno USD, **SLP**

Murzyn, Mrs Barbara Klabunde 812 Marian Way, Chicago Heights, IL 60411, (312) 758-4754, BS 56 Univ of WI - Madison; OM 78 Governors St Univ; Sp-Lang Path, Consol Sch of Sauk-Village, **SLP**

Musa, Mrs Judith F 5708 Covehaven Street, Dallas, TX 75252, (214) 380-0243, BA 63 Trenton St Coll; ME 65 Lesley Coll; **SLP**

Musalo, Sylvia C 1789 Sexas Drive, Land O'Lakes, FL 33539, **SLP**

Musante, Elizabeth Ann 16 Aldrich Street, Northampton, MA 01060, (413) 584-1347, BA 68 Univ of MA - Amherst; ME 69 PA St Univ - Univ Park; Sp/Lang Path, Northampton Publ Schs, **SLP**

Muscasella, Carol Frances 175 North Iowa Avenue, North Massapequa, NY 11758, **SLP**

Muse, Diane P O Box 1649, Laconia, NH 03247, (603) 528-4842, BA 77 Northeast LA Univ; MS 81 Rutger's St Univ - Douglas Coll; Sp-Lang Path, Private Practice, **SLP**

Musetti, Margaret C 230 North 10th, Pocatello, ID 83201, (208) 234-0777, BA 62 Coll of Notre Dame; MS 80 ID St Univ; **SLP**

Musgrave, Teresa L W 2669 Broad Oaks Place, Raleigh, NC 27603, (919) 783-8492, BS 75 East Carolina Univ; ME 77 Univ of NC - Greensboro; 88–Dir of Rehab Svcs, MedTherapy Inc, **SLP**

Musher, Mrs Karol Katz 4903 Heatherglen, Houston, TX 77096, (713) 791-4298, BS 65 Northwestern Univ; MA 66 Northwestern Univ; Sp/Lang Path, Chldns Hosp, **SLP**

Musial-Slowey, Vera J 1764 Wash Valley Road, Martinsville, NJ 08836, (201) 356-5242, BS 75 Seton Hall Univ; MA 79 Seton Hall Univ; Director, Improve Therapeutics Inc, **SLP**

Musiek, Dr Frank E Lyme Road, Hanover, NH 03755, (603) 646-5158, BS 68 Edinboro Univ of PA; MA 71 Kent St Univ; PH 75 (NS) Case Western Reserve Univ; Dir of Aud, Dartmouth-Hitchcock Med Cen, **A F**

Musin, Mrs Charlotte 326 North Yellowstone Dr, Madison, WI 53705, (608) 836-7371, BS 47 Univ of WI - Madison; MS 70 Univ of WI - Madison; Sp-Lang Path, Middleton Area Sch, **SLP**

Musket, Mrs Carolyn H 916 Beechwood Drive, Richardson, TX 75080, (214) 905-3107, BA 57 Univ of Denver; MA 59 Northwestern Univ; 79–Aud, Univ of TX at Dallas, **A ACE**

Musko, Sally E S 2363 Fosgate Avenue, Santa Clara, CA 95050, (408) 244-6473, BA 77 San Francisco St Univ; MS 80 San Francisco St Univ; Aud, Palo Alto Med Cl, **A**

Mussa, Laraine 30 Belknap Street, Arlington, MA 02174, **SLP**

Musselwhite, Dr Caroline R 83 Keesler Road, Asheville, NC 28805, (704) 274-7554, BA 73 Univ of NC - Chapel Hill; MS 75 Univ of NC - Chapel Hill; ED 82 (NS) WV Univ; SLP, Irene Wortham Cen, **SLP**

Mussen, Dr Ethel F 120 Hill Road, Berkeley, CA 94708, (415) 841-6330, BA 51 Univ of CA - Los Angeles; MA 52 OH St Univ; PH 54 (NS) OH St Univ; Owner/Pres, E Bay Aud & Sp Path Serv Inc, **SLP A LM**

Mussler, J James 12 Cedar Lane, Norwich, CT 06360, (203) 886-5500, Aud, Hearing Aid & Audiology Assoc, **A**

Mussman, Mrs Jill Marie 3155 Observatory, Cincinnati, OH 45208, (513) 559-4628, BS 64 Univ of IL - Urbana; MA 65 Northwestern Univ; Aud, Cincinnati Cen Dev Dis, **A**

Musson, Nan Denise 155 Sunrise Drive #2-C, Key Biscayne, FL 33149, (305) 361-0565, BA 80 Univ of Central FL; MA 82 Univ of Central FL; Sp-Lang Path, Miami VA Med Ctr, **SLP**

Mustain, Teresa B 4005 Coleman Court, Kansas City, KS 66102, (913) 321-0217, BS 77 Univ of KS; MA 78 Univ of KS; Sp/Lang Path, Wyandotte Dev Pre-Sch, **SLP**

Mustain, Vivian Burke 615 Bradbury Road, Monrovia, CA 91016, (213) 357-4751, **SLP**

Mustain, Dr William D Communicative Disorders Lab, U Of Mississippi Medical Cntr, 2500 North State, Jackson, MS 39216, (601) 984-4550, BA 71 Coll of William & Mary; ME 73 Univ of VA - Charlottesville; PH 78 (NS) Univ of VA - Charlottesville; Asst Prof and Aud, U of MS / Med Ctr, **A**

Musto, Lisa M 217 Smokeywood Drive, Pittsburgh, PA 15218, (412) 241-5177, BS 84 Marywood Coll; MA 86 Univ of Pittsburgh - Pittsburgh; **SLP**

Mutch, P Jane 324 N W 29th Street, Gainesville, FL 32607, (904) 392-3611, BA 72 Marietta Coll; MA 76 Univ of FL; 78–Sp-Lang Path, U of FL, **SLP**

Mutchler, Sharon Louise 623 Warren Avenue, Kingston, PA 18704, (717) 824-9742, BS 81 Bloomsburg Univ of PA; MS 82 Bloomsburg Univ of PA; SLP, Wilkes-Barre Sp & Lang Cl, **SLP**

Mutchler-Mathias, Karen Sue 2710 Ardsley Lane, Madison, WI 53713, (608) 247-4339

Muth, Mrs Lisa A P HCR 1 Box 620, Galilee, PA 18415, (914) 292-7500, BS 79 SUNY - Center at Albany; MS 80 WV Univ; 81–Sp-Lang Path, Sullivan Co BOCES, **SLP**

Muth, Sharon S 207 Drexel Avenue, Ventura, CA 93003, **SLP**

Muting, Elaine Kallas 9136 South Richmond, Evergreen Park, IL 60642, (312) 424-5351, BA 80 Saint Xavier Coll; MS 81 Marquette Univ; Sp-Lang Path, Southwest Cook Co Coop, **SLP**

Muto-Coleman, Mrs Dorothy E A R Services, 17800 Talbot Road South, Renton, WA 98055, (206) 228-8880, BA 76 San Jose St Univ; MA 78 San Jose St Univ; Aud / Owner, Private Practice, **A**

Mutterer, Mrs Carol Jean 249 N W 18th Street, Ontario, OR 97914, (503) 889-2362, BA 70 Univ of OR; MA 71 Univ of OR; Dir, Malheur Ed Serv Dist, **SLP**

Mutz, Laurie Fisher RD 4 Box 455, Canastota, NY 13032, (315) 697-2027, BS 79 SUNY - Coll at Geneseo; MA 80 Bowling Green St Univ; 85–Sp-Lang Path, Canastota Cent Schs, **SLP**

Muzelak, Mrs Kimberly Ann Booth 10481 Butterfield Street, #33, Manassas, VA 22110, (703) 330-1393, MA 88 Univ of FL

Muzzarelli, Robert A Speech-Lang & Auditory Path, School Of Allied Health Sciences, East Carolina University, Greenville, NC 27858-4353, (919) 757-6961, BA 63 Trenton St Coll; MA 68 Temple Univ; Assoc Prof Chair, E Caro U, **SLP A**

Myatt, Mrs Kelley Pipkin 133 Oak Lane, Cadiz, KY 42211, (502) 924-5306, MS 88 Murray St Univ; SLP, Hopkins Co Schl Sys

Myerow, Barbara G 16 Standish Circle, Wellesley, MA 02181, (617) 565-9598, BS 72 Univ of WI - Madison; MS 75 Boston Univ; Aud, VA Outpat Cl, **A**

Myers, Mrs Barbara Jean Route 13 Box 1098, Hattiesburg, MS 39401, MS 83 Univ Southern MS-Hattiesburg; 86–Sp-Lang Path, Petal Sch Sys, **SLP**

Myers, Mrs Barbara L 3801 West Gilbert, Muncie, IN 47304, (317) 285-8615, BA 62 Ball St Univ; MA 72 Ball St Univ; Asst Prof of SLP, Ball State U-Burris Lab Sch, **SLP**

Myers, Mrs Bernita A 400 South Homewood Avenue, Pittsburgh, PA 15208, (412) 242-2723, BA 77 Univ of Pittsburgh - Pittsburgh; MA 79 Univ of Pittsburgh - Pittsburgh; Sp/Lang Path, **SLP**

Myers, Mrs Betty B Route 16, 64 Woodland Square, Hattiesburg, MS 39401, (601) 582-5154, Univ Southern MS-Hattiesburg; Hattiesburg Public Schools, **SLP**

Myers, Corine C South Carolina State College, P O Box 1553, Orangeburg, SC 29117, **SLP ACE**

Myers, Mrs Donna L 4943 Sr 73-W, Wilmington, OH 45177, (614) 335-1810, BA 55 Bowling Green St Univ; MA 71 Univ of Cincinnati; SLP, Wash Court House Cty Sch, **SLP**

Myers, Dorothy E 4 Todd Circle #D, Carlisle, PA 17013, BS 32 PA St Univ - Univ Park; ME 52 PA St Univ - Univ Park; **SLP LM**

Myers, Elizabeth Ann 2513 South Harvard Place, Apartment 18-B, Tulsa, OK 74114, (918) 592-6000, **SLP**

Myers, Dr Florence L Department Of Speech Arts & Comm Disorders, Harvey Hall, Adelphi University, Garden City, NY 11530, (516) 228-7430, BA 68 Univ of MD - College Park; MS 72 PA St Univ - Univ Park; PH 76 (NS) PA St Univ - Univ Park; Chairperson Dept Comm Dis, Adelphi Univ, **SLP**

Myers, Mrs Gail S 9726 Boxford Way, Louisville, KY 40242, BS 74 Purdue Univ - West Lafayette; MS 75 Purdue Univ - West Lafayette; **SLP**

Myers, Mrs Gladys I 227 Minot Avenue, Chula Vista, CA 92010, (619) 422-5628, OB 56 San Diego St Univ; **SLP LM**

Myers, Jane F 3608 Elmley Avenue, Baltimore, MD 21213, (301) 243-3800, BA 76 Loyola Coll; MS 78 Loyola Coll; 85–Coor Parent-Infant Toddler Prg, Hrng & Sp Agcy/Metro Balto Inc, **SLP**

Myers, Mrs Jean T 2390 Clubview Circle, Yazoo City, MS 39194, (601) 746-6602, BS 71 Univ Southern MS-Hattiesburg; MS 72 Univ Southern MS-Hattiesburg; Sp-Lang Path, Yazoo Cty Mun Sep Sch Dist, **SLP**

Myers, Jeanette Marie 510 College Street, Lake Mills, WI 53551, (608) 222-8142, BS 83 Univ of WI - Madison; MS 84 Marquette Univ; 87–Sp-Lang Path, CES 5, **SLP**

Myers, Mrs Karen Beecher 3811 West 136th Street, Cleveland, OH 44111, MA 84 Cleveland St Univ; BA 82 Baldwin-Wallace Coll; Sp-Lang Path, Parma City Sch Dist, **SLP**

Myers, Mrs Karen Elizabeth Audiology & Speech/SGHSOS, Wilford Hall Medical Center, Lackland AFB, TX 78236, (512) 670-5437, BS 73 Southwest TX St Univ; MA 84 Our Lady Lake Univ-San Anton; 86–Sp-Lang Path, US Air Force, **SLP ACE**

Myers, Kathleen Kub 12 Lewis Drive, Medway, MA 02053, (617) 533-5126, SLP, Avon Public Schools, **SLP**

Myers, Laura J 14 Fay Street, Lynn, MA 01902, (617) 324-7300, BA 77 Univ of CT; MA 79 Univ of CT; Sp-Lang Path, Tri-City Early Intervention, **SLP**

Myers, Leslie Susan 4300 Rustic Road, Sand Springs, OK 74063, (918) 241-3476, BS 85 Univ of Tulsa; MA 87 Univ of Tulsa; **SLP**

Myers, Lisa Nanette P O Box 1233, Livingston, TX 77351, (409) 327-4019, BS 83 Stephen F Austin St Univ; ME 86 Stephen F Austin St Univ; 83–Sp-Lang Path, Livinston ISD

Myers, Margaret A 1351 West Lincoln Blvd, Freeport, IL 61032, (815) 966-3141, MA 53 MI St Univ; MS 64 Univ of WI - Madison; Sp-Lang Path, Rockford Public School 205, **SLP**

Myers, Mary Jane 608 North West Street, Ebensburg, PA 15931, (814) 472-9821, BS 58 Saint Francis Coll; MS 64 PA St Univ - Univ Park; Superv Sp & Hrng, Appalachia Inter Ut 08, **SLP**

Myers, Melissa P HC 70 Box 257, Limington, ME 04049-9616, (207) 764-3319, BS 78 SUNY - Coll at Geneseo; MA 82 Univ of ME - Orono; Sp-Lang Path, Aroostook Ment Hlth Cen, **SLP**

Myers, Mindy Fae 624 Boyer Road, Cheltenham, PA 19012, (215) 342-7660, BA 78 Temple Univ; MA 80 Temple Univ; Asst to Sp Prog Coord, Counseling or Referral Assist, **SLP**

Myers, Mrs Nadynne A Albuquerque Public Schools, District Diagnostic Center, 2700 Arizona Avenue N E, Albuquerque, NM 87110, (505) 883-9116, MS 69 Univ of NM; BA 68 Univ of NM; Coordinator Diagnostic Servs, Albuquerque Public Schools, **SLP**

Myers, Mrs Nancy McGlynn 632 Witmer Road, Horsham, PA 19044, (215) 628-9161, BS 75 West Chester Univ of PA; MA 79 West Chester Univ of PA; 86–Sp-Lang Path, Montgomery County Intermediate Unit, **SLP**

Myers, Penelope S 4425 Chatsworth Street, Shoreview, MN 55126, (612) 484-5328, BA 70; MA 74 George Washington Univ; **SLP**

Myers, Raymond Dan 18 Hazelwood Ct, Watsonville, CA 95076, (408) 728-2711, MA 75 CA St Univ - Long Beach; **SLP**

Myers, Robin Lynn 11475 Quivas Way, Northglenn, CO 80234-2620, (312) 665-8195, MA 85 Northern IL Univ - De Kalb; **SLP**

Myers, Roxanne Elizabeth 619 Longfellow Avenue, Hermosa Beach, CA 90254, (213) 374-3650, BA 82 Univ of Southern CA; MA 84 Whittier Coll; Sp-Lang Path, Bay Harbor Rehab Ctr, **SLP**

Myers, Sally A 31 Girad Avenue, Chatham, NJ 07928, **SLP**

Myers, Mrs Sara W 2599 Bahns Drive, Beaver Creek, OH 45385, (513) 429-5660, MS 87 Miami Univ - Oxford; 72–Sp-Lang Path, Kettering Bd of Educ, **SLP**

Myers, Mrs Tracy D 709 East Main, Blytheville, AR 72315, (501) 763-3776, **SLP**

Myers, Virginia C 6529 Esther N E, Albuquerque, NM 87109, (505) 821-1810, BA 74 Univ of NM; MS 77 Univ of NM; SLP, Albuquerque Pub Sch, **SLP**

Myers-Brashear, Mrs Melissa Box 224, Ramona, OK 74061, (918) 536-3175, BS 80 Phillips Univ; MA 83 OK St Univ; 88–Sp-Lang Path, Commun Dis Svc of Bartlesville, **SLP**

Myers-Schultz, Mrs Cheryl 1324 Overhill Road, Columbia, MO 65203, (314) 445-1411, OB 69 Drake Univ; MA 72 Auburn Univ - Auburn; Sp-Lang Path, Columbia Pub Sch, **SLP**

Myhre, Dr Steven J P O Box 9181, Savannah, GA 31412, (912) 651-7278, BA 73 Univ of South FL; MS 75 Univ of South FL; Aud, Savannah-Chatham Bd of Ed, **A**

Myland, Debra Jay 827 Ashby Street S W, Atlanta, GA 30310, (405) 624-1732, BS 85 IA St Univ; MA 87 OK St Univ

Myland, Jackie 7290 Samuel Dr, Denver, CO 80221, (303) 426-4373, Sp-Lang Path, Private Practice, **SLP**

Myles-Zitzer, Catherine A 796 Juniper Walk #A, Goleta, CA 93117, BA 77 Univ of WI - Milwaukee; MA 78 Univ of WI - Milwaukee; Tchr Asst, U of CA-Santa Barbara, **SLP**

Myres, Wendy A Indiana University Medical Center, Riley Hospital Suite A-56, 702 Barnhill Drive, Indianapolis, IN 46223, (317) 274-8868, BS 74 IN Univ - Bloomington; MA 76 IN Univ - Bloomington; Asst Prof Aud, IN U Med Cen, **A**

Myrick, Celia B 139 Brycewood Circle, Hattiesburg, MS 39401, (601) 266-5223, **SLP**

Myrick, Dean Kent 3221 Plymouth Place, New Orleans, LA 70131, (504) 393-2647, BS 60 LA St Univ - Baton Rouge; MS 66 Tulane Univ; 66–Sp-Lang Path, Private Practice, **SLP**

Myrick, Lisa Drummond 1005 S E 4th Street, Boynton Beach, FL 33435, (305) 943-8055, BS 83 FL St Univ; MS 86 FL St Univ

Myron, Susan J 67 Marion Street #11-C, Hillsdale, MI 49242, (517) 437-2778, BA 77 Univ of MI - Ann Arbor; MS 78 Univ of MI - Ann Arbor; 87–Sp-Lang Path, Hillsdale Co Inter Sch Dist, **SLP**

Myruski, Janet 4-Overhill Road, Middletown, NY 10940, (914) 342-4709, BS 77 SUNY - Coll at Geneseo; MA 84 Montclair St Coll; 78–Sp-Lang Path, Middletown PS, **SLP**

Mysak, Dr Edward D 106 Morningside Drive, New York, NY 10027, (212) 678-3892, BA 54 CUNY - Brooklyn Coll; MA 55 CUNY - Brooklyn Coll; PH 58 (Sp Path & Aud) Purdue Univ - West Lafayette; Prof SLP Chair Dept, Tchrs Coll Columbia Un, **SLP A F**

Myska, Mrs Carol B D 17 Jamaica Lane, Nashua, NH 03063, MA 77 Univ of ME - Orono; **SLP**

Mysliwy, Julie Thiel 3764 East Mallory Avenue, Cudahy, WI 53110, (414) 383-4490, BS 81 Univ of WI - Madison; MS 83 Univ of WI - Milwaukee; 88–Sp-Lang Path, Sacred Heart Rehab Hosp, **SLP**

Mytych, Mrs Mary Beth 808 Yorktown Street, Lansdale, PA 19446, BS 78 Western MI Univ; MA 79 Eastern MI Univ; Sp-Lang Path, Private Practice, **SLP**

N

Naab, Mrs Jennifer Slagle 4845 Avon Road, Plainfield, IN 46168, (419) 423-5308, BS 80 Miami Univ - Oxford; MA 81 OH St Univ; SLP, **SLP**

Naas, Dr James F Brescia Coll Speech & Hrng Clinic, Brescia College, 718 Allen Street, Owensboro, KY 42301, (502) 686-4233, BS 71 Central MI Univ; MA 72 MI St Univ; PH 80 (Sp-Lang Path) OH Univ - Athens; 81–Dir, Brescia Coll Sp & Hrng Cl, **SLP**

Nabelek, Dr Anna K Dept Audiology & Speech Path, University Of Tennessee, Knoxville, TN 37996, (615) 974-1806, BS 55; MS 59; PH 66 (NS); Research Prof, U of Tenn

Nabity, Mrs Regina M 3371 Mantilla Drive, Lexington, KY 40513, (606) 278-0540, BA 77 Univ of NE - Lincoln; MA 79 Univ of NE - Lincoln; Sp-Lang Path, Child Dev Cen of the Bluegrass, **SLP**

Naccarato-Gage, Mrs Susan Lyn 7008 Latham Circle, Saugerties, NY 12477, (914) 338-9320, BS 82 Nazareth Coll of Rochester; MS 85 SUNY - Coll at New Paltz; 85–Sp-Lang Path, UCP of Ulster County Children's Rehab Ctr, **SLP**

Naccari, Angela Pumilia 1418 Clermont Drive, Birmingham, AL 35209, (205) 251-7169, BS 77 Univ of AL-Tuscaloosa; MS 82 Univ of AL- Tuscaloosa; MS 82 Univ of AL- Tuscaloosa; Aud, Dennis G Pappas MD Pc, **A**

Nachbar, Mrs Charlotte 32 Back River Road, Bedford, NH 03102, MS 68 Rivier Coll; Sp-Lang Path, City of Manchester, **SLP**

Nachmias, Pamela G 103-10 Queens Boulevard, Apartment 5A, Forest Hills, NY 11375, (516) 481-8616, BS 77 SUNY - Center at Albany; MS 78 Adelphi Univ; SLP, NY Cty Bd of Ed, **SLP**

Nacht, Andrea B 8500 N W 2nd Manor, Coral Springs, FL 33071, (305) 755-7467, BA 75 Univ of Miami; MA 76 Univ of Miami; Sp-Lang Path, Speech Pathology Inc, **SLP**

Nachtigall-Harley, Aline 277 Chesnut Street, Fredonia, NY 14063, (716) 679-1718, BS 74 SUNY - Coll at Buffalo; MA 76 SUNY - Center at Buffalo; 86–Sp-Lang Path, Lake Shore Central Schs, **SLP**

Nackashi, Mrs Cynthia N P O Box 18133, Macon, GA 31209-8133, (912) 746-1041, BA 64 Univ of FL; MA 68 Univ of South FL; 84–Sp-Lang Path, Private Practice, **SLP ACE**

Nadeau, Gail Brenda Forest Pond Road, RFD 1 Box 321C, Ashland, NH 03217, (603) 279-5828, BA 71 Univ of NH; MS 85 Univ of NH; Dept Head/Sp-Lang Path, Laconia Developmental Svcs, **SLP**

Nadeau, Mrs Karen L G 2 Kyle Road, Merrimack, NH 03054, BA 64 Univ of CO - Boulder; MS 80 Univ of NH; Sp-Lang Path, Amherst Sch Dist, **SLP**

Nadeau, Leon N Audiology And Hearing Inst, 194 Pleasant Street, Suite 2, Concord, NH 03301, (603) 224-3346, MA Univ of MA - Amherst; 87–Aud, Aud & Hearing Inst of NH Inc, **A**

Nadel, Jill S 9-23 Westmoreland Avenue, Fair Lawn, NJ 07410, (201) 539-5636, BS 85 Ithaca Coll; MS 87 Northeastern Univ; 88–Sp-Lang Path, Morris Co Soc for Chld & Adults, **SLP**

Nadell-Siegel, Ellen 440 East 79th Street #3K, New York, NY 10021, (212) 737-2559, BS 77 Boston Univ; MA 79 Case Western Reserve Univ; **SLP**

Nadkarni, Mrs Kausalya Sunil 19 Bunker Hill Drive, Howell, NJ 07731, (201) 244-3100, SLP, Garden State Rehab Hosp, **SLP**

Nadler, Mrs Alexis Rauch Lima Memorial Hospital, 1001 Bellefontaine Avenue, Lima, OH 45805, (419) 331-5940, BS 85 Bowling Green St Univ; MS 86 Bowling Green St Univ; Aud, Lima Mem Hosp, **A**

Nadler, Amy 168 Acrebrook Drive, Florence, MA 01060, (413) 586-8473, BS 85 FL St Univ; MA 87 Univ of MA - Amherst; 88–Sp-Lang Path, So Deerfield Schs, **SLP**

Nadler, Mrs Susan L 10 Brittany Road, Montville, NJ 07045, **A**

Nadler, Mrs Suzanne Smith 5429 Donnefield Drive, Charlotte, NC 28212, (704) 545-4556, BS 80 Appalachian St Univ; MA 81 Appalachian St Univ; Sp-Lang Path, Charlotte/Mecklenburg Schools, **SLP**

Nadolski, Mark W 3829 North 55th Street, Milwaukee, WI 53216, (414) 442-4029, BS 76 Univ of WI - Milwaukee; MS 78 Marquette Univ; Sp-Lang Path, Milwaukee Public Schools, **SLP**

Nadoolman, Joanna PO Box #2, Gardiner, NY 12525, (914) 255-0441, BS 84 1541; MA 86 CUNY - Hunter Coll; Sp-Lang Path, The Early Educ Ctr, **SLP**

Naeser, Dr Margaret A Aphasia Research, 116-B VA Hospital, 150 South Huntington Avenue, Boston, MA 02130, (617) 232-9500, BA 66 Smith Coll; PH 70 (NS) Univ of WI - Madison; SLP, Boston VA Med Cen, **SLP**

Naf, Mrs Jane H 4384 Palm Place, Fort Myers, FL 33905, (813) 332-4124, BS 74 FL St Univ; MS 75 FL St Univ; **SLP**

Naffziger, Diane J D P O Box 384, Pennington, NJ 08534, (215) 757-0227, ME 72 Trenton St Coll; 72–Sp-Lang Path, Bucks County Intermed Unit 22, **SLP**

Nafman, Cheryl Sacks 6 Roberta Lane, Commack, NY 11725, (516) 499-2897, BA 75 CUNY - Queens Coll; MA 77 Hofstra Univ; Sp/Lang Path, Long Island Dev Cen, **SLP**

Naftol-Levitch, Mrs Linda 16 Winthrop Road, Plainview, NY 11803, (718) 539-2830, BS 79 SUNY - Center at Albany; MS 81 Columbia Univ Teachers Coll; SLP, NY Bd of Ed, **SLP**

Nagai, Mrs Jeanette F 4118 Trailcrest Drive, Moorpark, CA 93021, (213) 855-6265, BA 80 Univ of Southern CA; MA 82 Whittier Coll; Sp-Lang Path, Cedars-Sinai Med Ctr, **SLP ACE**

Nagami, Pamela S 658 East Puente, Covina, CA 91722, (213) 861-2891, BA 76 Univ of Redlands; MS 77 Univ of Redlands; SLP, LA Co Supt of Schs, **SLP**

Nagaraja, Girija 41 Taylor Street, Hillsdale, NJ 07642, **SLP A**

Nagasawa, Dr Taiko National Research Institute, For Special Education, 2360 Nobi Yokosuka, Kanagawa, Japan 239, BA 60 Meiji-Gakuin Univ; MA 64 Wichita St Univ; OD 70 (Health Science) Univ of Tokyo - Japan; Sp-Lang Path, National Inst of Sp Ed

Nagdeman, Mrs Kathryn J 7841 Northcote Avenue, Hammond, IN 46324, (815) 740-3196, BA 72 Coll of Saint Francis; MA 73 Univ of IL - Urbana; Sp-Lang Path, Joliet Pub Sch Dist #86, **SLP**

Nagel, Ann E 32 1/2 Carmel Road, Wheeling, WV 26003, (304) 242-1390, BS 78 Indiana Univ of PA; MS 86 PA St Univ - Univ Park; 86–Sp-Lang Path, Easter Seal Rehab Ctr, **SLP**

Nagel, Helen Moran 1413 32nd Street N E, Cedar Rapids, IA 52402, (319) 398-2273, BA 77 Univ of Northern IA; MA 78 Univ of Northern IA; Sp/Lang Path, Grant Wood AEA, **SLP**

Nagel, Dr Robert F 7116 East Port Au Prince, Tucson, AZ 85710, (602) 885-0337, BA 47 Univ of IL - Urbana; MS 54 Univ of IL - Urbana; PH 56 (Aud) Univ of IL - Urbana; **SLP A LM**

Nagel-Niehl, Patricia 2708 Old Quarry Road, Missoula, MT 59802, (406) 549-4902, BA 79 WA St Univ; MA 80 WA St Univ; Sp-Lang Path, Bitterroot Speech Ctr, **SLP**

Nager, Mrs Deborah F 10019 Inwood Drive, Houston, TX 77042, (713) 784-1177, BS 74 Miami Univ - Oxford; MA 76 Univ of KS; **A**

Nagey, Caroline 1903 White Star Drive, Diamond Bar, CA 91765, (818) 918-6652, BA 48 Stanford Univ; MA 74 CA St Univ - Fullerton; SLP, Los Angeles Supt of Sch, **SLP**

Naggatz, Kay Lynn Route 3 Box 51-E, North Branch, MN 55056, (612) 674-8709, BS 83 Univ of MN - Duluth; MS 85 Univ of WI - Stevens Point; 85–Aud, Minneapolis Otol PA, **A**

Naggi, Elaine J 322 Arcadia Drive, Vacaville, CA 95687, (707) 449-9006, BA 76 San Jose St Univ; MA 77 San Jose St Univ; 77–SLP, Solano Co Supt of Sch, **SLP**

Nagim, Mrs Denise H Metairie Lang & Learning Ctr, 4201 Saxon Street, Metairie, LA 70006, BS 75 Saint Mary's Dominican Coll; OM 77 LA St Univ - N O Medical Ctr; Dir/Pres, Metairie Lang & Hrng Cen, **SLP**

Nagle, Janice Oja 14150 Hillcrest, Livonia, MI 48154, BA 78 Univ of MI - Ann Arbor; MA 79 Western MI Univ; Tchr, Northville PS, **SLP**

Nagle, Kim Marie 508 Lincoln Avenue, Erie, PA 16502, (814) 453-5602, BS 81 CA Univ of PA; MS 83 CA Univ of PA; Sp-Lang Path, Lake Erie I of Rehab, **SLP**

Nagle, Mary Carlin 1023 East Villa Rita Drive, Phoenix, AZ 85022, (602) 275-2611, BA 78 WV Univ; MS 80 IN St Univ - Terre Haute; Sp-Lang Path, Deer Valley USD, **SLP**

Nagle, Maureen Elizabeth 39 Downer Avenue, Scarsdale, NY 10583, (914) 668-6580, BA 70 Mercy Coll; MA 86 CUNY - Lehman Coll; 70–Sp-Lang Path, Mt Vernon Bd of Educ, **SLP**

Nagle, Patricia 2007 Cedarbrook Court, Columbia, SC 29210, (803) 781-3347, BS 69 Miami Univ - Oxford; MA 73 Univ of Akron; **SLP**

Nagler, Mrs Janie D 20 Mario Drive, Higganum, CT 06441, (203) 345-8216, BS 69 Emerson Coll; MS 72 SUNY - Center at Albany; 74–Dir/Sp-Lang Path, Sp-Lang Pathology Associates, **SLP**

Nagle-Weible, Nancy Ann 814 Conestoga, St Louis, MO 63021, (314) 391-8179, BS 83 Southeast MO St Univ; MA 86 Southeast MO St Univ

Nagy, Mrs Denise E 6414 East Oak Street, Scottsdale, AZ 85257, (602) 839-7156, BS 79 IL St Univ - Normal; MS 82 AZ St Univ; Sp-Lang Path, Tempe Elementary School Dist 3, **SLP**

Nagy, Mrs MaryJo 842 Upton Road, Youngstown, OH 44509, (216) 797-2847, BS 80 Bowling Green St Univ; MA 82 OK St Univ; 82–Sp-Lang Path, Mahoning Co Bd of Men Ret & DD, **SLP**

Nagy, Mrs Regina L 2137 Crestwood Street, Rancho Palos Verdes, CA 90732, (213) 514-5385, BA 69 Duke Univ; MA 76 CA St Univ - Los Angeles; Sp-Lang Path, San Pedro Peninsula Hosp, **SLP**

Nagy-Greenberg, Janet Star Route Box 1141, Milford, PA 18337, (717) 491-5463, **SLP**

Nahin, Melinda J 111 Las Ondas Court, Santa Cruz, CA 95060, (408) 429-8631, BA 78 CA St Univ - Sacramento; MA 81 CA St Univ - Sacramento; Sp-Lang Path, Santa Cruz City Schs, **SLP**

Nahmias, Mrs Gail A 7702 20th Avenue, Brooklyn, NY 11214, (718) 946-9700, BS 84 SUNY - Coll at Brockport; MA 86 Long Island U - CW Post Ctr; 88–SLP, Brooklyn Schl for Spec Chldrn

Nahrwold, Mrs Marcia A Box 45, Bouck Island Road, Fultonham, NY 12071, (518) 827-5235, BS 81 Coll of Saint Rose; MS 82 Coll of Saint Rose; SLP, Nys Assoc Ret Chldn, **SLP**

Nailor, Audrey P O Box 202, College Place, WA 99324, MS; **LM**

Najac, John W 483 Emerald Avenue, San Carlos, CA 94070, **SLP**

Najaka, Elizabeth Hodovance 415 Keystone Avenue, Peckville, PA 18452, (717) 288-9386, BS 63 Bloomsburg Univ of PA; ME 75 Trenton St Coll

Nakai, Anne I 36386 Shelley Court, Newark, CA 94560, **SLP**

Nakamura, Patricia Shigetomi 3651 Mt Ariane Drive, San Diego, CA 92111, OB 74 San Diego St Univ; MA 82 San Diego St Univ; SLP, San Diego USD, **SLP**

Nakanishi, Laurel Ann 1511 Hidden Terrace Court, Santa Cruz, CA 95062, BA 82 Stetson Univ; MA 86 Stetson Univ; **SLP**

Nakasato, Mrs Jean M 849 Papalalo Place, Honolulu, HI 96825, (808) 261-3234, BS 72 Univ of HI - Manoa; OM 74 Univ of WA; Sp-Lang Path, Dept of Ed Windward Dist, **SLP**

Nakasone, Dr Hirotaka 1810 Harding Avenue, Altadena, CA 91001-3610, (213) 946-7147, BA 76 Univ of SC - Columbia; MA 79 MI St Univ; PH 84 (NS) MI St Univ; 85–Director of Research, Natl Forensic Voice & Acou Lab

Nakayama, Mrs Pat 45-106 Alina Place, Kaneohe, HI 96744, BS 70 Univ of HI - Manoa; MS 71 Univ of HI - Manoa; **SLP**

Nakles, Karen Oleyar 124 Lexington Avenue #4, Pittsburgh, PA 15215, (412) 363-0451, BA 83 Indiana Univ of PA; MA 86 Univ of Pittsburgh - Pittsburgh; 86–Sp-Lang Path, VA Med Ctr, **SLP**

Naliboff, Mrs Ellen C 6114 Madra Avenue, San Diego, CA 92120, (619) 583-0826, BS 51 Univ of Southern CA; MA 67 San Jose St Univ; BA San Jose St Univ; Sp-Lang Path, Ellen Naliboff, **SLP ACE**

Nalipinski, Mrs Paige McLarnon 15 Carlton Street #1, Salem, MA 01970, (215) 631-9300, BA 83 Univ of RI; MA 86 Temple Univ; 86–Sr Clin, InSpeech Inc, **SLP**

Nalitz, Mrs Noreen A G 204 West Fair Meadows, Canonsburg, PA 15317, (412) 394-5815, BS 71 Carlow Coll; MA 73 Univ of KS; SLP, Allegheny Intermediate Unit, **SLP**

Nall, Patricia Louise 1429 Robin Road, Owensboro, KY 42301, (812) 346-4401, BS 75 Brescia Coll; MS 85 Western KY Univ; **SLP**

Nallenweg, Mrs Mary K 1239 Redbud, Chesterton, IN 46304, (219) 926-2186, BS 80 Western MI Univ; MA 81 MI St Univ; SLP, Porter County Special Ed Coop, **SLP**

Nalls, Joseph C, II 4939 Laurel Canyon, Unit C, North Hollywood, CA 91607, (818) 985-3116, BA 82 CA St Univ - Los Angeles; MA 85 CA St Univ - Los Angeles; SLP, InSpeech Inc, **SLP**

Nalty, Lily Neumann 119 West Court, Columbia, SC 29212, (803) 758-4123, BS 76 Univ of TX - Austin; MA 82 Univ of TX - Austin; Unit Dir, Midlands Center, **SLP**

Namm, Rosanne Bishop 400 East 71st Street #12D, New York, NY 10021, (212) 737-2147, BS 74 PA St Univ - Univ Park; MA 78 NY Univ; OM 88 Fordham Univ; Sp-Lang Path, NY City Bd Educ, **SLP**

Namson, Mrs Sandra Kohn 2700 Bitternut Circle, Simi Valley, CA 93065, (805) 584-1227, BA 76 CA St Univ - Northridge; MA 78 CA St Univ - Northridge; SLP, LA USD, **SLP**

Nance, Dr Anita L 12736 St Andrews Terr, Oklahoma City, OK 73120, (405) 272-9876, BA 68 Abilene Christian Univ; MS 70 Univ of OK Medical Center; PH 79 (NS) Univ of OK Medical Center; Sp-Lang Path, VA Med Cen, **SLP**

Nance, Georgie C 11308 Marlee Avenue, Clinton, MD 20735, (703) 670-8126, BA 64 Univ of MD - College Park; MA 68 Univ of MD - College Park; Aud, Washington Hrng & Sp Soc, **A**

Nance, Mrs Rita F Carpenter 3 Julian Drive, Wonder Hills, Athens, OH 45701, (614) 593-3823, MA 88 OH Univ - Athens; 88–Sp-Lang Path, South Cent Ohio Sp & Hearing Ctr

Nandur, Srinivaskumar Udyavar 563 Peck Avenue, Fort Myers, FL 33919, (813) 694-2151, BS 74 All India Inst of Sp & Hrng; MS 76 All India Inst of Sp & Hrng; 86–Sp-Lang Path/Aud, Gulf Coast Center, **SLP A**

Nangle, Martha Barry 35 Cumberland Street, Yarmouth, ME 04096, (207) 775-4000, BA 82 Clark Univ; MS 87 Boston Univ; **SLP**

Nanna, Mrs Patricia McGuire 1446 Bridgedale Road, Crystal Lake, IL 60014, (312) 529-7281, BS 84 Northern IL Univ - De Kalb; MS 87 Marquette Univ; 88–Sp-Lang Path, Woodstock Comm Sch Dist 200

Nanni-Zacher, Deborah 39 Red Leaf Road, Moorestown, NJ 08057, (609) 722-1563, BA 76 Montclair St Coll; MA 83 Trenton St Coll; 88–Sp-Lang Path, Private Practice, **SLP**

Nantau, Judy L Speech And Language Clinic, Valparaiso University, Valparaiso, IN 46383, (219) 465-7806, BA 73 Valparaiso Univ; MA 74 Western MI Univ; Assoc Prof, Valparaiso Univ, **SLP**

Napier, Deborah L 969 Paradrome #101, Cincinnati, OH 45202, (513) 872-4241, BS 74 Univ of Cincinnati; MA 76 Univ of KY; Asst Prof of Otolaryngology, Univ of Cincinnati Med Cen, **SLP**

Napier, Julie Denise 1109 Columbia Avenue, Glasgow, KY 42141-3305, (502) 678-1671, **SLP**

Napier, Marcia Language & Learning Concepts, Oak Park Professional Bldg, 1910 Nacogdoches Rd Ste 4, San Antonio, TX 78209, (512) 824-0067, BA 73 Emory Univ; MA 77 Univ of TX - Austin; Sp/Lang Path, Lang & Learning Concepts, **SLP**

Napieralski, Linda Moore 4411 West Grange Avenue, Greenfield, WI 53220, (414) 421-7922, BS 71 Univ of WI - Milwaukee; MS 86 Univ of WI - Milwaukee; 88–Sp-Lang Path, Children's Hosp of WI, **SLP**

Naple, Mrs Ann M 3212 South 126th Avenue, Omaha, NE 68144, (712) 366-0503, BS 71 Univ of NE - Omaha; MS 72 Univ of NE - Omaha; Sp-Lang Path, Loess Hills AEA, **SLP**

Naples, Mrs Christy G 141 Troy Road, Delaware, OH 43015, (614) 224-5385, BS 75 Ashland Coll; MA 77 Case Western Reserve Univ; Aud, Barry S Hillman MD, **A**

Naples, Guy M 141 Troy Road, Delaware, OH 43015-5138, (614) 369-3650, OB 68 OH Univ - Athens; MA 74 OH Univ - Athens; Exec Dir, De Sp & Hrng Cen, **SLP A**

Napoli, Dennis M 4012 Winterhaven Street, Yorba Linda, CA 92686, (714) 973-0944, BA 75 Chapman Coll; MA 77 CA St Univ - Stanislaus; Sp-Lang Path, Private Practice, **SLP ACE**

Napoli, Mrs Janet Alviani 18604 Mandan Street, Canyon Country, CA 91351, (805) 251-9560, BA 78 CA St Univ - Northridge; MA 80 CA St Univ - Northridge; Sp-Lang Path, Los Angeles USD, **SLP**

Napoli, Janet H 11156 Whispering Oaks Drive, E, St Louis, MO 63136, (314) 664-6500, BS 76 Northern IL Univ - De Kalb; MA 79 Northern IL Univ - De Kalb; Aud, Incarnate Word Hosp, **A**

Napolitano, Patricia Ann 327 Clayton Road, Hillside, IL 60162, (312) 547-8399, BA 69 Loyola Univ of Chicago; MA 75 Western IL Univ; 87–Sp-Lang Path, U-SPEAC

Napp, Mrs Ann P 1101 Pheasant Ridge Drive, Lake Zurich, IL 60047, (312) 234-5600, BS 80 Northwestern Univ; MA 81 Northwestern Univ; Aud, Micheal Reese Hospital, **A**

Nappi, Claire A 104 Townsend Avenue, Pelham Manor, NY 10803, (212) 584-7679, BA 55 Coll of New Rochelle; MA 57 NY Univ; 84–Sp-Lang Path, Mt St Ursula Sp Ctr, **SLP**

Nappo, Cheryl Ann 1522 North Thompson Drive, Bay Shore, NY 11706, (516) 928-6655, BA 83 Adelphi Univ; MS 84 Adelphi Univ; Sp-Lang Path, BOCES III, **SLP**

Naranjo, Lucina A 10712 Shellyfield Rdoad, Downey, CA 90241, (213) 923-2934, BA 81 Univ of the Pacific; MA 83 Univ of Redlands; SLP, Montebello USD, **SLP**

Narburgh, David H 3412 Beaumont Road, Woodbridge, VA 22193, (703) 670-8126, BS 68 SUNY - Coll at Fredonia; ME 71 Univ of VA - Charlottesville; Sp-Lang Path, Prince William Speech/Hrng Ctr, **SLP**

Nardi, Mrs Deborah Jenene 337 Lyndon Road, Fairport, NY 14450, (716) 325-2255, BS 80 SUNY - Center at Buffalo; MA 82 SUNY - Center at Buffalo; Sp-Lang Path, Rochester City Schools, **SLP**

Naremore, Rita C Speech And Hearing Center, Indiana University, Bloomington, IN 47401, (812) 335-4156, BA 65 LA St Univ - Baton Rouge; MA 67 Univ of WI - Madison; PH 69 (Sp Communication) Univ of WI - Madison; Prof, Indiana Univ, **F**

Narkiewicz, Patricia Ann 7910 Coleman, Dearborn, MI 48126, (313) 832-1100, **SLP**

Narlock, Sr Marcella Mount Saint Clare, Speech And Hearing Center, Clinton, IA 52732, (319) 242-4070, BS 67 Marquette Univ; MS 69 Marquette Univ; Dir-Sp & Hrng Cen, Mount St Clare Coll, **SLP**

Naron, Clyde Allen 119 Windridge, West Monroe, LA 71291, (318) 396-6579, BS 78 Eastern WA Univ; MS 80 AR St Univ; 87–Sp-Lang Path, Monroe City Schs, **SLP**

Narotam, Ruksha 8450 Cambridge #3181, Houston, TX 77054, (713) 797-1466, MA 88 OH Univ - Athens; 88–Aud, MacGregor Med Ctr

Narsiah, Ravindra Enjaty 109 Elm Avenue, Takoma Park, MD 20912, (301) 270-8623, **SLP**

Narun, Mrs Linda R S 12410 Seaswept Drive, Houston, TX 77071, (713) 791-4298, BA 66 Witwatersrand Univ S Africa; MA 77 Witwatersrand Univ S Africa; Sp-Lang Path, TX Children's Hosp, **SLP**

Nasca, Michele Jasinski 90 Brigham Road # C-14, Fredonia, NY 14063-1025, (716) 672-4371, BS 76 SUNY - Coll at Geneseo; MA 81 Ball St Univ, Sp-Lang Path, Erie 2-BOCES, **SLP ACE**

Nasca, Vincent P 117 Old McHenry Road, Hawthorn Woods, Lake Zurich, IL 60047, (312) 631-8331, BS 66 Loyola Univ of Chicago; MA 69 De Paul Univ; 70–Sp-Lang Path, Chicago Bd of Educ, **SLP ACE**

Naseman, Suzanne Laborde 1840 Stall Drive, Harvey, LA 70058, (504) 367-3120, BA 79 Univ of Southwestern LA; OM 81 LA St Univ - N O Medical Ctr; Sp/Lang Path, Jefferson Parish Pub Sch Syst, **SLP**

Nash, Cynthia Lynne 1625 Saint Louis Drive, Honolulu, HI 96816, (808) 732-3608, BS 79 Univ of TN - Knoxville; MS 85 Univ of HI - Manoa; **A**

Nash, Deborah Jo 200 Maitland Avenue #119, Altamonte Springs, FL 32701, BA 75 Univ of FL; MS 76 FL St Univ; SLP, Seminole County Schools, **SLP**

Nash, Dr Dennis B 617 Sunset Boulevard, Stevens Point, WI 54481, (715) 346-2351, BA 62 Adams St Coll; MS 67 CO St Univ; PH 70 (NS) Univ of KS; Professor In Sch of Commun Dis, Univ of Wisconsin Stevens Pt, **SLP**

Nash, Mrs Georgia E 895 Brandywine Drive, Roselle, IL 60172-2806, (312) 837-3737, BA 70 Wheaton Coll; MA 73 Northern IL Univ - De Kalb; Sp-Lang Path, Schaumburg Sch Dist #54, **SLP**

Nash, Mrs Janice P 3410 Ensign Court, Arlington, TX 76017, MS 75 KS St Univ; **SLP**

Nash, Karen Erickson 24 Bennett Street, Phillipsburg, NJ 08865, (201) 689-2421, BA 78 Montclair St Coll; MA 86 Trenton St Coll

Nash, Kimberly Rene 1801 Mount Pisgah Lane #13, Silver Spring, MD 20903, (202) 877-1440, BS 85 Univ of NC - Greensboro; MA 87 George Washington Univ; 88–Sp-Lang Path, Natl Rehab Hosp, **SLP**

Nash, Maria L 10 Crestwood Drive, Narragansett, RI 02882, (401) 792-9652

Nash, Oliver A P O Box 1145, Cambridge, OH 43725-6145, (614) 439-3577, BA 74 Baldwin-Wallace Coll; MA 77 Cleveland St Univ; Sp-Lang Path, Guernsey Co Hlth Dept, **SLP**

Nash, Shirley B 473 Tharp Drive, Moraga, CA 94556, (415) 376-5799, BS 58 Univ of IA; MS 81 San Francisco St Univ; SLP, San Lorenzo USD, **SLP**

Nashban-Murphy, Mrs Janell P 1280-31 Sharon Park Drive, Menlo Park, CA 94025, (415) 854-1739, BS 47 Univ of WI - Madison; MS 69 Univ of WI - Milwaukee; Sp/Lang Path, San Carlos School District, **SLP**

Nasim, Abdo G 123 West View Road, Shrewsbury, PA 17361, (301) 592-7001, BS 64 CA Univ of PA; ME 70 Loyola Coll; 64–Sp-Lang Path, Baltimore Co Bd of Ed, **SLP**

Nason, Alice T Windlow Drive Roadsend, Otis, OR 97368, (503) 994-2921, BS 31 Northwestern Univ; ME 48 Saint Louis Univ; **SLP LM**

Nason, Mrs Janet F 106 Ashley Drive, Fairhope, AL 36532, (205) 943-2781, BS 74 Auburn Univ - Auburn; MS 81 East Carolina Univ; 86–Sp-Lang Path, InSpeech Inc, **SLP**

Nason, Mary Virginia University Of Mississippi, P O Box 2261, University, MS 38677, (601) 236-1346, BS 84 MS Univ for Women; MS 86 Univ of MS; **SLP**

Nasralla, Mrs Karen K 1422 Hydetown Road, Titusville, PA 16354, (814) 827-6499, BS 77 PA St Univ - Univ Park; MA 81 Ball St Univ; Sp-Lang Path, **SLP**

Nass, Mrs Susan Simpson 110 Pine Hill Avenue #2, Stamford, CT 06906, (203) 967-8737, BA 83 Loyola Coll; MS 84 Loyola Coll; Sp-Lang Path, St Agnes Hosp-Children's Rehab Ctr, **SLP ACE**

Nassar, Kim Ann 44 Mary Avenue, Poughkeepsie, NY 12603, (914) 564-6052, BA 81 SUNY - Coll at Cortland; MS 83 Boston Univ; Sp/Lang Path, Newburgh Dev Learn Ctr, **SLP**

Nassau-Taxon, Christy Ann 2107 Prosser Avenue, Los Angeles, CA 90025, (213) 470-5962, BS 72 Purdue Univ - West Lafayette; MA 75 CA St Univ - Northridge; MA 80 CA St Univ - Northridge; Sp-Lang Path, LA USD, **SLP**

Nassberg, Joan 11728 Wilshire #B-609, Los Angeles, CA 90025, (213) 997-2352, BA 61 CUNY - Brooklyn Coll; MS 62 Univ of WI - Madison; Audiologist, Los Angeles USD, **A**

Nastas, Laurie S 10006 Auburndale, Livonia, MI 48150, BA 79 MI St Univ; MA 81 Wayne St Univ - Sch of Med; Aud, Private Practice, **A**

Nat, Leba Y 75-27 169th Street, Flushing, NY 11366, (718) 969-9618, **SLP**

Nat, Mrs Melinda Fisk 151 Ragan Way, Grass Valley, CA 95945, **SLP**

Natale, Christine Clarino 31 Macarthur Avenue, Lodi, NJ 07644, (201) 472-7953, **SLP**

Natale, Janet Sue 250 Danbury Road #74, New Milford, CT 06776, (203) 797-4761, **SLP**

Natale, Kelly D 6 Coatbridge Court, Olney, MD 20832, (202) 541-6718, BS 79 WV Univ; MA 81 3346; Aud, Washington Hosp/Cen, **A**

Natale, Marianne Irene 8244 Daisy Field Path, Clay, NY 13041, (315) 488-2951, BA 82 Boston Coll; MS 84 Syracuse Univ; Sp-Lang Path, St Camillus Health/Rehab Ctr, **SLP**

Natale, Mrs Patricia G 39 Vlei Road, Rhinebeck, NY 12572, (914) 876-3796, BA 59 Univ of ME - Orono; MS 62 Univ of MI - Ann Arbor; 72–Sp-Lang Path, Hyde Park Public Schools, **SLP**

Natalicchio, Stefanie 4 Carol Court, East Brunswick, NJ 08816, (201) 321-7063, BA 86 Rutgers St Univ -N Brunswick; MS 88 Univ of AZ

Nathan, Colette 9 James Street, Shenton Park, West Australia, Australia 6008, **SLP**

Nathan, Debra E 5333 Knoxville Avenue, Lakewood, CA 90713, (203) 261-2072, BA 78 Univ of CA - Los Angeles; MA 81 CA St Univ - Northridge; Sp-Lang Path, **SLP**

Nathan, Mrs Diane Z 18449 Homewood Avenue, Homewood, IL 60430, (312) 672-2643, MA 82 Western IL Univ; Sp-Lang Path, Crete-Monee Sch Dist #201-U, **SLP**

Nathan, Jane E Rural Route 1 Box 451, Jericho, VT 05465, (802) 879-0411, MA 78 Univ of Denver; Audiological Consultant, Private Practice, **A**

Nathan, Mrs Jeanette 8915 North Bayside Drive, Milwaukee, WI 53217, (414) 692-2463, OB 71 0188; BA 68 1189; MS 79 Marquette Univ; Sp-Lang Path, Easter Seal Society, **SLP**

Nathan, Mrs Linda L 10828 East Crestridge Circle, Englewood, CO 80111, (303) 694-4736, BA 69 Univ of MO - Columbia; MA 71 Univ of CO - Boulder; Sp-Lang Path, Private Practice, **SLP**

Nathan-Gruber, Mrs Ellen 103 Lawrence Avenue, Highland Park, NJ 08904, (201) 247-6003, BA 80 CUNY - Queens Coll; MA 82 CUNY - City College; Sp/Lang Path, Robert Wood Johnson Univ Hosp, **SLP ACE**

Nathanson, Barbara 8764 Airport Road, Middleton, WI 53562-4107, (608) 798-4711, BS 79 Northern IL Univ - De Kalb; MS 81 Univ of IL - Urbana; Sp-Lang Path, University/Wisconsin Hos & Cl, **SLP**

Nathanson, Janis K 2790 West 5th Street #19E, Brooklyn, NY 11224, (212) 373-0364, BA 70 CUNY - Brooklyn Coll; MA 71 NY Univ; SLP, N York City Bd Ed Sp Serv Unit, **SLP**

Nathanson, Mrs Julie O'Connor 1524 East Madison, South Bend, IN 46617, (219) 284-7418, BS 74 Ball St Univ; MS 79 Univ of South FL; Clinical Mgr Neurolog Rehabil, Memorial Hospital of S Bend, **SLP**

Nathanson, Mrs Karen L 9 Moulton Road, Peabody, MA 01960, (617) 535-2788, BS 72 Boston Univ; MS 75 Boston Univ; **SLP**

Nathanson, Susan 27 Bayside Drive, Great Neck, NY 11023, (516) 741-7800, BA 63 Adelphi Univ; MA 66 CUNY - Brooklyn Coll; Sp-Lang Path, Herricks Pub Sch, **SLP**

Nathanson, Dr Susan N 227 East Walton Place #3E, Chicago, IL 60611, (312) 795-3415, BS 61 Northwestern Univ; MS 62 Northwestern Univ; PH 69 (NS) Northwestern Univ; 88–Dir, MacNeal Hosp, **SLP**

Nathanson, Yale S 2048 Pine Street, Philadelphia, PA 19103, (215) 732-2762, BS 23 Univ of PA; MA 24 Univ of PA; PH 30 (NS) Univ of PA; Private Practice, **SLP F LM**

Nation, Alta G RR 3 Box 450, Colorado City, TX 79512, BS 62 Hardin-Simmons Univ; MA 69 TX Woman's Univ; **SLP LM**

Nation, Dr James E 2600 Skyline Drive #19, Tucson, AZ 85718, (602) 577-1602, BS 59 IL St Univ - Normal; MA 60 Univ of WI - Madison; PH 64 (NS) Univ of WI - Madison; Sp-Lang Path, Tucson USD, **SLP F**

Natkin, Mrs Karen L 12602 Alcacer Del Sol, San Diego, CA 92128, (619) 532-3473, BA 70 Whittier Coll; ME 71 Boston Univ; 87–Educ Spec, Naval Educ/Training Support Ctr Pacific, **SLP**

Natoci, Mrs Karen Musselman 418 Village Green Boulevard, Apartment 107, Ann Arbor, MI 48105, (313) 572-2744, BA 81 Univ of MI - Ann Arbor; MS 82 Univ of MI - Ann Arbor; Sp/Lang Path, St Joseph Mercy Hospital, **SLP**

Natteford, Mary S 810 North Poplar, Manteca, CA 95336, (209) 823-1526, BA 49 Univ of Pittsburgh - Pittsburgh; MA 53 Univ of IA; SLP, Stockton USD, **SLP**

Nattkemper, Mrs Laurie L 109 Challis Court, Goose Creek, SC 29445, (803) 569-3240, BA 80 OH St Univ; MA 82 OH St Univ; **A**

Nau, Elaine B 2644 Shillington Road, Sinking Spring, PA 19608, (215) 378-0481, BS 77 Edinboro Univ of PA; MA 78 Edinboro Univ of PA; Sp-Lang Path, Berks Vn-Hha, **SLP**

Nau, Pamela R 255 Waller Street, San Francisco, CA 94102, BS 74 Ithaca Coll; MA 75 Univ of Denver; Sp-Lang Path, San Leandro USD, **SLP**

Naughton, Barbara M 191 North Road, Kingston, RI 02881, (401) 737-3300, BA 72 Univ of RI; MS 73 Univ of RI; Sp/Lang Path, Warwick Sch Dept, **SLP**

Naughton, Marie A 77 Circuit Road, Dedham, MA 02026, (617) 326-9330, OB 76 Emerson Coll; MA 77 IN Univ - Bloomington; Corp Mgr, Curtis-Newton, **SLP**

Naukam, Mrs Beth King 326 Fairport Road, East Rochester, NY 14445, (716) 232-2310, BA 81 SUNY - Center at Buffalo; MA 83 SUNY - Center at Buffalo; Sp-Lang Path, Rochester City Sch Dist, **SLP ACE**

Nauman, Suzanne W 9936 S W 37th Avenue, Portland, OR 97219, (503) 246-2131, BS 71 CO St Univ; MA 72 Univ of Northern CO; 88–Sp-Lang Path, Vancouver Sp Path, **SLP**

Naunton, Dr Ralph F Director CDP-NINDCS, NIH Federal Bldg #1C-11, 7550 Wisconsin Avenue, Bethesda, MD 20892, MD 45 (NS) Univ of London - England; Dir/Comm Dis Prgm, Natnl Inst of Hlth, **A F**

Nauseda, Bonnie F 141 East Street, Oxford, MI 48051, (313) 333-7870, BA 77 MI St Univ; MA 79 MI St Univ; **A**

Navarro, Mrs Jacquelyn 1327 North Marquette, Walnut, CA 91789-1255, (213) 726-1225, BS 78 KS St Univ; MA 80 KS St Univ; SLP, Montebello USD, **SLP**

Navarro, Dr M Richard 5250 Villla Verde #N-2, Reno, NV 89523, (702) 784-4887, BS 70 Western MI Univ; MA 71 Western MI Univ; PH 77 (NS) Vanderbilt Univ; Associate Professor, University of NV-Reno, **A**

Navia, Marilyn King Faisal Specialist Hosp, Dept Of Surgery, P O Box 3354, Riyadh, Saudi Arabia 11211, (305) 226-2305, MS 85 Univ of South FL; **A**

Navich, Michelle Ann 801 Spring Street, Moosic, PA 18507, (717) 737-6728, BS 84 Bloomsburg Univ of PA; MS 85 Bloomsburg Univ of PA; **SLP**

Navone, Michelle L 1701 Windjammer Court, Lodi, CA 95242, (209) 339-8841, BA 75 CA St Univ - Chico; Sp-Lang Path, Private Practice, **SLP**

Navratil, Shirley Ann 8929 Ellingham Street, San Diego, CA 92129-2109, (612) 522-4343, BA 82 Univ of MN - Minneap-St Paul; MA 86 Univ of MN - Minneap-St Paul; **A**

Navrotski, Darlette Sue 317 Elm Street, Westfield, NJ 07090, (201) 654-6847, BA 79 Univ of Pittsburgh - Pittsburgh; MA 86 Univ of Pittsburgh - Pittsburgh; Reg Consultant, Prentke Romich, **SLP**

Naylor, Dr Rex V 9910 Holmhurst Road, Bethesda, MD 20817, (301) 530-2340, BA 42 WV Wesleyan Coll; MA 52 OH St Univ; PH 55 (Sp Path) OH St Univ; Retired, Nav Med Cen Natl Capitol Reg, **SLP LM**

Naylor-Shelabarger, Mrs Barbara Ann 623 East Chestnut, Mason City, IL 62664, (217) 482-3002, BS 80 IL St Univ - Normal; MS 82 IL St Univ - Normal; Sp-Lang Path, Mason City Comm Ut Sch, **SLP**

Nayor, Mrs Rhoda A Audiology & Hearing Aid Serv, 30 Prospect Street, Ridgefield, CT 06877, (203) 438-9641, BS 65 Syracuse Univ; MA 66 Syracuse Univ; Aud, Jeffrey Monroe ENT, **A**

Neading, Mrs Diana Loechel 203 18th Street N W, Canton, OH 44703, (216) 453-3562, BS 76 Kent St Univ; MA 79 Kent St Univ; Sp-Lang Path, Canton City Sch, **SLP**

Neal, Julie A Route 6 Box 132-A, Marietta, OH 45750, (614) 374-1582, BS 80 WV Univ; MS 81 WV Univ; 86–Aud, Marietta Memorial Hosp, **A**

Neal, Mrs Marjorie Solliday 7074 Hites Cove Road, Mariposa, CA 95338-9640, (209) 742-6207, BA 51; BA 62 Pepperdine Univ - Los Angele; MA 65 Pepperdine Univ - Los Angele; Special Education Substitute, Huntington Beach High School, **SLP**

Neal, Mary R Route 15 Box 32, Cookeville, TN 38501, (615) 432-4421, BS 78 Univ of TX Med - Galveston; MS 82 Univ of MO - Columbia; 86–Sp-Lang Path, Putnam County Schs, **SLP**

Neal, Ronald Eugene P O Box 633, Halfway, OR 97834, (503) 523-5801, BA 79 Eastern WA Univ; MS 81 Eastern WA Univ

Neal, Vicki K 330 Sanchez, Santa Fe, NM 87501, (505) 984-1015, BA 76 Univ of KY; MA 78 Univ of TN - Knoxville; 88–SLP, Educ Assessment Sys Inc, **SLP**

Neal, Dr W Ray, Jr University Of Georgia, 570 Aderhold, Athens, GA 30602, (404) 542-1685, BA 55 Mercer Univ - Macon; ME 58 Univ of GA; ED 66 (Sp Path) Univ of GA; Assoc Prof SLP/Aud, U of GA, **SLP A F**

Neale, Mrs Tawana M 3000 7th Street N E #227, Washington, DC 20017, (202) 529-2707, BS 59 Univ of the DC; Sp/Lang Path, Dc Board of Ed, **SLP**

Neale-Tobener, Mrs Elisa PO Box 1231, Melrose, FL 32666-1231, (904) 475-2534, BA 84 Univ of FL; MA 85 Univ of TN - Knoxville; **SLP**

Neary, Mary Elizabeth 4256 Douglas Street, Omaha, NE 68131, (402) 551-7338, **SLP**

Nebel, Mrs Barbara Lynn 4508 50th Street, Des Moines, IA 50310, (515) 253-9417, BA 83 Univ of Northern IA; MA 85 Univ of Northern IA; Sp-Lang Path, Central Speach Rehab, **SLP**

Nebel, Cheryl Lehr 113 S Fair Street, Otsego, MI 49078, (616) 388-3468, BS 83 Western MI Univ; MA 85 Western MI Univ; **SLP**

Nebel-Gould, Mrs Amy Sue 8025 S W 107th Avenue #116, Miami, FL 33173, (305) 279-3560, BA 82 Univ of Toledo; BA 82 Univ of Toledo; MS 83 Miami Univ - Oxford; Sp/Lang Path, Jackson Memorial Hosp, **SLP**

Neben, Mrs Susan J 90 Quail Hill Place, Oroville, CA 95966, (916) 534-0423, BA 70 WA St Univ; MA 75 WA St Univ; Sp-Lang Path/Tchr, Butte Co Supt of Sch, **SLP**

Nebera, Rebecca Annette 3105 Cottage Oaks Court, Midlothian, VA 23113, (804) 321-6666, **SLP**

Nebuda, Marlene F 3321 Pierce Street, Sioux City, IA 51104, (712) 258-5523, BA 65 Briar Cliff Coll; MA 71 Univ of NE - Lincoln; Head Sp-Lang Path, Siouxland Er Sl So, **SLP**

Neck, Wayne Walter 825 Church Street S E, Gainesville, GA 30501, (803) 785-3900, BS 84 Central MI Univ; MA 85 Central MI Univ; Sp-Lang Path, Gainesville Physical Ther, **SLP**

Neckrich, Jaclyn S 8002 Valley Manor Road, Apartment 2-A, Owings Mills, MD 21117, (301) 356-6283, MS 77 Towson St Univ; Sp-Lang Path, Baltimore Cty Pub Sch, **SLP**

Nedbalsky, Anna M 69-53 229th Street, Bayside, NY 11364, (718) 224-9809, MA 76 NY Univ; Sp-Lang Path, NYC Bd of Ed, **SLP**

Nedberg, Patricia J 8126 East Buena Terrace Way, Scottsdale, AZ 85253, (602) 345-2011, BS 79 ND St Univ; MS 80 Univ of ND; SLP, AZ Sp Path, **SLP**

Nedelka, Anne M 59-31 161st Street, Flushing, NY 11365, (718) 463-4541, BA 76 CUNY - Queens Coll; MA 86 CUNY - Queens Coll; 86–Sp-Lang Path, Long Island Jewish Med Ctr, **SLP**

Neeb, Mrs Amy Warden 312 Copperleaf, Austin, TX 78734, (512) 385-2787, BS 85 Baylor Univ; MS 87 TX Christian Univ; 87–Sp-Lang Path, Del Valle Ind Sch Dist

Neece, M Maxine 2107 14th Street, Greeley, CO 80631, BA 49 Univ of CO - Boulder; MA 68 Univ of Northern CO; Sp-Lang Path, Weld BOCES, **SLP**

Neeck, Catherine Elizabeth 35 Ashford Avenue, Dobbs Ferry, NY 10522, (212) 379-5020, BS 82 Marywood Coll; MA 84 OH Univ - Athens; Sp-Lang Path, Hebrew Hosp for Chronic Sick, **SLP**

Needham, Alan C 8 Green Meadow Drive, Bloomfield, CT 06002, (203) 243-9510, BS 71 SUNY - Coll at Geneseo; MA 76 SUNY - Coll at Geneseo; Owner, Private Practice, **A**

Needham, Ellen C 1940 Palisades Drive, Appleton, WI 54915, (414) 735-6260, BA 66 Wittenberg Univ; MA 69 OH St Univ; Sp-Lang Path, Appleton Public Schools, **SLP**

Needham, Mrs Leslie F 61 Carleon Avenue, Larchmont, NY 10538, (914) 834-5278, BS 64 Univ of VA - Charlottesville; MA 66 Case Western Reserve Univ; **SLP**

Needham, Thyria H 1577 Maplewood Drive, Slidell, LA 70458, (504) 643-4418, MS; **SLP LM**

Needle, Lynn Ms Sp/Path -Sp/Hring Inst, Univ Of Texas - Health Sci, C - 1343 Moursund, Houston, TX 77030, (713) 792-4500, BA 84 Univ of MD - College Park; MS 85 Boston Univ; **SLP**

Needleman, Betty Unger 9 Woodfern Street, Edison, NJ 08820, (201) 769-7498, BA 76 SUNY - Center at Buffalo; MA 79 OH Univ - Athens; Aud, Barry Skobel MD, **A**

Needleman, Harriet L 86 Richardson Drive, Needham, MA 02192, (617) 444-2776, BA 70 Rutger's St Univ - Douglas Coll; ME 73 Boston Univ; Sp-Lang Path, Private Practice, **SLP**

Needles, Marita Riener 243 Friendship Drive, Paoli, PA 19301, (215) 891-3371, MS 87 Hahnemann Univ Grad Sch; 88–Chief Sp-Lang Path, Riddle Mem Hosp, **SLP**

Neeley, Cynthia H 385 Talbot #12, Pacifica, CA 94044, (415) 355-3950, BS 73 IL St Univ - Normal; MS 76 IL St Univ - Normal; 88–Sp-Lang Path, San Francisco USD, **SLP**

Neeley, Lambert W 1453 West Clair Street, Ontario, CA 91761-4713, (213) 868-9979, BA 52 CA St Univ - Chico; MA 55 CA St Univ - Los Angeles; Sp-Lang Path, CA Youth Authority, **SLP**

Neeley, Mrs Phyllis Miles PO Box 3719, State University, AR 72467, (501) 932-3799, OB 76 AR St Univ; OM 77 AR St Univ; 88–Sp-Lang Path, Cottage of Hope, **SLP**

Neeley, Richard A 3518 Bess Drive, Jonesboro, AR 72401, (501) 932-3799, OB 76 AR St Univ; OM 77 AR St Univ; Graduate Teaching Assistant, University of Tennessee, **SLP**

Neeley, Mrs Velma L 1453 Clair Street, Ontario, CA 91761, BA 76 CA St Univ - Fullerton; MS 82 Univ of LA Verne; SLP, San Bernardino County Schools, **SLP**

Neeley-Marshall, Vangie 2910 North Patterson Street, Valdosta, GA 31602, (912) 244-2562, BS 80 FL St Univ; MS 81 FL St Univ; 82–Aud, ENT & Allergy Associates of Valdosta, **A**

Neely, Ann N N Ju Kevil MH MR Center, South 10th Street Extended, Mayfield, KY 42066, (502) 247-5396, BS 75 Murray St Univ; MS 76 Murray St Univ; 78–Dir Sp-Lang Path, JuKevil MHMR Cen, **SLP**

Neely, Kathleen R Parroquia Santa Angela Marici, Morales Duarez 1048, Carmen DE La Legua, Sucursal 10, Callao, Peru 3, BA 65 Bellarmine Coll; ME 80 Spalding Coll; 88, Private Practice, **SLP**

Neeriemer, William R 10 Rolling Oaks Estates, Asheville, NC 28806, (704) 274-2400, BA 70 FL St Univ; OM 74; MS 79 East TN St Univ; Director, Thoms Rehabilitation Hospital, **SLP**

Neering, Diane Towns 121 Kipling Boulivard, Lansing, MI 48912, (313) 977-8988, BA 79 MI St Univ; MA 81 Wayne St Univ; 81–Aud, Macomb Aud Svcs, **A**

Neff, Dr Donna Lynn Boys Town Natl Institute, 555 North 30th Street, Omaha, NE 68131, (402) 498-6702, BS 76 Univ of NE - Omaha; MA 79 Univ of NE - Omaha; PH 83 (Experimental Psychology) Univ of NE - Lincoln; 88–Coord-Psychoacoustics Lab, Boys Town Natl Inst

Neff, Mrs Marilyn Gennarelli 8214 Black Oak Court, Fort Wayne, IN 46825, (219) 425-3053, BA 75 SUNY - Center at Buffalo; MA 77 OH St Univ; 88–Sp-Lang Path, St Joseph Med Ctr, **SLP**

Neff, Mrs Rachel Lynn P O Box 804, Seabrook, TX 77571, (817) 573-3791, BS 81 Univ of North TX; MS 81 Univ of North TX

Neff, Richard Wayne 315 Juniper Street, Mahtomedi, MN 55115, (612) 429-2088, BS 77 Mankato St Univ; MS 82 ID St Univ; Aud, 916 Spec Inter Sch Dist, **A**

Neff, Scott R P O Box 1152, Roswell, NM 88202, (505) 625-8200, BA 81 MI St Univ; MA 82 MI St Univ; Sp-Lang Path, Roswell ISD, **SLP**

Neff, Sue Ann 6415 Stumph Road #101, Parma Heights, OH 44130, (216) 842-0302, BS 77 Kent St Univ; MA 80 Cleveland St Univ; Sp/Lang Path, Private Practice, **SLP**

Neft, Mrs Beth Weinstock 23418 W Darcy Lane, Newhall, CA 91321, (805) 255-6665, BA 73 CA St Univ - Northridge; MA 75 CA St Univ - Northridge; SLP, Gardner-Manzella Assoc, **SLP**

Negrin, Jane D 4 Falcon Court, Livingston, NJ 07039, (201) 227-2021, BS 76 Montclair St Coll; MS 77 Columbia Univ Teachers Coll; **SLP**

Negron-Marrero, Sonia Ivette I 306 Condominium River Pk, Bayamon, PR 00619, (809) 798-2930, BA 83 Univ of PR - San Juan; MS 85 Univ of PR - San Juan; **SLP**

Negrotto, Mrs Carol Anne Route 4 Box 28WN, Folsom, LA 70437, (504) 892-0257, **SLP**

Neher, Mrs Winifred 848 Porter, Wichita, KS 67203, (316) 689-4820, BA 65 Wichita St Univ; MA 76 Wichita St Univ; Sp-Lang Path, St Joseph Med Cen, **SLP**

Nehls, Luanne 840 Tepic Drive, El Paso, TX 79912, (913) 648-2859, **SLP**

Nehlsen, Kerri Savage 136 Wilcox Court, Matawan, NJ 07747, (201) 583-3123, BA 83 Saint John's Univ - Jamaica; MS 85 CUNY - Brooklyn Coll; 84–Sp-Lang Path, League Sch, **SLP**

Neidecker, Elizabeth 911 Lambert Drive, Bowling Green, OH 43402, (419) 352-8047, BS 51 OH St Univ; MA 56 Case Western Reserve Univ; **SLP LM**

Neidenthal, Mrs Julie Schraeder 12400 North 64th Street, Riley, KS 66531-9607, (913) 485-2569, **SLP**

Neidich, Jay S 1520 Richmond, Arlington Heights, IL 60004, (312) 334-6290, BA 75 CUNY - City College; MA 79 Univ of Pittsburgh - Pittsburgh; Sp-Lang Path, Rehab Med Clin, **SLP**

Neidich, Mrs Robin B 1520 Richmond, Arlington Heights, IL 60004, (312) 878-8200, BA 76 Univ of WI - Madison; MA 78 Univ of Pittsburgh - Pittsburgh; OM 86 Loyola Univ of Chicago; Dir/Sp-Lang Path, Sweish Covenant Hosp, **SLP**

Neidlinger, Mrs Susan C 5955 North 83rd Street, Scottsdale, AZ 85253, (602) 375-1403, BS 62 Miami Univ - Oxford; MA 76 AZ St Univ; 74–Sp/Lang Path, Dept of Econ Sec, **SLP**

Neier, Mrs Kathryn R 399 Hotchkiss Road, Bay City, MI 48706, BS 79 Central MI Univ; MA 80 Central MI Univ; 86–Sp-Lang Path, Bay-Arenac Intermed Sch Dist, **SLP**

Neighbors, Mrs Victoria Ruth 1721 Highland, Northbrook, IL 60062, (312) 623-0021, MA 84 Northwestern Univ; Sp-Lang Path, Spec Ed Dist of Lake City, **SLP**

Neihardt, Carol Vilseck American School, Box 504, APO New York, NY 09112, BA 75 CA St Univ - Northridge; MA 79 CA St Univ - Northridge; Sp/Lang Path, Dept of Defense Dep Schs, **SLP**

Neil, Mrs Debra Campbell Rd #1 Box 182 A, Grindstone, PA 15442, (412) 439-1444, BS 81 CA Univ of PA; MS 86 CA Univ of PA; 88–Asst Dir of Sp Svcs, SG Rehab Inc, **SLP**

Neil, Gilbert G 2070 N W 47th Avenue, Lauderhill, FL 33313, (305) 981-5450, BA 57 Gordon Coll; MS 68 Emerson Coll; Sp Lang Cl, Broward Co Sch Bd, **SLP**

Neil, Mrs Linda Sue 1715 Seventh Avenue, Belvidere, IL 61008, (815) 522-3335, BS 78 Southern IL Univ-Edwardsvill; MA 81 Northern IL Univ - De Kalb; SLP, Hiawatha Comm Unit Dist #426, **SLP**

Neilitz, Mrs Frances Glowienka 918 Phasianus, Green Bay, WI 54311, (414) 436-7641, BA 76 Univ of WI - Eau Claire; MS 77 Univ of WI - Stevens Point; ME 83 Univ of WI - Oshkosh; Sp-Lang Path, Green Bay Area Pub Schs, **SLP**

Neill, Janet F 2026 South Village Lane, Bolivar, MO 65613, (417) 326-5247, BS 67 Central MO St Univ; MS 70 Central MO St Univ; Sp/Lang Path, Bolivar R-1 Pub Schs, **SLP**

Neill, Michele Caroline 3905 Nancy Court #5, Champaign, IL 61820, (217) 283-6661, **SLP**

Neill, Rebecca Ann 470 20th Avenue N E, Hickory, NC 28601, (704) 328-6557, BS 84 Appalachian St Univ; MA 86 Appalachian St Univ; Sp-Lang Path, Hickory PS, **SLP**

Neill, Mrs Sara Lee 4287 Monroe Boulevard, Ogden, UT 84403, (801) 625-2080, BA 65 Hiram Coll; MA 76 Univ of Northern CO; Director Sp-Lang Path Dept, Stewart Rehabilitation Center, **SLP ACE**

Neils, Dr Jean Rankin Dept Of Communication Disorder, Room 331 Braunstein Hall, University Of Cincinnati, Cincinnati, OH 45221, (513) 475-4883, BS 77 PA St Univ - Univ Park; MA 79 Case Western Reserve Univ; PH 84 (Sp Path) Case Western Reserve Univ; Sp/Lang Path, Univ of Cincinnati, **SLP**

Neils, Mrs Lynn Reimers 1452 Oak Avenue, #2-N, Evanston, IL 60201, (312) 869-4529, BS 73 IL St Univ - Normal; MA 83 Univ of IL - Urbana; Sp-Lang Path, Phd Student, **SLP**

Neilsen, Amy Marie 2957 Bonito Lane, Grand Junction, CO 81504, (303) 244-6158, BS 77 CO St Univ; MS 80 CO St Univ; 80–Sp-Lang Path, Hilltop Rehab Hosp, **SLP**

Neiman, Dr Gary S Sch Of Speech Path & Audiology, Kent State University, A104 Music & Speech Center, Kent, OH 44242, (216) 672-2672, BS 69 Univ of IL - Urbana; MA 71 Univ of IL - Urbana; PH 73 (NS) Univ of IL - Urbana; Dir Sch of SLP & Aud, Kent State U, **SLP**

Neiman-Diamond, Abby B 26 Kirkwood Street, Long Beach, NY 11561, (516) 889-4970, BA 79 SUNY - Center at Buffalo; MS 81 Columbia Univ Teachers Coll; Sp/Lang Path, Visiting Therapy Assoc, **SLP**

Neis, Kimberly Kae 7814 Unity Avenue West, Brooklyn Park, MN 55443, (612) 561-3090, MS 88 Univ of WI - Stevens Point

Neislar, Susan Kaye 12201 Banyan Lane, Oklahoma City, OK 73132, (405) 271-4214, BA 70 Univ of OK - Norman; MS 71 CO St Univ; Asst Professor/Clinical Supvr, Univ Oklahoma Health Sci Ctr, **SLP**

Nelcamp, Valerie Grace 1100 Snider Road #57, Mason, OH 45040, (606) 581-1253, BS 81 Univ of Cincinnati; MA 83 Univ of Cincinnati; Sp-Lang Path, Brookside, **SLP**

Neldon, Mrs Gayle B Route 10 Box 1-B, Morgantown, WV 26505-8818, (304) 599-3959, BA 77 West Liberty St Coll; MS 79 WV Univ; **A**

Nellany, Kim Ann 39 Atlas Avenue #2, San Jose, CA 95126, (408) 448-4357, BA Univ of CA - Santa Barbara; MA 84 San Jose St Univ

Nelles, Mrs Teresa M 411 Flett Drive, Airdrie, AB, Canada T4B 1N1, (403) 274-2749, BS 76 Univ of Western Ontario; OM 78 Univ of Western Ontario; Sp-Lang Path, Alberta Chldn's Prov Hosp, **SLP**

Nellhaus, Susan L 137 Aspen Road, Swampscott, MA 01907, BS 76 Ithaca Coll; MA 77 Central MI Univ; 85–Sp-Lang Path, Cohen Hillel Academy, **SLP**

Nelli, Jean Marie 2245 Cresent Avenue, Charlotte, NC 28207, (704) 333-8071, **SLP**

Nellis, Robert A Waisman Center, 1500 Highland Avenue Room 157, Madison, WI 53705-2280, (608) 263-5804, BA 67 St Mary of the Lake; MA 70 De Paul Univ; Supvr-Aud Sec, Waisman Cne-Cl Serv Ut, **A**

Nellist, Susan Gay P O Box 524, Lyons, CO 80540, (303) 441-0437, BA 72 WA St Univ; BA 84 Univ of CO - Boulder; MA 86 Univ of CO - Boulder; 86–Sp-Lang Path, Memorial Hosp-Boulder, **SLP**

Nellum-Davis, Dr Priscilla 3218 Dartmouth Court, Little Rock, AR 72204, (501) 569-3155, BS 67 Memphis St Univ; MA 72 Memphis St Univ; PH 81 (NS) SUNY - Center at Buffalo; Assoc Prof-SLP, U of AR-Little Rock, **SLP**

Nelly, Mrs Christine Kay 803 NE 98th Court, Vancouver, WA 98664, (206) 256-6022, BA 82 WA St Univ; MA 84 WA St Univ; Sp-Lang Path, Evergreen School District, **SLP**

Nelmes, Dale A 650 Oakview Drive, Algonquin, IL 60102-2049, **SLP**

Nelsen, Ann S 1701 Lincoln, Cozad, NE 69130, (308) 784-2416, 88 Kearney St Coll

Nelsen, Mrs Kristine Kay 714 N W 175th Place, Beaverton, OR 97006, BS 77 OR St Univ; MS 84 Western OR St Coll; **SLP**

Nelsen, Mrs Lynn E 447 Locust Street, Laguna Beach, CA 92651, (714) 494-1253, BA 65; ME 66 PA St Univ - Univ Park; 87–Sp-Lang Path, Private Practice, **SLP**

Nelson, Alexandra 2754-B Novato Boulevard, Novato, CA 94947, (415) 897-4269, BA 75 Sonoma St Univ; BA 79 Humboldt St Univ; MA 81 Humboldt St Univ; SLP, Novato USD, **SLP**

Nelson, Mrs Allison Leigh P O Box 722, Denton, TX 76202, (817) 382-8420, BA 74 Midwestern St Univ; MS 76 Baylor Univ; Director, Nelsons Clinic-Trtmnt-Comm Dis, **SLP**

Nelson, Mrs Ann Letitia 24 Marvin Street, Montpelier, VT 05602, (802) 223-6120, MS 83 Univ of VT; Sp-Lang Path, Montpelier Pub Schs, **SLP**

Nelson, Barbara A Route 1 Box 15-A, Stanton, IA 51573, (712) 829-2785, BS 75 Northwest MO St Univ; MS 77 Univ of NE - Omaha; SLP, Green Valley AEA, **SLP**

Nelson, Barbara Gail 185 Crago Avenue, Waynesboro, PA 15370, (412) 852-2529, BS 73 Indiana Univ of PA; ME 76 Indiana Univ of PA; 87–Sp-Lang Path, Monongalia Co Bd of Educ, **SLP**

Nelson, Barbara H 328 South 5th Street, Geneva, IL 60134, (313) 271-7170, BS 74 Univ of MI - Ann Arbor; MS 75 Univ of MI - Ann Arbor; Sp-Lang Path, Comp Commun Serv, **SLP**

Nelson, Mrs Barbara L 3502 Bentley Drive, Spring Valley, CA 92077, (619) 463-9227, BA 74 San Diego St Univ; MA 77 San Diego St Univ; Program Specialist, La Mesa-Sprng Valley Sch Dist, **SLP**

Nelson, Mrs Barbara Mills 14083 South 40th Street, Phoenix, AZ 85044, (602) 839-7156, BA 82 Univ of CA - Santa Barbara; OM 84 AZ St Univ; Sp-Lang Path, Tempe Elementary School Dist, **SLP**

Nelson, Beth V 4308 Rockport Lane, Bowie, MD 20715, (301) 677-7013, BS 83 WV Univ; MA 85 George Washington Univ; 87–Aud, DOD-Kimbrough Army Comm Hosp, **A**

Nelson, Betty E 1791 Little Fawn Trail, Conyers, GA 30207, (404) 363-1971, BS 78 Univ of GA; ME 79 Univ of GA; 88–Sp-Lang Path, Clayton Co Bd of Educ, **SLP**

Nelson, Beverly K 5623 West 157th Street, Overland Park, KS 66223, (913) 681-3966, BS 74 Univ of KS; MA 75 Univ of KS; Sp-Lang Path, Children's Ctr of Vis Imp, **SLP**

Nelson, Dr C Donald Oregon Health Science Univ, P O Box 574, Portland, OR 97207, (503) 279-8359, BS 53 Univ of UT; MS 56 Univ of UT; PH 67 (Sp Path) Univ of WA; Sp-Lang Path, Or Hlth Sci U, **SLP F**

Nelson, C Van 648 Rosemere Circle, Orlando, FL 32811-4424, (407) 351-8500, BA 80 Univ of Central FL; MA 82 Univ of Central FL; Sp-Lang Path, Orlando Reg Med Cen, **SLP ACE**

Nelson, Carol A 29005 Saddlebrook, Agoura, CA 91301, (805) 492-3565, BA 72 Univ of MI - Ann Arbor; MA 80 CA St Univ - Northridge; Sp-Lang Path, Conejo Valley USD, **SLP**

Nelson, Carol Ann 120-17 Alcott Place #17-G, Bronx, NY 10475, (315) 423-2251, BS 84 Syracuse Univ; MS 86 Columbia Univ Teachers Coll; **SLP**

Nelson, Carol L S 8410 45th Street West, Tacoma, WA 98466, (206) 627-3839, BS 70 SUNY - Coll at Geneseo; MS 73 SUNY - Coll at Geneseo; Sp-Lang Path, Tacoma Speech and Hearing, **SLP**

Nelson, Mrs Cathy Ann 55355 Elder Road, Mishawaka, IN 46545, (219) 256-9265, BS 83 Bowling Green St Univ; MA 87 Western MI Univ; 88–Sp-Lang Path, Sch City of Mishawaka

Nelson, Charles T Audiology & Speech Path Serv, 521 6th Street # A, Oakmont, PA 15139, (412) 363-0451, BS 75 WV Univ; MS 76 WV Univ; Aud, VA Med Ctr, **A**

Nelson, Chelie Ann 999 N Silver Springs Blvd, Apartment 1204, Wichita, KS 67212, (316) 262-8271, BA 84 Wichita St Univ; MA 85 Wichita St Univ; 86–Sp-Lang Path, I of Logopedics, **SLP**

Nelson, Cheryl Dee 332 East Leah Lane, Gilbert, AZ 85234, (602) 497-0844, BS 73 Univ of ND; MS 86 ID St Univ; 87–Sp-Lang Path, Gilbert PS, **SLP**

Nelson, Claudia P 1508 Laurel Hill Road, Vienna, VA 22180, (703) 691-2171, BS 51 Univ of IL - Urbana; MS 53 Univ of IL - Urbana; Prog Spec Sp-Lang, Fairfax Co Pub Sch, **SLP**

Nelson, Colleen Ann 500 N E Chipman Road #10, Lee's Summit, MO 64063, (303) 775-2342, BS 83 KS St Univ; MS 85 Fort Hays St Univ; **SLP**

Nelson, Crystal 5000 North 1 1/2 Street, Apartment 173, Mc Allen, TX 78504, (512) 632-4919, **SLP**

Nelson, Cynthia L 191 East Fairmount Avenue, Whitefish Bay, WI 53217, (414) 963-3951, BA 74 Univ of WI - Eau Claire; MS 75 Univ of WI - Eau Claire; Sp-Lang Path, Whitefish Bay Pub Sch, **SLP**

Nelson, Dr David A 2630 University Avenue S E, Minneapolis, MN 55414, (612) 627-4693, BA 63 Saint Olaf Coll; MA 66 Univ of MN - Minneap-St Paul; PH 70 (Hearing Science) Univ of MN - Minneap-St Paul; Prof, U of MN

Nelson, David G 1705 3rd Street S E, Minot, ND 58701, (701) 838-3945, PH 70 (Aud) Univ of KS; 73–Dir-Educ of the Deaf, Minot State Univ, **A**

Nelson, DeeAnn B 8708 Carole Circle #11, Des Moines, IA 50322, (515) 993-4596, BS 83 Northwest MO St Univ; MA 84 Northeast MO St Univ; 84–Sp-Lang Path, Heartland AEA 11, **SLP**

Nelson, Denise Smith 100 Brentway Circle #63, Knoxville, TN 37909, (615) 971-1349, BS 85 East TN St Univ; MA 86 Univ of TN - Knoxville; 88–Aud, Fort Sanders Regional Med Ctr, **A**

Nelson, Diana L G Ridge Road, St Anton Star Route, Nederland, CO 80466, (303) 444-2387, BA 74 Univ of CO - Boulder; MA 76 Univ of Northern CO; Sp/Lang Path, Boulder Educ & Ther Serv, **SLP**

Nelson, Elizabeth Ann 3918 Oneida Place, Hyattsville, MD 20782, (202) 745-5600, BA 81 Augustana Coll; MA 83 Univ of KS; Sp-Lang Path, Mid-MO Ment Hlth Cen, **SLP**

Nelson, Mrs Eudora P 8123 Cacus Street, Spring Valley, CA 92077, (619) 690-1334, BA 64 Univ of NE - Lincoln; MA 68 Univ of AR - Pine Bluff; Sp-Lang Path, Ch Lang Spec Day Class, **SLP**

Nelson, Mrs Evelyn Mae 1109 South 36th Street, Omaha, NE 68105, (402) 331-4700, BS 79 Univ of NE - Omaha; MS 80 Univ of NE - Omaha; **SLP**

Nelson, Gloria B 5103-E Backlick Road, Annandale, VA 22003, (703) 941-7544, BA 64 KS St Univ; MS 67 Univ of MI - Ann Arbor; 78–Dir, Gloria Bartholomew Nelson Assoc, **SLP ACE**

Nelson, Howard D Box 449, Cokato, MN 55321, (612) 286-2128, BA 54 Augustana Coll; BS 68 Mankato St Univ; MS 74 Saint Cloud St Univ; SLP, Passel-Cokato Sch, **SLP**

Nelson, Mrs Hunter McCorkle 121 Musket Drive, King, NC 27021, (919) 983-6395, BS 81 James Madison Univ; MS 82 James Madison Univ; Sp/Lang Path, **SLP**

Nelson, Iris Ripley 2434 Bella Coola, Kamloops, BC, Canada U2E 1T7, (604) 372-7788, BA 69 Dalhousie Univ - Nova Scotia; MA 71 Kent St Univ; Sp/Lang Path, Sch Dist of Kamloops, **SLP**

Nelson, James A 945 Appletree Lane, Brookfield, WI 53005-6833, (414) 782-3910, BS 65 Bradley Univ; MS 72 Univ of WI - Milwaukee; 72–Sp-Lang Path, Elmbrook Sch Dist, **SLP**

Nelson, Jane E T 10101 Waltham Drive, Richmond, VA 23223, (606) 573-4520, BS 78 East TN St Univ; MA 80 Univ of TN - Knoxville; **A**

Nelson, Janet L 408 North Cherry Street, Eudora, AR 71640, (318) 428-4791, OB 77 AR St Univ; OM 78 AR St Univ; Sp-Lang Path, West Carroll Parish Schools, **SLP**

Nelson, Janet R W 701 Carol Lynn Drive, Little Chute, WI 54140, **SLP**

Nelson, Dr Jeniece E Dept Of Comm Disorders, 110 Moore Bldg, Penn State Univ, University Park, PA 16802, (814) 863-1624, BS 77 Towson St Univ; MS 78 Towson St Univ; ED 88 (Administrative Leadership-HRD) Vanderbilt Univ; 88–Asst Prof, Penn State Univ, **SLP**

Nelson, Jill Annette 1124 First Street West #1, Dickinson, ND 58601, (701) 225-5715, BS 82 Moorhead St Univ; MS 85 Minot St Univ; 82–Sp-Lang Path, Dickinson PS, **SLP**

Nelson, Joan 7343 East Thornwood Drive, Scottsdale, AZ 85251, (602) 423-1332, OM 87 AZ St Univ; 88–Sp-Lang Path, InSpeech Inc, **SLP**

Nelson, Joanna Boettcher 538 East Ninth Street, Davis, CA 95616, (916) 753-2506, BA 86 San Francisco St Univ; MS 88 San Francisco St Univ; 88–Sp-Lang Path, InSpeech Inc

Nelson, Jodi E 407 2nd Avenue Place #10, Coralville, IA 52241, (319) 354-5617, MA 88 Univ of IA

Nelson, John Patrick 711 W Camino Real #202, P O Box 1877, Arcadia, CA 91006, (818) 574-0437, BA 72 Univ of CA - Berkeley; MA 80 CA St Univ - Los Angeles; Aud, VA Outpatient Clinic, **A**

Nelson, Joy I 229 North Russel, Denver, IA 50622, (319) 984-6072, BS 77 Univ of IA; MA 80 Univ of IA; Aud, Keystone AEA, **A**

Nelson, Mrs Joy Kiersted 8012 Hill Trail North, Lake Elmo, MN 55042, (612) 770-4750, BA 63 Univ of SD - Vermillion; MA 77 Univ of WI - River Falls; Sp/Lang Path, Maplewd No St Paul Oakdale Sch, **SLP**

Nelson, Karen D'Amico South 21 W27412 Kame Terr, Waukesha, WI 53188, (414) 549-4938, BA 83 Univ of WI - Eau Claire; OM 85 Univ of WI - River Falls; **A**

Nelson, Mrs Katherine Van Opens 1107 Russet Street, Racine, WI 53405, (414) 632-9790, BS 79 Marquette Univ; MS 80 Marquette Univ; Sp-Lang Path, Racine USD, **SLP**

Nelson, Mrs Kathryn M 25643 Gap Road, Brownsville, OR 97327, (503) 343-5861, BS 63 Univ of WI - Madison; MS 72 Univ of OR; Sp-Lang Path, Eugene Sch Dist 4J, **SLP**

Nelson, Mrs Kay E S 4047 Pine Ridge Court, Dousman, WI 53118, (414) 965-2171, BA 69 Univ of WI - Madison; MA 72 Univ of WI - Milwaukee; 80–Sp-Lang Path, Sch Dist of Kettle Moraine, **SLP**

Nelson, Mrs Kerri Rykal Telex Communications Inc, 9600 Aldrich Avenue South, Minneapolis, MN 55420, (612) 884-7430, BS 82 Univ of WI - Stevens Point; MS 84 Univ of WI - Stevens Point; Product Specialist, Telex Communication Inc, **A**

Nelson, Kimberly Wood Route 3 Box 33, Milrose, MN 56352, (612) 837-5892, **SLP**

Nelson, Kristin K 508 Minnequa #2, Pueblo, CO 81003, (719) 561-1439, BS 84 Moorhead St Univ; MA 86 Northeast MO St Univ; SLP, St Marys Corwin Hosp, **SLP**

Nelson, Dr Lauren K 4673 Greentree #D, Columbus, OH 43220, (614) 292-8207, BS 77 Northern MI Univ; MA 78 Central MI Univ; PH 84 (NS) Memphis St Univ; Asst Professor, Ohio State Univ, **SLP**

Nelson, Laurie 424 W Center #14, Bountiful, UT 84010-7015, (801) 467-0332, BS 84 UT St Univ; MS 86 Univ of UT; **A**

Nelson, Laurie Ellen 2723 N W 55th Street, Fort Lauderdale, FL 33309, (305) 735-4270, BS 84 Univ of TX - Dallas; MS 86 Univ of TX - Dallas; Aud, **A**

Nelson, Linda C P O Box 43, Harrisburg, IL 62946, BA 68 Northeastern OK St Univ; MS 71 Southern IL Univ -Carbondale; Assistant Director, Wabash Ohio Valley Sp Ed Dist, **SLP**

Nelson, Mrs Linda L 18 Underwood Drive, Lewisburg, WV 24901, (304) 645-6515, BA 70 Marshall Univ; MA 75 Marshall Univ; SLP/Aud, Greenbrier Co Bd of Ed, **SLP**

Nelson, Linda Lee 25317 1/4 Cypress, Lomita, CA 90717, (213) 517-3940, BA 80 Univ of CA - Santa Barbara; OM 83 Univ of WA; Aud, Kaiser Permanente, **A**

Nelson, Mrs Lisa L 17 Ledum Run Road, West Grove, PA 19390, (302) 998-8090, BS 77 West Chester Univ of PA; MA 80 West Chester Univ of PA; 88–Reg Dir of Therapy, Easter Seal Soc of Del Mar Inc, **SLP**

Nelson, Loetitia M 14114 Exmoor, San Antonio, TX 78217, (512) 657-5571, BS 78 Southwest TX St Univ; ME 79 Southwest TX St Univ; Resource Teacher/Sp-Lang Path, Alamo Heights ISD, **SLP**

Nelson, Dr Lois A Dept Communicative Disorders, University Of Wisconsin, 1975 Willow Drive, Madison, WI 53706, (608) 262-3951, BS 54 Univ of WI - Madison; MA 55 Western MI Univ; PH 60 (Speech) Univ of WI - Madison; Prof, U of WI-Madison, **SLP F**

Nelson, Mark I 6 Second Avenue, Warren, PA 16365, (814) 723-3930, BS 75 Syracuse Univ; MS 76 SUNY - Coll at Fredonia; Sp-Lang Path Consult, Sp and Hrng Inc, **SLP**

Nelson, Marlene Shapiro 23 Cedar Street, Eugene, OR 97402, (503) 942-8602, BS 83 Univ of OR; MS 87 Univ of WA; 87–Sp-Lang Path, Abel Ctr, **SLP**

Nelson, Mrs Mary F 115 Fairview Avenue, Painted Post, NY 14870, (607) 936-4486, BA 70 Russell Sage Coll; MS 82 Ithaca Coll; Sp-Lang Path, Corning Sch Dist, **SLP ACE**

Nelson, Mrs Maureen Quealy 6043 East 56th Street, Tulsa, OK 74135, (918) 622-5120, BS 79 OK St Univ; MS 81 CO St Univ; Aud, Eastern Oklahoma ENT Inc, **A**

Nelson, Dr Max Dept Of Speech Communication, California State Univ, Fullerton, CA 92634, (714) 773-3617, BA 41 Univ of Akron; MA 47 Univ of MI - Ann Arbor; PH 50 (NS) Univ of MI - Ann Arbor; Professor, Cal State Univ - Fullerton, **SLP A F LM**

Nelson, Mrs Michele 38682 Huntington Circle, Fremont, CA 94536, (415) 794-3728, BA 84 Humboldt St Univ; 86–Sp-Lang Path, CA Sch for the Deaf-Fremont, **SLP**

Nelson, Nancy B 1729 East Saginaw #204, Lansing, MI 48912, (517) 487-0933, BA 74 MI St Univ; MA 75 MI St Univ; Aud, Private Practice, **A**

Nelson, Dr Nickola W 225 Brush Road, Niles, MI 49120, (616) 387-8058, BA 68 Wichita St Univ; MA 69 Wichita St Univ; PH 73 (Logopedics) Wichita St Univ; Assoc Prof, Western MI Univ, **SLP F**

Nelson, Patricia E 1717 North 10th, Paducah, KY 42001, **SLP**

Nelson, Mrs Patricia M 3053 Mellow Woods Drive, North Pole, AK 99705, (907) 372-3258, BS 63 Minot St Univ; MS 69 Minot St Univ; Sp/Lang Path, Fairbanks N Star Borough Sch, **SLP**

Nelson, Mrs Patricia S 4 Cobbler's Mill Road, Sandy Hook, CT 06482, (415) 829-1780, BS 78 CA St Univ - Hayward; MA 79 Univ of the Pacific; **SLP**

Nelson, Peggy Bull 2107 Browning, Manhattan, KS 66502-1997, (913) 532-6879, BA 74 Saint Olaf Coll; MA 82 KS St Univ; Instructor, Ks State U Sp & Hrng Cen, **A**

Nelson, Penny O 106 North 3rd Street, Humboldt, IA 50548, (515) 576-7434, BS 76 Moorhead St Univ; MS 77 Moorhead St Univ; Supvr Cl Sp & Lang Serv, Arrowhead AEA, **SLP**

Nelson, R David 513 1st Avenue East, Spencer, IA 51301, (712) 262-7774, BA 62; MA 70 Univ of IA; Audiologist, Nelson Hearing Aid Service, **A**

Nelson, R Elizabeth P O Box 419, Redwood Falls, MN 56283, (507) 637-8393, BS 79 Univ of WI - River Falls; MS 80 Univ of WI - River Falls; Sp/Lang Path, Redwood Falls Sp Path Servs, **SLP**

Nelson, Rachelle Louise 965 Berryman #D, Pocatello, ID 83201, (208) 234-0120, BA 84 Humboldt St Univ; MS 86 ID St Univ; 88–Aud, Sch Dist 25

Nelson, Dr Robert G 8123 Cacus Street, Spring Valley, CA 92077, (714) 475-4411, BA 67 Univ of NE - Lincoln; MA 68 Univ of NE - Lincoln; PH 85 (NS) Columbia Pacific Univ; Sp-Lang Path, San Ysidro School District, **SLP A**

Nelson, Robert W, Jr 420 Autumn, Eugene, OR 97404, (503) 687-3496, BS 75 Univ of OR; MS 77 ID St Univ; SLP, Eugene Public Schools, **SLP ACE**

Nelson, Roberta Lynn 925 Lincoln Street, Superior, WI 54880, (218) 726-5584, BA 81 Univ of WI - Eau Claire; MS 82 Univ of WI - Eau Claire; 86–Therapy Patient Care Coord, St Luke's Hosp, **SLP**

Nelson, Mrs Sally M Olmos Speech & Language Clinic, 359 East Hildebrand, San Antonio, TX 78212, (512) 828-5583, BS 68 Kent St Univ; MA 79 Univ of CT; Sp-Lang Path, Olmos Sp Lang & Lrng Clinic, **SLP**

Nelson, Sharon S 4159 Wedgmont Circle South, Fort Worth, TX 76133, (817) 370-0729, BA 71 LA St Univ - Baton Rouge; MA 77 LA St Univ - Baton Rouge; **SLP**

Nelson, Sharon Woodcock P O Box 12575, St Louis, MO 63141-0075, **SLP**

Nelson, Sigfred A Ecorse Public Schools, 27385 West Outer Drive, Ecorse, MI 48229, (313) 382-1201, BA 50 Wayne St Univ; MA 55 Wayne St Univ; 53–Sp-Lang Path, Ecorse Public Schools, **SLP**

Nelson, Mrs Stephanie Broom Clinical Audiologist, 318 North Madison, Litchfield, IL 62056, (217) 324-2433, BA 80 Bradley Univ; MS 83 Bradley Univ; Aud, Private Practice, **A**

Nelson, Susan B P O Box 1531, Cumberland, MD 21501, (301) 777-2204, BA 66 Univ of MD - College Park; ME 67 PA St Univ - Univ Park; SLP, Brandenburg Cen, **SLP**

Nelson, Susan H 1958 N Sheffield, Chicago, IL 60614, (312) 633-5737, BA 68 Denison Univ; MA 73 Northwestern Univ; Sp/Lang Path, Cook Co Hosp, **SLP**

Nelson, T Russell P O Box 414, Bay Pines, FL 33504, (813) 398-9395, BA 68 Central WA Univ; ME 70 PA St Univ - Univ Park; PH 79 (NS) Case Western Reserve Univ; Sp-Lang Path, VA Med Cen-Bay Pines, **SLP**

Nelson, Mrs Tammie Lou 3095 Disney Drive, Idaho Falls, ID 83404, (208) 524-1651, MA 84 Univ of Northern CO; Director Audiological Services, Bonneville School District 93, **A**

Nelson, William H 18 Underwood Drive, Lewisburg, WV 24901, (304) 647-7515, BA 68 West Liberty St Coll; MA 75 Marshall Univ; Rehab Couns Deaf, WV Div Voctnl Rehab, **SLP**

Nelson, William R U S A Aeromed Research Lab, Box 577, Fort Rucker, AL 36362, (205) 255-6823, BS 66 UT St Univ; MS 72 UT St Univ; Audiologist, US Army Aeromed Research Lab, **A**

Nelson-Barber, Dr Sharon S 303 Edgewood Road, Redwood City, CA 94062, (415) 725-1228, BA 74 Mount Holyoke Coll; MS 77 Univ of VT; ED 85 (Human Development) Harvard Univ; 87–Research Associate, Stanford University, **SLP**

Nelson-Barlow, Nancy L Boys Town National Institute, 555 North 30th Street, Omaha, NE 68131, BS 79 Bowling Green St Univ; MS 82 Univ of WI - Madison; Aud, Boys Town National Institute, **A**

Nelson-Drake, Janice K 8402 Hartford Avenue, Silver Spring, MD 20910, (303) 320-6137, BA 71 Case Western Reserve Univ; MA 76 CA St Univ - Los Angeles; Audiologist, Kaiser Permanente, **A**

Nelson-Lehman, Mrs Susan L 38688 North Cedar Avenue, Zion, IL 60099-3408, (312) 336-1894, BA 78 Univ of WA; MA 80 Univ of WA; Sp-Lang Path, Zion Elem Sch, **SLP**

Nelson-Picrenpaugh, Mrs Susan Jane 262 Alumwood Drive, Westerville, OH 43081, (614) 891-2956, BA 76 Univ of Akron; ME 81 Old Dominion Univ; Sp-Lang Path, Affiliated Audiology Sp Path, **SLP**

Nemcik, Lawrence E Route 1, St Johns, MI 48879, **SLP**

Nemec, Elizabeth Kathryn 31 Pleasant Avenue, Bergenfield, NJ 07621-3125, (201) 596-3931, BA 83 Montclair St Coll; MS 85 Columbia Univ Teachers Coll; **A**

Nemec, Richard R Speech Pathology & Audiology, California State Univ, California, PA 15419, (412) 938-4176, BS 65 CA Univ of PA; MS 67 WV Univ; Assoc Prof, CA U of Pa, **SLP**

Nemergut, Joy C 51 Grand Street, Reading, MA 01867, (617) 944-8178, BA 72 Univ of CT; MS 73 Southern CT St Univ; Sp-Lang Path, Wakefield Pub Schs, **SLP**

Nemeth, George 245 East 19th Street, New York, NY 10003, (212) 777-4368, BA 54 Long Island U - Brooklyn Ctr; MA 60 CUNY - Brooklyn Coll; 88–Sp-Lang Path, Baruch College

Nemetz, Tobyann 415 Hawthorne Avenue, Yonkers, NY 10705, (914) 963-8834, BA 65 Univ of WA; MA 71 NY Univ; Sp-Lang Path, Spec Commun Services, **SLP**

Nemky, Martha T 151 Fennel, San Antonio, TX 78213, (512) 680-2923, BA 75 TX Lutheran Coll; MA 78 Univ of TX - Austin; 82–Sp-Lang Path, Northside ISD, **SLP ACE**

Nemmer, Mrs Ruthe L 85 Woodmere Drive, Tonawanda, NY 14150, **SLP**

Nens, Mrs Diane D 4225 Smoke Rise Drive, Stow, OH 44224, (216) 492-2844, BS 85 Clarion Univ of PA; MA 87 Univ of Akron; **A**

Nepo, Mrs Hellaine Drucker 11817 Rosalinda Drive, Potomac, MD 20854, (301) 762-0632, BA 58 CUNY - Brooklyn Coll; MA 61 CUNY - Brooklyn Coll; OM 64 Boston Univ; Sp-Lang Path, Montgy Co Pub Sch, **SLP**

Nepote, Mrs Karen A 11 Timber Ridge Court, Sayville, NY 11782, (516) 589-5100, BA 73 Hofstra Univ; MA 78 Hofstra Univ; Sp-Lang Path, Sayville Pub Sch, **SLP**

Nerbonne, Dr G Patrick Dept Communication Disorders, Univ Of Massachusetts, Arnold House, Amherst, MA 01003, (413) 545-0131, BS 59 Central MI Univ; MA 63 MI St Univ; PH 67 (NS) MI St Univ; Assoc Prof, U of MA, **SLP F**

Nerbonne, Dr Michael A Dept Communication Disorders, Central Michigan Univ, Mount Pleasant, MI 48859, (517) 774-3904, BA 66 MI St Univ; MA 67 MI St Univ; PH 70 (Aud) MI St Univ; Dir Aud, Central MI U, **A F**

Neri, Lorraine M 46 Stanavage Road, Colchester, CT 06415, (203) 282-3364, MA 84 Western MI Univ; Sp-Lang Path, E Hartford Bd of Educ, **SLP**

Nericcio, Mary Anne 2509 Toulouse, Austin, TX 78748, (512) 280-4321, BS 74 Univ of TX - Austin; MA 80 Univ of TX - Austin; Sp-Lang Path, Austin ISD, **SLP**

Nering, Gayle N 3100 14th Street S W #18, Minot, ND 58701, BS 76 Mayville St Coll; MS 86 Minot St Univ; 86–Sp-Lang Path, Souris Valley Spec Svcs, **SLP**

Nerison, Anne H 1006 Southeast 4th Avenue, Rochester, MN 55904, (612) 332-4337, BA 79 Univ of Northern IA; MA 80 Univ of Northern IA; MA 85 Univ of Northern IA; 86–Aud, Telex Communications, **SLP A**

Nerone, Mrs Michelle M 6290 Hamm Road, Lockport, NY 14094, (716) 631-4885, BS 69 SUNY - Coll at Buffalo; MS 73 SUNY - Coll at Buffalo; SLP, Williamsville Central Schools, **SLP ACE**

Nesbeda, Christina 390 Commercial Street, Braintree, MA 02184, (617) 848-5353, BS 77 Univ of MA - Amherst; MA 79 Univ of CT; 82–Sp-Lang Path, Braintree Hosp, **SLP**

Nesbit, Linda C 336 Bay Park Drive, Brandon, MS 39042, **SLP**

Nesdill, Mrs Judith Michele 54 Rope Ferry Road #141, Waterford, CT 06385, (203) 579-6906, **SLP**

Nesheim, Carolyn C 302 South Conrey, Knoxville, IA 50138, (515) 842-7197, BS 76 Northern St Coll; MS 78 Univ of WY; 88–Aud, Audiological Services Inc, **A**

Ness, Amber Cordahl 4631 South Park Drive, Savage, MN 55378, (612) 887-7246, BS 80 Moorhead St Univ; MA 81 Univ of MN - Duluth; Sp-Lang Path, Burnsville Sch, **SLP**

Ness, Joe A Box 1818, Bismarck, ND 58501, (701) 222-5396, BS 74 ND St Univ; MS 75 Minot St Univ; Aud, Quain & Ramstad Cl, **A**

Ness, Michanne Alexis 9-402 Royal Palm Way, Boca Raton, FL 33432, (407) 482-7877, MS 85 Univ of South FL; Reg Clin Coor, Family Hrng Cntrs, **A**

Ness, Vicki Lynn 3700 Bobwhite Lane, Rolling Meadows, IL 60008, (312) 394-9043, BA 83 Elmhurst Coll; MA 85 Univ of IL - Urbana; 88–Sp-Lang Path, Kildeer Countryside Sch Dist #96, **SLP**

Nessel, Mrs Jo Ann M 3 Cora Lane, Wilton, CT 06897, (203) 544-8861, BA 76 Univ of CT; MA 78 Univ of CT; Sp-Lang Path, Wilton Pub Sch, **SLP**

Nesseth, Virginia Marie Box 719, Hatch, NM 87937, (505) 267-4364, BA 75; MA 76; ES 78; 88–Sp-Lang Path, Hatch Valley Municipal Schs, **SLP ACE**

Nester, Mrs Ann A Jackson County Schools, Ripley, WV 25271, (304) 372-9231, BS 75 WV Univ; MS 76 WV Univ; Sp-Lang Path, Jackson Co Bd of Ed, **SLP**

Nestler-Faccini, Mrs Heidi Marie 8 Pauchogue Avenue, East Islip, NY 11730, (516) 581-5289, BA 83 SUNY - Coll at Plattsburgh; MA 86 Long Island U - CW Post Ctr; 87–Sp-Lang Path, BOCES III of Suffolk Co, **SLP**

Nestor, Andrea Faye 3027 Carriage Trail, Jonesboro, GA 30236-6835, (404) 968-0235, BS 78 Univ of WI - Whitewater; ME 81 GA St Univ; Sp-Lang Path, Clayton Co Bd of Ed, **SLP**

Netherland, Sherry 464 North Hobart Boulevard #2, Los Angeles, CA 90004, (213) 664-1896, MA 77 SUNY - Center at Buffalo; Aud, Centinela Hosp Med Ctr, **A**

Netsell, Ronald Boys Town Institute, 555 North 30th Street, Omaha, NE 68131, (402) 498-6753, BA 60 Linfield Coll; MA 65 Univ of IA; PH 69 (NS) Univ of IA; Staff Scientist, Boys Town, **SLP**

Netterville, Nancy L S 8770 Bienville, Beaumont, TX 77706, (409) 296-2980, BS 75 Lamar Univ; MS 77 Lamar Univ; Sp-Lang Path, East Chambers ISD, **SLP**

Nettling-Snyder, Mrs Peggy Eileen R-3410 Old Berwick Road, Bloomsburg, PA 17815, (717) 271-6379, BS 84 Bloomsburg Univ of PA; MS 85 Bloomsburg Univ of PA; Sp-Lang Path, Geisinger Med Ctr, **SLP**

Neu, Mrs Barbara J 4227 Palmyra, New Orleans, LA 70119, (509) 488-7650, BS 78 LA St Univ - Baton Rouge; OM 80 LA St Univ - N O Medical Ctr; Sp-Lnag Path, West Jefferson Gen Hosp, **SLP**

Neu, Mrs Jean H 4225 91st N E, Bellevue, WA 98004, (206) 455-5221, BA 72 Univ of WA; MS 76 Univ of UT; **SLP**

Neu, Mrs Patricia B 18 Kensington Terrace, Maplewood, NJ 07040, (201) 376-3600, BS 55 Newark St Coll; MA 61 Newark St Coll; **SLP**

Neubauer, Christine A 4841 35th Street, San Diego, CA 92116, (619) 281-5167, MS 88 Univ of Redlands; 88–Sp-Lang Path, Childrens Hosp & Health Ctr

Neuburger, Marilyn F Box 124-A, Seven Valleys, PA 17360, (717) 428-3490, BS 75 SUNY - Coll at Geneseo; MS 77 Southern IL Univ -Carbondale; Sp-Lang Path, Private Practice, **SLP**

Neuburger, Sandra Ileen P 3015 N E 17th Street, Portland, OR 97212, (503) 220-8262, MS 83 Portland St Univ; BS 78 Portland St Univ; Sp-Lang Path, Portland VA Med Cen, **SLP ACE**

Neuder, Cynthia I 42 Woodedge Avenue #5, Edison, NJ 08817, BA 69 CUNY - Brooklyn Coll; ME 70 PA St Univ - Univ Park; Tchr, Hrng Ed Serv/NYC Bd of Ed, **SLP**

Neufeld, Rebecca A 2011 11th Street, Reedley, CA 93654, (209) 638-3124, BA 75 Biola Univ; MA 79 Wichita St Univ; Sp-Lang Path, Irwin Lehroff and Associates, **SLP**

Neufer, Mrs Susan L 1429 Jackson, Selma, CA 93662, (209) 896-7135, BA 78 Univ of OR; MA 79 Univ of OR; Sp-Lang Path, Fowler Unified Schl Dist, **SLP**

Neugebauer, Freda W Rural Delivery 2, West Alexander, PA 15376, MS; **SLP LM**

Neuhart, Julee M 1526 East Mc Graw, Seattle, WA 98112, (206) 281-6943, BA 69 Western WA Univ; OM 75 Univ of WA; Sp-Lang Path, Seattle Sch Dist, **SLP**

Neuhaus, Anne Rachel 911 Willowbrook Road, Staten Island, NY 10314, BS 76 Towson St Univ; MA 78 Hofstra Univ; Sp-Lang Path, Private Practice, **SLP**

Neuman, Dr Arlene C 334 Barr Avenue, Teaneck, NJ 07666, (201) 692-1456, BS 72 Univ of Bridgeport; MA 75 CUNY - Hunter Coll; PH 82 (Aud Hrng Science) CUNY - Grad Sch & Univ Cntr; 82–Research Assoc, Grad Sch CUNY, **A**

Neuman, Faye J 25-03 Fairlawn Avenue, Fair Lawn, NJ 07410, (201) 796-8428, BA 74 CUNY - Hunter Coll; MA 76 CUNY - City College; Sp-Lang Path, Yorktown Central Schools, **SLP**

Neuman, Nilda M Calle Pensamientos #39, Colonia Ciudad Jardin, Mexico DF, Mexico, BS 69 Univ of PR - Rio Piedras; MS 71 Univ of PR - San Juan; Aud, Hrng & Sp Cen, **A**

Neumann, Brenda T 23081 Bittersweet Lane, Southfield, MI 48034, (313) 245-3678, BS 61 Wayne St Univ; MA 81 Wayne St Univ; SLP, Detroit Publ Schs, **SLP**

Neumann, Grace Ellen 1467 West Key Parkway Apartment 5C, Frederick, MD 21701, (301) 662-5924, BA 84 Loyola Coll; MS 85 Loyola Coll; Sp-Lang Path, Frederick County Bd of Educ, **SLP**

Neumann, Mrs Jacqueline Denise P O Box 347, Rugby, ND 58368, (701) 776-2108, BS 77 Minot St Univ; MS 83 Minot St Univ; **SLP**

Neumann, Marie Olin P O Box 121, Westhope, ND 58793, (701) 228-3743, BS 64 Minot St Univ; MA 82 Minot St Univ; Sp-Lang Path, Peace Garden Multi-Dist Coop, **SLP**

Neumann, Mrs Suzanne Marie 2414 Kohler Memorial Drive, Sheboygan, WI 53081, (414) 457-4461, BS 76 Univ of WI - Stevens Point; MS 77 Univ of WI - Stevens Point; Aud, Sheboygan Clinic, **A**

Neumeier, Marianne 1125 6th Street #2, Santa Monica, CA 90403, BA 79 CA St Univ - Northridge; MA 81 CA St Univ - Northridge; Sp-Lang Path, Los Angeles USD, **SLP**

Neumeyer, Jerry W P O Box 171, State University, AR 72467, (501) 236-6439, BS 78 AR St Univ; MS 79 AR St Univ; SLP, Greene Co Tech Sch Dist, **SLP**

Neuner, Mrs Sharon A 15409 Cousteau Drive, Florissant, MO 63034, (314) 838-3961, BS 79 Saint Louis Univ; MA 80 Saint Louis Univ; 80–Sp/Lang Path, St Louis Co Spec Sch Dist, **SLP**

Neupert, Catherine Cangelosi 2048 Lafitte Drive, La Place, LA 70068, (504) 652-9250, BA 82 Southeastern LA Univ; OM 85 LA St Univ - N O Medical Ctr; **SLP**

Neuroth-Gimbrone, Cindy 5 Maple Terrace, Cold Spring, NY 10516, (914) 949-7310, BS 81 SUNY - Coll at Fredonia; MS 87 Syracuse Univ; 86–Sp-Lang Path, New York Sch for the Deaf, **SLP**

Neuschotz, Carmen Kowalski 145 Elmira Loop #3-B, Brooklyn, NY 11239, (718) 642-3124, BA 71 CUNY - Hunter Coll; MA 73 NY Univ; 83–Sp-Lang Path, NYC Bd of Educ PS 158, **SLP ACE**

Neuss, Deirdre 168 Goulburn Avenue, Ottawa, ON, Canada K1N 8E2, (613) 737-2378, BA 71 McGill Univ - Quebec; MA 77 Case Western Reserve Univ; 87–Sp-Lang Path, Ottawa Separate Sch Bd, **SLP A**

Neustadt, Gail K 516 Harrogate Road, Pittsburgh, PA 15241, (412) 854-5368, BA 66 Case Western Reserve Univ; MA 67 Univ of MI - Ann Arbor; Sp-Lang Path, Negley House, **SLP**

Neuvirth, Debra Lynn 32450 Olde Franklin Drive, Farmington Hills, MI 48018, (313) 851-1731, BA 84 Univ of MI - Ann Arbor; MA 86 Wayne St Univ; **SLP**

Neuwald, Kathleen Marie 31430 Sherwood Road, Fort Bragg, CA 95437, (707) 961-2875, BA 72 Humboldt St Univ; MA 74 Humboldt St Univ; 86–Coord of Spec Educ, Fort Bragg USD, **SLP**

Nevala, Betty Hill 3811 Knollwood Drive, Anniston, AL 36201, (919) 642-5168, BA 74 Auburn Univ - Auburn; MS 75 Vanderbilt Univ; Aud, Anniston Ear Nose & Throat PC, **A**

Nevdahl, Martin Ted 8301 161st Avenue NE Suite 304, Redmond, WA 98105, (206) 882-4347, BS 82 Univ of WA; MS 84 Univ of WA; Sp-Lang Path, Evergreen Speech & Hearing, **SLP**

Nevers, Maxine Lorraine 765 Warburton Avenue, Yonkers, NY 10701, (212) 939-8700, MS 82 Columbia Univ Teachers Coll; ED 84 (NS) Columbia Univ Teachers Coll; **A**

Neves, Mrs Gail M 14 Doneraile Street, London, England SW6 6EN, BS 69 Ithaca Coll; MA 71 Columbia Univ Teachers Coll; **SLP**

Neville, Mrs Elizabeth 2700 Jerusalem Road, Kingsville, MD 21087, (301) 256-6218, BS 74 Towson St Univ; MS 76 Towson St Univ; Sp-Lang Path, Balt Co Bd of Ed, **SLP**

Neville, Mrs Katherine McGoldrick 5521 N 23rd Street, Arlington, VA 22205, (703) 237-9734, **SLP**

Neville, Mrs Lynn Bertino 119 John Street, Dwight, IL 60420, (815) 467-2900, BA 73 Coll of Saint Francis; ME 81 Northern IL Univ - De Kalb; MS 76 Eastern IL Univ; 85–Coord-Comm Dev Prog, Resa, **SLP**

Neville, Margaret M 109 Westminster Place, Flemington, NJ 08822, (201) 879-5022, BA 74 Rutger's St Univ - Douglas Coll; MA 76 Montclair St Coll; Comm Prog Spec, St of NJ-Div Ment Ret, **SLP**

Nevin, Mrs Barbara Anne 3610 Armstrong Avenue, Dallas, TX 75205, (214) 522-2960, BA 74 KS St Univ; MS 75 Wichita St Univ; 86–Sp-Lang Path, Dean Learning Ctr, **SLP**

Nevin, Nancy Patricia 11 Stonemark Court #9, Owings Mills, MD 21117, (301) 356-5380, BA 85 Loyola Coll; MS 86 Loyola Coll; **SLP**

Nevins, Mrs Arniel F 460 Willow Street, West Barnstable, MA 02668, (617) 945-0589, BA 63 Univ of MA - Amherst; MA 64 Univ of NE - Omaha; Sp-Lang Path, Chatham Pub Sch, **SLP**

Nevitt, Amanda L 5000 Woodview Avenue, Austin, TX 78756-2531, (512) 929-1356, BS 75 Univ of TX - Austin; MA 79 Univ of TX - Austin; 87–Aud, Educ Svc Ctr Region XIII, **A**

Nevitt, Susan G 3009 Driscoll Drive, San Diego, CA 92117, MA; **SLP**

Nevlud, Gail New 7704 Chimney Corners, Austin, TX 78731, (512) 444-4835, BS 79 Univ of TX - Austin; MA 81 Univ of Houston - Univ Park; Sp-Lang Path, Health Care Rehab Ctr, **SLP ACE**

New, Janie Cirlot 103 City Park Circle, Hattiesburg, MS 39401, (601) 266-5216, SLP, Univ of S MS, **SLP**

Newbauer, Mrs Alisa J 6024 S W 146th Court, Miami, FL 33183, (305) 374-4606, MS 71 Univ of South FL; SLP, Private Practice, **SLP**

Newberg, Michael R Country Life Farm, P O Box 107, Bel Air, MD 21014, (301) 879-1952, **SLP**

Newberg, Nanette L 5902 South 1560 East, Salt Lake City, UT 84121, (801) 521-1680, BA 69 Chadron St Coll; MS 81 Univ of UT; Aud, Primary Children's Med Cen, **A**

Newberger, Jeanne Ellen 150 So Ocean Avenue #2-M, Freeport, NY 11520, (516) 826-6200, BA 51 Adelphi Univ; MS 55 SUNY - Coll at New Paltz; MS 82 Adelphi Univ; **SLP**

Newberry, Dr George W 8758 Sturdy Drive, Crestwood, MO 63126, (314) 658-2939, BA 56 Univ of Denver; MA 58 Univ of Denver; PH 72 (NS) Saint Louis Univ; Associate Professor Comm Dis, St Louis University, **SLP**

Newbery, Mrs Rosemary Motley 3819 Northumberland Drive, Louisville, KY 40223, (502) 896-4155, BA 80 Catawba Coll; MA 82 Univ of TN - Knoxville; Aud, Louisville Hearing Ctr, **A**

Newburger, Dr Doris S Timber Trail, Rye, NY 10580, (914) 967-4011, BS 46 NY Univ; MA 49 NY Univ; PH 67 (NS) NY Univ; Prof Sp Commun, Borough of Manhattan Comm Coll, **SLP**

Newby, Mrs Bonita Perkins 8932 Lincolnwood, Evanston, IL 60203, (312) 492-7854, BA 78 Univ of NC - Chapel Hill; MS 81 Southern CT St Univ; 87–Sp/Lang Path, Sch Dist 65, **SLP**

Newby, Dr Hayes A 1780 Deborah Drive #12, Punta Gorda, FL 33950, (813) 639-4330, BA 35 OH Wesleyan Univ; MA 39 Univ of IA; PH 47 (Aud & Sp Path) Univ of IA; **SLP A F H LM**

Newby, Mrs Kathleen K 312 Montrose Avenue, Syracuse, NY 13219, (315) 473-5050, BS 78 SUNY - Coll at Geneseo; MS 80 Ithaca Coll; Sp-Lang Path, St Camillus Health & Rehab Ctr, **SLP**

Newcom, Mrs Mary Ann P O Box 398, Aspon, WY 83110, (701) 225-6736, BS 76 ID St Univ; MS 77 ID St Univ; Sp-Lang Path, Lincoln Uinta Chld Dev Assoc, **SLP**

Newcom, Robert D 16 Blackberry Lane, Herrin, IL 62948, (618) 993-3198, BS 67 Southern IL Univ -Carbondale; MS 73 Southern IL Univ -Carbondale; Aud, Sn IL Ed Serv Cen, **A**

Newcomb, Mrs Kathy A 1221 W Santa Cruz, San Pedro, CA 90732, (213) 519-8172, BA 80 Humboldt St Univ; MA 82 Univ of CA - Santa Barbara; 87–Aud, Private Practice, **A**

Newcomb, Sandra S 187 Goodhue, Akron, OH 44313, (216) 867-4137, BA 78 Univ of Akron; MA 82 Univ of Akron; Aud, Hay I Norin Assoc, **A**

Newcombe, Lorna H P O Box 6837, Portland, OR 97228-6837, **SLP**

Newcomer, Mrs Jill Lyerla 1468 Cheyenne Court, Stone Mountain, GA 30087, (404) 921-3809, ME 84 Univ of GA; Sp-Lang Path, DeKalb County Schs, **SLP**

Newcomer, Mrs Juleen S 1222 Madison Street, Rochester, IN 46975, (219) 223-4837, BS 76 Purdue Univ - West Lafayette; MA 78 Western MI Univ; 87–Sp-Lang Path, Rochester Community Schs, **SLP**

Newell, Mrs Kathleen Pierson 8218 Columbia Drive, Rowlett, TX 75088, (214) 226-9465, BA 78 Univ of WI - Eau Claire; MA 80 Northern MI Univ; Sp-Lang Path, Plano ISD, **SLP**

Newell, Mrs Mary Jo Shapland R R #1 Box 200, Dodge City, KS 67801, (316) 227-8002, BA 84 Fort Hays St Univ; MS 85 Fort Hays St Univ; 85–Sp-Lang Path, SW KS Area Coop #613, **SLP**

Newell, Sharon Lynn 513 Bayside Road, Bellingham, WA 98225, (206) 734-9922, MA 88 Western WA Univ; 88–Sp-Lang Path, Educ Service Dist 189

Newett, Norma J 7609 White Post Way, Louisville, KY 40220, (502) 636-7188, BA 70 Univ of KY; ME 76 Univ of Louisville; Aud/Sp-Lang Path, Private Practice, **SLP A**

Newhart, Mrs Patricia Hassan 811 Solana Drive, Lafayette, CA 94549, (415) 877-8801, MA 82 Univ of CA - Santa Barbara; Sp-Lang Path, S San Francisco USD, **SLP**

Newhoff, Dr Marilyn Hamiter Professional Bldg, Suite #305, 801 Gaines Avenue, Gadsden, AL 35903, (205) 543-4651, BA 66 Univ of AL- Tuscaloosa; MA 70 Univ of AL- Tuscaloosa; PH 78 (NS) Memphis St Univ; Sp-Lang Path, Sp-Lang Path Assoc, **SLP**

Newhouse, Susan J Plantation Oaks, 2225 Ashley River Rd #233, Charleston, SC 29414, (803) 889-6561, BS 85 Ball St Univ; MA 86 Ball St Univ; 86–Sp-Lang Path, Charleston County PS, **SLP**

Newirth, Jill Ann 301 Conestoga Way #A5, Norristown, PA 19403, (215) 277-0660, Dept Chair SLP, Pathway School, **SLP**

Newkirk, Mrs Alice B W Route 1, Mount Carmel, IL 62863, (618) 262-4587, OB 41 Eastern IL Univ; MA 48 Univ of IL - Urbana; **SLP LM**

Newkirk, Mrs Carol Stelting 16213 West 136th, Olathe, KS 66062, (314) 991-5259, BS 80 Univ of KS; MA 83 Univ of KS; **SLP**

Newland, Mrs Donna L M 624 Rosenberg, Galveston, TX 77550, (409) 763-0749, BS 78 Univ of TX - Austin; MA 80 Univ of Houston - Univ Park; Sp-Lang Path, Galveston Co Comm & Learing Svcs, **SLP**

Newland, Stephanie Ann 112 Rue Fontaine, Decatur, GA 30038, (404) 981-9710, BA 78 Univ of CO - Boulder; MS 82 Washington Univ; 88–Aud, Douglas County Schs, **A**

Newlin, Rhonda T 3104 Rockaway Road, Atlanta, GA 30341, (404) 493-6393, BA 71 Columbia Coll; OM 76 Univ of SC - Columbia; **SLP**

Newman, Ann 36 Hurricane Street, Marina Del Rey, CA 90292, **SLP**

Newman, Ann Birns Acoustic Hearing Services, 57 West 57th Street, Suite 1204, New York, NY 10019, (212) 421-0613, BA 67 CUNY - Queens Coll; MA 76 CUNY - Queens Coll; Owner/Aud, Acoustic Hrng Sers, **A ACE**

Newman, Barbara 2131 Hollywood Boulevard, Suite 204, Hollywood, FL 33020, (305) 922-TALK, BA 70 Temple Univ; MA 71 Temple Univ; Sp-Lang Path, Sp Path Inc, **SLP**

Newman, Mrs Barbara K 9 Courter Avenue, Maplewood, NJ 07040, (201) 434-7855, BA 61 Temple Univ; MA 63 Temple Univ; Sp-Lang Path, Hudson Unit Assoc Ret Citizens, **SLP**

Newman, Mrs Cindy Karesky 860 N W 86th Avenue, Apartment 607, Plantation, FL 33324, (305) 476-9438, BA 83 Univ of FL; ME 85 Univ of FL; SLP, **SLP**

Newman, Connie Meyer 2113 Pine Needle Dr West, Mobile, AL 36609, (205) 661-6760, BS 74 Northwestern Univ; MS 75 Vanderbilt Univ; **SLP**

Newman, Mrs Cora Sandra 178 Rolling Hills Green, Staten Island, NY 10312, (718) 317-8249, BA 71 CUNY - Brooklyn Coll; MS 76 CUNY - Brooklyn Coll; MS 80 CUNY - Brooklyn Coll; 79–Sp-Lang Path, Citywide Speech Unit NYC Bd of Educ, **SLP**

Newman, Dr Craig W Audiology/Otolaryngology, Henry Ford Hospital, 2799 West Grand Blvd, Detroit, MI 48202, (313) 876-3159, BS 75 Bowling Green St Univ; MA 77 Bowling Green St Univ; PH 82 (NS) Case Western Reserve Univ; 88–Aud, Henry Ford Hosp, **A**

Newman, Dr Denis G Department Of Speech & Hearing, University Of Queensland, 6 Rock Street, St Lucia, Brisbane, Queensland, Australia Q1 4067, BS 65 Univ of OR; MS 66 Univ of OR; PH 81 (Sp Path Child Health) Univ of Queensland - Australi; 78–Sp-Lang Path, Univ of Queensland, **SLP**

Newman, Diana 56 Frances Boulevard, Holtsville, NY 11742, (516) 736-4953, BA 79 Long Island U - CW Post Ctr; MA 80 Long Island U - CW Post Ctr; Sp-Lang Path, Private Practice, **SLP**

Newman, Mrs Diana B 231 East Opal Drive, Glastonbury, CT 06033-1455, (203) 659-9661, BA 73 CUNY - Lehman Coll; MS 74 SUNY - Center at Albany; 84–Sp-Lang Path, Consolidated Sch Dist of New Britain, **SLP**

Newman, Mrs Diane J 15 Chin Hill Road, Westerly, RI 02891, (401) 397-3771, BS 74 Univ of RI; MS 77 Univ of RI; 79–Sp/Lang Path, Exter-W Greenwich Sch Dept, **SLP**

Newman, Donald D 708 S E 6th Street, Forest Lake, MN 55025, (612) 623-5288, BS 62 Eastern Montana Coll; MS 69 Saint Cloud St Univ; 66–Hrng/Vision Consult, Minnesota Dept Hlth, **SLP**

Newman, Mrs Gail D 9504 Sea Turtle Drive, Plantation, FL 33324, (305) 472-0411, BA 72 Temple Univ-Tyler Sch of Art; MA 74 Temple Univ-Tyler Sch of Art; Sp/Lang Path, Pembroke Pines Gen Hosp, **SLP**

Newman, Mrs Geraldine Gerson 411 Darlington Road N E, Warren, OH 44484, (216) 856-4645, BA 67 Univ of Pittsburgh - Pittsburgh; MA 68 Case Western Reserve Univ; **SLP**

Newman, Gloria Ann 700 El Paseo, Denton, TX 76205-8318, **SLP**

Newman, Mrs Jill Hess 4017 St Germaine Court, Louisville, KY 40207, (502) 896-0586, **SLP**

Newman, Joanne Jacobs 1695 Lake Cook Road #233, Highland Park, IL 60035, (312) 831-4163, BA 83 Tulane Univ; MA 85 Northwestern Univ; Sp-Lang Path, Skokie School District 72, **SLP**

Newman, Mrs Jody Vanderdonc P O Box 12, Siasconset, MA 02564, (617) 228-3671, BS 82 Kent St Univ; MA 82 Kent St Univ; **SLP**

Newman, Mrs Judith C 18 Overlook Drive, Chelmsford, MA 01824, (617) 256-4363, BS 66 NY Univ; MA 68 NY Univ; Sp/Lang Path, Lowell Gen Hosp, **SLP**

Newman, Mrs Judith H 37 Twin Wells Court, Middletown, NY 10940, (914) 343-0791, BS 69 Northwestern Univ; MA 72 NY Univ; Dev Disabilities Prog Spec, Letchworth Village Dev Cen, **SLP**

Newman, Mrs Kristen Elizabeth 836 Bancroft Road, Walnut Creek, CA 94598, (415) 945-7605, BA 85 Univ of the Pacific; MA 86 Univ of the Pacific; 87–Sp-Lang Path, Veronica Harris Sp Lang Path, **SLP**

Newman, Leslie Suzanne 5000 Western Avenue #1708, Knoxville, TN 37921, (615) 971-1349, SLP, Fort Sanders Reg Med Ctr, **SLP**

Newman, Dr Linda Lee Univ Of Wisconsin Milwaukee, Dept Of Sp Path & Audio, 845 Enderis Hall, Milwaukee, WI 53201, (414) 229-6398, BS 81 Univ of WI - River Falls; MS 82 Univ of WI - River Falls; PH 86 (Sp Path and Aud) Univ of IA; 87–Asst Prof, Univ of Wisconsin-Milwaukee, **SLP**

Newman, Mrs Linda Vaughan 816 West Olive Avenue, Monrovia, CA 91016, (213) 483-9930, BA 82 Univ of Northern CO; MA 85 Univ of Northern CO; 86–Aud, Otologic Med Grp, **A**

Newman, Lisa A 18 Powell Street, West Roxbury, MA 02132, (617) 353-5640, BS 73 Northwestern Univ; MA 74 Northwestern Univ; Sp-Lang Path, Mass General Hospital, **SLP ACE**

Newman, M Jeanne 848B Cardinal Creek Blvd, Norman, OK 73072, (405) 271-7505, BS 63 Bradley Univ; MA 67 Bradley Univ; Sp-Lang Path, Dept of Human Serv, **SLP**

Newman, Mary Katherine 12375 Abrams Road #826, Dallas, TX 75243, (214) 385-6445, BS 86 TX Tech Univ; MS 88 TX Tech Univ

Newman, Dr Parley W Brigham Young University, 328 MCKB, Provo, UT 84602, (801) 378-4932, BS 50 UT St Univ; MS 51 UT St Univ; PH 54 (NS) Univ of IA; Dept Chair, Brigham Young U, **SLP F**

Newman, Peggy H 24 Cottonwood Drive, Commack, NY 11725, (516) 271-3931, BA 71 SUNY - Coll at Buffalo; MA 73 NY Univ; Sp-Lnag Path, Offi of Ment Ret & Dev Disabl, **SLP**

Newman, Dr Ruth Ann 205 North Pine, Vermillion, SD 57069, (605) 677-5474, OB 76 OK City Univ; MS 78 Univ of OK Medical Center; PH 84 (NS) Univ of OK Medical Center; Asst Prof, Univ of South Dakota, **SLP ACE**

Newman, Sandra G 2905 North East 59 Terrace, Kansas City, MO 64119, (816) 455-1818, SLP, Private Practice, **SLP**

Newman, Sandra Lee 5173 Canoga Street #7, Montclair, CA 91763, (714) 624-3663, BA 81 CA St Univ - Fullerton; MA 84 CA St Univ - Los Angeles; SLP, Sandra L Newman, **SLP**

Newman, Mrs Sheree L RR5 Frost MH #41, Carbondale, IL 62901, (618) 457-5916, MS 88 Southern IL Univ -Carbondale

Newman, Mrs Susan Howe Monroe County Boces #1, 41 Oconnor Road, Fairport, NY 14450, (716) 377-4660, MA 85 OH Univ - Athens; Aud, Monroe County BOCES #1, **A**

Newman, Suzanne M 334 Evanston Drive, East Windsor, NJ 08520-5310, (609) 426-1033, BA 83 Rutger's St Univ - Douglas Coll; MS 87 Rutgers St Univ -N Brunswick; 88–Sp-Lang Path, Mercer Co Spec Svcs Sch Dist, **SLP**

Newman, Valerie Lynne 113 Gilmer Street #1, Bluefield, WV 24701, (304) 327-5262, BS 82 Howard Univ; MS 85 Howard Univ; **A**

Newman, Wendy 10330 East Jewell Avenue, Unit 66, Denver, CO 80231, (303) 751-6011, BS 83 CO St Univ; MS 85 CO St Univ; Sp-Lang Path, Aurora Public Schools, **SLP**

Newmann, Mrs Melody L 329 South Wacouta, Praire Du Chien, WI 53821, (608) 348-2648, BA 86 Coll of Saint Teresa; MS 87 Univ of WI - Eau Claire

Newman-Teubl, Mrs Margaret 4015 Kirtland Road, Willoughby, OH 44094, (216) 946-9532, BA 78 John Carroll Univ; MA 80 Cleveland St Univ; Sp-Lang Path, P T Serv Inc, **SLP ACE**

Newquist, Mrs Cathy Robinson 5804 Highlander Street, Bakersfield, CA 93306, (805) 871-0921, BA 73 Univ of WA; MS 86 Portland St Univ; Sp-Lang Path, Bakersfield City Sch Dist, **SLP**

Newsome, Cheryl Ann 71 12th Avenue, Shalimar, FL 32579, (904) 432-6121, BS 85 FL St Univ; MS 86 FL St Univ; 88–Sp-Lang Path, Okaloosa County Schs, **SLP**

Newsome, Linda A 18 Winchester Drive, Califon, NJ 07830, BA 69 Montclair St Coll; MA 71 CUNY - City College; Sp/Lang Path, Welkind Rehab Hosp, **SLP**

Newsome, Peggy W Box 66, Cobbs Creek, VA 23035, (804) 725-3721, BA 71 Wichita St Univ; MA 72 Wichita St Univ; Sp-Lang Path, Middlesex Co Pub Sch, **SLP**

Newton, Mrs April Woodward 930 East 700 North, Provo, UT 84601, (801) 375-2205, BS 82 UT St Univ; MS 84 IN St Univ - Terre Haute; Sp-Lang Path, Provo Sch Dist, **SLP**

Newton, Mrs Ingeborg B 7321 Granby Drive, Hudson, OH 44236, (216) 656-1132, BA 61 OH St Univ; **SLP**

Newton, Mrs Judy Prather P O Box 3 Branch Street #2, Goodman, MS 39079, (601) 472-2279, BS 70 MS Univ for Women; MS 73 MS Univ for Women; Sp-Lang Path, Private Practice, **SLP**

Newton, Karen R Rural Route 2 Box 2-A, Connersville, IN 47331, (317) 825-1495, BS 79 Purdue Univ - West Lafayette; MA 85 Miami Univ - Oxford; MS 81 Purdue Univ - West Lafayette; 82 Dir of Sp-Lang Path, Fayette Mem Hosp, **SLP A**

Newton, Mrs Kathryn K 230 Rogers Avenue, Milford, CT 06460, (203) 874-7487, BS 51; MA 52 NY Univ; **SLP LM**

Newton, Mrs Kimberly Kahler 11 Alvena Avenue, Suite 1, Cortland, NY 13045, (607) 753-3368, BS 77 Ithaca Coll; MS 78 Syracuse Univ; Aud, Private Practice, **A**

Newton, Dr Lauren Principal Deaf-Blind School, Texas School For The Blind, 1100 West 45th Street, Austin, TX 78756, (512) 454-8631, BS 66 Washington Univ; MA 72 Univ of MT; PH 82 (NS) Univ of TX - Austin; Principal, TX School for the Blind, **SLP A**

Newton, Mrs Lori J 112 Bracelle Drive, Selma, AL 36701-7207, (205) 875-8002, BA 77 Auburn Univ - Auburn; MA 78 Univ of TN - Knoxville; Chief Sp-Lang Path, W Ctrl Al Rehab Cen, **SLP**

Newton, Margaret 368 Sherman Avenue, Arnold, MD 21012, **SLP**

Newton, Dr Mariana University Of North Carolina, 300 Arts And Sciences, Greensboro, NC 27412, (919) 334-5939, BA 60 Univ of Redlands; MA 63 Univ of Redlands; PH 69 (Commun Dis) Northwestern Univ; 76–Assoc Prof, U of NC-Greensboro, **SLP F ACE**

Newton, Pamela Kay 10S710 Lilac Lane #209, Hinsdale, IL 60521-6706, (312) 895-5966, BS 84 Eastern IL Univ; MS 86 Marquette Univ; **SLP**

Newton, Patricia 2231 East 4th Street, Duluth, MN 55812, **SLP**

Newton, Mrs Renee Pryor 5117 Cambridge Avenue, Kansas City, MO 64129, (816) 221-7565, BS 77 Univ of KS; MA 78 OH St Univ; **SLP**

Newton, Mrs Sonna K 3806 Cottage Grove, Des Moines, IA 50311, (319) 266-2424, BS 73 Univ of IA; MA 74 Univ of IA; Coord/Speech-Language Services, Educationl Resource Associates, **SLP**

Newton, Susan Mary 16 Rocco Drive, East Northport, NY 11731, (516) 368-3831, BA 81 SUNY - Coll at Plattsburgh; MS 85 Adelphi Univ; Sp-Lang Path, Huntington Hrng & Sp Ctr, **SLP**

Ney, Elise 4000 Tunlaw Road N W, Apartment 1021, Washington, DC 20007, (202) 244-4420, MA 84 George Washington Univ; Aud, Wash Hearing & Speech Society, **A**

Ney, William I 524 Buckingham Drive, Indianapolis, IN 46208, (317) 283-9359, BS 58 Butler Univ; MS 66 Butler Univ; MA 77 Ball St Univ; Sp-Lang Path, Butler University, **SLP**

Neyhus, Dr Arthur I 2858-C West Touhy, Chicago, IL 60645, (312) 996-5650, BA 45 Harvard Univ; OM 52 Boston Univ; PH 62 (NS) Northwestern Univ; Assoc Prof, U of IL / College of Ed, **A**

Neyland, Mrs Ann K 107 Cinnamon Oak, Houston, TX 77079, (713) 785-6760, BS 65 TX Tech Univ; MA 66 TX Tech Univ; 88–Sp-Lang Path, Sp and Lang Remediation Ctr, **SLP**

Neyman, Charles E 12-1675 Thayer Court, Kelowna, BC, Canada V1Y 8M2, (604) 762-3390, BA 64 ID St Univ; MS 70 ID St Univ; 88–Aud-Owner, The Hearing & Audiology Group, **SLP A**

Neymeyer, Nancy R 801 4th Avenue, Box H, Parkersburg, IA 50665, (319) 232-4529, BA 65 Wartburg Coll; MA 70 Univ of IA; Aud, AEA #7, **A**

Nezelek, Karen Lee 106 Victoria Place, Syracuse, NY 13210, (315) 475-7610, BA 65 SUNY - Center at Binghamton; MS 69 Syracuse Univ; Research Asst, Syracuse Univ, **SLP**

Ng, Mildred Y B 2333 Kapiolani Boulevard, Apartment 414, Honolulu, HI 96826, BS 74 Univ of HI - Manoa; MS 76 Univ of WI - Madison; Sp-Lang Path, Rehab Hosp/Pacific, **SLP ACE**

Nguyen, Mrs Kathie Rae 1206 4th Street, Stevens Point, WI 54481, (715) 346-2034, BA 76 Univ of WI - Eau Claire; MS 77 Univ of WI - Stevens Point; Sp-Lang Path, Stevens Point Area Schools, **SLP**

Niblack, Mrs Yolonda C 529 East 86th Street, Chicago, IL 60619, (312) 723-3135, BA 73 Saint Xavier Coll; OM 86 Governors St Univ; Sp-Lang Path, Chicago PS

Niccum, Mrs Mary Rose 4503 Fillingame Drive, Chantilly, VA 22021, (703) 378-7083, BS 80 FL St Univ; MS 81 FL St Univ; Sp-Lang Path, **SLP**

Niccum, Dr Nancy Ellen 10440 114th Street North, Stillwater, MN 55082, (612) 439-2748, BS 73 Univ of WI - River Falls; MS 74 Univ of WI - Milwaukee; PH 78 (Sp & Hrng Science) Univ of MN - Minneap-St Paul; 83–Res Assoc, U of MN

Nicely, Dr James E Dept Communication Disorders, Radford University, Radford, VA 24142, (703) 831-5453, BS 60 IN Univ - Bloomington; MA 68 IN Univ - Bloomington; PH 75 (Speech Science) Univ of IL - Urbana; Prof & Chrmn Dept Commun Dis, Radford U, **SLP**

Nicholas, Dr Jo Ann 13 Sherwood Ridge Road, Suffern, NY 10901, (914) 294-5441, BA 72 Montclair St Coll; MS 74 Columbia Univ Teachers Coll; ED 77 (Aud) Columbia Univ Teachers Coll; Assoc Prof Aud, Mercy Coll, **A**

Nicholas, Mrs Leslie Denise 10535 N W Routt Way, Broomfield, CO 80020, (303) 429-4031, **SLP**

Nicholas, Linda Elmore 4727 27th Avenue South, Minneapolis, MN 55406, (612) 725-6767, BS 69 Central MI Univ; MA 75 Univ of CO - Boulder; Sp-Lang Path, VA Med Cen of Minneapolis, **SLP**

Nicholas, Marjorie L 51 Hillside Avenue, Arlington, MA 02174, (617) 232-9500, BA 78 Brown Univ; MS 85 Boston Univ; 86–Sp-Lang Path, Boston VA Med Ctr, **SLP**

Nicholas, Marlee W 1859 Ellison Creek Road, Clemmons, NC 27012, (919) 945-4459, MA 74 Univ of FL; Sp-Lang Path, Upjohn Home Health, **SLP**

Nicholas, Patricia Kay 4816 N Sheffield Avenue, Whitefish Bay, WI 53217, (414) 332-2524, **SLP**

Nicholas, Rosalind H 131 Wabash Avenue, Carthage, IL 62321, (217) 357-2230, MA 68 Western IL Univ; BA 32; **SLP LM**

Nicholls, Gloria H Rural Free Delivery, Williamsburg, MA 01096, **SLP**

Nichols, Dr Alan C 4103 Loma Riviera Lane, San Diego, CA 92110, (619) 594-4177, OB 53 Bowling Green St Univ; MA 57 OH St Univ; PH 59 (Sp & Hrng Science) OH St Univ; Professor, San Diego State Univ, **SLP**

Nichols, Ann Pryor 3709 Huntington Street N W, Washington, DC 20015, (202) 994-3631, BS 81 PA St Univ - Univ Park; MA 82 George Washington Univ; Asst Dir SLP/Aud, GWU Med Ctr, **SLP**

Nichols, Anne Christine 1100 Mayfair Terrace #A-6, Florence, SC 29501, (803) 669-8891, BS 77 Univ of ME - Farmington; OM 83 Auburn Univ - Auburn; 87–Sp-Lang Path, Health South Rehab Ctr, **SLP**

Nichols, Anne E 4902-37th Street #1212, Red Deer, AB, Canada T4N 6M9, (403) 346-2708, BA 70 Univ of WA; MA 71 Univ of WA; Sp-Lang Path, Red Deer Regional Hosp Ctr, **SLP**

Nichols, Mrs Brenda Jean 19913 Beach Boulevard #278, Huntington Beach, CA 92648-3705, BA 81 CA St Univ - Long Beach; MA 83 CA St Univ - Long Beach; SLP, Long Beach USD, **SLP**

Nichols, Clare M 1000 Palm Trail #10, Delray Beach, FL 33444, (305) 737-7300, BS 51 Northern IL Univ - De Kalb; MA 53 Univ of AL- Tuscaloosa; Sp-Lang Path, Palm Beach Co Sch Dist, **SLP**

Nichols, Mrs Cynthia Dawson 2502 Stafford Avenue, Raleigh, NC 27607, (919) 834-2298, BA 77 Univ of MD - Baltimore CO; MS 80 Loyola Coll; 86–Sp-Lang Path, Wake County PS, **SLP**

Nichols, Cynthia Gay 2548 Beverly Drive, Birmingham, AL 35223, (205) 871-1606, BA 82 Univ of AL- Tuscaloosa; MS 84 Univ of AL- Tuscaloosa; Sp-Lang Path, Birmingham City Sch Sys, **SLP**

Nichols, Cynthia Marie 4185 West Medow #2295, Colorado Springs, CO 80906, (303) 576-3420, OB 83 Univ of NE - Lincoln; OM 84 Univ of NE - Lincoln; **SLP**

Nichols, Mrs Cynthia Zender 1071 Grasmere Avenue, Mansfield, OH 44906, (419) 755-5520, MA 83 Univ of Akron; SLP, Richland Co Bd of Ed, **SLP**

Nichols, Dean G 300 East Church Street, Apartment 1010, Orlando, FL 32801, (305) 254-1033, BA 28 Univ of WY; MA 31 Univ of WY; PH 38 (NS) Univ of MI - Ann Arbor; **SLP LM**

Nichols, Deborah H 4041 East Olive Road #383, Pensacola, FL 32514, BS 80 Univ of South AL; MS 77 Univ of FL; Clin Supvr, InSpeech Inc, **SLP**

Nichols, Diane E 7005 Maple Tree Lane, Springfield, VA 22152, (703) 644-0298, BS 73 Southwest MO St Univ; MA 79 Univ of TX - Austin; 87–Sp-Lang Path, Fairfax Co PS, **SLP**

Nichols, Elizabeth 204 Pine Street, Knightdale, NC 27545, (919) 832-8301, BS 66 East TN St Univ; MA 73 East TN St Univ; Sp-Lang Path, Rehab Serv of Wake Co Inc, **SLP**

Nichols, Mrs Elizabeth Gillingham Route 6 Box 541, Conway, AR 72032, (501) 329-6688, BS 86 Univ of Central AR; MS 87 Univ of Central AR; 87–Sp-Lang Path, N Hills Svc for the Hndcpd, **SLP**

Nichols, Jill H 633 Hampshire Drive, Mendota Heights, MN 55120, BA 76 Univ of MN - Minneap-St Paul; MA 78 Univ of MN - Minneap-St Paul; Homemaker, **SLP**

Nichols, Mrs Kathleen M 5911 Ayleshire Road, Baltimore, MD 21239, BA 77 Loyola Coll; MS 78 Loyola Coll; **SLP**

Nichols, Kathy Lynn 407 Hamby Avenue, Dawson Springs, KY 42408, (502) 797-2991, **SLP**

Nichols, Kim E 1705 Texas Avenue #8, Cookeville, TN 38501, (615) 526-9777, BS 79 TN Tech Univ; OM 82 Auburn Univ - Auburn; 83–Sp/Lang Path, Putnam Cty Sch Syst, **SLP ACE**

Nichols, Mrs Laura Rypkema 156 Cosman Street, Washington Township, NJ 07675, (914) 947-3000, BS 84 William Paterson Coll; MS 86 William Paterson Coll; Sp-Lang Path, Helen Hayes Hosp, **SLP**

Nichols, Mrs Lisa K 1112 Wildplum Drive, Lee's Summitt, MO 64063, (816) 524-2406, BS 80 Central MO St Univ; MS 87 Central MO St Univ; 83–Sp-Lang Path, Lee's Summit PS

Nichols, Lucinda 2517 24th Street, Meridian, MS 39301, (601) 634-0835, BS 77 MS St Univ - MS State; OM 81 Univ of MS; Sp/Lang Path, Private Practice, **SLP**

Nichols, Lynn Wagner 2936 Queen Bee Lane, St Louis, MO 63129, (314) 569-8310, BS 79 Southeast MO St Univ; MS 80 Fontbonne Coll; Sp-Lang Path, Spec Sch Dist St Louis Co, **SLP**

Nichols, Marie A PCI Incorporated, PO Box 242, Mount Prospect, IL 60056, (312) 394-5903, BS 74 SUNY - Center at Buffalo; MS 76 Purdue Univ - West Lafayette; OM 78 IN Univ - Gary; President, Direct Marketing, **A**

Nichols, Mrs Marilyn Casey R R #2 Box 154, Sullivan, IN 47882, (618) 563-4812, BS 75 IN St Univ - Terre Haute; MS 80 IN St Univ - Terre Haute; 86–Sp-Lang Path, Hutsonville Unit Sch Dist #1 and #3, **SLP**

Nichols, Mary Ploumis 1054 Hypoluxo Road, Lantana, FL 33462, (407) 588-0501, BA 77 Western KY Univ; MA 79 Western KY Univ; Sp-Lang Path, Private Practice, **SLP**

Nichols, Maureen T 1321 Newton Street N E, Washington, DC 20017, (202) 651-5018, BA 59 Univ of MI - Ann Arbor; MA 62 Stanford Univ; Sp/Lang Path, Gallaudet, **SLP**

Nichols, Murdayne A 3230 T C U Boulevard, Orlando, FL 32817, (305) 831-6700, BA 70 FL St Univ; MS 76 FL St Univ; SLP, Seminole Co Sch Sys, **SLP**

Nichols, Mrs Shari A 1019 Francis Drive, Apartment 3, Champaign, IL 61820, (217) 443-5276, BS 67 Eastern IL Univ; MS 72 Eastern IL Univ; Sp-Lang Path, United Samaritans Med Ctr, **SLP**

Nichols, Teresa Jane 304 Old Haw Creek, Asheville, NC 28805, (704) 669-3162, BS 80 Central MO St Univ; MA 82 Central MO St Univ

Nichols, Wanada Lorraine 722 Sagebrush Trail S E, Albuquerque, NM 87123, (505) 243-8030, BS 64 TX Woman's Univ; MS 85 San Francisco St Univ; Aud, New Mexico Ear & Vertigo, **A ACE**

Nichols-Klocke, M Sue 4267 Sayoko Circle, San Jose, CA 95136, (408) 266-8121, BA 62 San Jose St Univ; Un Sch Dist, **SLP**

Nicholson, Mrs Allison W 401 Taylor Lane, Kennett Square, PA 19348, (609) 467-0859, MS 76 Univ of South FL; Sp/Lang Path, Logan Township Sch Dist, **SLP**

Nicholson, Anne T P O Box 282, Webster, NC 28788, (704) 586-2819, BS 76 Western Carolina Univ; ME 78 Univ of NC - Greensboro; SLP, Jackson Co Pub Schs, **SLP**

Nicholson, Cynthia C 365 Lindsay Lane S E, Cedar Rapids, IA 52403-1093, (319) 399-6700, BA 72 Univ of IA; MA 74 Univ of IA; Sp-Lang Path, Grant Wood AEA, **SLP**

Nicholson, Cynthia Jane 47 Ranchwood Crescent, London, ON, Canada N6G 3A1, (519) 681-4820, BS 78 Univ of Western Ontario; OM 83 Univ of Western Ontario; 87–Sp-Lang Path, Bd of Educ City of London, **SLP**

Nicholson, Mrs Deborah Lynne 6149 Willis, Groves, TX 77619, (409) 983-1651, **A**

Nicholson, Jane Ann 7734 S E 21st Street, Portland, OR 97202, (503) 255-1841, BS 74 Purdue Univ - West Lafayette; MS 83 Portland St Univ; SLP, Multnomah Educ Serv District, **SLP**

Nicholson, Mrs June D Rd 1 Box 835, Arlington, VT 05250, (802) 375-6409, BS 63 Abilene Christian Univ; MS 80 Univ of VT; Sp/Lang Path, Arlington Pub Sch, **SLP**

Nicholson, Mrs Nancy Gregory 3450 Scott Street, San Francisco, CA 94123, (415) 931-7645, ME 85 Univ of GA; Audiologist, Ear Medical Group, **A**

Nicholson, Mrs Sandra 617 North 5th Avenue, St Charles, IL 60174, (312) 377-3601, **SLP**

Nicholson, Sandra E 403 South Armstrong, Litchfield, MN 55355, (612) 693-2436, BS 75 Moorhead St Univ; MS 77 Saint Cloud St Univ; 86–Sp-Lang Path, Meeker-Wright Spec Educ Coop, **SLP**

Nicholson-Barcal, Nancy K 3375 Ensenada, San Ramon, CA 94583, (415) 794-5155, BS 78 Bradley Univ; MA 80 Northern IL Univ - De Kalb; Director, Bay Area Sp-Hrng Cl, **SLP**

Nickel, George John, Jr 127 Rues Lane, East Brunswick, NJ 08816, (201) 390-9412, MS 88 CUNY - Brooklyn Coll

Nickels, Janet K 846 Wesley #2, Oak Park, IL 60302, (312) 386-3214, BA 83 Bradley Univ; MS 85 Rush Univ; **A**

Nickey, Jeryl M 1640 Harbert, Memphis, TN 38104, (901) 795-3930, BA 71 Memphis St Univ; MA 73 Memphis St Univ; Sp-Lang Path, Memphis City Schools, **SLP**

Nickey, Mrs Lynn M 109 Choctaw Trail, Madison, AL 35758, (205) 721-9926, BA 78 MI St Univ; MA 82 Wayne St Univ; Sp-Lang Path, Madison County Sch Sys, **SLP**

Nicklawsky, Lisa Mary 1075 North Miller Road, Apartment 234, Scottsdale, AZ 85257, (602) 990-7781, BA 84 Univ of ND; MS 85 Minot St Univ; 87–Sp-Lang Path, Synergos Neurological Ctr, **SLP**

Nickles, Dr Aleki C 4420 Drifton Drive, Columbus, OH 43227, (614) 861-2374, BS 50 Bloomsburg Univ of PA; MS 52 Univ of Pittsburgh - Pittsburgh; PH 70 (Sp & Hrng Science) OH St Univ; **SLP**

Nickles, Deborah L 31632 Waltham, Birmingham, MI 48009, **SLP**

Nickman, Stephanie Ann Box 236 Nickman's Plaza, Lemont Furnace, PA 15456, (412) 437-3276, BS 79 CA Univ of PA; MS 82 PA St Univ - Univ Park; 86–Aud, Private Practice, **A**

Nickols, Mrs Linda S 3303 West Cypress, Visalia, CA 93277, (209) 625-6698, BA 77 Humboldt St Univ; MA 78 Humboldt St Univ; SLP, Visalia USD, **SLP**

Nicks, Mrs Judith A B Route 3 Box 322, Amherst, VA 24521, (804) 441-5277, BS 68 Univ Southern MS-Hattiesburg; MA 75 Univ of San Diego; **SLP**

Nicodemus, Barbara 209 West Glenwood, Knoxville, TX 37917, (615) 521-7193, BS 77 Lamar Univ; MS 78 Lamar Univ; 88–Aud, Univ of IN, **A**

Nicol, Mrs Lori Sue 757 Townsend Avenue, New Haven, CT 06510, (303) 522-7384, BA 83 Augustana Coll; MA 85 Univ of Denver; 88–Sp-Lang Path, Stratford PS, **SLP**

Nicola, Sharon F 1180 Auborne, Adrian, MI 49221, (517) 265-2297, BS 77 Western MI Univ; MA 81 Eastern MI Univ; Sp-Lang Path, Saline Area Sch, **SLP**

Nicols, Joseph C, Jr 3107 Santa Monica Drive, Austin, TX 78741, (512) 444-4835, BA 71 Univ of TX - Austin; MA 81 Univ of TX - Austin; Sp-Lang Path, Brown Schs-Ranchtreat Cen, **SLP**

Niebel, Susan K P O Box 1096, Pine Bush, NY 12566-1096, (717) 275-8525, **SLP**

Niebuhr, Mrs Diane Dooley 415 Fifth Avenue, Iowa City, IA 52240, (319) 335-8736, BS 80 Univ of IA; MA 82 Univ of IA; Aud, Wendell Johnson Sp & Hrng Clinic, **A**

Nieburgs, Dr Tamara R 177 East 75th Street, New York, NY 10021, (212) 988-4800, BA 48 CUNY - Queens Coll; MS 62 Yeshiva Univ; PH 86 (Special Education) Columbia Pacific Univ; 76–Consultant, Private Practice, **SLP**

Niederhauser, Mrs Diane Lynn 4943 S Murray Blvd #Y24, Salt Lake City, UT 84123-2651, (801) 263-1841, BS 78 Mount Holyoke Coll; MS 82 SUNY - Coll at Fredonia; SLP, Dev Dis Inc, **SLP**

Niederjohn, Dr Russell J Department Of Elect Compt & Biomed Engineering, Marquette University, 1515 West Wisconsin Avenue, Milwaukee, WI 53233, (414) 224-6820, BS 67 Univ of MA - Amherst; MS 69 Univ of MA - Amherst; PH 71 (Electrical Engineering) Univ of MA - Amherst; Prof/Dept Chmn, Marquette U

Niederkohr, Mrs Carolyn H 4330 N W 19th Avenue, Gainesville, FL 32605, (904) 376-5057, BA 76; ME 77 Univ of FL; SLP, Littlewood Elementary School, **SLP**

Niederkorn, Terry Lynn 2217 Holly Avenue, Kennett, MO 63857, (314) 757-6615, BS 76 AR St Univ; MS 80 AR St Univ; Sp-Lang Path, Pemiscot Co Spec Sch Dist, **SLP**

Niedringhaus, Mrs Jacquelyn D 1822 Amherst Court, Rock Hill, SC 29730, (803) 366-9829, BS 75 Univ of GA; ME 76 Univ of GA; MA 79 Univ of SC - Columbia; 84–Aud/Sp-Lang Path, Central Carolina Aud Ctr, **SLP A**

Niedringhaus, Richard 108 S Washington Street, Norton, MA 02766, (617) 285-9763, BS 71 Univ of Cincinnati; MA 72 Northwestern Univ; Sp-Lang Path, Taunton Pub Schs, **SLP**

Nieds, Barbara G 210 Ahwahnee Road, Lake Forest, IL 60045, (312) 234-5600, BS 64 Marquette Univ; MA 65 Northwestern Univ; Aud, Lake Forest Hosp, **SLP A**

Nielsen, Mrs Barbara Jean 1137 Le Conte Drive, Riverside, CA 92507, (714) 784-0404, BA 71 Univ of CA - Riverside; BA 75 CA St Coll - San Bernardino; MA 84 CA St Univ - Fullerton; 85–Sp-Lang Path, Advocate Schs, **SLP**

Nielsen, Carol Sue 840 South 32nd, Lincoln, NE 68510, (402) 489-7102, **SLP**

Nielsen, Mrs Cathleen L 1435-E 140 South, Pleasant Grove, UT 84062, (801) 374-4925, BA 73 Brigham Young Univ; MA 75 Brigham Young Univ; Sp-Lang Path, Provo School District, **SLP**

Nielsen, Dr Donald W House Ear Institute, 256 South Lake Street, Los Angeles, CA 90057, (313) 876-1016, BA 63 Univ of Cincinnati; MA 67 Wayne St Univ; PH 68 (NS) Wayne St Univ; 86–Exec VP/Res, House Ear Institute

Nielsen, Mrs Elise E 685 East Valley Hills Dr, Heber, UT 84032, BS 73 Univ of UT; MS 74 Univ of UT; SLP, Wasatch Co Sch Dist, **SLP**

Nielsen, Elizabeth Ann 833 Shoshone Street N #103, Twin Falls, ID 83301, (208) 733-8456, BS 88 ID St Univ; MS 87 ID St Univ

Nielsen, Ellen S 625 N E Laurelhurst Place, Portland, OR 97232, (503) 967-8822, BA 58 Univ of WY; MS 79 Western OR St Coll; SLP, Esd 112, **SLP**

Nielsen, Jan K P 9 Water Way, Irvine, CA 92714, (213) 868-0871, BA 73 Univ of CA - Los Angeles; MA 78 CA St Univ - Northridge; SLP, LA County Supt Schs, **SLP**

Nielsen, Kris T Box 74, Gonvick, MN 56644, (218) 487-5742, BA 73 Saint Cloud St Univ; MS 75 Saint Cloud St Univ; Sp-Lang Path, Red Lake PS, **SLP**

Nielsen, Lucille T 170 East Chestnut Avenue, Metuchen, NJ 08840, **SLP**

Nielsen, Lynn 11 North 1650 West, Cedar City, UT 84720, (801) 586-6516, BS 50 UT St Univ; MS 57 Univ of UT; SLP, Iron Co Sch Dist, **SLP**

Nielsen, Mrs Nancy 220 South Vermont, Mason City, IA 50401, (515) 423-8996, BA 78 Univ of Northern IA; MA 79 Univ of Northern IA; SLP, Nn Trails AEA, **SLP**

Nielsen, Patricia P 806 Treehouse Lane, Sacramento, CA 95864, (916) 485-4872, BA 58 Univ of CA - Berkeley; MA 79 CA St Univ - Sacramento; Sp-Lang Path, San Juan USD, **SLP**

Nielsen, Susan E 148 Pine Street, Portland, ME 04102, (207) 772-1352, BA 64 Case Western Reserve Univ; MA 66 Case Western Reserve Univ; Sp-Lang Path, Portland Pub Sch, **SLP**

Nielsen, Mrs Susan McGuckin 710 Westchester, Bolingbrook, IL 60439, (312) 852-0600, BS 75 IL St Univ - Normal; MS 77 IL St Univ - Normal; 79–Sp/Lang Path, Downers Grove South HS, **SLP**

Nielsen-Ziegler, Mrs Michelle A 2401 N E Dexter, Gresham, OR 97030, (503) 666-5779, MS 87 Portland St Univ

Nielson, Dr Harriet R 2759 Commonwealth Avenue, Salt Lake City, UT 84109, (801) 487-4830, BS 62 Univ of UT; MA 64 De Paul Univ; PH 83 (Sp-Lang Path) Univ of UT; Sp-Lang Path, Private Practice, **SLP**

Nielson, Dr Melvin A 680 East Oaklane Circle, Kaysville, UT 84037, (801) 399-9631, BS 52 Univ of UT; MS 54 Univ of UT; PH 67 (Hrng) Univ of UT; 64–Aud/Admissions, UT Sch for Deaf & Blind, **SLP A**

Nielson, Mrs Sheila G Box 42 TLRB, BYU, Provo, UT 84602, (801) 378-6462, BA 78 Brigham Young Univ; OM 80 Brigham Young Univ; Cl Supvr Commun Dis, Brigham Young U, **SLP**

Niemann, Mrs Mary Kay 5207 Sprucewood Drive, Louisville, KY 40291, (502) 239-4760, BS 83 Eastern KY Univ; MS 85 Univ of Louisville; 86–Sp-Lang Path, Easter Seals H & S Ctr, **SLP**

Niemeyer, Judith Mary 1 Brook Road #7, Salem, NH 03079, (603) 894-5515, BS 84 Emerson Coll; MS 86 Univ of NH; **SLP**

Niemitz, Mrs Ann F RFD 1 Box 166, Brimfield, MA 01010, (203) 429-6316, BA 78 Univ of CT; MA 80 Univ of CT; 87–Sp-Lang Path, Stafford PS, **SLP**

Niemtzow, Patricia 1705 Lombard Street, Philadelphia, PA 19146, (215) 448-7698, **SLP**

Nienhueser, Mrs Kathleen E 1805 Dorwart Drive, Sidney, NE 69162, (308) 254-3642, BA 71 Creighton Univ; MS 75 CO St Univ; SLP, Sidney Pub Sch, **SLP**

Nienow, Patricia M Rural Route, Mapleton, MN 56065, (507) 524-3245, BS 63 SUNY - Coll at Geneseo; MS 64 SUNY - Coll at Geneseo; SLP, Le Sueur Co Dac, **SLP**

Nies, Linda Ann 772 Sapphire, San Diego, CA 92109, (619) 541-3088, BA 84 Chapman Coll; MS 85 Univ of Redlands; Sp-Lang Path, Childrens Hosp/Sharp Rehab Ctr, **SLP**

Niewoehner, Debra K 14323 Sunswept Park Court, #108, Florissant, MO 63033, (314) 569-6175, BS 80 Univ of ND; MS 81 Minot St Univ; Aud, St John's Mercy Med Ctr, **A**

Niezgorski, Mrs Angela 90 Budding Ridge, Southington, CT 06489, (203) 237-7835, BS 80 Northeastern Univ; MS 82 Southern CT St Univ; Sp/Lang Path, Bristol Bd of Ed, **SLP**

Niggemann, Debra J 1635 Concord Drive, Elgin, IL 60120, (312) 697-6167, MS 88 Univ of WI - Stevens Point

Nightengale, Mary Finan 1052 Cynthia Lane, San Jose, CA 95129, (408) 255-7498, BS 78 Univ of North TX; MA 79 Our Lady Lake Univ-San Anton; Sp/Lang Path, Neuro Care, **SLP**

Nightingale, Mrs Lorie Marie 15501 Bruce B Downs Blvd, Apartment 2107, Tampa, FL 33647, (813) 272-4530, BS 83 Eastern IL Univ; MS 84 Eastern IL Univ; Sp-Lang Path, Hillsborough Co Sch, **SLP**

Nigro, Carolyn Griffith 11392 Grassy Trail Drive, San Diego, CA 92127, (619) 588-3075, BA 82 Univ of CA - Santa Barbara; MA 85 San Diego St Univ; **SLP**

Nigro, Jill Lewis Hudson State Service Center, 501 Ogletown Road, Newark, DE 19711, (302) 368-6790, BA 82 Rutger's St Univ - Douglas Coll; MS 86 Hahnemann Univ Grad Sch; 86–Sp-Lang Path, Delaware Public Health, **SLP**

Nigro, Mrs Kerri F 6701 9th Avenue, Sacramento, CA 95820, (916) 451-5566, BA 75 CA St Univ - Sacramento; MA 77 CA St Univ - Sacramento; SLP, Sacramento City USD, **SLP**

Nigro, Louis J 97 Coolidge Avenue, Carteret, NJ 07008, (201) 541-5452, BS 51 Seton Hall Univ; MA 65 Seton Hall Univ; Dir/Sp-Lang Path, Carteret Bd of Ed, **SLP**

Niizawa, Judy J 834 Gary Avenue, Sunnyvale, CA 94086, (415) 856-1622, BA 66 San Jose St Univ; MA 70 San Jose St Univ; 70–Sp-Lang Path, Palo Alto USD, **SLP ACE**

Nikjeh, Mrs Deborah Adams 3545 Landmark Trail, Palm Harbor, FL 34684, (813) 462-7031, BS 78 WV Univ; MS 79 WV Univ; Sp-Lang Path, Morton F Plant Hosp/Barrett Ctr, **SLP ACE**

Niklaus, Phyllis Marie Exceptional Family Services, 546 General Dispensery, APO New York, NY 09086, BS 74 LA St Univ - Baton Rouge; 81 LA St Univ - N O Medical Ctr; 88–Sp-Lang Path, Dept of Defense, **SLP**

Nikodem, Caroline 23 Woods Road, Islip Terrace, NY 11752, (516) 758-1000, BS 84 SUNY - Coll at Fredonia; MS 86 Adelphi Univ; **SLP**

Nikodym, Deanna L 3339 La Mesa, San Carlos, CA 94070-4216, (415) 991-1285, BA 77 CA St Univ - Fresno; MA 79 CA St Univ - Fresno; 87–Sp-Lang Path, Jefferson Sch Dist, **SLP**

Nikoomanesh, Mrs Susan M Amini 205 Dunbeath Court, Lutherville, MD 21093, (301) 396-8987, MS 87 Towson St Univ

Nileshwar, Ramgopal S 200 Crestwood Street, Lake Charles, LA 70605, (318) 478-6987, **A**

Nilo, Dr Ernest R Ohio St Univ Medical Center, Univ Hosp Audiology Clinic, Room 4024, Columbus, OH 43210, (614) 293-8065, BS 53 Univ of WI - Madison; MA 57 Univ of MD - College Park; PH 65 (Aud) OH St Univ; Dir/Hrng Ser, OH St U-Coll/Med Dept Otol, **A**

Nilsen, Barbara S 459 East Fairmount Avenue, State College, PA 16801, (814) 237-8713, BA 69 PA St Univ - Univ Park; MS 75 PA St Univ - Univ Park; **SLP**

Nilsen, Dr Jill F Eastern Illinois University, Speech And Hearing Clinic, Charleston, IL 61920, (217) 581-2712, BS 74 Eastern IL Univ; MS 75 Eastern IL Univ; PH 83 (Supervision) Univ of IL - Urbana; Associate Professor, Eastern IL U, **SLP**

Nilson, Mrs Holly M 4 Village Way, Medfield, MA 02052, (508) 359-5338, BA 75 Univ of MA - Amherst; MA 80 WA St Univ; Sp-Lang Path, **SLP**

Nilson, Mrs Mary S M 2324 Canterbury Road, University Heights, OH 44118, (216) 321-1923, BS 73 Univ of Tulsa; MS 75 Univ of NM; Sp-Lang Path, Mt Sinai Med Cen, **SLP**

Niman, Mrs Barbara A 35 Wexford Green, Collinsville, IL 62234, (618) 288-7008, MS 88 Southern IL Univ-Edwardsvill

Nimelstein, Mrs Ruth L c/o Amoseas Rumbai, P O Box 237, Orchard Point Post Office, Singapore, Singapore 9123, BS 77 SUNY - Coll at Fredonia; MS 81 CO St Univ; Sp-Lang Path, Bakersfield City Schools, **SLP**

Nimmo, Mrs Debra Ryan 2 Nicholas Court, Bethpage, NY 11714, (516) 931-2625, BA 82 SUNY - Center at Stony Brook; MA 86 CUNY - Queens Coll; **SLP**

Nimmo, Mrs Regina E 8729 Hudson River Circle, Fountain Valley, CA 92708, (714) 968-1120, BA 63 PA St Univ - Univ Park; MA 79 CA St Univ - Long Beach; 79–Sp-Lang Path, Fountain Valley School Dist, **SLP**

Nimmons, Bonnie W 210 South Mission, Enid, OK 73703, (405) 233-6322, BS 84 FL St Univ; MA 86 Abilene Christian Univ; 88–Sp-Lang Path, Hedges Comm Sp/Hrng Clinic, **SLP**

Nimmons, Mrs Ellen Marie 727 Plankway, Belleville, IL 62221, (618) 234-2120, BA 83 Auburn Univ - Montgomery; OM 85 Auburn Univ - Auburn; 88–Sp-Lang Path, St Elizabeth's Hosp, **SLP**

Nimocks, Mrs Carla Morehead 468 Calvert, Forrest City, AR 72335, (501) 633-8494, BS 84 AR St Univ; OM 85 AR St Univ; **SLP**

Nimtz, Mrs Janet Marie 7108 Alexandria Place, Stockton, CA 95207-1504, (209) 477-0917, BA 66 Univ of CA - Berkeley; MA 85 Univ of the Pacific; **SLP**

Niner, David K Route 1 Box 206-G, Albany, IN 47320, (317) 747-3368, BS 76 Muskingum Coll; MA 78 Case Western Reserve Univ; 87–Dir Rehab Svcs, Ball Memorial Hosp, **SLP**

Niner, Mrs Holly Lee Route 1 Box 206-G, Albany, IN 47320, (317) 288-8761, BS 78 SUNY - Center at Albany; MA 80 Univ of CT; **SLP**

Ninneman, Mrs Margaret Sue P O Box 18-1706, Coronado, CA 92118, (619) 491-2438, BA 78 CA St Univ - Fullerton; MA 82 CA St Univ - Stanislaus; 84–Sp-Lang Path, San Diego USD, **SLP**

Nipp, Mrs Suzanne S 221 Green Springs Drive, Worthington, OH 43235, (614) 436-4400, BS 55 OR St Univ; MS 71 Portland St Univ; Sp-Lang Path, Worthington City Schools, **SLP**

Nipple, Mrs Donna Alligood 600 Snow Hill Street, Ayden, NC 28513, (919) 559-5133, BS 78 East Carolina Univ; MS 80 East Carolina Univ; Clin Mgr, Caswell Cen, **SLP ACE**

Nippold, Dr Marilyn A Speech Pathology & Audiology, University Of Oregon, Clinical Services Bldg, Eugene, OR 97403, (503) 686-3591, BA 72 Univ of CA - Los Angeles; MA 76 CA St Univ - Long Beach; PH 82 (NS) Purdue Univ - West Lafayette; Assoc Prof, Univ of OR, **SLP**

Nir, Talma 14 Williams Lane, Chappaqua, NY 10514, (914) 238-8749, BA Hebrew Univ-Jerusalem Israel; MA 86 CUNY - Queens Coll; 87–Sp-Lang Path, Lexington Hrng & Sp Ctr, **SLP**

Niren, Mrs Carol Snyder 1228 Beechwood Boulevard, Pittsburgh, PA 15206, (412) 422-1122, BA 77 Univ of Pittsburgh - Pittsburgh; ME 79 Northeastern Univ; **SLP**

Nisbet, Mrs Jean Boling 2415 Van Ness Avenue #304, San Francisco, CA 94109-1881, (415) 928-4941, BS 64 Southwest TX St Univ; ME 66 Southwest TX St Univ; 74–Dir Sp-Lang Path, Lettermn Army Med Cen, **SLP ACE**

Nisenboom, Jean M 1192 Elmwood Avenue, Mayfield Heights, OH 44124, (216) 231-8787, BS 79 Miami Univ - Oxford; MS 80 Miami Univ - Oxford; Sp-Lang Path Clinical Inst, Cleveland Hrng & Speech Center, **SLP**

Nishikawa, Mrs Dianne Haruye 991 Rock Canyon Circle, San Jose, CA 95127, (408) 251-6686, BA 81 San Jose St Univ; MS 83 San Jose St Univ; 83–Sp-Lang Path, Alum Rock USD, **SLP**

Nishikawa, Lynne K Lynne K Nishikawa & Assoc, 825 Smallwood Drive, Colton, CA 92324, (714) 824-0704, BS 78 Loma Linda Univ - Riverside; MS 80 Loma Linda Univ - Loma Linda; Owner/Dir Sp-Lang Path, Private Practice, **SLP**

Nishimitsu, Holly T 5696 Kula Mauu Street, Kapaa Kauai, HI 96746, (808) 822-7022, BS 76 Univ of HI - Manoa; MS 78 Univ of HI - Manoa; SLP, Dept of Ed, **SLP**

Nishizaki, Mrs Debra J 1015 Lakewood Drive, Lodi, CA 95240, (209) 369-7320, BA 78 CA St Univ - Sacramento; MA 80 CA St Univ - Sacramento; Sp-Lang Path, Lodi USD, **SLP**

Nisivaco, Mrs Julie Caulfield 10324 South Whipple, Chicago, IL 60655, (312) 238-2540, BS 81 Western IL Univ; MA 82 Western IL Univ; Tchr, Chicago Board of Education, **SLP**

Nispel, Cheri L 14565 41th Avenue North, Minneapolis, MN 55446, (612) 781-6571, OB 81 Univ of MN - Duluth; MS 82 Univ of WI - Eau Claire; Sp-Lang Path, Northridge Care Center, **SLP**

Nissan, Kathleen B Speech Therapist, 4186 Keefer Road, Chico, CA 95926, (916) 534-9222, BS 70 Univ of IL - Urbana; MS 71 Bradley Univ; MA 77 Governors St Univ; 87–Sp-Lang Path, Butte Co Schs, **SLP**

Nissen, Mrs Janet Siddens 13538 West Montana Place, Lakewood, CO 80228, (303) 279-6012, BA 74 Univ of Northern CO; MA 75 Univ of Northern CO; Sp-Lang Path, Jefferson Co Pub Sch, **SLP**

Nissen, Sheryl E 38 Livermore Road, Belmont, MA 02178, **SLP**

Nissenfeld-Sells, Mrs Lisa Rachel 36 Parkview Place, Baldwin, NY 11510, (516) 789-7796, BA 85 Adelphi Univ; MS 86 Adelphi Univ; 87–Sp-Lang Path, Brunswick Hosp Ctr Inc, **SLP**

Niswander, Dr Paul S Ohio State University, 1581 Dodd Drive, Columbus, OH 43210, (614) 292-9605, BS 63 OH St Univ; MA 64 MI St Univ; PH 68 (NS) MI St Univ; Assoc Prof, Ohio St U, **A**

Niswonger, Donna L 29047 Van Horn, New Boston, MI 48164, (313) 284-2400, BS 78 Eastern MI Univ; MA 79 Eastern MI Univ; Sp/Lang Path, Wyandotte Gen Hosp, **SLP**

Nitishin, Mrs Leah G Speech And Language Center, 327 Earl Garrett, Suite 103, Kerrville, TX 78028, (512) 896-7707, BA 77 Univ of Houston - Univ Park; MA 79 Univ of Houston - Univ Park; 83–Sp-Lang Path Dir, Sp & Lang Ctr, **SLP**

Nitschke, Terilynn 18345 W Bolter Lane, Brookfield, WI 53005, (414) 384-2000, BS 86 Marquette Univ; MS 87 Marquette Univ; 88–Sp-Lang Path, VA Med Ctr

Nitterauer, Richard A 7324 Kingsway Drive, Fort Wayne, IN 46819, BS 62 Purdue Univ - West Lafayette; ME 66 Southern IL Univ -Carbondale; Sp-Lang Path, Ft Wayne Comm Sch, **SLP**

Nittrouer, Dr Susan N Boys Town National Institute, 555 North 30th Street, Omaha, NE 68131, (402) 498-6720, BS 74 West Chester Univ of PA; ME 75 Smith Coll; PH 85 (NS) CUNY - Grad Sch & Univ Cntr; Staff Sci, Boys Town Natl Inst

Nitzke, Anne E 2701 Brunswick Avenue North, Minneapolis, MN 55422, (612) 541-0107, OB 79 Univ of Northern IA; MA 81 Northeast MO St Univ; Sp-Lang Path, Minneapolis PS, **SLP**

Nitzken, Syl J, Jr Department Of University Relations, Spalding University, 851 South Fourth Avenue, Louisville, KY 40203, (502) 585-9911, BS 50; MA 51; 88–Dir-Capital Campaign, Spalding Univ, **SLP**

Nitzsche, Deborah S 33 Schwartz Drive, Ottumwa, IA 52501, (515) 682-8635, BS 73 Southern IL Univ -Carbondale; MA 75 Northeast MO St Univ; 86–Sp-Lang Path, Southern Praire AEA 15, **SLP**

Nix, Anita L 1301 Vivan Drive, Carmel, IN 46032, Medical Search Specialist, Midwest Medical Consultants, **SLP**

Nix, Tonya L 101 Ferdinand Avenue, Glen Burnie, MD 21061, (301) 341-6448, BS 84 Towson St Univ; MS 86 Towson St Univ; 87–Sp-Lang Path, Prince George's Hosp Ctr, **SLP**

Nixon, M Colleen 744 Wall Road, Spring Lake, NJ 07762, (717) 763-7070, Professional Associate, InSpeech Inc, **SLP**

Nixon, Margaret Foster 5705 East 400 North, Greenfield, IN 46140, (317) 353-5429, BS 81 Purdue Univ - West Lafayette; MA 83 Ball St Univ; Sp-Lang Path, Comm Hospital of Indianapolis, **SLP**

Nixon, Melodee Annette 2114 Colorado, Kingsville, TX 78363, (512) 443-6282, MA 88 Southwest TX St Univ

Nixon, Pamela H 3447 Bleckley Drive, Lithonia, GA 30058, **SLP**

Nixon, Tani M Royal Victoria Hospital, 76 Ross Street, Barrie, ON, Canada L4N 1G4, (705) 728-9802, OB 75 Univ of Western Ontario; OM 76 Univ of Western Ontario; 87–Dir Sp-Hrng Svcs, Royal Victoria Hosp, **A**

Niziak, Kathleen J 21 Otis Avenue, Dedham, MA 02026, **SLP**

Noah, Mrs Deborah S 1701 Bedford Oaks Court, Bedford, TX 76021, (817) 283-4345, BS 76 Univ of North TX; MS 78 Univ of North TX; SLP, Hurst Independent School Dist, **SLP**

Nober, Dr E Harris 211 Heatherstone Road, Amherst, MA 01002, (413) 545-0131, BA 54 CUNY - Brooklyn Coll; MA 55 CUNY - Brooklyn Coll; PH 57 (NS) OH St Univ; Prof Commun Dis, Dept of Commun Dis U Ma, **SLP A F**

Nober, Dr Linda W 211 Heatherstone Road, Amherst, MA 01002, (413) 568-3311, BA 60 Adelphi Univ; MS 61 Adelphi Univ; ED 72 (NS) Univ of MA - Amherst; 87–Assoc Dean for Academic Aff, Westfield State Coll, **SLP**

Nobiensky, Wynne 3511 Paseo Salamoner, La Mesa, CA 92041, (619) 461-2611, BA 74 San Diego St Univ; MA 76 San Diego St Univ; Sp-Lang Path, La Mesa Spring Valley Sch Dist, **SLP**

Noble, Bart E 12308 Dellrey Drive #8, Austin, TX 78758-2501, (512) 458-2333, BS 73 United States Air Force Acad; MA 76 Saint Mary's Univ; Aud, A & B Hrng Aid & Audio Cen, **A**

Noble, Mrs Deborah Lynn 912 Pebble Creek Lane, Walnut, CA 91789, (213) 942-1500, BA 81 CA St Univ - Long Beach; MA 84 CA St Univ - Long Beach; SLP, El Rancho USD, **SLP**

Noble, Dennis R 1309 East Market Street, Searcy, AR 72143, (501) 268-0260, BA 70 Harding Univ; MA 73 Memphis St Univ; **A**

Noble, Mrs Leslie Steckbeck 4529 Ringgold Lane, Plano, TX 75075, (214) 423-7880, BA 80 IN Univ - Bloomington; MS 86 Univ of TX - Dallas; **SLP**

Noble, Mrs Lynn 13244 North 100th Place, Scottsdale, AZ 85260, (602) 391-3634, MA 88 Univ of Redlands

Noble, Marilyn L 267 Kennebec Avenue, Long Beach, CA 90803-5721, (213) 927-0341, BA 73 CA St Univ - Los Angeles; MS 81 Western OR St Coll; Aud, Marina Prof Sers, **A**

Noble, Nancy A 7727 Castle Ridge Circle, Indianapolis, IN 46256, (317) 845-9225, BS 67 Ball St Univ; MA 70 Ball St Univ; SLP, Msd WA Twsp, **SLP**

Noble, Paula L 315 Franklin Street, Middletown, OH 45042, (513) 424-2111, MS 80 Univ of North TX; Aud, Middletown Regional Hosp, **A**

Nobleman, Mrs Francie Robins 9023-139 Street, Edmonton, AB, Canada T5R 0G9, (403) 476-3823, BS 78 Univ of Alberta - Alberta; MA 80 Univ of MN - Minneap-St Paul; Sp/Lang Path, Edmonton Public School Board, **SLP**

Noble-Olson, Deborah A Box 129, Hawthorne, WI 54842, (715) 374-2391, BA 84 Univ of MN - Duluth; MA 85 Univ of MN - Duluth; 86–Sp-Lang Path, InSpeech Inc, **SLP**

Nobles, Mrs Penelope M 1 Fairview Lane, Bennettsville, SC 29512, (803) 758-5672, BA 74 Columbia Coll; OM 76 Univ of SC - Columbia; Sp-Lang Path Supervisor, S Carolina Dept Hlth/Envir Ctl, **SLP**

Noblin, Mrs Katherine Marie 311 Burberry Lane, Spring Hill, FL 33526, (215) 631-9300, BS 82 Southern IL Univ -Carbondale; OM 85 Governors St Univ; **SLP**

Nocito, Mrs Catherine B 1400 South Covenant Lane, Appleton, WI 54915, (919) 495-1322, BA 81 Univ of NC - Greensboro; ME 83 Univ of NC - Greensboro; Sp-Lang Path, Appleton Area School District, **SLP**

Nock, Mrs Janet Lynn 6390 Walnut Creek Drive, East Amherst, NY 14051, (716) 741-9780, BS 60 Carlow Coll; **SLP**

Noda, Ann Box 2384, APO New York, NY 09224, MS 73 Univ of South FL; SLP, Dept of Defense Dep Sch, **SLP**

Noda, Denise D 4168 S 900 E, Salt Lake City, UT 84107, (801) 581-2260, BS 83 Univ of UT; OM 85 Univ of UT; 88–Sp-Lang Path, Univ of UT Med Ctr, **SLP**

Nodar, Dr Richard H Head Communicative Disorders, The Cleveland Clinic A-71, 9500 Euclid Avenue, Cleveland, OH 44195-5034, (216) 444-6693, BS 62 SUNY - Coll at Geneseo; MS 64 Purdue Univ - West Lafayette; PH 67 (NS) Purdue Univ - West Lafayette; 75–Hd, Sec Commun Dis, The Cleveland Cl, **A F ACE**

Nodurft, Judith B 4703 Baccich Street, New Orleans, LA 70122, **SLP**

Nodzo, Ellen B 14 Silver Avenue, Auburn, NY 13021, **SLP**

Noe, Mrs Beth J 898 Watertown Street, West Newton, MA 02165-2108, (617) 965-7877, BS 74 Emerson Coll; ME 77 Northeastern Univ; Sp/Lang Path, Cambridge Pub Schs, **SLP**

Noe, Elizabeth Ann Route 2 Box 27, Harrisburg, AR 72432, (501) 578-5420, BS 66 AR St Univ; MS 85 AR St Univ; 85–Sp-Lang Path, East AR Reg Mental Hlth Ctr, **SLP**

Noe, Lana C P O Box 1144, Somerset, KY 42501-6044, (606) 679-7439, BA 70 Univ of KY; MA 71 Univ of KY; MA 72 Univ of KY; Sp-Lang Path, Lana Noe Sp-Lang Path, **SLP ACE**

Noehr, Mrs Bonnie B 17445 Pleasant View Avenue, Monte Sereno, CA 95030, (408) 354-3223, BS 68 PA St Univ - Univ Park; MA 69 Western MI Univ; Sp-Lang Path, Santa Clara Co Supt of Sch, **SLP**

Noel, Helen Patricia 4745 West Braddock Road, Apartment 101, Alexandria, VA 22311, (703) 845-3792, BS 78 CA Univ of PA; ME 81 Univ of Pittsburgh - Pittsburgh; MS 86 CA Univ of PA; 87–Sp-Lang Path, Fairfax County PS, **SLP**

Noel, Mrs Kristine Karen 705 West 8th, Silver City, NM 88061, (505) 537-3378, BA 83 Carroll Coll; MS 86 Univ of Redlands; SLP, Cobre Schl Dstr, **SLP**

Noel, Penny Kay 518 North Lindsey Avenue, Miamisburg, OH 45342, (513) 866-0369, BS 73 Miami Univ - Oxford; MS 87 Miami Univ - Oxford; 74–Sp-Lang Path, Beavercreek Schs, **SLP**

Noell, Elizabeth 7013 Ridge #1W, Chicago, IL 60645, (312) 441-9300, BS 72 Saint Louis Univ; MA 74 Saint Louis Univ; PH 80 (Learning Disabilities) Northwestern Univ; 84–Dir, Cove Sch, **SLP**

Noeth, Mrs Carolyn Frances 1849 Walnut Circle, Northbrook, IL 60062, (312) 272-6171, BA 63 Case Western Reserve Univ; ME 72 Univ of IL - Urbana; 84–Sp-Lang Path, Early Retiree Prog, **SLP ACE**

Nofal, Mrs Charlotte 6201 South Narragansett, Chicago, IL 60638, (312) 229-1016, BA 77 Coll of Saint Francis; MS 78 Bradley Univ; Sp-Lang Path, J Sterling Morton High, **SLP**

Noffsinger, Dr P Douglas 2814 Lambert Drive, Hollywood Hills, CA 90068-2323, (213) 824-3100, BA 64 Univ of Northern CO; MA 65 Northwestern Univ; PH 68 (Aud) Northwestern Univ; Ch Aud/Sp-Lang Path, VA Med Cen W La, **A**

Nofrey, Mrs Linda R 180 Brandt Street, Oak View, CA 93022, (805) 649-9771, BA 64 San Jose St Univ; SLP, Ventura USD, **SLP**

Noga, Alicia S 1902 Talon, Friendswood, TX 77546, (713) 996-7946, BS 75 Stephen F Austin St Univ; MS 77 Univ of North TX; Sp-Lang Path, Clear Creek ISD, **SLP**

Noh, Judy L 98-1072 Iliee Street, Aiea, HI 96701, (808) 488-9653, BA 79 Univ of CO - Boulder; MS 81 Western OR St Coll; Sp-Lang Path, **SLP**

Noha, Martha H P O Box 914, Eldridge, CA 95431, (707) 938-6472, BA 80 San Francisco St Univ; MS 81 San Francisco St Univ; Aud, Sonoma Developmental Center, **A**

Nojiri, Mrs Georgianne Hirota 4901 Chase, Downers Grove, IL 60515, (312) 448-6520, BS 79 Univ of IL - Urbana; MS 80 Univ of IL - Urbana; Sp-Lang Path, Lt Jos P Kennedy Sch Except Ch, **SLP**

Nolan, Barbara L 6877 Highland Road, Loomis, CA 95650, (916) 652-5228, BA 73; MS 79; **SLP**

Nolan, Brian Christophe Rd 1 Box 1379, Stroudsburg, PA 18360, (717) 424-5531, BS 70 Gannon Univ; ME 74 Bloomsburg Univ of PA; Owner-Aud, Private Practice, **A**

Nolan, Mrs Carol H 442 South Bennett, Palatine, IL 60067, (312) 934-0788, BA 72 Creighton Univ; MA 73 Univ of IL - Urbana; Sp-Lang Path, Private Practice, **SLP**

Nolan, Joan T c/o Pocono Medical Center, 206 East Brown Street, East Stroudsburg, PA 18301, (717) 421-4000, BS 75 East Stroudsburg Univ of PA; MS 77 Univ of WI - Madison; ME 83 East Stroudsburg Univ of PA; Sp-Lang Path, Private Practice, **SLP**

Nolan, Judith Anne 3636 West Eighty First St, Chicago, IL 60652, (312) 735-3040, BA 84 Saint Xavier Coll; OM 86 Governors St Univ; **SLP**

Nolan, Mrs Laurie Jean 209 East Washington Street, Carlinville, IL 62626, (217) 436-2442, BS 82 Western IL Univ; MA 83 Western IL Univ; Sp-Lang Path, Northwestern Elem Sch, **SLP**

Nolan, Lori A 204 5th Avenue North, Yorkton, SK, Canada S3N 0Z6, (306) 786-1609, BA 85 Minot St Univ; OM 86 Minot St Univ; **SLP**

Nolan, Steven C 6877 Highland Road, Loomis, CA 95650, (916) 973-7995, BA 73 CA St Univ - Fresno; MA 75 CA St Univ - Fresno; Aud, Kaiser Foundation Hosp, **A**

Nold, Anna M 96 Bradwood Road, Buffalo, NY 14224

Nold, Mrs Sally Smith 1281 Borough Court, Wheaton, IL 60187, (312) 668-8065, BS 70 CO St Univ; MS 72 Univ of Denver; **SLP**

Nolen, Bonnie Lynn UAB Audiology Service, Surgery Outpatient Clinic, 1813 Sixth Avenue South, Birmingham, AL 35294, (205) 934-9782, BS 83 Univ of Montevallo; MS 85 Univ of Montevallo; 86–Aud, Univ of AL Birminham, **A**

Nolen, Mrs Cynthia Alice 223 Palm Drive, Marlin, TX 76661, (817) 883-5819, BS 83 OK St Univ; MA 85 OK St Univ; 88–Sp-Lang Path, Marlin ISD, **SLP**

Nolen, Dr Jo Carol 205 Belle Meade Boulevard, Thibodaux, LA 70301, (504) 446-8111, BS 67 Stephen F Austin St Univ; MA 69 Memphis St Univ; PH 77 Univ of OK Medical Center; Assoc Prof, Nicholls State U, **SLP**

Nolin, Martha J 715 31st Street, Phenix City, AL 36867, (205) 297-8482, BS 80 Auburn Univ - Auburn; MS 82 Auburn Univ - Auburn; Sp-Lang Path, Phenix Cty Bd of Ed, **SLP**

Nolin, Mrs Traci E F 4280 Via Arbolada #318, Los Angeles, CA 90042, (818) 894-4588, BA 82 Univ of CA - Santa Barbara; MA 86 San Diego St Univ; 86–Aud, Auditory Vestibular Ctr

Noll, Heather Alise 825 South High Street, West Chester, PA 19382, (215) 696-1279, BA 78 Univ of Pittsburgh - Pittsburgh; MA 81 Univ of Pittsburgh - Pittsburgh; Sp-Lang Path, Neuro-Care Consultants, **SLP**

Noll, Dr J Douglas Purdue University, Audiology & Speech Science, West Lafayette, IN 47907, (317) 494-3823, BS 52 Univ of IL - Urbana; MA 56 Univ of IA; PH 60 (Sp Path) Univ of IA; 62–Prof, Prudue Univ, **SLP F ACE**

Noll, Paula Jodoin P O Box 664, 12 Fairview Avenue, Nassau, NY 12123, (518) 325-4471, BS 84 Coll of Saint Rose; ME 86 Coll of Saint Rose; 85–Sp-Lang Path, Copoke-Taconic Hills Cen Sch Dist, **SLP**

Nollau, Mrs Michaela K 638 South Berry Road, St Louis, MO 63122-4857, BS 75 Univ of MO - Columbia; MS 77 Fontbonne Coll; Sp-Lang Path, Pediatric Neurology, **SLP**

Nollkamper, Linda K 1470 Flintridge Court, Eugene, OR 97401, (913) 383-9014, BA 75 Univ of NE - Lincoln; MA 78 Univ of KS; **SLP**

Nondorf, Sandra B 12201 Quail Creek Road, Oklahoma City, OK 73120, (405) 751-9141, BA 70 Univ of OK - Norman; MA 71 Univ of OK - Norman; **SLP**

Nonis, Mrs Carol J 148 Wildflower Drive, Cranston, RI 02920, (401) 943-5593, BA 72 Boston Coll; MS 74 Univ of RI; Sp-Lang Path, Cranston Cen for Ret Citzns, **SLP**

Nonnenkamp, Lucy 2232 Northeast Flanders, Portland, OR 97232, (503) 233-5631, BS 72 Saint Louis Univ; MA 73 Saint Louis Univ; Res Assoc, Kaiser Permanente Hlth Care, **SLP**

Noodell, Marcy Anne 7415 Grant , Apt #12, Omaha, NE 68134, (402) 391-1328, OB 85 Univ of KS; MS 87 Univ of NE - Lincoln; 87–Sp-Lang Path, Sp Rehab Services PC, **SLP**

Noon, Gary C Head & Neck Surgical Assoc, 6724 Troost, Suite 200, Kansas City, MO 64131, (816) 333-6996, BS 70 ND St Univ; MA 71 OH Univ - Athens; Aud, Head Neck Surg Assoc, **A**

Noonan, Catherine L 342 Mira Flores, Camarillo, CA 93010, (805) 526-0200, BA 70 Univ of Redlands; ME 73 San Jose St Univ; Sp-Lang Path, Simi Valley USD, **SLP**

Noonan, Mrs Krista Weinhold 3537 West Mandalay Lane, Phoenix, AZ 85023, (602) 994-9321, MA 84 Saint Louis Univ; BA 80 Valparaiso Univ; SLP, Palo Alto Presch, **SLP**

Noonan, Mrs Mary Beth 6204 Chowen Avenue South, Edina, MN 55410, (612) 922-3385, BA 70 Saint Cloud St Univ; MA 76 Mankato St Univ; **SLP**

Noonan, Mary Katherine 55 Bartlett Avenue, Pittsfield, MA 01201, (802) 773-1940, BS 78 Univ of MA - Amherst; MS 81 Columbia Univ Teachers Coll; Sp/Lang Path, Pittsfield School System, **SLP**

Noone, Mrs Romney M 215 La Fayette Street, Harrisburg, PA 17109, BS 78 SUNY - Coll at Geneseo; MA 83 Bowling Green St Univ; Sp/Lang Path, Homer Cen Sch, **SLP**

Nooney, Mary-Jo 323 Dumbarton Road, Baltimore, MD 21212, (301) 363-2758, BA 78 Loyola Coll; MS 79 Loyola Coll; Sp-Lang Path, Rosewood Cen MD, **SLP**

Noplock, Marie L 115 Fulford Avenue, Bel Air, MD 21014, (301) 836-8159, BA 70 Loyola Coll; ME 71 Univ of VA - Charlottesville; Pvt Prac Dir, Speech Path & Rehab Ctr, **SLP ACE**

Norbash, Mrs Sherrie L Ear Nose & Throat Clinic, 4255 Venetian Lane, Fayetteville, AR 72703, (501) 521-1238, BS 79 Univ of TX - Austin; MS 81 Univ of North TX; 81–Aud, ENT Cl, **A**

Norberg, Diane 628 34th Avenue N E, Great Falls, MT 59404, BA 83 Univ of ND; MS 84 Minot St Univ; Sp-Lang Path, Grand Rapids PS, **SLP**

Norbury, Aaron William 4185 Smoke Tree Way, Waterford, MI 48095, (313) 623-9451, BA 39 Wayne St Univ; MA 41 Wayne St Univ; **SLP LM**

Nordahl-Aldape, Carol A 2011 Crucero Avenue, San Pablo, CA 94806, (415) 237-7257, MS 88 CA St Univ - Hayward; 88–Sp-Lang Path, Contra Costa Co Off of Educ

Nordell, Christine Allen 35 Hearthside Lane, Proctor, MN 55810, (218) 722-6343, BA 69 Univ of Redlands; MS 70 Univ of WI - Madison; Sp-Lang Path, Duluth Pub Sch, **SLP**

Nordheim, Mrs Lee T 1164 Roycott Way, San Jose, CA 95125, (408) 266-7649, BA 62 San Jose St Univ; **SLP LM**

Nording, Lori J 1808 East Wood Place #303, Shorewood, WI 53211, (414) 342-8255, BS 77 Univ of WI - Madison; MS 79 Univ of WI - Madison; Aud, Drs Fox Friedman & Kleiner, **A**

Nordlinger, Vivian M 222 Barclay Circle, Cheltenham, PA 19012, **SLP**

Nordloh, Mrs Sharon J Route 3 Box 235-1A-107, Calvert City, KY 42029, (502) 395-5278, BS 85 Eastern KY Univ; MA 87 Univ of Cincinnati; 88–Sp-Lang Path, Cane Creek Ctr/Rebound Inc, **SLP**

Nordman, Donna Lee 617 Sky Circle, Altus, OK 73521, (405) 482-2007, BA 84 Univ of OK - Norman; MS 86 Univ of North TX; 86, Dr Foster, **SLP**

Nordmeyer, Valerie Marie 821 Lebanon Street Upper, Aurora, IL 60505, (312) 844-0929, BS 82 Bradley Univ; MS 84 Bradley Univ; 87–Sp-Lang Path, Excellcare Rehab Inc, **SLP**

Nordquist, Carol L 705 Grant, Iowa City, IA 52240, (319) 353-6169, BA 54 Grinnell Coll; MA 59 Univ of IA; 72–Sp-Lang Path, U of Iowa Hosp & Clinics, **SLP**

Nordsiek, Mrs Sari Biddle 13 Oak Glen Drive, Frazer, PA 19355, (215) 296-8455, BS 80 WV Univ; MS 81 WV Univ; Aud, ENT Assoc of Wayne, **A**

Nordstrom, Mrs Judy A 937 West Southern Avenue, South Williamsport, PA 17701, (718) 323-8441, BS 77 Bloomsburg Univ of PA; MS 78 Bloomsburg Univ of PA; Sp-Lang Path, Blast Iu #17 Williamsport, **SLP**

Nordstrom, Patricia Torri Professional Hearing Services, 8803 North Meridian Street, Suite 220, Indianapolis, IN 46260, (317) 844-8127, BS 72 Northern IL Univ - De Kalb; MA 73 Northern IL Univ - De Kalb; Aud, Professional Hearing Services, **A**

Nordstrom, Vereen Ann 1629 West Foster Avenue, Chicago, IL 60640, (312) 831-9152, BA 64 Augustana Coll; MA 69 Northwestern Univ; OM 81 Nat'l Coll of Ed - Evanston; Sp-Lang Path/On-Site Coord, North Surburban Spec Ed Dist, **SLP**

Norfleet, Mrs Michele M 1721 Logwood Circle, Richmond, VA 23233, (804) 741-6157, BS 70 Southern IL Univ -Carbondale; MS 71 Southern IL Univ -Carbondale; SLP, Henrico Co Schs, **SLP**

Norfleet, Sheila G 818 Echo Bridge Drive, Louisville, KY 40243, (502) 245-0141, BS 85 Western KY Univ; MS 87 Univ of Louisville; 87–Sp-Lang Path, Easter Seal Hrng & Sp Ctr

Norin, Mrs Helene S R 2872 West Market Street, Akron, OH 44313, (216) 253-2221, BS 57 Case Western Reserve Univ; MA 80 Univ of Akron; Aud, Jay Norin & Assoc, **A**

Norland, Betty M 6001 Truxtun Avenue, Suite 240, Bakersfield, CA 93309, (805) 861-8255, BA 66 ID St Univ; MA 71 Univ of CA - Los Angeles; 78–Pres/Dir, Marjean Norland Speech Pathology Inc, **SLP**

Norlin, Peter F 403 Five Farms Lane, Timonium, MD 21093, (301) 494-5167, MA 74 Northwestern Univ; MS 83 Johns Hopkins Univ; PH 76 (NS) Northwestern Univ; 85–Consult, Blue Cross/Blue Shield of MD, **SLP**

Norman, Mrs Carol A 125 Wildwood Drive, Boardman, OH 44512, (216) 652-4929, BS 76 Edinboro Univ of PA; MA 81 Kent St Univ; Sp/Lang Path, Niles City Schs, **SLP**

Norman, Mrs Carol Slingerland 143 Laurel Avenue #7, Northport, NY 11768, (516) 754-0432, BS 82 SUNY - Coll at Fredonia; MS 86 Adelphi Univ; 82–Sp-Lang Path, Suffolk BOCES III, **SLP**

Norman, Elaine Marie 886 Lacon Drive, Newport News, VA 23602, (804) 826-8746, BS 77 Old Dominion Univ; MS 81 Old Dominion Univ; **SLP**

Norman, Janell B 526 East Maple, River Falls, WI 54022, (612) 293-8875, BS 68 Univ of WI - River Falls; MA 73 Northern IL Univ - De Kalb; Sp-Lang Path, St Paul Public Schools, **SLP**

Norman, Mrs Kitzi Colbert 3801 24th Avenue, Meridian, MS 39305, MS 82 Univ of MS; Sp-Lang Path, Lauderdale Co Schs, **SLP**

Norman, Laurie Ann 8142 Valley View Drive, Ypsilanti, MI 48198, (313) 782-3005, **SLP**

Norman, Michael C 210 Bragg Street, New Orleans, LA 70124, (504) 363-2299, BA 72 Nicholls St Univ; OM 76 LA St Univ - N O Medical Ctr; Prog Dir, F Edward Hebert Hosp, **SLP**

Norman, Natasha 3167 Victory Boulevard, Apartment 2-C, Staten Island, NY 10314, (814) 726-0951, BS 83 Univ of MD - College Park; MS 86 Howard Univ

Norman, Opal Jean Route 2 Box 792, Moultrie, GA 31768, (912) 324-2140, OB 82 Univ of GA; ME 83 Univ of GA; Sp-Lang Path, Colquitt Cty Bd of Educ, **SLP**

Norman, Peggy L Route 2 Box 27D, Sunman, IN 47041, (812) 654-2922, BS 79 Univ of Cincinnati; MA 81 Ball St Univ; Sp/Lang Path, Milan Comm Sch, **SLP**

Normand, Mrs Debra Ann R R 3 Box 369, North Scituate, RI 02857-9546, (401) 438-0860, BA 82 Univ of RI; MS 84 Univ of RI; SLP, Paul A Deaver State School, **SLP**

Normandeau, Ann Renee 1510 Richardson Drive, Anchorage, AK 99504, (907) 337-3875, BA 83 Univ of MT; MS 85 Univ of AZ; 88–Sp-Lang Path, SE Reg Resource Ctr, **SLP**

Norman-Murch, Dr Trudi N 5091 North Quail Run Road, Paradise Valley, AZ 85253, (602) 266-5976, BA 67 Swarthmore Coll; MA 69 Univ of Pittsburgh - Pittsburgh; PH 82 (NS) Univ of Pittsburgh - Pittsburgh; 87–Dir-Sp/Lang Svcs, Southwest Human Development, **SLP**

Norod, Mrs Carol N 5 Hamilton Avenue, Scituate, MA 02066, (617) 732-5601, MA; **A**

Noronha, Mrs Barbara Louise 2031 Fuerte Lane, Escondido, CA 92026, (619) 746-6425, BA 74 San Diego St Univ; MA 86 San Diego St Univ; 87–Sp-Lang Path, Escondido Union Elem Sch Dist, **SLP**

Noroski, Mrs Susan E 960 Hazelwood Road, Toms River, NJ 08753, (201) 240-2121, BA 75 William Paterson Coll; MA 79 Trenton St Coll; Sp-Lang Path/Superv, Early Intervention Prog Inc, **SLP**

Norris, Cathi D Box 511, Osburn, ID 83849, (208) 752-8815, BS 83 ID St Univ; MS 86 Univ of North TX; **A**

Norris, Cynthia Ferguson 300 Napoleon Road #A-5, Bowling Green, OH 43402, (419) 385-5771, OB 76 Bowling Green St Univ; MA 84 Bowling Green St Univ; SLP, Lucas Bd of Mr/Dd, **SLP**

Norris, Dia Vee 1224 SE Malden, Portland, OR 97202, (503) 283-1267, **SLP**

Norris, Mrs Diane L 617 Brian Avenue, Schaumburg, IL 60194, (312) 843-0180, BS 75 IL St Univ - Normal; MS 76 IL St Univ - Normal; **SLP**

Norris, Dr Jane C 4054 Solona Drive, Palo Alto, CA 94306, (415) 725-0616, MS 64 Univ of AZ; PH 83 (Auditory Neurophysiology) Stanford Univ; 84–Consult, Stanford U, **A**

Norris, Dr Janet A 366 Stoney Creek, Baton Rouge, LA 70808, (504) 388-3937, BA 75 Univ of NE - Lincoln; MA 76 Univ of NE - Lincoln; PH 85 (NS) Univ of NE - Lincoln; Asst Prof, Louisiana State Univ, **SLP**

Norris, Mrs Janice Sue 228 North Noble, Riley, KS 66531-9606, (913) 485-2302, **SLP**

Norris, Mrs Linda F 704 6th Avenue West, Lemmon, SD 57638-1708, (605) 374-3251, BA 76; MA 78; Teacher, Lemmon Schl Dstr, **SLP**

Norris, Mrs Marcia M 1210 Alder Tree Way #179, Sacramento, CA 95831, (916) 429-7412, BA 72 Univ of AL-Tuscaloosa; MA 76 San Jose St Univ; Comptr Tech, California Comm Coll, **SLP**

Norris, Mrs Mary P 2005 Pine Street, Harlan, IA 51537, BS 78 Univ of NE - Lincoln; MA 79 Univ of NE - Lincoln; SLP, **SLP**

Norris, Mary Velvet 2205 Dawns Pass, Knoxville, TN 37919, (615) 974-5453, BA; MS 85 Univ of TN - Knoxville; 85–Sp-Lang Path, Univ of Tennessee, **SLP**

Norris, Marylee K Miller Speech & Hearing Clinic, Texas Christian University, 5728 Wedgworth Road, Fort Worth, TX 76133, (817) 921-7620, OB 45 Univ of TX - Austin; MA 70 TX Christian Univ; Asst Prof, Miller Sp & Hrng Cl, **SLP**

Norris, Michael L 3129 Widgeon Avenue, Louisville, KY 40213, (502) 636 7188, BA 69 Memphis St Univ; OM 72; MS 80 Univ of Louisville; Aud, Private Practice, **A**

Norris, Michelle Marie 12 Blackwood Street #B-8, Boston, MA 02115, (617) 593-2727, BS 84 Univ of CA - Berkeley; MS 86 Boston Univ; **SLP**

Norris, Mrs Patricia Brown 3672 South Wedgewood Road, Salt Lake City, UT 84106, (801) 262-0550, BS 76 Univ of UT; MS 87 Univ of UT; 88–Sp-Lang Path, Granite Sch Dist

Norris, Paulette B 6733 South Crandon, Chicago, IL 60649, (312) 667-3488, BA 70 Southern IL Univ -Carbondale; MA 75 Governors St Univ; Sp-Lang Path, Chicago Bd of Ed, **SLP**

Norris, Dr Thomas W 8601 West Dodge Road #18, Omaha, NE 68114-3495, (402) 391-3982, BA 52 Fairmont St Coll; MA 57 WV Univ; PH 62 (Aud) Wayne St Univ; President, Private Practice, **SLP A**

Norris, Wendy Elaine 14030 Morrison St, Sherman Oaks, CA 91423, (818) 990-0859, BA 78 Univ of CA - Santa Barbara; MA 80 Univ of CO - Boulder; 88–Sp-Lang Path, Carondelet Rehab Centers of America, **SLP**

Norrix, James M 14 Bedford Court, Delmar, NY 12054, (518) 439-5361, BS 53 Western MI Univ; MS 58 Univ of UT; **SLP LM**

Norsigian, Mrs Deirdre Doran 13 Kimberly Court, Twin Lake, Clifton Park, NY 12065, (518) 584-0578, BS 86 Worcester St Coll; MA 87 Ball St Univ; 88–Aud, Saratoga Speech Hrng Ctr, **A**

North, Elise Ann Rd #1 Box 92, Fallentimber, PA 16639, (412) 349-2445, BS 84 Indiana Univ of PA; ME 86 James Madison Univ; **A**

North, Janice Carol P O Box 10, Brandon, MS 39042, (601) 939-8640, BS 84 Univ Southern MS-Hattiesburg; MS 86 Univ Southern MS-Hattiesburg

North, Mrs Kay Smith 1532 West Orchid Lane, Phoenix, AZ 85021, (602) 944-7486, BS 54 Washington Univ; MA 57 Washington Univ; Sp-Lang Path, Phoenix Un Hs Dist, **SLP A**

North, Susan Deary Route 3 Box 206, Brattleboro, VT 05301, (802) 257-0621, BA 75 CT Coll; ME 78 Northeastern Univ; Sp-Lang Path, Keene New Hampshire Sch Dis, **SLP**

Northcutt, Jana L H 1332 North Gow, Wichita, KS 67213, (316) 263-8733, BA 81 Wichita St Univ; MA 82 Wichita St Univ; Sp-Lang Path, Private Practice, **SLP**

Northern, Dr Jerry L Univ Colorado Health Sciences, Box B-210 4200 East 9th, Denver, CO 80262, (303) 270-7856, MS 63 Gallaudet Coll; MA 64 Univ of Denver; PH 66 (Aud) Univ of CO - Boulder; 70–Head Aud Div, U of CO Hlth Sci Cen, **A F**

Northern, Mrs Sandra W 1904 Fox Trail, Benton, AR 72015, (501) 778-1778, BA 79 Univ of AR - Little Rock; MS 81 Univ of AR - Little Rock; Sp-Lang Path, Private Practice, **SLP**

Northfield, Mrs Jeanne S R 1044 Loraine, Enumclaw, WA 98022, (206) 825-4844, BA 74 Univ of MT; MA 76 Univ of MT; **SLP**

Northrup, Barbara K 779 South Cassingham Road, Columbus, OH 43209, (614) 294-6403, BS 75 OH St Univ; MA 78 OH St Univ; SLP Prog Dev Spec, Columbus Sp & Hrng Cen, **SLP**

Northrup, Mrs Briseida D Callier Center, 1966 Inwood Road, Dallas, TX 75235, (214) 905-3000, BS 75 Bradley Univ; MS 77 Bradley Univ; 79–Aud, Callier Cen, **A**

Northrup, Peggy Oevering 1265 2nd Street S W, Huron, SD 57350, (605) 352-3005, MA 87 Univ of SD - Springfield; Sp-Lang Path, Huron PS, **SLP**

Northway, Nancy Ann 26160 West 12 Mile #C26, Southfield, MI 48034, (313) 541-0100, BA 80 Univ of MI - Ann Arbor; MS 83 Univ of MI - Ann Arbor; 83–Aud, ENT Surgical Assoc, **A**

Norton, Claire Margaret 227 Church Street, Mountain View, CA 94041, (415) 948-6834, BA 85 Univ of CA - Santa Barbara; MS 88 San Francisco St Univ

Norton, Darryl E 14946 Wellwood Road, Silver Spring, MD 20904, (301) 384-5483, BS 67 Southern IL Univ -Carbondale; MS 69 Southern IL Univ -Carbondale; PH 73 (NS) Univ of Pittsburgh - Pittsburgh; Sp-Lang Path, Commun Skills Consultants Inc, **SLP**

Norton, Heidi Lynn 35 Pinewood Drive, P O Box 276, Cumberland Center, ME 04021, (207) 829-6286, MA 88 OH Univ - Athens

Norton, Jennifer Salka 3327 Bryden Court, Lewiston, ID 83501, (208) 746-0838, BA 80 Univ of the Pacific; MS 82 ID St Univ; 87–Sp-Lang Path, Private Practice, **SLP ACE**

Norton, Kathleen Marie 5037 Chippewa, St Louis, MO 63109, (314) 946-6546, BS 82 Saint Louis Univ; MA 84 Saint Louis Univ; 86–Coord-SLP, United Services Inc, **SLP**

Norton, Kathryn A J 109 Espana Park, Waveland, MS 39576, (604) 865-3030, BA 76 Humboldt St Univ; MS 86 Univ Southern MS-Hattiesburg; Sp-Lang Path, Sun Coast Ctr for Rehab, **SLP**

Norton, Mrs Lynette A North 15320 Sheridan St, Mead, WA 99021-9562, (509) 455-4927, MS 87 Eastern WA Univ; Sp-Lang Path, Sacred Heart Medical Center, **SLP**

Norton, Mrs Margaret S Hearing Speech & Language Serv, 1044 Smithfield Avenue, Lincoln, RI 02865, (401) 725-5798, BA 73 Univ of VA - Charlottesville; ME 74 Univ of VA - Charlottesville; Vice Pres, Hrng Sp & Lang Serv, **SLP**

Norton, Dr Max C 5766 Stoddard Road, Modesto, CA 95356, BA 52 Univ of the Pacific; MA 55 Univ of the Pacific; PH 62 (NS) Univ of Denver; Total Learning & Counselng Cen, **SLP LM**

Norton, Mrs Nan C 446 North Hambden Street, Chardon, OH 44024, (216) 286-6131, BA 67 Elmira Coll; ME 70 SUNY - Coll at Geneseo; Sp-Lang Path, Private Practice, **SLP**

Norton, Norma Bain 5433 Shirley Avenue, Tarzana, CA 91356, (818) 342-4341, BA 54 Univ of CA - Los Angeles; MA 59 Univ of CA - Los Angeles; Consult, Aural Rehab Consultn, **SLP A**

Norton, Mrs Pamela G 1105 Jalna #1108, London, ON, Canada N6E 2S9, (519) 451-1990, BA 74 Northern MI Univ; MA 76 Northern MI Univ; Sp/Lang Path, Bd of Educ for City of London, **SLP**

Norton, Mrs Patricia R PO Box 144, Marion Junction, AL 36759, (205) 874-1625, BA 61 Vanderbilt Univ; MS 84 Univ of Montevallo; Sp-Lang Path, Bd of Ed-Selma, **SLP**

Norton, Robert Gerard 1044 Smithfield Avenue, Lincoln, RI 02865, (401) 725-5798, BA 72 Univ of MA - Amherst; MS 73 Univ of WI - Madison; 78–Dir President Aud/Sp-Lang Path, Hrng Sp & Lan Serv, **SLP A**

Norton, Mrs Robin Kellogg 1409 Lion Road, St Joseph, MO 64506, (816) 364-4502, BS 78 Northwest MO St Univ; MA 79 Univ of IL - Urbana; Sp/Lang Path, Private Practice, **SLP**

Norton, Mrs Sherri Lynnette P O Box 9, Carney, OK 74832-0009, (405) 649-2585, BS 83 Central St Univ; MA 86 OK St Univ; **SLP**

Norton, Dr Susan Joy Univ Of Kansas Medical Center, Dept Of Hearing & Speech, 326 HC Miller Bldg, Kansas City, KS 66103, (402) 449-6599, BA 71 Univ of Denver; MS 73 Purdue Univ - West Lafayette; PH 82 (NS) Univ of WA; Assistant Professor, University of Kansas, **A**

Norton-Darr, Sally Box 441, Mine Road, Asbury, NJ 08802, (201) 735-4031, BS 74 PA St Univ - Univ Park; MS 77 PA St Univ - Univ Park; Sp-Lang Path, Hunterdon Dev Cen, **SLP**

Norton-Kavanaugh, Carol Eye And Ear Clinic, 600 Orondo, P O Box 3027, Wenatchee, WA 98801, (509) 662-7143, BA 74 Western WA Univ; MA 78 Western WA Univ; Aud, Eye & Ear Cl of Wenatchee, **A**

Norvell, Beth Ann Frisk 2709 Floyd Avenue, Richmond, VA 23220, (804) 358-3224, BS 84 Univ of VA - Charlottesville; MA 85 George Washington Univ; 88–Sp-Lang Path, Virginia Rehab Svcs Inc, **SLP**

Norvid, Gail S 9645 Baymeadows Road #916, Jacksonville, FL 32216, (813) 586-6622

Norwood, Mrs Ann M Cheyenne Center For Comm Dis, 1801 Logan Avenue, Cheyenne, WY 82001, (307) 637-8281, BS 74 CO St Univ; MS 76 CO St Univ; Sp-Lang Path Dir, Cheyenne Cen Commun Dis, **SLP**

Norwood, Elena D 6102 East Joan de Arc, Scottsdale, AZ 85254, (602) 996-4965, **SLP**

Norwood, Phyllis Lloyd 2346 Stone Street Extension, Mebane, NC 27302, (919) 229-4893, BS 84 Univ of NC - Greensboro; MA 85 Univ of NC - Greensboro; Sp-Lang Path, Alamance Health Services, **SLP**

Norwood, Reed 100 West 4th Street, Cookeville, TN 38501, (615) 528-1575, BS 76 Eastern NM Univ; MA 79 Univ of TN - Knoxville; Aud, Upper Cumberland Otol Cl, **A**

Norwood, Thomas J Evergreen Speech & Hearing Clinic, 12034 N E 130th Lane, Suite 203, Kirkland, WA 98034, (206) 821-3747, BA 75 Univ of WA; OM 76 Univ of WA; President /Aud, Evergreen Sp & Hrng Cl, **A**

Noska, Mrs La Vonne I 1 Heritage Drive, Springfield, IL 62704, (217) 525-3060, BS 67 Univ of NE - Lincoln; MA 69 Univ of NE - Lincoln; Dept Head Sp-Lang Path, Springfield Pub Sch Dist 186, **SLP**

Notarianni, Julia 8125-A Lawson Loop, Fort Meade, MD 20755, (301) 242-9010, BS West Chester Univ of PA; MS Old Dominion Univ; 86–Sp-Lang Path, UCP Central MD Inc, **SLP**

Notbohm, Heidi L 641 Piper Drive, Madison, WI 53711, (608) 271-7527, BS 79 Univ of WI - Madison; MS 81 Univ of WI - Madison; 85–Sp-Lang Path, Waunakee Pub Schs, **SLP**

Notestine, Patricia Eireen 110 South Shore Drive, Clear Lake, IA 50428, (515) 357-6125, **SLP**

Notestine, Mrs Patricia I 1420 Wreath, Manhattan, KS 66502, (913) 539-4341, BA 57 Univ of IL - Urbana; MA 72 Univ of MO - Columbia; 74–Sp-Lang Path, USD #383, **SLP**

Notor, Nancy Schell 1548 Arata Court, San Jose, CA 95125, (408) 947-8635, BA 73 Univ of CA - Santa Cruz; MS 80 Univ of AZ; Aud, Ear Medical Clinic, **A**

Nott, Mrs Jane Richards 1609 Briarcrest Road, Bryan, OH 43506, (419) 636-4517, BS 62 Western MI Univ; Sp-Lang Path, Maumee Valley Sp & Hrng, **SLP**

Notte, Mrs Michele T Fredonia State College, Thompson Hall, Fredonia, NY 14063, (716) 673-3203, BS 66 SUNY - Coll at Fredonia; MS 71 SUNY - Coll at Fredonia; Cl Coord, NY St U Coll-Fredonia, **SLP**

Notton, Mrs Janet M 580 South Wall Street, Kankakee, IL 60901, (815) 939-3651, BA 79 Univ of Northern IA; MA 81 Univ of Northern IA; Sp-Lang Path, AR Spec Ed Co-Op, **SLP**

Nousak, Jo Manette K 47 East 3rd Street #6, New York, NY 10003, (718) 780-1498, BA 75 Cleveland St Univ; MA 76 Memphis St Univ; 86–Supvr-Hearing Aid Dispensary, L I College Hosp, **A**

Novack, Evelyn B 410 Noble Street 1st Floor, Souderton, PA 18964, (215) 539-8550, BA 78 Temple Univ-Tyler Sch of Art; MA 81 West Chester Univ of PA; SLP, Montgy Co Inter Unit #23, **SLP ACE**

Novack, Dr Harry S 124 Blackstone Boulevard, Providence, RI 02906, (401) 421-8536, BA 48 Emerson Coll; MA 53 Northwestern Univ; PH 58 (Ed Psych) Syracuse Univ; Retired, **SLP LM**

Novack, Lesley L 28 Sellers Avenue, Lexington, VA 24450, **SLP**

Novak, Barbara A 6986 Cimarron Drive S E, Grand Rapids, MI 49506, (616) 942-2109, BA 76 Univ of CO - Boulder; MA 79 Wichita St Univ; Sp-Lang Path, Mary Free Bed Hosp, **SLP**

Novak, Constance W 10152 Dreyfus, Scottsdale, AZ 85260, (313) 762-2362, BA 67 MI St Univ; OM 84 Central MI Univ; MA 68 MI St Univ; **SLP**

Novak, Denise Foss Carle Clinic Assoc, 602 West University Avenue, Urbana, IL 61801, (217) 337-3130, OB 71 OH St Univ; MA 85 Univ of IL - Urbana; Aud, Carle Cl Assoc, **A**

Novak, Ellen Sue 754 Stonegate Drive, Highland Park, IL 60035, (312) 890-8000, BS 84 Univ of WI - Madison; MA 85 Northwestern Univ; **SLP**

Novak, Mrs Janet Eaton 214 North Bierman, Villa Park, IL 60181, (312) 531-3771, BA 80 Elmhurst Coll; MS 82 Rush Univ; Sp/Lang Path, McGaw Hosp/Loyola U, **SLP**

Novak, Mrs Janet Lynn W Meddac Wurzburg, Box 213, APO New York, NY 09801, BS 79 James Madison Univ; MS 80 James Madison Univ; **SLP**

Novak, Mrs Karen R J 7809 Laurel Leaf Drive, Potomac, MD 20854, BA 70 Univ of KY; ME 76 GA St Univ; Sp-Lang Path, Montgomery Co Pub Sch, **SLP**

Novak, Marie M 1407 Windermere Road, Windsor, ON, Canada N8Y 3G1, (519) 255-7018, BA 73 Univ of Windsor - Ontario; MA 77 Wayne St Univ; 85–Sp-Lang Path, Children's Achievement Ctr, **SLP**

Novak, Robert E 7497 Gorge View Terrace, San Diego, CA 92120, PH (NS); **A**

Novak, Mrs Tranette M 1360 Hollyview Drive, Vermillion, OH 44089, (216) 967-8687, BA 77 OH St Univ; MA 79 OH St Univ; **SLP**

Novak, William Michael 16 Powderview Court, Baltimore, MD 21236, (301) 488-5915, BA 85 Loyola Coll; MS 87 Loyola Coll; 87–Sp-Lang Path, Baltimore County PS, **SLP**

Novakoski, William E 8 South Wynwyd Drive, Newark, DE 19711, (301) 398-0400, BS 73 Clarion Univ of PA; ME 74 Clarion Univ of PA; ES 81 Indiana Univ of PA; 81–Psychologist, Bd of Ed-Cecil Co, **SLP**

Novakovich, Harriet V 180 Fleetwood Terrace, Silver Spring, MD 20910, (301) 649-0223, BS 57 Southern IL Univ -Carbondale; MS 58 Southern IL Univ -Carbondale; OM 88 Johns Hopkins Univ; Computer Spec, Ivymount Sch, **SLP**

Novak-Szarek, Mrs Jean M 554 26th Avenue #4, San Francisco, CA 94121, (415) 221-0193, BA 78 CA St Univ - Fresno; MA 80 CA St Univ - Fresno; 87–Lecturer, San Fran State Univ, **SLP**

Novegrod, Mrs Marcia Kessert 20 Sycamore Creek, Irvine, CA 92715, (714) 833-8984, BA 67 CUNY - Hunter Coll; MA 68 NY Univ; **SLP**

Novell, Kathleen McGann 1978 Midlothian Drive, Altadena, CA 91001, (818) 359-5598, BA 81 Whittier Coll; MA 86 Whittier Coll; **SLP**

Novelli, Janine H 18345 Outer Drive, Dearborn, MI 48128, (313) 832-1100, MA 79 Eastern MI Univ; Sp-Lang Path, Detroit Inst for Chldrn, **SLP ACE**

Novelli, Patsy Grissom Studio 124-Audiology, 124 E Tennessee Street, Florence, AL 35630, (205) 764-4327, BA 67 Univ of Northern AL; MA 70 Univ of AL- Tuscaloosa; Aud, Studio 124, **A**

November, Mrs Ronni 150 Hartford Lane, Newtown, PA 18940, (609) 896-9500, BA 78 Univ of MA - Amherst; MA 80 George Washington Univ; Sp-Lang Path, St Lawerence Rehab Cen, **SLP**

Novetsky, Paula Rosner 21210 Potomac, Southfield, MI 48076, (313) 352-2650, BA 74 OH St Univ; MS 76 Univ of MI - Ann Arbor; Audiologist, Seth Cohen MD P C, **A**

Novina, Joan 8327 South Strub Avenue, Whittier, CA 90605, (213) 803-8324, BA 52 William Jewell Coll; MA 61 Whittier Coll; Consultant, LA Cty Supt Schs, **SLP**

Novinska, Mrs Deirdre A N5002 Ball Park Drive, Medford, WI 54451, (715) 748-5572, BA 82 Univ of WI - Eau Claire; MS 83 Univ of WI - Eau Claire; 85–Sp-Lang Path, Medford Public School District, **SLP**

Novosel, Lorna M 809-610 Lake Street, St Catharines, ON, Canada L2N 5T1, (416) 937-4961, BA 76; OB 77; OM 82 Univ of Western Ontario; 86–Sp-Lang Path, Lincoln Co Bd of Educ, **SLP**

Novotny, Ann Marie 1925 Bonnie Lane, #407, Waukesha, WI 53188, (414) 691-2100, BS 82 Marquette Univ; MS 83 Marquette Univ; Sp-Lang Path, Lake Country Excep Educ Coop, **SLP**

Novy, Fred John 4608 East Piedmont Road, Phoenix, AZ 85044, (602) 264-6139, BA 75 Univ of IA; MS 79 Univ of WI - Stevens Point; Owner/Audiologist, Phoenix Hearing Aid Center Inc, **A**

Nowak, Gwen F 941 Avenue E N W, Great Falls, MT 59404, BA 81 Univ of SD - Vermillion; MA 82 Univ of SD - Vermillion; Sp-Lang Path, Great Falls Pub Sch, **SLP ACE**

Nowak, Michele A 3607 49th Street N W #201, Calgary, AB, Canada T3A 2H3, (403) 229-7060, BS 78 Univ of WI - Stevens Point; MS 80 CO St Univ; Sp/Lang Path, Alberta Chldn's Hosp, **SLP**

Nowak, Mrs Patricia L Rd 2 Box 264, Stony Ford Road, Campbell Hall, NY 10916, (914) 294-8390, BA 70 Temple Univ; MS 72 William Paterson Coll; **SLP**

Nowalk, Barbara Covert 26 Reler Lane #C, Somerset, NJ 08873, (201) 821-4570, BS 79; MA 80 Montclair St Coll; Sp-Lang Path, Bryn Mawr Rehab Hosp, **SLP**

Nowell, Kathy Jean Route 2 Box 1032, Laurel, MS 39440, (601) 649-1805, BA 82 Univ Southern MS-Hattiesburg; MS 85 Univ Southern MS-Hattiesburg; 87–Sp-Lang Path, Jones County Sch Sys, **SLP**

Nowell, Dr Richard C Special Ed & Clinical Services, Davis Hall, Indiana, PA 15705, (412) 357-5678, BA 68 Georgetown Coll; MA 69 NY Univ; ED 76 (NS) Univ of Rochester; Asst Prof, IN U of Pa, **A**

Nowell, Mrs Susan Polk 839 Chestnut Street, Indiana, PA 15701, (814) 536-1222, BA 77 Point Park Coll; OM 81 Univ of NC - Chapel Hill

Nowikowski, Kayte 40 Citrus Court, Palm Harbor, FL 34683, (813) 784-3474, BS 71 PA St Univ - Univ Park; MS 72 PA St Univ - Univ Park; Sp-Lang Path, Private Practice, **SLP**

Nowinski, Mrs Hazel Y 1422 Vine Street, Union Grove, WI 53182, MS; **SLP LM**

Nowland, Margaret F 7232 San Diego Avenue #3, St Louis, MO 63121, (314) 867-0955, BS 68 Saint Louis Univ; MS 78 Southern IL Univ-Edwardsvill; SLP, St Louis Co Spec Sch Dist, **SLP**

Nowlin, Dr Joy O 1518 Garner Field Road, Apartment 1201, Uvalde, TX 78801, (512) 278-1823, BA 70 Our Lady Lake Univ-San Anton; MA 71 Our Lady Lake Univ-San Anton; ED 81 (Ed Psychology) Brigham Young Univ; 83–Asst Prof, Sul Ross State University, **SLP**

Noxsel, Mrs Jennifer Lee 10225 Hickory Valley Drive, Harrison, OH 45030, (513) 742-2200, BS 79 Miami Univ - Oxford; MS 81 Miami Univ - Oxford; **SLP**

Noyce, Betsy Ann P O Box 74, Lewisburg, PA 17837, (717) 742-2571, OM 87 Auburn Univ - Auburn; **SLP**

Noyer, Zama Helene P O Box 117, Ranchester, WY 82839, (307) 655-9541, BS 83 CO St Univ; MA 86 Western WA Univ; 86–Aud, Sheridan Sch Dist #1, **A**

Noyes, Joanne Gislason 1103 South Spring Street, Northfield, MN 55057, (507) 663-0670, BS 64 Univ of MN - Minneap-St Paul; OM 87 Univ of WI - River Falls; **SLP**

Noyes, Mrs MaryLou 6014 La Salle Avenue, Oakland, CA 94611, (415) 537-3000, BA 57 Univ of CA - Berkeley; MA 76 San Francisco St Univ; 73–Sp-Lang Path, Castro Valley USD, **SLP**

Nozaki, Joanne M 26105 Frampton Avenue D, Harbor City, CA 90710, BA 76 Univ of CA - Santa Barbara; MA 78 Univ of WA; SLP, LA Co Supt of Sch, **SLP**

Nozza, Robert J Childrens Hosp Of Pittsburgh, Division Of Audiology, One Childrens Place, Pittsburgh, PA 15213, (412) 647-5580, BA 68 Rutgers St Univ - Newark; MA 74 Seton Hall Univ; PH 81 (Aud) Univ of WA; 85–Dir of Aud, Chldn's Hosp of Pitt, **A**

Nuanes, Ladean 9151 East Eastman Avenue, Denver, CO 80231, (303) 755-8710, BA 67 Univ of OK - Norman; MA 70 Univ of OK - Norman; SLP, Denver Pub Sch, **SLP**

Nuck, Martha Ellen 3540 Stettinius Avenue #3, Cincinnati, OH 45208, (513) 220-2066, MA 84 Miami Univ - Oxford; 86–Sp-Lang Path, Miami Valley Hosp, **SLP**

Nuckels, Patricia M 7004 Copeleigh Road, Baltimore, MD 21212, (301) 825-0090, BA 68 Towson St Univ; MS 72 Loyola Coll; Sp-Lang Path, Balto Co Pub Schs, **SLP ACE**

Nuckols-Currence, Margaret 9543 Oldhouse Drive, Richmond, VA 23233, (804) 786-0207, BS 73 Radford Univ; ME 77 Univ of VA - Charlottesville; 86–Sp-Lang Path, Medical College of Virginia, **SLP**

Nudleman, Mrs Elisa Mitrani 8403 Manderville #1108, Dallas, TX 75231, (214) 750-1015, MS 84 Univ of TX - Dallas; **SLP**

Nudo, Dr Lawrence A 2420 North Knoxville #5, Peoria, IL 61604, (309) 693-5274, BS 54 Univ of IL - Urbana; MS 56 Univ of IL - Urbana; PH 67 (NS) Univ of IL - Urbana; Dir-Hrng & Sp Serv, G A Zeller Men Hlth Cen, **SLP A**

Nuelle, Kathleen M P O Box 342, Milford, PA 18337, (717) 296-9261, BA 78 Univ of CT; MA 80 Univ of IA; Dir of Progs, Head Injury Recovery Center, **SLP**

Nuffer, Mrs Patricia 1303 East Stone, Brenham, TX 77833, (409) 836-1580, BA 68 Valparaiso Univ; MS 75 Baylor Univ; Dir, Brenham Sp-Lang Cen, **SLP**

Nugent, Mrs Lynn B 184 Catherine Street, Lafayette, LA 70503, (318) 232-7710, MS 88 Univ of Southwestern LA

Nugent, Margaret Jo 23 Fisk Place, Avon, NY 14414, (716) 442-8580, BA 82 IN Univ - Bloomington; MS 84 Rush Univ; **SLP**

Nugent, Therese M 701 Monterey #3, Hermosa Beach, CA 90254, (213) 673-3490, BS 84 Loyola Marymount Univ; MA 87 San Diego St Univ; Sp-Lang Path, Lennox Sch Dist

Nullman, Mrs Susan L 9077 S W 117th Street, Miami, FL 33176, (305) 252-8469, BA 73 SUNY - Center at Buffalo; MA 75 SUNY - Center at Buffalo; **SLP**

Numer, Linda Jane 301 East Ogle Street #29, Ebensburg, PA 15931, (814) 472-7350, **SLP**

Nunemaker, Kathy L P O Box 12323, Boulder, CO 80303, (303) 449-8896, **SLP**

Nunez, Mrs Kaysea Copeland Route 2 Box 166-A, Picayune, MS 39466, (601) 798-9286, BA 79 Univ of Southwestern LA; OM 81 LA St Univ - N O Medical Ctr; 88–Sp-Lang Path, Picayune Sch Dist, **A**

Nunez, Lilliam 7 Lang Street #1, New Bedford, MA 02745, (508) 997-1515, BA 85; MA 88 Univ of MA - Amherst; 88–Sp-Lang Path, St Luke's Hosp

Nunez, Loretta M 3500 Hunter's Crossing Drive, Stow, OH 44224, (216) 672-2672, BA 76 OH St Univ; MA 78 OH St Univ; Instr of Aud, Kent St U, **SLP A**

Nunn, Mrs Carolyn M 6902 North Kimberly, Peoria, IL 61614, (309) 672-6557, BS 76 Bradley Univ; MS 77 Bradley Univ; Sp-Lang Path, Peoria Pub Sch Dist 150, **SLP**

Nunn, Mary P 881 North 10th Street, Apartment N, Coos Bay, OR 97420, (503) 267-5788, BS 69 OH St Univ; MS 70 Univ of MI - Ann Arbor; 85–Sp-Lang Path, Coos Co Ed Serv Dist, **SLP**

Nunn, Will Ann 1032 Eagle Drive, De Soto, TX 75115-5447, (214) 905-3033, MS 65 Hardin-Simmons Univ; OM 67 Univ of OK Medical Center; Sp-Lang Path, U of TX-Dallas, **SLP**

Nunnery, Betty D 1513 Field Cove, Plano, TX 75023, (214) 596-2300, BS 66 LA St Univ - Baton Rouge; MS 81 Univ of TX - Dallas; Sp-Lang Path, Plano ISD, **SLP**

Nunnery, Mrs Karen B 102 Fawn Trail, Lake Jackson, TX 77566, (409) 297-6932, BA 66 Our Lady Lake Univ-San Anton; MA 67 Our Lady Lake Univ-San Anton; Sp-Lang Path, Brazosport Independ Sch Dist, **SLP**

Nunn-Krieger, Barbara J 636 Lakeview, Birmingham, MI 48009, (313) 642-9593, BS 68 Univ of MI - Ann Arbor; MS 69 Univ of MI - Ann Arbor; Sp-Lang Path, Private Practice, **SLP**

Nunziata, Gale Margaret 2451 Brickell Avenue #5-G, Miami, FL 33129, (305) 285-1534, OB 82 Univ of FL; MA 84 Univ of FL; Sp-Lang Path, Dade Co Pub Schs, **SLP**

Nurick, Dr Etta-Lee K 2024 Wisteria Lane, Lafayette Hill, PA 19444, (215) 233-9559, BS 61 Temple Univ; MA 66 Temple Univ; ED 85 (NS) Temple Univ; Sp-Lang Path Superv, Montgy Co Inter Ut #23, **SLP ACE**

Nurin, Marabeth W P O Box 80, Redding Ridge, CT 06876, (802) 775-3264, BA 71 Mary Washington Coll; ME 72 Univ of VA - Charlottesville; Sp/Lang Path, Rutland S Supervisory Un, **SLP**

Nuru, Dr Njeri 1330 Geranium Street N W, Washington, DC 20012, (202) 651-5150, BA 69 Howard Univ; MA 71 Howard Univ; PH 75 (NS) Univ of MD - College Park; 87–Dean Sch of Comm, Gallaudet Univ, **A F**

Nusbaum, Mrs Gloria Shoemaker 1415 McGirr Road, Franklin Grove, IL 61031, (815) 625-0400, BS 71 Toccoa Falls Coll; BA 83 Northern IL Univ - De Kalb; MA 84 Northern IL Univ - De Kalb; **SLP**

Nusbaum-Hollenback, Mrs Janis 1865 North Sherry Drive, Atlantic Beach, FL 32233, (904) 399-6821, BS 72 Western KY Univ; MS 79 Old Dominion Univ; 83–Dir-Sp-Lang Path, Mem Reg Rehab Cen, **SLP**

Nussbaum, Mrs Debra 1403 Catlyn Place, Annapolis, MD 21401-4207, (202) 651-5274, BA 75 George Washington Univ; MA 76 George Washington Univ; Aud, Kendall Sch/Gallaudet Coll, **A**

Nussbaum, Jo Rural Route 1, Yankee Flats Road, Salmon Arm, BC, Canada V1E 4M1, (604) 228-2319, BA 67 Austin Coll; MA 72 IN Univ - Bloomington; 88–Visiting Sessional Lecturer, Univ of British Columbia, **SLP**

Nussbaum, Mary Kirby 95 Perry Street, Harrisonburg, VA 22801, (703) 433-5726, BS 80 Emerson Coll; MS 82 6839; **SLP**

Nussbaum, Rhoda Kahn 21 Lantern Lane, Weston, MA 02193, (617) 891-4992, BS 70 NY Univ; MS 78 Emerson Coll; Sp/Lang Path, Charmss Collaborative, **SLP**

Nussbaum, Mrs Susan Martin 6318 Pershing Avenue, St Louis, MO 63130-4703, (314) 821-0008, **SLP**

Nussbaumer, Mrs Carol W 1108 Martin Court, Loveland, CO 80537, (303) 669-4925, BA 67 CO St Univ; MA 83 Univ of Northern CO; Sp-Lang Path, Longmont Lrng Cen, **SLP**

Nusser, Mrs Michele J 9221 Collett Street, Sepulveda, CA 91343, (805) 947-7798, BA 74 CA St Univ - Northridge; MA 78 CA St Univ - Northridge; SLP, Los Angeles Co Supt of Sch, **SLP**

Nutley, Mrs Mandy Hubner 940 Van Buren, Dyer, IN 46311, (219) 933-2004, BS 83 Northern IL Univ - De Kalb; OM 85 Governors St Univ; 86–Sp-Lang Path, St Margaret Hosp, **SLP ACE**

Nutt, Mrs Lucille C 2856 Lamer Trace, Marietta, GA 30066, (404) 926-8136, BS 76 Univ of GA; MS 78 Univ of AL- Tuscaloosa; Sp-Lang Path, Fulton County Sch System, **SLP**

Nutt, Margaret Elizabeth 904 Pecan Street, Crosett, AR 71635, (501) 562-3040, MS 88 Univ of AR - Little Rock

Nuttall, Dawn M D 285 Shadow Lake Drive, Lilburn, GA 30247, (404) 925-9705, OB 76 Univ of GA; ME 79 GA St Univ; Sp-Lang Path, Gwinnett Co Sch Syst, **SLP**

Nuttall, Dr Edmund C Department Of Communication, University Of Oklahoma, Norman, OK 73019, (405) 325-3111, BA 50 San Diego St Univ; MA 52 Univ of Southern CA; PH 59 (NS) Univ of Southern CA; Prof, U of OK, **SLP**

Nutter, Mrs Marilyn M 110 Elk Ridge Drive, Forest, VA 24551, (804) 525-8229, OB 68 Northern IL Univ - De Kalb; MA 70 Univ of MD - College Park; Asst Prof, Liberty University, **SLP ACE**

Nutter, Mrs Susan Botts 3382 Buckhorn Drive, Lexington, KY 40515, (606) 272-5719, **SLP**

Nutter-Will, Mrs Debra Jean Rt 1 Box 163, Dallas, NC 28034, (704) 333-7107, BS 83 Appalachian St Univ; MS 84 Univ of NC - Chapel Hill; Sp-Lang Path, St Mark's Ctr-Dev Day Care, **SLP**

Nuytkens, Pamela Ann 56 Brentwood Drive, Pleasantville, NY 10570, (914) 769-5255, BS 84 Northwestern Univ; MA 85 Northwestern Univ; Sp-Lang Path, Crippled Childrens Society, **SLP**

Nuzum-Terjeson, Mrs Laurie Patricia Rt 1 Box 53, Helix, OR 97835, (503) 457-2703, BA 80 Eastern WA Univ; MS 82 Eastern WA Univ; 88–Sp-Lang Path, Umatilla Educ Svc Dist

Nyberg, Ruth M 18762 Salem #102, Lansing, IL 60438, BA 79; MS 81 IL St Univ - Normal; SLP Tm Ldr, S Metropltn Assoc, **SLP**

Nychka, Helen B 810 West Johnson Street, Raleigh, NC 27605, (919) 821-3897, BS 79 Miami Univ - Oxford; MS 82 Univ of WI - Whitewater; Sp-Lang Path, State of Norht Carolina, **SLP**

Nydam, Marion R 449 Hillsdale Avenue, Syracuse, NY 13206, (315) 437-7992, BA 71 SUNY - Center at Binghamton; MS 75 Syracuse Univ; SLP, Syracuse City School District, **SLP**

Nye, Dr Chad Dept Of Speech Pathology, Northern Arizona Univ, Box 15045, Flagstaff, AZ 86011, BA 69 Point Loma Nazarene Coll; MS 71 Eastern WA Univ; PH 84 (NS) Univ of CA - Riverside; 84–Prof, Northern Arizona Univ, **SLP**

Nye, Denita Scott 827 Jennifer Drive East, Tuscaloosa, AL 35404, (205) 345-3520, BA 82 Univ of AL- Tuscaloosa; MS 85 Univ of AL- Tuscaloosa; **SLP**

Nyenhuis, Sharon K 216 North Dellrose, Wichita, KS 67208, (316) 681-0611, BA 64 Wichita St Univ; Sp-Lang Path/Cl, Sp & Lang Serv, **SLP**

Nyer, Mrs Rochelle Rubin 5561 Kilbourne Drive, Lyndhurst, OH 44124, (216) 529-4218, BS 72 Kent St Univ; MA 84 Cleveland St Univ; Sp-Lang Path, Lakewood City Sch, **SLP**

Nygard, Joni Lea 4800 St James Drive #3, Sioux Falls, SD 57106, (605) 361-6361, BS 84 Moorhead St Univ; MS 85 Moorhead St Univ; 87–Sp-Lang Path, Crippled Childrens Hosp and Sch, **SLP**

Nyland, Mrs Christylee Kinkaid 10467 Sierra Crest Way, Rancho Cordova, CA 95670, (916) 369-2543, BA 84 CA St Univ - Chico; MA 87 CA St Univ - Chico; 88–Sp-Lang Path, Sacramento City USD, **SLP**

Nyman, Darlene Patricia 190-C Park Lake Circle, Walnut Creek, CA 94598, (415) 933-5363, BA 73 CA St Univ - Northridge; MA 83 CA St Univ - Northridge; Sp/Lang Path, Mt Diablo School District, **SLP**

Nyman, Marilyn S Communication Skills Inc, 1241 Cox Road, Rydal, PA 19046, (215) 886-2244, BA 71 George Washington Univ; ME 72 Northeastern Univ; Pres, Communication Skills Inc, **SLP**

Nyman, Mrs Peggy Graham 5526 Sylvia Avenue, Tarzana, CA 91356-3120, (818) 783-2204, BS 77 Bowling Green St Univ; MA 84 CA St Univ - Northridge; SLP, Montebello School District, **SLP**

Nypaver, Virginia Ireen 650 South Main Street #206, Oconto Falls, WI 54154, (414) 567-1133, BS 83 Towson St Univ; MS 85 Clarion Univ of PA; **SLP**

Nystrom, Dr Clarence L 919 Santa Rosa, Wheaton, IL 60187, BA 25 Greenville Coll; MA 29 Univ of IA; PH 32 (NS) Univ of IA; Retired, **SLP LM**

Nystrom, Mrs Rita Visceto Fort Hill Road, Oxford, MA 01540, (617) 764-8591, BA 73 Worcester St Coll; MS 80 Worcester St Coll; Sp-Lang Path, Southbridge Pub Sch, **SLP**

Nystrom, Mrs Sharon W 139 Donation Road, Greenville, PA 16125, (412) 588-6309, BA 73 Thiel Coll; MS 75 Univ of Pittsburgh - Pittsburgh; **SLP**

O

Oakes, Deborah K 1000 Olive Drive #38, Bakersfield, CA 93308, (805) 323-4591, BA 76 Northwestern Univ; MS 77 Univ of MI - Ann Arbor; Sp-Lang Path, Affiliated Speech Pathology, **SLP**

Oakley, Judith L 6720 N Damen Avenue #1-F, Chicago, IL 60645, (312) 878-8200, BS 84 Northwestern Univ; MA 85 Northwestern Univ; **SLP**

Oakley, Mrs Mary Ann 187 West Prospect Avenue, Pittsburgh, PA 15205, (412) 937-1125, BS 83 Marywood Coll; MA 85 Univ of Pittsburgh - Pittsburgh; 88–Research Assoc, Western Psych Inst and Clinic, **SLP**

O'Anna, Lisa Anne 1726 Slocum Street, Hewlett, NY 11557, BS 84 SUNY - Coll at Fredonia; MA 86 Hofstra Univ; 88–Sp-Lang Path, Little Village Sch, **SLP**

Oar, Judy Lee 351 South 400 East #12, St George, UT 84770, BS 83 Purdue Univ - West Lafayette; MS 85 Purdue Univ - West Lafayette; **SLP**

Oare, Katherine Adele c/o Florida Hearing Care Centers, 269 South Federal Highway, Deerfield Beach, FL 33441, (305) 426-2500, BS 79 FL Southern Coll; OM 82 Auburn Univ - Auburn; 88–Aud, Florida Hearing Care Ctrs, **A**

Oas, Mrs Donna Billington 308 Madison Street, Paw Paw, MI 49079, (616) 387-8059, BA 51 Univ of MI - Ann Arbor; MA 66 Western MI Univ; Assoc Prof, Dept Sp Path/Aud-Wn Mi U, **SLP ACE**

Oates, Kim Victoria RFD 2 Box 36-B, York, ME 03909, (207) 363-3613, MS 84 Univ of NH; 88–Sp-Lang Path, York Co Presch Svcs, **SLP**

Oates, Margaret Ann 415 East 78th Street, Apartment 4D, New York, NY 10021, (212) 605-3740, BA 80 Univ of VT; MS 82 Columbia Univ Teachers Coll; 87–Aud, Manhattan ENT, **A**

Obando, Nancy Moreno 134 Maynard Street, Glendale, CA 91205, (818) 244-4740, BS 74 Loma Linda Univ - Riverside; OM 86 Pepperdine Univ - Malibu; 74–Sp-Lang Path, LA County Office of Educ, **SLP**

O'Banion, Mrs Kathryn Lou 54 East Mistybreeze Circle, The Woodlands, TX 77381, (713) 298-1906, BA 79 Sam Houston St Univ; MA 83 Univ of CO - Boulder; Learning Disability Specialist, Conroe ISD, **SLP**

Obenberger, Nancy Ann 1026 Davenport Road #4, Plymouth, WI 53073, (505) 842-6727, BS 82 Univ of WI - Stevens Point; MS 83 Univ of WI - Whitewater; Sp-Lang Path, Sheboygan Co, **SLP**

Ober, Mrs Gail Silber 8220 North 2nd Drive, Phoenix, AZ 85021, (602) 944-5139, BA 73 Eastern MI Univ; MA 76 Univ of MI - Ann Arbor; Sp-Lang Path, Private Practice, **SLP**

Oberle, Mrs Barbara S Box 415, Kingston, RI 02881, BA 76 CUNY - Brooklyn Coll; MS 78 Univ of RI; Sp-Lang Path, Richmond School, **SLP**

Oberle, Kristina Lynn 3785 East 11th Street, Apt #103, Long Beach, CA 90804, (213) 674-7050, MS 84 Univ of IL - Urbana; BS 82 Univ of IL - Urbana; SLP, Inst Phys Medicine & Rehab, **SLP**

Oberlin, Melissa Waller Callier Cen For Comm Disorders, 1966 Inwood Road, Dallas, TX 75235, (214) 905-3000, BS 82 Southern Methodist Univ; MS 84 Univ of TX - Dallas; Aud, Callier Ctr, **A**

Obermann, C Esco 1735 Noe, San Francisco, CA 94131, PH; **SLP LM**

Oberndorfer, Adrienne P 145 West 67th Street #8D, New York, NY 10023, BS 64 OH St Univ; MS 68 Adelphi Univ; SLP, Speech Services Unit, **SLP**

Oberstein, Mrs Lori Andra 80 Village Green Way, Hazlet, NJ 07730, (718) 851-0685, BA 80 CUNY - Brooklyn Coll; MS 84 CUNY - Brooklyn Coll; SLP, New York City Bd of Education, **SLP**

Obert, Allan Dale 3300 South Tamarac Drive, Apartment D-312, Denver, CO 80231, (303) 752-1094, BA 76 Univ of Northern CO; MA 77 Univ of Northern CO; 88–Neuro Physiologist, Craig Hosp, **A**

O'Bert, Pamela A 32 South John Street, Pittsfield, MA 01201, (413) 443-6438, BS 77 East TN St Univ; MA 78 Ball St Univ; Aud, John F Burton MD, **A**

Oberweis, Susan P 43 Tall Oaks Drive, East Brunswick, NJ 08816, MS 78 CUNY - Brooklyn Coll; Sp-Lang Path, Private Practice, **SLP**

Oblak, Mrs Susan B 10318 15th Avenue N W, Seattle, WA 98177, (206) 782-6423, BA 72 Univ of WA; MS 73 Univ of WA; 74–Lecturer, Univ of Washington, **SLP**

Oblander, Catherine Miller 918 West 10th, Holland Center, Topeka, KS 66604, (913) 272-1944, BS 78 KS St Univ; MA 80 KS St Univ; Aud, USD 501 Topeka Publ Sch, **A**

Obler, Dr Loraine K CUNY Graduate Center, Dept Of Speech & Hrng Sci, 33 West 42nd Street, New York, NY 10036, (212) 790-4586, PH 75 (NS) Univ of MI - Ann Arbor; Associate Professor, CUNY

Obley-Kilborn, Nancy N 14933 Trinidad Drive, Rancho Murieta, CA 95683, (916) 323-4755, BS 69 Univ of KS; MA 70 Univ of KS; MA 76 San Francisco St Univ; Ed Admin, CA Dept of Ed, **SLP**

O'Boyle, Mrs Louise M Steinstrasse 61 5300, Bonn, West Germany 2, (412) 653-0156, BA 78 Univ of MD - College Park; MA 80 Northwestern Univ; **SLP**

O'Bray, Lynnann Susan 48 Ridge Road, Smithtown, NY 11787, (516) 329-1917, BA 84 Adelphi Univ; MS 86 Adelphi Univ; **A**

O'Brien, Mrs Alice Hargens 7825 North Michigan, Kansas City, MO 64118, (816) 454-3991, BS 81 IA St Univ; MA 83 Univ of KS; Sp-Lang Path, Ks City Ks Sch Dist #500, **SLP**

O'Brien, Ann Dorsey 19810 Deer Hollow Lane, Lutz, FL 33549, (813) 949-8766, BS 79 Northwestern Univ; MA 80 Northwestern Univ; 86–Sp-Lang Path, Skotko & Assoc, **SLP**

O'Brien, Dr Audrey Sp Path Aud & Ed Of Hrng Imp, Trenton State College, Hillwood Lakes CN4700, Trenton, NJ 08650-4700, (609) 771-2321, BA 42 CUNY - Hunter Coll; MS 43 Fordham Univ; PH 60 (Sp Science) Columbia Univ Teachers Coll; 67–Prof and Chairperson, Trenton St Coll, **SLP LM**

O'Brien, Bennie Kay 3309 Morrison Avenue, Tampa, FL 33609, **SLP**

O'Brien, Mrs Carol Powell 1547 Midland Road, Bay City, MI 48706, (517) 686-4410, Sp-Lang Path, Bay-Arenac Intermed Sch Dist, **SLP**

O'Brien, Colleen K 321 Roselawn Boulevard, Green Bay, WI 54301, (414) 336-9295, BA 85 Univ of WI - Eau Claire; MS 87 Univ of WI - Stevens Point

Obrien, Dr Denise P 80-50 189th Street, Jamaica, NY 11423, (212) 898-5962, BS 68 Saint John's Univ - Jamaica; ME 70 Univ of VA - Charlottesville; PH 78 (NS) NY Univ; Dir, Lexington Hrng & Sp Cen, **SLP**

O'Brien, Diane Lynn 555 27th Street, Niagara Falls, NY 14301, (716) 837-2441, BA 72 SUNY - Center at Buffalo; MA 74 SUNY - Center at Buffalo; 86–Sp-Lang Path, Language Dev Program, **SLP ACE**

O'Brien, Mrs Ellen M 5752 West Windsor, Chicago, IL 60630, (312) 749-2324, BA 79 Mundelein Coll; MS 80 Marquette Univ; Sp/Lang Path, Berwyn Sch Dist 100, **SLP**

O'Brien, Jane Asprinio 590 Toll Gate Road, Warwick, RI 02886, (401) 738-7004, BA 83 Univ of RI; MS 85 Univ of RI; Aud/Pres, Private Practice, **A**

O'Brien, Karen S 1022 Randall Avenue, Rhinelander, WI 54501, (715) 369-3311, BS 65 IL St Univ - Normal; MA 69 Univ of IL - Urbana; Asst Vp Rehabil Services, Sacred Heart St Marys Hosp Inc, **SLP**

O'Brien, Mrs Kathleen Sue 2200 Pine Island Road, Minnetonka, MN 55343, (612) 221-2066, BA 75 Carleton Coll; MA 85 Univ of MN - Minneap-St Paul; **SLP**

O'Brien, Mrs Kathryn S Route 1 Box 63-A, Concord, AR 72523, (501) 668-3265, BA 79 Univ of MS; MS 81 Univ of MS; 88–Sp-Lang Path, Batesville PS, **SLP**

O'Brien, Linda Ann 237 Wildwood Drive, Youngstown, OH 44512, (216) 726-8956, BS 77 Kent St Univ; MA 81 Kent St Univ; Sp-Lang Path, Private Practice, **SLP**

O'Brien, Mrs Lorraine K 4849 North 7th Street #M, Fresno, CA 93726-0844, (209) 441-3328, BA 73 CA St Univ - Fresno; MA 74 CA St Univ - Fresno; Sp/Lang Path, Fresno USD, **SLP**

O'Brien, Mrs Martha J Speech Language Pathologist, 110 North Main Street, Southside Rehab Inc, Farmville, VA 23901, (804) 392-9981, OB 75 Univ of Toledo; MA 79 Kent St Univ; Sp-Lang Path, Private Practice, **SLP**

O'Brien, Mrs Marti Marianne 8110 Liberty Avenue, Parma, OH 44129, (216) 351-3529, **SLP**

O'Brien, Mary Ann Monroe County Board Of, Cooperative Ed Services #1, 41 O'Connor Road, Fairport, NY 14450, (716) 377-4660, BS 57 Nazareth Coll of Rochester; MS 73 SUNY - Coll at Geneseo; OM 83 SUNY - Coll at Brockport; Dir Commun Serv, Monroe Co BOCES #1, **SLP**

O'Brien, Mrs Mary Borsari 369 Seekell Street, East Taunton, MA 02718-1420, (617) 822-4526, BS 79 Univ of MA - Amherst; Sp-Lang Path, Commonwealth of MA, **SLP**

O'Brien, Mary E 39 Thatcher, River Forest, IL 60305, (312) 366-2815, **SLP**

O'Brien, Mary E 1836 South 22nd Avenue, Maywood, IL 60153, (312) 629-8900, BA 85 MI St Univ; MA 87 Western MI Univ

O'Brien, Mary Rita 86-15 Broadway #5I, Elmhurst, NY 11373, BS 52 CUNY - City College; MS 65 Fordham Univ; SLP, New York City Board of Educ, **SLP LM**

O'Brien, Dr Maureen S 16103 Kenny Court, Laurel, MD 20707, (301) 490-2972, BS 62 PA St Univ - Univ Park; ME 64 PA St Univ - Univ Park; PH 87 (NS) Univ of MD - College Park; 88, **SLP**

O'Brien, Nancy L 1550 DeBenedetti Court, Benicia, CA 94510, (415) 458-6599, BA 71 Univ of CA - Santa Barbara; MA 74 San Diego St Univ; Resource Spec, Mt Diablo USD, **SLP**

Obrien, Mrs Nancy Lou Rhoads 452 South Feathering Road, Media, PA 19063, (215) 566-3212, BS 53 Bloomsburg Univ of PA; Sp-Lang Path, Chester Co Intermed Unit #24, **SLP**

O'Brien, Renee McMullen 1836 Sixty Oaks Lane, Vero Beach, FL 32966, (813) 262-0928, BS 81 Ball St Univ; MA 84 Ball St Univ; Aud, **A**

O'Brien, Mrs Valerie Lee 34990 Beacon Road, Livonia, MI 48150, (313) 572-3565, OB 83 Univ of Toledo; BA 83 Univ of Toledo; MS 86 Univ of MI - Ann Arbor; 86–Sp-Lang Path, St Joseph Mercy Hosp, **SLP**

O'Brien-Fallon, Mrs Maureen E 40 Markham Drive, Long Valley, NJ 07853, (201) 876-5292, BS 79 West Chester Univ of PA; MS 80 Univ of SC - Columbia; Sp-Lang Path, Private Practice, **SLP ACE**

Obrock, Ellen L 334 South 8th, Quincy, IL 62301, (217) 222-4180, BA 78 Augustana Coll; MS 79 Eastern IL Univ; Sp-Lang Path, Private Practice, **SLP**

O'Bryan, Mrs Anne L 2139 North Stratford Drive, Owensboro, KY 42301, (502) 685-5737, BA 73 Brescia Coll; MS 74 Purdue Univ - West Lafayette; **SLP**

Ocampo, Graciela M 513 South Bishopthorpe St, Bethlehem, PA 18015, (215) 867-8733, BS 74 West Chester Univ of PA; MA 85 Temple Univ-Tyler Sch of Art; 86–Sp-Lang Path, St Luke's Hosp, **SLP**

O'Carroll, Mrs Karen Gerber 2417 Rosewood Lane, Havertown, PA 19083, (215) 284-8570, BS 85 SUNY - Coll at Geneseo; MS 87 Coll of Saint Rose; 88–Sp-Lang Path, Delaware County Mem Hosp, **SLP**

Ocarz-Krumpak, Susan L 330 Wildwood Drive, Youngstown, OH 44512, (216) 782-5606, BS 77 Coll of Saint Rose; ME 78 Coll of Saint Rose; Sp/Lang Path, Vstng Nrse Assoc Gr Youngstown, **SLP**

Ochipa, Cynthia 3415 Southwest 24th Street, Apartment 9, Gainesville, FL 32608-2818, (904) 374-4140, MA 85 Univ of FL; Research Assistant, VA Medical Center, **SLP**

Ochoa, Bella Linda L Rt 2 Box 78-0, Mission, TX 78572, (512) 585-8381, BA 77 Our Lady Lake Univ-San Anton; MA 80 Univ of Houston - Univ Park; 82–Sp-Lang Path, SW Spec Ed Coop, **SLP**

Ochs, Dr Marleen G Vanderbilt University School Of Medicine, Wilkerson Hearing & Speech Center, 1114 19th Avenue South, Nashville, TN 37212, (615) 320-5353, BA 74 WA St Univ; MA 76 WA St Univ; PH 83 (Hrng & Speech Sciences or Aud) Vanderbilt Univ; Assistant Professor, Vanderbilt Univ, **A**

Ochsendorf, Mrs Karen L B 600 S E 24th Street, Willmar, MN 56201, (612) 231-5100, BS 75 Moorhead St Univ; MS 78 Saint Cloud St Univ; 77–SLP, Willmar Reg Treatment Ctr, **SLP**

Ochsner, Dr Glenda J 5900 Bluestem Place, Oklahoma City, OK 73132, (405) 271-4214, BA 63 Univ of OK - Norman; MS 67 Univ of OK Medical Center; PH 68 (NS) Univ of OK Medical Center; Prof, U of OK/Hlth Sci Cen, **SLP F**

Ochsner, Patricia Cady 1300 30th Street #A1-23, Boulder, CO 80303, (303) 786-4290, BA 68 San Diego St Univ; MA 70 San Diego St Univ; **SLP**

Ocmond, Wilbert J, Jr 4 Hickory, La Place, LA 70068, (504) 652-6536, BA 71 Nicholls St Univ; MA 73 Tulane Univ; Sp-Lang Path, St John the Baptist School Bd, **SLP**

O'Connell, Christine J D 7 Gilbert Place, White Plains, NY 10604, (212) 519-7000, BS 74 Bloomsburg Univ of PA; MS 78 Bloomsburg Univ of PA; Sp-Lang Path, The NY Institute for Spec Educ, **SLP**

O'Connell, Mrs Mary Lou 27 Beckwith Terrace, Rochester, NY 14610, BS 55 Nazareth Coll of Rochester; MS 64 SUNY - Coll at Geneseo; 55–Sp-Lang Path, BOCES, **SLP**

O'Connell, Mrs Marybeth O 401 Cedar Spring Road, Bel Air, MD 21014, (301) 836-8349, BA 76 Loyola Coll; MS 77 Loyola Coll; Sp-Lang Path, Harford Co Bd Ed, **SLP**

O'Connell, Maureen Ann 5755-A Harwich Court, Alexandria, VA 22311, (703) 971-9203, Sp-Lang Path, Fairfax Co Ps, **SLP**

O'Connell, Maureen Ann 5363 Mississippi Bar Drive, Orangevale, CA 95662-5434, (916) 927-3137, BA 80 TX Tech Univ; MA 83 CA St Univ - Sacramento; Aud, North Area ENT, **A**

O'Connell, Dr Pamelia F 6355 Westerly Terrace, Jamesville, NY 13078, (607) 756-5423, BA 52 Goucher Coll; MA 56 Univ of AL- Tuscaloosa; PH 74 (NS) Syracuse Univ; 86–Sp-Lang Path, SUNY Cortland, **SLP**

O'Connell, Mrs Susan D 354 Hillhurst Avenue, New Britain, CT 06053, (203) 224-8802, BA 73 Univ of CT; MS 74 Southern CT St Univ; Sp-Lang Path, Bd of Ed, **SLP**

O'Connell-Goodfellow, Eileen Mary 16 Wisteria Drive, Leominster, MA 01453, (617) 787-3390, BS 81 Univ of OR; MS 83 Boston Univ; Sp/Lang Path, Greenery Rehab Center, **SLP**

O'Connell-Halloway, Maureen 3810 North 36th Street, Tacoma, WA 98407, (206) 593-6814, BA 77 Gonzaga Univ; MS 79 Eastern WA Univ; SLP, Tacoma Pub Sch, **SLP**

O'Connell-Hanifan, Anne M 21 Hillside Avenue, Medford, MA 02155, (617) 396-6780, BS 76 Northeastern Univ; MS 80 Northeastern Univ; Sp/Lang Path, Malden Pub Schs, **SLP**

O'Connor, Alma Elizabeth 3200 Fernandina Road, #F-2, Columbia, SC 29210, (803) 731-9465, BA 76 Columbia Coll; MS 84 Univ of VT; 88–Sp-Lang Path, Saluda Co Dist #1, **SLP**

O'Connor, Anita M 3643 Dawes Avenue S E, Grand Rapids, MI 49508, (616) 241-9919, BS 78 Western MI Univ; MA 80 Western MI Univ; Sp-Lang Path, Private Practice, **SLP**

O'Connor, Ann Monsor P O Box 400, Tuba City, AZ 86045, (312) 633-8691, BS 81 Northwestern Univ; MA 82 Northwestern Univ; Sp/Lang Path, Private Practice, **SLP**

O'Connor, Anna 28-14 Crescent Street, Astoria, NY 11102, (212) 677-5800, BA 75 CUNY - Hunter Coll; MA 77 CUNY - City College; **SLP**

O'Connor, Mrs Anne Elizabeth 128 Heather Dale Circle, Henrietta, NY 14467, (716) 271-0680, BS 78 Nazareth Coll of Rochester; MS 80 Nazareth Coll of Rochester; 82–Sp/Lang Path, Hrng & Sp Cen of Rochester Inc, **SLP**

O'Connor, Annette Marie 512 South 18th, Parsons, KS 67357, (316) 421-6550, BS 82 KS St Univ; MA 83 Wichita St Univ; 87–Parapro Training Coord, Southeast Kansas Educ Svc Ctr, **SLP**

O'Connor, Mrs Barbara Ann 26 Willow Road, Glens Falls, NY 12801-1238, (518) 793-7721, Sp-Lang Path, **SLP**

O'Connor, Carol J 119 South Grant Street, Clinton, IL 61727, (217) 935-5707, BS 71 Univ of IA; MA 72 Univ of IA; Sp-Lang Path, Clinton Comm Sd #15, **SLP**

O'Connor, Cathleen A 900 Fairway Drive, Apartment 104, Naperville, IL 60540, (312) 416-3579, BS 83 Bradley Univ; MS 85 Rush Univ; 88–Dir of Aud, Chicago Otology Group Ltd, **A**

O'Connor, Constance North Anguilla Road, Pawcatuck, CT 06379, (203) 535-2732, BA 65; MS 80 Univ of RI; Owner, Private Practice, **SLP**

O'Connor, Deborah Ann 11433 Arbor Street #103, Omaha, NE 68144, (402) 334-8636, MS 87 Kearney St Coll; **SLP**

O'Connor, Mrs Elizabeth 64 Forest, Providence, RI 02906, (401) 273-7100, BS 63 Univ of WI - Madison; MA 70 Coll of Saint Rose; Sp-Lang Path, VA Medcen, **SLP**

O'Connor, Jean-Ann Nelson 4499B Via Marisol #219, Los Angeles, CA 90042, (818) 795-6981, BA 79 SUNY - Coll at Plattsburgh; MA 85 CA St Univ - Los Angeles; **SLP**

O'Connor, Jeanne A Dunn 174 Friends Lane, Westbury, NY 11590-6507, (516) 378-2000, BS 78 PA St Univ - Univ Park; MA 81 NY Univ; Sp-Lnag Path, UCP-Nassau, **SLP**

O'Connor, Mrs Judy L A 204 East Skyview, San Antonio, TX 78228, (512) 432-3138, BA 73 Univ of Rochester; MA 78 Our Lady Lake Univ-San Anton; **SLP**

O'Connor, Kathleen 1560 North Sandburg Terr, Apartment 2411, Chicago, IL 60610, (312) 883-5866, BS 72 Mundelein Coll; MS 73 Marquette Univ; Dir/SLP & Audiology, Columbus Hospital, **SLP**

O'Connor, Larry 2275 Calle Cacique, Santa Fe, NM 87501, (505) 983-5095, BA 72 Univ of Northern CO; MA 73 Univ of Northern CO; ED 79 (NS) Univ of Northern CO; Dir of Pupil Pers Serv, New Mexico School Deaf, **A**

O'Connor, Mrs Linda Basile S-4940 Clifton Parkway, Hamburg, NY 14075, (716) 662-0135, BS 80 SUNY - Coll at Fredonia; MS 85 1533; **SLP**

O'Connor, Lisa C 2134 Redcliff Street, Los Angeles, CA 90039, (213) 343-4690, BA 73 CA St Univ - Los Angeles; MA 75 CA St Univ - Los Angeles; Sp-Lang Path, CA St U-La, **SLP ACE**

O'Connor, Mrs Lisa M 4163 Hinsdale, South Euclid, OH 44121, (216) 951-7272, BS 82 Kent St Univ; MA 82 Kent St Univ; Sp-Lang Path, InSpeech Inc, **SLP**

O'Connor, M Catherine 855 Echo, Los Altos, CA 94022, (408) 646-4070, BA 75 Humboldt St Univ; MA 76 Humboldt St Univ; SLP, Mesa Comm Coll, **SLP**

Oconnor, Mrs Mary Gerilyn Rd 3 Box 219-C, Englishtown, NJ 07726, (201) 842-3514, BA 81 Montclair St Coll; MA 82 Montclair St Coll; **SLP**

O'Connor, Maureen M 845 Oak Grove Avenue #110, Menlo Park, CA 94025, (415) 324-0648, BS 69 Univ of WI - Stevens Point; MS 70 Purdue Univ - West Lafayette; 88–Sp-Lang Path, Private Practice, **SLP**

O'Connor, Patricia Mary 19 Winn Street Apt R-1, Woburn, MA 01801, BS 81 Saint Mary-of-the-Woods Coll; ME 87 Univ of VA - Charlottesville; 87–Sp-Lang Path, New England Rehab Hosp, **SLP**

O'Connor, Mrs Pearl May Route 2 Box 553, Chapin, SC 29036, BS; **SLP LM**

O'Connor, Sheila Leahy 3909 Robertson Boulevard, Alexandria, VA 22309, MS 78 SUNY - Coll at Buffalo; MS 82 Canisius Coll; **SLP**

O'Connor, Mrs Suzanne S 8256 Kimlough Drive, Indianapolis, IN 46240, (317) 844-5656, BA 82 IN Univ - Bloomington; MA 83 IN Univ - Bloomington; 84–Aud, Northside ENT Inc, **A**

O'Connor, Thomas E 2350 Mc Dowell Street, Augusta, GA 30904-4449, (404) 791-6689, BA 78 MI St Univ; MA 80 MI St Univ; Aud, Hitchcock Rehabilitation Ctr, **A**

O'Connor, Thomas M 10715 North Fairview Road, Spokane, WA 99207, (509) 467-5350, BA 75 Gonzaga Univ; MS 77 Purdue Univ - West Lafayette; OM 79 Univ of WA; Audiologist, Spokane Public Schools #8, **A**

O'Connor, Mrs Tommie Lou 909 East Main, West Point, MS 39773, (601) 494-6051, BS 51 Univ Southern MS-Hattiesburg; MS 58 Univ Southern MS-Hattiesburg; Sp-Lang Path, West Point Municipal Ssd, **SLP**

O'Connor-Beringer, Mrs Patricia Anne Route 3 Box 50, Montgomery City, MO 63361, (314) 882-1571, BS 84 Univ of WI - Stevens Point; MA 85 Northwestern Univ; 88–Aud, Univ of Missouri Columbia Med Ctr, **A**

O'Connor-Hodgdon, Eileen M 127 Garth Road #6-H, Scarsdale, NY 10583, (914) 472-9037, BS 76 Seton Hall Univ; MS 79 Columbia Univ Teachers Coll; Sp-Lang Path, NYC Bd of Ed Comm Sch Dist 2 Sp Prog, **SLP**

O'Connor-McManamon, Mrs Erin 414 16th Street, Huntingdon, PA 16652, (412) 325-1500, **SLP**

O'Connor-Putman, Maureen 613 F Street, Colma, CA 94014, (415) 997-0199, BA 68 Saint Mary's Dominican Coll; MA 70 Univ of CO - Boulder; 68–SLP, Private Practice, **SLP**

Oda, Mrs Susan Idell 501 Newford Drive, Bellefontaine, OH 43311, (513) 592-1201, BS 80 Miami Univ - Oxford; MS 81 Miami Univ - Oxford; 88–Sp-Lang Path, Tri-Co Head Start, **SLP**

Odabashian, Eileen 59 Williams Street, North Easton, MA 02356, (617) 784-6254, BA 72 Univ of MA - Amherst; MA 73 Univ of MA - Amherst; Sp-Lang Path, Sharon PS, **SLP**

O'Day, James Marshall 34 Pinewood Drive, Somersworth, NH 03878, (603) 335-4880, BS 75 Univ of MD - College Park; BS 77 Univ of MD - College Park; MA 82 Univ of MD - College Park; Aud, Private Practice, **A**

O'Day, Marlene Jankowski 2 Macclarey Way, Worcester, MA 01602, (617) 885-4842, BS 76 Worcester St Coll; MS 81 Worcester St Coll; Sp/Lang Path, Spencer Sch Dept, **SLP**

Oday, Paula A 312 West Carpenter Lane, Philadelphia, PA 19119, (215) 782-7543, BA 67 Catholic Univ of America; MA 71 Temple Univ-Tyler Sch of Art; PH 88 (Linguistics) Temple Univ; **SLP**

O'Dea-Dooley, Kathleen 8339 Church Street, Suite 110, Gilroy, CA 95020, (408) 847-5376, **SLP**

Odegard, Thomas B 1805 Cooks Hill Road, Centralia, WA 98531, (503) 738-8463, **A**

Odell, Brent C 5408 Main Street, McFarland, WI 53558, (608) 266-1783, BS 71 Univ of WI - Milwaukee; MS 74 Univ of WI - Milwaukee; OM 78 Univ of WI - Milwaukee; Sp-Lang Path, WI Dept of Pub Instruction, **SLP**

O'Dell, Mrs Elizabeth Ward 2804 Cahawba Trail, Birmingham, AL 35243, (205) 871-3878, **SLP**

O'Dell, Evelyn S P O Box 1635, La Porte, IN 46350, (219) 362-2074, BS 70 MS Univ for Women; ME 71 Univ of GA; Sp-Lang Path, South Bend Community Schools, **SLP**

Odell, Katharine Hobart 2110 Vilas Avenue, Madison, WI 53711, (608) 267-6000, **SLP**

Odell, Lee M 3140 S W Mitchell Court, Portland, OR 97201, BS 71 Portland St Univ; MS 74 Portland St Univ; Admin Accountant, Multnomah Sch of the Bible, **A**

O'Dell, Mrs Nancy Smith 4121 Williamsburg Ct #201, Glenview, IL 60025, (312) 390-6454, MA 87 Univ of IL - Urbana; 87–Sp-Lang Path, Libertyville Schs Dist #70, **SLP**

Odell, Mrs Ruth M 5408 Main Street, McFarland, WI 53558, (608) 873-7257, BS 73 Univ of WI - Milwaukee; MS 74 Univ of WI - Milwaukee; Sp-Lang Path, Stoughton Area Schs, **SLP**

Odell, Mrs Teresa Gail 440 West Highland Avenue, Redlands, CA 92373, (714) 381-1160, MS 85 Univ of Redlands; **SLP**

O'Dell-Doiron, Mary Catherine 1375 Chaney Avenue, Carpinteria, CA 93013, (805) 485-1442, BA 81 Univ of CA - Santa Barbara; MA 83 Univ of CA - Santa Barbara; Sp-Lang Path, Rio School District, **SLP**

Oden, Lorin Star 1614 Tree House Lane, Plano, TX 75023-7432, (214) 934-2961, BS 83 Univ of IA; MA 85 Univ of Denver; Aud, Omni Hearing Systems, **A**

Oden-Greenberg, Sandra E 6751 St Ives Court, Fort Myers, FL 33912, (813) 768-3507, BS 76 Univ of VA - Charlottesville; MA 78 Vanderbilt Univ; **SLP**

Odessa, Susan Iris 99 Pind Avenue #812-D, Brookline, MA 02146, (617) 739-3918, BA 79 Clark Univ; MS 81 Boston Univ; Sp/Lang Path, UCP-Infant-Toddler Dev Prog, **SLP**

Odlaug, Mrs Patricia B 1321 Greenleaf Blvd, Elkhart, IN 46514, (219) 262-0548, BA 73 Univ of MO - KS City; MA 75 Univ of MN - Minneap-St Paul; Sp-Lang Path, **SLP**

Odom, Mrs Amelia M Route 2 Box 94, Eufaula, AL 36027, (205) 687-7495, BS 77 Univ of Montevallo; MS 79 Univ of Montevallo; **SLP**

Odom, Amy C 1600 Sunrise, Norman, OK 73071, (405) 321-4830, BS 77 Murray St Univ; MS 80 Murray St Univ; 83–Sp-Lang Path, Jd McCarty Cen/Hndcpd Chldn, **SLP**

Odom, Mrs Glenna L 3808 Heywood Avenue, Fort Worth, TX 76109, (817) 924-7859, BA 53 TX Christian Univ; MS 54 Univ of WI - Madison; 74–Sp-Lang Path/Owner, Westcliff Speech & Lang Center, **SLP ACE**

Odom, Mrs Joyce R Route 1 Box 293, Pontotoc, MS 38863, (601) 489-4973, MS 72 Univ of IL - Urbana; 85–Sp-Lang Path, Pontotoc City Schs, **SLP**

Odom, Terria Lee 503 Hannon Avenue, Monterey, CA 93940-1562, (408) 375-4625, BA 81 San Jose St Univ; MA 83 San Jose St Univ; Sp/Lang Path, Monterey Peninsula C, **SLP**

Odom, Tina A P O Box 234, Rockwell, NC 28138, (704) 279-6164, BS 81 Appalachian St Univ; MA 82 Appalachian St Univ; Sp-Lang Path, Rowan Co Schs, **SLP**

Odom-Winn, Danni S 2306 18th Avenue, Columbus, GA 31901, (404) 324-6250, BA 73 Univ of AL- Tuscaloosa; MS 80 Univ of Montevallo; ES 86 Columbus Coll; Preschool Coord, Woodhall Psychoeducational Ctr, **SLP**

O'Donnell, Brian David 886 South Franklin St, Wilkes-Barre, PA 18702, (717) 822-6279, MS 87 Bloomsburg Univ of PA

O'Donnell, Connie C 1987 Midwick Drive, Altadena, CA 91001, (818) 791-3923, BS 70 Georgetown Univ; MA 77 George Washington Univ; SLP, LA Co Olive View Med Cen, **SLP**

O'Donnell, Constance Martello 11309 Dunleith Drive, Raleigh, NC 27614, (919) 684-5513, BS 80 Coll of Saint Rose; MS 85 SUNY - Coll at New Paltz; Sp-Lang Path, Duke Univ Med Ctr, **SLP**

O'Donnell, Mrs Cynthia 535A Fort Baker, Sausalito, CA 94965, (312) 447-6203, BA 78 Univ of Denver; MS 79 Univ of IL - Urbana; **SLP**

O'Donnell, Mrs Darlene Kay 706 South New Street, West Chester, PA 19380, BA 78 Clarion Univ of PA; MA 82 Edinboro Univ of PA; SLP, Assn for Ret Ctzs-Chester Co, **SLP**

O'Donnell, Georgette 44 No Murray Avenue, Ridgewood, NJ 07450, (201) 825-3388, BS 70 Rutger's St Univ - Douglas Coll; MS 73 Columbia Univ Teachers Coll; Sp-Lang Path, NM Highlands Reg Hs, **SLP**

O'Donnell, Grace B 4725 N W 5 Ct, Plantation, FL 33317, (305) 587-9386, ME 88 FL Atlantic Univ

O'Donnell, Jody Sue 305 South Johnson, Pocatello, ID 83204, (208) 226-5203, BA 77 IA St Univ; MS 83 ID St Univ; 78–Sp-Lang Path, American Falls Sch Dist, **SLP**

O'Donnell, Linda J 400 Avenue K, Matamoras, PA 18336, (914) 856-8033, BS 61 Syracuse Univ; MS 66 IN Univ - Bloomington; Sp-Lang Path, Port Jervis Bd of Ed, **SLP**

O'Donnell, Michael B 1709 West Fair, Marquette, MI 49855, (906) 228-9440, BS 72 Central MI Univ; MA 74 Central MI Univ; Aud, Marquette General Hospital, **A ACE**

O'Donnell, Patricia L 337 Fayette Avenue, Kenmore, NY 14223, (716) 694-9627, BA 85 SUNY - Center at Buffalo; MS 87 SUNY - Coll at Buffalo; **SLP**

O'Donnell, Sheila 812 West Altgeld #2, Chicago, IL 60614, (312) 525-3788, BS 84 Univ of IL - Urbana; MS 86 Univ of IL - Urbana; **SLP**

O'Donnell, Susan I Regional Memorial Hospital, Audiology Department, 66 Baribeau Drive, Brunswick, ME 04011, (207) 729-0181, BS 79 Univ of RI; MS 81 Gallaudet Coll; 88–Aud, Regional Memorial Hosp, **A**

O'Donovan, Mary W 8392 Knollwood Drive, Allison Park, PA 15101, (412) 366-3257, MS 76 Northwestern Univ; Sp-Lang Path, Easter Seal Society, **SLP**

O'Dornan, Sharon Theresa 202-2425 Alma Street, Vancouver, BC, Canada V6R 3R6, (604) 222-0821, BA 84 Western WA Univ; MA 86 Western WA Univ; 88–Sp-Lang Path, Vancouver Sch Bd, **SLP**

Oehler, Susan Marie 39 Charlton Avenue East, Hamilton, ON, Canada L8N 1Y3, (416) 522-0306, MA 86 Univ of Cincinnati; Aud, Self Employed, **A**

Oeky, Deborah F Conway Road, South Deerfield, MA 01373, (413) 538-5068, MA 72 Univ of MA - Amherst; Sp-Lang Path, South Hadley Public Schools, **SLP**

Oelker, Colleen Sue 304 East Gambier Street, Mount Vernon, OH 43050, (614) 633-3751, BA 78 OH St Univ; MA 81 OH St Univ; SLP, Mt Vernon Developmental Center, **SLP**

Oelschlaeger, Dr Mary L 1600 Highland Park Road, Denton, TX 76201, (214) 696-7983, BS 69 Southern IL Univ -Carbondale; MS 71 Southern IL Univ -Carbondale; PH 73 (NS) Southern IL Univ -Carbondale; Director, Dept of SLP, Presbyterian Hospital Ofdallas, **SLP**

OeltjenbrunsLindblad, Patricia Ann 12660 Panola Drive, Lindstrom, MN 55045, (612) 689-3632, BA 80 Univ of MN - Duluth; MS 83 Saint Cloud St Univ; 85–SLP & ECSE Coord, Rum River Spec Educ Cooperative, **SLP**

Oerther, Patricia L 15 War Admiral Lane, Media, PA 19063, (215) 565-1471, BS 67 Bloomsburg Univ of PA; MA 77 West Chester Univ of PA; Sp-Lang Path, Delaware Co Inter Ut, **SLP**

Oertli, Julene May 9900 Blundou Drive #103, Silver Spring, MD 20902, (301) 253-7000, MA 80 WA St Univ; Sp-Lang Path, Montgomery County Pub Schools, **SLP**

Oeser, Julie Ann 2413 Casa Bona, Belmont, CA 94002, (415) 668-1000, BA 80 Univ of the Pacific; MA 81 Univ of the Pacific; Rehab Supervisor, Care Point Industries, **SLP**

Oestreicher, Mrs Nancy K 8515 Wilkesboro Lane, Potomac, MD 20854, (301) 983-9255, BA 69 Dickinson Coll; MA 74 NY Univ; Sp-Lang Path, Montgomery County Pub Schools, **SLP**

Oettinger, Tambrey C 202 Hillcrest Road, Raleigh, NC 27605, (919) 966-3325, BA 74 Meredith Coll; MS 79 Univ of NC - Chapel Hill; Aud, Nc Mem Hosp, **A**

Oetzel, Mrs Judith Yohman 3382 Big Horn Court, Cincinnati, OH 45211, (513) 921-5419, BS 82 Univ of Cincinnati; MA 83 OH St Univ; Sp-Lang Path, Cincinnati Public Schools, **SLP**

O'Fallon, Mrs Celia M K 3 Apple Hill Lane, York, PA 17402, (717) 757-1572, BA 79 Univ of MD - College Park; MS 80 WV Univ; 88–Sp-Lang Path, Pvt Contractor, **SLP**

O'Farrell, Deirdre Ann 14118 52nd West, Edmonds, WA 98020, (307) 455-2323, BA 81 Univ of CA - Santa Barbara; MS 84 San Francisco St Univ; Sp-Lang Path, Dubois Sch District

Ofcharka, Carol Ann 6301 Stevenson Avenue #1117, Alexandria, VA 22304, (703) 941-7544, MS 84 Clarion Univ of PA; Sp-Lang Path, The Nelson Ctr, **SLP**

Off, C Elizabeth 3330 Sepulveda Blvd, Apartment 10, Los Angeles, CA 90034, (213) 312-0707, BA 80 William Paterson Coll; MS 88 Montclair St Coll; 88–Sp-Lang Path, InSpeech Inc

Offenbacher, Barbara Levine 2411 Avenue #T, Brooklyn, NY 11229-2445, (718) 645-5847, BA 74 CUNY - Brooklyn Coll; MS 79 CUNY - Brooklyn Coll; OM 82 CUNY - Brooklyn Coll; Sp-Lang Path, NYC Bd of Ed-Sp Serv Ut, **SLP**

Offeney, Sharon L 7 Lewis Drive, Fairfield, CT 06432, (203) 795-6075, BA 75 Southern CT St Univ; MS 78 Southern CT St Univ; Sp-Lang Path, Foundation Sch Inc, **SLP**

Offerle, Mrs Melanie Reszel 347 West Berry, Suite 102, Fort Wayne, IN 46802, (219) 426-8117, BA 80 IN Univ - Bloomington; MA 82 Ball St Univ; Aud, ENT Assn Inc, **A**

Offill, Mrs Elinor B 320 Pinehurst Trace Drive, Pinehurst, NC 28374, BA 40 Chatham Coll; MS 65 Univ of Pittsburgh - Pittsburgh; **SLP LM**

Offsay, Mrs Pamela S 4419 Conchita Way, Tarzana, CA 91356, (818) 881-1398, BA 75 SUNY - Center at Buffalo; MA 77 CUNY - Hunter Coll; Sp-Lang Path, Private Practice, **SLP**

Offstein, Lois 815 South Serenade Avenue, West Covina, CA 91790, (818) 960-9737, BA 70 William Paterson Coll; MA 75 CA St Univ - Los Angeles; Sp-Lang Path, InterComm Med Ctr, **SLP ACE**

Offutt, Pamela Gene 5443 Timber Post, San Antonio, TX 78250, (512) 680-0650, BA 72 Sam Houston St Univ; MA 80 Our Lady Lake Univ-San Anton; SLP, Northside ISD, **SLP**

Offutt, Suzanne Hear-Say Commun Disorders Spec, Route 3 Box 192, Berkeley Springs, WV 25411, (304) 258-4730, BS 72 WV Univ; MS 74 WV Univ; Sp-Lang Path, Hear-Say Commun Dis Spec, **SLP**

Ofield, Mrs Mary C 550 Crahen N E, Grand Rapids, MI 49506, (616) 942-5448, BS 71 Marquette Univ; MS 78 Western MI Univ; SLP, Mary Free Bed, **SLP**

O'Flaherty, Dr Kevin Paul 40 Washington Drive, Cranbury, NJ 08512, (212) 288-7307, BA 70 Boston Coll; MA 72 NY Univ; PH 79 (NS) NY Univ; Aud, Manhattan Aud Srvcs, **A**

Ofrichter, Marjorie A 926 North Arch Street, Allentown, PA 18104, (215) 437-5222, BS 77 Univ of Pittsburgh - Pittsburgh; OM 79 Hahneman Medical Coll; 83–Sp-Lang Path/Aud, John D Harwick MD, **SLP A**

Oftedahl, Mrs Geraldine Ann 100 Sagamore Drive, Rochester, NY 14617, (716) 266-2266, BA 62 Mundelein Coll; MA 64 Northwestern Univ; **SLP**

O'Gallagher, Elizabeth F 7528 Shadow Bay Drive, Panama City, FL 32404, (904) 785-9500, MA 85 Univ of CT; **A**

Ogan, Donna G P O Box 1616, Guymon, OK 73942, (316) 626-6126, BA 75 Univ of CO - Boulder; MA 78 Univ of CO - Boulder; Sp/Lang Path, USD #8, Guymon, Ok, **SLP**

Ogan, Susan S 28 Ocean Avenue, Marblehead, MA 01945, (617) 631-1707, BS 75 Univ of MA - Amherst; MS 78 Boston Univ; Aud, N Shore Chldns Hosp, **A**

O'Gara, Mary M 3515 Central Road, Glenview, IL 60025, (312) 266-5957, BA 75 Loyola Univ of Chicago; MA 80 Northwestern Univ; Cl Coord/Sp-Lang Path, Northwestern Univ, **SLP ACE**

O'Gara, Susan Curran 519 25th Avenue North, St Petersburg, FL 33704-2823, (813) 898-2344, BA 68 FL St Univ; MS 70 FL St Univ; 87–SLP, Pinellas Co Sch Bd, **SLP**

Ogas, Mrs Teresa O 225 Wittwer Court, Los Lunas, NM 87031, (505) 864-2215, BA 78 NM St Univ; MA 80 NM St Univ; **SLP**

Ogawa, Mrs Diana K 894 Vista Grande, Millbrae, CA 94030, (415) 348-8834, BA 66 San Jose St Univ; MA 66 San Jose St Univ; SLP, San Mateo Un H S Dist, **SLP**

Ogawa, Patricia Mary 4671 Belmont Drive, Macungie, PA 18062, (201) 222-4741, MS 84 Rutgers St Univ -N Brunswick; Sp-Lang Path, UCP, **SLP**

Ogawa, Mrs Toshiko O 2886 Poelua, Honolulu, HI 96822, (808) 737-2321, BA 57 Univ of HI - Manoa; SLP, Dept of Ed, **SLP**

Ogborn, Laurinda L 3843 Belker Court, Richmond, VA 23234, (804) 323-2613, BS 79 KS St Univ; MA 86 Univ of KS; 82–Sp-Lang Path, Dept of Correctional Educ

Ogden, Mrs Brenley A 4828 Carousel Drive, Charlotte, NC 28212, (704) 372-7790, BA 77 Univ of ND; MA 79 Saint Louis Univ; Sp-Lang Path, Cen for Human Dev, **SLP**

Ogden, Dr Christine E Head And Neck Surgery Assoc, 40 North Grand Avenue, Fort Thomas, KY 41075, (606) 781-4900, BS 74 Univ of MO - Columbia; MA 75 Univ of MO - Columbia; PH 86 (Aud) Univ of Cincinnati; 84–Dir Aud, Head & Neck Surgery Associates, **SLP A**

Ogden, Helen Vaughan 4237 Beulah Drive, La Canada, CA 91011, (818) 790-5605, MA 83 CA St Univ - Northridge; 79–Sp-Lang Path, Los Angeles USD, **SLP**

Ogden, Patricia 5704 Regency Court South, Mobile, AL 36609, (205) 341-1117, BS 73 IN Univ - Bloomington; OM 74 IN Univ - Bloomington; **SLP**

Ogden, Ruth A 203 Sycamore Drive, Paducah, KY 42001, (502) 443-5141, BA 71 Univ of KY; ME 78 Univ of Louisville; **SLP**

Oggel, Mrs Linda Lou Shearer 650 Blakeston Drive, Richmond, VA 23236, (804) 794-8135, BS 60 Kent St Univ; MA 65 Northwestern Univ; **SLP**

Ogle, Mrs Mary E 19 Dunmore Road, Baltimore, MD 21228, (301) 486-5518, BA 68 Fairleigh Dickinson U-Teanec; ME 70 PA St Univ - Univ Park; Sp-Lang Path, Baltimore Co Bd of Ed, **SLP**

Ogle, Mrs Sharon Kay 618 Illinois Avenue, Green Lake, WI 54941, MS 88 Univ of WI - Oshkosh; 88–Sp-Lang Path, BOCES Agency #6

Oglesby, Barbara B 4114 Oak Hollow Road, Claremont, CA 91711, **SLP**

Oglesby, Carole S 113 Knob Avenue, New Albany, IN 47150, (502) 583-8303, BS 72 Eastern IL Univ; MS 73 Eastern IL Univ; 88–Sp-Lang Path, Univ Sp Path Assoc, **SLP**

Oglesby, Margo Ann 3527 Winsor Place, Crown Point, IN 46307, (219) 464-9607, BA 83 IN Univ - Bloomington; OM 84 IN Univ - Bloomington; 85–Sp-Lang Path, Porter County Spec Educ Coop, **SLP**

Ogletree, Billy Townsend 1327 Hancock Street, Tallahassee, FL 32304-2131, **SLP**

Ogletree, Nancy Cureton 392 Fairlane Drive, Spartanburg, SC 29302, (803) 594-4440, BA 74 Columbia Coll; ME 75 Univ of GA; Sp-Lang Path, Spartanburg Cty Sch Dist #7, **SLP**

Ogline, Mrs Kathy Harrington Somerset Habilitation Center, P O Box 631, Somerset, PA 15501, (814) 445-6501, BS 77 Clarion Univ of PA; MS 81 Indiana Univ of PA; Sp-Lang Path, Somerset Hab Cen, **SLP**

Ognibene, Rocco James 136 Edgeworth Street, Valley Stream, NY 11581, (516) 701 5018, BA 84 CUNY - Queens Coll; MA 86 CUNY - Queens Coll; 87–Sp-Lang Path, Sunshine Developmental Sch, **SLP**

O'Grady, Gwendolyn M 7941 Shadyglade, North Hollywood, CA 91605, (213) 669-2137, Aud, Childrens Hosp of La, **A**

O'Grady, Kathleen A 96 Parker Street, Norwell, MA 02061-1427, (617) 848-5353, BS 78 IL St Univ - Normal; MS 80 Univ of NC - Chapel Hill; 85–Sp/Lang Path, Braintree Hosp, **SLP**

Ogrodnick, Patricia Ann 9666 Brentwood Way #302, Westminster, CO 80020, (303) 322-1871, BA 83 0500; MA 85 Univ of CO - Boulder; **SLP**

Ohanian, Dr Edward P O Box 1392, Pebble Beach, CA 93953, (408) 624-6880, BA 47 Univ of Southern CA; MA 50 Univ of Southern CA; PH 52 Univ of Southern CA; Sp-Lang Path, Private Practice, **SLP LM**

Ohanian, Rosemary C 115 Cypress Drive, East Windsor, NJ 08520, (609) 443-1474, BA 70 CUNY - Lehman Coll; MS 74 Columbia Univ Teachers Coll; **SLP**

O'Hanlon, Mrs Angela M 52 South Julia Street, Mobile, AL 36604, (205) 432-1149, BA 74 Univ of South AL; MA 76 LA St Univ - Baton Rouge; **SLP**

Ohanyan, Regina E 220 Monroe Avenue, River Edge, NJ 07661, **SLP**

O'Hara, Anne 710 Reflections Circle, Apartment 108, Casselberry, FL 32707, (305) 645-2081, BA 83 Univ of Central FL; MS 85 FL St Univ; Sp-Lang Path, Orlando Pedia Multi-Ther Clin, **SLP**

O'Hara, Daniel S 51290 Sunnyhill, Utica, MI 48087, (313) 263-7400, BA 78 MI St Univ; MA 80 Wayne St Univ - Sch of Med; Aud, Lakeshore ENT Center PC, **A**

O'Hara, Mrs Diane A 2104 Sherwood Avenue, Bakersfield, CA 93304, (805) 397-8737, BS 77 Clarion Univ of PA; ME 79 Clarion Univ of PA; 88–Sp-Lang Path, Bakersfield City Sch Dist, **SLP**

O'Hara, James J 3672 Roselawn Avenue, San Diego, CA 92105, **A**

O'Hara, Jane M 18 Rolling Lane, Needham, MA 02192, (617) 364-4850, BA 78 Boston Coll; MA 79 George Washington Univ; Director Sp-Lang & Hrng, New England Sinai Hospital, **SLP**

O'Hara, Nancy Lee 65 French Street, Quincy, MA 02171, (902) 429-4180, MS 80 Univ of TX - Dallas; 85–Aud, Burton Jaffe MD, **A**

O'Hara, Virginia R 1466 Tenbury Drive, Lynchburg, VA 24501, (804) 528-6993, BS 81 WV Univ; MS 82 Radford Univ; Sp-Lang Path, Central Virginia Training Ctr, **SLP**

O'Hara-Taylor, Mrs Patricia A 10 Wildwood Road #21A, Hartsdale, NY 10530, (201) 355-9316, **SLP**

O'Hare, Nancy J 604 Misty Lane, Friendswood, TX 77546, (713) 585-3349, BS 63 Univ of TN - Knoxville; MS 64 Vanderbilt Univ; Sp/Lang Path, Alvin ISD, **SLP**

O'Hare, Dr Nancy K 322 Rainbow Drive, Staunton, VA 24401, (703) 433-6440, BA 54 Seton Hill Coll; ME 56 Univ of Pittsburgh - Pittsburgh; PH 73 (NS) Univ of VA - Charlottesville; Prof, James Madison U, **SLP A F ACE**

Ohde, Ralph N 4509 Belmont Park Terrace, Nashville, TN 37215, (615) 320-5353, BA 66 Carthage Coll; ME 68 Univ of VA - Charlottesville; PH 78 (NS) Univ of MI - Ann Arbor; 81–Assoc Prof, Vanderbilt Univ School of Med, **SLP**

O'Hearn, Karen L 257 Rosebud, Corpus Christi, TX 78404, (512) 887-6784, BA 73 Southwest TX St Univ; ME 78 Southwest TX St Univ; SLP, Self Employed, **SLP**

O'Hearn, Victoria Moluse 276 Compton Ridge, Cincinnati, OH 45215, (513) 451-1544, BS 77 Bowling Green St Univ; MS 79 Univ of WI - Stevens Point; Aud, Western Hills Hearing Ctr, **A**

Ohl, Jacqueline Z 708 Hanover Manor #D-107, Carlisle, PA 17013, (717) 782-4350, BS 86 Bloomsburg Univ of PA; MS 87 Bloomsburg Univ of PA; 88–Sp-Lang Path, Polyclinic Med Ctr

Ohler, Elizabeth D 2713 South Surrey Drive, Carrollton, TX 75006, (817) 565-2262, BA 66 Winthrop Coll; MS 74 Southern Methodist Univ; 78–Superv Sp-Lang Path, Univ of N Texas, **SLP ACE**

Ohlin, Doug W U S Army Environmental Hygiene, Bio-Acoustics Division, Aberdeen Proving Ground, MD 21010-5422, (301) 671-3797, BS 67 Towson St Univ; MA 68 OH St Univ; PH 72 (Sp & Hrng Science) OH St Univ; Prog Mgr Hrng Conserv, US Army Environmental Agcy, **A**

Ohlweiler, Sr Zita 116 North A Street, Monmouth, IL 61462, (309) 734-6327, BS 66 Univ of IL - Urbana; MA 70 Univ of IL - Urbana; **SLP LM**

Ohnsman, Sharon Anne P O Box 65, Harriman, NY 10926, (914) 634-4648, BA 83 SUNY - Center at Binghamton; MS 86 Rutgers St Univ -N Brunswick; SLP, Rockland Co Ctr for Phys Hndcp, **SLP**

O'Hollaren, Mrs Colleen Marie 3515 SW Veterans Hospital Road, Portland, OR 97201, (503) 228-6479, BS 77 OR St Univ; MS 85 CA St Univ - Hayward; 85–Sp-Lang Path, Portland Ctr for Hrng & Sp, **SLP**

Ohree, Mrs Nathlyn B P O Box 2037, Rocky Mount, NC 27802, BA 78 Univ of NC - Chapel Hill; MA 80 Ball St Univ; Sp-Lang Path, Nash County Board of Education, **SLP**

Ohta, Debra Ann K 1455 Hoohaku Street, Pearl City, HI 96782, (808) 622-4123, BS 74 Univ of HI - Manoa; MA 76 CA St Univ - Los Angeles; MA 79 Univ of San Francisco; Sp-Lang Path, Dept of Ed St of Hawaii, **SLP**

Ohtaka, Mrs Keiko H 15 Cathy Road, Hillsdale, NJ 07642, **SLP**

Oistad, Mrs Georgia M 2802 11th Avenue East, Seattle, WA 98102, (206) 433-2576, BA 61 Univ of WA; BA 80 Univ of WA; OM 82 Univ of WA; SLP, Highline Sch Dist, **SLP**

Oja, Gregory Lawton Bemidji Regional Hrg Ctr, 403 4th St N W, Bemidji, MN 56601, (218) 751-0543, BA 81 Moorhead St Univ; BS 81 Moorhead St Univ; MS 83 ID St Univ; Aud, Self Employed, **A**

Ojakangas, Catherine Lee 3126 W Calhoun Pkwy #408, Minneapolis, MN 55416, (612) 624-7929, OB 79 Univ of MN - Duluth; BS 79 Univ of MN - Duluth; MS 81 Boston Univ; SLP, Univ of MN Doctoral Student, **SLP**

Okamura, Kay Emiko 2235-A Aulii Street, Honolulu, HI 96817, (808) 544-3333, BS 82 Univ of HI - Manoa; MS 84 Univ of HI - Manoa; Sp-Lang Path, Sr Francis Home Care, **SLP**

O'Kane, Mrs Florence K 260 Champion Way, Sewell, NJ 08080-1647, (609) 582-7062, **A**

Okanes, Mrs Barbara Marcus 870 Clarewood Court, Concord, CA 94518, (415) 432-3811, BA 48 Univ of RI; MA 55 CA St Univ - Los Angeles; SLP, Pittsburg USD, **SLP**

Okarski, Kim J 6937 Cloister, Toledo, OH 43617, (419) 841-4151, BA 75 MI St Univ; MA 76 MI St Univ; **A**

Okawachi, Pearl K 3103 Sea Gull Lane, Stockton, CA 95209, (209) 473-7539, BA 75 Univ of CA - Berkeley; MA 80 Univ of the Pacific; Sp-Lang Path, Stockton USD, **SLP**

O'Keefe, Bernard Michael 10 Vairo Boulevard #201-B, Box 224, State College, PA 16803, (814) 865-0971, BS 64 Emerson Coll; MS 70 Emerson Coll; Assoc Prof, U of Toronto, **SLP**

O'Keefe-La Pratt, Nancy J 18239 North 40th Street, Unit 142, Phoenix, AZ 85032, (602) 482-1150, BS 76 Marquette Univ; MS 78 Marquette Univ; Sp-Lang Path, Paradise Valley USD #69, **SLP**

O'Keeffe, Kathleen Noonan c/o Capt John S O'Keeffe, 9th Medical Detachment, APO New York, NY 09176, 011-49-7131-577211, BA 79 Gonzaga Univ; MS 81 Portland St Univ; Sp-Lang Path, **SLP**

O'Keeffe-Blue, Lisa Brooks 8760 Preston Place, Chevy Chase, MD 20815, (301) 424-5200, BS 83 Ithaca Coll; MA 85 NY Univ; Sp-Lang Path, The Rockville Treatment Ctr, **SLP**

Okeke, Irene N 8 Boyden Avenue, Maplewood, NJ 07040, (201) 761-7423, BA 78 Newark St Coll; MA 80 Montclair St Coll; **A**

Oken, Cheryl Lynn 44-20 Douglaston Parkway, Apartment 7C, Douglaston, NY 11363, (516) 466-2155, BA 80 SUNY - Center at Buffalo; MS 82 Univ of WI - Madison; Sp-Lang Path, Therapies Unlimtd, **SLP**

Oker, Susan Lynn 1209 Basswood, Naperville, IL 60540, (312) 420-7000, BS 86 Eastern IL Univ; MS 87 Eastern IL Univ; **SLP**

Okin, Mrs Deborah Fletcher 2329 Heron Hill Place, Lynchburg, VA 24503, (804) 845-4927, BS 76 Univ of VA - Charlottesville; ME 77 Univ of VA - Charlottesville; 88–Sp-Lang Path, Ctr for Rehab & Dev, **SLP**

Okonek, Ann Martha 3415 West Foster, Chicago, IL 60625, (312) 583-4249, BA 81 Mundelein Coll; MS 83 Rush Univ; Speech Language Pathologist, Chicago Board of Education, **SLP**

Okonek, Barbara J S 11625 Wilder Drive, Apt #317, Eden Prairie, MN 55344, (612) 339-7296, BS 81 Univ of WI - Stevens Point; MA 82 Northern IL Univ - De Kalb; Aud, Minneapolis ENT Clinic, **A**

Okoomian, Mrs Phyllis N 142 Glezen Lane, Wayland, MA 01778, (508) 358-7746, BA 51 Boston Univ; ME 52 Boston Univ; 70–Sp-Lang Path, Wayland Public Schools, **SLP**

Okrainec, Mrs J Alexa 256 Scotia Street, Winnipeg, MB, Canada R2V 1V9, (204) 338-9724, BS 74 Univ of Manitoba - Winnipeg; OM 77 Univ of Western Ontario; Sp-Lang Path, Seven Oaks Gen Hosp, **SLP ACE**

Okrent, Mrs Kathleen Mary 644 Lacrosse, Wilmette, IL 60091, (312) 251-2861, BS 83 Univ of IL - Urbana; MA 84 Northwestern Univ; 85–Aud, Oak Park Sp & H Center, **A**

Okun, Denise Riley 14 Cedar Drive, Canton, MA 02021, (617) 947-9295, BS 78 Emerson Coll; ME 80 Northeastern Univ; Coord/Commun Sers, Neurologic Cen at Forest Manor, **SLP**

Okun, Mrs Sue Kneler 13465 North 91st Place, Scottsdale, AZ 85260, (602) 391-9646, BS 78 Ithaca Coll; MS 80 AZ St Univ; Sp-Lang Path, Scottsdale Speech Pathology Associates, **SLP**

Olanoff, Rachel 253 Foxwood Lane, Marlton, NJ 08053, (609) 596-9442, BA 76 Univ of Pittsburgh - Pittsburgh; OM 78 Hahnemann Medical Coll; Aud Consult, Private Practice, **A**

Olarte, Dr Gerardo 991 N E 73rd Street, Miami, FL 33138, (305) 758-4003, MA 76 Univ of Northern IA; MA 77 Univ of Northern IA; PH 85 (Sp Path) Univ of FL; 85–Sp-Lang Path, Private Practice, **SLP**

Olarte, Mary P H 991 N E 73rd Street, Miami, FL 33138, (904) 378-0104, BA 74 Univ of Northern IA; MA 75 Univ of Northern IA; SLP, Private Practice, **SLP**

Olasker, Kathleen M 17 Bocock Place, St Albert, AB, Canada T8N 2K3, **SLP A**

Olasker, William Bruce 17 Bocock Place, St Albert, AB, Canada T8N 3K3, (403) 473-5616, BS 79 Univ of Alberta - Alberta; MA 83 Wichita St Univ; SLP, Edmonton Pub Sch Bd, **SLP**

Olberding, Debra L 811 E Jackson Street, Medford, OR 97504, (503) 773-6611, BA 77 CA St Univ - Chico; MS 79 Univ of OR; Super Commun Dis Dept, Providence Hosp, **SLP**

Olberding, Mrs Lucynda R 10510 Luzon, San Antonio, TX 78217, (512) 646-8432, BS 76 Univ of Tulsa; MA 78 Univ of Tulsa; **SLP**

Olday, Mrs Linda Jean RFD 1 Box 124A, Cherryfield, ME 04622, (207) 546-2424, BS 62 Emerson Coll; ME 72 Univ of MA - Amherst; Sp/Lang Path, Msad 37 Pub Sch Dist, **SLP**

Olde, Karen Leslie Box 1199, McCall, ID 83638, (208) 634-2219, **SLP**

Olden, Mrs Clara E 13906 Ramona Drive, Whittier, CA 90605, (213) 696-0625, MA 77 CA St Univ - Fullerton; Sp-Lang Path, Whittier Speech-Language Cen, **SLP**

Oldenburg, Lynda S 2929 Avila Bay Place, Davis, CA 95616, (916) 758-3290, BS 70 Univ of MN - Duluth; MA 71 Case Western Reserve Univ; 88–Sp-Lang Path, American River Hosp, **SLP**

Oldham, Mrs Elizabeth Belle 3293 Majestic Prince, Owensboro, KY 42303-2436, (502) 685-3161, BA 78 Univ of KY; MA 80 Eastern KY Univ; SLP, Daviess County Schools, **SLP**

Oldham, Jackson D 3601 3rd Avenue, Port Arthur, TX 77642, (409) 983-1651, BA 59 Univ of North TX; MA 65 Univ of TX - Austin; 74–Exec/Dir, Capland Cen for Commun Dis, **SLP ACE**

Oldknow, Wendy K 1466 East Ramon Road #259, Palm Springs, CA 92264, (619) 323-9203, MA 88 CA St Univ - Chico; 88–Sp-Lang Path, Palm Springs USD

Olds, Mrs Leesa Kae R R #3 Box 108, Morgantown, IN 46160, (812) 372-8211, **SLP**

Olds, Robert E, Jr 9470 Doty Drive, Beaumont, TX 77707, (409) 866-9590, BS 58 OH St Univ; ME 65 SUNY - Coll at Buffalo; Sp-Lang Path, Robert E Olds, **SLP**

Oldt, Lucy Altersitz Box 237-C Rd 2, High Hill Road, Swedesboro, NJ 08085, (609) 467-1635, BS 74 Univ of MD - College Park; MA 75 Trenton St Coll; Director/Owner, Joy of Learning Preschool, **SLP**

Oleaga-Labriola, Mrs Josephine 47-29 190th Street, Flushing, NY 11358, (718) 357-7099, BA 76 Hofstra Univ; MA 78 Hofstra Univ; Sp-Lang Path, West Islip Public Schools, **SLP**

Olean, Elizabeth P O Box 9, Hope Valley, RI 02832, **SLP**

O'Leary, Ann H K 2438 Billiton Court, Columbus, OH 43220, (614) 442-0860, BS 77 Miami Univ - Oxford; MS 78 Univ of MI - Ann Arbor; Sp-Lang Path, Franklin Ct Board MR/DD, **SLP**

O'Leary, Mrs Barbara L 13119 Amiot Drive, St Louis, MO 63146, (314) 569-8231, BS 63 Saint Louis Univ; MA 75 Saint Louis Univ; Area Coord, Spec Sch Dist of St Louis Co, **SLP**

O'Leary, Christine Marie 1020 North 29th, Billings, MT 59101, (406) 657-7945, BA 78 Univ of MT; OM 80 Univ of MT; Sp/Lang Path, St Vincent Hosp, **SLP ACE**

O'Leary, Debra M 2204 West Wall, Janesville, WI 53545, (414) 674-2840, BA 78 Univ of WI - Eau Claire; MS 79 Univ of WI - Eau Claire; SLP, Fort Atkinson Pub Sch, **SLP**

O'Leary, Dr Emmett L 1716 Comanche Road, Pueblo, CO 81001, (719) 549-2122, BA 63 Adams St Coll; MA 64 Central MI Univ; PH 72 (NS) Univ of NE - Lincoln; Sp-Lang Path, Univ of Southern Colorado, **SLP**

O'Leary, Georgia A 5553 Pine Lane Drive, Jackson, MS 39211, **SLP**

O'Leary, Mrs Geraldine 1860 Ala Moana #1903, Honolulu, HI 96815, (808) 947-1061, BS 70 Univ of NE - Omaha; MS 75 Univ of HI - Manoa; Sp-Lang Path, Doe Hi, **SLP**

Oleary, Mrs Joanne 10 Overlook Drive, Easthampton, MA 01027, (413) 586-3960, BA 64 Univ of MA - Amherst; Sp-Lang Path, Hampshire Reg Sch Dist, **SLP**

O'Leary, Jody B 623 Cortland Drive, Lake Zurich, IL 60047, **SLP**

O'Leary, Karen Schultz 1136 Maryland, Birmingham, MI 48009, (313) 540-6484, MA 80 Wayne St Univ; SLP, Sinai Hospital, **SLP**

O'Leary, Lauren Jean 8308 Shelter Creek Lane, San Bruno, CA 94066, (415) 921-0249, BA 78 San Francisco St Univ; MA 84 Univ of San Francisco; SLP, San Francisco USD, **SLP**

O'Leary, Mary Bridget 3823 West 51st Street, Chicago, IL 60632, (312) 582-5153, BA 80 Saint Xavier Coll; MS 82 Marquette Univ; Sp/Lang Path, Comm Consol Sch Dist 168, **SLP**

Oleary, Mrs Roberta M 449 2nd Avenue, San Francisco, CA 94118, (415) 664-1580, BA 38 Univ of MI - Ann Arbor; MA 70 San Francisco St Univ; **SLP LM**

O'Leary, Mrs Stephanie J S HCR #145, Richmond, VT 05477, (802) 878-1380, BA 80 Univ of VT; MS 81 Univ of VT; Sp-Lang Path, Chittenden Central Sch Dist, **SLP**

O'Leary, Virginia Marie 15 Hatfield Road, West Newton, MA 02165, (617) 964-2431, BA 82 Boston Coll; MS 84 Emerson Coll; SLP, Westwood Public Schools, **SLP**

Oleen, Cornelia J 4333 Brackenwood Court, Sarasota, FL 33582, (813) 365-0399, BS 73 SUNY - Coll at Buffalo; MS 78 Univ of South FL; SLP, Sarasota Co Sch Bd, **SLP**

Oleksiak, Colleen P 308 Atlantic Avenue, Massapequa Park, NY 11762, (516) 795-1467, BS 79 Univ of TN - Knoxville; MA 81 Univ of TN - Knoxville; Aud, Dr's Goodman Levy Stern BOCES, **A**

Oleksiuk, Adriana B Tierra Pines Convalescent Center, 7625 Ulmerton Road, Largo, FL 33540, (813) 535-9833, BA 71 Hofstra Univ; MA 73 CUNY - Queens Coll; 88–Sp-Lang Path, InSpeech Inc, **SLP ACE**

O'Leksy-Villarruel, Mrs Gail Anne 6047 Horizon, East Lansing, MI 48823, (517) 351-1668, MS 75 Univ of WI - Stevens Point

Olender, Mrs Rosemary 214 Cambridge Street, Syracuse, NY 13210, (315) 672-5228, BS 70 SUNY - Center at Albany; MA 74 Syracuse Univ; Tchr of Deaf/Sp-Lang Path, Orondaga Madison BOCES, **SLP**

Olenick, Gail M 1465 Geneva Loop, Brooklyn, NY 11239, (718) 385-2893, BA 79 CUNY - Brooklyn Coll; MS 82 CUNY - Brooklyn Coll; 81–Sp-Lang Path, NYC Bd of Ed, **SLP**

Oleski, Mrs Theresa Ann Rural Delivery 3, Box 3, Rome, NY 13440, (315) 336-4317, BS 78 Marywood Coll; MS 83 Ithaca Coll; Sp-Lang Path, UCP, **SLP**

Oleson, Susan H 21594 Birchwood, Farmington Hills, MI 48024, (313) 344-8460, OB 73 Miami Univ - Oxford; MA 79 Eastern MI Univ; SLP, Northville Publ Schs, **SLP**

Olexa-Smith, Mrs Sandra Kaye 516 Callen Avenue, Morgantown, WV 26505, (304) 366-2070, BS 82 WV Univ; MS 84 WV Univ; Sp-Lang Path, Marion County Schs, **SLP**

Olges, Kathleen N P O Box 16, Harrodsburg, IN 47434, (812) 279-6651, BS 77 IN Univ - Bloomington; MA 77 IN Univ - Bloomington; SLP, N Lawrence Comm Schs, **SLP**

Olicker, Mrs Charlene L 1940 N W 85th Way, Pembroke Pines, FL 33024, (305) 621-0509, BA 71 CUNY - Queens Coll; MS 72 Columbia Univ Teachers Coll; ES 87 Barry Univ; Sp-Lang Path, Dade Cty Publ Schs, **SLP ACE**

Oligschlaeger, Mrs Elayne Joy 6105 W 82nd Drive, Arvada, CO 80003, BS 82 Purdue Univ - West Lafayette; MS 84 Univ of WI - Madison; Sp-Lang Path, Mercy Med Ctr/Beth Israel Pavillon, **SLP**

Olin, Geraldine 3109 McMahan Boulevard, Louisville, KY 40220, (502) 245-4121, BA 67 Berea Coll; MA 72 Univ of KY; Sp-Lang Path, Cen State Hosp, **SLP**

Oliva, Constance 269 Covina #A, Long Beach, CA 90803, (714) 826-2140, BA 76 CUNY - Queens Coll; MA 78 Univ of Denver; Dir/Sp-Lang-Hrng Servs, College Hospital, **SLP**

Oliva, Deborah B 94 Old Mill Road, Harvard, MA 01451, (508) 772-7431, BA 74 Univ of ME - Orono; MS 76 Emerson Coll; 86–Sp-Lang Path, Judith Wisnia and Assoc, **SLP**

Olive, Debra A 27 Penwood Drive, Murray Hill, NJ 07974, (201) 233-3720, BS 80 Montclair St Coll; MA 81 NY Univ; Sp-Lang Path, Children's Specialized Hosp, **SLP**

Oliveira, Dr Robert J 225-In-12 3M Center, St Paul, MN 55144-1000, (612) 733-8128, BS 64; MS 67 Univ of MA - Amherst; PH 70 (Biochemistry) IA St Univ; Venture Director, Health Care Specialties

Oliver, Mrs Barbara J 500 N W 22nd Street, Wilton Manors, FL 33311, (305) 792-8772, BA 70 Univ of NC - Greensboro; ME 72 Univ of NC - Greensboro; Sp-Lang Path, Easter Seal Society of Broward Co, **SLP**

Oliver, Cynthia 3901 Indian School N E, #D-301, Albuquerque, NM 87110, (505) 764-2012, BA 82 Point Loma Nazarene Coll; MS 84 TX Tech Univ; SLP, Educ Assessment Systems Inc, **SLP**

Oliver, Mrs Cynthia Robinson 18630 Bonnie Lane, Brookfield, WI 53005, (414) 786-3929, BS 56 Univ of WI - Madison; MS 84 Marquette Univ; Sp-Lang Path, Racine Co, **SLP**

Oliver, Mrs Jean G Van Ness North #920, 3001 Veazey Terrace N W, Washington, DC 20008, (202) 363-0651, BA 50 OH Univ - Athens; MA 53 Univ of AL- Tuscaloosa; Retired, Offi of the Dir Nih, **SLP F**

Oliver, Kathryn Venaas 809 Adams Avenue, Eveleth, MN 55734, (218) 741-4772, BA 73 Univ of MN - Duluth; MS 81 Univ of WI - Eau Claire; SLP, ISD, **SLP**

Oliver, Mrs Kathy D 3716 44th Street Court N W, Gig Harbor, WA 98335, (206) 857-6171, BA 75 Univ of WA; OM 76 Univ of WA; Sp-Lang Path, Peninsula Sch Dist, **SLP**

Oliver, Mrs Kristina Weiskittle 229 West Highland Avenue, Ada, OH 45810, (419) 634-3465, BS 86 Miami Univ - Oxford; MS 87 Miami Univ - Oxford; **SLP**

Oliver, Mrs Leslie Blackwell 362 Blue Bonnet Boulevard, San Antonio, TX 78209, (512) 826-2650, BS 80 Southern Methodist Univ; MA 81 Our Lady Lake Univ-San Anton; 88–Sp-Lang Path, Our Lady of the Lake Univ, **SLP**

Oliver, Lisa Michele 3105 Barnsley Lane, Raleigh, NC 27604, (919) 876-8125, MA 88 Appalachian St Univ

Oliver, Lydia Tussey 2816 Mockingbird Drive, Williamsburg, VA 23185, (804) 220-3894, ME 76 Univ of VA - Charlottesville; 86–Sp-Lang Path, Child Development Resources, **SLP A**

Oliver, Nancy L 6121 36th Street, Lubbock, TX 79407, BA 81 TX Tech Univ; MA 86 TX Tech Univ; **SLP**

Oliver, Dr Paxton E Route 3 Box 84-C, Jonesboro, LA 71251, (318) 342-3057, BA 68 Northeast LA Univ; MA 75 LA Tech Univ; PH 81 (Sp Path) Univ Southern MS-Hattiesburg; 80–Coord-Grad Externs, Northeast La Univ, **SLP**

Oliver, Sara Ruth Ann 12937 N W Newberry Road, Portland, OR 97231, (503) 289-3845, MS 87 Portland St Univ

Oliver, Terrey A 1011 St John, Pearland, TX 77584, (713) 790-5913, BA 79 IN Univ - Bloomington; MS 83 Purdue Univ - West Lafayette; Aud, Baylor Coll of Med, **A**

Oliver, Vincent T 3001 Veazey Terrace N W, Apartment 920, Washington, DC 20008, BS 51 Central St Univ; MA 68 Kent St Univ; Retired, Private Practice

Oliver, William C 809 Adams Avenue, Eveleth, MN 55734, (218) 741-0150, BA 75 Univ of MN - Duluth; MA 76 Univ of MN - Duluth; Sp-Lang Path, East Range Clinics Ltd, **SLP**

Oliver-Hoge, Mrs Patricia D 3210 Montebello Terrace, Baltimore, MD 21214, (301) 687-1713, BS 80 Towson St Univ; MS 81 Towson St Univ; Sp/Lang Path, Baltimore Co Pub Sch Syst, **SLP**

Oliver-Hurt, Susan Kay 2965 Tuxedo Place, Santa Rosa, CA 95405, (707) 571-1890, BA 81 CA St Univ - Fresno; MS 86 CA St Univ - Sacramento; 86–Aud, Oakland Children's Hosp, **A**

Oliveri, Geraldine 409 Panorama Drive, Laguna Beach, CA 92651, (714) 497-1369, BA 55 Univ of CA - Santa Barbara; MA 79 Chapman Coll; **SLP**

Oliveri, Paula Jean 832 1/2 South Walnut, Springfield, IL 62704, BS 81 Western IL Univ; MA 86 Northern IL Univ - De Kalb; **SLP**

Oliverio, Alexis Matko Victoria Street #30, Windsor, CT 06095, BS 85 WV Univ; MS 86 WV Univ; **SLP**

Oliver-Padilla, Dr German P 804 Montevideo Street, Las Americas, Rio Piedras, PR 00921, (809) 751-6015, MS 71 Univ of PR - Rio Piedras; MD 57 (Pediatrics); Cleft Palate Team Dir, U of Puerto Rico, **SLP**

Ollinger, Mary Beth 950 Union Street #B, Platteville, WI 53818, (608) 348-2611, BA 83 Univ of WI - Eau Claire; MS 84 Univ of WI - Eau Claire; 84–Sp-Lang Path, Sch Dist of Platteville, **SLP**

Ollinger, Mrs Pamela L 509 Indian Lane, Salisbury, MD 21801, (301) 742-6599, BA 78 Depauw Univ; MS 83 Loyola Coll; Sp-Lang Path, Wicomico Co Bd of Ed, **SLP**

Olliver, Jodie Eileen 685 Hulls Hill Road, Southbury, CT 06488, (203) 264-3120, BS 82 Western KY Univ; MS 83 Western KY Univ; Sp-Lang Path, Southbury Trng Sch, **SLP**

Ollman, Jeffrey J 916 4th Avenue N E, Austin, MN 55912, (501) 433-0954, BS 72 Mankato St Univ; MA 78 Mankato St Univ; 78–Sp-Lang Path, Austin PS Dist 492, **SLP**

Olmstead, Mrs Mary J 300 Royal Palm Way, Palm Beach, FL 33480, (305) 655-7268, BA 82 Univ of FL; MA 84 Univ of FL; 84–Sp-Lang Path, Rehab Ctr for Child and Adults Inc, **SLP**

Olmstead, Mrs Patricia J P O Box 774462, Eagle River, AK 99577, (907) 694-3238, BA 74 Univ of AK - Fairbanks; MS 78 Univ of MT; Sp-Lang Path, Private Practice, **SLP**

Olness, Mrs June Birkelbach 530 Hall Street, Bridgeport, WV 26330, (304) 624-3300, **SLP**

Olney, Charlotte Anne 849 Webster, Traverse City, MI 49684, (616) 947-8765, MA 84 Central MI Univ; Sp-Lang Path, South Metro Assoc

Olofsson, Mrs Sheila Michaels 1928 West 102nd Street, Chicago, IL 60643, (312) 942-3700, BA 81 Saint Xavier Coll; MS 83 Rush Univ; Consult/Owner, Private Practice, **A**

O'Lowney, Mrs Patricia M 308 Dolphin Drive, Oceanside, CA 92054, (714) 651-9104, BS 73 SUNY - Coll at Geneseo; MA 76 SUNY - Coll at Geneseo; 88–Sp-Lang Path, San Maros USD, **SLP**

Olree, Mrs Kathy S 3942 Fillmore Avenue, St Louis, MO 63116-3116, (314) 968-4710, OB 82 Univ of MO - Columbia; MA 87 Eastern MI Univ; 88–Sp-Lang Path, St Louis Hrng-Sp Ctr, **SLP**

Olroyd, Dr Marie Hiern 525 Teddy Avenue, Slidell, LA 70458, (504) 643-2326, BS 63 LA St Univ - Baton Rouge; MA 65 LA St Univ - N O Medical Ctr; PH 72 (NS) LA St Univ - N O Medical Ctr; Aud, New Orleans Sch Bd, **SLP A**

Olscamp, Ruth P 625 Hillcrest, Bowling Green, OH 43402, (419) 372-2515, BA 70 Heidelberg Coll; MA 72 OH Univ - Athens; Asst Prof, Bowling Green St U, **SLP**

Olsen, Mrs Amy R 3272 Evergreen Drive, Wheatfield, NY 14120, (716) 282-1836, BS 84 SUNY - Coll at Fredonia; MA 85 Bowling Green St Univ; 88–Sp-Lang Path, Millard Fillmore Sub Rehab Ctr, **SLP**

Olsen, Mrs Betty 2815 Hermosita Drive, Glendale, CA 91208, **SLP LM**

Olsen, Dr Bruce D Dr F T Hill Ctr For Comm Dis, Mid Maine Med Ctr Seton Un, Chase Avenue, Waterville, ME 04901, (207) 872-4383, BA 62 Univ of RI; MA 64 MI St Univ; PH 72 (NS) Univ of Denver; Dir, Mid Maine Med Cen, **SLP A ACE**

Olsen, Dr Clifford C VA Medical Center, Audiology And Speech Pathology, 2615 East Clinton Avenue, Fresno, CA 93703, (209) 225-6100, BA 73 San Jose St Univ; MA 74 Univ of KS; PH 76 (Hrng Science) Univ of KS; 88–Aud, VA Med Ctr, **A**

Olsen, Cynthia Kathleen 901 North Curtis Road Suite 401, Boise, ID 83706, (208) 378-3320, BS 81 Brigham Young Univ; OM 83 Brigham Young Univ; 87–Aud, VA Med Ctr, **A**

Olsen, Mrs Elizabeth Field 1901 Berkeley Avenue, St Paul, MN 55105, (612) 698-5917, BA 84 Univ of WI - Eau Claire; MS 85 Univ of WI - Stevens Point; 86–Sp-Lang Path, St Paul PS #625, **SLP**

Olsen, Karel McSween 1778 Hoopes Avenue, Idaho Falls, ID 83404, (208) 523-6064, BS 85 Brigham Young Univ; OM 86 Brigham Young Univ; 88, **SLP**

Olsen, Kathryn Mary 4975 North Diversey Blvd, Milwaukee, WI 53217, (414) 963-9815, BA 79 Univ of WI - Madison; BA 81 Univ of WI - Madison; MS 83 Univ of WI - Madison; Audiologist, Milwaukee Medical Clinic, **A**

Olsen, Lylis E Alaska Treatment Center, 3710 E 20th Avenue, Anchorage, AK 99508, (907) 272-0586, BS 83 Mankato St Univ; MS 87 Univ of WA; **A**

Olsen, Pamela M 291 Valley Street, Pembroke, MA 02359, **SLP**

Olsen, Randall R 9218 Pleasant Lake Blvd, Parma, OH 44130, (216) 886-1333, BA 72 Cleveland St Univ; MA 74 Cleveland St Univ; Owner/Aud, Olsen Hearing Service, **A**

Olsen, Dr Richard H 1455 West Court Street, Kankakee, IL 60901, (815) 939-2024, BS 64 Univ of WI - River Falls; MA 66 Northern IL Univ - De Kalb; PH 70 (NS) Univ of Denver; Aud, Richard H Olsen Ph & Assoc Inc, **A**

Olsen, Sue King 3331 Briarwood Circle, Safety Harbor, FL 33572, (813) 535-3462, BA 76 Univ of FL; MS 81 Univ of South FL; SLP, Pinellas Co Sch Bd, **SLP**

Olsen, Dr Wayne O Dept Of Otorhinolaryngology, Mayo Clinic, Rochester, MN 55901, (507) 284-2577, BS 60 Univ of WI - Milwaukee; MA 62 Northwestern Univ; PH 65 (NS) Northwestern Univ; Consult/Aud, Mayo Clinic, **A F**

Olshin, Judith M 1418 Wynnemoor Way, Fort Washington, PA 19034, (215) 643-1157, MS; **SLP**

Olson, Mrs Alice Jane 9620 Ximines Lane North, Maple Grove, MN 55369, (612) 425-2024, BS 72 Mankato St Univ; MS 80 Univ of WI - Eau Claire; Sp/Lang Path, Osseo, **SLP**

Olson, Andrea B 523 Crestridge Road, Omaha, NE 68154, (402) 333-2325, BS 72 Univ of NE - Lincoln; MA 73 Univ of NE - Lincoln; 88–Sp-Lang Path, Omaha Hearing Sch, **SLP**

Olson, Anne Desmarais 3535 Randolph Road #100, Charlotte, NC 28211, (704) 364-4541, BA 81 Univ of FL; MA 85 Univ of TX - Austin; 87–Aud, Randolph Road ENT Assoc, **A**

Olson, Ardell E 1221 South 7th Street, Fargo, ND 58103, (701) 237-2441, BS 71 ND St Univ; MA 73 IN Univ - Bloomington; Aud, Fargo Cl Ltd, **A**

Olson, Carol Jean 155 Kathleen Drive, Elgin, IL 60123, (312) 888-5078, BS 64 IN Univ - Bloomington; MA 66 IN Univ - Bloomington; Sp-Lang Path, School District U-F6, **SLP**

Olson, Charlene Marie 1013 Howbert Avenue S W, Roanoke, VA 24015, (703) 981-1140, BA 84 Univ of ND; MS 86 James Madison Univ; 86–Sp-Lang Path, Pro Ther of Roanoke Inc, **SLP**

Olson, Mrs Christine C J Box 29 Rimrock West, Bend, OR 97701-9068, (503) 382-5874, BS 72 Univ of OR; MS 76 Western OR St Coll; Sp-Lang Path, Bend-LaPine Admin Sch Dist #1, **SLP**

Olson, Cindy L 460 5th Avenue North #406, Hopkins, MN 55343, (612) 835-4400, BS 77 Minot St Univ; BS 77 Minot St Univ; MS 78 Minot St Univ; Mktg/Sls Mgr, Maico Hrng Instruments, **A**

Olson, David Ray 3280 West Owasso Boulevard, St Paul, MN 55126-4137, (715) 386-9321, MS 83; Sp-Lang Path, River Ridge Rehabilitation, **SLP**

Olson, Dolores M 700 East Barrel Springs Road, Palmdale, CA 93550, (805) 273-5052, 85–Sp-Lang Path, Palmdale Sch Dist, **SLP**

Olson, Dr Don A 345 East Superior Street, Chicago, IL 60611, (312) 649-6179, BS 52 Univ of WI - Madison; MS 55 Northwestern Univ; PH 60 (NS) Northwestern Univ; 69–Dir, Rehab Inst of Chicago, **SLP F**

Olson, Mrs Donna K 732 North Lake Drive, Du Quoin, IL 62832, BS 70 Southern IL Univ -Carbondale; MS 74 Southern IL Univ -Carbondale; Sp/Lang Path, **SLP**

Olson, Dorothy M 1002 Buckingham Drive, Stevens Point, WI 54481, (715) 346-3588, BS 74 Univ of WI - Stevens Point; MS 75 Univ of WI - Stevens Point; Prof, U of WI-Stevens Point, **SLP**

Olson, Douglas M 411 1st Avenue, Audubon, IA 50025, (712) 563-2336, BA 80 Univ of Northern IA; MA 83 Univ of Northern IA; MA 83 Univ of Northern IA; Aud, Heartland AEA, **A**

Olson, Mrs Gail Lynn 13815 Riker, Chelsea, MI 48118, (313) 994-2318, BS 64 Eastern MI Univ; MA 78 Eastern MI Univ; Sp-Lang Path, Ann Arbor Publ Schs, **SLP**

Olson, Mrs Joan Abrahamson 830 West Way N W, Bemidji, MN 56601, (218) 759-1887, BS 63 Univ of MN - Duluth; ME 86 Univ of MO - Columbia; Sp-Lang Path, Bemidji PS, **SLP**

Olson, Joan R 5333 N Santa Monica Blvd, Milwaukee, WI 53217, (414) 351-0450, BS 63 Marquette Univ; MS 66 Purdue Univ - West Lafayette; Sp-Lang Path, Shared Therapeutic Serv of WI, **SLP**

Olson, Joni L 6205 Whitley Court, Bakersfield, CA 93309, BA 80 CA St Univ - Los Angeles; MA 81 CA St Univ - Chico; SLP, Bakersfield Cty Sch Dist, **SLP**

Olson, Joyce A M Route 2 Box 200, Agusta, WI 54722, BA 76 Univ of WI - Eau Claire; MS 77 Univ of WI - Eau Claire; Unit Director, Harborview Developmental Cen, **SLP**

Olson, Judith Buell 2 South 271 Oakwood Court, Wheaton, IL 60187, (312) 510-0766, MA 73 Northern IL Univ - De Kalb; OB 71 Northern IL Univ - De Kalb; Sp-Lang Path

Olson, Karin Elizabeth 10904 Southeast 254th St, Apartment A102, Kent, WA 98031, (206) 852-6060, BA 85 WA St Univ; MA 86 WA St Univ; **SLP**

Olson, Mrs Kathryn S 1832 North Adams Street, South Bend, IN 46628-1416, (219) 284-7134, BS 76 East Carolina Univ; MA 78 OH Univ - Athens; 87–Sp-Lang Path, Rehab Tech Ctr, **SLP**

Olson, Kimberly Kaye 4294 North Hughes Avenue, Apartment 176, Fresno, CA 93705, BS 84 Northern AZ Univ; MS 85 Northern AZ Univ; **SLP**

Olson, Mrs Laurel 8742 West Athens Street, Peoria, AZ 85345, (602) 972-1018, BS 85 Northern IL Univ - De Kalb; MA 87 Northern IL Univ - De Kalb; 88–Aud, Heskett Hearing Aid Center, **A**

Olson, Leila M 814 Stanford Road, Grand Forks, ND 58201, (701) 746-2230, BS 50 Minot St Univ; MA 69 Univ of ND; 71–Sp-Lang Path, Grand Forks Public Schools, **SLP**

Olson, Linda B 1262 1st Street, Los Osos, CA 93402, (805) 528-3852, MA 86 CA St Univ - Stanislaus; Sp-Lang Path, San Luis Coastal USD, **SLP**

Olson, Mrs Linda Kay 1806 Brittania Court, Chesterfield, MO 63017, (314) 569-8100, MS 82 Southern IL Univ-Edwardsvill; 83–Sp-Lang Path, St Louis Special Sch Dist, **SLP**

Olson, Lori Bastness Box 1630, Morden, MB, Canada R0G 1J0, (306) 882-2633, MS 85 Minot St Univ; Sp-Lang Path, Child Care & Dev Dept of Educ, **SLP**

Olson, Lynn M 15 Olympus Drive #3-A, Naperville, IL 60540, (312) 420-6385, BA 68 Augustana Coll; MA 77 Northern IL Univ - De Kalb; Sp-Lang Path, Naperville Pub Sch, **SLP**

Olson, Marilyn R N-84 W 15920 Menomonee Avenue, Menomonee Falls, WI 53051, (414) 255-2220, BA 66 Univ of IA; MA 67 Univ of IA; 88–Aud, MJ Therapy WCTC, **A**

Olson, Marla Lee 904 N W 36th Terrace #2, Oklahoma City, OK 73118-7129, BS 83 LA St Univ - Baton Rouge; MS 85 Univ of OK Medical Center; **SLP**

Olson, Mary Christine 3029 Long Meadow Circle, Bloomington, MN 55420, (612) 854-8803, BS 83 Univ of WI - River Falls; OM 85 Univ of WI - River Falls; 88–Sp-Lang Path, Minneapolis PS, **SLP**

Olson, Mrs Mary Crollard 5423 65th Avenue West, Tacoma, WA 98467, BA 79 Western WA Univ; MA 81 Western WA Univ; Aud, **A ACE**

Olson, Mary Ellen 17 Sanford Street, Bangor, ME 04401-6129, (207) 945-9670, BA 74 Univ of CO - Boulder; MA 85 Univ of CO - Boulder; **SLP**

Olson, Mary L 418 South Midpark Drive, Appleton, WI 54915, (414) 735-9642, BS 78 Northern MI Univ; MS 80 Northern MI Univ; Sp-Lang Path, **SLP**

Olson, Mrs Mary S 415 Peachtree Road, Orlando, FL 32804, (305) 423-1303, BA 57 MI St Univ; MA 61 MI St Univ; **SLP**

Olson, Nancy Elizabeth 4337 Southwind Drive, Raleigh, NC 27612, (919) 876-1401, BS 82 Univ of TN - Knoxville; MA 84 Memphis St Univ; Sp-Lang Path, Tammy Lynn Center, **SLP**

Olson, Patricia 3055 Hall Road, Kelowna, BC, Canada V1W 2R5, (604) 861-4727, BA 69; MA 73 MI St Univ; 86–Aud, Okanagan Hearing Clinic, **A**

Olson, Patricia A 21 Country Road, Lewisburg, PA 17837, BS 74 Indiana Univ of PA; MS 76 Indiana Univ of PA; Sp-Lang Path, Snyder Union Mifflin Child Dev Inc, **SLP**

Olson, Mrs Patricia Lynn 3620 Spencer Boulevard, Sioux Falls, SD 57103, (605) 339-4030, BS 78 Univ of IA; MA 84 Univ of IA; Sp-Lang Path, Sioux Falls Sch Dist, **SLP**

Olson, Paulette Marie D 3122 North 8th, Fargo, ND 58102, (218) 483-4516, BA 76 6876; MA 79 Univ of ND; Sp-Lang Path-Presch Spec Needs, Lake Agassiz Spec Ed Coop, **SLP**

Olson, Robert D Speech And Hearing Center, Marshall University, Huntington, WV 25701, (304) 696-3640, BA 50 Lewis-Clark St Coll; MA 55 OH Univ - Athens; PH 65 (NS) Northwestern Univ; Prof, Marshall Univ, **SLP F**

Olson, Romaine A 1944 Harris Avenue, Richland, WA 99352, **SLP ACE**

Olson, Rosalind 364 Ridge Circle Drive, Grand Junction, CO 81503, (303) 243-5236, MA Southern Methodist Univ; SLP, Mesa Cty Publ Sch Dist 51, **SLP**

Olson, Sandy L 6131 Power Drive, Dallas, TX 75227, (214) 690-8774, BS 78 Univ of North TX; MS 80 Southern Methodist Univ; Sp-Lang Path, Richardson ISD, **SLP**

Olson, Saundra L Special Education Department, Elgin Public Schools, Elgin, IL 60120, (312) 888-5078, BS 61 Univ of IL - Urbana; MA 73 Univ of IL - Urbana; Sp-Lang Path, Elgin Public Schools, **SLP**

Olson, Susan Hewitt 16475 South Manor Road, Eden Prairie, MN 55346, (612) 546-5411, BA 80 Univ of WI - Eau Claire; MS 81 Univ of WI - Stevens Point; 87–Regd Dir, Achievement Rehab Corp, **SLP**

Olson, Mrs Sylvia E L C-8 Oakwood, Indian Creek, IL 60060, (312) 362-0240, BS 77 Western IL Univ; MA 78 Western IL Univ; Sp-Lang Path, Libertyville District #70, **SLP**

Olson, Mrs Teri Daw 738 May Street, Waterloo, IA 50701-4342, (319) 234-4495, BA 84 Univ of Northern IA; MA 85 Univ of Northern IA; **SLP**

Olson, Mrs Terry Lee 1089 North Driftwood Avenue, Rialto, CA 92376-3950, (714) 820-9908, BA 80 Univ of LA Verne; MS 83 Univ of LA Verne; 86–Sp-Lang Path, San Bernardino County Sch, **SLP**

Olson, Thomas J Camp Merrill, HCR4 Box 228, Phillips, WI 54555, (715) 332-5255, BS 71 Univ of WI - Eau Claire; MS 72 Univ of WI - Eau Claire; Sp-Lang Path, Northwoods Rehabilitation Assoc, **SLP**

Olson, Mrs Valerie S 819 South Grand, Bozeman, MT 59715, (406) 388-4215, BA 62 Univ of MT; MA 67 Univ of MT; Sp/Lang Path, Belgrade Pub Schs, **SLP**

Olson-Silva, Mrs Sandra 322 Hilton Drive, Lexington Park, MD 20653, (301) 862-2417, BA 76 Temple Univ; MA 78 Trenton St Coll; Sp-Lang Path, St Mary's County Schs, **SLP**

Olson-Thomsen, Margaret 17291 Round Lake Road, Eden Prairie, MN 55346, (612) 933-9370, BA 75 Univ of MN - Minneap-St Paul; MA 78 Saint Cloud St Univ; Sp-Lang Path, Hopkins Pub Sch, **SLP**

Olsson, Robert J 5025 Laurel Street, San Diego, CA 92105, (619) 425-6830, MA 83 San Diego St Univ; Aud, Private Practice, **A**

Olswang, Dr Lesley B Department Of Speech & Hearing Sciences, JG-15, University Of Washington, Seattle, WA 98195, (206) 545-2997, BS 69 Northwestern Univ; MA 71 Univ of IL - Urbana; PH 78 (NS) Univ of WA; Assoc Prof, Univ of Washington, **SLP**

Olthoff, Mary Jo 1888 Olde Village Run, Dunwoody, GA 30338-5114, (404) 396-6224, BA 69 Fontbonne Coll; MA 70 Saint Louis Univ; Sp-Lang Path, Gwinnett Cen Family Couns, **SLP**

Oltman, Mrs Barbara Jean 4243 Pixie Avenue, Lakewood, CA 90712, (213) 673-3490, MA 83 CA St Univ - Long Beach; Sp-Lang Path, Lennox School District, **SLP**

Oltman, Mrs Shirley G R R 1 Box 228, Rosebud, MO 63091, (314) 764-2652, BS 49 Bradley Univ; MA 67 Saint Louis Univ; **SLP**

Oltmann, Mrs Donna Sandquist 802 West Kilarea, Mesa, AZ 85202, (602) 820-6708, BS 79 AZ St Univ; MS 82 AZ St Univ; SLP, Marilyn Hawker & Associates, **SLP**

Oltzik-Ladin, Mrs Barbara 150 Townhouse Road, Hamden, CT 06514, (203) 288-7293, BS 78 SUNY - Coll at Buffalo; MS 79 PA St Univ - Univ Park; Sp-Lang Path, Asl Sp & Lang Serv, **SLP**

Olvera-vonRabenau, Franz D 446 Lake Park Drive, Grand Prairie, TX 75051, (214) 372-7013, BA 62 Saint Mary's Coll; BA 77 Univ of MN - Minneap-St Paul; OM 79 Univ of WI - River Falls; 84–Aud, Dallas VA Med Cen, **A**

Olynick, Mrs Miriam Smoot 5800 Shadow Creek Road, Charlotte, NC 28226, (704) 543-1451, BA 82 Univ of NC - Greensboro; MS 83 Univ of NC - Chapel Hill; 84–Aud, Charlotte Sp & Hrng, **A**

Omafray, Mary Jo 8901 Grant Street #1622, Thornton, CO 80229, (303) 776-7417, BS 81 SD St Univ; MA 86 Univ of CO - Boulder; 87–Sp-Lang Path, St Vrain Early Intervention Ctr, **SLP**

O'Malley, Mrs Carol E L 18491 Durfee Circle, Villa Park, CA 92667, **SLP**

O'Malley, Mrs Colleen Corbett 4721 Lawsher Drive, Syracuse, NY 13215, (315) 469-8073, BS 74 SUNY - Coll at Fredonia; MS 79 Syracuse Univ; Sp-Lang Path, Jamesville Dewitt Cntrl Sch, **SLP**

O'Malley, Dr Honor Columbia Univ Teachers College, Box 145, 525 West 120th Street, New York, NY 10027, (212) 678-3893, BA 71 Manhattan Coll; MS 73 Purdue Univ - West Lafayette; PH 77 (Psychoacoustics) Purdue Univ - West Lafayette; Assoc Prof, Tchrs Coll, Columbia U

O'Malley, Mrs Janet B 431 Wood Shadow, San Antonio, TX 78216-1637, (512) 496-5487, BS 74 Saint Louis Univ; MA 75 Univ of KS; **SLP**

O'Malley, Marguerite Theresa 47 Old Fuller Road Ext, Blue Bird Acres Park, Chicopee, MA 01020, (413) 592-6111, BS 72 Nazareth Coll of Rochester; MS 86 Worcester St Coll; **SLP**

O'Malley, Mrs Nancy S 27726 Marquette Boulevard, North Olmsted, OH 44070, (216) 779-1747, BA 71 Cleveland St Univ; MA 72 Cleveland St Univ; Sp-Lang Path, Private Practice, **SLP**

Oman, Mrs Linda N 125 Whisperwood Lane, Battle Creek, MI 49017, (616) 979-2704, BS 62 Bowling Green St Univ; **SLP**

O'Meara, Patricia A 3822 N E 66th, Portland, OR 97213, (503) 280-5710, BS 77 Portland St Univ; MS 79 Portland St Univ; Sp/Lang Path, Portland PS Regional Programs, **SLP**

Omer, Mrs Elaine Okonek 228 W Rogers Street, Hartford, WI 53027, (414) 352-3100, MS 86 Univ of WI - Stevens Point; **A**

Omer, Mrs Jane Lewis 8031 Pawnee, Shawnee Mission, KS 66208, (913) 649-1542, BS 35 Univ of KS; MS 63 Univ of KS; **A LM**

Omiecinski, Mrs Mary K 2405 Tammeron Drive, Marietta, GA 30064, (404) 424-6493, BA 73 Univ of FL; ME 74 Univ of FL; **A**

Ominsky, Mrs Karen Fults 1200 Villa Isle Court, Pasadena, MD 21122, (301) 437-9241, **A**

Omiya, Grace Michiyo 3232 W Alpine Avenue, Stockton, CA 95204, (209) 463-2567, BA 81 Univ of the Pacific; MA 85 CA St Univ - Stanislaus; **SLP**

Omlin, Cynthia Joy H 6924 North Adams, Spokane, WA 99208, (509) 353-3747, BA 79 Gonzaga Univ; MS 81 Eastern WA Univ; Sp-Lang Path, Spokane PS, **SLP**

Omo, Mrs Patricia H 1901 Bay Oaks Court, Fort Worth, TX 76112, (817) 460-5621, BS 72 OK St Univ; MS 75 Univ of North TX; Sp-Lang Path, Arlington ISD, **SLP**

O'Neal, Carol M 77 Waverly, Clarendon Hills, IL 60514, (312) 968-3026, BA 56 Univ of IA; MS 79 IL St Univ - Normal; SLP, **SLP**

O'Neal, Elaine 5505 Adelina Court, Agoura Hills, CA 91301, (805) 498-6748, BA 78 CA St Univ - Northridge; MA 80 CA St Univ - Northridge; 86–Tchr, Conejo Valley USD, **SLP**

O'Neal, Harriett 8511 Marathon, Universal City, TX 78148, (512) 659-3186, OB 71 Univ of Central AR; MA 75 Our Lady Lake Univ-San Anton; **SLP**

O'Neal, Joy P 12504 Echo Cove, Buda, TX 78610, (512) 471-3841, BA 65 OK Baptist Univ; OM 69 Southern Methodist Univ; 81–Aud, Univ of Texas Spch & Hrng Cen, **A**

O'Neal, Linda M 24 Sweet Bay Lane, Hilton Head, SC 29926, (803) 681-5150, BS 60 Purdue Univ - West Lafayette; MA 65 Univ of CT; 88–Sp-Lang Path, Beaufort County Schs, **SLP ACE**

O'Neil, Denise C 1016 North Liberty Street, Arlington, VA 22205, (202) 363-7032, BA 77 Univ of RI; MS 80 Univ of RI; 87–Sch Prog Dir, St Johns Chld Dev Cen, **SLP**

O'Neil, Ellen Mary 8 Highland Street, Norwood, MA 02062, (617) 769-0854, BS 82 Marquette Univ; MA 84 Univ of MA - Amherst; Aud, Bay Colony Hearing Instruments, **A**

O'Neil, Mrs Lynn Scroggs 10244 West 80th #212, Overland Park, KS 66204, (913) 621-5155, BS 83 Univ of IA; MA 85 Univ of KS; Sp-Lang Path, Kansas City KS Sch Dist, **SLP**

O'Neil, Meghan Reardon 7 Burnham Road, Lexington, MA 02173, (617) 484-1469, BS 63 Boston Univ; ME 79 Northeastern Univ; Sp-Lang Path, Town of Belmont, **SLP**

O'Neil, Mrs Patricia M 3507 Sherwood Drive, Pascagoula, MS 39567, (601) 769-6305, BS 60 Auburn Univ - Auburn; 79–Sp-Lang Path, Chldn's Med Cen, **SLP ACE**

O'Neil, Therese M 36 Greenwood Street, Amesbury, MA 01913, (617) 388-1544, BS 79 Worcester St Coll; ME 81 Northeastern Univ; 88–Asst Dir-Sp Dept, Spaulding Rehab Hosp, **SLP**

O'Neil-Kayal, Jennifer Mary 200 Captain's Row #101, Chelsea, MA 02150, (617) 267-4730, BS 83 Worcester St Coll; MS 86 Univ of AR - Medical Sci; 86–Aud, Boston Guild for the Hard of Hearing, **A**

O'Neill, Mrs Andrea Bonchonsky 15 Little Plains Court, Huntington, NY 11743, (516) 673-1624, Coordinator Sp-Lang Services, South Huntington School Dist, **SLP**

O'Neill, Clare Elizabeth 1339 Alward Street, Prince George, BC, Canada V2M 2G4, (604) 564-1792, BA 80 Coll of Saint Francis; MS 81 Murray St Univ; 88–Sp-Lang Path/Dept Coord, Child Development Ctr, **SLP**

O'Neill, Mrs Ellen Kester 1052 McAllister Drive, New Kensington, PA 15068, (412) 335-9705, BS 80 Indiana Univ of PA; MA 82 Univ of IL - Urbana; **SLP**

O'Neill, Mrs Ellen R 231 Avalon Drive, Rochester, NY 14618, (716) 377-4660, BS 70 SUNY - Coll at Geneseo; MS 75 Nazareth Coll of Rochester; 75–Sp-Lang Path, BOCES 1 Monroe County, **SLP**

O'Neill, Janet J 3489 Beaver Ford Road, Woodbridge, VA 22192, (703) 590-6887, BA 70 Univ of Northern CO; MA 86 Miami Univ - Oxford; 88–Sp-Lang Path, Facquier County Schs VA, **SLP**

O'Neill, John J Speech And Hearing Clinic, University Of Illinois, 901 South 6th Street, Champaign, IL 61820, (217) 333-2230, BS 47 OH St Univ; PH 51 (NS) OH St Univ; Prof, U of IL, **SLP A F H**

O'Neill, Kerri R 3308 Janwood, Garland, TX 75042-2640, (214) 840-0294, BS Univ of TX - Austin; MS 79 Univ of TX - Dallas; **SLP**

O'Neill, Mrs Laura Lee 10570 Apple Grove, Rancho Cordova, CA 95670, (916) 985-9916, MA 83 CA St Univ - Fresno; Sp-Lang Path, Folsom-Cordova USD, **SLP**

Oneill, Margaret M 21 Plaske Drive, Schenectady, NY 12309, MA 79 SUNY - Center at Buffalo; Audiologist, Sunnyview Hospital, **A**

O'Neill, Mark A Rd 2 Route 44, Jersey Shore, PA 17740, **SLP ACE**

O'Neill, Pamela Jean 1414 Gesna Drive, Hanover, MD 21076, (301) 972-0202, BS 82 WV Univ; MS 84 Gallaudet Coll; **A**

O'Neill, Patricia Ilene 301 South G Street, Lompoc, CA 93436, (805) 735-8199, BS 84 Western MI Univ; MA 81 Western MI Univ; Sp-Lang Path, Private Practice, **SLP**

O'Neill, Patricia M 259-04 81st Avenue, Floral Park, NY 11004, (718) 343-0437, BA 79 CUNY - Queens Coll; MA 83 CUNY - Queens Coll; Sp-Lang Path, Brookdale Hospital, **SLP**

O'Neill, Peter 555 West Cornelia #1804, Chicago, IL 60657, **SLP**

O'Neill, Rosanna Marie 32126 20th Lane S W #124, Federal Way, WA 98023, (206) 572-5252, BA 81 Western WA Univ; MS 83 Univ of WA; 84–Sp-Lang Path, Multicare Medical Center, **SLP**

O'Neill-Baker, Mary Catherine 75 Myrtle Street, Watertown, MA 02172, MS 81 Boston Univ; 88–Sp-Lang Path, Charmss Collaborative, **SLP**

O'Neill-Fox, Barbara J 190 Bywater Way, Hillsborough, NJ 08876, (201) 731-3600, BA 76 Caldwell Coll; MA 80 Montclair St Coll; Sp-Lnag Path, Kessler Inst for Rehab, **SLP**

O'Neil-McCabe, Mrs Jana 95 Deer Ridge Drive, Barrington, NH 03825, (603) 749-5379, BS 80 Univ of NH; MS 85 Univ of NH; **SLP**

Ongley, Leena Marianna 5325 South Harper #3, Chicago, IL 60615-4506, (312) 239-0200, MA 83 Western MI Univ; 87–Aud, Management Planning Inst, **SLP A**

Onstine-Dill, Joanne 34541 Knox Butte Road E, Albany, OR 97321, (503) 967-4608, BA 71 Univ of CA - Santa Barbara; MA 74 Univ of CA - Santa Barbara; Sp-Lang Path, Gtr Albany Pub Sch, **SLP**

Onstott, Mrs Karla Cummings 2402 Roselawn, Wichita Falls, TX 76308, (817) 767-6835, BS 83 Univ of North TX; MS 86 Univ of North TX; 88–Sp-Lang Path, Burkburnett Indpt Sch Dist

Onufrak, Mrs Betty J 14 Westerly Drive, Fredonia, NY 14063, (716) 672-2336, MS 69 SUNY - Coll at Geneseo; Sp-Lang Path, Private Practice, **SLP**

Onufrak, Dr John A 14 Westerly Drive, Fredonia, NY 14063, (716) 673-3203, BS 66 SUNY - Coll at Geneseo; MS 69 SUNY - Coll at Geneseo; PH 73 (NS) SUNY - Center at Buffalo; Assoc Prof/Sp-Lang Path, SUNY/Fredonia, **SLP**

Onufrock, Mrs Elizabeth Hamm 2221 East Newton Avenue, Shorewood, WI 53211, (414) 639-0749, MA 83 Marquette Univ; Sp-Lang Path, Racine USD, **SLP**

Oolie, Marjorie R 26 East Greenbrook Road, North Caldwell, NJ 07006, (201) 226-7924, BS 59; ME 61; **SLP**

Opatrny, Gay 2316 Palos Verdes Drive W, Number 2, Palos Verdes Estates, CA 90274, (213) 377-0495, BS 74 Purdue Univ - West Lafayette; MS 76 Purdue Univ - West Lafayette; **A ACE**

Opauski, Marsha Kay Route 1 Box 376, Terlton, OK 74081, (918) 865-3078, MS 85 Gallaudet Coll; **A**

Opfer, Nanci B 1617 West 14th, Sedalia, MO 65301, (816) 836-8100, BA 75 William Jewell Coll; MS 81 Central MO St Univ; SLP, Indep Sanitarium & Hosp, **SLP**

Opie, Jane Maria Audiology & Hearing Impairment, Northwestern University, 2299 Sheridan Road, Evanston, IL 60201, (212) 532-2005, BA 83 SUNY - Center at Buffalo; MA 84 Northwestern Univ; **A**

Oppenheim, Mrs Carol Maple 12370 Valley Vista Drive, Chesterland, OH 44026, (216) 729-8035, BA 78 Univ of MI - Ann Arbor; MA 84 CA St Univ - Northridge; Sp-Lang Path, Cleveland Hearing-Speech Ctr, **SLP**

Oppenheim, Mrs Debra L 4852 Haskell, Encino, CA 91436, (818) 990-5715, BS 79 Univ of AZ; MA 81 CA St Univ - Los Angeles; Sp-Lang Path, Private Practice, **SLP**

Oppenheimer, Barbara B 116 Waverly Avenue, Newton, MA 02158, (617) 884-8300, BA 76 IN Univ - Bloomington; MA 78 Northwestern Univ; Adjunct Clinical Instructor, Boston U, **SLP**

Oppenheimer-Eidlin, Marsha 17 Highland Drive, Pembroke, MA 02359, (508) 580-7527, BS 75 SUNY - Center at Albany; MS 77 Columbia Univ Teachers Coll; 87–Team Facilitator, Brochton PS, **SLP**

Oppenheim-Errera, Gabrielle 57 Princeton Avenue, Princeton, NJ 08540, MS; **LM**

Oppfelt, Glenn R Bellevue Public School, P O Box 90010, Bellevue, WA 98009-9010, (206) 455-6077, BA 52 Univ of Denver; MA 53 Univ of Denver; Superv/Spec Serv, Bellevue Sch Dist, **SLP A**

O'Pry, Mrs Judy 101 Fanny Street, Lafayette, LA 70508, (318) 231-6869, BA 65 SUNY - Center at Buffalo; MA 68 Bradley Univ; Sp-Lang Path, Iberia School Board, **SLP**

Opsal, Cynthia R 1004 St Paul Avenue, St Paul, MN 55116, MS 79 Univ of WI - Stevens Point; Sp-Lang Path, ISD-196, **SLP**

Oquist, Mrs Kerstin 4419 234th Street N E, Arlington, WA 98223, (206) 435-9419, MS 69 UT St Univ; 87–Sp-Lang Path, Sultan Sch Dist, **SLP**

Oramas, Consuelo 429 B West Virginia Avenue, Morgantown, WV 26505, (304) 292-8772, BS 75 Universidad Nacional DE Colombia; MS 85 WV Univ; Aud, Morgantown ENT Clinic, **A**

Orange, Mrs Tina Tettenburn 3609 Juneau Road #98-G, Columbia, SC 29210, (803) 731-0976, BS 85 WV Univ; MA 86 Univ of SC - Columbia; Aud, Nu-Ear Hearing Aid Ctr, **A**

Oratio, Dr Albert R 41 West Central Avenue, Maywood, NJ 07607, (201) 595-2208, BA 72 Montclair St Coll; MA 73 Montclair St Coll; PH 77 (NS) Bowling Green St Univ; **SLP**

Oratio, Mrs Suzanne Lange 41 West Central Avenue, Maywood, NJ 07607, BA 72 Rutger's St Univ - Douglas Coll; MA 73 Montclair St Coll; SLP, Hackensack Pub Sch, **SLP**

Orchik, Dr Daniel J Hearing SVC MPHS, P O Box 17987, Memphis, TN 38187-0987, (901) 761-9729, BS 66 Clarion Univ of PA; MS 68 SUNY - Coll at Buffalo; PH 73 (Aud) MI St Univ; Chief of Aud, The Shea Cl&Deafness Found, **A**

Orcholski, Emil R 11330 North Glenwood Drive, Mequon, WI 53092-3709, BS 77 Univ of WI - Milwaukee; MS 78 Univ of WI - Milwaukee; 78–Sp-Lang Path, Milwaukee PS, **SLP**

Orcutt, Anne Witt Speech Pathology Service Inc, P O Box 85, 2007 Skyline Drive, Stoughton, WI 53589, (608) 873-4784, BS 63 Northwestern Univ; Pres, Sp Path Serv Inc, **SLP**

Ordona, Heather Ann Mississippi Bend Area Education Agency, 729 21st Street, Bettendorf, IA 52722, (319) 359-1371, BS 77 IA St Univ; MA 81 Univ of IA; 82–Sp-Lang Path, MS Bend AEA, **SLP**

Ordonez, Mrs Joan F 17161 Kristopher Lane, Huntington Beach, CA 92647, (213) 437-2851, MS 79 Marquette Univ; **SLP**

Ordower, Elaine L 132 Maple Avenue, Highland Park, IL 60035, (312) 433-9222, BS 75 Univ of MI - Ann Arbor; MS 76 Univ of MI - Ann Arbor; **SLP**

O'Reagan, Margaret Mary 600 East 8th #709, Kansas City, MO 64106, (816) 276-4023, BA 79 Univ of KS; MS 81 Southern Methodist Univ; Sp-Lang Path, Research Medical Ctr, **SLP**

O'Reilly, Ana Santos 3410 S W 6th Street, Miami, FL 33135, (305) 581-0530, BA 82 Univ of Northern CO; MA 84 Univ of Northern CO; 85–Aud, Sch Bd of Broward Co, **A**

O'Reilly, Mrs Ann E 132 Ocean Avenue, Amityville, NY 11701, (516) 321-3259, BA 79 SUNY - Coll at New Paltz; MA 85 Long Island U - CW Post Ctr; SLP, N Babylon Union Free Schl Dstr, **SLP**

O'Reilly, Mrs Sandra B 38 Turkey Lane, Cold Spring Harbor, NY 11724, (516) 757-3050, BA 76 Saint John's Univ - Jamaica; MA 78 CUNY - Queens Coll; Sp-Lang Path, **SLP**

O'Reilly, Mrs Victoria Guerrieri 6911 Waterfall Place, Downers Grove, IL 60516, (312) 325-6133, BS 82 Marquette Univ; MA 84 Northern IL Univ - De Kalb; 85–Aud, Sound Resources Inc, **A**

O'Reilly-Rao, Christine R R 1 Box 6-G, Fishkill, NY 12524, **A**

Orel, Sylvia P 719 Kings Croft, Cherry Hill, NJ 08034, (609) 267-1316, BA 61 Temple Univ; MS 78 Rutgers St Univ -N Brunswick; 70–Sp-Lang Path, Hainesport Bd of Ed, **SLP**

O'Relley, E Annette 3425 Par Street N E, Fargo, ND 58102, (701) 241-4898, BS 65 Maryville Coll; MA 70 Univ of TN - Knoxville; Sp-Lang Path, Fargo Public Schools, **SLP**

Orem, Mrs Ann P 2411 Crystal Spring Avenue S W, Roanoke, VA 24014, (703) 387-6522, BA 71 Loyola Coll; OM 76 Univ of SC - Columbia; Sp-Lang Path, Roanoke Co Sch, **SLP**

Oremland, Betty J 1048 N W 110th Lane, Coral Springs, FL 33065, (305) 482-5233, BA 76 Hofstra Univ; MA 77 Hofstra Univ; Aud, W Boca Hrng Cen, **A**

O'Renick, Pamela Sue 6536 West 91st #83, Overland Park, KS 66212-6017, (913) 648-3637, OB 84 Univ of MO - Columbia; OM 85 Univ of MO - Columbia; 87–Sp-Lang Path, Meadowbrook Hosp, **SLP**

Orf, Mrs Peggy A 4814 Middle Falls, Kingwood, TX 77345, (713) 360-8261, MS 78 Univ of North TX; BA 77 Univ of North TX; **A**

Organ, Dairlis Jane Monroe County Boces #1, 41 O'Connor Road, Fairport, NY 14450, (716) 377-4660, BA 83 MI St Univ; MA 84 MI St Univ; 85–Aud, Monroe County BOCES #1, **A**

Orgera-Mandey, Rena A P O Box 3019, Santa Clara, CA 95055, (415) 968-5602, BA 74 CUNY - Lehman Coll; MA 75 CUNY - Lehman Coll; Sp-Lang Path, Orgera-Mandey, **SLP**

Ori, Mrs Katherine P 822 Birch Street, Downers Grove, IL 60515, (312) 968-4182, BS 85 Northern IL Univ - De Kalb; MA 87 Northern IL Univ - De Kalb; 87–Sp-Lang Path, SW Cook Co Coop Assn for Spec Educ, **SLP**

Orichowskyj, Rose Marie 108 Old Orchard Road, Cherry Hill, NJ 08003, (609) 273-9343, BA 80 Rutger's St Univ - Douglas Coll; MS 82 PA St Univ - Univ Park; 88–Sp-Lang Path, Lourdes Rehab Svcs, **SLP**

Orion, Dr Gertrude 1 5th Avenue, New York, NY 10003, (212) 228-4536, BA 61 CUNY - Brooklyn Coll; MA 67 CUNY - Queens Coll; ED 76 (NS) Nova Univ; 67–Prof, Queensborough Comm Coll, **SLP LM**

Orlando, Ann-Marie 4945 South Arden Terrace, Inverness, FL 32650, (904) 336-2711, MS 87 Univ of South AL

Orlando, Mrs Joann Margaret 590 Rutter Avenue, Kingston, PA 18704, (717) 287-5388, BS 81 Bloomsburg Univ of PA; MS 82 Bloomsburg Univ of PA; Asst Director Sp-Lang Path Aud, John Heinz I of Rehab Medicine, **SLP**

Orlando, Mark Stephen 8601 15th Avenue North East, Apartment 101, Seattle, WA 98115, (206) 522-0627, BS 84 SUNY - Coll at Buffalo; MS 86 PA St Univ - Univ Park; **A**

Orlando, Nicholas A 15 Wadsworth Street, Geneseo, NY 14454, (716) 475-6258, BS 63 SUNY - Coll at Geneseo; MS 68 SUNY - Coll at Geneseo; Sp-Lang Path, Rochester I of Tech, **SLP ACE**

Orlando, Rosanna Marie 6 Lucille Drive, Syosset, NY 11791, (516) 921-7059, BS 85 Long Island U - CW Post Ctr; MA 87 CUNY - Queens Coll; 88–Sp-Lang Path, North Shore Univ Hosp, **SLP**

Orlando-Hayes, Carol 201 Rosewood Drive, Fort Pierce, FL 34947-3423, (305) 879-1222, BA 74 West Chester St Coll; MA 76 OK St Univ; Sp-Lang Path, InSpeech Inc, **SLP ACE**

Orlandoni, Nancy J 982 North Adams Road #6, Birmingham, MI 48009, (313) 548-2089, BS 72 MI St Univ; MA 74 MI St Univ; Sp-Lang Path, Ferndale Sch Dist, **SLP**

Orlesh, Mrs Dianne P 213 Norland Avenue, New Orleans, LA 70114, (504) 363-5329, BA 62 Saint Mary's Dominican Coll; MS 68 Tulane Univ; Sp-Lang Path, Jefferson Parish Sch Syst, **SLP**

Orlikoff, Dr Robert F Dept Of Audiology And Speech, Memphis State University, 807 Jefferson Avenue, Memphis, TN 38105, (901) 525-2682, BA 81 Rutgers St Univ -N Brunswick; MS 83 Columbia Univ Teachers Coll; PH 87 (Sp Science) Columbia Univ Sch of Gen St; 88–Asst Prof, Memphis State Univ, **SLP**

Orloff, Donna P 4465 Douglas Avenue #1K, Riverdale, NY 10471, (212) 737-2124, BA 68 George Washington Univ; MA 69 Columbia Univ Teachers Coll; Sp-Lang Path, Private Practice, **SLP**

Orloff, Wendy L 1225 N Louise, Glendale, CA 91207, (818) 545-8035, BS 73 Univ of OR; MS 77 Portland St Univ; Instructor, French Amer School, **SLP**

Orlowski, Michalynn 4648 North Elm Tree Road, Milwaukee, WI 53209, BS 76 Univ of WI - Milwaukee; MS 77 Univ of WI - Milwaukee; SLP, Milwaukee Pub Schs, **SLP**

Orman, M Jane 1229 8th Avenue, Fulton, IL 61252, (319) 242-6454, BA 64 Univ of IA; MA 79 Western IL Univ; Head-Testing Div, Linguisystems, **SLP**

Ormandy, Dr Roderick B 295 Thornell Road, Pittsford, NY 14534, (716) 381-6027, BA 49 Emerson Coll; MA 52 Northwestern Univ; PH 62 (NS) Northwestern Univ; Sp-Lang Path, Private Practice, **SLP**

Orme, Cheryl L 1379 31st Street, Ogden, UT 84403, (801) 394-9807, BA 75 UT St Univ; MS 76 UT St Univ; Sp-Lang Path, Private Practice, **SLP**

Ormiston, Sharon Jean 3413 Cheraz Road N E, Albuquerque, NM 87111-4638, (505) 298-3768, BS 75 Purdue Univ - West Lafayette; MA 82 Ball St Univ; Sp-Lang Path, CES, **SLP**

Ormond, Mary Frances 197 Hickory Pass, Bedford, NY 10506, **SLP**

Ormsby, Catherine Sarah 527 Newport Drive, Naperville, IL 60565, (312) 369-5929, BS 79 Governors St Univ; MS 82 Univ of WI - Oshkosh; 82–Sp-Lang Path, Chicago Bd of Ed, **SLP**

Ormsby, Rose A G 6720 Cameron Road, Rd 1 City Route 10, Bath, NY 14810, (607) 776-6770, MS 78 SUNY - Coll at Geneseo; Sp-Lang Path, BOCES-Early Intervention, **SLP**

Ormson, Kerry D Hearing Health Care Practice, 1901 Medi Park Place #1059, Amarillo, TX 79106, (806) 352-2321, BS 73 West TX St Univ; MS 75 Brigham Young Univ; Owner, Hrng Hlth Care Practice, **A ACE**

Ormson, Mary Frances Route 3 Box 972, 10508 North Russell Road, Maricopa, AZ 85239, (602) 568-2198, **A**

Ornelas, Myrna Joy 8602 Croydon Loop, Austin, TX 78748, (512) 353-2660, BS 81 Univ of TX - Austin; MS 86 Southwest TX St Univ; **SLP**

Ornstein, Mrs Amy Fleisher 345 East 86th Street #8B, New York, NY 10028, (212) 831-1086, BA 80 Univ of FL; MA 82 Memphis St Univ; Sp-Lang Path, Private Practice, **SLP**

Ornstein, Mrs Mary A 6075 Brighton Lane, Anaheim, CA 92807, (714) 558-5881, BA 73 CA St Univ - Fullerton; MA 80 CA St Univ - Fullerton; Sp-Lang Path, Santa Ana USD, **SLP**

Ornstein, Myrna 312 West 89th Street, New York, NY 10024, **SLP**

Orona, Mrs Kathryn Marie 1036 N Chester Avenue, Pasadena, CA 91104, (818) 791-8661, BS 77 CA Poly St Univ-San Luis Obi; MA 83 CA St Univ - Los Angeles; **SLP**

O'Rourk, Catherine 15348 Dale Road, Chagrin Falls, OH 44022, **SLP**

O'Rourke, Mrs Betty L 120 East 17th Street, Holland, MI 49423, (616) 392-8236, BS 74 Central MI Univ; MS 78 Central MI Univ; 88–Prog Supvr, Ottawa Co Comm Ment Hlth, **SLP**

O'Rourke, CarolAnn 659 Tobin Drive #102, Inkster, MI 48141, (313) 876-3280, BA 83 Butler Univ; MA 87 Wayne St Univ - Sch of Med; 88–Aud, Henry Ford Hosp, **A**

O'Rourke, Eileen P 15 Lincoln Avenue, Milltown, NJ 08850, (201) 846-6096, BA 78 Rutgers St Univ -N Brunswick; MS 79 Tulane Univ; Coord of Sp-Lang Path, UMDNJ-Ctr for Cognitive Rehab, **SLP**

O'Rourke, Mrs Margaret 1369 Bannister Drive, Naperville, IL 60565, BS 74 IL St Univ - Normal; MS 76 IL St Univ - Normal; Sp-Lang Path, SW Cook Co Coop Assn for Spec, **SLP**

O'Rourke, Maureen Rose 4613 Kaiser Peak Court, Bakersfield, CA 93304, (805) 837-2313, BA 83 Humboldt St Univ; **SLP**

O'Rourke, Mrs Melanie Z 425 North Westwood Drive, Wheaton, IL 60187, (312) 665-1547, BA 71 Univ of CT; MA 72 Univ of IL - Urbana; 88–Sp-Lang Path, Sherman Hosp, **SLP**

O'Rourke, Patricia Herrmann 58 Grand Street, Croton on Hudson, NY 10520, (914) 737-3300, BA 72 Le Moyne Coll; MS 74 Syracuse Univ; Sp/Lang Path, Peekskill Cty Sch, **SLP**

Orozco, Patricia 1216 West Washington St, Milwaukee, WI 53204, **SLP**

Orozco, Mrs Susan Elizabeth 4014 Carrie Bee Court, North Highlands, CA 95660, (916) 786-3574, BA 85 WA St Univ; MA 87 WA St Univ; **SLP**

Orr, Cynthia Sue 4567 Burnham Drive, Hoffman Estates, IL 60195, (312) 705-8240, BA 82 Augustana Coll; MS 84 IL St Univ - Normal; Sp-Lang Path, Com Consolidated Schl Dstr 93, **SLP**

Orr, Mrs Helen Bohn 2640-B Merrick, Fort Worth, TX 76107, (817) 534-5731, OB 64 TX Christian Univ; MS 75 Univ of North TX; SLP, Ft Worth ISD, **SLP**

Orr, Mrs Katie C 3835 Willow Run, Westlake, OH 44145, (216) 734-8525, BS 69 Purdue Univ - West Lafayette; MA 71 Northwestern Univ; **A**

Orr, Mrs Linda Dean RFD 2 Box 818, Bethel, VT 05032, (802) 234-9818, BA 76 Univ of VT; MS 77 Univ of VT; Sp-Lang Path, Windsor NW Superv Union, **SLP**

Orr, Lisa Ann 815 Dunes Way, Alpharetta, GA 30201, (404) 751-2631, BS 86 Univ of GA; ME 87 Univ of GA; 88–Sp-Lang Path, North Fulton Regional Hosp, **SLP**

Orraca, Neysa Idalia P O Box 504, Bayamon, PR 00619, (809) 780-2890, BA 79 Univ of PR - Rio Piedras; MS 81 Univ of PR - Rio Piedras; MS 85 Columbia Univ Teachers Coll; 88–Instr, Univ of Puerto Rico, **A**

Orrick, Sue S 9 Jordan, Montpelier, VT 05602, BS 68 Emerson Coll; MS 70 SUNY - Center at Albany; 88–Sp-Lang Path, Montpelier Sch Sys, **SLP**

Orringer, Mrs Maxine Katz 5629 Wilkins Avenue, Pittsburgh, PA 15217, (412) 421-4371, **SLP**

Orsak, Janice L 1300 Roma N W, Albuquerque, NM 87102, (505) 623-4389, BA 79 NM St Univ; MS 83 Univ of NM; Sp-Lang Path, Roswell ISD, **SLP**

Orsini, Mrs Barbara D 5 Alton Drive, Dudley, MA 01570, (508) 764-6611, BS 76 Worcester St Coll; MS 83 Worcester St Coll; Sp-Lang Path, Town of Southbridge, **SLP**

Orsini, Terri Ann 2-47 Columbia Gardens Apts, Cohoes, NY 12047, (518) 233-1586, BS 80 Coll of Saint Rose; ME 81 Coll of Saint Rose; Sp-Lang Path, Alby-Scnect-Schrt Co Bd Cop Ed, **SLP**

Orsten, Marguerite M 909 Oakhorn Drive, Harbor City, CA 90710, (714) 952-0971, BA 74 Univ of WA; MA 76 Univ of WA; Sp-Lang Path, Private Practice, **SLP**

Ort, Marlee P O Box 3277, La Vale, MD 21502, (301) 722-7850, BS 77 James Madison Univ; MS 80 James Madison Univ; Treas, Ort's Inc, **SLP**

Ort, Ruth G 2357 Riverside Avenue, Jacksonville, FL 32204, (904) 384-3600, BA 60 CUNY - Brooklyn Coll; ME 80 Univ of North FL; Private Practice, **SLP**

Ortega-Hillyer, Nereida I 8750 Georgia Avenue #326A, Silver Spring, MD 20910, (202) 636-6711, BS 69 Bradley Univ; MS 71 Bradley Univ; **SLP ACE**

Ortenberg, Celia Louise 821 Aspen Circle, Oxnard, CA 93030, (805) 984-8089, MA San Diego St Univ; 87–Sp-Lang Path, Oxnard Elem Sch Dist, **SLP**

Orth, Mrs Kay M 4633 St Roch Avenue, New Orleans, LA 70122, (504) 279-9944, BS 75 LA St Univ - Baton Rouge; OM 77 LA St Univ - N O Medical Ctr; Sp-Lang Path, Rufin Sp-Lang Ctr, **SLP**

Orth, Susan J 10794 Las Lunitas, Tujunga, CA 91042, (818) 352-4845, BA 66; MA 69 Univ of WA; Sp-Lang Path, Kaiser, **SLP**

Orthel, Susan D 2561 Terry Avenue, Longview, WA 98632, (206) 636-4801, BS 74 Univ of ID; MA 76 WA St Univ; Sp-Lang Path, Private Practice, **SLP ACE**

Ortiz, Ivette 1965 Schieffelin Avenue, Apartment 3-A, Bronx, NY 10466, (212) 881-1282, MS 88 PA St Univ - Univ Park

Ortiz, J Dennis Wyoming School For The Deaf, 539 South Payne, Casper, WY 82609, (307) 237-3634, BS 56 9404; BA 56 Coll of Santa Fe; MS 57 Univ of KS; Curricular Service Representv, Wyoming Dept of Education, **A**

Ortize, Nancy M 5421 Covey Creek Circle, Stockton, CA 95207, **SLP**

Orton, Clodagh P O Box 707, Stinson Beach, CA 94970, (415) 221-4810, MA 61; MA 73 San Francisco St Univ; Audiologist, VA Hosp San Francisco, **A**

Ortscheid, Mrs Cynthia Morris 1436 Heritage Landing #310, St Charles, MO 63303, (314) 831-2700, BA 79 Augustana Coll; MS 80 Northeast MO St Univ; 88–Sp-Lang Path, Sch Dist of St Louis, **SLP**

O'Ryan-Fox, Irene R 4732 Wolf Road, Western Springs, IL 60558, (312) 690-8580, BA 80 Saint Xavier Coll; MS 82 Marquette Univ; Sp-Lang Path, Therapeutic Systems, **SLP**

Orzechowski, John, Jr 39 Tawney Drive, Bethany, CT 06525, **SLP**

Orzechowski, Kathleen M 39 Tawney Drive, Bethany, CT 06525, MS; **SLP**

Orzell, Lisa O 617 Montrose Avenue, Solvay, NY 13219, (315) 488-3659, MS 87 Syracuse Univ

Osacho, Jennifer Marie 345 Lyall Avenue, West Covina, CA 91790, (818) 915-4201, MA 85 CA St Univ - Fullerton; SLP, Fullerton Union High Sch Dist, **SLP**

Osada, Diane G 2304 Falling Water Court, Santa Clara, CA 95054, (408) 988-2595, BA 82 San Jose St Univ; MA 85 San Jose St Univ; Aud, Csg Hrng Services, **A**

Osawa, Fumiko 2-6-1 Mejirodai, Hachioji, Tokyo, Japan 193, 045-473-0666, MA 85 San Jose St Univ; Sp-Lang Path, Yokohama Rehab Ctr

Osbahr, Tracy C 7 Bray Court, Pelham, MA 01002, (413) 586-8692, BA 69 Elmira Coll; MA 72 Univ of CT; Dir, The Reach Prog, **SLP**

Osbakken, Bonnie Rochelle 1259-A Fairview Court, Ojai, CA 93023, (805) 646-9092, Sp-Lang Path, **SLP**

Osberger, Dr Mary J Riley Hospital A-56, 702 Barnhill Drive, Indianapolis, IN 46223, (317) 274-4915, BS 69 Univ of Cincinnati; MS 71 Gallaudet Coll; PH 78 (NS) CUNY - City College; Assoc Prof, IN Univ Sch of Medicine, **A**

Osborn, Courtney D 2615 Cove Cay Drive #304, Clearwater, FL 34620, (813) 536-0288, BA 36 Wichita St Univ; MA 39 Wichita St Univ; **A F LM**

Osborn, Debra K 2567 North 89th Street, Wauwatosa, WI 53226, (414) 649-7647, BA 74 Univ of MA - Amherst; MA 76 MI St Univ; Sp-Lang Path, St Lukes Hosp, **SLP**

Osborn, Mrs Diana Dickens P O Box 1334, Florence, AL 35631, BS 80 Southern Methodist Univ; MS 82 Univ of TX - Dallas; SLP, Dallas ISD, **SLP**

Osborn, Mrs Emma Lou 201 Bartonwood Drive, Lebanon, TN 37087, (615) 444-5250, BA 39 Cumberland Univ; MA 62 G Peabody Coll-Vanderbilt U; Retired, Wilson Co Bd of Ed, **SLP LM**

Osborn, Joan H 4245 Pasadena Avenue, Sacramento, CA 95821, (916) 929-2277, BA 51 George Washington Univ; MA 54 Northwestern Univ; Co-Owner, Sutter Hrng/Sp Cen, **SLP**

Osborn, Mrs Katherine Vahey 1601 Aldrich Avenue, Wichita Falls, TX 76302, (817) 761-4069, BA 80 TX Tech Univ; MS 82 Univ of TX - Dallas; SLP, **SLP**

Osborn, Laura W 147 Hopkins Street #20, Battle Creek, MI 49017, (606) 269-2289, BA 85 Univ of KY; MS 87 Univ of KY; 88–Sp-Lang Path, Constance Brown Hearing Sp Ctr, **SLP**

Osborn, Richard Joseph 4245 Pasadena Avenue, Sacramento, CA 95821, (916) 929-2277, BS 58 Purdue Univ - West Lafayette; MA 60 Univ of MD - College Park; CEO, Sutter Hrng & Sp Ctr, **A**

Osborn, Mrs Sandra R 118 Northmoor Road, Casselberry, FL 32707, (407) 422-3200, BS 59 FL St Univ; MS 63 FL St Univ; Sr Admin, Orange Co Pub Sch

Osborne, Anne Stewart 1818 N Simpson, Portland, OR 97217-4659, (503) 280-4403, BS 82 Univ of WY; MS 87 ID St Univ; 84–Sp-Lang Path, Emanuel Hosp & Hlth Ctr, **SLP**

Osborne, Carmela Bari Nuernberg Es, APO New York, NY 09696, BS 79 Univ of IL - Urbana; MS 80 Univ of IL - Urbana; 87–Sp-Lang Path, Dept of Def Dependents Schs, **SLP**

Osborne, Charles Arno 7502 Mott Avenue, Orlando, FL 32810, (305) 422-3200, **SLP**

Osborne, Dr George S InSpeech-Oak Park, 6557 West North Avenue, Oak Park, IL 60302, (312) 848-9750, MS 65 Southern IL Univ -Carbondale; DD 72 Univ of IL - Chicago; PH 68 Southern IL Univ -Carbondale; Area Mgr, InSpeech Inc, **SLP A ACE**

Osborne, Jane A 143 East Muriel Street, Orlando, FL 32806, (407) 898-6997, BS 81 Southwest MO St Univ; MS 84 Central MO St Univ; Aud, Orange Co PS, **A**

Osborne-Hurley, Mrs Julie E 1763 Appleton Road, Menasha, WI 54952, (414) 735-9977, BS 85 Univ of WI - Stevens Point; MS 87 Univ of WI - Stevens Point; 87–Sp-Lang Path, Gmeiner Cl-Commun Dis/Lrng Dis, **SLP**

Osbourn, B Neil P O Box 135, Avon, CT 06001, (203) 236-4369, BA 54 Univ of Northern CO; MA 57 Univ of Northern CO; **SLP**

Osbourn, Patricia S 5851 Lost Dutchman N E, Albuquerque, NM 87111, (505) 299-9340, MS 78 CA St Univ - Los Angeles; SLP, Private Practice, **SLP**

Osburn, Catherine 1707 Hampton Knoll Drive, Akron, OH 44313-4862, (216) 929-0914, BS 61 OH St Univ; MA 71 Kent St Univ; Supvr, Stark County Schs, **SLP A**

Osburn, Cynthia H 1404 Eastridge Street, Clovis, NM 88101, (505) 482-3492, MS 76 Eastern NM Univ; 82–Sp-Lang Path, Texico Municipal Sch, **SLP**

Osenga-Manolovits, Diana L 809 1/2 N Michigan, La Porte, IN 46350, (312) 736-7000, BS 81 Northern IL Univ - De Kalb; MA 83 Northern IL Univ - De Kalb; Aud, Consultants In Neurology, **A**

Osenkowski, Carolyn Ann 15 Britto Lane, North Scituate, RI 02857, (508) 679-7026, BS 81 Boston Univ; MA 83 OH St Univ; Aud, Charlton Memorial Hospital, **A**

Oser, Carla Kay 2109 Lincoln Way East, Massillon, OH 44646, (213) 726-8348, BS 71 Ashland Coll; MS 73 AZ St Univ; 88–Sp-Lang Path, Strasburg-Franklin Local Schs, **SLP**

Oser, Mrs Tamara S 1505 Iron Liege Road, Indianapolis, IN 46217, (317) 882-4288, BS 78 Ball St Univ; MA 79 Ball St Univ; Aud, Indianapolis Otol Assoc Inc, **A**

Osgood, Mrs Cheryl Renee 2150 Sunrise Way, Jamison, PA 18929, (215) 539-8550, BS 79 Bloomsburg Univ of PA; MS 80 Bloomsburg Univ of PA; Sp-Lang Path, Mont Co Inter Ut, **SLP**

Osgood, Eleanor 4224 Lincoln Avenue, Culver City, CA 90232, (213) 876-1783, BA 67 Univ of CA - Berkeley; MA 77 CA St Univ - Los Angeles; Sp-Lang Path, LA County Schs, **SLP**

Osgood, Everett Clark 8610 Fernwood Drie, Rancho Cucamonga, CA 91730, (714) 988-8511, BA 80 CA St Univ - Fresno; MA 83 CA St Univ - Fullerton; 84–Sp-Lang Path, Chaffy Joint Union HS Dist, **SLP**

O'Shaughnessey, Mrs Mary Susan VA Medical Center, Audiology & Speech Pathology Service, 2215 Fuller Road, Ann Arbor, MI 48105, (313) 769-7100, BA 68 OH St Univ; MS 69 Univ of MI - Ann Arbor; 81–Aud, VA Med Ctr, **A**

O'Shaughnessy, Mrs Nina E 710 South Osage, Okmulgee, OK 74447, (918) 756-9211, BA 74 Univ of OK - Norman; MS 76 Univ of OK Medical Center; Sp Serv Superv, George Nigh Rehab Inst, **SLP**

O'Shea, Beverly M 903 28th Avenue South, Grand Forks, ND 58201, (701) 780-2447, BS 72 Univ of ND; MS 75 Univ of ND; 75–Sp-Lang Path, Medical Center Rehab Hospital, **SLP**

O'Shea, Mrs Julie B 416 Hinman Place, Mamaroneck, NY 10543, (212) 722-8100, BS 78 CUNY - Brooklyn Coll; MS 80 Columbia Univ Teachers Coll; Audiologist, New York League/Hard of Hearng, **A**

Oshiro, Susan Ruth P O Box 1149, Wahiawa, HI 96786, (808) 622-5809, BA 84 Univ of CO - Boulder; MS 86 Univ of HI - Manoa; **SLP**

Oshrin, Dr Stephen E Dept Of Speech & Hearing Sci, U Of Southern Mississippi, Southern Station Box 5092, Hattiesburg, MS 39406, (601) 266-5216, BA 72 SUNY - Coll at Plattsburgh; MA 73 OH Univ - Athens; PH 78 (Aud) OH Univ - Athens; Assoc Prof/Chair, Univ of Southern MS, **A**

Osika, Michele M 31 Gilbert Drive, Hyde Park, NY 12538, BS 83 SUNY - Coll at Geneseo; MA 86 Univ of MA - Amherst; 86–Sp-Lang Path, Rehabilitation Programs Inc, **SLP**

Osinski, Rose Marie 407-3420-50 Street NW, Calgary, AB, Canada T3A 2E1, (403) 268-9590, MS 86 Minot St Univ; 88–Sp-Lang Path, Calgary Gen Hosp, **SLP**

Osman, Ruth Folkman 76 Richter Road, Tabernacle, NJ 08088, (609) 268-0336, BS 75 Indiana Univ of PA; MA 77 Trenton St Coll; Sp-Lang Path, Springfield Township Sch Dist, **SLP**

Osmon, Mrs Jennifer E 5975 North Shoreland, Whitefish Bay, WI 53217, (414) 225-8135, BS 73 Northern IL Univ - De Kalb; MA 75 Northern MI Univ; Supervisor of Speech Pathology, St Mary's Hosp, **SLP**

Osredkar, Mark M 1932 Albee Street, Eureka, CA 95501, (707) 445-0609, MA 86 Humboldt St Univ; 87–Dir, Coastal Care Ctrs, **SLP**

Ossorio-Henriquez, Flor Del R Calle 21 S-24 Las Rosas, Rio Piedras, PR 00926, (809) 755-3193, 87–Sp-Lang Path, Hospital Pediatrico RCM, **SLP**

Osta, Norma Kalil 401 Westwood Road, Suite F5, Stamford, CT 06902, (203) 359-4431, BA 69 Albertus Magnus Coll; ME 70 Boston St Coll; OM 74 Southern CT St Univ; Sp-Lang Path Dir, Fairfield Co Sp & Hrng Cen, **SLP**

Ostarello, Denise R 18452 Francisco, Homewood, IL 60430, **SLP**

Ostby, Karen J Meetinghouse Village, Yale Avenue #63-02, Meriden, CT 06450, (203) 237-4239, BS 68 Ithaca Coll; MA 69 Western IL Univ; Sp-Lang Path, Regional Sch Dist #13, **SLP**

Ostendorf, Joseph C 5662 Lumberjack Lane, Tallahassee, FL 32303, (904) 562-5691, MS 83 Univ of WI - Milwaukee; 85–Sp-Lang Path, Tallahassee Mem Reg Med Ctr, **SLP**

Ostergaard, Sue Ann 1346 E Randolph Court #C, Milwaukee, WI 53212, (414) 289-3818, BS 77 Univ of WI - Milwaukee; MS 79 Washington Univ; Aud, N Point Med Group, **A**

Ostergren, Daniel Eugene, Jr P O Box 8066, Fort Collins, CO 80526, (303) 226-1837, BS 83 Univ of MN - Minneap-St Paul; MS 85 Univ of WY; Aud, Aud Resources, **A**

Ostergren, Patricia G 10480 Palmershein Drive, Hales Corners, WI 53130, BA 59 Carroll Coll; MA 72 Northern MI Univ; Sp-Lang Path, Sn WI Cen/Develop Dis, **SLP**

Osterhout, Cheryl A 46-5 Woodlake Rd, Albany, NY 12203-4108, (518) 452-0424, MS 81 Bowling Green St Univ; Sp-Lang Path, UCP-Schenectady, **SLP**

Osterkamp, Mrs Kaye A 3641 W 101st Avenue, Westminster, CO 80030, (303) 469-6127, BS 79 Univ of ID; MS 83 AZ St Univ; Sp/Lang Path, Adams Co School District 12, **SLP**

Osterling, Ann M Carle Clinic Assoc, Department Of Pediatrics, 602 West University, Urbana, IL 61801, (217) 337-3100, BS 75 Purdue Univ - West Lafayette; MA 78 Univ of IL - Urbana; 78–Sp-Lang Path, Carle Cl Assoc, **SLP ACE**

Osterloh, Patricia O'Neal Coastal Bend Speech And Language Associates, 3006 South Alameda, Corpus Christi, TX 78404, (512) 888-7020, BS 76 Univ of TX - Austin; MA 78 Our Lady Lake Univ-San Anton; 88–Sp-Lang Path, Coastal Bend Sp & Lang Assoc, **SLP**

Osth, Jodi A 18 Summit Avenue, Dundee, IL 60118, BA 85 Augustana Coll; MA 86 Western MI Univ; **SLP**

Ostlund, Nancy 3481 East Finger Rock Road, Tucson, AZ 85718, OH Univ - Athens; **SLP**

Ostop, Mrs Janet L PO 4874, Woodland Park, CO 80866, (303) 635-6350, BS 73 Univ of NE - Omaha; MS 74 Univ of NE - Omaha; Sp/Lang Path, Co Sprgs Sch Dist #11, **SLP**

Ostrander, Elizabeth Larimer 140 West Oak, Lake Mills, WI 53551, (608) 252-8123, BS 84 Bradley Univ; MS 86 Univ of WI - Madison; 86–Aud, Dean Med Ctr, **A**

Ostreicher, Harvey J 2630 Hampden Court #201, Chicago, IL 60614, PH 75 Univ of MI - Ann Arbor; MS 69 Case Western Reserve Univ; **SLP**

Ostro, Mrs Gayle Patrice 6633 Navajo, Lincolnwood, IL 60646, (312) 675-6363, BA 78 OH St Univ; MA 80 Saint Louis Univ; SLP, **SLP**

Ostrom, Mrs Kay Ann F 203 Bel Air, Mascoutah, IL 62258, (618) 224-9411, BS 70 Southern IL Univ -Carbondale; MS 72 Southern IL Univ -Carbondale; SLP, Wesclin Unit Dist #3, **SLP**

Ostrom, Mrs Sara W Anne Arundel Cnty Pub Schools, 2644 Riva Road, Annapolis, MD 21401, (301) 224-5477, BA 51 Univ of AL- Tuscaloosa; MA 57 Univ of AL- Tuscaloosa; Coord Speech and Hearing, Anne Arundel Cnty Pub Schools, **SLP**

Ostrosky, Mrs Pamela Ann 31005 Fernwood, Westland, MI 48185, (313) 722-5403, MA 82 Eastern MI Univ; SLP, **SLP**

Ostrovsky, Steven N Vta Management Services Inc, 1270 East 19th Street, Brooklyn, NY 11230, (718) 377-5090, BA 72 CUNY - Brooklyn Coll; MS 73 Adelphi Univ; Chief Executive Officer, Private Practice, **SLP**

Ostrow, Rhona E Houston Ear Nose & Throat, 820 Memorial Hosp Prof Bldg, 7777 Southwest Freeway, Houston, TX 77074, Aud, Houston Ear Nose & Throat, **A**

Ostrowski, Audrey A 959 Willowleaf Drive #2702, San Jose, CA 95128, (408) 947-7431, BS 76 Edinboro Univ of PA; MS 77 PA St Univ - Univ Park; Sp-Lang Path, Alum Rock School District, **SLP**

Ostroy, Zipora P 310 Hollowood Drive, West Lafayette, IN 47906, (317) 497-7710, BS 64 Case Western Reserve Univ; MA 66 Case Western Reserve Univ; Academic Advisor, Purdue University, **SLP**

Ostuni, Elizabeth 9 Hampton Downes Road #3, Newton, NJ 07860, (201) 989-3122, BA 59 Univ of KS; MA 72 Univ of KS; Dir Sp & Aud Servs, Dover Gen Hosp & Med Cen, **SLP ACE**

O'Sullivan, Avril PH#1 9737-112 Street, Edmonton, AB, Canada T5K 1L3, (403) 482-2869, BS 66 Northwestern Univ; MA 67 Northwestern Univ; 88–Sp-Lang Path, Glenrose Rehab Hosp, **SLP**

O'Sullivan, Mary E 63 Presidential Drive #5, Quincy, MA 02169, (617) 479-4503, BA 74 Univ of MA - Amherst; ME 79 Northeastern Univ; Sp/Lang Path, Cty Boston Pub Sch, **SLP**

O'Sullivan, Mary K 2462 North 64th Street, Wauwatosa, WI 53213, (414) 964-6682, BS 67 Spalding Coll; MS 71 Marquette Univ; Sp/Lang Path, Milwaukee Publ Sch, **SLP**

Osumi, Joy Lynne 4451 North Winery, Fresno, CA 93726, (209) 292-6945, BA 80 CA St Univ - Long Beach; MA 83 CA St Univ - Fresno; 83–Sp-Lang Path, Kings Canyon USD, **SLP**

Oswald, Mrs Beth A 23 Fenton Wood Drive, Sterling, VA 22170, (703) 444-6318, BS 82 East Stroudsburg Univ of PA; MS 84 Bloomsburg Univ of PA; 88–Sp-Lang Path, No VA Sp & Lang Ctr, **SLP**

Oswald, Sharon H University Of Chicago Medical Center, 5841 South Maryland, Box 412, Chicago, IL 60637, (312) 702-1864, BA 80 Creighton Univ; MS 84 Univ of NE - Omaha; MS 87 Vanderbilt Univ; 88–Aud, Univ of Chicago Med Ctr

Oswalt, Mrs Jan L 7855 South 66th E Avenue, Tulsa, OK 74133, MS 77 AR St Univ; Sp-Lang Path, Tulsa Cnty Sch Developmntl Ctr, **SLP**

Oswalt, Lisa H 4532 Providence Place, New Orleans, LA 70126, (504) 482-5742, **SLP**

Oswalt, Lora S 6409 Vickery Boulevard, Dallas, TX 75214, (214) 821-3998, BA 70 Univ of AR - Fayetteville; MS 72 Univ of OK Medical Center; Sp-Lang Path, Private Practice, **SLP**

Oswalt, M Jill 1330 South Belcrest, Springfield, MO 65804, (417) 887-6522, BS 75 Southwest MO St Univ; MA 79 Northeast MO St Univ; Sp/Lang Path, Sp-Lang Serv of SW MO, **SLP**

Oteri, Stephen E 671-5 Pleasant Street, Weymouth, MA 02189, BS 78 Univ of MA - Amherst; MA 80 Univ of MA - Amherst; Sp-Lang Path, Private Practice, **SLP**

Otero, Jane Hanich 2833 Hitchcock Mill Run, Marietta, GA 30068, (404) 973-5740, BS 76 Coll of Saint Rose; MA 78 Catholic Univ of America; **SLP**

Otey, Mrs Linda L 12206 S E 31 Place #114, Milwaukie, OR 97222-6886, (503) 653-3665, BS 74 Univ of OR; MS 79 Western OR St Coll; 79–Sp-Lang Path, N Clackcomas Sch Dist, **SLP**

Othold, Becky Jean P O Box 4911, Little Rock, AR 72214, (501) 565-3254, BS 77 LA St Univ - Baton Rouge; MA 81 LA St Univ - Baton Rouge; 88–Aud/Coord

Otis, Lindsay Ann 841 West Rose Street, Stockton, CA 95203, (209) 466-5471, **SLP**

Otlin, Mrs Jo-Ann F 19 Salvia Road, Milford, MA 01757, (617) 473-4670, BS 70 Boston Univ; MA 79 Marshall Univ; **SLP**

Otness, Mrs Martha A M 3956 South Nucla Street, Aurora, CO 80013, MA 79 Univ of Denver; **SLP**

Otness, Shirley M 405 Whispering River Lane, Farmington, MN 55024, (612) 463-7193, BS 59 Univ of MN - Minneap-St Paul; Sp/Lang Path, ISD #192, **SLP**

Otomo, Kiyoshi 4-18-1-607, Nerima Nerimaku, Tokyo, Japan 176, BA 80 Int'l Christian Univ - PR; MA 84 Univ of IL - Urbana; PH 88 (Sp Lang Science) Univ of WA

O'Toole, Mrs Dale L 6748 Luther Street, Niagara Falls, NY 14304, (716) 633-0330, BS 77 SUNY - Coll at Geneseo; MA 79 SUNY - Center at Buffalo; 85–Sp-Lang Path, Ctr for Hndcpd Chldrn, **SLP**

O'Toole, Dr Thomas J 217 Rolling Road, Gaithersburg, MD 20877, (301) 279-3135, BA 56 Bloomsburg Univ of PA; ME 59 Univ of Pittsburgh - Pittsburgh; ED 69 (Human Dev & Special Ed) Univ of MD - College Park; Dir Dept of Sp Ed&Related Serv, Montgomery Co Pub Sch, **SLP F**

O'Toole-Granberry, Mrs Cynthia O 1212 Lexington Way #3, Rockford, IL 61108, (815) 987-7956, BS 73 Western IL Univ; MA 74 Western MI Univ; Sp-Lang Path, State of Illinois Dmh-Dd, **SLP ACE**

Otsuka-Davis, Evelyn 1228 West 63rd Street, Kansas City, MO 64113, (816) 276-4023, BS 72 Western IL Univ; MA 75 Univ of IL - Urbana; **SLP**

Ott, Mrs Diane M 1138 Lake Shore Road, Grafton, WI 53024, (414) 358-0560, BS 76 Univ of WI - Madison; MS 77 Univ of WI - Milwaukee; Sp-Lang Path, Cedar Lake Home, **SLP**

Ott, Mrs Elizabeth Gayle 3501 West 10th Terrace, Lawrence, KS 66044, (913) 841-4876, BA 83 Wichita St Univ; MA 84 Wichita St Univ; Sp-Lang Path, USD 497, **SLP**

Ott, Jeanne Carolyn P O Box 1074, Southwest Harbor, ME 04679, (207) 244-5119, BA 76 Univ of ME - Orono; MA 86 Univ of ME - Orono; 76–Sp-Lang Path, Sch Union #98, **SLP**

Ott, Kimberly K 100 Gale Drive, Fairview Heights, IL 62208, (618) 397-5495, BS 79 Southern IL Univ-Edwardsvill; MS 81 Southern IL Univ-Edwardsvill; 86–Aud, Educ Dev Ctr, **A**

Ott, Penelope A 133 Townhouse Briarcrest, Hershey, PA 17033, (717) 367-1161, BA 80 Western CT St Univ; MS 82 Univ of AL- Tuscaloosa; Director Sp-Lang Path, Elizabethtown Hosp & Rehab Ctr, **SLP**

Ottaviani, Roberta M 4 West College Avenue, Poughkeepsie, NY 12601, (914) 471-9200, BA 58 SUNY - Center at Albany; MA 59 Univ of NE - Lincoln; Sp-Lang Path/Tchr of Deaf, Dutchess Co BOCES, **SLP**

Ottaway, Ruth 4360 Ryeland Drive, Broadview Heights, OH 44147-2758, (814) 454-0782, BS 40 Edinboro Univ of PA; MS 48 PA St Univ - Univ Park; **SLP LM**

Otte, Mrs Catherine Ann 6418 El Capitan Circle, Stockton, CA 95210, (209) 466-9460, BA 83 Univ of the Pacific; MA 84 Univ of the Pacific; 86–Sp-Lang Path, InSpeech Inc, **SLP**

Otten, Mrs Lysbeth M 2130 North 72nd Street, Wauwatosa, WI 53213, (414) 546-5554, BS 58 Univ of WI - Milwaukee; MS 80 Univ of WI - Milwaukee; Sp-Lang Path, W Allis/W Milwaukee Sch Dist, **SLP**

Ottenweller, Mrs Laura Hagedorn 6514 Hillsboro Lane, Fort Wayne, IN 46835, (219) 485-8951, MA 85 Ball St Univ; Sp-Lang Path, Ft Wayne Dev Ctr, **SLP**

Otterholt, Janelle 4902 S W Charlestown, Seattle, WA 98116, (206) 838-9994, BS 79 Univ of WA; MS 81 Univ of WA; Sp-Lang Path, Samaritan Hosp Rehab Cen, **SLP**

Otterson, Patricia Ann 2307 Tanager Trail, Madison, WI 53711, (414) 877-3049, BS 84 Univ of WI - Whitewater; MS 85 Univ of WI - Whitewater; 86–Sp-Lang Path, Cambridge Comm Schs, **SLP**

Otterstrom, David C 120 North Birmingham, Tulsa, OK 74110, **SLP**

Otterstrom, Elizabeth 120 North Birmingham, Tulsa, OK 74110, MS; **SLP**

Otting, Victoria Louise 1685 Portola Avenue #18, Livermore, CA 94550, (415) 935-4657, BS 83 CA St Univ - Hayward; MS 85 CA St Univ - Hayward; 88–Sp-Lang Path, Synergos Neurological Ctr, **SLP**

Otting-Blaine, Julia A 8200 Kroll Way #83, Bakersfield, CA 93311, (805) 322-3971, BA 76 Univ of Northern IA; MA 77 Univ of Northern IA; OM 82 CA St Coll - Bakersfield; Director Sp-Lang Path, Affiliated Speech Path, **SLP**

Ottinger, Mrs Mariann F 5725 Imperial Key, Tampa, FL 33615, (813) 886-2753, BA 70 Univ of Akron; MA 73 Univ of Akron; Sp-Lang Path, Hillsborough County Sch Board, **SLP**

Ott-Jones, Lori Kay 53 Lakeside Drive, Hamilton, OH 45013, (513) 563-5000, OB 83 Miami Univ - Oxford; MS 84 Miami Univ - Oxford; 85–Sp-Lang Path, Lockland City Sch Dist, **SLP**

Ottley, Melanie Dawn 620 Sheridan Street #502, Hyattsville, MD 20783, (202) 722-2914, BS 83 Andrews Univ; MA 85 Univ of MD - College Park; **A**

Ott-Milisits, Lavonne E 835 Greenfield Avenue, Pittsburgh, PA 15217, (412) 647-5580, MS 78 PA St Univ - Univ Park; 79–Aud, Chldn's Hosp of Pittsburg, **A**

Otto, Catherine Communications Reconsruction, 450 Park Avenue, New York, NY 10022, (212) 355-7111, BS 73 Univ of CT; MS 78 Southern CT St Univ; Dir, Commun Reconstruction Cen, **SLP**

Otto, Frances M Box 493, Nocona, TX 76255, (817) 825-3832, BS 73 TX Tech Univ; MS 75 TX Tech Univ; Sp-Lang Path, Montague Co Spec Cl Coop, **SLP**

Otto, Judith A 512 Missouri Avenue Circle Apartment C, McCook, NE 69001, (308) 345-1841, BS 71 Univ of NE - Lincoln; MS 78 Univ of NE - Omaha; SLP, McCook City Schs, **SLP**

Otto, Karen D 4003 North Greenview, Chicago, IL 60613, (312) 528-9401, BA 77 Augustana Coll; MS 79 Univ of WI - Madison; Sp-Lang Path, Rehab I of Chicago, **SLP**

Otto, Kay Anne S 119 Fairview, Ann Arbor, MI 48103, (313) 995-2771, MA 79 Eastern MI Univ; Sp-Lang Path, St Joseph Mercy Hosp, **SLP**

Otto, Mrs Lucia Marie 21375 Aberdeen Road, Rocky River, OH 44116, (216) 333-4960, BA 60 Univ of IA; MA 81 Cleveland St Univ; Sp-Lang Path, Parma Comm Gen Hosp, **SLP**

Otto, Patricia Ann 807 South Matthias Street, Appleton, WI 54915, (414) 733-3560, BS 79 Univ of WI - Madison; MS 81 Univ of WI - Madison; Sp-Lang Path, Appleton Schools, **SLP**

Otto, Mrs Peggie Ann 4903 Fite Drive, Imperial, MO 63052, (314) 479-3629, MS 85 Fontbonne Coll; 87–Prog Dir, Children's Learning and Rehab Center, **SLP**

Otto, Steven R House Ear Institute, 256 South Lake Street, Los Angeles, CA 90057, (213) 483-4431, BA 71 Grinnell Coll; MA 75 Univ of IA; 87–Aud, House Ear Inst Sensory Devices Resch, **A**

Otto, Dr Walter C, Jr 470 Arthur Avenue, Shreveport, LA 71105, (318) 674-6269, BS 74 Brigham Young Univ; MS 75 Brigham Young Univ; PH 79 (NS) Univ of UT; Asst Prof, LA St U Med Sch, **A**

Ottoel, Chris Ann 1317 Edgewood Avenue #5, Grafton, ND 58237, (701) 352-2140, BA 80 Univ of ND; MS 83 Univ of ND; Sp-Lang Path, Grafton State School, **SLP**

Otwell, Freda Williams 3004 West Northern Lights Boulevard 10-C, Anchorage, AK 99517, BS 77 FL St Univ; MS 79 FL St Univ; 88–Sp-Lang Path, Private Practice, **SLP**

Ouellette, Amelia Wittwer 8301 S W 56th Avenue, Portland, OR 97219, (503) 229-3533, BA 84 Univ of OR; MS 86 Portland St Univ; 86–Sp-Lang Path, Newberg Sch Dist 29JT, **SLP**

Ouellette, Mrs Anita 8 Simpson Road, Wayland, MA 01778, (617) 872-7280, BA 64 Merrimack Coll; MS 77 Boston Univ; Sp-Lang Path, Private Practice, **SLP**

Ouellette, Donna I 19203 North 29th Avenue, Apartment 424, Phoenix, AZ 85027, (602) 581-1807, BS 77 Northeastern Univ; MA 78; Clinical Rehabil/Dispensng Aud, Private Practice, **A**

Ouellette, Dr Eugene G 1350 Elizabeth Street, Redlands, CA 92373, (714) 793-2121, BA 57 Univ of Redlands; MA 58 Univ of Redlands; PH 60 (NS) Univ of WA; Prof, U of Redlands, **SLP A**

Ouellette, Marlene M Pine Tree Society, P O Box 518, Bath, ME 04530, (207) 443-3341, BS 68 Syracuse Univ; MA 69 Syracuse Univ; Director Speech & Hearing Serv, Pine Tree Society, **SLP**

Ough, Dwight S 36 Edith Avenue, St John, NB, Canada E2J 1P1, (506) 648-6741, OB 76 St Mary's Univ - Ns; MA 78 Univ of Northern CO; Dept Head-Aud, St John Reg Hosp, **A**

Oungst, Carmen Dee 21392 Town Lakes Drive, Apartment 10-23, Boca Raton, FL 33486, (305) 392-5294, BA 85 Univ of WI - Eau Claire; MS 87 FL St Univ; 87–Sp-Lang Path, Rehab Works, **SLP**

Ourand, Mrs Patricia Regina 2301 Argonne Drive, Baltimore, MD 21218, (301) 554-3118, BA 78 Loyola Coll; MS 79 Loyola Coll; OM 87 Johns Hopkins Univ; Sp-Lang Path, Maryland Rehabilitation Center, **SLP**

Ouren, Mary J Trevilla Of Robbinsdale, 3130 Grimes Avenue North, Minneapolis, MN 55422, (612) 588-0771, BA 67 Augustana Coll; MA 73 Univ of KY; Dir Sp-Lang Path Dept, Trevilla of Robbinsdale, **SLP**

Ousse, Anne M 505 South David Street, Church Point, LA 70525, BA 79 Univ of Southwestern LA; MS 86 Univ of Southwestern LA; 80–Sp-Lang Path, St Landry Parish Sch Bd, **SLP**

Outman, Richard R Diablo Valley Sp & Lang Clinic, 1844 San Miguel, Suite 308A, Walnut Creek, CA 94596, (415) 938-4722, BA 70 Univ of CA - Berkeley; MA 74 San Francisco St Univ; Dir, Diablo Valley Sp Lang Cl, **SLP**

Ouwens, Nel S Box 2608, Drumheller, AB, Canada T0J 0Y0, (403) 823-3341, BS 77 Univ of Alberta - Alberta; MS 78 Univ of WI - Madison; Mgr of Sp-Lang Path, Drumheller Health Unit, **SLP**

Ou-Young, Lai-Shyang Melody 1818 E Michigan Avenue, Apartment #711, Los Angeles, CA 90033, (213) 268-5000, MS 84 Southern IL Univ -Carbondale; Sp-Lang Path, White Memorial Medical Center, **SLP**

Ouzts, Mrs Florence L 811 South Court Street, Cleveland, MS 38732, (601) 843-4838, BA 66 Adrian Coll; ME 78 Delta St Univ; MA 68 OH St Univ; Dir Sp & Lang Serv, Delta St U Sp & Hrng Cl, **SLP**

Ouzts, Dr James W Delta State University, Box 3372, Cleveland, MS 38733, (601) 846-1897, BS 60 Delta St Univ; MA 63 Univ of MS; PH 67 (SH Sci-Psy) OH St Univ; Coord & Prof Aud/SLP, Delta State U, **A**

Ovadia, Mrs Joanne Ps 206, Avenue V & East 22nd St, Brooklyn, NY 11235, BS CUNY - Brooklyn Coll; MS Purdue Univ - West Lafayette; SLP, NYC Bd of Ed, **SLP**

Ovca, Nancy H 14326 Lake Tahoe Drive, Chesterfield, MO 63017, **SLP**

Over, Mrs Sandra Kay 1809 S E 9th Street, Moore, OK 73160, (405) 946-5563, BS 82 OK St Univ; MS 84 Univ of OK Medical Center; Audiologist, Otologic Medical Clinic, **A**

Overall, Mary Ann 1427 East 8th Streeet, Tulsa, OK 74120, (918) 587-8979, Area Mngr, Dept of Human Services, **SLP**

Overbay, Carolyn H 606 Crestview Drive, Johnson City, TN 37601, (615) 282-1700, BS 61 East TN St Univ; MA 65 East TN St Univ; Instr, Private Practice, **SLP**

Overbey, William F 613 East Street South, Talladega, AL 35160, **A**

Overchuk, Cynthia Lynne 468 Grace Trail, Orange, CT 06477, (203) 795-4907, BA 85 Univ of CT; MA 87 Univ of CT

Overhiser, Mrs Sandra T 7 Douglas Street, Cortland, NY 13045, (607) 753-9301, BA 81 SUNY - Coll at Cortland; MS 82 Ithaca Coll; Sp-Lang Path, Onondaga-Cortland-Madison BOCES, **SLP**

Overholt, Mrs Suzanne Welch 16 Oakwood Road, Huntington, WV 25701-4129, BA 79 Marshall Univ; MA 80 Marshall Univ; Sp-Lang Path, Cabell Co Sch, **SLP**

Overland, Mrs Lori L 46 Breeds Hill Place, Wilton, CT 06897, (516) 663-1003, BA 80 Hofstra Univ; MS 81 Adelphi Univ; Sp-Lang Path, Adelphi University, **SLP**

Overley, Mrs Cheryl Morton 24041 Gallery View, Winter Park, FL 32792, BS 81 Univ of GA; ME 82 Univ of GA; Sp-Lang Path, Cobb County Public Schools, **SLP**

Overly, Mrs Patricia Hargett 105 Clay Street, Cary, NC 27511, (919) 832-3909, BA 83 Univ of DE; MA 86 IN Univ - Bloomington; Sp-Lang Path, Tammy Lynn Ctr, **SLP**

Overman, Dr Carol Ann 7019 Churchill Road, Mc Lean, VA 22101, (202) 373-7374, BA 63 Coll of Saint Francis; MS 64 Univ of MI - Ann Arbor; PH 78 (NS) Univ of MD - College Park; Sp-Lang Path, CMHS St Elizabeths Hosp, **SLP**

Overman, Mrs Virginia S 1656 Rhonda Drive, Middleburg, FL 32068, (904) 272-4676, BA 80 Univ of MD - College Park; MA 82 Memphis St Univ; Aud, **A**

Overmann, Susan M 4413 Dublin Road, Marcellus, NY 13108, (315) 685-8351, BS 74 Univ of KS; MS 79 Coll of New Rochelle; Product Manager, Welch Allyn Inc

Overmyer, Mrs Claire Lee 6607 Hideaway Road, Ooltewah, TN 37363, (615) 778-7916, BS 78 Univ of TN - Knoxville; MA 80 Univ of KS; Sp-Lang Path, Erlanger Med Ctr, **SLP**

Overson, Joan Sandra W 1935 North 62nd Avenue, Eau Claire, WI 54701, (715) 289-4211, BA 76 Univ of WI - Eau Claire; MS 78 Univ of WI - Eau Claire; Sp-Lang Path, Sch Dist-Cadott, **SLP**

Overstake, Carol H 6120 Croyden Circle, Wichita, KS 67220, (316) 687-5000, BA 65 Wichita St Univ; MA 68 Wichita St Univ; 88–Sp-Lang Path, Wichita Speech Science Lab, **SLP**

Overstake, Dr Charles P 6120 Croyden Circle, Wichita, KS 67220, (316) 686-7367, BA 49 Wichita St Univ; MA 52 Wichita St Univ; PH 70 (Logopedics) Wichita St Univ; 72–Owner-Dir, Wichita Sp Science Lab, **SLP**

Overstreet, Paige Alise 1878 E Nine Mile Road, Eden Crosiin #503, Pensacola, FL 32514, (205) 665-5122, MS 87 Univ of Montevallo

Overton, Elaine Cecilia Box 3472, APO New York, NY 09057, BS 80 Univ of SD - Springfield; MS 81 Univ of SD - Springfield; 83–Sp-Lang Path, Dept of Defense Dependent Schs

Overton, Lynda L 525 Rutgers Avenue, Swarthmore, PA 19081, (215) 891-2210, BS 71 Auburn Univ - Auburn; MA 72 Univ of AL- Tuscaloosa; Sp/Lang Path, Elwyn Institutes, **SLP**

Overton, Rebecca Lynn 1014 W Gemini, Edmond, OK 73034, (405) 949-3280, BA 84 Univ of Northern IA; MS 86 Univ of OK Medical Center; 88–Sp-Lang Path, Baptist Med Ctr, **SLP**

Overton, Vivian F 4210 Mathewson Drive N W, Washington, DC 20011, **SLP A**

Oviatt, Carol C 2806 Heatherway, Ann Arbor, MI 48104, BA 75 McGill Univ - Quebec; MS 77 Univ of British Columbia; OM 82 Boston Univ; Market Researcher, Group Hlth Coop, **A**

Oviatt, Dana L 2806 Heatherway, Ann Arbor, MI 48104, BS 75 Saint Lawrence Univ; MS 77 Boston Univ; U of WI, **A**

Owaroff, Carol R 24 Lakeview Gardens #610, Natick, MA 01760-2630, (617) 332-6743, **SLP**

Owen, Mrs Barbara E R R 1-N Box 43, Oriska, ND 58063, (701) 845-0440, BS 77 OK St Univ; MA 79 OK St Univ; Sp/Lang Path, Sp & Hrng Serv Inc, **SLP**

Owen, Cynthia B 6299 South Iola Way, Englewood, CO 80111, **A**

Owen, Elizabeth A 68 Victoria Road, New Britain, CT 06052, (203) 747-6831, BS 84 Marywood Coll; MA 86 Univ of ME - Orono; 86–Sp-Lang Path, Wheeler Clinic Inc, **SLP**

Owen, Geraldine Box 569A, Kennebunkport, ME 04046, (207) 799-3309, BS 57 Univ of IL - Urbana; MS 68 Univ of IL - Urbana; MA 77 Univ of IL - Urbana; SLP, Cape Elizabeth Sch Syst, **SLP**

Owen, John R 466 Dogwood Road, Winchester, VA 22601, (703) 667-7200, BA 69 Alderson-Broaddus Coll; MA 72 Marshall Univ; Aud, ENT Consultants Inc, **SLP A ACE**

Owen, Mrs Karen Whisenhunt 5912 Old Rural Hall, Winston-Salem, NC 27105, (919) 760-5770, BS 80 Western Carolina Univ; MA 81 Western Carolina Univ; Sp-Lang Path, **SLP**

Owen, Laurie Moeller 2776 North Westfield Place, Claremont, CA 91711-1818, (714) 626-2013, MS 80 Univ of MI - Ann Arbor; Sp-Lang Path, Private Practice, **SLP**

Owen, Melanie Jean 580 South Pear Orchard Rd, Apartment 104, Ridgeland, MS 39157, (601) 922-5530, BA 83 MS Coll; MS 85 Univ Southern MS-Hattiesburg; **SLP**

Owen, Peggy M P O Box 101056, Pittsburgh, PA 15237, (412) 366-3167, MS 87 Univ of Pittsburgh - Pittsburgh

Owen-Garber, Diane P 3753 Druck Valley Road, York, PA 17402, (717) 771-2562, BA 74 Allegheny Coll; MS 76 Columbia Univ Teachers Coll; Dir/Phys Med & Rehab Dept, York Hosp, **SLP**

Owens, Mrs Alana Howard 326 Cate Road, Sevierville, TN 37862, (615) 428-2645, MA 81 Univ of TN - Knoxville; BS 80 Univ of TN - Knoxville; **SLP**

Owens, Mrs Alice Risley 63 Ragan Drive, Alexandria, LA 71303, (318) 473-0010, BA 79 Northeast LA Univ; MA 83 Northwestern St Univ; 87–Sp-Lang Path, VA Med Ctr, **SLP**

Owens, Aljean H 93 Holland Lane, East Hartford, CT 06118, BS 73 IN St Univ - Terre Haute; ME 77 Univ of Louisville; **SLP**

Owens, Alma D 6750 Ridge Moore Drive, Doraville, GA 30360, (404) 329-5520, BS 69 Middle TN St Univ; MS 70 Vanderbilt Univ; Sp/Lang Path, Emory U Hosp, **SLP**

Owens, Mrs Bonnie L 7440 S W Hunziker Suite D, Tigard, OR 97223, (503) 639-1229, BS 62 Saint Louis Univ; MS 76 Portland St Univ; 82–Sp-Lang Path, Private Practice, **SLP ACE**

Owens, Byron Chief Aud & Speech Path Services, VA Hospital, 2300 Ramey Street, Fayetteville, NC 28301, (919) 488-2120, BA 68 Univ of AL- Tuscaloosa; MA 70 Univ of AL- Tuscaloosa; ME 73 Univ of GA; Ch/Sp-Lang and Aud Serv, VA Med Cen, **SLP A**

Owens, Catherine Elaine 5547 Summerhill Drive, Los Angeles, CA 90043, (213) 290-1051, BA 84 CA St Univ - Northridge; MA 85 CA St Univ - Northridge; **SLP**

Owens, Cynthia Kay 1376 Lincoln Street, Salt Lake City, UT 84105, (801) 565-7482, BA 80 Univ of CA - Santa Barbara; MS 83 UT St Univ; 83–Sp-Lang Path, Jordan School District, **SLP**

Owens, Dr Earl R Northwest Nazarene College, 623 Holly Street, Nampa, ID 83651, (208) 467-8256, BA 52 Univ of CA - Santa Barbara; MA 56 Stanford Univ; ED 70 (NS) Univ of Northern CO; Head Dept of Sp Commun, NW Nazarene Coll, **SLP**

Owens, Prof Elmer Audiology And Speech, Univ Of Calif Medical Ctr, 400 Parnassus, San Francisco, CA 94143, (415) 666-2769, PH 59 (NS) Univ of Pittsburgh - Pittsburgh; Prof, U Cal San Fran, **SLP A F**

Owens, Gary W Cutler Army Community Hospital, U S A Meddac Audiology Clinic, Fort Devens, MA 01433, (617) 796-6815, BS 75 East TN St Univ; MA 77 East TN St Univ; Chief of Audiology Clinic, USA Meddac Cutler Army Hosp, **A**

Owens, Gloria J Box 66, 72 By Pass, Chester, SC 29706, (803) 385-3173, BA 72 Winthrop Coll; MS 74 Winthrop Coll; Sp-Lang Path, Chester Co Schls

Owens, Jerry Lee 1453 Elliott Street S E, Grand Rapids, MI 49507, BS 73 Western IL Univ; MA 76 Northern IL Univ - De Kalb; Audiologist, Private Practice, **A**

Owens, Mrs Karen E I 1333 Timberwood Trail, New Braunfels, TX 78132, (512) 379-2003, BS 73 Southwest TX St Univ; ME 74 Southwest TX St Univ; 88–Sp-Lang Path, Seguin ISD, **SLP**

Owens, Katharine 393 Ocean Avenue, Stratford, CT 06497, MS; **SLP LM**

Owens, Mrs Leslie H 28 West Belmeadow Lane, South Russell, OH 44022, (216) 338-5331, BS 75 Purdue Univ - West Lafayette; MA 77 Ball St Univ; 88–Sp-Lang Path, Orange Sch Dist, **SLP**

Owens, Robert E, Jr Dept Speech Path & Audiology, State Univ Of New York, Geneseo, NY 14454, (716) 245-5331, BA 66 Univ of DE; MA 68 Univ of DE; PH 78 (NS) OH St Univ; Assoc Prof, SUNY, **SLP**

Owens, Mrs Sandra Lee 505 North Court Street, Crown Point, IN 46307, (219) 663-3364, BS 76 Purdue Univ - West Lafayette; MS 78 Univ of KY; Sp-Lang Path, NW In Spec Ed Coop, **SLP**

Owens, Mrs Sarah J 11 Mars Road North Star, Newark, DE 19711, MS 78 West Chester Univ of PA; Sp-Lang Path, Red Clay School District, **SLP**

Owens, Shirley E 6829 Alpine Avenue, Cincinnati, OH 45236, (513) 891-0910, BA 78 MI St Univ; MS 79 PA St Univ - Univ Park; Aud, Chldn's Hosp Med Cen, **A**

Owens, Susan C 181 Hunt Valley Circle, Berwyn, PA 19312, (215) 565-4880, BS 64 Univ of KS; MA 66 Univ of KS; Mgt Spec, De Co Inter Unit, **SLP**

Owens, Susan M 4997 Tholozan, St Louis, MO 63109, (314) 353-1520, BS 85 Saint Louis Univ; MA 86 Saint Louis Univ; **SLP**

Owensrson, Mrs Teresa Kay 4143 Springbrook, Odessa, TX 79762, (915) 366-4177, BS 83 Univ of TX - Austin; MS 85 Univ of North TX; Aud, Permian Basin Rehab Cen, **A**

Owings, Dr Nathaniel 74 East San Francisco St, Santa Fe, NM 87501, (406) 994-5225, BS 68 CO St Univ; MS 72 Univ of WI - Madison; PH 76 (NS) Univ of WI - Madison; Associate Professor, Montana State University, **SLP**

Ownby, Mrs Jenifer C 2410 Watrous Avenue, Tampa, FL 33629, BA 77 Univ of FL; ME 78 Univ of FL; **SLP**

Ownby, Robert L Western Hills AEA 12, 1520 Morningside Avenue, Sioux City, IA 51106, (712) 274-6021, BS 71 Western IL Univ; MA 72 Western IL Univ; Supvr, Western Hills AEA-12, **A**

Owre, Mrs Deanne Marquerite Rural Free Delivery 1, Taber Hill Road, North Smithfield, RI 02895, (401) 568-3301, BA 65 Univ of WY; MS 85 Worcester St Coll; Sp-Lang Path, Burrillville PS Sys, **SLP**

Owsley, Robert Michael Newport Harbor Otology Inc, 2011 Westcliff Drive, Suite 5, Newport Beach, CA 92660, (714) 645-2520, BA 81 Mercer Univ - Macon; MS 84 Univ of WA; Aud, Private Practice, **A**

Oxendale, James Box 157, Arthur, IA 51431, **SLP**

Oxendine, Karen Ellis 1621 South 9th Street #2, Terre Haute, IN 47802, (812) 232-2011, BS 78 IN St Univ - Terre Haute; MS 79 IN St Univ - Terre Haute; SLP, Union Hospital, **SLP**

Oxenhandler, Gail H 9677 North West 28th Court, Coral Springs, FL 33065, BS 80 FL St Univ; MS 81 FL St Univ; Sp-Lang Path, Atlantic West Elem, **SLP**

Oxman, Barbara Louise Hunting Heights Drive, Apt #6 Washington Bldg, Storrs, CT 06268, (203) 429-4698, BS 83 Univ of NH; MS 85 Northeastern Univ; Sp-Lang Path, Southeastern CT Sp-Hrng Center, **SLP**

Oxman, Emily K 3730 Glenhurst, Minneapolis, MN 55416, (612) 920-1487, BS 42 Univ of MN - Minneap-St Paul; Retired, Private Practice, **SLP LM**

Oyama, Mrs Katherine Ann 400 Fort Pickens Road, Pensacola Beach, FL 32561, (904) 932-5949, MA 83 IN Univ - Bloomington; Sp-Lang Path, Palmetto Speech Pathology, **SLP**

Oyer, Dr Herbert J Speech & Hearing Science, 1430 London Drive, Columbus, OH 43221, (614) 422-8207, BA 43 Bluffton Coll; MS 49 Bowling Green St Univ; PH 55 (NS) OH St Univ; Prof Emeritus, The Ohio State Univ, **SLP A F H LM**

Oye-Shipp, Mrs May Mitsuko 108 Melissa Crescent, Whitby, ON, Canada L1N 8G4, (204) 586-9651, BA 76 Univ of Winnipeg - Manitoba; MA 80 Univ of TX - Austin; Sp-Lang Path, Durham Bd of Educ, **SLP**

Oyler, Anne L 1421 E Lee Street, Tucson, AZ 85719, (602) 621-7070, BS 80 Univ of IA; MA 82 Western IL Univ; Clinical Instructor, University of Arizona, **A**

Oyler, Robert F 1421 East Lee, Tucson, AZ 85719, (602) 881-3222, BS 70 NM St Univ; MA 74 NM St Univ; **SLP A**

Oyler-Russell, Mary Elizabeth 4212 Kensington Avenue, Richmond, VA 23221, (804) 359-2888, BS 69 Radford Univ; ME 72 Univ of VA - Charlottesville; Sp-Lang Path, **SLP**

Oza, Kalindi Uttam 4761 Mallard Common, Fremont, CA 94536, (408) 262-2100, **A**

Ozburn, Mrs Flora C Rural Route 13, Thunder Bay, ON, Canada P7B 5E4, (807) 622-9122, OB 80 Lakehead Univ - Ontario; MA 82 Univ of MN - Duluth; Sp-Lang Path, Lakehead Dist Catholic Sch Bd

Ozley, Mrs Carleen F 700 Stonehaven Road, Birmingham, AL 35226, (205) 979-5346, BS 73 Auburn Univ - Auburn; MS 76 Univ of Montevallo; 76–Sp/Lang Path, VA Med Cen Birmingham Al, **SLP**

Ozsvath, Nancy Lynn 256 Paseo Madero, Anaheim, CA 92807, (714) 787-0204, BA 81 CA St Univ - Long Beach; MA 84 CA St Univ - Long Beach; 88–Mgr of Clin Svcs, Team Rehab, **SLP**

P

Paarmann, Dr Larry Dean Drexel University, Ece Department, Philadelphia, PA 19104, (215) 895-2218, BS 70 Northern IL Univ - De Kalb; MS 77 Univ of IL - Urbana; PH 83 (Electrical Engineering) IL Inst of Tech; 83–Asst Prof, Drexel Univ

Paas, Deborah T 2079 North Chestnut #3, Fayetteville, AR 72703, (501) 521-8872, MS 88 Univ of AR - Fayetteville

Paasch, Elaine K 1134 East Beverly Way, Bountiful, UT 84010, (801) 298-8322, BS 76 Univ of WI - Madison; MS 77 Univ of WI - Madison; Sp/Lang Path, Davis Cty Sch Dist, **SLP**

Paasch, Kathryn Ann 23 Village West Court #302, Washington, MO 63090-1954, SLP, Depaul Hospital, **SLP**

Paatalo-Nelson, Heidi E 1442 Ryan Avenue West, Roseville, MN 55113, (612) 642-9429, OB 77 Univ of MN - Duluth; MA 78 Univ of Northern IA; SLP, St Paul Pub Schs, **SLP**

Paccioretti, Mrs Lorraine A 120 Harrington Road, Clifton, NJ 07012, (201) 423-6495, BA 78 Montclair St Coll; MA 80 Montclair St Coll; 81–Sp/Lang Path, Hawthorne Bd of Ed, **SLP**

Pace, Carlynn Marie P O Box 242, Hilmar, CA 95324, (209) 634-3886, MA 86 Northwestern Univ; **SLP**

Pace, Karmen Suzette 417 N E Shady Lane, Gladstone, MO 64118, (816) 454-9351, BS 79 Southwest MO St Univ; MS 86 Central MO St Univ; 80–Sp-Lang Path, No Kansas City Sch Dist, **SLP**

Pace, Mrs Melanie B 2620 Gladiolus Street, New Orleans, LA 70122, (504) 948-7782, BS 76 Saint Mary's Dominican Coll; OM 79 LA St Univ - N O Medical Ctr; SLP, Jefferson Parish Pub Sch Bd, **SLP**

Pace, Melissa J 116 Harmon Avenue, Winston-Salem, NC 27106, (919) 945-5163, BS 74 Appalachian St Univ; MA 76 Appalachian St Univ; Sp-Lang Path, Winston-Salem/Forsyth Co Schs, **SLP**

Pace, Salvatore Anthony 9 Wildwood Road, Lexington, MA 02173, (617) 862-7500, ME 61 Boston Univ; BS 61 Boston Univ; SLP, Town of Lexington, **SLP**

Pacelli, Monica M 13 Leverwood, The Woodlands, TX 77381, (713) 440-0734, BS 76 Southern IL Univ -Carbondale; MS 78 Baylor Coll of Medicine; Aud, Orl Assoc, **A**

Pacer, Sally A 1421 Monterey, Schaumburg, IL 60172, BS 78 De Paul Univ; MA 85 Northern IL Univ - De Kalb; Sp-Lang Path, District 88, **SLP**

Pacha, Sandra J R R 1 Box 155, Richland, IA 52585, (319) 694-3850, OB 80 Northeast MO St Univ; MA 81 Northeast MO St Univ; Sp-Lang Path, **SLP**

Pacheco, Christophr John 2133 Oakdale Avenue, Glenside, PA 19038, (215) 783-6010, BA 79 Univ of CT; MS 81 PA St Univ - Univ Park; Regional Dir, InSpeech Inc, **SLP**

Pachino, Judith L 3404 Slade Avenue, Baltimore, MD 21208, **SLP**

Pachtman, Prof Ruth Solow 368 Pitcher Terrace, Union, NJ 07083, (201) 547-3023, MA 65 Kean Coll of NJ; Assoc Prof Spec Ed, Jersey Cty St Coll, **SLP**

Pachura, Mrs Cristie W 1505 Highland Trail, Cary, NC 27511, (715) 536-9600, BS 78 Univ of WI - Eau Claire; MS 79 Univ of WI - Stevens Point; **SLP**

Pacifico, Daneen A 1122 Market Street, PO Box 2081, Parkersburg, WV 26102, (304) 428-2403, BS 75 WV Univ; MS 76 WV Univ; Aud/Owner, Audiology Services, **A**

Pacini, Mrs Claudette A 9209 Camino Cometa N E, Albuquerque, NM 87111, (505) 299-1402, BS 58 Northern IL Univ - De Kalb; MA 71 Univ of NM; ES 84 Univ of NM; 88–Asst Prin/Spec Ed, Albuquerque Pub Sch, **SLP**

Pacior, Brenda E 217 North Roosevelt Avenue, Fort Collins, CO 80521, (303) 226-2345, BS 81 Edinboro Univ of PA; MA 82 Kent St Univ; Foothills Gateway Rehab Cen In, **SLP**

Paciulli-MacAluso, Mrs Loretta 211 Walnut Street, East Rochester, NY 14445, (716) 385-6962, SLP, Hrng & Sp Cen of Rochester, **SLP**

Pack, Nancy J 190 Corona, Red Bluff, CA 96080-2130, (916) 527-5811, BA 75 CA St Univ - Chico; MA 77 CA St Univ - Chico; 88–CH Tchr, Tehama Co Dept of Educ, **SLP**

Packard, Debra M 1530 McNutt Drive, Wooster, OH 44691, (216) 262-3067, BA 74 Univ of Akron; MA 76 OH St Univ; Sp-Lang Path, Wooster City Sch, **SLP**

Packer, Karen Alane Route 1 Box 348-P, Lincolnton, NC 28092, (701) 433-2754, **SLP**

Packet, Linda L Box 5262, Ketchikan, AK 99901, (907) 225-8933, BS 73 Univ of MO - Columbia; MA 75 Univ of MO - Columbia; SLP, SE Island School District, **SLP**

Packford, Kathy Jean 5 Lovatt Place, St Albert, AB, Canada T8N 3X6, (403) 471-2262, BS 78 Dalhousie Univ - Nova Scotia; MS 80 Dalhousie Univ - Nova Scotia; Aud, Glenrose Rehab Hosp, **A**

Packman, Ellen R 2611 York Road, Swanendael Acres, Lewes, DE 19958, (302) 645-2345, BS 78 Trenton St Coll; MS 79 PA St Univ - Univ Park; 87–Sp-Lang Path, Cape Henlopen Sch Dist, **SLP**

Packness, Louise 865 West End Avenue #14-A, New York, NY 10025, (212) 864-2207, MA 87 CUNY - Hunter Coll; **SLP**

Packwood, Gary L 55 Barrett Road #139, Berea, OH 44017, (216) 726-8855, BA 65 Northwestern OK St Univ; MA 71 OH Univ - Athens; OM 81 Baldwin-Wallace Coll; Professor, Baldwin-Wallace Coll, **SLP**

Paczkowski, Mrs Patricia M 1400 Edwin Street, Marinette, WI 54143, (312) 887-8677, BS 80 IL St Univ - Normal; MS 81 IL St Univ - Normal; Sp/Lang Path, **SLP**

Padberg, Anne Montgomery 3526 Pestalozzi Street, St Louis, MO 63118-1114, (314) 577-5671, BS 79 Saint Louis Univ; MS 80 Southern IL Univ-Edwardsvill; Aud, Cardinal Glennon Mem Hosp, **A**

Padden, James Vincent 1603 Dundalk Avenue, Baltimore, MD 21222, (301) 328-2419, BA 83 Loyola Coll; MS 84 Loyola Coll; Sp-Lang Path, MIEMSS, **SLP**

Paddock, Jody Lynne 7286 Burke Hill Road, Perry, NY 14530, (716) 237-3264, BS 85 Nazareth Coll of Rochester; MS 86 Nazareth Coll of Rochester; 87–Sp-Lang Path, BOCES Holcomb Ctr, **SLP**

Paden, Dr Elaine P 2112 South Race Street, Urbana, IL 61801, (217) 244-2544, BA 37 Sioux Falls Coll; MA 39 Univ of IA; PH 43 (NS) Univ of IA; Assoc Prof Emerita, U of IL, **SLP F LM**

Paderewski, Ilyse 195 North Village Avenue, Rockville Centre, NY 11570, (516) 599-8653, BA 77 CUNY - Queens Coll; MA 79 CUNY - Queens Coll; Aud, Dennis Draizin MD, **A**

Padgett, Ann Midkiff 910 East Ocean View Avenue, #21, Norfolk, VA 23503, (804) 398-2402, BS 77 Old Dominion Univ; MS 85 Old Dominion Univ; SLP, Maryview Medical Center, **SLP**

Padgett, Mrs Carolynn J 5600 N E 7th Street, Ocala, FL 32671, (904) 351-7225, BA 80 Univ of FL; ME 82 Univ of FL; 87–Sp-Lang Path, Munroe Regional Med Ctr, **SLP ACE**

Padgett, Karen L 519 Missouri, Cincinnati, OH 45226, (513) 533-3714, BS 82 Univ of Cincinnati; MA 86 Univ of Cincinnati; 84–Sp-Lang Path, Cincinnati Pub Sch, **SLP**

Padilla, Belinda Hazel 3026 Hatton Drive, San Antonio, TX 78237, (512) 673-0980, BS 84 Baylor Univ; MS 86 Baylor Univ; 86–Sp-Lang Path, Northside ISD Educ Cody Elem, **SLP**

Padilla, Teresa C 1321 West Drew Street, Fort Worth, TX 76110, (915) 534-5731, BA 82 Univ of TX - El Paso; MS 83 TX Christian Univ; **SLP**

Padilla, Teresa Melendez P O Box 2251, Guaynabo, PR 00657-7006, (809) 787-5151, OB 83 Univ of PR - Rio Piedras; OM 85 Univ of PR - San Juan; 88–Sp-Lang Path, Domenech Coll, **SLP**

Padin-Soto, Rafaela P O Box 1670, Dorado, PR 00646, (809) 796-3706, BA 80 Univ of PR - Rio Piedras; MS 83 TX Christian Univ; 88–Sp-Lang Path, Department of Educ, **SLP**

Padish, Gail R 421 West Barry #405, Chicago, IL 60657-5566, (312) 747-4000, BS 80 IN Univ - Bloomington; MA 82 IN Univ - Bloomington; Aud, South Metropolitan Assoc, **A**

Padley, Susan Kay 19105 West Trowbridge Road, Martin, OH 43445, (419) 691-3459, BA 75 Bowling Green St Univ; MA 80 Bowling Green St Univ; Sp-Lang-Hrng Spec, Toledo Bd of Ed, **SLP**

Padnuk, Andrew S 1436 Royal Palm Square Blvd, Suite 2, Fort Myers, FL 33919, (813) 939-4114, BS 75 Loyola Coll; MS 76 Loyola Coll; Admin/Sp-Lang Path, Assoc In Sp-Path, **SLP**

Paesani, Andrew, Jr Dept Of Communication Sci U-85, University Of Connecticut, Storrs, CT 06268, (203) 486-2628, BA 54 West Liberty St Coll; MA 58 Univ of IA; PH 64 (NS) Univ of IA; Assoc Prof, U Ct, **SLP F**

Paff, Patricia Lee 9844 Pippin Road, Cincinnati, OH 45231, (513) 825-4192, BS 84 Univ of Cincinnati; MA 85 Northeast MO St Univ; **SLP**

Pafitis, Irene A 10810 Margate Road, Silver Spring, MD 20901, (202) 745-5600, BA 85 Univ of MD - College Park; MA 86 George Washington Univ; 87–Aud, Children's Hosp National Med Ctr, **A**

Pafunda, Mrs Katherine C Watson Clinic, 1600 Lakeland Hills Boulevard, Lakeland, FL 33804, (813) 680-7195, BA 76 Univ of FL; MS 82 Univ of South FL; 87–Aud/Sp-Lang Path, Watson Clinic, **A**

Pagano, Janice Ameen 24495 Simmons Drive, Novi, MI 48050, (313) 577-3337, BA 78 OH St Univ; MA 80 Cleveland St Univ; **SLP**

Pagano, Mrs Janie E 369 Brookwood Drive, Downingtown, PA 19335, (215) 873-1083, BS 76 SUNY - Center at Albany; MA 77 Hofstra Univ; SLP, Montgy Co Inter Unit, **SLP**

Pagano, Mrs Julie Anna 371 Westside Lane, Torrington, CT 06790, (203) 496-1802, BA 80 Saint Joseph Coll; MA 85 SUNY - Coll at Plattsburgh; 86–Sp-Lang Path, Litchfield CT PS, **SLP**

Pagano-Piacente, Geraldine 522 Shore Road #2KK, Long Beach, NY 11561, (718) 738-6200, OM 84 Adelphi Univ; MA 79 Hofstra Univ; Sp/Lang Path, Fineson Dev Cen, **SLP**

Page, Mrs Christy Ann 1722 West Sunshine, Springfield, MO 65807, (417) 864-3800, BS 79 Southwest MO St Univ; MA 85 Southwest MO St Univ; Sp-Lang Path, Springfield R-12 Schools, **SLP**

Page, Dr Edwin R Nu-Ed-Ventures Incorporated, Consultation Services, 11000 McClumpha Road, Plymouth, MI 48170, (313) 453-9319, BS 60 Western MI Univ; MS 62 OH Univ - Athens; PH 70 OH Univ - Athens; 86–Pres, Nu-Ed-Ventures Inc, **SLP**

Page, Mrs Gwendolyn M 14607 S E 267th Street, Kent, WA 98042, (206) 859-7513, BA 53 Univ of WA; OM 72 Univ of WA; 67–Sp-Lang Path, Kent Sch Dist #415, **SLP**

Page, Mrs Jane Bickerton 325 7th Street, Whitehall, PA 18052, (215) 866-8092, BA 62 CUNY - Hunter Coll; MS 64 Univ of MI - Ann Arbor; 84–Asst Prof & Dir Sp-Hrng Clinic, East Stroudsburg University, **SLP A**

Page, John Clifford Navy Environmental Hlth Ctr, Bldg X-353, Naval Station, Norfolk, VA 23511, (804) 444-4657, BA 73 LA Tech Univ; MA 74 Memphis St Univ; Aud, Navy Environ Hlth Cen

Page, Dr John McCue 325 7th Street, Whitehall, PA 18052, (215) 776-4795, BS 63 Univ of Cincinnati; MS 64 Univ of MI - Ann Arbor; PH 70 (NS) IN Univ - Bloomington; 75–Dir/Sp and Hrng, Sacred Heart Hosp, **A**

Page, Joseph M 304 Kh Exed Sucb, 1300 Elmwood Avenue, Buffalo, NY 14222, (716) 878-4639, MS 56 Univ of WI - Madison; **SLP A**

Page, Dr Judith L University Of Kentucky, Dept Of Special Education, 229 Taylor Education Bldg, Lexington, KY 40506, BS 71 Univ of MN - Minneap-St Paul; MA 72 Univ of IL - Urbana; PH 81 (NS) Purdue Univ - West Lafayette; Associate Professor, University of Kentucky, **SLP**

Page, Kathleen E 12 Pennsylvania Avenue, 2nd Floor, Long Beach, NY 11561-1620, (212) 239-1796, BA 77 Univ of FL; MA 79 Univ of FL; 86–Aud, New York City Dept of Health, **A**

Page, Leslie Ann 11062 Berrypick Lane, Columbia, MD 21044, (202) 651-5000, MA 85 Univ of IL - Urbana; **A**

Page, Mrs Linda J 2460 Harmony Drive, Charlottesville, VA 22901, (804) 979-7339, BA 70 Univ of North TX; MA 74 Univ of North TX; **SLP**

Page, Margaret R 1716 N W 27th Terrace, Gainesville, FL 32605, (904) 376-6986, MA 88 Univ of FL

Page, Michael Don 22 South 900 East, Salt Lake City, UT 84102, (801) 364-8692, BS 83 Brigham Young Univ; OM 84 Brigham Young Univ; 84–Aud, Audiology Assoc of SLC, **A**

Page, Olga H 724 Hawthorne Street, Memphis, TN 38107, (901) 369-4615, BS 71 MS Univ for Women; OM 85 Memphis St Univ; 85–Dir Prod Dev, Eastwood Hosp, **A**

Page, Mrs Ruth M 5221 Quarry Lane, Virginia Beach, VA 23464, (804) 497-7511, BS 69 MS Univ for Women; MA 72 LA Tech Univ; Sp-Lang Path, VA Beach Cty Pub Sch, **SLP**

Page, Suzanne 5611 Smoke Rise Lane, Fairfax Station, VA 22039, (703) 250-0002, BA 77 Univ of NC - Greensboro; MA 79 Univ of TN - Knoxville; Sp/Lang Path, **SLP**

Page, Mrs Yvonne 4534 Black Oak Woods, San Antonio, TX 78249, (512) 493-2418, BS 82 Univ of TX - Austin; ME 84 Southwest TX St Univ; **SLP**

Pagel, Mrs Janice Ruth 3870 Townsend Boulevard, Jacksonville, FL 32211-2260, (904) 768-3221, BS 81 Univ of WI - Madison; MS 83 Univ of WI - Stevens Point; SLP, Duval Co Sch Bd, **SLP**

Pagliaroli, Mrs Michele Terese 461 Lakewood Parkway, Snyder, NY 14226, (716) 839-2312, BS 82 SUNY - Coll at Fredonia, MA 83 Bowling Green St Univ; 86–Sp-Lang Path, Erie 1 BOCES, **SLP**

Pagnanelli, Jacqueline 2627 Santa Barbara Drive, Bethel Park, PA 15102, BS 82 Indiana Univ of PA; MA 84 Univ of Pittsburgh - Pittsburgh; Sp-Lang Path, Allegheny Intermed Unit, **SLP**

Pahel, Carey W 1207 Heathrow Drive, Greensboro, NC 27410, (919) 272-1721, BA 72 Catawba Coll; ME 75 Univ of NC - Greensboro; Dir, Cw Pahel Aud Serv, **A**

Pahl, Mrs Cynthia Rachel 1068 Schanock, Green Bay, WI 54303-4565, (414) 497-3886, BA 76 Univ of MN - Duluth; MA 77 Western MI Univ; Sp-Lang Path, Green Bay Pub Sch, **SLP**

Pahle, William F 30 East Elm Street, Chicago, IL 60611, (312) 890-8659, BS 54 Univ of WI - Milwaukee; MA 55 Northwestern Univ; Coord-Hs Prog for Hrng Imp, Chicago Bd of Ed, **SLP A**

Paier, Susan Barbara 44 St Mihiel Drive, Hamden, CT 06514, (203) 387-0190, BS 83 Northeastern Univ; MS 85 Northeastern Univ; Aud, New England Rehab Hosp, **A**

Paige, Gretchen Marie 7491 Hickory Log Circle, Columbia, MD 21045-5005, (301) 381-6926, BA 82 MI St Univ; MS 84 Purdue Univ - West Lafayette; Aud, Hearing Resources, **A**

Paige, Patricia Ann R 6301 Clearspring Road, Baltimore, MD 21212, (301) 435-8360, BA 74 Univ of CA - Santa Barbara; MS 76 AZ St Univ; **SLP**

Pailet, Mrs Janet Joseph 818 IDA Place, New Orleans, LA 70119, (504) 484-7413, BS 80 Univ of TX - Austin; OM 82 LA St Univ - N O Medical Ctr; Sp-Lang Path, Orleans Parish Sch Bd, **SLP**

Paine, Pamela J 33 Baxter Road, Unit 2-E, West Willington, CT 06279, (203) 486-2629, BS 74 PA St Univ - Univ Park; MS 76 PA St Univ - Univ Park; Aud, U of CT Sp/Hrng Cl, **A**

Paine, Sherry Lindsey Tiergartenweg 1 7000, Stuttgart, West Germany 1, **SLP**

Paine, Mrs Wendy Luecker 4317 Cassell Boulevard, Prince Frederick, MD 20678, (301) 535-1211, **SLP**

Painter, Lee Mariano 205 Fairmount Avenue, Philadelphia, PA 19123, (215) 221-7020, MA 84 Temple Univ; Sp-Lang Path, Temple University Hospital, **SLP**

Painton, Dr Stephen W School/Public & Allied Health, Dept/Comm Disorders, East Tennessee State Univ, Johnson City, TN 37614, (615) 929-5253, BA 69 Northwestern OK St Univ; MS 70 Univ of OK Medical Center; PH 75 (NS) Univ of OK Medical Center; Aud, East Tennessee University, **A**

Paisley, John M 800 8th Avenue, Cumberland, WI 54829, (715) 822-8252, BS 75 Mankato St Univ; MS 79 Mankato St Univ; 88–Sp-Lang Path, Northern Pines United Services, **SLP**

Paivanas, Susan M K 5813 Torington Drive, Springfield, VA 22152, BS 77 SUNY - Coll at Geneseo; MS 80 PA St Univ - Univ Park; SLP, Fairfax Co Pub Schs, **SLP**

Pajak, Nancy Hartman 1823 Chestnut, Everett, WA 98201, (206) 259-2476, BS 75 Univ of ND; MA 79 CO St Univ; Aud, Edmonds Schl Dstr, **A**

Pajares, Toni Mancuso 96 Greenwich Drive, Mount Holly, NJ 08060, (609) 267-7317, BA 79 Saint Mary's Dominican Coll; BS 79 Saint Mary's Dominican Coll; OM 80 LA St Univ - N O Medical Ctr; **SLP**

Pakosta, Judith Lynn 325 East 3rd Street #2, Alton, IL 62002, (618) 465-3261, BS 81 IL St Univ - Normal; MS 83 IL St Univ - Normal; Sp-Lang Path, Spec Sch Dist of St Louis Co, **SLP**

Pakosz, Elizabeth H 7151 Oak Hill Drive, Sylvania, OH 43560, (419) 882-0555, BS 70 Bowling Green St Univ; MA 77 Bowling Green St Univ; Sp-Lang Path, Sylvania Cty Sch, **SLP**

Pakula, Cynthia Ann 11012 Tam O Shanter Drive, Carmel, IN 46032, (317) 844-4929, BA 68 IN Univ - Bloomington; MA 84 Butler Univ; Sp-Lang Path, Private Practice, **SLP**

Palacios, Judith Tuck 8005 Algarve Street, Mc Lean, VA 22102, (703) 356-1339, BA 51 CUNY - Brooklyn Coll; MA 55 CUNY - Brooklyn Coll; Offi Mgr, Private Practice, **SLP**

Palangio, Judy 5 Elmhurst Avenue, Providence, RI 02908, (401) 331-8733, MS 87 Northeastern Univ

Palaski, Mrs Dorothy 132 10th Street, Seal Beach, CA 90740, (213) 832-3056, BA 71 CA St Univ - Northridge; MA 73 CA St Univ - Northridge; Sp-Lang Path, Los Angeles USD, **SLP**

Palasz, Richard W 163 Pier Court, Naperville, IL 60565, (312) 629-8900, BS 83 Bradley Univ; MS 84 Bradley Univ; 85–Mgr of Field Oper, MTS Assoc Inc, **A**

Palazzo, Mrs Jill Gannon 24381 Orchard Lake Road, Suite A, Farmington Hills, MI 48018, (313) 423-1881, BS 79 Central MI Univ; MA 80 Central MI Univ; Dir, Palazzo Sebring & Assoc, **SLP ACE**

Palcich, William Joseph 96 Shoshone Street, Flagstaff, AZ 86001, (602) 338-4848, BA 72 Coll of St Thomas; MS 82 Northern AZ Univ; MA 76 Northern AZ Univ; Dist Sp-Lang Path, Whiteriver PS, **SLP**

Palella, Marietta C 225 Lake Boulevard, Unit 516, Buffalo Grove, IL 60089, (312) 882-5811, BA 71 Northern IL Univ - De Kalb; MS 75 Southern IL Univ -Carbondale; 82–Director Speech Services, Northwest Sp Path Assoc Ltd, **SLP**

Palen, Dr Chester 7710 Windy Hill Drive, Kent, OH 44240, (216) 672-2672, BS 51 Bowling Green St Univ; MS 53 Bowling Green St Univ; PH 72 (NS) OH St Univ; Dir Sp & Hrng Cl, Kent St U, **SLP**

Palen, Sharon B 203 Darwin Drive, Snyder, NY 14226-4861, BS 71 IN Univ - Bloomington; MA 72 Purdue Univ - West Lafayette; **SLP LM**

Paleski, Tanya Elizabeth 1807 Remington, Fort Collins, CO 80525, (303) 482-2584, BS 71 Northern AZ Univ; MS 85 CO St Univ; 88–Sp-Lang Path, Poudre Valley Hosp, **SLP**

Palfrey, Cheryl C 1842 Oakwood Avenue, Arcadia, CA 91006, (818) 355-4700, MS 76 Univ of MI - Ann Arbor; BS 75 Univ of MI - Ann Arbor; 87–Aud, Los Angeles USD, **A**

Palfy, Susan Bieger 213 Allenwood Drive, Statesboro, GA 30458, (912) 764-9426, BS 77 FL St Univ; MS 78 FL St Univ; Indep Contractor, Private Practice, **SLP**

Palgutta, Renea Elaine 2528-3B Belmont Terrace, Fredericksburg, VA 22401, BS 82 CA Univ of PA; MS 85 CA Univ of PA; 88–Sp-Lang Path, Bowling Green Co PS

Palin, Sue Johnston 4234 Hacienda Drive Suite 210, Pleasanton, CA 94566, (415) 847-9666, BS 76 OK St Univ; MA 78 OK St Univ; 88–Dir Sp-Lang Path Svcs, Theapy Mgmt-Innovations, **SLP ACE**

Palitz, Marsha E 22 Woodlake Drive, Port Orange, FL 32019, (904) 255-4568, BA 69 Univ of PA; ME 75 Univ of FL; Developmental Therapist, Volusia Er Sl Cen, **SLP**

Pall, Roberta Granke 28005 Inkster, Farmington Hills, MI 48018, (313) 757-5520, BA 67 Marygove Coll; MA 76 Wayne St Univ; **SLP**

Pallanck, Patricia Gregorio 2 Forest Road, Stafford Springs, CT 06076, (203) 727-1318, BA 81 Univ of CT; MA 83 Univ of CT; Aud, American School for the Deaf, **A**

Palleja, Mrs Mary M 2168 Larch Street, Wantagh, NY 11793, (516) 783-0170, BA 74 CUNY - Hunter Coll; MA 77 CUNY - Hunter Coll; Sp-Lang Path, Mary M Palleja, **SLP**

Pallett, Stephen B 518 Oakham Court, Severna Park, MD 21146-1727, (301) 944-3100, MS 79 Towson St Univ; Audiologist, Audiology Associates, **A**

Pallotto, Michele Louise Saint Margaret Hospital, Department Of Communication Disorders, 5454 Hohman Avenue, Hammond, IN 46320, (219) 933-2004, BS 85 Northern IL Univ - De Kalb; MA 87 Northern IL Univ - De Kalb; 87–Sp-Lang Path, St Margaret Hosp, **SLP**

Palm, Dr David E Department Of Audiology, Gunderson Clinic Ltd, La Crosse, WI 54601, (608) 782-7300, BA 63 Univ of MI - Dearborn; MS 68 Wayne St Univ; PH 72 (NS) Univ of OK Medical Center; Aud, Gundersen Cl, **A**

Palmateer, Nadine Smith 6785 Cooper Hollow Road, Monmouth, OR 97361, (503) 588-6677, BS 74 OR St Univ; MA 78 OR St Univ; Aud, Mid or Regional Prgm, **A**

Palmberg, Colleen Marie 4910 Thomas Avenue North, Minneapolis, MN 55430, (612) 337-4302, BS 82 Mankato St Univ; MA 83 Univ of MN - Duluth; Sp-Lang Path, Riverside Med Ctr, **SLP**

Palmer, Mrs Anita Marie 717 Anderson Street, Manchester, IA 52057, (319) 927-6943, BS 86 Univ of IA; MA 87 Western IL Univ; SLP, AEA 1

Palmer, Mrs Barbara Weisburd 19700 Michaels Court, Castro Valley, CA 94546, (415) 886-1414, BS 59 Univ of MN - Minneap-St Paul; MA 64 CA St Univ - Hayward; Sp-Lang Path, Private Practice, **SLP**

Palmer, Carole C 533 North Patterson, Santa Barbara, CA 93111, (805) 683-1327, BA 63 Univ of Denver; MA 64 Stanford Univ; SLP, Goleta Union Sch Dist, **SLP**

Palmer, Catherine Vea 927 Forest Street #W-1, Evanston, IL 60201, (312) 491-3164, BS 84 Univ of MA - Amherst; MA 85 Northwestern Univ; Audiologist, Northwestern Univ, **A**

Palmer, Cheryl B 1408 8th Avenue #14, San Francisco, CA 94122, (415) 750-5950, BS 79 Univ of NH; MS 81 Southern CT St Univ; Chief Sp-Lang Pathologist, St Marys Hospital & Med Center, **SLP**

Palmer, Mrs Christine 919 Lynwood Court, Mars, PA 16046, (412) 761-6062, BS 78 Clarion Univ of PA; MA 80 Univ of Pittsburgh - Pittsburgh; Sp-Lang Path, Rehab Spec Inc, **SLP**

Palmer, Clarence 111 Camelot, Hot Springs, AR 71913, (501) 624-5422, MS 77 Phillips Univ; Aud, Hot Springs Clinic of Otolaryn, **A**

Palmer, David E 1350 North Huron River Dr, Ypsilanti, MI 48197-1615, BA 48 Univ of MI - Ann Arbor; MA 52 Univ of MI - Ann Arbor; Retired, En Michigan U, **SLP**

Palmer, Mrs Deborah Ann Rt 2 Box 40, Elkhorn, WI 53121, (414) 728-4760, BS 78 Univ of WI - Stevens Point; MS 79 Univ of WI - Whitewater; Sp-Lang Path, Homecare Network, **SLP**

Palmer, Mrs Deborah Hill PO Box 215, Dugger, IN 47848-0026, (812) 847-8651, BS 74 IN St Univ - Terre Haute; MA 81 Ball St Univ; 88–Sp-Lang Path, Linton-Stockton Sch Corp, **SLP**

Palmer, Diane Carol 16-1 San Gabriel Avenue, Chico, CA 95926, (916) 893-4205, BA 83 San Jose St Univ; MA 86 San Jose St Univ; **SLP**

Palmer, Mrs Floris N 701 1st Street, Liverpool, NY 13088, (315) 451-1723, BS 71 PA St Univ - Univ Park; MS 72 Syracuse Univ; Sp-Lang Path, N Syracuse Central School Dist, **SLP**

Palmer, Mrs Gail L Box 3, Syracuse, NE 68446, (402) 269-2381, MS 77 Miami Univ - Oxford; Sp-Lang Path, Educational Serv Unit 4, **SLP**

Palmer, Dr John M University Of Washington Jg-15, Speech/Hrng Sciences Dept, 1417 N E 42nd Street, Seattle, WA 98195, (206) 543-0095, BA 47 Univ of WA; MA 50 Univ of WA; PH 52 (NS) Univ of MI - Ann Arbor; Professor, University of Washington, **SLP A F LM**

Palmer, Dr Julia Rountree Rt #3 Ponderosa Drive, Swainsboro, GA 30401, (912) 237-6704, BA 70 Emory Univ; ME 72 Univ of GA; ED 80 (NS) Univ of GA; Sp-Lang Pathg Path, Southeast Rehab Servs, **SLP**

Palmer, Karen Joyce Upstate Home/Children, Rd 1 Box 155, Oneonta, NY 13820-9753, (607) 432-6936, BA 83 Univ of IA; MA 85 SUNY - Coll at Geneseo; **SLP**

Palmer, Mrs Kim Kokus 8824 Lea Place, Maineville, OH 45039, (513) 677-0316, MS 87 Univ of SC - Columbia; 88–Sp-Lang Path, Sp Path, **SLP**

Palmer, Kimberly Ann 2020 Wallace Street, Philadelphia, PA 19130, (518) 399-9377, BS 85 Ithaca Coll; MA 87 George Washington Univ; **SLP**

Palmer, Lee D Hot Springs Speech & Lang Ctr, 111 Camelot Lane, Hot Springs, AR 71913, (501) 767-5140, BA 72 Henderson St Univ; MS 77 Phillips Univ; Sp-Lang Path, Hot Spgs Sp & Lang Cen, **SLP ACE**

Palmer, Mrs Linda Oltman Natl Tech Inst For The Deaf, One Lomb Memorial Drive, Bldg 60 #3125, Rochester, NY 14623, (716) 475-6263, BA 73 Univ of IL - Chicago; MA 79 Northern IL Univ - De Kalb; Audiologist, NTID, **A**

Palmer, Mrs Lorraine M 1685 Aple Drive, Troy, MI 48098, (313) 689-6000, BA 84 MI St Univ; MA 85 MI St Univ; Sp-Lang Path, Troy School District, **SLP**

Palmer, Margaret L 408 Durand Street, East Lansing, MI 48823, BA 59 MI St Univ; MA 67 MI St Univ; Retired, Ingham Intermediate Sch Dist, **SLP**

Palmer, Mrs Maria R 2063 North 63rd Street, Philadelphia, PA 19151, (215) 879-5195, BA 72 Howard Univ; MS 73 Columbia Univ Teachers Coll; 87–Sp-Lang Path, Comm Child Dev Ctr, **SLP**

Palmer, Marjorie M Rancho San Julian, Star Route, Lompoc, CA 93436, (805) 736-6792, BA 67 Elmira Coll; MA 69 CA St Univ - Long Beach; Sp-Lang Path, Private Practice, **SLP**

Palmer, Mary A 155 Highspire Road, Richboro, PA 18954, **SLP**

Palmer, Michele Tullier 2254 Heather Road, Homewood, IL 60430-3612, (312) 957-2367, **SLP**

Palmer, Phyllis Mary 337 Garcia N E, Albuquerque, NM 87123, (505) 291-8896, BA 82 SUNY - Coll at New Paltz; MS 84 Emerson Coll; Sp-Lang Path, Univ of New Mexico Hosp, **SLP ACE**

Palmer, 1Lt Richard Lee Department Of ENT-Audiology Section, Fitzsimons Army Medical Center, Aurora, CO 80045-6300, (303) 361-3124, BS 83 Univ of UT; MS 86 Univ of UT; 88–Aud, US Army, **A**

Palmer, Mrs Susan A 35 Wolfe Avenue, Mansfield, OH 44907, (419) 756-1133, BA 76 Loyola Coll; MS 78 Loyola Coll; Sp-Lang Path, Richland City Board of Mr/Dd, **SLP**

Palmer, Yolanda 6115 Lynnhaven, Lubbock, TX 79413, (806) 796-0570, BA 77 TX Tech Univ; MA 78 TX Tech Univ; **SLP**

Palmeri, Daniel J P O Box 4625, Fort Lauderdale, FL 33338, **SLP**

Palmeri, Janine M 6157 Midnight Pass #G-11, Sarasota, FL 34242, (813) 924-7681, BS 76 Univ of Miami; MS 77 FL St Univ; 88–Aud, Doctors Hrng Ctr, **A**

Palmquist, Cheryl Louise 215 Sandercock, San Luis Obispo, CA 93401, (805) 541-8492, BA 80 Humboldt St Univ; MA 82 Humboldt St Univ; SLP, Mendocino Middle Sch, **SLP**

Palmquist, Mrs Pamela Louise P O Box 506, Cedar Crest, NM 87008, (505) 281-5951, BA 85 Univ of FL; MS 88 Univ of NM; 87–Sp-Lang Path, Moriarty Municipal Schs, **SLP**

Palombaro, Mary Mason 10 Beethoven Street, Binghamton, NY 13905, BA 80 SUNY - Center at Buffalo; MA 81 SUNY - Center at Buffalo; Sp-Lang Path, BOCES Binghamton NY Broome, **SLP**

Pals, Catherine L Vankka 408 Stratchcona Mews S W, Calgary, AB, Canada T3H 1W4, (403) 249-8224, BA 81 Univ of WA; OM 82 Univ of WA; Sp/Lang Path, Cariboo Hlth Unit, **SLP**

Pals, Mrs Marjorie E Box 10, Dumont, CO 80436, (303) 567-2820, BA 57; MA 68 Univ of Denver; Retired, **SLP LM**

Paluszek, Suzanne F 80-24 Cowles Court, Middle Village, NY 11379, BA 78 CUNY - Queens Coll; MA 80 CUNY - Queens Coll; Tchr, Japanese Sch of NY, **SLP**

Pamula-Murray, Mrs Karen Rural Route 1, Box 287K, Pittsboro, IN 46167, (317) 892-3958, BS 72 Bowling Green St Univ; MA 76 Cleveland St Univ; **SLP**

Panagos, Dr John M Oklahoma State University, Speech Pathology, 120 Hanner Hall, Stillwater, OK 74078, MA 65 WA St Univ; PH 69 (NS) OH Univ - Athens; Prof & Dept Head, OK St U, **SLP F**

Panasci, Mrs Nancy E 5610 South Kingston Way, Englewood, CO 80111, (303) 771-1190, BS 76 CO St Univ; MA 79 Catholic Univ of America; SLP, Littleton Public School Dist, **SLP**

Pandori, Joann 46432 Snowbird Drive, Mount Clemens, MI 48044, (313) 791-6300, BS 77 Wayne St Univ; MA 79 Wayne St Univ; 87–Sp-Lang Path, Clintondale Com School, **SLP**

Pane, Kimberly M 6148 North Karlov, Chicago, IL 60646, (312) 282-0630, MA 87 Univ of IL - Urbana

Panebianco, Marcia Lee 1614 Linden Street, Scranton, PA 18510, (717) 348-1321, BS 64 PA St Univ - Univ Park; MA 67 Syracuse Univ; Asst Dir Dept SLP & Aud, Allied Services Fr Handicapped, **SLP**

Panels, Mrs Floria G 4899 Yeaworth Lane, Manlius, NY 13104, (315) 682-6793, BA 76 Allegheny Coll; MS 77 Syracuse Univ; 86–Sp-Lang Path, East Syracuse-Minoa Cen Schs, **SLP**

Pang, Denise K 2504 Tantalus Drive, Honolulu, HI 96813, (808) 845-4663, MS 77 Gonzaga Univ; Sp-Lang Path, Dept of Education, **SLP**

Pang-Ching, Dr Glenn K 107 Kekaha Place, Honolulu, HI 96825, (808) 948-8279, BA 57 CA St Univ - Los Angeles; MS 58 Purdue Univ - West Lafayette; PH 66 (Aud) Univ of Southern CA; Prof Aud & SLP, U of HI, **A**

Pangori, Mrs Theresa Michele 30033 Gloria, St Clair Shores, MI 48082, (313) 294-0623, BS 83 Indiana Univ of PA; MA 84 MI St Univ; Sp-Lang Path, MacOmb ISD, **SLP**

Panichella, Amy G 9011 Andora Drive, Miramar, FL 33025, (305) 435-2358, BA 76 Univ of Miami; MA 77 Univ of Miami; SLP, School Board of Broward County, **SLP**

Panitch, Adine R 300 East Gittings Avenue, Baltimore, MD 21212, MS 73 CA St Univ - Sacramento; Sp-Lang Path, Jemicy Sch, **SLP**

Pankey, Mrs Catherine Norwood 544 Sabal Palm Drive, Lake Park, FL 33403, (407) 694-7359, BA 74 Palm Beach Atlantic Coll; MA 76 Univ of FL; Sp-Lang Path, Palm Beach County Schs, **SLP**

Pankiewicz, Shelley Maria 1111 South Nevada Street, Seattle, WA 98108, (206) 243-1473, BA 80 Univ of WA; OM 83 Univ of WA; Audiologist, Kent School District, **A**

Panko, Mrs Alice L 5605 Sweetwater, El Paso, TX 79924, (915) 821-9419, BA 85 Univ of TX - El Paso; MS 87 Univ of TX - El Paso; 87–Sp-Lang Path, Gadsden ISD, **SLP**

Pankow, Deanna K 1032 Walker, Oakland, CA 94610, (415) 835-3579, BA Towson St Univ; MS OH St Univ; Tchr, Canyon Sch Dist, **SLP**

Pankratz, Mrs Judy M 7478 Whitehall Circle, West Chester, OH 45069, (319) 779-1637, BS 75 Northern IL Univ - De Kalb; MA 76 Northern IL Univ - De Kalb; 86–Sp-Lang Path, Mason Schs, **SLP**

Pankratz, Lori Dee 307 S E College Complex, Wahpeton, ND 58075-3384, (701) 671-3076, BA 84 Univ of ND; MS 85 Minot St Univ; 88–Sp-Lang Path, Wahpeton PS Sch Sys, **SLP**

Pankratz, Nancy Stone 2318 Emerson, Wausau, WI 54401, (715) 848-2934, BA 62 Univ of CO - Boulder; MS 76 Univ of WI - Stevens Point; Dir Sp-Lang Path Serv, Wausau Sch Dist, **SLP**

Pankuch, Ann L 1441 Apple Circle A-184, Mechanicsburg, PA 17055, (717) 691-3835, BS 86 Indiana Univ of PA; MS 87 WV Univ; 88–Sp-Lang Path, Rehab Hosp in Mechanicsburg

Pannbacker, Mary Dirickson LSU Medcial Center, P O Box 33932, Shreveport, LA 71130, (318) 227-5156, BA 63 Univ of Science & Arts of OK; OM 64 Univ of OK Medical Center; PH 72 (NS) SUNY - Coll at Buffalo; Prof & Prog Dir, LA St U Med Cen, **SLP F**

Pannier, Mrs Audrey Forster 1245 Daubenberger Road, Turlock, CA 95380, (209) 667-0637, BA 70 Univ of WI - Eau Claire; MA 83 CA St Univ - Stanislaus; Sp-Lang Path, Turlock USD, **SLP**

Pannullo, Theresa A 110 South Centre Street, South Orange, NJ 07079, (201) 233-0691, BS 75 Seton Hall Univ; MA 77 Seton Hall Univ; Sp-Lang Path, Mt Carmel Guild, **SLP**

Pantano, Marilyn J 3143 Queens Chapel Road, Apt 202, Mount Rainer, MD 20712, (301) 927-5442, BS 75 Nazareth Coll of Rochester; MS 77 SUNY - Coll at Fredonia; 88–Sp-Lang Path, Private Practice, **SLP**

Panther, Mrs Kathy M 2139 Woodbourne Avenue, Louisville, KY 40205, (502) 582-2231, BA 76 Univ of KY; MS 81 Univ of Louisville; Director Sp-Lang Dept, Frazier Rehab Cen, **SLP ACE**

Panush, Robert Marc 6878 Glen Mawr, El Cerrito, CA 94530, (415) 836-8228, BA 83 Univ of CA - Berkeley; MS 84 CA St Univ - Hayward; **SLP**

Panyard, Vickie Lynn 6263 Beach Road, Fremont, MI 49412-9235, **A**

Panzarella, Linda Theresa 13 Margate Road, Lutherville, MD 21093, (301) 321-7396, BA 80 Loyola Coll; MS 81 Loyola Coll; Sp-Lang Path, Baltimore City Public Schools, **SLP**

Paolicelli, Catherine A 157 Bay Street Apartment D, Glens Falls, NY 12801, (518) 761-0659, BA 86 SUNY - Center at Buffalo; MA 88 SUNY - Center at Buffalo; 88–Sp-Lang Path, Glens Falls Hosp

Paolini, Barbara A 5443 West Crestwood Drive, Crestwood, IL 60445, (312) 496-8713, BS 78 Western MI Univ; MS 80 Purdue Univ - West Lafayette; 87–Sp-Lang Path, Indian Springs Sch Dist 109, **SLP**

Paolini, Elizabeth Anne 415 Lock Road #24, Deerfield Beach, FL 33442, (305) 480-8967, MS 84 SUNY - Coll at Buffalo; **SLP**

Paolini, Mrs Sheila Incorvati 1724 Sterigere Street, Norristown, PA 19401, (215) 631-1317, ME 78 2467; Sp-Lang Path, **SLP**

Paolino, Mrs Camille Marie 32 Colgate Road, Maplewood, NJ 07040, (201) 956-0529, BA 79 2358; MA 84 Montclair St Coll; 87–Sp-Lang Path, Totowa PS, **SLP**

Paolino, Donna S 4617 Fieldbrook Drive, Kannapolis, NC 28081, (704) 932-0490, BA 72 Catholic Univ of America; MS 74 Gallaudet Coll; 88–Aud, Audio-Prosthetics/Rowan Co Sch, **A**

Paolucci, Annita Louise 3830 Olentangy River Road, Columbus, OH 43214, (614) 459-8402, BS 81 Bowling Green St Univ; MA 84 Saint Louis Univ; Speech Language Pathologist, Riverside Neur Rehab Ctr, **SLP**

Paone, Charles A Dept Of Speech And Hearing, St Josephs Hospital #1512, 555 East Market Street, Elmira, NY 14902, (607) 733-6541, BS 72 OH Univ - Athens; MA 73 Bowling Green St Univ; **SLP**

Paonessa-Loftus, Carole L 1791 Stanley Road, Cazenovia, NY 13035, (315) 425-4555, BS 76 SUNY - Coll at Buffalo; MS 78 SUNY - Coll at Buffalo; Sp-Lang Path, Syracuse City School District, **SLP**

Papa, Elaine Marie 55 Grovers Avenue, Winthrop, MA 02152, (617) 846-3330, BA 85 Bridgewater St Coll; MS 87 Northeastern Univ; **SLP**

Papador, Amalia A 148 Woodland Lane, Oconomowoc, WI 53066, (414) 569-9616, BS 75 Univ of WI - Milwaukee; MS 77 Univ of WI - Milwaukee; Sp-Lang Path, Temporary Therapy Services, **SLP**

Papale, Mrs Lynda P 10327 Nakema Drive West, Jacksonville, FL 32257, (904) 262-4052, BA 71 Univ of CT; MS 73 Southern CT St Univ; **SLP**

Papangelou-Kakouris, Marina Elvira 4737 Creekbend, Houston, TX 77035, (713) 723-6084, BA 84 CUNY - Queens Coll; MS 86 San Francisco St Univ; 87–Sp-Lang Path, Houston ISD

Papanicolaou, Irene 15 Lynde Street #22, Salem, MA 01970-3449, (617) 744-7265, BS 78 PA St Univ - Univ Park; MA 81 Univ of Pittsburgh - Pittsburgh; Sp-Lang Path, Landmark Sch, **SLP**

Papczynski, Mrs Janice L 12022 Lupine Lane, Granger, IN 46530, (219) 282-4128, BS 72 IN Univ - Bloomington; ME 73 IN Univ - Bloomington; Sp-Lang Path, S Bend Comm Sch Corp, **SLP**

Pape, Robin A Dansville Hearing Center, 168 Main Street, Dansville, NY 14437, (716) 335-5724, BA 77 SUNY - Coll at Cortland; MA 79 SUNY - Coll at Geneseo; Aud, Craig Dev Cen, **A**

Pape, Mrs Sue M 3405 La Salle, St Charles, MO 63301, (314) 947-1356, BS 81 Southeast MO St Univ; MA 82 Southeast MO St Univ; Sp-Lang Path, St Charles Public Schools, **SLP**

Pape, Mrs Theresa Bender 34591 Aquarius #D, Sterling Heights, MI 48310, (313) 939-2354, MA 86 Western MI Univ; **SLP**

Papel, Mrs Leslie Bellah 48 Tudor Court, Lutherville, MD 21093, (301) 561-0487, BS 80 Univ of GA; MS 82 Boston Univ; 87–Aud, Hearing Assessment Ctr, **A**

Papilla, Mrs Minerva Windham 1879 South Winona Court, Denver, CO 80219, (303) 232-0404, BS 52 TX Woman's Univ; ME 66 Midwestern St Univ; Sp-Lang Path, Jefferson Co Sch R-1, **SLP**

Papillon, Nadjia Marie 633 South Plymouth Court, Apartment 409, Chicago, IL 60605-2032, (312) 955-5520, BS 78 Southern IL Univ -Carbondale; MS 82 Southern IL Univ -Carbondale; Coord-Resource Dev, Chi Bd of Ed, **SLP**

Papir, Wendy Hope 19 East 95th Street, New York, NY 10128, (212) 683-6970, OB 69 CUNY - Lehman Coll; MS 71 CUNY - Queens Coll; **SLP**

Papoutsakis, Catherine Christine 878 East 14th Street, Brooklyn, NY 11230, (718) 377-7031, BA 77 CUNY - Brooklyn Coll; MS 78 Columbia Univ Teachers Coll; ME 83 Columbia Univ Teachers Coll; Sp-Lang Path, Private Practice, **SLP**

Papp, Mrs Nancy E 7 Hartfield Lane, Farmington, CT 06032, (203) 268-8913, BA 75 Univ of CT; MS 77 Southern CT St Univ; SLP, Private Practice, **SLP**

Pappafava, Mrs Kathryn B 524 Chester Drive, Lower Burrell, PA 15068, (412) 339-2859, BS 67 Edinboro Univ of PA; ME 68 PA St Univ - Univ Park; **SLP LM**

Pappas, Cathryn Jean 7380 Chaparral Road, Worthington, OH 43085, BA 85 Univ of KY; MA 87 OH St Univ

Pappas, Chrissi 258 North Country Road, Miller Place, NY 11764, BS 76 SUNY - Coll at Brockport; MS 82 Adelphi Univ; 78–Sp-Lang Path, BOCES III, **SLP**

Pappas, Frances O LSU Medical Center, Dept Commun Disorders, 1900 Gravier Street, New Orleans, LA 70112, (504) 568-4348, BS 72 Tulane Univ; MA 73 Northwestern Univ; Coord/Sp-Lang Path, Lsu Med Cen, **SLP**

Pappas, Mrs Kristy K 3007 South 2515 West, West Valley City, UT 84119, (801) 966-8534, BA 80 Univ of UT; MS 82 Univ of UT; Aud, Jon Richard Aoki MD ENT, **A**

Pappas, Lisa Marie 110 Wyatt Road, Garden City, NY 11530, (516) 741-3567, BA 84 Adelphi Univ; MS 85 Adelphi Univ; **SLP**

Pappas, Mrs Michele Rebecca 9941 Whitehurst #2105, Dallas, TX 75243, (214) 343-4166, BS 81 Southern Methodist Univ; MS 84 Univ of TX - Dallas; Sp-Lang Path, Plano ISD, **SLP**

Pappas, Dr Nicholas James 216 East Wadena Street, Duluth, MN 55803, (218) 724-7811, BA 60 Univ of MN - Duluth; MS 61 Univ of WI - Madison; PH 67 (NS) Northwestern Univ

Pappas, Ranae Tone 13616 North 43rd Street, Apartment 252, Phoenix, AZ 85032, (602) 867-5115, BA 82 Univ of Northern CO; OM 84 AZ St Univ; Sp-Lang Path, Paradise Valley Sch Dist, **SLP**

Papper, Margaret A 1224 Jay Street, Boulder, CO 80302, (303) 772-6649, BA 73 Univ of CO - Boulder; MA 75 Univ of Denver; Sp-Lang Path, St Urain Valley Pub Schs, **SLP**

Papso, Catherine F 255 West Squire, Apt 5, Rochester, NY 14623, (716) 275-4852, BS 86 Boston Coll; MA 88 PA St Univ - Univ Park; 88–Aud, Univ of Rochester Med Ctr

Papuga, Susan Kathryn 10363 Aderman Avenue, San Diego, CA 92126, (619) 286-3577, BA 83 Boston Coll; MA 85 San Diego St Univ; **SLP**

Paquette, Mrs Michelle K 11215 Newcomb Avenue, Whittier, CA 90603, (213) 943-5413, BS 76 Purdue Univ - West Lafayette; MA 78 OH Univ - Athens; Sp-Lang Path, Los Alamitos USD, **SLP**

Paquette, Mrs Sharon Ann Murray P O Box 51, South Ashburnham, MA 01466, (508) 597-6914, BS 81 Coll of Saint Rose; MA 83 Univ of MA - Amherst; 85–Sp-Lang Path, No Middlesex Reg Sch Dist, **SLP**

Paquin, Denise A 21 Berwyn Street, South Hadley, MA 01075, (413) 781-9100, BS 83 Univ of MA - Amherst; MS 85 Northeastern Univ; Sp-Lang Path, Reg Rehab Ctr-Mercy Hosp, **SLP**

Paquin, Roger Lyle 1010 Baker Avenue, Mankato, MN 56001, (507) 389-2501, BS 62 Univ of MN - Minneap-St Paul; MS 72 Mankato St Univ; SLP, St Peter State Hosp, **SLP**

Parada, Mrs Luann Ulmann 200 Mc Grede, Longview, TX 75601, (214) 663-0652, BA 79 LA Tech Univ; MA 83 Northwestern St Univ; SLP, Marshall ISD, **SLP**

Parady, Susan K 1944 East Citation Lane, Tempe, AZ 85284, (602) 239-4755, BS 77 AZ St Univ; MS 79 AZ St Univ; 86–Sp-Lang Path, Good Samaritan Med Ctr, **SLP ACE**

Paranjpe, Meenakshi Anand 1930 Jasper Court, Coquitlam, BC, Canada V3J 2B3, (604) 941-3451, MA 65 0500; MA 70 Simon Fraser Univ - Bc; MA 83 Western WA Univ; 84–Sp-Lang Path, Ministry of Health, **SLP**

Paras, Teresita A 21084 Beacon Road, Metamora, IN 47030, (812) 934-5452, BS 84 Coll of Mount Saint Joseph; MA 87 Ball St Univ; 88–Sp-Lang Path, Good Samaritan Hosp, **SLP**

Parasnis, Dr Ila Dept Of Comm Research, Ntid At Rit, One Lomb Memorial Drive, Rochester, NY 14623, (716) 475-6708, BA 69; MA 72; PH 80 (Psychology) Univ of Rochester; Assoc Prof, NTID at RIT

Pardo, Patricia A 9 Cerqua Street, Woburn, MA 01801, (617) 727-7231, **SLP**

Pardon, Donna M Audiology Clinic, Silas B Hays Army Community Hospital, Fort Ord, CA 93941, (408) 242-4964, BS 79 Central MI Univ; MA 81 Central MI Univ; 82–Civilian Aud, Hays Army Comm Hosp, **A**

Pardy, Mrs Crystal Wendt 1014 Cedar #10, Yankton, SD 57078, (605) 665-6339, BS 85 Univ of SD - Vermillion; MA 87 Univ of SD - Vermillion; **SLP**

Paredes, Mrs Genoveva Cautino San Salvados, 981 Urb Las Americas, Rio Piedras, PR 00921, (809) 764-8684, BA 75; MS 79 Univ of PR - Rio Piedras; Head Start Guaynabo Pr, Genoveva Cautino-Paredes

Parent, Dawn E 8514 North Highland Road, Baileys Harbor, WI 54202, (414) 839-2259, BA 78 MI St Univ; MA 79 MI St Univ; Sp/Lang Path, Private Practice, **SLP**

Parente, Renee Freiman 19 Westwind Drive, Caribou, ME 04736, (207) 498-3111, BA 75 CUNY - Lehman Coll; MA 77 CUNY - Lehman Coll; 77–Sp-Lang Path, Aroostook Mental Health Center, **SLP**

Parenti, Mrs Margaret An 1108 Timber Top, Rogers, AR 72756, (501) 636-3581, BS 70 AR St Univ; MS 85 Univ of AR - Fayetteville; SLP, Bentonville Sch, **SLP**

Parete, Rose Marie 58 Elizabeth Street, Kingston, NY 12401, (914) 331-3154, BS 78 SUNY - Coll at Geneseo; MS 81 Coll of Saint Rose; **SLP**

Parham, Dr Janet S 1908 Heiman Street, Nashville, TN 37208, (615) 262-6670, BS 74 TN St Univ; MA 76 Univ of IA; ED 88 (Educational Administration) Vanderbilt Univ; Sp-Lang Path, Metro-Nashville Board of Educ, **SLP**

Parham, Mrs Lisa L PO Box 88, Buffalo, SC 29321, (803) 427-3905, BA 84 Columbia Coll; MS 85 Univ of SC - Columbia; 88–Sp-Lang Path, Union County Schs, **SLP**

Paris, Deanne R 36 Tennyson Drive, Short Hills, NJ 07078, (201) 379-9147, BS 64 Emerson Coll; MA 66 Columbia Univ Teachers Coll; **A**

Paris, John N Hearing And Speech Center, 1000 Elmwood Avenue, Rochester, NY 14620, (716) 271-0680, BA 51 Hobart-William Smith Coll; MA 66 Syracuse Univ; Exec Dir, Hearing and Speech Center, **SLP**

Paris, Melvin J 125 73rd Avenue N #214, St Petersburg, FL 33702, (813) 521-2899, BA Case Western Reserve Univ; MA 71 Case Western Reserve Univ; Sp-Lang Path, Private Practice, **SLP**

Paris, Vasilikie Sophia 29 Chittenden Avenue, New York, NY 10033, (212) 920-5445, BA 73 CUNY - Hunter Coll; MA 84 CUNY - Hunter Coll; 85–Sp-Lang Path, Montefiore Med Ctr, **SLP ACE**

Pariser, Karen G 175 Danbury Circle South, Rochester, NY 14618, (716) 338-4307, BA 68 CUNY - Hunter Coll; ME 69 Boston Univ; SLP, Rochester Gen Hosp, **SLP**

Parish, Deborah Clymer P O Box 355, Hartsville, SC 29550, (803) 383-3144, BS 71 Purdue Univ - West Lafayette; MA 78 Northwestern Univ; SLP, Darlington County Schools, **SLP**

Parish, Mrs Janine Diaz Route #1 Box 367, Brimley, MI 49715, (906) 478-7931, MA 76 MI St Univ; Sp-Lang Path, Rudyard & Brimley Area Sch, **SLP**

Parish, Robbin 11059 Timberline, Houston, TX 77043, (713) 467-3911, BA 66 Univ of TX - Austin; MA 67 Our Lady Lake Univ-San Anton; 72–Dir/Owner, Sp Path Assoc-the Parish Sch, **SLP**

Parish, Susan P 566 Mount Del Drive, Clayton, CA 94517, (415) 672-7115, Sp-Lang Path, Mount Diablo USD, **SLP**

Parisi, Frances Ellen 1104 Scott Drive, Valley Stream, NY 11580, (516) 561-0869, BA 86 Adelphi Univ; MS 88 Adelphi Univ; Sp-Lang Path, Nassau Ctr for the Developmentally Disabled

Parisi, Mrs Sharon A 37 Norroway Avenue, Randolph, MA 02368, (617) 963-8150, BA 75 Hofstra Univ; MA 77 Hofstra Univ; 84–Teacher, Boston School for the Deaf, **SLP**

Park, Charles R 311 Garlow Drive, Pittsburgh, PA 15235, (412) 795-1515, BA 52 Univ of Pittsburgh - Pittsburgh; MS 54 Univ of Pittsburgh - Pittsburgh; SLP, Penn Hills School District, **SLP**

Park, Kathleen Sarah 7700 East Thirteenth #84, Wichita, KS 67206, (316) 833-2780, BA 61 Wichita St Univ; MA 68 Univ of KS; Sp-Lang Path, USD 259, **SLP**

Park, Kay D 3939 Magnolia Avenue #A, St Louis, MO 63110, (314) 454-6171, BA 78 MI St Univ; MS 80 Washington Univ; Aud, Washington U, **A**

Park, Marilyn L 680 Hawley Road, Mason, MI 48854, (517) 789-6138, BA 83 MI St Univ; MA 86 MI St Univ; 86–Sp-Lang Path, Jackson PS, **SLP**

Park, Martha G 1231 Hope Street, Fayetteville, AR 72701, (501) 442-9381, BA 57 Univ of TN - Knoxville; MA 63 Univ of WI - Madison; MS 81 Univ of AR - Fayetteville; Sp/Lang Path, Northwest Psychology Group, **SLP ACE**

Park, Mary J 15 Sunnyside Lane, St Paul, MN 55118, **SLP**

Park, Michele A 11632 Northwest 11th St, Pembroke Pines, FL 33026, (305) 475-7075, BA 79 Univ of Miami; MS 81 Univ of South FL; Coord of Clin Practicum, Nova Univ, **SLP ACE**

Park, Patricia 7703 Queen Street, Wyndmoor, PA 19118-2032, (215) 456-9302, BS 73 West Chester Univ of PA; MS 74 Purdue Univ - West Lafayette; **SLP**

Park, Mrs Victoria L 121 Johnson Street, Little Rock, AR 72205, (501) 834-0217, BA 78 Univ of AR - Fayetteville; MA 79 Univ of AR - Fayetteville; SLP, Little Rock Pub Sch Dist, **SLP**

Park, William B 7300 N Mona Lisa Road, #8246, Tucson, AZ 85741, (602) 325-2547, BS 86 OR St Univ; MA 87 Northwestern Univ; Aud, Tucson Aud Ins

Parke, Mrs Sandra 5757 West Hefner Road #515, Oklahoma City, OK 73132, (405) 271-2791, BS 85 OK St Univ; MS 87 Univ of OK - OK City; 87–Aud, OK City Clinic, **A**

Parker, Aimee Bennett 221 N 25th Street, Wilmington, NC 28405, (919) 343-7218, BA 78 Stephens Coll; MS 86 Univ of NC - Chapel Hill; 86–Aud, New Hanover Memorial Hosp, **A**

Parker, Ann Orlando 148 Deerhurst Park Blvd, Kenmore, NY 14217, (716) 835-0417, BS 75 SUNY - Coll at Buffalo; MS 81 SUNY - Coll at Buffalo; 85–Sp/Lang Path, Cantelician Ctr, **SLP**

Parker, Anna L 2027 Greenway Avenue, Charlotte, NC 28204-3315, (803) 286-1961, BA 80 Univ of NC - Greensboro; MA 81 Univ of TN - Knoxville; 86–Prog Dir, Rebound Inc, **SLP**

Parker, Anna M L 908 Bluebird, Manchaca, TX 78652, (512) 282-5458, BS 74 IL St Univ - Normal; MS 75 IL St Univ - Normal; Sp-Lang Path, Eanes ISD, **SLP**

Parker, Anne Whitney 518 Sand Dollar Court, Fort Collins, CO 80525, (303) 669-3940, MS 84 CO St Univ; 84–Sp-Lang Path, Thompson R2-J School District, **SLP ACE**

Parker, Barbara D Rural Route 1, Nevada, IA 50201, (515) 382-6952, BS 73 Univ of IA; MA 74 Univ of IA; Sp-Lang Path, Heartland AEA, **SLP**

Parker, Barbara J 547 Emerald Street #A-11, Iowa City, IA 52240, (319) 335-8673, BS 79 Univ of North TX; MS 81 Univ of North TX; Research Asst, Univ of Iowa, **SLP A ACE**

Parker, Mrs Beverly Route 5, 2126 Swedish Drive, Anoka, MN 55304, **SLP**

Parker, Bobbie H 1604 Eastmoreland, Memphis, TN 38104, (319) 234-5920, MA 81 Univ of Northern IA; SLP, AEA #7, **SLP**

Parker, Bruce David 1312 Pheasant Hollow Way, Manteca, CA 95336, **SLP**

Parker, Carmen K 1470 Rue Paradise, El Centro, CA 92243, (619) 352-2877, BA 76 San Diego St Univ; MA 80 CA St Univ - Long Beach; Dir, Scottish Rite Chldhd Lang Dis, **SLP**

Parker, Mrs Carol Louise 1504 Honeysuckle Lane, Champaign, IL 61821, (217) 337-3130, BS 79 SUNY - Coll at Fredonia; MA 83 Univ of IL - Urbana; **A**

Parker, Mrs Caroline J 125 Highland Avenue, Jersey City, NJ 07306, (201) 434-4906, BA 74 Jersey City St Coll; MA 75 Montclair St Coll; Prof, Hudson Co Commun Coll, **SLP**

Parker, Catherine Spadaro 703 South Tyler Street, Suite A, Covington, LA 70433, (504) 893-4323, BA 77 LA Tech Univ; MS 78 Univ Southern MS-Hattiesburg; Dir/SLP, Covington Speech & Lang Cntr, **SLP**

Parker, Dr Charles D University Of Montana, Speech Path & Audiology, Missoula, MT 59801, BA 49 Univ of MT; MA 52 Univ of IA; PH 53 (NS) Univ of IA; Prof Emeritus, U of Montana, **SLP A F**

Parker, Cheryl 1230 Highway 17 By-Pass, Mount Pleasant, SC 29464, (803) 881-8666, BA 71 Vanderbilt Univ; ME 74 Univ of VA - Charlottesville; Director of Aud Services, McPherson Hosp, **A**

Parker, Christine 21 Huckleberry Hill Road, Avon, CT 06001, (203) 232-9525, BA 74 Univ of CT; MA 76 Univ of CT; **SLP**

Parker, Mrs Claire V 507 North Churton Street, Hillsborough, NC 27278, (919) 493-7002, BA 70 SUNY - Center at Buffalo; MS 71 Ithaca Coll; **SLP**

Parker, Colette Albritton 2304 Corey Court, Kinston, NC 28501, MS 84 Univ of NC - Chapel Hill; Sp-Lang Path, Caswell Center, **SLP**

Parker, Mrs Cynthia Foxwell 519 North Pine Street, Seaford, DE 19973, (302) 422-3311, BS 81 Towson St Univ; MA 83 Wichita St Univ; Aud, Milford Memorial Hosp, **A**

Parker, Diane Vanessa 4219 Colborne Road, Baltimore, MD 21229, (301) 566-4957, BA 80 Univ of MD - College Park; ME 82 NC Central Univ; Sp-Lang Path, InSpeech Inc, **SLP**

Parker, Dianne L 306 Brookmeade Drive, Statesville, NC 28677, (704) 873-5554, BA 68 Columbia Coll; MA 86 Appalachian St Univ; 71–Sp-Lang Path, Iredell County Schs, **SLP**

Parker, Dr Ellen 39 Roxbury Road, Port Washington, NY 11050, (516) 560-5656, BA 55 CUNY - Brooklyn Coll; MA 64 CUNY - Brooklyn Coll; PH 76 (Sp Science) CUNY - Grad Sch & Univ Cntr; Assoc Prof/Dir Sp&Hrng Cen, Hofstra U, **SLP**

Parker, Frances Jennings 348 South Austin Blvd, #3E, Oak Park, IL 60304, (312) 383-8219, OB 84 Univ of NC - Chapel Hill; MS 85 Univ of NC - Chapel Hill; Sp-Lang Path, Hawthorne Rehab Serv, **SLP**

Parker, Dr Frank P 2205 Myrtle Avenue, Baton Rouge, LA 70806, (504) 343-5511, BA 71 Univ of Houston - Univ Park; MA 73 Purdue Univ - West Lafayette; PH 76 (NS) Purdue Univ - West Lafayette; 84–Professor, LA St U

Parker, Mrs Glenda Chambers 7th Street Elementary, 7th And Beeech, North Little Rock, AR 72114, (501) 758-4660, BS 81 Univ of Central AR; OM 85 Univ of Central AR; Sp-Lang Path, North Little Rock Pub Schools, **SLP**

Parker, Hazel 2703 Messina Avenue, Orlando, FL 32811-5527, (305) 841-4576, BA 80 Univ of Central FL; MA 83 Univ of Central FL; Sp-Lang Path, UCP, **SLP**

Parker, Hugh G 2593 North Chipman, Owosso, MI 48867, (517) 723-7053, BA 65 Eastern MI Univ; MA 66 MI St Univ; ED 78 (NS) Eastern MI Univ; Sp-Lang Path, Shiawassee ISD, **SLP**

Parker, J Whitney 2002 Convent Place #5, Nashville, TN 37212, MA 88 Vanderbilt Univ

Parker, Mrs Janet Gallant P O Box 585, York, ME 03909, (207) 363-4870, BS 77 Northeastern Univ; MA 78 MI St Univ; 85–Sp-Lang Path, York PS, **SLP ACE**

Parker, Jayne H 70 Marvin Avenue, Los Altos, CA 94022, BS; **SLP LM**

Parker, Mrs Jeanette Luce Rt 3 Box 90, Carthage, TX 75633, (214) 947-6482, BS 84 Stephen F Austin St Univ; ME 87 Stephen F Austin St Univ

Parker, Jo Ann M Roscoe 313 2nd Street N W, Mayville, ND 58257, (414) 729-5800, BS 75 Univ of WI - Stevens Point; MS 77 Univ of WI - Stevens Point; Sp-Lang Path, Cen WI Rehab Associates Inc, **SLP**

Parker, Judith A 500 South Sonya, Anaheim, CA 92802, (213) 864-3071, BS 78 NM St Univ; MA 80 NM St Univ; SLP, Norwalk-Lamirada USD, **SLP**

Parker, Mrs Kathleen Diane 9336 Mabry N E, Albuquerque, NM 07109, (505) 821-7739, BA 82 Univ of NM; MS 85 Univ of NM; Sp-Lang Path, Albuquerque Public Schools, **SLP**

Parker, Mrs Kay Bruno 100 Ante Bellum Road, Carencro, LA 70520, (318) 942-4892, BA 82 Univ of Southwestern LA; MS 84 Univ of Southwestern LA; SLP, St Landry Parish Schools, **SLP**

Parker, Kenneth C Audiology Serv Of Chattanooga, Metropolitan Hospital, 511 McCallie Avenue, Chattanooga, TN 37402, (615) 267-9316, BA 72 David Lipscomb Coll; ME 74 Univ of GA; Audiologist, Audiology Services, **A**

Parker, Kristine J 550-101 Milton Court, Long Beach, CA 90803, (213) 807-6512, BA 75 Univ of MA - Amherst; MA 76 Western MI Univ; Sp-Lang Path, Kaiser Permanente Hosp, **SLP**

Parker, Mrs Leanne M 8407 Ashlawn Drive, Houston, TX 77083, (713) 496-9128, BS 80 Delta St Univ; MS 81 Univ Southern MS-Hattiesburg; SLP, Ft Bend ISD, **SLP ACE**

Parker, Mrs Lois M 113 Greenbrook Road, North Plainfield, NJ 07060, (201) 722-8222, MA 83 Kean Coll of NJ; Teacher of the Handicapped, The Midland School, **A**

Parker, Lucy L 3525 Sawtelle Boulevard, Los Angeles, CA 90066, (213) 337-1820, BA 64 SUNY - Center at Albany; MA 65 MI St Univ; Sp-Lang Path, InSpeech Inc, **SLP**

Parker, Mrs Margaret A 1717 Oak Drive, Bainbridge, GA 31717, (912) 228-2821, BS 80 FL St Univ; MS 81 FL St Univ; Sp-Lang Path, Decatur Co Schs, **SLP**

Parker, Mrs Maria Elena 2283 Washington Street, Canton, MA 02021, (617) 580-7241, MS 84 Northeastern Univ; Sp-Lang Path, Brockton Public Schools, **SLP**

Parker, Maria Guttentag 988 Warfield Avenue, Oakland, CA 94610, BA 70 Univ of CA - Berkeley; OM 78; MS 81 San Francisco St Univ; Sp-Lang Path, Private Practice, **SLP**

Parker, Marilyn F 1609 East 31th Street, Brooklyn, NY 11234, (718) 998-4298, BA 74 CUNY - Brooklyn Coll; MS 77 CUNY - Brooklyn Coll; Sp-Lang Path, NYC Bd of Educ, **SLP**

Parker, Martha V Medical Park #8, Morehead City, NC 28557, (919) 726-0658, BS 79 Western Carolina Univ; MA 80 Western Carolina Univ; Sp/Lang Path, Private Practice, **SLP**

Parker, Mary Catherine 2508 41st Avenue East, Apartment 352, Seattle, WA 98112, **SLP**

Parker, Mary D Rt 4 Box 308, Summerville, GA 30747, BS 69 Univ of GA; ES 73 Univ of GA; 88–Sp-Lang Path, Rome City Schs, **SLP**

Parker, Mrs Mary Semrick 103 Jones Avenue, Hueytown, AL 35023, (205) 491-4917, BS 83 Univ of Montevallo; MS 85 Univ of Montevallo; 87–Sp-Lang Path, Jefferson Co Bd of Ed, **SLP**

Parker, Nancy J 2921 E 92nd Place S #605, Tulsa, OK 74137, (918) 298-5512, MS 72 Southern Methodist Univ; BS 71 Southern Methodist Univ; Aud, Tulsa Otolaryngology, **A**

Parker, Dr Ron M 1425 West Spruce, Fresno, CA 93711, (209) 294-4221, BS 69; MS 72; PH 79 (Aud) Wichita St Univ; Prof, CA St U Fresno, **A**

Parker, Ruth N 1013 Dartbrook, Plano, TX 75075, BS 69 Univ of WI - Stevens Point; MA 84 Western MI Univ; 88–Sp-Lang Path, VNA-Collin County, **SLP**

Parker, Sharon Lynn 6255 Beechmont Avenue #21, Cincinnati, OH 45230, (513) 232-9650, MS 88 Miami Univ - Oxford

Parker, Mrs Sheryl H 404 Franklin Street, Remington, VA 22734, (703) 439-8885, BA 67 Tulane Univ; ME 75 Univ of VA - Charlottesville; 83–Sp-Lang Path, Consultant With Home Health Agencies, **SLP**

Parker, Mrs Susan C 5131 Arthur Court, Oakwood, GA 30566, (404) 536-3969, BS 74 Univ of GA; ES 80 Univ of GA; 86–Child Serve Coord, GA Learning Resources Sys-N GA Ctr, **SLP**

Parker, Mrs Susan M 1610 Huguenot Court, Chesterfield, MO 63017, BS 76; MA 79 Univ of MA - Amherst; **SLP**

Parker, Mrs Suzanne H Munson Speech And Hearing, 6th And Madison, Traverse City, MI 49684, (616) 922-9455, BA 77 Univ of MI - Ann Arbor; MA 79 Wayne St Univ; Sp-Lang Path, Munson Medical Center, **SLP**

Parker, Tammy Stevens 3814 Esters Road #502-li, Irving, TX 75038, (214) 252-8781, BS 82 Univ of Cincinnati; MA 85 Univ of Cincinnati; 86–Sp-Lang Path/Dept Head, Centre for Neuro Skills, **SLP**

Parker, Tommie Corbett 4583 Stella Drive N W, Atlanta, GA 30327, (404) 252-2591, BS 54 GA Southern Coll; ME 56 Emory Univ; Sp-Lang Path, Schenck Sch, **SLP**

Parker, Vicki S 7900 Creekwood Court, Alto, MI 49302, (616) 776-2034, BA 80 MI St Univ; MA 81 OH St Univ; 86–Sp-Lang Path Supvr, Butterworth Hosp, **SLP ACE**

Parker, Virginia W 6019 Jacobs Ladder, Columbia, MD 21045, (301) 490-3200, BA 67 Univ of AZ; MS 72 Univ of HI - Manoa; Sp-Lang Path, Howard Co Pub Sch, **SLP A**

Parker, Dr William L Parker Hearing And Speech Inst, 4201 Torrance Blvd, Suite 140, Torrance, CA 90503, (213) 540-HEAR, BA 69 CA St Univ - Los Angeles; MA 70 CA St Univ - Los Angeles; PH 73 (NS) Univ of FL; Aud/Dir, Wm L Parker & Assoc, **A**

Parker-Bright, Mrs Kimberly D 214 Waverly Place, Ridgeland, MS 39157, (601) 856-9304, BA 81 Temple Univ; MA 84 Temple Univ; 88–Adjunct Asst Prof, Univ of Mississippi, **A**

Parker Chapman, Mrs Susan B Route 6 Box 341C, Boone, NC 28607, (704) 264-0182, BS 75 Appalachian St Univ; MA 77 Appalachian St Univ; 87–State Coord, LOGOS-Sp and Lang Svcs Inc, **SLP**

Parkes, Mrs Barbara Joan 437 Center Street, Solvay, NY 13209, (315) 487-9122, MS 84 Marquette Univ; Sp-Lang Path, ENABLE UCP Assn, **SLP**

Parkes, Jo Anne S 1320 South Josephine St, Denver, CO 80210, (303) 690-9050, BA 76 CA St Univ - Long Beach; MA 79 Univ of Denver; Sp-Lang Path, Cherry Creek Sch, **SLP**

Parkhurst, Dr Barbara G 40 East 9th Street, New York, NY 10003, BA 60 CUNY - Brooklyn Coll; MS 62 Univ of MI - Ann Arbor; PH 71 (NS) CUNY - Grad Sch & Univ Cntr; **SLP**

Parkhurst, Mrs Connie H 69 Seeley Drive, Midland, MI 48640, (517) 774-3905, BS 75 Western MI Univ; MA 82 LA St Univ - Baton Rouge; 88–Aud, Dr Nicholas Redfield, **A**

Parks, Mrs Janet Elizabeth 5915 Mountainclimb Drive, Austin, TX 78731, (512) 331-0266, BS 79 Univ of TX - Austin; MA 85 Univ of TX - Austin; 84–Sp-Lang Path, Leander ISD, **SLP**

Parks, Mrs Kathleen Schneider 37 Matterhorn Drive, Glen Carbon, IL 62034, (618) 288-5461, BS 80 Southern IL Univ-Edwardsvill; MS 81 Southern IL Univ-Edwardsvill; 82–Sp-Lang Path, S IL Speech/Hearing Assoc, **SLP**

Parks, Linda Anne 28 Lincoln Avenue, Marblehead, MA 01945, (617) 387-9705, OM 83 Northeastern Univ; Sp-Lang Path, Judith Wisnia and Associates, **SLP**

Parks, Mrs Mary Dean 3747 Peachtree Road #416, Atlanta, GA 30319-3910, (301) 268-8097, MS 30 Univ of WI - Madison; **SLP LM**

Parks, Michael F 423 East Webster, Cuba City, WI 53807, (608) 744-2948, BA 79 Univ of Northern IA; MA 76 Univ of Northern IA; Sp-Lang Path, Shullsbury Pub Sch, **SLP**

Parks, Robin S P O Box 1676, Gate City, VA 24251, (703) 386-6912, MA 88 Univ of TN - Knoxville

Parks, Mrs Susan W 3425 Murphy Drive, Bedford, TX 76021, (817) 685-8597, BA 66 IN Univ - Bloomington; MS 67 Univ of WI - Madison; Sp-Lang Path, Hurst-Euless-Bedford ISD, **SLP**

Parks, Theresa M C 16910 N E 27th Street, Bellevue, WA 98008-2214, (206) 867-9783, BA 82 Creighton Univ; MS 83 Univ of OR; Sp/Lang Path, Vna & Rehab Serv, **SLP**

Parks, Virginia W 1038 Dearborn, Aurora, CO 80011, (303) 343-4215, MS 77 CO St Univ; Sp-Lang Path, Adams School District 12, **SLP**

Parlato, Mrs Patricia L 1175 Old Woodbine Road, Atlanta, GA 30319, (404) 451-2762, BS 67 Northwestern Univ; MA 71 Univ of TN - Knoxville; Clinical Dir/Sp-Lang Path, Childrens Therapy Services, **SLP**

Parlen, Mrs Marilyn J 29013 Old Carriage Court, Agoura Hills, CA 91301, MA; **SLP**

Parlet, Mrs Rebecca Jane 4825 Templeton Park Circle, Apartment 494, Colorado Springs, CO 80917, (719) 574-0843, BA 80 Creighton Univ; MS 82 Univ of NE - Omaha; Sp-Lang Path, Black Hills Rehab Hosp, **SLP**

Parlet, Mrs Theresa Rita 15 Rolling Meadows Way, Penfield, NY 14526, (716) 377-2028, MS 82 Nazareth Coll of Rochester; Sp-Lang Path, MacEdon Elementary School, **SLP**

Parmelee-Regittko, Mrs Luann Mary Route 5 Box 538, Lenoir, NC 28645, (704) 758-1243, BA 83 Univ of MI - Ann Arbor; MS 86 PA St Univ - Univ Park; SLP, Communicare Inc, **SLP**

Parmely, Janet C Drs Freeman & Cotton, 3725 Broadway, Kansas City, MO 64111, (816) 931-2606, BA 70 Univ of IA; MA 72 Univ of IA; Aud, Drs Freeman & Cotton, **A**

Parmenter, Mrs Wendy I 25457 Via Escovar, Valencia, CA 91355, (818) 997-2357, BA 73 CA St Univ - Northridge; MA 77 CA St Univ - Northridge; Sp-Lang Path, Los Angeles USD, **SLP**

Parmiter-Jacobs, Linda J 1339 Pin Oak Circle, Wichita, KS 67230-9245, (316) 262-8271, BA 72 Wichita St Univ; MA 74 Wichita St Univ; Super/Aud, I of Logopedics, **A**

Parnell, Dr Martha M Speech & Hearing Clinic, Univ Missouri Columbia, 125 Parker Hall, Columbia, MO 65211, (314) 882-4278, BA 71 Drury Coll; MS 73 Central MO St Univ; PH 77 (Sp-Lang Path) Univ of MO - Columbia; Assoc Professor Comm Disorders, University of Missouri, **SLP**

Parobek, Susan Elizabeth 6 Fieldstone Court, Arden, NC 28704, (704) 255-5001, BS 84 Miami Univ - Oxford; MA 86 OH Univ - Athens; 88–Sp-Lang Path, Asheville Cty Schs, **SLP**

Parodi, Louis M P O Box 30991, 65th Infantry Stat, Rio Piedras, PR 00929

Parolie, Mrs Donna O 6 Clover Court, White House Station, NJ 08889, (201) 534-6682, BA 75 Jersey City St Coll; MA 80 Montclair St Coll; **SLP**

Parolini, Mrs Pauline F 2931 West Zeering Road, Turlock, CA 95380, (209) 634-9556, BA 73 CA St Univ - Stanislaus; MA 74 CA St Univ - Stanislaus; Sp-Lang Path, Modesto City Sch Dist, **SLP**

Parolini, Richard J 1340 22nd Avenue South #7, Wisconsin Rapids, WI 54494, (715) 421-4529, BS 79 Northern MI Univ; MA 80 Western MI Univ; Sp-Lang Path, Private Practice, **SLP**

Parr, Enid A 241 Bluebird Lane, Oceanside, CA 92056, (619) 757-0912, BA 64 CA St Univ - Fullerton; MA 70 CA St Univ - Fullerton; Sp/Lang Path, Private Practice, **SLP**

Parr, Mrs Kristy Sjogren 1555 Hanford Street, Redlands, CA 92374-2697, (714) 793-7582, BA 84 CA St Univ - Fullerton; MS 85 Univ of Redlands

Parr, Mrs Patricia Tipton St Francis Hospital, 5959 Park Avenue, Memphis, TN 38119, (901) 765-2230, BS 69 Southeast MO St Univ; MS 81 AR St Univ; 88–Sp-Path Supvr, St Francis Hosp, **SLP**

Parra, Mrs Anne Sullivan 1916 Westheimer Drive, Clemmons, NC 27012, (919) 924-2451, BS 76 Regis Coll; MS 80 Univ of WY; Sp-Lang Path, Winston Salem Forsyth Co Pub S, **SLP**

Parratore, Mrs Christine Larsen 2021 Queensbury Court, Lombard, IL 60148, (312) 985-3797, BA 75 Augustana Coll; MS 76 Eastern IL Univ; 88–Sp-Lang Path, Woodridge Sch Dist 68, **SLP**

Parris, Mary 24 Beacon Hill Road, Ardsley, NY 10502, (914) 693-7510, BA 60 CUNY - City College; MS 62 Adelphi Univ; Sp-Lang Path, Ardsley Public Schools, **SLP**

Parris, Rachel K 19201 S St Andrews Drive, Country Club Of Miami, Miami, FL 33015, (305) 825-6737, BS 66 Jacksonville St Univ; MA 70 Univ of AL Tuscaloosa; Sp/Lang Path, Univ Miami, **SLP ACE**

Parrish, Joy Lea Route 2 Box 393-C, Jenks, OK 74037, **SLP**

Parrish, Mary Anne 64 Beverly Road # 22, Asheville, NC 28805, (704) 298-3225, BS 85 East Carolina Univ; OM 86 Auburn Univ - Auburn; **SLP**

Parrish, Mrs Patrice Weimert Speech Pathology Services, 280 South Pine Street, Spartanburg, SC 29302, (803) 583-1857, BS 74 Southern Methodist Univ; MA 75 Univ of TN - Knoxville; 75–Sp-Lang Path, Sp Lang Path Svc, **SLP**

Parrish, Shauna Lori 216 Richards Avenue, Clearwater, FL 34615, (813) 441-8944, BS 80 Brandon Univ - Manitoba; MS 83 Univ of ND; 85–Sp-Lang Path, Pinellas County School Board, **SLP**

Parrish, Mrs Sheryl Bruns 3819 Jones Street, Omaha, NE 68105, (402) 978-7316, BA 72 Kearney St Coll; MA 74 KS St Univ; 76–Sp-Lang Path, Omaha PS, **SLP**

Parrish, Mrs Susan Christine S9 W31682 Glacier Pass, Delafield, WI 53018, (414) 968-4642, BS 74 PA St Univ - Univ Park; MS 75 TX Tech Univ; **SLP**

Parrish, William C, Jr 2000 Camden Avenue, Parkersburg, WV 26101-5605, (304) 295-3316, BS 80 WV Univ; MS 81 WV Univ; Aud, Private Practice, **A**

Parrott, Dr Jean O Speech And Language Services, 909 Dairy Ashford #203, Houston, TX 77079, (713) 496-9128, BA 71 Univ of Houston - Univ Park; MA 72 Univ of Houston - Univ Park; ED 85 (Educational Psychology) Univ of Houston - Univ Park; Dir, Speech & Language Servs, **SLP**

Parrott, Mrs Margaret E 217 Brocton Drive, Victoria, TX 77904, (512) 575-5374, BA 70 McMurry Coll; MS 75 Washington Univ; 84–Aud, HEAR Foundation of Texas, **A ACE**

Parrucci, Mrs Regina Lucia 13211 Chestnut Drive, Bowie, MD 20715, (301) 390-6672, BA 78 Univ of MD - College Park; MA 83 Univ of MD - College Park; Sp-Lang Path, Pg Co Sp-Lang Presch Prog, **SLP**

Parry, Iola M J 1509 Turner, Allentown, PA 18102, (215) 432-1170, MA 52; Sp-Lang Path, Cedarbrook-Fountain Hill Annex, **SLP LM**

Parry, Laurie J 5102 Tocora Lane, Madison, WI 53711, (305) 645-3211, BA 83 SUNY - Center at Buffalo; MA 85 SUNY - Coll at Geneseo; **SLP**

Parsley, Alicia 20 Laurel Hill Drive, South Burlington, VT 05401, (802) 527-0565, BS 68 Central St Univ; MS 69 CO St Univ; Sp-Lang Path, Franklin Central Supv Union, **SLP**

Parsley, Debbie Barnett 769 Peachtree Lane, Bowling Green, KY 42101, (502) 781-8566, BS 79 Middle TN St Univ; MS 86 Western KY Univ; 88–Spec Educ Tchr SLP, Sumner County Bd of Educ, **SLP**

Parsly, Mrs Cinthia Rae 396 Fairfield Avenue, Columbiana, OH 44408, (216) 424-9591, BS 83 Kent St Univ; MA 83 Kent St Univ; Sp-Lang Path, Columbiana County Board of Ed, **SLP**

Parson, Cynthia Jean 149 Oakville Drive, Apartment 2B, Pittsburgh, PA 15220, (304) 242-1390, BA 86 Univ of PA; MA 87 Univ of PA; 88–Sp-Lang Path, Easter Seal Rehab Ctr

Parsons, Dr Carl L Lincoln School Of Health Sciences, 625 Swanston Street, Carlton, Victoria, Australia 3053, BS 72 SUNY - Coll at Geneseo; MS 73 SUNY - Coll at Geneseo; PH 81 (NS) Southern IL Univ -Carbondale; 80–Prof, Lincoln Sch of Hlth Sci, **SLP**

Parsons, Carla Ann 10612 Dorchester Road, Savannah, GA 31406, (912) 927-8931, Hilton Rehab Center, **SLP**

Parsons, Charlotte 101 Oakwood Lane, Ithaca, NY 14850, (607) 273-9467, BS 42 Syracuse Univ; BA 39 Syracuse Univ; **SLP LM**

Parsons, Deborah Ann 130 Moreland Avenue, Laurens, SC 29360, (803) 476-3174, BS 75 Univ of TN - Knoxville; MA 84 Univ of TN - Knoxville; SLP, Spartanburg District 4, **SLP**

Parsons, Helene Herzfeld 6 Loma Vista, Monterey, CA 93940, (408) 375-9466, BA 42 Univ of MI - Ann Arbor; MA 62 Univ of San Francisco; Sp/Lang Path, Pacific Sch Dist, **SLP LM**

Parsons, Mrs Jennifer G 219 Pineview, Irvine, CA 92720, (714) 544-8505, BA 82 Univ of Southern CA; MA 85 CA St Univ - Long Beach; **SLP**

Parsons, Mrs Joanna Dickerman Professional Health Services, 2120 Highland Avenue, Knoxville, TN 37916, (615) 525-4131, BS 70 Ithaca Coll; MA 72 Univ of IL - Urbana; 78–Sp-Lang Path, Pro Health Svcs, **SLP**

Parsons, Julie Marie 4426 Wickfield Drive, Flint, MI 48507, (313) 353-0310, BA 86 MI St Univ; MA 87 MI St Univ

Parsons, Sarah S 5166 Orangewood, Memphis, TN 38134, (501) 823-5577, BA 72 IN Univ - Bloomington; MA 80 Memphis St Univ; SLP, AR Pub Sch, **SLP**

Parsons, Sharon D 914 Bow Creek, Duncanville, TX 75116, **SLP**

Parsons, Steven Taylor Physical Therapy & Rehab Clin, 1797 Old Moultrie Road #12, St Augustine, FL 32086, (904) 824-3361, **SLP**

Parthasarathy, Dr Teralandur K 11142 Sierra Vista Pkwy #8, St Louis, MO 63138, (314) 741-6243, MS 80 Univ of Salford - England; PH 87 (Aud) Univ of TX - Dallas; 87–Asst Prof of Aud, So Illinois Univ, **A**

Partnow, Susan L 6737 Sycamore N W, Seattle, WA 98117, (206) 789-8697, MA 76 Northwestern Univ; Independant Consultant, Private Practice, **SLP**

Partridge, Kathleen Jones P O Box 126, 241 Water Street, Bolivar, OH 44612, (216) 438-2554, BS 77 Bowling Green St Univ; MA 79 Kent St Univ; Aud, Canton City Sch, **A**

Partridge, Lyman M California State University, Long Beach, CA 90840, PH (NS); **SLP LM**

Partridge, Mrs Marcia 47 Dock Lane, Wantagh, NY 11793, (516) 781-1947, MS 88 Adelphi Univ; 88–SLP, Nassau Co Board of Coop Educ Svcs

Partyka, Bernadette 70 Berdine Court, Colonia, NJ 07067, (201) 388-0469, BA 85 Kean Coll of NJ; MA 87 Montclair St Coll; 88–Audiologist, John F Kennedy Med Ctr, **A**

Partyka, Cynthia Marie 2013 Porte DE L'Eau Court, Apartment 204, Highland, IN 46322, (312) 862-6484, BS 79 Eastern IL Univ; MA 80 Northern IL Univ - De Kalb; Sp-Lang Path, Chicago Assoc Rehab Ed Serv, **SLP A ACE**

Parulekar, Dr Leela S Hearing Heights, P O Box 1244, Corbin, KY 40701, (606) 528-1234, PH 74 (NS) Coll of Saint Rose; **A**

Paruzynski, Thad F 10000 West Conrad Street, Hales Corners, WI 53130, (414) 425-3572, 49 Marquette Univ; MS 51 Marquette Univ; PH (NS); Sp-Lang Path, Amer Cancer Society Milw Div, **SLP F**

Paryl, Anita Bell 2873 East 89th St South, Tulsa, OK 74137, (918) 224-2028, BS 77 IN Univ - Bloomington; MA 78 Ball St Univ; Sp-Lang Path, Sapulpa Pub Schls, **SLP**

Parzivand, Harriet J 31 Oak Bluff Circle, East Longmeadow, MA 01028, (413) 567-3387, BA 70 Emerson Coll; MS 79 William Paterson Coll; Sp-Lang Path, Longmeadow PS, **SLP**

Pascatore, Linda Concetta Rd 3 Box 52, Jamestown, NY 14701, (716) 484-7562, BS 84 SUNY - Coll at Fredonia; MS 85 SUNY - Coll at Fredonia; **SLP**

Paschall, Mrs Frances Gulley 215 Walnut Street, Greenville, OH 45331, (513) 548-9495, BS 84 Ball St Univ; MA 87 Ball St Univ; 87–Sp-Lang Path, Western Ohio Therapy Associates, **SLP**

Pascoe, Dr David P Central Institute For The Deaf, 818 South Euclid Avenue, St Louis, MO 63110, (314) 652-3200, BS 51 George Williams Coll; MS 57 Washington Univ; PH 74 (NS) Washington Univ; Aud, Ctrl Inst for Deaf, **SLP A**

Pascual, Lydia 8400 S W 133rd Avenue Road, Apartment 322, Miami, FL 33183, (305) 547-6745, **SLP**

Pascu-Godwin, Victoria 1394 Bryden Drive, Akron, OH 44313, (216) 434-1661, BA 73 Univ of Akron; MA 74 OH Univ - Athens; Sp-Lang Path, Akron Public Schools, **SLP**

Pasek, Mrs Jill H 9280 University Avenue N W, Apartment 358, Coon Rapids, MN 55433, (612) 784-9596, MA 87 Univ of SD - Vermillion; 88–Sp-Lang Path, River Ridge Rehab

Pashek, Gail V 302 1/2 West Street, Wilkinsburgh, PA 15217-3341, (412) 828-1300, BA 77 Univ of MN - Minneap-St Paul; MA 79 Univ of MN - Minneap-St Paul; 85, The Rehab Institute of Pittsburgh, **SLP**

Pasierb, Meridith C 19 Springvale Road, Croton on Hudson, NY 10520, (914) 245-2700, BS 78 Mercy Coll; MA 85 CUNY - Lehman Coll; **SLP**

Pasikov, Renee G 380 Washington, Glencoe, IL 60022, (312) 838-2221, MA 70 Northwestern Univ; Sp-Lang Path, Glencoe Pub Sch Dist #35, **SLP**

Pasinkoff, Mrs Maureen M 2355 Bell Blvd #2H, Flushing, NY 11360-2049, (212) 596-3548, BA 78 San Francisco St Univ; MA 79 Hofstra Univ; SLP, NY Cty Bd of Ed Spec Serv Ut, **SLP**

Pasker, Julie Kay 216 2nd Street S E, Oelwein, IA 50662, (319) 283-4218, BA 85 Univ of Northern IA; MA 86 Univ of Northern IA; 87–Sp-Lang Path, Keystone AEA #1, **SLP**

Pasker, Ruthann W 129 Andrea Drive, Richboro, PA 18954, (215) 357-7154, BS 68 Emerson Coll; MS 69 Adelphi Univ; 86–Sp-Lang Path/VP, Desa Inc, **SLP**

Paskevich, Jeanne B 56 Arthur Avenue, Manchester, NH 03104, (603) 623-8088, BA 70 Univ of VT; MS 72 Univ of VT; SLP, Sch Admin Unit 19, **SLP**

Paskiet, Clare Ann 1117 Michael, Lockport, IL 60441, (815) 469-4977, BA 67 Univ of IL - Urbana; MA 69 Univ of IL - Urbana; 86–Sp/Lang Path, S/W Cook Co Coop Assoc for Spec Educ, **SLP**

Pasko, Dr Stanley J 7727 West Jarvis, Chicago, IL 60648, (312) 775-8453, MA 73 Loyola Univ of Chicago; MA 78 Northwestern Univ; PH 77 (Experimental Psychology) Loyola Univ of Chicago; Sp-Lang Path, Chicago Bd of Ed, **SLP**

Paskowitz, Pamela A 375 Homeland South Way #3B, Baltimore, MD 21212-4143, (301) 288-4515, BA 70 Loyola Coll; OM 71 Smith Coll; PH 82 (NS) OH Univ - Athens; Special Education Teacher, Baltimore County Board of Educ, **SLP**

Pasmore, Ronald R 1220 West 42nd Street So, Apartment 2, Wichita, KS 67217, (316) 221-1200, BA 75 Univ of CO - Boulder; MA 77 Wichita St Univ; Project Dir, Serendipity Spec Purpose Sch, **SLP**

Pasnak, Laurie A 382 Queenston Street #103, St Catharines, ON, Canada L2P 2X9, (416) 732-6111, MA 87 SUNY - Coll at Geneseo; **SLP**

Pasqualetto, Morgan 2449 Diamond Drive, Chino Hills, CA 91709-3537, (714) 620-4194, **SLP**

Pass, Barbara B 115 Valencia, Universal City, TX 78148, (512) 658-6329, BA 61 Southwest TX St Univ; ME 65 Southwest TX St Univ; Resource Teacher, Judson ISD, **SLP**

Passacantando, Mrs Janice Elaine 25 Sturbridge Road, Marlborough, CT 06447, (203) 295-0181, BA 81 Univ of CT; MA 84 Univ of CT; SLP, Private Practice, **SLP**

Passarella, Mrs Rosanne G 667 Longview, Antioch, IL 60002, (312) 395-0636, BA 68 CO St Univ; MS 69 Univ of IL - Urbana; Sp-Lang Path, Private Practice, **SLP**

Passaro, Mrs Nancy J 62 Ten Coat Lane, Shelton, CT 06484, (203) 729-6819, BA 69 Coll of William & Mary; MA 73 IN Univ - Bloomington; Sp-Lang Path, BOCES, **SLP**

Passley, Mrs Bonnie Jean Route 2 Box 61, Camp Point, IL 62320, (217) 223-8700, BS 72 Western IL Univ; MA 74 Western IL Univ; 75–Aud, Quincy Public Schools, **A**

Passman, Beth S 702 NW 102 Way, Plantation, FL 33324, (305) 749-0300, BS 79 Univ of KS; MA 81 Univ of KS; Dir Head Trauma Prog, Sunrise Rehab Hosp, **SLP**

Passmore, Susan Whiteley R R 4 Box 347-A, Macomb, IL 61455, (309) 833-4101, BS 64 Univ of IL - Urbana; MA 83 Western IL Univ; Sp-Lang Path, McDonough Dist Hosp, **SLP**

Pasta, Albert Stephen Apartment 140, 10720 Lakewood Boulevard, Downey, CA 90241, (213) 923-9322, BA 78 Univ of UT; BS 72 ID St Univ; MS 75 Miami Univ - Oxford; Sp-Lang Path, LAX Sch Dist, **SLP**

Pasternack, Barbara 720 East 19th Street, Brooklyn, NY 11230-1806, (718) 434-7051, BS 55 Long Island U - Brooklyn Ctr; MA 57 IN Univ - Bloomington; Associate Professor/Chair, Long Island Univ, **SLP**

Pasternack, Karen Franco South Miami Hospital, Sp Path Dept Rehab Serv, 7400 S W 62nd Avenue, Miami, FL 33143, (305) 662-8169, BA 78 Univ of FL; MA 80 Univ of FL; Sp-Lang Path, S Miami Hosp, **SLP ACE**

Pasternack, Lisa G 611 South Beaver Hill, Jenkintown, PA 19046, (215) 887-9535, BS 80 Syracuse Univ; MA 82 IN Univ - Bloomington; 88–Sp/Lang Path, Montgomery Co Intermed Unit, **SLP**

Pasternak, Judith A 465 Grover Cleveland Hwy, Eggertsville, NY 14226, (716) 833-1245, **SLP**

Pastor, Mrs Lois 1150 Lexington Drive, Bartlett, IL 60103, (312) 462-3180, BS 75 Northern IL Univ - De Kalb; MS 77 IL St Univ - Normal; Sp-Lang Path, U-SPEAC, **SLP**

Pastore, Mrs Caterina Anne 506 Whittier Avenue, Syracuse, NY 13204, (315) 472-0196, BS 85 SUNY - Coll at Fredonia; MA 87 SUNY - Center at Buffalo; 87–Sp-Lang Path, Oswego County BOCES, **SLP**

Pastore, Marc 1230 Via La Ranchita, San Marcos, CA 92069, **SLP**

Pastovic, Cora A 2731 Bedford Street, Johnstown, PA 15904, (814) 266-7902, BS 76 PA St Univ - Univ Park; MS 80 Indiana Univ of PA; 83–Sp-Lang Path, Private Practice, **SLP**

Patchen, Mrs Laura Gerardi 1142 Udall Road, Bay Shore, NY 11706, (516) 243-1765, BS 83 SUNY - Coll at Geneseo; MS 85 Univ of North TX; 88–Sp-Lang Path, Private Practice, **SLP**

Patchoski, Philip E Veterans Administration Medical Center, 1111 East End Boulevard, Wilkes-Barre, PA 18711, (717) 824-3521, BS 84 Marywood Coll; MS 85 Bloomsburg Univ of PA; **A**

Pate, Louise Ann 274 Hudson Court, Holland, PA 18966, (201) 234-0011, BS 79 PA St Univ - Univ Park; MS 82 Boston Univ; Sp-Lang Path, Matheny Sch, **SLP**

Pate, Robyn Jo 2303 Reese Road, Columbus, GA 31907, (404) 561-0417, BA 81 Columbus Coll; ME 83 Columbus Coll; **SLP**

Pate, Suzanne M The Learning Lab, 311 East Main Street, Suite 1, Hendersonville, TN 37075, (615) 822-5890, BS 58 Northwestern Univ; MS 60 Vanderbilt Univ; 86–Dir Sp-Lang Path, The Learning Lab Inc, **SLP**

Pate, Terri Lynn Cedar Rapids Hearing Evaluation Center, 860 2nd Avenue SE, Cedar Rapids, IA 52403, (319) 365-4857, BS 84 Northern IL Univ - De Kalb; MA 86 Northern IL Univ - De Kalb; 86–Aud, Drs Flynn & Grandon, **A**

Patel, Mrs Sonal R 1946 Crescent Court, Hoffman Estates, IL 60194, (312) 882-0571, BS 78 Bombay Univ - India; MS 81 Emerson Coll; Sp-Lang Path, **SLP**

Pater, John R 10164 South Bannerhill, Sandy, UT 84092, (801) 966-6203, BS 69 IN St Univ - Terre Haute; MA 72 MI St Univ; Aud, Private Practice, **A**

Paterno, Melissa Anne 6 Allston Road, Newington, CT 06111, (203) 666-6275, MS 88 Southern CT St Univ; 88–Sp-Lang Path, Wallingford PS

Paternoster, Debra L G 12 Penn Drive, Sewell, NJ 08080, **SLP**

Paternostro, Mrs Jennifer F 3005 Kingman Street #M, Metairie, LA 70006, (504) 785-6289, BA 84 Southeastern LA Univ; OM 87 LA St Univ - N O Medical Ctr

Paterson, Mrs Heather L 25 Tutt Avenue, Kingswood, South Australia, Australia 5062, 8-272-8929, BS 72 Dalhousie Univ - Nova Scotia; MS 75 McGill Univ - Quebec; **SLP**

Pathak, Bhama P 1800 Town Center Parkway, Suite 315, Reston, VA 22090, (703) 481-1234, MA 72 Howard Univ; Aud, Prof Hrng Aid Serv, **A**

Patick, Madelyne K 5632 East Silver Street, Tucson, AZ 85712, (602) 294-4471, BA 71 CUNY - Lehman Coll; MS 73 Univ of AZ; Spch-Lang Path - Dept Manager, Kino Community Hospital, **SLP**

Paticoff, Mrs Ellen Sara 11 Edwards Street #3-B, Roslyn Heights, NY 11577, (516) 588-0530, BA 83 Clark Univ; MA 86 Hofstra Univ; 87–Sp-Lang Path, Cleary Sch for the Deaf, **SLP**

Patigalia, Mrs Barbara S 9217 Wooden Bridge Road, Potomac, MD 20854, (301) 424-7282, BA 63 CUNY - Queens Coll; ME 66 CUNY - Queens Coll; Sp-Lang Path, Montgomery Co Pub Sch, **SLP**

Patnode, Margaret Mary N 65 W24062 Poplar Avenue, Sussex, WI 53089-2748, (414) 246-3324, BS 74 Univ of WI - Whitewater; MS 82 Univ of WI - Whitewater; Sp-Lang Path, Lutheran Social Services, **SLP**

Patrick, Linda 373 Rotary Street, Morgantown, WV 26505, (304) 599-5112, BS 73 WV Univ; MS 75 WV Univ; Sp-Lang Path, Monongalia Co Sch, **SLP**

Patrick, Polly S 5128 N W 27th, Oklahoma City, OK 73127, (405) 272-9876, BA 62 Southeastern OK St Univ; MS 70 Univ of OK Medical Center; 88–Aud, VA Med Ctr, **A**

Patrick, Sandra Lynn 1650 La Veta, 252 West Danbury Court, Grand Junction, CO 81503, (303) 242-8980, **SLP**

Patrick, Susan B 2906 Hickory Leaf Way, Silver Spring, MD 20904, (301) 454-6916, BA 71 Univ of KY; MA 75 OH Univ - Athens; Inst, U MD, **SLP**

Patrick, Mrs Theresa A Rd 3 Box 457, Shamrock Drive, Putnam Valley, NY 10579, (914) 666-9553, BA 71 Nazareth Coll of Rochester; MS 76 SUNY - Coll at Buffalo; Sp-Lang Path, NW Westchester Cen for Sp Dis, **SLP**

Patrick, Mrs Velva V Rural Delivery 3, 155 Leffler Drive, Johnstown, PA 15904, (814) 266-4119, BS 75 Indiana Univ of PA; ME 79 Indiana Univ of PA; Sp/Lang Path, Private Practice, **SLP**

Patrzykont-Horning, Patricia Jo 222 North Washington St, Council Grove, KS 66846-1522, (316) 343-2302, **SLP**

Patterson, Mrs Barbara A 3220 Otha Street, Carson City, NV 89701, (702) 329-5108, BS 71 Univ of NV - Reno; MS 81 Univ of NV - Reno; Sp-Lang Path, Nevada Comm Svcs, **SLP**

Patterson, Mrs Catherine Swift Good Samaritan Hospital, Speech Pathology, 5601 Loch Raven Boulevard, Baltimore, MD 21239, (301) 532-3740, BS 82 James Madison Univ; MS 84 James Madison Univ; Sp/Lang Path, Good Samaritan Hosp, **SLP**

Patterson, Dana Hall 2335 Federal Drive #D-5, Dyersburg, TN 38024, (901) 286-6703, BA 85 Univ of MS; MS 87 Univ of MS; 88–Sp-Lang Path, Communi-Care Inc

Patterson, Mrs Diane M 59 Rector St, East Greenwich, RI 02818-3312, (401) 737-3300, BA 77 Univ of RI; MS 79 Univ of RI; SLP, Warwick City Schls, **SLP**

Patterson, Mrs Elizabeth McCleave 509 170th Place S W, Lynnwood, WA 98037, (206) 742-9265, BA 80 Gonzaga Univ; MS 82 Eastern WA Univ; 86–Sp-Lang Path, Dept of Soc & Health Svcs, **SLP**

Patterson, Mrs Ellen Emilia 7020 Glendora Lane, El Paso, TX 79912, (915) 542-6561, BA 82 Univ of TX - El Paso; MA 83 Univ of TX - El Paso; **SLP**

Patterson, Janet L 4713 Haines N E, Albuquerque, NM 87110, (505) 277-4453, BA 77 Univ of CA - Santa Barbara; MS 79 Univ of NM; 88–Clin Supvr, Univ of NM, **SLP**

Patterson, Janet P 3581 Marcella Avenue, Stow, OH 44224, (216) 687-6987, BS 73 OH Univ - Athens; MA 82 Kent St Univ; 86–Instr, Cleveland State Univ, **SLP**

Patterson, Mrs Janet R 1233 Bristlecone Place, Loveland, CO 80538, (303) 669-3468, BS 65 CO St Univ; MS 66 CO St Univ; **SLP**

Patterson, Janice E P O Box 37166, Montara, CA 94037, (415) 728-7282, MS

Patterson, Jean Kraege Speech Pathology (126), VA Hospital, 7400 Merton Minter Boulevard, San Antonio, TX 78284, (512) 694-5209, BS 65 Southwest TX St Univ; MS 67 Univ of WI - Madison; Sp-Lang Path, Audie Murphy Mem VA Hosp, **SLP ACE**

Patterson, Jeanne M 5851 Old Scottsville Road, Alvaton, KY 42122, (502) 843-3156, MA 84 Eastern KY Univ; BS 83 Eastern KY Univ; Sp-Lang Path, Cardinal Health Care, **SLP**

Patterson, Jennifer A Waisman Center Room 399, 1500 Highland Avenue, Madison, WI 53706, (608) 263-9262, **A**

Patterson, Mrs Julie Neeley 754 South Ironwood Drive, South Bend, IN 46615, (219) 234-5495, BS 85 Purdue Univ - West Lafayette; MA 87 Ball St Univ; 88–Sp-Lang Path, Sch City of Mishawaka, **SLP**

Patterson, Mrs Julie S 4635 Reagan, Beaumont, TX 77706, (409) 899-1459, BS 76 Lamar Univ; MS 77 Lamar Univ; Sp-Lang Path, Port Arthur ISD, **SLP**

Patterson, Dr Karen A Central Missouri State University, Department Of Speech Pathology & Audiology, Warrensburg, MO 64093, (816) 429-4993, BS 70 TX Christian Univ; MS 73 Univ of North TX; PH 88 (College Teaching of Communication Disorders) Univ of North TX; Asst Prof, Ctrl MO St U, **SLP A ACE**

Patterson, Mrs Kathryn K 2741 Patton Drive, Speedway, IN 46224, (317) 924-3251, BS 76 Purdue Univ - West Lafayette; MS 77 Purdue Univ - West Lafayette; Sp-Lang Path, Crossroads Rehab Cen, **SLP**

Patterson, Mrs Kathy Coleman 315 Cherokee Street, New Orleans, LA 70118, (504) 483-7690, **SLP**

Patterson, Linda Jean 1660 South Cornwell, Clare, MI 48617, BS 75 Central MI Univ; MA 83 Central MI Univ; Sp-Lang Path, Clare-Gladwin ISD, **SLP**

Patterson, Mrs Linda Lee 1704 Foxhollow Road, Greensboro, NC 27410, (919) 379-4120, MA 86 Univ of NC - Greensboro

Patterson, Dr M Dean 628 Cascade Road, Pittsburgh, PA 15221, (412) 683-3000, OB 60 OH Univ - Athens; MA 61 OH Univ - Athens; PH 70 (Audiology) Univ of Pittsburgh - Pittsburgh; Ch Aud & SLP Serv, VA Med Cen, **SLP A**

Patterson, Margaret J 914 River Haven Circle, Hoover, AL 35244, (205) 491-4831, SLP, Jefferson County Schools, **SLP**

Patterson, Margaret K 39 Sydney Street, Willoughby, New South Wales, Australia 2068, **SLP**

Patterson, Dr Mary A Patterson Sp & Lang Services, 1503 South Spring, Sioux Falls, SD 57105, (605) 336-3230, BA 51 Sioux Falls Coll; MA 52 Univ of NE - Lincoln; PH 80 (NS) Univ of CO - Boulder; Chief Aud & Sp-Lang Path, Royal C Johnson VA Hosp, **SLP A ACE**

Patterson, Mary Louise 18150 S W Rosa Road #27, Beaverton, OR 97007, (503) 357-6171, BA 78 OR St Univ; OM 80 Univ of WA; Sp-Lang Path, Forest Grove School Dist 15, **SLP**

Patterson, Mrs Merry Watson Post Office Box 1816, Albemarle, NC 28001, (919) 572-3489, OB 83 Appalachian St Univ; OM 87 Appalachian St Univ

Patterson, Mrs Molly G P O Box 482, Blytheville, AR 72316, (501) 763-6639, BS 68 Memphis St Univ; MS 87 AR St Univ; 79–Sp-Lang Path, Armorel PS, **SLP**

Patterson, Nancy Elaine 8603 Holiday Drive, Sherwood, AR 72116, (501) 835-5622, BA 82 Ouachita Baptist Univ; MA 86 Memphis St Univ; 86–Sp-Lang Path, North Little Rock PS, **SLP**

Patterson, Pamela J 157 North Oak Street, London, OH 43140, (614) 878-0022, BS 73 OH St Univ; MA 76 Kent St Univ; 84–Pres/Aud, Micro Hrng Systs Inc, **A**

Patterson, Pamela J 406 Kesselring Avenue, Dover, DE 19901, (302) 422-3311, BS 76 Howard Univ; MS 78 Columbia Univ Teachers Coll; 84–Aud Dept Head, Milford Memorial Hospital, **SLP A ACE**

Patterson, Patricia Ann 208 Sunnyside Avenue, Toronto, ON, Canada M6R 2P6, (416) 531-7339, BA 77 Carleton Coll; OM 81 Univ of Toronto - Ontario; Sp/Lang Path, Mt Sinai Hosp, **SLP**

Patterson, Patti L 2450 Oarfish Lane, Oxnard, CA 93035, (805) 985-6884, BA 76 Univ of CA - Santa Barbara; MA 78 CA St Univ - Northridge; Sp-Lang Path, Oxnard School District, **SLP**

Patterson, Dr Ramelle F 8800 Staghorn Drive, Louisville, KY 40242, (502) 429-5659, BS 46 Univ of KY; MA 59 Univ of KY; PH 68 (NS) Univ of KY; 87–Sp-Lang Path, Jefferson County PS, **SLP A F**

Patterson, Robert E 201 Lakeside Drive #25, New Concord, OH 43762-1164, PH (NS); **SLP LM**

Patterson, Mrs Sheila Ann B 4800 Sheridan Avenue, Metairie, LA 70002, BS 76 LA St Univ - Baton Rouge; MA 81 Tulane Univ; SLP, Jefferson Parish School Board, **SLP**

Patterson, Shirley Sue 801 Randy Lane, Columbia, MO 65201, (314) 882-4278, BS 57 TX Woman's Univ; MA 69 Univ of MO - Columbia; Clinical Supervisor, University of Missouri, **SLP**

Patterson, Mrs Susan A P 105 Snapper Cove, Georgetown, TX 78628, (512) 259-5103, BS 67 Univ of TX - El Paso; MA 74 Univ of TX - El Paso; 84–Sp-Lang Path, Leander ISD, **SLP**

Patterson, Mrs Terri Loo 7777 SW Freeway Suite 820, Houston, TX 77074, (713) 776-2211, BA 80 Univ of FL; MA 83 Univ of FL; Aud, Houston ENT Clinic, **A**

Patterson-Waters, Jann P O Box 788, Fort Bragg, CA 95437, (707) 964-5645, BA 78 Humboldt St Univ; MA 80 Humboldt St Univ; Spec Ed Tchr, Ft Bragg USD, **SLP**

Pattillo, Mrs Janis S 1115 Point Of The Pines, Colorado Springs, CO 80907, (512) 657-2881, BS 75 Univ of TX - Austin; MA 77 Our Lady Lake Univ-San Anton; SLP, Pikes Peak Board of Coop Serv, **SLP**

Pattison, Darcy S 3707 Ridge Road, North Little Rock, AR 72116, (501) 758-6414, BA 74 Univ of AR - Fayetteville; MA 76 KS St Univ; **A**

Patton, Beverly Elaine 6300 Manchester Lane, Bakersfield, CA 93309, (805) 834-2436, BA 77 CA St Univ - Fullerton; MA 79 CA St Univ - Fullerton; 84–Sp-Lang Path, Private Practice, **SLP**

Patton, Mrs Carolyn D 82 Tree View Lane #C, Lithonia, GA 30038, (404) 593-4144, BA 82 Univ of Southwestern LA; MS 83 Lamar Univ; Sp-Lang Path, Fulton Co Sch Bd, **SLP**

Patton, Mrs Eleanor Miller 8901 South Sun Lakes Blvd, Sun Lakes, AZ 85248, BS 40 Northwestern Univ; MA 64 AZ St Univ; **SLP LM**

Patton, Gail D 5629 88th Street, Lubbock, TX 79424, (806) 744-3134, BS 71 TX Tech Univ; MS 75 TX Tech Univ; 86, Private Practice, **SLP**

Patton, Jennifer Sallman 257 Cabot Street, Newton, MA 02160, (617) 964-1502, BS 79 Univ of MN - Minneap-St Paul; MA 81 Univ of MN - Minneap-St Paul; **SLP**

Patton, Joseph A Chief, 9807 Mill Run Drive, Great Falls, VA 22066, BS 55; MS 64; Chief/SLP/Aud, Dc Govt, **SLP**

Patton, Mrs Kathryn M 5410 Williston Road, Minnetonka, MN 55343-4737, (612) 933-9385, BA 72 Univ of SD - Vermillion; MA 73 Univ of SD - Vermillion; Coord of Non-Public Spec Educ, School District #270, **SLP**

Patton, Mrs Laura Lee 108 Tammy Drive, Garner, NC 27529, (919) 934-3452, BS 82 OH Univ - Athens; MA 85 Montclair St Coll; SLP, Tammy Lynn Cntr, **SLP**

Patton, Lynda Rolan Rt 10 Box 770, Lubbock, TX 79404, (806) 741-0777, BS 85 TX Tech Univ; MS 87 TX Tech Univ; 88–Sp-Lang Path, Sp-Lang-Hearing Ctr

Patton, Mrs Mary Sabo 582 College Gardens, Kutztown, PA 19530, (215) 777-7615, ME 87 SUNY - Coll at Fredonia; **SLP**

Patton, Mrs Melinda Jane 701 Yucca, Mc Allen, TX 78504, (512) 631-4755, **SLP**

Patton, Mrs Patricia A 2664 Fairmont Road, Montgomery, AL 36111, (205) 288-0220, BA 59 Vanderbilt Univ; MA 73 Auburn Univ - Auburn; Admin Superv-Sp/Hrng Serv, State Crippled Chldn Serv, **A**

Patton, Susan A 3653 Larry Lane, Chattanooga, TN 37412-1811, (615) 266-5532, **SLP**

Pattullo, Anne Cox 2717 Roanoke Lane, Tyler, TX 75701, (214) 566-0729, BS 67 Univ of IA; MA 69 Univ of IA; Sp-Lang Path, Tyler ISD, **SLP**

Patty-Schwab, Dixie R 1325 Urban Avenue, Dayton, OH 45429, **SLP**

Patzelt, Rebecca S C c/o Alberta Childrens Hopt, 1820 Richmond Rd S W, Calgary, AB, Canada T2T 5C7, (403) 229-7225, MA 88 Western WA Univ

Pauker, Mrs Gail G 12 Yorke Drive, Freehold, NJ 07728, (201) 462-8413, BS 75 Ithaca Coll; MA 74 Trenton St Coll; SLP Coord, Prov Chld Mercer Co Spec Serv, **SLP**

Paukstis, Mrs Patricia F 19 Water Street, New Philadelphia, PA 17959, (717) 277-6966, BA 58; **SLP**

Paul, Alesia Renee 19107 Creek Drive, Dallas, TX 75252, (214) 964-3806, BA 84 Wichita St Univ; MA 85 Wichita St Univ; 88–Sp-Lang Path, Plano ISD, **SLP**

Paul, Mrs Barbara Weller 28 Aldrich Street, Gowanda, NY 14070, (716) 532-5328, BS 75 SUNY - Coll at Geneseo; MS 82 SUNY - Coll at Fredonia; 79–Sp-Lang Path, League for the Handicapped Inc, **SLP**

Paul, Mrs Bernice E 303 Alexander, Duncanville, TX 75116, MA 72 Southern Methodist Univ

Paul, Beth 516 6th Street N E, Massillon, OH 44646, (216) 438-2551, BS 68 Kent St Univ; ME 72 Kent St Univ; SLP, Canton City Schools, **SLP**

Paul, Christine Broadway East Hearing Center, 1170 East Broadway, Suite 200A, Louisville, KY 40204, (502) 581-1797, BS 73 Marquette Univ; MA 76 Wayne St Univ; Owner, Private Practice, **A**

Paul, Mrs Christine Drescher 231 Mar Vista Drive, Monterey, CA 93940, (408) 384-0255, BS 76 OH Univ - Athens; MA 85 San Jose St Univ; 80–Sp-Lang Path, Monterey Peninsula USD, **SLP**

Paul, Mrs Cindy L 294 Bristol, Northfield, IL 60093, (312) 251-2295, BS 78 Northwestern Univ; MA 79 Northwestern Univ; Sp-Lang Path, Wilmette Public School Dist 39, **SLP**

Paul, Mrs Clara D 721 Hilltop Drive, New Cumberland, PA 17070, (717) 737-6728, BA 52 Carlow Coll; ME 55 PA St Univ - Univ Park; 75–Superv Dept of Commun Dis, Capital Area Intermediate Unit, **SLP ACE**

Paul, Constance L 2783 Chateau Circle, Columbus, OH 43221, (614) 486-4510, BA 51 OH St Univ; MA 63 OH St Univ; 65–Aud, Osu Coll of Med, **A**

Paul, Cynthia G 3413 Marquette, Dallas, TX 75225, **SLP**

Paul, Donald W 44 Baltic Avenue, P O Box 312, North Easton, MA 02356, (508) 238-9904, BS 73 Boston Univ; MS 75 Boston Univ; Aud, Private Practice, **A**

Paul, Dr John E 221 Tyler Brooks Drive, Williamsburg, VA 23185, (804) 229-6621, BS 47 Eastern IL Univ; MS 48 Purdue Univ - West Lafayette; PH 51 (NS) Purdue Univ - West Lafayette; Retired, **SLP LM**

Paul, Kelly S 6311 Analii Street, Bay St Louis, MS 39520, (205) 759-7305, BS 86 Univ Southern MS-Hattiesburg; MS 88 Univ Southern MS-Hattiesburg; 88–Sp-Lang Path, DCH Speech & Hearing Clinic

Paul, Dr L Dixon 2539 Simpson Avenue, Salt Lake City, UT 84109, (801) 582-1565, BS 57 Univ of UT; MS 63 Univ of UT; PH 76 (NS) Stanford Univ; Sp/Lang Path, VA Med Cen, **SLP ACE**

Paul, Linda L Rural Route 6, Carolyn Lane, Vincentown, NJ 08088, (609) 726-1000, BS 76 Montclair St Coll; MA 80 Rutgers St Univ - Newark; SLP, New Lisbon Dev Cen, **SLP**

Paul, Miriam Beth 3532 Birchwood Trail, Shellville, GA 30278, (404) 767-0549, BA 83 George Washington Univ; MA 85 Univ of MD - College Park; **SLP**

Paul, Mrs Pamela Dudley 2301 Cortland, Charleston, IL 61920, (217) 345-2282, **SLP**

Paul, Patricia Ann 110 Eaton Avenue, Trenton, NJ 08619, (609) 989-2765, BS 79 Trenton St Coll; MA 83 Trenton St Coll; Sp-Lang Path, Trenton Board of Ed, **SLP**

Paul, Dr Rhea Department Of Speech, Portland State University, PO Box 751, Portland, OR 97207, (503) 464-3533, BA 71 Brandeis Univ; ME 75 Harvard Univ; PH 81 (Com Dis) Univ of WI - Madison; Prof, Portland State U, **SLP**

Paul, Dr Robert G Audiology Speech Pathology Ser, VA Medical Center, 508 Fulton Street, Durham, NC 27705, (919) 286-6961, BA 62 Vanderbilt Univ; MS 64 Vanderbilt Univ; PH 69 (Aud) Univ of OK Medical Center; 69–Ch,Aud/Sp-Path Serv, VA Med Ctr, **A**

Paul, Robert L 4894 Moonglow, Troy, MI 48098, PH (NS); **A**

Paul, Roger D 601 Indiana, Valparaiso, IN 46383, (219) 465-7821, BS 68 Univ of ME - Farmington; MS 70 Purdue Univ - West Lafayette; Instr/Aud, Valparaiso Univ, **A**

Paul, Mrs Susan P 434 Linden Place, Lafayette Hill, PA 19444, (215) 825-1521, BA 83 Temple Univ; MA 85 Temple Univ; 87–Sp-Lang Path, Sp Path Consultants, **SLP**

Paul, Wendy 3422 Hunter Blvd South, Seattle, WA 98144, (206) 258-7311, BA 71 WA St Univ; OM 73 Univ of WA; Sp-Lang Path, Pedia Diag & Treat Cen, **SLP**

Paul, Zoe Lillian 31-83 45th Street, Astoria, NY 11103, (914) 666-9553, BA 75 CUNY - City College; MA 77 NY Univ; **SLP**

Paulauskis, Mrs Jana L 138 Lower River Road, Great Falls, MT 59405-8203, (406) 727-4472, BS 76 Pacific Union Coll; MA 79 CA St Univ - Chico; Sp/Lang Path, N Ctrl Lrng Resource Cen, **SLP**

Paul-Bramer, Lisa Ann 5212-D Regency Drive, Toledo, OH 43615, (419) 536-1632, BS 81 Bowling Green St Univ; MA 82 Bowling Green St Univ; Sp-Lang Path, Rehab Spec Inc, **SLP**

Paul-Brown, Dr Diane National Institute Of Dyslexia, TRI-Services Inc, 3200 Woodbine Street, Chevy Chase, MD 20815, (301) 652-0942, BA 78 OH St Univ; MA 78 OH St Univ; PH 84 (Child Lang Dev and Disorders) Univ of MD - College Park; 86–Research Assoc, National Institute of Dyslexia, **SLP**

Paul-Cohen, Rhona S 107 Ramblewood Road, Moorestown, NJ 08057, (901) 578-5602, BS 78 Univ of MD - College Park; MS 81 Towson St Univ; Sp-Lang Path, Sinai Hosp of Balt Inc, **SLP**

Paul-Evenden, Renee A P O Box 96, Pattersonville, NY 12137, (518) 783-1644, BS 80 Coll of Saint Rose; MS 81 Ithaca Coll; Sp-Lang Path, SUNY Albany Research Found, **SLP**

Pauley, Mrs Nancy Maxwell Eugene Hearing & Speech Center, 1202 Almaden Street, Eugene, OR 97402, (503) 485-8521, BS 76 Portland St Univ; MS 78 Portland St Univ; Aud, Eugene Hrng & Sp Cen, **A**

Paullo, Ronald D 227 Lake Street, Vernon, CT 06066, (203) 647-1347, BS 65 Indiana Univ of PA; MA 66 Univ of CT; Sp-Lang Path, Newington Public Schools, **SLP**

Pauloski, Dr Barbara Roa 1104 Davison Street, Joliet, IL 60433, (312) 491-3066, BS 82 Northwestern Univ; MA 83 Northwestern Univ; PH 87 (Normal & Disordered Voice) Northwestern Univ; 87–Prog Proj Coord, Northwestern Univ

Paulsen, Larae J 1549 Rainbow Drive, Waterloo, IA 50701, (319) 232-9663, **SLP**

Paulson, Mrs Christine Ellen 3984 Reservoir Boulevard, Columbia Heights, MN 55421, (612) 484-5553, BA 79 Univ of WI - Eau Claire; MS 80 Univ of WI - Eau Claire; 81–Sp-Lang Path, Island Lake Elem, **SLP**

Paulson, Dana M 7 Pomfret Walk, Pleasant Hill, CA 94523, (415) 935-6558, BA 72 Univ of WA; MA 75 Western WA Univ; Resource Spec, Antioch Unified Schs, **SLP**

Paulson, Mrs Janet Elizabeth 1052 18th Street Apt B, Santa Monica, CA 90403, MA 81 CA St Univ - Northridge; Sp-Lang Path, Santa Monica-Malibu USD, **SLP**

Paulson, Mrs Jill Marie Route 1 Box 248, River Falls, WI 54022-9127, (715) 425-5362, BS 75 Mankato St Univ; MA 77 Univ of MN - Duluth; Sp-Lang Path, Hudson Public Schools, **SLP**

Paulson, Joan Marie 1394 Englewood Avenue, St Paul, MN 55104, (612) 222-3671, BS 73 Univ of WI - Madison; MS 81 Univ of WI - River Falls; SLP, St Paul Pub Sch, **SLP**

Paulson, Mrs Lucy H Box 873, Mt City Route, Clancy, MT 59634, (406) 442-6440, BS 79 Univ of IL - Urbana; MS 80 Univ of IL - Urbana; 80–Sp-Lang Path, Helena Pub Sch Dist #1, **SLP**

Paulson, Margaret Rose 123 North Paul Street, Appleton, MN 56208, (612) 564-4081, BS 83 Moorhead St Univ; MS 84 Kearney St Coll; Sp-Lang Path, Minnesota Vall Coop Ctr, **SLP**

Paulson, Mrs Shelley Baker 6621 Sheltor Lane, Las Vegas, NV 89103, BS 79 CA St Univ - Long Beach; MS 83 Univ of NV - Reno; Sp/Lang Path, Southern NV Mem Hosp, **SLP**

Paulus, Janet Eileen 3002 Main Street, Eureka, CA 95501, (707) 444-0418, BA 69 San Jose St Univ; MS 71 San Jose St Univ; MA 86 Humboldt St Univ; Sp-Lang Path, Coastal Assessment Ther Svcs, **SLP**

Pauly, Cathie A 7600 Terrace Avenue, Suite 201, Middleton, WI 53562, (608) 836-6855, BS 73 Univ of WI - Madison; MS 77 Univ of WI - Madison; Sp-Lang Path, Private Practice, **SLP**

Paustian, Glenn R Childrens Memorial Hospital, 2300 Childrens Plaza, Chicago, IL 60614, (312) 880-3430, BS 72 Loyola Univ of Chicago; MA 75 Northwestern Univ; 82–Sp-Lang Path, Chlds Mem Hosp, **SLP**

Pautler, Rosemary D 661 South Sherman, Denver, CO 80209-4034, (716) 862-2687, BS 66 Purdue Univ - West Lafayette; MA 70 SUNY - Center at Buffalo; Sp-Lang Path, Sisters of Charity Hosp, **SLP**

Pavelle, Mrs Anne D P 23 Berkshire Drive, Winchester, MA 01890, (617) 729-3746, BA 64 Rutger's St Univ - Douglas Coll; MA 67 Case Western Reserve Univ; Sp/Lang Path, Speech Language House, **SLP**

Paver, Stacey Ann 2291-D Washington Street, Newton Lower Falls, MA 02162, (617) 894-3600, BA 82 SUNY - Coll at Potsdam; MS 84 Northeastern Univ; 87–Sp-Lang Path, W E Fernald State Sch, **SLP**

Pavey, Carol Elaine 34 Homewood Avenue, Hamilton, ON, Canada L8P 2M2, (416) 521-7951, BA 82 IN Univ - Bloomington; MA 83 Univ of TN - Knoxville; Aud, Chedoke-McMaster Hospitals, **A**

Pavlakos, Dr Chris M 2600 Far Hills Avenue, Suite 19, Dayton, OH 45419, (513) 293-3574, BA 70; MA 75 Univ of Cincinnati; PH 78 (NS) Univ of Cincinnati; Pres/Dir, Cen Comm Dis/Aud Serv, **A**

Pavlik, Loriann 2519 Windwood Court, Atlanta, GA 30360, (404) 394-5338, BS 84 Univ of GA; ME 85 Univ of GA; 86–Sp-Lang Path, Bartow Co Bd of Educ, **SLP**

Pavloff, Patricia E 427 Willowbrook Drive, North Brunswick, NJ 08902, (201) 422-1929, MA 69 NY Univ; MA 75 Univ of WA; PH 88 (Doctorate of Jurisprudence); 88–Municipal Ct Liason, Middlesex Cty, **SLP**

Pavlovic, Dr Chaslav V Speech & Hearing Center, University Of Iowa, Iowa City, IA 52242, (319) 353-5139, BS 73; MS 79; PH 82 (NS) Wichita St Univ; Associate Prof, U of IA, **A**

Pavona, John T 8700 25th Avenue #7P, Brooklyn, NY 11214, (212) 780-5114, BA 70 CUNY - Brooklyn Coll; MS 69 CUNY - Brooklyn Coll; Dir Weekend College Asst Prof, Brooklyn College, **SLP**

Pawlas, Annette Arnone 1800 N McCord Road #158, Toledo, OH 43615, (419) 471-4398, BA 81 George Washington Univ; MA 83 Univ of CO - Boulder; 87–Sp-Lang Path, The Toledo Hosp, **SLP ACE**

Pawlesh, Mrs Marina M 298 Rainbow Drive, Clairton, PA 15025, (412) 469-5020, OB 78 CA Univ of PA; ME 82 CA Univ of PA; Sp-Lang Path, S Hills Hlth Syst, **SLP**

Pawlick, Mrs Judy Ann 21 Linda Lane, Waterford, NY 12188, (315) 895-7781, BA 84 SUNY - Coll at Plattsburgh; MS 85 Ithaca Coll; SLP, Frankfort-Schyler School, **SLP**

Pawliczek, Catherine 25 Flintlock Road, Lexington, MA 02173, (617) 692-2378, BA 69 Univ of MA - Amherst; MA 71 Univ of MA - Amherst; Sp-Lang Path, Westford Pub Sch, **SLP**

Pawling, Helen M P O Box 512, Lewisburg, PA 17837-0512, BS; **LM**

Pawlowski-Vincer, Mrs Karen 14004 Evans Lane, Sturtevant, WI 53177, (414) 886-8504, BS 75 Univ of WI - Madison; MS 79 Univ of WI - Whitewater; Sp-Lang Path, Racine USD, **SLP**

Pawluk, Michael Francis 3750 Wood Road, Lansing, MI 48906-1773, (517) 482-9660, MA 81 MI St Univ; 84–CEO, Family Hearing Care Inc, **A**

Paxson, Mrs Carmel Dowd 208 South Derbyshire Lane, Arlington Heights, IL 60004, (312) 448-4267, BS 76 Bradley Univ; MS 77 Bradley Univ; **SLP**

Paxson, Traci Meadows 14 Old University Drive, Chapel Hill, NC 27514, (919) 663-2221, BA 79 Westminster Coll; MS 87 Univ of NC - Chapel Hill

Paxton, Mrs Alice H 693 Cielo Vista Way, Sonora, CA 95370, (209) 532-6597, BA 63 San Jose St Univ; MA 84 Univ of San Francisco; Sp-Lang Path, Tri-Co Consort-Calaveras Schs, **SLP**

Paxton, Anita T Lloyd Noland Hospital, ENT Clinic, 701 Ridgeway Road, Fairfield, AL 35064, (205) 783-5644, BS 78 Univ of Montevallo; MS 80 Univ of Montevallo; Aud, Lloyd Noland ENT Cl, **A**

Paxton, Judith Lynn 9884 Menaul N E #H-25, Albuquerque, NM 87112, (505) 294-3713, BS 84 IL St Univ - Normal; MS 85 IL St Univ - Normal; 86–Sp-Lang Path, Albuquerque PS, **SLP**

Paxton, Kelli Lynne 1484 Joshua Run Road, Columbus, OH 43232, (614) 863-6157, BA 85 OH St Univ; MA 87 OH St Univ; Affiliated Aud & Sp P

Paxton, Kenneth Lowell 308 North Prairie #304, Champaign, IL 61820, (217) 384-3616, BS 83 Univ of IL - Urbana; MS 85 Univ of IL - Urbana; Sp-Lang Path, Urbana School District 116, **SLP**

Paxton, Mrs Martha Wilder 8621 Jordan Drive, Lubbock, TX 79423, (806) 793-5744, BS 72 Miami Univ - Oxford; MA 73 Kent St Univ; 86–Aud, Texas Tech Univ, **A**

Payan, Karen S 17 East Railroad Street, Nesquehoning, PA 18240, (717) 669-6439, BS 84 Bloomsburg Univ of PA; MS 86 Bloomsburg Univ of PA; 87–Aud, Lehigh Valley Easter Seal Society, **A**

Payerl, Mrs Christine A 2732 South Quincy Avenue, Milwaukee, WI 53207, (414) 873-9196, BS 83 Univ of WI - Milwaukee; MS 86 Univ of WI - Milwaukee; 86–Sp-Lang Path, Kenosha USD, **SLP**

Payerl, Douglas Gene 2732 South Quincy, Milwaukee, WI 53207, (414) 242-1050, BA 76 Univ of WI - Milwaukee; MS 86 Univ of WI - Milwaukee; Sp-Lang Path, Racine USD, **SLP**

Payne, Amy J 1307-A S W 61st Terrace, Gainesville, FL 32607, (904) 395-0174, OB 85 Univ of FL; MA 88 Univ of FL; **SLP**

Payne, Brenda Wildermuth 9803 Smokefeather, Dallas, TX 75243, (214) 241-3464, BS 76 Murray St Univ; OM 78 Univ of MS; SLP, Carrollton Fb ISD, **SLP**

Payne, Carey Meredith, III 3729 West 9th Street, Waterloo, IA 50702, (319) 291-3336, BA 75 Univ of MS; OM 77 Univ of MS; Sp-Lang Path, Covenant Med Cen, **SLP**

Payne, Dolores Y 1223 Trevanion Avenue, Pittsburgh, PA 15218, (412) 373-1151, BA 76 Univ of Pittsburgh - Pittsburgh; MA 77 Univ of Pittsburgh - Pittsburgh; 79–Aud, Pittsburgh Otological Assn, **A**

Payne, Mrs Edna Koonce 1504 West Terrace Circle, Apartment 6, Teaneck, NJ 07666, MS 72 Univ of the DC; OM 85 William Paterson Coll; 86–Sp-Lang Path, Hackensack Med Ctr-Inst Child Dev, **SLP**

Payne, Mrs Eva L T 14111 South Grace, Robbins, IL 60472, (312) 933-5523, BA 73 Governors St Univ; MA 75 Governors St Univ; Sp/Lang Path, Chicago Bd of Ed, **SLP**

Payne, James Sanford, Jr #7 Jefferson Drive, Rome, GA 30161, (404) 295-6076, ME 77 Univ of GA; Aud, The Hearing Center of Rome, **A**

Payne, Dr John A 3016 Windy Hill Lane, Tallahassee, FL 32308, (904) 644-5034, BS 70 FL A & M Univ; MS 71 FL St Univ; PH 81 (Sp Science) FL St Univ; 88–Assoc Prof, Coll of Comm FL St Univ

Payne, Joyce S P O Box 38, Tarpon Springs, FL 34688, (813) 934-2657, **SLP**

Payne, Dr Kay T 1101 3rd Street S W #702, Washington, DC 20024, **SLP ACE**

Payne, Mrs Kimberly Ann 361 E 800 S #E 215, Section 10 Box 11, Salt Lake City, UT 84111, (801) 565-7100, BS 84 Univ of WY; MS 87 Univ of UT; Sp-Lang Path, Roswell ISD, **SLP**

Payne, Mrs Linda 21 Fair Street, Nunda, NY 14517, (607) 734-0582, BS 76 SUNY - Coll at Geneseo; MA 78 SUNY - Coll at Geneseo; Instructor, State University Coll Geneseo, **SLP**

Payne, Linda C 22 Sidney, Independence, KY 41051, (606) 491-1171, BS 74 Eastern KY Univ; MA 78 OH Univ - Athens; Sp/Lang Path, North Kentucky Easter Seal Ctr, **SLP**

Payne, Lonnie Mark 8795 La Riviera Drive #174, Sacramento, CA 95826, (916) 966-5055, BS 83 CA St Univ - Hayward; MS 87 CA St Univ - Sacramento

Payne, Lynette Smith 8211 Ruidoso Road N E, Albuquerque, NM 87109, (505) 821-6550, MA 87 Univ of NM; **SLP**

Payne, Melitta H 2915 North Sheffield Drive, Indianapolis, IN 46229, (317) 894-3098, BS 69 Purdue Univ - West Lafayette; MS 70 Purdue Univ - West Lafayette; **SLP**

Payne, Mrs Nancy R Route 3 Box 420, Stillwater, OK 74074, MS 75 OK St Univ; Sp-Lang Path, Stillwater Public Schools, **SLP**

Payne, Neva R 8125 Azalea Avenue, Oklahoma City, OK 73132, (405) 737-4846, BS 70 OK St Univ; MA 72 OK St Univ; SLP, Mid-Del Sch System, **SLP**

Payne, Pamela C 21 College Avenue, Upper Montclair, NJ 07043, **SLP**

Payne, Mrs Patricia Garnsey S 3602 Jefferson Drive, Spokane, WA 99203, (509) 455-7979, BA 70 WA St Univ; MS 85 Eastern WA Univ

Payne, Dr Peter D Usl Box 43170, Lafayette, LA 70504, (318) 231-6721, BS 59 Indiana Univ of PA; MS 65 WV Univ; ED 68 (SLP-Aud) WV Univ; Prof, Univ of SW LA, **SLP A F**

Payne, Robert H 350 East New York, Suite 290, Indianapolis, IN 46204, (317) 637-1303, BS 67 IN Univ - Bloomington; MS 72 Boston Univ; Dir Aud, John H Payne Assoc,Inc, **A**

Payne, Robin L 806 Tullahoma Drive, Auburn, AL 36830, (205) 821-3609, OM 87 Auburn Univ - Auburn

Payne, Rose M 3911 S E 147th Avenue, Portland, OR 97236, (503) 232-2458, BA 62 Creighton Univ; MA 72 Portland St Univ; Sp-Lang Path, Portland Public Schools, **SLP**

Payne, Mrs Ruth T 411 South Ithan, Bryn Mawr, PA 19010, (215) 527-8557, BS 66 Western MI Univ; MA 67 Western MI Univ; OM 75 MI St Univ; Dir, Speech & Learning Assoc, **SLP**

Payne, Susan Clair R R 3 Box 189-A, Warrenton, VA 22186, (703) 788-4056, BA 74 Mary Washington Coll; ME 78 Univ of VA - Charlottesville; Sp-Lang Path, **SLP**

Payne, Mrs Virginia Anne 309 Country Club Blvd, Slidell, LA 70458, OM 81 LA St Univ - N O Medical Ctr; Sp-Lang Path, Communication Development Cen, **SLP ACE**

Payne, Mrs Virginia Mason 2122 Meharry Boulevard, Nashville, TN 37208, BS 42 TN St Univ; MS 55 Univ of TN - Knoxville; **SLP LM**

Payne-Blanton, Rebecca L 1655 North Pelham Road, Atlanta, GA 30324, (404) 325-9618, BA 72 Marshall Univ; MA 73 Marshall Univ; **SLP**

Payne-Johnson, Dr Joan C 7415 Blair Road N W, Washington, DC 20012, (202) 636-6711, BA 68 Howard Univ; MA 69 OH St Univ; PH 76 (NS) Howard Univ; Grad Assoc Prof, Howard University, **SLP**

Payne-Stikes, Lynda Denise 1001 East High Street B1, Springfield, OH 45505, (513) 324-2081, MS 88 Univ of Louisville; 88–Sp-Lang Path, W Cen Ohio Hearing & Sp Ctr

Paynter, Dr Earlene T 1022 Spent Wing, San Antonio, TX 78213, (512) 434-6711, BA 64 Our Lady Lake Univ-San Anton; MA 66 Our Lady Lake Univ-San Anton; PH 70 (Sp Path & Aud) Univ of KS; Prof & Dir, Our Lady of the Lake U, **SLP F ACE**

Payton, Mrs Laurie A 4-E Windsor Terrace, Freehold, NJ 07728, (201) 431-0857, BS 84 Kutztown Univ of PA; MS 86 Univ of North TX; 87–Sp-Lang Path, Tinton Falls Sch Dist, **SLP**

Payton, Mrs Rebecca Z Choate-Symmes Health Serv Inc, Symmes Hospital Division, Hospital Road, Arlington, MA 02174, (617) 646-1500, OB 76 IN Univ - Bloomington; MA 79 IN Univ - Bloomington; Chief Sp-Lang Path, Choate-Summes Hlth Serv Inc, **SLP**

Payton-Parr, Pamela 6706 Falcon Pointe Road, Wilmington, NC 28405, (919) 343-7218, MA 75 Univ of NE - Lincoln; Sp/Lang Path, New Hanover Mem Hosp, **SLP**

Paz, Christine Mary 2176 Highland Parkway, St Paul, MN 55116, (612) 699-8534, BA 81 San Jose St Univ; MA 83 San Jose St Univ; 88–Sp-Lang Path, St Paul PS

Pazak, Kathleen A 617 W Commercial Street, Appleton, WI 54911, (612) 430-1972, BS 80 Marquette Univ; MS 86 Marquette Univ; SLP, River Ridge Rehab, **SLP**

Pazornik, Sheri Robyn 3 Sugarloaf Court #101, Baltimore, MD 21209, (301) 653-2743, **SLP**

Peach, Mrs Cherylin J 1500 Ambridge Road, Centerville, OH 45459, (513) 436-1353, BA 72 Loma Linda Univ - Riverside; MA 74 Western MI Univ; Sp-Lang Path, Kettering Med Ctr, **SLP**

Peach, Dr Richard K Department Of Communication Sciences And Disorders, University Of Georgia, 556 Aderhold Hall, Athens, GA 30602, (404) 542-4604, BA 74 Univ of FL; MA 77 Memphis St Univ; PH 83 (Sp-Lang Path) Northwestern Univ; 87–Asst Prof, University of Georgia, **SLP**

Peacher, Dr Georgiana M 720 Greenwich Street #1D, New York, NY 10014, (212) 989-9180, BS 42 Syracuse Univ; MS 43 Syracuse Univ; PH 46 (NS) Northwestern Univ; Sp-Lang Path, CUNY-John Jay Coll, **SLP LM**

Peacher, William G 6152 Hawarden Drive, Riverside, CA 92506, (714) 788-6255, MA 48 Syracuse Univ; BA 35 Syracuse Univ; MD 38 (NS) Syracuse Univ; Neurosurgeon, Private Practice, **SLP F**

Peachey, Galen L 6700 Emerald Street, Boise, ID 83704, (208) 376-3591, BA 68 Eastern WA Univ; ME 69 Eastern WA Univ; Dir, Boise Sp & Hrng Cl, **SLP**

Peacock, Ann C 439 Elm Street, Clarksdale, MS 38614, **SLP**

Peacock, Mrs Deborah T 3939 Briggs Avenue #4, Erie, PA 16504, (814) 899-0651, BS 85 SUNY - Coll at Geneseo; MA 87 SUNY - Coll at Geneseo; 87–Sp-Lang Path, InSpeech Inc, **SLP**

Peacock, Elizabeth 301 Brady Point Road, Signal Mountain, TN 37377, **SLP**

Peacock, Mrs Judy H P O Box 147, Abington, CT 06230, (203) 974-3423, MS 71 Univ of OR; 88–Sp-Lang Path, Coventry PS, **SLP**

Peacock-Pearse, Mrs Mary E 14593 Big Timber Lane, Chesterfield, MO 63017, (314) 851-2934, BA 74 Univ of CO - Boulder; MS 81 Washington Univ; Aud, Hrng Assoc of St Louis Ltd, **A**

Peak, Cynthia E 909 Chadron Avenue, Chadron, NE 69337, BA 70 Kearney St Coll, MS 81 CO St Univ; Sp-Lang Path, **SLP**

Peak, Denise M Route 1 Box 131, Greenville, IN 47124-9707, (506) 361-6703, BS 78 Eastern KY Univ; MS 82 Univ of Louisville; Sp-Lang Path, Ss Mary & Elizabeth Hosp, **SLP**

Peak, Margaret F Audiology & Speech Path (126), VA Hospital, St Louis, MO 63125, (314) 894-4672, BS 59 Maryville Coll; MA 61 Saint Louis Univ; PH 75 (NS) Columbia Univ Teachers Coll; Aud, VA Med Cen, **A**

Peak, Patricia S 2525 N W 42nd, Oklahoma City, OK 73112, (405) 947-3435, OB 63 Wichita St Univ; BA 63 Wichita St Univ; MS 66 Univ of OK Medical Center; Sp-Lang Path, Private Practice, **SLP**

Peake, Mrs Mary L 607 West Delware, Tahlequah, OK 74464, MS; **SLP LM**

Peaks, S Darlene 107 Meadowview Drive, Cross Lanes, WV 25313, (304) 768-8861, BS 70; MS 72 WV Univ; SLP / Aud, WV Div of Voc Rehab, **SLP**

Peale, Janet L 7443 Jellico Avenue, Van Nuys, CA 91406, (818) 996-3739, BA 76 Univ of Southern CA; MA 79 CA St Univ - Fullerton; Sp-Lang Path, Beverly Hills USD, **SLP**

Peaper, Ruth E Rd 1 Box 113, Jericho, VT 05465-9711, (802) 656-3861, BA 70 Bellarmine Coll; ME 72 Univ of VA - Charlottesville; Director E M Luse Center, University of Vermont, **SLP**

Pearce, Beth Anne 975 Waterbury, Cheshire, CT 06410-2790, (617) 924-3434, OB 79 Univ of MN - Duluth; MA 80 Univ of MN - Duluth; Sp-Lang Path, Cumberland Hosp, **SLP**

Pearce, Carol Susan 3423 Shore Avenue, Everett, WA 98203, (206) 353-5717, BA 73 Univ of WA; OM 78 Univ of WA; SLP, Mukilteo School District, **SLP**

Pearce, Mrs Jeanne K 317 Euclid Avenue, Haddonfield, NJ 08033, (609) 428-9314, BA 47 Univ of PA; MA 64 Temple Univ; Aud, Private Practice, **A ACE**

Pearce, Margaret C 136 2nd Street, Pacific Grove, CA 93950, (408) 375-5565, BS 40 Univ of MN - Minneap-St Paul; **SLP LM**

Pearce, Mrs Margaret Muraik 106 Shale Place, Charlottesville, VA 22901, (804) 293-5332, BA 79 Univ of CO - Boulder; ME 82 Univ of VA - Charlottesville; **SLP**

Pearce, Patsy Steig Alberta Childrens Hospital, 1820 Richmond Road, Calgary, AB, Canada T2T 5C7, (403) 229-7048, BS 72 East Carolina Univ; MS 71 PA St Univ - Univ Park; Sp-Lang Path Superv, Alberta Chldn's Hosp, **SLP**

Pearce-Hopper, Mrs Lezlie Kaye 2065 Law Lane, Eugene, OR 97401, (503) 485-8672, BS 76 Portland St Univ; MS 78 Portland St Univ; Sp/Lang Path, Eugene Hearing and Speech, **SLP**

Pearcy, Mrs Altha B 308 Elizabeth Street, Walterboro, SC 29488, (803) 549-5739, BS 53 Northwestern Univ; MA 54 Univ of IA; Sp-Lang Path, Private Practice, **SLP**

Pearl, Bonnie P H B Speech-Lang & Hearing Ctr, 17552 Beach Boulevard, Suite 208, Huntington Beach, CA 92647, (714) 841-5551, BS 64 Purdue Univ - West Lafayette; MA 80 CA St Univ - Long Beach; Sp-Lang Path Dir, Hb Sp, Lang, Hrng Cen, **SLP**

Pearl, Mrs Ellen G 10 Meadowbrook Road, Randolph, NJ 07869, BS 75 Rutger's St Univ - Douglas Coll; MS 76 Columbia Univ Teachers Coll; **SLP ACE**

Pearl, Meredith E 17 Pilgrim Run, East Brunswick, NJ 08816, **A**

Pearl, Sharon K 221 Avon Road, Cherry Hill, NJ 08034, (609) 428-5618, BA 73 CUNY - Queens Coll; MA 74 CUNY - Queens Coll; Sp/Lang Path, Haddonfield Sp & Hrng Cen, **SLP**

Pearl, Susan Z 16 Aventura Court, Randallstown, MD 21133, (301) 521-4272, BA 75 Univ of MD - College Park; MA 76 Univ of MD - College Park; Sp-Lang Path, Sub Sp & Lang Assoc, **SLP**

Pearlman, Mrs Ilene G 600 Madison Place, Jericho, NY 11753, (516) 933-8891, MS 77 Hofstra Univ; SLP, Home Health Care, **SLP**

Pearlman, Peter Michael Louisville Hearing Aid Ctr Inc, 1169 Eastern Parkway, Suite G-9, Louisville, KY 40217, (502) 456-5831, BS 80 Univ of Louisville; MS 83 Univ of Louisville; Aud, Louisville Hrng Aid Cen Inc, **A**

Pearlman, Dr Ronald C School Of Communication, Howard University, Washington, DC 20059, (202) 554-2338, BA 67 Long Island U - CW Post Ctr; MS 70 Long Island U - CW Post Ctr; PH 74 (NS) Univ of MO - Columbia; Aud, Drs Aud Serv, **SLP A ACE**

Pearlstein, Meryl R 1168 East 56th Street, 2nd Floor, Brooklyn, NY 11234, (212) 698-2900, BA 78 Adelphi Univ; MA 80 Long Island U - CW Post Ctr; **SLP**

Pearlstein, Ruth Conis 1316 Texas Avenue, Grand Junction, CO 81501, (303) 243-5236, BS 82 Univ of GA; MS 84 CO St Univ; 86–Sp-Lang Path-ECP, Mesa County Sch Dist #51, **SLP**

Pearlstine, Mrs Edelu G 4134 East Buchanan Drive, Columbia, SC 29206, **SLP LM**

Pearman, Sophia Lee 1609 Elwood, Pomona, CA 91768, MS; **SLP LM**

Pearsall, Mrs Debra Ann 7426 West Tuckey Lane, Glendale, AZ 85303, OB 81 Univ of MN - Duluth; MS 84 Univ of South FL; Sp-Lang Path, **SLP**

Pearsall, Valerie 6401 Kenwood Road, Little Rock, AR 72207, BA 70 Agnes Scott Coll; ME 85 GA St Univ; SLP, North Little Rock School Sys, **SLP**

Pearse-Storey, Mrs Marla A PSC 1 Box 27418, APO, San Francisco, CA 96230, MA 85 Northern AZ Univ; 86–Sp-Lang Path, Dept of Defense Dep Schs, **SLP**

Pearson, Barbara A 6017 51st Avenue N W, Gig Harbor, WA 98335, (907) 562-2211, OB 76 Eastern WA Univ; MS 77 Eastern WA Univ; Coord Sp-Lang Path, Providence Hospital, **SLP**

Pearson, Mrs Beth R 1831 West Daisy Lane, Glendale, WI 53209, (414) 351-0021, BS 79 Univ of WI - Madison; MS 81 Univ of WI - Milwaukee; **SLP**

Pearson, Mrs Christina Zavrotny 1535 Pensacola Street, Apt 1000, Honolulu, HI 96822, (808) 537-3807, BS 81 Marywood Coll; MS 83 PA St Univ - Univ Park; Sp-Lang Path, Rehab Hosp of the Pacific, **SLP**

Pearson, Mrs Debra Ann 1825 Prior Drive, St Louis, MO 63136, (314) 869-9437

Pearson, Mrs Diana Johnson 13 Jodar Lane, Hot Springs Village, AR 71909, (501) 767-2301, OM 82 LA St Univ - N O Medical Ctr; Sp-Lang Path, Garland Co Spec Educ Coop, **SLP**

Pearson, Gwendolyn Marie 404 Angus Blvd, Warner Robins, GA 31088, BA 78 Valdosta St Coll; ME 81 GA St Univ; MS 84 Fort Valley St Coll; SLP, Housten County School System, **SLP**

Pearson, Mrs Helen R 105 Brynwood Drive, Easton, PA 18042, (215) 861-5350, BA 44 Cedar Crest Coll; MA 78 West Chester Univ of PA; ME 84 Lehigh Univ; Couns, Northampton Comm Coll, **SLP**

Pearson, Mrs Jane S 13174 Avenida Grande, San Diego, CA 92129, (619) 538-1466, BS 77 Ball St Univ; MS 78 Bradley Univ; Sp-Lang Path, Pacific Sp & Lang Ctr, **SLP ACE**

Pearson, Judith E St Paul Hearing Clinic, 280 North Smith Avenue #701, St Paul, MN 55102, (612) 227-0824, BS 76 Univ of WI - Madison; MS 78 Univ of WI - Stevens Point; Aud, St Paul Hearing Clinic, **A**

Pearson, Mrs Karen 24 East Scott, Chicago, IL 60610, (312) 522-2010, BA 78 MI St Univ; MA 79 MI St Univ; Dir, Schwab Rehab Cen, **A**

Pearson, Mrs Karen L 180 Shoddymill Road, Glastonbury, CT 06033, (203) 659-1226, BS 69 Syracuse Univ; MA 71 Univ of CT; Sp-Lang Path, Marlborough Sch Syst, **SLP**

Pearson, Mrs Lisa M 2862 North Ellis Street, Chandler, AZ 85224, (602) 820-7950, BA 85 Pacific Univ; MS 87 Univ of WI - Stevens Point; 87–Sp-Lang Path, Kyrene Sch Dist #28, **SLP**

Pearson, Lynn R 2267 East 6th, Long Beach, CA 90814-2116, (213) 420-1033, BA 67 Northern IL Univ - De Kalb; MA 72 Univ of IL - Urbana; SLP, LA Co Supt of Schs, **SLP**

Pearson, Margaret D Box 22, Sparta, TN 38583, (615) 836-3385, BS 44 G Peabody Coll-Vanderbilt U; MA 50 G Peabody Coll-Vanderbilt U; MS 54 Univ of TN - Knoxville; **F LM**

Pearson, Marilyn M 5000 Green Meadow Drive, Helena, MT 59601, (406) 458-5731, BS 64 Univ of WI - Madison; MA 67 Univ of MT; Sp-Lang Path, Mt Off of Pub Instr, **SLP**

Pearson, Mrs Marilyn M 3873 Canter Glen Lane, Eagan, MN 55123, (612) 457-8245, BS 71 Univ of OR; MS 74 Univ of OR; 88–Sp-Lang Path, Dakota Co ISD #917, **SLP**

Pearson, Mrs Mary G Usdlo Box 10, U S Consulate-Hong Kong, FPO San Francisco, CA 96659, BS 71 ND St Univ; ME 75 Univ of VA - Charlottesville; **SLP**

Pearson, Michele L 256 Andover Drive #7-F, Valparaiso, IN 46383, (219) 464-9607, BS 79 Ball St Univ; MA 80 Ball St Univ; Sp-Lang Path, Porter Co Spec Ed Coop, **SLP**

Pearson, Mrs Patricia C 205 Mourning Dove Lane, Goldsboro, NC 27530, (919) 237-2450, BS 75 East Carolina Univ; MS 76 East Carolina Univ; Director, Eastern Nc School for the Deaf, **A**

Pearson, Mrs Patricia Hanrahan 6170 Valley Glen Drive, San Jose, CA 95123, (408) 225-2635, BA 64 CA St Univ - Long Beach; MA 88 San Jose St Univ

Pearson, Mrs Susan Kay R R 1 Box 1237A, Spooner, WI 54801, (715) 234-1515, BS 79 Northern IL Univ - De Kalb; MA 81 Northern IL Univ - De Kalb; Sp-Lang Path, Lakeview Med Ctr, **SLP**

Peart, Mrs Joan T 319 East College Street, Covina, CA 91723, (818) 967-3215, BA 52 Univ of IA; MA 72 Northwestern Univ; Sp-Lang Path, Private Practice, **SLP**

Peart, Mrs Trixine Ratliff 848 Kern Street, Chico, CA 95928, (916) 893-9047, BA 78 CA St Univ - Chico; MA 86 CA St Univ - Chico; Sp-Lang Path, Red Bluff Elem Dist, **SLP**

Pease, Mrs Cathy Treer 42 Glencove Avenue, Bangor, ME 04401, (207) 942-7487, BS 81 IN St Univ - Terre Haute; MA 83 Univ of TN - Knoxville; 87–Sp-Lang Path, Private Practice, **SLP**

Pease, Francine Route 2, Whitewater, WI 53190, (414) 642-7361, BS 62 Univ of WI - Madison; MS 74 Univ of WI - Madison; Sp-Lang Path, Wchceb, **SLP ACE**

Pease, Mrs Leane E 407 West Main Street, Millbury, MA 01527, (508) 865-5241, BS 65 Worcester St Coll; MS 85 Worcester St Coll; 85–Sp-Lang Path, Millbury School District, **SLP**

Pease, Susan Noble 13667 N Dry Fork Canyon, Vernal, UT 84078, (801) 789-3702, 88–Sp-Lang Path, Unitah Schl Dstr, **SLP**

Peaster, Mrs Monica Soldevila 267 South Main, Apt 302, Memphis, TN 38103, (901) 526-0955, MS 88 Univ of MS

Peat, Mrs Melinda Myhres 120 Meadowcrest Street, Suite 200, Gretna, LA 70056, (504) 391-7650, BS 77 Saint Mary's Dominican Coll; OM 78 LA St Univ - N O Medical Ctr; 84–Aud, Dr E B Ross J R M D, **A**

Peavie, Linda Fairchild Mini Oak South, 580 Oak Hill Road, Somerset, KY 42501, (606) 679-4887, BS 83 Eastern KY Univ; MA 86 Eastern KY Univ; SLP, Pulaski Co Bd of Ed, **SLP**

Peavy, Angela McCall P O Box 724, Butler, GA 31006, (912) 862-3100, BS 85 Univ of GA; ME 86 Columbus Coll; 86–Sp-Lang Path, Taylor Co Sch Sys, **SLP**

Peca, Margaret B 26 Sweet Briar Lane, Glen Falls, NY 12801, (518) 793-8539, BS 73 Nazareth Coll of Rochester; MS 74 SUNY - Coll at Geneseo; 88–Sp-Lang Path, UCP Ctr of Tri Counties Inc, **SLP**

Peccon, Mrs Sharon Ugolini Box 212, Star Junction, PA 15482, (412) 736-2641, BS 76 CA Univ of PA; ME 81 CA Univ of PA; 77–Sp-Lang Path, Intermediate Unit #1, **SLP**

Pechan, Paula P 1136 Crystal Drive, Virginia Beach, VA 23451-3850, **A**

Peck, Mrs Ann Agnes 1290 Manor Drive, Warminster, PA 18974, (215) 441-5268, BS 71 Shippensburg Univ of PA; ME 86 Trenton St Coll; 86–Sp-Lang Path, Bucks County IU #22, **SLP**

Peck, Anne Rouleau 2210 Beech Street, St Paul, MN 55119, (612) 227-0824, BA 74 MI St Univ; MA 75 MI St Univ; Aud, St Paul Hrng Cl, **A**

Peck, Mrs Cynthia Reynolds Rural Delivery 5, 4 Pin Oak Lane, Hockessin, DE 19707, (312) 893-0110, BS 77 Northwestern Univ; MS 79 Vanderbilt Univ; **SLP**

Peck, Dr James E Communicative Disorders, Univ Mississippi Med Ctr, 2500 North State Street, Jackson, MS 39216, (601) 987-4550, BA 64 Univ of CT; MA 67 Univ of CT; PH 72 (NS) Vanderbilt Univ; 81–Assoc Dir, U of MS Med Cen, **A**

Peck, Jillian B 3718 Wilshire, San Mateo, CA 94403, (415) 578-9950, BA 76 San Francisco St Univ; MS 78 San Francisco St Univ; Sp-Lang Path, UCSF/Child Study Unit, **SLP**

Peck, Lois Robyn Pt Washington Speech Ctr, 191 Main St, Port Washington, NY 11050, (516) 883-9224, MA 83 Hofstra Univ; 86–Sp-Lang Path, Pt Washington Sp Lang & Hrng Ctr, **SLP**

Peck, Mrs Luann English 204 East Highview Drive, Mequon, WI 53092, (312) 358-3455, **SLP**

Peck, Ronald F 534 East Rarkway North, Apartment 2, Memphis, TN 38112, (901) 323-8554, BS 77 Bradley Univ; MS 79 Purdue Univ - West Lafayette; Research Asst/Clinical Instr, Memphis Speech & Hearing Ctr, **A**

Peck, Sandra L 115 S Thomas Street #2, Bellefonte, PA 16823, (717) 248-5411, BS 82 KS St Univ; MA 85 KS St Univ; **SLP A**

Peckarsky, Mrs Lori S 11408 Stonewood Lane, Rockville, MD 20852, (301) 468-2019, BS 73 Univ of WI - Madison; MS 74 Univ of WI - Madison; 87–Sp-Lang Path, Montgomery County Pub Schs, **SLP**

Peckins, Susan Tracey 39-24 212th Street, Bayside, NY 11361, (718) 631-7290, BS 83 Purdue Univ - West Lafayette; MA 86 Univ of Denver; **A**

Pecora, Mrs Grace A 56 Lantern Road, Hicksville, NY 11801, (516) 385-2700, BA 78 Saint John's Univ - Jamaica; MS 79 Adelphi Univ; Sp-Lang Path, Humanistic Consultants, **SLP**

Pecora, Jolanta M 30 Bank Street, New Britain, CT 06050, **A**

Pecora, Marian W 904 Old Hickory Road, Mount Lebanon, Pittsburgh, PA 15243, **SLP**

Pecora, Roberta L 1140 North Linden, Oak Park, IL 60302, **SLP**

Pecorelli, Mrs Judith A 3405 New Castle Road, Virginia Beach, VA 23452, (804) 463-9592, BS 74 Kent St Univ; MA 75 Kent St Univ; 87–Sp-Lang Path, The Easter Seal Soc Trumbull Co, **SLP**

Pecsok, Janet A 1432 Highlands Way, Hixson, TN 37343, (615) 238-4204, BA 77 Univ of NC - Chapel Hill; MA 79 Univ of TN - Knoxville; 82–Sp-Lang Path, Hamilton Co Bd of Ed, **SLP**

Pecyna Rhyner, Dr Paula M Dept Speech Path & Audiology, University Of Wisconsin, P O Box 413, Milwaukee, WI 53201, (414) 963-4025, BS 76 Clarion Univ of PA; MA 77 Kent St Univ; PH 84 (Sp Path) Kent St Univ; Asst Prof, U of WI, **SLP**

Pedersen, Mrs Elizabeth Dickson 271 Betts Branch Road, Bryson City, NC 28713, (704) 488-6693, **SLP**

Pedersen, Judy Elizabeth 2353 Pima Lane, Ventura, CA 93001, (805) 643-7742, BS 82 Saint Cloud St Univ; MA 84 Univ of IA; SLP, Burnwall Clinic, **SLP**

Pedersen, Klaudia M 3100 East Rosser Avenue #6, Bismarck, ND 58501, (701) 221-3490, BA 78 Minot St Univ; MS 79 Minot St Univ; 79–Sp-Lang Path, Bismarck Pub Sch Becep, **SLP**

Pedersen, Sarah G 578 South Hillcrest Drive, Verona, WI 53593, (608) 845-7878, MS 77 CO St Univ; **SLP**

Pedersen, Sharon L 623 Belle Avenue, Apartment 202, Mankato, MN 56001, (507) 345-8388, BS 83 Moorhead St Univ; MS 85 Univ of WI - Stevens Point; 87–Audiologist, Mankato Clinic Ltd, **A**

Pederson, Alane Kay 1322 Stanley, Missoula, MT 59802, (406) 728-4100, BA 85 Univ of ND; MA 87 Univ of Northern CO; **SLP**

Pederson, Mrs Deborah A P O Box 186, Mantorville, MN 55955, (507) 634-2881, BA 78 Univ of WI - Eau Claire; MS 79 Univ of WI - Eau Claire; Sp/Lang Path, Kasson-Mantorville Sch, **SLP**

Pederson, Dr Olen T Box 10050 Lamar Station, Beaumont, TX 77710, (409) 880-8153, BS 56 Univ of Houston - Univ Park; MS 63 East TX St Univ - Commerce; PH 69 (Aud) Univ of OK Medical Center; 88–Chair-Dept of Comm, Lamar U, **SLP A**

Pedicini, Kathryn A 2452 Calamonga Lane, Sarasota, FL 33579, (813) 755-2557, BA 79 Univ of FL; MS 81 FL St Univ; Sp-Lang Path, Southside Elementary School, **SLP**

Pedigo, Lois Verjean 609 North Howard #306, Montebello, CA 90640, (213) 674-7050, MA 85 CA St Univ - Los Angeles; 88–Sp-Lang Path, Neuro Care Inc, **SLP**

Pedinoff, Cara Susan 107 Wellington Place, Aberdeen, NJ 07747, (201) 566-5879, **SLP**

Pedro, Mrs Judite Vida 52 Soundview Avenue, White Plains, NY 10606, (212) 677-7400, BA 82 Iona Coll; MS 86 Columbia Univ Teachers Coll; **SLP**

Peebles, Mary Jane Delauter 6212 Chenoweth Run Road, Louisville, KY 40299-5154, (502) 245-3597, **SLP**

Peechatka, Barbara Jane 145 New Street Road #A-18, Millersville, PA 17551, (717) 291-8017, **A**

Peek, Barbara F Veterans Administration Hosp, 1310 24th Avenue South, Nashville, TN 37203, BA 65 Hanover Coll; MA 68 Northwestern Univ; PH 82 (NS) Vanderbilt Univ; Audiologist, Veterans Administration Hosp, **A**

Peek, Emily Francis 3121 Park Avenue, Richmond, VA 23221, (804) 358-1896, BS 82 WV Univ; ME 86 Univ of VA - Charlottesville; 88–Aud, Otol Assoc of Richmond, **A**

Peek, Mrs Michelle S 340 West 100 North 57, Hurricane, UT 84737, (801) 635-4586, BS 86 Brigham Young Univ; MA 87 Brigham Young Univ; **SLP**

Peel, Gretchen L 17128 Weaver Lake Drive, Maple Grove, MN 55369, (612) 425-4131, BS 72 Saint Cloud St Univ; MS 76 Saint Cloud St Univ; Sp-Lang Path, Osseo Sch Dist, **SLP**

Peel, Laurie Welsh 6226 South Acacia Avenue, Whittier, CA 90601, (213) 868-8241, BA 84 Whittier Coll; MA 86 Whittier Coll; 88–Sp-Lang Path, Little Lake City Sch Dist, **SLP**

Peele, Vicki Noeth 5963 Honeycomb Lane, Pfafftown, NC 27040, (919) 748-3103, MA 84 Univ of Akron; Sp-Lang Path, NC Baptist Hosp, **SLP**

Peelle, Louise M 807 Jones, Ann Arbor, MI 48105, (313) 764-8440, BA 61 Mount Holyoke Coll; MA 63 Univ of MI - Ann Arbor; Sp-Lang Path, Univ of MI Comm Dis Cl, **SLP**

Peer, Donna L 512 South Brodhead Road, Aliquippa, PA 15001, (412) 728-7000, BS 63 Indiana Univ of PA; ME 66 PA St Univ - Univ Park; 87–Sp-Lang Path, The Med Ctr of Beaver PA, **SLP**

Peercy, Martha W 7504 Pickard N E, Albuquerque, NM 87110, (505) 884-3849, BA 70 NM St Univ; MS 72 WV Univ; Sp-Lang Path, Albuquerque Pub Schs, **SLP**

Peery, Mrs Peggy C 3711 Mountain Way Cove, Lithonia, GA 30058, (404) 922-0666, BS 77 Univ of GA; ME 78 Univ of GA; Sp-Lang Path, Rockdale Co Bd of Ed, **SLP**

Peete, Brenda Carol 1845 Rt 245 Box 50, Naples, NY 14512, (315) 789-5271, BS 82 SUNY - Coll at Brockport; MS 85 Nazareth Coll of Rochester; 87–Sp-Lang Path, Private Practice, **SLP**

Peets, Mrs Ruth Du Puis 1521 South Franklin, Seaside, OR 97138, (503) 738-5697, BS 50 Lewis-Clark St Coll; MS 52 Univ of OR; **SLP A F LM**

Peffley, Mrs Mara S 1515 Fernwood Drive, Slidell, LA 70458, (504) 643-3514, BS 69 Purdue Univ - West Lafayette; MS 76 FL St Univ; **SLP**

Pegram, Nancy Metcalf 1931 Mango Street N E, Palm Bay, FL 32905, (305) 723-2664, BS 58 CA Univ of PA; **SLP**

Pegram, Tamara V 190 North Moore #1023, Coppell, TX 75019, (214) 920-2000, BA 78 Loyola Coll; MS 79 Loyola Coll; Sp-Lang Path, Intervention S/Pact Inc, **SLP**

Pehde, Mrs Harriet L 12801 Meadowlark Avenue, Granada Hills, CA 91344, (818) 362-2390, BA 76 CA St Univ - Northridge; MA 77 CA St Univ - Northridge; SLP, Los Angeles County USD, **SLP**

Pehringer, James L 10433 Vincent Avenue South, Bloomington, MN 55431, (612) 931-0291, BS 80 Univ of WI - Stevens Point; MS 82 CO St Univ; Aud, Williams Sound Corp, **A**

Pehrson, Julie J Wilmington Audiology Services, 2300 Pennsylvania Avenue, Wilmington, DE 19806, BS 76 Univ of VA - Charlottesville; ME 77 Univ of VA - Charlottesville; Aud, Wilmington Aud Serv, **A**

Peigelbeck, Will Gary P O Box 804, Wakefield, RI 02879, (401) 789-1906, BA 70 Univ of RI; MS 74 Univ of RI; Owner, S Co Hrng Serv, **A**

Peiler, Mrs Suzanne Giglio 1265 Nottingham, Beaumont, TX 77706, (409) 866-4850, BS 81 Lamar Univ; MS 85 Lamar Univ; **A**

Peimer, Mrs Fran Lavovitch 746 Windsor Place, Wallingford, PA 19086, (215) 872-8776, BS 77 Trenton St Coll; MA 82 Trenton St Coll; 87–Sp-Lang Path, Improve

Peins, Dr Maryann 5 Christie Street, Edison, NJ 08820, (201) 932-9335, MA 60 NY Univ; PH 58 (NS) PA St Univ - Univ Park; Sp-Lang Path/Aud, Rutgers St U of Nj, **SLP A F**

Peirce, Dr Henry B, Jr 218 Alpine Drive, Amherst, MA 01002, (413) 545-0551, BA 50 Univ of MA - Amherst; MA 55 Univ of MI - Ann Arbor; ED 70 (NS) Boston Univ; Assist Prof, Univ of MA, **SLP**

Peirce, Mrs Terrilee Los Angeles County School Dist, 2800 227th, Torrance, CA 90505, (213) 533-4444, BA 73 CA St Univ - Long Beach; MA 77 CA St Univ - Long Beach; SLP, Los Angeles County School Dist, **SLP**

Peirolo-Alt, Mrs Corine 2202 Goff Street, Tifton, GA 31794, (912) 386-4568, BS 75 Indiana Univ of PA; MS 76 WV Univ; 86–Sp-Lang Path, Tift Co Bd of Educ, **SLP**

Peirson, Mrs Lorelei 116322 Groveland Avenue, Whittier, CA 90604, (213) 943-4574, BA 81 Biola Univ; MA 85 CA St Univ - Fullerton; **SLP**

Peiser, Mrs Libby M 41 Wingate Road, Providence, RI 02906, (401) 272-4755, BA 71 Tufts Univ; ME 73 Boston Univ; **SLP**

Peitso, Mrs Lorraine A Route 5 Box 243, River Falls, WI 54022, (715) 425-1810, BS 66 Univ of MN - Duluth; MA 81 Univ of WI - River Falls; Sp-Lang Path, River Falls Pub Sch, **SLP**

Peitzer, Mrs Wendy Sarner 10 Berry Lane, Randolph, NJ 07869, (201) 584-8588, BS 78 SUNY - Coll at Oswego; MS 83 Winthrop Coll; 87–Sp-Lang Path, Randolph Township Schs, **SLP**

Peizer, Elaine Rosenstock 2720 53rd Avenue S W, Seattle, WA 98116, (206) 932-2274, BS 73 Northwestern Univ; MA 75 Northwestern Univ; 84–Sp-Lang Path, Providence Med Ctr, **SLP**

Pekler, Mrs June M 147 80th Street, Brooklyn, NY 11209, (212) 745-1782, BA 71 CUNY - Lehman Coll; MS 72 Eastern IL Univ; Sp-Lang Path, Private Practice, **SLP**

Pekny, Marvin 241 Pickardy Lane, Council Bluffs, IA 51503, (712) 322-8393, BS 66 Univ of NE - Lincoln; MS 68 CO St Univ; 88–Aud, Audiology Services, **A**

Pekny, Sharlene Clark 421 Pickardy Lane, Council Bluffs, IA 51503, (712) 322-8393, BS 67 CO St Univ; MS 68 CO St Univ; Aud, Aud Serv, **A**

Peksa, Paul E, Jr 706 South 2nd Street, Denton, MD 21629, (301) 758-2403, BS 71 Western MD Coll; MS 76 Gallaudet Coll; Aud, Mid-Shore Spec Educ Consortium, **A**

Peksa, Robin R 706 South 2nd Street, Denton, MD 21629, MS 76 Univ of CO - Boulder; Aud, Wicomico County Board of Educ, **A**

Pelc, Michael 848 Central Street, Framingham, MA 01701, (617) 875-4559, BA 68 Allegheny Coll; ME 70 Univ of GA; 85–Aud, The Lrng Ctr for Deaf Chldn, **SLP A**

Pelissier, Mrs Paula Ann 170 Cedarwood Road, Hanover, MA 02339, (617) 878-8336, BA 79 Bridgewater St Coll; MS 81 Boston Univ; Sp/Lang Path, Rockland Publ Schs, **SLP**

Pell, Florene P O Box 272, Waianae, HI 96792, **SLP**

Pell, Robert Joseph 603 Patricia Boulevard, Timmons, ON, Canada P4N 6Z4, (705) 267-1472, OM 81 Univ of Western Ontario; 88–Aud, Timmins Audiology Clinic, **A**

Pelland, Mrs Carmen M 6819 Fortuna Road, Goleta, CA 93117, (805) 968-0789, BA 69 Univ of SD - Vermillion; MA 75 Univ of SD - Vermillion; Sp-Lang Path, Santa Barbara Co Schs, **SLP**

Pellegrino, Joann McInnis 13712 Marianna Drive, Rockville, MD 20853, (301) 424-5200, BS 76 G Peabody Coll-Vanderbilt U; MS 79 Univ of WI - Madison; Sp-Lang Path, The Treatment Cen, **SLP**

Pellegrino, Mrs Mary M 3708 Foxford Circle, Tallahassee, FL 32308, (904) 893-3348, BA 75 Immaculata Coll; MA 77 Catholic Univ of America; Private Practice, **SLP**

Pellegrino, Patricia Ann 1650 Cardinal Drive, Coatesville, PA 19320, (215) 384-2261, MA 88 OH Univ - Athens

Peller, Barbara F 20005 Octavia Court, Gaithersburg, MD 20879, (301) 933-2661, BA 66 Newark St Coll; MA 68 Newark St Coll; Sp-Lang Path, Mont Co Pub Schs, **SLP**

Pellerin, Robert J 1207 Pioneer Drive, Richmond, TX 77469, (713) 342-4131, BS 74 Wayne St Univ - Sch of Med; MA 77 Wayne St Univ - Sch of Med; Territory Manager, Cilco, **A**

Pelletier, Cathy A The Neurologic Center At Cortland, 28 Kellogg Road, Cortland, NY 13045, (607) 753-9631, BS 77 SUNY - Coll at Geneseo; MS 78 PA St Univ - Univ Park; Sp-Lang Path, The Neurologic Ctr at Cortland, **SLP**

Pelletier, Dr Louis P, Jr Midcoast Speech & Hrng Center, 108 Elm Street, Camden, ME 04843, (207) 236-8381, BA 64 Univ of ME - Orono; ME 65 Boston Univ; OD 75 (Aud) Boston Univ; Dir/Aud, Mid Coast Sp & Hrng, **SLP**

Pelletier, Mark C Rd 3 Country Club Road, Brandon, VT 05733, (802) 247-5757, BS 81 Eastern MI Univ, MA 81 Eastern MI Univ; Tchg Principal, Sudbury Country Sch, **SLP**

Pelletier, Mary Anne Old Country Club Road, RR 3 Box 3748, Brandon, VT 05733, (802) 773-1990, BS 72 Western MI Univ; MA 81 Eastern MI Univ; 81–Sp/Lang Path, Rutland Cty Pub Sch, **SLP**

Pellett, Faith Susan 11900 White Bluff Road, Somerset Wharf #605, Savannah, GA 31419, (912) 927-5479, OM 85 Auburn Univ - Auburn; **A**

Pelley, Mrs Karen S 12909 Thraves Road, Garfield, OH 44125, (216) 476-7104, BA 77 Cleveland St Univ; MA 78 Cleveland St Univ; 80–Sp/Lang Path, Fairview General Hosp, **SLP**

Pellichero, Mrs Patricia 365 North Main Street, Milltown, NJ 08850, (201) 321-6800, BS 74 Trenton St Coll; MS 75 Rutgers St Univ - Newark; Sp-Lang Path, Roosevelt Hosp, **SLP**

Pelliciari, Thomas A 214 Willow Springs, New Milford, CT 06776, (203) 355-8749, BA 76 Iona Coll; MA 78 Long Island U - CW Post Ctr; Sp-Lang Path, Danbury Public Schools, **SLP**

Pellico, Mrs Janice Barbara 31 Eastshore, Irvine, CA 92714, (714) 786-6943, **SLP**

Pellinen, Mrs Sandra P Rd 1 Box 486-1, Voluntown, CT 06384, (203) 564-4086, MA 71 Univ of CT; BS 68 Emerson Coll; 88–Sp-Lang Path, Griswold Bd of Ed, **SLP**

Pellini, Mrs Jo Ann 3245 West Kristal Way, Phoenix, AZ 85027, (602) 869-6816, BS 75 Western IL Univ; MS 76 IL St Univ - Normal; Sp-Lang Path, Private Practice, **SLP**

Pellino, Phyllis Ann 3151 Cochise Way #32, Fullerton, CA 92633, (714) 994-6635, BA 70 Univ of CA - Santa Cruz; BA 80 CA St Univ - Fullerton; MA 82 CA St Univ - Fullerton; Sp/Lang Path, Beatty Ele Sch, **SLP**

Pellman, Alton A 921 East Maple Street, Annville, PA 17003, (717) 867-1369, ME 66 PA St Univ - Univ Park; BS 59 Bloomsburg Univ of PA; Sp-Lang Path, Lancaster-Lebanon I U 13, **SLP**

Pellosie, Mrs Elizabeth 4417 North Landmark Drive, Orlando, FL 32817, (512) 423-9293, BA 76 William Paterson Coll; MS 77 William Paterson Coll; Sp-Lang Path, Orange County PS, **SLP**

Pelman, Kathleen Grace 36W628 Oak Ridge Lane, St Charles, IL 60174, (815) 338-7411, BS 82 Univ of IL - Urbana; MS 84 Univ of IL - Urbana; 84–Sp-Lang Path, Spec Ed Dist of McHenry Co, **SLP**

Pelone, Carolyn R 146 Nelson Avenue, Saratoga Springs, NY 12866, BA 68 SUNY - Center at Albany; MS 71 Montclair St Coll; Sp-Lang Path, Private Practice, **SLP**

Pelowitz, Helene M 2301 Kings Highway, Brooklyn, NY 11229, (718) 338-6746, BA 82 CUNY - Brooklyn Coll; MS 85 CUNY - Brooklyn Coll; 82–Sp-Lang Path, Private Practice, **SLP**

Pelson, Dr Rodney O 7405 S W Beveland Road, Tigard, OR 97223, (503) 279-8356, BS 67 Portland St Univ; MS 69 Portland St Univ; PH 72 (Aural Rehab) Univ of WA; Assoc Prof Aud, Or Hlth Sci U - Crpld Chldn Dv, **A**

Pelsor, Jeanell Catherine 1208-C Ortiz S E, Albuquerque, NM 87108, (505) 841-5387, BA 83 Univ of NM; MS 85 Univ of NM; 85–Aud, Los Lunas Hosp & Training Sch, **A**

Pelszynski, Mrs Patricia A 52 Fen View Road, Gillette, NJ 07933, (201) 647-0033, 78 Rutgers St Univ -N Brunswick; Sp-Lang Path, **SLP**

Pelton, Marcia G 10913 Ralston Road, Rockville, MD 20852, (301) 493-6212, BS 78 Boston Univ; MA 80 George Washington Univ; Sp-Lang Path, Private Practice, **SLP**

Peltonen, Charles D 3600 10th Street, Vernon, BC, Canada V1T 6S9, (604) 442-8258, BA 74 Univ of WI - Milwaukee; MS 75 Univ of WI - Milwaukee; **SLP**

Pelts, Mrs Carol P P O Box 68, Kennett, MO 63857, (314) 888-9474, BA 76 AR St Univ; MA 79 Memphis St Univ; Sp/Lang Path, Kennett Pub Schls, **SLP**

Peltz, Beverly R 3219 Coachman Road, Wilmington, DE 19803, (302) 429-4421, BA 64 Wichita St Univ; MA 66 Univ of KS; Sp-Lang Path, Brandywine Sch Dist, **SLP**

Pelunis, Jill Dee P O Box 401, Derry, NH 03038, (603) 434-2438, BS 71 Boston Univ; ME 72 Boston Univ; Superv Sp/Lang Path, Reading Pub Sch, **SLP**

Pena, Mrs Cheryl Swaim 3411 Old Vineyard Road, #E-12, Winston-Salem, NC 27103, (919) 768-9090, BA 86 Univ of NC - Chapel Hill; MA 88 Western Carolina Univ; 88–Sp-Lang Path, Speech Pathology Associates

Pena, Elizabeth D 5432 Fulton Street, San Francisco, CA 94121, (415) 285-4050, BA 82 Univ of Redlands; MS 84 San Francisco St Univ; Sp-Lang Path, Access Speech & Language, **SLP**

Pence, David C Speech Hearing & Learning Ctr, 8-11 Pendleton Street, 9-11 Medical Court, Greenville, SC 29601, (803) 235-9689, BA 74 Univ of AR - Little Rock; MA 75 Univ of AR - Fayetteville; Dir of SLP, Sp Hrng Learning Ctr, **SLP ACE**

Pence, John R Columbus Hospital, 500 15th Avenue South, P O Box 5013, Great Falls, MT 59403, (406) 727-3333, BA 78 Eastern WA Univ; MS 79 Eastern WA Univ; Sp-Lang Path, Columbus Hosp, **SLP ACE**

Pence, Mrs Kimberly Lynne 4142 Sandpiper Lane West, Columbus, IN 47203, (812) 376-9091, OM 82 IN Univ - Bloomington; **SLP**

Pendarvis, 8167476713 I 64 Walnut Way, Warrensburg, MO 64093, (816) 747-6713, BS 69 KS St Univ, MA 71 KS St Univ; Sp-Lang Path, Private Practice, **SLP**

Pender, Mrs Elizabeth A RD 5 Box 532, Boyertown, PA 19512, (215) 233-9550, BS 83 West Chester Univ of PA; MS 85 Bloomsburg Univ of PA; 86–Sp-Lang Path, MCIU #23, **SLP**

Pender, Mrs Evelyn H 1257 Ivanhoe Drive, East Lansing, MI 48823, MA 57 Univ of MI - Ann Arbor; Tchr, Okemos Public Schools, **SLP**

Pender, F William Route 2 Box 100AA, Cambridge, MD 21613, (301) 228-4747, BA 74 9276; MS 78 Towson St Univ; **SLP**

Pendergast, Mrs Carmela T 1254 Vina Del Mar Avenue, Placentia, CA 92670, BA 71 Univ of CA - Santa Barbara; MA 74 CA St Univ - Los Angeles; **SLP**

Pendergast, Mrs Kathleen K 3816 East Madison Street, Seattle, WA 98112, (206) 322-3544, BA 41 Central WA Univ; MA 51 Univ of WA; **SLP F LM**

Pendergast, Laurie G 9909-104th Street #2008, Edmonton, AB, Canada T5K 2G5, (403) 471-2262, BS 77 Univ of AZ; MS 79 Univ of AZ; SLP, Edmonton Public Schools, **SLP**

Pendergast, Mrs Terri Miller 2036 Hild Burns Place, Lithonia, GA 30058, (404) 361-8650, BS 83 Univ of Montevallo; MS 84 Univ of Montevallo; Sp-Lang Path, Joseph H Huie Elem Sch, **SLP**

Pendergrass, Merrie Gibson 646 Oneonta, Shreveport, LA 71106, (318) 865-4761, BS 71 LA St Univ - Baton Rouge; MA 87 LA Tech Univ; **SLP**

Pendlebury, Mrs Marianne F 602 Truman Circle, Vienna, VA 22180, SLP, Montgomery Primary Achievement, **SLP**

Pendleton, Anne Zenobia 6320 Babson Way, Virginia Beach, VA 23464, (804) 424-4331, MS 88 Howard Univ

Pendleton, Jewel A 30 South Portola, Laguna Beach, CA 92677, (714) 854-7002, **SLP**

Pendleton, Mrs Juliene R Rural Route 1 Box 35, Bloomingdale, IN 47832, (812) 238-7577, MS 77 Univ of IL - Urbana; Sp-Lang Path, Union Hospital, **SLP**

Pendleton, Suzanne McDavid 158 Bobwhite Road, Royal Palm Beach, FL 33411, (305) 562-6877, BS 80 FL St Univ; MS 81 FL St Univ; Sp-Lang Path, Bethesda Mem Hosp, **SLP**

Pendley, Ann Louise 229 Whedbee, Fort Collins, CO 80524-2937, (303) 482-8267, OB 77 CA St Univ - Long Beach; BA 77 CA St Univ - Long Beach; MS 81 CO St Univ; Sp-Lang/Rehab Hlth Serv, Mckee Med Ctr, **SLP**

Pendley, Rosemary Verner 3400 Aspen Drive, Evansville, IN 47711, (812) 473-4016, BA 78 IN Univ - Bloomington; MS 81 Western KY Univ; Sp-Lang Path, Private Practice, **SLP**

Pendrak, Mrs Rose M 616 Campbell Street, Scranton, PA 18505, (717) 343-8624, BS 76 East Stroudsburg Univ of PA; MS 80 Bloomsburg Univ of PA; Sp-Lang Path, North East Speech Associates, **SLP**

Pendry, Dr Barry L All Childrens Hospital, 801 6th Street South, St Petersburg, FL 33701, (813) 892-4141, MS 72 Univ of South FL; PH 83 (Social-Educ Change) Walden Univ - Minneapolis; Dir, Al Chldns Hos Sp-Lang-Hrng Cen, **SLP**

Pendry, Margaret M 3907 West Deleon, Tampa, FL 33609, (813) 933-4753, MA 70 Univ of South FL; Sp-Lang Path, Private Practice, **SLP**

Pengelly, Michael H 2nd General Hospital, Box 52, APO New York, NY 09180, MS 75 East Stroudsburg Univ of PA; ME 76 Bloomsburg Univ of PA; Audiologist, US Army, **A ACE**

Pengilly, Kathryn Ann 3046-B Jackson Street, San Francisco, CA 94115, (415) 563-6541, BS 86 Univ of CA - Santa Barbara; MA 88 Northwestern Univ; 88–Sp-Lang Path, St Mary's Hosp & Med Ctr

Pengress, Mrs Tanya Kay 115 Evergreen, Anna, IL 62906, (618) 833-5161, BS 79 Southern IL Univ -Carbondale; MS 84 Southern IL Univ -Carbondale; SLP, Anna Men Hlth & Develpmntl Ctr, **SLP**

Penko, Mrs Maureen 321 Centennial Street, Winnipeg, MB, Canada R3N 1P6, (204) 787-2740, BA 75; MS 77 Minot St Univ; Sp-Lang Path, Hlth Sci Centre Sp/Hrng Cl, **SLP**

Penland, Mrs Amy K 501 Shumaker Drive, Statesville, NC 28677, (704) 876-1194, BA 75 Univ of NC - Greensboro; MA 76 Univ of NC - Greensboro; Sp-Lang Path, Statesville Cty Sch, **SLP**

Penland, Mrs Jennifer Eaton 3008 Kelsey Drive, Edmond, OK 73034, BS 81 OK St Univ; MS 83 Univ of OK Medical Center; Sp-Lang Path, Edmond Pub Sch, **SLP**

Penn, Mrs Erta V 9155 North 12th Avenue, Hanford, CA 93230, (916) 674-1823, BA 31 CA St Univ - Fresno; MA 61 CA St Univ - Fresno; **SLP LM**

Penn, Dr Jacques P Lewis Road, Irvington, NY 10533, (212) 879-1540, BA 32 CUNY - City College; MA 33 Columbia Univ Teachers Coll; PH 52 (NS) NY Univ; Private Practice, **A LM**

Penn, Kathryn L 398 Noe-Bixby Road, Columbus, OH 43213, (216) 297-0811, MA 87 Kent St Univ; **SLP**

Penn, Nancy E 15 Lake Street #2B, White Plains, NY 10603, (212) 584-7679, BS 75 SUNY - Coll at Geneseo; MS 77 Syracuse Univ; Sp-Lang Path, Blythedale Childrens Hosp, **SLP**

Penna, Mrs Joan Urniezus 35 Renee Court, Cheshire, CT 06410, (203) 223-2761, BS 79 Southern CT St Univ; MS 85 Southern CT St Univ; 87–Sp-Lang Path, New Britain Mem Hosp, **SLP**

Pennefeather, Ann 2101 Shore Line Drive #485, Alameda, CA 94501, (415) 836-8228, BS 59 Univ of WI - Madison; SLP, Oakland USD, **SLP**

Pennell, Connie R Cedar Grove #5-D, 17 Coram Road, Shelton, CT 06484, (203) 385-4225, BS 58 Bowling Green St Univ; ME 67 Southern CT St Univ; OM 78 Southern CT St Univ; 63–Head Sp-Lang Path, Stratford Pub Sch, **SLP**

Penner, Kandace A 214 S W 40th Street, Gainesville, FL 32607, (904) 336-2841, BS 68 Univ of TX - Austin; MA 70 Univ of TX - Austin; 79–Sp-Lang Path, Alachua County Sch Bd, **SLP**

Penner, Dr Merrilynn J Psychology Department, University Of Maryland, College Park, MD 20742, BS 66 Howard Univ; PH 70 (Psychophysics) Univ of CA - San Diego

Penner, Dr Sharon Gail 75 East Golden Lake Road, Circle Pines, MN 55014, (612) 786-7789, BS 76; MA 79 Univ of MN - Minneap-St Paul; PH 85 (NS) Univ of MN - Minneap-St Paul; Sp-Lang Path, Minn PS, **SLP**

Pennesi, Kathleen 270 Hazel Drive, Pittsburgh, PA 15228, (412) 531-1521, BS 76 Indiana Univ of PA; MA 80 Univ of Pittsburgh - Pittsburgh; SLP, Private Practice, **SLP**

Penney, Christine Ann 105 Greenway Blvd, Churchville, NY 14428, (716) 325-4560, BS 77 SUNY - Coll at Geneseo; MS 80 Nazareth Coll of Rochester; SLP, City School Dist of Rochester, **SLP**

Penney, Mary Louise P O Box 2241, Rawlins, WY 82301, (307) 324-7739, BA 77 Western St Coll of CO; MS 82 Univ of WY; SLP, Carbon Cnty Sch Dist 1, **SLP**

Pennigton, Mrs Denise Amedee 17764 Nine Oaks Avenue, Baton Rouge, LA 70817, (504) 923-1140, OB 82 Univ of Southwestern LA; MA 84 LA St Univ - Baton Rouge; Sp-Lang Path, Sp Pathology Ctr, **SLP**

Penning, Dr Marge S 3688 Lake Drive S E, Kentwood, MI 49506, (616) 949-9531, BA 71 Calvin Coll; MA 73 Univ of KY; PH 86 (Reading) MI St Univ; 78–Sp-Lang Path, Psychi Consult Serv, **SLP**

Pennington, Mrs Carolyn D 490 Dartmoor Drive, Eugene, OR 97401, (503) 344-9328, BS 69 Univ of OR; MA 71 Univ of TX - Austin; 85–Sp-Lang Path, Ctr for Neuro Educ Therapies, **SLP**

Pennington, Mrs Dixie Freydberg 2916 Fort Point Lane, Carrollton, TX 75007, (214) 245-2016, BS 84 Univ of North TX; MS 86 Univ of North TX; 88–Sp-Lang Path, Carrollton-Farmers Branch ISD, **SLP**

Pennington, Mrs Elisabeth Bulla 71 Baker Drive, Country Homes Estates, Haw River, NC 27258, (919) 578-2327, BA 80 NC St Univ at Raleigh; ME 83 Univ of NC - Greensboro; Dir, Alamance Health Svcs, **SLP**

Pennington, Mrs Gloria T 5807 Lenlock Circle, Huntsville, AL 35802, (205) 883-8854, BA 42 Univ of AL-Tuscaloosa; MA 49 Univ of AL- Tuscaloosa; **SLP**

Pennington, Gwendolyn 1408 North Carlton, Liberal, KS 67901, (316) 624-4560, BS 32 OK St Univ; ME 38 Phillips Univ; **SLP LM**

Pennington, Mrs Janet K 3409 Baker Boulevard, Altoona, PA 16602, (814) 946-2356, BA 74 Temple Univ; MS 75 PA St Univ - Univ Park; Sp-Lang Path, Altoona Hosp, **SLP**

Pennington, John C Mountain Region Sp & Hearing, 330 Broad Street, Kingsport, TN 37660, (615) 246-4600, BS 75 East TN St Univ; MA 77 Univ of TN - Knoxville; Sp-Lang Path, Mt Reg Sp & Hrng Cen, **SLP**

Pennington, Mrs Patricia Louise 3645 Blue Jacket Drive, Lee's Summitt, MO 64064, (816) 373-1680, BA 75 Univ of MO - KS City; MS 76 Central MO St Univ; Sp-Lang Path, Research Med Cen, **SLP**

Pennington, Penny P 228-12 Arnold Street, West Lafayette, IN 47907, BA 68 Univ of SD - Springfield; MA 77 Univ of SD - Springfield; Doctoral, Prudue Univ, **SLP**

Pennington, Dr R Corbin 777 Saturn Drive, Colorado Springs, CO 80906, (719) 632-8501, BS 27 Columbia Univ Sch of Gen St; MA 29 Columbia Univ Sch of Gen St; PH 39 (Sp) Columbia Univ Sch of Gen St; **LM**

Pennington, Mrs Ruth M 2916 Gilmore Avenue, Pittsburgh, PA 15235, (412) 243-9035, BA 64 Geneva Coll; MA 68 Univ of KS; 88–Sp-Lang Path, CA Univ of PA, **SLP**

Pennington, Mrs Sharon Alicia 248 Fire Tower Road, Mill Spring, NC 28756, (704) 894-3237, BA 74 Otterbein Coll; MA 76 Bowling Green St Univ; Sp/Lang Path, Private Practice, **SLP**

Pennington, Mrs Valerie Joan 719 Foerster, San Francisco, CA 94127, (415) 337-1276, BA 74 Univ of NM; MS 77 Univ of NM; Sp-Lang Path, **SLP**

Pennino, John Arthur 1690 University Avenue, Suite 430, St Paul, MN 55104, (612) 644-1718, MS 74 Univ of WY; Owner, Sp/L Stuttering Clinic, **SLP**

Penno, Catherine 27101 La Feunte, Mission Viejo, CA 92692, (714) 364-1830, OB 79 Univ of MN - Duluth; MS 81 Purdue Univ - West Lafayette; Sp-Lang Path, Newport Lang Sp/Aud, **SLP ACE**

Penny, Mrs Lynn B 1173 La Via, Sparks, NV 89431, (702) 359-0418, BS 69 Brigham Young Univ; MS 71 Brigham Young Univ; SLP, Washoe Co Sch Dist, **SLP**

Penrod, Alison Dawn 602 Cherry Street, Windber, PA 15963, (814) 535-5508, BS 81 Indiana Univ of PA; MS 84 Indiana Univ of PA; 81–Director/Sp-Lang Pathology, Easter Seal Society-Cambria Co, **SLP**

Penrod, Dr John P 223 East Washington Street, Quincy, FL 32351, (904) 627-3100, BA 67 Univ of FL; MA 68 Univ of FL; PH 76 (NS) FL St Univ; Aud, Audiology Assoc of No FL, **A**

Pensa, Mrs Donna Anne 569 Fruit Hill Avenue, North Providence, RI 02911, (401) 438-9500, MS 83 Univ of RI; SLP, Meeting Street School, **SLP**

Pensack, Irwin 104 Primrose Drive, Longwood, FL 32779, (305) 849-6520, BS 48 NY Univ; MS 77 William Paterson Coll; Aud, Orange Hrng Aid Cen, **A**

Pentenburg, Ellen Kay 891 Pimlico Drive #1-B, Centerville, OH 45459, (513) 436-9087, BS 85 Bowling Green St Univ; MA 87 Ball St Univ; 87–Sp-Lang Path, St Elizabeth Med Ctr, **SLP**

Pentz, Dr Arthur L, Jr Dept Speech Path & Audiology, Oklahoma State University, 120 Hanner, Stillwater, OK 74078, (405) 744-6021, BS 67 Bloomsburg Univ of PA; ME 71 Bloomsburg Univ of PA; PH 82 (NS) PA St Univ - Univ Park; Assoc Prof, OK St U, **SLP**

Penza, Allison M 6312 North First Street Apartment 106, Fresno, CA 93710-5441, (209) 435-7736, MA 87 CA St Univ - Fresno; 87–Sp-Lang Path, Selma USD, **SLP**

Penzi, Lori M 575 Armory Road, Whitefish, MT 59937, (406) 755-7619, BS 74 Univ of IA; MS 76 CO St Univ; Sp-Lang Path, Kalispell Pub Schs, **SLP**

Peoples, Nancy Velma 4083 Sunbeam Road #2302, Jacksonville, FL 32217, (904) 721-0088, **SLP**

Pepe, Tara Lynn 72 Orchard Road, Maplewood, NJ 07040, BS 81 Mercy Coll; MS 84 Rutgers St Univ -N Brunswick; Sp-Lang Path, UCP of North Jersey, **SLP**

Pepe-Caffrey, Christine E St Barnabas Medical Center, Old Short Hills Road, Livingston, NJ 07039, (201) 533-5786, BS 86 SUNY - Coll at Geneseo; MA 88 SUNY - Coll at Geneseo; 88–Sp-Lang Path, St Barnabas Med Ctr

Pepitone, Celeste C 5302 East Abbeyfield St, Long Beach, CA 90815-3023, (213) 597-0577, BA 80 CA St Univ - Long Beach; MS 83 Univ of LA Verne; Sp-Lang Path, Private Practice, **SLP**

Peppard, Ann Baker 502 Mira Vista Avenue, Oakland, CA 94610, (415) 685-1960, BA 69 Univ of CA - Berkeley; MA 72 Univ of the Pacific; Sp-Lang Path, Mt Diablo U S D, **SLP**

Peppard, Mrs Annette Rhoda 787 Stonington Place, Macon, GA 31210, (912) 474-9440, BA 70 Univ of Chicago; MA 84 Wayne St Univ; MA 74 Univ of MN - Minneap-St Paul; 88–Aud, Bibb Co PS, **A**

Peppard, Robert C 13 Sherman Terrace #6, Madison, WI 53704, BA 70 Cleveland St Univ; MA 72 Bowling Green St Univ; Research Assistant, Univ of Wisconsin-Madison, **SLP**

Perachio, Jey J 975 Providence Road, Springfield, PA 19064, (215) 461-7878, BS 75 West Chester Univ of PA; MA 78 West Chester Univ of PA; 86–VP, Keystone Rehab Sys, **SLP**

Peraino, Antoinette 20 Willow Street, Beverly, MA 01915-2249, BS 79 Wayne St Univ; MA 80 Western MI Univ; 87–Sp-Lang Path, Gr Lynn Ment Hlth & Ret Assoc, **SLP**

Peraino, Madonna Katherine 123 Blackman Road, Ridgefield, CT 06877, (203) 438-0520, BS 74 SUNY - Coll at Geneseo; MA 76 San Jose St Univ; 84–Sp-Lang Path, Ridgefield PS, **SLP**

Percell, Lisa Michele P O Box 5, Camden Point, MO 64018-0005, (816) 445-3471, MS 86 Northwest MO St Univ; 88–Sp-Lang Path, Rehab Institute, **SLP**

Perchacz, Teresa J 862 South Beech Street, Lakewood, CO 80228, (303) 452-8922, BA 72 Univ of Northern CO; MA 73 Univ of Northern CO; Sp-Lang Path, Adams Co Sch Dist #12, **SLP**

Percia, Valerie C 46 Kendall Hill Road, Sterling Junction, MA 01564, (617) 422-6793, BA 72 Saint John's Univ - Jamaica; ME 75 Bridgewater St Coll; 80–Sp-Lang Path, H Lipton Comm Ment Hlth Cen, **SLP**

Perdeus, Melanie 210 East Ross Street, Lancaster, PA 17602, (717) 569-7331, BS 81 Indiana Univ of PA; MS 82 Indiana Univ of PA; SLP, Lancaster-Lebanon Iu 13, **SLP**

Perdomo, Celia F P O Box 34, Descanso, CA 92016, (619) 588-3053, OB 50 Univ of MO - Columbia; ME 54 Univ of VA - Charlottesville; Prog Spec, Cajon Valley Sch Dist, **SLP**

Perdue, Mrs Annette P 1901 Landau Drive, Phenix City, AL 36867, (404) 327-2213, BA 61 Univ of AL- Tuscaloosa; OM 77 Auburn Univ - Auburn; Sp-Lang Path, Sp Path Serv, **SLP ACE**

Perdue, Nancy E 3802 Mitchell Circle, New Bern, NC 28562, (919) 633-0775, BS 78 East Carolina Univ; MS 80 East Carolina Univ; 80–Sp-Lang Path, Dev Evaluation Cen/Nc St, **SLP**

Perdue, Susan W Route 36 Box 269-2, Beattyville, KY 41311, (606) 464-8111, BS 84 Eastern KY Univ; MA 85 Eastern KY Univ; 85–Sp-Lang Path, Shearon & Associates, **SLP**

Perella, Karen D 219 Fallen Timber Road, Hendersonville, NC 28739, (704) 692-7068, BS 74 Kent St Univ; ME 80 Western Carolina Univ; Sp-Lang Path, Private Practice, **SLP**

Perenchio, Mrs Jan 1807 Country Club Drive, Redlands, CA 92373, (714) 792-0847, BA 59 Emerson Coll; MS 86 Univ of LA Verne; 80–Sp-Lang Path, Redlands USD, **SLP**

Perens, Margaret 1317 Via Gabriel, Palos Verdes Estates, CA 90274, (213) 533-2760, BA 65 Univ of CA - Los Angeles; MS 67 Univ of Southern CA; Cl Coord Sp-Lang Path, Harbor-UCLA Med Cen, **SLP**

Perera, Patricia M 2061 Shadow Wood Drive, Marietta, GA 30066, (404) 971-5850, BS 69 Univ of TN - Knoxville; ME 70 Univ of GA; 70–Sp-Lang Path, Cobb Co Pub Sch, **SLP**

Peretsman, Debora Russo 1233 York Avenue Apartment 12N, New York, NY 10021, (212) 861-5556, BS 77 Emerson Coll; MA 79 CA St Univ - Long Beach; **SLP**

Perez, Mrs Aldana S 1435 Bedford #6-N, Stamford, CT 06905, (203) 348-9388, BA 36 Univ of Chicago; MS 66 Southern CT St Univ; **SLP**

Perez, Mrs Carmen A Avenue DE La Pesadilla #64, Urb Fuente Del Fresno, San Sebastian DE Los Reyes, Madrid, Spain 28708, MA 70 Syracuse Univ; Audiologist, Chicano Community Health Ctr, **A**

Perez, Daisy 91 Marion Street, Paterson, NJ 07522, (201) 790-1360, MA 88 Montclair St Coll

Perez, Mrs Denice Gordon Head & Neck Surgery Box 69, M D Anderson Cancer Center, 1515 Holcombe, Houston, TX 77030, (713) 792-6523, BS 80 IA St Univ; MA 82 Northeast MO St Univ; Sp/Lang Path, U of TX Med Branch, **SLP ACE**

Perez, Dr Dennis M Box 64, 58 Highland Avenue, Brocton, NY 14716, (716) 673-3169, BS 68 SUNY - Coll at Geneseo; MS 69 Purdue Univ - West Lafayette; PH 75 (Doctor of Philosophy (Sp-Lang Path)) SUNY - Center at Buffalo; 77–Assoc Prof, St U Coll of NY-Fredonia, **SLP**

Perez, Elisa 7029 Verdure Way, Elk Grove, CA 95624-4912, (916) 684-1091, BA 83 CA St Univ - Sacramento; MA 84 Univ of the Pacific; 87–Sp-Lang Path, Mercy Gen Hosp, **SLP**

Perez, Dr Emilio Arkansas State University, P O Box 2763, State University, AR 72467, (501) 972-3106, BA 66 Univ of South FL; MA 67 Univ of South FL; PH 71 (NS) OH St Univ; Assoc Prof/Dir of Comm Disorders, AR St U, **SLP ACE**

Perez, Frank Joseph 2910 La Chiquita Avenue, Tucson, AZ 85715, (602) 298-0585, BA 71 Univ of CA - Los Angeles; MA 78 CA St Univ - Los Angeles; 86–Sp-Lang Path, Tucson USD, **SLP**

Perez, Mrs Josephine Rivas 898 North Chester Avenue, Pasadena, CA 91104, (818) 445-3102, BS 79 Univ of AZ; MS 81 4232; Sp-Lang Path, SW Human Dev, **SLP**

Perez, Juan M 358 A Wethersfield Avenue, Hartford, CT 06114-1414, (203) 246-3986, BA 72 Univ of PR - Rio Piedras; MS 77 Southern CT St Univ; Sp-Lang Path, Hartford Bd of Ed, **SLP**

Perez, Mrs Linda Maurine 1010 West MacArthur Boulevard #85, Santa Ana, CA 92707, (714) 966-2601, MA 88 CA St Univ - Fullerton; 88–Sp-Lang Path, Santa Ana USD

Perez, Margaret Manley 3552 Suncrest Drive, Lake Worth, FL 33467, (407) 659-2894, BA 79 Univ of NC - Chapel Hill; MS 81 Univ of NC - Chapel Hill; Sp-Lang Path, The Sch Bd of Palm Beach Co FL, **SLP**

Perez, Nilsa Rubin 1130 Pelham Parkway South, Apartment 4-F, Bronx, NY 10461, (212) 920-7583, BA 79 CUNY - Queens Coll; MS 81 Columbia Univ Teachers Coll; SLP, Rose F Kennedy Center-Cerc, **SLP ACE**

Perez, Mrs Randa A 6208 Pine Needle Drive, South, Mobile, AL 36609, (512) 576-5840, BA 75 Univ of South AL; MA 76 Univ of AL- Tuscaloosa; Sp/Lang Path, Private Practice, **SLP**

Perfect, Jolene A 982 Providence Road, Newtown Square, PA 19073, (215) 565-4085, BS 69 Ball St Univ; MS 73 Towson St Univ; Sp-Lang Path, De Co Iu #25, **SLP**

Perfect, Mrs Joni Boysen 1001 West Oraibi Drive, Phoenix, AZ 85027, (602) 866-5245, BS 77 Northeast MO St Univ; MA 78 Northeast MO St Univ; Sp-Lang Path, Washington Sch Dist #6, **SLP**

Pergande, Mrs Krisann S 2815 North 61st Street, Milwaukee, WI 53210-2112, (414) 445-4514, BS 77 Univ of WI - Milwaukee; MS 78 Univ of WI - Milwaukee; Sp-Lang Path, Milwaukee Pub Sch, **SLP**

Pergler, Harold R 425 Medical Drive, Suite 203, Bountiful, UT 84010, (801) 295-9644, BS 77 Brigham Young Univ; OM 79 Brigham Young Univ; 80–Owner & Aud, Bountiful Hrng Cen, **A**

Perica, Ellen G 6 Eyers Place, Somerdale, NJ 08083, President, Speech-Language Consultants, **SLP**

Perich, Audrey Hare 6993 Alabaster Court, Middletown, MD 21769, (301) 694-1466, BA 73 Northeastern OK St Univ; MA 74 Univ of OK - Norman; Sp-Lang Path, Frederick County PS, **SLP**

Pericozzi, Mrs Alice T L 129 Cedar Lane, Groton, NY 13073, (315) 473-6914, BS 76 SUNY - Center at Buffalo; MS 78 SUNY - Coll at Fredonia; Sp-Lang Path, NYS-Syr Dev Ctr, **SLP**

Perigoe, Christina Barris 3510 Connaught Avenue, Montreal, PQ, Canada H4B 1X3, (514) 488-9667

Perilman, Ross M 1428 Inverness, Pittsburgh, PA 15217, **SLP**

Periman, Mrs Peggy Gish 4101 Pinnacle Pines Court, Hephzibah, GA 30815, (404) 737-7310, BA 77 Univ of AZ; MS 84 Univ of HI - Manoa

Perin, Mrs Trina Ann 3563 Erie Avenue, Cincinnati, OH 45208, (513) 321-3774, BS 79 Univ of Cincinnati; MA 81 Univ of Cincinnati; Sp-Lang Path, Private Practice, **SLP**

Perini, Mrs Susan Guddie 1711 Holly Lane, Grafton, WI 53024, (414) 459-3677, SLP, Sheboygan Public Schools, **SLP**

Perkett, Vicki Ramee 2449 Cavitt Creek Road, Glide, OR 97443, (503) 249-3288, BA 80 CA St Univ - Long Beach; **SLP**

Perkins, Ann N G 4061 Richland Avenue, Louisville, KY 40207, (502) 583-8303, BS 76 Murray St Univ; MS 77 Univ of Louisville; Sp/Lang Path, Oldham Co Bd of Ed, **SLP**

Perkins, Mrs Charlotte 3309 Kenmore Street, Greensboro, NC 27408, (919) 282-1521, MA 38 LA St Univ - Baton Rouge; Retired, **SLP LM**

Perkins, Cynthia B Route 3, 100 Shenandoah Drive, Spartanburg, SC 29301, (803) 576-4212, BS 75 Northern IL Univ - De Kalb; MA 77 Northern IL Univ - De Kalb; Sp-Lang Path, Spartanburg Co Pub Sch Dist 6, **SLP**

Perkins, Denice Jane 257 Rozelle, Memphis, TN 38104, (901) 528-6511, BS 82 Western MI Univ; MA 84 Memphis St Univ; 84–Sp-Lang Path, University of Tennessee, **SLP**

Perkins, Denise Kay 550 Orange Avenue #313, Long Beach, CA 90802, (213) 435-0645, BS 83 Univ of CA - Santa Barbara; MA 86 Univ of TX - Austin; **SLP**

Perkins, Dorothy Rose 8323 South Vernon, Chicago, IL 60619, (312) 723-0953, BA 82 Saint Xavier Coll; MS 84 Governors St Univ; **SLP**

Perkins, Ellen U Rural Route 1, Long Pond Road, Wading River, NY 11792, **SLP**

Perkins, Geneva 106 Brookdale, Glasgow, KY 42141, (502) 651-6757, BS Western KY Univ; MA 64 Univ of KY; Sp-Lang Path, Glasgow Bd of Ed, **SLP**

Perkins, Giovanna Frittelli 601 1/2 Pine Street, Madison, WI 53715, (608) 255-4671, BA 82 Univ of VT; MS 85 Univ of WI - Madison; 88–Sp-Lang Path, Leader Nursing & Rehab Center, **SLP**

Perkins, James Patrick Route 7 Box 411-A, Abingdon, VA 24210, (703) 628-4900, **SLP**

Perkins, Mrs Jeanne P 538 Hobby Avenue, Frankfort, IL 60423-1110, (312) 702-1864, BA 79 Catholic Univ of America; MA 80 Western MI Univ; 82–Sp-Lang Path, U of Chicago Med Cen, **SLP A**

Perkins, Judy Marie 1990 Commonwealth Avenue #4, Brighton, MA 02135, (617) 720-6771, MA 85 Univ of Houston - Univ Park; 88–Sp-Lang Path, Spaulding Rehab Hosp, **SLP**

Perkins, Lana L 315 Springwood Lane, San Antonio, TX 78216, (512) 656-3227, BS 68 OH St Univ; MA 75 Temple Univ-Tyler Sch of Art; Sp-Lang Path, The Psychological Corp, **SLP**

Perkins, Mrs Marlene M 4921 South 67th Street, Lincoln, NE 68516, BA 60 Univ of IA; Sp-Lang Path, Seward Pub Sch, **SLP**

Perkins, Richard Alan 14774 Pioneer Blvd, Norwalk, CA 90650, (213) 868-1441, BA 77 CA St Univ - Fullerton; MA 82 CA St Univ - Fullerton; Self Employed, **SLP**

Perkins, Scott Tucker 7107 Ming Avenue #20, Bakersfield, CA 93309, (805) 872-3408, BS 85 Univ of OK - Norman; MS 87 Univ of OK - OK City; **SLP**

Perkins, Shawna Ann 6750 North Pennsylvania, Kansas City, MO 64118, (816) 436-4817, BS 85 Univ of AZ; MS 87 Gallaudet Coll; Audiologist, **A**

Perkins, Sheila R 15232 Elk Run Road, Chantilly, VA 22021, (703) 378-0784, BS 77 LA St Univ - Baton Rouge; MS 78 Univ of AL- Tuscaloosa; **SLP**

Perkins, Susan S 45-08 169th Street, Flushing, NY 11358, **SLP**

Perkins, Dr William H 5425 Weatherford Drive, Los Angeles, CA 90008, (213) 292-1624, BS 43 Southwest MO St Univ; MA 49 Univ of MO - Columbia; PH 52 (Sp Path) Univ of MO - Columbia; 52–Prof Emeritus, USC, **SLP F H LM**

Perl, Diane 3413 37th, Lubbock, TX 79413, (806) 799-7632, BA 78 Univ of CA - Santa Barbara; MS 81 TX Tech Univ; Sp-Lang Path, Sp-Lang-Hrng Cen, **SLP**

Perl, Mrs Ilene E 49 Far Brook Drive, Short Hills, NJ 07078, (201) 376-0745, BA 68 Rutger's St Univ - Douglas Coll; MA 69 Univ of IL - Urbana; **SLP**

Perl, Mrs Marlene Ruth 1382 East 49 Street, Brooklyn, NY 11234, (718) 258-0185, MS 87 CUNY - Brooklyn Coll; 88–Sp-Lang Path, Brooklyn Childhood Center

Perl, Sarah Miriam 2444 Main Street Suite 160, Fresno, CA 93721, (209) 442-6425, MS 81 Univ of NC - Chapel Hill; 86–Clin Supvr/Sp-Lang Path, Neurological Retraining Center, **SLP ACE**

Perla, Mrs Christine 25684 Hidden Acres Drive, Westlake, OH 44145, (216) 892-2888, BS 72 Bowling Green St Univ; MA 77 Cleveland St Univ; Sp-Lang Path, **SLP**

Perlewitz, Jo Ann 42236 Blacow Road, Fremont, CA 94538, (415) 794-2009, BA 68 San Jose St Univ; Sp-Lang Path, Newark USD, **SLP**

Perlich, Catherine Ann Univ Of The Virgin Islands, St Thomas, VI 00802, (809) 776-5593, BA 77 Brock Univ - Ontario; OB 78 Brock Univ - Ontario; ES 80 Brock Univ - Ontario; Dir of Testing, Univ of the Virgin Islands, **SLP**

Perlin, Ilene Gail 233 Cuba Hill Road, Huntington, NY 11743-4805, (718) 939-8700, **SLP**

Perlman, Abel 511 South Shore Drive, Madison, WI 53715, (608) 256-1145, BA 73 Univ of WI - Madison; MS 74 Univ of WI - Madison; 88–Independent Consult, Private Practice, **SLP**

Perlman, Dr Adrienne L Audiology-Speech Pathology Ser, VA Medical Center, Iowa City, IA 52240, (319) 354-9090, BA 63 Univ of IA; MA 76 Univ of Northern IA; PH 85 (NS) Univ of IA; Sp-Lang Path, VA Med Cen, **SLP**

Perlman, Mrs Cathy A 39 Kenwood Drive, Cherry Hill, NJ 08034, (609) 428-9235

Perlman, Eve S 11911 23rd Avenue North, Plymouth, MN 55441, (612) 472-1600, BS 71 Univ of MN - Minneap-St Paul; MA 75 Univ of MN - Minneap-St Paul; Sp-Lang Path, Westonka Sch Dist, **SLP**

Perlman, Mrs Gail Brenner 7419 Elizabeth Road, Melrose Park, PA 19126, (215) 928-8897, BA 78 Univ of MD - College Park; MA 79 Hofstra Univ; Aud, Thomas Jefferson U Hosp, **A**

Perlmutter, Deborah Judith 4607 Horizon Circle #104, Baltimore, MD 21208, (301) 484-7387, **A**

Perlmutter, Marilyn Bowling Green State University, Dept Of Commun Disorders, Bowling Green, OH 43403, (419) 372-7187, BA 55 Brandeis Univ; MA 56 Univ of Denver; 72–Asst Prof/Commun Dis, Bowling Green St U, **SLP**

Perlmutter, Robert Bennett 554 Blue Ridge Drive, Medford, NY 11763, (516) 266-5291, BA 54 IL Wesleyan Univ; MS 63 Adelphi Univ; SLP, Commack Pub Sch, **SLP**

Perlov, Betty Rd 2 Box 196, Prospect Road, Monroe, NY 10950, **SLP**

Perlow, Steven 64 Hunters Lane, Williamsville, NY 14221, (716) 873-7790, BA 77 SUNY - Center at Buffalo; MA 79 SUNY - Center at Buffalo; Audiologist, Accura Consultants, **A**

Perlow, Susan R 64 Hunters Lane, Williamsville, NY 14221, (716) 876-4242, BA 76 SUNY - Center at Buffalo; MA 78 SUNY - Center at Buffalo; Sp-Lang Path Instructor, SUNY College at Buffalo, **SLP**

Perlroth, Mrs Lynn Block 2 Whisperwood Court, Rockville, MD 20852, (301) 454-6906, BS 63 IN Univ - Bloomington; MA 64 Stanford Univ; 85–Audiology, University of Maryland College Park, **A**

Perlstein, Marie Maffeo 1311 Northeast 174 Street, North Miami Beach, FL 33162, MS

Perlwitz, Mrs Renee S 7931 43rd Avenue, Kenosha, WI 53142, (414) 694-5625, BS 83 Univ of WI - Whitewater; MS 85 Univ of WI - Whitewater; 87–Sp-Lang Path, Kenosha Hosp & Med Ctr, **SLP**

Pernick, Andrea Dale 3631 North Prospect Drive, Miami, FL 33133, (305) 531-0472, MA 76 Univ of FL; 85–Pres/Owner, S Miami Aud & Hrng Aid Ctr, **A**

Pernick, Mrs Dina Mae 19210-C 64th Avenue #1-A, Flushing, NY 11365-2719, (718) 454-7426, SLP, **SLP**

Pernikoff, Naomi Stilman 157 Mineral Spring Avenue, Passaic, NJ 07055, (201) 777-4131, BS 83; MS 85 CUNY - Brooklyn Coll; 83–Sp-Lang Path, Debbie Sussman c/o Bais Ezra

Pero, M Theresa 9150 S W 87th Avenue #103, Miami, FL 33176, (305) 595-1530, BS 81 FL St Univ; MS 82 FL St Univ; Aud, Aud & Vestbular Cen, **A**

Peros-Paone, Mariann 814 West 3rd Street, Elmira, NY 14905, BA 74 CUNY - Queens Coll; MA 75 OH Univ - Athens; **SLP**

Perotti, Diane Marie 1120 McArthur Drive #1004, Carrollton, TX 75007, (214) 824-1620, BA 80 CA St Univ - Chico; MA 82 CA St Univ - Chico; 84–Sp-Lang Path, Dallas ISD, **SLP**

Perozzi, Dr Joseph A Speech And Hearing Center, University Of Texas, El Paso, TX 79968, (915) 747-5250, BA 65 Univ of NV - Reno; MA 67 Univ of WA; PH 69 (Sp-Lang Path) Univ of WA; 71–Prof, U of TX-El Paso, **SLP**

Perrault, Sara Jeanne 950 Temple Hills Drive, Laguna Beach, CA 92651, (714) 494-5096, BA 81 Univ of CA - Santa Barbara; MS 84 Univ of Redlands; **SLP**

Perreault, Marilyn 48 Raymond Circle, Agawam, MA 01001, (508) 755-1391, BS 81 Univ of MA - Amherst; MA 83 Univ of MA - Amherst; 83–Aud, Central Hearing Instr Inc, **A**

Perreca, Mrs Dorothy 805 Aster Boulevard, Rockville, MD 20850, (301) 593-5237, BA 58 Allegheny Coll; MA 63 Univ of MD - College Park; 87–Proj Mgr, National Geographic Society, **SLP A**

Perretta, Mrs Rosemarie 80 Kingsberry Drive, Somerset, NJ 08873, (201) 735-7916, BA 74 Montclair St Coll; MA 77 Seton Hall Univ; Sp-Lang Path, Clinton Twp Pub Sch, **SLP**

Perriello, Elizabeth M 173 Lakemere Drive, Southbury, CT 06488, (203) 272-0335, MS Southern CT St Univ; Sp-Lang Path, Cheshire Ct Pub Sch Syst, **SLP**

Perriello, Mrs Miriam A 126 Raccoon Way, Gibsonia, PA 15044, (412) 443-1374, BS 76 Clarion Univ of PA; MS 77 WV Univ; 88–Sp-Lang Path, Compton P-ESL Prog, **SLP ACE**

Perrin, Mrs Karen I 10030 Scenic View Terrace, Vienna, VA 22180, BS 68 Bowling Green St Univ; MS 73 Columbia Univ Teachers Coll; 88–Sp-Lang Path, Fairfax Co PS, **SLP**

Perrin, Dr Kenneth L Tanglewood, 100 East Rosedale Avenue, West Chester, PA 19382, (215) 436-2471, BA 59 Occidental Coll; MA 64 CA St Univ - Long Beach; PH 69 (Sp & Hrng Sciences) Stanford Univ; Pres, West Chester U, **SLP F**

Perrine, Anne W 6320 Secret Drive, Raleigh, NC 27612, (919) 848-8410, BA 77 Kent St Univ; BS 80 Kent St Univ; MA 80 Kent St Univ; Sp-Lang Path, Murdoch Center, **SLP**

Perrine, Helen J 801 Jamestown Drive, Miamisburg, OH 45342, (513) 867-6460, BS 75 OH Univ - Athens; MA 78 OH Univ - Athens; Aud, Mercy Hosp-Hamilton, **A**

Perrine, Mrs Linda Rouhan 21737 North Center, Northville, MI 48167, (313) 540-5712, BS 72 Wayne St Univ; MA 76 Eastern MI Univ; Sp-Lang Path, Bloomfield Hills Schs, **SLP**

Perrine, Mrs Rita Kass RD 4, 286 Schoolhouse Road, Jamesburg, NJ 08831, (201) 533-5786, BA 82 Rutger's St Univ - Douglas Coll; MS 87 Rutgers St Univ -N Brunswick; 87–Sp-Lang Path, Saint Barnabas Med Ctr, **SLP**

Perron, Gale L 22 Liberty Road, Hingham, MA 02043, (617) 837-1311, BS 71 CUNY - City College; ME 79 Northeastern Univ; **SLP**

Perrone, Rosemary Petrovic 3314 Scathelocke Road, Pittsburgh, PA 15235, (412) 281-7244, BA 75 Univ of Pittsburgh - Pittsburgh; MS 76 Syracuse Univ; Sp-Lang Path, Er Sl So of Allegheny Co, **SLP**

Perrott, Emily H 2004 Eastridge Drive N E, Albuquerque, NM 87112, (505) 299-5574, BS 59 Univ of TX - Austin; ME 77 Tarleton St Univ; Sp/Lang Path, Albuquerque Publ Schs, **SLP**

Perrott, Karen Margaret 2552 Lynn Lake Circle S #D, St Petersburg, FL 33712, (813) 867-9205, BS 79 FL St Univ; MS 80 FL St Univ; **SLP**

Perrotta, Brigitte 1 Horizon Road #G-7, Fort Lee, NJ 07024, (201) 886-1141, MS 87 Columbia Univ Teachers Coll; 88–Aud, Newark Beth Israel Med Ctr

Perry, Mrs Alberta H 317 East Barber Avenue, Woodbury, NJ 08096, (609) 845-2846, BA 48 Glassboro St Coll; ME 55 Temple Univ-Tyler Sch of Art; **SLP LM**

Perry, Mrs Barbara Ann Rd 2 Box 92-A, Schaghticoke, NY 12154, (518) 274-0311, MA 81 Univ of Denver; Audiologist, James Fernbach MD, **A**

Perry, Mrs Beth Walker 8930 Kenilworth Drive, Burke, VA 22015, (703) 425-5756, BS 72 Indiana Univ of PA; MA 83 San Diego St Univ; 86–Sp-Lang Path, Fairfax Co PS, **SLP**

Perry, Mrs Carolyn S 421 Farmington Woods Drive, Cary, NC 27511, MS 78 Univ of NC - Chapel Hill; SLP, Wake County Health Dept, **SLP**

Perry, Cassandra Eve 1 Prescott Street Unit 306, East Boston, MA 02128, (617) 773-6100, BS 78 Marquette Univ; ME 80 Northeastern Univ; Sp-Lang Path, Quincy City Hosp, **SLP**

Perry, Cecyle K 120 Deer Creek, Rose Hill, KS 67133, (316) 776-0635, BS 73 Fort Hays St Univ; MS 75 Fort Hays St Univ; Instr, Ft Hay St U, **SLP**

Perry, Mrs Connie Bone Special Education, 440 East Ponce de Leon Avenue, Decatur, GA 30030, (404) 373-5809, BS 72 OK St Univ; MS 74 Univ of OK Medical Center; 88–Sp/Lang Path, City Sch of Decatur, **SLP**

Perry, Mrs Denise L Rural Free Delivery 1, Breezy Hill Road, St Johnsbury, VT 05819, (802) 748-5127, BA 73 Univ of NH; MS 74 Canisius Coll; MS 78 Ithaca Coll; 78–Aud, Robert Jauch MD, **A**

Perry, Dennis Robert 212 West John Beers Road, Stevensville, MI 49127, (616) 429-1989, BA Central MI Univ; MA 82 Central MI Univ; 88–Sp-Lang Path, Perry's Speech Svcs, **SLP**

Perry, Mrs Donna Marie 212 West John Beers Road, Stevensville, MI 49127, (616) 429-1989, BS 79 Trenton St Coll; MA 81 Central MI Univ; Sp-Lang Path, Perry's Speech Services, **SLP**

Perry, Isabelle 4 Sarah Drive, Princeton Junction, NJ 08550, (609) 275-6936, BA 74 Elmira Coll; MS 75 Univ of MI - Ann Arbor; 87–Sp-Lang Path, Cranbury Bd of Ed, **SLP ACE**

Perry, Jana Timm 22 West Pinehurst Circle #103, Glendale Heights, IL 60139, (312) 620-4433, BS 83 Northwestern Univ; MA 84 Northwestern Univ; 86–Aud, DuPage Easter Seal Rosalie Dold Ctr for Children, **A**

Perry, Julie 830 Oak Street #C, Brockton, MA 02401, (508) 583-2290, BS 80 Northeastern Univ; ME 82 Northeastern Univ; Aud, ENT Specialists Inc, **A**

Perry, June A 580 West Ravenswood Circle, Waukesha, WI 53186, (414) 475-8137, BS 44 Univ of WI - Milwaukee; ME 47 Univ of WI - Milwaukee; Lecturer Dept Sp-Lang Path, Univ of WI, **SLP A**

Perry, Karen F 2672 Beacon Hill Drive, Apartment 102, Auburn Hills, MI 48057, (313) 762-2362, BS 75 Boston Univ; MA 76 Wayne St Univ; Dir of Sp & Hrng, McLaren Gen Hosp, **SLP ACE**

Perry, Karen Sue 117 Richland Drive West, Mandeville, LA 70448, (504) 897-8563, BA 74 Univ of Northern IA; MA 75 Univ of Northern IA; SLP, Touro Inf, **SLP**

Perry, Linda Gail P O Box 91, Cleveland Street, Taylor, AR 71861-0091, (501) 694-5681, OB 82 Southern AR Univ; BA 85 LA Tech Univ; MA 87 LA Tech Univ; **SLP**

Perry, Maureen Mooney 7301 East Papago Drive, Scottsdale, AZ 85257, (602) 994-0252, BS 80 Marquette Univ; MS 82 AZ St Univ; Sp/Lang Path, Scottsdale Sch Dist, **SLP**

Perry, Mrs Natalie Colleen 854 West Spring Meadow Ct, Edgewood, MD 21040, (301) 676-4489, MS 84 Loyola Coll; Sp-Lang Path, Harford Co Pub Sch, **SLP**

Perry, Mrs Pamela J 127 Westwood Drive, Park Forest, IL 60466, (312) 748-5800, BA 76 Governors St Univ; MS 80 Governors St Univ; 83–Sp-Lang Path, Rich Twsp High Sch Dist #227, **SLP**

Perry, Paul J 2519 13th Avenue South, Great Falls, MT 59405, (406) 727-3115, BA 68 Univ of MT; MS 69 Univ of WI - Madison; Aud, Montana Med Aud, **A**

Perry, Mrs Ruthie L 11644 Captain Rhett Lane, Fairfax, VA 22039, BA 67 CA St Univ - Los Angeles; MA 69 CA St Univ - Los Angeles; Sp-Lang Path, Accotink Academy, **SLP**

Perry, Mrs Susan M 8444 Capricorn Way Apt 18, San Diego, CA 92126, (619) 297-4145, BS 84 Kent St Univ; MA 85 Kent St Univ; **A**

Perry, Mrs Susan Saulters 1010 North 29th Avenue, Hattiesburg, MS 39401, (601) 268-6561, BS 81 Univ Southern MS-Hattiesburg; MS 87 Univ Southern MS-Hattiesburg; 88–Sp-Lang Path, Lamar Co Schs, **SLP**

Perry, Terri Lynn 217-D Bull Run, Norman, OK 73071, (405) 364-9988, BA 83 Univ of OK - Norman; MS 85 Univ of OK Medical Center; 88–Sp-Lang Path, Norman PS, **SLP**

Perry, Dr William D 805 Virginia Avenue, Suite 27, Fort Pierce, FL 33482, (305) 464-4243, BA 65 LA St Univ - Baton Rouge; MS 67 6573; PH 70 (NS) Univ of FL; **A**

Perryman, Hugh Bryant 3708 Grier Avenue, Columbus, GA 31909, (404) 324-5661, ME 85 Columbus Coll; 82–Sp-Lang Path, Muscogee Co Sch Dist, **SLP**

Perry-Wilock, Linda L 7251 Emerson Avenue, Westminster, CA 92683, (714) 893-6571, BA 73 CA St Univ - Northridge; MA 75 CA St Univ - Northridge; Sp-Lang Path, Marina Hs, **SLP**

Perschetz, Babs H 176 East 77th Street #8F, New York, NY 10021, (212) 879-6630, BA 76 Univ of MD - College Park; MA 78 NY Univ; Aud, Carlyle Lab Inc, **A**

Perschon, Nancy 5527 West Agatite, Chicago, IL 60630, (312) 545-3620, OB 85 Univ of WI - Whitewater; MS 86 Univ of WI - Whitewater; 87–Sp-Lang Path, Schiller Park Sch Dist #81, **SLP**

Persell, Evelyn S 117 East 51st Street, San Bernardino, CA 92404, (714) 874-1127, BA 62 Univ of CT; MA 64 Stanford Univ; SLP, County of San Bernardino, **SLP**

Persenaire, L Ann 103-3 Chancery Court, Louisville, KY 40222, (812) 284-2626, BS 86 Northwestern Univ; MA 87 Northwestern Univ; 87–Aud, Louisville Hrng Aid Ctr, **A**

Pershey, Monica Gordon 116 Nesmith Street #4, Lowell, MA 01852, (617) 937-7283, BA 78 Cleveland St Univ; MA 85 Montclair St Coll; Sp-Lang Path, Methuen PS, **SLP**

Persiani, Mrs Nancy Hank 630 Kirkshire Drive, Perrysburg, OH 43551, (419) 874-6149, BS 78 Bowling Green St Univ; MA 79 Bowling Green St Univ; Sp-Lang Path, Toldeo Hrng & Sp Cen, **SLP**

Persico, Dena 143 Adelaide Road, Manchester, CT 06040, (203) 647-3487, BA 81 Univ of CT; MA 83 Univ of CT; SLP, Manchester Pub Sch Sys, **SLP**

Person, Beth A 5807 Warm Springs, Houston, TX 77035, BS 64 Southwest TX St Univ; ME 76 Stephen F Austin St Univ; MA 81 Univ of Houston - Univ Park; Spec Ed Coord, Stafford Msd, **SLP**

Person, Dr Carolyn J 1976 Cedar Avenue, Bronx, NY 10453, (212) 617-6707, **SLP**

Person, Cheryl L 8348 Traford Lane Suite 302, Springfield, VA 22152, (703) 451-5880, BS 73 Miami Univ - Oxford; MA 78 Univ of Cincinnati; Sp-Lang Path, Private Practice, **SLP ACE**

Person, J Brayton 4395 East Orchard Drive, Tucson, AZ 85712, (602) 325-4427, **SLP A**

Person, Joanne Tierney 725 Wagner Road, Glenview, IL 60025, (312) 729-2740, **SLP**

Pertile, Traci Lee Springdale ENT & Hearing Clin, 713 Quandt Avenue, Springdale, AR 72764, (501) 750-2080, MS 87 Univ of OK Medical Center; 87–Aud, Springdale ENT & Hrng Cl, **A**

Perttula, Betty S 501 Orizaba Avenue, Long Beach, CA 90814, (714) 581-2800, BA 78 CA St Univ - Long Beach; MA 81 CA St Univ - Long Beach; Sp-Lang Path, Private Practice, **SLP**

Perugino, Melissa C 2309 South Irvington, Tulsa, OK 74114, (918) 486-3675, BA 75 Montclair St Coll; MA 78 Univ of Tulsa; Sp-Lang Path, Coweta Public Schools, **SLP**

Perz, Catherine 3818 Shenandoah Drive, Crystal Lake, IL 60014, (815) 344-3954, BA 75 Eastern IL Univ; MS 76 Eastern IL Univ; Sp-Lang Path, McHenry Co Spec Ed Dist, **SLP**

Pesavento-Braun, Gail Jean 14715 Hoya Court, Houston, TX 77070, (713) 320-9471, BS 82 Univ of IL - Urbana; MA 84 Univ of Houston - Univ Park; Sp-Lang Path, Assoc Speech Lang Learning Inc, **SLP**

Pescevich, Lucille M 884 Country Club Road, Bridgewater, NJ 08807, (201) 725-5389, BA 57 CUNY - Hunter Coll; MS 80 William Paterson Coll; Sp/Lang Path, Private Practice, **SLP ACE**

Peschong, Elizabeth Johns 1228 Albany Drive, Bismarck, ND 58501, (701) 258-1503, BS 79 Northern St Coll; MS 82 Moorhead St Univ; 88–Sp-Lang Path, Mandan Sch Dist, **SLP**

Pesek, Mrs Elizabeth Ann 3645 South Libal, Green Bay, WI 54301, (414) 337-9988, BS 81 Univ of WI - Madison; MS 83 Univ of WI - Madison; Sp-Lang Path, Green Bay Area PS, **SLP**

Pesetski, Loretta S 49677 Stillmeadow Lane, Oakhurst, CA 93644, (805) 683-4842, BA 70 CA St Univ - Long Beach; MA 74 CA St Univ - Los Angeles; 84–Sp-Lang Path, Madera Co Supt of Schs, **SLP ACE**

Peshel, Mrs Cynthia A 15360 Strader Road, East Liverpool, OH 43920, (216) 385-7200, BS 78 Kent St Univ; MA 78 Kent St Univ; Sp-Lang Path, East Liverpool City Hosp, **SLP ACE**

Pesick, Paul I 5115 Bantry Drive, West Bloomfield, MI 48322, (313) 644-9300, BS 65 Eastern MI Univ; MA 67 Eastern MI Univ; 69–Sp-Lang Path, Private Practice, **SLP**

Pessis, Michelle G 370 Carriage Way, Deerfield, IL 60015, (312) 945-5187, BS 74 Northern IL Univ - De Kalb; MS 75 Univ of WI - Madison; Private Practice, **SLP**

Pessis, Paul 370 Carriage Way, Deerfield, IL 60015, (312) 433-5555, BS 74 Northern IL Univ - De Kalb; MS 75 Univ of WI - Madison; 76–Aud-Dir, Northshore Audio-Vestibular La, **A**

Pesti, Emily Conrad 8947 Centerway Road, Gaithersburg, MD 20879, (301) 840-1577, BA 71 Univ of MD - College Park; MA 74 Univ of MD - College Park; 75–Sp-Lang Path, Mont Co Pub Sch, **SLP**

Pestone, Robin Ross 12324 Chalford Lane, Bowie, MD 20715, (301) 593-5237, BA 73 Catholic Univ of America; MS 75 Gallaudet Coll; Aud, Mont Co Hlth Dept, **A**

Pestrong, V Monica 1764 Marco Polo Way, Burlingame, CA 94010, (415) 697-8924, MA 63 Stanford Univ; Dir/Sp-Lang Path Dept, Easter Seal Society-San Mateo, **SLP**

Peter, Frederick F 1057 North Colling Road, Caro, MI 48723, (517) 673-7224, BS 74 Central MI Univ; MA 81 Central MI Univ; Sp-Lang Path, Caro Comm Schs, **SLP**

Peter, Judith Herz 5 Swallow Lane, Huntington, NY 11743, (212) 920-9722, BA 75 CUNY - City College; MA 77 CUNY - City College; Aud, Misericordia Hosp, **A**

Peter, Laurie Ann 8552 California Avenue, Whittier, CA 90605, (213) 693-8383, 88 Whittier Coll

Peter, Mrs Marcia J R 3 Independence Drive, East Brunswick, NJ 08816, (201) 257-8300, BA 74 Rutger's St Univ - Douglas Coll; MA 77 Trenton St Coll; Sp-Lang Path, E Brunswick Pub Sch, **SLP ACE**

Peter, Tracy A 990 Foxcroft, Grand Island, NY 14072, (716) 773-2472, BS 86 SUNY - Coll at Fredonia; MS 87 SUNY - Coll at Fredonia; 88–Sp-Lang Path, DeGraff Mem Hosp, **SLP**

Peterein, Judy Lynne 6047 Grand Marnier, St Louis, MO 63129, (314) 362-7489, MS 83 Central MO St Univ; Audiologist, Washington U School of Med, **A**

Peterman, Cheryl Stewart 105 Newcombe Court, Dothan, AL 36301, (205) 793-6163, SLP, Sp & Lang Cntr, **SLP**

Peterman, Mrs Vicki Vaughn R R #3 Box 60-B, Sherman, IL 62684, (217) 525-3000, BS 84 Western IL Univ; MA 85 Western IL Univ; Sp-Lang Path, Springfield School Dist 186, **SLP**

Petermann, Mrs Patricia Marie Allenmore Medical Center, South 19th & Union #B2007, Tacoma, WA 98405, (206) 272-7614, BS 82 Bradley Univ; MS 85 Univ of HI - Manoa; 87–Aud, Drs Ritchie Spangler & Prewitt, **A**

Peters, Adrienne K 3803 Irvington Avenue, Miami, FL 33133, ME 76 Univ of FL; 87–Sp-Lang Path, Private Practice, **SLP**

Peters, Mrs Alice A 2611 Interlachen Drive, Stillwater, MN 55082, (612) 439-5160, BS 68 Univ of MN - Minneap-St Paul; MA 70 Univ of MN - Minneap-St Paul; Sp-Lang Path, ISD #834 Stillwater, **SLP**

Peters, Alma D Therapy Associates, 1516 West Mequon Road, Mequon, WI 53092, (414) 241-4240, BS 75 Marquette Univ; MS 76 Marquette Univ; Reg VP, Therapy Associates, **SLP**

Peters, Mrs Anne Hains 1502 Lucerne Terrace, Orlando, FL 32806, (407) 841-3620, BA 77 Univ of Central FL; MA 78 Univ of TN - Knoxville; Aud, Anne Hains Peters MA, **A ACE**

Peters, Barbara C 315 Spring Drive, Huddleston, VA 24104, (703) 981-2867, BS 77 Radford Univ; MS 81 Radford Univ; Sp-Lang Path, Private Practice, **SLP**

Peters, Mrs Becky S 2631 South Longmore, Mesa, AZ 85202, (602) 839-7160, BA 79 Univ of Northern IA; MA 81 Univ of Northern IA; Sp/Lang Path, Tempe Elem Dist, **SLP**

Peters, Brenda W 718-2 Zlotkin Circle, Freehold, NJ 07728, (201) 409-2977, BA 82 Univ of NC - Chapel Hill; MS 84 Univ of NC - Chapel Hill; 86–Sp-Lang Path, Private Practice, **SLP**

Peters, Mrs Cathy W 312 Tutwiler Drive, Trussville, AL 35173-1248, (205) 655-8429, BS 77 Univ of Montevallo; MS 78 Univ of Montevallo; Sp-Lang Path, Jeff Co Bd of Ed, **SLP**

Peters, Cindy L 1250 South Harbor City Boulevard, Melbourne, FL 32901, (407) 676-1431, BS 84 Southwest MO St Univ; MA 86 Southwest MO St Univ; 86–Sp-Lang Path, Brevard Sp & Lang Ctr, **SLP**

Peters, Colleen Kay 8905 West 4th Avenue, Lakewood, CO 80226, (303) 279-1571, BA 71 Univ of Northern CO; MA 72 Univ of Northern CO; SLP, Jefferson Co Schs, **SLP**

Peters, Debra N 136 South Highland, New Ulm, MN 56073, (507) 794-7905, BS 80 Univ of MN - Minneap-St Paul; MA 81 Univ of MN - Minneap-St Paul; Sp-Lang Path, Public Schools District 88, **SLP**

Peters, Donna Lee 1424 Bishop, Grosse Pointe Park, MI 48230, (313) 469-4406, BA 85 Loyola Coll; MS 87 Loyola Coll; 87–Sp-Lang Path, Samaritan Health Ctr, **SLP**

Peters, Dorothy M Research Center, PO Box 1111, Osprey, FL 34229, (813) 966-5497, BS 38 Syracuse Univ; MA 54 Case Western Reserve Univ; ED 64 Wayne St Univ; Sp-Lang Path, Self Employed-Research Center, **SLP LM**

Peters, Elaine Claire 2322 Turner Lane, Bel Air, MD 21014, (301) 396-6994, BA 81 Towson St Univ; MS 83 Purdue Univ - West Lafayette; Audiologist, Baltimore City Public Schools, **A**

Peters, Ellen B 420 Flicker Drive, Fort Collins, CO 80526, (303) 482-7420, BS 54 Coll of William & Mary; MS 65 CO St Univ; SLP, Poudre R-1 Sch Dist, **SLP**

Peters, Felicia A 1011 New Hope Street #67A, Norristown, PA 19401, (215) 272-7793, BS 85 Bloomsburg Univ of PA; MS 86 Bloomsburg Univ of PA; **SLP**

Peters, Dr Gilmour M 48660 Chambury Court, Allen Park, MI 48170, (313) 562-6000, BS 65 Eastern MI Univ; MS 66 Univ of MI - Ann Arbor; PH 74 (NS) Wayne St Univ; Aud Superv, VA Med Cen, **SLP A**

Peters, Mrs Harriet J 1827 South Armstrong St, Bartlesville, OK 74003, (918) 336-1218, BA 52 Wichita St Univ; Sp-Lang Path, Bartlesville Public Schools, **SLP**

Peters, Mrs Heidi Sawall 324 West Pleasant Hill, Palatine, IL 60067, (312) 358-3824, BS 85 Baylor Univ; MA 87 Northwestern Univ; 88–Sp-Lang Path, NW Suburban Special Educ Org, **SLP**

Peters, James L 2881 Eisenhower Parkway, Ann Arbor, MI 48104, **SLP**

Peters, Jane Marie 3226 Via Ensenada, San Luis Obispo, CA 93401-6966, (805) 543-1248, BA 79 CA St Univ - Stanislaus; MA 81 CA St Univ - Stanislaus; Sp-Lang Path, Pam Suess & Assoc, **SLP**

Peters, Mrs Janet A 52 Glocester Road, Massapequa, NY 11758, (516) 798-6362, BA 76 Adelphi Univ; MS 78 Adelphi Univ; 77–Sp-Lang Path, Massapequa School District 23, **SLP**

Peters, Jo E 4724 Davenport #9, Omaha, NE 68132, (402) 498-6672, BA 73 OK St Univ; MS 76 Purdue Univ - West Lafayette; Sp-Lang Path, Boys Town National I, **SLP**

Peters, Judy Woodall 407 Fox Hill Drive, Baiting Hollow, NY 11933, BA 82 Univ of NC - Chapel Hill; MS 86 Northeastern Univ; **SLP**

Peters, Mrs Kathleen M 1447 Hill Drive, Los Angeles, CA 90041, (213) 578-7062, BA 52 Univ of CA - Santa Barbara; MA 63 CA St Univ - Los Angeles; Sp-Lang Path, Pasadena City College, **SLP**

Peters, Kristine Louise 7354 East 75th Street, Tulsa, OK 74133, (418) 245-5911, BS 85 Univ of Tulsa; MA 87 Univ of Tulsa; 88–Sp-Lang Path, Dept of Human Services Hissom Mem Ctr, **SLP**

Peters, Dr Leslie J 3011 Rolling Green Drive, Churchville, MD 21028, (301) 278-5977, BA 68 Univ of FL; MA 73 Univ of FL; PH 86 (Industrial Aud); Aud, Human Engineering Lab US Army, **SLP A ACE**

Peters, Mrs Linda D 908 West Fulton, Seattle, WA 98119, (206) 282-8064, BA 63 Univ of WA; MA 71 Univ of WA; SLP, Northwest Speech & Hrng Center, **SLP**

Peters, Maryrita D 630 Michigan, Evanston, IL 60202, (312) 880-3430, BS 65 Marquette Univ; MS 67 Univ of MI - Ann Arbor; 78–Sp-Lang Path, Chldn Mem Hosp Dept Commun Dis, **SLP**

Peters, Maureen Ann 37 Pearl Street, Lewiston, ME 04240, (207) 345-3381, BS 74 Univ of ME - Farmington; MS 82 Univ of NH; 74–Sp-Lang Path, Mechanic Falls, **SLP**

Peters, Melissa R 5338 Williard Road, Oak Ridge, NC 27310, (919) 548-6075, BA 80 Univ of NC - Greensboro; ME 82 Univ of NC - Greensboro; Sp-Lang Path, Madison-Mayodan Cty Sch, **SLP**

Peters, Mrs Patricia Myers 3526 Penn Forest Blvd S W, Roanoke, VA 24018, (703) 982-3689, BS 76 Univ of VA - Charlottesville; ME 77 Univ of VA - Charlottesville; Sp-Lang Path, Rehab Serv of Roanoke, **SLP**

Peters, Regina C 1624 Dawnbreak, St Charles, MO 63303, (314) 947-3687, MA 78 Saint Louis Univ; MA 78 Saint Louis Univ; Sp-Lang Path, St Charles City Sch Dist, **SLP**

Peters, Robert M 1827 South Armstrong St, Bartlesville, OK 74003, (918) 336-1218, MA 63 Wichita St Univ; BA 46 Wichita St Univ; Retired, Bartlesville Public Schools, **SLP LM**

Peters, Robert W Div Speech & Hearing Sciences, Univ Of North Carolina, Chapel Hill, NC 27514, (919) 966-1006, BA 48 Univ of MN - Minneap-St Paul; MA 50 OH St Univ; PH 53 OH St Univ; Prof Sp&Hrng, U of NC-Chapel Hill, **SLP A F LM**

Peters, Dr Theodore J Dept Communication Disorders, Univ Of WI-Eau Claire, Eau Claire, WI 54701, (715) 836-4841, BS 61 Western MI Univ; MA 64 Western MI Univ; PH 67 (NS) MI St Univ; Prof, U of WI-Eau Claire, **SLP**

Petersdorf, Susan Hewitt 9747 Broadmoor Drive, San Ramon, CA 94583, (415) 687-1700, BA 74 Univ of FL; ME 75 Univ of FL; Spec Day Cl Tchr, Mt Diablo USD, **SLP**

Petersen, Mrs Brenda D 1106 Penoak, Euless, TX 76040, (817) 565-2262, BA 67 Univ of North TX; MA 69 Univ of North TX; Instr/Superv, Univ of North Texas, **SLP A ACE**

Petersen, Christine Kay 404 Knollglen, Irvine, CA 92714, (714) 733-9480, **SLP**

Petersen, Mrs Cynthia A 920 Edgehill Drive, Johnstown, PA 15905, (814) 533-0949, BS 69 Edinboro Univ of PA; MS 71 PA St Univ - Univ Park; Sp-Lang Path, Lee Hosp, **SLP**

Petersen, David R 920 Edgehill Drive, Johnstown, PA 15905, (814) 255-5881, BS 65 Edinboro Univ of PA; ME 66 PA St Univ - Univ Park; Superv of Sp and Hrng Serv, Hiram G Andrews Rehab Cen, **SLP**

Petersen, Daylene Patricia 2312 Valley High Drive N W, Rochester, MN 55901, (608) 252-8414, BS 72 Univ of WI - LA Crosse; MS 83 Univ of WI - Madison; 88–Aud, Bud Freeman Hrng Aid Sales & Svc, **A**

Petersen, Donna L 93 Duryea Lane, Nanuet, NY 10954, (914) 623-3828, BA 74 SUNY - Coll at Cortland; MA 77 Hofstra Univ; Sp-Lang Path, Rockland Co BOCES, **SLP**

Petersen, Mrs Donna V 1938 Kenilworth Avenue, Wilmette, IL 60091, (312) 251-4909, BA 68 Northwestern Univ; MA 70 Northwestern Univ; Private Practice, **SLP**

Petersen, Eugenia Kay 1800 Watrous Avenue #54-J, Des Moines, IA 50315, (816) 271-7577, MA 82 Northeast MO St Univ; SLP, Heartland Hospital West, **SLP**

Petersen, Florence M 124 Colgate Avenue, Somerdale, NJ 08083, (215) 893-2462, BA 67 Temple Univ-Tyler Sch of Art; MA 69 Temple Univ-Tyler Sch of Art; Aud, Grad Hosp Phila Pa, **A**

Petersen, Mrs Jacqueline 3004 Raven, Iowa City, IA 52240, (319) 399-6701, BA 72 Northern IL Univ - De Kalb; MA 76 Univ of IA; SLP, Grant Wood AEA, **SLP**

Petersen, Kate 1254 North 4th Street, Fargo, ND 58102, (701) 234-5119, BS 75 Moorhead St Univ; MS 87 Moorhead St Univ; **SLP**

Petersen, Mary Lou 16th Street, Plum Island, Newbury, MA 01950, (508) 465-5995, BS 80 New Hampshire Coll; MA 82 Northeastern Univ; 88–Sp-Lang Path, Private Practice, **SLP**

Petersen, Mrs MaryJoan Donahue Box 763, Colstrip, MT 59323, (406) 748-3190, BS 77 SD St Univ; MA 87 Univ of SD - Vermillion; 78–Sp-Lang Path, Colstrip Sch Dist #19, **SLP**

Petersen, Mrs P Diane 5728 East Sharon Drive, Scottsdale, AZ 85254, (602) 255-3183, BS 65 OK St Univ; MA 67 IN Univ - Bloomington; Deputy Assoc Superintendent, Ariz Dept Ed, **SLP**

Petersen, Mrs Pam R 1189 4050 Road, Paonia, CO 81428, (303) 527-6290, BA 71; MS 83 CO St Univ; Aud, Private Practice, **A**

Petersen, Tracy Wesbrook 2428 Second Street S W, Cedar Rapids, IA 52404, (319) 364-9134, BS 82 Univ of IA; MA 85 Univ of IA; Sp-Lang Path, Grant Wood AEA, **SLP**

Peters-Johnson, Dr Cassandra 14928 Hydrus Road, Silver Spring, MD 20906, (301) 598-4495, ME 71 Northeastern Univ; MA 80 Howard Univ; PH 83 (NS) Howard Univ; 88–Supvr, Mont Co Pub Sch, **SLP**

Peterson, Alicia Ruth 280-H Patriot Lane, Williamsburg, VA 23185, (804) 565-3099, ME 84 Northeastern Univ; 88–Aud, Riverside Rehab Institute, **A**

Peterson, Ann Marie 6205 Castleton Street, Bakersfield, CA 93309, (805) 589-4242, BS 74 UT St Univ; MS 75 UT St Univ; SLP, Kern Co Supt of Schools, **SLP**

Peterson, Mrs Annamary Section Audiology #L5, Mayo Clinic, Rochester, MN 55905, (507) 284-2577, BA 66 Albion Coll; BA 66 Albion Coll; MA 68 Western MI Univ; Aud, Mayo Cl, **A**

Peterson, Anne K 260 Weldon, Redding, CA 96001, (916) 243-5282, BA 66 Univ of CA - Berkeley; MA 86 CA St Univ - Chico; 88–Sp-Lang Path, Shasta Co Ofc of Educ, **SLP**

Peterson, Belinda F 61 Bradford Way, West Berlin, NJ 08091, (609) 429-0010, BA 76 CA St Univ - Northridge; MA 80 Trenton St Coll; Sp-Lang Path, Bancroft Sch, **SLP**

Peterson, Mrs Beverly H 1429 Northwestern Road, Longmont, CO 80501, (303) 447-1010, MA 70 Univ of Northern CO; SLP, Boulder Valley Public Schools, **SLP**

Peterson, Mrs Carole W 3009 Walnut, Grand Forks, ND 58201, (701) 772-7189, BS 59 Minot St Univ; MS 66 Univ of ND; SLP, Grand Forks Pub Schs, **SLP**

Peterson, Catherine E 249 East Walnut Street, Oneida, NY 13421, (315) 363-9496, MS 87 Syracuse Univ; **SLP**

Peterson, Catherine H 8021 East Osborn Road, Apartment 209A, Scottsdale, AZ 85251, (602) 990-7781, BS 80 Northern IL Univ - De Kalb; MA 82 Northern IL Univ - De Kalb; 87–Dir Sp-Lang Path, Synergos Neurological Center, **SLP**

Peterson, Mrs Cathi S 1924 Norma Road N E, Tacoma, WA 98422, (206) 952-6602, BA 73 WA St Univ; OM 77 Univ of WA; Sp-Lang Path, Federal Way Sch Dist, **SLP**

Peterson, Mrs Colleen E Murphy 9522 Caboose Court, Columbia, MD 21045, (301) 328-2419, BS 82 Worcester St Coll; MS 86 Worcester St Coll; 87–Sp-Lang Path, MIEMSS, **SLP**

Peterson, Colleen O'Brien 134 Grover Lane, Walnut Creek, CA 94596, (415) 685-1962, BA 77 Holy Names Coll; MA 78 MI St Univ; Aud, Mt Diablo U S D, **A**

Peterson, Dr David D Audiology/Speech Pathology Service (126), Veterans Administration Medical Center, Temple, TX 76504, (817) 778-4811, BS 65 Bemidji St Univ; MA 69 Saint Cloud St Univ; PH 73 (NS) Univ of NM; Ch, Aud/SLP Serv, Olin E Teague Vets Cen, **SLP**

Peterson, Mrs Debby L 2 Bontecou Lane, New City, NY 10956, (914) 634-5225, BS 73 SUNY - Coll at Buffalo; MA 74 Univ of Denver; **SLP**

Peterson, Deborah Ann 1007 Washington Avenue SE #11C, Bemidji, MN 56601, (218) 759-2056, BS 85 Moorhead St Univ; MS 87 Moorhead St Univ; **SLP**

Peterson, Dennis A 306 7th Street Ext, Patterson Hgts, Beaver Falls, PA 15010, (412) 774-6494, BS 73 Indiana Univ of PA; MS 75 WV Univ; Aud, Private Practice, **A**

Peterson, Donna M 2152 Aspenwood Court, San Bernardino, CA 92404, (714) 884-9279, BA 71 Univ of NH; MS 72 PA St Univ - Univ Park; SLP, San Bernardino Cty USD, **SLP**

Peterson, Douglas Scott 4331 N E 24th Avenue, Portland, OR 97211, (503) 284-9505, BA 79 Univ of OR; MS 81 Portland St Univ; 88–Prog Mgr, Good Samaritan Hosp & Med Ctr, **SLP**

Peterson, Mrs Eileen M RFD 2 Box 227, Merrill Road, Freeport, ME 04032, (207) 865-4348, BS 73 Syracuse Univ; MS 74 Syracuse Univ; Aud, Gov Baxter Sch for Deaf, **A**

Peterson, Mrs Elizabeth R InSpeech Inc, 448 Oakmoor, Bay Village, OH 44140, (216) 892-1977, BS 78 Miami Univ - Oxford; MS 79 Miami Univ - Oxford; Area Client Rel Mgr, InSpeech Inc, **SLP**

Peterson, Mrs Gail A H 905 Southern View, Ada, OH 45810, (419) 634-9719, BS 73 Northern IL Univ - De Kalb; MA 74 Northern IL Univ - De Kalb; **SLP**

Peterson, Gwen 8411 N E 54th Street #17, Vancouver, WA 98662, (206) 254-7923, **SLP**

Peterson, Dr Harold A Hearing And Speech Center, University Of Tennessee, Knoxville, TN 37996, (615) 974-5451, BS 58 Minot St Univ; MA 62 Univ of IA; PH 67 (NS) Univ of IL - Urbana; Prof/De Aud&SLP&Dir/Sp Cen, U of TN, **SLP F**

Peterson, Harry J Gundersen Clinic Ltd, 1836 South Avenue, La Crosse, WI 54601, (608) 782-7300, BS 69 Univ of WI - Stevens Point; MS 71 Univ of WI - Stevens Point; Aud, Gunderson Cl Ltd, **A**

Peterson, Mrs Ila C , Wildrose, ND 58795, (701) 539-2251, BS 61 Minot St Univ; **SLP LM**

Peterson, Jacqueline Kay 787 Northeast 68th Terrace, Gladstone, MO 64118, (816) 468-5470, BS 84 Univ of NE - Lincoln; MA 86 Northeast MO St Univ; **SLP**

Peterson, Mrs Jane Carol 5507 Pine Harbor, Houston, TX 77066, BS 64 Univ of NE - Lincoln; MA 69 Univ of NE - Lincoln; Sp-Lang Path, Klein ISD, **SLP**

Peterson, Mrs Jane Long 3617 North Birchwood, Davenport, IA 52806, (319) 391-8850, BS 83 Univ of IA; MS 86 Southern CT St Univ; Sp-Lang Path, Easter Seals Foundation, **SLP**

Peterson, Jeanette Marie 601 North Weber #1, Marshfield, WI 54449, (715) 462-3900, MS 83 Univ of WI - River Falls; BS 81 Univ of WI - River Falls; SLP, Lac Courte Oreilles Sch Syst, **SLP**

Peterson, Joan M 243 N Cleveland-Massillon, Akron, OH 44313, (216) 452-5938, BS 76 West Chester Univ of PA; MA 78 Kent St Univ; Sp-Lang Path, Tri-County Easter Seal Soc, **SLP**

Peterson, John L Dept Communicative Disorders, University Of Wisconsin, 1975 Willow Drive, Madison, WI 53706, (608) 262-3951, BA 51 Grinnell Coll; MA 52 Case Western Reserve Univ; PH 59 (Aud) Northwestern Univ; 75–Prof, U of WI-Madison, **A**

Peterson, Julia Gail 2512-B North Gordon Court, Milwaukee, WI 53212, (414) 259-1414, BS 83 Marquette Univ; MS 85 Marquette Univ; Sp-Lang Path, Curative Rehab Cntr, **SLP**

Peterson, Julie Lynn 7215 Glenwood Avenue North, Olden Valley, MN 55427, (612) 544-3736, BS 80 Moorhead St Univ; MS 83 Moorhead St Univ; Sp-Lang Path, Methodist Hospital, **SLP**

Peterson, June M 3892 Delmont Avenue, Oakland, CA 94605, (415) 638-5906, MA 86 Univ of San Francisco; **SLP**

Peterson, Mrs Katherine Garity 6752 Conrad North West, Albuquerque, NM 87120, (505) 899-8119, BS 69 Mankato St Univ; MA 74 Northeast MO St Univ; Sp-Lang Path, Albuquerque PS, **SLP**

Peterson, Mrs Kathleen Evans 7858 East Pecos Lane, Scottsdale, AZ 85253, (602) 820-3910, BA 74 Adelphi Univ; MA 76 Univ of IL - Urbana; Aud, Aud & Hrng Aid Serv Inc, **A**

Peterson, Kathleen Q 142 Brandon Road, Baltimore, MD 21212, (301) 828-1441, BA 68 Univ of MD - College Park; MS 78 Loyola Coll; Sp-Lang Path, Ridge Sch Baltimore County, **SLP**

Peterson, Kathleen Shanahan 7002 Healy Road, Cheyenne, WY 82009, (307) 635-1802, BS 73 Univ of NE - Lincoln; MA 78 Univ of Northern CO; SLP, Laramie Co Sch Dist #1, **SLP**

Peterson, Mrs Kay E 3233 S W 10th Avenue #S, Portland, OR 97201, (503) 226-2120, BS 76 Univ of IL - Urbana; MS 78 Northern IL Univ - De Kalb; SLP, Clarkston Sch Dist, **SLP**

Peterson, Kimberly Jeanne 2001 Connecticut G-4, Joplin, MO 64804, (417) 782-0208, MA 88 Southwest MO St Univ; 88–Sp-Lang Path, Seneca PS

Peterson, Laura Ide c/o Mark E Peterson, C Co, 547 ENGR Bn, APO New York, NY 09175, BS 80 Southwest TX St Univ; MS 85 Univ of MO - Columbia; 86–Sp-Lang Path, Frankfurt HS, **SLP**

Peterson, Dr Laura N 2725 Rockbridge Road, Tyler, TX 75701, BS 75 SUNY - Coll at Geneseo; MA 76 SUNY - Coll at Geneseo; ED 85 (Psychological Develop) Univ of Rochester; 88–Sp-Lang Path, Tyler ISD, **SLP**

Peterson, Laurie Denning P O Box 235, Stanton, IA 51573, (712) 623-3488, BA 76 Kearney St Coll; MS 78 Kearney St Coll; SLP, Green V AEA #14, **SLP**

Peterson, Linda A 2101 Illinois Road, Northbrook, IL 60062, (312) 520-9850, BS 75 Univ of Tulsa; MS 76 Vanderbilt Univ; 84–Dir/Supportive Svcs, Excellcare Inc, **SLP ACE**

Peterson, Linda Ann 175 1/2 River Street, Waltham, MA 02154, (617) 485-0883, BS 83 Ithaca Coll; MA 84 Bowling Green St Univ; Sp-Lang Path, Kennedy Mem Hosp, **SLP**

Peterson, Linda B R R 1 Box 75, Milmine, IL 61855, (617) 358-2293, BS 64 Univ of IL - Urbana; MA 69 Univ of IA; Dir, Hear Better Inc, **SLP A**

Peterson, Mrs Linda Moyer 739 Virginia Street, El Segundo, CA 90245, (213) 640-0600, BA 82 CA St Univ - Northridge; MA 84 CA St Univ - Northridge; 88–Sp-Lang Path, Private Practice, **SLP**

Peterson, Lori Lee 1509 Goodbar Avenue, Memphis, TN 38104, (901) 278-5447, BA 80 Memphis St Univ; MA 82 Memphis St Univ; 88–Sp-Lang Path, Mid-South Sp Path Group, **SLP**

Peterson, Mrs Lynn J 1601 First Avenue, Sterling, IL 61081, (815) 625-0400, BA 79 Univ of WI - Oshkosh; MA 80 Northern IL Univ - De Kalb; Admin Dir SLP Aud, Comm Gen Hosp, **SLP ACE**

Peterson, Mrs Marshalita Sims 8506 Korea Drive, St Louis, MO 63130, (314) 569-8226, BA 78 Spelman Coll; MS 80 Fontbonne Coll; **SLP**

Peterson, Marty F 223 South 3rd Street, Sauk Rapids, MN 56379, (612) 252-0233, BA 78 Univ of ND; MA 79 Univ of NE - Lincoln; Aud, St Cloud ENT Cl Pa, **A**

Peterson, Mrs Mary B 1615 Ladd Street, Silver Spring, MD 20902, (301) 649-3668, BA 36 Syracuse Univ; MA 39 Columbia Univ Teachers Coll; **SLP LM**

Peterson, Mrs Mary McC Route 3, Mentor Road, Louisville, TN 37777, (615) 856-3004, BA 67 Univ of TN - Knoxville; MA 71 Univ of TN - Knoxville; Sp-Lang Path, Blount Co Sch, **SLP**

Peterson, Dr Miles E California State Univ/La, Dept Of Comm Disorders, 5151 State University Dr, Los Angeles, CA 90032, (206) 545-7400, BS 80 UT St Univ; MA 82 UT St Univ; PH 87 (Aud) Univ of WA; 87–Asst Prof, Calif State Univ/LA, **A ACE**

Peterson, Nancy E 180 South Yarmouth Road, Dennis, MA 02638, (617) 267-4730, BS 73 Emerson Coll; ME 74 Northeastern Univ; Aud, Boston Guild for Hoh, **A ACE**

Peterson, Nancy Marie 3433 McIvor Street, Eau Claire, WI 54701-0266, (715) 835-2238, BS 85 Univ of WI - River Falls; MA 86 Univ of MN - Duluth

Peterson, Nancy Mary 1075-D Court Drive, Duluth, GA 30136, (404) 279-0634, BS 82 SUNY - Coll at Buffalo; ME 84 SUNY - Coll at Buffalo; Sp-Lang Path, Gwinett Cty Public Schools, **SLP**

Peterson, Nina E 3226 129th NE, Bellevue, WA 98005, (206) 881-8116, ME 78 Univ of WA; OM 75 Univ of WA; Sp-Lang Path, Bellevue Public Schools, **SLP**

Peterson, Paula Smead 916 17th Street, Gothenburg, NE 69138, (308) 537-7178, BS 84 Univ of NE - Lincoln; MS 85 Univ of NE - Lincoln; 88–Sp-Lang Path, Gothenburg PS, **SLP**

Peterson, Perry Jo 550 East Fairbrook Court, Boise, ID 83706, **SLP**

Peterson, Mrs Roberta Kuhns 111 Ridgeway Street, East Stroudsburg, PA 18301, (717) 296-9261, BS 83 Bloomsburg Univ of PA; MS 84 Bloomsburg Univ of PA; Sp-Lang Path, Hd Injury Recovery Ctr, **SLP**

Peterson, Rochelle C 22640 Twyckingham, Southfield, MI 48034, (313) 354-3956, MS; **SLP**

Peterson, Rosanne B P O Box 232, Gilman, WI 54433, (715) 447-8653, BS 73; MS 74 Univ of WI - Eau Claire; 78–Sp-Lang Path, Gilman Area Sch, **SLP**

Peterson, Sally Ann Route 3 Box 98-A, River Falls, WI 54022, (612) 430-1972, BS 77 Univ of WI - River Falls; MS 84 Univ of WI - River Falls; Sp-Lang Path, River Ridge Rehab, **SLP**

Peterson, Sue Ellen Cox Eliza Street, Darlington, WI 53530, (608) 776-4021, Sp-Lang Path, Darlington School District, **SLP**

Peterson, Susan B 5165 Keith Drive, Richton Park, IL 60471, (312) 863-3803, BA 69 Univ of WI - Madison; MS 70 Univ of WI - Madison; 87–Admin, Seguin Svcs Inc, **SLP**

Peterson, Mrs Susan Evans Mid Valley Speech And Hrng Ctr, 950 Southwest 29th Avenue, Albany, OR 97321, (503) 926-8092, BS 79 Univ of NE - Lincoln; MS 84 UT St Univ; 88–Aud, Midvalley Sp Hrng Ctr, **A**

Peterson, Susan K 7003 Cedar Street, Wauwatosa, WI 53213, (414) 423-0585, BS 72 Univ of WI - Milwaukee; MS 75 Univ of WI - Milwaukee; Sp-Lang Path, Greendale Public Schools, **SLP**

Peterson, Susan Kathryn Apple Computer Incorporated, 20525 Mariani Avenue #38-I, Cupertino, CA 95014, (408) 973-4840, BS 87 Baylor Univ; MS 87 Baylor Univ; 87–Area Assoc, Apple Computer Inc

Peterson, Teri Kaminski 900 Pontiac Lane, Chanhassen, MN 55317, (612) 541-1844, BS 83 Moorhead St Univ; MS 85 Moorhead St Univ; Sp-Lang Path, Rehabilitation Specialists Inc, **SLP**

Peterson, Theodore L 1005 East 157th Street, Burnsville, MN 55337, (507) 663-0690, BS 70 Univ of MN - Duluth; MS 73 Saint Cloud St Univ; SLP, Northfield Pub Sch, **SLP**

Peterson, Wayne Charles R R 2 Box 302, 817 17th Street, Windom, MN 56101, (507) 831-4600, BA 69 Moorhead St Univ; MA 72 Mankato St Univ; MS 77 Moorhead St Univ; Sp-Lang Path, Ed Coop Serv Ut, **SLP**

Peterson-Combs, Mary E Comprehensive Audiologic Servs, 570 Ten Mile Road N E, Rockford, MI 49341, (616) 866-9540, BS 84 Western MI Univ; MA 86 Western MI Univ; 87–Aud, Comprehensive, **A**

Peterson-Falzone, Dr Sally J Center For Craniofacial Anomalies, 747-S Medical Sciences, Univ Of California, San Francisco, CA 94143-0442, (415) 476-2271, BS 64 Univ of IL - Urbana; MA 65 Univ of IL - Urbana; PH 71 (Sp Path) Univ of IA; Prof, U of CA, **SLP F ACE**

Peterson-Schroeder, Dr Janet M Westphalia Family And, Obstetrical Health Center, 105 South Willow, Westphalia, MI 48894, (517) 587-4899, BA 72 MI St Univ; MA 73 MI St Univ; OD 82 (NS) MI St Univ; Physician, Westphalia Family & Ob Hlth Ct, **SLP**

Petigna, Lucrezia E 7586 High Drive, Prairie Village, KS 66208, (816) 353-4616, BS 81 Univ of KS; MS 83 Central MO St Univ; 84–Sp/Lang Path, Consolidated Sch Dist #2, **SLP**

Petit, Marcia Yvette 4412 Elmsgrove Drive, Austin, TX 78721, (512) 926-3567, BS 84 Univ of North TX; MS 86 Univ of North TX; 87–Sp-Lang Path, Manor ISD

Petitte, Mrs Janet J 11 Lakeview Drive, Morgantown, WV 26505, (304) 293-4241, BS 73 WV Univ; MS 74 WV Univ; Clinical Supervisor, West Virginia University, **A**

Petiya, Nancy Philips 1055 S Miller Way, Lakewood, CO 80226, (303) 452-4139, BA 72 Columbia Univ Sch of Gen St; MA 84 Univ of CO - Boulder; **SLP**

Peton, Eileen D 1605 Littlejohn Circle Dr, Apartment 12, Council Bluffs, IA 51503, (712) 322-1109, BS 77 Univ of SD - Vermillion; MA 78 Univ of SD - Vermillion; Sp-Lang Path, AEA 13, **SLP**

Petote, Cynthia Anne 163 Wood Smoke Lane, Rochester, NY 14612, (716) 232-2310, BS 76 SUNY - Coll at Geneseo; MS 77 Nazareth Coll of Rochester

Petrarca, Marilyn A 19 Bev Circle, Cranston, RI 02920, (401) 943-6889, BS 74 Emerson Coll; MS 80 Univ of RI; Intinerant Sp-Lang Path, Warwick Sch Dept, **SLP**

Petras, Dru Anne 1311 West Henderson #2-W, Chicago, IL 60657, (219) 836-5800, OB 78 Millikin Univ; MS 81 IL St Univ - Normal; Aud, Hammond Cl, **A**

Petras, Mrs Gail E 321 South Leitch, La Grange, IL 60525-2164, (312) 780-2486, BS 76 Western IL Univ; MA 77 Western IL Univ; 77–Sp-Lang Path, Lyons Sch Dist #103, **SLP**

Petrash, Marian Elizabeth 130 Landon Road, Ithaca, NY 14850, (607) 753-1145, MS 87 Ithaca Coll

Petrauskas, Mrs Geralyn M 1531 Lighthouse Drive, Naperville, IL 60565, (312) 983-6485, BS 80 Miami Univ - Oxford; MA 81 Univ of IL - Urbana; Sp-Lang Path, Private Practice, **SLP**

Petrella, Christine Ann 457 North Eden Drive, Bolivar, OH 44612, (216) 874-3829, BA 82 OH St Univ; MA 83 OH St Univ; Sp-Lang Path, Stark Co Bd of Mr/Dd, **SLP**

Petrey, Susan L Rd 2 Box 88, Morgantown, PA 19543, (215) 378-6904, BS 76 Clarion Univ of PA; MA 79 Univ of FL; Aud, Reading Hospital & Medical Cen, **A**

Petri, Pamela S 6920 Galena Road, Bristol, IL 60512, (312) 859-1687, SLP, Kendall County Special Ed, **SLP**

Petric, Roberta Lands 3900 Laurel Lane, Bedford, TX 76021, (714) 831-7511, BA 73 Univ of Redlands; MS 77 Univ of Redlands; Pres, Petric & Assoc Inc, **SLP**

Petrini, Mary E T 3820 Old Pine Trail, Midland, MI 48640, (517) 631-8485, MS 76 Univ of MI - Ann Arbor; BA 74 Univ of MO - Columbia; Sp-Lang Path, Private Practice, **SLP**

Petro, Mrs Gail Lynn 923 Dunton Avenue, Arlington Height, IL 60004, (312) 358-5510, BS 81 Southern Methodist Univ; MA 83 Univ of IA; SLP, Little City Foundation, **SLP**

Petro, Geraldine South Hills Health System, Home Health Agency, 1800 West Street, Homestead, PA 15120, (412) 464-6006, BA 77 Univ of Pittsburgh - Pittsburgh; MA 79 Univ of Pittsburgh - Pittsburgh; Sp-Lang Path, South Hills Hlth Syst, **SLP**

Petronchak, Mrs Joann V 14 Park Place, Little Falls, NJ 07424, (201) 785-0823, BA 81 William Paterson Coll; MS 83 Columbia Univ Teachers Coll; 87–Sp/Lang Path, St Joseph's Hosp, **SLP**

Petronio, Mrs Martha Jo 5502 Stull Avenue, Orlando, FL 32810, (305) 897-1927, MS 78 Kent St Univ; SLP, Florida Hospital, **SLP**

Petrosino, Dr Linda A Dept Of Communicative Disorder, Bowling Green State Univ, Bowling Green, OH 43403, (419) 372-7165, BS 77 Ithaca Coll; MS 78 Ithaca Coll; PH 83 (Sp Path) OH Univ - Athens; Asst Prof, **SLP**

Petrov, Susan Ann 5244 Zurich Place N E, Albuquerque, NM 87111, (801) 485-9169, BS 74 857; MS 81 UT St Univ; Aud/Sp-Lang Path, Albuquerque Public Schools, **SLP A**

Petrovic, Mrs Kathleen K 7100 Williams Creek Drive, Indianapolis, IN 46240, MS 75 IN Univ - Bloomington; Sp-Lang Path, Rise Special Services, **SLP**

Petrovich, Mrs Leslie Kirchoff 201 South Anita Street, Suite 101, Orange, CA 92668, (714) 385-3560, BA 80 Central MI Univ; MA 81 Central MI Univ; 86–Owner, Ameri-Corp Speech & Hearing, **SLP**

Petrovich-Larwood, Lou Yvonne 571 Madrona Avenue, Felton, CA 95018, BA 83 San Jose St Univ; MA 86 San Jose St Univ; 86–Sp-Lang Path, Pajaro Valley USD

Petru, Mrs Janis Ann M 5918 South Kolmar, Chicago, IL 60629, (312) 354-5730, BA 79 Saint Xavier Coll; MS 80 Bradley Univ; Sp-Lang Path, Lagrange Area Dept of Spec Ed, **SLP**

Petrucci, Mary E 67 Fuller Street #2, Waltham, MA 02154, **SLP**

Petrucci-Coley, Teresa M 1752 Harold, Houston, TX 77098, (409) 762-6661, BA 79 MI St Univ; MA 80 Eastern MI Univ; Sp-Lang Path, Transitional Learning Comm, **SLP**

Petrucelli, Lauren A 49 Surplus Street, Duxbury, MA 02332, (617) 631-7718, BA 74 Univ of RI; MA 76 Catholic Univ of America; **SLP**

Petruk, Mrs Marilyn Harris 23 Morrison Court, Little Rock, AR 72212, (501) 371-2554, BA 76 Univ of AR - Fayetteville; MA 77 Univ of AR - Fayetteville; 88–Sp-Lang Path, Ark Presch Network, **SLP**

Petruzzelli, Mrs Patricia Graf 905 William Penn Court, Pittsburgh, PA 15221, (412) 941-4434, BA 83 Univ of MI - Ann Arbor; MS 86 Rush Univ

Petruzzi, Pia M 2 Liberty Street, Ossining, NY 10562, (914) 941-0606, BA 83 LA St Univ - Baton Rouge; MA 85 LA St Univ - Baton Rouge; Sp-Lang Path, N Westchester Ctr Spch Disords, **SLP**

Petry, Susan M 3013 Vista Street, Philadelphia, PA 19152, (215) 739-7381, BS 79 West Chester St Coll; MA 87 Temple Univ; 80–Sp-Lang Path, Sch Dist of Philadelphia, **SLP**

Petschauer, Mrs Rosemarie S 5921 69th Avenue, Ridgewood, NY 11385, (212) 374-7882, BA 79 CUNY - Queens Coll; MA 81 CUNY - Queens Coll; Aud, Gouverneur Hosp, **A**

Pettas, Dr Mary 31-85 Crescent Street, Long Island, NY 11106, (212) 932-3996, BA 41 CUNY - Queens Coll; MA 42 Columbia Univ Teachers Coll; PH 63 (NS) Univ of FL; Professor Emeritus, New York University, **SLP**

Pettijohn, Mrs Kathy A 1601 South I Street, Elwood, IN 46036, BS 68 IN St Univ - Terre Haute; MA 78 Ball St Univ; SLP, Arcadia Childrens Home, **SLP**

Pettijohn, Mrs Susan 29 Fulmar Drive, Voorhees, NJ 08043, (803) 572-1551, BA 78 Temple Univ-Tyler Sch of Art; MA 80 Temple Univ-Tyler Sch of Art; Sp-Lang Path, Charleston Sp & Hrng Cen Inc, **SLP**

Pettit, Alyse Edwards P O Box 215, Westport, CA 95488, (707) 964-1393, BA 74 Humboldt St Univ; MA 75 Humboldt St Univ; 86–Sp-Lang Path, Alyse Pettit MA CCC, **SLP**

Pettit, Betty C Elm Street, P O Box 63, Winterport, ME 04496, (207) 827-6091, BS 53 Univ of Cincinnati; MA 63 OH St Univ; Sp/Lang Path, Old Town Sch Dept, **SLP**

Pettit, Dr John M Conley Speech & Hearing Center, University Of Maine, Orono, ME 04473, (207) 581-2008, BS 58 Univ of IL - Urbana; MA 62 OH St Univ; PH 69 (Sp Path) Purdue Univ - West Lafayette; Prof/Coord Clinical Services, University of Maine, **SLP ACE**

Pettit, Reba R 361 East Mayes Street, Jackson, MS 39206, (601) 982-6317, BA 64 MS St Univ - MS State; MA 72 Memphis St Univ; Sp-Lang Path, Counciling/ A Growing Place, **SLP**

Petty, Sr Alice G 84 Junest, Worcester, MA 01602, (617) 852-5966, BA 58 Anna Maria Coll; ME 61 Boston Univ; Sp-Lang Path, Catholic Charities -Mercy Cen, **SLP**

Petty, Anne M 340 Via Vista Drive, Redlands, CA 92373, (714) 881-2535, BA 65 Univ of UT; MS 81 Univ of Redlands; Tchr Presch, San Bernadino Co Supt of Schs, **SLP**

Petty, Nancy A Petty Schrager & Winslow Pa, 6100 S W 34th Street, Miami, FL 33155, (305) 653-0351, BA 68 Southern Methodist Univ; MA 73 TX Tech Univ; Director/Sp-Lang Pathology, Miami Heart Institute, **SLP**

Pettygrove, Laura Ann 1270 Coronado #7, Sunnyvale, CA 94086, (415) 941-4010, BA 82 San Jose St Univ; MS 84 CO St Univ; 86–Sp-Lang Path, Los Altos Elem Sch Dist, **SLP**

Peura, Robin Elayne 337 Garcia Northeast, Albuquerque, NM 87123-1114, (505) 299-4424, BS 82 Bowling Green St Univ; MA 83 Bowling Green St Univ; Sp/Lang Path, Albuquerque Publ Sch, **SLP**

Pevey, Mrs Jo Rhea B 2023 Birch Ridge, Baton Rouge, LA 70816, (504) 275-7543, BS 71 Stephen F Austin St Univ; ME 73 Stephen F Austin St Univ; Sp-Lang Path, Private Practice, **SLP**

Pevsner, Janet H 441 North Lombard, Oak Park, IL 60302, (312) 622-4830, BS 78 Northern IL Univ - De Kalb; MA 79 Northern IL Univ - De Kalb; 83–Sp-Lang Path, Chicago Bd of Ed, **SLP**

Pex, Carol M 914 Beach Park Boulevard, Apartment 73, Foster City, CA 94404, (415) 573-4026, BA 73 Humboldt St Univ; MA 74 Humboldt St Univ; 76–SLP, San Mateo Co Sch, **SLP**

Peyser, Barbara Truax 219 Augusta, Oak Park, IL 60302, (312) 383-2592, BA 69 Univ of OK - Norman; MS 71 Univ of OK Medical Center; Sp-Lang Path, Private Practice, **SLP**

Peyton, Mrs Bonnie Neukircher 5101 51st Way, West Palm Beach, FL 33409, (305) 626-3676, BS 80 ND St Univ; MS 87 Mankato St Univ; **SLP**

Peyton, Eileen M 27 Pond Street, Amesbury, MA 01913, (617) 388-0822, BS 77 Univ of MA - Amherst; MS 79 Univ of MI - Ann Arbor; Dir Communicatn Disorders Dept, Whittier Rehabilitation Hosp, **SLP**

Peyton, Katharine Taylor 147 Dawn Lauren Lane, Tallahassee, FL 32301, (904) 681-5160, BS 80 FL St Univ; MS 81 FL St Univ; 85–Sp-Lang Path, Tallahassee Mem Reg Med Center, **SLP**

Pezzano, Mrs Diane B 1871 Meadowlark, Niles, OH 44446, (216) 392-4400, BS 68 Kent St Univ; ME 74 Kent St Univ; 84–Supervisor, Trumbull County Board of Educ, **SLP**

Pezzano, Garry Richard 6 Sherwood Terrace, Glendora, NJ 08029, (215) 783-6010, **SLP**

Pezzelle, Mrs Sheryl Sue 1047 South Toltec, Mesa, AZ 85204, (602) 831-0814, BA 77 David Lipscomb Coll; OM 84 AZ St Univ; SLP, Kyrene Sch Dist 28, **SLP**

Pezzo, Donna Lee 617 Whistler Drive, Rochester, PA 15074, (412) 941-4434, 88–Sp-Lang Path, Crossroads Sp & Hrng Inc, **SLP**

Pfaff, Kurt T 9723 Dellford Court, Burke, VA 22015, (703) 536-1666, BS 76 Univ of Tulsa; MA 77 Central MI Univ; Aud, Arlington Fairfax Hrng-Sp Cen, **A**

Pfahler, Mrs Lorene A 6175 St Andrews, Canfield, OH 44406, (216) 743-1151, BS 73 Bowling Green St Univ; MA 76 Kent St Univ; Sp-Lang Path, Youngstown Cty Sch, **SLP**

Pfalzgraf, Beth 13393 Southshore Drive, Apartment 307, Sterling Heights, MI 48077, (313) 288-8085, BS 78 WV Univ; MA 80 Wayne St Univ; Sp/Lang Path, William Beaumont Hosp, **SLP**

Pfannebecker, Annette Eleanor Baker Lane, South Deerfield, MA 01373, (413) 665-7950, BS 67 Wayne St Univ; MA 76 Univ of MA - Amherst; Sp/Lang Path, Amherst Sch Syst, **SLP**

Pfannenstiel, Mrs Gloria L Rt #2 P O Box 73-P, Chapman, KS 67431-9998, (913) 922-6996, BS 72 Fort Hays St Univ; MS 73 Fort Hays St Univ; Sp-Lang Path, Private Practice, **SLP**

Pfannenstiel, Mrs Karen Stinson 2443 West 229th Street, Torrance, CA 90501, (213) 515-3008, BA 62 Univ of CA - Los Angeles; Sp-Lang Path, Los Angeles Cty USD, **SLP**

Pfannenstiel, Michael C P O Box 312, Ness, KS 67560, (913) 798-3888, **SLP**

Pfau, Mrs Margaret Klym 715 Regan Street, Rockford, IL 61107, (815) 229-1100, BS 72 ND St Univ; MA 74 Univ of Northern CO; SLP, Rockford Pub Sch Dist 205, **SLP**

Pfeffer, Ellen B 287 Main Street, Millburn, NJ 07041, (212) 741-7678, BS 81 SUNY - Coll at Geneseo; MA 83 CUNY - Hunter Coll; Aud, NY League for the Hd of Hrng, **A**

Pfeffer, Mrs Lynette S 19261 Montgomery Village, Suite G21, Gaithersburg, MD 20879, MA 70 NY Univ; Private Practice, **SLP**

Pfeifer, Mrs Christina Hunter 3603 Lotus Drive, San Diego, CA 92106, (619) 277-1914, SLP, Muray Associates, **SLP**

Pfeifer, Helen K 8 Beechwood Drive, Hillsdale, NJ 07642, **SLP**

Pfeifer, Patricia Ann 2321 Mellow Court, Baltimore, MD 21209, (301) 486-3855, BS 80 PA St Univ - Univ Park; MS 85 Towson St Univ; 85–Sp-Lang Path, Howard County PS, **SLP**

Pfeifer, Dr Rosemary C 19 Newcomb Boulevard, New Orleans, LA 70118, (504) 865-7138, BS 49 Boston Coll; MA 50 Boston Univ; ED 58 (Sp-Lang Path) Boston Univ; **SLP**

Pfeiffer, Mrs Bonnie McClellan 541 Glenwood Street S W, North Canton, OH 44720, (216) 375-3883, BA 79 Univ of Akron; MA 83 Univ of Akron; 85–Sp-Lang Path, Akron City Hosp, **SLP**

Pfeiffer, Debra A P O Box 772248, Steamboat Springs, CO 80477, (303) 879-4236, BA 78 Southwest TX St Univ; ME 79 Southwest TX St Univ; Sp-Lang Path, Horizons for the Handicapped, **SLP**

Pfeiffer, Mrs Laya Alyssa 904 Seagirt Boulevard, Far Rockaway, NY 11691, (718) 327-2515, BA 85 CUNY - Queens Coll; MA 87 CUNY - Queens Coll; 88–Sp-Lang Path, Private Practice, **SLP**

Pfeiffer, Mary P 1537 West Wagner Drive, Gilbert, AZ 85234, (602) 892-7015, **SLP**

Pfeiffer, Rebecca Rupley 52 Liberty Terrace, Buffalo, NY 14215, (716) 827-9726, BS 77 Ithaca Coll; ME 81 SUNY - Coll at Buffalo; Sp-Lang Path, Olv Infant Home Nursery Sch, **SLP**

Pfeil-McGlynn, Mrs Marsha A 10 North Grandview Terrace, Voorheesville, NY 12186, (203) 777-1482, BS 80 SUNY - Coll at Brockport; MA 81 Bowling Green St Univ; Aud, New Haven Hrng Sp Cen, **A**

Pferdehirt, Evelyn R 587 Old Leechburg Road, Pittsburgh, PA 15239, (412) 795-0660, BS 75 Univ of Pittsburgh - Pittsburgh; MA 79 Univ of Pittsburgh - Pittsburgh; 79–Sp-Lang Path, Plum Borough Sch Dist, **SLP**

Pflieger, Eunice A 21990 King Arthurs Court, Brookfield, WI 53005, (414) 781-2710, BS 75 Univ of WI - Milwaukee; MS 76 Univ of WI - Milwaukee; Sp-Lang Path, Hamilton Sch Dist, **SLP**

Pflug-Maslowski, Mrs Susan I 2530 North 88th Street, Wauwatosa, WI 53226, (414) 258-7972, BS 77 Marquette Univ; MS 78 Marquette Univ; **SLP**

Pfohl, Ann Marie Catherine 222 Fancher Avenue, Buffalo, NY 14223-1821, (716) 833-3807, MA 88 SUNY - Center at Buffalo

Pfrang, Mrs Cynthia L 1422 North Ambrosia, Mesa, AZ 85205, (602) 833-5566, BS 77 Univ of WI - Stevens Point; MS 78 Univ of WI - Milwaukee; Sp-Lang Path, Mesa Public Schools, **SLP**

Phares, Mrs Georgette Statham 304 Jerome Drive, Hammond, LA 70403, (504) 345-8912, OM 86 LA St Univ - N O Medical Ctr; 86–Sp-Lang Path, CM Fagan Special Svc Ctr, **SLP**

Phares, Mrs Meredith M 1637 Burnside Avenue, Hagerstown, MD 21740, (301) 842-2211, MS 78 Towson St Univ; Sp/Lang Path, Bd of Ed-Wash Co, **SLP**

Phares, T Michael Victor Cullen Center, 6000 Cullen Drive, Sabillasville, MD 21780, (301) 241-3131, MS 78 Towson St Univ; Sp-Lang Path, State of Maryland, **SLP**

Pharo, William R Melbourne Ear Clinic, 1208 S Harbor City Blvd, Melbourne, FL 32901, (305) 722-0955, BS 76 FL St Univ; MS 77 FL St Univ; Aud, Melbourne Ear Cl, **A**

Phatate, Dr Darlynne Devenny 70 West 95th Street #27A, New York, NY 10025, BA 64 Univ of British Columbia; MS 68 McGill Univ - Quebec; PH 87 (NS) CUNY - City College; 88–Psych, NY State Inst for Basic Res, **SLP A**

Phelan, Anna M 7618 Farmgate Way, Citrus Heights, CA 95610, (916) 624-3502, MA 71 CA St Univ - Sacramento; Coordinator of Instruction, North Sacramento School Dist, **SLP**

Phelan, Charlene A 38 Park Vista Circle, Sacramento, CA 95831, (707) 446-6991, BS 76 Univ of IA; MA 78 Univ of IA; 79–Sp-Lang Path, Solano Co Supt of Schs, **SLP**

Phelan, Mrs Elizabeth L 2445 Long Avenue, Beaumont, TX 77702, (409) 899-4099, BS 70 LA St Univ - Baton Rouge; MA 71 Baylor Univ; 74–Sp-Lang Path, Sp & Lang Assoc Inc, **SLP**

Phelan, James G 2261 North Street, Beaumont, TX 77701, (409) 832-9421, OB 71 Lamar Univ; MA 84 Lamar Univ; 83–Pres/Aud, Phelan Hearing Aid Center, **A**

Phelan, Katherine A 221 Mile Creek Road, Old Lyme, CT 06371, **SLP**

Phelan, Mark Dufner 2261 North Street, Beaumont, TX 77701, (409) 832-9421, BS 80 Lamar Univ; MS 83 Lamar Univ; 83–Aud, Phelan Hearing Aid Ctr

Phelan, Mrs Shannon B 8725 Gowan Court, Redwood Valley, CA 95470, (707) 485-8875, BA 77 CA St Univ - Chico; MA 81 CA St Univ - Chico; 88–Sp-Lang Path, Susan Pollesel Sp Pathology Inc, **SLP**

Phelan-Latimer, Mrs Barbara K 8418 Bud King Road, Knoxville, TN 37920, (615) 573-2778, BS 78 Boston Univ; MS 80 PA St Univ - Univ Park; 88–Sp-Lang Path, Blount County Sch Sys, **SLP**

Phelps, Bridgit Helene 3301 South Creek Drive S E, #202, Kentwood, MI 49508, (616) 940-6065, BA 86 MI St Univ; MA 87 MI St Univ

Phelps, Mrs Cathen H 29489 Via Las Colinas #128, Temecula, CA 92390, (619) 485-8490, BS 83 Pacific Union Coll; MA 85 San Diego St Univ; 86–Sp-Lang Path, Sp Hrng & Neurosensory Ctr, **SLP**

Phelps, Mrs E Patrice 432 Princeton Way N E, Atlanta, GA 30307, (404) 296-7101, BA 77 Univ of MS; ME 83 GA St Univ; OM 78 Univ of MS; Presch Classroom Tchr, Atlanta Area Sch for Deaf, **SLP**

Phelps, Mrs Elizabeth Waller 11932 Cherry Street, Los Alamitos, CA 90720, (213) 861-2891, BS 70 IN Univ - Bloomington; MA 72 Ball St Univ; Sp-Lang Path, Los Angeles County Bd of Educ, **SLP**

Phelps, Gail Z 12812 West 55th Street, Shawnee, KS 66216, (913) 631-0404, BA 78 Univ of IA; MA 80 Univ of KS; Sp-Lang Path, Private Practice, **SLP**

Phelps, Laura Beth 420 Ruddiman Road, North Muskegon, MI 49445, **A**

Phelps, Mrs Mary Anderson 12140 Whispering Woods Dr, Dunlap, IL 61525, (309) 243-5193, OB 59 Southeast MO St Univ; MS 65 Univ of IL - Urbana; **SLP**

Phelps, Mrs Pamela Bernadette 1842 Oak Bluff Way, Sacramento, CA 95833-1508, (916) 925-8437, BA 81 CA St Univ - Stanislaus; MS 87 CA St Univ - Sacramento; 86–Aud, Woodland Hearing Aid Services, **A**

Phelps, Richard Allan 827 East 25th, McMinnville, OR 97128-2236, (503) 472-7901, PH (NS); **SLP**

Phelps-Lindsay, Lucy 101 Norwalk Court, Vacaville, CA 95687, (707) 446-6858, BS 76 IN Univ - Bloomington; OM 77 IN Univ - Bloomington; Sp-Lang Path, Solano Co Supt Sch, **SLP**

Phifer, Mrs Cynthia Ann 799 Sandra Lane, Norristown, PA 19403, (215) 270-2400, BS 81 Bloomsburg Univ of PA; MS 82 Bloomsburg Univ of PA; 86–Dir of Sp-Lang Path, Montgomery Hosp, **SLP ACE**

Philbin, Erin Declan 2039 Noble Street, Pittsburgh, PA 15218, (412) 941-4434, BS 84 Marywood Coll; MA 86 Univ of Pittsburgh - Pittsburgh; **SLP**

Philip, Beverly Siegel 55 Sierra Court, Hillsdale, NJ 07642, (201) 666-0105, BA 57 CUNY - Brooklyn Coll; MS 60 Purdue Univ - West Lafayette; 80–SLP, Allendale Bd of Educ, **SLP**

Philips, Dr Betty Jane 227 North 118th Street, Omaha, NE 68154, (402) 498-6680, BS 46 CA Univ of PA; ME 47 PA St Univ - Univ Park; ED 51 (Sp Path) PA St Univ - Univ Park; Dir-Spec Cl Prog, Boys Twn Natl Inst, **SLP F ACE**

Phillabaum, Leeann Sue 102 Graceford Drive, Aberdeen, MD 21001, (301) 272-0306, BS 86 Towson St Univ; MS 88 Towson St Univ; 88–Aud, Towson State Univ

Phillips, Anne H Route 5 Box 401, Warrenton, VA 22186, (703) 347-3201, BA 78 Boston Coll; MA 79 George Washington Univ; Sp/Lang Path, Fauquier Co Pub Sch, **SLP**

Phillips, Mrs Arlene 10 Monroe Boulevard, Long Beach, NY 11561, (516) 889-9794, BA 62 CUNY - Brooklyn Coll; MS 65 CUNY - Brooklyn Coll; Private Practice, **SLP**

Phillips, Brenda Beck 921 Redwood Drive, Forrest City, AR 72335, (501) 633-5266, BS 74 AR St Univ; MS 85 AR St Univ; 85–Sp-Lang Path, St Francis Area Develop Ctr, **SLP**

Phillips, Carol Halpert 291 School Street, West Hempstead, NY 11552, (516) 485-6457, BA 78 CUNY - Queens Coll; MS 80 Adelphi Univ; 88–Sp-Lang Path, Ltle Village Sch Dev Dis Chldn, **SLP**

Phillips, Carol Marie 1919 South Wolf Road #314, Hillside, IL 60162, (312) 455-5299, BS 81 Northern IL Univ - De Kalb; MA 83 Northern IL Univ - De Kalb; MA 88 Northeastern IL Univ; Sp-Lang Path, InSpeech Inc, **SLP**

Phillips, Cathy Sue Hawkins 8613 East 106th Street S, Tulsa, OK 74133, (918) 369-1595, Sp-Lang Path, Tulsa Rehabilitation Center, **SLP**

Phillips, Dana M P O Box 111365, Pittsburgh, PA 15238, BS 66 Univ of MI - Ann Arbor; MS 67 Univ of MI - Ann Arbor; OM 84 Northwestern Univ; Prog Ofcr, Heinz Endowments, **SLP**

Phillips, Daniel E 412 Cliff Place, Homewood, AL 35209, (205) 226-8117, BA 73 Auburn Univ - Auburn; MA 75 Memphis St Univ; Dir/Sp-Hrng Cl, Lakeshore Birm Rehab Ctr, **SLP**

Phillips, Dena A 59585 Longbow Drive, Mishawaka, IN 46544, (219) 282-4128, BA 68 IN Univ - Bloomington; MA 73 IN Univ - Bloomington; Sp-Lang Path, S Bend Comm Sch Corp, **SLP**

Phillips, Dorothy C 4607A Kahala Avenue, Honolulu, HI 96816, BA 60 Univ of IL - Urbana; ME 63 Boston Univ; **SLP**

Phillips, Edgar W 7108 Mignonette Street, Bakersfield, CA 93308, (805) 392-9224, BA 60 CA St Univ - Fresno; MS 71 Western OR St Coll; 88–Sp-Lang Path, Kern Co Superintendent of Schs, **SLP A**

Phillips, Mrs Elizabeth Marie 5316 Mesquite Road, Memphis, TN 38119, BA 81 Hendrix Coll; MA 84 Memphis St Univ; **SLP**

Phillips, Mrs Erva J 2462 23rd Avenue, Columbus, NE 68601, (402) 563-2093, BS 56 Univ of NE - Lincoln; MA 65 Univ of NE - Lincoln; **SLP LM**

Phillips, Frances Carol 18328 Nob Hill Drive, Triangle, VA 22172, (703) 898-1433, **SLP**

Phillips, Gayle A 106 Clinton Hill Drive, Belleville, IL 62221, (618) 234-2120, BS 76 Fontbonne Coll; MS 77 Fontbonne Coll; Superv/Sp-Lang Path & Aud Dept, St Elizabeth's Hosp, **SLP**

Phillips, Gene B 2501 Laurelhurst Road, University Heights, OH 44118, (216) 932-9170, **SLP**

Phillips, Mrs Gwendolyn Hoff 669 Tahoe Circle, Stone Mountain, GA 30083, (404) 393-7260, ME 82 GA St Univ; Sp-Lang Path, Georgia Dept Human Resources, **SLP**

Phillips, James W R P O Box 342, Euless, TX 76039, (817) 382-1352, BA 71 TX Tech Univ; MA 74 TX Tech Univ; **A**

Phillips, Jane Marie 1846 South 11th Street, Apartment 3-C, Kalamazoo, MI 49009-1725, (517) 790-0130, BS 83 Central MI Univ; MA 86 Central MI Univ; 87–Aud, Constance Brown Sp & Hrng Ctr, **A**

Phillips, Janet Cheryl 3202 Panama Drive, Melbourne, FL 32935, (407) 254-7049, BA 83 Univ of Central FL; MS 85 FL St Univ; 88–Aud, Brevard County Sch Bd, **A**

Phillips, Mrs Janet Lynn 1770 Craig Drive, North Huntingdon, PA 15642, (412) 521-9000, BS 83 PA St Univ - Univ Park; ME 85 Univ of VA - Charlottesville; 86–Sp-Lang Path, The Rehab Inst of Pittsburgh, **SLP**

Phillips, Janice A 66 Laurence Parkway, Laurence Harbor, NJ 08879, (201) 566-4618, BA 83 Montclair St Coll; MS 85 PA St Univ - Univ Park; 85–Sp-Lang Path, JFK Med Ctr, **SLP**

Phillips, Janice Kay 4001 South Watt Avenue #64, Sacramento, CA 95826, (916) 686-7716, BA 74 CA St Univ - Chico; MA 85 CA St Univ - Chico; Sp-Lang Path, Elk Grove USD, **SLP**

Phillips, Janice Lynn 7503 Yellow Bluff Road, Panama City, FL 32404-5908, MS 73 FL St Univ; SLP, Dept of Defense Dependent Sch, **SLP**

Phillips, Jean M 80 Mt Pleasant Avenue, Gloucester, MA 01930, (508) 283-9878, BS 79 Univ of MA - Amherst; MA 80 MI St Univ; Sp-Lang Path, The Visit Nurse Assoc of N Shore, **SLP**

Phillips, Mrs Judy 1558 N W 12th Court, Gresham, OR 97030, (503) 666-2747, BS 70 Portland St Univ; MS 72 Portland St Univ; **SLP**

Phillips, Mrs Kathleen 358 N E 101st Street, Miami Shores, FL 33138, (305) 751-9901, BS 77 FL St Univ; MS 78 FL St Univ; Sp/Lang Path, Dade Co Pub Sch, **SLP**

Phillips, Kathleen C 12 Stoutenburgh Drive, Hyde Park, NY 12538, (914) 431-8801, BA 71 Mary Washington Coll; MS 77 VA Commonwealth Univ; MA 76 NY Univ; SLP, St Francis Hosp, **SLP**

Phillips, Kathleen Morris 560 Fisher Road, Winter Springs, FL 32708, BA 79 Univ of FL; ME 81 Univ of FL; **SLP**

Phillips, Mrs Kathy D Boulevard Extended, Lexington, MS 39095, (601) 353-4968, BS 78 Univ of MS; MA 81 Univ of MS; Sp-Lang Path, Jackson Sp & Hearing Clinic, **SLP**

Phillips, Kay S 3200 Durant, Midland, TX 79705, (915) 332-9151, BS 65 West TX St Univ; MA 71 Univ of Tulsa; Sp-Lang Path, Reg Day Sch Prog for the Deaf, **SLP ACE**

Phillips, Laura L 6504 Pineburr Court, Orangevale, CA 95662, BS 75 Brigham Young Univ; OM 77 Brigham Young Univ; **SLP**

Phillips, Leigh A Route 4 Box 48-A, Hillsville, VA 24343, (703) 728-3764, BS 77 Radford Univ; MS 81 Radford Univ; 87–Sp-Lang Path, Private Practice, **SLP**

Phillips, Lisa Kay 8125 Golden Rod Court, Indianapolis, IN 46219, (317) 898-2731, BA 84 Butler Univ; MA 86 Butler Univ; **SLP**

Phillips, Mrs Loretta A 3578 Brook Street #3, Lafayette, CA 94549, (415) 947-5300, BS 78 CA St Univ - Hayward; MS 80 Univ of WA; Sp-Lang Path, John Muir Med Ctr, **SLP ACE**

Phillips, Mrs Lorey House 3901 S W 5th Avenue, Ocala, FL 32674, (904) 732-7179, BA 65 Univ of FL; OM 67 Univ of FL; 88–Coord of Exceptional Stu Educ, Marion Co Sch Bd, **SLP**

Phillips, Lynn Bjork 801 6th Avenue S W, Rochester, MN 55902-6124, (405) 478-5110, BS 80 OK St Univ; MS 82 Univ of OK Medical Center; Sp/Lang Path, Edmond Publ Schs, **SLP**

Phillips, Marie 4 Park Lane #3C, Mount Vernon, NY 10552, (914) 632-9000, BA 78 SUNY - Coll at Plattsburgh; MS 80 PA St Univ - Univ Park; Sp-Lang Path, City Sch Dist of New Rochelle, **SLP**

Phillips, Martha A 546 Ashford Avenue, Ardsley, NY 10502, (914) 693-8376, BA 80 CUNY - Queens Coll; MA 82 CUNY - Queens Coll; Aud, Bellevue Hosp Cen, **A**

Phillips, Mrs Martha Zarzour 5306 Coldbrook Drive, Mantua, OH 44255, (216) 543-9722, BS 69 Bowling Green St Univ; MA 74 Bowling Green St Univ; Sp-Lang Path, Kenston Schs, **SLP**

Phillips, Merle A 1714 West Cherokee, Enid, OK 73701, (405) 946-5563, BS 57 OK St Univ; MA 61 Wichita St Univ; Aud, Otologic Med Clin, **SLP A**

Phillips, Nancy Marie 320 Elgin, Apt 3 North, Forest Park, IL 60130, (312) 366-1921, BA 83 MI St Univ; MA 84 MI St Univ; Area Mktg Mgr, InSpeech Inc, **SLP**

Phillips, Nevis C 6842 South Chappel Street, Chicago, IL 60649, (312) 288-3891, BS Northwestern Univ; MA Northwestern Univ; Sp-Lang Path, Chicago Board of Education, **SLP**

Phillips, Patricia A 2858 Liveoak Circle, Salt Lake City, UT 84117, (801) 277-7597, BS 62 Auburn Univ - Auburn; MS 87 Univ of UT

Phillips, Mrs Paula Brady 104 Heartwood Drive, Grimesland, NC 27837-9702, (919) 638-6519, BS 78 East Carolina Univ; MS 80 East Carolina Univ; SLP, Howell's Child Care Cen, Inc, **SLP**

Phillips, Dr Phyllis Route 2, Old Rome Pike, Lebanon, TN 37087, (615) 444-4148, BS 61 Auburn Univ - Auburn; ME 62 Auburn Univ - Auburn; ED 66 (NS) Auburn Univ - Auburn; Retired, Auburn Univ, **SLP**

Phillips, Mrs Phyllis A 1714 West Cherokee, Enid, OK 73701, (405) 722-5560, BA 60 Wichita St Univ; MS 68 Phillips Univ; Sp-Lang Path, Putnam City Schs, **SLP**

Phillips, Renee Jean 306 West 78th Street, Apt 1-A, New York, NY 10024, (212) 606-1226, BS 81 CUNY - Hunter Coll; MA 83 Columbia Univ Teachers Coll; Sp-Lang Path, Hospital for Special Surgery, **SLP**

Phillips, Rita H 10011 77th Street S W, Tacoma, WA 98498, (206) 582-5431, BA 75 Univ of MD - College Park; MA 76 Univ of MD - College Park; Aud, VA Med Cen, **A**

Phillips, Mrs Sally M 1102 Willow Run Drive, Opelika, AL 36801, (205) 298-6689, BS 69 Auburn Univ - Auburn; MA 76 Auburn Univ - Auburn; SLP, Lee Co Sch, **SLP**

Phillips, Sandra Lea 2201 Piper Place, Apt #5, Burlington, IA 52601, (319) 753-6561, BS 81 Northern IL Univ - De Kalb; MA 82 Northern IL Univ - De Kalb; Aud, AEA #16, **A**

Phillips, Stacia White 1505 Long Shadow Lane, Mesquite, TX 75149, (214) 563-1772, BS 79 Baylor Univ; MS 86 Univ of Central AR; 88–Sp-Lang Path, Denton State Sch, **SLP**

Phillips, Mrs Susan D 54 Hillside Avenue, Short Hills, NJ 07078, (201) 376-4255, BA 58 Middlebury Coll; MA 59 Northwestern Univ; **SLP**

Phillips, Suzanne K 2724 Acorn Drive, Kettering, OH 45419, (513) 222-8913, BS 81 Univ of Central AR; MA 82 Bowling Green St Univ; Aud, Dayton Pub Schools, **A ACE**

Phillips, Mrs Sylvia Dean Box 248, Medina, WA 98039, BA Cornell Univ; **SLP LM**

Phillips, Mrs Trevelyn Mosher 1303 Creekbend Street, White Oak, TX 75693, (214) 297-7469, BS 84 Baylor Univ; MS 85 Baylor Univ; Sp-Lang Path, Longview ISD, **SLP**

Phillips-Arthur, Sandra H 308 Bayside Drive, Baltimore, MD 21222, (301) 765-2130, BS 77 Towson St Univ; MA 79 Univ of MD - College Park; Admin, Westinghouse Elec Sys Group, **SLP**

Phillips-Littrell, Mrs Mary Ann 129 1/2 West John Street, Maumee, OH 43537, (419) 241-6219, BA 81 Coll of Wooster; MA 83 Case Western Reserve Univ; Aud, Toledo Speech and Hearing Cen, **A**

Phillips-Springer, Lisa Ann 235 Second Street, St James, NY 11780, BS 82 SUNY - Coll at Geneseo; MS 85 Adelphi Univ; 82–SLP, BOCES III Suffolk, **SLP**

Philp, Sandrya M 24 Wakefield Drive N E, Atlanta, GA 30309, (404) 436-4293, BS 68 Kent St Univ; ME 64 Kent St Univ; 88–Sp-Lang Path, Northwest Rehab Ctr, **SLP**

Philpot, Mrs Terri Lynn Miller 100 Springer Drive, Lawrenceburg, TN 38464, (615) 762-3282, BA 80 Univ of MS; OM 81 Univ of MS; 85–Sp-Lang Path, Speech Language & Learning Ctr, **SLP**

Phipps, Mrs Janet T 8000 S W 56th Avenue, Gainesville, FL 32608, (904) 338-1286, BA 74 Rutger's St Univ - Douglas Coll; MS 75 Columbia Univ Teachers Coll; Sp-Lang Path, M Jensen and Associates, **SLP**

Phipps, Mrs Linda M 3527 Nikki Lynn, Bossier City, LA 71112, (318) 742-1049, BA 78 LA St Univ - Shreveport; OM 81 LA St Univ - Shreveport; Sp-Lang Path, Assoc Ret Citz, **SLP**

Phipps, Mrs Mary Elizabeth 608 Illinois Street, Bicknell, IN 47512, (812) 735-3571, BS 82 IN St Univ - Terre Haute; MS 83 IN St Univ - Terre Haute; Sp-Lang Path, Union Hospital, **SLP**

Phipps, Mrs Pamela P 2201 Whilden Court, Charlotte, NC 28211, (704) 332-4834, BS 69 Univ of NC - Chapel Hill; ME 71 Univ of GA; OM 71 Univ of GA; Sp-Lang Path, Chld & Fam Dev Assoc, **SLP**

Phipps-Kauder, Mrs Tamara 2016 Oakmont Avenue, Havertown, PA 19083, (804) 468-3140, BA 82 Old Dominion Univ; MA 84 Hampton Univ; SLP, Coll of Sp Therapists, **SLP ACE**

Phoebus, Barbara M 4320 Cottington Road, Baltimore, MD 21236, (301) 256-0166, BS 71 Towson St Univ; MS 74 Towson St Univ; Sp-Lang Path, Private Practice, **SLP**

Phoebus, Brenda Lee 1631 Hyland Greens, Grapevine, TX 76051, (817) 336-9371, **SLP**

Phoebus, Maudie P 201 North Flagler Drive, Apartment 501, West Palm Beach, FL 33401, (305) 655-8423, BS 54 FL St Univ; BS; **SLP LM**

Phoenix, Mrs Lynann V C 1099 Gordon Road, Lyndhurst, OH 44124, BS 77 SUNY - Coll at Brockport; MS 79 PA St Univ - Univ Park; Sp-Lang Path, South Euclid Boe, **SLP**

Phoenix, Mary Lydon 3205 18th Street, Eureka, CA 95501, (916) 623-2861, MA 81 Humboldt St Univ; **SLP**

Phon, Gilbert Audiology Center Of St Peters, 4200 North Clover Leaf Dr, St Charles, MO 63303, (314) 441-7470, BS 73 SUNY - Coll at Brockport; MA 75 Hofstra Univ; Audiologist, Audiology Center of St Peters, **A**

Photos, Maria 330 South Hazel Drive, Schaumburg, IL 60193, (312) 869-8700, BS 84 Northwestern Univ; MA 85 Northwestern Univ; **A**

Phythian, Carla Andrews 9123 Westport, Wichita, KS 67212, (316) 689-3289, BA 84 Wichita St Univ; MA 86 Wichita St Univ; **SLP**

Piacenti, Mrs Terri 6310 Pemberton Drive, Dallas, TX 75230, (214) 368-0614, BA 73 Baylor Univ; MA 74 Vanderbilt Univ; **SLP**

Piacentine, Mrs Marjorie Hipp 222 Shady Oaks Circle, Lake Mary, FL 32746, (407) 321-5919, BA 68 FL St Univ; MS 69 Vanderbilt Univ; **SLP**

Pianin, Alissa M 617 South Connecticut, Royal Oak, MI 48067, (313) 548-1980, BS 80 MI St Univ; MS 81 Univ of MI - Ann Arbor; Aud, Dr Alter Dr Salama Dr Belf Dr Nowak, **A**

Piascik, Laura Catherine 562 7th Street #14, Brooklyn, NY 11215, (718) 854-3737, MS 84 Columbia Univ Teachers Coll; Sp-Lang Path, NY Childhood Ctr, **SLP**

Piasecki, Charlene P 22724 Cavalier Street, Woodland Hills, CA 91364, (213) 621-6582, BS 71 Marquette Univ; MS 72 Marquette Univ; Account Rep, IBM, **SLP**

Piatek, A 1850 Route 23 North, West Milford, NJ 07480, (201) 492-0416, BA 78 William Paterson Coll; MS 83 William Paterson Coll; Sp-Lang Path, Newark Board of Education, **SLP**

Piazza, Mrs Candice S 4330 Homesteaden, Wilsonville, OR 97070, (503) 638-6378, BS 69 OR St Univ; MS 74 Portland St Univ; **SLP**

Piazza, Carol Ann 1649 35th Street, Sacramento, CA 95816, (916) 348-3242, BA 81 Humboldt St Univ; MA 85 Humboldt St Univ; Sp-Lang Path, Petoluma City School District, **SLP**

Picago, Stanley T 1321 Bradley Avenue, Eau Claire, WI 54701, (715) 832-3218, OB 51 Marquette Univ; MS 63 Univ of WI - Milwaukee; **SLP**

Picantine, Jayna Lynn 500 110th Avenue N #201, St Petersburg, FL 33716, (813) 576-1923, BA 84 LA Tech Univ; MA 86 LA Tech Univ; Sp-Lang Path, InSpeech Inc, **SLP**

Picard, Mrs Marianne T 11604 Sansbury Court, Potomac, MD 20854, (301) 762-1010, BS 77 Univ of WI - Madison; MS 78 Syracuse Univ; Sp-Lang Path, Private Practice, **SLP**

Piccardo, Nancy J 6521 Cow Pen Road #G-208, Miami Lakes, FL 33014, (305) 891-8850, BA 71 George Washington Univ; MS 74 Univ of Pittsburgh - Pittsburgh; 88–Sp-Lang Path, Bon Secours Hosp, **SLP**

Piccillo-Stokes, Mrs Lois D 9122 Old Lakeshore Road, Angola, NY 14006, (716) 549-1699, BS 71 SUNY - Coll at Buffalo; MS 74 SUNY - Coll at Buffalo; 71–Sp-Lang Path, Buffalo Bd of Ed, **SLP**

Piccirilli, Mrs Mary Schmitt 12817 Willowyck, St Louis, MO 63146, BS 78 Fontbonne Coll; MA 80 Univ of KS; Sp-Lang Path, Jewish Hosp of St Louis, **SLP**

Piccolomini, Marion Marie 404 Continental Drive, Towamencincen Condominium, Harleysville, PA 19438, (215) 362-8635, BS 78 WV Univ; MS 84 PA St Univ - Univ Park; Sp-Lang Path, Lehigh Valley Hosp Ctr, **SLP**

Piccora, Mrs Rose Rocco 809 William Thomas Drive, Kennett Square, PA 19348, (215) 347-0249, BS 77 Saint John's Univ - Jamaica; MA 83 Kean Coll of NJ; Sp-Lang Path, **SLP**

Picek, Mrs Mary Colleen 230 South 2nd Street, Box 340, West Branch, IA 52358, (319) 399-6700, BA 68 Univ of IA; MA 70 Univ of IA; SLP, Grantwood AEA, **SLP**

Piche, Mrs Leslie Donelan 12714 East Asbury Circle, Apartment V-102, Aurora, CO 80014, (303) 573-7575, BS 79 CO St Univ; MS 80 PA St Univ - Univ Park; Sp/Lang Path, Visiting Nurse Assn of Denver, **SLP**

Picheny, Barbara M 6388 Ivarene Avenue, Los Angeles, CA 90068, **SLP**

Pichler, Cindy Beth CARC, 1640 West Roosevelt Road, Chicago, IL 60608, (312) 829-7716, BS 84 Northern IL Univ - De Kalb; MA 86 Univ of KS; 86–Aud, Chicago Assoc for Ret Citizens, **A**

Pichurko, Joann J 3032 Vancouver Avenue, San Diego, CA 92104, (619) 222-0411, BA 75 Saint John's Univ - Jamaica; MS 77 SUNY - Center at Albany; Sp/Lang Path, Sharp-Cabrillo Hosp, **SLP**

Pickens, Susan Alexander 8023 Willys Court, Sacramento, CA 95828, (916) 689-6516, BS 78 SUNY - Coll at Geneseo; MS 83 Ithaca Coll; **SLP**

Pickering, Mrs Joanna Hayes 7645 Danu Court, Orlando, FL 32822, (305) 896-4050, BA 81 Univ of Central FL; MA 85 Univ of Central FL; **SLP**

Pickering, John Edmund, Jr M-3 Millstreet Apartment, Athens, OH 45701, (614) 593-1415, BA 81 Univ of ME - Orono; MA 83 Univ of ME - Orono; **SLP ACE**

Pickering, Mrs Joyce 1733 Pine Harrier Circle, Sarasota, FL 33581, (813) 922-0002, BS 59 LA St Univ - Baton Rouge; MA 78 VA Polytechnic Inst St Univ; SLP/Aud, Sarasota School Dstr, **SLP**

Pickering, Dr Marisue 34 Forest Avenue, Orono, ME 04473, (207) 581-1512, BA 59 OH Univ - Athens; ME 62 Boston Univ; ED 79 (Humanistic & Behavioral Studies) Boston Univ; Assoc Prof, U of Maine, **SLP**

Pickering, Mrs Mary Fletcher 6 Chaffee Lane, Unionville, CT 06085, (203) 673-3609, **SLP**

Pickett, Donna L 14 Avellino, Irvine, CA 92714, (714) 447-7745, BA 76 CA St Univ - Fullerton; MA 82 CA St Univ - Fullerton; Sp-Lang Path, Fullerton Sch Dist, **SLP**

Pickett, Mrs Gloria Oakes Route 1 Box 56, Fitzpatrick, AL 36029, (205) 271-9025, MA 84 Auburn Univ - Auburn; ME 88 Auburn Univ - Auburn; Aud, Montgomery Co Bd of Educ, **A**

Pickett, Mrs Iris H Route 2 Box 129B, Trenton, SC 29847, (803) 637-5420, BA 70; ME 72; Dir of Spec Serv, The Sch Dist of Edgefield Co, **SLP**

Pickett, Dr James M Gallaudet College, Scrl Mtb B-5, Washington, DC 20002, (202) 651-5440, BA 43 Oberlin Coll; PH 51 (NS) Brown Univ; Gallaudet Coll

Pickett, Larry R Rt 1 Box 120F, Alexander, AR 72002, (501) 794-3503, BA 74 Univ of AR - Fayetteville; MA 75 Univ of AR - Fayetteville; Director, Learning Frontiers, **SLP**

Pickett, Len W 905 Bluff Avenue, Kingsford, MI 49801, (906) 774-4936, BS 70 Northern MI Univ; MA 72 Univ of NM; Superv Sp-Lang Path, VA Med Ctr, **SLP**

Pickett, Maureen Duane 10 Russell Road, Albany, NY 12203-2925, (518) 458-7277, BS 85 Coll of Saint Rose; MS 87 Coll of Saint Rose

Pickett, Owena Alston P O Box 431, Southmont, NC 27351, (704) 249-1926, **SLP**

Pickett, Trenna Jo 8917-A Trone Circle, Austin, TX 78758, (512) 926-6635, BS 67 Culver-Stockton Coll; ME 76 Southwest TX St Univ; Sp-Lang Path, Austin ISD, **SLP**

Pickford, Susan Kay 607 8th Street #9, Fort Madison, IA 52627, (319) 753-3551, BA 86 Univ of Northern IA; MA 87 Western IL Univ; Audiologist, Burlington Medical Center, **A**

Picking, Mrs Caroline Cumbie P O Box 460, Andalusia, AL 36420, (205) 222-7571, BA 70 Birmingham-Southern Coll; MS 72 Vanderbilt Univ; Aud, Aud Serv-Covington Co Bd of Ed, **SLP A**

Pickle, Patricia A 605 Conser Avenue, Poteau, OK 74953, (918) 963-2218, BS 76 OK St Univ; MS 87 Univ of AR - Fayetteville; 78–Sp-Lang Path, Panama PS, **SLP**

Pickrell, Kerry K 7643 Tophill Lane, Dallas, TX 75248, **SLP**

Pickton, Mrs Alice Monosmith 3283 Theresa Lane, Lafayette, CA 94549, (415) 794-3832, MA 82 San Jose St Univ; Sp-Lang Path, CA Sch for the Blind, **SLP**

Pickus, Mrs Francine S 20 Barnum Street, North Babylon, NY 11703, (516) 587-9099, BA 78 CUNY - Queens Coll; MS 81 CUNY - Brooklyn Coll; Sp-Lang Path, Private Practice, **SLP**

Picon, Edith J 5 Pheasant Way, Florham Park, NJ 07932, (201) 377-6316, BS 80 Ithaca Coll; MA 81 Montclair St Coll; Sp/Lang Path, Private Practice, **SLP**

Picone, Mrs Janet E 132 Rodgers Drive, Lower Burrell, PA 15068, (412) 337-9515, BA 72 Univ of Pittsburgh - Pittsburgh; MS 73 Univ of Pittsburgh - Pittsburgh; Aud, Paul E Antalik MD Pc, **A**

Pidek, Catherine Monica 1500 Robin Circle Apt 303, Hoffman Estates, IL 60195, (312) 885-0561, BS 76 Western MI Univ; MA 81 OH Univ - Athens; Sp-Lang Path/Consult, Communication Concepts, **SLP**

Piech, Mrs Sharon C 120 Woodland Drive, Havelock, NC 28532, (919) 447-5059, BS 76 OH Wesleyan Univ; MA 81 OH Univ - Athens; **SLP**

Piechna, Linda Lee 9959 South 86th Terrace Apartment 314, Palos Hills, IL 60465, (312) 756-0100, BS 85 Northern IL Univ - De Kalb; MA 86 Northern IL Univ - De Kalb; 87–Aud, Suburban Heights Med Ctr, **A**

Piechnik-Briggs, Diane C Rural Delivery 2, Maltbie Drive, Amsterdam, NY 12010, (518) 842-3100, BS 73 SUNY - Coll at Fredonia; MS 74 FL St Univ; Admin, Amsterdam Memorial Hospital, **SLP**

Piede, Mrs June E W 25 Valley View Drive, Frewsburg, NY 14738, (716) 664-3893, BS 75 SUNY - Coll at Fredonia; MA 77 SUNY - Coll at Geneseo; Sp-Lang Path, Chautaugua Co Resource Cen, **SLP**

Piede, Robert M 25 Valley View Drive, Frewsburg, NY 14738, (716) 487-0141, BS 75 SUNY - Coll at Fredonia; MA 76 SUNY - Coll at Geneseo; Dir of Sp and Hrng, Womens Chrishan Assoc Hosp, **A**

Piedt, Diane O 3344-A S Delaware Avenue, Milwaukee, WI 53207, **SLP**

Piehl, Mrs Ann G 43 Wyngate, Simsbury, CT 06070, (919) 727-1935, BA 64 Univ of IA; MA 66 Univ of IA; **A**

Piehler, Mrs Margaret Forbes 4367 Schenley Farms Terr, Pittsburgh, PA 15213, (412) 624-6571, BA 62 Randolph-Macon Woman's Coll; MA 76 Carnegie-Mellon Univ; MA 81 Univ of Pittsburgh - Pittsburgh; Research Assoc, Wn Psych I An Dcl, **SLP**

Pieras, Dr Guillermo J 423 Atlantic Avenue #2C, Brooklyn, NY 11217, (718) 780-5186, MS 74 CUNY - Brooklyn Coll; MD 64 Univ Santiago Compeste Spain; Assistant Prof, Brooklyn Coll/CUNY, **SLP**

Pierce, Alesia J 369 East 400 North, Logan, UT 84321, (318) 365-2341, BS 82 LA St Univ - Baton Rouge; MS 85 Univ of Southwestern LA; **SLP**

Pierce, Dr Bruce R 4625 Jamerson Creek Drive, Marietta, GA 30066, (404) 591-8818, BA 54 Univ of CA - Los Angeles; MA 55 Univ of CA - Los Angeles; PH 62 (Sp Path) Northwestern Univ; **SLP F**

Pierce, Mrs Christine W 626 Park Avenue, Kent, OH 44240, (216) 678-3218, BS 73 PA St Univ - Univ Park; MS 74 PA St Univ - Univ Park; Sp-Lang Path, Private Practice, **SLP**

Pierce, Mrs Claudia Grooms 40 S W 12th Street, Suite 202, Ocala, FL 32671, (904) 732-5666, OB 64 Univ of FL; OM 70 Univ of FL; 87–Sp-Lang Path, Munroe Reg Med Ctr, **SLP**

Pierce, Mrs Edwina S G 1320 Tumbleweed Way, Sacramento, CA 95834, (916) 454-8189, BA 59 Adelphi Univ; MS 61 Hofstra Univ; 85–Sp-Lang Path, Sacramento USD, **SLP**

Pierce, Jennifer Lynn 1-80 Patterson Avenue, Ottawa, ON, Canada K1S 1Y3, (802) 654-3861, BS 80 KS St Univ; MS 86 Univ of VT; **SLP**

Pierce, Mrs Jill Walker 1730 North Clark #2406, Chicago, IL 60614, (312) 337-3567, BS 81 Baylor Univ; MS 82 Baylor Univ; Sp-Lang Path, **SLP**

Pierce, Mrs Karen Dawn 3611 Jetton Avenue, Tampa, FL 33629, (813) 251-1113, BS 78 James Madison Univ; MS 84 Radford Univ; **SLP**

Pierce, Linda J 1501 Sunnyside Drive, Columbia, TN 38401, (615) 433-1561, BA 68 Lycoming Coll; MS 78 Univ of NV - Reno; 86–Sp-Lang Path, Lincoln Regional Hosp, **SLP**

Pierce, Linda Kite P O Box 2802, Staunton, VA 24401, (703) 337-0037, BS 71 James Madison Univ; MS 79 James Madison Univ; SLP, Staunton City Sch, **SLP**

Pierce, Mrs Lorraine M 4224 N W 20th Terrace, Gainesville, FL 32605, (904) 336-2710, BS 81 East Stroudsburg Univ of PA; MS 84 Univ of NV - Reno; 85–Sp-Lang Path, Sch Bd of Alachua County, **SLP**

Pierce, Mrs M Lynn 58 Overlook Drive, Danville, PA 17821, (717) 275-5112, MS 87 CA Univ of PA; 87–Sp-Lang Path, S G Rehab Agency Inc, **SLP**

Pierce, Nancy Broo 2315 Baxter Road, Chesterfield, MO 63017-7720, (314) 962-1876, BA 75 Univ of HI - Manoa; MS 79 Univ of HI - Manoa; MS 83 Washington Univ; Aud/SLP, St Louis Hrng & Sp Cen, **SLP A**

Pierce, Patricia D 1010 Samuel Street, Louisville, KY 40204, **SLP**

Pierce, Robert F 5406 Juniata Street, Duluth, MN 55804, (218) 726-8203, OB 42 Northern IL Univ - De Kalb; OM 47 Univ of WI - Madison; PH 53 (NS) Univ of WI - Madison; **SLP F LM**

Pierce, Dr Robert S 626 Park Avenue, Kent, OH 44240, (216) 672-2672, BS 72 Northwestern Univ; MA 73 Northwestern Univ; PH 79 (Sp Path) Univ of IA; Assoc Prof, Kent State U, **SLP**

Pierce, Mrs Roberta B Lakeshore Rehabilitation Center, 316 Longwood Drive, Huntsville, AL 35801, (205) 534-6421, BS 66 Univ of TN - Knoxville; MA 67 Univ of FL; Dir Sp Dept, Lakeshore Rehab Ctr, **SLP ACE**

Pierce, Dr Sharalee P O Box 60228, San Angelo, TX 76906, (915) 942-9393, BS 69 TX Tech Univ; MS 70 TX Tech Univ; ED 75 (NS) TX Tech Univ; **SLP**

Pierce, Shonna Medell 100 Chadell Road, Bogalusa, LA 70427, (504) 381-6520, MS 87 Baylor Univ

Pierce, Sondra Michelle 1091 N E 209th Terr, Miami, FL 33179, (305) 654-9557, BA 80 Univ of Miami; MS 85 Nova Univ; **SLP**

Pierce, Mrs Thelma Hilton 83 Day Street #3, Jamaica Plain, MA 02130, (617) 524-7636, BS 74 Suffolk Univ; ME 77 Suffolk Univ; 75–Sp-Lang Path, Boston PS, **SLP**

Pierce, Tina D 133 Hawthorne Avenue, Baltimore, MD 21208, (301) 396-0876, BS 73 Trenton St Coll; MS 79 Loyola Coll; Sp-Lang Path, Balt Cty Pub Sch, **SLP**

Piercy, Mrs Susan K 992 Devon Drive, West Lafayette, IN 47906, (317) 463-1502, BA 70 Wake Forest Univ; ME 71 Univ of SC - Columbia; Sp/Lang Path, Indiana Veterans Home, **SLP**

Pierdon, Laurie E 2810 Fawnwood Circle, Valdosta, GA 31602, (912) 559-5153, BS 79 Univ of GA; ME 81 Univ of GA; Sp-Lang Path, Lowndes Co Bd of Ed, **SLP**

Pierini, Mrs Carolyn Kuhn 10663 East Maplewood Drive, Englewood, CO 80111, (303) 771-0506, BA 78 Univ of OK - Norman; MS 80 Univ of OK Medical Center; Sp-Lang Path, AMI Presbyterian/St Lukes Hosp, **SLP**

Pierini, Sr M Paul Francis Villa Maria Del Mar, 2-1918 East Cliff Drive, Santa Cruz, CA 95062, (408) 475-1236, BA 44 Holy Names Coll; MA 53 Stanford Univ; Author, **SLP LM**

Piernick, Sherry Melinda 432 East Davis Boulevard, Tampa, FL 33606, (718) 240-6425, BS 79 SUNY - Coll at New Paltz; MS 85 Univ of South FL; **A**

Piersall, Mrs Marcia C 4379-C Willow Pond Road, West Palm Beach, FL 33417, (407) 471-1297, BS 83 FL St Univ; MS 85 FL St Univ; Sp-Lang Path, Palm Bch Co Sch Bd, **SLP**

Piersol, Barbara L 206 Primrose Drive, Blacksburg, VA 24060, **SLP**

Pierson, Mrs Blair Alison West Surburban Hospital, Erie At Austin, Oak Park, IL 60302, (312) 383-6200, BA 82 Valparaiso Univ; MA 84 Northwestern Univ; SLP, West Surburban Hosp, **SLP**

Pierson, Mrs Jan Latta 5717 Laurel Canyon Blvd, #211, North Hollywood, CA 91607, (213) 201-0731, BS 85 Univ of WY; MS 87 Univ of WY; **A**

Pierson, Janet E Rural Delivery 1 532-B, Gardiner, NY 12525, (914) 471-0176, MA 83 Northwestern Univ; SLP, Rehabilitation Programs Inc, **SLP**

Pierson, Joanne Marttila 1718 Weaver Drive, Portage, MI 49081, (616) 343-2601, BS 78 Western MI Univ; MS 85 Univ of MI - Ann Arbor; **SLP**

Pierson, John R 901 South Wildwood Avenue, Kankakee, IL 60901, (815) 937-2082, BS 76 Southern IL Univ-Edwardsvill; MS 77 Southern IL Univ-Edwardsvill; Dir/SLP & Audiology, St Marys Hospital, **SLP**

Pierson, Capt Linda Davis 2915 Whitefield Road, Churchville, MD 21028, (301) 671-3797, BA 76 SUNY - Coll at Plattsburgh; MA 80 NY Univ; Aud, Bio-Acoustics Div US Army Env Hygiene Agency, **A ACE**

Pierson, Nancy Bush Casa Felicidad, Lot 69 Sandy Lane, St James, Barbados, (809) 432-2330, BA 79 Colgate Univ; MS 84 Emerson Coll; Sp-Lang Path, Private Practice, **SLP**

Pierson, Patricia M 124 Hemlock Drive, East Greenwich, RI 02818, (401) 885-1887, BA 70 SUNY - Center at Buffalo; MS 71 SUNY - Center at Albany; 88–Tchr, Happy Hearts Learning Center, **SLP**

Pierson, Mrs Robin M M 8552 Hazel Crest Court, Elk Grove, CA 95624, (916) 366-2727, BS 75 CA St Univ - Sacramento; MA 77 CA St Univ - Sacramento; Prog Administrator Spec Educ, Sacramento County Office of Ed, **SLP**

Pierson, Sandra Kay 2201 Cedar Crest, Abilene, TX 79601, (915) 677-2553, BS 75 Abilene Christian Univ; MA 85 Abilene Christian Univ; 88–Sp-Lang Path, Abilene ISD, **SLP**

Pierucci, Dr Rita A 505 Redondo Court, Bakersfield, CA 93309-1762, (805) 398-3807, BS 75 FL St Univ; MA 76 FL St Univ; ED 85 (NS) Brigham Young Univ; Sp-Lang Path, Kern Co Supt of Schools, **SLP**

Pietrafesa, Barbara Jane 25 Jewett Pl, Utica, NY 13501, (315) 732-5845, BS 83 SUNY - Coll at Geneseo; MS 85 Coll of Saint Rose; **SLP**

Pietrafesa, Christina Inez 249 St Lawrence Avenue, North Buffalo, NY 14216, (315) 733-3221, **SLP**

Pietranton, Arlene Arrigan George Washington University, Medical Center Room 2357N, 901 23rd Street N W, Washington, DC 20037, (202) 994-3631, BA 74 George Washington Univ; MA 76 George Washington Univ; Dir SLP & Aud Serv, Geo WA U Med Cen, **SLP**

Pietrick, Julie A 1329 Farrington Drive, Knoxville, TN 37923, (615) 693-4788, BA 86 Univ of TN - Knoxville; MA 87 Univ of TN - Knoxville; **SLP**

Pietrowski, Mrs Ann Peyser 10133 N E 202nd Street, Bothell, WA 98011-2444, (206) 524-3118, BA 80 Western WA Univ; MS 83 Univ of WA; SLP, NW Sp/Hrng Cen, **SLP**

Piette, Catherine Mary 9955 Russell Avenue North #11, Brooklyn Park, MN 55444, (612) 533-1951, BA 85 Univ of WI - Eau Claire; MS 86 Univ of WI - Eau Claire; 86–Sp-Lang Path, Hnoka-Hennepin Sch Dist #11, **SLP**

Piette, Mrs Jean Ross 320 Forest Court, Auburn, CA 95603, (916) 823-4844, BA 75 CA St Univ - Sacramento; MA 81 CA St Univ - Sacramento; 85–Coord-Spec Educ, Placer County Ofc of Educ, **SLP**

Piette, Joe Northwest Rehabilitation Center, 7800 West Fond Du Lac Avenue, Milwaukee, WI 53218, (414) 464-9976, BA 73 Univ of MN - Duluth; MA 74 Univ of MN - Duluth; 88–Assoc Prog Dir, Northwest Rehab Center of Milwaukee, **SLP**

Piette, Sharon Louise 17205 Kinloch, Reford, MI 48240, (313) 534-0703, BA 81 MI St Univ; MS 86 Univ of MI - Ann Arbor; **SLP**

Pigage, Mrs Martha Jacqueline 3323 Southgate Drive, Hopkinsville, KY 42240, (502) 885-7285, BA 78 Harding Univ; MS 83 Univ of KY; Sp/Lang Path, Christian Co Sch Bd, **SLP**

Pigg, Mrs Sue Ann 4008 Kirchling Road, Hamilton, OH 45013, (513) 868-2000, BS 75 Miami Univ - Oxford; MS 82 Miami Univ - Oxford; Sp-Lang Path, Hamilton City Schools

Piggott, Susan L Metairie Park County Day School, Metairie, LA 70005, (504) 837-5204, BS 70 Miami Univ - Oxford; MA 75 Northwestern Univ; Sp-Lang Path, Metairie Park Country Day Sch, **SLP**

Pigott, Janice F 205 Avondale Drive, Augusta, GA 30907, (404) 860-1328, BA 75 Baylor Univ; MS 76 Baylor Univ; 83, Richmond Co Bd Educ, **SLP**

Pihl, Karen L 2435 East Southern, Suite 6, Tempe, AZ 85282, (602) 967-3703, BS 74 Univ of AZ; MS 76 Univ of AZ; Cl Dir, Ariz Sp Path Assoc, **SLP**

Piirainen, Paulette 2200 Heights Avenue, Lansing, MI 48912, (517) 887-1780, BS 65 Northern MI Univ; MA 72 MI St Univ; Sp-Lang Path, Lansing Sch Dist, **SLP**

Pike, Connie Moore 243 Summerfield Lane, Cordova, TN 38018, (901) 755-4070, BS 81 Auburn Univ - Auburn; MA 83 LA St Univ - Baton Rouge; Sp-Lang Path, Germantown Sp and Hrng Clinic, **SLP**

Pike, Debbie Lynn 13444 Telluride Drive, Chino Hills, CA 91709, (818) 967-2806, BA 81 San Diego St Univ; MA 86 CA St Univ - Los Angeles; 86–Sp-Lang Path, Los Angeles Co Ofc of Educ, **SLP**

Pike, Mrs Diane Jones 1953 Hillcrest Drive, Coshocton, OH 43812, (614) 622-9416, BA 62 1125; MA 64 Case Western Reserve Univ; 87–Sp-Lang Path, Hopewell Sch, **SLP**

Pike, Gayle Lancaster 4601 East Sandra Terrace, Phoenix, AZ 85032, **SLP**

Pike, Harriet H P O Box 111, Ashfield, MA 01330, MS; **A F LM**

Pike, Janet Marie 499 West Center Street, West Bridgewater, MA 02379, **SLP**

Pike, Lisa T 3 Beech Hills Drive, Tuscaloosa, AL 35404, **SLP**

Pike, Marilyn J 67 Harris Park Drive, Scarborough, ON, Canada M1L 3A8, (416) 965-4068, BA 70 Univ of Toronto - Ontario; OM 72 Univ of Toronto - Ontario; MA 78 SUNY - Center at Buffalo; Aud Consult, Ministry of Labor, **A**

Pike, Patricia A 1608 Cherry, Denver, CO 80220, (303) 837-7021, BA 62 Western WA Univ; MA 70 Univ of CT; 70–Dir of Neurodiag Cen, Saint Joseph Hosp, **SLP**

Pike, Sandra M 1154 North 45th Street, Milwaukee, WI 53208, **SLP**

Pike, Sheryl Kay 2869 Santiago Apt H, Florissant, MO 63033-5524, (618) 656-1530, BS 85 Northeast MO St Univ; MS 86 Southern IL Univ-Edwardsvill; **SLP**

Pike, Susan R 402 Mineral Point Court, Janesville, WI 53545, (608) 756-8317, BS 79 James Madison Univ; MS 87 Eastern IL Univ; 88–Sp-Lang Path, Sch Dist of Janesville

Pike, Vicki Jean 1465 N E 121st Street, Greenwich Apts #B110, North Miami, FL 33161, (215) 631-9300, BS 85 Brescia Coll; MS 86 Western KY Univ

Pikscher, Barbara A 8282 Lake Ridge Drive, Burr Ridge, IL 60521, BS 69 Ithaca Coll; MA 73 MI St Univ; 85–Sp-Lang Path, Private Practice, **SLP**

Pikul, Mrs Angela R 5 Wood Street, Whitesboro, NY 13492, BS 70 SUNY - Coll at Fredonia; MS 71 SUNY - Coll at Fredonia; Sp-Lang Path, Mohawk Ctr Sch Dist, **SLP**

Pikus, Mrs Anita 8808 Quiet Stream Court, Potomac, MD 20854, (301) 496-5368, BA 60 CUNY - Hunter Coll; MA 65 Temple Univ; 78–Ch, Aud, NIH, **A**

Pilati, Mrs Eleanor M 326 Niles-Vienna Road, Vienna, OH 44473, (216) 856-1519, BS 76 Kent St Univ; MA 79 Kent St Univ; Sp-Lang Path, M-P Services In Sp Pathology, **SLP**

Pilberg, Rochelle 8243 Toll House Road, Annandale, VA 22003, (703) 978-7894, BA 66 CUNY - Brooklyn Coll; MS 68 Univ of Pittsburgh - Pittsburgh; Speech Language Pathologist, Private Practice, **SLP ACE**

Pilcher, Beverly Michele 2401 Girard Avenue South #5, Minneapolis, MN 55405, (312) 328-3775, BS 84 Univ of WI - Madison; MA 87 Northwestern Univ; **SLP**

Pilcher, Mrs Ellen Elizabeth 709 Glenwood Lane, Glenview, IL 60025, BS 83 Southern Methodist Univ; ME 85 Southwest TX St Univ; **SLP**

Pile, Donna K Hughes 202 North Kenyon, Albany, MO 64402, (816) 726-5652, BS 75 Northwest MO St Univ; MS 78 Central MO St Univ; SLP, Albany R-III Sch Dist, **SLP**

Pile, William L 2138 Wantland, Klamath Falls, OR 97601, (503) 863-6934, BS 71 Humboldt St Univ; MA 72 Humboldt St Univ; SLP, Winston-Dillard Sch Dist #116, **SLP**

Pilelsky, Rhoda Gail 2060 Winner's Circle, North Lauderdale, FL 33068, (305) 583-4420, BS 81 Boston Univ; MA 83 Northwestern Univ; Sp-Lang Path, Speech Pathology Inc, **SLP**

Pilewski, Mrs Denise Ellen 1074 Lorimer Street, Brooklyn, NY 11222, (718) 389-1939, **SLP**

Piliero, Mrs Mildred H 18 Kayeton Road, Allendale, NJ 07401, (201) 934-1089, BA 49 CUNY - Hunter Coll; MA 65 Kean Coll of NJ; Retired, Paramus Pub Sch, **SLP**

Pillion, Dr Joseph Paul 6508 Loch Hill Road, Baltimore, MD 21239, (301) 522-5450, BA 72 Western MI Univ; MA 78 OH St Univ; PH 81 (Sp and Hrng Science) OH St Univ; Aud, Kennnedy Institute, **A**

Pillow, A Hart 7819 Hill Ridge, San Antonio, TX 78250, (512) 684-7857, OM 75 LA St Univ - N O Medical Ctr; SLP, Private Practice, **SLP**

Pillow, Gary L Alleghany Highlands Hrng & Sp, Emmett Medical & Surg Clin, Route 696 & I64, Low Moor, VA 24457, (703) 862-6688, BS 77 East TN St Univ; MA 75 East TN St Univ; Owner/Aud, Alleghany Highlands Hrng&Sp Ce, **A**

Pillsbury, David C 2631 Greencrest Drive, Winston-Salem, NC 27106, (919) 748-3103, BA 63 Randolph-Macon Coll; MA 73 Northwestern Univ; Dir/Dept Hrng & Sp, Nc Baptist Hosp, **A**

Pilsner, Judith Ann 209½ East Market Street, Center, ND 58530, BA 78 Univ of WI - Stevens Point; MS 81 Univ of WI - Stevens Point; MS 86 Univ of WI - River Falls; 88–SLP, Oliver-Mercer, **SLP**

Pilson, Mrs Susan C M 11426 Ortega Drive, St Louis, MO 63138, (314) 741-7878, BS 73 Southern IL Univ-Edwardsvill; MS 74 Southern IL Univ-Edwardsvill; 80–Sp-Lang Path, Reg Ill-Spec Ed, **SLP**

Piltch, Michelle Ann 3 Tilden Drive, Novato, CA 94947, (415) 897-0610, BA 81 Humboldt St Univ; MS 83 CO St Univ; 87–Aud, Petaluma Valley Hearing Services, **A**

Pimental, Dr Patricia Ann 211 East Ohio #2323, Chicago, IL 60611, (312) 906-7210, BS 78 Northwestern Univ; MA 79 Northwestern Univ; OD 87 (Clinical Psychology) Chicago Sch of Professional Psychology; 87–Asst Prof, Univ of IL/Coll of Med, **SLP**

Pimentel, Elizabeth Anne 789 Almond Drive, Clovis, CA 93612, BA 78 CA St Univ - Fresno; MA 80 CA St Univ - Fresno; Resource Spec Tchr, Clovis USD, **SLP**

Pinborough, Judith A 288 No 1460 W, P O Box 16650, Salt Lake City, UT 84116-0650, (801) 538-6165, BS 74 Univ of UT; MS 76 Univ of UT; Sp-Lang Path, Utah Dept of Hlth, **SLP**

Pinch, Diane Kathleen 380 Stannard Avenue, Victoria, BC, Canada V8S 3M4, (604) 598-0757, BA 80 Univ of Victoria - Bc; MS 82 Univ of British Columbia; Sp-Lang Path, Gorge Road Hospital, **SLP**

Pincombe, Mrs Jane Elizabeth 47 Springbank Drive, London, ON, Canada N6J 1E4, (519) 434-7351, OM 87 Univ of Toronto - Ontario; 87–Sp-Lang Path, Thames Valley Children's Ctr

Pincus, Mrs Clara F 809 Dumaine Street, New Orleans, LA 70116, (504) 523-2055, BA 46 Augustana Coll; MA 52 Northwestern Univ; **SLP**

Pincus, Mrs Karen Bernstein 12 Greenfield Lane, Commack, NY 11725, (516) 493-0799, BA 79 SUNY - Center at Buffalo; MA 81 SUNY - Center at Buffalo; 87–Sp-Lang Path, Hicksville PS, **SLP**

Pincus-Clatterbuck, Laurie 37 Summit Avenue, Salem, MA 01970, (508) 745-2709, BA 76 Fairleigh Dickinson U-Teanec; MS 81 Boston Univ; Sp-Lang Path, Winthrop PS, **SLP**

Pinder, Gay L 116 N E 77th, Seattle, WA 98115, (206) 523-7630, BA 68 Hollins Coll; ME 72 Boston Univ; Sp-Lang Path, Chldn Ther Cen, **SLP**

Pindzola, Dr Rebekah Hand Dept Communication Disorders, 1199 Haley Center, Auburn, AL 36849, (205) 826-5545, BS 75 East Carolina Univ; MS 76 East Carolina Univ; PH 79 (NS) Univ of TN - Knoxville; 79–Assoc Prof, Auburn U/Dept Commun Dis, **SLP**

Pine, Mrs Anne Danetz 625 Gramatan Avenue #6C, Mount Vernon, NY 10552, (914) 738-3434, BS 61 Boston Univ; MA 64 Columbia Univ Teachers Coll; Sp-Lang Path, Pelham Pub Sch, **SLP**

Pine, Bernard 2665 South Hewlett Avenue, Merrick, NY 11566, (516) 541-7400, BA 52 CUNY - Brooklyn Coll; 55–Retired, BOCES of Nassau County, **SLP A**

Pine, Rhoda Zucker 1946 West Riverview, Decatur, IL 62522, (217) 877-3410, BS 46 Univ of WI - Madison; MS 52 Northwestern Univ; 88–Sp-Lang Path, Meyer Mental Hlth Dev Ctr, **SLP**

Pine, Dr Shirley J Dept Communicative Disorders, Ualr-Uams, 2801 South University Avenue, Little Rock, AR 72204-1001, (501) 569-3155, BA 52 Univ of CO - Boulder; MA 66 Univ of AR - Fayetteville; PH 70 (NS) Univ of FL; Professor, University of Arkansas, **SLP**

Pine-Brandwein, Mrs Shefra T 2392 Via Camino Avenue, Carmichael, CA 95608, (916) 483-4118, BA 65 CA St Univ - Sacramento; MA 70 CA St Univ - Sacramento; **SLP**

Pinelli, Mrs Pamela Sears 1684 McBain Avenue, San Jose, CA 95125, (408) 998-6330, BA 76 CA St Univ - Chico; MA 81 San Jose St Univ; Sp-Path, San Jose USD, **SLP**

Piner, Mrs Andrea Winters 10126 Reseda Boulevard, Apartment 118, Northridge, CA 91325, BA 83 Univ of CA - San Diego; MA 86 CA St Univ - Northridge; 87–Sp-Lang Path, Los Angeles USD, **SLP**

Piner, Bruce D 16311 Ventura Boulevard #560, Encino, CA 91436, (818) 981-7464, BA 85 CA St Univ - Northridge; MA 87 CA St Univ - Northridge; 87–Aud, Private Practice, **A**

Pinerman, Eileen 2101 Burdock Road, Baltimore, MD 21209, (301) 396-0780, BS 61; Sp-Lang Path, Baltimore City Publ Schs, **SLP**

Pinero, Iris M R R #6 Box 9228, Rio Piedras, PR 00928, (809) 754-3621, BS 66 Univ of PR - Rio Piedras; MA 68 1599; OM 81 Univ of PR - Rio Piedras; Pr Hlth Dept, **SLP**

Pines, Patricia L 9611 Page Avenue, Bethesda, MD 20814, (703) 437-5300, BA 70 Elmira Coll; MA 78 Univ of MN - Minneap-St Paul; V-President for Communications, National Grocers Association, **SLP**

Pinette, Judy D 99 Webster Avenue, Bangor, ME 04401, (207) 945-7365, BS 82 Univ of ME - Farmington; MA 84 Univ of ME - Orono; 85–Sp-Lang Path, Eastern Maine Medical Center, **SLP**

Pinhas, Dr Joan Speech Pathology, SUNY Geneseo, Geneseo, NY 14454, (716) 245-5326, BA 74 SUNY - Center at Buffalo; MS 75 Ithaca Coll; PH 84 (Psychology) Cornell Univ; Assistant Professor, Suc Geneseo, **SLP**

Pinheiro, Marilyn L 3021 Frampton Drive, Toledo, OH 43614, (419) 385-9618, BA 45 Boston Univ; MA 57 Case Western Reserve Univ; PH 69 Case Western Reserve Univ; Retired, Med Coll of Ohio at Toledo, **A F LM**

Pinkerton, Mrs Hope Leeger 614 Yalesville Road, Cheshire, CT 06410, (203) 574-8171, BS 50 SUNY - Coll at Buffalo; MS 63 Southern CT St Univ; OM 75 Southern CT St Univ; Supervisor of Special Educatn, Waterbury Board of Education, **SLP ACE**

Pinkerton, Mrs Judith A 1630 East Choctaw Drive N W, London, OH 43140, (614) 481-8507, BS 53 OH Univ - Athens; MA 68 OH Univ - Athens; Owner, Private Practice, **SLP**

Pinkerton, Susan Joy 1475 West Shaw, Fresno, CA 93711, (209) 225-0148, BA 82 CA St Univ - Northridge; MA 84 CA St Univ - Fresno; Aud, Private Practice, **A**

Pinkin-Troyk, Mrs Marianne 6027 Capulina Avenue, Morton Grove, IL 60053, (312) 966-2381, BS 81 WV Univ; MS 83 Syracuse Univ; Aud, Cook County Hospital, **A**

Pinkley, Mrs Frances Clare 7 Estates Lane East, Edwardsville, IL 62025, **SLP ACE**

Pinkney, Mrs Ruth G 34148 Schulte, Farmington Hills, MI 48024, (313) 437-1761, BA 74 Univ of MI - Ann Arbor; MS 75 Univ of MI - Ann Arbor; Sp-Lang Path, South Lyon Comm Sch, **SLP**

Pinkowski, Jodi Lynne 1545 Leisure Drive, Florissant, MO 63031, (314) 821-0008, BS 83 Southeast MO St Univ; MA 84 Southeast MO St Univ; 87–Sp-Lang Path/Aud, Professional Rehab Center Inc, **SLP A**

Pino-Merriam, Mrs Barbara K N7744 Sandy Beach Road, Fond Du Lac, WI 54935, (414) 922-5788, BS 70 Univ of WI - Oshkosh; MS 79 Univ of WI - Madison; Sp/Lang Path, Campbellsport Dist Sch, **SLP**

Pinsky, Mrs Debra Chetlin 250 Mark Trail, Atlanta, GA 30328, (404) 252-7585, MA 76 OH Univ - Athens; Sp-Lang Path, Fulton Co Bd of Ed, **SLP**

Pinter, Mrs Ann R 2509 A South 70th Street, Milwaukee, WI 53219, (414) 321-7893, BS 84 Univ of WI - Milwaukee; MS 86 Univ of WI - Milwaukee; 86–Sp-Lang Path, Milwaukee PS, **SLP**

Pinter, Naomi L 1250 East 22 Street, Brooklyn, NY 11210, (718) 377-0455, BA 73 CUNY - Brooklyn Coll; MS 76 CUNY - Brooklyn Coll; Sp-Lang Path, Cen for Spec Ed, **SLP**

Pinter, Shaindy 1783 East 9th Street, Brooklyn, NY 11223, (212) 627-9066, BS 76 CUNY - Brooklyn Coll; MS 78 Columbia Univ Teachers Coll; Lect Sp/Lang Path, Touro Coll Private Practice, **SLP**

Pioli, Elizabeth 307 North Loraine Avenue, Glendora, CA 91740, (818) 409-8023, BA 72 IN Univ - Bloomington; MA 73 IN Univ - Bloomington; Director Commun Disorders, Glendale Adventist Medical Cen, **SLP**

Piotrowski, Patricia Norford Lake Road, Thetford, VT 05075, (802) 785-4962, BS 74 Central MI Univ; MA 75 Central MI Univ; Sp-Lang Path, Private Practice, **SLP**

Pipek, Merrie Rural Route 2, Staples, MN 56479, SLP / Aud, Southeast Human Serv Cen, **SLP**

Pipenur, Denise R 104 Stonybrook Road, Fairfield, CT 06430, **SLP**

Piper, Mrs Elizabeth 611 County Line Road, Highland Park, IL 60035, (312) 432-1221, BA 67 IN Univ - Bloomington; MA 69 De Paul Univ; Private Practice, **SLP**

Piper, Mrs Jocelyn Ann 219 Gila Way, Placentia, CA 92670, (714) 996-2550, BA 60 Miami Univ - Oxford; MS 85 Chapman Coll; 88–Sp-Lang Path, Placentia USD, **SLP**

Piper, Mrs Lisa C S 21256 Washington Street, Walnut, CA 91789, (818) 331-3371, BA 78 Whittier Coll; MA 80 Whittier Coll; 79–Sp-Lang Path, Los Angeles Office of Ed, **SLP**

Piper, Mrs Rebecca Ann Rural Route 5, Vincennes, IN 47591, BA 76 Brescia Coll; OM 77 IN Univ - Bloomington; Sp-Lang Path, Comm Unit Sch Dist #20, **SLP**

Piper, Mrs Sara Faith 706 West Main Street, Watertown, WI 53094, (414) 674-3200, BS 75 Univ of WI - Oshkosh; ME 77 Univ of WI - Oshkosh; Home Health Sp-Lang Path, Jefferson County, **SLP**

Piper, Mrs Teresa Kathryn 8 Alan Circle, Londonderry, NH 03053, (603) 434-6500, **SLP**

Pipes, Marilyn Anne 1650 East Roger Road, Tucson, AZ 85719, (602) 621-1969, BS 81 Northeastern Univ; MS 83 Univ of AZ; 86–Clin Instr, Univ of AZ, **SLP ACE**

Pippert, Mrs Linda K 1704 West Chapman Avenue, Fullerton, CA 92633, (714) 870-4158, BS 75 Saint Cloud St Univ; MA 87 CA St Univ - Fullerton; **SLP**

Pippes, Mrs Mary Kay 502 East Yerby, Marshall, MO 65340, (816) 886-8515, BS 70 Southwest MO St Univ; MS 81 Central MO St Univ; Sp-Lang Path, Marshall Pub Schs, **SLP**

Pippin, Mrs Jane B 615 Williams Avenue, Natchitoches, LA 71457, (318) 932-4616, BA 69 Univ of Southwestern LA; MA 79 Northwestern St Univ; Sp-Lang Path, Natchitoches Par Sch Syst, **SLP**

Pippin, Kerry Rae 10 Marietta #2, Fairbanks, AK 99701, (213) 625-4183, MA 84 CA St Univ - Northridge; **SLP**

Pipski, Mary Ann 800 Fairview Road, Pittsburgh, PA 15238, (412) 784-4026, **SLP**

Pires, Mrs Helen Marshall 413 Walker Road, West Orange, NJ 07052, (201) 736-5736, BA 84 Kean Coll of NJ; MA 87 Kean Coll of NJ

Pirhofer, Lenore Anne 207 Quapaw Street, Santa Fe, NM 87501, (505) 983-2273, BS 83 Marquette Univ; MS 85 Marquette Univ; 88–Sp-Lang Path, InSpeech Inc, **SLP ACE**

Pirnot, Dennis V Rd 3 Box 358, Danville, PA 17821, (717) 271-6377, BS 69 PA St Univ - Univ Park; ME 70 PA St Univ - Univ Park; 70–Aud, Geisinger Med Ctr, **A**

Piroli, James Robert 1020 Edgewood Avenue N E, Atlanta, GA 30307, (404) 325-6646, BS 75 Eastern MI Univ; MA 78 Eastern MI Univ; Instructor-Severe Language Imp, St Charles Parish Pub Sch, **SLP**

Pirone, Kim Cheryl 4028-A Koko Drive, Honolulu, HI 96816, (808) 531-3511, BS 82 TX Christian Univ; MS 85 Univ of TX - Dallas; Sp-Lang Path, Rehab Hosp of Pacific, **SLP**

Pirreca, Mrs Marcia S Viscount Medical Complex, 9398 Viscount #1-F, El Paso, TX 79925, (915) 592-4184, BA 70 9318; MA 72 NM St Univ; Sp-Lang Path, Private Practice, **SLP**

Pirrone, Mrs Elisa Golley 960 South Lincoln Avenue, Monterey Park, CA 91754, (818) 332-2001, BA 81 CA St Univ - Long Beach; MS 85 Univ of Redlands; **SLP**

Pirruccello, Kathleen H PO 95, Westminster, VT 05158, (802) 463-9958, BA 76 George Washington Univ; MS 79 Univ of VT; Prog Dir-Sp-Lang Dept, Windham NE Superv Un, **SLP ACE**

Pirttima, Elizabeth Furney S 4622 Bates Street, Spokane, WA 99206, (509) 928-6022, BA 80 Univ of South FL; MS 85 Eastern WA Univ; **SLP**

Pisa, Mrs Lisa G 7724 Breakwater Drive, New Orleans, LA 70124, (504) 283-0324, BS 82 LA St Univ - Baton Rouge; ME 87 Southeastern LA Univ; **SLP**

Pisacano, Margaret S 181-40 Tudor Road, Jamaica, NY 11432, MS; **SLP ACE**

Pisakov, Mrs Nesta 309 Barryknoll Street, Anaheim, CA 92807, (714) 535-6001, BA 53 Occidental Coll; MA 55 Occidental Coll; Sp-Lang Path, Anaheim Cty Sch, **SLP**

Pisarek-Freatman, Susan 4313 Beach Ridge Road, North Tonawanda, NY 14120, (716) 439-6169, BS 77 SUNY - Coll at Buffalo; MS 78 SUNY - Coll at Buffalo; Sp/Lang Path, Niagara Co Sp-Hrng/Lang Cen, **SLP**

Piscitelli, Mrs Maureen A M 3 Virginia Road, Tyngsboro, MA 01879, (508) 649-9767, BS 77 SUNY - Center at Albany; MS 82 Univ of South FL; 87–Sp-Lang Path, AGH Associates Inc, **SLP**

Piscotty, Michael A P O Box 348, Fairview Village, PA 19409, (215) 265-4404, BA 74 Univ of Notre Dame; MA 76 Memphis St Univ; Aud, Hearing Care Ctr, **A**

Piskator, Mrs Tara Mullins 1600 Buena Vista Road, Apt 245, Columbus, GA 31906, (404) 596-9623, BA 86 Boston Coll; MS 88 Northeastern Univ; 88–Aud, Roosevelt Warm Springs Inst for Rehab

Piske, Kathleen L S 3464 Timothy Lane, East Aurora, NY 14052, (716) 883-2607, OB 77 SUNY - Coll at Buffalo; MA 78 Kent St Univ; Sp-Lang Path, Buffalo Bd of Educ, **SLP**

Pistono, Dr Kathleen Susan 20811 Madison, St Clair Shores, MI 48081, (313) 286-8800, BA 65 MI St Univ; MA 68 Northwestern Univ; PH 80 (Communicative Disorders) Northwestern Univ; 83–Consult-Sp-Lang Path, Macomb ISD

Pistrang, Judith A 81 Adams Avenue, Haworth, NJ 07641, (201) 327-4401, BA 46 CUNY - Brooklyn Coll; MS 71 William Paterson Coll; SLP, Upper Saddle River Sch Syst, **SLP**

Pitarque, Patricia A 11408 Farmland Drive, Rockville, MD 20852, (301) 770-6318, MS 87 Ithaca Coll; **SLP**

Pitcher, Cindy L 3660 North Lake Shore Dr, Apartment #2607, Chicago, IL 60613-4745, (312) 696-6274, BS 78 Coll of Saint Rose; MS 80 Syracuse Univ; Sp/Lang Path, Lutheran Gen Hosp, **SLP**

Pitcher, Mrs Deborah S 1320 Hanson Drive, Normal, IL 61761, (309) 454-3858, BS 75 Miami Univ - Oxford; MS 81 East TN St Univ; Aud, Dr Thomas Ocheltree, **A**

Pitcher, Mrs Mary M 140 Elm Street #2, Cortland, NY 13045, (607) 753-3142, BS 79 SUNY - Coll at Geneseo; MA 81 SUNY - Coll at Geneseo; Sp-Lang Path, Special Childrens Cen Inc, **SLP**

Pitcher, Michael Joseph 140 Elm Street #2, Cortland, NY 13045, (607) 753-0785, BS 81 SUNY - Coll at Geneseo; MS 85 Ithaca Coll; **A**

Pitcher-Fisher, Donna 9270 West 9th Avenue, Lakewood, CO 80215, (303) 238-5691, MS 74; Aud, Private Practice, **A**

Pitman, Mrs Rosamond M 1517 12th Street, Bedford, IN 47421, BS 48; MS 53 IN Univ - Bloomington; **LM**

Pitre, Derek Jerome 4927 Gambier Street, Los Angeles, CA 90032, (213) 582-7358, BS 83 Pacific Union Coll; MA 85 CA St Univ - Northridge; **SLP**

Pitre, Retha White 19660 Crystal Springs Ct, Newhall, CA 91321, (805) 251-2901, BS 64 Univ of TX - El Paso; MS 70 Univ of OK Medical Center; Spec Day Class Tchr, Los Angeles Co Supt of Schs, **SLP**

Pitt, Laurel Ann H 3817 Lynbrook Lane, Arlington, TX 76015, (817) 460-6022, BS 80 Univ of North TX; MA 81 Univ of North TX; SLP, Arlington ISD, **SLP**

Pittaway, Carmel I 578 Maidstone Lane, Clemmons, NC 27012, (919) 766-0650, BA 70 Marywood Coll; MA 73 Memphis St Univ; **SLP**

Pittelkow, Lynne Hebert 206 North Main Street, Wayland, MI 49348, (616) 962-9529, BS 84 Western MI Univ; MA 86 Western MI Univ; **SLP**

Pittenger, Anne M 12-D St Albans Avenue, Newtown Square, PA 19073, (215) 692-3636, BS 81 West Chester Univ of PA; MA 82 Bowling Green St Univ; Sp-Lang Path, Keystone Rehab Sys East, **SLP**

Pittenger, Mrs Gail S 2427 South Allison Way, Lakewood, CO 80227, (303) 797-0851, BA 69 George Washington Univ; MA 71 George Washington Univ; SLP, Jefferson Co Sch Sys, **SLP**

Pitti, Mary John 11 Heritage Road, Quincy, MA 02169, (617) 471-4210, BS 86 Ithaca Coll; MS 87 Ithaca Coll; Sp-Lang Path, Speech-Language Hearing Assoc

Pittman, Mrs Angela Sadler 7910 Cahill Drive, Austin, TX 78729, (512) 444-4835, BS 83 Southwest MO St Univ; MA 84 Southwest MO St Univ; 87–Sp-Lang Path, Healthcare Rehab Ctr, **SLP**

Pittman, Barbara Ann 4763-B Capital Circle SE, Tallahassee, FL 32301, (904) 488-7526, BS 74 FL St Univ; MS 75 FL St Univ; 78–Sp-Lang Path, Leon Co Sch Bd, **SLP**

Pittman, Cecilia L 21 East Market Street #3, Rhinebeck, NY 12572, (914) 876-3075, BS 74 SUNY - Center at Albany; MS 75 SUNY - Center at Albany; Sp-Lang Path, Rhinebeck Cen Sch, **SLP**

Pittman, Mrs Charlotte Leigh P O Box 298, Turpin, OK 73950, (405) 778-3333, BS OH St Univ; ME 88 Central St Univ; 88–Sp-Lang Path, Turpin PS

Pittman, Mrs Frankie L Route 1 Box 332, Bailey, NC 27807, (919) 235-4264, BA 71 Univ of NC - Greensboro; MA 72 Univ of NC - Greensboro; 84–Sp-Lang Path, Nash Co Sch, **SLP**

Pittman, Jimmy D 1308 Bayou Drive, Ocean Springs, MS 39564, (601) 872-2808, MS; 83–Aud, Keesler Med Ctr, **A**

Pittman, Mrs Laura M 1591 Hawthorne Avenue, Chico, CA 95926, (916) 343-1032, BA 59 CA St Univ - Chico; MA 73 CA St Univ - Chico; **SLP LM**

Pittman, Mrs Mary Lou 1966 Imperial Glf Crs Blvd, Naples, FL 33942, (813) 598-1235, BA 67 Univ of FL; MS 70 FL St Univ; 88–Sp-Lang Path, Naples Comm Hosp, **SLP**

Pittman, Mrs Susan K 221 South 6th, Terre Haute, IN 47807, (812) 232-0564, BS 82 Purdue Univ - West Lafayette; MS 85 Purdue Univ - West Lafayette; 85–Aud, A P & S Clinic, **A**

Pitts, Mrs Christine 3786 Heritage, Billings, MT 59102, (406) 657-6970, BA 77 Univ of MN - Minneap-St Paul; SLP, Indian Hlth Serv, **SLP**

Pitts, Dawna Gail 4814 Capitol Avenue #3, Omaha, NE 68132, (402) 554-6080, BS 82 Univ of NE - Lincoln; MS 84 Univ of NE - Lincoln; 84–Sp-Lang Path, Omaha Public Schools, **SLP**

Pitts, Mrs Deborah Dailey 921 South College, Tyler, TX 75701, (214) 597-0075, BA 80 Univ of TN - Knoxville; MA 83 Memphis St Univ; **SLP**

Pitts, Mrs Geraldine Mae 3266 East Scarborough Road, Cleveland Heights, OH 44118, (216) 265-3030, BA 79 Cleveland St Univ; MA 81 Cleveland St Univ; 86–Sp-Lang Path, Cuyahoga County Bd MR/DD, **SLP**

Pitts, Janice K 12401 East La Salle Place, Aurora, CO 80014, (303) 364-7657, BS 71 Northwestern Univ; MA 72 Univ of Northern CO; Sp-Lang Path, Cherry Creek Sch Dist #5, **SLP**

Pitts, William M 3266 East Scarborough Road, Cleveland Heights, OH 44118, (216) 459-3164, BA 62 Case Western Reserve Univ; MA 65 Case Western Reserve Univ; **SLP LM**

Pitts, Dr Willis N, Jr P O Box 257, 165 Washington Street, Sherborn, MA 01770, MA 41 Univ of MI - Ann Arbor; MA 42 Univ of MI - Ann Arbor; PH 52 (NS) Univ of MI - Ann Arbor; **SLP LM**

Pitz, Mrs Maria Anna 14 Louise Bay, Selkirk, MB, Canada R1A 0C7, (204) 467-5100, BS 80; MS 84 Univ of ND; 88–Sp-Lang Path, Interlake Sch Division #21, **SLP**

Pitzer, Mrs Carol Woodruff 4668 Edenfield Avenue, Covina, CA 91722, (213) 498-6626, BA 82 CA St Univ - Fullerton; MA 83 CA St Univ - Los Angeles; **A**

Pitzonka, Linda J 111 Scamridge Curve, Williamsville, NY 14221, (716) 686-2082, **SLP**

Pivor, Nadine R 1170 Ocean Parkway, Brooklyn, NY 11230, **SLP**

Piza, Maria E Menfias C-3, Villas DE Cupey, Rio Piedras, PR 00928, MS; **SLP**

Pizarro, Shea A Box 190, 10 Oak Street, Eufaula, OK 74432, (918) 689-9387, **A**

Pizer, Sherry H 12289 Arabian Place, Lake Ridge, VA 22192, (703) 690-2790, BA 72 IN Univ - Bloomington; MA 80 Univ of MD - College Park; Sp-Lang Path, Private Practice, **SLP**

Pizzano, Theresa Marie 4120 Helene Street, Simi Valley, CA 93063-2930, (805) 581-9353, BA 78 CT Coll; MA 84 CA St Univ - Northridge; **SLP**

Pizzi, Mrs Lisa Marie 527 Laurel Hill Avenue, Cranston, RI 02920, (401) 946-5533, MA 88 Univ of MA - Amherst

Pizzo, Mrs Bonnie Jean 67 Village Green, Princeton, WV 24740, (304) 487-8153, BS 82 Bloomsburg Univ of PA; MS 83 Bloomsburg Univ of PA; Sp-Lang Path, Southern Hills/Reg Rehab Hos, **SLP**

Pizzolato, Gene W 112 Main Street, Wareham, MA 02571, (617) 291-1333, BS 75 OH Univ - Athens; MS 77 Columbia Univ Teachers Coll; Clin Dir, In House Hrng Svcs, **SLP**

Pizzuti, Mary R 897 Woodmere Drive, Cleveland, OH 44147, (216) 526-6727, BA 70 Cleveland St Univ; MA 73 Cleveland St Univ; **SLP**

Pizzuti-Almazan, Annamaria 25 Archer Road, West Hempstead, NY 11552, (516) 483-1678, BA 77 Queens Coll; MS 79 Adelphi Univ; 79–Sp-Lang Path, NYC Bd of Educ, **SLP**

Place, Patti J 477 Brentwood, Kent, OH 44240, (216) 633-2055, MA 87 Kent St Univ; 88–Coord Tech Training, Children's Hosp Med Ctr of Akron, **SLP**

Placek, Susan Gale 5806 Independence #1E, Oak Forest, IL 60452, (312) 687-7647, **SLP**

Placko, Mrs Judith Ryan 309 Superior, Genoa, OH 43430, (419) 855-4223, BS 63 Miami Univ - Oxford; Sp-Lang Path, Benton-Carroll-Salem Bd of Ed, **SLP**

Plager, Mrs Sara S 7711 S W 136 Avenue, Miami, FL 33183, (305) 595-8232, BA 79 Univ of FL; ME 81 Univ of FL; Sp/Lang Path, Learning Workshop, **SLP**

Plain, Maureen O 12 Denton Avenue, Middletown, NY 10940, (914) 692-2748, BS 77 Loyola Coll; MS 79 Rutgers St Univ - Newark; Sp-Lang Path, Private Practice, **SLP**

Plaisance, Cynthia L 4535 Murietta Avenue #6, Sherman Oaks, CA 91423, (818) 986-9231, MA 80 CA St Univ - Northridge; Sp-Lang Path, Private Practice, **SLP ACE**

Plake, Terri L 5805 Lenz Court, Bakersfield, CA 93307, (714) 826-1025, BA 77 Brigham Young Univ; OM 78 Brigham Young Univ; SLP, Centre for Neuro Skills, **SLP**

Plakke, Dr Bruce L Dept Communicative Disorders, Univ Of Northern Iowa, Cedar Falls, IA 50614, (319) 273-3695, BA 71 Western MI Univ; MA 72 Western MI Univ; PH 78 (Aud major Statistics minor) Memphis St Univ; 78–Asst Prof of Aud, Dept Commun Dis U of Nn IA, **A**

Plamondon, Emily Ann 8650 W Peoria Avenue #1085, Peoria, AZ 85345, (602) 878-2432, **SLP**

Plamondon, Keith Allen 8650 W Peoria Avenue #1085, Peoria, AZ 85345, (602) 849-9060, Aud, Hrng Care 2000, **A**

Plank, Mrs Karlen Tilus 138 Lee Ann Lane, Chandler, OK 74834, (405) 258-2640, BS 77 Univ of Cincinnati; MS 78 Miami Univ - Oxford; 82–Sp-Lang Path, Lincoln Co Hlth Dept, **SLP**

Plant, Susannah 2839 Santa Cruz Drive, Rock Springs, WY 82901, MA 71 Kent St Univ; 81–Sp-Lang Path, Sweetwater Co Sch Dist 1, **SLP**

Plante, Amy Solomon P O Box 155, West Nottingham, NH 03291, (603) 692-4411, BS 80 Univ of NH; MS 82 Univ of NH; Sp-Lang Path, Stafford Lrng Cen, **SLP**

Plante, Elena Margaret 1611 North Mountain Avenue, Tucson, AZ 85719, (602) 795-7493, BA 84 Loyola Coll; MS 85 Loyola Coll; **SLP**

Plante, Theresa Clark 16 Quail Run, Hampstead, NH 03841, (603) 424-6211, BS 77 Univ of NH; ME 82 Northeastern Univ; **SLP**

Plapinger, Dr Donald S 1470 N W 124th, Portland, OR 97229, (503) 225-8356, ED 85 (Aud) Univ of Cincinnati; Asst Prof Sp-Lang Path & Aud, The Oregon Health Sciences Uni, **A**

Plass, Mrs Beverly Goodrich 16 New Haven, Irvine, CA 92720, (714) 496-1215, BA 81 CA St Univ - Fullerton; MA 85 CA St Univ - Long Beach; **SLP**

Plasterer, Lisa Rose 3816 S Lamar Blvd Apt 2019, Austin, TX 78704, (512) 447-7251, BS 84 Purdue Univ - West Lafayette; MA 86 Memphis St Univ; 86–Sp-Lang Path, InSpeech Inc, **SLP**

Plastino, Mrs Sue Ellen 238 Maple Hill Road, Gladwyne, PA 19035, (215) 642-0532, BS 76 SUNY - Coll at Geneseo; MS 78 PA St Univ - Univ Park; **SLP**

Platenberg, Lynn Route 2 Box 211, Marthasville, MO 63357, (314) 433-2691, BS 77 Northwest MO St Univ; MS 85 Northwest MO St Univ; 88–Sp-Lang Path, Sch Dist of WA, **SLP**

Platis, Dr Dean Salt Lake Hearing & Speech Center, 1377 East 3900 South, Suite 201, Salt Lake City, UT 84124, (801) 272-1232, BA 69 Univ of UT; MA 73 Univ of UT; PH 80 (NS) Univ of UT; Director/Sp-Lang Path & Aud, Salt Lake Hrng & Sp Cen, **SLP A**

Platt, Cindy Lyn 4775 Oakridge Drive, North Royalton, OH 44133, BS 78 OH Univ - Athens; **A**

Platt, Felice Ruth 507 Birch Drive, Cherry Hill, NJ 08003, BA 50 Univ of PA; MA 64 Temple Univ; Sp-Lang Path, Kingsway Learning Center, **SLP**

Platt, Dr James H 3313 Rhone Dr, Ceres, CA 95307, (209) 537-1286, BA 40 Bowling Green St Univ; MA 46 Univ of IA; PH 54 (Communication Methodologies) Univ of Denver; 66–Sp-Lang Path, Calif State Univ Stanislaus, **SLP LM**

Platt, Janelle Renee 6032-A 35th Avenue N E, Seattle, WA 98115, (206) 524-9028, BA 84 Univ of OR; MS 88 Univ of WA; 87–Sp-Lang Path, Sp Lang & Hrng Svcs, **SLP**

Platt, Mrs Judy Lynn 10170 South Seeley, Chicago, IL 60643, (312) 371-6340, BS 75 Southern IL Univ -Carbondale; OM 80 Governors St Univ; Sp/Lang Path, S Metropolitan Assoc, **SLP**

Platt, Mrs Mary F 1641 Banks, Houston, TX 77006, (713) 862-1796, BA 39 TX Woman's Univ; MA 40 TX Woman's Univ; MA 67 Univ of Houston - Univ Park; Retired, **SLP LM**

Platt, Roberta S 39 Wensley Drive, Great Neck, NY 11021, (212) 736-1100, BA 55 Adelphi Univ; MA 58 Columbia Univ Teachers Coll; **SLP**

Platt, Robin Dale 47 1/2 East 7th Street #Bb, New York, NY 10003, (212) 533-1440, BS 82 SUNY - Coll at Oneonta; MA 87 NY Univ

Platte-Worth, Mrs Susan Marie 735 West Duarte Road #305, Arcadia, CA 91006, (818) 967-4428, BA 79 CA St Univ - Los Angeles; MA 82 CA St Univ - Los Angeles; SLP, Foothill Sp-Lang & Hrng Cen, **SLP**

Platz, Janet A RFD 2, Skinner Hill Road, Coventry, CT 06238, (203) 647-3495, **SLP**

Plaut, Joyce Felice 793 McLean Avenue, Yonkers, NY 10704, (914) 277-3399, BS 78 SUNY - Center at Albany; MS 80 Columbia Univ Sch of Gen St; 80–Sp-Lang Path, Somers Cent Sch Dist, **SLP**

Plawecki, Mrs Lynne Myers 1358 Fairfield Court, Naperville, IL 60540, (312) 932-5200, BS 84 Purdue Univ - West Lafayette; MS 85 Purdue Univ - West Lafayette; 87–Sp-Lang Path, Coop Assoc for Spec Educ, **SLP**

Player, Mrs Kim Williams Box 132, Cleveland, UT 84518, (801) 653-2440, BS 76 UT St Univ; MS 77 UT St Univ; Sp-Lang Path, Emery County School District, **SLP**

Player, Mrs Marian Gray 7409 Wedgestone Court, Raleigh, NC 27615, (919) 733-0763, BA 70 Univ of NC - Greensboro; MS 83 East Carolina Univ; Dir of Sp-Lang Path, Dorothea Dix Hosp, **SLP**

Plaza, Yvonne S 627 Mountain Road, Hamburg, NJ 07419, (201) 827-3105, MA 88 Montclair St Coll

Pleasant, Kelly J 197 West Kemper Road, Cincinnati, OH 45246, (513) 867-6460, BS 85 Eastern IL Univ; MS 86 Miami Univ - Oxford; SLP, Mercy Hosp, **SLP**

Pleasonton, Dr Anna 1000 Adams Street, New Orleans, LA 70118, BA 58 CUNY - Hunter Coll; MA 59 Northwestern Univ; PH 68 (NS) LA St Univ - N O Medical Ctr; SLP, Orleans Parish Sch Bd, **SLP A**

Pleckaitis, Carolyn D 18 Main Street, Woodbridge, CT 06525, (203) 389-2920, BS 70 Central CT St Univ; MS 74 Southern CT St Univ; Sp/Lang Path, Project Learn, **SLP**

Pleiss, Claire W 3181 Stoneybrook Circle, Antioch, TN 37013, (615) 360-3758, BS 76 Marquette Univ; MS 77 Univ of WI - Milwaukee; **SLP**

Plenge, Teresa F 1192 Woodleigh Road, Marietta, GA 30064, (404) 436-9504, BA 75 Univ of TN - Knoxville; MA 77 Univ of TN - Knoxville; Sp-Lang Path, Cobb County Schools, **SLP**

Pleskac, Mrs Claudia L 7001 Huntington Avenue, Lincoln, NE 68507, (402) 464-2014, BS 72 Univ of NE - Lincoln; MA 75 Univ of NE - Lincoln; Aud, Lincoln Ear Nose & Throat, **A**

Pleskus, Mrs Judy Lynn 11022 Yarmouth Avenue, Granada Hills, CA 91344-6431, (213) 625-4138, BA 83 CA St Univ - Northridge; MA 85 CA St Univ - Northridge; **SLP**

Plevan, Mrs Janet C 13 Cornell Road, New Fairfield, CT 06812, (203) 796-1836, BA 63 CUNY - Queens Coll; MS 66 CUNY - Queens Coll; Sp-Lang Path, New Fairfield Bd of Ed, **SLP**

Plevin, Francine S 870 East El Camino Real #521, Sunnyvale, CA 94087, (415) 948-6834, BA 85 San Francisco St Univ; MS 87 San Francisco St Univ; 88–Sp-Lang Path, The Morgan Ctr, **SLP**

Pliskin, Mrs Doris K 4021 Estes, Lincolnwood, IL 60646, (312) 463-1884, MA 85 Northeastern IL Univ; Sp-Lang Path, Chicago Bd of Ed, **SLP**

Pliszka, Katherine Lynn 4867 Oak Knoll Avenue, Newton Falls, OH 44444, (216) 856-2107, BS 82 Kent St Univ; MA 83 Kent St Univ; Sp-Lang Path, Childrens Rehabilitation Cen, **SLP**

Ploch, Janice Ann C 15985 Huff, Livonia, MI 48154, (313) 582-6171, BS 73 Western MI Univ; MA 78 Eastern MI Univ; Sp-Lang Path, Dearborn Pub Sch, **SLP**

Plonsker, Leslie Schmidt 43 Vansant Road Apartment A, New Hope, PA 18938, (215) 598-0894, 88–Sp-Lang Path, The Wood Schools, **SLP**

Plost, Debra L 3459 South Florence Place, Tulsa, OK 74105, **SLP**

Plotkin, Mrs Donna B 15 Princeton Drive, Syosset, NY 11791, (516) 681-3963, BA 76 CUNY - Queens Coll; MA 77 Hofstra Univ; Sp-Lang Path, Pp/Horizon Sch Percept Dev, **SLP**

Plotkin, Dr William H 5451 N E River Road #1011, Chicago, IL 60656, (312) 483-0900, BA 50 Roosevelt Univ; MA 51 Northwestern Univ; PH 57 (Sp Path) Northwestern Univ; 80–Sp-Lang Path, Private Practice, **SLP F**

Plotnick, Charlotte B 3432 Bayfront Drive, Baldwin, NY 11510, (516) 378-2000, BA 56 CUNY - Brooklyn Coll; MS 84 Adelphi Univ; Sp-Lang Path, UCP of Nassau Co, **SLP**

Plotnick, Cheryl H 230 East 87th Street, New York, NY 10028, (718) 403-8431, BA 78 CUNY - Queens Coll; MA 80 CUNY - Queens Coll; Aud, Brooklyn Hosp Sp & Hrng Cen, **A**

Plourde, Lynn M P O Box 168, Anson, ME 04911, (207) 696-3331, BA 76 Univ of ME - Orono; MA 78 Univ of ME - Orono; Sp-Lang Path, Private Practice, **SLP**

Plous, Mrs Helen C 8575 43rd Avenue, Kenosha, WI 53142, (414) 656-2209, BS 65 Univ of WI - Madison; MS 67 Univ of WI - Madison; 69–Sp-Lang Path, Kenosha Hosp & Med Ctr, **SLP**

Plucker, Paul R L Doerfler Audiology Assoc, Central Medical Arts Bldg, Rural Delivery 7, Greensburg, PA 15601, (412) 539-3750, BS 73 Univ of WI - Stevens Point; MS 74 Univ of WI - Stevens Point; Aud, L Doerfler Audio Assoc, **A**

Plucknett, Janet F Boulder Drive, Peekskill, NY 10566, (914) 736-6504, BA 77 Pace U -NY City; MA 86 NY Univ; 85–Sp-Lang Path, NYC Bd/Ed-City Sp Svcs Unit, **SLP**

Plum, Sandra R 1254 Dayton Avenue, St Paul, MN 55104, (612) 879-2823, BS 83 Bradley Univ; MA 86 Univ of MN - Minneap-St Paul; 87–Sp-Lang Path, Ebenezer Caroline Ctr, **SLP**

Plumb, Kathleen B 1539 South Gillette, Tulsa, OK 74104, (918) 622-7064, BS 78 Southern Methodist Univ; MS 79 Southern Methodist Univ; Sp-Lang Path, Tulsa Scottish Rite Chldhd Cen, **SLP**

Plumb, Norma Hansen 1252 Brookview Station Rd, Castleton on Hudson, NY 12033, (518) 732-2450, BS 49 Univ of NE - Lincoln; MA 52 Univ of NE - Lincoln; **SLP LM**

Plumer, Elizabeth H P O Box 4403, Riverside, CA 92514, (714) 684-3491, BS 63 Bowling Green St Univ; Real Estate Analyst, Arlington Investments, **SLP**

Plumley, G Joyce Dade Home Health Care Services, 5959 Blue Lagoon Drive, Suite 230, Miami, FL 33126, MS 78 Univ of South FL; Administrator, Dade Home Health Care Services, **SLP**

Plumley, Jeffrey Lew Walker Road, Long Lake, NY 12847, (518) 624-2961, BA 81 SUNY - Coll at Plattsburgh; MA 84 SUNY - Coll at Plattsburgh; **A**

Plumley, Mrs Vickie Lynn Walker Road, Long Lake, NY 12847, (518) 359-3311, BA 81 SUNY - Coll at Plattsburgh; MA 84 SUNY - Coll at Plattsburgh; **SLP**

Plummer, Dr Bonnie A Soland County Office Of Educ, 655 Washington Street, Fairfield, CA 94533, (707) 429-6418, BA 66 Western MI Univ; ME 67 PA St Univ - Univ Park; PH 83 (Sp & Hrng Science) San Francisco St Univ; Dir Instr Support Svcs, Solano Co Off Ed, **SLP**

Plummer, Mrs Hazel M 11019 Blenheim Drive, Oakton, VA 22124, (703) 698-3653, BA 60 Rutger's St Univ - Douglas Coll; MA 80 George Washington Univ; 87–Chief-Sp & Hrng, Fairfax Hospital, **SLP**

Plummer, Sally Ann 1796 Kenny Road, Columbus, OH 43212, (614) 461-2440, BA 62 Hiram Coll; MA 64 OH St Univ; PH 72 (NS) OH St Univ; Audiologist, Columbus Childrens Hospital, **A**

Plummer, Susan Lynn 1315 South Maple Street, Sioux City, IA 51106, (712) 276-6656, MA 88 Univ of SD - Vermillion

Plumridge, Mrs Teri Salter 12346 Capri Circle North, Treasure Island, FL 33706, MA 84 Univ of FL; 88–Sp-Lang Path, Lashley & Associates Inc, **SLP**

Plung, Debbie 401 Amberson Avenue #241, Pittsburgh, PA 15232, (412) 622-3862, Supervisor, Pittsburgh-Mt Oliver Inter Unt, **SLP**

Plunket, Jane M 1010 Monroe Street #11G, Grenada, MS 38901, (601) 236-4474, BA 76 Univ of MS; MS 77 Univ of MS; 87–Sp-Lang Path Psychometrist, Mississippi State Dept of Educ, **SLP**

Plyler, Juliana Gibbs 4566 Mustang Road, Melbourne, FL 32935-2459, (407) 723-2566, BS 83 Univ of Montevallo; ME 85 GA St Univ; 88–Sp-Lang Path, Brevard Cty Sch Sys, **SLP**

Plymale, Mrs Judy D 4200 Ellinwood Drive, Apex, NC 27502, (919) 755-6560, MS 78 Univ of NC - Chapel Hill; **SLP A**

Poag, Linda J 5501 Dolores Avenue, Baltimore, MD 21227-2728, (301) 247-3843, BS 71 Auburn Univ - Auburn; MA 73 Univ of MD - College Park; Sp-Lang Path, Bd of Ed-Baltimore Co, **SLP**

Poage, Mrs Diane Louise 8806 Dome Circle, Eagle River, AK 99577, (907) 274-4582, BS 81 OR St Univ; MS 85 Western OR St Coll; 88–Sp-Lang Path, Anchorage Sch Dist, **SLP**

Poane, Mrs Lydia Luttrell 131 Beechtree Drive, Toms River, NJ 08753, (201) 341-9200, BA 71 Montclair St Coll; MA 75 Montclair St Coll; Sp/Lang Path, Toms River Bd of Ed, **SLP ACE**

Pobjecki, Donna Pauline 921 Grand Boulevard, Westbury, NY 11590, (516) 293-7826, **SLP**

Poburka, Bruce J 3513 Timber Tr, Little Suamico, WI 54141-8263, (414) 434-2617, MS 86 Univ of WI - Oshkosh; **SLP**

Poch, Nancy E Ms Hershey Medical Center, P O Box 850, Hershey, PA 17033, (717) 531-8904, BS 77 Univ of NH; MS 82 Bloomsburg Univ of PA; Aud, MS Hershey Med Cen, **A**

Pochant, Marylou Boots 1140 23rd Street, Minot, ND 58701-7205, (701) 839-1540, BS 78 Minot St Univ; MS 86 Minot St Univ; **SLP**

Pochily, Mrs Barbara Mahone 311 Wilson Avenue, Endwell, NY 13760, (607) 773-3105, MS 85 Ithaca Coll; **SLP**

Pochtar, Mrs Linda S 6 Putnam Avenue, Jericho, NY 11753, (516) 933-0963, BA 77 Hofstra Univ; MA 78 Hofstra Univ; **SLP**

Pocoroba, Mrs Catherine Mary 78 Scudder Avenue, Copiaque, NY 11726, (516) 933-6541, BA 80 Hofstra Univ; MA 82 Hofstra Univ; Sp-Lang Path, Hicksville Pub Schs, **SLP**

Podbelski, Mrs Susan Novak 5640 Deerpath Lane, Downers Grove, IL 60516, (312) 969-1518, BS 71 IL St Univ - Normal; MS 72 IL St Univ - Normal; Sp/Lang Path, Private Practice, **SLP**

Podesta, Mindy T 21 Seafield Lane, Bay Shore, NY 11706, **SLP**

Podewils, Mrs Jacqueline Ann 669 North 72nd Street, Wauwatosa, WI 53213, (414) 281-8777, BS 81 Univ of WI - Madison; MS 83 Univ of WI - Madison; Sp-Lang Path, St Luke's Hosp, **SLP**

Podhajski, Dr Blanche R Center For Language And, Learning, 81 West Canal Street, Winooski, VT 05404, (802) 655-2332, BS 67 Boston Univ; MS 69 Univ of VT; PH 80 (NS) Northwestern Univ; Dir, Cen Lang & Cerebral Func, **SLP**

Podleski, Jane P 1045 North Lafayette St, Florissant, MO 63031, (314) 838-1925, BA 71 Fontbonne Coll; MA 72 Saint Louis Univ; Sp-Lang Path, Spec Sch Dist of St Louis Co, **SLP**

Podol, Mrs Joanne C 923 Metz Avenue, State College, PA 16801, (814) 231-1076, BA 65 Univ of PA; MS 75 PA St Univ - Univ Park; SLP, St Coll Area Sch Dist, **SLP**

Podolsky, Vivian W 893 Webster Street, Needham, MA 02192, (617) 449-3666, BA 83 Boston Univ; MS 86 Boston Univ; Sp-Lang Path, Boston P S, **SLP**

Podvin, Julie A 2029 Greenway Cross #4, Madison, WI 53713-3018, (608) 252-8219, BS 82 Univ of WI - Stevens Point; MS 84 Univ of WI - Stevens Point; Aud, ENT Professional Assoc Sc, **A**

Podwall, Dr Arthur Syosset Speech & Hearing Ctr, 175 Jericho Turnpike, Syosset, NY 11791, (516) 364-1234, BA 66 Adelphi Univ; MS 70 Long Island U - CW Post Ctr; PH 84 (Sp-Lang Path & Aud) Columbia Pacific Univ; 70–Dir, Syosset Sp & Hrng Cen, **SLP A**

Podwall, Marcia Sue Syosset Speech & Hearing Ctr, 175 Jericho Turnpike, Syosset, NY 11791, (516) 364-1234, BA 68 CUNY - Queens Coll; MS 72 CUNY - Queens Coll; 72–Asst Dir, Syosset Sp & Hrng Cen, **SLP**

Podyma, Mrs Noreen Susan 160 King Road, Churchville, NY 14428, (716) 594-0685, BS 84 SUNY - Coll at Geneseo; MA 86 SUNY - Center at Buffalo; **SLP**

Poe, Mrs Esther F 12 Stoner Drive, West Hartford, CT 06107, (203) 525-9326, BA 60 Univ of VT; MA 61 Univ of CT; 74–Sp-Lang Path, Hartford Bd of Ed, **SLP**

Poels, Kathleen M 1512 Walls Street, Green Bay, WI 54304, BS 77 Univ of WI - Madison; MS 79 Univ of WI - Madison; Sp-Lang Path, Green Bay Bd of Ed, **SLP**

Poen, Beth D 963 Mallard Drive, Bradley, IL 60915, (815) 933-2546, BS 79 Western IL Univ; MA 81 Western IL Univ; SLP, Lasalle Co Ed Alliance-Spec Ed, **SLP**

Poeppelman, Lisa Louise Speech Pathology Services, 1402 Wagner Avenue, Greenville, OH 45331, (513) 549-9495, BS 83 Univ of Cincinnati; MS 84 Miami Univ - Oxford; 86–Dir, Speech Pathology Services, **SLP**

Poepping, Mrs Kathleen Marie 13937 Drommond Trail, Apple Valley, MN 55124, (612) 566-4780, BS 81 Saint Cloud St Univ; MA 87 Univ of Northern CO; Sp-Lang Path, InSpeech Inc, **SLP**

Poertner, Mrs Luanne Conrad 1328 Creamer Road, Norfolk, VA 23503, (804) 446-5939, BA 80 Mary Washington Coll; ME 82 Univ of VA - Charlottesville; Sp-Lang Path, E Virginia Ctr Commun Disordrs, **SLP ACE**

Poffenbarger, Kathryn L 105 Mohawk Court, Anderson, IN 46012, BS 69 Ball St Univ; MS 76 Univ of HI - Manoa; Sp-Lang Path, Anderson Community Schools, **SLP**

Poggi, Karen J 8 Oakside Lane, Peekskill, NY 10566, (203) 358-4922, BA 73 Mercy Coll; MS 76 Long Island U - CW Post Ctr; Sp/Lang Path, Stamford Pub Schs, **SLP**

Pogroszewski, Janis M 22727 Middle Camp Road, Twain Harte, CA 95383, (209) 586-1326, MA 84 CA St Univ - Stanislaus; Sp-Lang Path, Private Practice

Pogue, Dr Elizabeth 222 Martling Avenue, Tarrytown, NY 10591, (914) 631-3547, BA 53 Manhattan Coll; ME 63 Fordham Univ; PH 77 (NS) NY Univ; Prof, Mercy Coll, **SLP**

Pohl, Mrs Anne M 2336 Bretton Drive, Cincinnati, OH 45244, (513) 369-4730, BS 72 OH St Univ; ME 77 Univ of Cincinnati; Superv of Sp-Lang Serv, Cincinnati Pub Sch, **SLP**

Pohl, Mrs Joan K Speech-Language Pathologist, P O Box 2451, Winter Park, FL 32790, (305) 628-4477, BA 75 Univ of Miami; MA 79 Univ of CA - Los Angeles; Private Practice, **SLP**

Pohlenz, Mrs Mary Lynn Route 1 Box 48-M, Towanda, KS 67144, (316) 778-1917, BA 68 Wichita St Univ; MA 74 Wichita St Univ; Sp-Lang Path, Private Practice, **SLP**

Pohlman, Janie Lynn 2350 South 8th Avenue, Apartment A211, Yuma, AZ 85364, (602) 782-6450, BA 81 Univ of Northern CO; MA 83 Univ of Northern CO; Sp-Lang Path, Crane Sch Dist 13, **SLP**

Pohlman, Mrs Virginia Bregar 4117 E Pasadena, Phoenix, AZ 85018, (602) 277-5551, BS 84 AZ St Univ; OM 87 AZ St Univ; **SLP**

Pohlmann, Karen Trissel 2511 New Lexington Drive, Bettendorf, IA 52722, (319) 383-1499, BS 84 IA St Univ; MS 85 Univ of WI - Stevens Point; SLP, Mercy Hosp, **SLP**

Pohlot, Mrs Nancy Elizabeth 26851 Via Grande, Mission Viejo, CA 92691, (714) 582-2324, BA 70 Saint Olaf Coll; MA 72 Univ of IA; 88–Sp-Lang Path, InSpeech Inc, **SLP**

Pohutsky, Mrs Joelyne C J Rural Delivery 1, Christopher Street, Stroudsburg, PA 18360, BS 75 East Stroudsburg Univ of PA; MS 81 Bloomsburg Univ of PA; Sp-Lang Path, Colonial Intermed Ut No 20, **SLP**

Poillon, Patricia 11 Ridge Court, Hauppauge, NY 11788, (516) 473-2800, BS 84 SUNY - Coll at Geneseo; MS 85 Univ of NC - Chapel Hill; Sp-Lang Path, St Charles Hosp, **SLP**

Poiset, Melissa L Scripps Memorial Hospital, 9888 Genessee, P O Box 27, La Jolla, CA 92037, (619) 452-0344, MS 76 Humboldt St Univ; Dir Sp-Lang Path, Scripps Mem Hosp, **SLP**

Poisson, Doris A 155 Railroad Street, Manville, RI 02838, (617) 883-6060, BS 79 Worcester St Coll; MA 83 Univ of MA - Amherst; Sp-Lang Path, Blackstone/Millville Sch, **SLP**

Poke, Mrs Lynn Washington 714 West Lenawee, Lansing, MI 48915, (517) 887-3057, BS 71 Western MI Univ; ME 76 Wayne St Univ; ES 84 (NS) Univ of Detroit; 87–Sp-Lang Path, Lansing Sch Dist, **SLP**

Poklepovic, Mrs Michel Stewart 5111 Longfellow Avenue, Tampa, FL 33629, (813) 837-5467, OB 64 Emory Univ; MA 69 Univ of FL; **A**

Pokorny, Ellen Brooke 115 Laurel Lane, Austin, TX 78705, (512) 479-0345, BS 82 Stephen F Austin St Univ; MS 84 Univ of TX - Dallas; Sp-Lang Path, **SLP**

Polakof, Isabel Box 326 USAHN, 98th General Hospital, APO New York, NY 09105-3501, BS 71 Trenton St Coll; MA 73 Trenton St Coll; 78–Sp-Lang Path, USA Meddac Nurnberg

Polan, Pam L 3220 Glen Iris Court, Milford, MI 48042, (313) 360-2885, BS 76 Eastern MI Univ; MA 77 Eastern MI Univ; Manager Community Relations, Vna, **SLP**

Poland, Robert M Easley Head & Neck Surgery, Hrng Serv-Individual/Indus, 109 Fleetwood Drive, Easley, SC 29640, (803) 855-2411, BS 68 Central MI Univ; MA 70 MI St Univ; MA 77 OH Univ - Athens; Aud, Easley Head & Neck Surgery Pa, **A**

Polangin, Arlene K 9806 Broad Street, Bethesda, MD 20814, (301) 530-1595, BS 61 PA St Univ - Univ Park; MA 69 Univ of MD - College Park; Sp-Lang Path, Montg Co MD Pub Sch, **SLP**

Polehna, Mrs Priscilla 4524 White Pine Drive N E, Cedar Rapids, IA 52402, (319) 399-6700, BA 75 Univ of Northern IA; MA 77 Western IL Univ; SLP, Grant Wood AEA, **SLP**

Polen, Dr Samuel B Dept Speech Path & Audiology, Western Washington Univ, 033 Parks Hall, Bellingham, WA 98225, (206) 676-3881, BS 66; MA 70; PH 73 (NS); Assoc Prof, Western Washington, **SLP**

Polen, William D, Jr 1000 East 3rd Street, Medical Towers Suite 102, Chattanooga, TN 37403, (615) 266-8618, BS 72 Univ Southern MS-Hattiesburg; MS 73 Univ Southern MS-Hattiesburg; Aud, Otologic Cen, **A**

Poleshuck, Deborah S 85 Walnut Street, Staten Island, NY 10310, MA 76 Montclair St Coll; SLP, New York City Board of Educ, **SLP**

Polgroszek, Mrs Beverly B 42 Parish Drive, Kensington, CT 06037, (203) 828-3553, BA 72 Central CT St Univ; MS 76 Southern CT St Univ; Sp-Lang Path, Wolcott Pub Schs, **SLP**

Poliak, Mrs Diana R W 1345 Bismarck Avenue, Oshkosh, WI 54901, (414) 685-2741, BS 79 Univ of WI - Oshkosh; OM 81 Univ of WI - Oshkosh; 81–Sp/Lang Path, Sch Dist of Omro, **SLP**

Polich, Laure Yakima Valley Hrng & Sp Center, 303 S 12th Avenue, Yakima, WA 98902, (509) 453-8248, MS 80 Eastern WA Univ; MS 87 Univ of WA; 88–Aud/Sp-Lang Path, Yakima Valley H & S Ctr, **SLP**

Polichar, Donna J 10320 Cresta Drive, Los Angeles, CA 90064, (213) 997-2330, BA 72 CA St Univ - Northridge; MA 74 CA St Univ - Northridge; SLP, LA USD, **SLP**

Polignano, Mrs Maria L 19 Byron Drive, Basking Ridge, NJ 07920, (201) 464-7625, BA 67 Trenton St Coll; MS 70 Rutger's St Univ - Douglas Coll; Sp-Lang Path, Morris Union Consortium, **SLP**

Polikowsky, Ann Wennblom 421 Sumter Avenue South, Golden Valley, MN 55426, (612) 541-1844, BS 84 Univ of MN - Minneap-St Paul; MS 85 Univ of WI - Eau Claire; Sp-Lang Path, Columbia Hgts Sch Dist, **SLP**

Poling, Mrs Cheryl Rene 211 Simmons Drive, Ripley, WV 25271, (304) 372-6447, MA 85 Marshall Univ; **SLP**

Polinsky, Mrs Debra Shapiro 8619 Brookshire #D, St Louis, MO 63132, (314) 993-1431, BS 86 Fontbonne Coll; MS 88 Fontbonne Coll; 87–Sp-Lang Path, Christian Hospital Northeast, **SLP**

Polishook, Pnina T 563 Heath Road, Merion, PA 19066, (215) 922-6177, BS 70 Long Island U - CW Post Ctr; MA 72 Temple Univ-Tyler Sch of Art; **SLP**

Polishook, Mrs Robin Paige 25 Mary Ellen Road, Waban, MA 02168, (617) 965-6374, BA 77 Univ of RI; MS 80 Columbia Univ Teachers Coll; Sp-Lang Path, Private Practice, **SLP**

Polizzi, Anne Maureen 226 Mabel Ann Avenue, Franklin Lakes, NJ 07417, (201) 881-6131, BA 83 William Paterson Coll; MA 86 Montclair St Coll; 87–Sp-Lang Path, City of Paterson Bd of Educ, **SLP**

Polk, Mrs Gloria H 18105 Fairfield, Detroit, MI 48221, (313) 927-7640, BA 66 Hampton Univ; MA 67 Western MI Univ; 85–Sp-Lang Path, Mt Carmel Mercy Hosp, **SLP ACE**

Polk, Jane Midkiff 543 Laketower #130, Lexington, KY 40502, (606) 268-4545, BA 53 Georgetown Coll; Executive Director, Lexington Hearing & Speech Cen

Polk, Katherine Elaine 1560 Mosaic #219, Stockton, CA 95207, (209) 944-4486, OB 73 Univ of the Pacific; BA 80 CA St Univ - Sacramento; MA 81 Univ of the Pacific; SLP, Stockton USD, **SLP**

Polk, Mrs Marian L 2418 East Edgedale Drive, Missouri City, TX 77489, (713) 438-1963, BA 78 Sam Houston St Univ; MA 80 Univ of Houston - Univ Park; Sp/Lang Path, Houston ISD, **SLP**

Polk, Pamela M R 13672 West 54th Avenue, Arvada, CO 80002, **SLP**

Polk, Teresa C 14111 Badger Avenue, Sylmar, CA 91342, (818) 997-2330, BA 76 CA St Univ - Northridge; MA 78 CA St Univ - Northridge; Sp-Lang Path, LA USD, **SLP ACE**

Polka, Linda 13133 North Twentieth, Apt 210, Tampa, FL 33612, (813) 974-3504, BA 80 Slippery Rock Univ of PA; MA 84 Univ of MN - Minneap-St Paul; 88–Research Asst, Univ of South Florida

Polkowski, Mrs Diane Patricia 312 Berkshire Road, Mechanicsburg, PA 17055, (717) 766-7957, BS 81 Bloomsburg Univ of PA; MS 82 Bloomsburg Univ of PA; 82–Sp-Lang Path, Capital Area I U 15, **SLP**

Poll, Mrs Karen Richler 1768 East 18th Street, Brooklyn, NY 11229, (718) 376-5114, BA 77; MS 79 Columbia Univ Teachers Coll; **SLP**

Pollack, Mrs Doreen M 14285 East Marina Drive, Aurora, CO 80014, (303) 755-3694, BA 61 Univ of Denver; OM 44; **SLP A LM**

Pollack, Mrs Dorothy H 212-09 16th Avenue, Bayside, NY 11360, (212) 780-5186, BA 63 CUNY - Brooklyn Coll; MA 68 CUNY - Queens Coll; Instr/Super, CUNY Brooklyn Coll, **SLP**

Pollack, Evelyn 405 East 82nd Street #3-F, New York, NY 10028, (212) 481-4464, BA 59 CUNY - Hunter Coll; MA 62 NY Univ; Sp-Lang Path, CUNY-Hunter Coll, **SLP**

Pollack, Dr Helen A 4710 Bethesda Avenue #916, Bethesda, MD 20814, (301) 654-8456, BA 69 Monmouth Coll; MS 74 Boston Univ; ED 84 (Instructional Media & Technology) Boston Univ; 87–Dir/Admin App of Tech, ASHA, **SLP**

Pollack, Janet Lynn Rd 1 Box 275, Dogwood Drive, Wading River, NY 11792, (516) 744-1600, BA 78 SUNY - Coll at Oneonta; MA 83 SUNY - Center at Buffalo; Sp-Lang Path, St Vincents Medical Center, **SLP**

Pollack, Dr Michael C 2180 Pinebrook Trail, Cuyahoga Falls, OH 44223, (216) 376-1221, BS 64 Emerson Coll; MS 66 AZ St Univ; PH 70 (NS) Univ of Southern CA; Aud, Professional Hearing Services, **A**

Pollack, Peggy Blum 4216 North Turnbull Drive, Metairie, LA 70002, (504) 885-3527, BS 72 Univ of TX - Austin; OM 75 LA St Univ - N O Medical Ctr; Clinical Instructor, Lsu Med Ctr, **A**

Pollack, Sharon R 4134 Minden, Memphis, TN 38117, **SLP**

Pollack, Sheri 1019 Reads Lane, Far Rockaway, NY 11691, (718) 946-9700, BA 79 SUNY - Coll at Cortland; MS 81 Adelphi Univ; Sp-Lang Path, Brooklyn Sch for Spec Chldrn, **SLP**

Pollack-Klein, Sandra R 179 Madison Road, Scarsdale, NY 10583, (212) 345-6410, **SLP**

Pollak, Mrs Renee 15500 Southwest 89th Avenue, Miami, FL 33157, (305) 235-5545, OB 67 Univ of Miami; MA 79 Univ of Miami; Sp-Lang Path, Dade Co Publ Schs, **SLP**

Pollard, Mrs Catherine 4404 South Marion Road, Sioux Falls, SD 57106, (605) 332-4762, BS 80 Univ of NE - Lincoln; MS 82 Univ of NE - Lincoln; SLP, Sioux Falls Public Schools, **SLP**

Pollard, Kenneth H P O Box 4508, Macon, GA 31208, (912) 743-8953, BS 65 Jacksonville St Univ; MA 71 Univ of AL- Tuscaloosa; Aud, ENT Med Gp, **A**

Pollard, Michele M 1039 Bishop Court, Palatine, IL 60067, BS 69 Boston Univ; MS 71 Univ of WI - Madison; **SLP**

Pollard, Stephanie Crum 15210 Hesta Street, Poway, CA 92064, (714) 532-3264, BA 84 Chapman Coll; MA 87 CA St Univ - Fullerton

Polledri, Mrs Diane M 349 Park Street, Upper Montclair, NJ 07043, (201) 743-4653, BA 78 Montclair St Coll; MA 83 Montclair St Coll; Sp-Lang Path, Private Practice, **SLP**

Pollens, Robin Dovitz 601 Egleston, Kalamazoo, MI 49001, (616) 372-2047, BA 77 Univ of MI - Ann Arbor; MS 78 Univ of MI - Ann Arbor; Sp-Lang Path, Constance Brown Hrng & Sp, **SLP ACE**

Pollesel, Susan S Box 1313, Ukiah, CA 95482, **SLP**

Pollett, Pamela A L 140 Eaton Drive, Lincoln, IL 62656, (217) 732-1079, MS 76 Southern IL Univ -Carbondale; Sp-Lang Path, Private Practice, **SLP**

Polley, Mrs Mary Ann Key 3975 Park Avenue, Fairfield, CT 06430, (203) 966-4506, BA 65 Catholic Univ of America; MA 66 Northwestern Univ; Sp-Lang Path, New Canaan Bd of Ed, **SLP**

Pollikoff, Francine 1000 Valley Forge Circle, Unit 316, King of Prussia, PA 19406, (215) 539-8550, BA 48 CUNY - Hunter Coll; MA 50 OH St Univ; Sp-Lang Path, Mont Co Inter Ut 23, **SLP**

Pollins, Mrs Judith L 19 Susquehanna Trail, Somerville, NJ 08876, BA 53 CUNY - Queens Coll; MA 56 CUNY - Brooklyn Coll; 87–Sp-Lang Path, Midland Sch, **SLP**

Pollnow, Rita K P O Box 2351, Davis, CA 95617, (916) 666-8710, MA 79 CA St Univ - Sacramento; SLP, Yolo County Office of Educ, **SLP**

Pollock, Mrs Carol R 228 Kings Way, Clemson, SC 29631, (404) 548-3550, BS 76; ME 77 Univ of GA; Sp-Lang Path, Private Practice, **SLP**

Pollock, Debra Kotelchuck 3822 Hendon Road, Randallstown, MD 21133, (301) 484-0209, BA 78 Univ of MD - College Park; MS 79 Loyola Coll; 73–Sp-Lang Path, Chldn's Sp & Lang Serv, **SLP ACE**

Pollock, Gail Lynn 939 East Jefferson, Morton, IL 61550, (309) 266-9949, BS 85 IL St Univ - Normal; MS 86 IL St Univ - Normal; 87–Aud, St Francis Med Ctr, **A**

Pollock, Dr Karen E Department Of Communicative Disorders, University Of Northern Iowa, Cedar Falls, IA 50614-0356, (319) 273-6806, BA 75 Univ of OR; MA 80 Univ of OR; PH 86 (Phonology/Language) Purdue Univ - West Lafayette; 86–Asst Prof, Univ of Northern Iowa, **SLP**

Pollock, Marianne M R-40 Atherholt Drive, Bunker Hill, Wyoming, PA 18644, (717) 288-1411, BS 82 Bloomsburg Univ of PA; MS 84 Bloomsburg Univ of PA; Sp-Lang Path, InSpeech Inc, **SLP**

Pollock, Mrs Marion C 32 Locksley Road, Newton Center, MA 02159, (617) 244-7289, BS 72 Ithaca Coll; MS 73 Ithaca Coll; Sp-Lang Path, Newton Public Schools, **SLP**

Pollock, Mrs Norma Haegg 825 Olive Street, Menlo Park, CA 94025, BA 49 Univ of IA; MA 52 Univ of IA; **SLP**

Pollock, Mrs Pamela K 96 Ashland, Buffalo, NY 14222, (716) 882-8951, BA 65 Stanford Univ; MA 66 Univ of WA; Sp-Lang Path, Buffalo PS, **SLP ACE**

Pollock, Pattie L 1048 W Rancho Road, Corona, CA 91720, (714) 683-6255, BA 78 Univ of Redlands; MA 80 CA St Univ - Los Angeles; Aud, Riverside County Schools, **A**

Pollok, Mrs Janice J 2109 Nottingham Drive, Omaha, NE 68123, (307) 291-1037, BA 77 Univ of CO - Boulder; MS 79 Minot St Univ; **SLP**

Pollom, Mrs Judy L 4814 Peachtree Avenue, Louisville, KY 40215, (502) 636-2084, BS 77 Spalding Coll; MS 79 Univ of Louisville; Sp-Lang Path, Louisville Deaf Oral Sch, **SLP**

Polmanteer, Mrs Kathryn N P O Box 1151, Brevard, NC 28712, (704) 884-3232, BS 74 FL St Univ; MS 75 FL St Univ; 88–Sp-Lang Path, Transylvania Co Sch Sys, **SLP**

Polmateer-McKnight, Mrs Carol R 1722 Kingston Avenue, Kalamazoo, MI 49001, (616) 674-8091, BA 78 MI St Univ; MA 80 Central MI Univ; Sp-Lang Path, Van Buren Intermed Sch Dist, **SLP**

Polniak, Alan Martin 217 West Broadway # D-6, Columbia, MO 65201, (314) 442-5670, BA 84 SUNY - Center at Buffalo; MA 86 Univ of Denver; 86–Aud, Harry S Truman VA Hosp, **A**

Polon, Mrs Marilyn B 2212 Fort Ward Place, Alexandria, VA 22304, (703) 379-4971, BA 66 Univ of MD - College Park; MA 67 Columbia Univ Teachers Coll; Sp-Lang Path, Private Practice, **SLP ACE**

Polonsky, Mrs Adrienne 8 North Green Acre Drive, Cherry Hill, NJ 08003, (609) 424-5113, BA 77 CUNY - Brooklyn Coll; MS 79 Hahneman Medical Coll; Sp-Lang Path, Private Practice/Consultant, **SLP**

Polonsky, Ronnie Jane 5545 Lawton Avenue, Oakland, CA 94618, **A**

Polow, Dr Nancy Gross 667 Brentwood Drive, South Orange, NJ 07079, (201) 761-1400, BS 67 NY Univ; MA 68 Seton Hall Univ; PH 74 (NS) Fordham Univ; Sp/Lang Path, Suburban Speech Center, **SLP**

Polsky, Marla R 4295 Nerissa Circle, Fremont, CA 94555, (408) 262-1780, **SLP**

Polson, Cynthia Brown 312 Wedgewood Lane North, Plymouth, MN 55441, (612) 457-7285, BS 79 Univ of MN - Minneap-St Paul; MA 81 Univ of MN - Duluth; Sp-Lang Path, North Memorial Med Ctr, **SLP**

Polson, Debra L 500 Emerson Avenue, Hamilton, OH 45013, (513) 863-6544, BS 75 Miami Univ - Oxford; MS 78 Miami Univ - Oxford; SLP, Lakota Local Schools, **SLP**

Polson, Joan C 4026 N E Davis, Portland, OR 97232, (503) 235-6963, BA 78 Portland St Univ; MS 80 Portland St Univ; **SLP**

Polson, Mrs Kathryn E 40 West Marble Street, Duluth, MN 55811, (218) 727-1616, OB 82 Univ of MN - Duluth; MA 83 Univ of MN - Minneap-St Paul; SLP, Superior Pub Schs, **SLP**

Polster, Mrs Cindy Miller 2845 Shakercrest Boulevard, Beachwood, OH 44122-2325, (216) 464-3398, BA 84 Cleveland St Univ; MA 86 Cleveland St Univ; **SLP**

Polston, Mrs Paula Denise 3532 Warwick Glen, Brownsville, TX 78521, (512) 546-3101, BS 71 Indiana Univ of PA; ME 82 Clarion Univ of PA; Sp-Lang Path, Brownsville ISD, **SLP**

Poluha, Patricia C Speech Pathology Department, St Marys Hospital, 35 Grosvenor Street, London, ON, Canada N6A 1Y6, (519) 439-3271, BA 73 Lakehead Univ - Ontario; MA 77 Univ of MN - Minneap-St Paul; Mgr Commun Dis, St Marys/St Josephs Hosp, **SLP**

Polys, Christine Meyer 1921 Windy Hill, Kirkwood, MO 63122, (314) 479-3029, BA 83 Fontbonne Coll; MS 86 Fontbonne Coll; **SLP**

Polzer, Mrs Kathleen R 5 Peter's Lane, Port Jefferson Station, NY 11776, (516) 924-0008, BA 77 CUNY - Queens Coll; MA 78 CUNY - Queens Coll; 86–Supvr Sp-Lang Path, Just Kids Early Childhood Learning Ctr, **SLP**

Polzin, Franklin Dow 18680 Gratiot, Merrill, MI 48637, (517) 776-0303, BS 69 Central MI Univ; MS 72 Univ of MI - Ann Arbor; Sp-Lang Path, Sch Dist of Saginaw, Mi, **SLP**

Pomaville, Mrs Frances Marian 55 West Bullard #284, Clovis, CA 93612, (209) 298-5036, BA 82 CA St Univ - Fresno; MA 84 CA St Univ - Fresno; Sp-Lang Path, Fresno USD, **SLP**

Pomeranc, Mrs Carol R 84 Mandon Drive, Wayne, NJ 07470, (201) 696-0414, BA 71 CUNY - City College; MA 73 Montclair St Coll; Sp-Lang Path, Private Practice, **SLP**

Pomerantz, Bonnie K 323 North Westfield Road, Buffalo, NY 14226, MS; **SLP LM**

Pomerantz, Harris I P O Box 18733, Tampa, FL 33679, (813) 251-2248, BA 53 Syracuse Univ; MS 54 Syracuse Univ; Aud, Harris I Pomerantz Ms, **SLP A**

Pomerantz, Jilda Colville Rural Free Delivery, Chelsea, VT 05038, (802) 479-0179, BS 66 Miami Univ - Oxford; MA 67 Miami Univ - Oxford; Sp-Lang Path, Barre City Sch, **SLP**

Pomerantz, Joan K 1700 N W 82th Avenue, Pompano Beach, FL 33065, (305) 721-3500, SLP, Sch Bd of Broward Co, FL, **SLP**

Pomeranz, Shira Tolwin 1102 South Rexford Drive, Apartment 3, Los Angeles, CA 90035, (213) 271-9416, BS 83 Univ of WI - Milwaukee; MS 86 Emerson Coll; **SLP**

Pomes, Mrs Leticia Flores 10160 Whitmore Street, El Monte, CA 91733, (818) 442-3599, BA 82 CA St Univ - Fullerton

Pomilio, Mrs Carole B Rd 3 Germantown Park, Morristown, PA 19403, (215) 539-0493, BS 84 Stockton St Coll; MS 85 Univ of MI - Ann Arbor; **SLP**

Pommerening, Mrs Connie E 7614 Shady Hollow, San Antonio, TX 78255, (512) 673-2111, BA 70 Saint Mary's Univ; MA 73 Our Lady Lake Univ-San Anton; Early Chldhood Tchr, Northside ISD, **SLP**

Pommers, Mrs Susan G 606 Old Stone Brook, Village Of Nagog Woods, Acton, MA 01718, (508) 369-9500, BS 69 SUNY - Coll at Geneseo; MS 72 SUNY - Center at Albany; Sp-Lang Path, Concord Public Schools, **SLP**

Pomper, Michael S 1403 Janet Circle, Adel, IA 50003, (515) 993-3782, BA 74 Drake Univ; MA 80 Univ of Northern IA; Sp-Lang Path, Pt & Rehabilitation Specialsts, **SLP**

Pomplun, Mrs Beverlee J 1305 Bradley Court, Princeton, NJ 08540, (609) 683-0224, BS 77 Ball St Univ; MA 82 Univ of IL - Urbana; 88–Sp/Lang Path, Private Practice, **SLP**

Poms, Mrs Lillian R 8955 S W 85th Terrace, Miami, FL 33173, (305) 274-3451, OB 60 Univ of FL; ME 61 Boston Univ; Executive Director, Hrng & Sp Cen of FL, **SLP ACE**

Pomy, Valerie A 1922 Penwood Drive, Knoxville, TN 37922, (615) 945-2908, BS 79 Univ of TN - Knoxville; MA 80 Univ of TN - Knoxville; Sp-Lang Path, Anderson Co Sch-Preschool, **SLP**

Pona, Rosemary 136 Jockey Hollow Way, Union, NJ 07083, (201) 687-8682

Ponche, Mrs Diane K 164 Fort Sumter Way, St Charles, MO 63303, (314) 447-6727, BS 79 Northeast MO St Univ; MA 80 Northeast MO St Univ; Sp/Lang Path, Francis Howell Sch Dist, **SLP**

Pond, Mrs Deneen Schneiter 476 Bringhurst Circle, Providence, UT 84332, (801) 753-6293, MS 85 UT St Univ; **SLP**

Poniatowski, Sonja M 5312 Andover Circle, Cross Lanes, WV 25313, (304) 768-8861, BS 72 Purdue Univ - West Lafayette; MA 78 Marshall Univ; **SLP**

Pons, Kevin C 1125 South Hill Drive, Waterloo, IA 50701, (319) 234-6881, BA 74 Univ of CT; MA 76 Univ of CT; Dir of Aud, ENT Assoc Pc, **A**

Pons, Shayna Karas 901 Gilbert Road, Rockville, MD 20851, (202) 877-1440, BS 83 Boston Univ; MS 85 Vanderbilt Univ; 88–Sp-Lang Path, Natl Rehab Hosp, **SLP**

Ponte, Mrs Colleen M 14218 Foch, Livonia, MI 48154, (313) 593-7725, BS 79 Eastern MI Univ; MA 81 Eastern MI Univ; Sp-Lang Path, Oakwood Hosp, **SLP**

Ponticello, Michelina Ann Hrng & Sp Ctr Of Rochester Inc, 1000 Elmwood Avenue, Rochester, NY 14620, (716) 271-0680, OB 68 Northern IL Univ - De Kalb; MA 70 Univ of MD - College Park; Asst Dir/Sp-Lang Path, Hrng & Sp Cen of Rochester, **SLP**

Ponticiello, Michelle Maria 40-1B Richmond Boulevard, Ronkonkoma, NY 11779, (516) 981-0727, MS 83 Univ of LA Verne; 82–Sp-Lang Path, William Floyd School District, **SLP**

Pontius, William L 1320 Watson Street, Williamsport, PA 17701, (717) 321-2700, BS 68 Bloomsburg Univ of PA; MS 71 WV Univ; Admin Dir of Sp/Lang Path/Aud, Williamsport Hosp, **A**

Pontorno, Deborah Rewee 10001 Greebelt Road #201, Lanham, MD 20706, (301) 794-6571, BS 80 Univ of WI - Whitewater; MS 81 Univ of WI - Whitewater; Sp/Lang Path, Private Practice, **SLP**

Pool, Grace Gismondi 11 Annie J Circle, Milford, MA 01757, BA 83 SUNY - Center at Buffalo; MA 85 SUNY - Center at Buffalo; SLP, Middlesex Cild Dev Ctr, **SLP**

Poole, Mrs Ann Taylor 102 Lancelot, Simpsonville, SC 29681, (803) 243-3171, BS 64 Univ of GA; ME 80 Converse Coll; SLP, Greenville County Schools, **SLP**

Poole, Mrs Anne P 3413 Judy Lane, Shreveport, LA 71119, (318) 636-3484, BA 72 LA Tech Univ; OM 81 LA St Univ - Shreveport; Sp-Lang Path, Caddo Parish Sch Syst, **SLP**

Poole, Mrs Jean O Route 1 Box 38, Axtell, NE 68924, (308) 743-2528, BS 71 CA St Univ - Northridge; MA 75 Univ of NE - Lincoln; 88–Resource Tchr, Axtell Comm Sch, **SLP**

Poole, Joann Neu 872 Atlanta Court, Claremont, CA 91711, **SLP**

Poole, Julia Ann 1001 Heartwood Lane, Lake Zurich, IL 60047, (312) 882-2780, BA 84 MI St Univ; MA 85 MI St Univ; Sp-Lang Path, Comm Concepts, **SLP**

Poole, Mrs Marilyn R 14 Rebecca Lane, Conway, AR 72032, (501) 371-3402, BS 53 Univ of North TX; ME 70 Univ of Central AR; MS 77 Univ of AR - Little Rock; Staff Dev Spec II, AR Dev Dis Serv, **SLP**

Poole, Mrs Pamela B 315 Shiloh Lane, Tuscaloosa, AL 35406, (205) 553-3760, BS 73 MS Univ for Women; MS 78 Univ of AL- Tuscaloosa; Aud, VA, **A**

Poole, Penny Jean 4576 Maj Sprague Street, El Paso, TX 79924, (915) 755-8596, BA 83 Univ of TX - El Paso; MS 85 Univ of TX - El Paso; Regis Therpist 1, El Paso St Cntr, **SLP**

Poole, Ronald D 112 Hawaiian Drive, Mankato, MN 56001, (507) 389-1414, BS 61 Mankato St Univ; MA 65 Univ of KS; OD 74 (NS) Univ of Denver; Assoc Prof, Mankato St U, **A**

Pooler, Shannon Gill 49388 Olson Road, Avondale, CO 81022, (303) 353-2085, MA 88 Univ of Northern CO

Pooley, Mrs Mary Ann Shurina 425 Marseille Drive, Hurst, TX 76054, (817) 498-2988, BS 62 Duquesne Univ; MS 67 WV Univ; Sp-Lang Path, VA Med Ctr Nrsng Home, **SLP**

Poolos, Mrs Hazel P P O Box 353, Richfield, NC 28137, (704) 463-7962, BA 57 Univ of GA; ME 80 Univ of NC - Greensboro; 84–Sp-Lang Path, Stanly Co Schs, **SLP**

Poor, Nancy 125 East 87th Street #10A, New York, NY 10128, (212) 369-0987, BS 83 Trenton St Coll; MS 85 Columbia Univ Teachers Coll; **SLP ACE**

Pooser, Mrs Polly B 1603 Seminole, Tallahassee, FL 32301, (904) 644-2238, MS 71 Univ of South FL; Sp-Lang Path, FL St U, **SLP**

Pope, Carol L Box 212, Rimforest, CA 92378, (714) 337-9318, MA 72 CA St Univ - Los Angeles; Sp/Lang Path, Sn CA Permanente Med Gp, **SLP**

Pope, Mrs Catherine Turner 1434 Crestview Avenue, Tallahassee, FL 32303-5814, (912) 246-0733, Audiologist, Audio Rehab Lab, **A**

Pope, Mrs Denise L 9 Kingston Street, Belmont, NC 28012, (704) 825-5905, BS 73 Appalachian St Univ; MS 74 Appalachian St Univ; Consultant, Private Practice, **SLP**

Pope, Gina Denise 2642 Forrister Court, Lithia Springs, GA 30057, (404) 949-2587, ME 88 West GA Coll; 88–Sp-Lang Path, Douglas Co Sch Sys

Pope, Kathy Ann 7 Railroad Street, Danville, PA 17821, (717) 621-5030, BS 79 East Stroudsburg Univ of PA; MS 82 Hahneman Medical Coll; 87–Dir of Sp-Lang Path, Pottsville Hosp/Warner Clinic, **SLP A**

Pope, Mrs Lois A 11536 S W 33rd Avenue, Portland, OR 97219, BA 65 Lewis & Clark Coll; MS 80 Western OR St Coll; Sp-Lang Path, **SLP**

Pope, Mary Anne L 20 Baron Court, Danville, IN 46122, (317) 264-8868, BA 71 IN Univ - Bloomington; MA 73 IN Univ - Bloomington; Aud, IN U Med Cen, **A**

Pope, Mrs Monica M 5390 Velo Court, Riverside, CA 92506, (714) 371-2109, BA 76 CA St Univ - Fullerton; MA 79 CA St Univ - Fullerton; SLP, Corona-Norco USD, **SLP**

Pope, Mrs Patricia L 1523 Homewood Avenue, High Point, NC 27260, (919) 884-4250, BA 83 Univ of NC - Chapel Hill; MS 85 Univ of NC - Chapel Hill; Sp-Lang Path, Guilford County Schools, **SLP**

Pope, Zandra M P O Box 5051, Augusta, GA 30906, **A**

Popeck, Mrs Gay Lounsberry 1139-B Bobo Avenue, MCAS, Yuma, AZ 85365, (602) 726-8341, BA 81 Univ of Southwestern LA; MS 84 Univ of Southwestern LA; Sp-Lang Path, Private Practice, **SLP**

Pope-Hartman, Florence 21 Bernard Drive, West Trenton, NJ 08628-2311, BS 75 Montclair St Coll; MS 79 Rutger's St Univ - Douglas Coll; **SLP**

Popejoy, Maurice E 7601 East Imperial Highway, Downey, CA 90242, (213) 940-7684, **A**

Popelka, Dr Gerald Raymond 21 Berkley Lane, St Louis, MO 63124, (314) 652-3200, BA 68 Kent St Univ; MA 70 Kent St Univ; PH 74 (Dr of Philosophy) Univ of WI - Madison; 80–Head of Aud, Cen I for the Deaf, **A F**

Popelka, Jean Sladek 108 Dianthus Street North, Manhattan Beach, CA 90266, (213) 836-7251, BS Northern IL Univ - De Kalb; MA Loyola Univ; MS Loyola Univ; Psych, Los Angeles Co Ofc of Educ, **SLP**

Popiel, Rebecca L 3421 Wallace, Grand Island, NY 14072, (716) 674-6300, BA 77 SUNY - Center at Buffalo; MA 79 SUNY - Center at Buffalo; Sp-Lang Path, West Seneca Developmental Cen, **SLP**

Popielec, Eugene A Henry Ford Hospital, 2799 West Grand Boulevard, Detroit, MI 48202, (313) 876-3286, BS 56 Bowling Green St Univ; MS 60 Wayne St Univ; 67–Sp-Lang Path, Henry Ford Hosp/Dept-Neurology, **SLP ACE**

Popovics, Alice M 6 Meadow Lane #10, Bridgewater, MA 02324-1899, (508) 824-6911, BS 75 Emerson Coll; MA 77 Hofstra Univ; Asst Dir/Sp-Lang Path, Morton Hosp & Med Ctr Inc, **SLP ACE**

Popowsky, Karen Rudnick 61-19 218th Street, Bayside, NY 11364, (212) 423-2217, BA 72 SUNY - Center at Buffalo; MA 74 Boston Univ; SLP, NYC Bd of Educ, **SLP**

Popowych, Daria Teresa 2249 West Iowa, Chicago, IL 60622, (312) 784-3277, BA 79 Univ of IL - Chicago; MS 83 Rush Presbyterian St Luke's Medical Center; 86–Owner, Northside Aud Group Inc, **A**

Popowych, Mrs Katherine 1708 Churchville Road, Bel Air, MD 21014, (301) 396-1397, BA 78 Loyola Coll; MS 79 Loyola Coll; Sp/Lang Path, Baltimore City Publ Schs, **SLP**

Popp, Sharon Ad 4665 55th Street, San Diego, CA 92115, **SLP**

Popp, Stephanie L 4622 Lake Valley #3-C, Lisle, IL 60532, (312) 357-5692, BS 78 Univ of AZ; MS 80 Univ of AZ; Sp-Lang Path, Spec Sch Dist of St Louis Co, **SLP**

Popp-Dipietro, Debra K 33 Log Pond Drive, Horsham, PA 19044, (215) 957-0226, BA 75 Wichita St Univ; MA 77 NY Univ; 87–Sp-Lang Path, Pathway School, **SLP**

Poppe, Carol RFD 2 Granger Hollow Road, North Bennington, VT 05257, (802) 442-2692, BS 72 OH St Univ; MA 74 OH St Univ; Sp-Lang Path, Southwest VT Supervisory Union, **SLP**

Poppe, Mrs Nancy I 804 West 12th Street, Spencer, IA 51301, (712) 262-7608, BA 81 Kearney St Coll; MS 82 Kearney St Coll; 88–Sp-Lang Path, Private Practice, **SLP**

Popper, Mrs Roberta Antell 6 Hickman Street, Syosset, NY 11791, (516) 922-9022, BA 63 CUNY - Brooklyn Coll; MS 78 CUNY - Brooklyn Coll; 86–Sp-Lang Path, Westbury Union Free Sch Dist, **SLP**

Popplewell, Deatra Ann Wood Co Office Of Education, 1 Courthouse Square, Bowling Green, OH 43402, (419) 354-9010, BS 82 Ball St Univ; MA 84 Ball St Univ; 84–Aud, Wood Co Ofc of Educ, **A ACE**

Porcaro, Mrs Susan C C 43 Liberty Lane, Petaluma, CA 94952, (707) 778-4614, BA 69 CA St Univ - Long Beach; ME 84 Sonoma St Univ; MA 73 Humboldt St Univ; Sp-Lang Path, Petaluma Cty Sch, **SLP**

Porcelan, Mindy Abrams 34 Comanche Avenue, Rockaway Township, NJ 07866, (201) 627-2123, BA 77 Rutger's St Univ - Douglas Coll; MS 82 Syracuse Univ; Sp-Lang Path, Rehabilitation Ctr for Hndcpd, **SLP**

Porcella, Nancy Weldon 813 1/2 North Harper Avenue, Los Angeles, CA 90046, (213) 885-8500, **SLP**

Porcelli, Mrs Janet J 1017 Prospect Ridge, Haddon Heights, NJ 08035, (215) 329-5715, BA 69 Rutger's St Univ - Douglas Coll; MA 73 Temple Univ-Tyler Sch of Art; Asst Dir-Cen/Commun Dis, Moss Rehab Hosp, **SLP**

Porch, Dr Bruce 713 Parkland Circle S E, Albuquerque, NM 87108, (505) 255-6901, BS 55 Wayne St Univ; ME 57 Wayne St Univ; PH 66 (NS) Stanford Univ; 68–Assoc Prof, Univ of New Mexico, **SLP F**

Porch, Meg 713 Parkland Circle S E, Albuquerque, NM 87108, (505) 255-6901, BA 59 Univ of NM; MA 60 Stanford Univ; 83–Sp-Lang Path, Ed Assessment Systems Inc, **SLP**

Porch, Mrs Robyn Bailey 6006 West Shore Drive, Pensacola, FL 32506, (904) 476-2021, BA 79 Pan American Univ; MS 82 Univ of AR - Little Rock; Sp/Lang Path, Escambia Sch Dist, **SLP**

Pore, Sally G Heritage Apartment #5, Summer Street, Peterborough, NH 03458, BA 70 Thiel Coll; ME 73 Northeastern Univ; 87–Sp-Lang Path, Easter Seal of NH, **SLP**

Porec, John Paul El Camino Medical Center, 8100 Constitution Place N E, Suite 4100, Albuquerque, NM 87110, (505) 888-4844, BS 72 WV Univ; MS 74 Univ of NM; PH 83 (NS) Univ of NM; Clinic Dir, Clinical Assoc Pc, **SLP**

Porras-Bagingito, Tina L 7400 Parkway Drive #20, La Mesa, CA 92042, (619) 466-9736, MA 88 San Diego St Univ; 87–Sp-Lang Path, La Mesa-Spring Valley Sch Dist

Porrazzo, Shirley 1927 Washburn Avenue North, Minneapolis, MN 55411, (612) 725-6767, BS 66 Univ of MN - Minneap-St Paul; MA 69 Univ of MN - Minneap-St Paul; Sp-Lang Path, VA Med Cen, **SLP**

Porreca, Rosemarie A 266 Highview Drive, Leola, PA 17540, (717) 656-8314, BS 80 Indiana Univ of PA; MA 88 West Chester Univ of PA; 84–Sp-Lang Path, S June Smith Ctr

Porreca-Mansilla, Mrs Patricia L 23 Cynthia Lane, Pittsfield, MA 01201, (413) 637-2834, BA 78 Anna Maria Coll; MA 82 Univ of MA - Amherst; **SLP**

Porrino, Mrs Andrea Mittleman 23 Kinder Drive, Bloomfield, NJ 07003, (201) 338-0602, SLP, Englewood Hospital, **SLP**

Porteous, Mrs Mary Jane 8643-D Rosecrans Avenue, Paramount, CA 90723, (213) 868-8241, BS 75 Western MI Univ; MA 78 Eastern MI Univ; Sp-Lang Path, Little Lake Cty Sch, **SLP**

Porter, Alicia K Route 7, 232 Scenic View Drive, Clinton, TN 37716, (615) 945-2222, BS 76 Univ of GA; MA 77 Univ of TN - Knoxville; 84–Sp-Lang Path, Anderson Co Schs, **SLP**

Porter, Belinda J 1806 Larch Place, Urbana, IL 61801, (217) 384-3551, BS 73 IL St Univ - Normal; MS 74 IL St Univ - Normal; 83–Sp-Lang Path, Urbana Sch Dist #116, **SLP**

Porter, Betty J 2005 Crown Avenue, Cincinnati, OH 45212, BS 79 Univ of Cincinnati; MA 81 Univ of Cincinnati; Aud, Dayton ENT Surgeons Inc, **A**

Porter, Mrs Carolyn T 428 Woodland Circle, Lynchburg, VA 24502, (804) 237-3874, BS 83 Longwood Coll; ME 85 Univ of VA - Charlottesville; SLP, Central Virginia Training Ctr, **SLP**

Porter, Mrs Christine 4119 Riverside Drive, Youngstown, OH 44511, (216) 743-1151, BS 58 Kent St Univ; MA 76 Kent St Univ; SLP, Youngstown Pub Sch, **SLP**

Porter, Mrs Claudia 110 Lake Top Court, Roswell, GA 30076, (404) 992-4006, BA 69 Occidental Coll; MA 70 Occidental Coll; Sp-Lang Path, Early Success Program, **SLP**

Porter, Donica T 76 Countryside Drive, Cumberland, RI 02864, (401) 765-2506, BA 68 Emmanuel Coll; MA 79 Univ of Pittsburgh - Pittsburgh, Fulton-Porter Assoc Inc, **A**

Porter, Donna S 106 Bayou Lane, Picayune, MS 39466, (601) 798-4182, BS 79 Univ Southern MS-Hattiesburg; MS 80 Univ Southern MS-Hattiesburg; Sp-Lang Path, Picayune Sch Sys, **SLP**

Porter, Dora Thea P O Box 564, Alamo, CA 94507, (415) 633-5269, MA 59 OH St Univ; Aud, Naval Hospital, **SLP A ACE**

Porter, Mrs Elaine A 6148 North 12th Road, Arlington, VA 22205, MA 74 Univ of Pittsburgh - Pittsburgh; Sp-Lang Path, Chldrns Sp-Lang Serv, **SLP**

Porter, Elizabeth Ann White 4222 Edinburgh Drive, Cincinnati, OH 45245, (513) 825-5454, BS 79 WV Univ; MS 81 WV Univ; Aud, Tri-County ENT, **A**

Porter, Elizabeth Mulligan 130-C Versailles Drive, Melbourne Beach, FL 32951, (407) 768-2931, BS 74 Bridgewater St Coll; MA 85 3515; Sp-Lang Path, **SLP**

Porter, James F P O Box 2, Templeton, CA 93465, (805) 238-6058, BA 69 Humboldt St Univ; BA 69 Humboldt St Univ; MA 70 Humboldt St Univ; Sp-Lang Path, San Luis Obispo Co Supt of Sch, **SLP**

Porter, Jane Boyd 7945 S W Churchill Way, Tigard, OR 97224, (503) 684-9248, Aud, Reg Prog For Hearing Imp, **A**

Porter, Jane W 800 West Airport Freeway, Suite 118A, Irving, TX 75062, (214) 438-9360, BS 68 Univ of TN - Knoxville; MA 70 Univ of TN - Knoxville; Owner, Private Practice, **A**

Porter, Kimberly Stickel P O Box 694, Man, WV 25635, (304) 583-6360, BS 82 WV Univ; MA 86 Marshall Univ; **SLP**

Porter, Lawrence A 6078-600 Avenue West, Oak Harbor, WA 98277, (206) 679-5809, BA 62 Central WA Univ; ME 68 Central WA Univ; 63–Sp-Lang Path, Oak Harbor Sch Dist, **SLP**

Porter, Linda I 1103 Stone Creek Drive, Blue Springs, MO 64015, (816) 228-5929, BA 73 Univ of MO - KS City; MA 75 Univ of KS; Sp-Lang Path, Blue Springs R-IV, **SLP**

Porter, Dr Lois S 18 Ashford Lane, Schenectady, NY 12309, (518) 869-3467, BA 66 Montclair St Coll; MA 67 Northwestern Univ; PH 77 (NS) Union for Experi Coll & Univ; Exec Dir, NYS Fed of Growers & Proc Inc, **A**

Porter, Mary S 17 Westwind Road, Louisville, KY 40207, (502) 895-3385, BA 67 Univ of KY; ME 71 Univ of KY; **SLP**

Porter, Dr Patricia B Mental Retardation/Developmental Disability Services, Department Of Human Resources, Albemarle Bldg Salisbury Street, Raleigh, NC 27611, (919) 733-3654, BA 71 Marshall Univ; MA 72 Marshall Univ; PH 80 (NS) Univ of NC - Chapel Hill; 88–Dep Dir for MR Svcs, Dept of Human Res North Carolina, **SLP**

Porter, Patricia L 611 Coronet, San Antonio, TX 78216, (512) 342-6378, BS 70 Southwest TX St Univ; ME 72 Southwest TX St Univ; St Andrew's Weekday Sch, **SLP**

Porter, Dr Robert J, Jr Department Of Psychology, University Of New Orleans, Lakefront, New Orleans, LA 70148, (504) 947-6641, BS 67; MA 69 Hollins Coll; PH 71 (NS) Univ of CT; Prof, U of New Orleans

Porter, Mrs Sandra P 13608 Pheasant Circle, Lockport, IL 60441, (815) 838-3588, BS 74 Univ of KS; MS 76 Southern IL Univ -Carbondale; Sp/Lang Path, Commun Sch Dist 218, **SLP**

Porter, Susan Swigart 170 Beech Avenue, Melrose, MA 02176, (617) 665-4165, BA 79 Allegheny Coll; MA 81 MI St Univ; Sp-Lang Path, **SLP**

Porter, Dr Thomas A 1106 Avalon, Olathe, KS 66062, (913) 764-1993, BS 62 Mankato St Univ; MS 66 Univ of KS; PH 71 (NS) Univ of KS; Director of Audiology, Kansas State School for Deaf, **A**

Porter, Todd H Irving Hearing Aid Dispensary, 800 West Airport Freeway, Suite 118A, Irving, TX 75062, (214) 438-9360, BS 68 Univ of TN - Knoxville; MA 70 Univ of TN - Knoxville; Owner, Irving Hearing Aid Dispensary, **A**

Porter, Wyne W 1907 Edison, Santa Ynez, CA 93460, (805) 688-3898, BA 48 Whittier Coll; MA 49 Whittier Coll; Aud, Private Practice, **SLP A LM**

Portera, Rosemary V 1201 Australian Avenue, Riviera Beach, FL 33404, (407) 842-3213, BS 85 FL St Univ; MS 86 FL St Univ; 87–Sp-Lang Path, Assoc for Retarded Citizens, **SLP**

Portera, Mrs Suzanne Haley 2009 Tidewater Lane, Madison, MS 39110, (601) 856-6461, OB 75 Univ of MS; OM 76 Univ of MS; Sp-Lang Path, Suzanne H Portera, **SLP**

Porter-Cope, Judith L 26944 Girard Street, Hemet, CA 93244, (714) 929-6338, BA 62 Univ of MN - Minneap-St Paul; MA 75 CA St Univ - Los Angeles; Sp-Lang Path, Riverside County Supt of Sch, **SLP**

Porter-Couto, Bonnie J 10 Maple Avenue, Chelmsford, MA 01824, (508) 250-1608, BA 83 Bridgewater St Coll; MS 85 Northeastern Univ; Sp-Lang Path, Hudson Public Schools, **SLP**

Porterfield, Mrs Janet L 534 Taft Court, Delaware, OH 43015, (614) 369-3101, BS 69 OH Univ - Athens; MS 72 Univ of RI; SLP, Marion City Schools, **SLP**

Porterfield, Wendy Sue c/o Modjeski, 3520 Merrick Drive, Lexington, KY 40502, **SLP**

Porter-Kanel, Mrs Robin 151 Country Farms Road, Marlton, NJ 08053, (609) 983-1800, BA 80 Tel Aviv Univ - Israel; MS 82 Syracuse Univ; 82–Sp-Lang Path, Evesham Twsp Bd of Ed, **SLP**

Portley, Rossanna S 9503 Red Willow Lane, Dallas, TX 75249, (214) 296-8147, BS 78 TX Woman's Univ; MS 85 Univ of TX - Dallas; **SLP**

Portnoy, Mrs Frances W 4 Alton Court, Merrick, NY 11566, (516) 921-5500, BA 70 Hofstra Univ; MA 72 Hofstra Univ; SLP, Syosset Pub Schs, **SLP**

Portnoy, Mrs Mary Regina 1114-A Ralph Terrace, St Louis, MO 63117, (314) 842-3050, BS 83 Fontbonne Coll; MS 84 Fontbonne Coll; Sp-Lang Path, Afton School District, **SLP**

Portnoy, Mrs Mona Semel 9 Lackawanna Court, Dayton, NJ 08810, (201) 873-2800, BS 74 Boston Univ; MA 77 Trenton St Coll; Sp-Lang Path, Franklin Twsp Pub Sch Syst, **SLP**

Portnoy, Robert A 12944 Frengate Lane, St Louis, MO 63141-6131, (314) 895-7005, **SLP**

Posch, Susan C 641 1/2 West 11th Street, Dubuque, IA 52001, (319) 588-8014, BA 71 Case Western Reserve Univ; MA 72 Case Western Reserve Univ; **SLP**

Posch-Baldy, Mrs Vickie L 729 Southern Avenue, Pittsburgh, PA 15235, (412) 394-5815, BS 79 Clarion Univ of PA; MS 80 WV Univ; Sp-Lang Path, Allegheny Intermed Ut, **SLP**

Posluns, Sandy Ellen 474 Oriole Parkway, Upper Duplex, Toronto, ON, Canada M5P 2H8, (416) 624-6526, BS 79 Univ of Western Ontario; MS 81 Univ of WI - Madison; SLP, Dufferm-Peel Rcss Board, **SLP**

Posner, Mrs Annette Chester 430 South Hanover Street, Baltimore, MD 21201, (301) 727-0052, MS 85 Towson St Univ; **SLP**

Posner, Carol Lynn 2301 Kings Highway #4F, Brooklyn, NY 11229, (212) 403-8431, BA 75 CUNY - Brooklyn Coll; MA 80 NY Univ; Sp-Lnag Path, The Brooklyn Hosp, **SLP**

Posner, Elizabeth H 431 Del Oro Avenue, Davis, CA 95616, (916) 927-3481, BA 76 Occidental Coll; MA 81 CA St Univ - Sacramento; Sp/Lang Path, Private Practice, **SLP**

Posner, Mrs Ellen S 9438 North 52nd Street, Paradise Valley, AZ 85253, (602) 945-4810, BS 65 NY Univ; MA 68 CUNY - Hunter Coll; Sp/Lang Path, Private Practice, **SLP**

Posner, Dr Judd E 120 Neptune Boulevard, Long Beach, NY 11561, (516) 542-3455, BA 60 CUNY - Queens Coll; MA 64 Columbia Univ Teachers Coll; ED 74 (NS) Columbia Univ Teachers Coll; Dir Sp & Hrng Ctr, Nassau Co Med Ctr, **SLP A**

Poss, David Robert 5008 Lake Riverside Estate, Thomasville, GA 31792, (912) 377-8441, BS 84 FL St Univ; MS 85 FL St Univ

Poss, Mrs Edith S 1665 Miller Road, Flint, MI 48503, (313) 767-4310, BS 47 Northwestern Univ; MA 67 Univ of KS; GISD-ICSI, **A**

Post, Gail-Susan F 12099 E Archer Place #117, Aurora, CO 80012, (303) 270-7798, MS 87 WV Univ; SLP, Univ of CO Hlth Sc Ctr

Post, Jimmy D 1905 Columbia Drive, Richardson, TX 75081, PH; **A**

Post, Kathryn N 6701 N W 30th Terrace, Gainesville, FL 32606, BA 76 Univ of FL; MA 77 Univ of FL; MS 83 Univ of FL; Supvr of Grad Cl, Univ of Fla Sp & Hrng Cl, **A**

Post, Mrs Kathy Milner 1410 West Block, El Dorado, AR 71730-4249, (501) 862-0819, OB 77 LA Tech Univ; MA 83 LA Tech Univ; Sp-Lang Path, Private Practice, **SLP**

Post, Lonni T 12 Marlan Court, Smithtown, NY 11787, **SLP**

Post, Lorena Ann 3403 East Dixon Avenue, Orange, CA 92669, (213) 595-2911, **SLP**

Post, Mrs Verna Ruth 1511 North Harmon, Tacoma, WA 98406, (206) 752-3527, BA 52 Central MI Univ; ME 70 Univ of Puget Sound; Tacoma Sch Dist 10, **SLP**

Posta, Elizabeth Anderson 2121 Briar Gate Drive, Montgomery, AL 36116, (804) 887-9226, BA 72 Univ of FL; MA 86 Hampton Univ; 88–Sp-Lang Path, InSpeech Inc, **SLP**

Postal, Mindy B 10 Tuckahoe Court, Gaithersburg, MD 20878, (301) 294-9095, BA 77 Univ of MD - College Park; MS 79 Univ of WI - Madison; 80–Sp-Lang Path, Pg Co Pub Schls Duckwrth Cen, **SLP**

Poster, Mrs Roberta F 17000 Cotter Place, Encino, CA 91436, (818) 708-7106, BA 71 Univ of CA - Los Angeles; MA 75 CA St Univ - Los Angeles; Sp-Lang Path, Roberta Fields Poster & Assoc, **SLP**

Post-Hyndman, Patricia M 4222 Hazelhurst, Fort Wayne, IN 46804, (219) 485-7554, BS 82 Ball St Univ; MA 84 Ball St Univ; Aud, Ft Wayne Sp St Dev Ctr, **A**

Postiglione, Dana M 1156 Brookwood Lane, Glenolden, PA 19036, (215) 532-7689, MA 88 OH Univ - Athens

Postle, Mrs Cleo B 36330 Bridgepointe Drive, Newark, CA 94560, (415) 967-7879, BA 61 Univ of MT; Sp/Lang Path, Whisman Elem Sch Dist, **SLP**

Poston, Alison Kirschner 5020 Columbia Circle, Hamilton, OH 45011, **SLP**

Poston, Mrs Allison Evans c/o Mrs Sally Evans, 3614 Hedrick Street, Jacksonville, FL 32205, BS 84 FL St Univ; MS 85 FL St Univ; **A**

Poston, Mary Baron 2342 Wofford Road, Charleston, SC 29407, (813) 577-5410, BA 79 Univ of FL; MS 80 FL St Univ; Sp-Lang Path, Charleston Sp & Hrng Cen, **SLP**

Postove, Mrs Mary A 1130 Van Ness North, 3001 Veazey Terrace N W, Washington, DC 20008, (202) 966-6894, BS 43 SUNY - Center at Buffalo; MA 59 Univ of MD - College Park; **A LM**

Potanos, Mrs Jenny Fritsch 144 West Road, Lombard, IL 60148, (312) 617-3197, BA 87 Elmhurst Coll; MA 87 Northern IL Univ - De Kalb; 88–Coord, Elmhurst Coll Speech Clinic, **SLP**

Potechin, Dr Gail Carol 233 Valley View Drive, Wilmette, IL 60091-3331, (312) 251-4509, BS 79 Univ of Western Ontario; MA 82 Emerson Coll; Sp-Lang Path, Private Practice, **SLP**

Poteet, Carol Elaine 11305 Tunnel Hill Way, Gold River, CA 95670, (916) 921-3660, BA 77 CA St Univ - Sacramento; MA 81 CA St Univ - Sacramento; 80–Sp-Lang Path, Grant Joint Union H Sc Dist, **SLP**

Poterek, Theresa Marie 4159 A Woods Edge Circle, Palm Beach Gardens, FL 33410, (305) 863-7717, BS 84 Western MI Univ; MA 86 Western MI Univ

Potesta, Karen L 2010 Beechwood Drive, South Charleston, WV 25303, (304) 348-2025, BS 74 WV Univ; MS 75 WV Univ; **SLP**

Potkay, Raymond J 1105 Plaza Place, Absecon, NJ 08201, (609) 465-3181, BA 64 Rutgers St Univ -N Brunswick; MA 72 Seton Hall Univ; SLP, Cape May Co Hlth Dept, **SLP**

Potoker, Dr David R 1611 Peach Street 290, Erie, PA 16508, (914) 866-3871, BA 65 Long Island U - Brooklyn Ctr; MA 66 Columbia Univ Teachers Coll; ED 75 (NS) Columbia Univ Teachers Coll; Sp/Lang Path, Private Practice, **SLP**

Potrocky, Dr Michael G Michael Gerard Inc, 2275 Swallow Hill Road, Bldg 1200, Pittsburgh, PA 15220, (412) 276-2865, BS 65 CA Univ of PA; MS 69 Univ of Pittsburgh - Pittsburgh; PH 77 (NS) Univ of Pittsburgh - Pittsburgh; President, Michael Gerard Inc, **SLP**

Potrykus, Rebecca A 1935 Galewood S W, Wyoming, MI 49509, (616) 942-1660, MA 88 Central MI Univ; 88–Aud, Comprehensive Audiologic Svcs

Pott, Mrs Evanne M 525 Hawthorne Place #2506, Chicago, IL 60657, (312) 525-0824, BA 86 MI St Univ; MA 87 Western MI Univ; Sp-Lang Path, Therapeutic Sys

Pottash, Karen W 6702 Chokeberry Road, Baltimore, MD 21209, (301) 486-2599, Sp-Lang Path, Associated Spch/Lang Services, **SLP**

Potter, Anne T M 10 Logan Road, Nashua, NH 03063-2214, **SLP**

Potter, Cilinda G 495 South Kipling, Lakewood, CO 80226, (303) 388-4801, SLP, Hope Center, **SLP**

Potter, Cyndy O 10954 Ash Circle, Thornton, CO 80233, BA 81 Univ of Northern CO; MA 82 Univ of Northern CO; **A**

Potter, David R 3304 Canterbury Avenue, Kalamazoo, MI 49007, (616) 674-8091, BS 57 Western MI Univ; MS 63 Univ of WI - Madison; Aud, Van Buren ISD, **A**

Potter, Deborah Shidler 357 Tidewater Circle East, Jacksonville, FL 32211, BS 81 Eastern MI Univ; MA 82 Eastern MI Univ; Sp-Lang Path, **SLP**

Potter, Mrs Donna J 8824 Winding Ridge Road, Indianapolis, IN 46217, (317) 872-4210, BA 81 IN Univ - Bloomington; MA 82 IN Univ - Bloomington; Asst Admin, St Vincent New Hope Inc, **SLP**

Potter, Elizabeth Walker 9095 Woodprint Lane, Mason, OH 45040, (513) 872-2481, BS 81 Univ of MN - Minneap-St Paul; MS 84 Univ of WI - Madison; Sp-Lang Path, Good Samaritan Hospital, **SLP**

Potter, Ellen L 211 Hampton, Summerville, SC 29483, **SLP**

Potter, Ellen Mittelman 12 Churchill Road, Rye Brook, NY 10573, (212) 362-8160, BA 78 Univ of PA; MS 80 Columbia Univ Teachers Coll; Sp-Lang Path, Greenwich Hosp, **SLP**

Potter, Frances T Route 1 Box 479-A, Vicksburg, MS 39180, (601) 634-6261, BS 75 Univ of GA; ME 76 Univ of GA; **SLP**

Potter, Lois S Department Of Teaching, Univ Of Northern Iowa, Cedar Falls, IA 50613, (319) 273-2546, BA 46; MA 50 Univ of IA; PH 59 (NS) Univ of WI - Madison; Prof/SLP, U of N IA, **SLP**

Potter, Marjorie E 7648 Robinwood Drive, Chesterfield, VA 23832, (804) 524-7331, BA 64 Mount Holyoke Coll; ME 65 Tufts Univ; MA 79 OH St Univ; Sp-Lang Path, Southside VA Trng Cen, **SLP**

Potter, Dr Robert E Department Of Speech, Washington State Univ, 201 Daggy, Pullman, WA 99164, (509) 335-4525, BA 54 Univ of MT; MA 58 Columbia Univ Teachers Coll; ED 63 (Sp Path) Univ of OR; Chair/Dept-Sp & Hrng Sci, WA St U, **SLP F**

Potter, Mrs Sallie J H Route 2, Bolckow, MO 64427, (816) 428-3962, BA 71 Georgetown Coll; MA 73 LA St Univ - Baton Rouge; Sp-Lang Path, Fillmore Sch Dist, **SLP ACE**

Potter, Susan Dale 6360 Surfside Way, Sacramento, CA 95831, (916) 392-6401, MA 84 CA St Univ - Sacramento; 87–Sp-Lang Path, Yolo Co Ofc of Educ, **SLP**

Potter, Mrs Susan W 2136 Dorchester, Birmingham, MI 48009, (313) 977-8988, BA 79 MI St Univ; MA 81 Wayne St Univ - Sch of Med; Aud, Macomb Aud Serv, **A**

Potter, Suzanne 26319 Dundee, Huntington Woods, MI 48070-1318, **SLP**

Potter-Manion, Ann M 5405 Blondo Street, Omaha, NE 68104, (402) 553-5026, BA 74 Creighton Univ; MS 79 Univ of NE - Omaha; ES 87 Univ of NE - Omaha; Sp-Lang Path, Omaha Pub Sch, **SLP ACE**

Potthoff, Mrs Patricia Tagler 2211 Woodscrest, Lincoln, NE 68502, (402) 476-9061, BS 81 Univ of NE - Lincoln; MS 82 Univ of NE - Lincoln; 88–Sp-Lang Path, Seward Pub Schools, **SLP**

Pottorf, Mrs Molly 1610 Culen, Wichita, KS 67206, (316) 833-2782, BS 74 Friends Univ; MA 76 Wichita St Univ; 77–Aud, USD 259 Wichita Public Schools, **SLP A**

Potts, AnnMarie Desandre 58-16 Garden View Terrace, East Windsor, NJ 08520, (609) 426-0205, BS 84 Trenton St Coll; MA 86 Trenton St Coll; 86–SLP, Washington Twp Bd of Educ, **SLP**

Potts, Mrs Ellen P H 904 North Pembroke, Effingham, IL 62401, (217) 342-3421, BS 53 Eastern IL Univ; MS 62 Univ of IL - Urbana; Retired, **SLP**

Potts, Mrs Linda A N 5859 Fredricks Road, Sebastopol, CA 95472, (805) 527-2271, BA 70 CA St Univ - Chico; ME 78 CA Lutheran Coll; SLP

Potts, Maryann Wenner 1325 Idaho Street, San Jose, CA 95126, (408) 249-5200, BS 83 Bloomsburg Univ of PA; MS 84 Bloomsburg Univ of PA; Dir Sp-Lang Path, Meadowbrook Neurologic Care Ctr, **SLP**

Potts, Paula L 8727 Falkstone Lane, Alexandria, VA 22309, BS 70 Univ of Houston - Univ Park; MS 75 Univ of WY; Director of Testing, Anglo-American School Moscow, **A**

Potts, Rebecca Kay 8171 Lewis Road, Birch Run, MI 48415, (517) 673-5200, BA 84 MI St Univ; MA 86 MI St Univ; Aud, Tuscola Intermediate Sch Dist, **A**

Potucek, Ann B 104 Idaho, Laredo, TX 78041, (512) 722-3938, BA 72 Cleveland St Univ; MA 73 Cleveland St Univ; Sp-Lang Path, Utd ISD, **SLP**

Potyka, Pamela Spencer 5800 Preston Oaks Road, Dallas, TX 75240, (214) 386-7140, BS 85 Baylor Univ; MS 86 Baylor Univ

Poulin, Cynthia Anne 32 Ledgeview Drive, Rochester, NH 03867, (603) 742-5252, BA 82 SUNY - Coll at Plattsburgh; MS 84 Syracuse Univ; Sp-Lang Path, Wentworth Douglas Hosp, **SLP**

Poulin, Doreen 15 Maple Street, Middlebury, VT 05753, (802) 655-4755, BS 78 SUNY - Coll at Geneseo; MS 82 Adelphi Univ; **SLP**

Poulin, Linda Lee RFD 1 Box 900, Weare, NH 03281, MS 84 Univ of RI; 85–Sp-Lang Path, Private Practice, **SLP**

Poulos, Thomas H 7455 E Overton Drive, Leesburg, FL 32788, (904) 728-4733, PH (NS); **A LM**

Poulsen, Barbara Frantz 8422 Aristotle, Universal City, TX 78148, (512) 659-8956, BS 72 OH Univ - Athens; MA 74 Univ of Denver; 87–Aud/SLP, Northeast Pediatric Assoc, **SLP A**

Poulton, Dr Karen T 516 Danbury Lane, Topeka, KS 66606, (913) 272-1053, BS 72 OH St Univ; MA 75 OH St Univ; PH 82 (NS) Univ of FL; **SLP**

Pound, Kathy Jo Parsons State Hosp & Trng Ctr, Speech And Hearing Dept, 2601 Gabriel, Parsons, KS 67357, (316) 421-6550, BA 78 Wichita St Univ; MA 80 Wichita St Univ; Sp-Lang Path, Parsons St Hosp & Trng Cen, **SLP**

Pound, Rebecca Walker 2224 Crawford, Parsons, KS 67357, 84–Sp-Lang Path, Private Practice, **SLP**

Pounds, Mrs Gayle Montrevil 27 Pipes Loop, Covington, LA 70433, (504) 626-8161, **SLP A**

Pourchot, Mrs Ann Marie 1711 Birch Road #5, Kenosha, WI 53140, (715) 341-2156, BS 82 Univ of WI - Stevens Point; MS 84 Univ of WI - Eau Claire; **SLP**

Pourkaveh, Faith Alison 6914 West Tucky Lane, Glendale, AZ 85303, (602) 943-2381, BS 82 Northern AZ Univ; MS 84 Northern AZ Univ; Sp-Lang Path, John C Lincoln Hosp, **SLP**

Poussart, Mrs Susan B 256 Peppermill Road, Berlin, NJ 08009, (609) 767-1578, BA 77 Temple Univ-Tyler Sch of Art; MA 79 Temple Univ-Tyler Sch of Art; **SLP**

Povanda, Elizabeth Ann 106 Clarkson Avenue, Jessup, PA 18434, (717) 296-9261, BS 83 Marywood Coll; MA 85 Univ of Pittsburgh - Pittsburgh; Sp-Lang Path, Head Injury Recov Cntr, **SLP**

Poveromo, Judith A G 244 Norwood Avenue, Northport, NY 11768, **SLP**

Powell, Amy J 3050 Kirklevington Drive, # 70, Lexington, KY 40502, (606) 276-5563, MA 87 IN Univ - Bloomington; **A**

Powell, Mrs Annette S 2907 Nashville Avenue, Nederland, TX 77627, (409) 722-3484, BS 70 Lamar Univ; MS 71 Lamar Univ; 77–Sp-Lang Path, Nederland ISD, **SLP**

Powell, Mrs Celia K 2615 Voorhees Avenue #5, Redondo Beach, CA 90278, (213) 371-1218, BS 73 Emerson Coll; OM 76 Southern CT St Univ; **SLP**

Powell, Colette Suzanne 7831 E Culver Street, Mesa, AZ 85207, (602) 986-3460, BS 80 AZ St Univ; OM 86 AZ St Univ; **SLP**

Powell, Constance 405 Skyview Drive, Clemson, SC 29631, BS 63 Purdue Univ - West Lafayette; 85–Sp-Lang Path, Sch Dist of Pickens Co, **SLP**

Powell, Mrs Cynthia 3601 Peggy's Place, Tyler, TX 75701, (214) 561-1754, BA 75 Univ of North TX; MA 76 Univ of North TX; **SLP**

Powell, Deborah Renee 2693 Darwin Street, Sacramento, CA 95821, (916) 927-3137, BA 83 Humboldt St Univ; MS CA St Univ - Sacramento; **A**

Powell, Diane J 119 Carolina Avenue, Cherry Hill, NJ 08003, (609) 662-8500, 82–Sp-Lang Path, Pennsauken PS, **SLP**

Powell, Mrs Donna J 466 Thomas Lane, Grand Blanc, MI 48439, (313) 762-1594, BA 51 Central MI Univ; MA 70 Central MI Univ; 53–Sp-Lang Path, Flint Bd of Ed, **SLP**

Powell, Mrs Donna Lynne 2028 Washington Street, Waco, TX 76701, (817) 460-4611, **SLP**

Powell, Mrs Edna M M 1994 McSwain, Merced, CA 95340, (209) 385-6623, BA 73 CA St Univ - Stanislaus; MA 75 CA St Univ - Stanislaus; 80–Sp-Lang Path, Merced City Sch Dist, **SLP**

Powell, Emily H 321 North Indiana Avenue, Watertown, NY 13601, (315) 788-7400, BS 85 Ithaca Coll; MS 87 Ithaca Coll

Powell, Mrs Gail C 2276 Fallen Tree Drive, Jacksonville, FL 32216, (904) 221-5521, BA 59 Vanderbilt Univ; **SLP**

Powell, Dr Harold Speech & Hearing Program, South Carolina State Coll, Orangeburg, SC 29117, (803) 536-8074, BA 61 SC St Coll; MS 63 PA St Univ - Univ Park; PH 66 (NS) PA St Univ - Univ Park; Department Chairman, S C State Coll, **SLP F**

Powell, James E Hearing Associates Inc, 8901 West 74th Street, Suite 150, Shawnee Mission, KS 66204, (913) 384-5880, BS 72 Univ of MO - KS City; MS 73 Central MO St Univ; Aud, Hrng Assoc Inc, **A**

Powell, Jane 12137 Calla Zagal N E, Albuquerque, NM 87111, (505) 298-5886, **SLP**

Powell, Mrs Janna Rhodes 4334 Putting Green Drive, San Antonio, TX 78217, (512) 657-0925, BS 84 Baylor Univ; MA 85 Our Lady Lake Univ-San Anton; 86–Sp-Lang Path, Easter Seal Rehab Ctr, **SLP**

Powell, Janna Y Hearing Associates Inc, 8901 West 74th Street, Suite 150, Shawnee Mission, KS 66204, (913) 384-5880, BA 72 Univ of MO - KS City; MS 73 Central MO St Univ; Industrial Audiometric Tech, Hearing Associates Inc, **SLP**

Powell, Mrs Jeanne Marie Route 2 Box 394, Ashland, MO 65010, (314) 657-4168, BA 80 Univ of MO - Columbia; MS 84 CO St Univ; **SLP**

Powell, Jeannette H Rt 5 Box 455 A, Lake City, FL 32055, (904) 755-5955, BA 85 Univ of FL; MA 87 Western Carolina Univ; **SLP**

Powell, Kathleen A 23599 Newcastle, Taylor, MI 48180, (313) 676-4200, BS 79 Eastern MI Univ; MA 80 Eastern MI Univ; Dir/SLP, Riverside Osteopathic Hosp, **SLP**

Powell, Mrs Kathy Rein 8116 Woodland Hills Lane, Fairfax Station, VA 22039, (301) 762-0632, **SLP**

Powell, Laura Marie 2034 Pamela Street, Corona, CA 91720, (714) 737-8208, BA 84 CA St Univ - Fullerton; MS 86 Univ of Redlands; **SLP**

Powell, Mrs Louise McGinnis P O Box 901, Carlisle, PA 17013, (717) 245-5332, BS 62 PA St Univ - Univ Park; MA 79 George Washington Univ; Sp/Lang Path, Carlisle Hosp, **SLP**

Powell, Lynn E 1945 Main Street, Glastonbury, CT 06033-2902, (203) 563-1362, BS 69 Ithaca Coll; MS 79 Southern CT St Univ; SLP, Wethersfield Board of Educ, **SLP**

Powell, Mrs Lynne S 22 Alan Road, Danbury, CT 06810, (203) 834-0325, BS 70 Rutger's St Univ - Douglas Coll; MS 78 Southern CT St Univ; Preschool Coord, Wilton Pub Sch, **SLP**

Powell, Mrs Marsha Stollings 167 Harmon Street, Stephens City, VA 22655, (703) 667-4253, BS 77 James Madison Univ; MS 82 James Madison Univ; Sp-Lang Path/City Coordinator, Winchester City Schools, **SLP**

Powell, Myrna T 6301 East Fordham Drive, Baltimore, MD 21215, MS; **SLP**

Powell, Mrs Orpha L 2823 Crescent Drive, Stillwater, OK 74075, (405) 372-1382, BS 38 OK St Univ; MS 64 OK St Univ; **SLP LM**

Powell, Paulette I 71 West 112th Street, New York, NY 10026, BS 75 NY Univ; MS 87 Columbia Univ Teachers Coll; ME 77 Columbia Univ Teachers Coll; 87–Aud, Woodhull Med & Mental Hlth Ctr, **A**

Powell, Ramona Kellie 2318 Middle Coff Drive, Gulfport, MS 39507, (601) 896-1278, BS 85 Univ Southern MS-Hattiesburg; MS 87 Univ Southern MS-Hattiesburg; 88–Aud, E B Ross Jr MD, **A**

Powell, Renee J 4223 Kahala Avenue, Honolulu, HI 96816, (808) 737-6035, BA 47 Muskingum Coll; MA 48 Northwestern Univ; SLP, UCP, **SLP**

Powell, Mrs Sharon S 7109 Stoney Ridge Road, Matthews, NC 28105, (704) 283-1537, BS 82 Kent St Univ; MA 82 Kent St Univ; Sp-Lang Path, Charlotte Speech/Hearing Ctr, **SLP ACE**

Powell, Sheila L 5057 Woodward Room 1028, Detroit, MI 48202, (313) 494-1643, BS 67 Wayne St Univ; ME 68 Wayne St Univ; 87–Supvr Comm Disorders, Detroit Pub Sch, **SLP ACE**

Powell, Mrs Teresa B 320 W Main Street, Worthington, IN 47471, BS 78 IN Univ - Bloomington; MA 79 IN Univ - Bloomington; **SLP**

Powell, Mrs Terren 1052 Hewitt Drive, San Carlos, CA 94070, (408) 379-9268, BA 77 Univ of the Pacific; MA 79 Univ of the Pacific; **SLP**

Powell, Thomas W 3709 Chadam Lane #2-C, Muncie, IN 47304, (317) 285-8164, BA 79 IN Univ - Bloomington; MA 82 IN Univ - Bloomington; 87–Asst Prof, Ball State Univ, **SLP ACE**

Powell, Mrs Vanessa Koonce 2715 Timberpeg Court, Conway, AR 72032, (501) 329-5773, BS 83 Univ of Central AR; MS 85 Univ of Central AR; 85–Sp-Lang Path, Conway Pub Sch, **SLP**

Powell-Todd, Gwendolyn 4 Honeysuckle Lane, San Carlos, CA 94070, (313) 927-7328, BA 69 Case Western Reserve Univ; MS 70 Univ of Dayton; **SLP**

Power, Leslie D West 1108 15th, Spokane, WA 99203, (509) 924-7795, BA 74 Elmira Coll; MS 76 Univ of WA; Supervisor Sp-Lang Path, St Lukes Memorial Hospital, **SLP**

Power, Mrs Lorraine Liput 2020 Fort Hill Road, Phelps, NY 14532, (315) 548-9411, BA 71 Duquesne Univ; MS 77 SUNY - Coll at Buffalo; Instr Severe Sp/Lang/Hrng Imp, Wayne-Finger Lakes Bd of Coop, **SLP**

Power, Mark 406 East Monroe Avenue, Orange, CA 92667-5730, BS 68 Saint Lawrence Univ; MA 73 CA St Univ - Long Beach; MA 75 CA St Univ - Long Beach; Director, Private Practice, **SLP**

Power, Mary S 2021 Ridge Avenue, Evanston, IL 60201, (312) 492-5958, BS 66 Bloomsburg Univ of PA; MS 69 Univ of OR; SLP, Dist 65, **SLP**

Power, Dr Maryann H 236 Grove Street, Paxton, MA 01612, (617) 793-8055, BA 62 Univ of MA - Amherst; ME 65 Salem St Coll; ED 85 (NS) Clark Univ; Asst Prof-Cl Dir, Worcester St C, **SLP**

Power, Paula A W 1845 Scott Avenue, Ventura, CA 93004, (805) 647-3785, MS 73 Univ of CA - Santa Barbara; **SLP**

Power, Mrs Peggy J Hudspeth Center, P O Box 127B, Whitfield, MS 39193, (601) 939-8640, BA 79 Univ of MS; MA 80 Univ of MS; 87–Dir Early Intervention Prog, Hudspeth Cntr, **SLP**

Powers, Alice G 311 Concord Drive, Fayetteville, NC 28301, (919) 485-5145, BS 80 East Carolina Univ; OM 82 Univ of SC - Columbia; Sp/Lang Path, Sen Sp/Hrng Serv Inc, **SLP**

Powers, Barbara Colbert 31 Beekman Avenue, Croton on Hudson, NY 10520-2556, (914) 271-2416, BA 75 CUNY - Lehman Coll; MS 77 Columbia Univ Teachers Coll; Sp-Lang Path, Westchester Assoc for Ret Cit, **SLP**

Powers, Mrs Bonnie R P O Box 537, Soldotna, AK 99669, BA 69 Eastern WA Univ; MA 74 WA St Univ; Sp-Lang Path, Kenai Peninsula Sch Dist, **SLP**

Powers, Cynthia Ann 509 Martin Drive N, Bellevue, NE 68005, (402) 291-3431, BA 60 MI St Univ; MS 83 Univ of NE - Omaha; **SLP**

Powers, Mrs Diane B 4495 Hunters Ridge Lane, Greenwood, IN 46142, (317) 782-2630, Vice President, Rehabilitative Health Services, **SLP**

Powers, Dr Gene R Prog In Communication Disorder, University Of Texas, Austin, TX 78712, (512) 471-7703, BA 49 TX Tech Univ; MA 58 Univ of IA; PH 60 (NS) Univ of IA; Prof, U of TX-Austin, **SLP F**

Powers, Jeri L 3710 East 20th Avenue, Anchorage, AK 99508, (907) 272-0586, MS 84 Western OR St Coll; Aud, AK Treatment Cen, **A**

Powers, Joyce S 404-D Fisher Park Circle, Greensboro, NC 27401, (919) 274-7079, BS 64 OH St Univ; MA 67 OH St Univ; 87–Sp/Lang Path, Guilford County Schs, **SLP**

Powers, Kenneth E 1900 West Wynnewood, Sulphur, OK 73086, (405) 332-6540, BS 68 Central St Univ; MA 75 Univ of Tulsa; Aud, Private Practice, **A**

Powers, Mrs Linda M 323 Madison Avenue, Cuyahoga Falls, OH 44221, (216) 794-9332, BS 83 Kent St Univ; MA 84 Kent St Univ; **A**

Powers, Mrs Myrna G 244 North Renn, Fresno, CA 93727, (209) 456-2520, MS 80 Univ of TX - Dallas; Sp-Lang Path, **SLP**

Powers, Mrs Rita Jackson 6904 Seat Pleasant Drive, Apartment 201, Capitol Heights, MD 20743, (202) 651-5031, MS 80 Howard Univ

Powers, Mrs Ruth M S 98 Winchester Road, Natchez, MS 39120, (601) 442-2531, BA 77 Northeast LA Univ; MA 78 Memphis St Univ; Sp-Lang Path, Cathedral Unit Sch, **SLP**

Powers, Sally L 541 Bondstone, Dallas, TX 75218, (214) 343-1416, BS 74 TX Christian Univ; MA 76 Univ of TX - Austin; 86–Sp-Lang Path, Irving Hosp, **SLP ACE**

Powers, Susan M 1282 Gladys Avenue, Lakewood, OH 44107, (216) 352-8993, BS 79 Miami Univ - Oxford; BA 79 Miami Univ - Oxford; MA 82 Humboldt St Univ; Dir/Dept Communicative Disordr, Lake County Soc Crippled Chldn, **SLP**

Powers, Dr Thomas A Siemens Hearing Instruments, 10 Corporate Place So, Piscataway, NJ 08854, (800) 345-0183, BS 71 SUNY - Coll at Geneseo; MA 75 OH Univ - Athens; PH 77 (NS) OH Univ - Athens; VP, Siemens Hearing Instruments, **A**

Powers, Vicki Stafford 910 Woodmont Boulevard, Apartment K-3, Nashville, TN 37204-3310, (615) 292-6748, **A**

Powers-Jakimo, Benay 59 Stuart Street, Syosset, NY 11791, (516) 496-2256, **SLP**

Powers-Rabideau, Debora L 8119 Rapallo Way, Clay, NY 13041, (315) 425-5311, MS; Sp-Lang Path, Seguin Community Services, **SLP ACE**

Powers-Richard, Vivian L 614 South McKinley Avenue, Arlington Heights, IL 60005, BA 76 SUNY - Coll at New Paltz; ME 80 Northern IL Univ - De Kalb; MS 82 Governors St Univ; Ed $ Spec Svcs Coord, Ccdi, **SLP**

Powers-Todt, Mrs Maureen F 3164 North 55th Street, Milwaukee, WI 53216, (414) 444-7848, BS 76 Univ of WI - Milwaukee; MS 79 Univ of WI - Milwaukee; 79–Sp-Lang Path, Milwaukee Pub Sch, **SLP**

Powley, Carl E 1613 Lakeview, St Joseph, MI 49085, (616) 471-9080, BS 53 Concordia Coll; MA 71 Western MI Univ; Aud, Hearing Ctr Berrien County, **A ACE**

Poynor, Robert E 1120 Eastwood Drive, Mount Pleasant, MI 48858, (517) 774-3471, BS 61 Central MI Univ; MA 63 Central MI Univ; MA 66 Western MI Univ; Assoc Prof-Dir Sp-Lang Path, Ctrl MI U-Dept of Commun Dis, **SLP ACE**

Poythress, Mrs Darla H 1180 Bellaire Drive, Atlanta, GA 30319, (404) 237-9286, BS 67 Univ of TX - Austin; MA 69 Univ of TX - Austin; Pre Sch Coord, Trinity Sch Inc, **SLP**

Pozza, Carrie Anne 2989 Hickory Lane, Ann Arbor, MI 48104, (313) 971-2172, MA 82 Wayne St Univ; Sp-Lang Path, Detroit Pub Sch, **SLP**

Pozza, Charlyn M 3129-A North 56th Street, Milwaukee, WI 53216, (414) 475-8137, BS 75 Marquette Univ; MS 77 Marquette Univ; Sp-Lang Path, Milwaukee Pub Sch, **SLP**

Pozza, Cynthia Ann 1553 North 116th Street, Milwaukee, WI 53226-3205, (414) 781-5491, **SLP**

Prabhudas, Jayne M 44 Strawberry Hill Avenue 11F, Stamford, CT 06902, (203) 325-1544, BA 83 Univ of CT; MA 85 Univ of CT; 85–Sp-Lang Path, Easter Seal Rehab Ctr, **SLP**

Praechter, Dawn Marie 11831 Eddie And Park Road, St Louis, MO 63126, (314) 942-2565, BS 83 Fontbonne Coll; MS 84 Fontbonne Coll; 87–Sp-Lang Path, Special Services Cooperative

Praefke, Mrs Marie H 728 Kensington Road, Neenah, WI 54956, (414) 722-2275, BS 71 Univ of WI - Milwaukee; MS 73 Univ of WI - Milwaukee; 88–Sp-Lang Path, Appleton Area Sch Dist, **SLP ACE**

Prager, Mrs Marlene Mitauer 145 West 58th Street, New York, NY 10019, (212) 307-0664, BA 63 CUNY - Hunter Coll; MS 71 CUNY - Hunter Coll; MA 87 CUNY - Hunter Coll; 86–SLP, NYC Bd of Educ

Prakup, Barbara R 4129 Sierra Circle, Medina, OH 44256, (216) 253-1161, BA 79 Cleveland St Univ; MA 81 Cleveland St Univ; 88–Sp-Lang Path, Litchfield Rehab Ctr, **SLP**

Prall, Josephine 332 Dupre Drive, Spartanburg, SC 29302, (803) 585-6394, BA 33 Elmira Coll; BS 36 Washington Univ; MA 52 Northwestern Univ; **A LM**

Pranikoff, Merle G 192 Meadowview Lane, Williamsville, NY 14221, MS

Prasad, Mrs Kamala R 4404 Lowell Rd Brandywine, Wilmington, DE 19802, (302) 421-6281, BA 65; MA 67; MA 72 Univ of MN - Minneap-St Paul; Sp-Lang Path, Terry Childrns Psychiatric Ctr, **SLP ACE**

Prascher, Elaine C 2320 Emerson, Brush, CO 80723, (303) 842-4270, BA 64 OH Wesleyan Univ; MA 68 Univ of Northern CO; Sp/Lang Path, Sp/Lang Path, **SLP**

Prasen, Patricia A 644 A Corkhill #703, Bedford, OH 44146, (216) 663-9476, BA 79 Cleveland St Univ; MA 81 Cleveland St Univ; Sp/Lang Path, P S I Associates Inc, **SLP**

Prater, Laura Chappell 800 Little Pine Drive, South Daytona, FL 32019, (305) 668-8641, BA 77 Clarion Univ of PA; MS 80 Clarion Univ of PA; SLP, Volusia Co Dept of Ed, **A**

Prater, Dr Rex Joe 3 Amberhill Court, Greensboro, NC 27405, (919) 379-5939, BS 70 OH St Univ; MS 72 OH St Univ; PH 75 (NS) OH St Univ; Assoc Prof, U of NC/Greensboro, **SLP**

Prather, Dr Elizabeth M 357 East Palm Lane, Phoenix, AZ 85004, (602) 965-2373, BS 52 Univ of NE - Lincoln; MA 57 Univ of IA; PH 60 (Sp Path & Aud) Univ of IA; Prof, Arizona St U, **SLP F**

Prather, Mrs Julia E C 1317 North Banner Avenue, Indianapolis, IN 46224, (317) 247-4983, BS 70 IN St Univ - Terre Haute; MS 73 IN St Univ - Terre Haute; Sp-Lang Path, Cold Spring Sch Indpls Pub Sch, **SLP**

Prather, Mrs Phyllis Crew 119 Holland Road, South Orange, NJ 07079, (201) 680-8500, BA 73 Montclair St Coll; MA 74 Montclair St Coll; 81–Sp-Lang Path, Bloomfield Bd of Educ, **SLP**

Prather, Dr William F 357 East Palm Lane, Phoenix, AZ 85004, (602) 222-6412, BA 53 Univ of CA - Berkeley; MA 58 Univ of IA; PH 60 (NS) Univ of IA; Chief-Aud & SLP Serv, VA Med Cen, **A F**

Pratt, Janet 968 First Colonial, Virginia Beach, VA 23454, (804) 481-4004, BA 82 Augustana Coll; MA 84 Univ of KS; Sp-Lang Path, InSpeech Inc, **SLP**

Pratt, Mrs Jeanne S 6904 Mainsgate, Wichita, KS 67226, (316) 833-2780, MA 78 Kent St Univ; BS 77 Kent St Univ; Sp-Lang Path, Wichita Public Schools, **SLP ACE**

Pratt, Judith E Center For Communicative Disorders, University Of Wisconsin, Stevens Point, WI 54481, (715) 346-4516, BA 60 Univ of CA - Los Angeles; MA 67 San Jose St Univ; PH 72 (NS) Univ of IL - Urbana; Prof, U of WI-Stevens Pt, **SLP**

Pratt, Mrs Kim Loraine 829 Madison Street, Port Townsend, WA 98368, (206) 683-7955, BS 79 Eastern KY Univ; MS 84 Univ of OR; Sp-Lang Path, Sequim School District, **SLP**

Pratt, Mrs Linda S 124 South Crawford Street, Millersburg, OH 44654, (216) 674-8045, BA 73 OH Wesleyan Univ; MA 76 OH Univ - Athens; Sp-Lang Path, Holmes Co Trng Cen, **SLP**

Pratt, Mrs Margaret Spinney 38 Sassafras Trail, Narragansett, RI 02882, (401) 738-6111, MS 84 Univ of RI; Aud, George J Jacewicz MD Inc, **A**

Pratt, Mrs Miriam Markowitz 651 Oriental Boulevard, Apartment 10-P, Brooklyn, NY 11235, (718) 934-4583, BA 85 CUNY - Hunter Coll; MS 87 CUNY - Brooklyn Coll; **SLP**

Pratt, Robert E, Jr 1738 Pine Street #3A, Philadelphia, PA 19103, (215) 662-6525, BA 77 Bob Jones Univ; MA 79 Northwestern Univ; Aud Lecturer/Superv, Northwestern U, **A**

Pratt, Roger Sayers 109 East Fellows Street, Dixon, IL 61021-2145, (815) 284-7722, BS 83 Northern IL Univ - De Kalb; MA 85 Northern IL Univ - De Kalb; **SLP**

Pratt, Dr Shelia Rose 2135 Hollister, Madison, WI 53705, (608) 262-6484, PH 88 (Aud/Sp Path) Univ of IA; 88–Research Assoc, Univ of Wisconsin, **SLP A**

Pratte, Catherine A 121 School House Road, Warren, RI 02885, (401) 351-8819, MA 74 Middlebury Coll; BA 70 Salve Regina - Newport Coll; MS 85 Univ of RI; Sp-Lang Path, Providence School Department, **SLP**

Prause, Mrs Jacqueline 3686 Lantern Lane, Port Huron, MI 48060, (313) 985-5434, BS 73 Northern MI Univ; MA 77 Wayne St Univ; Sp-Lang Path, Marysville Pub Sch, **SLP**

Pravda, Mrs Linda Friedman 12306 Secretariat Court, Houston, TX 77071, (713) 777-2162, BA 73 Univ of Houston - Univ Park; MA 76 Univ of Houston - Univ Park; Sp/Lang Path, Private Practice, **SLP**

Pravda, Mrs Lynn F 22 Salem Drive, Scarsdale, NY 10583, (914) 698-6677, BS 67 NY Univ; MA 68 NY Univ; Sp-Lang Path, Eastchester Bd of Ed, **SLP**

Prax, Mary Louise 403 1/2 East 3rd Street N, Melrose, MN 56352, (612) 256-3617, BS 79 Saint Cloud St Univ; MS 84 Saint Cloud St Univ; 80–Sp-Lang Path, Melrose ISD #740, **SLP**

Pray, Mrs Rita S 526 60th Street, Des Moines, IA 50312, (515) 279-5659, OB 81 Univ of NE - Omaha; MA 83 Univ of IA; Sp-Lang Path, Des Moines Hrng & Sp Cen, **SLP**

Prebys, Paul T P O Box 360, El Cajon, CA 92020, (619) 441-9781, BS 72 Portland St Univ; MS 74 Eastern WA Univ; SLP, Mountain Empire School Distric, **SLP**

Prechowski, Catherine Anne 10414 Tamryn Boulevard, Holly, MI 48442, (313) 762-2362, BA 79 MI St Univ; MA 82 Western MI Univ; SLP, McLaren Gen Hosp, **SLP**

Preciado-Lumsden, Mrs Eva Maria 2304 Lake Park Court, Martinez, CA 94553, (415) 798-4078, MA 88 San Jose St Univ; 86–Sp-Lang Path, Mt Diablo USD

Pred, Dr Lynne B Pediatric Therapy Institute, 720 Kipling, Suite 17, Lakewood, CO 80215, (303) 239-6535, BA 67 Montclair St Coll; MA 69 Univ of Denver; PH 77 (NS) Univ of CO - Boulder; SLP, Pediatric Therapy Institute, **SLP**

Preece, Dr John P Audiology-126, Veterans Administration Medical Center, 5901 East Seventh Street, Long Beach, CA 90822, (213) 494-5414, BS 74 Northwestern Univ; MA 76 Northwestern Univ; PH 85 (Aud) Univ of IA; 85–Aud, VA Med Ctr, **A**

Preer, Vicki Marie 12129 Thicket Green, #955, Houston, TX 77035, (713) 729-8550, MA 83 Univ of Houston - Univ Park; BS 79 Western MI Univ; SLP, Houston Sch Dist, **SLP**

Preheim, Michaelene Weidemann Box 252, Parker, SD 57053-9999, (605) 297-3127, BA 78 SD St Univ; MA 80 SD St Univ; Sp-Lang Path, Corn Belt Educ Coop, **SLP**

Prehm, Mrs Katherine T 3401 West Lincoln Avenue, Yakima, WA 98902, (509) 965-2080, BA 64 Western WA Univ; ME 66 Western WA Univ; Sp-Lang Path, W Valley Sch Dist #208, **SLP**

Preisman, Mrs Barbara 1286 Windemere Court, Schenectady, NY 12309, BA 63 SUNY - Center at Albany; MA 64 SUNY - Center at Albany; MS 82 Coll of Saint Rose; 84–Sp-Lang Path, St Peters Hosp, **SLP**

Preis-O'Brennan, Janet 8531 Morven Road, Baltimore, MD 21234, (301) 882-4928, BS 82 Towson St Univ; MS 85 Towson St Univ; **SLP**

Preisser, Debra A 2816 Sue Lane N W, Cedar Rapids, IA 52405, (319) 398-2273, BS 71 Eastern IL Univ; MS 74 Eastern IL Univ; PH 83 (Sp Path) Univ of IL - Urbana; Sp-Lang Path, Grant Wood AEA, **SLP**

Prejean, Barbara A 206 Rhett Place, Gray, LA 70359, (504) 868-4267, BA 71 Nicholls St Univ; OM 82 LA St Univ - N O Medical Ctr; Sp-Lang Path, Terrebonne Parish Sch Bd, **SLP**

Prejean, Marsha J 638 Port Street, New Orleans, LA 70117, (504) 834-4744, BS 79 Univ of North TX; MS 81 Univ of North TX; Dir, Communication & Learning Ctr, **SLP**

Prejean, Mrs Sheila Duplechain 200 Steeple Chase Drive, Lafayette, LA 70506, (318) 783-3664, **SLP**

Prekker, Janet Erren 2401 Silver Lane N E, St Anthony, MN 55421, (612) 788-4719, MA 88 Univ of MN - Minneap-St Paul

Prelock, Dr Patricia A 11415 Terwilliger's Valley, Cincinnati, OH 45249, (513) 489-9716, BS 76 Kent St Univ; MA 77 Kent St Univ; PH 83 (NS) Univ of Pittsburgh - Pittsburgh; Clinical Super, U of Pitts, **SLP ACE**

Preminger, Jill 110 Grant, Apartment 8-A, Minneapolis, MN 55403, BS 80 Boston Univ; MS 82 Univ of WI - Madison; Aud, Univ of MN, **A**

Prem-Stein, Jutta W 3520-B 24th Avenue, Vernon, BC, Canada V1T 1L8, (604) 542-6999, BS 75 Univ of Victoria - Bc; BA 77 Univ of MT; MA 80 Univ of MT; Sp/Lang Path/Consult, Sch Dist #57, **SLP**

Prendergast, Sandra Kay 10106 Headley Hill Road, Louisville, KY 40223, (502) 425-7380, **SLP**

Prendergast, Susan G 1515 East Olive, Bloomington, IL 61701, (812) 479-1411, BS 69 Univ of IL - Urbana; MS 74 Southern IL Univ -Carbondale; Lecturer, Il State U, **A**

Prendeville, Jo-Anne 7158 Anderson Woods Drive, Cincinnati, OH 45244-3260, (513) 232-4116, BA 69 MI St Univ; MA 78 Univ of Cincinnati; SLP, Self Employed, **SLP**

Prenovost, Annette Louise 2721 Via Casa Loma, San Clemente, CA 92672, (213) 328-3611, BA 80 CA St Univ - Long Beach; MA 83 CA St Univ - Long Beach; SLP, Switzer Cen, **SLP**

Prentice, Dr Abbie Shuford 6711 Sunnyslope Avenue, Van Nuys, CA 91401, (818) 846-7121, BA 73 CA St Univ - Los Angeles; MA 75 CA St Univ - Los Angeles; PH 86 (Education) Claremont Graduate Sch; Sp-Lang Path, Burbank USD, **SLP**

Prentice, Charlotte Henninger 916 Evans Road, Nashville, TN 37204, (615) 361-3219, MS 85 Vanderbilt Univ; **A**

Presbitero, Mrs Michele Marie 9222 Virginia Court, Orland Park, IL 60462, (219) 243-5600, MA 84 Northern IL Univ - De Kalb; 86–Aud, Hammond Clinic, **A**

Prescod, Dr Stephen V College Of Applied Med Science, King Saud University, P O Box 10219, Rizadh, Saudi Arabia 11433, (604) 545-0651, BA 67 Andrews Univ; MA 74 Western MI Univ; PH 82 (NS) SUNY - Center at Binghamton; Chief Audiologist, Ministry of Health, **A**

Prescott, Hope 29 Winfield Road, Providence, RI 02906, **SLP**

Prescott, Karen Annette 2534A S Harvard Place, Tulsa, OK 74114, (918) 744-2350, BS 82 Baylor Univ; MA 83 Univ of Tulsa; 86–Sp-Lang Path, St John Med Ctr, **SLP**

Prescott, Marian H P O Box 760, Exeter, NH 03833, BS 82 Univ of NH; MS 86 Univ of NH; 86–Sp-Lang Path, Exeter Hosp, **SLP**

Prescott, Maj Richard 115 Dupont Way, Afb, Wright Patterson, OH 45433, (513) 256-9569, BS 67 Phillips Univ; MA 74 Univ of Tulsa; Chief-Hrng Conservation Ctr, US Air Force, **A ACE**

Prescott, Dr Thomas E 2695 South Gilpin, Denver, CO 80210, (303) 393-2871, BA 60 Mankato St Univ; MA 63 Univ of KS; PH 70 (NS) Univ of Denver; Chief Audiology/Speech Service, VA Medical Center, **SLP**

Preshaw, Linda Sue 6767 South Broadway, Littleton, CO 80122, (303) 795-5891, BA 74 Univ of CO - Boulder; MA 78 Univ of San Diego; Sp-Lang Path, Private Practice, **SLP**

Preski, Jeanne 938 Jefferson Avenue, Waynesboro, VA 22980, (703) 942-5299, BA 73 Univ of RI; MS 75 Univ of IL - Urbana; 87–Sp-Lang Path, Virginia Rehab Agency Inc, **SLP**

Preslan, Mrs Jacque Schmidt 7502 South Cove Circle, Littleton, CO 80122, (303) 798-5458, **SLP**

Preslar, Joyce W 1008 Beecher Road, Winston-Salem, NC 27104, (919) 768-5991, BA 72 Wake Forest Univ; MA 73 Univ of NC - Greensboro; Sp-Lang Path, Private Practice, **SLP**

Presley, Emelia Elizabeth 1618 Babs, Memphis, TN 38116, (901) 346-1185, BS 84 Lambuth Coll; MA 86 Memphis St Univ; 88–Aud, Mid South Ear Nose & Throat Assoc, **A**

Presley, Karen June 164 West Spain, Sonoma, CA 95476, (707) 643-0341, BS 73 FL St Univ; MS 74 FL St Univ; Sp-Lang Path, Vallejo County USD, **SLP**

Presnell, Eileen Kanczak 3460 Millcrest Drive, Lake Orion, MI 48035, (313) 493-6315, BA 81 Univ of Pittsburgh - Pittsburgh; MS 83 Purdue Univ - West Lafayette; 86–Sp-Lang Path, Sinai Hospital of Detroit, **SLP**

Press, David 347 5th Avenue, Room 1207, New York, NY 10016, (212) 481-1717, BS 60 Emerson Coll; MS 64; Pres, Audio Dispensary Corp, **SLP A**

Press, Mrs Ivy L 7701 Bay Parkway, Brooklyn, NY 11214, (212) 780-1755, BS 77 SUNY - Coll at Brockport; MS 80 CUNY - Brooklyn Coll; Aud, Long Island Coll Hosp, **A**

Press, Mrs Joy A 9213 West 115th Terrace, Overland Park, KS 66210, (913) 451-4714, BA 76 Univ of MO - Columbia; MS 77 Central MO St Univ; Aud, Prime Hlth, **A**

Press, Mrs Judy Reed 1132 57th Street, Sacramento, CA 95819, (916) 454-8387, BA 73 CA St Univ - Sacramento; MA 75 CA St Univ - Sacramento; Sp/Lang Path, Sacdo Cty USD, **SLP**

Press, Mrs Linda Corrie 27 Glendale Drive, Melville, NY 11747, (516) 293-6050, MS 85 Adelphi Univ; SLP, BOCES Nassau Co, **SLP**

Press, Steven E 9213 West 115th Terrace, Overland Park, KS 66210, (913) 782-3377, PH 80 (Aud) Univ of KS; 88–Aud, Bruce Zimmerman MD PA, **A**

Pressel, Gene 530 East Mohawk Road, West Hempstead, NY 11552, PH (NS); **SLP F**

Pressley, Glenda Earline 2033 50th Avenue, Sacramento, CA 95822, (916) 364-8364, BS 76 Univ of Science & Arts of OK; ME 81 Central St Univ; **SLP**

Pressman, Dr D Elaine Childrens Hosp Of East Ontario, Speech Pathology Dept, 401 Smyth Road, Ottawa, ON, Canada K1H 8L1, (613) 737-2373, BA 66 Univ of Manitoba - Winnipeg; MA 69 OH St Univ; PH 71 (NS) OH St Univ; Assoc Prof, Univ of Ottawa, **SLP**

Pressman, Hilda T 59 Edgewood Avenue, West Orange, NJ 07052, (201) 268-8140, BA 63 CUNY - Queens Coll; MA 74 Seton Hall Univ; 87–Dir-Hrng & Sp Ctr, United Hosp Med Ctr, **SLP ACE**

Pressman, Mrs Karla S 32 Winshaw Road, Swampscott, MA 01907, Principal/Dir of Special Educ, Georgetown Public Schools, **SLP**

Pressnell, Dr Lucille M 1500 North Decatur Road N E, Atlanta, GA 30306, (404) 373-7288, BS 66 Washington Univ; MS 67 Washington Univ; PH 70 (Sp-Lang Path) Northwestern Univ; 72–Dir, The Davison School Inc, **SLP**

Preston, Donna M Community Health Services Inc, 3918 Dickerson Road, Nashville, TN 37207, (615) 865-7400, BS 74 Middle TN St Univ; MA 78 Univ of TN - Knoxville; Sp/Lang Path, Commun Hlth Serv Inc, **SLP**

Preston, Mrs Gwenn E 22771 Foxborough Way, El Toro, CA 92630, (714) 558-5591, BA 75 Univ of MA - Amherst; MA 77 Memphis St Univ; Sp-Lang Path, Santa Ana USD, **SLP**

Preston, Mrs Janet Kowalsky 12729 Willowyck Drive, Creve Coeur, MO 63146, (314) 344-6460, BA 77 SUNY - Center at Buffalo; MA 79 Kent St Univ; Aud, De Paul Hlth Cen, **A**

Preston, Jodi Weber 1917 2nd Street East, Menomonie, WI 54751, (715) 835-5845, BA 85 Univ of WI - Eau Claire; MS 86 Univ of WI - Eau Claire; **SLP**

Preston, Stuart R 1909 White Hollow Drive, Greenville, NC 27858, (919) 355-5815, BS 77 East Carolina Univ; MS 79 East Carolina Univ; Sp-Lang Path, Pitt Co Mem Hosp, **SLP**

Preston-Krackenfels, Joan 109 Grove Street, Wilkes-Barre, PA 18702, (717) 829-6306, BS 79 Bloomsburg Univ of PA; MS 80 Bloomsburg Univ of PA; 85–Sp-Lang Path, Wilkes-Barre Sp & Lang Clin Inc, **SLP**

Pretsfelder, Loreen Horowitz 5212 Kaitlyn Court, Laurenceville, NJ 08648, (609) 799-2000, BS 78 SUNY - Center at Albany; OM 80 Hahneman Medical Coll; Sp-Lang Path, Princeton Winsor Sp Assoc, **SLP ACE**

Prettner, Laurie K 3757 Harriet Avenue South, Apartment 7, Minneapolis, MN 55409, (612) 824-5982, BS 84 Univ of WI - Madison; MS 86 Univ of WI - Madison; Aud, Allied Hrng Svcs, **A**

Pretzloff, Mrs Lucia Kowalski 6701 Grandview Drive, Independence, OH 44131, (216) 575-0965, BA 86 Cleveland St Univ; MA 87 Cleveland St Univ; 88–Sp-Lang Path, PSI-Affiliates Inc

Preuss, Jodie R Rd 6 Box 432, Sylvan Lake Road, Hopewell Junction, NY 12533, **SLP**

Preuss, Mrs Kathleen M 232 South Woods Mill Road, Chesterfield, MO 63017, (314) 434-1500, BS 78 Saint Louis Univ; OM 82 Webster Univ; MA 80 Saint Louis Univ; 87–Ch Sp-Lang Path, St Luke's Hosp, **SLP**

Prevatte, Beverly Elizabeth 1709 #11 Chambers Drive, Matthews, NC 28105, (704) 283-3724, BS 83 Appalachian St Univ; ME 86 Univ of NC - Greensboro; **SLP**

Prevett, Mrs Donna K 3046 Teller Avenue, Grand Junction, CO 81504-5862, (303) 244-6153, BA 79 CA St Univ - Fresno; MA 82 CA St Univ - Fresno; 87–Sp-Lang Path, Hilltop Rehabilitation Hosp, **SLP**

Previtera, Mrs Susan Leaman 3109 Parklane N W, Canton, OH 44709, (216) 497-9781, BS 79 Kent St Univ; MA 80 Kent St Univ; Sp-Lang Path, Private Practice, **SLP**

Prevo, Mrs Cheryl Allen Route 3 Box 649, Thomasville, NC 27360-9328, (704) 352-2777, BS 83 Univ of NC - Greensboro; ME 84 Univ of NC - Greensboro; Sp-Lang Path, Randolph County Schools, **SLP**

Prevost, Mrs Susan P O Box 305, Mahopac Falls, NY 10542, (914) 628-4945, BA 74 CUNY - Brooklyn Coll; MA 75 Univ of Northern CO; Sp/Lang Path, Private Practice, **SLP ACE**

Prewitt, Deborah F 6500 East 4th Avenue, Gary, IN 46403, **SLP**

Prezant, Fran Pollock 303 South 6th Street, Indiana, PA 15701, (412) 357-8945, BA 74 CUNY - Queens Coll; ME 75 Northeastern Univ; Sp-Lang Path, IN Univ of Pa, **SLP**

Pribic, Mrs Mary Lou Brinker P O Box 1, Martins Creek, PA 18063, (215) 866-5555, BA 71; MA 73 Univ of Northern CO; 88–Aud, Professional Hrng Assoc, **SLP A**

Pribilsky, Todd A 215 1900 Richmond Avenue, Victoria, BC, Canada V8R 4R2, (604) 592-9911, BS 79 Univ of WA; MS 81 Univ of WA; 88–Aud, West Coast Hrg Ctr, **A**

Pribnow, Signe Hagen 3857 16C Wolverine St N E, Salem, OR 97305, (503) 588-1039, BA 72; MS 83 Western OR St Coll; Aud, Salem Audiology Clinic, **A**

Pribyl, Julianne L 2720 North 53rd Street, Omaha, NE 68104, (402) 572-2295, BA 73 Univ of NE - Omaha; MS 78 Univ of NE - Omaha; 78–Sp-Lang Path, Immanuel Med Ctr, **SLP**

Price, Mrs Alyson Duffie 532 C Avenue, West Columbia, SC 29169, (803) 794-5621, MS 88 Univ of SC - Columbia; 88–Sp-Lang Path, Lexington Sch Dist #2

Price, Barbara 2157 Evansdale, Toledo, OH 43607, (419) 245-4150, BA 73 OH Wesleyan Univ; MS 74 Vanderbilt Univ; Aud, Lucas Co Off Ed, **A**

Price, Mrs Barbara J 521 Avila Road, San Mateo, CA 94402, (415) 697-8924, BS 54 Univ of MN - Minneap-St Paul; MA 58 Stanford Univ; Sen Sp-Lang Path, Er Sl So, **SLP**

Price, Dr Carol M 13223 Greenmount Avenue, Beltsville, MD 20705, (301) 572-7796, BA 63 Marietta Coll; MA 64 OH St Univ; PH 66 (Sp & Hrng Path) OH St Univ; 66–Sp-Lang Path, Private Practice, **SLP**

Price, Mrs Claudia S 669 Morwood Road, Telford, PA 18969, (215) 721-9251, BA 71 Univ of Southern CA; MA 73 Univ of Southern CA; **SLP ACE**

Price, Cynthia Lee 820 Lindh Road #117, Gulfport, MS 39501, (601) 896-4365, **SLP**

Price, Deborah 5477 Glen Lakes Drive, Suite 106, Dallas, TX 75231, (214) 987-4114, BS 78 Univ of TX - Dallas; MS 80 Univ of TX - Dallas; Pres, Hearing Prof Cen, **A ACE**

Price, Mrs Dee Ann Route 4 Box 81, Arkadelphia, AR 71923, (501) 246-5110, BA 75 FL St Univ; MA 78 Univ of FL; Sp-Lang Path, Arkadelphia PS Dist, **A**

Price, Mrs Denise Faye 104 S 50th Court, West Des Moines, IA 50265, (515) 223-7227, BA 83 MI St Univ; MA 86 MI St Univ; Sp-Lang Path, Des Moines PS, **SLP**

Price, Mrs Dorothy M 4757 South Ridge Terrace, Fort Worth, TX 76133, (817) 534-8123, BA 49 Univ of Northern IA; MA 71 TX Christian Univ; Superv, Ft Worth ISD, **SLP**

Price, Georgianna La Rocque 47-D Scarborough Lane, Wappingers Falls, NY 12590, (914) 297-0179, **SLP**

Price, Harold A InSpeech Inc, P O Box 928, Valley Forge, PA 19482, (215) 631-9300, BS 71 Memphis St Univ; MA 73 Memphis St Univ; Vice President-Field Operation, InSpeech Inc, **SLP**

Price, Jean Albert 8119 South 77th East Avenue, Apartment 202, Tulsa, OK 74133, (918) 455-3535, BA 80 OH St Univ; MA 82 OH St Univ; 87–Sp-Lang Path, Broken Arrow Med Ctr, **SLP**

Price, Mrs Jeanne Virginia 1809 Midcrest, Plano, TX 75075, (214) 423-2224, MS 88 Univ of TX - Dallas; 88–Sp-Lang Path, Princeton ISD

Price, Jenny Brown 2702 Jetton Avenue, Tampa, FL 33629, BS 83 Auburn Univ - Auburn; MS 84 Auburn Univ - Auburn; **SLP**

Price, Joanne 228 West Birch, Walla Walla, WA 99362, (509) 525-2759, BS 70 OR St Univ; MA 75 OR St Univ; Aud, Private Practice, **A**

Price, Judith Kalan 104 Crosshill Road, Philadelphia, PA 19151, (215) 642-1849, BS 74 Northeastern Univ; MA 78 West Chester Univ of PA; Sp-Lang Path, Sch Dist of Phila, **SLP**

Price, Mrs Juneanne Downs 105 Oakridge Cove, Maumelle, AR 72118, **SLP**

Price, Karen Jo 24 Taymil Road, New Rochelle, NY 10804, (212) 222-6051, BA 72 CUNY - Hunter Coll; MS 73 Univ of IL - Urbana; SLP, BOCES of So Westchester, **SLP**

Price, Karen M 83 Perkins Street, Jamaica Plain, MA 02130, (617) 726-2755, BA 78 Univ of MI - Ann Arbor; MA 79 Western MI Univ; Sp-Lang Path, Massachusetts General Hospital, **SLP**

Price, Mrs Karen S 636 Westwood Avenue, River Vale, NJ 07675, (201) 666-5115, BA 75 Pace U -NY City; MS 87 William Paterson Coll; 88–Sp-Lang Path, Private Practice, **SLP**

Price, Kathleen Gerianne 5657 Golf Ridge Drive #E, St Louis, MO 63128, (314) 962-0235, BS 75 Southeast MO St Univ; MA 76 Memphis St Univ; 82–Sp-Lang Path, Spec Sch Dist of St Louis Co, **SLP**

Price, L Denise D 3034 Chimney Rock, Abilene, TX 79606, (915) 672-4321, BS 74 Univ of North TX; MS 75 Univ of North TX; Dir-Humana Hrng & Sp Cen, Humana Hosp, **A**

Price, Mrs Lee A 4792 Barkshire Drive, Memphis, TN 38115, (901) 362-8261, MS 85 Univ of South FL; 88–Sp-Lang Path, Professional Health Services, **SLP**

Price, Lynda McCann 6239 East Twin Peak Circle, Anaheim, CA 92807, (714) 736-3308, BA 84 CA St Univ - Fullerton

Price, Margaret J 3409-B West Barcelona St, Tampa, FL 33629, BS 76 Indiana Univ of PA; MS 77 WV Univ; 84–Sp-Lang Path, Hillsborough Co PS, **SLP**

Price, Margaret Mary Route 7 Box 91-B, Russellville, AR 72801, (501) 968-3315, BS 81 Univ of Central AR; MA 87 Univ of Central AR; 88–Sp-Lang Path, Russellville Sp & Lang Clinic, **SLP**

Price, Mary Beth McCreery 8328 North Mount Tabor Rd, Ellettsville, IN 47429, (812) 335-6251, BS 78 IN St Univ - Terre Haute; MA 82 IN Univ - Bloomington; Instr, Indiana Univ Speech & Hrng Ctr, **SLP**

Price, Mary Jo 413 West First Street, Elmira, NY 14901, BS 80 Elmira Coll; MS 85 Ithaca Coll; **SLP**

Price, Mrs Maryjo Anna HCR 1 Box 23, Douglas, ND 58735, (701) 529-4887, BA 82 Univ of ND; MS 83 Minot St Univ; Sp-Lang Path, Souris Valley Spec Serv, **SLP**

Price, Peggy Gayle 816 Drake, Centerville, IA 52544, BS 82 Northeast MO St Univ; MA 85 Northeast MO St Univ

Price, Roslyn R 4110 Cannon Crest Road W, San Ramon, CA 94583, (415) 866-8637, BA 61 Univ of MD - College Park; MA 66 Univ of MD - College Park; Sp-Lang Path, **SLP**

Price, Sandra Wayne 2924 Lewis Street, Birmingham, AL 35243, (205) 323-3683, BS 84 Univ of Montevallo; MS 85 Univ of Montevallo; Sp-Lang Path, Assn for Retarded Citizens, **SLP**

Price, Sharon R 2326 South 24th #12101, Kansas City, KS 66106-4348, (913) 362-2945, OB 83 Univ of KS; MA 85 Univ of KS; 86–Sp-Lang Path, St Luke's Hosp, **SLP**

Price, Susan Crain 6108 N W 77th Street, Kansas City, MO 64151, (816) 587-4488, MS 84 Univ of SD - Vermillion; Sp-Lang Path, Yankton Public Schools, **SLP**

Price, Mrs Susan M P O Box 280, Norton, MA 02766, (508) 285-6357, BS 69 Bowling Green St Univ; MA 78 Univ of CO - Boulder; 86–Sp-Lang Path, Norton PS, **SLP**

Price, Teresa Clark Route 2 Box 207, Magnolia, MS 39652, (601) 783-6194, **SLP**

Price, Tobianne 24575 Melrose Place, Elkhart, IN 46517, (219) 875-8517, BA 69 Western MI Univ; MA 70 Western MI Univ; 84–Sp-Lang Path, Concord Comm Schs, **SLP**

Price, Mrs Vickie H 79 Woodgreen, Belden, MS 38826, (601) 842-1891, BS 77 East TN St Univ; MA 79 Memphis St Univ; Sp-Lang Path, North Mississippi Medical Ctr, **SLP**

Price-Goldman, Mrs Wendi 38 Park Street #12C, Florham Park, NJ 07932, (201) 822-8315, BS 80 Ithaca Coll; MA 82 Montclair St Coll; **SLP**

Price-Larson, Marilyn 3386 East Birch Circle, Salt Lake City, UT 84124, BS 74; MA 76 UT St Univ; SLP, Murray School District, **SLP**

Priceman, Lorraine R 5417 Ellenvale Avenue, Woodland Hills, CA 91367, (818) 883-1381, BA 68 Wichita St Univ; MA 70 Wichita St Univ; Sp/Lang Path, Cen for Commun Dis, **SLP**

Prichard, Carole J 602 Hickory Road, Woodstock, IL 60098, (815) 455-3101, BS 56 Univ of IL - Urbana; MA 75 Northern IL Univ - De Kalb; Sp-Lang Path, Commun Disorders Serv, **SLP ACE**

Prichard, Cheryl L Route 6 Box 231-C, Cherry Hill, Morgantown, WV 26505, (304) 293-4242, BS 70 WV Univ; MS 76 WV Univ; Asst Prof, WV U-Dept Sp Path & Aud, **SLP**

Prichard, Mrs Deborah Gray 1404 F Paegelow, Scott AFB, IL 62225, (618) 746-4020, BA 81 Ouachita Baptist Univ; MS 84 Minot St Univ; Sp-Lang Path, Midwest Sp Path, **SLP**

Prickett, Mrs Anita Louise Bear Hill Road, Chichester, NH 03263, (603) 269-5161, BA 78 Univ of AL- Tuscaloosa; MS 84 Univ of NH; 88–Sp-Lang Path, Barnstead Sch, **SLP**

Prickett, John M Route 5 Box 602, Scottsboro, AL 35768, (205) 574-2004, BA 72 Univ of AL- Tuscaloosa; MA 74 Univ of AL- Tuscaloosa; Sp-Lang Path, Jackson Co Schs, **SLP**

Priebe, Florence M 8115 Langbrook Road, Springfield, VA 22152, (703) 591-7553, BA 63 Southern Methodist Univ; OM 72 Tulane Univ; SLP, Fairfax Co Pub Schs, **SLP**

Priest, Mrs Linda Wadsworth 10 Stanford Drive, Homer, NY 13077, (315) 473-6916, **SLP**

Prieston, Mrs Cathy M G 203 Madison Avenue, Hamilton, VA 22068, BS 75 WV Univ; MS 76 WV Univ; SLP, Loudoun County School Board, **SLP**

Prietto, Anita L 1343 Moursund, Houston, TX 77030, (713) 792-4500, 78 Univ of CA - Irvine; 83 Univ of CA - Santa Barbara; Aud, Univ of TX Sp & Hrng Ins, **A**

Prieve, Beth Anne Wendell Johnson Sp & Hrng Ctr, Hawkins Drive, University Of Iowa, Iowa City, IA 52242, (319) 353-4816, **A**

Prill, Pamela Renae Route 1 Box 285, Lucedale, MS 39452, (601) 947-7757, MS 82 Univ of South AL; SLP, George County Schools, **SLP**

Prillwitz, David Charles Rehabilitation Institute Of Or, Good Samaritan Hospital, 1040 N W 22nd Avenue, Portland, OR 97210, (503) 229-7151, BS 82 Univ of WI - Stevens Point; MS 84 Univ of WI - Madison; 85–Sp-Lang Path, Good Samaritan Hosp & Med Ctr, **SLP**

Prime, Mrs Donna Harris 4332 Collingswood Drive, Chesterfield, VA 23832-8723, (804) 780-0666, BS 79 Longwood Coll; ME 81 Univ of VA - Charlottesville; Aud, Randall Dalton MD, **A**

Prime, Karen Anne 34 Colony Drive East, West Orange, NJ 07052, (201) 533-5786, MA 87 Montclair St Coll; 88–Sp-Lang Path, St Barnabus Med Ctr, **SLP**

Primeau, Richard L 4872 West Rosebay, Tucson, AZ 85741, (602) 792-1450, BS 78 Central MI Univ; MA 79 Central MI Univ; Aud, VA Med Ctr, **A**

Primiano, Christine R 388 East Foster Street, Melrose, MA 02176, (617) 935-5050, BA 74 Univ of MA - Amherst; MS 75 Univ of MI - Ann Arbor; Administrator Ambulatory Care, New England Rehabilitation Hos, **SLP**

Primley, Alice A 2455 F Street S E #78, Auburn, WA 98002, BS; **SLP LM**

Primus, Dr Michael A Dept Of Sp Path & Audiology, University Of Wyoming, P O Box 3311, 30 Ross Hall, Laramie, WY 82071, (307) 766-6426, BA 69 Univ of MN - Minneap-St Paul; MS 75 CO St Univ; PH 84 (Aud) Univ of WA; 84–Assistant Professor, University of Wyoming, **A**

Prince, Annette J P O Box 59671, Chicago, IL 60659, (312) 566-9180, BA 80 Northwestern Univ; MA 82 Northwestern Univ; SLP, Spec Ed Dist/Lake Co, **SLP**

Prince, David C 114 Tazewell Avenue, Tazewell, VA 24651, (703) 988-7879, BS 86 Lamar Univ; MS 87 Radford Univ; 88–Pres, Associated Hrng & Diag

Prince, Mrs Elizabeth Dent P O Box 325, Douglasville, GA 30133-0325, (404) 949-9095, **SLP**

Prince, Jane B 921 Fairway Circle, Jonesboro, AR 72401, (501) 450-3176, BS 72 Univ Southern MS-Hattiesburg; MS 76 Univ Southern MS-Hattiesburg; PH 81 (Aud) Univ Southern MS-Hattiesburg; 88–Aud, Arkansas Audiometrics, **A**

Prince, Mrs Joyce Ann RFD 4 Box 43, Fairbury, NE 68352, (402) 729-5755, BS 52 Northwestern Univ; MA 57 Univ of NE - Lincoln; Sp-Lang Path, Fairbury Pub Sch, **SLP**

Prince, Mrs Karen Janes 666 West Eldorado Street, Decatur, IL 62522, (217) 877-8121, BS 81 IL St Univ - Normal; MS 83 IL St Univ - Normal; 83–Sp-Lang Path, Decatur Mem Hosp, **SLP**

Prince, Linda Price 5177 Goldmar Drive, Birmingham, AL 35210-2807, **SLP**

Prince, Mrs Nada 1898 White Chapel Circle N W, Uniontown, OH 44685, (216) 830-8024, BA 66 OH Univ - Athens; MA 70 Kent St Univ; Sp-Lang Path, Jackson Local School District, **SLP**

Principe, Donna L 2546 Westlake Avenue, Oceanside, NY 11572, (516) 536-2193, MA 86 CUNY - Hunter Coll; **SLP**

Principe, Sharon A 27 North Ritters Lane, Owings Mills, MD 21117, (301) 396-0013, BA 78 Loyola Coll; MS 79 Loyola Coll; Sp-Lang Path, Baltimore City Public Schools, **SLP**

Prindiville, Rita Ann 3323 Dutch Bottom Road, Arnold, MO 63010, (314) 296-7568, BS 83 Univ of MO - Columbia; MA 84 Northeast MO St Univ; SLP, Marceline R-V School, **SLP**

Prine, Amy Pratt 613 Willow Heights Drive, Atlanta, GA 30328, (318) 325-3963, BA 86 LA Tech Univ; MA 87 LA Tech Univ; **SLP**

Pringle, Mrs Emily Porter 790 Beaver Branch Road, Pennsylvania Furnace, PA 16865, (303) 238-7985, BA 75 MI St Univ; MA 77 Univ of CO - Boulder; 88–Sp-Lang Path, St Coll Area Sch Dist, **SLP**

Prins, Dr David 13130 N E 31st Place, Bellevue, WA 98005, (206) 543-7974, BA 52 Central Univ of IA; MA 57 Univ of MI - Ann Arbor; PH 61 (NS) Univ of MI - Ann Arbor; Prof, U of WA, **SLP**

Prinsket, Donnamarie H 1418 Sellers Street, Philadelphia, PA 19124, (215) 671-5078, MS 78 Bloomsburg Univ of PA; 84–Dir Spch/Lang/Hearing Services, Temple Univ Woodhaven Center, **SLP**

Prinz, Dr Philip M Program In Communication Disorders, Department Of Special Education, San Francisco State Univ, 1600 Holloway Avenue, San Francisco, CA 94132, (415) 338-1161, MS 72 Northwestern Univ; MS 74 Boston Univ; ED 78 (NS) Boston Univ; 88–Prof of Commun Dis, San Francisco St Univ, **SLP**

Prislupski, Mrs Denise T Globe Hearing Aid Center, 119 Wyoming Avenue, Scranton, PA 18501, (717) 344-7271, BS 79 Marywood Coll; MS 81 Bloomsburg Univ of PA; Aud, Globe Hearing Aid Center, **A**

Pristo, Ellen 9046 North 123th Street, Scottsdale, AZ 85259, (602) 967-0286, BS 70; MS 75 Univ of ND; Sp-Lang Path, Professional Association, **SLP**

Pritchard, Annette D 616 Huff Avenue, Manville, NJ 08835-2430, **SLP**

Pritchett, Mrs Joy W Aud Speech & Hearing Aid Ctr, Suite 8 Lafayette Sqaure, Milledgeville, GA 31061, (912) 452-0578, BS 77 Auburn Univ - Auburn; MS 78 Auburn Univ - Auburn; Aud, Est Medical Group, **A**

Pritchett, Mrs Judy G 1303 Panorama Drive, Chattanooga, TN 37421, (615) 899-1085, BA 70 David Lipscomb Coll; MS 73 Murray St Univ; Sp-Lang Path, Boyd Buchanan Sch, **SLP**

Pritz-Mullin, Christina 7272 Cinnamon Woods Drive, West Chester, OH 45069-1074, (304) 665-7893, **SLP**

Privratsky, Mrs Kathy I 1101 Boulder Run, Harker Heights, TX 76543, (817) 699-9556, BA 69 Eastern WA Univ; MS 73 Eastern WA Univ; 86–Sp/Lang Path, Killeen Independent Sch Dist, **SLP**

Prizant, Dr Barry M Communication Disorders Department, Bradley Hospital, 1011 Veterans Memorial Pky, East Providence, RI 02915, (401) 434-3400, BA 72 SUNY - Center at Binghamton; MA 75 SUNY - Center at Buffalo; PH 78 (Communication Disorders and Sciences) SUNY - Center at Buffalo; 84–Dir/Communication Disorders, Bradley Hospital, **SLP ACE**

Pro, Mrs Melissa Le Ann 4511 Graves Drive, Odessa, TX 79762, (915) 368-7937, BS 82 Eastern NM Univ; MS 84 TX Tech Univ; Sp-Lang Path, Ector Cty ISD, **SLP**

Probst, Angela Sanders 85 East Street, Rutland, VT 05701, BS 84 Bloomsburg Univ of PA; MS 85 Bloomsburg Univ of PA; 88–Sp-Lang Path, Vermont Achievement Center

Probst, Dianne Marie 1101 Buford Court, Chesapeake, VA 23320, (919) 436-3724, BS 84 Appalachian St Univ; MS 86 Old Dominion Univ; Sp-Lang Path, Communi-Care Inc, **SLP**

Probst, Gretchen E 7547 Penn Bridge Court, Pittsburgh, PA 15221, (412) 647-5580, BA 66 IN Univ - Bloomington; OM 68 IN Univ - Bloomington; Audiologist, Chldns Hosp of Pittsburg, **A**

Prochaska-Charf, Mrs Mary Jane 5330 South 37th, Lincoln, NE 68516, (402) 423-0548, BS 73 Univ of NE - Lincoln; MS 80 Kearney St Coll; Sp-Lang Path, Educational Serv Unit 9, **SLP**

Prochazka, Katherine Marie 5315 Fredericksburg Road, Apartment 1122, San Antonio, TX 78229, (512) 341-7623, BA 84 Our Lady Lake Univ-San Anton; MA 86 Our Lady Lake Univ-San Anton; **SLP**

Procopi, Nickolas 1412 North Laurel Avenue, Apartment 21, Los Angeles, CA 90046, (213) 222-8090, BA 82 Hofstra Univ; MS 86 Columbia Univ Teachers Coll; 88–Sp-Lang Path, Diog Ctr for Neur Hndcpd Chldn, **SLP**

Procopio, Mrs Karen A Teeling 29 Pasture Lane, Poughkeepsie, NY 12603, (914) 462-6182, BS 85 SUNY - Coll at Geneseo; MA 87 Univ of MA - Amherst; 87–Sp-Lang Path, St Francis Hosp, **SLP**

Proct, Mrs Marlene P 2149 Isabelle Court, North Bellmore, NY 11710, (516) 663-5773, BA 68 Hofstra Univ; MA 70 Hofstra Univ; Sp-Lang Path, Patterson Home Dept of Soc Ser, **SLP**

Proctor, Dr F Adele 133 Park Street #1002, Brookline, MA 02146, (617) 437-2492, BA 66 Morgan St Univ; MS 68 PA St Univ - Univ Park; OD 79 (NS) Johns Hopkins Univ; Assoc Prof, Northeastern U, **SLP**

Proctor, Jaclin K 1879 Sycamore Court, Crown Point, IN 46307, (219) 738-2528, BA 72 IN Univ - Bloomington; MA 73 IN Univ - Bloomington; Aud, Southlake Sp & Hrng Ctr Inc, **A**

Proctor, Mrs Linda McCormick 827 West Plata, Mesa, AZ 85210, (602) 272-4010, BS 81 Eastern MI Univ; MA 83 Eastern MI Univ; 88–Sp-Lang Path, Mesa Public Schools, **SLP**

Proctor, Mrs Lorraine DeStefano 2202-D Mandalay Drive, Richmond, VA 23224, (804) 745-7532, BS 81 IA St Univ; MA 84 Western MI Univ; Sp-Lang Path, Sheltering Arms Rehab Hosp, **SLP**

Proctor, Marlene Koscak 1016 Oak Way, Rock Springs, WY 82901, (307) 382-2474, BS 75 Univ of WY; MS 82 Univ of WY; SLP, Sweetwater Co Sch Dist #1, **SLP**

Proctor, Minnie B P O Box 41, Montauk, NY 11954, (516) 668-2036, BA 34 CUNY - Brooklyn Coll; Private Practice, **SLP LM**

Proctor, Nancy H 1311 Westchester Drive, Baton Rouge, LA 70810, (504) 261-4093, BS 74 Saint Mary's Dominican Coll; OM 75 LA St Univ - N O Medical Ctr; SLP, E Baton Rouge Parish Sch Bd, **SLP**

Proctor, Roy E 302 Glendening, Orange Park, FL 32073, (904) 355-3403, BS 68 Memphis St Univ; MA 69 Memphis St Univ; Sp-Lang Path, Sp & Hrng Cen, **SLP**

Profant, Deborah Susan K 5434 Park Vista Court, Stow, OH 44224, (216) 666-8815, BA 79 Eastern WA Univ; MA 81 Kent St Univ; Sp-Lang Path, Bd of Ment Ret & Dev Disabl, **SLP**

Profet, Sharon Beth c/o Fairmont Elementary School, 5241 Fairmont Boulevard, Yorba Linda, CA 92686, (714) 996-2550, MA; 80–Sp-Lang Path, Placentie USD, **SLP**

Proffitt, Kimberly G 6607 Tottenham, Louisville, KY 40207, BA 81 Bellarmine Coll; MS 82 Univ of Louisville; Sp-Lang Path, Private Practice, **SLP ACE**

Progar-Borowy, Mrs Pamela J 5377 Broadview Road, Gahanna, OH 43230, (614) 461-2420, SLP, Children's Hospital, **SLP**

Progebin-Graffe, Barbara L 7 Welbourn Lane, Coram, NY 11727, (516) 331-7884, BA 70 Hofstra Univ; MA 71 Hofstra Univ; Sp-Lang Path, The New Interdisciplinary Sch, **SLP**

Proger, Laura Ellen 14614 Bauer Drive #3, Rockville, MD 20853, (301) 762-1015, BA 80 Univ of MD - College Park; MS 82 Gallaudet Coll; Aud, The Audiology Ctr, **A**

Prohaska, Ann M Uniyed States Air Force, Usafh/Sgpma, Tinker AFB, OK 73145, (405) 734-3309, BS 77 Univ of WI - Milwaukee; MS 78 Univ of WI - Stevens Point; Chief Audiology, United States Air Force, **A ACE**

Prohaska, Mrs Denise I 10317 South Mason, Oak Lawn, IL 60453, (312) 424-0216, BA 73 Saint Xavier Coll; MS 75 Bradley Univ; 77–Sp-Lang Path, Palos Consol Dist 118, **SLP**

Prohl, Mrs Maureen Foy PO Box 1541, Burpee Hill, New London, NH 03257-0078, (603) 526-2143, BA 73 Univ of Cincinnati; MA 74 Northwestern Univ; 88–Sp-Lang Path, Sch Admin Unit #24, **SLP**

Prokes, Jerry E 207 N San Marco Avenue, St Augustine, FL 32084, (904) 824-1654, BA 55 OH Univ - Athens; MA 57 Case Western Reserve Univ; Director Child Study Center, Florida Sch for Deaf & Blind, **A**

Prokes, Mrs Kim C 7820 Banks, Justice, IL 60458, (312) 598-0515, BS 73 Western IL Univ; MA 74 Western IL Univ; SLP, School District 111 S Stickney, **SLP**

Prokop, Beverly Jo Box 401, Plap, MB, Canada R1N 3B7, BS 64 Univ of NE - Omaha; MA 68 Univ of NE - Omaha; **SLP**

Prokop, Mrs Terry Hall 18 Giles Road, Grafton, OH 44044, (216) 748-3017, BA 77 Univ of Akron; MA 81 Univ of Akron; SLP, Brunswick City Sch, **SLP**

Pronovost, Dr Wilbert 65 Burleigh Street, Waterville, ME 04901, (207) 873-2000, BA 35 Univ of ME - Orono; MA 37 Univ of IA; PH 39 (Sp & Hrng Science) Univ of IA; Retired, **SLP A F LM**

Proper, Marcia Lee 4597 Meadow Circle, Avon, NY 14414, (716) 245-5688, BS 84 SUNY - Coll at Geneseo; MA 85 SUNY - Coll at Geneseo; 86–Sp-Lang Path, Livingston-WY ARC Chldrn Svcs, **SLP**

Prosek Phd, Robert A Army Audiology & Speech Center, Walter Reed Army Med Ctr, Washington, DC 20307, PH (NS)

Prosnitz, Gabrielle C 3 Gerald Circle, Acton, MA 01720, (508) 897-5960, BA 76 Univ of CT; MS 78 Syracuse Univ; Sp-Lang Path, Private Practice, **SLP**

Proteau, Dawn Agnes 32777 Grand River #305, Farmington Hills, MI 48024, BA 54 Mercy Coll of Detroit; ME 58 Wayne St Univ; SLP, Detroit Bd of Ed, **SLP**

Prothero, Emily Diane 6940 White Pine Place, Albuquerque, NM 87109, (505) 298-5009, BA 82 Depauw Univ; MA 84 Northern IL Univ - De Kalb; Sp-Lang Path, Albuquerque PS, **SLP**

Prothro, Jana K 241 Settlers Park, Shreveport, LA 71115, (318) 227-4527, BA 80 Northeast LA Univ; MA 87 LA Tech Univ; 88–Sp-Lang Path, Schumpert Med Ctr, **SLP**

Proto, Josephine 251 Noble Avenue #4, Pittsburgh, PA 15205, BS 77 Indiana Univ of PA; MA 79 Univ of Pittsburgh - Pittsburgh; Sp-Lang Path, Allegheny Inter Ut, **SLP**

Protti-Patterson, Mrs Elizabeth 50 Battery Hill Drive, Voorhees, NJ 08043, (215) 284-8579, BS 70 Indiana Univ of PA; MS 72 Univ of OK Medical Center; Director of Clinical Services, Speech & Hearing Network Inc, **A**

Proudfoot, Mrs Penny Ann 550 Westmount Drive, London, ON, Canada N6K 1X8, (519) 471-0606, BA 54 Univ of Western Ontario; OM 79 Univ of Western Ontario; Sp-Lang Path, Private Practice, **SLP**

Proust, Janice 347 Doone Road, Fairless Hills, PA 19030, (609) 586-1597, SLP, Mercer Co Spec Srvs Schl Dstr, **SLP**

Prout, Nancy A 9630 South 252nd Street, Apartment D-105, Kent, WA 98031-6384, (206) 852-0941, BS 78 Univ of WA; MA 80 WA St Univ; 87–Sp-Lang Path, Kent Sch Dist 415, **SLP**

Prouty, Sharon W 81 Ryder Road, Briarcliff Manor, NY 10510, (914) 428-8319, BA 78 Rutger's St Univ - Douglas Coll; MS 80 Columbia Univ Teachers Coll; Sp-Lang Path, Westchester Assoc for Ret Citz, **SLP**

Prouty, Mrs Vicki L 7880 Meadowbrook Drive, Frisco, TX 75034, (214) 596-3618, BS 77 Univ of North TX; MS 80 Univ of North TX; Sp/Lang Path, Plano ISD, **SLP**

Provenzale-Buono, Judith 16 Franklin Drive, Voorhees, NJ 08043, (609) 770-1328, MS 84 Hahnemann Univ Grad Sch; Sp-Lang Path, Lourdes Reg Rehabilitation Ctr, **SLP**

Provenzano, Nora 14 Foothills Drive, South River, NJ 08882, (201) 388-7900, MA 82 Trenton St Coll; Sp-Lang Path, Clark Bd of Ed, **SLP**

Providence, Christophr Alan 5436 Harpers Farm Road #C1, Columbia, MD 21044, (301) 396-1370, BA 78 Hampton Univ; MA 80 Univ of Pittsburgh - Pittsburgh; Sp/Lang Path, Great Oaks Cen, **SLP**

Provo, Deborah K 15114 Weeks Drive, La Mirada, CA 90638-1245, **SLP**

Prucha, Mrs Kathleen Barnum 2109 Neyrey Drive, Metairie, LA 70001, (504) 889-0467, BS 79 SUNY - Coll at Fredonia; ME 80 Univ of VA - Charlottesville; **SLP**

Prucy, Nancy Ann 35 1/2 South Goodman St, Rochester, NY 14607, (716) 461-5160, BS 84 Clarion Univ of PA; MS 85 Clarion Univ of PA; **A**

Prudhomme, Maria R 9019 Winthrop Drive, Cincinnati, OH 45249, PH (NS); **SLP**

Pruet, Mrs Mary Montera Porter Memorial Hospital, Dept/Speech & Hearing, 2525 South Downing Street, Denver, CO 80210, (303) 778-1955, MS 84 Eastern NM Univ; Sp-Lang Path, Porter Memorial Hosp, **SLP**

Pruett, Paula M 503 Auburn Avenue, Monroe, LA 71201, (318) 396-6300, OB 67 Univ of AR - Monticello; MA 69 Univ of AR - Fayetteville; Sp-Lang Path, Js Clark Elementary, **SLP**

Pruett, Mrs Ruby Toliver P O Box 274, Huron, IN 47437, (812) 279-3581, BS 47 IN Univ - Bloomington; MS 57 IN Univ - Bloomington; 73–Sp-Lang Path, Bedford Med Center Headstart, **SLP LM**

Pruiett, Mrs Mary Clift P O Box 29, Farmersburg, IN 47850, (812) 696-2893, BS 84 Purdue Univ - West Lafayette; MS 86 IN St Univ - Terre Haute; 86–Sp-Lang Path, Daviess Martin Special Ed Coop

Pruitt, Chris W Aaron's Hearing Aid, 8317 Whitesburg Way #808, Huntsville, AL 35802-3466, (205) 882-2766, BS 74 Auburn Univ - Auburn; MS 76 Auburn Univ - Auburn; Director/ Owner, Aarons Family Hearing Aid Ctr, **A**

Pruitt, Debra Michelle Route 1 Box 523, Marianna, FL 32446, (305) 841-5111, BA 85 Univ of FL; ME 87 Univ of FL; **SLP**

Pruitt, Jeanine Blake 6501 Fannin #NA-200, Houston, TX 77030, (713) 790-5913, BA 83 Wake Forest Univ; OM 85 LA St Univ - N O Medical Ctr; 87–Aud, The Methodist Hosp, **A**

Pruitt, Mrs Joy 1636 Waianuenue Avenue, Hilo, HI 96720, (808) 961-2148, BA 66 American Univ; MA 69 NY Univ; Sp-Lang Path, Private Practice, **SLP ACE**

Pruitt, Mrs Joyce D 148 Edgecombe Road, Spartanburg, SC 29302, (803) 579-0052, BA 58 Univ of MO - Columbia; Sp-Lang Path, Spartanburg School District 5, **SLP**

Pruitt, Mrs Lisa Hendrix Route 8 Box 631, North Wilkesboro, NC 28659, (919) 667-8149, MA 85 Appalachian St Univ; Sp-Lang Path, Wilkes County Public Schools, **SLP**

Pruitt, Mary Eliz 3027 Niles Buchanan Road, Buchanan, MI 49107, (616) 695-3851, MA 72 IN Univ - Bloomington; Dir of Rehab, Visitors Hosp, **SLP**

Pruitt-Shough, Mrs Ann L 6035 West Metropolitan Plz, Los Angeles, CA 90036, (818) 997-2330, BA 66 MI St Univ; MA 67 MI St Univ; MA 71 Eastern MI Univ; SLP, USD, **SLP**

Prusslin, Gail F 2736 Independence Avenue, Apartment 2-B, Riverdale, NY 10463-4651, (415) 931-1972, **SLP**

Prust, Jeanette Hickey 513 North Oak, Gordon, NE 69343, (605) 867-5174, BS 83 Moorhead St Univ; MS 85 Moorhead St Univ; 88–Sp-Lang Path, Shannon County PS, **SLP**

Pruszenski, Malea Anne 3102 Cove View Blvd #B-101, Galveston, TX 77554-8025, (412) 232-7773, BA 82 Univ of MD - College Park; MA 83 George Washington Univ; Aud, U of TX, **A**

Prutting, Carol Ann Speech And Hearing Center, University Of California, Santa Barbara, CA 93106, (805) 682-1994, PH (NS); **SLP F**

Pruyne, Karen Ziemba 92 Breckwood Boulevard, Springfield, MA 01109, (413) 283-3411, BS 76 Univ of MA - Amherst; MA 82 Trenton St Coll; Sp/Lang Path, Monson Devel Cen, **SLP**

Pruzansky, Mrs Karen I 141-27 72nd Drive, Flushing, NY 11367, (718) 268-3781, BS 80 NY Univ; MA 84 NY Univ; **SLP**

Pry, Mrs Erlene B 802 Palm Grove Circle, Sugar Land, TX 77478, BS 72 Southwest TX St Univ; ME 73 Southwest TX St Univ; Sp-Lang Path, **SLP**

Pryble-Dattalo, Susan M 506 Andy Drive, Melrose Park, IL 60160, (213) 237-1181, BA 74 Elmhurst Coll; MA 75 Northwestern Univ; Sp-Lang Path, Chicago Board of Education, **SLP**

Pryby, Mrs Helen Nessmith 11 Wilson Avenue, Ozark, AL 36360, (701) 727-6424, OB 84 Minot St Univ; MS 85 Minot St Univ

Pryce, Jane Watson 217 Cooper Lane, Coventry, CT 06238, (203) 429-6451, BS 83 Elmira Coll; MA 85 OH Univ - Athens; **A**

Pryor, Mrs Dana Richmond Route 3 Box 568, Austin, AR 72007, (501) 843-2919, BA 76 Harding Univ; MS 82 Univ of AR - Little Rock; Sp-Lang Path, Bryant Pub Sch, **SLP**

Pryor, Laura Ann 401 North 40th Avenue, Yakima, WA 98902, (208) 678-4070, BA 85 Eastern WA Univ; MS 86 Eastern WA Univ; **SLP**

Pryor, Maryann S P O Box 802, Vienna, VA 22180, (703) 893-4099, BS 74 Radford Univ; MA 78 Catholic Univ of America; Assoc-SLP, Fairfax Co Pub Sch, **SLP**

Prystalski, Sharon M Naples American High School, Box 15 Usna, FPO New York, NY 09521, (312) 735-0377, BS 78 Univ of IL - Urbana; MS 79 IL St Univ - Normal; MS 85 Univ of IL - Chicago; SLP, Dept of Defense Sch, **SLP**

Prytula, Sandra Joanne 27130 Grandmont, Roseville, MI 48066, (313) 779-0428, BA 84 MI St Univ; MA 86 Wayne St Univ - Sch of Med; **A**

Przybycien, Mrs Julianne MacFadden 181 Steele Road, West Hartford, CT 06119, (203) 653-7445, BS 65 Univ of CT; MS 78 Southern CT St Univ; 70–Sp-Lang Path, Granby & East Granby Pub Schs, **SLP**

Przybylinski, Donna G 1950 Highway 11, Burlington, WI 53105-9066, (414) 723-5292, BS 78 Univ of WI - Stevens Point; MA 79 Western MI Univ; Dir/Speech Pathology, **SLP**

Przybylski, Sandra M H 3302 Broad Lawn Drive, Kirksville, MO 63501, (816) 665-8536, BS 68 Univ of IA; MA 71 Univ of IL - Urbana; Sp-Lang Path, La Plata R-II Sch, **SLP**

Przywara, Mrs Kathy I 39 Butternut Drive, Meriden, CT 06450, (203) 289-7411, BA 80 Southern CT St Univ; MA 82 Univ of MA - Amherst; Sp-Lang Path, East Hartford Public Schools, **SLP**

Psalidas, Mrs Joyce Y 2600 Pine Creek Court, Raleigh, NC 27612, (914) 876-1401, OB 77 Univ of GA; ME 79 Univ of GA; Sp-Lang Path / Teacher, Shelley Child Dev Ctr, **SLP**

Psaltis, Mrs Cynthia Doyen 7539 East Pinewood Place, Tucson, AZ 85715, (602) 885-8334, BS 71 Northwestern Univ; MS 83 Univ of AZ; 88–Sp-Lang Path/Instr, Univ of Arizona, **SLP**

Ptak, Lori Avends 2658 McKinley Street N E, Minneapolis, MN 55418, BS 79 Moorhead St Univ; MA 80 Univ of WI - Eau Claire; SLP, Rosemount School District, **SLP**

Puccio, Linda M 914 Elsie Drive, Melrose Park, IL 60160, (312) 681-2427, BA 85 Elmhurst Coll; MA 87 Univ of IL - Urbana

Puchalski, Maureen A 117 Darrah Lane, Lawrenceville, NJ 08648, (609) 883-2600, BS 74 PA St Univ - Univ Park; MA 77 MI St Univ; Aud, Katzenbach Sch for the Deaf, **A**

Pucillo, Mrs Joan M 350 Lisle Street, Braintree, MA 02184, (617) 843-8457, BA 80 Bridgewater St Coll; MS 82 Boston Univ; Sp-Lang Path, Boston PS, **SLP**

Puckett, Mrs Linda J 21672 Flamenco, Mission Viejo, CA 92692, (714) 496-6151, BS 72 OK St Univ; MA 73 Univ of IA; Sp-Lang Path, Capistrano USD, **SLP**

Puckey, Roberta M 7277 Long Springs Butte, Littleton, CO 80127, (303) 973-0225, BA 70 Univ of Akron; MA 73 Univ of Akron; Parent Family Specialist, Douglas County School District, **SLP**

Pudas, Marilynn A 122 N W 5th Avenue, Magee, MS 39111, (601) 849-3463, **SLP**

Pudish-Holland, Mrs Elizabeth 5 Westmore Lane, Cortland, NY 13045, (607) 753-9301, BS 77 SUNY - Coll at Geneseo; MA 78 SUNY - Coll at Geneseo; Sp-Lang Path, Cortland-Madison BOCES, **SLP**

Pudlo, Linda Mainiero 1533 Stonegate Road, La Grange Park, IL 60525, (312) 831-4930, BS 73 Bradley Univ; MS 74 Bradley Univ; Sp-Lang Path, Stratford Sch, **SLP**

Pudup, Mrs Kathleen M 164 Merrick Street, Rochester, NY 14615, (716) 325-4560, BS 76 SUNY - Coll at Brockport; MA 78 SUNY - Coll at Geneseo; Aud/Sp-Lang Teac, Cty Sch Dst-NY, **SLP A**

Puett, Valerie King 1126 Carolina, Shreveport, LA 71104, (318) 227-5156, BS 80 Univ of MO - Columbia; MS 81 Central MO St Univ; Asst Prof, Louisiana State U Med Cen, **SLP ACE**

Puffenberger, Beth Larue Route 12 Box 190, Chapel Hill, NC 27514, (919) 489-7931, BS 79 WV Univ; MS 85 Univ of NC - Chapel Hill; 86–Aud, McPherson Hosp, **A**

Puffenberger, Mrs Janice K 101 North Will Scarlet Ln, Williamsburg, VA 23185, (804) 229-4889, BA 50 Univ of MI - Ann Arbor; Retired, York Co Pub Schs, **SLP**

Pufnock, Mrs Joyce Gatlin 2021 Meadows Drive, Woodstock, GA 30188, (404) 924-7812, BS 85 Univ of GA; ME 86 Univ of GA; **SLP**

Pufpaff, Marcia Ward 305 West Orchard Avenue, Shepherd, MI 48883, (517) 773-6956, BA 76 Alma Coll; MA 83 Central MI Univ; 78–Sp-Lang Path, Gratiot-Isabella ISD, **SLP**

Pugh, Bradley Keith St Louis University Medical Center, Department Of Otolaryngology, 3660 Vista Suite 312, St Louis, MO 63110, (314) 577-6110, BS 82 OK St Univ; MS 84 CO St Univ; 87–Aud, St Louis University Med Ctr, **A**

Pugh, Gaylen S 9621 Seligman Avenue N E, Albuquerque, NM 87109, (505) 823-9725, BA 70 Huntingdon Coll; MA 71 Univ of AL- Tuscaloosa; 86–SLP, Educ Assessment Systems Inc, **SLP**

Pugh, Natalie Jean Rd 1 Box 474, Chester, WV 26034, (304) 387-2638, BS 85 WV Univ; MS 86 WV Univ; **SLP**

Pugh, Sallie Jeanette 1365 Felder Avenue, Montgomery, AL 36106, (205) 263-3526, BS 85 Univ of South AL; MS 87 Auburn Univ - Auburn; **SLP**

Pugh, Mrs Wilhelmina Scott 9707 Antioch Street, Upper Marlboro, MD 20772, (301) 843-8745, BA 78 NC A & T St Univ; MA 79 Bowling Green St Univ; 80–Sp-Lang Path, Charles Co Bd of Educ, **SLP**

Puglisi, Dr Elizabeth Antonia Apdo 1-2045, Guadalajara, Jalisco, Mexico, BA 35 Univ of MI - Ann Arbor; MS 46 Univ of MI - Ann Arbor; OD 54 (NS) Univ of MI - Ann Arbor; **LM**

Puglisi-Creegan, Santina V 4688 North 68th Street, Milwaukee, WI 53218, (414) 463-6376, BS 79 Marquette Univ; MS 80 Marquette Univ; Sp/Lang Path, Therapy Assoc, **SLP**

Puhak, Mary Louise 525 School Street #7B, Collegeville, PA 19426, (215) 539-8550, BS 82 Bloomsburg Univ of PA; MS 83 Bloomsburg Univ of PA; Sp-Lang Path, Montgomery Co Intermed Unit, **SLP**

Puhl, Janice Lee 8 Magnolia Drive, Belleville, IL 62221, (314) 362-2355, BS 83 Southern IL Univ-Edwardsvill; MS 85 Fontbonne Coll; 88–Sp-Lang Path, Washington Univ Med Ctr, **SLP**

Puich, Virginia L Speech And Hearing Center, University Of The Pacific, Stockton, CA 95204, (209) 946-2381, BA 52 San Diego St Univ; MS 57 Univ of OR; 69–Assoc Prof, University of the Pacific, **SLP**

Pulcifer, Maj Donald E 9354 Lamerton, San Antonio, TX 78250, (512) 670-5422, Aud, Air Force, **SLP A**

Pulda, Marianne 1824 Miller Street #D, West Bend, WI 53095, (414) 626-2740, BS 73 Central MI Univ; MA 78 Central MI Univ; SLP, Kewaskum Pub Sch, **SLP**

Puleo, Shirley Bragg 6 Noonan Drive, Batavia, NY 14020, (716) 344-2205, BS 77 SUNY - Coll at Geneseo; MA 82 SUNY - Coll at Geneseo; Sp-Lang Path, Elba Central Sch, **SLP**

Pulford, Laureen Rizzo 1505 Arborview, Ann Arbor, MI 48103, (313) 286-8400, BA 81 Boston Coll; MS 83 ID St Univ; SLP, Dept/Mental Health-State/Mich, **SLP**

Pulice, Sally A 825 Russell Street, Annville, PA 17003, (717) 867-4225, BS 72 WV Univ; MS 75 WV Univ; Sp/Lang Path, Lancaster-Lebanon Inter Unit 13, **SLP**

Pulikowski, Mrs Gail Ponte 542 North Kramer, Lombard, IL 60148, (312) 932-7321, BA 77 Elmhurst Coll; MS 79 Univ of WI - Madison; **SLP**

Pullen, Catherine N 312 Fruitwood Lane, Knoxville, TN 37922, (615) 482-7698, BS 79 Auburn Univ - Auburn; MA 81 Univ of TN - Knoxville; 87–Sp-Lang Path, Ctr for Outpatient Rehab Ltd, **SLP**

Pullen, Mrs Cynthia P 408 Florida Grove Road, Keasbey, NJ 08832, (201) 442-5413, BA 83 NC St Univ at Raleigh; MS 88 Rutger's St Univ - Douglas Coll; 88–Sp-Lang Path, United Hosp Med Ctr

Pulley, Dawn A 1402 Kessler Boulevard East Drive, Indianapolis, IN 46220, (317) 842-8838, BS 83 Purdue Univ - West Lafayette; MS 85 Purdue Univ - West Lafayette; 85–Aud, The Ear Institute of Indiana, **A**

Pulliam, Bonnie L 32 Kingsbury Court, Chico, CA 95926, (916) 345-8585, MA 83 CA St Univ - Chico; 83–Sp-Lang Path, Butte Co Super of Sch, **SLP**

Pulliam, Diana E 15 Pine View Road, West Nyack, NY 10994, **SLP**

Pulliam, Louis L 894 Maple Street, Pacific Grove, CA 93950, (408) 375-7427, BA 49 Univ of Denver; MA 51 Univ of Denver; **SLP LM**

Pullin, Cheryl Ann 3902 Furneaux Lane, Carrollton, TX 75007, (214) 492-5110, BS 82 Midwestern St Univ; MS 84 Univ of North TX; 85–Sp-Lang Path, ENT Med Ctr of TX, **SLP**

Pullins, Mrs Mary Ann M 810 Parkway, Bluefield, WV 24701, (304) 325-6513, BA 75 Marshall Univ; MS 76 WV Univ; **SLP**

Pullins, Mrs Vickie H Box 40, Craigsville, WV 26205, (304) 742-3974, OB 74 Marshall Univ; MA 75 Marshall Univ; Coord/Sp-Lang Services, Nicholas County Board of Educ, **SLP**

Pullman, Pamela K 2601 Colvin Boulevard, Tonawanda, NY 14150, (716) 692-3018, MS 87 SUNY - Coll at Buffalo; **SLP**

Puls-Grzybowski, Mrs Beth D 15541 Mosscove, Dallas, TX 75248, (214) 233-1559, BA 79 MI St Univ; MA 80 MI St Univ; Sp-Lang Path, Plano ISD, **SLP**

Pulver, Maija G 840 North Haddow Avenue, Arlington Heights, IL 60004, (303) 493-5449, BS 85 Univ of IA; MS 87 CO St Univ; **SLP**

Pulvino, Patricia Jeanne 9233 Acuff Lane, Lenexa, KS 66215, (913) 681-2866, BS 83 Univ of WI - Stevens Point; MS 85 Univ of WI - Stevens Point; SLP, Blue Valley School Dstr, **SLP**

Puma, Michelle A 1707 Meadowbrook Dr #9, Syracuse, NY 13224, (315) 445-8757, BS 86 SUNY - Coll at Buffalo; MS 87 SUNY - Coll at Buffalo; 88–Sp-Lang Path, Syracuse City Sch Dist, **SLP**

Pumphrey, Mrs Debra Lehman 1128 West Clarion Drive, Torrance, CA 90502, (213) 602-6916, **SLP**

Pumphrey, Mrs Leslie G 115 Wyndmoor Road, Springfield, PA 19064, (215) 328-9650, BA 66 Rutger's St Univ - Douglas Coll; ME 67 PA St Univ - Univ Park; MA 83 Univ of PA; Sp-Lang Path, Private Practice, **SLP**

Puncar, Josephine Anselmo 116 Texas Avenue, Bronxville, NY 10708, (718) 423-7300, BA 81 Iona Coll; MA 83 CUNY - Queens Coll; Sp-Lang Path, Stepping Stone Day School, **SLP**

Punch, Dr Jerry L Nicolet Instrument Corp, Audiodiagnostics Div, PO Box 7010, Madison, WI 53707, (608) 271-3333, BA 65 Wake Forest Univ; MS 67 Vanderbilt Univ; PH 72 (Aud) Northwestern Univ; Aud, Nicolet Instrument Corp, **A**

Punt, Mrs Ruth B 424 22nd Street, Santa Monica, CA 90402, (213) 458-2019, BA 71 Univ of CA - Santa Barbara; MA 74 CA St Univ - Los Angeles; SLP, Santa Monica USD, **SLP**

Puntil, Jo A P O Box 3169, Laguna Hills, CA 92654, (213) 595-2411, BS 81 IL St Univ - Normal; MS 82 IL St Univ - Normal; Sp-Lang Path, Newport Lang-Mem Med Cen, **SLP**

Punzi, Lucille M 26-12 166th Street, Flushing, NY 11358, (718) 461-9226, MA 85 CUNY - Queens Coll; Sp-Lang Path, Queens College, **SLP**

Puopolo, Edward C 401 Ferry Street, Everett, MA 02149, (617) 389-7950, BS 75 Salem St Coll; ME 77 Northeastern Univ; SLP, Everett Public Sch, **SLP**

Pupulidy, Susan Ann 226 Fort Pleasant Avenue, Springfield, MA 01108, (413) 589-9161, BS 83 Boston Univ; MS 84 Boston Univ; 87–Sp-Lang Path, Children's Lang Inst, **SLP**

Purcell, Debra A St Lukes Regional Medical Cntr, 190 East Bannock, Boise, ID 83706-3650, (208) 344-1582, BA 76 Univ of Northern CO; MA 79 Univ of Northern CO; Sp/Lang Path, St Luke's Reg Med Cen, **SLP**

Purcell, Jackie Lianne 1301 North Water Street, Ellensburg, WA 98926, (509) 925-7884, BA 78 Central WA Univ; MS 85 Eastern WA Univ; **SLP**

Purcell, Mrs Laura Kelley 29 Pine Drive, New Milford, CT 06776, (203) 354-0145, BA 74 SUNY - Coll at Plattsburgh; MS 81 Univ of AR - Fayetteville; 88–Sp-Lang Path, **SLP**

Purcell, Orland 5203 Lavaca, Midland, TX 79707, BS 79 Eastern NM Univ; MS 81 Univ of OK Medical Center; Aud, Audio Acoustics, **A**

Purcell, Rita Marie 115 Casmar Street, Vienna, VA 22180, (703) 327-6343, BS 78 James Madison Univ; MS 80 PA St Univ - Univ Park; 87–Sp-Lang Path, Loudoun County Schs, **SLP**

Purcell, Roberta L 2344 Western Meadows, Flushing, MI 48433, (313) 664-1838, BA 73 Central MI Univ; MA 74 Central MI Univ; Supervisor of Special Educ, Lapeer Co Inter Sch Dist, **SLP**

Purcell, Sherry L 6155 West 78th Street, Los Angeles, CA 90045, (203) 974-1184, BS 71 SUNY - Center at Albany; MA 80 Univ of CT; **SLP ACE**

Purcell, Mrs Sheryll R 5203 Lavaca, Midland, TX 79707-3127, (915) 697-8836, BS 78 Eastern NM Univ; MS 79 Eastern NM Univ; **SLP**

Purdy, Barbara Elaine 8 Homestead Lane, Lincoln Park, NJ 07035, (201) 694-8600, BA 76 Montclair St Coll; MA 82 Montclair St Coll; 76–Sp-Lang Path, Wayne Bd of Educ, **SLP**

Purdy, Carol A 6526 Vanderbilt, Dallas, TX 75214, (214) 826-7030, BA 77 Univ of MO - Columbia; MA 78 Univ of MO - Columbia; Dir-SLP, Baylor I for Rehab, **SLP**

Purdy, Daryl A 5210 Buena Vista Drive, Belgrade, MT 59714, (406) 586-8211, BS 73 CO St Univ; MS 75 Univ of UT; Sp/Lang Path, Boreman Pub Sch Sys, **SLP**

Purdy, Mrs Dianne Ella 7863 Glenda Court, Apple Valley, MN 55124, (612) 431-3350, BS 85 Univ of MN - Minneap-St Paul; OM 87 Univ of WI - River Falls

Purdy, Julie Kay 1412 East Kensington Avenue, Salt Lake City, UT 84105, (801) 364-8692, BS 83 Brigham Young Univ; MA 85 Brigham Young Univ; 87–Aud, Audiology Assoc of SLC Inc, **A**

Purdy, Lori Ebling 4225 Neely Road, Elida, OH 45807, (419) 226-9019, BA 78 Univ of KY; MS 80 Purdue Univ - West Lafayette; Aud, St Ritas Medical Cente, **A**

Purdy, Mrs Mary Harlin 88 Robbins Drive, Wethersfield, CT 06109, (203) 269-3344, BS 81 Northwestern Univ; MS 84 Southern CT St Univ; **SLP ACE**

Purdy, Richard H 804 Magnolia Drive, Radcliff, KY 40160, (502) 351-0777, BA 65 Univ of Northern CO; MS 67 CO St Univ; Audiologist, US Army, **A**

Purdy, Rosemary Mallor 1082 Carter Drive, Grand Island, NY 14072-2657, (716) 773-5548, BS 60 Syracuse Univ; MS 67 SUNY - Coll at Buffalo; 88–Sp-Lang Path, Buffalo PS, **SLP A**

Purinton, Laural Wolfe 5320 Manitowac Drive, Palos Verdes Peninsula, CA 90274, (213) 373-6425, MA 85 CA St Univ - Long Beach; 87–Aud, Harbor UCLA Med Ctr, **A**

Purkett, Joseph C 219 South Bozeman, Bozeman, MT 59715, MA 75 Southeast MO St Univ; Sp-Lang Path, Livingston School District, **SLP**

Purn, Janet M 3379 Route 46 #18-H, Parsippany, NJ 07054, **A**

Pursglove, Janet T 5201 Longrifle Road, Westerville, OH 43081, (614) 891-3001, BS 72 Miami Univ - Oxford; MS 73 Univ of WI - Milwaukee; 86–Sp-Lang Path, Private Practice, **SLP ACE**

Pursley, Martha Elaine 842 Crosscourt Drive, Augusta, GA 30909, (404) 738-9028, BS 82 Univ of GA; ME 84 Univ of GA; Sp-Lang Path, Richmond Co Bd of Ed, **SLP**

Purswell, Jeralyn K 7915 South Monaco Court, Englewood, CO 80112, (303) 694-1202, BS 69 CO St Univ; MS 72 Univ of WY; Sp-Lang Path, **SLP**

Purver, Jessica A 11 Champlin Avenue, East Islip, NY 11730, (516) 277-5038, BA 75 Hofstra Univ; MA 76 Hofstra Univ; SLP, Center Moriches Sch, **SLP**

Purvis, Dr George O'Neill Department Of Audiology, VA Medical Center, 800 Zorn Avenue, Louisville, KY 40202, (502) 895-3401, BA 68 Univ of Louisville; MS 70 Washington Univ; PH 73 (Aud) Univ of KS; 84–Chief Aud & SLP, VA Med Cen, **A ACE**

Purvis, Mrs Judie W 149 Pine Drive, Poca, WV 25159, (304) 348-7760, BS 64 Univ of TN - Knoxville; MS 66 Vanderbilt Univ; Sp-Lang Path, Kanawha Co Schs, **SLP A**

Pusakulich, Kay M VA Hospital (126), 1030 Jefferson Avenue, Memphis, TN 38104, (901) 523-8990, BS 78 AR St Univ; MA 80 Memphis St Univ; Aud, VA Med Cen, **A**

Pusey, Mrs Kim Karla 32 Corthell Road, North Billerica, MA 01862, (508) 670-2330, BS 83 Univ of MA - Amherst; MS 87 Northeastern Univ; Sp-Lang Path, Judith Wisnia & Assoc

Puskaric, Nada Jane 6600 Alpha Drive #234, Kent, OH 44240, (216) 673-2877, BA 82 Allegheny Coll; MS 85 Clarion Univ of PA; Doctoral, Kent State University, **SLP**

Puskas, Rene R 3022 Pecan Circle, Fairfield, CA 94533, (707) 426-0531, BA 78 Univ of Akron; MA 79 Cleveland St Univ; **SLP**

Putman, Donna Manning 2025 Crest Lane, Birmingham, AL 35226, (205) 822-4013, BS 64 Univ of AL- Tuscaloosa; MA 65 Univ of AL- Tuscaloosa; 85–Sp-Lang Path, Chilton County Board of Educ, **SLP**

Putnam, Christina Rena Saint John's Hospital, 139 North Penn, Salina, KS 67401, (913) 823-4382, MA 87 Wichita St Univ; 87–Sp-Lang Path, St John's Hosp, **SLP**

Putney, Mrs Jill Isler 7300 Andorra Place, Boca Raton, FL 33433, (305) 368-1391, BA 74 Long Island U - CW Post Ctr; MS 80 Adelphi Univ; Sp-Lang Path, Palm Beach Co PS, **SLP**

Putter, Phyllis S 170 East 77th Street #3-F, New York, NY 10021, (212) 734-9588, BS 67 Boston Univ; MA 71 CUNY - Queens Coll; OM 81 NY Univ; SLP, Private Practice, **SLP**

Putty, Mrs Patricia Isabel 57 Nasturtium Court, Lake Jackson, TX 77566, (409) 297-7631, BS 79 CO St Univ; MS 81 CO St Univ; SLP, Brazosport ISD, **SLP**

Putz, Janine Lynette 488 Larkspur Street, Ann Arbor, MI 48105-1125, (313) 467-2700, BA 82 MI St Univ; MA 83 MI St Univ; Aud, Westland Med Ctr, **A**

Putz, Randee I 509 Rutgers, Swarthmore, PA 19081, (215) 561-2546, BA 63 CUNY - Brooklyn Coll; ME 64 Boston Univ; 84–Aud, Drs Wolfson & Marlowe, **A**

Putzier, Patrick Vincent 626 S Santa Fe, Salina, KS 67401, (913) 823-7225, BS 80 Univ of NE - Lincoln; MS 82 Univ of NE - Lincoln; Aud, Central KS ENT Assoc, **A**

Puzel, Vicki Renken 3818 Santiago Street, Sebring, FL 33872, (813) 382-1121, BA 84 Saint Cloud St Univ; MS 86 Saint Cloud St Univ

Pyatak, Patricia Suzanne 4204 Brookfield Dr, Kensington, MD 20895, (301) 424-5200, BA 83 Univ of MD - College Park; MS 84 Syracuse Univ; Sp-Lang Path, Treatment & Learning Centers, **SLP**

Pybus, Edith Connor 8789 Susquehanna Street, Lortonx, VA 22079, (703) 558-2848, BS 83 James Madison Univ; ME 85 Univ of GA; **SLP**

Pyers, Mrs Marilyn J 10611 Northwest 20th St, Pembroke Pines, FL 33026, (305) 431-2386, MS 87 Nova Univ; 88–Sp-Lang Path, Broward Co Sch Bd-North Fork Elem

Pyke, Mrs Arlene May 6330 Trotwood, Portage, MI 49081, (616) 674-8091, BS 81 Western MI Univ; MA 83 Western MI Univ; Sp-Lang Path, Van Buren ISD, **SLP**

Pyle, Karla J 205 W Montgomery Cross Rds, Apartment 205, Savannah, GA 31406, (912) 351-3030, BS 85 Auburn Univ - Auburn; OM 87 Auburn Univ - Auburn; **A**

Pyle, Marilyn W 11507 Hemlock, Overland Park, KS 66210, (913) 451-1974, BA 70 MI St Univ; MS 72 Washington Univ; 88–Sp-Lang Path, USD #233 Olathe PS, **SLP**

Pynckel, Lori Danette 605 13th Place, Kenosha, WI 53140, (414) 656-3390, BA 75 Augustana Coll; MA 75 Univ of IL - Urbana; Sp-Lang Path, St Catherines Hospital, **SLP**

Pyne, Katharine Dyer 42 Surprenant Circle, Brunswick, ME 04011, (207) 865-6051, BA 81 Univ of ME - Farmington; MA 86 Univ of CT; 87–Sp-Lang Path, Freeport PS, **SLP**

Pyontek, Alaina May 273 Allentown Road, Parsippany, NJ 07054, (201) 334-4854, BA 78 William Paterson Coll; MS 80 William Paterson Coll; **SLP**

Pytel, Mrs Linda Lee-Kolasa 22375 Rygate Road, Woodhaven, MI 48183, (313) 295-5763, BS 79 Wayne St Univ; MA 80 Wayne St Univ; Sp-Lang Path, Taylor Pub Sch, **SLP**

Q

Quaglia, Mrs Margo Grace 71 Homestead Lane, Attleboro, MA 02703, (508) 226-1777, BA 81 Bridgewater St Coll; MS 86 Worcester St Coll; 84–Sp-Lang Path, Bi-Co Collaborative (BICO)

Quain-Krukowski, Mrs Elizabeth J Rd 4 Box 485B, Oak Hill Road, Binghamton, NY 13901, (607) 724-1306, BA 82 SUNY - Coll at Cortland; MS 83 Ithaca Coll; Sp-Lang Path, Chenango Valley Cen Sch Dist, **SLP**

Qualiardi, Virginia Pangburn 125 Fern Road, Lake Zurich, IL 60047, BA 78 Univ of OK - Norman; MS 80 Univ of OK - OK City; Sp/Lang Path, **SLP**

Qualley, Michael David 8738 25th Avenue, Brooklyn, NY 11214, (718) 266-1372, BA 84 SUNY - Coll at Cortland; MS 86 Adelphi Univ; **A**

Qualls, Dr Pamela Hammett 5909 Gloucester Avenue, Springfield, VA 22150-3713, (703) 866-1563, BS 73 Univ of GA; ME 74 Univ of GA; ED 83 (Sp Path) Univ of GA; **SLP**

Qualls, Tamara Jo 12202 Jill Sue Court, Austin, TX 78750, (512) 335-1068, BA 81 TX Tech Univ; MS 83 TX Tech Univ; Sp-Lang Path, Round Rock ISD, **SLP**

Quam, Mrs Colleen Ann 1422 Houser Street, Muscatine, IA 52761, (319) 263-8476, OB 83 Univ of MO - Columbia; MA 85 Univ of IA; Sp-Lang Path, Mississippi Bend AEA, **SLP**

Quan, Karyn Lynne Hollanale Apartment #41M, Clifton Park, NY 12065, (518) 383-4576, BA 82 Univ of CA - Berkeley; MS 86 San Francisco St Univ; **SLP**

Quane, Patricia G 1115 South Home Avenue, Oak Park, IL 60304, (312) 848-7830, BS 75 Northern IL Univ - De Kalb; MS 77 Northern IL Univ - De Kalb; Sp-Lang Path, Chicago Bd of Ed, **SLP**

Quante, Cheryl L 1240 Visitation, St Louis, MO 63125, (314) 544-1355, BA 78 Saint Louis Univ; BS 78 Saint Louis Univ; MA 80 Saint Louis Univ; Sp-Lang Path, Spec Sch Dist of St Louis Co, **SLP**

Quantz-Ratliff, Patricia 6934 Fallen Timber Drive, Dublin, OH 43017, (614) 761-2029, BS 75 Univ of Cincinnati; MA 77 Univ of Cincinnati; Sp/Lang Path, Hilliard City Sch, **SLP**

Quaranta, Jolene L 1301 Grant Avenue South, Apartment E-103, Renton, WA 98055, (509) 334-7881, MA 87 WA St Univ

Quarfot, Laney Jean 1006 Harvard Street, Rochester, NY 14610, (716) 271-0680, BS 84 SUNY - Coll at Geneseo; MA 86 SUNY - Coll at Geneseo; **SLP**

Quarterman, Pamela H 3112 Southwestern Boulevard, Dallas, TX 75225, (214) 361-5695, BA 75 Hollins Coll; MS 78 Emory Univ; 88–Sp-Lang Path, Oak Hill Academy, **SLP**

Quarto, Nick J 1380 Anna Avenue, Muskegon, MI 49445, (616) 744-2233, BS 53 Western MI Univ; MA 57 Western MI Univ; Retired, **SLP**

Quattlebaum, Patricia D 504 Chatham Avenue, Columbia, SC 29205, (803) 359-7387, BA 76 Univ of SC - Conway; OM 78 Univ of SC - Columbia; Sp-Lang Path, Easter Seal Rehab Ctr/Comm Svcs, **SLP**

Quattrini, Debra Jacobson RD 1 Box 187W, Ava, NY 13303, (315) 336-6751, BA 84 SUNY - Center at Buffalo; MA 86 SUNY - Center at Buffalo; 88–Aud, SUNY-Hlth Science Ctr, **A**

Qudsi, Laila 2134 North 89th Street, Seattle, WA 98103, (206) 527-9767, MS 88 Univ of WA

Quebedeaux, Darla Rochelle 5201 Summerhill # 1410, Texarkana, TX 75501, (214) 838-0576, BS 85 Lamar Univ; MS 87 Lamar Univ; 88–Sp-Lang Path, Taxarkana ISD, **SLP**

Queen, Elizabeth Ann 1008 Ponderosa Lane, Alexander City, AL 35010, (205) 234-5074, BS 59 Univ of Montevallo; MA 67 Univ of AL- Tuscaloosa; Coord/Prog Except Stud, Alexander City Bd of Ed, **SLP**

Queen, Laurie Ann 1013 Turtle Creek Drive, Asheville, NC 28803, (704) 274-5638, BS 83 Western Carolina Univ; MA 84 Western Carolina Univ; 85–Sp-Lang Path, Henderson County Schools, **SLP**

Queen, Marlene S 11316 East 62nd Street, Raytown, MO 64133-4408, (816) 353-0113, BS 77 Central MO St Univ; MS 78 Central MO St Univ; Aud, Old Westport Med Assn, **A**

Queen, Sharon L 132 Moss Court, Pittsburgh, PA 15237, (402) 592-1337, BS 77 Bowling Green St Univ; MA 78 Kent St Univ; SLP, Omaha Pub Sch, **SLP**

Queen, Sheila M 107 Lewis O Gray Drive, Saugus, MA 01906, (617) 581-9200, BS 78 Univ of MA - Amherst; MS 80 Univ of WI - Madison; 84–Aud, Atlanticare Med Cen, **A**

Queene, Lisa Annette P O Box 60081, Washington, DC 20039-0081, (202) 576-6550, BA 80 Hampton Univ; MA 83 Hampton Univ; **SLP**

Quenelle, C P 24 Point View Drive, East Greenbush, NY 12061, (518) 462-3311, BA 75 SUNY - Coll at Potsdam; MA 81 SUNY - Coll at Plattsburgh; Aud, VA Med Cen Albany, **A**

Quercia, Mrs Cindy Harvey 1502 Liberty Avenue, Ogden, UT 84404, (801) 394-4034, BA 79 CA St Univ - Chico; MA 82 CA St Univ - Chico; SLP, Weber School District, **SLP**

Querry, Mrs Patricia H 36 Oakglade Drive, Hummelstown, PA 17036, (717) 564-4841, BS 58 PA St Univ - Univ Park; MS 68 Univ of Pittsburgh - Pittsburgh; 88–Asst Dir of Spec Svcs, Capital Area Inter UT #15, **SLP F ACE**

Quesal, Mrs Donna Livingston 1-A Sandra Avenue, Plattsburgh, NY 12901, (518) 563-9634, BA 69 Univ of Northern IA; MA 82 Univ of IA; 84–Sp-Lang Path, JCEO Clinton Co Head Start, **SLP**

Quesal, Dr Robert W Dept Of Hearing & Speech Science, State University Of New York At Plattsburgh, Plattsburgh, NY 12901, (518) 564-2170, BA 76 IN Univ - Bloomington; MA 77 IN Univ - Bloomington; PH 84 (Sp Path) Univ of IA; 86–Asst Prof, State Univ of NY at Plattsburgh, **SLP**

Quesnel, Leah Kayrin 1600 LaSalle Drive #B107, Sherman, TX 75090, (214) 463-1130, MS 88 Univ of Southwestern LA; 88–Aud, Dr W F Looney

Quick, Deborah A 2207 Wade Hampton Blvd, Apartment B-310, Greenville, SC 29615, (803) 242-6450, BS 84 Univ of IL - Urbana; MS 85 Miami Univ - Oxford; 86–Sp-Lang Path, The Sch Dist of Greenville Co, **SLP**

Quick, Gloria G 1326 Elmira Avenue, Durham, NC 27707, (919) 688-7497, BA 69 Columbia Coll; MS 71 Vanderbilt Univ; SLP, Chapel Hill-Carraboro Schls, **SLP**

Quick, Margaret M 2310 Kelly Road, Bellingham, WA 98226, (206) 424-9573, BA 76 Western WA Univ; MA 78 Western WA Univ; Sp-Lang Path, Esd 189, **SLP**

Quick, Victoria Ann 3209 Merida Avenue, Fort Worth, TX 76109, (817) 626-0321, BS 76 TX Christian Univ; MS 80 TX Christian Univ; 80–Sp-Lang Path, Ft Worth ISD, **SLP**

Quicksell, Mrs Joanne Scully 46 Blooming Grove Turnpike, New Windsor, NY 12550, (914) 534-8333, BA 80 William Paterson Coll; MS 85 William Paterson Coll; 87–Sp-Lang Path, Cornwall Central Sch Dist, **SLP**

Quigley, Mrs Anne Sonsmith 1297 Pine Burr Drive, Lugoff, SC 29078, (803) 438-2256, BA 64 Marygove Coll; ME 69 Marygove Coll; Sp-Lang Path, Private Practice, **SLP**

Quigley, Dr Stephen P 4341 N Camino DE Carrillo, Tucson, AZ 85715, (217) 344-5179, BA 53 Univ of Denver; MA 54 Univ of IL - Urbana; PH 57 (NS) Univ of IL - Urbana; Prof/Ed-Sp&Hrng Sci, U of IL-Urbana-Champaign, **F**

Quigley, Mrs Suzanne Marion 1029 Springbrook Road, Lake Stevens, WA 98258, (206) 545-7489, BA 83 George Washington Univ; MS 84 Columbia Univ Teachers Coll; 87–Aud, Univ of Washington, **A**

Quiles-Contreras, Sara Yleana 3715 Avenue I, Brooklyn, NY 11210, (718) 645-8515, BA 82 CUNY - Brooklyn Coll; MS 86 CUNY - Brooklyn Coll; **SLP**

Quillian, Sally L 2610 NW Expressway Suite E, Oklahoma City, OK 73117, (405) 947-4327, BS 70 Lindenwood Coll; MS 79 Univ of OK Medical Center; Aud, Private Practice, **A**

Quilligan, Donna H 14220 Adios Pass, Carmel, IN 46032, (317) 844-7881, BA 76 Bellarmine Coll; MS 80 Univ of Louisville; **SLP**

Quin, Paul E 599 Stony Hill Road, Wilbraham, MA 01095, (413) 589-9161, BS 71 Syracuse Univ; MS 73 Portland St Univ; Ed Dir, Chldn's Lang I, **SLP ACE**

Quine, Doris Meacham 22555 Cranbrooke Drive, Novi, MI 48050, (313) 273-3446, BA 55 Boston Univ; ME 58 Boston Univ; **SLP LM**

Quinette, Karen Sue 120 South Wilcox #201, Rochester, MI 48063, (313) 656-1888, BA 83 Univ of WI - Eau Claire; MS 85 Univ of WI - Madison; **SLP**

Quinlan, Karen Marie 24 Dublin Road, Peabody, MA 01960, (617) 388-4407, BS 79 Univ of WI - Stevens Point; MS 84 Univ of WI - Madison; SLP, Amesbury Public Schools, **SLP**

Quinlan, Mrs Lorraine W 21 Oak Tree Road, Monmouth Junction, NJ 08852, (201) 821-8447, BA 74 Univ of CT; MA 76 Univ of CT; **SLP**

Quinlan, Mrs Maureen Patrice 1702 Roneys Corner Road, Oxford, PA 19363, (215) 384-7711, BA 80 Univ of SC - Columbia; MA 82 Univ of SC - Columbia; Sp-Lang Path, Coatesville Vet Med Ctr, **SLP**

Quinn, Allison Mary 8823 Holly Drive #A-206, Everett, WA 98208, (206) 339-5441, BS 82 CO St Univ; MS 84 CO St Univ; Aud, The Everett Clinic, **A**

Quinn, Barbara K 5231 South Kenneth, Chicago, IL 60632, (312) 496-0500, BS 62 Marquette Univ; 62–Sp/Lang Path, Burbank Sch Dist #111, **SLP**

Quinn, Bernadette Mary 130 Adams Street, Keene, NH 03431, (603) 357-7411, BS 83 Worcester St Coll; MS 85 Syracuse Univ; Aud, Keene Clinic, **A**

Quinn, Janet M P O Box 386, Hancock, NH 03449, (603) 525-4977, BS 59 SUNY - Coll at Geneseo; MA 75 Univ of Houston - Univ Park; Retired, Private Practice, **SLP**

Quinn, Mrs Joanne S 46752 Houghton Drive, Utica, MI 48087, BA 71 Rutger's St Univ - Douglas Coll; MA 72 Montclair St Coll; Sp-Lang Path, Clintondale Comm Sch, **SLP ACE**

Quinn, Katherine C 2009 Lost Lake Place, Martinez, CA 94553, (415) 685-1960, BS 77 Western Carolina Univ; MA 80 Univ of FL; Sp-Lang Path, Mt Diablo USD, **SLP**

Quinn, Dr Kathleen S 1710 Gregory, Ypsilanti, MI 48197, (313) 487-4412, BS 61 Washington Univ; MA 68 Eastern MI Univ; PH 86 (NS) Univ of MI - Ann Arbor; 68–Assoc Prof, Eastern Michigan Univ, **SLP A**

Quinn, Linda B 14 Robin Hood Road, Morris Plains, NJ 07950, (201) 540-8815, BS 73; MS 74 Seton Hall Univ; **SLP**

Quinn, Mrs Margaret F Route 3 Box 54, Hastings, NE 68901, (402) 463-8566, BA 76 Univ of NE - Lincoln; MA 77 Univ of NE - Lincoln; Aud, Foote & Beck Otol Cl, **A**

Quinn, Marion 1226 Knox Road, Wynnewood, PA 19096, (215) 895-5500, BA 72 CUNY - Queens Coll; MA 73 NY Univ; Assistant Director, Elwyn Institutes Natl Rehab Cr, **SLP**

Quinn, Mary K 21322 Lopez Street, Woodland Hills, CA 91364, (818) 888-8862, BA 66 Univ of CA - Santa Barbara; MA 80 CA St Univ - Northridge; Sp-Lang Path, Conejo USD, **SLP**

Quinn, Maureen A 12415 Rock Ridge Road, Herndon, VA 22070, **SLP**

Quinn, Michelle A Boys Town National Institute, 555 North 30th Street, Omaha, NE 68131, BA 78 Univ of Notre Dame; MA 83 Univ of IA; Supvr, Boys Town National Institute, **SLP**

Quinn, Rhonda Rougelot 7796 Beachcomber Drive, Huntington Beach, CA 92648, (714) 969-7479, BS 81 Univ of UT; MA 82 Univ of thc Pacific; **SLP**

Quinn, Rosemary 1527 Spruce Street #20 B, Philadelphia, PA 19102, BS 77 CUNY - Hunter Coll; MA 87 Temple Univ; 88–Sp-Lang Path, Med Ctr, **SLP**

Quinn, Ruth Marie 136 Wildwood, Cincinnati, OH 45216, (606) 331-0880, MA 84 Univ of Cincinnati; Sp-Lang Path, Redwood School Rehabilitation, **SLP**

Quinn, Shirley B 271 Lincoln Avenue, Rockville Centre, NY 11570, (516) 678-1200, BA 42 CUNY - Queens Coll; MA 56 NY Univ; Retired, Oceanside Pub Sch, **SLP**

Quinn, Wendy M 1020-E Rolling Glen Drive, Harrisburg, PA 17109, (717) 540-1377, BA 85 Thiel Coll; MA 87 Edinboro Univ of PA; **SLP**

Quinn-Padron, Maura Marshfield Clinic, 1000 North Oak Avenue, Marshfield, WI 54449, (715) 387-5128, BS 84 Univ of WI - Madison; MS 86 Univ of WI - Madison; 86–Sp-Lang Path, Marshfield Clinic, **SLP**

Quinoa, Joanne T 4 Donovan Drive, Huntington, NY 11743, (516) 883-4000, BA 75 Hofstra Univ; MA 76 Hofstra Univ; Sp-Lang Path, Port Washington Public Schools, **SLP ACE**

Quinones-Nitsch, Mrs Wilma D P O Box 871, North Bay, ON, Canada P1B 8G6, (705) 776-7835, BA 79 Univ of PR - Mayaguez; MS 82 Univ of PR - Rio Piedras; 88–Sp-Lang Path, Nipissing Bd of Educ, **SLP**

Quinones-Perez, Aracelis 129 Yaguez Street, Urb Rio Piedra Heights, Rio Piedras, PR 00926, (809) 751-9916, BA 84 Univ of PR - Rio Piedras; MS 86 Univ of PR - San Juan; **SLP**

Quint, Janice H 3403 34th Avenue Southwest, Seattle, WA 98126, (206) 932-8019, BA 75 Univ of WA; MS 78 Univ of WA; 88–Sp-Lang Path, Northshore Sch Dist #417, **SLP**

Quintana, Mrs Marilyn Miller Good Samaritan Medical Center, Speech-Lang Path Dept #AT1, 1111 East McDowell Road, Phoenix, AZ 85006, (602) 239-4755, BA 58 Univ of Denver; MA 68 Univ of Denver; Sp-Lang Path, Good Samaritan Med Cen, **SLP ACE**

Quintanilla, Jerilyn B 3157 Entrada Drive, Ventura, CA 93003, (805) 648-5391, BA 76 CA St Univ - Northridge; MA 80 CA St Univ - Northridge; Sp-Lang Path, Ventura USD, **SLP**

Quinter, Valerie Elise 3137 Brooksvalley Street, Memphis, TN 38119, (901) 754-0507, BS 83 East Carolina Univ; MS 84 East Carolina Univ; Sp-Lang Path, Communi-Care Inc, **SLP**

Quinton, Janice #1105 290 Main Avenue, Halifax, NS, Canada B3M 3V3, (902) 798-5580, BA 63 Univ of London - England; MS 86 Dalhousie Univ - Nova Scotia; 88–Sys Consult, Hants W Dist Sch Bd, **SLP**

Quirico, Dorothy 7536 South Penrose Court, Littleton, CO 80122, (303) 837-1000, BA 49 Univ of Denver; MA 53 Univ of Denver; MA 67 Univ of Denver; SLP, Denver Public Schools, **SLP**

Quiring, Lillian D 1222N Calhoun, Liberal, KS 67901, (316) 624-3791, BS 72 Univ of KS; MA 74 Univ of KS; ES 79 Wichita St Univ; 85–Sp-Lang Path, USD #480 Liberal, **SLP**

Quirk-McGloin, Mrs Jennifer Marie 28 Gorden Place, Merrick, NY 11566, (516) 543-5100, BA 82 Adelphi Univ; MS 84 Adelphi Univ; Sp-Lang Path, CES, **SLP**

Quirk-Stauch, Kathleen A 4601 West 72nd Street, Prairie Village, KS 66208, (913) 782-8950, BS 76 Univ of KS; MS 78 Fort Hays St Univ; 87–Sp-Lang Path, Olathe PS #233, **SLP**

Quirolo, Mrs Josephine 24 Woods End Lane, Hartsdale, NY 10530, (914) 337-5600, MA 72 CUNY - Hunter Coll; Sp/Lang Path, Bronxville Pub Schs, **SLP**

Quist, Dr Raymond W Indiana State University, Dept Of Comm Disorders, School Of Education, Terre Haute, IN 47809, (812) 237-2804, BA 57 Hamline Univ; MA 67 Univ of MN - Minneap-St Paul; PH 71 (NS) Univ of MN - Minneap-St Paul; Dept Chair, Indiana State U, **SLP**

Qvammen, Brian Dale 3906 Simonview Court, Grand Forks, ND 58201, (701) 780-2447, BS 78 Univ of ND; MS 79 Minot St Univ; Aud, Med Ctr Rehab Hosp, **A**

R

Raab, Eileen W 12205 Northwood Drive, Upper Marlboro, MD 20772, BA 62 Univ of MT; MS 74 Univ of the DC; Sp-Lang Path, Prince Georges County Bd of Ed, **SLP**

Raab, Katherine Anne 6335 Windharp Way, Columbia, MD 21045, (301) 593-3797, BS 85 Towson St Univ; MS 87 Towson St Univ

Raabe, Mrs Ann Hammond 601 Access Road, New Lisbon, WI 53950, BS 83 Univ of WI - Madison; MS 85 Univ of WI - Madison; **A**

Raabe, Christine Nitschke 1080 Hawthorne Ridge Drive, Waukesha, WI 53186, (414) 797-9476, BS 75 Univ of WI - Stevens Point; MS 76 Univ of WI - Stevens Point; **SLP**

Raack, Catherine Brown 26 W 155 Mayflower Place, Wheaton, IL 60187, BA 76 Valparaiso Univ; BS 78 Eastern IL Univ; MA 80 OH Univ - Athens; Exec Dir, Community Therapy Services, **SLP**

Raad, Mrs Mary Gorman 40 Carstairs Road, Valley Stream, NY 11581, (212) 741-7673, MS 82 Adelphi Univ; 87–Aud, The NY League for the Hard of Hrng, **A**

Raade, Dr Adele Suzanne Dept Of Comm Disorders, Univ Of Western Ontario, Elborn College, London, ON, Canada N6G 1H1, (519) 661-2001, BS 78 Western MI Univ; MA 82 Northwestern Univ; PH (Sp-Lang Path) Univ of FL; 87–Lecturer, Univ of W Ontario Dept Com Dis, **SLP**

Raarup, Beth Bellgowan 408 Southeast 12th Avenue, Forest Lake, MN 55025, (612) 464-1539, OB 85 Univ of MN - Duluth; MA 86 Univ of MN - Duluth; 86–Sp-Lang Path, North Branch PS, **SLP**

Rabassa-Thompson, Mrs Ana Maria 300 Ridgewood Drive, Key Biscayne, FL 33149, (305) 549-6397, BS 83 Univ of FL; MS 85 Vanderbilt Univ; Sp-Lang Path, Jackson Mem Hosp, **SLP**

Rabbitt, Barbara Jill 5201 Sutton Place Ext, Wexford, PA 15090, (412) 366-3471, BS 83 Clarion Univ of PA; MS 84 Clarion Univ of PA; Aud, Metro ENT Assoc, **SLP A**

Rabe, Maureen R 238 5th Avenue, Troy, NY 12180-1019, (518) 233-0290, BA 82 SUNY - Coll at Plattsburgh; MA 83 SUNY - Coll at Plattsburgh; Sp-Lang Path, Private Practice, **SLP**

Rabeau, Nancy Christine 8239 East Rawhide Trail, Tucson, AZ 85715, (602) 325-1571, BS 84 Northern AZ Univ; MS 85 Northern AZ Univ; **SLP**

Raber, Mrs Maya Gerkina 3619 Bedford Avenue #6-B, Brooklyn, NY 11210, (718) 258-8327, OB 57 The Kiev's State Pedagogical Inst; ME 81 CUNY - Brooklyn Coll; OD 72 (Logopedics Sp-Lang Path) The Academy of Pedagogical Science Research Inst of Defectology; 86–Sp-Lang Path, New York City Bd of Educ, **SLP**

Rabidoux, Paula C 2412 Deming, Columbus, OH 43202, **SLP**

Rabidoux, Mrs Susan W 2615 Harper Road, Mason, MI 48854, (517) 676-1051, BA 69 MI St Univ; MA 62 MI St Univ; 74–Sp-Lang Path, Ing Intermediate Schools, **SLP**

Rabin, Mrs Elizabeth Ahrenbeck 8510 SW 102nd Avenue, Miami, FL 33173, (305) 274-4902, BA 84 Univ of FL; MS 87 Univ of AZ; **A**

Rabin, Mrs Sandra C 2103 Fairway Lane, Harrisburg, PA 17112, (717) 540-5477, BA 77 Cleveland St Univ; MA 78 Cleveland St Univ; 88–Aud, InSpeech Inc, **A**

Rabin, Susan L 4256 Mary Ridge Drive, Randallstown, MD 21133, (301) 521-4635, BA 75 Univ of MD - College Park; MS 77 Loyola Coll; Sp-Lang Path, Balto Co Bd of Ed, **SLP**

Rabine, Mrs Nina P 139 Driftwood Lane, Trumbull, CT 06611, (203) 375-0732, BA 74 CUNY - Lehman Coll; MA 76 CUNY - Hunter Coll; **SLP**

Rabinovitz, Mrs Jane Ena 66 Canavan Circle #F, Needham, MA 02192-1127, (617) 449-1672, BS 70 Univ of Cincinnati; ME 71 Boston Univ; Neurman Assoc, **SLP**

Rabinowitz, Allan Jay 26 Sylvia Lane, Plainview, NY 11803, (718) 361-8220, BA 71 Long Island U - Brooklyn Ctr; MA 78 NY Univ; Sp-Lang Path, Sp Serv UT-Bd of Ed NYC, **SLP**

Rabinowitz, Christine 9 Noreen Drive, Bedford, MA 01730, (617) 484-8700, BA 72 Northern IL Univ - De Kalb; MA 74 Northern IL Univ - De Kalb; 87–Aud, Audiology Svcs Inc, **A**

Rabinowitz, Marcia G 400 Central Park West, New York, NY 10025, (212) 866-0604, BA 32 CUNY - Hunter Coll; MA 37 CUNY - Hunter Coll; MA 68 CUNY - Hunter Coll; **A LM**

Rabin-Posner, Mrs Debra Sue 15427 Camarillo Street, Sherman Oaks, CA 91403, (818) 907-0301, OM 76 Univ of CA - Los Angeles; Sp-Lang Path, Private Practice, **SLP**

Rabner, Mrs Hilary Feig 13 Stevens Terrace, West Orange, NJ 07052, (201) 267-2642, BA 81 Rutger's St Univ - Douglas Coll; MS 83 Rutgers St Univ -N Brunswick; Sp-Lang Path, Early Childhood Lrng Cen, **SLP**

Rabon, Mrs Donna Switzer 7128 Sythe Court, Charlotte, NC 28226, (704) 541-6511, MS 82 Univ of SC - Columbia; Sp-Lang Path, Charlotte Mecklenburg SCHOOLS8, **SLP**

Rabon, John Davis Route 1 Box 244-D, Ash Flat, AR 72513, (501) 994-2161, BA 73 FL Atlantic Univ; OM 83 AR St Univ; **SLP**

Rachek, Patricia A Psc 1 Box 23347, Apo, San Francisco, CA 96230, BA 72 Univ of MD - College Park; MS 77 Loyola Coll; Sp-Lang Path, Dept of Def Dependents Sch, **SLP**

Rachek, Mrs Sally Anne 4510 Lilac Road, South Euclid, OH 44121, (216) 476-7104, **A**

Rachford, Sharon L 2426 Ransdell Avenue, Louisville, KY 40204, (502) 454-8300, BA 74 Bellarmine Coll; MA 78 Ball St Univ; Sp-Lang Path, Jefferson Co Pub Sch, **SLP**

Rachlin, Holly Fiebert 301 North Wolf Road, Hillside, IL 60162-1409, (312) 547-8810, **SLP**

Rachlin, Paul 5229 Outerview Drive, Springfield, OH 45502, (513) 324-5874, BA 72 SUNY - Coll at Plattsburgh; MA 73 OH Univ - Athens; Pres, Indust Testing Serv, **A**

Rachow, Roger L 6106 South 91st Avenue, Omaha, NE 68127, (712) 328-6474, BA 69 Univ of NE - Omaha; MA 73 Univ of NE - Omaha; SLP, AEA 13, **SLP**

Racinowski, Mrs Darlene H 7505 West Garfield Avenue, Wauwatosa, WI 53213, (414) 224-3137, BA 58 Univ of WI - Milwaukee; Supervisor, Marquette University, **SLP**

Rackliffe, Roberta A 22 Flint Ridge Drive, Mableton, GA 30059, (703) 437-3888, **SLP**

Racoosin, Mrs Lauren Schoenfeld 10120 Ashwood Drive, Kensington, MD 20895, (202) 745-8270, BA 83 Univ of MD - College Park; MA 85 George Washington Univ; Audiologist, VA Medical Center, **A**

Racoosin, Mrs Suzanne D 6109 Plainview Road, Bethesda, MD 20817, (301) 229-1330, BA 54 Univ of MD - College Park; MA 65 George Washington Univ; SLP, Mont Co Pub Sch, **SLP ACE**

Racosky, Janice D 25888 Juniper, Loma Linda, CA 92354, BA 66 Univ of Houston - Clear Lake; MA 70 Univ of Houston - Clear Lake; Sp-Lang Path, San Bernardino City USD, **SLP**

Raczynski, Mrs Sharon M 5416 Albia Road, Bethesda, MD 20016, MA 63 Catholic Univ of America; **SLP**

Radaich, Susan J 3862 Toland Avenue, Los Alamitos, CA 90720, (213) 596-9507, BA 84 CA St Univ - Fullerton; MA 87 CA St Univ - Fullerton; **SLP**

Radbel, Mrs Shelley Jacovsky 32-25 91st Street #309, Jackson Heights, NY 11369, (718) 672-0818, BA 77 SUNY - Center at Buffalo; MS 80 CUNY - Brooklyn Coll; Teacher, New York City Board of Educ, **SLP**

Radcliff, Kendrea D'Lyn 301 North 7th, Petersburg, IN 47567-1215, (812) 354-8175, BS 84 IN St Univ - Terre Haute; MA 85 Ball St Univ; **SLP**

Radcliffe, Wendy E 8110 Sonnet Drive, #101, Austin, TX 78759, (512) 451-2931, BS 82 Univ of KS; **SLP**

Rade, Susan J 3 Tanglewylde Avenue #5D, Bronxville, NY 10708, (914) 761-5055, BA 78 CUNY - Queens Coll; MA 79 Hofstra Univ; Tchr for Ed/Sp & Hrng Hndcpd, BOCES/Sn Wchester, **SLP**

Rademacher, Mrs Ann D 1429 North Shore Drive, Gaylord, MI 49735, (517) 732-4616, BA 80 MI St Univ; MA 81 MI St Univ; 84–Sp-Lang Path, COPISD, **SLP**

Rademaker, Mrs Barbara K 801 East Lake Shore Drive, Wausau, WI 54401, (715) 693-2810, OB 68 Univ of WI - Whitewater; MA 69 OH Univ - Athens; 86–Sp-Lang Path, Mosinee PS, **SLP**

Rademaker, Mrs Nancy M 14-A Havens Street, San Francisco, CA 94133, (415) 499-5807, BA 72 CA St Univ - Fresno; MA 75 San Francisco St Univ; 75–Sp-Lang Path, Marin Co Off of Ed, **SLP**

Rader, Mrs Krista L 2405 House Avenue, Cheyenne, WY 82001, (307) 638-9430, BS 77 Univ of WY; MS 83 Univ of WY; Sp-Lang Path, Laramie Co Sch Dist #1, **SLP**

Rader, Suzanne 30 Shelton Road, Trumbull, CT 06611, **SLP**

Rader, Thomas W 514 West Main Street, Silverton, OR 97381, (503) 371-6486, BS 65 OR St Univ; MS 67 Western OR St Coll; Sp-Lang Path, Salem Sp Lang Cen, **SLP**

Radich, Diane E 747 Highland Drive, Apartment # 65, Medford, OR 97504, (503) 776-8552, BA 81 Humboldt St Univ; MA 84 Humboldt St Univ; Sp-Lang Path, Jackson Education Service Dist, **SLP**

Radin, Mrs Hyla Beth 78 Concord Drive, Rocky Hill, CT 06067, (203) 223-2761, BA 84 Tulane Univ; MS 86 Univ of South FL; 86–Sp-Lang Path, New Britain Memorial Hosp, **SLP**

Radin, Nona S P O Box 5816, 12366 S E 41st Lane, Bellevue, WA 98006, (206) 641-7633, BS 75 Syracuse Univ; MS 76 Univ of WA; Northwestern Div Mgr, Rexton Inc, **A**

Radke, Jean M 115 South 1100 East #713, Salt Lake City, UT 84102, (801) 521-1680, BS 73 Kent St Univ; MA 76 Kent St Univ; Aud, Primary Chldns Med Cen, **A**

Radke, Mary C Popp 8416 Derby Court, Springfield, VA 22151, (808) 624-4303, BS 69 ND St Univ; OM 71 Univ of WA; **SLP**

Radke, Mrs Michelle Lee W355N5865 Bridle Lane, Oconomowoc, WI 53066, (414) 567-9646, BS 83 Marquette Univ; MS 84 Marquette Univ; Cl Supvr, Omni Therapy, **SLP**

Radley, Mrs Janine G 1783 East Cornwall Court, Sandy, UT 84092, (801) 487-0342, BS 78 Univ of UT; MS 76 Univ of UT; Sp-Lang Path, Granite School District, **SLP**

Radner, Susan Rebecca 100 Highpoint Drive, Apartment 410, Hartsdale, NY 10530, (914) 948-5812, BA 84 SUNY - Center at Buffalo; MA 87 CUNY - Queens Coll; **SLP**

Radtke, Judith W 15605 West Mark Drive, Brookfield, WI 53005, (414) 786-2849, BS 76 Marquette Univ; MS 77 Marquette Univ; **SLP**

Radus, Dr Libby 130 Woods Road, Newport News, VA 23601, (804) 596-7998, BA 50 Univ of Denver; MA 51 Univ of Denver; PH 65 (NS) Univ of FL; Coord, Peninsula Crani Anomal Cl, **SLP F LM**

Radziewicz, Dr Christine 169 Kilburn Road, Garden City, NY 11530, (516) 228-7993, BA 67 Catholic Univ of America; MA 72 Hofstra Univ; OD 85 (NS) Adelphi Univ; 85–Clin Dir, Adelphi University, **SLP**

Radzimanowski, Kathryn Anne 4223 Windrift #3-B, Aurora, IL 60504-5009, (312) 820-2365, BS 84 Western IL Univ; MA 85 Western IL Univ; **SLP**

Raecker, Shirley H 120 Norfolk Road, Waterloo, IA 50701, (319) 235-3860, MA 76 Univ of Northern IA; SLP, Allen Memorial Hosp, **SLP**

Raeder, Celia R 615 Eastern Parkway, Brooklyn, NY 11216, **SLP**

Rafalak, Susan Laura 144 Sixth Street, Scotia, NY 12302, (518) 783-1644, BS 74 SUNY - Coll at Fredonia; MA 82 SUNY - Coll at Geneseo; SLP, Wildwood School, **SLP**

Rafenski, Janet G PO Box 372, Bethpage, NY 11714, (516) 931-0401, BA 73 CUNY - Queens Coll; MS 80 Emerson Coll; Sp-Lang Path, **SLP**

Raff, Mrs Joan Warrick 408 Logan Drive, Rensselaer, IN 47978, (219) 866-8212, BS 74 Purdue Univ - West Lafayette; MS 77 Purdue Univ - West Lafayette; 80–Sp-Lang Path, Rensselaer Cen Sch Corp, **SLP**

Raff, Michael J 1501 Larkspur, Mc Allen, TX 78501, (512) 630-4327, BA 77 Columbia Univ Teachers Coll; MS 81 Adelphi Univ; Aud, Private Practice, **A**

Raff, Nina Zahn 1501 Larkspur, Mc Allen, TX 78501, (512) 630-1067, BA 79 SUNY - Center at Buffalo; MA 80 Hofstra Univ; Sp-Lang Path, Private Practice, **SLP**

Rafferty, Richard A 174 Colonial Road, Summit, NJ 07901, (201) 747-5300, BA 70 Curry Coll; MA 81 Montclair St Coll; Aud, Otolaryngology Associates, **A**

Raffin Phd, Dr Michael J M Mass Eye & Ear Infirmary, 243 Charles Street, Audiology Clinic Service, Boston, MA 02114, (617) 573-3266, PH 76 (NS) Univ of IA; 87–Dir-Aud Cl, Mass Eye and Ear Infirmary, **A ACE**

Raffo, Christine M Madison Hearing Center Inc, 747 Madison Avenue, Albany, NY 12208, (518) 465-6585, BS 77 Bloomsburg Univ of PA; MS 79 Bloomsburg Univ of PA; Dir, Madi Hear Cen Inc, **A**

Raffoni, Mrs Theresa Beller 67 Blackbird Lane, Levittown, NY 11756, (516) 277-4994, BA 82 Hofstra Univ; MA 84 Hofstra Univ; **SLP**

Rafkin, David 626 Arenas Street, La Jolla, CA 92037, (619) 454-0539, BA 55 Syracuse Univ; MA 73 CA St Univ - Northridge; Owner, Private Practice, **SLP**

Rafkind, Mrs Shirley M 14144 Dickens Street #207, Sherman Oaks, CA 91403, (818) 760-3460, BS; **SLP LM**

Raforth, Donna F 6351 Glenmoor Road, Boulder, CO 80303, (303) 447-1010, BS 71 Univ of WY; MA 76 Univ of CO - Boulder; SLP, Boulder Valley Pub Sch, **SLP**

Rafter, Kristine Olson 313 Barry Lane, Wallingford, PA 19086, (215) 662-2784, BA 77 Univ of Rochester; MA 79 Northwestern Univ; Aud, Hosp of the U of Pa, **A**

Rafuse, Mrs Donna W 124 Lafayette Court, Trappe, PA 19426, (215) 539-8550, BS 81 Bloomsburg Univ of PA; MS 82 Bloomsburg Univ of PA; Sp-Lang Path, Montgomy Cnty Intermed Unit 23, **SLP**

Ragan, Mrs Anita Louise 5620 Oxford Street, New Orleans, LA 70114, (704) 392-6380, BS 80 WV Univ; MA 83 WV Univ; Sp-Lang Path, Jefferson Parish Schools, **SLP**

Ragan, Mrs Judith Logan 5524 Central, Kansas City, MO 64113, (312) 352-2693, BA 66 Fontbonne Coll; MS 70 Washington Univ; **SLP ACE**

Ragen, Lauren M 1 Geyerwood Lane, Frontenac, MO 63131, (314) 965-1813, BS 81 Central MO St Univ; MS 83 Central MO St Univ; 88–Aud, Cardinal Glennon Child Hosp, **A**

Raggio, Marcia Eve 5005 Palmetto Avenue #57, Pacifica, CA 94044, (415) 994-7470, **A**

Raghavendra, Parimala Dept Of Aus Heavilon Hall, Purdue University, West Lafayette, IN 47907, (317) 494-6423, BS 75 All India Inst of Sp & Hrng; MS 77 All India Inst of Sp & Hrng

Ragland, Donald Elliott 520 Indian Hill Boulevard, Apartment 204, Claremont, CA 91711, (714) 626-7830, BA 82 San Francisco St Univ; MS 85 Univ of WI - Milwaukee; Sp-Lang Path, Lanterman Dev Ctr, **SLP**

Ragland, Pamela D 4516 Forestgate Circle, Arlington, TX 76017, (817) 467-1300, BS 83 TX Christian Univ; MS 85 Univ of TX - Dallas; **SLP**

Ragland, Mrs Rebecca Raye 367 North Winsome, Lake Mary, FL 32746, (407) 321-2253, MS 87 Southern IL Univ-Edwardsvill; 88–Sp-Lang Path, Deltona Lakes Elem Sch

Ragonese, Maria Theresa 13520 West Dakota Street, New Berlin, WI 53151, (517) 774-5929, 87 Central MI Univ

Ragosin, Mrs Edria M 2513 Rowland Avenue N E, Canton, OH 44714, (216) 454-3962, BS 68 Kent St Univ; MA 71 Kent St Univ; Sp-Lang Path, Private Practice, **SLP**

Ragovin, Lori E 30 Arvin Road, Old Bridge, NJ 08857, BA SUNY - Coll at Cortland; MA 79 NY Univ; Sp-Lang Path, Private Practice, **SLP**

Ragsdale, Elizabeth 1020 Fincastle Road, Lexington, KY 40502, (606) 277-1949, BA 74 Univ of KY; MA 75 Univ of TN - Knoxville; **SLP**

Rahe, Frederick A 201 N W 82nd Avenue, Suite 103, Plantation, FL 33324, (305) 472-1212, OB 75 Univ of FL; MA 76 Univ of FL; Aud, Private Practice, **A ACE**

Rahill, Mrs Valerie Zehnder 11501 Stone Avenue North, Apartment C-217, Seattle, WA 98133, (206) 367-4562, BA 82 WA St Univ; MA 84 WA St Univ; Sp-Lang Path, Shoreline School Dist, **SLP**

Rahilly-Coviello, Sandra J 8 Cortland Drive, Greenland, NH 03840, (603) 436-7100, BA 72 Central MI Univ; MA 76 Eastern MI Univ; Sp-Lang Path, Portsmouth Public Schools, **SLP**

Rahman, Mrs Persephone 26 Treeview Drive, Melville, Long Island, NY 11746, BA 54 Adelphi Univ; MA 56 CUNY - Brooklyn Coll; SLP, Half Hollow Hills Sch Dist, **SLP**

Rahman, Sahara 2300 Bouck Avenue, Bronx, NY 10469, (718) 270-7099, BA 78 CUNY - Lehman Coll; MA 80 CUNY - Lehman Coll; 88–Chief of Sp-Lang Path & Aud, Maimonides Med Cen, **SLP**

Rahn, Dawn Renee 4C Clintwood Drive, Rochester, NY 14620, (716) 442-3302, BS 85 Nazareth Coll of Rochester; MA 86 SUNY - Center at Buffalo; 87–Aud, Park Ridge Hearing Center, **A**

Raibley, Ann B Welborn Clinic, 421 Chestnut, Evansville, IN 47713, (812) 426-9202, BS 74; OM 75 IN Univ - Bloomington; Aud, Welborn Cl, **A**

Raica, Anthony N Conroe ENT Associates, 333 North Rivershire Drive, Conroe, TX 77304, (409) 756-5593, BS 73 CO St Univ; MS 74 CO St Univ; Sp-Lang Path, Conroe Ear Nose Throat, **A**

Raichle, Ruth Ann 501 Cherry Hill Drive, Poughkeepsie, NY 12603, (914) 485-8269, BS 84 Coll of Saint Rose; MA 87 Univ of TX - Austin; 87–Sp-Lang Path, St Francis Hosp, **SLP**

Raiford, Dr Carolyn Ann Speech And Hearing Clinic, University Of Arkansas, 410 Arkansas Avenue, Fayetteville, AR 72701, (501) 575-4509, BA 58 Univ of North TX; MA 61 Univ of TX - Austin; PH 69 (NS) Purdue Univ - West Lafayette; Assoc Prof, U of AR-Fayetteville, **A**

Raifsnider, Mrs Jacquie S 703 Kilbourne Street, Bellevue, OH 44811, (419) 483-2184, BS 86 Bowling Green St Univ; MA 87 Bowling Green St Univ

Raimondis, Nina M 2620 Elden #B-3, Costa Mesa, CA 92627, MS; **SLP**

Rain, Keirsten 291 Sterling Place, Brooklyn, NY 11238, (718) 789-7085, BS 80 Hood Coll; MA 86 CUNY - Lehman Coll; 87–Sp-Lang Path, St Francis de Sales Sch for the Deaf, **SLP**

Rainbolt, Harry R Kansas State Univ, Speech & Hearing Center, 107 Leasure Hall, Manhattan, KS 66506, PH (NS); **A**

Rainbolt, Mrs Rebecca M 132 Greenwood Court, Coppell, TX 75019, (214) 247-7153, BA 79 TX A & I Univ; ME 80 Southwest TX St Univ; Sp-Lang Path, Carrollton-Farmers Branch ISD, **SLP**

Rainbolt, Mrs Rosella T 1408 Nichols Street, Manhattan, KS 66502, MS; **SLP**

Rainer, Mrs Deborah F PO Box 1404, Bruceville, TX 76630, (817) 755-2567, BS 81 Baylor Univ; MS 82 Baylor Univ; Cl Superv, Baylor U, **SLP**

Rainey, Barbara J Trost 749 Euclid Avenue, Long Beach, CA 90804, (213) 439-3566, BS 78 Northern AZ Univ; MS 80 ID St Univ; SLP, Marina Professional Services, **SLP**

Rainey, Cheryl Lee 2116 Hobbs Road, Unit E-6, Nashville, TN 37215, (615) 298-5436, BA 86 Harding Univ; MS 88 Vanderbilt Univ; Sp-Lang Path, Bill Wilkerson Hrng & Sp Ctr

Rainey, Chris A 1086 Pacific Avenue, Coos Bay, OR 97420, **SLP A**

Raino-Hoglund, Mrs Kimberly P O Box 366, Minooka, IL 60447-2050, (815) 744-3500, BA 80 Coll of Saint Francis; MS 81 Bradley Univ; Sp-Lang Path, U C P of Will Co, **SLP**

Rains, E Bobbie 6355 East Skelly Drive, Tulsa, OK 74135, (918) 622-7064, BS 69 Univ of TX - Austin; MA 70 Univ of OK - Norman; Dir, Tulsa Scottish Rite Clin, **SLP**

Rains, Jennifer Lee 10023 14th Street N #105, St Petersburg, FL 33716, (813) 576-5010, BA 82 Univ of FL; MA 84 Univ of FL; 84–Sp-Lang Path, Pinellas County Sch Bd, **SLP**

Rainsford, Evangelyon Holmes 16 Savage Street, Charleston, SC 29401, (803) 723-6302, **SLP**

Rainville, Mrs Marilyn 6291 Occoquan Forest Drive, Manassas, VA 22110, (703) 670-6107, BA 77 Hofstra Univ; MS 80 Rutgers St Univ - Newark; SLP, Prince William Co Sch, **SLP**

Rainwater, Mrs Jenny Hook 806 Pandora Street, Lafayette, LA 70506, (318) 265-5322, BA 79 Northeast LA Univ; MS 82 Univ Southern MS-Hattiesburg; 87–Aud, State of LA/Dept-Hlth & Hosp, **A**

Rainwater-Ross, Janet P O Box 90, Benton, AR 72015, (501) 778-6355, BS 78 Huron Coll; MA 80 Univ of AR - Fayetteville; Sp-Lang Path, Russellville Pub Sch, **SLP**

Raisner, Susan J 38 Brookside Drive, Cranston, RI 02910, (401) 277-3840, BA 69 Northeastern Univ; ME 71 Northeastern Univ; OM 75 Univ of RI; Ed Spec II Spec Ed Supp Srv Ut, Ri Dept of Elem/Sec Ed, **SLP**

Rajala, James S Route 10 Box 414, Hayward, WI 54843, (612) 689-5209, BA 73 Saint Cloud St Univ; MS 74 Saint Cloud St Univ; Sp-Lang Path, Private Practice, **SLP**

Rajnic, Alexine M 10 West Phillip Street, Coaldale, PA 18218, (215) 777-7615, Sp-Lang Path, Reading Rehabilitation Hosp, **SLP**

Rajotte, Margaret 29 November Trail, Weston, CT 06883, (203) 454-9679, BS 72 Nazareth Coll of Rochester; MS 73 Univ of MI - Ann Arbor; 88–Dir of Rehab, New Medico, **SLP**

Rakay, Cynthia J 2 Westminster Drive, Annandale, NJ 08801, (201) 735-6208, BA 76 Rutger's St Univ - Douglas Coll; MS 80 Rutger's St Univ - Douglas Coll; **SLP**

Rakestraw, Rebecca C 238 Tonti Avenue, South Bend, IN 46617, (219) 284-7312, BA 78 Jyoti Nivas Coll - Bangalore, India; BS 80 B.M. Inst - Gujerat, India; MA 83 Case Western Reserve Univ; 84–Sp-Lang Path, Memorial Hosp of South Bend, **SLP**

Rakfeldt, Mrs Kristi R 43 Willard Street, New Haven, CT 06515, BA 75 Univ of CT; MS 77 Southern CT St Univ; Sp-Lang Path, West Haven PS, **SLP**

Rakovic, Patricia A 59 Wildwood Road, Narragansett, RI 02852, (401) 751-3113, BA 77 CUNY - Lehman Coll; MA 79 NY Univ; Dept & Head Sp-Lang & Aud, Sargent Rehab Ctr, **SLP**

Rakowitz, Mrs Julie C 237 Strawberry Hill Avenue #9, Stamford, CT 06902, (203) 359-9200, BA 77 Southern CT St Univ; MS 78 Univ of AL- Tuscaloosa; 87–Pers Ofcr, Charter Federal Savings&Loan, **SLP**

Ralabate, Mrs Patricia Kelly 90 South King Street, Danbury, CT 06811, (203) 797-4744, BS 72 SUNY - Coll at Fredonia; MA 77 Univ of MA - Amherst; 84–Sp-Lang Path, Danbury Bd of Ed, **SLP**

Raleigh, Mrs Louise Ferguson 2519 Glen Burnie Drive, Greensboro, NC 27406, (919) 621-0631, **SLP**

Ralen, Mrs Sally Rigelhaupt 24 Strawberry Hill Road, Natick, MA 01760, (508) 358-2120, MS 85 Worcester St Coll; 84–Sp-Lang Path, Wayland Pub Sch, **SLP**

Ralph, Dawn Marie 1900-7 Tryon Drive, Fayetteville, NC 28303, (919) 488-2120, BS 81; MS 82; Sp-Lang Path, VA Med Ctr, **SLP**

Ralph, Luwana Diane 115 Madison Creek Road, Goodlettsville, TN 37072, (606) 324-0465, BS 82 Western KY Univ; MS 84 Western KY Univ; Sp-Lang Path, Geiger Easter Seal Sp-Hrng Cen, **SLP**

Ralph, Michael Ray 526 Fountain Drive, Seymour, IN 47274, (502) 456-5831, BS 85 Purdue Univ - West Lafayette; MS 87 Purdue Univ - West Lafayette; Aud, Louisville Hearing Aid Ctr

Ralph, Mrs Valerie C Route 1 Box 502-A, Webb Lake, WI 54830, (715) 259-3900, BS 52 Univ of MN - Minneap-St Paul; MA 76 Mankato St Univ; Sp-Lang Path, Hopkins Pub Schs, **SLP**

Ralstin, Robert H 3745 Circle Drive, Wichita, KS 67218, (316) 682-1112, BA 52 Wichita St Univ; MA 67 Wichita St Univ; 68–Sp-Lang Path, Private Practice, **SLP**

Ramage, Mrs Margaret McClure 526 Grand Avenue, Hackettstown, NJ 07840, (201) 852-2218, BS 79 Murray St Univ; MS 81 Murray St Univ; Sp-Lang Path, **SLP**

Ramakrishnan-Rothe, R K 5959 Meadow Drive, Lisle, IL 60532, (815) 740-7110, BA 75; MS 78 IL St Univ - Normal; SLP, Private Practice, **SLP ACE**

Rambo, Elizabeth J 638 Gleason Circle, East Rochester, NY 14445, (716) 424-7442, BS 84 Nazareth Coll of Rochester; MA 86 SUNY - Coll at Geneseo; 86–Sp-Lang Path, Assoc for Ret Citizens, **SLP**

Rambo, Mrs Mary H B 8928 49th Avenue West, Mukilteo, WA 98275, (206) 364-0300, BA 74 CA St Univ - Northridge; MA 76 CA St Univ - Northridge; Sp-Lang Path, Dept/Soc & Hlth Ser-Frcrst Sch, **SLP**

Rambow, Mary W 655 Royal Abbey Drive, Stone Mountain, GA 30088, (404) 469-5768, BA 72 Columbia Coll; MA 79 Univ of KS; Sp-Lang Path, Private Practice, **SLP**

Rambusch, Mrs Nancy-Jo Geiger 73 Highland Avenue, Rowayton, CT 06853, (203) 854-6650, BS 65 Nazareth Coll of Rochester; MS 66 Univ of MI - Ann Arbor; 88–Sp-Lang Path, Norwalk Schs, **SLP**

Ramedia, Mary A c/o Dauphin Deposit, P O Box 190, Carlisle, PA 17013-0190, (717) 766-0048, BA 48 PA St Univ - Univ Park; ME 40 PA St Univ - Univ Park; **SLP LM**

Ramer, Deborah S 50 Floral Avenue, Cortland, NY 13045, (607) 753-6061, BS 76 SUNY - Coll at Geneseo; MS 81 Ithaca Coll; Sp-Lang Path, O-C-M BOCES, **SLP**

Ramey, Anna M C 4133 Purdue, Dallas, TX 75225, (214) 521-3168, BA 59 Univ of OK - Norman; MS 69 Univ of OK - Norman; Assist Dir Child Dev Div, TX Scottish Rite Hosp/Crpld Ch, **SLP**

Ramey, Mrs Rita C Gray 8900 Copper Oaks Lane, Fort Smith, AR 72903, (501) 452-2942, BS 76 AR St Univ; MS 81 AR St Univ; Sp-Lang Path, Private Practice, **SLP**

Ramig, Dr Lorraine Olson Dept Of Comm Dis & Speech Sci, University Of Colorado, Campus Box 409, Boulder, CO 80309, (303) 492-6446, BS 72 Univ of WI - Oshkosh; MS 75 Univ of WI - Madison; PH 80 (Sp Path) Purdue Univ - West Lafayette; Assoc Prof, Dept Comm Dis & Sp Sci U Co, **SLP**

Ramig, Dr Peter R Dept Of Comm Dis & Speech Sci, University Of Colorado, Campus Box 409, Boulder, CO 80309, (303) 492-5375, BS 72 Univ of WI - Oshkosh; MS 75 Univ of WI - Madison; PH 79 (NS) Purdue Univ - West Lafayette; Professor, University of Colorado, **SLP**

Ramirez, Aurora Parreno 686 San Antonio Court, Merced, CA 95348, (209) 385-5651, BA 83 CA St Univ - Stanislaus; MA 85 CA St Univ - Stanislaus

Ramirez, Cynthia Anne 8782 Treasure Avenue, Walkersville, MD 21793-7779, (304) 263-0811, BS 73 Towson St Univ; OM 78 Hood Coll; MS 85 Towson St Univ; **SLP**

Ramirez, Irma Leticia 59 Addington Road #5, Brookline, MA 02146, (617) 732-5613, BA 73 Our Lady Lake Univ-San Anton; MA 74 Western MI Univ; OM 87 Boston Coll; 88–Dir Med Staff Aff, Brigham & Women's Hosp, **SLP**

Ramirez, Jennifer Thompson 785 Islay Street, San Luis Obispo, CA 93401, (805) 541-2755, BA 84 CA St Univ - Northridge; MA 86 CA St Univ - Northridge; 86–Sp-Lang Path, Lucia Mar USD, **SLP**

Ramirez, Julie Ann 1031 Stonegate Cove Drive, Porterville, CA 93257, (209) 782-7099, BA 81 San Jose St Univ; MA 87 San Jose St Univ

Ramirez, Susan Gayle 2301 S Millbend #2415, Woodlands, TX 77380, (713) 790-8100, BA 82 Univ of Houston - Univ Park; MA 87 Univ of Houston - Univ Park; 88–Sp-Lang Path, Med Ctr Hosp Del Oro Inst/Rehab, **SLP**

Ramirez, Mrs Toni G 16106 Seahorse Drive, Houston, TX 77062, **SLP**

Ramirez-Krambs, Mrs Olga V 2021 N Street, Suite 201, Sacramento, CA 95814, (916) 447-5468, BA 73 San Diego St Univ; MA 75 San Diego St Univ; SLP, Olga Ramirez Assoc, **SLP**

Ramm, Elaine 321 Sunrise Boulevard, Buffalo, NY 14221, BA 60; MS 75 SUNY - Coll at Buffalo; Sp-Lang Path, Clarence Central Schools, **SLP**

Ramos, Luz Martina Calle 18 N-O 1352, Puerto Nuevo, San Juan, PR 00920, (809) 782-7017, BS 74 Univ of PR - San Juan; MS 85 Univ of HI - Manoa; 86–Aud, Sp & Hrng Ctr of San Juan

Ramos, Rosalva A 714 West 181st Street #32, New York, NY 10033, (212) 927-8743, BS 74 Loyola Coll; ME 77 Seton Hall Univ; Sp-Lang Path, Private Practice, **SLP**

Ramos-Pizarro, Carmen Ana Quintas DE Cupey Garden, Apartment A-202, Rio Piedras, PR 00926, (809) 758-2525, BS 81 Univ of PR - Rio Piedras; MS 83 Univ of PR - San Juan; 83–Instructor, University of Puerto Rico, **SLP**

Rampey, Robin Sue 12472 Elmwood, Garden Grove, CA 92640, (308) 234-5351, MS 87 Kearney St Coll

Rampp, Dr Donald L Dept Communication Disorders, LSU Medical Center, 1900 Gravier Street, New Orleans, LA 70112, (504) 568-4348, BA 53 Northeastern OK St Univ; MA 58 OH St Univ; PH 67 (Sp Path Cleft Palate) Univ of OK Medical Center; Dept Head & Prof, Lsu Med Cen, **SLP F**

Rampulla, Mary Louise 8 W High Street, Nazareth, PA 18064, (215) 776-3270, BA 81 Thiel Coll; MA 84 West Chester Univ of PA; **SLP**

Ramsay, Carolyn M 191 Village Circle Way, Apartment #2, Manchester, NH 03102, (603) 623-8863, BA 83; OB 84; MA 86 Univ of ME - Orono; 87–Sp-Lang Path, Easter Seal Rehab Ctr, **SLP**

Ramsayer, Mrs Carolyn B 309 Ruth Street, Bay Village, OH 44140, (216) 871-6339, BA 80 Cleveland St Univ; MA 82 Cleveland St Univ; Sp-Lang Path, Private Practice, **SLP**

Ramsberger, Dr Gail 2805 Kenyon Circle, Boulder, CO 80303, (303) 441-0437, BA 77 Univ of CO - Boulder; MA 79 Univ of CO - Boulder; OD 86 (Communication Disorders) Boston Univ; Dir Sp-Lang Path & Aud, Mem Hosp-Boulder, **SLP ACE**

Ramsdell, Rebecca Sue 2990 Dove Street, Redding, CA 96001, (916) 244-4600, BA 76 CA St Univ - Chico; MA 83 CA St Univ - Chico; **SLP**

Ramser, Mrs Angelique Thacker 1507 Honor Drive, Richmond, VA 23228-3364, (804) 321-7474, BS 82 Longwood Coll; ME 84 Univ of VA - Charlottesville; Sp-Lang Path, Chldrns Hosp, **SLP**

Ramsey, Mrs Barbara A 295 Woodland Hills, Southbury, CT 06488, **SLP**

Ramsey, Belinda R 1850 Raymond Place, Bloomfield Hills, MI 48013, (313) 756-9800, BA 82 MI St Univ; MA 85 Wayne St Univ; 88–Dir, Neurological Recovery Sys, **SLP**

Ramsey, Deborah J 5092 Hutchins Street, Winston-Salem, NC 27106, (919) 748-3103, BA 75 Univ of FL; MA 76 Univ of FL; Aud, North Carolina Baptist Hosp, **A**

Ramsey, Gale Mayhew 350 Old Highway 2570, Marshall, NC 28753, (704) 253-9992, BA 72 Western Carolina Univ; MA 80 Western Carolina Univ; Sp-Lang Path, Buncombe Co Pub Sch Syst, **SLP**

Ramsey, K Judith Celebration Point, 15515 Miami Lakeway North, Apartment 105, Miami Lakes, FL 33014, (305) 891-8850, BA 51 Univ of IA; MA 63 Univ of IA; Sp-Lang Path, Bon Secours Rehab Hosp, **SLP ACE**

Ramsey, Mrs Mary Lindsay 20384 West Geer Avenue, Hilmar, CA 95324, (209) 668-8081, **SLP**

Ramsey, Myra G PO Box 8844, Columbia, SC 29202, (803) 737-5318, BA 75 Winthrop Coll; MS 77 Univ of SC - Columbia; Dir of Rehab Services, C M Tucker Jr Human Resouces, **SLP**

Ramsey, Mrs Pamela Davis 237 Ridgewood, Village, Auburn, AL 36830, (205) 864-9343, BS 85 Auburn Univ - Auburn; OM 87 Auburn Univ - Auburn; **SLP**

Ramsey, Sidney L 2612 57th Street, Des Moines, IA 50310, (515) 283-6344, BS 74 Univ of IA; MA 75 Univ of IA; 86–Dir-SLP & Aud, IA Methodist Med Cen, **A**

Ramsey, Mrs Wendy H 815 Cordova Street, Dallas, TX 75223-1229, (214) 596-2707, BS 78 Univ of North TX; MS 79 Univ of North TX; **SLP**

Ramspacher, Mrs Kathryn K 2028 Oak Avenue, Hatfield, PA 19440, (215) 539-8550, BS 77 PA St Univ - Univ Park; MA 79 Trenton St Coll; SLP, Mont Co Inter Ut, **SLP**

Ramstad, Mrs Margaret R 4272 Persimmon Path, Liverpool, NY 13090, (315) 593-3856, BS 79 Univ of IL - Urbana; MA 81 Univ of IL - Urbana; Aud, Central Hearing Consultants, **A**

Ranck, Mrs Sheryl Ann Rd 2 Box #391, Montoursville, PA 17754, (717) 435-0504, BS 85 Bloomsburg Univ of PA; MS 86 Bloomsburg Univ of PA; 86–Aud, Dr Geeta Krishnan MD, **A**

Rand, Mrs Diane J P O Box 127, Hampstead, NC 28443, (919) 455-2211, BA 82 Univ of NC - Chapel Hill; MA 85 Univ of TN - Knoxville; 87–Sp-Lang Path, Onslow County Schs, **SLP**

Rand, Marilyn A 11 Robert Best Road, Sudbury, MA 01776, (508) 443-6536, BS 75 Boston Univ; MA 77 Hofstra Univ; Sp-Lang Path, Assabet Valley Reg Voc HS, **SLP**

Rand, Shann 2420 South Union, Suite 100, Tacoma, WA 98405, (206) 756-8707, BA 72 United States Int'l Univ; MA 76 CA St Univ - Fresno; Aud, Head & Neck Surg Assoc, **A**

Randall, Carol G 12500 Riviera Place N E, Seattle, WA 98125, (206) 361-4252, BA 58 Univ of WA; ME 66 Univ of WA; MS 69 Chaminade Univ of Honolulu; Prog Mgr for Hrng Imp, Shoreline Pub Sch, **SLP A**

Randall, Joellen M 1820 Westmoreland Street, Mc Lean, VA 22101-5101, BS 74 Longwood Coll; ME 75 Univ of VA - Charlottesville; Sp/Lang Path, Duval Cty Sch Bd, **SLP**

Randall, Kurt D 1206 North 150 East, Layton, UT 84041, (801) 626-3645, BS 70 Univ of UT; ME 71 Univ of UT; MS 76 Vanderbilt Univ; Aud, Utah Department of Health, **A**

Randall, Mrs Linda Mallick 20 Highknoll Drive, South Berwick, ME 03908, (207) 384-2293, **A**

Randall, Rebecca Sue 1901 South Center Street, Terre Haute, IN 47802-2311, (812) 232-4125, BS 83 IN St Univ - Terre Haute; MS 85 IN St Univ - Terre Haute; Sp-Lang Pathologist, Union Hospital, **SLP**

Randall, Yolaine G 25 Central Park West #2-R, New York, NY 10023, BA 65 Univ of Miami; MA 69 CUNY - Hunter Coll; Sp-Lang Path, Private Practice, **SLP ACE**

Randant, Mrs Barbara F 1520 Oak Street, Highland, IL 62249-2219, (618) 654-5533, BS 80 Southern IL Univ-Edwardsvill; MS 81 Southern IL Univ-Edwardsvill; SLP/Aud, St Elisabeth's Hosp, **SLP A**

Randel, Dr Elizabeth G 380 Euclid Street #303, Pasadena, CA 91101, (818) 962-3311, BS 80 Univ of NE - Lincoln; MS 82 Univ of NE - Lincoln; Sp-Lang Path, Wahoo Pub Sch, **SLP**

Randel, Roberta Malat 8436 N W 52nd Place, Coral Springs, FL 33067, (305) 972-1600, BA 78 CUNY - Queens Coll; MA 80 Univ of CT; 87–Aud, Children & Infant Diag Ctr, **A**

Randle, Bonnie 12524-C East Pacific Circle, Aurora, CO 80014, (303) 750-1150, BA 75 Univ of MO - KS City; MS 77 Univ of AZ; Sp-Lang Path, Cherry Creek Sch Dist #5, **SLP**

Randle, Mrs Kathleen Miller 919 73rd Street, Kenosha, WI 53140, (414) 652-7333, BS 84 Univ of WI - Madison; MS 86 Univ of WI - Madison; 88–Sp-Lang Path, Western Racine County, **SLP**

Randle, Mrs Mary Ann 290 Fondulal Drive, East Peoria, IL 61611, (309) 699-5709, BS 73 IL St Univ - Normal; MS 75 IL St Univ - Normal; Sp/Lang Path, Peoria Publ Schs, **SLP**

Randles, Susan M 1835 S W Runnion Place, Pendleton, OR 97801, (503) 276-7363, BA 69 Western WA Univ; MA 75 Univ of SD - Vermillion; 76–Sp-Lang Path, Umatilla Ed Serv Dist, **SLP ACE**

Rando, Carolyn E M P O Box 0983, Ocean Gate, NJ 08740, (201) 269-9252, BS 85 Stockton St Coll; MA 87 OH Univ - Athens; **SLP**

Randolph, Beverly 119 Fountain View, Shreveport, LA 71118-2948, (318) 686-1754, BA 65 Northwestern St Univ; MA 79 Northwestern St Univ; Sp-Lang Path, Caddo Parish Sch Bd, **SLP A**

Randolph, Dr Karin M P O Box 438, 95 Puddin Lane, Mansfield Center, CT 06250, (203) 742-5039, BA 64 Principia Coll; MA 68 Boston Univ; Early Childhood Coord, Coventry Pub Sch, **SLP**

Randolph, Dr Kenneth J 95 Puddin Lane, P O Box 438, Mansfield Center, CT 06250, (203) 486-3289, BA 64 IN Univ - Bloomington; MS 67 IN Univ - Bloomington; PH 69 (NS) IN Univ - Bloomington; Assoc Prof of Aud, U of Connecticut, **A**

Randolph, Laddie A 2954 Coloma Street, Placerville, CA 95667, (916) 453-4923, BA 78 Univ of the Pacific; MA 81 Univ of the Pacific; Sp-Lang Path, Mercy Gen Hosp, **SLP**

Randolph, Loren J P O Box 354, Magna, UT 84044, (801) 581-8915, BA 72 Univ of ID; MS 79 ID St Univ; Cl Superv, Univ of Utah ENT Associates, **A**

Rane, Dr Robert L 7950 Floyd Curl #509, San Antonio, TX 78229, (512) 696-4541, BS 71 Brigham Young Univ; MS 73 Brigham Young Univ; PH 78 (NS) Kent St Univ; Aud, Med Cen ENT, **A**

Raney, Judith Kellogg 1009 Arrow Court, Bowling Green, KY 42101-4664, (502) 782-0391, BS 65 Kent St Univ; MS 86 Baylor Univ; Sp-Lang Path, Home Health/Preschool, **SLP**

Raney, Melissa Lynne P O Box 1084, Hampton, AR 71744, (501) 863-6995, BA 78 AR St Univ; BS 80 Henderson St Univ; MS 82 Univ of AR - Little Rock; Audiologist, R C Pillsbury MD, **A**

Raney, Sandra Lee Box 304, Hubbard, IA 50122, (515) 864-2229, BS 79 IA St Univ; MA 81 Northeast MO St Univ; Sp-Lang Path, AEA 6, **SLP**

Rankell, Gail E 603 N Howard Street #401, Alexandria, VA 22304, (301) 375-7444, BS 76 Ithaca Coll; MA 78 Hofstra Univ; Sp-Lang Path, Charles Co Boed, **SLP**

Rankin, Mrs Deena W Box 221, Ashkum, IL 60911, (815) 698-2028, BS 76 Eastern IL Univ; MS 77 Eastern IL Univ; **SLP**

Rankin, Julie H 5128 Manning Drive, Bethesda, MD 20814, (202) 745-5600, BA 83 Univ of VT; MA 85 George Washington Univ; 86–Sp-Lang Path, Chldn Hosp Natl Med Ctr, **SLP**

Rankin, Kristin Lee 8370 West 38th Avenue, Apartment 102-B, Wheatridge, CO 80033, (303) 425-0449, BA 82 Univ of Northern CO; MA 83 Univ of Northern CO; **A**

Rankin, Lorna Janet 4288 Victoria Avenue, Port Alberni, BC, Canada V9Y 7L1, (604) 723-3744, OB 73 Univ of British Columbia; MA 83 Western WA Univ; Sp-Lang Path, School District #70, **SLP**

Rankin, Lynn J 44 Hennig Drive, Pittsburgh, PA 15236, (412) 521-9000, BS 81 Baylor Univ; MA 83 Univ of Pittsburgh - Pittsburgh; Sp-Lang Path, The Rehab I of Pittsburgh, **SLP**

Rankin Coffin, Robin L 211 South 37th Avenue, Yakima, WA 98902, (509) 965-3946, BA 74 Western WA Univ; MA 77 Western WA Univ; 87–Sp-Lang Path, Yakima Sch Dist, **SLP**

Rankinen, Lynn M 57 Inner Drive #D9, St Paul, MN 55116, (612) 627-2750, BS 79 Univ of WI - Madison; MS 81 Univ of WI - Madison; 81–Sp-Lang Path, Minneapolis Pub Sch, **SLP**

Rankins, Scott D 5700 Rivermill Circle, Portsmouth, VA 23703, (804) 483-6601, BS; MS 88 Old Dominion Univ; 88–Sp-Lang Path, Portsmouth PS

Rankovic, Christine Marie 3538 South Fremont Avenue, Apartment 1, Minneapolis, MN 55408, (206) 364-0500, **A**

Rann, Patti Elfreda 3105 Clearwater Drive, Cleveland, TN 37311, (615) 476-4713, BS 80 Middle TN St Univ; MA 85 Univ of TN - Knoxville; Aud, Cleveland Head & Neck Clinic, **A**

Rannard, Elizabeth Joan 6750 Beadnell Way #7, San Diego, CA 92117, (619) 340-4566, MS 86 UT St Univ; 87–Aud, Desert Ear Nose & Throat

Ranney, Mrs Elizabeth Anne 191-4 Oko Street, Kailua, HI 96734, (808) 235-3416, BS 79 SUNY - Coll at Geneseo; ME 85 Columbus Coll; Sp-Lang Path, Windward Dept of Educaton, **SLP**

Ranney, Dr J Buckminster NIH NINCDS CDP, Federal Bldg #1C11, 7550 Wisconsin Avenue, Bethesda, MD 20892, (301) 496-1804, BA 46 NY Univ; MA 47 NY Univ; PH 57 (Speech) OH St Univ; Health Scientist Admin, NIH, **SLP A F**

Ranochak, Patricia 4902 Christiana Campbell, Fort Wayne, IN 46804, **SLP**

Ransaw, Mrs Anna K 829 South 40th Street, Louisville, KY 40211, (502) 778-7145, BA 39 KY St Univ; MS 51 IN Univ - Bloomington; Sp-Lang Path, **SLP LM**

Ransom, Kathleen M 415 North 38th Street, Omaha, NE 68131, BS 70 IA St Univ; MS 74 Univ of NE - Omaha; Sp-Lang Path, Omaha Pub Schs, **SLP**

Ransom, Mrs Nina D 460 Glenwood, Satellite Beach, FL 32937, (305) 777-1687, BS 59 Purdue Univ - West Lafayette; MS 61 Purdue Univ - West Lafayette; Sp/Lang Path, Sch Bd Brev Co, **SLP A**

Ranton, Debra Beth 1213 Devlin Court, Arcata, CA 95521, (707) 445-3261, BA 79 Sonoma St Univ; MA 85 Humboldt St Univ; **SLP**

Rao, Mrs Martina M 12 Elkwood Court, Catonsville, MD 21228, (301) 744-8933, BA 70 Catholic Univ of America; MA 71 Catholic Univ of America; Sp-Lang Path, Balto Co Hlth Dept, **SLP**

Rao, Dr Paul Richard 12 Elkwood Court, Catonsville, MD 21228, (202) 877-1440, BA 68 Saint Vincent Coll; MA 71 Catholic Univ of America; PH 85 (Hrng & Sp Science) Univ of MD - College Park; Dir Sp-Lang Path, National Rehab Hosp, **SLP**

Raphael, Dr Lawrence J 6 Longview Place, Great Neck, NY 11021, (212) 960-8400, BA 59 CUNY - Queens Coll; MA 65 CUNY - Queens Coll; PH 70 (Speech Science) CUNY - Grad Sch & Univ Cntr; Prof, Herbert H Lehman Coll

Raphael, Mrs Rachel Aaron 108 Strongwood Road, Owings Mills, MD 21117, (301) 356-9758, BA 85 Univ of MD - College Park; MA 87 George Washington Univ; 88–Aud, Dr Alan E Oshinsky MD PA, **A**

Rapinchuk, Mrs Laurie E 17243 Inverness, Tinley Park, IL 60477-7371, (312) 974-3300, BS 80 IL St Univ - Normal; MS 81 IL St Univ - Normal; Sp-Lang Path, Consolidated Hs District #230, **SLP**

Rapkin, Mrs Enid S 307 Sharpley Road, Wilmington, DE 19803, (302) 571-1563, BS 68 PA St Univ - Univ Park; MA 70 Temple Univ-Tyler Sch of Art; Sp-Lang Path, Private Practice, **SLP**

Rapkin, Judy 603 Clinton Avenue, Toronto, ON, Canada M6G 2Z8, (416) 630-4764, BA 74 McGill Univ - Quebec; MS 76 McGill Univ - Quebec; Head/Sp/Lang Servs, Adventure Place, **SLP**

Rapkin-Berger, Mrs Ellen 175-06 Devonshire Road, Jamaica, NY 11432, (718) 423-4904, BS 74 NY Univ; MA 75 NY Univ; Sp-Lang Path, Utd Cp of NYC, **SLP**

Rapp, Mrs Amy L 533 South Pershing, Wichita, KS 67218-2307, (316) 682-0596, BA 83 Wichita St Univ; MA 84 Wichita St Univ; Sp-Lang Path, Wichita PS USD 259, **SLP**

Rapp, Deborah E 2419 East Sandpebble Lane, Brea, CA 92621, BA 76 Univ of Redlands; MS 77 Univ of Redlands; Sp-Lang Path, LA Co Super of Schs, **SLP**

Rapp, Gail M P O Box 13732, Portland, OR 97213, (503) 233-5925, BA 79 Univ of OR; MS 81 Purdue Univ - West Lafayette; Aud, Portland Otologic Clinic, **A**

Rapp, Mrs Kathleen Wilks 98 Alicante Aisle, Irvine, CA 92714, (714) 756-9323, BA 83 Loyola Coll; MS 84 Loyola Coll; Sp-Lang Path, Santa Ana USD, **SLP**

Rapp, Sharon Beall 205 Haywood Drive, Fort Worth, TX 76126, (817) 921-7620, BS 80 CO St Univ; MS 82 CO St Univ; Aud, TX Christian U, **A**

Rappaport, Dr Bruce Z Audiology & Speech Pathology Service, VA Medical Center, 2100 Ridgecrest Drive SE, Albuquerque, NM 87108, (505) 265-1711, BA 68 Northern MI Univ; MA 69 Univ of WA; PH 76 (Aud) Univ of MI - Ann Arbor; 88–Chief-Aud & SLP Svc, Albuquerque VA Med Cen, **A**

Rappaport, Margery F 1700 York Avenue #6F, New York, NY 10128, (212) 996-9355, OB 65 Boston Univ; MA 70 Columbia Univ Teachers Coll; Sp/Lang Path, Private Practice, **SLP**

Rappaport, Michele Coy 5629 Sierra Avenue, Richmond, CA 94805, (415) 237-3920, MS 85 San Francisco St Univ; Sp-Lang Path, Aaron Sp Path Inc, **SLP**

Rappe, Elizabeth Medlock 4824 Lafayette, Fort Worth, TX 76107-3726, (817) 738-5888, BS 80 Univ of Houston - Univ Park; MA 84 Univ of Houston - Univ Park; Sp-Lang Path, Ft Worth ISD, **SLP**

Rappold, Patrick Wynn 16635 Tiger Bend Road, Baton Rouge, LA 70817-4832, BS 85 LA St Univ - Baton Rouge; OM 83 LA St Univ - N O Medical Ctr; **A**

Rapport, Karlyn I 711 West Magnetic, Marquette, MI 49855, (906) 228-9440, BA 57 OH St Univ; MA 69 Northern MI Univ; **SLP**

Raquer, Linda A 517 North 60th, Seattle, WA 98103, (206) 545-2529, BA 76 Univ of MI - Ann Arbor; MA 77 Western MI Univ; Sp-Lang Path, Univ of Washington, **SLP**

Rasche, Laura Baggett 950 North Street #7, Jackson, MS 39202-2617, (601) 939-8640, SLP, Hudspeth Retardation Cntr, **SLP**

Rash, Mrs Joni Louise 11912 Springmeadow Lane, Goshen, KY 40026-9529, **SLP**

Rash, Mrs Robin Zachow 15002C SE 179th Street, Renton, WA 98058, (206) 235-8923, BA 80 WA St Univ; MA 81 WA St Univ; Sp-Lang Path, Renton Sch Dist, **SLP**

Rashok, Katherine P O Box 4466, Crestline, CA 92325, MS

Rasin, Mrs Judy Warshaver 32 Arbor Road, Roslyn Heights, NY 11577, (212) 445-1400, MA 70 CUNY - Queens Coll; Aud, Lawrence Deutch, **A**

Raskin, Mrs Carol Wolitzky 520 East 76th Street #4C, New York, NY 10021, (212) 899-8800, BA 65 Adelphi Univ; OM 75 Columbia Univ Teachers Coll; MA 68 NY Univ; SLP, Lexington Sch for the Deaf, **SLP**

Raskin, Cynthia Landis 12309 Woodbine Road, Minnetonka, MN 55343, (612) 936-0096, BS 80 Northwestern Univ; MA 82 Univ of MN - Minneap-St Paul; 87–Sp-Lang Path Dir, The Caroline Ctr, **SLP**

Raskind, Linda Ann 6425 City West Parkway #3212, Eden Prairie, MN 55344, (612) 941-6401, **A**

Raskin-Holmes, Mrs Wendy Fae Sturbridge Meadow, 90 Hall Road, Apartment 46, Sturbridge, MA 01566, (203) 564-4086, BS 83 Univ of MA - Amherst; MS 85 Boston Univ; Sp-Lang Path, Plainfield CT PS, **SLP**

Rasley, Alexis Gray 604 South Lombard, Oak Park, IL 60304, (312) 908-8035, BA 79 IL St Univ - Normal; MA 86 Northwestern Univ; Sp-Lang Path, Northwestern Univ Med School, **SLP**

Rasmus, Dr Ward 1761 Carmel Drive #205, Walnut Creek, CA 94596, (415) 934-7425, BA 32 Whitman Coll; MA 40 Univ of WA; PH 55 (NS) Stanford Univ; **SLP LM**

Rasmussen, Catherine Ann 2222 West Michelle Drive, Phoenix, AZ 85023, BS 75 Univ of OR; MS 77 UT St Univ; Sp-Lang Path, Paradise Valley School Dist, **SLP**

Rasmussen, Mrs Delia Graham 6 Crestwood Drive, Ava, NY 13303, (315) 336-1406, BA 83 CA St Univ - Chico; MA 84 CA St Univ - Chico; **SLP**

Rasmussen, Louise A 1260 McKendne Street, San Jose, CA 95126, **SLP**

Rasmussen, Mrs Louise Pearl 17022 Northeast 100th Pl, Redmond, WA 98052, (206) 867-0222, BA 78 Chapman Coll; MS 80 Chapman Coll; Sp-Lang Path, Snoqualmie Valley Sch Dist #410, **SLP**

Rasmussen, Marjorie R 901 Carlson Drive, Brea, CA 92621, (714) 529-5611, BA 50 Bradley Univ; MA 86 CA St Univ - Fullerton; 87–Sp-Lang Path, Private Practice, **SLP**

Rasmussen, Mary Janet 618 E Milwaukee Street, Janesville, WI 53545-3159, (608) 755-2984, **SLP**

Rasmussen, Randall L 610 Barrie Street, Fort Atkinson, WI 53538, (414) 563-7811, BA 73 Univ of WI - Madison; BA 78 Univ of WI - Eau Claire; MS 79 Univ of WI - Eau Claire; 80–Sp-Lang Path, Ft Atkinson Pub Sch, **SLP**

Rasmussen, Rosalie P 5904 Cherry Creek, Austin, TX 78745, **SLP**

Rasmussen, Mrs Susan Gayle R R 3 Box 279, Jefferson, IA 50129, (515) 386-8188, BA 82 Univ of Northern IA; MA 83 Northeast MO St Univ; 83–Sp-Lang Path, Arrowhead AEA, **SLP**

Rasmussen Noble, Shelly Rae 1043 North Mollison, Apt I, El Cajon, CA 92021, (619) 442-5283, BS 86 SD St Univ; MA 87 Univ of SD - Vermillion; 87–Sp-Lang Path, Eloise R Johnston and Assoc, **SLP**

Rasner, Mrs Janine Dee 8112 Chestnut Ridge Drive, Charlotte, NC 28215, (704) 536-0643, MS 88 Univ of TX - Dallas; 88–Sp-Lang Path, Charlotte/Mechlenburg Sch Dist

Rasnick, Catherine Sue 305 West Valley Street, Abingdon, VA 24210, (703) 889-1389, BS 78 Appalachian St Univ; MS 84 Radford Univ; **SLP**

Raso, Susan D 1217 Foothill Drive, Champaign, IL 61821, (217) 351-3815, BS 75 Univ of IL - Urbana; MS 76 Univ of IL - Urbana; Sp-Lang Path, Champaign Unit 4 Sch, **SLP**

Rasor, Mrs Glynn H 517 Pebblecreek, Garland, TX 75040, (214) 239-1724, BS 81 TX A & M Univ; MS 83 Univ of TX - Dallas; Sp-Lang Path, Richardson ISD, **SLP**

Rassi, Judith A 435 Ridge Road #403, Wilmette, IL 60091, (312) 491-3165, BS 61 IL St Univ - Normal; MA 63 Northwestern Univ; 82–Dir, Northwestern Univ, **A F ACE**

Rassiga, Malinda Ann 523 Raintree Court, Harrodsburg, KY 40330, (606) 276-5563, BA 80 Univ of KY; MS 84 Univ of KY; **SLP ACE**

Rassiga, Nancy Diane 1422 Julia Avenue, Mc Lean, VA 22101, BS 72 SUNY - Coll at Buffalo; MS 75 Columbia Univ Teachers Coll; 87–Dir, Sp & Lang Ctr of No Virginia, **SLP**

Rassmann, Diane L 104 South Interlachen #315, Winter Park, FL 32789, (305) 645-4019, SLP, Tampa Gen Hosp, **SLP**

Rastatter, Dr Mary Doyle 808 Duke Street, Alexandria, VA 22314, (202) 373-7374, OB 62 OH Univ - Athens; ME 63 Univ of VA - Charlottesville; ED 70 (NS) Univ of VA - Charlottesville; Ch SLP & Aud Branch, St Elizabeths Hosp, **SLP A**

Rastatter, Dr Michael P 370 North Ridge, Perrysburg, OH 43551, (419) 372-8242, BS 72 Clarion Univ of PA; MS 75 SUNY - Coll at Fredonia; PH 80 (Comm Dis) Bowling Green St Univ; Assoc Professor & Assoc Dean, Bowling Green State University, **SLP**

Rastetter, Mrs Marcelle T 1216 Timber Hawk Terrace, Spring Valley, OH 45370, (513) 885-3483, BS 70 Kent St Univ; ME 78 Central St Univ; 88–Sp-Lang Path, Creene County Bd of Educ, **SLP**

Raszler, Diane W Doctors Clinic Of Bremerton, 2512 Wheaton Way, Bremerton, WA, (206) 377-8561, BA 82 CA St Univ - Sacramento; MS 85 CA St Univ - Sacramento; 88–Dir-Aud Dept, Doctor's Clinic of Bremerton, **A**

Ratcliff, Mrs Alice 1501 Flamingo, Arlington, TX 76012, (817) 265-9339, BS 77 Baylor Univ; MS 78 Baylor Univ; **SLP**

Ratcliff, Ann E Department Of Speech-Language Pathology And Audiology, School Of Allied Health Professions, Loma Linda University, Loma Linda, CA 92350, (714) 824-4998, BA 72 Univ of Redlands; MS 73 Univ of Redlands; PH 87 (Childhood Lang Augmentative Comm) Univ of WI - Madison; 81–Asst Prof, Loma Linda U, **SLP**

Ratcliff, Mrs Brenda S 1333 Clover, Angleton, TX 77515, (409) 848-1098, BS 77 Southwest TX St Univ; ME 78 Southwest TX St Univ; 87–Resource Tchr, Angleton Independent Sch Dist, **SLP**

Ratcliff, L Gay 710 East Bella Vista St, Lakeland, FL 33805, (813) 686-3189, BS 67 WV Univ; MS 73 Univ of South FL; Exec Dir, Ctrl FL Sp & Hrng Cen, **A ACE**

Ratcliff-Fais, Mary Beth 3545 Olentangy River Road, Suite 525, Columbus, OH 43214, (614) 267-2587, BA 75 OH St Univ; MA 77 OH St Univ; Aud, ENT Head & Neck Surg Inc, **A**

Ratelle, Constance Briscoe 4733 3rd Avenue South, Minneapolis, MN 55409, (612) 932-5496, BA 78 Case Western Reserve Univ; MA 80 Saint Louis Univ; Sp/Lang Path, Ebenezer Caroline Center, **SLP**

Rater, Rae J 1006 W 9th Street, Hastings, NE 68901, (402) 463-5611, BA 85 Univ of Northern IA; MA 87 Univ of Northern IA; 87–Sp-Lang Path, Educ Svc Unit #9, **SLP**

Rath, Mrs Antoinette Petrillo 156 East Browning Road, Belmar, NJ 08031, (609) 933-1346, BS 81 West Chester Univ of PA; MA 85 West Chester Univ of PA; SLP, **SLP**

Rath, Jessica Lynn 29-33 Bell Boulevard, Bayside, NY 11360, (516) 338-4204, BA 80 SUNY - Center at Binghamton; MA 84 CUNY - Hunter Coll; Sp-Lang Path, North Shore Univ Hosp, **SLP**

Rath, Roger J 1616 South Carolina, Harlingen, TX 78550, (512) 428-4221, BA 69 SD St Univ; MA 75 Univ of SD - Vermillion; MA 82 Univ of SD - Vermillion; 82–Aud, Gerald J Collins MD PA, **SLP A**

Rathbone-Meeks, Nancy L 719 N W 90th Street, Seattle, WA 98117, (206) 433-2557, BS 77 Univ of OR; OM 79 Univ of WA; SLP, Highline Sch Dist, **SLP**

Rathbun, Evelyn Kowalysyn 66 River View Avenue, Noank, CT 06340, (201) 536-9477, BS 56 Purdue Univ - West Lafayette; MS 76 Southern CT St Univ; Coord/Sp-Lang Path, Ledyard Board of Education, **SLP**

Rathge, Mrs Karen Maureen 9105 Lagrima DE Oro N E, Albuquerque, NM 87111, (505) 848-8000, BA 79 CA St Univ - Long Beach; MA 82 Univ of NM; MS 82 Univ of NM; Sp-Lang Path, St Joseph's Hospital, **SLP**

Rathhaus, Mrs Coralita 7618 Amber Way, Stockton, CA 95207, (209) 944-4308, BA 55 Univ of the Pacific; Sp-Lang Path, Stockton USD, **SLP**

Rathke, Maj John J EENT Clinic, Darnall Army Community Hospital, Fort Hood, TX 76544-5063, (817) 288-8490, BS 71 Morningside Coll; MS 73 AZ St Univ; 87–Chief-Aud, Darnall Army Hosp, **A**

Ratiner, Sharon Paula 2 River Road #16, Highland Park, NJ 08904, (201) 846-2136, MA 83 Montclair St Coll; BA 80 Montclair St Coll; Sp-Lang Path, Private Practice, **SLP**

Ratkiewicz, Brenda J 40 South Hess, Golden, CO 80401, (303) 238-5566, MA 85 Univ of CO - Boulder; **A**

Ratliff, Mrs Janet Hall 2813 Pleasant Drive, Muncie, IN 47302, (317) 358-3324, BS 75 IN St Univ - Terre Haute; MA 82 Ball St Univ; 88–Pres, Hall-Ratliff Consulting, **SLP**

Ratliff, Janis Lynn 1426 Garden Street #15, Santa Barbara, CA 93101, (805) 965-2417, BA 84 CA St Univ - Sacramento; MA 86 Univ of CA - Santa Barbara; **SLP**

Ratliff, Patricia Ann P O Box 73, Ona, WV 25545, (304) 733-3000, BA 74 Marshall Univ; MA 75 Marshall Univ; 88–Sp-Lang Path, Cabell County PS, **SLP**

Ratliff, Dr Sandra Sue 2141 Fox Hunt Drive, Gastonia, NC 28054, (704) 866-2167, BS 61; MA 62 Bowling Green St Univ; PH 72 (NS) Bowling Green St Univ; Mgr-Sp & Hrng Cen, Gaston Mem Hosp Inc, **SLP A**

Ratliff, Susan L H Route 2 Box 456, Waynesboro, VA 22980, **SLP**

Ratner, Mrs Barbara M 11421 Great Meadows Drive, Reston, VA 22091, (703) 435-1612, BS 71 SUNY - Center at Buffalo; ME 75 Univ of VA - Charlottesville; SLP, Fairfax Co Pub Sch, **SLP**

Ratner, Mrs Ellen J 318 Costello Drive, Los Altos, CA 94022, (415) 948-7714, BA 67 San Jose St Univ; MA 68 San Jose St Univ; Sp-Lang Path, Private Practice, **SLP**

Ratner, Dr Nan E Bernstein 9907 Wildwood Road, Kensington, MD 20895, (301) 454-6912, BA 74 Tufts Univ; MA 76 Temple Univ; ED 82 (Applied Psycholinquistics) Boston Univ; 82–Asst Prof, U of MD/Dept Hrng & Sp Sci, **SLP**

Ratner, Mrs Roberta E P O Box 867, Waterville, ME 04901, (207) 873-3801, BA 73 CUNY - Brooklyn Coll; MS 74 Univ of MI - Ann Arbor; Sp/Lang Path, Private Practice, **SLP**

Ratnofsky-Reiss, Selma Esther 209-39 23rd Avenue #3H, Bayside, NY 11360, (212) 591-6889, BA 77 CUNY - Queens Coll; MA 79 Hofstra Univ; 84 CUNY - Queens Coll; Sp-Lang Path, Speech Services Unit, **SLP**

Rattiner, Rochele G 11 Wilshire Lane, Plainview, NY 11803, (516) 681-4657, BA 82 CUNY - Queens Coll; MA 84 CUNY - Queens Coll; Sp-Lang Path, East Williston School District, **SLP**

Rattmann, Janet M 120 South Bird Street, Sun Prairie, WI 53590-4824, (414) 262-0507, BS 84 Univ of WI - Whitewater; MS 85 Univ of WI - Whitewater; 86–Sp-Lang Path, Bethesda Lutheran Home, **SLP**

Rattner, Dr Bonnie G 249 Selby Lane, Atherton, CA 94025, (415) 593-1661, MA 63 Stanford Univ; MA 75 Univ of Santa Clara; ED 81 (NS) Univ of San Francisco; Sp-Lang Path, Private Practice, **SLP**

Ratto, Mrs Lorene Lynne 717 Crossway Road, Burlingame, CA 94010-3704, (415) 723-6818, BS 82 AZ St Univ; MS 84 AZ St Univ; Aud, Stanford Univ, **A**

Ratto-Joy, Mrs Elsie M 639 St Frances, Pleasanton, CA 94566-7927, (415) 846-7462, BA 77 Univ of the Pacific; MA 78 Univ of the Pacific; 88–Sp-Lang Path, Childrens Hosp, **SLP**

Rattray, Mrs Kathryn Jean 308 Garfield Street, Fort Atkinson, WI 53538, (414) 563-9521, BS 72 Univ of WI - Oshkosh; MS 86 Univ of WI - Whitewater; **SLP**

Ratusnik, Dr David L 1681 Oneco Avenue, Winter Park, FL 32789, (305) 275-2121, BS 71 Northwestern Univ; MA 72 Northwestern Univ; PH 74 (NS) Northwestern Univ; Prof, University of Central Florida, **SLP**

Rau, Charlene E 12049 Phoenix Drive, Cerritos, CA 90701, (818) 575-2318, BA 65 San Diego St Univ; MA 76 CA St Univ - Long Beach; Sp-Lang Path, LA Co Supt of Sch, **SLP**

Rau, Mrs Dale Pruim 925 Santiago Drive, Placentia, CA 92670, (714) 558-5591, BA 78 CA St Univ - Fullerton; MA 80 CA St Univ - Fullerton; Sp-Lang Path, Santa Ana USD, **SLP**

Rau, Mrs Elaine K 306 North Emerson Street, Mount Prospect, IL 60056, (312) 550-3724, BA 68 Barnard Coll; MS 71 Washington Univ; **SLP ACE**

Rau, Dr Marie Costa 3610 S W Alice Street, Portland, OR 97219, (503) 220-8262, BA 58 Marygove Coll; MS 62 Univ of MI - Ann Arbor; PH 86 (Urban Studies/Gerontology) Portland St Univ; Sp-Lang Path, Portland VA Med Cen, **SLP**

Raubicheck, Letitia E 120 East Hartsdale Avenue, Hartsdale, NY 10530, **SLP F LM**

Rauch, Rita A 915 Harrison, Lincoln Park, MI 48146, (313) 582-6128, BA 73 Central MI Univ; MA 76 Central MI Univ; MA 79 Eastern MI Univ; Sp-Lang Path, Dearborn Public Schools, **SLP**

Rauch, Mrs Roberta J 3111 Warrington Road, Shaker Heights, OH 44120, (216) 761-4224, BA 63 Ursinus Coll; MA 80 Case Western Reserve Univ; 82–Sp-Lang Path, Meridia Huron Hosp, **SLP ACE**

Rauchle, Mrs Judith Lee 12505 Hornbeam Drive, Dallas, TX 75243, (214) 231-0718, BA 70 Memphis St Univ; MS 71 Memphis St Univ; 86–Sp-Lang Path, Richardson ISD, **SLP**

Rauch-Mahoney, Christine 10692 Riviera Place N E, Seattle, WA 98125, (206) 323-5770, BS 78 Univ of WA; MS 80 Univ of WA; Aud, Wash Otology Neurology Group, **A**

Rauchwerk, Mrs Starling Mara 4 Willow Road, Holmdel, NJ 07733, (201) 946-2632, BA 76 Rutger's St Univ - Douglas Coll; MS 81 Columbia Univ Teachers Coll; 87–Sp-Lang Path, Monmouth Rehab, **SLP**

Rauh, Linda A N85 W17948 Ann Avenue #6, Menomonee Falls, WI 53051, (414) 255-9303, BS 83 Univ of WI - Milwaukee; MS 85 Univ of WI - Madison; 86–Sp-Lang Path, St Joseph's Hosp, **SLP**

Raupp, Mrs Colleen Campbell 1611 Gateway Street, Middleton, WI 53562, (414) 544-8820, BS 77 Marquette Univ; MS 79 Univ of WI - Madison; SLP, Waukesha Sch Dist, **SLP**

Rausch, Mrs Kathleen S 1796 Kinglet Court, Costa Mesa, CA 92626, (714) 751-4762, BS 73 Univ of AZ; MS 75 Univ of AZ; **SLP**

Rausch, Dr Marie A 5295 South Moorland Road, New Berlin, WI 53151, (414) 422-1556, BS 66 Marquette Univ; MA 68 Univ of WI - Milwaukee; PH 75 (NS) Univ of CO - Boulder; **SLP**

Rausch, Shelia Marc-Aurel 151 Lanipo Drive, Kailua, HI 96734-3228, (808) 262-4203, **SLP**

Rauscher, Mrs Ann Wall 7225 South Hampton Road, Lincoln, NE 68506, (402) 489-4148, BS 69 Univ of NE - Lincoln; MA 70 Univ of NE - Lincoln; **SLP**

Rauscher, Debra Lynn 18 Clamshell Road, Clinton, MA 01510-4211, (508) 562-9144, BS 79 Worcester St Coll; MS 83 Worcester St Coll; ME 87 Fitchburg St Coll; 80–Sp/Lang Path, Hudson Pub Schs, **SLP**

Rauss, Laura C 10800 Rose Avenue #20, Los Angeles, CA 90034, (213) 829-6592, BS 68 OH St Univ; MS 69 Univ of MI - Ann Arbor; Clin Assessor, NeuroCare Inc, **SLP**

Rauterkus, Mrs Mary Beth 511 West 7th Street, Red Wing, MN 55066, (612) 388-7303, BS 80 Univ of WI - River Falls; MS 81 Univ of WI - River Falls; SLP, Anoka-Hennepin Ind Sch Dist, **SLP**

Ravalli, Susan Linda 866 Lancaster Street, Albany, NY 12203, BS 84 Coll of Saint Rose; MS 86 Coll of Saint Rose; 86–Sp-Lang Path, Sp & Reading Improvement Ctr Inc, **SLP**

Ravens, Eleanor I 115 South Kansas Avenue, Marceline, MO 64658, **SLP**

Raver, Mrs Cynthia Litman 6585 N Cortlawn Circle, Golden Valley, MN 55426, (612) 545-5363, BS 59 Univ of MN - Minneap-St Paul; MA 85 Univ of MN - Minneap-St Paul; 85–Aud, MN Otolaryngology, **A**

Ravin, Judith Barbara 116 Woodhollow Drive, Marlton, NJ 08053, (717) 287-8649, BS 82 Syracuse Univ; MA 85 Temple Univ-Tyler Sch of Art; **A**

Ravlin, Mrs Susan A Route 4 Box 203, Christiansburg, VA 24073, (703) 639-9639, BA 72 MI St Univ; MA 73 MI St Univ; Sp-Lang Path, Home Link, **SLP**

Ravski, Barbara 11 Milan Road, Woodbridge, CT 06525, (203) 397-8869, BA 70 CUNY - City College; MS 71 PA St Univ - Univ Park; Supervisor Clinical Services, **SLP**

Ravsten, Mrs Mildred T Brigham Young University, 129 Tlrb, Provo, UT 84602, (801) 378-6458, BA 52 Brigham Young Univ; MS 71 Brigham Young Univ; Asst Prof Ed Psy, Brigham Young Univ, **SLP**

Rawiszer, Steven J 129 Cerrito Drive, Folsom, CA 95630, (916) 322-2950, BA 77 A321; MA 79 CA St Univ - Fresno; Aud, CA St Dept of Hlth Serv, **A**

Rawlings, Diane Lynne 5200 Desoto Parkway, Sarasota, FL 34234, (813) 355-7637, BA 81 OH St Univ; MA 83 OH St Univ; SLP, Happiness House Rehabilitation, **SLP**

Rawlings-Boyd, Joan 3081 Whitbeck Boulevard, Eugene, OR 97405, (503) 686-7085, BS 74 ID St Univ; MA 78 WA St Univ; 88–Sp/Lang Path, Eugene Hearing and Speech Ctr, **SLP**

Rawlins, J'Lene 227 1/2 North 400 East, Logan, UT 84321, (801) 399-3748, BS 79 UT St Univ; MS 83 UT St Univ; 81–Sp/Lang Path, Utah Sch for the Blind, **SLP**

Rawson, Craig Allen 11611 Nelson Street, Loma Linda, CA 92354, (714) 796-5745, BS 75 Loma Linda Univ - Riverside; MS 84 Univ of Redlands; Aud, Private Practice, **A**

Rawson, Mark L 132 North Serrano Avenue, Los Angeles, CA 90004, (213) 388-6661, BA 70 Univ of CA - Los Angeles; MA 71 Univ of CA - Los Angeles; SLP, Los Angeles USD, **SLP**

Ray, Mrs Amy Sue 3750 Quaker Ridge Drive, Meridian, ID 83642, (208) 888-3406, BA 82 Eastern WA Univ; MS 83 Eastern WA Univ; Sp-Lang Path, Malheur Co Ed Serv Dist, **SLP**

Ray, Beverly N P O Box 3444, Brookhaven, MS 39601, (601) 833-8363, BS 71 Univ Southern MS-Hattiesburg; MS 72 Univ Southern MS-Hattiesburg; Sp/Lang Path, Sp Path Assoc, **SLP**

Ray, Cathy Coldren 1915 Monticello Place, Edwardsville, IL 62025, (618) 656-7834, BS 80 Southern IL Univ-Edwardsvill; MS 81 Southern IL Univ-Edwardsvill; Sp-Lang Path, Spec Sch Dist of St Louis Co, **SLP**

Ray, Mrs Deidre Wright 148 Toyon Drive, Vallejo, CA 94590, (707) 553-9254, BA 86 CA St Univ - Long Beach; MA 88 CA St Univ - Long Beach; 88–Sp-Lang Path, Fairfield-Suisun USD

Ray, Mrs Gayle C 13639 Garner Lane, Chico, CA 95926, (916) 891-2793, BA 68 Montclair St Coll; MA 74 CA St Univ - Chico; SLP, Butte County Supt of Schools, **SLP**

Ray, Georgine Haines Saint Joseph's Hospital, Children's Rehabilitative Services, 124 West Thomas Road, Phoenix, AZ 85013, (602) 263-7140, BS 79 AZ St Univ; MS 83 AZ St Univ; Coord-Sp/Hrng Dept, St Joseph's Hosp, **A**

Ray, Mrs Janice K 5104 Cinderella Drive, Oklahoma City, OK 73129, (405) 737-4461, BA 77 Univ of OK - Norman; MS 79 Univ of OK - OK City; SLP, Mid-Del Sch Syst, **SLP**

Ray, Joan P 8529 Dresden Drive, Knoxville, TN 37923, (615) 917-1349, BA 79 Univ of FL; MA 81 Univ of TN - Knoxville; Sp/Lang Path, Ft Sanders Reg Med Cen, **SLP ACE**

Ray, John G 316 Beach Plum Court, Tuckerton Meadows, Tuckerton, NJ 08087, (201) 244-3100, BA 70 Parsons Coll; MS 74 Auburn Univ - Auburn; MA 80 Trenton St Coll; Aud, Garden St Rehab Hosp, **A ACE**

Ray, Judy C 279 Lustrosos Street, Oceanside, CA 92056, (619) 721-0142, BA 57 Univ of Denver; MA 75 Univ of MT; Supv/SLP, Sd Chldn Hosp Hlth, **SLP**

Ray, Mrs Kristin Elaine 1222 Settle Avenue, San Jose, CA 95125, (408) 998-2370, MA 80 San Jose St Univ; **SLP**

Ray, Lorie Renee 5104 N E Mallory Avenue, Portland, OR 97211, (503) 280-5860, **SLP**

Ray, Mrs Marsha W 121 10th Avenue, Huntington, WV 25701, (304) 525-9460, BA 64 Marshall Univ; MA 73 Marshall Univ; SLP, Cahell Co Pub Sch, **SLP**

Ray, Nancy J P O Box 130, Cisne, IL 62823, (618) 673-2701, BS 78 Southern IL Univ -Carbondale; MS 81 Eastern IL Univ; Sp-Lang Path, Greenview Christian Sch, **SLP**

Ray, Mrs Susan Jordan 1710 East 24th #1, Hutchinson, KS 67502, (316) 663-2761, BS 83 Ball St Univ; MA 84 Ball St Univ; Sp-Lang Path, Reno Co Educ Cooperative, **SLP**

Raycraft, Mrs Laura Beth 644 Magnolia, Chatham, IL 62629, BS 84 IL St Univ - Normal; MS 85 IL St Univ - Normal; 86–Sp-Lang Path, Memorial Med Ctr, **SLP**

Raycraft, Melissa Lee 4111 Northeast Davidson Rd, Apartment 390, Kansas City, MO 64116, (517) 792-5693, BS 85 Western MI Univ; MA 86 Western MI Univ; **A**

Raye, Mrs Janine Solkov 13 Joan Avenue, Novato, CA 94947, (415) 892-4746, BS 78 Kent St Univ; MS 87 Northern AZ Univ; SLP, Team Rehab, **SLP**

Rayel, Doreen Ann 404 Woodtick Road 1-R, Waterbury, CT 06705, (203) 754-6971, BA 84 Univ of CT; MS 86 Southern CT St Univ; 86–Sp-Lang Path, Waterbury PS, **SLP**

Raykovics, Patricia Marie 8741 Harperpoint Drive #C, Cincinnati, OH 45249-2415, (513) 489-3140, BS 82 Edinboro Univ of PA; MS 84 Indiana Univ of PA; **SLP**

Rayman, Naomi Sinai 16 Sherwood Court, Kentfield, CA 94904, (415) 454-5756, **SLP**

Raymer, Mrs Anastasia Moynihan 5437 Brockie Street, Virginia Beach, VA 23464, (301) 454-6918, BS 80 Univ of WI - Madison; MA 82 Univ of FL; Superv, U of MD-Sp & Hrng Cl, **SLP**

Raymer, Anne Church 15827 Haynes Road, Laurel, MD 20707-3305, (301) 441-8928, BS 73 IA St Univ; MA 82 Univ of MD - College Park; Sp-Lang Path, Private Practice, **SLP**

Raymon, Mrs Ruth R 13 Merrymount Drive, North Dartmouth, MA 02747, (617) 992-7345, BS 74 Boston Univ; MA 75 Univ of Denver; Sp/Lang Path, St Vincents Home, **SLP**

Raymond, Mrs Carol A 1111 Fieldgate Road, Lawrenceville, GA 30244, (404) 297-5516, BS 71 Univ of GA; ME 73 Univ of GA; SLP/Aud, Dekalb Gen Hosp, **SLP ACE**

Raymond, Charlean 2512 Chellwood Park Dr N E, Albuquerque, NM 87112, (505) 268-4592, BA 79 San Diego St Univ; MS 81 Univ of NM; Project Aud, **A**

Raymond, Mrs Debra Sue 25 Pleasant Drive, Niantic, CT 06357, (203) 739-3218, BS 81 SUNY - Coll at Geneseo; MS 83 Southern CT St Univ; Sp-Lang Path, Southeastern Conn Hrng & Sp Ctr, **SLP**

Raymond, Henry A Audiology & Speech Pathology Services, Veterans Administration Medical Center, 1481 West 10th Street, Indianapolis, IN 46202, (317) 635-7401, BS 64 Purdue Univ - West Lafayette; MS 74 Purdue Univ - West Lafayette; Aud, VA Med Cen, **A**

Raymond, Jennifer Carniglia 712 Canyon Drive, Pacifica, CA 94044, (415) 282-2551, Sp-Lang Path, Mills Mem Hosp, **SLP**

Raymond, John W 800 Washington #3, Woodstock, IL 60098, (815) 338-5221, **SLP**

Raymond, Marie E 7719 Redding, Houston, TX 77036, (713) 497-7600, BA 64 Mount Holyoke Coll; MA 65 Syracuse Univ; MA 66 Univ of MA - Amherst; Sp-Lang Path, Houston ISD, **SLP**

Raymond, Mrs Maryann Perugino 277 Fieldboro Drive, Lawrenceville, NJ 08648, (609) 394-2255, BS 81 Bloomsburg Univ of PA; MS 82 Bloomsburg Univ of PA; 86–Sp-Lang Path, The Newgrange Sch, **SLP**

Raymond, Sandra L Speech & Language Associates, 5 Walnut Avenue, Suite 2, Stoughton, MA 02072, (617) 344-6502, BA 73 Univ of MA - Amherst; MS 78 Univ of RI; Co-Dir, Sp/Lang Assoc, **SLP**

Raymond, Susan Benjamin 2910 E Laurel Lane, Phoenix, AZ 85028, (602) 971-3319, BA 83 IN Univ - Bloomington; MA 84 Case Western Reserve Univ; 88–Sp-Lang Path, Southwest Human Dev, **SLP ACE**

Raymond, Susan J C 14576 Vintage Drive, San Diego, CA 92129, (612) 871-8011, BA 66 Univ of MN - Minneap-St Paul; MA 75 Univ of MN - Minneap-St Paul; SLP, San Diego Public Schools, **SLP**

Raymonda, Mrs Barbara Jean 409 North Bellinger Street, Herkimer, NY 13350, (315) 866-1977, BS 81 SUNY - Coll at Geneseo; MS 86 Coll of Saint Rose; **SLP**

Raymonds-Sharp, Marianne 3511 Tricklewood Drive S E, Grand Rapids, MI 49506, (616) 455-7300, BS 76 Marquette Univ; MS 77 Marquette Univ; Dir Brain Inj Ch Care Prog, Butterworth Hosp, **SLP**

Raysby, Cheryl A 3712 South Terry #302, Sioux Falls, SD 57106, (605) 336-1840, BA 80 Univ of SD - Vermillion; MA 81 Univ of SD - Vermillion; SLP, Crippled Childn's Hosp & Sch, **SLP**

Raysby, Julie L 807 West Street Apartment 13, Yankton, SD 57078, (605) 665-6820, MA 88 Univ of SD - Vermillion; 88–Aud, Yankton Ear Nose & Throat

Raz, Dr Israel Bio-Logic Systems Corp, One Bio-Logic Plaza, Mundelein, IL 60060, (312) 949-5200, BA 72 Tel Aviv Univ - Israel; MA 74 Tel Aviv Univ - Israel; PH 77 (NS) Univ of KS; Dir of Applications, Bio-Logic Systems Corp, **A**

Razum, Cheryl A 1644 Waterbury Road, Lakewood, OH 44107, (216) 221-0260, BA 77 Cleveland St Univ; MA 78 Cleveland St Univ; Sp-Lang Path, Lake Co Bd Ment Retard, **SLP**

Rdzanek, Irena R 190 Estrellita Drive, Fort Myers Beach, FL 33931, (813) 261-7116, BS 76 SUNY - Coll at Geneseo; MA 78 SUNY - Coll at Geneseo; Aud, Miracle Ear Hearing Aid Ctr, **A**

Rea, Dr James R College Of Wooster, Wishart Hall, Wooster, OH 44691, (216) 263-2541, BA 53 Otterbein Coll; MA 68 OH St Univ; PH 78 (NS) OH Univ - Athens; Professor Speech Communication, College of Wooster, **SLP ACE**

Rea, Renee Riley 3032 Jarrard, Houston, TX 77005, (713) 664-0981, BA 84 Baylor Univ; MA 86 Univ of Houston - Univ Park; **SLP**

Rea, Sharon Patricia 340 North 5th Avenue, Des Plaines, IL 60016, (312) 399-7360, MA 83 Northern IL Univ - De Kalb; SLP, Park Ridge Sch Dist 64, **SLP**

Reach, Lynn 313 East Chestnut Street, Second Floor, Coatesville, PA 19320, (215) 384-5504, BS 79 West Chester Univ of PA; OM 86 Hahneman Medical Coll; **SLP**

Read, Allison L 5848 North Main Street, Sylvania, OH 43560, (517) 263-8931, BA 75 Eastern MI Univ; MA 76 Eastern MI Univ; Supvr of Spec Educ, Lenawee Inter Sch Dist, **SLP**

Read, Mrs C Renee Goodin 104 Brycewood Circle, Hattiesburg, MS 39402, (601) 264-3545, BA 85 Southeastern LA Univ; MS 87 Univ Southern MS-Hattiesburg

Read, Mrs Laurie Smith 132 Wildflower Avenue, Vallejo, CA 94591, (707) 642-9518, BA 77 CA St Univ - Sacramento; MA 83 San Diego St Univ; Sp-Lang Path, Vallejo City School District, **SLP**

Read, Mrs M Margaret 139 Day Street, Auburndale, MA 02166, (617) 862-7500, BS 58 Western MI Univ; MS 61 Univ of WI - Madison; Sp-Lang Path, Lexington PS, **SLP A**

Reade, Mrs Robin L 448 Fall Mountain Road, Bristol, CT 06010, (203) 584-9236, BS 72 Univ of Bridgeport; MS 74 Southern CT St Univ; Sp-Lang Path, Bristol Bd of Ed, **SLP**

Readecker, Alece A Center Director, Timbre Hear & Sp Ctr Inc, 13520 J East 40 Highway, Independence, MO 64055, (816) 478-4040, BS 76 Central MO St Univ; MS 77 Central MO St Univ; 86–Dir, Timbre Hearing & Speech Ctr, **A**

Readhead, Donna Geralyn 7755 North 19th Avenue, Phoenix, AZ 85021, (602) 870-1309, BS 83 Northern AZ Univ; MS 85 Northern AZ Univ; **SLP**

Reading, Patricia 10153 Parkwood Drive #3, Cupertino, CA 95014, (408) 866-5204, BA 66 Univ of IA; MA 67 Univ of IA; Sp-Lang Path, Private Practice, **SLP**

Reagan, Mrs Deborah A 3305 19th Street N W, Washington, DC 20010, (301) 341-6448, **SLP**

Reagan, Mrs Sharon S 2110 Timber Creek, Manhattan, KS 66502, (913) 539-6377, BS 67 Univ of Tulsa; MA 71 Univ of Tulsa; Sp-Lang Path, USD #383, **SLP**

Reagan, William G 17538 Covello Street, Van Nuys, CA 91406, (818) 896-2474, BA 73 CA St Univ - Northridge; MA 75 CA St Univ - Northridge; Sp-Lang Path, Hathaway Children Service, **SLP A**

Reagor, Terrylea M 117 Greenwood, Helena, MT 59601, **SLP**

Real, Mrs Karen K 701 Coventry Lane, Phoenixville, PA 19460, (215) 546-6050, BA 70 Temple Univ-Tyler Sch of Art; MA 72 Temple Univ-Tyler Sch of Art; Aud, Locust Audiology, **A**

Realy, Janice Scully Route 33 Box 3, Stanardsville, VA 22973, (804) 296-9161, ME 79 Univ of VA - Charlottesville; Aud, Pediatric Associates, **A**

Reams, Kenneth L 1119 Polk Boulevard, Des Moines, IA 50311, (515) 255-2173, BA 58 Univ of IA; MA 62 Univ of IA; Aud, VA Med Cen Des Moines, **SLP A**

Reams, Virginia F 5 Rocky Brook Drive, North Easton, MA 02356, (617) 824-5881, BA 74 Mount Saint Mary Coll; MA 76 NY Univ; Superv of Sp & Hrng, Com of Mass-Dever St Sch, **SLP**

Reams, Mrs Virginia K 810 17th Street, Fairbury, NE 68352, (402) 729-2921, BS 62 Univ of KS; MA 64 Univ of KS; **SLP**

Reanier, Mrs Carol Cook 15514 64th N E, Bothell, WA 98011, BA 64; MA 69; SLP, Seattle Pub Sch, **SLP**

Reap, Anne Roussel 15 Purchase Street #1-A, Rye, NY 10580, (914) 967-1098, BS 84 Univ of NH; ME 86 Univ of VA - Charlottesville; **A**

Rearden, Eileen Marie Rd #2 Box 2539, Fleetwood, PA 19522, (215) 779-7111, BS 80 West Chester Univ of PA; MA 86 West Chester Univ of PA; 81–Sp-Lang Path, Berks Co Intermediate Unit, **SLP**

Reardon, Mrs Catherine 908 Gay Street, Phoenixville, PA 19460, (215) 935-2913, BA 74 Temple Univ-Tyler Sch of Art; MA 76 Temple Univ-Tyler Sch of Art; Aud, Private Practice, **A**

Reardon, John J M 5078 Carriage Lane, Lockport, NY 14094, (716) 439-6169, BA 75 SUNY - Coll at Oneonta; MA 77 Northern IL Univ - De Kalb; Dir, Niagara Co Sp-Hrng-Lang Cen, **SLP**

Reardon, Mrs Nina A Route 1 Box 11, 2858 East 29th Road, Seneca, IL 61360-9705, (815) 357-8153, BS 82 IL St Univ - Normal; MS 87 IL St Univ - Normal

Rearic, Betsy Jane 109-C Josephine Street, Minersville, PA 17954, BA 82 Duquesne Univ; 88–Sp-Lang Path, Private Practice, **SLP**

Rearick, Mrs Sarah Whitsett 9016 Piney Grove Drive, Fairfax, VA 22031, (703) 494-6677, BA 75 Univ of NC - Greensboro; MA 77 Univ of NC - Greensboro; SLP, Prince William County Schools, **SLP**

Reaser, Mrs Ann R 221 Shenandoah Trail, Warner Robins, GA 31088, (912) 929-8434, BA 56 Univ of AL-Tuscaloosa; 87–Sp-Lang Path, Houston Speech Sch, **SLP**

Reasonover, Patricia Dianne 901 Princeton Road, Apt 1403, Madisonville, KY 42431, (502) 821-7469, BS 80 Western KY Univ; ME 84 0184; **A**

Reath, Mrs Lisa Ann 320 East River #12, Grand Ledge, MI 48837, (517) 627-8675, BA 85 MI St Univ; MA 87 MI St Univ

Reber, Mrs Clarice K Speech And Hearing Clinic, Indiana University Of Pa, Indiana, PA 15705, (412) 357-2451, BS 65 Northwestern Univ; MS 66 Univ of MI - Ann Arbor; Asst Prof, IN U of Pa, **SLP A**

Reber, Mrs Mary Katharine 2500 Elizabethtown Road, Elizabethtown, PA 17022, (717) 367-8488, BS 80 Bloomsburg Univ of PA; MS 81 Bloomsburg Univ of PA; Sp-Lang Path, Private Practice, **SLP**

Reboli, Jean O 16818 160th Court SE, Renton, WA 98058, (206) 235-7939, BA 82 Univ of OK - Norman; MS 85 Univ of OK Medical Center; 88–Sp-Lang Path, Univ of Washington

Rebstock, Therese E 4204 Eureka #D, Metairie, LA 70001, (504) 456-9538, BS 82 LA St Univ - Baton Rouge; OM 87 LA St Univ - N O Medical Ctr; Sp-Lang Path, Jefferson Paris School, **SLP**

Recchia, Mrs Audrey T 13209 Silver Saddle Lane, Poway, CA 92064, (619) 487-1180, BS 73 SUNY - Center at Albany; MA 76 San Diego St Univ; 76–SLP, Poway Unif Sch Dist, **SLP**

Recchia, Jayne 62 Jamaica Street, Jamaica Plain, MA 02130, (617) 787-0566, BA 71 CUNY - Lehman Coll; ME 72 Northeastern Univ; **A**

Rech, Karl H Ear Nose & Throat Associates, OF Oneonta Pc, 41-45 Dietz Street, Oneonta, NY 13820, (607) 432-1355, BA 77 SUNY - Coll at Plattsburgh; MS 79 Syracuse Univ; Clin Rehab Aud, ENT Assoc of Oneonta, **A ACE**

Reck, Joelene S 4425 Meadow View East, Brookfield, WI 53005, (414) 251-8140, MS 74 Univ of WI - Milwaukee; Sp-Lang Path, School Dist of Menomonee Falls, **SLP**

Reckell, Mrs Barbara J 2960 Cherithbrook Drive, Mason, MI 48854, (517) 887-3235, BS 72 Northern MI Univ; MA 74 MI St Univ; SLP, Lansing School District, **SLP**

Reckord, Catherine Elizabeth 1316 Cedarcroft Road, Baltimore, MD 21239, (301) 522-5450, BS 83 OH Univ - Athens; MS 85 PA St Univ - Univ Park; 86–Sp-Lang Path, Hearing & Speech Agency of Metro Balto Inc, **SLP**

Records, Mrs Bobbye R 6521 Chilton, North Richland Hills, TX 76180, (817) 481-5575, BS 74 Univ of TX - Austin; MS 75 Univ of North TX; Sp/Lang Path, Grapevine-Colleyville ISD, **SLP**

Records, Nancy L 374 Westgate Street #2, Iowa City, IA 52240, (319) 351-4100, BS 75 OH Univ - Athens; MS 76 Univ of WI - Milwaukee; **SLP**

Rector, Kathryn L 1541 Red Fern Drive, Pittsburgh, PA 15241, (412) 941-4434, BS 70 OH Univ - Athens; MA 73 Kent St Univ; Dir/Pres, Crossroads Sp & Hrng Inc, **SLP**

Rector, Mrs Susan Ann 620 Forest Avenue, St Louis, MO 63135, (314) 521-7456, BS 78 Southeast MO St Univ; MA 80 Southeast MO St Univ; Sp-Lang Path, Wentzville Sch Dist, **SLP**

Redd, Mrs Jill 4651 Forest Avenue S E, Mercer Island, WA 98040-4306, (206) 236-1298, **SLP**

Redd, Phillip M Audiology Service 126, VA Hospital, 1201 N W 16th Street, Miami, FL 33125, (305) 324-3148, MS 72 Univ of South FL; **A**

Reddan, Patricia M 123-11 5th Avenue, College Point, NY 11356, (718) 353-6378, BA 86 CUNY - Queens Coll; MA 88 CUNY - Hunter Coll; 88–Sp-Lang Path, Hospital for Joint Diseases Orthopaedic Inst, **SLP**

Reddell, Dr Rayford C 1234 Divisadero Street, San Francisco, CA 94115, (415) 921-7658, PH 63 (NS) Stanford Univ; Exec Dir, San Francisco Hrng/Sp Cen, **A**

Redden, Camille Josephine 124 Laguadia Avenue, Staten Island, NY 10314, (718) 680-2042, BA 79 CUNY - Hunter Coll; MA 81 CUNY - Hunter Coll; Sp-Lang Path, Seaview Hosp & Home, **SLP**

Redden, Mrs Joan R 25 Congress Terrace, Milford, MA 01757, (617) 473-1097, BS 66 Boston Coll; ME 69 Northeastern Univ; Exec VP, Gr Milford Chamber of Commerce, **SLP**

Redden, Dr Robert B 25 Congress Terrace, Milford, MA 01757, (617) 473-2646, BS 64 Northeastern Univ; ME 69 Northeastern Univ; ED 73 (NS) Boston Univ; 88–Sp-Lang Path, Northeastern Univ, **A**

Redden, William J 912 North Zeyn #2, Anaheim, CA 92805, (714) 533-9693, MA 86 CA St Univ - Fullerton; 87–Sp-Lang Path, B A Landes PhD & Assoc, **SLP**

Redder, Alice T 37 Coral Tree Court, Society Hill, Lawrenceville, NJ 08648, (609) 896-9500, BA 73 CUNY - Queens Coll; MA 75 Univ of MD - College Park; Sp-Lang Path, St Lawrence Rehab Cen, **SLP**

Reddick, Genevieve Nottingham 4354 Hiawatha Street, Jacksonville, FL 32210, (904) 384-8235, BA 76 Tulane Univ; MS 78 FL St Univ; Sp-Lang Path, Duval County Schs, **SLP**

Reddin, Mrs Marcelle Cherry 14378 S W 97th Terrace, Miami, FL 33186, (305) 654-9557, BS 85 LA St Univ - Baton Rouge; MA 87 LA St Univ - Baton Rouge; Sp-Lang Path, ABC Speech & Language Therapy, **SLP**

Redding, Mrs Marguerite S 14215 Peacan Park Lane #8, El Cajon, CA 92021, (619) 561-5706, BA 62 2908; MA 64 2908; **A LM**

Redding, Mrs Sandra Lea 29838 Quail Hollow Lane, Valley Center, CA 92082, (619) 749-1631, BA 81 San Diego St Univ; MA 83 San Diego St Univ; Sp-Lang Path, Valley Center Union Sch Dist, **SLP**

Reddington, Christine Ann 1300 Crown Point Avenue, Apartment 24, Norman, OK 73072, (405) 793-8738, BA 83 Univ of OK Medical Center; MS 85 Univ of OK Medical Center; **SLP**

Redeker, Mrs Janet Wollangk W 9177 Lake Emily Road, Waupun, WI 53963, (414) 324-3288, BS 79 Univ of WI - Oshkosh; OM 80 Univ of WI - Oshkosh; SLP, CES #6, **SLP**

Redenbaugh, Margaret Ann 11001 S E 24th Place, Bellevue, WA 98004, (206) 455-2198, BA 81 Univ of WA; MS 84 Univ of WA; Sp-Lang Path, Private Practice, **SLP ACE**

Redfearn, Barbara 314 Buckner Drive, Wilmington, NC 28403, (919) 343-7218, BA 66 FL St Univ; ME 76 Univ of FL; Cl Dir, New Hanover Mem Hosp, **SLP**

Redfearn, Mrs Deborah P 1670 Woodside Drive, East Lansing, MI 48823, (517) 353-8780, BA 78 MI St Univ; MA 79 MI St Univ; Sp-Lang Path Supvr, MI State Univ, **SLP**

Redfield, Susan Stewart 6A Denise Drive, Latham, NY 12110, (518) 827-4117, BA 78 SUNY - Coll at Plattsburgh; MA 83 SUNY - Coll at Geneseo; Sp-Lang Path, BOCES, **SLP**

Redington, Mrs Barbara L 421 Nottingham Drive, Northumberland, PA 17857, (717) 286-3725, BS 73 Edinboro Univ of PA; MS 77 Bloomsburg Univ of PA; SLP, Csiu 16, **SLP**

Redington, Mrs Mary O 13309 Locksley Lane, Silver Spring, MD 20904, (301) 924-4041, BA 62 Univ of IA; MA 63 Univ of IA; SLP, Mont Co Pub Sch, **SLP**

Redington-Gilroy, Mrs Eileen Marie 304 Doyleson Avenue, Endwell, NY 13760, (607) 798-5255, BS 82 Marywood Coll; MS 84 PA St Univ - Univ Park; Sp-Lang Path, Lourdes Hosp, **SLP**

Redino, Michelle A 11 Huntleigh Circle, Amherst, NY 14226, MS 80; Sp-Lang Path, Cantalician Cen for Learning, **SLP**

Redler, Sherry P 28 Lockwood Circle, Fairfield, CT 06430, (203) 384-0344, BA 54 Adelphi Univ; MS 71 Southern CT St Univ, OM 79 Southern CT St Univ; Aud, Fairfield Pub Sch, **SLP A**

Redmerski, Mrs Christina Murdza 95 Liberty Street, Trenton, NJ 08611, (609) 387-2200, BS 77 Trenton St Coll; MA 82 Trenton St Coll; Sp-Lang Path, Beverly Bd of Educ, **SLP**

Redmon, Melinda A 16550 Shady View Lane, Los Gatos, CA 95030, (408) 288-7777, BA 77 Univ of CA - Santa Barbara; MA 79 Univ of MA - Amherst; Aud, Ear Med Cl, **A**

Redmond, Mrs Beatrice Myers 5957 Brown Bark Drive, Orlando, FL 32822, (407) 898-6997, BA 79 Univ of Northern CO; MA 80 Univ of TN - Knoxville; 81–Aud, Orange Co Pub Sch, **A ACE**

Redmond, Jacquelyn Ann 2700 Fifth Avenue #3, Stevens Point, WI 54481, (715) 341-8443, MS 88 Univ of WI - Stevens Point

Redmond, Mrs Janice Munday 270 Clinton Street, Watertown, NY 13601, (919) 484-2454, BS 62 Univ of CO - Boulder; MS 64 CO St Univ; **SLP**

Redmond, Kathleen J 1711 West Jarvis #1F, Chicago, IL 60626, (312) 508-0733, BA 74 Univ of WI - Milwaukee; MA 77 Univ of MN - Minneap-St Paul; 85–Sp-Lang Path, Univ of IL Coll of Medicine, **SLP**

Redmond, Mrs Linda D P O Box 72, Calais, VT 05648, (802) 476-6617, BA 70 Univ of VT; MS 72 Univ of VT; Sp/Lang Path, Barre Town Elem Sch, **SLP**

Redmond, Mary Catherine 40 Dietz Court, Kingston, NY 12401, (914) 331-0066, MS 86 SUNY - Coll at Plattsburgh; MA 85 SUNY - Coll at Plattsburgh; 87–Aud, NYU Med Ctr, **A**

Redmond-Tillotson, Barbara 6427 Quimby Road, Dalzell, SC 29040, (803) 499-2328, BS 78 Univ of IL - Urbana; MS 79 Univ of IL - Urbana; **SLP**

Redmon-Trame, Mrs Billie 6242 Shagbark, Loveland, OH 45140, (513) 625-5478, BS 79 Bowling Green St Univ; MS 84 Miami Univ - Oxford; Sp-Lang Path, Clermont Northeastern Schools, **SLP**

Redstone, Fran 640 Mapleton Avenue, Boulder, CO 80301, (201) 337-7842, BA 67 CUNY - Hunter Coll; MA 72 CUNY - Hunter Coll; Sp-Lang Path, Private Practice, **SLP**

Redwine, Linda Simpson 2686 South Sable Way, Aurora, CO 80014, (303) 869-2257, BS 69 TX Tech Univ; MA 79 Univ of CO - Boulder; Supervisor SLP & Audiology, St Lukes Hospital, **SLP A ACE**

Redwine, Ruth W 2510 Glenhaven Drive #B, Midwest City, OK 73110, BA 26 Univ of OK - Norman; MA 41 Northwestern Univ; **SLP LM**

Redwood-Pilgrim, Mrs Rosemary 718 Downing Street, Parlin, NJ 08859, (201) 525-9638, BA 84 Hofstra Univ; MA 88 CUNY - Brooklyn Coll; 86–Sp-Lang Path, Newark Bd of Educ

Reeb, Paul R R R 4 Box 352, Muscatine, IA 52761, (319) 264-2899, BS 65 Northeast MO St Univ; MA 74 Northeast MO St Univ; SLP, AEA #9, **SLP**

Reece, Joann M 5132 Penn Avenue South, Minneapolis, MN 55419, **SLP**

Reece, Paul A 7009 Santa Rita Court, Fort Worth, TX 76133, (817) 346-3247, MS 75 TX Christian Univ; President, Self Employed, **SLP**

Reece, Richard E 5132 Penn Avenue South, Minneapolis, MN 55419, **SLP**

Reece, Teryl Lyn 2634 South 10th, Abilene, TX 79605, (915) 691-7300, BS 78 OK St Univ; MS 80 Univ of OK Medical Center; 80–Sp/Lang Path, W Tx Rehab Cen, **SLP**

Reed, Agnes Faye 10440 Irvington Street, Commerce City, CO 80022, (303) 654-0522, MS 82 UT St Univ; Sp-Lang Path, **SLP**

Reed, Mrs Alice N 4270 Keim Road, Lisle, IL 60532, (312) 654-1391, BS 74 Miami Univ - Oxford; MA 77 Northern IL Univ - De Kalb; Aud, Auditory Serv Inc, **A**

Reed, Andrea Brown Cigna Health Plan, 10861 Cherry Street, Los Alamitos, CA 90720, (213) 594-9531, BA 76 Pacific Oaks Coll; MA 80 CA St Univ - Los Angeles; Aud, Cigna Hlth Plans Inc, **A**

Reed, Mrs Anne Free Rt 5 Box 950, Dahlonega, GA 30533, (404) 754-2118, BS 81 Univ of GA; ME 84 Univ of GA; SLP, Habersham County Board of Educ, **SLP**

Reed, Mrs Betty Lou 4155 Mountain Avenue, San Bernardino, CA 92404, (714) 876-4116, BS 74 Univ of Redlands; MS 76 Univ of Redlands; Sp-Lang Path, Colton Joint USD, **SLP**

Reed, Dr Charles G 2254 26th Avenue, San Francisco, CA 94116, (415) 221-4810, BS 66 Northeast MO St Univ; MA 67 Northeast MO St Univ; PH 73 (NS) Univ of KS; Sec Chief, VA Med Cen, **SLP**

Reed, Charlotte 115 Overlook Road, Arlington, MA 02174, PH 73 (NS) Univ of Pittsburgh - Pittsburgh; Research Associate, MIT

Reed, Cynthia Ann 824 North 123rd Court, Omaha, NE 68154, (402) 895-0387, BS 83 Univ of NE - Lincoln; MS 85 Univ of NE - Omaha; **SLP**

Reed, De Etta Marie 810 North 15th Street, Blair, NE 68008, (402) 426-2610, BA 81 Kearney St Coll; MS 84 Univ of NE - Omaha; Sp-Lang Path, Blair Comm Schs, **SLP**

Reed, Mrs Donna M 1104 West Daniel, Champaign, IL 61821, (217) 351-3860, BS 70 IL St Univ - Normal; MA 77 Western KY Univ; Sp-Lang Path, Champaign Ut 4 Sch, **SLP**

Reed, Mrs Dora Ruskin 7 Woodlawn Avenue, Albany, NY 12208, (518) 482-6110, BA 34 CUNY - Brooklyn Coll; MA 39 Columbia Univ Teachers Coll; **SLP LM**

Reed, Gail A 6837 Havenhurst Drive, Sacramento, CA 95831, (916) 391-8522, BA 74 CA St Univ - Sacramento; MA 75 Humboldt St Univ; **SLP**

Reed, Mrs Gayle Lynette 507 Elm Trail, Belton, TX 76513, (817) 780-2034, BS 85 Univ of South AL; MS 87 Baylor Univ; **SLP**

Reed, Georgeanna 4862 South 1710 East, Salt Lake City, UT 84117, ME 70 Univ of UT; MS 78 Univ of UT; Sp-Lang Path, Granite School District, **SLP**

Reed, Harriet S 162 6th Street, Providence, RI 02906, (401) 277-3525, BS 73 Emerson Coll; ME 81 Providence Coll; MA 75 Univ of CT; Sp-Lang Path, Ri Sch for Deaf, **SLP**

Reed, Mrs Jane Elizabeth PO Box 33, Metaline Falls, WA 99153, (509) 442-3725, BA 83 WA St Univ; MA 84 WA St Univ; 84–Sp-Lang Path, Educational Service Dist 101, **SLP**

Reed, Mrs Jane M 2254 26th Avenue, San Francisco, CA 94116, (415) 877-8738, BS 68 Kent St Univ; MA 69 Univ of Denver; Sp-Lang Path, San Francisco USD, **SLP**

Reed, Kristi Holzheimer So 101 Neyland #3, Liberty Lake, WA 99019, (509) 255-6029, BA 83 Univ of WA; MS 85 Univ of WA; **A**

Reed, Dr L Deno 4329 Verplanck Place N W, Washington, DC 20016, (202) 732-1193, BS 51 PA St Univ - Univ Park; OD 59 Johns Hopkins Univ; Res Sci, Natl I of Hndcpd Res, **SLP A F**

Reed, Lauren C 2046 East Young Place, Tulsa, OK 74110, (918) 425-3687, BS 72 IA St Univ; MS 74 Univ of OK Medical Center; **SLP**

Reed, Linda L 150 Erie Street, Tiffin, OH 44883-1635, (419) 448-9701, BS 86 Bowling Green St Univ; MS 87 Bowling Green St Univ; 88–Sp-Lang Path, PT Services Inc, **SLP**

Reed, Lisa Carriker 3100 Sweetwater Road #108, Lawrenceville, GA 30244, (404) 923-1140, BS 77 Stephen F Austin St Univ; ME 80 Stephen F Austin St Univ; **SLP**

Reed, Mrs Lynn J 215 Ashley Circle, Martinez, GA 30907, (404) 868-5715, BS 77 SUNY - Coll at Buffalo; MS 80 SUNY - Coll at Buffalo; Sp-Lang Path, Columbia Co Spec Serv, **SLP**

Reed, Marilyn Nadine c/o Good Samaritan Hospital, 407 14th Avenue S E, Puyallup, WA 98372, (206) 848-6661, BS 68 Northwestern Univ; MS 85 Univ of WA; **SLP**

Reed, Marlene J 42211 Toddmark Lane, Mount Clemens, MI 48044, (313) 293-5100, BS 67 Clarion Univ of PA; ME 73 Wayne St Univ; SLP, Fraser Pub Sch, **SLP**

Reed, Mrs Martha K 6288 White Oaks Drive, Anderson, IN 46013, (317) 778-4171, BS 45 Ball St Univ; MA 48 Ball St Univ; **SLP LM**

Reed, Nancy J 440 Tavara Place, San Diego, CA 92106, (619) 223-9044, **SLP**

Reed, Nancy L Route 2 Box 299, Chassell, MI 49916, (906) 482-1122, BA 75 Univ of MI - Ann Arbor; MA 79 Western WA Univ; Aud, Portage View Hosp, **A**

Reed, Dr Nancy Larkin 37 North Benton Street, Palatine, IL 60067, (312) 617-3555, BA 66 Univ of MI - Ann Arbor; MA 67 Northwestern Univ; PH 87 (Comm Sci & Dis-Lrng Dis) Northwestern Univ; 78–Asst Prof/Clinic Dir, Elmhurst Coll, **SLP**

Reed, Mrs Nikki Doreen 5N702 Chambellen Box 452, Wayne, IL 60184-0452, **SLP**

Reed, Mrs Pamela Pickering 1503 North 1st Avenue, Upland, CA 91786, (714) 653-6114, BA 76 Univ of Redlands; MS 83 Univ of LA Verne; Sp-Lang Path, Bonita USD, **SLP**

Reed, Mrs Patricia George 15215 Ringfield Drive, Houston, TX 77084, (713) 469-7320, BS 79 Central MI Univ; MA 85 Univ of Houston - Univ Park; **SLP**

Reed, Paula L 3306 Water Oak, Farmers Branch, TX 75234, (214) 241-2046, BA 76 Univ of North TX; MA 77 Univ of North TX; Sp-Lang Path, Carrollton Branch Ind Sch Dist, **SLP**

Reed, Penelope D 1329 Lake Shore Drive, Muskegon, MI 49441, (616) 722-2302, BS 70 Western MI Univ; MA 77 Western MI Univ; 70–Sp-Lang Path, Mercy Hosp, **SLP**

Reed, Robbin C 811 Papalalo Place, Honolulu, HI 96825, (808) 531-7498, BA 68 Univ of CO - Boulder; MS 75 Univ of HI - Manoa; Sp-Lang Path, State of HI Dept of Education, **SLP**

Reed, Sherry Y 3617 North Cleveland, Kansas City, MO 64117-0000, (816) 453-4639, BS 79 Northwest MO St Univ; MS 80 Northwest MO St Univ; Dir, Northland Sp & Hearing Services, **SLP**

Reed, Susanne 3332 Angel Drive, Stockton, CA 95209, (209) 953-8540, BA 79 Eastern WA Univ; MS 81 Eastern WA Univ; Resource Spec, Lodi USD, **SLP**

Reed, Dr Vicki A Cumberland College Of Health Sciences, PO Box 170, Lidcombe, New South Wales, Australia 2141, (02) 646-6447, BS 68 Northwestern Univ; MA 69 Univ of Denver; ED 78 (Special Education) Univ of Northern CO; 87–Dir, Cumberland Col of Health Scs, **SLP**

Reed, Mrs Wanda B 95-3450 Road, R R#1 Rural Box #47, Crawford, CO 81415, (303) 921-3275, BA 68 Humboldt St Univ; MA 69 Humboldt St Univ; 87–Retired, Napa Valley USD, **SLP**

Reed-Curbow, Mrs Linda 3454 West Wayland, Springfield, MO 65807, (417) 887-9900, BS 80 Nazareth Coll of Rochester; MS 81 Ithaca Coll; Aud, ENT Cl Inc, **A**

Reeder, Ruth M Central Assoc For Special Educ, ICBD, 51 East Gerty Drive, Champaign, IL 61820, (217) 333-7023, BS 73 IL St Univ - Normal; MA 81 Univ of IL - Urbana; Aud, Central Assoc for Spec Ed, **A**

Reed-Musto, Mrs Barbara 5233 Hickory Lane, Stockton, CA 95212, (209) 931-5768, BS 73 Univ of HI - Manoa; MA 75 Univ of Akron; SLP, Lincoln USD

Reedy, Debra Strawhun 5598 Coronado Way, Rocklin, CA 95677, (916) 624-2064, BA 77 Sonoma St Univ; MS 81 AZ St Univ; Sp-Lang Path, Rio Linda Sch Dist, **SLP**

Reeh, Mrs Hilary L Center For Aud & Speech, University Of Texas, Medical Branch, Galveston, TX 77550, (409) 761-2711, BS 77 Old Dominion Univ; MA 79 Univ of MD - College Park; 84–Aud, Univ of Texas Medical Branch, **A**

Reel, Mrs Carla Jean 77 Meadow Drive, Tijeras, NM 87059, (505) 281-5953, MA 84 Clarion Univ of PA; 87–Sp-Lang Path, St Joseph Hosp, **SLP**

Reel, Mrs Evelyn E 313 Constance Drive, Chesapeake, VA 23320, (804) 547-0153, BS 45; ME 53 Univ of VA - Charlottesville; Superv, Chesapeake Pub Sch, **SLP**

Reel, Kathryn Elizabeth 661 East Michigan Avenue, #206, Grass Lake, MI 49240, (517) 787-1468, MA 83 MI St Univ; Sp-Lang Path, Jackson Sp & Hrng Clinic, **SLP**

Reel, Sharon Marie 580 Coles Mill Road, Haddonfield, NJ 08033, (609) 795-8552, SLP, Winona Ps, **SLP**

Rees, Deidre G 5 Francis Wyman Road, Burlington, MA 01803, **SLP A**

Rees, Marjorie Addie 2748 West Highcliff Drive, Tucson, AZ 85745-3547, (602) 294-1411, BS 79 Univ of AZ; MS 81 Univ of AZ; Sp-Lang Path, Sunnyside Sch Dist #12, **SLP**

Rees, Mrs Muriel 22777 S W 65th Terrace, Boca Raton, FL 33428, (305) 482-5929, BA 43 2893; MA 54 2893; Sp-Lang Path, Private Practice, **SLP LM**

Rees, Dr Norma S 120 Beaconsfield Road, Brookline, MA 02146, (617) 727-7785, BA 52 CUNY - Queens Coll; MA 54 CUNY - Brooklyn Coll; PH 59 (NS) NY Univ; Vice Chancellor/Acad Affairs, Brd of Regents of Higher Ed, **SLP A F H**

Rees, Dr Thomas S Department Of Otolaryngology, Harborview Medical Center, 325 Ninth Avenue, Seattle, WA 98104, (206) 223-3231, BA 68 Univ of Redlands; MA 69 Univ of Redlands; PH 72 (Aud) Univ of WA; 72–Asst Prof of Otol, U of WA Sch of Med, **A**

Reese, Bertrand 4753 So Hemingway Circle, Margate, FL 33063, (305) 771-8000, BS 61 PA St Univ - Univ Park; MS 65 PA St Univ - Univ Park; Dir, Bertrand S Reese Ms Inc, **SLP**

Reese, Carol Doerfler 612 S E 7th, Pendleton, OR 97801, (503) 276-6616, BS 81 OR St Univ; MS 85 Eastern WA Univ; 81–Sp-Lang Path, Umatilla Co Educ Svc Dist, **SLP**

Reese, Gaylen L 4937 West Larkspur Drive, Phoenix, AZ 85304, (602) 277-5551, BS 66 UT St Univ; MS 68 UT St Univ; Aud, VA Med Cen, **A ACE**

Reese, Janice C 7340 Skillman #108, Dallas, TX 75231, **SLP**

Reese, Katherine Thomas 1101 East 1st Street, Tustin, CA 92680-3814, (714) 633-7400, BA 80 Oberlin Coll; MA 84 OH Univ - Athens; Sp-Lang Path, Riverview Hearing Spch & Lang, **SLP**

Reese, Lynn Marie 6208 Butte Street, Boise, ID 83704, (208) 377-0901, BS 84 ID St Univ; MS 87 ID St Univ; 86–Aud, Idaho State Univ, **A**

Reese, Martha M 905 N E 7th Avenue, Delray Beach, FL 33483, (305) 243-8104, BA 75 OH St Univ; MA 77 OH St Univ; Director Private Practice, M M Reese Sp-Lang Path Serv, **SLP**

Reese, Mary Landry P O Box 426, Filkins Hill Road, East Berne, NY 12059, (518) 434-4103, BS 79 SUNY - Center at Albany; MS 80 SUNY - Coll at Buffalo; 88–Sp-Lang Path, Private Practice, **SLP**

Reese, Robert C, Jr 814 Philadelphia Avenue, Reading, PA 19607, (215) 779-7111, BS 67 Bloomsburg Univ of PA; ME 70 Bloomsburg Univ of PA; 87–Supvr, Berks Co I U, **SLP**

Reese, Scott J 1011 2nd Avenue S W, Austin, MN 55912, (507) 433-1886, BS 72 IA St Univ; MS 75 Univ of WY; 84–Sp-Lang Path, Austin Pub Sch, **SLP**

Reese, Mrs Sharon H 4310 Adams Avenue, Des Moines, IA 50310, (515) 277-6311, BA 53 Univ of OR; MS 74 Northeast MO St Univ; Sp-Lang Path, Des Moines Indep Comm Sch Dist, **SLP**

Reese, Sheryl 931 Stagecoach Road, Santa Fe, NM 87501, (817) 387-7502, BS 73 Univ of North TX; MS 75 Univ of North TX; Sp-Lang Path, **SLP**

Reeser, Mrs Judith P 14909 Emory Lane, Rockville, MD 20853, (301) 460-5842, BA 60 Univ of MD - College Park; MA 65 Univ of MD - College Park; Sp-Lang Path, Montgomery Co Pub Sch, **SLP**

Reesor, Myrna Diane 806 Sugar Place, Lakeland, FL 33801, (813) 665-7253, BA 81 Univ of TN - Knoxville; MS 82 Univ of TN - Knoxville; Sp-Lang Path, Polk County Schools, **SLP**

Rees Phd, Dr Maryjane 2312 Lloyd Lane, Sacramento, CA 95825, PH; Prof, CSU, **SLP F**

Reetz, Mrs Deborah K 1448 Sunset Drive, St Charles, MN 55972, (507) 452-5038, BS 70 Univ of WI - River Falls; MS 75 Univ of WI - Stevens Point; SLP, Winona Public Schools, **SLP**

Reeve, Mrs Leighton M R R 11 Box 89, Brazil, IN 47834, (812) 448-2052, MS 74 Univ of GA; ME 75 Univ of GA; **A**

Reeve, Dr Rolland Ralph 7923 Bobbyboyar Avenue, Canoga Park, CA 91304, (213) 885-2858, BA 51 Univ of Southern CA; MA 53 Univ of Southern CA; PH 64 (NS) Univ of Southern CA; **SLP**

Reeves, Mrs Charlene Baird 2006 Denfield Lane, Childress, TX 79201, (817) 937-6528

Reeves, Mrs Cindy W 217 Romany Road, Lexington, KY 40502, (606) 269-3576, MS 87 Univ of KY; 88–Sp-Lang Path, Swigert & Associates Inc

Reeves, Cintealia Paige 607 Garden Ridge Circle, Birmingham, AL 35244, (205) 988-0103, BA 79 Univ of MS; MS 87 Univ of Montevallo; 80–Sp-Lang Path, Shelby Co Bd of Educ, **SLP**

Reeves, Deborah A 8730 Jack Bean, San Antonio, TX 78240, (512) 567-2777, OB 79 Central MO St Univ; MS 81 Central MO St Univ; Aud, UTHSC-SA, **A**

Reeves, Gwenlynn Diann 3721 William Dehaes, #1708, Irving, TX 75038, (214) 255-2151, BS 84 Univ of North TX; MS 85 Univ of North TX; SLP, Irving ISD, **SLP**

Reeves, Mrs Jerri Jo 193 Woodvale Circle, Slidell, LA 70461, (318) 948-3657, BA 80 Southeastern LA Univ; MS 84 Univ of Southwestern LA; **SLP**

Reeves, Lisa Ann 917 2nd Avenue, Saraland, AL 36571, (205) 675-3110, BS 84 Univ of South AL; MS 86 Univ of South AL; 87–Aud, AL Dept of Mental Hlth, **A**

Reeves, Mrs Marilyn Ziton 16938 Dearborn Street, Sepulveda, CA 91343, (818) 894-0833, BA 82 CA St Univ - Northridge; MA 86 CA St Univ - Northridge

Reeves, Mrs Marsha M 2475 Tronjo Circle, Pensacola, FL 32503, (904) 433-3456, BS 76 Univ of GA; MA 77 Univ of TN - Knoxville; Sp-Lang Path, Pro Health Svcs, **SLP**

Reeves, Martha 3017 9th Street N E, Great Falls, MT 59404, (406) 791-2270, BA 71 ND St Univ; MA 73 KS St Univ; Great Falls Pub Sch, **SLP**

Reeves, Ossie R 900 Homestead Boulevard, Gautier, MS 39553, (601) 497-3398, BA 60 Univ of Southwestern LA; MA 67 LA St Univ - Baton Rouge; Sp/Lang Path, Pascagoula Schs, **SLP**

Reeves, Paula J 22 Regency Drive, Windsor, CT 06095, (203) 688-0322, MS 88 Southern CT St Univ

Reeves, Rebecca Fulghum 225 Brenda Drive, Shreveport, LA 71115, (318) 797-7668, BS 74 LA St Univ - Baton Rouge; OM 78 LA St Univ - Shreveport; SLP, Caddo Parish Sch Bd, **SLP**

Reeves, Mrs Rebecca K 3529 Hunters Hill Drive, Lithonia, GA 30058, (404) 656-6317, BA 71 SC St Coll; MA 72 Univ of IL - Urbana; Consult Sp Lang Dis Prog, GA Dept of Ed, **SLP ACE**

Reeves, Mrs Rita P O Box 4069, Carson City, NV 89702, (702) 246-5000, BA 64 CA St Univ - Fullerton; MA 71 Univ of IL - Urbana; 86–Sp-Lang Path, Lyon County Sch Dist, **SLP**

Reeves, Mrs Sheri Kaye P O Box 33-Sbc, Walnut Ridge, AR 72476, (501) 886-6755, BS 82 TX Christian Univ; MS 83 TX Christian Univ; **SLP**

Reeves, Mrs Susan D West Texas Rehabilitation Ctr, 3001 South Jackson, San Angelo, TX 76901, (915) 949-9535, BA 77 Southwest TX St Univ; ME 78 Southwest TX St Univ; Ch SLP, W Tx Rehab Cen, **SLP**

Reeves, Toni Ann 101 Civic Center Lane, Lake Havasu City, AZ 86403, (602) 855-8181, MA 86 Univ of OK - OK City

Reeves-Lamson, Sharon 2111 Murray Circle, Wichita, KS 67212, **SLP**

Refkin, Ilene M I M Speech/Language Associates, 6 Lenbar Circle, New City, NY 10956, (914) 638-4480, BA 79 NY Univ; MA 81 CUNY - Lehman Coll; Dir, Im Sp-Lang Assoc, **SLP**

Regal, Darah J 2628 Pleasant View Road, Richmond, IN 47374, (317) 288-8821, BS 84 Andrews Univ; MA 86 Ball St Univ; **A**

Regal, Jeffrey D 2628 Pleasant View Road, Richmond, IN 47374, BS 84 Andrews Univ; MA 86 Ball St Univ; **A**

Regalado-Robb, Mrs Sharon F 323 Lowell Avenue, Mill Valley, CA 94941, (415) 928-7727, BA 70 San Francisco St Univ; MA 71 San Francisco St Univ; Sp-Lang Path, San Francisco USD, **SLP**

Regan, Dr J Barry Route 1, Rise-N-Sun Drive, Hope, RI 02831, (401) 277-5485, BA 53 Emerson Coll; MA 54 Emerson Coll; ED 67 (Aud) Boston Univ; 58–Dir, Hrng Sp Cen, Ri Hosp, **SLP A ACE**

Regan, James M 414 Beverly Drive, Erie, PA 16505, (814) 453-7967, BS 77 SUNY - Coll at Geneseo; MS 79 Syracuse Univ; Clinical Supervisor, InSpeech Inc, **SLP**

Regan, Jeanette N 3536 Edgemont Road, Troy, MI 48084, (313) 649-1902, BA 75 OH St Univ; MA 77 OH St Univ; 87–Sp-Lang Path, Madison Heights PS, **SLP**

Regan, Mrs Kathy Ossi 3125 Bridlewood Lane, Jacksonville, FL 32257, (904) 731-8531, BS 79 FL St Univ; MS 80 FL St Univ; 88–Sp-Lang Path, Private Practice, **SLP**

Regan, M Clare 514 DE Soto Avenue, Inverness, FL 32650, (904) 344-0985, BA 43 Emerson Coll; ME 45 IN Univ - Bloomington; **SLP LM**

Regan, Mrs Margaret Brady 918 East Neadow Place, Milwaukee, WI 53217, MS 80 Marquette Univ; Sp-Lang Path, Therapy Assoc, **SLP**

Regan, Margaret Elizabeth Speech And Hearing Center, 1601 St Julian Place, Middleburg Office Park, Columbia, SC 29204, BA 81 SUNY - Coll at Plattsburgh; MA 85 Univ of CT; Instructor, Univ of SC, **A**

Regan, Mrs Mary M 4420 Canterbury Lane, Davenport, IA 52806, (608) 274-5803, SLP, Mississippi Bend AEA, **SLP**

Regan, Mary Margaret S 57 Chamberlain Road, Wethersfield, CT 06109, (203) 721-7936, BA 81 Univ of MD - College Park; MA 83 George Washington Univ; 88–Aud, The Gaylord Hosp, **A**

Regan, Peggy Anne 190 Stonehenge Terrace, Clark, NJ 07066, (201) 789-8591, BA 74 Rutger's St Univ - Douglas Coll; MA 77 Kean Coll of NJ; **SLP**

Regan-Burton, Laurie P 174 Guindon Boulevard, Fond Du Lac, WI 54935, (414) 241-5530, **SLP**

Regas-Yutzy, Mrs Mary A 415 Beech Street, Berea, OH 44017, (216) 845-1382, MA 80 Univ of Akron; Sp-Lang Path, Parma City Sch Dist, **SLP**

Reggio-Seng, Donna Regina 36 Jeanne Avenue, Port Jefferson, NY 11776, (516) 929-3833, BA 84 Adelphi Univ; MS 85 Adelphi Univ; 88–Sp-Lang Path, PreSch Place for Lrng, **SLP**

Regina, Mrs Jane McNamara 2411 Aberdeen Street, East Meadow, NY 11554, (516) 794-6549, BA 77 Hofstra Univ; MA 78 Hofstra Univ; Sp-Lang Path, NYC Bd of Ed - Sp Serv Ut, **SLP**

Regler, Fred, Jr 2221 Pelham Avenue, Baltimore, MD 21213, Sp-Lang Path, Baltimore City Pub Sch, **SLP**

Regnell, Mrs Joan Roddy 11502 Farmland Drive, Rockville, MD 20852, (202) 994-7111, BA 56 George Washington Univ; MA 60 George Washington Univ; Assoc Prof, Gco Wash U, **SLP**

Regner, Jennifer C 4305 North 88th Street, Milwaukee, WI 53222, (414) 463-7116, BS 82 Univ of WI - Madison; MS 84 Univ of WI - Madison; SLP, Milwaukee Public Schools, **SLP**

Regoord, Sally 46 San Marie Drive, Rochester, NY 14622, (716) 325-4560, BS 75 Ithaca Coll; MS 76 SUNY - Coll at Fredonia; Sp-Lang Path, Rochester City Schl Dist, **SLP**

Rehberg, Barbara Foos 810 West Main Street, Somerset, PA 15501, (814) 443-1990, BA 74 Coll of William & Mary; MA 77 Univ of Pittsburgh - Pittsburgh; 85–Sp-Lang Path, Comm Nursing Svc, **SLP**

Rehder, Douglas E Rehder Hearing Clinic, 1537 Avenue D, Suite 360, Billings, MT 59102, (800) 227-3181, BA 73 Univ of MN - Duluth; MA 74 Univ of MN - Duluth; Aud/Sp-Lang Path, Rocky Mt Hrng/Sp Serv, **SLP A**

Rehling, Mrs Jan D 6192 Wilder Court, Parker, CO 80134, (303) 841-8318, BA 72 Univ of CT; ME 74 Univ of VA - Charlottesville; SLP, Douglas Co PS, **SLP**

Rehor, Linda S 847 Hazelwood, Jackson, MI 49203, (517) 787-9769, BS 74 Eastern MI Univ; MA 76 Eastern MI Univ; Sp-Lang Path, Jackson Co ISD, **SLP**

Reibetanz, Dr Karen R 201 Castille Avenue #4, Madison, WI 53713, (608) 274-8060, BS 64 Univ of WI - Madison; MS 65 Univ of WI - Madison; PH 75 (Behavioral Disab (Mental Retard)) Univ of WI - Madison; Exec Dir, Madison Oppty Cen Inc, **SLP**

Reice, Mrs Jeanne B 11808 Lipsey Road, Tampa, FL 33618, (813) 879-6207, BS 76 West Chester Univ of PA; OM 79 Hahneman Medical Coll; 83–Instr, Univ South Florida, **A ACE**

Reich, Dr Alan Richard Dept Of Speech & Hearing Sci, University Of Washington, Seattle, WA 98195, (206) 543-7888, BA 67 Univ of CT; MA 69 Univ of CT; PH 75 (NS) Univ of IA; Assoc Prof, U of WA Dept of Sp & Hrng Sci, **SLP**

Reich, Mrs Arlene E 377 Buckingham Road, Cedarhurst, NY 11516, (516) 295-4569, BA 74 George Washington Univ; MS 75 Univ of MI - Ann Arbor; Sp-Lang Path, Private Practice, **SLP**

Reich, Denise Michele 25 Oliver Street #4-E, Brooklyn, NY 11209, (718) 854-3737, BA 83 SUNY - Center at Binghamton; MS 85 Columbia Univ Teachers Coll; Sp-Lang Path, New York Childhood Center, **SLP**

Reich, Mrs Janet E 59 Farrand Drive, Parsippany, NJ 07054, (201) 335-0271, BA 76 Rutger's St Univ - Douglas Coll; MA 77 Hofstra Univ; **SLP**

Reich, Mrs Janet Riggan 366 Forest Street, Hamden, CT 06518, (203) 287-0883, BA 76 Marygove Coll; MA 84 Eastern MI Univ; Sp-Lang Path, New Haven Public Schools, **SLP**

Reich, Rita Daum 2 Bay Club Drive #20W, Bayside, NY 11360, (212) 423-5777, BA 60 Adelphi Univ; MA 61 NY Univ; Full Prof, Queensborough Com Coll of CUNY, **SLP A**

Reich, Susan B 3254 Pebblebrook Lane, Cincinnati, OH 45251, (513) 385-9231, BS 72 OH Univ - Athens; MS 78 Miami Univ - Oxford; Sp-Lang Path, Hamilton Co Off Ed, **SLP**

Reich, Tamara J 9020 Lamon Avenue, Apartment Ground East, Skokie, IL 60077, (312) 498-3830, BS 81 Univ of IL - Urbana; MS 82 Univ of IL - Urbana; Sp-Lang Path, Northbrook Sch Dist 27, **SLP**

Reichard, Mrs Cheryl Lynn 7 Wodenshire Lane, Danville, PA 17821, (717) 286-7121, BS 80 Bloomsburg Univ of PA; MS 81 Bloomsburg Univ of PA; Sp-Lang Path, InSpeech Inc, **SLP**

Reichard, Mrs Joan M 1074 Wenston Court, Kettering, OH 45429, (513) 293-2917, BS 74 Loma Linda Univ - Riverside; MS 77 Loma Linda Univ - Loma Linda; **SLP A**

Reichardt, Mrs Margaret Meyer 122 Estberg, Waukesha, WI 53186, (414) 363-7151, BS 78 Univ of WI - Stevens Point; MS 79 Univ of WI - Eau Claire; Sp-Lang Path, Munkwonago Area Sch, **SLP**

Reichenbach, Mrs Valerie C 108 Park Circle, Elkton, MD 21921, (301) 398-1441, BS 76 Towson St Univ; MS 80 Towson St Univ; Sp-Lang Path, Cecil Co Pub Sch, **SLP**

Reichert, Judith A 5728-4 North Monte, Fresno, CA 93711, (209) 441-3328, BA 73 CA St Univ - Fresno; MA 76 CA St Univ - Fresno; SLP, Fresno USD, **SLP**

Reichle, Patti S A District 917 Special Educ, 1400 Thompson Avenue, South St Paul, MN 55075, **A**

Reichlin, Holly 1522 55th Street, Brooklyn, NY 11219, (718) 851-7646, **SLP**

Reichman, Julie 2500 East Calle Sin Contro, Tucson, AZ 85718-1260, (602) 621-7070, BA 73 Goucher Coll; MS 75 Vanderbilt Univ; Aud, U of AZ, **A**

Reichmann, Shelly Snow 7705 South 2250 West, West Jordan, UT 84084, (801) 533-3830, BA 84 Univ of UT; MA 86 Univ of UT; 86–Sp-Lang Path, Therapy Management, **SLP**

Reichmuth, Sara 507 North Cemter, Clay Center, NE 68933, (402) 463-5611, BS 85 Univ of NE - Lincoln; MS 86 Univ of NE - Lincoln; Sp-Lang Path, Educ Ser Unit #9, **SLP**

Reid, Annie Kathleen 11 South Buena Vista, Redlands, CA 92373, (714) 874-0404, BA 84 CA St Univ - Chico; MS 87 Univ of Redlands; Sp-Lang Path, San Bernardino Co Supt of Schs, **SLP**

Reid, Carol A 10640 West 46th Avenue, Wheat Ridge, CO 80033, (303) 425-0449, BS 83 Ithaca Coll; MA 85 Univ of Northern CO; Aud, Western Otolaryngology, **A**

Reid, Mrs Dorothy F RFD 1 Box 218, Fisher Road, Northfield, MA 01360, (413) 498-5044, BA 51 Grinnell Coll; MS 52 Purdue Univ - West Lafayette; Sp-Lang Path, VA Med Cen-Northampton, **SLP**

Reid, Mrs Gloria Ann 9859 Geyser Avenue, Northridge, CA 91324, (818) 349-8316, BA 63 CA St Univ - Northridge; MA 70 CA St Univ - Northridge; Asst Prof, CA St U, **SLP**

Reid, Mrs Janell D 222 West 5th Street, Santa Ana, CA 92701, (714) 543-3941, BA 74 CA St Univ - Northridge; MA 75 CA St Univ - Northridge; Aud, Burton Assoc, **A**

Reid, Jeffrey Bruce 9859 Geyser Avenue, Northridge, CA 91324, (818) 349-8316, MA 84 CA St Univ - Northridge; Aud, Hearing Health Svc, **A**

Reid, Karyn A P O Box 22458, Flagstaff, AZ 86023, (602) 779-6460, BA 73 Univ of NM; MS 74 Univ of NM; Sp-Lang Path, Flagstaff Public Schools, **SLP**

Reid, Louise 11 Valerie Circle, Rural Route 2, Ashburnham, MA 01430, (617) 827-5750, BA 61 Bates Coll; MS 75 Boston Univ; SLP, Ashburnham-Westminster Sch Dis, **SLP**

Reid, Mary Elizabeth 1744 Speyer Lane, Redondo Beach, CA 90278, (213) 832-8130, BA 77 San Francisco St Univ; MS 81 San Francisco St Univ; 81–SLP, Los Angeles USD, **SLP**

Reid, Dr Philip 9859 Geyser, Northridge, CA 91324, (818) 885-2852, BA 57 CA St Univ - Los Angeles; MA 60 Univ of Southern CA; PH 66 (NS) Univ of Southern CA; Chmn, Dept of Commun Dis, CA State U, **SLP A F**

Reid, Mrs Sheryl Guest 1546 Red Fern Drive, Farmington, NY 14425, (716) 544-1240, BS 84 SUNY - Coll at Geneseo; MA 86 Univ of CT; 87–Aud, Rochester Sch for the Deaf, **A**

Reidenbach, Elizabeth 1635 Timothy Drive, Charleston, SC 29407, **SLP**

Reidenbach, John 3811 Riverhills Drive, Tampa, FL 33604, (813) 988-5492, MS 73 Univ of South FL; Sp-Lang Path, Private Practice, **SLP**

Reidlich, Mrs Carole E 45 Empress Pines Drive, Ronkonkoma, NY 11779, (516) 345-2767, BA 62 CUNY - Queens Coll; MS 67 CUNY - Queens Coll; Sp-Lang Path, Longwood Central Schs, **SLP**

Reid-Malleck, Linda 11 Lenox Street, Edison, NJ 08817, (201) 932-9335, BA 75 Rutger's St Univ - Douglas Coll; MA 76 Univ of MO - Columbia; 88–Insr Sp-Lang Path, Rutgers Univ, **SLP**

Reidy, Jeanne S 15 West 256 Harvard, Elmhurst, IL 60126, **SLP**

Reierson-Griffith, Karen J 2190 Santa Cruz Drive, Atwater, CA 95301, (209) 358-8390, BS 81 Minot St Univ; MS 83 Minot St Univ; Sp-Lang Path, **SLP**

Reif, Mrs Tamara Kay 443 Winston Lane, Chicago Heights, IL 60411, (312) 361-2121, BS 80 LA St Univ - Baton Rouge; MA 82 Northern IL Univ - De Kalb; Sp-Lang Path, Sertoma Cen for Commun Dis, **SLP**

Reiff, Donald Gene 131 Astor Drive, Rochester, NY 14610, (716) 263-2850, MA 59 Univ of WI - Madison; MA 62 Univ of MI - Ann Arbor; PH 63 (Linguistics) Univ of MI - Ann Arbor; 85–Sp-Lang Path, Private Practice, **SLP**

Reiff, Mrs Janice Roper 8390 N W 25th Court, Sunrise, FL 33322, (305) 741-2126, MS 73 Univ of South FL; Sp-Lang Path, Alpha-Omega Rdg-Sp Center Inc, **SLP**

Reiff, Patricia Hartnett Associates In Hearing Incorporated, The Hearing Aid Specialists, 300 Century Plaza Bldg, Lansdale, PA 19446, (215) 855-4217, BS 79 PA St Univ - Univ Park; MS 81 Hahnemann Medical Coll; 85–Aud, Assoc in Hearing Inc, **A**

Reiff, Sharyn Lachman 8341 North Keystone, Skokie, IL 60076, (312) 674-3740, BS 75 Northern IL Univ - De Kalb; MA 77 Northern IL Univ - De Kalb; 85–Sp/Lang Path, Private Practice, **SLP**

Reigle, Carol A 1778 Arcadia, St Joseph, MI 49085, **SLP**

Reihing, Terri Marie 509 Springfield Street, Pittsburgh, PA 15220, (412) 922-1945, BS 83 CA St Coll - Bakersfield; MS 84 Clarion Univ of PA; **SLP**

Reilly, Mrs Camille Acquaviva Rd 4 Box 190, Milford, NJ 08848, (201) 735-5580, BA 78 Rutgers St Univ -N Brunswick; MS 86 Rutgers St Univ -N Brunswick; Sp-Lang Path, Clinton Public Schools, **SLP**

Reilly, Cathleen Reap 1982 Rush Mendon Road, Rush, NY 14543, (716) 461-2800, BA 79 SUNY - Coll at Potsdam; ME 81 SUNY - Coll at Buffalo; SLP, Monroe Developmental Center, **SLP**

Reilly, Mrs Ida Pedergnana 1773 Acorn Drive, Sinking Spring, PA 19608, BS 82 Bloomsburg Univ of PA; MS 83 Bloomsburg Univ of PA; Sp-Lang Path, Capital Area Inter Ut, **SLP ACE**

Reilly, Mrs Katherine 234 Madrone Avenue, Larkspur, CA 94939, (415) 461-9444, BA 68 San Francisco St Univ; MA 69 San Francisco St Univ; Dept Manager Hrng and Sp Dept, Marin General Hospital, **A**

Reilly, Kathleen 25 Northgate Road, Mendham, NJ 07945, (201) 526-4918, BA 70 Rutger's St Univ - Douglas Coll; MA 71 Univ of MD - College Park; **SLP**

Reilly, Margaret Hoover 4400 Horizon Hill, Apartment 3203, San Antonio, TX 78229, (512) 525-1859, Sp-Lang Path, Coastal Sp & Hrng Clinic, **SLP ACE**

Reilly, Marilyn E 760 South Washburn Suite 4A, Corona, CA 91720, (714) 736-1630, BS 67 Northern IL Univ - De Kalb; MA 76 CA St Univ - Long Beach; Aud, Private Practice, **A**

Reilly, Mary C RR1 Box 195-A, Pawling, NY 12564, **SLP**

Reilly-Sardegna, Gerri M 82 Longview Avenue, Rocky Point, NY 11778, (516) 744-7354, BA 75 Hofstra Univ; MA 76 Hofstra Univ; OM 82 Long Island U - CW Post Ctr; Sp-Lang Path, Sachem Public Schools, **SLP**

Reimbold, John 806 North Billy Bryan, Carbondale, IL 62901, (618) 457-0457, BS 77 Northern IL Univ - De Kalb; MS 82 Southern IL Univ -Carbondale; Aud, Pearlman M H Co, **A**

Reimer, Faith Forman 7529 West Isham, Chicago, IL 60631, (312) 631-4528, BS 74 Cornell Univ; MA 77 Northwestern Univ; Sp-Lang Path Supervisor, Excellcare Rehabilitation, **SLP**

Reimer, Patricia Thompson 10600 4th Street North, Mc Gregor Place #416, St Petersburg, FL 33716, (813) 577-5065, OB 85 Univ of KS; MA 87 Univ of KS; 87–Sp-Lang Path, InSpeech Inc, **SLP**

Rein, Mrs Lorraine C 347 Fern Street, South Hempstead, NY 11550, (212) 990-3832, BA 78 Hofstra Univ; MA 79 Hofstra Univ; Aud, Long Island Jewish Med Ctr, **A**

Rein, Mrs Sheila G 246-22 51st Avenue, Douglaston, NY 11362, (718) 423-5292, BA 56 CUNY - Hunter Coll; MA 70 CUNY - Hunter Coll; Tchr, NY Cty Bd of Ed Sp Serv Unit, **SLP**

Rein, Mrs Susan Lee Cuba 246 East 68th Street, New York, NY 10021, (212) 596-5742, BA 59 CUNY - Brooklyn Coll; MS 61 CUNY - Brooklyn Coll; OM 77 CUNY - Brooklyn Coll; Sp-Lang Path, NYC B of Ed, **SLP**

Reinecke, Mrs Joy G 147 Sand Pine Road, Indialantic, FL 32903, ME 68 Emory Univ; 79–Sp-Lang Path, Brevard Co Sch Bd, **SLP**

Reineking, Mrs Mary B R R 1 Box 46, Almond, WI 54909, (715) 346-3731, BS 72 Univ of WI - Stevens Point; MS 73 Univ of WI - Stevens Point; SLP, Stevens Point Area Pub Schs, **SLP**

Reiner, Dr Barbara J 11243 Bybee Street, Silver Spring, MD 20902, (301) 649-2374, BS 50 PA St Univ - Univ Park; MA 70 Univ of MD - College Park; PH 77 (Sp-Lang Path) Univ of MD - College Park; 87–Sp-Lang Path, Speech Works Associates, **SLP ACE**

Reiners, Cheryl Joy 8384 Mississippi Blvd N W, Coon Rapids, MN 55433, (612) 784-7225, MS 84 Saint Cloud St Univ; Sp-Lang Path, ISD 16, **SLP**

Reinfrank-Dedo, Mrs Susan Ann 14601 Country Creek Lane, Gaithersburg, MD 20878, BS 74 Northwestern Univ; MA 75 Northwestern Univ; Aud, U of MI Hosp, **A**

Reinhardt, Donna RFD 5 Box 22, Laconia, NH 03246, (603) 524-8822, BS 82 Univ of NH; MA 87 Univ of Northern CO

Reinhardt, Lynn K K 9 Walnut Avenue, Pompton Plains, NJ 07444, (201) 835-4042, BS 74 William Paterson Coll; MA 75 William Paterson Coll; SLP, Private Practice, **SLP**

Reinhardt, Mary A 2400 North Dustin, Farmington, NM 87401, (701) 252-5179, BA 79 Univ of NM; MA 81 Univ of SD - Vermillion; 88–Sp-Lang Path, San Juan Reg Med Ctr, **SLP**

Reinhardt, Susan E 36 Jefferson Road, Chestnut Hill, MA 02167, (617) 739-6565, BA 68 Univ of RI; MS 72 Emerson Coll; SLP, Needham Pub Schs, **SLP**

Reinhart, Mrs Daren Deslatte 6629 Golf Club Drive, Bay St Louis, MS 39520, (601) 467-4466, BA 82 Univ of Southwestern LA; MS 85 Lamar Univ; 88–Sp-Lang Path, Hancock County Schs-Gulfview Elem, **SLP**

Reinhart, Janet B 6201 Sneed Cove #922, Austin, TX 78744, (512) 444-4835, BS 64 Univ of TX - El Paso; MA 77 Univ of TX - Austin; Sp-Lang Path, Healthcare Rehab Ctr, **SLP**

Reinhart, Kimberly Kay 312 Leatherbark Drive, Mars, PA 16046, (412) 776-5427, BS Clarion Univ of PA; MS 83 Clarion Univ of PA; 85–Aud, John A Straka MD Inc, **A**

Reinhart, Lori Ann 421 Confer Avenue, Hamburg, PA 19526, (215) 378-8353, BS 84 Kutztown Univ of PA; MS 85 Bloomsburg Univ of PA; **SLP**

Reinhart, Mrs Rae L 2184 Hyde Shaffer Road, Bristolville, OH 44402, (216) 841-3700, BS 84 Kent St Univ; MA 85 Kent St Univ; Sp-Lang Path, Hillside Hospital, **SLP**

Reinhartsen, Debra A Route 11 Box 313, Burlington, NC 27215, (919) 222-6480, BA 79 Sophia Univ - Japan; ME 81 Univ of NC - Greensboro; Sp-Lang Path, Alamance-Caswell Mental Health, **SLP**

Reinheimer, Rita K 409 South 3rd Avenue West, Newton, IA 50208, (515) 792-4870, BA 72 Univ of Northern IA; MA 74 Univ of Northern IA; Sp-Lang Path, Heartland AEA II, **SLP**

Reinholt, Lisa Ann 3954 Wind Drift Drive East, Apartment 3-B, Indianapolis, IN 46254, (317) 298-4905, BS 85 Purdue Univ - West Lafayette; MS 87 Purdue Univ - West Lafayette; **A**

Reinick, Mrs Lynn P 1275 North 118th Street, Milwaukee, WI 53226, (414) 548-0000, BS 78 Univ of WI - Madison; MS 80 Univ of WI - Milwaukee; SLP, Waukesha Pub Sch, **SLP**

Reining, Penny 9807 Zimmer Drive, Algonquin, IL 60102, (312) 658-4807, BA 76 Augustana Coll; MA 77 Western IL Univ; 88–Sp-Lang Path, Spec Educ Dist of McHenry Co, **SLP**

Reinis, Belinda Jane 4951 Cherry Avenue #222, San Jose, CA 95118, (408) 267-4356, **SLP**

Reinitz, Mrs Francine Lynn S 434 Carlton Road, Wyckoff, NJ 07481, (201) 891-3996, BS 77 SUNY - Coll at New Paltz; MA 81 CUNY - Hunter Coll; Sp-Lang Path, JCC on the Palisades, **SLP**

Reinman, Miriam K 1075 East 26th Street, Brooklyn, NY 11210, (718) 951-9541, BA 78 CUNY - Brooklyn Coll; MS 81 CUNY - Brooklyn Coll; SLP, Sp Serv UT, **SLP**

Reinthal, S Heidi 1218 Grand Avenue, Parsons, KS 67357, (316) 724-6281, BS 76 WV Univ; MS 78 WV Univ; 88–Aud, Southeast KS Educ Svc Ctr, **A**

Reis, John W Route 1 Box 64, Ogden, IA 50212, (515) 294-6582, SLP, Iowa State University, **SLP**

Reis, Kathy S P O Box 27214, Denver, CO 80227, (303) 394-8606, BA 75 Univ of CO - Boulder; MA 77 Univ of Denver; Sp-Lang Path, J F K Child Dev Ctr, **SLP**

Reis, Mrs Michelle Ann 17528 West Windslow Drive, Grayslake, IL 60030, (312) 680-7348, BS 80 Purdue Univ - West Lafayette; MA 81 Northern IL Univ - De Kalb; SLP, Fairview Sch Dist #72, **SLP**

Reisbaum, Margaret L 4415 Gainsborough Avenue, Los Angeles, CA 90027, (213) 287-5223, BA 63 Univ of CA - Los Angeles; MS 70 Univ of Southern CA; MS 83 Univ of LA Verne; SLP, LA Co Office of Ed, **SLP ACE**

Reisberg, Debra R 3323 Kings Highway #6-H, Brooklyn, NY 11234-2639, (212) 338-4724, BA 76 CUNY - Brooklyn Coll; MA 80 NY Univ; Sp-Lang Path, Life Skills Sch Ltd, **SLP**

Reisberg, Marni H 652 Ridgeview Court, Toms River, NJ 08753, (201) 240-8000, BS 76 Boston Univ; MS 78 Rutger's St Univ - Douglas Coll; Dir Sp-Lang Path, Comm Mem Hosp, **SLP ACE**

Reisberg, Mrs Susan Scalise 881 Somerset Avenue, Davie, FL 33325, (305) 390-0700, BA 79 Univ of FL; MS 82 WV Univ; 82–Sp-Lang Path, School Board of Broward County, **SLP**

Reisch, Mrs Beryl Stanley 117 East Bodley Avenue, Apartment B-4, St Louis, MO 63122-4465, BS 56 Saint Louis Univ; MA 60 Stanford Univ; **SLP**

Reisch, Sandy J 4314 San Gabriel Drive, Dallas, TX 75229-4130, (214) 357-5990, **A**

Reisdorf, Mrs Jean Marie 773 Audubon, Jackson, MI 49203, (517) 784-8501, BA 68 Wheaton Coll; MA 85 MI St Univ; 87–SLP, Jackson PS, **SLP**

Reisen, Patricia D RD 3 Box 682, Newton, NJ 07860, (201) 948-7733, BA 68 Newark St Coll; MS 78 William Paterson Coll; **A**

Reiser, Lawrence A 119 North Castle Drive, Dunlap, IL 61525, (309) 672-6716, BS 74 Bradley Univ; MS 76 Bradley Univ; Aud, Peoria Pub Sch, **A**

Reiser, Mrs Trude M 119 North Castle Drive, Dunlap, IL 61525, (309) 672-6716, BS 75 Saint Louis Univ; MA 77 Wayne St Univ - Sch of Med; Aud, Peoria Pub Sch, **A**

Reisfeld, Mrs Lora Schachter 2287 Johnson Avenue #7-A, Riverdale, NY 10463, (212) 496-8400, BA 81 George Washington Univ; MA 84 NY Univ; Sp-Lang Path, **SLP**

Reisinger, Mrs Joan H 10178 S W 53rd Court, Cooper City, FL 33328, (305) 434-7676, BA 71 FL St Univ; MS 80 Univ of Miami; Sp-Lang Path, Dade Co Pub Sch, **SLP**

Reisler, Laura M 152 Prospect Park West, Brooklyn, NY 11215, (212) 780-4670, BA 73 CUNY - City College; MS 74 Columbia Univ Teachers Coll; Sp-Lang Path, Private Practice, **SLP**

Reiss, Debra Elizabeth 66 Atwood Street #16, Plainville, CT 06062, (203) 282-3110, BA 81 Adams St Coll; MA 82 Adams St Coll; **SLP**

Reiss, Dorothy 520 East 76th Street #6-G, New York, NY 10021, (212) 734-6458, BS 63 Syracuse Univ; MS 64 Univ of MI - Ann Arbor; **SLP A**

Reiss, Evelyn P 3245 Pawnee Place, Sioux City, IA 51104, (712) 279-2692, BS 60 Boston Univ; MA 80 Univ of SD - Vermillion; Supervisor Sp/Lang Path, Marian Health Center, **SLP**

Reiss, Mrs Judith D 74 Westvelt Place, Passaic, NJ 07055, (212) 694-2961, BS 79 SUNY - Coll at Buffalo; MA 81 Univ of Pittsburgh - Pittsburgh; Sp-Lang Path, Columbus Presbyterian Med Cen, **SLP**

Reiss, Mrs Kathleen A 619 Magee Avenue, Rochester, NY 14613, (716) 352-2400, BA 80 SUNY - Center at Buffalo; MA 82 SUNY - Center at Buffalo; 82–Sp-Lang Path, BOCES #2 Monroe-Orleans Co, **SLP**

Reiss, Phyllis Hochberg 215 Washington Avenue, Edison, NJ 08817, (718) 330-9333, BA 80 CUNY - Brooklyn Coll; MS 84 CUNY - Brooklyn Coll; SLP, Board of Education, **SLP**

Reister, Gaye McKinnon 10910 SE 238th Street, Apartment 2G-201, Kent, WA 98031, (206) 852-7614, BA 84 WA St Univ; MA 87 WA St Univ; 87–Sp-Lang Path, Puyallup School District

Reitema, Gordon Harrison Rd #1 Box 75, Interlaken, NY 14847, (607) 869-3111, BA 71 SUNY - Coll at Oneonta; MS 76 Ithaca Coll; 83–Sp-Lang Path, NYS Office of Mental Hygiene, **SLP**

Reiter, Dr Levi A 885 Montgomery Street, Brooklyn, NY 11213, (212) 778-9749, BA 70 CUNY - Hunter Coll; MA 74 CT Coll; PH 78 (NS) Univ of Rochester; Asst Prof-Aud & Hrng Sci, Hofstra U-Dept of Sp & Hrng, **A**

Reiter, Linda Jo 10716 Waco Drive, Upper Marlboro, MD 20772, (202) 745-5600, BA 79 Univ of MD - College Park; MA 87 Univ of MD - College Park; 88–Aud, Children's Hosp Natl Med Ctr, **A**

Reithal, Kathryn Frances 22125 Ridgeway Avenue, Richton Park, IL 60471-1425, (815) 667-4417, BS 81 IL St Univ - Normal; MS 83 IL St Univ - Normal; Sp-Lang Path, Streator Elem School Dist #45, **SLP**

Reither, Mrs Linda P 1702 East Bullard Suite 100, Fresno, CA 93710, (209) 432-5805, BA 78 CA St Univ - Fresno; MA 80 CA St Univ - Fresno; Sp-Lang Path, Private Practice, **SLP A**

Reitman, Gail S 8 Ivory Road, Bloomfield, CT 06002, (203) 242-7739, BA 65 Univ of CT; MA 67 Univ of CT; Sp-Lang Path, Bloomfield Pub Sch, **SLP**

Reitnour, Melissa Adsit 106B North Main Street, Spring City, PA 19475, (215) 948-0808, BS 82 WV Univ; MA 84 Temple Univ; Aud, Coatesville Veteran's Admin Hosp, **A**

Reitter-Turner, Mrs Becky Lee 11405 S W 90th, Tigard, OR 97223, (503) 230-6195, OB 77 Univ of MN - Duluth; MS 82 Univ of MN - Duluth; 84–Sp-Lang Path, Providence Med Cen, **SLP**

Reitz, Ellen Christine 8046 West Manor Circle, Milwaukee, WI 53223-6228, (414) 545-6403, BS 76 Univ of WI - Milwaukee; MS 79 Univ of WI - Milwaukee; MS 83 Marquette Univ; SLP, W Allis-W Milwaukee Pub Sch, **SLP**

Reitz, Janet L S 7855 Stonehouse Road, Centerville, OH 45459, (513) 299-2004, BA 75 OH St Univ; MA 77 OH St Univ; Aud, Springham Aud Inc, **A**

Reitz, Mary Lou D 124 East 1825 North, Centerville, UT 84014, (801) 295-4219, BS 80 Univ of UT; MS 82 Univ of UT; Aud, Ogden Clinic, **A**

Reitz, Mrs Patricia Schrodt 7840 Stonehurst Drive, Indianapolis, IN 46256, (317) 274-8868, BA 79 IN Univ - Bloomington; MA 81 IN Univ - Bloomington; Aud, Indiana Univ Medical Center, **A**

Reiz, Mrs Zelda L 10200 Bond, Overland Park, KS 66214, (913) 631-3700, MA 70 Univ of KS; SLP, Shawnee Mission Sch Dist 512, **SLP LM**

Rejc, Cheryl S 17167 West Woodland Drive, Grayslake, IL 60030, (312) 367-3214, BS 78 Western IL Univ; MS 79 Marquette Univ; Sp/Lang Path, Hawthorn Sch Dist 73, **SLP**

Rejzer, Alexandra A P O Box 444, Kahului, HI 96732, (808) 244-7467, BS 77 CA Univ of PA; MS 78 WV Univ; 87–Exec Dir, Society for Crippled Children, **SLP**

Rekart, Dr Deborah Marie 2041 Highland Drive, State College, PA 16803, (814) 234-0188, BA 72 Univ of Dayton; MA 74 Univ of Rochester; PH 85 (Sp Science) LA St Univ - Baton Rouge; 86–Asst Prof, Pennsylvania State Univ

Rella, Anthony Robert 484 Caldwell Avenue, Belford, NJ 07718, (718) 351-8113, BA 78 Kean Coll of NJ; MA 79 Kean Coll of NJ

Rella, Mrs Marguerite Sheridan 41 Stratford Lane, Mount Laurel, NJ 08054, (609) 795-5878, BS 78 Trenton St Coll; MA 81 Trenton St Coll; Sp-Lang Path, Private Practice, **SLP**

Relojo, Mrs Patricia Lira 3860 Hyde Park Avenue, Cincinnati, OH 45209, (513) 351-1639, BS 79 Univ of Cincinnati; MA 81 Univ of Cincinnati; 86–Sp-Lang Path, Cincinnati Ctr for Dev Dis, **SLP**

Relph, Mrs Theresa Lynne 4102 Horseshoe Drive, Cedar Falls, IA 50613-4807, (319) 266-0028, BA 84 Univ of Northern IA; MA 85 Univ of Northern IA; Sp-Lang Path, Spring Valley Public Schools, **SLP**

Relyea, Linda A 11 Laurel Drive, Little Silver, NJ 07739, **SLP**

Relyea-Conklin, Mrs Rhonda 4475 Pembrook Village Dr, Alexandria, VA 22309, (703) 664-7190, MS 82 Purdue Univ - West Lafayette; Sp/Lang Path, Mt Vernon Hosp, **SLP ACE**

Rembe, Raymond R 7116 Munford Road, Baltimore, MD 21207, (301) 298-4179, BS 62 SUNY - Coll at Fredonia; ME 64 SUNY - Center at Buffalo; Aud, Private Practice, **A**

Rembisz, Linda S 23 Cypress Neck Road, Lincroft, NJ 07738, (201) 741-8073, BS 68 Ithaca Coll; MA 69 MI St Univ; Dir Sp-Lang Path, Speech Therapy Service, **SLP**

Remegio-Loges, Lorilee Mariko 5248 Saratoga Court N W, Albuquerque, NM 87120, (505) 247-4224, BA 82 Univ of Northern CO; MA 83 Univ of Northern CO; Audiologist, Albuquerque Hrng & Spch Center, **A**

Remelius, Fae Ellen 319 Worcester Road, Westminster, MA 01473, (617) 355-2055, BA 65 Elmira Coll; MS 83 Worcester St Coll; Sp-Lang Path, Quabbin Reg Sch Dist, **SLP**

Remenick, Mrs Deedee 52 Chesapeake Landing, Annapolis, MD 21403, (301) 262-8680, BA 63 Univ of MD - College Park; ME 76 Bowie St Coll; Sp-Lang Path, Prince Georges County Pub Sch, **SLP**

Remensnyder, Linda S Hearing Associates PC, 1105 West Park Avenue, Suite 3B, Libertyville, IL 60048, (312) 680-7580, BA 69 Northern IL Univ - De Kalb; MA 73 Northern IL Univ - De Kalb; Aud, Hearing Assoc PC, **A**

Remillaro, Susan Marie 614 West 114th Street, New York, NY 10025, (212) 280-3062, BA 83 Lawrence Univ; MA 87 Columbia Univ Teachers Coll; MS 87 Columbia Univ Teachers Coll

Remmel, Dr Kerri Simpson P O Box 4864, Shreveport, LA 71104, (318) 868-4338, BS 76 LA St Univ - Baton Rouge; MA 79 LA St Univ - Baton Rouge; PH 85 (NS) LA St Univ - Baton Rouge; Sp-Lang Path, Private Practice, **SLP**

Remmers, Page Peters 131 Wilson Avenue, Waukesha, WI 53186, (414) 351-0352, BS 83 Bradley Univ; MS 85 Southern IL Univ -Carbondale; Sp-Lang Path, St Francis Childrens Center, **SLP ACE**

Rempel, Susan Anne 52 Penfound Drive, Bowmanville, ON, Canada L1C 3K1, (416) 623-7706, BS 84 Miami Univ - Oxford; MA 85 Bowling Green St Univ; **SLP**

Remsberg, Cheryl Ann 5409 South Rocheblave, New Orleans, LA 70125, (504) 821-2775, BS 70 Susquehanna Univ; OM 82 LA St Univ - N O Medical Ctr; Asst Dir, Sp & Lang Svcs, **SLP**

Remsburg, Mrs Rebecca K 613 West Main, Lake City, IA 51449, (712) 297-8913, BS 74 Northwest MO St Univ; MA 75 Northeast MO St Univ; Sp-Lang Path, Arrowhead AEA, **SLP**

Remsperger, Annette Jackson ENT Clinic, 2585 Spring Arbor Road, Suite 600, Jackson, MI 49203, (517) 787-0039, BA 77 Univ of MI - Ann Arbor; MA 79 MI St Univ; Aud, Jackson ENT Cl, **A**

Remus, Ruth Outer Drive Hospital, Speech-Rehabilitation Med, 26400 West Outer Drive, Lincoln Park, MI 48146, (313) 594-6110, BA 69 Marygove Coll; MA 83 Wayne St Univ; 83–Supvr-SLP/Aud, Pcha-Outer Drive Hospital, **SLP**

Remy, Mrs Darlene Robert R R #1 Box 1122, Ludlow, VT 05149, (802) 228-4907, BS 79 Worcester St Coll; MS 86 Worcester St Coll; **SLP**

Renaud, Mrs Joyce Rita 116 South Main, Perryville, MO 63775, (314) 547-2124, **SLP**

Renberg, Gay Scott 2470 North 91st Street, Wauwatosa, WI 53226, (414) 931-4065, BS 70 Northern IL Univ - De Kalb; MS 79 IL St Univ - Normal; 87–Sp-Lang Path, Children's Hosp of Wisc, **SLP**

Renck, Gene B Aud & Eng Ctr Of Orange Co, 1801 West Romneya Drive, Suite 205, Anaheim, CA 92801, (714) 956-2881, MA 64 CA St Univ - Los Angeles; Aud, Private Practice, **A**

Rende, Barbara 3575 28th Street #202, Boulder, CO 80301, (303) 426-9666, BA 74 Seton Hall Univ; MS 81 Univ of AZ; Sp/Lang Path, Boulder Mem Hosp, **SLP**

Rende, Mrs Sharon Sue 43 Mercedes Drive, Rochester, NY 14624, (716) 271-0680, BS 82 WV Univ; MA 84 OH Univ - Athens; 87–Aud, The Hearing Center Inc, **A**

Rendleman, Mrs Gail Anne 309 Boeing Drive, New Lenox, IL 60451, (815) 467-2900, BS 82 IL St Univ - Normal; MS 84 IL St Univ - Normal; 84–Sp-Lang Path, Reg Educ Svc Agency, **SLP**

Rendon, Anita S 5568 Avenida Adobe, Yorba Linda, CA 92686, (714) 535-6001, BA 76 Our Lady Lake Univ-San Anton; MA 78 Our Lady Lake Univ-San Anton; Sp-Lang Path, Anaheim Cty Sch Dist, **SLP**

Rendon, Kristine Lois 7008 Finn, Houston, TX 77022, (713) 699-4992, BS 81 Univ of Houston - Univ Park; MA 86 Univ of Houston - Univ Park; **SLP**

Renfandt, Mrs Paula E 521 18th Street N W, Minot, ND 58701, (701) 838-7268, BS 73 Univ of ND; MS 77 Minot St Univ; **SLP**

Renfro, Mrs Elizabeth M 1103 Buckboard Boulevard, Papillion, NE 68046, (402) 331-9270, BS 73 Marquette Univ; MS 75 Marquette Univ; Sp-Lang Path, Omaha PS, **SLP**

Renfro-Lesley, Rachel Pozniak 6311 Tally Gate, San Antonio, TX 78240, (512) 522-1057, MA 70 Our Lady Lake Univ-San Anton; Sp-Lang Path, Private Practice, **SLP**

Renge, Joyce Lynn 19610 Ronald Avenue, Torrance, CA 90503, (213) 371-2483, BA 74 Univ of CA - Santa Barbara; MA 81 CA St Univ - Long Beach; SLP, LA Co Supt of Schls, **SLP**

Renie, Tamara Ann 1106 Bon Air Drive, Augusta, GA 30907, (404) 721-6009, OM 87 Auburn Univ - Auburn; Aud, The Med Col of GA

Renier, Michelle P 2418 East Fourth Street, Duluth, MN 55812, (218) 724-2558, OB 87 Univ of MN - Duluth; MA 87 Univ of MN - Duluth

Renken, Susan Marie 2520 Elmwood Avenue #3, Kenmore, NY 14217, (716) 876-0463, BS 82 Syracuse Univ; MA 84 SUNY - Center at Buffalo; **SLP**

Renner, Mrs Carol M 89 Amsterdam Road, Rochester, NY 14610, (716) 482-2000, BS 78 SUNY - Coll at Geneseo; MS 80 Ithaca Coll; 80–Sp-Lang Path, City Sch Dist, **SLP**

Renner, Lisa A 3700 Madera, Columbia, MO 65203, (314) 442-3567, BA 77 Stephens Coll; MA 79 Univ of MO - Columbia; Coord of Aud Svc, Truman VA Hosp, **A ACE**

Renner, Mrs Sherlyn S 247 E 73rd Street, Kansas City, MO 64114, (816) 523-5176, BA 73 Univ of MO - Columbia; MA 74 Univ of MO - Columbia; Director/SLP & Audiol, Medical Center of Independence, **SLP**

Rennick, Patricia Ann 120 Fieldwood Avenue, Seekonk, MA 02771, (617) 336-7558, BS 83 Univ of MA - Amherst; ME 85 Univ of VA - Charlottesville; Sp-Lang Path, Seekonk Special Needs Dept, **SLP**

Rennick, Sydelle 32706 Via Palacio, Rancho Palos Verdes, CA 90274, (213) 377-1924, BA 83 CA St Univ - Long Beach; MA 86 CA St Univ - Long Beach; Sp-Lang Path, Speech & Hearing Services, **SLP**

Rennie, Mrs Kathleen A R R 2 Box 149K, Yorktown, IN 47396, (317) 847-2595, BS 71 Edinboro Univ of PA; MA 86 Ball St Univ; 87–Sp-Lang Path, East Central Spec Svcs, **SLP**

Renshaw, Julia J 6328 Watercrest Way, Indianapolis, IN 46278, (317) 274-8868, BA 80 IN Univ - Bloomington; MA 82 IN Univ - Bloomington; Aud, Riley Hosp, **A**

Rensin, Mrs Katherine 15221 Centergate Drive, Silver Spring, MD 20904, (301) 384-7814, BS 63 Vanderbilt Univ; MA 64 Syracuse Univ; Sp-Lang Path, Private Practice, **SLP**

Rentschler, Fred W 148 Columbia Avenue, Wheeling, WV 26003, (304) 242-5355, BA 74 Capital Univ; MS 79 WV Univ; Sp-Lang Path, Brooke Co Wv Dd of Ed, **SLP**

Rentschler, Dr Gary J Portland Ctr Hearing & Speech, 3515 S W Veterans Hospital, Portland, OR 97201, (313) 764-4493, BA 69 Baldwin-Wallace Coll; MA 72 SUNY - Center at Buffalo; PH 77 (NS) SUNY - Center at Buffalo; Executive Director, Portland Hrng & Speech Ctr, **SLP**

Rentschler, Nancy S 5521 Belpine Trail, Birmingham, AL 35210, (205) 655-3221, BS 74 Univ of AL- Tuscaloosa; MS 79 Univ of Montevallo; SLP, Jefferson Bd of Ed, **SLP**

Rentschler, Mrs Pamela Jo 1325 Colmar Drive, Plano, TX 75023, (214) 517-2969, BS 84 Central MI Univ; MS 86 Univ of MI - Ann Arbor; 88–Sp-Lang Path, Visiting Nurse Association, **SLP**

Rentschler, Paula C 155 Barrington Street, Apt 1, Rochester, NY 14607, (716) 442-5148, MA 87 SUNY - Coll at Geneseo; **SLP**

Renza, Geraldine 35 Olde Country Village, Londonderry, NH 03053, (617) 372-8000, BS 80 Mercy Coll; MS 82 Boston Univ; Sp-Lang Path & Assistant Dir, Northeast Reahb Hospital, **SLP**

Repa, Donna Bromiel Route 2 Box 211 E-3, Yadkinville, NC 27055, (919) 679-2600, BS 78 Univ of IL - Urbana; MS 80 Univ of IL - Urbana; 87–Sp-Lang Path, Yadkin Valley Sp Therapy Svcs, **SLP**

Repass, Mrs Grace S 315 Burlage Circle, Chapel Hill, NC 27514, (703) 981-2867, BS 61 Univ of VA - Charlottesville; MS 81 Radford Univ; 86–Sp-Lang Path, Chapel Hill-Carrboro Schs, **SLP**

Repka, Donna L 7-E Williamsburg East, Greensburg, PA 15601, (412) 836-3292, BS 69 Indiana Univ of PA; MA 74 IN Univ - Bloomington; Sp-Lang Path, Westmoreland Inter Ut 7, **SLP**

Repp, Mrs Lora E E 412 South Lombard Street, Muncie, IN 47304, (317) 642-0201, BS 75 Bowling Green St Univ; MA 76 Western MI Univ; Sp-Lang Path, Hopewell Center, **SLP**

Reppa, Cathleen Joan 2022 North Clifton Avenue, Chicago, IL 60614, (312) 348-4080, BS 84 Purdue Univ - West Lafayette; MS 86 Rush Univ; **SLP**

Resager, Mrs Barbara W 10199 Arrow Point Drive N E, Bainbridge Island, WA 98110, (213) 440-5458, BA 77 CA St Univ - Los Angeles; MA 74 CA St Univ - Los Angeles; **SLP**

Resau, Christine 4145 Henhawk Court, Ellicott City, MD 21043, (301) 569-5537, BA 67 Western MD Coll; MS 78 Loyola Coll; Sp-Lang Path, Anne Arundel Co Schs, **SLP**

Resener, Mrs Ann M 67 Lincoln Avenue, Elgin, IL 60120, (312) 888-5088, MA 75 IN Univ - Bloomington; Sp-Lang Path, Elgin School District U-46, **SLP**

Reses, Nina Arkin 909 Clinton Street #2-A, Philadelphia, PA 19107, (215) 625-8648, BA 85 Franklin & Marshall Coll; MA 87 Tel Aviv Univ - Israel; 88–Sp-Lang Path, The Bancroft Sch

Resnick, Mrs Cynthia B 94-11 59th Avenue, Suite A7, Rego Park, NY 11373, (718) 592-4568, BA 76 Marymount Coll; MS 78 Columbia Univ Teachers Coll; Sp-Lang Path-Consult, Private Practice, **SLP**

Resnick, Dr David M 1620-Earlham Avenue, Crofton, MD 21114, (202) 877-6779, BA 52 Univ of MD - College Park; MA 57 Univ of MD - College Park; PH 66 (Hrng & Sp Science) Univ of MD - College Park; Dir Hrng & Sp, Wash Hosp Cen Hrng & Sp Cen, **SLP A F ACE**

Resnick, Mrs Fern Phillips 9 Joseph Court, Syosset, NY 11791, (516) 681-0225, BA 74 SUNY - Coll at New Paltz; MS 77 Adelphi Univ; Sp-Lang Path, Nassau BOCES, **SLP**

Resnick, Mrs Robin Ellen P O Box 1371, Westhampton Beach, NY 11978, (516) 288-9599, **SLP**

Resnick, Dr Steffi B Resnick & Spencer Inc, 103 East Read St, Baltimore, MD 21202, (301) 234-0007, BA 67 Univ of IA; MS 69 Univ of IA; PH 73 (Aud) Univ of OK Medical Center; 86–Dir of Aud, Resnick & Spencer Inc, **A F ACE**

Resnick, Mrs Sylvia 23-45 Bell Boulevard, Apartment 4G, Bayside, NY 11360, (718) 631-1341, BA 63 CUNY - Brooklyn Coll; MA 68 CUNY - Brooklyn Coll; PH 88 (Sp & Lang) New York Univ; Sp-Lang Path, Private Practice, **SLP**

Resnik, Jane I 2409 Greshan Court, Arlington Heights, IL 60004, (312) 255-1315, BA 77 SUNY - Coll at Cortland; MA 79 Northwestern Univ; **SLP**

Resnik, Mrs Kathleen Collins 3909 Log Trail Way, Reisterstown, MD 21136, BS 75 Northwestern Univ; MA 76 Northwestern Univ; **SLP**

Resnitzky, Lauren Cwenar 51 Ireland Place #8, Amityville, NY 11701, (516) 378-2000, BA 82 Saint John's Univ - Jamaica; MA 84 CUNY - Queens Coll; Sp-Lang Path, UCP, **SLP**

Respess, Joyce Ann 16226 Remuda Trail, Buda, TX 78610, (512) 295-2357, BS 75 Southwest TX St Univ; ME 77 Southwest TX St Univ; Sp-Lang Path, Austin ISD, **SLP**

Ressler, Jane E 81 Bishop Lane, Madison, CT 06443, (203) 245-4561, BS 72 Syracuse Univ; MS 78 Southern CT St Univ; Sp-Lang Path, Madison Bd of Educ, **SLP**

Rest, Mrs Deborah C 425 Sherwood Road, Bristol, VA 24201, (703) 466-6841, BS 72 Longwood Coll; ME 75 Univ of VA - Charlottesville; 88–Sp-Lang Path, Mt Rogers Sp & Lang Path, **SLP**

Restifo, Cheryl Ann Geneseo Heights, Bldg 3 Apartment 11, Geneseo, NY 14454, (716) 243-5223, BS 81 SUNY - Coll at Geneseo; MA 83 SUNY - Coll at Geneseo; 84–Sp-Lang Path, Mt Morris Central Sch, **SLP**

Restivo, Mrs Susan Marold 310 Virginia Drive, Wauseon, OH 43567, (419) 267-3331, BS 75 Edinboro Univ of PA; MA 81 Bowling Green St Univ; SLP, Four County Joint Vocatnl Sch, **SLP**

Restrepo, Maria Adelaida 94 Old Goshen Road, Williamsburg, MA 01096, (413) 534-2508, BA 83 Univ of FL; MA 85 Univ of MA - Amherst; 87–Sp-Lang Path, Holyoke Hosp, **SLP**

Restum, Dr William H 20300 Pollyanna, Livonia, MI 48152, (313) 493-6314, BS 69 Western MI Univ; MA 70 Western MI Univ; PH 78 (NS) Wayne St Univ; Admin Dir Dept of Rehabilitatn, Sinai Hospital of Detroit, **SLP**

Retherford-Stickler, Dr Kristine Sue Dept Communicative Disorders, University Of Wisconsin, Eau Claire, WI 54701, (715) 836-4905, MS 75 Univ of WI - Madison; PH 80 (NS) Univ of WI - Madison; Asst Prof, U of WI, **SLP**

Rethlefsen, Lola L 4187 Ramona Place S E, Albany, OR 97321, (503) 928-2288, MS 84 Univ of WI - Whitewater; Sp-Lang Path, Outpatient Rehab Inst, **SLP**

Reticker, Mrs Aleyda De Jesus 935 West Cornelia #1-A, Chicago, IL 60657, (312) 880-8161, BS 84 Univ of PR - San Juan; MA 86 Northwestern Univ; 86–Sp-Lang Path, Chicago Bd of Educ, **SLP**

Retish, Mrs Esther S 66 Penfro Drive, Iowa City, IA 52240, (319) 354-4211, MA 66 PA St Univ - Univ Park; Esl Tchr, Iowa Cty Sch Dist, **SLP**

Retseck, Mrs Kathleen Kuzydym 0481 North 700 West, La Porte, IN 46350, (219) 879-2411, BS 76 Purdue Univ - West Lafayette; MA 79 IN Univ - Bloomington; Sp Lang Cl, Michigan Cty Area Sch, **SLP**

Rettgers, Bonnie J Second General Hospital, Audiology, P O Box 52, APO New York, NY 09180-3460, BS 74 East Carolina Univ; MS 80 CO St Univ; 86–Aud, US Dept of the Army, **A**

Rettig, Nancy D Communication Plus Inc, P O Box 1454, Bellevue, WA 98009-1454, (206) 453-0233, BA 67 Univ of WA; MS 71 Syracuse Univ; Sp-Lang Path, Private Practice, **SLP**

Retzer, Mrs Chare N 123 North Haven Drive, Kalispell, MT 59901, (406) 755-3669, BA 69 Loma Linda Univ - Riverside; MA 71 CA St Univ - Fullerton; Sp-Lang Path, Private Practice, **SLP**

Retzlaff, Suellen S 2714 Bayshore Drive, La Crosse, WI 54603, (608) 784-1697, BS 74 Univ of WI - Madison; MS 76 Univ of WI - Madison; Sp-Lang Path, Sch Dist of Lacrosse, **SLP ACE**

Retzlaff, Wesley 127 West Lincoln Avenue, Barrington, IL 60010, MS; **SLP LM**

Reuben, Eileen R 2583 Ashford Road N E, Atlanta, GA 30319, (404) 451-7484, BS 71 Univ of MO - Columbia; ME 75 GA St Univ; 76–Sp-Lang Path, American Home Health, **SLP**

Reuben, Gail D 9 Barberry Road, Convent, NJ 07961, (201) 539-2825, BA 62 Rutger's St Univ - Douglas Coll; MA 64 Seton Hall Univ; Aud Consult, Lake Dr Sch/Hrng Imp Chldn, **A**

Reuler, Mrs Ellen S 7529 S E 28th Avenue, Portland, OR 97202, (503) 777-4327, BA 72 Northwestern Univ; MA 73 Northwestern Univ; Instr, Portland State Univ, **SLP**

Reuler, Peggy R Beaverton School District #48, P O Box 200, Beaverton, OR 97075, (503) 649-0241, BS 71 Univ of IL - Urbana; MA 72 Northwestern Univ; Sp-Lang Path, Beaverton School District #48, **SLP**

Reuse, Alison Foote P O Box 687, Urbanna, VA 23175, (804) 758-2496, BS 85 Univ of WI - Stevens Point; MS 86 Univ of WI - Eau Claire; 87–Sp-Lang Path, Middlesex Co PS, **SLP**

Reuter, Catherine 300 Spring Street, Thiensville, WI 53092, **SLP**

Reuter, Mrs Ellen R 97 Sheffield Road, Cranston, RI 02920, (401) 944-7094, BS 69 Boston Univ; MS 84 Univ of RI; 85–Sp-Lang Path, Burrillville RI Sch Sys, **SLP**

Reuter-Donato, Cathleen Anne 11 Katherine Avenue, Passaic, NJ 07055, (201) 778-2703, BA 76 William Paterson Coll; MA 80 Ball St Univ; Sp-Lang Path, Wyckoff Day Training Center, **SLP**

Reutter, Susan L 865 Donovan Court, Davis, CA 95616, (916) 753-8718, BA 82 Univ of CA - Davis; MS 84 San Francisco St Univ; 88–Sp-Lang Path, Davis Med Ctr, **SLP**

Reveron, Dr Wilhelmina Communication Sciences, 916 G Street N W, Washington, DC 20001, (202) 727-2636, BS 75 Boston Univ; MA 76 OH St Univ; PH 79 (NS) OH St Univ; Asst Prof Sp-Lang Path, Univ of District of Columbia, **SLP**

Revis, Margret F 108 Lafayette Lane, League City, TX 77573-1934, (713) 332-3080, OB 28 Baylor Coll of Medicine; BA 28 Baylor Coll of Medicine; MA 43 Univ of North TX; Retired, **SLP LM**

Revis-Fax, Mrs Andrea Michelle 831 Rio Grande, Pasadena, CA 91104, (213) 938-1033, BA 80 Univ of CA - Santa Barbara; **SLP**

Revit, Lawrence Jay c/o Frye Electronics Inc, 9826 SW Tigard Street, Tigard, OR 97223, (503) 620-2722, OB 79 Univ of Miami; MA 87 Northwestern Univ; 88–Aud, Frye Electronics Inc

Revling-Kreb, Roberta A 17281 88th Avenue North, Maple Grove, MN 55369, (612) 781-6571, BA 74 Univ of MN - Minneap-St Paul; MS 76 Saint Cloud St Univ; 87–Dir of Mktg & Research, Achievement Rehab Corp, **SLP H ACE**

Revoile, Dr Sally G Gallaudet University, CASS-MT Bldg, Washington, DC 20002, (202) 651-5460, BA 62 Univ of MD - College Park; MA 65 Univ of MD - College Park; PH 70 (Hrng Science) Univ of MD - College Park; 87–Dir/Prof of Auditory Res, Gallaudet Univ, **A**

Revoir, Katherine Elaine 1650 Holden Avenue #215, Orlando, FL 32809, BA 84 Univ of Central FL; MA 86 Univ of Central FL; **SLP**

Revord, Marceia Joyce Route 7 Box 481, Columbus, MS 39701, (601) 327-3648, BS 84 MS Univ for Women; MS 86 Univ Southern MS-Hattiesburg; 86–Sp-Lang Path, West Point PS, **SLP**

Revucky, Mrs Mary C 1201 Delaware Lane, Downingtown, PA 19335, (215) 383-5463, BA 63 Temple Univ-Tyler Sch of Art; MA 66 Temple Univ-Tyler Sch of Art; Sp/Lang Path, Hm Hlth Serv, **SLP**

Rew, Mrs Christy Jackson 1534 Lahotan Way, Las Vegas, NV 89110, (803) 499-9019, BA 81 LA Tech Univ; ME 84 Univ of NV - Las Vegas; MA 85 LA Tech Univ; **SLP**

Rexroth, Donna Louise 248 Reindollar Avenue, Marina, CA 93933, (408) 384-3069, BA 85 CA St Univ - Long Beach; MA 88 CA St Univ - Fresno; 88–Sp-Lang Path, Hollister USD

Rey, Mrs Janice Whitehead 881 Northwest 67th Avenue, Plantation, FL 33317, (305) 926-0940, BA 75 Rutger's St Univ - Douglas Coll; MS 76 Rutgers St Univ -N Brunswick; 87–Asst Prin, Broward Dist Schools, **SLP**

Reyell, Joan K Box 369 Rd 1, Trudeau Road, Saranac Lake, NY 12983, (518) 891-2026, **SLP**

Reyes, Mrs Belinda Alvarado 505 Green Oaks Court #1034, Arlington, TX 76006, (817) 275-7901, BS 81 Baylor Univ; MS 84 Univ of TX - Dallas; Sp-Lang Path, University of Texas, **SLP**

Reyes, Jacqueline G 78 Autumn Avenue, Cypress Hills, NY 11208, (718) 235-5022, BA 85 CUNY - Hunter Coll; MS 86 Ithaca Coll; **SLP**

Reyna, Mrs Diane S 48 Dupont Terrace, Wayne, NJ 07470, (201) 628-1638, BA 75 William Paterson Coll; MS 86 William Paterson Coll; **SLP ACE**

Reyna, Gaila Denise 4940 Shadowbend Drive, Corpus Christi, TX 78413, (512) 991-9690, BS 76 Univ of Central AR; MS 85 Univ of Central AR; 88–Sp-Lang Path, Rehab Hosp of So TX, **SLP**

Reyna, Karen Ann 311 South 8th Street, West Helena, AR 72390, (501) 572-5975, BS 70 Univ of ND; OM 86 AR St Univ; **SLP**

Reyneke, Mrs Judith Ann Long 2872 Metolius Drive, Eugene, OR 97401, (503) 345-8642, BS 75 OR St Univ; MS 77 Univ of OR; 86–Sp/Lang Path, Lowell PS, **SLP**

Reynolds, Anne T 203 Hartwell Road, Silver Spring, MD 20901, (207) 622-9351, BA 73 Univ of ME - Orono; MS 76 Univ of VT; Sp-Lang Path, The Treatment & Learning Centers, **SLP**

Reynolds, Beverly A 95 Center Street, Rutland, VT 05701, (802) 775-2395, MA 81 Bowling Green St Univ; 88–Sp-Lang Path, Vermont Achievement Ctr, **SLP**

Reynolds, Mrs Beverly R 232 Evans Avenue, Missoula, MT 59801, (406) 243-4131, BS 56 Univ of WI - Madison; MS 61 Univ of WI - Madison; Asst Prof, U Mt, **SLP ACE**

Reynolds, Dr Brian W Dept Communication Disorders, University Of North Dakota, PO Box 8040, Grand Forks, ND 58202, (701) 777-3232, BS 74 Brigham Young Univ; MS 75 Brigham Young Univ; PH 80 (NS) Purdue Univ - West Lafayette; 81–Assoc Prof of Aud, U of ND, **A**

Reynolds, Bruce E PO Box 1160, Captain Cook, HI 96704, (808) 328-9158, BA 76 Univ of HI - Manoa; MA 82 Univ of Northern CO; Sp-Lang Path, Private Practice, **SLP**

Reynolds, Carol Suzanne Route 3 Box 121, Smithsburg, MD 21783, (301) 824-2158, MS 87 Loyola Coll; **SLP**

Reynolds, Mrs Catherine 240 Chasse Circle, St Charles, IL 60174, (312) 232-0883, BS 70 Western IL Univ; MA 79 Western IL Univ; 85–Sp-Lang Path, Geneva School District 304, **A**

Reynolds, Charla L 1076 Oaklawn Drive, Culpeper, VA 22701, (703) 825-1987, BA 72 Univ of MS; ME 73 Univ of VA - Charlottesville; Sp-Lang Path, Culpeper Mem Hosp, **SLP**

Reynolds, Mrs Colette Bartlinski 5679 Rayburn Avenue, Alexandria, VA 22311, (202) 745-5600, BA 78 Wilson Coll; MA 82 George Washington Univ; 87–Coord Sp-Lang Path Svcs, Chldn Hosp Hrng & Sp Cen, **SLP**

Reynolds, Mrs Danielle Helen 25-A Ted Street, St Catharines, ON, Canada L2N 1E6, (416) 937-0803, BA 71 Univ of Toronto - Ontario; MA 85 SUNY - Coll at Buffalo; 85–Sp-Lang Path, Niagara Peninsula Rehab Ctr, **SLP**

Reynolds, Dean E 74 Walden, Burnsville, MN 55337, (612) 293-7621, BA 60 Augustana Coll; 65–Facilitator, St Paul Pub Schs, **SLP**

Reynolds, Deb S 3300 Eveningside #12, Topeka, KS 66614, (913) 232-0597, BS 80 KS St Univ; MA 83 KS St Univ; 88–Sp-Lang Path, Topeka Assoc for Ret Citizens, **SLP**

Reynolds, Deborah A 3403 Bayshore Drive, Doraville, GA 30340, (404) 938-8403, BS 75 PA St Univ - Univ Park; ME 76 Univ of GA; **SLP**

Reynolds, Deborah L 2912 Manhattan Boulevard, Unit 135, Harvey, LA 70058, (504) 341-3437, BA 77 Tulane Univ; OM 79 Univ of MS; Sp/Lang Path, Jefferson Parish Pub Sch Syst, **SLP**

Reynolds, Diana Lynn 3 Clint Court #B, Little Rock, AR 72205, (501) 661-2320, BS 84 Univ of Central AR; MS 87 Univ of AR - Little Rock; 87–Sp-Lang Path, AR Dept of Health, **SLP**

Reynolds, Mrs Eileen Kahl 521 South Dupont Highway, Smyrna, DE 19977, (302) 454-7234, BS 82 Towson St Univ; MS 84 Towson St Univ; Aud, Christiana Med Ctr, **A**

Reynolds, Ellen B 1012 Darrow Avenue, Evanston, IL 60202, (312) 492-3840, BA 57 Howard Univ; MS 59 Gallaudet Coll; Dir of Spec Ed, Evanston Twsp Hs

Reynolds, Dr Garnet L 10725 S W 128th Terrace, Miami, FL 33176, (305) 666-7613, BS 60 CA Univ of PA; MS 67 FL St Univ; PH 77 (NS) FL St Univ; Dir, A Positive Comm Image Inc, **SLP**

Reynolds, Mrs Jennifer Elaine Route 2 Box 2150, Burley, ID 83318, (208) 678-3911, BS 82 Brigham Young Univ; MS 83 Brigham Young Univ; 87–Sp-Lang Path, Minidoka Co Schs Dist 331, **SLP ACE**

Reynolds, Mrs Jerri Bolling 321 South Elm Street #201, Greensboro, NC 27401, (919) 275-9437, BS 83 Appalachian St Univ; MS 85 Univ of NC - Chapel Hill; **SLP**

Reynolds, Judith L 2601 Woodhaven Drive, Ashland, KY 41101, **SLP**

Reynolds, Mrs Judith T 1705 Haggin Grove Way, Carmichael, CA 95608, **SLP**

Reynolds, Julia Winifred P O Box 0397, Oak Harbor, WA 98277, BA 85 Univ of Central FL; MA 87 Univ of Central FL; **A**

Reynolds, Linda Estelle 753 Janice Drive, Columbia, SC 29210-7825, (803) 798-9184, BA 72 Univ of MI - Ann Arbor; MS 74 Univ of MI - Ann Arbor; ES 83 East TN St Univ; SLP, East Midlands Home Health, **SLP**

Reynolds, Lisa C 4532 Westchester, Louisville, KY 40211, (502) 454-8348, BA 77 Univ of KY; MA 79 Univ of IA; SLP, Jefferson Co Bd of Ed, **SLP**

Reynolds, Louise 36 Oxford Street, Claremont 7700, Cape Province, South Africa T100, BS 85 Univ of Capetown - S Africa; 88–Sp-Lang Path/Aud, Private Practice

Reynolds, Marilyn Ostrowski 225 Podunk Road, Sturbridge, MA 01566, (508) 765-9771, BS 78 Ithaca Coll; MA 81 Univ of MA - Amherst; Aud, Harrington Memorial Hosp, **A**

Reynolds, Mary D Dir Of Aud Prof Hearing Consit, Mo Baptist Diagnostic Ctr, 3009 N Ballas Rd Suite 201, St Louis, MO 63131, (314) 567-6741, BS 74 AZ St Univ; MA 76 Univ of IL - Urbana; Dir-Aud/Hrng Aid Serv Mgr, Christie Clinic, **A**

Reynolds, Mrs Mary E 214 11th Avenue, Huntington, WV 25701, (606) 836-8186, BA 73 Univ of KY; MA 77 Marshall Univ; Sp-Lang Path, Russell ISD, **SLP**

Reynolds, Mary J 1810 Commonwealth Avenue, Apt #21, Brighton, MA 02135, (617) 647-6564, MS 84 Cleveland St Univ; Sp-Lang Path, Waltham Weston Hosp, **SLP**

Reynolds, Mrs Mary Patricia 66 Miriam Street, Valley Stream, NY 11581, (516) 223-8100, **SLP**

Reynolds, Mrs Marylou F 22533 Imperial Drive, Richton Park, IL 60471, (312) 481-1574, BS 77 Radford Univ; MA 78 Trenton St Coll; Sp/Lang Path, Good Shephard Cen Flossmoor, **SLP**

Reynolds, Mrs Nancy B 513 Homestead Avenue, Metairie, LA 70005, (504) 835-8439, BA 72 Univ of MS; MA 72 Tulane Univ; 73–Sp-Lang Path, Jeff Parish PS Sys, **SLP**

Reynolds, Patricia Ann 15 Cotton Street, Leominster, MA 01453, (617) 537-6443, BS 76 Worcester St Coll; MS 85 Northeastern Univ; **A**

Reynolds, R Eric 4300 Rosemeade #428, Dallas, TX 75252, (214) 946-6085, BS 85 TX Tech Univ; MS 86 TX Tech Univ; **A**

Reynolds, Mrs Rebecca Birsner 1216 Twilight, Midwest City, OK 73110, (405) 733-7106, BS 78 Univ of Tulsa; MS 83 Univ of OK - OK City; Sp-Lang Path, Mid-Del Pub Sch, **SLP**

Reynolds, Robert B, Jr 106 Pollasky Street Ste 3, Clovis, CA 93612, (209) 299-3566, BA 69 CA St Univ - Fresno; MA 71 CA St Univ - Fresno; Audiologist, Private Practice, **A**

Reynolds, Mrs Rosemary P O Box 28, Absarokee, MT 59001, (406) 322-5372, BS 71 MT St Univ; MS 73 Univ of OK Medical Center; Sp/Lang Path, Stillwater/Sweetgrass Coop, **SLP**

Reynolds, Sandra Gayle 679 University Drive, Prestonsburg, KY 41653, (606) 886-9200, BA 84 Univ of KY; MS 86 Univ of KY; 87–Sp-Lang Path, Johnson Co Bd of Educ, **SLP**

Reynolds, Susan Marie 4420 San Mateo, Mc Kinney, TX 75070, (214) 540-1800, BS 84 Univ of TX - Dallas; MS 87 Univ of North TX; 87–Aud, ENT Surgical Assoc, **A**

Reynolds, Toni A 69 Westminster Road, Rochester, NY 14607, (716) 271-0680, BA 84 SUNY - Center at Buffalo; MA 86 SUNY - Center at Buffalo; 87–Aud, Hrng & Sp Ctr of Rochester, **A**

Reyor, Lea J B Star Rt Box 25B, 31C Hoel Pond Road, Saranac Lake, NY 12983, (518) 891-3693, MA 83 SUNY - Coll at Plattsburgh; Sp-Lang Path, Private Practice/FEH BOCES, **SLP**

Rezabek, Mrs Barbara Campbell 125 Kedzie Street #2, Evanston, IL 60202, (312) 869-9204, BA 82 Univ of IA; MA 85 Univ of IA; Aud, Chicago Bd of Ed, **A**

Rezai, Mrs Terry F Box 53, Bloomfield, IA 52537, (515) 664-3488, BS 71 Northeast MO St Univ; MA 72 Northeast MO St Univ; Sp-Lang Path, Sn Pr AEA, **SLP**

Rezen, Dr Susan V 207 Lovell Road, Holden, MA 01520, (617) 793-8055, BA 69 SUNY - Center at Albany; MS 71 Purdue Univ - West Lafayette; PH 80 (Aud) Syracuse Univ; 80–Prof, Worcester St Coll, **A ACE**

Reznicek, Virginia L Route 2 Box 2950, Hartsburg, MO 65039, (314) 876-7309, BS 65 Univ of MO - Columbia; MA 66 Univ of MO - Columbia; 66–Director Sp-Lang Services, Woodhaven Learning Center, **SLP**

Rhame, Leland W P O Box 1515, Morganton, NC 28655, (704) 433-7452, BA 72 Wofford Coll; ME 74 Univ of SC - Columbia; Aud, Blue Ridge Aud Hrng Aid Svc, **A**

Rhatigan, Rebecca J 423 North Terrace, Wichita, KS 67208, (316) 682-6878, MA 88 Wichita St Univ

Rhea, Melinda Kaye 7109-A Tanager Court, Chattanooga, TN 37412, (615) 267-5641, BS 86 Univ Southern MS-Hattiesburg; MS 87 Univ Southern MS-Hattiesburg

Rhein, Alice Laster 203 North Lafayette #202, Royal Oak, MI 48067, (313) 465-5501, BA 84 Univ of MI - Ann Arbor; MS 86 Univ of MI - Ann Arbor; Sp-Lang Path, St John Hosp Macomb Ctr, **SLP**

Rhein, Mrs Catherine T 23 Karnell Drive, Piscataway, NJ 08854, (201) 463-7644, BS 72 Trenton St Coll; MA 75 Trenton St Coll; Sp-Lang Path, Piscataway Bd of Ed, **SLP**

Rhein, Ingeborg 6109 Dunleer Court, Bethesda, MD 20817, (301) 279-8490, BA 76 Univ of MD - College Park; MA 78 Univ of MD - College Park; 79–Sp-Lang Path, McPs, **SLP**

Rhein, Stephanie A 2136 Muren Boulevard, Belleville, IL 62221, (618) 398-7222, BS 78 Southern IL Univ-Edwardsvill; MS 79 Southern IL Univ-Edwardsvill; **SLP**

Rheingold, Gail 170 South Manning Blvd, Albany, NY 12208, (518) 828-9493, BA 61 Wells Coll; MS 65 Coll of Saint Rose; MA 70 Columbia Univ Teachers Coll; Sp/Lang Path, Hudson City Sch Dist, **SLP**

Rhicard, Ellen 97 Gillette Avenue, Springfield, MA 01118-1519, (413) 533-7318, BA 66 Univ of MA - Amherst; MA 68 Univ of MD - College Park; Sp-Lang Path, Springfield Mass Pub Sch, **SLP**

Rhoades, Inez B 3045 Terrace Drive #303E, Las Cruces, NM 88001, (505) 522-2268, BA 28 Huron Coll; MA 42 Univ of Denver; OD 54 (NS) Univ of Northern CO; **SLP LM**

Rhoades, Mrs Jeanne C 351 East Main, Du Quoin, IL 62832, BS 45 Fontbonne Coll; MS 74 Southern IL Univ -Carbondale; 88–Sp-Lang Path, Private Practice, **SLP**

Rhoades, Mrs Lynn Margaret 1480 U S Highway 46 #160B, Parsippany, NJ 07054, (201) 906-2929, BA 83 SUNY - Coll at Cortland; MS 85 Southern CT St Univ; 88–Sp-Lang Path, JFK Med Ctr, **SLP**

Rhoads, Mrs Lynn T 1010 Pilot Avenue, Cherokee, IA 51012, (712) 225-2568, BS 67 Western IL Univ; MA 79 Univ of SD - Vermillion; SLP, Wn Hills AEA 12, **SLP**

Rhoads, Mrs Marjorie J 1101 Morrow Avenue, Nashville, TN 37204, (615) 259-8702, BS 64 Central MI Univ; MS 72 Vanderbilt Univ; Sp-Lang Path, Metro Nashville Public Schools, **SLP**

Rhoads-Leslie, Janet 54 Peach Tree Lane, Mount Sinai, NY 11766-9130, (516) 467-3440, BS 74 SUNY - Coll at Geneseo; MA 75 Hofstra Univ; Sp-Lang Path, Sachem Cen Sch Dist, **SLP**

Rhode, Kathy Lyn 34 Rainbow Drive, Humboldt, IA 50548, (515) 332-3024, BS 82 IA St Univ; MS 83 Univ of NE - Lincoln; 85–Sp-Lang Path, Arrowhead AEA, **SLP**

Rhodehamel, Mrs Susan E 1255 North Fairfield Road, Beaver Creek, OH 45432, (513) 429-1064, BS 58 OH St Univ; MA 80 Univ of Cincinnati; Sp-Lang Path, Beavercreek Sp Cen, **SLP**

Rhodes, Alice E 240 East 35th Street #11-K, New York, NY 10016, (212) 686-8732, BA 48 Syracuse Univ; MA 68 NY Univ; Private Practice, **SLP**

Rhodes, Catherine Anne 2922 North Hills Drive, Atlanta, GA 30305, (404) 233-4157, BA 81 Univ of AL- Tuscaloosa; MS 83 Univ of AL- Tuscaloosa; 88–Sp-Lang Path, Associated Health Focus, **SLP**

Rhodes, Cheryl D 1114 Burlington, Flint, MI 48503-2935, (313) 743-2474, MA 78 Eastern MI Univ; Sp-Lang Path, McLaren Gen Hosp, **SLP A**

Rhodes, Diane I 6226 Lake Aral Avenue, San Diego, CA 92119, (619) 292-9931, BA 67 San Diego St Univ; MS 68 Univ of MI - Ann Arbor; 84–Sp-Lang Path, San Diego Speech & Rehab Serv, **SLP**

Rhodes, Don E 12711 Blue Mt Crescent, R R #4, Maple Ridge, BC, Canada V2X 8X8, (604) 467-1101, BA 71 Western WA Univ; MA 73 WA St Univ; Sp-Lang Path, Sch Dist #42, **SLP**

Rhodes, Franklin E 5670 Deerfield Place, Kennesaw, GA 30144, (404) 426-6330, BS 60 Kent St Univ; MA 65 Kent St Univ; Administrator, Self Employed, **SLP**

Rhodes, Mrs Janice Lynne 292 Sandy Run, Melbourne, FL 32940, (305) 254-1337, **SLP**

Rhodes, Mrs Jean 1112 Newman Street, Winnsboro, LA 71295, (318) 435-5408, BA 76 LA Tech Univ; ME 81 Northeast LA Univ; MA 85 Northeast LA Univ; **SLP**

Rhodes, Mrs Jerilyn Deboer 5214 Brookfield Lane, Sylvania, OH 43560, (419) 666-5180, ME 80 Univ of Toledo; MA 83 Bowling Green St Univ; Aud/Sp-Lang Path, Toledo Pub Sch, **A**

Rhodes, Linda T 19 Walnut Farms Road, Farmington, CT 06032, (203) 674-9461, BS 77 Bradley Univ; MS 78 Adelphi Univ; **SLP**

Rhodes, Lynne S Forrest General Hospital, Hattiesburg, MS 39401, (601) 264-4386, BA 69 Univ of WY; MS 70 Univ of WY; Sp-Lang Path, Commun & Acoust Conslt, **SLP**

Rhodes, Mrs P Joyce 1216 Allison Lane, Schaumburg, IL 60194, (312) 934-2883, BS 62 Southern IL Univ -Carbondale; MA 73 Sangamon St Univ; Sp-Lang Path, Ccsd #15 Palatine Il, **SLP**

Rhodes, Rebecca Sue 30 Bungay Road Apartment 3, Seymour, CT 06483, (203) 888-1610, BA 86 Central MI Univ; MA 87 MI St Univ; Sp-Lang Path, InSpeech Inc, **SLP**

Rhodes, Dr Robert C 104 Redbud Lane, Hattiesburg, MS 39402, (601) 266-5216, BS 61 CO St Univ; MS 65 Univ of CO - Boulder; PH 68 (NS) Univ of Pittsburgh - Pittsburgh; Prof, U So Mississippi, **SLP**

Rhubart, Myla Ann 583 Maurice River Parkway, Vineland, NJ 08360, (609) 794-5709, BA 77 Rutger's St Univ - Douglas Coll; MA 82 Trenton St Coll; Sp-Lang Path, Vineland Dev Cen, **SLP ACE**

Rhyne, Mrs Lauren Clarkson Box 779, Bermuda Run, Advance, NC 27006, (704) 872-6552, BA 82 NC St Univ at Raleigh; ME 84 Univ of NC - Greensboro; 84–Sp-Lang Path, Iredell Co Hlth Dept, **SLP**

Rhyne, Mrs Tina M 11 Brookside Road, Darien, CT 06820, (203) 655-6109, BA 81 Lenoir-Rhyne Coll; MS 86 Southern CT St Univ; **SLP**

Rhyner-Saulnier, Mary 1410 Westover Road, Austin, TX 78703, (512) 480-1999, BS 74 Southern Methodist Univ; MS 75 Southern Methodist Univ; 85–SLP, Brackenridge Hosp, **SLP**

Ribbeck, Karen S 1587 Assumption #4, Windsor, ON, Canada N9A 3E2, (519) 254-7937, BA 85 Augustana Coll; MA 86 Western MI Univ; 88–Sp-Lang Path, Windsor Western Hosp Ctr, **SLP**

Ribbler, Mrs Nancy S 580 Bucknell #M, Claremont, CA 91711, (714) 596-7733, BA 80 Univ of MI - Ann Arbor; MA 83 CA St Univ - Fresno; Sp-Lang Path, Casa Colina Rehab Hosp, **SLP**

Ribera, John E 5026 El Capitan, San Antonio, TX 78233, (512) 221-5636, BA 69 Brigham Young Univ; OM 80 Brigham Young Univ; Assistant Chief Aud, US Army, **A**

Riccardi, Linda M P O Box 238, Humarock, MA 02047, (617) 837-0024, ME 83 Northeastern Univ; 86–Sp-Lang Path, Norwell PS, **SLP**

Ricci, Carol Lisa 2650 North Lakeview #3004, Chicago, IL 60614, (312) 525-2132, BA 76 Univ of CO - Boulder; MA 81 Univ of Miami; Aud, **A ACE**

Ricci, Paula Ann P O Box 295, Guilford, CT 06437, (203) 484-0485, BA 80 Univ of RI; MS 84 Southern CT St Univ; **SLP**

Ricci, Mrs Rosanne Palermo 128 Kaywood Drive, Rochester, NY 14626, (716) 325-4560, BS 78 Nazareth Coll of Rochester; MS 83 Nazareth Coll of Rochester; SLP, Rochester City School District, **SLP**

Ricciardi, Mrs Geraldine Dunaway P O Box 68235, Grand Rapids, MI 49516-8235, (616) 940-9877, BS 83 Stephen F Austin St Univ; ME 85 Stephen F Austin St Univ; SLP, Sabine Independent School Dist

Ricciardi, John G Manor Care, Nursing & Rehabilitation, Mountainside, NJ 07092, (201) 654-0020, BA 73 Fairleigh Dickinson U-Madisn; MS 78 Seton Hall Univ; 88–Sp-Lang Path, Manor Healthcare Corp, **SLP**

Ricciardi, Karen M 1149 Appian Drive, Webster, NY 14580, (716) 872-1971, BS 80 SUNY - Coll at Fredonia; MS 81 Bloomsburg Univ of PA; Sp-Lang Path, Private Practice, **SLP**

Ricci-Braum, Diane 9961 Darrow Park Drive, Apartment 131-D, Twinsburg, OH 44087, (216) 487-0916, BS 75 PA St Univ - Univ Park; MS 76 PA St Univ - Univ Park; Sp-Lang Path, Brunswick City Schools, **SLP**

Riccio, Susan E 60 Knolls Crescent, Bronx, NY 10463, (914) 668-6580, BA 82 SUNY - Coll at Cortland; MA 84 CUNY - Lehman Coll; Sp-Lang Path, Mt Vernon Board of Education, **SLP**

Riccobono, Mrs Pina Tosca 10 Sherwood Avenue, Brunswick, NJ 08816, (201) 390-7632, BA 78 CUNY - Brooklyn Coll; MA 85 Kean Coll of NJ

Rice, Barbara D 7311 Fairington Circle, Hixson, TN 37343, (615) 877-8313, BA 62; MS 74 Boston Univ; Sp-Lang Path, Hamilton Co Schs, **SLP**

Rice, Mrs Cheryl E 2141 Silentree Drive, Vienna, VA 22180, (703) 481-4242, BA 69; MS 71 CO St Univ; 85–Aud, Fairfax Co Hlth Dept, **A**

Rice, Donna Marie P O Box 4696, Salem, OR 97302, (303) 597-2230, MA 84 Univ of Northern CO; Sp-Lang Path, Latch School, **SLP**

Rice, Gale Borkowski 3932 Connecticut, St Louis, MO 63116, (314) 889-1407, BS 76 Bradley Univ; MS 77 Bradley Univ; Clinic Director, Fontbonne College, **SLP**

Rice, Mrs Janet G 13512 Greenleaf Drive, Tampa, FL 33613, (813) 972-7529, BS 77 Southern IL Univ-Edwardsvill; MS 78 Southern IL Univ-Edwardsvill; 86–Sp-Lang Path, James A Haley VA Med Ctr, **SLP**

Rice, Dr Mabel L Department Of Speech - Language - Hearing, Room 2101 Haworth Hall, University Of Kansas, Lawrence, KS 66044, (913) 864-4570, BA 78 Univ of KS; MA 67 Univ of Northern IA; PH 66 (NS) Univ of Northern IA; Prof, U of KS, **SLP**

Rice, Mrs Marcia E 3331 Eden Hollow Place, Carmel, IN 46032, (317) 846-5613, BA 62 IN Univ - Bloomington; MS 63 Univ of WI - Madison; **SLP A**

Rice, Mary W T 2081 Linden Avenue, Memphis, TN 38104, (901) 272-0804, **SLP**

Rice, Mrs Nancy J M 2311 Brentwood Lane, Billings, MT 59102, (406) 656-1713, BA 82 Univ of ND; OM 86 Univ of MT; 87–Sp-Lang Path, Private Practice, **SLP**

Rice, Pat M Minnesota State Academy / Deaf, P O Box 308, Faribault, MN 55021, (507) 332-3350, BA 65 Saint Cloud St Univ; MA 66 Northwestern Univ; Aud, MN State Dept of Health, **A**

Rice, Robyn R 420 South Main Street, Hebron, IN 46341, **A**

Rice, Sally J 20 Main Street, Shelburne Falls, MA 01370, (413) 625-2963, BS 85 Univ of MA - Amherst; MA 88 IN Univ - Bloomington; 88–Sp-Lang Path, Mohawk Trail Reg Sch Dist

Rice, Mrs Shannon L 8226 Running Creek Court, Springfield, VA 22153, (703) 938-7743, BS 73 Old Dominion Univ; MA 75 George Washington Univ; SLP, Fairfax Co Public Sch, **SLP**

Rice, Teresa Denese 801 West Loomis Street, Ludington, MI 49431, (616) 845-1940, BA 83 Univ of Northern CO; MA 84 Univ of Denver; **SLP**

Rice, Mrs Vicki Colliver 4211 Levee Road, Mount Sterling, KY 40353, (606) 498-3793, BS 76 Western KY Univ; MA 78 Univ of KY; Sp-Lang Path, **SLP**

Rice, Vickie Diann 801 Sandycreek Drive, Allen, TX 75002, (214) 727-4227, BS 82 Univ of TX - Dallas; MS 85 Univ of TX - Dallas; **A**

Rice-Fenstermaker, Mrs Claire 193 Whitman Street, East Bridgewater, MA 02333, (508) 824-6911, BS 80 Worcester St Coll; MA 81 SUNY - Coll at Geneseo; 84–Sp/Lang Path, Morton Hospital, **SLP ACE**

Rich, Mrs Gay Dingman 37 Cedar Drive, North Stonington, CT 06359, (315) 628-5056, BA 70 9245; Sp-Lang Path, New London Public Schools, **SLP**

Rich, Mrs Janice Smithbauer 42263 Greenwood Drive, Canton, MI 48187, (313) 745-8903, BA 84 MI St Univ; MS 86 Univ of MI - Ann Arbor; **A**

Rich, Mrs Joan Pedersen 6641 South Magnolia Court, Englewood, CO 80111, (303) 861-6800, BA 64 Grinnell Coll; MA 66 Univ of WI - Madison; Sp/Lang Path, The Children's Hosp, **SLP**

Rich, Mrs Lori A 15 Crescent Square, Newton Corner, MA 02158, (617) 969-4304, BS 85 Elmira Coll; MS 86 Univ of MI - Ann Arbor; 88–Sp-Lang Path, Mass Gen Hosp, **SLP**

Rich, Rita Dushman 7626 Harshmanville Road, Huber Heights, OH 45424, (513) 276-5007, BA 71 CUNY - Brooklyn Coll; MA 73 Univ of IA; Sp-Lang Path, Private Practice, **SLP**

Rich, Rose Rubel 5446 Marcia Avenue, New Orleans, LA 70124, (504) 482-9627, BA 64 Tulane Univ; MS 66 Tulane Univ; Sp-Lang Path, **SLP**

Rich, Wanda M 119 Ridge Road, Summerville, SC 29485, (803) 571-2868, BS 81 Radford Univ; MS 82 Radford Univ; Dir Speech Therapy Dept, Associated Healthfocus, **SLP**

Richard, Dr Gail J Communication Disorders & Sciences, Eastern Illinois University, Charleston, IL 61920, (217) 581-2712, BA 76 Augustana Coll; MS 77 Eastern IL Univ; PH 87 (Comm Disorders & Sciences) Southern IL Univ -Carbondale; 81–Assoc Prof, Eastern IL Univ, **SLP ACE**

Richard, Mrs Holly B 14710 Acorn Ridge Place, Midlothian, VA 23113, (804) 745-0827, BA 77 Miami Univ - Oxford; MS 78 Miami Univ - Oxford; Sp-Lang Path, Chesterfield County Schools, **SLP**

Richard, Isabel 902-1120 Beach Drive, Victoria, BC, Canada V8S 2N1, MS; **SLP LM**

Richard, Mrs Mimi Barry 250 Rosewood Drive, Metairie, LA 70005, (504) 392-0172, BS 80 Southern Methodist Univ; MA 82 Northwestern Univ; 88–Sp-Lang Path, Therapy Assoc of LA, **SLP**

Richard, Dr Nancy B 2640 Dole Street #D-5, Honolulu, HI 96822, (808) 948-7740, BA; MS; PH 87 (Special Education) Univ of WA; 86–Proj Dir, Univ of Hawaii, **SLP**

Richard, Mrs Sharon Smith 938 St Johns Wood Drive, Richmond, VA 23225, (804) 323-1676, **SLP**

Richard, Mrs Twana S 610 S W 88th Terrace, Gainesville, FL 32607, (904) 332-9678, BA 74 Asbury Coll; MA 81 OK St Univ; SLP, Self Employed, **SLP**

Richard-Edwards, Deborah A Speech & Hearing Department, 2100 Pontiac Lake Road, Pontiac, MI 48054, (313) 858-1924, BA 77 MI St Univ; MS 78 Univ of MI - Ann Arbor; Aud, Oakland Sch Sp & Hrng Clin, **A**

Richards, Dr Alan M 28 Melby Lane, East Hills, NY 11576, (212) 722-8100, BA 66 CUNY - Queens Coll; MA 68 CT Coll; PH 71 (NS) CUNY - Grad Sch & Univ Cntr; Assoc Prof, Cty U of NY, **A**

Richards, Dr Allan L Dept Communication Disorders, Baylor University, Neil Morris Hall, Waco, TX 76798, (817) 755-2567, BA 53 Univ of ND; MS 55 Purdue Univ - West Lafayette; PH 66 (Aud) Univ of WI - Madison; Prof, Baylor Univ, **A**

Richards, Amy Briner 1644 Beaconshire Road, Houston, TX 77077, (713) 589-1461, BS 83 Univ of IA; MA 86 Univ of Houston - Univ Park; **SLP**

Richards, Bruce L 409 Parkwood Drive, Mars, PA 16046, (412) 625-1588, BS 74 Clarion Univ of PA; ME 77 Clarion Univ of PA; MS 83 Clarion Univ of PA; Sp-Lang Path, Mars Area Sch Dist, **SLP**

Richards, Mrs Carol Schmidt 1215 Fern, New Orleans, LA 70118, (504) 866-2414, BS 64 Univ of IL - Urbana; MA 65 MI St Univ; SLP-Aud, Private Practice, **SLP A**

Richards, Dana Williams Anchorage Apartment, 451 Constellation #1610, League City, TX 77573, (713) 792-4500, MA 85 Univ of TX - Austin; 88–Sp-Lang Path, Univ of TX Health Science Ctr, **SLP**

Richards, Darlene Marie 4300 Woodley Square, Apartment 103-A, Montgomery, AL 36116, (205) 288-6098, BS 85 Auburn Univ - Auburn; OM 86 Auburn Univ - Auburn; 87–Sp-Lang Path, AL Health Related Svcs, **SLP**

Richards, Deborah J 147 Spring Street, Willimantic, CT 06226, (203) 456-3261, BA 77 Univ of CT; MS 80 Univ of OR; Sp-Lang Path, Eastconn, **SLP**

Richards, Denise S 196 Station Hospital, EFMD, APO New York, NY 09055, BA 74 Univ of ME - Orono; MS 75 Ithaca Coll; 84–Sp-Lang Path, Dept of Army, **SLP ACE**

Richards, Dr Doris M 1310-B Kingsridge Court, Normal, IL 61761, (309) 452-2244, BA 46 Univ of MI - Ann Arbor; MS 48 Univ of MI - Ann Arbor; PH 75 (Sp Science Voice) Case Western Reserve Univ; **SLP A LM**

Richards, Dorothy J 9508 East 29th Street, Independence, MO 64052, (816) 221-7565, BS 49 Central MO St Univ; MS 65 Central MO St Univ; SLP, Kansas City Mo Pub Sch, **SLP**

Richards, Douglas 1114 Tustin Pines Way, Tustin, CA 92680, (714) 581-2800, BA 73 CA St Univ - Stanislaus; MA 76 CA St Univ - Fullerton; Aud, Newport Lang-Sp & Aud Cen, **A**

Richards, Grace Marcum 5116 Parklawn Terrace #103, Rockville, MD 20852, (301) 468-0603, BS 84 WV Univ; MS 86 CUNY - Brooklyn Coll; 88–Aud, Treatment & Learning Centers, **A**

Richards, Dr Griffith G 810 Gonzalez Drive #3-B, San Francisco, CA 94132, BA 57 Univ of CA - Berkeley; MA 59 Stanford Univ; PH 70 (NS) Stanford Univ; Prof, San Fran St U, **SLP**

Richards, Jacqueline J 1203 Louden Lane, Imperial Beach, CA 92032-3240, (619) 233-2241, BS 68 Northern MI Univ; MA 69 Univ of AZ; Aud, Naval Hosp San Diego Ca, **A**

Richards, Mrs Janice M 416 South High Street, Belleville, IL 62221, (314) 892-2250, BA 78 Augustana Coll; MS 79 Eastern IL Univ; Sp-Lang Path, Special Sch Dist St Louis Co, **SLP**

Richards, Jerome F 2 Roxbury Road, Rockville Centre, NY 11570, (516) 678-6669, BA 55 Saint John's Univ - Jamaica; MA 56 Columbia Univ Teachers Coll; 58–Sp-Lang Path, Private Practice, **SLP**

Richards, Mrs Julia Ficek RR 3, Streator, IL 61364, (815) 673-2311, BS 80 Eastern IL Univ; MS 81 Eastern IL Univ; Sp/Lang Path, St Mary's Hosp, **SLP ACE**

Richards, Mrs Karen Ann 15907 Mesa Gardens Drive, Houston, TX 77095, (713) 550-0128, BS 81 Southwest TX St Univ; MA 84 Univ of Houston - Univ Park; SLP, **SLP**

Richards, Karen B 1131 Rainbow Circle, Elmer, NJ 08318, (609) 358-0440, BA 75 Glassboro St Coll; MA 80 OH Univ - Athens; Proprietor-Administrator, Tri-County Speech Rehabilitatn, **SLP ACE**

Richards, Kathleen L 348 South Spring Street, Blairsville, PA 15717, (412) 254-4332, BS 77 Indiana Univ of PA; MS 84 Indiana Univ of PA; Sp-Lang Path, Arin Inter Unit

Richards, Maribeth J 10 Houston Drive, Mechanicsburg, PA 17055, (717) 691-7727, MS

Richards, Mrs Marilyn M 9219 Lewis Avenue, Kansas City, MO 64138, BA 69 Lambuth Coll; MS 73 Murray St Univ; Sp-Lang Path, Marillac Cen for Chldn, **SLP**

Richards, Mrs Maureen M 18 All Point Terrace, Holbrook, NY 11741, (516) 736-4667, BA 72 Adelphi Univ; MS 74 Adelphi Univ; Tchr, Middle Co Sch Dist, **SLP**

Richards, Melonie Sauceda 10945 Evans Street, Loma Linda, CA 92354, (714) 825-3832, BS 83 Pacific Union Coll; MS 86 Loma Linda Univ - Riverside; **SLP**

Richards, Michael R 802 17th Street, Cody, WY 82414, (307) 587-9269, BS 67 UT St Univ; MS 69 UT St Univ; Coord-Dept of Spec Servs, Cody Pub Schs, **SLP**

Richards, Mrs Nancy C 3985 Brindlewood Lane, Elgin, IL 60120, (312) 464-5206, BS 53 SUNY - Coll at Buffalo; MA 85 Northern IL Univ - De Kalb; **SLP**

Richards, Mrs Natalie Ann 965-C Berryman, Pocatello, ID 83201, (208) 238-1977, BA 85 Northwest Nazarene Coll; MS 87 ID St Univ

Richards, Nelda S 1605 Dublin Road, Charlottesville, VA 22903, (317) 259-8105, BA 76 George Washington Univ; MS 77 Univ of IL - Urbana; SLP, Indianapolis Sp/Hrng Cen, **SLP**

Richards, Pamela R 242 Highland Creek Parkway, Baton Rouge, LA 70808, (504) 687-6845, BS 77 LA St Univ - Baton Rouge; MA 79 LA St Univ - Baton Rouge; 79–Sp & Hrng Path, Iberville Parish Sch Bd, **SLP**

Richards, Mrs Patricia Hartigan Waltham Weston Hosp & Med Ctr, Center For Speech Language & Hearing, Hope Avenue, Waltham, MA 02254, (617) 647-6418, BA 76 Saint Joseph's Coll; MA 78 NY Univ; 82–Dir SLP & Aud, Waltham Weston & Med Ctr, **SLP**

Richards, Richard Mark 2847 Baltimore Boulevard, Finksburg, MD 21048, (301) 528-6101, BS 83 ID St Univ; MS 85 ID St Univ; **SLP**

Richards, Roberta D 43 Pennsylvania Avenue, Newton, MA 02164, (617) 455-0466, BS 69 SUNY - Coll at Buffalo; MA 71 SUNY - Center at Buffalo; 78–Sp/Lang Path, Needham Pub Sch, **SLP**

Richards, Robin Beth **SLP**

Richards, Ruth Marie N114 W15927 Sylvan Circle, Apartment 14, Germantown, WI 53022, (414) 358-1000, BS 81 Marquette Univ; MS 82 Marquette Univ; SLP, Sen WI Med & Social Serv, **SLP**

Richards, Sarah Lee 3822 Parkdale, Cleveland Heights, OH 44121, (216) 291-1553, MA 83 Cleveland St Univ; 88–Sp-Lang Path, Lake Hosp Sys Inc, **SLP**

Richards, Sharol L 6419 Harper Drive N E, Albuquerque, NM 87109, (505) 344-1647, BS 78 Eastern NM Univ; MS 79 Eastern NM Univ; Sp-Lang Path, Albuquerque Pub Sch, **SLP**

Richards, Theodora Rinck 7651 West F Avenue, Kalamazoo, MI 49009, (616) 349-7447, BS 67 San Jose St Univ; MA 68 Western MI Univ; Sp/Lang Path, Private Practice, **SLP**

Richardson, Dr Alice P 6906 Shumard Circle, Austin, TX 78759, (512) 471-3841, BA 68 Emory Univ; ME 70 Emory Univ; PH 80 (Lang Disorders) Univ of TX - Austin; 74–Sp-Lang Path, Univ of Texas, **SLP**

Richardson, Beverly Anne 14255 Preston Road #436, Dallas, TX 75240, (214) 824-1620, **SLP**

Richardson, Carol M 2816 Lombardy, Memphis, TN 38111, (901) 452-3781, BA 76 Baylor Univ; MA 77 Vanderbilt Univ; **SLP ACE**

Richardson, Cherie M Rt 5 Box 312, Murray, KY 42071, (502) 436-5580, BA 68 Central WA Univ; MS 72 Central WA Univ; 86–Asst Prof, Murray State Univ, **SLP**

Richardson, Claretta C 3301-C Regents Park Lane, Greensboro, NC 27405, (919) 288-1779, BA 65 Wichita St Univ; MA 68 Wichita St Univ; Sp-Lang Path, Greensboro Publ Schs, **SLP A**

Richardson, Mrs Connie D 705 Orchard Lane, Monticello, IN 47960, (219) 583-3660, BS 74 Purdue Univ - West Lafayette; MS 59 Purdue Univ - West Lafayette; 87–Sp-Lang Path, White County Memorial Hosp, **SLP**

Richardson, D E 2196 Schaefer Road, Abington, PA 19001, (215) 597-7167, BA 74 Univ of VT; MA 76 Saint Louis Univ; Sp/Lang Path, VA Admin/MC/ACC, **SLP**

Richardson, Darlene Marie 133B Loma Lane, San Clemente, CA 92672, (714) 492-5878, BA 83 Univ of CA - Santa Barbara; MA 85 CA St Univ - Long Beach; **SLP**

Richardson, Deborah Young Medical Hearing Aid Associates, 3500 Broadway, Fort Myers, FL 33901, (813) 936-0721, BA 81 SUNY - Coll at Plattsburgh; MA 84 SUNY - Center at Buffalo; Aud, Ear Nose Throat Associates, **A**

Richardson, Mrs Debra Heramb Rt 2 Box 113, Bristol, WV 26332, (304) 782-1571, BS 79 IN St Univ - Terre Haute; MS 81 IN St Univ - Terre Haute; 88–Sp-Lang Path, Speech Language Svcs, **SLP**

Richardson, Mrs Debra Lee 6351 Meadow Crest Circle, Reno, NV 89509, (702) 827-3644, BS 76 IL St Univ - Normal; MS 77 IL St Univ - Normal; Sp-Lang Path, Sierra Rehab Svcs, **SLP ACE**

Richardson, Mrs Elizabeth Bressler 12 Bradford Street #1, Boston, MA 02118-2119, (617) 787-3390, BS 79 Ithaca Coll; MA 81 MI St Univ; Clinical Supervisor, Greenery, **SLP**

Richardson, Elton 225 East 72nd Street #702, New York, NY 10021, (212) 861-2381, MA 71 Grand Canyon Coll; **SLP**

Richardson, Joyce C Route 2, Stewart Hollow Road #7, Gurley, AL 35748, **SLP A**

Richardson, Mrs Karen Hill 29 Green Avenue #A-2-2, Madison, NJ 07940-2522, (202) 636-6990, BS 79 Univ of Cincinnati; MA 81 Univ of MD - College Park; Cl Superv Aud, Howard U, **A**

Richardson, Kari Sandvig 2086 Wealdwood, Kirkwood, MO 63122, (314) 849-1654, BS 81 Univ of MN - Minneap-St Paul; MS 86 Southern IL Univ-Edwardsvill; **SLP**

Richardson, Mrs Kelli Taylor 509 South Euclid, St Louis, MO 63110, (314) 362-2355, BA 81 Univ of NC - Chapel Hill; MS 83 Univ of NC - Chapel Hill; 86–Sp-Lang Path, Washington Univ Med Cntr, **SLP**

Richardson, Mrs Linda S 3705 South 3100 East, Salt Lake City, UT 84109-3718, (801) 278-3654, BA 72 Univ of Pittsburgh - Pittsburgh; OM 78 Brigham Young Univ; Houseparent, Proj Turn, **SLP**

Richardson, Lisa G 9041 Westglen, Dallas, TX 75228, (214) 324-0864, MS 87 6987

Richardson, Lisa Marie 2751 Atkinson Street, Regina, SK, Canada S4N 3Y2, (306) 949-6667, BA 84 Minot St Univ; MS 85 Minot St Univ; 87–Aud, Regina Hrng Svcs Inc, **A**

Richardson, Marcelle R 4323 Canterbury Road, La Mesa, CA 92041, (619) 588-3249, BA 76; MA 80; SLP, Cajun Vy Un Sch Dist, **SLP**

Richardson, Mrs Margaret R 5732 Antonio Lane, Hixson, TN 37343, (615) 825-7276, BA 76 IN Univ - Bloomington; MA 78 IN Univ - Bloomington; 86–Sp-Lang Path, Chattanooga PS, **SLP**

Richardson, Mrs Melissa A Rd 6 Box 636, Bedford, PA 15522, (814) 623-1390, BS 75 Clarion Univ of PA; ME 81 Clarion Univ of PA; Sp-Lang Path, Appalachia Inter Unit 08, **SLP**

Richardson, Mrs Melissa Ann 4938 Caldwell Mill Lane, Birmingham, AL 35243-3638, (205) 325-5217, BA 81 Univ of MS; MS 85 Univ of Montevallo; **A**

Richardson, Methlee E 7 Legare Street #B, Charleston, SC 29401, (803) 577-5410, BS 72 Univ of SC - Columbia; OM 80 Univ of SC - Columbia; Clinical Supervisor, Charleston Speech&Hearing Ctr, **SLP ACE**

Richardson, Mrs Natalie 2317-1/2 Teviot Street, Los Angeles, CA 90039, (213) 662-3611, BA 69 CA St Univ - Los Angeles; MA 71 CA St Univ - Los Angeles; Sp-Lang Path, Amer Eng Enhancement Ctr, **SLP**

Richardson, Penny Wan Audiology Associates, 1915 State Street, Nashville, TN 37203, (615) 327-0555, BS 75 Middle TN St Univ; MA 76 Univ of TN - Knoxville; Aud/Owner/Mgr, Aud Assoc Inc, **A**

Richardson, Sharon A 1417 Brookside Drive #B-2, Munster, IN 46321, (219) 924-9923, BA 71 MI St Univ; MA 74 MI St Univ; Aud, Trade Winds Rehab Cen, **A**

Richardson, Sharon L 1601 Ronald, Missoula, MT 59801, (406) 728-4000, BA 54 Univ of KY; MA 70 9489; Sp-Lang Path, Missoula Sch Dist I, **SLP**

Richardson, Mrs Sharon M Star Route 1 Box 448, Spring Branch, TX 78070, (512) 885-7403, BA 67 Baylor Univ; OM 69 Southern Methodist Univ; Sp-Lang Path, Comal ISD, **SLP**

Richardson, Mrs Soundra Thomason 6303 S Old Village Road, Columbia, MO 65203, (314) 581-1760, OB 85 Univ of MO - Columbia; OM 87 Univ of MO - Columbia

Richardson, Mrs Susan R Speech And Hearing Clinic, Oklahoma State University, 120 Hanner, Stillwater, OK 74078, (405) 744-8939, BA 50 TX Christian Univ; MA 68 OK St Univ; Instr, OK S U, **SLP ACE**

Richardson, Dr Sylvia O 4141 Bayshore Boulevard, Apartment 1701, Tampa, FL 33611, (813) 974-2006, BA 40 Stanford Univ; MA 42 Columbia Univ Teachers Coll; MD 48 (NS) McGill Univ - Quebec; Prof, U of S FL, **SLP F H LM**

Richardson, Mrs Virginia Ratliff 2051 New Orleans Drive, Lexington, KY 40505, (606) 278-4574, **SLP**

Richardson, Wanda Arlene P O Box 117, Garberville, CA 95440, (707) 923-2386, BA 80 Univ of CA - Santa Barbara; MA 83 CA St Univ - Northridge; SLP, **SLP**

Richardson, Wendy J 10585 S W 109 Court #207, Miami, FL 33176, (305) 274-7883, BA 74 Univ of Miami; MA 75 Univ of Miami; Dir, Kendall Sp & Lang Cen, **SLP**

Richardson-Zizi, Mrs Pamela A 1251 NE 108th #507, Miami, FL 33161, (305) 895-4449, MS 86 Univ of South FL; 87–Sp-Lang Path, Easter Seal Soc of Dade Co, **SLP**

Richert, Daniel R PO Box 68, Bethany, MO 64424, (816) 425-7140, BS 74 Western IL Univ; MA 75 Western IL Univ; **SLP A**

Richert, Dr M Jeanne Rt 1 Box 991, Laurel, MS 39440, (601) 649-1334, BA 78 Univ of Southwestern LA; MS 80 Univ of Southwestern LA; PH 87 (NS) Univ of MS; 88–Sp-Lang Path, Jones County Schs, **SLP**

Richesin, Kathy Nash 3201 E Tenaya, Fresno, CA 93710, (209) 229-9600, MA CA St Univ - Fresno; **A**

Richeson, Mrs Denice Elaine D 7310 Goldfinch Court S E, Lacey, WA 98503, (206) 458-5731, BA 75 WA St Univ; MA 76 WA St Univ; SLP, Yelm Sch Dist #2, **SLP**

Richey, Mrs Cheryl Merdgen 15400 Belgrade Street, Apartment 20, Westminster, CA 92683, (714) 775-7293, BA 84 CA St Univ - Long Beach; MA 86 CA St Univ - Long Beach; **SLP**

Richey, Mrs Lisa C 703 Fernwood, Benton, AR 72015-0687, (501) 776-1277, BA 83 Ouachita Baptist Univ; MS 87 Univ of AR - Little Rock; 87–Aud, Benton Hearing Clinic, **A**

Richey, Mrs Vera Crow 317 Ashland Court, Gainesville, TX 76240, BS 66 East TX St Univ - Commerce; MS 70 East TX St Univ - Commerce; 85–Sp-Lang Path, Gainsville ISD, **SLP**

Richie, Dr Dolores J 5833 Tellefson Road, Culver City, CA 90230, PH (NS); **SLP**

Richilson, Mary Jane 47 Mallard Drive, Avon, CT 06001, (203) 673-6092, BA 76 Hofstra Univ; MA 77 Hofstra Univ; Sp-Lang Path, Bristol Pub Sch Syst, **SLP**

Richins, Jon C ENT Associates, 1605 East Capitol Avenue, Bismarck, ND 58501, (701) 258-6556, BA 78 Brigham Young Univ; MS 79 Brigham Young Univ; Aud, E N T Assoc Ltd, **A**

Richlie, Mary D 428 West 16th Avenue, Spokane, WA 99203, **SLP**

Richman, Mrs Ann R 3936 Enfield, Skokie, IL 60076, (312) 774-8211, BS 62 Northwestern Univ; MA 76 Northeastern IL Univ; Sp-Lang Path, Private Practice, **SLP**

Richman, Mrs Eileen K 8790 Matthew Street North, Seminole, FL 33542, (813) 393-6430, MS 74 Univ of South FL; SLP, Pinellas Co Sch Bd, **SLP**

Richman, Harriet U 160 Harvest Avenue, Akron, OH 44313, (216) 666-6364, **SLP**

Richman, Mrs Kim S 4492 Groveland, University Heights, OH 44118, (216) 371-7230, BS 78 Miami Univ - Oxford; MA 79 OH St Univ; SLP, Cleveland Hts-U Hts Bd of Ed, **SLP**

Richman, Linda G 5 Cherry Brook Lane, East Windsor, NJ 08520, (609) 890-2922, BA 80 Montclair St Coll; MS 82 Syracuse Univ; Sp-Lang Path, Mercer Co Sp Sers Sch Dist, **SLP**

Richman, Mrs Nancy S 1108 East Maple, Columbus, KS 66725, (316) 429-1181, **SLP**

Richmond, Dr Allen M Buffalo Hearing & Speech Ctr, 325 Summer, Buffalo, NY 14222, (716) 836-3150, BS 58 SUNY - Coll at Geneseo; ME 61 PA St Univ - Univ Park; PH 65 (NS) OH Univ - Athens; SLP, Buffalo Hearing & Speech Ctr, **SLP**

Richmond, Deserie J 239 Pebbleview Drive, Rochester, NY 14612, (716) 352-2400, BS 79 SUNY - Coll at Buffalo; MS 83 Nazareth Coll of Rochester; 79–Sp/Lang Path, BOCES II-Monroe/Orleans Co, **SLP**

Richmond, Mrs Donna Porterfield Route 2 Box 366, Osceola, AR 72370, (501) 475-2632, OM 88 AR St Univ; 87–Sp-Lang Path, East Poinsett Co Sch

Richmond, Jessica Jane 8907 Greylock Road, Baltimore, MD 21208, (301) 662-4159, BA 85 Univ of MD - College Park; MS 88 Loyola Coll; **SLP**

Richmond, Mrs Prudence Rd 1 Box 186, Red Hook, NY 12571, (914) 338-9320, BS 84 Coll of Saint Rose; MS 85 Coll of Saint Rose; 85–Sp-Lang Path, UCP Assoc, **SLP**

Richmond, Thomas E, Jr 133 Crandon Circle, Beaver, PA 15009, (412) 775-5408, BS 49 OH St Univ; MA 51 OH St Univ; Aud, Beaver Valley Inter Ut, **SLP A LM**

Richner, Mrs Susan Mayes 1026 31st Street N W, Washington, DC 20007, (202) 333-3624, BA 83 MI St Univ; MA 84 MI St Univ; 85–Sp-Lang Path, Montgomery Co PS, **SLP**

Richter, Ellen M Route 4 Box 1720, Palatka, FL 32077, (904) 328-1110, BS 65 PA St Univ - Univ Park; ME 66 PA St Univ - Univ Park; Sp-Lang Path, Lawrence J Richter MD, **SLP**

Richter, Mrs Ellen Wilcox 6400 Snowbird Lane, Charlotte, NC 28212, (704) 376-1342, BA 71 Elmira Coll; MA 76 Univ of TN - Knoxville; **SLP**

Richter, Mrs Judy Kathryn 2034 East Mimosa, Springfield, MO 65804, BS 77 Central MO St Univ; MA 80 Central MO St Univ; **SLP**

Richter, Katherine 232 East Palatine Road, Palatine, IL 60067, BS; **SLP LM**

Richter, Mrs Theresa Webber 5469 South Dorchester, Chicago, IL 60615, (312) 241-6361, BA 69 MI St Univ; MS 84 Governors St Univ; 84–Sp-Lang Path, South Metro Assoc for Handicapped, **SLP**

Richter-McEathron, Virginia Strohmeyer 6005 South 149th Street, Omaha, NE 68137, (402) 896-3310, BS 74 Univ of WI - River Falls; MS 78 Univ of WI - River Falls; 86–Sp-Lang Path, Nebraska Sch for the Deaf, **SLP**

Richtner, Ulla E M 1602 N W 35th Way, Gainesville, FL 32605, (904) 376-6543, MA 72 Univ of Stockholm - Sweden; MS 75 Univ of South FL; PH 86 (Cleft Palate) Univ of FL; **SLP**

Richvalsky, Stephanie 1 Saint Phillips Drive, Clifton, NJ 07013, (201) 384-5450

Rickarby, Janet H 23 Haven Avenue, Chicopee, MA 01013, BA 48 Emmanuel Coll; MA 65 Univ of MA - Amherst; SLP, Springfield Pub Schs, **SLP**

Rickard, Lisa K 6032 35th Avenue N E, Seattle, WA 98115-7313, (206) 543-4011, BS 85 Univ of AZ; MS 87 Univ of WA

Rickard, Lisa R 224 E King Street #201, Lancaster, PA 17602, (717) 394-6508, BS 81 PA St Univ - Univ Park; MA 86 Hahnemann Medical Coll; Aud, Dr David Rosenfeld, **A**

Ricke, Dianna M RR 13 Box 2-A, Topeka, KS 66610, (913) 232-0551, BA 76 Wichita St Univ; MA 78 Wichita St Univ; Sp-Lang Path, USD #501, **SLP**

Rickenbaker, Mrs Joyce Brown 2823 Wilton Road, West Columbia, SC 29169, (803) 794-1551, BA 77 Presbyterian Coll; MA 83 SC St Coll; Sp-Lang Path, Orangeburg District 5 Schools, **SLP**

Ricker, Lynn Marie 3210 Saddlebrook Avenue, Tampa, FL 33618, (813) 870-3560, MS 82 Univ of South FL; 88–Aud, Tampa Sp & Hearing Ctr Inc, **A**

Ricker, Margaret M 104 Mount Auburn Street, Watertown, MA 02172, (617) 573-3266, BS 86 Univ of MA - Amherst; MS 88 PA St Univ - Univ Park; 88–Aud, MA Eye/Ear Infirmary

Ricker, Nancy P 1624 NW Trenton Avenue, Bend, OR 97701, (503) 388-7727, BS 59 Central MO St Univ; MA 65 Case Western Reserve Univ; Sp/Lang Path, Private Practice, **SLP ACE**

Ricker, Stephanie Anne 3314 Melrose Road Suite 105, Fayetteville, NC 28304, (919) 323-1250, BS 83 East Carolina Univ; MA 85 Univ of TN - Knoxville; Aud, Aud Clinic Inc, **A**

Ricker, Mrs Susan Klingbell 2034 Shady Lane, Green Bay, WI 54304, MS 81 Univ of NC - Chapel Hill; Audiologist, Drs Randolph Larsen & Bell Sc, **A**

Rickert, Mary T 2570 Madison Road #15, Cincinnati, OH 45208, (513) 423-9496, SLP, Dogy House of Midletown, **SLP**

Rickert, Nancy E W 20819 114th Place S E #6, Kent, WA 98031-2188, (206) 575-4718, BS 74 Univ of WY; MS 78 Univ of WY; Supvr Sp & Hrng, Valley Med Cen, **SLP**

Ricketts, Mrs Kristyn Jean 208 Edwards Drive, Normal, IL 61761, (309) 452-8481, BS 86 Eastern IL Univ; MS 87 Eastern IL Univ; 87–Sp-Lang Path, Hammitt Sch-The Baby Fold, **SLP**

Rickey, Mrs Carol Edna 10331 Brooks-Carroll Road, Waynesville, OH 45068, (513) 897-9140, BS 77 Univ of Cincinnati; MS 83 Miami Univ - Oxford; 87–Sp-Lang Path, Lakota Public Schools, **SLP**

Rickey, Mrs Lola Ann 8993 Scotia Road, Newport, WA 99156, (509) 292-2223, BA 79 WA St Univ; MS 81 Eastern WA Univ; 86–Sp-Lang Path, Newport Sch Dist, **SLP**

Ricklefs, Sheila 901 East Michigan, Apartment 35, Hobbs, NM 88240, (505) 393-9062, BS 85 Univ of WI - Stevens Point; MS 87 Univ of WI - Stevens Point

Rickler, Irwin 40 Revere Road, Ardsley, NY 10502, (914) 835-3300, BA 51 CUNY - Brooklyn Coll; MA 49 Columbia Univ Teachers Coll; **SLP LM**

Rickoff, Mrs Michelle Ann 5021 Mill Creek Road, Dallas, TX 75244, (214) 358-8336, BS 80 Univ of TX - Austin; MA 82 Univ of Houston - Univ Park; Sp-Lang Path, Dallas Rehabilitation Institute, **SLP**

Rickoff, Mrs Olga Feldman 790 Loridans Drive, Atlanta, GA 30342, (404) 237-5625, BA 77 Tulane Univ; OM 79 Emory Univ; **SLP**

Rickon, Sandra 3120 Goldsmith Street, San Diego, CA 92106, (619) 223-0737, MS 85 Chapman Coll; Sp-Lang Path, Orange USD, **SLP**

Ricks, Mrs Barbara G 2676 Highland Village Lane, Miamisburg, OH 45342, (513) 439-5249, BA 76 Coll of Mount Saint Joseph; MA 78 Marshall Univ; 80–Sp-Lang Path, Middletown County Schools, **SLP**

Ricks, Melissa Ann 1103 Forest Hills, Gladewater, TX 75647, (214) 236-2090, BS 82 Stephen F Austin St Univ; ME 84 Stephen F Austin St Univ; **SLP**

Ridarelli, Susan L 63-F Briarwood Lane, Branford, CT 06405, (203) 481-2890, BA 77 Univ of MI - Ann Arbor; MA 78 Western MI Univ; Sp-Lang Path, The Foundation Sch Inc, **SLP**

Riddell, S Frances 2834 Woodcrest, San Antonio, TX 78209, (512) 820-0442, BS 72 Southwest TX St Univ; ME 74 Southwest TX St Univ; MS 76 Univ of North TX; 86–Sp-Lang Path/Aud, Private Practice, **SLP A**

Ridder, Mrs Jane 13662 Falmouth Drive, Tustin, CA 92680, (714) 838-4039, BA 75 Wichita St Univ; MS 76 Wichita St Univ; Sp-Lang Path, **SLP**

Riddle, Laura S 800 No Smith Road #21Z, Bloomington, IN 47401, (812) 331-7201, BA 74 Univ of AR - Fayetteville; MS 76 Univ of OK Medical Center; **SLP**

Riddle, Peggy Denise 1702 Crow Valley Road #205, Dalton, GA 30720, (205) 937-6281, BS 84 Univ Southern MS-Hattiesburg; MS 86 Univ Southern MS-Hattiesburg; **A**

Riddle, Rebecca Elaine 107 North Elmhurst Avenue, Mount Prospect, IL 60056-2420, (219) 462-6388, MA 86 Northern IL Univ - De Kalb; **SLP**

Riddle, Sherri Lynne 169 Dogwood Drive, Weaverville, NC 28787, (704) 255-5369, BS 84 Univ of NC - Greensboro; MA 86 Univ of NC - Greensboro; 86–Sp-Lang Path, Asheville City Schs, **SLP**

Ride, Kristen Jane 2610 G Paces Place, Atlanta, GA 30339, (404) 433-2740, BS 85 Univ of GA; ME 86 Univ of GA; **SLP**

Ridenhour, Michael W 122 Mountain Avenue,S W, Roanoke, VA 24016, (703) 345-7821, BA 71 Univ of VA - Charlottesville; ME 73 Univ of VA - Charlottesville; Aud, Private Practice, **A**

Ridenour, Ellen H 3401 Firefly Court, Columbus, OH 43220, (614) 878-4403, BS 77 Minot St Univ; MS 78 Minot St Univ; SLP, Cty Sch, **SLP**

Ridenour, Mrs Melanie Bridgforth 1915 West Jefferson, Lovington, NM 88260, (505) 396-4311, BS 77 Eastern NM Univ; MS 82 Eastern NM Univ; Sp-Lang Path, Lovington Pub Sch, **SLP**

Rider, Mrs Janice Lynn 36241 Panorama Drive, Yucaipa, CA 92399, (714) 797-1772, BA 78 Univ of Redlands; MS 80 Univ of Redlands; SLP, San Bernardino City USD, **SLP**

Rider, John Milton 24 Oteen Park Place, Asheville, NC 28805-2528, (504) 355-0388, **SLP**

Rider, Dr Larry P Speech Clinic, University Of Redlands, Redlands, CA 92373, (714) 793-2121, BA 68 Winona St Univ; MS 70 CO St Univ; PH 79 (NS) Univ of WI - Madison; 73–Prof, U of Redlands, **SLP**

Rider, Mrs Molly Carlson 534 McClure Avenue, Elgin, IL 60123, (312) 529-7166, BS 81 Univ of IL - Urbana; MS 82 Univ of IL - Urbana; Sp-Lang Path, Cook Co Sch Dist #54, **SLP**

Ridge, Denecia Dodson 203 Morningside Drive, Mexia, TX 76667, (817) 562-6032, BS 82 Stephen F Austin St Univ; ME 83 Stephen F Austin St Univ; Sp-Lang Path, Mexia State School, **SLP**

Ridge, Ellen M 12 Wampatuck Road, Quincy, MA 02169, (617) 963-8150, BA 79 Univ of MA - Boston; ME 82 Northeastern Univ; Sp/Lang Path, Quincy Pub Sch, **SLP**

Ridge, Mrs Holly Share 2629 Byron Avenue, Louisville, KY 40205, (502) 583-6531, **SLP**

Ridge, Michelle Manyak 883 Sandalwood East, Perrysburg, OH 43551, (419) 381-4012, BA 77 Bowling Green St Univ; MA 78 Bowling Green St Univ; Dir Sp and Hring, Med Coll of OH Hosp, **SLP**

Ridgley, Tami Michelle 811 Unetta Avenue, Baltimore, MD 21229, (301) 494-3210, BA 82 Loyola Coll; MS 84 Loyola Coll; Sp-Lang Path, Frederick Co Health Dept, **SLP**

Ridgway, Alice Emily 295 Temple Street Unit 101, Boston, MA 02132-3752, (617) 469-5288, BA 83 Depauw Univ; MS 85 Boston Univ; 85–Sp-Lang Path, Southwest Boston Comm Svcs, **SLP**

Riding, Mrs Nancy Campbell 2333 East Southern Avenue, Apartment 1039, Tempe, AZ 85282, (602) 898-7873, BA 63 Univ of CT; MS 82 AZ St Univ; Aud, Mesa USD, **A**

Ridky, Dr Joseph R 7103 Forbes Boulevard, Seabrook, MD 20706, (301) 794-4443, BS 63 SUNY - Coll at Geneseo; MS 64 SUNY - Coll at Geneseo; PH 75 (NS) GA St Univ; Psychol, Montgy Co Sch, **SLP**

Ridl, Mrs Jane E O 1017 Campbell Drive, Grand Forks, ND 58201, (701) 772-4638, BS 85 ND St Univ; MS 87 Minot St Univ; **A**

Ridley, Donna Ridley & Fill Sp & Lang Assoc, 4909 Hampden Lane, Suite One, Bethesda, MD 20814, (301) 652-8997, OB 66 Univ of VA - Charlottesville; ME 68 Univ of VA - Charlottesville; Sp-Lang Path, Ridley & Fill Sp-Lang Assoc, **SLP**

Rieck, Cynthia A 618 South Lake Street, Neenah, WI 54956, (414) 729-6980, BA 75 Univ of WI - Eau Claire; MS 76 Univ of WI - Eau Claire; Sp-Lang Path, Neenah Jt Sch Dist, **SLP**

Riecken, Frances B 4100 Cathedral Avenue N W, Washington, DC 20016, BS 39 Univ of MN - Minneap-St Paul; MS 53 Univ of MN - Minneap-St Paul; **SLP**

Ried, Dr Stephanie 2829 Timmons Lane, Houston, TX 77027, (713) 791-4297, MA 74 Western MI Univ; MD 86 (NS) Univ of MI - Ann Arbor; Physician, Baylor College of Medicine, **SLP**

Riede, Carol Wentworth 2925 S E Carlton, Portland, OR 97202, (503) 774-3573, BA 72 OR St Univ; ME 73 Smith Coll

Riedel, Mrs Barbara 4651 Hamlet Drive South, Saginaw, MI 48603, (517) 776-0401, BS 61 Northwestern Univ; MS 64 Univ of MI - Ann Arbor; Teacher Early Chldhd Spec Educ, Saginaw City School System, **SLP**

Riedel, Dr Karen L 145 East 15th Street #3, New York, NY 10003, (212) 340-6027, BA 64 Eastern MI Univ; MS 65 Univ of MI - Ann Arbor; PH 80 (NS) CUNY - Grad Sch & Univ Cntr; Asst Dir, Inst Rehab Med-Nyu, **SLP**

Riedel, Mary Ellen 14743 Kenton #1-C, Midlothian, IL 60445, (312) 687-0900, BS 77 IL St Univ - Normal; MA 79 Univ of IL - Urbana; SLP, SW Cook Co Coop for Spec Ed, **SLP**

Riedell, Gail M 10 Barrett Drive, Hopewell Junction, NY 12533, (914) 831-7300, BS 71 SUNY - Coll at Buffalo; MS 75 Univ of WI - Madison; SLP, Dutchess Co Dept of Mntl Hygn, **SLP**

Rieder, Katharine Ann 8193 Alpine Lane #L-405, Crown Point, IN 46307-1364, (219) 736-9443, **SLP**

Riederer, Renee A 1339 West Packard Street, Appleton, WI 54914, BA 69 Univ of WI - Oshkosh; MS 71 Univ of WI - Milwaukee; Real Estate Investor, Self Employed, **SLP**

Riedinger, Vicki Lynn 1405 15th Avenue East, West Fargo, ND 58078, (701) 237-6424, BS 78 Moorhead St Univ; MA 81 Moorhead St Univ; 86–Gen Mgr, Human Communication Associates Ltd, **SLP**

Riedl, Patricia 2480 West Scheibe Drive, Brookfield, WI 53005, (414) 797-8236, BS 78 Univ of WI - Stevens Point; MS 79 Marquette Univ; **SLP**

Riedl, Patricia L 388 Sussex Road, East Meadow, NY 11554, **SLP**

Riedler, Valerie L 511 Gardendale Road, Encinitas, CA 92024-1950, **SLP**

Riedman, Dr Richard M Dept Communication Disorders, San Diego State University, San Diego, CA 92182, (619) 265-6774, BA 55 Univ of Redlands; MA 56 Univ of Redlands; PH 62 (NS); Prof, San Diego St U, **SLP A**

Riedner, Dr Erwin D 7656A Belair Road, Baltimore, MD 21236, (301) 668-3434, BS 64 Univ of WI - Madison; MA 68 Univ of MI - Ann Arbor; OD 77 (NS) Johns Hopkins Univ; Pres, Private Practice, **A**

Riegel, Marsha Fay 42 Murdock Street, Huntington Station, NY 11746, (516) 562-4679, BA 83 Adelphi Univ; MS 85 Adelphi Univ; 87–Tech, North Shore Univ Hosp

Rieger, Mrs Pearl H 4950 Chicago Beach Drive, Chicago, IL 60615, (312) 241-5592, BA 48 Univ of MI - Ann Arbor; MA 73 Univ of Chicago; Psychoed Diagnostician, Private Practice

Riegler, Mrs Marilyn G 1849 Syracuse, Naperville, IL 60565, BS 64 Univ of Akron; Sp-Lang Path, Frances Howell School District, **SLP**

Rieker, Carole Sue 3442 North 41st Street, San Diego, CA 92105, (619) 297-4145, MA 80 Univ of Northern CO; **A**

Rielle, Mrs Judith L 12 Holt Road, Hyde Park, NY 12538, (914) 431-8800, BS 58 OH St Univ; MS 79 Coll of Saint Rose; Sp-Lang Path, St Francis Hosp, **SLP**

Riely, Mrs Joann Edwards P O Box 65007, Baton Rouge, LA 70896, (504) 923-3420, BA 69 Northwestern St Univ; ME 76 Southeastern LA Univ; 78–Sp-Lang Path, United Way Cerebral Palsy Ctr

Rieman, Mrs Deirdre Ann 2560 Lisa Drive #2, Cape Girardeau, MO 63701-2363, (314) 625-8962, BS 81 Southeast MO St Univ; MA 83 Southeast MO St Univ; SLP, Spec Sch Dist of St Lewis Cty, **SLP**

Riemer, Gayle P 883 Fawn Hill Drive, Covington, KY 41017-9647, (513) 559-4236, BS 74 Univ of Cincinnati; MA 78 Univ of Cincinnati; Aud, Chldns Hosp Med Cen, **A**

Riemer, Vernon Dale 165 Edgewood Street, Wheeling, WV 26003, (304) 242-3164, BA 48; MA 50 Northwestern Univ; Chm Dept of Oral Commun, West Liberty St Coll, **SLP**

Riemma, Angela Z 2800 Gerken Place, Oceanside, NY 11572, BA 76 CUNY - Queens Coll; MS 77 Adelphi Univ; Aud, Li Jewish Hrng & Sp Cen, **A**

Riensche, Dr Linda Communicative Disorders Unit, University Of New Mexico, 901 Vassar N E, Albuquerque, NM 87131, (505) 277-4453, BS 70 Univ of NE - Lincoln; MA 75 Univ of NE - Lincoln; PH 78 (Sp-Lang-Hrng Science) Memphis St Univ; Assoc Prof, U of New Mex, **SLP**

Rierson, Mrs Patricia Louise 353 Bahamaloop, Fayetteville, NC 28304, (206) 535-0950, MA 84 Univ of Northern IA; **SLP**

Rierson, Mrs Terrie Stanley 3217 Kayenta Court, Orlando, FL 32829, (407) 423-9293, MS 82 Univ of Central FL; 86–Sp-Lang Path, Orange County PS, **SLP**

Ries, Dr Julie E 825 Evesham Avenue, Baltimore, MD 21212, (301) 321-3096, BS 65 Towson St Univ; MA 68 Univ of Pittsburgh - Pittsburgh; OD 78 (Communicative Sciences) Johns Hopkins Univ; Assoc Prof, Towson St U/Dept Comm Sci & Disorders, **SLP**

Riese, Mrs Diane Hinkley 8039 Pickett Lane, Clay, NY 13041, (315) 652-0215, BS 81 SUNY - Coll at Geneseo; MS 85 Syracuse Univ

Riess, Richard L 2611 Sandelwood, College Station, TX 77840, (409) 268-3300, BS 63 Central MI Univ; OM 64 Univ of OK Medical Center; PH 72 (NS) Univ of UT; 86–Aud, Scott & White Clinic-Coll Station, **A**

Rietta, Mrs Katrina Hamilton 10630 Greenock Way, Duluth, GA 30136, (404) 476-3846, BS 70 Univ of AL-Tuscaloosa; MA 72 Univ of AL- Tuscaloosa; Sp-Lang Path, **SLP**

Riffkin, Constance B 48-10 43rd Street, Apt 5-H, Woodside, NY 11377, (718) 723-7200, BA 84 Adelphi Univ; MS 87 Columbia Univ Teachers Coll; Sp-Lang Path, Samuel Field Sch, **SLP**

Riffle, Paige A 650 Via Hierba, Santa Barbara, CA 93110, (805) 683-3788, BA 80 Univ of CA - Santa Barbara; MA 82 Univ of CA - Santa Barbara; Sp-Lang Path, Rehab Inst at Santa Barbara, **SLP**

Rifkind, Mrs Susan Huck 33 Forrest Place, Amityville, NY 11701, (516) 922-4100, **SLP**

Rigano, Paula Jeanne Austine Evaluation Center, 120 Maple Street, Brattleboro, VT 05301-3014, (802) 254-4571, BS 85 Ithaca Coll; MA 87 Univ of MA - Amherst; 87–Aud, Austine Sch for Deaf & Hard of Hrng Children, **A**

Rigas, Lucinda Luhman 3550 Deephaven Avenue, Wayzata, MN 55391, BS 65 Saint Cloud St Univ; MA 87 Univ of MN - Minneap-St Paul

Rigatti, Carol F 903 East McMurray Road, Venetia, PA 15367, (412) 941-6558, BA 73 CA Univ of PA; ME 78 CA Univ of PA; Self Employed, **SLP**

Rigby, Denise Frances 20 Roxbury Street, South Huntington, NY 11746, BS 84 Northeastern Univ; MS 86 Northeastern Univ; **SLP**

Rigby, Susan P 114 Scenic Way, Wimberley, TX 78676, (512) 478-2581, BS 80 CA Univ of PA; MA 84 Univ of TX - Austin; Prog Coord, Capital Area Easter Seal Rehab, **SLP**

Rigg, M Leslie 10162 Springdale Court, Boise, ID 83704, (208) 344-4012, BA 75 San Jose St Univ; MS 81 Central MO St Univ; Sp-Lang Path, Adaptive Therapeutic Systems-Wheelchair Co, **SLP**

Riggi, Mrs Cynthia L 10 Sleepy Hollow Drive, Clifton Park, NY 12065, (518) 371-1641, BS 76 Coll of Saint Rose; MS 77 Coll of Saint Rose; SLP, NY Assn for Lrng Disabl, **SLP**

Riggin Springstead, Mary Catherine 55 Varden Crescent, Barrie, ON, Canada L4M 4P4, (705) 728-9802, BS 80 Univ of Western Ontario; OM 84 Univ of Western Ontario; 84–Sp-Lang Path, Royal Victoria Hosp of Barrie, **SLP**

Riggs, Mrs Kristy 1072 San Antonio Avenue, Fullerton, CA 92635, (714) 255-1710, BA 73 Univ of CA - Santa Barbara; MA 75 CA St Univ - Long Beach; 88–Tchr, Bellflower USD, **SLP**

Riggs, Mrs Sandra Fritz 1528 Channel Court, Fort Wayne, IN 46825, (219) 482-1015, BA 65 IN Univ - Bloomington; MA 67 IN Univ - Bloomington; Sp-Lang Path, Ft Wayne Comm Schs, **SLP**

Riggs, Mrs Shelli D 2200 South 52nd, Lincoln, NE 68506, (402) 489-7102, BS 86 Univ of SD - Vermillion; MA 88 Univ of SD - Vermillion; 88–Sp-Lang Path, Madonna Centers

Riggs-Stites, Mrs Kathy Marie 1623 Shady Leaf Drive, Valrico, FL 33594, (215) 945-1730, BS 80 West Chester Univ of PA; MA 83 Trenton St Coll; SLP, Private Practice, **SLP**

Righetti, Dennis 101 Clark Street #12-B, Brooklyn Heights, NY 11201, (718) 780-3231, BA 69 Montclair St Coll; MS 70 Adelphi Univ; Director/Sp&Aud, The Methodist Hosp, **SLP**

Righter, Mrs Amanda Kirman 7301 Onate Court N E, Albuquerque, NM 87109, (505) 821-2455, BS 81 Univ of AZ; OM 84 AZ St Univ; Sp-Lang Path, **SLP**

Rigler, Mrs Caryl R 27882 Mazagon, Mission Viejo, CA 92692, BS 54 Univ of WI - Madison; MA 83 United States Int'l Univ; Sp-Lang Path, Newport-Mesa USD, **SLP**

Rigler, Cheryl C 1734 N W 101st Street, Clive, IA 50322, (515) 223-7833, SLP, Des Moines Public Schools, **SLP**

Rigney, Kathleen M 25 Rutland Street, Warwick, RI 02888, (401) 463-9091, MS 88 Univ of RI

Rigo, Dr Thomas G Department Of Communicative Disorders, University Of Southwestern Louisiana, PO Box 43170, Lafayette, LA 70504-3170, (904) 231-6721, PH 84 (Aud) FL St Univ; 84–Asst Prof of Aud, Univ of Southwestern LA, **A**

Rigoni, Mrs Karen E 11109 Daniel Trail, Mokena, IL 60448, (312) 246-7678, BS 78 Eastern IL Univ; MS 79 Eastern IL Univ; SLP, La Grange Dept Sp Ed, **SLP**

Rigrodsky, Dr Seymour 12 York Drive, New City, NY 10956, (212) 678-3890, BA 52 CUNY - Brooklyn Coll; MA 55 CUNY - Brooklyn Coll; PH 59 (NS) Purdue Univ - West Lafayette; Prof Sp-Lang Path, Tchrs Coll Columbia U, **SLP F**

Rigsby, Mrs Donna Brock 5100 N E 4th Street, Ocala, FL 32671, (904) 622-5213, BS 81 Appalachian St Univ; MA 82 Appalachian St Univ; Sp-Lang Path, Marion Co Sch Syst, **SLP**

Rike, Mrs Ruth University Of Tennessee-Memphis, 711 Jefferson Avenue, Memphis, TN 38105, (901) 528-6511, BA 60 Vanderbilt Univ; MA 63 Northwestern Univ; Asst Prof/Chief SLP & Aud, U of TN Memphis, **SLP A**

Riley, Anita Marcott 23401 Middlebelt Road, Farmington Hills, MI 48018, (313) 421-3363, BA 71 West Liberty St Coll; MA 75 Eastern MI Univ; SLP, Garden Cty Pub Sch, **SLP**

Riley, Mrs Cindra Lee 155 East Main Street, Norwalk, OH 44857, (419) 668-9556, MA 83 Bowling Green St Univ; SLP, Christie Lane School Workshop, **SLP**

Riley, Cynthia J Route 2 Box 478, Crestview, FL 32536, (904) 682-2501, BS 86 FL St Univ; MS 87 FL St Univ; SLP, Okaloosa Sch Bd, **SLP**

Riley, Daniel S 4632 Westway, Toledo, OH 43612, (419) 245-4150, BA 76 Miami Univ - Oxford; MA 82 Bowling Green St Univ; Aud, Lucas County Office of Educ, **A**

Riley, Deborah Schwied 2754 South Quince Street, Denver, CO 80231, (303) 337-7737, **SLP**

Riley, Dorlas L 407 Weldon Drive, York, PA 17404, (717) 741-3891, BA 71 Towson St Univ; MS 72 Towson St Univ; 73–Sp-Lang Path, Easter Seal Society of York Co, **SLP**

Riley, Elizabeth 215 Calle Diaz, Anaheim, CA 92807, (213) 920-6674, BA 79 Whittier Coll; MA 80 Whittier Coll; SLP, Kaiser Permante, **SLP**

Riley, Dr Glyndon D 17400 Irvine Blvd, Suite K, Tustin, CA 92680-3030, BA 52 Pepperdine Univ - Los Angele; MA 59 Pepperdine Univ - Los Angele; PH 63 (NS) FL St Univ; Prof of Commun Dis, CA St U Fullerton, **SLP F**

Riley, Mrs Janet A H 14014 S W 107th Terrace, Miami, FL 33186, (305) 387-9037, BS 68 OH St Univ; MS 69 Univ of MI - Ann Arbor; Sp-Lang Path, Private Practice, **SLP**

Riley, Janeva S 11014 Ambergate Drive, Humble, TX 77338, ME 76 Southwest TX St Univ; Ech Teacher, Houston ISD, **SLP**

Riley, Dr Jeanna N 17400 Irvine Boulevard, Suite K, Tustin, CA 92680-3030, (714) 731-7331, BA 67 CA St Univ - Fullerton; MA 71 CA St Univ - Fullerton; Dir, Private Practice, **SLP**

Riley, John Scott 768 78th Place South, Birmingham, AL 35206, **A**

Riley, Judi Carey 3828 South Berkley, Cincinnati, OH 45236, BS 83 Miami Univ - Oxford; MS 85 Miami Univ - Oxford; SLP, Clermont County Bd Men Retardn, **SLP**

Riley, Mrs Karen L Route 5 Box 885, Abilene, TX 79605, (915) 677-2746, BS 71 Hardin-Simmons Univ; MA 76 Abilene Christian Univ; SLP, Abilene ISD, **SLP**

Riley, Kathleen J 21C6 Capano Drive, Newark, DE 19702, (302) 454-2062, BS 81 Bloomsburg Univ of PA; MS 82 Bloomsburg Univ of PA; Aud, Sterck Sch for Hrng Imp, **A**

Riley, Kathryn S 841 Village Parkway, Waterville, OH 43566, (419) 878-8096, BS 78 Bowling Green St Univ; MS 87 Bowling Green St Univ; **SLP**

Riley, Leslie Denise 9311 Iowa Street, Livonia, MI 48150-3834, (313) 745-9721, BA 83 MI St Univ; MA 85 0685; 86–Sp-Lang Path, Rehab Inst, **SLP**

Riley, Mrs Linda Pitner Route 6 Box 121, Denton, TX 76205, (817) 382-9313, BA 65 TX Woman's Univ; MA 70 TX Woman's Univ; SLP, Denton ISD, **SLP**

Riley, Loy Dona 7 Winchester Avenue, Auburn, MA 01501, (617) 832-5522, BA 74 Univ of RI; MA 79 Univ of RI; Sp-Lang Path, Harrington Mem Hosp, **SLP**

Riley, Mrs Lyanne 306 Cumberland, Columbia, MO 65203-3036, BS 72 KS St Univ; MA 73 KS St Univ; PH 88 (NS) Univ of MO - Columbia; Sp-Lang Path, VA Memorial Hosp, **SLP**

Riley, Mrs Peggy Jo 5709 Saddle Rock Road, Manhattan, KS 66502, (913) 776-4861, BS 74 KS St Univ; MA 76 KS St Univ; 77–Sp-Lang Path, USD #383 Manhattan, **SLP**

Riley, Dr Russell V 265-D West El Pintado Road, Danville, CA 94526-2512, (415) 837-7343, BA 68 Univ of Northern IA; MA 69 Univ of Northern IA; ED 81 (Educational & Counseling Psychology) Univ of the Pacific; 70–Sp-Lang Path, Newark USD, **SLP**

Riley, Sherri B G Germantown Speech & Hearing Clinic, 2028 Exeter Road Suite 2, Germantown, TN 38138, (901) 756-4499, BA 78 Univ of AR - Fayetteville; MA 79 Univ of AR - Fayetteville; 87–Sp-Lang Path, Germantown Sp & Hrng Clinic, **SLP**

Riley, Susan K P 7 Spencer Street, Orono, ME 04473, (207) 581-7872, **SLP**

Riley-Blazina, Mrs Roberta J 1900 East 30th Street #401, Cleveland, OH 44114, (216) 621-0578, **SLP**

Rill, Kathryn Elizabeth 445 West 39th Street Apartment A, San Pedro, CA 90731, (714) 525-4664, BA 81 Univ of Redlands; MS 85 Univ of Redlands; 88–Sp-Lang Path, Los Angeles USD, **SLP**

Rilla, Mrs Donna C 7 Cheverly Circle, Cheverly, MD 20785, (202) 675-7324, BA 67 Catholic Univ of America; MA 69 Catholic Univ of America; Sp-Lang Path, Dc Dept of Human Serv, **SLP**

Rillston, Mrs Mary J 4709 Carleton-Rockwood Rd, South Rockwood, MI 48179, (313) 283-9200, BA 78 Univ of MI - Ann Arbor; MA 80 Wayne St Univ; Sp-Lang Path, Southgate Reg Cen, **SLP**

Rimac, Dr Robert T PO Box 3002, Laramie, WY 82071, (307) 766-6185, BS 77 Northwestern Univ; MS 79 Univ of WY; PH 85 (Sp-Lang Path) Northwestern Univ; 88–Prof, Univ of Wyoming, **SLP**

Rimas, Mrs Ramune V U S Embassy, P O Box 5000, Ogdensburg, NY 13669-0430, BA 65 CUNY - Queens Coll; MA 67 CUNY - Queens Coll; **SLP**

Rimbert, Mrs Susan Lynn 6500 Lamy Street N W, Albuquerque, NM 87120, (505) 898-6451, BS 83 Southeast MO St Univ; ME 84 Central St Univ; Sp-Lang Path, Chldrns Psychiatric Hosp, **SLP**

Rinaldi, Donna M 11 Myrtle Avenue, Caldwell, NJ 07006, (201) 226-1325, BA 77 Montclair St Coll; MA 82 Seton Hall Univ; 87–Sp/Lang Path, Verona Bd of Educ, **SLP**

Rinaldi, Marilyn L 6741 50th Avenue, Kenosha, WI 53142, (414) 654-7217, BS 71 Marquette Univ; MS 79 Marquette Univ

Rinaldi, Rosa A Five Counties Chldrn Centre, 872 Dutton Road, Peterborough, ON, Canada K9H 7G1, BS 80 Univ of Western Ontario; OM 84 Univ of Western Ontario; 80–Sp-Lang Path, Five Counties Children's Centre, **SLP**

Rindo, Mrs Ellen Sue 3833 No Oakland Avenue #7, Shorewood, WI 53211, (414) 332-0372, BS 82 Univ of WI - Milwaukee; MS 84 Univ of WI - Milwaukee; Sp-Lang Path, Racine Co Opportunity Ctr, **SLP**

Rine, Helen E 61 Par Court, Pennsauken, NJ 08109, (609) 663-2723, BA 62 Marietta Coll; MA 69 9940; OM 80 Eastern Baptist Theological Seminary; Sp-Lang Path, Memorial Hosp of Burlington Co, **SLP**

Rinehard, Jean M Tibbitts Road, New Hartford, NY 13413, (315) 737-8092, BS 69 Coll of Saint Rose; ME 70 Northeastern Univ; Sp-Lang Path, Private Practice, **SLP**

Rinehart, Gaye Michelle 815 Middle River Drive #318, Fort Lauderdale, FL 33304, (305) 481-5755, BA 82 KS St Univ; MS 84 TX Tech Univ; 86–Sp-Lang Path, Broward County Schs, **SLP**

Rinehart, Monica Joy 2008-H Falcon Wood Court, Winston-Salem, NC 27127, (919) 768-0886, MS 88 Radford Univ; Aud, Forsyth Hd & Neck Assoc

Rinehart, Phyllis M 27 Sawmill Road, Brick, NJ 08723, **SLP**

Riner, Mrs Elaine Bottari 1120 South Dean Street, Woodstock, IL 60098, (815) 385-8810, BS 77 Bradley Univ; MS 79 Bradley Univ; Sp-Lang Path, McHenry Consol Sch Dist #15, **SLP**

Riner-Costantino, Patricia Collleen 4250 Pennyslvania Avenue, Suite 102B, La Crescenta, CA 91214, (818) 957-2766, BA 76 CA St Univ - Los Angeles; MA 78 CA St Univ - Los Angeles; Private Practice, **SLP**

Ring, Mrs Cosette Laurie P O Box 1593, Longview, WA 98632-0149, (707) 425-8451, MA 82 CA St Univ - Chico

Ring, Mrs Karen Overby Route 1 Box 210, Danbury, NC 27016, (919) 593-8146, BS 80 Western Carolina Univ; MA 81 Univ of TN - Knoxville; Sp-Lang Path, Stokes County Board of Educ, **SLP**

Ring, Mrs Ngareta E 5420 Repecho Drive Apartment S-109, San Diego, CA 92124, (619) 278-8459, BA 63; OB 67; Sp-Lang Path, Fallbrook Union Elem Sch Dist, **SLP**

Ringdahl, Marian M 555 North May Street #7, Mesa, AZ 85201, (602) 271-5401, BS 72 AZ St Univ; MS 74 AZ St Univ; Aud, Cigna Health Plan of AZ, **A**

Ringel, Dr Robert L Young Graduate House, Purdue University, West Lafayette, IN 47907, (317) 494-2604, BA 59 CUNY - Brooklyn Coll; MS 60 Purdue Univ - West Lafayette; PH 62 (Sp Sciences) Purdue Univ - West Lafayette; 86–VP/Dean, Prudue Univ/Grad Sch, **SLP F**

Ringenberg, Dr Carol Watson 601 Highland Avenue #2, Waterbury, CT 06708, (203) 595-1696, BA 69 Eastern KY Univ; MA 71 OH St Univ; PH 76 (Sp & Hrng Science) OH St Univ; 87–Sp-Lang Path, InSpeech Inc, **SLP**

Ringer, Mrs Kayleen Mulford 2002 Leighton Avenue, Anniston, AL 36201-3272, (205) 237-9125, BS 82 Univ of GA; ME 84 Univ of GA; Aud/Sp-Lang Path, Anniston City Schs, **A**

Ringers, Mrs Barbara B 1436 Kenwood Lane, Charlottesville, VA 22901, BS 76 Ithaca Coll; MS 80 Gallaudet Coll; **A**

Ringger, Joy M 620 East Amherst Avenue, Englewood, CO 80110, (303) 861-6800, BS 83 Univ of IL - Urbana; MA 85 Univ of IL - Urbana; 85–Aud, Childrens Hosp, **A**

Ringle-Bartels, Janet E 2813 Abbott, Midland, MI 48640, (517) 631-1100, BS 77 Univ of KS; OM 79 Univ of WA; 86–Sp-Lang Path, Head Injury Ther Svcs Inc, **SLP ACE**

Ringler, Dr Norma M 3721 Lytle Road, Shaker Heights, OH 44122, (216) 991-0932, BA 45 Case Western Reserve Univ; MA 45 Case Western Reserve Univ; PH 73 (NS) Case Western Reserve Univ; Research Cons, Rainbow Babies Children, **SLP**

Ringsby, Mrs Sandra Lynn 6079 Hammett Road, Modesto, CA 95351, (209) 545-1075, **SLP**

Ringwalt, Sharon S Division Of Speech & Hearing, 76 Wing D Medical School, UNC-CH CB 7190, Chapel Hill, NC 27599-7190, (919) 966-1006, BA 74 Univ of NC - Chapel Hill; MS 76 Vanderbilt Univ; 81–Sp-Lang Path, Div-Sp & Hrng Sci Unc-Ch, **SLP ACE**

Rini, Mrs Denise L 420 Norton Parkway, New Haven, CT 06511, (203) 397-4569, BS 71 Boston Univ; MA 72 Case Western Reserve Univ; 85–Cl Superv, Sn CT St U, **SLP**

Rini, Mrs Kathleen S PO Box 596, Great Falls, VA 22066, (703) 759-5985, BA 69 Case Western Reserve Univ; MA 70 Case Western Reserve Univ; Sp-Lang Path, Fairfax PS, **SLP**

Rink, Dr Timothy L 94 Northwoods Boulevard, Worthington, OH 43085-4414, (614) 885-2997, BA 68 Capital Univ; MA 71 OH St Univ, PH 73 (NS) OH St Univ; Pres, HTI Inc, **A**

Rinker, Nancy C Route 2 Box 252, Stephens City, VA 22655, (703) 665-0825, BS 76 James Madison Univ; ME 77 Univ of VA - Charlottesville; Consult, American Red Cross, **A**

Rinko, Mrs Ferris D Forman 1604 Heard Drive, Maple Glen, PA 19002, (215) 643-9713, BA 77 Temple Univ; ME 81 Trenton St Coll; SLP, Er Sl So, **SLP**

Rinschler, Roger Jay Psc Box 1074, APO New York, NY 09293, BS 67 Emerson Coll; MS 75 Southern CT St Univ; 78–Sp-Lang Path, DOD Overseas Schs, **SLP**

Rintelmann, Joan 2512 Westwood Drive, Racine, WI 53404, (414) 634-0583, BS 71 OH Univ - Athens; MA 72 Univ of MA - Amherst; SLP, Racine USD, **SLP**

Rintelmann, Mary J 1467 Stonegate, East Lansing, MI 48823, (517) 676-3201, BS 55 Bradley Univ; MA 56 Univ of KS; **SLP**

Rintelmann, Dr William F Audiology Department, Wayne State University, 4201 St Antonie #5-E, Detroit, MI 48201, (313) 577-1393, BS 52 AZ St Univ; MA 57 IN Univ - Bloomington; PH 60 (Aud & Sp Path) IN Univ - Bloomington; Prof & Chmn, Dept of Aud Wayne St U, **SLP A F**

Rintoul, Mrs Dorothy Blake 3811 Central Avenue, Great Falls, MT 59405, BS 58 Portland St Univ; MA 64 Bradley Univ; SLP, Montana Sch for Deaf and Blind, **SLP LM**

Riolo, Mrs Eva Banham 200 North Village Avenue, Apt 3H, Rockville Centre, NY 11570, (516) 678-0694, BA 79 CUNY - Queens Coll; MA 81 CUNY - Queens Coll; SLP, New York City Board of Educ, **SLP**

Riordan, Ann R 14603 West 89th Street, Lenexa, KS 66215, **SLP**

Riordan, Anne E 242 Talcottville Road #305, Vernon, CT 06066, (203) 872-4731, BS 83 Univ of TN - Knoxville; MS 86 Purdue Univ - West Lafayette; 86–Research Asst, Univ of Conn, **A**

Riordan, Barbara Baldwin 8907 Bobrader Court, Louisville, KY 40299, (502) 267-8643, BA 76 Bellarmine Coll; MA 80 IN Univ - Bloomington; 80–Sp-Lang Path, Jefferson Co Pub Sch, **SLP**

Riordan, Mrs Jean E 3400 South Dahlia, Denver, CO 80222, (303) 693-8770, 68 Duke Univ; 76 Univ of CO - Boulder; 77–Sp-Lang Path, Cherry Creek Sch Dist 5, **SLP**

Riordan, Mrs Jeanine W 3033 Silver Bow, St Louis, MO 63129, (314) 846-5555, BS 76 Univ of MO - Columbia; MS 77 TX Tech Univ; 82–Sp-Lang Path, Private Practice, **SLP**

Riordan, Mrs Karin Salline 14 Yerks Lane, Ossining, NY 10562, (212) 920-5445, BS 73 Ithaca Coll; MA 74 NY Univ; 79–Sp-Lang Path, Montefiore Med Cen, **SLP**

Riordan, Patricia Martin 140 West Church Street, Wauconda, IL 60084-1812, BS 82 Univ of Evansville; MA 85 Northern IL Univ - De Kalb; **SLP**

Riordan, Peg 310 Whittier Avenue, Joliet, IL 60435-6926, BS 76 IL St Univ - Normal; MS 78 IL St Univ - Normal; SLP, Restorative Hlth Syst, **SLP ACE**

Ripich, Dr Danielle N Case Western Reserve Univ, 11206 Euclid Avenue, Cleveland, OH 44106, (216) 368-2384, BA 76 Cleveland St Univ; MA 77 Cleveland St Univ; PH 82 (NS) Kent St Univ; Exec Officer, Case Wn Reserve U, **SLP**

Ripinsky, Sharon 151-20 82 Street, Howard Beach, NY 11414, (212) 904-2677, BA 83 CUNY - Queens Coll; MA 85 CUNY - Queens Coll; **A**

Ripkin, Mindy Perlman 1244 Imperial Road, Rydal, PA 19046, (215) 884-3933, BS 78 SUNY - Center at Albany; MA 81 Temple Univ-Tyler Sch of Art; Sp-Lang Path, Northwest Center, **SLP**

Ripley, Mrs Barbara Deville 103 North Marshall Blvd, Bunkie, LA 71322, (318) 443-8275, BS 76 LA St Univ - Baton Rouge; MA 81 Northwestern St Univ; 88–Pres/Sp-Lang Path, Crossroads Rehab Assoc Inc, **SLP**

Ripley, Bethann Weiss 3020 Staten #7, Lansing, MI 48910, (517) 349-5471, BA 84 MI St Univ; MA 87 MI St Univ; 87–Sp-Lang Path, Tamarack Inc, **SLP**

Ripley, Mrs Julie Margaret 9278 Angus Place, Philadelphia, PA 19114, MA 81 Trenton St Coll; SLP, Pass Program, **SLP**

Riplinger, Patricia S 801 East Garden, Coeur d'Alene, ID 83814, (208) 743-9553, BA 76 Eastern WA Univ; MS 77 Eastern WA Univ; Sp-Lang Path, Lewiston Public Schools, **SLP**

Ripple, James Michael 5600 West Alexis Road #335, Sylvania, OH 43560, (419) 241-6219, MA 85 Eastern MI Univ; 87–Sp-Lang Path, Toledo Hearing and Speech Ctr, **SLP**

Rippy, James V 3629 McCain Boulevard Suite 230, North Little Rock, AR 72116, (501) 753-8444, BA 78 Univ of AR - Little Rock; MS 80 Univ of AR - Medical Sci; Aud, Jerry Potts MD, **A**

Rippy, Mrs Janice Gail 101 Gilbert Drive, Little Rock, AR 72205, (501) 227-2118, **SLP**

Riquelme, Luis F 57 Gates Avenue, Brooklyn, NY 11238, (718) 857-3899, BA 84 Long Island U - Brooklyn Ctr; MS 86 Columbia Univ Teachers Coll; 86–Sp-Lang Path, Internatl Ctr for the Dis, **SLP**

Risbrough, Ned P Eugene Hearing & Speech Center, 1500 West 12th, P O Box 2087, Eugene, OR 97402, (503) 485-8521, BS 61 Univ of OR; MS 62 Univ of OR; 62–Exec Dir, Eugene Hrng & Sp Cen, **SLP A**

Rischall, Mrs Cindy E 64 Lavender Lane, Rocky Hill, CT 06067, (203) 529-3328, BA 76 Adelphi Univ; MS 78 Boston Univ; 88–Sp-Lang Path, Rocky Hill PS, **SLP**

Risen, Anne Dachel 505 South Barstow #205, Eau Claire, WI 54701, (715) 672-8919, MS 87 Univ of WI - Eau Claire; 88–Sp-Lang Path, Durand USD

Risey, John A, Jr 9405 Dante Court, River Ridge, LA 70123, (504) 833-6562, BA 73 Univ of MS; OM 82 LA St Univ - N O Medical Ctr; Aud, Private Practice, **A**

Risher, Mrs Barbara E 297 Edgemere Drive, Annapolis, MD 21403, (301) 255-1394, BA 55 Univ of HI - Manoa; MS 57 PA St Univ - Middletown; 88–Sp-Lang Path, Anne Arundel Co Bd of Educ, **SLP**

Risher, Timothy B Ahs S-8-C22, Fort Sam Houston, TX 78234, BS 80 Brigham Young Univ; OM 81 Brigham Young Univ; Aud, US Army, **A**

Risi, Mrs Laurie 312 Main Street #4-E, White Plains, NY 10601, (914) 285-8189, BA 84 SUNY - Coll at Cortland; MA 87 NY Univ; 87–Sp-Lang Path, Westchester County Med Ctr, **SLP**

Risinger, Lois Ann 12702 South 81st Court, Palos Park, IL 60464, (312) 448-9420, BA 71 CO St Univ; MA 86 Northwestern Univ; 87–Sp-Lang Path, Elim Christian Sch

Riski, Dr John E Box 3887, Durham, NC 27710, (919) 684-3859, MS 71 Univ of South FL; PH 76 (NS) Univ of FL; Asst Prof, Duke U Med Cen, **SLP**

Risler, Susan Stinson 355 Brookstone Drive, Athens, GA 30605, (404) 549-0157, BS 83 Univ of GA; ME 84 Univ of GA; Sp-Lang Path, Clarke County School District, **SLP**

Risley, Mrs Laura Dreiman 855 B Pinewood Drive, Plainfield, IN 46168-0009, (317) 839-5542, BS 77 Purdue Univ - West Lafayette; MS 78 Univ of WY; **A**

Riso, Mrs Claire A 47 Barlow Lane, Rye, NY 10580, (914) 937-3800, BS 76 Mercy Coll; MA 78 NY Univ; 79–Sp/Lang Path, UCP Westchester Co, **SLP**

Rissman, Mrs Marlene S 7804 Lake Tahoe Avenue, San Diego, CA 92119, (619) 576-5878, BS 67 McGill Univ - Quebec; MS 69 McGill Univ - Quebec; Sp-Lang Path, Chldn Hosp & Hlth Cen, **SLP**

Ristau, Mrs Elizabeth S 50 Nursey Street, Norwalk, CT 06850, (203) 854-4000, BA 58 Hofstra Univ; MS 61 Adelphi Univ; Sp-Lang Path, Norwalk Bd of Ed, **SLP**

Ritchey, Gilbert G Ritchey Hearing Lab Inc, 731 North Fielder, Arlington, TX 76012, (817) 265-1466, BA 61 East TX St Univ - Commerce; ME 64 Univ of Houston - Univ Park; Owner/Dir, Ritchey Hrng Lab Inc, **A**

Ritchey, Mrs Lisa Ann 950 Mesa Terrace, Katy, TX 77450, (713) 392-8455, BA 83 Univ of Houston - Univ Park; MA 85 Univ of Houston - Univ Park; SLP, Cypress ISD, **SLP**

Ritchey, Rebecca Anne 118 W Colorado Blvd #7, Monrovia, CA 91016, (818) 359-1624, BA 83 San Jose St Univ; MS 85 San Francisco St Univ; **A**

Ritchie, Dr Betty C 4332 North Sheffield, Shorewood, WI 53211, (414) 963-5076, BS 50 LA St Univ - Baton Rouge; MA 51 LA St Univ - Baton Rouge; PH 64 (NS) Northwestern Univ; Chairpers, U of WI-Milwaukee, **SLP A ACE**

Ritchie, Bruce W Box 512, 1212 A Avenue, Vinton, IA 52349, (319) 472-5218, BA 71 Univ of Northern IA; MA 73 Univ of Northern IA; Investment Rep, Edward D Jones & Co, **SLP**

Ritchie, Mrs Joyce L 126 Stage Road, Newport News, VA 23606, (804) 599-5730, BS 77 Univ of VA - Charlottesville; ME 79 Univ of VA - Charlottesville; 87–Aud, Henry Hecker, **A**

Ritchie, Kathryn L 1222 East Boyd, Norman, OK 73071-2609, (405) 872-5943, **SLP**

Ritchie, Mrs Lynda C Genesee Intermediate School District, Center For Autism, 2413 West Maple Road, Flint, MI 48507, (313) 768-4485, BA 81 MI St Univ; MA 83 MI St Univ; 87–Sp-Lang Path, Genesee ISD, **SLP**

Ritgert, Barbara A 3008 Rueckert Avenue, Baltimore, MD 21214, BA 78 Towson St Univ; MA 79 Wichita St Univ; Sp-Lang Path, U of MD / Dept of Neurology, **SLP**

Ritschl, Nancy V Speech Pathology Department, 1000 Carondelet Drive, Kansas City, MO 64114, **SLP**

Rittenberg, Mrs Susan Vincent 5907 East Jamison Lane, Englewood, CO 80112, (303) 837-7021, BA 73 Univ of CO - Boulder; MA 77 Univ of CA - San Diego; Sp Lang Path, Saint Joseph Hosp, **SLP**

Rittenhouse, Sharon S 26728 Sheringham, Perrysburg, OH 43551, (419) 698-7615, BA 78 MI St Univ; MA 79 Bowling Green St Univ; 83–Sp-Lang Path, St Charles Hospital, **SLP**

Ritter, Mrs Becky A 124 West Summit Avenue, West Grove, PA 19390, (215) 383-5862, BS 74 West Chester Univ of PA; MA 79 West Chester Univ of PA; **SLP**

Ritter, Dawn Ranee 106 South Cottage, Normal, IL 61761, (309) 454-4652, BS 84 IL St Univ - Normal; MS 85 IL St Univ - Normal; **SLP**

Ritter, Dona H 22 Darwin Drive, Snyder, NY 14226, (716) 636-3410, BA 71 SUNY - Center at Buffalo; MS 72 Univ of WI - Madison; Cl Asst Prof, St Univ of NY - Buffalo, **SLP ACE**

Ritter, Dr E Gene 511 Staats Drive, Bloomington, IN 47408, (812) 335-4156, BA 50 William Jewell Coll; MA 53 Univ of MO - Columbia; PH 62 (Sp Path) Univ of MO - Columbia; Assoc Prof, IN U Dept Sp&Hrng Scs, **SLP F**

Ritter, Mrs Juliann V 7346 Creek View, West Bloomfield, MI 48322, (313) 851-2874, BA 74 Univ of MI - Ann Arbor; MA 76 Wayne St Univ; Ch Sp-Lang Path, Providence Hosp, **SLP**

Ritter, Mrs Lynn E 9 Parliament Drive, New City, NY 10956, MS 78 Purdue Univ - West Lafayette; SLP, Clarkstown School District, **SLP**

Ritter, Lynne M G 139 Mill Spring Place, Ormond Beach, FL 32074, (904) 673-6070, BA 78 CUNY - Queens Coll; MS 80 CUNY - Brooklyn Coll; Aud, Morton Hosp/Sp Lang Hrng Cen, **A**

Ritter, Michaela J 9407 Wildflower, Waco, TX 76712, (817) 666-7309, BS 73 Hardin-Simmons Univ; ME 77 Univ of Louisville; Sp/Lang Path Superv, McLennan Cty Coop, **SLP**

Ritter, Dr Patricia P O Box 1012, Ogdensburg, NY 13669-0476, (613) 744-3082, BS 74 Bowling Green St Univ; MA 78 Univ of TX - El Paso; PH 87 (NS) OH Univ - Athens; Sp-Lang Path, Childrens Hospital/Eastern Ont, **SLP**

Ritter, Dr Ronald L 5918 Pineway, San Antonio, TX 78247, (512) 653-1856, BA 64 9416; MA 66 Northern IL Univ - De Kalb; PH 78 (NS) Univ of Denver; 79–Aud, South Texas Aud Assoc, **A**

Ritterman, Dr Stuart I 181 Ellerbee Road, Wesley Chapel, FL 34249-4202, (813) 974-2006, BA 59 NY Univ; PH 68 (NS) Case Western Reserve Univ; Prof, Univ South FL, **SLP**

Rittgarn, Mrs Gwendolyn 1661 Otoe Street, Lincoln, NE 68502, (402) 464-9423, BS 74 Univ of NE - Lincoln; MA 75 Univ of NE - Lincoln; Sp-Lang Path, Speech Assoc, **SLP**

Ritthaler, Christophr R 3012 Rosewood, Parsons, KS 67357, (405) 237-1027, BS 71 Univ of Science & Arts of OK; MS 73 Univ of NM; Sp/Lang Path, Dept Human Serv, **SLP**

Rittmanic, Dr Paul A 5721 Elaine Drive, Rockford, IL 61108, (815) 399-9515, BS 52 Univ of IL - Urbana; MA 53 Northwestern Univ; PH 61 (Aud) Univ of OK Medical Center; Dir, Midwest Sp & Hrng Assoc, **SLP A F**

Rittore, Carol B 637 East Pintail Circle, Fresno, CA 93710, (209) 441-3328, Sp-Lang Path, Prog Spec, **SLP**

Ritz, Mrs Susan C Village Speech & Hearing Serv, 8209 North Dovin Gates Rd, Muncie, IN 47302, (317) 288-4796, BS 69 Ball St Univ; MA 71 Ball St Univ; Pres, Private Practice, **SLP A**

Rivard, Mrs Joan M 83 Dearwood Way, Folsom, CA 95630, BA 75 Univ of ME - Orono; MA 76 Univ of ME - Orono; Sp-Lang Path, Maine School Admin District #6, **SLP**

Rivas, Jeanne 5614 Netherland Avenue, Apartment 3-B, Bronx, NY 10471, MS 84 Columbia Univ Teachers Coll; **SLP**

Rivas, Mary S 4120 Rio Bravo Suite 311, El Paso, TX 79902, (915) 542-0463, BA 76 Univ of TX - El Paso; MA 79 Univ of TX - El Paso; Sp-Lang Path, Private Practice, **SLP**

Rivas, Monica 227 North Olive Avenue #2, Alhambra, CA 91801, (818) 570-0039, BA 83 Univ of Southern CA; MA 86 CA St Univ - Long Beach

Rivera, Brenda 5848 South Staples, Corpus Christi, TX 78413, (512) 992-4815, BA 76; MS 82; 87–Sp-Lang Path, Assoc Health Focus, **SLP**

Rivera, Enid M 4601 63rd Street #20, San Diego, CA 92115, (619) 576-5837, MA 88 San Diego St Univ

Rivera, Izel Marice 810 Washington Avenue Apartment 1017, Memphis, TN 38105, (901) 527-4473, MA 88 Univ of FL

Rivera, Mary Lou 115 Frontera Road, El Paso, TX 79922, **A**

Rivera, Sunshine Lynda 942 Bertrand Street, Houston, TX 77088, (713) 448-3236, BA 81 Univ of Houston - Univ Park; MA 87 Univ of Houston - Univ Park; 81–Sp-Lang Path, Aldine Ind Sch Dist, **SLP**

Rivera, Mrs Theresa Ann 937 Forest Creek Drive #1012, Garland, TX 75043, (214) 240-8132, BS 84 CO St Univ; ME 86 Univ of VA - Charlottesville; **A**

Rivera, Velma L 1075 Grand Concourse #4-G, Bronx, NY 10452, BA 81 CUNY - Lehman Coll; MA 83 CUNY - Lehman Coll; SLP, Bd of Ed, **SLP**

Rivers, Dr David L Dept Communication Disorders, Baylor University, Waco, TX 76798, (817) 755-2567, BS 66 Univ of KY; MS 68 Purdue Univ - West Lafayette; PH 77 (Sp-Lang Path) Vanderbilt Univ; Assoc Professor Commun Disord, Baylor University, **SLP ACE**

Rivers, Esther 7241 Sheila Turn, Clinton, MD 20735, (301) 856-2677

Rivers, Jill 2731 Loyola, Davis, CA 95616, (916) 322-4636, BA 64 San Jose St Univ; MS 72 Univ of HI - Manoa; Sp-Lang Path, CA Community Coll, **SLP**

Rivers, Mrs Paula R 10537 Tolling Clock Way, Columbia, MD 21044, BA 59 Univ of CT; MA 64 CUNY - Brooklyn Coll; ED 88 (Reading & the Hrng Impaired) Univ of MD - College Park; 75–Sp-Lang Path, Howard Co Pub Schools, **SLP**

Rivers, Susan W 228 Amberjack Drive #27, Fort Walton Beach, FL 32549, (904) 678-4812, BS 80 Univ Southern MS-Hattiesburg; MS 82 Univ Southern MS-Hattiesburg; Sp-Lang Path, Okalossa County Schools, **SLP**

Rivers, Tracy Irene 2706 Cheatham Street, Richmond, VA 23234, (804) 233-7967, BS 85 Ithaca Coll; MA 87 MI St Univ

Rives, Cheryl R 23621 Nottingham Court, Southfield, MI 48034, (313) 338-0361, BS 70 Wayne St Univ; MA 72 MI St Univ; Tchr for Autistic Impaired, Oakland Schs, **SLP**

Rives, Mrs Mary E B 711 Lamar, Winters, TX 79567, (915) 653-5981, BA 74 Univ of MO - KS City; MS 76 Central MO St Univ; Sp-Lang Path, Small Schools Cooperative, **SLP**

Rivette-Smith, Mrs Patricia Walker 9620 Creekwood Road, Louisville, KY 40223, (502) 228-1839, BA 73 Univ of KY; MA 78 Western KY Univ; 85–Sp-Lang Path, Oldham Co Bd of Educ, **SLP**

Rivetti, Denise Marie 315 Monahan Street, Aliquippa, PA 15001, (412) 378-3779, BS 83 CA Univ of PA; MS 87 CA Univ of PA; 84–Sp-Lang Path, Laurel Sch Dist, **SLP**

Rivier, Susan Hamilton 2190 Goldcrest Circle, Pleasanton, CA 94566, (415) 846-6646, 88–Sp-Lang Path, Lafayette Sch Dist, **SLP**

Rivkin, Gail R 2171 East 19th Street, Brooklyn, NY 11229, (718) 615-5200, BA 83 Hofstra Univ; MS 85 Columbia Univ Teachers Coll

Rivkin, Mrs Harriet B 303 Oakley Street, Cambridge, MD 21613, (301) 228-4747, BA 71 Univ of Pittsburgh - Pittsburgh; MA 73 CUNY - City College; Sp-Lang Path, Dor Co Bd of Ed, **SLP**

Rivkind, Sheryl W 2001 Marina Drive #513, Marina Bay, MA 02171, (617) 479-7503, BS 78 Boston Univ; ME 80 Northeastern Univ; Aud, Aud Assoc Inc, **A**

Rixon, Mrs Shelley Eckels 1030 Borst Avenue N E, North Bend, WA 98045, (206) 888-3232, BS 77 Univ of MN - Minneap-St Paul; OM 81 Univ of WA; **SLP**

Rizner, Constance B Speech-Language Pathologists, 2061 Dundee Drive, Winter Park, FL 32792, (407) 644-0666, BS 62 Univ of TN - Knoxville; MA 66 Univ of TN - Knoxville; Owner/Dir, Private Practice, **SLP ACE**

Rizzo, Anne Marie 133 Wabash Street, Kenmore, NY 14217, (716) 875-9129, BS 85 SUNY - Coll at Buffalo; MS 86 SUNY - Coll at Fredonia; 87–Sp-Lang Path, Children's Hosp of Buffalo

Rizzo, Crystal S 414 West Avenue, Northvale, NJ 07476, (201) 784-0955, Sp/Pathologist, Letchworth Village, **SLP**

Rizzo,, Dr Stephen R, Jr P O Box 1818, Chillicothe, OH 45601, PH 80 (NS) Bowling Green St Univ; Sp-Lang Path, Veterns Admin Medical Center, **A**

Rizzo, Mrs Valerie Jp 274 Sweeney Street, North Tonawanda, NY 14120, (716) 878-7371, BS 85 SUNY - Center at Buffalo; MS 86 SUNY - Coll at Fredonia; 88–Sp-Lang Path, Early Childhood Prog-Chldn Hosp of Buffalo

Rizzo, Wendy Suzanne 1847 Kirts #220, Troy, MI 48084, (313) 252-1355, BA 81 Univ of MI - Ann Arbor; MA 83 Wayne St Univ - Sch of Med; Super of Aud, Metro Med Group, **A**

Rizzuto, Frances Pauline 10 Park Hill Drive, New Windsor, NY 12550, (914) 562-6891, BA 83 SUNY - Coll at Plattsburgh; MS 86 SUNY - Coll at New Paltz; **SLP**

Roach, April S 56 Fairview Avenue, Morrisville, PA 19067, (215) 295-6453, BA 68 Boston Univ; MA 78 Temple Univ; 85–Sp-Lang Path, Moss Rehab Hosp, **SLP**

Roach, Beth Anne 855 Bader Street, Green Bay, WI 54302, (414) 498-1545, BA 85 Coll of Saint Teresa; MS 86 Univ of WI - Eau Claire; **SLP**

Roach, Mary Jane 420 Sand Creek Road, Bldg 1 #606, Albany, NY 12205, (518) 768-2318, MS 79 SUNY - Coll at Geneseo; 88–Sp-Lang Path, Bethlehem Cen Schs, **SLP**

Roach, Robert A Box 1177, Loma Linda, CA 92354, BA 48 Southern Coll of S D A; OM 70 Loma Linda Univ - Loma Linda; MA 67 Univ of Redlands; Sp-Lang Path, Private Practice, **SLP LM**

Roach, Dr Robert E 5316 8th Avenue South, Birmingham, AL 35212, (205) 592-8057, BA 36 IL Coll; MA 40 Columbia Univ Teachers Coll; PH 52 (Aud) Northwestern Univ; Retired, DNA, **A F LM**

Roach, Sharla B Route 2, 35 Elkins Lane, Roanoke, TX 76262, (817) 577-1560, **A**

Roach, Virginia A 5236 Muirhouse Place, San Jose, CA 95136, (408) 629-6850, BS 78 Marquette Univ; MA 81 Whittier Coll; **SLP**

Roat, Mrs Shirley E Renner 1297 Wilson Road, Macedon, NY 14502, (716) 377-4660, BS 79 Nazareth Coll of Rochester; MS 81 Nazareth Coll of Rochester; Sp/Lang Path, BOCES #1 Monroe County, **SLP**

Robandt, Mrs Theresa L P O Box 549, Darlington, SC 29532, (803) 393-2586, BS 80 Western MI Univ; MA 82 Western MI Univ; Sp-Lang Path for Hrng Imp, Except Ed Serv Proj Share, **SLP**

Robb, Delores A P O Box 342, Preemption, IL 61276, (319) 359-1325, BS 86 Western IL Univ; MA 87 Western IL Univ; 88–Aud, Audiology Consultants Inc

Robb, Mrs Edith C 1114 Bishop Walsh Drive, Cumberland, MD 21502, (301) 724-0267, BS 74 Univ of MD - College Park; MS 77 Towson St Univ; **SLP**

Robb, Dr Michael Paul University Of Hawaii, Division Of Sp & Aud, 1410 Lower Campus Drive, Honolulu, HI 96822, (808) 948-8279, BS 79 Western MI Univ; MS 83 Syracuse Univ; PH 88 (Sp Path) Syracuse Univ; Asst Prof, Univ of HI, **SLP**

Robb, Mrs Tommye L S Illinois Easter Seal Society, P O Box 3249, Carbondale, IL 62901, (618) 457-3333, MS 71 Southern IL Univ -Carbondale; Exec Dir, S Il Er Sl So, **SLP**

Robbie, Marguerite Pryor 214 Apt F Falls Street, Morganton, NC 28655, (704) 433-6149, BS 85 Appalachian St Univ; MA 86 Univ of SC - Columbia; 86–Sp-Lang Path, Logos, **SLP**

Robbin, Barbara Lee 4837 Stern Avenue, Sherman Oaks, CA 91423, (818) 995-7489, BA 67; OM 74 Pacific Oaks Coll; MS 83 CA St Univ - Los Angeles; Consultant, Private Practice, **SLP**

Robbins, Amy McConkey Rielly ENT, A-56, 702 Barnhill Drive, Indianapolis, IN 46223, (317) 274-8868, BA 77 Hollins Coll; OB 77; MS 79 Purdue Univ - West Lafayette; Slpr/Cochlear Implant Team, IN U Med Cen, **SLP**

Robbins, Christine 714 Merrimac Place, Danville, CA 94526, (415) 838-2329, BA 73 Univ of MI - Ann Arbor; MA 77 Cleveland St Univ; Sp-Lang-Hrng Spec, Murray Sch Dist, **SLP**

Robbins, Christine 94 Burning Tree, Chesterfield, MO 63017, (314) 469-1859, BA 74 Univ of MN - Minneap-St Paul; MA 79 Mankato St Univ; **SLP**

Robbins, Colleen 1000 Ainsworth, Suite 100, Prescott, AZ 86301, (602) 445-1303, BS 74 Northern AZ Univ; MS 79 Univ of OK - Norman; Sp/Lang Path, Prescott Rehabilitation Assoc, **SLP ACE**

Robbins, Deborah Cameron 726 Elizabeth Drive, Crown Point, IN 46307, (312) 210-2300, MS; 80–Sp-Lang Path, Assoc for Low-Incidence Handicaps, **SLP**

Robbins, Mrs Janice Schwenk 249 Kensington Drive, Delaware, OH 43015, (614) 369-8761, BA 67 Lycoming Coll; ME 69 Univ of VA - Charlottesville; 78–Sp-Lang Path, Delaware Co Schs, **SLP**

Robbins, Dr Joanne Neurology Service B6/052, WM S Middleton VA Hospital, 2500 Overlook Terrace, Madison, WI 53705, (608) 262-3951, BA 72 Temple Univ-Tyler Sch of Art; MS 73 Univ of WI - Madison; PH 82 (NS) Northwestern Univ; 87–Assoc Sci, U of WI, **SLP**

Robbins, Maxine G F-13 235 37th Street East, Tuscaloosa, AL 35405, (205) 553-3760, OB 73 Univ of NC - Chapel Hill; OM 74 Univ of GA; MS 83 Univ of AL-Tuscaloosa; Aud, VA Med Cen, **A**

Robbins, Dr Myra G 70 Centre Street, Woodmere, NY 11598, (516) 569-4744, BA 51 CUNY - Brooklyn Coll; MA 52 CUNY - Brooklyn Coll; PH 71 (NS) CUNY - Grad Sch & Univ Cntr; Sp-Lang Path, Private Practice, **SLP A**

Robbins, Nancy V 1 Hampstead Road, Jamaica Plain, MA 02130, (617) 727-5106, ME 59 Boston Univ; BA 55 Radcliffe Coll; Special Asst for Planning, MA Office of Deafness, **A**

Robbins, Mrs Rosalyn J 3306 Albermarle, Greensboro, NC 27410, (919) 299-8156, BA 69 Univ of MI - Ann Arbor; MA 71 Case Western Reserve Univ; Sp-Lang Path, Greensboro Pubsch, **SLP**

Robbins, Sharon Bowen 405 El Greco Drive, Brandon, FL 33511, (813) 272-4530, MS 74 Univ of South FL; 88–Sp-Lang Path, Hillsborough County Schs, **SLP**

Robbins, Wendy M 8956 West Sample Road, Coral Springs, FL 33065, (305) 786-3713, MA 83 Trenton St Coll; 87–Sp-Lang Path, Pompano Beach Elem, **SLP**

Robenalt, Kathleen S 2601 Winterlake, Carrollton, TX 75006, (214) 416-9190, BS 78 Univ of Cincinnati; MA 80 Auburn Univ - Auburn; PH 85 (Sp Path) Univ of MI - Ann Arbor; Sp-Lang Path, **SLP**

Roberson, Mrs Carolyn J 3835 McMahon Avenue, Anchorage, AK 99516, BS 50; MA 56; Retired, Anchorage Borough Sch Dist, **SLP**

Roberson, Mrs Janet Gary 2012 West Ohio Street, Midland, TX 79701, (915) 683-2521, BA 82 TX Tech Univ; MS 84 TX Tech Univ; 84–Aud, Midland Aud Assoc, **A**

Roberson, Joan Lee 918 Wesley Court, Jonesboro, AR 72401, (501) 972-3106, BA 60 Univ of AR - Fayetteville; MA 75 Univ of AR - Fayetteville; Instructor/Clinical Supervisor, Arkansas State University, **SLP**

Roberson, Mrs Judith E 3314 Tunison Drive, Wilmington, DE 19810, (302) 478-9393, BS 69 Purdue Univ - West Lafayette; MA 71 IN Univ - Bloomington; Sp-Lang Path, Speech Therapeutics Inc, **SLP ACE**

Roberson, Kendel E 3726 East 36th Place, Tulsa, OK 74135, (918) 745-6800, BS 80 Univ of Tulsa; MA 82 Univ of Tulsa; Sp-Lang Path, Tulsa Pub Sch, **SLP**

Roberson, Mrs Terri Hill 13614 Bell Drive, San Antonio, TX 78217-1478, (512) 657-3383, BS 82 Baylor Univ; MS 84 Univ of TX - Dallas; Aud, A & B Hearing Aid & Audiol Cen, **A**

Robert, Alice C 192 Redwood Road, Manchester, CT 06040, (203) 647-3367, BS 67 Univ of CT; MA 71 Univ of CT; Sp/Lang Path/Spec Ed, Manchester Board of Ed, **SLP**

Robert, Mrs Betty Swanick Calle Reina Isabel 177, La Villa DE Torrimar, Guaynabo, PR 00657, (809) 764-8096, BS 64 Saint Louis Univ; MS 76 Univ of PR - Rio Piedras; Sp-Lang Path, Villa Nevarez Sp & Hrng Cen, **SLP**

Robert, Mrs Carolyn A 5901 Woodcliff Drive, Midland, MI 48640, (517) 776-0286, BS 69 Marygove Coll; MS 71 Purdue Univ - West Lafayette; Sp-Lang Path, Saginaw Pub Sch Syst, **SLP**

Robert, Jan M 503 East Guidry, Covington, LA 70433, (919) 748-0269, BS 76 Saint Mary's Dominican Coll; OM 78 LA St Univ - N O Medical Ctr; Consul Sp/Lang Path, Chld Guidance Cl, **SLP**

Robert, Mrs Margaret Thompson 4806 Fern Street, Bellaire, TX 77401, (713) 667-0105, BS 80 LA St Univ - Baton Rouge; MA 81 LA St Univ - Baton Rouge; 88–Sp-Lang Path, InSpeech Inc, **SLP**

Roberts, Barbara Ann 1107 Lennon Way, San Jose, CA 95125, (408) 867-3404, BS 75 Northwestern Univ; MS 76 Univ of Redlands; **SLP**

Roberts, Barbara Kubasta 11200 S W 70th Avenue, Miami, FL 33156, (305) 661-8263, BA 74 Colgate Univ; MA 79 Univ of MA - Amherst; Private Practice, **SLP**

Roberts, Cathryn L Dynamic Communication Inc, 4200 Lake Otis Pkway #304, Anchorage, AK 99508, (907) 563-3175, BA 72 CA St Univ - Northridge; MA 74 CA St Univ - Northridge; President, Dynamic Commun Inc, **SLP**

Roberts, Cheri T 581 West Tropical Way, Plantation, FL 33317, (305) 791-2372, BA 72 West TX St Univ; MS 77 TX Christian Univ; **SLP**

Roberts, Christina Lee 1614 Donovan Place, Longmont, CO 80501, (303) 651-3361, BA 83 CA St Univ - Long Beach; MA 85 Univ of CO - Boulder; SLP, **SLP**

Roberts, Cindy Abbott 521 Surrey Circle, Irving, TX 75061, (214) 358-8335, BS 78 Bloomsburg Univ of PA; MA 81 Univ of Pittsburgh - Pittsburgh; 86–Sp-Lang Path, Dallas Rehab Inst, **SLP**

Roberts, Mrs Deborah I 12 Temple Avenue, Hackensack, NJ 07601, **SLP**

Roberts, Deborah Morris 1603 John Orr Drive, Tifton, GA 31794, (912) 386-4646, BA 74 Univ of FL; ME 83 Valdosta St Coll; Sp-Lang Path, Medivance Rehab Serv Inc, **SLP**

Roberts, Mrs Debra V 2489 Bunker Hill, Ann Arbor, MI 48105, (313) 769-7100, **SLP**

Roberts, Mrs Elise R 235 Garth Road #C2B, Scarsdale, NY 10583, (914) 941-9513, BA 75 Adelphi Univ; MA 76 Univ of IL - Urbana; Sp-Lang Path, Assoc Ment Ill Chldn of Wstctr, **SLP**

Roberts, Elizabeth 11155 Citrus Drive #60, Ventura, CA 93004, BA 78 Univ of RI; MA 81 CA St Univ - Long Beach; Tchr, Oxnard Sch Dist, **SLP**

Roberts, Mrs Gail Forman 3732 Arborlawn Drive, Fort Worth, TX 76109, (201) 238-6877, BA 82 Rutger's St Univ - Douglas Coll; MS 84 Emory Univ; **SLP**

Roberts, Gay W 4080 Ashmore Place, Pensacola, FL 32503, (904) 433-2829, BS 63 Univ of TN - Knoxville; MA 69 Memphis St Univ; Sp-Lang Path, Escambia Co Sch, **SLP**

Roberts, Dr Jan Avent 1479 Brian Court, Milpitas, CA 95035, (408) 263-1135, MA 79 Univ of KS; PH 88 (NS) Univ of CA - San Francisco; Sp-Lang Path, **SLP**

Roberts, Janet Lynne 35-1/2 Orchard Place, Forty Fort, PA 18704, (717) 824-9742, BS 81 Bloomsburg Univ of PA; MS 82 Bloomsburg Univ of PA; Sp-Lang Path, Wilkes-Barre Sp-Lang Clinic, **SLP**

Roberts, Joan Elizabeth 7660 Lakeside Drive, Riverside, CA 92509, (714) 685-6996, BA 82 Univ of Redlands; MS 83 Univ of Redlands; SLP, Riverside USD, **SLP**

Roberts, Dr Joanne Erwick 207 Stagecoach Road, Chapel Hill, NC 27514, (919) 966-4121, BA 71 PA St Univ - Univ Park; MA 73 Trenton St Coll; PH 81 (NS) IN Univ - Bloomington; Investigator In Child Dev, U of NC, **SLP A**

Roberts, Mrs Joanne S 9760 Northwest 10th Street, Pembroke Pines, FL 33024, (305) 432-6584, BA 81 SUNY - Center at Buffalo; MA 84 Univ of FL; Aud, Dade Co Pub Sch, **A**

Roberts, Mrs Juanita Dundon 6000 Romaine Drive, Dayton, OH 45415, (513) 222-5597, BS 61 Kent St Univ; MS 83 Miami Univ - Oxford; 84–Coord, Hearing & Speech Center of Metropolitan Dayton, **SLP**

Roberts, Judith L 137 Quail Run, Boise, ID 83709, (801) 561-2269, BS 80 Brigham Young Univ; OM 81 Brigham Young Univ; Sp-Lang Path, Jordan Sch Dist, **SLP**

Roberts, Julia L 1003 South 46th Street, Philadelphia, PA 19143, (215) 387-6674, BS 69 WV Univ; MS 78 Emerson Coll; Sp/Lang Path, Private Practice, **SLP**

Roberts, Mrs Karen Aicher 18 Lovewell Street, Nashua, NH 03060, (603) 883-2900, BS 81 Bloomsburg Univ of PA; MS 82 Bloomsburg Univ of PA; Sp/Lang Path, Northeast Rehab Hospital, **SLP**

Roberts, Karen Ann P O Box 8182 S I, Christiansted, St Croix, VI 00823, (809) 778-3063, MS 84 Univ of VT; 87–Sp-Lang Path, Virgin Islands Dept of Educ, **SLP**

Roberts, Mrs Karen F 2409 Country Way, Fayetteville, AR 72703, (501) 443-1496, BS 72 Ouachita Baptist Univ; MA 74 Univ of AR - Fayetteville; SLP, Fayetteville Phys Ther Cl, **SLP ACE**

Roberts, Kathleen Ann 2455 Jefferson, Eugene, OR 97405, **A**

Roberts, Mrs Kathleen B 210 Crystal Court, Little Rock, AR 72205, (501) 661-0486, BS 71 Univ of AR - Fayetteville; MS 73 Univ of OK Medical Center; Sp-Lang Path, Sp-Lang Path Consults, **SLP**

Roberts, Kathryn L 201 Brunswick Court, Lansdale, PA 19446, (215) 855-2821, 88–Sp-Lang Path, Holy Redeemer Hosp & Med Ctr, **SLP**

Roberts, Mrs Kathylene 2107 Hailstone Circle, Kings Point, Sun City, FL 33570, MA 50 IA St Univ; Sp-Lang Path, **SLP LM**

Roberts, Dr Kenneth R Coordinator Lang Develop Lab, Boys Town National Inst, 555 North 30th Street, Omaha, NE 68131, (402) 498-6750, BA 71 Univ of KS; MS 73 Univ of OK Medical Center; PH 79 (Child Lang Acquisition) Univ of KS; 88–Coord Lang Dev Lab, Boys Town Natl Inst, **SLP**

Roberts, Keyenna 70 Booth Street, Needham Heights, MA 02194, (617) 449-4249, Private Practice, **SLP**

Roberts, Mrs Kim Meyer 421 North Huron, Pierre, SD 57501, (605) 224-2906, BA 78 SD St Univ; MA 83 Univ of SD - Springfield; Sp-Lang Path, Pierre Pub Schs, **SLP**

Roberts, Laura Montgomery 233 Merriman Street, Rochester, NY 14607, (716) 473-0399, MS 84 Univ of NC - Chapel Hill; **SLP**

Roberts, Mrs Leticia A 3425 San Joaquin Road, Covina, CA 91724, BA 75 Univ of Redlands; MS 76 Univ of Redlands; Sp-Lang Path, Los Angeles County Sup Schools, **SLP**

Roberts, Mrs Linda D 9 West 22nd, Hutchinson, KS 67501, (316) 665-2130, BS 77 Univ of KS; MA 79 Univ of KS; Dir of Sp Dept, Hutchinson Hosp Corp, **SLP**

Roberts, Linda J 8205 South Oswego, Tulsa, OK 74137, (918) 481-5138, BA 72 Univ of Tulsa; MA 74 Univ of Tulsa; Sp-Lang Path, Private Practice, **SLP**

Roberts, Linda Sobel Denver General Hospital, 8th Avenue & Cherokee, Denver, CO 80204, (303) 893-7494, BA 73 Univ of Denver; MA 74 Univ of Denver; Sp/Lang Path, Denver Gen Hosp, **SLP**

Roberts, Mrs Lynn 27762 Autumn Court, Hayward, CA 94542, (415) 469-6217, BS 73 CA St Univ - Hayward; MA 77 San Francisco St Univ; Sp-Lang Path, Diag Sch Neuro Hand Chld, **SLP**

Roberts, Marcy Diane 5923 Cedar Fern Court, Columbia, MD 21044, (301) 720-1013, BA 82 Loyola Coll; MS 83 Loyola Coll; 86–Sp-Lang Path, UCP of Central MD, **SLP**

Roberts, Dr Margaret Mills Childrens Hospital, Sp Path & Audiology Dept, 700 Childrens Drive, Columbus, OH 43205, (614) 461-2420, BA 62 OH St Univ; MA 63 OH St Univ; PH 66 (Sp & Hrng Science) OH St Univ; Director SLP & Aud Dept, Chlds Hospital, **SLP**

Roberts, Marilyn Baugham Rt 1 Box 20A, Blanch, NC 27212, BS 71 NC Central Univ; ME 77 NC Central Univ; 88–Sp-Lang Path, Caswell County Schs, **SLP**

Roberts, Mary Ann K Speech Language Pathology, 5800 Monroe Street, Bldg F, Sylvania, OH 43560, (419) 885-3666, BA 80 Univ of Toledo; MA 81 Bowling Green St Univ; 86–Sp-Lang Path, Private Practice, **SLP**

Roberts, Mary C K 501 Blueberry Lane, Syracuse, NY 13219, (315) 635-3941, BS 74 SUNY - Coll at Geneseo; MS 76 SUNY - Coll at Buffalo; Sp-Lang Path, Baldwinsville Ctrl Sch Dist, **SLP**

Roberts, Mary D 9049 Autumn Woods Drive, Apartment 1-C, Indianapolis, IN 46250, (317) 353-5949, BS 83 Purdue Univ - West Lafayette; MS 85 Purdue Univ - West Lafayette; 88–Sp-Lang Path, Community Hosp Indianapolis, **SLP**

Roberts, Mary Elizabeth 25 A Northwood Hills Drive, Gulfport, MS 39503, (601) 832-0596, BS 73 Henderson St Univ; MS 85 Univ of Central AR; **SLP**

Roberts, Mrs Maxine J 1902 Plum Creek Lane, Lexington, NE 68850, (308) 324-5929, BS 63 Univ of NE - Lincoln; SLP, Ed Serv Unit 10, **SLP**

Roberts, Nancy E 320 Ferry Road #1104, Galveston, TX 77550, (409) 765-5472, BA 62 Univ of IA; MA 74 Univ of Northern IA; Sp/Lang Path, Univ Texas/Medical Branch-Dir, **SLP**

Roberts, Mrs Nancy Kaye 1893 Bear Path Trail, Eagan, MN 55122, (612) 941-1655, BA 80 Univ of WI - Eau Claire; MS 81 Univ of WI - Eau Claire; Sp-Lang Path, Edina PS, **SLP**

Roberts, Mrs Noreen Hubbard 2536 East Woodland Drive, Ogden, UT 84403, (801) 479-6374, BA 56 Brigham Young Univ; SLP, Private Practice, **SLP**

Roberts, Mrs Patricia Jean S 1934 Strathaven Road, Winter Park, FL 32792, (305) 740-8357, BA 75 Western IL Univ; MS 76 Western IL Univ; 86–Sp-Lang Path, Orange County PS, **SLP**

Roberts, Mrs Patricia Leigh P O Box 804, Quitman, GA 31643, (912) 333-8505, BS 80 Univ of GA; ME 81 Univ of GA; Sp-Lang Path, Valdosta City Schs, **SLP**

Roberts, Patricia M St Vincent Hospital, 60 Cambridge Street North, Ottawa, ON, Canada K1R 7A5, (613) 782-2748, BA 77 Queens Univ - Ontario; MA 80 FL St Univ; 88–Sp-Lang Path, St Vincent Hosp, **SLP**

Roberts, Paul E 257 North Sergeant, Buckley, WA 98321, (206) 829-1111, BA 61 Univ of WA; MA 81 Western WA Univ; SLP, Aud, Dept of Social & Health Svcs, **SLP**

Roberts, Robbie Dethelia 3956 S Street S E, Washington, DC 20020, (202) 583-0303, **A ACE**

Roberts, Roland James 8064 Martingrove Road, Woodbridge, ON, Canada L4L 4B5, (416) 438-6128, BS 83 Howard Univ; MS 85 Howard Univ; 88–Aud, Scarborough Gen Hosp

Roberts, Mrs Roselyn C 110 Tandy Trace, Fayetteville, GA 30214, (404) 767-5546, BS 76 GA St Univ; ME 78 Univ of GA; Sp-Lang Path, Fulton County Board of Educ, **SLP**

Roberts, Rosemarie Stavros 421 Piper Road, Haslett, MI 48840, (517) 339-0751, BA 84 MI St Univ; MA 85 MI St Univ; 86–Sp-Lang Path, Tamarack Inc, **SLP**

Roberts, Ruth Ellen 403 Village Green Blvd, Gallatin, TN 37066, (615) 865-3586, BA 75 Univ of KY; MA 76 Univ of TN - Knoxville; Sp/Lang Path, Self Employed, **SLP**

Roberts, Sandra E 8328 Sunflower Court, Jacksonville, FL 32244, BS 79 FL St Univ; MS 80 FL St Univ; **SLP**

Roberts, Mrs Sharon L 6107 Morningview Drive, Anaheim, CA 92807, (213) 263-5106, BA 73 CA St Univ - Fullerton; MS 76 Univ of Redlands; ED 88 (Organizational Leadership) Univ of Southern CA; 87–Prin/Admin Asst, Los Angeles Co Schs, **SLP**

Roberts, Dr Stephen D Valley Childrens Hospital, 3151 North Millbrook, Fresno, CA 93703, (209) 225-3000, BA 74 CA St Univ - Sacramento; MS 76 Univ of UT; PH 79 (NS) Wayne St Univ - Sch of Med; 79–Dir of Sp-Lang Path & Aud, Valley Chldn Hosp, **A**

Roberts, Susan 4245 Manteca Lane, Bridgeton, MO 63044, (314) 968-4710, Audiologist, St Louis Hearing and Spch Ctr, **A**

Roberts, Mrs Susan M 0N 521 Willow Road, Wheaton, IL 60187, (312) 668-5930, BS 68 Univ of IL - Urbana; MA 70 Univ of IL - Urbana; Sp/Lang Path, Comm Nursing Assoc of Dupage, **SLP**

Roberts, Tamra Sarita 7401 New Hampshire Avenue, Apartment 703, Hyattsville, MD 20783, (301) 439-6647, BA 81 Hampton Univ; MA 83 Univ of IL - Urbana; Aud, Washington Hospital Center, **A**

Roberts, Terry Lynn Center For Audiology, 3914 Parliament Drive, Alexandria, LA 71303, (318) 442-9707, BA 76 LA Tech Univ; MA 78 LA Tech Univ; Aud, Private Practice, **A**

Roberts, Valeria A 1601 15th Avenue South, Nashville, TN 37212, (615) 320-5353, BS 83 TN St Univ; ME 86 TN St Univ; **A**

Roberts, Mrs Wanda T Route 2 Box 85, Murray, KY 42071, (502) 753-9776, BS 72 Murray St Univ; MS 75 Murray St Univ; Sp-Lang Path, Calloway County Schools, **SLP ACE**

Roberts, Dr William H 2024 Yorkshire Drive, Winter Park, FL 32792, (407) 671-0333, BA 53 Univ of FL; MA 54 Univ of FL; PH 70 (NS) OH Univ - Athens; Private Practice, **SLP A LM**

Robertshaw, Mrs Kristan Kulch 88 Walnut Hill Road, Derry, NH 03038, (603) 434-1031, BS 76 Rutger's St Univ - Douglas Coll; MS 78 Rutgers St Univ -N Brunswick; Sp/Lang Path, Private Practice, **SLP**

Robertson, Mrs Cecilia Dianne 3 Waterford Road, Salisbury, NC 28144, (704) 633-6325, BA 77 Univ of TN - Knoxville; MA 81 Univ of TN - Knoxville; 87–Sp-Lang Path, Rowan County Schs, **SLP**

Robertson, Mrs Cheryl A K 241 Pin Oak Drive, Geneseo, IL 61254, (309) 944-2520, BA 78 Augustana Coll; MA 79 Univ of Northern IA; SLP, Henry Stark Co Special Ed Coop, **SLP**

Robertson, Christine E 5400 Langdale Drive, Racine, WI 53402, (414) 786-7330, BS 62 Eastern IL Univ; ME 84 Marquette Univ; 88–Assoc Dir for Human Res, Archdiocese of Milwaukee, **SLP**

Robertson, Darlene M 2736 South Hiwan Drive, Evergreen, CO 80439, (303) 674-7470, BS 53 Univ of NE - Lincoln; MA 62 Columbia Univ Teachers Coll; SLP Orofacial Myologist, Private Practice, **SLP**

Robertson, Eugene L, Jr 2207 Park Avenue, St Louis, MO 63104, (314) 772-4553, BS 79 Fontbonne Coll; MS 80 Fontbonne Coll; 80, Private Practice, **SLP**

Robertson, Mrs Helen 566 Pierce Avenue, Baton Rouge, LA 70806, (504) 926-5631, BA 55 Univ of Southwestern LA; Sp-Lang Path, Private Practice, **SLP LM**

Robertson, James B 35 Llanberris Road, Bala-Cynwyd, PA 19004, (215) 897-6845, BA 70 Univ of KS; MA 72 Univ of KS; 86–Hearing Conservationist, Basil Health Systems, **A**

Robertson, Jana Renee 9506 Estate Lane, Dallas, TX 75238, (214) 341-0609, BS 83 East TX St Univ - Commerce; MS 85 East TX St Univ - Commerce; Sp-Lang Path, InSpeech Inc, **SLP**

Robertson, Jane Ann 3054 Buttrick Avenue S E, Ada, MI 49301, (616) 243-6926, BA 68 Western MI Univ; MA 69 Western MI Univ; Sp-Lang Path, Grand Rapids Board of Educ, **SLP**

Robertson, Jeanne Sheldon 160 Cottage Road, Sydney, NS, Canada B1P 2E6, (902) 564-5414, BA 78 Univ of ME - Orono; MA 80 Western WA Univ; 84–Sp-Lang Path, Nova Scotia Hrg and Sp Clin, **SLP**

Robertson, Kiz W 2010 Sumac Drive, Champaign, IL 61821, (217) 356-8254, MA 88 Univ of IL - Urbana

Robertson, Mrs Lois A 4006 Boxelder Drive, Brecksville, OH 44141, (216) 526-9571, BS 75 Miami Univ - Oxford; MA 76 Kent St Univ; Sp-Lang Path, Private Practice, **SLP**

Robertson, Lynne Farrar 549 Indian Lake Road, Hendersonville, TN 37075, (615) 865-3741, BA 83 Univ of MS; MA 85 Memphis St Univ; 87–Dir Sp-Lang Path, Nashville Memorial Hospital, **SLP**

Robertson, Margaret Alexandra 61 Warren Avenue, Mystic, CT 06355, (203) 536-7133, Sp-Lang Path, Norwich Board of Ed, **SLP**

Robertson, Mark Lawrence Box 249, East Silkirk, MB, Canada R0E 0M0, (204) 482-6997, BA 84 Univ of Winnipeg - Manitoba; MS 86 Univ of ND; 88–Sp-Lang Path, InSpeech Inc, **SLP**

Robertson, Mary Lu Oakland Schools Speech Clinic, 2100 Pontiac Lake Road, Pontiac, MI 48054, BS 54 IL St Univ - Normal; MA 59 Univ of MI - Ann Arbor; Sp-Lang Path, Oakland Schools, **SLP F**

Robertson, Patricia Rita 721 Kendall Drive, Birmingham, AL 35226, (205) 823-6207, BA 70 Indiana Univ of PA; MS 82 Clarion Univ of PA; 87–Aud, Univ of Montevallo, **A**

Robertson, Penny S 28 Westmoreland, Naperville, IL 60540, (312) 961-1117, BA 65 Univ of NE - Lincoln; MA 71 Univ of NE - Lincoln; **SLP**

Robertson, Dr Ronald McDonald 1128 Candlewood Circle, Pensacola, FL 32514, (904) 452-6456, PH 68 (Aud & Sp Science) Purdue Univ - West Lafayette; 85–Head-Aud Div, Naval Hosp, **A**

Robertson, Mrs Shari Brand 5120 Beechnut Drive, Kewaskum, WI 53040, (414) 338-5478, BS 80 Western MI Univ; MA 82 Central MI Univ; Sp-Lang Path, West Bend Jt Sch Dist #1, **SLP**

Robertson, Mrs Valerie H 1501-E Villa Drive, Butler, PA 16001, BS 78 Indiana Univ of PA; MS 80 WV Univ; Sp-Lang Path, **SLP**

Robertson, Virginia R 4634 South Gary Place, Tulsa, OK 74105, (918) 747-7952, BA 72 Southern Methodist Univ; MS 79 Univ of TX - Dallas; 86–Sp Svcs Supvr, Tulsa Child Dev & Reg Guid Ctr, **SLP**

Robertson-Soriano, Mrs Kristie 1 Compton Court, Basking, NJ 07920, (201) 334-5000, BA 81 Montclair St Coll; MS 82 Boston Univ; Sp-Lnag Path, JFK Med Cen, **SLP**

Roberts-Yuen, Sharon 2306 Park Boulevard, Oakland, CA 94606, (415) 893-3527, OB 69 Cornell Coll; MS 86 Univ of HI - Manoa; 87–Sp-Lang Path, Richmond USD, **SLP**

Robey, Dr Randall R Southern Illinois University, Dept Of Comm Disorders &, Sciences, Carbondale, IL 62901, (618) 453-4301, BA 75 Marshall Univ; MA 76 Marshall Univ; PH 85 (Sp-Lang Path) OH Univ - Athens; Assistant Professor, Southern Illinois University, **SLP**

Robier, Therese Clarke Army Audiology & Speech Center, Walter Reed Army Med Ctr, Washington, DC 20307-5001, (202) 576-1646, BS 83 Towson St Univ; MS 84 Towson St Univ; 87–Aud, US Army, **A**

Robin, Mrs Constance 11251 Riverview Way, Houston, TX 77042, (818) 360-0530, BA 58 Univ of KY; MA 78 CA Lutheran Coll; Los Angeles Esd Spec Ed

Robin, Dr Donald A Department Of Sp Path & Aud, Univ Of Iowa, Iowa City, IA 52242, (319) 335-8727, BA 76 Boston Univ; MS 81 Univ of Redlands; PH 84 (Communication Sciences) Case Western Reserve Univ; Asst Prof, Univ of Iowa, **SLP**

Robin, Lois L 607 Burns Avenue, Aptos, CA 95003, (408) 662-2950, BA 52 Univ of CA - Los Angeles; MA 67 Univ of CA - Santa Barbara; Sp/Lang Path, Lois Robin, **SLP**

Robin, Peggy T J 16963 Bosque Drive, Encino, CA 91436, **SLP**

Robinette, Connie C 224 Fox Run Drive, Hopkins, SC 29061, (803) 776-3228, Coord Fostr Grandprt Progrm, Council On Aging Midlands, **A**

Robinette, Dr Martin S Mayo Clinic Audiology L-5, Rochester, MN 55905, (507) 284-2577, BS 65 Univ of UT; MS 67 Univ of UT; PH 70 (NS) Wayne St Univ; Dept Chair, U of UT, **A**

Robins, Arlene G 31 Locke Drive, Pittsford, NY 14534, (716) 248-9457, **SLP**

Robins, Mrs Laurie Galey 5992 Brookmont Drive, Yorba Linda, CA 92686, (714) 996-1921, BA 83 CA St Univ - Fullerton; MA 86 CA St Univ - Fullerton; 86–Sp-Lang Path, Placentia USD, **SLP**

Robinson, Alice Jean 1903 Bataan Road #13, Redondo Beach, CA 90278, (213) 374-8699, BA 76 Univ of CA - Berkeley; MS 83 San Francisco St Univ; Sp Lang Path, LA City Un Schl Dst, **SLP**

Robinson, Barbara B 7000 Channel Village Court, Apartment 202, Annapolis, MD 21403, (301) 263-3140, **A**

Robinson, Carol Ann Rural Delivery 4, Box 167, Birdsboro, PA 19508, (215) 779-7111, BA 69 Davis & Elkins Coll; ME 73 Univ of VA - Charlottesville; MA 87 Temple Univ; 73–Tchr Consult-Deaf Educ, Berks County Intermed Unit, **A**

Robinson, Mrs Carol M 420 Thompson Boulevard, Buffalo Grove, IL 60089, BA 77 Tulane Univ; MS 79 Tulane Univ; **SLP A**

Robinson, Mrs Carol Mauney 7625 Fayver Avenue, Norfolk, VA 23505, (804) 441-2891, BS 84 Old Dominion Univ; MS 87 Old Dominion Univ; 85–Sp-Lang Path, Norfolk PS

Robinson, Mrs Carolyn C 3612 Westcliff Road N, Fort Worth, TX 76109-2123, (817) 921-4334, MS 75; BS 74 TX Christian Univ; Sp/Lang Path, Fort Worth ISD, **SLP**

Robinson, Catherine Ono 1338 Zimmerman Road, Carlisle, PA 17013, (717) 697-2366, BS 77 WV Univ; MS 79 WV Univ; 79–Sp-Lang Path, Prof Home Hlth Care Agcy, **SLP**

Robinson, Charlene 977 N W 109th Terrace, Coral Springs, FL 33071, (305) 772-5303, BA 71 Newark St Coll; MA 72 Newark St Coll; 86–VP, InterPay Inc, **SLP**

Robinson, Cheryl B Route 9 Box 96, Evansville, IN 47712, **SLP**

Robinson, Cindy L Route 1 Box 80-E, McCall, ID 83638, (206) 634-2762, BS 72 WA St Univ; MS 77 Eastern WA Univ; SLP, Private Practice, **SLP**

Robinson, Dale H 5918 North 110th Plaza, Omaha, NE 68164, (402) 572-7866, BA 72 Univ of Northern CO; MA 74 Univ of Northern CO; 86–Aud, Millard PS, **A**

Robinson, Dr Dale Omar 1033 Kennesaw Avenue, Birmingham, MI 48009, (313) 577-1393, BA 62 Western MI Univ; MA 65 Univ of Northern CO; PH 70 (NS) Wayne St Univ - Sch of Med; Assoc Prof, Wayne St U, **SLP A ACE**

Robinson, Dana Karol 1518 Hamlin Valley, Houston, TX 77090, (713) 444-7112, BS 85 TX Christian Univ; MS 86 TX Christian Univ; **SLP**

Robinson, Debra L 14100 Montfort Drive #3224, Dallas, TX 75240, BS 77 Univ of North TX; MS 78 Univ of North TX; Sp-Lang Path, Frisco ISD, **SLP**

Robinson, Deirdre 622 Eastwood Court, Altamonte Springs, FL 32714, (305) 423-9293, BS 84 Oakwood Coll; MA 86 Univ of KS

Robinson, Mrs Diana Asner 1212 Westchester Drive, Oklahoma City, OK 73114, (405) 272-5545, BS 82 Univ of OK - Norman; MS 84 Univ of OK - OK City; Sp-Lang Path, Oklahoma City Public Schools, **SLP**

Robinson, Diane C 2104 Michael Lane, Smithfield, NC 27577, BA 74 Univ of NC - Greensboro; ME 78 Univ of NC - Greensboro; **SLP**

Robinson, Dr Donald L Speech Pathology Services Inc, 751 East 63rd Street, Suite 278, Kansas City, MO 64110-3358, (816) 523-5993, MA 64 San Francisco St Univ; MA 66 Univ of IA; PH 69 (Sp-Lang) Univ of OR; 79–Dir, Sp Path Serv Inc, **SLP**

Robinson, Dorothy Polite 18 Berry Hill Road 27-G, Columbia, SC 29210, (803) 731-5108, BA 82 SC St Coll; MS 88 SC St Coll; 87–Dir of SLP Svcs, Associated Healthfocus Inc, **SLP**

Robinson, Elizabeth Prudence 3637 Parker Avenue, West Palm Beach, FL 33405, (305) 582-2539, BA 78 Univ of FL; MA 83 Univ of FL; Dept Head, Palm Beach Co School Bd, **SLP**

Robinson, Evelyn B 14100 46th Street North, Apartment N-20, Tampa, FL 33613, (813) 973-2791, MS 74 Univ of South FL; Sp-Lang Path, Dist Co Sch Bd of Pasco, **SLP**

Robinson, Frank B 6141 Torrington, Kalamazoo, MI 49009, (616) 375-9409, **SLP F LM**

Robinson, Gayle R 1386 Lewiston Drive, Sunnyvale, CA 94087, (415) 573-2323, BA 69 Whittier Coll; MA 72 TX Tech Univ; Sp-Lang Path, San Mateo Co Off of Ed, **SLP**

Robinson, Mrs Helaine Winakor 120 Applegate Lane, East Brunswick, NJ 08816, (201) 656-1000, BA 84 CUNY - Brooklyn Coll; MS 87 CUNY - Brooklyn Coll; **A**

Robinson, Jacqueline 9801 Golf Course Road N W, Albuquerque, NM 87114, (505) 836-4911, BS 71 Eastern NM Univ; BS 71 Eastern NM Univ; MS 73 Eastern NM Univ; SLP, Albuquerque Pub Sch, **SLP**

Robinson, Dr Jane E 3727 Greenleaf Circle #109, Kalamazoo, MI 49008, (616) 673-2167, OB 68 Univ of MI - Ann Arbor; ME 74 Wayne St Univ; PH 84 (Commun Dis & Sciences) Wayne St Univ; 88–Sp-Lang Path, Allegan Cty Intermediate Sch Dist, **SLP**

Robinson, Janet A 42 Leonard Street, Buffalo, NY 14215, (716) 837-4107, BA 78 SUNY - Center at Buffalo; MA 80 SUNY - Center at Buffalo; Sp-Lang Path, Buffalo Board of Education, **SLP**

Robinson, Mrs Janet E RFD 3-84D, Stonington, CT 06378, (203) 444-2111, **SLP**

Robinson, Joan Nancy 7364 Haskell Street, Kansas City, KS 66109, (913) 334-0257, BS 81 KS St Univ; MA 84 KS St Univ; SLP, USD 500, **SLP**

Robinson, Joe Ann 1836 Metzerott Road #1026, Adelphi, MD 20783-3475, (301) 279-9040, BS 70 Southern IL Univ -Carbondale; MS 71 Southern IL Univ -Carbondale; Sp/Lang Path, Mont Cty Publ Sch, **SLP**

Robinson, John E 1503 Ellis Avenue, Hammond, LA 70402, PH; **SLP LM**

Robinson, Mrs Kaloha Lloyd 390 Maple Drive, Rexburg, ID 83440, (208) 356-6300, BS 74 ID St Univ; MS 76 ID St Univ; 88–Sp-Lang Path, Private Practice, **SLP**

Robinson, Karen Lynn 5000 Western Avenue #1300, Knoxville, TN 37921, (615) 971-1349, BA 86 Abilene Christian Univ; MA 87 Univ of TN - Knoxville

Robinson, Kathleen 337 Greenhills Drive, Saline, MI 48176, **SLP**

Robinson, Mrs Kathleen L Illinois State Bd Of Education, 100 North 1st Street, Springfield, IL 62777, (217) 782-6601, BS 57 IL St Univ - Normal; MS 73 IL St Univ - Normal; Special Educ Spec, Il St Bd of Ed, **SLP**

Robinson, Kathryn A 3455 Countryside Boulevard, Apartment 71, Clearwater, FL 33519, (813) 577-6712, BS 77 Bowling Green St Univ; MA 80 Bowling Green St Univ; Sp-Lang Path, Er Sl Rehab Cen, **SLP**

Robinson, Kristi Ellice 11637 100th Northeast #1B, Kirkland, WA 98034, (206) 455-6077, BA 83 WA St Univ; MA 84 WA St Univ; SLP, Bellevue Sch Dist, **SLP**

Robinson, Leslie K 2134 Vestridge Court, Birmingham, AL 35216, (205) 868-2369, BS 78 Univ of Montevallo; MS 80 Univ of Montevallo; 88–Sp-Lang Path, Lakeshore Rehab Facility, **SLP**

Robinson, Mrs Leslie Susan 4971 Kensington Drive, San Diego, CA 92116, (619) 691-5595, BA 76 San Diego St Univ; MA 84 San Diego St Univ; **SLP**

Robinson, Lillian E 1488 C Willow Lake Drive, Atlanta, GA 30329, (404) 455-3916, BS 84 Xavier Univ; MA 88 Southern CT St Univ; 88–Sp-Lang Path, Dekalb County PS, **SLP**

Robinson, Linda Louise 2425 Cromwell Circle #1406, Austin, TX 78741, (512) 476-7111, SLP, St Davids Hospital, **SLP**

Robinson, Mrs Lynn D 1509 S E Blvd, Evansville, IN 47714, (812) 477-6527, BS 72 Eastern KY Univ; ME 80 Univ of VA - Charlottesville; Aud, Deaconess Service Corp, **A**

Robinson, Martha P P O Box 855, Mount Juliet, TN 37122, (615) 754-4160, BS 76 G Peabody Coll-Vanderbilt U; MA 78 Vanderbilt Univ; SLP, Metro Nashville Pub Sch, **SLP**

Robinson, Maureen C 1794 South Gilpin Street, Denver, CO 80210, (303) 425-2425, BA 71 Univ of MN - Duluth; MA 72 Univ of Northern CO; Sp-Lang Path, Darrel L Teter & Assoc Inc, **SLP**

Robinson, Michael E Pacific Hearing Services, 270 East 7th Street #1C, Upland, CA 91786, BA 75 CA St Univ - Fullerton; MS 77 Univ of Redlands; Owner-Aud, Pacific Hrng Serv, **A**

Robinson, Michael T 5225-A Penrith Drive, Durham, NC 27713, (919) 544-3057, BA 74 CUNY - City College; MA 84 Univ of Pittsburgh - Pittsburgh; SLP, **SLP**

Robinson, Mrs Michelle Kimberly 695 Pineloch Drive #1012, Webster, TX 77598, (713) 422-9605, BS 86 Univ of Houston - Univ Park; MA 88 Univ of Houston - Univ Park; 88–Sp-Lang Path, Bay Area Rehab Ctr

Robinson, Mrs Myrna B 14 Peaceable Street, West Redding, CT 06896, **SLP**

Robinson, Mrs Norma Lou 11 Oakwilde Drive, Asheville, NC 28803, (704) 298-7911, BA 53 Miami Univ - Oxford; MS 54 Vanderbilt Univ; 72–Sp-Lang Path, VA Med Ctr, **SLP ACE**

Robinson, Pauline Katherine 631 Woodcrest Avenue, Ardmore, PA 19003, (215) 525-7735, BA 75 Univ of TN - Knoxville; MA 82 Univ of TN - Knoxville; Aud, Mainline Audiology Consultants, **A**

Robinson, Raymond A, II Rural Route 3, Centerville, IA 52544-9803, (515) 856-6102, SLP, Southern Prairie AEA, **SLP**

Robinson, Rhonda M 510 South Lea Avenue, Roswell, NM 88201, (505) 625-8191, MS 87 Fort Hays St Univ; 87–Sp-Lang Path, Roswell ISD

Robinson, Richard Mark 9-C Queen Victoria Way, Chester, MD 21619, (301) 643-7037, BA 83 Loyola Coll; MS 84 Loyola Coll; 86–Sp-Lang Path, RMR Inc, **SLP**

Robinson, Robin Lee 889 McKinley Road, Chelsea, MI 48118, (313) 475-1311, MA 83 OH Univ - Athens; Sp-Lang Path, Chelsea Comm Hosp, **SLP**

Robinson, Mrs Robin Maines Aspen Right Of Way Rt 219, Ellicottville, NY 14731, (716) 699-2991, BS 78 SUNY - Coll at Fredonia; MS 81 SUNY - Coll at Buffalo; Sp-Lang Path, BOCES, **SLP**

Robinson, Rosanne Theresa 12 Charles Lane, Apartment #2D, Pomona, NY 10970, (914) 354-7116, BA 81 Dominican Coll of Blauvelt; MA 83 Montclair St Coll; 85–Sp-Lang Path, Rockland BOCES, **SLP**

Robinson, Sandra Sue 6565 Demoss, Suite 123, Houston, TX 77074, (713) 778-2623, BA 79 Univ of NC - Chapel Hill; MS 81 Univ of NC - Chapel Hill; Director of Aud, ENT Assoc, **A**

Robinson, Sarah Barham 4-D Street Croix Place, Greensboro, NC 27410, (919) 299-8571, BA 79 Univ of NC - Greensboro; ME 85 Univ of NC - Greensboro; **SLP**

Robinson, Sheila Caleria 575 South 72nd Avenue #3, Pensacola, FL 32506, (904) 452-3302, Audiologist, Michael Wood MD, **A**

Robinson, Shelley Elizabeth 2908 Atlantic Avenue, Penfield, NY 14526, (315) 524-2811, BS 80 SUNY - Coll at Geneseo; MS 84 Nazareth Coll of Rochester; **SLP**

Robinson, Sherry A 1517 S W 66th, Portland, OR 97225, (503) 244-6111, BA 60 San Jose St Univ; MA 65 San Jose St Univ; 88–Assoc Dean Stu Dev, Portland Community College, **SLP**

Robinson, Sheryl K 815 N E Eads, Newport, OR 97365, **SLP**

Robinson, Stephanie Elaine 63 Kings Ferry Road, Montrose, NY 10548, (914) 739-0161, BA 84 SUNY - Center at Buffalo; MA 85 SUNY - Center at Buffalo; Audiologist, Sonatone, **A**

Robinson, Susan Marie 5609 Bjelde Lane #A, Madison, WI 53716, (608) 221-4683, BS 82 Univ of WI - Madison; MS 84 Univ of WI - Madison; SLP, Jefferson School District, **SLP**

Robinson, Mrs Susan Mulder 11170 Poplar #C, Loma Linda, CA 92354, (714) 788-7460, BS 86 Loma Linda Univ - Riverside; MS 87 Loma Linda Univ - Loma Linda; 88–Tchr, Riverside USD

Robinson, Mrs Sylvia L 6730 Lost Valley Drive, Austin, TX 78745, (512) 454-0341, BA 71 Whittier Coll; MS 73 Gallaudet Coll; 73–Aud, Austin Otological Assoc, **A**

Robinson, Thomas W Univ Texas Austin, Dept Speech Communication, Austin, TX 78712, (512) 471-3841, BA 73 Univ of FL; MA 74 Univ of FL; 86–Research Asst, Univ of Texas at Austin, **SLP**

Robinson, Tommie L 4406 South Dakota Avenue N E, Washington, DC 20017-2750, (202) 745-5600, BA 84 Univ of MS; MS 86 Univ of MS; 87–Sp-Lang Path, Children's Hosp Natl Med Ctr, **SLP**

Robinson, Valerie 4042 Pawnee Drive, Liverpool, NY 13090, (315) 488-2951, MA 70 Syracuse Univ; Aud, St Camillus Health & Rehab Ctr, **A**

Robinson-Murphy, Jennifer 5490 California Avenue, Long Beach, CA 90805, (213) 422-2197, **SLP**

Robison, Connie June 2200 Montgomery Park Blvd, Partment 1009, Conroe, TX 77304, (409) 539-6480, MA 83 TX Woman's Univ; Sp-Lang Path, Public Schools, **SLP**

Robison, Mrs Jan M 1001 Grand Tree Court, Fenton, MO 63026, (314) 768-5336, BA 72 Fontbonne Coll; MA 74 Saint Louis Univ; Dir-Speech Pathology Dept, SSM Rehabilitation Institute, **SLP ACE**

Robison, Mrs Lynn Bruckner 70-B Turtleback Road, Califon, NJ 07830, (201) 876-9211, BS 65 Purdue Univ - West Lafayette; MS 68 Emerson Coll; Sp-Lang Path, Washington Twsp Bd of Ed, **SLP**

Robison, Myrna Kay 7316 East Parkway, Sacramento, CA 95823, (916) 454-8183, BA 54 Univ of OR; MA 78 CA St Univ - Sacramento; MA 83 Univ of San Francisco; Sp-Lang Path, Sacramento USD, **SLP**

Robl, Gwen S 326 Orchard Drive, Madison, WI 53705, (608) 849-8191, BS 71 Univ of WI - Eau Claire; MS 79 Univ of WI - Madison; Sp-Lang Path, Waunakee Pub Sch, **SLP**

Robl, Mrs Janet T 10310 Alamo Court, Wichita, KS 67212, (316) 722-2125, BA 73 Univ of KS; MA 74 Univ of KS; **A**

Roblee, Mrs Lorraine A 470 Village Place, Apt 118-D, Longwood, FL 32779, (407) 862-4780, OB 35; MA 37; Consultant, I for Aud Verbal Commun & Res, **SLP A LM**

Robman, Jolie D Century City Medical Plaza, 2080 Century Park East, Suite 108, Los Angeles, CA 90067, (213) 201-0717, BA 75 Univ of CA - Los Angeles; MA 78 CA St Univ - Los Angeles; Dir of Aud, Otosurgical Group Med Cl, **A**

Robottom, Mrs Natalie Claire 364 St Andrewws, La Place, LA 70068, (504) 536-1106, BA 81 Univ of Southwestern LA; MA 85 LA St Univ - Baton Rouge; SLP, St Johns School Bd, **SLP**

Robson, Mrs Nancy L 1505 Double Oaks, Greensboro, NC 27410, (513) 777-0841, BS 74 Univ of WI - Madison; MA 75 Northwestern Univ; **SLP**

Robson-Brandi, Carol Ann 124 Patterson Avenue, Carnegie, PA 15106, (412) 521-9000, BS 82 Carlow Coll; MA 84 Univ of Pittsburgh - Pittsburgh; 85–SLP, Rehabil Institute Pittsburgh, **SLP**

Robuck, Mrs Sally J 1011 Carol, Jefferson City, MO 65101, (314) 636-4213, BS 63 Univ of MO - Columbia; **SLP**

Rocchio, Catherine 2823 Forest Glen Drive, Baldwin, MD 21013, (301) 679-5395, BS 73 Towson St Univ; MS 79 Towson St Univ; Sp-Lang Path, Private Practice, **SLP**

Rocco, Mrs Cynthia R 28 Wood Avenue, Patchogue, NY 11772, (516) 654-2058, BS 77 SUNY - Coll at Geneseo; MS 78 Ithaca Coll; Sp-Lang Path, Private Practice, **SLP**

Rocco, Mrs Marcia M 80 Cobbles Drive, Penfield, NY 14526, (716) 381-0590, BA 75 Towson St Univ; MA 76 Case Western Reserve Univ; SLP, **SLP**

Rocco, Pamela Jean 5371 Southside Road, Hollister, CA 95023, (408) 758-9825, BA 82 San Jose St Univ; MA 85 San Jose St Univ; 86–SLP, Salinas City Sch Dist, **SLP**

Rocconi, Carol Ann 4444 Tena, Memphis, TN 38128, (901) 794-6152, BS 68 LA St Univ - Baton Rouge; MA 70 LA St Univ - Baton Rouge; Sp-Lang Path, Memphis Cty Schls, **SLP**

Roche, Mrs Ada Iris Calle Benavente, 524 Purple Tree Cupey Bajo, Rio Piedras, PR 00926, (809) 763-5750, BA 73 Univ of PR - Rio Piedras; MS 82 Univ of PR - Rio Piedras; **SLP**

Roche, Lorraine M 34 Tiverton Avenue, Toronto, ON, Canada M4M 2L9, (416) 393-0644, BA 72; MA 76 NY Univ; ME 80; Program Coordinator, Toronto Bd of Ed, **SLP**

Roche, Mrs Luella 784 Willive Drive, Decatur, GA 30033, (404) 727-5520, BS 68 FL St Univ; MS 69 Univ of TN - Knoxville; Asst Dir, Commun Dis Emory U Hosp, **SLP**

Roche, Maryjo 10524 South Kedzie Avenue, Chicago, IL 60655, (312) 445-9325, **SLP**

Roche, Rosanne V Flower Memorial Healthplex, 5200 Harroun Road, Sylvania, OH 43560, (419) 885-1444, BS 72 Clarion Univ of PA; MA 76 Kent St Univ; 86–Sp-Lang Path, Flower Mem Lake Prk Hosp, **SLP ACE**

Roche, William J R R 2 P O Box 483, Highland Lakes, NJ 07422, (201) 977-2435, BS 73 SUNY - Coll at Oneonta; MS 75 Columbia Univ Teachers Coll; SLP, St Joseph's Hosp & Med Cen, **SLP ACE**

Rochet, Dr Anne Putnam Dept Speech Path & Audiology, University Of Alberta, 400-11044 82nd Avenue, Edmonton, AB, Canada T6G 0T2, (403) 432-5990, BA 68 Hollins Coll; MS 71 Purdue Univ - West Lafayette; PH 73 (Sp Physiology) Purdue Univ - West Lafayette; Assoc Prof, U of Alberta, **SLP**

Rochlen, Mrs Libby Beth 39-12 211th Street, Bayside, NY 11361, (718) 423-8611, BS 82 Boston Univ; MS 84 Emory Univ; Sp-Lang Path, VA Med Cen, **SLP**

Rochlin, Gail D Az School For The Deaf & Blind, Box 5545, Tucson, AZ 85703, (602) 628-5427, BS 74 Univ of AZ; MS 75 Univ of AZ; ME 81 Univ of AZ; Aud/Spvsr, AZ Sch Deaf/Blind, **A**

Rochon, Carol Joyce 3119 Royal Gable Drive, Dallas, TX 75229, (214) 358-8339, BS 78 Central MO St Univ; MS 80 Fontbonne Coll; 88–Sp-Lang Path, Dallas Rehab Inst, **SLP**

Rock, Deborah M 3255 Gateway Street #224, Springfield, OR 97477, **SLP**

Rock, Mrs Jo Ann L 11 Welwyn Road #1G, Great Neck, NY 11021, (212) 470-8910, BA 69 SUNY - Center at Albany; MA 72 SUNY - Center at Buffalo; Sp-Lang Path, L Island Jewish Medical Center, **SLP**

Rock, Katherine Ann 17 Todd Court, Huntington Station, NY 11746, (516) 922-4100, BA 82 SUNY - Coll at Cortland; MA 86 Long Island U - CW Post Ctr; 83–Sp-Lang Path, Mill Neck Manor Sch for the Deaf, **SLP**

Rock, Marian V Hastings Way #203A, Mount Laurel, NJ 08054, (609) 261-7030, BA 80 Duquesne Univ; MS 82 WV Univ; 84–Sp-Lang Path, Memorial Hospital of Burl Co, **SLP**

Rockafellow, Susan S Rehab Works Inc, 5567 West 73rd Street, Indianapolis, IN 46268-2162, (317) 297-2273, BA 70 Univ of MI - Ann Arbor; MS 72 Univ of OK Medical Center; Admin, Rehab Works Inc, **SLP**

Rockett, Mrs Leda Watson 903 Tarreyton Drive, Ruston, LA 71270, (318) 251-3433, BA 83 LA Tech Univ; MA 85 LA Tech Univ; Sp-Lang Path, Sp Path Assoc, **SLP**

Rockfield, Naomi M 635 Nutley Place, North Woodmere, NY 11581, (516) 791-8182, BA 75 CUNY - Brooklyn Coll; MA 76 Hofstra Univ; Sp-Lang Path, Hewlett-Woodmere School Dist, **SLP**

Rockhold, Mrs Thayne Hamilton 1024 Leycester, Baton Rouge, LA 70808, (504) 769-1090, BS 67 LA St Univ - Baton Rouge; MA 74 LA St Univ - Baton Rouge; 88–Aud, ENT Med Ctr, **A**

Rockman, Dr Barbara Karp 363 Jersey, San Francisco, CA 94114, (415) 550-8255, BS 64 WV Univ; MA 66 Case Western Reserve Univ; PH 83 (Sp and Hrng Sciences) IN Univ - Bloomington; 84–Clin Coord, CA State U Hayward, **SLP**

Rockoff, Carrie Ellen 2662 Fresno Street, Santa Cruz, CA 95062, (408) 443-7216, BA 81 CA St Univ - Northridge; MA 83 CA St Univ - Northridge; 83–Sp-Lang Path, Santa Rita Union Sch Dist, **SLP**

Rockwell, Mrs Amy White 3565 Shore Lane, Matthews, NC 28105-7434, (912) 346-3830, BS 82 Valdosta St Coll; ME 84 Univ of GA; Sp-Lang Path, Rock Hill Schools, **SLP**

Rockwell, Mrs Jackie M 519 North Main Street, P O Box 379, Seven Mile, OH 45062, (513) 829-6300, BS 73 Miami Univ - Oxford; MS 75 Miami Univ - Oxford; Sp-Lang Path, Butler Co Easter Seal Soc, **SLP**

Rockwell, Sharon Sue 22 Maple Avenue, Gloversville, NY 12078, (518) 725-6894, MA 86 KS St Univ; **SLP**

Rockwood, Mrs Judith D 7599 Vogels Way, Springfield, VA 22153, **SLP**

Roda, Vicki A C 41 Flamingo Drive, Halifax, NS, Canada B3M 1S8, **SLP**

Rodal, Mrs Jacquelyn Egger 849 S W 18th Street, Richmond, IN 47374, (317) 966-1521, BS 78 Miami Univ - Oxford; MA 82 Ball St Univ; Sp-Lang Path, Richmond Comm Schs, **SLP**

Rodd-Marks, Jane J 211 Frontier, Mulvane, KS 67110, **SLP**

Rodel, Michael J The Audiology Group, 1032 Luke Street, Fort Collins, CO 80524, (303) 482-5700, BS 73 IN Univ - Bloomington; MA 74 IN Univ - Bloomington; 84–Aud, The Audiology Group, **A**

Rodemack, Mrs Kayleen Hawker 460 Old Town Road #9-K, Port Jefferson Station, NY 11776, (516) 474-3813, BS 84 ID St Univ; MS 86 ID St Univ; 88–Sp-Lang Path, St Charles Hosp & Rehab Ctr, **SLP**

Rodenbuecher, Nancy Marie 1644 Via Estrella, Pomona, CA 91768-4104, (714) 629-2498, BS 73 SUNY - Coll at Buffalo; MA 81 CA St Univ - Los Angeles; SLP, Corona-Norco USD, **SLP**

Roderick, Mrs Barbara A 26 Grant Drive, St Peters, MO 63376, (314) 569-8100, BS 82 Southern IL Univ-Edwardsvill; MS 83 Southern IL Univ-Edwardsvill; Sp-Lang Path, Francis Howell Sch Dist, **SLP**

Roderick, Janice Mattei 536 Arundel Boulevard, Crownsville, MD 21032, (301) 923-2932, BA 71 Saint Mary's Coll; ME 82 Bloomsburg Univ of PA; **SLP**

Rodgers, Mrs Brigitte E 2734 Corte Bandera, Pleasanton, CA 94566, (408) 262-2100, BS 80 CA St Univ - Hayward; MA 81 Univ of the Pacific; SLP, Agnew Residential Facility, **SLP**

Rodgers, Dwight Carew 1628 Roys Avenue, Elkhart, IN 46516, (219) 294-4930, BA 72 Milligan Coll; MS 80 East TN St Univ; Sp-Lang Path, Elkhart Community Schools, **SLP**

Rodgers, Julie Ann 2602 Fairview Drive, Monroeville, PA 15146, (412) 856-2695, BA 81 Allegheny Coll; MS 83 PA St Univ - Univ Park; 88–Sp-Lang Path, Greater Pittsburgh Rehab Hosp, **SLP**

Rodgers, Mrs Mary Sue 2710 North Hackett Avenue, Milwaukee, WI 53211, (414) 964-7147, BA 72 Western WA Univ; MA 74 LA St Univ - Baton Rouge; Sp-Lang Path, Milwaukee Pub Schs, **SLP**

Rodgers, Patricia L Rt 9 Box 72E, Poplar Bluff, MO 63901, (314) 785-0101, BS 68 Sch of the Ozarcks; MA 86 Southeast MO St Univ; 87–Sp-Lang Path, Poplar Bluff Reg Ctr, **SLP**

Rodgers, Mrs Theresa H 41106 Galvez Avenue, Prairieville, LA 70769, (504) 644-2181, BS 76 LA St Univ - Baton Rouge; MA 79 LA St Univ - Baton Rouge; SLP/Aud, Ascension Parish Sch Bd, **SLP**

Rodie, Mrs Sharon Marie 15753 East Gunnison Place, Aurora, CO 80017, (303) 751-7470, BS 77 Univ of Southern CO; MS 81 CO St Univ; Sp-Lang Path, Aurora Public Schools, **SLP**

Rodin, Dr Alan 1225 Ocean Parkway #3-F, Brooklyn, NY 11230, (718) 252-7309, BA 73 CUNY - Brooklyn Coll; MA 75 Northwestern Univ; OD 79 (NS) 9321; Self Employed, **SLP**

Roditi, Mrs Denise Sher 18 August Drive, Framingham, MA 01701, (508) 329-1800, BA 77 SUNY - Coll at Cortland; MS 78 PA St Univ - Univ Park; Sp-Lang Path, Dedham Pub Sch, **SLP**

Rodman, Mrs Martha Fitzsimmon 2205 New Garden Road #4309, Greensboro, NC 27410, (919) 288-6835, BA 78 Univ of NC - Greensboro; MA 79 Univ of NC - Greensboro; SLP, Greensboro PS Sys

Rodman, Melissa 2978 Sunridge Drive, Santa Rosa, CA 95405, (707) 523-4009, BA 85 Univ of CA - Los Angeles; MS 88 San Francisco St Univ; 88–Sp-Lang Path, Harris & Associates

Rodney, Mrs Patricia Barone Rural Delivery 2, Sunset Road, Moscow, PA 18444, (717) 969-8188, BA 64 Carlow Coll; MA 65 Univ of WI - Madison; Sp-Lang Path, Frank Di Simoni PhD, **SLP**

Rodrigues, Mrs Barbara 206 East Steuben Street, Bath, NY 14810, (607) 776-2111, BS 69 SUNY - Coll at Geneseo; MS 70 SUNY - Coll at Geneseo; Sp-Lang Path, Bath VA Med Cen, **SLP**

Rodriguez, Barbara Salazar 909 Ortiz S E, Albuquerque, NM 87108, (505) 266-5783, BA 85 Univ of NM; MS 86 Univ of NM; **SLP**

Rodriguez, Carol Shade 6930 Candlish Drive, Reynoldsburg, OH 43068, (614) 422-9920, BA 80 OH St Univ; MA 82 OH St Univ; Sp-Lang Path, Columbus Sp & Hrng Cen, **SLP**

Rodriguez, Mrs Carroll Jane 97 West 41st Avenue, San Mateo, CA 94403, (415) 349-7357, BS 80 Univ of OR; MA 86 San Jose St Univ; 86–Sp-Lang Path, Laguna Salada Sch Dist

Rodriguez, Mrs Debra Jean 402 Stagecoach Circle, Salado, TX 76571-9528, (809) 780-1257, **SLP**

Rodriguez, Gary P 3502 Kilkenny Drive East, Tallahassee, FL 32308-3111, (904) 644-2238, BS 78 FL St Univ; MS 79 FL St Univ; PH 86 (NS) Univ of FL; Asst Prof, Florida State Univ, **A**

Rodriguez, Mrs Joan E 2711 Woodside Drive, Duluth, GA 30316, (404) 263-8147, BA 78 Univ of MD - College Park; MS 79 PA St Univ - Univ Park; 87–Aud, DeKalb Co Health Dept, **A**

Rodriguez, Dr Joyce M 276 Funston Avenue, San Francisco, CA 94118, BA 72 Univ of PR - Rio Piedras; MS 75 Columbia Univ Teachers Coll; PH 81 (NS) Columbia Univ Teachers Coll; Aud, Private Practice, **A**

Rodriguez, Judith T 3931 Park Avenue, Coconut Grove, FL 33133, (305) 661-4410, BS 66 Univ of NE - Lincoln; MA 67 Univ of NE - Lincoln; **SLP**

Rodriguez, Lisa Zimmerman 169 West Street, Brockton, MA 02401-4132, (617) 745-2100, **SLP**

Rodriguez, Marcia Weaver 3029-A Kelsey Creek Road, Spartanburg, SC 29302, (803) 585-7711, BA 81 SUNY - Coll at Plattsburgh; MS 84 Univ of SC - Columbia; Sp-Lang Path, Sc School for Deaf & Blind, **SLP**

Rodriguez, Mrs Maria I G 7934 Golondrina Drive, Houston, TX 77083, (713) 277-3998, BA 80 Univ of PR - Rio Piedras; MS 82 Univ of PR - Rio Piedras; 87–Sp-Lang Path, InSpeech Inc, **SLP**

Rodriguez, Mary Ruth 241 East French, San Antonio, TX 78212, (512) 736-4361, BA 76 Our Lady Lake Univ-San Anton; MA 77 Our Lady Lake Univ-San Anton; SLP, Edward C Gooze & Assoc, **SLP**

Rodriguez, Pamela Hoffman 109 Beechwood Circle, Daphne, AL 36526, (205) 626-9751, BS 81 Univ of South AL; MS 85 Univ of South AL; Sp-Lang Path, Baldwin Co Bd of Ed, **SLP**

Rodriguez, Mrs Sandra Lynn 100 Village Green Blvd, Apartment 1012, Gallatin, TN 37066, (615) 452-3721, BS 85 CO St Univ; MS 88 Univ of AZ; 88–Sp-Lang Path, Rebound Inc

Rodriguez, Terry J 7642 Parfet Court, Arvada, CO 80005, (303) 837-1000, BA 67 Univ of Northern CO; MA 80 Univ of Northern CO; SLP, Denver Pub Sch, **SLP**

Rodriguez-Bravo, Leticia P O Box 163, Missouri City, TX 77459, (713) 623-2500, BS 76 Catholic Univ Puerto Rico; ME 79 Univ of FL; SLP Superv, Twelve Oaks Hosp, **SLP**

Rodriquez, Mrs Hilda Velez E-14 5th Street, Villas San Agustin, Bayamon, PR 00619, (809) 754-4064, BA 73 Univ of PR - Rio Piedras; MS 85 Univ of PR - San Juan; 86–Aud, Head-Start Program, **A**

Rodriquez, Linda Iris 64-77 84th Street, Middle Village, NY 11379, (718) 636-4573, **SLP**

Rodriquez, Rebecca Angeli 1110 Dardel Drive, Wilmington, DE 19803, (302) 478-3635, MS 87 PA St Univ - Univ Park

Rodriquez, Rubina Rueda 11360 Bob Mitchell, El Paso, TX 79936, (915) 591-4198, BA 74 Univ of TX - El Paso; MS 77 Univ of TX - El Paso; Sp-Lang Path, Ysteta ISD, **SLP**

Rodriquez, Sara R 6902 Geneva Drive, Austin, TX 78723, (803) 771-4588, BS 73 Eastern WA Univ; OM 78 Univ of SC - Columbia; **SLP**

Rodwell, Mary C 815 First Street S W, Apt 3, Rochester, MN 55902, (507) 284-2577, BS 85 Univ of WI - Oshkosh; MA 87 Univ of TN - Knoxville; 88–Aud, Mayo Clinic

Roe, Barbara W 4608 Forestview, Midland, MI 48640, **SLP**

Roe, Mrs Joan L 160 Penfield, Dundee, MI 48131, (313) 269-3605, BS 68 Eastern MI Univ; MA 72 Eastern MI Univ; Sp-Lang Path, Ida Public Schools, **SLP**

Roe, Rochelle Williams 26766 Trasmiras, Mission Viejo, CA 92692, BS 72 Middle TN St Univ; MA 73 Univ of TN - Knoxville; Audiologist, Private Practice, **A**

Roe, Susan G 108 South Spruce, Hope, AR 71801, (501) 777-8064, BS 85 Henderson St Univ; MS 86 Univ of Central AR; 86–Sp-Lang Path, Hope PS, **SLP**

Roebuck, Marsha Roberta 3915 Liberty Heights Avenue, Apartment B-9, Baltimore, MD 21207, (301) 396-0612, BS 72 CA Univ of PA; MS 76 Howard Univ; **SLP**

Roedema, Mrs Laurie Frances 690 13th Avenue, Union Grove, WI 53182, (414) 878-3717, BS 68 Miami Univ - Oxford; MS 81 Univ of WI - Whitewater; Sp-Lang Path, Racine Co Hndcpd Chldn Bd, **SLP**

Roeder, Kathleen Ventre 28043 New Bedford Drive, Farmington Hills, MI 48018, (313) 288-8085, BA 73 Wayne St Univ; MA 74 Wayne St Univ; Coord Inpatient Svc, Wm Beaumont Hospital, **SLP**

Roeder, Mrs Melissa Jane 44 Central Boulevard, Merrick, NY 11566, (516) 378-3900, BS 81 Ithaca Coll; MA 82 Hofstra Univ; 83–Tchr, Merrick Union Free Sch Dist, **SLP**

Roeder, Mrs Sharon L 102 Hawks Nest Circle, Middletown, CT 06457-1514, (203) 347-5317, BA 77 Univ of CT; MA 79 Univ of CT; Sp-Lang Path, Wheeler Cl, **SLP**

Roedner, Doris C 78 High Street, Saco, ME 04072, (207) 284-6420, BS 84 Univ of NH; MS 86 ID St Univ; Sp-Lang Path

Roegiers, Jane Michelle 207 Woodside Drive, Iowa City, IA 52240, (319) 337-9514, BS 84 Univ of IA; MS 86 Univ of WI - Stevens Point; **SLP**

Roehrig, Sharon A Route 1 Box 22BA, Owingsville, KY 40360, (606) 674-2321, BA 73 Bellarmine Coll; OM 81 IN Univ - Bloomington; 85–Sp-Lang Path, St Claire Medical Center, **SLP ACE**

Roelfs, Mrs Donna S 1290 Peterson Drive, Omaha, NE 68130, (402) 289-3433, BS 73 KS St Univ; MA 74 KS St Univ; Sp/Lang Path, Elkhorn Public Schools, **SLP**

Roemer, Mrs Janet DeGrazia 655 Westgate Road, Deerfield, IL 60015, (312) 945-7164, BA 61 Mundelein Coll; MA 62 Northwestern Univ; Sp-Lang Path, Private Practice, **SLP**

Roesch, Mrs Margaret Anne 2244 Iris Way, Fort Myers, FL 33905, (813) 693-2185, BS 80 CA Univ of PA; MS 85 CA Univ of PA; **SLP**

Roesch, Pauline Jean 244 South Camden Drive, Beverly Hills, CA 90212, (213) 394-3244, SLP, Northridge Hosp, **SLP**

Roese, Mrs Constance 1823 Dunwoody Road, Parkville, MD 21234, (301) 477-2960, BS 70 SUNY - Coll at Buffalo; MS 72 SUNY - Coll at Buffalo; Sp-Lang Path, Baltimore Co Pub Sch, **SLP**

Roeser, Dr Ross J Callier Center, 1966 Inwood Road, Dallas, TX 75235, (214) 783-3036, BS 66 Western IL Univ; MA 67 Northern IL Univ - De Kalb; PH 72 (NS) FL St Univ; Actg Dir/Prof, Callier Cen/Utd, **A F**

Roeske, Christine Ann 559-A Somers Point Road, Mays Landing, NJ 08330-9801, BS 81 Univ of WI - River Falls; MS 82 Univ of WI - River Falls; 87–Sp-Lang Path, UCP, **SLP ACE**

Roesle, Sue A 5301 Faraon Street #160, St Joseph, MO 64506, (816) 364-3277, BS 77 Central MO St Univ; MS 78 Central MO St Univ; Aud, Dr Sidney Christiansen, **A**

Roesler, Mrs Cynthia P 905 Franklin Avenue, Franklin Lakes, NJ 07417, (201) 441-2165, BA 79 Loyola Coll; MS 80 Loyola Coll; Sp-Lang Path, Hackensack Med Cen-l Chld Dev, **SLP ACE**

Roesler, Mary L 2712 Taiesin Drive, Kalamazoo, MI 49008, (616) 381-0180, BA 71 Nazareth Coll; MA 74 Western MI Univ; Aud, Locklin-Roesler-Milko, **A**

Roesser, Mrs Sheryl L 3608 Maple Forge Lane, Gainesville, GA 30501, (404) 536-2858, BS 72 WV Univ; MS 79 WV Univ; 86–Sp-Lang Path, Hall County Sch Sys, **SLP**

Roessler, Lisa Beth 37 Mt View Street, West Orange, NJ 07052, (201) 285-4529, BS 82 Ithaca Coll; MA 85 Kean Coll of NJ; 85–Sp-Lang Path, Morristown Memorial Hosp, **SLP ACE**

Roethe, Lynn A 4301 Mohawk Drive, Madison, WI 53711, (608) 263-5766, BS 78 Univ of WI - Madison; MS 80 Univ of WI - Madison; Sp-Lang Path, Univ of Wisconsin-Madison, **SLP**

Roettger, Ruby W 320 Watt Road, Knoxville, TN 37922, (615) 966-6297, BS 68 East TN St Univ; MA 71 Univ of TN - Knoxville; **A**

Roffman, Mrs Carol A 2100 N W 105 Lane, Coral Springs, FL 33065, (305) 753-0455, BS 74 Ithaca Coll; MA 75 MI St Univ; **A**

Rogal, Mrs Carol J 2507 Indian Ridge Drive, Glenview, IL 60025, BA 73 Univ of IL - Urbana; MS 74 Univ of IL - Urbana; **SLP**

Rogalla, Leonard T 2291 North Roberts Road, Muskegon, MI 49445, (616) 744-9747, BS 80; MA 82; 88–Sp-Lang Path, Muskegon Reg Ctr, **SLP**

Rogalla, Susan A P O Box 1843, Ruidoso, NM 88345, (505) 257-4744, BA 80 NM St Univ; MA 82 NM St Univ; 88–Sp-Lang Path, Tularosa Municipal Schs, **SLP**

Rogalski, Dr Lois A P O Box 1242, Scarsdale, NY 10583, (914) 723-6721, BA 68 CUNY - Brooklyn Coll; MA 69 Univ of MA - Amherst; PH 75 (Psycholinguistics) NY Univ; Sp-Lang Path, Private Practice, **SLP**

Rogan, Ellen Walsh 152 Collins Avenue, Williston Park, NY 11596, (516) 435-2215, BA 79 Long Island U - CW Post Ctr; MS 82 Adelphi Univ; 79–Tchr, Brentwood PS, **SLP**

Rogan, Jane Elizabeth 1601 Barton Road #1501, Redlands, CA 92373, (714) 799-3343, MS 83 Univ of WA; Aud, Loma Linda Med Grp, **A**

Rogan, Susan Denise 41 Crabtree Drive, Westmont, IL 60559, (312) 325-6133, BA 78 Marquette Univ; MS 81 Purdue Univ - West Lafayette; Aud, Sound Resources Inc, **A**

Rogatz, Linda B 2655 South Bayshore Drive, Apartment 310, Miami, FL 33133, (305) 635-7505, BA 71 Univ of Miami; ME 74 Univ of Miami; SLP, Dade Co Pub Sch, **SLP**

Rogero, Mrs Elaine A 506 South 28th Street, Escanaba, MI 49829, (906) 789-1489, BS 71 Saint Louis Univ; MA 72 Saint Louis Univ; Sp-Lang Path, Private Practice, **SLP**

Rogers, Alpha S 37 Elm Street, Park Forest, IL 60466, **SLP**

Rogers, Amy H 24865 Wood Ridge Dr #310, Farmington Hills, MI 48018, SLP, Total Therapy Management, **SLP**

Rogers, Mrs Anastasia Maria 14 Virginia Circle, Randolph, MA 02368, (617) 848-5353, ME 82 Northeastern Univ; Sp-Lang Path, Braintree Hospital, **SLP**

Rogers, Mrs Ann E 624 Willow Grove Avenue, Glenside, PA 19038, (215) 885-0532, BS 70 Western MI Univ; MS 76 Trenton St Coll; Sp-Lang Path, Private Practice, **SLP**

Rogers, Annette Piscopo 115 Albert Avenue, Cranston, RI 02905, (401) 277-5485, BA 75 SUNY - Center at Buffalo; MS 76 FL St Univ; SLP, Hode Island Hospital, **SLP**

Rogers, Beth Ann 8110 E Speedway Boulevard, Apartment 6364, Tucson, AZ 85710, (602) 722-5259, BS 83 Northern AZ Univ; MS 85 Northern AZ Univ; **SLP**

Rogers, Carla Jean 9883 Heath Avenue, Cottage Grove, MN 55016, (612) 423-8202, **SLP**

Rogers, Caroline I 1298 Priory Road, Eau Claire, WI 54701, (715) 597-3196, BA 60 Denison Univ; BS 80 Univ of WI - Eau Claire; MS 81 Univ of WI - Eau Claire; SLP, Osseo-Fairchild Schs, **SLP**

Rogers, Carolyn L 459 Belanger, Grosse Pointe, MI 48236, (313) 881-2319, SLP, Beaumont Hosp, **SLP**

Rogers, Cathy Sue 12351 North Lakeview, Baton Rouge, LA 70810, (504) 383-5055, BS 85 Bloomsburg Univ of PA; MS 86 Bloomsburg Univ of PA; SLP, Renaissance Rehab, **SLP**

Rogers, Cheryl Ann 44 Manchester Place, Buffalo, NY 14213, (716) 633-4440, BS 70 SUNY - Coll at Buffalo; MA 71 SUNY - Center at Buffalo; Sp/Lang Path, U C P Assn of W New York, **SLP**

Rogers, Cheryl Ann 11 Pearl Street, Clifton Springs, NY 14432, (716) 394-9510, BS 82 SUNY - Coll at Fredonia; MS 83 Nazareth Coll of Rochester; 85–Sp-Lang Path, Finger-Lakes United Cere Palsy, **SLP**

Rogers, Mrs Cheryl W 1946 Mitchell Avenue, Clovis, CA 93612, (209) 439-0282, BA 74 CA St Univ - Fresno; MA 75 CA St Univ - Fresno; Sp-Lang Path, Clovis USD, **SLP**

Rogers, Crystal F Route 1 Box 355-A, Waco, TX 76710, (817) 848-4906, BS 75 Baylor Univ; MS 77 Baylor Univ; **SLP**

Rogers, Donna B G 1973 Sheridan Avenue South, Minneapolis, MN 55405, **SLP**

Rogers, Evelyn M RD1 Box 159 #2, Oneonta, NY 13820, BS 74 SUNY - Coll at Fredonia; MS 76 SUNY - Center at Albany; Sp-Lang Path, Northern Catskills BOCES, **SLP**

Rogers, Gail Karen 3532 Pierce Street, San Francisco, CA 94123, (415) 579-2071, BA 83 Univ of the Pacific; MS 85 CA St Univ - Hayward; **SLP**

Rogers, Janet Alma 722 Dargan St Health South, 600 Stoneybrook Lane, Florence, SC 29501, (803) 669-3816, SLP, Bamberg School Dist #1, **SLP**

Rogers, Janice R 2703 Woodmont Trail, Fort Worth, TX 76133, (817) 534-4831, BA 75 Elmira Coll; MS 76 Univ of North TX; Sp-Lang Path, Ft Worth State Sch, **SLP**

Rogers, Jean A 417 Beach 120th Street, Rockaway Park, NY 11694, **A**

Rogers, Jodi A 3332 Arawak Place, Dallas, TX 75234, (214) 956-9164, BA 70 Univ of Denver; MS 83 Univ of TX - Dallas; Aud, Dallas Neuroscience, **A**

Rogers, Julianna C Ohio State University Hospital, 472 West 8th Avenue, Columbus, OH 43210, (614) 421-3818, MA 74 OH St Univ; Sp-Lnag Path, Ohio State U Hosp, **SLP ACE**

Rogers, Julie F 534 West 2nd Street, Lansdale, PA 19446, (215) 333-1711, BS 70 Bloomsburg Univ of PA; MS 76 Ithaca Coll; Sp-Lang Path, Philadelphia Sch Dist, **SLP**

Rogers, Kerrilyn Kaye 116 Gulpha, West Monroe, LA 71291, (318) 728-5964, BA 83 Northeast LA Univ; MA 86 Northeast LA Univ; **SLP**

Rogers, Mrs Linda Phifer 353 Coventry Road, Decatur, GA 30030, (303) 861-5881, **SLP**

Rogers, Linda S 4880 County Road #11, Rushville, NY 14544, (315) 536-4431, BS 73 SUNY - Coll at Geneseo; MA 77 SUNY - Coll at Geneseo; Sp-Lang Path, Soldiers & Sailors Mem Hosp, **SLP ACE**

Rogers, Mrs Lisa B P O Box 402, Cross Hill, SC 29332, (803) 223-4862, BA 76 Univ of Akron; MA 78 Univ of Akron; 85–Coord-Aud Svcs, St Nicholas Sp/Hrng, **A**

Rogers, Mrs Lucille Volk 136 Roadrunner Drive, Ponca City, OK 74604, (405) 762-9752, BS 75 Towson St Univ; MS 79 Towson St Univ; Sp-Lang Path, Private Practice, **SLP**

Rogers, Mrs Margaret A 211 Highland Drive, Iowa City, IA 52240-3049, (319) 338-6399, BA 79 Grinnell Coll; MS 84 Univ of IA; **SLP**

Rogers, Mrs Margaret Denise 501 E Orangethorpe, #53 Orange, Anaheim, CA 92801, (714) 992-0997, MA 88 CA St Univ - Fullerton; 88, La Habra Rehab Assoc

Rogers, Mariann 7324 Skilman #1308, Dallas, TX 75231, (214) 343-4733, **SLP**

Rogers, Mrs Marilyn B 8309 Bowling Green Drive, Austin, TX 78758, (512) 451-9335, BS 75 Univ of IL - Urbana; MA 87 Univ of TX - Austin; 87–Sp-Lang Path, Austin ISD

Rogers, Martha E 3333 North 100th Street, Milwaukee, WI 53222, (414) 259-1414, MS 79 Univ of WI - Whitewater; BS 69 Marquette Univ; Sp-Lang Path, Curative Rehab Cen, **SLP**

Rogers, Mrs Mary Ann 2811 Lombardy Court, Augusta, GA 30909, (404) 738-8421, BA 64 Northeastern OK St Univ; ME 82 Columbus Coll; Sp/Lang Path, Columbia County Schs, **SLP**

Rogers, Mercedes #9 El Camino Real, Wimberley, TX 78676, (512) 847-2449, BA 83 Fort Hays St Univ; MS 84 Fort Hays St Univ; Sp-Lang Path, San Marcos Treatment Ctr, **SLP**

Rogers, Mrs Patricia A 6911 Richmond Highway, Alexandria, VA 22306, (703) 765-3857, BA 71 Univ of Northern CO; MA 73 Saint Louis Univ; Director, Chesapeake Speech Center, **SLP**

Rogers, Mrs Rebecca A 4393 Levelside Avenue, Lakewood, CA 90712, (714) 595-1261, BS 78 AZ St Univ; MA 81 CA St Univ - Long Beach; Sp-Lang Path, Walnut Valley USD, **SLP**

Rogers, Robert Kimsey 13110 Creek View Drive, #101, Garden Grove, CA 92644, (714) 636-7471, Navy-Long Beach, **A**

Rogers, Robert R 115 Albert Avenue, Cranston, RI 02905, (401) 331-4444, BA 74 Bridgewater St Coll; MS 76 FL St Univ; **A**

Rogers, Ronald M 1520 King George Court, Ann Arbor, MI 48104-6927, **A**

Rogers, Sheila Kathleen 105 Heather Lane, Goldsboro, NC 27530, (919) 751-1462, BA 79 IN St Univ - Terre Haute; ME 81 Univ of VA - Charlottesville; Sp-Lang Path, Cerebral Palsy of Phila, **SLP**

Rogers, Shelley D Highland Lakes Hrng & Sp Ctr, 1718 Highway 1431 West, Marble Falls, TX 78654, (512) 693-7020, BS 73 TX Tech Univ; MS 76 TX Tech Univ; Dir/Aud, Private Practice, **A**

Rogers, Mrs Sheryl Robinson R R 1 Box 66, McCracken, KS 67556, (316) 227-8002, BS 79 Fort Hays St Univ; MS 80 Fort Hays St Univ; Sp-Lang Path, SW KS Area Cooperative Dist #613, **SLP**

Rogers, Stacy Leigh 1024 North Olive Street, Santa Ana, CA 92703, (714) 558-7069, BA 85 CA St Univ - Long Beach; MA 86 CA St Univ - Los Angeles; 88–Aud, S L Rogers & Associates Inc, **A**

Rogers, Mrs Susan E 4004 Bayberry Drive, Hamilton, OH 45011, (513) 683-2820, BS 83 Miami Univ - Oxford; MS 84 Miami Univ - Oxford; Sp-Lang Path, Kings Local Sch Dist, **SLP**

Rogers, Mrs Susan Fulmer 2814 Oak Drive, Pawleys Island, SC 29585, (803) 237-2849, BA 81 Columbia Coll; MS 83 Univ of SC - Columbia; 86–Sp-Lang Path, Georgetown Co PS, **SLP**

Rogers, Mrs Susan G 187 Greenvale Drive, Springfield, OR 97477, (503) 747-5346, BS 67 OR St Univ; MS 87 Univ of OR

Rogers, Susan H 14570-C Growler Circle, Bangor, WA 98315, (206) 779-6326, **SLP**

Rogers, Therese M 1201 Alcott, Wichita, KS 67204, BA 77 Wichita St Univ; MA 79 Wichita St Univ; Sp-Lang Path, I of Logopedics, **SLP**

Rogers-Brunner, Cindy L 5404 Laurelwood Place, Sarasota, FL 33582, OB 77 Univ of FL; ME 78 Univ of FL; SLP, Mem Hosp Sarasota, **SLP**

Rogers-Jordan, Mrs Jana Kaye 2316 Chapel Hill Road, Ponca City, OK 74604-1666, (405) 762-9252, BS 83 OK St Univ; MS 85 Univ of OK Medical Center; **A**

Rogers-Leimbach, Mrs Julie Ann 4443 Casa Grande Circle, Apartment 161, Cypress, CA 90630, (213) 826-3199, BA 82 CA St Univ - Fullerton; MA 85 CA St Univ - Long Beach; Sp-Lang Path, Norwalk USD, **SLP**

Rogerson, Brenda S 261 Hungington Avenue, Buffalo, NY 14214, (716) 836-3199, BS 76 OH Univ - Athens; MA 78 OH St Univ; 87–Sp-Lang Path, People Inc, **SLP**

Roggatz, Karyn Joan 5150 West Cornelia, Chicago, IL 60641, (312) 545-0097, BS 82 Northern IL Univ - De Kalb; MS 85 Rush Univ; Chicago-Reed Mental Health Ctr, **A**

Rogister, Stephanie 1408 Dellwood Drive, Raleigh, NC 27607, (919) 781-0107, BA 72 Univ of NC - Chapel Hill; MS 75 Univ of NC - Chapel Hill; Sp/Lang Path, Sp & Lang Services of Raleigh, **SLP**

Rogovin, Karen Susan 30 Marlin Lane, Port Washington, NY 11050, (516) 883-6789, BA 82 SUNY - Center at Buffalo; MA 84 SUNY - Center at Buffalo; Sp-Lang Path, Sp Svcs Unit-Bd of Educ, **SLP**

Rohde, Mrs Ruthann 35382 Wisconsin Avenue, Oconomowoc, WI 53066, (414) 786-9606, BS 75 Univ of WI - Milwaukee; MS 76 Univ of WI - Milwaukee; SLP, Elmbrook Sch Dist, **SLP**

Rohe, Susan Westervelt 4338 Melody Lane #205, Madison, WI 53704, (608) 244-0618, BA 83 Univ of WI - Eau Claire; MS 86 Univ of WI - Madison; **SLP**

Rohl, Mrs Nancy Dee 3233 Creekwood, Lawrence, KS 66044, (913) 841-8463, BS 82 Northeast MO St Univ; MA 84 Northeast MO St Univ; Sp-Lang Path, Lawrence PS, **SLP**

Rohland, Pamela A 159 Julian First, Providence, RI 02909, (401) 421-1292, BS 75 Univ of TX - Austin; MA 77 Univ of TX - Austin; 87–Indep Consult, Private Practice, **A**

Rohlf, Jo Ann 319 East 18th #3, Carroll, IA 51401, (712) 792-3529, BS 84 IA St Univ; MS 86 Univ of WI - Stevens Point; **SLP**

Rohm, Mrs Cathy S 748 Southview Drive, Landisville, PA 17538, (717) 624-4616, BS 78 CA Univ of PA; MS 81 Towson St Univ; Sp-Lang Path, Lincoln Independent Unit 12, **SLP**

Rohm, Susan Marie 710 Executive Center Drive, Apartment 728, West Palm Beach, FL 33401, (407) 659-6901, BS 85 Northern IL Univ - De Kalb; MA 87 Northern IL Univ - De Kalb; 88–Aud, Palm Bch Ear Nose Throat Assoc, **A**

Rohn, Cheri L 122 Schiller Avenue, Syracuse, NY 13203, (315) 470-3260, BS 80 SUNY - Coll at Geneseo; MA 81 Bowling Green St Univ; Sp-Lang Path, N Syracuse Ctrl Sch, **SLP**

Rohovsky, Mrs Karen A 41 Glen Drive, Doylestown, PA 18901, (215) 348-1424, BS 64 OH St Univ; MA 65 OH St Univ; Sp-Lang Path, Private Practice, **SLP**

Rohr, Mrs Elaine H 1424 Spruce Street, South Pasadena, CA 91030, BA 65 Baylor Univ; MA 68 CA St Univ - Los Angeles; Sp/Lang Path, Elaine H Rohr, **SLP**

Rohr, Mrs Kari Vj 4143 Rosewood Place, Riverside, CA 92506, (714) 781-1771, BA 84 Univ of Redlands; MA 87 CA St Univ - Fullerton

Rohr, Mrs Linda J 1211 Hillsboro, Batavia, IL 60510, (312) 406-9285, BS 73 Northern IL Univ - De Kalb; MA 83 Northern IL Univ - De Kalb; 88–Sp-Lang Path, Dist 129 West Aurora Schs, **SLP**

Rohrbach, Kay E 2249 S W 33rd Way, Fort Lauderdale, FL 33312, BS 63 OH St Univ; MS 86 Nova Univ; 86–Sp-Lang Path, Broward County Schs, **SLP**

Rohrbacher, Mrs Susan H 761 Las Palmas Drive, Vista, CA 92083, (619) 945-3263, BA 72 CA St Univ - Northridge; MA 74 CA St Univ - Northridge; SLP, **SLP**

Rohrbaugh, Mrs Christine Ann 11977 Gadwell Drive, Cincinnati, OH 45246, (513) 671-7446, BS 84 West Chester Univ of PA; MS 86 PA St Univ - Univ Park; 88–Sp-Lang Path, Tri-County Speech Associates Inc, **SLP**

Rohrecker, Allison Clare 21 Nathan Hale Drive #39B, Huntington, NY 11743, (516) 928-0085, BA 84 Villanova Univ; MA 86 Hofstra Univ; Sp-Lang Path, Volz Amato Li Ctr for Com Dis, **SLP**

Rohren, Linda Michele 1829 Vienna Court #2, Pekin, IL 61554, (309) 346-4590, BS 85 Western IL Univ; MA 86 Western IL Univ; 86–Sp-Lang Path, Forman CUSD #124, **SLP**

Rohrer, Rosemary Elizabeth 4395 West Fisher Road, Winton, CA 95388, (209) 357-1222, BA 84 Holy Names Coll; MA 86 CA St Univ - Stanislaus; 86–Sp-Lang Path, Sp-Lang Path Hearing Clinic, **SLP**

Rohs, Mrs Carol M W215 N10228 Hickory Drive, Colgate, WI 53017, (414) 251-1931, BS 63 OH Univ - Athens; 86–Sp-Lang Path, Luthern Social Services, **SLP**

Rohsler, Maria Susan 276 Marlboro Road, Wood Ridge, NJ 07075, (201) 546-2813, MS 78 William Paterson Coll, BA 76 William Paterson Coll; Sp-Lang Path, Pre-K Hand River Vale Boe, **SLP**

Rohweder, Deborah Lynn 100 John Street, Washington, IN 47501, (812) 254-1530, BS 85 Southern IL Univ-Edwardsvill; MS 86 Southern IL Univ-Edwardsvill; 88–Sp-Lang Path, Daviess-Martin Spec Educ Coop, **SLP**

Roice, Mrs Susan E 12121 S E Skyline Drive, Santa Ana, CA 92705, (714) 351-9336, BS 66 Univ of CO - Boulder; MS 68 Univ of Pittsburgh - Pittsburgh; 87–Coord-Spec Educ, Alvord USD, **SLP**

Rokaitis, Mrs Beth Lorraine 2224 Quebec Court, Modesto, CA 95350, (209) 529-0490, BA 84 Augustana Coll; MA 86 CA St Univ - Fresno; 87–Sp-Lang Path, Sylvan Union Sch Dist, **SLP**

Roland, Mrs Adrienne Chavers 6484 Brickleigh Court, Alexandria, VA 22310, (703) 360-8000, BS 80 Miami Univ - Oxford; MS 81 Miami Univ - Oxford; SLP, Mt Vernon Hosp, **SLP**

Roland, Mrs Barbara Ann 289 Gertrude Avenue, Warwick, RI 02886, (401) 421-8826, BA 80 Univ of RI; MS 83 Univ of RI; Dispensing Aud, Aud Corp/America, **A**

Roland, Margaret G 20911 National Lane, Huntington Beach, CA 92646-6545, **SLP**

Roland, Nancy M L 515 Toddville Road, Charlotte, NC 28214, (704) 399-6979, BS 73 Winthrop Coll; MS 76 Winthrop Coll; SLP, Charlotte Mecklenburg Schools, **SLP**

Role, Ellen B 35 O'Neil Street, Hudson, MA 01749, (508) 793-8055, BA 80 SUNY - Coll at Cortland; MA 81 Western MI Univ; 86–Sp-Lang Path, Worcester State College, **SLP**

Rolfe, Brenda Smith 110th Med Dept Vs, 97th Gen Hosp Box 3, APO New York, NY 09757-5000, (209) 723-5395, BS 83 KS St Univ; MA 85 KS St Univ; **A**

Rolff, Susan B 3398 16th Street, San Francisco, CA 94114, (415) 225-1819, BA 65 CA St Univ - Northridge; MA 76 Humboldt St Univ; Sp-Lang Path, Easter Seals/Marin County, **SLP**

Roll, Julia B 1762 North Clark #2-N, Chicago, IL 60614, (212) 299-7600, BA 81 Boston Coll; MS 83 Columbia Univ Teachers Coll; Sp-Lang Path, Kingsbrook Jewish Medical Cen, **SLP**

Rolle, Mrs Jean T 22 Roger Road, St Cloud, MN 56301, (612) 251-1322, BA 55 Luther Coll; MS 77 Saint Cloud St Univ; Sp-Lang Path, St Cloud MN Sch Dist #742, **SLP**

Roller, Rena Paulette 2615 57th Street East, Bradenton, FL 33508-9556, (813) 729-8233, **SLP**

Rollert, Linda Cooper 5337 South Truckee Court, Aurora, CO 80015, (303) 693-8325, BS 79 CO St Univ; MS 81 Univ of Denver; Sp-Lang Path, Communication Disorders Spec, **SLP**

Rollhaus, Mrs Gila 147-24 75th Avenue, Flushing, NY 11367, (718) 793-6231, BA 77 CUNY - Queens Coll; MA 79 CUNY - Queens Coll; Aud, Lexington Hrng/Sp Cen, **A**

Rollin, Dr Walter J 579 Cedarberry Lane, San Rafael, CA 94903, BA 54 Queens Coll; MS 58 Univ of Pittsburgh - Pittsburgh; PH 62 (NS) Wayne St Univ; Prof Commun Dis In Spec Ed, San Francisco St U, **SLP**

Rollins, Dr David T Rehab Consulting Services Corp, P O Box 02355, Portland, OR 97202, (503) 777-4884, BS 64 Univ of ND; MS 65 Canisius Coll; PH 71 Univ of OR; Exec Dir, Rehab Consult Serv, **A**

Rollins, Mrs Kara M 11148 Boeger Court, Westchester, IL 60153, (312) 420-6575, BA 85 Elmhurst Coll; MS 86 Marquette Univ; 86–Sp-Lang Path, Naperville Dstr 203, **SLP**

Rollins, Laurel D 1814 North Dayton, Chicago, IL 60614, (312) 644-7705, BS 75 Univ of IL - Urbana; MS 76 Univ of IL - Urbana; 87–Provider Rel Consult, Equicor-Equitable HCA Corp, **SLP**

Rollins, Pamela Rosenthal 141 Spruce Street #2, Watertown, MA 02172, (617) 783-3141, **SLP**

Rollins, Mrs Rebecca Pinedo 40 North Sprague #5, Pittsburgh, PA 15202, (412) 734-3757, **SLP**

Rollins, Mrs Teresa A 2917 East Magill, Fresno, CA 93710, (209) 297-7322, BA 85 CA St Univ - Fresno; MA 87 CA St Univ - Fresno; 87–Sp-Lang Path, Clovis USD, **SLP**

Rollins-Bellows, Joan C Baudhuin Oral School, 3375 SW 75th Avenue, Fort Lauderdale, FL 33314, (305) 475-7325, BS 55 IA St Univ; MS 57 Univ of WI - Madison; ED 88 (Early Childhood) Nova Univ; Dir Hrng Impr Prog, Baudhuin Oral Sch, **SLP**

Rollinson, Mrs Frances M 63 Bellevue Street, Willimantic, CT 06226, (203) 642-7593, BA 83 Univ of CT; MA 85 Univ of CT; Sp-Lang Path, Town of Lebanon, **SLP**

Rollison, Larry L 2302 Memorial Parkway, Portland, TX 78374, (512) 888-5301, BS 72 Univ Southern MS-Hattiesburg; MS 78 Univ Southern MS-Hattiesburg; Aud, Corpus Christi State Sch, **A**

Rollman, Mrs Cynthia R 11513 Oak Knoll Drive, Austin, TX 78759, (512) 454-4869, BA 73 Southwest TX St Univ; ME 75 Southwest TX St Univ; Sp-Lang Path, Austin ISD, **SLP**

Rolls, Denise Patricia 15639 View Ridge Lane, Granada Hills, CA 91344, (805) 296-8611, BA 84 CA St Univ - Northridge; MA 86 CA St Univ - Northridge; Sp-Lang Path, Saugus Schl Dstr, **SLP**

Rolnick, Dr Michael I Dir Speech & Language Path, William Beaumont Hospital, 3601 West 13 Mile Road, Royal Oak, MI 48072, (313) 288-8085, BA 64 Wayne St Univ; ME 65 Wayne St Univ; PH 69 (Sp-Lang Path) Wayne St Univ; Dir/Sp-Lang Path, William Beaumont Hosp, **SLP ACE**

Rolph, Teresa K 15110 Mira Vista, Houston, TX 77083, BA 77 Denison Univ; MA 79 Univ of Cincinnati; SLP, Lamar School District, **SLP**

Rolzin, Mrs Elaine A 947 Anton Road, Plymouth, WI 53073, (414) 892-4353, BS 67 Northern MI Univ; MS 69 Univ of WI - Stevens Point; Sp-Lang Path, Plymouth Sch Dist, **SLP**

Rom, Mrs Anita Block 22 Edward Avenue, Woodmere, NY 11598, (516) 295-5568, BA 73 Tel Aviv Univ - Israel; PH 79 (Sp-Lang Path) Wayne St Univ; 87–Asst Prof, C W Post Long Island Univ, **SLP**

Rom, Patricia 108 Garrison, Wilmette, IL 60091, (312) 256-3913, BA 73 Mundelein Coll; MA 74 Northwestern Univ; Sp-Lang Path, Private Practice, **SLP**

Romack, Carolee A 5109 Westpark Drive, North Hollywood, CA 91601, (818) 763-5446, BS 57 Eastern IL Univ; MA 72 CA St Univ - Northridge; SLP, Los Angeles USD, **SLP**

Roman, Allison Sedey 5313 Brody Drive #202, Madison, WI 53705, (608) 231-6957, BA 82 CA St Univ - Northridge; MA 84 CA St Univ - Northridge; 88–Research Asst, Univ of Wisconsin-Madison, **SLP A**

Roman, Mrs Ann C 153 Butternut Road, 7 Midway Manor, Shavertown, PA 18708-9645, (717) 287-9681, BS 72 PA St Univ - Univ Park; MS 73 PA St Univ - Univ Park; **SLP**

Roman, Mrs Barbara Johnson 2955 Windy Hill Road, Allentown, PA 18103, (215) 820-9883, MS 84 Boston Univ; BA 82 Univ of CT; Sp-Lang Path, Easter Seal Soc Broward County, **SLP**

Roman, Elfriede 8071-B Puritan Drive, Mentor, OH 44060, (216) 255-7411, BA 76 Cleveland St Univ; MA 78 Cleveland St Univ; 88 Cleveland St Univ; 88–Dir of Human Resources, Deepwood Cen, **SLP**

Roman, Mrs Virginia P Virginia P Roman Inc, 246 Maple Avenue East, Vienna, VA 22180, (703) 281-2722, BS 51 Indiana Univ of PA; ME 52 1873; Sp-Lang Path, Private Practice, **SLP**

Romanelli, Constance Ann 1998 Hazel, Birmingham, MI 48008, (313) 857-8580, BS 69 Kent St Univ; MA 76 Eastern MI Univ; Sp/Lang Path, Sch Dist City of Pontiac

Romanelli, Mrs Maryann 1809 North 26th Street, Broken Arrow, OK 74012, (918) 682-5501, BS 85 Northern IL Univ - De Kalb; MA 87 OK St Univ; **SLP**

Romaniello, Mrs Diane 4 Brookstone Drive, Voorhees, NJ 08043, (609) 751-7216, BA 76 Montclair St Coll; MA 79 Trenton St Coll; Sp/Lang Path, Gloucester Cty Pub Sch, **SLP**

Romanin, Kay E B 1827 Edwards Avenue, Cedar Falls, IA 50613, (319) 266-1824, BS 67 Kent St Univ; MS 73 Southern IL Univ -Carbondale; SLP, AEA #7/ U of Nn IA, **SLP**

Romaniszak, Vivian Marie 1500 E Avenue NW, Apartment #3A, Cedar Rapids, IA 52405, (319) 363-7352, BS 83 Southern IL Univ -Carbondale; MS 86 Southern IL Univ -Carbondale; 87–Aud, Dr J Spoden, **A**

Romano, Alex T 509 Berard Street, Breaux Bridge, LA 70517, (318) 237-7744, MA 69 Univ of South FL; PH 80 Univ of VA - Charlottesville; Dir Area Agency On Aging, Cajun Area Agency on Aging, **SLP**

Romano, Grace Mary 220 Clark Avenue, Branford, CT 06405, (203) 488-6216, BA 68 Cardinal Cushing Coll; MS 71 Southern CT St Univ; OM 74 Southern CT St Univ; 70–Sp-Lang Path, New Haven PS, **SLP**

Romano, Mrs Jacqulyn 509 Berard Street, Breaux Bridge, LA 70517, (318) 332-5698, BA 74 Univ of Southwestern LA; MS 80 Univ of Southwestern LA; Sp-Lang Path, PsyCog Assoc Inc, **SLP**

Romano, Mrs Lois J 195 Oakmont Drive, Deerfield, IL 60015, (312) 940-8820, MA 74 Univ of Denver; **SLP**

Romano, Mary Anne McMahon 3016 E Cheryl Drive, Phoenix, AZ 85028, (602) 266-9315, BS 65 Syracuse Univ; MS 86 AZ St Univ; 86–Sp-Lang Path, Judith Meyer Certified Sp Path Inc, **SLP**

Romano, Tina Lisa 989 South Emerson, Denver, CO 80209-4329, (303) 698-0533, MS 86 CO St Univ; 86–Aud, CO Ear Clinic, **A**

Romanow, Judith Lynn 6505 Bella Vista #201, Rockford, MI 49341, (616) 874-6270, BA 78 Univ of MI - Ann Arbor; MS 80 Columbia Univ Teachers Coll; 88–Sp-Lang Path, New Port Hosp/Vanderbilt Rehab, **SLP**

Romas, Mrs Debra B P O Box 534, Mount Vernon, OH 43050, (614) 397-4548, BA 71 Catawba Coll; MA 73 OH St Univ; Sp-Lang Path, Debra B Romas & Assoc Inc, **SLP**

Rombakis Crawford, Mrs Georgia 8918 Bissonnet #107, Houston, TX 77074-2432, (713) 933-6000, BS 79 Univ of IA; ME 81 Southwest TX St Univ; Sp-Lang Path, Belle Park Hosp, **SLP**

Rombro, Nancy Block 6317 Green Meadow Parkway, Baltimore, MD 21209, (301) 396-3245, BA 67 Univ of MD - College Park; MS 80 Towson St Univ; Sp-Lang Path, Baltimore City Pub Sch, **SLP**

Rome, Mrs Deborah K 16944 Ventura Boulevard, Encino, CA 91316, (818) 783-6633, BS 74 Univ of Southern CA; MS 76; MS 76 Columbia Univ Teachers Coll; Sp/Lang Path, Private Practice, **SLP**

Romeo, Mrs Teri Louise 5280-A Tamarus, Las Vegas, NV 89119, (702) 739-7664, BS 84 Univ of NV - Reno; MS 86 Univ of NV - Reno; **SLP**

Romer, Susan O'Day 2B Cumberland Street #2, Boston, MA 02115, (617) 426-5555, MS 86 Northeastern Univ; 88–Sp-Lang Path, VNA of Boston, **SLP**

Romereim, Beverly May 822 North Belmont, Wichita, KS 67208, (316) 685-2221, OB 81 Wichita St Univ; MA 85 Wichita St Univ; Aud, VA Medical Center, **A**

Romero, Mrs Jeannie G 816 San Mateo Boulevard S E, Albuquerque, NM 87108, (505) 268-0565, BS 72 Kent St Univ; MA 76 Kent St Univ; Sp-Lang Path, Dance & Fitness Place, **SLP A**

Romesburg, Jocelyn 2100 Rebsamen Park Road, Apartment 316, Little Rock, AR 72202, (501) 372-4601, BA 83 Ouachita Baptist Univ; MS 85 Univ of AR - Little Rock; **SLP**

Romine, Mrs Linda K P 27589 Bittersweet Lane, Elkhart, IN 46514, (219) 264-6828, BA 71 Bethel Coll; OM 73 IN Univ - Bloomington; Sp-Lang Path, Private Practice, **SLP**

Romine, Mark Laurence 1112 E Lake Place, Fort Collins, CO 80524, (303) 482-3569, BA 86 Univ of Northern CO; MA 87 Univ of Northern CO; 88–Aud, Cheyenne Hearing Cl

Romm, Marcia K Mevo Hapartizanim #306, Apartment 5 French Hill, Jerusalem, Israel, **A**

Romolino, Diane Duk 2144 Knollwood Drive, Martinez, CA 94553, (415) 370-0749, BS 81 Eastern MI Univ; MA 82 Eastern MI Univ; Sp-Lang Path, Private Practice, **SLP**

Romoser, Mrs Mechthild A Worester Road, Eliot, ME 03903, (603) 692-4411, MS 86 Univ of NH; **SLP**

Romoser, Patricia R 9909 Harford Road, Baltimore, MD 21234, **SLP**

Rompa, Kathleen Patricia 6617 Alexander, Hammond, IN 46323, (312) 947-9695, BA 74 San Diego St Univ; MS 81 Purdue Univ - West Lafayette; Aud, Sound Resources, **A**

Rompala, David J 7912 West 172nd Place, Tinley Park, IL 60477, (312) 532-3810, BS 72 Western IL Univ; MA 73 Baylor Univ; Dir, Sertoma Cen, **SLP A**

Romski, Dr Maryann Language Research Center, Department Of Psychology, Georgia State University, Atlanta, GA 30303, (404) 243-8286, BA 74 CUNY - Hunter Coll; MA 75 SUNY - Coll at Geneseo; PH 81 (NS) Univ of KS; 81–Assoc Prof, Georgia St U, **SLP**

Romuld, Kathy Sue Kiewel 1712 Beech Street, St Paul, MN 55106, **SLP**

Ron, Ann Creamer 15306 Windy Cove Drive, Houston, TX 77095, (713) 855-0732, BS 80 Univ of TX - Austin; MA 82 Univ of KS; Sp/Lang Path, Private Practice, **SLP**

Ronan, Mrs Gail A 29 Madeline Street, Brighton, MA 02135, (617) 653-7113, BA 76 Boston Coll; ME 78 Northeastern Univ; Sp Lang Cl, Natick Pub Sch, **SLP**

Ronayne, Liza Ann Gingras 208 21st Avenue North East, Aberdeen, SD 57401, (703) 825-9153, **SLP**

Ronci, Eileen Stanton 2225 South 110th Street, Omaha, NE 68144, (219) 289-4831, BS 80 Purdue Univ - West Lafayette; MA 82 Univ of TN - Knoxville; Sp-Lang Path, Council for Ret/St Joseph Co, **SLP**

Ronck, Sharon B Route 4 Box 39, Enid, OK 73701, (405) 233-9692, BA 73 Univ of OK - Norman; MS 75 Univ of OK Medical Center; Sp/Lang Path, Private Practice, **SLP ACE**

Ronczkowski, Mrs Mary Ann 530 Lakeside Circle, Sunrise, FL 33326, (305) 389-1582, BS 84 Elmhurst Coll; MS 86 Univ of South FL; 87–Sp-Lang Path, Hollywood Mem Hosp, **SLP**

Rondinelli, Michelle L 832 Continental, Waterville, OH 43566, (419) 784-1414, BA 83 OH St Univ; MS 86 Bowling Green St Univ; 86–Aud/Sp-Lang Path, The Defiance Clinic, **SLP A**

Rondino, Joyce A 26 Francis Street, East Hartford, CT 06108, (203) 528-7411, BA 67 Coll of New Rochelle; MA 69 Columbia Univ Teachers Coll; SLP, East Hartford Bd of Ed, **SLP**

Rone, Mrs Kathleen L 1327 West Avenue South, La Crosse, WI 54601, (608) 785-0940, BA 71 Univ of WI - Eau Claire; MS 72 Univ of WI - Eau Claire; Sp-Lang Path, **SLP**

Rone, Mrs Linda H 19 Roland Road, Jamestown, NY 14701, (716) 487-0141, BS 70 SUNY - Coll at Fredonia; MS 85 SUNY - Coll at Fredonia; 85–Sp-Lang Path, WCA Hosp, **SLP ACE**

Rones, Mrs Cynthia Nothan 5105 Old Chestnut Court, Woodstock, GA 30188, (404) 926-0283, ME 87 Univ of GA; SLP, Cherokee Co Bd of Ed, **SLP**

Rongstad, William Alver Comm Disorders Program, Northern Regional Office, 1020 Barnett Street, Fairbanks, AK 99701, (907) 452-6291, **A**

Roninson, Olga Z 818 South Laflin, Chicago, IL 60607, (312) 666-8611, BS 78 Moscow Pedagogical Inst-Ussr; MS 82 Boston Univ; 85–Sp-Lang Path, Cook County Hospital, **SLP**

Ronken, Mrs Donna M Ongalo Box 205, Lake Park, MN 56554, (218) 238-5916, BA 72 Saint Cloud St Univ; MS 81 Moorhead St Univ; Sp-Lang Path, Lake Park Pub Sch, **SLP**

Ronneberg, Mrs Gail V 5561 Huntington Drive, Santa Barbara, CA 93111, (415) 254-3058, MA 72 San Francisco St Univ; BA 70 San Francisco St Univ; **SLP**

Ronnei, Mrs Eleanor C c/o Clark, 3 Ridgewood Circle, Wilmington, DE 19809, MS; **A LM**

Ronning, Mrs Nina M 1006 Nunn Avenue #5, Rice Lake, WI 54868, (715) 924-3136, MA 87 Univ of MN - Duluth; 87–Sp-Lang Path, Chetek PS, **SLP**

Ronowski, Laura J 3100 West Howard #14, Milwaukee, WI 53221, (414) 282-0243, BS 84 Univ of WI - Milwaukee; MS 86 Marquette Univ; **SLP**

Ronquillo, Yazmin J 3021 Villa Sur Trail, Dallas, TX 75228, (214) 946-2671, BS 76 Trenton St Coll; MS 80 Southern Methodist Univ; SLP, Dallas ISD, **SLP**

Ronson, Dr Irwin 70 Lasalle Street, Apartment #20C, New York, NY 10027-4747, (212) 749-0338, BA 53 CUNY - City College; MA 54 Columbia Univ Teachers Coll; PH 74 (NS) CUNY - Grad Sch & Univ Cntr; Prof, Bronx Com Coll-Cuny, **SLP**

Ronzani, Mrs Judith M 1904 Arbor Vitae Lane, Plover, WI 54467, (715) 344-7963, BA 69 MI St Univ; MS 71 Univ of WI - Stevens Point; Sp-Lang Path, Mosinee Comm Schs, **SLP**

Rood, Mrs Leah Berman 1291 N W 91st Avenue, Coral Springs, FL 33065, (305) 752-0053, **SLP**

Rood, Dr Stewart R University Of Pittsburgh, Eye & Ear Hospital, Dept Of Otolaryngology, Pittsburgh, PA 15213, (412) 647-2110, BA 67 CUNY - Brooklyn Coll; OM 82 Univ of Pittsburgh - Pittsburgh; PH 72 (Biocommunications) Univ of Pittsburgh - Pittsburgh; 76–Assoc Prof, U of Pitts, **SLP A**

Rook, Mrs Judith Ann Morrison 9926 Devonshire, Omaha, NE 68114, BA 63 Univ of AZ; MA 64 Northwestern Univ; **SLP A**

Rook, Paul D Fort Sanders Prof Hearing Serv, 501 20th Street, Suite 202, Knoxville, TN 37916, (615) 522-0630, BA 68 Univ of South FL; MS 74 Univ of South FL; Aud, Ft Sanders Prof Hrng Serv, **A**

Rooks, Mrs Mary P 452 Sparrow Drive, Satellite Beach, FL 32937, (407) 723-1055, BA 57 Catholic Univ of America; MS 76 Adelphi Univ; Sp/Lang Path, Palm Bay Elem Sch, **SLP**

Rooney, Barbara Ann 100 Parkway Road Apartment 2C, Bronxville, NY 10708, (914) 337-5722, MS 84 Columbia Univ Teachers Coll; 84–Aud, Hackensack Med Ctr, **A**

Rooney, Mrs Bridget Knowles 1999 Stanford Drive, Naperville, IL 60565, (312) 961-0025, BA 81 IN Univ - Bloomington; MA 82 IN Univ - Bloomington; 85–Sp-Lang Path, Southern Will Co Coop, **SLP**

Rooney, Joan Franzese 29 Raymond Street, Rockville Centre, NY 11570, (516) 223-7574, BA 71 Adelphi Univ; MA 73 Columbia Univ Teachers Coll; Sp-Lang Path, Private Practice, **SLP**

Rooney, Lisa E 8922 South Hoyne, Chicago, IL 60620, (219) 933-2004, BS 85 Univ of Miami; MS 87 Rush Univ; 87–Sp-Lang Path, Saint Margaret Hosp, **SLP**

Rooney, Nancy 1100 Transcas Street Suite 206, PO Box 2099, Napa, CA 94558, (707) 255-6293, BA 70 San Francisco St Univ; MA 72 San Jose St Univ; MA 70 San Jose St Univ; Admin/Owner, Napa Valley Speech Ctr, **SLP**

Rooney, Robin Theresa 666 Edgewater Boulevard, Apartment 302, Foster City, CA 94404-2851, MA 85 San Jose St Univ; **SLP**

Roope, Mrs Jane E 3209 Oakridge Drive, Bakersfield, CA 93306, (805) 398-3799, BS 77 Kent St Univ; MA 78 Kent St Univ; Sp-Lang Path, Kern Co Supt of Sch, **SLP**

Roos, Sharon Williams 4405-A Fieldgreen Rd, Baltimore, MD 21236, BS 74 Towson St Univ; MA 78 Wayne St Univ - Sch of Med; Aud, Oticon Corporation, **A ACE**

Roosa, Kelly Ann R R 1, Box 197, Stone Ridge, NY 12484, (914) 687-7021, BA 85 Univ of CT; MA 87 Univ of CT; 87–Sp-Lang Path, UCP of Ulster Co Inc, **SLP**

Roos-Marr, Ellen Juhl 42 Laiki Place, Kailua, HI 96734, (808) 261-4184, BA 72 Hobart-William Smith Coll; MS 82 Univ of HI - Manoa; Sp-Lang Path, Windword Spec Svc/Dept Educ, **SLP**

Root, Karen L 3435 MacNichol Trail, West Bloomfield, MI 48033, (313) 626-3471, BS 73 SUNY - Center at Buffalo; MS 74 Univ of MI - Ann Arbor; **A**

Root, Mrs Linnea S 887 Brentwood Drive, Crystal Lake, IL 60014, (312) 658-2540, BS 60 Univ of IL - Urbana; MA 62 Northwestern Univ; 79–Sp-Lang Path, Comm Unit Sch Dist #300, **SLP**

Root, Mrs Lynn E 3309 Stockholm Drive, Shaker Heights, OH 49120, BA 85 MI St Univ; MA 87 Wayne St Univ - Sch of Med; 88–Sp-Lang Path, Cleveland Sp and Hrng Ctr, **A**

Root, Susan D P O Box 3514, Grand Rapids, MI 49501, (616) 242-0426, BA 77 MI St Univ; MA 78 MI St Univ; Sp-Lang Path, Mary Free Bed Rehabilitatn Ctr, **SLP ACE**

Ropek, Renee Marilyn 6515 North Kenton, Lincolnwood, IL 60646, (312) 239-2191, BA 84 Northern IL Univ - De Kalb; MA 86 Northern IL Univ - De Kalb; **SLP**

Roper, Julie Marie 514 Bethlehem Park, Fort Washington, PA 19034-2107, (215) 646-3797, BS 85 PA St Univ - Univ Park; MA 87 Temple Univ; 87–Aud, Intercounty Audiology, **A**

Roper, Linda Joyce 411 East 76th Street, Los Angeles, CA 90003, (213) 758-8064, BA 72 Univ of Redlands; MS 73 Univ of Redlands; SLP, Los Angeles USD, **SLP**

Rophie, Mrs Sharon Slaughter 487 Winding Willow Drive, Palm Harbor, FL 34683, (813) 785-5045, BA 79 IN Univ - Bloomington; MA 80 Memphis St Univ; **A**

Roppolo, Mrs Cynthia M 300 Rosa Avenue, Metairie, LA 70005, (504) 830-4424, BS 71 Univ of Southwestern LA; OM 72 Tulane Univ; Sp-Lang Path, Jefferson Parish Sch Bd, **SLP**

Roquemore, Leslie C 3127 Heather Glynn, Mulberry, FL 33860, (813) 425-2074, MS 80 Univ of South FL; Sp-Lang Path, Florida Medical Systems, **SLP**

Rorie, Beverly Lewis 2215 Clapboard Hill, Little Rock, AR 72207, (817) 573-7121, BS 81 Southeast MO St Univ; MA 85 Southeast MO St Univ

Rosa, Janice Ann 46 Theroux Drive #3-B, Chicopee, MA 01020, (413) 534-2508, BS 84 Boston Univ; MS 85 Boston Univ; 85–Sp-Lang Path, Holyoke Hosp Sp & Hrng Ctr, **SLP**

Rosado, Mrs Maria L 22936 Kingsbury Avenue #B, Bayside, NY 11364-3127, (718) 793-7078, MS 78 Columbia Univ Teachers Coll; SLP, Quick Start Head Start Program, **SLP**

Rosage, Kristine B 185 Woodin Road, Clifton Park, NY 12065, (518) 371-1613, BS 72 SUNY - Coll at Geneseo; MA 76 Coll of Saint Rose; 87–Sp-Lang Path, Saratoga-Warren Co BOCES, **SLP**

Rosaly, Maria DeLourdes 470 Second Avenue, New York, NY 10016, (212) 685-7795, BA 81 CUNY - Hunter Coll; MA 85 CUNY - Hunter Coll; 84–Teacher, New York City Board of Educ, **SLP**

Rosano, Anne 4018 Richmond Avenue, Staten Island, NY 10312, (201) 750-4660, BA 78 CUNY - Brooklyn Coll; MA 84 Kean Coll of NJ; **A**

Rosa-Reed, Clare M 506 Balmoral Circle, New Windsor, NY 12550, (914) 431-8800, BA 79 Saint John's Univ - Jamaica; MS 81 Syracuse Univ; Sp/Lang Path, St Francis Hosp, **SLP**

Rosati, Juliann Marie 138 Newton Road #23, Plainstow, NH 03865-2411, (603) 382-1797, BS 82 Worcester St Coll; MA 84 MI St Univ; Sp-Lang Path, Boston Center for Blind Chldn, **SLP**

Rosato, Lynne A 815 Stonybrook Drive, Norristown, PA 19403, (215) 275-2770, MS 83 Bloomsburg Univ of PA; 88–Sp-Lang Path, Montgomery Assoc for Retarded Citizens, **SLP**

Rosato-Ziggas, Mrs Diane M 6 Hutchman Road, Mars, PA 16046, (412) 828-1300, BA 77 Duquesne Univ; MA 78 Central MI Univ; Sp-Lang Path, Harmarville Rehab Cen, **SLP**

Roschwalb, Adena 32 Birch Drive, Plainview, NY 11803, (516) 931-3621, **SLP**

Roscoe, Barbara Wais 235 Norway Road, Bangor, ME 04401-5820, BA 75 SUNY - Coll at Brockport; MA 78 SUNY - Center at Buffalo; 88–Sp-Lang Path, Sch Admin #63 Holden, **SLP ACE**

Roscoe, Mrs Lauren Route 5 Box 303, Anderson, SC 29621, (803) 224-8575, BA 65 AR St Univ; MA 69 Vanderbilt Univ; Aud, Robert Jordan MD, **A**

Rose, Mrs Bonnie Mae P O Box 88, Sudlersville, MD 21668, (301) 438-3164, BS 74 Edinboro Univ of PA; MA 75 Edinboro Univ of PA; 83–Sp-Lang Path, Queen Anne's Co Bd of Educ, **SLP**

Rose, Mrs Carol Ann 125 Louden Road, Saratoga Springs, NY 12866, (518) 587-8459, BS 78 SUNY - Coll at Geneseo; MA 79 SUNY - Coll at Geneseo; Sp-Lang Path, Warren-Washington Co BOCES, **SLP**

Rose, Carol Maj 23 Timbercrest Circle, Anniston, AL 36206, (205) 820-2469, BS 76 TX Tech Univ; MA 77 Univ Southern MS-Hattiesburg; 88–Sp-Lang Path, Private Practice, **SLP**

Rose, Carolyn Estelle 6878 Glen Mawr, El Cerrito, CA 94530, (408) 378-6131, MS 84 CA St Univ - Hayward; Sp-Lang Path, Herrick Hospital & Health Ctr, **SLP**

Rose, Mrs Corie H 9570 Mamota Way, Cypress, CA 90630, (213) 493-5428, BA 75 Univ of Redlands; MS 76 Univ of Redlands; Sp-Lang Path, Los Alamitos USD, **SLP**

Rose, Mrs Darlene 17540 Redvere Drive, Brookfield, WI 53005, (414) 781-3412, BA 64 Briar Cliff Coll; MS 66 Marquette Univ; Sp-Lang Path, Rehab Assoc, **SLP**

Rose, Dr Darrell Eugene 2476 Peg Leg Road, Jacksonville, FL 32224, (904) 223-2217, BS 60 Brigham Young Univ; MS 61 Southern IL Univ -Carbondale; PH 65 (NS) Univ of OK - Norman; Dir of Aud, Mayo Cl-Jacksonville Florida, **A F**

Rose, Darryl R 11270 30 Mile Road, Romeo, MI 48065, (313) 778-1492, BS 67 Wayne St Univ; ME 72 Wayne St Univ; SLP, Fraser Pub Sch, **SLP**

Rose, Deborah L 107 Acorn Drive, Bridgeport, IL 62417, **SLP**

Rose, Denise Fisher P O Box 1831, Kill Devil Hills, NC 27948, (919) 441-0339, BS 77 SUNY - Coll at Brockport; MA 78 Bowling Green St Univ; Sup, Alta Petens Inc, **SLP**

Rose, Mrs Eileen A 1718 Linden Place, North Merrick, NY 11566, (516) 486-5825, BS 79 Saint John's Univ - Jamaica; MA 81 CUNY - Queens Coll; Sp/Lang Path, Nassau BOCES Hearing Impaired, **SLP**

Rose, Mrs Emily S 4728 Deerfield Place, Binghamton, NY 13903, (607) 722-5308, BS 74 Syracuse Univ; MS 75 Syracuse Univ; Sp-Lang Path, Rehab Services Inc, **SLP**

Rose, Heidi Fleck 2700 Ocean Drive #300, Vero Beach, FL 32963, (407) 567-7165, BA 85 OH St Univ; MA 87 Case Western Reserve Univ

Rose, John S 1268-B Timberlane Road, Tallahassee, FL 32308, (904) 893-8743, BS 72 FL St Univ; MS 73 FL St Univ; Sp-Lang Path, Private Practice, **SLP**

Rose, Karen 3350 Redwood Avenue, Los Angeles, CA 90066, **SLP**

Rose, Mrs Karen Marie 20 Walnut Street, Stony Point, NY 10980, (914) 429-4502, MA 84 Montclair St Coll; SLP, N Rockland Sch Dist, **SLP**

Rose, Lauraine Sara 69 Glen Avenue, Apartment 206, Oakland, CA 94611, (415) 658-4634, BA 73 Beloit Coll; MS 83 Columbia Univ Teachers Coll; Sp-Lang Path, Childrens Hospital Oakland, **SLP**

Rose, Leah Z 17-2 Pond Way, Manorville, NY 11949, (516) 874-4151, BS 77 SUNY - Center at Albany; MS 78 Adelphi Univ; Sp-Lang Path, Brentwwod Ps, **SLP**

Rose, Linda B 5409 Marigny Street, New Orleans, LA 70122, (504) 826-2400, BA 76 LA St Univ - Baton Rouge; OM 80 LA St Univ - N O Medical Ctr; SLP/Audio Mgr, Dept Hhr Commun Dis Sec, **A**

Rose, Margaret A 300 Sunburst, Flushing, MI 48433, **SLP**

Rose, Myrna F 25 Clover Lane, Randolph, NJ 07869, (201) 543-7107, BS 55 CUNY - City College; MA 73 Kean Coll of NJ; 72–Sp-Lang Path, Mendham Twp Schs, **SLP**

Rose, Mrs Opal L 720 Corhell, Oakley, KS 67748, (913) 672-4288, BS 28 Fort Hays St Univ; MS 70 Fort Hays St Univ; **SLP LM**

Rose, Pamela S Box 165, Anna, IL 62906, BS 76 Southern IL Univ -Carbondale; MS 78 Southern IL Univ -Carbondale; 85–Research, Kenneth D Rose Atty at Law, **SLP**

Rose, Mrs Patricia Ann 2906 University Drive, Lawrence, KS 66044, (913) 842-0761, BS 70 SUNY - Coll at Geneseo; MS 72 CUNY - Queens Coll; 77–Sp/Lang Path, Rehab Act Ser Inc, **SLP**

Rose, Patricia M 9410 South 79th Court #2SW, Hickory Hills, IL 60457, **SLP**

Rose, Mrs Rochelle Honig 2816 Rosebud Avenue, Merrick, NY 11566, (516) 623-6379, BS 58 Adelphi Univ; MS 66 Adelphi Univ; Sp-Lang Path, Levittown Un Free Sch, **SLP**

Rose, Shannon E 51 Maple Ridge Lane, Asheville, NC 28806, (704) 251-6091, BA 80 Northwestern St Univ; MA 85 Northwestern St Univ; 88–Sp-Lang Path, Asheville Dev Evaluation Ctr, **SLP**

Rose, Mrs Sheila Kaye 916 Harold Drive, Midwest City, OK 73110, (405) 737-4461, BS 76 Central St Univ; ME 86 Central St Univ; 85–Sp-Lang Path, Midwest City-Del City Schs, **SLP**

Rose, Mrs Susan A 322 Burleigh Avenue, Norfolk, VA 23505, (804) 440-9835, BS 74 Bowling Green St Univ; MA 76 Univ of TN - Knoxville; Sp-Lang Path, InSpeech Inc, **SLP**

Roseberry, Celeste Arleen Department Of Education, Ca State University-Chico, Chico, CA 95929-0222, (916) 895-4652, BA 80 CA St Univ - Fresno; MA 82 CA St Univ - Fullerton; PH 87 (Sp Path Lang & Cognition) Northwestern Univ; Lecturer/Asst Prof, California State University, **SLP ACE**

Roseberry, Sherry Kay P O Box 473, Purvis, MS 39475, (601) 584-6311, BS 73 Univ Southern MS-Hattiesburg; MS 76 Univ Southern MS-Hattiesburg; Sp/Lang Path, Hattiesburg Pub Schs, **SLP**

Rosedale, Mrs Judith B 2069 Fargo Avenue, Des Plaines, IL 60018, (312) 255-9700, BA 76 Elmhurst Coll; MA 77 Northern IL Univ - De Kalb; SLP, High Sch Dist #214, **SLP**

Rosedale, M Yvonne 45 Duncott Road, Fairport, NY 14450, PH (NS); **SLP**

Rosedale, Michelle 174-A Cedar Lane, Highland Park, NJ 08904, (212) 448-9775, BA 76 Temple Univ; MS 78 Rutgers St Univ -N Brunswick; Sp/Lang Path, Staten Is Ment Hlth Soc, **SLP**

Rosegger, Mrs Leslie K 1723 Moose Drive, Lakeland, FL 33801, (813) 666-5633, BS 83 James Madison Univ; ME 85 James Madison Univ; Aud, Central FL Sp/Hrng Ctr, **A**

Rose-Jones, Kathleen A 376 Normandy Drive, Norwood, MA 02026, (617) 848-6250, **SLP**

Rose-Kroll, Mrs Deborah 2746 Suwanee Way, Marietta, GA 30067, (404) 952-4114, BA 83 Univ of FL; MA 85 George Washington Univ; **A**

Roselle, Mrs Rebecca S 2010 Wolftrap Oaks Court, Vienna, VA 22180, (716) 488-9450, BS 71 Kent St Univ; MA 72 Univ of Cincinnati; Sp/Lang Path, Private Practice, **SLP**

Roseman, Marcia H Sunnyhill Road, Dover, NJ 07801, (201) 361-5931, BS 56 CUNY - Brooklyn Coll; MA 73 Seton Hall Univ; Sp-Lang Path, Private Practice, **SLP ACE**

Roseman, Marcia L 8 Five Oaks Court, Owings Mills, MD 21117, (301) 323-2200, BS 75 Univ of MD - College Park; MS 76 Univ of MI - Ann Arbor; Sp-Lang Path, Private Practice, **SLP**

Rosen, Adrienne Z 11 Thornwood Road, Armonk, NY 10504, (914) 273-9559, BA 74 SUNY - Center at Buffalo; MA 77 SUNY - Center at Buffalo; Sp/Lang Path, Private Practice, **SLP**

Rosen, Mrs Annie Rebecca 1142 49th Street, Brooklyn, NY 11219, (718) 854-4354, BA 83 Yeshiva Univ; MA 85 CUNY - Queens Coll; Sp-Lang Path, **SLP**

Rosen, Arlene S 2323 Schiller, Wilmette, IL 60091, (312) 256-1375, BS 56 Univ of IL - Urbana; MA 61 Northwestern Univ; Sp-Lang Path, Private Practice, **SLP LM**

Rosen, Mrs Barbara L B R Audiology & Counseling Ctr, 165 North Village Avenue, Suite 117, Rockville Centre, NY 11570, (516) 764-2094, BS 69 Syracuse Univ; MA 71 NY Univ; Aud, Drs Steinberg & Arnold, **A**

Rosen, Carol 355 Bard Avenue, Staten Island, NY 10310, (718) 390-1480, BA 59 Adelphi Univ; MS 61 Adelphi Univ; 70–Admin Dir, St Vincent's Med Ctr, **SLP**

Rosen, Cynthia D 14 Eucalyptus Road, Berkeley, CA 94705, MS 84; SLP, Hayward USD, **SLP**

Rosen, Mrs Debra L 539 Hoffman Drive, Bryn Mawr, PA 19010, (215) 527-4824, **A**

Rosen, Mrs Ella Zittrer 61 Arcadia Drive, Tuscaloosa, AL 35404, (205) 556-2058, BA 66 Univ of FL; MS 70 FL St Univ; MS 87 Univ of AL- Tuscaloosa; **SLP**

Rosen, Gale Goodman 4344 Stoneycroft, Okemos, MI 48864, (517) 337-1646, BA 70 CUNY - Queens Coll; MS 72 PA St Univ - Univ Park; Head Sp-Lang Path, Lansing Gen Hosp, **SLP**

Rosen, H Fabrien 67 Oliver Street, Watertown, MA 02172, (617) 899-4709, MA 82 Univ of San Francisco; Private Practice, **SLP**

Rosen, Dr Jack 6628 Pontchartrain Blvd, New Orleans, LA 70124, (504) 486-9236, BA 51 Stanford Univ; MA 53 Stanford Univ; PH 62 (Sp Path & Aud) Stanford Univ; Retired, Private Practice, **SLP A F LM**

Rosen, Dr Jeanette K 11 Jendi Avenue, Bayview, New South Wales, Australia 2104, 2-477-9216, OB 59; MA 70 San Francisco St Univ; PH 77 (NS); Hd/Dept of Aud, Hornsby & Kuringai Hosp, **SLP A**

Rosen, Mrs Karen P 15 Tacoma Circle, Nashua, NH 03062, BA 79 Southern CT St Univ; ME 81 Northeastern Univ; Sp/Lang Path, MA Easter Seal Soc, **SLP**

Rosen, Dr Linda M 2111 Latham Street #307, Mountain View, CA 94040-1649, (415) 852-3251, BS 68 Northwestern Univ; MS 70 Univ of Pittsburgh - Pittsburgh; PH 77 (Aud/Sp Path) Univ of Pittsburgh - Pittsburgh; 86–Sp-Lang Path, Palo Alto VA Med Ctr, **SLP**

Rosen, Penny A 46 Remsem Street, Brooklyn Heights, NY 11201, (212) 875-3077, BA 70 Boston Univ; MA 80 NY Univ; Sp/Lang Path, Private Practice, **SLP**

Rosen, Perry Alan 10656 Caminito Chueco, San Diego, CA 92126, (619) 583-3111, BS 79 Univ of WI - Madison; MS 80 Univ of WI - Milwaukee; 88–Sp-Lang Path, Leir of San Diego, **SLP ACE**

Rosen, Rebecca G 77 Glendale Avenue, Albany, NY 12208-3121, (518) 445-4526, BA 75 Coll of Saint Rose; MA 76 Coll of Saint Rose; Sp-Lang Path, Commun Dis Cen Albany Med Cen, **SLP**

Rosen, Robert Gerald 29275 Northwestern Highway, Suite 208, Southfield, MI 48034, (313) 353-0310, BS 64 Wayne St Univ; ME 67 Wayne St Univ; 70–Sp-Lang Path, Rehabilitation Network, **SLP**

Rosen, Roberta A 3170 Val Verde Avenue, Long Beach, CA 90808, (714) 821-9440, BS 53 Univ of Rochester; MA 76 CA St Univ - Long Beach; SLP, Anaheim Union HS Dist, **SLP**

Rosen, Mrs Robin L 243 Hemlock Road, Wynnewood, PA 19096, (215) 275-6153, BA 73 Case Western Reserve Univ; MA 73 Case Western Reserve Univ; Aud, ENT Associates, **A**

Rosen, Sherrill S 70 Waterford Park, Williamsville, NY 14221, **SLP**

Rosen, Shirley Rona 1655 Flatbush Avenue, Apartment B1611, Brooklyn, NY 11210, (212) 270-2049, BA 60 CUNY - Brooklyn Coll; MA 63 CUNY - Brooklyn Coll; 66–Superv Sp/Lang Path, Downstate, **SLP**

Rosen, Mrs Stacey Jill 74 Bermuda Street, Atlantic Beach, NY 11509, (516) 371-1445, MS 85 Adelphi Univ; 87–Sp-Lang Path, Little Village Sch, **SLP**

Rosenbauer, Diane D 312 West North Street, Butler, PA 16001, (412) 282-6215, BS 75 Univ Southern MS-Hattiesburg; MS 76 Univ Southern MS-Hattiesburg; Sp-Lang Path, Private Practice, **SLP**

Rosenbaum, Alane A 8750 Point Park Drive, #1806, Houston, TX 77095, (713) 469-2152, BS 86 Baylor Univ; MS 87 Baylor Univ; 87–Sp-Lang Path, Cypress-Fairbanks ISD, **SLP**

Rosenbaum, Cynthia L 109 Denison Avenue, Elyria, OH 44035, (216) 322-8621, BA 77 OH St Univ; MA 79 OH St Univ; **SLP**

Rosenbaum, Mrs Elise Rosen 11 Putnam Avenue, Jericho, NY 11753, (516) PE1-8820, BA 73 Hofstra Univ; MA 74 Hofstra Univ; Sp-Lang Path, Bethpage Sp & Hrng Cen, **SLP**

Rosenbaum, Mrs Kathleen Margaret 2209 Hunt Club Drive, Castleton, NY 12033, (518) 479-4017, BS 79 SUNY - Center at Albany; MS 83 Coll of Saint Rose; **SLP**

Rosenbaum, Mrs Mary R 19214 Lomond Boulevard, Cleveland, OH 44122-5108, MA 77 Cleveland St Univ; Aud, Cleve Hearing & Speech Ctr, **A**

Rosenbaum, Robert Lee 71-49 Harrow Street, Forest Hills, NY 11375, (718) 520-7358, BA 52 Univ of IA; MA 53 Univ of IA; Assoc Dir Coord Grad Stu, Queens Coll CUNY, **SLP A**

Rosenbaum, Dr S Steve 11 Putnam Avenue, Jericho, NY 11753, (718) 470-8912, BA 49 CUNY - Brooklyn Coll; MA 57 Univ of MD - College Park; ED 76 (Aud) Columbia Univ Teachers Coll; Dir/Aud & SLP, Long Island Jewish Med Cen, **SLP A**

Rosenbek, John C VA Hospital, 2500 Overlook Terrace, Madison, WI 53705, (608) 256-1901, BA 66; MS 69; PH 70 (NS); Chief Aud & SLP, VA Hosp, **SLP F**

Rosenberg, Arthur L 8000 Oakdell Way, #10043, San Antonio, TX 78240, (512) 692-0935, BS 66 Towson St Univ; MS 73 Univ of Pittsburgh - Pittsburgh; Sp-Lang Path, Private Practice, **SLP**

Rosenberg, Barbara C 219 Lombardy, Sugar Land, TX 77478, (713) 494-2668, BS 68 Univ of TX - Austin; MA 70 Univ of Houston - Univ Park; **SLP**

Rosenberg, Mrs Barbara C 3730 North 32nd Terrace, Hollywood, FL 33021, (305) 963-3439, BS 70 Syracuse Univ; MA 71 NY Univ; **SLP**

Rosenberg, Edward S 41 Choir Lane, Westbury, NY 11590, (718) 470-8916, BA 81 SUNY - Center at Buffalo; MA 84 SUNY - Center at Buffalo; Aud, Long Island Jewish Med Ctr, **A**

Rosenberg, Gail Gegg 5465 Creeping Hammock Dr, Sarasota, FL 33581, (813) 922-0002, BS 70 Southeast MO St Univ; MS 78 Univ of South FL; 74–Aud, Sarasota Co Sch Bd, **A**

Rosenberg, Jacqueline 86 Vista Drive, Easton, CT 06612, (203) 852-9868, BA 49 CUNY - Brooklyn Coll; MA 62 CUNY - Brooklyn Coll; Sp-Lang Path, Norwalk Bd of Ed, **SLP**

Rosenberg, Jeanette 4917 41st Street N W, Washington, DC 20010, (202) 576-1348, BS 76 Univ of VA - Charlottesville; MS 77 Univ of MI - Ann Arbor; SLP, Private Practice, **SLP**

Rosenberg, Joan M 70 Riverside Drive, Apt 3-D, New York, NY 10024, (212) 947-5770, BA 74 SUNY - Coll at New Paltz; MS 76 Columbia Univ Teachers Coll; 85–Sp-Lang Path, UCP Assn of NYS, **SLP**

Rosenberg, Mrs Karen J 313 Hermleigh Road, Silver Spring, MD 20902, (301) 593-9008, BA 74 CUNY - Queens Coll; MA 75 Univ of Houston - Univ Park; Cl Superv, U of MD, **SLP**

Rosenberg, Mrs Lillian R 8700 S W 54th Avenue, Miami, FL 33143, (305) 666-6511, BA 77 Univ of Miami; MA 78 Univ of Miami; 88–Sp-Lang Path, Miami Chldn's Hosp, **SLP ACE**

Rosenberg, Lynn 3275 Victory Boulevard, Staten Island, NY 10314, (718) 761-2250, MS 87 2358; UCP, **SLP**

Rosenberg, Margo H 5017-5 Green Mountain Circle, Columbia, MD 21044, (301) 730-3314, BS 79 Ithaca Coll; MA 80 George Washington Univ; Sp/Lang Path, Private Practice, **SLP**

Rosenberg, Marion W 53 Starling Court, Roslyn, NY 11576, **SLP**

Rosenberg, Marylynn 9621 Reach Road, Potomac, MD 20854, (301) 279-0350, BA 73 SUNY - Center at Buffalo; MA 75 SUNY - Center at Buffalo; **SLP**

Rosenberg, Michaelle 119 Hards Lane, Lawrence, NY 11559, MS 86 Adelphi Univ; **A**

Rosenberg, Mrs Nancy Anne 7504 Brenish Drive, Gaithersburg, MD 20879, (301) 990-1324, BS 82 Univ of Hartford; MA 84 George Washington Univ; Sp-Lang Path, Montgomery County Public Schls, **SLP**

Rosenberg, Pamela H 3580 Castlehill Court, Tucker, GA 30084, **SLP**

Rosenberg, Robin 15 Briar Lane, Jericho, NY 11753, (516) 935-2462, BA 74 CUNY - City College; MS 80 Adelphi Univ; Sp-Lang Path, Private Practice, **SLP**

Rosenberg, Mrs Sandra M 8030 Hampton Boulevard, Apartment 211, North Lauderdale, FL 33068, BA 59 CUNY - Hunter Coll

Rosenberg, Sara W 704 John Barry Drive, Bryn Mawr, PA 19010, (215) 527-1342, BS 73 Syracuse Univ; MA 74 Case Western Reserve Univ; SLP, Elwyn Inst, **SLP**

Rosenberg, Mrs Taube Shiffman 34 Pool Drive, Roslyn, NY 11576, (516) 938-5400, MA 63 CUNY - Brooklyn Coll; SLP, Plainview Sch, **SLP**

Rosenberg, Terri Godlas 136 North Seventh Avenue, Highland Park, NJ 08904, (201) 572-4822, BA 75 Univ of CA - Los Angeles; MA 78 Univ of CA - Santa Barbara; Sp-Lang Path, Private Practice, **SLP ACE**

Rosenberg, Terry C 198 Winding River Road, Wellesley, MA 02181, (617) 431-7866, BS 72 Boston Univ; MA 74 NY Univ; **SLP**

Rosenberg, Trudy Lorraine 772 Yuba Street, Richmond, CA 94805, (415) 235-7000, BA 65 Univ of MI - Ann Arbor; MA 67 San Francisco St Univ; 76–Sp-Lang Path, Brookside Hosp/Doctors Hosp, **SLP**

Rosenberg-Alpert, Mrs Beth 4060 Santa Nella, San Diego, CA 92130, (619) 272-9023, BS 76 Northwestern Univ; MS 78 Emory Univ; Sp-Lang Path, San Diego City Schs, **SLP**

Rosenberg-Arps, Joanne R Box 46, West Newbury, VT 05085, (802) 429-2365, BS 63 Boston Univ; MA 68 Temple Univ; Consult for Hrng Impaired, State of Vermont, **A**

Rosenberg-Levi, Mrs Meta 240 West 98th Street #6H, New York, NY 10025, (212) 864-0070, BA 71 CUNY - City College; MS 72 Columbia Univ Teachers Coll; 87–Sp-Lang Path, Cooke Foundation for Spec Educ, **SLP**

Rosenberg-Stein, Mrs Jan 11252 S W 91 Terrace, Miami, FL 33176, (305) 279-1149, Sp-Lang Path, **SLP**

Rosenblat, Mrs Bonnie Smith 128 West Central, Titusville, PA 16354, (814) 827-3637, MS 84 Clarion Univ of PA; Aud, Dhr Diagnostics Inc, **A**

Rosenblatt, Mrs Ellen S 10430 S W 115th St, Miami, FL 33176, (305) 233-5545, OB 67 Univ of FL; ME 68 Univ of FL; Aud, Drs Cohen Harris Goldberg, **SLP**

Rosenblatt, Enid S 934 Ardis Drive, Fort Wayne, IN 46819, (219) 484-6636, BS 69 Univ of IL - Urbana; MS 71 Univ of MI - Ann Arbor; Asst Dir Rehab SLP, Parkview Mem Hosp, **SLP**

Rosenblatt, Mrs Erica W 2418 Gough Street, San Francisco, CA 94123, (415) 771-9168, BA 67 CUNY - Queens Coll; MA 71 SUNY - Center at Buffalo; OD 79 (NS) 4712; Attrny, Law Offices of John C Suttle, **SLP**

Rosenblatt, Janet Two Hawthorne Place, Boston, MA 02114, (617) 625-6600, BS 68 Emerson Coll; ME 73 Northeastern Univ; Sp-Lang Path, City of Somerville Sch Dept, **SLP**

Rosenblatt, Judith E 160 West Washington Street, #F4, Forestville, CT 06010, (203) 283-8787, BA 77 CUNY - Lehman Coll; MA 79 CUNY - Lehman Coll; Sp-Lang Path, Plymouth Pub Sch, **SLP**

Rosenblatt, Mrs Judith M 6060 Neddy Avenue, Woodland Hills, CA 91367, (213) 625-4183, MA 84 CA St Univ - Los Angeles; SLP, Los Angeles USD, **SLP**

Rosenblatt, Michael P 1409 Pennsylvania Avenue N, Minneapolis, MN 55427, (800) 328-0626, BA 75 Univ of CT; MA 76 MI St Univ; Mgr/Prof Serv, Dahlberg Electronics, Inc, **A**

Rosenblit-Braunstein, Lori Beth 888 North Beechwood Street, Philadelphia, PA 19130, (215) 236-9483, BS 85 Syracuse Univ; MA 87 George Washington Univ; 88–Sp-Lang Path, Mediplex Rehab Camden, **SLP**

Rosenbloom, Mrs Anita G 2823 Baneberry Court, Baltimore, MD 21209, (301) 358-7098, BS 73 Towson St Univ; MS 74 Towson St Univ; Sp-Lang Path, Baltimore Co Bd of Ed, **SLP**

Rosenblum, Judith Fiestal 3300 S W Evergreen Lane, Portland, OR 97201, (503) 225-1963, BA 71 NY Univ; MS 74 Portland St Univ; Cl Practicum Supvr, Portland St U, **SLP**

Rosenblum, Melanie R 1099 Bridlewood Trail, Oakville, ON, Canada L6M 2L1, (416) 847-3521, MS 86 McGill Univ - Quebec; 88–Sp-Lang Path, St Joseph's Hosp, **SLP**

Rosenblum, Mrs Michele 1211 East Broadway #C11, Hewlett, NY 11557, (718) 945-7100, BA 79 CUNY - Queens Coll; MA 81 CUNY - Queens Coll; Aud, Peninsula Hosp Cen, **A**

Rosendahl, Pamela DePonty 2728 37th Street N W, Gig Harbor, WA 98335, (206) 543-8799, BA 72 Univ of WA; MS 75 Univ of WA; Sp-Lang Path, U of WA, **SLP**

Rosenfeld, Carol Dee 3016 Romaric Court #G, Baltimore, MD 21209, (301) 683-3240, BA 65 CUNY - Brooklyn Coll; MS 66 Univ of MI - Ann Arbor; Sp-Lang Path, Baltimore Co Bd of Ed, **SLP**

Rosenfeld, Mrs Cathy Ann 27 Andrews, Cheektowaga, NY 14225, (716) 894-3825, BS 84 SUNY - Coll at Buffalo; MS 86 SUNY - Coll at Buffalo; 85–Sp-Lang Path, Erie I BOCES, **SLP**

Rosenfeld, Mrs Diane S 3521 Singers Glen Drive, Olney, MD 20832, (301) 774-1930, BA 70 Univ of MD - College Park; MA 74 Catholic Univ of America; 88–Sp-Lang Path, Mont Primary Ach Ctr, **SLP**

Rosenfeld, Laura S 720 Paseo Potrerro, Green Valley, AZ 85614-9740, (602) 625-6540, BA 39 CUNY - Hunter Coll; MA 40 Univ of IA; **SLP LM**

Rosenfeld, Mrs Miriam Siegel Montgomery Speech & Lang Serv, 12501 St James Road, Rockville, MD 20850, (301) 340-0360, BA 71 Univ of MD - College Park; MA 72 Univ of MD - College Park; 84–Director, Montgomery Speech & Lang Serv, **SLP ACE**

Rosenfeld, Mrs Rene Gail 143 Truman Road, Newton, MA 02159, (617) 969-2595, BS 81 Univ of MA - Amherst; MS 83 Boston Univ; Sp-Lang Path, Medfield Public Schools, **SLP**

Rosenfeld, Ronni J 4545 Niagara Avenue, San Diego, CA 92107, (619) 588-3053, BA 70 Univ of TX - El Paso; MA 72 Univ of TX - El Paso; Sp-Lang Path, Cajon Valley Sch Dist, **SLP**

Rosenfield, David B Stuttering Center, Department Of Neurology, Baylor Coll Of Medicine, Houston, TX 77030, MS

Rosenfield, Helaine W 185 Winslow Drive, Stoughton, MA 02072, **SLP**

Rosenfield, Dr Irma B 6 Lamson Place, Cambridge, MA 02139, (617) 358-7401, BS 64 PA St Univ - Univ Park; MA 68 Temple Univ; ED 87 (Applied Psycholinguistics) Boston Univ; Sp-Lang Path, Wayland Public Schools, **SLP**

Rosengarten, Amy 39-2B Richmond Boulevard, Ronkonkoma, NY 11779, (516) 588-7886, BS 86 Ithaca Coll; MS 87 Columbia Univ Teachers Coll; 88–Sp-Lang Path, Frank Volz & John Amato Ctr for Comm Disorders

Rosengarten, Robert E Ctr For Hearing Services, 7714 Bay Parkway, Brooklyn, NY 11214, (718) 236-0010, BA 69 SUNY - Center at Albany; MA 76 CUNY - Brooklyn Coll; Aud, Cen for Hrng Servs, **A**

Rosengarten, Mrs Susan H Center For Hearing Services, 7714 Bay Parkway, Brooklyn, NY 11214, (718) 236-0010, BA 73 CUNY - Brooklyn Coll; MS 78 Adelphi Univ; Aud, Cen for Hrng Servs, **A**

Rosenkranz, Diane F 12 Hartford Lane, White Plains, NY 10603, (914) 592-4417, BA 76 CUNY - Lehman Coll; MA 78 CUNY - Lehman Coll; Sp-Lang Path, Ruth Taylor I-Hawthorne NY, **SLP**

Rosenman, Dr Patricia 3425 Garrison Street N W, Washington, DC 20008, (202) 966-8740, BA 56 Univ of MI - Ann Arbor; MA 59 Stanford Univ; PH 82 (NS) American Univ; **SLP**

Rosenmeyer, Debra D 75 Knightsbridge Road #2-E, Great Neck, NY 11021, (718) 470-7551, BS 73 Boston Univ; MA 75 Hofstra Univ; Aud, LI Jewish Med Ctr/ENT, **A**

Rosenquist, Mrs Teresa Davis 3954 60th #79, San Diego, CA 92115, (619) 583-6166, BS 79 Abilene Christian Univ; MA 81 Univ of KS; Sp-Lang Path, Sp Path Services, **SLP**

Rosen-Rudin, Robin Amy 6540 North 7th Avenue #45, Phoenix, AZ 85013, (602) 246-2158, BA 80 Long Island U - CW Post Ctr; OM 84 AZ St Univ; Sp-Lang Path, Private Practice, **SLP**

Rosenshein, Sandra 20 Caveswood Lane, Owings Mills, MD 21117, **SLP A**

Rosenstein, Mrs Beverly B 32 Saddlewood Drive, Hillsdale, NJ 07642, (201) 599-7262, BA 43 CUNY - Hunter Coll; 68–Sp-Lang Path, River Dell Reg Sch Dist, **SLP LM**

Rosenstein, Dr Joseph 332 M Street S W, Washington, DC 20024, (202) 732-1176, BS 55 Washington Univ; MA 56 Washington Univ; PH 59 (NS) Washington Univ; Ed Prog Spec, US Dept of Ed, **A**

Rosenstein, Mrs Tamara P 624 West Upsal Street, Philadelphia, PA 19119, (215) 848-7659, BS 68 Univ of WI - Madison; MA 70 Univ of CT; **SLP**

Rosenstock, Mrs Arlene S 1323 East 24th Street, Brooklyn, NY 11210, (212) 252-9818, BA 74 CUNY - Brooklyn Coll; MS 77 CUNY - Brooklyn Coll; Sp-Lang Path, Jewish Ctr for Spec Educ, **SLP**

Rosenthal, Amy Lynne 3980 South East Francis, Portland, OR 97202, (503) 280-5757, BS 74 Univ of TX - Austin; MA 75 Univ of KS; Aud, Prof for Deaf/Portland Pub Sch, **A**

Rosenthal, Mrs Carolyn M 39 Joelson Court, Albany, NY 12209, (518) 462-6222, BA 47 CUNY - Queens Coll; MS 61 SUNY - Coll at Buffalo; Superv Sp-Lang Path, Capital Area Sp Cen Inc, **SLP**

Rosenthal, Felice Marsha 1386 Edcris Road, Yorktown Heights, NY 10598, BS 62 Emerson Coll; MS 68 NY Univ; SLP, Southern Westchester BOCES, **SLP**

Rosenthal, Judee Anne 9702 Cisco Street, Los Angeles, CA 90034, (213) 838-4857, **SLP**

Rosenthal, Mrs Laurie Shcolnek 4115 Winterset Lane, West Bloomfield, MI 48033, (313) 851-3309, BA 70 Univ of MI - Ann Arbor; MS 71 Univ of MI - Ann Arbor; Sp-Lang Path, Private Practice, **SLP**

Rosenthal, Mrs Loren B 32-11 Rosalie Street, Fair Lawn, NJ 07410, (201) 891-8099, BA 75 William Paterson Coll; MA 78 Montclair St Coll; SLP, Wyckoff Board of Education, **SLP**

Rosenthal, Mrs Lori Sternig 23 Percheron Lane, Roslyn Heights, NY 11577, (212) 390-9470, MA 77 NY Univ; BA 76 Case Western Reserve Univ; Aud, Staten I Hosp, **A**

Rosenthal, Marjorie Hodes 49 Carleton Street, Newton Corner, MA 02158, (617) 332-8336, BA 78 Univ of CA - Santa Barbara; MA 82 Case Western Reserve Univ; **SLP**

Rosenthal, Mary D 18206 Spellbrook Drive, Houston, TX 77084, (713) 463-3584, BS 78 Univ of GA; ME 79 Univ of GA; **SLP**

Rosenthal, Michael J 21742 Fernleaf Drive, El Toro, CA 92630, (714) 261-2123, BA 75 Univ of Rochester; MA 77 Northwestern Univ; Sp Prog Man, Texas Instruments Inc, **SLP**

Rosenthal, Phyllis H 112 East 84th Street, New York, NY 10028, (212) 288-6262, BA 74 CUNY - Brooklyn Coll; MS 76 CUNY - Brooklyn Coll; Aud, Private Practice, **A**

Rosenthal, Robin Shari 505 East 82nd Street #1-J, New York, NY 10028, (212) 650-6153, MS 86 FL St Univ; SLP, Mt Sinai Hospital, **SLP**

Rosenthal, Dr Ruth Dorothy 77 7 Avenue Apartment 15M, New York, NY 10011, (212) 725-3184, BA 66 CUNY - Brooklyn Coll; MS 67 CUNY - Brooklyn Coll; PH 72 (NS) CUNY - Grad Sch & Univ Cntr; Assoc Prof, Baruch Coll Cuny, **SLP A**

Rosenthal, Stephen M 594 Ramapo Road, Teaneck, NJ 07666-1804, (212) 920-5690, BA 75 CUNY - Brooklyn Coll; MS 76 CUNY - Brooklyn Coll; 87–Dir-Prog Dev, Montefiore Med Ctr, **A**

Rosenthal, Susan J Wheaton Plaza, South Annex, 11160 Viers Mill Road, Wheaton, MD 20902, (301) 949-8070, BA 79 Univ of MD - College Park; MA 82 Univ of MD - College Park; 88–Sp-Lang Path, The Hearing Ctr, **SLP**

Rosenthal, Susan Richards 14900 Dinsdale Drive, Silver Spring, MD 20906, (301) 598-9245, BA 84 Univ of MD - College Park; MS 85 Univ of NC - Chapel Hill; 87–Sp-Lang Path, M C PS, **SLP**

Rosenthal, Dr William Sidney Dept Comm Science & Disorders, California State Univ, Hayward, CA 94542, (445) 881-3233, BA 61 Univ of Chicago; MA 66 George Washington Univ; PH 70 (Sp & Hrng Science/Psychology) Stanford Univ; Prof, CA St U-Hayward, **SLP**

Rosenthal-Tanzer, Mrs Jo 7935 SW Willowmere Drive, Portland, OR 97225, (503) 228-6479, BS 76 Portland St Univ; MA 77 Univ of the Pacific; 84–Director/Sp-Lang Path, Portland Cen for Hrng & Sp, **SLP**

Rosenwasser, Linda Tucker 3383 Swan Drive, Vineland, NJ 08360, (609) 696-6757, BA 74 Univ of MD - College Park; MA 77 Trenton St Coll; Sp-Lang Path, Vineland Dev Cen Hosp, **SLP**

Rosenwasser, Marian Bellevue Psychiatric Hospital, PS106 21st Floor, 1st Avenue & 27th Street, New York, NY 10016, (212) 865-4269, BA 54 CUNY - Brooklyn Coll; MA 61 CUNY - Brooklyn Coll; Sp-Lang Path, NYC Bd of Ed, **SLP**

Rosenwinkel, Deborah A P O Box 2007, Kearney, NE 68847, (308) 237-5927, BA 74 Kearney St Coll; MS 77 Kearney St Coll; MA 78 Univ of Northern CO; Aud/Sp-Lang Path, Ed Serv Unit #10, **SLP A**

Rosenzweig, Betsy J 1822 East 3RDSTREET, Duluth, MN 55812, (715) 394-0630, OB 77 Univ of MN - Duluth; MS 78 Univ of WI - Stevens Point; Sp-Lang Path, Superior Public Sch, **SLP**

Rosenzweig, Lisa P 14-35 212 Street, Bayside, NY 11360, (718) 428-5975, BA 81 SUNY - Coll at Oneonta; MS 84 CUNY - Brooklyn Coll; 88–Sp-Lang Path/Consult, United Odd Fellow & Rebekah Home, **SLP**

Rosenzweig, Luann B 81 Sylvan Hills Road, Guilford, CT 06437, (203) 624-3140, BS 74 SUNY - Coll at Fredonia; MS 81 Southern CT St Univ; Sp-Lang Path, Gaylord/Yale New Haven Rehab Center, **SLP**

Rosenzweig, Mrs Margaret C 3511 Green Fields, Sugar Land, TX 77479, MA 70 Univ of Houston - Univ Park; Sp-Lang Path, Fort Bend ISD, **SLP**

Rosenzweig, Meri Sue 1531 Meadows Circle West, Boynton Beach, FL 33462, (407) 736-5447, BA 81 Univ of FL; MA 84 Univ of FL; 87–Sp-Lang Path, Bethesda Memorial Hosp, **SLP ACE**

Rosenzweig, Mrs Sue D 5522 Kuldell, Houston, TX 77096, (713) 771-2461, BA 60 Vanderbilt Univ; MA 66 Univ of Houston - Univ Park; Co-Dir, Southwest Sp, **SLP A**

Rosete, Mrs Louise 48-50 188th Street, Flushing, NY 11365, (212) 430-0479, BA 75 CUNY - Queens Coll; MA 77 Hofstra Univ; Sp-Lang Path, Bronx Dev Serv, **SLP**

Rosher, Ellen M 5900 East Thomas #E121, Scottsdale, AZ 85251, (602) 267-0055, BS 76 Univ of AZ; MS 78 Univ of AZ; Sp-Lang Path, Scottsdale USD, **SLP**

Rosica, Lenore M 4855 East Avenue, Clarence, NY 14031, (716) 759-6875, BA 44 Coll Misericordia; MA 51 Northwestern Univ; Sp-Lang Path, Private Practice, **SLP**

Rosica, Sebastian Joseph St Marys School For The Deaf, 2253 Main Street, Buffalo, NY 14214, (716) 834-7200, BS 48 Canisius Coll; ME 50 SUNY - Center at Buffalo; MA 51 Northwestern Univ; Dir/Aud Servs, St Marys Sch for the Deaf, **SLP A**

Rosin, Margaret Mary 1515 Vilas Avenue, Madison, WI 53711, (608) 262-6471, BS 71 Marquette Univ; MS 74 Univ of WI - Madison; Sp-Lang Path, Univ of WI/Dept of Commun Dis, **SLP**

Rosinski, Joyce E HC 79 Box 263, Orland, ME 04472, (207) 469-3266, MS 70 Univ of IA; SLP, Bucksport Ele Schl, **SLP**

Rosinski, Mrs Patrice Ann 3432 Indian Peak Drive, Lake Havasu City, AZ 86403, (602) 855-3891, MA 83 CA St Univ - Chico; Dir Sp-Lang Path, Havasu Regional Hosp, **SLP**

Roskin, Mrs Lessa C 1 Avizohar, Beit Hakaram, Jerusalem, Israel 96267, BS 64 Northwestern Univ; 85–Sp-Lang Path, Alyn Rehab Ctr for Hndcpd Chld, **SLP**

Rosko, Mrs Sue A 313 Ferguson Road, Marshall, MI 49068, (616) 781-4707, BS 72 Western MI Univ; MA 76 Western MI Univ; Sp-Lang Path, Children's Therapy Ctr-Battle Ck Health Sys, **SLP**

Rosner, Sharon E 226 East 29th Street, New York, NY 10016, (212) 724-2800, **A**

Rosoff, Nancy E 20 Florence Circle, Medway, MA 02053, Director, Little Peoples School, **A**

Rosoff-Foster, Mrs Beverly 1730 Chelsea Way, Roseville, CA 95661, (916) 783-9168, BA 78 CA St Univ - Sacramento; MA 80 Univ of the Pacific; **SLP**

Rosowski, Mrs Jean Trelawny Audiology Services Inc, 90 Concord Avenue, Belmont, MA 02178, (617) 484-8700, BS 75 SUNY - Coll at Geneseo; MS 77 Gallaudet Coll; Aud, Audiology Services Inc, **A**

Rospenda, Mrs Sharon 3264 South 93rd Street, Milwaukee, WI 53227, (414) 464-8230, BS 76 Marquette Univ; MS 77 Marquette Univ; Sp-Lang Path, Milwaukee Pub Schs, **SLP**

Ross, Amanda M 9863 Belleford Court, Cincinnati, OH 45242, (607) 432-7230, BS 81 Bowling Green St Univ; MA 82 Bowling Green St Univ; Sp-Lang Path, Mercy Hosp, **SLP**

Ross, Anne Louise Box 434, Garibaldi Hi, BC, Canada V0N 1T0, (604) 898-4439, BA 75 Univ of WA; MA 77 Univ of WA; SLP, Bc Ministry of Health, **SLP**

Ross, Barbara Ann 916 East 4th Street, Dover, OH 44622, (216) 823-4640, BA 84 Southern CT St Univ; MA 86 Kent St Univ; Sp-Lang Path, Tuscarawas Co Hlth Dist, **SLP**

Ross, Becky L 5018 Presidio, Garland, TX 75043, (214) 285-8901, BS 74 Univ of North TX; MS 75 Univ of North TX; Sp-Lang Path, Dallas ISD, **SLP**

Ross, Brenda K 4228 Chess Drive, Anchorage, AK 99508-5631, **SLP**

Ross, Carol Frances 6845 Southwest Ventura Dr, Tigard, OR 97223, (503) 245-6842, BA 60 Univ of WA; MS 85 Portland St Univ; Sp-Lang Path, Good Samaritan Hosp, **SLP A**

Ross, Cindy A 89 Live Oak Avenue, Fairfax, CA 94930, (415) 459-3134, BA 78 San Francisco St Univ; MS 82 San Francisco St Univ; Aud, Kaiser Permanent Med Cen, **A**

Ross, Clara Murch RR 1 Box 201, Casco, ME 04015, (207) 345-3093, BA 77 Univ of ME - Orono; MA 79 Univ of ME - Orono; Dir Spec Educ, Sch Union 29, **SLP**

Ross, Cynthia Marie 3325 NW 52nd Terrace, Gainesville, FL 32606, (904) 376-4780, BS 81 CO St Univ; MA 83 MI St Univ; Aud, U of FL-Shands Tchng Hosp, **A**

Ross, Mrs Dana 3075 Woodland Hills Drive, Apartment 613, Colorado Springs, CO 80918, BS 83 Eastern NM Univ; MS 86 Eastern NM Univ; **SLP**

Ross, David Hugh 41 Werner Road, Clifton Park, NY 12065, (518) 664-6396, BS 71 SUNY - Coll at Buffalo; MS 74 SUNY - Center at Albany; 81–Exec Dir, Helping Hands Sch Sp Lang & Hrng Cl

Ross, Debbie Faye 250 Vilma Drive, Oakville, ON, Canada L6L 3J7, (416) 878-2851, BS 81 Boston Univ; MA 83 SUNY - Center at Buffalo; Aud, Ernest C Drury Sch-Hrng Hndcpd, **A**

Ross, Deborah 825 Forest, Evanston, IL 60202, (312) 492-9862, BS 75 Univ of IA; MA 76 Western MI Univ; 88–Reach Rehab Program Director, Manor HealthCare Corp, **SLP**

Ross, Mrs Deborah G 170 Sotoyome, Suite B, Santa Rosa, CA 95405, (707) 575-1468, MS 75 CA St Univ - Sacramento; 85–Dir, Ross and Assoc, **SLP**

Ross, Diane B 110 Highland, Flemingsburg, KY 41041, (606) 845-7531, BA 73 Western MI Univ; MS 74 Vanderbilt Univ; Sp-Lang Path, Fleming County Schs, **SLP**

Ross, Diane C Nevada Communication Dis Serv, 505 South Arlington, Suite 206, Reno, NV 89509, (702) 329-5108, BS 71 Univ of NV - Reno; MS 75 Univ of NV - Reno; Dir, Nevada Communication Svcs, **SLP ACE**

Ross, Dona R P O Box 625, Metlakatla, AK 99926, (907) 886-7492, BA 72 Univ of Northern CO; MA 73 Univ of Northern CO; SLP, Annette Island Schools, **SLP**

Ross, Mrs Dorothy E 3530 Ferry Street, Eugene, OR 97405, BA 42 1332; MA 45 Syracuse Univ; **SLP LM**

Ross, Elva Ann 6519 Jesse Jackson Avenue, Hillsdale, MO 63121, (314) 434-7924, BA 77 IN Univ - Bloomington; MS 79 Univ of Louisville; Sp-Lang Path, Normandy Sch Dist, **SLP**

Ross, Dr Florence 1871 San Pedro Avenue, Berkeley, CA 94707, (415) 798-7466, BA 57 CUNY - Hunter Coll; MS 60 PA St Univ - Univ Park; ED 82 (NS) Univ of San Francisco; Sp/Lang Path, Contra Costa Co Offi of Ed, **SLP**

Ross, Francie 3116 Roberta Drive N W, Atlanta, GA 30327, (404) 233-5332, BA 45 Univ of IA; MA 47 Univ of IA; Sp-Lang Path, Atlanta Sp Sch Inc, **SLP**

Ross, Mrs Francine C 3442 Attica Road, Olympia Fields, IL 60461, (312) 748-5644, BS 72 SUNY - Center at Albany; MA 76 SUNY - Center at Buffalo; 87–Sp-Lang Path, Southlake Sp & Hrng Ctr Inc, **SLP ACE**

Ross, Dr Frona S 30 Tucker Creek Road, Conway, AR 72032, (501) 327-1510, BA 73 CUNY - Brooklyn Coll; MS 74 Rutgers St Univ - Newark; PH 83 (NS) FL St Univ; Asst Prof, **SLP**

Ross, Gail 3120 Oakdell Lane, Studio City, CA 91604, (213) 654-0770, BA; MA 75; SLP, Private Practice, **SLP**

Ross, Harriet Pearlston 1425 Stanford Street #7, Santa Monica, CA 90404, (213) 453-5424, BA 64 Univ of CA - Los Angeles; MA 79 CA St Univ - Northridge; Sp-Lang Path, Los Angeles Co Supt of Sch, **SLP**

Ross, Mrs Helen 9 Thomas Drive, Storrs, CT 06268, (203) 429-9391, BA 58 CUNY - City College; MA 60 Stanford Univ; 81–Sp-Lang Path, Willington Bd of Ed, **SLP**

Ross, Ilene Simon 3930 North Pine Grove, Apartment 2213, Chicago, IL 60613, BS 72 Univ of IL - Urbana; MS 73 PA St Univ - Univ Park; Sp-Lang Path, Chicago Bd of Ed, **SLP**

Ross, Dr Irwin 1103 North Bellevue, Hastings, NE 68901, (402) 463-5611, BS 62 Western MI Univ; MA 67 Univ of WI - Madison; ED 73 (NS) Univ of IL - Urbana; Sp-Lang Path, Ed Serv Unit #9, **SLP**

Ross, Jean C 92 Edgerton Street, Rutland, VT 05701, (802) 773-7301, BS 32 Syracuse Univ; MA 37 Univ of IA; **SLP LM**

Ross, Jennifer Ruth 210 N W 201st Street, Seattle, WA 98177-2012, (213) 625-4183, MS 81 Univ of WA; SLP, LA USD, **SLP**

Ross, Jill B 19454 Edinburgh, South Bend, IN 46614, (219) 284-7312, BS 68 IN Univ - Bloomington; MS 70 Emerson Coll; Sp-Lang Path, Mem Hosp, **SLP**

Ross, Jo-Ann F 337 Stevens Street, Lowell, MA 01851, (617) 458-1411, BA 70 Temple Univ; MA 72 Temple Univ; Sp/Lang Path, Private Practice, **SLP**

Ross, Mrs Joann Horner 1305 22 Street West, Williston, ND 58801-3138, (701) 572-6757, BS 74 Minot St Univ; MS 77 Minot St Univ; Sp-Lang Path, Wilmac Spec Educ, **SLP**

Ross, Karen Pontius 211 Fox Street, Sidney, NY 13838, (607) 432-8860, BA 80 SUNY - Coll at Cortland; MS 81 Ithaca Coll; Sp/Lang Path, Otsego Regl Cen, **SLP**

Ross, Mrs Karen Young 618 Clemmer Avenue, Cincinnati, OH 45219, (513) 421-6792, BS 78 Miami Univ - Oxford; MA 86 Miami Univ - Oxford; 85–Sp-Lang Path, Hamilton Co Bd of MR/DD, **SLP**

Ross, Kate D Rd 3 Box 57, Montpelier, VT 05602, (802) 223-5656, BS 78 Bowling Green St Univ; MS 87 Univ of VT; 87–Sp-Lang Path, Worcester Elem Sch, **SLP**

Ross, Mrs Lajuana Dee 669 Dutchmans Drive, Hermitage, TN 37076, BS 75 Univ of North TX; MS 77 Univ of North TX; Sp-Lang Path, Nashville Metro Schs, **SLP**

Ross, Linda Jane 107 Westminster, St Clairsville, OH 43950, (304) 242-3430, BS 82 Univ of Houston - Univ Park; MA 85 Univ of Houston - Univ Park; Sp-Lang Path, Ohio County Schools, **SLP**

Ross, Lori Linwood 8413 Westmont Terrace, Bethesda, MD 20817, (301) 469-0424, BA 84 George Washington Univ; MA 85 Kean Coll of NJ; 88–Sp-Lang Path, Ridley & Fill Sp & Lang Assoc, **SLP A**

Ross, Lori Louise 307 S Hoover Avenue, Louisville, CO 80027, (303) 427-8484, BA 82 Augustana Coll; MA 86 Univ of CO - Boulder; **SLP**

Ross, Mrs Lynn E 71 Pheasant Run Drive, Nepean, ON, Canada K2J 2R3, (613) 737-2372, BS 78 Univ of Western Ontario; OM 81 Hahneman Medical Coll; 84–Sp-Lang Path, Childrens Hosp of En Ontario, **SLP**

Ross, Dr M Gerlene 84 Brookline Avenue, Albany, NY 12203, (518) 747-3949, BA 65 SUNY - Center at Albany; MA 69 SUNY - Center at Albany; PH 73 (NS) Univ of Pittsburgh - Pittsburgh; Ch Bureau of Res & Innovation, NY St Ed Dept, **SLP**

Ross, Mrs Margaret M 39 Capitolian Boulevard, Rockville Centre, NY 11570, (516) 796-6608, BA 77 CUNY - Queens Coll; MA 78 Hofstra Univ; Sp-Lang Path, Manhasset Pub Sch, **SLP**

Ross, Dr Mark 9 Thomas Drive, Storrs, CT 06268, (203) 425-6688, BA 57 CUNY - Brooklyn Coll; MA 58 CUNY - Brooklyn Coll; PH 62 (Aud) Stanford Univ; Consult Adj Prof Aud, City Univ of NY, **A F**

Ross, Mary Anne 2338 Admiral Street, Aliquippa, PA 15001, (412) 787-2350, BA 84 Loyola Coll; MA 86 Univ of Pittsburgh - Pittsburgh; **SLP**

Ross, Michele Ilene 93 LEXINGTON Street, Waltham, MA 02154, (617) 891-9521, BS 76 Ithaca Coll; MS 81 Emerson Coll; Sp-Lang Path, Framingham Public Schools, **SLP**

Ross, Mrs Nancy D 6100 Fairlane Drive, Clarence Center, NY 14032, 87–Sp-Lang Path, Lang Dev Prog, **SLP**

Ross, Mrs Nancy M 13 Sunset Boulevard, Massapequa, NY 11758, (516) 541-1535, BA 74; MA 75 Hofstra Univ; Sp-Lang Path, Private Practice, **SLP**

Ross, Mrs Pamela P 1405 Pinehurst, Edmond, OK 73034, (405) 348-9645, BS 72 Univ of NM; SLP, Moore Public Schools, **SLP**

Ross, Rebecca Gould Speech And Hearing Center, P O Box 4384, Fort Walton Beach, FL 32549, (904) 243-8741, BA 76 Auburn Univ - Auburn; MS 77 Auburn Univ - Auburn; Dir, Sp & Hrng of Ft Walton Bch, **SLP ACE**

Ross, Mrs Rhonda E 853 Victoria Place, Glendale, MO 63122, (314) 965-4157, BA 76 Univ of MO - Columbia; MA 78 Univ of MO - Columbia; **SLP**

Ross, Rhonda F 2 Birch Road, Staten Island, NY 10301, **SLP**

Ross, Mrs Rita Waltz R R 3 Box 10-A, Vevay, IN 47043, (812) 537-1738, BS 85 Purdue Univ - West Lafayette; MS 87 Purdue Univ - West Lafayette; **SLP**

Ross, Mrs Sharon Elser #6 Sedgefield, Conway, AR 72032, (501) 743-2011, OB 78 Univ of Central AR; MS 82 Univ of AR - Little Rock; Sp-Lang Path, Conway Schools, **SLP**

Ross, Susan K 9020 Clipper Court North, Indianapolis, IN 46256, (317) 842-7580, MS 77 IN St Univ - Terre Haute; Sp-Lang Path, Msd of Warreu Township, **SLP**

Ross, Suzanne L 997 Beacon Street, Newton Center, MA 02159, (617) 969-2142, BA 64 Univ of CT; MS 65 Univ of WI - Madison; OM 78 Boston Univ; 87–Sp-Lang Path, Brookline PS, **SLP**

Ross, Teresa Annette 413-D Honey Locust Lane, Birmingham, AL 35209, BS 84 Murray St Univ; MS 85 Murray St Univ; Sp-Lang Path, The Children's Hosp of Alabama, **SLP**

Ross, Theresa L 735 Bitterroot, Pocatello, ID 83201, (208) 234-0777, BS 79 ID St Univ; MS 81 ID St Univ; 84–Sp-Lang Path, Pocatello Reg Med Cen, **SLP**

Ross, Vicki K HHC 6ASG, Box 414, APO New York, NY 09154-3345, BS 64 Univ of KS; MA 81 Western MI Univ; Sp/Lang Path, Except Family Member Serv, **SLP ACE**

Rossa, Denise Marie 11455 Nava Place, Norwalk, CA 90650, (714) 595-1221, BA 81 CA St Univ - Los Angeles; MS 86 Univ of Redlands; **A**

Rossborough, Meredith Morgan 5 South Hill Circle, Rochester, NY 14606, (716) 271-0680, BS 81 Elmira Coll; MA 82 SUNY - Coll at Geneseo; 84–Sp-Lang Path, Hrng & Sp Ctr of Rochester, **SLP**

Ross-Brennan, Laurie 1705 Camino Gusto N W, Albuquerque, NM 87107, (505) 345-0030, BA 80 Univ of NM; MS 81 Univ of NM; Sp-Lang Path, Private Practice, **SLP ACE**

Ross-Crabtree, Mrs Vicki L 3535 North 49th Street, Milwaukee, WI 53216, (414) 871-0406, BS 74 Bowling Green St Univ; OM 83 Univ of WI - Milwaukee; MA 75 Bowling Green St Univ; 87–Sp-Lang Path, Anew Health Care Assoc, **SLP**

Rosseel, Lorraine 21 Free Street, Hingham, MA 02043, **SLP**

Rossetti, Mrs Colleen Sneddon 94 Park Avenue, Flemington, NJ 08822, (201) 638-6702, BA 80 Univ of VT; MA 85 Trenton St Coll; Sp-Lang Path, Highbridge School Dist, **SLP**

Rossetti, Dr Louis M Speech & Hearing Clinic, Arts & Communication Ctr, Univ Of WI Oshkosh, Oshkosh, WI 54901, (414) 424-2421, BA 70 Northern MI Univ; MA 72 Northern IL Univ - De Kalb; PH 78 (NS) Southern IL Univ -Carbondale; Coor of Com Dis Program, Univ of WI Oshkosh, **SLP**

Rossetti, Marybeth 3905 West Grove Avenue, McHenry, IL 60050, (815) 344-5000, **A**

Rossettie, Kathleen Santilli 203 Pritchard Avenue, Corning, NY 14830, (607) 962-6930, MA 85 SUNY - Coll at Geneseo; **SLP**

Rossi, Mrs Bernice Liberatore 23 Dresser Avenue, Dedham, MA 02026, (617) 326-3699, **SLP**

Rossi, Carla Anne 801 83rd Avenue North #107, St Petersburg, FL 33702, (813) 576-7796, BS 85 IL St Univ - Normal; MS 87 IL St Univ - Normal; 88–Sp-Lang Path, Bayfront Med Ctr

Rossi, Carolyn S 251 E Lk Samn Shorelane N E, Redmond, WA 98052, (206) 821-3388, BA 77 Univ of the Pacific; MS 79 Univ of WA; SLP, Childhaven, **SLP**

Rossi, Edith A 304 East 62nd Street, New York, NY 10021, BA 70 Marymount Coll; MA 73 CUNY - Hunter Coll; Sp-Lang Path, NYC Bd Ed, **SLP**

Rossi, Mrs Leisha Moyer 127 Victoria Lane, Wyomissing, PA 19610, (717) 393-0425, BS 82 PA St Univ - Univ Park; MS 84 Purdue Univ - West Lafayette; Sp-Lang Path, Easter Seal Rehabilitation Ctr, **SLP**

Rossi, Louise F 4215 Nez Perce, Coeur d'Alene, ID 83814, (208) 773-1508, BS 69 Univ of ID; MA 76 WA St Univ; Sp-Lang Path, Post Falls Sch Dist #273, **SLP**

Rossio-Edwards, Mrs Patricia A 4670 Braeburn S E, Grand Rapids, MI 49506, (616) 242-0425, BA 80 MI St Univ; MA 81 MI St Univ; 87–Clin Coord, Mary Free Bed Hosp & Rehab Cen, **SLP**

Rossman, Harry Richard 7610 Penn Avenue South, Apartment 201, Richfield, MN 55423, (612) 884-2499, BA 68 San Francisco St Univ; MS 84 Univ of WI - River Falls; **A**

Rossman, Mrs Katharine Crews 3122 Northway Drive, Baltimore, MD 21234-7825, (301) 288-7088, BS 84 Towson St Univ; MS 85 Towson St Univ; 86–Sp-Lang Path, Balt Co PS, **SLP**

Rossman, Reva N 1315 Murdoch Road, Pittsburgh, PA 15217, (213) 825-6147, BA 72 SUNY - Center at Buffalo; MS 74 Univ of MI - Ann Arbor; **A**

Rossman, Robin A c/o Rossman Antiques, 425 Boehmian Way, Freestone, CA 95472-9579, (415) 461-1519, BS 74 CA St Univ - Hayward; MA 76 Univ of Denver; Sp-Lang Path, Private Practice, **SLP**

Rossman, Mrs Terri L 6 Horizen Road #1106, Fort Lee, NJ 07024, (201) 224-2807, BS 79 Ithaca Coll; MS 82 Boston Univ; Sp-Lang Path, Private Practice, **SLP**

Rossmeisl, Mrs Kathryn L 1022 Maryland Avenue, Schenectady, NY 12308, (518) 462-6222, BA 72 SUNY - Coll at New Paltz; MA 73 Hofstra Univ; Sp-Lang Path, Schenectady City Schs, **SLP**

Rosso, Audrey P 2909 N W 65th Avenue, Margate, FL 33063, (305) 972-4698, BA 77 FL Atlantic Univ; MS 81 Univ of South FL; 81–Sp-Lang Path, Sch Bd of Broward County, **SLP**

Rosso, Dr Louis J Dept Of Speech, Winthrop College, Rock Hill, SC 29733, (803) 323-2379, BS 67 Kent St Univ; MA 68 Kent St Univ; PH 71 (Sp-Hrng Science) OH St Univ; 71–SLP, Winthrop Coll, **SLP**

Rosson, Grace L 1400 Geary Boulevard #2009, San Francisco, CA 94109, MS; **SLP LM**

Rost, Alan John Audie L Murphy VA Hospital, Audiology & Speech Path, 7400 Merton Minter Blvd, San Antonio, TX 78284, (512) 696-9660, MA 58; Aud, Audie L Murphy VA Hosp, **A**

Rost, Mrs Mara L 1712 Bancroft Street, San Diego, CA 92102, (619) 233-0143, MA 87 San Diego St Univ

Rost, Michele P 118 Pearl Drive N E, Rio Rancho, NM 87124, (505) 344-3927, BS 79 Northeastern Univ; MS 81 Univ of NM; Sp-Lang Path, Albuquerque Pub Sch Syst, **SLP**

Rostolsky, Mrs Maureen D 505 Randolph Drive, Lititz, PA 17543, (717) 569-8453, MS 71 PA St Univ - Univ Park; Sp-Lang Path, Lanc Cleft Palate Clinic, **SLP**

Roston, Amanda R 3555 Keystone Avenue #201, Los Angeles, CA 90034, (213) 838-5321, BA 55 Univ of Southern CA; MA 76 Whittier Coll; Sp-Lang Path, Supt of Sch-Los Angeles Co, **SLP**

Rotches, Meryl 64-45 213th Street, Bayside, NY 11364, (718) 229-8392, BA 85 Adelphi Univ; MS 86 Adelphi Univ; 88–Sp-Lang Path, St Mary's Hosp for Children, **SLP**

Rote, Ronda Route 106 P O Box 14, North Leeds, ME 04263, (207) 524-3281, BS 77 Univ of ME - Farmington; MA 80 Univ of ME - Orono; Sp/Lang Path, Private Practice, **SLP**

Rotert, Teresa Marie 3266 South Little, Flagstaff, AZ 86001, (602) 774-3137, BS 83 Central MO St Univ; MS 84 Central MO St Univ; SLP, Prescott USD, **SLP**

Roth, Mrs Barbara Edeson 11 Green Avenue, Rye, NY 10580, (914) 921-0529, BS 76 PA St Univ - Univ Park; MA 78 Kent St Univ; Sp-Lang Path, Private Practice, **SLP**

Roth, Dr Carole R 9985 Union Terrace Lane, Maple Grove, MN 55369, (612) 255-2200, BA 76 Univ of CA - Santa Barbara; MA 78 CA St Univ - Los Angeles; PH 86 (Sp Path) Univ of CO - Boulder; 88–Asst Prof, St Cloud St Univ-Minn, **SLP**

Roth, Mrs Christine L 1426 Terrance Drive, Naperville, IL 60565, (312) 983-6210, BA 75 Univ of IA; MA 76 Northeast MO St Univ; **SLP**

Roth, Cicely Anne 3618 Clarington Avenue #4, Los Angeles, CA 90034, (213) 202-1448, MA 83 CA St Univ - Northridge; Sp-Lang Path, Los Angeles USD, **SLP**

Roth, Mrs Deborah Darling 1720 Beechwood Boulevard, Pittsburgh, PA 15217, (412) 521-7799, BS 70 Univ of Pittsburgh - Pittsburgh; ME 72 Northeastern Univ; 86–Sp-Lang Path, Pittsburgh Mt Oliver Inter Ut, **SLP**

Roth, Mrs Diane Renee 25 Manigault Court, Florence, SC 29501, (803) 669-3661, BS 82 Purdue Univ - West Lafayette; MA 85 Univ of TN - Knoxville; SLP, Pee Dee Mental Retardation Ctr, **SLP**

Roth, Donald E 481 N W 44th Avenue, Plantation, FL 33317, (305) 926-0890, BA 66 Univ of MO - Columbia; MS 67 Univ of MI - Ann Arbor; Sp-Lang Path, Broward Co Sch, **SLP**

Roth, Mrs Francine Feder 71 Kensington Terrace, Passaic, NJ 07055, (201) 471-2231, BA 67 Rutger's St Univ - Douglas Coll; MS 68 Univ of MI - Ann Arbor; **SLP**

Roth, Dr Froma P 2 Drake Court, Rockville, MD 20853, (301) 454-6902, BA 70 CUNY - Hunter Coll; MA 73 CUNY - Queens Coll; PH 80 (NS) CUNY - Grad Sch & Univ Cntr; Assoc Prof, U of MD, **SLP**

Roth, Mrs Harriet T 266 Shelter Rock Road, Stamford, CT 06903, (203) 358-4390, BA 57 Tufts Univ; MS 72 Southern CT St Univ; 72–Sp-Lang Path, Stanford Health Dept, **SLP**

Roth, Mrs Hazel F 520 Fifth Street, Apartment #6, Catasauqua, PA 18032, (215) 264-3534, BS 55 Kutztown Univ of PA; ME 58 Temple Univ-Tyler Sch of Art; **SLP LM**

Roth, Mrs Janet E 700 Alter Drive, Mount Pleasant, IA 52641, (319) 385-9005, BS 59 IA St Univ; MA 62 Ball St Univ; 69–Sp-Lang Path, Great River AEA 16, **SLP**

Roth, Jill G G 32597 Buffalo Park Road, Evergreen, CO 80439, (303) 466-1791, BA 77 Univ of CO - Boulder; MA 79 Univ of Denver; Sp-Lang Path, Adams Co Dist 12, **SLP**

Roth, Jill Kathleen 1741 Park Village, Worthington, OH 43085, (614) 267-5128, BA 82 OH St Univ; MA 84 OH Univ - Athens; Aud, Audiology & Hearing Aid Serv, **A**

Roth, Judith A 1108 South Elm, Champaign, IL 61820, (217) 356-9176, BS 60 Northwestern Univ; MA 63 Syracuse Univ; SLP, Eastern Illinois Assn Spec Ed, **SLP**

Roth, Mrs Judith S 907 West Fullerton, Chicago, IL 60614, (312) 337-3728, BA 61 Univ of MI - Ann Arbor; MS 62 Univ of MI - Ann Arbor; 83–Aud, Chicago Bd of Ed, **SLP A**

Roth, Mrs Julie Ann 2213 Saratoga #2, Springfield, IL 62704, (217) 525-3006, BS 80 Bradley Univ; MA 81 Univ of IL - Urbana; Sp-Lang Path, Springfield Sch Dist 186, **SLP**

Roth, Mrs Linda Louise 5321 Crowndun Drive, St Louis, MO 63129, (314) 296-1413, BS 69 Southeast MO St Univ; MS 85 Fontbonne Coll; Sp-Lang Path, C-6 Consolidated School Dist, **SLP**

Roth, Mrs Lori L 8 Beaver Ridge Road, Morris Plains, NJ 07950, (301) 974-0925, BA 72 George Washington Univ; MA 74 Catholic Univ of America; Sp-Lang Path, Private Practice, **SLP**

Roth, Mrs Mary Hawkins 946 Vernon Road, Columbus, OH 43209, (614) 236-8524, BA 70 Univ of Cincinnati; MA 72 Univ of Cincinnati; 86–Sp-Lang Path, Franklin Co Bd of MR/DD, **SLP**

Roth, Nancy K 15 Sumner Street, Colorado Springs, CO 80906, (719) 520-0130, MS 80 Univ of OK - OK City; Sp-Lang Path, Transitions Head Injury Recovery Ctr, **SLP**

Roth, Patrick T 2816 S E 58th, Portland, OR 97206, (503) 777-0217, BS 76 Univ of OR; MA 79 Western WA Univ; Sp-Lang Path, Portland Public Schools, **SLP**

Roth, Ronal Rock Run Road, Star Route, Pottstown, PA 19464, (215) 935-6188, BS 61 PA St Univ - Univ Park; ME 71 Clarion Univ of PA; SLP, Pennhurst Cen Comm of Pa Dpw, **SLP**

Roth, Mrs Sue E 88 Clover Hill Road, Colts Neck, NJ 07722, (201) 946-3433, BS 77 NY Univ; MA 79 NY Univ; **SLP**

Roth, Susan Peio 2972 Asbury Court, Miamisburg, OH 45342-4433, (513) 435-0507, BS 85 Miami Univ - Oxford; MA 87 Univ of Cincinnati

Roth, Mrs Tammy Buss 1039 South Parker Road, Apartment I-8, Denver, CO 80231-2532, (303) 752-0435, BS 82 UT St Univ; MA 84 SUNY - Center at Buffalo; 87–Sp-Lang Path, Developmental Pathways, **SLP**

Roth, Werner Roland 855 Eighth Avenue SW #204, Calgary, AB, Canada T2P 3P1, (403) 261-0687, MS 83 CO St Univ; Aud, T H Moore Aud Consultants Ltd, **A**

Roth, William Russell 5 Panorama Lane, Hanover, PA 17331, (717) 632-5899, **SLP**

Rothaar, Thomas S 824 Pine Run Road, Mobile, AL 36609, (205) 471-1716, BS 70 Miami Univ - Oxford; MA 72 Univ of TN - Knoxville; Dir, Sertoma Club of Mobile, **SLP**

Rothaug, Mrs Wendy Wallach 419 Lemarc Street, Fremont, CA 94539, (415) 794-5155, BA 77 San Diego St Univ; MA 85 San Diego St Univ; 87–Sp-Lang Path, Bay Area Sp & Hrng Cl

Rothbard, Mrs Elise L 1 Rolleston Road, Marblehead, MA 01945, (617) 223-2084, BA 69 Univ of WI - Madison; MA 71 George Washington Univ; Aud, VA, **A**

Rothberg, Mrs Caryl R 1012 Crest Park Drive, Silver Spring, MD 20903, (301) 439-7338, BS 74 Univ of MD - College Park; MA 75 Univ of MD - College Park; Sp-Lang Path, Montgomery Co Public Schools, **SLP**

Rothberg, Susan Lori 5209 North 25th Place, Phoenix, AZ 85016, (602) 955-5993, MS 87 Marquette Univ; 87–Sp-Lang Path, Mesa PS Dist

Rothberg, Suzanne G 5012 N W 86 Way, Coral Springs, FL 33067-1970, (305) 344-2866, BA 79 Univ of FL; MA 81 Univ of Miami; SLP, Broward County School System, **SLP**

Rothblum, Mrs Alice G 5 Tanglewood Lane, Freeport, NY 11520, (516) 623-7088, BA 51 Adelphi Univ; MA 73 Adelphi Univ; **SLP**

Rothchild, Fred H 49793 Thornberry Road 420, Coarsegold, CA 93614, (209) 877-2215, BA 74 CA St Univ - Chico; MA 77 CA St Univ - Chico; Sp-Lang Path, Chawanakee Joint Union Sch Dist, **SLP**

Rothchild, Mrs Rita R 49793 Thornberry Road 420, Coarsegold, CA 93614, (209) 877-2215, BA 74 CA St Univ - Chico; MA 77 CA St Univ - Chico; Sp-Lang Path, Madera Co Supt Offi, **SLP**

Rothenberg, Mrs Carol E 6303 Leafy Screen, Columbia, MD 21045, (301) 762-0632, BA 69 Univ of MD - College Park; MA 73 Catholic Univ of America; Sp-Lang Path, Baltimore Co Pub Schs, **SLP**

Rothenberg, Dr Martin Dept Of Electrical And Computer Engineering, Syracuse University, Link Hall, Syracuse, NY 13244, (315) 443-4402, BS 59 Univ of MI - Ann Arbor; MA 63 Univ of MI - Ann Arbor; PH 66 (NS) Univ of MI - Ann Arbor; 76–Prof, Syracuse U

Rothenberg, Meredith H 3 Jacobs Lane, Westfield, NJ 07090, (201) 232-8841, BA 72 Franklin & Marshall Coll; MA 80 Kean Coll of NJ; 86–Aud, The Hearing Center, **A**

Rothenstein, Amy Jill 57 Falkland Street, Brighton, MA 02135, MS 82 Univ of South FL; Sp/Lang Path, Lawrence & Mem Hosp, **SLP**

Rother, Judy R 4632 West 11th Avenue, Vancouver, BC, Canada V6R 2M7, (604) 731-1131, BS 72 Univ of Toronto - Ontario; MS 74 Syracuse Univ; SLP/Aud, Vancouver Sch Bd, **SLP**

Rothermel, Mrs Barbara Armor 287 Franklin Drive, Pittsburgh, PA 15241, (412) 941-4518, BS 81 Indiana Univ of PA; MA 83 Kent St Univ; Sp-Lang Path, Comprehensive Therapy Svcs, **SLP**

Rothermel, Mrs Carol N 228 Woodhaven Drive, Bridgeville, PA 15017, (412) 349-9652, BS 80 PA St Univ - Univ Park; MA 81 Kent St Univ; Sp/Lang Path, South Hills Health Sys, **SLP**

Rothfeld, Diddy L 174 Southerd Avenue, Rockville Centre, NY 11570, (516) 764-6170, BA 73 SUNY - Coll at Plattsburgh; MA 76 Hofstra Univ; Sp/Lang Path, Northport Ufsd, **SLP**

Rothfuss, Martha J 80 Monmouth Road, Oakhurst, NJ 07755, (212) 870-5067, BS 79 Elmira Coll; MS 81 Univ of NC - Chapel Hill; Sp-Lang Path, Monmouth Med Ctr, **SLP ACE**

Rothhammer, Mrs Carma L CS Box AO 276, Oklahoma City, OK 73162, (405) 728-0404, BA 81 Wichita St Univ; MS 83 Univ of OK Medical Center; Sp-Lang Path, **SLP**

Rothlein, Laurie Goodman 1 Filomena Court, Dix Hills, NY 11746, (516) 326-5621, BA 78 SUNY - Center at Buffalo; MA 80 Univ of MD - College Park; Sp-Lang Path, Private Practice, **SLP**

Rothman, Mrs Ann R 1215 Adams Drive, Midland, MI 48640, (517) 631-5421, MA 71 MI St Univ; **SLP**

Rothman, Frederick 72 Shore Drive, Waterford, CT 06385, (203) 443-4507, BS 51 SUNY - Coll at Buffalo; MA 58 Univ of CT; OM 64 Univ of Bridgeport; School Psychologist, Groton Public Schools, **SLP LM**

Rothman, Mrs Gayle Hannah 62 Akbar Road, Stamford, CT 06902, (212) 679-0100, BA 82 CA St Univ - Northridge; MA 84 New York Univ; Sp-Lang Path, Intl Ctr for Disabled, **SLP**

Rothman, Dr Howard B University Of Florida, Iascp ASB51, Gainesville, FL 32611, (904) 392-2046, BA 61 CUNY - City College; MA 64 NY Univ; PH 71 (NS) Stanford Univ; Assoc Prof, Dept Sp, U FL

Rothman, Mrs Ralle K 21861 Stratford, Oak Park, MI 48237, (313) 494-2201, BA 52 Univ of MI - Ann Arbor; MA 71 Wayne St Univ; Aud, Detroit Pub Sch Sp & Hrng Cl, **SLP A**

Rothman, Mrs Ruth Agert 905-A N W 29th Avenue, Delray Beach, FL 33445, (407) 276-6108, OM 71 New York Univ; BA 61 Kean Coll of NJ; MA 65 Kean Coll of NJ; **SLP LM**

Rothman, Mrs Ruth S 15651 Dickens Street #106, Encino, CA 91436, MS 78 CA St Univ - Los Angeles; SLP, Los Angeles USD, **SLP**

Rothman, Mrs Sandra W 86-75 Midland Pky #3-J, Jamaica Estates, NY 11432, (718) 297-5957, BS 77 SUNY - Center at Albany; MS 79 Columbia Univ Teachers Coll; Sp-Lang Path, Private Practice, **SLP**

Rothman-Hazard, Mrs Loree Gay 2 Market Street, Peabody, MA 01960, (617) 631-0960, **SLP**

Rothschild, Devera R 144 Windham Court, Newtown, PA 18940, (215) 968-7928, MA 76; Sp-Lang Path, Family Guidance Ctr, **SLP**

Rothschild, Jane Lowenthal 25 Concord Road, Longmeadow, MA 01106, (413) 567-3802, BA 79; MA 82 George Washington Univ; Sp-Lang Path, Valley Infant Dev Service, **SLP**

Rothschild, Laurie 5858 East Molloy Road, Suite 155, Syracuse, NY 13211, (315) 455-7548, BS 81 SUNY - Center at Buffalo; MS 83 Columbia Univ Teachers Coll; **SLP**

Rothschild, Mrs Linda Rothenstei 83-77 116th Street, Kew Gardens, NY 11418, (718) 846-2419, BA 74 CUNY - Queens Coll; MA 76 CUNY - Hunter Coll; Sp-Lang Path, Private Practice, **SLP**

Rothschild, Patricia K 24 Brook Lane, Maplewood, NJ 07040, (201) 762-6171, BA 72 Rutger's St Univ - Douglas Coll; MA 74 CUNY - City College; Sp-Lang Path, NY League for Hd of Hrng, **SLP**

Rothschild, Mrs Suellen Blum 7224 Hillwood, Dallas, TX 75248, MS 81 Univ Southern MS-Hattiesburg; SLP, Private Consultant, **SLP**

Rothschild-Goldman, Mrs Lynn 6 Clipper Court, New Port Richey, FL 34652, (813) 938-1529, BS 81 Towson St Univ; MS 82 Towson St Univ; Sp-Lang Path, Pinellas Co Sch, **SLP**

Rothstein, Mrs Carole Gray 250 River Road, Millington, NJ 07946, (201) 647-1202, MA 76 Fairleigh Dickinson U-Teanec; MS 67 Kean Coll of NJ; 66–Sp-Lang Path, Passaic Township Bd Educ, **SLP**

Rothstein, Evelyn 105 Flagstaff Road, Philadelphia, PA 19115, (215) 676-0897, BS 75 PA St Univ - Univ Park; MA 77 Trenton St Coll; 86–Sp-Lang Path, NE Communication Specialists, **SLP ACE**

Rothstein, Mrs Jean Cofsky 220 Brentwood Road, Havertown, PA 19083, (215) 446-7755, BA 72 George Washington Univ; MS 73 Univ of MI - Ann Arbor; Sp/Lang Path, Private Practice, **SLP**

Rothstein, Lisa Ilene 48-49 47th Street #3-F, Woodside, NY 11377, (718) 729-5940, BA 82 SUNY - Coll at Cortland; MA 87 CUNY - Lehman Coll; 88–Tchr, NYC Bd of Educ

Rothstein, Mrs Lori J 3021 Gloss Avenue, Cincinnati, OH 45213, (513) 872-2481, BS 79 Purdue Univ - West Lafayette; MA 80 Bowling Green St Univ; Sp/Lang Path, Good Samaritan Hosp, **SLP**

Rothstein, Marilyn C 7103 Bremerton Court, Dallas, TX 75252, **SLP**

Rothstein, Michael J 131 Kelvin Avenue, Staten Island, NY 10306-3743, (718) 983-5406, BA 81 CUNY - Lehman Coll; MA 82 CUNY - Lehman Coll; Sp-Lang Path, SIDDSO

Rothstein, Rabbi S c/o Trz, 17655 Devonshire St, Worthridge, CA 91325, (213) 475-1625, MA 58 Columbia Univ Teachers Coll; OD 82; Rabbi, Temple Ramat Zion, **SLP**

Rothstein, Mrs Roberta Arlene 7005 Wandermere Drive, San Diego, CA 92119, (619) 691-7123, BA 68 San Diego St Univ; MA 73 San Diego St Univ; Sp-Lang Path, Bay Hospital Medical Cen, **SLP**

Rothstein, Mrs Sharon H 538 West Fransee Lane, Glendale, WI 53217, BS 61 Univ of WI - Madison; MS 74 Univ of WI - Milwaukee; Teacher, Shorewood Public Schools, **SLP**

Rothwax, Helen Frances 3520 Fillmore Avenue, Brooklyn, NY 11234, (718) 627-4044, BA 75 CUNY - Brooklyn Coll; MS 81 Adelphi Univ; MS 83 Adelphi Univ; Sp-Lang Path, NYC Bd of Ed, **SLP**

Rothwell, Mrs Gail W 5119 South Angeline Street, Seattle, WA 98118, (206) 593-6814, BA 71 Central WA Univ; MA 74 Western WA Univ; SLP, Tacoma Sch Dist, **SLP**

Rothwell, Karen R 74 Lakepines, Irvine, CA 92720, BA 75 Univ of the Pacific; MS 76 Univ of Southern CA; MA 79 Univ of Denver; Aud, Private Practice, **A ACE**

Rotman, Mrs Iris Kline 81 Kingsbury Street, Wellesley, MA 02181, (617) 237-9410, BS 58 Boston Univ; ME 60 Boston Univ; Sp-Lang Path, Private Practice, **SLP**

Rotman, Mrs Linda Carole 405 East Creekside Circle, Apartment F, Murray, UT 84107, (801) 565-7100, BS 83 Univ of MA - Amherst; MS 85 PA St Univ - Univ Park; **SLP**

Rotondi, Paula E 422 Ridge Place NE, Albuquerque, NM 87106, (505) 256-2733, BS 72 Univ of MA - Amherst; MS 76 Univ of NM; Aud, VA Med Ctr, **A**

Rott, Mrs Betty Baker 2031 Nantucket Place, Tustin, CA 92680, (714) 832-1041, BS 73 Univ of the Pacific; MS 75 CO St Univ; **SLP**

Rottenberg, Paula A 225 Peyton Avenue, Haddonfield, NJ 08033, (609) 429-5873, BA 72 Univ of Pittsburgh - Pittsburgh; MA 73 Univ of Pittsburgh - Pittsburgh; Sp-Lang Path, Private Practice, **SLP**

Rotter, Margaret A 1302 Fenwick, Lynchburg, VA 24502, **SLP A**

Rotter, Dr Paul 218 Pearsall Place, Woodmere, NY 11598, (516) 295-3813, BS 47 Columbia Univ Teachers Coll; MA 47 Columbia Univ Teachers Coll; ED 59 (NS) Columbia Univ Teachers Coll; Consult Spec Ed & Adm, Self Employed, **A LM**

Rottersman, Judy E 411 West End Avenue, New York, NY 10024, (212) 724-9895, BA 66 CUNY - Brooklyn Coll; MS 67 Univ of MI - Ann Arbor; Sp-Lang Path, Private Practice, **SLP**

Rotunno, Rosemarie 411 27th Street, San Francisco, CA 94131, (415) 852-3251, BA 77 CUNY - Brooklyn Coll; MS 79; 87–Aud, VAMC-Palo Alto, **A**

Rotz, Mrs Marian Babbitt 1756 Altland Avenue, York, PA 17404, (717) 843-8091, BS 53 PA St Univ - Univ Park; SLP, Private Practice, **SLP**

Rotz, Sandra W 42 Elm Street, Rutland, VT 05701-4121, (802) 775-0071, BS 80 PA St Univ - Univ Park; MS 82 PA St Univ - Univ Park; Sp/Lang Path, Addison Rutland Superv Un, **SLP**

Roueche, James Richard 711 Stanton Young Blvd, Suite 601, Oklahoma City, OK 73104, (405) 271-6876, Dir-Dept of Neuropsychology, Presbyterian Hos Dept Cl N-P, **SLP**

Rouleau, Mary L 1507 East Saveland, Milwaukee, WI 53207, (414) 482-0123, BS 71 Univ of WI - Milwaukee; MS 72 Univ of WI - Milwaukee; Sp-Lang Path, Milwaukee Public Schools, **SLP**

Roulo, Rosemary A 3531 East 84th, Anchorage, AK 99507, (907) 344-3219, BS 72 Northern MI Univ; MA 75 Northern MI Univ; Sp-Lang Path, Anchorage Sch Dist, **SLP**

Roumel, Maria H 9224 Orchard Brook Drive, Potomac, MD 20854, (301) 340-0718, BS 68 George Washington Univ; MA 70 George Washington Univ; Sp-Lang Path, Private Practice, **SLP ACE**

Rounds, Anne E 151 Thornhill Crescent, Chatham, ON, Canada N7L 4M2, (519) 354-0520, BA 66 Univ of RI; MA 85 MI St Univ; **SLP**

Rounds, Brenda Cook 28 Pond Hill Avenue, Warwick, NY 10990, (914) 294-5431, BS 65 Syracuse Univ; MS 85 William Paterson Coll; **SLP**

Roundtree-Newell, Janice 207-B Parris Street, Jacksonville, AL 36265, (205) 435-8660, BS 83 Jackson St Univ; MA 86 SC St Coll; 88–Sp-Lang Path, Med Therapy-Rehab Svc Inc, **SLP**

Rounsefell, Nancy L S Australian Coll Advanced Ed, School Of Speech Pathology, Sturt Road, Bedford Park, South Australia, Australia 5042, (08) 275-5310, BA 64 Univ of North TX; MA 66 TX Woman's Univ; 88–Clin Supvr, So Australian Coll Advanced Educ, **SLP**

Roupe, Mrs Karla Kay Koch 1625 Ann Dossy Court, Crowley, TX 76036, (817) 294-8408, BS 79 Univ of IA; ME 81 Southwest TX St Univ; Sp/Lang Path, Private Practice, **SLP**

Rouse, Mrs Ann T 2380 West Hill Drive, Madison, WI 53711, (608) 873-7257, BS 69 Univ of WI - Eau Claire; MS 71 Univ of WI - Madison; 71–Sp-Lang Path, Stoughton Pub Sch, **SLP**

Rouse, Mrs Carolyn B 1112 Willow Springs Drive, Louisville, KY 40242, (502) 425-9382, BS 76 Eastern KY Univ; MA 79 Eastern KY Univ; SLP, Cumberland River Comp Care Cen, **SLP**

Rouse, Geraldine Rodriguez 2814 Rio Vista Court S W, Albuquerque, NM 87105, (505) 294-5061, BA 69 Univ of NM; MS 76 Univ of NM; 85–Sp-Lang Path, Therapeutic Horsemanship of NM, **SLP ACE**

Rouse, Mrs Jean L B 1235 Arthur Avenue, Racine, WI 53405, (414) 634-4526, BA 77 Univ of WI - Eau Claire; MS 78 Univ of WI - Eau Claire; Sp-Lang Path, Racine USD, **SLP**

Rouse, Mrs Lucy W 895 Texas Avenue, Grand Junction, CO 81501, (303) 243-6695, BA 56 Adams St Coll; MA 63 Univ of Denver; **SLP LM**

Rouse, Mrs Marie T 134 Cumings Lane, Neenah, WI 54956, (414) 729-6046, BS 74 Univ of WI - Whitewater; MS 81 Univ of WI - Whitewater; Sp-Lang Path, University of Wisconsin, **SLP**

Rouse, Mrs Radyne P 3637 Snell Road, Space 391, San Jose, CA 95136, (408) 225-2554, MA 88 San Jose St Univ

Rouser, Mrs Holly Elaine 8913 So Blackstone Avenue, Chicago, IL 60619, (312) 890-8345, BS 81 Univ of IL - Urbana; MS 85 Governors St Univ; 85–Sp-Lang Path, Chicago Bd of Educ, **SLP**

Rousey, Dr Carol H 921 Garfield, Suite 2, Topeka, KS 66606, (913) 357-0953, BS 55 Central MO St Univ; MA 58 Univ of KS; PH 76 (NS) Univ of KS; Sp-Lang Path, Drs Rousey & Rousey Ltd, **SLP ACE**

Rousey, Dr Clyde L Drs Rousey & Rousey Ltd, 921 Garfield, Topeka, KS 66606, (913) 357-0953, BA 51 Ottawa Univ; MA 52 Northwestern Univ; PH 55 (NS) Northwestern Univ; Sp-Lang Path/Aud, Rousey & Rousey Ltd, **SLP A F**

Rousey, Mrs Juliet S 1103 Apache Pass, Anniston, AL 36206, (205) 820-2420, BS 69 Syracuse Univ; ME 86 West GA Coll; 85–Sp-Lang Path, Ft McClellan Elem Sch, **SLP**

Roush, Mrs Betty Michie 23400 South Western Avenue, Apartment D, Harbor City, CA 90710, (714) 978-6226, BA 78 CA St Univ - Long Beach; MA 82 CA St Univ - Long Beach; Sp-Lang Path, Craig & Ford Inc, **SLP**

Roush, Dr Jackson 108 Braswell Road, Chapel Hill, NC 27516, (919) 967-1006, BS 75 Western MI Univ; MA 76 Western MI Univ; PH 81 (Speech & Hrng Sciences) Univ of MI - Ann Arbor; Asst Prof, Univ of NC-Chapel Hill, **A**

Roush, Mrs Mary Renee 12423 St Joe Road, Grabill, IN 46741, (219) 627-3140, BS 83 Purdue Univ - West Lafayette; MS 84 Purdue Univ - West Lafayette; **SLP**

Roush, Patricia A 108 Braswell Road, Chapel Hill, NC 27516, (919) 967-1770, BA 75 Univ of MA - Amherst; MA 76 Univ of IA; **A**

Roush, Ted L 310 Liberty Street, Pella, IA 50219, (515) 223-6620, BA 75 Univ of Northern IA; MA 76 Univ of Northern IA; Sp-Lang Path, Med Rehab Agency, **SLP**

Rousse, Valerie M 32 Summit Avenue, Somerville, MA 02143, (808) 689-0553, BA 74 Univ of MI - Ann Arbor; MA 80 MI St Univ; Sp-Lang Path, Methuen Public Schools, **SLP**

Rousseau, Frank E Physicians' Office Bldg, J C Blair Memorial Hospital, Warm Springs Avenue, Huntingdon, PA 16652, (814) 643-6320, BS 66 CA Univ of PA; MS 67 WV Univ; Aud/Sp-Lang Path, Private Practice, **SLP A**

Roussi, Lisa Ann 116 Joanmoor Drive, Tonawanda, NY 14150, (716) 837-2441, BA 85 SUNY - Center at Buffalo; MA 87 SUNY - Coll at Geneseo

Roussos, Catherine Athena 123 Hawthorn Street, New Bedford, MA 02740, (617) 997-4511, BA 84 Bridgewater St Coll; MS 86 Northeastern Univ; 87–Sp-Lang Path, New Bedford PS

Roussos, Dr Christine Strike Department Of Communication Disorders, California State University Northridge, 18356 Plummer Street, Northridge, CA 91330, (818) 885-2852, BA 74 Northwestern Univ; MA 75 Northwestern Univ; PH 88 (Clinical Supervision/Phonology) IN Univ - Bloomington; 88–Asst Prof, California State Univ, **SLP ACE**

Routenberg, Linda P 2130 Six Branches Drive, Roswell, GA 30076, (404) 993-5294, BA 71 Univ of KY; ME 76 GA St Univ; Sp/Lang Path, Private Practice, **SLP**

Routman, Frank Joseph P O Box 18867, Cleveland Heights, OH 44118, (216) 368-2470, BS 58 Case Western Reserve Univ; MA 68 Case Western Reserve Univ; Instr/Coord of Sp & Hrng Serv, Case Western Reserve Univ, **SLP**

Routson, Margueite Elaine 2655 Monroe, Laramie, WY 82070, (307) 721-4436, BS 75 Univ of WY; MS 83 Univ of WY; Sp-Lang Path, Albany County Sch Dist #1, **SLP**

Roux, Mrs Pam J L 621-A Kentucky Street, Columbia, SC 29201, 80-377-9214, MA 88 Univ of SC - Columbia

Roverts, Mrs Diana Lynn 7510 Armand Circle, Tampa, FL 33634-2902, (813) 882-0580, BA 81 Univ of CT; MA 83 Univ of FL; Sp-Lang Path, **SLP**

Rovezzi, Mrs Susan C Hahnemann Rehab Center, 535 Lincoln Street, Worcester, MA 01605, (617) 792-8500, BS 79 Worcester St Coll; MA 81 Univ of MA - Amherst; Aud, Hahnemann Rehab Cen, **A**

Rovig, Glen W Box 65-1624, U S Naval Hospital, FPO Seattle, WA 98765-1600, 0468-26-1911, BA 71 Univ of WI - Madison; MA 75 Western IL Univ; Operational Aud Officer, U S Navy, **A**

Rovito, Mrs Guadalupe M 212 Temona Drive, Pleasant Hills, PA 15236, (412) 222-4300, BA 79 OH St Univ; MA 81 OH St Univ; Sp/Lang Path, Private Practice, **SLP**

Row, Sandra M 7730 East Sheridan, Scottsdale, AZ 85257, (602) 834-1211, BS 71 ID St Univ; MS 73 AZ St Univ; Director Sp-Lang Path, John C Lincoln Hospital, **SLP ACE**

Rowan, Mrs Cynthia Lee 1768 Willowhurst Avenue, San Jose, CA 95125, (408) 842-3135, BA 78 San Jose St Univ; MA 81 San Jose St Univ; Sp-Lang Path, Gilroy USD, **SLP**

Rowan, Mrs Eleanor J 7100 South Villa, Oklahoma City, OK 73159, (405) 737-7025, BS 68 Univ of OK - Norman; MA 69 Univ of OK - Norman; Sp/Lang Path, Mid-Del Pub Sch, **SLP**

Rowan, Karen A 1 Riverside Street, Danvers, MA 01923, BS 76 Northeastern Univ; MS 77 Ithaca Coll; Aud, Krown Hrng Svcs Inc, **A**

Rowan, Mrs Lydia A 353 Briar N E, North Canton, OH 44720, (216) 375-3882, BS 76 Ashland Coll; MA 79 Univ of Akron; 81–Aud, Akron City Hosp-Comm Disord, **A**

Rowan, Dr Lynne E Speech & Hearing Science, University Of Illinois, 901 South 6th Street, Champaign, IL 61820, (217) 244-2543, BS 68 Kent St Univ; MA 72 Univ of CT; PH 82 (Sp-Lang Path) Purdue Univ - West Lafayette; 84–Asst Prof, University of Illinois, **SLP**

Rowe, Mrs Barbara Munnerlyn 104 Sedgefield Drive, Goldsboro, NC 27530, (919) 778-8827, BA 77 SC St Coll; MA 78 SC St Coll; 88–Sp-Lang Path, Logos Inc, **SLP**

Rowe, Colleen M 6014 44th Avenue N W, Gig Harbor, WA 98335, (206) 857-6171, BA 74 Western WA Univ; MA 75 Western WA Univ; Sp-Lang Path, Peninsula Sch Dist, **SLP**

Rowe, Mrs Karen A 495 West Sample, Fresno, CA 93704, (209) 439-0176, BA 73 CA St Univ - Fresno; MA 77 CA St Univ - Fresno; Sp-Lang Path, Clovis USD, **SLP**

Rowe, Katherine Liann 13506 209th Avenue SE, Issaquah, WA 98027, (206) 226-3826, MA 87 Northwestern Univ; Sp-Lang Path, **SLP**

Rowe, Linda Jo 5639 Pony Court, Oceanside, CA 92056, (619) 277-5160, BS 63 Univ of Southern CA; MA 67 Univ of Southern CA; Tchr, San Diego USD, **A**

Rowe, Dr Margaret L 139 South 26th Street Dr, Terre Haute, IN 47803, (812) 235-2326, BA 32 Univ of Evansville; MA 39 Northwestern Univ; ED 55 (Sp Path/Ed Psychology) IN Univ - Bloomington; **SLP LM**

Rowe, Mrs Marjean S 604 Vinson Street, Little Rock, AR 72205, (501) 776-2337, BA 80 Univ of AR - Little Rock; MS 85 Univ of AR - Medical Sci; 85–Sp-Lang Path, Harmony Grove PS, **SLP**

Rowe, Mary Grace 2215 Wood Trail Drive, Milton, WI 53563, (608) 868-7086, BS 81 Univ of WI - Whitewater; MS 83 Univ of WI - Whitewater; 83–Sp-Lang Path, Milton Sch Dist, **SLP**

Rowe, Mrs Mary K 8922 Arbor View Court, Fort Wayne, IN 46835-8848, BA 69 Coll of Saint Francis; OM 71 IN Univ - Bloomington; Sp-Lang Path, Fort Wayne Comm Sch Cord, **SLP**

Rowe, Nancy 627 NE 17th Avenue, Fort Lauderdale, FL 33304, (305) 524-4251, BS 68 NY Univ; MS 70 Washington Univ; Aud, Auditory-Verbal Therapy Inc, **A**

Rowe, Mrs Susan E 18 Windy Hill Road, Glen Arm, MD 21057, (301) 592-6043, BA 71 Univ of MD - College Park; MS 82 Towson St Univ; Sp-Lang Path, Stella Maris Hospice, **SLP**

Rowe, Mrs Susan E B 1605 Field Road, Sarasota, FL 34231, (813) 924-4243, BA 74 Eastern MI Univ; MA 75 Eastern MI Univ; Sp-Lang Path, Sarasota Co Sch Bd, **SLP**

Rowe, Mrs Tammy De Boer 384 Brookgreen Ln, Helena, AL 35080, (205) 985-0217, **A**

Rowell, Rebecca E 234 Brockinton Drive, St Simons Island, GA 31522, (912) 264-3141, BS 76 Univ of GA; ME 77 Univ of GA; Cen Dir & Hd SLP, Er Sl Sp & Hrng Cen, **SLP**

Rowell, Mrs Tommye S 4412 Willow Bend Road, Decatur, AL 35603, (205) 353-7601, OM 85 MS St Univ - Meridian; Sp-Lang Path, **SLP**

Rowen, Jane F 2743 West Central Avenue, Toledo, OH 43606, (419) 471-2553, BS 69 Univ of Cincinnati; MA 70 Univ of Cincinnati; Aud, Toledo Otolary Ngology, **A**

Rowinsky, Mrs Wendy Sue 14 Dyson-Dan Ct, Reisterstown, MD 21336, (301) 526-4463, BS 78 OH Univ - Athens; MA 80 OH Univ - Athens; **SLP**

Rowland, Anne Bigelow 11205 51st Avenue No, Plymouth, MN 55442, (612) 520-5614, BA 80 MI St Univ; MA 81 Memphis St Univ; SLP, North Memorial Med Cntr, **SLP**

Rowland, Cynthia Jane 280 West Center, Logan, UT 84321, (801) 257-3413, OB 78 Westmont Coll; BS 80 Univ of CA - Santa Barbara; MS 84 UT St Univ; 85–Clin Instr, Utah St Univ, **SLP**

Rowland, Mrs Debra Spencer 810 3rd Avenue East, Spencer, IA 51301, (712) 362-7295, BS 76 Clarion Univ of PA; MA 78 Univ of IA; Aud, Lakeland AEA #3, **A**

Rowland, Elizabeth Jane 668 22nd Avenue, San Francisco, CA 94121-3703, (415) 931-7023, BA 82 IN Univ - Bloomington; MA 84 IN Univ - Bloomington; Sp-Lang Path, San Francisco USD, **SLP**

Rowland, Mrs Lillian K Rd 5 Box 209, Carlisle, PA 17013, (717) 737-6728, BS 64 SUNY - Coll at Buffalo; ME 65 PA St Univ - Univ Park; Sp-Lang Path, Capital Area Iu, **SLP ACE**

Rowland, Mrs M Annette 6909 47th Avenue North, Minneapolis, MN 55428, (612) 871-0666, BS 61 Mankato St Univ; MA 73 Univ of MN - Minneap-St Paul; Admin, St Ann Residence & Grp Home, **SLP**

Rowland, Rebecca R 206 Sipes Street, Nashville, AR 71852, **SLP**

Rowland, Dr Roy C Audiology Laboratory, 2610 N W Expressway, Suite E, Oklahoma City, OK 73112, (405) 947-4327, MA 60 Stanford Univ; PH 66 Univ of OK - Norman; OD 79 (NS) OK City Univ; Assoc Prof, Cen St U, **SLP A**

Rowlett, Mrs Karen L 3522 Marlin Drive, Louisville, KY 40299-3531, (502) 267-4889, BS 78 Eastern KY Univ; MA 80 Univ of Cincinnati; 86–Sp-Lang Path, Private Practice, **SLP**

Rowlett, Lisa Kathleen 28 Homestead Avenue, Port Jefferson Station, NY 11776-1432, (818) 445-3102, **SLP**

Rowlette, Sandra M 706 West Broadway, Decorah, IA 52101, **SLP**

Rowley, Mrs Anne Toolan 7 Silverside Lane, Latham, NY 12110, (518) 783-7571, BA 73 Saint John's Univ - Jamaica; MA 75 Catholic Univ of America; Sp-Lang Path/Adjunct Prof, Coll of St Rose, **SLP**

Rowley, Carla Jean 14514 Foxglove Drive, Chino, CA 91709, (714) 591-3682, BA 80 Univ of LA Verne; MS 84 Univ of LA Verne; 87–Sp-Lang Path, Chino USD, **SLP**

Rowley, Mrs Cindy Jo 4325 172nd Street S W, Lynnwood, WA 98037, (206) 743-3498, BA 80 Biola Univ; OM 83 Univ of WA; 86–Sp-Lang Path, Little Red Sch House, **SLP**

Rowley, Elaine M P O Box 27, 68 Institute Street, Frewsburg, NY 14738, **SLP**

Rowley, Melody 1715 Shirley Street, Merced, CA 95340, BA 74 CA St Univ - Stanislaus; MA 82 CA St Univ - Stanislaus; SLP, Office Merced Co Sch, **SLP**

Rowley, Dr Rodney Ray 409 Arrowview Drive, Redlands, CA 92373, (714) 796-2525, BS 59 Brigham Young Univ; MA 61 Univ of MD - College Park; PH 65 (NS) Univ of OK Medical Center; Aud, Loma Linda Aud Cen, **A**

Rowley, Thomas William 1010 Avenue G, Powell, WY 82435, (307) 754-5181, BA 76 Geneva Coll; MA 78 Western MI Univ; 80–Sp-Lang Path, Park Co Sch Dist #1, **SLP**

Rowsey, Linda Margaret 7068 Ashlawn Drive, Brecksville, OH 44141, (216) 526-5494, MA 84 Cleveland St Univ; Aud, Cleveland State U, **A**

Rowsey, Lisa Renae 11601 4th Street N #3108, St Petersburg, FL 33702, (813) 545-0996, BS 84 Auburn Univ - Auburn; OM 85 Auburn Univ - Auburn

Roy, Beverly J Box 142, Fort Shaw, MT 59443, **SLP**

Roy, Linda McCarty P O Box 533, Nome, AK 99762-0533, (417) 885-3282, BS 78 Southwest MO St Univ; MS 80 Central MO St Univ; SLP, St John's Reg Hlth Cen, **SLP**

Roy, Louise Michele 500 Springbank Drive #511, London, ON, Canada N6J 4G6, (519) 472-0959, OM 85 Univ of WI - Madison

Roy, Melissa Passaro 16 Hudson Avenue, Spotswood, NJ 08884, (201) 251-1054, BA 84 Montclair St Coll; MS 85 Columbia Univ Teachers Coll; SLP, Kesler Ins for Rehab, **SLP**

Roy, Melody Bakos 770 Lester Lane, Auburn, CA 95603, (916) 663-2096, BA 77 Univ of CA - Santa Barbara; MS 79 Univ of Redlands; Sp-Lang Path, Placer Co Off Ed, **SLP**

Roy, Patricia V 2101 Evergreen Lane, Point Pleasant, NJ 08742, (201) 321-7063, BS 63 Syracuse Univ; MA 70 IN Univ - Bloomington; Dir of Sp/Hrng, JFK Med Cen, **SLP**

Roy, Susan Holly 21746 Lanar, Mission Viejo, CA 92692, (714) 951-1611, BS 80 Ithaca Coll; MS 82 Purdue Univ - West Lafayette; Sp-Lang Path, **SLP**

Roy, Susan Jane 1969 Lowell Lane, Merrick, NY 11566, (212) 831-5160, BS 64 CUNY - Brooklyn Coll; MS 67 CUNY - Hunter Coll; OM 73 CUNY - Hunter Coll; Asst Prin Day Sch for Deaf, Bd of Ed of Cty of NY, **SLP**

Royal, Caroline Anne 1406 Northwest 19th Street, Oklahoma City, OK 73106, (405) 236-3131, BS 80 Univ Southern MS-Hattiesburg; MS 81 Univ Southern MS-Hattiesburg; 88–Sp-Lang Path, Health South Rehab Ctr, **SLP ACE**

Royal, Verne G 31182 Claymore, Farmington Hills, MI 48018, (313) 493-6315, MA 74 Univ of AL-Birmingham; MA 75 Univ of AL-Birmingham; MA 81 Wayne St Univ; Sp-Lang Path, Sinai Hosp of Detroit, **SLP**

Royall, Julia B 3302 Ridgecrest Court, Raleigh, NC 27607, (919) 684-3859, BS 75 Hollins Coll; MS 80 Univ of NC - Chapel Hill; Sp-Lang Path, Duke Univ Med Ctr, **SLP**

Royals, Mrs Waverlyn Jones 112 Farmhouse Place, Greenville, NC 27834, (919) 551-4448, BA 79 Univ of NC - Greensboro; MS 81 Univ of AZ; 85–Sp-Lang Path, Pitt County Memorial Hospital, **SLP**

Roybal, Bernadette Trujillo 2615 Via Caballero Del Nor, Santa Fe, NM 87505, (505) 471-7721, BA 83 NM St Univ; MS 85 Univ of NM; 85–Sp-Lang Path, Santa Fe PS, **SLP**

Royer, Patricia A 2250 Piccardo Circle, Stockton, CA 95207, (209) 944-4235, BS 52 McPherson Coll; MA 80 Univ of the Pacific; **SLP**

Roysdon, Valisa Jean 1119 Needles Drive, Indianapolis, IN 46217, (317) 630-7418, BS 77 Ball St Univ; MA 79 Ball St Univ; Aud, Mem Hosp, **A**

Royse, Catherine L P O Box 582, Laveen, AZ 85339, (602) 237-3800, BS 75 AR St Univ; MS 77 Univ of OK - OK City; Sp-Lang Path, Cartwright School District 83, **SLP**

Royster, Dr Julia Doswell 4706 Connell Drive, Raleigh, NC 27612, (919) 782-1624, BA 72 Univ of NC - Chapel Hill; MS 75 Univ of NC - Chapel Hill; PH 81 (Psychology) NC St Univ at Raleigh; Pres, Environ Noise Consultants Inc, **SLP A**

Roza, Diane M 209 South Drive, Bridgewater, MA 02324, (617) 697-3938, BS 69 Emerson Coll; ME 70 Boston Univ; 79 Boston Univ; Sp-Lang Path, Bridgewater Pub Schs, **SLP**

Roza, Robert T 7343 West Archer Avenue, Summit, IL 60501, BA 78 Saint Xavier Coll; MS 80 Marquette Univ; **SLP**

Rozak, Mrs Deanna Podhorn 56 Hawthorne Avenue, Cheshire, CT 06410, (203) 272-6053, BS 83 Univ of IL - Champaign; MS 85 Southern CT St Univ; **SLP**

Rozelle, Anne M M 222 Mockingbird Trail, Palm Beach, FL 33480-3118, (407) 844-6393, BS 78 Marquette Univ; MS 79 Marquette Univ; Sp/Lang Path, Private Practice, **SLP**

Rozen, Mrs Audrey L 4055 Lindenwood Lane, Northbrook, IL 60062, (312) 272-5947, BS 75 Univ of IL - Urbana; MS 76 Univ of IL - Urbana; 85–Sp-Lang Path, West Northfield Dist 31, **SLP**

Rozen, Charlotte Riverside Towers, 5 Riverside Drive #603, Binghamton, NY 13905, (607) 724-3818, BS 56 Ithaca Coll; ME 58 PA St Univ - Univ Park; Retired, Sch Dist of Philadelphia, **SLP ACE**

Rozestraten, Mrs Elizabeth D 101 Carverdale, Rochester, NY 14618, (716) 482-9290, MS 79 Nazareth Coll of Rochester; Sp-Lang Path, **SLP**

Rozier, Mrs Judith Ann 501 Terrace Avenue, Alexandria, LA 71303, (318) 443-4572, **SLP**

Rozzi, Mrs Mary Ruth 259 Stoopville Road, Newtown, PA 18940, (215) 348-2940, BS 59 CA Univ of PA; MA 62 WV Univ; SLP, Bucks Co Inter Ut, **SLP**

Ruah, Catarina Korn 301 S Shelard Parkway #108, St Louis Park, MN 55426, (612) 893-0117, BS 85 Northeastern Univ; MS 86 Northeastern Univ; Aud/Ofc Mgr, Miracle Ear, **A**

Ruane, Mrs Ruth Schalk 7119 Wessynton Drive, Charlotte, NC 28226, (704) 541-9044, BA 76 Geneva Coll; MA 78 Univ of KS; **SLP**

Ruane, Thomas Joseph 1543 Wyoming Avenue, Scranton, PA 18509, (717) 421-5123, MS 83 Rutgers St Univ -N Brunswick; Sp-Lang Path, Logopedic Assoc, **SLP**

Rubano, Mrs Bernedette 302 Neill Drive, Watertown, CT 06795, (203) 274-5606, BA 75 Southern CT St Univ; MS 78 Southern CT St Univ; Sp-Lang Path, Sp & Lang Therapy Serv, **SLP**

Rubano, Dennis P 910 Crestwood Drive, Brookfield, OH 44403, (216) 747-4340, BS 73 Edinboro Univ of PA; MS 78 Clarion Univ of PA; Sp/Lang Path, Youngstown Hrng & Sp Cen, **SLP**

Rubano, Mrs Nancy G 504 Laning Street, Southington, CT 06489, (203) 584-7740, OB 61 Duquesne Univ; MS 73 Southern CT St Univ; SLP, Cty of Bristol Bd of Ed, **SLP**

Rubbelke, Mrs Cynthia M 219 Sheila Drive, Beulah, ND 58523, (701) 748-6383, BA 78 Univ of ND; MA 79 Univ of ND; Sp-Lang Path, Oliver-Mercer Special Ed Unit, **SLP**

Rube, Jean R Crotched Mountain Rehabilitation Center, Greenfield, NH 03047, (603) 547-3311, BS 81 Ithaca Coll; ME 83 Northeastern Univ; 83–Dir of Comm, Crotched Mountain Rehab Ctr, **SLP**

Ruben, Dr Robert J Chairman Dept Of Otorhinolary, Montefiore Medical Center, 111 East 210 St (Vca-4), Bronx, NY 10467, (212) 920-2992, BA 55 Princeton Univ; MD 59 (NS) Johns Hopkins Univ; Prof & Chmn, Montefiore Hosp & Med Cen

Rubenacker, Kenneth W 624 Moore Avenue, Sikeston, MO 63801-2123, (314) 471-7264, BS 77 Southern IL Univ -Carbondale; MS 81 Southern IL Univ -Carbondale; Aud, Wabash Ohio Valley Spec Ed, **A**

Rubendunst, Mrs Marilyn L 906-C Montevideo, Lansing, MI 48917, (517) 887-1780, BA 74 MI St Univ; MA 75 MI St Univ; 86–Sp-Lang Path, Lansing Sch Dist, **SLP**

Rubenstein, Dr Joyce 75 Brook Court North, New Hyde Park, NY 11040-2203, (212) 403-8431, BA 74 Hofstra Univ; MA 75 Hofstra Univ; PH 82 (NS) NY Univ; Admin-Rehab Svcs, Brooklyn Hosp, **SLP A**

Rubenstein, Merilyn B 633 West Evergreen Court, Milwaukee, WI 53217, (414) 351-1517, BS 54 Univ of WI - Milwaukee; **SLP**

Rubin, Alanna 6005 Freud Avenue, Cote St Luc, PQ, Canada H4W 3A8, (514) 598-6210, BS 75 McGill Univ - Quebec; MS 77 McGill Univ - Quebec; Sp-Lang Path, Montreal Catholic Sch Cmsn, **SLP**

Rubin, Arlene Faye 712 80th Street, North Bergen, NJ 07047, (201) 854-6056, BA 80 Montclair St Coll; MA 82 NY Univ; Dir/Sp-Lang Path, Good Talking People, **SLP ACE**

Rubin, Arlene S 4212 West 73rd Terrace, Prairie Village, KS 66208, (816) 556-3198, BA 76 Univ of MO - Columbia; MA 78 Northern IL Univ - De Kalb; Aud, Truman Med Cen, **A**

Rubin, Audrey S 12 Rose Glen Drive, Andover, MA 01810, (508) 475-6335, BS 72 Univ of WI - Madison; MS 74 Emerson Coll; Sp-Lang Path, Andover Sp Path, **SLP**

Rubin, Barbara R 61-24 228th Street, Bayside, NY 11364, (718) 279-9248, BA 76 CUNY - Queens Coll; MA 78 CUNY - Queens Coll; 88–Prog Coord, H G Birch Early Chldhd Cen, **SLP**

Rubin, Bonnie R 5 Holland Avenue, North Tarrytown, NY 10591, (914) 939-5190, BA 77 Rutger's St Univ - Douglas Coll; MA 78 George Washington Univ; Aud, Drs Solomon & Jamal, **A**

Rubin, Cynthia B 2471 McIntosh Way, Maitland, FL 32751, (407) 628-5585, BA 68 CUNY - Queens Coll; MA 83 Univ of Central FL; SLP, Orange Co, **SLP**

Rubin, Deborah 67-87 Booth Street #3-G, Forest Hills, NY 11375, (718) 997-0132, BA 76 CUNY - Queens Coll; MA 78 CUNY - Queens Coll; 79–Sp-Lang Path, New York City Board of Educ, **SLP**

Rubin, Denise J 164 Caswell Street, Narragansett, RI 02882, (401) 792-9426, BS 73 CUNY - Lehman Coll; MS 76 Univ of RI; Sp-Lang Path, Narragansett Sch Dept, **SLP**

Rubin, Mrs Gail 115 Central Park West, New York, NY 10023, (212) 787-0750, BA 56 Mount Holyoke Coll; MA 57 Columbia Univ Teachers Coll; Retired, **SLP**

Rubin, Mrs Harriet Levinson 93 Lambert Place, Paramus, NJ 07652, (201) 652-2737, BA 54 Emerson Coll; 56–Sp-Lang Path, Private Practice, **SLP**

Rubin, Mrs Helen Leser 1760 54th Street, Brooklyn, NY 11204, (718) 256-6845, BA 71 CUNY - Brooklyn Coll; MS 76 CUNY - Brooklyn Coll; **SLP**

Rubin, Dr Herbert Communication Department 1117CL, University Of Pittsburgh, Pittsburgh, PA 15260, (412) 624-6765, BA 51 CUNY - Queens Coll; MA 55 CUNY - Brooklyn Coll; PH 59 (NS) Harvard Univ; 72–Prof/Assoc Dean, U of Pittsburgh, **SLP F**

Rubin, Dr Hyla 185 Poyntz Avenue, Willowdale, ON, Canada M2N 1J5, (416) 978-8331, BA 71 Univ of CT; MS 72 Univ of VT; PH 84 (NS) Univ of CT; 84–Asst Prof, Univ of Toronto, **SLP**

Rubin, Julie K 117 Griggs Road, Brookline, MA 02146, (617) 536-7255, BS 78 Univ of MA - Amherst; MS 80 Purdue Univ - West Lafayette; 88–Aud, Emerson Coll, **A**

Rubin, Marsha J 175 Maple Avenue #5F, Westbury, NY 11590, **SLP**

Rubin, Martha Chickering 1432 Sunnyslope Avenue, Belmont, CA 94002, (415) 369-1411, SLP, Sequoia Union H S District, **SLP**

Rubin, Dr Martha Teichholtz 750 Park Avenue #2C, New York, NY 10021, (212) 249-0550, BA 44 CUNY - Hunter Coll; MA 45 Columbia Univ Teachers Coll; ED 69 (Aud) Columbia Univ Teachers Coll; 88–Research Associate, Bruner Foundation, **A F**

Rubin, Mrs Maxine S 10 Sheldon Road, Marblehead, MA 01945, (617) 631-0754, BS 63 Simmons Coll; ME 65 Boston Univ; **SLP A**

Rubin, Nan P 20 Pinckney Street, Boston, MA 02114, (617) 735-2073, BA 74 George Washington Univ; MS 75 Univ of MI - Ann Arbor; Sp-Lang Path, Beth Israel Hosp, **SLP ACE**

Rubin, Mrs Phyllis B 229 North Taylor Avenue, Oak Park, IL 60302, (312) 450-2100, BA 65 Univ of MD - College Park; MA 69 De Paul Univ; Sp/Lang Path, Proviso Area for Except Chldn, **SLP**

Rubin, Rona B 127 Morningside Drive, Longmeadow, MA 01106, (413) 567-6007, BA 78; MA 76; SLP, Lower Pioneer Val Ed Coll, **SLP**

Rubin, Sharon Tepfer 18 Cortland Road, Monsey, NY 10952, (914) 354-7633, MS 87 CUNY - Brooklyn Coll

Rubin, Mrs Shellie G 1439 Wakefield Court East, Columbus, OH 43209, (614) 491-4100, BS 80 IN Univ - Bloomington; ME 82 IN Univ - Bloomington; Sp-Lang Path, Hamilton Local Sch, **SLP**

Rubin, Sylvia 8099 N W 71 Court, Tamarac, FL 33321, (305) 735-9630, BA 58 CUNY - Brooklyn Coll; MA 71 Hofstra Univ; Sp-Lang Path, Broward County Schools, **SLP**

Rubin-Flukman, Ellen D 313 William St, Scotch Plains, NJ 07076, (201) 889-8226, MS 86 CUNY - Brooklyn Coll; **SLP**

Rubin-Haskell, Mrs Hinda P 14 John Poulter Road, Lexington, MA 02173, (617) 863-0339, BA 71 Univ of Hartford; MA 73 NY Univ; SLP, **SLP**

Rubinoff, Mrs Laura A 10216 Garden Way, Potomac, MD 20854, (301) 986-8747, BS 74 Northwestern Univ; MS 75 Univ of MI - Ann Arbor; 85–Sp-Lang Path, Private Practice, **SLP**

Rubinowitz, Linda 1211 Dobson, Evanston, IL 60602, **SLP A**

Rubins, Mrs Merry Sumner 734 Topaz, New Orleans, LA 70124, (504) 833-5865, BS 82 LA St Univ - Baton Rouge; MA 84 LA St Univ - Baton Rouge; SLP, St Bernard Parish Schl Bd, **SLP**

Rubins, Sherry R 16004 Fernway Road, Shaker Heights, OH 44120, (216) 991-7837, BS 69 OH St Univ; MS 71 Miami Univ - Oxford; Sp-Lang Path, Cleveland Hrng & Sp Cen, **SLP**

Rubins, Mrs Sue G 1 Gable Lane, Lafayette, CA 94549, (415) 283-7106, BS 67 Univ of VT; MA 80 Our Lady Lake Univ-San Anton; Dir, Clear Sp & Commun, **SLP**

Rubinstein, Adrienne 8 Dogwood Drive, Staten Island, NY 10312, (212) 780-5186, BA 73 CUNY - City College; MA 76 CUNY - City College; OM 83; Instructor, Brooklyn College, **A**

Rubinstein, Carrie M 245 Golden Oak Drive, Portola Valley, CA 94025, (415) 573-4010, BA 75 Northwestern Univ; MS 76 Univ of WI - Madison; Aud, San Mateo Office of Ed, **A**

Rubinstein, Julie A 515 East 83rd Street, New York, NY 10028, (212) 517-9321, BA 78 SUNY - Center at Buffalo; MA 80 NY Univ; Sp-Lang Path, Private Practice, **SLP**

Rubio, Mrs Linda P Speech Pathology Associates, 907 2nd Avenue, P O Box 2557, Opelika, AL 36801, (205) 749-0146, BA 77 Auburn Univ - Auburn; OM 79 Auburn Univ - Auburn; 81–Dir, Sp Path Assoc, **SLP**

Ruble, Cynthia E 5605 Delora Avenue, Cleveland, OH 44144, (216) 749-4952, BS 80 Northern MI Univ; MA 82 MI St Univ; Sup Sp-Lang Path, Broadview Dev Cntr, **SLP**

Ruble, Marilou Gerhardt Professional Audiological Serv, 245 Bailliere Drive, Martinsville, IN 46151, (317) 342-9394, BS 74 Purdue Univ - West Lafayette; MS 75 Univ of WI - Stevens Point; **A**

Ruby, Josephine R 234 Fountain Street #1-B, New Haven, CT 06515, BS 52 Southern CT St Univ; MS 58 Southern CT St Univ; **SLP**

Ruby, Trena G c/o Good Samaritan Medical Center, 1111 East McDowell Road, Phoenix, AZ 85006, (602) 239-4577, MS 87 Univ of WY; 88–Aud, Good Samaritan Med Ctr, **A**

Rucci-Zimmer, Susan 1665 Garcia, Atascadero, CA 93422, (805) 481-2528, BA 77 Univ of CA - Santa Barbara; MA 81 Univ of TX - El Paso; Sp-Lang Path, Newport Lang Speech & Audiology Ctr, **SLP**

Ruch, Shirley Ann 399 Parkway Drive, Sag Harbor, NY 11963, (516) 725-9347, BS 79 Miami Univ - Oxford; MA 84 OH St Univ; Sp-Lang Path, Private Practice, **SLP**

Rucho, Patricia Ann 38 Paul Street, Auburn, MA 01501, (617) 832-7696, BS 78 Worcester St Coll; MS 86 Worcester St Coll; **SLP**

Ruchti, Lynda Lee 4217 Beverly Road, Madison, WI 53711, (608) 273-5900, BS 83 Univ of WI - Madison; MS 86 Univ of WI - Madison; **SLP**

Rucker, Mrs Brenda M 830 Oak Hill Avenue, Endicott, NY 13760, (607) 797-1271, BA 70 Montclair St Coll; MS 73 Ithaca Coll; Sp-Lang Path, Binghamton City Sch Dist, **SLP**

Rucker, Mrs Emily Gressette 201 Chestnut Street, St Matthews, SC 29135, (803) 874-3314, BA 66 Columbia Coll; MA 85 SC St Coll; Sp-Lang Path, Calhoun Sch Dist, **SLP**

Rucker, Leigh-Ann 949 Northfield Court, Harrisonburg, VA 22801, (703) 434-5910, BS 81 Purdue Univ - West Lafayette; ME 83 James Madison Univ; Teacher of Hearing-Impaired, Harrisonburg City Schools, **A**

Rucker, Lila 21700 West McNichols #8, Detroit, MI 48219, (517) 355-2197, BA 74 Univ of AL- Tuscaloosa; MA 78 Wayne St Univ - Sch of Med; **A**

Rucker, Mrs Merrie Dee 1209 C E King, Excelsior Springs, MO 64024, (913) 686-3393, OB 82 Univ of KS; **SLP**

Rucker, Mrs Sandra A 3017 Gilmore Avenue, Pittsburgh, PA 15235, (412) 371-7200, OB 66; MS 72 Univ of Pittsburgh - Pittsburgh; SLP, Vna-Allegheny Co, **SLP**

Rucklos, Kimberly Dawn 526 Lavina Avenue, Sandpoint, ID 83864, (208) 267-3146, BA 82 Humboldt St Univ; MA 84 Humboldt St Univ; **SLP**

Ruckriegel, Linda Anne 6613 Styles Street, Fort Worth, TX 76114, (817) 782-4450, BA 81 Univ of South FL; MS 84 East Carolina Univ; Chief Aud, USAF, **A ACE**

Rucksdashel, Mrs Sharon V R R 1 Box 34, Aplington, IA 50604, (515) 456-4882, BS 60 Univ of NE - Lincoln; MA 72 Univ of NE - Lincoln; SLP, Northern Trails AEA, **SLP**

Ruda, Linda C 55 Airport Road, Dudley, MA 01570, (508) 987-3347, BA 68 Anna Maria Coll; MS 82 Worcester St Coll; Sp-Lang Path, Dudley-Charlton Reg Sch Dist, **SLP**

Rudd, Amy Key 7000 West Markham Street, Little Rock, AR 72205, PH (NS); **A**

Rudder, Marynell H 3410 54th Street, Lubbock, TX 79413, **SLP**

Rudder, Nancy L P O Box 63, Plainfield, IN 46168, BA 84 IN Univ - Bloomington; MA 85 IN Univ - Bloomington; Audiologist, John H Payne Associates Inc, **A**

Ruddle, Eugenia Marie P O Box 1091, Kamuela, HI 96743-1091, (808) 885-6238, BA 76 Humboldt St Univ; MA 77 Humboldt St Univ; Sp-Lang Path, Calif-Hi Elks Major Project, **SLP**

Ruddock, Mrs Gay L R R #52 Box 52, Terre Haute, IN 47805, (812) 237-7577, BS 85 IN St Univ - Terre Haute; MS 86 IN St Univ - Terre Haute; **SLP**

Ruddock, Jane Levine 92 Town Farm Road, New Boston, NH 03070, (603) 487-2211, BS 80 Syracuse Univ; MS 82 Columbia Univ Teachers Coll; Sp-Lang Path, New Boston Central Sch, **SLP**

Ruddock, Lisa Jean 1308 Wayland Street, Beaver Dam, WI 53916, (608) 854-2216, MS 84 Marquette Univ; BS 82 Marquette Univ; **SLP**

Rudeen, Lori L 1008 Square Terrace, Green Bay, WI 54313, (414) 497-3891, BS 82 Western IL Univ; MA 83 Western IL Univ; Sp-Lang Path, Green Bay Area Sch Dist, **SLP**

Rudel, Debra L 7980 Northwest 3rd Place, Plantation, FL 33324, (305) 473-9323, BS 84 OH Univ - Athens; MA 86 NY Univ; 87–Sp-Lang Path, Sunrise Rehab Hosp, **SLP**

Ruder, Charlotte 212 Country Club Lane, Carterville, IL 62918, **SLP A**

Ruder, Dr Kenneth F Dept Communication Dis & Sci, Southern Illinois Univ, Carbondale, IL 62901, (618) 453-4301, BA 62 Fort Hays St Univ; MS 64 Univ of WI - Madison; PH 69 (Comm Sciences) Univ of FL; Prof, S Il U Carbondale Dept Dis & S, **SLP**

Ruder, Larry Lee 4801 Cliff Avenue Suite 212, Independence, MO 64055, (816) 478-3555, BS 64 Fort Hays St Univ; MA 66 Univ of KS; Dir of Aud, Frederick W Hahn Jr MD, **A**

Ruderman, Mrs Lois Grebelsky 18 Geiger Lane, Warren, NJ 07060, (201) 271-1386, BA 76 Rutger's St Univ - Douglas Coll; MS 77 Adelphi Univ; Sp-Lang Path, Edison Twp Bd of Ed, **SLP**

Ruderman, Mrs Ruth S 24 Belknap Drive, Andover, MA 01810, (617) 862-7500, BA 67 Univ of MI - Ann Arbor; MS 68 Univ of MI - Ann Arbor; SLP, Lexington Pub Sch, **SLP**

Rudge, Nancy Joan 3710 Homewood Road, Cincinnati, OH 45227-3611, (513) 683-4200, BS 75 Bowling Green St Univ; MS 80 Miami Univ - Oxford; Sp/Lang Path, Loveland City Schs, **SLP**

Rudin, Bonnie L 420 East 72nd Street #12-B, New York, NY 10021, (212) 794-8883, BS 75 Emerson Coll; MS 76 Columbia Univ Teachers Coll; Sp/Lang Path, Overlook Hosp, **SLP**

Rudin, Steffi W 1077 Superba, Venice, CA 90291, **A**

Rudisill, D Kay 6206 Briar Rose, Houston, TX 77057, (713) 780-1085, BS 68 Stephen F Austin St Univ; MA 70 Southern Methodist Univ; Sp-Lang Path, Private Practice, **SLP**

Rudisill, Mrs Harlene C 15 East Aberdeen Road, P O Box 923, Ocean City, NJ 08226, BA 39 Wilson Coll; MA 67 Montclair St Coll; SLP, **SLP LM**

Ruditsky, Sherry Lynn 726 Chantry Circle, Simi Valley, CA 93065, (805) 526-7435, BA 85 CA St Univ - Northridge; MA 87 CA St Univ - Northridge; 87–Sp-Lang Path, Ventura Co Supt of Schs Ofc, **SLP**

Rudkin, Jean M Daniel Jorgensen MD PC, 920 Grand Avenue, Spencer, IA 51301, (712) 262-8120, BA 81 Univ of WI - Eau Claire; MS 83 Univ of WI - Stevens Point; Audiologist, Daniel Jorgensen MD, **A**

Rudman, Mrs Cynthia M 133 Rosemont Court, Walnut Creek, CA 94596, (415) 825-0144, BA 67 0187; MA 75 San Francisco St Univ; Sp-Lang Path, Mt Diablo USD Diag Cen, **SLP**

Rudnick, Marcia E 1114 Garfield Avenue, Wyomissing, PA 19610, (215) 378-0481, BS 72 Ithaca Coll; MA 75 Univ of MD - College Park; Sp-Lang Path, Berks VNA Inc, **SLP**

Rudnick, Sherry J 1420 Ocean Parkway, Apartment 3H, Brooklyn, NY 11230, (718) 636-4573, BA 78 CUNY - Brooklyn Coll; MS 81 CUNY - Brooklyn Coll; 79–Sp-Lang Path, St Frances de Sales Sch, **SLP**

Rudock, Michele Gabriele 311 West 3rd Street, Mount Carmel, PA 17851, (717) 339-3016, BS 85 Clarion Univ of PA; MS 86 Clarion Univ of PA; **A**

Rudolph, Ann Elizabeth 39 Hilton Street, Pequannock, NJ 07440, (201) 941-4011, BA 83 Montclair St Coll; MA 87 Montclair St Coll; 86–Sp-Lang Path, ECLC of NJ, **SLP**

Rudolph, Mrs Carolyn R 5815 Ropes Drive, Cincinnati, OH 45244, (513) 232-9007, BS 69 Univ of DE; ME 72 Univ of SC - Columbia; 88–Sp-Lang Path, Clermont County Bd of MRDD, **SLP**

Rudolph, Mrs Catherine Louise 15385 Inlet Place, Dumfries, VA 22026, (703) 878-0654, BS 80 Univ of MO - Columbia; MA 82 George Washington Univ; Sp-Lang Path, Private Practice, **SLP**

Rudolph, Deborah A 6 Powderhorn, Little Rock, AR 72212, (501) 663-8331, BA 71 Univ of AR - Fayetteville; MA 72 Univ of IA; Dir Outp Chdn Serv, Easter Seal Rehab Cen, **SLP**

Rudolph, Donna Ellen 1517 Brick Road, Cherry Hill, NJ 08003, (609) 267-0700, BA 83 Rutger's St Univ - Douglas Coll; OM 85 Hahneman Medical Coll; **SLP**

Rudolph, Mrs Judith C 1447 N W 12th Street, Corvallis, OR 97330, (503) 967-4617, BA 52 Univ of Cincinnati; MA 54; MA 71 IN Univ - Bloomington; Sp/Lang Path, Albany Pub Sch Dist, **SLP**

Rudolph, Mrs Patricia Marguerite 23 Continental Drive, West Milford, NJ 07480, (312) 447-7902, **SLP**

Rudrauff, Sally Ann 2416 Yorktown #378, Houston, TX 77056, (713) 723-9623, BS 83 Univ of TX - Austin; MA 85 Univ of TX - Austin; Sp-Lang Path, Houston ISD, **SLP**

Rudy, Jane Hunter Hearing And Speech Center, 730 Valley Street, Dayton, OH 45403, (513) 222-5597, BS 73 Miami Univ - Oxford; MA 74 Univ of MD - College Park; Aud, Hrng/Sp Cen of Metro Dayton, **A**

Rudy, Mrs Janice 20 Heritage Drive, Lexington, MA 02173, (617) 259-8342, BS 69 Emerson Coll; MS 71 Emerson Coll; 83–Sp-Lang Path, Carroll Sch, **SLP**

Rudy, John Michael 29 Henry Street, East Brunswick, NJ 08816, (201) 821-7748, BA 84 Kean Coll of NJ; MA 86 Kean Coll of NJ

Rudy, Susan Kay 312 Dogwood Lane, Hillsville, VA 24343, (703) 728-3549, **SLP**

Rudy, V Susan 1321 West 36th Street, Erie, PA 16508, BS 68 Edinboro Univ of PA; MS 69 CO St Univ; 88–Sp-Lang Path, Sch Dist-City of Erie, **SLP**

Rue, Hazel May 11220 N E Morris Street, Portland, OR 97220, (503) 254-0971, BS 57 Portland St Univ; ME 59 Univ of OR; **SLP LM**

Rue, Ken 1018 Durango, Great Falls, MT 59401, (406) 452-0480, BS 72 Moorhead St Univ; MA 75 Univ of MT; SLP, Great Falls Pub Schs, **SLP**

Rue, Mrs Patricia A 4830 Pembroke, Reno, NV 89502-9715, (702) 789-3268, BS 76 Keene St Coll; MS 81 Univ of NV - Reno; SLP, St Marys Hosp Reno Nv, **SLP**

Ruebl, Celeste Burnett Avenue 1287 Donald Drive, Woodruff, WI 54568, (715) 479-6479, BA 75 Univ of WI - Eau Claire; MS 80 Univ of WI - River Falls; SLP, CES #9, **SLP**

Ruebush-Gonzales, Lynn N 1145 Heaven Hill Road, Sonoma, CA 95476, **SLP**

Ruef, Carolyn Larson 154 East Briar Lane, Green Bay, WI 54301, (414) 822-3191, BA 65 Univ of WI - Madison; BS 83 Univ of WI - Stevens Point; MS 85 Univ of WI - Stevens Point; Sp-Lang Path, Pulaski Community Schools, **SLP**

Ruehle-Kumar, Karen 1502 Holly River, Houston, TX 77077, (713) 496-3497, BS 81 Baylor Univ; MA 84 Univ of TX - Austin; Sp-Lang Path, Private Practice, **SLP**

Ruelle, Mrs Martha L 5802-D Torington Drive, Springfield, VA 22152, (703) 323-1317, MS 74 CUNY - Brooklyn Coll; Sp-Lang Path, Fairfax Co Pub Sch, **SLP**

Ruff, Jacqueline 2118 9th Avenue, Bloomer, WI 54724, (507) 454-2930, BA 77 Univ of WI - Eau Claire; MS 78 Univ of WI - Eau Claire; Asst Prof/Cl Coord, Coll of St Teresa, **SLP**

Ruffen, Frederick 30 Roosevelt Street, Glen Cove, NY 11542, (516) 759-0008, BA 69 Hofstra Univ; MA 71 CUNY - Queens Coll; Private Practice, **A**

Ruffin, Margaret A 712 St Thomas Street, Lafayette, LA 70506, (318) 233-5079, BS 77 LA St Univ - Baton Rouge; MS 80 Univ of Southwestern LA; Sp-Lang Path, Private Practice, **SLP**

Ruffin, Mrs Patricia Dean 3196 Vista Circle, Macon, GA 31204, (912) 474-6536, BS 75 Auburn Univ - Auburn; MS 77 Auburn Univ - Auburn; Sp/Lang Path, Bibb Co Publ Sch, **SLP**

Ruffner, Mrs Michele A 30 Bay Avenue, Hampton Bays, NY 11946, (516) 728-9298, BS 82 Marywood Coll; MA 83 Hofstra Univ; 86, Private Practice, **SLP**

Ruffolo, Mrs Linda P 2820 Chichester Lane, Fort Wayne, IN 46815, (219) 485-0846, BA 63 Univ of WI - Madison; MS 66 IL St Univ - Normal; **SLP**

Rufin, Virginia Dare Rufin Speech And Language Ctr, 900 Beverly Garden Drive, Metairie, LA 70002, (504) 835-9654, BA 58 Southern Methodist Univ; MS 64 Tulane Univ; Dir, Rufin Sp & Lang Cen, **SLP A**

Ruflin, Joan Marie 213 Chartwell Court, Rochester, NY 14618, (716) 442-0922, MA 87 SUNY - Coll at Geneseo; **SLP**

Ruge, Mrs Mary E 6121 Old Brentford Court, Alexandria, VA 22310-4347, (703) 971-8842, BS 78 Northern MI Univ; MA 81 Northern MI Univ; 85–Sp-Lang Path, Prince William County, **SLP**

Rugg, Mrs Joanne D 80 Mohawk Trail, Buffalo Grove, IL 60089, (312) 255-1233, BS 73 Northern IL Univ - De Kalb; MA 74 Northern IL Univ - De Kalb; SLP, Mount Prospect Sch Dist 57, **SLP**

Ruggiero, Mrs Gina Marchese 73-T Farm Road, Hillsborough, NJ 08876, BA 81 Rutger's St Univ - Douglas Coll; MS 83 Columbia Univ Teachers Coll; Sp-Lang Path, Overlook Hosp, **SLP**

Ruggiero, Mrs Judith Lynn 2415 Wingedfoot Drive, Westlake, OH 44145, (216) 331-4904, **SLP**

Rugh, Caroline Lee RD 4 Box 171, Greensburg, PA 15601, (412) 281-1122, BS 85 WV Univ; MA 86 Univ of Pittsburgh - Pittsburgh; 87–Aud, Hearing Unlimited Inc, **A**

Ruguleiski, Michelle Anne 36 Argonne Street, West Quincy, MA 02169, (617) 770-0514, MA 84 Univ of MT; **A**

Ruhaak, Linda Ellen 6205 West 10th Street, Sioux Falls, SD 57107, (605) 333-6665, BS 85 SD St Univ; MA 86 Univ of Northern IA; **SLP**

Ruhalter, Fern Gayle 211-10 18th Avenue #3-G, Bayside, NY 11360, (516) 746-5575, **SLP**

Ruhalter, Wendy Baer 506 Lindsley Drive, Morristown, NJ 07960, (201) 233-6384, **SLP**

Ruhl, A Connie (Kuhrt) 2030 Baker Terrace, Olympia, WA 98501, (206) 357-3339, BA 64 Univ of WA; MS 71 Portland St Univ; 88–Sp-Lang Path, Private Practice, **SLP**

Ruhl, Mrs Kelly Sue 1127 North Street, Logansport, IN 46947, (219) 563-7438, BS 82 Ball St Univ; MA 83 Ball St Univ; 84–Sp-Lang Path, Metropolitan Sch Dist of Wabash Co, **SLP**

Ruhland, Carol A 8255 North Cedarburg Road, Brown Deer, WI 53209, (414) 377-6030, BS 59 Marquette Univ; MA 68; Sp-Lang Path, Cedarburg Sch, **SLP**

Ruhland, Mrs Robin Kay N6786 Jonathan Drive, Pardeeville, WI 53954, (715) 723-0756, MA 84 Univ of WI - Eau Claire; SLP, Portage Comm Sch, **SLP**

Ruhlin, Amy Noggle 426 S Kirkwood Rd Unit J, St Louis, MO 63122, (314) 966-3521, BA 84 LA St Univ - Baton Rouge; MA 86 LA St Univ - Baton Rouge; **SLP**

Ruhlin, Mrs Susan U 3089 State Road, Medina, OH 44256, (216) 375-3882, MA 78 Univ of Denver; BA 75 Denison Univ; Sp-Lang Path, Akron City Hosp, **SLP**

Ruhm, Dr Howard B Audiology & Speech Pathology, VA Hospital, 3350 La Jolla Village Dr, San Diego, CA 92161, (619) 453-7500, BA 55 George Washington Univ; MA 56 Univ of MD - College Park; PH 59 (NS) Northwestern Univ; Ch, Aud & Sp - Lang Path, VA Med Cen - San Diego, **A F**

Ruiter, Irma Divera 73 Graystone Crescent, Welland, ON, Canada L3C 6G6, (416) 732-2284, BA 77 Ryerson Polytech Inst - On; MA 84 SUNY - Coll at Buffalo; 84–Sp-Lang Path, Niagara Assess & Prog Svcs, **SLP**

Ruiz, Cesar E 2250 Holly Hall #262, Houston, TX 77054, (713) 790-5916, BS 86 Saint Louis Univ; MA 88 Saint Louis Univ

Ruiz, Judith H 1745 Northridge, Hurst, TX 76053, (817) 460-3591, BS 76 Univ of North TX; MS 78 Univ of North TX; Sp-Lang Path, Arlington ISD, **SLP**

Ruiz, Victor G 9860 Adolfo Court, Rancho Cucamonga, CA 91730, (714) 945-2006, MA CA St Univ - Fullerton; Sp-Lang Path, Lanterman Development Center, **SLP**

Ruiz, Willie 2727 Old Alice Road #39, Brownsville, TX 78521, (512) 544-0640, BS 83 Univ of TX - Austin; MS 86 Univ of NM; **A**

Rukin, Sharon Faye 4529 West Columbia, Lincolnwood, IL 60646, (312) 677-1282, BS 78 Tel Aviv Univ - Israel; MS 81 Univ of WI - Milwaukee; Northwestern Univ; **SLP**

Rukstalis, Kathleen Grace 97 Slocum Street, Apartment 2, Forty Fort, PA 18704, (717) 342-8379, BS 83 King's Coll; MS 86 PA St Univ - Univ Park; Sp-Lang Path, St Joseph Center, **SLP**

Rule, Karley Dona 11824 S W Windmill Drive, Beaverton, OR 97005, (503) 626-6609, BA 84 Eastern WA Univ; MS 85 Eastern WA Univ; **SLP**

Rulon, Mrs Kristi J 2508 East 12th Street, Cheyenne, WY 82001, (307) 638-7741, BS 86 Univ of WY; MS 88 CO St Univ; 88–Sp-Lang Path, Cheyenne Ctr Comm Dis

Rumack, Mrs Nancy Berg 2421 South Standage, Mesa, AZ 85202, (602) 838-8175, BA 75 Purdue Univ - West Lafayette; MA 77 Northwestern Univ; Sp-Lang Path, Private Practice, **SLP**

Rumbaugh, Mrs Lisa Schubert 2576 Wilma Drive, Wooster, OH 44691-1917, (216) 263-8243, BS 83 Bowling Green St Univ; MA 84 Bowling Green St Univ; 86–Sp-Lang Path, Wooster Com Hosp, **SLP**

Ruminski, Mrs Marion G 20 Lost Brook Lane, Wallingford, CT 06492, (203) 265-3020, BA 64 William Paterson Coll; MA 67 Columbia Univ Teachers Coll; Sp-Lang Path, Area Coop Ed Serv, **SLP**

Rummel, Mrs Veronica Kadala Route 1 Box 1103, Newberry, FL 32669, (904) 472-4035, BA 78 Univ of FL; ME 87 Univ of FL

Rummelhart, Patricia D 20 Gant Circle #F, Streamwood, IL 60107, (312) 893-7995, BS 76 Northern IL Univ - De Kalb; OB 83 Governors St Univ; MS 86 Governors St Univ; 86–Sp-Lang Path, Comm Therapy Svcs, **SLP**

Rumping, Mrs Jane Bles 416 Donnelly, De Soto, MO 63020, (314) 937-3633, MA 83 Southeast MO St Univ; BS 81 Southeast MO St Univ; SLP, MD State Schs for Sev Hndcpd, **SLP**

Runa-Hencley, Mrs Cynthia 3013 Thunder Bay Road, Little Canada, MN 55117, (612) 779-8506, BS 82 Moorhead St Univ; MS 83 Saint Cloud St Univ; Sp-Lang Path, Spec Intermdt Sch Dist 916, **SLP**

Runbeck, Mrs Robyn Goddard 3342 East Yucca, Phoenix, AZ 85028, (602) 952-0157, BA 80 Univ of Redlands; OM 82 Univ of WA; Sp-Lang Path, Scottsdale Pub Sch, **SLP**

Rundbaken, Ann E 914 South Avenue #C-8, Secane, PA 19018, (215) 876-5555, BS 77 PA St Univ - Univ Park; MS 78 Univ of MI - Ann Arbor; Sp-Path, Delaware Co Home Health Ser, **SLP**

Rundbaken, Sol Savannah Speech & Hearing Ctr, 1206 East 66th Street, Savannah, GA 31404, (912) 355-4601, BA 55 Univ of GA; ME 60 Univ of GA; PH 66 (Sp & Hrng Science) MI St Univ; Dir, Savannah Sp/Hrng Cen, **SLP A**

Rundberg, Elizabeth Ann 3601 Greenwood Avenue, Los Angeles, CA 90066, (213) 372-0852, BA 57 Univ of IA; MA 65 Univ of Southern CA; SLP, Los Angeles Co Supt of Sch, **SLP**

Runfola, Rosanne M 16 Hartlawn Road, West Roxbury, MA 02132, ME 75 Northeastern Univ; Sp-Lang Path, Woburn Public Schools, **SLP**

Runge, Cheryl A Southwest Audiology Inc, 3104 East Indian School #100, Phoenix, AZ 85016, (602) 224-5970, BS 78 Univ of CA - Santa Barbara; MS 80 Univ of AZ; Aud/Pres, Southwest Audiology Inc, **A**

Runge, Mrs JoAnn Kay Box 153, Unity, WI 54488, (715) 659-4211, BA 70 Univ of WI - Eau Claire; MS 73 Univ of WI - Stevens Point; Sp-Lang Path, Spencer Schools, **SLP**

Runion, Dr Howard L 18616 N 99th Avenue, Sun City, AZ 85373, (602) 977-6507, BA 31 Univ of MI - Ann Arbor; MA 32 Univ of MI - Ann Arbor; PH 36 (NS) Univ of MI - Ann Arbor; **SLP LM**

Runnels-Contee, Cathy 806 Gregorio Drive, Silver Spring, MD 20901, BA 73 Chapman Coll; MS 75 Syracuse Univ; Coordinator Language Classes, Montgomery Co Pub Schs, **SLP**

Runner, Sandra J 4910 Pleasant Street #13, West Des Moines, IA 50265, (515) 283-6344, BS 73 IA St Univ; MS 75 Univ of WY; Sp-Lang Path, IA Methodist Med Cen, **SLP**

Runyan, Dr Charles M 306 Fairway Drive, Harrisonburg, VA 22801, (703) 568-3870, BA 62 Grove City Coll; MA 72 Univ of KY; PH 75 (NS) Purdue Univ - West Lafayette; Prof, Jame Madison U, **SLP**

Runyan, Mrs Kathryn A 595 Coachman Drive #5, Troy, MI 48083, (313) 756-9800, BA 87 MI St Univ; MA 87 MI St Univ; 88–Sp-Lang Path, Neurological Recovery Sys, **SLP**

Runyan, Laura Kathleen 13130 West 88th Court #98, Lenexa, KS 66215, (816) 932-3262, BS 83 IA St Univ; MA 85 Western MI Univ; McFarland Clinic, **A**

Runyan, Sara Elizabeth 306 Fairway Drive, Harrisonburg, VA 22801, (703) 568-3873, MA 70 Univ of KY; Assoc Prof, James Madison U, **SLP ACE**

Runyon, Mrs Jill Lynn 319 East Voltaire Avenue, Phoenix, AZ 85022, (602) 993-4349, BS 75 Univ of WI - Stevens Point; MS 76 Marquette Univ; Sp/Lang Path, Private Practice, **SLP**

Runyon, Mrs Phyllis J 1620 East Pine Avenue, Lompoc, CA 93436, (805) 934-2526, BA 76 Humboldt St Univ; MA 77 Humboldt St Univ; Sp-Lang Path, Orcutt Union Sch Dist, **SLP**

Runyon, Mrs Ramona G 8 Maple Drive, Huntington, WV 25705, (304) 696-3640, BA 76 Marshall Univ; MA 78 Marshall Univ; Clinical Coordinator/Supervisr, Marshall Univ Sp/Hrng Center, **SLP**

Rupard, Mrs Robyn Chandler 510 Dorado Drive, Mandeville, LA 70448, (504) 626-5225, ME 87 Southeastern LA Univ; 84–Sp-Lang Path, St Tammany Parish Sch Bd, **SLP**

Rupert, Mrs Catherine 908 East Euclid, Peoria Heights, IL 61614, (309) 693-5350, BA 77 Augustana Coll; MA 78 Univ of IL - Urbana; 86–Sp-Lang Path, Div Svc for Crippled Chldrn, **SLP**

Rupert, Sandra 5029 Chuckleberry Lane, Westerville, OH 43081, (614) 345-9891, BS 75 OH St Univ; MA 76 Kent St Univ; Sp-Lang Path, Newark Cty Sch, **SLP**

Ruplinger, Kathleen A 2676 Four Mile Road, Marathon, WI 54448, (715) 443-2402, **SLP**

Rupp, Diana Susan 4210 East 53rd #1321, Odessa, TX 79762, (915) 366-3793, BS 86 Baylor Univ; MS 87 Baylor Univ; 88–Sp-Lang Path, Permian Basin Rehabilitation Ctr

Rupp, Dr Ralph R 1004 West Cross, Ypsilanti, MI 48197, (313) 487-4411, BA 51 Univ of MI - Ann Arbor; MA 52 Univ of MI - Ann Arbor; PH 64 (NS) Wayne St Univ; Coord of Aud, Eastern Michigan Univ, **SLP A F**

Rupp, Shayne D Y 515 East 2nd Street, Brooklyn, NY 11218, BA 74 CUNY - Brooklyn Coll; MS 77 CUNY - Brooklyn Coll; **SLP**

Rupp, Susan K 1005 Robertson #B-1, Fort Collins, CO 80524, (303) 491-1961, BS 70 KS St Univ; MS 82 Fort Hays St Univ; **SLP**

Rupp, Mrs Virginia H 5416 Tomahawk Trail, Fort Wayne, IN 46804, (219) 432-7259, MA 77 Univ of MT; BA 74 Univ of MT; Sp-Lang Path, Dillingham Cty Sch Dist, **SLP**

Ruprecht, Audrey J 163 Upper Lea Lane, Long Lake, MN 55356, (612) 477-5838, BS 76 Univ of IA; MA 77 Univ of IA; Sp-Lang Path, Rockford ISD #883, **SLP**

Ruscello, Dr Dennis M West Virginia University, 805 Allen Hall, P O Box 6122, Morgantown, WV 26506, (304) 293-4241, BS 69 CA Univ of PA; MS 72 WV Univ; PH 77 (Sp Path) Univ of AZ; 86–Prof, West Virginia University, **SLP F**

Rusch, Mrs Catherine Rea 3520 Nashville Avenue, New Orleans, LA 70125, (504) 897-8563, BS 79 Vanderbilt Univ; MS 81 Purdue Univ - West Lafayette; 86–Sp-Lang Path, Touro Infirmary, **SLP ACE**

Ruscio, Mrs Denise R 109 Waterford Road, Island Park, NY 11558, (516) 432-6971, MS 87 Adelphi Univ; 83–Sp-Lang Path, NYC Bd of Educ, **SLP**

Ruscito, Mary Ann 18 Donna Terrace, Hyde Park, MA 02136, (617) 361-7537, BA 75 Boston Coll; MA 77 Central MI Univ; 87–Sp-Lang Path, Canton PS, **SLP**

Ruse, Susan Dankovich 969 Fife Avenue Apartment 9, Wilmington, OH 45177, (513) 393-1904, BS 74 CA Univ of PA; MS 87 CA Univ of PA; 88–Sp-Lang Path, Clinton Co Bd of Educ, **SLP**

Rush, Carol Schaffer 128 Marine Avenue #6L, Brooklyn, NY 11209, BS 76 Northeastern Univ; MS 79 Paterson St Coll; Sp-Lang Path, Private Practice, **SLP**

Rush, Dathan D 10608 Flamingo Avenue, Oklahoma City, OK 73162, (405) 427-8651, BS 83 Central St Univ; MA 85 OK St Univ; Sp-Lang Path, OK City-County Health Dept, **SLP**

Rush, Mrs Debra Shelton Box 5326, APO New York, NY 09012, BS 78 MS Univ for Women; MS 80 MS Univ for Women; 80–Sp-Lang Path, Lamar County Pub School System, **SLP**

Rush, Mrs Elizabeth S 424 Bywood Drive, Durham, NC 27712, (919) 575-7908, BA 67 Univ of NC - Greensboro; MA 68 OH Univ - Athens; Dir Dept Sp/Lang/Hrng Serv, Murdoch Cen, **SLP**

Rush, Mrs Judith I 20301 Maplewood Drive, Edmonds, WA 98020, (206) 774-2788, BA 62 Univ of WA; MA 72 CA St Univ - Los Angeles; **SLP**

Rush, Mrs Juliann Finegan 1646 Peregrine Point Drive, Sarasota, FL 34231, (813) 924-9221, MS 82 Univ of South FL; Aud, Self Employed/Dispensing Aud, **A**

Rush, Mrs Lisa B 5910 North San Bernardo, Apartment 175, Laredo, TX 78041, (512) 722-2431, **SLP**

Rush, Mrs Mary B 1681 Berry Lane, Snellville, GA 30278, (404) 985-0825, BS 73 OH Univ - Athens; ME 78 GA St Univ; Sp-Lang Path, Metro Area Sp & Lang Svcs, **SLP**

Rush, Mrs Patricia A Hearing And Speech Services, 1038 River Oaks Drive, Flowood, MS 39208, (601) 939-0547, BA 73 Univ of MS; OM 74 Univ of MS; Aud, Hrng/Sp Serv, **SLP A**

Rush, Mrs Sandra L 2045 South Hillcrest, Springfield, MO 65807, (417) 886-7416, **SLP**

Rushfeldt, Mrs Betty Jane , Oberon, ND 58357, Minot St Univ; Chapter I Remedial Rdng Tchr, Oberon Pub Sch, **SLP**

Rushing, Mrs Karen C 2920 Ruskin Court, Abingdon, MD 21009, (301) 676-2455, BS 71 G Peabody Coll-Vanderbilt U; MS 73 Vanderbilt Univ; Sp-Lang Path, Private Practice, **SLP**

Rushing, Robert O, Jr 327 Meadowlark Circle, Statesboro, GA 30458, (912) 489-8601, BA 75 Auburn Univ - Auburn; OM 77 Auburn Univ - Auburn; Aud, First Dist Coop Ed Ser Agcy, **A**

Rushing, Robin Ann 11 Plantation Gates, Hilton Head Island, SC 29928, (803) 686-4879, BS 85 Western KY Univ; MS 86 Western KY Univ; Sp-Lang Path, InSpeech Inc, **SLP**

Rushing, Susan Yvonne 1581 Roxbury Court, Palm Bay, FL 32905, (305) 777-1373, BA 82 Univ of Central FL; MA 83 Univ of Central FL; Sp-Lang Path, Brevard County Schools, **SLP**

Rusignola, Kathryn Sosnicky 536 Valley Road, Watchung, NJ 07060, (201) 756-4121, BA 71 Catholic Univ of America; MA 72 Montclair St Coll; **SLP**

Rusk, Bobbie Leigh 3428 Cove View Boulevard, Apartment 832, Galveston, TX 77554, (409) 744-8322, BS 82 Northwest MO St Univ; MS 84 Northwest MO St Univ; Sp-Lang Path, Mainland Center Hospital, **SLP**

Ruskey, Debra Ann 1686 Carman Mill, St Louis, MO 63011, (314) 644-7804, BS 79 Southern IL Univ -Carbondale; MA 81 Southeast MO St Univ; SLP, St Louis Dev Deabl Treat Cen, **SLP**

Rusnak, Elaine M 4907 Kinley Avenue, Pittsburgh, PA 15207, (412) 751-6769, BA 78 Univ of Pittsburgh - Pittsburgh; MA 80 Univ of Pittsburgh - Pittsburgh; SLP, Allegheny I U, **SLP**

Rusnak, Julianna 4643 South Francisco, Chicago, IL 60632, (312) 890-0529, BA 84 Saint Xavier Coll; OM 86 Governors St Univ; **SLP**

Russ, Mrs Diane Mendelsohn 1621 South Boulevard, Evanston, IL 60202, (312) 657-7560, BA 67 CUNY - Brooklyn Coll; MA 84 Northwestern Univ; 86–Sp-Lang Path, Comm Care Ctr Ltd, **A**

Russ, Lugene A 805 Old Metairie Drive, Metairie, LA 70001, (504) 885-6633, BA 78 Univ of Southwestern LA; OM 80 LA St Univ - N O Medical Ctr; Owner, Russ Semmes & Assoc Inc, **SLP**

Russel, Mrs Gina P 11951 Fairway Circle North Dr, Indianapolis, IN 46236, (317) 845-9259, BS 81 Ball St Univ; MA 86 Ball St Univ; **SLP**

Russel, Mark 5123 East 69th Street, Indianapolis, IN 46220, (219) 284-7134, BA 76 Eastern WA Univ; MS 79 Eastern WA Univ; Sp-Lang Path, Mem Hosp of South Bend, **SLP**

Russell, Mrs Andrea I P 1005 Westerly Drive, Marlton, NJ 08053, (609) 547-1322, BA 71 CUNY - Brooklyn Coll; MA 77 Trenton St Coll; Sp-Lang Path, Haddon Heights Pub Sch, **SLP**

Russell, Ann Faith 1613 West Lock Raven Road, Champaign, IL 61821, (217) 352-7724, BA 76 Univ of South Africa; BA 80 Witwatersrand Univ S Africa; MS 86 Washington Univ; 87–Research Asst, Univ of Illinois, **A**

Russell, Belinda Brooks 919 North 5th Street, Grand Junction, CO 81501, (303) 244-6531, BA 78 Univ of AL- Tuscaloosa; MS 79 Univ of AL- Tuscaloosa; SLP, Hilltop Rehab Hosp, **SLP**

Russell, Mrs Charleen G 2875 Fox Hill Road, Aurora, IL 60505-5906, BS 76 Northern IL Univ - De Kalb; MA 77 Northern IL Univ - De Kalb; Sp-Lang Path, Aurora E Sch Dist #131, **SLP**

Russell, Mrs Cheryl Winchester 25285 Randolph Road, Bedford Heights, OH 44146, (216) 651-3219, BS 76 Saint Louis Univ; MA 82 Cleveland St Univ; Sp/Lang Path, Cleveland Pub Sch Syst, **SLP**

Russell, Cynthia A 3518 Williamsburg Lane N W, Washington, DC 20008, (202) 966-4420, BS 69 Univ of OK - Norman; MA 70 Univ of OK - Norman; Dir-SLP & Aud, Rehab I of W FL, **SLP**

Russell, Cynthia Ramsey 3226 West Fox Farm Road, Manistee, MI 49660, (616) 757-3716, BS 76 Central MI Univ; MA 81 Central MI Univ; Sp-Lang Path, Mason-Lake Inter Sch Dist, **SLP**

Russell, David F 149 Pakachoag Street, Auburn, MA 01501, (508) 792-8500, BA 66 Marietta Coll; MA 68 OH Univ - Athens; 71–Dir Sp-Lang Path, Hahnemann Rehab Cen, **SLP**

Russell, Dawn 139 Dean Street, Norwood, MA 01062, (617) 769-2597, BS 82 Northwestern Univ; MA 83 Northwestern Univ; Sp-Lang Path, Comm Ther Svcs, **SLP ACE**

Russell, Diane B 185 Covington Street, Oakland, CA 94605, (415) 638-9595, BA 73 Univ of CA - Santa Barbara; MS 76 AZ St Univ; 81–Sp-Lang Path, Livermore Jt Unif Sch Dist, **SLP**

Russell, Elizabeth 1250 Bailey Road, Naperville, IL 60565, (312) 420-1570, BA 73 Saint Xavier Coll; MA 76 Northern IL Univ - De Kalb; Dept Hd - Sp - Lang Path, Americana Healthcare, **SLP**

Russell, Mrs Glennae Anderson 15 Rockledge Place, Maumelle, AR 72118, (501) 851-3292, OB 78 Univ of Central AR; MS 83 Univ of AR - Little Rock; Sp-Lang Path, Private Practice, **SLP**

Russell, Jamie Sue 33 South Fairview, Liberty, MO 64068, (816) 472-0545, MS 84 Fontbonne Coll; BS 82 Fontbonne Coll; SLP, Lexington R-V Sch Dist, **SLP**

Russell, Jan Elaine 1500 North Bowman, Danville, IL 61832, (217) 446-4390, BS 86 IN St Univ - Terre Haute; MS 87 IN St Univ - Terre Haute; 88–Sp-Lang Path, Oakwood Comm USD #76, **SLP**

Russell, Jean Westfall 504 Carnation Drive, Clarks Summit, PA 18411, BA 77 MI St Univ; MA 78 MI St Univ; **SLP**

Russell, Joanne Marie 706 Hood Road, Swarthmore, PA 19081, (215) 876-9229, BS 75 PA St Univ - Univ Park; MA 81 West Chester Univ of PA; Sp-Lang Path, Delaware Co Inter Ut, **SLP**

Russell, Kimberly K 620 1st Street, Mounds, IL 62964, (618) 745-6227, MS 88 Murray St Univ; 88–Sp-Lang Path, Illinois Center for Autism, **F**

Russell, Mrs Leigh Ann 2219 Kings Lake Blvd, Naples, FL 33962, (813) 262-1171, BS 79 Clarion Univ of PA; MA 81 Kent St Univ; 84–Aud, Dr Raymond L Pfister MD, **A**

Russell, Linda Kay 1730 Penfield Road #64, Penfield, NY 14526, (716) 271-0761, BS 80 SUNY - Coll at Geneseo; MS 82 Nazareth Coll of Rochester; Sp-Lang Path, Mary Cariola Childrens Center, **SLP**

Russell, Dr Lorraine H 1315 Barton Drive, Fort Washington, PA 19034, (215) 787-1876, BS 59 Syracuse Univ; MA 62 Western MI Univ; PH 77 (NS) CUNY - Grad Sch & Univ Cntr; Associate Professor, Temple University, **SLP**

Russell, Mrs Luanne S 425 Whiteheath Road, Louisville, KY 40243, (502) 245-5661, BS 76 Univ of Louisville; MS 79 Univ of Louisville; **SLP**

Russell, Marcus Randall 10753 N W 21st Street, Coral Springs, FL 33065, (305) 845-2800, **A**

Russell, Dr Marilyn Margaret W26308 Drumheller Road, Cheney, WA 99004, (509) 359-6624, BS 79 Clarion St Coll; ME 80 Clarion St Coll; PH 86 (Anatomy) Univ of NC - Chapel Hill; 87–Asst Prof, Eastern Washington Univ, **SLP**

Russell, Mary C 521 East 24th Street, Brooklyn, NY 11210, BA 64 Sioux Falls Coll; MS 79 Coll of Saint Rose; SLP, NYC Bd of Ed, **SLP**

Russell, Mrs Mary Jo Burns Route 2 Box 1470, Atlanta, MI 49709, (517) 786-2253, BA 73 Central MI Univ; MA 78 Central MI Univ; OM 82 MI St Univ; Sp-Lang Path, Speech Pathology Services, **SLP**

Russell, Mrs Mary M 8815 N W Lake Crest Avenue, Vancouver, WA 98665, (206) 687-5171, BA 66 Central WA Univ; MS 73 Portland St Univ; Sp-Lang Path, Battleground Sch Dist, **SLP**

Russell, Dr Nancy K SUNY - College At Buffalo, Speech Language Pathology & Audiology K217, 1300 Elmwood Avenue, Buffalo, NY 14222, (716) 878-5306, BA 76 Univ of MN - Minneap-St Paul; MA 78 Univ of NE - Lincoln; PH 86 (NS) SUNY - Center at Buffalo; Asst Prof, SUNY-Buffalo, **SLP**

Russell, Randy P 3112 East 21st Street, Odessa, TX 79761, (915) 563-0323, BA 71 Hardin-Simmons Univ; MA 73 Memphis St Univ; President, Audio Acoustics Inc, **SLP A**

Russell, Rebecca R 510 South Extension #1021, Mesa, AZ 85210, (602) 967-2426, BA 85 Univ of MN - Duluth; MA 86 Univ of MN - Duluth; 88–Sp-Lang Path, Develop Svcs Ctr Inc, **SLP**

Russell, Mrs Sandra L 7737 Bellaire Avenue, North Hollywood, CA 91605, (818) 764-4148, BA 75 San Jose St Univ; MA 79 CA St Univ - Northridge; 78–SLP, LA Cty USD, **SLP**

Russell, Shari L 438 Ridge Road #8, Greenbelt, MD 20770, (301) 474-2725, BA 85 Univ of MD - College Park; MA 87 Univ of MD - College Park; 87–Sp-Lang Path, Anne Arundel Co Bd of Educ, **SLP**

Russell, Mrs Sharon A 3312 Eisenhower Lane, Plano, TX 75023, (913) 541-1208, BS 76 Southeast MO St Univ; MA 79 Northeast MO St Univ; SLP, Blue Valley Sch Dist, **SLP**

Russell, Mrs Susan 3120 Crabtree Lane, Elkhart, IN 46514, (219) 533-2141, BS 73 IN St Univ - Terre Haute; MS 74 IN St Univ - Terre Haute; Sp-Lang Path, Goshen General Hosp, **SLP**

Russell, Susan 10749 East 29th Place, Tulsa, OK 74129, (918) 663-6361, BA 77 SUNY - Center at Buffalo; MA 79 Univ of Tulsa; Sp-Lang Path, Private Practice, **SLP**

Russell, Susan Jeanne MHMR-Infant Stimulation, 3701 North Big Spring, Midland, TX 79705, (915) 683-5591, BA 79 Stephen F Austin St Univ; MS 84 TX Tech Univ; 88–Sp-Lang Path, Permian Basin Com Ctr for MHMR, **SLP**

Russell, Susan Moore 20307 Hellenic, Olympia Fields, IL 60461, (815) 740-3196, BS 80 MacMurray Coll; MS 85 Vanderbilt Univ; 86–Aud, Regional Educ Service Agency, **A**

Russell, Mrs Susan Scanlan 7210 Kingwood, Little Rock, AR 72207, (501) 664-8125, BS 77 Univ of North TX; MS 85 Univ of AR - Little Rock; 85–Sp-Lang Path, Arkansas Children's Hosp, **SLP**

Russell, Mrs Vicki R 810 Highland Drive East, Altamonte Springs, FL 32701, (305) 862-6304, MA 82 Univ of Central FL; Sp-Lang Path, Douglas Sq Ther, **SLP**

Russell-Marquard, Erin Marie 432 Dewey, Royal Oak, MI 48067, (313) 398-7657, BA 84 MI St Univ; MA 86 MI St Univ

Russini, Teri-Anne 653 Madson Avenue, Lindenhurst, NY 11757, (516) 957-5222, BS 86 SUNY - Coll at Geneseo; MS 88 Univ of MI - Ann Arbor

Russinko, Mrs Valerie Louise 40 Wilson Avenue East, Riverdale, NJ 07457, (201) 697-1700, BA 79 William Paterson Coll; MS 82 William Paterson Coll; Sp-Lang Path, W Milford Bd of Ed, **SLP**

Russo, Arlyne E 1481 Fairfield Beach Road, Fairfield, CT 06430, (203) 255-5604, BA 67 Manhattanville Coll; MA 69 Univ of CT; Sp-Lang Path, Private Practice, **SLP**

Russo, Barbara P 2065 South Tropical Trail, Merritt Island, FL 32952, (407) 453-0884, BA 68 Univ of FL; ME 69 Univ of FL; 88–Sp-Lang Path, Sch Bd of Brevard County, **SLP**

Russo, Mrs Barbara Stafura 301 Center Avenue, Charleroi, PA 15022, (412) 483-8552, BS 72 CA Univ of PA; ME 81 CA Univ of PA; Sp-Lang Path, South Hills Health System, **SLP**

Russo, Mrs Deborah Piehler 910 Mulford Court S E, Grand Rapids, MI 49507, (616) 532-7958, BA 75 1485; MA 76 MI St Univ; Sp/Lang Path, Jenison Public Schools, **SLP**

Russo, Jo-Ann B 59 Vernon Street, Waltham, MA 02154, (617) 899-4709, BS 78 SUNY - Coll at Geneseo; MA 79 SUNY - Coll at Geneseo; 84–Sp-Lang Path, Comm Health Care Assoc Inc, **SLP**

Russo, Kathryn 1508 South Iseminger St, Philadelphia, PA 19147, **SLP**

Russo, Lorraine A Daniels Hearing Center, Boston Univ Medical Center, 720 Harrison Avenue Suite 601, Boston, MA 02118, (617) 536-3220, BA 77 CUNY - Lehman Coll; MS 79 Boston Univ; Dir Aud, Boston U Med Cen Daniels Hrng, **A**

Russo, Maryhelen West Road #F-29, Country Commons, Pleasant Valley, NY 12569-9316, (914) 635-1741, BS 86 Coll of Saint Rose; MS 87 Coll of Saint Rose; 87–Sp-Lang Path, Wassaic Developmental Center, **SLP**

Russo, Mrs Michelle 2205 Winding Way, Broomall, PA 19008, (215) 353-3369, BA 74 Temple Univ; MA 75 Temple Univ; 83–Dir, Sp Path Serv, **SLP**

Russo, Robert L 404 East 75th Street #1A, New York, NY 10021, (212) 694-2961, BA 69 Montclair St Coll; MA 74 Montclair St Coll; Super of Aud, Columbia-Pres Med Cen, **A**

Russo, Sharon H John A Straka MD, 1099 Ohio River Boulevard, Sewickley, PA 15143, (412) 741-5670, BS 78 Duquesne Univ; ME 80 Univ of VA - Charlottesville; 80–Aud, Sewickley Hrng Aids & J A Straka MD, **A**

Russo, Sheila D 939 Arbor Lane, Jacksonville, FL 32207, ME; 88–Sp-Lang Path, Duval Co Sch Bd, **SLP**

Russon, Mrs Karen Vincent 5489 W 10180 N, Highland, UT 84003, (801) 571-7394, BS 82 Brigham Young Univ; OM 83 Brigham Young Univ; SLP, Intermountain Health Care, **SLP**

Rust, Mrs Lyann Louise 809 Seacove, Pascagoula, MS 39567, (601) 762-7036, BS 79 ND St Univ; MS 81 UT St Univ; SLP, **SLP**

Rust, Roxanna Lou 359 Calle Alcazar, Walnut, CA 91789, (714) 983-9501, BS 71 CO St Univ; MA 82 CA St Univ - Fullerton; **SLP**

Rust, William L Nebo School District, 350 South Main Street, Spanish Fork, UT 84660, (801) 798-8651, BS 57 Brigham Young Univ; MS 67 Brigham Young Univ; Director Pupil Services, Nebo School District

Rust-Miron, Mrs Jana Elizabeth 2423 Chestnut Ridge Place, Birmingham, AL 35216, (205) 988-3742, BA 85 Marshall Univ; MA 86 Marshall Univ; 88–Sp-Lang Path, Med Therapy Inc, **SLP**

Rutberg, Barbara L 41 Indian Ridge Road, South Natick, MA 01760, (508) 620-1442, BS 68 Emerson Coll; ME 71 Boston Univ; Prgm Coord, Middlesex Child Dev Cen, **SLP**

Rutenberg, Mrs Judith B 2411 Clapboard Hill, Little Rock, AR 72207, (501) 225-7878, BS 69 OH Univ - Athens; ME 72 Kent St Univ; SLP, Geyer Sprng 1st Baptist Chrch, **SLP ACE**

Rutenberg, Mrs Kirsten V 2820 N W 31st Terrace, Gainesville, FL 32605, (904) 372-0568, BA 70 Univ of FL; MA 75 Univ of FL; 88–Clin Supvr, Univ of Florida, **SLP ACE**

Ruth, Kelley Grace 116 Twin Oaks Drive, Nashville, TN 37211, (615) 832-6518, BA 84 Middle TN St Univ; MA 85 Univ of TN - Knoxville; Sp-Lang Path, Speech Pathology Associates, **SLP**

Ruth, MaryLee 1560 Thurston Avenue #1101, Honolulu, HI 96822, (808) 537-2211, BS 78 PA St Univ - Univ Park; MS 82 PA St Univ - Univ Park; Aud, The Honolulu Med Gp, **A**

Ruth, Dr Roger A Department Of Otolaryngology HNS, Box 430, University Of VA Medical Center, Charlottesville, VA 22908, (804) 924-2050, BS 73 OH St Univ; MA 74 OH St Univ; PH 77 (NS) OH St Univ; Assoc Prof/Dir of Aud, Uva Med Cen, **A**

Rutherford, Berneice R 5223 Vincent Avenue South, Minneapolis, MN 55410, MS; **SLP F LM**

Rutherford, David R Dept Communication Disorders, Northwestern University, 2299 Sheridan Road, Evanston, IL 60201, (312) 492-5074, BA 53 Univ of OK - Norman; MA 54 Univ of OK - Norman; PH 58 (NS) Northwestern Univ; Professor Sp-Lang Path, Northwestern University, **SLP F**

Rutherford, Gorin 2804 Prairie Road, Topeka, KS 66614, (913) 272-4456, BA 48 Abilene Christian Univ; MA 65 Univ of MO - Columbia; Retired, Ks Dept Hlth Envr, **SLP LM**

Rutherford, Dr Karen M 7452 Brian Lane, La Palma, CA 90623, (213) 922-8258, BS 78 East TN St Univ; MS 80 East TN St Univ; Audiologist, Rancho Los Amigos Hospital, **A**

Rutherford, Pamela 56 South Wade Avenue, Washington, PA 15301, (304) 242-1390, BS 83 CA Univ of PA; MS 85 CA Univ of PA

Rutigliano, Cynthia J 30-11 Parsons Blvd, Apt 3D, Flushing, NY 11354, (718) 762-3420, BA 84 CUNY - Queens Coll; MA 86 CUNY - Queens Coll; **SLP**

Rutkowski, Mrs Kristine Arlene 964 Floyd, Birmingham, MI 48009, (313) 362-4299, **SLP ACE**

Rutkowski, Mrs Leanne H 323 West Asher Street, Culpeper, VA 22701, (703) 825-1760, BA 72 SUNY - Center at Buffalo; MA 74 SUNY - Center at Buffalo; **SLP**

Rutland, Mrs Kjaeren Aleece 33 Wells Drive, Loring AFB, ME 04751, (207) 328-9213, OB 69 TX Christian Univ; MS 71 Univ of OK - OK City; 88–Sp-Lang Path, Limestone Sch Dist, **SLP**

Rutledge, Cynthia Lynn 9511 Willow Ridge Road 3C, Charlotte, NC 28210, (704) 371-4137, BA 80 Clemson Univ; ME 86 Univ of VA - Charlottesville; 88–Sp-Lang Path, Presbyterian Hosp, **SLP**

Rutledge, Mrs Shelby Mullins 1708 Chelmsford Drive, Lexington, KY 40505, (606) 299-8877, BS 79 Eastern KY Univ; MA 82 Eastern KY Univ; **SLP**

Rutledge, Wynne Sutter 10 Holman Road, Moberly, MO 65270, (816) 263-4304, BS 57 Univ of MO - Columbia; ME 62 Univ of MO - Columbia; Sp/Lang Path, Private Practice, **SLP**

Rutnik, Margaret Mary 17 Stewart Street, Amsterdam, NY 12010, (518) 842-0060, BS 78 Coll of Saint Rose; MS 79 Coll of Saint Rose; Sp-Lang Path, Montgomery Co Arc, **SLP**

Rutstein, Irving T 9 Downing Circle, Bloomfield, CT 06002, (203) 529-2571, BS 38 CUNY - City College; MA 49 Columbia Univ Teachers Coll; Sp/Lang Path, St of CT Veterans Home & Hosp, **SLP LM**

Rutt, Diane E 49 Randolph Avenue #33, Meriden, CT 06450, (203) 238-3258, MS 88 Southern CT St Univ; Sp-Lang Path, Pomperaug Sch Dist 15

Rutt, Marjorie North 146 South Babylon Turnpike, Merrick, NY 11566, (516) 379-4118, BA 67 CUNY - Hunter Coll; OM 69 CUNY - Hunter Coll; MA 82 Adelphi Univ; SLP, Visiting Ther Assoc, **SLP**

Rutter, Vicki 1455 Quail Ridge Drive, Gering, NE 69341, (308) 436-3228, BA 82 Univ of Northern CO; MA 83 Univ of Northern CO; Sp-Lang Pathologist, Educational Service Unit 13, **SLP**

Rutz, Terry A Hearing Center Of Delray, 250 Dixie Boulevard #201, Delray Beach, FL 33444, (407) 276-2254, BA 74 SUNY - Center at Buffalo; MA 75 Bowling Green St Univ; Aud, Hearing Center of Delray, **A ACE**

Ruud, Elizabeth McKee 106 Millstone Drive, Verona, VA 24482-9548, (703) 885-9370, BS 78 James Madison Univ; MS 81 James Madison Univ; Sp-Lang Path, St of VA-Wn St Hosp, **SLP**

Ruvane, Anne B The Gab Lab, 29 Huron Drive, Chatham Township, NJ 07928, BS 56 PA St Univ - Univ Park; MA 78 Montclair St Coll; Dir, The Gab Lab, **SLP**

Rux, Mrs Dawn Whites 524 North First, Aberdeen, SD 57401, (605) 225-3162, BA 84 Northern St Coll; MA 88 Moorhead St Univ; **SLP**

Ruybal, Alfredo E 41167 McDowell, Hemet, CA 92343, (714) 657-1720, MS 73 Eastern WA Univ; SLP, Riverside Co Supt of Sch, **SLP**

Ruymann, Mrs Marilyn Q 2614 N E 15th Street, Fort Lauderdale, FL 33304, (305) 561-1418, BS 67 Univ of MD - College Park; ME 72 Univ of MD - College Park; MS 87 Nova Univ; 88–Sp-Lang Path, Broward Co PS, **SLP**

Ruzicka, Mrs Tamyra L 815 East Grovers, Villa 67, Phoenix, AZ 85022, (602) 971-8558, MS 88 Northern AZ Univ; 88–Sp-Lang Path, Good Samaritan Med Ctr

Ryal, Mary Kay 8418 Vicksburg Avenue, Westchester, CA 90045, BS 68 Northern IL Univ - De Kalb; MA 69 Univ of IL - Urbana; SLP, Los Angeles USD, **SLP**

Ryall, Judy Lynn 430 South Caldwood, Beaumont, TX 77707, (409) 866-2752, BS 83 Lamar Univ; MS 86 Lamar Univ

Ryalls, Dr John Herman Dept Of Speech & Hrng Sci, S C Indiana University, Bloomington, IN 47405

Ryals, Dr Brenda Morgan Audiology & Speech Path 126, VA Medical Center, Richmond, VA 23249, (804) 230-1326, BS 71 East Carolina Univ; MA 73 Univ of TN - Knoxville; PH 81 (Aud) Univ of VA - Charlottesville; Aud, VA Med Ctr, **A**

Ryals, Karen E 4514 Beachway Drive, Tampa, FL 33609, (813) 239-1179, BA 77 Univ of FL; MS 79 FL St Univ; Sp-Lang Path&Dir of Prog Serv, UCP of Tampa, **SLP**

Ryan, Mrs Alesia Houston 825 Edgewood Drive, Lexington, KY 40503, (606) 273-4112, BA 83 Univ of KY; MS 85 Univ of KY; **SLP**

Ryan, Barbara V 5416 Oleta Street, Long Beach, CA 90815, MS; **SLP**

Ryan, Bruce P Dept Of Communicative Disorder, California State Univ, Long Beach, CA 90840, (213) 498-4583, BS 53 Southern OR St Coll; MS 57 Western MI Univ; PH 64 (NS) Univ of Pittsburgh - Pittsburgh; Prof,Sp-Lang Path, CA St U Long Beach, **SLP F**

Ryan, Mrs Caryl Thomas 1925 19th Street, Cuyahoga Falls, OH 44223, (216) 928-8733, BS 77 Indiana Univ of PA; MA 79 Kent St Univ; SLP, Summit Co Bd Ment Ret & Dev Di, **SLP**

Ryan, Cathy Elizabeth 15919 Alsace, San Antonio, TX 78232, (512) 691-0737, BS 79 Univ of WI - Madison; MA 82 Northern IL Univ - De Kalb; 87–Prog Dir, Rehab Inst of San Antonio, **SLP**

Ryan, Mrs Cecilia H 97 Cambridge Avenue, Holbrook, NY 11741, (516) 585-1496, BA 74 Hofstra Univ; MA 76 Hofstra Univ; Tchr of Deaf & Sp & Hrng Imp, Sachem Ctrl Sch Dist, **SLP**

Ryan, Constance M P O Box 994, Meredith, NH 03253, (603) 279-7343, BS 76 Nazareth Coll of Rochester; MA 78 SUNY - Center at Buffalo; Assistant Clinical Director, Laconia St Sch-Train Cen, **SLP**

Ryan, Cynthia Bird 6836 Granada Road, Prairie Village, KS 66208, (816) 276-8225, BS 80 Univ of VA - Charlottesville; MS 82 James Madison Univ; Sp-Lang Path, Menorah Med Ctr, **SLP**

Ryan, Mrs Elizabeth 210 Heady Avenue, Louisville, KY 40207, (502) 895-7503, BA 77 Murray St Univ; MS 79 Univ of KY; SLP, Jefferson Co Bd of Ed, **SLP**

Ryan, Mrs Elizabeth MacKle 5424 Haymeadow Lane #Th-1, Peoria, IL 61615, (309) 347-5164, BS 84 Western IL Univ; MA 86 Western IL Univ; **SLP**

Ryan, Helen Rose 4715 Sabre Lane, Manlius, NY 13104, (315) 682-8930, BS 77 PA St Univ - Univ Park; MA 79 Hofstra Univ; 87–Sp-Lang Path, Fayetteville Manlius Sch Dist, **SLP**

Ryan, Janis C 502 Pacific Avenue, Salona Beach, CA 92075, (619) 554-8998, BS 71 Miami Univ - Oxford; MS 76 San Diego St Univ; Head of Aud, Scripps Cl & Research Found, **A**

Ryan, Jodell Newman 944 Cherokee Trail, Plano, TX 75023, (214) 517-4632, BS 77 OH St Univ; BA 81 OH St Univ; MA 83 OH St Univ; Aud, White Rock Otolaryngology, **A**

Ryan, Joelyn V 693 Brookside Drive, Danville, CA 94526, (415) 837-6779, BS 76 CA St Univ - Hayward; MS 78 San Francisco St Univ; Sp-Lang Path, Private Practice, **SLP**

Ryan, John P Route #1, Valparaiso, NE 68065, (402) 784-6591, BA 60 Univ of Northern IA; MA 76 Western IL Univ; Aud, Private Practice, **SLP A ACE**

Ryan, Karen Maria 3521 Sitio Baya, Carlsbad, CA 92009, (619) 723-7036, MA 86 San Diego St Univ; **SLP**

Ryan, Kathryn Riedlinger 11220-23B Avenue, Edmonton, AB, Canada T6J 4Z6, (403) 352-3337, BA 77 Wilfrid Laurier Univ - On; OM 81 Univ of Western Ontario; 85–Supvr-Sp-Lang-Hrng Prog, Wetoka Health Unit, **SLP**

Ryan, Kelly Marie 1311 Avenue Road, Toronto, ON, Canada M5N 2G8, (416) 487-0774, MA 88 Case Western Reserve Univ

Ryan, L Margaret 6 South Easton Road #3, Glenside, PA 19038, (215) 576-6954, BS 85 Bloomsburg Univ of PA; MS 86 Bloomsburg Univ of PA; 88–Aud, Associates in Hearing, **A**

Ryan, Mrs Lavonne B 49 Thorndale Road, Slingerlands, NY 12159, (518) 459-1333, BS 54 SUNY - Coll at Buffalo; MA 63 Coll of Saint Rose; Sp-Lang Path, S Colonie Sch Dist, **SLP**

Ryan, Mrs Lori A P O Box 1676, El Granada, CA 94018, (415) 726-5442, BA 78 Univ of CA - Santa Barbara; MS 79 Eastern WA Univ; Tchr, San Mateo Co Supt of Sch, **SLP**

Ryan, Lori F 8430 Timber Creek Drive, Memphis, TN 38134, (901) 754-4891, BA 81 Univ of AR - Fayetteville; MS 82 Univ of NC - Chapel Hill; Sp-Lang Path, **SLP**

Ryan, Mrs Marcia Leslie 113 South Church Street, Watertown, WI 53094, (414) 261-8534, BA 79 Pacific Univ; MS 85 Univ of WI - Oshkosh; 88–Sp-Lang Path, Private Practice, **SLP**

Ryan, Maryann H 5906 Cove Landing Road, Unit 203, Burke, VA 22015, (703) 323-4026, BS 80 Towson St Univ; MS 82 Towson St Univ; SLP, Fairfax County Pub Sch, **SLP**

Ryan, Mrs Mona Boydston 900 North Klein, Oklahoma City, OK 73106, (405) 272-5545, BS 82 OK St Univ; MS 85 Univ of OK Medical Center; 85–Sp-Lang Path, Oklahoma City Public Schools, **SLP**

Ryan, Patrice M 119 North Cliff, Willow Springs, IL 60480, (312) 839-1340, BS 79 IL St Univ - Normal; MS 82 Governors St Univ; Sp-Lang Path, Marian Joy Rehab Ctr HS Dist 230, **SLP**

Ryan, Mrs Patricia M 6427 West Evans Drive, Glendale, AZ 85306, (602) 978-1100, BS 77 Northeastern Univ; ME 80 Northeastern Univ; Sp-Lang Path, Peoria USD #11, **SLP**

Ryan, Remy Karen P O Box 2075, Carmel, CA 93921, (408) 625-1244, BS 71 Minot St Univ; MS 83 Minot St Univ; Sp-Lang Path, Carmel USD, **SLP**

Ryan, Mrs Rosemary E 417 Park Ridge, Bellingham, WA 98225, (206) 671-7801, BS 64 Clarion Univ of PA; MA 82 Western WA Univ; Director/Owner, Whatcom Speech and Language, **SLP**

Ryan, Mrs Sandra Lee 17532 Fairlie Road, San Diego, CA 92128, (619) 485-7396, **SLP**

Ryan, Mrs Sara Daly 4706 Mt Zion Road, Frederick, MD 21701, (301) 992-4159, **A**

Ryan, Stephan B Medical College Of Wisconsin, Department Of Audiology, 8700 West Wisconsin Avenue, Milwaukee, WI 53226, (414) 257-5866, BS 73 Univ of WI - Madison; MS 74 Univ of WI - Madison; Cl Instr, Med Coll of WI, **A**

Ryan, Stephenie Pickering 100 Brown Street, Little Rock, AR 72205, (501) 666-3301, BS 79 Radford Univ; MS 83 Univ of AR - Little Rock; Resource Assoc, New Medico, **SLP**

Ryan, Teresa Ann Pickwick Apartment, Apartment R-7, Maple Shade, NJ 08066, (609) 273-1309, BS 85 Bloomsburg Univ of PA; MS 86 Bloomsburg Univ of PA; 87–Sp-Lang Path, PREP Presch Hndcpd Program, **SLP**

Ryan, Victoria Ganz 1375 Taft Place, Hamilton, OH 45013, (513) 868-2000, BS 75 Miami Univ - Oxford; MS 84 Miami Univ - Oxford; Sp-Lang Path, Hamilton City Schools, **SLP**

Ryan-Carpenter, Sheila M 8370 Jackies Drive, Cincinnati, OH 45239-4232, (513) 522-0661, BA 78 Univ of Dayton; MA 80 Univ of Cincinnati; Sp-Lang Path, Hamilton Co Education Office, **SLP**

Ryan-Hammon, Patricia Ann 310 Westlind Road, Syracuse, NY 13219-1318, (714) 673-4975, **A**

Ryan-Rivers, Michelle M 23 Osborne Road, Colonie, NY 12205, (518) 458-9545, BS 76 Coll of Saint Rose; MS 78 Coll of Saint Rose; 87–Sp-Lang Path, Parsons Child & Family Ctr, **SLP**

Ryback-Cohen, Mrs Rachelle 811 Sturgis Place, Baltimore, MD 21208, (301) 484-7976, BA 76 SUNY - Center at Buffalo; MS 79 Columbia Univ Teachers Coll; **SLP**

Rybacki, Mary-Jean 21 Englewood Drive, East Haven, CT 06513, **SLP**

Ryberg, Wendy Sue 108 East Skillman Avenue, Maplewood, MN 55117, BS 85 Univ of WI - River Falls; OM 86 Univ of WI - River Falls; **SLP**

Ryburn, Mrs Charlotte Ferguson P O Box 547, Mena, AR 71953, (501) 637-2454, BS 77 Henderson St Univ; MS 78 AR St Univ; Sp-Lang Path, Waldron PS Sys, **SLP**

Rychnowski, Sharon L 801 Prospect Avenue, Buffalo, NY 14213, (716) 822-2676, BS 77 SUNY - Center at Buffalo; MS 80 SUNY - Center at Buffalo; Tchr, Buffalo Bd Ed, **SLP**

Rycyna, Mrs Mary E 114 Morris Avenue, Buffalo, NY 14214, (716) 838-5312, BS 75 Ithaca Coll; MS 77 Miami Univ - Oxford; **SLP**

Rydarowski, Mrs Lisa Neff 3418 Cranborne Chase, Marietta, GA 30062, (404) 565-2982, MS 74 OH Univ - Athens; Sp-Lang Path, Sc Sch for the Deaf & Blind, **SLP**

Rydell, Patrick J 5935 Tangeman Terrace, Lincoln, NE 68505, (402) 466-0976, BA 79 Univ of NE - Lincoln; MS 81 Southern IL Univ -Carbondale; **SLP**

Ryden, Mrs Karen Lawson 3 Plainfield Road, Pepperell, MA 01463, BA 82 Univ of VT; MS 83 Univ of VT; 86–Sp-Lang Path, North Middlesex Reg Sch Dist, **SLP**

Ryder, Joyce P 7700 West 99th Street, Bloomington, MN 55438, (612) 933-9343, BS 71 Univ of MN - Minneap-St Paul; MS 78 Saint Cloud St Univ; Sp/Lang Path, Hopkins Sch Dist, **SLP**

Ryder, Mrs Susan Klann 1213 29th Avenue Court, Moline, IL 61265, (319) 359-1371, BS 78 Western IL Univ; MA 79 Western IL Univ; 79–Sp-Lang Path, Mississippi Bend AEA, **SLP**

Rydgig, Kathleen Ann 3546 Olds Road, Oxnard, CA 93033, (805) 252-9580, BA 78 CA St Univ - Northridge; MA 80 CA St Univ - Northridge; 80–Sp-Lang Path, Los Angeles Co Office of Educ, **SLP**

Ryding, Melanie C 5985 Dearborn #306, Mission, KS 66202, (913) 362-0135, BA 66 Wichita St Univ; MA 70 Univ of Tulsa; Sp-Lang Path, Shawnee Misson Med Cen, **SLP**

Rye, Carol V 6 Pine Forest Drive, Maumelle, AR 72118, (800) 367-0806, BS 71 Univ of IA; MA 72 Univ of IA; 87–Aud, Dahlberg Inc, **A**

Ryerson, Wayne Scott 14 Hinchman Avenue, Dover, NJ 07801, (201) 328-7682, BA 74 Long Island U - Brooklyn Ctr; MA 78 NY Univ; Sp/Lang Path, Commun Lrng Inst, **SLP**

Ryker, Angela M 31 Seaview Drive South, Rolling Hills, CA 90274, 13-541-0380, MA 88 CA St Univ - Fullerton

Ryks, Joan Gilbertson 1918 East 3rd Street, Apt 8, Duluth, MN 55812, (218) 724-8032, OB 86 Univ of MN - Duluth; MA 87 Univ of MN - Duluth

Ryland, Mark Gordon 1936 Summit Road, Kent, OH 44240, (216) 297-0811, BS 85 Kent St Univ; MA 86 Kent St Univ; 86–Supvr of Aud & Neurology, Robinson Memorial Hosp, **A**

Rylander, Robert E Vancouver Schools, 605 North Devine Road, Vancouver, WA 98661, (206) 896-7256, MA 63 WA St Univ; Coord/Sp-Lang Path, Vancouver Pub Sch, **SLP**

Ryll, Carolyn M Memorial Hospital, 3301 Johnson Street, Hollywood, FL 33021, (305) 987-8007, BS 69 FL St Univ; MS 70 FL St Univ; Sp/Lang Path, Mem Hosp, **SLP**

Rynar, Mrs Susan G 21 Puddingstone Way, Florham Park, NJ 07932, (201) 377-8658, BS 76 Boston Univ; MS 77 Boston Univ; **SLP**

Rynes, Dr Edward J VA Medical Center, Audiology Service - 126W, 10701 East Boulevard, Cleveland, OH 44106, (216) 421-3047, BS 52 OH Univ - Athens; MA 57 LA St Univ - Baton Rouge; PH 69 (NS) Case Western Reserve Univ; Aud, VA Med Cen, **SLP A**

Rysberg, Mrs Linda M P O Box 411, Okemos, MI 48864, (517) 349-5868, BA 71 MI St Univ; MA 74 1415; SLP, Dewitt Public Schools, **SLP**

Rysticken, Noreen Ann 17 Cinder Road, Timonium, MD 21093, (301) 252-2784, BA 66 Loyola Coll; ME 70 Loyola Coll; 86–Sp-Lang Path, Private Practice, **SLP**

Rzadkiewicz, Joan K 132 Fordham Drive, Buffalo, NY 14216, (716) 842-3154, BS 74 SUNY - Coll at Buffalo; MS 77 SUNY - Coll at Buffalo; SLP, Cty of Buffalo Pub Schs, **SLP**

Rzepnick, Adrienne 165 North Myrtle, PO Box 170, Tustin, CA 92680, (714) 832-9200, BS 78; MA 80 San Diego St Univ; Administrator, Western NeuroCare Center, **SLP**

S

Sa, Theresa Rene 5182 West Sussex Way, Fresno, CA 93722, (209) 298-5458, BA 82 CA St Univ - Fresno; MA 85 CA St Univ - Fresno; **SLP**

Saari, Mrs Kay Ann W 740 East Woodward Street, Lakeland, FL 33803, (813) 686-3189, BS 77 FL St Univ; MS 79 Emory Univ; Sp-Lang Path, Polk County School Board, **SLP**

Saario, Mrs Laurie Box 26, Amasa, MI 49903, (906) 822-7812, BS 66 Eastern MI Univ; MA 71 Univ of TN - Knoxville; MS 88 Univ of WI - Stevens Point; 88–Aud, Tri-County Comm Svcs, **SLP**

Saathoff, Neva M Route 1 Box 119, Overton, TX 75684, (214) 895-2234, BS 73 Southwest TX St Univ; ME 75 Southwest TX St Univ; Sp-Lang Path, Rusk Co Plan A Co-Op, **SLP**

Saathoff, Mrs Susan L S 0571 County Road #130, Glenwood Springs, CO 81601, (303) 945-9183, BA 76 Univ of Northern CO; MA 78 Univ of Northern CO; Sp-Lang Path, Roaring Fork Sch Dist Re-1, **SLP**

Sabado, Mrs Diane Duclos 11540 Clover Avenue, West Los Angeles, CA 90066, BS 66 Univ of OR; MA 83 CA St Univ - Northridge; SLP, LA USD, **SLP**

Sabah, Mrs Debra Brim 15137 Hesby Street, Sherman Oaks, CA 91403, (213) 667-4661, BS 81 AZ St Univ; MA 83 Univ of CA - Santa Barbara; Aud, Kaiser Permanente, **A**

Sabanos, Mrs Debra Tiffany 3 Cork Place, Huntington, NY 11743, (516) 351-1739, BA 79 Adelphi Univ; MA 81 Hofstra Univ; Sp-Lang Path, Variety Preschool Workshop, **SLP**

Sabatini, Joyce A 5820 West 83rd Street, Burbank, IL 60459, (312) 423-7882, BA 79 Saint Xavier Coll; MS 81 Governors St Univ; Director Speech Pathology, Americana Healthcare Center, **SLP**

Sabella, Darleen Sue 318 Columbus Parkway, Mineola, NY 11501, (516) 352-2580, BA 84 Adelphi Univ; MS 85 Adelphi Univ; 85–Sp-Lang Path, Sch for Lang & Commun Dev, **SLP**

Saber, Mrs Diana Powell 2131 Funston Avenue, San Francisco, CA 94116, (415) 661-6296, BA 81 San Diego St Univ; MA 83 Univ of San Francisco; Sp-Lang Path, Western Med Ctr-Santa Ana, **SLP**

Sabers, Mrs Rhonda Kaye Box 253, 210 North Hill, Salem, SD 57058, (605) 425-3155, MA 88 Univ of SD - Vermillion

Sabia, Mrs Sharon A 217 Haviland Road, Stamford, CT 06903, (203) 637-0150, BA 73 Southern CT St Univ; MS 75 Southern CT St Univ; 79–Sp-Lang Path, Greenwich Bd of Ed, **SLP**

Sabia-Peters, Toni M 7 Country Squire Ct, Dix Hills, NY 11746-5307, (516) 462-1017, BA 82 SUNY - Coll at Cortland; MS 83 Adelphi Univ; Sp-Lang Path, Three Village Central Sch, **SLP**

Sabin, George Alfred 5050 East 5th Street, Apartment E4, Tucson, AZ 85711, (602) 571-1596, BS 81 Northern AZ Univ; MS 82 Northern AZ Univ; Sp-Lang Path, Tuscon Med Center, **SLP**

Sabin, Mrs Joanne M 19504 Dubarry Drive, Brookeville, MD 20833, (301) 774-2247, BS 64 Kent St Univ; MA 71 George Washington Univ; Dir/Owner, Sp/Lang Cen of Olney, **SLP ACE**

Sabino, Ann Marie 4229 West 217th Street, Fairview Park, OH 44126, (216) 356-2469, BA 83 OH St Univ; MA 85 OH St Univ; 87–Sp-Lang Path, Lorain Comm Hosp, **SLP**

Sable, Mrs Randye Hoffman 9200 Bustleton Avenue, Apartment 1912, Philadelphia, PA 19115, (215) 548-4010, BA 75 Temple Univ-Tyler Sch of Art; MA 77 Temple Univ-Tyler Sch of Art; Sp-Lang Path, School Dist of Philadelphia, **SLP**

Sablove, Audrey B 1493 Lakeridge Lane, El Cajon, CA 92020, (619) 448-3100, BA 73 CUNY - Queens Coll; MA 74 George Washington Univ; SLP, San Diego USD, **SLP**

Sabo, Ana M Calle 2 D-4 Urb, Colinas Verdes, Rio Piedras, PR 00924, (809) 758-2525, BS 78 Univ of PR - Rio Piedras; MS 80 Univ of PR - Rio Piedras; Sp/Lang Path, Med Sci Campus Rio Piedras, **SLP**

Sabo, Denise R 7115 Society Drive, Claymont, DE 19703, (609) 825-5840, BA 74 Univ of KY; MS 75 Southern IL Univ -Carbondale; Sp-Lang Path, Private Practice, **SLP**

Sabo, Diane L 300 Grant Avenue, Carnegie, PA 15106, (412) 647-5580, BA 76 Univ of Pittsburgh - Pittsburgh; MA 78 Univ of Pittsburgh - Pittsburgh; Sp-Lang Path, Childrens Hosp of Pittsburgh, **A**

Sabo, Mrs Karen King 7792 Oak Creek, Pleasanton, CA 94566, (415) 846-7078, BS 64 Purdue Univ - West Lafayette; MA 67 Miami Univ - Oxford; **SLP**

Sabo, Mrs Marilyn E 678 14th Street, Lakewood, NJ 08701, (201) 363-1900, BS 58 Rutger's St Univ - Douglas Coll; MS 76 Rutgers St Univ -N Brunswick; Dir Sp-Lang Path, Kimball Medical Center, **SLP**

Sabo, Michael P Director Of Audiology, Good Samaritan Hospital, 1111 East McDowell Road, Phoenix, AZ 85006, (602) 239-4577, BA 66 SUNY - Coll at Plattsburgh; MS 74 Ithaca Coll; 86–Dir, Samaritan Health Services, **A**

Sabo, William Joseph 7862 Raglan Drive N E, Warren, OH 44484, (216) 841-2321, **SLP**

Sabol, Barbara Ann 1940 3rd Street #1, Cuyahoga Falls, OH 44221, MA 85 Univ of MA - Amherst; Sp-Lang Path, Edwin Shaw Hosp, **SLP**

Sabol, Laura R 354 Atkins Avenue, Lancaster, PA 17603, (717) 393-0425, BA 76 Mary Washington Coll; ME 78 Univ of VA - Charlottesville; Sp-Lang Path, Lancaster General Hospital, **SLP ACE**

Sabourin, Mrs Theresa Mitchell 173 Mary Avenue, London, ON, Canada N6J 3L8, (416) 388-0240, BA 79 SUNY - Coll at Oswego; MA 83 SUNY - Center at Buffalo; Sp-Lang Path, Chedoke-McMaster Hospitals, **SLP**

Sabrowsky, Norman J Route 4 Box 88, Princeton, MN 55371, (319) 422-5678, BS 66 Saint Cloud St Univ; MS 71 Saint Cloud St Univ; SLP, Aal, **SLP**

Sacca, Janet S 47-01 Hunters Glen Drive, Plainsboro, NJ 08536, (201) 788-6424, BA 74 CUNY - Queens Coll; MA 76 CUNY - Queens Coll; 87–Aud, Hunterdon Med Ctr, **A**

Sacco, Mrs Adrienne G 116 Main Street, Mount Morris, NY 14510, (716) 243-5480, BS 78 SUNY - Coll at Geneseo; MA 79 SUNY - Coll at Geneseo; Aud, Craig DDSO, **A**

Sacco, Deborah J 9 East Marie Street, Hudson, NY 12534, **SLP**

Sacco, Linda J 306 Windebank Lane, Minoa, NY 13116, (315) 656-2278, BS 73 SUNY - Coll at Plattsburgh; MA 74 Syracuse Univ; 86–Sp-Lang Path, E Syracuse-Minoa Cen Schs, **SLP**

Sacco, Lynne M 43 Baxter Boulevard, Portland, ME 04101, (207) 775-6381, BS 85 Worcester St Coll; MS 87 CO St Univ; 87–Aud, Maxwell Roediger & Knowland MD PA, **A**

Sacco, Pat Richard 116 South Main Street, Mount Morris, NY 14510, (716) 245-5332, BS 63 SUNY - Coll at Geneseo; MA 65 IN Univ - Bloomington; Dir,Sp Cen, St Univ Coll-Geneseo, **SLP ACE**

Sacco, Robert C 8358 South 3580 West, West Jordan, UT 84088, (801) 561-4614, BA 76 Univ of UT; MS 79 Univ of UT; Audiologist, Wasatch Audiology Assoc, **A**

Sacco-Andree, Maryann 1 Wiseman, Peabody, MA 01960, BS 77 Northeastern Univ; ME 79 Northeastern Univ; Sp/Lang Path, Middlesex Home Health Care Inc, **SLP**

Sachau, Beth Ann 2296 Foothill Drive #309-D, Salt Lake City, UT 84109, (801) 974-8307, BA 82 Univ of Northern IA; MS 86 Univ of UT; 85–Sp-Lang Path, Salt Lake City Sch Dist, **SLP**

Sacher, Martin H 7501 Tuscola Drive, Trotwood, OH 45426, Sp-Lang Path, Al-Mar Speech Clinic Inc, **SLP**

Sachs, Mrs Anne Quinn 221 South Southwood Avenue, Annapolis, MD 21401, (301) 269-6751, **SLP A**

Sachs, Lori Weisberger 99 Gibson Blvd, Valley Stream, NY 11581, (516) 791-3704, BS 84 Ithaca Coll; MS 85 Adelphi Univ; 87–Sp-Lang Path, Lawrence PS, **SLP**

Sachs, Michelle Anne 65 New Road #38, Rumford, RI 02916, (302) 738-9756, BA 80 Univ of DE; MA 82 OH Univ - Athens; Sp-Lang Path, Pro Home Hlth Agcy, **SLP**

Sachs, Sharon Ann 1011 Willsie, Rapid City, SD 57701, (605) 348-0020, BS 82 Univ of WY; MS 84 Univ of WY; Aud, Gary L Carlson MD Pc, **A**

Sachs, Shirley A 6100 West 79 Street, Prairie Village, KS 66208, (913) 642-2650, BA 54 Coe Coll; MS 68 Univ of NE - Omaha; Sp-Lang Path, Shawnee Mission Sch Dist 512, **SLP**

Sacia, Jane A 8776 Paisley Drive N E, Seattle, WA 98115, (206) 527-8350, MA 80 Univ of MT; **SLP**

Sack, Dr Leo P 2248 Shannon Drive, South San Francisco, CA 94080, (415) 589-9021, BA 50 Univ of CA - Berkeley; MA 52 San Francisco St Univ; PH 68 (NS) Univ of CA - Los Angeles; SLP, Leo P Sack, **SLP LM**

Sack, Dr Sara H Parsons State Hospital & Training Center, 2601 Gabriel, Parsons, KS 67357, (316) 421-6550, MA 74 Univ of KS; MA 86 Univ of KS; PH 88 (Developmental Psychology) Univ of KS; 84–Dir of Sp & Hrng, Parsons St Hosp & Trng Ctr, **SLP ACE**

Sack, Theresa O Wausau Hospital Center, Communicative Disorders, 333 Pine Ridge Boulevard, Wausau, WI 54401, (715) 847-2826, BS 68 Saint Louis Univ; MA 69 Univ of MO - Columbia; Dir Communicative Disorders, Wausau Hospital Center, **SLP**

Sackett, Karen M 722 Bingham Place, Lake Mary, FL 32746, BS 67 Univ of Tulsa; MS 74 FL St Univ; 76–Sp-Lang Path, Seminole Co Sch Board, **SLP**

Sackler-Feldblum, Cynthia 782 Stern Avenue, Palo Alto, CA 94303, (415) 856-0786, BA 84 San Francisco St Univ; MS 85 San Francisco St Univ; Sp-Lang Path, **SLP**

Sacks, Cheryl L 8317 Charwood, Kalamazoo, MI 49002, (616) 327-6320, BS 75 Purdue Univ - West Lafayette; MS 76 Purdue Univ - West Lafayette; **SLP**

Sacks, Gail Karen Society Hill Towers, 9E South, 220 Locust Street, Philadelphia, PA 19106, (215) 427-5466, BA 68 Temple Univ; MA 70 Temple Univ; Sp-Lang Path, St Christophers Hosp Children, **SLP**

Sacks, Mrs Jo-Anne 516 Belle Pointe, Nashville, TN 37221, (615) 297-3939, MS 88 Vanderbilt Univ; 88–Aud, Miracle Ear Ctr

Sacks, Leslie S 6747 Surreywood Lane, Bethesda, MD 20817-1567, (301) 365-1232, BS 80 NY Univ; MA 84 NY Univ; Sp-Lang Path, Er Sl So, **SLP**

Sacks, Linda Nancy 1800 Camden Avenue #209, Los Angeles, CA 90025, (213) 681-4641, BA 80 San Diego St Univ; MA 83 San Diego St Univ; Sp-Lang Path, Culver City USD, **SLP**

Sacks, Pamela Enid 515 East 82nd Street #3-A, New York, NY 10028-7166, (212) 288-8042, BA 80 Univ of CT; MA 83 Univ of CT; Coord of Sp-Lang Path Serv, Mt Sinai Hosp, **SLP**

Sacks, Stephen W 943 West Santa Ana, Fresno, CA 93705, (209) 573-6051, BS 74 Univ of CA - Berkeley; MA 79 CA St Univ - Fresno; Sp-Lang Path, Madera Co Dept of Ed, **SLP**

Sackschewsky, Louise B 5479 Seneca Place, Boulder, CO 80303, (303) 499-9317, BA 70 Univ of CO - Boulder; MA 73 Univ of CO - Boulder; SLP, Boulder Valley Sch Dist, **SLP**

Sadarangani, Karin Lee 632 Palmer Road #7-C, Yonkers, NY 10701, (914) 359-1000, MS 88 Nazareth Coll of Rochester; 88–Sp-Lang Path, Rockland Psych Ctr

Sadasivan, Mangala Gowri Michigan State University, Audiology & Speech Sci, East Lansing, MI 48825, (517) 353-9206, BA 78 George Washington Univ; MA 81 MI St Univ; Tchng Asst, Michigan State U, **SLP**

Saddler, Karen B 7510 Hampton Oaks, Portage, MI 49002, (616) 323-8502, BS 77 Purdue Univ - West Lafayette; MS 78 Purdue Univ - West Lafayette; **SLP**

Saddler, Mrs Yvonne N Department Of Human Services, Western Carolina Univ, Cullowhee, NC 28723, (704) 227-7310, BS 69 Univ of GA; ME 71 Univ of GA; ES 72 Univ of GA; 72–Asst Prof, Wn Carolina U, **SLP**

Sadick, Robert H 80 Pickwick Drive, Rochester, NY 14618, (716) 288-8008, BS 62 SUNY - Coll at Geneseo; MA 71 SUNY - Coll at Geneseo; 62–Sp-Lang Path, Rochester City Sch Dist, **SLP**

Sadigh-Behzadi, Mrs Marianne Morrisey 14960 Lanark Street, Van Nuys, CA 91402, (818) 908-1297, BA 84 CA St Univ - Northridge; MA 86 CA St Univ - Northridge; **SLP**

Sadinsky, Priscilla Mount Sinai Hospital, Speech Pathology Dept, 600 University Avenue, Toronto, ON, Canada M5G 1X5, (416) 586-5035, BS 73 Univ of Toronto - Ontario; OM 75 Univ of Toronto - Ontario; Sp-Lang Path, Mount Sinai Hosp, **SLP**

Sadja-Thompson, Lynn 6244 Nagle Avenue, Van Nuys, CA 91401, (213) 393-6538, BA 68 San Francisco St Univ; MA 73 CA St Univ - Northridge; SLP, LA USD, **SLP**

Sadler, Mrs Dorothy O 260 East Chestnut Street, Chicago, IL 60611, (312) 337-4013, BS 35 Northwestern Univ; MA 39 Univ of MN - Minneap-St Paul; **SLP LM**

Sadler, Laura L 86 Overlook Place, Bedford, OH 44146, (216) 439-2838, BS 79 Kent St Univ; MA 80 Kent St Univ; 87–Aud, E B Brown Opticians, **A**

Sadler, Mrs Rebecca Eggers 8248 Toll House Road, Annandale, VA 22003, (703) 698-7500, BA 66 Ball St Univ; MA 82 Univ of MD - College Park; 83–Sp-Lang Path, Fairfax Co Pub Sch-Head Start, **SLP ACE**

Sadler, Mrs Suzanne M 2106 Murfield, League City, TX 77573, (713) 334-1076, BA 78 MI St Univ; MA 79 MI St Univ; SLP, Clear Crk ISD, **SLP**

Sadonis, Cynthia 205 Bookerdale Road #29, Waynesboro, VA 22980, (703) 943-3088, SLP, Augusta County Schools, **A**

Sadownik, Sharyn M 5201 Ernie Lane, Frederick, MD 21701, (301) 845-2529, BA 76 CUNY - Queens Coll; MS 78 Loyola Coll; Program Developer, Vicksburg Public Schools, **SLP**

Sadowski, Teresa Buckley 133 Pleasant #3, North Andover, MA 01845, (617) 686-6472, BS 83 Eastern MI Univ; MA 84 Eastern MI Univ; SLP, Anne Sullivan Center, **SLP**

Sadowsky, Mrs Sara L 203 Fox Glen Road, Fredonia, WI 53021, (414) 692-2401, BS 76 Univ of WI - Milwaukee; MS 77 Univ of WI - Milwaukee; Sp-Lang Path, Northern Ozaukee Sch Dist, **SLP**

Saenz, Amparo Aida 314 Westhill, San Antonio, TX 78201, (512) 732-4100, MA 88 Our Lady Lake Univ-San Anton

Saenz, Belinda M 7308 Wellcrest Drive, Dallas, TX 75230, (214) 824-1620, MS 84 Univ of TX - Dallas; Sp-Lang Path, Dallas ISD, **SLP**

Saenz, Terry I 315 South 45th Street #3-I, Philadelphia, PA 19104, (215) 387-1856, BA 74 Univ of CA - Los Angeles; MA 79 Univ of Denver; 87–Sp-Lang Path, **SLP**

Safer, Deborah Griffin 10115 Siegen Lane #B, Baton Rouge, LA 70810, (504) 647-5473, BS 83 LA St Univ - Baton Rouge; MA 86 LA St Univ - Baton Rouge; 83–Sp-Lang Path, Ascension Parish Sch Bd, **SLP**

Saferstein, Sharon 3844-A Stepes Court, Falls Church, VA 22041, MS

Saffer, Mrs Eva Kinsey P O Box 8327, Knoxville, TN 37996, (806) 372-4197, BS 76 TX Tech Univ; MS 79 TX Tech Univ; Aud, U of TN, **A**

Saffer, Susan K 22 Hunts Point Road, Cape Elizabeth, ME 04107, (207) 799-7339, BA 69 Elmira Coll; MA 70 Columbia Univ Teachers Coll; Sp/Lang Path, Cape Eliz Sch Dept, **SLP**

Safian, Marilyn 3 Lowe Circle, Framingham, MA 01701, (617) 877-2641, BA 61 CUNY - Queens Coll; ME 64 Boston Univ; Sp-Lang Path, Framingham Sp & Hrng Cl, **SLP**

Safir, Mrs Irene J 251-31 61st Avenue, Little Neck, NY 11362, (718) 821-2062, BA 76 CUNY - Queens Coll; MS 77 Ithaca Coll; Aud, Otolaryngologist's Office, **A**

Safran, Valerie 20 Waterside Plaza #20-G, New York, NY 10010, (212) 523-8539, MS 84 Columbia Univ Teachers Coll; Sp/Lang Path, Roosevelt Hosp, **SLP ACE**

Sage, Annette Marie 846 North Tuxedo, Indianapolis, IN 46201-2547, (317) 636-8280, MA 88 Ball St Univ

Sagendorph, Mrs Lynn Legate 1305 Ansley Court, Mundelein, IL 60060, (312) 623-0021, BA 84 IL St Univ - Normal; MS 85 IL St Univ - Normal; SLP, Special Ed Dist of Lake County, **SLP**

Sager, Mrs Gwen Hahn 395 20th Avenue, Brick, NJ 08724, (201) 928-1500, **SLP**

Sager, Mrs Lois Gibbons 4 Old Tree Farm Road, Mattapoisett, MA 02739, (508) 758-9417, BA 75 Univ of Denver; MA 76 Univ of Denver; 81–Sp-Lang Path, Private Practice, **SLP ACE**

Sagharichi, Mahmoud 2503 Lucylee Parkway, Poplar Bluff, MO 63901, (913) 236-4642, OB 81 Univ of KS; MA 83 Univ of KS; **A**

Sahaj, Erika Loring 1105 Sterling Ridge Drive, Augusta, GA 30909, (404) 868-5433, BS 81 Old Dominion Univ; MS 87 Old Dominion Univ; 88–Sp-Lang Path, Richmond Co Bd of Educ, **SLP**

Sahlberg, Richard A 2421 West 227th Street #41, Torrance, CA 90501, (213) 530-7627, BS 51 Bridgewater St Coll; ME 56 Boston Univ; Sp-Lang Path, Los Angeles USD, **SLP**

Sahley, Tony L 4663A Rishell Court East, Concord, CA 94521, (415) 674-9058, MA 82 Bowling Green St Univ; MA 84 Bowling Green St Univ; Doctoral Fellow, U of CA San Francisco

Sahlie, Elizabeth 3949 Montclair Road, Birmingham, AL 35213, (615) 320-5353, BS 82 Auburn Univ - Auburn; MS 84 Vanderbilt Univ; Sp-Lang Path, Bill Wilkerson Hrng & Sp Ctr, **SLP**

Saichek, Susan Lynn 2405 Eastmoreland Avenue, Apt 10, Rockford, IL 61108, (815) 397-3508, BS 85 Northern IL Univ - De Kalb; MA 86 Northern IL Univ - De Kalb; Sp-Lang Path, Harlem Consolidated Schs, **SLP**

Saidel, Joan Fox 2414 Henslowe Drive, Potomac, MD 20854, (301) 294-0565, BS 72 Cornell Univ; MS 76 SUNY - Center at Albany; Sp-Lang Path, Private Practice, **SLP**

Saidel, Susan M R Rural Free Delivery 1, Collinsville, CT 06022, **SLP**

Saiki, Kenneth J 2855 West Berwyn Avenue, Chicago, IL 60625, (312) 784-2950, MA 87 Univ of IL - Urbana

Sailer, Mrs Sarah B Rd 1 Box 43-A, Glen Gardner, NJ 08826, (201) 537-2636, BA 78 Univ of MT; OM 81 Univ of MT; Sp-Lang Path, Alexandria Township Schools, **SLP**

Sailors, Stephanie Gaye 2627 Park Avenue, Laramie, WY 82070, (307) 742-6374, BS 81 ID St Univ; MS 83 Univ of WY; Sp-Lang Path, Developmental Preschool, **SLP**

Sainio, Seija B 471 East 200 North, Provo, UT 84601, (801) 756-6022, BS 73 Brigham Young Univ; MS 74 Brigham Young Univ; Sp-Lang Path, UT Trng Sch, **SLP**

Saint Blancard, Carol Ann 223 Skylark Drive, Rockford, IL 61107, (815) 226-9527, BA 84 Univ of IL - Urbana; MA 86 Univ of IL - Urbana

Saives, Christine Ann 3030 Eastland Blvd, Imperial Oaks Apt 101, Clearwater, FL 34621, BA 85 SUNY - Coll at Plattsburgh; MA 86 SUNY - Coll at Plattsburgh

Sajwaj, Mrs Eva M 4256 Greenacres Drive, Ooltewah, TN 37363, (404) 226-8961, BA 71 Univ of MS; OM 72 Univ of MS; Clin Serv Coord, Looper Sp & Hrng Cen, **SLP**

Sak, Carla A 8341 Bridle Court, Mentor, OH 44060, (216) 255-4444, BS 71 Kent St Univ; MA 75 Kent St Univ; Sp-Lang Path, Mentor Exempted Village Sch, **SLP**

Sakada, Mrs Janet P 1275 Waterwyck Trail, Spring Valley, OH 45370, (513) 433-8841, BS 61 Bowling Green St Univ; Sp-Lang Path, Centerville Cty Sch, **SLP**

Sakadales, M Susanne 520 Estates Drive, Athens, OH 45701, (614) 698-8831, OB 59 OH Univ - Athens; ME 60 Gallaudet Coll; Tchr for Talented & Gifted, Alexander Local Sch Dist, **SLP**

Sakaguchi, Mrs Linda M 3804 Debsom Way, Louisville, KY 40241, (812) 945-5287, BS 77 Purdue Univ - West Lafayette; MS 79 Purdue Univ - West Lafayette; Sp-Lang Path, Silvercrest Chldrns Devel Ctr, **SLP**

Sakai, Connie Sayo 2602 Northeast 87th Street, Seattle, WA 98115, (206) 543-5230, BA 76 San Francisco St Univ; MA 78 Univ of WA; Aud, University of Washington, **A**

Sakai, Grace M 1737 South Beretania St, Apartment 403A, Honolulu, HI 96826, (808) 422-4077, BS 77 Univ of HI - Manoa; MS 79 Univ of HI - Manoa; Sp-Lang Path, Dept of Ed-Cen Oahu Dist, **SLP**

Sakata, Mrs Karen Shigezumi 101 Bountiful Court, Danville, CA 94526, (415) 685-3533, BA 73 Univ of CA - Berkeley; MA 76 San Jose St Univ; Prog Spec/Spec Educ, Mt Diablo USD, **SLP**

Sakelaris, Patricia G 3469 Skyline Boulevard, Reno, NV 89509, (702) 359-1980, BS 75 Univ of NV - Reno; MS 77 Univ of NV - Reno; Aud/Owner, Hearing Plus, **A**

Sakellakis, Tessie Jean 300 Wood Street #A-8, Mansfield, OH 44902, (419) 756-1133, MA 84 Cleveland St Univ; 84–Sp-Lang Path, Rehab Svc of N Central OH, **SLP**

Saken, Toby J Route A1 Box 92, Cobden, IL 62920, (618) 684-5844, BS 65 Southern IL Univ -Carbondale; MS 66 Southern IL Univ -Carbondale; MA 73 Southern IL Univ -Carbondale; Assoc Dir, Shawnee Hlth Serv & Dev Corp, **SLP**

Sakover, Mrs Patricia E 5934 Ordway Street, Riverside, CA 92504, BA 68 Saint Xavier Coll; MS 78 Loma Linda Univ - Riverside; SLP, Desert Hosp, **SLP**

Sakovich, Linda Marie 1406 Applewood Acres, Clarks Summit, PA 18412, (914) 794-1400, BS 82 Marywood Coll; MS 84 Ithaca Coll; Sp-Lang Path, Brd of Coop Educ Serv, **SLP**

Sakurada, Faith A 3242 Y Street, Lincoln, NE 68503-1945, (402) 466-3880, MS 87 Univ of NE - Lincoln

Salamander, Philip Box 403, Painted Hills, Martinsville, IN 46151, (812) 332-5633, BS 65 IN Univ - Bloomington; MA 71 Ball St Univ; 80–Aud, Private Practice, **A**

Salamon, Judy T 1975 Anderson Drive, Las Cruces, NM 88001, (505) 523-5884, BA 76 NM St Univ; MA 77 NM St Univ; Sp-Lang Path, Las Cruces Pub Sch, **SLP**

Salamone, Lisa Gail 26 Circle Wood Road, Rochester, NY 14625, (716) 586-5210, BS 85 SUNY - Coll at Geneseo; MA 88 Nazareth Coll of Rochester

Salamy, Dr Alan University Of California, Lpi Box F, San Francisco, CA 94143, (707) 938-4701, BA 68 Univ of HI - Manoa; PH 72 (NS) Univ of OK - OK City; Adjunct Prof, Res Psychol, U of CA San Francisco

Salamy, Jacque Spalding Rehabilitation Center, 1919 OGDEN Street, Denver, CO 80218, (303) 861-0504, BS 67 OK St Univ; MS 69 Univ of OK Medical Center; Dir/Sp-Lang Sers, Spalding Rehab Hosp, **SLP**

Salas, Carmen Cecilia Box 784, Arecibo, PR 00613, (809) 854-5115, BS 82 Univ of PR - Rio Piedras; MS 84 Univ of PR - San Juan; **SLP**

Salas-Provance, Marlene B R R 2 Box 34, Urbana, IL 61801, (217) 367-8145, BA 73 NM St Univ; MA 74 NM St Univ; Sp-Lang Path, Carmichael Sp Path, **SLP**

Salata, Bonnie J 633 Squireel Hill, Boardman, OH 44512, (216) 726-8855, MA 84 Univ of Cincinnati; MS 86 Miami Univ - Oxford; Sp-Lang Path, Youngstown Hearing & Sp Ctr, **SLP**

Salata, Linda T 147-27 72nd Avenue, Flushing, NY 11367, (718) 380-3000, BA 68 CUNY - Queens Coll; MA 70 CUNY - Queens Coll; 80–Superv Sp-Lang Dept, UCP Queens, **SLP**

Salata, Marie E 25 Tanglewood Drive, Danbury, CT 06810, (203) 748-1739, BS 77 Nazareth Coll of Rochester; MS 80 Nazareth Coll of Rochester; SLP, Danbury Bd of Ed, **SLP**

Salazar-Jaffe, Renee 58 Royal Oak Circle, Lake Jackson, TX 77566, (713) 422-9605, **SLP**

Salazer, D Rosine 376 Wharncliffe Road North, London, ON, Canada N6G 1E6, (519) 452-2041, BS 74 Univ of IA; MA 78 Univ of FL; Sp-Lang Path, Bd of Ed Cty of London, **SLP**

Salciccia, Cathy E 121-G Old Tous Farm Road, Peterborough, NH 03458, (603) 924-4150, BA 76 Rutger's St Univ - Douglas Coll; MS 80 Columbia Univ Teachers Coll; Dir of Sp & Hrng, Crotched Mt Rehab Ctr, **SLP**

Sale, Mrs Cheryl C 1710 Devers Road, Richmond, VA 23226, (804) 282-6367, BS 86 Univ of VA - Charlottesville; ME 87 Univ of VA - Charlottesville; 88–Aud, Pratt Medical Center, **A**

Salee, Mrs Susan Elizabeth 2929 Cimarron Trail, Apartment 1, Madison, WI 53719, (608) 276-9134, BA 82 IN Univ - Bloomington; OM 83 IN Univ - Bloomington; Sp-Lang Path, **SLP**

Saleeby, Nancy C W 2423 Rosewood Court, Chapel Hill, NC 27514, (919) 929-4008, BA 64 St Andrews Presbyterian Coll; MA 69 Appalachian St Univ; MS 76 Univ of NC - Chapel Hill; Sp-Lang Path, Chapel Hill Lang-Lrng Services, **SLP**

Saleem, Naheed 5 Holliday Court, Columbia, SC 29223, (803) 788-3040, MA 86 Univ of SC - Columbia; 87–Aud, SC Dept of Mental Retardation

Saleem-Brodsky, Laura Fern 172 Chestnut Street, Albany, NY 12210, (518) 462-8119, BA 75 CUNY - Queens Coll; MS 86 Adelphi Univ

Saleh, Mrs Florence B 56 Spring Run Road, Freeville, NY 13068, (607) 844-4500, BA 74 SUNY - Coll at Buffalo; MA 76 Kent St Univ; Sp-Lang Path, Dryden Central Schs, **SLP**

Saleh, Michele J 1996 Grandview, Seaside, CA 93955, (408) 755-6433, BA 73 CA St Univ - Fresno; MA 75 CA St Univ - Fresno; MA 81 Chapman Coll; Director Special Education, Monterey Co Office of Educ, **SLP**

Salemi, Joseph 745 Lakeview, Schaumburg, IL 60194, **SLP**

Salemi, Kelly Joseph, Jr East Carroll Parish School Bd, Special Educational Serv, 203 Schneider Lane, Lake Providence, LA 71254, (318) 559-3770, BA 63 Univ of Southwestern LA; MA 65 LA St Univ - Baton Rouge; Spec Ed Superv, E Carroll Parish Sch Bd, **SLP**

Salerno, Linda L 7941 Madison Street, Burr Ridge, IL 60521, (312) 323-6446, BA 71 Elmhurst Coll; OM 82 Governors St Univ; 75–Sp-Lang Path, Gower Dist #62, **SLP**

Salerno, Margaret Gilbreath 81 John Mardon Lane, Oroville, CA 95966, (916) 538-7241, BS 74 CA St Univ - Hayward; MA 77 San Francisco St Univ; Sp-Lang Path, Butte Co Supt of Sch, **SLP**

Salerno-Reed, Mrs Marianne 235 Lovering Avenue, Buffalo, NY 14216, (716) 878-7370, BS 75 SUNY - Coll at Buffalo; MS 76 SUNY - Coll at Buffalo; 87–Sp-Lang Path, Children's Hosp of Buffalo, **SLP**

Sales, Debra B 11430 Red Jade Court, Upper Marlboro, MD 20772, (301) 248-2456, BS 81 Towson St Univ; MA 83 George Washington Univ; Sp-Lang Path, Commun Skills Consult Inc, **SLP**

Salesin, Mrs Susan S 5123 Corners Drive, West Bloomfield, MI 48033, BA 62 Univ of MI - Ann Arbor; ME 66 Wayne St Univ; Sp-Lang Path, Communication Disorders Inc, **SLP**

Salick, Mrs Gloria 175 North Bentley Avenue, Los Angeles, CA 90049, BA 65 Occidental Coll; MA 69 CA St Univ - Northridge; **SLP**

Salih, Mrs Ursula Fulcher 400 Cozine Avenue 7L, Brooklyn, NY 11207, BA 78 CUNY - City College; MA 80 CUNY - City College; 87–Supervisor of Sp-Lang Path, Wishing Well Preschool, **SLP**

Saline, Jerry W 27403 Ynez Road #107, Temecula, CA 92390, BA 81 Univ of Redlands; BS 79 Univ of Redlands; MS 82 Univ of Redlands; Audiologist, Private Practice, **A**

Saline, Jocelyn Barnstead R R #1 Box 85, Dahinda, IL 61428, (309) 852-5696, BS 70 Western IL Univ; MA 73 Western IL Univ; Aud, Henry Stark Spec Ed, **A**

Saling, Reanna L 10200 El Ventoso Court, Louisville, KY 40291, (502) 454-8295, BS 79 Murray St Univ; MS 81 Murray St Univ; 81–Sp-Lang Path, Jefferson Co Bd of Ed, **SLP**

Salinger, Roberta Lynn 909 South 5th Street, 318 Sherman Hall, Champaign, IL 61820, (217) 332-4690, MA 88 Univ of IL - Urbana

Salisbury, Mrs Dawn 1515 Sonoma, Albany, CA 94706, (415) 222-2161, BA 56 Univ of MN - Minneap-St Paul; Sp-Lang Path, Richmond USD, **SLP**

Salisbury, Jean T John Tracy Clinic, 806 West Adams Boulevard, Los Angeles, CA 90007, (213) 748-5481, BA 71 Univ of CA - Berkeley; MA 74 Univ of Southern CA; PH 87 (Special Education) Univ of CA - Los Angeles; 87–Aud, John Tracy Clinic, **A**

Salisbury, Joan L 4209 Allott Avenue, Sherman Oaks, CA 91423, (818) 789-8381, BS 75 SUNY - Coll at Fredonia; MS 78 Eastern IL Univ; **SLP**

Salisbury, John A 194 Avenue 64, Pasadena, CA 91105, (213) 484-3234, BA 74 CA St Univ - Los Angeles; Aud Dir, Cigna Hlth Plans Inc, **A**

Salisbury, John R 30 Fallingbrook Road, Fairport, NY 14450, (315) 462-9561, BA 75 SUNY - Center at Buffalo; ME 77 Coll of Saint Rose; MS 78 Syracuse Univ; Aud, Private Practice, **A ACE**

Salisbury, Mrs Lynda L 8037 Kolb, Allen Park, MI 48101, (313) 582-5253, BA 59 MI St Univ; MA 63 MI St Univ; 76–Sp-Lang Path, Dearborn Bd of Ed/Pub Sch, **SLP**

Salisbury, Patricia Christoff J-8 27 East Central Avenue, Paoli, PA 19301, (215) 444-1601, BS 81 Bloomsburg Univ of PA; MS 82 Bloomsburg Univ of PA; Sp-Lang Path, Team Rehab Inc, **SLP**

Salisbury, Toni Ann 67 Prospect Avenue #6, Wickford, RI 02852, (401) 294-4561, BS 76 SUNY - Coll at Oneonta; MS 82 Univ of RI; Sp-Lang Path, Ladd Ctr, **SLP**

Salisch, Sandra L 971 Garrison Avenue, Teaneck, NJ 07666, (212) 488-1204, BA 69 Pace U -NY City; MS 71 Long Island U - CW Post Ctr; Assist Prof, Pace Univ, **SLP**

Salitan, Mrs Kathleen Joanne 3479 Woodlands Circle, Macedon, NY 14502, (315) 986-9864, BA 80 Coll of Saint Rose; MS 81 Nazareth Coll of Rochester; 86–Aud/Sp-Lang Path, Associated Comm Professionals, **SLP A**

Salitsky, Maureen E 10343 Arrowhead Drive, Jacksonville, FL 32217, (904) 262-5685, **A**

Salkas, Mrs Theresa Melican 9321 South Richmond, Evergreen Park, IL 60642, (312) 997-3600, BA 82 Elmhurst Coll; MS 84 IL St Univ - Normal; SLP, Chicago Board of Education, **SLP**

Salkaus, Joan T 38 Carey Avenue #8, Watertown, MA 02172, Aud, Middlesex County Hosp, **A**

Salkeld, Mrs Virginia L 1125 Sheerer Avenue, Waterloo, IA 50701, (319) 234-5920, BS 75 Edinboro Univ of PA; MA 82 Univ of Northern IA; 82–Sp-Lang Path, AEA 7, **SLP**

Salkovitch, Mrs Barbara L Dept Of Communication Disorder, Baycrest Hospital, 3560 Bathurst Street, Toronto, ON, Canada L4J 3B9, (416) 785-2377, BS 72 Towson St Univ; MS 73 PA St Univ - Univ Park; Superv SLP, Baycrest Hosp, **SLP**

Salkowitz, Bobbe Banks 118 North Croft Avenue, Los Angeles, CA 90048, (213) 655-6839, BA 51 Hartwick Coll; MA 68 CA St Univ - Northridge; Sp/Lang Path, Private Practice, **SLP**

Sallack, Mrs Hilda W 1500 Kings Row, Denton, TX 76201-1237, (601) 234-1476, BS 80 Univ of MS; MS 82 Univ of MS; Sp-Lang Path, Denton State Sch, **SLP**

Sallas, Victoria Ann 2538 S Christiana Avenue, Chicago, IL 60623, (312) 690-8580, **SLP**

Sallee, Mrs Gayle A D 1040 Taranto Drive, San Diego, CA 92107, (619) 692-3044, BA 70 LA St Univ - Baton Rouge; MA 71 Univ of FL; 80–Sp-Lang Path, Private Practice, **SLP**

Sallet, Mrs Lauren Lazeroff 152 Beverly Road, Chestnut Hill, MA 02167, BS 70 Syracuse Univ; ME 71 Northeastern Univ; ME 76 Northeastern Univ; 71–Sp-Lang Path, Brockton Pub Sch, **SLP**

Sallis, Judith L P 110 Old Orchard Road, Saco, ME 04062, **SLP**

Sallmann, Nancy Ann 2225 Wharf Drive #1008, Woodridge, IL 60517, (312) 968-1168, BS 78 IL St Univ - Normal; MS 79 IL St Univ - Normal; 81–Sp-Lang Path, Cass Sch Dist #63, **SLP**

Salmon, Mrs Jeannette Wernette 5413 Merrell, The Colony, TX 75056, (214) 442-2264, BS 77 TX Tech Univ; MA 84 TX Woman's Univ; Sp-Lang Path, Collin Co Spec Ed Coop, **SLP**

Salmon, Kimberly Ann 12-B Red Fox Drive, Albany, NY 12205, (518) 382-4550, BS 77 SUNY - Center at Albany; MS 82 Coll of Saint Rose; **SLP**

Salmon, Paul N 1844 8th Avenue North, Fort Dodge, IA 50501, (515) 576-7434, BS 69 Central MO St Univ; MS 73 Central MO St Univ; Super Hrng Serv, Arrowhead AEA, **A**

Salmon, Rita A 841 South Wilder St #1, St Paul, MN 55116, (612) 698-5779, BS 51 Univ of Denver; MS 53 Univ of Denver; 88–Sp-Lang Path /Phys Therapist, Private Practice, **SLP**

Salmon, Dr Shirley J Speech Pathology, VA Hospital, 4801 Linwood Boulevard, Kansas City, MO 64128, (816) 861-4700, BA 55 Huron Coll; MA 61 Univ of IA; PH 65 (NS) Univ of IA; 72–Sp-Lang Path, Ks Cty VA Med Cen, **SLP F ACE**

Salo, Ladonna P O Box 8043, La Jolla, CA 92038, (619) 470-4300, MA 74 CA St Univ - Los Angeles; 88–Dir of Sp-Lang Path, Paradise Valley Hosp, **SLP**

Salo, Rhonda Lee 2226 South Marion Street, Denver, CO 80210, (303) 861-6800, BS 79 Univ of WY; MA 83 Univ of Denver; Sp-Lang Path, The Children's Hosp, **SLP**

Salomon, Amy G 1249 Evergreen Drive, Cardiff, CA 92007-1035, (619) 576-2960, BS 76 Emerson Coll; MA 78 Univ of CO - Boulder; Sp/Lang Path/Commun Consult, Private Practice, **SLP**

Salomon, Mrs Bethany Chaitoff 3794 Warrendale Road, South Euclid, OH 44118, (216) 261-2900, BS 72 Cleveland St Univ; MA 74 Cleveland St Univ; Sp-Lang Path, Euclid Public Schools, **SLP**

Salomon, Joanna L 17180 Nadora, Southfield, MI 48076, BA 84 MI St Univ; MA 86 Wayne St Univ; **SLP**

Salomon, Mrs Judith Zalmanott 9043 Richmond Hill, San Antonio, TX 78250, (512) 647-2100, BS 69 SUNY - Coll at Buffalo; MA 86 Our Lady Lake Univ-San Anton; **SLP**

Salomon-Friedmann, Regina Ana Calz Al Desierto, D L Leones 4036-1-401, Mexico DF, Mexico 01790, (905) 515-6898, BA 79 0500; MS 81 Washington Univ; **A**

Salser, Bobbie C 18806 Walnut Drive, Gretna, NE 68028, (712) 366-0505, BS 71; MS 72 Univ of NE - Omaha; Sp-Lang Path, AEA 13, **SLP**

Salter, Mrs Charlotte 110 Alta Avenue, Piedmont, CA 94611, (415) 420-3682, BS 61 Univ of NV - Reno; MS 80 San Francisco St Univ; 78–Sp-Lang Path, Piedmont USD, **SLP**

Salter, Kathryn Meyer 95 Heritage Road, Hannibal, MO 63401, (314) 221-0414, MA 84 Northeast MO St Univ; 88–Sp-Lang Path, Hannibal Reg Hlthcare Sys Inc, **SLP**

Salter, Lorraine Zaisser 56 Pearl Street, Reading, MA 01867, (617) 828-2440, BS 82 Emerson Coll; MS 85 Emerson Coll; Sp-Lang Path, Massachusetts Hospital School, **SLP**

Saltman, Norva G 1220 Hiawatha Drive N E, Albuquerque, NM 87112, (505) 299-1402, BS 71 Central MI Univ; MA 75 Central MI Univ; Sp-Lang Path, Albuquerque Pub Sch, **SLP**

Saltness, Mrs Lori Jo 205 East 8th Street, Battle Ground, WA 98604, (206) 686-3202, BS 75 ND St Univ; MS 83 Moorhead St Univ; SLP, Battle Ground Sch District, **SLP**

Saltsman, Robert H, Jr Saltsman & Assoc Audiology Ctr, York Place Suite 29-B, 1205 York Road, Lutherville, MD 21093, (301) 825-9580, BA 79 Towson St Univ; MS 81 Towson St Univ; Aud, Saltsman & Assoc Aud Cen, **A ACE**

Saltysiak, Mrs Elaine B 6604 Loch Raver Boulevard, Baltimore, MD 21239, (301) 323-1010, BA 49 Coll of New Rochelle; MA 50 Columbia Univ Teachers Coll; 88–Asst Prof, Loyola Coll, **SLP**

Saltzman, Dorothy Jeanne Dept Of Speech & Hrng Sci, Indiana University, Bloomington, IN 47405, (812) 335-6251, BA 46 CUNY - Hunter Coll; MA 48 Johns Hopkins Univ; Staff Psychologist, Indiana Univ

Saltzman, Galen Dean 1315 Elida Street, Janesville, WI 53545, (608) 752-7413, BS 60 Univ of NE - Lincoln; MA 70 Univ of NE - Lincoln; SLP/Aud, Janesville Bd of Ed, **SLP**

Salus, Dr Mary W 377 Santa Clara Avenue, Oakland, CA 94610, (415) 893-6872, OM 72 Univ of Toronto - Ontario; MA 75 San Diego St Univ; ED 82 (Applied Psycholinguistics) Boston Univ; Sp-Lang Path, Timothy Murphy Sch, **SLP**

Salutsky, Rita Gale 1259 Wavery Place, Apt 2-L, Elizabeth, NJ 07208, (201) 351-6094, BA 84 IN Univ - Bloomington; MA 86 Memphis St Univ; 87–Sp-Lang Path, Kessler Inst for Rehab, **SLP**

Salva, Caroline Teresa 800 Sunset #2E, Manhattan, KS 66502, (913) 532-6879, BA 84 CUNY - Queens Coll; MA 86 KS St Univ; 87–Instructor, Kansas St Univ, **SLP**

Salva, Lora Lei 11105 Burton, Sugar Creek, MO 64054, (816) 252-4571, BS 85 Central MO St Univ; MS 86 Central MO St Univ; 87–Sp-Lang Path, The Rehab Inst, **SLP**

Salvatore, Dr Anthony Paul 1906 Princeton Drive, Columbia, MO 65203, BS 67 Emerson Coll; MS 69 Emerson Coll; PH 76 (Sp-Lang Path) Univ of Pittsburgh - Pittsburgh; Aud, Univ of MO Hosp & Clinics, **SLP**

Salvatore, Carol A 46 Henderson Street, Paterson, NJ 07501, (201) 345-9311, BA 78 William Paterson Coll; MS 86 William Paterson Coll; Sp-Lang Path, Paterson Bd of Educ, **SLP**

Salvi, Dr Richard J Hearing Research Lab, 215 Parker Hall, Buffalo, NY 14260, (716) 636-3400, BS 68 ND St Univ; PH 75 (NS) Syracuse Univ; 87–Prof, SUNY Univ of Buffalo

Salvin, Bernice Y 3408 Northampton Drive, Greensboro, NC 27408, **SLP**

Salvione, Lisa Angela 5 Ingalls Road, Jaffrey, NH 03452, (603) 532-4290, BA 81 SUNY - Coll at Plattsburgh; MS 85 Univ of RI; 88–Sp-Lang Path, Crotched Mountain Rehab Ctr, **SLP**

Salvo, Mrs Donna Arthur 293 Penns Way, Basking Ridge, NJ 07920, (201) 926-1193, BA 79 Kean Coll of NJ; MA 82 Kean Coll of NJ; 80–Sp-Lang Path, Bruce St Sch for the Deaf, **SLP**

Salwach, Deborah Lynn 111 Eldred #6, Wausau, WI 54401, (715) 847-2827, BS 81 Univ of WI - Stevens Point; MS 83 Univ of WI - Stevens Point; 87–Sp-Lang Path, Wausau Hosp Ctr, **SLP**

Salwin, Mrs Nancy K 10 Sunnymeade Court, Potomac, MD 20854, (301) 251-4742, BS 74 Univ of WI - Madison; MS 75 Univ of WI - Madison; Sp-Lang Path, Private Practice, **SLP**

Salyer, Betty Jean H Rt Box 252, Whittier, NC 28779, (704) 497-7680, BA 69 IN Univ - Bloomington; MA 73 Univ of Louisville; Sp/Lang Path, Jackson Co Sch, **SLP**

Salyer, Gregory W 103 Ashville Highway, Sylva, NC 28779, (704) 586-7477, BA 69 Univ of Louisville; MS 71 Univ of Louisville; Aud, Salyer Hrng Ctr, **A**

Salyer, Mrs Karen S 908 West 10th, McCook, NE 69001, (308) 345-2650, BS 74 Univ of NE - Lincoln; MS 78 Kearney St Coll; Sp-Lang Path, Commun Hosp, **SLP ACE**

Salzbank, Sharon L 28 Brentwood Street #9, Allston, MA 02134, (617) 587-2121, BA 75 SUNY - Center at Buffalo; MA 77 MI St Univ; Sp-Lang Path, Needham PS, **SLP**

Salzbank-Barron, Mrs Shelley 80 Hanson Road, Newton, MA 02159, BS 76 SUNY - Center at Albany; MA 77 MI St Univ; Sp-Lang Path, Wakefield Pub Sch, **SLP**

Salzberg, Mrs Arlene M 800 Johnston Drive, Watchung, NJ 07060, (201) 668-0500, BA 61 CUNY - Brooklyn Coll; MA 62 Columbia Univ Teachers Coll; Sp-Lang Path, Private Practice, **SLP ACE**

Salzberg, Beth Friedman 22 Woodhaven Drive, Simsbury, CT 06070, (203) 561-2345, BS 78 SUNY - Coll at New Paltz; MS 83 CUNY - Brooklyn Coll

Salzbrenner, Mrs Lynn G 1282 Cleveland Hts Blvd, Cleveland Heights, OH 44121, (216) 231-8787, BA 79 Cleveland St Univ; MA 81 Cleveland St Univ; 82–Aud, Cleveland Hrng & Sp Cen, **A**

Salzman, Gilbert M 3179 North D Street, San Bernardino, CA 92405, **SLP**

Salzman, Lenore R 10508 Gainsborough Road, Potomac, MD 20854, (301) 871-8074, BA 53 CUNY - Brooklyn Coll; MA 71 Univ of MD - College Park; 70–Sp-Lang Path, Montg Co Pub Schs, **SLP**

Salzman, Virginia H 717 North 1st, Temple, TX 76501, (817) 774-3950, BS 77 Baylor Univ; MS 78 Baylor Univ; Sp-Lang Path, Scott & White Clinic, **SLP ACE**

Salzmann, Mrs Mary Anne 45783 Cheyenne Place, Fremont, CA 94539, (415) 651-5617, BS 62 Nazareth Coll of Rochester; MS 64 Syracuse Univ; Sp-Lang Path, Fremont USD, **SLP**

Samalot, Diana Isabel 5820 Oakwood Drive #4-L, Lisle, IL 60532, (312) 462-4220, BA 81 Univ of PR - Rio Piedras; MS 84 PA St Univ - Univ Park; Sp-Lang Path, Marionjoy Rehab Ctr, **SLP**

Samar, Dr Vince Joseph Dept Of Communication Research, Ntid, Rochester, NY 14623, (716) 475-6338, BA 73 Univ of Rochester; MA 80 Univ of Rochester; PH 81 (NS) Univ of Rochester; Asst Prof, NTID

Samartin, Mrs Lucille P 1211 Timber Court, Southlake, TX 76092, (817) 481-1285, BA 63 Kean Coll of NJ; MS 69 Univ of OK Medical Center; **SLP**

Samelson, Mrs Vicki Weiss 917 Shabbona Trail, Batavia, IL 60510, (312) 406-9545, BS 76 IL St Univ - Normal; MA 78 Northern IL Univ - De Kalb; Sp-Lang Path, **SLP**

Samet, Julie B 7412 Central #11, Westland, MI 48185-2554, (313) 353-0310, BA 83 MI St Univ; MA 84 MI St Univ; **SLP**

Samfield, Barbara A 212 East Rainbow Ridge Circle, The Woodlands, TX 77381, (713) 363-9061, BS 74 Univ of TX - Austin; MA 75 Univ of Houston - Univ Park; 87–Sp-Lang Path, Speech and Language Svcs, **SLP**

Sammeth, Dr Carol Anne c/o Vanderbilt University, 1114 19th Avenue South, Nashville, TN 37211, (608) 233-9427, BA 81 Univ of CO - Boulder; MS 83 Univ of OK Medical Center; PH 86 (NS) Univ of OK Medical Center; 88–Asst Prof, Vanderbilt Univ, **A**

Sammis, Barbara G 7226 Cobblestone Court, Cincinnati, OH 45244, (513) 221-0527, BS 70 Kent St Univ; MA 76 West Chester Univ of PA; 88–Coord, Cincinnati Sp & Hrng Ctr, **SLP**

Sammis, Mrs Suzanne M 5 Corte Gracitas, Greenbrae, CA 94904, (415) 461-0648, BA 68 Univ of CA - Santa Barbara; MS 69 Univ of MI - Ann Arbor; SLP, Private Practice, **SLP**

Sampat, Jyoti D 905 Queensbury Court, Naperville, IL 60540, (319) 359-1317, BS 68; MS 71 Vanderbilt Univ; Aud, MS Bend AEA, **A**

Sample, Mrs Mary Henderson 4 Forestwood Cove, Little Rock, AR 72212, (501) 778-1111, MS 85 Univ of AR - Little Rock; BS 83 Univ of AR - Little Rock; Sp-Lang Path, HealthCare Plus-Sp Path Svcs, **SLP**

Sample, Pamela A UCSD, Ophthalmology M018, La Jolla, CA 92093, BA 73 IN Univ - Bloomington; MA 75 IN Univ - Bloomington; PH 88 (Psychology) Univ of CA - San Diego; 88–Research Fellow, Ophthalmology UCSD, **A**

Sample, Mrs Walterine Britt 111 Peck Boulevard, Lafayette, LA 70508, (318) 988-3027, BA 81 Univ of Southwestern LA; OM 83 LA St Univ - N O Medical Ctr

Samples, David M 18 Drexel Drive, Rome, GA 30161, (404) 295-6389, BA 72 Auburn Univ - Auburn; OM 73 Auburn Univ - Auburn; Sp-Lang Path, NW Georgia Regional Hospital, **SLP**

Samples, Dianne L 4725-B Hoen Avenue, Santa Rosa, CA 95405, (707) 542-1154, BS 74 CA St Univ - Hayward; MA 77 San Jose St Univ; Sp-Lang Path, Santa Spch & Lang Services Inc, **SLP**

Samples, Dr John Mar 4725B Hoen Avenue, Santa Rosa, CA 95405-7862, (707) 542-1154, OM 85 Golden Gate Univ; MA 63 Univ of CO - Boulder; PH 77 (Special Education) Univ of CA - Berkeley; 79–Dir, Santa Rosa Sp & Lang Ser, **SLP**

Samples, Sheila Carol 2655 Shoreline Drive #A-18, Akron, OH 44314, BA 85 OH Univ - Athens; MA 87 OH Univ - Athens; **A**

Sampson, Mrs Arlene F 22 Robin Hill Road, Holliston, MA 01746, (617) 429-5512, BA 66 Univ of MA - Amherst; MS 74 Boston Univ; **SLP A**

Sampson-Lester, Alice M 33 Gotham Hill Drive, Marshfield, MA 02050, BS 81 Worcester St Coll; MS 83 Boston Univ; Sp-Lang Path, North River Collaborative, **SLP**

Sams, Mrs Helen V 838 Burton Road, Georgetown, KY 40324, (606) 234-1001, BA 63 Georgetown Coll; MA 84 Eastern KY Univ; Sp-Lang Path, Harrison Co Boe, **SLP**

Sams, Mrs Lois Buchanan 10403 Zerlee Street, Baton Rouge, LA 70807, (504) 387-0476, BS 61 Southern Univ - Baton Rouge; MA 63 LA St Univ - Baton Rouge; Sp-Lang Path Consult, E Baton Rouge Parish Sch Bd, **SLP**

Samsky, Jay G 45 Briary Road, Dobbs Ferry, NY 10522, (914) 761-6000, BA 56 CUNY - City College; MA 59 NY Univ; Sp-Lang Path, Greenburg Cen 7 Sch Dist, **SLP**

Samson, Beth 3812 El Prado Blvd, Apartment B, Tampa, FL 33629, (813) 839-4198, BS 84 LA St Univ - Baton Rouge; MA 86 Memphis St Univ; Sp-Lang Path, InSpeech Inc, **SLP**

Samson, Molly 15 Spinney Creek Road, Eliot, ME 03903-2220, (207) 439-5414, BA 73 Beloit Coll; ME 76 Univ of VA - Charlottesville; Sp-Lang Path, Private Practice, **SLP**

Samson, Sarla Wyn 314 East Mill Street, Mount Holly, NJ 08060, (609) 261-3683, BS 67 Syracuse Univ; MA 71 Adams St Coll; MA 83 Trenton St Coll; Sp-Lang Path, NJ Dept of Human Svcs, **SLP ACE**

Samuel, Mrs Sheran L 18693 Samuel Road, Zachary, LA 70791, (504) 654-4724, BS 83 LA St Univ - Baton Rouge; MS 87 LA St Univ - Baton Rouge; 84–Sp-Lang Path, East Baton Rouge Parish Sch Bd

Samuel, Susan Candler 5977 New England Woods Dr, Burke, VA 22015, (703) 250-0019, BA 70 Auburn Univ - Auburn; MS 85 Univ of NC - Chapel Hill; SLP, Child Development Ctr, **SLP**

Samuelian, Mrs Charlene J 5250 North Pleasant, Fresno, CA 93711, (209) 488-3325, BA 68 CA St Univ - Fresno; MA 71 CA St Univ - Fresno; Coord of Sp-Lang Path, Fresno Co Office of Educ, **SLP**

Samuels, Barbara A Ctr For Communication Dis, 7349 Topanga Canyon Blvd, Canoga Park, CA 91303, (818) 883-1381, BA 71 CA St Univ - Northridge; MA 72 CA St Univ - Northridge; 74–Dir, Cen for Commun Dis, **SLP ACE**

Samuels, Mrs Carole c/o Carole Samuels, East Orleans Radiology, 6010 Bullard Avenue Suite 107, New Orleans, LA 70128, (313) 493-6315, BS 64 Univ of MI - Ann Arbor; MA 78 Wayne St Univ; **SLP**

Samuels, Mrs Cynthia R 122 Washington Street, Arlington, MA 02174, (617) 729-3094, BS 81 CO St Univ; MS 84 Emerson Coll; Sp-Lang Path, Waltham Weston Hosp Med Center, **SLP**

Samuels, Devorah Yoshpe 501 E 87th Street #3E, New York, NY 10128, BA 79 Univ of CA - Santa Barbara; MA 83 CUNY - Hunter Coll; Sp-Lang Path, **SLP**

Samuels, Ellen M 1 Lake Shore Drive, Lake Isle, New Rochelle, NY 10804, (914) 576-2079, BS 68 SUNY - Coll at Buffalo; MS 70 SUNY - Coll at Buffalo; Sp/Lang Path, Private Practice, **SLP**

Samuels, Jessica R 1201 South Scott Street, Arlington, VA 22204, (804) 520-5480, BS 70 FL A & M Univ; ME 73 Univ of VA - Charlottesville; Assist Prof/Dir Sp Clinic, VA State U, **SLP**

Samuels, Paula M 916 Old Metairie Drive, Metairie, LA 70001, (504) 838-3900, BS 71 LA St Univ - Baton Rouge; MA 72 OH Univ - Athens; Sp-Lang Path, Ochsner Cl, **SLP ACE**

Samuels, Ruth F 1515 North Flagler Drive, West Palm Beach, FL 33401, (305) 629-2266, BS 68 Ithaca Coll; MS 70 Syracuse Univ; 79–Aud, Palm Beach ENT Assoc, **A**

Samuelsen, Ruth A 4531 South Glen Place, Rapid City, SD 57702, (605) 343-8500, BA 65 Univ of SD - Vermillion; MS 68 CO St Univ; Sp/Lang Path, Black Hills Rehab Hosp, **SLP**

Samuelson, Virginia C 4011 Belle Avenue, Davenport, IA 52807, (319) 355-5065, BS 69 Univ of IA; MA 70 Univ of IA; **SLP**

Samuels-Rojo, Linda 3477 Savage Avenue, Pinole, CA 94564, (415) 758-3909, BA 76 CA St Univ - Northridge; MA 84 CA St Univ - Los Angeles; SLP, Richmond USD, **SLP**

Sanagorski-Phillips, Mrs Susan Beth 25 Winter Street #4, Weatherville, ME 04901, (207) 872-2867, BS 84 Univ of ME - Farmington; MS 85 Syracuse Univ; **SLP**

Sanborn, Barbara A 3263 South Ivy Way, Denver, CO 80222, (303) 399-1800, BA 78 MI St Univ; MA 80 Memphis St Univ; Sp-Lang Path, Sewall Rehab Cen, **SLP**

Sanborn, Dr E Sue 8910 Inverness Drive N E, Seattle, WA 98115, (808) 261-7002, BA 65 Univ of WA; MA 67 Univ of WA; PH 70 (NS) Univ of WA; Associate Professor, George Washington University, **A**

Sanborn, Mrs Pamela H 2510 Lakeside Court, Palm Harbor, FL 34684, (813) 787-1949, BA 70 Univ of MA - Amherst; ME 74 Northeastern Univ; **SLP**

Sanches, Jean Elizabeth 5014 South Murray Boulevard, Apartment D-3, Murray, UT 84123, (801) 565-7450, BA 83 WA St Univ; MS 85 Eastern WA Univ; 88–Sp-Lang Path, Jordon Sch Dist, **SLP**

Sanchez, Mrs Linda 10742 Avenue L, Chicago, IL 60617, (312) 890-8349, BA 83 IN Univ - Bloomington; MA 84 IN Univ - Bloomington; SLP, The Chicago Board of Education, **SLP**

Sanchez, Mrs Mary E P O Box 234, Grants, NM 87020, (505) 552-6907, BS 77 Radford Univ; MS 79 Purdue Univ - West Lafayette; Cl Coord, Indian Chldrn's Prog, **SLP**

Sanchez, Rachel Lara 4605 Tobago Cove, Austin, TX 78749, (512) 280-1642, BS 83 Univ of TX - Austin; ME 85 Southwest TX St Univ; **SLP**

Sanchez-Boyce, Michele L 206 Gifford Way, Sacramento, CA 95864, (916) 482-5254, BA 77 CA St Univ - Sacramento; MA 79 CA St Univ - Sacramento; Sp-Lang Path, Elk Grove USD, **SLP ACE**

Sancibrian, Cheryl L 9208 Flint, Lubbock, TX 79423, (806) 742-3908, BS 77 TX Tech Univ; MS 78 TX Tech Univ; 84–Clinic Director, Texas Tech University, **SLP**

Sancilio, Susan Lisa 78-12 35th Avenue #3-K, Jackson Heights, NY 11372, (212) 741-7698, BS 83 Univ of VA - Charlottesville; ME 86 Univ of VA - Charlottesville; **SLP**

Sand, Mrs Nancy L 5430 Rosebriar Court, Lincoln, NE 68516, (402) 423-5896, BS 77 Univ of NE - Lincoln; MA 78 Univ of NE - Lincoln; Sp-Lang Path, Lincoln Pub Schools, **SLP**

Sandage, Michelle R 112 North 22nd Street, Maltoon, IL 61938, (217) 235-0551, MA 84 Northern IL Univ - De Kalb; Aud, Central Assoc for Spec Educ, **A**

Sandahl, Maureen Darin 303 Wight Street, St Johns, MI 48879, (517) 224-6319, BA 75 Denison Univ; MA 76 Western MI Univ; Sp/Lang Path, Private Practice, **SLP**

Sandberg, Deborah Tavalaro 54 School Road, Colchester, CT 06415, (203) 537-5862, BA 76 Boston Coll; MS 77 Syracuse Univ; Sp-Lang Path, Columbia Pub Sch Sys, **SLP**

Sande, Caren D 472 18th Street, West Babylon, NY 11704, (516) 921-7650, BS 78 SUNY - Coll at Fredonia; MS 81 Adelphi Univ; Sp/Lang Path, Nassau Cen/Developmentally Dis, **SLP**

Sande, Laninda Arisa 2132 Longview, Tallahassee, FL 32303, (904) 562-8452, BS 85 FL St Univ; MS 86 FL St Univ; 88–Sp-Lang Path, Gadsden Co Sch Sys

Sande, Susan Tourdot 282 Cottage Avenue, Fond Du Lac, WI 54935, (414) 923-1495, BA 84 Univ of WI - Eau Claire; MS 85 Univ of WI - Eau Claire; Sp-Lang Path, ARC Early Ed Program, **SLP**

Sandefur, Mrs Dona Rae 2728-A Pali Highway, Honolulu, HI 96817, (808) 595-8297, **SLP**

Sander, Mrs Cindy Lee 13024 Winding Trail Lane, Des Peres, MO 63131, (314) 966-8462, BS 77 Central MO St Univ; MS 80 Southern IL Univ-Edwardsvill; Sp-Lang Path, Spec Sch Dist, **SLP**

Sander, Mrs Diane Quam 244 Circle Hills Drive, Grand Forks, ND 58201, (701) 746-2275, BS 70 Minot St Univ; MS 81 Univ of ND; Sp-Lang Path, Grand Forks Pub Schs, **SLP**

Sander, Prof Eric Kurt Department Of Speech, Cleveland State University, Cleveland, OH 44115, (216) 687-3805, BS 56 Marquette Univ; MA 59 Univ of IA; PH 64 (NS) Case Western Reserve Univ; Prof of Sp & Hrng, Cleveland St U, **SLP**

Sanderford, Patricia Murphy 5607 NW Raintree, Parkville, MO 64152, (816) 587-3521, BS 82 Black Hills St Coll; MA 86 Univ of SD - Vermillion; 88–Aud, Earth Dental Lab Inc, **A**

Sanders, Albert G, III 203 Foxridge Road, Orange Park, FL 32065, (804) 272-6761, BS 74 Murray St Univ; MA 75 Memphis St Univ; 80–Aud, US Navy, **A**

Sanders, Aliceann C 652 North Williams Drive, Palatine, IL 60067, (312) 358-6222, BA 51 Vanderbilt Univ; MA 54 Univ of KY; 72–Sp/Lang Path, Township H S Dist 211, **SLP**

Sanders, Mrs Andrea S Route 4 Box 180, Gallatin, TN 37066, (615) 452-8567, BA 71 Carleton Coll; MA 76 Univ of IA; 87–Sp-Lang Path, Rebound Inc, **SLP**

Sanders, Ann C 3913 Candlewick Court, Bedford, TX 76021, **SLP**

Sanders, Bettina D 518 Royal Greens Drive, Temple Terrace, FL 33617, (813) 972-7529, MS 77 Univ of South FL; Aud, VA Hosp, **A**

Sanders, Mrs Cynthia A 1121 Western Hills, Sherman, TX 75090, (214) 893-2459, BA 71 Baylor Univ; MS 73 Baylor Univ; Private Practice, **SLP**

Sanders, Mrs Deanna Dear 1690 Oaken Bucket Drive, Cordova, TN 38018, (901) 756-9894, BA 84 Univ of MS; MS 86 Univ Southern MS-Hattiesburg; 88–Sp-Lang Path, Baptist Mem Hosp, **SLP**

Sanders, Deborah Eve One Montgomery Avenue, Apartment 108, Bala-Cynwyd, PA 19004, (609) 342-7600, BA 83 Univ of CO - Boulder; MS 85 Columbia Univ Teachers Coll; 86–Sp-Lang Path, Mediplex-Rehab-Camden, **SLP**

Sanders, Mrs Deborah P 8326 Babe Ruth, San Antonio, TX 78240, (512) 674-0131, BA 64 Wichita St Univ; ME 70 Southwest TX St Univ; Sp-Lang Path, Northside ISD, **SLP**

Sanders, Dr Derek A Dept Communicative Dis & Sci, State Univ Of New York, 4226 Ridge Lea Road, Buffalo, NY 14226, (716) 839-4148, BA 56 West End Hosp-London England; MS 58 Syracuse Univ; PH 61 (NS) Royal Victoria Univ -England; Aud, St U NY at Buffalo, **SLP A F**

Sanders, Elizabeth C 111 Pilgrim Road, Lynchburg, VA 24502, (804) 947-6870, BA 74 Mary Washington Coll; ME 75 Univ of VA - Charlottesville; Sp-Lang Path & Aud Dir, Ctrl VA Trng Cen, **SLP**

Sanders, Mrs Elizabeth G 6848 Sauterne Cove, Memphis, TN 38115-5341, (901) 767-7750, BS 80 AR St Univ; MA 84 Memphis St Univ; Aud, Shea Hubbard & Futrell, **A**

Sanders, Mrs Elizabeth M 908 Station Avenue, Haddon Heights, NJ 08035, (609) 546-1880, BA 80 Univ of AL-Tuscaloosa; MS 81 Univ of AL- Tuscaloosa; Dir-SLP Servs, Care Enterprises, **SLP**

Sanders, Mrs Irene M 1164 Ollerton Road, West Deptford, NJ 08066, (609) 848-8268, **SLP**

Sanders, Mrs Jana S 3118 Rustlewood Lane SE, Port Orchard, WA 98366, (206) 876-1399, BA 66 Univ of KS; MA 71 CA St Univ - Northridge; Sp-Lang Path, South Kitsap School Dist #402, **SLP**

Sanders, Jay W Bill Wilkerson Hrng & Sp Ctr, 1114 19th Avenue South, Nashville, TN 37212, (615) 320-5353, BA 50 Univ of NC - Chapel Hill; MA 51 Columbia Univ Teachers Coll; PH 57 (Sp & Hrng) Univ of MO - Columbia; 87–Prof Emeritus, Vanderbilt U Sch of Med, **SLP A F**

Sanders, Jeannine Meyer 1810 Gordon Avenue, Lansing, MI 48910, (517) 353-8780, **SLP**

Sanders, Johnny Lee 700 Waugh Drive, Houston, TX 77019, (713) 520-0066, BS 73 Univ of Houston - Univ Park; MA 74 Univ of Houston - Univ Park; Pres, Hlth Testing Inc, **A**

Sanders, Mrs Karen S 27220 Old Edgewood Road, Weed, CA 96097, (916) 938-3795, BA 82 Humboldt St Univ; MA 84 Humboldt St Univ; 88–Sp-Lang Path, Siskiyou Co Dept of Educ, **SLP**

Sanders, Mrs Kathryn L 2808 Windy, Commerce, TX 75428, (214) 785-4521, BS 68 West TX St Univ; MS 80 East TX St Univ - Commerce; Clinic Supervisor/Instructor, East Texas State University, **SLP**

Sanders, Mrs Linda B 12323 Chesterbrook, Houston, TX 77031, (713) 498-8948, BS 69 Stephen F Austin St Univ; MA 70 Stephen F Austin St Univ; **SLP**

Sanders, Mrs Lisa Carolyn 6 Jardin Court Apt #1, Collinsville, IL 62234, (314) 865-3333, BS 80 Southern IL Univ-Edwardsvill; MS 81 Southern IL Univ-Edwardsvill; 81–Aud/Sp-Lang Path, Alexian Bros Hosp, **SLP A**

Sanders, Dr Lois Joan 1501 Delmont Court #2, Urbana, IL 61801, (217) 328-2911, BA 48 Ripon Coll; MS 50 Univ of WI - Madison; PH 63 (Sp-Lang Path) Northwestern Univ; 87–Retired, Univ of Illinois, **SLP**

Sanders, Mrs Marla Watson 409 Ray Avenue N W #C, New Philadelphia, OH 44663, (216) 343-2924, MA 88 Kent St Univ

Sanders, Patricia Mary 112 Abbott Street, North Massapequa, NY 11758, (516) 783-7523, BA 83 Adelphi Univ; MA 84 Adelphi Univ; Sp-Lang Path, Sch for Lang & Comm Dev, **SLP**

Sanders, R Richard 38 Creeley Road, Belmont, MA 02178, (617) 489-5607, BA 75 Univ of NC - Chapel Hill; MS 80 Boston Univ; Sp-Lang Path, Private Practice, **SLP**

Sanders, Mrs Rachel Johnson 419 6th Street, Suite 322, Juneau, AK 99801, (907) 586-5794, BA 82 Univ of NC - Chapel Hill; MS 84 Univ of NC - Chapel Hill; Sp-Lang Path, St Jude Ctr Inc, **SLP**

Sanders, Richard Route 4 Box 180, Gallatin, TN 37066, (615) 452-8567, BA 71 Carleton Coll; MA 75 Univ of IA; 87–Aud, Rebound Incorporated, **A**

Sanders, Dr Sara B 5656 Buxbriar Avenue, Memphis, TN 38119, (901) 683-1693, BA 61 Univ of AR - Fayetteville; MA 73 Memphis St Univ; PH 81 (NS) Memphis St Univ; Chief SLP Sect, VA Med Cen, **SLP ACE**

Sanders, Mrs Sarah Mullaney 1012 Wagner Avenue, Louisville, KY 40217, (502) 584-9781, BS 82 Eastern KY Univ; MS 86 Univ of Louisville; 87–Sp-Lang Path, Easter Seal Hearing & Sp Ctr, **SLP**

Sanders, Stephen Jeffrey 34022 Zarzito Drive, Dana Point, CA 92629, (714) 768-3536, BS 76 Univ of CA - Irvine; MA 86 Univ of CO - Boulder; 88–Aud, Head & Neck Assoc of Orange Cty, **A**

Sanders, Mrs Terri T 6464 West Stones Crossing, Greenwood, IN 46143, (317) 929-3311, BS 75 Purdue Univ - West Lafayette; MA 77 Ball St Univ; Sp/Lang Path, Indiana Home Health Services, **SLP**

Sandersen, Marsha Becker Yakima Valley Hearing & Speech, 303 South 12th Avenue, Yakima, WA 98902, (509) 453-8248, BS 66 IN Univ - Bloomington; MA 68 IN Univ - Bloomington; Ex Dir, Yakima Valley Hrng & Sp Cen, **SLP**

Sanders-Jackson, Elaine Route 1 Box 788, Santee, SC 29142, (803) 665-4820, **SLP**

Sanders-Lofaso, Mrs Jamie Sue 7 Milady Road, Weston, ON, Canada M9L 2H7, (416) 743-1210, BS 80 IN Univ - Bloomington; MA 82 IN Univ - Bloomington; SLP, Bethesda Home, **SLP**

Sanders-Mascari, Mrs Aviva 26 New York Avenue, Hawthorne, NJ 07506, (201) 423-1781, OM 81 Univ of Bridgeport; BA 75 Hofstra Univ; MA 76 Univ of IL - Urbana; Sp-Lang Path, Northern Valley Reg High Sch Dist, **SLP**

Sanderson, Mrs Deborah Briggs 209 Lark Street, Rochester, NY 14613, (716) 271-0680, BS 81 SUNY - Coll at Geneseo; MA 82 SUNY - Coll at Geneseo; Aud, Hrng & Sp Ctr, **A ACE**

Sanderson, Laurie B 129 Peachtree Road, Cheektowaga, NY 14225, (716) 854-6886, BA 84 SUNY - Center at Buffalo; MA 86 SUNY - Center at Buffalo; **SLP**

Sanderson, Pamela M 7061-B Appian Drive, San Diego, CA 92139, (619) 295-3141, BS 70 Loma Linda Univ - Riverside; MS 80 Loma Linda Univ - Riverside; Aud, Bruce Sanderson MD Med Cl, **A**

Sanderson, Paul Daniel 610 West Cavour, Fergus Falls, MN 56537, (218) 739-3592, BS 79 Moorhead St Univ; MS 80 Univ of WI - Stevens Point; Aud, Fergus Falls Med Group, **A**

Sanderson, Robert G 64 Halifax Street, Jamaica Plain, MA 02130, (617) 437-1036, BS 66 Auburn Univ - Auburn; MA 68 Auburn Univ - Auburn; 84–Dir, Boston Hrng Serv, **A**

Sanderson, Mrs Sandra A 11013 North Tall Oaks, Peoria, IL 61615, (309) 672-6788, BA 61 Augustana Coll; MA 65 Case Western Reserve Univ; Sp-Lang Path, Peoria Pub Sch Dist #150, **SLP**

Sanderson, Tanya B 420 Redondo #209, Long Beach, CA 90814, BA 72 MI St Univ; MA 79 Whittier Coll; SLP, Los Angeles Co Supt of Schools, **SLP**

Sanderson, Virginia S Somesville, Mount Desert, ME 04660, (207) 244-3808, OB 18 Univ of CA - Berkeley; MS 20 Univ of CA - Berkeley; PH 28 (Psych & Speech) OH St Univ; Prof-Psych, Ohio State Univ, **SLP LM**

Sandhofer, Jean S Naples Elementary School, Box 39, FPO New York, NY 09521-0005, BS 79 Old Dominion Univ; OM 81 Univ of SC - Columbia; Sp-Lang Path, Dept of Defense Dependent Schs, **SLP**

Sandifer, Henri D Speech & Language Services, P O Box 2008, Orangeburg, SC 29116, (803) 536-6355, BA 70 Columbia Coll; MA 76; Dir, Sp & Lang Serv, **SLP**

Sandler, Eileen B 5050 Garford #52, Long Beach, CA 90815, (213) 438-9781, BA 77 San Diego St Univ; MA 79 San Diego St Univ; 86–Sp-Lang Path, Villa Serena Tran Living Ctr, **SLP**

Sandler, Janet L 800 Palisade Avenue #1205, Fort Lee, NJ 07024, (201) 224-4777, OB 75 Univ of Miami; MA 76 Univ of Miami; Pres, Janet Sandler Ma & Assoc, **SLP**

Sandler, Mrs Judith A 3755 Arrowood Lane, Plymouth, MN 55441, (612) 474-5448, BA 72; MA 75 Univ of MN - Minneap-St Paul; Sp-Lang Path, Minnetonka Schools, **SLP**

Sandler, Mrs Judith G 337 Taylors Mill Road, Manalapan Township, NJ 07726, (201) 462-8412, BA 71 Univ of MA - Amherst; MA 72 Kean Coll of NJ; 87–Aud, The Hearing Ctr, **A**

Sandler, Mrs Louise Gilles 1441 Jaywood Drive, St Louis, MO 63146, (314) 878-7427, BA 65 Univ of IA; MS 85 Fontbonne Coll; 88–Sp-Lang Path, Special Sch Dist, **SLP**

Sandler, Mrs Marcia G 55 Chestnut Lane, Woodbury, NY 11797-4806, (516) 364-3196, **SLP**

Sandler, Mrs Marilyn 2853 West Glenlake, Chicago, IL 60659, (312) 338-2907, BA 74 Rutgers St Univ - Camdem; MS 76 William Paterson Coll; Sp-Lang Path, Rimland Sch, **SLP ACE**

Sandler, Ronna 11932 Canfield Road, Potomac, MD 20854, **A**

Sandler, Steven J 8 S Barn Hill Road, Bloomfield, CT 06002, (203) 282-3362, BA 75 CUNY - Queens Coll; MS 77 Eastern IL Univ; 80–Sp-Lang Path, East Hartford Publ Schs, **SLP**

Sandlin, Dr Robert E 1920 Estela Drive, El Cajon, CA 92020, (619) 442-0413, BA 50 San Diego St Univ; MA 54 Wayne St Univ; PH 61 (NS) Wayne St Univ; Aud, Re Sandlin Phd & Assoc Inc, **SLP A**

Sandlin, Vicki L P O Box 463, Bentonville, AR 72712, (501) 273-1810, BA 80 Univ of AR - Fayetteville; MA 81 Univ of AR - Fayetteville; Sp-Lang Path, Benton County Sunshine Sch, **SLP**

Sandman, Sharon Elizabeth 14 Chesnut Lane, Ledyard, CT 06339, (203) 572-8385, BS 78 Eastern CT St Coll; MA 86 Univ of CT; **SLP**

Sandness, Mrs Beret S 1703 East 7th Street, Duluth, MN 55812, (218) 724-6593, BA 81 Univ of MN - Duluth; MS 82 Univ of WI - Eau Claire; Sp/Lang Path, ISD #710, **SLP**

Sandness, Dr Donald L 1025 Barnett Way #33, Madera, CA 93637-8840, (209) 673-4709, BS 61 Valley City St Coll; MA 65 Univ of MN - Minneap-St Paul; PH 73 (NS) Univ of UT; Asst Prof, Nd St U, **SLP**

Sandness, Serena Marie 31000 Ruth Hill Road, Squaw Valley, CA 93675, (209) 338-2511, BS 83 ND St Univ; MS 85 Univ of ND; 87–Sp-Lang Path, Kings Canyon USD, **SLP**

Sandor, Mrs Susan S 1505 Hickory Heights Drive, Waverly, IA 50677, (319) 352-4366, BS 74 Northern IL Univ - De Kalb; MA 75 OH Univ - Athens; Sp-Lang Path, Private Practice, **SLP**

Sandore, Lisa M 4326 Villa #12, Cincinnati, OH 45242, (513) 872-2481, BA 78 OH St Univ; MA 80 Univ of Cincinnati; 87–Sp-Lang Path, Good Samaritan Hosp, **SLP**

Sandoval-Pugh, Cheryl Ann 1043 Menlo, Clovis, CA 93612, (209) 298-1683, MS 84 Univ of NV - Reno; BS 82 Univ of NV - Reno; SLP, Kings Co Schl Dstr, **SLP**

Sandquist, Mrs Mary Anne 22 El Dorado Road, Cannon Falls, MN 55009, BA 63 Briar Cliff Coll; Sp-Lang Path, St Paul Pub Sch, **SLP**

Sandretto, Gary Charles 8911 Blackpool Drive, St Louis, MO 63123, (314) 621-1462, BS 79 Southeast MO St Univ; MS 84 Fontbonne Coll; 80–Sp-Lang Path, St Louis PS, **SLP**

Sandridge, Dr Sharon A Dep Of Communicative Disorders, Northern Illinois Univ, De Kalb, IL 60115, (815) 753-1484, BA 83 Univ of Akron; MA 84 Univ of Akron; PH 88 (Aud) Univ of FL; 88–Asst Prof, Northern Illinois Univ, **A ACE**

Sands, Denise M M 808 Blue Gate Lane, Sinking Spring, PA 19608, (215) 777-3085, BS 75 Bloomsburg Univ of PA; MS 78 Bloomsburg Univ of PA; Sp-Lang Path, InSpeech Inc, **SLP**

Sands, Dr Elaine S 101 Soundview Drive, Port Washington, NY 11050, (516) 294-8700, BA 60 CUNY - Brooklyn Coll; MS 61 Univ of MI - Ann Arbor; PH 77 (NS) NY Univ; Prof, Adelphi U, **SLP F**

Sands, Leslie Leigh 922 Cedar Grove Road, Broomall, PA 19008, (215) 596-9125, MS 87 PA St Univ - Univ Park; **A**

Sands, Sindy 3904 Clark Avenue, Vancouver, WA 98661, (206) 256-6022, BA 74 WA St Univ; MA 77 Univ of OR; Sp-Lang Path, Evergreen Sch Dist, **SLP**

Sandusky, Kathryn A 374 Stratford Drive, Lexington, KY 40503, (606) 278-9434, **A**

Sandy, Don Glen Post Box 621, Funchal, Portugal 09008, BS Boston Univ; ME 60 Boston Univ; ED 65 (NS) Boston Univ; **SLP**

Sanek, Gregory Paul 2130 Green Road, Cleveland, OH 44121, (216) 687-3803, BA 82 Oberlin Coll; MA 86 Cleveland St Univ; 87–Aud, Betty Jane Rehab Ctr, **A**

San Filippo, Jane Wicks 57 Country Lane, Penfield, NY 14526, (716) 385-1148, BS 72 SUNY - Coll at Brockport; MS 86 Nazareth Coll of Rochester; **SLP**

Sanford, Carol Ann 113 Taos, Edmond, OK 73034, (215) 783-6010, BS 73 Southeast MO St Univ; MS 83 Univ of TX - Dallas; Sp-Lang Path, Oklahoma City Public Schools, **SLP ACE**

Sanford, Catherine Izzi P O Box 96, Still River, MA 01467, **SLP**

Sanford, Mrs Elizabeth Boozer 7400 Fannin, Suite 900, Houston, TX 77054, (713) 792-4746, BS 83 Auburn Univ - Auburn; OM 85 Auburn Univ - Auburn; Aud, Univ of Texas, **A**

Sanford, Mrs Helen J 9113 H Derbyshire Road, Richmond, VA 23229, (804) 741-8701, BA 68 VA Commonwealth Univ; MA 71 Univ of VA - Charlottesville; Sp-Lang Path, Chesterfield Sch Bd, **SLP**

Sanford, Mrs Jill T 925 Oronoke Road #18-F, Waterbury, CT 06708, (203) 574-8000, MA 77 Western CT St Univ; MS 87 Southern CT St Univ; MS 87 Southern CT St Univ; **SLP**

Sanford, Karl R 1304 Hamilton Boulevard, Hagerstown, MD 21740, (301) 791-4415, BS 69 SUNY - Coll at Geneseo; MA 73 Western MI Univ; Dir, Commun Dis Serv, Wn Maryland Hosp Cen, **SLP**

Sanford, Marie 509 Lake Street, Fall Haven Apts #D-5, Ithaca, NY 14850, (607) 274-3248, BS 73 SUNY - Center at Albany; MS 74 Ithaca Coll; Clinical Super, Ithaca College, **SLP ACE**

Sanford, Mark Joseph 25315 Arriba Del Mundo, Carmel, CA 93923, (408) 624-1680, BA 84 Univ of the Pacific; MS 86 Univ of TX - Dallas; Audiologist, Dr William McAfee, **A**

Sanford, Mildred M 50 Oak Meadows Drive, Alexander, AR 72002, (501) 847-4124, BS 84 Univ of AR - Little Rock; MS 86 Univ of AR - Medical Sci; 87–Aud, Arkadelphia Human Development Ctr, **A**

Sanford, Tracey 5101 Sweetbriar #123, Tyler, TX 75703, (214) 531-8190, BS 83 Univ of TX - Austin; MA 86 Univ of TX - Austin; **SLP**

Sanft, Mrs Suzanne B 19206 Pires Avenue, Cerritos, CA 90701, (213) 926-5566, BA 72 CA St Univ - Long Beach; MA 74 CA St Univ - Long Beach; 88–Sp-Lang Path, ABC School District, **SLP**

Sang, Ruth Gooden 2 Kings Mews, Kingston, Jamaica 10, (809) 926-5489, BA 85 Kean Coll of NJ; MA 86 Kean Coll of NJ

Sanger, Dr Dixie D 1611 Horseshoe Drive, Ashland, NE 68003, (402) 477-4566, BA 67 Univ of NE - Lincoln; MA 70 CA St Univ - Long Beach; PH 81 (NS) Univ of NE - Lincoln; Assoc Prof, U of NE-Lincoln, **SLP**

Sanginario-Victor, Mrs Jeanne Marie 2 West Park Drive, Huntington Station, NY 11746-2417, (516) 689-9600, SLP, BOCES 2, **SLP**

Sanginiti, Janette Christine 1110 Livingston Street, Turnersville, NJ 08012, (609) 784-2102, BA 76 Glassboro St Coll; MA 83 Trenton St Coll; **SLP**

Saniga, Dr Richard D Box 5092 Southern Station, Hattiesburg, MS 39401, (601) 266-5216, BS 67 Indiana Univ of PA; MS 68 Univ of OK Medical Center; PH 80 (NS) Southern IL Univ -Carbondale; Associate Professor, U of Southern MS, **SLP ACE**

Sankey, Carole J 3916 Rigel Avenue, Lompoc, CA 93436, (805) 736-2371, BS 64 Northwestern Univ; MS 73 Univ of Houston - Univ Park; SLP, Lompoc USD, **SLP**

Sankin, Susan J P 50 Frame Road, Briarcliff Manor, NY 10510, **SLP**

San Martin-Edmunds, Mrs Mary P 11510 West Kenny Lane, Wichita, KS 67212, (316) 721-5475, **SLP**

San Martino, Mrs Alice Pauline 37 Maple Street, Malden, MA 02148, (617) 321-9062, BS 83 Univ of CA - Santa Barbara; MS 84 Boston Univ; **SLP**

San Miguel, Sonia Calle 9 D-30 Valparaiso, Bayamon, PR 00949, (809) 787-5151, BA 74 Univ of PR - Rio Piedras; MS 82 Univ of PR - San Juan; **SLP**

Sanner, Mrs Joan Ella 148 Brightwood, San Antonio, TX 78209, (602) 899-6006, BA 78 San Diego St Univ; MS 83 CO St Univ; SLP, Mesa Pub Sch, **SLP**

Sans, Mrs June Gordon 24 Stone Bridge Lane, Princeton, NJ 08540, (609) 452-1697, BA 76 Rutger's St Univ - Douglas Coll; MS 77 Adelphi Univ; Aud, Aud & Hrng Aid Dispensing Assc, **A**

Sansalone, Teresa Nievez 1153 North 78th, Seattle, WA 98103, (206) 442-7124, BS 77 OK St Univ; MS 79 Univ of NM; Aud, US Pub Hlth Serv, Ind Hlth Ser, **A**

Sansbury, Dr Russell J 719 Sunset Road, Ann Arbor, MI 48103, (313) 349-3000, BA 57 Manchester Coll; MA 61 Eastern MI Univ; PH 77 (NS) Univ of MI - Ann Arbor; Dir-Lang Cl, Hawthorn Cen, **SLP**

Sansone, Dr Frank E, Jr Southern Ct State University, 501 Crescent Street, New Haven, CT 06515, (203) 397-4571, MA 63 Univ of AL- Tuscaloosa; OM 86 Southern CT St Univ; PH 69 (Communication Disorders) Univ of OK Medical Center; Chair Dept Comm Dis, Southern Connecticut St Univ, **SLP**

Sansted, Phyllis H 49 St Germain Circle, Lake St Louis, MO 63367, **SLP**

Santa, Daphne A 3101 South Manchester St, Apartment 621, Falls Church, VA 22044, (703) 827-0980, BA 78 Loyola Coll; MS 80 Loyola Coll; Sp/Lang Path, Speech Path Serv, **SLP**

Santagato, Mrs Jeannette M 10822 Lawnbrook Drive, St Louis, MO 63123, (314) 942-3484, BS 81 Fontbonne Coll; MS 84 Fontbonne Coll; Sp-Lang Path, Northwest R-1 Sch Dist, **SLP**

Santalone, Marianne T 656 Veterans Hwy 24, Hauppauge, NY 11787, (516) 473-2800, BA 77 Hofstra Univ; MA 80 NY Univ; SLP, UCP of NY, **SLP**

Santana, Altagracia A 591 Prospect Place, Brooklyn, NY 11238, (718) 965-4800, BA 80 Univ of Rochester; MS 85 Columbia Univ Teachers Coll; **SLP**

Santana, Mrs Elizabeth 7324 Skillman, Apartment #1204, Dallas, TX 75231, (214) 340-7843, BA 81 MI St Univ; MA 82 MI St Univ; Sp-Lang Path, **SLP**

Santana, Mery Luz H 614 Mountain Road, Kinnelon, NJ 07405-2129, (803) 785-3900, SLP, Speech Language Proffesionals, **SLP**

Santangelo, Mrs Gretchen L 55 Evergreen Drive, Rochester, NY 14624, (716) 594-2336, BS 69 SUNY - Coll at Geneseo; MS 70 SUNY - Coll at Geneseo; **SLP**

Santaniello, Jean L 285 Carroll Street, Brooklyn, NY 11231, (718) 596-7051, BA 85 CUNY - Hunter Coll; MA 87 CUNY - Hunter Coll; 87–Sp-Lang Path, UCP of NYC, **SLP**

Santella-Johnson, Mary Elizabeth Box 22, McGregor, ND 58755, (701) 546-4771, BS 72 Univ of Northern CO; MS 76 Univ of WI - Eau Claire; 79–Sp-Lang Path, Tioga PS

Santiago, Nydia I Sky Towers I #12B, Rio Piedras, PR 00926, (809) 764-6035, BS 72 Univ of PR - Rio Piedras; MS 74 Univ of PR - Rio Piedras; Asst Prof, Upr, **A**

Santiago, Vilma A P O Box 1344, Arecibo, PR 00613, (809) 878-3535, BS 77; MS 81 TX Christian Univ; SLP, Arecibo Dist Hosp, **SLP**

Santisi, Rosemarie 556 4th Street, Brooklyn, NY 11215, (212) 498-6902, **SLP**

Santivasi, Jill G 1558 South Josephine, Denver, CO 80210, (303) 986-1555, BA 74 Univ of Denver; MA 75 Univ of Denver; 79–Sp-Lang Path, Jefferson Co Sch Dist, **SLP**

Santo, Daniel J 4140 Workman Mill Road, Apartment 272, Whittier, CA 90601, (213) 941-2251, BA 85 Whittier Coll; MA 87 Whittier Coll; Sp-Lang Path, Calif Phys Therp at Med Ctr of La Mirada, **SLP**

Santo Pietro, Dr Mary Jo Cook 25 High Street, Metuchen, NJ 08840, (201) 932-9335, BA 67 Catholic Univ of America; MA 70 Columbia Univ Teachers Coll; PH 79 (NS) Columbia Univ Teachers Coll; Asst Prof/Dir of Grad Prog, Rutgers U, **SLP**

Santora, Paula S 1809 Coachman Drive, Camarillo, CA 93010, (805) 484-3661, BS 77 WV Univ; MS 79 WV Univ; Sp-Lang Path, Camarillo St Hosp, **SLP**

Santore, Frances C 3900 Gretstone Avenue #61D, Riverdale, NY 10463, (212) 543-2869, **SLP**

Santoro, Mrs Elizabeth 695 Bryant Avenue, Roslyn, NY 11576, (516) 354-5412, BS 58 Kent St Univ; MS 71 Long Island U - CW Post Ctr; 88–Sp-Lang Path, Private Practice, **SLP**

Santoro, Mrs Judy S 5 Tide Mill Lane, Nissequogue, NY 11780, (516) 281-3020, BA 75 Hofstra Univ; MA 81 Hofstra Univ; Sp-Lang Path, Wm Floyd Sch Dist, **SLP**

Santoro, Mary Anne Memorial Medical Center, 27450 Schoenherr, Warren, MI 48093, (313) 445-6850, BA 79 MI St Univ; MA 81 Wayne St Univ - Sch of Med; Aud, Mem Med Cen, **A ACE**

Santoro, Mrs Susan Foglia 2449 Westley Road, Westbury, NY 11590, (516) 997-8327, BA 78 SUNY - Coll at Cortland; MS 79 Adelphi Univ; Sp-Lang Path, BOCES-III, **SLP**

Santos, Mrs Bonita B 1429 Fernview Drive, Modesto, CA 95355, (209) 869-3633, BA 70 CUNY - Brooklyn Coll; MA 74 CA St Univ - Los Angeles; Prin, Riverbank Elem Sch Dist, **SLP**

Santos, Maria Emilia Lab Estudos DE Linguage, Cntro DE Estud Egas Moniz, Hosp DE Santa Maria, Lisbon, Portugal 1600, MS

Santostefano, Joyce A 91 Holman Street, Laconia, NH 03246, (603) 668-3545, BA 76 Montclair St Coll; MS 78 Columbia Univ Teachers Coll; 88–Coord-Sp-Lang Svcs, Catholic Med Ctr, **SLP**

Santucci, Gayle M 2309 Hilton Avenue, St Louis, MO 63144, (314) 388-8000, OB 73 Univ of KS; MA 75 Univ of KS; Aud, Private Practice, **A**

Santucci, Michael Joseph 1255 N Sandburg Terrace, Apartment 1712, Chicago, IL 60610, (312) 988-4822, BA 75 Univ of IA; MS 79 IL St Univ - Normal; **A**

Sanvi, Mrs Jennifer R 5564 Mark Court S E, Salem, OR 97301, (503) 581-0909, BS 71 Saint Louis Univ; MA 73 Univ of IL - Urbana; 87–Sp-Lang Path, Private Practice, **SLP**

Sanz, Karen Leslie 320 S E Richland, Corvallis, OR 97333, (503) 451-7378, BS 83 OR St Univ; MS 86 Western OR St Coll; 84–Sp-Lang Path, Lebanon PS, **SLP**

Sapharas, Barbara A 2310 South Overlook Road, Cleveland Heights, OH 44106, (216) 475-7066, BA 75 Cleveland St Univ; MA 76 Cleveland St Univ; Sp-Lang Path, Cuyahoga Co Bd of Men Ret, **SLP**

Saphier, Marlene P O Box 833, Cambria, CA 93428, (805) 927-8858, BA 62 CUNY - Hunter Coll; MA 69 Univ of Southern CA; Sp-Lang Path, Marlene Saphier, Ma/Ccc, **SLP**

Sapienza-Crowley, Mrs Patricia 212 Calvert Boulevard, Tonawanda, NY 14150, (716) 852-1519, **SLP**

Sapinkopf, Mrs Ellen F 10815 Stockbridge Lane, Cincinnati, OH 45249, (513) 489-3182, BA 74 SUNY - Center at Buffalo; MA 76 Univ of MD - College Park; 82–Sp/Lang Path, Private Practice, **SLP**

Sapir, Dr Shimon Dept Of Comm Sciences And Disorders, Northwestern University, 2299 Sheridan Road, Evanston, IL 60208, (312) 491-2416, BA 75 Univ of WA; MS 78 Univ of WA; PH 82 (Sp and Hrng Sciences) Univ of WA; 87–Asst Prof, Northwestern Univ, **SLP**

Sapiro, Mrs Vivian A 2220 West Kendall Avenue, Milwaukee, WI 53209, (414) 475-8137, BS 73 Univ of WI - Milwaukee; MS 74 Univ of WI - Milwaukee; Sp-Lang Path, Milwke Pub Sch, **SLP**

Saponaro, Patricia P 848 West State Street, Trenton, NJ 08618, (609) 989-1205, BA 81 Univ of NC - Chapel Hill; MS 82 Univ of NC - Chapel Hill; 85–Sp-Lang Path Supvr, Med Ctr at Princeton, **SLP ACE**

Sapora, Mrs Laurie M 205 3rd Avenue #6-H, New York, NY 10003, (212) 533-7519, OB 69 Univ of Miami; MS 70 Adelphi Univ; OM 74 Yeshiva Univ; Sp/Lang Path, NYC Bd of Ed, **SLP**

Saporito, Karen Ann 64 Bidlack Street, Forty Fort, PA 18704, (412) 341-5599, BS 82 Marywood Coll; MS 84 PA St Univ - Univ Park; Sp-Lang Path, John Heinz Rehab Institute, **SLP**

Saportin, Charlene T 109 Kaye Vue Drive #2P, Hamden, CT 06514, (203) 932-5711, BA 73 Univ of CT; MS 78 Southern CT St Univ; Sp-Lang Path, Monroe BOCES, **SLP**

Sapovits, Mrs Cynthia Roddy 558 South Coventry Lane, West Chester, PA 19382, (215) 692-9931, BS 79 West Chester Univ of PA; MA 81 West Chester Univ of PA; SLP, De Co Iu, **SLP**

Sapp, Ann Christine 8298 South Argenta Drive, West Jordan, UT 84084, BA 75 Univ of UT; MA 80 Univ of UT; Sp-Lang Path, Dod Depend Schs, **SLP**

Sapp, Mrs Helen D 58 North Fawn Drive, Terre Haute, IN 47802, (812) 237-2804, BS 52 Southern IL Univ -Carbondale; MS 55 Univ of IL - Urbana; 63–Assoc Prof, Indiana St Univ, **SLP**

Sapp, Mrs Sally Sue 12828 North 72 Avenue, Peoria, AZ 85345, (602) 866-5629, **SLP**

Sappol, Davida W 134-31 58th Road, Flushing, NY 11355, (914) 632-9000, BA 67 CUNY - Queens Coll; MS 69 CUNY - Queens Coll; OM 77 CUNY - Queens Coll; Sp-Lang Path, New Rochelle Cty Sch Dist, **SLP ACE**

Saraceno, Mrs Maria Panico 3500 East Fletcher Avenue, Suite 121, Tampa, FL 33613, (813) 971-7466, 84–Aud, Private Practice, **A**

Saras, Loline J Center For Communication Disorders, 146 Old Main, Kutztown University, Kutztown, PA 19530, (215) 683-4293, BS 77 Bloomsburg Univ of PA; MS 78 Bloomsburg Univ of PA; 88–Asst Prof, Kutztown Univ, **SLP**

Sarason, Linda A Rd 5 Box 237-C, Jackson, NJ 08527, (201) 363-0227, **SLP ACE**

Saravay, Mrs Elizabeth Schiller 7 Dogleg Lane, Roslyn Heights, NY 11577, BA 59 CUNY - Brooklyn Coll; MS 79 Adelphi Univ; SLP, Nassau Co BOCES, **SLP**

Sarb, Mrs Eileen Ayres 1044 West State Street, Mason City, IA 50401-2838, (515) 424-1926, BS 76 OH Univ - Athens; MA 81 Univ of Cincinnati; Aud, Univ of Michigan Hospital, **A**

Sardynski, Susan Q Rural Delivery 1, 266-A Miller Road, East Greenbush, NY 12061, (518) 477-8984, BS 76 Coll of Saint Rose; MS 77 Coll of Saint Rose; Sp-Lang Path, Columbia Co ARC, **SLP**

Sarfeld, Evelyn A 21 Hector Avenue, Toronto, ON, Canada M6G 3G2, (416) 296-7577, BA 77; OM 82 Univ of Western Ontario; Sp-Lang Path, Scarborough Bd of Ed, **SLP**

Sargent, Barbara J Pediatric Therapy Services, 1601 West Koenig Lane, Austin, TX 78756, (512) 453-0037, MS 77 Univ of TX - Houston; Sp-Lang Path, Pediatric Therapy Services, **SLP**

Sargent, Mrs C I 397 Bramans Lane, Portsmouth, RI 02871, (401) 847-2483, BS 67 Bowling Green St Univ; MA 70 Univ of MD - College Park; SLP, **SLP**

Sargent, Mrs Irene 462 Firetown Road, Simsbury, CT 06070, BA 70 Jersey City St Coll; MA 71 MI St Univ; Sp-Lang Path Consultant, Capitol Region Educ Council, **SLP**

Sargent, Kenneth John 332 South Cayuga Street, Ithaca, NY 14850, (607) 535-2745, BS 84 Ithaca Coll; MS 85 Ithaca Coll; **SLP**

Sargent, Laura Elizabeth 411 Callan Avenue #A, Evanston, IL 60202, (312) 864-5035, BS 86 Northwestern Univ; MA 87 Northwestern Univ; 87–Sp-Lang Path, Des Plaines Sch Dist 62, **SLP**

Sargent, Mrs Ruth S 11120 Saffold Way, Reston, VA 22090, (703) 481-6855, BA 54 Bates Coll; MA 57 Univ of IA; 74–Aud, Colorado Otolaryngology PC, **A**

Sargent, Mrs Shanone Kaye 5-A 259 South Wymount Terr, Provo, UT 84604, (801) 374-4955, MS 85 ID St Univ; Sp-Lang Path, Granite School District, **SLP**

Sarginger, Kathryn Steinbach 1809 East Kathleen, Phoenix, AZ 85022, (814) 834-2535, BS 78 Indiana Univ of PA; MS 80 Indiana Univ of PA; Supervisor Sp-Lang Path Dept, Phoenix General Hospital, **SLP**

Sarginger, Maryrose Sharkey 701 Timberset Court, Lutz, FL 33549, (813) 785-5545, BS 78 Ithaca Coll; MS 86 Univ of South FL; **SLP**

Sargisson, Lisa J 8800 Aquarius Avenue, Elk Grove, CA 95624, (916) 482-6954, OB 62 Mount Holyoke Coll; MA 84 Chapman Coll; MA 70 Univ of Northern CO; SLP, Elk Grove USD, **SLP**

Saricks, Dr Margaret C Byrne 2552 Arkansas Street, Lawrence, KS 66046, (913) 843-4858, BA 39 Univ of Pittsburgh - Pittsburgh; MA 45 Northwestern Univ; PH 58 (Sp Path) Northwestern Univ; Professor Emeritus, University of Kansas, **SLP F H LM**

Sarill, Debra Beth 9 Quail Court, Marlboro, NJ 07746, (201) 780-9883, **SLP**

Sarkis, Joanna L 302-5 Diamond Village, Gainesville, FL 32603, (904) 377-9563, BS 73 Eastern MI Univ; MA 78 Wayne St Univ; 86–Adjunct Instructor, Hillsborough Comm Coll, **A**

Sarmanian, Mrs Donna S 32 Tamarack Terrace, Stoneham, MA 02180, BS 76 Univ of MA - Amherst; MS 78 Boston Univ; Sp-Lang Path, Arlington Public Schools, **SLP**

Sarmento, Nidia B 7 Running Deer Road, North Dartmouth, MA 02747, (617) 997-1515, BS 85 Univ of MA - Amherst; MA 87 Univ of MA - Amherst; Sp-Lang Path, St Lukes Hosp, **SLP**

Sarmir, Mrs Wendy L 13 Mamopa Court, Reisterstown, MD 21136, (301) 429-1941, BS 77 Miami Univ - Oxford; MS 78 Southern Methodist Univ; Sp-Lang Path, Private Practice, **SLP**

Sarnecky, Dr Ellen A 5225 Pooks Hill Road #907S, Bethesda, MD 20814, (301) 897-5700, ME 69 Univ of VA - Charlottesville; ME 70 Univ of VA - Charlottesville; PH 82 (Special Education Administration) Gallaudet Coll; Dir Membership & Career Dev, ASHA, **A**

Sarnes, Ann E Route 1 Box S-33, West Salem, WI 54669, (608) 785-0940, BA 73 Alma Coll; MA 78 Eastern MI Univ; Dir of SLP, St Francis Med Ctr, **SLP**

Sarnes, Mrs Diane Bea 9121 Beachway Lane, Springfield, VA 22153, (703) 573-7139, BA 64 CUNY - Hunter Coll; MA 83 George Washington Univ; 83–Sp-Lang Path, Fairfax County Public Schools, **SLP ACE**

Sarno, Martha Taylor Rusk Institute Of Rehab Med, NYU Medical Center, 400 East 34th Street, New York, NY 10016, (212) 340-6025, BA 49 MI St Univ; MA 54 NY Univ; 50–Dir Sp-Path Serv, NYU Med Ctr, **SLP F**

Sarofeen, Carole Bishop 133 South Street, Auburn, NY 13021, (315) 255-2746, BA 77 SUNY - Coll at Cortland; MS 82 Ithaca Coll; Sp-Lang Path, E Johns Gavras Cen/Ucpa, **SLP**

Saroli-Taylor, Mrs Diane Antoinette 11482 Bradley, Jerome, MI 49249, BA 82 MI St Univ; MA 83 Central MI Univ; Sp-Lang Path, Emma L Bixby Hosp, **SLP**

Sarosi, Mrs Nancy G P 1561 East Mitchell, Petoskey, MI 49770, (616) 347-0115, BA 75 Univ of MI - Ann Arbor; MA 77 Wayne St Univ; **SLP**

Sarpa, Mrs Nancy Needham 21663 Flanders, Farmington Hills, MI 48024, (313) 288-8085, OM 84 IN Univ - Bloomington; Sp-Lang Path, Beaumont Hosp, **SLP**

Sarr, Mrs Jean Bills 139 North Mildred, Dearborn, MI 48128, BS 67 Eastern MI Univ; MA 71 Eastern MI Univ; Sp-Lang Path, Southfield Public Schools, **SLP**

Sarradet, Valerie K 12860 Tan Oak Lane, Beaumont, TX 77713, (409) 753-1477, BS 84 Univ of TX - Austin; MS 87 Univ of North TX; 87–Aud, David W Granitz PhD & Assoc, **A**

Sarrat, Larry J 10 Charlotte Drive, New Orleans, LA 70122, (504) 288-6660, OB 73 Loyola Univ; OM 76 LA St Univ - N O Medical Ctr; **SLP**

Sarrett, Mrs Elizabeth G 2334 N W 15th Place, Gainesville, FL 32605, (904) 378-0104, OB 76 Univ of FL; ME 77 Univ of FL; Sp-Lang Path, Michelle Jensen PhD, **SLP**

Sarris, Mrs Melanie L 2055-D Lake Park Drive, Smyrna, GA 30080, (404) 843-1893, BS 78 MS Univ for Women; MS 80 MS Univ for Women; 88–Sp-Lang Path, Adaptive Lrng Ctr for Infants/Chldn, **SLP**

Sarro, Mrs Victoria Anne 12050E Little Patuxent Parkway, Columbia, MD 21044-2778, (301) 740-4133, BS 79 SUNY - Coll at Geneseo; MS 84 Nazareth Coll of Rochester; Sp-Lang Path, Howard County PS, **SLP**

Sarrow, Mrs Anne M 9 Samuel Court, Lincoln Park, NJ 07035, (201) 6633-3175, BS 79 Bloomsburg Univ of PA; MA 81 Seton Hall Univ; 81–Sp-Lang Path, Wayne Board of Education, **SLP**

Sarte, Mrs Pamela Lois 3115 Lisbon Avenue, Toms River, NJ 08753, (609) 726-1000, **SLP**

Sarvela, Mrs Junia L 666 72nd Street, Wauwatosa, WI 53213, (414) 281-7200, BA 58 Augsburg Coll; MA 69 Northern MI Univ; Dir/SLP, Mt Carmel Nrsng Home, **SLP**

Sarvey, Mrs Sally H 922 South Center, Casper, WY 82601, (307) 237-2663, BA 67 Univ of WY; MA 68 Western MI Univ; Sp-Lang Path, Natrona Co Mem Hosp, **SLP**

Sasaki, Mrs Elaine Kaoru 1919 Golf Road, Turlock, CA 95380, (209) 632-2641

Sasala, John C 412-A Deer Trail Hill, Lake Barrington, IL 60010, (312) 304-1922, MS 75 OH Univ - Athens; Midwestern Area Mgr, Bio-Logic Systems, **A**

Sasano, Lynn A 15342 Yorkshire Lane, Huntington Beach, CA 92647, (714) 964-3339, BA 85 Univ of the Pacific; MA 86 Univ of the Pacific; 88–Sp-Lang Path, West Orange Co Consortium/Spec Educ, **SLP**

Sasanuma, Dr Sumiko 34-10 2-Chome Amanuma, Suginami-Ku, Tokyo, Japan 167, BA 53 Tsuda Coll - Japan; MA 59 Univ of IA; PH 68 (NS) Univ of IA; Dir Dept of Rehab Res, Tokyo Metro I of Gerontology

Saslow, Katherine 2608 Regal Oaks Lane, Lutz, FL 33549, (813) 977-3075, BS 71 PA St Univ - Univ Park; MS 74 Univ of Pittsburgh - Pittsburgh; Aud, Uniphy Diagnostic Ctr, **A**

Sasnett, Wendy C 49 Bowen Street, Pawtucket, RI 02861, (401) 727-1852, BS 76 Univ of MA - Amherst; MS 86 Univ of RI; **SLP**

Sass, Margaret M 469 Greenwood S E, Grand Rapids, MI 49506, (616) 459-7111, BS 84 Central MI Univ; MA 85 Central MI Univ; 86–Aud, Mc Donald Aud & Hrng Health

Sasser, Elizabeth K 23208 Lake Roesiger Drive, Snohomish, WA 98290, (206) 568-1041, BA 84 Eastern WA Univ; MS 85 Eastern WA Univ; 88–Sp-Lang Path, Pacific Hearing & Speech Svcs Inc, **SLP**

Sasser, Mrs Mercedes P 1770 Wilson Road, Huntingtown, MD 20639, (301) 535-1211, BS 62 Univ of Southwestern LA; SLP, Calvert Co Bd of Ed, **SLP**

Sasserath, Richard J 89 Ridge Street, Nesquehoning, PA 18240, (215) 759-7600, BA 72 Pace U -NY City; MA 73 NY Univ; SLP, Col Nhampton Int Ut, **SLP**

Sasso, Anne Vickery 3519 North Leavitt Street, Chicago, IL 60618, (312) 908-6134, BS 74 Northwestern Univ; MA 75 Northwestern Univ; 86–Clin Supvr, Rehab Inst Chicago, **SLP**

Sasso, Laraine M 38-02 Trafford Street, Meriden, CT 06450, (203) 223-2761, BA 75 Boston Coll; MA 81 Univ of CT; Ch Sp-Lang Path, New Britain Mem Hosp, **SLP**

Sataloff MD, Joseph 1530 Locust Street #6-A, Philadelphia, PA 19103, (215) 735-0205

Satell, Mrs Margaret Cox 1158 West Valley Road, Wayne, PA 19087, (215) 964-9208, BA 69 Mount Holyoke Coll; MA 71 Northwestern Univ; **SLP ACE**

Satin, Sally J 35-24 78th Street, Jackson Heights, NY 11372, (718) 458-2502, BA 82 Univ of FL; MA 86 Univ of FL; 87–Sp-Lang Path, The Hugh MacMillan Med Ctr, **SLP**

Satin, Terry L 6304 Friars Road #133, San Diego, CA 92108, (619) 747-1040, BA 79 San Diego St Univ; Sp-Lang Path, Escondido USD, **SLP**

Satir, Mrs Roxana E 2270 Edna Court, Baldwin, NY 11510-3104, (718) 728-1459, BS 85 Saint John's Univ - Jamaica; MS 88 Adelphi Univ

Sato, Mrs Karen S K 1810 Hoomalolo, Pearl City, HI 96782, (808) 456-9222, BS 75 Univ of HI - Manoa; MS 77 Univ of HI - Manoa; SLP, Department of Education, **SLP**

Sato, Mrs Sharon K 98-121 Naalii Place, Aiea, HI 96701, (808) 486-0455, BA 77 Univ of the Pacific; MA 79 Saint Louis Univ; Aud, Dept of Hlth, **A**

Satorhelyi, Mrs Donna Gail 10419 Lee Drive, Eden Prairie, MN 55344, (612) 926-0901, **A**

Sattem, Karen Ann 7427 Tempest Court #C, Baltimore, MD 21237, (301) 668-0080, BA 69 Loyola Coll; ME 70 Loyola Coll; Sp-Lang Path, Hearing & Speech Agency, **SLP**

Satter, Mrs Susan Ann 858 North Burritt, Buffalo, WY 82834, (307) 684-7872, BA 59 OH Univ - Athens; MS 62 Gallaudet Coll; 86–Sp-Lang Path, Washakie Co Sch Dist #2, **SLP**

Satterfield, Cindy Lee 4058 Hinsdale Road, Cleveland, OH 44121-2702, (216) 442-6606, BA 80 OH St Univ; MA 82 Cleveland St Univ; Sp-Lang Path, Cleveland Hrng-Sp/Ctr - K/Perm, **SLP**

Sattinger, Karen 770 N E 199th Street #F-207, North Miami Beach, FL 33179, (305) 556-0121, BA 72 IN Univ - Bloomington; MA 76 IN Univ - Bloomington; Sp-Lang Path, Private Practice, **SLP**

Sattui, Melanie Anne 4 Stowe Lane, Menlo Park, CA 94025, (408) 923-1935, BA 78 San Jose St Univ; Sp-Lang-Hrng Spec, Berryessa Un Sch Dist, **SLP**

Satuloff, Mrs Marilyn B 20305 Tulsa Street, Chatsworth, CA 91311, (213) 907-7944, BA 75 Univ of CA - Los Angeles; MA 79 CA St Univ - Northridge; **SLP**

Saturday-Rollet, Mrs Kelly Lynne 630 East 74th Terrace, Kansas City, MO 64131, (816) 276-4023, BA 85 IN Univ - Bloomington; OM 86 IN Univ - Bloomington; 88–Sp-Lang Path, Research Med Ctr, **SLP**

Sauber, Mrs Kitty F 12 East 86th Street #621, New York, NY 10028, (212) 535-0974, BA 56 CUNY - Hunter Coll; MA 59 Columbia Univ Teachers Coll; SLP, Hosp for Spec Surg Rehab Med, **SLP**

Saucier, Mrs Linda Jill 711 West 1st Street #E-205, Santa Ana, CA 92701, (213) 860-3378, BS 76; MA 79; 88–SLP, ABC USD, **SLP**

Sauder, Frank D 505 Fletcher Street, Roanoke, IL 61561, (309) 923-7161, BA 79 Univ of IL - Urbana; MS 81 Univ of IL - Urbana; Sp-Lang Path, Mercy Hosp, **SLP**

Sauer, Jacquelyn Ann 1303 Jackson Street #32, La Crosse, WI 54601, (608) 785-0646, OM 86 Univ of WI - River Falls; 87–Sp-Lang Path, St Francis Med Ctr, **SLP**

Sauer, Margaret Lois 81 Middlesex Road, Chestnut Hill, MA 02167, (617) 277-4535, BA 83 Univ of CO - Boulder; MS 85 CO St Univ; 86–Sp-Lang Path, Children's Hosp, **SLP**

Sauer, Richard C 575 Harvest Lane, Verona, WI 53593, (608) 255-7878, BS 72 Univ of WI - Stevens Point; MS 73 Univ of WI - Stevens Point; Dir, Madison Med Ctr Hrng Serv, **A**

Sauers, Mrs Judith F 311 Ponce DE Leon Blvd, Clearwater, FL 34616, (813) 581-6470, BA 62 FL St Univ; MS 88 Univ of FL; 88–Sp-Lang Path, Pinellas Co Schs, **SLP**

Saul, Barbara J 2310 Dover, Fort Lauderdale, FL 33326-2324, (305) 370-1660, BA 75 Northeastern IL Univ; MS 77 Southern IL Univ -Carbondale; Sp-Lang Path, School Board of Broward County, **SLP**

Saul, Jonathan O Naval Medical Clinic, 6500 Hampton Boulevard, Norfolk, VA 23508, (804) 444-3163, BS 79 Univ Southern MS-Hattiesburg; MS 81 Univ Southern MS-Hattiesburg; Operational Aud, US Navy, **A**

Saul, Mrs Nancy Q 3841 North Chesterbrook Rd, Arlington, VA 22207, (703) 358-6650, BA 72 George Washington Univ; MA 75 George Washington Univ; Sp-Lang Path, Arlington Public Schools, **SLP**

Saul, Dr Richard S 1201 NW 16th Street, Miami, FL 33125, (305) 324-3148, BA 73 FL Atlantic Univ; MA 76 Univ of FL; PH 83 (Aud) SUNY - Center at Buffalo; 87–Coord Aud, VA Med Ctr, **A**

Saulles, Mrs Lisa Kanagur 1630 Waltham, Ann Arbor, MI 48103, (313) 769-5542, BA 80 MI St Univ; MA 81 MI St Univ; Aud, Providence Hosp, **A**

Sauls, Lauri Ann 816 Dahlia Lane, Vero Beach, FL 32963, (305) 567-7111, BS 85 FL St Univ; MS 86 FL St Univ; **A**

Saunders, Mrs Anne Z Emory University Clinic - ENT, 1365 Clifton Road N E, Atlanta, GA 30322, (404) 321-0111, BA 49 Duke Univ; ME 70 Emory Univ; Administrative Assistant, The Emory Clinic, **A**

Saunders, Barbara Gray 215 Jordan Drive, Smithfield, VA 23430, (919) 684-3859, BS 73 East Carolina Univ; MA 74 Univ of TN - Knoxville; Aud, J Parker Cross MD Otology, **A**

Saunders, Mrs Deborah Lynn 15370 Tropic Court #8, San Leandro, CA 94579, (415) 483-1254, BA 85 San Francisco St Univ; MS 87 San Francisco St Univ; 87–Sp-Lang Path, San Lorenzo USD, **SLP**

Saunders, Elizabeth Lynne 55 Frazer Road #D-32, Malvern, PA 19355, (215) 640-3070, BS 86 Bloomsburg Univ of PA; MS 87 Bloomsburg Univ of PA; Sp-Lang Path, Bryn Mawr Rehab Hosp, **SLP**

Saunders, Elizabeth O 7700 NW 11th Place, Plantation, FL 33313, (305) 985-3070, ME 81 Old Dominion Univ; Sp-Lang Path, Quest Ctr Broward Co Sch Sys, **SLP**

Saunders, Mrs Joyce E 6500 Telephone Road #2501, Ventura, CA 93003, (805) 644-4923, BA 78 Univ of CA - Santa Barbara; MS 80 Univ of AZ; **SLP**

Saunders, Mrs Kathleen Duerr 616 W Lynn Shores Circle, Virginia Beach, VA 23452, (804) 340-9372, BS 80 James Madison Univ; MS 83 Towson St Univ; Sp-Lang Path, Chesapeake Pub Sch, **SLP**

Saunders, Mrs Mary N 426 Brewers Creek Lane, Carrollton, VA 23314, (804) 238-2778, BS 81 James Madison Univ; ME 83 Old Dominion Univ; 85–Sp-Lang Path, Chesapeake PS, **SLP**

Saunders, Mrs Nedra J 160 Sequoia Avenue, Carlsbad, CA 92008, (619) 729-3103, BA 64 San Diego St Univ; MA 66 Stanford Univ; **SLP**

Saunders, Steven James Route 2 Box 540, Blanchard, ID 83804, (509) 455-4927, BS 76 Univ of ID; MS 82 Univ of OR; 86–Sp-Lang Path, Sacred Heart Med Ctr, **SLP**

Saunders, Mrs Wilma W Box 228B, Mayville, NY 14757-9802, (716) 789-3124, BA 49 SUNY - Center at Albany; MS 78 SUNY - Coll at Fredonia; Retired, Erie County Bd Coop Ed Serv 2, **SLP**

Saunders, Zane G Newington Childrens Hospital, 181 East Cedar Street, Newington, CT 06111, (203) 667-5320, BS 59 Kent St Univ; MA 66 Kent St Univ; Dir SLP & Aud, Newington Chldn Hosp, **SLP**

Saunders-Culp, Mrs Karen T 282 Rich Road, Park Forest, IL 60466, (312) 481-2500, BS 76 FL A & M Univ; MA 77 Western MI Univ; 87–Sp-Lang Path, Private Practice, **SLP**

Sauter, Mrs Gail Louise 1177 North 600 East, Orem, UT 84057-2770, (801) 785-1617, BS 74 CA Univ of PA; OM 85 Brigham Young Univ; 80–Sp-Lang Path, Alpine Sch Dist, **SLP**

Sautner, Mrs Elaine Marie Box 178 Rd 4, Middleburg, PA 17842, (717) 837-0726, BS 81 East Stroudsburg Univ of PA; MS 85 Bloomsburg Univ of PA; **SLP**

Savad, Mrs Libby 1492 East 9th Street, Brooklyn, NY 11230, (212) 258-8230, BA 68 CUNY - Brooklyn Coll; MS 72 CUNY - Brooklyn Coll; Superv/Adj Lect, Brooklyn Coll Sp & Hrng Cen, **SLP**

Savage, Mrs Barbara A 441 Sayre Drive, Princeton, NJ 08540, (201) 297-3400, **SLP**

Savage, David H 1333 Pembrook Court, Montgomery, AL 36109, (205) 288-0220, BA 73 Harding Univ; MS 77 Auburn Univ - Auburn; Sp-Lang Path, Crippled Chldrn Serv, **SLP**

Savage, Diane J 939 Western Road #D7, London, ON, Canada N6G 1G3, (519) 673-3885, OM 88 Univ of Western Ontario

Savage, Dr Hallie E 1265 West Arndale, Stow, OH 44224, (216) 762-5425, BA 71 Baldwin-Wallace Coll; MA 72 Cleveland St Univ; PH 84 (Cleft Palate/Voice) Kent St Univ; 85–Dir of Sp-Lang Path, Blick Clinic, **SLP**

Savage, Mrs Judy A 7717 Laurel Ridge, Louisville, KY 40219, (502) 454-8285, BS 80 Eastern KY Univ; MA 81 Eastern KY Univ; SLP, Jefferson Co Bd of Ed, **SLP**

Savage, Linda Amalia P O Box 1313, Marina, CA 93933-1313, (408) 649-1455, BA 82 Humboldt St Univ; MA 85 San Diego St Univ; 85–Sp-Lang Path, Monterey Penin Unif Sch Dist, **SLP**

Savage, M Martha 3289 Hostetter Road, San Jose, CA 95132, (408) 251-6482, BA 77 CA St Univ - Fresno; MA 80 San Jose St Univ; Teacher, Metropolitan Adult Ed Program, **SLP**

Savage, Mary Jo 626 Sheridan Road, Evanston, IL 60202, (312) 689-1438, BS 82 OH Univ - Athens; MA 84 Northwestern Univ; Sp/Lang Path, N Chicago Sch Dist #64, **SLP**

Savage, N Leslie 6909 East Paradise Parkway, Scottsdale, AZ 85251, (602) 994-3443, BA 61 Univ of CA - Santa Barbara; MA 81 Northern AZ Univ; 87–Sp-Lang Path, Scottsdale Public Schools, **SLP**

Savage, Roberta A 2559 Plaze Del Amo #310, Torrance, CA 90503-7318, (213) 320-9528, BS 70 Case Western Reserve Univ; MA 72 Univ of Southern CA; 83–Prin, Offi of LA Co Supt of Sch, **SLP**

Savage, Sandra McEwen 217 Charlemagne Way, Modesto, CA 95350, (209) 521-5573, BA 70 Univ of CA - Davis; MA 86 CA St Univ - Stanislaus; 88–Sp-Lang Path, Modesto City Sch Dist, **SLP**

Savage, Mrs Trudy H 3 Cropley Court, Melville, NY 11747, (516) 491-1839, **SLP**

Savarese, Sharon Jean 119 W 25th Avenue, North Wildwood, NJ 08260, (609) 729-5808, BS 81 Bloomsburg Univ of PA; MA 84 Trenton St Coll; SLP, Wildwood Crest School District, **SLP**

Savasten, Patricia T 325 Hickory Knoll, Birmingham, AL 35226, (205) 348-7131, BS 77 Univ of Montevallo; MS 78 Univ of AL- Tuscaloosa; 87–Sp-Lang Path, Tuscaloosa City Schs, **SLP**

Savela, Kay Dianne 440 11th Street South, Wisconsin Rapids, WI 54494, BS 81 Northern MI Univ; MA 83 Northern MI Univ; **SLP**

Savell, Mrs Mildred S 6479 Keena Court, North Port, FL 34287, (813) 426-1292, BA 31 9979; MA 37 Duke Univ; **SLP LM**

Savell, Paula E 3818 Drexel, Port Arthur, TX 77642, (409) 735-3555, BS 74 Lamar Univ; MS 75 Lamar Univ; Sp-Lang Path, Bridge City ISD, **SLP**

Savery, Janice S 2 Meadowbrook Road, Sherborn, MA 01770, (617) 655-5884, BS 78 Univ of MA - Amherst; ME 80 Northeastern Univ; Sp-Lang Path, Private Practice, **SLP**

Savia, Karen 6920 Hovingham Court, Centreville, VA 22020, (703) 830-2339, BS 75 James Madison Univ; MS 77 James Madison Univ; **SLP**

Savich, Dr Patricia A California State University LA, Dept Communication Disorders, 5151 State University Dr, Los Angeles, CA 90032, (213) 438-6562, BS 67 Northern IL Univ - De Kalb; MA 71 Univ of IL - Urbana; PH 80 (Lang & Learning Disability Comm Dis) Univ of CO - Boulder; Assoc Prof, CA State Univ/LA, **SLP**

Saville, Mrs Sharon Drysdale 3491 Huntington Lane, St Charles, MO 63303, (314) 928-5279, BS 75 Northeast MO St Univ; MA 80 Saint Louis Univ; **SLP**

Savitsky, Mrs Sheila Krute 21 Silver Birch Road, Waban, MA 02168, (508) 667-8300, BA 58 Emerson Coll; 59–Supvr, Billerica PS, **SLP**

Savitt, Mrs Amy E P 3505 Knightsbridge Close, Worcester, MA 01609, (508) 752-0961, BA 79 Univ of Rochester; MS 81 Washington Univ; Aud, **A**

Savitz, Deborah R 75-74 199th Street, Flushing, NY 11366, (718) 470-8910, BA 86 Hofstra Univ; MA 87 Hofstra Univ; Aud, L I Jewish Med Ctr

Savitz, Lynne Dept Of Human Communcation, Pennsylvania Hospital, 8th And Spruce Streets, Philadelphia, PA 19107, (215) 829-5182, BA 69 Temple Univ-Tyler Sch of Art; MA 71 Temple Univ-Tyler Sch of Art; 78–Sp-Lang Path, Pennsylvania Hospital, **SLP**

Sawallisch, Mrs Mary Beth P O Box 52, Marengo, IL 60152-0052, (815) 568-7019, BS 85 Marquette Univ; MS 88 Marquette Univ; 88–Sp-Lang Path, Spec Educ Dist of McHenry County

Sawan, Denise M Language Learning Associates, 71 Baker Boulevard #102, Akron, OH 44313, (216) 864-4990, BS 78 Kent St Univ; MA 78 Kent St Univ; Owner Sp-Lang/Path, Language Learning Assoc, **SLP**

Sawyer, Mrs Diana I Southern Station, Box 5092, Hattiesburg, MS 39406, (601) 266-5232, BA 74 Our Lady Lake Univ-San Anton; MA 75 Our Lady Lake Univ-San Anton; 84–Sp-Lang Path, Univ of Southern MS, **SLP**

Sawyer, Mrs Judith Cooper 4815 West 63rd South, Wichita, KS 67215, BA 69 Wichita St Univ; MA 82 Wichita St Univ; SLP, Wichita Public Schools, **SLP**

Sawyer, Linda Delgado 110 Balboa Avenue, Stuart, FL 34994, (407) 286-9398, BA 82 Univ of FL; MS 85 Univ of Montevallo; **A**

Sawyer, Lori Elizabeth 3920 N W 60th Avenue, Virginia Gardens, FL 33166, (305) 634-8883, BS 81 Southern Coll of S D A; MA 87 Univ of FL; 87–Sp-Lang Path, Baptist Hosp of Miami, **SLP**

Sawyer, Mrs Marie Y 256 N E 56th Court, Newport, OR 97365, (503) 336-5123, BA 75 Western WA Univ; MA 77 Western WA Univ; 80–Sp-Lang Path, Lincoln Co Sch Dist, **SLP**

Sawyer, Mary E 405 Linda, Keller, TX 76248, **SLP**

Sawyer, Sarah A 27 Cadman Drive, Williamsville, NY 14221, (716) 626-5924, **SLP**

Sawyer-Woods, Linda M 658 Apollo Way, Navan, ON, Canada K4A 1A4, BA 72 Univ of Toronto - Ontario; MA 76 SUNY - Center at Buffalo; Sp-Lang Path, Ottawa Civic Hosp, **SLP**

Sax, Eva Helene 1839 Spruce Street, Berkeley, CA 94709, (415) 849-0578, BA 73 San Diego St Univ; MS 79 CA St Univ - Hayward; Sp-Lang Path, Richmond USD, **SLP**

Sax, Mrs Mary R 31320 Woodside, Franklin, MI 48025, (313) 626-1481, BA 47 MI St Univ; MA 49 Univ of MI - Ann Arbor; **SLP**

Saxe, Mrs Kathryn S 3113 Englewood Drive, Stow, OH 44224, (216) 543-9722, BS 76 Bowling Green St Univ; MA 77 Kent St Univ; SLP, Kenston Local Schools, **SLP**

Saxman, Dr John H 114 White Heron Circle, Fayetteville, NY 13066-9667, (315) 443-2506, BA 60 San Diego St Univ; MS 63 Purdue Univ - West Lafayette; PH 65 (NS) Purdue Univ - West Lafayette; 88–Assoc Dean for Acad Prog, Syracuse University

Saxman, Rosalie G 12071 Beatrice Street, Culver City, CA 90230-6212, (818) 997-2357, MA 80 CA St Univ - Los Angeles; Aud, Los Angeles USD, **A**

Saxton, Anne E 185 McKee Street, Aliquippa, PA 15001, (412) 457-0961, MA 87 Univ of Pittsburgh - Pittsburgh; **SLP**

Say, Mrs Frances P 126 Leeds Road, Mount Laurel, NJ 08054, (609) 261-7030, BA 70 PA St Univ - Univ Park; MA 80 Memphis St Univ; Supvr Sp-Lang Path, Memorial Hosp Burlington Co, **SLP**

Saya, Mrs Nancy Cabana 4994 Lincklaen Road, Cuyler, NY 13050, (315) 655-3444, BS 80 SUNY - Coll at Fredonia; MS 84 Syracuse Univ; Sp-Lang Path, Cazenovia Central Sch District

Sayers, Elizabeth S R R 4 Box 284, Knoxville, IA 50138, (515) 828-5007, BS 64 MS Univ for Women; MA 65 Univ of AR - Fayetteville; MA 80 Northeast MO St Univ; 80–Sp-Lang Path, VA Med Cen, **SLP**

Sayers, Mrs Leigh Camp 2641 Indian Hill Road, Auburn, AL 36830, (205) 821-8819, BS 78 Auburn Univ - Auburn; OM 82 Auburn Univ - Auburn; Sp-Lang Path, Chambers Co Schs, **SLP**

Sayers, Patricia J 2047 North Racine Avenue, Chicago, IL 60614, (312) 929-7784, MA Univ of Cincinnati; BS Univ of Cincinnati; Indep Contr-Sp-Lang Path, Private Practice, **SLP**

Sayler, Julie Ann 334 Pearl Street #5, Alpine Apartment, Cadillac, MI 49601, (616) 775-1607, BS 85 Central MI Univ; MA 86 Central MI Univ; 87–Sp-Lang Path, Wexford Missaukee ISD, **SLP**

Sayler, Mrs Mary Ellen Route 2 McKinney Road, Blaine, TN 37709, (615) 544-3610, BA 83 Univ of TN - Knoxville; MA 85 Univ of TN - Knoxville; 86–Sp-Lang Path, Knox Co Sch Sys, **SLP**

Sayler, Sherri Lynn 1708 East 80th, Bloomington, MN 55425, (612) 927-3250, BS 83 Minot St Univ; MS 85 Univ of WA; 87–Aud, Park Nicollet Med Ctr, **A**

Sayles, Adriane Hope 11106 Webbwood Court, Largo, MD 20772, (301) 725-1323, BA 71 Howard Univ; MA 72 Univ of MD - College Park; Training Coordinator, Psi Associates Inc, **SLP**

Saylor, Mrs Diane Patricia 682 Eugenie Street East, Windsor, ON, Canada N8X 2Y4, (519) 966-4137, BS 83 Northern MI Univ; MA 86 Northern MI Univ; **SLP**

Saylor, Suzanne P 27015 S E 160th Street, Issaquah, WA 98027, (206) 392-0723, BA 68 Univ of WA; MA 72 Univ of WA; SLP, Issaquah Sch Dist, **SLP**

Saylor-Connell, Deborah Sue P O Box 122, Herrin, IL 62948, (618) 942-2921, BS 82 Southern IL Univ -Carbondale; MS 85 Southern IL Univ -Carbondale; Consult, Private Practice, **SLP**

Sayre, Mrs Vivien L North East Systems Associates, P O Box 67, Acton, MA 01720, BS 74 Boston Univ; ME 75 Northeastern Univ; Co-Own Bus Man, NE Systems Assoc, **SLP**

Sayward, Catherine 901 Henselin Road, Grand Rapids, MN 55744, BS 76 Univ of NH; MS 78 Univ of CT

Sazama, Carol Lee Repensky 4014 McCulloch Street, Duluth, MN 55804, (218) 726-6152, BS 73 IL St Univ - Normal; MA 76 Univ of MN - Duluth; Sp-Lang Path, U of MN, **SLP**

Sazama, Melissa D 721 Granite, Florence, CO 81226, (303) 275-1007, **SLP**

Sbaschnig, Kristine V Wayne State University, 563 Manoogian Hall, Detroit, MI 48202, (313) 577-3337, BA 69 Wichita St Univ; MA 70 Wichita St Univ; Coordinator of Clinical Serv, Wayne State University, **SLP**

Scafa, Gina A 38 West Road, Burlington, VT 05401, (802) 864-8463, BS 75 Ithaca Coll; MS 76 Ithaca Coll; Sp-Lang Path, Burlington Sch Dept, **SLP**

Scafe, Mrs Darnell Holler 3937 Quail Lane North, Chattanooga, TN 37415, (615) 698-8981, MA 82 Univ of TN - Knoxville; 83–Aud, Chattanooga ENT Assoc, **A**

Scaglione, Matthew Paul 163 Lindell Boulevard, Long Beach, NY 11561, BA 79 Jersey City St Coll; MA 81 Hofstra Univ; Sp-Lang Path, Long Beach Sch Dist, **SLP**

Scales, Kim D 5601 Loch Raven Boulevard, Baltimore, MD 21239, (301) 532-3740, BS 81 Northwestern Univ; MS 86 Purdue Univ - West Lafayette; 87–Sp-Lang Path, Good Samaritan Hosp of MD, **SLP**

Scales, Phyllis Z 17191 Cherrylawn, Detroit, MI 48221, **SLP**

Scalione, Patricia 3225 Wisconsin Street, Oakland, CA 94602, (415) 667-3586, BS 75 SUNY - Coll at Brockport; MS 84 San Jose St Univ; 86–Sp-Lang Path, San Leandro Unified Sch Dstr, **SLP**

Scalo, Marilyn 43 Washington Place, Hasbrouck Heights, NJ 07604, BA 76 Montclair St Coll; MA 79 Montclair St Coll; 87–Sp-Lang Path, UCP of Northern NJ, **SLP**

Scalzi, Karen W 39 Fitchett Street, Poughkeepsie, NY 12601, (914) 473-2121, BS 83 Bloomsburg Univ of PA; MS 85 Bloomsburg Univ of PA; **SLP**

Scalzone, Mrs Diane Boehler 5815 Scenic Edge Boulevard, Dublin, OH 43017, (614) 764-7837, BS 85 Bowling Green St Univ; MS 86 Bowling Green St Univ; 88–Sp-Lang Path, Fisher-Titus Med Ctr, **SLP**

Scampini, Mrs Deanna L 2511 North 95th Street, Wauwatosa, WI 53226, (414) 342-3356, BS 75 Marquette Univ; MS 78 Marquette Univ; Sp-Lang Path, Milwaukee Pub Schools, **SLP**

Scandlyn, Kay B 308 W Heritage Drive, Knoxville, TN 37922, (615) 966-3561, MA 84 Univ of TN - Knoxville; BS 82 Univ of TN - Knoxville; Audiologist, Knoxville City Schools, **A**

Scanga, Connie C Rear 310 North 7th Street, Indiana, PA 15701, (412) 465-8345, BS 75 Indiana Univ of PA; MS 78 Indiana Univ of PA; Sp-Lang Path, Arin Iu #28, **SLP**

Scanio, Dr Tom S 3007 West Broad Street, Tampa, FL 33614, (813) 398-9395, BA 66 Univ of South FL; MA 68 Univ of South FL; PH 72 (Sp Path) Bowling Green St Univ; 80–Sp-Lang Path, VA Med Ctr, **SLP**

Scanlan, Mrs Carol S Rural Delivery 3, 306 Laurel Brook Road, Ebensburg, PA 15931, BS 68 PA St Univ - Univ Park; MA 70 Univ of AZ; Sp-Lang Path, Inter Unit 8, **SLP**

Scanlan, Mrs Crista C 142 Fox Hollow Way, Manchester, NH 03104, (603) 647-7127, MS 87 Ithaca Coll

Scanlan, Margaret 1437 East Drachman, Tucson, AZ 85719, (602) 326-1465, MS 88 Univ of AZ

Scanlon, Mrs Louise 105 Cordoba Circle, Universal City, TX 78148, (512) 271-7611, BA 64 Our Lady Lake Univ-San Anton; MA 74 Our Lady Lake Univ-San Anton; 74–Erly Chldhd Consult/Hndcpd, Ed Serv Cen Reg 20, **SLP**

Scanlon, Dr Patrick J 113 Woodview Drive, Horseheads, NY 14845, (607) 734-3911, BS 70 Univ of WI - Oshkosh; MA 71 OH Univ - Athens; Assoc Prof, Elmira Coll, **A**

Scanlon, Dr Stanley L 5581 West Avenue, Edinboro, PA 16412, (814) 732-2444, BS 57 Indiana Univ of PA; MS 66 Univ of KS; PH 71 (NS) Univ of KS; Prof, Edinboro U of Pa, **SLP A**

Scantlin, Dorothy L Route 14, Lyons Bend Road, Knoxville, TN 37919, MS; **SLP LM**

Scarboro, Mrs Kim Schirrman Route 7 Box 11, Wilbrook Drive, Thomasville, NC 27360, (919) 476-7134, BS 78 Appalachian St Univ; MA 83 Appalachian St Univ; SLP, Davidson County School System, **SLP**

Scarborough, Sarah Catherine 52 White Circle, Athens, GA 30605, (404) 354-3025, BS 79 Univ of SC - Columbia; MA 86 Univ of TN - Knoxville; 88–Sp-Lang Path, St Mary's Hosp/Home Hlth Care, **SLP**

Scarborough, Sheri Lynn 2018 9th Street, #H, Berkeley, CA 94710, (415) 548-5529, BS 79 CA St Univ - Long Beach; MS 81 Univ of HI - Manoa; 87, **SLP**

Scarbrough, Mrs Elizabeth 212 5th Street, Marks, MS 38646, (601) 326-8178, BS 73 Delta St Univ; OM 74 Univ of MS; Prog Dev for Hndcpd, Quitman Cty Schs, **SLP**

Scarcella, Mrs Lori S 15779 Buena Vista Drive, Derwood, MD 20855, (301) 840-1207, BS 79 Ithaca Coll; MS 80 Southern Methodist Univ; Sp/Lang Path, Montgomery Cty Publ Schs, **SLP**

Scardino, Virginia J Mayo Clinic, Neurology Department, Speech Pathology Section, Rochester, MN 55904, (507) 284-3112, BS 76 SUNY - Coll at Geneseo; MA 78 Hofstra Univ; 88–Sp-Lang Path, The Mayo Clinic, **SLP ACE**

Scariano, Mrs Rebecca Ratliffe 1933 Chestnut Grove Road, Knoxville, TN 37932, (615) 694-2003, BA 77 Emory & Henry Coll; MA 80 Univ of TN - Knoxville; 85–Sp-Lang Path, W Knoxville Neurological Assn, **SLP**

Scarinzi-Owen, Dr Ann University Of Oklahoma Health Sciences Center, Dept Of Communication Disorders, PO Box 26901 825 NE 14th Street, Oklahoma City, OK 73190, (405) 271-4214, BA 73 Newark St Coll; MA 75 TX Woman's Univ; PH 81 (Sp-Lang Path) Univ of OK Medical Center; 85–Asst Prof, U of OK-Hlth Sci Ctr, **SLP**

Scarlett, Mrs Deborah S 25 Sagamore Lane, Greenville, SC 29607, (803) 277-3793, BA 76 Columbia Coll; OM 77 Univ of SC - Columbia; SLP, Sch Dist of Greenville Co, **SLP**

Scarpa, Gaye A 1401 Cocoanut Road, Boca Raton, FL 33432, (305) 368-5853, BA 76 Kean Coll of NJ; MS 86 Nova Univ; 79–Sp-Lang Path, Palm Beach Co Sch Bd, **SLP**

Scarpellino, Susan 148 Robertson Way, Lincoln Park, NJ 07035-1137, (201) 456-3466, BA 77 Montclair St Coll; MA 79 Montclair St Coll; Sp-Lang Path, U of Med/Dentistry of Nj, **SLP**

Scarpino, Christiane Jane 59 Church Street #2, Leominster, MA 01453, (508) 534-0157, BA 77 Rutger's St Univ - Douglas Coll; MS 79 Purdue Univ - West Lafayette; 86–Sp-Lang Path, Private Practice, **SLP ACE**

Scarpulla, Margaret Ciak 175 Wilkinson Road, Fairport, NY 14450, (716) 425-2917, BS 84 Nazareth Coll of Rochester; MS 85 Nazareth Coll of Rochester; Sp-Lang Path, Wayne Finger Lakes BOCES, **SLP**

Scarr, Mrs Gail A 240 Alhambra Street, Salinas, CA 93906, (408) 449-6053, BA 76 CA St Univ - Fresno; MA 78 CA St Univ - Fresno; **SLP**

Scarry-Larkin, Marna Kathryn 366 Corrida Drive, San Luis Obispo, CA 93401, BA 80 Loyola Coll; MA 82 San Diego St Univ; Sp-Lang Path, Language Learing & Sp Ctr, **SLP**

Scates, Mrs Penny Barham ENT Medical Centers Of Texas, 1521 Northwest Highway, Garland, TX 75041, (214) 271-0516, BS 82 Univ of TN - Knoxville; MS 84 Univ of North TX; 84–Aud, ENT Med Ctrs of Texas PA, **A**

Scavuzzo, Annebelle 877 Beacon Street, Boston, MA 02215, (617) 267-8990, BA 71 Univ of MA - Amherst; MS 75 Minot St Univ; Sp-Lang Path, Private Practice, **SLP**

Scelfo, Rosemarie Babylon Speech & Language Serv, 469 French Avenue, North Babylon, NY 11703, (516) 667-7085, BA 78 Adelphi Univ; MS 79 Adelphi Univ; Sp/Lang Path, Babylon Sp & Lang Servs, **SLP ACE**

Scerri, Janice M L 3811 S W 11th Street, Fort Lauderdale, FL 33312, (305) 583-8287, BA 79 CUNY - Brooklyn Coll; MS 81 CUNY - Brooklyn Coll; Sp/Lang Path, **SLP**

Schaack, Anita L 708 Remington #4, Fort Collins, CO 80524, (303) 482-5305, BA 85 Univ of WI - Eau Claire; MS 88 CO St Univ

Schaaf, Mrs Jeanne Dolph 100 Rogers Lake Trail, Old Lyme, CT 06371, MA 80 San Jose St Univ; Sp-Lang Path, Project Learn, **SLP**

Schaaf, Joan Annette 605 N E Windrose Court #E, Bldg 7, Kansas City, MO 64155, (816) 436-1666, MS 87 Univ of NE - Lincoln; 87–Aud, Aud Svcs Inc, **A**

Schaal, Patricia Ann 522 Seminole Drive, Erie, PA 16505, (814) 453-7661, **SLP**

Schaan, Mrs Linda L Box 64, Berthold, ND 58718, (701) 453-3131, BS 86 Minot St Univ; MS 87 Minot St Univ; **SLP**

Schaap, Mrs Joni Martin 3110 Federal Avenue, Los Angeles, CA 90066, (213) 398-3173, BA 81 CA St Univ - Northridge; MA 82 CA St Univ - Northridge; Sp-Lang Path, Kaiser Permanente, **SLP**

Schaare-Denio, Regina RFD 2 Box 290, Barnes Point, South Harpswell, ME 04079, (207) 781-3165, BA 70 Univ of ME - Orono; MA 71 Univ of ME - Orono; Dir-Spec Svcs, Governor Baxter Sch f/t Deaf, **SLP**

Schabel, Mrs Diana Phyllis 11549 Tomarsue Drive, Marilla, NY 14102, (716) 837-2441, BA 71 SUNY - Center at Buffalo; MS 73 SUNY - Coll at Buffalo; **SLP**

Schabo, Kathleen K 380 Highland Way, Worthington, OH 43085, **SLP**

Schachner, Janet Smallberg 8855 S W 118th Street, Miami, FL 33176, (305) 232-3909, BA 67 Hofstra Univ; MA 69 Hofstra Univ; **SLP**

Schachter, Alison Donna 32 Camberwell Road, Toronto, ON, Canada M6C 3E8, (416) 782-0904, BA 71 0209; MS 74 Univ of WI - Madison; **SLP**

Schachterle, Bruce D Communication Associates Of, Colorado, 1550 South Potomac #305, Aurora, CO 80012, (303) 789-3327, BS 69 CO St Univ; MS 71 CO St Univ; VP, Comm Assoc of Colorado Inc, **A**

Schachtschneider, Mrs Marietta Sobocinski 1237 Natchez Trace Circle, Naperville, IL 60540, (312) 961-3604, BS 72 PA St Univ - Univ Park; MS 73 Auburn Univ - Auburn; 87–Sp-Lang Path, Naperville Sch Dist #203, **SLP**

Schack-Hanson, Nancy 34 Duggan Drive, Leominster, MA 01453, (508) 534-3012, BA 77 CUNY - Queens Coll; BA 77 CUNY - Queens Coll; MA 79 Univ of MA - Amherst; 82–Sp-Lang Path, N Middlesex Reg Schs, **SLP**

Schacter, Chedva 1768 46 Street, Brooklyn, NY 11204, (718) 853-4695, BA 85 CUNY - Brooklyn Coll; MS 87 CUNY - Brooklyn Coll; 86–Sp-Lang Path, Hebrew Inst for Deaf Children, **SLP**

Schade, Mrs Kristine 825 Nicolet Avenue, Oshkosh, WI 54901, (414) 424-0167, BA 75 Univ of WI - Eau Claire; MS 76 Univ of WI - Stevens Point; Sp/Lang Path, Oshkosh Area School, **SLP**

Schade, Mary Beth 3553 Camino Mira Costa, San Clemente, CA 92672, (714) 240-7070, BA 72 SUNY - Coll at Cortland; MA 74 Coll of Saint Rose; Dir-Sp/Hrng Serv, Family Hearing and Speech, **SLP**

Schade, Mrs Paula M 2035 West Relations, Safford, AZ 85546, (602) 428-2950, BA 68 Univ of AZ; MA 69 Univ of AZ; 87–Sp-Lang Path, Safford USD, **SLP**

Schade, William A Family Hearing And Speech, 3553 Camino Miracosta, San Clemente, CA 92672, (714) 240-7070, BS 72; MA 74 Coll of Saint Rose; Aud-Owner, Family Hrng/Sp, **A**

Schadelbauer, Margaret J 55 Sycamore Street, Belmont, MA 02178, (617) 894-3600, BA 71 CUNY - Lehman Coll; ME 72 Boston Univ; Sp/Lang Path, We Fernald State Sch, **SLP**

Schaefer, Amy Beth UCLA Dept Head & Neck Surgery, 32-24 Rehabilitation Bldg, Los Angeles, CA 90036, (213) 825-3037, BS 78 NY Univ; MA 80 Northwestern Univ; Staff Research Associate, Univ of California-Los Angeles, **A**

Schaefer, Mrs Ellen L 1836 Baldwin Drive, Mc Lean, VA 22101, (301) 320-3366, BA 62 Univ of MD - College Park; MA 68 Univ of MD - College Park; Sp-Lang Path, Montgy Co Pub Sch, **SLP**

Schaefer, James B 13202 N E Village Green Dr, Vancouver, WA 98684-6866, (206) 254-7314, BA 72 WA St Univ; MS 74 Eastern WA Univ; SLP, Evergreen School District, **SLP**

Schaefer, Linda Dell P O Box 56502, Riverside, CA 92517, (714) 824-4401, BA 81 CA St Univ - Fullerton; MA 83 CA St Univ - Fullerton; SLP, Loma Linda Univ Med Cntr, **SLP**

Schaefer, Linda K 12074 Burdette Circle, Omaha, NE 68164, (402) 559-4069, BS 71 Univ of NE - Lincoln; MS 76 Univ of NE - Omaha; SLP, U of NE Med Cen, **SLP**

Schaefer, Lynn A P O Box 9957, South Lake Tahoe, CA 95731, (916) 694-2238, BA 73 Univ of Redlands; MA 77 San Diego St Univ; SLP, Alpine Co USD, **SLP**

Schaefer, Mrs Mary K 905 Meadowlark Drive, O'Fallon, IL 62269, MA 80 Wichita St Univ; BA 79 Creighton Univ; Sp-Lang Path, Alief ISD, **SLP**

Schaefer, Mrs Patricia 738 East Becker Lane, Phoenix, AZ 85020, (602) 944-9382, BS 65 Southern IL Univ -Carbondale; MA 74 Western MI Univ; Sp-Lang Path, Paradise Valley USD, **SLP**

Schaefer, Dr Ronald D Special Education Dept, Northeastern State Univ, Tahlequah, OK 74464, (918) 456-5511, BS 72 OK St Univ; MS 74 Univ of OK Medical Center; PH 85 (NS) Univ of OK Medical Center; Asst Prof, Northeastern State, **SLP**

Schaefer, Shirley 225 West Park Street, Jackson, MO 63755, (314) 887-3244, BS 73 Southeast MO St Univ; MA 81 Southeast MO St Univ; Sp/Lang Path, Scott Co Sch Dist R-2, **SLP**

Schaefer, Susan Brown 966 Clarkson Court, Denver, CO 80229, (303) 287-2728, BS 82 Brigham Young Univ; MA 84 Univ of MN - Duluth; Sp-Lang Path, Private Practice, **SLP**

Schaefer-Norris, Christine 3900 Hillgrove Way, Carmichael, CA 95608, (916) 944-3679, BA 75 San Jose St Univ; MA 77 San Jose St Univ; Spec Day Class Tchr, Los Altos Elem Sch Dist, **SLP**

Schaeffer, Cheryl A 1805 Sybil Court, St Louis, MO 63125, (314) 894-5400, BS 80 Saint Louis Univ; MA 81 Saint Louis Univ; Sp/Lang Path, St Louis Dev Disabled Tr Cen, **SLP**

Schaeffer, Kathleen 3829 Benedict Canyon Drive, Sherman Oaks, CA 91423, (213) 836-7000, BA 75 George Washington Univ; MA 77 Catholic Univ of America; Chief/Commun Dis, Brotman Med Cen, **SLP A**

Schaeffer, Mrs Lynne Guggenheim Route 2 Box 967, Lacombe, LA 70445, (504) 893-4323, BA 83 Southeastern LA Univ; OM 85 LA St Univ - N O Medical Ctr; 85–Sp-Lang Path, Covington Sp & Lang Cen, **SLP**

Schaeffer, Mindy I 2537 East Parker Court, Visalia, CA 93291, (209) 625-4955, BS 74 CUNY - Queens Coll; MS 79 East Carolina Univ; Sp-Lang Path, Sonoma Developmental Center, **SLP**

Schaeffer, Natalie G 141-10 82nd Drive #335, Briarwood, NY 11435, (212) 870-6373, BS 73 NY Univ; MS 76 Adelphi Univ; SLP, St Lukes Hospital, **SLP**

Schaeffer, Remle Sue 44 Golfview Court, Rotonda West, FL 33947, (813) 697-4272, BS 84 WV Univ; MS 85 WV Univ; 85–Sp-Lang Path, Assoc Rehab Svcs, **SLP**

Schaen, Nancy R F 64 Cannonade Drive, Marlboro, NJ 07746, (201) 431-4557, BA 73 CUNY - Brooklyn Coll; MS 74 Boston Univ; **SLP**

Schaenman, Helene K 1341 Colonial Court, Mamaroneck, NY 10543, **A**

Schaetz, Doreen 791 East Summit Avenue, Memorial Hospital At Oconomowoc, Oconomowoc, WI 53066, (414) 367-3412, BS 66 Univ of WI - Madison; MA 73 Univ of IA; Sp-Lang Path, Memorial Hosp at Oconomowoc, **SLP**

Schaetzel, Mrs Anne Nottingham 17814 137th Drive, Sun City West, AZ 85375, BS 52 Univ of MN - Duluth; MA 57 Univ of Southern CA; Sp-Lang Path, Private Practice, **SLP**

Schafer, David J 4358 East Old Mill Road, Tucson, AZ 85712, (602) 296-3211, BA 79 ND St Univ; MS 87 CO St Univ; 88–Sp-Lang Path, Carondelet Health Services, **SLP**

Schafer, Deborah Ann 1371 East Sudbury Avenue, Sandy, UT 84093, (801) 565-7440, BS 78 Univ of WI - Oshkosh; MS 82 UT St Univ; 88–Sp-Lang Path, Jordan Sch Dist, **SLP**

Schafer, Diane S 1709 Edgewater Avenue, Fort Wayne, IN 46805, (219) 484-6636, BS 76 Eastern MI Univ; MA 77 Eastern MI Univ; Sp/Lang Path, VA Medical Center, **SLP**

Schafer, Dr Judy D 4700 Davenport Street N W, Washington, DC 20016, (202) 745-8270, BA 72 Loyola Coll; MS 73 Loyola Coll; PH 79 (NS) Univ of MD - College Park; Aud, VA Med Cen, **A**

Schafer, Mrs Karen S 50 Fairfax Drive, Chagrin Falls, OH 44022, (512) 250-0677, BS 70 OH Univ - Athens; MA 72 OH St Univ; Doctoral, U of TX - Austin, **SLP**

Schafer, Mrs Linda M 3797 West Parks Road, St Johns, MI 48879, BS 79 Central MI Univ; MA 80 MI St Univ; Private Practice, **SLP**

Schafer, Nancy Neilan 7252 Rene, Shawnee, KS 66216, (913) 831-1900, **SLP**

Schafer, Stuart 26116-K Narbonne, Lomita, CA 90717, (313) 285-0730, BS 83 Univ of MI - Flint; BA 77 Univ of MI - Ann Arbor; MS 78 Univ of MI - Ann Arbor; **A**

Schafer, Susan Ashley 10535 East Main Street, Stoutsville, OH 43154, (614) 421-2880, BA 76 Univ of KY; MA 85 OH St Univ; **A**

Schafer, Susan Mary 7865 Red Hill Court, Worthington, OH 43085, (513) 644-8836, BA 70 OH St Univ; MA 72 OH St Univ; Sp-Lang Path, InSpeech Inc, **SLP**

Schaffer, Mrs Carolyn S 795 East 36th Place, Eugene, OR 97405, (503) 485-8521, BA 80 Univ of OR; MS 82 Univ of OR; Sp-Lang Path, Eugene Hearing and Speech Cen, **SLP**

Schaffer, Mrs Elizabeth Willen 129 El Capitan Drive, Stevensville, MT 59870, (406) 363-2280, BS 77 Boston Univ; MA 78 Saint Louis Univ; Sp-Lang Path, Bitterroot Valley Spec Educ Coop, **SLP**

Schaffer, Dr Elliott J 208 Lambert Avenue, Fredonia, NY 14063, (716) 679-1482, BA 50 Univ of Pittsburgh - Pittsburgh; MS 51 Univ of Pittsburgh - Pittsburgh; PH 58 (Sp Path & Aud) Syracuse Univ; 81–Retired, **SLP A LM**

Schaffer, Mrs Kay N 608 Elkins Avenue, Elkins Park, PA 19117, (215) 348-2940, BS 73 Bloomsburg Univ of PA; ME 74 Bloomsburg Univ of PA; SLP, Bucks Co Iu #22, **SLP**

Schaffer, Lori Foster 8 Oak Street, Blackwood, NJ 08012, (609) 757-3947, BA 82 Stockton St Coll; BS 82 Stockton St Coll; MA 84 Temple Univ; 85–Sp-Lang Path, Our Lady of Lourdes Med Ctr, **SLP ACE**

Schaffer, Mary Ann c/o Wilkerson Center, 1114 19th Avenue South, Nashville, TN 37212, (615) 320-5353, MS 82 Univ of WI - Stevens Point; BS 78 Mankato St Univ; Coord, Bill Wilkerson Hrng & Sp Cen, **SLP**

Schaffer, Mrs Rochelle N 3257 Westwood Drive, Doraville, GA 30340, (404) 945-5735, BA 78 Univ of GA; ME 79 Univ of GA; Sp-Lang Path, Gwinnett Co Sch Syst, **SLP**

Schaffer, Susan Renee 1705 South Cutler Drive, Apartment 7D, Tempe, AZ 85281, (602) 968-1013, BS 79 Western MI Univ; MS 82 AZ St Univ; Sp-Lang Path, Tempe Ele Schl Dstr, **SLP**

Schaffer-Cohen, Mrs Phyllis Beth 154 Queen Anne Road, Bogota, NJ 07603, (212) 605-3740, BA 84 CUNY - Brooklyn Coll; MS 86 CUNY - Brooklyn Coll; 87–Aud, Manhattan ENT Hosp, **A**

Schaffmeyer, Mrs Mary Jeanne 44 7th Street, Berlin, NH 03570, (603) 752-1410, BA 72 2343; MA 76 CUNY - Lehman Coll; SLP, North Country Ed Servs, **SLP**

Schaffner, Elaine Merkley 441 South State #24, Orem, UT 84058, (801) 225-1612, BS 84 Brigham Young Univ; OM 85 Brigham Young Univ; **SLP**

Schaible-McArdle, Helen F 192 North Magnolia Street, Pearl River, NY 10965, (914) 735-7814, BA 78 Univ of MD - College Park; MS 80 Columbia Univ Teachers Coll; 80–SLP & Aud Prog Coord, Offi of Mr and Devel Disablts, **SLP**

Schain, Mrs Judith W 182 Cook Road, Prospect, CT 06712, (203) 758-4181, BA 80 Univ of CT; MS 83 Southern CT St Univ; Sp-Lang Path, Dept of Ment Ret, **SLP**

Schairer, Mrs Loretta Martin 304 Perry Court, Sycamore, IL 60178, (815) 338-1707, BS 79 Univ of WI - Whitewater; MS 81 Univ of WI - Whitewater; Sp/Lang Path, **SLP**

Schalick, Nadine H 707 White Pine Circle, Lawrenceville, NJ 08648, (215) 750-2225, BA 77 Bucknell Univ; MS 85 Boston Univ; 88–Sp-Lang Path, St Mary Hosp, **SLP ACE**

Schalk-Russell, Dr Mary C Cincinnati Board Of Education, 230 East Ninth Street, Cincinnati, OH 45202, (513) 369-4726, BS 59 Daemen Coll; MA 67 OH St Univ; PH 70 (Sp Path) OH St Univ; 83–Superv Sp/Lang Serv, Cincinnati Bd of Ed, **SLP**

Schall, Cheryl Castellana 2421 Lake In The Woods Blvd, Apartment 697, Ypsilanti, MI 48198, (313) 764-8440, BS 86 SUNY - Coll at Fredonia; MS 87 SUNY - Coll at Fredonia; 87–Sp-Lang Path, Univ of Michigan Residential Aphasia Prog

Schall, Mrs Wendy Rosenthal 922 Teakwood Road, Los Angeles, CA 90049, (213) 472-6691, BA 79 Univ of MD - College Park; MA 81 Northwestern Univ; Sp-Lang Path, Centilena Hosp, **SLP**

Schallenkamp, Dr Kay K Chadron State College, Chadron, NE 69337, (308) 432-6203, BS 72 Northern St Coll; MA 73 Univ of SD - Vermillion; PH 82 (NS) Univ of CO - Boulder; 88–Provost, Chadron State Coll, **SLP**

Schaller, Sheran M 3439 Innsbruck Lane, Crete, IL 60417, **SLP**

Schall-Krokosky, Charlotte Route 2, Broadway Drive, Appleton, WI 54915, (414) 735-6214, BS 75 Univ of WI - Stevens Point; MS 76 Univ of WI - Stevens Point; Sp-Lang Path, Appleton Area Sch Dist, **SLP**

Schall-Woodley, Dr Joann 2208 South Catarina Drive, Mesa, AZ 85202, (602) 838-4102, BS 70 AZ St Univ; MS 71 AZ St Univ; ED 80 (NS) AZ St Univ; Preschool Coord, Arizona State Dept of Educ, **SLP**

Schandl, Kathleen Marie Gallaudet University, P O Box 2476, Washington, DC 20002, (314) 843-9652, BS 81 Southeast MO St Univ; MS 83 Southern IL Univ-Edwardsvill; Sp-Lang Path, Ranken Jordan, **SLP**

Schaning, Helen D 1040-A South 30th, Milwaukee, WI 53215, (414) 383-4490, BA 77 Metropolitan St Coll; MA 79 Univ of Denver; Clinical Supervisor, Sacred Heart Rehabilitatn Hosp, **SLP**

Schantz, Deborah Lyn P O Box 20818, Oakland, CA 94620-0818, (503) 775-6781, BA 80 Univ of OR; MS 84 Central WA Univ; Sp-Lang Path, San Francisco USD, **SLP**

Schantz, Elizabeth R 344 North Dillwyn Road, Windy Hills, Newark, DE 19711, (302) 429-4062, BS 52 Manchester Coll; MS 56 Univ of Denver; Colonial Sch Dist-John G Leach, **SLP**

Schanzenbach, Nancy R 86 Drummer Lane, Wayne, PA 19087, (215) 327-1195, BS 71 Syracuse Univ; MS 75 Indiana Univ of PA; Sp-Lang Path, Devereux Foundation, **SLP**

Schaper, Mrs Nan D 10515 Quail Ridge Drive, Olathe, KS 66061, (913) 829-9604, BS 74 OK St Univ; MA 75 Wichita St Univ; Sp-Lang Path, Nan D Schaper Ma & Assoc, **SLP**

Schapire, Irene Sue 6045 28th Avenue N E, Seattle, WA 98115, (206) 587-5150, BA 75 Goddard Coll; MA 81 Univ of CO - Boulder; SLP, Seattle Sch Dist, **SLP**

Schapiro, Mrs Dorris B 65 La Rue Drive, Huntington, NY 11743, (516) 427-3450, BS 36 NY Univ; MA 40 NY Univ; **SLP LM**

Schappell, Linda 1914 Belleview Drive, Whitehall, PA 18052, (215) 820-3775, **SLP**

Scharber, Robert J 556 West Laguna Azul, Mesa, AZ 85210, (602) 969-3775, BS 76 Trenton St Coll; MS 79 AZ St Univ; Aud, Brent Sanders MD Pc, **A**

Schardein-Smith, Mrs Carolyn Lee 2954 Weatherly Drive, Howell, MI 48843, (313) 353-0310, BS 82 GA St Univ; ME 84 GA St Univ; 86–SLP, Rehab Network, **SLP**

Scharein, Edna Ward 6428 Forward Pass Trail, Tallahassee, FL 32308, (904) 668-1779, BS 81 5919; MS 83 5919; SLP, Thomas Co Schools, **SLP**

Scharenbroch, Mary Schanock 2227 Moreland, Janesville, WI 53545-0154, (608) 756-5409, BS 78 Univ of WI - Stevens Point; MS 79 Univ of WI - Stevens Point; 85–Sp-Lang Path, **SLP**

Scharfenaker, Sarah Koehne 681 South Clarkson Street, Denver, CO 80209, (303) 399-1800, BA 79 Univ of MT; MA 81 Univ of MT; 88–Sp-Lang Path, The Children's Hosp, **SLP**

Scharff, Laury Gold 616 Sudbrook Road, Baltimore, MD 21208, (301) 486-6908, BS 84 Univ of VT; MS 87 Loyola Coll; 87–Sp-Lang Path, Carroll Co Bd of Educ

Scharlack, Gaby Ray E 121 Twinleaf Lane, San Antonio, TX 78213, (512) 735-9505, BA 59 Trinity Univ; SLP, San Antonio Sp Lang Hrng Serv, **SLP**

Scharrer, Mrs Ann F 1530 North 10th, Sheboygan, WI 53081, BS 80 Central MI Univ; MA 81 Central MI Univ; Sp-Lang Path, Sheboygan Area School District, **SLP**

Scharrer, Breena Lynn Cedarwood Medical Center, 820 Lester Avenue, St Joseph, MI 49085, (616) 983-0571, BS 82 Western MI Univ; MA 85 Western MI Univ; 88–Aud, Cedarwood Med Ctr, **A**

Scharver, Mrs M Candice 5202 Autumn Drive, Durham, NC 27712, (919) 477-1063, BS 69 Bowling Green St Univ; MA 70 Bowling Green St Univ; Sp-Lang Path Consult, Durham VA Med Ctr, **SLP**

Schary, Mrs Varda Feinsilber 14 Inverness Road, Trumbull, CT 06611, (203) 268-2617, BS 72 Queens Coll, MS 76 Syracuse Univ; Audiologist, ENT Assoc, **A**

Schatz, Joan Ann 13 Thomas Drive, Rome, NY 13440, (315) 337-0308, BA 69 SUNY - Center at Buffalo; MS 70 Univ of WI - Madison; 84–Sp-Lang Path, Rome City Public Schools, **SLP**

Schatz, Kenneth H 2333 Jonathan Court, Ann Arbor, MI 48104, (313) 971-3539, BS 85 Eastern MI Univ; MA 86 Eastern MI Univ; **SLP**

Schatz, Nancy Troxel 424 St Francis Drive, Danville, CA 94526, (415) 820-5779, BS 60 Univ of NE - Lincoln; MS 83 CA St Univ - Hayward; **SLP**

Schatz, Susan A 909 Padre Drive, Salinas, CA 93901, (408) 757-8400, BS 71 Univ of IL - Urbana; MA 73 Univ of CA - Santa Barbara; Dir, Ctrl Coast Sp & Hrng - Cen, **SLP A**

Schaub, Dr Janette M 9571 Oxborough Curve, Bloomington, MN 55437, (612) 831-8250, BA 74 Univ of MN - Minneap-St Paul; MA 76 Univ of MN - Minneap-St Paul; PH 85 (NS) Univ of MN - Minneap-St Paul; Psychologist & Sp/Lang Path, Hennepin Co Med Cen, **SLP**

Schaub, Mrs Lisa J 2501 Riverfront #G-104, Little Rock, AR 72207, (501) 224-3045, BA 82 Ball St Univ; MA 83 Univ of KY; Sp-Lang Path, Arkansas School for the Blind, **SLP**

Schaub, Mrs Mary T 1305 Concart, Hattiesburg, MS 39401, (601) 266-5216, BA 68 Univ of WY; MS 69 Univ of WY; Asst Prof-Sp-Lang Path, U Sn MS, **SLP**

Schaub, Michele Mary 5229 Little Cedar Lane, West Bend, WI 53095, (414) 241-5530, BS 84 Univ of WI - Oshkosh; MS 86 Univ of WI - Oshkosh; **SLP**

Schauben-Fuerst, Renna S 10 Norfolk Avenue, Swampscott, MA 01907, (617) 592-9119, BA CA St Univ - Northridge; MS 79 Southern CT St Univ; **SLP**

Schaubert, Mrs Lynn M 5112 Twin Mound Drive N E, Cedar Rapids, IA 52402, (319) 399-6842, BS 79 ND St Univ; MS 81 ID St Univ; Aud, Grant Wood AEA, **A**

Schaude, Mrs Bonnie A S 5349 Forest Springs Drive, Dunwoody, GA 30338, (215) 750-2225, BA 74 WV Univ; MA 76 Univ of Pittsburgh - Pittsburgh; Sp-Lang Path, Emory University Sch of Med, **SLP**

Schauer, Mrs Glenda M P O Box 1054, Choteau, MT 59422, (406) 466-5394, BS 79 Moorhead St Univ; MS 82 Moorhead St Univ; 82–Sp/Lang Path, Choteau Pub Schs, **SLP ACE**

Schauer, Mrs Paula C 2502 Ebony Road, Baltimore, MD 21234, (301) 664-0533, MS 87 Towson St Univ; Aud/Clin Supvr, Hrng Res/Towson State Univ, **A**

Schaulis, Susan Ann 1540 5th Avenue NE, Rochester, MN 55904, (507) 281-6107, BS 84 Univ of NE - Lincoln; MS 86 Univ of NE - Lincoln; 88–Sp-Lang Path, Rochester ISD #535, **SLP**

Schay, Mrs Nancy Lambdin 4903 West Grace Street, Richmond, VA 23230, (804) 288-3364, BS 77 Old Dominion Univ; MA 78 Univ of TN - Knoxville; Dir of Aud, Fred T Shaia M-D, **A**

Schechter, Dr Martin A 5005 S W Miles Street, Portland, OR 97219, (503) 220-8262, BA 73 CUNY - Brooklyn Coll; MS 76 CUNY - Brooklyn Coll; PH 81 (NS) Univ of MI - Ann Arbor; 80–Aud, VA Med Ctr, **A**

Schechter-Stein, Elaine 412 Ocean Avenue, Sea Bright, NJ 07760, (212) 390-9470, BA 66 Kean Coll of NJ; MA 67 Kean Coll of NJ; Admin, Statin Is Hosp Sp/Hrng Cen, **SLP**

Scheckel, Joanne C 15010 Fernway Avenue, Cleveland, OH 44111, (216) 795-7100, BA 73 John Carroll Univ; MA 75 Cleveland St Univ; Dir of Sp/Lang Path, Soc Crpld Chldn/Cuyahoga Co, **SLP**

Schectman, Mrs Barbara L 1816 Cliffe Hill Way, Potomac, MD 20854, (301) 762-9220, BA 72 Univ of TN - Knoxville; MA 74 Univ of TN - Knoxville; Sp-Lang Path, Montgomery County Pub Schools, **SLP**

Schee, Jon Erik 301 Mercy Health Care Center, Coon Rapids, MN 55433, (612) 421-3400, BA 83 Univ of WI - Eau Claire; OM 85 Univ of WI - River Falls; 87–Aud, Audiometrics, **A**

Scheel, Joan M 342 Withington, Ferndale, MI 48220, MA 55 Ball St Univ; SLP, Royal Oak Schools, **SLP**

Scheer, Becky R 12904 Burlingame, Oklahoma City, OK 73120, (405) 755-8592, BS 75 Univ of NE - Lincoln; MA 77 Univ of NE - Lincoln; Sp-Lang Path, Med Contract Svcs Inc, **SLP**

Scheer, Debra Ann 1833 Preble Avenue #3, Green Bay, WI 54935, (414) 433-8263, BS 84 Univ of WI - Oshkosh; MS 85 Univ of WI - Oshkosh; SLP, St Vincent Hospital, **SLP**

Scheer, Mrs Judith A 1814 9th Street S E, Puyallup, WA 98372, (206) 593-6814, BS 62 Purdue Univ - West Lafayette; SLP, Tacoma Pub Sch, **SLP**

Scheer, Paula 326 Blue Ledge Drive, Roslindale, MA 02131, BA 73 Brandeis Univ; MS 77 Columbia Univ Teachers Coll; OD 83 (NS); Sp-Lang Path, Boston Public Schools, **SLP**

Scheerer, Jennifer J 9730 Wenonga, Leawood, KS 66206, **SLP**

Scheerhorn, Mrs Cindy Dykstra 478 Fourth Street, Harbor Springs, MI 49740, (616) 526-5161, BS 80 Western MI Univ; MA 82 Western MI Univ; Sp-Lang Path, Westview Corp, **SLP**

Scheffler, Mrs Frances Vandenburg West Circle, Bedford, NY 10506, (914) 234-9644, BS 68 SUNY - Center at Albany; MS 74 Columbia Univ Teachers Coll; Sp/Lang Path, Flv Vandenburg, **SLP**

Scheib, Donna S 11729 College View Drive, Wheaton, MD 20902, (301) 933-2717, BS 68 SUNY - Coll at Buffalo; MS 70 Univ of MI - Ann Arbor; 88–Dir Sp-Lang Path, Metro Rehab Associates, **SLP**

Scheib, Rebecca L 3253 Calle DE Molina, Santa Fe, NM 87505, (505) 988-5504, BS 72 Univ of WY; MS 79; 80–Sp-Lang Path, Santa Fe Pub Sch, **SLP**

Scheibe, Peter H 324 Greenwood Place, Syracuse, NY 13210, (315) 425-4386, BA 72 SUNY - Center at Binghamton; MS 77 Univ of WI - Madison; **SLP**

Scheibel, Mrs Mary C 15640 92nd, Florissant, MO 63034, (314) 821-0008, BS 84 Saint Louis Univ; MA 85 Saint Louis Univ; SLP, Prof Rehab Cntr Inc, **SLP**

Scheid, Sandra Lee 1201 106 Lane N W, Coon Rapids, MN 55433, (612) 566-4780, BS 81 Univ of WI - Madison; MS 83 Univ of WI - Madison; Sp-Lang Path, Northside Therapy Services, **SLP**

Scheidhauer, Karen Elizabeth 5002 Crestwood Drive, Colorado Springs, CO 80918, (719) 593-1676, BS 81 CA Univ of PA; BA 81 CA Univ of PA; MS 83 Loyola Coll; **SLP**

Scheidt, Mrs Susan Vae 1518 Calvert Ct, Fort Wayne, IN 46845, (219) 489-3936, BS 83 Purdue Univ - West Lafayette; MS 85 Purdue Univ - West Lafayette; **SLP**

Scheinberg, Dr Judith C 13614 Mar Scenic Drive, Del Mar, CA 92014, (619) 758-8770, MA 71 CUNY - Queens Coll; MA 73 Univ of CA - San Diego; PH 88 (NS) CUNY - Grad Sch & Univ Cntr; 83–Aud, Aud Serv of North Co, **A**

Scheinberg, Mrs Louise G 9 Oak Lane, Scarsdale, NY 10583, (212) 430-2441, BA 50 Univ of MI - Ann Arbor; MA 78 NY Univ; 87–Sp-Lang Path, Rose F Kennedy Ctr, **SLP**

Scheinfeld, Debra B 401 East 74th Street #12K, New York, NY 10021, (212) 288-0958, BA 76 OH St Univ; MS 78 Boston Univ; Sp-Lang Path, Andover Pub Sch, **SLP**

Scheinman, Brenda Robin 245-35 149th Avenue, Rosedale, NY 11422, (516) 921-7650, **SLP**

Schein-Sokolow, Adrian 5749 Hudson Bay Drive, Anaheim, CA 92807, (619) 323-6175, MA 78 CA St Univ - Fresno; **SLP ACE**

Schell, Mrs Kathy G 1118 Southeast 36th Street, Cape Coral, FL 33904, (813) 542-7341, BS 74 Eastern IL Univ; MS 75 Eastern IL Univ; 86–Sp-Lang Path, Lee Co Schs, **SLP**

Schellack, Carol B RR 2 Box 29, Park Rapids, MN 56470, (218) 732-1141, BA 73 Univ of MN - Minneap-St Paul; MA 76 Mankato St Univ; 88–Sp-Lang Path, Sebeka PS, **SLP**

Schellenberg, Mrs Carol Faye 1704 Witt Road, Lebanon, IN 46052, BS 76 Purdue Univ - West Lafayette; MS 79 Southern IL Univ-Edwardsvill; Audiologist, Wditham Memorial Hospital, **A**

Scheller, Mrs Lorrie Drake 2343 Arthur Street N E, Minneapolis, MN 55418, (612) 823-0793, BS 78 CO St Univ; MS 79 Univ of WI - Stevens Point; Field Audiologist, Cochlear Corporation, **A**

Schellinger, Mrs Debra D 60 Rt 47 South, Cape May Court House, NJ 08210, (609) 465-2721, BS 79 Trenton St Coll; MA 80 Univ of IL - Urbana; Sp-Lang Path, Cape May Co Spec Serv Sch Dist, **SLP**

Schellman, Mary Jeanne L 9933 Hampstead Court, Cincinnati, OH 45241-3648, (513) 745-1240, BA 71 Fontbonne Coll; MA 72 Univ of MO - Columbia; Sp-Lang Path, Bethesda North Hosp, **SLP**

Schellschmidt, Joyce 5063 Sprucewood Court, Sylvania, OH 43560, (419) 474-2612, BS 72 IN Univ - Bloomington; OM 73 IN Univ - Bloomington; **SLP**

Schemanske, Judith A 2164 E Bellevue Road, Merced, CA 95340, (209) 385-8445, SLP, Merced Co Bd of Ed, **SLP**

Schemm, Donna Kay 519 Fourth Avenue, Eau Claire, WI 54703, (715) 836-4186, BA 81 Univ of WI - Eau Claire; MS 82 Univ of WI - Eau Claire; 88–Clin Supvr/Lecturer, Univ of WI, **SLP**

Schemmel, Mrs Phyllis J 434 Woodview Drive, Springfield, OH 45504, (513) 324-2081, BS 70 Bowling Green St Univ; MS 71 Univ of MI - Ann Arbor; Sp-Lang Path, W Central Oh Hrng Sp Cen, **SLP**

Schempp, Mrs Nancy F Route 7 Box 793, Murray, KY 42071, (502) 753-4182, BA 72 Murray St Univ; MS 74 Murray St Univ; Sp-Lang Path, Calloway Co Sch Syst, **SLP**

Schenasi, Mrs Carol L 2300 Maple Avenue, Unit 165, Torrance, CA 90503, (213) 320-6658, BA 78 CA St Univ - Fresno; MA 80 CA St Univ - Fresno; Sp-Lang Path, CA Dept Ed Diag Sch, **SLP**

Schenck, Betty Jo 3613 N W 30th Boulevard, Gainesville, FL 32601, (904) 373-5192, ME 73 Univ of FL; Dir Except Stud Ed, Alachua Co Sch Bd, **SLP**

Schend, Mary B 1102 Nambe Street, Hobbs, NM 88240, (505) 397-2828, BA 74 Univ of MN - Duluth; MA 75 Univ of MN - Duluth; Sp/Lang Path, Hobbs Muncp Sch, **SLP**

Schendel, Laurel L 328 Cortez Street, Tallahassee, FL 32303, (914) 644-2238, BA 39 North Central Coll; MA 47 Northwestern Univ; PH 59 (NS) Northwestern Univ; Prof, FL St U, **SLP F LM**

Scheneman, Mrs Mary A 2513 Plymouth Street, Blacksburg, VA 24060, (703) 953-1693, BS 73 Univ of MO - Columbia; ME 74 Univ of VA - Charlottesville; 88–SLP, Private Practice, **SLP**

Schenkein, Lisa C P O Box 1022, Red Lodge, MT 59068, (406) 662-3588, BS 75 Univ of KS; MA 77 Univ of IA; Sp-Lang Path, Yellowstone-W/Carbon Co Coop, **SLP ACE**

Schenkel, Lynne B 13 Macopin Drive, Livingston, NJ 07039, (201) 740-0849, BA 73 Univ of CT; **SLP**

Schenker, Roz 2800 Quebec Street N W #745, Washington, DC 20008, (202) 363-8429, **A**

Schepers, Christine M 305 Hickory Street, Chaska, MN 55318, (218) 726-6094, BS 85 Univ of MN - Duluth; MS 86 Univ of WI - Eau Claire; 88–Sp-Lang Path, Minnesota River Valley Spec Educ Coop, **SLP**

Scheps, Amy Heller 296 Eliot Street, Newton, MA 02164, (617) 527-6464, BS 85 Ithaca Coll; MS 87 Boston Univ; **SLP**

Scher, Mrs Stephanie B 20 Holly Court, Owings Mills, MD 21117, (301) 356-1930, BS 74 Univ of MD - College Park; MS 78 Towson St Univ; Sp-Lang Path, Baltimore City Public Schools, **SLP**

Scherber, Mrs Connie J 3512 North Shore Drive, Clear Lake, IA 50428, (515) 357-6125, BA 76 Univ of Northern IA; MS 77 Univ of WI - Stevens Point; Sp-Lang Path, Northern Trails AEA, **SLP**

Scherbert, Thomas G 6030 West Armour Avenue #7, Greenfield, WI 53220, (414) 281-3345, BS 84 Univ of WI - Madison; MS 87 Univ of WI - Milwaukee; Sp-Lang Path, St Joseph Hosp, **SLP**

Scherer, Dr Nancy J 10041 Dewey Drive, Garden Grove, CA 92640, (714) 639-4990, BS 71 Univ of WI - Madison; MS 72 Univ of WI - Madison; PH 80 (NS) Univ of WA; Dir Clin Svcs, Providence Spec & Hea Cen, **SLP**

Scherer, Dr Ronald C Denver Ctr For Performing Arts, Research & Recording Ctr, 1245 Champa Street, Denver, CO 80204, (303) 893-4000, BS 68 Kent St Univ; MA 72 IN Univ - Bloomington; PH 81 (NS) Univ of IA; Res Sci, Denver Cen for Perform Arts

Scherich, Dayl L 1707 Brackenridge, Austin, TX 78704, (512) 476-6461, BS 74; MA 77; Dir of Aud, Brackenridge Hospital, **A**

Scherker, Mrs Dorothy Sholin P O Box 523704, Miami, FL 33152-3704, (305) 262-2664, BA 52 CUNY - Brooklyn Coll; ME 72 Univ of Miami; Private Practice, **SLP**

Schermer, Anita Dorn 2129 Eleanor Avenue, St Paul, MN 55116, (612) 693-2441, **SLP**

Schermer, Sheryl Lynn 3278 South Springfield, Milwaukee, WI 53207, (414) 483-4180, MS 87 Univ of WI - Stevens Point; **SLP**

Schermerhorn, Carol Costa 1887 Shirley Drive, Benicia, CA 94510, (707) 745-6604, BA 77 Univ of Denver; MA 79 Univ of Denver; Sp-Lang Path, Solano Co Supt of Sch, **SLP**

Schermerhorn, Mark Charles 553 So 1000 East, Salt Lake City, UT 84102, (801) 364-4607, BS 76 Univ of Redlands; MS 82 Univ of Redlands; **SLP**

Schermerhorn-Grossman, Mrs Siobhan 1550 Woodlynne Boulevard, Linwood, NJ 08221, (609) 347-6150, BS 82 Boston Univ; MA 84 Northwestern Univ; Sp-Lang Path, Children's Seashore House, **SLP**

Scherr, Charlene K 11111 Lamplighter Lane, Potomac, MD 20854, **A**

Scherr, Daun Willoughby 633 St Georges Station Rd, Reisterstown, MD 21136, (301) 526-7643, BS 82 Towson St Univ; MS 85 Loyola Coll; 85–Sp-Lang Path, Carroll County PS, **SLP**

Scherr, Pia Sadowsky 12 Darewood Lane, Valley Stream, NY 11581, (516) 239-6400, BA 85 CUNY - Brooklyn Coll; MS 87 CUNY - Brooklyn Coll; **A**

Scherr, Dr Robert 1208 Orchard Circle, Salisbury, MD 21801, (301) 749-7804, BA 66 Univ of MD - College Park; MA 70 Univ of MD - College Park; ED 83 (Education) Univ of MD - College Park; 70–Sp-Lang Path, Private Practice, **SLP**

Schery, Teris Kim 137 West 8th Street, Claremont, CA 91711, (714) 626-6533, BA 65 Stanford Univ; MA 66 Stanford Univ; PH 80 (Child Development) Claremont Graduate Sch; 81–Professor, California State University, **SLP F**

Scherz, Julie W 2323 North Woodlawn #309, Wichita, KS 67220, (316) 689-3240, BA 69 Wichita St Univ; MA 71 Wichita St Univ; 84–Clinical Supervisor, Wichita State University, **SLP**

Schessler, Mrs Carol J 25 Spring Garden Drive, Madison, NJ 07940, (201) 822-2202, BA 66 Marymount Coll; MA 69 CUNY - Hunter Coll; 86–Sp-Lang Path, Assn for Retarded Citizens, **SLP**

Schetter, Jacqui L 209 Delta Oaks, Sacramento, CA 95831, (916) 421-9880, BA 76 CA St Univ - Sacramento; MA 78 CA St Univ - Sacramento; Aud, **A**

Schettler, Mrs Jamie Rae 1709 4th Street SW #4, Minot, ND 58701, (701) 838-5669, BS 86 Minot St Univ; MS 87 Minot St Univ; 86–Sp-Lang Path, Minot Voc Adjustment Workshop, **SLP**

Schetz, Mrs Katherine 607 Rainbow Ridge, Blacksburg, VA 24060, (703) 552-9201, MS 81 Radford Univ; MS 77 VA Polytechnic Inst St Univ; Sp-Lang Path, Mont Co Sch Syst, **SLP**

Scheuerle, Dr Jane F University Of South Florida, Department Of Communication Sciences & Disorders, CBA 255, Tampa, FL 33620, (813) 974-2006, MS 58 Univ of Louisville; MA 68 Univ of South FL; ED 75 (Human Behavior) Nova Univ; 75–Prof, U S FL, **SLP**

Scheuerman, Martha A 3224 Marvin Drive, Adrian, MI 49221, (419) 882-4622, BS 85 Central MI Univ; MA 86 Central MI Univ; **SLP**

Scheuerman, Sandi L 10015 Stevenson Drive, Temperance, MI 48182, (419) 422-6121, BS 84 Western MI Univ; MA 86 Eastern MI Univ; **SLP**

Schewitz, Mrs Sheila 53 Warrington Court, Lake Bluff, IL 60044, (312) 234-4775, BA 50; MS 76; Sp-Lang Path, **SLP**

Schiano, Ilene Lieberman 33 Spruce Street, Top Apartment, Great Neck, NY 11021, (516) 562-4600, BS 69 SUNY - Coll at Buffalo; MS 71 SUNY - Coll at Buffalo; Chief SLP / Aud Serv, N Shore U Hosp, **SLP**

Schiano, Maria Angela 3 Derby Lane, New City, NY 10956, (914) 359-7179, BS 85 Coll of Saint Rose; MS 87 CUNY - Brooklyn Coll; **SLP**

Schiaroli, Kathryn Ada 200 Alden Avenue #7, New Haven, CT 06515, (203) 389-8413, MS 87 Southern CT St Univ

Schiavetti, Dr Nicholas Dept Speech Path & Audiology, St University Of New York, 314 Sturges Hall, Geneseo, NY 14454, (716) 245-5328, BA 65 Cornell Univ; MA 67 Columbia Univ Teachers Coll; PH 69 (NS) Columbia Univ Teachers Coll; Prof, SUNY, **SLP A**

Schiavone, Diane Adele Rd 2 Neck Road, Burlington, NJ 08016, (609) 386-0144, Private Practice, **SLP**

Schiavone, Diane C 2712 East 65th Street, Brooklyn, NY 11234, **SLP**

Schiavone, James Robert 2712 East 65th Street, Brooklyn, NY 11234, (718) 531-8221, **SLP**

Schibel, Mrs Linda Grossman 16862 Edgar, Pacific Palisades, CA 90272, (213) 459-3391, BS 63 Boston Univ; MA 66 Univ of MN - Minneap-St Paul; Sp/Lang Path, Pac Palisades Except Chldn Cl, **SLP**

Schicht, Michele Keys Speech & Hearing Center, Health Sci Ctr Univ Of Ok, 825 N E 14th, Oklahoma City, OK 73104, (405) 271-4214, BA 67 Fontbonne Coll; MS 69 Univ of OK Medical Center; Asst Prof, Univ of Oklahoma Hlth Sci Cen, **SLP**

Schick, Dr Brenda S Boys Town National Institute, 555 North 30th Street, Omaha, NE 68131, (402) 498-6691, BS 73 Purdue Univ - West Lafayette; MS 76 Univ of WA; PH 87 (Language Acquisition) Purdue Univ - West Lafayette; 88–Coord-Sign Lang Lab, Boys Town Natl Inst

Schicker, Mrs Patricia L 3715 Mormon Street, Omaha, NE 68112, (402) 572-2279, BA 68 Creighton Univ; MS 69 Univ of NE - Omaha; SLP, Immanuel Med Cen, **SLP**

Schickler, Judy Sobel 3222 Horton Avenue, San Diego, CA 92103, **SLP**

Schiebel-Knox, Mrs Cynthia Diane 1303 Rosemont, Amarillo, TX 79106, (806) 371-5737, BS 75 West TX St Univ; MA 78 West TX St Univ; ME 88 West TX St Univ; 87–Sp-Lang Path, Amarillo ISD, **SLP**

Schieber, Cindy C 1835 Winding Hills Road, Apt 1412, Davenport, IA 52807, BS 80 Northwest MO St Univ; MS 81 Northwest MO St Univ; SLP, Ed Agcy 13, **SLP**

Schiefelbusch, Dr Richard L Bureau Of Child Research, University Of Kansas, 2045 Haworth Hall, Lawrence, KS 66045, (913) 864-4295, BS 40 Pittsburg St Univ; MA 47 Univ of KS; PH 51 (NS) Northwestern Univ; Dir-Bureau of Chld Res, U of KS, **SLP F H**

Schiefer, Penelope B Box 964, Havre, MT 59501, (406) 265-4356, MS 78 Nazareth Coll of Rochester; Sp-Lang Path, Havre Pub Sch 16A, **SLP**

Schiemann, Mrs Winifred W 5551 Canalino Drive, Carpinteria, CA 93013, (805) 684-3078, BA 49 Univ of CA - Santa Barbara; Sp-Lang Path, Santa Barbara County Schools, **SLP**

Schienberg, Steven Emanuel Rehabilitation Ctr, 3001 N Gantenbien Avenue, Portland, OR 97227, (503) 280-3808, BA 77 CUNY - Queens Coll; MA 79 Memphis St Univ; SLP, Emanuel Rehab Ctr, **SLP**

Schier, Mrs Dianne W 1198 Cherry Lane, Calimesa, CA 92320, (714) 849-4786, BA 80 Univ of Redlands; MS 82 Univ of Redlands; Sp-Lang Path, Banning USD, **SLP**

Schierwagen, Mrs Karin Ann P O Box 697, Miller Place, NY 11764, (516) 928-7758, BA 75 CUNY - Queens Coll; MA 77 Hofstra Univ; SLP, Commack Public Schools, **SLP**

Schiesser-Manser, Mrs Pamela Susan 4373 Stoneybrook Drive S E, Warren, OH 44484, (216) 841-2240, **SLP**

Schifalacqua, Christine Victoria 816 Old Wyomissing Road, Reading, PA 19611, (215) 372-8269, BS 79 East Stroudsburg Univ of PA; MA 81 Hahneman Medical Coll; Aud/Sp-Lang Path, InSpeech Inc, **SLP A ACE**

Schiffer, Mrs Judith Mason 7210-B Eden Brook Drive, Apartment 104, Columbia, MD 21046, (301) 381-4436, BS 81 Northwestern Univ; MS 82 Columbia Univ Teachers Coll; Sp-Lang Path, Montgomery County PS, **SLP**

Schiffler, Linda P 5 South 066 Pebblewood Ln, Apartment 8A, Naperville, IL 60540, (312) 531-3821, BS 71 Southern IL Univ -Carbondale; MS 72 Southern IL Univ -Carbondale; Aud, Private Practice, **A**

Schiffmacher, Pamela W 2254 Gaviota Avenue #6, Signal Hill, CA 90806-3653, (818) 584-4888, BA 68 Univ of the Pacific; MA 69 Univ of the Pacific; 87–Reg Oper Dir, Neuro Care Inc, **SLP**

Schiff-Myers, Dr Naomi B 25 Nimitz Place, Old Greenwich, CT 06870, (201) 893-4226, BA 60 Barnard Coll; MA 64 Columbia Univ Teachers Coll; PH 76 (NS) Columbia Univ Teachers Coll; Assoc Prof, Montclair St Coll, **SLP**

Schiff-Pasekoff, Mrs Deanna 1288 Firwood Drive, Mount Lebanon, PA 15243, (412) 276-0840, BA 75 Univ of Pittsburgh - Pittsburgh; MA 76 Univ of Miami; Sp-Lang Path, **SLP**

Schild, Mrs Pamela K 2109 130th Place S E, Bellevue, WA 98005, (206) 643-1676, BS 70 Western OR St Coll; MS 75 Western OR St Coll; Instr, Beaverton Sch Dist, **SLP**

Schilder, Theresa D 305 Fox Run Trail, Dothan, AL 36303, (205) 792-8730, BA 70 Seton Hall Univ; MA 73 Seton Hall Univ; 87–Sp-Lang Path, Steensland Ctr for Sp Path, **SLP**

Schildkraut, Mrs Roberta H 1 Scholar Court, East Northport, NY 11731, (516) 261-6784, BA 66 CUNY - Brooklyn Coll; MA 83 Long Island U - CW Post Ctr; Sp-Lang Path, Huntington USD #3, **SLP**

Schildwachter, Mrs Allison St C 2662 Jefferson Park Circle, Charlottesville, VA 22903, (804) 979-7966, BS 75 Univ of VA - Charlottesville; MA 76 Vanderbilt Univ; **SLP**

Schilke, Mrs Margaret L 4 Hempshire Court, Scotia, NY 12302, (518) 346-6005, BS 66 Kent St Univ; ME 69 Kent St Univ; SLP, **SLP**

Schill, Dr Herman Allan P O Box 547, Sharon, MA 02067, (617) 565-9598, BA 53 CUNY - Brooklyn Coll; MA 59 CUNY - Brooklyn Coll; PH 62 (Aud) Univ of Pittsburgh - Pittsburgh; 85–Chief-Audiology Sec, US VA, **A**

Schill, Mrs Mary Jo S 1009 Belmont Road, Grand Forks, ND 58201, (701) 777-3232, BS 70 Univ of ND; MA 71 IN Univ - Bloomington; 77–Sp-Lang Path, U of ND, **SLP**

Schiller, Dr Newton M 142 Lee Road, Scarsdale, NY 10583, (914) 997-1344, BA 50 IN Univ - Bloomington; MA 53 IN Univ - Bloomington; ED 77 (NS) Columbia Univ Teachers Coll; Sp-Lang Path, Private Practice, **SLP**

Schilling, Mrs Edda Acosta Crisantemo 165, Rio Piedras, PR 00927, MS 64 PA St Univ - Univ Park; Sp-Lang Path, Vamroc, **SLP A**

Schilling, Karen Marie 130 1/2 N Wacouta, Praire Du Chien, WI 53821, (608) 326-4637, MS 87 Univ of WI - Eau Claire; **SLP**

Schilling, Mrs Kristin Mary 1607 East Carlton, Springfield, MO 65804, (417) 836-0400, BS 83 Univ of NE - Lincoln; MS 84 Univ of NE - Lincoln; 84–Sp-Lang Path, Dept of Mental Health, **SLP**

Schilling, Marcia M 12700 Reata, Anchorage, AK 99516, (907) 345-5629, BA 71 Wellesley Coll; BA 74 Univ of MN - Minneap-St Paul; MA 76 Univ of MN - Minneap-St Paul; Sp-Lang Path, AK Treat Cen, **SLP**

Schilling, Rhonda Ann 2630 Bissonnet #158, Houston, TX 77005-1335, (713) 859-6600, BS 72 LA St Univ - Baton Rouge; MA 77 Northwestern St Univ; Sp-Lang Path, Cypress Fairbanks ISD, **SLP**

Schillinger, Karen M 29-28 Ditmars Boulevard, Astoria, NY 11105, (718) 721-9894, BA 78 CUNY - Queens Coll; MS 80 CUNY - Brooklyn Coll; Private Practice, **SLP**

Schillio, Mrs Vivian Burness 2425 Anderson, Saginaw, MI 48603-3821, (517) 790-8687, BA 76 MI St Univ; MA 77 Central MI Univ; Sp-Lang Path, **SLP**

Schillne, Sheryl Marie 111 East 35th Street #8, Davenport, IA 52806, (319) 391-1218, BA 83 Saint Mary's Coll; MA 87 Western MI Univ

Schilp, Mrs Carol D 225 Lenox Avenue, Albany, NY 12208, (518) 482-9132, BA 56 Univ of OR; MA 76 Coll of Saint Rose; Sp-Lang Path, Private Practice, **SLP**

Schimel, Mrs Alison B 3706 Pebble Beach, Northbrook, IL 60062, MA 73 Oakland City Coll; **SLP**

Schimke, Mrs Jean G R 2619 Marilyn Drive, Eau Claire, WI 54701, BS 59 Minot St Univ; MA 62 Univ of Northern CO; MS 78 Univ of WI - Eau Claire; **SLP**

Schimmel, Mrs Ellen S 35 Hidden Lake Drive, North Brunswick, NJ 08902, (201) 821-7271, BS 76 Emerson Coll; MS 78 Boston Univ; Sp-Lang Path, Private Practice, **SLP**

Schimmel, Mrs Judith M 1456 Hazelwood Lane, Bethlehem, PA 18018, (215) 759-7600, BS 70 PA St Univ - Univ Park; MS 87 Bloomsburg Univ of PA; 70–SLP, Colonial-Northampton IU #20, **SLP**

Schimmelpfenneg, Nancy Leigh 3422 A-1 S Stafford Street, Arlington, VA 22206, (301) 336-0071, BS 83 Central MI Univ; MA 85 MI St Univ; Sp-Lang Path, Prince Georges Co Schools, **SLP**

Schimnich, Kaye M 701 5th Avenue North #2, St Cloud, MN 56303, (612) 259-8737, BA 83 Coll of Saint Benedict; MA 87 Univ of MN - Minneap-St Paul; 87–Sp-Lang Path, Dist 742 Comm Schs, **SLP**

Schindelman, Maxine Rd 5 Box 137, Binghamton, NY 13905, (607) 770-8895, BA 73 SUNY - Center at Binghamton; MS 77 Ithaca Coll; 82–Sp-Lang Path, Broome Developmental Services, **SLP ACE**

Schindler, Susan Kahalas 13138 Broadmore Road, Silver Spring, MD 20904, (301) 989-0038, MS 84 Towson St Univ; **SLP**

Schindler-Reich, Mrs Wendy 198-08 53rd Avenue, Flushing, NY 11365, (718) 631-8180, BA 76 CUNY - Lehman Coll; MA 77 Univ of Miami; SLP, **SLP**

Schindler-Wale, Barbara 18 Old Country Lane, Fairport, NY 14450, (716) 271-0660, BS 75 SUNY - Coll at Geneseo; MA 78 SUNY - Coll at Geneseo; 87–Asst Exec Dir, Monroe Co Assn for Retard Citz, **SLP**

Schinske, Dr Erhart A 214 South Garden Street, Bellingham, WA 98225, (206) 733-1383, BA 40 Hamline Univ; MA 52 Univ of MN - Minneap-St Paul; PH 60 (Sp Path) Univ of MN - Minneap-St Paul; 57–Retired, Western Washington Univ, **SLP LM**

Schinsky, Mrs Lorraine B 3926-A Dover Place, St Louis, MO 63116, (314) 752-3285, BA 67 Fontbonne Coll; MA 71 Saint Louis Univ; SLP, St Louis VA Medical Center, **SLP**

Schipper, Mrs Beverly Lynn 3303 Acorn Lane, Jeffersonville, IN 47130, (812) 283-7908, BS 69 OH Univ - Athens; MS 84 Univ of Louisville; 86–Sp-Lang Path, Easter Seal Hearing & Sp Ctr, **SLP**

Schipper, Mrs Catherine 711 Kokomo Lane, Indianapolis, IN 46241, (317) 924-3251, BA 78 IN Univ - Bloomington; ME 79 IN Univ - Bloomington; Sp/Lang Path, Crossroads Rehab Cen, **SLP**

Schippits, Sandra Renee 656 13th Avenue N W, New Brighton, MN 55112, (612) 636-1248, BA 63 Elmhurst Coll; MS 83 Univ of WI - River Falls; SLP, Minneapolis Pub Sch, **SLP**

Schirber, Carol M Minn Ear Head & Neck Clinic, 701 25th Avenue South, Minneapolis, MN 55410, (612) 339-2836, BS 83 ND St Univ; MS 84 ID St Univ; Aud, Minn Ear Head Neck Clinic, **A**

Schiro, Mrs Suzanne Y 3321 Calvano Drive, Grand Island, NY 14072, (716) 837-2441, BS 69 SUNY - Coll at Geneseo; ME 73 SUNY - Coll at Geneseo; 85–Sp-Lang Path, Language Development Program, **SLP**

Schissel, Mrs Ann 214 Tudor Road, Ithaca, NY 14850, (501) 521-3029, BA 70 Eastern Coll; MS 74 PA St Univ - Univ Park; Speech-Language Pathologist, Ithaca Pub Schs, **SLP**

Schissel, Dr Richard J Dept Of Speech Pathology And, Audiology, Ithaca College, Ithaca, NY 14850, (607) 274-3248, BS 70 Univ of WI - Whitewater; MS 71 PA St Univ - Univ Park; PH 75 (NS) PA St Univ - Univ Park; Dept Chrmn Sp-Lang Path, Ithaca College, **SLP**

Schlabach, Sheryl L 2802 Firecrest Drive, Austin, TX 78748, (512) 450-1177, BA 76 Sam Houston St Univ; MA 79 Univ of TX - Austin; 88–Sp-Lang Path, Austin ISD, **SLP**

Schlader, Susan Stuedemann 2626 4th Avenue North, Fort Dodge, IA 50501, (515) 576-7434, BA 81 Univ of Northern IA; MA 82 Univ of Northern IA; Sp-Lang Path, Arrowhead AEA, **SLP**

Schlager, Mrs Sandra 3048 Newport Court, Troy, MI 48084, (313) 445-4443, BS 66 MI St Univ; MA 67 MI St Univ; Sp-Lang Path, E Detroit Pub Sch, **SLP**

Schlagheck, Mrs Grace Judith Schubertstrasse 32 6911, Malsch, West Germany, 011-49-7253-25213, BS 81 Eastern MI Univ; MA 84 Wayne St Univ - Sch of Med; 84–Aud, **A**

Schlais, Mrs Susan Elaine 2749 East 400 South, Kokomo, IN 46902, (317) 452-8285, BS 83 Univ of WI - Madison; MS 85 Univ of WI - Madison; Sp-Lang Path, Psi Iota Xi Sp Clin, **SLP**

Schlaman, Suzanne Marie 26140 Regency Club Drive #5, Warren, MI 48089, (313) 772-3685, MA 88 MI St Univ; 88–Sp-Lang Path, Lakeshore ENT Ctr PC

Schlanger, Dr Bernard B 143 Coventry Place, Palm Beach Gardens, FL 33418, (407) 626-4058, BA 37 Univ of WI - Madison; MA 39 Univ of WI - Madison; PH 52 (NS) Univ of WI - Madison; Prof Emeritus, The City College (Cuny), **SLP F LM**

Schlanger, Mrs Phoebe H 143 Coventry Place, Palm Beach Gardens, FL 33418, (407) 626-4058, BA 43 CUNY - Brooklyn Coll; MA 44 Univ of WI - Madison; Asst Prof Emeritus, Herbert H Lehman Co, **SLP F LM**

Schlanser, Mrs Theresa Dianne 3718 Quail Hollow Drive, Columbus, OH 43228, (614) 272-1907, BS 85 Eastern KY Univ; MA 86 Eastern KY Univ; 88–Sp-Lang Path, Communication Disorders Institute, **SLP**

Schlappi, Mrs Carole Rayline 2240 East Belmont Avenue, Phoenix, AZ 85020, (602) 861-1606, MS 80 Univ of OR; 84–Sp-Lang Path, Private Practice, **SLP**

Schlecht, Mrs Kathleen Marie 4878 S96TH Street, Greenfield, WI 53228, (414) 786-1330, MS 84 Univ of WI - Madison; Sp-Lang Path, New Berlin Pub Schs, **SLP**

Schlegel, Rita A 21 Wildwood Road, Kennebunkport, ME 04046, (207) 967-2625, BA 83 Univ of ME - Orono; MS 87 Emerson Coll; 86–Sp-Lang Path, York Co Counseling Svcs Inc, **SLP**

Schleicher, Melaine Ann 10084 Cliffwood Court, Cincinnati, OH 45241, (414) 383-4490, BS 81 Bowling Green St Univ; MS 83 Univ of WI - Stevens Point; Sp-Lang Path, Sacred Heart Rehab Hosp, **SLP**

Schleifer, John Gary 123 Vinsant, Brooks AFB, TX 78235-5000, (512) 536-2909, MA 75 SUNY - Center at Buffalo; 86–Ch Hrng Conserv Registry, US Air Force, **A**

Schleifer, Nancy I 7507 Constitution Drive, Cincinnati, OH 45215, (513) 872-2481, BS 76 SUNY - Center at Albany; MA 78 Univ of CT; 87–Sp-Lang Path, Good Samaritan Hosp, **SLP**

Schleifer, Patricia H Box 561, Stoneboro, PA 16153, (412) 376-3772, BS 79 Clarion Univ of PA; MA 82 Kent St Univ; SLP, InSpeech Inc, **SLP**

Schleifer, Randi 11 Suttonwood Drive, Commack, NY 11725, **SLP**

Schlein, Charles M 203 Inglewood Drive, Morganton, NC 28655, (704) 433-2746, BS 71 Appalachian St Univ; MA 72 Appalachian St Univ; Sp-Lang Path, Child Spec Hlth Svcs, **SLP**

Schlein, Mrs Elizabeth Golden 70 Dane Street, Beverly, MA 01915, (617) 927-8977, BS 82 MI St Univ; MS 84 Boston Univ; Sp/Lang Path, Private Practice, **SLP**

Schleis, Beth Ann 2013 Orrie Lane, Green Bay, WI 54304, (414) 494-9349, MS 86 Univ of WI - Whitewater

Schlemper, Mrs Kathie Laraine Route 5 Box 464, Rolla, MO 65401, (314) 364-4746, BS 83 Minot St Univ; MS 85 Minot St Univ; **SLP**

Schlender, Margaret Mary 653 Ravenswood Drive, Green Bay, WI 54302-4253, (414) 497-3905, BS 83 Univ of WI - Stevens Point; MS 84 Univ of WI - Stevens Point; SLP, Green Bay Area PS, **SLP**

Schleser, Marilyn Melis Rd 2 Box 210C, Doll Road, Bloomingburg, NY 12721, (914) 294-5431, BA 75 William Paterson Coll; MS 78 William Paterson Coll; 84–Sp-Lang Path, Orange-Ulster BOCES, **SLP**

Schlesinger, Fern Winkler 4829 S W Stonebrook Court, Portland, OR 97201, (503) 246-3533, BA 73 Univ of WA; MA 74 Univ of WA; Sp-Lang Path, Portland Pub Sch, **SLP**

Schlessinger, Amy Joan 6958 Laguna Place #C, Cucamonga, CA 91730, (714) 983-9501, BA 80 Univ of CA - Santa Barbara; MS 83 Univ of LA Verne; SLP, Ontario-Montclair School Dist, **SLP**

Schlett, Carolyn Elizabeth 313 Fremont Avenue, Sandusky, OH 44870, **SLP**

Schlicher, Karen S 131 East Onota, Munising, MI 49862, (906) 387-2103, BA 75 Lake Superior St Coll; MA 79 Northern MI Univ; SLP, Munising Pub Sch, **SLP**

Schliesser, Barbara H 6325 Eastshore Drive, Lincoln, NE 68516, (402) 471-2471, BS 58 Univ of NE - Lincoln; MA 61 Univ of IA; Admin, State Dept Ed-NE, **SLP**

Schliesser, Dr Herbert F 6325 Eastshore Drive, Lincoln, NE 68516, (402) 472-2071, BS 54 Univ of NE - Lincoln; MA 60 Univ of NE - Lincoln; PH 65 (NS) Univ of IA; Prof Sp-Lang Path, U of NE, **SLP**

Schlievert, Mary Ellen 6198 Wildacre Road, Curtice, OH 43412, (419) 836-7762, BA 83 Mount Union Coll; MA 85 OH Univ - Athens; **SLP**

Schlisselberg, Dr Gloria F 212-10 69th Avenue, Bayside, NY 11364, (516) 560-5656, BA 72 SUNY - Center at Stony Brook; MA 74 CUNY - Queens Coll; PH 88 (Sp/Hrng Sciences) CUNY - Grad Sch & Univ Cntr; Cl Superv, Hofstra U, **SLP**

Schlitt, Mary M A 1886 Verlin Road, Apt 10, Green Bay, WI 54302, (414) 465-0965, BS 83 Univ of WI - Milwaukee; MS 85 Univ of WI - Milwaukee; 85–Sp-Lang Path, Brown County, **SLP**

Schlitt, Robert #4 Sandy Lake Drive, Hampton, VA 23666, (804) 766-3824, MA 54 CUNY - Brooklyn Coll; **SLP F**

Schloesser, Mrs Mary Patricia 13207 Ladybonklane, Herndon, VA 22071, (202) 562-7112, **SLP**

Schloff, Laurie 4 Chiswick Road #35, Brookline, MA 02146, (617) 739-3330, BA 73 Rutger's St Univ - Douglas Coll; MS 75 Columbia Univ Teachers Coll; Consult, Speech Improvement Co Boston, **SLP**

Schloff, Mary J 5729 10th Avenue South, Minneapolis, MN 55417, (612) 627 2339, OM 88 Univ of WI - River Falls; 76–Sp-Lang Path, Spec Sch Dist #1

Schloff, Sandra Joan 35749 Terrace Court, Farmington Hills, MI 48331, (313) 684-8040, BA 80 MI St Univ; MS 83 Univ of MI - Ann Arbor; 86–Sp-Lang Path, Huron Valley Schs, **SLP**

Schlofner, Denise Barsella 808 West Thomas, Arlington Heights, IL 60004, (312) 354-6929, BA 85 Bradley Univ; MS 86 Marquette Univ; 88–Sp-Lang Path, Helping Hand Rehab Ctr, **SLP**

Schloss, Cynthia Diane 3127-A North 54th Street, Milwaukee, WI 53216, (414) 461-2322, BS 81 Univ of WI - Milwaukee; MS 83 Univ of WI - Milwaukee; Sp-Lang Path, Milwaukee Pub Sch, **SLP**

Schloss, Sharon Merker 31 Woods Run, Farmington, CT 06032, (203) 674-8468, BS 84 Ithaca Coll; MS 86 PA St Univ - Univ Park; Sp-Lang Path, New Britian Sch Dist, **SLP**

Schlossberg, Mrs Pamela Mitchell 23 Elmwood Avenue, Rye, NY 10580, (914) 921-0929, BA 81 Chapman Coll; MS 83 Chapman Coll; Sp-Lang Path, Midpoint Assoc Practitioners Inc, **SLP**

Schlosser, Mrs Barbara F 4054 Roger Drive, Encino, CA 91436, (818) 784-4643, BS 56 Univ of Southern CA; MS 74 CA St Univ - Northridge; SLP, Los Angeles USD, **SLP**

Schlosser, Diane K 7861-C North 60th, Milwaukee, WI 53223, (414) 355-0275, BS 76 Univ of WI - Whitewater; MS 77 Univ of WI - Whitewater; Sp-Lang Path, Greenfield Pub Schs, **SLP**

Schlosser, Dr Frances D 7914 Donzee, San Diego, CA 92123, (619) 569-1252, BA 52 IN Central Univ; MA 54 Northwestern Univ; PH 71 (NS) Univ of Southern CA; Dir, Private Practice, **SLP LM**

Schlosser, Joan E 2849 Mead Street, Yorktown Heights, NY 10598, (914) 245-6640, BA 69 Univ of CT; MA 76 CUNY - Lehman Coll; Sp-Lang Path, Yorktown Ctrl Sch Dist, **SLP**

Schlosser, Valerie Ashman 1434 Bywood Avenue, Upper Darby, PA 19082, (215) 688-8777, BS 81 Southern IL Univ -Carbondale; MS 85 Univ of MS; 87–Aud, ENT Associates Wayne PA, **A**

Schlosser, Wendy Lynn 495 Windermere Avenue, Mount Arlington, NJ 07856, (201) 398-8969, BA 84 Rutgers St Univ -N Brunswick; MA 86 Montclair St Coll; 87–Sp-Lang Path, Kessler Institute for Rehab, **SLP**

Schlueter, Sandra S 6711 South Clayton Way, Littleton, CO 80122, **SLP**

Schmaelzle, James G 5408 North Sapulpa Avenue, Oklahoma City, OK 73112, (405) 271-4477, BA 66 OK City Univ; OM 67 Univ of OK Medical Center; 88–Asst Prof/Aud Svcs Supvr, Oklahoma State Dept of Health, **A**

Schmalz, Mary J 65 St George Street #20, Brantford, ON, Canada N3R 1V2, (519) 752-7871, BA 73; MA 75 Western MI Univ; Dir/Dept of Sp-Lang Path & Aud, Brantford Gen Hosp, **SLP**

Schmalzer, Mrs Nancy 512 Alden Street, Baltimore, MD 21225, (301) 969-7078, BS 77 Towson St Univ; MS 78 Towson St Univ; Sp/Lang Path, Anne Arundel Co Pub Schs, **SLP**

Schmanski, Karen M 28111 East Jefferson, St Clair Shores, MI 48081, BS 76 Eastern MI Univ; MA 77 Eastern MI Univ; Sp-Lang Path, Bon Secours Hospital, **SLP**

Schmauss, Cheryl L 10607 Vickers Drive, Vienna, VA 22180, (703) 281-4737, **SLP**

Schmeltz, Leslie R Catch Clinic, 1208 East High Street, Davenport, IA 52803, (319) 326-2131, BS 65 Northern MI Univ; MS 71 Univ of WI - Stevens Point; Head/Catch Clinic, MS Bend AEA 9, **A**

Schmeltzer, Marguerite 1049 Buckskin Lane, Carol Stream, IL 60188, (312) 289-8130, BS 71 Northern IL Univ - De Kalb; MA 83 Northern IL Univ - De Kalb; Sp-Lang Path, Kenneyville Sch Dist 20, **SLP**

Schmelz, Mrs Janice S K 6008 Hinsdale Lane, Fort Wayne, IN 46815, BS 74 IL St Univ - Normal; MS 75 IL St Univ - Normal; SLP, East Noble Schools, **SLP**

Schmelzer, Mindy Sue 112 East 84 Street, New York, NY 10028, (212) 288-6262, MS 82 AR St Univ; 88–Aud, Private Practice, **A**

Schmid, Mrs Kathleen A 2709-D Laclede Station Rd, Maplewood, MO 63143, (314) 645-5412, BS 74 Southern IL Univ -Carbondale; MS 77 Southern IL Univ-Edwardsvill; Sp-Lang Path, Special School District, **SLP**

Schmida, Milton Joseph Gundersen Clinic Limited, 1836 South Avenue, La Crosse, WI 54601, (608) 783-7300, BS 85 Univ of IA; MA 87 Univ of Northern IA; 88–Aud, Gundersen Clinic, **A**

Schmidbauer, Judith A 2080 Quingate Place #322, Halifax, NS, Canada B3L 4R9, (902) 625-3100, BA 79 SUNY - Center at Buffalo; MA 81 SUNY - Center at Buffalo; Sp/Lang Path, Nova Scotia Hrng & Sp Cl, **SLP**

Schmidbauer, Lawrence M 65 St Francis Avenue, Tiffin, OH 44883, (419) 447-9811, BA 78 Univ of Toledo; BA 78 Univ of Toledo; MA 79 Bowling Green St Univ; Asst Dir Sp-Lang-Hrng/Aud, Betty Jane Rehab Cen, **A**

Schmidt, Mrs Anita M 5608 Winter Garden Court, St Louis, MO 63129-5904, (314) 487-4432, BS 80 Northeast MO St Univ; MA 81 Northeast MO St Univ; Sp-Lang Path, St Louis Co Spec Sch, **SLP**

Schmidt, Ann Eliz 12310 Skyline Drive, Jenks, OK 74037, (918) 299-6518, BA 72 Univ of Pittsburgh - Pittsburgh; MA 73 Univ of Pittsburgh - Pittsburgh; **SLP**

Schmidt, Mrs Ann W 36558 Nichols Avenue, Fremont, CA 94536, (408) 288-7777, BA 75 CA St Univ - Sacramento; BA 75 CA St Univ - Sacramento; MA 76 CA St Univ - Sacramento; Audiologist, Ear Medical Clinic, **A**

Schmidt, Barbara M 405 Davis Court #807, San Francisco, CA 94111, (415) 472-4110, BA 55 San Jose St Univ; MA 69 San Francisco St Univ; 78–Sp-Lang Path, Marin Co Offi of Ed, **SLP**

Schmidt, Mrs Barbara Teresa 32 Jackson Avenue, Rockville Centre, NY 11570, (516) 764-3440, BA 75 Adelphi Univ; MS 84 Adelphi Univ; Sp-Lang Path, Private Practice, **SLP**

Schmidt, Mrs Carol S 2921 North Shepard Avenue, Milwaukee, WI 53211, (414) 449-2422, BS 64 Univ of WI - Milwaukee; MS 68 Univ of WI - Milwaukee; Superv Sp/Lang Disabl Prog, Milwaukee Pub Sch, **SLP**

Schmidt, Catherine 10 West Spors, Le Center, MN 56057, (507) 389-1414, BS 74 Mankato St Univ; MA 77 Mankato St Univ; Early Childhood Special Lneeds, Waterville District 395, **SLP**

Schmidt, Mrs Danielle D c/o Darby, Box 494, Billings, MT 59101, (406) 252-5246, BA 64 MT St Univ; MA 65 CO St Univ; **SLP**

Schmidt, Mrs Diana Ferga 40 Park Circle Drive, Fairport, NY 14450, (315) 462-3216, BS 80 Nazareth Coll of Rochester; MS 84 Nazareth Coll of Rochester; SLP, Monroe Cnty Bd Coop Ed Serv 1

Schmidt, Mrs Donna Gail Route 1 Box 165-A, Ramsey, IN 47166, (812) 347-2161, BS 79 IN St Univ - Terre Haute; MS 85 Univ of Louisville; 79–Sp-Lang Path, East Washington Sch Corp

Schmidt, Edith W 1700 Ben Franklin Parkway, Apartment 714, Philadelphia, PA 19103, (215) 587-3203, BA 48 Depauw Univ; ME 58 Temple Univ; 58–Dir Sp-Lang Path, Magee Rehab Hosp, **SLP**

Schmidt, Elizabeth Anne 85-14 86 Street, Woodhaven, NY 11421, (718) 441-7508, BA 85 Saint John's Univ - Jamaica; MS 87 Columbia Univ Teachers Coll; **SLP**

Schmidt, Mrs Ellen D 2005 Lakeside Court, Champaign, IL 61821, (217) 352-2211, BS 74 Univ of IL - Urbana; MS 75 Univ of IL - Urbana; **SLP**

Schmidt, Janet C 219 Mansfield #2, Norton, MA 02766, BA 78 Allegheny Coll; MA 80 OH Univ - Athens; 88–Sp-Lang Path/Tchr, Walpole PS, **SLP**

Schmidt, Mrs Janet K V R R 2 Box 299, Valley Falls, KS 66088, (913) 863-2919, BS 70 Fort Hays St Univ; MS 74 Saint Cloud St Univ; SLP, Atchison-Jefferson Educ Coop, **SLP**

Schmidt, Janice O 146 McGehee Drive, Baton Rouge, LA 70815, **SLP**

Schmidt, Dr Jean W 226 Parsonage Hill Road, Short Hills, NJ 07078, (201) 376-3600, BS 55 Newark St Coll; MS 58 Kean Coll of NJ; PH 72 (Sp-Path) NY Univ; Principal, Millburn Twp Bd of Ed, **SLP**

Schmidt, John H 551 Pacific Avenue, Plymouth, MI 48170, BS 61 Central MI Univ; MA 67 Eastern MI Univ; Sp-Lang Path, Farmington Public Schools, **SLP**

Schmidt, Kathryn Jean P O Box 9062, Gillette, WY 82716, (307) 687-0596, BS 83 Univ of WY; MS 85 Univ of WY; **A**

Schmidt, Dr Marilynn Jo 409 10th Street, Warrensburg, MO 64093, BS 54 Bob Jones Univ; MA 60 Univ of Denver; PH 72 (Articulation Disorders) Univ of Denver; Prof of Sp-Lang Path, Central Missouri State U, **SLP**

Schmidt, Marjorie Thorn 221 Gus Rallis Drive, El Paso, TX 79932, (505) 589-1180, BS 68 PA St Univ - Univ Park; ME 69 Boston Univ; 88–Sp-Lang Path, Gadsden PS, **SLP**

Schmidt, Mrs Melissa Ann 809 Layton, Olathe, KS 66061, (816) 221-7565, BS 82 IA St Univ; MA 86 Univ of Northern IA

Schmidt, Mrs Nan Norton Route 2 Box 74L, Mc Gregor, TX 76657, **SLP**

Schmidt, Nancy A 255 East Golden Lane, Oak Creek, WI 53154, (414) 654-7714, BA 83 Univ of WI - Eau Claire; MS 85 Univ of WI - Milwaukee; 85–Sp-Lang Path, Dev Disabilities Svc Ctr, **SLP**

Schmidt, Mrs Pamela S 1812 Cedar Hill Road, Norman, OK 73072-3153, (405) 364-2614, BA 76 Phillips Univ; MS 78 Univ of OK Medical Center; **SLP**

Schmidt, Richard J, Jr P O Box 763, Montrose, CA 91020, (818) 705-0507, BA 73 Univ of Southern CA; MA 77 CA St Univ - Los Angeles; Sp-Lang Path, Private Practice, **SLP**

Schmidt, Richard P 806 5th Avenue North, Glasgow, MT 59230, (406) 228-9520, MS 66 Univ of Southern CA; SLP/Aud, Glasgow Sch Dist, **SLP A**

Schmidt, Robert K 730 Valley Street, Dayton, OH 45404, (513) 222-5597, BS 56 Kent St Univ; MA 67 Kent St Univ; 60–Exec Dir, Hrng & Sp Cen for Chldn/Adults, **SLP A**

Schmidt, Mrs Sandra Jeanne 1772 West Arrow Highway #206, Upland, CA 91786, (714) 624-9041, BA 84 CA St Univ - Fullerton; MA 86 CA St Univ - Fullerton; Sp-Lang Path, Claremont USD, **SLP**

Schmidt, Mrs Susan Todd 122 West Main Street, Norwalk, OH 44857-2031, (419) 639-2626, BS 82 Henderson St Univ; MS 84 Purdue Univ - West Lafayette; Sp-Lang Path, Sr Francis Rehab Hosp, **SLP**

Schmidt, Valerie J 6 Munroe Street, Woburn, MA 01801, (617) 787-3390, BA 83 SUNY - Coll at Plattsburgh; MA 85 SUNY - Coll at Plattsburgh; Sp-Lang Path, New England Rehab Hosp, **SLP**

Schmiechen, Susan Elizabeth 2011 40th Place, Des Moines, IA 50310, (303) 778-7622, OB 84 Univ of WI - Whitewater; MA 86 Univ of Denver; **A**

Schmiel, Mrs Katherine Elizabeth R R 2 Box 2490, Cramer Ridge Road, Lake George, NY 12845-9656, (216) 923-4535, **SLP**

Schmierer, Mrs Kimberly Marie 714 Vine Street, West Lafayette, IN 47906, (317) 447-6811, **A**

Schmierer, Merri S 75 Gibson Boulevard #1-C, Valley Stream, NY 11581-2007, (516) 825-1013, BA 80 George Washington Univ; MA 82 Hofstra Univ; Aud, Instrumentation Inc, **A**

Schmincke, Janet Lee 1202 1st Street, Northfield, NJ 08225-1918, (609) 652-7000, MA 85 Kent St Univ; Aud, Betty Bacharach Rehab Hospital, **A**

Schmit, Pamela S 1814 Mary Catherine Drive, Louisville, KY 40216, (502) 624-2345, OM 82 IN Univ - Bloomington; Sp-Lang Path, Ft Knox Ky Sch, **SLP**

Schmit, Mrs Sharon A 3234 Moraine Road, Cazenovia, NY 13035, (315) 445-0709, BS 70 SUNY - Center at Albany; MS 71 Syracuse Univ; Sp-Lang Path, Onondaga Madison BOCES, **SLP ACE**

Schmitke, Mrs Linda K 1424 Hawthorne Street, Grants Pass, OR 97526, (503) 476-6831, BA 73 San Diego St Univ; MA 75 San Diego St Univ; Sp/Lang Path, Private Practice, **SLP**

Schmitt, Dr John F 800 Monmouth Road, Tuscaloosa, AL 35406, (205) 348-7131, BA 71 Univ of Akron; MA 73 Univ of Akron; PH 79 (NS) Wichita St Univ; Assoc Prof, U of AL Dept of Commun Dis, **SLP**

Schmitt, Mrs Joyce Beckey 8812 Candelaria N E, Albuquerque, NM 87112, (505) 881-9722, BS 71 UT St Univ; MA 72 Univ of AZ; Sp-Lang Path, Albuquerque Pub Schs, **SLP**

Schmitt, Lane S 800 Monmouth Road, Tuscaloosa, AL 35406, (205) 877-6498, BA 74 Univ of AL- Tuscaloosa; MA 76 Univ of AL- Tuscaloosa; OM 88 Univ of AL- Tuscaloosa; 86–Mgr, Oxmoor House, **SLP**

Schmitt, Lisa L 154 1st Street, Hicksville, NY 11801, (516) 385-2872, BA 74 SUNY - Center at Buffalo; MA 76 NY Univ; Sp-Lang Path, Private Practice, **SLP**

Schmitt, Dr Philip J Dept Of Ed Fowler Hall 308, Gallaudet College, 800 Florida Avenue N E, Washington, DC 20002, (202) 651-5400, BS 54 Univ of WI - Milwaukee; MA 60 Northwestern Univ; PH 69 (NS) Univ of IL - Urbana; Prof Dept of Ed, Gallaudet Coll, **A**

Schmitt, Sharon P 2256 Loch Haven Drive, Roanoke, VA 24019, (703) 563-8732, BS 77 James Madison Univ; MS 78 James Madison Univ; SLP, **SLP**

Schmitt-Chan, Mrs Christine 2035 Lucerne Avenue, Stockton, CA 95203, (209) 944-4559, BA 79 Univ of CA - Santa Barbara; MA 83 UT St Univ; SLP-Spec Day Class-Ch, Stockton USD, **SLP**

Schmittgens, Jane T 75 Peters Circle, Southington, CT 06489, (203) 756-7843, SLP, UCP of Grtr Waterbury, **SLP**

Schmitz, Mrs Carol A W 1841 Sparling, Milford, MI 48042, (313) 360-2834, BA 77 MI St Univ; MA 79 Eastern MI Univ; Sp/Lang Path, Priv Pract, **SLP ACE**

Schmitz, Dr Henry D 1441 Avocado, Suite 208, Newport Beach, CA 92660, (714) 640-5702, BA 58 OH Northern Univ; MA 60 OH Univ - Athens; PH 68 (NS) Case Western Reserve Univ; 78, Private Practice, **A**

Schmitz, Mrs Judy C 5915 Patterson Drive, Troy, MI 48098, (313) 689-6000, BS 64 Eastern MI Univ; Sp-Lang Path, Troy Pub Sch, **SLP**

Schmitz, Julianne O 1326 Baltimore, Waterloo, IA 50704, (319) 277-3321, BA 66 Univ of Northern IA; MA 75 Univ of Northern IA; Sp-Lang Path, AEA 7, **SLP**

Schmitz, Marlies Waldstrasse 8-B 5202, Hennef, West Germany, **SLP**

Schmitz, Mrs Nancy J 3615 North 47th Street, Milwaukee, WI 53216, (414) 645-8035, BS 64 Univ of MN - Duluth; MS 71 Univ of WI - Milwaukee; Sp-Lang Path, Milwaukee Pub Sch, **SLP**

Schmitz, Mrs Nancy Wicker Route 1 Box 466, Perham, MN 56573, (218) 346-6500, BS 78 Univ of MN - Minneap-St Paul; MS 80 Saint Cloud St Univ; SLP, Perham Public Schools, **SLP**

Schmitz, Sarah E 902 8th Street, Las Vegas, NM 87701, (619) 579-2054, BA 64 San Diego St Univ; MA 74 GA Southern Coll; Sp-Lang Path, NW Nm Rehab Center, **SLP ACE**

Schmucker, Sheryl E 3970 Sabal Drive, Oviedo, FL 32765, (407) 831-6700, BA 76 FL St Univ; MS 79 FL St Univ; Sp-Lang Path, Seminole Co Schs, **SLP**

Schmunk, Mrs Linda M 84 Baylor Drive, Longmont, CO 80501, (303) 651-2172, 82–Aud, St Vrain Sch Dist, **A**

Schnabel, Beverly S 2222 N W Lovejoy, Suite 315, Portland, OR 97210, (503) 229-8455, BS 77 Portland St Univ; MS 79 Portland St Univ; 80–Aud, Private Practice, **A**

Schnabel, Corinne V 8 Pony Circle, Roslyn Heights, NY 11577, BA 75 CUNY - Queens Coll; MA 77 CUNY - Queens Coll; 88–Sp-Lang Path, NYC Bd of Educ, **SLP ACE**

Schnabel, Mary Frances 1176 Topaz Avenue, San Jose, CA 95117, (408) 248-1991, MA 88 San Jose St Univ; 88–Sp-Lang Path, Berryessa USD

Schnack, Lori Rae 325 Coronado Street, Balboa, CA 92661, (714) 673-1985, BA 75 Bethel Coll; MA 85 CA St Univ - Fullerton; **SLP**

Schnack, Mrs Susan Guthrie 818 18th Street NW Suite 520, Washington, DC 20006, (202) 466-4270, BS 85 WV Univ; MA 87 George Washington Univ; 87–Aud/Mgr, Audiphone Washington Co Inc, **A**

Schnaittacher, Mrs Esther Kimberg 55 Walthery Avenue, Ridgewood, NJ 07450, (516) 764-4567, **SLP**

Schnebelen, Cheryl H 1916 Frazer Avenue N W, Canton, OH 44709, **SLP**

Schnee, Mrs Karen Fern 10731 Belmar Avenue, Northridge, CA 91326, (818) 368-3543, BA 74 Univ of CA - Berkeley; MA 77 CA St Univ - Northridge; MA 80 CA St Univ - Northridge; Sp-Lang Path, Private Practice, **SLP**

Schneeberger, Jeanne Professional Hearing Serv Inc, 2354 Hassell Road, Hoffman Estates, IL 60195, (312) 490-1670, BA 76 Univ of Denver; MA 78 Univ of Denver; Aud, Prof Hrng Serv Ltd, **A**

Schneider, Barbara Ann 541 Church Avenue, Woodmere, NY 11598, (516) 295-4149, BA 83 Adelphi Univ; MS 85 Adelphi Univ; **SLP**

Schneider, Beth Ellen 3359 Cochise Drive, Pittsburgh, PA 15241, (412) 835-4757, BS 83 Purdue Univ - West Lafayette; MS 85 Purdue Univ - West Lafayette; **A**

Schneider, Bonnie S Newington Childrens Hospital, 181 East Cedar Street, Newington, CT 06111, (203) 667-5320, BS 73 SUNY - Center at Buffalo; MS 74 Columbia Univ Teachers Coll; Supvr, Newington Chldns Hosp, **A**

Schneider, Carol Ruth 10818 Whiterim Drive, Potomac, MD 20854, (301) 762-6606, BA 77 Univ of MD - College Park; MA 84 George Washington Univ; Sp-Lang Path, Montgomery Co Pub Sch, **SLP**

Schneider, Daniel C Genesee Hearing Services, 61 Wehrle Drive, Buffalo, NY 14225, (716) 837-6213, BA 71 SUNY - Center at Buffalo; MA 77 SUNY - Center at Buffalo; Aud, Genesee Hearing Svcs, **A**

Schneider, Mrs Deborah L 3207 Catesby Street, St Charles, MO 63301, (314) 925-2750, BS 76 Northeast MO St Univ; MA 77 Northeast MO St Univ; **SLP**

Schneider, Debra Ann 104 Lenox Avenue, Lynbrook, NY 11563, (516) 663-1084, **SLP**

Schneider, Diana Rose 5610 S E Flavel Street, Portland, OR 97206, (503) 230-1111, BS 80 Univ of OR; MS 85 Portland St Univ; Sp-Lang Path, Providence Med Cen, **SLP ACE**

Schneider, Mrs Donna Segal 36-06 Raven Crest Drive, Plainsboro, NJ 08536, (609) 799-8352, BA 83 IN Univ - Bloomington; MS 85 Purdue Univ - West Lafayette; Audiologist, **A**

Schneider, Dorothy E 215 Hanford Drive, Fairfield, CT 06430, (203) 254-2391, BS 71 OH Univ - Athens; MS 75 Columbia Univ Teachers Coll; Sp-Lang Path, Fairfield Board of Education, **SLP**

Schneider, Mrs Elaine Dolgin 699 West 239th Street Apt 1T, Riverdale, NY 10463, (212) 549-7166, BA 78 SUNY - Center at Buffalo; MA 80 Hofstra Univ; Sp-Lang Path, Private Practice, **SLP**

Schneider, Dr Elaine Fogel Antelope Valley Language, Movement & Sp Therapy Ctr, 727 West Lancaster Blvd, Lancaster, CA 93534, (805) 945-7878, MA 69 CUNY - Queens Coll; MA 77 NY Univ; PH 85 (Psychology) CUNY - Queens Coll; 81–Exec Dir, Antelope Valley Sp Lang Cen, **SLP**

Schneider, Mrs Eve 259 West Johnson Street, Apartment E-2, Philadelphia, PA 19144, (215) 951-8915, BA 66 Boston Univ; MA 80 Temple Univ; Aud, Germantown Hosp & Med Cen, **A**

Schneider, Grace E 83 Mohican Road, Blairstown, NJ 07825, (201) 362-9505, BA 63 William Paterson Coll; 86–Sp-Lang Path, Newton Memorial Hosp, **SLP**

Schneider, Mrs Harriet Shapiro 49 Jefferson Avenue, Short Hills, NJ 07078, (201) 564-7572, BA 78 William Paterson Coll; MS 79 William Paterson Coll; Sp-Lang Path, Private Practice, **SLP**

Schneider, Helene Mary Dales's Barclay Apts #5, Barclays Street, Saugerties, NY 12477, (914) 338-9320, BS 81 SUNY - Coll at Geneseo; MA 83 Univ of IL - Urbana; 83–Supervisor SLP Dept, UCP of Ulster Co Inc, **SLP**

Schneider, Mrs Ilene F 8519 Victory Lane, Potomac, MD 20854, (301) 279-9040, BA 65 CUNY - Queens Coll; ME 68 CUNY - Queens Coll; Sp-Lang Path, Montgomery City Pub Schs, **SLP**

Schneider, Mrs Kathryn J 240 Ash Street, Oregon City, WI 53575, (608) 835-7443, BS 73 Univ of WI - Stevens Point; MS 77 Univ of WI - River Falls; 87–Sp-Lang Path, Stoughton Area Sch, **SLP**

Schneider, Kathy Elaine 4057 South 70th Street, Milwaukee, WI 53220, BS 77 Univ of WI - Milwaukee; MS 78 Univ of WI - Milwaukee; 79–Sp-Lang Path, Elmbrook Sch Dist, **SLP**

Schneider, Kerri Dee 909 Avenue E, Powell, WY 82435, (307) 754-9763, BA 84 Univ of WY; MS 86 Univ of WY; 86–Sp-Lang Path, Absaroka Head Start, **SLP**

Schneider, Mrs Lianne P 118 Cherry Hill Road, De Witt, NY 13214, (315) 446-2292, BA 67 Univ of Toronto - Ontario; MS 69 Syracuse Univ; Sp-Lang Path, Jamesville School District, **SLP LM**

Schneider, Mrs Linda R Holbrook Speech & Hearing Clinic, 24 Middle Lane, Jericho, NY 11753, (516) 681-8961, BA 72 Montclair St Coll; MA 73 CUNY - City College; Sp Reahab Consult, Holbrook Sp-Hrng Cl, **SLP**

Schneider, Dr Marie J 2534 Mountain Drive, Upland, CA 91786, (714) 982-3849, BA 55; MA 65 Univ of CA - Los Angeles; PH 75 (NS); **SLP LM**

Schneider, Marsha Jolene 221 Wintergreen Drive, Noblesville, IN 46060-8895, (317) 773-9264, BS 82 Southern IL Univ-Edwardsvill; MS 84 Southern IL Univ-Edwardsvill; 88–Sp-Lang Path, Hancock-South Madison Svcs, **SLP**

Schneider, Mrs Mary Jane 445 3rd Avenue, Jasper, IN 47546, (812) 482-5714, BS 60 Saint Louis Univ; **SLP**

Schneider, Mrs Mary Walters 4330 Timberbrook Drive, Canfield, OH 44406, (216) 788-2481, BS 75 Kent St Univ; MA 87 Kent St Univ; 79–Sp-Lang Path, Mahoning Co Ofc of Educ

Schneider, Megan Allen 24 Maple Road, Longmeadow, MA 01106, (413) 567-3055, BA 73 Univ of MA - Amherst; MA 75 Univ of MA - Amherst; Consult, Private Practice, **A**

Schneider, Michael D 4401 Dorthea Street, Yorba Linda, CA 92686-2625, MS

Schneider, Nancy 592 Stratford Road, Union, NJ 07083, (201) 456-4967, BA 81 Montclair St Coll; MA 83 Univ of MD - College Park; 87–Aud, Audiology Service, **A ACE**

Schneider, Mrs Paula 1412 Woodvale, Bedford, TX 76021, (817) 571-0086, BA 72 Univ of Houston - Univ Park; MA 74 Univ of Houston - Univ Park; **SLP**

Schneider, Paula Kathleen 22585 Maywood Court, Farmington Hills, MI 48024, (313) 745-8903, BA 79 Ball St Univ; MA 84 Wayne St Univ; Aud, Children's Hosp of Michigan, **A**

Schneider, Dr Phillip A 3935 Blackstone Avenue, Apartment 7-B, Riverdale, NY 10471, (212) 543-2111, BA 71 CUNY - City College; MA 74 CUNY - Queens Coll; ED 80 (Sp Science) Columbia Univ Teachers Coll; Sp-Lang Path, Private Practice, **SLP**

Schneider, Sandra L 4660 Ocean Boulevard #Q-2, Sarasota, FL 34242, (813) 349-8236, BS 73 Western MI Univ; MS 75 Vanderbilt Univ; Sp-Lang Path, Sarasota Co Sch, **SLP**

Schneider, Mrs Sandra S 174 Krawski Drive, South Windsor, CT 06074, (203) 688-6401, BS 73 SUNY - Center at Albany; MA 83 Saint Joseph Coll; Sp-Lang Path, Hampden Pub Sch, **SLP**

Schneider, Mrs Sandra V 3318 East Sample, Fresno, CA 93710, (209) 441-3040, BA 71 Vanderbilt Univ; MA 73 CA St Univ - Fresno; Tchr, Fresno USD, **SLP**

Schneider, Susan B 3751 Pebble Beach Road, Northbrook, IL 60062, (312) 498-1962, BA 73 Washington Univ; MA 75 Northwestern Univ; Sp-Lang Path, Susan B Schneider, **SLP**

Schneider, Susan L 825 8th Street, Ames, IA 50010, (515) 232-7583, BA 77 Univ of NE - Lincoln; MA 78 Univ of NE - Lincoln; Sp-Lang Path, Heartland AEA, **SLP**

Schneiderman, Dr Carl Royce Valley Children's Hospital, 3151 North Millbrook, Fresno, CA 93703, (209) 225-3000, BA 65 Willamette Univ; MS 66 Western OR St Coll; PH 69 (Sp-Lang Path) SUNY - Center at Buffalo; Admin-Rehab Svcs, Valley Chlrns Hosp, **SLP**

Schneiderman, Dr Jeffrey R 9604 Cortez Road West, Unit 336, Bradenton, FL 34210, (813) 746-5171, BA 68 Upsala Coll; MA 72 Newark St Coll; PH 78 (NS) FL St Univ; 87–Exceptional Stu Educ Coord, Sch Bd of Manatee County, **SLP**

Schneiders, Marie H 405 Hurley Avenue, Rockville, MD 20850, (301) 340-1932, BA 70 Chestnut Hill Coll; MS 79 Univ of the DC; Sp-Lang Path, Private Practice, **SLP**

Schneier, Mrs Charlene M 1007 Fraser Road, Philadelphia, PA 19118, (215) 233-5218, BS 61 Boston Univ; MS 62 Univ of WI - Madison; 79–Sp-Lang Path, Sch Dist of Phila, **SLP**

Schneier, Mrs Dorothy B 36 Woodmere Road, North Brunswick, NJ 08902, (609) 466-2989, BS 64 Emerson Coll; MS 81 Rutgers St Univ - Newark; Sp-Lang Path, The Rock Brook School, **SLP**

Schnell, Roxanne 8203 South Strub Avenue, Whittier, CA 90602, (213) 726-1225, BA 76 Whittier Coll; MA 79 Whittier Coll; Prgm Spec, Montebello USD, **SLP**

Schneller, Carol Ann 336 South Palouse Street, Apartment 2, Walla Walla, WA 99362, (509) 525-3320, BA 70 WA St Univ; MS 71 Univ of OR; Sp-Lang Path, St Mary Med Cen, **SLP ACE**

Schneller, Mrs Wendy D 31 Glover Road, Needham, MA 02194, BS 70 Boston Univ; MS 71 Adelphi Univ; Sp-Lang Path, Wellesley PS, **SLP**

Schnider, Mrs Evelyn H 111 Hamlet Hill Run #1302, Baltimore, MD 21210, (301) 661-2800, BS 65 Towson St Univ; MA 71 Univ of MD - College Park; Sp-Lang Path, Bd of Ed Baltimore Co, **SLP**

Schnieders, Mrs Susan S Rural Route 2, West Branch, IA 52358, (319) 351-2510, BS 69 Univ of IA; MA 70 Univ of IA; SLP, Grant Wood AEA, **SLP**

Schnip, Barbara S 205 Wightman Avenue, Norwich, CT 06360, (203) 887-9355, BS 71 Boston Univ; ME 72 Boston Univ; Sp/Lang Path, Private Practice, **SLP**

Schnipper, Philip D 204 East Dean Street, Freeport, NY 11520-2421, (516) 884-4670, MS 73 Bradley Univ; **SLP**

Schnitzer, Dr Marc L Universidad de Puerto Rico, Box B-G, Ingles-Humanidades, Rio Piedras, PR 00931, (809) 731-9215, BA 68 Cornell Univ; MA 70 Univ of Rochester; PH 71 (Linguistics) Univ of Rochester; 88–Dir-Programa de Linguistica, U of Puerto Rico, **SLP**

Schnitzer, Ruth Ellen 1529 P Street N W #3, Washington, DC 20005, (202) 265-8526, MS 88 Gallaudet Coll

Schnob, Carol A RFD #1 Box 80-A, Morrisonville, NY 12962, BA 74 SUNY - Coll at Plattsburgh; MA 86 SUNY - Coll at Plattsburgh; **SLP**

Schnoebelen, Judy Shackman 5121 Luverne Avenue, Minneapolis, MN 55419, BS 83 Univ of WI - Madison; MS 85 Univ of WI - Madison; **SLP**

Schnorbus, Ann Elizabeth 27 Lake Street, Apt #1, Fort Wright, KY 41011, (606) 371-6366, **SLP**

Schnorr, John R 200 South Orchard, Northfield, MN 55057, (507) 645-8866, BA 78 Saint Cloud St Univ; MS 81 Univ of TX - Dallas; Sp/Lang Path, Northfield PS, **SLP**

Schnugg, Jill Taylor 1840 White Oak Drive, Menlo Park, CA 94025, (415) 821-8014, BS 71 Univ of CA - San Diego; MS 80 Purdue Univ - West Lafayette; Sp-Lang Path Dept Coord, San Francisco General Hosp, **SLP**

Schnur, Mrs Jane R 25 Laurel Leaf Drive, Gales Ferry, CT 06335, (203) 739-2922, BS 60; Sp/Lang Path, East Lyme Bd of Ed, **SLP**

Schnur, Dr Marvin R 25 Laurel Leaf Drive, Gales Ferry, CT 06335, (203) 447-3056, BA 55 OH St Univ; MS 63 Long Island U - Brooklyn Ctr; ED 71 (Aud Perception Sp-Lang Path) Columbia Univ Teachers Coll; Dept Head Sp-Lang Hrng, New London Publ Schs, **SLP**

Schnurr, Ruth Glesne 6793 Deepwater Point Road, Williamsburg, MI 49690, (616) 938-1318, MA 66 Univ of IA; 87–Sp-Lang Path, Traverse Bay Area In Sch Dist, **SLP**

Schober-Peterson, Debra Lynn 1003 South Mattis Avenue, Apartment 1-1, Champaign, IL 61821, (217) 333-2230, BS 82 IL St Univ - Normal; MA 85 Univ of IL - Urbana; PH 88 (Language Development) Univ of IL - Urbana; 88–Visiting Asst Prof, Univ of IL-Urbana, **SLP**

Schoch, Candace J 103 Stony Way, Norristown, PA 19403, (215) 272-5155, BS 74 Marquette Univ; MS 75 Marquette Univ; Supervisor Sp-Lang Path & Aud, New Medico, **SLP**

Schock, Mrs Diane M 821 Greenwood Drive, Lodi, CA 95240, (209) 944-4756, BA 78 CA St Univ - Stanislaus; MA 80 CA St Univ - Stanislaus; SLP, Stockton USD, **SLP**

Schock, Pamela Lynn 1158 Marion Street #10, Denver, CO 80218-2049, (303) 894-0745, BS 82 Northern AZ Univ; MS 84 Northern AZ Univ; **SLP**

Schockow, Mrs Tammy Anne 280 Palmer Road, Churchville, NY 14428, (716) 352-2440, BS 81 Nazareth Coll of Rochester; MS 83 Nazareth Coll of Rochester; Tchr, Monroe-2 Orleans BOCES, **SLP**

Schoder, Mrs Debra J 6376 Marina Drive, Prospect, KY 40059, (502) 228-2057, BS 76 SUNY - Coll at Geneseo; MS 80 Southern CT St Univ; Sp-Lang Path, **SLP**

Schodorf, Dr Jean Kurtis 11303 West Alderny, Wichita, KS 67212, (316) 722-2714, BA 72 Univ of NM; MS 73 Univ of NM; PH 81 (NS) Wichita St Univ; Consultant Sp-Lang Path, Kansas Elks Training Cen, **SLP**

Schoeberle, Leesa Jones 504 Bethel Road, Apartment 906, Morganton, NC 28655, (704) 438-9302, BA 83 Univ of NC - Chapel Hill; MS 85 Univ of NC - Chapel Hill; 87–Sp-Lang Path, Western Carolina Ctr, **SLP**

Schoen, Constance M 2832 Sugar Pine Circle, Northbrook, IL 60062, (312) 932-4599, BA 75 Univ of MN - Minneap-St Paul; MS 77 Univ of WI - Madison; 86–Sp-Lang Path, Private Practice, **SLP**

Schoen, Madelyn K 412 36th Street, West Des Moines, IA 50265, (515) 255-0483, BS 74 Univ of IA; MA 75 MI St Univ; Sp-Lang Path, IA Methodist Med Cen, **SLP**

Schoen, Mrs Mary Stephanie 621 Oak Street, East Hartford, CT 06118, BA 75 Univ of CA - Santa Barbara; MA 78 Univ of CT; 79–Sp-Lang Path, Glastonbury PS, **SLP**

Schoen, Paula Hollins 3413 Tezcucco Drive, Baton Rouge, LA 70820, (504) 767-2262, **SLP**

Schoen, Rosanne Z 138-10 Franklin Avenue #5K, Flushing, NY 11355, (516) 579-9120, BA 68 CUNY - Brooklyn Coll; MA 70 NY Univ; 79–Sp-Lang Path, E Meadow Un Fr Sch Dist, **SLP**

Schoenagel, Mrs Alyce Tomiko 1411 Kahoe Road, Forest Hill, MD 21050, (301) 836-9358, BS 78 Bloomsburg Univ of PA; MS 79 Bloomsburg Univ of PA; Sp-Lang Path, Harford Co Pub Sch, **SLP**

Schoenberg, Barbara 1120 Barcroft Court, Naperville, IL 60540, BS 69 Univ of WI - Madison; MS 71 Univ of WI - Madison; ME 82 Northern IL Univ - De Kalb; 88–Sp-Lang Path, Il Dist #203, **SLP**

Schoenberg, Mrs Marlene C 411 South Warwick Street, St Paul, MN 55105, (612) 699-9233, BA 72 CUNY - City College; ME 73 Boston Univ; 87–Dir, Ethnic Communication Arts, **SLP**

Schoenberg, Mrs Rena Dreskin 3386 Heathcliff Lane, Jacksonville, FL 32217, (904) 731-5038, BS 77 Vanderbilt Univ; MA 79 Univ of FL; Sp-Lang Path, S Allen Smith Clinic, **SLP**

Schoenbrodt-Myers, Mrs Lisa Ann 4089 Old Columbia Pike #A, Ellicott City, MD 21043-5412, (301) 461-8683, BA 82 Univ of MD - College Park; MS 84 James Madison Univ; Sp-Lang Path, Allied Sp Path Svcs, **SLP ACE**

Schoenfeld, Debra 612 North Maple Drive, Beverly Hills, CA 90210, (213) 859-2922, BA 76 CA St Univ - Northridge; MA 78 CA St Univ - Northridge; Sp-Lang Path, Wilshire Hrng & Sp Cen, **SLP**

Schoenfeld, Julie T 929 South Main, Shawano, WI 54166, (715) 526-5258, BS 85 Univ of WI - Milwaukee; MS 87 Marquette Univ; 87–Sp-Lang Path, CESA #8, **SLP**

Schoenfeld, Sidney L 9038 Watsonia Court, Olivette, MO 63132, (314) 569-8100, BS 53 Washington Univ; MS 58 Washington Univ; Area Coord, Spec Sch Dist, **A**

Schoenfelder, Gail L 100 Kay Street, Ithaca, NY 14850, (607) 257-6831, BA 67 MacAlster Coll; MS 74 Saint Cloud St Univ; Sp-Lang Path, Spec Chldn Ctr-Head Start Site, **SLP**

Schoenhofer, Deborah Heidi 570 Cathcart Street, Winnipeg, MB, Canada R3R 0S6, (204) 261-3305, BA 82 Univ of Manitoba - Winnipeg; MS 85 Univ of ND; 88–Sp-Lang Path, Child Care & Dev Branch, **SLP**

Schoenleber, Gloria Jean 305 Madison NE, Albuquerque, NM 87108, (505) 884-8282, BA 83 Duquesne Univ; MA 85 George Washington Univ; Sp-Lang Path, Assessment Systems Inc, **SLP**

Schoenmakers, Steve Dell 1626 Cliffdale, Pueblo, CO 81006, (719) 546-4220, **SLP**

Schoen-Rene, Mrs Patricia Anne 8 Harlowe Street, Rockville, CT 06066, BS 81 Ithaca Coll; MS 83 PA St Univ - Univ Park; SLP, Corning-Pp Area Sch Dist, **SLP**

Schoeny, Dr Zahrl G University Of Virginia, Speech Language Hearing Ce, 132 Emmet Street Box 9022, Charlottesville, VA 22906-9022, (804) 924-4620, BS 61 Northern IL Univ - De Kalb; MA 64 Univ of KS; PH 68 (NS) Northwestern Univ; Associate Professor, U of VA-Dept Sp Pat & Aud, **SLP A**

Schoepf, Thomas J Route 1 Box 28, Little Falls, MN 56345, (612) 632-2921, BA 74 Univ of MN - Duluth; MS 78 Univ of WI - Eau Claire; Spec Ed Coord, Mid-St Ed Agcy, **SLP**

Schoepflin, Janet Reath 18 Stuyvesant Oval #6H, New York, NY 10009, (212) 254-9868, BA 71 PA St Univ - Univ Park; MA 80 Temple Univ; **A ACE**

Schoepp, Mrs Donna J 118 Carley Drive, West Sayville, NY 11796, (516) 567-7386, BS 76 SUNY - Coll at Buffalo; MA 78 Hofstra Univ; Sp/Lang Path, Eastport Public Schools, **SLP**

Schoeppner, Mrs Carol T 2938 Majestic Terrace, Las Cruces, NM 88001, (505) 522-0980, BS 83 Eastern NM Univ; MA 85 NM St Univ; 87–Sp-Lang Path, InSpeech Inc, **SLP**

Schoer, Felicia E 28 Colorado Court, Syosset, NY 11791, (516) 364-9437, BA 77 CUNY - Brooklyn Coll; MA 78 Hofstra Univ; Sp-Lang Path, Private Practice, **SLP**

Schofer, Mrs Joan W 16127 Deer Lake Road, Derwood, MD 20855, (313) 341-1353, BS 76 Univ of IL - Urbana; MS 78 PA St Univ - Univ Park; Audiologist, Montgomery County Health Dept, **A**

Schohl, Mrs Betty Jane 1721 Bonita Drive, Knoxville, TN 37918, (615) 579-2454, BA 75 Univ of MI - Ann Arbor; MS 76 Univ of MI - Ann Arbor; 88–Aud, Tenn Sch for the Deaf, **A**

Scholer, Sally E 2832 Redwing Road, Fort Collins, CO 80525, BS 72 CO St Univ; MS 73 CO St Univ; Aud, Thompson Sch Dist R2-J, **A**

Scholl, Dr Hannah H 1 Half Moon Isle, Port Liberte, Jersey City, NJ 07305, (201) 915-4285, BA 48 CUNY - Hunter Coll; MA 49 Columbia Univ Teachers Coll; PH 59 (Sp-Lang Path) Columbia Univ Teachers Coll; Sp-Lang Path, Private Practice, **SLP**

Scholl, Dr Harold M 1 Half Moon Isle, Port Liberte, Jersey City, NJ 07305, (201) 435-4100, OB 46 CUNY - Bernard M Baruch Coll; OM 49 CUNY - Bernard M Baruch Coll; ED 57 (Sp Path) Columbia Univ Teachers Coll; Sp-Lang Path, Private Practice, **SLP A F ACE**

Scholl, Mrs Kay L Amarillo Speech Hearing & Lang, 1300 Wallace Boulevard, Amarillo, TX 79121, (806) 359-7681, BS 61 Univ of NE - Lincoln; ME 73 West TX St Univ; Sp-Lang Path, Amarillo Sp/Hrng/Lang Cen, **SLP**

Scholten, Mrs Connie Lynn 1612 Silver Creek Circle, Sioux Falls, SD 57106, (605) 361-7211, MA 87 Univ of SD - Vermillion; 87–Sp-Lang Path, Cornbelt Educ Coop

Scholz-Raben, Mrs Jane J 412 Palmor, Ottawa, IL 61350, (612) 421-9250, **SLP**

Schon, Terry D 201 West 89th Street, New York, NY 10024, (201) 893-4227, BS 55 Bowling Green St Univ; MA 64 CUNY - Hunter Coll; PH 68 (NS) Syracuse Univ; Assoc Prof, Montclair State Coll, **A ACE**

Schonberger, Eve B 249 John Street, South Amboy, NJ 08879, (201) 727-3090, BA 80 Rutger's St Univ - Douglas Coll; MA 81 Kean Coll of NJ; Sp-Lang Path, South Amboy Board of Education, **SLP**

Schonbrun, Les Edward 174 Williamsburg Lane, Lakewood, NJ 08701, (201) 367-4467, BS 68 Ithaca Coll; MS 71 Rutger's St Univ - Douglas Coll; Sp-Lang Path, Plumsted Twsp Sch, **SLP ACE**

Schonbrun, Mrs Vita 9754 West 115th Terrace, Overland Park, KS 66210, (913) 897-2381, BS 72 Bradley Univ; MS 74 Bradley Univ; Sp-Lang Path & Teacher, Blue Valley School District, **SLP**

Schons, Barbara R Rural Route 1, Stoney Point, Storm Lake, IA 50588, (712) 732-2257, BA 71 Saint Cloud St Univ; MS 72 Saint Cloud St Univ; Sp Lang Cl, Arrowhead AEA, **SLP**

School, Grace M 120 East Harris Street, P O Box 2019, Appleton, WI 54913, (414) 735-6111, **SLP**

Schoolcraft, Mary C 2026 Anchor #4, San Antonio, TX 78213, (512) 494-3172, BS 77 Southwest TX St Univ; ME 78 Southwest TX St Univ; Sp-Lang Path, N E ISD-Coker Element, **SLP**

Schooling, Mrs Margaret Goldbach 1596 New Danville Pike, Lancaster, PA 17603, (215) 232-1475, BS 79 Bloomsburg Univ of PA; MS 80 Bloomsburg Univ of PA; 88–Sp-Lang Path, Lancaster Sch Dist, **SLP ACE**

Schoonover, Priscilla A 7376 Brooken Staff, Columbia, MD 21045, (301) 381-0048, BS 73 PA St Univ - Univ Park; MS 74 PA St Univ - Univ Park; Sp-Lang Path, MIEMSS, **SLP**

Schopfer, Kathryn Humphreys 6835 Woodland Drive, Dallas, TX 75225, (214) 363-4049, BS 83 Univ of TX - Dallas; MS 85 Univ of TX - Dallas; **SLP**

Schopman, Nancy Graham 14 Sandown Road, Audubon, PA 19403, (215) 539-8550, BS 84 PA St Univ - Univ Park; MA 87 Temple Univ; 87–Sp-Lang Path, Montgomery Co Interm Unit, **SLP**

Schopmeyer, Betty B 3009 Homewood Parkway, Kensington, MD 20895, (301) 469-0223, BA 70 OH St Univ; MA 74 Univ of MD - College Park; Sp-Lang Path Supvr, Ivymount Sch, **SLP**

Schor, Ronnie M 328 West 86th, New York, NY 10024, **SLP**

Schorn-Bellows, Marilyn T 4000 Gillionville Rd #109, Albany, GA 31707, (912) 439-7061, BA 79 MI St Univ; MA 80 MI St Univ; 87–Aud, Easter Seal Rehab Cntr, **A**

Schorrman, Dorothy 80 East End Avenue #10C, New York, NY 10028, (718) 470-8910, BA 71 CUNY - Queens Coll; MA 73 Hofstra Univ; 73–Sp-Lang Path, Long Isl Jewish Med Ctr, **SLP**

Schory, Maria Emmi 129 Breezewood Common, East Amherst, NY 14051, (716) 688-2497, BA SUNY - Coll at Buffalo; ME 77 SUNY - Coll at Buffalo; 77–Sp-Lang Path, Buffalo Bo of Ed, **SLP**

Schosheim, Joanne Katz Speech Associates Of Boca Raton, 2499 West Glades Road Suite 301, Glades-Saint Andrews Professional Center, Boca Raton, FL 33431, (407) 368-3700, BA 79 Hofstra Univ; MS 86 Nova Univ; 88–Sp-Lang Path, Private Practice, **SLP**

Schotland, Henrietta L 1206 Birks Court, Birks Court, La Grange, IL 60525, (312) 996-7202, BA 51 CUNY - Brooklyn Coll; MA 53 Univ of IA; Cl Coord, U Il-Cen Hndcp Chldn, **SLP**

Schott, Deborah M 1156 McFarlane Avenue, Spring Hill, FL 33526, (914) 795-1033, BS 78 WV Univ; MA 79 Kent St Univ; Sp-Lang Path, Private Practice, **SLP**

Schott, Mrs Kim S 3162 Baker Drive, Concord, CA 94519, (415) 682-4292, MS 87 CA St Univ - Hayward; Sp-Lang Path, Pittsburgh USD, **SLP**

Schott, Marcella K 2820 Graysby Avenue, San Pedro, CA 90732, **SLP**

Schott-Evans, Mrs Diane M Route 3, Flowery Trail #86, Chewelah, WA 99109, (509) 935-4043, BA 74 Briar Cliff Coll; MS 76 Washington Univ; **SLP**

Schottler, Laura D 15413 West 80th Place, Lenexa, KS 66219, (913) 831-1900, BS 82 Central MO St Univ; MA 83 KS St Univ; **SLP**

Schou, Mrs Linda Ann 2012 North 45th Rd, Leland, IL 60531, (815) 495-9338, BA 78 Purdue Univ - West Lafayette; MS 81 Purdue Univ - West Lafayette; Sp-Lang Path, Leland Comm Ut Sch Dist 1, **SLP**

Schow, Ronald L Dept Speech Path & Audiology, Idaho State University, Pocatello, ID 83209, (208) 236-2853, BS 67 UT St Univ; MS 69 UT St Univ; PH 74 (NS) Northwestern Univ; Professor, ID State Univ, **A**

Schrader, Clarence H Air Force Village #1630, 4917 Ravenswood Drive, San Antonio, TX 78227, PH (NS); **SLP LM**

Schrader, Margaret A P O Box 44148, Tucson, AZ 85733, (602) 887-3516, BS 75 Univ of AZ; MS 77 Univ of AZ; Sp/Lang Path, Private Practice, **SLP ACE**

Schrader, Patricia F 5335 N Black Canyon, Phoenix, AZ 85015, (602) 242-0685, OM 84 AZ St Univ; **SLP**

Schraeder, Patricia B 317 West Fountain, Dodgeville, WI 53533, (608) 348-2611, BA 74 Univ of WI - Madison; MS 75 Univ of WI - Madison; Sp-Lang Path, Platteville Pub Sch, **SLP**

Schrager, Mrs Brenda D 728 Spring Mill Lane, Indianapolis, IN 46260, (317) 257-2295, BA 81 IN Univ - Bloomington; MA 84 IN Univ - Bloomington; Aud, John H Payne Associates Inc, **A**

Schrager, Mrs Rhea H Bon Secours Rehab Hospital, 1050 N E 125th Street, North Miami, FL 33161, (305) 891-8850, BA 57 CUNY - Hunter Coll; MS 82 Nova Univ; Superv SLP Dept, Bon Secours Hosp, **SLP**

Schram, Geraldine Elaine 200 Bay Street South #1409, Hamilton, ON, Canada L8P 4S4, (416) 526-7864, BS 78 Univ of Western Ontario; OM 80 Univ of Western Ontario; 87–Sp-Lang Path, Chedoke-McMaster Hosp Cereb Pal Ctr, **SLP**

Schram, Judith R 7433 Franklin Court, Franklin, MI 48025, (313) 855-5088, BA 72 Univ of MI - Ann Arbor; MS 74 Univ of MI - Ann Arbor; Sp-Lang Path, Private Practice, **SLP**

Schram, Mrs Susan Lex 29 Kohleen Drive, Mc Kees Rocks, PA 15136, (304) 564-3411, BS 79 Edinboro Univ of PA; MS 87 CA Univ of PA; 80–Sp-Lang Path, Hancock Co Schs, **SLP**

Schramm, Britta J 2409 Arbutus Street, Los Angeles, CA 90049, (213) 647-6274, BA 68 Temple Univ; MA 76 West Chester Univ of PA; SLP, Benchmark Sch, **SLP**

Schramm, Molly Jean 32 Split Rail, Painted Post, NY 14870, (607) 936-3700, BS 84 Kutztown Univ of PA; MA 88 SUNY - Coll at Geneseo; 84–Sp-Lang Path, Corning-Painted Post Sch Dist

Schramm, Sara Ann 522 East Chestnut, Bloomington, IL 61701, (217) 735-2361, BS 83 IL St Univ - Normal; BS 84 IL St Univ - Normal; Sp-Lang Path, Lincoln Dev Ctr, **SLP**

Schramm, Mrs Teresa Natale 26 Turtle Dove Court, Gaithersburg, MD 20879, (301) 990-0298, BS 75 Bloomsburg Univ of PA; ME 76 Bloomsburg Univ of PA; Sp-Lang Path, Delaware Co Inter Ut, **SLP**

Schranz, Mrs Nancy M 183 Georgia Avenue, North Kingstown, RI 02852, (401) 295-2421, BS 79 SUNY - Coll at Fredonia; MS 81 SUNY - Coll at Buffalo; SLP, Hearing Speech & Lang Services, **SLP**

Schraub, Stacy 255-25 149th Avenue, Rosedale, NY 11422, (718) 528-5754, BA 86 Adelphi Univ; MS 87 Adelphi Univ; Sp-Lang Path, Herbert G Birch Early Childhood Ctr

Schreck, Byron L 31 Farmhouse Lane, Camp Hill, PA 17011, (717) 737-6728, BS 73 CA Univ of PA; MS 78 Univ of WY; Sp-Lang Path, Capital Area Intermed Unit #15, **SLP ACE**

Schreck, Karen Tulin 1231 Northover Drive, Bloomfield Hills, MI 48013, (313) 642-3734, BA 66 Univ of MD - College Park; MS 67 Univ of IL - Urbana; Sp-Lang Path, Private Practice, **SLP**

Schreffler, Amy E 168 Medway Street, Providence, RI 02906, (401) 331-6767, BA 78 Univ of Pittsburgh - Pittsburgh; MA 81 Univ of MD - College Park; Sp-Lang Path, Private Practice, **SLP**

Schreiber, Betsy C 9 Bridle Lane, Glen Cove, NY 11542, (516) 671-2073, BA 75 Emory Univ; MS 76 Emory Univ; Sp-Lang Path, Private Practice, **SLP**

Schreiber, Dale L 46 Broadview Drive, Clayton, MO 63105, (314) 727-2742, BA 70 SUNY - Center at Buffalo; MA 72 SUNY - Center at Buffalo; **A**

Schreiber, Marie Kathryn 1616 Alta Vista Avenue, Wauwatosa, WI 53213, (414) 258-7014, BA 82 Univ of WI - Eau Claire; MA 84 Univ of IL - Urbana; Sp-Lang Path, Sacred Heart Rehab Hosp, **SLP**

Schreiber, Meryl A 590 Sylvan Place, Haworth, NJ 07641, (201) 501-0742, BS 76 SUNY - Coll at New Paltz; MA 80 Montclair St Coll; 76–Sp-Lang Path, East Ramapo School, **SLP**

Schreiber, Rebecca Cronin Battles Road, Gates Mills, OH 44040, (216) 423-1121, **A**

Schreiber, Sue G 6300 Queens Drive, Apartment 3, Lincoln, NE 68516, (402) 423-0839, BS 61 Univ of NE - Lincoln; MA 71 Univ of NE - Lincoln; Sp-Lang Path, Norris Pub Sch, **SLP**

Schreiner, Mrs Elaine Holbrook 6905 White Road, Conesus, NY 14435, (716) 658-2291, BS 77 SUNY - Coll at Geneseo; MA 88 Nazareth Coll of Rochester; 88–Sp-Lang Path, BOCES, **SLP**

Schreiner-Stotz, Mrs Dee Ann P O Box 5087, Canyon Lake, CA 92380, (714) 982-5542, Aud, Professional Hearing Services, **SLP**

Schrenko, Mrs Joanna C Strickly Speaking, Stonehill At Marblehead, 33 Gerald Road, Marblehead, MA 01945, (617) 631-9565, BS 75 SUNY - Center at Albany; MS 76 SUNY - Center at Albany; Sp-Lang Path, Private Practice, **SLP**

Schrenzel, Jane R 29 Eucalyptus Drive, Irvine, CA 92715, (714) 639-4990, BA 76 Univ of CA - Santa Barbara; MA 78 Univ of WA; 86–Audiologist, Providence Speech and Hearing, **A**

Schrepfer, Mrs Betty P Route 15 Box 1930, Lake Charles, LA 70601, **SLP**

Schrepfer-Mekemson, Sheryl 202 Ashland Court, Vernon Hills, IL 60061, (312) 362-2744, MA Univ of Northern IA; **SLP**

Schreter, Beatrice 420 East 72nd Street #20-E, New York, NY 10021, (212) 472-6050, BA 73 CUNY - Lehman Coll; MA 75 CUNY - Queens Coll; 84–SLP, New York Hospital Cornell Univ, **SLP**

Schreuder, Mary Sue 1353 Van Auken SE, Apt C, Grand Rapids, MI 49508, (616) 246-5173, MA 84 Western MI Univ; 84–Aud, Grand Rapids Pb Schs, **A**

Schreurs, Kevin K 2038 26th Avenue N W, Rochester, MN 55901, (507) 284-2577, BA 61 Univ of Northern IA; MA 65 Univ of Northern IA; Audiologist, Mayo Clinic, **SLP A**

Schrimper, Mrs Patricia Beilhart 3434 Maxim Drive, Fort Wayne, IN 46815, (219) 482-1334, BS 70 Old Dominion Univ; MA 75 Eastern MI Univ; Sp/Lang Path, Allen Co Soc for Crippled Children & Adults, **SLP**

Schripsema, Lois Elaine 996 Kenwood Drive, Holland, MI 49423, (616) 857-2139, BS 81 Central MI Univ; MA 82 Central MI Univ; 83–Sp-Lang Path, Saugatuck Pub Sch, **SLP**

Schrock, Mrs Adeleen S 610 Luzerne Street, Johnstown, PA 15905, (814) 536-5096, BS 38 Northwestern Univ; SLP, Childrens Development Center, **LM**

Schrock, Kathleen C 2240 West Sunset Drive, Inverness, IL 60067, (312) 259-2189, BS Muhlenberg Coll; MS Marquette Univ; **SLP**

Schrock, Laura L 506 West Sandusky Street, Findlay, OH 45840-3224, (419) 423-5308, BA 81 Heidelberg Coll; MS 86 Bowling Green St Univ; 86–Sp-Lang Path, Betty Jane Memorial Rehab Ctr, **SLP**

Schrock, Patricia Bradley 5405 Baltimore Drive #46, La Mesa, CA 92041-2779, (619) 274-9871, **SLP**

Schroder, Mrs Karen K 3630 Tanglewood Drive N W, Atlanta, GA 30339, (404) 432-0822, BA 71 Emory Univ; MS 74 Emory Univ; **SLP**

Schroder, Thomas L 4066 Oregon Trail, Martinez, GA 30907, (404) 860-3512, BS 73 Fort Hays St Univ; MA 74 Wichita St Univ; 88–Aud, Augusta Hearing Institute, **A**

Schroeder, Mrs Ann Lawrence 7360 Coffman Road, Indianapolis, IN 46268, (317) 299-2911, BA 80 IN Univ - Bloomington; MA 82 IN Univ - Bloomington; Sp-Lang Path, Methodist Hosp, **SLP**

Schroeder, Mrs Brenda Brownlee 312 Deerfield, Irvine, CA 92714-7606, (714) 638-6384, BS 82 UT St Univ; MS 84 UT St Univ; 85–Sp-Lang Path, Garden Grove USD, **SLP**

Schroeder, Mrs Catherine 411 3rd Street, Wakefield, NE 68784, (402) 287-2061, BA 77 Univ of ME - Orono; MA 78 Memphis St Univ; Sp-Lang Path, Esu #1, **SLP**

Schroeder, Mrs Catherine Route 1 Box 99, Plymouth, NE 68424, (402) 729-2418, BS 80 Univ of NE - Lincoln; MS 81 Univ of NE - Lincoln; Sp/Lang Path, Fairbury Pub Sch, **SLP**

Schroeder, Elaine 3630 Austin Street, Corpus Christi, TX 78411, (512) 241-9026, BS 71 Univ of TX - Austin; MA 76 Our Lady Lake Univ-San Anton; Sp-Lang Path, Tuloso-Midway ISD, **SLP**

Schroeder, Ellen K 3900 Bailey Avenue #7-J, Bronx, NY 10463, (212) 543-2506, **SLP**

Schroeder, Karen Elizabeth 523 Robert E Lee, New Orleans, LA 70124, (504) 595-6153, MS 87 Univ Southern MS-Hattiesburg

Schroeder, Katherine Marie 802 South Belgrade Road, Silver Spring, MD 20902, (301) 649-1775, MS 88 Towson St Univ

Schroeder, Linda L 9209 Fletcher Drive, La Mesa, CA 92041, (619) 438-6653, BA 60 4689; MA 68 4689; MA 79 4689; Audiologist, San Diego City Schools, **A**

Schroeder, Marjorie A 8116 Clear Brook Drive, Raleigh, NC 27609, (919) 755-3021, BA 78 Univ of FL; ME 79 Univ of FL; Sp/Lang Path, Rex Hosp, **SLP**

Schroeder, Mrs Nancy H 805 Ralston Avenue, Defiance, OH 43512, (419) 352-6531, BS 64 Univ of KY; MS 67 Vanderbilt Univ; Aud, Wood Co Off of Ed, **A ACE**

Schroeder, Scott C 3111 N E 57th Street, Portland, OR 97213, (503) 230-1111, BS 78 Portland St Univ; MA 81; Sp-Lang Path, Good Samaritan Hosp, **SLP**

Schroeder, Susan Hill 352 Roxbury Street, Keene, NH 03431, (603) 357-2221, BS 70 Mount Holyoke Coll; MS 83 Univ of AL- Tuscaloosa; 84–Sp-Lang Path, Keene School District, **SLP**

Schroeder, Mrs Tamara P 227-07 64th Avenue, Bayside, NY 11364, (212) 224-1425, BA 45 CUNY - Brooklyn Coll; MA 46 Northwestern Univ; **SLP LM**

Schroeder, Virginia Marie 303 Charlesworth, Dearborn Heights, MI 48127, BA 80 MI St Univ; MA 82 Wayne St Univ - Sch of Med; **A**

Schroeder-Oswalt, Ann 3932 Carlton Avenue, Columbus, OH 43227, (614) 231-6721, BS 83 Univ of WI - Madison; MA 84 Case Western Reserve Univ; **SLP**

Schrott, Mrs Ruth G 2304 Rosedown Drive, Reston, VA 22091, (703) 273-5389, BA 62 Baylor Univ; SLP, Fairfax Co Pub Sch, **SLP**

Schruntek, Dr Agnes M 21 Hastings Drive, Fort Salonga, NY 11768, (516) 261-4400, BS 60 Saint John's Univ - Jamaica; MS 62 Saint John's Univ - Jamaica; Sp-Lang Path, St Charles Hosp, **SLP ACE**

Schuber, Mrs Suzanne Perez 110 Chamale Cove, Slidell, LA 70460, (504) 641-8752, Aud, Dr Trail, **A**

Schubert, Annegret 429 Tompkins Street, Syracuse, NY 13204, (315) 422-2761, BA 76 SUNY - Center at Buffalo; MA 78 SUNY - Center at Buffalo; Sp-Lang Path, Syracuse Sch Dist, **SLP**

Schubert, Dr George W University Of North Dakota, P O Box 8026, Grand Forks, ND 58202, (701) 777-3531, BS 62 Univ of WI - LA Crosse; MS 65 Univ of WI - Madison; PH 72 (Sp Path) Univ of WA; Prof Sp-Lang Path, Univ of ND, **SLP F**

Schuchard, Susan E 12550 Whittington #1018, Houston, TX 77077, (713) 785-6760, BS 75 Univ of TX - Austin; MA 77 Southwest TX St Univ; SLP, Sp-Lang Remediation Cen, **SLP**

Schuchman, Dr Gerald I 2227 Forest Glen Road, Silver Spring, MD 20910, BA 66 CUNY - Queens Coll; MS 68 Univ of Pittsburgh - Pittsburgh; PH 76 (NS) Univ of Pittsburgh - Pittsburgh; Aud, VA Med Cen, **A**

Schuckers, Dr Gordon Howard Louisiana St Univ Medical Ctr, Kings Highway, Shreveport, LA 71130, (318) 674-6800, BS 58 CA Univ of PA; MA 64 Univ of IA; PH 70 (Sp Sci) Univ of IL - Urbana; 86–Assoc Dean, Lsu Med Cen, **SLP F**

Schuckers, Mrs Rita Carole 1164 Runningbrook Drive, Shreveport, LA 71118, (318) 424-8263, BS 59 CA Univ of PA; MA 61 Univ of IA; Sp-Lang Path, Caddo Parish Sch Bd, **SLP**

Schuddeboom-Kelley, Mrs Joan 2804 Tahoe Drive, Merced, CA 95340, (209) 385-7000, SLP, Private Practice, **SLP**

Schudrich, Brynna Joy 1126 Commonwealth Avenue, Apartment 2, Allston, MA 02134, (301) 649-6414, **SLP**

Schuele, Clare Melanie 100 Rock Creek Drive, Apt M-302, Carrboro, NC 27510, (919) 966-4713, BS 81 Miami Univ - Oxford; MA 85 Univ of TX - Austin; 88–Sp-Lang Path, Univ of NC-Chapel Hill, **SLP**

Schuelke, Sandra H 4139 Scone, Houston, TX 77084, (713) 463-6456, BS 74 Univ of TX - Austin; MA 76 Univ of TX - Austin; Sp-Lang Path, Speech-Language Services, **SLP**

Schuerger, Karen Stafford P O Box 3143, Ketchikan, AK 99901, (907) 225-3358, BA 77 Univ of WA; OM 78 Univ of WA; 88–Sp-Lang Path, Ketchikan Gateway Sch Dist, **SLP**

Schuett, Mrs Carmen Bernice 1041 Carey Avenue, Clovis, CA 93612, (206) 299-0642, BA 80 Western WA Univ; MA 84 Western WA Univ; Sp-Lang Path, **SLP**

Schuettler, Mrs Susan Scheaffer 341 Coal Street, Port Carbon, PA 17965, (717) 622-6786, BS 78 PA St Univ - Univ Park; MS 83 Bloomsburg Univ of PA; Sp-Lang Path, Pottsville Hosp & Warne Cl, **SLP**

Schuetze, Bronwyn L 1901 Arapahoe Drive, Longmont, CO 80501, (303) 776-2914, BS 68 CO St Univ; MS 69 CO St Univ; Dir, Longmont Lrng Cen, **SLP**

Schugar, Linda R P O Box 536, Lake Forest, IL 60045, **SLP**

Schuh, Mrs Mary Joanne 3917 Bent Grass Road, Jacksonville, FL 32210, (904) 786-4878, BA 81 Univ of FL; MS 82 FL St Univ; Aud, A Sp Hrng & Stress Cl, **A**

Schuhmacher, Mrs Anita Hood 558 Schuyler Way, Union, NJ 07083, (201) 687-3019, BA 60 Newark St Coll; MA 61 Northwestern Univ; Sp-Lang Path, Cerebral Palsy League of Union County, **SLP**

Schukraft, Nancy V 1108 Sunnyside Drive, Hagerstown, MD 21740, (301) 797-1758, **SLP**

Schuldt, Marlo E P O Box 1599, Orem, UT 84057, (801) 224-2014, BS 72 Brigham Young Univ; OM 74 Brigham Young Univ; VP, Harding & Harris Inc, **SLP**

Schuleman, Mrs Barbara Ann 5751 Jason Street, Houston, TX 77096, (713) 774-5777, BA 58 Univ of MI - Ann Arbor; MA 62 Univ of MI - Ann Arbor; **SLP**

Schuler, Adriana L Dept Of Special Education, San Francisco State Univ, 1600 Holloway, San Francisco, CA 94133, (415) 932-4156, **SLP**

Schuler, Eileen 160 East 84th Street #3K, New York, NY 10028, (212) 734-8906, BA 66 CUNY - Brooklyn Coll; MS 68 CUNY - Brooklyn Coll; SLP, NYC Bd of Ed-Sp-Serv Ut, **SLP**

Schuler, Gail Lynn P O Box 326, Hazel Green, WI 53811, (608) 854-2558, BS 84 KS St Univ; OM 86 KS St Univ; 88–Sp-Lang Path, Comp P T Rehab Agency, **SLP**

Schuler, Janice M 5949 N Kilpatrick Avenue, Chicago, IL 60646, (312) 272-6158, Tchr of Phy Hndcpd, N Sub Spec Ed Dstr, **SLP**

Schuler, Kay A 65 Walnut Street, East Providence, RI 02914, (401) 438-6859, BS 85 Marquette Univ; MS 87 Marquette Univ; **SLP**

Schuler, Susan L Speech Pathology Department, 5073 Rum Creek Court S E, Kentwood, MI 49508, (617) 455-7300, BA 78 Albion Coll; MA 80 Western MI Univ; Sp/Lang Path, Private Practice, **SLP**

Schuler-Volger, Maria 447 Bunning Drive, Downers Grove, IL 60516, BA 77 IN Univ - Bloomington; MS 78 IN Univ - Bloomington; Systems Analyst, Continental Bank, **A**

Schulist, Carol 2606 Everglade Street, Santa Ana, CA 92704, (714) 545-4114, MA 88 Northwestern Univ

Schulkin, Mrs Florence P 5736 Wallis Lane, Woodland Hills, CA 91367, (818) 883-0322, BA 50 Univ of MI - Ann Arbor; MA 72 CA St Univ - Northridge; **SLP**

Schulman, Jill Theise 7 Ginger Court, Newtown, PA 18940, (215) 860-5584, MA 84 Trenton St Coll; BA 82 Long Island U - CW Post Ctr; **SLP**

Schulman, Linda S 1201 Hillgrove Place, Beverly Hills, CA 90210, **SLP**

Schulman-Heffley, Mrs Sharon 3113 Waterside Lane, Alexandria, VA 22309, (703) 780-0412, BA 70 Univ of Pittsburgh - Pittsburgh; MA 72 Univ of Pittsburgh - Pittsburgh; 87–Pvt Prac, Accent Modification Center of No VA, **SLP**

Schulstad, Lorie Jean 510 Jackson Street, Hutchinson, MN 55350-9076, (612) 587-2860, BS 72 Moorhead St Univ; MS 77 Univ of WI - Stevens Point; ES 86 Saint Cloud St Univ; Director of Special Ed, Crow River Special Ed Coop, **SLP**

Schulte, Edward J 617 West 27th Place, Lawrence, KS 66046, (913) 841-8723, BA 78 Kearney St Coll; MS 80 Kearney St Coll; Area Mgr, Communicare Inc, **SLP**

Schulte, Luanne 6570 West 51st Street, Mission, KS 66202, (913) 262-3683, BS 74 Fort Hays St Univ; MS 75 Fort Hays St Univ; Private Practice, **SLP**

Schulte, William Charles W63 N14334 Washington Avenue, #2, Cedarburg, WI 53012, (414) 542-8036, BS 86 Univ of WI - Whitewater; MS 87 Univ of WI - Whitewater

Schulten, Mrs Margaret 11012 Old Landing Road, Kingsville, MD 21087, (301) 592-2039, BS 70 WV Univ; MS 74 Loyola Coll; Sp-Lang Path, Balto Co Board of Educ, **SLP**

Schultz, Adeline R 305 Westmont Avenue, Haddonfield, NJ 08033, (215) 928-7445, BA 66 Rutger's St Univ - Douglas Coll; ME 67 PA St Univ - Univ Park; Ch Sp-Lang Path, Thomas Jefferson U Hosp, **SLP ACE**

Schultz, Mrs Cheryl Ann 32224 26th Avenue SW, Federal Way, WA 98023, (206) 433-2557, BS 73 Portland St Univ; MS 76 Portland St Univ; MS 86 Portland St Univ; Sp-Lang Path, Highline PS, **SLP**

Schultz, Mrs Colleen Mary 10113 South St Louis St, Evergreen Park, IL 60642, (312) 687-0900, BA 84 Saint Xavier Coll; MA 85 Northwestern Univ; Sp-Lang Path, Southwest Cook Cnty Coop Assn, **SLP**

Schultz, Cynthia Bishop Route 1 Box 218, New Ulm, MN 56073, (507) 359-8490, BA 78 Central MI Univ; MS 81 Central MI Univ; 88–Sp-Lang Path, New Wm Sch Dist #88, **SLP**

Schultz, Cynthia Lynn 13850 North 19th Avenue, Apartment 217, Phoenix, AZ 85023, (602) 272-4010, BA 81 Univ of Denver; MA 85 Univ of Northern CO; 88–Sp-Lang Path, Samuel Gompers Rehab Ctr, **SLP**

Schultz, Deborah 195 Bennett #4-H, New York, NY 10040, (201) 441-2161, Hackensack Medical Center, **A**

Schultz, Janet Marie 1029 Ransom Road, Grand Island, NY 14072, (716) 837-2441, BA 82 SUNY - Center at Buffalo; MA 84 SUNY - Center at Buffalo; MA 85 SUNY - Center at Buffalo; **SLP**

Schultz, Jean M 11825 N E 172nd Street, Bothell, WA 98011, (206) 488-1396, BA 69 Columbia Univ Teachers Coll; MS 72 Columbia Univ Teachers Coll; Sp-Lang Path, Private Practice, **SLP**

Schultz, Jean S 12303 Remington Drive, Silver Spring, MD 20902, (301) 593-4948, BA 65 Univ of NC - Greensboro; MA 67 Case Western Reserve Univ; Sp-Lang Path, Montgomery Co Pub Sch, **SLP**

Schultz, Mrs Jeanie Barry 2575 Devonshire Road, Ann Arbor, MI 48104, (313) 973-9782, OM 65 Univ of GA; OM 72 Univ of FL; **SLP**

Schultz, Joanne M 1925 Kalakaua Avenue #2602, Honolulu, HI 96815, (415) 835-2131, BS 78 IA St Univ; MS 80 Univ of WI - Stevens Point; 86–Chief of Sp-Lang Path, Private Practice, **SLP**

Schultz, Mrs Karen Marie R R 3 Box 224, Moorhead, MN 56560, (218) 233-4671, BS 81 Moorhead St Univ; MS 84 Univ of WI - Eau Claire; 85–Dir, Speech & Language Services, **SLP**

Schultz, Mrs Katherine Clark 1549 Slaterville Road, Ithaca, NY 14850, (607) 273-9100, BS 80 SUNY - Coll at Buffalo; MS 85 SUNY - Coll at Buffalo; Sp-Lang Path, Special Children's Ctr, **SLP**

Schultz, Mrs Kathy Jo 615 Brockton Lane, Florence, SC 29501, (803) 664-9613, BS 84 IN St Univ - Terre Haute; MS 86 IN St Univ - Terre Haute; SLP, Florence Pub Schl Dis #1, **SLP**

Schultz, Laura Lee 17778 Kent Road, Dundee, MI 48131, (313) 529-2827, MS 88 Univ of MI - Ann Arbor

Schultz, Lynette C 3410 John Speier, San Antonio, TX 78217, BS 74 Univ of KS; MA 78 Univ of Houston - Univ Park; SLP Coord, Home Nursing & Therapy Service, **SLP**

Schultz, Lynette Lee 517 St Charles, Rapid City, SD 57701, (605) 341-6508, BA 83 Univ of SD - Vermillion; MA 85 Univ of SD - Vermillion; Sp-Lang Path, Black Hills Special Svc Coop, **SLP**

Schultz, Mrs Marilyn C 1224 South Main Street, Findlay, OH 45840, (419) 448-2134, BA 56 Univ of IA; ME 67 Univ of MO - Columbia; Prof of Education, Heidelberg College, **SLP**

Schultz, Dr Martin C Southern Il University, Dept Of Comm Disorder Sci, Carbondale, IL 62901, (618) 453-4301, BA 50 Temple Univ; MA 52 Univ of MI - Ann Arbor; PH 55 (NS) Univ of IA; 86–Prof, Southern IL U, **A**

Schultz, Mrs Mary Lee C 1300 Military Road, Jacksonville, AR 72076, (501) 771-6153, BA 79 Univ of AR - Little Rock; MS 81 Univ of AR - Little Rock; Sp-Lang Path, North Little Rock School Dist, **SLP**

Schultz, Michael A 2130 University Avenue, Apartment 129, Madison, WI 53705, (608) 238-4884, MS 88 Univ of WI - Madison

Schultz, Mimi Dryce 408 Frankel Boulevard, Merrick, NY 11566, (516) 489-7980, BA 79 Univ of MI - Ann Arbor; MS 81 Univ of MI - Ann Arbor; Sp-Lang Path, W Hempstead Union Free Sch, **SLP**

Schultz, Moritz L Foxwood Estates, 4900-B Alder Drive, West Palm Beach, FL 33417, (305) 684-5151, BS 59 Bloomsburg Univ of PA; ME 63 PA St Univ - Univ Park; Aud, Sch Bd of Palm Beach Co, **A**

Schultz, Nancy Ruth Route 3 Box 10, Wells, MN 56097, (612) 454-2732, BS 82 Saint Cloud St Univ; MA 84 Univ of Northern CO; Sp-Lang Path, Dakota Inc, **SLP**

Schultz, Norman R 2320 Marjorie Lane, Clio, MI 48420, **SLP**

Schultz, Pamela A N8077 Highway Q, Watertown, WI 53094, (414) 648-5797, MS 85 Univ of WI - Eau Claire; **SLP**

Schultz, Robert E 57 Belmont Avenue, Ottawa, ON, Canada K1S 0V2, (613) 235-0469, BS 69 Bloomsburg Univ of PA; MA 74 Temple Univ-Tyler Sch of Art; Aud, Private Practice, **A**

Schultz, Sara Joanne 2225 Churchill Drive, Ann Arbor, MI 48103, (313) 665-0496, BA 85 Univ of MI - Ann Arbor; MS 87 Univ of WI - Madison; 88–Aud, Jackson Sp & Hearing Cl

Schultz, Susan E 509 Van Dyke Avenue, Ripon, WI 54971, BA 77 Univ of WI - Eau Claire; MS 78 Univ of WI - Eau Claire; SLP, Ripon Public Schools, **SLP**

Schultz, Susan Schaner P O Box 589, 422 East Second Street, Perry, MI 48872, (517) 625-7939, BA 75 MI St Univ; MA 78 MI St Univ; 78–Sp-Lang Path, Swartz Creek Comm Sch, **SLP**

Schultze, Dr Betty Robb 3849 Hermitage Lane, St Charles, MO 63303, (314) 533-3366, BS 54 Central MO St Univ; MA 76 Saint Louis Univ; ED 79 (NS) Univ of TX - El Paso; Assistant Professor, Harris-Stowe State College, **SLP**

Schultze, Laura J 345 Field Street, Rochester, NY 14620, (716) 271-0680, BA 76 SUNY - Coll at Potsdam; MS 77 Ithaca Coll; Sp/Lang Path, Hrng/Sp Cen of Rochester, **SLP**

Schulz, Mrs Elizabeth Ruth E-9689 Valley View Court, Wisconsin Dells, WI 53965, (608) 254-8667, BS 77 Eastern KY Univ; MA 78 Western MI Univ; **SLP**

Schulz, Geralyn Marie Speech Pathology Unit-N I H, 9000 Rockville Pike, Bldg 10/5N226, Bethesda, MD 20892, (301) 496-9365, MA 82 SUNY - Center at Buffalo; SLP, Christy Ludlow Phd Ccc-Sp, **SLP**

Schulz, Mrs Mary E 1560 Belle Avenue, Lakewood, OH 44107, (216) 529-4201, BA 75 Bowling Green St Univ; MA 78 Cleveland St Univ; Sp-Lang Path, Lakewood Cty Sch, **SLP**

Schulz, Nancy A 49 Pemberton Road, Nashua, NH 03063, **SLP**

Schulz, Ronald E 609 Raritan Avenue, Perth Amboy, NJ 08861, (201) 870-5067, BA 69 Newark St Coll; MA 72 Kean Coll of NJ; Director Aud Sp-Lang Path, Monmouth Medical Center, **SLP**

Schulz, Capt Theresa Yarber USAF Clinic McClellan, SGPMH, McClellan AFB, CA 95652-5300, (916) 646-8452, BS 81 Univ of TX - Austin; MA 83 Univ of TX - Austin; Chief-Aud, USAF, **A ACE**

Schulze, Barbara Gay 500 Medical Center Boulevard, Suite 340, Conroe, TX 77304, (409) 539-4700, BS 81 Lamar Univ; MS 83 Lamar Univ; 85–Aud, Affiliated ENT Clinic, **A**

Schulze, Mrs Gaynelle Babb 9121 Pinewood Drive, Dallas, TX 75243, (214) 348-5965, BA 58 Univ of North TX; MA 61 Univ of TX - Austin; Director, Private Practice, **SLP A**

Schulze, Mrs P Marilyn 826 Rivercrest Street, Abilene, TX 79605, (915) 677-7372, BS 63 Abilene Christian Univ; MA 65 Univ of NE - Lincoln; 88–Sp-Lang Path, Abilene ISD, **SLP**

Schulze, Theresa Wulff 630 South 126th Street, Omaha, NE 68154, BS 75 Univ of NE - Omaha; MS 76 Univ of NE - Omaha; Sp/Lang Path, Dist 46 Springfield Sch Syst, **SLP**

Schulze, Victoria Lynne 24 Blossom Lane, Merrimack, NH 03054, (603) 429-0478, BS 85 Univ of MA - Amherst; MS 86 Univ of MI - Ann Arbor; 86–Sp-Lang Path, Nashua Mem Hosp, **SLP**

Schum, Dr Donald Joseph 1425 Topaz Drive, Mount Pleasant, SC 29464, (803) 792-7975, BS 82 Univ of IL - Urbana; MA 84 Univ of IA; PH 88 (Aud) LA St Univ - Baton Rouge; 88–Asst Prof, Med Univ SC, **A**

Schum, Judith A 13203 Nickleson Drive, Dale City, VA 22193, (312) 748-9453, **SLP**

Schum, Lorianne Katherine Amplimed Inc, Suite 300 315 Calhoun Street, Charleston, SC 29401, (803) 722-8387, BS 81 Univ of IL - Urbana; MA 83 Univ of IL - Urbana; 88–Aud, Amplimed Inc, **A**

Schum, Dr Robert L 116 Shc, University Of Iowa, Iowa City, IA 52242, (319) 335-8736, BS 72 Univ of IA; MA 74 Univ of Denver; PH 83 (Clinical Psychology) Univ of Denver; 77–Clin Psych, Dept Sp Path & Aud Univ of Iowa

Schumacher, Dawn M 24789 Broadmore Avenue, Hayward, CA 94544, BA 81 San Francisco St Univ; MS 86 CA St Univ - Hayward

Schumacher, Edith Kathryn 2565 Browncroft Blvd, Rochester, NY 14625, (716) 482-9290, BS 78 Nazareth Coll; MS 81 Nazareth Coll; Rochester City School District, **SLP**

Schumacher, Gretchen Klopf 116 Volusia Avenue, Dayton, OH 45409, (513) 226-7877, BA 79 Wright St Univ; MS 80 Miami Univ - Oxford; 84–Dir/Sp-Lang Path, Aud and Sp Assoc, **SLP**

Schumacher, James Gregory VA Medical Center, Speech Pathology Section, 54th St And 48th Avenue South, Minneapolis, MN 55417, (612) 725-2000, BS 82 Univ of WI - Milwaukee; MS 86 Univ of WI - Madison; 87–Sp-Lang Path, VA Med Ctr, **SLP**

Schumacher, Janis Lynn 806 Bear Valley Parkway, Escondido, CA 92025, (619) 438-6634, **SLP**

Schumacher, Mrs Jerelyn Wodill 3421 Miller Street, Eau Claire, WI 54701, (715) 834-3448, BA 84 Univ of WI - Eau Claire; MS 86 Univ of WI - Stevens Point; 87–Aud, ENT Cl of Eau Claire, **A**

Schumacher, Joyce Ann 808 West Main Street, Little Chute, WI 54140, (815) 625-0400, BS 82 Univ of WI - Oshkosh; MS 83 Univ of WI - Stevens Point; Sp-Lang Path, Holy Family Medical Center, **SLP**

Schumacher, Mrs Kimberly Renee P O Box 6283, Toledo, OH 43614, (419) 531-6660, MA 87 Eastern MI Univ

Schumacher, Marilyn E 1015 Pomona Avenue, Albany, CA 94706, (707) 425-4633, BA 74 Sonoma St Univ; MA 82 Western WA Univ; Sp-Lang Path, Fairfield-Suisun USD, **SLP**

Schumacher, Mary Martha 4309 Oregon Avenue North, New Hope, MN 55428, (612) 533-4530, BA 85 Univ of WI - Eau Claire; MS 87 Univ of WI - Stevens Point; 88–Sp-Lang Path, Robbinsdale PS Dist, **SLP**

Schumacher, Walter C 895 Sutter Street #302, San Francisco, CA 94109, (415) 775-2181, BA 27; Sp-Lang Path, Private Practice, **SLP LM**

Schumaier, Dr Daniel R 209 East Unaka Avenue, Johnson City, TN 37601, (615) 928-5771, BS 61 Southeast MO St Univ; MA 69 Washington Univ; PH 72 (Aud) MI St Univ; Owner, Private Practice, **A**

Schumaker, Anita Drost 100 Flint Street, Trumbull, CT 06611, BS 77 MI St Univ; MA 78 MI St Univ; Sp-Lang Path, Trumbull Pub Sch, **SLP**

Schuman, Gayle 1920 Carriage Hill, Lisle, IL 60532, (312) 416-8420, BA 76 Augustana Coll; MS 77 Bradley Univ; 84–Sp-Lang Path, Sch Dist 89, **SLP**

Schuman, Leslie E 1029 Bernice Street, St Louis, MO 63122, (314) 965-4684, **SLP**

Schuman, Mrs Linda L Steiner 4132 Willmar Drive, Palo Alto, CA 94306, BA 72 Stanford Univ; MA 74 Univ of the Pacific; SLP, Mt View Elem Sch Dist, **SLP**

Schuman, Lois J 48 Markwood Road, Ardsley, NY 10502-2008, BS 70; MA 76; Sp-Lang Path, Yonkers Bd of Ed, **SLP**

Schuman, Ronda Lynn 35 0AKLAND Avenue, Second Floor, Warwick, NY 10990, (914) 986-4620, BS 76 Univ of GA; ME 83 Univ of VA - Charlottesville; **A**

Schumann, Gretchen Rosemond 2513 Morning Star, Corpus Christi, TX 78410, (512) 241-7396, BS 85 Baylor Univ; MS 86 Baylor Univ; 87–Sp-Lang Path, Corpus Christi ISD, **SLP**

Schumann, Mrs Nancy 2000 Apricot Glen, Austin, TX 78746, (512) 477-1771, BS 73 Univ of TX - Austin; MS 74 Univ of South FL; Sp-Lang Path, Austin ISD, **SLP**

Schumann, Nancy V 6 Kennedy Drive, Denville, NJ 07834, (201) 383-1900, BS 80 Clarion Univ of PA; MA 82 Montclair St Coll; Sp-Lang Path, Newton Child Study Team, **SLP**

Schunk, Marlene Joanne 8951 Meadowbrook Way, Buena Park, CA 90621, BA 83 CA St Univ - Fullerton; MA 86 CA St Univ - Fullerton; 88–SLP, Norwalk-La Mirada USD, **SLP**

Schupbach, Joanne E 312 Memory Lane, #18-4, Westmont, IL 60559, (312) 787-7631, MS 79 Eastern IL Univ; MA 82 Northern IL Univ - De Kalb; 88–Dir of Aud, Neurotology Inc, **SLP A**

Schur, Mrs Karen G 421 Ronnie Drive, Buffalo Grove, IL 60090, (312) 634-1088, BS 76 Univ of WI - Madison; MS 78 IL St Univ - Normal; SLP, Waukegan Pub Sch Dist 60, **SLP**

Schur, Mrs Lenora Singer 2655 West Balmoral Street, Chicago, IL 60625, (312) 728-1368, BS 50 Northwestern Univ; MA 67 Northeastern IL Univ; Sp/Lang Path, Chicago Bd of Ed, **SLP ACE**

Schur, Wendy Broker 3830 Victoria Street, Minnetonka, MN 55345, (612) 451-1331, BA 81 Univ of WI - Madison; MS 83 Univ of IL - Urbana; Sp-Lang Path, Dakot Inc, **SLP**

Schurman, Gary W 2136 Laurel Lane, Allison Park, PA 15101, (412) 784-4025, BA 73 Newberry Coll; MS 75 Newberry Coll; Pres, Noise & Hrng Constultants Inc, **A**

Schurmann, Deborah Jean 415 7th Avenue East #4, Alexandria, MN 56308, (218) 236-3269, BS 83 Moorhead St Univ; MS 85 Moorhead St Univ; **SLP**

Schurr, Margaret S 14371 East Carolina Drive, Aurora, CO 80012, BS 69 Univ of ND; MA 71 Univ of Denver; Aud, Cherry Creek Schools, **A**

Schurrer, Judy S 106 Northwest Lane, Charlottesville, VA 22901-8419, (715) 425-8004, BA 74 Univ of SD - Vermillion; MA 78 Univ of CO - Boulder; Cl Supvr, U of WI-River Falls, **SLP ACE**

Schussler, Elizabeth 240 Maple, PO Box 919, Woodruff, WI 54568, (715) 356-4413, BS 73 Univ of WI - Stevens Point; MS 74 Univ of WI - Stevens Point; Sp-Lang Path, Northwoods Rehab Assoc, **SLP**

Schust, Judith Ann 1823 West Granville #4A, Chicago, IL 60660, BA 53 Montclair St Coll; MA 68 Northwestern Univ; Coord Academic Skills Prog, Harold Washington Coll, **SLP**

Schuster, Mrs Bette 2308 Chesterton Drive, Walnut Creek, CA 94596, MA 70; **SLP**

Schuster, Carolyn Susan 3437 North 49th Drive, Phoenix, AZ 85031, (602) 247-8196, BA 84 Grand Canyon Coll; MA 86 Grand Canyon Coll; **SLP**

Schuster, Cheryl Jahn 3508 Captain's Court, Rockford, IL 61109, (815) 544-9851, BS 81 Northern IL Univ - De Kalb; MS 86 Northern IL Univ - De Kalb; **SLP**

Schuster, Lauren K 8211 West Eastwood Avenue, Norridge, IL 60656, **SLP**

Schuster, Martha Lee 12011 East Harvard Avenue, Apartment 12-104, Aurora, CO 80014, (303) 837-1000, BS 54 Univ of NE - Lincoln; Sp-Lang Path, Denver Public Schools, **SLP**

Schuster, Mrs Renee M #1 Rosebrook Drive, Florissant, MO 63031, (314) 837-4776, BS 78 Univ of MO - Columbia; MA 79 Univ of MO - Columbia; 87–Sp-Lang Path, Private Practice, **SLP**

Schutt, Carol Jean 1324 Apple Ridge Court, Edgewood, MD 21040, (301) 578-8600, BA 82 Loyola Coll; MS 83 Loyola Coll; 87–Sp-Lang Path, Mt Washington Pediatric Hosp, **SLP ACE**

Schutte, Mrs Kris Dykstra 8131 Pennington Drive, Huntington Beach, CA 92646, (714) 536-9616, MA 88 CA St Univ - Long Beach; Sp-Lang Path, Santa Ana USD

Schutte, Mrs Melissa W 9528 Chatterleigh Drive, Richmond, VA 23233, (804) 780-8636, BA 74 Mary Washington Coll; ME 75 Univ of VA - Charlottesville; **SLP**

Schutz, Mrs Barbara J McLemore 5350 Jornada Road South, Las Cruces, NM 88001, (505) 523-5504, BS 71 NM St Univ; MA 74 NM St Univ; 76–Sp-Lang Path, Las Cruces Pub Schs, **SLP**

Schutza, Mrs Patricia Frances 927 Fisher Road, Grosse Pointe, MI 48230, (313) 573-5123, BA 74 Univ of MI - Ann Arbor; MA 76 Wayne St Univ; 86–Sp-Lang Path, Macomb Hosp Ctr, **SLP**

Schutzbank, Myrna P RFD #1 Birch Road Box 159, Yorktown Heights, NY 10598, (718) 423-7300, BA 73 Temple Univ-Tyler Sch of Art; MA 75 Temple Univ-Tyler Sch of Art; 85–Sp-Lang Path, Stepping Stone Day Sch, **SLP**

Schutzel, Elizabeth A 3317 Bridgmanor Drive, Kansas City, MO 64137, (913) 362-3095, MA 88 Univ of KS

Schutzenhofer, Tom 4657 Bridlewood Terrace, St Louis, MO 63128, (314) 569-8168, BS 73 Southern IL Univ-Edwardsvill; MS 74 Southern IL Univ-Edwardsvill; **SLP**

Schutzer, Barbara M 201 East 83rd Street, Apt 3-A, New York, NY 10028, (212) 294-0464, **SLP**

Schwab, Constance 5363 Brookway #6, Columbia, MD 21044, MS; **SLP LM**

Schwab, Ingrid Ursula 2400 Bethards Drive #279, Santa Rosa, CA 95405, (707) 542-2771, BS 82 CA St Univ - Hayward; MS 84 CA St Univ - Hayward; Sp-Lang Path, Santa Rosa Sp-Hrng Center, **SLP**

Schwabe, Annette Marie 65 3rd Place, Brooklyn, NY 11231, (718) 630-7425, BS 80 Mankato St Univ; MS 84 Univ of WA; Sp-Lang Path Consultant, Private Practice, **SLP**

Schwaber, Donna K G 118 Chatsworth Drive, Nashville, TN 37215, (904) 384-8088, BA 77 Auburn Univ - Auburn; MS 78 Auburn Univ - Auburn; Aud, Private Practice, **A**

Schwaid-Antin, Sandra 3199 Amelia Drive, Mohegan Lake, NY 10547, (914) 245-3705, BA 75 Adelphi Univ; MS 76 Adelphi Univ; Sp-Lang Path, Lakeland Sch Dist, **SLP**

Schwake, Mrs Eileen M 4517 Washburn Avenue South, Minneapolis, MN 55410, (612) 922-5799, MS 78 Univ of MN - Duluth; Sp-Lang Path, Sr Kenny Institute, **SLP**

Schwalbach, Mrs Diane Mc Coy 100 Meadow Street, Bethel Academy, Warrenton, VA 22186, (703) 347-0505, BS 81 James Madison Univ; ME 85 James Madison Univ; Aud, J L Manwaring MD, **A**

Schwallie, Mrs Lora L 25682 Cresta Loma, Laguna Niguel, CA 92677, (714) 364-6310, MA 88 Univ of Cincinnati; 88–Aud, Otologic Medical Group

Schwan, Mrs Sabina A 702 University, Grosse Pointe, MI 48230, (313) 745-4651, OB 70; MA 72 MI St Univ; Cl Coord-Aud Serv, Harper Hosp, **A ACE**

Schwander, Teresa Jane 123 Washington Avenue, Matawan, NJ 07747, (212) 790-4318, BS 77 Clarion Univ of PA; MS 78 Clarion Univ of PA; Aud, CUNY Grad Sch Sp/Hrng Sci, **A**

Schwandes, Jean K 63 Botany Drive, Asheville, NC 28805, (704) 252-8600, BS 63 Univ of WI - Milwaukee; MS 86 Western Carolina Univ; 87–Sp-Lang Path, Haywood Co Hosp, **SLP**

Schwanger, Joan W 229 Arch Street, Carlisle, PA 17013, (717) 243-4064, BA 81 SUNY - Coll at New Paltz; MS 87 Coll of Saint Rose; 88–Sp-Lang Path, Easter Seal Soc, **SLP**

Schwanke, Mrs Janet L H 950 Brookside, Deerfield, IL 60015, (312) 948-5914, BA 74 Univ of IA; MA 75 Univ of IA; Sp/Lang Path, Private Practice, **SLP**

Schwartz, Janet Rector Route 2 Box 330-A, Lubbock, TX 79415, (806) 799-2927, BS 80 Univ of North TX; MS 82 Univ of North TX; SLP, Great Plains Home Hlth Agency, **SLP**

Schwartz, Mrs Alice E 7716 Delafield Place, Alexandria, VA 22306, (703) 765-9299, BS 65 NY Univ; ME 67 SUNY - Center at Buffalo; MA 78 George Washington Univ; Sp/Lang Path, Alexandria Hosp, **SLP**

Schwartz, Mrs Amy Bruckner 11 Bernard Street, Great Neck, NY 11023, (718) 591-6717, BA 79 Queens Coll; MA 80 Hofstra Univ; Sp-Lang Path, Boe of New York City, **SLP**

Schwartz, Anita B 117 East 89th Street, New York, NY 10028, MA 81 NY Univ; Sp-Lang Path, Kateri Residence, **SLP**

Schwartz, Anna S P O Box 384, Apo, San Francisco, CA 96555-0008, **SLP**

Schwartz, Arlene Randy 188 Cold Spring Street, Apartment 5, New Haven, CT 06511, (203) 284-2880, BA 81 CUNY - Queens Coll; MA 85 Univ of CT; 88–Sp-Lang Path, Gaylord Hosp, **SLP**

Schwartz, Mrs Arlene Susan 69 Camino Arroyo Place, Palm Desert, CA 92260, (619) 346-3582, BA 70 MI St Univ; ME 74 Wayne St Univ; 88–Sp-Lang Path, Desert Hosp, **SLP**

Schwartz, Dr Arthur H Dept Speech & Hearing Mc-430, Cleveland State University, Cleveland, OH 44115, (216) 687-6990, BS 65 Indiana Univ of PA; MA 66 Case Western Reserve Univ; PH 72 (NS) Vanderbilt Univ; Professor and Chairperson, Cleveland State University, **SLP F**

Schwartz, Barbara R 876 Tam O'Shanter, Las Vegas, NV 89109, (702) 383-2239, BA 76 CA St Univ - Los Angeles, MA 85 Univ of Northern CO; Sp-Lang Path, Univ Med Cntr, **SLP**

Schwartz, Mrs Camilla M 45 Sparta Road, Stanhope, NJ 07874, (201) 579-8602, BA 71 Marshall Univ; MA 72 Seton Hall Univ; Dir of Sp/Lang/Aud, Newton Memorial Hospital, **SLP**

Schwartz, Mrs Caren S 92 Francis Place, Spring Valley, NY 10977, (201) 670-0707, BS 79 Ithaca Coll; MA 81 Hofstra Univ; Sp-Lang Path, Communication Therapy Ctr Inc, **SLP**

Schwartz, Caryl H 1 Haven Court #S2A, Nyack, NY 10960, (914) 592-7555, BA 71 SUNY - Center at Buffalo; MS 73 Columbia Univ Teachers Coll; 88–Sp-Lang Path, Blythedale Childrens Hosp, **SLP**

Schwartz, Dr Daniel M Otorhinolary & Human Comm, Univ Of Pa Sch Of Medicine, 34th & Spruce Streets, Philadelphia, PA 19104, (215) 662-3696, BS 70 Old Dominion Univ; MA 71 Central MI Univ; PH 74 (NS) Vanderbilt Univ; Assoc Prof, Hosp of U of Pa, **A F**

Schwartz, Mrs Deborah F 2 Robinhood Road, White Plains, NY 10605, (914) 381-4485, BA 68 Syracuse Univ; MS 69 Syracuse Univ; **SLP**

Schwartz, Mrs Debra Goldzweig 414 Elmwood Avenue, Brooklyn, NY 11230, (718) 258-0656, MS 86 CUNY - Brooklyn Coll; **A**

Schwartz, Dr Edith M 165 Seafare, Laguna Niguel, CA 92677, (714) 495-2709, BA 60 CA St Univ - Los Angeles; MA 63 CA St Univ - Los Angeles; PH 76 (Human Bahavior) United States Int'l Univ; **SLP A LM**

Schwartz, Elisa F 110 Tekening Drive, Tenafly, NJ 07670, (201) 569-4492, BS 75 NY Univ; MA 77 NY Univ; **SLP**

Schwartz, Ellen R 2401 Pennsylvania Avenue, 1st Floor, Philadelphia, PA 19130, (215) 236-2160, BA 67 George Washington Univ; MA 69 Temple Univ; Sp/Lang Path, Private Practice, **SLP ACE**

Schwartz, Mrs Ellen S 44 McClellan Avenue, Amsterdam, NY 12010, (518) 843-1748, BS 77 Ithaca Coll; MS 78 Syracuse Univ; Sp-Lang Path, Private Practice, **SLP**

Schwartz, Fmdr Elsie Newman 171 Fox Run, Poughkeepsie, NY 12603, BA 79 CUNY - Queens Coll; MA 82 CUNY - Queens Coll; Sp-Lang Path, St Francis Hosp, **SLP**

Schwartz, Mrs Estelle N 76-25 269th Street, New Hyde Park, NY 11040, (212) 598-6676, BA 73 CUNY - Hunter Coll; MA 75 Hofstra Univ; OM 78 Long Island U - CW Post Ctr; 79–Admin Dir, Hospital for Joint Diseases, **SLP**

Schwartz, Florence P O Box 66973, Suite 137, Houston, TX 77006, BA 45 Univ of TX - Austin; MA 51 Univ of Houston - Univ Park; **SLP**

Schwartz, Gail E 6651 Edinborough, West Bloomfield, MI 48322, **SLP**

Schwartz, Mrs Gail S 903 Brentwood Lane, Silver Spring, MD 20902, **SLP**

Schwartz, Mrs Harriett 5 Rydal Drive, Lawrenceville, NJ 08648, (609) 882-1503, BA 62 Univ of MD - College Park; MS 64 Purdue Univ - West Lafayette; Pres, Private Practice, **SLP**

Schwartz, Dr Howard D 6 South 114 Lakewood Drive, Naperville, IL 60540, BA 72 SUNY - Coll at New Paltz; MA 74 MI St Univ; PH 84 (Sp Path) Syracuse Univ; Asst Prof, Northern IL Univ, **SLP**

Schwartz, Mrs Illeane Epstein 980 Mountain Drive, Deerfield, IL 60015, (312) 782-0029, BS 60 Northwestern Univ; MS 83 Rush Univ; Sp/Lang Path, Private Practice, **SLP**

Schwartz, Joyce K 1017 Fernwood Avenue, Pleasantville, NJ 08232, **SLP**

Schwartz, Mrs Joye R 623 Elkins Avenue, Elkins Park, PA 19117, (215) 635-4363, BA 74 Univ of Denver; MA 76 Univ of Denver; Dispensing Audiologist, Herb & Associates Inc, **A**

Schwartz, Mrs Judith M 1811 East D, North Platte, NE 69101, (308) 534-9310, BA 74 Kearney St Coll; MS 78 Kearney St Coll; Coord/Sp-Lang-Hrng Svcs, Great Plains Regional Med Ctr, **SLP**

Schwartz, Dr Judith Stockheim 115 Round Hill Road, Armonk, NY 10504, (212) 532-1460, BA 64 CUNY - Queens Coll; MA 69 NY Univ; PH 83 (NS) NY Univ

Schwartz, Katharine 24 Craig Drive, Reading, PA 19606, BS 77 Northwestern Univ; MA 79 Vanderbilt Univ; 88–Sp-Lang Path, St Joseph Hosp, **SLP**

Schwartz, Katherine L 17210 N W Valsetz Court, Beaverton, OR 97006, (503) 645-4242, BA 77 Univ of OR; MS 78 Univ of OR; Sp-Lang Path, Washington Co Ed Serv Dist, **SLP**

Schwartz, Laurie I 324 Post Avenue #4K, Westbury, NY 11590, (516) 997-8700, BA 77 SUNY - Coll at Cortland; MA 78 Long Island U - CW Post Ctr; Educational Spec, NY Dept of Educ, **SLP**

Schwartz, Mrs Leanne Greenwald 715 Empire Avenue, West Lawrence, NY 11691, (718) 327-6118, BA 75 CUNY - Brooklyn Coll; MS 76 CUNY - Brooklyn Coll; 81–Sp-Lang Path, NYC Headstart Prog, **SLP**

Schwartz, Leslie P O Box 218, East Northport, NY 11731, 72–Aud, Northport VA Hosp, **SLP A**

Schwartz, Linda Route 3 Box 237, Osseo, WI 54758, (715) 538-4316, BA 75 Univ of WI - Eau Claire; MS 76 Univ of WI - Eau Claire; Regional Service Specialist, Cesa #4, **SLP**

Schwartz, Linda Raskin 2520 Batchelder Street #6M, Brooklyn, NY 11235, (718) 648-1545, BS 73 Univ of WI - Madison; MA 76 NY Univ; Sp-Lang Path, Private Practice, **SLP**

Schwartz, Lorene M 7667 Whitewater Drive, Huntington Beach, CA 92648, (714) 841-1008, BA 76 SUNY - Center at Buffalo; MA 77 Western MI Univ; Sp-Lang Path, Sp-Lang Dev Cen-Duena Pk, **SLP**

Schwartz, Lori Ann N2754 Highway 22, Clearwater Hts #5, Waupaca, WI 54981, (608) 462-8242, BS 84 Univ of WI - Stevens Point; MA 85 Univ of MN - Duluth; **SLP**

Schwartz, Mrs Lorna T 443 Wyldhaven Road, Rosemont, PA 19010, (215) 739-9360, MA 77 Temple Univ; OM 79 Temple Univ; Sp-Lang Path, School District of Phila, **SLP**

Schwartz, Lynn Thomas 61 Babcock Street, Brookline, MA 02146, (617) 731-0963, BA 76 SUNY - Coll at Oswego; MS 86 Northeastern Univ; **A**

Schwartz, Marsha S 14123 Weeping Willow Dr, Apartment 22, Silver Spring, MD 20906, (301) 871-7978, BA 72 CUNY - Hunter Coll; MS 73 PA St Univ - Univ Park; PH 79 (Aud) SUNY - Center at Buffalo; **A**

Schwartz, Dr Melvin J 8381 S W 91st Terrace, Miami, FL 33156, (305) 274-0632, BA 54 Univ of Miami; ME 56 Wayne St Univ; PH 67 (NS) Wayne St Univ; Prof, Miami Dade Commun Coll, **SLP**

Schwartz, Mrs Michelle L Route 2 Box 182, Jefferson, GA 30549, (404) 367-8486, BS 79 Univ of GA; ME 80 Univ of GA; Sp-Lang Path, Clarke County School District, **SLP**

Schwartz, Mona Serotta 88 Oakwood Drive, Wayne, NJ 07470, (201) 694-5045, BA 80 OH St Univ; MA 82 OH St Univ; 86–Sp-Lang Path, Hackensack Med Ctr, **SLP**

Schwartz, Dr Nancy Z 15 Trail's End Road, Weston, CT 06883, (203) 226-5328, BA 70 CUNY - Queens Coll; MA 72 CUNY - Queens Coll; PH 77 (Communication Disorders) CUNY - Grad Sch & Univ Cntr; Sp-Lang Path, Private Practice, **SLP**

Schwartz, Mrs Paula Carol 2091 N W 103 Terrace, Coral Springs, FL 33071, (305) 752-4273, BS 83 SUNY - Coll at Potsdam; MS 86 Nova Univ

Schwartz, Mrs Pearl E 93 Luyster Street, Huntington Station, NY 11746, (516) 427-6512, BA 78 CUNY - Queens Coll; MA 80 Hofstra Univ; Sp/Lang Path, Sch for Lang & Comm Dev, **SLP**

Schwartz, Dr Ralph J Assoc Prof Of Sp Path & Aud, Univ Of Northern Iowa, Cedar Falls, IA 50614, (319) 273-2549, BS 41 Northwestern Univ; MA 48 Marquette Univ; PH 58 (Sp Path and Aud) Purdue Univ - West Lafayette; 63–Assoc Prof/SLP & Aud, U of N IA, **SLP A LM**

Schwartz, Rebecca Levine 25 Dierauf Street, Staten Island, NY 10312, MS 86 CUNY - Brooklyn Coll; **SLP**

Schwartz, Dr Richard G Dept Of Audiology & Speech Sci, Purdue University, Heavilon Hall, West Lafayette, IN 47907, (317) 494-3824, MS 74 Univ of South FL; PH 78 (Sp-Lang Path) Memphis St Univ; Assoc Prof, Prudue Univ, **SLP**

Schwartz, Roberta Maryland Instit Emergency Med, University Of MD At Balt, 22 South Greene Street, Baltimore, MD 21201, (301) 328-6101, BA 73 Loyola Coll; ME 74 Univ of VA - Charlottesville; Sp-Lang Path, U of MD-Baltimore, **SLP**

Schwartz, Robin N 260 N W 19th Street #3, Boca Raton, FL 33432, (407) 391-8812, BA 77 Univ of FL; OM 78 Univ of TN - Knoxville; MA 79 Univ of Miami; 86–Sp-Lang Path & Aud, Pinecrest Rehab Hosp, **SLP A ACE**

Schwartz, Mrs Sally Yevette 2 Peach Street, Nanuet, NY 10954, (914) 735-1276, BA 81 SUNY - Center at Albany; MA 84 CUNY - Hunter Coll; **SLP**

Schwartz, Sandi 573 Plymouth Street, Holbrook, MA 02343, (617) 767-2094, BA 81 Montclair St Coll; MS 86 Rutgers St Univ - Newark; 88–Sp-Lang Path, Braintree Hosp, **SLP**

Schwartz, Sandra Levine 2022 Rowley Road, Ballston Spa, NY 12020, (518) 587-2778, BA 65 SUNY - Center at Buffalo; MA 66 SUNY - Center at Albany; Sp-Lang Path, Saratoga Springs City Schs, **SLP**

Schwartz, Scott E 3637 Milano Court #7, Middleton, WI 53562, BA 80 SUNY - Coll at New Paltz; MA 82 OH Univ - Athens; Univ of WI, **SLP**

Schwartz, Mrs Sharon Salzman 4020 Hemlock Circle, Orange Village, OH 44122, (216) 831-3881, MA 83 Cleveland St Univ; Sp-Lang Path, Psi Affiliates, **SLP**

Schwartz, Mrs Shawnee K 10617 North 37th Avenue, Phoenix, AZ 85029, (602) 866-5107, BS 75 AZ St Univ; MS 79 AZ St Univ; Sp-Lang Path, WA District Elementary Schools, **SLP**

Schwartz, Mrs Sherry F 2411 Margolin Lane, Clearwater, FL 34624-7517, (813) 536-4691, BS 64 NY Univ; MA 65 NY Univ

Schwartz, Mrs Susan 1681 Longbow Lane, Clearwater, FL 33546, (813) 535-6086, BA 74 George Washington Univ; MS 75 Columbia Univ Teachers Coll; **SLP**

Schwartz, Mrs Susan R 5531 West 84th Street, Shawnee Mission, KS 66207, BA 69 Univ of KY; MA 71 Saint Louis Univ; Sp-Lang Path, **SLP**

Schwartz, Dr Sybil J 2177 Lincoln #11, Montreal, PQ, Canada H3H 1J2, (514) 934-4491, BS 56 McGill Univ - Quebec; MA 57 Univ of IA; PH 75 (NS) McGill Univ - Quebec; Sp/Lang Path, Montreal Chldns Hosp, **SLP**

Schwartz, Teresa M 416 Second Street, Encinitas, CA 92024, (619) 588-3053, BA 82 Univ of CO - Boulder; MA 87 San Diego St Univ; **SLP**

Schwartz, Virginia Anne 912 North 64th Street, Philadelphia, PA 19151, (215) 358-6643, BS 76 West Chester Univ of PA; MA 83 West Chester Univ of PA; **SLP**

Schwartzberg, Gary David 325 Kennedy Memorial Drive, Waterville, ME 04901, (207) 873-7191, BS 82 Stockton St Coll; MS 84 Univ of VT; Aud, William H Diehl Jr MD PA, **A**

Schwartzbord, Carolyn 572 Seahorse Lane, Redwood City, CA 94065, (415) 494-1200, BA 71 Univ of CA - Berkeley; MA 75 NY Univ; Sp-Lang Path, San Mateo Co Bd of Educ, **SLP**

Schwartzkroin, Gail M 14 Willow Brook Drive, Glastonbury, CT 06033, (203) 633-5231, BS 70 Univ of MA - Amherst; MA 74 Univ of CT; 74–Sp/Lang Path, Glastonbury Pub Sch, **SLP**

Schwartz-Reitzel, Dr Joyce 22 Tudor Court, Timonium, MD 21093, (301) 321-3098, BS 63 OH St Univ; MA 65 OH St Univ; PH 79 (Communicative Sciences) Johns Hopkins Univ; Prof, Towson St Univ, **SLP**

Schwartz Rostker, Mrs Jill 23940 Middlebelt Road, Apartment 4102, Farmington Hills, MI 48024, (313) 478-6672, BS 79 MI St Univ; MS 81 Univ of MI - Ann Arbor; Sp-Lang Path, William Beaumont Hospital, **SLP**

Schwarz, Diane 269 Rutland Avenue, Teaneck, NJ 07666, (201) 461-9100, BA 54 CUNY - Hunter Coll; MA 81 Montclair St Coll; Sp-Lang Path, Leonia Board of Education, **SLP ACE**

Schwarz, Gail Cahn 1021 N W 167th Street, Seattle, WA 98177, (206) 546-3887, BA 67 CUNY - Hunter Coll; MA 67 Columbia Univ Teachers Coll; 85–Sp-Lang Path, Northwest Sp & Hrng Ctr, **SLP ACE**

Schwarz, Dr Ilsa Ellen Dept Speech Path & Audiology, University Of Oregon, 901 East 18th Street, Eugene, OR 97403, (503) 686-3591, BS 78 Univ of OR; MS 79 Univ of OR; PH 82 (Sp Path/Spec Educ) Univ of OR; Asst Prof, Univ of OR, **SLP**

Schwarz, Mrs Sheryl Lynn 16 Tammy Terrace, Wayne, NJ 07470, (201) 731-3600, BA 77 CUNY - Brooklyn Coll; MA 78 NY Univ; Sp-Lang Path, Private Practice, **SLP**

Schwarzbaum, Mrs Elisa M 10 Lakeview Drive, West Orange, NJ 07052, (201) 268-8187, BA 82 CUNY - Brooklyn Coll; MS 84 CUNY - Brooklyn Coll; **SLP**

Schwarzberg, Rona Sheryl 51 West 86th Street #201, New York, NY 10024, (212) 561-3564, MS 81 Columbia Univ Teachers Coll; 81–Sp-Lang Path, Bellevue Hosp, **SLP**

Schwarz-Cordier, Mrs Jean Marie Box 4103, APO Miami, FL 34001, (507) 264-3059, BS 84 PA St Univ - Univ Park; MS 86 PA St Univ - Univ Park; 88–Sp-Lang Path, Gorgas Army Hosp, **SLP**

Schwarzrock, Lorraine 3928 24th Avenue So, Minneapolis, MN 55406, (612) 293-8845, BA Univ of MN - Minneap-St Paul; MA Univ of MN - Minneap-St Paul; Sp-Lang Path, St Paul PS, **SLP**

Schwarzwalder, Mrs Susan D 106 Van Riper Lane, Woodcliff Lake, NJ 07675, **SLP**

Schwebach, Lee Ann Star Route Box 89, Sandia Park, NM 87047, (505) 281-9341, BS 81 Univ of SD - Vermillion; MA 82 Univ of SD - Vermillion; SLP, CES, **SLP**

Schwebel, Rochelle Feifer 1723-48th Street, Brooklyn, NY 11204, (212) 782-0064, BA 72 CUNY - Brooklyn Coll; MS 74 CUNY - Brooklyn Coll; SLP, Jewish Cen for Spec Ed, **SLP**

Schweber, Mrs Susan Baer 58 Pleasant Street, Sharon, MA 02067, (617) 784-6807, BA 74 Univ of MA - Amherst; MS 75 Boston Univ; **SLP**

Schwebke, Steven Paul Day One East, 3903 West Lisbon Avenue, Milwaukee, WI 53208, (414) 342-8777, BS 78 Univ of WI - Whitewater; MS 79 Univ of WI - Whitewater; 84–SLP, Bell Therapy Inc, **SLP**

Schweiger, Mrs Barbara Reese 934 Monarch Drive, Virginia Beach, VA 23462, (804) 481-4004, BS 83 Miami Univ - Oxford; MA 84 Bowling Green St Univ; **SLP**

Schweiger, Mrs Linda Ann 1116 Winslow, Richland, WA 99352, (509) 943-3720, MS 84 ID St Univ; SLP, Kennewick School Dstr, **SLP**

Schweigert, Mrs Ruth Annette 85 East Strasma Drive, Kankakee, IL 60901, (815) 933-4313, BA 85 Ball St Univ; MA 86 Ball St Univ; 87–Sp-Lang Path, Herscher Comm Sch Dist #2, **SLP**

Schweihs, Mrs Karen Mascolo 9 Laurel Street, Melrose, MA 02176, (617) 665-2967, MA 74 Univ of CT; SLP, Massachusetts Easter Seal, **SLP**

Schweitzer, Lisa A 6115 Vine Park Drive, Salt Lake City, UT 84121, BA 82 Minot St Univ; MS 83 Minot St Univ; Sp-Lang Path, Holy Cross Hospital, **SLP**

Schweitzer, Maureen Cassidy P O Box 11, 586 Cheyney Road, Thornton, PA 19373, BA 79 IN Univ - Bloomington; MA 84 West Chester Univ of PA; **SLP**

Schwellenbach, Julie Ann 443 Farnham #3, Marshall, WI 53559, (414) 261-6061, MS 83 Univ of WI - Whitewater; Sp-Lang Path, Watertown USD, **SLP**

Schwerin, Barbara Jean 341 Outwater Lane, Saddle Brook, NJ 07662, (201) 967-4040, BA 81 Montclair St Coll; MS 83 Boston Univ; Sp-Lang Path, Bergen Pines Co Hosp, **SLP ACE**

Schwieder, Jane 427 Grand Avenue, South Pasadena, CA 91030, (213) 682-1581, BA 68 Eckerd Coll; MA 70 Eckerd Coll; Substitute Teacher, Pasadena USD, **SLP**

Schwin, Evelyn Boyle 1804 Villanova Drive, Naperville, IL 60565, (312) 369-1642, BS Purdue Univ - West Lafayette; MS WV Univ; Aud, Sound Resources Inc, **A**

Schwitzgebel, Rita A 5807 Griffith Avenue N W, North Canton, OH 44720, **SLP**

Schwolow, Rhoda Jacobs 565 Upper Mountain Avenue, Montclair, NJ 07043, (201) 783-5221, BA 66 Univ of FL; ME 68 Univ of FL; Sp-Lang Path, Private Practice, **SLP ACE**

Sciackitano, Gwenn 5798 Ellsworth Street, Merrillville, IN 46410, (219) 769-4000, BS 71 IN Univ - Bloomington; MA 72 IN Univ - Bloomington; Superv Commun Dis, NW In Sp Ed Co-Op, **SLP**

Sciarappa, Jaryl Ann 5 Lafayette Street, 2nd Floor, Fairhaven, MA 02719, (617) 990-3603, BA 83 George Washington Univ; MA 85 George Washington Univ; **SLP**

Sciarrino, Sr Maralynn Mount Mercy Speech Center, 625 Abbott Road, Buffalo, NY 14220, (716) 826-6192, BA 61 Medaille Coll; MA 69 Catholic Univ of America; Dir/Sp-Lang Path, Mount Mercy Speech Center, **SLP**

Scifo, Marianne Conrad 500 Potter Boulevard, Brightwaters, NY 11718, (516) 654-3200, BS 79 SUNY - Coll at Buffalo; MS 82 SUNY - Coll at Buffalo; 84–Adjunct Faculty Member, St Josephs College, **SLP**

Scigliano, Vikki S 23 Cedar Drive, Massapequa, NY 11758, (516) 783-9515, BA 75 Hofstra Univ; MA 76 Hofstra Univ; 88–Sp-Lang Path, Wantagh PS, **SLP ACE**

Scipior, Joan Marie 2823 Garfield Street N E, Minneapolis, MN 55418, (612) 227-8471, BS 77 Univ of WI - Stevens Point; MA 78 Western MI Univ; Sp/Lang Path, St Paul Rehab Cen, **SLP**

Sciplin, Mrs Camille L 1445 South Cove Boulevard, Toledo, OH 43606, (419) 471-2061, BA 75 Fisk Univ; MA 77 OH St Univ; 88–Sp-Lang Path, The Toledo Hosp, **SLP**

Sclar, Judith 23634 Decoroh Road, Diamond Bar, CA 91765, (714) 397-4700, BS 52 Syracuse Univ; MS 76 Univ of LA Verne; Sp-Lang Path, Pomona USD, **SLP**

Scobell, Lynnette 100 Lanark Road #7, Brookline, MA 02146, (617) 734-6661, BS 82 WV Univ; MA 84 Kent St Univ; 88–Sp-Lang Path, Private Practice, **SLP**

Scoffone, Mrs Diane M 5 Blacksmith Road, Cumberland, RI 02864, BA 76 Rutger's St Univ - Douglas Coll; MS 79 Southern CT St Univ; 85–Sp-Lang Path, AGH Associates, **SLP**

Scofield, Michelle Renee 1607 Main Street #303, Springfield, MA 01103, (413) 781-9100, BA 84 SUNY - Coll at Cortland; MS 86 2923; Mercy Hospital, **A**

Scogg, Mrs Renee Ann 3420 Pine Ridge Parkway, Apartment 304, Grand Rapids, MI 49505, (517) 773-4356, BS 85 Central MI Univ; MA 86 Central MI Univ; 87–Sp-Lang Path, Stride Inc, **SLP**

Scolaro, Celeste P 1732 Sunnyside Circle, Northbrook, IL 60062, (312) 272-3297, BA 73 Saint Mary's Coll; MS 77 Univ of WA; **SLP**

Scollard, Blaise D 5305 S E 41st, Portland, OR 97202, **SLP**

Scollins, Beth Anne 121 Magnolia Drive, Westwood, MA 02090, (617) 581-9200, BS 80 Univ of NH; MS 81 Univ of NC - Chapel Hill; Dir-Comm Disorders, AtlantiCare Med Ctr, **SLP**

Sconfietti, Sandra C 19 Modelane, Rochester, NY 14618, **SLP**

Scoones, Mark Howard Hearing Systems Northwest, 3005 Simpson Avenue, Hoquiam, WA 98550, (206) 533-0633, BA 82 Univ of Northern CO; MS 84 Univ of WY; Aud, Hearing Systems Northwest, **A**

Scopp-Liegel, Elizabeth Ann 1826 North 53rd Street, Milwaukee, WI 53208, (414) 447-2208, BS 77 Univ of WI - Eau Claire; MS 81 Univ of WI - Milwaukee; Sp-Lang Path, St Joseph's Hospital, **SLP**

Scorse, Denise 802 West Iowa, Holbrook, AZ 86025, (602) 524-3921, BA 73 Brigham Young Univ; OM 79 Brigham Young Univ; 87–Sp-Lang Path, Holbrook Sch Dist, **SLP**

Scott, Allan Dill Lane, Poughkeepsie, NY 12601, (914) 877-6821, BS 72 SUNY - Coll at New Paltz; MS 80 Coll of Saint Rose; 86–Coord of Prof Svcs, NY St Off Ment Ret/Wassaic Dvc, **SLP**

Scott, Mrs Anne C 2522 Berwyck Road S E, East Grand Rapids, MI 49506, (616) 774-2702, BA 58 MI St Univ; ME 64 Wayne St Univ; Sp-Lang Path, Visiting Nurse Service, **SLP**

Scott, Mrs Anne Marie 18723 Barn Swallow Terrace, Gaithersburg, MD 20879, (301) 963-4059, BS 81 Towson St Univ; MS 83 Univ of SC - Columbia

Scott, Mrs Atheria C 1748 Hampton Drive, Harvey, LA 70058, (504) 362-4232, BS 76 Univ of GA; ME 77 Univ of GA; Sp-Lang Path, Jefferson Parish Sch Syst, **SLP ACE**

Scott, Mrs Brenda Mueller 5215 Tamerlane Road, Louisville, KY 40207, (502) 459-6005, BA 69 Miami Univ - Oxford; ME 71 Univ of KY; Sp/Lang Path, Private Practice, **SLP**

Scott, Brian Lee 1111 Willow Springs Drive, Denton, TX 76205, (817) 382-9421

Scott, C Rex Aud Assoc Of Salt Lake City, 22 South 900 East, Salt Lake City, UT 84102, (801) 364-8692, BS 65 Brigham Young Univ; MS 70 Brigham Young Univ; Private Practice, **A**

Scott, Dr Carl H 13280 Skyline, Woodside, CA 94062, (415) 324-4200, BA 56 Univ of Southern CA; MA 65 Univ of Southern CA; PH 70 (NS) Wayne St Univ; Private Practice, **SLP**

Scott, Mrs Carol S 14331 River Forest, Houston, TX 77079, (713) 493-0806, BA 65 MI St Univ; MS 66 Vanderbilt Univ; Sp-Lang Path, **SLP**

Scott, Mrs Carol Virginia 226 Beverly, Missoula, MT 59801, (406) 549-7950, BA Univ of MT; MA 85 Univ of MT; **A**

Scott, Dr Cheryl M Department Speech Language Pathology & Audiology, Oklahoma State University, 120 Hanner, Stillwater, OK 74078, (405) 744-8947, BS 65 Purdue Univ - West Lafayette; MA 66 Northwestern Univ; PH 70 (NS) Purdue Univ - West Lafayette; 78–Assoc Prof, OK St U, **SLP F**

Scott, Mrs Christie Miller 1163 Lakepointe, Grosse Pointe Pk, MI 48230, (313) 823-6708, BA 81 OH Univ - Athens; MA 84 OH Univ - Athens; Sp-Lang Path, Interpointe Sp & Lang Serv, **SLP**

Scott, Colleen Gail 170 Fifth Street, Providence, RI 02906, (401) 861-9874, BA 83 Univ of RI; MS 86 Univ of RI; 88–Sp-Lang Path, J Arthur Trudeau Memorial Ctr, **SLP**

Scott, David Michael 1497 Channel Lane, Mount Vernon, WA 98273, (206) 466-4156, BA 76 Univ of CA - Berkeley; MA 81 Western WA Univ; **SLP**

Scott, Davis A Department Of Speech, Moorhead State University, Moorhead, MN 56560, (218) 236-2286, BA 50 Grinnell Coll; MA 53 IN Univ - Bloomington; PH 67 (NS) IN Univ - Bloomington; Prof, Moorhead St U, **SLP**

Scott, Diane M Dept Of Aud & Sp Sciences, Michigan State Univ, East Lansing, MI 48824-1212, (517) 355-7628, BS 78 Univ of VA - Charlottesville; ME 80 Univ of VA - Charlottesville; PH 86 (Aud) Vanderbilt Univ; 86–Asst Prof in Aud, Michigan State Univ, **A**

Scott, Mrs Donna Jean 205 Brookdale Drive, Jamestown, NC 27282, (919) 885-8722, BA 83 Univ of NC - Chapel Hill; MA 86 Univ of NC - Greensboro; **SLP**

Scott, Duncan R 404 Peniel Road, Columbus, NC 28722, (704) 894-3958, BA 46 Univ of Chicago; MA 49 Northwestern Univ; **SLP A LM**

Scott, Mrs Elizabeth P O Box 665, St Charles, MO 63301, MS; **A LM**

Scott, Homer W 12 Huckleberry Lane, West Hartford, CT 06110, (203) 521-7294, MA 48 Harvard Univ; Sp-Lang Path, Hartford Bd of Educ, **SLP**

Scott, Mrs Jacquelyn S 2208 41st Street, Meridian, MS 39305, (601) 693-0948, BS 71 MS Univ for Women; MS 72 Univ Southern MS-Hattiesburg; Sp-Lang Path, Meridian PS, **SLP**

Scott, James E 14 Weinel Drive, Fairview Heights, IL 62208, (314) 362-7489, BA 71 Southern IL Univ-Edwardsvill; MS 81 Southern IL Univ-Edwardsvill; Aud, Washington U Med Sch, **A**

Scott, Mrs Jane R 8234 Litchfield Drive, Mentor, OH 44060, (216) 256-8484, BS 51 Kent St Univ; ME 62 Kent St Univ; Super-Consult, Mentor Exempted Sch/E Shore, **SLP**

Scott, Janet C 181 Cherovan Drive S W, Calgary, AB, Canada T2V 2P4, (403) 229-7044, OB 74 Univ of Western Ontario; MS 80 Ithaca Coll; Sp/Lang Path, Alberta Chldn's Hosp, **SLP**

Scott, Mrs Karen Heckman 133 Dorr Drive, Rutland, VT 05701, (802) 775-1990, BS 81 Northwestern Univ; MA 84 Univ of IA; 86–Sp-Lang Path, Rutland City Piblic Schools, **SLP**

Scott, Karen M 125 Regal Drive, Santa Maria, CA 93454, (805) 541-1790, MA 71 Univ of CA - Santa Barbara; Aud, Private Practice, **SLP A**

Scott, Mrs Kathleen Ann 3194 West Fremont Avenue, Fresno, CA 93711, (209) 441-3089, BA 73 CA St Univ - Fresno; MA 75 CA St Univ - Fresno; Special Education Teacher, Fresno USD, **SLP**

Scott, Mrs Kathleen Ann R 78 Country Corner Lane, Fairport, NY 14450, (716) 223-3155, BS 79 Nazareth Coll of Rochester; MS 81 Nazareth Coll of Rochester; Sp-Lang Path, Rochester Sch for Deaf, **SLP**

Scott, Kathleen L 4253 Still Meadow Lane, West Bloomfield, MI 48033, (313) 851-2982, **SLP**

Scott, Kathy P 880 Wildwood Boulevard S W, Issaquah, WA 98027, (206) 455-4042, BA 75 WA St Univ; MA 76 WA St Univ; Sp-Lang Path, Group Hlth Coop, **SLP**

Scott, Kimberly Rae Wilford Hall Medical Center, Speech And Hearing Department/SGHS05, Lackland AFB, TX 78236, (512) 670-5420, BS 83 Univ of WY; MS 85 Univ of AR - Little Rock; Sp-Lang Path, US Air Force, **SLP**

Scott, Laura M 399 Warren Wright Road, Belchertown, MA 01007, (413) 253-2235, MS 87 Univ of MA - Amherst; **SLP**

Scott, Laurie Louise 7 Relmar Road #1, Toronto, ON, Canada M5P 2Y4, (416) 425-6220, BA 85 Univ of ND; MS 86 Univ of MI - Ann Arbor; **SLP**

Scott, Lawrence C, Jr Natl Tech Inst For The Deaf, 1 Lomb Memorial Drive, Rochester, NY 14623, (716) 475-6790, BS 75 SUNY - Coll at Geneseo; MS 76 Southern IL Univ -Carbondale; Aud/Asst Prof, NTID, **A**

Scott, Lewis Henry, Jr Ames Elementary School, 1760 Ames Place, St Paul, MN 55106, (612) 293-8970, BS 73 Moorhead St Univ; MA 77 Coll of St Thomas; MS 83 Univ of WI - River Falls; 75–Sp-Lang Path, St Paul Pub Sch, **SLP**

Scott, Dr Lorel M Department Of Communication, Saint Louis University, 3733 West Pine Boulevard, St Louis, MO 63108, (314) 658-3191, BS 72 Univ of Southwestern LA; MS 74 Univ of Southwestern LA; PH 84 (Sp Communication) Univ of TX - Austin; 88–Prof, St Louis Univ, **SLP**

Scott, Mrs Mary Anne S 20 Spindlewick Drive, Nashua, NH 03062, (603) 888-5870, BA 74 Boston Coll; MA 76 NY Univ; Sp/Lang Path, Leonard Morse Hosp, **SLP**

Scott, Mrs Pamela S Green Acres Trailer Park, 1 Henry Street, Kinston, NC 28501, (919) 527-6690, BA 80 Marshall Univ; MA 81 Marshall Univ; Sp-Lang Path, Private Practice, **SLP**

Scott, Pamela Sue B 496 Colonial Avenue, Worthington, OH 43085, (614) 228-5523, BA 80 Ball St Univ; MA 81 Ball St Univ; Sp-Lang Path, Easter Seals Rehab Cen, **SLP**

Scott, Paulette 2413 S E 45th, Oklahoma City, OK 73129, (405) 672-0552, MS 88 Univ of OK Medical Center

Scott, Rosemary 1808 Gillette Crescent, South Pasadena, CA 91030, (213) 258-5566, BA 75 Univ of Redlands; MA 78 CA St Univ - Los Angeles; SLP, Rosemary Scott Ma-Ccc, **SLP**

Scott, Mrs Ruth P O Box 26, Hampton Falls, NH 03844, BA 72 Univ of MD - College Park; MA 73 Univ of MD - College Park; **SLP**

Scott, Saralynn 7575 Cambridge, Apartment 3303, Houston, TX 77054, (713) 792-4500, BA 73 Queens Univ - Ontario; MS 75 Eastern IL Univ; 84–Sp-Lang Path, University of Texas S/H Inst, **SLP**

Scott, Susan C 4508 Cobblers Lane, Dallas, TX 75252, (817) 565-2262, BS 76 Southern Methodist Univ; MS 77 Southern Methodist Univ; Cl Supv, North TX St U, **SLP**

Scott, Mrs Susan M 5600 Lake Resort Terrace, Apartment 419J, Chattanooga, TN 37415, (615) 757-1880, BS 68 Purdue Univ - West Lafayette; MS 69 Purdue Univ - West Lafayette; Sp-Lang Path, Hamilton Co Sch, **SLP**

Scott, Susan Scoggins 1109 Rambler, Waco, TX 76710, (817) 774-4442, BS 81 Univ of TX - Austin; ME 84 Southwest TX St Univ; 88–Sp-Lang Path, Scott & White Hosp-Clinic, **SLP**

Scott, Susanne Manzi 5845 North 21st Street, Arlington, VA 22205, (202) 651-5960, BS 78 Bloomsburg Univ of PA; MS 80 Gallaudet Coll; Aud, Model Secondary/Gallaudet Coll, **A**

Scott, Wallace G 1387 Crown Drive, Alameda, CA 94501, (415) 769-8188, BA 51 Walla Walla Coll; MS 52 Univ of OR; President, Aaron Associates Inc, **SLP**

Scott, William C 30 Pinehurst Circle, Arden, NC 28704, (704) 684-6312, BA 66 Univ of South FL; ME 73 Western Carolina Univ; Sp-Lang Path, Buncombe Co Schs, **SLP**

Scott-Casucci, Mrs Robin J 2290 Galloway Road D-13, Bensalem, PA 19020, (215) 295-1155, BS 85 East Stroudsburg Univ of PA; MS 87 Temple Univ; 87–Sp-Lang Path, Valley Day Sch

Scotti, Mrs Amy B 1927 Fowker Avenue, Bronx, NY 10462, (212) 792-4134, BA 80 CUNY - Queens Coll; MS 81 Adelphi Univ; **SLP**

Scotti, Mark R 506 Windsor Court, Somerville, NJ 08876, (201) 647-0180, BS 68 Fordham Univ; MA 71 SUNY - Coll at Geneseo; Spec Assistant to the Director, VA Med Center, **SLP**

Scoufis, Margaret R 1211 Milwaukee Street, Delafield, WI 53018, (414) 327-6670, **SLP**

Scow, Mrs Cecilia H Route 1 Box 415, Chassell, MI 49916-9726, (517) 821-6308, BA 76 Univ of MI - Ann Arbor; MA 78 Eastern MI Univ; Sp-Lang Path, McKennan Hospital, **SLP**

Scram, Jeanette Ballard Rd 1, 344 Dir Road, Hickory, PA 15340-9801, (412) 257-2960, MS 80 Univ of NC - Chapel Hill; Program Coord, Crossroads Sp-Lang & Hrng Inc, **SLP**

Scramlin, Mrs Cheryl D Route 2 Box 221, Hillman, MI 49746, (616) 238-9394, BS 75 Central MI Univ; MA 80 Central MI Univ; Sp-Lang Path, Cheboygan-Otsego-Presque Isle, **SLP**

Scranton, Mrs Judith Whitacre 3 Rocky Point Drive RFD 12, Concord, NH 03301, (603) 224-3951, OB 63 OH Univ - Athens; **SLP**

Screen, Dr Robert Martin Hampton University, Box 6633, Hampton, VA 23668, (804) 727-5435, BA 53 Hampton Univ; MA 54 NY Univ; PH 68 (NS) MI St Univ; Prof & Chair/Dept Commun Dis, Hampton Univ, **SLP F**

Scrima-Castelli, Mrs Lisa Marie 15 Elm Court, Sayville, NY 11782, (516) 567-8016, BA 77 CUNY - Hunter Coll; MA 80 NY Univ; Sp-Lang Path, Suffolk Hrng & Sp Ctr, **SLP**

Scrimshire, Linda B 850 Congdon #19, Elgin, IL 60120, (312) 888-5262, BS 64 IL Wesleyan Univ; MS 73 IL St Univ - Normal; Sp-Lang Path, School District U-46, **SLP**

Scriven, Mrs Louise M 22412 Pico Street, Grand Terrace, CA 92324, (714) 783-0369, BA 53 Univ of CA - Berkeley; MS 81 Loma Linda Univ - Riverside; Sp-Lang Path, Private Practice, **SLP**

Scroggie, Everett, Jr 2100 S W 79th Drive, Gainesville, FL 32607, (904) 373-5507, BS 58 Univ of TN - Knoxville; MA 63 Univ of TN - Knoxville; Pres, Audio Hrng Serv, **A**

Scroggin, Mrs Deborah K 4149 Briar Hill, Grand Prairie, TX 75052, (817) 565-1845, BS 78 TX Woman's Univ; MA 80 TX Woman's Univ; Sp-Lang Path, Communication Disorders Clinic, **SLP**

Scroggs, Dana J 40 A Broadview Court, Columbia, MO 65201, (314) 882-6988, OB 81 Univ of MO - Columbia; OM 82 Univ of MO - Columbia; 85–Sp-Lang Path, Univ Missouri Hosp & Clinics, **SLP**

Scruggs, Susan Dianne P O Box 427, Mars Hill, NC 28754, (704) 689-4238, **SLP**

Scruggs, Theresa Babinsky 4626 Allegheny, San Antonio, TX 78229, (512) 692-1555, BS 76 Univ of TX - Austin; MA 79 Our Lady Lake Univ-San Anton; Sp-Lang Path, San Antonio ISD, **SLP**

Scudder, Dr Rosalind Department Of Communicative Disorders, Wichita State University, Wichita, KS 67208-1595, (316) 689-3289, BA 64 Wichita St Univ; MA 72 Wichita St Univ; PH 78 (Sp-Lang Path) Wichita St Univ; Asst Prof & Cl Dir, Wsu Sp-Lang-Hrng Cl, **SLP ACE**

Scukanec, Gail Patricia 321 South Summit Street, Bowling Green, OH 43402-3018, (419) 353-0038, BA 73 MI St Univ; MA 86 Central MI Univ; 88–Tchg Fellow, Bowling Green State Univ, **SLP**

Scull, Janet Loeper 3326 Earl Street, Laureldale, PA 19605, (215) 921-9879, BS 82 East Stroudsburg Univ of PA; MS 83 Bloomsburg Univ of PA; Sp/Lang Path, Berks Co Intermed Unit, **SLP**

Scully, Martha S 10923 Wickshire Way, Rockville, MD 20852, **SLP**

Scully-Burch, Julie Ann 608 Laverne Place, Macon, GA 31204, (912) 742-6333, BS 77 Armstrong St Coll; MS 80 Univ of KY; Sp-Lang Path, Central State Hosp, **SLP**

Sculnick, Mrs Gloria Nevard 24 Fanton Hill Road, Weston, CT 06883, BA 43 Ithaca Coll; MS 75 Adelphi Univ; **SLP**

Scurfield, Mrs Jerri L 739 California St, Alma, MI 48801, (517) 463-8582, MA 88 Central MI Univ

Scurlock, Mrs Margaret L 140 2nd Avenue, Burlington, ND 58722, BS 66 KY St; MS 68 Minot St Univ; **SLP**

Scurr, Deborah D 5143 28th Avenue North, St Petersburg, FL 33710, (813) 327-0079, BS 77 Ball St Univ; MA 79 Case Western Reserve Univ; Sp-Lang Path, 16th St Middle Sch, **SLP**

Scurry, Donna Jean 706 North Patton, Arlington Heights, IL 60004, (312) 577-7349, BS 82 Univ of IL - Urbana; MS 83 Univ of IL - Urbana; SLP, Lutheran General Hosp, **SLP ACE**

Scygiel, Sr M Dominica St Joseph Medical Center, 333 North Madison Street, Joliet, IL 60435, (815) 725-7133, BA 64; MS 71 Marquette Univ; Dir SLP, Saint Joseph Hospital, **SLP**

Sea, Louise Marie 1505 S W Broadway, Albany, OR 97321, (503) 370-8990, BS 78 Northern MI Univ; MS 81 Univ of MT; 87–Speech/Lang Pathologist, Mid-Valley Children's Guild, **SLP**

Seabeck, Mrs Diana J 2533 Park Avenue, Laramie, WY 82070, (307) 721-4460, BA 69 Univ of AZ; MS 76 Univ of WY; Case Mgr, Albany Co Sch Dist #1, **SLP**

Seabourn, Mrs Beverly Jolene 4120 Selene Drive, Denton, TX 76201, (817) 382-2736, BS 77 Univ of North TX; MS 81 Univ of North TX; 86–Sp-Lang Path, Jolene Seabourn, **SLP**

Seacrist, Anne M 5809 North Lindenwood Dr, #2606, Peoria, IL 61615, (309) 692-6558, MS 87 IL St Univ - Normal; 88–Sp-Lang Path, Speech & Language Rehab Svcs

Seaford, Nancy I 7800 Touch ME Not Lane, Concord, NC 28025, (704) 782-3519, BS 72 Appalachian St Univ; MA 73 Appalachian St Univ; Sp/Lang Path, Private Practice, **SLP**

Seagren, Mrs Jill C 250 Ogden Street, Denver, CO 80218, (303) 322-1871, BA 74 CA St Univ - Northridge; MA 75 CA St Univ - Northridge; 79–Mgr of Aud Svcs, Cen for Hrng Sp & Lang, **A**

Seal, Mrs Brenda C Route 2 Box 232, Bridgewater, VA 22812, (703) 568-3876, BS 72 Appalachian St Univ; MA 75 Appalachian St Univ; Dir-Sp & Hrng Ctr, JMU/Dept of Sp-Path and Aud, **SLP ACE**

Seal, Mrs Joy M 4303 Woodlynne Lane, Orlando, FL 32812, (407) 855-2806, BS 71 OK St Univ; MS 73 Univ of OK Medical Center; Sp-Lang Path, Orange Co Pub Sch, **SLP**

Seal, Mrs Nelda C 363 Windermere Boulevard, Apartment 109, Alexandria, LA 71303, (504) 735-9540, BA 57 Southeastern LA Univ; OM 61; MS 72 Univ Southern MS-Hattiesburg; Sp-Lang Path, Speech Pathology Services, **SLP**

Seal, Mrs Sharon B 1817 Heatherhill Drive, Trenton, MI 48183, (313) 284-4900, BS 69 Univ of MI - Ann Arbor; MS 70 Univ of MI - Ann Arbor; Aud, Hrng Serv Ltd, **A**

Seale, Linda Ruth 500 North Metro Boulevard #2007M, Chandler, AZ 85226, (602) 345-0964, BS 81 Univ of AZ; MS 83 Univ of AZ; Aud, Gordon E Genta MD PC, **A**

Seals, Mrs Jody Lynn Route 1 Box 562 C-93, Country Road, Texarkana, TX 75502, (214) 794-2705, **A**

Seals, Sharon Skrivanos 7575 Katy Freeway #16, Houston, TX 77024, (713) 680-8576, BS 70 Centenary Coll of LA; MS 79 Univ of AR - Little Rock; Sp-Lang Path, Sharon Seals-Sp & Lang Path, **SLP**

Sealy, Lynn 7 Lyon Crescent, Sayville, NY 11782, (516) 567-8087, BA 71 Hofstra Univ; MA 72 Hofstra Univ; Sp-Lang Path, Sayville Pub Schs, **SLP**

Seaman, Bruce D 11 Johnson Road, Lawrenceville, NJ 08648, (609) 443-5334, MA Trenton St Coll; Seaman Associates, **SLP**

Seaman, Constance R R 1 Box 152, Papaikou, HI 96781, (808) 935-1455, BA 63 Stanford Univ; MA 73 Univ of TX - El Paso; Sp-Lang Path, **SLP**

Seaman, Don P Box 1539, Salmon Arm, BC, Canada VOE 2T0, (604) 832-5157, BS 84 Northern AZ Univ; MS 86 Northern AZ Univ

Seaman, Karen Ricketts 5957 East 72nd St South, Apartment 2006, Tulsa, OK 74136, BS 82 Northern IL Univ - De Kalb; MA 83 Northern IL Univ - De Kalb; Sp-Lang Path, OK Dept Human Svcs Dev Dis, **SLP**

Seaman, Mrs Linda S 12 The Poplars, Roslyn Estates, NY 11576, (516) 883-4000, BA 59 CUNY - Brooklyn Coll; MA 79 Hofstra Univ; SLP, Port Wash Pub Sch Dist, **SLP**

Seaman, Mrs Michelle Gardner P O Box 1539, Salmon Arm, BC, Canada V0E 2T0, (604) 387-2663, BS 85 Northern AZ Univ; MS 86 Northern AZ Univ

Seaman, Victoria Ann 785 Virginia Avenue, North Bellmore, NY 11710, (516) 921-7171, BA 82 SUNY - Coll at Cortland; ME 84 Univ of GA; **SLP**

Seamens, John B P O Box 58, Lakeland, FL 33802, (813) 644-6070, BS 64 East TN St Univ; MA 66 Univ of TN - Knoxville; Dist Mgr, Unitron Indust Inc, **SLP A ACE**

Seamons-Lindquist, Carla 1510 North 260 East, North Logan, UT 84321, (801) 753-6456, MS 88 UT St Univ; 88–Aud, Utah Valley Reg Med Ctr

Seanor, Suzann 30 Greenview Drive, Jeanette, PA 15644, (412) 837-7187, BS 86 Clarion Univ of PA; MS 87 Clarion Univ of PA; 88–Aud, Allegheny Hearing Aid Ctr

Searcy, Deborah A 11963 Canyon Court, Louisville, KY 40229, **SLP**

Searcy, Karyn Lewis 18811 Dixie Highway, Suite 102, Homewood, IL 60430, (312) 798-6988, BA 75 Elmhurst Coll; MA 76 Univ of IL - Urbana; Owner / Asst Prof, Private Practice / Elmhurst Coll, **SLP**

Searer, Wilbur G 203 East Douglas Street, Fort Wayne, IN 46802, (219) 425-7463, BS 49 Manchester Coll; MA 51 Univ of Denver; 65–Superv of Sp/Lang Path, Fort Wayne Commun Sch, **SLP**

Seargent, Mrs Janice W 602 Main Street, Murray, KY 42071, (502) 753-5022, BS 78 Murray St Univ; MS 79 Murray St Univ; Sp-Lang Path, Murray ISD, **SLP**

Searle, Linda Lee 106 Church Street, Waltham, MA 02154, (617) 529-7711, BS 82 Univ of MA - Amherst; MS 86 Worcester St Coll

Searles, Mrs Carol L P 136 Dumbarton Road, Baltimore, MD 21212, (301) 823-3385, MS 78 Loyola Coll; **SLP**

Searles, Linda M 6252 South Elmira Circle E, Englewood, CO 80111, (303) 741-0781, BA 63 Univ of MI - Ann Arbor; **SLP**

Sears, Carolyn Jean UT Southwestern Medical Center, Department Of Otolaryngology, 5323 Harry Hines Boulevard, Dallas, TX 75235, (214) 688-4757, BS 85 TX Tech Univ; MS 87 Univ of TX - Dallas; 87–Aud, UT Southwestern Med Ctr, **A**

Sears, Cathy L 707 Francis Drive, Lafayette, CA 94549, (415) 372-9484, BA 82 CA St Univ - Sacramento; MS 84 San Francisco St Univ; 84–Sp-Lang Path, Vallejo City USD, **SLP**

Sears, Cynthia Hooker 3031 Green Fields, Sugar Land, TX 77479, (713) 342-6415, BA 79 Univ of MS; MA 81 Univ of MS; Aud, Brazoria-Fort Bend Coop, **A**

Sears, Lillian Wright 11 Dewey Street, Manhasset, NY 11030, (516) 883-4000, BA 80 Saint John's Univ - Jamaica; MA 82 CUNY - Queens Coll; Sp-Lang Path, Port Washington Un Fr Sch Dist, **SLP ACE**

Sears, Loie P 107 Vestavia Hills, Northport, AL 35476, (205) 758-3970, BA 68 Univ of South FL; MA 69 Univ of South FL; Dir, Alabama Hlth-Related Serv, **SLP**

Sears, Richard B 3257 Parker Street, Dearborn, MI 48124, (313) 562-6631, BS 78 Eastern MI Univ; MA 79 Eastern MI Univ; Sp-Lang Path, Oakwood Hosp, **SLP**

Sears, Mrs Sara P Route 1 Box 23, Edgefield, SC 29824, (803) 279-0606, BS 58 Univ of GA; ME 63 Univ of GA; Sp-Lang Path, Aiken Co Sch Sys, **SLP ACE**

Sears, Valerie Ann 127 Main Street, Bondsville, MA 01009, (413) 283-8547, BS 84 Univ of MA - Amherst; MS 87 Worcester St Coll

Sears-Bode, Deborah 95 Poiniciada #108, Brownsville, TX 78521, (512) 542-8504, BS 74 OK St Univ; MA 75 Western MI Univ; Executive Director, Brownsville Soc Crippled Chldn, **SLP**

Seaton, Jane B 680 Kings Road, Athens, GA 30606, (404) 742-8292, BS 63 Northwestern Univ; MS 64 Univ of MI - Ann Arbor; Aud, NE GA RESA, **SLP A**

Seaton, Mrs Joanne C 7901 Brown Road, Richmond, VA 23235, (804) 272-1414, BS 71 James Madison Univ; ME 72 Univ of VA - Charlottesville; Audiologist, Dr Wm L Wilkes, **A**

Seaton, Kay P 3301-C Regents Park Lane, Greensboro, NC 27405, (919) 288-1779, BA 63 Wichita St Univ; MA 68 Central MI Univ; SLP, Greensboro City Pub Sch, **SLP**

Seaton, Stewart S 1754 South Mountain Avenue, Apartment C, Ontario, CA 91761, (714) 595-1221, BA 76 San Diego St Univ; MA 79 San Diego St Univ; SLP, Lanterman Developmental Center, **A**

Seaton, Dr William H School Of Hearing And Speech, Ohio University, 201 Lindley Hall, Athens, OH 45701, (614) 593-1407, BS 71 Univ of IL - Urbana; MS 73 Univ of IL - Urbana; PH 76 (NS) Univ of IL - Urbana; Assoc Prof/Dir, OH U, **A**

Seaver, Earl J Dept Communicative Disorders, Northern Illinois Univ, De Kalb, IL 60115, BS 69 Western MI Univ; MA 70 Western MI Univ; PH 79 (NS) Univ of IA; 75–Assoc Prof/Dir Cl Svc, Nn IL U, **SLP**

Seavertson, Dr John M 12607 West 101st Street, Lenexa, KS 66215, (816) 861-4700, BA 72 San Jose St Univ; MA 76 Univ of KS; PH 81 (NS) Univ of KS; Aud, VA Medical Center, **A**

Seavy, Mrs Dorothy J Hoyt 3015 Oakcrest Drive N W, Salem, OR 97304, (503) 581-7251, BA 67 CA St Univ - Northridge; MA 75 CA St Univ - Northridge; MA 83 Western OR St Coll; 88–Sp-Lang Path, D Seavy's Sp & Lang Cen, **SLP ACE**

Seavy, Judith L 22 Clauss Road, Clark, NJ 07066, (201) 388-2944, BS 76 West Chester Univ of PA; MA 78 Seton Hall Univ; Aud, Newark Beth Israel Med Ctr, **A**

Seay, Lela Jane Salem Pines, 1904 East Mulberry #702, Angleton, TX 77515, (409) 849-2447, **SLP**

Sebastian, Judith Jackson 3000 Reynwest Court, Tobaccoville, NC 27050, (919) 924-9309, BS 81 Radford Univ; MS 83 James Madison Univ; 87–Sp/Lang Path, Stokes Cty Schs, **SLP**

Sebastian, Mrs Karen D 3712 Shiloh Road, Kennesaw, GA 30144, (404) 926-6169, BS 72 Eastern MI Univ; MA 75 Eastern MI Univ; Sp-Lang Path, Cobb Co Pub Schs, **SLP**

Sebastian, Linda Lee 631 Leona Street, Sharpsville, PA 16150-1629, (216) 746-7211, BA 83 Kent St Univ; MA 83 Kent St Univ; Sp-Lang Path, St Elizabeth Hosp Med Center, **SLP**

Sebby-Hornbruch, Mrs Ingrid 10 Kepler, Irvine, CA 92715, (213) 515-3084, BA 75 San Diego St Univ; MA 80 CA St Univ - Northridge; SLP, Irvine USD, **SLP**

Sebetka, Mrs Patricia M 2545 N Avenue N W, Cedar Rapids, IA 52405, (319) 399-6874, BS 72 Univ of IA; MS 73 Univ of IA; Early Childhood Sp-Lang Path, Grant Wood AEA, **SLP**

Sebian, Sr Mary Ann St Elizabeth Hosp Med Center, 1044 Belmont, P O Box 1790, Youngstown, OH 44501, (216) 746-7211, BS 63 Nazareth Coll of Rochester; MA 72 Kent St Univ; 78–Sp-Lang Path, St Elizabeth Hosp Med Ctr, **SLP**

Sechler, Mrs Linda 8320 Monclova Road, Monclova, OH 43542, (419) 245-4150, BS 78 Bowling Green St Univ; MA 79 Bowling Green St Univ; 84–Sp-Lang Path, Lucas Co Office of Ed, **SLP**

Seckinger, M Suzanne Tomlinson 1036 Cedar Ridge Court, Annapolis, MD 21403, (412) 622-4484, BA 76 Mansfield Univ of PA; MA 85 Univ of Pittsburgh - Pittsburgh; Sp-Lang Path, **SLP**

Secondino, Kathryn Susan 2430 North Eustis Drive, Indianapolis, IN 46229, (317) 898-9635, BS 84 Purdue Univ - West Lafayette; MS 85 IN St Univ - Terre Haute; 87–Sp-Lang Path, Hendricks Comm Hosp, **SLP**

Secor, Julianna Louise 5901 Poso Court, Bakersfield, CA 93309, (805) 325-3329, BA 84 CA St Univ - Northridge; MA 86 CA St Univ - Northridge; SLP, Kern County Superv of Schools, **SLP**

Secor, Virginia M 7 Greenbriar Way, East Greenbush, NY 12061, (518) 235-1410, BS 75 SUNY - Center at Albany; MS 77 SUNY - Center at Albany; SLP, Highgate Manor/New Medico, **SLP**

Secord, Dr Wayne A 4875 Widner Street, Columbus, OH 43220, (419) 372-6031, BS 71 OH St Univ; MA 77 OH St Univ; PH 80 (NS) Univ of Cincinnati; Chair-Dept of Comm Disorders, Bowling Green St Univ, **SLP**

Secrest, Mrs Mary Miller 1308 Gray Hawk Road, Lexington, KY 40502, (606) 269-8068, MS 87 Univ Southern MS-Hattiesburg; 87–Sp-Lang Path, Swigert and Associates, **SLP**

Secrest, Molly 48 Oak Drive, Upton, MA 01568, (508) 791-6351, BA 79; MA 82 Portland St Univ; 88–Sp-Lang Path, Fairlawn Rehab Hosp, **SLP**

Secunda, Lynne G 102 Plush Mill Road, Wallingford, PA 19086, (215) 565-8779, BA 67 PA St Univ - Univ Park; MA 80 West Chester Univ of PA; Sp/Lang Path, Taylor Hosp Rehab Ut, **SLP**

Seda, Mrs Susan Tavernia 405 Fox Avenue, Yonkers, NY 10704, (914) 776-6507, BA 80 CUNY - Queens Coll; MA 83 CUNY - Queens Coll; 86–Sp-Lang Path, Young Adult Institute, **SLP**

Sedat, Nancy A 8861 Alcott #2, Los Angeles, CA 90035, (213) 674-7050, BA 68 San Francisco St Univ; MS 73 Univ of OK Medical Center; Cl Spec, Daniel Freeman Hosp, **SLP**

Sederburg, Mrs Claudette N 1175 Office Park Road, Apartment 300, West Des Moines, IA 50265, (515) 226-0861, MA 88 CA St Univ - Fullerton; 88–Sp-Lang Path, Central Rehab

Sederholm, Steven Daniel 1210 Route 10, Dover, NJ 07801, (201) 328-9039, BA 84 Jacksonville Univ; MA 88 Univ of FL; 88–Aud, The Hrng Lab Inc, **A**

Sedge, Dr Roy Kenneth 6261 Cardinal Lane, Columbia, MD 21044, (301) 663-7301, BS 63 Central MI Univ; MA 65 MI St Univ; PH 70 (Aud) Univ of WA; Dir, US Army Med R & D Command, **A F**

Sedgwick, Linda S 832 Fondulac Drive, East Peoria, IL 61611, **A**

Sedlacek, Virginia 6759 West Cheryl Drive, Peoria, AZ 85345, (602) 486-8601, **A**

Sedlak, Mrs Ginnie Deangelis 208 Hilltop Lane, Sleepy Hollow, IL 60118, (312) 428-0925, BS 81 Northern IL Univ - De Kalb; MA 82 Northern IL Univ - De Kalb; Sp-Lang Path, Medinah Elem Sch Dist #11, **SLP**

Sedlik, Mrs Bernice M 18070 Boris Drive, Encino, CA 91316, (213) 344-0335, BA 79 CA St Univ - Northridge; MA 83 CA St Univ - Northridge; Sp-Lang Path, Language & Speech Associates, **SLP**

Sedory, Susan Elaine Natl Institute Of Health, Bldg 10/5N226, Bethesda, MD 20892, (301) 496-9365, BS 84 Indiana Univ of PA; MA 86 Univ of MD - College Park; 86–Sp-Lang Path, NIH, **SLP**

Sedota, Anthony R 184 Water Street, Fredonia, NY 14063, (716) 673-1182, BS 55 SUNY - Coll at Fredonia; MS 61 SUNY - Coll at Fredonia; Retired, BOCES Chautauqua Co, **SLP**

Sedovsky, Donna Cheryl 118 Crooked Hill Road, Huntington, NY 11743, BA 83 Hofstra Univ; MA 86 Hofstra Univ; **SLP**

See, Lavonne E 25 South Shore Drive, Canyon, MN 55717, (218) 741-4772, BS 68 Univ of MN - Duluth; MA 76 Univ of MN - Duluth; Sp Coord, St Louis Co Sch, **SLP**

Seed, Mrs Pamela F 177 Gunstock Hill Road, Gilford, NH 03246, (603) 524-6733, MS 82 Seton Hall Univ; 87–Sp-Lang Path, Granite State Sp-Lang Services, **SLP**

Seedman, Mrs Jamie Chalfon 5 Carl Court, Spring Valley, NY 10977, (914) 352-6369, BA 72 CUNY - Queens Coll; MA 74 CUNY - Queens Coll; Sp-Lang Path, Private Practice, **SLP**

Seefeldt, Mrs Ellen Homann 15 Spiros Way, Menlo Park, CA 94025, (415) 323-4944, BS 59 Univ of IL - Urbana; MA 60 Stanford Univ; Sp-Lang Path, Cupertino Union Sch Dist, **SLP**

Seefeldt, Mariel D 6010 16th Street #201, Racine, WI 53406, (414) 886-3343, BS 75 Univ of WI - Eau Claire; MS 77 Univ of WI - Stevens Point; Sp-Lang Path, Racine USD, **SLP**

Seeger, Cynthia S Box 205, West Sand Lake, NY 12196, **SLP**

Seehorn, Mrs Terry E P O Box 3002, Lake City, FL 32056, (904) 752-5323, BA 86 Univ of FL; ME 87 Univ of FL; 88–Sp-Lang Path, InSpeech Inc

Seekamp, Sandra J 495 West End Avenue, New York, NY 10024, (212) 920-5445, BA 67 Emmanuel Coll; MA 81 CUNY - Hunter Coll; 88–Dir, Seekamp Associates, **SLP**

Seeker, Tamara J 2510 E Johnson Street, Madison, WI 53704, (608) 241-9054, BS 80 Univ of WI - Madison; MS 86 Univ of WI - Whitewater; **SLP**

Seeley, Joyce Irene #130 8051B Ryan Road, Richmond, BC, Canada V7A 2E4, (604) 939-9201, BA 78 Carleton Univ - Ontario; MA 87 Western WA Univ; 88–Sp-Lang Path, Coquitlam Sch Dist #43, **SLP**

Seelig, Mrs Karen S Speech-Path & Audiology Dept, Western Michigan Univ, Kalamazoo, MI 49008, (616) 387-8060, BA 64 Western MI Univ; MA 67 Northwestern Univ; Assoc Prof, Sp Path & Aud Dept/Wn MI U, **SLP**

Seelig, Mrs Renee Cohen 27 Urban Street, Stamford, CT 06905, (203) 977-4474, BS 76 Univ of North TX; MS 78 Univ of North TX; Sp-Lang Path, Stamford Pub Sch, **SLP**

Seelinger, Janet W 11 Kittiwake, Orinda, CA 94563, (415) 944-1774, BA 55 Univ of MI - Ann Arbor; MA 59 Bowling Green St Univ; Sp-Lang Path, San Ramon Valley Unif Sch Dist, **SLP**

Seely, Kathleen W RD #1 Box 253, Deansboro, NY 13328, (315) 841-8537, BA 67 SUNY - Center at Albany; MS 71 SUNY - Center at Albany; 74–Sp-Lang Path, Private Practice, **SLP**

Seelye, Dr Barbara J Route 1 Box 192, Walpole, NH 03608, (603) 352-1909, BS 52; MA 55 Univ of Denver; PH 67 (NS) Univ of Denver; Pres, Keene State Coll, **SLP**

Seery, Joyce Bowen 626 South Pascack Road, Spring Valley, NY 10977, (914) 735-3268, BA 80 Montclair St Coll; MS 82 PA St Univ - Univ Park; Sp-Lang Path, Private Practice, **SLP**

Seeto, Debra Ann 46 Porter Road, Natick, MA 01760, BA 81 Boston Coll; MA 83 Northwestern Univ; Sp-Lang Path, Framingham PS, **SLP**

Seewald, Dr Richard C Communication Disorders, Elborn/Uwo, London, ON, Canada N6G 1H1, (519) 661-2001, BS 69 Ithaca Coll; MA 74 Univ of MN - Minneap-St Paul; PH 81 (Aud) Univ of CT; 86–Asst Prof, Univ of Western Ontario, **A**

Sefcik, Mrs Jan B 490 Middlesex Court, Buffalo Grove, IL 60089, (312) 835-2238, BA 71 Univ of IL - Urbana; MA 75 Northwestern Univ; Sp-Lang Path, No Suburban Spec Ed Dist, **SLP**

Seff, Jane 890 West End Avenue, New York, NY 10025, (212) 679-0100, BA 59 2950; MA 79 CUNY - Hunter Coll; 84–Asst Dir Sp & Hrng, Internatl Cen for the Disabled, **SLP**

Seffinger, Debra 23680 Village House Dr N, Apartment 5B, Southfield, MI 48034, (313) 357-2047, BS 78 Wayne St Univ; MA 79 Wayne St Univ; SLP, Prof Ther Staffing, **SLP**

Segal, Alan I Rt 1 Box 216-J, Davisville, WV 26142, (304) 424-4277, BS 73 Univ of Pittsburgh - Pittsburgh; MS 75 Univ of Pittsburgh - Pittsburgh; Dir Aud Dept, St Joseph Hosp, **A**

Segal, Mrs Andrea Sue 16 Canterbury Road #1D, Great Neck, NY 11021, (516) 623-2534, BS 82 Boston Univ; MS 83 Columbia Univ Teachers Coll; 84–Sp-Lang Path, N Merrick Union Free Sch Dist, **SLP**

Segal, Mrs Beverly D 1174 East 22nd Street, Brooklyn, NY 11210, (212) 253-3465, BA 54 CUNY - Brooklyn Coll; MS 78 CUNY - Brooklyn Coll; **SLP**

Segal, Mrs Beverly E 15002 Cobre Valley Drive, Houston, TX 77062, (713) 488-2544, BS 50 Northwestern Univ; MA 52 Northwestern Univ; Sp-Lang Path, Private Practice, **SLP**

Segal, Dr Denise Erica 5 Regent Road, Belmont, MA 02178, BA 76 0500; MA 80 0500; PH 86 (Psycholinguistics) South Africa Rhodes Univ; 87–Research Assoc, Boston Univ Sch of Educ, **SLP**

Segal, Judy Marilyn 13010 Debby Street, Van Nuys, CA 91401, (213) 873-2227, BA 68 CA St Univ - Los Angeles; MA 82 CA St Univ - Los Angeles; Doctoral, Univ of California Los Angeles, **SLP**

Segal, Lauren Kirsch 9 Tree Bark Lane, Holland, PA 18966, (215) 860-9642, BS 79 PA St Univ - Univ Park; OM 81 Hahneman Medical Coll; 81–Mgr of Natl Aud Oper, InSpeech Inc, **SLP A**

Segal, Lesley E 230 North Street #C-34, Buffalo, NY 14201-1407, (716) 886-4039, **A**

Segal, Mrs Renee R 740 Chaucer Way, Buffalo Grove, IL 60089, (312) 634-6547, BS 72 Univ of VA - Charlottesville; ME 73 Univ of VA - Charlottesville; **SLP**

Segal, Sharon 4306 Jason, Houston, TX 77096-1705, (713) 552-1626, BS 84 Univ of TX - Austin; MA 86 Univ of Houston - Univ Park; **SLP**

Segal, Mrs Teri B 2485 Wendling Drive, Akron, OH 44313, (216) 867-0115, BA 73 Southern CT St Univ; MS 75 Southern CT St Univ; 88–Sp-Lang Path, PSI Affiliates, **SLP**

Segall, Linda Susan 1369 Argyle Way, Bensalem, PA 19020, (215) 245-6544, 87 Hahnemann Univ Grad Sch

Segalowitz, Mrs Bernice S 15 Canterbury Road, Suite A-1, Great Neck, NY 11021, (516) 773-3298, BA 76 CUNY - Queens Coll; MA 78 Hofstra Univ; Sp/Lang Path, Segalowitz & Mostel, **SLP**

Segel, Cheri Buck 11861-15 Mile Road #2-A, Sterling Heights, MI 48077, (313) 264-7402, BS 86 Central MI Univ; MA 87 Central MI Univ; **SLP**

Segel, Mrs Holly Ann 4098 Verona Road, South Euclid, OH 44121, (216) 444-4961, BS 79 Bowling Green St Univ; MA 82 Case Western Reserve Univ; 88–Sp-Lang Path, Cleveland Clinic Found, **SLP**

Segel, Mitchell 11861 15 Mile Road #2-A, Sterling Heights, MI 48077, (313) 745-1152, BA 84 MI St Univ; MA 86 Central MI Univ; 87–Sp-Lang Path, Rehabilitation Inst, **SLP**

Segel, Philip Allen 4098 Verona Road, South Euclid, OH 44121, (216) 382-7918, BA 81 Case Western Reserve Univ; MA 83 Case Western Reserve Univ; Aud, Cleveland Cl Fndt, **A**

Segelman, Sheera T 41 Colonel Drive #21, Weymouth, MA 02189, (508) 790-2700, BA 84 Univ of MA - Amherst; MS 86 Northeastern Univ; 88–Sp-Lang Path, Braintree Hosp, **SLP**

Seger, Dr Cheryl A D 3313 South 91st Street, Omaha, NE 68124, (402) 331-6388, BS 75 Univ of NE - Omaha; MS 76 Univ of NE - Omaha; Sp-Lang Path, Papillion Public Schools, **SLP**

Segers, Mrs Vicki Ann 9750 Beryl Street N W, Canal Fulton, OH 44614, (216) 854-2635, BA 84 Univ of Akron; MA 85 Univ of Akron; 87–Sp-Lang Path, Akron City Hosp, **SLP**

Segmond, Andrea M The Newark DDSO, 703 East Maple Avenue, Newark, NY 14513, (315) 331-1700, **A**

Segress, Mrs Carla Jo 9712 South 227th East Avenue, Broken Arrow, OK 74014, (918) 266-6333, BS 82 Univ of Tulsa; MA 83 Univ of Tulsa; 86–Sp-Lang Path, Verdigris PS, **SLP**

Segriff, Carla Helene 416 Unique Drive, Burnsville, MN 55337, (612) 894-4959, BS 83 Univ of IA; MA 86 Northern IL Univ - De Kalb; 87–Aud, Audiometrics Inc, **A**

Seher, Donald Matthew 2609 Capistrano Court N, Arlington, TX 76015, (817) 548-9059, OB 80 Hardin-Simmons Univ; MA 84 TX Woman's Univ; Sp-Lang Path, Arlington ISD, **SLP**

Seiber, James L 3217 216th Court S E, Issaquah, WA 98027, (206) 392-0791, BA 67 Western WA Univ; MA 73 Univ of WA; Coord/Commun Dis Ser, Issaquah Sch Dist, **SLP**

Seibert, Mrs Pamela J 1501 Beam Street, Chesterton, IN 46304, (219) 464-8611, BS 74 Purdue Univ - West Lafayette; OM 77 IN Univ - Bloomington; Sp-Lang Path, Speech Dynamics, **SLP**

Seich, Diane Marie 4945 Quincy Street N W, Canton, OH 44708, (216) 477-1065, BA 85 Univ of Akron; MA 86 Univ of Akron; **SLP**

Seid, Jill B 20421 Hemmingway Street, Canoga Park, CA 91306, (818) 709-4599, MA 78 CUNY - Queens Coll; Sp-Lang Path, Private Practice, **SLP**

Seid, Phyllis H 4036 26th Street, San Francisco, CA 94131, (415) 349-9922, BS 69 Boston Univ; MA 71 NY Univ; Sp-Lang Path, San Mateo Cty Sch Dist, **SLP**

Seidel, Mrs Susan J 720 Providence Road, Towson, MD 21204, (301) 828-2142, BA 59 Univ of KY; MA 63 IN Univ - Bloomington; Aud, Gtr Baltimore Med Cen, **A**

Seideman, Mrs Avonne P 154 Weston Road, Weston, CT 06883, (203) 255-8318, BA 62 CUNY - Hunter Coll; MA 64 Case Western Reserve Univ; Sp-Lang Path, Fairfield Pub Sch, **SLP**

Seidemann, Dr Michael F Hearing And Speech Center, EENT Hospital, 2626 Napoleon Avenue, New Orleans, LA 70115, (504) 896-1170, BS 68 Old Dominion Univ; MS 69 Old Dominion Univ; PH 73 (Aud) FL St Univ; 85–Dir of Sp-Lang Path, Eye Ear Nose & Throat Hospital, **A F**

Seiden, Mrs Bucky Rogers Box 1152, Plattsburgh, NY 12901, (518) 643-9431, BS 74 SUNY - Coll at Brockport; MA 86 SUNY - Coll at Plattsburgh

Seiden, Lea F 811 Swed Circle, Yorktown Heights, NY 10598, (914) 528-0950, BA 68 SUNY - Center at Albany; MS 72 Adelphi Univ; Sp-Lang Path, Lakeland Sch, **SLP**

Seidenberg, Karen Hedia 226 Little Falls Street, Falls Church, VA 22046, (703) 941-7704, BS 72 Ithaca Coll; MS 73 Ithaca Coll; Sp-Lang Path, Sch for Contemporary Ed, **SLP**

Seidenberg, Susan B 152 Norwalk Avenue, Buffalo, NY 14216, (716) 878-7371, BS 69 SUNY - Center at Buffalo; MS 71 SUNY - Center at Buffalo; MS 81 Canisius Coll; **SLP**

Seidl, Dennis M R R 3 Box 229, Stanley, WI 54768, (715) 644-2425, BA 86 Univ of WI - Eau Claire; MS 87 Univ of WI - Eau Claire; **SLP**

Seidler, Ann G Montclair State College, Upper Montclair, NJ 07043, (201) 893-4217, BA 46 NY Univ; MA 51 NY Univ; PH 67 (NS) Smith Coll; Professor, Montclair State College, **SLP**

Seidman, Mrs Arleen B 12 Mohawk Street, Sharon, MA 02067, BS 77 Univ of MA - Amherst; MS 79 Boston Univ; Sp-Lang Path, Dedham Public Schools, **SLP**

Seidman, Jill W 4609 Wellington Drive, Bensalem, PA 19020, (215) 752-4662, BA 77 Temple Univ; MA 78 Trenton St Coll; Sp-Lang Path, Barc, **SLP**

Seidman, Joyce H 10101 Grosvenor Place, Apartment 1005, Rockville, MD 20852, (301) 295-2202, BA 74 Univ of MD - College Park; MA 79 Catholic Univ of America; OM 85 National Univ; Head Aud Div, US Navy, **A**

Seidman, Kathryn Allison 681 Hamlet Road, Auburn Hills, MI 48057, BS 85 CO St Univ; MS 87 CO St Univ; 87–Sp-Lang Path, William Beaumont Hosp, **SLP**

Seidman, Mrs Marlene Dymant 414 North Midland Avenue, Apartment A-1, Saddle Brook, NJ 07662, (201) 794-7311, BA 79 Hofstra Univ; MS 82 William Paterson Coll; 86–Sp-Lang Path, Kessler Institute for Rehab, **SLP**

Seidman, Marsha R 2401 Penn Avenue #8A1, Philadelphia, PA 19130, BA 70 Univ of Pittsburgh - Pittsburgh; MS 72 Emerson Coll; Aud, Sch Dist of Phila, **SLP**

Seidmon, Mrs Nancy Friedman 2400 Honey Run Roadns, Ambler, PA 19002, (215) 643-5524, BS 72 Boston Univ; MA 74 CUNY - Hunter Coll; Sp-Lang Path, Main Line Sp Consult, **SLP**

Seidner, Roslyn F J 184 Hollywood Avenue, Albany, NY 12209, (518) 489-4516, BA 53 SUNY - Center at Albany; MA 54 CUNY - Brooklyn Coll; Sp-Lang Path, Sch Dist of Troy, **SLP**

Seifarth, Mrs Victoria W 1548 Walthall Court N W, Atlanta, GA 30318, (404) 355-3027, BA 52 Vanderbilt Univ; MS 54 Vanderbilt Univ; Sp-Lang Path, Atlanta Pub Schs, **SLP**

Seifer, Patricia J 616 Grey Avenue, Evanston, IL 60202, (312) 869-5471, BS 71 Northwestern Univ; MA 72 Northwestern Univ; Sp-Lang Path, Private Practice, **SLP**

Seifert, Elizabeth Dean 10 Barclay Street, Poughkeepsie, NY 12601, (904) 229-9290, MA 78 NY Univ; Sp-Lang Path, Wappingers Central Schools, **SLP**

Seifert, Janet L 55 Mill Plain Road 31-14, Danbury, CT 06811, (203) 790-1682, MS 87 PA St Univ - Univ Park

Seiferth, Ellen Walk 5802 Guilford Avenue, Indianapolis, IN 46220, (317) 924-3251, BS 75 Ithaca Coll; MA 77 IN Univ - Bloomington; Aud, Crossroads Rehab Cen, **A**

Seifferth, Susan Kay 220 Southbrook Drive, Dayton, OH 45459, (513) 461-3000, **SLP**

Seigel, Mrs Laurie B 17 Clairmont, Longmeadow, MA 01106, (203) 741-3551, BA 76 CUNY - Queens Coll; MS 77 Ithaca Coll; 86–Sp-Lang Path, Enfield PS, **SLP**

Seiger, Mrs Lynann Louise RD2 Box 67, Birdsboro, PA 19508, (215) 582-1323, BS 83 Bloomsburg Univ of PA; MS 84 Bloomsburg Univ of PA; Sp-Lang Path, InSpeech Inc, **SLP**

Seigle, Melanie N 8319 Braesdale, Houston, TX 77071, (713) 621-3072, BA 65 IN Univ - Bloomington; MA 66 OH St Univ; SLP, The Battin Clinic, **SLP**

Seikel, John A Department Speech & Hearing Sciences, Washington State University, Pullman, WA 99164-2420, (509) 335-0111, BS 79 Phillips Univ; MA 81 Wichita St Univ; PH 88 (Sp & Hrng Sciences) Univ of KS; Prof, Washington State U, **SLP**

Seiler, Mrs Amy A 2007 Oregon Avenue, Rockford, IL 61108, (815) 229-4230, BS 80 Univ of WI - Madison; MS 81 Univ of WI - Whitewater; 85–Sp-Lang Path, Rockford Public Schools, **SLP**

Seiler, Elizabeth Holly Cross Hospital, 2701 West 68th Street, Chicago, IL 60629, (312) 471-5632, BA 77 Saint Xavier Coll; MA 79 Northern IL Univ - De Kalb; 79–Mgr Dept Commun Dis, Holy Cross Hosp, **SLP**

Seiler, Mrs Nancy E 1589 Fulmar Drive, Delray Beach, FL 33444, (305) 481-5757, BS 70 Nazareth Coll of Rochester; MS 71 Syracuse Univ; Sp-Lang Path, Sch Bd of Broward Co, FL, **SLP**

Seiler, Roberta S 32 Mills Road, Needham, MA 02194, (617) 668-5400, BS 74 Trenton St Coll; MA 76 Trenton St Coll; Sp/Lang Path, Walpole Pub Sch, **SLP**

Seiler, Mrs Sheri Elyse 110-45 71st Road #7-K, Forest Hills, NY 11375, (516) 783-7523, MA 85 Long Island U - CW Post Ctr; BA 82 SUNY - Coll at Cortland; SLP, School for Lang & Comm Devel, **SLP**

Seiler, Susan 3326 North 3rd Avenue, Phoenix, AZ 85013, (602) 264-4834, BS 70 AZ St Univ; MS 74 AZ St Univ; Aud, ENT Assoc Ltd, **A**

Seilo, Dr Michael T Dept Speech Path & Audiology, Western Washington Univ, Parks Hall #39, Bellingham, WA 98225, (206) 676-3881, BA 63 Northern MI Univ; MA 67 Univ of AZ; PH 70 (Aud) OH Univ - Athens; 70–Prof of Aud, Western Washington Univ, **SLP A**

Seip, Mrs Jodi A 311 Lightstreet Road, Bloomsburg, PA 17815, (717) 389-4444, BS 84 Bloomsburg Univ of PA; MS 85 Bloomsburg Univ of PA; Sp-Lang Path, Cent Susquehanna Int Unit, **SLP**

Seipkes, Pamela Elizabeth P O Box 266, Staples, MN 56479, (218) 894-2438, BS 80 ND St Univ; MS 85 Moorhead St Univ; SLP, Freshwaters Spec Ed Coop, **SLP**

Seipp, Patsy Leigh East 24th Liberty, Spokane, WA 99207, (509) 456-3948, MS 81 Eastern WA Univ; Consultant SLP, **SLP**

Seipp, William S 217 Melanchton Avenue, Lutherville, MD 21093, (301) 760-4327, BA 72 Univ of MD - College Park; MS 73 Loyola Coll; President, Applied Conservation Tech, **SLP A**

Seitel, Dr Alan L 13723 Marylebone, Houston, TX 77034, (713) 794-4040, BA 70 SUNY - Center at Albany; MA 71 Univ of FL; PH 75 (Psycholinguistics-Communication Disorders) Univ of TX - Austin; 83–Assoc Prof, U of TX Hlth Sci Cen, **SLP**

Seither, Mary Regan 4 Lemore Circle, Rocky Hill, NJ 08553, (609) 924-5924, BS 79 Boston Univ; MS 81 Emory Univ; **SLP**

Seitsinger, Mrs Merrisue L 109 South Orchard Lane, Stillwater, OK 74074, (405) 377-2724, BS 79 OK St Univ; MA 82 Wichita St Univ; **A**

Seitter, Mrs Rebecca 4916 Quail Hollow Lane, Waldo, OH 43356, (614) 387-3300, BA 74 Univ of Louisville; MA 76 Univ of Cincinnati; Sp-Lang Path, Marion County Schools, **SLP**

Seitz, Andrew Joseph, Jr 141 Waldorf Drive, Akron, OH 44313, (216) 499-5531, BS 75 Univ of Akron; MA 85 Univ of Akron; **A**

Seitz, Mrs Christine Schrock 16303 Alladin Way, Tampa, FL 33624, (813) 962-2976, BS 74 OH Univ - Athens; MS 78 Univ of South FL; Sp/Lang Path, Private Practice, **SLP**

Seitz, Mrs Gail Metta 21601 Sunnyside, St Clair Shores, MI 48080, (313) 526-3409, BA 33 Wayne St Univ; BA 33 Wayne St Univ; OM 36 Wayne St Univ - Sch of Med; Dir-SLP for Foreign Adults, Internatl I, **SLP LM**

Seitz, Jay D 4422 Wesley, Corpus Christi, TX 78412, (505) 842-1656, MS 84 Northern AZ Univ; Aud, Affilated Aud Assoc, **SLP**

Seitz, Mrs Laura L 19910 Bolton Bridge Lane, Humble, TX 77338, (713) 795-7492, BA 77 FL St Univ; MA 79 Vanderbilt Univ; Aud, VA Hosp, **A**

Seitz, Dr Michael R 14617 Carlson Street, Poway, CA 92064, (619) 265-6774, BA 67 Univ of WA; MA 70 Univ of WA; PH 72 (NS) Univ of WA; 85–Prof, San Diego State U /Commun Dis, **SLP F**

Seitz, Sandra L 230 14th Street, Buffalo, NY 14213, (716) 838-5980, BA 86 SUNY - Coll at Buffalo; MA 88 SUNY - Coll at Buffalo

Seitzinger, Joanne R 2807 Heritage Drive, Champaign, IL 61821, (217) 333-6528, BS 80 Univ of IL - Urbana; MS 81 Univ of IL - Urbana; 87–SLP/Aud, Univ of IL-DSCC, **SLP ACE**

Seitzman, Sheila D 3400 Winterberry, Orchard Lake, MI 48033, **SLP**

Sekel, Patricia P 15218 La Paloma, Houston, TX 77083, (713) 879-1823, BS 75 OH Univ - Athens; MA 79 OH Univ - Athens; Sp-Lang Path, Alief ISD, **SLP**

Sekely, Mrs Bonnie Ann 9411 David Andrew Way, Centerville, OH 45458, (513) 885-4211, BA 68 Allegheny Coll; MA 70 Case Western Reserve Univ; Consult SLP, Maria Joseph Liv Care Cen, **SLP**

Sekhon, Mrs Laura Jane 7221 Bucknell Drive, Dallas, TX 75214, (214) 341-0537, BS 83 Univ of North TX; MS 85 Univ of North TX; 88–Sp-Lang Path, Pediatric Therapy Assoc, **SLP**

Sekine, Dennis T 98-919A Kaonohi Street, Aiea, HI 96701, (808) 471-8115, BS 68 Univ of HI - Manoa; MS 71 Univ of HI - Manoa; OM 82 Univ of HI - Manoa; Aud, Naval Med Cl, **A**

Selb, Louise Kathryn 5013 Queen Avenue South, Minneapolis, MN 55410, (612) 920-0449, BA 73 Univ of MN - Minneap-St Paul; MA 87 Univ of MN - Minneap-St Paul; 88–Sp-Lang Path, Special Sch Dist #1, **SLP**

Selber, Stephen M 2710 North 47th Street, Philadelphia, PA 19131, (215) 595-6000, BS 70 Temple Univ; MA 81 West Chester Univ of PA; Sp-Lang Path, Taylor Hosp, **SLP**

Selbst, Andrea K 634 Ashbourne Road, Elkins Park, PA 19117, (215) 635-6410, BS 74 Goucher Coll; MS 76 Columbia Univ Teachers Coll; **SLP**

Selby, Elizabeth 1781 S E 9th Street, Fort Lauderdale, FL 33316, (305) 522-4036, **SLP**

Selby, Mrs Karen J Box 245, Waynetown, IN 47990, (317) 234-2328, BS 76 IN St Univ - Terre Haute; MA 78 IN St Univ - Terre Haute; Sp/Lang Path, Psi Iota Xi Summer Sp Cl, **SLP**

Selck, Mrs Faye A 6839 West Wellauer Drive, Wauwatosa, WI 53213, (414) 276-4370, BS 66 Univ of MN - Minneap-St Paul; MS 71 Univ of WI - Milwaukee; 87–Dir-Sp-Lang Path, Cedar Haven Rehab Agency, **SLP ACE**

Selden, Beverly L 4229 Portland Court, Orchard Lake, MI 48033, (313) 858-1912, BS 56 Western MI Univ; MA 65 Western MI Univ; Consul Sp & Lang, Oakland Sch, **SLP**

Selden, Mrs Deborah Holston 225 Colony Road, New Haven, CT 06511, (203) 397-4569, BA 68 Univ of Science & Arts of OK; MS 81 Southern CT St Univ; Sp-Lang Path/Cl Superv, Sn CT St V, **SLP**

Selden, Kathleen E 315 Radcliffe Drive, Claremont, CA 91711, **SLP**

Selden, Mrs Louise M 30 Sheila Drive, Hauppauge, NY 11788, (516) 361-6088, BA 78 CUNY - Hunter Coll; MA 80 CUNY - Hunter Coll; Sp-Lang Path, Private Practice, **SLP**

Seldin, Lila Bergman 2005 Vera Court, Simi Valley, CA 93063-3748, (805) 584-0175, BA; MS; Sp-Lang Path, Los Angeles USD, **SLP**

Selesnick, Mrs Randy L 6634 Acacia Court, Davis Gardens, Miami, FL 33143, (305) 661-2055, BS 80 Northwestern Univ; MA 81 Northwestern Univ; **SLP**

Seletsky, Mrs Marcia Gail 15 Harrison Street, Newton Highlands, MA 02161, (617) 552-7678, **SLP**

Self, Mrs Deborah L 1108 West Lillie Boulevard, Madill, OK 73446, (405) 564-3035, BA 75 East Central OK St Univ; MS 77 Univ of OK Medical Center; Sp-Lang Path, Madill Pub Sch, **SLP**

Self, Mrs Jennifer Nass 12421 Bears Den Court, Jacksonville, FL 32258, (904) 262-4194, BA 80 Univ of FL; ME 82 Univ of FL; 84–Sp-Lang Path, St Johns County School Board, **SLP**

Self, Mrs Lana C C 4565 Brockland Drive, Morristown, TN 37813, (615) 587-0779, BA 77 Univ of TN - Knoxville; MA 78 Univ of TN - Knoxville; 87–Sp-Lang Path, Hamblen County Schs, **SLP**

Self, Michele Lynn 2722 Trader Court, Bldg #17, South Bend, IN 46628, (219) 272-3594, BS 85 IN St Univ - Terre Haute; MS 87 Ball St Univ; 86–Clin Supvr, InSpeech Inc, **SLP**

Self, Mrs Trisha Lynn 7211 Suncrest, Wichita, KS 67212, (316) 721-4093, BA 84 Wichita St Univ; MA 85 Wichita St Univ; Sp-Lang Path, Newton Special Ed Coop, **SLP**

Selger, Donna J 17 Warren Street, Lowell, MA 01852, (508) 454-1966, BA 73 Elmira Coll; MA 74 Univ of Denver; 86–Aud, Audio Hearing Ctr, **A**

Selgrad, Mrs Carol Cinnick 1007 Deerfield Road #224, Deerfield, IL 60015-4150, (312) 689-8150, BS 80 Bradley Univ; MA 82 Northwestern Univ; Sp-Lang Path/Dept Coord, Bd of Educ Chicago, **SLP**

Selig, Mrs Gertrude Zanar 1319 Keller Lane, Seguin, TX 78155, (512) 379-6521, BA 53 CUNY - Hunter Coll; ME 79 Southwest TX St Univ; Sp/Lang Path, Private Practice, **SLP**

Seligman, Darlene 1414 Cambridge Road, San Marino, CA 91108, (213) 449-2660, BS 56 Northwestern Univ; MA 59 Northwestern Univ; OD 79 (NS) Loyola Marymount Univ; Attorney at Law, Private Practice, **SLP**

Seligman, Daryl A 3123 31st Way, West Palm Beach, FL 33407, (407) 478-0290, BA 78 Univ of CO - Boulder; MS 80 Univ of NM; Sp-Lang Path, Palm Beach Co Sch Bd, **SLP**

Seligman, Dawn L 21 Midland Crescent #84, Nepean, ON, Canada K2H 8P6, (613) 237-5660, BA 80 McGill Univ - Quebec; MS 82 Boston Univ; Sp/Lang Path, Chldn Hosp/En Ontario, **SLP**

Seligman, Denise M 4505 N E Alemeda, Portland, OR 97213, **SLP**

Seligman, Mrs Lillian O 5811 Glen Park Road, Louisville, KY 40222, (502) 895-3401, BA 67 IN Univ - Bloomington; MA 68 IN Univ - Bloomington; Sp-Lang Path, VA Med Cen, **SLP**

Selikowitz, Jeanne E 15 Franklin Place, Glen Rock, NJ 07452, BA 70 Oakland Univ; MS 75 Rutgers St Univ -N Brunswick; SLP, Wyckoff Pub Sch, **SLP ACE**

Selin, Mrs Ann Bulmash 444 West Fullerton Parkway, Apartment 304, Chicago, IL 60614, (312) 348-3449, MA 72 Univ of IL - Urbana; **SLP**

Seline, Gloria Ellen 810 NE 94th, Seattle, WA 98115, (206) 524-6537, MS 84 Saint Cloud St Univ; 88–Sp-Lang Path, Ballard Comm Hosp, **SLP**

Selinger, Dr Marilyn 1111 Humbaldt Street, Denver, CO 80218, (303) 831-0641, BS 73 Northeastern Univ; MA 74 Univ of Denver; PH 82 (NS) Univ of Denver; SLP, VA Medical Center, **SLP**

Seliskar, Jeanne R 793 West State Street, Columbus, OH 43222, (614) 225-5761, BS 75 Miami Univ - Oxford; MA 76 Kent St Univ; Dir of Sp-Lang Path, Mt Carmel Med Ctr, **SLP**

Selker-Adams, Judith M 16772 Coral Cay Lane, Huntington Harbor, CA 92649, (213) 420-5140, ME 71 Clarion Univ of PA; **SLP**

Sell, Susan Stewart 2818 Blue Sage, Woodward, OK 73801, (405) 256-5028, BS 79 Phillips Univ; MA 81 OK St Univ; Sp-Lang Path, CES, **SLP**

Selland-Lichter, Sandra 815 Campbell Drive, Grand Forks, ND 58201, (701) 780-2447, BS 77 ND St Univ; MS 82 Moorhead St Univ; Sp/Lang Path, Med Cen Rehab Hosp, **SLP**

Sellar, Barbara Gail P O Box 462, Dayton, WY 82836, (307) 655-9541, MS 84 San Francisco St Univ; Sp-Lang Path, Sheridan Cnty Sch Dist 1-West, **SLP**

Sellars, Carole A 536 Jonalyn Circle, Minneapolis, MN 55416, (612) 291-2848, BA 60 Univ of WI - Madison; MS 69 FL St Univ; Superv-Sp-Lang Path, Gillette Children Hosp, **SLP**

Seller, Mrs Carole C 5863 Northumberland Street, Apartment #2, Pittsburgh, PA 15217, (412) 281-1375, BS 64 PA St Univ - Univ Park; ME 66 PA St Univ - Univ Park; Sp-Lang Path, Allegheny General Hosp, **SLP**

Sellers, Anita Barbee 12531 East 20th, Tulsa, OK 74128, (405) 948-1661, BS 84 OK St Univ; MS 86 Univ of OK Medical Center; **SLP**

Sellers, Clarence Route 7 Box 109, Concord, NC 28025, (704) 786-9163, BA 67 Univ of NC - Chapel Hill; MA 74 Univ of NC - Greensboro; MA 75 Univ of NC - Greensboro; SLP, Division of Youth Services, **SLP A**

Sellers, Dr Daniel E Speech & Hearing Ctr Humb 69, Univ Of South Alabama, Mobile, AL 36688, (205) 460-6327, BS 62 Univ of AL- Tuscaloosa; MA 64 Univ of AL-Tuscaloosa; PH 72 (NS) FL St Univ; Assoc Prof of Aud, U of South AL, **A**

Sellers, Mrs Kathryn Brabec Lake Serene, Box 533-B, Hattiesburg, MS 39401, (601) 268-5670, BA 82 Univ of MS; MS 83 Univ Southern MS-Hattiesburg; Aud, Hattiesburg Clin, **A**

Sellig, Sara G 18 Webster Avenue, Glens Falls, NY 12801, (518) 793-7914, MA 65 Northwestern Univ; Sp-Lang Path, Warren Wash Co Pub Hlth Assoc, **SLP**

Sells, Mrs Janet P Naval Hospital, Audiology Clinic, Newport, RI 02841, (401) 841-2158, BS 79 Univ of RI; MA 81 Univ of RI; Aud, Newport Naval Hospital, **A**

Sells, Mrs Susan Elizabeth 602 Greentree, Rolla, MO 65401, (314) 341-2155, OB 82 Northeast MO St Univ; MA 83 Northeast MO St Univ; Sp-Lang Path, Rolla Pub Sch District, **SLP**

Sells-Rabold, Mrs Denise E 962 Norway Drive, Columbus, OH 43221, (614) 451-4337, BA 80 OH St Univ; MA 82 OH St Univ; 84–Sp-Lang Path, Rehabilitation Psychology Inc, **SLP**

Selman, Mrs Elsie M 134 South Fenwick Street, Arlington, VA 22204, (703) 455-2100, BA 51 NY Univ; MA 70 George Washington Univ; 81–Sp-Lang Path, Fairfax County Public Schools, **SLP**

Selmar, John W 12232 Fremont Avenue North, Seattle, WA 98133, (206) 362-6936, BA 51 Univ of Dubuque; MA 54 Univ of IA; Sp-Lang Path, Private Practice, **SLP**

Seltz, Ann Eleanor Park Nicollet Medical Center, 5000 West 39th Street, Minneapolis, MN 55416, (612) 927-3407, BS 55 Univ of MN - Minneap-St Paul; MA 67 Univ of MN - Minneap-St Paul; 74–Aud, Park Nicollet Med Cen, **A F ACE**

Seltzer, Dr Herbert N P O Box 90026, Pittsburgh, PA 15224, (412) 369-0109, BS 64 CUNY - Brooklyn Coll; MS 67 CUNY - Brooklyn Coll; PH 73 (NS) Univ of Pittsburgh - Pittsburgh; 83–Dir, W Penn Sp & Lang, **SLP**

Semach, Diane L 301 Smoketree Terrace, Richmond, VA 23236, (804) 379-0513, BA 74 Cleveland St Univ; MA 75 Cleveland St Univ; SLP, Er Sl So-VA, **SLP**

Semanchik, Karen 1510 North Kenilworth St, Arlington, VA 22205, (202) 651-5961, BS 74 Georgetown Univ; MS 78 Columbia Univ Teachers Coll; **SLP**

Semanko, Gay E 917 East Chestnut, Bloomington, IL 61701-3307, (701) 438-5264, BS 73 Univ of WI - Whitewater; MS 76 Univ of WI - Whitewater; 82–Instr, Il St U, **SLP**

Semans, Susan L 1944 Janet Avenue, San Jose, CA 95124, (408) 559-4734, BA 71 Northeast LA Univ; MA 79 Northwestern St Univ; Sp-Lang Path, Campbell Union Sch Dist, **SLP**

Sember, Margaret D 188 Chipman Street Ext, Waterbury, CT 06708, (203) 574-8053, BA 75 Southern CT St Univ; MS 76 Southern CT St Univ; Sp-Lang Path, Bd of Ed City of Waterbury, **SLP**

Semel, Donna R 54 Knob Hill Street, Sharon, MA 02067, (617) 965-8379, BS 78 FL St Univ; MA 80 Emerson Coll; Sp-Lang Path, Newton Pub Sch, **SLP**

Semel, Dr Eleanor 905 Commonwealth Avenue, Newton, MA 02159, (617) 353-3252, BS 50 NY Univ; MA 53 NY Univ; ED 73 (NS) Boston Univ; Professor, Boston U

Semela, Jacob J M Ne 1540-A Spartan Village, East Lansing, MI 48823, (312) 633-7168, Research Asst, Aud & Sp Sciences, **A ACE**

Sementelli, Catherine Ann 2227 16th Street, Boulder, CO 80302, (303) 444-1156, MA 88 Univ of CO - Boulder; 88–Sp-Lang Path, Children's Hosp Denver CO

Seminara, Dr Gloria F 281 Benedict Road, Staten Island, NY 10304, (212) 987-8553, BA 56 CUNY - Brooklyn Coll; MA 59 CUNY - Brooklyn Coll; PH 85 (Sp-Lang Path) Columbia Univ Sch of Gen St; 85–Sp-Lang Path, Private Practice, **SLP**

Semmes, Joan L Russ Semmes, 5036 Yale Street Ste 201, Metairie, LA 70006, (504) 885-6633, BA 78 Univ of Southwestern LA; MA 80 Case Western Reserve Univ; SLP, Russ, Semmes, **SLP**

Semmes, Dr Marilyn Beverly 7104 Arrowood Road, Bethesda, MD 20817, (301) 496-9223, BA 53 Univ of AR - Fayetteville; MA 67 Univ of MD - College Park; PH 72 (NS) Univ of MD - College Park; Sp-Lang Path/Aud, NIH, **SLP A**

Semon, Diane Leiman 2000 Linwood Avenue #23-A, Fort Lee, NJ 07024, (201) 670-0707, BA 76 CUNY - Brooklyn Coll; MS 78 Emerson Coll; 86–Sp-Lang Path, Communication Therapy Center, **SLP**

Semow, Shirley P 14435 Benefit Street #3, Sherman Oaks, CA 91403, (818) 986-0811, MA 76; BA 68; Sp-Lang Path, Los Angeles USD, **SLP**

Semper-Veith, Mrs Cynthia Ann 70 Law Street, Valley Stream, NY 11580, (516) 285-7528, **SLP**

Semple, Jean Elizabeth 3590 Kaneff Crescent, Apartment #404, Mississauga, ON, Canada L5A 3X3, (416) 279-1826, BA 48 Univ of British Columbia; BA 55 Univ of WA; MA 64 Northwestern Univ; 80–Retired, **SLP A LM**

Semrad, Sherry Noel 5044 East Regency Circle S, Tucson, AZ 85711, (602) 798-2649, BS 85 TX Tech Univ; MS 87 Univ of AZ; 87–Sp-Lang Path, Tucson USD

Sena, Nancy 1661 Frederick, San Luis Obispo, CA 93401, (805) 543-5025, BS 73 TX Tech Univ; MS 75 Univ of OK Medical Center; Sp-Lang Path, Private Practice, **SLP**

Sender, Dina L 679 West 239th Street #5D, Bronx, NY 10463, (212) 601-3392, BS 81 Univ of GA; ME 82 Univ of GA; Sp-Lang Path, **SLP**

Senders, Pamela C 3733 S W Chehalem Avenue, Portland, OR 97201, (503) 228-5073, BS 73 Univ of OR; MA 77 Portland St Univ; Sp-Lang Path, Portland Pub Sch, **SLP**

Seneca, Eileen Coyle 18 Council Place, Harrington Park, NJ 07640, (914) 358-3540, BA 64 Loyola Coll; MA 71 Montclair St Coll; 64–Dept Hd-Sp/Hrng Serv, Clarkstown Cen Sch Dist, **SLP**

Seneker, Jeannie Lytton 2203 Londonderry Drive, Murfreesboro, TN 37130, (901) 423-2251, **A**

Senf, Linda K R R 1 Box 278, Montrose, IA 52639, (319) 524-2682, BA 68 Briar Cliff Coll; MA 70 Univ of MO - Columbia; Sp-Lang Path, Great River AEA, **SLP**

Sengbusch, Mrs Diane Kittsley 8005 South 77th Street, Franklin, WI 53132, (414) 639-4400, BS 78 Univ of WI - Madison; MS 79 Univ of WI - Madison; Sp-Lang Path, Racine USD, **SLP**

Senick, Denise Ann 9 Youngs Place, Latham, NY 12110, (518) 785-5469, BS Coll of Saint Rose; MS 86 Coll of Saint Rose

Senio, Mrs Judith E 100 Pleasant Way, Penfield, NY 14526, Sp-Lang Path, Penfield Central Schools, **SLP**

Senne, Allen John 2164 La Canada Crest #3, La Canada, CA 91011, (213) 483-9930, BS 82 San Diego St Univ; MA 84 San Diego St Univ; Aud, Otologic Med Gp, **A**

Senne, Mrs Catherine Ann 2164 La Canada Crest #3, La Canada, CA 91011, (818) 248-0801, BA 82 San Diego St Univ; MA 84 San Diego St Univ; Aud, Aud Vestibular Ctr, **A**

Sennett, Mrs Holly Ann 9627 Ohio Street, Omaha, NE 68134, (402) 572-2277, BS 81 Univ of NE - Omaha; MS 82 Univ of NE - Omaha; Sp/Lang Path, Immanuel Med Cen, **SLP**

Sennett, Susan Jank 353 Sunset Court, Rochester, NY 14618, (716) 352-2440, BS 79 SUNY - Coll at Geneseo; MS 84 Nazareth Coll of Rochester

Sennett, William Fitzgerald Department Of Speech, St Xavier College, 3700 W 103rd Street, Chicago, IL 60655, (312) 779-3300, BA 79 Univ of MI - Ann Arbor; MA 82 MI St Univ; Asst Prof, St Xavier Col

Sens-Azara, Mary Catherine 18 Broadmoor Drive, Lincroft, NJ 07738, (201) 530-4968, BS 72 Kent St Univ; MA 76 Kent St Univ; **SLP**

Sepe, Mrs Barbara C 4 Castle Court, Woodbury, NY 11797, (516) 541-6600, BA 74 Hofstra Univ; MA 76 Hofstra Univ; OM 82 Hofstra Univ; Supv of Elem Spec Ed, Massapequa Pub Sch, **SLP**

Seplow, Mrs Marilyn K Camelback Communication Center, 4300 North Miller Road, Suite 132, Scottsdale, AZ 85251, (602) 945-3530, BS 72 AZ St Univ; MS 73 AZ St Univ; Dir, Camelback Commun Cen, **SLP ACE**

Seplowe, Mrs Robin Lori 51 N Strathmore St, North Woodmere, NY 11581, (516) 791-6362, BS 77 Boston Univ; MA 80 CUNY - Queens Coll; 80–Sp-Lang Path, Sch Dist, **SLP**

Seppmann, Jody Lee Route 9 Box 173, Mankato, MN 56001, (507) 726-2320, BS 83 Mankato St Univ; MS 85 Mankato St Univ; 83–Sp-Lang Path, ISD #70 Lake Crystal PS, **SLP**

Serabin, Margaret 17168 Falmouth Drive, Strongsville, OH 44136, (216) 572-3688, BS 68 Kent St Univ; MA 72 Univ of Denver; SLP, Cleveland Board of Education, **SLP**

Sera-Budney, Kathryn K 919 North Cedar, Colorado Springs, CO 80903-2719, (303) 635-5513, BS 75 CO St Univ; MS 76 CO St Univ; Aud, ENT Clinic, **A**

Serafin, Mary M 1300 East Hickory Lane, Orange, CA 92666-1207, (714) 581-8048, BA 76 Univ of MI - Ann Arbor; MS 79 Univ of WI - Madison; 88–Supvr-Ped Prog, Newport Lang Sp & Aud Ctr Inc, **SLP**

Seraydarian, Fredi Diamond 2211 Fox Hills Drive, Los Angeles, CA 90064, (213) 553-1423, BA 78 Univ of CA - San Diego; MS 83 San Diego St Univ; 86–Sp-Lang Path, Los Angeles USD, **SLP**

Serber, Rhonda L 22 Broadfield Road, New Rochelle, NY 10804, (914) 235-4047, BA 72 CUNY - City College; MA 75 CUNY - Lehman Coll; 79–Sp-Lang Path, Westchester Co Med Cen, **SLP**

Serdar, Mrs Marla Joy 51 North McAree Road, Waukegan, IL 60085-4541, (312) 623-5422, MA 84 1159; 88–Sp-Lang Path, North Chicago Sch Dist #64, **SLP**

Sergeant, Dr Russell L 68 Shore Avenue, Groton Long Point, CT 06340, (212) 481-4464, BA 53 George Washington Univ; MA 58 Univ of MD - College Park; PH 62 (NS) OH St Univ; Assoc Prof, Hunter Coll & Grad Cen Cony, **SLP F**

Serota, Mrs Cynthia J 2709 Altadena Lake Road, Birmingham, AL 35243, (205) 967-6084, BS 75 Auburn Univ - Auburn; MS 78 James Madison Univ; Sp-Lang Path, Private Practice, **SLP**

Serpanos, Yula Cherpelis 53-17 250th Street, Little Neck, NY 11362, (718) 470-8910, BA 84 Saint John's Univ - Jamaica; MS 85 Columbia Univ Teachers Coll; 86–Aud, Long Isl Jewish Hrng & Sp Ctr, **A**

Serra, Marilyn Frances 53 Ward Avenue, Westerly, RI 02891, (401) 751-3113, BA 67 Univ of RI; MS 72 Boston Univ; President, Sargent Rehab Cen, **SLP**

Serrano, Maria A 8891 S W 142nd Avenue 8-34, Miami, FL 33186-4900, (305) 595-1530, BA 83 Univ of TN - Knoxville; MA 87 Univ of TN - Knoxville; **A**

Serrano-Flaisher, Mrs Enid 5532 Dunmore Drive, West Bloomfield, MI 48032, (313) 737-1832, BA 73 Univ of Miami; MS 75 Univ of PR - Rio Piedras; Sp/Lang Path, Metro Home Hlth Care, **SLP**

Sershen, Elizabeth 194 Kathleen Drive, West St Paul, MN 55118, (612) 681-2311, BS 54 Univ of MN - Duluth; MS 79 Univ of WI - River Falls; Sp-Lang Path, ISD 197, **SLP**

Servedio, Dominick 203 Coachlight Square, Montrose, NY 10548, (212) 722-8100, BA 84 CUNY - Lehman Coll; MA 86 CUNY - Lehman Coll; 87–Aud, Madison Audiology Assoc, **A**

Servedio, Mrs Kathleen 203 Coachlight Square, Montrose, NY 10548, (914) 736-1103, BA 82 CUNY - Lehman Coll; MA 84 CUNY - Lehman Coll; 86–Sp-Lang Path, BOCES, **SLP ACE**

Serventi, Edwina R 6260 Chesapeake Circle, Stockton, CA 95209, (209) 946-2381, BA 75 Univ of the Pacific; MA 76 Univ of the Pacific; **SLP**

Serventi, Gail W 158 West Buffalo Street, Warsaw, NY 14569, (716) 786-8611, BA 72 Ithaca Coll; MA 76 SUNY - Coll at Geneseo; 88–Supvr, SUNY Geneseo, **SLP**

Servetter, Miriam 12247 Caminito Mira Del, San Diego, CA 92130-2305, BS 79 Univ of Toronto - Ontario; MA 81 SUNY - Center at Buffalo; Sp-Lang Path, Lemon Grove School District, **SLP**

Servos, Mrs M Virginia 108 Amherst Road, Pelham, MA 01002, (413) 253-9934, BA 73 CUNY - Hunter Coll; MA 75 Univ of MD - College Park; **SLP**

Serwe, Mrs Ann Schmitz 1737 Underwood Avenue, Wauwatosa, WI 53213-2233, (414) 453-1122, BS 78 Marquette Univ; MS 80 Marquette Univ; Sp-Lang Path, S Milwaukee Pub Schs, **SLP**

Serwin, Gaynol N 231 Pines Lake Drive East, Wayne, NJ 07470, (201) 835-2615, BA 75 William Paterson Coll; MS 76 William Paterson Coll; Sp-Lang Path, Pequannock Township Bd of Ed, **SLP**

Sescourka, DeAnna M 2166 Grissom Drive N E, Warren, OH 44483, (216) 372-3415, BS 85 Eastern MI Univ; MA 87 Eastern MI Univ; 88–Sp-Lang Path, Children's Rehab Ctr

Sessions, Mrs Jan A 1127 East New Boston Road, Nash, TX 75569, (214) 794-2705, BS 85 Univ of AR - Little Rock; MS 87 Univ of AR - Little Rock; **SLP**

Sessions, Mrs Judith M PO Box D365, Kalb American Elementary School, APO New York, NY 09696-0005, BA 66 Univ of IA; MA 70 Univ of IA; Teacher, Dept Defense Dependnts Schools, **SLP**

Sessler, Patricia L 16089 Top-O-Hill Drive, New Berlin, WI 53151, (414) 786-7068, BA 75 Univ of WI - Madison; BS 80 Univ of WI - Milwaukee; MS 82 Univ of WI - Milwaukee; 87–Sp-Lang Path, St Mary's Hosp, **SLP**

Sessoms, Mrs Melody Ann 1267-B East Parkway, Rantoul, IL 61866, (217) 892-4309, BA 74 Murray St Univ; MS 84 Minot St Univ; Aud, Audiology of Central Illinois, **A**

Setchell, Cherryl Mae 99 Innisfil St, Barrie, ON, Canada L4N 3E3, (705) 728-9802, BS 84 Brigham Young Univ; MS 85 Brigham Young Univ; 85–Sp-Lang Path, Royal Victoria Hosp, **SLP**

Settele, Mrs Alison L Bradbury 702 Mount Alban Drive, Annapolis, MD 21401, BS 81 East Stroudsburg Univ of PA; OM 83 Hahneman Medical Coll; 88–Aud, Children's Hosp National Med Ctr, **SLP**

Settles, Mrs Gloria Harvin 3040 Mink Point Boulevard, Beaufort, SC 29902, (803) 525-7404, BA 73 SC St Coll; MA 79 SC St Coll; Program Coordinator, Coastal Speech-Hearing Clinic, **SLP**

Settle-Strain, Lisa Ann Route 2 Box 2644, Boerne, TX 78006, (512) 696-3841, BS 82 Univ of TX - Austin; MA 85 Our Lady Lake Univ-San Anton; Sp-Lang Path, San Antonio ISD, **SLP**

Setzen, Sheryl D 44 Spring Hollow, Roslyn, NY 11576, **SLP**

Setzman, Mrs Lynn H 82 Kara Lane, Feasterville, PA 19047, (215) 757-0227, BA 69 Temple Univ; MA 70 Temple Univ; 73–Sp-Lang Path, Bucks Co Inter Ut #22, **SLP**

Sever, Joseph C, Jr Child Study Center, Old Domimion University, Norfolk, VA 23508, PH (NS); **A**

Severance, Mrs Maria Dispenzier 93-19 93rd Avenue, Woodhaven, NY 11421, (718) 847-6552, BA 85 CUNY - Queens Coll; MA 88 CUNY - Hunter Coll

Severino, Mrs Elissa W 7476 Rhoads Street, Philadelphia, PA 19151, (215) 431-8153, BA 75 Univ of MA - Amherst; MA 77 Univ of Pittsburgh - Pittsburgh; Sp-Lang Path, The Devereux Found, **SLP**

Severinsen, Mrs Rosalie H 103 Penny Lane, Macomb, IL 61455, BS 72 Western IL Univ; MA 75 Western IL Univ; Sp-Lang Path, Knox-Warren Sp Ed Dist, **SLP**

Severns, Mrs Jennifer Renee' 102 North 18th Street, Murray, KY 42071, (502) 442-1899, BS 83 Murray St Univ; MS 85 Murray St Univ; 88–Sp-Lang Path, Kentucky Comm for Handi Children, **SLP**

Severns, Mrs Patty Dorann 3752 Concomly Road South, Salem, OR 97306, (503) 773-6281, MA 73 WA St Univ; Sp-Lang Path, Private Practice, **SLP**

Severson, Debra D 20 Roberts Street #5, Brookline, MA 02146, (617) 421-1120, BS 74 Moorhead St Univ; MS 75 Univ of WI - Stevens Point; 87–Coord of Aud & Sp Svc, Harvard Comm Health Plan, **A**

Seville, Mrs Diane Tofini 770 North 7th Street, Laramie, WY 82070, (307) 766-6183, BA 79 Kutztown Univ of PA; MS 87 Univ of WY; 88–Sp-Lang Path, Univ of WY, **SLP**

Seward, Mrs Helen M Rural Delivery 5, Hammondtown Road, Amsterdam, NY 12010, (518) 843-3180, BS 73 SUNY - Coll at Fredonia; MS 75 SUNY - Center at Albany; MS 78 Coll of Saint Rose; SLP, Gtr Amsterdam Sch Dist, **SLP**

Seward, Linda H 117 Rhone Street, Aiken, SC 29801, (404) 863-6393, BA 71 Univ of Southern CA; MA 73 Univ of Southern CA; Aud, Auburn ENT Cl, **A**

Sewell, Mrs Jill N 2304 West 21st Street, Panama City, FL 32405-2424, (904) 769-9481, BA 77 Indiana Univ of PA; MS 79 Univ of Pittsburgh - Pittsburgh; SLP, Bay County School Board, **SLP**

Sewell, Dr John C Speech Pathology Associates, 2131 Elm Hill Pike, Suite C-67, Nashville, TN 37210, (615) 885-5232, BA 53 David Lipscomb Coll; MS 56 Vanderbilt Univ; PH 79 (NS) Baptist Christian Coll; Director, Speech Pathology Associates, **SLP ACE**

Sewell, Natalie B 150 Oak Ridge Place #2-M, Greenville, SC 29615, (803) 585-7711, BS 76 VA Commonwealth Univ; ME 78 Clarion Univ of PA; Sp-Lang Path, Sc Sch for Deaf/Blin/& Muti Ha, **SLP**

Sexton, Barbara M 55 Bay View Avenue, South Portland, ME 04106, (207) 799-5914, BA 68 Univ of ME - Orono; MA 70 Univ of CT; Sp-Lang Path, Private Practice, **SLP**

Sexton, Mrs Florence E 16265 Bowline Street N W, Bokeelia, FL 33922, (813) 694-2151, BA 67 Univ of IL - Urbana; MS 68 FL St Univ; 84–Residential Svcs Dir, Gulf Coast Cen at Ft Myers, **SLP**

Sexton, Janet D 1104 Jenks Avenue, St Paul, MN 55106-3310, (612) 770-4675, BS 81 Univ of WI - River Falls; MS 82 Univ of WI - River Falls; Early Childhood Sp-Lang Clin, N St Paul Indepen Sch Dist 622, **SLP**

Sexton, Mrs Jill D 10 Humes Court, Stratham, NH 03885, (603) 772-7126, BS 74 Northeastern Univ; ME 75 Northeastern Univ; **SLP**

Sexton, Johnnie E 3806 Kirby Drive, Greensboro, NC 27403-1026, (919) 854-0705, BS 77 East Carolina Univ; MS 79 East Carolina Univ; Pres, Carolina Hearing & Sp Svcs Inc, **A**

Sexton, Joyce Forrester HC 79 Box 6438, Chugiak, AK 99567, (907) 274-4582, BS 79 Purdue Univ - West Lafayette; MA 81 Univ of MT; 88–Aud, Private Practice, **SLP A**

Sexton, Sandra Sue P O Box 578603, Chicago, IL 60657-8603, (312) 942-2497, BA 73 Elmhurst Coll; MA 74 Saint Louis Univ; Sp-Lang Path, Cty of Chicago Dept of Hlth, **SLP**

Sexton, Mrs Susan M 3580 Crestwood Drive, Lapeer, MI 48446, (313) 664-5917, BS 78 Western MI Univ; MA 82 Eastern MI Univ; Sp/Lang Path, Lapeer Co Inter Sch Dist, **SLP**

Sexton, Mrs Valerie Anne 59 Winding Brook Trail, Vernon, CT 06066, (203) 875-6042, BS 73 Lamar Univ; MS 77 Univ of Southwestern LA; Spec Educ Tchr, Vernon ISD, **SLP**

Seyfried, Deborah Ann University Of Iowa, WJ Speech & Hearing Center, Iowa City, IA 52240, (319) 351-6965, **A**

Seymore, Mrs Charla Belle 1485 Manchester, McPherson, KS 67460, (316) 241-5499, MA 87 Wichita St Univ; 87–Sp-Lang Path, Hope Preschool USD #418, **SLP**

Seymour, Mrs Bonnie Lee P O Box 1203, Kings Beach, CA 95719, (916) 546-4474, BA 70 San Jose St Univ; ME 71 San Jose St Univ; 77–Sp/Lang Path, Placer Co Offi of Ed, **SLP**

Seymour, Dr Charlena Moten 37 Grantwood Drive, Amherst, MA 01002, (413) 545-0298, BA 65 Howard Univ; MA 67 OH St Univ; PH 71 (Communication Disorders) OH St Univ; 71–Assoc Prof, U of MA Dept of Commun Dis, **SLP F**

Seymour, Deborah T 601 2nd Street, Golden, CO 80401, (303) 279-1796, BA 74 Columbus Coll; MA 76 Vanderbilt Univ; SLP, Denver Public Schools, **SLP**

Seymour, Dr Harry N 37 Grantwood Drive, Amherst, MA 01002, (413) 545-0298, BA 64 Howard Univ; MA 68 OH St Univ; PH 71 (NS) OH St Univ; Assoc Prof, U of MA, **SLP F**

Seymour, Patricia Jean-Anne 4750 Sepuiveda Blvd #107, Sherman Oaks, CA 91403, (714) 526-4527, BA 82 CA St Univ - Fullerton; MA 85 CA St Univ - Fullerton; **SLP**

Sforza, Suzanne 27 W 94th Street #1, New York, NY 10025, (212) 864-0310, BS 82 SUNY - Coll at Geneseo; MA 86 SUNY - Center at Buffalo; Sp-Lang Path, N Central Bronx Hosp, **SLP**

Shaban, Helen 2117 Clover Street, Simi Valley, CA 93065, **A**

Shaber, A David 1550 California Street #6216, San Francisco, CA 94109, (415) 561-9023, BA 67 CUNY - Brooklyn Coll; MA 70 San Francisco St Univ; Dir, Sp & Lang Cen, **SLP**

Shablow, Mrs Denise Conroy 5646 Chatsworth Street, Shoreview, MN 55126, (612) 422-5650, MS 83 Univ of ND; 86–Sp-Lang Path, Anoka-Hennepin Ind Sch Dist #11, **SLP**

Shachar-Hill, Susan Cogan 96 Livingston Street #37, New Haven, CT 06511, (203) 624-1710, **SLP**

Shackelford, Allen El 8573 Buena Tierra Place, Buena Park, CA 90620, (213) 644-4478, BA 65 Whittier Coll; ME 70 Whittier Coll; Prin-Spec Ed, LA Co Office of Ed, **SLP**

Shackelford, Mrs Anne Rushton Route 1 Box 278, Keswick, VA 22947, (804) 973-1693, BS 79 WV Univ; ME 82 Univ of VA - Charlottesville; Sp-Lang Path, VA Er Sl So, **SLP**

Shackelford, Mrs Helen Carolyn 2078 Weymouth Circle West, Jacksonville, FL 32216, (904) 642-1392, BA 77 Meredith Coll; ME 87 Univ of North FL; **SLP**

Shackelford, Mrs Kathleen J P O Box 1232, Talladega, AL 35160, (205) 362-6959, BS 73 Henderson St Univ; MA 74 OH Univ - Athens; 84–Sp-Lang Path, Alabama Public School for Deaf, **SLP ACE**

Shackelford, Mary E P O Box 422, Webbers Falls, OK 74470, (918) 464-2885, BS 70 OK St Univ; MA 72 OK St Univ; Sp-Lang Path, Checotah Pub Sch, **SLP**

Shadd, Nancy Griffin 30 Pioneer Drive, Fairport, NY 14450, (716) 265-4057, BS 64 Nazareth Coll of Rochester; MS 68 SUNY - Coll at Geneseo; 88 SUNY - Coll at Brockport; Sp-Lang Path, BOCES #1 Monroe County NY, **SLP**

Shadden, Dr Barbara B Speech And Hearing Clinic, University Of Arkansas, 410 Arkansas Avenue, Fayetteville, AR 72701, (501) 575-4509, BA 69 Oberlin Coll; MS 73 Southern CT St Univ; PH 79 (NS) Univ of TN - Knoxville; Assoc Prof, U of AR-Fayetteville, **SLP**

Shade, Mrs Teresa Ellis 3222 Oxford Drive, Durham, NC 27707, (703) 528-3646, BA 72 Univ of MS; OM 75 Univ of MS; SLP, Merdock Center, **SLP ACE**

Shadid-Wray, Robin P 13529 Inverness, Oklahoma City, OK 73120, **SLP**

Shadowens, Dr Melvin R 12910 Bandera Road PO 669, Helopes, TX 78023, (512) 695-9432, BS 68 Southern IL Univ -Carbondale; MS 70 Southern IL Univ -Carbondale; PH 79 (NS) Kent St Univ; Dir Audio Vestibular Lab, Private Practice, **A**

Shafer, James L 133 Hummel Avenue, Lemoyne, PA 17043, (717) 761-4348, MA 84 Temple Univ-Tyler Sch of Art; BS 79 PA St Univ - Univ Park; **A**

Shafer, Joyce T Star Route Box 815, Corrales, NM 87048, **SLP**

Shafer, Margaret Payne 593 Witmer Road, Horsham, PA 19044, (215) 576-2160, BS 75 PA St Univ - Univ Park; MA 76 Case Western Reserve Univ; Sp-Lang Path, Abington Memorial Hosp, **SLP**

Shafer, Margaret Sorenson 26 Windbrooke Court, Gaithersburg, MD 20879, MA 67 SUNY - Center at Albany; BA 64 SUNY - Center at Albany; Sp-Lang Path, Mont Co Pub Sch, **SLP**

Shafer, Mrs Mary B North 21420 Pease Hill Rd, Colbert, WA 99005, (509) 276-8168, BA 73 Gonzaga Univ; MS 75 Eastern WA Univ; 84–Sp-Lang Path, Spokane Sch Dist, **SLP**

Shaffer, Chester M 125 Pine Street, Petersburg, WV 26847, (304) 257-4956, BA 35 Glenville St Coll; ME 42 Univ of TN - Knoxville; **A LM**

Shaffer, Dr Deborah J 400 East Randolph #2612, Chicago, IL 60601, (312) 597-6300, BS 71 Northwestern Univ; MA 75 Governors St Univ; ED 84 (NS) Vanderbilt Univ; Sp/Lang Path, Comm H S Dist #218, **SLP**

Shaffer, George 1305 Palmer Drive #212, West Lafayette, IN 47906, (317) 463-5844, BA 36 PA St Univ - Univ Park; MS 38 Univ of IA; PH 50 (Aud) Purdue Univ - West Lafayette; Retired, Purdue, **SLP A F LM**

Shaffer, Lori J 4021 Etter Road, Mogadore, OH 44260, (216) 743-1168, BA 83 Univ of Akron; MA 85 Univ of Akron; **SLP**

Shaffer, Norma L W 1344 Lost Creek Boulevard, Austin, TX 78746, (512) 444-4835, BA 71 Univ of South AL; MA 73 Univ of Houston - Univ Park; Dir of Sp-Lang Path, Brown Sch Healthcare Reh Ctr, **SLP**

Shaffer, Mrs Paula P 1806 Wesley Avenue, Evanston, IL 60201, (312) 498-7970, BS 65 Shippensburg Univ of PA; MA 67 Northwestern Univ; Sp-Lang Path, Comm Consolidated Dist 65, **SLP ACE**

Shaffer-Bartley, Susan 90 Valley View, Suffield, CT 06078, (203) 668-7733, BS 70 SUNY - Coll at Potsdam; MA 83 Univ of MA - Amherst; Sp-Lang Path, Suffield Pub Sch, **SLP**

Shafland, Karen J 460 Oak Run Drive #12, Bourbonnais, IL 60914, (815) 933-0720, BA 73 Bethel Coll; MS 75 Univ of IL - Urbana; Sp-Lang Path, Kankakee Sch Dist #111, **SLP ACE**

Shafton, Mrs Judith H 22550 Liberty Bell Road, Woodland Hills, CA 91364, (818) 997-2357, BA 63 Univ of CA - Los Angeles; MA 77 CA St Univ - Northridge; SLP, LA USD, **SLP ACE**

Shahak, Antoinette E 77 West Norman Avenue, Arcadia, CA 91006, (818) 986-1977, BA 79 SUNY - Center at Buffalo; MA 84 CA St Univ - Los Angeles; Dir of SLP, South Pacific Rehab, **SLP**

Shahbazpour, Mrs Karin-Lyn 2193 Surreywood Drive, Dublin, OH 43017, (614) 766-0176, BS 79 WV Univ; MS 80 WV Univ; 87–Sp-Lang Path, Columbus Sp/Hearing Ctr, **SLP**

Shaiman, Dr Susan Kresge Hearing Research Lab, Louisiana State University Medical Center, 2020 Gravier Street, New Orleans, LA 70112, (504) 568-4785, BA 78 Univ of Pittsburgh - Pittsburgh; MS 80 Columbia Univ Teachers Coll; PH 88 (Sp Physiology) Univ of WI - Madison; Kresge Hring Research Lab, **SLP**

Shaker, Catherine Shriver 1905 East Iron Street, Milwaukee, WI 53207, (414) 447-2208, BS 76 Marquette Univ; MS 77 Marquette Univ; Dir-SLP Svcs, St Josephs Hosp, **SLP**

Shaklee, Janet H 3000 South Elm Place, Broken Arrow, OK 74012, (918) 455-3535, BS 78 Phillips Univ; MA 80 Wichita St Univ; 87–Sp-Lang Path, Broken Arrow Med Ctr, **SLP ACE**

Shalda, Susan L 1182 Hidden Ridge, Toledo, OH 43615, (419) 473-3561, BA 77 MI St Univ; MA 78 MI St Univ; 80–Aud, Toledo Clin, **A**

Shalek, Sara E 1515 S W Boulevard #19-G, Tulsa, OK 74107, (918) 599-0458, MS 88 Univ of Tulsa

Shalhoub, Amy Jo 829 Doty Street, Green Bay, WI 54301, (414) 435-7312, MS 88 Univ of WI - River Falls; 84–Sp-Lang Path, Denmark Pub Schs

Shallant, Mrs Robin Blackman 1007 North Terrill Street, Alexandria, VA 22304, (703) 358-6041, BS 75 Boston Univ; MA 77 SUNY - Center at Buffalo; Sp-Lang Path, Arlington Co Pub Sch, **SLP**

Shaller, Randy Lynn 9 Vanderbilt Way, North Woodmere, NY 11581-2346, (516) 543-5100, BA 80 Emory Univ; OM 82 Emory Univ; Sp-Lang Path, UCP Assoc of Greater Suffolk, **SLP**

Shalley, Mrs Carol J 9 Hennessy Drive, Huntington, NY 11743-3823, (516) 549-7972, BS 79 Hofstra Univ; MS 81 Adelphi Univ; Sp-Lang Path, Private Practice, **SLP**

Shallop, Dr Jon K 203 Pine Tree Lane, Boulder, CO 80302, (303) 442-2125, BS 61 Edinboro Univ of PA; MA 63 Kent St Univ; PH 65 (NS) OH St Univ; Aud/SLP, Private Practice, **SLP A F**

Shallow, Mrs Lisa Kundinger 8741 S Country Drive #204, Oak Creek, WI 53154, (414) 383-3699, BS 84 Marquette Univ; MS 86 Univ of WI - Milwaukee; 87–Sp-Lang Path, InSpeech Inc, **SLP**

Shamasko, Ellenor K 12630 Monte Vista #208, Poway, CA 92064, (619) 743-4343, BS 64 Northwestern Univ; MA 66 Univ of KS; Chief/SLP Services, Palomar Momerado Hosp District, **SLP**

Shambelan, Michele Ruth 2500 Clarendon Boulevard #732, Arlington, VA 22201, (703) 569-1031, BA 84 Montclair St Coll; MA 86 George Washington Univ; 86–Sp-Lang Path, Fairfax County Health Dept, **SLP**

Shamel-Pertuso, Karen Lee 1309 Quincy Street, Alexandria, VA 22303, (203) 787-3853, BS 80 Central MI Univ; MA 84 Memphis St Univ; Special Agent, FBI, **SLP**

Shames, Dr George H University Of Pittsburgh, Dept Of Communication, 1117 Cathedral Of Learning, Pittsburgh, PA 15260, (412) 624-6103, BS 48 Univ of Pittsburgh - Pittsburgh; MS 49 Univ of Pittsburgh - Pittsburgh; PH 52 (Sp Path & Psychol) Univ of Pittsburgh - Pittsburgh; Prof/Coor Div Commun Disorders, University of Pittsburgh, **SLP F ACE**

Shames, Mrs Joan Kramer 216 Gladstone Road, Pittsburgh, PA 15217, (412) 682-4009, BA 52 Univ of Pittsburgh - Pittsburgh; MS 56 Univ of Pittsburgh - Pittsburgh; Sp-Lang Path, Private Practice, **SLP A**

Shamey, Lenore T 1308 Westgate Center Drive, Winston-Salem, NC 27103, (919) 768-7946, BA 77 Rutger's St Univ - Douglas Coll; MS 78 Univ of NC - Chapel Hill; Sp/Lang Path, Private Practice, **SLP**

Shamoo, Mrs Joan H Columbia Speech/Language Cntr, 6328 Amherst Anenue, Columbia, MD 21046, (301) 730-0579, MS 74 CUNY - Hunter Coll; Dir, Columbia Speech & Language Ctr, **SLP**

Shampain, Lisa Plattner 721 Piedmont Avenue, Rocky Mount, NC 27803, (919) 443-8730, BS 80 Univ of MA - Amherst; MS 82 Columbia Univ Teachers Coll; Sp/Lang Path, Nash General Hospital, **SLP**

Shanahan, Mrs Denise Kotyk 16 Alder Lane, Rural Route 3, Sandy Hook, CT 06482, (203) 735-3864, **SLP**

Shanahan, James H 730 Gypsy Lane, Pittsburgh, PA 15228, (412) 683-3000, BS 75 PA St Univ - Univ Park; MS 77 PA St Univ - Univ Park; Aud, U Drive Vamc Pittsburgh Pa, **A**

Shanahan, Mrs Mona Aida 176 College Street, Thunder Bay, ON, Canada P7A 5J7, (807) 622-9122, BA 79 Univ of ND; MA 81 Univ of MN - Minneap-St Paul; Sp-Lang Path, Thunder Bay Home Care Prog, **SLP**

Shanahan, Patrick E 176 College Street, Thunder Bay, ON, Canada P7A 5J7, (807) 345-6473, **SLP**

Shander, Mrs Sari G 16112 Howard Landing Drive, Gaithersburg, MD 20878, (301) 977-2045, BA 74 Univ of CT; MS 76 Southern CT St Univ; **SLP**

Shandler, Phyllis 3001 Trinity Road, Glen Ellen, CA 95442, (707) 996-9324, BA 73 Univ of CA - Berkeley; MS 83 CA St Univ - Hayward; 88–Sp-Lang Path, NAPA Co of Educ, **SLP**

Shandor, Judith A Sparks 3305 Caleo Court, Plano, TX 75023, (702) 673-5827, MS 73 Univ of WI - Stevens Point; BS 71 Univ of WI - Stevens Point; SLP, Alpha Sch, **SLP**

Shane, Carole J 05534 Lakeshore Road, Boyne City, MI 49712, (616) 547-9947, BS 75 Central MI Univ; MA 80 Central MI Univ; Sp-Lang Path, Charlevoix-Emmet Sch Dist, **SLP**

Shane, Mrs Esther McGeoch 440 School Street, Indiana, PA 15701, (412) 357-2453, BA 59 Westminster Coll; MS 68 WV Univ; Director Speech & Hrng Clinic, Indiana University of Pa, **SLP**

Shane, Dr Howard C The Childrens Hospital, 300 Longwood Avenue, Boston, MA 02115, PH (NS); **SLP**

Shanebeck, Mrs Camilla Diane Communications Disorders Dept, Biola University, 13800 Biola Avenue, La Mirada, CA 90639, (213) 944-0351, BA 56 Asbury Coll; MA 69 CA St Univ - Long Beach; Assoc Prof, Biola U

Shanin, Sandra J 5444 Corteen Pl #3, North Hollywood, CA 91607, (818) 289-3691, BA 76 Univ of CA - Santa Barbara; MA 80 CA St Univ - Los Angeles; SLP, San Marino USD, **SLP**

Shank, Jean W P O Box 368, 737 Pinehurst, Port Orford, OR 97465, (503) 332-2712, BA 80 Humboldt St Univ; MA 82 Humboldt St Univ; 82–Sp-Lang Path, Curry Co Ed Serv Dist, **SLP**

Shank, Julie E 6272 Meridian Avenue, San Jose, CA 95120, (916) 487-0628, BA 85 San Jose St Univ; MS 87 CA St Univ - Sacramento; Sp-Lang Path, Easter Seal Society, **SLP**

Shank, Kathleen Ryan 20 Barbara Circle, Rumford, RI 02916, (401) 438-4298, BA 70 Wells Coll; MA 76 San Francisco St Univ; Sp-Lang Path, **SLP ACE**

Shank, Dr Kennon H 6410 East Bender Road, Bloomington, IN 47401, (812) 335-3251, BA 42 Simpson Coll; MA 47 Univ of Denver; PH 54 (NS) Univ of Denver; Professor, Indiana University, **SLP F LM**

Shank, Patricia T 105 Phillips Lane, Mc Kees Rocks, PA 15136, (412) 869-2755, BS 78 Indiana Univ of PA; MS 80 WV Univ; Aud, The Hearing Labortory, **A**

Shank, Sandra J 1596 Peck Street, Muskegon, MI 49441, (517) 723-5323, MA 88 MI St Univ

Shanklin-Shay, Mrs Donna Ruth 512 Quail Valley, Princeton, WV 24740, (304) 487-7000, BS 81 WV Univ; MS 82 WV Univ; 85–Sp-Lang Path, Princeton Aud-Sp-Path Clinic, **SLP**

Shanks, Carolyn A P O Box 27, Weston, OR 97886, (503) 566-3715, BA 66 CA St Univ - Sacramento; MS 75 WA St Univ; Sp-Lang Path, Private Practice, **SLP**

Shanks, Dr James C, Jr 1908 Orlando Street, Indianapolis, IN 46208, (317) 630-8979, BA 43 MI St Univ; MA 49 Univ of Denver; PH 57 (NS) Northwestern Univ; Prof Emeritus Sp-Lang Path, IN U Sch of Med, **SLP F LM**

Shanks, Janet E Audiology 126, VA Medical Center, 5901 East 7th Street, Long Beach, CA 90822, (213) 494-5414, BS 71 Western MI Univ; MA 73 Univ of NM; PH 79 (Aud) Univ of IA; Aud, VA Med Ctr, **A**

Shanks, Mrs Karen L 56 Braemar Avenue, Winnipeg, MB, Canada R2H 2K3, (201) 786-7841, MA 79 Univ of ND; BA 77; Sp-Lang Path, Chld Guid Cl, **SLP**

Shanks, Mrs Paulette Willie 5107 Whites Creek Pike, Whites Creek, TN 37189, (615) 320-5353, BS 73 Univ of WI - River Falls; MA 76 Univ of KS; Sp/Lang Path Clinical Super, Billwilkerson Hrng-Sp Clinic, **SLP**

Shanks, Rosemarie Ann W 151 S7043 Cornell Circle, Apartment 6, Muskego, WI 53150, (414) 383-4490, BS 82 Univ of WI - LA Crosse; MS 87 Marquette Univ; 87–Sp-Lang Path, Sacred Heart Rehab Hosp, **SLP**

Shanks, Dr Susan 5330 North Colonial #101, Fresno, CA 93704, (209) 294-2634, OB 57 Univ of Toledo; MA 60 Bowling Green St Univ; PH 66 (Sp) LA St Univ - Baton Rouge; Prof Commun Dis, CA St U Fresno, **SLP**

Shanley, Valerie J R R 1 Box 506, Creamery Road, Stanfordville, NY 12581, (914) 877-6821, MA 77 SUNY - Coll at Geneseo; Sp-Lang Path, Wassaic Dev Cen, **SLP**

Shannon, Mrs Claudia J 3125 S W 20th, Topeka, KS 66604, (913) 232-0551, BS 75 Univ of MO - Columbia; MA 76 KS St Univ; 78–Sp-Lang Path, Topeka Public Schools, **SLP**

Shannon, Donna Jo 3828 W 154th Place, Markham, IL 60426, (312) 672-2670, BA 82 Saint Xavier Coll; OM 86 Governors St Univ; **SLP**

Shannon, Dr Dorothy A 9936 Whitworth Way, Ellicott City, MD 21043, (301) 578-5602, BA 65 Montclair St Coll; MS 66 PA St Univ - Univ Park; PH 73 (Aud/Sp-Lang Path) Univ of MD - College Park; 73–Chief Aud, Sinai Hosp of Baltimore, Inc, **SLP A**

Shannon, Janet Louise 715 Esther Way, Redlands, CA 92373, (714) 829-6993, BS 81 Univ of Redlands; BS 81 Univ of Redlands; MS 82 Univ of Redlands; Sp/Lang Path Coordinatoar, Kaiser Permanente Med Cen, **SLP ACE**

Shannon, Jeanette Manning 323 Richmond Road, Salisbury, NC 28144, (704) 633-1454, BS 67 Univ of MN - Minneap-St Paul; MA 71 MI St Univ; Sp-Lang Path, Rowan County Schs, **SLP**

Shannon, Mrs Michelle Renee 17410 N 15th Street #2053, Phoenix, AZ 85022, (602) 266-5976, MA 83 Northeast MO St Univ; Sp-Lang Path, Southwest Human Dev, **SLP**

Shannon, Robert V Boys Town National Institute, 555 North 30th Street, Omaha, NE 68131, (402) 449-6700, BA 71 Univ of IA; MS 75 Univ of CA - San Diego; PH 75 (Psychology) Univ of CA - San Diego; Aud, Boys Town Natl Inst

Shapanka, Judith M 16 Country Squire Lane, Holmdel, NJ 07733, (201) 946-9180, **SLP**

Shapero, Sheldon O Comprehensive Comm Develop Ctr, 2100 West Magnolia Blvd, Burbank, CA 91506, (818) 843-0502, BA 55 Wayne St Univ; MA 61 Univ of CA - Los Angeles; Owner/Dir, Comprehensive Commun Dev Cen, **SLP**

Shapiro, Arnold 3 Azalea Drive, Nanuet, NY 10954, (212) 650-6153, BA 72 CUNY - Hunter Coll; MA 71 CUNY - Hunter Coll; 72–Dir-Comm Disorders, Mount Sinai Med Cen, **SLP**

Shapiro, Mrs Barbara B 16 Via Maria Theresia, Manitou Springs, CO 80829, (303) 636-5186, BA 63 Univ of AZ; MA 64 Univ of Denver; 85–Sp-Lang Path, Colorado Springs Sch Dist #11, **SLP**

Shapiro, Betty Pollack 8808 Revere Street, Philadelphia, PA 19152, (215) 677-0303, BS 73 Northern IL Univ - De Kalb; MA 78 Temple Univ; Sp-Lang Path, Private Practice, **SLP**

Shapiro, Mrs Carole L 89 Melrose Avenue, Needham, MA 02192, (617) 455-0736, BS 80 Boston Univ; MA 82 Univ of CT; Sp-Lang Path, CASE Collaborative, **SLP**

Shapiro, Carrie Janine 8797 21st Avenue, Brooklyn, NY 11214, (718) 403-8431, BA 85 CUNY - Brooklyn Coll; MS 87 CUNY - Brooklyn Coll; 88–Aud, Brooklyn Hosp Sp & Hrng Ctr

Shapiro, Caryn L 1415 Pontiac Trail #2, Ann Arbor, MI 48105, (313) 662-7465, BA 83 Univ of MN - Minneap-St Paul; MS 86 Univ of NM; 87–Sp-Lang Path, Manchester Comm Schs, **SLP**

Shapiro, Dr David A Western Carolina Univer, Human Services Killian, Cullowhee, NC 28723, (704) 227-7310, BA 76 SUNY - Center at Albany; MS 77 Univ of VT; PH 84 (Sp-Lang Path (The Supervisory Process Childhood Lang & Lang Disorders)) IN Univ - Bloomington; Assistant Professor, Western Carolina University, **SLP**

Shapiro, Deborah Ann 4724 N W 76th, Oklahoma City, OK 73132, (405) 732-8288, BA 86 Univ of OK - Norman; MS 88 Univ of OK Medical Center; 88–Sp-Lang Path, Oklahoma City-County Health Dept, **F H**

Shapiro, Elizabeth De Ritter 2 Flower Lane, Jericho, NY 11753, (516) 924-5583, **SLP**

Shapiro, Gail Andrea 2021 Randolph Road, Apartment 102, Silver Spring, MD 20906, (301) 933-7269, BA 85 George Washington Univ; MA 86 George Washington Univ; Sp-Lang Path, Mont Co PS, **SLP**

Shapiro, Gertrude G 15 Hamilton Avenue, Cranford, NJ 07016, (201) 276-2648, BS Kean Coll of NJ; MA Columbia Univ Teachers Coll; **SLP LM**

Shapiro, Dr Holly Rose 655 Le Parc Circle, Buffalo Grove, IL 60089, (312) 459-8810, BS 82 Univ of IL - Urbana; MS 83 Univ of IL - Urbana; PH 88 (Learning Disabilities) Northwestern Univ; 88, Private Practice, **SLP**

Shapiro, Dr Irving 5294 Vista Del Sol, Cypress, CA 90630, (213) 517-4736, BS 58 Western MI Univ; MA 60 Syracuse Univ; PH 64 (Aud) Case Western Reserve Univ; Aud, Private Practice, **A ACE**

Shapiro, Mrs Janet R 1555 Fescue Court, Reno, NV 89509, (702) 786-4240, BA 76 CA St Univ - Northridge; MA 77 CA St Univ - Northridge; 87–Clin Coord-Comm Dis, Nevada Communications Services, **SLP**

Shapiro, Jeanne Kantauskis 37 Lanark Drive, Westwood, MA 02090, (617) 543-2542, BS 74 Univ of ME - Orono; ME 82 Northeastern Univ; Sp-Lang Path, Kennedy-Donovan Cen, **SLP**

Shapiro, Joyce A 115 Millwood Street, Framingham, MA 01701, **SLP**

Shapiro, Mrs Joyce Reich 2800 Crystal Court, Coconut Grove, FL 33133, (305) 667-8804, BS 75 PA St Univ - Univ Park; MA 76 Univ of Miami; SLP, Edd Ann Freeman & Ass, **SLP**

Shapiro, Karen 47 Forest Drive, Holden, MA 01520, (617) 829-5460, ME 80 Northeastern Univ; 88–Sp-Lang Path, Clinton Hosp, **SLP**

Shapiro, Lawrence S 15 Cottonwood Avenue, Port Jefferson, NY 11776, (516) 665-7772, BA 66 CUNY - Queens Coll; MS 68 Adelphi Univ; Sp-Lang Path, Suffolk Hrng & Sp Cen, **SLP**

Shapiro, Lori S 4623 Anza Street, San Francisco, CA 94121, (415) 565-9000, BA 85 Univ of NM; MS 87 Univ of NM

Shapiro, Mrs Marian C 1319 Forest Avenue, Evanston, IL 60201, MA 68 Columbia Univ Teachers Coll; Sp-Lang Path, Private Practice, **SLP**

Shapiro, Mark J 3620 Floradale Court, Thousand Oaks, CA 91306, (805) 498-3608, BA 68 Colgate Univ; MS 73 SUNY - Center at Buffalo; SLP, Conejo Vallay USD, **SLP**

Shapiro, Mrs Melissa Malis 23-55 Bell Boulevard #5B, Bayside, NY 11360, (718) 225-1146, BA 77 CUNY - Queens Coll; MA 79 CUNY - Queens Coll; 79–Aud, Helen Keller Nat Cen, **A**

Shapiro, Nancy H 220 Palisade Street, Memphis, TN 38111, (901) 761-1500, BA 75 Univ of Bridgeport; MA 80 Memphis St Univ; MS 87 Memphis St Univ; 79–Aud/Consulting Tchr, Memphis City Schs, **A**

Shapiro, Robert B 15 Wild Rose Drive, Andover, MA 01810, **SLP**

Shapiro, Mrs Ruth Wagner 4880 Northwest 72 Terrace, Lauderhill, FL 33319, (305) 741-3773, BA 79 Univ of FL; MS 81 Boston Univ; Sp-Lang Path, Private Practice, **SLP ACE**

Shapiro, Mrs Susan G 106 Burlington Road, Murray Hill, NJ 07974, (201) 464-9465, BS 60 Syracuse Univ; MA 63 NY Univ; Sp-Lang Path, Private Practice, **SLP**

Shapiro, Susan L 3121 S E 35th Street, Gainesville, FL 32601, (904) 486-4550, BA 68 CUNY - Brooklyn Coll; ME 69 Boston Univ; **SLP**

Shapiro, William H 23-55 Bell Boulevard #5B, Bayside, NY 11360, (718) 225-1146, BA 77 CUNY - Brooklyn Coll; MA 78 CUNY - Queens Coll; Dir, Park West Hrng Cen, **A**

Shapley, Dr James 1253 23rd Avenue East, Seattle, WA 98112, (206) 764-2404, BA 47 Univ of WA; MA 51 Univ of WA; PH 54 (NS) Univ of IA; **A LM**

Sharbaugh, Donna P 1101 Springdale Road, Atlanta, GA 30306, (404) 377-1565, BS 71 PA St Univ - Univ Park; MS 78 Emory Univ; **SLP A**

Sharer, Anita Marie 385 West Side Drive #301, Gaithersburg, MD 20878, (301) 963-2053, BA 85 Univ of MD - College Park; MA 87 George Washington Univ; **A**

Sharf, Dr Donald J 8917 Windtree, Boca Raton, FL 33434, BA 51 Wayne St Univ; MA 52 Wayne St Univ; PH 57 (NS) Univ of MI - Ann Arbor; Prof Emeritus, U of MI

Shargel, George M 2145 Randall Lane, Bloomfield Hills, MI 48013, MS

Shariff, Kelly Bur 2623 B Summit Road, Columbia, MO 65203, (314) 445-0045, BS 83 Univ of WI - Madison; MS 84 Univ of WI - Eau Claire; SLP, **SLP**

Sharkey, Laurie Ann 3544-D Creekside Road, Port Orange, FL 32019, (904) 767-8552, BS 78 SUNY - Coll at Plattsburgh; MA 83 Univ of TN - Knoxville; 87–Sp-Lang Path, Rehab Works Inc, **SLP**

Sharp, Angela Helen 4145 Crisfield Lane, Pleasanton, CA 94566, (415) 828-2551, BA 77 0175; MA 79 Univ of Philippines; **SLP**

Sharp, Carol Ann 109 Highland, Charles City, IA 50616, (515) 228-7564, BA 73 Univ of Northern IA; BA 82 Univ of Northern IA; MA 84 Univ of Northern IA; **SLP**

Sharp, Carrie J 56 N W Wallula, Gresham, OR 97030, (503) 775-4366, BS 71 OR St Univ; MS 77 Western OR St Coll; OM 78 Western OR St Coll; Assistant Prof Early Child Ed, Warner Pacific College, **SLP**

Sharp, Mrs Cheryl S 23549 Broadway Boulevard, Elkhart, IN 46516, (217) 351-1243, BS 80 Ball St Univ; MA 81 Ball St Univ; Audiologist, Christie Clinic, **A**

Sharp, Mrs Deborah C 7710 Ensley Drive, Huntsville, AL 35802, (205) 883-1072, BS 83 Southwest MO St Univ; MA 85 Memphis St Univ; 88–Sp-Lang Path, Ctr for Sp and Lang Path, **SLP**

Sharp, Deena S 944 6th Street #7, Santa Monica, CA 90403, **SLP**

Sharp, Mrs Dolores S 1838 7th Street, Astoria, OR 97103, (503) 325-2862, BA 55 Univ of Northern IA; MS 73 Western OR St Coll; 68–Sp-Lang Path, Clatsop Ed Serv Dist, **SLP ACE**

Sharp, Dr Florence A 133 North Mariposa Avenue, Los Angeles, CA 90004, PH 49 (NS) Univ of Southern CA; **SLP LM**

Sharp, Jack R 3008 Milford Lane, Virginia Beach, VA 23452, (804) 340-4863, BS 74 CA Univ of PA; ME 78 Old Dominion Univ; Sp/Lang Path, VA Beach Pub Sch, **SLP**

Sharp, Mrs Janet Sue 923 Bonita, Hitchcock, TX 77563, (409) 938-0185, BS 77 Univ of TX - Dallas; MS 78 Southern Methodist Univ; 88–Sp-Lang Path, Private Practice, **SLP**

Sharp, Karen Link 500 North Sunnyside Avenue, Sierra Madre, CA 91024, (213) 793-2000, BA 79 CA St Univ - Los Angeles; MA 81 CA St Univ - Los Angeles; SLP, Pasadena USD, **SLP**

Sharp, Mrs Linda Gayle 2008 Tulane, Gainesville, TX 76240, (817) 665-1390, BS 81 OK St Univ; MS 83 Univ of North TX; Sp-Lang Path, Washington Elem, **SLP**

Sharp, Margaret Ann 3500 Paradise, Vernon, TX 76384, (817) 553-1896, BS 75 Univ of TX - Austin; MA 85 TX Woman's Univ; **SLP**

Sharp, Mary Christian 11069 Strayhorn Drive, Dallas, TX 75228, (214) 270-6611, BA 69 East TX St Univ - Commerce; MS 70 East TX St Univ - Commerce; Coor, Mesquite ISD, **SLP**

Sharp, Patricia Ann 713 Stratford Place, Blue Springs, MO 64015, (816) 229-8389, **SLP**

Sharp, Mrs Patricia Stone 2413 Chinaberry Drive, Bedford, TX 76021-5211, BS 79 Univ Southern MS-Hattiesburg; MS 80 Univ Southern MS-Hattiesburg; Sp-Lang Path, **SLP**

Sharp, Mrs Sherrie Lynn 1501 Pecan Street, Weatherford, OK 73096, (405) 772-8144, MS 81 Univ of Central AR; Sp-Lang Path, Southwestern Oklahoma St Univ, **SLP**

Sharp, Mrs Sheryl Fursteneau 23 West Erie, Tempe, AZ 85282, (602) 839-7172, BS 66 Minot St Univ; MS 69 Minot St Univ; Assistant Principal, Tempe District 3 Frank School, **SLP**

Sharpe, Julie Vaughan 199 Base Line Road East, London, ON, Canada N6C 2N6, BS 77 Univ of Western Ontario; MA 78 Western MI Univ; Sp-Lang Path, Thames Vy Chln Cen, **SLP**

Sharpless, Mrs Clair 1 Drumlin Road, West Simsbury, CT 06092, (203) 658-0562, BS 60 Northwestern Univ; MA 66 Univ of FL; **SLP**

Sharron, Anna Carol Route 2 Box 24, Lindale, TX 75771, (214) 531-8190, MS 84 Univ of South FL; **A**

Sharrow, Margaret F 3080 Princess Street, Corvallis, OR 97330, (503) 838-1220, BA 73 TX Tech Univ; MA 75 TX Tech Univ; Asst Prof, Wn or St Coll, **SLP**

Shasserre, Mrs Mary L 421 Orchard Avenue, St Louis, MO 63119, (314) 962-7250, BS 64 Saint Louis Univ; MA 65 Saint Louis Univ; **SLP**

Shatford, Jill C 73 Dogwood Place, Regina, SK, Canada S4S 5A1, (306) 586-3423, BA 84 Minot St Univ; MS 85 Minot St Univ; 86–Sp-Lang Path, Community Hlth Svcs, **SLP**

Shatto, Donna Leta 465 East Norman, Orange, TX 77630, (409) 838-8179, BS 75 Lamar Univ; MS 77 Lamar Univ; Audiologist, David W Granitz Phd, **A**

Shatto, Mrs Kathleen C Route 4 Box 4078, Pearland, TX 77581, (713) 485-8279, BS 77 Univ of Houston - Univ Park; MS 79 Univ of TX - Houston; Sp-Lang Path, Pasadena ISD, **SLP**

Shatz, Mrs Karen S 29 Montrose Road, Scarsdale, NY 10583, (212) 870-6372, BA 67 Sarah Lawrence Coll; MS 69 Columbia Univ Teachers Coll; 86–Consult Sp-Lang Path, Isabella Geriatric Center, **SLP A**

Shatz, Mrs Phyllis Goldstein 1383 Fisher Hawk, Sunnyvale, CA 94087, (408) 738-3060, BA 60 Univ of IA; Sp-Lang Path, South Peninsula Heb Day School, **SLP**

Shaughnessy, Dale H P O Box 507, 1762 Main Street, West Chatham, MA 02669, (617) 945-4555, BA 74 Boston Coll; MS 76 Washington Univ; 78–Sp-Lang Path, Rehab Assoc of Cape Cod, **SLP**

Shaughnessy, Mrs Margaret Ann 93 Minnesota Avenue #2, Buffalo, NY 14214, (716) 674-6300, BS 82 Nazareth Coll of Rochester; MA 84 SUNY - Center at Buffalo; 85–Aud, West Seneca Developmental Ctr, **A**

Shaul, Mrs Cynthia Shock 544 Appalachian Avenue, Mechanicsburg, PA 17055, (717) 763-9501, BS 78 Indiana Univ of PA; MS 79 Indiana Univ of PA; Sp-Lang Path, Capital Area Iu, **SLP**

Shaver, Mrs Cinda King Route 3 Box 84, Weston, WV 26452, (304) 269-4585, BS 71 WV Univ; MS 87 WV Univ; 88–Sp-Lang Path, Lewis County PS

Shaver, Robert S 2506 Crosby Street, Rockford, IL 61107, (815) 389-2311, BS 80 Central MI Univ; MA 81 Central MI Univ; Sp-Lang Path, S Beloit Pub Sch, **SLP**

Shaw, Mrs Ann E 1303 Navaho Trail, Richardson, TX 75080, (214) 248-6300, BS 65 Univ of TX - Austin; MA 68 Univ of TX - Austin; Sp-Lang Path, Developmental Lrng Material, **SLP**

Shaw, Anne E 328 Huron Street, Decatur, GA 30030, (404) 233-5332, BA 65 Vanderbilt Univ; MA 67 Univ of IA; OM 78 Northwestern Univ; 88–Sp-Lang Path, Atlanta Speech Sch, **SLP**

Shaw, B Dennis Speech/Hearing Aid Services, 3370 Hermitage Square Professional Bldg, Hermitage, PA 16148, (412) 347-7005, BS 67 Clarion Univ of PA; ME 69 Clarion Univ of PA; Owner/Dir, Private Practice, **SLP**

Shaw, Barbara K 189 Norwood Avenue, Buffalo, NY 14222, (716) 882-5574, BS 85 SUNY - Coll at Fredonia; MS 85 SUNY - Coll at Fredonia; 87–Sp-Lang Path, Kenmore Mercy Hosp, **SLP**

Shaw, Carla Market R R 4 Box 263, Rockville, IN 47872, (317) 569-5363, BS 81 IN St Univ - Terre Haute; MS 82 IN St Univ - Terre Haute; Sp-Lang Path, Rockville Comm Schs, **SLP**

Shaw, Mrs Debra Young 56 Brainard Road, Wilbraham, MA 01095, (413) 599-1642, BS 78 Bridgewater St Coll; MS 82 Univ of MA - Amherst; 81–Sp-Lang Path, Somers Pub Sch, **SLP**

Shaw, Elizabeth 5599 Fenwick Street, NS Hearing & Sp Cl, Halifax, NS, Canada B3H 1R2, (902) 423-7354, OB 73 Univ of Queensland - Australi; MS 82 FL St Univ; 83–Sp-Lang Path, Nova Scotia Hrng & Sp CL, **SLP**

Shaw, Dr Irwin R P O Box 9002, Mercaz Nafati, Ashkelon, Israel, BS 57 SUNY - Coll at Geneseo; MA 58 Univ of Denver; PH 66 Wayne St Univ; Psych and SLP, City of Ashkelon, **SLP**

Shaw, Jill D 680 N W 10th Court, Boynton Beach, FL 33426, (305) 734-4756, MS 79 Univ of South FL; Sp-Lang Path, Sch Bd of Palm Beach Co, **SLP ACE**

Shaw, Joan Kain 6941 Hunters Ridge, Dallas, TX 75248, (214) 980-8912, BA 50 Rockford Coll; MS 54 Univ of WI - Madison; **SLP**

Shaw, John D 129 Dale Avenue, San Carlos, CA 94070, (415) 573-2109, **SLP**

Shaw, Mrs Karen A 16239 North 67th Place, Scottsdale, AZ 85254, (602) 971-5356, BA 75 Univ of SD - Vermillion; MA 76 Univ of SD - Vermillion; **SLP**

Shaw, Kathie J 1802 Barb Drive, Norman, OK 73071, (405) 794-1591, BA 77 Univ of OK - Norman; MS 79 Univ of OK Medical Center; Sp-Lang Path-Sp Serv Superv, Okla St Dept of Hlth, **SLP**

Shaw, Linda 1838 Mc Kelvey Road, Maryland Heights, MO 63043-2819, (314) 629-3637, **SLP**

Shaw, Mrs Marian Watts 4031 Hillandale Drive, Gautier, MS 39553, (601) 769-7780, **SLP**

Shaw, Nancy L 126 West Ridgeway, Clifton Forge, VA 24422, (703) 862-7124, BA 76 Univ of AR - Fayetteville; MA 78 Univ of AR - Fayetteville; Sp-Lang Path, **SLP**

Shaw, Rebecca E 1021 Hickory Lane S W, Rochester, MN 55902, (507) 281-2645, BA 79 Univ of IA; MA 80 Univ of IA; 87–Sp-Lang Path, Stanley Jones & Assoc, **SLP**

Shaw, Tonya J 2619 Cloverlane Drive, Wheelersburg, OH 45694-9037, (614) 574-5796, MA 83 OH Univ - Athens; 88–Sp-Lang Path, Greenup Co Schs, **SLP**

Shaw, Wendy H 5708 Glenwood Road, Bethesda, MD 20817, (301) 656-4889, BA 71 Simmons Coll; BA 76 Univ of MN - Minneap-St Paul; MA 78 Univ of MD - College Park; **SLP**

Shaw-Holmes, Mrs Faith Suzanne 8713 Contee Road #202, Laurel, MD 20708, (301) 735-1515, BS 83 Towson St Univ; MS 84 Towson St Univ; **SLP**

Shawron, Mrs Virginia Miller 6101 Janes Street, Downers Grove, IL 60516, (312) 971-8494, BS 80 Western IL Univ; MA 81 Western IL Univ; Sp-Lang Path, **SLP**

Shawver, Katrina L Rd 1 Box 327, New Bloomfield, PA 17068, (717) 692-4350, BS 83 Indiana Univ of PA; MS 85 PA St Univ - Univ Park; Sp-Lang Path, Central PA Rehabilitation, **SLP**

Shawver-Stearns, Heidi Ann 700 Stoney Mill Court #B, Cockeysville, MD 21030, (301) 667-4265, MS 87 PA St Univ - Univ Park; 87–Sp-Lang Path, Lewistown Hosp, **SLP**

Shay, Donna M 2290 Grape Avenue, Boulder, CO 80302, (303) 447-1010, BS 52 Univ of KS; MA 73 Univ of CO - Boulder; SLP, Boulder Valley Sch Dist Re-2, **SLP**

Shay, Mrs Lynne Mason 1301 Wyncrest, Ballwin, MO 63011-4413, (314) 432-4110, BS 78 MacMurray Coll; MA 80 Univ of IL - Urbana; Aud, Washington U Med Sch, **A**

Shay, Mrs Margaret Irene 6051 Harrison Street, Merrillville, IN 46410, (219) 980-5575, **SLP**

Shayne, Ava B 3114 Isabella Street, Evanston, IL 60201-2775, (312) 833-1400, **SLP**

Shea, Ann Kathleen 3020 Meadowbrook Drive, Rapid City, SD 57702-5028, (605) 348-6697, BA 83 Univ of SD - Vermillion; MA 85 Univ of SD - Vermillion; 85–Sp-Lang Path, Douglas Sch Sys, **SLP**

Shea, B David 47 Round Hill Road, Northampton, MA 01060, (413) 584-3450, BS 80 Univ of MA - Amherst; BS 80 Univ of MA - Amherst; MA 82 Univ of CT; Aud, Clarke Sch for Deaf, **A**

Shea, Mrs Catherine Ann 3054 Cranberry, Wichita, KS 67226-1209, (316) 833-3410, BS 77 0500; MA 79 Wichita St Univ; Sp-Lang Path, Levy Spec Ed Ctr, **SLP**

Shea, Deborah Longaker 1951 West Oak Shadows Circle, Memphis, TN 38119, (901) 763-3530, BA 81 Univ of GA; MA 84 Univ of SC - Columbia; Aud, **A**

Shea, Dr John J P O Box 17987, Memphis, TN 38187-0987, (901) 523-2122, MD 47 (NS) Harvard Univ; Pres, Shea Clinic

Shea, Mrs Judith Orrill 68 Drummer Trail, South Down Shores, Laconia, NH 03246, (603) 528-2647, BA 74 Univ of CT; MA 76 Case Western Reserve Univ; Sp-Lang Path/Aud, The Laconia Clinic, **SLP A**

Shea, Kathleen L 37 Myers Farm Road, Hingham, MA 02043, (617) 749-2349, BA 68 Trinity Coll; Aud, Plymouth Hearing Service, **A**

Shea, Patricia A 8768 North Old Sr 37, Bloomington, IN 47401, (812) 339-1991, BS 74 IN Univ - Bloomington; MA 76 IN Univ - Bloomington; Aud, **A**

Shea, Dr William L 1429 Alegriano, Coral Gables, FL 33146, (305) 661-6756, BA 37; MA 41 MI St Univ; PH 57 (Sp Path Aud) Univ of FL; Professor Emeritus, University of Miami, **SLP LM**

Sheaffer, David Bryan 2504 Capitol Avenue, Sacramento, CA 95816, (916) 736-3399, Audiologist, Sacramento Ear Nose & Throat, **A**

Sheafor, Mrs Patricia F 228 Blenheim Road, Baltimore, MD 21212-1703, (301) 396-1387, BS 60 Phillips Univ; MA 63 MI St Univ; 84–Sp-Lang Path, Balt Cty Pub Sch, **SLP**

Shealy, Candler Leslie 105 South Ocean Blvd, Myrtle Beach, SC 29577, (803) 448-2913, BA 85 Columbia Coll; MA 86 Univ of SC - Columbia; 87–Aud, Pee Dee Sp & Hrng Ctr, **A**

Shearer, Cynthia Ann 6821 East Baker Street, Tucson, AZ 85710, BS 82 Univ of AZ; MS 84 Univ of AZ; **SLP**

Shearer, Dale C 8501 Shakespeare, Orange, TX 77630, (409) 886-2263, BS 77 Southwest TX St Univ; ME 78 Southwest TX St Univ; 84–Director, Sp-Lang Services of SE TX, **SLP**

Shearer, Mrs Janet L 416 East 17th Street, Portales, NM 88130, (505) 356-8007, MS 87 Univ of NM

Shearer, Paulette B 269 Regal Street, Louisville, CO 80027, (303) 441-0493, BS 77 Edinboro Univ of PA; MA 82 Univ of CO - Boulder; Sp-Lang Path, Boulder Mem Hosp, **SLP**

Shearer, Robert R P O Box 567, Concord, CA 94522-0567, (415) 687-7546, BA 50 San Francisco St Univ; Dir, Private Practice, **SLP ACE**

Shearer, Dr William M Speech And Hearing Clinic, Northern Illinois Univ, De Kalb, IL 60115, (815) 753-6516, BA 51 IN Univ - Bloomington; MA 54 Western MI Univ; PH 58 (NS) Univ of Denver; Professor, Northern Illinois University, **SLP A**

Shearn, Nancy Weaver 3123 Iron Stone Lane, San Antonio, TX 78230, (512) 492-7180, BA 73 Trinity Univ; MA 76 Univ of TX - Austin; Sp-Lang Path / Aud, Private Practice, **SLP A**

Shearon, Lynn B 210 St George Street Suite 201, Richmond, KY 40475, (606) 624-1597, BS 66 Univ of KY; ME 82 Univ of VA - Charlottesville; Sp/Lang Path, Private Practice, **SLP ACE**

Shearon, Mrs Mary E 1501 Sierra Drive, Visalia, CA 93291, (209) 732-3206, MS 69 CA St Univ - Long Beach; **SLP**

Shearon, Mrs Nancy P 6908 Russwood Lane, Mabelvale, AR 72103, (501) 888-2313, BS 71 SUNY - Coll at Geneseo; MS 73 CUNY - Coll of Staten Island; MS 81 Univ of AR - Little Rock; Sp-Lang Path, Private Practice, **SLP**

Shebesta, Mrs Jann K 283 East Miramar, Claremont, CA 91711, **SLP**

Shebly, Sharon K 11639 23rd Avenue S W, Seattle, WA 98146, (206) 339-4335, BA 75 Univ of WA; OM 76 Univ of WA; SLP, Everett Sch Dist, **SLP**

Sheckman, Iris Ettelman 11400 S W 82nd Terrace, Miami, FL 33173, (305) 279-6725, OB 73 Univ of Miami; ME 74 Univ of Miami; Sp-Lang Path, Dade Co Pub Sch, **SLP**

Shediac, Mrs Julie M Speech And Hearing Department, Yarmouth Regional Hospital, Yarmouth, NS, Canada B5A 2P5, (902) 742-3541, BA 68 Mercy Coll of Detroit; MA 72 Ball St Univ; Sp-Lang Path, Wn Reg Hlth Cen, **SLP**

Sheehan, Charlene Cox 684 Lock E Road, Cadiz, KY 42211, (502) 924-5510, BS 79 Murray St Univ; MS 86 Murray St Univ; 83–Sp-Lang Path, Trigg County Schs, **SLP**

Sheehan, Eileen Marie 3372 Coolidge Highway #072, Royal Oak, MI 48072-2854, (313) 474-0390, BS 84 Western MI Univ; MA 86 1998; **SLP**

Sheehan, Mrs Kimberly Jowers P O Box 1553, Ruston, LA 71270, (318) 251-2205, BS 82 LA Tech Univ; MA 83 LA Tech Univ; Sp-Lang Path, Bienville Parish Sch Bd, **SLP**

Sheehan, Linda S 14 Forest View Way, Ormond Beach, FL 32074, (904) 677-4392, BA 69 Muhlenberg Coll; Sp-Lang Path, Easter Seals, **SLP**

Sheehan, Dr Marian 602 36th Avenue, Seattle, WA 98122, (206) 323-8126, BA 74 Univ of MN - Minneap-St Paul; MA 78 Univ of MN - Minneap-St Paul; PH 81 (Communication Disorders) Univ of MN - Minneap-St Paul; 87–Sp/Lang Path, Childrens Hospital & Med Ctr, **SLP**

Sheehan, Mary T 510 South Extension, Apartment 2033, Mesa, AZ 85210, (602) 962-0780, BS 81 Univ of AZ; MS 83 Univ of AZ; SLP, Highland Park School District, **SLP**

Sheehan, Vivian Mowat 416 21st Place, Santa Monica, CA 90402, (213) 393-2382, BA 38 Adrian Coll; MA 42 Univ of MI - Ann Arbor; Sp-Lang Path, Private Practice, **SLP F**

Sheehy, Bruce Frank 733 East Palmaire, Phoenix, AZ 85020, (602) 994-9667, **A**

Sheehy, Judith M 140 West Wood #212, Palatine, IL 60067, (312) 927-1616, **SLP**

Sheehy, Mrs Kathleen 3683 W North Wood Lake Dr, Columbus, IN 47201, (812) 342-6491, BA 72 Univ of WA; MS 75 AZ St Univ; Sp-Lang Path, Bartholomew Cty Hospital, **SLP**

Sheehy, Loretta M 1467 Birch Road, Homewood, IL 60430, (312) 868-1870, BA 73 Saint Xavier Coll; MS 79 Governors St Univ; Sp/Lang Path, S Dist #149, **SLP**

Sheeks, Debra Sue 21131 Chubasco Lane, Huntington Beach, CA 92646, (714) 667-3397, BA 84 Chapman Coll; MS 85 Univ of Redlands; **SLP**

Sheeler, Betty Ward 604 Hundred Oaks, Ruston, LA 71270, (318) 255-7041, BA 70 Univ of AR - Little Rock; MA 72 Memphis St Univ; Asst Prof, Louisiana Tech Univ, **SLP**

Sheeley, Mrs Elizabeth Ann 110 Gray Rock Drive, Rome, GA 30161, (404) 235-5847, OB 81 Baylor Univ; MS 83 TX Christian Univ; Sp-Lang Path, Floyd Co Bd of Educ, **SLP**

Sheeley, Dr Eugene C University Of Alabama, PO Box 870242, Tuscaloosa, AL 35487, (205) 348-7131, BA 54 Heidelberg Coll; MA 55 Case Western Reserve Univ; PH 64 (Aud) Univ of Pittsburgh - Pittsburgh; Prof, U of AL, **A**

Sheese, Mrs Rebecca J 12837 Framingham Court, Herndon, VA 22071, (703) 860-3500, BA 72 CA St Univ - Fresno; MA 75 Trenton St Coll; 80–Sp-Lang Path, Fairfax Co Pub Sch, **SLP**

Sheetreet, Mrs Pamela B 5527 Oakwood Avenue, Montreal, PQ, Canada H4W 2A8, (514) 482-9579, BA 78; MS 80 McGill Univ - Quebec; 86–Sp-Lang Path, Montreal Neurological Hosp

Sheets, Mrs Cheryl C 2140 Prather Drive, Nancy, KY 42544, (606) 636-6960, BS 67 OH St Univ; MA 79 Western KY Univ; 87–Sp/Lang Path, Pulaski County Schs, **SLP ACE**

Sheets, Gregory B Yakima Valley Hrng & Sp Center, 303 South 12th Avenue, Yakima, WA 98902, (509) 453-8248, BS 78 AZ St Univ; MS 80 AZ St Univ; Director of Audiology, Yakima Valley Hrng & Spch Cen, **A**

Sheets, Mrs Loretta W 6710 Marcia Lane, Lincoln, NE 68505, (402) 466-9040, BS 61 KS St Univ; MA 64 Univ of KS; Sp-Lang Path, Lincoln Pub Sch, **SLP**

Sheets, Mrs Pamela M 3410 West Country Club, Apartment 291, Irving, TX 75038, (214) 255-3304, MA 87 OH St Univ

Sheff, Martha I 4986 Esplanade Street, Bonita Springs, FL 33923, (813) 261-4592, MS 77 Univ of South FL; Sp-Lang Path, Rehabilitation Associates Inc, **SLP**

Shefferman, Ileen S 6460 Madison Court, Mc Lean, VA 22101, (703) 821-3261, BA 62 Univ of MD - College Park; MA 79 Antioch Coll; Instructional Aide, Fairfax Co Pub Sch, **SLP**

Sheffey, Ronald Carl 188 Forrest Retreat, Hendersonville, TN 37075, (615) 327-1500, BS 75 East TN St Univ; MA 77 East TN St Univ; Aud, US Hearing Centers Inc, **SLP**

Sheffield, Leslie Elaine 501 Brettonwood Drive #308, Knoxville, TN 37919, (615) 691-2225, BA 78 Univ of TN - Knoxville; BS 78 Univ of TN - Knoxville; MA 86 Univ of TN - Knoxville; **SLP**

Sheffield, Mrs Priscilla Jo 10 Aladdin, Lumberton, TX 77656, (409) 755-2724, BS 75 Stephen F Austin St Univ; MS 77 Lamar Univ; 84–Sp/Lang Path, Hardin Jefferson ISD, **SLP**

Shefield, Cynthia N 721 Cobblestone, Shreveport, LA 71106, (318) 424-8263, BA 71 Northwestern St Univ; MA 82 LA St Univ - Shreveport; Tchr, Caddo Parish Sch, **SLP**

Shehabi, Mrs Pamela Lou 14 Timothy Lane, Battle Creek, MI 49015, (616) 964-9426, BS 80 Central MI Univ; MS 82 IL St Univ - Normal; Sp-Lang Path, Doris Klaussen Dev Ctr, **SLP**

Sheiffele, Wendy Ann 531 Empire Avenue, North Babylon, NY 11704, (516) 673-1624, BS 81 Ithaca Coll; MA 83 Hofstra Univ; Sp-Lang Path, Cold Spring Harbor Schs, **SLP**

Sheil, Mrs Francine Fister 3120 Miles Avenue N W, Canton, OH 44718, (216) 478-5155, BS 80 WV Univ; MS 81 WV Univ; Aud, Rosedale & Pickett Mds Inc, **A**

Sheimo, Mrs Diane L Route 6, Fond Du Lac, WI 54935, (414) 922-7725, BS 70 Winston-Salem St Univ; MS 87 Univ of WI - Oshkosh; 87–Sp-Lang Path, Therapy and Support Svcs Inc, **SLP**

Shekim, Dr Lana O George Washington University Medical Center, Speech Pathology & Audiology Service, 901 23rd Street NW, Washington, DC 20037, (202) 994-3631, BA 75 Univ of MO - Columbia; MA 76 Univ of MO - Columbia; PH 83 (NS) Univ of FL; Sp-Lang Path, George Washington Univ Med Ctr, **SLP ACE**

Shelby, Ronald J 6550 1st Avenue North, St Petersburg, FL 33710, (813) 343-2180, BA 65 2322; MA 71 Univ of OK - Norman; PH 85 (NS) Walden Univ; Cl Dir, A Speech Hrng & Stress Cl, **SLP A**

Shelby, Theresa M 719 South Pantano Parkway, Tucson, AZ 85710, (602) 748-1356, BS 72 Bowling Green St Univ; MA 73 Bowling Green St Univ; SLP, Tucson USD, **SLP**

Shelby, Mrs Tracie Lathram 2210 Turf Club Drive, Arlington, TX 76107, (817) 467-5838, BS 84 Baylor Univ; MS 85 Baylor Univ; Sp-Lang Path, Arlington ISD, **SLP**

Sheldon, Mrs Alexis H 14121 Picasso Court, Irvine, CA 92714, (714) 558 5591, BS 78 Univ of HI - Manoa; MS 79 Univ of HI - Manoa; 87–Sp-Lang Path, Santa Ana USD, **SLP**

Sheldon, Mrs Dorothy L 1403 Maplewood Court, De Witt, IA 52742, (319) 242-6454, BA 76 Univ of Northern IA; MA 77 Univ of Northern IA; Sp-Lang Path, Mississippi Bend AEA 9, **SLP**

Sheldon, Dr Neil Director Sp & Hrng Program, CW Post Center, Long Island University, Greenvale, NY 11548, (516) 299-2436, BA 52 Carnegie-Mellon Univ; MA 59 NY Univ; PH 63 (NS) NY Univ; Assoc Prof/Prog Dir, Lng Isl U-CW Post, **SLP F**

Sheldon, Sandra M 3925-H Valley Court, Sherwood West, Winston-Salem, NC 27106, (919) 727-2343, BS 70 East Carolina Univ; ME 71 East Carolina Univ; Sp-Lang Path, W-S Forsyth Co Sch, **SLP**

Sheldon, Shelly A 25043 Summit Creek, San Antonio, TX 78258, (512) 655-3021, BS 78 Southern Methodist Univ; ME 79 Southwest TX St Univ; Sp-Lang Path, NE ISD, **SLP**

Shelfer, Janet S 1708 Riggins Road, Tallahassee, FL 32308, (904) 878-7228, BS 75 FL St Univ; MS 76 FL St Univ; Aud, Aud Rehab Lab Inc, **A**

Sheline, Linda M 834 North Harlem Avenue, River Forest, IL 60305, (312) 366-6692, BA 79 MI St Univ; MA 80 Western MI Univ; Sp-Lang Path Dir, Westlake Comm Hosp, **SLP**

Shell, Mrs Claire L F 1809 Hobkirk Court, Camden, SC 29020, (803) 425-5305, BA 78 Columbia Coll; MA 79 Univ of SC - Columbia; **SLP**

Shell, Mrs Melanie Peacock Shell Comm Disorders Center, 2535 Lafayette Plaza Drive, Suite C, Albany, GA 31707, (912) 435-1313, BS 79 Univ of GA; ME 80 Univ of GA; Sp-Lang Path, Private Practice, **SLP**

Shell, Shirley J 31315 West Rutland, Birmingham, MI 48009, BS 63 Wayne St Univ; **SLP**

Shellenberger, Sharon L T 1542 Monmouth Drive, San Diego, CA 92109, (619) 221-6000, BA 78 San Diego St Univ; MA 81 San Diego St Univ; Sp-Lang Path, Kaiser Permanente, **SLP**

Shelley, Mrs Erin E 2811 Warford, Perry, IA 50220, (515) 465-2984, MA 86 Western IL Univ; **SLP**

Shelley, Mrs Gina Lee 8 Shadow Lane, St Peters, MO 63376, (314) 441-3035, BS 83 Southeast MO St Univ; MA 84 Southeast MO St Univ; Sp-Lang Path, Assoc Rehab Services, Inc, **SLP**

Shelley, Suzanne Rosenast 51 Munson Court, Melville, NY 11747, (516) 789-7342, BA 84 Adelphi Univ; MS 85 Adelphi Univ; 86–Sp-Lang Path, Brunswick Hosp Ctr Inc, **SLP**

Shellner, Mrs Jacqueline 1210 Park Lane, Brandenburg, KY 40108, (502) 422-4931, OB 70 Univ of Miami; MS 73 Vanderbilt Univ; 76–Sp/Lang Path, Meade Co Bd of Ed, **SLP**

Shelor, Mrs Joan White 1050 White Oak Lane, Christiansburg, VA 24073, (703) 382-4559, BS 83 Radford Univ; MS 87 Radford Univ; **SLP**

Shelquist, Darleen M 78 River Woods Lane, Burnsville, MN 55337, (612) 890-0034, BS 73 Univ of ND; MA 78 WA St Univ; 78–SLP, ISD 196, **SLP**

Shelton, Mrs Carole W San Francisco Hrng & Sp Center, 1234 Divisadero Street, San Francisco, CA 94115, (415) 921-7658, BA 66 Univ of AR - Fayetteville; MA 64 Temple Univ-Tyler Sch of Art; Aud, San Francisco Hrng & Sp Cen, **A**

Shelton, Dale Sandusky 1010 South Main Street, Somerville, TN 38068, (901) 465-9861, BS 75 Baylor Univ; MA 77 Memphis St Univ; Sp/Lang Path, Professional Health Services, **SLP**

Shelton, Mrs Diane Welsh 9930 Bella Marche Drive, Charlotte, NC 28212, BA 84 Univ of NC - Chapel Hill; MA 85 Univ of NC - Chapel Hill; SLP, Charlotte-Mecklenburg Schools, **SLP ACE**

Shelton, Dr Doris H 1330 Doyal Drive, Morristown, TN 37814, (615) 639-2131, BA 64 East TN St Univ; MA 65 Univ of TN - Knoxville; PH 76 (NS) Univ of TN - Knoxville; Dir Sp & Hrng Dept, Greene Valley Dev Cen, **SLP**

Shelton, Ivy L 1332 Union City Road, Richmond, KY 40475, BS 77 Univ of WI - Eau Claire; ME 79 Univ of WI - LA Crosse; MS 83 Univ of WI - Eau Claire; Sp-Lang Path, Private Practice, **SLP**

Shelton, Dr June Ford 628 Mimosa, Denton, TX 76201, (214) 357-4714, BS 58 Univ of OK - Norman; PH 65 (NS) Univ of OK - Norman; Exec Dir Emeritus, Shelton Sch & Evolution Cen, **SLP**

Shelton, Mrs Kathleen Mary 4505 Carrie Circle, Lexington, KY 40503, (606) 272-2412, BA 79 Univ of KY; MS 85 Univ of KY; 87–Sp-Lang Path, Jessamine Co Bd of Educ, **SLP**

Shelton, Mrs Lesa L Gray ACRE Center Incorporated, 18 Loudoun Street S E, Leesburg, VA 22075, (703) 777-8181, BS 79 James Madison Univ; MS 80 James Madison Univ; Director, Acre Center Inc, **SLP**

Shelton, Madelyn L Box 313, Clay, WV 25043, (304) 587-4266, BS 55 Univ of Charleston; MS 66 WV Univ; Retired, Clay Co Sch, **SLP LM**

Shelton, Maura Vaughn 5391 Pecan Grove Lane, Memphis, TN 38119, (901) 683-8010, **SLP**

Shelton, Dr Ralph L, Jr University Of Arizona, Speech Bldg, Tucson, AZ 85721, (602) 621-1489, BS 52 Univ of UT; MS 56 Univ of UT; PH 59 (Sp Path) Univ of UT; Prof, U of AZ, **SLP F**

Shelton, Shirlene Matthews 15411 Pond Woods Drive W, Tampa, FL 33618, (801) 752-1811, BS 69 UT St Univ; MS 71 UT St Univ; Professional Associate, InSpeech Inc, **SLP**

Shelton, Mrs Susan N 4445 Denver Drive, Plano, TX 75075, (214) 596-0009, BS 75 Univ of TX - Austin; MA 78 Univ of TX - Austin; Sp-Lang Path, Galand ISD, **SLP**

Shelton, Mrs Vicki Diane 122 Jackson Place #1-B, Martinsburg, WV 25401, (304) 229-5757, BS 84 WV Univ; MS 85 WV Univ; **SLP**

Shendge, Mrs Valerie Carroll P O Box 358, Scottdale, PA 15683, (412) 941-4434, BS 84 Indiana Univ of PA; MS 86 James Madison Univ; 87–Sp-Lang Path, Crossroads Sp & Hrng Inc

Shenesky, Della Butcher 213 Emerson Drive, Zelienople, PA 16063, (412) 728-3730, MA 70 Bowling Green St Univ; BA 68 Geneva Coll; Sp-Lang Path, Beaver Valley ISD 27, **SLP**

Shenk, Amy L 4 Matthew Drive, Littleton, MA 01460, (508) 937-6403, BA 71 SUNY - Center at Buffalo; MA 73 Univ of MA - Amherst; Sp-Lang Path, Lowell Gen Hosp, **SLP**

Shenk, Kalomyra C 1151 East 5730 South, Salt Lake City, UT 84121, (801) 967-0310, BS 80 Univ of WY; MS 82 Univ of WY; Sp/Lang Path, Primary Childrens Med Cen, **SLP**

Shenker, Mrs Basi Krasnow 1006 Neilson Street #30, Far Rockaway, NY 11691, (718) 498-2500, BS 85 CUNY - Queens Coll; MS 87 CUNY - Brooklyn Coll

Shenker, Joan Buchman 17 Valley Road, Kinnelon, NJ 07405, (201) 956-1200, MA 85 OH Univ - Athens; **A**

Shenkler, Mrs Barbara Effron 3 Cherry Hill Court, Hillsdale, NJ 07642, (201) 684-2445, BS 71 OH Univ - Athens; MA 72 OH Univ - Athens; Sp-Lang Path, Private Practice, **SLP**

Shenuski, Doris Marie 2916 California Street N E, Albuquerque, NM 87110, (505) 881-4670, BA 80 Univ of NM; MS 83 Univ of NM; **SLP**

Shepard, Carole Spolar 9061 Pine Heights Place, Pittsburgh, PA 15237, (412) 856-2400, BS 78 Northwestern Univ; MS 80 PA St Univ - Univ Park; 88–Prog Dir-Head Injury Prog, Greater Pittsburgh Rehab Hosp, **SLP**

Shepard, Dale R 4 Station Lane, Philadelphia, PA 19118-2939, (215) 750-2226, SLP, St Mary Hosp, **SLP**

Shepard, Janice Tucker 3319 Laurel Lane, Hazel Crest, IL 60429, (312) 723-8969, **SLP**

Shepard, Linda J 5611K Hornaday Road, Greensboro, NC 27409, BS 78 East Carolina Univ; MS 81 East Carolina Univ; SLP, Guilford County Dept Pub Hlth, **SLP**

Shepard, Dr Neil T 5425 Salburg Court, Ann Arbor, MI 48103, BS 72 Univ of KY; MS 74 MA Inst of Tech; PH 79 (NS) Univ of IA; Dir-Vestibular Testing Ctr, Dept of ENT-Univ of MI Hosp, **A**

Shepard, Shari Ann RR 1 Box 1355, Poestenkill, NY 12140, (518) 274-3684, BA 83 SUNY - Coll at Plattsburgh; MA 84 SUNY - Coll at Plattsburgh; Sp-Lang Path, Pinewoods Center, **SLP**

Shephard, Mrs Cheryl Lynn 599 Georgia Road, Otto, NC 28763, (704) 369-7599, BA 76 Wayne St Univ; MA 77 Wayne St Univ; Administrator, Smoky Mountain Comp Hlth Care, **SLP**

Shepherd, Carrie Lynn 2100 Broadway, Hannibal, MO 63401-3103, (314) 221-6002, BS 84 Western IL Univ; MA 85 Western IL Univ; 87–Sp-Lang Path, Hannibal Regional Ctr, **SLP**

Shepherd, Mrs Cynthia Skurner 6126 Aragon Drive, Fort Wayne, IN 46818, (219) 489-2001, BS 80 Ball St Univ; MA 84 Ball St Univ; Sp-Lang Path, Smith-Green Comm Schs, **SLP**

Shepherd, Dr David C 1013 Silver Palm Way, Sabal Key, Apollo Beach, FL 33570, PH (NS); **A F**

Shepherd, Janet C 11111 East Cortez Street, Scottsdale, AZ 85259, (602) 285-3473, MA 71 Univ of IL - Urbana; 88–Sp-Lang Path, St Joseph Hosp, **SLP**

Shepherd, Mrs Jennifer Felts 535 S Mesa Hills Drive, El Paso, TX 79912, (915) 544-8484, BA 86 IN Univ - Bloomington; MA 87 Western IL Univ

Shepherd, Mrs Laurie Barr 154 Barcelona Avenue, Westerville, OH 43081, (614) 794-0864, BS 81 Ball St Univ; MA 82 Ball St Univ; Sp-Lang Path, **SLP**

Shepherd, Suzanne C 151 N Michigan Avenue #2007, Chicago, IL 60601, (312) 782-9153, BA 64 MI St Univ; MA 65 MI St Univ; Manager, Dr Dane Shepherd, **SLP**

Sheppard, Angela Dawn 1001 Ewell Road, Virginia Beach, VA 23455, (804) 481-4003, BS 86 Radford Univ; MS 87 Radford Univ; 87–Aud, Virginia Audiology Associates, **A**

Sheppard, Douglas R 5201 V Street, Sacramento, CA 95817, **SLP**

Sheppard, Dr Justine Joan 111 Chincopee Road, Lake Hopatcong, NJ 07849, (201) 663-3630, BA 59 NY Univ; MA 64 Columbia Univ Teachers Coll; PH 79 (NS) Columbia Univ Teachers Coll; 68–Consult Sp-Lang Path, Private Practice, **SLP ACE**

Sheppard, Sr Mary F 61-16 Maspeth Avenue, Maspeth, NY 11378, (212) 492-1800, BA 63 Brentwood Coll; MA 70 CUNY - Hunter Coll; MS 77 Adelphi Univ; 88–Sp/Lang Path, Brooklyn Diocesan Offi, **SLP**

Sheppard, Shirley Jean 8730 Raven Oaks Drive, Omaha, NE 68152, (402) 978-7078, BA 81 Univ of Northern IA; MA 83 Univ of Northern IA; Sp-Lang Path, Omaha Public Schools, **SLP**

Sheppard, Susan Elizabeth 6510 Brint Road #301, Sylvania, OH 43560, (800) 331-3058, BA 84 OH St Univ; ME 86 Univ of VA - Charlottesville; SLP, Aprn, **SLP**

Sheppard, Susan Saynt 1360 77th Street North, St Petersburg, FL 33710, (813) 868-6800, BS 75 Univ of Montevallo; MS 76 Univ of Montevallo; Dir Comm Dis, Bayfront Med Ctr, **SLP**

Sheppard-Nene, Karen 412 Walnut Street, Erie, PA 16507, (814) 734-5610, BS 80 Edinboro Univ of PA; MA 84 Edinboro Univ of PA; SLP, NE Tri-Co Iu #5, **SLP**

Shepro, Wendy J 6-4 Christopher Drive, Easton, MA 02375, (617) 238-8472, BA 83 Clark Univ; MA 86 Univ of MA - Amherst; SLP, The Neurologic Center, **SLP**

Sher, Diane Davis 8011 Berger Place, Playa Del Rey, CA 90293, (213) 823-7316, BA CA St Univ - Los Angeles; MA CA St Univ - Los Angeles; **SLP**

Sheran, Christina Pietro 35 University Court, Viking Terrace, Mankato, MN 56001, (507) 387-1364, BS 75 Creighton Univ; MS 77 Mankato St Univ; Instr/Cl Superv, Commun Dis Dept/Mankato Stu, **SLP**

Sherbecoe, Robert L Memphis Speech And Hearing Center, 807 Jefferson Avenue, Memphis, TN 38105, (901) 525-2682, BS 78 Davidson Coll; MA 83 Memphis St Univ; 82–Research Assist, Memphis St U

Sherbin, Charles S 624 Main Road, Hanover Green, Wilkes-Barre, PA 18702, (717) 829-2244, BS 69 Bloomsburg Univ of PA; ME 71 Bloomsburg Univ of PA; Sp-Lang Path, Luzerne Inter Ut #18, **SLP**

Sherbin, Mrs Lillian K 30875 Lincolnshire East, Birmingham, MI 48010, (313) 832-6400, BA 71 Wayne St Univ; MS 73 Wayne St Univ; SLP, Detroit Pub Sch, **SLP**

Sherick-Bennett, Dana 50384 Barcus Circle, Coarsegold, CA 93614, (209) 673-6051, BA 78 CA St Univ - Chico; MA 81 CA St Univ - Stanislaus; SLP, Madera Co Dept of Ed, **SLP**

Sheridan, Mrs Amelia P 10739 Northgate Avenue, Culver City, CA 90230, (213) 836-3889, BA 70 Adelphi Univ; MA 71 Hofstra Univ; SLP, Private Practice, **SLP**

Sheridan, Anne P 7900 Keswick Drive, Austin, TX 78745-5954, (512) 448-3221, BS 82 Southwest TX St Univ; MS 83 Univ of North TX; Sp-Lang Path, Del Valle Integrated Sch Dist, **SLP**

Sheridan, Catherine 14000 Burning Bush Lane, Silver Spring, MD 20906, (301) 871-3768, BA 80 Harding Univ; MS 84 Nazareth Coll of Rochester; 88–Research Assoc, Power Intl Inc, **SLP**

Sheridan, Mrs Joanne M A 719 Fairview Avenue, Westbury, NY 11590-4933, BA 78 Saint John's Univ - Jamaica; MA 79 Hofstra Univ; Sp-Lang Path, Levittown Union Free Sch Dist, **SLP**

Sheridan, Mrs Maria G 121-57 237th Street, Rosedale, NY 11422, BA 42 CUNY - Hunter Coll; MA 45 Columbia Univ Teachers Coll; **SLP**

Sheridan, Patricia A 559 Laurel Road, Ridgewood, NJ 07450, (201) 444-6084, BA 76 William Paterson Coll; MS 80 William Paterson Coll; Sp-Lang Path, Region I-Presch Spec Prog, **SLP**

Sheridan, Patricia E 22 Brookwood Drive, South Burlington, VT 05403, (802) 482-2106, BA 70 Regis Coll; MS 82 Univ of VT; 82–SLP, Chittenden South Sch Dist, **SLP ACE**

Sheridan, Susan M 3566 Val Verde Avenue, Long Beach, CA 90808, (213) 430-5851, BS 66 Marquette Univ; ME 78 Northeastern Univ; 86–Sp-Lang Path, LA Cty Ofc of Educ, **SLP**

Sheridan-Schell, Patricia Louise 8237 Jordan Road, Melvin, MI 48454, (517) 635-7425, BS 77 Central MI Univ; MA 82 Central MI Univ; 78–Sp-Lang Path, Marlette Community Schools, **SLP**

Sherin, Krista 414 Pearl Street, Sparta, WI 54656, **SLP**

Sherman, Ann Cheryl 169 Portsmouth St #111, Concord, NH 03301, (603) 623-8863, BS 83 FL St Univ; MS 87 Univ of South FL; **SLP**

Sherman, Arleen Abzug 15 Lake Shore Drive, Watervliet, NY 12189, BA 60 CUNY - Hunter Coll; MA 71 CUNY - Hunter Coll; Sp-Lang Path, Wildwood School, **SLP**

Sherman, Barbara C RFD 4 Box 266, Pelham, NH 03076, BA 69 Brown Univ; MS 75 Boston Univ; Sp-Lang Path, Dracut Pub Sch, **SLP**

Sherman, Mrs Bernadette G J11 Shirley Lane, Lawrenceville, NJ 08648, (201) 725-4000, BA 80 SUNY - Coll at Fredonia; MS 82 Purdue Univ - West Lafayette; Sp-Lang Path, Drs Woods Blake & Witter, **SLP**

Sherman, Cynthia Jean 1942 Deepark Drive #54, Fullerton, CA 92631, (714) 524-1581, BA 82 CA St Univ - Long Beach; MA 84 CA St Univ - Los Angeles; Aud, Long Beach Naval Hosp, **A**

Sherman, Deborah Murtaugh 345 East 86th Street #15F, New York, NY 10128, (212) 722-8034, BA 73 Hofstra Univ; MS 74 Columbia Univ Teachers Coll; Tchr, E Meadow Sch Dist, **SLP**

Sherman, Debra Lynne 26 Starhauen Avenue, Middletown, NY 10940, (914) 634-4648, BA 85 SUNY - Coll at Cortland; MA 87 SUNY - Center at Buffalo; **A**

Sherman, Dr Dorothy 4 Oak Park Court, Iowa City, IA 52246, (319) 337-4516, BA 31 Univ of IA; MA 38 Univ of IA; PH 51 (Sp Path/Aud) Univ of IA; Prof Emeritus, U of IA, **SLP F H LM**

Sherman, Eileen R 5819 Norththumberland Str, Pittsburgh, PA 15217, (412) 422-0710, BA 74 Univ of Pittsburgh - Pittsburgh; MS 75 Bradley Univ; Sp-Lang Path/Consult, Private Practice, **SLP**

Sherman, Ellen Sue 730 Terrill Road, Plainfield, NJ 07061, (201) 755-3933, BA 79 Miami Univ - Oxford; MA 85 Kean Coll of NJ; 86–Sp-Lang Path, St Barnabas Med Ctr, **SLP**

Sherman, Janine Buehling 3609 Gillham, Alton, IL 62002, (618) 465-0105, **SLP**

Sherman, Kathie J 21 Channing Road, Watertown, MA 02172, (617) 924-6025, BS 76 Eastern NM Univ; MS 85 Univ of NM; **SLP**

Sherman, Mrs Leann A 5757 Terrace, Rocklin, CA 95677, (815) 223-2036, BS 76 Univ of North TX; MS 78 Univ of North TX; **SLP**

Sherman, Mrs Lorene H 649 Hanford Place, Westfield, NJ 07090, (201) 233-3720, BA 60 Univ of MD - College Park; MA 78 Kean Coll of NJ; 88–Sp-Lang Path, Private Practice, **SLP**

Sherman, Mrs Lynn W 3200 Broadway Suite 190, Garland, TX 75043, (214) 278-9685, BS 54 Northwestern Univ; MA 55 Northwestern Univ; Sp-Lang Path, Private Practice, **SLP**

Sherman, Patricia M 790 Gilbert Stuart Road, Saunderstown, RI 02874, (401) 277-5485, BA 72 Univ of RI; MS 75 Univ of RI; 79–Aud, Ri Hosp-Hrng/Sp Cen, **A**

Sherman, Dr Randi S 14 Bayberry Lane, Rye Brook, NY 10573, (914) 337-0018, BA 69 CUNY - Queens Coll; MA 72 2780; PH 85 (NS) Columbia Univ Teachers Coll; Director of Audiology, Montefiore Med Ctr, **A**

Sherman, Roslyn S 107 Fitz Court #104, Reisterstown, MD 21136, (301) 282-7173, BA 83 Univ of MD - College Park; MS 86 Towson St Univ; Aud, Hearing Lab, **A**

Sherman, Mrs Saundy C 1006 Red Cliff Drive, Austin, TX 78758, (512) 478-2581, BS 69 Univ of TX - Austin; MA 71 Univ of TX - Austin; Sp/Lang Path, Capital Area Rehab Cent, **SLP**

Sherman, Sura J 17 Plugat Hakotel, Old City Jewish Quarter, Jerusalem, Israel 97500, (02) 280-068, BA 84 CUNY - Queens Coll; MA 88 CUNY - Queens Coll; 88–Sp-Lang Path, Israeli Govt Sch Sys, **SLP**

Sherman, Susan L 11645 Chispa Creek Drive, Corpus Christi, TX 78410, (512) 241-6915, BS 78 Hardin-Simmons Univ; MS 81 Univ of WY; **SLP**

Sherman, Susan L 8310 Hamlin, Skokie, IL 60076, (312) 824-4375, BS 81 Univ of IL - Urbana; MS 83 Washington Univ; Aud, Audiological Laboratory Ltd, **A**

Sherman-Proehl, Dr Laurabelle 5324 Jennifer Drive, Pleasant Hill, IA 50317, (515) 265-7536, BS 79 Northwest MO St Univ; MS 81 Northwest MO St Univ; PH 87 (Sp-Lang Path Phonological disorders and clinical supervision) Univ of KS; 87–Sp-Lang Path, Des Moines PS, **SLP**

Sheroff, Rita J 8280 Sunrise Lakes Blvd, Apartment 312, Sunrise, FL 33322, (305) 749-1083, BA 76 CUNY - Queens Coll; ME 78 Northeastern Univ; Sp-Lang Path, Sunrise Hospital, **SLP**

Sherrard, Mrs Kyla C 101 Winston Circle, Ozark, AL 36360-1157, (205) 774-9033, BA 76 Baylor Univ; MS 77 Baylor Univ; Sp-Lang Path, Dothan City Schs, **SLP**

Sherrets, Mrs Trish Anne 12742 Cryer Avenue, Omaha, NE 68144-2608, (402) 333-1344, BS 73 Univ of NE - Omaha; MS 82 Univ of NE - Omaha; Sp-Lang Path, Millard Public Schools, **SLP**

Sherretta, Mrs Carrie Hirschhorn 73 Rossmore Avenue, Bronxville, NY 10708, (914) 337-6544, BS 77 PA St Univ - Univ Park; MA 87 NY Univ; 88–Sp-Lang Path, Alcott Preschool, **SLP**

Sherrill, Dr Donald D Lincoln Public Schools Dist #1, P O Box 82889, Lincoln, NE 68501, (402) 475-1081, BA 54 Kearney St Coll; MA 58 Univ of NE - Lincoln; ED 66 (NS) Univ of NE - Lincoln; Dir/Spec Ed, Lincoln Pub Schs Dist #1, **SLP**

Sherrill, Mrs Vonnie K 623 Antietam Drive, Stone Mountain, GA 30087, (404) 879-0072, BS 79 Univ of GA; ME 81 Univ of GA; Sp-Lang Path, Decatur County Schools, **SLP**

Sherrin, Mrs Janet R 731 Norfolk Lane, Langhorne, PA 19047, (215) 364-0161, BS 78 Boston Univ; MA 79 NY Univ; Sp-Lang Path, SPIN, **SLP**

Sherris, Capt Cari Ann 5315 Gawain #1422, San Antonio, TX 78218, (512) 536-2909, BA 72 Concord Coll; ME 76 Univ of NC - Greensboro; ME 79 Univ of MD - College Park; Aud, US Air Force, **SLP A**

Sherrod, Barbara W 8 Loch Haven, St Louis, MO 63011, **SLP**

Sherrod, Mrs Lynn R 2811 Steven Drive, Johnson City, TN 37604, (615) 928-1821, BS 73 East TN St Univ; MA 74 Univ of TN - Knoxville; Sp-Lang Path, Private Practice, **SLP**

Sherry, Linda W 1370 Sheldon, St Paul, MN 55108, (612) 770-4750, BS 75 Univ of MI - Ann Arbor; MS 77 Univ of WI - Madison; SLP, School District 622, **SLP**

Sherry, Mrs Melinda Lewis Columbus Speech & Hearing Ctr, 4110 North High Street, Columbus, OH 43214, (614) 294-6403, BS 77 Kent St Univ; MA 79 Kent St Univ; 88–Exec Dir, Columbus Speech & Hearing Ctr, **SLP**

Shervanian, Anna Ethel 130 Nutmeg Lane #314, East Hartford, CT 06118, (203) 569-7113, BS 60 Boston Univ; **SLP**

Shervanian, Chris C 5500 North St Louis Avenue, Chicago, IL 60625, (312) 583-4050, BS 49 Boston Univ; MA 51 Northwestern Univ; PH 59 (NS) Univ of Pittsburgh - Pittsburgh; Prof/Psych & SLP, Northeaster Il U, **SLP F**

Shervin, Mrs Cheri Jeannette 5538 Hawthorne Place N W, Washington, DC 20016, (202) 466-8579, BA 82 VA Polytechnic Inst St Univ; MA 86 Univ of MD - College Park; Aud, Dr Feldman-Hausfeld, **A**

Sherwood, Dr Karen Heerse 9030 Midland Trail Drive, Apartment C-14, Ashland, KY 41101, BA 80; MA 82 Univ of Cincinnati; PH 84 (NS) Univ of Cincinnati; 86–Aud, Our Lady of Bellefonte Hosp, **A**

Sherwood, Patricia 805-C6 West Aaron Drive, State College, PA 16803, (814) 231-0933, BA 79 Adelphi Univ; MS 80 Adelphi Univ; 88–Clin Supvr/Instr, Penn St Univ, **SLP ACE**

Sheterom, Mrs Helen Ronke 7145 Southmeadow Drive, Painesville, OH 44077, (216) 357-6121, BS 61 Miami Univ - Oxford; MA 65 Kent St Univ; Sp-Lang Path, Painesville Cty Sch, **SLP**

Shetler, Susan K 197 West Lawrence Street, Albany, NY 12203, (518) 438-5604, BS 76 SUNY - Center at Albany; MS 79 Coll of Saint Rose; Sp-Lang Path, **SLP**

Sheviakov, Mrs Carole K 30 Oakwood Avenue, San Anselmo, CA 94960, (415) 499-5807, BS 64 PA St Univ - Univ Park; MA 66 Stanford Univ; Sp-Lang Path, Marin Co Offi of Ed, **SLP**

Shevin-Finck, Eileen Carol 22639 Heatherwood, Novi, MI 48050, (313) 857-7361, BA 75 MI St Univ; MA 79 MI St Univ; **A**

Shevitz, Stephen D 8220 Canning Terrace, Greenbelt, MD 20770, (301) 345-9191, BA 65 Univ of MD - College Park; MA 69 Univ of MD - College Park; Dir/Owner, Communication Associates, **SLP**

Shewan, Dr Cynthia M 12301-201 Village Sq Terr, Rockville, MD 20852, (301) 897-5700, BA 65 McGill Univ - Quebec; MA 67 Northwestern Univ; PH 69 (Sp-Lang Path) Northwestern Univ; Director Research Division, ASHA, **SLP F ACE**

Sheward, Douglas John 3952 Clark, Kansas City, MO 64111, (913) 384-5808, BS 74 Pittsburg St Univ; MA 76 Pittsburg St Univ; MA 86 Univ of KS; 88–Sp-Lang Path, Doug Sheward Speech Svcs, **SLP**

Sheward, Lois Ellen W 1416 Douglas Lane, Anderson, IN 46011, (317) 778-2161, BA 74 Ball St Univ; MA 78 Ball St Univ; Sp-Lang Path, Greenfield Ctrl Serv Ut, **SLP**

Shick, Karen Zamberlan 2330 North Oliver #1211, Wichita, KS 67220, (316) 221-1200, BS 64 Kent St Univ; MA 87 Wichita St Univ; 88–Sp-Lang Path, Winfield St Hosp & Trng Ctr

Shicotte, Cynthia Louise 925 South Washington, Park Ridge, IL 60068, (312) 275-8822, BS 80 Northern IL Univ - De Kalb; MA 81 Northern IL Univ - De Kalb; Asst Dir, Sp-Lang Rehab Cen, **SLP**

Shidlovsky, Cathy M 47 East Street, Claremont, NH 03743, (603) 742-7429, BS 79 Ithaca Coll; MA 80 Bowling Green St Univ; Sp-Lang Path, Valley Regional Hospital, **SLP**

Shiebler, Karen Merullo 38 Endicott Road, Stoneham, MA 02180, (617) 279-1099, BA 78 Univ of MA - Boston; MS 83 Rutgers St Univ -N Brunswick; Sp-Lang Path, Private Practice, **SLP**

Shield, Mrs Lea Anne 1006 East Miami, McAlester, OK 74501, (918) 423-9042, BS 79 OK St Univ; MS 81 Univ of OK Medical Center; Sp-Lang Path, McCurtain Co Guid Cen, **SLP**

Shields, Anne Ruppe 1125 State Street, Lafayette, IN 47905, (317) 494-3789, BS 84 Purdue Univ - West Lafayette; MS 86 Purdue Univ - West Lafayette; Grad, Purdue Univ, **A**

Shields, Mrs Dianne T 43 Williamsburg Road, Evanston, IL 60203, (312) 679-6718, BS 66 Purdue Univ - West Lafayette; MA 67 Northwestern Univ; PH 72 (Learning Disabilities) Northwestern Univ; Ed Spec, Evanston Hosp, **SLP**

Shields, Dorothy D 6477 Knox Road, Norfolk, VA 23513, MS; **SLP LM**

Shields, Mrs Karen F 117 Orchard Ridge, Hillsdale, MI 49242, (517) 537-4055, BS 75 Western MI Univ; MA 77 Eastern MI Univ; SLP, Hillsdale Co ISD, **SLP**

Shields, Lynne W 3218 Portis Avenue, St Louis, MO 63116, (314) 889-1407, BS 75 Univ of IL - Urbana; MA 76 Univ of TN - Knoxville; Asst Prof, Fontbonne Coll, **SLP**

Shields, Mrs Michele K 5 Linda Lane, Schenectady, NY 12309, (518) 370-7336, BA 75 Elmira Coll; MA 76 George Washington Univ; 86–Aud, Oswald D Heck Dev Center, **A**

Shields, Richard W 1296 Tod Place N W, Suite 203, Warren, OH 44485, **SLP**

Shields, Sarah E 502 William Street, Jackson, MS 39209-5145, (601) 948-6620, BS 69 Jackson St Univ; MS 71 Univ of WI - Madison; SLP, MS Action for Progress Inc, **SLP**

Shields, Mrs Susan Sinnamon 3413 Timber Trail, Antioch, TN 37013, (615) 367-2651, BA 80 SUNY - Coll at Plattsburgh; MS 81 TX Christian Univ; 87–Sp-Lang Path, Prospect Child Develop Ctr, **SLP**

Shields-Cole, Mrs Sara L 5496 Hyde Park Blvd #601, Chicago, IL 60615, (312) 413-1486, BS 80 Bradley Univ; MS 81 Bradley Univ; 84–Sp-Lang Path, Il Ins for Dev Dis, **SLP**

Shiffler, Therese Anstead 115 Fremont Street, Caro, MI 48723, (517) 673-7162, BS 83 Central MI Univ; MA 86 Central MI Univ; **SLP**

Shifflett, Martha Ellen 958 Georgetown Street #2, Staunton, VA 24401, (703) 885-9370, BS 77 Old Dominion Univ; ME 81 James Madison Univ; Aud, Div of Behav Med/West St Hosp, **A**

Shiffman, Mrs Elizabeth 144 Thornbush Drive, West Lafayette, IN 47906, (317) 494-3792, MS 61 Purdue Univ - West Lafayette; Sp-Lang Path, Purdue University, **SLP**

Shiffman-Sacks, Susan Lee 22815 Malaga Way, El Toro, CA 92630, (714) 458-9427, BS 83 AZ St Univ; MA 86 CA St Univ - Long Beach; 88–Aud, International Hearing Aids, **A**

Shifman, Suzanne K 1474 Inwoods Circle, Bloomfield Hills, MI 48013, (313) 858-3111, BA 53 Wayne St Univ; MA 73 Wayne St Univ; Aud, Private Practice, **A**

Shifrin, Rosalyn Davis 189 Middlesex Avenue, Iselin, NJ 08830, (201) 725-2828, BS 73 Trenton St Coll; MS 76 Rutger's St Univ - Douglas Coll; Sp-Lang Path, Branchburg Twsp Pub Sch, **SLP**

Shifrin, Susan 9700 Dee Road, Des Plaines, IL 60016, (312) 299-8412, BS 84 Bradley Univ; MA 87 Univ of WI - Madison; **SLP**

Shigemoto, Joan Hamatake 5037 Maunalani Circle, Honolulu, HI 96816, (808) 622-2269, **SLP**

Shikany, Susan Dye 1072 South Roanoke, Springfield, MO 65807, (417) 865-2766, BS 78 Univ of Science & Arts of OK; MA 80 OK St Univ; Sp-Lang Path/Cl Dir, Missouri Crippled Child Serv, **SLP**

Shikiar, Karen A 296 Elliot Street, Newton Upper Falls, MA 02164, (617) 527-6464, BS 83 Ithaca Coll; MS 85 Emerson Coll; **SLP**

Shikowitz, Mrs Sheila Marilyn 9 Mount Rainier Avenue, Farmingville, NY 11738, (516) 698-1242, MS 73 CUNY - Brooklyn Coll; Sp-Lang Path, Contemporary Sp & Lang Service, **SLP**

Shiland, Mrs Sybil B Box 252 Lower Main Street, Cornish, ME 04020, (207) 642-2480, BA 74 SUNY - Coll at Plattsburgh; MA 77 SUNY - Center at Buffalo; Sp-Lang Path, ME Sch Admin Dist #6, **SLP**

Shilling, Mrs Noel Sue 467 Village Drive East, Carmel, IN 46032, (317) 353-5429, BS 72 Indiana Univ of PA; MA 74 Kent St Univ; 86–Dir/Aud & Sp, Commun Hosp of Indpls, **SLP**

Shilling, Samuel P 443 East Butler Street, Mercer, PA 16137, (412) 376-7911, BS 53 PA St Univ - Univ Park; MS 54 PA St Univ - Univ Park; Sp-Path, Mid Wn Iu, **SLP A**

Shillingburg, Mrs Nancy Freese 2619 N W Roanoke Street, Portland, OR 97210, (503) 222-5465, **SLP**

Shimek, Mrs Barbara B Rural Delivery 3 Box 291, Conneautville, PA 16406, (814) 587-2984, BS 60 Edinboro Univ of PA; ME 68 Kent St Univ; Supvr-Educ Svcs, Edinboro Univ of PA, **SLP**

Shimer, Mrs Linda L 415 Fort Street, Marietta, OH 45750, (614) 373-7550, BA 72 WV Wesleyan Coll; MA 75 OH Univ - Athens; Sp-Lang Path, Self Employed, **SLP**

Shimizu, Mrs Carol A 2 Park Avenue #4-C, Eastchester, NY 10709, (914) 779-5794, BS 78 Southeast MO St Univ; ME 79 Southeast MO St Univ; Sp/Lang Path, **SLP**

Shimizu, Dr Hiroshi Department Of Otolaryngology, Johns Hopkins Hospital, Baltimore, MD 21205, (301) 955-6151, MD 49 (NS); Sp-Lang Path, The John Hopkins Univ, **A F**

Shimon, Debra Ann P O Box 434, Mazomanie, WI 53560, (608) 252-8219, BS 76 Univ of WI - Madison; MS 79 Univ of WI - Madison; Aud, Dean Med Cen, **A**

Shimotakahara, Joanne N 79 Glenforest Road, Toronto, ON, Canada M4N 2A1, (416) 890-1221, BA 68 Univ of Toronto - Ontario; OM 75 Univ of Toronto - Ontario; Sp/Lang Path, Dufferin-Peel R C Separate Sch, **SLP**

Shin, Moonja 40-152 3KA Hankang-Ro, Yongsan-Ku, Seoul, Korea 140, BA 83 Wayne St Univ; MA 80 Ewha Womans Univ; MA 85 MI St Univ; 85–Sp-Lang Path, Seoul National Univ Hosp

Shinder, Mrs Anne 934 Ann Arbor, Ventura, CA 93003, (805) 251-8316, BA 60 Univ of CA - Los Angeles; MA 76 CA St Univ - Los Angeles; SLP, Osai USD, **SLP**

Shinder, Mrs Jane F 2 Oak Court, Madison, NJ 07940, (201) 731-3600, BA 78 Montclair St Coll; MA 82 Kean Coll of NJ; Sp-Lang Path, Mt Kemble Rehab, **SLP**

Shindler, Andrea Gellin Michael Reese Hospital, Department Of Neurology, 31st Street & Lakeshore Dr, Chicago, IL 60616, (312) 248-5929, BA 73 Adelphi Univ; MA 74 Northwestern Univ; Research Associate, Michael Reese Hospital, **SLP**

Shine, Dr Richard E Speech-Language Auditory Path, School Allied Health Sciences, East Carolina University, Greenville, NC 27858-4353, (919) 757-6961, BA 60 Univ of Northern CO; MA 61 Univ of Northern CO; ED 69 (NS) PA St Univ - Univ Park; Prof Sp-Lang Path, E Carolina U, **SLP**

Shinn, Dr Joyce A 5921 Oakbrook, Long Beach, CA 90815, BA 71 CA St Univ - Long Beach; ED 86 (Computer Education) United States Int'l Univ; Tchr of Sdc/Ch, Sausd, **SLP**

Shinn, Dr Roy E, Jr Western Kentucky University, College Of Education, Room 117, Bowling Green, KY 42101, (502) 745-4299, BS 82 Edinboro Univ of PA; MS 84 Univ of OK - OK City; PH 87 (Aud) Univ of OK - OK City; Asst Prof Aud, Western Kentucky Univ, **A**

Shinn, Mrs Susan 3783 San Ramon Drive Apartment #248, Oceanside, CA 92056, (619) 229-6200, BS 78 Bradley Univ; MS 79 Bradley Univ; 86–Sp-Lang Path, InSpeech Inc, **SLP**

Shinn, Wanda L 432-A Collingswood Street, San Francisco, CA 94114, (415) 565-9000, BA 53 San Francisco St Univ; SLP, San Francisco USD, **SLP**

Shinner, Deborah B Dickenson Road, Leverett, MA 01054, BA 72 Marymount Coll; MA 74 Univ of CT; **A**

Shinner, Glenn T Dickenson Road, Leverett, MA 01054, (413) 586-9572, BS 72 Columbia Univ Sch of Gen St; MA 74 Univ of CT; Aud, Hampshire Hrng Serv, **A**

Shintani, Janice S 94-201 Mahapili Street, Mililani Town, HI 96789, (808) 947-8511, BS 72 Univ of HI - Manoa; MS 74 Univ of HI - Manoa; Sp/Lang Path, Kapiolani-Chldrns Med Cen, **SLP**

Shinto, Marilyn M 348 Stannard Avenue, Victoria, BC, Canada V8S 3M4, (604) 595-8195, BS 74 CO St Univ; MA 75 Univ of Northern CO; Dir-Sp & Hrng Br, BC Govt Ministry of Health, **A**

Shiplett, Mrs Laura J 16181 Logarto Lane, Lakeville, MN 55044, (612) 892-1147, BS 81 Kent St Univ; MA 82 Kent St Univ; Aud, Maico of Cleveland Inc, **A**

Shipley, Janet L 233 South Orchard Drive, Park Forest, IL 60466, (312) 748-3822, BA 72 Northern IL Univ - De Kalb; MS 81 Governors St Univ; **SLP**

Shipley, Jean E P O Box 2231, Woodland, CA 95695, (916) 666-1631, BS 67 Univ of CA - Davis; MA 79 CA St Univ - Sacramento; SLP, Private Practice, **SLP**

Shipley, Kathryn Hendrick 8085 West Geddes Avenue, Littleton, CO 80123, (417) 836-0400, BS 84 Univ of NE - Lincoln; MS 85 Univ of NE - Lincoln; **SLP**

Shipley, Dr Kenneth G 2735 East Fremont Avenue, Fresno, CA 93710, (209) 294-2423, BA 72 CA St Univ - Los Angeles; MA 74 CA St Univ - Los Angeles; PH 77 (Communicative Sciences & Disorders) Wichita St Univ; 80–Prof, California State Univ-Fresno, **SLP**

Shipley, Larry B P O Box 192, Grenloch, NJ 08032, (609) 228-4393, BS 69 East TN St Univ; MA 72 Univ of TN - Knoxville; President, Private Practice, **A**

Shipley-Brown, Frances Hawpe 1035 30th Street NW, Washington, DC 20007, (202) 965-2235, MS 86; 86–Sp-Lang Path, Private Practice, **SLP**

Shipman, Linda Marie 1270 Sterling Avenue #208, Palatine, IL 60067, (312) 991-1267, BA 83 Augustana Coll; MA 84 Western MI Univ; **SLP**

Shipp, Polly Moore P O Box 15073, Gainesville, FL 32604, (904) 392-2041, MA 84 Univ of FL; 85–Graduate Teaching Assistant, University of Florida, **A**

Shipp, Mrs Susan S Bad Aibling Station #757, APO New York, NY 09098-4812, (301) 730-3662, BS 77 West Chester Univ of PA; MS 82 Loyola Coll; Sp-Lang Path, Baltimore Cty Pub Sch, **SLP**

Shipp, Dr Thomas Speech Research Lab (126), VA Medical Center, San Francisco, CA 94121, (415) 221-4810, BA 50 Stanford Univ; PH 63 (NS) Stanford Univ; Sp-Lang Path, VA Med Cen, **SLP F**

Shippee, Frank H 2022 Jaques Road, Palm Springs, CA 92262, (619) 327-4404, BA 51 Univ of Redlands; MA 61 Univ of Redlands; **SLP LM**

Shipstead-Cox, Mrs Nancy Jean 4236 Del Mar Avenue, San Diego, CA 92107, (619) 588-3087, MA 84 San Diego St Univ; SLP, Cajon Valley Union School Dist, **SLP**

Shirar, Lynda C 1447 Descanso Street, San Luis Obispo, CA 93401-6116, MS 74 1119

Shirek, Mrs Paula G The Better Speech Clinic, 631 Bourne Place, Orlando, FL 32801, (305) 855-4884, BA 78 Univ of FL; MS 80 Univ of South FL; Sp/Lang Path, Hjelm & Shirek PA, **SLP**

Shirk, Charles F 329 East California Blvd, Apartment 4, Pasadena, CA 91106, (213) 443-0173, BA 68; BS 56 West Chester Univ of PA; ME 61 Temple Univ-Tyler Sch of Art; Sp-Lang Path, Rosemead Sch Dist, **SLP**

Shirk, Mrs Sandra Potts 149 East Highland Road #3, Johnson City, TN 37601, (615) 461-6981, BS 85 Univ of TN - Knoxville; MA 87 Univ of TN - Knoxville; 87–Rehab Sp-Lang Path, Johnson City Med Ctr Hosp, **SLP**

Shirkey, Dr Edward A Department Of Communicative Disorders, University Of New Mexico, 901 Vassar N E, Albuquerque, NM 87131, (505) 277-4453, BS 67 Western MI Univ; MS 74 Univ of WI - Eau Claire; PH 82 (Sp Path) Memphis St Univ; 83–Prof, U of NM, **SLP**

Shirley, Beth Ann 552 River Road, Chatham, NJ 07928, (201) 635-4830, BA 80 Rutger's St Univ - Douglas Coll; MS 86 Rutgers St Univ -N Brunswick; 88–Sp-Lang Path, No Westchester Ctr for Sp Dis, **SLP**

Shirley, Mrs Ellen M 11 Marc Terrace, Monroe, NY 10950, BS 72 SUNY - Coll at New Paltz; MA 80 Univ of AR - Fayetteville; SLP, UCP, **SLP**

Shirley, Jeanette M Box 145, Elkader, IA 52043, (319) 245-1480, BS 75 Eastern IL Univ; MS 76 Eastern IL Univ; 77–Sp-Lang Path, Keystone AEA, **SLP**

Shirley, Dr Judith G Audiology & Spch Pathology SVC, VA Medical Center, Allen Park, MI 48101, (313) 562-6000, BA 61 Wayne St Univ; MA 66 Wayne St Univ; PH 79 (Sp-Lang Path) Wayne St Univ; 74–Sp/Lang Path, VA Med Cen, **SLP**

Shirley, Mrs Maureen Kluegel 2716 Stearns Way, St Cloud, MN 56303, (612) 259-0825, BS 80 Moorhead St Univ; MS 81 Saint Cloud St Univ; Sp-Lang Path, Kimball Sch Dist, **SLP**

Shirley, Sue A 17350 F M 149, Suite 149, Houston, TX 77064, (713) 955-9545, BS 64 Univ of TX - Austin; MA 81 Univ of Houston - Univ Park; Sp/Lang Path, Private Practice, **SLP ACE**

Shiroma, Charlene E Department Of Education, Windward Oahu District, Special Services, 46-169 Kamehameha Highway, Kaneohe, HI 96744, (808) 235-2343, BS 74 Univ of HI - Manoa; MS 79 Univ of UT; 80–Sp-Lang Path, Dept of Educ/Windward Oahu Dist, **SLP**

Shisler, Mrs Wendy S 223 Sweetman Road, Ballston Spa, NY 12020, (518) 382-4550, MS 74 Purdue Univ - West Lafayette; 88–Sp-Lang Path, Private Practice, **SLP**

Shively, Larry E 9918 East Limberlost Trail, Fort Wayne, IN 46825, BA 66 Ball St Univ; MA 70 Ball St Univ; Sp-Lang Path, Ft Wayne Commun Sch, **SLP**

Shively, Louise Ann 701 Walnut Street #3, Mifflinburg, PA 17844, (717) 966-3646, Sp-Lang Path, Geisinger Med Ctr, **SLP**

Shively, Mrs Patricia D Route 1 Box 486, Cooper Road, Eden, MD 21822, (301) 742-6195, BA 70 Univ of MD - College Park; MA 73 Univ of MD - College Park; Sp-Lang Path, Wicomic Co Bd of Ed, **SLP**

Shively, Philip Thomas 1114 4th Street Apartment C, Aurora, NE 68818, (402) 694-6707, BS 79 Univ of North TX; MS 81 Univ of North TX; 81–Sp-Lang Path, Educational Service Unit #9, **SLP ACE**

Shlaes, Toni E 3916-1/2 Huron Avenue, Culver City, CA 90230, (213) 657-6422, **SLP**

Shneider, Mrs Carole A 3521 River Falls Drive, Northbrook, IL 60062, (312) 564-0567, BS 63 Univ of IL - Urbana; MS 64 Univ of WI - Madison; **SLP**

Shnider, Dr Arline 5180 S W 17th Court, Plantation, FL 33317, (305) 431-8666, BS 69 FL St Univ; MA 71 Univ of MD - College Park; ED 80 (NS) Nova Univ; Aud, Hearing Health Care Ctr, **A**

Shnider, Mrs Doris Fern 105 Nob Hill Drive South, Gahanna, OH 43230, (614) 471-7093, BS 65 OH St Univ; MA 66 OH St Univ; **A**

Shoaf, Mrs Betsy Barber Route 5 Box 158, Lexington, NC 27292, (704) 787-5171, MA 83 Appalachian St Univ; Sp-Lang Path, Davidson Co Schools, **SLP**

Shober, Mrs Gerarda A Box 191-3 Rd #2, Reinholds, PA 17569, (215) 484-1213, BS 81 West Chester Univ of PA; MA 85 West Chester Univ of PA; Sp-Lang Path, Lancaster/Lebanon IU #13, **SLP**

Shock, Charles A, Jr P O Box 1894, South Bend, IN 46634, (800) 521-5400, BS 67 Ball St Univ; MA 72 Ball St Univ; MA 73 Ball St Univ; Dist Manager, Unitron Industries, **A**

Shockey, Kathleen M 1411 Grandview Avenue #103, Pittsburgh, PA 15211, (412) 481-2063, BS 80 Baylor Univ; MA 82 Univ of Pittsburgh - Pittsburgh; Sp-Lang Path, Robinson Developmental Center, **SLP**

Shockley, Suzanne H Route 2 Box 6, Middletown, IN 47356, (317) 747-3386, BS 74 Purdue Univ - West Lafayette; MA 80 Ball St Univ; Dept Hd of Aud, Ball Mem Hosp, **SLP A**

Shoemaker, Barbara Knapp 514 South 2nd Street, Wilmington, NC 28401, (919) 251-1811, BS 79 Ithaca Coll; MA 83 Univ of FL; 87–Aud, Shoemaker Hearing Care Ctr, **A**

Shoemaker, Jeffrey R 333 East Willow, Detroit Lakes, MN 56501, (218) 847-1810, MA 78 Univ of MN - Duluth; Sp-Lang Path, Private Practice, **SLP**

Shoemaker, Sheela 202 Sayre Drive, Princeton, NJ 08540, (609) 987-8885, BA; MA; Sp-Lang Path, Communication Success Inc, **SLP ACE**

Shoemaker-Scott, Debra 2108 Kirby N E, Albuquerque, NM 87112, (505) 298-6752, BA 79 Univ of NM; MS 81 Univ of NM; Sp-Lang Path, Albuquerque Pub Sch, **SLP**

Shoen, Cathy Jo 486 Clay Road #C, Rochester, NY 14623, (716) 461-8680, BA 79 SUNY - Coll at Potsdam; MA 80 SUNY - Coll at Geneseo; Aud, Monroe Developmental Center, **A**

Shoenut, Dr Blanca M 1638 Santa Brigida Street, Rio Piedras, PR 00926, (809) 761-5155, BS 47 Univ of PR - Rio Piedras; MA 63 G Peabody Coll-Vanderbilt U; PH 67 (Aud) IN Univ - Bloomington; 72–Retired, San Juan Veterans Admn Med Ctr, **SLP A**

Shoham, Andrea B 10121 Wendover Drive, Vienna, VA 22180, (703) 281-9246, BS 70 Emerson Coll; MA 72 NY Univ; **SLP**

Shohet-Hamel, Francine L 8420 S W 133rd Avenue Road, Apartment 2-419, Miami, FL 33183, MS; ED 87 (Early Childhood Ed) Nova Univ; Dir/Owner, Hamel Sch, **SLP**

Shoji, Leslie Shawn 202 South Vancouver, Los Angeles, CA 90022, (213) 589-4852, **A**

Sholar, Joanne Franck Route 2 Box 507, Floyd, VA 24091, (703) 745-2734, BA 79 Univ of WA; OM 81 Univ of WA; Sp-Lang Path, **SLP**

Sholes, Gertrude Jozefowicz 737 Namquid Drive, Warwick, RI 02888, (401) 331-5511, BA 72 Univ of RI; MS 75 Univ of RI; Audiologist, G J Sholes Audiology Assoc, **A**

Sholly, Ralph G 1726 North Keim Street, Pottstown, PA 19464, **SLP**

Shomberg, Mrs Jane Ellen 564 Sunset Drive, Woodmere, NY 11598, (516) 295-0495, BA 80 Long Island U - CW Post Ctr; MA 82 Hofstra Univ; Sp/Lang Path, Herb Birch Sch for Except Chdn, **SLP**

Shomo, Mrs Barbara Patterson P O Box 1118, 142 Oakland Drive, Pulaski, VA 24301, (703) 980-0563, OB 73 Radford Univ; MS 81 Radford Univ; Sp-Lang Path, Sp-Lang Services SW Virginia, **SLP**

Shonbrun, Susan H 10115 North 14th Street, Tampa, FL 33612, (813) 974-3570, MS 79 Univ of South FL; Sp-Lang Path, UCP, **SLP**

Shonce, Jan Doughty 6890 Yorkdale Court, Westland, MI 48185, **SLP**

Shonrock, Cynthia M 270 East Highland Avenue #226, Milwaukee, WI 53202, (414) 276-5584, BA 73 Univ of Northern IA; MA 74 Univ of Northern IA; **SLP**

Shoobs, Mrs Diane S Naiman 10 Wedgewood Drive, West Paterson, NJ 07424, (201) 451-9000, BS 77 Boston Univ; MA 79 NY Univ; Sp-Lang Path, Jewish Hosp/Rehab Cen/Nj, **SLP**

Shook, Mrs Anita Mobley Children's Center, 310 North Madison Terrace, Montgomery, AL 36107, (205) 262-4850, BA 83 Auburn Univ - Montgomery; OM 84 Auburn Univ - Auburn; BS 88 Auburn Univ - Montgomery; 88–Sp-Lang Path, Montgomery PS, **SLP**

Shook, Mrs Ellen Stephens 1307 North 12th, Garden City, KS 67846, (316) 275-8016, BA 59 Univ of Northern CO; MA 64 Univ of MO - Columbia; Sp-Lang Path, USD 457, **SLP**

Shook, Mrs Jane Ellen 2507 Tisinger, Dallas, TX 75228, (214) 821-9083, **SLP**

Shook, Janelle B 2140 Fort Harrods Drive, Apartment 40, Lexington, KY 40513, (203) 655-7520, BS 74 Univ of GA; MA 76 Univ of TN - Knoxville; Sp-Lang Path, **SLP**

Shook, Janice Victoria 107 E Hightower Street, Sardis, MS 38666, (601) 563-9361, OB 74 MS St Univ - MS State; MS 86 Univ of MS

Shook, Sharon J 4909 Casey Court, Independence, MO 64055, (816) 373-9533, BS 78 Univ of MO - Columbia; MA 79 Univ of MO - Columbia; 79–Sp-Lang Path, Sch Dist of Indep, **SLP**

Shoom, Mrs Lauren Ann 300 Antibes Drive #1806, Willowdale, ON, Canada M2R 3N8, (416) 667-1653, BS 83 Northeastern Univ; MS 85 Boston Univ; Sp-Lang Path, Randolph Ma Public Schools, **SLP**

Shoop, Deborah H 5920 West Monte Cristo Avenue, Glendale, AZ 85306, (602) 939-9583, BA 76 Univ of Redlands; MS 83 AZ St Univ; 88–Sp-Lang Path, Private Practice, **SLP**

Shoop, Mrs Kathryn Kight 69 Jadwin #16, Richland, WA 99352-4626, (509) 796-4727, BA 83 Eastern WA Univ; MS 84 Eastern WA Univ; Sp-Lang Path, Private Practice, **SLP ACE**

Shope, Marie D J 712 SE 37th, Hillsboro, OR 97123, (503) 648-3127, BA 76 Portland St Univ; MS 78 Portland St Univ; 78–Sp-Lang Path, Hillsboro Elem Sch Dist #7, **SLP**

Shopwin, Dr Charles D Schip Vios, Stadhouderskade T/O 86A, Amsterdam, Netherlands 107388, BA 51 CA St Univ - Los Angeles; MA 54 Univ of Southern CA; PH 58 (NS) Univ of Southern CA; Retired, **SLP LM**

Shore, Gretchen Lubov 314 Fairview Road #4, Asheville, NC 28803, (704) 274-7955, BS 82 Appalachian St Univ; MA 84 IN Univ - Bloomington; 88–Sp-Lang Path, Buncombe Co PS, **SLP**

Shore, Mrs Jeanne B Route 2 Box 106-A, Trinity, NC 27370-9802, (919) 434-6656, BA 75 Univ of NC - Greensboro; ME 80 Univ of NC - Greensboro; SLP, Davidson County Schools, **SLP**

Shore, Mrs Karen M 136 Thornhill Road, Cherry Hill, NJ 08003, (609) 424-2659, BA 79 Univ of WI - Eau Claire; MS 80 Univ of WI - Eau Claire; Sp-Lang Path, **SLP**

Shore, Linda Suzanne 1034 Koelle Boulevard, Secaucus, NJ 07094, (718) 987-9400, MS 84 Emerson Coll; **SLP**

Shore, Susan Lee 126 Braemar Avenue, Toronto, ON, Canada M5P 2L4, (416) 481-2729, BS 82 Univ of Alberta - Alberta; MS 84 Univ of VT; 87–Sp-Lang Path, Peel Bd of Educ, **SLP**

Shore-Rushfeldt, Bette H 2358 Bay Village Court, Lake Park, FL 33410, (305) 626-9365, OB 73 Univ of Miami; ME 78 Northeastern Univ; Sp-Lang Path, Private Practice, **SLP**

Shores, Mrs Ann Christine 10424 Floral Drive, Adelphi, MD 20783, (301) 937-5818, BA 78 Univ of MD - College Park; MS 80 Loyola Coll; Sp/Lang Path, Prince Georges Cty Schs, **SLP**

Shores, Linda Sue 15161 Security Way, Aurora, CO 80011, (303) 344-2933, BA 84 Metropolitan St Coll; MA 86 Univ of Denver

Shorey, Mrs Carrie Elizabeth 922 North Princeton, Arlington Height, IL 60004, (312) 275-8822, BS 82 Univ of WI - Madison; MS 84 Univ of WI - Madison; **SLP**

Shorn-Fletcher, Amy M 2262 Soledad Rancho Road, San Diego, CA 92109, **SLP**

Shorr, Dr David N Central Washington Univ, 801 Southwest 174th Street, Seattle, WA 98166, (206) 433-8045, BA 73 CA St Coll - San Bernardino; PH 80 (NS) Univ of WA; Asst Prof of Early Child Educ, Central Washington University

Shorr, Mrs Wendy E 1511 Susan Drive, Lansdale, PA 19446, (215) 362-1572, BA 74 Temple Univ-Tyler Sch of Art; MA 76 Temple Univ-Tyler Sch of Art; Sp-Lang Path, Visting Nurse Assoc, **SLP**

Short, Cynthia Anne 505 Elm Street, Rome, NY 13440, (315) 733-5083, BA 81 SUNY - Coll at Plattsburgh; OM 84 Coll of Saint Rose; OM 85 SUNY - Coll at Plattsburgh; Sp-Lang Path, Rome Developmental Center, **SLP**

Short, Cynthia Jo Audio/Vestibular Lab, 899 Madison, Suite 400M, Memphis, TN 38146, (901) 522-5651, MS 83 Univ of South FL; 85–Aud, Baptist Memorial Hospital, **A**

Short, Deborah L 3815 Brotherton Road #15, Cincinnati, OH 45209, (513) 561-7853, BS 84 Miami Univ - Oxford; MA 85 MI St Univ; 86–Aud, N KY Head & Neck Spec, **A**

Short, Gaylord R 2601 Fremont Street #121, Bakersfield, CA 93304, (805) 398-3855, BA 67 San Jose St Univ; MA 80 San Jose St Univ; Aud, Aurally Exceptional Cen, **A**

Short, Mrs Judith H 3305 Cardinal, Woodstock, IL 60098, BS 63 Univ of IL - Urbana; MA 67 De Paul Univ; 86–Aud, David S Hemmer MD SC, **A**

Short, Julie A 30-80 32nd Street, Astoria, NY 11102, (212) 679-0100, BS 76 Ball St Univ; MA 81 NY Univ; Sp-Lang Path, Internatl Center for Disabled, **SLP**

Short, Mrs Mary Ann Marik 101 South Edgewood Avenue, La Grange, IL 60525, (312) 579-1454, BA 81 Augustana Coll; MA 82 Northwestern Univ; Sp-Lang Path, Restorative Health Management, **SLP**

Short, Mrs Mary Garrity 8 Col Christopher Green, Portsmouth, RI 02871, (401) 847-2992, BA 68 Loyola Coll; MA 70 MI St Univ; Sp-Lang Path, Portsmouth Sch Syst, **SLP**

Short, Shirley Crandall 4915 Herndon Circle, Colorado Springs, CO 80920, (918) 224-5527, BS 79 Phillips Univ; MA 81 OK St Univ; **SLP**

Short, Susan 8 Doe Court, Gillette, WY 82716, (307) 686-2214, BA 74; MS 76 Southern IL Univ -Carbondale; Sp-Lang Path, Private Practice, **SLP**

Shortall, Mrs Ann L 10415 Carry Back Place, Dallas, TX 75229, (214) 247-7153, BS 76 Univ of North TX; MS 77 Univ of North TX; **SLP**

Shortino, Mrs Margaret Denise 2713 Club Meadow, Garland, TX 75043, (214) 494-8308, **SLP**

Shortridge, Mrs Judith C 112 South Benton Street, Waynesville, MO 65583, BS 78 Eastern IL Univ; MS 79 Eastern IL Univ; Sp-Lang Path, Waynesville R Vi Sch Dist, **SLP**

Shortsleeve, Mary 12 Chapel Place #1, Danbury, CT 06810, (203) 791-8356, BA 77 Univ of FL; MA 79 Univ of FL; MA 86 CUNY - Hunter Coll; SLP, **SLP**

Shotland, Dr Lawrence U Of Northern Colorado, Dept Of Comm Disorders, Greeley, CO 80639, (303) 351-1589, BA 76 San Diego St Univ; MA 79 Western WA Univ; PH 86 (Aud-Noise) Univ of UT; 88–Asst Prof of Aud, Univ of Northern Colorado, **A**

Shotland, Mrs Rochelle C 18 Colby Avenue, Rye, NY 10580, (914) 948-0050, BA 64 CUNY - City College; MA 79 Hofstra Univ; Aud, Burke Rehab Cen-Dept/Sl & A, **A**

Shotwell, Cherrie L 1015 Laakea Place, Honolulu, HI 96818-2365, (808) 422-9063, BA 73 Univ of Redlands; MS 75 Univ of Redlands; Sp-Lang Path, Honolulu Com Action Prog-Headstart, **SLP**

Shotwell, Mrs Jeannette 18414 99th Drive, Sun City, AZ 85373, (602) 974-4359, BA 39 Grinnell Coll; MA 40 Univ of IA; **SLP LM**

Shotwell, Mrs Rochelle 68 Springwood, Northfield Center, OH 44067, BS 72 Kent St Univ; MA 74 Kent St Univ; Sp-Lang Path, Marymount Hospital, **SLP**

Shotwell, Sue Christense 11581 Rabaul Drive, Cypress, CA 90630, (714) 892-5128, ME 86 CA St Univ - Long Beach

Shoup, Nancy L Route 5 Box 88, Brenham, TX 77833, BS 54 Univ of Houston - Univ Park; MA 72 Univ of Houston - Univ Park; 86–Tchr, Brenham ISD, **SLP**

Shouse, Sherry W 1005 Girard Drive, Louisville, KY 40222, (502) 361-6703, BA 74 Univ of KY; MS 75 Murray St Univ; Sp-Lang Path, Sts Mary & Elizabeth Hosp, **SLP**

Shovan, Diane R 602 Market Street, Algonac, MI 48001, (313) 725-2801, BS 71 Indiana Univ of PA; MA 72 Western MI Univ; SLP, Sch Dist, **SLP ACE**

Shovlin, Deborah Anne 106 Leslie Lane, Pittston, PA 18640, (717) 654-7141, BS 75 Marywood Coll; MS 79 Bloomsburg Univ of PA; SLP, Luzerne Inter Unit, **SLP**

Shovlin, Rose Ann 281 Burnt Mill Road, Somerville, NJ 08876, (201) 725-3496, BA 80 Hofstra Univ; MS 82 PA St Univ - Univ Park; 85–Consultant Audiologist, Private Practice, **A ACE**

Show, Mrs Sandra Dickinson 2806 Eastwood Drive, Iowa City, IA 52245, (319) 351-7744, BA 75 SUNY - Coll at Buffalo; MA 77 Univ of IA; 77–Sp-Lang Path, Grant Wood AEA, **SLP**

Showalter, Maria R T 4785 Marjorie Drive, Lockport, NY 14094, (716) 439-6169, BS 77 Purdue Univ - West Lafayette; MS 78 SUNY - Coll at Geneseo; Sp-Lang Path, Niagara Co Sp/Hrng/Lang Cen, **SLP**

Showalter, Robert G Audiology And Speech Sciences, Purdue University, Lafayette, IN 47907, (317) 494-3793, BS 52 Ball St Univ; MA 57 Ball St Univ; Prof, Prudue Univ, **SLP A F ACE**

Showers, Mrs Drusilla Ramsay 1313 Rothes Road, Cary, NC 27511, (919) 683-2591, MS 83 Univ of NC - Chapel Hill; Sp-Lang Path, Durham Regional Hrng Imp Prog, **SLP**

Showman, Rebecca N P O Box 786, Morganton, NC 28655, (704) 433-2921, BS 75 East TN St Univ; MS 78 East TN St Univ; Sp-Lang Path, Nc Sch for the Deaf, **SLP**

Shown, Suzanne 1301 Waverly Place, Owensboro, KY 42301, (502) 685-3141, BS 78 Brescia Coll; MS 84 Western KY Univ; Sp-Lang Path, InSpeech Inc, **SLP**

Shows, Dennis L 1818 Shadow Lane, Montgomery, AL 36106, (205) 567-8471, BA 66 Huntingdon Coll; MA 74 Univ of AL- Tuscaloosa; ME 72 Amer Int'l Coll; SLP/Aud, J S Tarwater Dev Cen, **SLP**

Shprintzen, Dr Robert J 3331 Bainbridge Avenue, Bronx, NY 10467, (212) 920-4781, BA 68 Univ of Rochester; MS 70 Univ of RI; PH 73 (NS) Syracuse Univ; Director, Montefiore Med Ctr, **SLP**

Shpritz, Mrs Ruth B 3 Hunt Meadow Court, Owings Mills, MD 21117, (301) 484-4842, BS 76 Loyola Coll; MS 78 Ithaca Coll; Sp-Lang Path, Carroll County Board of Educ, **SLP**

Shrack, Mrs Amy J R R 2 Box 220, Muncie, IN 47302, (317) 482-2700, BA 80 IN Univ - Bloomington; MA 82 Ball St Univ; Aud, St Johns Medical Center, **A**

Shrader, Jean 13900 180th Avenue N E, Redmond, WA 98052, (913) 492-0647, BA 73 WA St Univ; MS 77 Loyola Coll; **SLP**

Shrader-Cory, Mrs Kathleen J S 2212 Manito Boulevard, Spokane, WA 99203, (509) 455-3711, BS 74 Univ of WY; MS 77 Univ of WY; SLP, Spokane Sch Dist 81, **SLP**

Shragg, Judith Metchik 2011 West Katella #72, Anaheim, CA 92804, (714) 535-5463, BA 80 Univ of PA; MS 82 Columbia Univ Teachers Coll; 88–Sp-Lang Path, Mem Med Ctr of Long Beach, **SLP**

Shreiber, Mrs Ida F 1917 North Oxford Avenue, Los Angeles, CA 90027, (213) 462-7875, BA 48 Univ of OK - Norman; MA 74 CA St Univ - Los Angeles; Retired, LA USD, **SLP**

Shrewsberry, Mrs Sonya E 711 Highland Avenue, Princeton, WV 24740, (304) 425-7946, BS 75 WV Univ; MS 81 Radford Univ; Sp-Lang Path, Mercer Co Bd of Ed, **SLP**

Shrewsbury, Dr Margaret E 933 Cromwell Bridge Road, Towson, MD 21204, (301) 494-4130, BA 57 WV Univ; MA 70 OH St Univ; PH 72 (Sp and Hrng Science) OH St Univ; 80–Superv, Baltimore Co Pub Sch, **SLP**

Shrewsbury, Rosemary G 308 53rd Street, Vienna, WV 26105, (304) 422-8612, BS 73 WV Univ; MS 75 WV Univ; SLP, Wood Co Bd of Ed, **SLP**

Shriberg, Dr Lawrence D University Of Wisconsin, 1975 Willow Drive, Madison, WI 53706, (608) 262-3951, BS 61 Syracuse Univ; ME 66 Boston Univ; PH 70 (NS) Univ of KS; Prof, U of WI-Madison, **SLP F**

Shriftman, Mrs Eileen C 31901 Foxmoor Court, Westlake Village, CA 91361, (818) 889-7872, BA 71 SUNY - Center at Albany; MS 72 SUNY - Center at Albany; SLP, Putnam Valley School District, **SLP**

Shrigley-Parker, Mrs Sandra Jo 1503 Foster Drive, Reno, NV 89509, (702) 348-0200, MS 83 Univ of NV - Reno; Sp-Lang Path, Washoe Co Sch Dist, **SLP**

Shriner, Jane Nemec 9040 SW 79th Avenue, Miami, FL 33156, (305) 595-7022, BS 66 Marquette Univ; MA 68 Univ of IL - Urbana; Sp-Lang Path Chairperson, Dade County Public Schools, **SLP**

Shrira, Lois R 5315 Zelzah Avenue #5, Encino, CA 91316-2267, (213) 625-4183, BS 64 OH St Univ; MA 65 OH St Univ; SLP, Los Angeles USD, **SLP**

Shriro, Dr Marjorie J 10355 Buglenote Way, Columbia, MD 21044, (301) 997-1599, BA 63 Barnard Coll; MA 65 Columbia Univ Teachers Coll; PH 80 (Sp Path) Univ of Pittsburgh - Pittsburgh; Sp-Lang Path, Private Practice, **SLP**

Shrive, Albert Precision Hearing Instruments, 1102 South Main Avenue, Scranton, PA 18504, (717) 343-1414, BS 73 East Stroudsburg Univ of PA; MS 80 Bloomsburg Univ of PA; Aud, Private Practice, **A**

Shriver, Carla Jean 13613-D East Yale Avenue, Aurora, CO 80014, (303) 745-7079, BS 84 Univ of WY; MS 86 CO St Univ; **SLP**

Shriver, Rebecca L 842 West Lincoln Boulevard, Freeport, IL 61032-4914, (815) 232-5069, BS 74 Univ of IL - Urbana; MS 75 Univ of IL - Urbana; Sp-Lang Path, Freeport Sch Dist #145, **SLP**

Shrull, Sharla Sue 3510 N E Independence, Lee's Summit, MO 64064, (816) 792-7197, **SLP**

Shrum, Dr William F 1264 Manzanita Avenue, Chico, CA 95926, (916) 895-5871, BA 52 PA St Univ - Univ Park; MS 60 PA St Univ - Univ Park; PH 67 (NS) Univ of IA; Sp-Lang Path, CA St U Chico Dept of Ed, **SLP**

Shrut, Mrs Jamisen S 1223 North Woodbine Avenue, Penn Valley, PA 19072, (215) 664-3592, BS 73 Ithaca Coll; MA 74 Temple Univ-Tyler Sch of Art; 85–Sp-Lang Path, Lower Merion Sch Dist, **SLP**

Shubach, Nancy K 112 Sandringham Road, Cherry Hill, NJ 08003, (609) 424-4785, BA 73 CUNY - City College; MA 77 CA St Univ - Sacramento; Sp-Lang Path, Moorestown High Sch, **SLP**

Shubat, Sally Jo 4129 Cambridge, Kansas City, KS 66103, (816) 234-3677, BS 77 IA St Univ; MA 80 Univ of MO - Columbia; Sp-Lang Path, Chldn Mercy Hosp, **SLP**

Shubitowski, Yvonne Densie 3454 Moretti Drive, Concord, CA 94519-2803, (415) 228-6800, BS 80 Univ of MI - Ann Arbor; MS 84 Univ of WI - Madison; Sp-Lang Path, VA Hosp, **SLP**

Shubow, Gerri Feuer 172 Lindbergh Avenue, Needham, MA 02194, (617) 735-6485, BS 72 OH Univ - Athens; MS 73 Univ of MI - Ann Arbor; Chief Aud, Chldn Hosp Boston, **A**

Shuck, Anna Marie 380 Platteview Drive, Springfield, NE 68059-9617, (402) 253-8284, OB 84 Univ of NE - Lincoln; OM 85 Univ of NE - Lincoln; **SLP**

Shudy, Mrs Jane M P 1022 Clara Street, Appleton, WI 54915, (414) 731-0600, BS 75 Univ of WI - Stevens Point; MS 76 Univ of WI - Stevens Point; **SLP**

Shue, Michelle Marie 1136 Yale Avenue, Billings, MT 59102, (406) 245-4687, BA 82 Univ of MT; OM 85 Univ of MT; 88–Sp-Lang Path, St Vincent's Hosp & Health Care Ctr, **SLP**

Shuey, Elaine M P O Box 356, Delaware Water Gap, PA 18327, (216) 672-2672, BS 78 Clarion Univ of PA; MA 80 Kent St Univ; Assistant Professor, East Stroudsburg University, **SLP ACE**

Shufer, Sylvia F 263 West End Avenue, Freeport, NY 11520, (516) 379-8025, BA 58 CUNY - Hunter Coll; MA 71 Hofstra Univ; 85–Sp-Lang Path, Remediation Ctr for Comm Dis, **SLP**

Shugars, Mrs Lori Ann 316 W Washington Boulevard, Apartment 1-R, Oak Park, IL 60302, (312) 547-3080, BA 84 Augustana Coll; MA 85 Northeast MO St Univ; 88–Sp-Lang Path, Proviso Area for Excep Children, **SLP**

Shugarts, Dawn Denise 9 Payne Road, Newton Highlands, MA 02161, (617) 720-6763, MS 86 Univ of WA; Sp-Lang Path, Spaulding Rehab Hosp, **SLP**

Shulak, Cynthia B 61 Winthrop Street, Newton, MA 02165, (617) 924-3434, BA 77 Univ of MI - Ann Arbor; MA 79 Univ of CA - Santa Barbara; Consultant, Private Practice, **SLP**

Shulenberger, Kayle A 1323 East College Way, Mount Vernon, WA 98273, (206) 424-8110, BA 73 Western WA Univ; MA 74 Western WA Univ; Dir/Owner, Island Sp & Hrng Cl, **SLP**

Shuler, Mrs Cleta J 5601 New Haven, Greenville, TX 75401, (214) 455-2112, BS 70 East TX St Univ - Commerce; MS 73 East TX St Univ - Commerce; Sp-Lang Path, Greenville ISD, **SLP**

Shuler, Glenda D 2385 North Forest Drive, Marietta, GA 30062, (404) 255-3616, BA 75 CA St Univ - Sacramento; MS 81 Univ of TX - Dallas; Sp-Lang Path, Fulton Co Bd of Ed, **SLP**

Shuler-Scott, Carolyn Anita 100 M Lofton Drive, Fayetteville, NC 28311, (919) 822-3543, MS 86 Univ of NC - Chapel Hill; 88–SLP, Logos Inc, **SLP**

Shuller, Janis C 8135 Glenmil Court, Cincinnati, OH 45242, (614) 222-6533, BS 76 Univ of VA - Charlottesville; MA 77 OH St Univ; Sp-Lang Path, Chldrns Hosp Med Cen, **SLP**

Shulman, Mrs Audrey 85 Old Smalleytown Road, Warren, NJ 07060, (201) 668-0005, BA 56 CUNY - Brooklyn Coll; MA 74 Kean Coll of NJ; PH 87 (Behavioral Science) Pacific Western Univ; Dir, New Jersey Stuttering Center, **SLP**

Shulman, Dr Brian B Dept Of Speech, City College Of New York, 138th St And Convent Avenue, New York, NY 10031, (212) 690-5377, BA 79 SUNY - Coll at Cortland; MA 81 Bowling Green St Univ; PH 83 (NS) Bowling Green St Univ; Associate Professor, City College of New York, **SLP**

Shulman, Carole 3601 Connecticut Avenue N W, Apartment 612, Washington, DC 20008, (703) 356-3200, **SLP**

Shulman, Dr Edward 25 Chatham Place, Glen Rock, NJ 07452, (201) 445-1025, BA 39 Western MI Univ; MS 40 Univ of MN - Minneap-St Paul; PH 44 (Psychology/Sp Path & Aud) Univ of IA; 55–Dir, Private Practice, **SLP A LM**

Shulman, Ellen L 70 Kansas Street, Rochester, NY 14609, (716) 288-2862, BS 79 SUNY - Coll at Buffalo; ME 80 SUNY - Coll at Buffalo; Sp-Lang Path, Rochester Cty Sch Dist, **SLP**

Shulman, Marc A 120 96th Street, Brooklyn, NY 11209, (212) 238-9673, BA 70 CUNY - City College; MS 76 CUNY - Brooklyn Coll; Sp-Lang Path Coord, Bronx Childrens Psy Center, **SLP**

Shulman, Marsha A 503 Hunters Run, Dobbs Ferry, NY 10522, (914) 693-9452

Shulman, Dr Martin D 14 Bernard Road, East Brunswick, NJ 08816, (201) 536-2292, BS 67 CUNY - Brooklyn Coll; PH 73 (NS) Univ of MN - Minneap-St Paul; 73–Coord/Sp & Hrng Prog, Kean Coll of Nj, **SLP**

Shulman, Susan C 12700 Hillcrest Road, Suite 258, Dallas, TX 75230, (214) 233-4660, BS 66 Univ of MS; MS 69 Univ of North TX; Sp-Lang Path, Private Practice, **SLP A ACE**

Shultz, Cathleen M 20 Rushmore Drive, Glen Carbon, IL 62034, (618) 288-3431, MS 77 Univ of IL - Urbana; 88–Sp-Lang Path, Alton Catholic Children's Home, **SLP**

Shultz, Mrs Diane Carol 3032 West Missouri Avenue, Phoenix, AZ 85017, (602) 933-3088, BS 62 CA St Univ - Los Angeles; MA 64 CA St Univ - Los Angeles; Aud, Sun City Aud & Hrng Aid Ctr, **A**

Shultz, Judith M 3798 Royal Avenue, Montreal, PQ, Canada H4A 2M2, (514) 937-6011, BA 76 McGill Univ - Quebec; MS 78 McGill Univ - Quebec; SLP, Montreal Gen Hosp, **SLP**

Shultz, Karla Jean 184 Maitland Avenue, Altamonte Springs, FL 32701, BS 83 Governors St Univ; MS 84 Governors St Univ; Sp-Lang Path, **SLP**

Shultz, Mrs Sharon L 28735 Summerwood, Farmington Hills, MI 48018-4627, BA 70 Univ of MI - Ann Arbor; MA 74 Eastern MI Univ; SLP, Clarenceville School District, **SLP**

Shultz, Tracy Ann 7504 Brighton Road #1, Pittsburgh, PA 15202, (412) 761-8171, BA 81 Univ of Pittsburgh - Pittsburgh; MA 86 Univ of Pittsburgh - Pittsburgh; 87–Sp-Lang Path, InSpeech Inc, **SLP**

Shumate, Mrs Lena Scurry 10 Birch Drive, Huntington, WV 25705-3219, (304) 522-8800, BS 81 James Madison Univ; ME 82 James Madison Univ; 83–Aud, Huntington Ear Clinic Inc, **A**

Shumate, Robert Bradley 10 Birch Drive, Huntington, WV 25705-3219, (304) 522-8800, BA 81 Univ of KY; ME 83 James Madison Univ; Aud, Huntington Ear Clinic Inc, **A**

Shumate-Houston, Mrs Stacie 1171 W Covered Bridge Road, Rt 3, Columbia, MO 65203, (314) 442-8915, BS 67 WV Univ; MA 70 Kent St Univ; 85–Sp-Lang Path, Private Practice, **SLP**

Shuminsky, Diane M 2301 McDonald, Sioux City, IA 51104, (712) 279-6040, MA 72 Univ of SD - Vermillion; SLP, Wn Hills AEA Xii, **SLP**

Shumway, Erma J 8415 North Calaveras, Fresno, CA 93711, (209) 291-9807, BA 73 CA St Univ - Stanislaus; MA 74 CA St Univ - Stanislaus; Sp/Lang Path, Fresno USD, **SLP**

Shumway, Sally Louise 2585-6 Woodlake Road S W, Wyoming, MI 49509, (616) 538-1789, BA 72 Central MI Univ; MA 79 Central MI Univ; Sp-Lang Path, Jenison PS, **SLP**

Shumway, Teresa J 7438 Schenck Road, Perry, NY 14530, (716) 245-5328, BS 78 SUNY - Coll at Fredonia; MA 86 SUNY - Coll at Geneseo; **A**

Shunfenthal, Sherri F 9037 Brook Ford Road, Burke, VA 22015, (703) 866-9729, BS 78 PA St Univ - Univ Park; MS 80 Indiana Univ of PA; SLP/Aud, Alexandria Rehab, **SLP**

Shunk, Mrs Laurel Sue 375 Silvervale, Rochester Hills, MI 48309, (605) 339-9990, **SLP**

Shupe, Dr Lewis K Wright State University, Colonel Glen Highway, Dayton, OH 45435, (513) 873-2145, BS 57 Univ of UT; MS 60 Univ of UT; PH 68 (NS) SUNY - Center at Buffalo; Prof Dept of Commun, Wright St U, **SLP**

Shur, Mrs Iris B 197 Holdenwood, Concord, MA 01742, (617) 369-1357, BA 61 SUNY - Center at Buffalo; MS 63 Univ of Pittsburgh - Pittsburgh; **A**

Shurer, Thomas E 413 West Market Street, West Chester, PA 19382, (215) 873-4918, BS 82 PA St Univ - Univ Park; MA 84 George Washington Univ; Sp-Lang Path, Thedevereux Foundation, **SLP**

Shurson, Tedd Dennis 2316 W Whitendale Suite A, Visalia, CA 93277, (209) 625-8960, BA 73 CA St Univ - Fresno; MA 75 CA St Univ - Fresno; 79–Aud, Shurson Hearing & Speech Ctr, **A**

Shurtleff, Mrs M'Liss Marler 11465 Spitfire Road, San Diego, CA 92126, (619) 549-3220, BS 83 Univ of UT; MS 86 Univ of UT

Shuster, Carol A 9 Hazelwood Drive, Norwood, MA 02062, (617) 647-6418, BS 74 PA St Univ - Univ Park; MS 77 Boston Univ; Sp-Lang Path, Waltham Weston Hosp & Med Ctr, **SLP**

Shuster, Cheryl 61 Cliffwood Road, Willowdale, ON, Canada M2H 3K3, (416) 225-8072, BS 75 McGill Univ - Quebec; MS 77 McGill Univ - Quebec; Sp-Lang Path, Centenary Hosp, **SLP**

Shuster, Lia 255 West 84th Street, New York, NY 10024, **A**

Shuster, Dr Linda I West Virginia University, 805 Allen Hall, Dept Of Speech Path & Aud, Morgantown, WV 26506-6122, (304) 293-4241, BA 76 Univ of MI - Ann Arbor; MS 78 Univ of MI - Ann Arbor; PH 86 (Sp Science) OH St Univ; 86–Asst Prof, West Virginia Univ, **SLP**

Shuster, Mrs Nancy Lite 1121 Johnson Ferry Rd, Suite 340, Marietta, GA 30068, (404) 565-4052, BA 78 Univ of MD - College Park; MS 80 Emory Univ; Aud, **A**

Shusterman, Mrs Joan S 211-35 23rd Avenue, Bayside, NY 11360, (516) 561-8686, BS 72 SUNY - Center at Albany; MS 76 CUNY - Hunter Coll; Tchr, Valley Stream Ctrl Hs Dist, **SLP**

Shusterman, Karen Lynn 531 Cynwyd Circle, Bala-Cynwyd, PA 19004, (215) 673-2312, BS 83 PA St Univ - Univ Park; MA 85 Temple Univ-Tyler Sch of Art; 86, Abington Sch Dist, **SLP**

Shute, Brian James 2518 South Grand Avenue, Spokane, WA 99203, (509) 332-7494, BA 84 WA St Univ; MA 86 WA St Univ; 86–Sp-Lang Path, Sacred Heart Med Ctr, **SLP**

Shute, Mary Julia 620 S 28th Avenue#302, Hattiesburg, MS 39402, (601) 264-3495, BS 62 MS Univ for Women; MS 65 Univ Southern MS-Hattiesburg; SLP, Hattiesburg P S, **SLP ACE**

Shutt, Mrs Elizabeth Anne Rt 2 Box 1485, Montpelier, VA 23192, (804) 749-4504, BS 73 Radford Univ; ME 78 Univ of VA - Charlottesville; Sp-Lang Path, Private Practice, **SLP**

Sibbald, Julie Monroe 139 Rochelle Avenue #3, Rochelle Park, NJ 07662, (201) 440-2782, BA 68 Boston Univ; MA 82 Montclair St Coll; Sp-Lang Path, South Hackensack Board of Educ, **SLP**

Sibbett, Kathy Sheridan 2068 Mango Circle, Fayetteville, NC 28304, (919) 485-5145, BS 78 WV Univ; MA 79 Univ of Northern IA; Sp-Lang Path, Sthen Sp and Hrng Serv, **SLP**

Sibille, Mrs Claudette B 229 Beverly Drive, Lafayette, LA 70503, (318) 235-5224, BA 57 Univ of Southwestern LA; Sp-Lang Path, Lafayette Parish Schools, **SLP**

Siblesz, Ana Maria Veterans Administration, Audiology And Speech Dep, 3350 La Jolla Village Drive, San Diego, CA 92161, (619) 453-7500, BA 83 Univ of FL; MA 85 FL St Univ; 88–Sp-Lang Path, VA Med Ctr, **SLP**

Sibley, Mrs Kathryn H 302 Rush Road, Fayetteville, NC 28305, (919) 485-6054, BS 42 Northwestern Univ; MA 43 Northwestern Univ; MA 70 Univ of AZ; Sp-Lang Path, Sibley Sp & Lang Serv, **SLP**

Sibley, Michele T 1353 Kensington Road, Grosse Pointe Pk, MI 48230, (203) 456-0575, BA 77 Univ of CA - Santa Barbara; MA 80 Univ of CT; **SLP**

Sibley, William C 12 Northwest Road, Westfield, MA 01085, (413) 568-9592, BA 69 Univ of MA - Amherst; MS 74 Ithaca Coll; Sp/Lang Path, Westfield Pub Sch, **SLP**

Sibon, Brenda Dice Kendall Co Special Ed, 2010 Heather Drive, Aurora, IL 60506, (312) 553-4383, BS 81 Univ of IL - Urbana; MS 83 IL St Univ - Normal; Early Childhood Tchr, Kendall County Special Ed Coop, **SLP**

Sicard, Lisa Anne 837 Combs Street, Jackson, MS 39204, (601) 371-4274, BS 81 Univ Southern MS-Hattiesburg; MS 87 Univ Southern MS-Hattiesburg; 83–Aud, Hinds ENT Surgical Assoc PA, **A**

Sichel, Mrs Ronnie N 23 Alton Road, Stamford, CT 06906, (203) 325-2865, BS 70 CUNY - Brooklyn Coll; MS 74 CUNY - Brooklyn Coll; Sp-Lang Path, Stamford Public Schools, **SLP**

Siciliano, Mrs Linda G 46 Deer Run Road, Brookfield, CT 06804-1723, (203) 775-6347, BA 74 CUNY - Brooklyn Coll; MA 78 NY Univ; Sp-Lang Path, Brookfield Publ Schls, **SLP**

Siciliano-Cagle, Anna M 328 Wilcrest, Houston, TX 77042, (713) 493-9015, BS 82 UT St Univ; MA 85 Univ of Houston - Univ Park; **SLP**

Sick, Steven Wesley 20 Willow Way, Canfield, OH 44406, (216) 533-3675, MA 88 Univ of South AL

Sickles, Robin E Speech Pathologist, 304 Surburban Drive, Toms River, NJ 08753, (201) 244-4953, BA 73 Rider Coll; ME 75 Trenton St Coll; MA 80 Glassboro St Coll; Sp/Lang Path, Private Practice, **SLP**

Sidak, Julie Ann 1225 Sandburg Drive, Bloomington, IL 61704, (309) 438-8641, BS 83 IL St Univ - Normal; MS 85 IL St Univ - Normal; 86–Lecturer, IL St Univ, **A**

Sidler, Mrs Mary E 709 Odana Lane, Madison, WI 53711, (608) 274-4714, BS 74 Univ of WI - Stevens Point; MS 75 Univ of WI - Stevens Point; **SLP**

Sidles, Mrs Sherry Elise 526 West Lane, Centerville, IA 52544, (515) 437-7083, BS 80 Univ of TX - Austin; MA 84 Northeast MO St Univ; Sp-Lang Path Research Assoc, University of Iowa, **SLP**

Sidman, Helene Ruth 2273 East Maple #301, Birmingham, MI 48008, (313) 649-6251, **SLP**

Sidoff, Mrs Chris Ellen Alexis 2900 State Road A1A #622, Atlantic Beach, FL 32233, (904) 246-9576, BS 84 Univ of WI - Milwaukee; MA 86 Our Lady Lake Univ-San Anton; 88–Sp-Lang Path, Duval Co PS Sys, **SLP**

Sidor, Paula M 632 Hill Street, Rochester, MI 48063-7547, **SLP**

Sidtis, Dr John J Department Of Neurology, Memorial Sloan-Kettering, 1275 York Avenue, New York, NY 10021, (212) 207-3279, BA 73 Columbia Univ Teachers Coll; MA Univ of Waterloo - Ontario; PH 78 (Psychology) SUNY - Center at Stony Brook; 87–Asst Psych, Memorial Sloan-Kettering Cancer Ctr

Siebenaler, Ginia K 3772 North Tillotson # 181, Muncie, IN 47304-1654, (317) 286-5724, MA 87 Ball St Univ

Siebers, Mrs Judith M K 2701 Ken Ray Drive, Quincy, IL 62301, (217) 224-0949, BS 76 Western IL Univ; MA 77 Western IL Univ; Sp-Lang Path, Quincy Sch Dist #172, **SLP**

Siebert, Susan Marie 116 Ventura Apartment A, Jefferson City, MO 65109, (314) 635-7141, MA 88 Saint Louis Univ; 88–Sp-Lang Path, Charles E Still Hosp

Sieck, Mrs Sharon 1630 North Murray #204, Colorado Springs, CO 80915, (817) 274-4541, BS 83 Stephen F Austin St Univ; MS 87 Univ of North TX; **SLP**

Sieczko, Christine Krys 2100 North Richmond, Chicago, IL 60647, (312) 278-9436, BA 74 Northeastern IL Univ; MA 76 Memphis St Univ; Consult, Private Practice, **SLP**

Siedenstrang, Mrs Lynn Littleton 3302 South Midland, Nampa, ID 83651-9083, (208) 322-2711, BS 84 ID St Univ; MS 87 ID St Univ

Siedleck, Teri Moser 21 Cedar Court #5, Vernon Hills, IL 60061, (312) 362-2900, BS Eastern IL Univ; MS 86 Eastern IL Univ; 87–Sp-Lang Path, Broy Speech Pathology Assoc, **SLP**

Siefert, Michael J 5480 Cascade Drive, Lisle, IL 60532, (312) 883-3711, BA 72 Lewis Univ; MA 74 Northern IL Univ - De Kalb; Sp-Lang Path, Grant Hosp of Chicago, **A**

Sieff, Dr Sherri L 255-11 Lucas Lane, Voorhees, NJ 08043, (609) 652-1776, BA 72 Case Western Reserve Univ; MA 74 Univ of Southern CA; PH 83 (Special Educ) Univ of Southern CA; 86–Assoc Prof, Stockton St Col, **SLP**

Siegal, Mrs Dorothy R 71 Pilgrim Road, Wellesley, MA 02181, (617) 237-5328, BA 58 Tulane Univ; MS 66 Emerson Coll; Spec Ed Asst Tchr, Wellesley Pub Sch, **SLP**

Siegel, Barbara G 520 West 92nd Street, Indianapolis, IN 46260, (317) 929-3311, BA 79 Lake Forest Coll; MS 81 Univ of MI - Ann Arbor; Sp-Lang Path, Methodist Hosp Indep In, **SLP**

Siegel, Cheryl Lester 2408 Beachwood Boulevard, Beachwood, OH 44122, (216) 382-7663, BS 66 OH St Univ; MA 82 Cleveland St Univ; Sp-Lang Path, Beachwood City Schools, **SLP**

Siegel, Mrs Christine Earle 6035 Valkeith, Houston, TX 77096, (713) 729-5218, BS 80 Southwest TX St Univ; ME 81 Southwest TX St Univ; Sp/Lang Path, Sp Path Assoc, **SLP**

Siegel, Constance 3652 Caminito Carmel Lndg, San Diego, CA 92130, (619) 440-1501, BA 76 CA St Univ - Northridge; MA 78 CA St Univ - Northridge; Sp-Lang Path, Grossmont Un Hs Dist, **SLP**

Siegel, Elaine S 138 Beacon Hill Drive, West Hartford, CT 06117, (203) 236-5294, BS 72 CT Coll; MS 75 Ithaca Coll; 86–Consult/Sp-Lang Path, Hebrew Academy of Greater Hartford, **SLP**

Siegel, Dr Gerald M Speech And Hearing Clinic, University Of Minnesota, 110 Shevlin Hall, Minneapolis, MN 55455, (612) 624-3322, BA 53 CUNY - Brooklyn Coll; MA 54 CUNY - Brooklyn Coll; PH 57 (Comm Disorders) Univ of IA; 61–Professor Communication Disord, University of Minnesota, **F**

Siegel, Harlan C 1 Deborah Drive, Latham, NY 12110, (518) 783-6629, BA 70 Univ of South FL; MA 73 Coll of Saint Rose; Sales Rep, Metropolitan Life Ins Co, **SLP**

Siegel, Mrs Heather B 6374 Northfield Road, West Bloomfield, MI 48322, (313) 851-5960, BS 56 Wayne St Univ; MA 78 Wayne St Univ; 84–Sp/Lang Path, Chldrns Hosp of Mi, **SLP ACE**

Siegel, Helen Lillian 40 Village Hill Drive, Dix Hills, NY 11746, **SLP**

Siegel, Ilene S 6425 North Washtensaw, Chicago, IL 60645, (312) 359-3100, BS 78 Univ of IL - Urbana; MS 79 Univ of IL - Urbana; Sp-Lang Path, Kirk Dev Cen, **SLP**

Siegel, Mrs Julie Regina 709-1 Zlotkin Circle, Freehold, NJ 07728, (201) 308-0125, BS 84 Ithaca Coll; MS 85 Adelphi Univ; Sp-Lang Path, Our Place School Inc, **SLP**

Siegel, Mrs Karen C 229 West Seaview Avenue, Linwood, NJ 08221, (609) 927-2244, BA 60 Stanford Univ; MA 62 Columbia Univ Teachers Coll; Aud, Aud & Assit Lstng Sys, **A ACE**

Siegel, Kim Stevens 332 Virginia Road, Excelsior Springs, MO 64024, (816) 356-3600, BS 82 Central MO St Univ; MS 86 Central MO St Univ; 82–Sp-Lang Path, Raytown Cons Sch Dist, **SLP**

Siegel, Marcia G 24402 Little Hollow Lane, Hidden Hills, CA 91302, **SLP**

Siegel, Mrs Marjory Ellen Marks 8 Richview Court, Potomac, MD 20854, (301) 762-3636, BA 78 Univ of MD - College Park; MA 80 Univ of IL - Urbana; Sp-Lang Path, Private Practice, **SLP ACE**

Siegel, Marshall H Box 452, Lansdale, PA 19446, BS 66 Bloomsburg Univ of PA; MA 72 Temple Univ; Program Dir/Speech-Hrng-Vision, Montgomery Cnty Intermed Unit, **SLP**

Siegel, Mary Ann 1 Deborah Drive, Latham, NY 12110, BS 71 Nazareth Coll of Rochester; MA 73 Coll of Saint Rose; **SLP**

Siegel, Robert B 1 Eves Drive Suite 111, Marlton, NJ 08053-3121, (609) 596-9670, BA 70 Monmouth Coll; MS 73 WV Univ; 84–Aud, Family Hrng Ctrs, **A**

Siegel, Mrs Rona N 38 Mohawk Drive, Springfield, NJ 07081, (201) 467-5425, BA 70 Rutger's St Univ - Douglas Coll; ME 74 Northeastern Univ; 84–Sp-Lang Path, Scotch Plains-Fanwood Sch, **SLP**

Siegel, Mrs Terri M 6007 Howard Road, Panama City, FL 32404, (904) 769-0278, BA 79 Tulane Univ; MS 81 Vanderbilt Univ; Aud, B Philip Cotton MD, **A ACE**

Siegel-Grieves, Cheryl M Director Audiology, St Elizabeth Medical Ctr, 2100 Madison Avenue, Granite City, IL 62040, (618) 798-3616, BA 72 Southern IL Univ-Edwardsvill; MS 77 Southern IL Univ-Edwardsvill; Dir of Aud, St Elizabeth Med Cen, **A**

Siegelman, Steven M 12675 North 79th Dr, Peoria, AZ 85345, (602) 486-1755, OB 71 CUNY - Bernard M Baruch Coll; MS 80 AZ St Univ; Sp-Lang Path, Alhambra Sch Dist, **SLP**

Siegenthaler, Dr Bruce M 126 West Maryln Avenue, State College, PA 16801, (814) 863-2009, BS 43 Bowling Green St Univ; MS 49 Univ of MI - Ann Arbor; PH 51 (NS) Univ of MI - Ann Arbor; 85–Prof/Sp-Lang Path, Penn St U, **SLP A F LM**

Sieger, Ann Parsons 9035 Saranac Drive, Richmond Heights, MO 63117, (314) 946-9499, BS 79 Purdue Univ - West Lafayette; MS 81 Washington Univ; **A**

Siegfried, Pamela N 721 Shady Lane, Pittsburgh, PA 15228, BS 65 Northwestern Univ; MA 66 Northwestern Univ; Sp-Lang Path, Easter Seal Soc/Allegheny Co, **SLP ACE**

Siegle, Diane H Department Of Speech & Hrng Science, University Of Illinois, 901 South 6th Street, Champaign, IL 61820, (217) 333-2230, BS 72 Purdue Univ - West Lafayette; MA 76 Northern IL Univ - De Kalb; Dir of Sp Clinic, Univ of IL, **SLP**

Siegle, Peggy 12 Landing Woods Lane, Falmouth, ME 04105, (207) 781-4230, BA 70 Allegheny Coll; MS 72 Univ of VT; Early Chldhood Consult, Proj Co-Step, **SLP**

Siehl, Georgiana Pacini 2344 Haisley Drive, Ann Arbor, MI 48103, (313) 994-1943, BA 70 9386; MA 71 Western MI Univ; 87–Sp-Lang Path, Lakewood Day Treatment Ctr, **SLP**

Siekmann, Susan N 715 Northbridge Lane, Worthington, OH 43085, (614) 888-4061, **SLP**

Sieling, Mary Margaret 54 Forest Street #214, Medford, MA 02155, (617) 246-3549, BS 84 Ball St Univ; MA 86 Ball St Univ; **SLP**

Sieminski, Dr Louis R 534 Wyoming Avenue, Kingston, PA 18704, (717) 287-8649, BS 69 WV Univ; MA 73 Temple Univ-Tyler Sch of Art; PH 75 (NS) Temple Univ-Tyler Sch of Art; Owner Aud, Aud Consults of NE Pa, **A**

Siems, Mrs Deborah A 9914 West 85th Way, Arvada, CO 80005-1204, (303) 423-1227, BA 77 Univ of CO - Boulder; MA 79 Univ of CO - Boulder; SLP, Jefferson County Schools, **SLP**

Siener, Mrs Mary Ellen Townsend Road, RFD, Groton, MA 01450, (617) 486-4166, **SLP**

Siepser, Mrs Zell A 265 Chadbourne Way, Oakland, CA 94619, (415) 530-3127, BA 75 Univ of CA - Berkeley; MA 77 Univ of the Pacific; 86–Sp-Lang Path, Faltz Associates, **SLP**

Sierra, Mrs Lynne Marie 111 Lathrop Road, South Hadley, MA 01075-1736, (413) 538-8182, BA 82 Univ of RI; MA 84 Univ of RI; **SLP**

Sierra-Irizarry, Benigno 5110 Cabin Lake, San Antonio, TX 78244, (512) 662-7005, BS 72 0169; MS 74 Univ of PR - Rio Piedras; Chief of Aud, U S Air Force, **A ACE**

Sierzega, Carol D 823 Oakridge Dr, Milton, WI 53563, (312) 349-4163, BS 77 Western IL Univ; MA 79 Univ of IL - Urbana; SLP, Aero Sp Ed Dist, **SLP**

Sieve, Patricia Ann 7544 Lovella, St Louis, MO 63117, (314) 645-8936, BS 82 Saint Louis Univ; MA 83 Saint Louis Univ; Sp-Lang Path & Classroom Tchr, Sp Sch Dist of St Louis County, **SLP**

Sievers, Frankie J 931 King Drive, Bartlesville, OK 74006, (918) 335-0588, BA 75 Southern IL Univ-Edwardsvill; MS 76 Southern IL Univ-Edwardsvill; Sp-Lang Path, Tri-Quad Sp Serv Coop, **SLP**

Sievert, Amy Jo 2925 Glenhurst Avenue #2, St Louis Park, MN 55416, (612) 474-2305, BS 84 Univ of WI - Stevens Point; MS 86 Univ of WI - Stevens Point; 87–Aud, West Metro Aud Spec, **A**

Sievert, Rosalind June 485 Bille Road, Paradise, CA 95969, (916) 534-0423, 88–CH Tchr, Butte Co Spec Educ, **SLP**

Siff, Mrs Jacqueline 11111 Hedwiglane, Houston, TX 77024, **SLP**

Siffrin, Sandra L 5504 Sycamore Avenue, Baltimore, MD 21227, (301) 396-0528, BS 68 Towson St Univ; MS 80 William Carey Coll; Sp-Lang Path, Balto Cty Pub Sch, **SLP**

Sigal, Beverly 1 Horizon Road #619, Fort Lee, NJ 07024, BA 67 Jersey City St Coll; MA 69 Gallaudet Coll; Chief Aud, Beth Israel Med Cen, **A**

Sigal, Mrs Paula Ellen B 124 Caroline Avenue, Somerset, MA 02725, (401) 245-7400, BA 78 Univ of RI; MS 80 Univ of RI; Sp-Lang Path, Barrington Pub Sch, **SLP**

Sigars, Judith Regina 110 Seeno Street, Monterey, CA 93940, (408) 649-4087, BS 72 CA St Univ - Hayward; MS 87 Nova Univ; 87–Sp-Lang Path, InSpeech Inc, **SLP**

Sigel, Mrs Meryl L 24 Lantern Lane, Newton, MA 02159, (617) 527-6977, BS 65 Boston Univ; ME 66 Boston Univ; Sp-Lang Path, Private Practice, **SLP**

Sigelman, Joye A 4006 Basswood Road, Minneapolis, MN 55416, (612) 942-9232, BS 64 Univ of IA; MA 66 Stanford Univ; Aud, Sales, Serv, Consult, Argosy Electronics, **A**

Sigl, Bonnie L 2612 South Judy Avenue, Sioux Falls, SD 57103-6321, (605) 371-2215, BS Univ of NE - Omaha; MS 84 Univ of NE - Omaha; **SLP**

Sigman, Myrna K 45 Shadetree Lane, Roslyn Heights, NY 11577, (516) 621-5440, OB 56; MS 68 Adelphi Univ; Dir-Cl Serv, Private Practice, **SLP**

Sigmund, Mrs Claudia J 601 Stewart Avenue, Grove City, PA 16127, (412) 458-7570, BS 72 Kent St Univ; MA 76 IN Univ - Bloomington; 81–Sp-Lang Path, Grove City Area Schools, **SLP**

Signoracci, Christine Jeanette 105 1/2 Columbia Street, Mansfield, OH 44902, (419) 264-2446, BA 1952; MA OH St Univ; Sp-Lang Path, Richland Therapy Service, **SLP**

Siguenza, Philippa M 731 Farmingdale Road, Lancaster, PA 17603, (717) 392-6076, BS 84 Bloomsburg Univ of PA; MS 85 Loyola Coll; **SLP**

Sigvardt, Mrs Dorothy 1440 Downington Avenue, Salt Lake City, UT 84105, (801) 328-7372, BA 74 Univ of UT; MA 76 Univ of UT; Consult, Salt Lake City Sch Dist, **SLP**

Sihler, Mrs Patricia C 1310 Chestnut Ridge, Naperville, IL 60540, (312) 355-4150, BA 70 Univ of KY; MA 72 Univ of KY; Sp-Lang Path, Easter Seal Cen, **SLP**

Sijan, Amy O 868 Creighton Drive, Fort Myers, FL 33907, (813) 936-1459, BA 72 Miami Univ - Oxford; MA 78 Bowling Green St Univ; Teacher, Lee County Schools, **SLP**

Sikes, Mrs Kelly Dowdle 106 Lone Pine, De Queen, AR 71832, (501) 584-4311, BS 82 Henderson St Univ; MS 85 Univ of AR - Fayetteville; 82–Sp-Lang Path, DeQueen PS, **SLP**

Sikes, Mrs Terri Eith 3102 W Roxboro Road N E, Atlanta, GA 30324, (404) 953-2223, BS 85 Univ of GA; ME 87 Univ of GA

Sikorski, Christine 101 Pepper Place, Charlottesville, VA 22901, **A**

Sikorski, Lorna D 11142 Wickford Drive, Santa Ana, CA 92705, (714) 838-6002, BA 74 Univ of CA - Davis; MA 80 CA St Univ - Long Beach; 87–Sp-Lang Path, LDS & Associates, **SLP**

Sikov, Mrs Elaine Linda 2701 Colby Avenue, Los Angeles, CA 90064, (213) 294-0031, BS 71 Wayne St Univ; MA 83 CA St Univ - Los Angeles; SLP, Los Angeles Cty Sch, **SLP**

Silbar, Jean C 3260 Bradford N E, Grand Rapids, MI 49506, (616) 241-2338, BA 74 MI St Univ; MA 76 MI St Univ; Exec Dir, Comp Therapy Ctr Inc, **SLP**

Silber, Kim Marie 5677-2 Carter Street, Fort Hood, TX 76544, (817) 532-7291, BA 83 Univ of Northern CO; MS 86 Baylor Univ; **SLP**

Silberberg, Rhonda L 12501 West 97th Terrace, Lenexa, KS 66215, (212) 519-7000, **SLP**

Silberg, Kathryn S 1409 Ashland Road #G, Columbia, MO 65201, (314) 442-5437, OB 86 Univ of MO - Columbia; OM 87 Univ of MO - Columbia; 88–Sp-Lang Path, Therapy for Kids, **SLP**

Silbergleit, Alice Klain University Of Michigan Medical Center, University Hospital-Department Of PM&R, Room 1H243, Ann Arbor, MI 48109-0050, (313) 936-7080, BA 81 MI St Univ; MA 83 Wayne St Univ; 86–Sp-Lang Path, Univ of MI Med Ctr, **SLP**

Silberman, Hilary Joy 235 West 102 Street 10E, New York, NY 10025, (212) 222-1823, BS 84 Ithaca Coll; MS 87 Columbia Univ Teachers Coll; 88–Sp-Lang Path, NY League for Hard of Hrng

Silberman, Mrs Judith 552 Choptank Cove Court, Annapolis, MD 21401, (301) 687-6500, BA 66 Univ of MI - Ann Arbor; MS 68 Univ of MI - Ann Arbor; OM 81 George Washington Univ; Ch Sp-Lang Hrng, Baltimore Co Dept of Hlth, **SLP**

Silberman, Judith R 4801 Chesapeake Street N W, Washington, DC 20016, **SLP**

Silbernagel, Mrs Melinda J 733 North Knox #81, Monmouth, OR 97361, (503) 838-3062, ME 88 Western OR St Coll

Silbernagle, Mary Jo 410 Pinal Avenue, Old Orcutt, CA 93455, MA 73 Humboldt St Univ; Sp-Lang Path, Private Practice, **SLP**

Silcox, Terry L 116 B Lester Road, Statesboro, GA 30458, (912) 764-8200, BS 79 Auburn Univ - Auburn; OM 82 Auburn Univ - Auburn; 88–Owner, Audiological Svcs, **A**

Siler, Mrs Kathy F 6521 Winifred Drive, Fort Worth, TX 76133, BS 74 TX Tech Univ; MS 74 TX Tech Univ; **SLP**

Siler, Mrs Rebecca S 6756 Moss Lake Drive, Hixson, TN 37343, (615) 870-0616, BS 63 East TN St Univ; MA 77 East TN St Univ; 66–Sp/Lang Path, Chatnga Pub Sch, **SLP**

Silio, Paula M 341 Holt Lane, Springfield, PA 19064, (215) 328-6257, BA 75 Catholic Univ of America; MA 81 West Chester Univ of PA; Sp/Lang Path, De Co Inter Ut, **SLP**

Silkensen, Mary P P O Box 947, Russellville, AR 72801, (501) 968-2527, BA 58 Univ of AR - Fayetteville; **SLP**

Silkwood, Valerie Gail 8454 Los Serranos Way, Citrus Heights, CA 95610, (916) 722-4616, BA 81 Univ of CA - Santa Barbara; MS 83 Univ of WY; 86–Sp-Lang Path, Olga Ramirez Assoc, **SLP**

Siller, Mrs Evelyn Anne 3336 S W 57th Place, Fort Lauderdale, FL 33312, (305) 961-4718, BA 76 CUNY - Brooklyn Coll; MS 79 CUNY - Brooklyn Coll; 88–Aud, Nova Univ Comm Dis Ctr

Silliman, Elaine R 4479 Vieux Carre Circle, Tampa, FL 33613, (813) 974-2006, BS 60 Syracuse Univ; PH 76 (NS) CUNY - Grad Sch & Univ Cntr; Prof & Dept Chair, Univ of S Florida, **SLP F ACE**

Sills, Audrey E 4481 Washington Square #2, Youngstown, OH 44515, (216) 793-4022, BS 67 Central MO St Univ; MS 71 Central MO St Univ; Sp-Lang Path, Austintown Sch Sys, **SLP**

Sills, Mrs Margaret S 28 Lakeside Drive, Guilford, CT 06437, (203) 453-8605, BA 60 Albright Coll; MA 62 Univ of CT; 88–Sp-Lang Path, New Haven Bd of Educ, **SLP**

Sills, Marsha H 16058 Haynes Bluff, Baton Rouge, LA 70816, **SLP**

Silman, Dr Shlomo 3123 Avenue P, Brookland, NY 11234, (201) 676-1000, BA 60; MS 71 Columbia Univ Teachers Coll; PH 77 (NS) NY Univ; Professor, City Univ of New York-Brooklyn, **A F**

Silny, D Elaine 14744 S W 71st Terrace, Miami, FL 33193, (305) 386-3634, BS 72 Skidmore Coll; MA 75 CUNY - Queens Coll; Sp/Lang Path, Dade Co PS, **SLP**

Siloac, Dr Kenneth T 285 Dorchester Road, Akron, OH 44313, (216) 375-7883, BS 62 Wayne St Univ; ME 68 Wayne St Univ; PH 71 (SLP) Wayne St Univ; 71–Assoc Prof, U of Akron, **SLP**

Silva, Deborah B 1 Sassafras Lane, Pittsford, NY 14534, BA 71 Univ of MA - Amherst; MA 73 Univ of CT; 87–Sp-Lang Path, Honeoye Falls-Lima Central Schs, **SLP**

Silva, Mrs Michele R Rd 2 Box 2695, 29 Birch Avenue, Lake George, NY 12845, (518) 668-3579, BS 75 Coll of Saint Rose; MS 77 Coll of Saint Rose; 82–Sp-Lang Path, UCP Cen of Tri-Co, Inc, **SLP**

Silva, Susan C 25 Newcomb Street, Haverhill, MA 01830, (617) 374-3440, BA 67 Univ of NH; MS 76 Univ of South FL; Coord-Spec Ed, Haverhill Pub Schs, **SLP**

Silver, Clara M 11518 Gauguin, Potomac, MD 20854, (301) 762-2607, BA 60 Univ of MD - College Park; MA 65 George Washington Univ; Sp-Lang Path, **SLP**

Silver, J Diane 16842 West 74th Avenue, Golden, CO 80403, (303) 288-0791, BA 75 CA St Univ - Northridge; MA 76 CA St Univ - Northridge; SLP, Adams Co Sch Dist #14, **SLP**

Silver, Jane 242 Stanford, Kensington, CA 94708, (415) 524-7010, SLP, Private Practice, **SLP**

Silver, Jane Ellen 783 English Road, Rochester, NY 14616, (716) 637-5303, BA 85 SUNY - Coll at Cortland; MA 86 SUNY - Coll at Geneseo; 86–Sp-Lang Path, Brockport Central Sch, **SLP**

Silver, Joy E 3 South Haddon Avenue Suite 6, Haddonfield, NJ 08033, (609) 428-5516, BA 73 Montclair St Coll; MA 76 Trenton St Coll; 87–Sp-Lang Path/Dir, Silver Speech Associates, **SLP ACE**

Silver, Lynn 4601 Eaton Ct, Plano, TX 75093, (214) 964-7806, **SLP**

Silver, Dr Marilyn B 95 West 95th Street #18-G, New York, NY 10025, (212) 430-5595, BA 54 CUNY - Hunter Coll; MA 60 CUNY - Brooklyn Coll; PH 76 (Sp & Hrng Sciences) CUNY - Grad Sch & Univ Cntr; Asst Prof, A Einstein Coll of Med, **SLP A**

Silver, Marsha A Childrens Health Council, 700 Sand Hill Road, Palo Alto, CA 94304, (415) 326-5530, BS 73 Syracuse Univ; MS 76 Univ of Redlands; Chief/Speech-Language, Childrens Health Council, **SLP**

Silver, Nancy Reguly 27621 Agrado, Mission Viejo, CA 92692, (714) 837-5689, BA 84 Univ of CA - Santa Barbara; MA 86 CA St Univ - Northridge; 88–Sp-Lang Path, Winways Trans Living Ctr, **SLP**

Silver, Roberta 5415 North Sheridan Road, Apartment 4809, Chicago, IL 60640, (312) 508-4136, BS 73 Northern IL Univ - De Kalb; MA 74 Northern IL Univ - De Kalb; Sp-Lang Path, Chicago Bd of Ed, **SLP**

Silver, Mrs Roberta A Lotreck 903 Naugatuck Avenue, Milford, CT 06460, (203) 385-4225, BS 77 Miami Univ - Oxford; MS 79 Coll of Saint Rose; Sp/Lang Path, **SLP**

Silver, Sharon Arlene 10511 N E 38th Court, Vancouver, WA 98686, (206) 573-0653, BS 79 OR Coll of Education; MS 84 Univ of WI - Stevens Point; 87–Sp-Lang Path, Emanuel Hosp, **SLP**

Silver, Mrs Susan A 1034 Bertram Avenue, Dayton, OH 45406, (513) 855-6581, BS 73 Univ of Cincinnati; MS 75 Indiana Univ of PA; SLP, Valley View Local Schools, **SLP**

Silver, Mrs Valeria Bonnette 205 Maple Drive, West Oaks, Summerville, SC 29483, (803) 873-3050, BA 75 SC St Coll; MA 79 SC St Coll; Sp-Lang Path, Summerville School District 2, **SLP**

Silver, Valerie 12111 Audelia #1914, Dallas, TX 75243, (214) 358-5261, BS 81 Univ of North TX; MS 82 Univ of North TX; Sp-Lang Path, Dallas Soc for Crippled Chldn, **SLP**

Silverberg, Barbara Sue 357-A Wrenfield Road, Florence, SC 29501, (803) 669-8891, BS 80 WV Univ; MS 81 WV Univ; 87–Sp-Lang Path, Hlth South Rehab Ctr, **SLP**

Silverberg, Mary H 111 Newington Road, West Hartford, CT 06110, (203) 827-2235, BA 70 Kean Coll of NJ; MS 79 Southern CT St Univ; 79–Sp-Lang Path, New Britain Pub Sch, **SLP**

Silverio, Albert P Audiologic Services, 238 West State Street, Jacksonville, IL 62650, (217) 243-5121, BA 68 Univ of IA; MA 73 Univ of IA; Owner/Mgr, Aud Serv, **A**

Silverman, Mrs Anita H Sir Mortimer B Davis-Jewish General Hospital, 3755 Cote St Catherine Road, Montreal, PQ, Canada H3P 1E2, (514) 342-8276, BA 69 McGill Univ - Quebec; ME 71 Boston Univ; 73–Sp-Lang Path, Davis-Jewish Gen Hosp, **SLP**

Silverman, Mrs Barbara K 7817 Beckwith, Morton Grove, IL 60053, (312) 966-2709, BS 67 Univ of WI - Madison; MS 68 Univ of WI - Madison; Sp/Lang Path, ABC Home Hlth of Illinois, **SLP**

Silverman, Dr Carol A 625 Main Street #338, New York, NY 10044, (212) 481-4464, BA 75 Wellesley Coll; MS 76 Columbia Univ Teachers Coll; PH 82 (Aud) NY Univ; 88–Assoc Prof of Aud, Hunter Coll City Univ of New York, **A**

Silverman, Mrs E Sara 6 Woodsyde Place, Owings Mills, MD 21117, (301) 356-9229, BA 71 CUNY - Queens Coll; MA 74 Cleveland St Univ; Sp-Lang Path, Madeline Fox Associates, **SLP**

Silverman, Mrs Eleanor T 347 West 57th Street #29C, New York, NY 10019, (212) 586-1191, BA 40 CUNY - Hunter Coll; MA 53 CUNY - Brooklyn Coll; Assoc Prof, NY U Coll of Dentistry, **SLP LM**

Silverman, Dr Ellen-Marie 3475 North Cramer, Milwaukee, WI 53211, (414) 962-4482, BS 64 Univ of WI - Milwaukee; MA 67 Univ of IA; PH 70 (NS) Univ of IA; Sp-Lang Path, Curative Rehab Ctr, **SLP F**

Silverman, Mrs Fran L 322 Raussell Place, Severna Park, MD 21146, (301) 263-3065, BA 77 CUNY - Queens Coll; MA 78 Univ of MD - College Park; SLP, Anne Arundel Co Pub Sch, **SLP**

Silverman, Dr Franklin H College Of Speech, Marquette University, Milwaukee, WI 53233, (414) 421-4254, BS 60 Emerson Coll; MA 61 Northwestern Univ; PH 66 (NS) Univ of IA; Prof of Speech, Marquette University, **SLP F**

Silverman, Henrietta C 11516 Lake Ridge Road, Tampa, FL 33618, (813) 872-2771, BA 65 CUNY - Queens Coll; MA 66 OH St Univ; Dir Sp-Lang Path, Hill Haven Inc, **SLP ACE**

Silverman, Dr Irving University Of Louisville, Department Of Pediatrics, Louisville, KY 40292, (502) 562-7710, BS 51 Univ of Pittsburgh - Pittsburgh; MS 55 Univ of Pittsburgh - Pittsburgh; PH 63 (Aud) Univ of WI - Madison; Dir Commun Dis Serv, Pedia Dept U of Louisville, **SLP A LM**

Silverman, Jan L 10 Elm Ridge Drive, Toronto, ON, Canada M6B 1A1, (416) 789-2212, BA 73 SUNY - Center at Buffalo; MA 75 SUNY - Center at Buffalo; Aud, Central Clinic, **A**

Silverman, Jane M 10 North Buckhout Street, Irvington, NY 10533-1809, (914) 591-9198, MA 75 Univ of Denver; Research Associate, Alan Guttmacher Institute, **SLP**

Silverman, Judith 73-22 192nd Street, Flushing, NY 11366, (516) 599-1393, BA 60 CUNY - Queens Coll; MA 61 Univ of WI - Madison; Sp-Lang Path, Lynbrook NY Bd of Ed, **SLP**

Silverman, Kathe F 84 Dover Street, Brooklyn, NY 11235, **SLP**

Silverman, Laurie A 3300 Third Avenue, San Diego, CA 92103, (619) 581-0051, BA 77 Univ of MD - College Park; MA 79 San Diego St Univ; 86–Dir of Sp-Lang Path, Laurie Silverman & Assoc, **SLP**

Silverman, Lenore A 47 Roselyn Terrace, San Francisco, CA 94118-4320, (415) 752-9134, **SLP**

Silverman, Mrs Melanie 521 Prescott Road, Merion, PA 19066, (215) 527-3005, BA 67 Rutger's St Univ - Douglas Coll; MA 68 Northwestern Univ; Aud, A J Woodring MD & M R Pugh MD, **A**

Silverman, Miriam Beth 607 Winterset Parkway, Marietta, GA 30067-6543, (205) 871-2495, OB 83 Univ of MO - Columbia; ME 85 Univ of GA; **SLP**

Silverman, Mrs Nancy E 2102 East Plumwood Lane, Santa Ana, CA 92701, (714) 996-5550, BA 72 CA St Univ - Los Angeles; MA 74 SUNY - Coll at Geneseo; Sp-Lang Path, Placentia USD, **SLP**

Silverman, Rita C 520 North Croft Avenue, Apartment 212, Los Angeles, CA 90048, (213) 936-2153, BA 76 CUNY - Queens Coll; MA 78 CUNY - Queens Coll; Sp-Lang Path, Scottish Rite Chldrn Lang Dis, **SLP**

Silverman, Robyn D 326 Kirkland Drive, Richmond, VA 23227, (804) 254-6071, BS 85 SUNY - Coll at Buffalo; MS 87 SUNY - Coll at Buffalo; 88–Sp-Lang Path, Sheltering Arms Rehab Hosp

Silverman, Dr S Richard 2510 N W 38th Street, Gainesville, FL 32605, (904) 377-2310, BA 33 Cornell Univ; MS 38 Washington Univ; PH 42 (Education) Washington Univ; **A F H LM**

Silverman, Sandra D 30030 Cheviot Hills Drive, Franklin, MI 48025, (313) 851-4670, BS 71 Northeastern IL Univ; MS 74 Southern CT St Univ; **SLP**

Silverman, Sheryl 401 Executive Center Drive, Apartment G206, West Palm Beach, FL 33401, (305) 478-5006, BS 85 McKendree Coll; MS 87 McKendree Coll; **SLP**

Silverman, Mrs Shirley 604-36 Washington Sq South, Apartment 2817, Philadelphia, PA 19106-4115, (215) 592-4069, BA 74 Temple Univ-Tyler Sch of Art; MA 75 Trenton St Coll; Sp-Lang Path, Sch Dist of Phila, **SLP**

Silverman, Shirley S 1354-D Sperber Road, Fair Lawn, NJ 07410, (201) 791-9577, BA 45 CUNY - Hunter Coll; MS 73 Paterson St Coll; **SLP**

Silverman, Dr Sidney I 80 Park Avenue, New York, NY 10016, (212) 697-5988, BS 34 CUNY - City College; DD 37 (Prosthodontics Geriatrics) NY Univ; Res Prof-Nyu Coll Dent, Private Practice, **LM**

Silvernail, Karen M 7478 Canford Court, Winter Park, FL 32792, ME 71 Univ of FL; SLP, Seminole Co Sch Bd, **SLP**

Silverstein, Aditi Eve Center For Rehabilitation & Development Incorporated, 1615 Franklin Road SW, Roanoke, VA 24016, (703) 343-2753, BA 68 Univ of MI - Ann Arbor; MA 69 Univ of IL - Urbana; 86–Pres/Dir, Ctr for Rehab & Dev Inc, **SLP**

Silverstein, Dr Bernard 7808 Sheffield Drive, Knoxville, TN 37919, (615) 974-4643, BA 49 PA St Univ - Univ Park; MA 51 Temple Univ; PH 53 (NS) Purdue Univ - West Lafayette; Prof, University of Tennessee, **SLP**

Silverstein, Cheryl Rita 118 Pepperidge Circle, Fairfield, CT 06430, (203) 255-7424, BA 83 Univ of CT; MS 85 Univ of MI - Ann Arbor; 85–Aud, Drs Gill & Levinson PC, **A**

Silverstein, Jan W 5989 South Wolff Court, Littleton, CO 80123, (303) 795-9859, BS 68 TX Tech Univ; MA 70 Univ of Denver; Sp-Lang Path, Private Practice, **SLP**

Silverstein, Mrs Lori Michele 2580 Oxford #A-5, Berkley, MI 48072, (313) 544-7681, BA 84 MI St Univ; MA 86 Wayne St Univ; **SLP**

Silverstein, Roberta J 1602 Endriss Drive, Martinez, CA 94553, (707) 643-8474, BA 72 Univ of MI - Ann Arbor; MS 73 Univ of MI - Ann Arbor; Special Education Teacher, Valleio USD, **SLP**

Silvertrust, Joanne E 214 First Street, Libertyville, IL 60048, (312) 367-3250, BS 78 Bradley Univ; MS 80 Bradley Univ; Sp-Lang Path, Hawthorn Dist 73, **SLP**

Silverwood, Pamela Army Audiology & Speech Center, Walter Reed Hospital, 6825 16th Street NW, Washington, DC 20307-5001, (202) 576-1677, BS 62 IL St Univ - Normal; MA 65 Western MI Univ; Sp-Lang Path, Walter Reed Army Med Cen, **SLP ACE**

Silvestain, Carol B 8129 South Corona Court, Littleton, CO 80122, (303) 893-4509, BA 82 Univ of KY; MA 85 Univ of Denver; 87–SLP, Denver Gen Hosp, **SLP**

Silvestri, Susan C 590 Doremus Avenue, Glen Rock, NJ 07452, (201) 427-0397, BS 72 Kent St Univ; MS 74 William Paterson Coll; Private Practice, **SLP**

Silvestro, Mrs Elizabeth Rice 227 Lark Circle, Clemson, SC 29631, BA 81 Case Western Reserve Univ; MA 83 Cleveland St Univ; SLP, Oconee Ps, **SLP**

Silvey, A Anne Box 396, Lancaster, MO 63548, (515) 682-8591, BS 68 Northeast MO St Univ; MA 69 Northeast MO St Univ; Sp-Lang Path, Southern Prairie AEA 15, **SLP**

Silvidi, Alfred C 4461 Salsbury Lane, Stow, OH 44224, (216) 650-7448, BS 64 Kent St Univ; MA 69 Kent St Univ; 86–Reg Vice President, Alltel Service Corp, **SLP**

Sima, Shannon Marie 1229 Pineview Street, Cheney, WA 99004, (509) 456-7086, BA 83 Eastern WA Univ; MS 84 Eastern WA Univ; 84–Sp-Lang Path, Educ Svc Dist 101, **SLP**

Sima-Eichler, Elizabeth 21 Hidden Creek Circle, Pittsford, NY 14534, (716) 334-7090, BS 75 SUNY - Coll at Geneseo; MS 77 Nazareth Coll of Rochester; Sp-Lang Path, Monroe Co BOCES #1, **SLP**

Siman, Dr Robin K 41899 Waterfall Road, Northville, MI 48167, (313) 348-1322, BA 73 Univ of MI - Ann Arbor; MS 74 Univ of MI - Ann Arbor; DD 84 (NS) Univ of MI - Ann Arbor; Dentist, Private Practice, **SLP**

Simancek, Gerald E Rrd 1 Box 13, Gouldsboro, PA 18424, (717) 348-1321, BS 72 East Stroudsburg Univ of PA; MA 75 Trenton St Coll; Dir SLP/Aud, Allied Serv Hndcpd Inc, **SLP**

Simanonis, Mrs Marcy Koonz 10010 Forest Lane #321, Dallas, TX 75243, (214) 343-2467, MS 88 Univ of TX - Dallas

Simasek, Mrs Mary Grace 108 Nina Circle, Williamsburg, VA 23185, (804) 565-0303, BS 77 WV Univ; MS 78 Indiana Univ of PA; Sp/Lang Path, Chld Dev Resources, **SLP**

Simek, Marlene Theresa 4601 Hartford, Abilene, TX 79605, (915) 692-1633, BA 82 TX Tech Univ; MS 84 Univ of TX - Dallas; Aud, West TX Rehab Cen, **A**

Simek, Sheryl L P O Box 7496, Glendale, CA 91205, (619) 327-1581, BS 80 Purdue Univ - West Lafayette; MS 82 Purdue Univ - West Lafayette; Sp-Lang Path, Los Angeles USD, **SLP**

Simenc, Bridget Garin 227 East 214th Street, Euclid, OH 44123, (216) 289-7251, BA 86 Cleveland St Univ; MA 87 Cleveland St Univ; 88–Sp-Lang Path, The Positive Educ Prog

Simison, Paul R 315 Ratley Road, West Suffield, CT 06093, (203) 561-2345, BS 73 Rensselaer Polytech Inst; OM 74 Smith Coll; MA 81 Univ of CT; Aud, Hearing Aid Servs, **A**

Simison, Mrs Victoria B 3486 Charlevoix Avenue, Windsor, ON, Canada N9E 3B1, (519) 253-2481, OB 74 Univ of Western Ontario; OM 75 Univ of Western Ontario; 82–Sp-Lang Path, Windsor Catholic Sep Sch Bd, **SLP**

Simko, Rita McWilliams 3330 Churn Creek Road #D-3, Redding, CA 96002, (916) 221-7380, BA 77 Humboldt St Univ; MA 80 Humboldt St Univ; Aud, Audiology Assoc of Redding, **A**

Simmering, Brenda D 403 Valley Drive, Pine Bluff, AR 71602, (501) 247-5040, BS 83 AR St Univ; MS 87 Univ of AR - Medical Sci; Sp-Lang Path, Sheridan Sch Dist, **SLP**

Simmie, Mrs Kathy Jo 2005 St Henry Avenue, Saskatoon, SK, Canada S7M 0P4, (306) 966-1320, BS 73 Minot St Univ; MS 74 Minot St Univ; 80–Sp/Lang Path, Saskatch Presch Aud Rehab Cen, **SLP**

Simmonds, Nancy G 5 Cambridge Drive, Annandale, NJ 08801, (201) 730-8878, BA 67 Rutger's St Univ - Douglas Coll; MS 69 Univ of HI - Manoa; SLP, Home Health Services, **SLP**

Simmons, Mrs A Ferrin 1313 Hammerhead Lane, Virginia Beach, VA 23464, BA 73 Univ of MS; OM 74 Univ of MS; **SLP**

Simmons, Beth H 3550-M Water Vistas Pkwy, Lawrenceville, GA 30244, (404) 483-9504, BS 74 Univ of GA; ME 75 Univ of GA; Sp-Lang Path, Rockdale Co Bd of Ed, **SLP**

Simmons, Bettie B 402 Medical Arts Tower, Jasper, AL 35501, (205) 221-4630, BS 74 Univ of TX - Austin; OM 76 LA St Univ - N O Medical Ctr; Audiologist, Jasper Eye and Ear Clinic, **A**

Simmons, Mrs Deborah A 3399 Eden Way Circle, Carmel, IN 46032, (317) 773-6579, BS 76 Univ of IL - Urbana; MA 77 Univ of IL - Urbana; 86–Aud, Northeast Otolaryngology, **A**

Simmons, Deborah S Box 4717 RR2, Bowdoinham, ME 04008, (207) 729-6751, BS 69 Kent St Univ; MA 71 Kent St Univ; Sp-Lang Path, Maine Sch Admin Dist #75, **SLP**

Simmons, Mrs Diana Strauss Bowling Green St Univ, 338 South Hall, Bowling Green, OH 43403, (419) 372-7185, BS 78 Northeastern Univ; MA 79 Case Western Reserve Univ; Supvr of Aud, Bowling Green State U, **A**

Simmons, Donna M Doctors Hearing Center Inc, 1950 Arlington Street, Suite 232, Sarasota, FL 34232, (813) 953-7097, BA 75 Tulane Univ; OM 76 LA St Univ - N O Medical Ctr; Aud/Owner, Doctors Hearing Center Inc, **A**

Simmons, Mrs Elizabeth Champe 2410 Woodland Avenue, South Charleston, WV 25303, (304) 348-6689, MA 84 Marshall Univ; Sp-Lang Path, Kanawha County Schools, **SLP**

Simmons, Dr Frederick 1421 South Orleans Avenue, Bowling Green, OH 43402, (419) 241-6219, BS 77 Edinboro Univ of PA; MA 79 Bowling Green St Univ; PH 82 (Aud) Bowling Green St Univ; 85–Policy Advisor, Blue Cross of NW Ohio, **A**

Simmons, Mrs Harriet A 202 Spyglass Drive, Eugene, OR 97401, (503) 686-0802, BS 53 Univ of OR; ME 62 Univ of OR; Retired, **SLP**

Simmons, Joanne 242 North Estelle, Wichita, KS 67214, (316) 683-4654, BA 51 Univ of IA; MA 55 Univ of IA; Sp-Lang Path, Wichita Pub Sch #259, **SLP**

Simmons, John R 101 Billings Drive, Edinboro, PA 16412, (814) 732-2432, BS 53 Eastern IL Univ; MS 55 PA St Univ - Univ Park; 67–Associate Professor, Edinboro University, **SLP**

Simmons, Johnny O Speech Pathology & Audiology, 1410 Lower Campus Drive, University Of Hawaii, Honolulu, HI 96822, (808) 948-8279, BS 71 East Carolina Univ; MA 72 East Carolina Univ; ED 83 (Sp-Lang Path) Univ of GA; 86–Asst Prof, Univ of Hawaii, **SLP**

Simmons, Juanita Faye 9117 Winton Road #2, Cincinnati, OH 45231-3845, (513) 522-8508, BA 67 IN Univ - Bloomington; OM 72 IN Univ - Bloomington; Sp-Lang Path, Cincinnati PS, **SLP**

Simmons, Judi I 65 Alden Avenue, Revere, MA 02151, **SLP**

Simmons, Kathryn M Dept Communicative Disorders, University Of Wisconsin, 1975 Willow Drive, Madison, WI 53706, (608) 262-3951, BS 62 Univ of WI - Madison; MS 70 Univ of WI - Madison; Cl Instr, Dept of Commun Dis U of WI, **SLP**

Simmons, Katrina June 1408 Chickasaw Road, Oxford, MS 38655, (601) 465-7436, **SLP**

Simmons, Laura Vanita 6932 Petworth, Memphis, TN 38119, (901) 756-0581, MA 87 Memphis St Univ; 80–Sp-Lang Path/Coord of Sp Therapy Svcs, Shelby County Schs

Simmons, Margaret E 3465 Tulipwood Drive, Paducah, KY 42001, (503) 443-3232, BA 65 Univ of KY; ME 67 Wayne St Univ; SLP, Private Practice, **SLP**

Simmons, Mrs Marie Vest 1308 Fairfax Drive, Raleigh, NC 27609-4706, (919) 693-4613, BS 85 East Carolina Univ; MS 86 Univ of NC - Chapel Hill; 86–Sp-Lang Path, Granville Co PS, **SLP**

Simmons, Mrs Mary E 302 Hillcrest Road, Franklin, KY 42134, (502) 586-8493, BA 76 Western KY Univ; MA 77 Western KY Univ; OM 81 Western KY Univ; Sp-Lang Path, Simpson Co Sch Syst, **SLP**

Simmons, Mrs Nanci W 6282 Occoquan Forest Drive, Manassas, VA 22111, (703) 450-4000, BS 79 Old Dominion Univ; OM 81 Univ of SC - Columbia; Sp-Lang Path, Prince William Public Schools, **SLP**

Simmons, Nina N 1347 Coliseum Street, New Orleans, LA 70130, (504) 897-8563, BA 69 LA St Univ - Baton Rouge; MS 75 Tulane Univ; Chief Sp-Lang Path, Touro Inf, **SLP**

Simmons, Mrs Patricia C 915 South Green Street, Glasgow, KY 42141, (502) 773-3671, BA 76 Western KY Univ; MA 77 Western KY Univ; Sp-Lang Path, Cauerna Indep Sch Syst, **SLP**

Simmons, Patrilla Sue 1024 Columbine, Wenatchee, WA 98801, (509) 662-9167, BA 79 CA St Univ - Northridge; MA 80 CA St Univ - Northridge; **SLP**

Simmons, Mrs Ruby Kelly Route 3 Box 147, Newport, NC 28570, (919) 223-4840, BA 36 East Carolina Univ; MA 67 Western Carolina Univ; **SLP LM**

Simmons, Mrs Sally D 120 Sunset Drive, Lot 8, Lodi, OH 44254-0251, (216) 948-2046, BA 85 Univ of Akron; MA 87 Univ of Akron; 87–Sp-Lang Path, InSpeech Inc, **SLP**

Simmons, Sheila 410 North 29th Street, Parsons, KS 67357, (316) 421-6550, BA 79 Univ of Northern IA; MA 80 Univ of Northern IA; 87–Direct Care Staff Training Coord, Southeast Kansas Educ Svc Ctr, **SLP**

Simmons, Wendy Margaret 75 Temple Boulevard West, Apartment 201, Lethbridge, AB, Canada T1K 5M2, (403) 381-8030, BS 84 CO St Univ; MA WA St Univ; 88–Sp-Lang Path, Chinook Health Unit, **SLP**

Simmons-Carr, Mrs Stephanie 1415 S California Avenue, Monrovia, CA 91016, (818) 795-6981, BA 77 CA St Univ - Los Angeles; MA 80 CA St Univ - Los Angeles; MA 82 Point Loma Nazarene Coll; 79–SLP, Pasadena USD, **SLP**

Simmons-Martin, Dr Audrey Ann 334 Geyer Forest, Kirkwood, MO 63122, (314) 965-5285, BS 41 Washington Univ; MS 45 Washington Univ; ED 63 (NS) Washington Univ; Retired, **A F LM**

Simmons-Miles, Rhonda Z P O Box 340, Ermine, KY 41815, (606) 633-2211, MS 82 Murray St Univ; BS 80 Murray St Univ; 84–Sp-Lang Path, Whitesburg Appalachian Reg Hos, **SLP**

Simms, Mrs Barbara O 4910 Snowmountain Road, Yakima, WA 98908, (509) 966-6529, BS 73 Spring Hill Coll; MA 74 Univ of FL; 80–Sp-Lang Path, Yakima Valley Hearing & Sp Ctr, **SLP**

Simnacher, L Sharon M 304 Sunland Drive, Clovis, NM 88101, (505) 762-1053, BS 70 Eastern NM Univ; MS 76 Eastern NM Univ; Sp-Lang Path, Clovis Municipal Schools, **SLP**

Simner, Mrs Phyllis Starnbach 191 Iroquois Avenue, London, ON, Canada N6C 2K9, (519) 471-2540, BS 64 Univ of Cincinnati; Sp-Lang Path, Cpri, **SLP**

Simon, Mrs Ann H 15 Strathmore Drive, Cherry Hill, NJ 08003, (609) 424-0782, BA 73 Univ of Akron; MA 75 Univ of Akron; Sp-Lang Path, Kingsway Learning Center, **SLP**

Simon, Anne E Ottawa General Hospital, Speech Language Disorders, 501 Smyth Road, Ottawa, ON, Canada K1H 8L6, (613) 737-8251, MS 86 Univ of Montreal - Quebec; Sp-Lang Path, Ottawa General Hospital, **SLP**

Simon, Mrs Bobbie L 116 Rosedown Street, Thibodaux, LA 70301, (504) 447-8181, MA 73 LA St Univ - Baton Rouge; Sp-Lang Path, Lafourche Parish Schl Bd, **SLP**

Simon, Bonita 317 Otis, Downers Grove, IL 60515, (312) 629-7272, BS 69 Northern IL Univ - De Kalb; MS 70 CO St Univ; MS 87 Loyola Univ of Chicago; 88–Admin-Pers/Diagnostics, Dupage/W Cook Reg Spec Ed Asso, **A**

Simon, Bonnie L 402 Pepper Road, Huntingdon Valley, PA 19006, MA 73 Temple Univ-Tyler Sch of Art; Sp-Lang Path, Private Practice, **SLP**

Simon, Candace A 19777 Hayes Court, Northville, MI 48167, (313) 476-5220, BS 76 Eastern MI Univ; MS 77 Eastern MI Univ; 82–Sp/Lang Path, Dalys Sp & Lang Ctr, **SLP**

Simon, Charlann S 5630 South Rocky Point Rd, Tempe, AZ 85283, (602) 839-2733, BS 61 Northwestern Univ; MA 69 Univ of KY; Sp-Lang Path, Tempe Elem Sch Dist, **SLP**

Simon, Cindy Ann South Miami Audiology Consultants, 6280 Sunset Drive, 2nd Floor, South Miami, FL 33143, (305) 663-0505, BA 77 SUNY - Center at Buffalo; MA 78 Wayne St Univ; 87–Ed Services, Private Practice, **A ACE**

Simon, Clara Rose 810 East Siebenmorgen Rd, Conway, AR 72032, (501) 329-6346, BS 81 Univ of Central AR; MS 83 Univ of Central AR; Sp-Lang Path, Conway Pub Sch Syst, **SLP**

Simon, Mrs Dana Lee 9 Stanford Court, Wantagh, NY 11793, (516) 785-0265, BA 83 SUNY - Center at Buffalo; MA 85 CUNY - Queens Coll; 87–Sp-Lang Path/Dept Co-Coord, Franklin Gen Hosp, **SLP**

Simon, Mrs Deborah Ann 510 Maple Avenue, Teaneck, NJ 07666, (201) 692-0986, **A**

Simon, Dee Ann M 205 Wilson Street, Ravenswood, WV 26164, (304) 273-2873, **SLP**

Simon, Elaine B 470-3M Raintree Court, Glen Ellyn, IL 60137, (312) 369-6767, BS 74 CA St Univ - Hayward; MA 77 Univ of IA; Sp/Lang Path, Indian Prarie Sch, **SLP**

Simon, Ellen Shapiro 6236 Mammoth Avenue, Van Nuys, CA 91401, (213) 681-4641, BS 78 Univ of MI - Ann Arbor; MS 79 Univ of MI - Ann Arbor; Dept Hd/Aud, Hear Cen, **A**

Simon, Gail Beth 25 Trinity Place #3-K, New Rochelle, NY 10805-2606, (914) 967-4949, BA 82 George Washington Univ; MA 85 Univ of MD - College Park; SLP, Burke Rehab Cntr, **SLP**

Simon, Geraldine 80 Van Cortland Park South, Apartment 7-H-32, Bronx, NY 10463, (212) 543-2553, BA 77 CUNY - Lehman Coll; MA 82 CUNY - Lehman Coll; SLP, Sp Serv NYC Bd of Ed, **SLP**

Simon, Dr Helen J 2232 Webster, c/o Smith-Kettlewell, San Francisco, CA 94115, (415) 561-1681, BS 62 Syracuse Univ; MA 63 Stanford Univ; PH 77 (Sp Hrng Science) CUNY - Grad Sch & Univ Cntr; Aud/Assoc Sci, Smith-Kettlewell Eye Res Inst, **SLP A**

Simon, Joanne Miller P O Box 546, Northboro, MA 01532, (617) 366-0596, BS 78 Univ of MA - Amherst; ME 80 Northeastern Univ; **SLP**

Simon, Mrs Joanne V 949 Edwards Boulevard, North Valley Stream, NY 11580, (718) 723-7200, BA 60 CUNY - Queens Coll; MA 82 Hofstra Univ; Sp-Lang Path, Samuel Field Sch, **SLP**

Simon, Julie Ann 1570 Response Road #1085, Sacramento, CA 95815-4859, (916) 925-1202, BA 83 CA St Univ - Chico; MA 86 San Jose St Univ; **SLP**

Simon, Mrs Linda J 189-04 64th Avenue #11-K, Fresh Meadows, NY 11365, (718) 454-1036, BA 75 CUNY - Queens Coll; MA 78 CUNY - Hunter Coll; Sp-Lang Path, New York City Board of Educ, **SLP**

Simon, Mrs Lisa McKay 11285 Secor Road, Temperance, MI 48182, (313) 856-8311, BS 83 Univ of Cincinnati; MA 85 Bowling Green St Univ; **SLP**

Simon, Mrs Marguerite Feeley 1835 North Hudson, Chicago, IL 60614, (312) 440-0872, MA 79 Northern IL Univ - De Kalb; Sp-Lang Path, Grant Hospital of Chicago, **SLP**

Simon, Mrs Marilyn C 34 Ann Drive, Bethany, CT 06525, (203) 393-3426, BA 54 Brown Univ; MS 74 Southern CT St Univ; 79–Sp-Lang Path, Naugatuck Bd of Ed, **SLP**

Simon, Marilyn F 190 Glenview Road, South Orange, NJ 07079, (201) 762-5600, BA 50 Upsala Coll; MA 70 Kean Coll of NJ; Spec Educ, Mplewd So Orange Bd of Ed, **SLP**

Simon, Mrs Michele B Olean Medical Group, 535 Main Street, Olean, NY 14760, (716) 372-0141, BA 80 SUNY - Center at Buffalo; MA 82 SUNY - Center at Buffalo; Aud, Olean Medical Group, **A**

Simon, Pamela J 105 Garfield Court, Olean, NY 14760, (716) 372-9321, BA 74 SUNY - Center at Buffalo; MA 75 SUNY - Center at Buffalo; 76–Sp-Lang Path & Consult, Private Practice, **SLP**

Simon, Susan Markowitz 875 University Avenue #6, Palo Alto, CA 94301, (415) 856-0877, BS 76 Northwestern Univ; MS 78 San Francisco St Univ; Sp-Lang Path, Palo Alto USD, **SLP**

Simon, Mrs Toby Lazar 428 Brook Avenue, Passaic, NJ 07055, (718) 745-6009, BS 77 CUNY - Brooklyn Coll; MS 80 CUNY - Brooklyn Coll; 85–Sp-Lang Path, NY League for Early Lrng, **SLP**

Simon, Vicki Jean 122 West Pershing Street, Santa Maria, CA 93454-6504, (805) 928-1415, BA 78 Univ of CA - Santa Barbara; BA 78 Univ of CA - Santa Barbara; MA 84 Humboldt St Univ; SLP, Santa Barbara Co Sch, **SLP**

Simone, Mrs Carol A K 144 Wood Street, Rutherford, NJ 07070, (201) 915-6020, BA 75 Montclair St Coll; MS 80 Columbia Univ Teachers Coll; 76–Sp-Lang Path, Jersey Cty Bd of Ed, **SLP**

Simone, Danielle 572 South Gaylord, Denver, CO 80209, (303) 425-2425, MS 84 Bloomsburg Univ of PA; OM 86 Hahneman Medical Coll; 86–Sp-Lang Path/Aud, D L Teter Assoc Inc, **SLP**

Simons, Barbara H 3325 Webber Woods Drive, Sarasota, FL 34240, (813) 924-1389, BS 60 Northwestern Univ; MS 78 Univ of South FL; SLP, Sarasota Co Pub Schs, **SLP**

Simons, Mrs Candace Rosenbaum 37863 Thames Drive, Farmington Hills, MI 48108, (313) 661-8204, BS 79 Wayne St Univ; MA 81 Wayne St Univ; Director/Sp-Lang Pathology, D&D Health Associates Inc, **SLP ACE**

Simons, Doris Ilene 5250 Las Verdas Circle, Apartment 112, Delray Beach, FL 33484, (407) 495-2743, BA 78 George Washington Univ; MA 82 George Washington Univ; 84–Sp-Lang Path, InSpeech Inc, **SLP ACE**

Simons, Janice L 3800 East Mabbie Peak, Tucson, AZ 85716, (503) 635-4548, BS 76 KS St Univ; MS 78 Portland St Univ; Rehab Superv, Sst of AZ Crpld Chldrn Svc, **SLP**

Simons, Lynn 4 Nantasket Avenue, Brighton, MA 02135, (617) 327-9264, BS 75 PA St Univ - Univ Park; MS 76 Indiana Univ of PA; Sp-Lang Path, Boston Sch Sys, **SLP ACE**

Simons, Monica Jean 2102 North West Street, Carroll, IA 51401, (712) 792-5703, BA 79 Briar Cliff Coll; MA 82 Univ of SD - Vermillion; Sp-Lang Path, Heartland AEA #11, **SLP**

Simons-McCandless, Marsha University Of Utah, 1201 Behavioral Science Bldg, Salt Lake City, UT 84112, (801) 581-6725, BS 69 Univ of IL - Urbana; MA 72 CA St Univ - Los Angeles; 88–Clinic Dir-Aud, Univ of UT, **A**

Simonson, Mrs Donna O 6233 South 89th E Avenue, Tulsa, OK 74133, (918) 250-7045, BS 69 OK St Univ; MA 70 OK St Univ; 84–Sp-Lang Path, Private Practice, **SLP**

Simonson, Faith Hiney 2542 West Country Club Dr, Fargo, ND 58103, (701) 241-4751, BS 81 Moorhead St Univ; MA 87 Univ of MN - Minneap-St Paul; **SLP**

Simonson, Josephine 4411 McKinney Avenue, Dallas, TX 75205, (214) 526-0492, BS 33 Univ of WI - Madison; MA 39 Univ of WI - Madison; **SLP F LM**

Simonton, Mrs Kamala Joy 1520 Fulton Court, Davenport, IA 52803, (319) 337-9514, BS 84 Univ of Northern IA; MA 85 Univ of Northern IA; **SLP**

Simonton, Mrs Martha Rae 6724 Panorama Drive, Riverbank, CA 95367, (209) 525-6600, BA 68 Univ of CO - Boulder; MA 86 CA St Univ - Stanislaus; Sp-Lang Path, Stanislaus Co Dept of Ed, **SLP**

Simos, Karen S 86 Demarest Avenue #4, West Nyack, NY 10994, (212) 519-2406, BA 77 SUNY - Coll at Cortland; MS 79 PA St Univ - Univ Park; 87–Sp-Lnag Path, New York League for Early Learning, **SLP**

Simpkins, Mrs Bernadine 647 Northbridge Court, Westerville, OH 43081, (614) 369-3650, BS 68 OH Univ - Athens; MA 70 OH Univ - Athens; Sp-Lang Path, Westerville City Schools, **SLP**

Simpkins, William T, Jr 10830 Childs Street, Silver Spring, MD 20901, (202) 593-5876, BA 55 Case Western Reserve Univ; MA 57 Case Western Reserve Univ; 66–Superv/Sp/Lang Path, Walter Reed Army Med Cen, **SLP**

Simpson, Alice Young 627 East 13th Street, Bowling Green, KY 42101, (502) 782-7771, BA 73 Western KY Univ; MA 80 Western KY Univ; Sp-Lang Path, Panorama Res-Care Inc, **SLP**

Simpson, Anne E P O Box 3101, Long Beach, CA 90803, (213) 602-6965, BA 71 CA St Univ - Long Beach; MA 82 Whittier Coll; Sp-Lang Path, Paramount USD, **SLP**

Simpson, Bessie C 1108 Scranton Place, Durham, NC 27713-1254, MS; **SLP LM**

Simpson, Brenda Gail 46 Monte Vista Road, Candler, NC 28715, (704) 667-2594, ME 87 Univ of NC - Greensboro; 88–Sp-Lang Path, Buncombe Co Bd of Educ

Simpson, Carol A P O Box 3211, Pineville, LA 71360, (318) 640-8590, BA 73 Univ of MO - Columbia; MS 80 MS Univ for Women; Asst Director Sp-Hrng Dept, Pinecrest State School, **SLP**

Simpson, Carolyn E P O Box 2776, Revelstoke, BC, Canada V0E 2S0, (604) 837-9338, MA 87 Western WA Univ; 88–Sp-Lang Path, Sch Dist #19 (Revelstoke)

Simpson, Carolyn S 1203 Oliver, Stuttgart, AR 72160, (501) 673-3561, BA 64 Univ Southern MS-Hattiesburg; MS 65 Univ Southern MS-Hattiesburg; Sp-Lang Path, Stuttgart Pub Sch, **SLP ACE**

Simpson, Mrs Catherine Norris 1510 South Farwell Street, Eau Claire, WI 54701-4010, (715) 839-4365, BS 83 Marquette Univ; MS 85 Marquette Univ; 87–Sp-Lang Path, Sacred Heart Hosp, **SLP**

Simpson, Mrs Claire R 96 Bank Street #3, St Albans, VT 05478, (802) 527-7117, BA 45 Univ of Cincinnati; MS 73 Univ of VT; Sp-Lang Path, Franklin Ctrl Superv Un, **SLP**

Simpson, Mrs Connie V 815 South Lemaster Road, Othello, WA 99344, (509) 488-5531, BA 79 WA St Univ; MS 81 Eastern WA Univ; Sp-Lang Path, Private Practice, **SLP**

Simpson, Mrs Diane Lynette 1011 North Oakland, Kirksville, MO 63501, (816) 665-2744, BS 84 Northeast MO St Univ; MA 85 Northeast MO St Univ; Sp-Lang Path, Southern Prairie AEA, **SLP**

Simpson, Edwin R 210 Crestmont Drive, Shippenville, PA 16254, (814) 226-2588, BS 52 Bloomsburg Univ of PA; MA 58 Univ of IA; Retired, Clarion Univ of Pa, **SLP**

Simpson, Elizabeth 10031 Burgandy, Waco, TX 76712, (817) 776-1400, BA 75 Baylor Univ; MA 76 Baylor Univ; **SLP**

Simpson, Mrs Elizabeth P O Box 426, 318 North Elm Street, Marshville, NC 28103, (704) 624-6411, BA 76 Univ of NC - Greensboro; MA 76 Univ of NC - Greensboro; Sp-Lang Path, Union County Schools, **SLP**

Simpson, Mrs Elizabeth Taylor 34 Boothby Drive, Mount Laurel, NJ 08054, (609) 267-8565, BS 78 Trenton St Coll; MA 82 Trenton St Coll; SLP, Westampton Board of Education, **SLP**

Simpson, Mrs Emily F 2 Laurel Place, Eastchester, NY 10709, (914) 779-8758, OB 67 Univ of NC - Greensboro; MS 71 Univ of NC - Chapel Hill; OM 85 Fordham Univ; Aud, City Sch Dist of New Rochelle, **SLP A**

Simpson, Jane L W Audiology Associates, 1010 Xray Drive, Gastonia, NC 28054, (704) 867-6442, OB 74 Lenoir-Rhyne Coll; MS 76 Univ of NC - Chapel Hill; Aud, Aud Assoc & Hrng Aid Cen, **A**

Simpson, Janet P Box 32, Grande Cache, AB, Canada T0E 0Y0, (403) 826-3381, BS 78 Univ of Western Ontario; MS 80 TN St Univ; Sp-Lang Path, Alberta W Central Health Unit, **SLP**

Simpson, Jeffrey M 6470 Longridge Way, Sacramento, CA 95831, (916) 424-2880, BA 73 Univ of CA - Davis; MA 80 San Jose St Univ; 79–Sp-Lang Path, Sacramento Co Office of Educ, **SLP**

Simpson, Joan Adele 178 South Dellrose, Wichita, KS 67218, (316) 681-1881, **A**

Simpson, Dr Joann Margaret 9727 Mill Court East, Palos Park, IL 60464, (312) 361-4705, MA 67 De Paul Univ; ME 81 Nat'l Coll of Ed - Evanston; ED 88 (Sp-Lang Path) Univ of VA - Charlottesville; 68–Sp-Lang Path, Chicago Bd of Ed, **SLP**

Simpson, Joanne C 718 North Maple Drive, Beverly Hills, CA 90210, (213) 274-7563, **SLP**

Simpson, Mrs Joanne Medeiros 3702 67th Street West, Bradenton, FL 34209, (813) 748-2181, MS 82 Univ of South FL; Sp-Lang Path, Manatee Co Sch Bd, **SLP**

Simpson, Joseph Gerard West 920 Westmont Way, Spokane, WA 99208, (509) 483-7337, BA 77 Univ of MT; MS 81 ID St Univ; Aud, ENT Assoc of Spokane, **A**

Simpson, Mrs Joyce B Rd 3 Box 3265, East Stroudsburg, PA 18301, (717) 424-3247, BA 69 Morgan St Univ; ME 72 PA St Univ - Univ Park; ED 88 (Educ Theory) Rutgers St Univ -N Brunswick; Assoc Prof, E Stroudsburg U, **SLP ACE**

Simpson, Karen Rademaker West 920 Westmont Way, Spokane, WA 99208, (509) 326-1651, BA 77 Univ of MT; MA 80 Univ of MT; SLP, Spokane Guilds Sch/Nrmslr Cen, **SLP**

Simpson, Kenneth O 125 9th Street N W, Mason City, IA 50401, (515) 357-6125, BS 74 Univ of SD - Vermillion; MA 79 Univ of SD - Vermillion; 79–Sp-Lang Path, Nn Trails AEA, **SLP**

Simpson, Leslie A 433 Timberlea #176, Rochester Hills, MI 48309, (313) 656-8142, BS 86 Central MI Univ; MA 87 Central MI Univ; 87–Sp-Lang Path, Medi-Speech Services Inc

Simpson, Linda Smith 11818 Freelan Drive 1, San Antonio, TX 78253, (512) 679-6302, MA 83 Univ of Northern CO; Aud, Wilford Hall USAF Med Ctr, **A**

Simpson, Mrs Marcia A 5690 South Maplewood Drive, South Ogden, UT 84405, (801) 476-0850, BA 78 Univ of Northern IA; MA 80 Univ of Northern IA; SLP, Ogden City Sch, **SLP**

Simpson, Marcia S 3004 Cornell Avenue, Iowa City, IA 52245, (319) 351-7590, BA 62 Univ of IA; Sp-Lang Path, Grant Wood AEA, **SLP**

Simpson, Mrs Marianne VA Medical Center 126, 5901 East 7th Street, Long Beach, CA 90822, MA 75 CA St Univ - Long Beach; Sp-Lang Path, VA Med Cen, **SLP**

Simpson, Dr Mark Louis 6730 Indianwood Trail, Birmingham, MI 48010, (313) 562-6000, BA 70 Wayne St Univ; MA 74 Wayne St Univ; PH 82 (NS) Wayne St Univ; Sp-Path, VA Med Cen, **SLP**

Simpson, Martha A 112 Tyborne Circle, Columbia, SC 29210, (803) 758-4427, BS 77 IN St Univ - Terre Haute; MA 78 IN St Univ - Terre Haute; Sp-Lang Path, Sc Dept of Ment Retard, **SLP**

Simpson, Mrs Mary E 6027 Walnut Grove Road, Suite 411, Memphis, TN 38119, (901) 767-7750, MS 65 Vanderbilt Univ; Office Manager, Shea Hubbard & Futrell E-N-T, **A**

Simpson, Mrs Mary P P O Box 67, Lockport, LA 70374, (504) 532-2233, BA 80 Nicholls St Univ; OM 81 Tulane Univ; Sp/Lang Path, Lafourche Parish Sch Bd, **SLP**

Simpson, Maryann S 29 Woodlane Road, Ithaca, NY 14850, BS 78 SUNY - Coll at Geneseo; MA 79 Bowling Green St Univ; 88–Sp-Lang Path, Private Practice, **SLP**

Simpson, Mike Alan 2328 Monroe, Topeka, KS 66605, (913) 232-0583, **SLP**

Simpson, Patricia J 249 Garfield Place, Brooklyn, NY 11215, **SLP**

Simpson, Richard Peerman 408 South Poplar Street Apartment 8, Carbondale, IL 62901, BA 79 Univ of TN - Knoxville; MS 84 Murray St Univ; **SLP ACE**

Simpson, Robert Kennedy 901 South 6th Street, Champaign, IL 61820, (217) 333-2230, BS 50 Eastern IL Univ; MS 55 Univ of IL - Urbana; PH 63 (Sp-Lang Path) Univ of IL - Urbana; 64–Assoc Prof, Dept of Sp & Hrng Sci-U of Il, **SLP**

Simpson, Rosemary 3102 Faith Lane, Tyler, TX 75703, (214) 663-1882, BS 70 Univ of North TX; MS 76 Univ of North TX; Aud, Private Practice, **A**

Simpson, Mrs Sally Herman P O Box 787, Smithfield, NC 27577-0787, (919) 934-7237, BS 79 Kent St Univ; MA 81 Univ of Akron; Sp-Lang Path, Caswell Center, **SLP**

Simpson, Mrs Sarah M 10158 Sandyglen, San Antonio, TX 78240, (512) 691-0056, BS 75 Univ of TX - Austin; MS 78 Univ of North TX; Sp-Lang Path, Sp-Lang Path Serv, **SLP**

Simpson, Susan K 9055 Windjammer Drive, Fort Mill, SC 29715, (803) 547-2053, BA 72 Pfeiffer Coll; MS 74 Winthrop Coll; Sp-Lang Path, Indian Land Sch Lnac Consult, **SLP**

Simpson, Dr Thomas Henry 1705 Lyons Avenue, Lansing, MI 48910, (517) 482-3934, MA 72 MI St Univ; PH 84 (NS) MI St Univ; **A**

Simpson, Mrs Vickie Myers 10231 North Scottsdale Road, Suite 109, Scottsdale, AZ 85253, (602) 998-6655, MA Univ of TN - Knoxville; Sp-Lang Path, Private Practice, **SLP**

Simpson, Victoria Lynn 4104 Orchardale Drive N W, Apartment A, Canton, OH 44709, (800) 362-6687, BA 83 Univ of Akron; MA 84 Univ of Akron; Aud, E Ctrl Ohio Spec Ed Resrce Cen, **A**

Simpson, William L, II 700 Levert Drive, Thibodaux, LA 70301, (504) 448-4586, BS 78 LA St Univ - Baton Rouge; OM 80 LA St Univ - N O Medical Ctr; Instr, Nicholls State U, **A**

Simpson-Sears, Marion June 9 Ocean Avenue, East Patchoque, NY 11772, (516) 758-2896, MA 85 Long Island U - CW Post Ctr; Private Practice, **SLP**

Simpson-Steele, Mrs Harriet K Suite 405, 890 Poplar Church Road, Camp Hill, PA 17011, (717) 761-6794, BS 54 Univ of WI - Madison; MS 76 Univ of MI - Ann Arbor; Director, Private Practice, **SLP**

Simrin, Shelley 216 Arlington Avenue, Kensington, CA 94707, (415) 881-3233, BA 72 Univ of CA - Berkeley; MA 76 San Francisco St Univ; Sp-Lang Path, Alta Bates Hosp, **SLP**

Sims, Mrs Alice M 4437 Drusilla Drive, Baton Rouge, LA 70809, (504) 926-2790, BA 55 Northeast LA Univ; MA 61 LA St Univ - Baton Rouge; ME 69 LA St Univ - Baton Rouge; **SLP**

Sims, Carole Latice 1502 Hillside Terrace, Pennsauken, NJ 08110, (609) 342-3060, BA 82 Univ of Pittsburgh - Pittsburgh; MA 84 Temple Univ-Tyler Sch of Art; **SLP**

Sims, Dr Donald George National Technical Institute For The Deaf, Rochester Institute Of Technology (60-3851), Rochester, NY 14623-0887, (716) 475-6285, BA 65 Univ of CO - Boulder; MS 66 Univ of Pittsburgh - Pittsburgh; PH 70 (Aud) Univ of Pittsburgh - Pittsburgh; Research Associate, NTID, **A**

Sims, Mrs Elizabeth Asbury 2408 Belmont Place, Plano, TX 75023, (214) 964-1083, BS 82 Baylor Univ; MS 85 Univ of NV - Reno; 87–Sp-Lang Path, Plano ISD, **SLP**

Sims, Elwin Lawson 13730 Broken Bridge Drive, Houston, TX 77085, (409) 983-1651, **SLP**

Sims, Mrs Frankie B 3701 68th, Lubbock, TX 79413, (806) 792-6135, BS 76 TX Tech Univ; MS 78 TX Tech Univ; Sp/Lang Path, Sp-Lang Hrng Cen, **SLP**

Sims, Mrs Gretha Burch 1301 Neelys Bend Road H-74, Madison, TN 37115, (615) 327-6316

Sims, Dr Juanita L P O Box 16666, Jackson, MS 39236, (601) 366-8309, BS 73 Univ Southern MS-Hattiesburg; MS 74 Univ Southern MS-Hattiesburg; ED 85 (Early Childhood Education) Jackson St Univ; 86–Asst Prof, Jackson State Univ, **SLP ACE**

Sims, Judy K 14618 East 36th Street, Tulsa, OK 74134, BS 75 Univ of TX - Austin; MA 86 Univ of Tulsa; **SLP**

Sims, Kathleen Dawn 2200 Garland Drive #29, Missoula, MT 59803, (406) 251-2797, BA 84 Univ of MT; MA 87 Univ of MT; **SLP**

Sims, Mrs Laura Whitman Route 11 Box 509, Athens, AL 35611, (205) 350-2041, **SLP**

Sims, Leslie Ellen 3278B Oakwood Village Lane, Chamblee, GA 30341, (404) 589-4679, BA 84 Emory Univ; OM 85 Emory Univ; Aud, Grady Memorial Hospital, **A**

Sims, Leslie Leanne 15022 Wycliffe Drive #24, Omaha, NE 68154, (402) 397-0670, BS 79 Univ of NE - Lincoln; MS 84 Univ of NE - Lincoln; Aud, Omaha Ear Head & Neck Spec, **A**

Sims, Mrs Nancy Monroe 1687 Willowspring Drive N, Encinitas, CA 92024, (619) 541-4415, BA 78 Wake Forest Univ; MA 82 Univ of CO - Boulder; **SLP**

Sims, Mrs Pamela M 145 Grand Castle Terrace, Battle Creek, MI 49017, BS 79 Central MI Univ; MA 80 Central MI Univ; Sp-Lang Path, Private Practice, **SLP**

Sims, Patricia A 8225 Bielby Road #6, Rome, NY 13440, (315) 336 2300, **SLP**

Sims, Sue E 3400 Faulkner Road, Little Rock, AR 72210, (501) 455-3110, BA 60 Univ of CO - Boulder; ME 68 Univ of OK - Norman; MS 79 Univ of AR - Little Rock; Sp-Lang Path, Pulaski Co Spec Sch Dist, **SLP**

Sims, Vicki J D 2508 West Koenig, Grand Island, NE 68801, (308) 382-3660, BA 76 Kearney St Coll; MS 78 Kearney St Coll; SLP, VA Med Cen, **SLP**

Sin, Yuen Ming 5635 Eagle Court, North Vancouver, BC, Canada V7R 4T9, (604) 968-6395, BA 83 Guilford Coll; MA 85 Univ of NC - Greensboro; Children's Hosp, **SLP**

Sinast-House, Linda 8304 Grayledge, Austin, TX 78753, (512) 834-2305, BS 66 6862; ME 68 Southwest TX St Univ; Sp/Lang Path, Private Practice, **SLP**

Sinatra, Kathleen S 1135 Ridgeley Drive, Campbell, CA 95008, (408) 371-4177, BS 71 Univ of Santa Clara; MA 73 Univ of NE - Lincoln; Private Practice, **SLP**

Sinclair, Beverly J 1733 Oakwood Drive, Anaheim, CA 92807, (714) 730-7360, Asst Prin, Tustin USD, **SLP**

Sinclair, Cynthia S 218 East 10th #1, Lamoni, IA 50140, (515) 784-6790, BS 85 Northeast MO St Univ; MA 86 Northeast MO St Univ; 88–Sp-Lang Path, Green Valley AEA, **SLP**

Sinclair, Mrs Janet K 1775 Longwood Drive, Sycamore, IL 60178, (815) 895-2045, BA 52 Cornell Coll; MA 67 Northern IL Univ - De Kalb; **SLP**

Sinclair, Mrs Jennifer Josik 11 Cambridge Square, Williamsville, NY 14221, (716) 634-1889, BA 80 SUNY - Center at Buffalo; MA 82 SUNY - Center at Buffalo; Sp-Lang Path, Lang Dev Prog of W NY, **SLP ACE**

Sinclair, Mrs Joan B 14 5th Artillery Road, Fort Leavenworth, KS 66027, (913) 651-3648, BA 77 Marywood Coll; MA 79 Temple Univ; **SLP**

Sinclair, Dr John Stephen 1701 Roosevelt Avenue, Altadena, CA 91001, (818) 885-2852, BA 69 Univ of Redlands; MS 74 Univ of Redlands; PH 80 (Hrng and Sp Science) Vanderbilt Univ; 80–Prof, Dept/Commun Dis Ca St U Nrdge, **A**

Sinclair, Kathleen E Foundation School, 719 Derby-Milford Road, Orange, CT 06477, (203) 795-6075, BA 65 Eastern MI Univ; MA 67 Northwestern Univ; Dir Lower Sch, Foundation Sch, **SLP**

Sinclair, Mrs Leona D 21 Coburn Street, Auburn, ME 04210, (207) 784-2968, BS 72 Univ of ME - Farmington; MS 80 Univ of OK Medical Center; Sp-Lang Path, Auburn Sch Dept, **SLP**

Sinclair, Mrs Margaret Lunnie 69 Belvedere Blvd, Toronto, ON, Canada M8X 1K5, (416) 393-0630, MS 87 Syracuse Univ; 88–Sp Resource Tchr, Toronto Bd of Educ, **A**

Sinclair, Mary Patrcia c/o Major C B Sinclair, Psc Box 9562, APO New York, NY 09012, 001-49-0631-536-7596, BA 81 TX Tech Univ; OM 86 AZ St Univ; 88–SLP, Dept of Defense Dependent Schs, **SLP**

Sinclair, Mrs Miriam N 4172 Winchester Road, Allentown, PA 18104, SLP, Private Practice, **SLP**

Sinclair, Mrs Nancy P 804 Timberoaks Drive, Azle, TX 76020, (817) 281-1201, BS 79 Univ of North TX; MS 80 Univ of North TX; Sp/Lang Path, Birdville ISD, **SLP**

Sinclair, Mrs Paula 626 21st Street, Huntington Beach, CA 92648-3319, (714) 840-9365, MS CUNY - Hunter Coll; Sp-Lang Path, **SLP**

Sinclair, Rose C Rural Route 4, Mount Brydges, ON, Canada N0L 1W0, BS 82 Univ of Western Ontario; OM 85 Univ of Western Ontario

Sinclair, Sally W 7221 Sheffield Drive, Knoxville, TN 37919-5367, (615) 521-2589, BS 72 Auburn Univ - Auburn; MA 73 Univ of TN - Knoxville; Superv Chapter I, Knox Co Sch, **SLP**

Sinclair-Weitzner, Leslie Victoria 2772 Nottingham Way, Hamilton, NJ 08619, (609) 987-0099, BS 83 Trenton St Coll; MA 84 Trenton St Coll; Sp-Lang Path, Eden Institute Inc, **SLP**

Sindel, Mrs Lisa Lynn 619 Wallach Drive, Eureka, MO 63025, (314) 569-6040, BA 85 Saint Louis Univ; MA 86 Saint Louis Univ; SLP, St Johns Mercy Med Ctr, **SLP**

Sinden, Nancy L 6972 Village Woods Place, Worthington, OH 43085, (614) 433-0446, BA 74 Univ of MA - Amherst; MS 79 Boston Univ; Sp-Lang Path, Phoenix Hudson Corp, **SLP**

Sineps, Mrs Diane Barber 2155 Pinehurst Avenue, St Paul, MN 55116, (612) 298-8288, BS 60 Univ of WI - Madison; MA 61 Marquette Univ; Dir Sp-Lang Path, Unit Hospital & St Pauls Childrn, **SLP ACE**

Siner, Cheryl B 150 Avenue B SE, Winter Haven, FL 33880, (813) 294-1429, BS 85 Radford Univ; MS 86 Radford Univ; Sp-Lang Path, Communication Specialists Inc, **SLP**

Siner, Kathleen Read 53 Central Street, Harrisville, RI 02830, (401) 942-2388, BA 80 Univ of RI; MS 85 Worcester St Coll; 85–Sp-Lang Path, Cranston Ctr, **SLP**

Sinett, Eileen N 610 Plainsboro Road, Plainsboro, NJ 08536, (201) 469-9070, BS 71 Emerson Coll; MA 74 Kean Coll of NJ; Sp-Lang Path/Commun Consult, Private Practice, **SLP**

Singer, Beth Renee 12121 Village Square Terrace #401, Rockville, MD 20852, (301) 651-5328, MS 84 Gallaudet Coll; 88–Aud, Gallaudet Univ, **A**

Singer, Janice L 77 Pomeroy Terrace, Northampton, MA 01060, (413) 737-7368, BS 78 SUNY - Center at Albany; MS 79 Columbia Univ Teachers Coll; 85–Sp-Lang Path, Western Mass Sp-Lang Serv Asso, **SLP**

Singer, Jay 11 Greenbriar Place, Kingston, RI 02881, (401) 792-5969, BA 70 CUNY - Brooklyn Coll; MA 72 Univ of FL; PH 76 (NS) Case Western Reserve Univ; Chmn Dept of Commun Disorders, University of Rhode Island, **A**

Singer, Dr Jeane Violon 501 Howard Avenue, Altoona, PA 16601, (814) 946-0721, BS 72 SUNY - Coll at Buffalo; MS 73 Ithaca Coll; PH 81 (Aud/Acoustical ENG) PA St Univ - Univ Park; Aud/Pres, Aud and Has, **A**

Singer, Louis 3930 Morrison Street N W, Washington, DC 20015, (202) 362-7581, BA 34 CUNY - Brooklyn Coll; MA 36 NY Univ; Sp-Lang Path & Consult, Private Practice, **SLP LM**

Singer, Mrs Mindy Z 2943 Joyce Lane, Merrick, NY 11566, (516) 379-1934, BS 78 SUNY - Center at Albany; MA 79 Hofstra Univ; Sp-Lang Path, Private Practice, **SLP**

Singer, Mrs Rivelle Feldman 209 McCarthy Street, Manchester, NH 03104, (603) 668-5716, BA 48 De Paul Univ; MS 69 Emerson Coll; ME 74 Harvard Univ; Sp-Lang Path Consult, Private Practice, **SLP**

Singer, Roberta N 11 Greenbriar Place, Kingston, RI 02881, (401) 294-4561, BA 76 Univ of Rochester; MS 78 Univ of RI; Chief of Audiology, Joseph Ladd Center, **A**

Singer, Rosalind D 4644-B South 36th Street, Arlington, VA 22206, (202) 373-7374, MA 73 Univ of MD - College Park; Sp-Lang Path, St Elizabeths Hosp, **SLP ACE**

Singer, Mrs Tina H 474 Cassin Road, Naperville, IL 60565, (312) 369-8905, BS 72 Northeastern Univ; MA 74 Northern IL Univ - De Kalb; Sp-Lang Path, Private Practice, **SLP**

Singer, Tina Marie 5109 Pleasant Avenue #103, Fairfield, OH 45014, (513) 896-5452, BS 82 Miami Univ - Oxford; MS 83 Miami Univ - Oxford; SLP, Hamilton Co Bd Men Ret/Dev Dst, **SLP**

Singerman, Mrs Susan H 1044 Ashland, Wilmette, IL 60091, (312) 251-6531, BS 71 Washington Univ; MA 74 Tulane Univ; Sp-Lang Path, Private Practice, **SLP**

Singerman-Berman, Beth M 118 Valley View Road, Irvington, NY 10533-1847, (914) 693-8500, BA 76 SUNY - Center at Buffalo; MA 78 NY Univ; Sp-Lang Path, Greenburgh 11 UFSD, **SLP**

Singh, Dr Davinder Annapolis Road Aud Ctr Inc, 5632 Annapolis Road, Suite 9, Bladensburg, MD 20710, (301) 779-6864, BS 58; MS 61; PH 75 (NS) Bowling Green St Univ; Aud/Owner, Annapolis Rd Aud Cen Inc, **SLP A**

Singh, Dr Sadanand 4284 41st Street, San Diego, CA 92105, PH (NS); **F**

Singletary, Mrs Floris F 5223 Damascus Road North, Jacksonville, FL 32207, (904) 244-2161, OB 73 Univ of FL; MS 74 PA St Univ - Univ Park; SLP, Okaloosa Co Sch Bd, **SLP**

Singletary, Louise J 101 Myer Circle, Goose Creek, SC 29445, (803) 553-9242, BS 73 Hampton Univ; MA 78 SC St Coll; Sp-Lang Path, Berkeley County Public Schools, **SLP**

Singletary, Mrs Theronne Burlison Univ Of Tennessee Medical Ctr, Knoxville, 1924 Alcoa Hwy Box U-52, Knoxville, TN 37920-6999, (615) 544-9151, BA 70 Baylor Univ; MS 71 CO St Univ; 72–Instr SLP, U of Tenn-Dept/Aud & Sp Path, **SLP**

Singleton, James M P O Box 4378, Mc Allen, TX 78501, (512) 686-6881, BA 70 CA St Univ - Fullerton; OM 73 Univ of WA; Aud/Dir, Beltone Hrng Aid Ser, **A**

Singleton, Karen Mary 52 Friends Street, Portsmouth, RI 02871, (401) 683-1863, BS 70 Univ of RI; MS 86 Univ of RI

Singleton, Mrs Linda W 510-D Tillman Place, West Point, NY 10996, (914) 446-0903, BS 79 East Carolina Univ; MA 80 Univ of TN - Knoxville; Sp-Lang Path, **SLP**

Singleton, Mary K L 110 East Avenue, Morganton, NC 28655-3126, (704) 433-4802, BS 75 Appalachian St Univ; MA 78 Appalachian St Univ; Sp/Lang Path, Commun Rehab Serv, **SLP**

Singleton, Mrs Mary Susan 80 Orchard, Irvine, CA 92714, (303) 660-9839, BS 84 CO St Univ; MS 86 CO St Univ; 88–Aud, Riverview Sp Lang & Hrng Ctr, **A**

Singleton, Sandra L 330 Bandini Place, Vista, CA 92083, (714) 676-3381, BA 75 William Paterson Coll; MS 82 Loma Linda Univ - Loma Linda; Sp-Lang Path, Private Practice, **SLP**

Singleton, Susan Kessler Lewis-Gale Hospital, 1900 Electric Road, Salem, VA 24153, (703) 989-4261, BS 85 Radford Univ; MS 86 Radford Univ; **SLP**

Singleton-Filio, Kimberly Faye 3884 Isabella Avenue, Cincinnati, OH 45209, (513) 351-7878, BS 79 OH Univ - Athens; MS 81 Miami Univ - Oxford; SLP, Speechpath, **SLP**

Singson, Maile Tanaka 40 Aulike Street Suite 311, Kailua, HI 96734, (808) 262-9222, BA 73; MS 75 Univ of HI - Manoa; Sp-Lang Path, Private Practice, **SLP ACE**

Sinha, Dr Narendra K 436 Hilton Drive, Madison, WI 53711, (414) 241-5530, MA 55 Patna Univ - India; MS 83 Bradley Univ; PH 63 (NS); **SLP**

Sininger, Dr Yvonne S House Ear Institute, 256 South Lake Street, Los Angeles, CA 90057, (213) 483-4431, BA 72 IN Univ - Bloomington; MA 73 IN Univ - Bloomington; PH 84 (Sp & Hrng Science) Univ of CA - San Francisco; Research Assoc, House Ear I, **A**

Sinnott, Jan Morris 27 Heritage Hills, Carbondale, IL 62901, (618) 529-3060, BS 80 Southern IL Univ -Carbondale; MA 84 Saint Louis Univ; 87–Supvr of Comm/Cognition Rehab, Ctr for Comprehensive Svcs Inc, **SLP**

Sinnott, Mary A 312 Sutherland, Bloomingdale, IL 60108, (312) 742-3264, BA 77 Mundelein Coll; MA 80 Northern IL Univ - De Kalb; SLP, Jayne Shover Rehab Cen, **SLP**

Sinopoli, Terese Adele 2480 South Downing Suite 200, Denver, CO 80210, (303) 698-0533, **A**

Sins, Mrs Bonnie T 1955 Henry Meiners Road, Mandeville, LA 70448, (504) 626-7416, BA 71 Nicholls St Univ; MA 73 Tulane Univ; **SLP**

Sinsley, Mrs Debbie M 3509 Empedrado Street, Tampa, FL 33629, (813) 832-3402, MS 85 Univ of TX - Austin; 88–Sp Lang Path, Tampa General Hosp, **SLP**

Sinteff, Elizabeth G 149 Washington Street, Pittsburgh, PA 15218-1351, (412) 521-9000, BS 78 CA Univ of PA; MS 81 Univ of NC - Chapel Hill; Sp-Lang Path, The Rehab Ins of Pittsburgh, **SLP**

Sipe, Mrs Linda J 608 Malen Road, Virginia Beach, VA 23454, (804) 539-0251, BA 68 Univ of FL; MA 69 Univ of FL; Aud, Lakeview Med Cen, **A**

Siperstein, Mira S 2669 Anthony Avenue, Bellmore, NY 11710, (516) 783-8746, BA 75 SUNY - Coll at New Paltz; MA 77 CUNY - Queens Coll; **SLP**

Siperstein, Mrs Mynde S 155 Weetamoe Drive, Warwick, RI 02888, (401) 722-6000, BS 78 Boston Univ; MS 80 Columbia Univ Teachers Coll; **SLP**

Sipp, Myrita Yvonne 2602 Cedar Avenue #185, Cleveland, OH 44115, (216) 382-9979, BS 83 Univ of Cincinnati; MA 85 Cleveland St Univ; **A**

Sipple-Wallace, Connie 1734 Promontory Drive, Florence, KY 41042-1180, (606) 491-1171, BS 83 Eastern KY Univ; ME 84 Eastern KY Univ; Sp-Lang Path, N Kentucky Easter Seal Ctr, **SLP**

Siragusa, Mrs Susan Marie 8301 Quarters Lane, Charlotte, NC 28212, (704) 545-2820, BS 84 SUNY - Coll at Geneseo; MS 85 Univ of SC - Columbia; Sp-Lang Path, Charlotte Rehab Hosp, **SLP**

Siref, Judith E 47 Wheeler Circle #156, Stoughton, MA 02072, (617) 848-4000, BS 81 Univ of NE - Omaha; MS 82 Univ of NE - Omaha; Sp/Lang Path, Braintree Pub Sch, **SLP**

Siren, Kathleen Ann 5815 West 78th Terrace, Prairie Village, KS 66208, (913) 648-6187, MA 87 Univ of KS

Siris, Teresa P 3 Revere Court, Upper Brookville, NY 11545, (516) 626-2470, BA 71 Vassar Coll; MA 86 Long Island U - CW Post Ctr; **SLP**

Sirk, Mrs Carolyn King 900 Riverside Drive, Holly Hill, FL 32017, (904) 258-8931, BA 71 WV Univ; MS 73 WV Univ; SLP, Volusia County Schools, **SLP**

Sirlin, Dr Mindy Wertheimer 216 Ronbru Drive, New Rochelle, NY 10804, (914) 633-2401, BA 73 CUNY - Queens Coll; MA 75 CUNY - Queens Coll; PH 85 (NS) CUNY - Grad Sch & Univ Cntr; Asst Prof, Iona Coll, **A**

Sirois, Diane Patricia 534 Willow Street, Waterbury, CT 06710-1318, (203) 754-7096, BS 75 Univ of MI - Ann Arbor; MA 87 Eastern MI Univ; 87–Sp-Lang Path, Waterbury Schs, **SLP**

Sirois, Doris Petrauskas 2 Buckingham Drive, Westford, MA 01886, (508) 448-6665, BA 74 Univ of MA - Amherst; MS 85 Worcester St Coll; Sp-Lang Path, Groton Public Schools, **SLP**

Siroky, Denise M 2820 Hazelwood, Apartment B-11, Nashville, TN 37212, (402) 543-2474, BA 85 Univ of NE - Lincoln; MS 87 Vanderbilt Univ

Sirota-Rosen, Lori 53 Sherman Avenue, North Merrick, NY 11566, (516) 379-4773, BA 82 Univ of MD - College Park; MS 84 Boston Univ; Sp-Lang Path, The Little Village School, **SLP**

Sirovatka, Anne Therese 85-40 Grand Avenue, Elmhurst, NY 11373, (212) 605-3740, BA 79 Catholic Univ of America; MS 85 Columbia Univ Teachers Coll; **SLP**

Sirovy, Mrs Karen Lynn 708 Hennepin, Marquette, MI 49855, (906) 226-6962, BS 82 IL St Univ - Normal; OM 84 Governors St Univ; SLP, **SLP**

Sirow, Dr Lynn W 45 West Creek Farms Road, Sands Point, NY 11050, (516) 883-9224, BA 72 Case Western Reserve Univ; MA 73 Case Western Reserve Univ; PH 78 (Aud) Columbia Univ Teachers Coll; Aud, Pt Wash Speech Lang & Hrng Ctr, **A**

Sischo, Luther W 303 West Avenue #C, Newberry, MI 49868, (906) 293-5121, BS 73 Northern MI Univ; MA 75 Northern MI Univ; Sp-Lang Path, State of MI, **SLP ACE**

Sisk, Mrs Belinda Kathleen C 4711 Willowmist Drive, Dayton, OH 45424, (513) 237-1590, BS 72 WV Univ; MS 75 Southern IL Univ-Edwardsvill; Sp-Lang Path, Private Practice, **SLP**

Sisk, Daina A Rt 2 Box 334, Galax, VA 24333, (703) 236-4060, ME 88 James Madison Univ

Sisk, E Diane 3610 Creek Mill Circle, Mobile, AL 36609, (205) 633-6996, BS 80 Talladega Coll; MS 85 Talladega Coll; **SLP**

Sisk, Mrs Lore A P O Box 16, Galata, MT 59444, (406) 432-3370, BA 80 Creighton Univ; MA 82 Univ of WA; SLP, Shelley Pub Sch, **SLP ACE**

Sisk, Michael V 791 Ashbury Street, San Francisco, CA 94117, (415) 577-1579, BA 74 Univ of MD - College Park; MA 77 Univ of MD - College Park; Director of Audiology, The Hearing Society, **A**

Sisneros, Lisa Therese 4700 Southern S E, Albuquerque, NM 87108, (505) 766-3034, BA 81 Univ of NM; MS 82 Univ of NM; Sp-Lang Path, Bia-Sn-Pueblos Agcy, **SLP**

Sisolak, Debra J 22 Elmwood Avenue, Edison, NJ 08837, (201) 549-9738, BA 84 Kean Coll of NJ; MA 85 Kean Coll of NJ; 86–Sp-Lang Path, Edison Township Bd of Educ, **SLP**

Sisskin, Vivian D 1577 East Braeburn Road, Altadena, CA 91001, (213) 993-9311, BA 74 Univ of CA - Los Angeles; MS 80 Chapman Coll; Sp-Lang Path, San Fernando Vly Child Guid Cl, **SLP**

Sisson, Elizabeth Marie 4217 West Lakeshore Drive, Moses Lake, WA 98837, (509) 765-3929, BA 82 Eastern WA Univ; MS 83 Eastern WA Univ; Sp-Lang Path, Moses Lake Sch Dist #161, **SLP**

Sisson, Susan Lynn 4748 Ironbridge Drive, Lexington, KY 40503, (502) 454-8236, BS 74 Murray St Univ; MS 83 Murray St Univ; **SLP**

Sisson-Alness, Julia A 4652 Munger Shaw Road, Saginaw, MN 55779-9509, **SLP**

Sisterhen, Mrs Christa C 3465 Stillridge Drive, Alpharetta, GA 30201, (404) 751-1713, BA 73 LA St Univ - Baton Rouge; OM 75 LA St Univ - N O Medical Ctr; **SLP**

Sisterhen, Dr Daniel H 3465 Stillridge Drive, Alpharetta, GA 30201, (404) 751-1713, MA 71 LA St Univ - Baton Rouge; PH 85 (NS) Univ of New Orleans; Aud, Biocommunity Serv Inc, **SLP A**

Sistrunk, Cathy Rawls 6623 Immokalee Road, Keystone Heights, FL 32656, (904) 473-7503, ME 72 Univ of FL; Sp-Lang Path, Putnam Co Schs, **SLP**

Sistrunk, Mrs Debra Ann Route 1 Box 855 #7, Mc Gaheysville, VA 22840-9727, (602) 839-7160, **SLP**

Sisul, Leonard A 1033 Patience, Florissant, MO 63034, (314) 854-6368, BA 74 Southern IL Univ-Edwardsvill; MA 76 Saint Louis Univ; 86–Sp-Lang Path, Metro Employment & Rehab Svc, **SLP**

Si-Tayeb, Betty G P O Box 1973, Porterville, CA 93258, (209) 782-2690, MA 83 CA St Univ - Chico; Sp-Lang Path, Porterville Developmental Ctr, **SLP**

Siter, Mrs Vicki Evans 1216 Bonaventure Drive, Melbourne, FL 32935, (804) 877-4084, BS 81 Phillips Univ; MS 82 Wichita St Univ; Sp-Lang Path, Hampton City Public Schools, **SLP**

Sitler, Barbara A Valley Park East #1967-B, Bethlehem, PA 18018, (215) 865-5286, BA 62 2279; MA 65 Univ of CT; SLP, Lehigh Valley Easter Seal Soc, **SLP**

Sitler, Dr Ronald W 75 St Helena Street, Perry, NY 14530, (716) 245-5328, BS 66 Bloomsburg Univ of PA; MS 68 Syracuse Univ; PH 72 Syracuse Univ; Prof and Chair, SUNY Geneseo, **A**

Sitler, Susan Elizabeth 3388 West 41st Street, Cleveland, OH 44109, (316) 678-7175, BS 80 Kent St Univ; MA 80 Kent St Univ; Sp/Lang Path, Akron Pub Sch, **SLP**

Sitman, Bonnie 220 Clearview Avenue, Huntingdon Valley, PA 19006, (215) 242-4320, BA 79 Clark Univ; MA 85 Temple Univ-Tyler Sch of Art; **SLP**

Sitton, Mrs Ann Bradshaw 3929 Woodlawn Drive, Nashville, TN 37205, (615) 377-0420, BA 60 Vanderbilt Univ; MS 61 Vanderbilt Univ; 85–Aud, Brentwood Hrng & Hrng Aid Cen, **A**

Sitts, Joanne P B 5405 Prado Court, San Bernardino, CA 92407, BA 78 Univ of Redlands; MS 81 Univ of Redlands; Sp-Lang Path, Cotton Joint USD, **SLP**

Sitver-Kogut, Marsha 244-09 73rd Avenue, Douglaston, NY 11362-2321, (718) 225-2229, BA 74 CUNY - Queens Coll; MS 75 Univ of MI - Ann Arbor; 87–Sp-Lang Path, Private Practice, **SLP**

Sitz, Janet M B P O Box 453, Cedarville, MI 49719, (906) 484-3990, BS 78 Fontbonne Coll; MS 79 Fontbonne Coll; 85–Sp-Lang Path, Eastern Upper Peninsula Interm Sch Dist, **SLP**

Sitzer, Nancy Jane 1210 Madison Avenue, Austin, TX 78757-1928, (512) 926-2410, MA 83 Univ of TX - Austin; Supervisor Rehabilitation Spec, Brackenridge Hospital, **SLP**

Siu, Tai Ling Wong 11 Preston Avenue, East Hanover, NJ 07936, (212) 238-7894, 81 Rutgers Coll; 84 Montclair St Coll; Aud, Gouverneur Hosp, **A**

Siva, Mrs Sue Ann 83-43 118th Street #2A, Kew Gardens, NY 11415, (718) 738-1800, BS 80 SUNY - Coll at Fredonia; MA 81 Bowling Green St Univ; Sp-Lang Path, Special Kids Intervention Prog, **SLP ACE**

Sives, Sheila Mae 1700 Butler Pike #33F, Conshohocken, PA 19428, (215) 539-8550, BS 82 PA St Univ - Univ Park; MA 84 Kent St Univ; Sp-Lang Path, Montg County Inter Unit, **SLP**

Siviski, Marsha T 77 Babbidge Road, Falmouth, ME 04105, (207) 797-0877, BA 78 Univ of ME - Orono; BA 78 Univ of ME - Orono; MA 80 Univ of ME - Orono; Sp-Lang Path, Private Practice, **SLP**

Siwek, Marilyn L 219 Woodland Terrace, Alexandria, VA 22302, (703) 684-6819, BS 74 Emerson Coll; MA 75 George Washington Univ; SLP, Fairfax Co Public Schools, **SLP**

Sizemore, Ramona P O Box 765, Manchester, KY 40962, (606) 598-7741, MA 88 Eastern KY Univ

Sizer, Mary K 1430 Holly Creek, Mansfield, TX 76063, (817) 473-3128, BS 75 Emporia St Univ; MA 80 Wichita St Univ; Sp-Lang Path, **SLP**

Sizer, Mary R A Route 2 Box 50, Todd, NC 28684, (704) 262-2185, BA 74 Columbia Coll; MA 75 Vanderbilt Univ; Aud, Appalachian St U, **A**

Sjoberg-Anderson, Cynthia 2102 Jane Court, Grand Haven, MI 49417, (616) 842-3571, BS 72 Western MI Univ; MA 74 Western MI Univ; 74–Sp/Lang Path, Grand Haven Pub Sch, **SLP**

Sjoli, Karen M 1097 Chilver Road, Windsor, ON, Canada N8Y 2K6, (519) 252-7281, BS 86 Minot St Univ; MS 87 Minot St Univ; 87–Sp-Lang Path, Children's Rehab Centre

Skaar, Mary George 640 McKinley Avenue, Geneva, IL 60134, SLP, Mid-Valley Special Education, **SLP**

Skaggs, Mrs Kyle Grenda 15270 Oakmont, Olathe, KS 66062, (913) 897-9485, BS 82 Ball St Univ; MA 84 Ball St Univ; Sp-Lang Path, Shawnee Mission Sch, **SLP**

Skalabrin, Theresa Ann The Mason Clinic, Neurotology, 1100 9th Avenue, Seattle, WA 98101, (206) 223-6393, BA 81 WA St Univ; MA 83 Univ of WA; Aud, The Mason Clinic, **A**

Skalbeck, Dr Gretchen 14865 N E Eugene Street, Portland, OR 97230, BS 52 Univ of MN - Minneap-St Paul; MA 55 Univ of WA; PH 63 (Aud/Sp Path) Univ of WA; **A**

Skapik, Gail S 587 Broadway #M-18, Menands, NY 12204, (518) 274-6200, BA 79 SUNY - Coll at Cortland; MS 79 Ithaca Coll; 84–Sp-Lang Path, Visiting Nurse Assoc of Cap Reg, **SLP**

Skarakis-Doyle, Dr Elizabeth School Of Human Comm Disorders, Dalhousie University, 5599 Fenwick Street, Halifax, NS, Canada B3H 1R2, (902) 424-7052, BA 74 Univ of CA - Santa Barbara; MA 76 Univ of CA - Santa Barbara; PH 82 (Communic Dison/Psycholing) Univ of CA - Santa Barbara; Asst Prof, Dalhousie U, **SLP**

Skarin, Dr Brenda Dudley 920 North Stoddard, Wheaton, IL 60187, (312) 279-4100, BA 76 IN Univ - Bloomington; MA 78 IN Univ - Bloomington; PH 84 (NS) Northwestern Univ; Assistant Professor, Elmhurst College, **SLP**

Skarphol, Katherine Rae 6635 South Staples Street, Apartment 1318, Corpus Christi, TX 78413, (512) 992-9682, BA 84 Univ of WI - Eau Claire; MS 86 Univ of WI - Stevens Point; 88–Sp-Lang Path, Corpus Christi ISD, **SLP**

Skarzynski, Mrs Shelly Elving 5219 West James Lane, Crestwood, IL 60445, (312) 396-1429, BS 84 Univ of IL - Urbana; MS 85 Univ of IL - Urbana; Sp-Lang Path, South Metro Assoc, **SLP**

Skeegan, Mrs Joan M 1093 N W 82nd Avenue, Coral Springs, FL 33071, (305) 755-7564, BS 72 OH St Univ; MA 74 Kent St Univ; Sp/Lang Path, Private Practice, **SLP**

Skeel, Mary L 1122 Peachcreek Road, Centerville, OH 45459, (513) 667-5238, **SLP**

Skeels, Kathleen Fujinaka 5209 Shippee Lane, Stockton, CA 95212, MA 79 Univ of the Pacific; Tchr, Stockton Devel Cen, **SLP**

Skeels, Susan F 171 West Hazeltine Avenue, Kenmore, NY 14217, (716) 875-1625, BS 76 SUNY - Coll at Brockport; MA 78 Ball St Univ; 86–Sp-Lang Path, Kenmore, **SLP**

Skelly, Mrs Alicia 529 North Howard Street, Moscow, ID 83843, (208) 882-3169, BS 82 Ithaca Coll; MS 83 Syracuse Univ; Sp-Lang Path, Warren Ctr Child Dev Prog, **SLP**

Skelly, Barbara Graves 4930 Yorktown Lane, Plymouth, MN 55442, (612) 627-2261, OB 79 Univ of MN - Duluth; MS 80 Saint Cloud St Univ; Sp-Lang Path, Minneapolis Public Schools 8, **SLP**

Skelly, Nancy 8611 Cushman Place, Alexandria, VA 22308, **SLP**

Skelly-Hakanson, Dr Madge Tower Grove Manor Suite 901, 2710 South Grand Boulevard, St Louis, MO 63118, (314) 771-4741, BA 24 Seton Hill Coll; MA 28 Duquesne Univ; PH 61 (NS) Saint Louis Univ; Prof Comm Med, St Louis Univ Sch of Med, **SLP F LM**

Skelton, Ann G Route 3 Box 7, Bailey Road, Senatobia, MS 38668, (601) 562-5301, **SLP**

Skelton, Mrs Kathy Carter 8604 Sargent Way, Bakersfield, CA 93311, (805) 398-3799, BA 80 CA St Univ - Fresno; SLP, Office of Kern Co Supt Sch, **SLP**

Skelton, Steven L 8604 Sargent Way, Bakersfield, CA 93311, (805) 398-3799, BA 77 CA St Coll - Bakersfield; MA 83 CA St Univ - Fresno; SLP, Kern Co Supt Sch, **SLP**

Skenes, Dr Linda Lilley VA Medical Center (126), 2460 Wrightsboro Road (10), Augusta, GA 30910, (404) 724-5116, BS 79 East Carolina Univ; MA 80 Univ of TN - Knoxville; PH 82 (NS) Univ of TN - Knoxville; Coordinator Sp & Lang Services, VA Medical Center, **SLP**

Skibinski, Mrs Diane K 2 Vista Drive, Scotia, NY 12302, (518) 381-9320, BS 81 SUNY - Coll at Geneseo; MS 82 Ithaca Coll; Sp-Lang Path, Private Practice, **SLP**

Skibinski, Stephanie J Saint Joseph Hospital, 172 Kinsley Street, Nashua, NH 03051, BS 75 Marquette Univ; MS 79 Univ of WI - Milwaukee; 88–Sp-Lang Path, St Joseph Hosp, **SLP**

Skidmore, Mrs Sydney H 11703 Tifton Drive, Potomac, MD 20854, (301) 299-6280, BA 65 San Francisco St Univ; MA 70 Univ of MD - College Park; Sp-Lang Path, Montgomery Co Pub Sch, **SLP**

Skiff, Pamela J P O Box 22946, Tampa, FL 33622-2946, (813) 677-8949, **SLP**

Skiftun, Annette Breider 824 2nd Avenue Apartment C-1, Devils Lake, ND 58301, (701) 662-5082, OB 72 Valley City St Coll; BS 76 ND St Univ; MS 77 Minot St Univ; 79–Aud, North Dakota Sch for the Deaf, **A**

Skillicorn, Mrs Jane E 8918 Woodstream Drive, Fort Wayne, IN 46804, (219) 432-3928, BS 67 Univ of IA; MA 80 Kean Coll of NJ; 87–Sp-Lang Path, Ft Wayne St Dev Ctr, **SLP**

Skillicorn, Patricia Lynn Learning Services Department, Santa Rosa Junior College, 1501 Mendocino Avenue, Santa Rosa, CA 95401, (707) 527-4278, BA 82 Sonoma St Univ; MS 85 San Francisco St Univ; 85–Sp-Lang Path, Santa Rosa Jr Coll, **SLP**

Skillings, Linda J 59 Boston Avenue, Worcester, MA 01604, (508) 792-2864, BS 85 Univ of ME - Farmington; MS 86 Syracuse Univ; 87–Sp-Lang Path, Harrington Mem Hosp, **SLP**

Skillion, Kim H 2303 Monroe #2, Memphis, TN 38104, (901) 278-7620, BS 78 Delta St Univ; MS 79 Univ of MS; Sp/Lang Path, Senatobia City Schl System, **SLP**

Skinner, Barbarba K 1617 South Co Road #5, Fort Collins, CO 80525, (307) 771-2148, BS 74 CO St Univ; MS 76 CO St Univ; ED 87 (Special Education Administration) Univ of Northern CO; 80–Aud, Laramie Co Sch Dist No 1, **A**

Skinner, Mrs Betty R 237 West 33rd Place, Panama City, FL 32405, (904) 763-8922, BS 67 FL Atlantic Univ; MS 70 FL St Univ; Sp-Lang Path, Private Practice, **SLP**

Skinner, Christina T 1654 19th Street, Cuyahoga Falls, OH 44223, **SLP**

Skinner, Mrs Dawn Viosca 732 Heavens Drive, Apartment 3D, Mandeville, LA 70448, (504) 845-4112, BS 85 LA St Univ - Baton Rouge; MA 87 LA St Univ - Baton Rouge; Sp-Lang Path, Jefferson Sp & Lang Ctr, **SLP**

Skinner, Diane L 214 Tioga St, Johnstown, PA 15905, (814) 472-9821, BS 75 Clarion Univ of PA; MS 79 Indiana Univ of PA; SLP, Appalachia Inter Ut 08, **SLP**

Skinner, Elaine 1951 Ticonderoga Drive, San Mateo, CA 94402, **A**

Skinner, Mrs Holly Katherine 15811 Crying Wind Drive, Tampa, FL 33624, (813) 963-1567, BA 83 Univ of FL; MS 85 Univ of South FL; 86–Aud, Pinellas County Public Sch, **A**

Skinner, Mrs Linda S 334 East Hillcrest Street, Altamonte Springs, FL 32701, (305) 260-5019, MA 83 Ball St Univ; Sp-Lang Path, Seminole Co Sch, **SLP**

Skinner, Dr Margaret W Director Of Audiology, Department Of Otolaryngology, 517 South Euclid, St Louis, MO 63110, (314) 362-7489, BA 56 Wellesley Coll; MA 60 Case Western Reserve Univ; PH 76 (NS) Washington Univ; Aud, Dept of Otol Wash U Med Sch, **A**

Skinner, Mrs Mary E 116 Timber Lane, Holden, MA 01520, (617) 852-2101, BS 78 Anna Maria Coll; MS 82 Worcester St Coll; Sp-Lang Path, Shrewsbury Public Schools, **SLP**

Skinner, Patricia F Dayton Public Schools, 348 West 1st Street, Dayton, OH 45402, (513) 461-3057, BA 50 Capital Univ; MA 74 OH Univ - Athens; Coord Sp/Lang/Aud, Dayton Pub Sch, **SLP**

Skipper, Sandra Lane The Inner Ear Hearing Clinic, 20 Memorial Medical Park, Greenville, SC 29605, (803) 269-0474, BS 80 Univ of SC - Columbia; MA 83 Univ of SC - Columbia; Aud, The Inner Ear Hearing Clinic, **A**

Skipton, Mrs Anne Broussard P O Box 175, Maurice, LA 70555, (318) 893-4978, BA 81 Univ of Southwestern LA; MS 85 Univ of Southwestern LA; SLP, Vermilion Parish School Board, **SLP**

Skladany, Leah Ann M J Dance Rehabilitation Center, Greater Baltimore Medical Center, 6701 North Charles Street, Baltimore, MD 21204, (301) 828-2087, BS 75 Univ of AZ; MS 85 Loyola Coll; 86–Sp-Lang Path, M J Dance Rehab Ctr, **SLP**

Sklar, Mrs Linda Ellen 423 49th NW, Canton, OH 44709, (216) 455-0022, Super Chldrns Serv, Bes-Mont Sp Ctr, **SLP**

Sklar, Dr Maurice 3553 Moore Street, Los Angeles, CA 90066, (213) 397-7222, BA 35 CUNY - City College; MS 54 Univ of Southern CA; PH 57 (NS) Univ of Southern CA; Consultant, **SLP A LM**

Sklare, Daniel A 6601 Greenspring Avenue, Baltimore, MD 21209, (301) 484-3072, BA 75 Yeshiva Univ; MA 78 NY Univ; Audiolgist, NIH, **A**

Sklarow, Mrs Mindy E 4940 McFarland Drive, Fairfax, VA 22032, (703) 425-9035, BS 80; MA 82; Sp-Lang Path, Kingsway Learning Center, **SLP**

Skoglund, Mrs Dianne Boutwell RFD 1 Box 467, Warner, NH 03278, (603) 225-7503, BS 79 Univ of NH; MS 83 Univ of NH; Sp-Lang Path, Concord School District, **SLP**

Skoler, Mrs Charlotte Cranberry Lane, Box 827, Eastham, MA 02642, (617) 255-4922, BS 56 Boston Univ; ME 60 Boston Univ; **A**

Skomski, Diane Csizmar 1370 Harvard Avenue, North Tonawanda, NY 14120, (716) 884-9437, BS 77 SUNY - Coll at Buffalo; MS 78 SUNY - Coll at Buffalo; Sp-Lang Path, Childrens Hospital of Buffalo, **SLP**

Skopp, Elaine R 4004 Bon Homme Road, Woodland Hills, CA 91364, (818) 884-1946, BA 79 CA St Univ - Northridge; MA 80 CA St Univ - Northridge; Sp-Lang Path, Private Practice, **SLP**

Skorney, Debra A 219 Milbank Avenue, Greenwich, CT 06830, (203) 629-8179, BS 77 Montclair St Coll; MS 79 Gallaudet Coll; 88–Aud, Hearing & Sp Assoc of Stamford, **A**

Skotko, Mrs Janet Y 722 West Buffalo Avenue, Tampa, FL 33603, (813) 224-0249, BS 69 Kent St Univ; ME 70 Boston Univ; Sp-Lang Path, Private Practice, **SLP**

Skoulikaris, Sonya 4221 North Ottawa, Norridge, IL 60634, (312) 450-2100, BS 83 Elmhurst Coll; MS 84 Eastern IL Univ; Sp-Lang Path, Proviso Area for Except Chldrn, **SLP**

Skov, Mrs Jinda Marie 813 Peregrine Drive, Norman, OK 73072, (405) 364-9029, BA 80 Univ of OK - Norman; MS 83 Univ of NE - Omaha; Sp-Lang Path, **SLP**

Skow, Mrs Marie L 72 Covered Bridge Road, Warwick, NY 10990, (914) 294-8161, BA 74 CUNY - Queens Coll; MS 76 CUNY - Brooklyn Coll; 78–Sp-Lang Path, Nysddso-Treat Cen, **SLP**

Skow, Mrs Nancy Lee 1180B Mount Vernon Court, Wheaton, IL 60187, (312) 260-9645, BA 82 Augustana Coll; MA 83 Western MI Univ; Sp-Lang Path, **SLP**

Skowron, Christine 550 Deep Woods Drive #3-I, Mundelein, IL 60060, MA 79 Northwestern Univ; Sp-Lang Path, Sch Dist #64, **SLP**

Skowronski, George J 2980 Heshbon Road, Williamsport, PA 17701, (717) 322-2483, BS 72 Mansfield Univ of PA; ME 74 Bloomsburg Univ of PA; Aud Consult, Private Practice, **A**

Skowronsky, Susan A 957-B Grayling Court, Port Orange, FL 32019, (904) 788-6408, BA 77 William Paterson Coll; MS 80 William Paterson Coll; SLP, Volusia Co Sch Bd, **SLP**

Skrabut, Diana H 260 East Haverhill Street, Apartment 12, Lawrence, MA 01841, **SLP**

Skramstad, Mrs Mary K 3035 Kimberly, Plymouth, MN 55447, (612) 475-4560, BS 67 Univ of ND; MS 68 Univ of ND; Sp-Lang Path, Wayzata Dist 284, **SLP**

Skrine, Mrs Rebecca A 600 Benton Street, Mountain Home, AR 72653, (501) 425-7932, BS 73 Univ Southern MS-Hattiesburg; MS 74 Univ Southern MS-Hattiesburg; SLP, **SLP**

Skrivan, Mary Anne 1302 Brixton Road, Baltimore, MD 21239, (301) 828-0351, BA 85 Loyola Coll; MS 86 Loyola Coll; 87–Sp-Lang Path, The Chimes Inc, **SLP**

Skrobacz, Mrs Margaret Mary 207 Page Avenue, Endicott, NY 13760, (607) 748-5044, MS 87 Ithaca Coll; **SLP**

Skrodzki, Mrs Cheryl T 9302 Many Flower Lane, Jessup, MD 20794, (301) 924-4503, BS 75 SUNY - Coll at Buffalo; MS 76 SUNY - Coll at Buffalo; Sp-Lang Path, Montgomery County Schs, **SLP ACE**

Skruck, Connie Belleville 36 Lexington Avenue, Manchester, NH 03104, (608) 622-7020, OB 65 OH Univ - Athens; MS 85 Univ of NH; **SLP**

Skrzypczak, Mrs Ann M 42 Worcester Road, Princeton, MA 01541, (617) 464-2737, BA 73 Manhattanville Coll; ME 77 Northeastern Univ; Sp-Lang Path, Quabbin Reg Sch Dist, **SLP**

Skutshek, Mrs Denise Lynne 335 Windyridge Glen, Escondido, CA 92026, (619) 432-6688, BA 79 Univ of Northern CO; MA 82 San Diego St Univ; Sp-Lang Path, Scripps Clinic, **SLP**

Skuza, Karen Ann 301 Hamilton Avenue, Apt #C, Coshocton, OH 43812, (614) 622-2032, SLP, **SLP**

Skvarla, AnneMarie 383 Leonard Drive, New Milford, NJ 07646, (201) 967-4040, BS 82 Seton Hall Univ; MA 85 Seton Hall Univ; 85–Sp-Lang Path, Bergen Pines Co Hosp, **SLP**

Skwarecki, Robert M 3617 Wayne Road, Munhall, PA 15120, (412) 622-4484, BS 74 Duquesne Univ; MS 77 Univ of Pittsburgh - Pittsburgh; 85–Sp/Lang Path, St Francis Med Ctr, **SLP**

Skydell, Mrs Sandra S 67-15 102nd Street, Forest Hills, NY 11375, (718) 261-4913, BA 76 Hofstra Univ; MA 78 Hofstra Univ; SLP, Summit School, **SLP**

Slabaugh, Gerri K Box 269, Cambridge, MN 55008, (612) 689-1670, BS 72 Moorhead St Univ; MA 74 Univ of KS; SLP, Cambridge-Isanti Sch Dist 911, **SLP**

Slaby, Mrs Robin Dale 66 Bay Wood Drive, Safety Harbor, FL 34695, (813) 725-1692, BS 77 Elmira Coll; MA 79 Bowling Green St Univ; Sp-Lang Path, Private Practice, **SLP**

Slack, Mrs Carol Dianne Western Arkansa ENT Clinic, 600 South 16th Street, Fort Smith, AR 72903, (501) 782-6022, BA 81 Univ of AR - Fayetteville; MS 83 Univ of AR - Little Rock; Aud, Wn AR ENT Cl, **A ACE**

Slack, Elizabeth Louise 1604 Rock Creek Drive #114, Sioux Falls, SD 57103, (605) 335-4153, BS 82 Univ of SD - Vermillion; MA 85 Univ of SD - Vermillion; **SLP**

Slack, Kay E 816 Walnut Creek Drive, Austin, TX 78753, (512) 339-6306, BA 82 Boston Univ; MA 87 Univ of TX - Austin; 87–Sp-Lang Path, Austin ISD, **SLP**

Slack, Mrs Kirsten Nielsen 846 Burlington Avenue, Ventura, CA 93004, (805) 488-3659, BA 79 CA St Univ - Long Beach; MA 80 CA St Univ - Long Beach; Sp-Lang Path, Ocean View Sch Dist, **SLP**

Slack, Mrs Linda J 69 Belmont Avenue, West Babylon, NY 11704, (516) 587-0729, BA 79 Adelphi Univ; MS 80 Adelphi Univ; Sp-Lang Path, Self Employed, **SLP**

Slack, Lisa Cheryl 442 East Kiowa #B, Colorado Springs, CO 80903, (303) 473-7492, BS 84 CO St Univ; MA 86 Univ of Northern CO; **SLP**

Slack, Mrs Martha P 4402 Shawnee Circle S E, Decatur, AL 35603, (713) 785-6760, BA 73 WV Inst of Tech; MA 75 Marshall Univ; Sp-Lang Path, Sp-Lang Learning Clinic, **SLP**

Slack, Mrs Mary Beth G American Embassy, Apo, San Francisco, CA 96301-0001, BS 77 Purdue Univ - West Lafayette; MA 78 Ball St Univ; Aud, Dept of the Army, **A**

Slack, Patti Jo 28650 Cork Oak Lane #3109, Hayward, CA 94544, (415) 278-0908, MS 88 CA St Univ - Hayward; 88–Spec Day Class Tchr, San Lorenzo USD

Slack, Mrs Rhonda Ivy 203 Enoch Drive, Tupelo, MS 38801, (601) 842-1891, BS 81 Univ Southern MS-Hattiesburg; MS 82 Univ Southern MS-Hattiesburg; Sp/Lang Path, **SLP**

Slade, Christina Louise 2200 South Gessner #1104, Houston, TX 77063, (713) 776-2211, BS 83 Baylor Univ; MS 85 Baylor Univ; Aud, Houston ENT, **SLP A**

Slade, Mrs Marilyn V 70 Clifton Hill, London, England NW8 Ojt, BS 76 Univ of MA - Amherst; ME 79 Northeastern Univ; SLP, National Health Service, **SLP**

Sladek, Mrs Brenda K 7906 Shady Arbor Lane, Houston, TX 77040, (713) 462-6192, BS 75 Southwest TX St Univ; ME 76 Southwest TX St Univ; Sp-Lang Path, Assoc in Sp Lang & Learning Inc, **SLP**

Slaff, Laurie Ann 4340 Tucker North Court, Tucker, GA 30084, (404) 941-2133, BA 81 Univ of FL; ME 85 Univ of GA; **A**

Slager, Sara 3735 Sacramento Avenue, Santa Rosa, CA 95405, (707) 527-2271, BA 77 Univ of CA - Santa Barbara; MA 80 Univ of CO - Boulder; Sp-Lang Path, Sonoma Co Offi of Ed, **SLP**

Slaine, Mrs Joan Shearer 74 Stanton Lane, Stamford, CT 06902, (203) 327-2343, BA 73 SUNY - Center at Buffalo; ME 77 Northeastern Univ; Sp-Lang Path, Norwalk Bd of Ed, **SLP**

Slana, Audrey Ann 833 Ridge #503, De Kalb, IL 60115, (815) 756-3397, MA 88 Northern IL Univ - De Kalb

Slaney, Maureen Lee 161 Rossmore Court, Pittsburgh, PA 15229, (412) 734-0946, BS 85 Clarion Univ of PA; MS 86 Clarion Univ of PA; Sp-Lang Path, Self Employed, **SLP**

Slanina-Orfei, Caroline Frances 4727 Lenore Lane, Eagan, MN 55122, (612) 452-6620, BS 83 Mankato St Univ; MA 84 Univ of MN - Duluth; 88–Sp-Lang Path/Spec Educ Tchr, South Wash Co Sch Dist, **SLP**

Slansky, Barry L 7722 Carrington Drive, Apartment D, Madison, WI 53719, (608) 833-7223, BS 81 Indiana Univ of PA; MS 82 Indiana Univ of PA; 85–Project Assistant, Univ of Wisconsin-Madison, **SLP**

Slansky, Pamela M 7722 Carrington Drive, Apartment D, Madison, WI 53719, (608) 258-6711, BS 80 Indiana Univ of PA; MS 81 Indiana Univ of PA; 88–Sp-Lang Path, St Mary's Hosp Med Ctr, **SLP**

Slapin, Mrs Anita E 3560 North 46th Avenue, Hollywood, FL 33021, (305) 966-3997, BA 68 CUNY - Brooklyn Coll; MS 70 CUNY - Brooklyn Coll; Co-Dir, FL Sp&Lng Cen, **SLP ACE**

Slapper, Mrs Beth W 14242 South 140th Place, Gilbert, AZ 85234, (602) 839-7156, BS 73 CO St Univ; MS 75 Univ of WI - Stevens Point; Sp/Lang Path, Tempe Elementary Sch Dist #3, **SLP**

Slate, Suzanne I 1540 N E 129th Street, North Miami, FL 33161, (305) 891-4760, BS 70 Ithaca Coll; MS 71 Ithaca Coll; **LM**

Slaten, Mrs Nancy J 9907 Golden Meadow, Houston, TX 77064, (713) 890-3648, BS 78 Southeast MO St Univ; MS 84 Lamar Univ; **SLP**

Slater, C Richard 103 Wildbrier Road, Guthriesville, PA 19335, ME 70 Clarion Univ of PA; Dir/Social Rehabilitation Serv, White Haven Center, **SLP**

Slater, Carol Ann P O Box #3, Hockingport, OH 45739, (614) 667-3210, BS 86 OH Univ - Athens; MA 87 OH Univ - Athens; 88–Sp-Lang Path, InSpeech Inc, **SLP**

Slater, Emma Lu 723 Beatty Avenue, Cambridge, OH 43725, (614) 439-1371, BA 81 Univ of Akron; MA 83 Univ of Akron; Dept Hd/Sp & Hrng, Cambridge Men Hlth Cen, **A**

Slater, Mrs Glenda Richmond 93 Winding Way, Fort Thomas, KY 41075, (606) 781-5051, MA 63 Univ of AL-Tuscaloosa

Slater, Mrs Laurie G 2674 SW Talbot Road, Portland, OR 97201, (503) 223-4521, BA 80 Univ of UT; MA 82 Univ of the Pacific; 88–Sp-Lang Path, Private Practice, **SLP**

Slater, Mary E 2607 Thomas Avenue North, Minneapolis, MN 55411, (612) 421-4670, BA 74 Univ of MN - Minneap-St Paul; MA 78 Univ of TX - Austin; Aud, Minnesota Ear-Head-Neck Clinic, **A**

Slater, Rebecca H 105 Lake Lynn Drive, Harvey, LA 70058, (504) 392-0172, BS 79 Univ of South AL; MS 81 Univ of South AL; Director of Sp & Hrng, Therapy Associates of La Inc, **SLP A**

Slater, Robyn L 420 South Madison #204, Pasadena, CA 91101-3339, **SLP**

Slater, Sandra Lanz Leflore County Guidance Center, P O Box 37, Poteau, OK 74953, (918) 647-8601, BA 76 Univ of AR - Fayetteville; MA 77 Univ of AR - Fayetteville; Sp-Lang Path, Leflore Co Guidance Cen, **SLP**

Slater, Sandra Lee 711 East University Street, Harvard, IL 60033, (815) 943-6081, MA 88 Northern IL Univ - De Kalb

Slaton, Mrs Teresa A P O Box 834, Springdale, AR 72764, (501) 273-3339, BA 75 LA St Univ - Baton Rouge; MA 77 LA St Univ - Baton Rouge; Sp/Lang Path, Springdale Pub Schools, **SLP**

Slattery, Janet Turrou Box 576, Elk Point, SD 57025, (712) 279-2690, BA 73 CO St Univ; MA 84 Univ of SD - Vermillion; **SLP ACE**

Slattery, Mrs Linda Carole 21 Sugar Toms Lane, East Norwick, NY 11732, (516) 922-4100, BS 65 Saint John's Univ - Jamaica; MS 81 Adelphi Univ; Sch Aud, Mill Neck Manor Luthern Sch, **A**

Slattery, Linda K 14794 West Plaza, Omaha, NE 68137, (402) 895-5314, BS 85 Univ of NE - Omaha; MS 86 Univ of NE - Omaha; 87–Sp-Lang Path, Omaha PS, **SLP**

Slattery, Margaret I 2015 9th Street, Charleston, IL 61920, (217) 348-7605, MS 88 Eastern IL Univ

Slattery, Timothy Michael 9970 Menaul Northeast #J18, Albuquerque, NM 87112, (505) 291-8756, BA 82 Univ of Akron; MA 83 Univ of Akron; 84–Sp-Lang Path, Albuquerque Pub Sch, **SLP**

Slaughter, Mrs Mary Lou P O Box 1056, Bend, OR 97709, (503) 389-8010, BA 67 Wichita St Univ; MA 68 Univ of IA; 88–Sp-Lang Path, Private Practice, **SLP**

Slaughter, Marylin M 7412 Tower Street, Falls Church, VA 22046, (703) 525-1898, BS 76 WV Univ; MS 78 WV Univ; Aud, Arlington Hrng Cen, **A**

Slaughter, Robert L 4036 Acacia Drive, Columbus, GA 31904, (404) 327-2213, BA 78; MA 81 Auburn Univ - Auburn; Sp-Lang Path, Heard County Schools, **SLP**

Slauson, Thomas Jay 2256 East Silver Street, Tucson, AZ 85719, (602) 327-5461, BA 83 Univ of CO - Boulder; MS 85 Univ of AZ; 88–Sp-Lang Path, Tucson Med Ctr, **SLP**

Slaven, Margaret 24 Highland Avenue, Demarest, NJ 07627, (201) 837-8070, BS 58 Shippensburg Univ of PA; MS 72 Paterson St Coll; Sp-Lang Path, The Community School, **SLP**

Slavik, Mrs Cynthia Ann 9220 Hunters Creek, Apartment D, Cincinnati, OH 45242, (513) 791-7059, BS 85 Univ of IL - Urbana; MA 87 Univ of IL - Urbana

Slavik-Moreau, Mrs Debra A 19 Lincoln Place #D, North Brunswick, NJ 08902, (201) 821-3299, BS 82 PA St Univ - Univ Park; MS 83 Syracuse Univ; 86–Sp-Lang Path, Linden Bd of Educ, **SLP**

Slavin, Dianne C 21 East 22nd Street, Apartment 7-L, New York, NY 10010, (212) 679-0100, BS 71 Boston Univ; MA 73 NY Univ; Dir-Sp & Hrng Dept, Internatl Cen for Disabl, **SLP**

Slavin, Laverne A The Professional Voice, 3550 Wilshire Boulevard, Suite 1406, Los Angeles, CA 90010, (213) 739-8510, BA 77 CUNY - Queens Coll; MA 79 Univ of Houston - Univ Park; Dir, The Professional Voice, **SLP**

Slavin, Sandra H 130 New Road #E-9, Parsippany, NJ 07054, (201) 672-7979, BA 70 Trenton St Coll; MA 74 Montclair St Coll; 83–Superv Instr/Sp Corp, Essex Co Ed Serv Cmsn, **SLP**

Slavitt, Mrs Stephanie 5 Mohawk Drive, Livingston, NJ 07039, (201) 994-9094, BS 69 NY Univ; MA 70 NY Univ; **SLP**

Slay, Matilda W 3949 Berkley Drive, Jackson, MS 39211, **SLP**

Slayden, Mitzie Michele 220 Stowe Avenue #14, Orange Park, FL 32073-5669, (904) 264-7472, BS 84 Murray St Univ; MA 86 Memphis St Univ; **A**

Sleasman, Mrs Katherine U-1 Richard Mine Road, Wharton, NJ 07885, (215) 631-9300, BA 80 SUNY - Coll at Plattsburgh; MS 81 Ithaca Coll; Sp-Lang Path, InSpeech Inc, **SLP**

Sledd, Mrs Lourie S 2303 Huntcliff Court, Richmond, VA 23229, (804) 266-4809, BS 77 Radford Univ; ME 79 James Madison Univ; Aud, Henrico Co Sch, **A**

Sledge, Mrs Kim L 104 King Circle, Louisburg, NC 27549, (919) 496-4015, BS 79 Appalachian St Univ; MS 82 Univ of NC - Chapel Hill; 85–Sp-Lang Path, Franklin County Schs, **SLP**

Sleek, James Edward One Freeport Place Unit#13, Holbrook Street, Freeport, ME 04032, (207) 797-5753, BS 74 PA St Univ - Univ Park; MS 86 TX Tech Univ; 87–Aud, Head & Neck Surgical Assoc, **A**

Slegman, Dorothy 1987 Goodrich Avenue, St Paul, MN 55105, (612) 627-3080, Sp-Lang Path, Minneapolis Public Schools, **SLP**

Sleight, Dr Christine C School Of Speech Path & Aud, Kent State University, Kent, OH 44242, (703) 731-5204, BA 72 Hofstra Univ; MS 73 SUNY - Center at Albany; PH 82 (NS) PA St Univ - Univ Park; Asst Prof, Kent State U, **SLP**

Sleight, Marsha A 339 Corral Path, Lansing, MI 48917, (517) 543-5500, SLP, Eaton Intermediate Schools, **SLP**

Sleight, Mrs Wendy Corrine S P O Box 69, Belfair, WA 98528, (206) 275-2863, BA 78 WA St Univ; MA 79 WA St Univ; SLP, North Mason School Dist 403, **SLP**

Slein, Joan Strassner 41 Rye Lane, St Louis, MO 63132, (314) 997-2552, BS 63 Washington Univ; MA 84 Saint Louis Univ; Sp-Lang Path, Private Practice, **SLP ACE**

Sleister, Cheryl A 2605 Springwood Drive, Augusta, GA 30904, (404) 722-1957, OB 80 Univ of GA; ME 81 Univ of GA; Aud, Hrng & Sp Cen of Augusta, **A**

Slentz, Patricia C 202 Orchard Avenue, Dover, DE 19901, BA 79 Glassboro St Coll; MA 85 West Chester Univ of PA; **SLP**

Slesinski, Carolyn A 5 Meadowbrook Lane, St Albans, VT 05478, (802) 527-7665, BA 70 Marymount Coll; MA 73 Univ of MA - Amherst; 81–Sp-Lang Path, Private Practice, **SLP**

Slette, Renee Downs 2120 Bert Kouns Ind Loop, Suite F, Shreveport, LA 71118, (318) 688-6706, BA 78 LA St Univ - Shreveport; OM 80 LA St Univ - N O Medical Ctr; Aud, Shreveport ENT Clinic, **A**

Sletteland, Hildegarde P O Box 1580, Evanston, IL 60204, BS 54 Northwestern Univ; MS 71 Northwestern Univ; 82–Interviewer-Research Proj, Private Practice, **SLP**

Slevin, Mrs Barbara J 417 West Oakwood Lane, Castle Rock, CO 80104, BA 68 Adelphi Univ; MA 81 Univ of CO - Boulder; SLP, Arapahoe Co Dist #6, **SLP**

Slevin, Mrs Elizabeth M 174 Montague Place, South Orange, NJ 07079, (201) 396-1020, BA 73 William Paterson Coll; MA 87 Kean Coll of NJ; **SLP**

Sleyster, Mrs Tina Shaffer 5050 Pine Street Loop, Sandpoint, ID 83864, (208) 263-3506, BA 81 Univ of CO - Boulder; MA 87 Univ of MT; SLP, Kootenai Med Ctr-Rehab, **SLP**

Sligh, Julie Elizabeth 2763 Cottage Pl, Greensboro, NC 27405-2349, (919) 288-6085, BA 78 Columbia Coll; ME 81 Univ of NC - Greensboro; Sp-Lang Path, Reidsville City/Co-op Rock, **SLP**

Slijepcevic, Jane E Box 196, Eleanor, WV 25070, (304) 586-3958, BA 78; MA 79; Sp-Lang Path, Putnam County Board of Educ, **SLP**

Slind, Mrs Margaret A 54-1415 Lameys Mill Road, Vancouver, BC, Canada V6H 3W1, (604) 731-1551, BA 34 Univ of Saskatchewan - Sask; MA 55 FL St Univ; **SLP LM**

Slingerland, Barbara M 100 Haven Avenue, Tower 3 #6-G, New York, NY 10032, (212) 568-7579, BS 84 SUNY - Coll at Geneseo; MA 85 SUNY - Coll at Geneseo; 88–Sp-Lang Path, Private Practice, **SLP**

Slingerland, Susan Carol 5107 S E Stark #B, Portland, OR 97215-1750, (503) 241-3475, BA 71 Saint Martin's Coll; MS 79 Western OR St Coll; Sp/Lang Path, Vna, **SLP**

Slipakoff, Mrs Ethel L 5234 Imogene, Houston, TX 77096, BS 36 TX Woman's Univ; MA 41 Northwestern Univ; Consultant, Private Practice, **SLP LM**

Slipski, Mrs Geralyn Balchak 1302 Woodledge Drive, Mineral Ridge, OH 44440, (216) 747-5668, BA 78 Univ of Akron; MA 80 OH Univ - Athens; Aud, Aud Assn Inc, **A**

Slivinski, Ann L 511 Normal Road Apartment 309, De Kalb, IL 60115, (312) 450-2053, BS 85 Southern IL Univ -Carbondale; MA 88 Northern IL Univ - De Kalb; 88–Sp/Lang Path, School District 89

Slizeski, Kimberly Ann 36 Moreland Street, Worcester, MA 01609-1023, (603) 926-7312, BA 79 Univ of CO - CO Springs; MA 84 OK St Univ; **SLP**

Sloan, Annette Virginia 1240 Saxon, Birmingham, MI 48009, (313) 646-0366, BA 68 Marygove Coll; MA 85 Wayne St Univ; **SLP**

Sloan, Debra Peacock 1102 West Pershing Avenue, Phoenix, AZ 85029, (602) 266-5976, BA 83 San Diego St Univ; MS 86 AZ St Univ; 88–Sp-Lang Path, Southwest Human Dev, **SLP**

Sloan, Ellen C 8 Gainsville Drive, Plainview, NY 11803, (718) 470-8920, BA 76 SUNY - Center at Buffalo; MS 78 Columbia Univ Teachers Coll; 86–Aud, Long Island Jewish Med Ctr, **A**

Sloan, Mrs Gayle Y 203 Lander Dr, Conway, SC 29526, (803) 347-1772, BA 75 Elmira Coll; MA 76 Univ of TN - Knoxville; Sp-Lang Path, Horry Co Sch, **SLP**

Sloan, Mrs Helen Ann 1619 Harvard, Clearwater, FL 33515, (813) 441-2854, **SLP**

Sloan, John M Loyola College Of Maryland, Speech & Hearing Center, 4501 North Charles Street, Baltimore, MD 21210, (301) 323-1010, MS 74 Towson St Univ; Clinic Administrator, Loyola College of Maryland, **SLP**

Sloan, Karla Ann 3839 Northampton Drive, Lexington, KY 40503, (502) 564-4970, BS 78 Western MI Univ; MA 81 Central MI Univ; 86–Consult, Kentucky Dept of Educ, **SLP ACE**

Sloan, Lisa Karen 7112 Gatewood, Tyler, TX 75703, (214) 581-7178, BS 81 Southwest TX St Univ; MS 83 Univ of TX - Dallas; 88–Sp-Lang Path, Allied Health Assoc of East Texas, **SLP**

Sloan, Nahum 277 Silver Birch Avenue, Toronto, ON, Canada M4E 3L6, (416) 820-7111, BA 66 Univ of CT; MS 76 Southern CT St Univ; 81–Dir, Erinoak, **SLP**

Sloan, Mrs Paula S Rural Route 2 Box 454, Mulkeytown, IL 62865, (618) 937-2464, BS 68 Univ of IL - Urbana; MA 77 Univ of IL - Urbana; Sp/Lang Path, Frankfort Unit Schs, **SLP**

Sloan, Rosemary Minogue 30 Maple Avenue, Ellenville, NY 12428-2141, (914) 647-6465, BS 77 Bloomsburg Univ of PA; MS 84 SUNY - Coll at Geneseo; Sp-Lang Path, The Childrens Annex, **SLP**

Sloan-Brown, Nancy 3609 Park East Drive #201, Beachwood, OH 44122, (216) 464-1760, BA 73 Univ of MI - Ann Arbor; MS 74 Univ of MI - Ann Arbor; Sp-Lang Path, Private Practice, **SLP**

Sloane, Deborah S 157 Richmond Avenue, Worcester, MA 01602, **SLP**

Sloane, Mrs Jeanine 550 Oxford Street #1201, Chula Vista, CA 92011, (619) 267-8440, BA 76 Univ of Denver; MA 80 San Diego St Univ; Dir of Aud, Audio Logic Associates, **A**

Sloane, Dr Neal A 560 Northern Boulevard, Suite 204, Great Neck, NY 11021, (516) 466-3266, BA 75 CUNY - Queens Coll; MA 77 OH Univ - Athens; PH 81 (Psychoacoustics) OH Univ - Athens; 85–Aud, Private Practice, **A**

Sloate, Mrs Carolyn Reid 3511 S W 100th Street, Gainesville, FL 32607, BA 79 Univ of FL; MA 82 Univ of FL; SLP, Alachua Co Sch Bd, **SLP**

Sloate, Mrs Meryl H 62 Hazel Street, South Windsor, CT 06074, (203) 282-3370, BA 75 CUNY - Queens Coll; MA 77 SUNY - Center at Buffalo; 78–Sp-Lang Path, E Hartford Pub Sch, **SLP**

Slobof, Maxine S 1016 James Court, Mendota Heights, MN 55118, (612) 347-8550, BA 64 Miami Univ - Oxford; MA 73 Ball St Univ; Sp/Lang Path, Hennepin Co Med Cen, **SLP**

Slocum, Barbara B Rural Delivery 1, Chenango Fork, NY 13746, (607) 648-8511, BS 66 SUNY - Coll at Buffalo; ME 67 PA St Univ - Univ Park; Sp-Lang Path, Chenango Forks Ctrl Sch, **SLP**

Slocum, Grace Ellen P O Box 1484, Chico, CA 95927, (415) 282-2551, BA 82 CA St Univ - Chico; MS 84 Univ of Redlands; **SLP**

Slominski, Thomas J 188 Pray Road, Gaylord, MI 49735, (517) 732-3866, BS 68 Central MI Univ; MA 72 Central MI Univ; Sp-Lang Path, Northern Speech Services Inc, **SLP ACE**

Slomovitz, Linda Faye 111 Summerview Road, Williamsville, NY 14221, (716) 835-0417, BA 69 Rutger's St Univ - Douglas Coll; MS 77 Rutgers St Univ -N Brunswick; Sp-Lang Path, Cantalician Ctr for Learning, **SLP**

Slone, Ann M 9624 Leebrook Drive, Cincinnati, OH 45231, (513) 742-2200, BS 75 Miami Univ - Oxford; MA 76 Miami Univ - Oxford; Sp-Lang Path, Hamilton County Office of Educ, **SLP**

Sloneker, Mrs Kathy R 3259 Sutherland Drive, Lexington, KY 40502, (606) 987-1550, BS 77 Eastern KY Univ; MA 83 Eastern KY Univ; Sp-Lang Path, Bourbon Co Bd of Ed, **SLP**

Sloniger, Diann Marie 13151 Lilly Street, Garden Grove, CA 92643, (714) 828-6248, BA 82 CA St Univ - Fullerton; MA 86 CA St Univ - Fullerton; 88–Sp-Lang Path, Savanna Sch Dist, **SLP**

Sloniker, Mrs Sheila J 3703 Yale Drive, Oceanside, CA 92056, (402) 734-2808, BS 72 San Diego St Univ; MA 74 CA St Univ - Long Beach; **SLP**

Slosberg, Marion G 5 Cliffweller Court, Owings Mills, MD 21117, **SLP**

Slosson, Cynthia Worth 526 351/2 Road, Palisades, CO 81526, (303) 723-4938, BA 78 Univ of CO - Boulder; MA 80 Univ of CO - Boulder; Sp-Lang Path, Private Practice, **SLP**

Slota, Mrs Ginger Route 6, Homestead Road, Eau Claire, WI 54701, (715) 834-9275, BA 73 Univ of WI - Eau Claire; MS 74 Univ of WI - Eau Claire; 85–Sp-Lang Path, Chippewa Falls PS, **SLP**

Slothower, Margaret G 61483 Longview Street, Bend, OR 97702, (503) 389-1499, BA 70 Lewis & Clark Coll; MA 74 IN Univ - Bloomington; Sp-Lang Path, Central Oregon Reg Prog, **SLP**

Slotnick, Karen Rochelle 46 West 88th Street, New York, NY 10024, (212) 420-2760, MA 85 CUNY - Hunter Coll; 86–Sp-Lang Path, Beth Israel Med Ctr, **SLP**

Slotnick, Phyllis Beth 7602 21st Avenue, Brooklyn, NY 11214, (718) 990-3832, BA 83 CUNY - Brooklyn Coll; MS 85 CUNY - Brooklyn Coll; **A**

Slott, Shelley H 515 Sabine Circle, Wynnewood, PA 19096, (215) 783-6010, BS 73 West Chester Univ of PA; MS 74 Ithaca Coll; **SLP**

Sloup, Patricia Lackovic Route 1 Box 25, Prague, NE 68050, BS 79 Univ of NE - Omaha; MS 80 Univ of NE - Omaha; Sp-Lang Path, Wahoo PS, **SLP**

Slovin, Mrs Loretta R 45 Brentwood Road, Eatontown, NJ 07724, (201) 449-3070, BA 63 Rutger's St Univ - Douglas Coll; MA 66 Kean Coll of NJ; Sp-Lang Path, Wall Township Bd of Ed, **SLP**

Slovin, Susan Colvin 619 Westbourne Street, La Jolla, CA 92037, **SLP**

Slowinski, Deidre E 245 George Urban Boulevard, Cheektowaga, NY 14225, (716) 759-6985, BA 76 SUNY - Center at Buffalo; MA 78 SUNY - Center at Buffalo; 80–Dir of Sp-Lang Path Serv, Brothers of Mercy Nursing & Rehab Ctr, **SLP**

Slowley, Jeanne I 34820 Eight Mile #204R, Farmington Hills, MI 48018, (313) 745-8903, BS 77 Wayne St Univ; MA 78 Wayne St Univ; Sp-Lang Path, Chldn's Hosp of MI, **SLP**

Slugaski, Mrs Nancy 324 Dogwood Drive, Union, NJ 07083, (201) 558-3237, BA 77 Univ of RI; MS 78 Ithaca Coll; Sp-Lang Path, Elizabeth Bd of Ed, **SLP**

Slusser, Janice Lee K Behavioral Prosthetics, 447 East 1st South, Salt Lake City, UT 84111, (801) 532-1955, BS 76 Univ of UT; MS 81 Univ of UT; Aud Owner, Behavioral Prosthetics, **A**

Slutsky, Marsha Joan 185 East 33rd Street, Paterson, NJ 07504, BA 60 Montclair St Coll; SLP, Paterson Board of Education, **SLP**

Slutsky, Dr Sidney S Cottman Professional Bldg, 1936 Cottman Street, Philadelphia, PA 19111, (215) 722-1404, BA 51 Temple Univ-Tyler Sch of Art; ME 54 Temple Univ-Tyler Sch of Art; ED 66 (NS) Temple Univ-Tyler Sch of Art; Sp-Lang Path & Cl Psychol, Private Practice, **SLP**

Sly, Joanne Ruth 1770 Spitler Drive, Decatur, IL 62521, (217) 428-5016, BA 83 Univ of IL - Urbana; Sp-Lang Path, Veterans Administration, **SLP**

Slye, Tracy Rice 33 Swantonstreet, Winchester, MA 01890, (508) 745-2100, BS 84 Ithaca Coll; MS 86 Northeastern Univ; 87–Sp-Lang Path, North Shore Children's Hosp, **SLP**

Smadbeck, Diana W 1468 Cherryvale Road, Boulder, CO 80303, (303) 444-1015, MA 80 Univ of CO - Boulder; SLP, Private Practice Peak Performance, **SLP**

Smaldino, James M 145 Glenridge Road, East Aurora, NY 14052, (716) 887-4635, BS 71 SUNY - Coll at Fredonia; MS 73 SUNY - Coll at Fredonia; 88–Dir of Sp-Lang Path, Millard Fillmore Hosp, **SLP**

Smaldino, Dr Joseph J Dept Communicative Disorders, Univ Of Northern Iowa, Cedar Falls, IA 50614-0356, (319) 273-2560, BS 67 Union Coll; MS 72 Univ of CT; PH 74 (Audition/Aud) Univ of FL; Dept Head, U of Northern Iowa, **A**

Smale, Mrs Ruth Box 259, Round Hill, VA 22141, (703) 777-2290, BS 72 Longwood Coll; ME 73 Univ of VA - Charlottesville; Sp-Lang Path, Loudoun Co Pub Sch, **SLP**

Small, Dr Anita Ruth 1213 Beacon Street #6, Brookline, MA 02146, (513) 475-4542, BS 79 Univ of Toronto - Ontario; MS 81 Dalhousie Univ - Nova Scotia; ED 85 (NS) Univ of Cincinnati; Coordinator Outpatient Clinic, Learning Center Deaf Children, **SLP**

Small, Dr Arnold M Dept Speech Path & Audiology, University Of Iowa, Iowa City, IA 52242, (319) 335-8734, BA 51 San Diego St Univ; MS 53 Univ of WI - Madison; PH 54 (Exp Psychology) Univ of WI - Madison; Professor, University of Iowa, **F**

Small, Mrs Audrey Gale 303 Emerson Drive, Lafayette Hill, PA 19444, (215) 825-9438, BA 82 Temple Univ; MA 84 Hahnemann Univ Grad Sch; 88–Aud, Atkins-Keane-Rowe Otolaryngic Assoc, **A**

Small, Jamie Ann 634 Longstaff, Missoula, MT 59801, (406) 728-3506, BA 82 Univ of MT; **A**

Small, Judith L 10714 Outpost Drive, Gaithersburg, MD 20878, (301) 294-6095, BA 80 Rutger's St Univ - Douglas Coll; MA 81 Trenton St Coll; 88–Sp-Lang Path, Natl Rehab Hosp, **SLP**

Small, Kristi Lynn Route 1 Box 612, Normangee, TX 77871, (409) 396-6925, BS 85 OK St Univ; MA 86 OK St Univ; **SLP**

Small, Dr Larry H Dept Of Comm Disorders, Bowling Green State Univ, Bowling Green, OH 43403, (419) 372-7182, BS 77 Kent St Univ; MA 77 Kent St Univ; PH 84 (NS) OH Univ - Athens; Asst Prof Aud, Bowling Green State U, **A**

Small, Mary Elizabeth 925 Whitmore #A-5, Detroit, MI 48203, (313) 864-5221

Small, Stacy A Thoms Rehabilitation Hospital, 1 Rotary Drive, Asheville, NC 28803, (704) 274-2400, BA 81 0500; MS 86 Western Carolina Univ; SLP, Thoms Rehab Hosp, **SLP**

Smallcomb, Kathleen 45 Moulton Street, West Newburg, MA 01985, (617) 774-6946, **SLP**

Smallets, Sharon Marie 230 Old Line Avenue, Laurel, MD 20707, (301) 454-6911, BA 80 Univ of MD - College Park; MA 82 Univ of MD - College Park; Audiologist, University of Maryland, **A**

Smalls, Jacquelyn Elaine 560 Brummel Court, Washington, DC 20012, (202) 291-4632, BA 68 Hampton Univ; MA 80 Howard Univ; PH 84 (NS) Howard Univ; SLP, Dc Pub Schs, **SLP**

Smallwood, Anita E 409 Darby, Sheffield, AL 35660, (615) 433-7026, BS 86 Auburn Univ - Auburn; MS 88 AL A & M Univ

Smanda, Debra S 1780 West 51st Street, Indianapolis, IN 46208, (317) 272-4859, BA 79 IN Univ - Bloomington; MA 81 IN Univ - Bloomington; Sp-Lang Path, Avon Comm Sch, **SLP**

Smarra, Mrs Paula Denise 6602 Brittany Park Lane, Houston, TX 77066, (713) 783-6220, BS 82 Indiana Univ of PA; MA 85 Univ of Pittsburgh - Pittsburgh; 87–Sp-Lang Path, T H Rogers, **SLP**

Smart, Mrs Mary L 50 Meadowbrook Road, Weston, MA 02193, (617) 893-0679, BA 69 CA St Univ - Los Angeles; MS 76 Univ of London - England; Sp-Lang Path, Waltham Weston Hospital, **SLP**

Smart, Mrs Nancy Sundahl Ear Nose And Throat Assoc, 209 South 12th Avenue, Yakima, WA 98902, (509) 575-1000, BS 74 ND St Univ; MS 76 Minot St Univ; 78–Aud, Ear Nose and Throat Assoc, **A**

Smartt, Joan D Route 3, McMinnville, TN 37110, (615) 728-2316, BS 52; MS 72 Vanderbilt Univ; Sch Psychol, Manchester City Sch, **SLP**

Smaston, Mrs Sharon 8812 Gelligum Drive, Charlotte, NC 28226, (704) 343-6422, BS 79 Central MI Univ; MA 81 Central MI Univ; 83–Sp-Lang Path, Charlotte-Mecklenburg Schools, **SLP**

Smathers, Jessica C 2570 Woodstock Place, Boulder, CO 80303, (303) 447-1010, OB 62 OH Univ - Athens; MA 68 OH Univ - Athens; SLP, Boulder Val Sch Dist, **SLP**

Smay, Karen J 396 Maryland Avenue, York, PA 17404, (717) 771-2380, BS 79 Bloomsburg Univ of PA; MS 80 Bloomsburg Univ of PA; Sp-Lnag Path, York Hosp, **SLP ACE**

Smayling, Mrs Lyda M 3430 List Place #506, Minneapolis, MN 55416, **SLP LM**

Smead, Kathleen 1013 Airport Boulevard, Pensacola, FL 32504, (904) 484-9292, BS 73 IN Univ - Bloomington; MS 74 East TX St Univ - Commerce; Dir, Sp & Lang Ctr of NW FL, **SLP**

Smead, Mrs Lucille J 205 Butler Avenue, St Simons Island, GA 31522, (912) 638-8570, BS 38 Longwood Coll; ME 59 Univ of VA - Charlottesville; **SLP F LM**

Smedal, Mrs Heidi Ann 715 Bickley Court, Stoughton, WI 53589, (608) 255-7878, BS 82 Univ of WI - Stevens Point; MS 84 Univ of WI - Stevens Point; Aud, Madison Med Ctr Hrng Serv, **A**

Smedley, Elaine Ann 38 Amherst Lane, Hicksville, NY 11801, (516) 293-0060, BA 82 Dowling Coll; MS 85 Adelphi Univ

Smedley, Mrs Elizabeth M 127 Crescent Drive, DE Cordora Bend Estates, Granbury, TX 76048, (817) 443-0256, BS 43 TX Woman's Univ; MA 54 TX Woman's Univ; **SLP**

Smedley, Dr Thayne C Isu Box 8116, Pocatello, ID 83209, (208) 236-3495, MS 64 UT St Univ; PH 69 (NS) Stanford Univ; Asst Prof, Idaho St U, **A**

Smedra, Carol Ann 506 South Plum Road, Grand Island, NE 68801, (402) 336-4457, **SLP**

Smeltzer, Mrs Joan E 972 Box Elder, Kirkwood, MO 63122, (314) 447-4142, BS 74 Eastern IL Univ; MS 75 Eastern IL Univ; Sp-Lang Path, Francis Howell Sch Dist, **SLP**

Smeraski, Joan Ellen 27 Lexington Drive, Medford, NJ 08055, MA 78 Temple Univ

Smetana, Wayne R 14804 Ashford Court, Laurel, MD 20707, (301) 497-9784, BS 82 Northwestern OK St Univ; MS 84 Univ of OK - OK City; Aud, Walter Reed Army Med Ctr, **A**

Smette, Mrs Alice Marie 1825 Park Boulevard, Fargo, ND 58103, (218) 233-4671, BS 76 6475; MS 85 Moorhead St Univ

Smider, Wilma J E 520 Sheridan Road #3-B, Evanston, IL 60202, (312) 835-2238, BS 60 Purdue Univ - West Lafayette; MS 61 Purdue Univ - West Lafayette; Sp-Lang Path, Northern Suburban Spec Ed Dist, **SLP**

Smiderski, Sarah J 1630 Leyden, Denver, CO 80220, **SLP**

Smidt, Janet C 235 Auburn Court, St Charles, IL 60174, (312) 529-5670, BS 73 Purdue Univ - West Lafayette; MA 75 Northern IL Univ - De Kalb; Sp-Lang Path, Sased, **SLP**

Smigo, Therese M Bradley 4418 Crossland Road, Philadelphia, PA 19154, (215) 563-1844, MA 84 Temple Univ; Sp-Lang Path, Communication Associates, **SLP**

Smiley, Ann M 17-B Brookwood Drive, Rocky Hill, CT 06067, (203) 721-1668, BS 82 RI Coll; MS 86 Univ of RI; **SLP**

Smiley, Mrs Deborah T 2514 Highland Drive, Palatine, IL 60067, (312) 934-2908, BS 72 Purdue Univ - West Lafayette; MS 73 Purdue Univ - West Lafayette; Sp-Lang Path, Comm Consoldtd Sch Dist 15, **SLP**

Smiley, Helen Nutter 2972 Courville Drive, Bloomfield Hills, MI 48013, (313) 628-1323, BA 76 Kutztown Univ of PA; MA 80 Wayne St Univ; Sp-Lang Path, Oxford Area Comm Sch, **SLP**

Smiley, Kathy H 60 Juniper Lane, West Hartford, CT 06117, (203) 232-8513, BS 74 Boston Univ; MS 75 Hofstra Univ; **SLP**

Smiley, Melinda E 84 Lidgerwood Parkway, Morristown, NJ 07960, (718) 987-9400, BA 85 Rutger's St Univ - Douglas Coll; MA 87 Univ of Houston - Univ Park; 87–Sp-Lang Path, Our PLACE Sch Inc, **SLP**

Smiley, Nancy Marie 5628 NW 87th Terrace #351, Kansas City, MO 64154, (816) 756-2250, BS 76 Fontbonne Coll; MS 77 Fontbonne Coll; Sp/Lang Path, The Rehabilitation Institute, **SLP**

Smiley, Rosemary 4000 Amberley Road, Montgomery, AL 36116, (205) 284-5304, **SLP**

Smiley-Slocum, Mrs Kimberly Marie 12 Sugarbush Road, Clifton Park, NY 12065, (518) 383-4732, BA 86 SUNY - Coll at Plattsburgh; MS 88 Coll of Saint Rose; 87–Sp-Lang Path, Wildwood Sch

Smit, Dr Ann B Speech Pathology Audiology Pro, Kansas State University, Manhattan, KS 66506-7061, (913) 532-6879, BA 66 Calvin Coll; MA 69 Univ of IA; PH 80 (Hrng & Sp Sciences) Univ of MD - College Park; 87–Asst Prof, Kansas State Univ, **SLP**

Smit, Beth G 1627 Sun Prairie Drive, St Joseph, MI 49085, (616) 429-2578, BA 71 Western MI Univ; MA 72 MI St Univ; **SLP**

Smit, Mrs Pamela Mills 1545 C Honey Grove Drive, Richmond, VA 23279, (804) 285-7086, BA 75 Univ of FL; MS 76 FL St Univ; Sp-Lang Path, Private Practice, **SLP**

Smith, Mrs Agatha 1345 Shenandoah Oval, Parma, OH 44134, BS 70 Bowling Green St Univ; MA 71 Bowling Green St Univ; Sp-Lang Path, Cleveland Public Schools, **SLP**

Smith, Alice B 95 Lovering Avenue, Buffalo, NY 14216, (716) 881-5400, BS 72 SUNY - Coll at Buffalo; MS 74 SUNY - Coll at Buffalo; 88–Uni Serv Rep, National Education Assoc, **SLP**

Smith, Mrs Alice E 287 Benton Avenue, Missoula, MT 59801, (406) 243-4131, BA 74 Mary Baldwin Coll; MS 77 Univ of NC - Chapel Hill; MA 87 Univ of MT; Instr, Univ of Montana, **SLP**

Smith, Mrs Alice V 901 Sierra Drive, Denton, TX 76201, (817) 382-1591, BS 71 TX Woman's Univ; MA 72 TX Woman's Univ; 88–Sp-Lang Path, Denton TX ISD, **SLP A**

Smith, Alison Kelford 1200 Royal York Road, Etobicoke, ON, Canada M9A 4B3, (416) 424-3805, BS 84 Univ of Toronto - Ontario; OM 86 Univ of Toronto - Ontario; 88–Aug Comm Consult, Hugh MacMillan Med Ctr

Smith, Allison Harmon 1821 Marshall #1, Houston, TX 77098, (713) 771-9966, BS 80 Baylor Univ; MA 83 Univ of TN - Knoxville; Sp-Lang Path, Houston Ear Research Fnd, **SLP**

Smith, Dr Andree Durieux Childrens Hosp Of East Ontario, 401 Smyth Road, Ottawa, ON, Canada K1H 8L1, (613) 737-2379, BS 64 McGill Univ - Quebec; MS 68 McGill Univ - Quebec; PH 74 (Sp Perception) McGill Univ - Quebec; Director of Audiology, Childrens Hosp of East Ontario, **A**

Smith, Ann L 17 Viewpoint Circle, Phillips Ranch, Pomona, CA 91766, MS; **SLP**

Smith, Anne Dept Aud & Speech Science, Heavilon Hall, Purdue University, West Lafayette, IN 47907

Smith, Anne Jaquette 1708 Kenmar Drive, Manhattan, KS 66502, (913) 532-6879, MS 84 Univ of WI - Madison; 88–Instr, Kansas State Univ, **SLP**

Smith, Mrs Anne Maven 495 Three Springs Road, Bowling Green, KY 42101, (502) 843-5816, BS 80 PA St Univ - Univ Park; MS 84 Univ of MS; Aud, Kentucky Comm for Hndcpd Chldn, **A**

Smith, Annette M 1315 Splice Circle, Okemos, MI 48864, (517) 787-8910, BS 66 Univ of MI - Ann Arbor; MA 72 MI St Univ; Sp-Lang Path, Jackson Cnty Intermed Sch Dist, **SLP A**

Smith, April Gayle 11815 Vance Jackson #2403, San Antonio, TX 78230-1457, (512) 699-1190, BA 83 CA St Univ - Stanislaus; MA 85 CA St Univ - Stanislaus; 87–Sp-Lang Path, Communication & Learning Svcs, **SLP**

Smith, Mrs Arlene Dawn Route 5 Box 631, Front Royal, VA 22630, (703) 636-6010, BA 82 Marshall Univ; MA 83 Marshall Univ; Sp-Lang Path, Warren Co School System, **SLP**

Smith, Arlene R 335 Daisy Farms Drive, Scarsdale, NY 10583, (212) 679-0100, BA 73 CUNY - Hunter Coll; MA 76 CUNY - Hunter Coll; Aud, Internal Cen for the Disabled, **A**

Smith, Audrey Lynn 430 Landing Boulevard, Inverness, FL 32650, (904) 726-8170, BS 86 Valdosta St Coll; ME 87 Valdosta St Coll; **SLP**

Smith, Mrs Barbara Berglund 108 Candee Lane, Marquette, MI 49855, (906) 228-9400, BA 75 Univ of MN - Duluth; MA 77 Northern MI Univ; 88–Sp-Lang Path, Marquette-Alger Inter Sch Dist, **SLP**

Smith, Barbara M 26 Swart Terrace, Nashua, NH 03060, (603) 885-4794, BS 48; ME 49 Boston Univ; **SLP LM**

Smith, Mrs Barbara Varkoly 376 Hillcrest, Grosse Pointe Farms, MI 48236, BS 79 Eastern MI Univ; MA 81 Eastern MI Univ; Sp-Lang Path, Out Wayne County Head Start, **SLP**

Smith, Becky Lee 1622 East Fairway Drive #9, Orange, CA 92666, (714) 997-9301, MS; 88–Aud, Centralia Sch Dist, **A**

Smith, Mrs Beth Ann 360 Cator Avenue, Jersey City, NJ 07305, (201) 385-4857, BS 79 Syracuse Univ; MA 84 Montclair St Coll; SLP, Bergen Ctr for Chld Dev, **SLP**

Smith, Mrs Betty A River Ridge Rehab Inc, 275 South 3rd Street, Suite 102, Stillwater, MN 55082, (612) 430-1972, BS 74 Univ of WI - River Falls; MS 80 Univ of WI - River Falls; Pres, River Ridge Rehab, Inc, **SLP ACE**

Smith, Betty Jo Royal York Apartment, 3955 Bigelow Blvd #403, Pittsburgh, PA 15213, (412) 231-6080, MS 65 Univ of Pittsburgh - Pittsburgh; SLP, Vna of Allegheny Co, **SLP**

Smith, Betty M 14 Mitchell Road, Port Washington, NY 11050, (516) 883-4000, BA 46 Univ of WI - Madison; MA 70 CUNY - Queens Coll; Dept Chairperson, Port Washington Pub Sch, **SLP**

Smith, Bettye H 3432 Ponce DE Leon, Jacksonville, FL 32217, (904) 282-5494, BA 56 Univ of AL- Tuscaloosa; ME 80 Univ of North FL; SLP, Clay County Sch Bd, **SLP**

Smith, Dr Bettye W 1300 Shadybrook Drive, Beverly Hills, CA 90210, BA 50 Univ of MD - College Park; MA 52 Univ of MD - College Park; PH 63 (NS) Univ of Southern CA; Retired, VA Outpatient Clin, **SLP A**

Smith, Mrs Beverly B Route 2 Box 205, Arlington, GA 31713, (912) 725-4985, BS 80 Auburn Univ - Auburn; OM 81 Auburn Univ - Auburn; Sp-Lang Path, Calhoun Co Sch, **SLP**

Smith, Dr Bonnie E 917 Ontario #E-3, Oak Park, IL 60302-1945, (312) 996-6520, BS 74 Syracuse Univ; MS 76 Purdue Univ - West Lafayette; PH 81 (Sp-Path) Purdue Univ - West Lafayette; Chmn Sp-Lang Path/Asst Prof, Univ Illinois College Medicine, **SLP**

Smith, Brian E 221 Glenridge Avenue #407, St Catharines, ON, Canada L2T 3J7, (416) 685-1551, BA 75 St Mary's Univ - Ns; MA 78 WA St Univ; Sp-Lang Path, Lincoln Co Bd of Ed, **SLP**

Smith, Dr Bruce L Communication Sciences & Disorders, Northwestern University, 2299 Sheridan Road, Evanston, IL 60208, (312) 491-5076, BA 72 Brigham Young Univ; MA 73 Brigham Young Univ; PH 76 (Linguistics) Univ of TX - Austin; 81–Assoc Prof, Northwestern U

Smith, Mrs Camille St Hilaire 105 Nettlecreek Drive, Fairport, NY 14450, (716) 223-6657, BA 78 Saint Mary's Coll; MA 80 George Washington Univ; Sp-Lang Path, UCPA Rochester, **SLP**

Smith, Mrs Carla Jamison 827 Buoy, Houston, TX 77062, (713) 487-3777, BA 78 Univ of Houston - Univ Park; MA 81 Univ of Houston - Univ Park; SLP, Pasadena ISD, **SLP**

Smith, Carleen Wendt Doe Special Education, Lower Base, Saipan, Mariana Islands 96950, (804) 481-4004, BS 82 Univ of WI - Madison; MS 84 Univ of WI - Madison; **SLP**

Smith, Carol A 19 Geoffrey Court, Chatham, NJ 07928, (201) 701-0253, BA 71 CUNY - City College; MA 73 CUNY - City College; Sp-Lang Path, Private Practice, **SLP**

Smith, Carol A 609 White Pine Circle, Lawrenceville, NJ 08648, (609) 883-0690, BS 79 Trenton St Coll; MA 80 Trenton St Coll; Sp-Lang Path, Hopewell Valley Reg Sch Dist, **SLP**

Smith, Mrs Caroline 1910 South Virginia, Hopkinsville, KY 42240, (502) 885-7023, BA 73 Hillsdale Coll; MS 74 Murray St Univ; Sp-Lang Path, Private Practice, **SLP ACE**

Smith, Carolyn Dana 1183 Haselton Road, Cleveland Heights, OH 44121, (216) 791-8363, BA 69 Coll of Wooster; MA 71 Case Western Reserve Univ; 71–Dir of Children's Prog, UCP Assoc, **SLP**

Smith, Carolyn Jo 195 Round Key Circle, Naples, FL 33962-5058, (813) 774-3460, BS 81 Western MI Univ; MA 83 Western MI Univ; Sp-Lang Path, Collier County Public Schools, **SLP**

Smith, Catherine 719 East Riverview Drive, Suffolk, VA 23434, (804) 539-8808, **SLP**

Smith, Catherine L 205 Harris Road, Charlottesville, VA 22901, (804) 973-6600, BS 75 VA Polytechnic Inst St Univ; MA 77 James Madison Univ; Sp-Lang Path, Albemarle County Pub Schools, **SLP**

Smith, Catherine M 541 Clarkson, Denver, CO 80218, (303) 789-8397, BS 79 West Chester Univ of PA; MA 85 Univ of CO - Boulder; 87–Sp-Lang Path, Craig Hosp, **SLP**

Smith, Catherine Patricia 214 Bloomsbury Avenue, Baltimore, MD 21228, (703) 691-2851, BS 82 Towson St Univ; MS 84 Towson St Univ; **SLP**

Smith, Mrs Charlotte Box 12, 503 Main, Flagler, CO 80815, (303) 765-4679, BS 73 CO St Univ; MA 73 Univ of Denver; Sp-Lang Path/Aud, E Central BOCES, **SLP**

Smith, Dr Cheryl 43 Countryside Drive, Essex Junction, VT 05452, (802) 656-3861, BS 69 Miami Univ - Oxford; MS 73 Emerson Coll; PH 85 (NS) Univ of CT; Sp-Lang Path, Private Practice, **SLP**

Smith, Christine Ann 5801 East Hawthorne, Tucson, AZ 85711, (602) 798-2558, BS 83 Univ of AZ; MS 85 Univ of AZ; 86–Sp-Lang Path, Tucson USD, **SLP**

Smith, Mrs Christine Buscaino Center For Comm Disorders, 101 Old Short Hills Road, Suite 211, West Orange, NJ 07052, (201) 731-6115, BA 78 Montclair St Coll; MA 80 Ball St Univ; Director of Audiology, Center for Communications, **A**

Smith, Dr Clarissa R Livingston Road Rd #7, Lake Carmel, NY 10512, (914) 225-7159, BS 45 Northwestern Univ; MA 62 CUNY - Hunter Coll; PH 72 (Sp & Hrng Science) CUNY - Grad Sch & Univ Cntr; **A LM**

Smith, Clyde G 137 Rawlins Run Road, Pittsburgh, PA 15238, (412) 647-5470, BA 68 Saint Vincent Coll; MS 73 Univ of Pittsburgh - Pittsburgh; Aud/Admin Coord, Chldn Hosp of Pittsburgh, **A**

Smith, Mrs Colleen Kroswek 4424 Indian Road, Toledo, OH 43615, (419) 536-4026, BS 83 Central MI Univ; MA 86 Central MI Univ; **A**

Smith, Connie J 12611 Sunset Boulevard, Los Angeles, CA 90049-3832, (213) 472-5124, **SLP**

Smith, Constance 74 Fair Oaks, St Louis, MO 63124, (314) 993-6420, BS 71 Purdue Univ - West Lafayette; MS 72 Purdue Univ - West Lafayette; Sp-Lang Path, Comm Sch, **SLP**

Smith, Constance Cheryl 100 Martin Drive, Raynham, MA 02767, (617) 644-2214, BS 80 Elmira Coll; MS 81 Ithaca Coll; Sp/Lang Path, Iddi/Crystal Springs School, **SLP**

Smith, Dr Curtis R P O Box 2278, Auburn, AL 36830, (205) 826-5545, BS 60 Univ Southern MS-Hattiesburg; MS 61 Univ Southern MS-Hattiesburg; PH 65 (NS) Univ Southern MS-Hattiesburg; 69–Prof of Aud, Auburn U, **SLP A**

Smith, Mrs Cynthia B 2003 Winston Avenue, Louisville, KY 40205, (502) 561-3349, BA 71 IN Univ - Bloomington; OM 72 IN Univ - Bloomington; Sp-Lang Path, Private Practice, **SLP ACE**

Smith, Mrs Cynthia Griffin 22 Day Street South, West Gramby, CT 06090, (203) 658-2251, BS 77; MS 79 Southern CT St Univ; Sp-Lang Path, Simsbury Pub Schs, **SLP**

Smith, D Wayne Aud & Sp Services Of Oakland, 77JACK London Square, Suite G, Oakland, CA 94607, (415) 451-8336, BA 49 Univ of Akron; MA 50 Case Western Reserve Univ; Dir, Aud & Sp Serv of Oakland, **SLP A LM**

Smith, Dale K P O Box 6348, Dunedin, New Zealand, (024) 740-999, BA 75 Depauw Univ; MA 81 Univ of MT; 87–Aud, Otago Area Health Bd, **A**

Smith, David L 14 Willoughby Avenue, Huntington, WV 25705, (304) 522-6388, BA 69 Marshall Univ; MA 74 Kent St Univ; Aud, Tri St Otol, **A**

Smith, Deborah Ann 201-08 43rd Avenue, Bayside, NY 11361, (718) 229-4423, MA 86 CUNY - Hunter Coll; **SLP**

Smith, Deborah L Route 1 Box 31, Ripley, WV 25271, (304) 372-9231, BA 77 Marshall Univ; MA 80 Marshall Univ; Sp/Lang Path, Jackson Co Bd of Ed, **SLP**

Smith, Deborah Lynn 966 Locust Drive #2E, Dundee, IL 60118, (312) 742-3264, BS 82 Bradley Univ; MS 84 Bradley Univ; 85–Aud, Jayne Shover Rehab Ctr, **A**

Smith, Mrs Deborah M 1206 Westway Circle, Killeen, TX 76542-1064, (817) 288-8513, BS 76 Southwest TX St Univ; ME 77 Southwest TX St Univ; Sp-Lang Path, Darnall Army Commun Hosp, **SLP**

Smith, Deborah Rowland 511 South 2nd Street, Walla Walla, WA 99362, (509) 527-3000, BA 76 WA St Univ; MS 78 Eastern WA Univ; Sp-Lang Path, Walla Walla Sch Dist, **SLP**

Smith, Mrs Deborah Shontz 22-Q Reading Road, Edison, NJ 08817, (800) 526-3921, BS 83 Clarion Univ of PA; MS 84 Clarion Univ of PA; 86–Aud, Oticon Corp, **A**

Smith, Debra Ann 60-40 Madison Street #B-8, Ridgewood, NY 11385, (718) 366-6424, BS 78 Marywood Coll; MS 83 Bloomsburg Univ of PA; 86–Sp-Lang Path, Visiting Therapists Associates, **SLP**

Smith, Debra Kay 30 Half Moon Lane, Tarrytown, NY 10591, (914) 631-7357, BA 79 Wichita St Univ; MA 80 Wichita St Univ; **SLP**

Smith, Mrs Debra L 13308 Mohler Road, Grand Rapids, OH 43522, (419) 592-6991, BA 74 Bowling Green St Univ; MA 79 Bowling Green St Univ; SLP, Napolean City Sch, **SLP**

Smith, Debra L 555 North 30th Street, Omaha, NE 68131, BA 79 Salem St Coll; MA 82 Univ of TN - Knoxville; 83–Aud, Boys Town Natl Inst, **A**

Smith, Mrs Denise Elliott 2376 Grant Place, Fairfield Plantation, Villa Rica, GA 30180, (404) 832-1336, BS 76 SUNY - Coll at Fredonia; ME 79 SUNY - Coll at Fredonia; 76–Sp-Lang Path, Carroll Co Bd of Ed, **SLP**

Smith, Denise Marie 2206 Covey Creek Court, Stockton, CA 95207-5367, (209) 944-4266, BS 73 Kent St Univ; MA 74 Kent St Univ; **SLP**

Smith, Diana Ep 2222 Marston, Flossmoor, IL 60422, (312) 799-5563, MA 88 Northern IL Univ - De Kalb

Smith, Mrs Diane E O P O Box 863, Elk Grove, CA 95624-0863, (209) 944-4262, MA 80 CA St Univ - Stanislaus; Sp-Lang Path, Stockton USD, **SLP**

Smith, Dr Dianna M 747 Shady Creek Place, Salt Lake City, UT 84106, (801) 582-1565, BA 68 San Diego St Univ; MA 69 San Diego St Univ; PH 72 (Aud) Univ of OK - Norman; Chief-Aud & Sp/Lang Path, VA Med Center, **A**

Smith, Mrs Dianne P 21 Yosemite, Kenner, LA 70065, (504) 466-8273, BA 76 Univ of Southwestern LA; OM 77 LA St Univ - N O Medical Ctr; **A**

Smith, Dinah K University Of Vermont, E M Luse Center, 461 Main Street, Burlington, VT 05405, (802) 656-3861, BA 70 IN Univ - Bloomington; MA 72 IN Univ - Bloomington; Intern Prog Coord, U of VT, **A**

Smith, Donna M 7461 South Harrison Way, Littleton, CO 80122, (303) 771-7165, BA 70 Baylor Univ; MS 71 Baylor Univ; Remediation Spec/Psychometrist, Hillel Academy, **SLP**

Smith, Donna Marie 3401 S Plaza Drive #N, Santa Ana, CA 92704, (714) 751-2040, BA 83 Chapman Coll; MA 87 San Diego St Univ; **A**

Smith, Donna W 121 Avenue Of Trees, Elon College, Burlington, NC 27244, BS 77 Baylor Univ; MS 78 Baylor Univ; Sp-Lang Path, Burlington PS, **SLP**

Smith, Dori Jean 1309 Partridge Road, Roslyn, PA 19001, (215) 657-2219, **SLP**

Smith, Doris J P O Box 386, Big Sur, CA 93920, (408) 667-2715, LA City School, **SLP**

Smith, Douglas M P O Box 245, Woodlawn, VA 24381, (703) 728-3121, BS 76 James Madison Univ; MS 79 James Madison Univ; Sp-Lang Path, Swn VA Trng Cen, **SLP**

Smith, Mrs Eileen F McAs Futenma, P O Box 786, FPO Seattle, WA 98772, BS 82 Bloomsburg Univ of PA; MS 83 Bloomsburg Univ of PA; **A**

Smith, Mrs Eileen Ward Route 2 Box 347, Fall Branch, TN 37656, (615) 348-6503, BS 83 Univ of GA; MS 87 Univ of SC - Columbia; 85–Sp-Lang Path, Mountain Reg Sp & Hrng Ctr, **SLP**

Smith, Mrs Elaine Ann 2117 East 154th Street, Olathe, KS 66062, (913) 782-7735, MA 84 Univ of KS; Sp-Lang Path, East Cent Kansas Cooperative, **SLP**

Smith, Mrs Elaine Genuardi 1820 Meredith Lane, Blue Bell, PA 19422, BS 71 PA St Univ - Univ Park; MA 73 Trenton St Coll; 87–Sp-Lang Path, Mont Cty Intermediate Unit, **SLP**

Smith, Elaine M 760 Los Pueblos, Los Alamos, NM 87544, (505) 662-4136, BS 65 Purdue Univ - West Lafayette; MS 67 Purdue Univ - West Lafayette; SLP, Los Alamos Schls, **SLP**

Smith, Mrs Eleanor Colby 680 Tierra Linda Court, Camarillo, CA 93010, (805) 527-2462, BA 83 CA St Univ - Northridge; MA 84 CA St Univ - Northridge; 87–Dir-Comm Dis Dept, Simi Valley Adventist Hosp, **SLP**

Smith, Elizabeth Helen 217 Mechanic Street, Cape May Court House, NJ 08210, (609) 861-6031, BS 77 Loyola Coll; MS 79 Loyola Coll; Dir Sp & Hrng Serv, Woodbine Dev Cen, **SLP**

Smith, Elizabeth Imle 4422 Pali Way, Boulder, CO 80301, (303) 530-3356, BA 65 Univ of TX - Austin; MA 67 Stanford Univ; 88–Sp-Lang Path, Front Range Educ Assoc, **SLP**

Smith, Mrs Elizabeth Kolski 105 Old Farm Drive, Pittsburgh, PA 15239, (412) 793-2126, BS 81 WV Univ; MS 82 WV Univ; Aud, Harmarville Rehabilitation, **A**

Smith, Mrs Elizabeth Mary 20625 Reid Lane, Saratoga, CA 95070, (408) 985-1050, BA 63 6687; MA 66 San Jose St Univ; Retired, Santa Clara USD, **SLP**

Smith, Mrs Ellen D Pssc Box 501, APO San Francisco, CA 96206, BA 68 Univ of MO - Columbia; MA 69 Univ of MO - Columbia; **SLP**

Smith, Elliott Gregory 1548 Aviators #D, New Orleans, LA 70122, (504) 568-4785, BA 84 Wichita St Univ; MS 86 Univ of AZ; Aud, Lsu Med Ctr-Kresge Hrng Labs, **A**

Smith, Eloise K P O Box 1061, Carrollton, TX 75006, (214) 492-1629, BA 75 GA Southern Coll; MS 82 Univ of TX - Dallas; **SLP**

Smith, Mrs Enid Dianne Discount Hearing Aids, 2500 Hillsboro Road, Suite 102, Nashville, TN 37212, (615) 385-3042, BA 81 Univ of GA; MS 84 Vanderbilt Univ; Aud, Discount Hearing Aids, **A**

Smith, Eric Lamont 914 Carvel Drive, Dover, DE 19901, (302) 674-3752, BA 80 Univ of MD - College Park; MS 83 Howard Univ; 86–Aud, ENT Associates, **A**

Smith, Mrs Esther Goldwasser 5839 North Drake Avenue, Chicago, IL 60659-4403, (312) 478-3979, **SLP**

Smith, Mrs Evelyn H 3510 44th Street, Lubbock, TX 79413, (806) 799-5882, BA 40 TX Tech Univ; ME 51 TX Tech Univ; **SLP LM**

Smith, Mrs Frances A 713 Dawley Avenue, West Covina, CA 91790, (213) 681-4681, BA 75 CA St Univ - Northridge; MA 80 CA St Univ - Northridge; SLP, Hear Center, **SLP**

Smith, Mrs Frances G 1539 Burton Court, Ogden, UT 84403, BA 34 Stanford Univ; **SLP LM**

Smith, Dr Frances S 230 Arlington Road North, Jacksonville, FL 32211, (904) 725-8972, BA 54 Univ of MS; MA 56 Univ of MS; PH 61 (NS) Purdue Univ - West Lafayette; Admin & Dir/Sp-Path Aud Ser, S Allen Smith Cl, **SLP A F**

Smith, Mrs Geraldine Jones 7220 Chadbourne Drive, New Orleans, LA 70126, (504) 246-2930, BA 68 Southern Univ - Baton Rouge; MA 69 Northwestern St Univ; 69–Sp-Lang Path, Southern Univ at New Orleans, **SLP**

Smith, Mrs Gina Lynne 3705 Sage Avenue, Charlotte, NC 28216, (704) 523-0363, BA 81 Univ of NC - Greensboro; ME 82 Univ of NC - Greensboro; SLP, Charlotte-Mecklenburg Schools, **SLP**

Smith, Glenn L 1044 Presidio Drive, Costa Mesa, CA 92626, (714) 546-4219, MA 56 Univ of Southern CA; **SLP LM**

Smith, Mrs Gloria M 376 Ridgedale Avenue, East Hanover, NJ 07936, BS 43 Newark St Coll; MA 47 Columbia Univ Teachers Coll; MA 76 Montclair St Coll; Sp-Lang Path, **SLP ACE**

Smith, Mrs Gregoria A 376 Ridge Road, West Milford, NJ 07480, (201) 456-5347, BA 76 William Paterson Coll; MS 78 William Paterson Coll; **SLP**

Smith, Harlie R 35998 Charter Crest Road, Farmington Hills, MI 48331, (517) 335-8958, BA 67 OH Wesleyan Univ; MS 68 Univ of MI - Ann Arbor; Aud, Michigan Dept of Public Health, **A**

Smith, Mrs Helen K 208 Gates Avenue, Montclair, NJ 07042, BA 51 Kalamazoo Coll; MA 76 Montclair St Coll; 80–Asst Director SLP & Aud, Kessler Institute for Rehab, **SLP**

Smith, Mrs Hilary C Y 733 Town Place, Hinsdale, IL 60521, (312) 655-1934, OD 58 0196; MA 62 Univ of Southern CA; 75–Sp-Lang Path, Schaumburg Dist #54, **SLP**

Smith, Jack H Harvey Road, Foxburg, PA 16036, (814) 226-2445, BS 52 Saint Cloud St Univ; MA 57 Univ of NE - Lincoln; Associate Professor-SLP, Clarion University of Pa, **SLP**

Smith, Jaclyn D S Western Hills AEA 12, 1520 Morningside Avenue, Sioux City, IA 51104, (712) 274-6040, MS 78 Baylor Univ; SLP, Western Hills AEA, **SLP**

Smith, Mrs Jamie Lynn 7500 Lincoln Avenue, Evansville, IN 47715, (812) 479-1411, BA 82 Ball St Univ; MA 83 Ball St Univ; Sp-Lang Path, Evansville Vanderburge Sch, **SLP**

Smith, Jane Anne 418 West Jefferson #4, Morton, IL 61550, (309) 266-5229, BS 85 IL St Univ - Normal; MS 86 IL St Univ - Normal; **SLP**

Smith, Jane Coe 5195 Buckskin Road, Pocatello, ID 83201, (208) 232-5841, BA 79 Western MI Univ; MA 81 Western MI Univ; 88–Sp-Lang Path, Private Practice, **SLP**

Smith, Mrs Janet Darchuk 6912 Lido Court, Parma, OH 44129, (216) 888-8632, BS 72 OH St Univ; MA 75 Bowling Green St Univ; Sp-Lang Path, Parma Cty Sch Dist, **SLP**

Smith, Janet G 3131 South Xeric Court, Denver, CO 80231, (303) 755-0323, BA 67 Univ of Denver; MA 78 Univ of CO - Denver; 88–Sp-Lang Path, Aurora PS, **SLP**

Smith, Janet K 826 N E 16th Street, Fort Lauderdale, FL 33304, **SLP**

Smith, Janet L 36 Farview Avenue Rear Apt, Danbury, CT 06810, (203) 743-4799, BS 77 SUNY - Coll at Geneseo; MA 78 MI St Univ; Sp-Lang Path, Danbury Ct Sch Dist, **SLP**

Smith, Mrs Janet Novella 4524 East Ashcroft, Fresno, CA 93726, (213) 273-8480, BA 81 CA St Univ - Fresno; MA 85 CA St Univ - Fresno; SLP, Irwin Lehroff and Associates, **SLP**

Smith, Janice A 3408 Lindsay Avenue, Bellingham, WA 98226, (206) 734-9210, BS 76 Univ of WA; MS 77 ID St Univ; Director Rehab Development, Visiting Nurse Home Health, **SLP**

Smith, Janice C 7240 Shirley Avenue #301, Reseda, CA 91335, (818) 701-1747, BA 72 Univ of the Pacific; MA 73 Univ of the Pacific; SLP, Los Angeles City Sch, **SLP**

Smith, Mrs Janlee E 2199 Sunrise Lane, Prineville, OR 97754, (208) 756-3684, BA 66 MI St Univ; MA 69 Humboldt St Univ; SLP, Larsen Learing Center, **SLP**

Smith, Jean D 313 East Lucas, Castalia, OH 44824, (419) 433-6343, BS 72 Bowling Green St Univ; MA 76 Bowling Green St Univ; Sp-Lang Path, Erie Co Bd of Ed, **SLP**

Smith, Jean McKernan Rochester Inst Of Technology, Ntl Tech Inst For The Deaf, One Lomb Memorial Drive, Rochester, NY 14623, (716) 475-6344, BS 66 Nazareth Coll of Rochester; MS 72 SUNY - Coll at Geneseo; 69–Sp-Lang Path, NTID, **SLP**

Smith, Jeanne A Route 1 Box 114E, Lexington Park, MD 20653, (314) 962-9324, **SLP**

Smith, Prof Jeanne K Department Of Otolaryngology, University Hospital, Iowa City, IA 52241, (319) 645-2525, BA 33 Univ of IA; MA 37 Univ of IA; **SLP A F LM**

Smith, Mrs Jeanne Lynn 2616 Westminister Drive, Wilson, NC 27893, (919) 537-0461, BS 81 East Carolina Univ; MS 83 East Carolina Univ; Sp-Lang Path, Roanoke Vlly Phys Ther Ctr, **SLP**

Smith, Jill Pierce 903 North Eugene Street, Greensboro, NC 27401, (919) 379-9296, BS 82 Appalachian St Univ; MA 86 Appalachian St Univ; 88–Sp-Lang Path, Greensboro City Schs, **SLP**

Smith, Mrs Jo Ellyn 1652 Central Avenue, Harrisonburg, VA 22801-2758, (703) 885-9080, BS 78 James Madison Univ; MS 79 Univ of WI - Madison; Clinical Super, James Madison U, **SLP ACE**

Smith, Joann 145 Watchung Avenue, Chatham, NJ 07928, (201) 635-1598, BS 76 Saint Louis Univ; MA 77 Saint Louis Univ; Sp/Lang Path, **SLP ACE**

Smith, Mrs Joann Caiola 523 Amderson Avenue, Woodridge, NJ 07075, (201) 933-9873, BA 76 Jersey City St Coll; MA 85 Montclair St Coll; **SLP**

Smith, Mrs Joanna T 11913 Maple Hollow Court, Oklahoma City, OK 73120, (405) 751-1705, BA 75 Univ of OK - Norman; MS 77 Univ of OK Medical Center; Child Serve Facilitator, OK Cty Pub Sch, **SLP**

Smith, Mrs Joanne Geraldine 62 Burnt Bridge Avenue, Bricktown, NJ 08724, (201) 244-3100, BS 74 Trenton St Coll; MA 80 Trenton St Coll; Asst Dir/Sp Dept, Garden St Rehab Hosp, **SLP**

Smith, Mrs Joanne Parsons 92 Graymoor Lane, Olympia Fields, IL 60461, (312) 747-4000, **SLP**

Smith, Jonette T 25 Horizon Drive, Council Bluffs, IA 51503, (712) 322-0164, BA 69 Univ of Northern IA; MA 71 IN Univ - Bloomington; Sp-Lang Path, Independent Contractor, **SLP**

Smith, Judith A Route 5 Box 1168, Hickory, NC 28601, (704) 433-2850, BS 74 Auburn Univ - Auburn; MS 75 Auburn Univ - Auburn; 87–Aud, Viewmont EENT Assoc, **A**

Smith, Mrs Judith Ann 1305 Ridgewood, Ames, IA 50010, (515) 233-1367, OM 85 Univ of Northern IA

Smith, Mrs Judith Michelle 485 Dartmouth Avenue, Buffalo, NY 14215, (716) 893-2641, BA 80 SUNY - Center at Buffalo; MA 83 SUNY - Center at Buffalo; SLP, Buffalo Bd of Ed, **SLP**

Smith, Judy G 2030 Connecticut #4, Joplin, MO 64804, (316) 663-7178, BS 69 KS St Univ; MA 72 Wichita St Univ; Sp/Lang Path, Reno Co Ed Coop, **SLP**

Smith, Mrs Judy K 1453 West 2nd Avenue, Columbus, OH 43212, (614) 486-1089, MA 87 Bowling Green St Univ

Smith, Mrs Judy Shaw Route 5 Box 491-S, Lincolnton, NC 28092, (704) 735-5251, BS 75 Appalachian St Univ; MA 76 Appalachian St Univ; 79–Sp-Lang Path, Lincoln Co Sch, **SLP**

Smith, Julie Tackabury 2615 N E 27th, Portland, OR 97212, (503) 280-6171, BA 78 Univ of Northern CO; MA 80 Univ of Northern CO; Sp-Lang Path, Portland Public Schools, **SLP**

Smith, K Roger 5646 New Meadow, Ypsilanti, MI 48197, (313) 481-0883, BA 74 Western MI Univ; MA 76 Western MI Univ; Audiologist/Manager, Beltone Hearing Aid Center, **A**

Smith, Mrs Karen Beth 59 Lora Lane, Hamilton, OH 45013, (513) 423-9496, MA 84 Miami Univ - Oxford; Sp-Lang Path, Doty House, **SLP**

Smith, Karen Denise 5700 Roper Street #015, East Ridge, TN 37412, BS 82 Auburn Univ - Auburn; MS 84 Auburn Univ - Auburn; Sp-Lang Path, Catoosa County Board of Ed, **SLP**

Smith, Mrs Karen E Box 12 CNFJ Code 012, FPO Seattle, WA 98762-0051, **SLP**

Smith, Karen Gregory 140 Hartwood Circle, Columbia, SC 29212, (803) 781-3592, BA 76 Columbia Coll; MS 77 Univ of SC - Columbia; 79–Sp-Lang Path, Lexington Co Sch Dist #5, **SLP**

Smith, Mrs Karen Iati 6881 Laurelton Avenue, Garden Grove, CA 92645, (714) 891-6710, BS 77 Nazareth Coll of Rochester; MS 83 Nazareth Coll of Rochester; SLP, Irvine USD

Smith, Mrs Karen Weller 4571 Bain Park Drive, Fairview Park, OH 44126, (216) 331-4822, BA 83 OH St Univ; MA 85 OH St Univ; Aud, ENT Group of Cleveland, **A**

Smith, Katherine Dunn 24432 Effingham Boulevard, Euclid, OH 44117, (216) 486-1302, MA 85 OH Univ - Athens; Sp-Lang Path, Deepwood Ctr, **SLP**

Smith, Katherine Virginia 1675 Shepard Mesa Lane, Carpinteria, CA 93013, (805) 648-5391, BA 77 San Jose St Univ; MA 80 CA St Univ - Northridge; SLP, Ventura USD, **SLP**

Smith, Kathleen Joan West 1527 13th Avenue, Spokane, WA 99204, (509) 927-1140, BA 77 Univ of ME - Orono; MA 83 WA St Univ; Sp-Lang Path, West Valley School District, **SLP**

Smith, Kathleen M 8508 20th N W, Seattle, WA 98117, (206) 543-3134, BA 66 Univ of WA; OM 71 Univ of WA; Sp-Lang Path, University Hosp, **SLP**

Smith, Kathleen McCullum 1417 Tennis Match Way, Encinitas, CA 92024, (619) 942-4055, BA 84 CA St Univ - Long Beach; MA 86 CA St Univ - Long Beach; **SLP**

Smith, Dr Kathryn J 5364 Graceland, Indianapolis, IN 46208, (317) 283-9492, BS 69 Ball St Univ; MA 71 Ball St Univ; PH 78 (NS) IN Univ - Bloomington; 81–Cl Super/Asst Prof, Butler U, **SLP**

Smith, Mrs Keith Ann 824 Glendale Avenue, South Charleston, WV 25303, **SLP A**

Smith, Mrs Kelly Hudspeth 4310 Woodcrest, Dallas, TX 75206, (214) 238-8111, BS 82 Baylor Univ; MS 83 Univ of North TX; Sp-Lang Path, **SLP**

Smith, Dr Kenneth E Hearing Associates Inc, 8901 West 74th Street, Suite 150, Shawnee Mission, KS 66204, (913) 384-5880, BA 65 Otterbein Coll; MA 67 OH Univ - Athens; PH 71 (NS) Univ of KS; Aud, Hrng Assoc, Inc, **A**

Smith, Keoni 2208 North 46th Street, Seattle, WA 98103, (206) 863-2201, BS 77 Loma Linda Univ - Riverside; MA 81 Univ of WA; Sp-Lang Path, E Pierce Co Spec Services Coop, **SLP**

Smith, Kristy Lynne 2020 Cheyenne Way #203, Modesto, CA 95356, (209) 838-3591, BS 85 Loma Linda Univ - Riverside; MA 87 CA St Univ - Stanislaus; 88–Tchr, Escalon USD

Smith, Lana Sue 12369 West Alabama Place, Lakewood, CO 80228, (303) 985-3423, BA 84 Metropolitan St Coll; MA 87 Univ of CO - Boulder; 88–Sp-Lang Path, Jefferson County Comm Ctr, **SLP**

Smith, Dr Laura Ann 642 Tommy Aaron Drive, Gainesville, GA 30506, (404) 864-3254, **SLP**

Smith, Laura Lee 1221 Waterside Cove #22, Midvale, UT 84047, (307) 265-5097, BS 83 Phillips Univ; OM 85 Univ of MT; Sp-Lang Path, Western Rehab Institute, **SLP**

Smith, Lauri Sue RR 2 Box 157B, Marysville, KS 66508, (913) 562-2943, BS 84 Central MI Univ; MA 85 Central MI Univ; Sp-Lang Path, USD #364, **SLP**

Smith, Laurie Ellen 329 East Penn Street, Long Beach, NY 11561, (513) 742-2200, BS 83 Univ of Cincinnati; MA 86 Univ of Cincinnati; **SLP**

Smith, Mrs Linda 42315 Edward Circle, Columbiana, OH 44408, (216) 726-8855, BS 73 Bowling Green St Univ; MS 74 Bowling Green St Univ; Sp-Lang Path, Youngstown Hrng/Sp Cen, **SLP ACE**

Smith, Linda Aldridge 203 West 29th, Lamberton, NC 28358, (919) 738-6071, BS 70 East Carolina Univ; MS 75 Univ of SC - Columbia; Sp-Lang Path, Private Practice, **SLP ACE**

Smith, Mrs Linda Ellen 133 Birch Terrace, Stoughton, MA 02072, (617) 993-1710, **A**

Smith, Mrs Linda Emrich 8625 South Meadowlark Circle, Highlands Ranch, CO 80126, (314) 361-4565, MA 84 Saint Louis Univ; Sp-Lang Path, St Louis State Hosp, **SLP**

Smith, Mrs Linda G 12 Heritage Lane, New Orleans, LA 70114, (504) 367-3120, BA 76 LA St Univ - Baton Rouge; OM 78 LA St Univ - N O Medical Ctr; Sp-Lang Path, Jefferson Parish Pub Schs, **SLP**

Smith, Linda Hicks 370 Dillon Lane, Swansea, MA 02777, (617) 679-5606, BS 79 Univ of NH; MS 80 Ithaca Coll; Sp/Lang Path, Swansea Pre Sch Speech Dept, **SLP**

Smith, Dr Linda Lou Michigan State University, Coll Of Comm Arts/Sciences, Dean's Office Rm 287, East Lansing, MI 48824-1212, (517) 355-3410, BA 68 Univ of KY; MS 71 Univ of WI - Madison; PH 72 (NS) Univ of WI - Madison; Asst Dean, Coll of Commun Art&Sci/Mi St U, **A F**

Smith, Linda Poppell Pediatric Therapies Of Savannah, C-131 Executive Court, 5105 Paulsen Street, Savannah, GA 31405, (912) 354-4774, BS 73 Univ of GA; ME 76 Univ of GA; Sp-Lang Path, Private Practice, **SLP**

Smith, Mrs Linda Skapura 2103 North Crescent Blvd, Yardley, PA 19067, (215) 493-1843, **SLP**

Smith, Mrs Linda T 4117 Ridgeway Lane, Knoxville, TN 37919, (615) 588-2677, BA 85 Univ of TN - Knoxville; MA 87 Univ of TN - Knoxville; 87–Sp-Lang Path, Anderson Co Schs, **SLP**

Smith, Lisa Jane 2034 Swallow Hill Road, Apartment 222, Pittsburgh, PA 15220, (216) 653-9738, **SLP**

Smith, Lisa Joan 254 West Slade Street #2W, Palatine, IL 60067, (312) 526-6671, MA 84 Northern IL Univ - De Kalb; **SLP**

Smith, Mrs Lisa K 112 Boston Commons Place, Roseville, CA 95678-7345, (916) 782-7367, BA 80 Humboldt St Univ; MS 81 Northern AZ Univ; Clin Supvr, InSpeech Inc, **SLP**

Smith, Mrs Lisa W 4205 Arbor Court #C, Kenner, LA 70065, (504) 467-7582, BS 86 FL St Univ; MS 87 FL St Univ; **SLP**

Smith, Mrs Lois Reiko 9880 S W Pimlico Terrace, Beaverton, OR 97005, (503) 591-8000, BA 81 CA St Univ - Northridge; MA 83 CA St Univ - Northridge; 88–Sp-Lang Path, Beaverton Sch Dist

Smith, Dr Loretta Wagner 207 Cedarwood Commons, La Bar Village, Stroudsburg, PA 18360, (717) 424-8581, BA 30; MA 32; PH 37 (Speech Path Clinical Psychology) Univ of IA; Prof Emerita, CUNY-Brooklyn Coll, **SLP LM**

Smith, Lori Denise 2227 South National, Springfield, MO 65804, (417) 883-5851, BS 83 Northwest MO St Univ; MA 84 Northeast MO St Univ; Sp-Lang Path, Developmental Ctr of the Ozarks, **SLP**

Smith, Lourie Elaine 148 Calle Vadito N W, Albuquerque, NM 87120, (505) 831-6017, MA 84 SUNY - Center at Buffalo; 87–Sp-Lang Path, Los Lunas Hosp & Training Sch, **SLP**

Smith, Mrs Lydia H P O Box 1764, Cross City, FL 32628, (904) 542-7818, BS 79 Univ of TN - Knoxville; MA 80 Univ of TN - Knoxville; 88–Sp/Lang Path, Dixie Co Schs, **SLP**

Smith, Mrs Lyna L 3151 Adirondack Avenue, Columbus, OH 43229-3121, (614) 891-0506, BA 74 Univ of Akron; MA 76 Univ of Akron; Cl Coord, Ohio St U Nisonger Cen, **SLP**

Smith, Lynn Goldberg 220 East Northport Road, Kings Park, NY 11754-2517, (516) 543-5100, BA 74 SUNY - Center at Buffalo; MS 77 Ithaca Coll; Sp-Lang Path, UCP of Greater Suffolk, **SLP**

Smith, Mrs Lynn Z 166-08 24th Avenue, Whitestone, NY 11357, (718) 352-8053

Smith, Mae Ann Levine 1811 Clinton Avenue, Alameda, CA 94501, (415) 769-1857, BA 75 Univ of NH; ME 76 Trenton St Coll; **SLP**

Smith, Mrs Maree Nipper 4504 Mellowood Circle, Knoxville, TN 37920, (615) 577-0159, BA 73 Univ of TN - Knoxville; MA 74 Univ of TN - Knoxville; **SLP**

Smith, Mrs Margaret Girton 7206 Winbert Drive, North Tonawanda, NY 14120, (716) 837-2441, BA 77 IN St Univ - Terre Haute; MS 74 IN St Univ - Terre Haute; Dir Sp-Lang-Hrng Program, Lan-Dev Prog Wn NY Inc, **SLP**

Smith, Margaret J 5801 Eubank Boulevard N E, Apartment 235, Albuquerque, NM 87111, (505) 828-1781, BA 83 Univ of OK - Norman; MS 85 Univ of OK Medical Center; **SLP**

Smith, Mrs Margo Schenck 178 North Pardee, Wadsworth, OH 44281, (216) 334-7895, BS 76 Miami Univ - Oxford; MA 78 Kent St Univ; **SLP**

Smith, Mark Allen 1185 Monroe Street #127, Salinas, CA 93906, (408) 633-4196, BA 82 CA St Univ - Sacramento; MA 84 CA St Univ - Sacramento; SLP, North Monterey Co Unif Sch Dis, **SLP**

Smith, Marlene Therese 105 Glenridge Lane, Schaumburg, IL 60193, (312) 885-6776

Smith, Mrs Marsha Burwell 2970 Borge Street, Oakton, VA 22124, (703) 830-8181, MS 78 James Madison Univ; SLP, Fairfax County Public Schools, **SLP**

Smith, Dr Marshall M 1315 Wilson Street #B, Eau Claire, WI 54701, (715) 836-9502, BS 70 Auburn Univ - Auburn; MS 72 PA St Univ - Univ Park; PH 81 FL St Univ; Asst Prof, Bradley U, **A**

Smith, Martha J 2404 Daphne Lane, Alexandria, VA 22306, (703) 664-7190, BA 69 Univ of WI - Madison; MS 70 Univ of MI - Ann Arbor; 85–Sp-Lang Path, Mt Vernon Hosp, **SLP**

Smith, Mrs Martha L 604 Willow Drive, Ayden, NC 28513, (919) 746-2121, BA 66 Meredith Coll; MS 81 East Carolina Univ; SLP, Pitt Co Bd of Ed, **SLP ACE**

Smith, Mary Ann 698 Curtiswood Drive, Key Biscayne, FL 33149, (305) 361-1996, BA 65 Univ of FL; ME 67 Univ of FL; SLP, Private Practice, **SLP**

Smith, Mary Beth 226 King Lane, Des Plaines, IL 60016-5906, (312) 837-2430, BS 85 Univ of IA; MA 87 Univ of IA; 88–Sp-Lang Path, Schaumburg Dist 54, **SLP**

Smith, Mrs Mary Brousseau 4657 Knight Drive, New Orleans, LA 70127, (504) 887-0470, BS 72 LA St Univ - Baton Rouge; MA 74 LA St Univ - Baton Rouge; Sp/Lang Path, Jefferson Parish Sch Bd, **SLP**

Smith, Mary C 13330 W 113th Street, Overland Park, KS 66210, (913) 469-9089, BA 73 Kearney St Coll; MS 76 Kearney St Coll; **SLP**

Smith, Mary E University Of Wisconsin, 1975 Willow Drive, Madison, WI 53706, (608) 262-3951, BS 63 Univ of WI - Madison; MA 66 Northwestern Univ; **SLP**

Smith, Mrs Mary E 1812 Concord, Denton, TX 76205, (817) 565-1976, BA 65 Univ of OK - Norman; MA 85 TX Woman's Univ; **SLP**

Smith, Mary E 103 East Seneca Street, Oswego, NY 13126, (315) 593-5550, BS 76 SUNY - Coll at Geneseo; MS 81 Bradley Univ; Sp-Lang Path, Fulton Consolidated Sch, **SLP**

Smith, Mary Ellen 109 South Lake Drive, Red Bank, NJ 07701, MA 76 Kean Coll of NJ; SLP, Litzelman and Schultz, **SLP**

Smith, Matthew W F 605 Burma Drive N E, Albuquerque, NM 87123, (505) 293-4327, BA 73 Univ of NM; MS 74 Univ of NM; Aud/Mgr, Family Hearing Ctr, **A**

Smith, Melanie 2728 N E 15th Street, Oklahoma City, OK 73117, **SLP**

Smith, Dr Michael Douglas Speech And Hearing Center, Communication Disorders, Western Carolina Univ, Cullowhee, NC 28723, (704) 227-7251, PH 75 (NS) Univ of KS; Chair, Wn Carolina U-Commun Dis, **SLP**

Smith, Michael Keith P O Box 347, Hamburg, AR 71646, (501) 853-5312, OM 84 AR St Univ; Sp-Lang Path, Drew Memorial Hosp, **SLP**

Smith, Michele 718 West 350 South, Orem, UT 84057, (801) 226-8996, BS 78 Brigham Young Univ; OM 80 Brigham Young Univ; Alpine Sch Dist, **SLP**

Smith, Mrs Michele Elizabeth 4384 Mackinaw, Saginaw, MI 48603-3110, (517) 793-0543, BS 78 Northern MI Univ; MS 82 Univ of MI - Ann Arbor; 86–Sp-Lang Path, Visiting Nurse Association, **SLP**

Smith, Mrs Michele G 1150 Bounty Boulevard, Vero Beach, FL 32963, (407) 234-8821, BA 78 Univ of FL; MA 80 Univ of FL; Sp-Lang Path, **SLP**

Smith, Michele L 290 Bedford Avenue, Buffalo, NY 14216, (716) 887-4422, BS 76 SUNY - Coll at Geneseo; MS 77 Columbia Univ Teachers Coll; 85–Sp-Lang Path, Millard Fillmore Hospital, **SLP**

Smith, Mischa Jerine 6208 Indian Canyon Drive, Austin, TX 78746, (512) 327-7237, BA 83 CA St Univ - Northridge; MA 85 CA St Univ - Northridge; 87–Sp-Lang Path, Brackenridge Hosp, **SLP**

Smith, Myron Dee 4722 S W 47th Avenue, Portland, OR 97221, (503) 229-7860, Aud, Good Samaritan Hos & Med Ctr, **A**

Smith, Mrs Nancy A 4219 Blueflax, Pueblo, CO 81001, (303) 543-1265, BS 73 CO St Univ; MS 75 CO St Univ; 88–Sp-Lang Path, Southern CO Dev Disabilities Svcs, **SLP**

Smith, Nancy A 9512 Catesby Lane, Richmond, VA 23233, (804) 266-1642, BA 76 Mary Washington Coll; ME 79 James Madison Univ; 79–Aud, Henrico Co Sch Richmond VA, **A**

Smith, Mrs Nancy B 414 West 3rd Street, Elmhurst, IL 60126, (312) 450-2100, BA 76 Augustana Coll; MA 77 Northern IL Univ - De Kalb; Sp/Lang Path, Proviso Area for Except Chldn, **SLP**

Smith, Mrs Nancy Brizzie 11210 Turnley Lane, Midlothian, VA 23113, (804) 320-0154, BS 73 East Carolina Univ; MS 77 East Carolina Univ; Sp-Lang Path, Henrico County Schools, **SLP**

Smith, Nancy Edwards 1617 Roseland Street, Greensboro, NC 27410, (919) 841-2137, BS 79 AR St Univ; MS 87 Univ of Central AR; 88–Sp-Lang Path, MedTherapy Inc

Smith, Nancy Jean 200 Evergreen Avenue, Apartment 1A, Hamden, CT 06518, (203) 785-2467, BA 82 Southern CT St Univ; MS 88 Southern CT St Univ; Sp-Lang Path/Aud, Yale New Haven Hospital, **SLP A**

Smith, Nancy L 805 Michigan Avenue #3, Evanston, IL 60202, (312) 328-1165, **SLP**

Smith, Nancy L 413 1st Avenue, Audubon, IA 50025, (712) 563-3176, BA 73 Univ of Northern IA; MA 74 Univ of Northern IA; Sp-Lang Path, Private Practice, **SLP**

Smith, Nancy S 4473 Maumee Drive, Okemos, MI 48864, **SLP**

Smith, Mrs Nancy Stecker 135 N W 171st, Seattle, WA 98177, (206) 542-4643, BA 64 Univ of KY; MA 66 Univ of WA; 76–Sp-Lang Path, Private Practice, **SLP**

Smith, Dr Nancy W 1229 Madison Street, Rochester, IN 46975, (317) 842-0000, BS 72 IN Univ - Bloomington; ME 73 IN Univ - Bloomington; ED 79 (NS) IN Univ - Bloomington; Dir of Ed Serv, McGuire & Shook Corp, **SLP**

Smith, Norbert E 10278 Leelanau Court, Traverse City, MI 49684, **A**

Smith, Dr Norma D 18 Rodney Street, Hartford, CT 06105, (203) 827-7582, BA 45 Univ of Southern CA; MA 51 Columbia Univ Teachers Coll; ED 75 (NS) Univ of MA - Amherst; Assoc Prof, Ctrl Ct St U, **SLP**

Smith, Norma J 1350 Third Avenue, San Francisco, CA 94122, BA 63 Andrews Univ; MA 65 MI St Univ; Sp-Lang Path, **SLP**

Smith, Mrs Pamela Kennette 4422 Wesley E, Corpus Christi, TX 78412, (505) 247-4224, BA 76 Univ of OK - Norman; MS 82 Northern AZ Univ; SLP, Albuquerque Hearing Sp Ctr, **SLP**

Smith, Mrs Pamela Z 1728 Maplewood, La Verne, CA 91750, (714) 593-9303, BA 74 Univ of LA Verne; MS 77 Eastern WA Univ; Sp-Lang Path, Southland Pediatrics, **SLP**

Smith, Mrs Patricia 708 Drywood Avenue, Fern Park, FL 32730, (407) 331-0832, BA 74 Univ of Central FL; MA 75 Univ of Central FL; Sp-Lang Path, Private Practice, **SLP**

Smith, Patricia A 1757 Thomas Avenue #6, St Paul, MN 55104-1727, (612) 674-7001, BS 72 Saint Cloud St Univ; MS 84 Univ of ND; Sp-Lang Path, North Branch Public Schools, **SLP**

Smith, Patricia Ann 716 Woodlawn, Joliet, IL 60435, BA 80 Coll of Saint Francis; MS 82 Bradley Univ; Sp-Lang Path, Regional Educ Service Agency, **SLP**

Smith, Patricia E 10103 Crestside Place, Spring Valley, CA 92077, (619) 698-8979, BA 69 Univ of CA - Santa Barbara; MS 78 Univ of HI - Manoa; **SLP**

Smith, Patricia Fennell 590 Three Mile Harbor Road, East Hampton, NY 11937, (516) 537-0271, BS 72 SUNY - Center at Albany; MA 76 Coll of Saint Rose; Sp-Lang Path/Ch Commit Hndcpd, Bridgehampton Un Fr Sch Dist, **SLP**

Smith, Patricia H 1525 Euston Road, San Marino, CA 91108, **SLP**

Smith, Mrs Patricia R 1040 Rose Circle, College Station, TX 77840, (409) 696-8052, BA 62 Univ of Southwestern LA; Sp-Lang Path, St Michaels Academy, **SLP**

Smith, Mrs Patricia S RFD 1 Box 155, Fairview, UT 84629, (801) 462-2485, BA 70 Brigham Young Univ; OM 71 Brigham Young Univ; Sp-Lang Path, No Sanpete Sch Dist, **SLP**

Smith, Patricia S 326 Drace Street, Rochester, MI 48063, (313) 652-1358, BA 79 MI St Univ; MA 80 MI St Univ; Sp/Lang Path, Michigan Allied Health Professionals Inc, **SLP**

Smith, Paula Susan 9132 Champlain Avenue, Niagara Falls, NY 14304, (716) 283-8303, BS 85 SUNY - Coll at Geneseo; MA 87 SUNY - Center at Buffalo; Aud, Niagara Co Sp Hrng & Lang Ctr, **A**

Smith, Dr Peter B, Jr Dept Of Speech And Hearing, Northern Michigan Univ, Marquette, MI 49855, (906) 227-2125, BA 62 San Diego St Univ; MA 64 San Diego St Univ; PH 67 (General) Univ of WA; Prof, Nn MI U, **SLP**

Smith, Randall D 22509 Bluejay Road, Morrison, CO 80465-4655, (301) 778-5645, BA 72 Northeast LA Univ; ME 75 McNeese St Univ; Acting Director, Porter Mem Hosp, **SLP**

Smith, Randall W 7315 Marcia Drive, Little Rock, AR 72209, BS 71 Southeast MO St Univ; MS 72 Univ Southern MS-Hattiesburg; Consultant/Commun Disorders, Private Practice, **SLP**

Smith, Rayma E 1155 S Yellowsprings St, Springfield, OH 45506, MS; **SLP**

Smith, Rebecca Dawn 7491 Old Dixiana Road, Pinson, AL 35126, (205) 681-9613, BA 85 Univ of AL- Tuscaloosa; MS 86 Univ of Montevallo

Smith, Mrs Regina Teresa 2198 Glenbury Avenue, Lakewood, OH 44107, (216) 521-5050, BA 83 Cleveland St Univ; MA 85 Cleveland St Univ; Sp-Lang Path, Achiev Ctr for Child, **SLP**

Smith, Reginald Robin 576 Bellflower Blvd #241, Long Beach, CA 90814, (213) 597-8940, BA 78 WA St Univ; MA 86 CA St Univ - Los Angeles; **SLP**

Smith, Renee J 555 Rosewood #1205, Camarillo, CA 93010, (805) 484-3661, BS 75 Northeast MO St Univ; MA 83 Southwest MO St Univ; Sp-Lang Path, Camarillo Developmental Ctr, **SLP**

Smith, Renee Lynne 1486 Dewberry Court N E #7, Grand Rapids, MI 49505, (616) 451-1918, BS 84 Central MI Univ; MA 85 Central MI Univ; 87–Sp-Lang Path, Lowell Public Schools, **SLP**

Smith, Richard M Rd 1 Box 208, Danville, PA 17821, (717) 275-7796, BS 62 Edinboro Univ of PA; MA 66 Temple Univ; Sp-Lang Path, Private Practice, **SLP**

Smith, Robert M 139 West Norman Street, Wernersville, PA 19565, (717) 272-6621, BS 61 Indiana Univ of PA; ME 65 PA St Univ - Univ Park; Ch/SLP & Aud, VA Medical Center, **SLP**

Smith, Roberta Leigh Rt 2 Box 16, Belhaven, NC 27810, (919) 964-4305, BS 83 NC St Univ at Raleigh; MS 85 Univ of NC - Chapel Hill; 88–Sp-Lang Path, Leigh Smith MS & Associates, **SLP**

Smith, Robinann S 38-B Farmland Road, Lowell, MA 01850, (617) 774-5000, BS 84 Northeastern Univ; MS 86 Northeastern Univ; 87–Aud, Alanticare Med Ctr, **A**

Smith, Mrs Roblyn Thompson 111 1st Street N E, Pryor, OK 74361, (918) 825-4224, BS 78 AR St Univ; OM 79 Univ of MS; Sp-Lang Path, Mayes County Guidance Clinic, **SLP**

Smith, Romayne A 4132 Sharp Road, Glenelg, MD 21737, (301) 854-6507, BA 75 Univ of NC - Charlotte; MA 79 Univ of NC - Greensboro; 84–Sp-Lang Path, Private Practice, **SLP**

Smith, Dr Rosalie H 11 West Ridge Drive, West Hartford, CT 06117, (203) 236-2929, MA 56 CUNY - Brooklyn Coll; MA 85 Columbia Univ Teachers Coll; ED 86 (Adult Ed) Columbia Univ Teachers Coll; 76–Pres, Dynamic Trng & Consult Serv, **SLP**

Smith, Rosemary B Hastings Regional Center, Apartment 22, Hastings, NE 68901, (402) 463-2471, BS 70 Univ of NE - Lincoln; MA 71 Univ of NE - Lincoln; Dept Head Sp & Hrng Serv, Hastings Reg Cen, **SLP A**

Smith, Mrs Rosemary Hanley 14429 Michael Drive, North Huntingdon, PA 15642, (421) 281-7244, BS 60 Carlow Coll; ME 63 Duquesne Univ; Sp-Lang Path, Er Sl So Pittsburgh, **SLP**

Smith, Dr Rosemary L 2008 Kanawha Boulevard, Charleston, WV 25311, (304) 344-0349, BS 73 WV Univ; MS 75 WV Univ; PH 87 (Clinical Psychology) FL Inst of Tech; 87–Psychologist, Charleston Psych Group Inc, **A**

Smith, Ruby D 409 Cameron Circle #902, Chattanooga, TN 37403, (615) 825-7269, BA 73 Univ of MS; MS 76 Univ Southern MS-Hattiesburg; Sp-Lang Path, Chattanooga Cty Sch, **SLP**

Smith, Mrs Ruth E 5 Cunningham Lane, Bella Vista, AR 72714, BS 75 Central St Univ; ME 79 Central St Univ; Sp-Lang Path, Decatur Public Schools, **SLP**

Smith, Ruth Joyce 915 2nd Street S E, New Philadelphia, OH 44663, (216) 339-6631, BA 60 OH Univ - Athens; MA 62 OH Univ - Athens; SLP, New Phila City Schs, **SLP**

Smith, Mrs Sandra B 6814 Los Tios, Houston, TX 77083, (713) 879-8498, BS 71 LA St Univ - Baton Rouge; MA 75 Univ of Houston - Univ Park; Sp/Lang Path, Alief ISD, **SLP**

Smith, Sandra Jean 147 Oak Grove Church Road, Mount Airy, NC 27030, (919) 386-8211, BS 85 Univ of NC - Greensboro; ME 86 Univ of NC - Greensboro; 88–Sp-Lang Path, Surry Co Sch, **SLP**

Smith, Mrs Sandra Kay 700 Hereford Court, Odessa, MO 64076, (816) 633-5334, BS 79 Central MO St Univ; MS 85 Central MO St Univ; **SLP**

Smith, Sarah Williston 6 Tara Drive #9, Weymouth, MA 02188, (716) 394-2626, BS 84 Ithaca Coll; MA 85 Bowling Green St Univ; SLP, Canandaigua City Schools, **SLP**

Smith, Sharon Elaine 945-#8 Falls Creek Lane, Charlotte, NC 28209, (704) 399-7489, BA 82 Appalachian St Univ; ME 84 Univ of NC - Greensboro; **SLP**

Smith, Sharon K 411 South 154th Street, Omaha, NE 68154, BS 79 Univ of NE - Omaha; MS 81 Univ of NE - Omaha; Sp-Lang Path, Millard Pub Sch, **SLP**

Smith, Sharon L Route 6 Box 26-J, Alexander City, AL 35010, (205) 329-1730, BS 74 Auburn Univ - Auburn; MS 77 Univ of AL- Tuscaloosa; Sp-Lang Path, Tallapoosa Co Bd of Ed, **SLP**

Smith, Sharon Marie 2213 Ridgewood, Sherman, TX 75090, (214) 494-8211, BS 85 TX Tech Univ; MS 87 TX Tech Univ

Smith, Mrs Sheila L 1912 East Riverside Blvd, Apartment 16, Rockford, IL 61111, (815) 654-9440, BS 85 Northern IL Univ - De Kalb; MA 86 Northern IL Univ - De Kalb; 88–Sp-Lang Path, Rockford PS Dist 205, **SLP**

Smith, Mrs Sherry Stewart 1625 West Pecos Avenue, Mesa, AZ 85202, (602) 730-9116, BS 83 Brigham Young Univ; OM 84 Brigham Young Univ; Aud, Private Practice, **A**

Smith, Mrs Sherry Sue 448 Cloverwood Drive, Mason, OH 45040, (513) 398-7947, BS 78 Miami Univ - Oxford; MS 82 Miami Univ - Oxford; Sp-Lang Path, Lakota Sch Dist, **SLP**

Smith, Shirley Cronin 306 Shamrock Place, Richardson, TX 75081, (214) 238-8526, BS 81 Univ of TX - Dallas; MS 83 Univ of TX - Dallas; Sp-Lang Path, Richardson ISD, **SLP**

Smith, Mrs Shirley Mayo 14 Crosswicks Ridge Road, Wilton, CT 06897, (203) 834-0442, **SLP**

Smith, Simalee Carol 8436 Reims Court, Stockton, CA 95209, (209) 946-3229, BS 76 Univ of WY; MA 82 Univ of the Pacific; 83–Instr/Clin Supvr, Univ of the Pacific, **SLP**

Smith, Sonja M 2 North Broadway, White Plains, NY 10601, BA 53 CUNY - Brooklyn Coll; MA 54 CUNY - Brooklyn Coll; SLP

Smith, Mrs Stacie Rubin 8020 S W 148 Drive, Miami, FL 33158, (305) 233-6683, BA 82 George Washington Univ; MS 84 Boston Univ; Sp-Lang Path, South Miami Hosp, **SLP ACE**

Smith, Mrs Stacy A 120 East Mesa Verde Drive, Yukon, OK 73099, (405) 376-2491, MS 82 Phillips Univ; Sp-Lang Path, Mustang Public Schools, **SLP**

Smith, Stephanie Stewart 108 Pebble Beach Drive, Georgetown, KY 40324, (502) 863-4533, BA 77 Western KY Univ; MS 80 Western KY Univ; Sp-Lang Path, Cardinal Hill Hosp, **SLP ACE**

Smith, Stephany Myatt 520 South 7th Avenue, Pocatello, ID 83201, (208) 785-2424, BA 71 ID St Univ; MS 79 ID St Univ; Sp-Lang Path, Sch Dist 55

Smith, Dr Stephen J 1729 Madison, Evanston, IL 60202, (312) 328-9049, BS 77 Southern IL Univ -Carbondale; MA 79 Northwestern Univ; PH 85 (NS) Northwestern Univ; SLP, School District 65, **SLP**

Smith, Mrs Sue McQuaig 6710 Audubon Drive, Columbus, GA 31909, (404) 563-6612, BA 78 Columbus Coll; ME 82 Columbus Coll; **SLP**

Smith, Susan Carol 9645 Old Placerville Road, Sacramento, CA 95827, (916) 364-8364, BA 81 MI St Univ; MA 82 MI St Univ; Clin Super, InSpeech Inc, **SLP**

Smith, Mrs Susan Harris 209 Royal Oak Drive, Wilmington, NC 28403-4757, ME 83 Univ of NC - Greensboro; Sp-Lang Path, Assoc Healthfocus, **SLP**

Smith, Mrs Susan Kalas 4923 Cypress Drive, Hillside, IL 60162, (312) 547-5037, BS 85 Univ of IL - Urbana; MA 86 Northwestern Univ; **A**

Smith, Mrs Susan L 62 Drexel Street, Worcester, MA 01602, (508) 754-3314, BA 60 Syracuse Univ; MA 61 Stanford Univ; Pub Relations Dir, Worcester Foothills Theatre Co, **A**

Smith, Mrs Susan Marie 231 Old North Road, Kingston, RI 02881, (401) 782-8147, BA 80 Univ of RI; MS 83 Univ of RI; Sp-Lang Path, Rhode Island Med Ctr Gen Hosp, **SLP**

Smith, Mrs Susan P 824 East Morningside Drive, Atlanta, GA 30324, (404) 963-6713, BA 67 Rutger's St Univ - Douglas Coll; MS 69 Rutgers St Univ -N Brunswick; ED 88 Univ of GA; SLP, Gwinnett Co Pub Sch, **SLP ACE**

Smith, Mrs Susan Vansant 156 Hillside Avenue, Arlington, MA 02174, (617) 884-0532, **SLP**

Smith, Suzanne Marie 4898 Sandstone Lane #206, West Palm Beach, FL 33417-8270, (305) 478-3661, MA 86 Western MI Univ; **SLP**

Smith, Mrs Suzanne Ryder 33491 Michele, Livonia, MI 48150, (313) 421-4194, BS 82 Eastern MI Univ; MA 84 Eastern MI Univ; 87–Sp-Lang Path, Wayne Comm Living Svcs, **SLP**

Smith, Mrs Sylvia Lee 4402 S W Flower Street, Portland, OR 97221, (503) 232-2458, BA 66 Lewis & Clark Coll; MS 72 ID St Univ; Sp-Lang Path, Portland Public Schools, **SLP**

Smith, Terrie Lynn 7400 Sepulveda Boulevard, Apartment 123, Van Nuys, CA 91405, (818) 787-6489, BA 84 Univ of the Pacific; MA 85 Univ of the Pacific; **SLP**

Smith, Theresa A Route 1 Box 120A, Battle Ground, IN 47920, (317) 463-6651, **A**

Smith, Theresa A 3413 North State Street, Jackson, MS 39216, (601) 359-1288, BA 79 Univ of MS; MA 81 Univ of MS; Dir-Div of Planning & Info, MS Dept of Mental Health, **SLP**

Smith, Thomas C 6022 Fabian Road, North Port, FL 34287, (813) 426-4484, BS 58 Kent St Univ; MA 64 Kent St Univ; 87–Sp-Lang Path, Venice Hosp, **SLP A**

Smith, Thomas D 6755 Filbro #D, Gilroy, CA 95020, (408) 637-3781, BA 79 Univ of Redlands; MS 81 Univ of Redlands; Sp-Lang-Hrng Spec, Hollister Elem Sch Dist, **SLP**

Smith, Mrs Tina Thompson South Carolina State College, P O Box 1943, Orangeburg, SC 29117, (803) 531-2461, **SLP**

Smith, Tracey S 3828 Diamond Head Road, Honolulu, HI 96816, BS 77 Gonzaga Univ; MS 79 Univ of HI - Manoa; SLP, Kapiolani Med Ctr, **SLP**

Smith, Mrs Valerie A P O Box 568, Lake Charles, LA 70602, (318) 433-1775, BS 48 LA St Univ - Baton Rouge; MA 57 LA St Univ - Baton Rouge; Sp-Lang Path, The Speech and Hearing Clinic, **SLP ACE**

Smith, Mrs Valerie Crawford 120 Pine Street, Wyoming, DE 19934, (302) 736-5597, BS 77 Bloomsburg Univ of PA; MS 78 Bloomsburg Univ of PA; 81–Sp-Lang Path, Capital Sch Dist, **SLP**

Smith, Vera D 1401 North Los Robles #20, Pasadena, CA 91104, (818) 358-1191, BS 76 Northwestern Univ; MS 78 Vanderbilt Univ; SLP, Los Angeles Co Supt Schs, **SLP**

Smith, Mrs Verna Elaine 9220 Arvada N E, Albuquerque, NM 87112, (505) 293-6721, BA 73 AZ St Univ; MS 82 Univ of NM; Sp-Lang Path, Albuquerque Pub Sch, **SLP**

Smith, Veronica Nadine 4280 Via Arbolada #110, Los Angeles, CA 90042, (213) 257-8085, BA 83 TX A & I Univ; MA 85 Univ of North TX; **SLP**

Smith, Virginia G 590 East Stanford Street, Bartow, FL 33830, (813) 533-2649, BA 47 FL St Univ; ME 75 Univ of VA - Charlottesville; Sp-Lang Path, Russel Co Sch Bd, **SLP**

Smith, Dr Wendell F P O Box 42, Montevallo, AL 35115, (205) 665-6717, OB 62 Southern Methodist Univ; MA 66 Southern Methodist Univ; PH 73 (NS) Univ of OK Medical Center; Prof & Dir Sp-Lang Path, U of Montevallo, **SLP**

Smith, William J 263 Acorn Ridge, Frankfort, IL 60423, (815) 469-1159, OM 87 Governors St Univ

Smith, Yolanda 17800 East Colima Road #88, Rowland Heights, CA 91748, (818) 965-2541, BA 76 Whittier Coll; MA 81 Whittier Coll; Sp-Lang Path, Rowland USD, **SLP**

Smitheal, Mrs Judith W Route 2 Box 70-M, Richmond, TX 77469, (713) 342-5521, BA 76 Univ of Houston - Univ Park; MA 79 Univ of Houston - Univ Park; **SLP**

Smitheimer, Dr Luella Sude 3 Harborview Road, Port Washington, NY 11050, (516) 883-9224, BA 50 Adelphi Univ; MS 67 Adelphi Univ; PH 80 (NS) NY Univ; Coor/Sp-Lang Path, Port Washington Sp-Lang Center, **SLP ACE**

Smither, Donna Lauber 4007 Longmoor Circle, Phoenix, MD 21131-2105, (301) 592-5262, BA 69 Towson St Univ; MS 74 Loyola Coll; Prin, Balto Co Bd of Ed, **SLP**

Smitheran, Judith R 3301 East Yorba Linda Blvd, Apartment 213, Fullerton, CA 92631, (714) 639-4990, BA 78 Univ of CO - Boulder; MS 80 Univ of AZ; Sp-Lang Path Clin Super, Providence Speech Hearing Cen, **SLP**

Smitherman, Mrs Arlene Palumbo 2743 Seneca Trail, Duluth, GA 30136, (404) 446-7475, BS 81 FL St Univ; MA 82 FL St Univ; **SLP A**

Smith-Eusebio, Mrs Falicia E 6691 East Abby Lane, Tucson, AZ 85715, (602) 722-8844, BA 83 Univ of the Pacific; MA 84 Univ of the Pacific; **SLP**

Smithey, Nancy T 2912 Tree Swallow Road, Roanoke, VA 24018, BA 62 Converse Coll; ME 63 Univ of VA - Charlottesville; Sp-Lang Path, Roanoke City Sch, **SLP**

Smith-Farach, Sheri 2425 Holly Hall #105, Houston, TX 77054, (713) 790-5913, BA 83 Univ of AR - Fayetteville; MS 85 Washington Univ; 85–Aud, Baylor Coll of Med, **A**

Smith-Fox, Lynn B P O Box 514, Dallas Center, IA 50063-0514, (515) 992-3139, ME 69 Univ of VA - Charlottesville; **SLP**

Smith-Greene, Mrs Joyce 45 Joyceton Way, Upper Marlboro, MD 20772, (301) 772-6611, BS 72 Univ of the DC; MS 73 Univ of the DC; Sp/Lang Path, BOCES, **SLP**

Smith-Koehler, Robin E Friedrich-Missler-Str 2A 2800, Bremen, West Germany 1, 0421-665767, MA 77 Western MI Univ; Sp/Lang Path, Smith-Koehler & Grabatsch, **SLP**

Smith-Lehmann, Rebecca 2111 Quail Ranch Court, Elverta, CA 95626, (916) 991-9527, BS 77 Northern MI Univ; MS 79 Univ of WI - Stevens Point; Sp-Lang Path, North Sacramento School Dist, **SLP**

Smithpeter, Mrs Joann V 3931 S W South Shore Blvd, Lake Oswego, OR 97035, (503) 636-6844, BA 58 Whittier Coll; MS 64 Univ of OR; 64–Sp-Lang Path, Private Practice, **SLP ACE**

Smith-Ray, Brenda J 10123 Bon Vista Court, San Jose, CA 95127, (408) 258-4923, BA 69 San Jose St Univ; MA 70 San Jose St Univ; Coord-Spec Serv, Alum Rock Union Elemen, **SLP**

Smithwick, Mrs Connie G 105 Forest Drive, Washington, NC 27889, (919) 946-0694, BS 73 East Carolina Univ; MS 74 East Carolina Univ; Sp-Lang Path, En Carolina Home Hlth Serv, **SLP**

Smithyman, Mrs Jennifer Ann 2121 University Avenue #4, Madison, WI 53705, (608) 238-0927, BS 86 Univ of WI - Madison; MS 88 Univ of WI - Madison; 88–Sp-Lang Path, Richland Sch Dist

Smithyman, Rosemary L 11 Knickernocker Drive, Belle Mead, NJ 08502, **SLP**

Smits, Mrs Millicent 15520 Oak Drive, Spring Lake, MI 49456, (616) 846-2699, BS 66 Western MI Univ; MA 69 Western MI Univ; Sp-Lang Path, Commun Cl Inc, **SLP**

Smock, Mrs Nancy E 52 Wilshire Park, Needham, MA 02192, (617) 444-7107, 69 OH Wesleyan Univ; 72 Univ of Pittsburgh - Pittsburgh; 87–Sp-Lang Path, Belmont PS, **SLP**

Smola, Kimberly Ann 261 Colgate Avenue, Elyria, OH 44035, (216) 323-8772, BS 83 Miami Univ - Oxford; MS 84 Miami Univ - Oxford; 86–Sp-Lang Path, Elyria City Schs, **SLP**

Smolaga, Mrs Deborah Jean 11 Hinchman Avenue, Dover, NJ 07801, (201) 852-1894, BA 77 Paterson St Coll; MS 79 Paterson St Coll; **SLP**

Smolak, Arlene 301-113 Market Avenue, Winnipeg, MB, Canada R3B 0P5, (204) 947-1561, BA 74; MA 77 Univ of ND; Sp-Lang Path, Child Guidance Clinic, **SLP**

Smolak, Lisa Hunter Minneapolis Neuro-Science Inst, Abbott N W Hospital, 800 East 28th Street, Minneapolis, MN 55407, (612) 863-3210, BA 83 Univ of MT; MA 85 Univ of Cincinnati; Aud, Minneapolis Nero-Science Instu, **A**

Smolar, Aimee L 525 Willow Knoll Drive, Marietta, GA 30067, (404) 952-2613, BA 74 Univ of TN - Knoxville; MA 77 Univ of TN - Knoxville; **SLP**

Smolek-Sharp, Mrs Joyce Ann 300 South 26th Street #7, Lincoln, NE 68510, (402) 477-7309, MS 88 Univ of NE - Lincoln; 88–Aud, Univ of NE Med Ctr

Smolensky, Mrs Terri Allyn 7001 Utica Avenue #908, Lubbock, TX 79424, (516) 484-6755, BA 83 CUNY - Queens Coll; MA 85 CUNY - Queens Coll; **SLP**

Smolin, Lori Kay Frankfurt High School, Box 30, APO New York, NY 09710, (516) 223-3850, BS 81 SUNY - Coll at Buffalo; MS 83 SUNY - Coll at Buffalo

Smolin, Louanne I 1443 Dartmouth Lane, Deerfield, IL 60015, (312) 787-3230, BS 77 Univ of IL - Urbana; MS 80 Southern IL Univ -Carbondale; Res & Trng Consult, Lis Consult Serv, **SLP**

Smolin, Mrs Shirlee J 3729 Silverwood Drive, York, PA 17402, (717) 845-8750, BA 49 Univ of IA; MS 76 William Paterson Coll; Sp-Lang Path, Lincoln Inter Ut #12, **SLP**

Smoller, Mrs Henny Perlmutter 105 South Orlando #301, Los Angeles, CA 90048, (213) 653-5291, BA 75 Univ of CA - Los Angeles; MA 82 CA St Univ - Los Angeles; Sp/Lang Path, Temple City USD, **SLP**

Smoly, Mrs Eleanor St Route 237, Aspen Woods, Vernon, NJ 07462, (201) 764-1700, BA 69 Montclair St Coll; MA 70 CUNY - City College; Sp-Lang Path, Vernon Township Pub Sch, **SLP**

Smoot, Mrs Karen Marty 70 South Sherwood Glen, Monument, CO 80132-8749, BS 74 CO St Univ; MS 76 CO St Univ; Sp-Lang Path, Private Practice, **SLP**

Smoot, Rikki J 9907 White Oak Avenue #117, Northridge, CA 91325, (213) 276-5322, BA 79 CA St Univ - Northridge; MA 82 CA St Univ - Northridge; 81–Sp-Lang Path, Beverly Hills USD, **SLP**

Smoski, Dr Walter J 30 Kenfield Circle, Bloomington, IL 61704, (309) 438-8643, BA 70 Benedictine Coll; MS 74 Southern IL Univ -Carbondale; PH 81 (Aud) Univ of IL - Urbana; Asst Prof for Aud, Illinois State University, **A**

Smothers, Celeste 905 Montgomery Street #D, Sikeston, MO 63801, (314) 471-7348, BS 86 Murray St Univ; MS 88 Murray St Univ; 88–Sp-Lang Path, Sikeston PS R-6

Smuckler, Karen J 1607 Montuale, Maryville, TN 37801, (615) 984-3143, BA 71 Univ of MD - College Park; MA 73 Univ of MD - College Park; **A**

Smyka, Richard Joseph 3156 East 5400 North, Liberty, UT 84310, (801) 399-9631, BA 82 Univ of Northern CO; MA 83 Univ of Northern CO; 87–Aud, Utah Schs for the Deaf and Blind, **A**

Smyke, Anna T 121 Magnolia Boulevard, Harahan, LA 70123, (504) 738-1076, BA 75 Coll of New Rochelle; MS 78 Gallaudet Coll; **A**

Smyth, Jill Flynn 1012 North Anderson Street, Bismarck, ND 58501, (404) 329-5520, BS 66 Univ of ND; MS 74 Emory Univ; Faculty Assoc, Emory U/Dept Commun Dis, **SLP**

Smyth, Thomas C 23001 Femes, Mission Viejo, CA 92692, (714) 586-7507, MA 52 CA St Univ - Sacramento; Aud, Private Practice, **SLP A**

Smyth, Troy 308 North Mesquite, Olathe, KS 66061, (913) 621-5155, BS 81 KS St Univ; MA 83 KS St Univ; Sp-Lang Path, Kansas City School System, **SLP**

Smythe, Linda T 83 Hardwick Road, Forestville, CT 06010, (203) 747-3314, BA 70 Central CT St Univ; MS 73 Southern CT St Univ; Sp-Lang Path, Plainville Bd of Ed, **SLP**

Snaidman, Mrs Patricia J 30 Fox Grove Drive, Hampton, VA 23664, (804) 825-4642, BS 74 Western Carolina Univ; ME 76 Western Carolina Univ; Rehabilitation Director, Commonwealth Health Care Inc, **SLP**

Snape, Cynthia A 24348 Eastwood Village Ct, Apartment 204, Mount Clemens, MI 48043, (313) 465-6100, BA 79 Western MI Univ; MA 80 Western MI Univ; Asst Prog Dir, Total Therapy Management, **SLP**

Snavely, Christophr R 1381 Oakdale Avenue, Rialto, CA 92376, (714) 737-4200, **A**

Snavely, Jan Allyson 811 Beaver Street, Santa Rosa, CA 95404, (213) 397-3157, BA 76 Holy Names Coll; MS 80 Univ of Redlands; Director, Private Practice, **SLP**

Snead, Colleen c/o Kresge Hearing Research, 1301 East Ann Street, University Of Michigan, Ann Arbor, MI 48109, (313) 964-8110, BS 73 CO St Univ; MS 77 Univ of AZ; Graduate Research Asst, U of MI, **A**

Snead, Linda J 217 South Clinton Street, East Orange, NJ 07018, (201) 429-8300, BA 73 Rutger's St Univ - Douglas Coll; MA 78 Montclair St Coll; Sp-Lang Path, Glen Ridge Pub Sch Dist, **SLP ACE**

Snead, Nancy A S 1565 Washington Avenue, Louisville, CO 80027, (303) 673-9280, BS 75 Univ of Alberta - Alberta; MA 76 Univ of KS; Sp-Lang Path, Private Practice, **SLP**

Snead, Sarah Ann Charlotte Eye Ear Nose & Throat Associates, 1600 East Third Street, Charlotte, NC 28204, (704) 372-3300, MS 88 Univ of NC - Chapel Hill; 88–Aud, Charlotte EENT Assoc

Snedden, Susan L 2015 Fairmount Avenue #2-F, Philadelphia, PA 19130, (302) 996-0900, BS 85 Bloomsburg Univ of PA; MS 87 Bloomsburg Univ of PA

Snedeker, Dr Leo W, Jr P O Box 3814, De Land, FL 32723, (305) 321-5368, BA 63 FL St Univ; MA 65 FL St Univ; PH 70 (NS) Univ of FL; Aud Conslt, Masters Hrng Aids, **SLP A LM**

Sneed, Mrs Donna Doss 12121 Audelia Road #2304, Dallas, TX 75243, (214) 783-4889, BS 78 Univ of Central AR; MS 83 Univ of AR - Little Rock; Sp-Lang Path, Richardson ISD, **SLP**

Sneider, Mrs Cecile D 6 Half Mile Road, Norwalk, CT 06851, (203) 847-0481, BA 53 Saint John's Univ - Jamaica; MS 74 Southern CT St Univ; SLP, Norwalk Board of Education, **SLP**

Snelgrove, Kathy A 10315 Orton Avenue, Los Angeles, CA 90064, (213) 515-3084, BA 71 Occidental Coll; MA 82 CA St Univ - Northridge; SLP, Los Angeles USD, **SLP**

Snell, Helen P 413 Dexter Avenue, Birmingham, AL 35213, (205) 871-9043, BA 37 Univ of GA; MA 56 Univ of AL- Tuscaloosa; **SLP LM**

Snell, Susan J Dept Of Special Education, Murray State University, Murray, KY 42071, (502) 762-2446, BS 73 Purdue Univ - West Lafayette; MA 78 Univ of IL - Urbana; Aud, Murray St U, **A ACE**

Snelling, Mrs Barbara Oberg 1615 Halfmoon Drive, Wharton, TX 77488, (409) 532-2284, **A**

Snelling, Theresa Marie Speech-Language Rehabilitation Section, Fitzsimons Army Medical Center, Aurora, CO 80045-5001, (303) 361-8120, BA 81 Univ of Northern CO; MA 84 Univ of Northern CO; 84–Sp-Lang Path, Fitzsimons Army Med Ctr, **SLP**

Snider, Bonita J 154 Arnold Avenue, Lancaster, OH 43130, (614) 653-4570, BS 78 Bowling Green St Univ; MA 79 Bowling Green St Univ; Sp/Lang Path, Lancaster Fairfield Comm Hosp, **SLP**

Snider, Elizabeth 9720 Chanelka Lane, Chesterfield, VA 23832, (804) 524-7561, BA 70 Emory Univ; ME 79 Old Dominion Univ; Sp-Lang Path, Southside Virginia Trng Center, **SLP**

Snider, Eunice A R R 3 Box 89, Charleston, IL 61920, (217) 345-2106, BS 61 Ball St Univ; MS 85 Eastern IL Univ; 86–Sp-Lang Path, Comm Unit Sch Dist #1, **SLP**

Snider, Judith L 115 Paseo DE La Playa #2, Redondo Beach, CA 90277, (213) 375-9626, BS 68 CA St Univ - Northridge; MA 69 CA St Univ - Northridge; Sp-Lang Path Spec, Supt of Sch-Los Angeles Co, **SLP**

Snider, Mrs Mary Ann 12465 N W Marshall, Portland, OR 97229, (503) 649-0357, BS 57 Carlow Coll; MA 59 Case Western Reserve Univ; Sp-Lang Path, Beaverton Sch Dist #48, **SLP**

Sniderman, Mrs Shirley G 4140 Hayvenhurst Avenue, Encino, CA 91436, (818) 789-0748, BA 60 CUNY - City College; MA 61 Columbia Univ Teachers Coll; SLP, Tarzana Speech & Lang Center, **SLP**

Snipes, Mrs Ann Rae 1675 South Quintero Way, Aurora, CO 80017, (303) 695-4411, BA 73 Univ of Denver; MA 74 Univ of Denver; 82–Sp-Lang Path, Cherry Creek Sch, **SLP**

Sniscak, Linda J 1082 Jeffrey Drive, Southampton, PA 18966, **SLP**

Snodgrass, R E R R 1 Box 156, Valley Center, KS 67147, (316) 744-0350, BS 32 Pittsburg St Univ; **SLP LM**

Snodgress, Kathleen L 1304 Park Avenue #B, Goldsboro, NC 27530, (919) 559-5371, BS 74 IN St Univ - Terre Haute; MS 75 IN St Univ - Terre Haute; Director Commun Serv, Caswell Cen, **SLP**

Snoek, Mrs Barbara B 46 Bancroft Road, Northampton, MA 01060, (413) 538-5077, BA 54 Univ of MI - Ann Arbor; MA 81 Univ of MA - Amherst; 88–Sp-Lang Path, Spec Ed Dept S Hadley, **SLP**

Snogans, Mrs Kathryn Laborioso 131 Park Avenue, Verona, NJ 07044, (201) 772-2600, MS 85 William Paterson Coll; Sp-Lang Path, Elks Cerebral Palsy Treatment, **SLP ACE**

Snook, Robert Winson 113 Landward Drive, Jupiter, FL 33477, (305) 744-8101, ME 83 Northeastern Univ; SLP, West Palm Beach Public Schools, **SLP**

Snope, Trudy L 10361 Barcan Circle, Columbia, MD 21044, (301) 897-5700, BA 68 Univ of MD - College Park; MA 72 Univ of MD - College Park; 83–Dir Prof Ed Br, ASHA, **SLP ACE**

Snorgrass, Mrs Cheryl J 2200 Barber, Kansas City, KS 66106, (816) 436-7747, BS 76 Univ of KS; MS 81 Univ of Montevallo; Sp-Lang Path, State of MO Schs for Severely Handicapped, **SLP**

Snow, Mrs Billie Reed 806 Grinnell, Richardson, TX 75081, (214) 235-8776, BS 66 East TX St Univ - Commerce; MS 71 Univ of North TX; Sp-Lang Path, Richardson ISD, **SLP**

Snow, David Page 3801 Brooklyn Avenue, Apartment B-1236, Seattle, WA 98105, (206) 634-2676, BA 81 CA St Univ - Long Beach; MA 86 CA St Univ - Fullerton; Grad, Univ of WA

Snow, Mrs Katherine L 3635 Kelway Avenue, Charlotte, NC 28210, (704) 563-6505, BA 77 Clemson Univ; ME 79 Univ of GA; Sp/Lang Path, Charlotte-Mecklenburg Sch, **SLP**

Snow, Linda B P O Box 1101, Gardiner, ME 04345, (207) 582-4000, BS 78 Northeastern Univ; MA 80 Univ of CT; Aud, Mid-Maine Medical Center, **A**

Snow, Mrs Marsha W 114 Sandpiper Lane, Venetia, PA 15367, (412) 664-2468, BA 79 IN Univ - Bloomington; OM 81 IN Univ - Bloomington; Sp/Lang Path, McKeesport Hosp, **SLP**

Snowden, Bruce Oswald 717 Oak Street, Burlington, IA 52601, (319) 752-9837, BA 83 Univ of MD - College Park; MS 86 Univ of OK - OK City; 86–Aud, Burlington Med Ctr, **A**

Snowden, Mrs Patricia Burke 2811 Janet Drive, Benton, AR 72015, (501) 778-1525, **SLP**

Snowden, Patricia H 2201 Matterhorn Lane, Austin, TX 78704, (512) 442-7821, OB Coll of Spch Therapists Eng; MA 65 Univ of TX - Austin; Consult to Phys Hndcpd - Aud, TX Sch for the Deaf, **SLP A**

Snyder, Ann Elizabeth Rd 2 Box 242, Hummelstown, PA 17036, (717) 533-5926, BS 85 PA St Univ - Univ Park; MS 87 Vanderbilt Univ; **SLP**

Snyder, Mrs Annemarie Luginbuhl 217 South Orange Avenue, Lodi, CA 95240, (209) 334-0479, BA 85 San Jose St Univ; MA 88 San Jose St Univ; **SLP**

Snyder, Mrs Beth Alaine 1041 Third Street, Second Floor, Whitehall, PA 18052, (215) 391-1111, BS 86 Bloomsburg Univ of PA; MS 87 Bloomsburg Univ of PA

Snyder, Mrs Beverly Jo 6520 Fairways Drive, Longmont, CO 80501, (303) 443-6802, BS 71; MS 76 Minot St Univ; Audiologist, **A**

Snyder, Carol Thurlow 30 Corliss Avenue, Greenwich, NY 12834, (518) 692-9307, OB 79 SUNY - Coll at Fredonia; OM 81 SUNY - Coll at Fredonia; Sp-Lang Path, Saratoga Co Bd of Coop Ed Svs, **SLP**

Snyder, Charles J, Jr 226 Pleasant Street, Ithaca, NY 14850, (607) 272-2984, OB Columbia Univ Teachers Coll; MA Syracuse Univ; Assoc Prof, Ithaca Coll, **SLP**

Snyder, Cheryl Ann 1401 Hennessey Street #73, Dodge City, KS 67801, (316) 225-3524, BA 86 Wichita St Univ; MA 87 Wichita St Univ

Snyder, Mrs Christine 1418 Wicklow Road, Boulder, CO 80303, (303) 447-1010, BA 75 Kent St Univ; MA 78 Kent St Univ; SLP, Boulder Valley Schs Dist RE2, **SLP**

Snyder, Deborah S Coastal Pediatric Speech Clinic, 180 Newport Center Drive, Suite 208, Newport Beach, CA 92660, (714) 759-3390, BA 75 Univ of MI - Ann Arbor; MS 76 Univ of MI - Ann Arbor; 79–Dir, Coastal Ped Sp Clinic, **SLP**

Snyder, Mrs Denise Nelson 4445 Slater Road, Eagan, MN 55122, (612) 887-9165, BA 76 Univ of MN - Minneap-St Paul; MA 80 Univ of WI - River Falls; SLP, Bloomington Pub Sch, **SLP**

Snyder, Diana A Box M, Kennett Square, PA 19348, (302) 995-8676, BS 71 Edinboro Univ of PA; MA 72 Bowling Green St Univ; Super-Office of Sp & Hrng, Dept of Health & Social Serv, **SLP**

Snyder, Elizabeth Ellen 1324 Park Avenue, Portsmouth, OH 45662, (614) 354-7896, BA 81 Univ of Southwestern LA; MA 84 OH Univ - Athens; Scioto Memorial Hosp, **A**

Snyder, Florence H 160 Snapfinger Drive, Athens, GA 30605, (404) 548-7581, BS 80 Univ of GA; ME 82 Univ of GA; Sp-Lang Path, St Marys Hosp, **SLP**

Snyder, Mrs Francesca Engler 8344 East Thoroughbred Tr, Scottsdale, AZ 85258, (602) 994-9390, BA 75 Hofstra Univ; MS 76 Adelphi Univ; Sp-Lang Path, Scottsdale Sp Path Assoc, **SLP**

Snyder, Gayle P Gayle P Snyder MA, 6314 Mojave Drive, San Jose, CA 95120, (408) 356-9465, BA 74 CA St Univ - Northridge; MA 75 CA St Univ - Northridge; Sp/Lang Path, Private Practice, **SLP ACE**

Snyder, Dr Jack M Dept Of Otolaryngology RL-30, School Of Medicine, University Of Washington, Seattle, WA 98195, (206) 543-5230, BA 53 Univ of MI - Ann Arbor; MA 56 Univ of MI - Ann Arbor; PH 71 (Aud) Univ of WA; 69–Prof & Dir of Aud, U WA Sch of Med, **SLP A**

Snyder, Janet Kaye F 6149 Valley Glen Drive, San Jose, CA 95123, **A**

Snyder, Jean RD 1 Box 222, Zion Grove, PA 17985, (717) 889-3253, BS 84 Marywood Coll; MS 85 Bloomsburg Univ of PA; 87–Sp-Lang Path, Carbon Pike Monroe, **SLP**

Snyder, Mrs Jill Marie 1676 Scheffer Avenue, St Paul, MN 55116, (612) 221-2066, BS 84 Mankato St Univ; MA 86 Univ of MN - Minneap-St Paul; 86–Sp-Lang Path, St Paul-Ramsey Med Ctr, **SLP**

Snyder, Joan S 3224 Ethan Allen Court, Bensalem, PA 19020, (215) 225-4437, BS 67 PA St Univ - Univ Park; MA 77 Trenton St Coll; 79–Sp-Lang Path, Sch Dist of Phila Pa, **SLP**

Snyder, John C, Jr 204 Memorial Drive, Bristol, TN 37620, (615) 968-2732, BA 74 Univ of TN - Knoxville; MA 76 Univ of TN - Knoxville; Aud, Otol Assoc Pc, **A**

Snyder, Kathleen Jean 3645 North Greenview, Apartment #3C, Chicago, IL 60613, (312) 337-5400, **SLP**

Snyder, Kimberly Sue 9514 E 65th Street #1404, Tulsa, OK 74133, (918) 254-0582, BA 84 Univ of OK - Norman; MS 86 Univ of OK - OK City; **SLP**

Snyder, Kristi S 1716 Chacoma Place S W, Albuquerque, NM 87104, **A**

Snyder, Mrs Kristi W Rd 5 Box 115-S, Selinsgrove, PA 17870, (717) 737-6728, BS 79 Bloomsburg Univ of PA; MS 80 Bloomsburg Univ of PA; Master Itinerant, Captial Area Intermed Ut, **SLP**

Snyder, Mrs Laura Ann 6009 Ken Avenue, Arlington, TX 76017, (817) 483-1650, BS 82 Baylor Univ; MS 84 Baylor Univ; **SLP**

Snyder, Lee Z 21 East 26th Street, Covington, KY 41014, (606) 491-1171, BS 72 PA St Univ - Univ Park; MS 73 CO St Univ; Executive Director, N Kentucky Easter Seal Center, **A**

Snyder, Linda Route 4 Box 60, Maquoketa, IA 52060, (319) 652-2474, BS 75 Northern IL Univ - De Kalb; MA 76 Northern IL Univ - De Kalb; Sp-Lang Path, Private Practice, **SLP**

Snyder, Mrs Linda Huber 6 Whittier Road, Clark, NJ 07066, (201) 688-1200, BA 68 Kean Coll of NJ; MA 71 Kean Coll of NJ; **SLP**

Snyder, Loretta S P O Box 523, Mableton, GA 30059, **SLP**

Snyder, Mrs Louise M 338 East Garfield Road, Coldwater, MI 49036, (517) 279-7524, BS 72 Western MI Univ; MA 72 Western MI Univ; SLP, Branch ISD, **SLP**

Snyder, Dr Lynn Sebestyen 12100 Montecito Road #141, Los Alamitos, CA 90720, (213) 985-4593, BA 64 Coll of New Rochelle; MA 66 Seton Hall Univ; PH 75 (NS) Univ of CO - Boulder; 88–Prof, California State Univ Long Beach, **SLP**

Snyder, Maripat Pyatok 5614 Baywater Drive, Tampa, FL 33615, (813) 854-3313, BS 81 Marquette Univ; MA 83 Montclair St Coll; 88–Sp-Lang Path, Hillsborough Co Sch Sys, **SLP**

Snyder, Mrs Nancy Bredbenner 1297 Kearney Drive, North Brunswick, NJ 08902, (201) 925-2390, BS 65 Bloomsburg Univ of PA; MA 86 Kean Coll of NJ; Sp-Lang Path, Kohler Child Dev Ctr, **SLP**

Snyder, Mrs Patricia D 360 Bernice Drive, East Meadow, NY 11554-4309, (516) 735-8845, BA 75 Adelphi Univ; MA 79 Hofstra Univ; Sp-Lang Path, Human Resources Sch-Albertson, **SLP**

Snyder, Paula M 335 East 22nd Street #3A, New York, NY 10010, (212) 563-7474, BS 78 CUNY - Brooklyn Coll; MS 80 CUNY - Brooklyn Coll; Supvr, Young Adult Inst, **SLP**

Snyder, Rebecca Ann 172 Wickham Avenue, Middletown, NY 10940, (914) 794-1400, BS 83 SUNY - Coll at Fredonia; MS 86 Bloomsburg Univ of PA; **A**

Snyder, Rebecca M 1617 North 60th Street, Omaha, NE 68104, (712) 322-7354, BS 67 Univ of IA; MA 69 Univ of IA; Sp/Lang Path, AEA 13, **SLP**

Snyder, Rosanne Marie 9645 Baymeadows Road #704, Jacksonville, FL 32256, (904) 730-2909, BS 86 Univ of Central AR; OM 87 Univ of Central AR; 88–Sp-Lang Path, Duval Co Sch Bd A Smith Clinic, **SLP**

Snyder, Mrs Ruth 18 Sherry Lane, Brownsburg, IN 46112-9218, (317) 852-2459, BS 72 Purdue Univ - West Lafayette; MS 73 Purdue Univ - West Lafayette; Sp-Lang Path, Brownsburg Comm Schs, **SLP**

Snyder, Mrs Shelley Henry 602 Danbury Street, Pittsburgh, PA 15214, (412) 681-7755, BA 77 Univ of Pittsburgh - Pittsburgh; MA 79 Univ of Pittsburgh - Pittsburgh; **A**

Snyder, Mrs Sue P 193 Parkerville Road, Southborough, MA 01772, (508) 485-8847, BA 65 Univ of CT; MA 66 Univ of WI - Madison; Aud, Fallon Cl, **A**

Snyder, Winona M Rd 1 Box 910-A, Evans Mills, NY 13637, (315) 788-2730, **SLP**

Snyder-McLean, Dr Lee K Univ Of Kansas/Parsons Res Ctr, Bureau Of Child Research, P O Box 737, Parsons, KS 67357, (316) 421-6550, BS 69 Syracuse Univ; ME 74 Univ of WA; PH 77 (NS) G Peabody Coll-Vanderbilt U; Research Associate, University of Kansas

Snyders, Cathryn Pearse 1820 Duke Of York Quay, Virginia Beach, VA 23454, (804) 628-7182, BS Univ of VA - Charlottesville; ME Univ of VA - Charlottesville; Sp-Lang Path, Chldn Hosp of King's Daughters, **SLP**

Snyder-Williams, Mrs Mary Ann 145 Youngstown Hubbard Rd, Apt #78, Hubbard, OH 44425, BS 67 Miami Univ - Oxford; MA 76 Kent St Univ; 67–Tchr/Cl, Youngstown Cty Sch, **SLP**

Snyderwine, Mrs Carol Hazlett 10350 Prouty Road, Painesville, OH 44077, (216) 531-9000, BS 83 Clarion Univ of PA; MA 84 Univ of Akron; Aud, Meridia Euclid Hosp, **A**

Soales, Madelyn G 8132 Irwin N E, Albuquerque, NM 87109, (505) 822-0476, BS 75 Kean Coll of NJ; MS 76 Rutgers St Univ -N Brunswick; 85–Sp-Lang Path, DLD Sch, **SLP**

Soares-Brown, Camille Pauline P O Box 508, McArthur, CA 96056, (916) 336-5551, MA 83 CA St Univ - Chico; Sp-Lang Path, Fall River USD, **SLP**

Soat, Lynn A 1303 Crossbow Drive, Stevens Point, WI 54481, (715) 344-2425, BS 70 Marquette Univ; MS 72 Univ of WI - Milwaukee; **SLP**

Sobchuk, Lucille H 24 Knox Street, Thomaston, ME 04861, **SLP**

Sobel, Catherine Mary 69 Brookside Drive West, Harriman, NY 10926, (914) 783-6618, BA 84 SUNY - Coll at Cortland; MA 86 Montclair St Coll; 88–Sp-Lang Path, St Dominic's Sch, **SLP**

Sobel, Paula R 8230 Forrest Avenue, Elkins Park, PA 19117, (215) 576-6948, BS 76 Temple Univ; MA 78 Temple Univ; 78–Sp-Lang Path, Private Practice, **SLP ACE**

Sobelson, Mrs Marna G 31 Meadow Woods Road, Great Neck, NY 11020, (516) 482-5279, BS 51 Syracuse Univ; MS 79 Adelphi Univ; **SLP**

Soberano, Mrs Carol A W 5838 Iva Drive, Akron, OH 44319, (216) 753-1025, BS 68 Kent St Univ; MA 80 Univ of Akron; Sp-Lang Path, Barberton Pub Sch, **SLP ACE**

Soby, Mrs Annette M 869 Alameda, Redwood City, CA 94061, (408) 998-6395, MA Case Western Reserve Univ; BA 60 Univ of MI - Ann Arbor; Sp/Lang Path, San Jose USD, **SLP**

Sochaczewski, Mrs Ruth W 3401 Shelburne Road, Baltimore, MD 21208, (301) 522-5450, **SLP**

Socha-Smith, Karen Marie 5037 Colonial Drive, Flower Mound, TX 75028, (214) 323-6621, BS 79 Wayne St Univ; MA 80 Wayne St Univ; Sp-Lang Path, Carrollton-Farmers Branch ISD, **SLP**

Sochocki, Mrs Rita Gail 6015 Sundance Trail, Brighton, MI 48116, (313) 547-7200, Sp-Lang Path, Berkley Sch, **SLP**

Sochrin, Mrs Phyllis L 51 Strawberry Lane, Shelton, CT 06484, (203) 735-4327, BA 59 Univ of CT; MA 60 Univ of CT; Dir, The Hrng Cen, **SLP A**

Socolof, Mrs Gale L 3808 Vicksburg Street, Plano, TX 75023, (214) 423-9664, BS 71 Univ of OK - Norman; MS 81 Univ of TX - Dallas; Sp-Lang Path, Plano ISD, **SLP**

Socolofsky, Ginger K 9 S 775 Clarendon Hills, Hinsdale, IL 60521, (312) 323-5505, BA 69 Depauw Univ; MA 72 Northern IL Univ - De Kalb; **SLP**

Soderberg-Stefanek, Mrs Beth E 312 Runaway Bay Circle, Apt 3-D, Mishawaka, IN 46545, (219) 258-0525, BA 85 MI St Univ; MA 86 MI St Univ; Childrens Therapy Services, **SLP**

Soderlind, Ann Hittner 5871 130th Street Court, Apple Valley, MN 55124, (612) 431-2919, BS 76 Saint Cloud St Univ; MS 77 Univ of WI - Eau Claire; Sp-Lang Path, **SLP**

Soderlind, Mrs Isabel M 8702 South Cedarwood Lane, Highlands Ranch, CO 80126-2136, (303) 791-2811, BA 76 Elmhurst Coll; MA 78 Northwestern Univ; **SLP**

Soelling, Mrs Carol Sue 2837 Marietta Street, Steilacoom, WA 98388, (206) 584-0060, BA 78 Western WA Univ; MA 82 Western WA Univ; **SLP**

Sofen, Linda N 4481 Rolfe Road, San Diego, CA 92117, (619) 581-9057, BA 82 Univ of CA - San Diego; MA 87 San Diego St Univ; 88–Sp-Lang Path, Children's Hosp

Soffin, Bonnie S Providence Hospital, Department Of Audiology, 16001 West 9 Mile Road, Southfield, MI 48037, (313) 424-3392, BA 71 Univ of MI - Ann Arbor; MS 72 Univ of MI - Ann Arbor; 79–Assoc Dir, Providence Hospital, **A**

Sofiak, Nancy T 1934 Jackson Lane, Daytona Beach, FL 32014-6631, (904) 788-4651, MA 78 IN Univ - Bloomington; 87–Aud, Veterans Administration, **A**

Sofley, Frances Eckel 319 Kilbourne Road, Columbia, SC 29205, (803) 252-2538, BS 78 Indiana Univ of PA; MS 80 Univ of AZ; 87–Sp-Lang Path, Palmetto Sp Path Assoc and Consultants, **SLP**

Soforenko, Rhonda A 57 Fernwood Drive, East Longmeadow, MA 01028-1302, **SLP**

Sofra, Mrs Brita Elina 305 Westover Drive #16-B, Hattiesburg, MS 39402, (601) 264-1705, BS 80 Kent St Univ; MA 83 Univ of Akron; 88–Sp-Lang Path, Forrest Co Sch Dist, **SLP**

Sofranko-Noto, Mary A Box 295-B Mt Bethel Road, Rd #1, Clarks Summit, PA 18411, (717) 348-3455, BS 77 Marywood Coll; MS 81 Bloomsburg Univ of PA; Sp-Lang Path, Scranton Sch Dist, **SLP**

Sogin, Ruth R 6312 Patton Street, New Orleans, LA 70118-5836, (504) 589-5266, MA 47 CUNY - Hunter Coll; MS 75 Tulane Univ; **SLP**

Sohl, Mrs Mary P 83 Elm Bank Gardens, Barnes, London, England SW1 30NX, (703) 250-8198, BS 76 IA St Univ; MA 78 Northern IL Univ - De Kalb; Clinical Coord Outpatient Serv, Mt Vernon Hospital, **SLP**

Sohlberg, McKay Moore 2112 East Shelby, Seattle, WA 98112, (206) 323-8711, MS 84 Univ of WA; Clinical Coordinator, Good Samaritan Hospital, **SLP**

Sohler, Rhonda A 1547 C Street, Lincoln, NE 68502, BS 84 Kearney St Coll; MS 88 Univ of NE - Lincoln; 88–Aud, Madonna Ctr Rehab Hosp

Sohn, Lucinda Anne 510 Sunvalley Drive, Farmington, MO 63640, (314) 756-3571, BS 82 Southeast MO St Univ; MA 84 Southeast MO St Univ; 84–Sp-Lang Path, Private Practice, **SLP**

Sohner, Linda L 637 South 3rd Street, Columbus, OH 43206, (614) 877-4361, MA 78 OH St Univ; ME 72 PA St Univ - Univ Park; Clinical Supervisor, OH St Univ Sp-Lang-Hrng Clinic, **SLP**

Soifer, Dr Lydia H 4901 Henry Hudson Parkway, Riverdale, NY 10471, (914) 472-7080, BA 71 CUNY - Brooklyn Coll; MS 72 PA St Univ - Univ Park; PH 86 (Sp Path & Aud) Columbia Univ Teachers Coll; 82–Dir, Total Learning Ctr, **SLP**

Soika, Tina M 118 Arch Avenue, Pittsburgh, PA 15202, (412) 766-1124, BS 77 CA Univ of PA; MS 81 WV Univ; Clinical Supervisor, InSpeech Inc, **SLP**

Soiles, Mrs Leslie Peterson 36 Enfield Street, Worcester, MA 01602, BA 82 Worcester St Coll; MA 85 Univ of MA - Amherst; Audiologist, Neri Holzer MD, **A**

Soisson, Dianne C 285 Glen Eagles Drive, Winston-Salem, NC 27104, (919) 768-6794, MS 88 Univ of North TX; 88–Sp-Lang Path, Forsyth Mem Hosp

Soisson, Margaret 5050 Oak Street #1017, Twin Oaks, Kansas City, MO 64112, (816) 753-6759, BA 28 Goucher Coll; MA 47 Univ of IA; **A LM**

Sokal, Mrs Rhoda H R 5035 Entrada Curta, Tucson, AZ 85718, (602) 622-5833, BA 68 CUNY - Queens Coll; MA 70 CUNY - Lehman Coll; **SLP**

Sokol, Mrs Betty Ann 455 Park Avenue, Leonia, NJ 07605, (201) 438-3070, BA 50 San Diego St Univ; MA 52 Univ of Southern CA; Sp-Lang Path, Davis Reg Cen, **SLP ACE**

Sokol, Christine Mallard 2915 N E Davis, Portland, OR 97232, (503) 233-0338, BA 75 Univ of CA - Santa Barbara; MS 77 Univ of OR; Sp-Lang Path, Portland PS, **SLP**

Sokol, Ellen R 137 Weeks Road, East Williston, NY 11596, (516) 467-2224, BA 74 Long Island U - CW Post Ctr; MS 76 Adelphi Univ; Sp-Lang Path, Sachem Sch Dist, **SLP**

Sokol, Heidi 69-09H 186 Lane, Flushing, NY 11365, (212) 591-0869, BA 77 CUNY - Queens Coll; MA 79 CUNY - Queens Coll; 86–Aud, St John's Univ, **A**

Sokol, Janice Lynn 401-71 Grand Avenue, London, ON, Canada N6C 1M1, (519) 438-7424, MA 87 Univ of MN - Duluth; 87–Sp-Lang Path, Thames Valley Chldn Ctr

Sokol, Mrs Mary G 11 Flora Lane, Oxford, CT 06483, (203) 888-5060, BS 73 Mankato St Univ; MS 78 Southern CT St Univ; Sp-Lang Path, Brookfield Bd of Ed, **SLP**

Sokol, Rose Taubenfeld 336 West End Avenue #1-A, New York, NY 10023, (212) 873-9613, BA 71 CUNY - Brooklyn Coll; MS 73 CUNY - Brooklyn Coll; Sp-Lang Pathologist, Private Practice, **SLP ACE**

Sokol-Cass, Helene M 8 Pride Crossing, Eliot, ME 03903, (617) 942-0886, BA 75 Rutger's St Univ - Douglas Coll; MS 76 PA St Univ - Univ Park; Sp-Lang Path, **SLP**

Sokol-Evans, Mrs Sandra A 181 Dehaven Road, Beaver Falls, Beaver Falls, PA 15010, (412) 843-1542, **SLP**

Sokolnicki, Alfred J College Of Speech, Marquette University, 1131 West Wisconsin Avenue, Milwaukee, WI 53233, (414) 224-3488, 42 Marquette Univ; MA 47 Marquette Univ; PH (NS); Dean Emeritus, Marquette U, **SLP F LM**

Sokoloff, Dr Martin A 32 Harwich Pines Way RR4, Harwich, MA 02645, (617) 432-3483, BA 47 CUNY - Brooklyn Coll; MA 50 NY Univ; PH 59 (Sp Path and Psychology) NY Univ; Prof Emeritus Sp & Psychology, Pace University, **SLP LM**

Sokoloski, Danette K 1550 East Germaine Street, Apartment 153, St Cloud, MN 56301-2126, (612) 252-0233, MA 87 Univ of IA

Sokoly, MD Judith Gootjes 1567 Peck Street, Muskegon, MI 49441, (616) 773-9161, BA 85 MI St Univ; MA 86 Western MI Univ; 87–Sp-Lang Path, Muskegon Reg Ctr for Developmental Disabilities, **SLP**

Solan, John Raymond 404 East Beatryce Street, Tempe, AZ 85281, (602) 941-0519, BA 77 SUNY - Coll at Plattsburgh; MS 87 AZ St Univ; 87–Aud, Audiology & Hearing Aids Inc, **A**

Solanas, Elizabeth 5353 Greenside Lane, Baton Rouge, LA 70806, **SLP**

Solberg, E Jane Box 187, #275 Glenwood Road, Whitefish, MT 59937, (406) 862-2850, BA 72 Univ of MT; MA 74 Univ of MT; Sp-Lang Path, Tamarack Clin Svcs, **SLP**

Solberg, Larry C 2099-A Rickards Road, Tallahassee, FL 32308-4821, (715) 758-4812, BA 79 Univ of WI - Eau Claire; MS 80 Univ of WI - Eau Claire; Dir of SLP, Lakeview Med Cen, **SLP**

Solecki, Janet M 325 Summer, Buffalo, NY 14222, (716) 885-8318, BS 79 Northwestern Univ; MS 82 Washington Univ; Aud, Buffalo Hearing & Speech Ctr, **A**

Soler, Mrs Sandra Gearhart Box 450-A Rd 1, Macungie, PA 18062-9744, (215) 845-2018, **SLP**

Solheim, Tammy Dee Box 31, Frankfort, SD 57440-0031, (605) 472-1877, MS 88 Moorhead St Univ

Soli, Dr Sigfrid D Biosciences Lab, Bldg 270-4S-11, 3M Center, St Paul, MN 55144, (612) 733-3312, BA 68 Saint Olaf Coll; BA 72 Univ of MN - Minneap-St Paul; PH 78 (Experimental Psychology) Univ of MN - Minneap-St Paul; SLP, Biosciences Lab 3M Cen

Soli, Sydney Jane 11105 North 115th St #2088, Scottsdale, AZ 85259, (602) 860-6404, MS 83 Univ of WI - Stevens Point; Sp-Lang Path, **SLP**

Soliman, Mrs Ann Hisley 10 Saray El-Gizera Street, Zamalek, Cairo, Egypt, BA 59 Western MD Coll; MA 64 Univ of MD - College Park; **SLP**

Soliman, Dr Salah M 10 Saray El-Gizera Street, Zamalek, Cairo, Egypt, MD 68; PH 59 (NS) Johns Hopkins Univ; Prof & Dir of Aud, Ain Shams University ENT Dept, **A F**

Solis-Cohen, Ellen 765 Arden Road, Jenkintown, PA 19046, (215) 576-7658, BS 74 NY Univ; MS 76 Columbia Univ Teachers Coll; Sp/Lang Path, Private Practice, **SLP**

Sollecito, Kathy Jeanne 4235 Colorado Street, Long Beach, CA 90814, (818) 962-4011, BS 78 SUNY - Center at Albany; OM 84 Univ of WA; 86–Mgr-Comm Dis & Occup Ther Depts, Queen of the Valley Hosp, **SLP**

Solodar, Mrs Helena Stern Audiological Consultants, 2550 Windy Hill Road #200, Marietta, GA 30067, (404) 953-2223, OB 73 Univ of GA; OM 75 Univ of SC - Columbia; Aud, Aud Consult of Atlanta Inc, **SLP A**

Soloff, Dr Hillary E 7250-D Eden Brook Drive, Apartment 204, Columbia, MD 21046, (301) 381-7345, BA 77 Univ of FL; MA 78 Univ of FL; PH 84 (Sp-Lang Path) Memphis St Univ; 85, Private Practice, **SLP**

Solomon, Anita K One Ascan Avenue #5, Forest Hills, NY 11375, **SLP**

Solomon, Dr Arthur L Department Of Speech, Western Washington Univ, Bellingham, WA 98225, BA 46 Antioch Coll; MA 47 Univ of NC - Chapel Hill; PH 60 (NS) Stanford Univ; Prof of Communication, Western Washington Univ, **SLP LM**

Solomon, Mrs Barbara S W Purdue University, Aus Heavilon Hall, West Lafayette, IN 47907, (317) 494-3820, BA 72 CUNY - City College; MA 74 CUNY - City College; 79–Superv Sp-Lang Path, Prudue Univ, **SLP**

Solomon, Beth I 150 West End Avenue #20-G, Lincoln Towers, New York, NY 10023, (212) 316-9344, BS 85 Univ of MA - Amherst; MS 87 Columbia Univ Teachers Coll; 87–Sp-Lang Path, Mem Sloan Kettering Can Ctr, **SLP ACE**

Solomon, Dr Beverly 924 North 33rd Street, Allentown, PA 18104, (215) 398-3958, BA 47 Wilson Coll; MS 57 PA St Univ - Univ Park; PH 65 (NS) PA St Univ - Univ Park; **SLP**

Solomon, Charles Mease Clinic, Dunedin, FL 34698, (813) 734-6563, BA 74 Univ of Central FL; MA 75 Univ of Central FL; Aud, Private Practice, **A**

Solomon, Mrs Elaine W Developmental Learning Center, 537 Albin Street, Teaneck, NJ 07666, (201) 836-8051, BS 51 Syracuse Univ; MA 52 Columbia Univ Teachers Coll; Dir, Dev Lrng Cen, **SLP**

Solomon, Mrs Estelle W 89 Baldwin Terrace, Wayne, NJ 07470, (201) 696-3928, BA 68 CUNY - Queens Coll; MS 70 CUNY - Queens Coll; SLP, **SLP**

Solomon, Mrs Greta N 5733 El Canon Avenue, Woodland Hills, CA 91367, BA 77 CA St Univ - Northridge; MA 80 CA St Univ - Northridge; SLP, LA USD, **SLP**

Solomon, James R 28484 Mission Boulevard #304, Hayward, CA 94544, (415) 538-9889, BA 63 Stanford Univ; MS 75 Univ of WI - Madison; PH 88 (Neurolinguistics) Univ of WI - Madison; 88–Consult Sp-Lang Path, Kaiser-Permanente Med Ctr, **SLP ACE**

Solomon, Mrs Jenny A 17440 N E 38th #A-304, Redmond, WA 98052-5716, (206) 881-6043, BA 79 Univ of Houston - Univ Park; MA 81 Univ of Houston - Univ Park; 87–Sp-Lang Path, Eastside Men Hlth Disabilities Prog, **SLP**

Solomon, Dr Linda Z Hearing And Speech Department, Menorah Meidcal Center, 4949 Rockhill Road, Kansas City, MO 64110, (816) 276-8225, BA 61 NY Univ; MA 63 Stanford Univ; PH 81 (NS) Univ of KS; Dir Hrng & Sp, Menorah Med Cen, **SLP**

Solomon, Loryn Maude 68-61 Yellowstone Boulevard, Forest Hills, NY 11375, (914) 723-5500, BS 76 Boston Univ; MS 78 Washington Univ; SLP, Scarsdale High Sch, **SLP**

Solomon, Mona Schechter 1036 East 5th Street, Brooklyn, NY 11230, (718) 252-5940, BA 73 CUNY - Hunter Coll; MA 75 Northwestern Univ; Sp-Lang Path, Chicago Pub Schls, **SLP**

Solomon, Mrs Nancy Pearl 250 North Arcadia Avenue #610, Tucson, AZ 85711, (602) 790-5957, BA 82 Univ of MD - College Park; MA 84 Univ of MD - College Park; Sp-Lang Path, University of Arizona, **SLP**

Solomon, Mrs Sandra P 26 Blair Road, Armonk, NY 10504-2526, (914) 273-8043, BA 60 Cornell Univ; MA 62 CUNY - Hunter Coll; Supervisor of Aud, Burke Rehab Cen, **A**

Solomon-Dworkin, Mrs Marsha 309 South Middletown Road, Media, PA 19063, (215) 565-4585, BA 73 Temple Univ-Tyler Sch of Art; MA 75 Temple Univ-Tyler Sch of Art; Career/Voc Coord for Hrng Imp, De Co Inter Ut, **SLP**

Solomon-Rice, Patti L 3206 Upper Lock Avenue, Belmont, CA 94002, (415) 593-1773, BS 77 Univ of WI - Madison; MA 80 Univ of MT; 86–Dir, Patti Solomon-Rice MA Assoc, **SLP ACE**

Solomonson, Barbara Ann 1116 Hill Street, Traverse City, MI 49684, BS 74 Central MI Univ; MS 80 Univ of South FL; 88–Sp-Lang Path, Traverse Bay Area ISD, **SLP**

Solon, Carol 945 Bell Lane, Maple Glen, PA 19002-3014, BA 75 1985; MA 77 Univ of Pittsburgh - Pittsburgh; Sp-Lang Path, Montgomery Co Intermediate Unit, **SLP**

Solon, Elizabeth M 114 East Keller Street, Rear Apartment, Mechanicsburg, PA 17055, (717) 737-6728, BA 81 Univ of CT; BS 85 Bloomsburg Univ of PA; Sp-Lang Path, Capital Area Intermediate Unit, **SLP ACE**

Solon, Laurel Frassinell 1517 Wells Street, Ann Arbor, MI 48104, (313) 475-1311, BS 75 WV Univ; MA 77 Memphis St Univ; 84–Sp-Lang Path, Chelsea Comm Hosp, **SLP**

Solot, Cynthia Beth 1828 Spruce Street, Philadelphia, PA 19103, (215) 596-9123, **SLP**

Solotoff, Mrs Barbara B 2 Spruce Street #1C, Great Neck, NY 11021, BA 78 CUNY - Queens Coll; MA 79 Hofstra Univ; 80–Sp-Lang Path, NYC Bd of Ed Dist 24, **SLP**

Solow, Dr Lawrence Valley Hearing Aid Center, 982 Park Row, Salinas, CA 93901, (408) 757-3589, BA 73 CA St Univ - Northridge; MA 75 CA St Univ - Northridge; PH 77 (NS); Owner Valley Hearing Aid Cen, Private Practice, **A**

Solties, Mrs Barbara Carter Rd #2 Box 289-1A, Finleyville, PA 15332, (304) 243-0300, BS 82 CA Univ of PA; MS 84 CA Univ of PA

Soltman, Shirley K 13 Maple Avenue, Wheeling, WV 26003, (304) 234-0544, BS 60 Eastern MI Univ; MA 67 Eastern MI Univ; Sp-Lang Path/Dept Mgr, Ohio Valley Med Ctr, **SLP**

Soman, Mrs Bonnie Commander 21 Wedgewood Lane, Wantagh, NY 11793, (516) 731-4314, BA 74 CUNY - Queens Coll; MS 75 Adelphi Univ; 87–Sp-Lang Path, Sch for Lang and Comm Dev, **SLP**

Soman, Bonnie L 14388 North 95th Street, Longmont, CO 80501, (303) 772-7700, BS 77 SUNY - Coll at Fredonia; MA 78 Univ of Northern CO; 84–Sp-Lang Path, St Vrain Valley Sch Dist Reij, **SLP**

Sombat, Margaret M 13054 Millstone, Chardon, OH 44024, BA 83 John Carroll Univ; MA 86 Cleveland St Univ; **SLP**

Somer, Ellen S 618 Ledgeview Park Drive, Louisville, KY 40206, (502) 588-5331, BS 72 Univ of MA - Amherst; MS 73 Univ of WI - Madison; Coord Prog Dev, Chld Eval Cen-U of Louisville, **SLP**

Somers, Mrs Andrea C 37 Belmont Street, Abington, MA 02351, BS 78 Univ of NH; ME 81 Northeastern Univ; Sp/Lang Path, Charmss Collaborative, **SLP**

Somers, Dr Janet M 1155 Eugenia Boulevard, New Smyrna Beach, FL 32069, (904) 427-5296, MA 83 Univ of Central FL; SLP, Volusia Co Sch, **SLP**

Somers, Louise Z 86 Tecumseh Drive, Hanover, MA 02339, (617) 335-1460, BA 54 Univ of WI - Madison; ME 79 Northeastern Univ; Sp/Lang Path, Weymouth Ma, **SLP**

Somerstein, Esther Deborah 137-18 71st Avenue, Flushing, NY 11367, (516) 560-8628, MA 84 CUNY - Queens Coll; Sp-Lang Path, Sewanhaka High Sch Dist, **SLP**

Somerville-Pedi, Rae Ann 214 Robertson Way, Lincoln Park, NJ 07035, (201) 587-8500, BS 85 Univ of NH; MS 87 Boston Univ; 87–Sp-Lang Path, Kessler Inst for Rehab, **SLP**

Somma, Christine A 209 11th Street, Brooklyn, NY 11215, (718) 963-8319, BS 83 SUNY - Coll at Plattsburgh; MA 86 Univ of CO - Boulder; **SLP**

Somma, Dolores R 1127 Meadowlark Drive, Pittsburgh, PA 15243, (412) 394-5766, BA 53 Carlow Coll; ME 67 Kent St Univ; Sp-Lang Path, Allegheny Inter Unit, **SLP**

Sommer, Anne Elizabeth 312 Hamilton Street, West Lafayette, IN 47906, (317) 423-6336, BS 83 Purdue Univ - West Lafayette; MS 85 Purdue Univ - West Lafayette; Aud, St Elizabeth Hosp, **A**

Sommer, Mrs Carol Galbany 8248 Mapleway Drive, Olmsted Falls, OH 44138, (216) 235-2328, MA 83 Cleveland St Univ; Aud, Northcoast Rehabilitation Ctr, **A**

Sommer, Mrs Deborah J 78 Heritage Drive, MacKinaw, IL 61755, BA 73 IA St Univ; MA 74 Western IL Univ; Sp-Lang Path, Schramm Educational Ctr, **SLP**

Sommer, Mrs Lillian S 5 Brevity Court, Binghamton, NY 13905, (607) 797-0812, BA 65 CUNY - Hunter Coll; ME 66 PA St Univ - Univ Park; Sp-Lang Path, Twin Tier Home Hlth, **SLP**

Sommer, Sue A 875 Lyman Avenue, Reno, NV 89509, MS 79 Univ of NV - Reno; **SLP**

Sommerer, Claudia Villanova 1064 Liberty Avenue, Union, NJ 07083, (201) 548-7610, BA 76 New Sch for Social Research; MA 84 Seton Hall Univ; 87–Sp-Lang Path, Ped Rehab Dept JFK Med Ctr, **SLP**

Sommerfield, Sandra Lee Milford Administration Bldg, 906 Lakeview Avenue, Milford, DE 19963, (302) 422-1600, BS 79 Edinboro Univ of PA; MA 81 Edinboro Univ of PA; 81–Sp-Lang Path, Milford School District, **SLP**

Sommers, Mrs Chandra D 114 Sherwood, Morris, IL 60450, (309) 833-4101, BS 66 IL St Univ - Normal; MA 69 Western IL Univ; **A**

Sommers, Lisa K Box 673, Skaneateles, NY 13152, (315) 488-2951, BS 85 Bowling Green St Univ; MA 87 Kent St Univ; 88–Sp-Lang Path, St Camillus Rehab Ctr, **SLP**

Sommers, Nancy Henrikson 5025 East 220th Street, Faribault, MN 55021, (507) 334-8751, BS 74 Mankato St Univ; MS 79 Univ of WI - Eau Claire; **SLP**

Sommers, Mrs Patricia A 2960 North 73rd Street, Milwaukee, WI 53210, (414) 352-3300, BS 78 Marquette Univ; MA 79 Western MI Univ; Sp-Lang Path, Amer Med Ser, **SLP**

Sommers, Rona S 2 Cornish Court, Dix Hills, NY 11746, (516) 369-1917, BA 79 SUNY - Center at Stony Brook; MA 82 Long Island U - CW Post Ctr; Aud, East End Hrng & Sp, **A ACE**

Sommers, Dr Ronald K Speech And Hearing Clinic, Kent State University, Kent, OH 44242, (216) 672-2672, BS 52 Kent St Univ; MA 53 Northwestern Univ; ED 61 (NS) Univ of Pittsburgh - Pittsburgh; Prof, Kent St U, **SLP A F**

Sommers, Tami Jo 1695 East County Road D #332, Maplewood, MN 55109, (612) 426-3214, OB 81 Univ of MN - Duluth; MS 82 Univ of WI - Eau Claire; 85–Sp-Lang Path, Mahtomedi Sch Dist, **SLP**

Sommerville, Patricia J 3313 Edward Street N E, Minneapolis, MN 55418, (612) 788-4597, **SLP**

Sommerville, Dr Suzanne Saginaw Valley Hearing Clinic, 3175 Christy Way, Saginaw, MI 48603, (517) 799-1611, BA 64 Baylor Univ; MS 67 Univ of OK Medical Center; PH 78 (NS) Purdue Univ - West Lafayette; Aud, Sag Valley Hrng Cl/Aud Vestlab, **A**

Sonday, Dr Francis L 7716 B Somerset Bay, Indianapolis, IN 46240, (317) 251-7822, BA 38 IN Univ - Bloomington; PH 57 (Aud) Northwestern Univ; **A F LM**

Sonderman-Thompson, Mrs Judith Clar 2750 Pike Drive, Napa, CA 94558, (707) 257-2858, BA 67 Univ of AZ; MS 69 Univ of Pittsburgh - Pittsburgh; PH 78 (NS) Univ of Pittsburgh - Pittsburgh; Dir of SLP, Irwin Lehroff PhD and Associates, **SLP**

Soneda, Mrs Rosaline Ong 7447 Terrace Drive, El Cerrito, CA 94530, (415) 222-2161, BA 76 Univ of CA - Berkeley; SLP, Richmond USD, **SLP**

Songer, Judy A 1967 Rollins Drive, Loveland, OH 45140, (513) 683-8267, BS 73 Eastern KY Univ; MS 81 Miami Univ - Oxford; Sp-Lang Path, Hamilton Co Office of Educ, **SLP**

Songster, Mrs Pamela J 5700 Mainsgate #2201, Wichita, KS 67220, (316) 682-2185, MS 87 Wichita St Univ

Songy, Cherie T Box 8, Oscar, LA 70762, (504) 627-5232, BS 80 LA St Univ - Baton Rouge; MA 81 LA St Univ - Baton Rouge; **SLP**

Sonies, Dr Barbara C 8826 Tuckerman Lane, Potomac, MD 20854, (301) 496-4733, BS 61 Univ of MN - Minneap-St Paul; MA 63 Stanford Univ; PH 81 (Hrng & Sp Sciences) Univ of MD - College Park; Sp-Lang Path, NIH, **SLP ACE**

Sonnenberg, Esther A P O Box 465, Carnelian Bay, CA 95711, (916) 546-2884, MS 87 Univ of NV - Reno; **SLP**

Sonnenberg, Joseph P 6479 Old Lakeshore Road, Derby, NY 14047, (716) 835-6009, BS 73 SUNY - Coll at Buffalo; MS 74 SUNY - Coll at Buffalo; Supvr/Sp-Lang Path, Buffalo Hrng & Sp Cen, **SLP**

Sonnenmeier, Rae M 64 Anderson Place, Buffalo, NY 14222, (716) 878-5306, BS 80 SUNY - Coll at Buffalo; MA 84 SUNY - Center at Buffalo; 87–Sp-Lang Path, SUNY Coll at Buffalo, **SLP**

Sonnenschein, Mrs Tamar G 169 Bonad Road, Chestnut Hill, MA 02167, (617) 344-2320, MS 77 Emerson Coll; Sp-Lang Path, Charmss Collaborative, **SLP**

Sonnichsen, Mrs Lucille B 108 Victory Lane, Bel Air, MD 21014, (301) 838-5563, BS 66 SUNY - Coll at Geneseo; MA 69 Columbia Univ Teachers Coll; Sp-Lang Path, **SLP**

Sonnier, Eileen R 7242 Seven Oaks Avenue, Baton Rouge, LA 70806, (504) 923-1233, BA 69 LA St Univ - Baton Rouge; MA 71 LA St Univ - Baton Rouge; Vp, Adv Consul Gr, **SLP**

Sonntag-Vucich, Mrs Karin Marie 707 Reamer Avenue, Carnegie, PA 15106, (412) 279-7183, BS 83 Marywood Coll; MS 85 Lamar Univ; Sp-Lang Path, Pittsburgh Hearing Sp & Deaf Svcs, **SLP**

Sonti, Lakshmi V 890 North Myrtle Avenue, Pomona, CA 91768, (714) 623-2389, BA 69 Univ of CA - Berkeley; BS 70 Western OR St Coll; MA 75 CA St Univ - Los Angeles; Aud, Dr A D Palmer, **A**

SooHoo, Leo Audiology And Speech Sciences, Purdue University, West Lafayette, IN 47907, (317) 494-3805, BS 78 IL St Univ - Normal; MA 82 MI St Univ; 88–Aud, Purdue Univ, **A**

Soo Hoo, Marianne White Memorial Otolarygology, 414 North Boyle Avenue, Suite 1047, Los Angeles, CA 90033, (213) 268-3352, MA 75 CA St Univ - Los Angeles; 79–Aud, White Mem Otol Foundation, **A**

Sook, Mrs Cynthia L Ciha 3808 Delahaut Street, Green Bay, WI 54301, (414) 336-3234, **SLP**

Soper, Donna Marie 305 Lindenhurst, Apartment #2061, Lexington, KY 40509, (606) 263-3141, BS 78 Eastern KY Univ; MA 80 Eastern KY Univ; Sp-Lang Path, Fleming County Board of Educ, **SLP**

Soper, Mrs Ellen A 27 Tyson's Ford Road, Newark, DE 19711, (302) 999-0702, BS 85 ND St Univ; MS 87 Moorhead St Univ; 88–Sp-Lang Path, The Speech Clinic, **SLP**

Soper, Mrs Heather L 3917 Gatewood Drive, Amarillo, TX 79109, (806) 355-9644, BS 72 NM St Univ; MA 74 NM St Univ; Sp/Lang Path, Amarillo ISD, **SLP**

Soper-Cotter, Sally J N34 W22217 Memory Lane, Pewaukee, WI 53072, **SLP**

Sopko, Heidi G 29 Windchime Drive, Mansfield, MA 02048-2933, (617) 339-0923, BS 78 Nazareth Coll of Rochester; MS 79 Miami Univ - Oxford; SLP, Kennedy-Donovan Center, **SLP**

Sopko, Mary Helen 10051 Deer Run, Brecksville, OH 44141, (216) 526-8054, MA 84 Case Western Reserve Univ; Sp-Lang Path, Private Practice, **SLP**

Sopp, Nancy Ruth Dodds Yokota East, Psc Box 838, Apo, San Francisco, CA 96293, (714) 688-6928, MA 83 CA St Univ - Northridge; **SLP**

Soraci, Mrs Lynne L 325 Garfield, Fort Collins, CO 80524, (303) 484-8300, BS 75 CO St Univ; MA 78 Univ of CO - Boulder; Sp-Lang Path, Fort Collins Youth Clinic, **SLP**

Sorbo, Joann E P O Box 913, Ridgecrest, CA 93555, (619) 375-4966, BA 49 San Jose St Univ; MA 71 CA St Univ - Northridge; SLP, Sierra Sands U S D, **SLP**

Sorell, Jeannie M Rural Delivery 9, Fair Street, Carmel, NY 10512, (914) 225-8729, BA 78 CUNY - Queens Coll; MA 81 CUNY - Hunter Coll; Sp-Lang Path, Private Practice, **SLP**

Sorensen, Dr David N 2260 Butte, Pocatello, ID 83201, (208) 236-3495, BS 70 Univ of UT; MS 71 Univ of UT; PH 80 (Sp-Lang Path) Purdue Univ - West Lafayette; Assoc Prof, Idaho State University, **SLP**

Sorensen, Eugenia R 684 Benicia Drive #6, Santa Rosa, CA 95405-3059, (415) 321-9325, BA 27 Univ of CA - Berkeley; MA 53 Stanford Univ; **A LM**

Sorensen, Nancy E 3 N 173 Woodcreek Lane, West Chicago, IL 60185, (312) 627-9250, BA 61 Bowling Green St Univ; MA 76 Northern IL Univ - De Kalb; Sp/Lang Path, Glenbard Twp Dis 87, **SLP**

Sorensen, Pamela M 3045 So Willow Street, Denver, CO 80231, BS 72 West Chester Univ of PA; MA 76 Univ of CO - Denver; Sp-Lang Path, Spalding Rehab Hosp, **SLP**

Sorenson, Brenda Ranee 1261 Honey Run Road, Chico, CA 95928, (916) 534-0423, BA 80 CA St Univ - Chico; MA 82 CA St Univ - Chico; Sp-Lang Path, Devereux Fndtn, **SLP**

Sorenson, Mrs Danita D 1755 9th Avenue, San Francisco, CA 94122, (415) 476-7246, BA 59 San Jose St Univ; MA 65 San Francisco St Univ; SLP, Ucsf Langley Porter I, **SLP**

Sorenson, Diane Lorene 1375 Country Lane Drive, Conyers, GA 30207, (404) 922-3931, BS 85 Univ of GA; ME 86 Univ of GA; **SLP**

Sorenson, Dr Fay D 134 Mokelumne River Drive, Lodi, CA 95240-7614, (916) 454-8387, BA 58 Our Lady Lake Univ-San Anton; MS 62 Baylor Univ; PH 69 (NS) Stanford Univ; Aud, Sacramento Cnty USD, **A**

Sorenson, Thomas A 675 Green Meadow Court, Northfield, MN 55057, (507) 663-0670, MA 73 ND St Univ; Sp-Lang Path, Northfield Public Schools, **SLP**

Sorge, Mrs Carol Nolan 267 Kingbird Court, Three Bridges, NJ 08887, (201) 788-8814, BS 84 Marywood Coll; MA 85 Montclair St Coll; **SLP**

Soria, Mrs Jeanne Marie 2824 58th Street, Lubbock, TX 79413, (806) 792-6301, BS 84 TX Tech Univ; MS 85 TX Tech Univ; Aud, Dr William Ullom, **A**

Soriano, Deborah Ann 392 State Street #8-H, North Haven, CT 06473, (203) 234-0303, BS 83 PA St Univ - Univ Park; MS 85 Southern CT St Univ; 88–Sp-Lang Path, ACES, **SLP**

Soriano, Mrs Lynn Friedlande 47 Oakrest Lane, North Babylon, NY 11703, (516) 543-5100, BS 86 Univ of MA - Amherst; MA 87 Hofstra Univ

Sorice, Mrs Diane Patricia 33-34 158th Street, Flushing, NY 11358, (212) 463-1850, BA 75 CUNY - Queens Coll; MS 76 Adelphi Univ; Sp-Lang Path, Private Practice, **SLP**

Sorice-Clark, Mary Jo 4416 Jacqueline Lane, Raleigh, NC 27604, (919) 878-0100, BS 75 Carlow Coll; MA 77 Kent St Univ; Sp-Lang Path, InSpeech Inc, **SLP**

Sorin, Riva Ann 145 Marlee Avenue, Apartment 1113, Toronto, ON, Canada M6B 3H3, (416) 549-6525, BS 83 McGill Univ - Quebec; OM 85 Univ of Toronto - Ontario; 88–Sp-Lang Path, Centenary Hosp, **SLP ACE**

Sorkowitz, Melvin J Royal Palm Hearing Aid Center, 209-B S E 1st Avenue, Boca Raton, FL 33432, (305) 395-4242, **A**

Soroky, Dr Doris L 6249 Randi Avenue, Woodland Hills, CA 91367, (818) 887-9266, BA 67 CA St Univ - Northridge; MA 70 CA St Univ - Northridge; ED 79 (NS) Univ of Northern CO; Coord Spec Ed, LA City Sch, **SLP**

Sorrell, Mrs Angela Fisher 4027 Heath Moor Court, Duluth, GA 30136, (404) 953-2223, BS 81 Univ of TN - Knoxville; MA 82 Univ of TN - Knoxville; 88–Sp-Lang Path, Aud Consult of Atlanta Inc, **SLP**

Sorrels, Lynne Walker 4709 West Brae Court, Fuquay-Varina, NC 27526, (919) 832-8301, BA 79 Univ of NC - Greensboro; MS 81 Univ of NC - Chapel Hill; SLP, Rehab Serv Wake Co, **SLP**

Sorrentino, Gayle E 196 Woods Avenue, Malverne, NY 11565, (718) 470-8910, BA 66 Ithaca Coll; MS 67 Ithaca Coll; Sp-Lang Path, Lng Is Jewish Hillside Med Cen, **SLP**

Sorrentino, Mrs Marie R 119 Idlewood Road, Rochester, NY 14618, BS 72 SUNY - Coll at Geneseo; MS 77 Nazareth Coll of Rochester; Sp-Lang Path, City Sch Dist of Rochester, **SLP**

Sorsby, Mrs Patricia Glass 3333 Knob Oak Drive, Grapevine, TX 76051, (817) 267-7545, BA 75 Univ of Akron; MA 83 Kent St Univ; SLP, Dallas ISD, **SLP**

Sorth, Mrs Mary Emma Rt 2 Box 2113, Blairsville, GA 30512, BS 53 PA St Univ - Univ Park; ME 57 PA St Univ - Univ Park; MA 70 Columbia Univ Teachers Coll; Retired, **SLP**

Sortini, Dr Adam J 1260 D Street, Merced, CA 95340, BS 49 Boston Univ; MA 51 Univ of IL - Urbana; ED 55 (NS) Boston Univ; Dir, Valley Hrng & Sp Cen, **SLP A**

Sortor, Kathryn E 550 North 1st Avenue, Upland, CA 91786, (714) 593-7521, BA 77 Stanford Univ; MA 80 Stanford Univ; MA 82 Northwestern Univ; Sp/Lang Path, Casa Colina Hospital, **SLP**

Soso, Verafran P O Box 50545, Washington, DC 20004-0442, Clinical Supervisor, University of Dist of Columbia, **SLP**

Sostarich, Mary Elizabeth 521 Barnett, Kansas City, KS 66101, (816) 765-7772, BS 79 Univ of NE - Lincoln; MS 81 Univ of WA; 87–Aud, Timbre Hearing & Sp Ctr, **A**

Sotelo, Mrs Judith Connolly 4228 East Indianola, Phoenix, AZ 85018, (602) 468-0458, BS 80 Miami Univ - Oxford; MS 81 Miami Univ - Oxford; Sp-Lang Path, AZ Inst Comm Cog Disorders, **SLP**

Sotelo, Kathy M 100 Overhill Road, Middletown, NY 10940, (914) 343-2233, BA 85 SUNY - Coll at New Paltz; MS 86 SUNY - Coll at New Paltz; 87–Sp-Lang Path, Middletown PS Sys, **SLP**

Sotile, Kathryn Marie 8 Ferry Road N E, Fort Walton Beach, FL 32548, (904) 243-3902, BS 81 Univ Southern MS-Hattiesburg; MS 83 Univ Southern MS-Hattiesburg; 86–Sp-Lang Path, Silver Sands Sch, **SLP**

Sotiropoulos, Peter D 4200 Roosevelt Street, Hollywood, FL 33021-4215, (305) 963-4819, BS 84 Vanderbilt Univ; MS 86 Northeastern Univ; 87–Reg Clin Dir, Family Hearing Centers, **A ACE**

Soto, Mrs Betty A 654 St Ann's Avenue, Brown, NY 10455, (212) 665-9808, MA 88 CUNY - City College; 88–Sp-Lang Path, Educational Speech Pathologists

Soucaze, Carole E 2021 Castleman Drive, Nashville, TN 37215, (615) 269-6640, BA 75 Rutger's St Univ - Douglas Coll; MS 76 Vanderbilt Univ; Exec Dir, High Hopes Inc, **SLP**

Souders, Kimberly Jenine 345 Sunset, Plymouth, MI 48170, (313) 455-9224, BA 84 MI St Univ; MA 86 Central MI Univ; **SLP**

Soukup, Connie Marie 1900 Solera Drive, Columbus, OH 43229, (614) 263-5151, BS 85 Kent St Univ; MA 85 Kent St Univ; 86–Sp-Lang Path, Colum Sp & Hrng Ctr, **SLP**

Soukup, Mrs Lisa Stipe Cerebral Palsy Inc, 2801 South Webster Avenue, Green Bay, WI 54301, (414) 337-1122, BA 80 Saint Norbert Coll; MS 85 Univ of WI - Oshkosh; 86–Sp-Lang Path, Cerebral Palsy Inc, **SLP**

Soukup, Mrs Nina R 5367 North 83rd, Milwaukee, WI 53218, (414) 461-7344, BA 75 Univ of WI - Eau Claire; MS 79 Marquette Univ; Sp-Lang Path, Therapy Associates, **SLP**

Sousa, Veronica M 3119 Kilo Avenue, San Jose, CA 95124, **SLP**

South, Laura L 5602 Bentbough Lane, Houston, TX 77088, (713) 792-4500, MA 76 Marshall Univ; 87–Sp-Lang Path, Sp & Hearing Inst UTHSC-H, **SLP**

Southall, Julia M 1303 West Cornwallis, Greensboro, NC 27408, (919) 378-1859, BA 63 Mary Washington Coll; ME 64 Univ of VA - Charlottesville; **SLP**

Southard, Mrs Laurie Jones 8214 Chancery Court, Alexandria, VA 22308, (703) 780-6983, BS 82 Univ of GA; ME 83 Univ of GA; Sp-Lang Path, **SLP**

Southard, Susan D 567 Seventh Street West, Sonoma, CA 95476, (707) 996-8445, BA 75 Univ of Redlands; MS 77 Univ of Redlands; SLP, Sonoma Valley USD, **SLP**

Southard, William Michael 567 Seventh Street West, Sonoma, CA 95476, (707) 433-0700, **A**

Souther, Mrs Nancy S 5010 Wagon Trail Drive, Littleton, CO 80123, BA 76 Univ of CO - Boulder; MA 77 Univ of Denver; SLP, Arapahoe Co Sch Dist 6, **SLP**

Southerland, Donna Jan 419 Woodland Avenue, Lexington, KY 40508, (606) 744-6922, **SLP**

Southerland, Mrs Patricia Elizabeth 4850 Medlock Bridge Road, Duluth, GA 30136, (404) 449-5089, BA 77 Univ of GA; ME 78 GA St Univ; Sp-Lang Path, Private Practice, **SLP**

Southern, Toni Jane 2467 Buckingham Drive, Windsor, ON, Canada N8T 2B4, (519) 945-3448, BA 79 Univ of Windsor - Ontario; OM 82 Univ of Western Ontario; 84–Sp-Lang Path, Windsor Western Hospital Ctr, **SLP**

Southwick, Renee E 203 Fairway Village, Leeds, MA 01053, (413) 586-5136, BS 76 Edinboro Univ of PA; MS 79 Vanderbilt Univ; Dir of Dev, AMS-Rehab Inc, **SLP**

Southwood, Mrs Jane W R R 9 Box 109-A, Warsaw, IN 46580-9257, (219) 269-3616, BS 73 Purdue Univ - West Lafayette; MS 75 Purdue Univ - West Lafayette; Sp-Lang Path, Private Practice, **SLP**

Sova, Mrs Carol Frances 200 North 13th Street, Suite 303, Reading, PA 19604, (215) 378-2031, BS 86 Bloomsburg Univ of PA; MS 87 Bloomsburg Univ of PA; 88–Aud, Saint Joseph Hosp, **A**

Sowar, Mrs Deborah Fessenden P O Box 184, Franklin, WV 26807, (304) 358-7937, BS 74 SUNY - Coll at Fredonia; MS 76 WV Univ; Sp-Lang Path, Speech and Language Service, **SLP**

Sowards, Mrs Ellen L R R 1 Box 225, Alum Creek, WV 25003, BA 77 Marshall Univ; MA 78 Marshall Univ; Sp-Lang Path, Lincoln Co Bd of Ed, **SLP**

Sowder, Sharon C 2417 South Porter, Joplin, MO 64804, (417) 624-0364, BA 85 Univ of Northern CO; MA 87 Univ of Northern CO; 87–Sp-Lang Path, St John's Regional Med Ctr, **SLP**

Sowell, Mrs Barbara Fitzpatrck 12 Sugar Creek Road, North Little Rock, AR 72116, BS 76 Univ of VA - Charlottesville; MS 78 WV Univ; Dir of Comprehensive/Neurological Prog, HealthSouth Rehab Ctr, **SLP**

Sowell, Mrs Janis Belkin 859 Natalie Drive, Windsor, CA 95492, (707) 838-2630, MA 87 CA St Univ - Chico; 87–Sp-Lang Path, Redwood Inst for Designed Educ, **SLP**

Sowell, Kathy Brakefield 5424 Mona Lane, Dallas, TX 75236, (214) 780-0619, BA 84 Northeast LA Univ; MS 86 Univ of TX - Dallas; SLP, Arlington ISD, **SLP**

Sowell, Michele McCord 12702 Shady Acres, Buda, TX 78610, (512) 295-4986, BS 82 Southwest TX St Univ; ME 84 Southwest TX St Univ; Sp-Lang Path, Austin ISD, **SLP**

Sowell, Thomas William 12 Sugar Creek Road, North Little Rock, AR 72116, BS 72 Univ of NE - Omaha; MS 74 Univ of NE - Omaha; Sp-Lang Path, VA Med Ctr, **SLP**

Sowinski, Christine 36141 Hardenburg, Farmington Hills, MI 48018, (313) 474-8570, BA 75 MI St Univ; MA 76 Wayne St Univ; 86–Director/Audiology & SLP, Oakwood Hospital, **SLP**

Sowinski, Mary B 2355 South 76th Street #3, West Allis, WI 53219, **SLP**

Sowle, Elizabeth Margaret 171 Highland Avenue #305, Taunton, MA 02780, (617) 824-5881, BS 82 Central MI Univ; MA 86 Central MI Univ; 85–Sp-Lang Path, Paul A Dever St Sch, **SLP**

Sowle, Karolyn Kay 1419 Walnut Hall, Memphis, TN 38119, (901) 523-8990, BS 84 AR St Univ; MA 86 Memphis St Univ; **A**

Soyez, Mrs Debbie D 4209 Shateau Boulevard, Apartment O, Kenner, LA 70065, (504) 466-2232, BA 73 LA St Univ - Baton Rouge; MA 75 LA St Univ - Baton Rouge; Sp/Lang Path, Jefferson Parish Schs, **SLP**

Spacagna, Robert A 6600 Bruceville Road, Sacramento, CA 95823-4691, (916) 686-2242, BA 75 CA St Univ - Sacramento; MA 77 CA St Univ - Sacramento; Aud, Kaiser Permanente, **A**

Spack, Cathy M #404-2945 Pembina Highway, Winnipeg, MB, Canada R3T 3R1, BA 75 Univ of Manitoba - Winnipeg; MA 77 Univ of ND; Sp/Lang Path, Child Guidance Clinic, **SLP**

Spadafore, Mary Jo 8649 East Royal Palm Road, Apartment 232, Scottsdale, AZ 85258, (602) 991-0157, OM 84 AZ St Univ; 84–Sp-Lang Path, Tempe Elementary Schools #3, **SLP**

Spadoni, Kimberly Anne 224 Seymour Road, Rochester, NY 14609, (716) 288-4576, BS 81 Nazareth Coll of Rochester; MS 84 Nazareth Coll of Rochester; Sp-Lang Path, Monroe BOCES 1, **SLP**

Spahr, Frederick T 6 Elmwood Court, Rockville, MD 20850, (301) 897-5700, BA 61 IN Univ - Bloomington; ME 63 Boston Univ; PH 68 (Sp Path) Univ of Southern CA; 80–Exec Dir, ASHA, **SLP F**

Spak, Constance Univ Of Michigan Hospital, Tc-1904, 1500 East Medical Center, Ann Arbor, MI 48109-0312, (313) 936-8013, BA 77 MI St Univ; MA 78 Central MI Univ; Asst Dir Aud, U of MI Hosp, **A**

Spalding, Mrs Catherine Lucas 1882 Princeton Drive #4, Louisville, KY 40205, (502) 454-5738, BS 84 Univ of AR - Fayetteville; MA 86 Memphis St Univ; **SLP**

Spalding, Jody L P 3022 Lexington, Ann Arbor, MI 48105-1481, (313) 662-5410, BS 75 Univ of IA; MA 78 Univ of IA; Aud, Mc Auley Aud Svcs, **SLP A**

Spalding, Kathleen J 527 Crowley, Arlington, TX 76012, (817) 795-6331, BS 79 Baylor Univ; MS 80 Baylor Univ; Aud, Mem Hosp, **SLP A**

Spalter, Mrs Joanne Belofsky 19514 Shinwood Drive, Humble, TX 77346, (713) 852-1462, BS 82 Boston Univ; MA 84 George Washington Univ; 85–Sp-Lang Path, HealthSouth Rehab Hosp, **SLP**

Spandet, Diane C 7854 Nan Drive, Roscoe, IL 61073, (815) 968-6861, BS 74; MS 76; 84–Sp-Lang Path, Rockford Memorial Hosp, **SLP**

Spaner, Vicki Joanne 8664 Cashio Street, Los Angeles, CA 90035, (213) 275-6378, BS 82 West Chester Univ of PA; MA 85 CA St Univ - Northridge; **SLP**

Spang, Peter J 1619 Wildwood Road, Toledo, OH 43614, (419) 385-4734, BS 54 Bowling Green St Univ; MA 67 Bowling Green St Univ; Retired, Maumee Board of Education, **SLP**

Spangenberg, Sheryl L 206½ Brookside Drive, Jacksonville, IL 62650, (217) 243-7329, BS 85 IL St Univ - Normal; MS 86 IL St Univ - Normal; 86–Sp-Lang Path, IL Sch for the Visually Impr, **SLP**

Spangler, Carol S 47 Hudson Avenue, Athens, OH 45701, (614) 662-4311, BA 75 Marshall Univ; MA 76 Marshall Univ; Sp-Lang Path/Title V1-B Coord, Fed Hocking Local Schl Dist, **SLP**

Spangler, Laurie Gail 116 Virginia Park Blvd, Fort Pierce, FL 33947, (305) 461-7370, BS 83 Eastern MI Univ; MS 85 Eastern MI Univ; Sp-Lang Path, St Lucy County Schools, **SLP**

Spangler, Nancy Rebecca 2-F Holly Court, Harrisonburg, VA 22801, (717) 367-3013, BS 80 Bloomsburg Univ of PA; MS 83 James Madison Univ; Sp/Lang Path, Woodrow Wilson Rehab Center, **SLP**

Spanier, Cynthia Ann Allegheny Neuro-Psy Inst, Speech Pathology Depart, 7777 Steubenville Pike, Oakdale, PA 15071, (412) 747-2006, BS 81 Marquette Univ; MS 82 Marquette Univ; Dir Sp /L Dept, Alleghany Neuropsy Imst, **SLP**

Spanier, Paul M 605 East 82nd Street, New York, NY 10028, **SLP**

Spankowski, Mrs Geralyn C 3745 South 56th Street, Greenfield, WI 53220, BS 77 Marquette Univ; MS 78 Marquette Univ; Sp Lang Cl, Greenfield Sch Dist, **SLP**

Spann, E Daniel 6108 Beaver Ridge Road, Knoxville, TN 37931, (615) 482-1086, BA 62 David Lipscomb Coll; MA 74 Univ of TN - Knoxville; Aud, Hear Servico Inc, **A**

Spann, Melanie H 5 Wactor Street, Sumter, SC 29150, (803) 775-1171, BA 80 Columbia Coll; MS 81 Univ of AL-Tuscaloosa; Sp-Lang Path, Toumey Hosp, **SLP**

Spanos, Mrs Katina 2299 Saddle Drive, Allison Park, PA 15101, (412) 741-6632, BS 71 OH St Univ; MA 72 Kent St Univ; SLP, Alegany Interm Unit, **SLP**

Sparker, Ann W 1821 Wroxton Road, Houston, TX 77005, (713) 797-4213, BA 76 Rice Univ; MS 80 Univ of KY; 80–Sp-Lang Path, U of TX Sp & Hrng Inst, **SLP**

Sparkman, Coleen Kelley 1518 Coffee Road, Suite C, Modesto, CA 95355, (209) 572-2505, BA 77 CA St Univ - Fresno; MA 79 CA St Univ - Fresno; Owner, Strand-Kelley Speech Path Inc, **SLP ACE**

Sparkman, James L 1285 Heights Avenue, Atwater, CA 95301, (209) 357-1222, BA 76 Univ of CA - Los Angeles; MA 80 CA St Univ - Stanislaus; Co-Director, Speech-Lang-Hearing Clinic, **SLP**

Sparkman, Linda L The Vistas, 4242 Medical Drive, Suite 1125, San Antonio, TX 78229, (512) 692-3434, BS 71 Southwest TX St Univ; ME 72 Southwest TX St Univ; Owner, Self Employed, **SLP**

Sparks, Diane Seydell 2067 Central Road, Everson, WA 98247, (604) 826-4736, MS 81 Western WA Univ; 76–Sp-Lang Path, School District #75, **SLP**

Sparks, Mrs Joni F 738 Best Way, San Antonio, TX 78260, (512) 532-8811, BA 80 TX Tech Univ; MS 82 TX Tech Univ; SLP, San Antonio ISD, **SLP**

Sparks, Joseph D 1031 N W 6th Street #D-2, Gainesville, FL 32601, (904) 375-1559, BA 76 Univ of FL; MA 78 Univ of FL; Aud, Private Practice, **A**

Sparks, Mrs Laurie Newell 1721 Wellman Court, St Louis, MO 63146, (314) 878-1682, BA 79 Univ of Rochester; MA 81 Northwestern Univ; **A**

Sparks, Mrs Sheldia Bishop 1412 Mount Rainier, Lexington, KY 40502, (606) 259-1411, BA 74 Univ of KY; MA 82 Univ of KY; **SLP**

Sparks, Mrs Shirley N 144 Waupakisco Beach, Battle Creek, MI 49015, (616) 387-8061, BS 55 Univ of IA; MS 71 Tulane Univ; Associate Prof, Western Michigan U, **SLP**

Sparnon, John R 6921 East Port Bay Road, Wolcott, NY 14590, BS 60 SUNY - Coll at Geneseo; MS 64 Syracuse Univ; Northrose-Wolcott Sch Dist, **SLP**

Sparr, Mrs Sandra B 5 Label Avenue, Portland, ME 04103, (207) 878-2576, BA 77 SUNY - Coll at Plattsburgh; MS 79 Emerson Coll; Sp-Lang Path, Cerebral Palsy Cen, **SLP**

Spatafore, Julie Lizanne 345 Sheridan Avenue, Apartment 415, Palo Alto, CA 94306, (415) 321-7424, BA 83 Univ of CA - San Diego; MA 86 Humboldt St Univ; **SLP**

Spates, Eleanor F 2780 Xerxes Avenue South, Minneapolis, MN 55416, BS; **LM**

Spath, Kathy B R R 1 Box 149, Petersburg, IL 62675, BS 78 Marquette Univ; MS 77 Marquette Univ; Sp/Lang Path, Springfield Sch Dist, **SLP**

Spatola, Glenn J 7028 17th Avenue N W, Seattle, WA 98117, (206) 277-3374, BA 68 Univ of MA - Amherst; ME 77 Northeastern Univ; Aud, Boeing Co, **A**

Spaulding, Mrs Kay H 2617 Delane, Waterloo, IA 50701, (319) 268-0487, BA 64 Univ of Northern IA; MA 83 Univ of Northern IA; Sp-Lang Path, AEA, **SLP**

Spaulding, Laura C 1283 West Parklane Blvd, Apartment 216, Chandler, AZ 85224, (602) 899-3223, BA 79 Saint Xavier Coll; MS 81 Southern IL Univ -Carbondale; **SLP**

Spaulding, Mary E 89 Ball Road #7, Syracuse, NY 13215, (315) 474-1561, BS 59 Nazareth Coll of Rochester; MA 63 Syracuse Univ; PH 79 (Sp-Lang Path) Syracuse Univ; 84–Dir-SLP Dept, James Square Hlth & Rehab Ctr, **SLP**

Spaulding, Mrs Rose Pesce 9 B Frye Drive, Cumberland, ME 04021, (207) 874-1065, BS 83 Northeastern Univ; MS 85 Northeastern Univ; 87–Aud, Northeast Hearing & Sp Ctr, **A**

Speake, Mrs Jennifer Araj 9191 136th Way North, Seminole, FL 34646, (813) 546-9897, BA 82 Univ of FL; MS 84 Univ of South FL; Sp-Lang Path, Pinellas County School Board, **SLP**

Speaker, Virginia K 402 Howard Road, West Chester, PA 19380, BS 47 Lock Haven St Coll; MA 68 Univ of CO - Boulder

Speakman, Dianne Melody 2-10 Liden Avenue, Apartment B-102, Haddonfield, NJ 08033, (201) 337-3866, BS 72 Fairleigh Dickinson U-Teanec; MA 75 Fairleigh Dickinson U-Teanec; MS 83 William Paterson Coll; SLP, Private Practice, **SLP**

Speaks, Dr Charles E 10440 North 114th Street, Stillwater, MN 55082, (612) 624-3322, BS 57 OH Univ - Athens; MA 58 OH Univ - Athens; PH 63 (Sp Path & Aud) Univ of MI - Ann Arbor; Prof and Chair, U of Minn, **F**

Speaks, Mrs Nancy Jo J 16 East Mable Street, Harrisburg, IL 62946, (618) 937-1412, BS 73 IL St Univ - Normal; MS 75 Southern IL Univ -Carbondale; Sp-Lang Path, Pub Sch Dist 168, **SLP**

Spear, Barbara H 860 Bear Creek, Costa Mesa, CA 92626, (714) 641-7575, BA 49 Univ of ME - Orono; MA 56 Northwestern Univ; Retired, Private Practice, **SLP LM**

Spear, Douglas James Holiday Apartment, Apartment 35, Harlan, KY 40831, (606) 573-6244, MA 87 Central MI Univ; 88–Aud, Daniel Boone Clinic, **A**

Spear, Rebecca Felton 333 Crossman Street, Jamestown, NY 14701, (716) 487-0497, OB 69 Univ of Cincinnati; OM 71 Univ of Cincinnati; MS 86 SUNY - Coll at Fredonia; 86–Sp-Lang Path, WCA Hosp, **SLP**

Spear, Susan Therese 4226 Eubank N E #2, Albuquerque, NM 87111, (505) 292-4087, BS 74 Worcester St Coll; MS 80 Univ of Albuquerque; Sp-Lang Path, Albuquerque Public Schools, **SLP**

Spears, Mrs Amy Beth 22 Fourth Street, 2nd Floor, Brooklyn, NY 11231, (718) 852-3220, BS 80 Murray St Univ; MS 83 Murray St Univ; **SLP**

Spears, Mrs Ann I 1825 River Street, Readville, MA 02136, (617) 254-3800, BS 84 Boston Univ; MS 86 Boston Univ; 87–Sp-Lang Path, Kennedy Mem Hosp for Chldn, **SLP**

Spears, Mrs Dale Anne 12707 Russell Avenue, Chino, CA 91710, (818) 287-5223, BA 72 CA St Univ - Sacramento; MA 74 CA St Univ - Sacramento; 85–Aud, Los Angeles Co Office of Ed, **SLP A**

Spears, Mrs Iris E 7002 East Calle Canis, Tucson, AZ 85710, (602) 745-5637, BA 80 Univ of TN - Knoxville; MA 81 Univ of Northern CO; Aud, **A**

Spears, Judy L 1109 Cherrytree Court, Woodstock, GA 30188, (404) 252-6241, **A**

Spears, Mark Thompson 844 Lake Terrace Drive, Dallas, TX 75218-2147, **A**

Spears, Mrs Mary Ann 105 West M Street, Jenks, OK 74037, (918) 299-4411, MA 83 Univ of Tulsa; Sp-Lang Path, Jenks Pub Sch, **SLP**

Spease, Wendy Kay Sugartown Mews, Bldg R640, 261 Poplar Avenue, Devon, PA 19333, (401) 421-4677, MS 86 Bloomsburg Univ of PA; 88–Aud, Valley Forge Facial Plastic Surgery Ear Nose & Throat Assoc Ltd, **A**

Specht, Mrs Sally R 8731 Niwot Road, Longmont, CO 80501, (303) 776-8674, BS 65 CO St Univ; MA 75 Univ of Northern CO; Aud, St Vrain Valley Pub Sch, **A**

Specterman, Paul 4240 Park Newport #304, Newport Beach, CA 92660, (714) 759-1491, BA NY Univ; MA NY Univ; Sp-Lang Path, Private Practice, **SLP**

Spector, Dr Cecile C 6 Green Hill Lane, Spring Valley, NY 10977, (914) 354-4418, BA 58 CUNY - Brooklyn Coll; MA 60 CUNY - Brooklyn Coll; PH 77 (Sp Path) NY Univ; Sp/Lang Path, N Rockland Sch Dist, **SLP**

Spector, Mrs Diane J c/o MCCA Inc, PO Box 2870, Estes Park, CO 80517, (813) 474-8528, BA 65 Fontbonne Coll; MA 67 Wichita St Univ; Sp-Lang Path, Private Practice, **SLP**

Spector, Mrs Judith K 4238 St Vincents Drive, Baltimore, MD 21215, (301) 484-8939, MS 88; 88–Sp-Lang Path, Baltimore City Schs, **SLP**

Spector, Lizabeth 8124 Roxburgh Apartment 1-E, Clayton, MO 63105, (314) 652-3200, MA 88 San Diego St Univ; 88–Sp-Lang Path, Central Inst for the Deaf

Spector, Mrs Sima 5709 River Oak Way, Carmichael, CA 95608, (916) 483-3725, BA 66 CUNY - Queens Coll; MA 72 CA St Univ - Sacramento; Sp-Lang Path, N Sacramento Sch Dist, **SLP**

Spector, Mrs Susan Naimark 19 Merryhill Lane, Pittsford, NY 14534, (716) 586-1377, BA 71 McGill Univ - Quebec; MS 73 McGill Univ - Quebec; **SLP**

Spector, Toby Rose 8124 SW 81st Place, Miami, FL 33143-6613, BA 77 CUNY - Hunter Coll; MA 80 CUNY - Hunter Coll; **A**

Specyal, Laura A 388 French Street, Bangor, ME 04401, (207) 947-7389, **SLP**

Speechly, Marla D 1128 West Fountain Way, Fresno, CA 93705, (209) 255-8318, BA 76 CA St Univ - Fresno; MA 78 CA St Univ - Fresno; Sp-Lang Path, Fresno USD, **SLP**

Speed, Marilynn E 22093 Stocklmeir Court, Cupertino, CA 95014, (408) 998-6099, BS 67 Western MI Univ; MA 79 San Jose St Univ; Prog Spec, San Jose USD, **SLP**

Speed, Peggy H 2807 Jefferson Drive, Hattiesburg, MS 39401, (601) 583-0960, BS 69 Univ Southern MS-Hattiesburg; MA 81 Univ Southern MS-Hattiesburg; Sp-Lang Path, Hattiesburg Pub Sch Syst, **SLP**

Speed, Mrs Tanya Jo Lennard 11236 Quail Run Road, Dallas, TX 75238, (214) 494-8379, BS 82 Southern Methodist Univ; MS 84 Univ of North TX; Sp/Lang Path, Garland ISD, **SLP**

Speeks, Emelda L 4869 Linden Street, Baton Rouge, LA 70805, (504) 929-5282, BS 74 Southern Univ - Baton Rouge; MA 75 Western MI Univ; Aud, E Baton Rouge Parish Sch, **SLP A**

Speer, Mrs Jessica Christine 7330 Marianne Avenue, Indianapolis, IN 46219, (317) 646-8411, BS 83 Ball St Univ; MA 85 Ball St Univ; 87–Aud, St John's Health Care Corp, **A**

Speer, Mrs Rebecca Baker 5215 Lichfield Road, Columbus, GA 31904, (404) 322-4148, BA 75 Univ of AL-Tuscaloosa; MA 86 Columbus Coll; 87–Sp-Lang Path, Muscogee Counth Sch Dist

Speerschneider, Jane Marie 1111 Post Oak Boulevard, Apartment 736, Houston, TX 77056, (713) 688-3431, BS 82 Univ of WI - Madison; MS 84 Univ of WI - Madison; Audiologist, NW Otolaryngology Assoc, **A**

Spees, Edgar Brian 1810 Peach Street, Wisconsin Rapids, WI 54494, (715) 886-3771, BS 78 Univ of WI - Eau Claire; MS 80 Univ of WI - Stevens Point; Sp-Lang Path, Nekoosa School District, **SLP**

Speier, Nancy E 201 Lake Road, Greenville, NC 27834, (919) 756-0685, BS 72 SUNY - Coll at Geneseo; MA 73 Bowling Green St Univ; Sp-Lang Path, Pitt Co Schs, **SLP ACE**

Speirs, Dr James A 665 Winslow Street, Long Beach, CA 90814, (213) 494-6498, BA 58 CA St Univ - Los Angeles; MA 64 Univ of Southern CA; PH 72 (NS) Univ of Southern CA; Sp-Lang Path, N Puget Sound Hrng & Sp Cen, **SLP**

Speirs, Jan Carol 249 South Gilpin, Denver, CO 80209, (303) 534-5968, MA 84 Univ of Northern CO; Sp-Lang Path, Craig Rehabilitation Hospital, **SLP**

Speirs, Louise Hope Box 1775, 664 Old Strawberry Hill Rd, Hyannis, MA 02601, (617) 771-0612, BS 73 Gettysburg Coll; MS 78 PA St Univ - Univ Park; Program Case Manager, New Medico Head Injury Center, **SLP**

Spellman, Mrs Sharon Wilson 2909 Parapet Ct, Chesapeake, VA 23323, (919) 335-3475, BS 80 Norfolk St Univ; MS 86 Univ of the DC; **SLP**

Spells-Greene, Mrs Ina Ruth 4327 Lacy Cove, Newport News, VA 23602, (804) 253-5403, BS 83 James Madison Univ; MS 84 James Madison Univ; Sp-Lang Path, Eastern State Hosp, **SLP**

Spells-Thompson, Mrs Vanessa R 949 East Golf Road, Apt 5, Arlington Height, IL 60005, (312) 439-7352, BA 77 Univ of TN - Knoxville; MA 79 Univ of TN - Knoxville; Human Resources Rep, InSpeech Inc, **SLP**

Spelman, Mrs Sylvia L K 2916 Date Street #12-A, Honolulu, HI 96816, (808) 547-6511, BS 81 Univ of HI - Manoa; MS 83 Univ of HI - Manoa; Sp/Lang Path, St Francis Home Health Care, **SLP**

Spence, Donna Joan 6009 Fountain Pointe #2, Grand Blanc, MI 48439, (313) 694-9322, BS 86 Central MI Univ; MA 87 MI St Univ

Spence, Elizabeth Ann Ft Hill Ctr For Commun Dis, Mid Maine Medical Ctr, Waterville, ME 04901, (207) 872-4383, MS 80 Purdue Univ - West Lafayette; SLP, Mid Maine Medical Ctr, **SLP**

Spence, Judith Ann 25 West Plumstead Avenue, Apartment 3, Lansdowne, PA 19050, (215) 871-2727, BA 72; MS 78; MA 84 George Washington Univ; Aud, Osteopathic Med Coll of PA, **SLP A**

Spence, Mrs Lee Ann M 26 Uncas Avenue, Quaker Hill, CT 06375, (203) 443-7758, BS 78 Marquette Univ; MS 79 Univ of WI - Stevens Point; Sp/Lang Path, Cty of New London Dept of Hlth, **SLP**

Spence, Marcia Gillcrist 28781 Naylor Drive, Solon, OH 44139, (216) 231-5757, BS 77 Towson St Univ; MA 80 George Washington Univ; Sp/Lang Path, Beachwood Bd of Ed, **SLP**

Spence, Mrs Mary E 6973 Bridgetown Road, Cincinnati, OH 45248, (513) 574-5163, BS 68 Univ of Cincinnati; MA 69 Univ of Cincinnati; Sp-Lang Path, Private Practice, **SLP**

Spence, Dr Nancy Long 325 N W 18th Street, Delray Beach, FL 33444, (305) 737-7733, BA 60 Baylor Univ; MS 73 Southern Methodist Univ; PH 83 (NS) Case Western Reserve Univ; Rehabilitation Coordinator, Bethesda Memorial Hospital, **SLP**

Spence, Scott W 75 South Saint Clair St, Painesville, OH 44077, (216) 231-5757, BA 78 Wittenberg Univ; MA 82 Case Western Reserve Univ; Territorial Mng, Oticon Corp, **A**

Spence, Dr Susan Durham P O Box 1589, Princeton, WV 24740, (304) 425-5846, BA 59 Univ of GA; ME 62 Univ of VA - Charlottesville; PH 76 (Psychology) Heed Univ; 88–Sp-Lang Path, InSpeech Inc, **SLP ACE**

Spencer, Amy 801 Peter Christopher Dr, West Chester, PA 19382, BA 75 Univ of DE; MA 78 George Washington Univ; **SLP**

Spencer, Denise Bradshaw 20 Pearl Street, Everett, MA 02149, (617) 598-0013, BS 82 Boston Univ; MS 84 Emerson Coll; **SLP**

Spencer, Mrs Donna Kent P O Box 806, Hanson, MA 02341, (617) 647-6418, BS 76 Univ of MA - Amherst; MA 78 Univ of MA - Amherst; 86–Coord of Aud, Waltham Weston Hosp & Med Ctr, **A ACE**

Spencer, Jodene 3079 West 34th Avenue, Denver, CO 80211, (303) 789-1322, BA 83 Metropolitan St Coll; MA 87 Univ of CO - Boulder; 87–Mgr-Echo Hrng Ctr, Sur-Hagen Inc

Spencer, Jody L 1615 South College Avenue, Tulsa, OK 74104, (918) 742-6767, BS 75 OK St Univ; MA 76 OK St Univ; 88–Prog Mgr Rehab Svcs, St John med Ctr, **SLP ACE**

Spencer, Kathleen M 209 Asylum Road, Warwick, RI 02886, (401) 739-6664, MS 88 Univ of RI

Spencer, Kathleen Mary 5557 Donald Street, Stevensville, MI 49127, (616) 695-9631, BA 77 MI St Univ; MA 83 Western MI Univ; Sp-Lang Path, Buchanan Sch Syst, **SLP**

Spencer, Leigh C 87 Stoney Hill Village, Brookfield, CT 06805, (203) 868-7377, **SLP**

Spencer, Dr Linda E 103 East Read Street, Baltimore, MD 21202, (301) 234-0007, BS 67 Southern IL Univ -Carbondale; MA 69 Northwestern Univ; PH 75 (Sp-Lang Path) Univ of OK Medical Center; 86–Dir Sp-Lang Path, Resnick & Spencer Inc, **SLP**

Spencer, Loretta B Summer Street, Portland, CT 06480, (203) 342-1896, MS 84 Central MO St Univ; SLP, Rockey Hill Public Schools, **SLP**

Spencer, Marilyn G 1108 McFarland, Stillwater, OK 74074, (405) 372-4606, BS 77 Brigham Young Univ; MS 78 Brigham Young Univ; Sp-Lang Path, Stillwater Pub Sch, **SLP**

Spencer, Mary E J 5627 North Chipman, Owosso, MI 48867, (517) 723-6784, BA 72 MI St Univ; MA 76 MI St Univ; Sp-Lang Path, Shiawassee Inter Sch Dist, **SLP**

Spencer, Mrs Mary-Jo Ferreira Barstow Street, Lakeville, MA 02346, (617) 878-2017, **SLP**

Spencer, Mrs Maryann M 26 Hillview Avenue, Rensselaer, NY 12144, (518) 472-1002, BA 75 SUNY - Coll at Plattsburgh; MA 77 Coll of Saint Rose; SLP, East Greenbush Central Schools, **SLP**

Spencer, Mrs Maureen M 8008 Jeanette Place, New Orleans, LA 70118, (504) 568-6511, BA 81 Univ of MS; MA 82 LA St Univ - N O Medical Ctr; Instr, Lsu Med Cen, **SLP**

Spencer, Nancy B 1330-15 Ephesus Church Rd, Chapel Hill, NC 27514, (919) 933-5171, BS 84 Miami Univ - Oxford; MS 85 Univ of NC - Chapel Hill; **SLP**

Spencer, Mrs Nancy Bolton 3440 Northstar Drive, Stockton, CA 95209, (209) 957-4462, BA 81 Univ of WI - Eau Claire; MS 83 CO St Univ; 88–Sp-Lang Path, Lincoln USD, **SLP**

Spencer, Nedra Elaine 331 Cocoanut Row #2, Palm Beach, FL 33480, (305) 655-9643, BS 74 MS Univ for Women; MS 78 MS Univ for Women; SLP, Palm Beach Co Schools, **SLP**

Spencer, Raymond E 741 Bowen Court, Sonoma, CA 95476, MA 77 CA St Univ - Sacramento; Aud, Private Practice, **A**

Spencer, Mrs Rena Elizabeth 4331 Shawn Drive, Traverse City, MI 49684, (616) 947-2324, BS 82 Central MI Univ; MA 83 Central MI Univ; Sp-Lang Path, Saginaw Community Hospital, **SLP**

Spencer, Sara 1808 Funston, San Francisco, CA 94116, **SLP**

Spencer, Sarah Lynne 2745 Bristol Drive Apartment 207, Lisle, IL 60532, (312) 462-4220, BS 83 Univ of IA; MA 84 Western MI Univ; 87–Sp-Lang Path, Marianjoy Rehab Ctr, **SLP**

Spencer, Stephanie 13110 Hugo Place, Silver Spring, MD 20906, (301) 949-7209, **SLP**

Spencer, Mrs Terri Lynn 7332 Parkcrest Drive, La Vista, NE 68128, (402) 572-2274, BS 79 Northwest MO St Univ; MS 81 Univ of NE - Omaha; **SLP**

Spenia, Lisa A 614 Radburn Drive, Indianapolis, IN 46224, (317) 745-3414, BS 81 WV Univ; MA 82 IN Univ - Bloomington; Sp-Lang Path, Methodist Hosp of Indiana, **SLP**

Spensko-Arellano, Kelly Sue 790 West Greenoaks Drive, Murray, UT 84123, (801) 565-7490, BS 81 Univ of UT; BS 82 Univ of UT; MS 85 Univ of UT; Sp-Lang Path, Jordan Schl Dstr, **SLP**

Sperberg, Mrs Holly Hofman 809 Michigan Avenue, Stevens Point, WI 54481, (715) 345-1061, BS 84 Univ of WI - Stevens Point; MS 86 Univ of WI - Stevens Point

Sperber-Halprin, Marilyn S 57 Cedar Lane, Closter, NJ 07624, (201) 768-2990, BA 76 CUNY - Lehman Coll; MS 77 Columbia Univ Teachers Coll; Research Assist, Res Found, **SLP**

Sperling, Andrew L 255 Main Street, Hackensack, NJ 07601, (201) 487-6860, BA 68 CUNY - City College; MS 76 Columbia Univ Teachers Coll; Aud, Private Practice, **A ACE**

Sperling, Mrs Deborah Lea 15 Old Pond Road, Rochester, NY 14625, (716) 377-4660, **SLP**

Sperling, Heidi 86 Gatehouse Lane Court, Apartment 10, Edison, NJ 08837, (201) 321-7063, BA 79 Rutgers Coll; MS 81 Columbia Univ Teachers Coll; Sp-Lang Path, Rahway Hospital, **SLP**

Sperling, Mrs Ilene 11 Elmwood Lane, Syosset, NY 11791, (718) 347-8030, BA 71 CUNY - Queens Coll; MA 73 CUNY - Queens Coll; 88–Sp-Lang Path, Dev Therapy Consult Inc, **SLP**

Sperling, Robin Sue 3343 Carroll Court, Bensalem, PA 19020, (215) 752-2974, BA 81 Temple Univ; MA 85 Temple Univ; 88–Sp-Lang Path, Warminster Gen Hosp, **SLP**

Sperling, Terri Bukaitz 17800 East Colima, Apartment 547, Rowland Heights, CA 91748, (818) 913-6258, BA 83 Univ of MD - College Park; MA 85 Whittier Coll; Sp-Lang Path, Private Practice, **SLP**

Sperry, Elizabeth Ellen 76 Gordon Street #16, Brighton, MA 02135, (617) 782-8026, BS 84 Kent St Univ; MA 85 Kent St Univ; **SLP**

Sperti, Mrs Karen Nancy 36 Glenwood Avenue, Glenwood, IL 60425, (312) 758-9267, OM 87 Governors St Univ; **SLP**

Spevak, Ronald E 208 Pinebrook Drive, Fort Myers, FL 33907, (813) 482-7270, BA 71 Univ of IA; MS 72 IL St Univ - Normal; Dir Sp-Lang Path, Dupage Co Convalescent Cen, **SLP**

Spice, James G 2155 West Edward Lane, Glendale, WI 53209, (414) 647-6270, BS 67 Univ of WI - Milwaukee; MS 73 Univ of WI - Milwaukee; SLP, Milwaukee Publ Schs, **SLP**

Spiceland, Joseph Cecil 227 Wilton Circle, Paducah, KY 42003, (502) 442-0770, BS 73 Murray St Univ; MS 76 Murray St Univ; **SLP**

Spicer, Elizabeth Ann 4663 20th Court South, Salem, OR 97302, (503) 378-5286, MS 87 Western OR St Coll; 88–Instr, Western OR State Coll

Spicer, Harry S 2260 East Langston Street, Springfield, MO 65804, (417) 881-3015, BA 64 Baylor Univ; MA 70 Baylor Univ; 85–Instr of Comm, Southwest Mo State U

Spicknall, Mrs Diane D 2209 Arizona, Iowa City, IA 52240, (319) 399-6700, BS 77 Univ of IA; MA 78 Univ of IA; SLP, Grant Wood AEA, **SLP**

Spiegel, Bernard B 3207 Vanfleet Parkway, Toledo, OH 43615, PH (NS); **SLP**

Spiegel, Mrs Donna R 27 Harvest Drive, Scarsdale, NY 10583, BA 68 NY Univ; MA 70 NY Univ; **SLP**

Spiegel, Elisa L 3 Sherman Court, Plainsboro, NJ 08536, (609) 275-0680, BS 77 SUNY - Coll at Geneseo; MS 79 CUNY - Brooklyn Coll; Educational Consultant, Discovery Toys, **SLP**

Spiegel, Hazel S 113 Forest Avenue, Vermillion, SD 57069, (605) 677-5311, OB 55 Univ of HI - Manoa; MA 58 Univ of HI - Manoa; ED 86 (School Psychology) Univ of SD - Vermillion; 80–Coord, Cen for Dev Disabl, **SLP**

Spiegel, Lisa Michelle 17632 Jordan Avenue #40-D, Irvine, CA 92715, (714) 859-5529, **SLP**

Spiegel, Susan L 222 Elleen Terrace #8A, Hackensack, NJ 07601, (201) 489-0289, BA 79 Kean Coll of NJ; MA 80 Kean Coll of NJ; Sp-Lang Path, Private Practice, **SLP**

Spiegelberg, Beverly Box 883, Mercer Island, WA 98040, (206) 226-6111, BS 66 Phillips Univ; MA 67 Western MI Univ; Sp-Lang Path, Hrng Sp & Deafness Ctr, **SLP ACE**

Spiegler-Gordon, Karin Ethel 2006 Sheldon Drive, Newark, DE 19711, BA 77 Earlham Coll; MA 87 Temple Univ-Tyler Sch of Art; Sp-Lang Path, DE Statewide Autistic Prog, **SLP**

Spielberg, Martin H Falls Church Medical Center, 6062 Arlington Boulevard, Falls Church, VA 22044, (703) 533-8020, BS 50 OH Univ - Athens; MA 51 Univ of AL-Tuscaloosa; Sp/Lang Path, Private Practice, **SLP**

Spielberg, Paula G 602 Washington Square S, Philadelphia, PA 19106, (215) 473-4101, BS 67 Temple Univ; ME 71 Temple Univ; MA 76 Temple Univ; Sp-Lang Path, Sch Dist of Phila, **SLP**

Spielman, Beth Ann 281 Forestcliff, Davis, IL 61019, (815) 248-2051, BS 85 Northern IL Univ - De Kalb; MA 86 Northern IL Univ - De Kalb

Spier, Susan Ann 1300 North Astor #23-B, Chicago, IL 60610, (312) 332-4242, BS 80 Univ of GA; ME 81 Univ of GA; Aud, Gordon Siegel MD, **A**

Spierer, Lili 200 East 16th Street #10K, New York, NY 10003, (212) 790-2711, MS 84 Boston Univ; 86–Sp-Lang Path, St Vincent's Hosp, **SLP**

Spiess, Mrs Gwen H 4606 Lakeshore Road, Port Huron, MI 48060, (313) 984-3101, BS 71 Univ of NE - Lincoln; MS 77 Univ of NE - Omaha; Sp-Lang Path, Port Huron Area Sch Dist, **SLP**

Spieth, Martha L 1617 Ann Street, East Lansing, MI 48823, (517) 887-3235, BA 70 MI St Univ; MA 71 MI St Univ; SLP, Lansing Sch Dist, **SLP**

Spiewak, Lauren N 945 Red Fox Road, Orange, CT 06477, (203) 795-6033, BA 70 Rutger's St Univ - Douglas Coll; MS 73 Columbia Univ Teachers Coll; **SLP**

Spigel, Francine B 1 Canterbury Road, Livingston, NJ 07039, (201) 992-3142, BA 64 Montclair St Coll; MA 75 Montclair St Coll; Sp-Lang Path, NJ Assn of Ret Citzns, **SLP**

Spigel, Mrs Susan G 27 Zephyr Terrace, Lyttelton Road #1, Governors Bay, New Zealand, BA 68 MI St Univ; MA 71 MI St Univ; **SLP**

Spigener, Laurie Toy Brandon Hall School, 1701 Brandon Hall Drive, Dunwoody, GA 30350, (404) 394-8177, BS 74 PA St Univ - Univ Park; MS 75 PA St Univ - Univ Park; 85–Dir of Academics, Brandon Hall Sch, **SLP**

Spigos, Mrs Janet C 330 Ravine Road, Hinsdale, IL 60521, (312) 323-1191, BA 83 Mundelein Coll; OM 85 Governors St Univ; 87–Sp-Lang Path, Cass Sch Dist 63, **SLP**

Spilar, Kathleen Therese 715 East 159th Street, Cleveland, OH 44110, (216) 932-4735, BA 81 Cleveland St Univ; MA 83 Cleveland St Univ; Audiologist, Maico of Cleveland, **A**

Spillane, Eileen M 303 South Midler Avenue, Syracuse, NY 13206, BS 81 SUNY - Coll at Fredonia; MA 85 Univ of Pittsburgh - Pittsburgh; Sp-Lang Path, North Syracuse Sch Dist, **SLP**

Spillane, Mrs Lisa Palazzolo 5794 Old Cumming Highway, Buford, GA 30518-4510, (404) 945-0550, BS 83 Univ of TN - Knoxville; MA 85 Univ of TN - Knoxville; Sp-Lang Path, Gwinnett County Public Schools, **SLP**

Spillers, Dr Cindy S 242 Montague Hall, University Of Minnesota Duluth, Duluth, MN 55812, (218) 726-7992, BA 77 OH St Univ; MA 79 OH St Univ; PH 83 (NS) Wichita St Univ; Asst Prof, U of MN, **SLP**

Spillers, Nancy Sansom 619 Harbor Walls Drive, Fort Wayne, IN 46819, (219) 747-5470, BS 79 Purdue Univ - West Lafayette; MA 81 Ball St Univ; Sp-Lang Path, Fort Wayne Commun Dis Cen Inc, **SLP**

Spillman, Denise Ann 409-1/2 North Evans, Tecumseh, MI 49286-1453, (313) 434-5466, BS 82 Eastern MI Univ; MA 83 Eastern MI Univ; **SLP**

Spillman, Donna Ellen 59 Sturgis Road, Edison, NJ 08817, (201) 549-5580, BA 84 Rutger's St Univ - Douglas Coll; MS 86 Rutgers St Univ - Newark; **SLP**

Spina, Mrs Nancy Claire 2015 Huntington Drive, Florissant, MO 63033-1225, (314) 838-5831, BS 83 Central MO St Univ; MS 85 Southern IL Univ-Edwardsvill; **SLP**

Spinale, Marilyn R 28 Fountain Lane #11, South Weymouth, MA 02190, (617) 824-6911, MS 84 Southern CT St Univ; Aud, Morton Hosp & Med Ctr, **A ACE**

Spindler, Kristine 117 Westview Avenue, Paramus, NJ 07652, (201) 438-0223, BS 75 Trenton St Coll; MA 78 Montclair St Coll; Sp/Lang Path, Bergen Co Spec Serv Sch Dist, **SLP**

Spinelli, Francesca M 2222 Westerland #130, Houston, TX 77063, (713) 782-5537, BS 74 Northwestern Univ; MA 76 Univ of IA; PH 82 (Child Lang) Univ of WI - Madison; **SLP**

Spiniello, Therese M 171 Dorchester Road, River Edge, NJ 07661, (201) 967-5263, BA 76 Montclair St Coll; MA 85 Montclair St Coll; 85–Sp-Lang Path, N Highlands Reg HS, **SLP**

Spinnato, Ann 730 Valley Street, Dayton, OH 45405, (513) 222-5597, BA 72 Bellarmine Coll; MA 73 Bowling Green St Univ; Sp-Lang Path, Hrng & Sp Cen for Chldn & Ad, **SLP**

Spinner, Ann Louise 1852 Wexford Road, Palmyra, PA 17078-9243, (717) 367-1161, BS 80 WV Univ; MS 82 Bloomsburg Univ of PA; 85–Sp-Lang Path, PA State U, **SLP**

Spinrad, Myrna Z 35 Edgemont Road, West Orange, NJ 07052, **SLP**

Spire, Mrs Victoria Ann 723 East 1st Street, Maryville, MO 64468, (816) 582-7628, BS 83 Northwest MO St Univ; MS 86 Northwest MO St Univ; 88–Sp-Lang Path, Jefferson C-123 Sch Dist

Spires, Diantha K 613 Truesdell Avenue, Altamonte Springs, FL 32701, MS 80; **SLP ACE**

Spires, Karen L 4951 Platt Springs Road, West Columbia, SC 29169, (803) 359-6101, BS 78 Murray St Univ; MS 79 Univ of SC - Columbia; Sp-Lang Path, Lexington Sch Dist #1, **SLP**

Spiser, Holly Kay 7434 Louis Pasteur, Suite 111, San Antonio, TX 78229, (512) 697-3555, MS 87 Univ of TX - Dallas; 83–Aud, Alamo Hearing Aid Svc, **A**

Spiser, Valarie L 8525 Floyd Curl #1901, San Antonio, TX 78240, (512) 342-1776, BA 76 Our Lady Lake Univ-San Anton; MA 77 Our Lady Lake Univ-San Anton; Sp-Lang Path, Communication & Learning Serv, **SLP**

Spittler, Janice 6810 Renfro, Richmond, TX 77469, (713) 232-6494, BS Lamar Univ; MS Lamar Univ; Sp-Lang Path, Angleton Independent Sch Dist, **SLP**

Spittler, Karen A 1010 Chestnut Street, Atlantic, IA 50022, (712) 243-1480, BS 72 Univ of IL - Urbana; MA 76 Univ of IL - Urbana; 76–Sp-Lang Path, Loess Hills AEA 13, **SLP**

Spitz, Diane E 517 Murray Hill Road, Binghamton, NY 13903, (602) 797-4943, BA 74 Univ of MI - Ann Arbor; MS 76 Univ of WI - Madison; Lect, **SLP**

Spitz, Mrs Roberta E 118 Gladys Drive, Normal, IL 61761, (309) 527-4405, BS 74 IL St Univ - Normal; MS 75 IL St Univ - Normal; Sp-Lang Path, El Paso Unit 375 Sch Dist, **SLP**

Spitz, Robin Leah 2443 North Seminary Avenue, Chicago, IL 60614, (312) 791-2900, BA 80 Univ of Pittsburgh - Pittsburgh; MA 82 Memphis St Univ; 87–Sp-Lang Path, Siegel Institute, **SLP**

Spitzenberger, Gail M 3207 West Mangold Avenue, Greenfield, WI 53217, (414) 878-3717, BS 79 Marquette Univ; MS 81 Univ of WI - Milwaukee; Sp-Lang Path, Racine County Sch Ofc, **SLP**

Spitzer, Dr Jaclyn Barbara Audiology & Sp Path Sect/117, VA Medical Center, West Spring Street, West Haven, CT 06516, (203) 932-5711, BA 72 CUNY - Brooklyn Coll; MS 73 Columbia Univ Teachers Coll; PH 78 (Aud) Columbia Univ Teachers Coll; Aud, VA Med Ctr, **A**

Spitzer, Linda 200 West 79th Street #15M, New York, NY 10024, (212) 874-7249, BA 76 SUNY - Center at Buffalo; MA 78 Hofstra Univ; Sp-Lang Path, Bd of Ed NYC/Sp Serv U, **SLP**

Spiva, Jane A 306 Dartbrook Drive, Rockwall, TX 75087, **SLP**

Spivak, Dr Lynn G Dept Hearing & Speech, Bellevue Hospital Center, 1st Avenue & 27th Street, New York, NY 10016, (212) 561-3564, BA 69 Hofstra Univ; MS 77 CUNY - Brooklyn Coll; PH 85 (Speech & Hearing Sciences) CUNY - Grad Sch & Univ Cntr; 86–Asst Dir, NYU Med Ctr-Bellevue Hosp, **A**

Spivey, Mrs Kay W 1101 Jones Drive, Montgomery, AL 36108, (205) 265-0933, BS 76 Auburn Univ - Auburn; BA 77 Auburn Univ - Auburn; MS 83 Auburn Univ - Auburn; Sp-Lang Path, Montgomery Pub Sch, **SLP**

Spivy, Rebecca Ellen S 5106 Nevada, Greenville, TX 75401, (214) 455-2112, BS 76 East TX St Univ - Commerce; MS 80 East TX St Univ - Commerce; Tchr, Greenville ISD-Sch F/T Deaf, **SLP**

Splain, Gay L 160 Walden Way, Imperial, PA 15126, (412) 279-7790, BS 70 Longwood Coll; ME 71 Univ of VA - Charlottesville; Sp-Lang Path, Allegheny Intermed Unit #3, **SLP**

Splattstoesser, Deanne J 2919 Westside Street, Grand Island, NE 68803, (308) 381-5931, MS 82 Kearney St Coll; Sp-Lang Path, Central NE Support Svcs Prog, **SLP**

Splawski-Roach, Jill L 1151 West Wrightwood #3, Chicago, IL 60614, (312) 929-7254, BS 83 IL St Univ - Normal; MS 85 IL St Univ - Normal; 88–Sp-Lang Path, Community Therapy Svcs, **SLP**

Spletzer-Cheetwood, Mrs Barbara 9204 Buck Road, Perrysburg, OH 43551, (419) 698-6004, BS 78 Univ of GA; MA 80 Univ of TN - Knoxville; Sp/Lang Path, Oregon Sch Dist, **SLP**

Spliedt, William J 5425 Council Street, Baltimore, MD 21227, (301) 552-1665, BA 76 Loyola Coll; MS 77 Loyola Coll; Sp/Lang Path, Prince Georges Co Bd of Ed, **SLP**

Splitter, Marianne 13585 S W 115th Terrace, Miami, FL 33186, (305) 274-8640, BA 72 Coll of Wooster; MA 80 George Washington Univ; 88–Sp-Lang Path, Miami Fluency Clinic, **SLP ACE**

Spogen, David Roy PO Box 369, South Bend, WA 98586, (206) 875-6439, 75–Supt, South Bend Sch Dist #118, **SLP**

Spohn-Grall, Kelly Jeanne 3300 South Tamarac Drive, Apartment #M102, Denver, CO 80231, (303) 750-0126, BA 84 Univ of OR; MA 86 Univ of Denver; 86–Sp-Lang Path, Denver PS, **SLP**

Spokane, Frances G 3327 Monogram Avenue, Long Beach, CA 90808, **SLP**

Sponseller, Karen S 23615 108th Place S E, Apartment 1L-306, Kent, WA 98031, (206) 854-6003, BA 82 WA St Univ; MA 83 WA St Univ; Sp-Lang Path, Bethel School District, **SLP**

Spooner, Mrs Ellen L 15 Chapman Street, Brewer, ME 04412, (207) 941-6290, BS 77 Univ of ME - Orono; MA 81 Univ of ME - Orono; 80–Sp-Lang Path, Bangor Sch Dept, **SLP**

Sporkman-Link, Mrs Ann Grace P O Box 152, West Point, IA 52656, (319) 753-3551, **SLP**

Sporleder, Jeannie A 6450 Temple City Boulevard, Temple City, CA 91780, (818) 447-8981, BA 83 Univ of LA Verne; MA 86 Whittier Coll; **SLP**

Sporn, Marcia W 82 North Dunning, Ventura, CA 93003, (805) 642-7419, MS 87 Univ of IL - Urbana; Sp-Lang Path, Burnwall Clinic, **SLP**

Spose, Mrs Beth Ann 15 Mansfield Road, North Haven, CT 06473, (203) 239-7407, BS 76 Wheelock Coll; MS 82 Columbia Univ Teachers Coll; **SLP**

Spoth, Mrs Elizabeth Segovia 3602 Beaver Ford Road, Woodbridge, VA 22192, (703) 590-6886, BA 78 Radford Univ; ME 84 Columbus Coll; **SLP**

Spottiswood, Lydia Lynne 5943 Westfall Road, Lake Worth, FL 33463, (305) 641-3072, BS 82 Northern IL Univ - De Kalb; MA 84 Northwestern Univ; **A**

Spradlin, Mrs Kelly T 2312 South 26th Street, Fort Smith, AR 72901, (501) 782-6022, BS 85 Univ of AR - Fayetteville; MS 88 Univ of AR - Medical Sci; 87–Aud, Western AR ENT Cl

Spradlin, Sally J 55715 Raintree Drive, Osceola, IN 46561, (219) 259-3763, BS 74 IN St Univ - Terre Haute; MA 81 Ball St Univ; Sp-Lang Path, Sch City of Mishawaka, **SLP**

Spradling, Mrs Janabeth W 2055 White Oak Circle, Wichita, KS 67207, (316) 685-1181, BA 78 TX Tech Univ; MS 79 TX Tech Univ; Sp-Lang Path, National Sp & Hrng, **SLP**

Sprague, Linda L 25106 West 8 Mile Road Apartment #810, Southfield, MI 48034, (313) 927-7000, MA 77 MI St Univ; BA 76 MI St Univ; Aud, Mount Carmel Mercy Hospital, **A**

Spratlin, Mrs Barbara P 9087 Farmoor Road, Germantown, TN 38138, OB 77 Univ of MS; MA 78 Memphis St Univ; **SLP**

Spremulli, Mary 111 Bayberry Lane, Bedford, OH 44146, (216) 721-5400, BA Cleveland St Univ; MA 79 Cleveland St Univ; Dir Dept of Comm Dis, Health Hill Hosp, **SLP**

Spretnjak, Maureen Lee 8450 Cambridge #3172, Houston, TX 77054, (713) 790-5913, BA 85 Saint Xavier Coll; MS 87 Rush Univ; 88–Aud, The Methodist Hosp

Spriestersbach, Mrs Bette Rural Route 6, River Heights, Iowa City, IA 52240, (319) 353-5488, BA 43 Univ of IA; MA 45 Univ of IA; 88–Retired, Chld Hlth Specialty Cl U of IA, **SLP F LM**

Spriestersbach, D C Graduate College, University Of Iowa, 201 Gilmore Hall, Iowa City, IA 52242, (319) 335-2132, OB 39 Winona St Univ; MA 40 Univ of IA; PH 48 (NS) Univ of IA; 65–Vp Ed Dev & Res/Dean Grad Coll, U of IA, **SLP F H**

Spriet, Mrs Sheryl Y 486 East 180 South, Smithfield, UT 84335, (801) 563-6118, MS 88 UT St Univ; 87–Aud, Logan Regional Hosp

Spriggs-Blair, Mrs Susan M 801 N Cleveland Bldg 801, Apartment 103, Sioux Falls, SD 57103-6066, (605) 334-8872, BA 76 Northwest MO St Univ; MA 78 Univ of SD - Vermillion; **SLP**

Spring, Karen A 14 Norman Avenue, Albany, NY 12203, **SLP**

Spring, Mrs Theresa M 72 West End Avenue, Binghamton, NY 13905, (607) 798-9980, BA 74 Elmira Coll; MS 75 Ithaca Coll; **SLP**

Springate, Nancy Leigh 2050 Versailles Road, Lexington, KY 40504, (606) 254-5701, BS 85 Central MI Univ; MA 86 Central MI Univ; 86–Sp-Lang Path, Cardinal Hill Hosp, **SLP**

Springer, Anita S 1502 Hawk Tree, College Station, TX 77840, (409) 822-0193, BA 71 Jacksonville St Univ; MS 77 Univ of Montevallo; Dir of Aud, Brazos Valley Rehab Cen, **A**

Springer, Clare S 6121 Ashburton Drive, San Jose, CA 95123, (408) 998-6000, BA 64 Univ of Northern CO; Sp/Lang Path, San Jose USD, **SLP**

Springer, Ira Steven 354 East Jericho Turnpike, Mineola, NY 11501, (516) 741-3000, MA 78 Long Island U - CW Post Ctr; President/Audiologist, Meadowbrook Hearing Aid Center, **A**

Springer, Mrs Leann Marie 4819 Freedom Avenue, Pocatello, ID 83202, (208) 254-3306, BS 81 ID St Univ; MS 83 ID St Univ; 83–Sp-Lang Path, Marsh Valley Jt Sch Dist #21, **SLP**

Springer, Mark T 3484 Pioneer Drive S E, Salem, OR 97302, (503) 399-3198, BS 72 Western OR St Coll; MS 73 Western OR St Coll; 73–Sp-Lang Path, Salem Pub Sch, Dist 24J, **SLP**

Springer-Hann, Patricia Box 3434, Soldotna, AK 99669, (907) 283-4826, BS 76 ID St Univ; MS 78 ID St Univ; SLP, Kenai Peninsula Borough Sch, **SLP**

Springfield, Mrs Amy P 1029 Drexel Drive, Birmingham, AL 35209, (205) 945-2957, BS 84 Auburn Univ - Auburn; MS 86 Vanderbilt Univ; 87–Sp-Lang Path, Birmingham City Schs, **SLP**

Springsted, Mrs Kim Ann R 206 Donald Street, Lanoka Harbor, NJ 08734, (609) 971-7427, BA 75 Catawba Coll; MA 79 Trenton St Coll; 82–Sp-Lang Path, Barnegat Sch Dist, **SLP**

Spring-Whiddon, Diane Rita 94 Chadduck Avenue, Buffalo, NY 14207, (716) 885-4128, BS 80 SUNY - Center at Buffalo; MS 82 SUNY - Center at Buffalo; SLP, Buffalo Bd of Ed, **SLP**

Sprinkle, Ruth S 3277-B Roswell Road #408, Atlanta, GA 30305, MA 72 Vanderbilt Univ; **A**

Sproles, Linda O 25 Shadowfield Drive, West Columbia, SC 29169, (803) 635-5594, BA 76 Univ of NC - Greensboro; MS 81 Univ of SC - Columbia; Sp-Lang Path, Fairfield Co Schs, **SLP**

Spruce, Wayne Vee 6520 Secrest Court, Tampa, FL 33625, (813) 961-0443, BA 68 Univ of South FL; MS 70 Univ of South FL; Consult, Wayne U Spruce Ms Inc, **SLP**

Spruell, Mrs Sheri L 503 East 5th, Mount Carmel, IL 62863, (618) 263-3876, BA 76 Western KY Univ; MA 78 Western KY Univ; Sp-Lang Path, School District 348, **SLP**

Sprung, Mrs Mindy Parmett 12 Northstar Road, Closter, NJ 07624, (201) 585-9182, BS 75 SUNY - Center at Albany; MA 78 Hofstra Univ; Sp-Lang Path, Private Practice, **SLP**

Sprung, Susan C 1 Debra Court, Wayside, NJ 07712, (201) 922-0808, BA 77 Lafayette Coll; MA 80 Temple Univ; Sp-Lang Path, Private Practice, **SLP ACE**

Sprunger, Margaret Liechty 7153 Stockley Road, Upper Darby, PA 19082, (215) 447-2428, BA 85 IN Univ - Bloomington; MA 86 IN Univ - Bloomington; 87–Sp-Lang Path, Crozer-Chester Med Ctr, **SLP**

Sprunk-Berlin, Holly Suzanne 208 Tacoma Avenue Apt 7, Tacoma, WA 98403, (206) 845-1755, BA 85 WA St Univ; MA 87 Western WA Univ; Sp-Lang Path, Good Samaritan Hosp, **SLP**

Sprute, Debra Bengoa 3221 Galaxy, Bossier City, LA 71112, (318) 631-5110, BA 81 Northeast LA Univ; MS 83 LA St Univ - N O Medical Ctr; 87–Sp-Lang Path, Caddo Parish School Board, **SLP**

Spry-Packard, Sheila M 308 West Quincy, Pittsburg, KS 66762, (316) 231-3870, BS 75 MO Southern St Coll; MS 78 Central MO St Univ; Sp-Lang Path, SE KS Spec Ed Co-Op, **SLP**

Spudie, Annette Ryerson Toledo Hearing & Speech Center, 1 Stranahan Square, Toledo, OH 43604, (419) 241-6219, BA 82 SUNY - Center at Buffalo; MA 85 Bowling Green St Univ; 85–Aud, Toledo Hearing & Speech Ctr, **A**

Spuehler, Dr H E 7916 Chelton Road, Bethesda, MD 20814, (202) 389-2008, BS 53 Purdue Univ - West Lafayette; MS 54 Purdue Univ - West Lafayette; PH 56 (NS) Purdue Univ - West Lafayette; Dir Aud & SLP Serv, VA Central Office, **F**

Spuhler, Barbara 293 Fulton Street, Redwood City, CA 94062, (415) 365-1550, MA 85 San Jose St Univ; Sp-Lang Path, Redwood City Sch Dist, **SLP**

Spuhler, Linde M P O Box 3434, Sparks, NV 89432-3434, (702) 789-3268, BS 78 Univ of CA - Los Angeles; MS 81 Univ of WY; 84–Supvr-Commun Dis Dept, St Mary's Reg Med Ctr, **SLP**

Spund, Ellen H 210 Atlantic Avenue, Lynbrook, NY 11563, BA 74 SUNY - Center at Buffalo; MA 76 CUNY - Queens Coll; Sp-Lang Path, NYC Bd of Ed, **SLP**

Spurgin, Tracy Gail 2515 Heather Brook Lane, Apartment 703, Arlington, TX 76006, (817) 649-1740, BS 85 TX Tech Univ; MS 87 TX Tech Univ

Spurlock, Shelley Lynn 2655 Keystone Avenue #4, Santa Clara, CA 95051, BA 82 CA St Univ - Chico; MA 84 CA St Univ - Chico; Sp-Lang Path, Santa Clara USD, **SLP**

Spurrier, Mrs Jean M A 114 Seminole Drive, Vincennes, IN 47591, (812) 886-0057, BS 66 Northeast MO St Univ; MA 69 Univ of MO - Columbia; **SLP**

Sputz, Carla Ann 420 East 79th Street, Apt 6-E, New York, NY 10021, (212) 988-7283, BA 83 Rutgers St Univ - Newark; OM 85 Hahneman Medical Coll; **SLP**

Spyker, Margaret Mary 17290 Van Wagoner, Spring Lake, MI 49456, (616) 777-2667, BS 73 Western MI Univ; MS 78 Western MI Univ; Sp-Lang Path, Muskegon Pub Sch, **SLP**

Squibb, Kevin Dexter Department Of Communication Disorders, S E Missouri University, 900 Normal Avenue, Cape Girardeau, MO 63701, (314) 651-2498, BS 83 East TN St Univ; MS 85 East TN St Univ; PH 88 (Communication Disorders) Bowling Green St Univ; 88–Prof, Southeast Missouri State Univ, **A**

Squier, Mrs Judith R 4113 Alpine, Portola Valley, CA 94025, (415) 851-8720, MA 68 Univ of IL - Urbana; **SLP**

Squier, Sheryl Lynn 9605 South 48th Street, Apt 1032, Phoenix, AZ 85044, (602) 893-0860, BS 86 Univ of WI - Oshkosh; MS 87 Marquette Univ; **SLP**

Squier, Victoria J 89 South Stanwood Road, Columbus, OH 43209, (614) 258-1160, MA 74 Univ of the Pacific; Sp-Lang Path, Sp Therapy-Voice Therapy, **SLP**

Squillante, Mrs Susan McHenry 28 Holloway Avenue, Coventry, RI 02816, (813) 343-2180, BA 80 Univ of RI; MS 83 Univ of RI; Sp/Lang Path, Exeter-W Greenwich Sch, **SLP**

Squire, Shauna K 7245 Apple Honey Lane #21, Midvale, UT 84047, (801) 562-5194, BS 83 Brigham Young Univ; MS 86 UT St Univ; Sp-Lang Path, **SLP**

Squires, Deborah Pershern 15 Bradley Drive, Shoreham, NY 11786, (516) 821-6191, BA 79 Cleveland St Univ; MA 80 Cleveland St Univ; Sp-Lang Path, Sachem School District, **SLP**

Squires, Mrs Gail Ann 14 Chennault Court, Mount Holly, NJ 08060, (609) 261-7177, BS 78 Trenton St Coll; MA 82 Trenton St Coll; 82–Sp-Lang Path, Private Practice, **SLP**

Squires, Mrs Laura Louise 1720 N E 107th Street, Seattle, WA 98125, (206) 365-0300, **SLP**

Squires, Mrs Regena H Speech & Hearing Services, 134 South Houston Street, P O Box 47, Wharton, TX 77488, (409) 532-8230, BS 72 Lamar Univ; ME 75 Lamar Univ; MS 78 Lamar Univ; Owner/Dir, Sp-Hrng Servs, **SLP A**

Squires, Richard L ENT Assoc Of Clarksburg, 125 North 6th Street, Clarksburg, WV 26301, (304) 623-6533, BS 73 WV Univ; MS 75 WV Univ; Aud/Offi Mgr, ENT Assoc of Clarksburg Inc, **A**

Squires, Ty Warren 1680 Cliffdale Lane, Pueblo, CO 81006, (719) 384-5412, BS 84; MS 86; 87–Aud, Private Practice, **A**

Squitieri, Elena 299 South Avenue, New Canaan, CT 06840, BS 45 Columbia Univ Teachers Coll; MS 71 Southern CT St Univ; Sp-Lang Path, Bd of Educ Greenwich CT, **SLP ACE**

Srb, Mrs Charlene J 11205 Martha Street, Omaha, NE 68144, (402) 390-3300, BS 54 Univ of NE - Lincoln; MS 72 Univ of NE - Omaha; Coord Prog/Hrng Imp, Westside Commun Sch Dist #66, **SLP**

Srbeny, Joy Brown 1 South 252 Stratford, Villa Park, IL 60181, (312) 450-2000, BS 81 Northwestern Univ; MA 82 Northwestern Univ; SLP, School District 89, **SLP**

Srinivasan, Mrs Pratibha Box 736 Peabody College, Nashville, TN 37203, (615) 320-5353, MS 87 Vanderbilt Univ; Aud, Bill Wilkerson Hrng & Sp Ctr, **A**

Sroda, Mrs Mary Ellen 7721 Via DE La Montana, Scottsdale, AZ 85258, (602) 991-1672, BA 62 Carlow Coll; **SLP**

Sroges, Cara Bianca 406 S Olive, Hammond, LA 70401, BA 80 Univ of New Orleans; ME 87 Southeastern LA Univ; **SLP**

Srsen, Mrs Paula M 7334 Dawn Place, Mentor, OH 44060, (216) 255-4444, BS 80 Kent St Univ; MA 80 Kent St Univ; Sp-Lang Path, Mentor Pub Sch, **SLP**

Staab, Marla Schmidt HC 39 Box 50, Hays, KS 67601, (913) 628-5366, BA 73 Fort Hays St Univ; MS 74 Fort Hays St Univ; Instr Cl Superv, Fort Hays St U/ Sp&Hrng Cl, **SLP ACE**

Staab, Dr Wayne J 512 East Canterbury Lane, Phoenix, AZ 85022, (602) 942-4939, BA 63 Fort Hays St Univ; MS 65 Univ of WI - Madison; PH 71 (Aud) MI St Univ; 88–VP Pro Svcs, Dahlberg Inc, **A**

Staaf, Susan J 260 5th Avenue, Roebling, NJ 08554-1304, (609) 499-0555, OB 78 Bloomsburg Univ of PA; MS 79 Bloomsburg Univ of PA; Sp-Lang Path, Cp Sch & Treat Cen-Camden Co, **SLP**

Staal, Donna J 5407 Ventana Place, Citrus Heights, CA 95610, (209) 442-6425, BA 78 Seton Hall Univ; MS 79 PA St Univ - Univ Park; Sp/Lang Path, Fresno Commun Hosp & Med Cen, **SLP**

Staats, Diane M 408 Evergreen Street, Hurst, TX 76054, (817) 354-1373, BS 78 Baylor Univ; MA 80 Univ of NE - Lincoln; **SLP**

Stach, Dr Brad A Baylor College Of Medicine, Department Of Oto, 1 Baylor Plaza, Houston, TX 77030, (713) 790-5913, BA 77 NM St Univ; MA 79 Vanderbilt Univ; PH 86 (Aud) Baylor Coll of Medicine; Aud, The Methodist Hosp, **A**

Stach, Carol Blossom 14600 Fonmeadow #1703, Houston, TX 77035, (713) 795-7492, BA 80 NM St Univ; MA 82 Memphis St Univ; Sp-Lang Path, VA Med Cen, **SLP**

Stachowiak, Linda Ann 220 Parker Avenue, Cheektowaga, NY 14206, (716) 832-5400, MS 83 SUNY - Coll at Buffalo; 84–SLP, Visiting Nursing Assn Inc, **SLP ACE**

Stachowiak, Shirley K 22241 N E 31st Street, Redmond, WA 98052, (206) 868-2993, BS 74 IN Univ - Bloomington; ME 75 IN Univ - Bloomington; Sp-Lang Path, **SLP**

Stachowicz, Karen Schultz 343 Tullamore Terrace, Matteson, IL 60443, (312) 720-0636, BA 85 Valparaiso Univ; MA 86 Western MI Univ; 88–Aud, Ingalls Memorial Hosp, **A**

Stachowski, Mrs Claudia C 5280 Goodrich Road, Clarence, NY 14031, (716) 741-2891, BS 72 SUNY - Coll at Buffalo; ME 78 Wayne St Univ; Sp-Lang Path, Clarence Central School Dist, **SLP**

Stachowski, David E 6820 West Lake Road, Conesus, NY 14435, (716) 243-5470, BS 74 SUNY - Coll at Geneseo; MS 80 UT St Univ; Sp-Lang Path, Liv-Ste-Wyo BOCES, **SLP**

Stack, Mrs Christine R 404 West Delaware Avenue, Urbana, IL 61801, (217) 586-4583, BS 73 Univ of IL - Urbana; MS 75 Univ of IL - Urbana; Sp/Lang Path, Unit 3 Sch Mahomet-Seymour, **SLP**

Stack, Frances M 11318 South Neenah, Worth, IL 60482, (312) 425-8000, BA 74 Saint Xavier Coll; MA 75 Univ of IL - Urbana; Superv, Christ Hosp, **SLP ACE**

Stack, Janet R 1720 Meadow Lane, Edwardsville, IL 62025, (618) 656-2888, BA 74 Southern IL Univ-Edwardsvill; MS 77 Southern IL Univ-Edwardsvill; 87–Sp-Lang Path, Prof Sp Lang Svcs, **SLP**

Stack, Jean H 138 Bodman Place, Apartment 12, Red Bank, NJ 07701, **SLP**

Stack, Mary F HCR 62 Box 203, Raton, NM 87740, (505) 445-9627, BS 72 Purdue Univ - West Lafayette; MS 78 Eastern NM Univ; Sp-Lang Path, High Plains Rcc, **SLP ACE**

Stack, Mrs Mary W 501 Nicklaus, Goshen, IN 46526, (219) 533-3151, BA 70 IN Univ - Bloomington; MA 77 Ball St Univ; Sp/Lang Path, Goshen & Middlebury Comm Sch, **SLP**

Stackhouse, Mrs Rhoda J 2023 Westwood Terrace, Vienna, VA 22180, (301) 649-8060, OB 61 OH Univ - Athens; MS 77 Fontbonne Coll; Sp-Lang Path, Montgy Co Pub Sch, **SLP**

Stack-McLaughlin, Mrs Eileen Marie 1524 Mayfair Terrace, Florence, SC 29501, (803) 667-6307, MA 84 Univ of Pittsburgh - Pittsburgh; SLP, Florence County Sch District, **SLP**

Stacy, Ann Rhoten 220-A Street Price Road, Lexington, KY 40511, (606) 255-6841, BA 85 Univ of KY; MS 86 Univ of Louisville; 87–Aud, Lexington Clinic, **A**

Stacy, Laurence W 203 3rd Street S E, Stewartville, MN 55976, (507) 533-4243, BA 74 Univ of Northern IA; MA 75 Univ of Northern IA; Sp-Lang Path, ISD #534, **SLP**

Stacy, Mrs Lisa Marie 722 Hampton Place, Joplin, MO 64801, (417) 649-7045, BS 81 Univ of North TX; MS 83 Univ of NM; 86–Sp-Lang Path, Carl Junction Schools, **SLP**

Stacy, Susan J 411 Stanford Southeast, Albuquerque, NM 87106, BA 72 Univ of MD - College Park; MS 78 Univ of NM; Sp-Lang Path, Albuquerque Pub Sch, **SLP**

Stadelmaier, Ann Elizabeth 20 Truesdale Road, Buffalo, NY 14223, (716) 883-6800, MA 84 SUNY - Center at Buffalo; Aud, Buffalo Otol Group Pc, **A**

Stadelman, Cindy M 2545 HE Nis Ra Lane, Green Bay, WI 54304-1771, (414) 494-8791, BS 77 Univ of WI - Madison; MS 78 Univ of WI - Stevens Point; Sp-Lang Path, Comm Serv Center, **SLP**

Stader, Mrs Cynthia E 7028 Red Arrow Highway, Coloma, MI 49038, (616) 468-2430, BS 86 Central MI Univ; MA 87 Central MI Univ; 88, Coloma Comm Sch

Stadjuhar-Watson, Mrs Karen G 568 West Sagebrush Court, Louisville, CO 80027, (303) 666-7615, BA 70 Univ of Denver; MA 72 IN Univ - Bloomington; MA 80 Univ of Northern CO; Special Education Teacher, Adams County School Dist #12, **SLP**

Stadler, Jacqueline C 917 Federal Street, Philadelphia, PA 19147, (215) 427-5590, BA 78 Univ of PA; MA 80 Temple Univ; 88–Sp-Lang Path/Consult, Early Childhood Eval Ctr, **SLP**

Stadler, Marie Alice 293 North Liberty Street, Delaware, OH 43015, (614) 363-1188, BS 73 Univ of WI - Eau Claire; MS 84 San Francisco St Univ; 87–Sp-Lang Path, Delaware City Schs, **SLP**

Stadnicki, Mrs Barbara A 4 Beechwood Drive, Morrisonville, NY 12962, (518) 563-2929, BS 73 Univ of MA - Amherst; MA 78 OK St Univ; Tchr, Saranac Cen School, **SLP**

Stadt, Vicki L 1099 Linde, New Braunfels, TX 78130, (512) 625-2718, BS 79 Univ of TX - Austin; **SLP**

Staehle, Mrs Gayle Hornbeck 11354 Bloomington Way, Dublin, CA 94568, (415) 829-1780, BA 74 Univ of CA - Santa Cruz; MS 83 CA St Univ - Hayward; SLP, Oakland Sch Dist, **SLP ACE**

Staffan, Kristin Ann 8540 N Central #20, Phoenix, AZ 85020, (602) 870-1012, BS 86 Northern AZ Univ; MA 87 MI St Univ; Sp-Lang Path, Tempe Elem Sch Dist #3

Staffin, Mrs Andrea Gross 301 Ward Court, Holland, PA 18966, (215) 860-8699, BA 79 Temple Univ; MA 81 Temple Univ; Sp-Lang Path, Private Practice, **SLP**

Stafford, Barbara S 7083 Saddle Creek Lane, Sarasota, FL 34241, (813) 371-1914, BS 70 SUNY - Coll at Brockport; MS 73 SUNY - Coll at Geneseo; Sp-Lang Path, Sarasota Co Bd of Ed, **SLP**

Stafford, Mrs Evelyn S 2017 West Westbrook Drive, Peoria, IL 61614, (309) 691-2200, OB 42 IL St Univ - Normal; MA 59 Bradley Univ; MA 64 Bradley Univ; George Zeller Ment Hlth Cen, **SLP**

Stafford, Joel Lindsey 5608 Eisenhower Drive, Lawton, OK 73505, (405) 353-0334, ME 87 Central St Univ; Sp-Lang Path, Lawton Public Schools

Stafford, Lucinda K 1400-B Vassar N E, Albuquerque, NM 87106, (505) 888-3535, MS 83 Univ of NM; 84–Sp-Lang Path, Albuquerque PS, **SLP**

Stafford, Mary F W 48 La Gue Lane, Barre, VT 05641, (802) 879-4918, BA 77 Univ of MI - Ann Arbor; MA 78 Central MI Univ; **SLP**

Stafford, Mrs Sally H 2215 Cherryleaf Lane, Silver Spring, MD 20906-5735, (301) 598-7533, BA 67 IN Univ - Bloomington; OM 68 IN Univ - Bloomington; Sp-Lang Path, Montgomery County PS, **SLP**

Stafford-Litton, Bonnie Jean 226 Village Square, Fillmore, CA 93015, (805) 524-0619, MA 83 CA St Univ - Chico; **SLP**

Stager, Mrs Sharlene M 226 Avenue C, San Manuel, AZ 85631, (602) 385-4341, BA 76 Univ of the Pacific; MA 77 Univ of the Pacific; Sp/Lang Path, Mammoth-San Manuel Pub Sch Dis, **SLP**

Stager, Dr Sheila V 261 Pleasant Street, Dartmouth, NS, Canada B2Y 3S1, (902) 424-7052, MS 80 Purdue Univ - West Lafayette; MS 83 Univ of TX - Dallas; PH 85 (NS) Univ of TX - Dallas; Research Fellow, NIH, **SLP**

Staggs, Mrs Susan F 3018 Valley Drive, Jeffersontown, KY 40299, (502) 267-0396, BS 75 Eastern KY Univ; MS 82 Univ of Louisville; **SLP**

Stagnaro, Mrs Phyllis C 233 Monterey Street, Santa Cruz, CA 95060, (408) 427-1904, BA 68 San Jose St Univ; MA 71 San Jose St Univ; Teacher Sdl Special Day Class, Santa Cruz City Schools, **SLP**

Stagnitti, Charles D P O Box 4076, Springfield, MA 01101, (413) 568-0152, BA 78 SUNY - Coll at Potsdam; MS 80 Syracuse Univ; Sp/Lang Path, East Mountain Cen, **SLP**

Stagray, James Ronald 847 Allerton Street, Kent, OH 44240-4586, (216) 678-2416, MA 85 MI St Univ; Grad, Kent State U, **A**

Stahelek, Mrs Linda M 94 Carver Street, Springfield, MA 01108, (413) 781-9100, MA 80 Northwestern Univ; Aud, Mercy Hospital, **A**

Stahl, John E P O Box 162, Flint, MI 48501, (313) 694-8615, BA 55 Univ of Akron; MS 61 Univ of MI - Ann Arbor; Owner, Private Practice, **SLP**

Stahl, Mrs Judith A 15331 South Lilac Court, Orland Park, IL 60462, (312) 429-2653, BS 68 Northern IL Univ - De Kalb; MA 74 Northern IL Univ - De Kalb; **SLP**

Stahl, Mrs Lisa Marie 2605 Orchard Run, Dayton, OH 45499, (419) 433-8841, BS 84 Bowling Green St Univ; MA 85 Miami Univ - Oxford; **SLP**

Stahl, Michael T 2050 Breton SE, Grand Rapids, MI 49506, (616) 949-5850, BS 65 IN St Univ - Terre Haute; MA 73 Central MI Univ; Aud, Private Practice, **A**

Stahl, Valerie J 6310 Gato Path, Austin, TX 78731, BA 71 Humboldt St Univ; MA 73 Humboldt St Univ; **SLP**

Stahl, Mrs Wendy B 2005 Riding Ridge Road, Columbia, SC 29223, (803) 788-6165, BS 73 Ithaca Coll; MS 75 Columbia Univ Teachers Coll; 83–Sp-Lang Path, Private Practice, **SLP**

Stahle, Mrs Carol Wimmer 626 East Wiltshire Drive, Wallingford, PA 19086, (215) 431-8112, BS 83 Bloomsburg Univ of PA; MS 84 Bloomsburg Univ of PA; 88–Sp-Lang Path, Delaware Co Interm Unit, **SLP**

Stahlecker, Sue Schoenrock 1464 Saratoga, Pocatello, ID 83201, (208) 684-3001, BS 82 Kearney St Coll; MS 84 ID St Univ; 85–Sp-Lang Path, Snake River Sch Dist, **SLP**

Stahr, Karen Coleman 1859 Chestnut Court, Crown Point, IN 46307, (219) 736-6474, BA 84 IN Univ - Bloomington; MA 86 Ball St Univ; Sp-Lang Path, Lakeport Rehab Svcs, **SLP**

Staiano, Dr Anthony V 5577 Wedge Lane, Wescosville, PA 18106, (215) 395-4912, BA 68 CUNY - Queens Coll; MA 70 Univ of IA; PH 85 (NS) Univ of KS; Private Practice, **SLP**

Staiger, Sharon J 2813 Westwood Drive N W, Olympia, WA 98502, (206) 866-1971, BA 67 CA St Univ - Hayward; MS 71 Lamar Univ; Sp-Lang Path, **SLP**

Stainken, Mrs Marie A O 1 Estel Place, Green Brook, NJ 08812, (201) 968-2458, BA 70 Rutger's St Univ - Douglas Coll; MA 80 Montclair St Coll; **SLP**

Stainsby, Leslie Michelle Box 755, Bella Coola, BC, Canada V0T 1C0, BA 73 Univ of Manitoba - Winnipeg; MS 78 Minot St Univ; Sp-Lang Path, Schs Consultant, **SLP**

Stalcup, Rebecca N Route 1 Box 51, Odem, TX 78370, (512) 368-2237, **SLP**

Staley, Anne 1434 West 10th Court, Panama City, FL 32401, (904) 769-1511, BS 78 FL St Univ; MS 80 FL St Univ; 83–Dir/Sp-Lang Path, Bay Med Cen, **SLP**

Staley, Mrs Barbara Kay 19425 Lemarsh, Northridge, CA 91324, (818) 997-2357, MA 82 CA St Univ - Northridge; 84–Sp-Lang Path, Los Angeles USD, **SLP**

Staley, Mrs Patricia C Broadmea Farm, Slaggy Fort, Carlisle Cumbria, England CA6 7NJ, (612) 854-7098, BA 84 Univ of MN - Duluth; MA 85 Western MI Univ; **SLP**

Stalgaitis, Mrs Kathleen Rural Delivery 1, 634 River Road, Upper Black Eddy, PA 18972, (201) 782-8313, BS 79 Trenton St Coll; MA 82 Trenton St Coll; 84–Sp-Lang Path, Flemington-Raritan Reg Sch, **SLP**

Stalker, Catherine Harriette 1920 Bloor Street West #1, Toronto, ON, Canada M6P 3K8, (416) 763-5073, OM 84 Univ of Western Ontario; 87–Sp-Lang Path, Joseph Brant Memorial Hosp, **SLP**

Stalker, Janet Sillman 419 Dufferin Street, Thunder Bay, ON, Canada P7B 1N7, (807) 343-2407, BA 76 Lakehead Univ - Ontario; MA 79 Univ of MN - Duluth; 82–Dir Sp/Lang Path, Thunder Bay, **SLP**

Stall, Robin C 50 Fleetwood Avenue #5A, Fleetwood, NY 10552, (914) 245-2700, BS 79 SUNY - Coll at Buffalo; MA 82 CUNY - Hunter Coll; Sp/Lang Path, Putnam/No Westchester BOCES, **SLP**

Stallcup, Thomas Allan 1909 Morning Side N E, Albuquerque, NM 87110, (505) 255-2682, BS 51 Southeast MO St Univ; MS 58 Univ of KS; Retired, Lovelace Med Cen, **A**

Staller, Dr Steven J Lochlear Corporation, 61 Inverness Drive East, Englewood, CO 80112, (303) 790-9010, BA 74 Univ of CA - Santa Barbara; MA 76 Univ of CO - Boulder; PH 81 (NS) Univ of CO - Boulder; Sp-Lang Path, Lochlear Corp, **A**

Stalletti, Mrs Amy Baxter 1605 Creed Road, Furlong, PA 18925-1337, (215) 348-2940, BS 82 Kutztown Univ of PA; MS 86 Trenton St Coll

Stalling, Judith E 1311 West Moss, Peoria, IL 61606, (309) 671-2950, BA 62 Northwestern Univ; MS 74 Bradley Univ; Lecturer, Illinois State Univ, **SLP**

Stalling, Paulette 12106 Red Stream Way, Columbia, MD 21044, (301) 465-9611, BA 70 Howard Univ; MS 72 Gallaudet Coll; Communications Coordinator/Aud, Maryland School for the Deaf, **A**

Stallings, Debra Marlene P O Box 3790, Venice, FL 34293, (813) 475-2859, MS 85 FL St Univ; 85–Sp-Lang Path, InSpeech Inc, **SLP**

Stallings, Mrs Melody Akers 1110 Five Point Road, Virginia Beach, VA 23454, (804) 481-9126, BS 81 James Madison Univ; MS 83 James Madison Univ; Sp-Lang Path, Richmond Public Schools, **SLP**

Stallings, Stephen Scott P O Box 597, Richmond, TX 77469, (409) 793-6052, MS 86 Baylor Univ; 87–Aud, Richmond State Sch, **A**

Staloff, Mrs Debbie C 205 3rd Avenue, New York, NY 10003, (212) 677-7400, BA 76 CUNY - Queens Coll; MS 77 PA St Univ - Univ Park; Sp-Path/Aud, UCP of NYC, **SLP**

Stalter, Margaret L 1586 Oakmount Road, South Euclid, OH 44121, (216) 382-7700, BS 80 Kent St Univ; MA 81 Kent St Univ; Sp/Lang Path, Lyndhurst Cty Sch, **SLP**

Stambaugh, Lora Kay Box 4575 R D 4, Spring Grove, PA 17362, (717) 845-2661, BS 84 Bloomsburg Univ of PA; MS 85 Bloomsburg Univ of PA; 88–Dir of Sp/Lang Path, Colonial Manor Nursing & Rehab, **SLP**

Stamm, Lenore K 391 Links Drive East, Oceanside, NY 11572, (516) 536-7164, BA 73 CUNY - Hunter Coll; MA 78 Hofstra Univ; 85–Supvr Sp-Lang Path, LI Infant Develop Prog, **SLP**

Stamos-Bushey, Elizabeth 1097-C Kirts, Troy, MI 48084, (313) 626-1200, BA 60 MI St Univ; MA 64 MI St Univ; Sp-Lang Path, Farmington Public Schools, **SLP**

Stamos-Owen, Mrs Lydia A 1655 Indian Hills Drive, Green River, WY 82935, (307) 382-6010, BS 72 UT St Univ; MS 74 UT St Univ; Prog Coord, Sweetwater Cnty Child Dev Cen, **SLP**

Stamp, Judith Long 14 Linkside Villas, Isle of Palms, SC 29451, (803) 886-2872, Aud, **A**

Stamps, Dennis Earl 490 Cameron Circle #2303, Chattanooga, TN 37403, BA 65 Univ Southern MS-Hattiesburg; MA 67 Univ of IL - Urbana; Aud/Asst Dept Head, Baptist Hosp Sp &Hrng Cl, **A**

Stamps, Patricia Lynn 524 Carol Court, Richardson, TX 75081, (214) 231-4190, BS 82 Baylor Univ; MS 85 Univ of TX - Dallas; 85–Sp-Lang Path, Richardson ISD, **SLP**

Stanage, Sally Ann P O Box 1005, Yankton, SD 57078, (605) 665-2484, BS 77 Univ of SD - Vermillion; MA 79 Univ of SD - Vermillion; Sp/Lang Path, Yankton Pub Schs 63-3, **SLP**

Stanaland, Joyce L 12003 Skipjack Court, Lakeridge, Woodbridge, VA 22192, (703) 497-0016, BA 70 MI St Univ; MA 71 MI St Univ; MA 82 Ball St Univ; 88–Consult/Sp-Lang Path, Sp Path Consult Svcs PC, **SLP**

Standarski, Susan M 210 McCullough Place, Rensselaer, NY 12144, (518) 283-0611, BS 78 Coll of Saint Rose; MS 80 Coll of Saint Rose; SLP, Montgy Co Assoc Ret Chldn, **SLP**

Standish, Claire Ann 1435 Kingwood, Ypsilanti, MI 48197, (313) 936-8013, **A**

Standley, Mrs Cathie H 330 Alturas Drive, Twin Falls, ID 83301-3241, (208) 734-0439, BS 81 UT St Univ; MS 83 UT St Univ; 87–Sp-Lang Path, Magic Valley Sp/Hrng Clinic, **SLP**

Standley, Mrs Christine A 3816 Fort Donelson Drive, Stockton, CA 95209, (209) 477-5304, BS 69 Univ of the Pacific; MA 70 Univ of the Pacific; Sp-Lang Path, Stockton USD, **SLP**

Standridge, Rebecca E 10642 East 18th Street, Tulsa, OK 74128, (918) 272-2204, BS 74 Univ of Tulsa; MA 79 Univ of Tulsa; Sp-Lang Path, Owasso Public Schools, **SLP**

Standring, Lorene Carver 444 North Pebble Beach Dr, Crescent City, CA 95531-8605, (707) 464-4445, BS 81 Brigham Young Univ; OM 83 Brigham Young Univ; 84–Sp-Lang Path, **SLP**

Stanek-Prats, Susan 1601 Folkstone Road N E, Atlanta, GA 30329, (404) 876-8540, BA 77 Univ of MD - College Park; MS 79 Gallaudet Coll; Audiologist, Hrng & Sp Ctr Inc, **A**

Stanfield, Dr Gordon Lee 440 Linda Drive, Biloxi, MS 39531, (601) 388-1376, BA 65 Depauw Univ; MA 67 IN Univ - Bloomington; PH 78 Univ Southern MS-Hattiesburg; Aud, Keesler Med Ctr, **A**

Stanford, Gary D Stanford-Roland Ltd, Hearing & Vision Assoc, 301 West 14th Street, Sioux Falls, SD 57102, (605) 338-6251, BS 76 Augustana Coll; MS 77 Minot St Univ; Aud-Owner, Stanford-Roland Ltd, **A**

Stanford, Linda Seestedt 930 South Crawford, Mount Pleasant, MI 48858, (517) 774-3904, BS 73 Central MI Univ; MA 74 Central MI Univ; Coor Hrng Cl, Ctrl MI U, **A**

Stanford, Marilyn Sachs 1634 Edison Drive, Maple Glen, PA 19002, (215) 643-2777, BS 71 OH Univ - Athens; MA 72 MI St Univ; Sp-Lang Path, Roxborough Mem Hosp, **SLP**

Stange, Wanda Jean 116 South Main Street, St Genevieve, MO 63670, (314) 883-5720, BS 73 Southeast MO St Univ; MA 84 Southeast MO St Univ

Stanger, Jessica Ann 1415 South K Street, Elwood, IN 46036, (317) 674-3321, BS 75 Purdue Univ - West Lafayette; MA 79 Ball St Univ; Sp-Lang Path, VA Med Cen Marion In, **SLP**

Stangler, Sharon Lynn 1 Devonshire Place #1015, Boston, MA 02109, (617) 331-0686, BS 85 Boston Univ; MS 87 Northeastern Univ; 87–Sp-Lang Path, Speech-Lang Hearing Associates

Stanifer, Mrs Jan Weller P O Box 511, New Tazewell, TN 37825, (615) 626-9502, BS 76 Southern Methodist Univ; MS 77 Southern Methodist Univ; Sp-Lang Path, Claiborne County School System, **SLP**

Stanifer, Mary Jo 1123 Lavender Street, Monroe, MI 48161, (313) 848-5595, BS 68 Eastern MI Univ; MA 71 Eastern MI Univ; Sp-Lang Path, Mason Consolidated Sch, **SLP**

Stanilonis, Daisy Nelson 1142 T-Square Court, Middleburg, FL 32068, (904) 272-8140, BS 73 FL St Univ; MS 79 FL St Univ; Sp-Lang Path, Clay Co Sch Bd, **SLP**

Stanis, Mrs Elizabeth 4 169th Street, Hammond, IN 46324, (219) 937-3668, BS 73 Northwestern Univ; MA 74 Northwestern Univ; Sp-Lang Path, Sch Dist 154.5, **SLP**

Stanislav, Monica L 5050 Tanglewood #2303, Odessa, TX 79762, (915) 366-4672, BS 85 Stephen F Austin St Univ; MS 87 Univ of North TX; **SLP**

Stankiewicz, Ann W 28 Brompton Lane, Cincinnati, OH 45218, (513) 825-5393, **SLP**

Stankoski, Mrs Mary Jean 412 Benner Road, Apt 202, Allentown, PA 18104, (215) 395-9182, BS 83 Bloomsburg St Coll; MS 84 Bloomsburg Univ of PA; 86–Sp-Lang Path, Good Shepherd Outpatient Serv, **SLP**

Stankov, Mary Anne 5916 Crandall Road, Howell, MI 48843, (313) 437-6322, BS 77 Eastern MI Univ; MA 79 Eastern MI Univ

Stankus, Mrs Marlene L 93 Terrapin Lane, Trenton, NJ 08619, (609) 896-9500, BS 74 Seton Hall Univ; MA 75 Montclair St Coll; Superv of Sp Serv, St Lawrence Rehab Cen, **SLP**

Stanley, Beverly A Taylor Education Bldg, University Of Kentucky, Room 229, Lexington, KY 40506, (606) 257-7924, BA 58 Univ of KY; MA 59 Univ of KY; 60–Assistant Professor, University of Kentucky, **SLP A**

Stanley, Dr Elnita O Box 6146, SFA Station, Nacogdoches, TX 75962, (409) 569-2906, BS 44 Northwestern Univ; MA 47 Columbia Univ Teachers Coll; ED 72 (Speech Path) Univ of Northern CO; 88–Prof, S F Austin St U, **SLP**

Stanley, Gay 199 Hess Street South, Hamilton, ON, Canada L2S 2H5, (416) 521-2100, MA 86 SUNY - Center at Buffalo; **SLP**

Stanley, Mrs Jane Tartre 45 West Acres Drive, Lunenburg, MA 01462, (617) 365-4531, BS 73 Ithaca Coll; MS 78 Syracuse Univ; Sp-Path Consult, Norht Central Human Serv, **SLP**

Stanley, Lee Ann 1880 South Wyoming, Salt Lake City, UT 84108, (801) 393-3411, BS 81 IL St Univ - Normal; MS 84 Eastern IL Univ; Sp-Lang Path, Weber Trng Ctr for the Hndcpd, **SLP**

Stanley, Linda H 356-D Whitestown Road, Butler, PA 16001, (412) 287-4781, BS 69 Univ Southern MS-Hattiesburg; MS 75 Univ Southern MS-Hattiesburg; Aud, VA Med Cen, **A**

Stanley, Mrs Margaret D 3201 East Oaklawn Drive, Muncie, IN 47303, (317) 747-5401, BA 52 Ball St Univ; MA 63 Ball St Univ; Sp/Lang Path, Muncie Comm Sch, **SLP**

Stanley, Renee L 1 Queensview Court, Dallas, TX 75225, (214) 368-1197, BS 75 Southern Methodist Univ; MS 77 Southern Methodist Univ; **SLP**

Stanley, Ruth J H 25 Lexington Park, Vienna, WV 26105, (304) 295-9509, BS 79 Stephen F Austin St Univ; ME 81 Stephen F Austin St Univ; Sp/Lang Path, ISD, **SLP**

Stanley, Mrs Sue L 3217 17th Street, Santa Monica, CA 90405, (213) 393-2785, MA 68 Univ of the Pacific; BS 67 Univ of the Pacific; **SLP**

Stanley, Mrs Susan Plaster Box 101 L-18, St Leonard, MD 20685, (301) 586-1251, BS 85 Univ of VA - Charlottesville; ME 87 Univ of VA - Charlottesville; Sp-Lang Path, St Marys Public Schools, **SLP**

Stanley, Susan Williams 14 Desoto Circle, Texarkana, TX 75703, (214) 793-5606, BS 76 Univ of AZ; MS 77 Univ of AZ; **SLP**

Stannard, Margaret K 4725 West Quincy #208, Denver, CO 80236, (303) 798-2811, BA 72 Univ of CO - Boulder; MA 74 Univ of CO - Boulder; ED 80 (NS) Univ of Northern CO; President, Comprehensive Learning Assoc, **SLP**

Stansberry, Gloria Bisson 6222 Brookside Drive, Cleveland, OH 44144, (216) 398-8226, BA 85 Cleveland St Univ; MA 86 Cleveland St Univ; 86–Sp-Lang Path, Cuyahoga Co Bd of Mental Ret, **SLP**

Stansbury, Mrs Carol Lee 22707 Susanna Avenue, Torrance, CA 90505-3220, (213) 545-5887, BA 77 CA Lutheran Coll; Sp-Lang Path, LA USD, **SLP**

Stansell, Dr Barbara J 6843 Fashion Hills Boulevard, San Diego, CA 92111, (619) 277-7738, BS 39 Washington Univ; MA 55 CA St Univ - Los Angeles; PH 69 (Communicative Disorders) Univ of Southern CA; Retired, Chapman Coll, **SLP LM**

Stanton, Dr Fred E E 1540 South Riverton, Spokane, WA 99207, (509) 535-6267, BA 40 Whitman Coll; MA 52 Gonzaga Univ; PH 62 (NS) WA St Univ; Prof Sp/Lang Path, Gonzaga U, **SLP LM**

Stanton, Karen M Dept Rehabilitation Medicine, University Of Washington, Rj-30, Seattle, WA 98195, (206) 545-7457, BS 76 Univ of OR; MS 79 Univ of WA; Sp-Lang Path, University of Washington, **SLP**

Stanton, Kay 448 Paseo Companeros, Chico, CA 95928-8857, (916) 893-4355, MA 74 CA St Univ - Northridge; Teacher, Glenn County Supt of Schools, **SLP**

Stanton, Lisa Ann 332 Commonwealth Avenue, Springfield, MA 01108, (413) 589-9161, BS 77 SUNY - Coll at Geneseo; MA 84 Univ of MA - Amherst; Sp-Lang Path / Teacher, Childrens Lang Inst, **SLP**

Stanton, Lydia Dawn 5503 Swift Current Court, Burke, VA 22015, MS 83 James Madison Univ; **SLP**

Stanush, Mrs Priscilla Diane Route 9 Box 113-A, Converse, TX 78109, (512) 672-6592, BS 83 Univ of TX - Austin; MA 85 Our Lady Lake Univ-San Anton; 85, Warm Springs Rehab Hosp, **SLP**

Stanzel, Laurel Strong Memorial Hospital, 601 Elmwood Avenue Box 629, Rochester, NY 14642, (716) 275-2501, BA 77 Univ of IA; MA 79 Univ of IA; Aud, Strong Mem Hosp, **A**

Stapell, Mrs Jamie Michele 7918 S W 13th Road, Gainesville, FL 32607, (904) 392-2041, BA 81 Univ of FL; MA 84 Univ of FL; **SLP**

Stapells, Dr David Richard Albert Einstein Coll Of Med, Kennedy Center Room 817, 1410 Pelham Parkway, Bronx, NY 10461, (212) 430-3147, BA 79 Simon Fraser Univ - Bc; PH 84 (Evoked Potentials) Univ of Ottawa - Ontario; Dir, Albert Einstein College of Med

Staples, Kimberly Anna 4733 N O'Connor Road #1059, Irving, TX 75062, (804) 798-7376, BA 84 Coll of William & Mary; MS 86 James Madison Univ; Clinician, **SLP**

Staples, Theresa O 3131 Waterton Drive, Midlothian, VA 23113, (804) 230-1388, BA 63 Greensboro Coll; ME 69 Univ of VA - Charlottesville; 69–Aud, VA Med Cen, **SLP A**

Stapleton, Eileen T 2-C Soundview Gardens, Port Washington, Elmont, NY 11050, (516) 542-3933, BS 69 Saint John's Univ - Jamaica; MA 72 CUNY - Queens Coll; Sp-Lang Path, Nassau Co Med Cen, **SLP**

Stapleton, Jenny 1111 Houghton Road #905, Katy, TX 77450, (713) 550-8282, BS 81 IL St Univ - Normal; MA 84 Univ of Houston - Univ Park; **SLP**

Star, Alice Jo 605 Rex Street, South Bend, IN 46616, (414) 372-0641, MS 74 IN St Univ - Terre Haute; Sp-Lang Path, United Health Services, **SLP**

Starch, Mrs Sandy Abolins 3615 Mountain View Drive, Rocklin, CA 95677-1920, (916) 791-7067, BA 81 Univ of WA; MS 82 Univ of WA; 87–Sp-Lang Path, Meadowbrook Rehab Group, **SLP**

Starck, MaryJo 9023 Barcelona Street, Naval Hospital, Oakland, CA 94605, (415) 633-0649, BA 81 Creighton Univ; MS 82 Marquette Univ; Sp-Lang Path, Private Practice, **SLP**

Stare, Mrs Tina M 2203 Briarwood Drive, Elizabeth Township, Mc Keesport, PA 15135, (412) 751-6305, BS 74 Shippensburg Univ of PA; MS 80 Rutgers St Univ -N Brunswick; **SLP**

Stark, Mrs Betsie Dillard 1347 Ewald S E, Salem, OR 97302, (503) 588-5124, BA 79 CA St Univ - Long Beach; **SLP**

Stark, Diane Elizabeth 3023 Puckett Road #17, Kansas City, KS 66103, (913) 621-5155, BA 78 Creighton Univ; MS 80 Central MO St Univ; Sp-Lang Path, Bd of Ed Sch Dist 500, **SLP**

Stark, Dr Earl W Scott And White Clinic, 2401 South 31st Street, Temple, TX 76508, (817) 774-2754, BA 57 Univ of UT; MA 58 OH St Univ; PH 63 (Aud) Univ of MN - Minneap-St Paul; 83–Aud & Ch: Aud Sect, Scott & White Cl, **A F**

Stark, Elizabeth A 723 North Pomeroy, Hill City, KS 67642, (417) 667-4528, BA 85 Wichita St Univ; MA 87 Wichita St Univ; 88–Sp-Lang Path, Develop Svc of NW KS, **SLP**

Stark, Mrs Irene Anstendig 9511 S W 6th Court, Pembroke Pines, FL 33025, (305) 765-6551, BA 76 CUNY - City College; MA 78 CUNY - City College; Sp-Lang Path, Private Practice, **SLP**

Stark, Dr Joel Program Director, Queens College, Flushing, NY 11367, (212) 520-7358, BA 50 Long Island U - Brooklyn Ctr; MA 51 Columbia Univ Teachers Coll; PH 56 (NS) NY Univ; Prof & Dir-Sp & Hrng Cen, Queens Coll of CUNY, **SLP F ACE**

Stark, Lois D 139 Ridge Park Avenue, Stamford, CT 06905, BS 77 Northwestern Univ; MS 78 Univ of WI - Madison; **SLP**

Stark, Mary Beth Van Osten 2301 Holmes Way, Schaumburg, IL 60194, (312) 843-8953, **SLP**

Stark, Dr Rachel E 1716 Fernleaf Drive, West Lafayette, IN 47906, (317) 494-3788, BA 46 0174; MA 61 Northwestern Univ; PH 65 (NS) Univ of OK Medical Center; 87–Dept Head Aud/Sp Sci, Purdue Univ, **SLP F**

Starkel, John Philip 3518 Cotillion, Plano, TX 75074, (214) 248-6300, BA 68 Hastings Coll; MS 75 Univ of KS; PH 78 (Learning Disabilities) Univ of KS; Editor In Ch, DLM Teaching Resources

Starkey, Mrs Aleecia A P O Box 5503, Jacksonville, AR 72076, (501) 370-1830, OB 73 AR St Univ; OM 77 AR St Univ; Sp-Lang Path, Dennis Dev Ctr Ark Children's Hosp, **SLP ACE**

Starkey, Mrs Cynthia Lynn 27476 Limones, Mission Viejo, CA 92691, (714) 828-0350, **SLP**

Starkey, Mrs Marta I Route 1 Box 415J, White Plains, MD 20695, (301) 934-4687, MS 79 WV Univ; 86–Sp-Lang Path, Charles Co Bd of Educ, **SLP**

Starkey, Mrs Martha Krisko 6837 Centennial Drive, Reynoldsburg, OH 43068, (614) 294-6403, BS 79 Univ of Toledo; BA 79 Univ of Toledo; MA 80 Bowling Green St Univ; Sp-Lang Path, Columbus Speech-Hearing Center, **SLP**

Starkey, Mary B 134 Pennbrook Avenue, Robesonia, PA 19551, BS 77 WV Univ; MS 79 WV Univ; MS 79 WV Univ; SLP/Aud, Reading Rehab Hosp, **SLP A**

Starkey, Mrs Shirley J Box 38, Institute, WV 25112, (304) 766-4873, BA 56 Tougaloo Coll; MS 57 CUNY - Hunter Coll; MA 60 Univ of IA; 86–Chief Sp-Lang Path, West Virginia Rehabilitatn Ctr, **SLP**

Stark-Nemon, Barbara A 1922 Day Street, Ann Arbor, MI 48104, (313) 662-4366, BA 71 Univ of MI - Ann Arbor; MS 77 Univ of MI - Ann Arbor; Sp-Lang Path, Ann Arbor Public Schools, **SLP**

Starks, Janet Marie 5244 West 126 Terrace, Leawood, KS 66211-3126, (913) 491-5553, **SLP**

Starks, Mary Alice 641 South 217th Street, Elkhorn, NE 68022, (402) 289-4080, BS 84 Univ of NE - Omaha; MS 86 Univ of OK Medical Center; **SLP**

Starkweather, Dr C Woodruff 457 Old Farm Road, Wyncote, PA 19095, (215) 886-0368, BA 61 Hamilton Coll; PH 70 (NS) Southern IL Univ -Carbondale; Prof, Temple Univ, **SLP F**

Starling, Mrs Julia Mary 1836 Busch Court, Fort Collins, CO 80525, (303) 482-7890, OB 71 Univ of London - England; MS 88 CO St Univ

Starliper, Deborah S 210 Orchard Drive, Purcellville, VA 22132, (703) 777-7421, BS 77 Univ of VA - Charlottesville; ME 78 Univ of VA - Charlottesville; Sp-Lang Path, Loudoun Co Pub Sch, **SLP**

Starll, Steven 18812 Martin Place, Woodhaven, MI 48183, (313) 562-6000, **SLP**

Starman, Christine Joy 35 Judith Drive, Danbury, CT 06811, (203) 797-4761, BS 82 Southwest TX St Univ; ME 84 Southwest TX St Univ; 88–Sp-Lang Path, Danbury PS, **SLP**

Starmer, Dr Garrett L Special Services Center, 1430 The Esplanade, Suite 16, Chico, CA 95926, (916) 891-6629, BA 40 Stanford Univ; MA 43 Stanford Univ; PH 53 (NS) Univ of UT; Owner, Spec Services Cen, **SLP**

Starn, Cynthia Jo 38 Bell Street, Chicopee, MA 01013, (413) 592-7855, BS 84 Northeastern Univ; MA 86 Univ of MA - Amherst; **A**

Starnes, Deborah Kaye 7800 Greenview, Detroit, MI 48228, (313) 494-2201, **A**

Starobin, Mrs Caryl W 1023 East Glenbrook Road, Milwaukee, WI 53217, (414) 354-7878, BS 53 Univ of WI - Madison; MS 70 Univ of WI - Milwaukee; Sp-Lang Path, Sch Dist of Brown Deer, **SLP**

Staron, Maryann 141 Barkley Avenue, Clifton, NJ 07011, (201) 234-0011, BA 76 Kean Coll of NJ; MA 85 Montclair St Coll; **SLP**

Starp, Carolyn Gail 6513 Gates Mills Boulevard, Mayfield Heights, OH 44124-4221, (216) 492-6180, BA 84 Case Western Reserve Univ; MA 85 Case Western Reserve Univ; 87–Sp-Lang Path, InSpeech Inc, **SLP**

Starr, Dr Clark D Communication Disorders, 115 Shevlin Hall, 164 Pillsbury Drive S E, Minneapolis, MN 55455, (612) 373-4116, BS 50 Hamline Univ; PH 56 (Sp Path) Northwestern Univ; Prof, Univ of Minn 1954, **SLP F**

Starr, Deborah H 4525 Sequoia Road, Memphis, TN 38117, (901) 761-1220, Aud, ENT Group, **A**

Starr, Kathleen M 12204 S E 31st Place #110, Milwaukie, OR 97222, (503) 654-6441, BS 76 Portland St Univ; MS 78 Portland St Univ; SLP, N Clackamas Sch Dist 12, **SLP**

Starr, Mrs Lee Anne M 6 Beech Drive, Apartment 5, Norwich, CT 06360, (203) 447-3106, BS 82 Worcester St Coll; MA 85 Univ of CT; New London Public School, **SLP**

Starr, Mrs Marilyn W A-4 St Marc Circle, South Windsor, CT 06074, (203) 289-3393, BA 75 SUNY - Coll at Cortland; MS 76 Ithaca Coll; 79–Sp-Lang Path, Manchester Pub Sch, **SLP**

Starr, Mrs Nancy E 14310 Citation, San Antonio, TX 78248, (512) 492-9494, BS 72 TX Tech Univ; MA 75 Our Lady Lake Univ-San Anton; Sp-Lang Path, NE ISD, **SLP**

Starr, Mrs Nancy S 7106 Blazier Court, Louisville, KY 40228, (502) 239-3061, BS 62 Eastern MI Univ; MS 80 Univ of Louisville; SLP, Jefferson Co Sch, **SLP**

Starr, Noreen 6 Donnamora Crescent, Thornhill, ON, Canada L3T 4K5, (416) 886-0262, BA 74 York Univ - Ontario; MS 76 Boston Univ

Starr, Sheryl Silver 5241 Meadowknoll Lane, Columbus, OH 43220, (614) 459-4066, BA 81 Univ of Miami; MA 85 OH St Univ; **A**

Starsoneck, Karen Ann 70 Follett Street, East Providence, RI 02914, (401) 277-5485, BA 80 Univ of RI; MA 81 Western MI Univ; Sp/Lang Path, RI Hosp, **SLP**

Stasiak, Mrs Vicki W 3276 Hampton Ridge Drive, Marietta, GA 30066, (404) 924-0561, BS 72 Northern IL Univ - De Kalb; MA 73 Northern IL Univ - De Kalb; SLP, Sedom, **SLP**

Stassen, Raymond A 35 Castle Heights Avenue, Tarrytown, NY 10591, (201) 456-4967, BA 52; MA 63 Univ of MN - Minneap-St Paul; Dir Aud Serv, U of Med & Dent of Nj, **A**

Stassi, Dr Eugene J 2412 Pressburg Street, New Orleans, LA 70122, (504) 568-5028, BA 58 Univ Southern MS-Hattiesburg; MS 65 Univ Southern MS-Hattiesburg; PH 68 (NS) Univ Southern MS-Hattiesburg; Admin, Dept of Hlth & Human Resources, **SLP**

Stastny, Mrs Gwynn S 3836 Homeward Road, Richmond, VA 23234, (804) 271-8690, BS 64 Univ of NE - Lincoln; **SLP**

Staten, Mrs Kathleen Ann 809 Yale, Edwardsville, IL 62025, MS 82 Fontbonne Coll; **SLP**

Statham, Sherri Lynn 2529 N W 61st, Oklahoma City, OK 73112, (405) 848-0920, BA 84 Univ of OK - Norman; MS 86 Univ of OK Medical Center; **A**

Stathis, Eileen 183 Beach 127 Street, Belle Harbor, NY 11694, (718) 318-1642, BA 83 SUNY - Coll at Cortland; MA 85 NY Univ; 88–Sp-Lang Path, Brooklyn Sp Lang Path Associates PC, **SLP**

Stathopoulos, Dr Elaine T Dept Communication Dis & Sci, State Univ Of New York, Park Hall Room 109, Buffalo, NY 14260, (716) 636-3400, BS 71 Univ of WI - Milwaukee; MS 73 Univ of WI - Madison; PH 80 (Sp Science) IN Univ - Bloomington; Assoc Prof, SUNY-Buffalo, **SLP**

Statkus, Donna Ahlert 9122 West 140th Street, Orland Park, IL 60462, (312) 349-3812, BA 81 Saint Xavier Coll; OM 85 Governors St Univ; 86–Chief Sp-Lang Path, Little Company of Mary Hosp, **SLP**

Statland, Alexandra 628 Somerset Drive, Indianapolis, IN 46260, SLP, **SLP**

Staton, Mrs Deborah P Rural Route 1, Versailles, IL 62378, (217) 225-3531, BS 76 Western IL Univ; MA 78 Western IL Univ; Sp/Lang Path, Brown Co Comm Sch Dist, **SLP**

Staton, Mrs Patricia A 7020 North Broad Street, Apartment C-6, Philadelphia, PA 19126, (215) 549-9309, MS 87 Clarion Univ of PA; 87–Sp-Lang Path, Robin Muller & Assoc

Staton, Robert N 3302 46th Court S E, Olympia, WA 98501, (206) 456-1122, BA 69 WA St Univ; MA 76 WA St Univ; 83–Aud, Memorial Clinic Ltd Ps, **A**

Staton, Mrs Yvonne Fauber 2708 Lakeside Drive, Lynchburg, VA 24502, (804) 528-0100, BS 81 Radford Univ; MS 82 Radford Univ; 88–Sp-Lang Path, Laurel Reg Sch, **SLP**

Staubach, Lynn Carol 7110 Captains Cove Court, Alexandria, VA 22310, (703) 922-0104, BA 83 Rutger's St Univ - Douglas Coll; MA 85 George Washington Univ; Sp-Lang Path, Self Employed/Contract-Cheryl Person & Assoc, **SLP**

Stauber, Mary Brudnicki 3 Falkirk Road, Hawthorne Woods, IL 60047, (312) 438-6319, MS 76 Univ of WI - Stevens Point; Administrator, Hawthorn Rehab Ser, **SLP**

Stauber, Ronald C 3105-X North Frontage Road, Arlington Height, IL 60004, (312) 632-0160

Stauber, Shoshana 4201 Torrance Blvd #140, Torrance, CA 90503-3711, (213) 540-4327, BS 82 San Diego St Univ; MS 84 Univ of Redlands; 86–Dir Sp/Lang Path, Parker Hearing & Speech Institute, **SLP**

Stauble, Ann-Marie Elizabeth 25728 Miramonte St, Redlands, CA 92373, (714) 796-2304, MS 83 Univ of Redlands; PH 81 (NS) Univ of CA - Los Angeles; Sp-Lang Path, Kaiser Permanente, **SLP**

Stauffer, Regis Jean 5702 Avondale Street, Duluth, MN 55804, (218) 726-7993, BS 82 Univ of MN - Duluth; MA 83 Univ of MN - Duluth; Instr/Clin Supvr, Univ of MN-Duluth, **SLP**

Staugler, Mrs Kathy M P O Box 432, Fort Recovery, OH 45846, (419) 586-6628, BS 72 Ball St Univ; MA 75 Ball St Univ; Sp-Lang Path, Mercer Co Bd of Educ, **SLP**

Stavolone, Patricia A 15 Old Pine Island Road, Newbury, MA 01950-4834, BS 75 Emerson Coll; MS 76 Columbia Univ Teachers Coll; 87–Dir-Clin Svcs, Easter Seal of NH, **SLP**

Stayer, Mrs Janet H 7633 Totman Road, North Syracuse, NY 13212, (315) 457-2889, BA 85 SUNY - Coll at Cortland; MS 87 Syracuse Univ; 88–Aud, SUNY Health Science Ctr, **A**

Steadham, Renee G 954 Coronado Drive, Gulf Breeze, FL 32561, (904) 474-8328, BA 80 Auburn Univ - Auburn; MS 81 Auburn Univ - Auburn; 86–Aud, Med Ctr Clinic PA, **A**

Steadman, Dorothy Bates 6317 Wildwood Trail #B, Myrtle Beach, SC 29577, (803) 272-2292, BS 82 East Carolina Univ; MS 84 East Carolina Univ; Aud, Hearing Centers of America Inc, **A**

Steadman, Maryanne R R 1 Box 217, Cummington, MA 01026, (413) 634-2174, MA 87 Univ of MA - Amherst; **SLP**

Steadman, Sharon K 1525 Gentry Boulevard, Gering, NE 69341, (308) 635-3696, BS 65 Chadron St Coll; MA 67 Univ of NE - Lincoln; 67–Consultant, Educ Service Unit No 13, **SLP**

Stearn, Mrs Diane M 5660 Buffwood Place, Agoura Hills, CA 91301, (818) 991-3787, BS 70 MI St Univ; MA 74 Eastern MI Univ; 88–Sp-Lang Path, Los Angeles USD, **SLP**

Stearns, Agnes T 15963 Viney Creek, Houston, TX 77095, (713) 855-9732, MA; **SLP**

Stearns, Mrs Cynthia Sims 1110 4th Avenue, Opelika, AL 36801, (404) 832-1488, BA 80 Auburn Univ - Montgomery; MS 81 Auburn Univ - Auburn; Aud, John Burson MD, **A**

Stearns, Martha R 1800 Old Meadow Road #713, Mc Lean, VA 22102, (703) 356-5199, BS 48 Univ of AR - Fayetteville; MA 62 Univ of KS; SLP, Fairfax Co VA Pub Sch, **SLP ACE**

Stearns, Mrs Phyllis Brusie 54 Calhoun Street, Torrington, CT 06790, (203) 482-8708, BA 78 Univ of CT; MS 80 Bloomsburg Univ of PA; Aud, **A**

Stearns, Terah Ann Martin Box 202 Route 4, Harrisburg, IL 62946-9431, (618) 252-8673, MS 80 Southern IL Univ -Carbondale; Sp-Lang Path, Harrisburg Pub Schs, **SLP**

Stebbins, Willard P P O Box 935, Manchester, CT 06040, **SLP**

Stec, Mrs Jonelle Irene 7444 Theisen, Dearborn, MI 48126, (313) 453-1300, **SLP**

Stechel, Barbara Gordon 110 East Rockaway Road, Hewlett, NY 11557, **SLP**

Stechel, Sandra S 79-36 214th Street, Oakland Gardens, NY 11364, **SLP**

Stecher, Catherine P O Box 522, Greenville, RI 02828-0522, (401) 949-4182, **SLP**

Steck, Cynthia Diane 32 Holly Court, Mercerville, NJ 08619, BA 85 Univ of MO - KS City; MS 87 Univ of Southwestern LA

Steck, Mrs Mary Theresa 205 East Irving Street, Normal, IL 61761, BS 84 Purdue Univ - West Lafayette; MS 86 IN St Univ - Terre Haute; **SLP**

Steck, Mrs Rosemary A 3377 Alderdale, Sterling Heights, MI 48310, (313) 651-6210, BA 79 MI St Univ; MA 80 MI St Univ; Sp-Lang Path, Rochester Comm Sch, **SLP**

Steckbeck, Mrs Pamela Meza 4187 Lodi-Way, San Diego, CA 92117, (619) 281-6644, BA 81 San Diego St Univ; MA 83 San Diego St Univ; Sp-Lang Path, San Diego USD, **SLP**

Steckel, Laura Ann 6266 Portage Street N W #6, North Canton, OH 44720, (215) 631-9300, BS 85 Univ of Akron; MA 87 Univ of Akron

Steckel, Mary Clare W200 S10715 East Shore Dr, Muskego, WI 53150, BS 74 Marquette Univ; MS 75 Marquette Univ; 87–Sp-Lang Path, Lutheran Social Services

Stecker, Kay E S 6843 Tuxedo Road, San Diego, CA 92119, **A**

Stecker, Dr Nancy A 29 Bentham Parkway, Amherst, NY 14226, (716) 636-3400, MS 77 SUNY - Coll at Buffalo; MA 79 SUNY - Center at Buffalo; PH 84 (Aud) SUNY - Center at Buffalo; Cl Asst Prof, SUNY-Buffalo, **SLP A**

Steckler, Jane F 132 North Ridgewood Place, Los Angeles, CA 90004, (213) 688-3850, BA 74 CUNY - Hunter Coll; MA 76 Univ of CA - Santa Barbara; Aud, Los Angeles VA Outpatient Cl, **A**

Steckler, Mrs Susan Elizabeth 12150 Pebblebrook Court, Indianapolis, IN 46236, (317) 823-1690, BS 78 IN Univ - Bloomington; MA 84 Ball St Univ; 85–Sp-Lang Path, Hancock-South Madison Jt Svcs, **SLP**

Steckley, J Lynn 110 Bayberry Lane, Watchung, NJ 07060, (201) 233-3720, BA 59 Montclair St Coll; MA 79 Trenton St Coll; SLP, Childrens Specialized Hosp, **SLP ACE**

Steckol, Dr Karen Faye 11608 Frank Avenue, Louisville, KY 40243, (502) 588-5274, BS 71 IN Univ - Bloomington; MA 72 Memphis St Univ; PH 78 (NS) Memphis St Univ; Assoc Prof, University of Louisville, **SLP ACE**

Steddum, Mrs Mary Y 2835 East 48th Street, Tulsa, OK 74105, (918) 749-2217, BA 70 Northeastern OK St Univ; MS 72 Central MO St Univ; Sp-Lang Path, Home Health Care Contract, **SLP**

Stedge, Mrs Patricia F 35 Major Andre Drive, Stony Point, NY 10980, (914) 947-1000, BS 73 Ashland Coll; MS 77 William Paterson Coll; Sp/Lang Path, Letchworth Village Dev Cen, **SLP**

Steeb, Carol L 1201 Westminster Row #733, Greenwood, IN 46142, (317) 888-2398, MS 87 Purdue Univ - West Lafayette; **A**

Steed, Susie F Susie F Steed Sp & Lang Rehab, 5 Lagrange Street #2, Newnan, GA 30263, (404) 251-3558, BS 71 Old Dominion Univ; ME 72 Univ of VA - Charlottesville; Owner, Susie F Steed Sp & Lang Rehab, **SLP**

Steege, Mrs Suzanne E 4402 Somerset Lane, Madison, WI 53711, (608) 884-9402, BA 65 Valparaiso Univ; MS 69 Southern CT St Univ; 78–Sp-Lang Path, Edgerton Commun Sch, **SLP**

Steel, Mrs Kelly N 203 Arriba Drive #2, Sunnyvale, CA 94086, (415) 968-5548, BS 85 Eastern IL Univ; MS 86 Eastern IL Univ; **SLP**

Steele, Mrs Connie Elaine 121 Pearl Street, Iowa City, IA 52245, (815) 589-2911, BS 67 Purdue Univ - West Lafayette; MS 70 Purdue Univ - West Lafayette; 88–Sp-Lang Path, River Bend Sch Dist, **SLP**

Steele, Mrs Dedra L Rehab Service Of N Ctrl Ohio, 270 Sterkel Boulevard, Mansfield, OH 44904, (419) 756-1133, BA 77 Bowling Green St Univ; MA 78 Kent St Univ; Sp-Lang Path, Rehab Serv N Cen Oh, **SLP**

Steele, Eileen R 240 Hanford Street, Columbus, OH 43206, (614) 444-5460, BS 84 Marywood Coll; MS 85 Clarion Univ of PA; 88–Sp-Lang Path, Affiliated Aud & Sp Path, **SLP**

Steele, Mrs Elizabeth 1458 Scalesville Road, Summerfield, NC 27358, (919) 349-4632, BA 67 Duke Univ; MS 74 Univ of NC - Chapel Hill; Sp-Lang Path, Reidsville Cty Sch, **SLP**

Steele, Judith M 8 Briargate Circle, Aurora, IL 60506, (312) 466-1534, BA 74 Vanderbilt Univ; MA 77 OH St Univ; **SLP**

Steele, Judy K P O Box 1103, Elk City, OK 73648, (405) 225-7722, BS 74 OK St Univ; MA 75 OK St Univ; 81–Sp/Lang Path, Elk City Publs Schs, **SLP**

Steele, Mrs Lisa E 17714 Surreywest Lane, Spring, TX 77379, (713) 376-3704, BA 79 Univ of NC - Chapel Hill; MS 81 Univ of Louisville; Coord of Sp & Hrng Serv, Wendell Foster Cen for Cp, **SLP**

Steele, Lynne Jeck 4709 Stoughton Court, Indianapolis, IN 46254, (317) 871-2270, BA 79 IN Univ - Bloomington; ME 81 Univ of VA - Charlottesville; 82–Aud, St Vincent Hosp & Hlth Care Ce, **A**

Steele, Merri L 3456 Donald Street, Eugene, OR 97405, BS 72 Western IL Univ; MA 73 Western IL Univ; SLP, Eugene School District, **SLP**

Steele, Michele Shelly PO Box 551, Janesville, CA 96114, (916) 253-3815, BA 85 CA St Univ - Chico; MA 87 CA St Univ - Chico; Sp-Lang Path, Lassen Co Sch Supt

Steele, Mrs Nancy R P O Box 7553, Incline Village, NV 89450, (702) 825-6006, BA 70 CA St Univ - Fresno; MA 72 CA St Univ - Fresno; Aud, Reno Hrng Ctr, **A**

Steele, Mrs Sandra Covell 217 Sunrise Drive, Rd #2, Irwin, PA 15642, (412) 394-5815, BS 76 Edinboro Univ of PA; ME 80 Clarion Univ of PA

Steele, Mrs Sandra D P O Box 602, Frankfort, MI 49635, (602) 879-6634, MA 85 Western WA Univ; **A**

Steele, William Fredrick 6426 Primrose Place, Richmond, VA 23225, (804) 353-9780, MS 84 Radford Univ; 88–Aud, Maico Hearing Aid Svc, **A**

Steelman, Mrs Anna A 109 Leslie Court, Advance, NC 27006, (919) 284-2581, BS 79 Appalachian St Univ; MA 80 Appalachian St Univ; Sp-Lang Path, Davie County PS, **SLP**

Steelman, Carol R P O Box 14484, Fort Lauderdale, FL 33302, **SLP**

Steelman, Mrs Mary L 4201 Lee Avenue, Little Rock, AR 72205, (501) 370-1652, OB 66 Henderson St Univ; MA 72 Univ of AR - Fayetteville; Coord/Sp-Lang Path, Little Rock Sch Dist, **SLP**

Steely, Brian Richard P O Box 1364, Sisters, OR 97759, (503) 549-8981, BA 71 Southern OR St Coll; MA 85 Univ of OR; Sp-Lang Path, Sisters School District 6, **SLP**

Steen, Cynthia A 4608 North Kenwood, Kansas City, MO 64116, (816) 356-0500, OB 74 Central MO St Univ; MS 76 Central MO St Univ; Aud, Dr Guy A Francis / Otor, **A**

Steen, Mrs Lisa Ann 35 Lexington Parkway, Rochester, NY 14624-4242, (716) 426-0059, BS 82 Elmira Coll; MA 84 SUNY - Coll at Geneseo; **SLP**

Steenbarger, Mrs Donna D 8230 Bishops Lane, Indianapolis, IN 46217, (317) 243-7559, BS 64 Purdue Univ - West Lafayette; MS 66 Ball St Univ; Sp-Lang Path, Rise Spec Serv-Indpls, **SLP**

Steenhausen, Joan M 883 Seminole #3, Elgin, IL 60120, (312) 426-1250, BS 74 Purdue Univ - West Lafayette; MA 76 Ball St Univ; Sp-Lang Path, Comm Ut Sch Dist 300, **SLP**

Steensland, Dianne D 2806 Briar Cliff Road, Dothan, AL 36301, (205) 793-5771, BA 73 Univ of AL- Tuscaloosa; MA 75 Univ of AL- Tuscaloosa; Sp-Lang Path Director, Steensland Ctr for Sp Path, **SLP**

Steenson, Juliet B 1540 Hoover Avenue, Eau Claire, WI 54701, MS 76 Univ of WI - Eau Claire; Sp-Lang Path, Fall Creek School System, **SLP**

Steer, Mrs Elizabeth (Betsy) L 5206 Olympia Fields, Houston, TX 77069, (713) 580-3277, **SLP**

Steer, Dr Mack David 342 Westview Circle, West Lafayette, IN 47906, (317) 494-3825, MA 33 Univ of IA; OD 57 Long Island U - Brooklyn Ctr; PH 38 (NS) Univ of IA; Dist Prof Emeritus, Prudue Univ, **SLP F H LM**

Steer, Ruth K 342 Westview Circle, West Lafayette, IN 47906, (317) 463-9471, BS Univ of WI - Madison; MS Purdue Univ - West Lafayette; **SLP LM**

Steeves, Nancy C R R 1 Box 435, Sebago Lake, ME 04075, (207) 874-1065, BA 72 Univ of ME - Orono; MS 85 Northeastern Univ; 86–Aud, Northeast Hrng & Sp Ctr Inc, **A**

Steeves, Sherri Lee P O Box 1123, Frisco, CO 80443, (303) 486-2603, BA 82 Univ of CO - Boulder; MS 84 Univ of VT; 87–Sp-Lang Path, Mtn Bd of Cooperative Services, **SLP**

Stefan, Loretta 760 Metro Lane N E, Albuquerque, NM 87123, (505) 864-2215, BS 78 NM St Univ; MA 80 NM St Univ; 81–Sp/Lang Path, Belen Consolidated Schs, **SLP**

Stefanakos, Karlene M 19202 Blount Road, Lutz, FL 33549, BA 70 WA St Univ; MA 80 Univ of NC - Greensboro; Dir, Forrest Oaks Sp/Lang Cl, **SLP**

Stefanini, Mrs Sally Butler 402 Bancroft Road, Liberty, MO 64068, (816) 781-6456, 88–Sp-Lang Path, Liberty MO Sch Dist, **SLP**

Stefankiewicz, Sabina P 646 44th Street, Brooklyn, NY 11220, **SLP**

Stefanski-Brown, Margaret Bridget 5006 West Placita DE Los, Vientos, Tucson, AZ 85745-9729, (602) 621-3727, BS 82 Univ of AZ; MS 84 Univ of AZ; Aud, Univ of Arizona, **A**

Steffan, Karen Anne 1940 Pacific Beach Dr #J, San Diego, CA 92109, (408) 899-7015, MA 83 CA St Univ - Sacramento; Sp-Lang Path, Natl City Schl Dstr, **SLP**

Steffan, Sharon H R R 3 Box 314, Montgomery City, MO 63361, (314) 849-4770, BS 77 Fontbonne Coll; MS 78 Fontbonne Coll; SLP, Spec Sch Dist-St Louis Co, **SLP**

Steffel, Sue Reedy 915 Barkstone Court S E, Salem, OR 97306, (503) 399-3138, BS 74 Univ of WI - Oshkosh; MS 83 AZ St Univ; Sp-Lang Path, Salem Keizer PS, **SLP**

Steffen, Mrs Catherine 1310 Roger Street, Stevens Point, WI 54481, (715) 345-5424, BS 71 Univ of WI - Stevens Point; MS 72 Univ of WI - Stevens Point; 72–Sp-Lang Path, Stevens Pt Area Bd of Ed, **SLP**

Steffen, Colette M 25075 8th Avenue, Los Molinos, CA 96055, (916) 384-1996, BS 72 Portland St Univ; MS 74 Portland St Univ; **SLP**

Steffen, Mrs Paula S 2276 Broken Horse Lane, St Louis, MO 63129, (314) 846-2335, BA 80 Univ of MO - Columbia; MA 87 Fontbonne Coll; 87–Sp-Lang Path, St Joseph's Hosp

Steffen, Susan Rae 1903 Willow Drive, Grand Forks, ND 58201, (701) 324-4811, BA 83 Univ of ND; MS 84 Minot St Univ; Sp-Lang Path, Lonetree Special Ed Unit, **SLP**

Steffens, April 1526 Solano N E, Albuquerque, NM 87110, **SLP**

Steffens, Janet S R R 1 Box 51, Acton, ME 04001, BA 67 SUNY - Center at Albany; MS 77 Boston Univ; SLP, Private Practice, **SLP**

Steffens, Michele Leigh The Mailman Ctr For Child Dev, Univ Of Miami Schl Of Med, P O Box 016820 (D-820), Miami, FL 33101, (305) 547-6350, BS 82 Western MI Univ; MS 85 Univ of South FL; **A**

Steffensmeier, Anne E 4013 Lexington Drive N E #B, Cedar Rapids, IA 52402, (319) 399-6855, BS 73 Northeast MO St Univ; MA 74 Northeast MO St Univ; Sp-Lang Path, Grantwood AEA, **SLP**

Stefka, Mrs Paulette Sue 1901 Cedarberry Road, North Platte, NE 69101, (308) 534-2416, **SLP**

Stefkovich, Donna M P O Box 915, Vernon, NJ 07462, (201) 764-4071, BA 77 Rutger's St Univ - Douglas Coll; MA 87 Montclair St Coll; 78–Sp-Lang Path, Vernon Township Bd of Educ, **SLP**

Steflik, Gary L 528 Avenue D, Fort Madison, IA 52627, BS 75 Northeast MO St Univ; MA 76 Northeast MO St Univ; SLP, Sn Prairie AEA, **SLP**

Steg, Mrs Katherine P O Box 1013, Ault, CO 80610, (303) 834-2239, BS 72 Kent St Univ; MA 75 Univ of Northern CO; Cl Superv, U Northern Colorado, **SLP ACE**

Stegeman, Susan 715 Farnum, Madison Heights, MI 48071, (313) 545-4732, MS 88 Eastern MI Univ

Steger, Nancy H 6915 Argonne Boulevard, New Orleans, LA 70124, (504) 282-6747, MS 87 LA St Univ - N O Medical Ctr; 88–Sp-Lang Path, Jefferson Parish Sch Sys, **SLP**

Stegman, Robin Eckstein 491 Raymond Street, Rockville Centre, NY 11570, (516) 877-2620, BA 74 Montclair St Coll; MA 76 Univ of CO - Denver; Audiologist, BOCES of Nassau Co, **A**

Stegmann, Nina Valente Box 145, Niverville, NY 12130, (518) 758-6931, BS 75 SUNY - Center at Albany; MS 81 Coll of Saint Rose; MS 85 Coll of Saint Rose; **SLP**

Stegner, Mrs Sandra N 5913 Vernons Oak Court, Burke, VA 22015, (703) 250-4225, BS 69 CO St Univ; MS 70 CO St Univ; Sp/Lang Path, Fairfax Co Pub Sch, **SLP**

Stehman, Helen E S 4350 North Pennsylvania, Indianapolis, IN 46205, **SLP**

Steichen, Mary L 15812 Dearborn, Overland Park, KS 66223, (913) 642-9592, BS 74 Univ of KS; MA 75 Univ of KS; SLP, Shawnee Mission Pub Schs, **SLP**

Steider, Patricia L 5 Beaver Branch Road, Pennsylvania Furnace, PA 16865, (814) 867-6600, BS 79 Univ of MN - Minneap-St Paul; MA 80 Univ of MN - Duluth; Sp-Lang Path, **SLP**

Steiger, Cynthia J 75 Sherwin Drive, Tonawanda, NY 14150, (716) 773-9100, BS 74 SUNY - Coll at Buffalo; ME 75 Canisius Coll; MS 81 SUNY - Coll at Buffalo; Sp-Lang Path, Grand Is Cen Sch Dist, **SLP**

Steighner, Richard Lee 3240 So Newland Street, Denver, CO 80227, (303) 778-5645, MA 80 Univ of CO - Boulder; 85–Aud, Phonic Ear Inc, **A**

Steigleder, Susan Mane P O Box 595, Chester, CT 06412, (203) 526-3779, BA 82 RI Coll; MS 87 Southern CT St Univ; **SLP**

Steih, Mrs Gail Marie 3390 Sherwood, Saginaw, MI 48603, (517) 790-8673, OB 85 Governors St Univ; OM 87 Governors St Univ; 88–Sp-Lang Path, St Mary's Med Ctr, **SLP**

Steiling, Mrs Margaret 3025 Crane Creek Road, Boise, ID 83702, BS 67 ID St Univ; MA 71 ID St Univ; Sp/Lang Path, Nampa School District 131, **SLP**

Steimel, Beth Ellen 557 Williamsburg Court, Suite E, Wooster, OH 44691, (216) 263-8244, BA 82; MS 84; Sp-Lang Path, Wooster Community Hosp, **SLP**

Steimer, Mrs Charlotte Jean 1136 Mike Reed Drive, Library, PA 15129, (412) 831-6391, BS 74 CA Univ of PA; ME 79 CA Univ of PA; Sp-Lang Path, Allegheny Inter Utd, **SLP**

Stein, Andrea Vallen Oakland Center, 950 McElvaney Lane, Lawrenceville, GA 30245, (404) 963-6713, MS 84 Emory Univ; Audiologist, Oakland Center, **A**

Stein, Barbara J 435 Cregennan Bae, Wales, WI 53183, (414) 544-9196, BS 70 Univ of WI - River Falls; MS 75 Univ of WI - Milwaukee; SLP, Waukeshau WI Pub Sch, **SLP**

Stein, Mrs Barbara Tepper 2456 5th Avenue, East Meadow, NY 11554, (516) 221-9489, BA 72 CUNY - Queens Coll; MA 74 CUNY - Queens Coll; Sp-Lang Path, Lifeline Ctr Child Develop, **SLP**

Stein, Mrs Beth I 290 Atlantic Avenue #245, East Rockaway, NY 11518, (516) 223-8100, BA 76 SUNY - Coll at New Paltz; MS 77 Adelphi Univ; Sp-Lang Path, Baldwin Pub Sch, **SLP**

Stein, Dr Cecile L 168 Greenridge Avenue, White Plains, NY 10605, (914) 725-2222, BA 65 CUNY - Hunter Coll; MA 66 Columbia Univ Teachers Coll; PH 83 (Sp-Lang Path) CUNY - Grad Sch & Univ Cntr; 88–Consult, Windward Sch, **SLP**

Stein, Mrs Cheryl Stern 302 Ridge Point Medical Bldg, 14050 Nicollet Avenue S, Burnsville, MN 55337, (612) 926-1867, BS 76 Western Carolina Univ; ME 77 Univ of NC - Greensboro; 87, Private Practice, **SLP**

Stein, Cyndi J 1018 East 22nd Street, Brooklyn, NY 11210, (212) 343-9348, BA 78 CUNY - Brooklyn Coll; MS 82 CUNY - Brooklyn Coll; College Assis, Brooklyn Coll Sp & Hrng Cen, **SLP**

Stein, Mrs Cynthia Hall 2208 Willivee Place, Decatur, GA 30033, (404) 294-7788, BA 76 Elmira Coll; OM 78 Emory Univ; Sp-Lang Path, Dekalb Co School System, **SLP**

Stein, Dr David W 211 Essex Knoll Drive, Coraopolis, PA 15108, (412) 647-8093, BS 75 Indiana Univ of PA; MA 76 Kent St Univ; PH 84 (Sp-Lang Path) Univ of Pittsburgh - Pittsburgh; 86–Assoc Dir Sp-Lang Path, Eye & Ear Hospital of Pitts, **SLP ACE**

Stein, Deborah 4 Camino DE Las Mananitas, Los Lunas, NM 87031, (505) 877-9718, BS 75 ID St Univ; MS 77 ID St Univ; Sp-Lang Path, Albuquerque Pub Sch, **SLP**

Stein, Debra J 230 Jay Street #5-H, Brooklyn, NY 11201, **SLP**

Stein, Dr Dorothy M 410 Mockingbird Valley Road #6, Louisville, KY 40207, (502) 897-0997, BS 67 Syracuse Univ; MA 69 Univ of Southern CA; PH 80 (NS) Univ of IA; 87–Exec Dir, KY Ofc of Business & TX, **A**

Stein, Felisha Glass 6511 Dunn, Waco, TX 76710, (817) 776-9090, BA 85 Baylor Univ; MA 86 Baylor Univ; **SLP**

Stein, Garie Morgonstem 64 Winifred, Worcester, MA 01602, (508) 799-2009, BS 72 Boston Univ; MS 74 Univ of WI - Madison; Sp/Lang Path, Private Practice, **SLP**

Stein, Mrs Gary Bonita P O Box 875663, Wasilla, AK 99687, (907) 373-3880, BA 77 Western WA Univ; OM 83 Univ of the DC; 86–Sp-Lang Path, Matanuska Susitna Sch Dist

Stein, Mrs Harlee A L 85-42 214th Street, Hollis Hills, NY 11427, (212) 776-1466, BA 71 Adelphi Univ; MS 72 Adelphi Univ; **SLP**

Stein, Mrs Helene F 27 Rabbits Run, Palm Beach Gardens, FL 33418-6809, BS 75 Northwestern Univ; MA 77 Northwestern Univ; **A**

Stein, Mrs Jacqueline A 811 Reiman Court, Fairmont, MN 56031, (507) 235-3640, BA 74 Univ of Pittsburgh - Pittsburgh; MA 77 Mankato St Univ; Sp-Lang Path, Martin Co Spec Ed Coop, **SLP**

Stein, Janet A 629 Oak Street, Suite 201, Cincinnati, OH 45206, (513) 961-7173, BA 73 Univ of CA - Los Angeles; MA 75 San Diego St Univ; Aud, Hrng&Bal Lab/S Geo Lesinski MD, **A**

Stein, Mrs Judith E 104 Majestic Drive, Dix Hills, NY 11746, (516) 499-5404, BA 75 SUNY - Coll at Cortland; MA 77 Hofstra Univ; SLP, N/Port-E N/Port Un Sch Dist, **SLP**

Stein, Mrs Karen Goltz 211 Essex Knoll Drive, Coraopolis, PA 15108, (412) 741-6600, BS 74 Edinboro Univ of PA; MA 75 Kent St Univ; Dir SLP Dept, Sewickley Valley Hosp, **SLP**

Stein, Karin 1117 North Ott Street, Allentown, PA 18104, (201) 232-0280, **SLP**

Stein, Kathie L 5 Brainerd Drive, Stony Point, NY 10980, (914) 634-4648, BS 75 Bowling Green St Univ; MA 77 Montclair St Coll; Aud, Rockland Co Cen Phys Hndcpd, **A**

Stein, Mrs Kathleen Noel 438 Overbrook Road, Baltimore, MD 21228, (301) 848-8280, BA 83 Loyola Coll; MS 85 Loyola Coll; **SLP**

Stein, Kristi Lynn 409 East Main #B, Brenham, TX 77833, (409) 836-4511, BA 80 Univ of WI - Eau Claire; MA 85 Univ of TX - Austin; 86–Sp-Lang Path, Brenham State Sch, **SLP**

Stein, Dr Laszlo K Siegel Inst Michael Reese Hosp, Lake Shore Dr At 31st St, Chicago, IL 60616, (312) 791-2910, BS 53 Northern IL Univ - De Kalb; MA 57 Northwestern Univ; PH 63 (Aud) Northwestern Univ; 68–Dir of the Siegel Inst, Siegel Inst Michael Reese Hosp, **A F**

Stein, Dr Leon 22250 Providence Drive, Suite 408, Southfield, MI 48075, (313) 569-5985, BS 58 Wayne St Univ; ME 67 Wayne St Univ; PH 72 (NS) Wayne St Univ - Sch of Med; Aud, D M Davis MD PC, **A**

Stein, Mrs Leslie G 20240 S W 92nd Avenue, Miami, FL 33189, (305) 238-7361, MS 76 Univ of South FL; **SLP**

Stein, Lindsay M 285 Compton Road, Cincinnati, OH 45215, (513) 761-0456, OM 71 Witwatersrand Univ S Africa; MA 81 Univ of Cincinnati; 86–Aud, Univ of Cincinnati Med Ctr, **A**

Stein, Mrs Louise I 104 Woodridge Drive, Stamford, CT 06905, (203) 322-4071, BA 71 Univ of CT; ME 72 Northeastern Univ; Private Practice, **SLP**

Stein, Margo E Rehab Care Corp, 688 J Tempo Trail Drive, St Louis, MO 63141, (314) 537-1288, BA 73 Case Western Reserve Univ; MS 74 Univ of WI - Madison; 85–Program Consultant, Rehab Care Corp, **SLP ACE**

Stein, Mrs Marilyn L 4343 Chevy Chase, La Canada, CA 91011, (818) 952-1021, BS 71 Univ of TX - Austin; MA 76 CUNY - Hunter Coll; Sp-Lang Path, Glendale Adventist Medical Cen, **SLP**

Stein, Mrs Marlene C 76 Shallmar Boulevard, Toronto, ON, Canada M6C 2J9, (416) 963-2234, BA 65; OM 67; SLP and Aud, Govt of On/Ministry Hlth

Stein, Pamela D 4211 West Concordia Avenue, Milwaukee, WI 53216, (414) 251-1000, BS 73 Univ of WI - Milwaukee; MS 74 Marquette Univ; 87–Sp-Lang Path, Rehab Care Unit-Comm Memorial Hosp, **SLP**

Stein, Mrs Sandra J 64 Carter Road, Princeton, NJ 08540, (609) 683-8414, BS 81 SUNY - Coll at Fredonia; MS 83 Univ of Pittsburgh - Pittsburgh; Sp/Lang Path, Medical Center of Princeton, **SLP**

Stein, Mrs Sandra Jean 4675 East Camino Rosa, Tucson, AZ 85718, (602) 295-4895, BS 54 Univ of WI - Madison; MS 61 Univ of WI - Madison; ME 81 Univ of AZ; 82–Pers Dev Rep, Hughes Aircraft Corp, **SLP**

Stein, Dr Seline 4098 Ellison Road, South Euclid, OH 44121, (216) 464-1695, BA 69 Cleveland St Univ; MA 71 Kent St Univ; PH 83 (NS) Case Western Reserve Univ; Sp/Lang Path, Cuyahoga Co Bd Men Ret, **SLP**

Stein, Sharon Bengel 444 East Vera Lane, Tempe, AZ 85284, (214) 730-9676, BA 74 Univ of MN - Minneap-St Paul; MA 75 Univ of MN - Duluth; 87–Sp-Lang Path, Tempe Sch Dist, **SLP**

Stein, Mrs Sharon P 1004 Princeton, Highland Park, IL 60035, (312) 831-0054, BA 74 Univ of IL - Urbana; MA 75 Univ of IL - Urbana; **SLP**

Stein, Mrs Shirley P 3202 Coquelin Terrace, Chevy Chase, MD 20815, BA 37 CUNY - Hunter Coll; MA 40 Columbia Univ Teachers Coll; Assoc Prof Commun Arts, Gallaudet College, **SLP A LM**

Steinau, Stanley J 4422 North Nelson Drive, Peoria, IL 61614, (309) 672-6527, BA 49 Bradley Univ; MA 51 Univ of IA; Sp-Lang Path, Peoria Public Schools, **SLP**

Steinauer, Judith A 1311 Harrison Blvd, Boise, ID 83702, (702) 329-1075, BS 80 Univ of NV - Reno; MS 81 Univ of NV - Reno; SLP, Assoc Sp Lang Path, **SLP**

Steinbaugh-Kristek, Jeanette Marie P O Box 208, Billings, MO 65610, (417) 744-2212, BS 78 Southwest MO St Univ; MS 84 Univ of WY; Sp-Lang Path, Greene County Spec Educ Coop, **SLP**

Steinberg, Caren L 4 Christopher Road, Randolph, MA 02368, (617) 963-7800, BA 75 Univ of MA - Amherst; MS 76 Boston Univ; Sp-Lang Path, Randolph Pub Sch, **SLP**

Steinberg, Mrs Ethel M 3344 Alignet Drive, Encino, CA 91436, (818) 783-2631, BS 70 Univ of NE - Omaha; MS 72 Univ of NE - Omaha; Sr Supvr, InSpeech Inc, **SLP**

Steinberg, Mrs Marcy Gail Rt HCR Box 109, Sand Lake, NY 12153-9713, (518) 674-2121, BA 74 SUNY - Coll at New Paltz; ME 81 SUNY - Coll at Plattsburgh; MA 83 OH Univ - Athens; Sp-Lang Path, Rensselaer Bd Coop Educ Serv, **SLP**

Steinberg, Marilyn A 9272 Oak Knoll CV, Cordova, TN 38018, (901) 761-1220, BA 77 Univ of TN - Knoxville; MA 81 Memphis St Univ; Aud, Ear Nose & Throat Group Inc, **A**

Steinberg, Mary D 51 Parker Boulevard, Monsey, NY 10952, (212) 377-6548, BA 79 CUNY - Brooklyn Coll; MS 81 CUNY - Brooklyn Coll; SLP, NY Cty Bd of Ed, **SLP**

Steinberg, Randee C 124-6 Kirkbride Road, Voorhees, NJ 08043, (609) 424-1505, BA 78 Temple Univ; MA 81 Univ of MD - College Park; Sp-Lang Path, Cherry Hill Bd of Ed, **SLP**

Steinberg, Mrs Randi Joy 1545 E 12th Street, Brooklyn, NY 11230, (718) 376-3324, BA 84 Adelphi Univ; MS 86 Adelphi Univ; 88–Aud, Ctr for Improved Commun, **A**

Steinberg, Mrs Virginia 113 Pierce Avenue, Cuyahoga Falls, OH 44221, (216) 467-0580, BS 72 Kent St Univ; MA 78 Kent St Univ; Sp-Lang Path, Nordonia Hill Cty Sch, **SLP**

Steinberger, Andrea R 256 Keith Avenue, Akron, OH 44313, (215) 735-1566, BA 76 Univ of Cincinnati; MA 78 Case Western Reserve Univ; **A**

Steinbuch, Mrs Debra Wolkoff 765 Vernon, Columbus, OH 43209, (614) 421-1204, BA 82 Case Western Reserve Univ; MA 83 OH St Univ; Sp-Lang Path, Private Practice, **SLP**

Steinburg, Susan Palmer 1319 North Van Doren, Alexandria, VA 22304, (703) 538-4400, BS 83 Brigham Young Univ; OM 84 Brigham Young Univ; **A**

Steinemann, Mrs Lorri C 49 Crestwood Drive, Elkton, MD 21921, (301) 398-8800, BA 75 SUNY - Coll at Cortland; MS 76 Univ of NC - Chapel Hill; 87–Sp-Lang Path, Laurelwood Nursing Center, **SLP**

Steiner, Debra Marie 217 Farmington Rd, Delran, NJ 08075, (609) 261-7030, OM 85 Hahnemann Univ Grad Sch; Aud, Mem Hosp Burlington Cty, **SLP A**

Steiner, Mrs Elissa Beth 513 East 75th Street, New York, NY 10021, (212) 744-2421, BA 78 CUNY - Queens Coll; MA 80 Hofstra Univ; **SLP**

Steiner, Mrs Linda M 9719 Ironmaster Drive, Burke, VA 22015, MA 73 OH Univ - Athens; Sp-Lang Path, **SLP**

Steiner, Dr Sylvia Department Of Communication Disorders, University Of Wisconsin-Eau Claire, Eau Claire, WI 54701, (715) 836-4186, BA 59 Baldwin-Wallace Coll; MS 63 Univ of IA; PH 64 (Sp and Hrng Science) Univ of IA; 83–Chair Dept Commun Disorders, University of Wisconsin-Eau Claire

Steinfeld, Mrs Marcia L P O Box 16810, Plantation, FL 33318, (305) 473-9745, BS 75 Northwestern Univ; ME 76 Univ of Miami; Sp-Lang Path, Private Practice, **SLP**

Steingold, Gail H 1648 C N Burling, Chicago, IL 60614, (312) 951-6040, BS 73 Univ of WI - Madison; MS 74 Univ of WI - Madison; Sp-Lang Path, Illinois Masonic Medical Ctr, **SLP**

Steinhart, Susan M 10045 East Calusa Club Dr, Miami, FL 33186, (305) 382-6860, BA 73; MA 76 SUNY - Center at Buffalo; 88–Sp-Lang Path, Private Practice, **SLP**

Steinhauser, Elizabeth R 1348 South Finley #1-D, Lombard, IL 60148, (312) 971-0840, BS 84 Northern IL Univ - De Kalb; MA 85 Northern IL Univ - De Kalb; **SLP**

Steinhauser, Mrs Michal Urban 741 Morninghome Road, Danville, CA 94526, (415) 838-2153, BA 64 Univ of TX - Austin; MS 71 Lamar Univ; Sp-Lang Path, Mount Diablo USD, **SLP ACE**

Steinhoff, Rin C 3125 North Racine, 1st Floor, Chicago, IL 60657, (312) 281-3832, **A**

Steinholz, Mrs Bonnie Fern 3329 Bayfield Blvd, Oceanside, NY 11572, (718) 241-1086, BA 79 SUNY - Coll at Cortland; MS 81 CUNY - Brooklyn Coll; Sp-Lang Path, New York City Bd of Educ, **SLP**

Steiniger, Mrs Peggy Carroll 652 Weybridge Ctace, Lake Mary, FL 32746, (407) 330-1869, BA 84 MI St Univ; MA 85 MI St Univ; Sp-Lang Path, Seminole Co Schs, **SLP**

Steinke, Mrs Clella J 4285 Del Rio Road, Atascadero, CA 93422, (805) 543-2010, BS 77 ID St Univ; MS 78 ID St Univ; Sp-Lang Path, Sanluis Coastal USD, **SLP**

Steinken, Terri L 3824 Springdale, Glenview, IL 60025, (312) 729-4721, BS 80 IL St Univ - Normal; MS 81 IL St Univ - Normal; **SLP**

Steinkohl, Mrs Sari H 330EAST Cordova Street, Apartment #165, Pasadena, CA 91101, (518) 869-7671, BA 78 SUNY - Center at Buffalo; MS 80 Syracuse Univ; Sp-Lang Path, Early Childhood Education Cen, **SLP**

Steinkraus, Susan I 146 Mell Street #2, Athens, GA 30605, (404) 354-1088, ME 88 Univ of GA

Steinkrauss, Mrs Barbara L 4 Old Wood Road, Framingham, MA 01701, (617) 872-4036, BA 67 MI St Univ; MA 68 MI St Univ; MA 69 MI St Univ; **SLP**

Steinmeyer, Mrs Christine K 3360 Longbow Court, Woodbridge, VA 22192, (703) 590-4712, BA 84 Univ of Northern IA; MA 85 Univ of Northern IA; 87–Sp-Lang Path, Arlington PS, **SLP**

Stein-Meyers, Anita Robin 3323 Kings Highway, Brooklyn, NY 11234, (212) 741-7650, BA 84 CUNY - Brooklyn Coll; MS 86 CUNY - Brooklyn Coll; 86–Aud, NY League for the Hard of Hrng, **A**

Steinpress, Rene J 1510 Vista Larga Court N E, Albuquerque, NM 87106, (505) 262-0393, BA 76 Univ of CA - Santa Barbara; MS 78 Univ of NM; OM 83 Univ of NM; Aud, **A**

Steinsapir, Carolyn Denise 9214-C Hunters Creek Drive, Cincinnati, OH 45242, (513) 475-4883, MA 85 Univ of Cincinnati; 85–Sp-Lang Path, Univ of Cincinnati, **SLP**

Steinwinter, Sheryl S B 7379 Brydon Road, La Verne, CA 91750, (714) 599-6787, BA 72 Univ of OK - Norman; MS 74 Univ of AZ; Sp-Lang Path, Bonita USD, **SLP**

Stelling, Kelly Ann 9308 George Williams Road, Knoxville, TN 37922, (615) 971-1349, BS 85 Univ of TN - Knoxville; MA 87 Univ of TN - Knoxville; **SLP**

Stelling, Martha D 5809 N Lindenwood Drive, Apartment 2604, Peoria, IL 61615, (309) 347-5121, BS 80 Southern IL Univ-Edwardsvill; MS 81 Southern IL Univ-Edwardsvill; Sp-Lang Path, Holiday Ctr Head Start, **SLP**

Stellini, Mrs Deborah A 24300 Genesee Village Road, Golden, CO 80401-9381, (303) 526-9233, BA 78 Univ of CO - Boulder; MA 81 Univ of Northern CO; 86–Sp-Lang Path, Private Practice, **SLP**

Stelmachowicz, Dr Patricia G Boys Town National Institute, 555 North 30th Street, Omaha, NE 68131, (402) 449-6522, BS 70 CO St Univ; MS 71 CO St Univ; PH 80 (NS) Univ of IA; Coord Aud Ser, Boys Town Natl I, **A**

Stelzer, Mrs Barbara M 1229 Hoffman Road, Ambler, PA 19002, (215) 646-6599, BA 66 Adelphi Univ; MS 69 SUNY - Center at Albany; Sp-Lang Path, Abington Mem Hosp, **SLP**

Stemach, Gerald J 7740 Sonoma Highway, Santa Rosa, CA 95409, (707) 833-2134, OB 68 9398; BA 68; MS 77 San Francisco St Univ; Sp-Lang Path, Sonoma County Schools, **SLP**

Stember, Lynn G 2722 South St Marks Avenue, Bellmore, NY 11710, (516) 781-4044, BA 67 CUNY - Brooklyn Coll; MS 68 Univ of MI - Ann Arbor; Sp/Lang Path, Rosemary Kennedy Cen-Nassau, **SLP**

Stemmelen, Maureen Therese 1421 Beaconsfield, Grosse Pointe, MI 48230, (313) 885-1346, BA 83 MI St Univ; MA 85 Wayne St Univ; Supvr of SLP, Rehab Network, **SLP**

Stemmerman, Mrs Anne Farley Physicians Audiological, 13910 Lakeshore Boulevard, Suite 110, Hudson, FL 34667, (813) 868-2113, MS 85 Univ of South FL; Aud, Humana Hospital, **A**

Stempien, Mrs Theresa L 1955 Baylis, Union Lake, MI 48085, (313) 363-5747, BA 76 MI St Univ; MA 77 Central MI Univ; Sp-Lang Path, Sinai Hospital of Detroit, **SLP**

Stemple, Dr Joseph C 601 Edwin C Moses Blvd, Dayton, OH 45408, (513) 229-6081, BS 73 Univ of Cincinnati; MA 75 Univ of Cincinnati; PH 77 (NS) Univ of Cincinnati; 88–Dir, Dayton Head and Neck Surgeons Inc, **SLP**

Stempler, Mrs Jacqueline Abbe 15 Elmary Place, Wayne, NJ 07470, (201) 694-5665, BS 69 Ithaca Coll; MS 72 William Paterson Coll; Sp/Lang Path, Maywood Board of Education, **SLP**

Stempler-Bloom, Susan 18 Sidney Lane, Wappingers Falls, NY 12590, (914) 947-1000, BS 80 SUNY - Coll at Fredonia; MS 82 Boston Univ; Aud, Letchworth Village Dev Cen, **A**

Stenberg, Margaret L 4319 North Dayton, Chicago, IL 60613, **SLP**

Stenehjem, Bonnie Buchanan 4024 S W Thistle, Seattle, WA 98136, (206) 937-9103, BA 78 Univ of Northern CO; MA 80 Univ of Northern CO; 87–Sp-Lang Path, Merrywood Sch, **SLP**

Stenerson, Mrs Cynthia Hemmens 11083 Beloit Road, Belvidere, IL 61008, (815) 547-4493, MA 77 Western IL Univ; Sp-Lang Path, Harlem Consolidated Sch Dist, **SLP**

Stengel, Mark L 8796 Pampa Street, La Mesa, CA 92042, (619) 697-0676, BS 74 SUNY - Center at Albany; MS 77 SUNY - Center at Buffalo; 88–Tchr, Lakeside Union Sch Dist, **SLP**

Stengel-Wittke, Mrs Patricia Ann 503 Swallow, Warrensburg, MO 64093-2835, (715) 232-2661, BS 81 Univ of WI - Eau Claire; MS 82 Univ of WI - Eau Claire; 85–Sp-Lang Path, Lafayette Co SD, **SLP**

Stenhouse, Sylvia T 8239 Copper Creek Drive, Louisville, KY 40222, (919) 477-9809, BA 48 Rockford Coll; MA 52 Northwestern Univ; SLP, Henry County Public Schools, **SLP**

Stennett, Mrs Nadine E 3221 Norris Avenue, Sacramento, CA 95621, (916) 481-9651, BA CA St Univ - Sacramento; MA 60 CA St Univ - Sacramento; Retired, **SLP LM**

Stenseth, Mrs Natalie W 8722 N E 142nd Street, Bothell, WA 98011, (206) 670-7212, BS 62 Tufts Univ; MA 65 Case Western Reserve Univ; Sp-Lang Path, Edmonds School Dist, **SLP**

Stenson, Mary Hartley 21 Forest Lane, Hingham, MA 02043, (617) 749-5999, BS 78 Univ of DE; MA 81 George Washington Univ; Sp-Lang Path, Duxbury PS, **SLP**

Stensrud, Kathryn Jo 9010 Firewood Trail, St Louis, MO 63126, (314) 842-0075, BS 84 Saint Louis Univ; MA 85 Saint Louis Univ; **SLP**

Stepak, Bryna C 2401 Pennsylvania Avenue, Apartment 10-B-22, Philadelphia, PA 19130, (215) 763-4133, BS 71 Ithaca Coll; MS 72 Syracuse Univ; Sp-Lang Path, Phila Bd of Ed, **SLP**

Stepanik, Mark J 28 Lexington Drive, Shrewsbury, PA 17361, (301) 528-2419, OB 76 Mansfield Univ of PA; BS 79 Bloomsburg Univ of PA; MS 80 Bloomsburg Univ of PA; Cl Superv, U of MD-Balt, **SLP**

Stephan, Mrs Jean M 3843 San Anseline Avenue, Long Beach, CA 90808, (213) 868-0431, BS 72 CA St Univ - Long Beach; MA 80 CA St Univ - Long Beach; Aud, Norwalk-Lamirada USD, **SLP**

Stephan, Mrs Roberta J 145A Bennington Road, Annandale, NJ 08801, (201) 788-6424, BA 67 Univ of CO - Boulder; ME 70 PA St Univ - Univ Park; Sp-Lang Path, Hunterdon Med Cen, **SLP**

Stephani, Mrs Lauren Fae 2341 Walden Lane, Arlington Height, IL 60004-7217, (312) 253-9839, BS 81 IL St Univ - Normal; MS 83 Rush Univ; SLP, Laremont School, **SLP**

Stephanie, Sandra G 1500 Carnegie Drive, Binghamton, NY 13903, (607) 729-2527, BS 67 Univ of IA; MA 69 Univ of IA; Aud, Private Practice, **A**

Stephans, Kathy Hurst 2703 Tanglewood Drive, Durham, NC 27705, (919) 575-7529, BA 80 Univ of NC - Chapel Hill; MS 82 Univ of NC - Chapel Hill; SLP/Aud, Murdoch Cen, **SLP**

Stephen, Frances Leslie R R 2 Box 79-A, Rochester, IN 46975, (219) 223-2333, BS 78 IN St Univ - Terre Haute; MS 85 IN St Univ - Terre Haute; **SLP**

Stephen, Mrs Patricia McShane 632 Norwich Road, Plainfield, CT 06374, (203) 464-8080, BS 81 Central CT St Univ; MS 83 Univ of RI; Sp-Lang Path, Ledyard Board of Education, **SLP**

Stephens, Mrs Christey H 902 Thomas, Redlands, CA 92373, (714) 874-1127, BA 77 Univ of Redlands; MS 78 Univ of Redlands; SLP, San Bernardino County Schools, **SLP**

Stephens, Mrs Christine Bender Box 283, Newark, NY 14513, (315) 331-1700, BS 74 Edinboro Univ of PA; MA 77 Adams St Coll; Sp-Lang Path, Newark Dev Ctr, **SLP**

Stephens, Mrs Constance Fiero 1709 Lakeshore Drive, Abilene, TX 79602, (915) 676-2507, BS 71 Univ of TX - Austin; MS 75 Univ of TX - Dallas; Aud, Abilene State Sch, **A**

Stephens, Cynthia 77-34 113th Street #2-D, Forest Hills, NY 11375, (212) 738-6200, BA 74 CUNY - City College; MA 77 CUNY - City College; SLP & Aud Prog Coord, Bernard Fiveson Dev Cen, **SLP**

Stephens, Gay 3650 Tates Creek Road #112, Lexington, KY 40502, (502) 695-4035, BA 75 Univ of KY; MA 76 Univ of TN - Knoxville; Sp-Lang Path, Franklin County Board of Educ, **SLP**

Stephens, Ginger R 2502 Heritage Circle, Statesville, NC 28677, (704) 872-3488, BS 63 TX Tech Univ; MA 82 Lenoir-Rhyne Coll; MA 87 Appalachian St Univ; 77–Sp-Lang Path, Iredell County Sch Sys, **SLP**

Stephens, Mrs Harriet Kennedy PO Box 545, Williston, SC 29853, (803) 266-3737, BA 74 Winthrop Coll; MA 77 SC St Coll; Sp-Lang Path, Williston Sch Dist #29, **SLP**

Stephens, James F 3314 Melrose Road, Suite 105, Fayetteville, NC 28304, (919) 323-1250, BA 72 SUNY - Coll at Plattsburgh; MA 74 OH Univ - Athens; Director, Audiology Clinic Inc, **A**

Stephens, Mrs Jane B Rt 12 Box 311, 806 West Whippoorwill Circle, Columbia, MO 65203, (314) 751-6246, BS 69 Northeast MO St Univ; MA 70 Northeast MO St Univ; Sp-Lang Path, Mo Crpld Chldn Serv, **SLP A**

Stephens, Jane M 2208 Hathway, Wichita, KS 67226, **SLP**

Stephens, Mrs Janet Sanborn P O Box 1136, Dubois, WY 82513, (307) 455-2488, BS 81 CO St Univ; MS 83 CO St Univ; Sp-Lang Path, Fremont Co Dstr 2, **SLP**

Stephens, Mrs Janice Clare 5154 Jason Street, Houston, TX 77096, (713) 522-4219, BA 55 Mary Baldwin Coll; MA 82 Univ of Houston - Univ Park; Sp-Lang Path, Houston ISD, **SLP**

Stephens, Mrs Jayne 3721 Brock Road, Chattanooga, TN 37421, (615) 622-8255, BS 79 Saint Mary's Dominican Coll; MA 81 Memphis St Univ; 84–Asst Dir Sp-Lang Path, Communication Clinic, **SLP**

Stephens, John Charles 842 Ridge Road, Lansing, NY 14882, (607) 533-4596, MS 82 Ithaca Coll; Aud, Ithaca Coll, **A**

Stephens, Louis M 132 Coffman Drive, Fort Oglethorpe, GA 30742, (615) 757-5811, BA 59 Harding Univ; MA 61 Univ of IA; Aud, MacK Stephens & Assoc, **A**

Stephens, Lynda Jean 1920 Gunbarrel Road #1618, Chattanooga, TN 37421, (615) 892-4718, BS 81 Univ of TN - Chattanooga; MA 83 Univ of TN - Knoxville; 84–Aud, Aud Svcs-Kenneth C Parker, **A**

Stephens, Mark J 880 San Ardo Way, Mountain View, CA 94043, (415) 592-9555, BA 77 CA St Univ - Long Beach; MA 79 CA St Univ - Long Beach; Sp-Lang Path, San Mateo Ofc of Ed, **SLP**

Stephens, Dr Mary Irene Department Of Communicative Disorders, Northern Illinois University, De Kalb, IL 60115, (815) 753-6517, BA 52 Depauw Univ; MS 56 OH St Univ; PH 72 (Developmental Psycholinguistics) Purdue Univ - West Lafayette; 77–Prof, N IL Univ, **SLP**

Stephens, Dr Myrna Mannila Audiology Consultants, 3319 Spring Street, Suite 104, Davenport, IA 52807, (319) 359-1325, BS 62 Univ of MN - Minneap-St Paul; MS 64 Univ of WI - Madison; PH 73 (NS) MI St Univ; Aud, Aud Consultants, **SLP A ACE**

Stephens, Nancy Jo 1775 E Lakewood, Springfield, MO 65807, (417) 887-8455, BS 77 Southwest MO St Univ; MS 85 Southwest MO St Univ; **SLP**

Stephens, Phyllis Kay 3909 Amherst, Dallas, TX 75225, (214) 783-3008, BS 67 Stephen F Austin St Univ; MS 87 Univ of TX - Dallas; **A**

Stephens, Robert William 157 Union Avenue #D14, Campbell, CA 95008, (408) 559-6298, MA 83 San Jose St Univ; Teacher Sdc & Commun Handicpd, San Jose USD, **SLP**

Stephens, Suzann K 7674 Wise Avenue #1-E, St Louis, MO 63117-1554, **SLP**

Stephens, Terirae 105 Normandy Road, Lafayette, LA 70503, **SLP**

Stephens, V Carole Audiology-Hearing Aid Association Inc, 2309 Atherholt Road, Lynchburg, VA 24501, (804) 528-4245, BA 75 Averett Coll; BA 78 Univ of VA - Charlottesville; ME 80 Univ of VA - Charlottesville; Aud, Aud Hrng Aid Assoc Inc, **A**

Stephens Brown, Mrs Sally Willis 17913 Elm Street, Fountain Valley, CA 92708, (714) 968-2659, 61 Columbia Coll; BS 63 Univ of NE - Lincoln; MA 75 CA St Univ - Long Beach; Sdl Tchr, Ocean View Sch Dist, **SLP**

Stephens-Johnson, Pamela S 2584 Camino Chueco, Santa Fe, NM 87505, (505) 471-1068, BS 75 Univ of NM; MA 76 Univ of Northern CO; **SLP**

Stephenson, Bonita K Route 3 Swiss Arms #9, Vevay, IN 47043, (812) 427-2268, BS 80 Coll of Mount Saint Joseph; MS 87 Miami Univ - Oxford; 87–Sp-Lang Path, Madison Consolidated Sch

Stephenson, Cathy Lynne 5400 Orange Suite 220, Cypress, CA 90630, (714) 826-0443, BA 82 Humboldt St Univ; MA 83 Univ of the Pacific; 87–Clin Supvr, InSpeech Inc, **SLP**

Stephenson, Mrs Eleanor Alice 1239 Avacado Summit Drive, El Cajon, CA 92019, (619) 449-1145, MA 84 Northwestern Univ; Sp-Lang Path, San Diego USD, **SLP**

Stephenson, Elizabeth Z 940 Poppleton, Birmingham, MI 48008, **SLP**

Stephenson, Heather Lucile 43317 Gadsen #547, Lancaster, CA 93534, (707) 822-8750, BA 85 Humboldt St Univ; MA 87 Humboldt St Univ

Stephenson, Kim Lambert St Joseph's Hosp And Health Ctr, Dept Of Speech Language Pathology & Audiology, 820 Clarksville St, Paris, TX 75460, (214) 737-3605, BS 79 East TX St Univ - Commerce; MS 84 East TX St Univ - Commerce; Dir Sp-Lang Path/Aud, St Joseph's Hosp, **SLP A**

Stephenson, Lydia Jane 45 North Pershing Street, Akron, OH 44313, BA 84 Marshall Univ; MS 85 WV Univ; **SLP**

Stephenson, Paul Gregory Dr Fred Owens, 3600 Gaston Avenue, Barnet Tower Ste 1103, Dallas, TX 75242, (214) 742-2194, BS 83 Midwestern St Univ; MS 85 Univ of North TX; Aud, Dr Owens, **A**

Stephenson, Ruthanne B 871 West Donna Drive, Merced, CA 95348-2212, (209) 722-0110, BA 64 ND St Univ; MA 86 CA St Univ - Stanislaus

Stephenson, William T 940 Poppleton, Birmingham, MI 48008, (313) 858-1924, BS 52 Wayne St Univ; ME 53 Wayne St Univ; ED 65 (Administration Special Education) Wayne St Univ; 66–Consult Sp & Hrng, Oakland Sch, **SLP A F**

Stephenson-Opsal, Deborah Graduate Hospital, 1800 Lombard Street, Philadelphia, PA 19146, (215) 893-7094, BA 82 Univ of MD - College Park; MA 86 Univ of MD - College Park; 86–Sp-Lang Path, Graduate Hosp, **SLP**

Stepkin, Richard L Enviromed, Patrick Bldg, 201 South Black Horse Pike, Blackwood, NJ 08012-2802, (609) 228-3353, BS 71 FL St Univ; MS 72 FL St Univ; Aud, Enviromed Corp, **A**

Stepp, Mrs Helen Elizabeth 2465 Granger Road, Medina, OH 44256, (216) 723-4192, **SLP**

Steppling, Mrs Mary Lou G 63 Main Street, Conyngham, PA 18219, (717) 788-1869, BS 71 Bloomsburg Univ of PA; ME 72 Bloomsburg Univ of PA; Sp-Lang Path, Private Practice, **SLP ACE**

Sterensis, Mrs Barbara G 8550 143rd Lane N, Seminole, FL 34646, (813) 391-1319, BS 73 Emerson Coll; ME 76 Northeastern Univ; 83–Pres & Sp-Lang Path, Speech Therapy Associates, **SLP**

Sterkel, Mrs Mary J K 9952 Kings Canyon Drive, Huntington Beach, CA 92646, (714) 963-8302, BA 75 CA St Univ - Fullerton; MA 79 CA St Univ - Fullerton; Retired, Huntington Beach City Sch Dist, **SLP**

Sterkens, Juliette P M 400 Ceape Avenue, Oshkosh, WI 54901, (414) 235-5326, MS 83 Univ of WI - Oshkosh; Aud, Private Practice, **A**

Sterling, Beverly A 3504 West Brookview Drive, Waco, TX 76710, (817) 562-2821, BS 79 Southwest TX St Univ; ME 80 Southwest TX St Univ; Sp-Lang Path, Mexia St Sch, **SLP**

Sterling, Debra G 928 South Paca Street, Baltimore, MD 21230, (301) 396-4461, BS 71 CUNY - City College; MA 73 Univ of CT; OM 81 Johns Hopkins Univ; Admin/School & Adolescent Hlth, Baltimore City Hlth Dept, **A**

Sterling, Doris A 5603 Pioneer Drive, Baltimore, MD 21214, (301) 426-9322, **SLP**

Sterling, Gail R 2801 West Wattles Road, Troy, MI 48098, (313) 876-3285, BA 70 Vanderbilt Univ; MS 71 Vanderbilt Univ; Aud, Henry Ford Hospital, **A**

Sterling, Mrs Tinette D 28 The Intervale, Roslyn Estates, NY 11576, (516) 593-3355, BS 50 NY Univ; MS 65 Adelphi Univ; Sp-Lang Path, Private Practice, **SLP A**

Stern, Adele Jones 360 Cabrini Boulevard #8E, New York, NY 10040, (212) 923-4556, BA 81 IN Univ - Bloomington; MS 84 Columbia Univ Teachers Coll; Sp/Lang Path, Albert Einstein Coll of Med, **SLP ACE**

Stern, Mrs Barbara J 1909 Narragansett Avenue, Bronx, NY 10461, BA 51 CUNY - Brooklyn Coll; MA 72 CUNY - Lehman Coll; SLP, Bd of Ed City of NY, **SLP**

Stern, Mrs Barbara K 1743 Tarrytown Avenue, Crofton, MD 21114, (301) 261-3477, BA 64 Univ of MD - College Park; Sp-Lang Path, Anne Arundel Co Bd of Ed, **SLP**

Stern, Cynthia Billian 190 Garden Street, Farmington, CT 06032, (203) 724-2651, BS 71 PA St Univ - Univ Park; MA 73 Temple Univ; SLP, Capitol Region Ed Council, **SLP**

Stern, Doris Rapisardi P O Box 1138, Montclair, NJ 07042, (201) 268-8140, MA 83 Montclair St Coll; Aud, United Hosp Med Cen, **A**

Stern, Elaine L 1301 Lees Drive, Las Cruces, NM 88001, BA 84 Grand Canyon Coll; MA 86 Grand Canyon Coll; **SLP**

Stern, Evelyn Frances 193 Everett St, East Boston, MA 02128, (617) 567-0585, ME 70 Boston Univ; ME 76 Lesley Coll; 84–Sp-Lang Path, Judith Wisnia and Associates, **SLP**

Stern, Howard J 18 Wyndham Place, Robbinsville, NJ 08691, (609) 691-4162, BA 81 Glassboro St Coll; MA 85 SUNY - Center at Buffalo; 87–Aud, Miracle Ear Hearing Centers, **A**

Stern, Jeane 619 Forest Court #103, St Louis, MO 63105, (314) 727-1211, BS 40 Washington Univ; MA 45 Columbia Univ Teachers Coll; Retired, **SLP A**

Stern, Lori Robbin 300 South Central Park Avenue, Apartment B-23, Hartsdale, NY 10530, (914) 949-1500, BA 81 Emerson Coll; MA 84 CA St Univ - Los Angeles; 87–Aud, Westchester Hrng Svcs, **A**

Stern, Lynn Davidow 8560 Aborcrest Drive, Cincinnati, OH 45236, (513) 791-8774, BA 66 Univ of GA; MA 82 Univ of Cincinnati; Aud, David Zipfel MD, **A**

Stern, Meryl J 6530 Road 28 1/2, Sterling, CO 80751, (303) 522-0122, MS 83 9075; 85–Sp-Lang Path, Sterling Regional Med Ctr, **SLP**

Stern, Susan Bette 1953 Flowering Tree Terr, Silver Spring, MD 20902, (301) 681-7253, BA 65 Univ of MD - College Park; MA 66 Univ of CO - Denver; BS 77 George Washington Univ; 78–Sp-Lang Path, Montgomery Co PS, **SLP**

Stern, Zina G 2323 Wyoming Avenue N W, Washington, DC 20008, (202) 234-7040, BA 56 CUNY - Queens Coll; MS 58 CUNY - Queens Coll; Sp-Lang Path, Prince Georges Co Pub Schs, **SLP**

Sternberg, Mrs Joan Fuertes 2899 Queens Way, Thousand Oaks, CA 91362, (805) 527-2349, BA 76 Chapman Coll; MS 81 Chapman Coll; Sp-Lang Pathologist, Hueneme School District, **SLP**

Sternberg, Mrs Lois W 2635 Pennington Road, Pennington, NJ 08534, **SLP**

Sternberg, Mrs Marsha L Smith 342 Church Avenue, Jasper, IN 47546, (812) 482-6661, BS 74 IN St Univ - Terre Haute; MS 81 IN St Univ - Terre Haute; Sp-Lang Path, Dubois-Spencer-Perry Chldn Coo, **SLP**

Sterne, Susan L 3921 Maybury Mall #2, Bloomington, IN 47401, BS 61 IN Univ - Bloomington; SLP, Reg Early Childhood Ed Prog, **SLP A**

Sternemann, Mrs Phyllis M 83-35 246th Street, Bellerose, NY 11426, (718) 347-7349, BA 81 CUNY - Queens Coll; MA 83 CUNY - Queens Coll; 84–Sp-Lang Path, Private Practice, **SLP ACE**

Sterner, Marcia Klein 33 East Lemon Street, Lancaster, PA 17602, (717) 733-0311, BA 78 Univ of Pittsburgh - Pittsburgh; MS 80 PA St Univ - Univ Park; Dir of SLP, Ephrata Community Hosp, **SLP**

Sterner, Teri Lee 1139 Arbor Vista Way, San Jose, CA 95126, (408) 286-1250, BA 76 Univ of Redlands; MS 77 Univ of Redlands; Sp-Lang Path, Santa Clara Co Off of Ed, **SLP**

Sternig, Pamela A 4710 North Habana Avenue, Suite 205, Tampa, FL 33614, BS 70 Syracuse Univ; MS 71 SUNY - Center at Albany; Dir Sp-Lang Path, Sp-Lang-Lrng Ctr, **SLP**

Sterns, Gladys M P O Box 20233, Braden River Branch, Bradenton, FL 34203, (813) 349-2829, BA 40 OH Wesleyan Univ; MA 52 NY Univ; **SLP**

Sternsdorff, Donna Lee Osterhotz Elementary School, APO New York, NY 09355, BS 84 KS St Univ; MA 86 KS St Univ; Sp-Lang Path, Dept of Defense Depend Sch, **A**

Stern-Weisman, Phyllis 301 Lakeview Drive, Buffalo Grove, IL 60089, (312) 981-3670, BS 75 Bradley Univ; MA 76 Northern IL Univ - De Kalb; Aud, Elk Grove Hrng Ctr, **A**

Sterrett, Mrs Mary Sue 1027 Bonnie Glen, Kingwood, TX 77339, (409) 539-3306, BS 70 Univ of Houston - Univ Park; MA 73 Univ of Houston - Univ Park; Ed Diagnstch, Humble ISD, **SLP**

Sterrett, Michael L 406 West 34th Street, Suite 410, Kansas City, MO 64111, (816) 531-4847, BS 71 Univ of KS; MA 74 Univ of KS; Aud, Impact Hrng Conserv, Inc, **A**

Sterry, Mrs Merri Lynne 6015 Rock Glen Drive #409, Baltimore, MD 21227, (301) 379-1922, BA 84 Univ of KY; MS 86 Univ of KY; 87–Sp-Lang Path, Carroll County Schs, **SLP**

Stetson, Mrs Joan Ruth 2455 Randy Lane, Bellmore, NY 11710, (516) 486-7711, BS 53 Syracuse Univ; MS 75 Adelphi Univ; SLP, Nassau BOCES-Hrng Imp Prog, **SLP**

Stetson, Mrs Roxanne E 20 Tahoe, Irvine, CA 92715, (714) 786-6899, BA 72 Univ of MI - Ann Arbor; MA 76 Univ of CA - Santa Barbara; SLP, Huntington Beach Sch Dist, **SLP**

Steuben, Nancy R 1010 Noyes #311, Evanston, IL 60201, (312) 866-5976, BS 77 Augustana Coll; MA 78 IN Univ - Bloomington; Sp-Lang-Path, St Francis Hosp of Evanston, **SLP**

Steur, Elizabeth 265 Culpepper Road, Williamsville, NY 14221, **A**

Steury, Marlyn Ligner 6775 Breckenridge Road, Lisle, IL 60532, (312) 420-5258, BS 75 Univ of IL - Urbana; MS 76 Univ of IL - Urbana; 88–Sp-Lang Path, Ped Sp and Lang Therapy Svcs Ltd, **SLP**

Steven, Rene Schwalbach 2569 South 66th Street, Milwaukee, WI 53219, (414) 541-0822, BS 84 Univ of WI - Milwaukee; MS 85 Univ of WI - Milwaukee; 86–Sp-Lang Path, St Mary's Med Ctr, **SLP**

Stevens, Anne Richardson 603 Essex Avenue, Gloucester, MA 01930, (617) 682-9750, BA 79 Beloit Coll; MS 84 Boston Univ; Sp-Lang Path, Lawrence School Department, **SLP**

Stevens, Bette J 9814 Homeland Avenue, Baltimore, MD 21234, (301) 444-5000, BS 76 Towson St Univ; MS 78 Gallaudet Coll; Supvr of Aud Svcs, MD Sch-Blind, **A**

Stevens, Debralea 2400 Arrowhead #192, Abilene, TX 79606-2857, (915) 465-4391, OB 82 Hardin-Simmons Univ; MS 84 Univ of TX - Dallas; Sp-Lang Path, San Angelo State School, **SLP**

Stevens, Mrs Donna Shuler 209 Loring Street, Spartanburg, SC 29302, (803) 583-0535, BA 81 Columbia Coll; ME 83 Converse Coll; OM 86 Univ of SC - Columbia; **SLP**

Stevens, Mrs Dorothy C 5908 Plainview Road, Bethesda, MD 20817, (301) 320-3449, BA 59 George Washington Univ; OM 68 George Washington Univ; Retired, **SLP**

Stevens, Mrs Elaine R 243 Main Street, P O Box 362, Waterville, ME 04901, (207) 873-7186, BA 68 Univ of ME - Orono; MA 71 Univ of Denver; Dir, Private Practice, **SLP**

Stevens, Ellen B 3201 Maryland Parkway S, Apartment 2, Las Vegas, NV 89109, **A**

Stevens, George H Illinois Department Of Public Health, 4302 North Main Street, Rockford, IL 61103, (815) 987-7865, BS 64 Northern IL Univ - De Kalb; MA 68 Northern IL Univ - De Kalb; Consult, IL Dept of Pub Hlth, **SLP ACE**

Stevens, Helen 166 East 200 South, Vernal, UT 84078, (801) 789-4479, BS 59 Univ of UT; MS 65 UT St Univ; SLP/Aud, UT St Dept of Hlth, **SLP A**

Stevens, Dr James H 605 Jinings Drive, Bellevue, NE 68005, (402) 559-3771, BA 65 Univ of FL; MA 68 Univ of FL; PH 76 (NS) Univ of KS; Manager Otoneurologic Serv, Bishop Clarkson Hosp, **A**

Stevens, Jamie H Box 903, Gig Harbor, WA 98335, (206) 373-7276, BA 66 Univ of KS; MS 73 Univ of Pittsburgh - Pittsburgh; Sp-Lang Path, Private Practice, **SLP ACE**

Stevens, Mrs Janeen Weyland 3679 Willow Canyon Drive, Sandy, UT 84092, (801) 535-7137, MA 84 Univ of UT; BA 80 Univ of UT; **SLP**

Stevens, Mrs Janetta Buchner Uassb-Wsb-Usmca, Box 405, APO New York, NY 09457-5000, MS 85 TN St Univ; 87–Sp-Lang Path, Dept of Defense Dependents Sch, **SLP**

Stevens, Mrs Joanne K 4351 Cleveland Road, Syracuse, NY 13215, (315) 682-9192, BS 73 SUNY - Coll at Geneseo; MA 76 SUNY - Coll at Geneseo; Sp-Lang Path, Fayetteville-Manlius Ctrl Sch, **SLP**

Stevens, Mrs Joanne M 4732 Loretta Way, Union City, CA 94587, (415) 471-1100, BS 76 CA St Univ - Hayward; MA 81 San Jose St Univ; SLP, New Haven USD, **SLP**

Stevens, Karen C 3933 Brighton Road, Nashville, TN 37205, (615) 297-6832, SLP, Metro Board of Ed, **SLP**

Stevens, Kathleen A 10616 South Sawyer, Chicago, IL 60655, (312) 779-6739, BA 69 Saint Xavier Coll; MA 79 NM St Univ; Sp-Lang Path, SW Cook Co Coop for Spec Educ, **SLP**

Stevens, Dr Linda B Route 1 Box 409, Guyton, GA 31312, (912) 728-3558, BS 57 Univ Southern MS-Hattiesburg; MS 66 Univ Southern MS-Hattiesburg; ED 79 (Sp Ed Adm) Univ of FL; 88–Asst Prin, Effingham County Schools, **SLP**

Stevens, Mrs Linda V P O Box 158, Westtown, NY 10998, BA 77 CUNY - Lehman Coll; MA 79 CUNY - Lehman Coll; Sp-Lang Path, NY Cty Bd of Ed, **SLP**

Stevens, Mrs Lizbeth 1922 Edgewood, Berkley, MI 48072, (313) 772-8380, BA 74 Univ of MI - Ann Arbor; MS 76 Univ of MI - Ann Arbor; 78–Sp-Lang Path, Warren Wood Pub Sch, **SLP ACE**

Stevens, Capt Marc J HSXB-K-D, CDR USA MEDDAC, Fort Benning, GA 31905, (404) 544-4450, BA 81 Univ of MD - College Park; MS 83 Gallaudet Coll; 88–Chief Aud, Martin Army Community Hosp, **A**

Stevens, Mrs Marcy Lynne 2908 Central Avenue, Kearney, NE 68847, (308) 995-8663, **SLP**

Stevens, Dr Merle 6 Linnaean Street, Cambridge, MA 02138, (617) 876-7274, BA 49 Univ of NC - Chapel Hill; MS 58 Vanderbilt Univ; PH 63 (NS) Univ of IA; Sp-Lang Path, Private Practice, **SLP**

Stevens, Nancy C Route 2 Box 1515, Sanger, TX 76266, (817) 627-3349, BS 58 Univ of IL - Urbana; MA 76 TX Woman's Univ; Sp-Lang Path, Wise Co Spec Classes, **SLP**

Stevens, Mrs Nancy J H 206 Parkview Drive, Bloomington, IL 61701, (309) 452-1170, BS 74 Univ of IL - Urbana; MS 75 Univ of IL - Urbana; Sp-Lang Path, The Baby Fold, **SLP**

Stevens, Pamela Thomas 1702 Mullburry Drive, Norfolk, NE 68701, (402) 379-2016, BS 85 OK St Univ; MS 86 Univ of NE - Lincoln; 87–Sp-Lang Path, Educ Svc Unit #1

Stevens, Patricia Hagan 6611 Falling Waters Drive, Spring, TX 77379, (713) 440-5858, **A**

Stevens, Mrs Patricia Kathleen 8080 Caribbean Way, Sacramento, CA 95826, (916) 381-0886, BA 81 CA St Univ - Sacramento; MA 82 Univ of the Pacific; SLP/Aud, Grant Jt Un Hs Dist, **SLP**

Stevens, Robin Lynn 743 Birchwood Street, Flora, IL 62839, (618) 662-2014, BS 82 IN St Univ - Terre Haute; MS 83 IN St Univ - Terre Haute; 83–Sp-Lang Path, Flora Commun Unit Dist #35, **SLP**

Stevens, Sharon F 1711 Adeline, Hattiesburg, MS 39401, (601) 736-5336, BS 79 Univ Southern MS-Hattiesburg; MS 80 Univ Southern MS-Hattiesburg; Sp-Lang Path, Columbia Sch Dist, **SLP**

Stevens, Mrs Sheila Rhodes 3601 St Joseph Street, Sanford, NC 27330, (919) 776-1822, BA 77 Univ of NC - Greensboro; MS 81 Winthrop Coll; 87–Sp-Lang Path, Lee County Bd of Educ

Stevens, Shelley L 52 Colborne Road, Brighton, MA 02135, (617) 789-4913, MA CUNY - Queens Coll; 87–Sp-Lang Path, Private Practice, **SLP**

Stevens, Susan M 171 Heather Lane, Mankato, MN 56001, (507) 345-4287, MA 86 Mankato St Univ; Sp-Lang Path, Dstr 77 Mankato Ps, **SLP**

Stevenson, Carol Ann Route 1 Box 1554, Las Vegas, NM 87701, (505) 454-2173, BA 65 Tulane Univ; MS 74 Purdue Univ - West Lafayette; 88–Dir Comm Disorder Dept, Las Vegas Med Ctr, **SLP**

Stevenson, Dedra Michelle 775 Mills Avenue, Baton Rouge, LA 70807, (504) 775-0224, BS 82 Southern Univ - Baton Rouge; ME 86 Southern Univ - Baton Rouge; 83–Sp-Lang Path, E Baton Rouge Par Sch Bd, **SLP**

Stevenson, Hideko 1543 Mansfield Court, Upland, CA 91786, (213) 960-3802, BA 65 IN Univ - Bloomington; MA 68 Western MI Univ; SLP, Los Angeles Co Supt Sch, **SLP**

Stevenson, J Marie Box 7, East Derry, NH 03041, (603) 434-0686, BA 63 Univ of MA - Amherst; MA 65 Univ of MA - Amherst; Special Education Director, Pinkerton Academy, **SLP**

Stevenson, Kristen K 210 Pfeiffer Avenue, Akron, OH 44312, (216) 733-5600, BA 84 Univ of Akron; MA 86 Univ of Akron; **A**

Stevenson, Linda L 5100 West Clearwater, H-3, Kennewick, WA 99336, (509) 946-2231, BS 66 IL St Univ - Normal; MS 73 ID St Univ; Sp-Lang Path, Certified Sp-Lang Servs Ps Inc, **SLP**

Stevenson, Marcia B 1509 18th Avenue East, Seattle, WA 98112, (206) 322-2024, BA 67 Middlebury Coll; BA 78 Univ of WA; MS 79 Univ of WA; 86–Sp-Lang Path, Seattle PS, **SLP**

Stevenson, Mrs Marina Lynch 103 Belmont Drive, Greenville, NC 27858, (919) 758-9950, MS 87 East Carolina Univ; 87–Sp-Lang Path, Pitt County Schs, **SLP**

Stevenson, Mrs Maureen Dempsey 225 Grant Street, Centerport, NY 11721, (516) 435-2215, BA 69 Hofstra Univ; MA 71 Hofstra Univ; SLP, Brentwood Public Schools, **SLP**

Stevenson, Michael H 8331 Fredericksburg #1302, San Antonio, TX 78229-3338, (512) 270-3505, MA 86 Univ of TX - Dallas; 86–Aud, Med Ctr Hosp, **A**

Stevenson, R Jeneine 62230 Charolais Drive, Montrose, CO 81401, (303) 249-5639, BA 73 Loma Linda Univ - Riverside; MS 78 Univ of Redlands; Sp/Lang Path, Uncompahgre Valley Spch & Lang, **SLP**

Stevenson, Rebecca Elliott Route 7 Fairway Drive, Lancaster, SC 29720, (803) 285-5612, BA 72 Furman Univ; MS 74 Winthrop Coll; 88–Sp-Lang Path, Private Practice, **SLP**

Stevenson, Mrs Sandra Jo Route 1 Box 69-S, Victoria, TX 77901, (512) 575-1085, BS 60 East TX St Univ - Commerce; MS 61 East TX St Univ - Commerce; **SLP**

Stevenson, Sarah A H 591-A Noe Street, San Francisco, CA 94114, (415) 665-5130, BA 73 Univ of Denver; MA 74 Univ of Denver; Sp-Lang Path, Ralph K Davies Medical Center, **SLP**

Stevenson, Susan Farr 3600 Hillsdale Road, Baltimore, MD 21207, (202) 483-6030, BA 65 CUNY - Hunter Coll; MS 71 Univ of Pittsburgh - Pittsburgh; Sp/Lang Path, Mt Washington Pediatric Hosp, **SLP**

Stevenson, Virginia E 4106 Yardley Court, Bowie, MD 20715, BS 64 Emerson Coll; MS 66 PA St Univ - Univ Park

Steventon, Bonnie M 6 Millbank Court, Voorhees, NJ 08043, (609) 772-1240, BS 79 PA St Univ - Univ Park; MS 80 Southern Methodist Univ; Sp-Lang Path, Voorhees School District, **SLP**

Stevick, Mrs Elaine M 19 Bernice Court, Petaluma, CA 94952, (707) 763-6419, BA 73 San Francisco St Univ; MA 75 San Francisco St Univ; Sp-Lang Path, Sp&Lang Serv of Marin-Sonoma, **SLP ACE**

Steward, Dr Noreen 1824 Druid Oaks NE, Atlanta, GA 30329, (404) 651-2310, BS 70 Univ of WI - Stevens Point; MS 72 Southern IL Univ -Carbondale; ED 81 Univ of GA; 88–Assistant Professor, Georgia State Univ, **SLP**

Stewart, Adele 7912 Jolliet Drive, Jacksonville, FL 32217, ME 80 Univ of North FL; MA 75 Univ of FL; Sp-Lang Path, Clay Co Schs, **SLP**

Stewart, Andrew P ELB & Associates Incorporated, 605 Eastowne Drive, Chapel Hill, NC 27514, (919) 967-2228, BA 65 Mount Saint Mary's Coll; MA 71 Univ of TN - Knoxville; 82–Dir of Aud Serv, ELB & Associates Inc, **A**

Stewart, Mrs Barbara J 399 Denrose Drive, Tonawanda, NY 14150, (716) 691-9367, BA 78 SUNY - Center at Buffalo; MS 80 AZ St Univ; 86–Aud, Lang Dev Prog of W NY, **A**

Stewart, Barbara Stewart 7591 Autumn Park, San Antonio, TX 78249, (512) 647-2100, BS 86 Stephen F Austin St Univ; ME 87 Stephen F Austin St Univ

Stewart, Dr Billie Ackerman ASHA, 10801 Rockville Pike, Rockville, MD 20852, (301) 897-5700, BA 57 Univ of TX - El Paso; MA 63 Univ of KS; PH 75 (Sp-Lang Path) Univ of MD - College Park; 78–Dir Ed Div, ASHA, **SLP ACE**

Stewart, Brenda Lou 5853-G Century Oaks Drive, Fayetteville, NC 28304, (919) 485-5145, BA 81 Univ of NC - Greensboro; ME 85 Univ of NC - Greensboro; **SLP**

Stewart, Carol C 59 Pierce Avenue, Lakeville, MA 02346, (617) 947-8530, BA 72 Bridgewater St Coll; MS 74 Univ of VT; Director Language Inter Prog, Reads Educational Collaboratn, **SLP**

Stewart, Mrs Carolyn H P O Box 7459, Silver Spring, MD 20910, (202) 636-6977, BA 37 WV St Coll; MA 40 Univ of IA; Consultant Commun Arts & Sci, Chs Sp-Lang Diag & Therapy, **SLP**

Stewart, Carolyn Rose Star Route 2, Box 126, Rison, AR 71665-9612, (501) 879-0065, **SLP**

Stewart, Mrs Catherine 951 Nepawin Lane, Scotch Plains, NJ 07060, (201) 889-7872, BS 72 Southern IL Univ -Carbondale; MS 76 Univ of WI - Madison; Sp-Lang Path, Bernards Twp Board of Ed, **SLP**

Stewart, Mrs Catherine M 2 Stewart Farm Road, Atkinson, NH 03811, (603) 362-5864, BS 83 Univ of NH; MA 85 Univ of CT; Sp-Lang Path, Northeastern Rehabil Hospital, **SLP**

Stewart, Catherine Yeakle Professional Hearing Consultan, 1729 East Saginaw, Suite 201, Lansing, MI 48912, BA 76 MI St Univ; MA 78 OH St Univ; Aud, Professional Hearing Consultan, **A**

Stewart, Celia F 529 West 42nd Street #3-C, New York, NY 10036, (212) 694-2961, BS 73 CO St Univ; MS 75 Phillips Univ; 83–Sp-Lang Path, Columbia Presbyterian Med Ctr, **SLP ACE**

Stewart, Cheri L 404 East 2nd Street, Dixon, IL 61021, (815) 284-6651, BS 78 IL St Univ - Normal; MS 80 IL St Univ - Normal; Sp-Lang Path, Lee Co Spec Ed Assoc, **SLP**

Stewart, Cheryl B 5 Tangerine Place, Kingston, Jamaica 10, (809) 926-0568, BA 76 CA St Univ - Los Angeles; MA 79 CA St Univ - Los Angeles; SLP/Aud, Speech Pathology Services, **SLP**

Stewart, Corinne Kelly 8100 West 89th Street, Hickory Hills, IL 60457, (312) 598-5864, BA 72 IL St Univ - Normal; MS 86 Governors St Univ; 86–Sp-Lang Path, New Medico-Rehab Svcs of Chicago, **SLP**

Stewart, Deborah C Mass Eye & Ear Infirmary, 243 Charles Street, Audiology Department, Boston, MA 02114, (617) 573-3266, BA 82 SUNY - Coll at Cortland; MS 84 Syracuse Univ; 86–Aud, Mass Eye & Ear Infirmary, **A**

Stewart, Deborah L 575 South Rengstorff Avenue, #173, Mountain View, CA 94040, (415) 965-1240, BA 79 OR St Univ; MS 81 Western OR St Coll; Aud, VA Hosp Palo Alto, **A**

Stewart, Denise Elissa 45 E Providence Road, Yeadon, PA 19050, (215) 895-5710, MS 83 PA St Univ - Univ Park; BS 77 West Chester Univ of PA; **A**

Stewart, Dianne B 211 Greendale Avenue, Cincinnati, OH 45220, (513) 761-3440, BA 72 Univ of Cincinnati; MA 75 Univ of Cincinnati; **SLP**

Stewart, Mrs Donna Smith 3126 Colony Lane, Plymouth Meeting, PA 19462, (215) 251-5432, BS 81 Indiana Univ of PA; MS 83 WV Univ; 86–Sp-Lang Path, Bryn Mawr Rehab Hosp, **SLP ACE**

Stewart, Eleanor K 5240 Myna Circle, Wilmington, NC 28403, (919) 763-6879, BA 49 Univ of MI - Ann Arbor; MA 66 Western MI Univ; Sp/Lang Path, Child Dev Cen, **SLP**

Stewart, Elizabeth Los Alamos Sp-Lang Consultants, 111 Piedra Loop, Los Alamos, NM 87544, (505) 672-1060, BS 66 Univ of TN - Knoxville; MS 69 Vanderbilt Univ; **SLP**

Stewart, Ellen W 312 Sunset Street, Longmont, CO 80501, (303) 772-8446, BS 59 Skidmore Coll; OB 76 CO St Univ; Sp-Lang Path, St Vrain Valley Sch Dist Re-lj, **SLP**

Stewart, Elton L 5488 S W Alger Avenue #4, Beaverton, OR 97005, (503) 644-6538, BA 51 Lewis & Clark Coll; MS 70 Portland St Univ; Sp-Lang Path, Private Practice, **SLP**

Stewart, Farrell Multnomah Education Serv Dist, 220 S E 102nd Street, Portland, OR 97216, (503) 255-1841, BS 62 Univ of UT; MS 68 Southern OR St Coll; Dir of Spec Ed, Multnomah Ed Serv Dist, **SLP**

Stewart, Gail P Box 413, Marshfield Hills, MA 02051, (800) 922-8290, BA 47 Radcliffe Coll; MA 81 Emerson Coll; Sp/Lang Path, MA Easter Seal Soc, **SLP**

Stewart, Gregory D 8411 Forest Hill Road, Dewitt, MI 48820, (517) 483-2750, BS 74 Univ of CO - Boulder; MS 76 Univ of AZ; Superv-Hrng & Sp Dept, Sparrow Hosp, **A**

Stewart, Mrs Helga J 3473 Woodstock Lane, Mountain View, CA 94040, (415) 965-9081, BS 72 Univ of Toronto - Ontario; MS 73 Syracuse Univ; **SLP**

Stewart, Irene E Northeast Rehabilitation Hospital, 70 Butler Street, Salem, NH 03079, (603) 893-2900, BS 84 SUNY - Coll at Geneseo; MS 88 Nazareth Coll of Rochester; 88–Sp-Lang Path, Northeast Rehab Hosp, **SLP**

Stewart, Dr James Monroe P O Box 278, Cookeville, TN 38503, (615) 372-3889, BA 70 Howard Univ; MA 71 Howard Univ; PH 76 (Hear & Spch Sciences) OH Univ - Athens; 85–Assoc Prof, Tenn Tech Univ

Stewart, Janet C Route 2 Box 159-A, Eddyville, KY 42038, (502) 388-2156, MS 87 Murray St Univ; 87–Sp-Lang Path, Sp Hrng Cnsl Services Inc

Stewart, Mrs Janice Ann 732 Arlington, Waco, TX 76712, (817) 776-4489, BA 71 Baylor Univ; MS 72 Baylor Univ; Sp-Lang Path, Midway ISD, **SLP**

Stewart, Jean L 1731 Halekoa Drive, Honolulu, HI 96821-1026, BS 63 Univ of TN - Knoxville; MA 64 Northwestern Univ; OM 77 Univ of HI - Manoa; 77–Aud/, Aud Assoc, **A**

Stewart, Joanne S 306 Hubbard, Elgin, IL 60123, (312) 888-5000, BS 70 Miami Univ - Oxford; MS 78 Northeastern IL Univ; 73–Sp-Lang Path, District U-46, **SLP**

Stewart, Judy 6451 South Lakeview Street, Littleton, CO 80120-3340, (303) 730-1044, BS 72 TX Christian Univ; MS 73 TX Christian Univ; 75–Sp-Lang Path, Jefferson County Schs R-1, **SLP**

Stewart, Judy Laverne 1606 Carryback Court, Annapolis, MD 21401, (301) 757-5692, BS 84 Towson St Univ; MS 85 Univ of NC - Chapel Hill; 88–Dir, Magic Years Childcare Ctr, **SLP**

Stewart, Karen Moran R R #1 Box 121, Oelwein, IA 50662, (319) 283-3907, BS 84 IA St Univ; MA 86 Univ of Northern IA; **A**

Stewart, Katherine Priddy 3831 East Van Norman Avenue, Cudahy, WI 53110, **SLP**

Stewart, Kimberly Jane 221 Parkway Drive, Bluefield, WV 24701, (304) 325-8174, BS 83 James Madison Univ; ME 85 James Madison Univ; 86–Aud, Dr Albert Paine MD Inc, **A**

Stewart, Mrs La Tricia Pritchard 1918 Deerfield, Bakersfield, CA 93312, BA 79 Wichita St Univ; MA 80 Wichita St Univ; 88–Sp-Lang Path, Kern County Schs, **SLP**

Stewart, Leslie Aurora Audiology Services, 425 Main Street, East Aurora, NY 14052, (716) 652-6464, BA 66 PA St Univ - Univ Park; MA 76 CA St Univ - Los Angeles; Aud, Aurora Audiology Services, **A**

Stewart, Linda Pennington Route 1 Box 460, Pocola, OK 74902, OB 79 Univ of Central AR; OM 83 Univ of Central AR; 88–Sp-Lang Path, Ft Smith PS, **SLP**

Stewart, Lynne Tsuchida Hawaii District Kona Annex, Box 689, Kealakekua, HI 96750, (808) 323-2743, BS 73 Univ of HI - Manoa; OM 77 San Jose St Univ; SLP, State of Hawaii, Dept of Ed, **SLP**

Stewart, Marianne 7969 Timberlake Drive, Melbourne, FL 32904, OB 72 Univ of FL; ME 73 Univ of FL; **SLP**

Stewart, Marjorie M 128 North Adelle Avenue, De Land, FL 32720, (904) 734-2410, BA 47 Stetson Univ; MA 69 OH Univ - Athens; 81–Sp Lang Cl, Sch Bd of Seminole Co, **SLP**

Stewart, Mary Jo G 2765 Ripple Way, Milford, MI 48042, (313) 685-1511, BA 77 Univ of MI - Ann Arbor; MA 79 Wayne St Univ; SLP, Huron Valley Schools, **SLP**

Stewart, Michael G Dept Audiology & Speech Sci, Michigan State University, East Lansing, MI 48824, **A**

Stewart, Michelle Rural Route 2 Box 129, Marion, NC 28752, (704) 738-4764, MA 84 IN Univ - Bloomington; Sp-Lang Path, Balck Mountain Center, **SLP**

Stewart, Myralyn A 10151 Curran #190-G, New Orleans, LA 70127, **SLP**

Stewart, Mrs Nancy L 29 Juncfield Avenue, Cincinnati, OH 45218, (513) 825-8340, MA 73 Wayne St Univ; Sp-Lang Path, Mt Healthy Cty Schs, **SLP**

Stewart, Mrs Pamula Faye 23 Indian Trail, Searcy, AR 72143, (501) 268-6929, BS 84 Univ of Central AR; MS 85 Univ of Central AR; 88–Sp-Lang Path, Searcy PS, **SLP**

Stewart, Sharon 855 Tremont Avenue, Lexington, KY 40502, (606) 255-5282, MS 72 Purdue Univ - West Lafayette; **SLP**

Stewart, Mrs Sharon S 29582 Teracina, Laguna Niguel, CA 92677, (714) 495-0475, BS 59 ND St Univ; MA 68 CA St Univ - Los Angeles; SLP, Ocean View School District, **SLP**

Stewart, Stacie Jo 12801 Indian School Rd N E, Apartment 2006, Albuquerque, NM 87112, MS 84 CO St Univ; Sp-Lang Path, Albuquerque Pub Sch, **SLP**

Stewart, Mrs Susan E B 724 Ruby Red, Mercedes, TX 78570, MS 78 TX Woman's Univ; Sp-Lang Path, McAllen ISD, **SLP**

Stewart, Susan R 3935 N E Hazelfern Place, Portland, OR 97232, (503) 229-7151, BS 75 Univ of OR; MS 76 Univ of MI - Ann Arbor; Sp/Lang Path, Good Samaritan Hosp/Med Cen, **SLP**

Stewart, Mrs Suzanne Johnson 6395 Vernon Woods Drive N E, Atlanta, GA 30328, (404) 255-7568, BA 48 Univ of GA; ME 64 Emory Univ; Sp-Lang Path, Atlanta Public Schools, **SLP**

Stewart, Suzette Marie 610 East Roosevelt Street, Appleton, WI 54911, (414) 788-3595, **SLP**

Stewart, Terri S Rt 1 Box 637 Sandy Road, Wichita Falls, TX 76301, (817) 855-0686, BS 74 Univ of GA; ME 76 Univ of GA; Sp-Lang Path, Ron Bender, **SLP**

Stewart, Vicki Eklund 6926 Lakeshore Drive, Dallas, TX 75214-3741, (214) 321-7568, BA 69 Wayne St Univ; MA 80 George Washington Univ; Aud, Child Study Ctr, **A**

Stewart, Wren Easter Seal Center, 333 S W 28th Street, Fort Lauderdale, FL 33315, (305) 962-7590, BS 75 Ithaca Coll; MS 77 Univ of OK Medical Center; Program Superv, Easter Seal Cen, **SLP**

Stewart-Muirhead, Gwyneth Eleanor 9632 74th Street, Edmonton, AB, Canada T6B 2B9, (403) 328-5571, BS 79 Dalhousie Univ - Nova Scotia; **SLP**

Stewman, W Denette Yarber VA Medical Center, 3400 Lebanon Road, Murfreesboro, TN 37130, (615) 893-1360, BA 78 Univ of MS; MS 79 Univ of MS; Sp-Lang Path, VA Med Ctr, **SLP**

St George, Dr Marilyn F McGill University, 1266 Pine Avenue West, Montreal, PQ, Canada H3G 1A8, MS 75; PH 85 PA St Univ - Univ Park; Asst Prof, McGill U, **A**

Stibora, Debra Ann 9920 Cedarwood, North Royalton, OH 44133, (216) 845-4620, BA 80 Cleveland St Univ; MA 76 Cleveland St Univ; Sp-Lang Path, Parma Cty Sch, **SLP**

Stice, Linda Sue 8023 E 63rd Place Ste 350, Tulsa, OK 74133-1212, (918) 250-1180, BS 69 Southwest MO St Univ; MS 73 Central MO St Univ; Sp-Lang Path/Consult, Private Practice, **SLP ACE**

Sticha, Lee Ann 7408 Concerto Curve N E, Fridley, MN 55432, (612) 533-2441, BS 79 Saint Cloud St Univ; MS 80 Saint Cloud St Univ; Sp/Lang Path, ISD #279, **SLP**

Sticher, Jenny Lee 6874 #28 Allen Circle, Norcross, GA 30093, (404) 439-1661, BS 84 Univ of South AL; ME 87 GA St Univ; 88–Sp-Lang Path, Emory Univ, **SLP**

Stick, Dr Sheldon L 3609 South 77th Street, Lincoln, NE 68506, (402) 472-5490, BA 60 Northeastern Univ; MA 66 Univ of KS; PH 72 (Aud & Sp-Lang Path) Univ of MI - Ann Arbor; Prof, U of NE-Lincoln, **SLP**

Stickels, Dorothy L V Central School, Roxana, IL 62084

Stickler, Nancy Sima 638 Bay Road, Stoughton, MA 02072, (617) 894-3600, BS 84 Univ of MA - Amherst; MA 85 George Washington Univ; **A**

Stickles, Judith Lee 11 Tamarack Terrace, Fredericton, NB, Canada E3B 2S3, (506) 453-5403, BA 79 Acadia Univ - Nova Scotia; MA 82 Univ of ME - Orono; SLP, Learning Center, **SLP ACE**

Stickney, Joyce Karen 135 Westland Avenue, Manchester, NH 03103, (603) 673-4411, BA 73 Univ of NH; MS 82 Univ of NH; **SLP**

Stickney, Lycia Lauka 4802 S Quintero Circle, Aurora, CO 80015, (303) 861-0504, BS 83 TX Woman's Univ; MA 84 TX Woman's Univ; 86–Sp-Lang Path, Spalding Rehab Hosp, **SLP**

Stidham, Mrs Patricia Joanne 5009 Ironwood Trail, Bartow, FL 33830, (813) 644-9935, SLP, Polk Co Schools, **SLP**

Stidworthy, Helen Lavora c/o Guadalupe Medical Center, 2430 West Pierce, Carlsbad, NM 88220, (505) 887-6633, BS 82 Mercy Coll; MS 84 Columbia Univ Teachers Coll; 86–Sp-Lang Path, Guadalupe Med Ctr, **SLP**

Stiebel, Hart Henry 13335 La Salle Avenue, Huntington Woods, MI 48070, (313) 548-1929, BS 48 Wayne St Univ; MA 53 Wayne St Univ; SLP, Hart Stiebel Associates Inc, **SLP LM**

Stiefel, Betty Jean Box 424, Victor, IA 52347, (319) 647-3513, BS 80 Univ of IA; MA 85 Univ of IA; 85–Sp-Lang Path, Grant Wood AEA, **SLP**

Stiegle, Mrs Melissa Elkins 414 Lyman Circle, Brunswick, OH 44212, (216) 225-0533, BS 78 Cleveland St Univ; MA 86 Cleveland St Univ; Sp-Lang Path, Medina Co Ach Ctr, **SLP**

Stiegler, Mrs Lillian Nielsen Route 1 Box 350, Covington, LA 70433-9719, (504) 893-2859, **SLP**

Stiemann-Brown, Mrs Kathleen T 3920 Central, Western Springs, IL 60558-1126, BS 80 IL St Univ - Normal; MS 81 IL St Univ - Normal; Sp-Lang Path, River Forest Public Schools, **SLP**

Stier, Arlene J 18234 Windsor Hill Drive, Olney, MD 20832, (301) 570-5091, BA 79 Univ of CA - Santa Barbara; MS 81 Univ of NC - Chapel Hill; Sp-Lang Path, Montgomery Co Public Schools, **SLP**

Stier, Mrs Carolyn Schaefer 8 Sieverwood Court, Streamwood, IL 60103, (312) 966-3530, BS 80 Univ of WI - Whitewater; MS 81 Univ of WI - Whitewater; Sp-Lang Path, N SSEO, **SLP**

Stieren, Angelika Janas 1436 Cresthill Drive, Tarpon Springs, FL 34689, (813) 937-7765, BS 73 Saint Louis Univ; MS 87 Univ of South FL; **A**

Stiernberg, Jeanne A 599-B Washington Street, Wellesley, MA 02181, (508) 230-3235, BS 72 Univ of WI - Oshkosh; MS 76 Univ of WI - Oshkosh; Sp/Lang Path, Easton Publ Schs, **SLP**

Stierwalt, Mrs Debra D 101 North Lake Summit Road, Zirconia, NC 28790, (704) 697-6231, BS 66 FL St Univ; ME 78 Univ of FL; Director, Debra D Steinwalt & Associates, **SLP**

Stifel, Judith L 3906 Byrd Road, Kensington, MD 20895, (202) 331-1011, BS 73 Univ of NH; MA 78 Univ of MD - College Park; 79–Aud, PA Coyne MD Pc, **A**

Stiff, Janet Maria 126 Elizabeth Avenue, Talladega, AL 35160, (205) 362-1500, BS 83 Univ of Montevallo; MS 84 Univ of Montevallo; Sp-Lang Path, Al Institute for Deaf & Blind, **SLP**

Stigora, Mrs Cynthia Marie 975 Jefferis Bridge Drive, West Chester, PA 19382, (215) 431-7891, MS 78 West Chester Univ of PA; Clin Dir, Council for Sp Dev, **SLP**

Stigora, Dr Joseph A 975 Jefferis Bridge Drive, West Chester, PA 19382, PH 73 (Sp Path) Bowling Green St Univ; Prof, West Chester U, **SLP**

Stiles, 524595 C Route 2 Box 122, Cedar Creek, TX 78612, MS; **SLP LM**

Stiles, Cynthia L 2027 Greenway Avenue, Charlotte, NC 28204-3315, (803) 286-1961, BS 74 Western Carolina Univ; MA 75 Western Carolina Univ; 88–Sp-Lang Path, Rebound Inc, **SLP ACE**

Stiles, Mrs Jean E 3779 Sheldon Drive, Ventura, CA 93003, (805) 642-6756, BA 70 Univ of Akron; MA 79 CA St Univ - Northridge; SLP, Ventura USD, **SLP**

Stiles, Mrs Sharon Kubacki 6320 East Vermont Street, Long Beach, CA 90803, (213) 868-0431, BA 73 Univ of Redlands; MA 74 Humboldt St Univ; 81–Sp-Lang Path, Norwalk-LaMirada-USD, **SLP**

Still, Mrs Deborah Beth 25 Liberty Circle, Carrollton, GA 30117, (404) 832-3588, BS 76 Kent St Univ; MA 80 Univ of Akron; Sp-Lang Path, Carroll Co Bd of Ed, **SLP**

Still, Mrs Linda L 5 Nantucket, Irvine, CA 92720, (714) 857-6165, BA 75 Univ of Southern CA; MA 78 CA St Univ - Long Beach; SLP, Ocean View Sch Dist, **SLP**

Still, Sheri Frances 2100 Heatherwood Drive B-6, Lawrence, KS 66046-2364, (913) 749-7355, BA 82 Fort Hays St Univ; MS 84 Fort Hays St Univ; Sp-Lang Path, Atchison-Jefferson Educ Coop, **SLP**

Stillerman, Fern 5115 Downy Lane #203, Richmond, VA 23228, (804) 230-0001, BA 71 Mary Washington Coll; ME 72 Univ of VA - Charlottesville; Sp-Lang Path, VA Admin Med Cen - Richmond, **SLP ACE**

Stillerman, Wendy 1255 North Sandburg Terr, Apartment 1501, Chicago, IL 60610, (312) 890-8349, BS 81 San Diego St Univ; MS 82 Boston Univ; **SLP**

Stilling, Catherine M 3310 West 2nd Avenue, McHenry, IL 60050, (815) 459-6070, BS 66 Northern IL Univ - De Kalb; MA 70 Northern IL Univ - De Kalb; Sp-Lang Path, Sch Dist #47, **SLP**

Stillman, Gail Y 110 North Street, Greenwich, CT 06830, (203) 661-0640, MA 70 Columbia Univ Teachers Coll; Sp-Lang Path, Sp & Lang Assoc, **SLP**

Stillman, Judy L 212 Olive Branch, Nashville, TN 37205, **SLP**

Stillman, Lori Ann 310 Market Street #C, New Cumberland, PA 17070-2157, (717) 782-5590, BS 82 SUNY - Coll at Fredonia; MS 84 Vanderbilt Univ; 84–Sp-Lnag Path, InSpeech Inc, **SLP**

Stillman, Nancy M 3120 Tiny Lanert, Roseville, CA 95678, (916) 771-0604, MA 80 Humboldt St Univ; **SLP**

Stillman, Dr Robert David University Of Texas At Dallas, Callier Center For Communication Disorders, 1966 Inwood Road, Dallas, TX 75235, (214) 905-3106, BS 64 Onion Coll; PH 69 (NS) Syracuse Univ; Prog Head, U of TX/Dallas

Stilwell, Catherine A 4329 Mt Vernon Mem Highway, Alexandria, VA 22309, (703) 360-3364, BS 86 James Madison Univ; MS 87 James Madison Univ

Stimatz-Elchesen, Marcia 1159 Killarney Street, Livermore, CA 94550, (415) 426-4293, BA 73 Gonzaga Univ; MA 75 Univ of MT; Sp/Lang Path, Pleasanton Sch Di, **SLP A**

Stimbert-Guck, Karen F 3611 South 116th Street, Omaha, NE 68144, BS 77 Univ of NE - Lincoln; MA 79 Univ of NE - Lincoln; Sp-Lang Path, Omaha Pub Sch, **SLP**

Stimley, Lisa L 412 Russell Street, West Lafayette, IN 47906, BS 79 Ball St Univ; MA 80 Ball St Univ; Sp-Lang Path, New Hope of In, **SLP**

Stimley, Mark A 412 Russell, West Lafayette, IN 47906, (317) 842-1095, BS 76 Purdue Univ - West Lafayette; MA 81 Ball St Univ; Superv Sp-Lang Path, Prudue Univ, **SLP**

Stimpert, Kevin Alan Route 5 Box 163A, Portsmouth, OH 45662, **SLP**

Stimpert, Terri Wuthrick 118 East New England Avenue, Worthington, OH 43085, (614) 369-8735, BS 80 Miami Univ - Oxford; MS 81 Miami Univ - Oxford; Sp-Lang Path, Buckeye Valley Sch De Co, **SLP**

Stimson, Linda C 14315 Troy Way, Magalia, CA 95954, (916) 877-3800, BA 72 CA St Univ - Fullerton; MS 75 Portland St Univ; Sp-Lang Path, Butte Co Supt Sch, **SLP**

Stimson, Mrs Linda D PO Box 350, Baldwinsville, NY 13027, (315) 622-1707, BS 70 Medaille Coll; MS 80 Syracuse Univ; 86–Sp-Lang Path, Private Practice, **SLP**

Stines, Elizabeth A 2884 East Paul Avenue, Fresno, CA 93710-4860, **SLP**

Stinnett, Elizabeth A/Simpson 8642 Grape Creek Road, San Angelo, TX 76901, (915) 949-9535, BS 82 Univ of TX - Austin; MA 85 Univ of TX - Austin; Sp-Lang Path, West Texas Rehab Ctr, **SLP ACE**

Stinnett, Joseph Michael Suite 106 1460 Pandosy Street, Kelowna, BC, Canada V1Y 1P3, (604) 861-7449, BS 72 Brescia Coll; ME 77 Univ of Louisville; 78–Aud, Min Hlth-S Okanagan Hlth Unit, **A**

Stinnett, Lisa Dawn 18269 Leman Lake Drive, Olney, MD 20832, (301) 570-8929, BS 85 East Carolina Univ; MA 87 George Washington Univ; 87–Sp-Lang Path, Mary E Carr & Associates PA, **SLP**

Stinson, Danita A 1682 University Terrace, Apartment 224, Ann Arbor, MI 48104, (313) 763-9475, BA 75 Augustana Coll; MS 77 Eastern IL Univ; SLP, Chicago Board of Education, **SLP**

Stinson, Dr Michael S Rochester Inst Of Technology, Ntl Tech Inst For The Deaf, Dept Educational Research, Rochester, NY 14623, (716) 475-6598, PH 72 (NS) Univ of MI - Ann Arbor; Res Assoc, NTID

Stinson, Mrs Myra Livingston 2209 Lake Forrest Drive, Weatherford, TX 76086, BA 68 East TX St Univ - Commerce; MA 69 East TX St Univ - Commerce; MA 72 TX Christian Univ; **SLP**

Stinson, Mrs Robin H 8005 Goodhurst Drive, Gaithersburg, MD 20879, (301) 997-7605, BA 69 Univ of MD - College Park; MS 74 CO St Univ; Aud, Howard Co Pub Schs, **A**

Stinson, Mrs Suzanne B Star Route Box 22, Castroville, TX 78009, (512) 538-2349, BS 78 Univ of TX - Austin; MA 80 Our Lady Lake Univ-San Anton; Sp-Lang Path, Wilford Hall USAF Med Ctr, **SLP**

Stinson, Mrs Sylvia Salinas 2003 Surrender Avenue, Austin, TX 78728, (512) 473-8382, BS 76 Univ of TX - Austin; MS 79 Univ of North TX

Stipe, Marsha M P O Box 38, Pendleton, OR 97801, (503) 276-6616, BA 69 Western WA Univ; MA 71 KS St Univ; Sp-Lang Path, **SLP**

Stirewalt, Tina Marie 55-C William & Mary Apts, 624 N Hamilton Street, High Point, NC 27262, (919) 882-3228, BA 83 Univ of NC - Chapel Hill; ME 86 Univ of NC - Greensboro; 86–Sp-Lang Path, Asheboro City Schs, **SLP**

Stiritz, Lori L 903 Norwalk Lane, Austin, TX 78703, (512) 478-2724, BA 81 Case Western Reserve Univ; MA 83 Case Western Reserve Univ; **A ACE**

Stitsinger, Gretchen 113 Hideaway Drive, Chapel Hill, NC 27514, **SLP**

Stitt, Barbara J 185 Beacon Street #3R, Boston, MA 02116, (617) 552-7680, BS 71 Syracuse Univ; MA 74 Northwestern Univ; Sp-Lang Path, City of Newton, **SLP**

Stitt, Mrs Cheryl Christine 16415 Seminole Road, Noblesville, IN 46060, (317) 773-5240, MA 83 Ball St Univ; Clinical Supervisor, Ball State University, **SLP**

Stitt, Dr Clyde L 2251 Cobblehill Place, San Mateo, CA 94402, (415) 573-8834, BS 49 Columbia Univ Teachers Coll; MA 50 Columbia Univ Teachers Coll; PH 61 (NS) Stanford Univ; Professor, San Francisco State U, **SLP LM**

Stitt, Signe Lynn 5874 Troy Villa Boulevard, Dayton, OH 45424, (513) 225-4610, BA 69 Heidelberg Coll; MA 71 Bowling Green St Univ; Coord of Sp-Lang Path Serv, Montgy Co Bd of Ed, **SLP**

Stivers, Ann B 11705 Little Lane, Anchorage, KY 40223, (502) 454-8274, BA 60 Univ of KY; ME 80 Univ of Louisville; SLP, Jefferson Co Bd of Ed, **SLP**

St Jacques, Mrs Patricia Bohac 7000 Cook, Apartment 807, Houston, TX 77072, (713) 568-6487, BS 83 Univ of North TX; MS 84 Univ of North TX; 88–Sp-Lang Path, Cypress-Fairbanks ISD, **SLP**

St Louis, Karen W 1357 Headlee Avenue #F, Morgantown, WV 26505, (304) 599-7342, BS 69 SUNY - Coll at Geneseo; MS 70 Univ of MI - Ann Arbor; Sp-Lang Path, Monongalia Co Bd of Educ, **SLP**

St Louis, Dr Kenneth O West Virginia University, 805 Allen Hall, P O Box 6122, Morgantown, WV 26506, (304) 293-4242, BS 66 CO St Univ; MS 70 Univ of MI - Ann Arbor; PH 73 (Communication Disorders) Univ of MN - Minneap-St Paul; Prof, West Virginia U, **SLP**

St Martin, Mrs Anne Griggs 19 Peacock Street, 4871, Trinity Beach Cairns, Queensland, Australia, 7-55 -6098, MA 84 CA St Univ - Los Angeles; **SLP**

Stobbs, Kathryn J 1604 Eva Street, Dayton, OH 45410, (513) 223-3175, BS 74 Miami Univ - Oxford; MA 75 Bowling Green St Univ; Teacher of Multihandicapped, Dayton Bd Ed, **SLP**

Stock, Sharon Nyquist 106 West 5th, Morris, MN 56267, (612) 589-1745, MS 87 Saint Cloud St Univ; 87–Sp-Lang Path, Morris PS, **SLP**

Stockbower, Martha L 3017 10th N W, Albuquerque, NM 87107, (803) 669-8891, BS 84 WV Univ; OM 86 Univ of SC - Columbia; SLP, Healthsouth, **SLP**

Stockbridge, Judith L 115 West 9th Street, Carroll, IA 51401, BS 77 IN Univ - Bloomington; OM 78 IN Univ - Bloomington; SLP, AEA #11, **SLP**

Stockdale, Marianne Elizabeth Governors Plaza Apt #305, 600 Pennsylvania, Denver, CO 80203, (303) 860-8402, MA 84 Univ of CO - Boulder; 88–Sp-Lang Path, Laradon Hall, **SLP**

Stockdell, Kenneth G 2714 Morgan Road, Murfreesboro, TN 37130, (615) 890-5160, BS 53 Purdue Univ - West Lafayette; MS 60 Vanderbilt Univ; Owner, Private Practice, **A**

Stocker, Mrs Beatrice 17 West 54th Street #6-E, New York, NY 10019, (212) 245-1985, BA 31 Barnard Coll; MA 37 Columbia Univ Teachers Coll; Director/Owner, Private Practice, **SLP A LM**

Stocker, Dr Harold S 3309 Wayland Drive, Fort Worth, TX 76133, (817) 292-8006, MA 63 Wayne St Univ; DD 43 Univ of Detroit; PH 70 (NS) Wayne St Univ; Sp-Lang Path, Private Practice, **SLP LM**

Stocking, Christina 93 Lamarck Drive, Snyder, NY 14226, (716) 636-3410, BS 78 Ithaca Coll; MA 80 SUNY - Center at Buffalo; 88–Aud, State of NY at Buffalo, **A**

Stockman, Diane S 2645 Folsom Avenue, Boulder, CO 80302, MA 88 Univ of CO - Boulder

Stockman, Ida Jones 326 Northlawn, East Lansing, MI 48823, PH (NS); **SLP**

Stockman, Lavonne S 5704 East Aire Libre Avenue, Unit 1041, Scottsdale, AZ 85254, (602) 971-0987, BS 60 ND St Univ; MS 77 IN St Univ - Terre Haute; Sp-Lang Path, Paradise Valley USD #69, **SLP**

Stocks, Christy Gail 13546 S E Stephens Place, Portland, OR 97233, (503) 253-5761, BS 85 Portland St Univ; MS 87 Portland St Univ

Stocksdale, Carla Portney 1674 Kirkwood Road, Baltimore, MD 21207, (301) 298-6010, BA 84 Univ of MD - College Park; MA 86 Univ of MD - College Park; 88–Sp-Lang Path, Howard Co PS Sys, **SLP**

Stockton, Charles R 9 Montclair Lane, Willingboro, NJ 08046, (609) 989-2591, MA 65 Temple Univ-Tyler Sch of Art; MA 70 Trenton St Coll; OD 75 (NS) Trenton St Coll; Learning Consultant, Trenton Board of Education, **SLP**

Stockton, Karen D 6 Arlington Heights, Norwich, CT 06360, (203) 889-5100, BA 73 Univ of CT; MA 78 Univ of CT; 88–Supvr/Parent Child Prog, American Sch for the Deaf, **A**

Stockton, Martha Stockton And Associates, 14651 South Bascom Avenue, Suite 260, Los Gatos, CA 95032, (408) 356-1400, BA 83 CA St Univ - Chico; MA CA St Univ - Chico; Sp Lang Path, Private Practice, **SLP**

Stockton, Nancy Miller 6862 Acacia Avenue, Garden Grove, CA 92645, (213) 436-9931, BA 71 CA St Univ - Long Beach; MA 80 CA St Univ - Long Beach; SLP, Long Beach USD, **SLP**

Stockwell, Dr Charles Warren Michigan Ear Institute, 27555 Middlebelt Road, Farmington Hills, MI 48018, (313) 476-4622, BA 64; MA 66; PH 68 (NS); 86–Dir of Vestibular Lab, Michigan Ear Inst

Stockwell, Dean A 1370 Altura Drive, Dubuque, IA 52001, (319) 588-0506, BS 72 IN St Univ - Terre Haute; MS 73 IN St Univ - Terre Haute; 85–Aud, Dubuque Otol, **A**

Stoddard, Jeanne Hagen Northwest Speech & Hearing Ctr, 1475 West Shaw Avenue, Fresno, CA 93711, (209) 225-0148, BA 80 Univ of CA - Santa Barbara; MA 83 CA St Univ - Fresno; Sp-Lang Path, Northwest Sp & Hrng Cen, **SLP**

Stoddard-Schneider, Mrs Mary 67 Dewey Avenue, Staten Island, NY 10308, (212) 596-3545, BA 75 Saint John's Univ - Jamaica; MA 80 Kean Coll of NJ; SLP, NYC Bd of Ed Spec Serv Unit, **SLP**

Stoddart, Mary B 131 Clyde #2-F, Evanston, IL 60202, BA 72 Wittenberg Univ; BS 75 Kent St Univ; MA 77 Kent St Univ; SLP, Home Hlth Agcys, **SLP**

Stoebner, Mrs Ronda Palmer 18640 Jamie Drive, Eagle River, AK 99577, (907) 694-5151, BS 75 Univ of SD - Vermillion; MA 76 Univ of SD - Vermillion; Parent/Infant Education, Focus Inc, **SLP**

Stoeckel, Mrs Ruth B 1410 N W 34th Street, Rochester, MN 55901-1451, (507) 285-0495, BS 77 Univ of IA; MA 80 Univ of MN - Minneap-St Paul; 80–Sp-Lang Path, ISD #535, **SLP**

Stoecklin, Mrs Judy L HCR69 Box 111, Sanbornton, NH 03269, (603) 286-4270, BA 80 MI St Univ; MS 82 Univ of WA; Sp-Lang Path, Private Practice, **SLP**

Stoehr, Roxanne Wright 102 Quandry Trail, Graham, NC 27253, **SLP**

Stoel-Gammon, Dr Carol University Of Washington, Speech & Hearing Sciences, (Jg-15), Seattle, WA 98195, (206) 545-7400, BA 65 Smith Coll; MA 68 Stanford Univ; PH 74 (NS) Stanford Univ; 87–Prof, University of Washington

Stoerzinger, Helen C 1540 North Pascal, St Paul, MN 55108, (612) 644-5127, **A**

Stoesz, Barbara 3824 Dutch Village Road, Apartment 54, Halifax, NS, Canada B3L 4G2, (902) 752-4507, BS 78 Univ of ND; MA 80 Univ of KS; Sp/Lang Path, Nova Scotia Hrng/Sp Cl, **SLP**

Stoever, Jean E 4688 Cliffside Drive, Riverside, CA 92506, (714) 788-7236, BA 72 Univ of Redlands; MS 73 Univ of Redlands; 77–Sp-Lang Path, Riverside USD, **SLP**

Stoff, Mrs Nancy L 182-37 Tudor Road, Jamaica Estates, NY 11432-1509, (718) 380-5486, MA 88 CUNY - Queens Coll; 88–Sp-Lang Path, UCP of Queens, **F**

Stoffregen, Tracey Ann 1116 West Weiland Lane, Appleton, WI 54911, BS 81 Univ of WI - Oshkosh; MS 83 Univ of WI - Oshkosh; Sp-Lang Path, New London Sch Dist, **SLP**

Stofle, Mrs Patricia Tewksbury P O Box 132, Mendocino, CA 95460-1135, (707) 937-4431, BA 56 Stanford Univ; Sp-Lang Path, Private Practice, **SLP**

Stogner, Mrs Barbara Pate 1808 Claiborne, League City, TX 77573, (713) 332-1907, BS 69 Univ of Houston - Univ Park; MA 70 Univ of Houston - Univ Park; Sp-Lang Path, Clear Crk ISD, **SLP**

Stogner, Cindy Smith 100 Hospital Drive, Tylertown, MS 39667, (601) 876-2122, BS 85 Univ Southern MS-Hattiesburg; MS 87 Univ Southern MS-Hattiesburg; 88–Sp-Lang Path, Outpatient Speech Lang Svcs, **SLP**

Stohr, Kathleen M 3451 Mountainside Drive, Colorado Springs, CO 80918, (719) 630-5205

Stohr, Pamela M 17210 N W 58th Avenue, Ridgefield, WA 98642, **SLP**

Stoia, Dr George 28 Denny Road, Chestnut Hill, MA 02167, BS 55 Boston Univ; ME 57 Boston Univ; ED 79 (Spec Ed Admin) Univ of Sarasota; **SLP**

Stoia, John 54 Shaker House Road, Yarmouth Port, MA 02675, MA 59 Boston Univ; **SLP A**

Stoia, Louis 599 Red Top Road Rd #1, Brewster, MA 02631, (617) 385-9012, BA 50 Emerson Coll; MA 51 Univ of Southern CA; ED 61 (NS) Columbia Univ Teachers Coll; Retired, **SLP A F LM**

Stoicheff, Dr Margaret L Rural Route 4, 144 Curtis Crescent, King City, ON, Canada L0G 1K0, (416) 978-6890, BA 55 Univ of Toronto - Ontario; MA 57 Univ of IA; PH 59 (Aphasia) Univ of IA; 72–Prof & Chrmn, University of Toronto, **SLP**

Stoioff, Madonna M 687 Greenwood Road, Northbrook, IL 60062, (312) 480-7682, BS 71; MA 72 Kent St Univ; Asst Prof-Aud, Rush/Presby-Med Cen, **A**

Stok, Mrs Vivian Kallus 1257 East 29th Street, Brooklyn, NY 11210, (718) 615-5200, MS 84 CUNY - Brooklyn Coll; **SLP**

Stoker, Dr Richard Glen Central Institute For The Deaf, 818 South Euclid Avenue, St Louis, MO 63110, (314) 652-3200, ME 73 Univ of UT; MS 77 Salford Univ - England; PH 80 (Aural Rehabilitation) McGill Univ - Quebec; Dir, Central Institute for the Deaf, **A**

Stokes, Ann Marie #3-306 1st Street East, Fort Frances, ON, Canada P9A 1K7, (807) 274-9384, BA 82 Univ of Western Ontario; MA 85 Northwestern Univ; Dir of Sp-Lang Path, Northwestern Home Care, **SLP**

Stokes, Anne Katherine 51-J South Avenue, Harrisonburg, VA 22801, (703) 433-3270, BS 79 James Madison Univ; MS 85 James Madison Univ; Program Coordinator SLP, Parent and Child Education, **SLP**

Stokes, Christine Montelone 94B Avon Circle, Rye Brook, NY 10573, (718) 935-7399, **SLP**

Stokes, Dorothy W 17995 Haskins Road, Bowling Green, OH 43402, **SLP**

Stokes, Martha A 2903 40th Avenue, Gulfport, MS 39501, **SLP**

Stokes, Mary Hug 10 Phelps Lane, Newark, DE 19711, (302) 731-8314, BS 78 WV Univ; MS 81 Towson St Univ; SLP, Private Practice, **SLP**

Stokes, Nona B 1611 Crittenden Street N W, Washington, DC 20011, **A**

Stokes, Orvil J 6879 North Highway 69, P O Box 147, Honeyville, UT 84314, (801) 621-1123, **SLP**

Stokes, Mrs Rosemary H 434 North Tampa Avenue, Orlando, FL 32805, (305) 422-3200, MA 73 Univ of Central FL; BA 47 Millsaps Coll; Consultant, Orange Co Sch

Stolarik, Gail A 711 Marshall Road, Vienna, VA 22180, (703) 941-7704, BS 74 Univ of IL - Urbana; MS 75 Univ of IL - Urbana; Sp-Lang Path, Sch for Contemporary Ed, **SLP**

Stoll, Bernard 400 Prospect Street, New Haven, CT 06511, PH (NS); **SLP**

Stoll, Julie Bethea 2221 Holbrook, Hamtramck, MI 48212, BS 79 Baylor Univ; MS 80 Baylor Univ; Sp-Lang Path, **SLP**

Stolle, Mrs Marcia Zieman 5801 Ogilby Drive, Hudson, OH 44236, (216) 656-3964, MA 84 Univ of Akron; 88–Sp-Lang Path, RehabCare Inc, **SLP**

Stolp, Lauren E 2347 Kenderton Avenue, Roslyn, PA 19001, (215) 885-2766, BA 47 Eastern WA Univ; MS 51 IN St Univ - Terre Haute; Sp-Lang Path, Private Practice, **SLP LM**

Stolpa, Mrs Rebecca T 1365 Forest Avenue, Palo Alto, CA 94301, (415) 327-1151, BS 72 Auburn Univ - Auburn; MA 80 San Jose St Univ; Sp-Lang Path, Private Practice, **SLP**

Stoltz, Mrs Terri Lynn 7109 Uranus Drive, Louisville, KY 40258, (502) 332-1658, BS 80 Western KY Univ; MS 85 Univ of Louisville; 88–Sp-Lang Path, Private Practice, **SLP**

Stolzberg, Mrs Hilary M 8218 Misty Ridge Lane, Houston, TX 77071, (713) 931-9433, BA 78 SUNY - Center at Buffalo; MA 80 IN Univ - Bloomington; 81–Sp-Lang Path, Klein ISD, **SLP**

Stom, Mrs Sylvia Thompson 1804 Tison, Brenham, TX 77833, (409) 836-4511, BS 77 Lamar Univ; MS 78 Lamar Univ; 88–Aud, Brenham State Sch, **A**

Stomackin, Karen M 617 Cross Street, Lewistown, PA 17044, (717) 248-4652, BS 77 West Chester Univ of PA; MA 79 Trenton St Coll; Sp/Lang Path, Tuscarora Iu, **SLP**

Stombaugh, Linda A 4330 Melis Street, Port Charlotte, FL 33948, **SLP**

Stomel, Mrs Andrea W 3402 Elderta Lane, Marlton, NJ 08053, BA 81 Rutger's St Univ - Douglas Coll; MS 83 Boston Univ; 87–Sp-Lang Path, St John of God Comm Svcs, **SLP ACE**

Stone, Anita T 6475 S W 92nd Street, Miami, FL 33156, (305) 666-1642, BS 72 Ball St Univ; MS 76 FL St Univ; **SLP**

Stone, Mrs Ann Marie 20711 Vista Del Sol, Yorba Linda, CA 92686, (714) 537-7661, BA 78 CA St Univ - Fullerton; MA 81 CA St Univ - Fullerton; SLP, Anaheim Cty Sch Dist, **SLP**

Stone, Barbara F 14928 Manor Lake Drive, Chesterfield, MO 63017, **SLP**

Stone, Beth V 20481 Royal Drive, Malibu, CA 90265, (213) 456-6066, BA 71 Univ of Miami; MA 72 George Washington Univ; Sp-Lang Path, Private Practice, **SLP**

Stone, Mrs Carole R 9931 South 67th East Avenue, Tulsa, OK 74133, (918) 299-6115, BA 57 Northwest Nazarene Coll; MA 64 Northwestern Univ; Dir, Lrng & Lang Spec, **SLP**

Stone, Carolyn 10415 Pagewood, Dallas, TX 75230, (214) 661-7643, BA 63 Southern Methodist Univ; MA 68 Southern Methodist Univ; Aud, Otol Labco, **A**

Stone, Charles R 6545 France Avenue South, Suite 614, Edina, MN 55435, (612) 929-0501, BS 70 Univ of WI - Stevens Point; MS 71 Univ of WI - Stevens Point; Pres, Allied Hrng Serv, **A**

Stone, Mrs Cynthia V 501 County Line Road, Albany, GA 31705, (912) 439-8162, ME 88 Valdosta St Coll

Stone, F Scott 360 Pearl Street #102, Box 3, Burlington, VT 05401, (802) 496-6221, BS 71 Emerson Coll; MS 78 Univ of VT; Sp-Lang Path, Washington W Supervisory Union, **SLP**

Stone, Mrs Harriet Cohen 8312 Kilbourn, Skokie, IL 60076, (312) 676-9280, BA 52 IN Univ - Bloomington; MA 56 IN Univ - Bloomington; Sp-Lang Path, Skokie Sch Dist 68, **SLP**

Stone, Mrs Hortense W 39 Eunice Drive, Longmeadow, MA 01106, (413) 567-0464, BA 50 Case Western Reserve Univ; SLP/Aud, Jewish Nursing Home of Wn Ma, **SLP**

Stone, Mrs Janet L 124 Scenery Drive, Morgantown, WV 26505, (301) 296-9237, MS 84 WV Univ; 84–Sp-Lang Path, Monogalia Co Sch, **SLP**

Stone, Jeannine 41 Upland Road, Great Neck, NY 11020-1133, **SLP**

Stone, Mrs Joan Marie 3330 Robin Road, Louisville, KY 40213, (502) 454-8222, MS 83 Univ of Louisville; **SLP**

Stone, Judith R 303 16th East #203, Seattle, WA 98112, (206) 543-5065, MA 87 7030; MA 77 Univ of IL - Urbana; PH 86 (Sp-Lang Path) Univ of WA; 86–Lecturer, University of Washington, **SLP**

Stone, Mrs Karen Ann 4317 Oak Lane, St Augustine, FL 32086, (904) 797-4978, BS 78 Central MI Univ; MA 79 Central MI Univ; Sp-Lang Path, InSpeech Inc, **SLP**

Stone, Mrs Katrinka L 917 Campbell Avenue, Hamilton, OH 45011, (513) 863-3951, BS 78 Miami Univ - Oxford; MS 81 Miami Univ - Oxford; Sp/Lang Path, Hamilton Co Off of Ed, **SLP**

Stone, Mrs Marilyn L 2539 New York Avenue, Melville, NY 11746, (516) 271-6263, BA 71 CUNY - Queens Coll; MS 75 Adelphi Univ; 78–Aud, Huntington Hrng and Sp Cen, **A**

Stone, Dr Mary Ann P O Box 1841, Goldsboro, NC 27533, (919) 734-6900, BA 69 Univ of MD - College Park; MA 72 Univ of MD - College Park; PH 78 (NS) Univ of TN - Knoxville; Aud/Sp-Lang Path, Private Practice, **SLP A**

Stone, Mary F 203 Trackers Rd, Cary, NC 27513, (919) 467-3388, BS 74 Indiana Univ of PA; MA 82 OH St Univ; Sp-Lang Path, **SLP**

Stone, Mrs Mary Pearsall Box 833, Daly City, CA 94017, (415) 574-5005, BS 57 Northwestern Univ; MA 59 Northwestern Univ; 74–Dir & Tchr, Mary Stone Sch, **SLP**

Stone, Mrs Maryalice 7 September Road, Storrs, CT 06268, (203) 423-8620, BS 73 SUNY - Coll at Oswego; MS 76 SUNY - Coll at Geneseo; Sp/Lang Path, Maryalice M Stone, **SLP**

Stone, Dr Maureen L 4219 Woodberry Street, University Park, MD 20782, (301) 496-4733, BA 69 CUNY - Queens Coll; MS 71 Boston Univ; PH 79 (NS) Univ of MD - College Park; Deputy Chief for Research, NIH, **SLP**

Stone, Nicola F R 9217 West 112th Terrace, Overland Park, KS 66210, **SLP**

Stone, Paula 8234 South Evans, Chicago, IL 60619, (312) 980-8366, **SLP**

Stone, Mrs Peggy L 4414 N W 41st Lane, Gainesville, FL 32605, (904) 395-0174, BA 73 Univ of FL; ME 74 Univ of FL; Sp-Lang Path, Fulton Co Board of Education, **SLP**

Stone, Rebecca Jane-Boyd 6045 Aspinwall Road, Oakland, CA 94611, (415) 748-2326, MS 83 San Francisco St Univ; BA 62 Kalamazoo Coll; Sp-Lang Path, Comm Coll Foundation, **SLP**

Stone, Dr Robert E, Jr Dept Of Otolaryngology, Vanderbilt Univ, Nashville, TN 37232, (317) 343-9630, BS 60 Whitworth Coll; ME 64 Univ of OR; PH 71 (NS) Univ of MI - Ann Arbor; Assoc Prof, Vanderbilt Univ Med Sch, **SLP F**

Stone, Robin Gayle 7900 La Riviera Drive #301, Sacramento, CA 95826, (916) 386-2387, MS 88 CA St Univ - Sacramento

Stone, Mrs Sharon Rala 59 Ivyhurst, Eggertsville, NY 14226, (716) 636-3410, BA 65 McGill Univ - Quebec; MA 74 SUNY - Center at Buffalo; Asst Prof, SUNY-Buffalo, **SLP ACE**

Stone, Sue Sherwood Family Hearing Center, 5106 Kingston Pike, Knoxville, TN 37919, (615) 588-3511, BA 75 Univ of FL; MA 76 Univ of TN - Knoxville; Aud, Family Hrng Cen, **A**

Stone, Mrs Sueann 331 Barton Place, Menlo Park, CA 94025, (415) 325-5883, BA 59 Temple Univ-Tyler Sch of Art; MS 83 San Francisco St Univ; Sp-Lang Path, Peninsula Chldrns Ctr, **SLP**

Stone, Mrs Susan B 2217 Cornwell Drive, Jeffersonville, IN 47130, (812) 282-5671, BS 82 Ball St Univ; MA 84 IN Univ - Bloomington; Sp-Lang Path, Greater Clark Co Sch, **SLP**

Stone, Terry A 12060 Stoneybrook Drive, Reno, NV 89511, **SLP**

Stone, Mrs Wanda Jean 302 Circle Dr, Decatur, TX 76234, (817) 627-5276, BS 80 TX Woman's Univ; MA 84 TX Woman's Univ; 88–Sp-Lang Path, Wise Co Spec Educ, **SLP**

Stone-Beasley, Stephanie 302 North Stonewall Street, Memphis, TN 38112, (901) 274-3772, BS 77 Univ of TN - Martin; MA 80 Memphis St Univ; Sp-Lang Path, Private Practice, **SLP**

Stonefield, Ross 87 Crestwood Terrace, Albany, NY 12203, (518) 456-9060, BA 68 SUNY - Center at Albany; MS 70 SUNY - Center at Albany; Sp-Lang Path, Alb-Schoh-Schen Bd Coop Ed Ser, **SLP**

Stone-Gross, Dale Ellen 25521 Via Heraloo, Valencia, CA 91355, (805) 254-0751, BS 76 SUNY - Center at Albany; MA 78 Hofstra Univ; Sp-Lang Path, Private Practice, **SLP**

Stoneham, Mrs Martha Transue 50 Winfield Drive, Tiffin, OH 44883, (419) 447-9811, BS 46 Bowling Green St Univ; MA 47; Sp-Lang Path, Betty Jane Rehab Cen, **SLP**

Stoneking, Brenda Jo 1492 Callie Road, Charleston, WV 25314, (304) 346-7821, BS 82 WV Univ; MS 83 WV Univ

Stoneman, Janice Green 3635 Wabeek Lake Dr West, Bloomfield Hills, MI 48013-1937, (313) 348-8000, BS 74 Wayne St Univ; MA 76 Wayne St Univ - Sch of Med; Aud, Woodland Medical Group, **A**

Stoneman, Mrs Mary Frances 5508 Cottonwood Drive N W, Lawton, OK 73505, (405) 357-7122, BA 80 Columbus Coll; ME 82 Columbus Coll; Sp-Lang Path, Lawton Pub Schs, **SLP**

Stoner, Mrs Janet Lynn 4405 Scott Carpenter, Jackson, MI 49201, (517) 787-2800, BS 76 Western MI Univ; MS 82 Eastern MI Univ; 77–Sp-Lang Path, Jackson Inter Sch Dist, **SLP**

Stoner, Mrs Julia B 1401 West Parkside Drive, Peoria, IL 61606, (309) 686-0548, MS 81 Bradley Univ; BS 79 Univ of Southwestern LA; **SLP**

Stoner, Susan Ballew 161 California Avenue K202, Palo Alto, CA 94306, (415) 321-3759, BS 84 Baylor Univ; MS 85 Baylor Univ; Sp-Lang Path, Stanbridge Academy

Stoner, Wynette Renae 7500 Bellerive #1805, Houston, TX 77036, (713) 791-7010, BA 86 Baylor Univ; MS 87 Baylor Univ; 87–Aud, Baylor Coll of Med, **A**

Stonestreet, Rebecca Vernon High Point Audiological Assoc, 624 Quaker Lane, Office 113 A, High Point, NC 27262, (919) 884-5929, BA 80 Univ of NC - Greensboro; ME 82 Univ of NC - Greensboro; Aud, Private Practice, **SLP A**

Stonestreet, Dr Ruth H 645 Baker, Rochester, MI 48063, (313) 286-8800, BS 69 MS Univ for Women; MS 71 MS Univ for Women; PH 86 (NS) Southern IL Univ -Carbondale; Sp-Lang Path, MacOmb ISD, **SLP**

Stong, Mont Edward 2550 El Camino Real, Mountain View, CA 94040, (415) 948-6700, BS 81 Southern Methodist Univ; MS 84 Univ of North TX; Aud, Hearing Aid Ctr, **A**

St Onge, Keith R 120 Bluffview, Collinsville, IL 62234, PH (NS); **SLP LM**

St Onge, Tracie Lee 2626 B Ocean Front Walk, San Diego, CA 92109, (619) 488-9710, 80 San Diego St Univ; MA 84 San Diego St Univ; **SLP**

Stoots, Mrs Sheri L 87 North Pond Street, Bristol, CT 06010, (203) 667-5320, BS 85 James Madison Univ; ME 87 James Madison Univ; Aud, Newington Children's Hosp, **A**

Stopol, Joy E 8550 Boulevard East, North Bergen, NJ 07047, (516) 921-7171, Sp-Lang Path, Yeshiva Univ/Therpeutc Nursery, **SLP**

Stoppenbach, Daniel T VA Hospital, Pass Road, Biloxi, MS 39531, (601) 388-5541, BA 78 Univ of WI - Madison; MS 80 Univ of WI - Madison; Aud, VA, **A**

Storch-Joiner, Mrs Kimberly Yvonne 100 Oak Knoll Way, Roswell, GA 30075-2354, (404) 475-3361, BS 82 Univ of GA; ME 84 Univ of GA; Aud, North Suburban Ear-Nose-Throat, **A**

Storer, Dr Paula Square Grad Dept Speech Pathology, University Of Toronto, 88 College Street, Toronto, ON, Canada M5G 1L4, (416) 978-2770, BS 70 Miami Univ - Oxford; MA 76 Kent St Univ; PH 81 (Sp-Lang Path) Kent St Univ; Associate Professor, Univ of Toronto, **SLP**

Storey, Julia Lynn 1275 Glendale Drive, Dunedin, FL 34698, (813) 733-9042, BA 85 Univ of FL; ME 87 Univ of FL; 87–Sp-Lang Path, Lashley & Assoc Inc, **SLP**

Storey, Mary F P O Box 255, Hunt, TX 78024, **SLP LM**

Stork, Mrs Kristine A 1011 Nevada, Columbia, IL 62236, (314) 454-7759, BS 81 Eastern IL Univ; MA 82 Saint Louis Univ; Sp-Lang Path, Jewish Hosp of St Louis, **SLP**

Storm, Mrs Florence R 20750 Edgewood, Big Rapids, MI 49307, (616) 689-6691, BA 42 CUNY - Queens Coll; MA 65 OR St Univ; **SLP LM**

Storm, Henry W, Jr 142 Fox Chapel Road, Henrietta, NY 14467, (716) 473-4080, BS 59; MS 70 SUNY - Coll at Geneseo; Supv SLP, Monroe Comm Hosp, **SLP**

Storm, Jill B Strullendorf Elem School, APO New York, NY 09139, BS 75 Univ of WI - Stevens Point; MS 76 Univ of WI - Stevens Point; Sp-Lang Path, Dept of Defense Dependent Sch, **SLP**

Storm, Mrs Pamela Adele 43 Chestnut Street, Lunenburg, MA 01462, (617) 368-8482, **SLP**

Storm, Patricia Grady 172 Whitehall Road, Hooksett, NH 03106, (603) 627-3084, BA 71 Univ of NH; MS 86 Univ of NH; 79–Sp-Lang Path, Manchester Program Hrng Imp, **SLP**

Storrs, Jack L 2934 Waverly Drive, Shingle Springs, CA 95682, (916) 677-4265, BA 78 CA St Univ - Sacramento; MA 79 Univ of the Pacific; Sp-Lang Path, El Dorado Co Offi of Ed, **SLP**

Storrs, Sheila A 306 East Rambo Street, Bridgeport, PA 19405, (215) 645-2210, BS 77 Bloomsburg Univ of PA; MS 78 Bloomsburg Univ of PA; 87–Chief Sp-Lang Path, Lankenau Hosp, **SLP**

Storrs, Sherrill Gonyea 23 Beman Street, Malone, NY 12953, (518) 483-7370, BA 68 Catholic Univ of America; MS 76 SUNY - Coll at Plattsburgh; MA 85 SUNY - Coll at Plattsburgh; 87–Sp-Lang Path, Franklin Co Nursing Svc, **SLP**

Storti, Dr Susan Learning & Lang Specialists, 1405 Lilac Drive, Suite 200, Minneapolis, MN 55422, (612) 545-7708, BS 64 Univ of MN - Minneap-St Paul; ME 66 Wayne St Univ; PH 71 (NS) Wayne St Univ; Sp-Lang Path, Lrng/Lang Spec, **SLP**

Storton, Deborah S 4514 3rd Street #20, La Mesa, CA 92041, (619) 449-6781, BA 73 Univ of San Diego; MA 75 Univ of San Diego; SLP, Santee Sch Dist, **SLP**

Story, Mrs Robin Seider Haskins Laboratories, 270 Crown Street, New Haven, CT 06510, (203) 359-2801, BA 77 SUNY - Coll at Brockport; MA 78 Bowling Green St Univ; Asst Sp-Lang Path, Haskins Laboratories, **SLP**

Story, Mrs Tamara Beazell 608 West Main Street, Midland, MI 48640, (517) 832-8914, BA 66 Case Western Reserve Univ; MA 68 Case Western Reserve Univ; 83–Pres, Head Injury Ther Svcs Inc, **SLP ACE**

Storz, Mrs Debra McClung Route 1 Box 81, Adams, NE 68301, (402) 223-2302, BS 80 Central MO St Univ; MS 87 Central MO St Univ; 88–Sp-Lang Path, Beatrice State Dev Ctr

Stosic, Mrs Patricia Waylonis 107 Village Drive, Pittsburgh, PA 15227, (412) 828-1300, BS 84 Indiana Univ of PA; MS 85 Indiana Univ of PA; 86–Sp-Lang Path, Harmarville Rehab Ctr, **SLP**

Stoskopf, Colette M 303 Greenwich Avenue Apartment A207, Warwick, RI 02886, (401) 331-8842, BA 80 Valparaiso Univ; MA 81 Western MI Univ; 86–Sp-Lang Path, Visiting Nurses of RI, **SLP**

Stoskopf, Mrs Sharon L 129 North Summit, El Dorado, KS 67042, (316) 321-4024, BS 73 Univ of KS; MA 74 Univ of KS; Sp-Lang Path, Butler County School Bd Couns, **SLP**

Stott, Beverly Liddicote 214 Felton Street, Highland Park, NJ 08904, (201) 321-7764, BA 82 Rutgers St Univ -N Brunswick; MS 84 PA St Univ - Univ Park; SLP, J F Kennedy Medical Center, **SLP**

Stotts, Janet Fay 409 Cameron Circle #2004, Chattanooga, TN 37403, (615) 622-8255, BS 81 Western KY Univ; MA 83 Univ of TN - Knoxville; Sp-Lang Path, Commun Cl-Bev Inman-Ebel, **SLP**

Stotz, Mrs Valorie 22 Jemison Road, Rochester, NY 14623, (716) 352-2440, BS 78 SUNY - Coll at Fredonia; MS 79 PA St Univ - Univ Park; 84–Sp-Lang Path, BOCES #2, **SLP**

Stotz, William Albert P O Box 5087, Canyon Lake, CA 92380, (714) 982-5542, BS 77 Pacific Union Coll; MS 84 Univ of Redlands; Aud, Professional Hearing Services, **A**

Stoudt, Dr Ralph J, Jr Speech And Hearing Center, 132 Emmet Street, P O Box 9022, Charlottesville, VA 22906-9022, (804) 924-4615, BA 50 Albright Coll; MA 59 Univ of VA - Charlottesville; PH 64 (Sp Path) Univ of MI - Ann Arbor; Assoc Prof, U of VA, **SLP**

Stouffer, Dr James L University Of Western Ontario, Elborn College, London, ON, Canada N6G 1H1, (519) 679-6465, BS 64 SUNY - Coll at Buffalo; MS 66 PA St Univ - Univ Park; PH 69 PA St Univ - Univ Park; Associate Professor, University of Western Ontario, **A**

Stouffer, Mrs Jodi L Communication Disorders Department, Pennsylvania State University, 3 G Moore, University Park, PA 16802, (814) 863-2008, BS 79 Indiana Univ of PA; MS 82 Indiana Univ of PA; Sp-Lang Path, **SLP**

Stouffer, John 2112 Commanche Road, Pueblo, CO 81001, (303) 545-4123, BA 62 Univ of Northern CO; MA 74; **SLP**

Stough, Mrs Susan Jane PG County Health Department, Division Speech And Audiology, 6490 Landover Road Suite E, Landover, MD 20785, (301) 772-0990, BA 85 Mary Washington Coll; ME 87 Univ of VA - Charlottesville; 87–Sp-Lang Path, Prince George's Co Hlth Dept, **SLP**

Stouppe, Mrs Marilyn Ann 109 Village Estates Drive, Lewisville, TX 75067, (817) 488-9588, MA 83 TX Woman's Univ; 81–Sp-Lang Path, Grapevine-Colleyville ISD, **SLP**

Stout, Mrs Carol Elizabeth P O Box 24, Mounds, IL 62964, (618) 745-6213, **SLP**

Stout, Connie E 5914 Paramount Drive, Oklahoma City, OK 73162, (405) 271-4477, BA 67 Univ of NM; MA 69 Univ of NM; Dir SLP/Aud, OK St Dept Hlth, **SLP**

Stout, Gayle 12 Woodstone, Houston, TX 77024, (713) 523-3633, BA 57 TX Christian Univ; MA 71 Southern Methodist Univ; Aud, Houston Sch for Deaf Chldn, **A**

Stout, Mrs Joann Cooper Rural Delivery 2, 102 Jonslea Lane, Moscow, PA 18444, (717) 383-0060, BS 60 PA St Univ - Univ Park; ME 61 PA St Univ - Univ Park; Sp-Lang Path, Nen Ed Inter Ut #19, **SLP**

Stout, Patricia E H 2764 NE Wiberg Lane, Portland, OR 97213, (503) 229-7151, BS 76 James Madison Univ; MS 78 James Madison Univ; 88–Asst Dir, Rehab Inst of Oregon, **SLP**

Stout, Mrs Tamara Worrell Summit Oaks, 1108 Montreal Road #109, Clarkston, GA 30021, BA 80 Auburn Univ - Auburn; MS 82 Vanderbilt Univ; **SLP**

Stout, Yvette C 375 Big Horn Ridge N E, Albuquerque, NM 87122, **SLP**

Stoutt, Tyleen Roe 1107 Old Harrods Creek Rd, Anchorage, KY 40223, (502) 245-5580, OB 79 Univ of Louisville; BS 64 Northwestern Univ; MS 65 Vanderbilt Univ; **SLP**

Stovall, Inger Benedikte 219 East 84th Street #6-E, New York, NY 10028, (212) 677-7400, BA 83 Boston Coll; MA 86 NY Univ; **SLP**

Stovall, Mrs Janice J c/o Mc Gehee, 77 Mid Oak Lane, Roseville, MN 55113, (612) 645-2993, BS 38 Univ of WI - Madison; MS 50 Univ of WI - Madison; **SLP A LM**

Stovall, Joan Cody 1182 Ottawa Avenue, West St Paul, MN 55118, (612) 423-9394, BS 79 ND St Univ; MA 81 Northern MI Univ; Sp-Lang Path, Apple Valley Rosemount, **SLP**

Stovall, Susan Marie 1966 Stanley Avenue, Santa Clara, CA 95050-5721, (408) 998-6255, MA 80 Humboldt St Univ; **SLP**

Stovall, Wanda W 4009 Inwood Road, Fort Worth, TX 76109, (717) 534-4871, BA 67 TX Christian Univ; MS 72 TX Christian Univ; SLP, Fort Worth ISD, **SLP**

Stover, Gale Lynn RR1 Box 377, Arcadia, IN 46030, (317) 844-5037, BS 82 Purdue Univ - West Lafayette; MA 87 Butler Univ; 87–Sp-Lang Path, Healthmark, **SLP**

Stover, Mrs Joan L P O Box 179, Middlesex, NY 14507, (716) 377-4660, BS 56 SUNY - Coll at Geneseo; MS 64 SUNY - Coll at Geneseo; Sp-Lang Path, BOCES #1, **SLP**

Stover, Joanne Elizabeth 890 Foxworth Blvd, #412, Lombard, IL 60148, (312) 932-4738, BA 85 MI St Univ; MA 87 Central MI Univ; 88–Aud, Sound Resources, **A**

Stover, Susan Eugena P O Box 388, Sylacauga, AL 35150, (813) 893-6703, MS 88 Auburn Univ - Auburn; 88–Sp-Lang Path, Bayfront Med Ctr, **F**

Stow, Mrs Carol Jean 11 Hartzel Court, Mount Laurel, NJ 08054, (609) 261-7030, OM 84 Hahnemann Univ Grad Sch; SLP, Memorial Hos/Burlington County, **SLP**

Stowell, Mrs Virginia Harrel Route 2 Box 35, Rising Sun, IN 47040, (812) 438-2026, BA 66 Univ of OK - Norman; MS 68 Univ of OK Medical Center; **SLP**

Stowers, Richard A 1582 Falda Del Cerro, El Cajon, CA 92020, (619) 462-7255, Sp/Lang Path, Lemon Grove Sch Dist, **SLP**

Stowers, Shirley Richard 1582 Falda Del Cerro, El Cajon, CA 92019, (619) 447-4721, BS 64 Univ Southern MS-Hattiesburg; MS 66 Univ Southern MS-Hattiesburg; Sp-Lang Path, Lemon Grove Sch Dist, **SLP**

Stoy, Mrs Mary Philipps 231 Hazelwood Drive, Washington, PA 15301, (412) 225-0194, BS 79 WV Univ; MS 80 WV Univ; 88–Sp-Lang Path, Allegheny Intermediate Unit #3, **SLP**

Stoyko, Mrs Donna Jane N 14502 Pinetree Drive, Spokane, WA 99208, (509) 466-0309, BA 74 Eastern WA Univ; MS 85 Eastern WA Univ; **SLP**

St Peter, Katherine A 167 Haverhill Street, Rowley, MA 01969, (617) 468-3713, BA 75 Univ of ME - Orono; ME 78 Northeastern Univ; Early Childhood Specialist, Hamilton-Wenham Public Sch, **SLP**

St Peters, Mary C 7301 Girard Avenue, Apt #302, San Diego, CA 92037, (619) 481-8802, BA 75 Univ of MO - Columbia; MS 77 Fontbonne Coll; Site Manager SLP, Childrens Hospital, **SLP**

St Pierre, Dianne Marie 86 Day Street, West Springfield, MA 01089, (413) 734-0871, BS 83 Springfield Coll; MA 85 Univ of MA - Amherst; **SLP**

St Pierre, Karrie A 21281 Harper #29, St Clair Shores, MI 48080, (313) 774-7419, BS 78 Central MI Univ; MA 79 Eastern MI Univ; ES 88 Wayne St Univ; 86–Sp-Lang Path, Warren Woods Sch Dist, **SLP**

St Pierre, Mrs Melissa P O Box 273, Bradford, NH 03221, (603) 938-5467, BS 78 Worcester St Coll; MA 79 Case Western Reserve Univ; Sp/Lang Path, Kearsarge Regional Sch Dist, **SLP**

St Pierre Hetz, Mrs Michelle Marie 13 Ashlor Drive, Middle Grove, NY 12850-9518, **SLP**

Stracci, Mary E 3288 Agar Place, Bronx, NY 10465, (212) 882-1477, BA 76 CUNY - Hunter Coll; MA 79 CUNY - Lehman Coll; Sp/Lang Path, Lavelle Sch Blind & Vis Imp, **SLP**

Strachn-Hunt, Josephine 62 Knob Hill Road, Hackettstown, NJ 07840, (201) 852-0216, BA 74 Rutger's St Univ - Douglas Coll; MA 79 San Jose St Univ; SLP, Mt Olive Schl Dstr, **SLP**

Strack, Mrs Alison Kay 12 Hillside Drive, Apalachin, NY 13732-9487, (607) 687-4550, BS 78 PA St Univ - Univ Park; MS 81 Ithaca Coll; Sp-Lang Path, Owego-Apalachin Ctrl Dist, **SLP**

Strader, Mrs Ann Teas 3580 Liberty Lane, Marietta, GA 30062, (404) 565-5551, BA 76 Hollins Coll; ME 79 Univ of VA - Charlottesville; Sp-Lang Path, Private Practice, **SLP**

Stradinger, Mrs Teresa Carpentier 408 Nadig Drive, Fort Atkinson, WI 53538, (414) 563-5210, **SLP**

Strahle, Jane C c/o Speakeasy Inc, 3414 Peachtree Road N E, Suite 800, Atlanta, GA 30326, (404) 261-4029, BS 66 Univ of GA; MA 72 Univ of GA; ME 78 GA St Univ; 81–Sp-Lang Path, Speakeasy, Inc, **SLP**

Strahle, Marjorie James 2020 Crooked Lane, Flint, MI 48503, **SLP**

Straight, Jenise Schroeder Route 1 Box 6, Shickley, NE 68436, (402) 463-5611, MS 84 Univ of NE - Lincoln; Sp-Lang Path, Ed Serv Unit 9, **SLP ACE**

Strain, Mrs Donna Spiers 113 Beau Pre Drive, Mandeville, LA 70448, (504) 845-8819, BS 79 LA St Univ - Baton Rouge; MS 82 LA St Univ - N O Medical Ctr; 87–Sp-Lang Path, St Tammany Parish Schs, **SLP**

Strain, Mary K 5916 North Ross, Oklahoma City, OK 73112, **SLP**

Strait, Marcia M 2610 Garfield Avenue South, Apartment 207, Minneapolis, MN 55408, (612) 861-8282, BA 70 MacAlster Coll; MA 75 Univ of MN - Minneap-St Paul; 75–Sp-Lang Path, Richfield Pub Sch, **SLP**

Strait, Mary Wells P O Box 151, 2201 Lexington Avenue, Ashland, KY 41105-0151, (606) 329-1746, BA 71 Marshall Univ; MA 72 Marshall Univ; Exec Dir, Geiger Er Sl Sp & Hrng Cen, **SLP ACE**

Strait, Mrs Rose 142 Melrose, Pueblo, CO 81004, (303) 545-4531, BA 49; MA 50; **SLP LM**

Straitman, Nina P 103 West Sutton Place, Wilmington, DE 19810, (302) 651-6054, BA 71 Chatham Coll; MS 76 PA St Univ - Univ Park; SLP, Alfred I Dupont Inst, **SLP**

Straka, Elizabeth A 661 Ruth Avenue, Idaho Falls, ID 83401, (208) 525-7236, BA 84 Univ of WI - Eau Claire; MS 86 Univ of WI - Eau Claire; Sp-Lang Path, Adult Child Dev Ctr, **SLP**

Straka, Mrs Elizabeth M 2210 Lelaray, Colorado Springs, CO 80909, (719) 633-9114, BA 78 Univ of CO - Boulder; MS 80 Phillips Univ; Sp-Lang Path, Lee & Straka Assoc, **SLP**

Stram, Sarah T 11 Chestnut Street, Dover, NH 03820, (603) 749-2446, BS 57 Univ of MD - College Park; MA 64 Univ of MD - College Park; MS 80 Univ of NH; Sp-Lang Path, Private Practice, **SLP ACE**

Strand, Dr Edythe A Department Of Communication Science & Disorders, Allen House, University Of Vermont, Burlington, VT 05405, (802) 656-3861, BA 72 Univ of the Pacific; MA 73 Univ of the Pacific; PH 87 (Communicative Disorders) Univ of WI - Madison; 88–Asst Prof, Univ of Vermont, **SLP**

Strand, Gayle Jean 103 East 16th, Yankton, SD 57078, (402) 287-2061, BA 84 Univ of SD - Vermillion; MA 85 Univ of SD - Vermillion; **SLP**

Strand, Joan Marie Owen-Withee Public Schools, P O Box 417, Owen, WI 54460, (715) 229-2151, BS 82 Univ of WI - Stevens Point; MA 83 Univ of MN - Duluth; SLP, Owen-Withee Pub Sch, **SLP**

Strand, Dr Kristine E 151 Tremont Street, Boston, MA 02111, (617) 254-3800, BS 67 Northwestern Univ; MA 68 Northwestern Univ; ED 82 (Psycholinguistics) Boston Univ; 86–Dir Sp-Lang-Hrng Serv, Kennedy Mem Hosp for Chldrn, **SLP**

Strand, Richard L Marshfield Clinic, Audiology 4A1, 1000 North Oak Street, Marshfield, WI 54449, (715) 387-5371, BS 59 Saint Cloud St Univ; MS 61 PA St Univ - Univ Park; 61–Aud, Marshfield Clinic, **A ACE**

Strand, Mrs Valerie Wilson 3219 S W Twilight Drive, Topeka, KS 66614, (913) 273-0245, BS 84 Univ of South AL; MS 86 Univ of South AL; **SLP**

Strandberg, Mrs Roberta Harnois 18 North Broadway #204, Tarrytown, NY 10591-3224, (914) 631-5100, **SLP**

Strand-Janicek, Mrs Michele Darlene 6901 West 8th Street #210, Bloomington, MN 55438, (612) 520-5616, BA 81 Univ of ND; MA 83 Univ of IA; 86–Sp-Lang Path, North Memorial Med Ctr, **SLP**

Strane, Kim K 1404 Woodlawn Boulevard #D, Austin, TX 78703, (512) 440-7083, BS 76 Univ of TX - Austin; MS 78 Baylor Coll of Medicine; Aud Consultant, Private Practice, **A**

Strange, Beth Arlene 11673 Hornsilver Mountain, Littleton, CO 80127-3235, (303) 499-2458, BA 83 Mary Washington Coll; MA 86 Univ of CO - Boulder; **SLP**

Strange, Karen W 3771 Northpoint Drive, Marietta, GA 30062, **SLP**

Strange, Kelley Harmon 4753 Naches Heights Road, Yakima, WA 98908, (509) 966-1553, BA 80 Univ of WA; OM 82 Univ of WA; 88–Sp-Lang Path, West Valley Sch Dist, **SLP**

Strange, Sheri Foshee 4252 Lady Slipper Lane, Memphis, TN 38115, (901) 795-7458, BA 81 Univ of MS; OM 83 Univ of MS; Sp-Lang Path, St Francis Hosp, **SLP**

Stranger, Linda Paine 6143 Davenport, Coeur d'Alene, ID 83814, (208) 772-7113, BS 77 Univ of ME - Farmington; MA 85 Eastern WA Univ; **SLP**

Strang-Wolf, Christina Mayer 100 Watchung Drive, Hawthorne, NJ 07506, (201) 676-1000, BA 85 Montclair St Coll; MS 86 Columbia Univ Teachers Coll; Sp-Lang Path, VA Med Ctr, **SLP**

Straquadine, Judith E T 1213 East 2750, Logan, UT 84321, (701) 223-3708, BA 77 NM St Univ; MA 79 NM St Univ; Aud & SLP, Private Practice, **SLP**

Strassberg, Mrs Miriam Anne 1441 Wilson Road, East Meadow, NY 11554, (516) 483-2290, BA 76 CUNY - City College; MA 79 Hofstra Univ

Strasser, Dr Delbert H Salt Lake Clinic, 333 South 900 East, Salt Lake City, UT 84102, (801) 535-8185, BA 68 Univ of UT; MA 69 Univ of UT; PH 75 (NS) Univ of UT; Aud, Salt Lake Cl, **A**

Strate, Shirlene S E 2121 Upriver Drive #22, Spokane, WA 99207, (509) 455-3765, BA 53 Univ of MT; ME 69 Eastern WA Univ; Sp-Lang Path, Spokane Sch Dist #81, **SLP**

Strattman, Mrs Kathy H 310 N Dellrose, Wichita, KS 67208, (316) 689-3240, BA 70 Midland Lutheran Coll; MA 71 Wichita St Univ; Inst & Cl Superv, Wichita St U, **SLP**

Stratton, Dr Cleavonne 200 Meadow Lake Drive, Bldg 12 #93-B, Downingtown, PA 19335, (215) 436-2132, BA 73 Miles Coll; BA 75 OH St Univ; PH 76 (NS) OH St Univ; Cl Coord, West Chester U, **SLP ACE**

Stratton, Constance Cutter On Call Communication Service, 423 Oaklawn Avenue, South Pasadena, CA 91030, (818) 799-5324, BA 65 Univ of CA - Berkeley; MA 80 CA St Univ - Fullerton; Sp-Lang Path, On Call Commun Serv, **SLP**

Stratton, Elizabeth 7765 West 91st Street, Apartment F-1111, Playa Del Rey, CA 90293, (213) 305-7297, BA 69 Univ of AZ; MA 81 CA St Univ - Northridge; Sp-Lang Path, Los Angeles USD, **SLP**

Stratton, June R R R 1 Box 126, Gilman, IL 60938-9801, (815) 265-4281, BS 60 IN St Univ - Terre Haute; OM 70 IN St Univ - Terre Haute; MS 86 IL St Univ - Normal; 88–Sp-Lang Path, Kankakee Area Spec Educ Co-op, **SLP**

Stratton, Terry L 395 Redding Road #240, Lexington, KY 40502, (606) 273-8745, BS 77 Eastern KY Univ; MA 78 Univ of TN - Knoxville; Sp-Lang Path, Cardinal Hill Hosp, **SLP**

Straub, Charles S Hearing Aid Center Of, Panama City Inc, 303 East 7th Street, Panama City, FL 32401, (904) 769-2705, BS 61 IN St Univ - Terre Haute; MA 68 Univ of IL - Urbana; Owner, Hrng Aid Cen/Panama Cty Inc, **A**

Strauch, Richard J 24 Walnut Street, Wellsboro, PA 16901, (717) 724-4042, BS 70 Bloomsburg Univ of PA; ME 73 Bloomsburg Univ of PA; Owner-Aud, Private Practice, **A**

Straus, Mrs Harriet D 106 Winding Way, Little Silver, NJ 07739, (201) 741-9214, BA 72 George Washington Univ; MS 73 PA St Univ - Univ Park; SLP, Red Bank Regional High School, **SLP**

Straus, Monica B W 184-12 Radnor Road, Jamaica Estates, NY 11432, (212) 380-1621, **SLP**

Strauss, Anne M 6 Puget Sound Court, Coram, NY 11727, BA 78 Long Island U - CW Post Ctr; MS 81 Adelphi Univ; Sp-Lang Path, BOCES-II, **SLP**

Strauss, Paul Karel 20th Support Group, Box 2753 Taegu Korea, Apo, San Francisco, CA 96218, BA 62 Univ of TX - Austin; MA 67 Univ of TX - Austin; Sp/Lang Path, US Army, **SLP A**

Strauss, Dr Raymond B 216 Engle Street, Englewood, NJ 07631, (201) 567-1616, BA 50 Washington Univ; MD 58 Case Western Reserve Univ; PH 56 (NS) Univ of FL; Otor, Private Practice, **SLP A**

Strautman, Susan 3346 East Lester, Tucson, AZ 85716, (602) 941-8128, BS 76 AZ St Univ; MS 78 Univ of AZ; Sp-Lang Path, Amphitheater Public Schools, **SLP**

Strawder, Veronica G 2001 McGraw Avenue, Bronx, NY 10462, BA 75 Columbia Univ Teachers Coll; MS 77 Columbia Univ Teachers Coll; 81–Sp-Lang Path, Private Practice, **SLP**

Strawley, Brenda Nelson Route 9 Box 222, Charlottesville, VA 22901, (804) 924-4621, BS 67 PA St Univ - Univ Park; MA 76 West Chester Univ of PA; PH 79 Univ of VA - Charlottesville; 77–Sp-Lang Path, U VA-Comm Disord Prog, **SLP ACE**

Strawn, Mrs Charlotte R 404 West Broadway, Columbia, MO 65203, (314) 449-5503, BS 78 Univ of MO - Columbia; OM 87 Univ of MO - Columbia; 87–Aud, Boone Clinic, **A**

Strayer, Lorna Schwab Strayer Fisher-Titus Med Ctr, 272 Benedict, Norwalk, OH 44857, (419) 668-8101, BA 82 OH St Univ; MA 83 OH St Univ; Dept Head-Comm Disorders, Fisher-Titus Med Ctr, **SLP**

Stream, Dr Kathryn S 2029 Pembrooke, Denton, TX 76205, (817) 455-2201, BA 60 Vanderbilt Univ; MA 61 Northwestern Univ; PH 82 (NS) Univ of TX Med - Galveston; Vice-Pres Clinical Services, Baylor Health Care System Inc, **A F**

Stream, Dr Richard W Division Of Communication Disorders, University Of North Texas, Denton, TX 76203, (817) 565-2262, BS 55 Univ of IL - Urbana; MS 60 Vanderbilt Univ; PH 64 (NS) Northwestern Univ; 80–Prof, Univ of North Texas, **A F ACE**

Streater, James A, Jr 2525 Monroe Street, Columbia, SC 29205-3153, (803) 777-7096, BA 71 Univ of SC - Columbia; ME 74 Univ of SC - Columbia; **A**

Streator, Rondi Elizabeth 96 Main Street, Colchester, VT 05446, (802) 878-5881, BA 81 Univ of VT; MS 85 Univ of VT

Stredwick, Laura Lee 3006 South Morain Place, Kennewick, WA 99337-2513, (509) 582-2500, MA 82 WA St Univ; BA 79 Eastern WA Univ; Sp-Lang Path, Kennewick School District, **SLP**

Streebel, Laurie Aileen 770 Lancer Court #B-3, Depew, NY 14043, (716) 795-3237, BS 83 SUNY - Coll at Fredonia; MS 84 SUNY - Center at Buffalo; Sp-Lang Path, Childrens Hospital, **SLP**

Street, Brenda Brehob Research Med Center, 2316 East Meyer Blvd, Comm Disorders Dept, Kansas City, MO 64132, (816) 276-4023, BS 79 Purdue Univ - West Lafayette; MS 81 Purdue Univ - West Lafayette; 86–Aud, Research Med Ctr, **A**

Street, Caroline 1524 Lynnwood, Logan, UT 84321, (801) 752-3925, BS 83 UT St Univ; MS 87 UT St Univ; **A**

Street, Mrs Nancy Anne 1103 Finney, College Station, TX 77840, (409) 693-5563, BS 77 Univ of TX - Austin; MA 80 Univ of TX - Austin; Sp-Lang Path, Private Practice, **SLP**

Street, Mrs Robin Webb 2509 Fain Street, Wichita Falls, TX 76308, (817) 767-6066, BS 76 Trinity Univ; MS 78 Univ of North TX; Coord Sp/Lang Hrng Serv, Wichita Falls State Hosp, **SLP**

Street, Sherry Lynn N 103 Rogers Road, Athens, GA 30605, (404) 548-7517, BA 84 IN Univ - Bloomington; MA 85 Memphis St Univ; Sp-Lang Path, Barrow County Board of Educ, **SLP**

Streeter, Amy Beth 1701 Sharp Road, Waterford, WI 53185, (414) 534-2301, MS 86 Univ of WI - Eau Claire; 87–Sp-Lang Path, New Medico Rehab Ctr of WI, **SLP**

Streeter-Discenzo, Mrs Suzanne Speech Pathology Associates, 2130 Academy Circle, Suite A, Colorado Springs, CO 80909, (303) 591-1933, BS 71 OK St Univ; MS 74 Univ of OK Medical Center; 83–Dir of Sp-Lang Path, Private Practice, **SLP**

Street-Speck, Mrs Diane M 3503 E Dragoon Avenue, Mesa, AZ 85204, (602) 832-1912, BS 80 Kearney St Coll; MS 84 Kearney St Coll; **SLP**

Streett, Mrs Sharon S 799 Long Corner Road, Mount Airy, MD 21771, (301) 694-1489, BS 77 James Madison Univ; MS 78 James Madison Univ; Sp-Lang Path, Frederick Co MD Bd of Ed, **SLP**

Streicher, John Paul 18 Willowood, Laguna Hills, CA 92656-2972, **SLP**

Streicker, Mrs Carol R 1231 Linden Avenue, Highland Park, IL 60035, (312) 441-6714, MA 71 Southern Methodist Univ; **SLP**

Streiler, Kathi 9 Royalty Court, Florissant, MO 63034, BA 68 Harris-Stowe St Coll; MA 75 Webster Univ; MA 78 Webster Univ; **SLP**

Streit, Mrs Ann Ralsten 7480 Terry Court, Golden, CO 80403-7920, (303) 467-9460, BA 76 CO St Univ; MA 81 Univ of CO - Boulder; Sp-Lang Path, Private Practice, **SLP**

Streit, Mrs Diane K 307 Campus Drive, Dodge City, KS 67801, (316) 225-1409, **SLP**

Streit, Gloria Jane 408 East 12th Street, Hobart, IN 46342, BA 84 IN Univ - Bloomington; MS 87 Univ of WI - Madison; **SLP**

Streit, Mrs Joanne M Box 393, Fort Benton, MT 59442, (406) 622-3721, BA 74 Univ of MT; MA 76 Univ of MT; 82–Sp-Lang Path, Fort Benton Sch Dist #1, **SLP ACE**

Stremsterfer, Mrs Jerry McIlvaney 11307 Key West Drive N E, Albuquerque, NM 87111, (505) 293-1178, BS 63 Southeast MO St Univ; MS 84 Univ of NM; Sp-Lang Path, Albuquerque Public Schools, **SLP**

Streng, Alice H Dept Speech Path & Audiology, University Of Wisconsin, P O Box 413, Milwaukee, WI 53201, (414) 962-5529, OB 33 Univ of WI - Milwaukee; MA 38 Columbia Univ Teachers Coll; OD 83 (NS) Univ of WI - Milwaukee; **A LM**

Strenkert, Dr Nancy T 180 Middle River Road, Danbury, CT 06811-2713, (203) 791-1233, **SLP**

Strennen, Mary Lou 2675 Richardson Street, Madison, WI 53711-5430, (815) 397-4327, BS 67 American Univ; MA 72 NM St Univ; 88–Aud, Miracle-Ear, **A**

Streu, Mrs Patricia Erickson 1113 Palma Sola Blvd, Bradenton, FL 34209, (813) 746-2133, BA 59 Univ of DE; ME 80 Univ of VA - Charlottesville; Sp-Lang Path, Manatee Co Public Sch Sys, **SLP**

Stribling, Mrs Catherine 75 Marsh Road, Hartwood, VA 22405, (703) 752-2516, BS 79 James Madison Univ; MS 77 James Madison Univ; SLP, Fauquier Co Schls, **SLP**

Stribling, Daulma Box 14, Dawn, TX 79025, (806) 258-7738, BS 53 TX Tech Univ; MS 55 TX Tech Univ; 88–Sp-Lang Path, Walcott Sch, **SLP**

Stricker, Mrs Maureen Jones 129 Rivergate Cove, Ridgeland, MS 39157, (601) 968-2426, BA 70 Southeastern LA Univ; OM 72 Univ of MS; Aud, Jackson St U, **A**

Strickland, Cynthia S 409 West 11th Street, Cozad, NE 69130, MS; **SLP**

Strickland, Elizabeth Ann 205 Elliott Hall, 75 East River Road, Minneapolis, MN 55455, (612) 624-3322, MS 84 IN Purdue Univ -Indianapolis; Univ of MN, **A**

Strickland, Mrs Kristie Jensen 2912 Fountainhead Dr, Plano, TX 75023, SLP, San Ramon Valley USD, **SLP**

Strickland, Margaret J 1420 Marengo, New Orleans, LA 70115, (501) 557-6351, **SLP**

Strickland, Mrs Martha R Box 128, South Haven, KS 67140, (316) 892-5506, BA 76 Wichita St Univ; MA 77 Wichita St Univ; 88–Sp-Lang Path, Blackwell PS Sys, **SLP**

Strickland, Sherrill Moll 40 Fairmont Street, Clinton, MA 01510, (617) 486-3959, BA 73 Clark Univ; MS 84 Worcester St Coll; Sp-Lang Path, Littleton Pub Sch, **SLP**

Strickler, Carol J 1130 Agatha Way, Sacramento, CA 95825, (916) 922-5958, MS 88 CA St Univ - Sacramento

Strickler, Karen G 13 Dix Circle, Dix Hills, NY 11746, **SLP**

Strickler, Mrs Ruth E 270 Sunrise Way, Vallejo, CA 94591, (503) 649-6032, BA 77 Northwest Nazarene Coll; MS 78 ID St Univ; SLP, Elk Grove USD, **SLP**

Stricklin, Mrs Delaine L 5708 Anniston, Shreveport, LA 71105, (318) 868-8911, BS 81 Univ Southern MS-Hattiesburg; MS 82 Univ Southern MS-Hattiesburg; 85–Sp-Lang Path, Willis-Knighton Med Ctr, **SLP**

Striegl, Mrs Janet W 581 Debbington Drive, Bay Village, OH 44140, (216) 871-7673, BA 73 Fontbonne Coll; MA 75 Tulane Univ; SLP, Psi Assoc Inc, **SLP**

Striffler, Nancy S 1293 Bartonshire Way, Rockville, MD 20854, (202) 687-8784, BA 63 2612; MS 64 Univ of MI - Ann Arbor; 73–Dir, Georgetown Univ Child Dev Ctr, **SLP**

Strikowsky, Shari D 45 Route 9W Roundtree, Piermont, NY 10968, (914) 359-6223, MA 84 Chengchi Univ; Sp-Lang Path, Burke Rehabilitation Center, **SLP**

Strimple, Kathleen P O Box 912, Santa Fe, NM 87504, (505) 982-5765, BA 72 Miami Univ - Oxford; MA 76 Univ of Cincinnati; Sp-Lang Path, Private Practice, **SLP**

Stringer, Gary K 5182 West Jerelyn Place, Milwaukee, WI 53219, (414) 449-2422, **SLP**

Stringer, Jerrie S 4162 East Canterbury Drive, San Diego, CA 92116, (619) 588-3123, BA 76 San Diego St Univ; MA 80 San Diego St Univ; Sp-Lang Path, Cajon Valley Union Sch Dist, **SLP**

Stringer, William E Hearing And Speech Center, University Hospital, Augusta, GA 30910, (404) 722-1957, BS 50 Kent St Univ; MA 63 Kent St Univ; Director, Hearing/Speech Ctr of Augusta, **SLP A**

Stringert, Terese Dunlavy 27 Verdosa Drive, Pueblo, CO 81005, (303) 630-5208, BS 78 Univ of WI - Stevens Point; MS 81 Univ of WI - Eau Claire; SLP, Mercy Med Cen, **SLP**

Stringfellow, Mrs Johannah Goodman P O Box 52, Newburgh, IN 47630, (812) 473-3598, BS 78 IN St Univ - Terre Haute; MS 79 IN St Univ - Terre Haute; Sp-Lang Path, Deaconess Hosp, **SLP**

Stringfellow, Mrs Verna W 4682 Ivanhoe Road, Jacksonville, FL 32210, (904) 725-8972, BS 59 Univ of WI - Madison; MA 64 Case Western Reserve Univ; Sp-Lang Path, S Allen Smith Cl, **SLP**

Stringham, Roxanne H 111 West Inglenook Drive, Apartment 2108, Midvale, UT 84047, (801) 533-6175, MA 81 Brigham Young Univ; 88–Sp-Lang Path, Utah St Dept of Health, **SLP**

Strobbe, Mrs Margaret Irene Box 89, East Glacier Park, MT 59434, (406) 338-2715, BS 76 Miami Univ - Oxford; MA 84 Univ of MT; Sp-Lang Path, Browning Public School Dist 9, **SLP**

Stroble, Susan Michele 6573 Mardel, St Louis, MO 63109, (314) 454-6171, BS 81 Marquette Univ; MA 84 Northwestern Univ; Aud, St Louis Chldrns Hosp, **A**

Strobridge, Mary Ann 2055 Balsam Drive, Boulder, CO 80302, (303) 443-4005, MA 66 Univ of CO - Boulder; PH 74 Univ of CO - Boulder; OD 78 (NS) Univ of CO - Boulder; SLP, Boulder Valley Sch, **SLP A**

St Rock, Kathleen A 2 Jessica Lane, Ledyard, CT 06339, (203) 536-7915, BA 77 Univ of CT; MS 79 Southern CT St Univ; Sp-Lang Path, UCP, **SLP**

Strock, William F Medford ENT Clinic, 19 Myrtle, Medford, OR 97504, (503) 779-7331, BS 69 Eastern NM Univ; MS 71 UT St Univ; Dir of Aud, Medford ENT Clinic, **A**

Strode, Robin M 20 Spendthrift, Frankfort, KY 40601-5832, (502) 695-1925, BA 72 Univ of KY; MA 73 Univ of KY; Sp-Lang Path, Private Practice, **SLP**

Stroebel, Rose Chervenak 109 Summerhill Lane, Trafford, PA 15085, (412) 373-2514, BS 81 John Carroll Univ; MA 83 Kent St Univ; SLP, Easter Seal, **SLP**

Stroer, Mrs Barbara S St Joseph Institute For Deaf, 1483 82nd Boulevard, St Louis, MO 63132, (314) 993-1507, BA 71 Fontbonne Coll; MA 74 Saint Louis Univ; 81–Aud, St Joseph I for the Deaf, **A**

Stroetzel, Deborah L 227 Barbara Street, Westfield, MA 01085, (413) 562-5350, MA 85 Univ of MA - Amherst; **A**

Strohfus, Brenda Kay 9955 Russel Avenue North #11, Brooklyn Park, MN 55444, (612) 422-5233, BA 83 SD St Univ; MS 86 Univ of WI - Eau Claire; SLP, Anoka Hennepin School Dstr, **SLP**

Strohmaier, Alison A 10009 Woodhill Road, Bethesda, MD 20817, (301) 365-0167, BS 73 SUNY - Center at Albany; MA 75 Univ of MD - College Park; Sp-Lang Path, Ivymount Sch, **SLP**

Strohmeyer, Karen Lynn 316 Dickinson Road, Apt 8, Springfield, IL 62704, (217) 546-6008, OB 79 Southern IL Univ-Edwardsvill; BS 79 Southern IL Univ-Edwardsvill; MS 87 Southern IL Univ-Edwardsvill; 88–Sp-Lang Path, Springfield Sch Dist #186

Strohmeyer, Linda J 29 Riverview Drive, Bridgeport, CT 06606, (203) 255-8389, BA 66 Nazareth Coll of Rochester; MS 70 SUNY - Center at Buffalo; Coord Sp-Lang Svcs, Fairfield Bd of Ed, **SLP**

Strojny, Mrs Linda A R R 1 Box 240, Moretown, VT 05660, (802) 656-4535, BA 78 Bridgewater St Coll; MS 80 Boston Univ; Dir of Aud, Surgical Assoc Foundation Inc, **A**

Strole, Mrs Christy O P O Box 225, Cerro Gordo, IL 61818, (217) 424-3230, BS 79 Eastern IL Univ; MS 80 Eastern IL Univ; 87–Sp-Lang Path, Decatur School District, **SLP**

Strollo, Janet Ann K 53 Blossum Street, Nashua, NH 03060, (603) 886-0902, BA 77 Boston Coll; MS 80 Rutgers St Univ - Newark; Sp-Lang Path, Ks Neur I, **SLP**

Strom, Mary Patrice 5305 Parview Drive, Charlotte, NC 28105, (704) 542-5790, MA 87 Univ of CO - Boulder; **SLP**

Strom, Mary T 147 West Sidney, St Paul, MN 55107, (612) 776-2791, BA 74 Southwest St Univ; MA 81 Univ of MN - Minneap-St Paul; SLP, St Paul Pub Sch, **SLP**

Stromberg, Eleanor M 9872 Butler Warren Road, Cincinnati, OH 45241, (513) 221-0527, BA 63 Univ of Northern IA; MA 81 Univ of SD - Vermillion; PH 88 (Aud) Univ of Cincinnati; Aud, Cincinnati Spch & Hearing Cen, **A**

Stromberg, Mrs Sadie G Route 2 Box 70, Lockhart, TX 78644, (512) 321-2546, BA 63 Univ of TX - Austin; ME 79 Southwest TX St Univ; Sp-Lang Path, Bastrop ISD, **SLP**

Stromer, Dr Jeffrey M 11245 Seaview Avenue, Bldg H6 #2C, Brooklyn, NY 11239, (212) 631-6284, BA 69 CUNY - Lehman Coll; MS 76 CUNY - Brooklyn Coll; OD 87 (Doctor of Arts Sp Path) Adelphi Univ; 74–Asst Prof/Dir of Rem Sp, CUNY Queensborough Comm Coll, **SLP**

Stromeyer, Katharina M c/o George Stromeyer, 40 Bowdoin Street, Medford, MA 02155, (617) 391-7245

Strominger, Ann Z 2030 Mass Avenue, Lexington, MA 02173, (617) 735-6479, OD 83 (NS) Boston Univ; Sp-Lang Path, The Children's Hosp, **SLP**

Strommer, Amy 5185 Luigi Terrace #43, San Diego, CA 92122, (619) 576-5838, MS 87 Univ of AZ; 87–Sp-Lang Path, Children's Hosp, **SLP**

Stromquist, Dagmar T 206 North 60th Avenue East, Duluth, MN 55804, **SLP**

Stromsta, Courtney 2323 Rambling Road, Kalamazoo, MI 49008, (616) 381-4890, BS 48 Western MI Univ; MA 51 OH St Univ; PH 56 (NS) OH St Univ; Retired, Western Michigan University, **SLP A F LM**

Stroney, Mrs Mary Q 600 West North Boulevard, Suite D, Leesburg, FL 32748, (904) 728-3000, MS 75 Univ of South FL; Dir of Sp-Lang Serv, FL Phys Ther & Rehab Serv, Inc, **SLP ACE**

Strong, Brian K 1148 Ontario Street Apt 1, Oak Park, IL 60302, (312) 848-9750, BA 77 CA St Univ - Fresno; MA 79 CA St Univ - Stanislaus; Co Dir, Sp-Lang Hrng Cl, **SLP**

Strong, Carol D 947 Sumac, Logan, UT 84321-4811, BA 71 UT St Univ; MA 72 Univ of IL - Urbana; Cl Asst Prof, Utah State U, **SLP**

Strong, Gail K P O Box 438, Waukesha, WI 53187, (414) 542-5301, BS 76 CO St Univ; MS 78 Minot St Univ; Consult-Aud, Aud Consult, **A**

Strong, Dr Jacqueline C 2628 Cottage Place, Greensboro, NC 27408, (919) 379-5939, OB 65 OH Univ - Athens; MA 72 Our Lady Lake Univ-San Anton; PH 77 (NS) PA St Univ - Univ Park; Assoc Prof of Commun Dis, U of North Carolina, **SLP**

Strong, Mrs Nancy A B 3117 Edgetone Drive, Raleigh, NC 27604, (919) 790-2500, BA 75 Univ of NC - Greensboro; MS 81 Univ of NC - Chapel Hill; Sp-Lang Path, Wake County PS, **SLP**

Strong, Rebecca Ann 9810 West Cory, Boise, ID 83704, (208) 343-2583, BS 83 ID St Univ; MS 85 ID St Univ; 85–Sp-Lang Path, Idaho Elk's Rehabilitation Hosp, **SLP**

Strother, Dorothy K 2007 York Drive, Columbia, SC 29204, (803) 765-6553, BA 73 Columbia Coll; OM 74 Univ of SC - Columbia; Industrial Marketing Rep, Doctor's Care, **SLP**

Strother, Mrs Jean Downey 10 Saddlewood Lane, Greenville, SC 29615, (803) 297-5360, BS 77 Western Carolina Univ; MS 80 Univ of AR - Fayetteville; Sp-Lang Path, Greenville Cty Sch, **SLP**

Strother, Mrs Rebecca Joy 2310-D Nantucket, Houston, TX 77057, (713) 780-5871, BA 81 Univ of TX - El Paso; MA 85 Univ of Houston - Univ Park; 87–Sp-Lang Path, Rosewood Med Ctr, **SLP**

Strother, Terry Lee 212 South Gunnison, Burlington, IA 52601, (319) 753-6561, MA 66 Western MI Univ; BA 65 Northeast MO St Univ; SLP, Gr River Area Ed Agency 16, **SLP**

Stroud, Mrs Janice W 9336 Springwater Drive, Dallas, TX 75228, (214) 521-2098, BA 71 Southern Methodist Univ; MS 72 Southern Methodist Univ; SLP, Highland Park ISD, **SLP**

Stroud, Linda Payne 429 Smith Avenue, Henderson, KY 42420, (502) 826-0313, BS 81 Murray St Univ; MS 82 Murray St Univ; Sp-Lang Path, Henderson Co Board of Ed, **SLP**

Stroup, Mrs Nancy R 3521 Corto Avenue, Fort Worth, TX 76109, (817) 336-8311, BS 75 TX Christian Univ; MS 77 TX Christian Univ; 77–Sp-Lang Path, Ft Worth ISD, **SLP ACE**

Strubbe, Esther O Avenue Mejico B-10 Parkville, Parkville Townhouse, Guaynabo, PR 00656, PH (NS); **SLP**

Struck, Richard E 5035 Aldrick Avenue South, Minneapolis, MN 55419, (612) 339-0304, BA 70 Metropolitan St Coll; MA 72 Univ of Denver; Aud, ENT Prof Assoc Ltd, **A**

Strudthoff, Jean Marie 833 South Atlantic, Dillon, MT 59725, (406) 683-4472, BA 74 Univ of Northern IA; MA 82 Univ of Northern IA; 88–Instr, Western MT Coll, **SLP**

Strueby, Mrs Laurie Culberson 2421 S Carrier Parkway, #3129, Grand Prairie, TX 75051, (214) 790-8505, BS 85 Univ of North TX; MS 87 Univ of North TX

Strugatch, Mrs Mindy K 17 Cooper Court, Freehold, NJ 07728, (201) 409-2546, BA 75 George Washington Univ; MA 76 George Washington Univ; Sp/Lang Path, Marlboro Township PS, **SLP**

Strumpf, Sylvia G 6212 Hollins Drive, Bethesda, MD 20817, (703) 591-7553, BS 63 CUNY - Hunter Coll; ME 70 Emory Univ; OM 86 Univ of MD - College Park; Coord, Fairfax Co Pub Schs, **SLP**

Strunin, Bonnie H 29 Ferris Avenue, Bldg 1 #10, Norwalk, CT 06854, (203) 625-7498, BA 80 Southern CT St Univ; MA 83 CA St Univ - Los Angeles; Sp-Lang Path, Greenwich Boe, **SLP**

Struntz, Brian Gerard 10401 46th Avenue #102, Beltsville, MD 20705, BA 83 Univ of MD - College Park; MA 85 Univ of MD - College Park; **SLP**

Struthers, Polly J 86 Old Mill Road, Shrewsbury, MA 01545, (508) 755-3327, BA 78 Univ of Denver; MA 80 Univ of Denver; Sp-Lang Path, Weston PS, **SLP**

Strutzel, Karla K 3550 West Dimond Boulevard, Apartment 315, Anchorage, AK 99515, (907) 276-8029, BA 77 Univ of WA; OM 78 Univ of WA; SLP, Anchorage Sch Dist, **SLP**

Stryk, Mrs Rebecca Phillips P O Box 1062, Portland, TX 78374, (713) 499-1559, BS 79 Univ of TX - Austin; MA 82 Univ of Houston - Univ Park; SLP, Fort Bend ISD, **SLP**

Stryker, Dr Stephanie Stephanie Stryker Phd & Assocs, 1688 Meridian Avenue, Suite 605, Miami Beach, FL 33139, (305) 534-3676, OB 62 Univ of Miami; MA 65 NY Univ; PH 82 (Sp-Lang Path) Pacific Western Univ; Sp-Lang Path, Private Practice, **SLP ACE**

Stryk-Longoria, Mrs Janice 410 Antietam, Victoria, TX 77904, (512) 575-8792, BA 78 Our Lady Lake Univ-San Anton; MA 80 Our Lady Lake Univ-San Anton; Sp-Lang Path, HEAR Foundation of Texas Inc, **SLP**

Strzelecki, Eve M Route 3 Highway 50, Box 461, Delavan, WI 53115, (414) 248-3145, BS 79 Marquette Univ; MS 82 Univ of WI - Whitewater; Sp-Lang Path, Therapy Assoc, **SLP**

Stuart, Carole Levinson 7198 Via Maria, San Jose, CA 95139, (408) 281-4010, BA 64 Univ of MD - College Park; MS 66 Univ of OK Medical Center; Sp-Lang Path, Santa Clara County Office Educ, **SLP**

Stuart, Carolyn M 761 Thayer, Northville, MI 48167, **SLP**

Stuart, Debra M 8839 North Awl Road, Parker, CO 80134, (303) 426-2151, BS 75 Auburn Univ - Auburn; MS 78 Univ of South AL; Sp/Lang Path, Spalding Rehabilitation Hosp, **SLP**

Stuart, Diana M 8664 Rebecca Drive, Williamsville, NY 14221, (716) 837-2441, BS 64 Daemen Coll; MA 78 SUNY - Center at Buffalo; Aud, Lang Dev Prog of W NY, **A**

Stuart, Mrs Elena A 210 Mansion House Drive, West Chester, PA 19382, (215) 436-3401, BA 61 Emerson Coll; MS 63 Purdue Univ - West Lafayette; 77–Asst Prof of Comm Diso, West Chester University, **SLP**

Stuart, Frank J Rd 1 Box 613, Liberty, NY 12754, (914) 794-4240, BS 52 Syracuse Univ; MS 58 Syracuse Univ; Audiologist, Monticello Central Schools, **SLP A**

Stuart, Keith 3104 Dixie Highway, Suite 204, Erlanger, KY 41018, **SLP ACE**

Stuart, Mrs Lesley A 98 Valleyridge Crescent, Waterloo, ON, Canada N2T 1X2, (519) 746-6342, **SLP**

Stuart, Mrs Loraine G 4222 Westlake Drive, Austin, TX 78746, (512) 459-0515, BS 77 Univ of TX - Austin; MS 78 Southern Methodist Univ; Aud-Sp/Lang Path, Private Practice, **SLP A**

Stuart, Sheela L 509 East Oak Street, Sioux Falls, SD 57105, (605) 336-1840, BS 77 Univ of SD - Vermillion; MA 78 Univ of SD - Vermillion; Superv SLP Dept, Crpld Chldn Hosp & Sch, **SLP**

Stubbe, Mrs Mary Bolgren 5219 Fjord Street, Cedar Falls, IA 50613, (515) 752-1578, MA 84 Univ of Northern IA; SLP, AEA 7, **SLP**

Stubbins, Sherry D Rd 3 Box 7952, Post Road Ext, Rutland, VT 05701, **SLP**

Stubblefield, Dr James H Sp & Hrng Ctr Sch Of Hlth Prof, Northern Arizona Univ, Box 15045, Flagstaff, AZ 86011, (602) 523-2522, BA 57 Univ of TX - Austin; MS 72 Western OR St Coll; PH 74 (NS) Purdue Univ - West Lafayette; Aud, Northern Arizona U, **SLP A**

Stubblefield, Lacinda Kaye 800 Post Oak #72, Houston, TX 77056, (713) 792-4500, BA 85 Univ of Houston - Univ Park; MA 87 Univ of Houston - Univ Park; 88–Sp-Lang Path, Univ of TX Sp & Hrng Inst, **SLP**

Stubbs, Stephanie A 2885 Dominique, Galveston, TX 77551, (409) 744-4935, BS 86 Univ of TX - Austin; MS 88 Univ of TX - Dallas; 88–Sp-Lang Path, Dallas ISD

Stublen, Mrs Greta Pilson 27342 Deep Creek Boulevard, Punta Gorda, FL 33983, (813) 624-4401, BS 80 WV Univ; MS 81 WV Univ; Sp-Lang Path, Charlotte Co Bd of Educ, **SLP**

Stuckey, Mrs Patricia A 615 Pemberton, Grosse Pointe Pk, MI 48230, (313) 875-5250, BS 67 Northwestern Univ; MS 69 Univ of MI - Ann Arbor; Aud, Detroit Pub Sch Sp & Hrng Cl, **A**

Stucki, Peter F K P O Box 911, Amherst, NS, Canada B4H 4E1, (902) 667-7491, BS 69 Univ of MD - College Park; MS 76 Loyola Coll; **SLP**

Stucky, Lynda R 4401 Campbell, Kansas City, MO 64110, (816) 756-3891, OB 84 Univ of KS; MA 86 Univ of KS; **SLP**

Stucky-Pirner, Angela Kay 1658 Garland, Wichita, KS 67217, (316) 261-6271, BA 85 Wichita St Univ; MS 86 Univ of KY; Sp-Lang Path, Wesley Med Ctr, **SLP**

Studebaker, Barbara Ann 1159 North Mayfair, Anaheim, CA 92801-2950, (714) 241-6540, **SLP**

Studebaker, Diane Joy 4521 Cavallo Real, Carmichael, CA 95608, (916) 366-8434, MA 84 CA St Univ - Sacramento; **SLP**

Studebaker, Dr Gerald A 807 Jefferson Avenue, Memphis, TN 38105, (901) 525-2682, BS 55 IL St Univ - Normal; MS 56 Syracuse Univ; PH 60 (Aud) Syracuse Univ; Prof, Memphis St U, **F**

Studley, Mrs Lisa Sharon 2 Bay Club Drive #4-C, Bayside, NY 11360, (718) 224-2620, BS 82 Boston Univ; MS 84 Columbia Univ Teachers Coll; **A**

Stuebe, Mrs Sara C 7757 S Louthan Street, Littleton, CO 80120, (303) 797-7871, BA 68 Ball St Univ; MS 69 SUNY - Coll at Geneseo; Sp-Lang Path, Douglas Co Pub Schs, **SLP**

Stuefen, Betty Watkins 110 Forest Avenue #101, Vermillion, SD 57069, (605) 339-7522, BA 75 Univ of SD - Vermillion; MA 85 Univ of SD - Vermillion; 88–Sp-Lang Path, McKennan Hosp, **SLP**

Stuhr, Fonda Carol 686 Buckhall Court, Mount Pleasant, SC 29464, (803) 884-9537, BA 84 Columbia Coll; MS 85 Univ of SC - Columbia; SLP, Charleston County Schools, **SLP**

Stukas, Natalie Latoza 4637 Downers Drive, Downers Grove, IL 60515, (312) 310-0220, BA 79 MacMurray Coll; MA 82 Northern IL Univ - De Kalb; Aud, Mobilear Inc, **A**

Stula, Mrs Trudy Jolene 4135 Knollcrest Circle, Martinez, GA 30907, (619) 452-9125, BA 79 Wichita St Univ; MA 83 San Diego St Univ; Sp-Lang Path, **SLP**

Stulberg, Ellen W 345 Tilbury Road, Birmingham, MI 48009, **SLP**

Stull, Mrs Mary Young 403 East Todd, Minden, LA 71055, (318) 377-7112, BA 60 Baylor Univ; MS 68 Phillips Univ; 87–Sp-Lang Path, Webster Parish Sch Bd, **SLP**

Stull, Mrs Sheila Ann 11037 South St Louis, Chicago, IL 60655, (312) 445-6124, BS 82 Western IL Univ; MA 85 Western IL Univ

Stuller, Mrs Arlene 1900 East Ocean Boulevard, Apartment 601, Long Beach, CA 90802, (213) 832-3056, BS 50 Univ of IL - Urbana; MA 71 CA St Univ - Northridge; SLP, Los Angeles USD, **SLP**

Stults, Karen Marie 1640 Corte Verano, Oceanside, CA 92056, (619) 945-7737, BA 82 Univ of Redlands; MA 85 San Diego St Univ; SLP, Encinitas USD, **SLP**

Stultz, Pamela Ann 5312 East Windsor, Phoenix, AZ 85008, (602) 982-1110, BS 80 Univ of AZ; MS 86 Northern AZ Univ; 80–Sp-Lang Path, Apache Junction Unified Schs, **SLP**

Stumacher, Mrs Sharon G 1400 Hillside Road, Wynnewood, PA 19096, (215) 893-7094, BS 71 Boston Univ; MS 73 Emerson Coll; 80–Sp-Lang Path, The Graduate Hospital, **SLP**

Stuman, Lillian Yvonne 1524 DE La Vina #A, Santa Barbara, CA 93101, **SLP**

Stump, Ann Howell 5614 Lorraine Avenue, Sioux City, IA 51106, (712) 274-6040, BS 59 Univ Southern MS-Hattiesburg; MA 60 OH St Univ; Sp-Lang Path, Western Hills AEA 12, **SLP**

Stump, Mrs Lynn Ahrenbeck 607 Thunder Trail, Maitland, FL 32751, (305) 830-9911, BA 78 Univ of FL; MS 80 Purdue Univ - West Lafayette; SLP, Sch Bd of Seminole Co, **SLP**

Stumpf, Sandra E 103 Hart Street, Bldg 4, #105, Taunton, MA 02780, (508) 676-3411, BS 83 Worcester St Coll; MS 85 Washington Univ; 85–Aud, R H Fitton Jr MD Inc, **A**

Stumpf, Mrs Teresa Flahive 617 Meadow Ridge Trail, Indianapolis, IN 46217, (317) 783-8661, BA 78 Wright St Univ; MA 80 Ball St Univ; Director of Sp-Lang Pathology, St Francis Hospital Center, **SLP**

Stunson, Mrs Da Fayne R 11 Overbrook Road, Painted Post, NY 14870, (607) 936-3700, BS 68 TN St Univ; MS 72 Murray St Univ; 78–Sp-Lang Path, Corning-Painted Post Sch Dist, **SLP**

Stupich, Michael C 148 Warren, Beaver Dam, WI 53916, (414) 885-9776, BS 77 Univ of WI - Stevens Point; MS 79 Univ of WI - Stevens Point; Aud, Private Practice, **A**

Sturges, Mrs Patricia Mazza 70 Riverside Drive, Ridgefield, CT 06877, BA 73 Elmira Coll; MA 76 IN Univ - Bloomington; Handicap Coordinator, Child Inc, **SLP**

Sturiale, Mrs Madeleine M 2122 Bay Street, San Francisco, CA 94123, (415) 685-1960, BA 74 San Francisco St Univ; Sp-Lang Path, Mt Diablo USD, **SLP**

Sturkey, Clare A P 332 Stephanie Lane, Rock Hill, SC 29730, (803) 323-2244, BA 60 Univ of AZ; MS 77 Winthrop Coll; 87–Coord Educ Serv, Winthrop Coll, **SLP**

Sturkie, Mrs Bernice Barrett 7236 Quorum Drive, Baton Rouge, LA 70817, (504) 291-0890, BS 81 Univ Southern MS-Hattiesburg; ME 87 Southeastern LA Univ; 82–Sp-Lang Path, East Baton Rouge Par Sch, **SLP**

Sturlaugson, Dr William R WM R Sturlaugson Phd & Assocs, 149 Walnut Avenue, Redlands, CA 92373, (714) 792-3223, BS 65 Univ of WI - Madison; MS 66 Univ of WI - Madison; PH 69 (NS) Univ of WI - Madison; Owner/Sp-Lang Path, Private Practice, **SLP**

Sturm, Andrea E 16-70 Bell Boulevard #113, Bayside, NY 11360, (212) 596-3548, BS 71 Boston Univ; MA 83 Hofstra Univ; SLP, New York City Board of Educ, **SLP**

Sturm, Mrs Mary C G 105 Jefferson Boulevard, Greenfield, IN 46140, (317) 462-9219, BS 73 Ball St Univ; MA 75 Ball St Univ; Dept Head-SLP, Hancock S Mad Jt Serv, **SLP**

Sturm, Mrs Mindy Robin 11 Tower Place, Smithtown, NY 11787, (516) 361-4970, BA 82; MS 83; Sp-Lang Path, Connetquot Central Sch Dist, **SLP**

Sturmak, Michael J 5180 Turret, Boise, ID 83703, (208) 343-2583, MS 87 ID St Univ; Aud, Idaho Elks Rehab Hosp, **A**

Sturm-Getchell, Joanne 298 Franklin Street, Braintree, MA 02184, (617) 849-1830, OB 75 SUNY - Coll at Buffalo; OM 77 SUNY - Coll at Buffalo; Sp-Lang Path, Freetown Lakeville Reg Sch Dis, **SLP**

Sturtevant, Arlene Frances 2408 Eastmoreland #3D, Rockford, IL 61108, (815) 226-7048, BS 83 Northern IL Univ - De Kalb; MA 85 Northern IL Univ - De Kalb; **SLP**

Sturtevant, Janet Evans 4654 Briarwood Drive, Charlottesville, VA 22901, (804) 924-2050, BA 78 Univ of VA - Charlottesville; ME 80 Univ of VA - Charlottesville; ME 81 Univ of VA - Charlottesville; 84–Aud, Univ of VA Hlth Sci Ctr, **A**

Sturtz, Robin E 1787 Washington Avenue, Seaford, NY 11783, (516) 562-4600, BA 75 Univ of CT; MA 77 Northwestern Univ; Aud, North Shore Hosp, **A ACE**

Stutz, Sue Ann 1080 East Lassen Avenue #25, Chico, CA 95926, (916) 894-5529, MA 86 CA St Univ - Chico; **SLP**

Stutzman, Mrs Anne Reidelberg 1708 Belvedere Street, Tallahassee, FL 32308-5205, (617) 552-7488, BA 72 Univ of FL; MA 74 Univ of FL; Interperter for the Deaf, **A**

Stuve, Mrs Carolyn S Manthei 1813 Windsor, Las Cruces, NM 88005, (505) 522-0909, BA 75 NM St Univ; MA 77 NM St Univ; Sp-Lang Path, Lascruces Sch Dist #2, **SLP**

Stuve, Mark K 1813 Windsor Place, Las Cruces, NM 88005, (505) 523-5884, BA 76 NM St Univ; MA 79 NM St Univ; Sp-Lang Path, Sch Dist, **SLP**

Stwarka, Mrs Jeanne Ann 3290 Brush Creek Road, Manchester, OH 45144, (513) 549-4009, BS 79 Univ of ME - Farmington; MA 83 Univ of Cincinnati; Sp-Lang Path, **SLP**

Stwora, Linda Swiatkowsk 9033 South 49th Avenue, Oak Lawn, IL 60453, (312) 687-7200, BA 79 Saint Xavier Coll; MA 80 Univ of IL - Urbana; Sp/Lang Path, Oak Forest Hosp, **SLP**

Styczynski, Celeste R 1757 73 Rd Street #2-R, Brooklyn, NY 11204, (718) 604-5378, BS 85 SUNY - Coll at Geneseo; MS 86 Columbia Univ Teachers Coll; Sp-Lang Path, Kingsbrook Jewish Med Ctr, **SLP**

Styer, Mrs Brenda McAfee 189 Berrywood Drive, Severna Park, MD 21146, (301) 544-7762, BS 78 Bloomsburg Univ of PA; MA 81 Wayne St Univ - Sch of Med; **A**

Styer, Mrs Jana K 120 Church Street South, Mohnton, PA 19540, (215) 779-7111, BS 74 Bloomsburg Univ of PA; MA 78 West Chester Univ of PA; Sp-Lang Path, Berks Co Inter Ut, **SLP**

Styer, Susan L 1536 Shadyside Road, Baltimore, MD 21218, (301) 687-6500, MS 81 Loyola Coll; Sp-Lang Path, Baltimore County Health Dept, **SLP**

Stylman, Randi L 595 Northfield Anenue, Apartment 59, West Orange, NJ 07052, (201) 731-3695, BA 81 SUNY - Coll at Cortland; MS 86 CUNY - Brooklyn Coll; **SLP**

Stypula, Mrs Roseann C 73 Pleasant View Road N E, Granville, OH 43023, (614) 443-9425, BA 73 OH St Univ; MA 74 OH Univ - Athens; Sp/Lang Path, Childhood Lgue Cen, **SLP**

Suarez, Janet Kalina 23-A East Prospect Street, Paramus, NJ 07652, (201) 447-8131, BA 80 CUNY - Queens Coll; MA 83 CUNY - Hunter Coll; 87–Sp-Lang Path, The Valley Hosp, **SLP**

Suarez, Mrs Mildred Martinez 10352 S W 14th Street, Miami, FL 33174, (305) 554-5431, BS 78 Eastern IL Univ; MS 79 Eastern IL Univ; Sp-Lang Path, Private Practice, **SLP**

Suarez-Marina, Maria Luisa Iturbide #1, Apdo #10, Coalcalco, Mexico 55700, (525) 874-2070, MA 86 Univ of CO - Boulder

Suber, Margaret C 2432 Algodones N E, Albuquerque, NM 87112, **SLP**

Suber, Mrs Patricia A 27 Intervale Road, West Peabody, MA 01960, **SLP**

Sublette-Sloan, Mrs Cynthia B 744 Periwinkle Turn, Bourbonnais, IL 60914, (815) 933-2233, BS 77 Southern IL Univ -Carbondale; MS 82 Governors St Univ; 87–Sp-Lang Path, Bradley Elem Sch Dist #61, **SLP**

Subrahmanyam, Mrs Carol Elizabeth 19 Holly Road, Southampton, PA 18966, (215) 750-4150, **SLP**

Subrizi, Laurie Perry 13 Cherry Lane, Pomona, NY 10970, (914) 693-4443, BA 77 SUNY - Coll at Cortland; MS 81 Rutger's St Univ - Douglas Coll; **SLP**

Subtelny, Dr Joanne D 72 South Main Street, Pittsford, NY 14534, (716) 586-6130, BS 47 Univ of PA; ME 50 PA St Univ - Univ Park; PH 56 (Sp-Lang Path) Northwestern Univ; Prof Sp-Lang Path-Comm Prog, NTID, **SLP F**

Succo, Peter Jay 1212 Bookcliff Avenue, Grand Junction, CO 81501, (303) 241-8255, OM 84 Brigham Young Univ; Aud, Private Practice, **A**

Suchow, Linda Beth 140 Hoyt Street #4B, Stamford, CT 06905, BA 85 SUNY - Coll at Plattsburgh; MA 86 SUNY - Coll at Plattsburgh; 88–Aud, Dr Edward Gaynor, **A**

Suchowiecki, Jill Ann 38 Bourbon Court, Perry Hall, MD 21234, (301) 676-8151, BS 78 Trenton St Coll; MS 80 Loyola Coll; Sp/Lang Path, Harford Co Pub Sch Syst, **SLP**

Sudak, Mrs Diane R Academic Consulting Service, 23811 Chagrin Boulevard, Space LI-46, Cleveland, OH 44122, (216) 464-3686, BS 56 Case Western Reserve Univ; MA 62 Case Western Reserve Univ; PH 78 (NS) Case Western Reserve Univ; Indep Ed Consult, Acad Consult Serv, **SLP**

Sudaka, Mrs Martha F 217 Greer Crest, Millbrook, NY 12545, (914) 723-8471, 31; BS 41 Columbia Univ Teachers Coll; MA 68 CUNY - Hunter Coll; **SLP LM**

Sudbrink, Pamela Dawn 728 Sherwood, Richardson, TX 75080, (214) 231-2467, MS 87 Univ of TX - Dallas

Suddath, Mrs Carol R Gordon 523 Lincoln Green Drive, West Carrollton, OH 45449, (513) 859-3272, BA 70; MA 79; Sp-Lang Path, Dayton Public Schools, **SLP**

Sudderberg, Mrs Jane Marie 1836 Oxford Street, Rockford, IL 61103, (815) 962-4967, MA 84 Univ of Northern IA; SLP, Freeport School System, **SLP**

Suddick, Mary 7 Basswood Hollow, Unionsville, ON, Canada L3R 3Z5, (416) 296-7577, BS 74 0222; MS 77 Clarion Univ of PA; **SLP**

Suder, Darlene Sue Rt 1 Box 704, Bluemont, VA 22012, (703) 821-8883, MS 83 Clarion Univ of PA; Sp-Lang Path, Yvonne Henry & Assoc, **SLP**

Suder, Mrs Nancy Higgs 1511 Fairmount Road, Hampstead, MD 21074, (301) 833-9300, MS 78 Loyola Coll; Sp-Lang Path, Timber Grove Elem, **SLP**

Sudler, William H 234 Davenport Avenue, Akron, OH 44312, MS 73 Kent St Univ; Sp-Lang Path, **SLP**

Sudlik, Susan Ruth 740 Indian Church Road, West Seneca, NY 14224, (716) 847-3154, BS 73 SUNY - Center at Buffalo; MS 76 SUNY - Center at Buffalo; **SLP**

Sudman, Mrs Joanne A 10619 Thistlewood Court, Cincinnati, OH 45242, (513) 489-4898, BS 68 Kent St Univ; MA 70 Kent St Univ; Sp-Lang Path, Private Practice, **SLP ACE**

Sudore, Mrs Deborah E 15 Marco Lane, Rochester, NY 14622, (716) 352-2440, BS 79 Nazareth Coll of Rochester; ME 83 Nazareth Coll of Rochester; Sp-Lang Path, BOCES II-W Monroe/Orleans Co, **SLP**

Suede, Mrs Diane Randie 1458 Ocean Parkway, Brooklyn, NY 11230, (718) 339-9269, BS 84 SUNY - Coll at Oneonta; MS 85 Adelphi Univ; Sp-Lang Path, **SLP**

Sueiro, Mrs Gladys V Greater Miami Hearing Inst, 777 East 25th Street, Suite 116, Hialeah, FL 33013, (305) 836-1416, BA 58 Spalding Coll; BS 58 Spalding Coll; MA 59 Northwestern Univ; Aud, Greater Miami Hrng Inst, **A**

Suematsu, Kikuyo McKinley Complex, 1486 Aala Street, Honolulu, HI 96817, BA 53 Univ of HI - Manoa; MA 56 IN Univ - Bloomington; Sp-Lang Path, Dept of Ed, **SLP A**

Suen, Arleen J Box 155, Blubber Bay, BC, Canada V0N 1E0, (604) 485-2768, BA 74 San Francisco St Univ; MA 78 San Francisco St Univ; Sp/Lang Path, Powell River Sch Dist #47, **SLP**

Suenaga, Patricia S Y 1017 Kikeke Avenue, Honolulu, HI 96816, (808) 235-2343, BS 78 Univ of HI - Manoa; MS 79 Univ of HI - Manoa; SLP, Dept of Ed Windward Spec Serv, **SLP**

Sue-O'Brien, Mrs Debora C 16046 E Sierra Pass Way, Hacienda Heights, CA 91745, (213) 743-2476, BA 73 CA St Univ - Long Beach; MA 76 Whittier Coll; Sp-Lang Path, U Southern CA, **SLP**

Suesse, Karen S 1141 Curtiss, Downers Grove, IL 60515, (312) 969-0442, BS 80 Marquette Univ; MS 82 IL St Univ - Normal; Sp-Lang Path, Joliet Pub Sch Dist 86, **SLP**

Sufana, Mrs Karen Kicho 1137 Azalea Drive, Munster, IN 46321, (219) 923-8308, BS 74 Purdue Univ - West Lafayette; MS 75 Purdue Univ - West Lafayette; Sp-Lang Path, Private Practice, **SLP ACE**

Suffolk, Mrs Debra R S 711 Fairway Road, State College, PA 16803, (814) 865-5414, BS 74 Purdue Univ - West Lafayette; MA 76 Univ of TN - Knoxville; Coord of Cl Exper, Penn State U, **SLP ACE**

Suffredini, Carol Roser 4132 Metauro Drive, Liverpool, NY 13090-6819, (716) 674-6781, SLP, Erie 1 BOCES, **SLP**

Suffredini, Doreen Elizabeth 651 Newton Square, Coraopolis, PA 15108-1050, (412) 741-9500, BS 79 Ithaca Coll; MA 84 SUNY - Coll at Geneseo; Sp-Lang Path, D T Watson Rehabilitation Hosp, **SLP**

Sugarman, Mrs June 51 Rockledge Drive, Livingston, NJ 07039, (201) 992-1806, BA 57 CUNY - Brooklyn Coll; MA 64 CUNY - Brooklyn Coll; **SLP**

Sugden, Mrs Frances B 55 Brier Street, Winnetka, IL 60093, (312) 446-1068, BS 45 Northwestern Univ; MA 46 Northwestern Univ; Retired, Evanston Sch Dist 65, **SLP**

Suggs, Laura G 1609 Oak Creek Lane #D, Bedford, TX 76022, (817) 283-4345, BS 80 TX Christian Univ; MS 81 TX Christian Univ; SLP, Hurst-Euless-Bedford ISD, **SLP**

Suggs, Shelly Jones 3245 Elm Swamp Road, Lebanon, IN 46052, (817) 275-5858, BS 84 TX Christian Univ; MS 86 Univ of TX - Dallas; **SLP**

Sugimura, Cathryn Michiko 6545 Delmonico Drive, Apartment 213, Colorado Springs, CO 80919, (719) 594-4226, MA 87 Univ of Northern CO; 88–SLP, Dist #20

Sugrue, Mrs Joan Coughlan 25602 Coltrane Drive, Damascus, MD 20872, (301) 253-1136, BA 82 Loyola Coll; MS 84 Loyola Coll; 86–Sp-Lang Path, State of MD-Rosewood Ctr, **SLP**

Suhadolnik, Sarah Jane 8263 South Franklin Road, Clinton, WA 98236, (206) 321-5265, BA 85 WA St Univ; MA 87 WA St Univ; 88–Sp-Lang Path, South Whidbey Sch Dist

Suick, Joan M 2802 King Place, Eau Claire, WI 54701, (715) 834-8104, BA 69 Univ of WI - Eau Claire; MS 73 Univ of WI - Eau Claire; Sp-Lang Path, Eau Claire Board of Education, **SLP**

Suire, Mrs Lisa T 215 Meadow Bend Drive, Baton Rouge, LA 70820, (504) 767-7612, BS 83 LA St Univ - Baton Rouge; MA 87 LA St Univ - Baton Rouge; 84–Sp-Lang Path, East Baton Rouge Parish Sch Bd, **SLP**

Suit, Kimberly A 2461 Brodalski Street, Atwater, CA 95301, (209) 357-6100, BA 77 CA St Univ - Stanislaus; MA 79 CA St Univ - Stanislaus; Sp-Lang Path, Atwater Sch Dist, **SLP**

Suite, Leslie P 66 Highland Avenue #9, Belleville, ON, Canada K8P 3R3, (613) 968-5511, BS 85 Howard Univ; MS 86 Howard Univ; 86–Sp-Lang Path, Belleville General Hosp

Sukernick, Gail Rubini 220 West Allendale Avenue, Allendale, NJ 07401, (914) 357-7783, MA 74 Trenton St Coll; Sp-Lang Path, Ramapo Central Schools, **SLP**

Sukoneck, Lenore L 2784 Calle DE Dalias, Tucson, AZ 85745, (602) 797-0274, BS 78 Auburn Univ - Auburn; ME 87 Univ of GA; **SLP**

Sukowske-Miles, Mrs Pauline G 864 East Pioneer Avenue, Redlands, CA 92374, BA 73 CA St Univ - Los Angeles; MS 74 Univ of Redlands; 86–Coord Spec Educ/Instruction, Colton Joint USD, **SLP**

Suleski, Mrs Nancy L 930 Lochmeath Way, Brookfield, Dover, DE 19901, (302) 736-5597, BS 68 CA Univ of PA; ME 73 CA Univ of PA; **SLP**

Sulkes-Segal, Mrs Marcia R 2302 Bourgoin Ville, St Laurent, PQ, Canada H4R 1M9, (514) 333-0488, **SLP**

Sullivan, Mrs A Constance 226 Wilson Avenue, Rumford, RI 02916, (401) 245-7400, BA 57 Coll of New Rochelle; ME 60 Boston Univ; Sp/Lang Path, Barrington Pub Sch Ri, **SLP**

Sullivan, Mrs Audrey Tichacek 13073 Winding Trail Lane, Des Peres, MO 63131, (314) 454-7875, BS 56 Saint Louis Univ; MA 65 Saint Louis Univ; Chief Sp-Lang Path, Jewish Hosp WA U Med Cen, **SLP ACE**

Sullivan, Barbara A 2614 Mountair Lane, Greeley, CO 80631, (303) 352-6168, BA 71 Univ of Northern CO; MA 72 Univ of Northern CO; Sp-Lang Path, Weld BOCES, **SLP**

Sullivan, Betty 265 South Walnut Street, Huntington, WV 25705, (304) 528-5175, BA 69 Marshall Univ; MA 72 Marshall Univ; Sp-Lang Path, Cabell County Schools, **SLP**

Sullivan, Burton H 6810 99th Avenue North, Pinellas Park, FL 33565, **SLP**

Sullivan, Mrs Carol A 50 Willow Street, Garden City, NY 11530, (516) 294-0253, BA 61; MS 71 Univ of HI - Manoa; Sp-Lang Path, Private Practice, **SLP**

Sullivan, Carol R 6824 South Lagoon Drive, Panama City Beach, FL 32407, (904) 769-1431, BS 74 Univ of MD - College Park; MA 77 Univ of Miami; Sp-Lang Path, Bay County Sch Bd, **SLP**

Sullivan, Danita Whitworth 1902 Fox Sterling Drive, Raleigh, NC 27606-6554, (919) 790-2489, BS 80 East Carolina Univ; ME 82 Univ of NC - Greensboro; Aud, Wake Co Pub Sch Syst, **SLP A**

Sullivan, Darcy Nordquist 570 West Sandhurst Drive, Apt#206, Roseville, MN 55113, (612) 779-5788, BS 84 Univ of MN - Minneap-St Paul; MS 86 Saint Cloud St Univ; 86–Sp-Lang Path, Northeast Metro Tech SD 916, **SLP**

Sullivan, Deborah W 10140 S W Paulina Drive, Tualatin, OR 97062, (503) 684-2145, BA 74 Univ of MT; MA 76 Univ of MT; Sp-Lang Path, Washington County Ed Serv Dist, **SLP**

Sullivan, Sr Declan Boston School For The Deaf, 800 North Main Street, Randolph, MA 02368, (617) 963-8150, BA 50 Regis Coll; MA 60 Boston Univ; MA 60 Boston Univ; Aud, The Boston Sch for the Deaf, **A**

Sullivan, Mrs Diane Riser 22 Willey Street, Brockton, MA 02401, (617) 587-1114, BS 84 WV Univ; MS 85 WV Univ; Sp-Lang Path, Brockton City Schools, **SLP**

Sullivan, Dorothy S 818 West Altgeld, Chicago, IL 60614, (312) 650-5800, BS 70 Univ of WI - Madison; MS 71 Univ of WI - Madison; Sp-Lang Path, Chicago Pub Schs, **SLP**

Sullivan, Mrs E Barbara 77 Russ Road, Trumbull, CT 06611, (203) 372-0835, BA 46 Wichita St Univ; MS 62 Southern CT St Univ; 84–Consultant, Speech Lang Hrng Therapy, **SLP**

Sullivan, Mrs Elizabeth Mascolo 3005 Thorn St, #8, San Diego, CA 92104, (619) 260-7161, BS 82 Boston Coll; MA 84 Northwestern Univ; Sp-Lang Path, Mercy Hosp Med Ctr, **SLP**

Sullivan, Gayla K 11808 Westmere, Houston, TX 77077, **A**

Sullivan, Glenda Moss 4128 Heath Road, Jacksonville, FL 32211, (904) 399-6704, MS 82 Univ of South FL; Sp-Lang Path, Memorial Reg Rehab Ctr, **SLP**

Sullivan, Mrs Helen A 24001 Muirland Boulevard, Space 82, El Toro, CA 92630, (714) 586-7458, BS 30 Univ of Southern CA; MA 30 Univ of Southern CA; **SLP LM**

Sullivan, Holly Le Blanc 12700 Hillcrest Suite 258, Dallas, TX 75230, (214) 385-0836, BS 75 LA St Univ - Baton Rouge; OM 76 LA St Univ - N O Medical Ctr; Sp-Lang Path, Private Practice, **SLP**

Sullivan, Holly Lynn 10415-L Hickory Ridge Rd, Columbia, MD 21044, (202) 363-7032, ME 79 Clarion Univ of PA; Sp-Lang Path, Michael Girard Inc, **SLP**

Sullivan, Mrs Jacqueline Jones P O Box 816, Windermere, FL 32786, (305) 422-3200, **SLP**

Sullivan, Dr James L 6824 South Lagoon Drive, Panama City Beach, FL 32407, (904) 769-1431, BS 51 FL St Univ; MS 66 FL St Univ; PH 76 (NS) FL St Univ; Audiologist, Bay Coounty School Board, **A**

Sullivan, Mrs Janet Kaminsky 1949 Michael Place, Charlottesville, VA 22901, (804) 973-4136, BS 59 Carlow Coll; MA 67 IN Univ - Bloomington; Sp-Lang Path, U of VA Dept of Sp Path & Aud, **SLP**

Sullivan, Jean A House Ear Institute, 256 South Lake Street, Los Angeles, CA 90057, (213) 483-4431, BS 77 Boston Univ; MA 78 MI St Univ; 86–Aud, House Ear Institute, **A**

Sullivan, Jean L 182 Federal Street, Salem, MA 01970, (508) 741-2794, BA 82 Univ of Northern CO; MS 84 CO St Univ; Slp, North Shore Childrens Hosp, **SLP**

Sullivan, Mrs Jeri Boudreaux 6380 Val, Groves, TX 77619, (409) 962-5541, BS 81 Lamar Univ; MS 87 Lamar Univ; **SLP**

Sullivan, Joanna K 811 East First Street, Madison, IN 47250, (812) 265-2382, BS 74 IN St Univ - Terre Haute; MS 75 IN St Univ - Terre Haute; Sp-Lang Path, Madison Consol Sch, **SLP**

Sullivan, Judy M 1210 Oak Grove Avenue #10, Burlingame, CA 94010, **SLP**

Sullivan, Mrs Karen A 16106 West 139th Street, Olathe, KS 66062, (913) 764-7488, BA 75 Univ of Northern IA; MA 76 Univ of Northern IA; Sp-Lang Path, Shawnee Mission Sch Dist, **SLP**

Sullivan, Karen E 23 Blauvelt Street, Nanuet, NY 10954, (914) 947-3000, BS 77 Emerson Coll; MS 80 Columbia Univ Teachers Coll; Sp-Lang Path, Helen Hayes Hosp, **SLP**

Sullivan, Karen L 104 Indian Drive, Clarendon Hills, IL 60514, (312) 333-7812, BS 80 Univ of IL - Urbana; MS 81 Univ of IL - Urbana; Parent/Infant Supvr, S Metro Assoc, **SLP**

Sullivan, Mrs Karen Schneider 46 High Street, Assonet, MA 02702, (508) 420-0302, BA 81 Bridgewater St Coll; MS 83 Boston Univ; Sp-Lang Path, Barnstable Public Schools, **SLP**

Sullivan, Kathleen E 11 Maple Glen Glen, Nesconset, NY 11767, (213) 745-2435, BA 77 SUNY - Coll at Plattsburgh; MA 78 SUNY - Coll at Geneseo; Coord-Sp/Lang Serv, Switzer Cen, **SLP**

Sullivan, Kathleen Elizabeth 227 Aspinwall Avenue, Brookline, MA 02146, (617) 734-5715, BS 84 Boston Univ; MS 86 Northeastern Univ; 86–Sp-Lang Path, WE Fernald State Sch, **SLP**

Sullivan, Kathleen K 15 Ives Street, Apt #25, Beverly, MA 01915, (617) 254-3800, MS 87 Purdue Univ - West Lafayette; 88–Sp-Lang Path, Kennedy Mem Hosp for Children, **SLP**

Sullivan, Kathleen M 7013 Slayton Court, Woodridge, IL 60517, (312) 964-4745, BA 75 John Carroll Univ; MS 78 Governors St Univ; Sp/Lang Path, Sch Assn for Spec Ed, **SLP**

Sullivan, Lori Chirnside 7054 Flower Lane, St Louis, MO 63129, (314) 441-3035, MA 82 Southeast MO St Univ; 85–Sp-Lang Path, Associated Rehab Services Inc, **SLP**

Sullivan, Mrs Lynn Stein 109 Susan Court, Clifton, NJ 07012, (201) 438-2217, BA 64 William Paterson Coll; MA 77 Montclair St Coll; Sp-Lang Path, E Rutherford Bd of Ed, **SLP**

Sullivan, Margaret Ann 341 West 24th Street, New York, NY 10011, (212) 924-1527, MA 87 CUNY - Hunter Coll; **SLP**

Sullivan, Margaret M 20 Granite Lane, Barnstable, MA 02630, (617) 362-2251, BA 73 Univ of MA - Amherst; MS 75 SUNY - Center at Albany; SLP, Plymouth Sch Dist, **SLP**

Sullivan, Maria A 632 88th Street, Brooklyn, NY 11228, BA 77 Pace U -NY City; MA 80 NY Univ; Sp-Lang Path, Private Practice, **SLP**

Sullivan, Mrs Marsha Dawn 9 Parkwood Circle, Council Bluffs, IA 51503, (402) 559-6460, BA 69 Univ of IA; MA 71 Univ of IA; Sp-Lang Path, U of NE Med Cent, **SLP**

Sullivan, Martha Anne 404 Highland Avenue, Winchester, MA 01890, (617) 828-2440, BS 84 Nazareth Coll of Rochester; MA 86 Univ of MA - Amherst; **SLP**

Sullivan, Mrs Martha M 40 Eliot Street, Jamaica Plain, MA 02130, (617) 522-6951, BS 66 Boston Univ; MA 77 Boston Univ; Sp-Lang Path, Boston Pub Sch, **SLP**

Sullivan, Mary Ann 427 West Century Avenue #101, Bismarck, ND 58501, (701) 224-6176, BA 64 Univ of ND; MA 65 Wayne St Univ; Dir Dept of Commun Dis, Medcenter One, **SLP**

Sullivan, Mary Jane 6 Hill Street, Stoneham, MA 02180, (617) 267-4730, Aud, North Shore Childrens Hospital, **A**

Sullivan, Mary Patricia 10838 Stone Canyon Road, Apartment 1427, Dallas, TX 75230, (817) 460-7211, BS 76 Univ of Houston - Univ Park; MS 78 Univ of TX - Dallas; Sp-Lang Path, Arlington ISD, **SLP**

Sullivan, MaryBeth 34 1st Avenue, Auburn, NY 13021, (315) 488-2951, BS 83 Nazareth Coll of Rochester; MS 86 Nazareth Coll of Rochester; 88–Sp-Lang Path, St Camillus Health & Rehab Ctr, **SLP**

Sullivan, Marybeth Bothmann 3815 Gentle Springs Drive, Arlington, TX 76017, (817) 483-0528, BS 74 Western IL Univ; MS 77 Bradley Univ; Sp-Lang Path, **SLP**

Sullivan, Melissa Stagg 105 Stoney Brook Drive, Carrollton, GA 30117, (404) 258-3322, BS 86 West GA Coll; ME 88 West GA Coll

Sullivan, Michael Patrick 3221 Fremont South #3, Minneapolis, MN 55408, BS 83 Univ of OR; MS 84 Univ of OR; SLP, North Fulton Medical Center, **SLP**

Sullivan, Mrs Mildred Alison Qtrs Si Nas North Island, Coronado, CA 92135, (619) 435-8279, **SLP**

Sullivan, Patricia Anne 1285 Richmond Road #2108, Ottawa, ON, Canada K2B 7Z4, (613) 829-4481, BS 81; MA 85 SUNY - Center at Buffalo; 87–Sp-Lang Path, Children's Hosp of E Ontario, **SLP**

Sullivan, Patricia C 916 7th Street South, Fargo, ND 58103, (218) 236-6400, BA 74 ND St Univ; MS 76 Moorhead St Univ; Sp/Lang Path, Moorhead Pub Sch, **SLP**

Sullivan, Dr Patricia M Boys Town National Inst For, Comm Disorders In Children, 555 North 30th Street, Omaha, NE 68131, (402) 498-6600, BA 68 Marycrest Coll; OM 77 Univ of IA; PH 78 (NS) Univ of IA; Dir, Boys Town National Inst

Sullivan, Paula A 13913 Village View Drive, Tampa, FL 33624, (813) 972-8449, MS 78 Univ of South FL; 76–Sp-Lang Path, H Lee Moffitt Can Ctr & USF Med Ctr, **SLP**

Sullivan, Mrs Rosemary 9732 Kent Village Drive, Charlotte, NC 28213, (704) 372-7790, BA 84 Saint John's Univ - Jamaica; MS 86 Adelphi Univ; 87–Sp-Lang Path, Ctr for Human Dev, **SLP**

Sullivan, Dr Roy F 50 Willow Street, Garden City, NY 11530, (516) 294-0253, BA 60 CUNY - Brooklyn Coll; MA 62 CUNY - Brooklyn Coll; PH 72 (NS) CUNY - Brooklyn Coll; Aud, Private Practice, **A F**

Sullivan, Susan W 264 South Walnut Street, Huntington, WV 25705, (304) 696-3640, BA 71 Marshall Univ; MA 72 Marshall Univ; Assistant Professor of Speech, Marshall University, **SLP**

Sullivan, Suzanne 222 South Front Street #3, Wormleysburg, PA 17043, (717) 761-3363, BS 82 Edinboro Univ of PA; ME 85 Univ of VA - Charlottesville; 87–Sp-Lang Path, InSpeech Inc, **SLP**

Sullivan, Theresa P 604 Hardscrabble Road, Chappaqua, NY 10514, (914) 747-1783, BA 76 CUNY - Queens Coll; MA 77 CUNY - Queens Coll; Sp-Lnag Path, Blythedale Chldn Hosp, **SLP**

Sullivan, Tyece L 203 Baltimore Way, Vancouver, WA 98664, (206) 693-7960, BA 79 WA St Univ; MA 80 WA St Univ; SLP, Evergreen School District, **SLP**

Sullivan, Wendy R 54 Amory Road, Marlboro, MA 01752, (508) 562-7819, BS 74 Worcester St Coll; MS 81 Worcester St Coll; Sp-Lang Path, Pub Schs, **SLP**

Sullivan, Mrs Wendy Sue 6926 Oak Circle, Centerville, MN 55038, (612) 422-5233, BS 82 Mankato St Univ; MS 84 Mankato St Univ; SLP, Anoka Hennepin Schl Dstr 11, **SLP**

Sullivan-Shepard, Karen Marie 16 Two Buck Ring, Burlington, CT 06013, (203) 574-6054, BA 81 Southern CT St Univ; MA 83 Univ of CT; Sp-Lang Path, St Mary's, **SLP**

Sullivan-Witmer, Deborah J 128 Elm Street, Minoa, NY 13116, (315) 470-3170, BS 78 SUNY - Coll at Brockport; MS 82 Ithaca Coll; Sp-Lang Path, North Syracuse Central Sch Dis, **SLP**

Sulprizio, Sandra L 1392 Sunset Loop, Lafayette, CA 94595-1061, (415) 428-3344, BA 75 Univ of WA; OM 76 Univ of WA; Sp-Lang Path, Chldn Hosp Med Cent, **SLP**

Sulsen, Mrs Katherine Lee P O Box 262, Van Buren, MO 63965, (314) 323-8336, BS 81 Southeast MO St Univ; MA 84 Southeast MO St Univ; Sp-Lang Path, Carter County Schools, **SLP**

Suman, Mrs Mary Katherine 1717 N E Clubhouse Drive, Apartment 301, North Kansas City, MO 64116, (816) 421-2917, BS 86 Southwest MO St Univ; MS 88 Central MO St Univ; 88–Sp-Lang Path, Park Hill Sch Dist

Sumida, Fay S M 98-644 Kuini Street, Aiea, HI 96701, (808) 423-2477, BS 77 Univ of OR; MA 79 WA St Univ; Sp-Lang Path, Dept of Ctrl Oahu Sch Dist, **SLP**

Sumithra, Mrs Radha Simhadri 3 Westminster, London Square, Clifton Park, NY 12065, (518) 899-2030, BA 74 0500; MS 77 0500; PH 86 (NS) Univ of TX - Dallas; Audiologist, SW Vermont Supervisory Union, **A**

Summa, Maureen E 88 Gorsline Street, Rochester, NY 14613, (716) 254-4700, BA 71; MA 75 Skidmore Coll; Aud, Delco Gm, **A**

Summars, Mrs Lisa Rains 3417 Lyric Street, Norman, OK 73071, (405) 387-5075, BA 81 Univ of OK - Norman; MS 83 Univ of OK - OK City; Sp/Lang Path, New Castle Schs, **SLP**

Summer, Sheila Jones 6508 Woodshire Place, Raleigh, NC 27612, (919) 733-6895, BS 80 East Carolina Univ; MS 82 East Carolina Univ; 83–Sp-Lang Path, Dev Evaluation Ctr-Sp & Hrng Clinic, **SLP**

Summerhayes, Elizabeth 557 Burger Place, Baldwin, NY 11510, (212) 347-5055, **SLP**

Summers, Mrs Anne C 2212 Fairmount Court, Bloomington, IN 47401, (812) 336-2246, BA 63 SUNY - Center at Buffalo; MS 65 Purdue Univ - West Lafayette; Sp/Lang Path, Monroe Co Commun Sch, **SLP**

Summers, Mrs Debbie Lynn 1647 S Florence Place, Tulsa, OK 74104, (918) 664-6422, BS 80 Univ of Tulsa; MA 82 Univ of Tulsa; SLP, Tulsa Co School Jones Dev, **SLP**

Summers, Mrs Donna Jo Route 13 Highway 96-E, Franklin, TN 37064, (615) 395-7046, BS 71 Samford Univ; OM 83 Auburn Univ - Auburn; **A**

Summers, Mrs Geniel Y 5625 South 1475 East #1-D, South Ogden, UT 84403, (801) 479-6500, BS 75 UT St Univ; MS 75 UT St Univ; Dir, Dept of Social Serv to Hndcpd, **SLP**

Summers, Mrs Janet T Mt Royal Towers Drive, Apartment 1021, Birmingham, AL 35209, (205) 879-3366, BA Univ of AL- Tuscaloosa; MA Univ of AL- Tuscaloosa; **SLP LM**

Summers, Jerry G Route 2 Box 221, Crofton, KY 42217, BA 68 Western MI Univ; MA 69 Western MI Univ; Sp-Lang Path, Private Practice, **SLP**

Summers, Mrs Juanita W 3610 Honeywood Drive, Johnson City, TN 37601, (615) 282-4540, BA 72 Columbia Coll; ME 73 Univ of SC - Columbia; **SLP**

Summers, Judith A 3250 Wing Street, San Diego, CA 92110, (619) 221-6000, BA 61 Univ of CA - Los Angeles; MA 82 San Diego St Univ; Sp-Lang Path, Kaiser Perm Mg, **SLP**

Summers, Kristine J Early Childhood Special Education, Meadow Lane School, 7300 Vine Street, Lincoln, NE 68505, (402) 464-3749, BS 75 Univ of NE - Lincoln; MA 83 Univ of Northern CO; MA 77 Univ of NE - Lincoln; Teamleader ECSE, Lincoln Public Schools, **SLP**

Summers, Mrs Mary R R 1 Box 188-A, Marshall, MN 56258, (507) 532-2582, BA 79 Univ of NE - Lincoln; MA 80 Univ of NE - Lincoln; Sp-Lang Path, Marshall PS Dist, **SLP**

Summers, Patricia 1571 Judson Drive, Boulder, CO 80303, (303) 447-1010, BA 75 Univ of CO - Boulder; MA 77 Univ of CO - Boulder; Special Educ Preschool Coord, Boulder Valley School District, **SLP**

Summers, Patricia Anne 1528 East Windsor, Denton, TX 76201, (817) 565-2262, BA 61 Southern Methodist Univ; OM 64 Univ of OK Medical Center; 67–Asst Prof, Univ Of North Texas, **SLP ACE**

Summers, Paula Elaine Route 2 Box 3200, Bowman, SC 29018, (803) 829-2478, BA 82 Columbia Coll; MA 84 SC St Coll; Sp-Lang Path, Anderson Sch Dist #5, **SLP**

Summers, Sharon H 3950 N Lake Shore Drive, Apartment 1002, Chicago, IL 60613, (312) 525-7879, BA 67 Univ of MO - Columbia; MS 72 Univ of HI - Manoa; MS 72 Univ of HI - Manoa; Sp-Lang Path, Chicago Bd of Ed, **SLP**

Summers, Steve R 2495 Northgate Avenue N E, Salem, OR 97303, (503) 378-5286, BA 69 4582; MS 77 Western OR St Coll; Coord Sp & Aud Serv, Fairview Trng Cen, **SLP A**

Summers, Mrs Victoria E 1209 Creekwood, Longview, TX 75602, (214) 236-4139, BS 73 TX Christian Univ; MS 75 East TX St Univ - Commerce; 88–Educ Diagnostician, Hallsville TX ISD, **SLP**

Summers-Johnson, Wendy 2400 California Avenue, Modesto, CA 95351, (209) 524-5181, BA 85 CA St Univ - Stanislaus; MA 85 CA St Univ - Stanislaus; **SLP**

Summerson, Deborah N 313 Park Shore East, Columbia, SC 29204, (803) 736-4367, **SLP**

Summitt, Diana Lynn 3525 Sawtelle #205, Los Angeles, CA 90066, (213) 337-1820, BA 81 CA St Univ - Northridge; MA 83 CA St Univ - Northridge; Sp-Lang Path, InSpeech Inc, **SLP**

Summy, Mrs Barbara Ann 9957 Halberns Blvd, Santee, CA 92017, (619) 258-8703, BA 79 Univ of Toronto - Ontario; MA 85 OK St Univ; 86–Sp-Lang Path, Pomerado Hosp Dist, **SLP**

Summy, Cynthia K 5625 Trishlyn Cove, Fort Wayne, IN 46835, (219) 486-4669, BA 77 Univ of OK - Norman; MS 79 Univ of OK Medical Center; **SLP**

Sumner, Ann Swensen 3947 Sherwood Drive, Provo, UT 84604, (801) 373-7850, BS 71 Brigham Young Univ; OM 72 Brigham Young Univ; Sp-Lang Path, Utah Valley Reg Med Cen, **SLP**

Sumner, Elizabeth 1 Gould Road, Bedford, MA 01730, (617) 264-4700, BS 75 Univ of MA - Amherst; MS 81 Boston Univ; Sp-Lang Path, Acton Pub Sch Syst, **SLP**

Sumner, Florence Greis Route 3 Box 429C, Sylva, NC 28779, (704) 586-5863, BA 36 Univ of NC - Greensboro; MA 61 Western Carolina Univ; OD 71 (NS) Univ of GA; **SLP LM**

Sumner, Jane E 16509 Branchwood Drive, Ellisville, MO 63011, (314) 868-5330, BS 76 Northwest MO St Univ; MA 78 Saint Louis Univ; Sp-Lang Path, Special School District, **SLP**

Sumner, Mrs Nancy C 4247 Charles Samuel Drive, Tallahassee, FL 32308, (904) 488-0167, BS 78 FL St Univ; MS 80 FL St Univ; SLP, Tallahassee Mem Reg Med Ctr, **SLP**

Sumner, Mrs Pamela J 1346 South Almond Circle, Mesa, AZ 85204, (602) 275-4457, BS 77 Fontbonne Coll; MS 78 Fontbonne Coll; SLP, Balsz Elem Sch Dist 31, **SLP**

Sumner, Theresa J 227 West Main Street, Meddletown, NY 10940, (914) 294-8806, Orange Co Cerebral Palsy Assoc, **SLP**

Sumter, Mrs Debra Gethers 1936 Sunnyvale Avenue, Charleston, SC 29407, (803) 763-4674, BA 80 SC St Coll; MA 81 SC St Coll; Sp-Lang Path, Charleston Co Sch, **SLP**

Sundar, Girija S 23 Horizon Drive, Succasunna, NJ 07876, (201) 989-3634, BA 71 Queen Mary's Coll - Madras, India; BA 76 William Paterson Coll; MS 77 William Paterson Coll; Aud, Private Practice, **A ACE**

Sunday, Deborah Lynne 2053 East Minton Drive, Tempe, AZ 85282, (602) 243-4866, BS 83 Brigham Young Univ; OM 84 Brigham Young Univ; 84–Sp-Lang Path, Roosevelt School District 66, **SLP**

Sundbeck, John J Audiology (126), VA Medical Center, 1111 East End Boulevard, Wilkes-Barre, PA 18711, BS 74 Central MI Univ; MA 76 Saint Louis Univ; Aud, VA Med Cen, **SLP A**

Sundberg, Mrs Darleen H 8945 Quigley Street, Westminster, CO 80030, (303) 429-6239, BA 61 Univ of AR - Fayetteville; MA 63 LA St Univ - Baton Rouge; **SLP**

Sundberg, Joan Aline 11610 South 98th East Avenue, Bixby, OK 74008-2219, (513) 661-5077, BS 84 Univ of Cincinnati; MA Univ of Cincinnati; SLP, Cincinnati P S, **SLP**

Sunderbruch, Roberta L 729 21st Street, Bettendorf, IA 52722, (319) 359-1370, BS 76 IN Univ - Bloomington; MA 77 IN Univ - Bloomington; SLP, MS Bend AEA 9, **SLP**

Sunderhaus, Mrs Erika Courlander 3241 Buell Road, Cincinnati, OH 45251, (513) 853-5055, BS 62 Northwestern Univ; MA 78 Univ of Cincinnati; Sp-Lang Path, Providence Hospital, **SLP**

Sunderland, Mrs Linda G 58 Quay Court #42, Sacramento, CA 95831, (309) 344-2138, BS 67 Univ of KS; MA 69 Univ of WA; Sp-Lang Path, Sacramento City USD, **SLP**

Sundstrom, Pat K 4057 East Windrose, Phoenix, AZ 85032, (602) 898-2951, BS 79 AZ St Univ; MS 85 AZ St Univ; Sp-Lang Path, Mesa Public Schools, **SLP**

Sundstrom, Susan Colleen 1502 Lincoln, Salt Lake City, UT 84105, (801) 582-1565, BS 78 Univ of UT; MS 81 Univ of UT; Aud, Veterans Administration, **A**

Sundt, Mrs Christi Morrow 2611 Crofthill, Auburn Hills, MI 48057, (313) 280-8400, BS 86 OH Univ - Athens; MA 88 Wayne St Univ

Sung, Dr Jing J 100 Woodgate Road, Pittsburgh, PA 15235, (412) 683-3000, MA 65 Univ of IA; PH 69 (NS) Univ of KS; 70–Aud, VA Med Cen, **A**

Sung, Dr Show Stu 100 Woodgate Road, Pittsburgh, PA 15235, (412) 232-7785, MA 65 Univ of IA; PH 69 (NS) Univ of KS; Aud, Private Practice, **A ACE**

Sunnquist, Ellen Catherine P O Box 101, Okawville, IL 62271, (618) 532-0005, BS 67 Southern IL Univ -Carbondale; MS 85 Southern IL Univ-Edwardsvill; 85–Sp-Lang Path, Kaskaskia Educ Ctr, **SLP**

Sunshine, Betty 110 Bowline Circle, Atlanta, GA 30328, (404) 255-3160, MA 75 George Washington Univ; Dir Commun Ther, St Francis Country House, **SLP**

Suozzi, Laura 15 Georgia Drive, Wayne, NJ 07470, (201) 461-9100, BA 79 Montclair St Coll; MA 81 Montclair St Coll; Sp-Lang Path, Leonia Bd of Ed, **SLP**

Supal, Connie Alane 2872 Anza Lane, Costa Mesa, CA 92626, (714) 957-0597, MA 81 MI St Univ

Super, Mrs Encie J 3642 Traynham Road, Shaker Heights, OH 44122, (216) 283-4141, BS 76 Ashland Coll; MS 81 Southern CT St Univ; Sp-Lang Path, Private Practice, **SLP**

Super, Margaret S 9 Westward Drive, Corte Madera, CA 94925, (415) 924-6232, BA 67 Temple Univ; MA 69 Temple Univ; Sp-Lang Path, The Breakthrough Group, **SLP**

Super, Sarah Lorraine 9309 North Redfox Lane, Tucson, AZ 85741, (602) 296-3211, BS 83 Univ of AZ; MS 85 Univ of AZ; 88–Aud, Carondelet Health Svcs Inc, **A**

Supercinski, Mrs Becky Reed 1105 Seminole Lane, Longview, TX 75601, (214) 663-1118, BA 64 Baylor Univ; ME 83 Univ of TX - Tyler; Tchr, Longview ISD, **SLP**

Superfine, Donald M 13901 N Florida Avenue #I127, Tampa, FL 33613, (813) 961-7996, BS 65 Northern IL Univ - De Kalb; MA 69 Roosevelt Univ; MA 77 Roosevelt Univ; 86–Sp-Lang Path, Hernando Co School Bd, **SLP**

Superior, Karen M 80 Beaumont Avenue, Newtonville, MA 02160, (617) 964-1025, BA 74 Simmons Coll; MA 77 Univ of Pittsburgh - Pittsburgh; Sp-Lang Path, McLean Hosp, **SLP**

Supler, Rebecca A 101 Fabiola, Lafayette, LA 70508, (318) 233-9345, BS 60 Carlow Coll; MS 65 Univ of Pittsburgh - Pittsburgh; Sp-Lang Path, Sp Dis Cen Inc, **SLP**

Suppa, Rosanna P 3915 Gideon Road, Brookhaven, PA 19015, (215) 447-2044, BS 72 Indiana Univ of PA; MA 74 Temple Univ; Chief/Aud, Crozer Chester Med Cen, **A ACE**

Suppan, Mrs Josephine 202 E Township Line Road, Exton, PA 19341, (215) 458-5992, BA 37 MacAlster Coll; MA 53 Columbia Univ Teachers Coll; **SLP LM**

Suppan, Vincent V 202 E Township Line Road, Exton, PA 19341, (215) 458-5992, BS 47 West Chester Univ of PA; MA 53 Columbia Univ Teachers Coll; Retired, **SLP LM**

Supple, Sr Maria Demontfort Sch Of Remedial Linguistics, 184 Pearse Street, Dublin, Ireland 2, OM 76; Director of Training, U of Dublin Trinity College, **SLP**

Surabian, Julia Ann 711 North State #2, Caro, MI 48723, BS 82 Central MI Univ; MA 83 Central MI Univ; Sp-Lang Path, Caro Regional Mental Hlth Ctr, **SLP**

Surace, Patricia 901 West Wrightwood #1, Chicago, IL 60614-2303, (312) 957-7014, **SLP**

Surbeck, Kathryn Silvis 214 West Bridgeport, White Hall, IL 62092, (217) 245-5141, MS 74 PA St Univ - Univ Park; Sp-Lang Path, Illinois Sch for the Deaf, **SLP**

Surber, Barbara Kaufman 4608 Sylvan Oak Drive, Dayton, OH 45426, (513) 837-6069, BA 65 Univ of IL - Urbana; MS 67 Southern IL Univ -Carbondale; Sp-Lang Path, VA Medical Center, **SLP**

Surbrook, Mrs Janet H 3922 N E 33rd Avenue, Portland, OR 97212, (503) 282-0279, BS 63 Univ of MN - Minneap-St Paul; MA 67 Univ of MN - Minneap-St Paul; Sp-Lang Path, Portland Pub Sch, **SLP**

Surch, Patricia Joyce 875 Stevens Avenue #2209, Solana Beach, CA 92075-2708, (619) 481-1241, **SLP**

Surell, Mrs Susan H 2308 Hanway Road, Baltimore, MD 21209, (301) 484-2556, BS 77 Univ of MD - College Park; MS 80 Loyola Coll; Dir, Private Practice, **SLP**

Surgers, Brenda J 150 Pearl #213, Oakland, CA 94611, (415) 237-1441, BS 79 Univ of NV - Reno; BA 71 Univ of Houston - Univ Park; Richmond Schs, **SLP**

Surkis, Eleanor 116 Pinehurst Avenue, New York, NY 10033, (212) 928-3263, BS 59 Boston Univ; MA 61 Columbia Univ Teachers Coll; Consultant In Aud, NY St Off/Hlth Systs Mgmt, **A**

Surowicz, Christal Maria 3108 Laurel Avenue, Cheverly, MD 20785, (301) 772-0264, BA 85 Univ of MD - College Park; MS 87 Gallaudet Coll; 87–Aud, Washington Hosp Ctr

Surowiecki, Mrs Patricia D 9 Weatherside Drive, Wallingford, CT 06492, (203) 238-1273, BA 72 Univ of Denver; MS 81 Southern CT St Univ; Sp-Lang Path, Meriden Pub Schls, **SLP**

Surowitz, Ellen 127 Princeton House, Clusters Of Lexton, Maple Shade, NJ 08052, (215) 331-6878, BA 78 SUNY - Center at Buffalo; MA 81 Temple Univ-Tyler Sch of Art; Aud, Dr Arnold King Brenman, **SLP A**

Surr, Mrs Rauna K Army Audiology & Speech Center, Walter Reed Army Med Ctr, Washington, DC 20307, (202) 576-1649, BA 63 Univ of CA - Riverside; MS 69 Gallaudet Coll; Aud, Walter Reed Army Med Cen, **A**

Survance, Mrs Cathi Ann 428 Green Oak Drive, Huntington, WV 25705, (304) 523-3417, MA 82 Marshall Univ; Sp-Lang Path, Cabell County Board of Educ, **SLP**

Survant, Mrs Maureen Connell 590 Alihi Place, Kailua, HI 96734, (808) 423-1356, **SLP**

Susca, Mary Alice Schiff 1640 Primrose Drive, El Cajon, CA 92020, (619) 588-4747, BA 73 Univ of CA - Los Angeles; MA 79 George Washington Univ; 88–Sp-Lang Path, San Diego Rehab Ins at Alvarado, **SLP**

Susca, Michael 1640 Primrose Drive, El Cajon, CA 92020, (619) 588-4747, BA 75 Univ of CA - Santa Barbara; MS 77 Univ of NM; Cl Superv Site Operations Mgr, Sp-Hrng & Neurosensory Cen, **SLP**

Susienka, Cindy Hasenzahl 1437 West Abbott Avenue, Milwaukee, WI 53221, (414) 282-0625, BS 81 Marquette Univ; MS 82 Marquette Univ; SLP Coord, Greenfield Rehab Agcy Inc, **SLP ACE**

Susmar, Ann E 2695 Trindad Circle, Melbourne, FL 32935, (407) 242-9100, BA 73 Univ of FL; MA 75 Our Lady Lake Univ-San Anton; 88–Sp-Lang Path, Devereux Hosp & Children's Ctr, **SLP**

Susnik, Jackie L 4747 Scarff Road, New Carlisle, OH 45344, (513) 253-4178, BA 78 Our Lady Lake Univ-San Anton; MA 80 Our Lady Lake Univ-San Anton; Sp-Lang Path, Mont Co Pub Sch, **SLP**

Suson, Karen Anne 3300 Wailea Alanui #27-C, Waialae Maui, HI 96753, (808) 244-7467, BA 80 Univ of CO - Boulder; MS 83 Univ of MI - Ann Arbor; Sp-Lang Path, IMUA Rehab-Soc for Crippled Children, **SLP**

Susser, Mrs Bonnie S 3309 Hillside Terrace, Fair Lawn, NJ 07410-4212, (201) 299-8358, BA 75 Univ of MD - College Park; MA 78 CUNY - Queens Coll; Sp/Lang Path, Private Practice, **SLP**

Susser, Robin D 3260 Lake Shore Drive #4A, Chicago, IL 60657, BA 78 IN Univ - Bloomington; MS 80 Univ of WI - Madison; Consult/Sp-Lang Path, **SLP**

Susskind, Mrs Cathy A 11636 Orange Blossom Lane, Boca Raton, FL 33433, (305) 523-8516, BS 80 IN Univ - Bloomington; MA 81 IN Univ - Bloomington; SLP, Er Sl So, **SLP**

Susslin, Margaret Ann 1515 Fifth Street, Slidell, LA 70458, (504) 641-0699, BA 84 Southeastern LA Univ; OM 86 LA St Univ - N O Médical Ctr; 86–Sp-Lang Path, St Tammany Parish PS, **SLP**

Sussman, Anita Jones 224 Ray Road, New Haven, CT 06515-2324, (615) 387-2337, BA 74 SUNY - Center at Buffalo; MS 79 Purdue Univ - West Lafayette; **SLP**

Sussman, Mrs Beryl M 294 Ewing Terrace, San Francisco, CA 94118, (415) 346-2776, BS 52 Wichita St Univ; MA 57 Wichita St Univ; Sp-Lang Path, San Fran USD, **SLP**

Sussman, Dr Joan E 515 Linwood Avenue, Buffalo, NY 14209, (716) 636-3400, PH 84 (NS) Purdue Univ - West Lafayette; Asst Professor Speech Sciences, State University of New York, **SLP**

Sussman, Karen A 940 Lawrence Court, North Bellmore, NY 11710, (516) 483-3836, BS 79 Hofstra Univ; MA 80 Hofstra Univ; 82–Sp-Lang Path, Lynbrook Un Fr Sch Dist, **SLP**

Sussman, Susan T 38 Summit Street, Hicksville, NY 11801, (516) 681-4886, BS 85 Univ of MA - Amherst; MA 86 Hofstra Univ; 88–Sp-Lang Path, The Ctr for Rehab-Merrick, **SLP**

Sustich, Linda LaBuda 1111 Rial Drive, Bethel Park, PA 15102, (412) 831-1809, BS 76 Univ of IL - Urbana; MS 77 Univ of IL - Urbana; **SLP**

Sutadisastra, Rozella J J1 Pinang Ii Kav 12, Pondok Labu, Cilandak, Jakarta, Indonesia 12450, **SLP**

Sutcliffe, Natalie M 308 West 105th Street #3B, New York, NY 10025, (212) 584-9000, BS 80 Univ of NH; MS 82 Columbia Univ Teachers Coll; Sp-Lang Path, Bronx VA Med Ctr, **SLP**

Suter, Dr Alice H 1501 Red Oak Drive, Silver Spring, MD 20910, (301) 588-3471, BA 59 American Univ; ME 60 Gallaudet Coll; PH 77 (NS) Univ of MD - College Park; Consult Industrial Aud, Sonus Company, **A**

Suter, Mrs Carole P 4250 Valley Crest Hills Dr, St Louis, MO 63128, (314) 846-8611, BS 59 Bradley Univ; ME 82 Univ of MO - Saint Louis; SLP, Spec Schl Dist of St Louis Co, **SLP**

Suter, Cherri A 414 North Lincoln, Jerome, ID 83338, (208) 324-2443, MS 78 ID St Univ; 84–Sp-Lang Path, Magic Valley Sp & Hrng Clinic, **SLP**

Suter, Laura Jane 7046 Copperwood Way, Columbia, MD 21046, (301) 290-9458, BA 84 Eastern WA Univ; MS 86 Eastern WA Univ; **SLP**

Sutherland, Alan C 10445 Tara Drive, Riverview, FL 33569, (813) 677-7048, MS 88 Univ of South FL

Sutherland, Ann Elizabeth Dr Bennett And Associates Incorporated, 5203 Magnolia Place, Fredericksburg, VA 22401, (703) 898-6146, BS 80 SUNY - Coll at Geneseo; MS 83 James Madison Univ; 84–Sp-Lang Path, Dr Bennett & Associates, **SLP**

Sutherland, Dee Mills Route 3 Box 19O, Dowdy Cemetery Road, Benton, KY 42025, (502) 527-7270, BA 61 Univ of KY; MA 63 G Peabody Coll-Vanderbilt U; 76–Sp-Lang Path, Marshall Co Bd of Ed, **SLP A**

Sutherland, Dr Dorothy F Columbus College, Speech Clinic, Jordan Hall, Columbus, GA 31993, (404) 568-2222, BA 66 Univ of GA; ME 70 Univ of GA; ED 86 (Special Education) Univ of AL- Tuscaloosa; Assoc Prof, Columbus Coll, **SLP**

Sutherland, Harrell C, Jr 229 Trails End, La Vernia, TX 78121, (512) 779-1701, BA 54 Southwest TX St Univ; ME 58 Southwest TX St Univ; Retired, USAF-Sch Aerospace Med, **A**

Sutherland, LaVerne Deel 2197 Homet Road, San Marino, CA 91108, MA 53 Univ of Southern CA; 53–Sp-Lang Path, Los Angeles City USD, **SLP LM**

Sutherland, Mrs Lindsey Martin 1153 Menlo, Clovis, CA 93612, (209) 299-8418, BA 83 CA St Univ - Fresno; MA 86 CA St Univ - Fresno

Sutherland, Mrs Marcia Evans 981 Summer Place, Pittsburgh, PA 15243, (412) 561-4791, BA 64 PA St Univ - Univ Park; MS 65 Vanderbilt Univ; Sp-Lang Path, Private Practice, **SLP**

Sutherland, Martin P O Box 313, St Anne, IL 60964, (815) 937-2082, BS 77 Southern IL Univ -Carbondale; MS 79 Southern IL Univ -Carbondale; Sp-Lang Path, St Marys Hosp, **SLP**

Sutor, Ann Crawford 36 Heath Avenue, Oakhurst, NJ 07755-1007, (201) 870-1708, BS 78 Seton Hall Univ; MA 80 Montclair St Coll; Sp/Lang Path, Private Practice, **SLP**

Sutter, Mrs Ann Marie 63 Wyandanch Avenue, Babylon, NY 11702, BS 81 Saint John's Univ - Jamaica; MS 82 Adelphi Univ; Sp/Lang Path, Nassau BOCES, **SLP**

Sutter, Jane C Route 1 Box 77, Lee, ME 04455, (207) 738-3293, BA 77 Ball St Univ; MA 78 Ball St Univ; Aud, Idaho State U, **A**

Sutter, Dr Judith Carol University Of Alberta, Dept Sp Pathology & Aud, 400-11044 82nd Avenue, Edmonton, AB, Canada T6G 0T2, (403) 432-5990, OB 74 Univ of Calgary - Alberta; MA 76 WA St Univ; PH 86 (Sp Path) Univ of IL - Urbana; 86–Asst Prof, Univ of Alberta, **SLP**

Sutton, Ann Colquhoun 49 50th Avenue, Lachine, PQ, Canada H8T 2T4, (514) 482-0500, BA 76 Univ of Toronto - Ontario; MA 79 Univ of Toronto - Ontario; MS 83 Boston Univ; SLP, MacKay Center, **SLP**

Sutton, Cheryl Anne 4903 17th Street, San Francisco, CA 94117, (415) 681-3211, MS 84 Univ of Redlands; **SLP**

Sutton, Cynthia F 3175 South Tenaya Way, Las Vegas, NV 89117, BA 75 Univ of FL; OM 76 Auburn Univ - Auburn; Sp/Lang Path, Nevada Easter Seal Soc, **SLP**

Sutton, Mrs Kathleen Johns 1922 Lakewood Circle South, Jacksonville, FL 32207, (904) 448-0564, BA 80 Columbia Coll; MA 85 Univ of GA; Sp-Lang Path, Duval County Schools, **SLP**

Sutton, Dr Lois 702 East 8-1/2 Street, Houston, TX 77007, (713) 795-7492, BS 67 Univ of IA; MA 69 Univ of IA; PH 79 (NS) Baylor Coll of Medicine; Aud, VA, **A ACE**

Sutton, Marjorie Alice 17623 Nassau Drive, Brookfield, WI 53005, (414) 463-0756, BS 59 Univ of WI - Madison; MS 86 Marquette Univ; **SLP**

Sutton, Sandra W 334 Courtney Place, Wexford, PA 15090, **SLP**

Sutton, Valerie S 16005 Mills Orchard Drive, Gaithersburg, MD 20878, (301) 589-6616, BS 74 Univ of MD - College Park; MS 76 Gallaudet Coll; Aud, Bruce Bloom MD, **A**

Sutton-Merritt, Mrs Rhonda Jean Route 5 Box 57, Mount Olive, NC 28365, (919) 731-2234, MA 85 East Carolina Univ; Sp-Lang Path, Eastern Assoc, **SLP**

Suty, Dr Karen A Dept Of Speech & Hearing, Cleveland State University, East 22nd & Euclid, Cleveland, OH 44115, (216) 687-3805, BA 72 MI St Univ; MS 74 Washington Univ; PH 82 (NS) Univ of TX - Dallas; Asst Prof, Cleveland State U, **A**

Suzuki, Deborah S 1106 Club Drive, Wahiawa, HI 96786, (808) 621-8337, BS 75 Univ of HI - Manoa; MS 76 Univ of WI - Stevens Point; Aud, Private Practice, **A**

Suzuki, Gwen Mitsuko 1379 Komohana Street, Hilo, HI 96720, (808) 961-7537, BS 80 CO St Univ; MA 83 Kent St Univ; 83–Sp/Lang Path, State of Hawaii Dept of Educ, **SLP**

Svagerko, James Michael 230 Courtland Avenue, Campbell, OH 44405, (216) 744-5550, MA 87 OH St Univ; **A**

Svarc-Hopkins, Joyce 2435H Presidential Way, West Palm Beach, FL 33401, (305) 478-2140, BA 76 McGill Univ - Quebec; MS 79 McGill Univ - Quebec; **SLP**

Svec, Mrs Mary Arnold 302 North Belt East, Belleville, IL 62221, (618) 234-5250, BS 79 Southern IL Univ-Edwardsvill; MS 80 Southern IL Univ-Edwardsvill; Audiologist & Sp-Lang Path, Alton Audiology Center, **SLP A**

Svendsen, Mrs Mary Lou 150 Crown Point Road, Springfield, VT 05156, BS 66 Carlow Coll; MA 67 Columbia Univ Teachers Coll; **SLP**

Svien, Leonard D Route 3 Box 205-A, Stephenville, TX 76401-9536, (817) 968-3054, BS 75 Abilene Christian Univ; MA 77 Abilene Christian Univ; 87–Dir MHMR Svcs, Pecan Valley MHMR Region, **SLP**

Svigals, Dolores J 6460 Shire Way, Long Beach, CA 90815, (213) 430-2704, BA 49 Bard Coll; MA 50 Columbia Univ Teachers Coll; 78–Sp-Lang Path, El Rancho-USD, **SLP**

Sviland, Carmen C 18025 Buckingham, Birmingham, MI 48009, **SLP**

Svingen, Julianne P Boystown National Institute, 555 North 30th Street, Omaha, NE 68131, (402) 498-6619, BS 80 IA St Univ; MA 82 Univ of KS; Sp-Lang Path, Boys Town National Institute, **SLP**

Svitko, Dr Carol Schnippert Ithaca College, 304 Smiddy, Ithaca, NY 14850, (412) 938-4175, BS 72 CA Univ of PA; MS 76 Univ of Pittsburgh - Pittsburgh; PH 87 (Communication Disorders) PA St Univ - Univ Park; 88–Asst Prof/Aud, Ithaca College, **A**

Svoboda, Mrs Cheryl L 2602 Avenue D, Scottsbluff, NE 69361, (308) 632-7146, BA 66 Univ of Northern CO; ME 69 Kent St Univ; Sp-Lang Path, Scottsbluff Pub Sch, **SLP**

Svoboda, James S 2409 Highland Drive, Scottsbluff, NE 69361, (308) 632-5226, BA 67 Kent St Univ; MA 69 Kent St Univ; 82–Sp/Lang Path, Private Practice, **SLP**

Svoboda, Kathleen D Route 1 Box 102-A, Bucyrus, KS 66013, (913) 642-9592, BS 74 Univ of KS; MA 76 Univ of KS; SLP, Shawnee Mission Pub Sch #512, **SLP**

Swafford, Katherine 1093 South Holland Street, Lakewood, CO 80226, BA 76 Univ of Northern CO; MA 78 Univ of Northern CO; Sp-Lang Path, Spalding Rehab Hosp, **SLP**

Swagemakers, Kimberly Anne Rd 2 Box 17, Route 31, Hudson, NY 12534, (518) 828-3890, BS 84 SUNY - Coll at Fredonia; MS 86 SUNY - Coll at Fredonia; **SLP**

Swailes, Winifred Louise 6335 Landover Road #303, Cheverly, MD 20785, (301) 773-2307, **SLP**

Swain, Beth Carver 6912 Hallet, Shawnee, KS 66216, MS 80 Univ of KS; Sp-Lang Path, Research Med Ctr, **SLP**

Swain, Dr Charles E, Jr 20 Woodbury Hill, Springfield, IL 62702, (217) 793-2763, MS 65 Southern IL Univ -Carbondale; PH 71 (NS) Univ of IL - Urbana; Aud, Springfield Cl, **SLP A**

Swain, Elizabeth Ann 649 Bending Bough Drive, Webster, NY 14580, (716) 271-0680, MS 88 Emerson Coll; 88–Sp-Lang Path, Hrg & Sp Ctr of Rochester

Swain, Joan Kasabach Dept Of Speech & Language Path, William Beaumont Hospital, 3601 West 13 Mile Road, Royal Oak, MI 48072, (313) 258-1090, BA 64 Univ of MI - Ann Arbor; MA 73 Wayne St Univ; 75–Sp-Lang Path, William Beaumont Hosp, **SLP**

Swain, Mrs Robin H P O Box 6104, South Lake Tahoe, CA 95729, (916) 541-6711, BA 52 Univ of CO - Boulder; MA 62 San Francisco St Univ; Innkeeper, Swains' Bed/Breakfast, **SLP**

Swallow, Barbara Center For Hearing Speech & Language, 4280 Hale Parkway, Denver, CO 80210, (303) 322-1871, BS 75 Purdue Univ - West Lafayette; MS 76 Purdue Univ - West Lafayette; Mgr Cl Serv, Cen for Hrng-Sp-Lang, **SLP**

Swallum, Mrs Alice 1209 Butts Avenue #3, Tomah, WI 54660, (605) 372-5396, BA 66; MA 67 Adams St Coll; 78–Sp-Lang Path, Sioux Vally Hosp, **SLP LM**

Swan, Mrs Cynthia S 1911 Healy Drive, Mobile, AL 36695, (205) 633-8458, BS 71 Univ of Montevallo; MS 74 Univ of Montevallo; Sp-Lang Path, Mobile Co Pub Sch Syst, **SLP**

Swander, Camille Grace P O Box 1056 Lakeview Rd, Windham, ME 04062, (207) 892-7242, BS 74 SUNY - Coll at Geneseo; MS 76 Univ of Southern ME; **SLP**

Swander, Donald E P O Box 1056 Lakeview Road, North Windham, ME 04062, (207) 892-7242, BS 60 Edinboro Univ of PA; MS 76 Univ of Southern ME; 74–Sp-Lang Path, Portland PS, **SLP**

Swanhorst, Lisa Carole 2832 Westcliffe Drive, Burnsville, MN 55337-6958, (605) 624-6723, BS 85 Univ of SD - Vermillion; MA 86 Univ of SD - Vermillion; **SLP**

Swanik, Mrs Nancy Jane 15 Robin Drive, Washington, PA 15301, (412) 222-4300, BS 68 CA Univ of PA; MS 84 CA Univ of PA; Sp-Lang Path, Keystone Rehab Sys, **SLP**

Swank, Mrs Jo-Ann B 4491 East Wembley Lane, Columbus, IN 47201, (812) 376-0798, BS 69 IN Univ - Bloomington; MA 70 Ball St Univ; Sp/Lang Path, Bartholomew Consol Sch Corp, **SLP**

Swank, Mrs Linda K 3310 Normandy Road, Hutchinson, KS 67502, (316) 662-4461, BA 74 Wichita St Univ; OM 79 Wichita St Univ; MA 75 Wichita St Univ; Sp-Lang Path, USD #308 Hutchinson, Ka, **SLP**

Swank, Phyllis M Route 10 Box 62, Chapel Hill, NC 27514, (919) 942-3627, BS 61 Western MI Univ; MA 85 Univ of NC - Greensboro; 88–Sp-Lang Path, Chapel Hill Carrboro Cty Sch, **SLP**

Swann, Maria T 1542 South Bedford Street, Los Angeles, CA 90035, (213) 278-1655, PH 85 (NS); Educational Programming Spec, Focus, **SLP**

Swanson, Allen F 5400 Mad River Lane, Columbia, MD 21044, (301) 997-0231, BA 70 Hiram Coll; MA 74 Kent St Univ; 74–Sp/Lang Path, Bd of Educ of Baltimore Co, **SLP**

Swanson, Ann Marie 215 Antelope Trail, Whitefish, MT 59937, (406) 752-5300, BA 77 Univ of MT; MA 84 Univ of MT; Sp/Lang Path, Flathead Co Spec Ed, **SLP**

Swanson, Mrs Barbara Izzett 108 Tanglewood Place, Parkersburg, WV 26101, (304) 485-7211, BS 63 Northwestern Univ; **SLP**

Swanson, Barbara L 8009 Delmar Boulevard #4, St Louis, MO 63130-3721, (314) 839-6170, BA 71 Elmhurst Coll; MS 72 IL St Univ - Normal; SLP, St Louis Co Spec Sch Dist, **SLP**

Swanson, Bonnelynn M 195 Frederick Boulevard, Jamestown, NY 14701, (716) 485-7080, BS 80 SUNY - Coll at Fredonia; MS 82 SUNY - Coll at Fredonia; SLP, Jamestown Publ Schs, **SLP**

Swanson, Brad Lauren 230 Stony Run Lane #5-H, Baltimore, MD 21210, (301) 528-2419, **SLP**

Swanson, Christine B 11131 East Daines Drive, Arcadia, CA 91006, (818) 448-4039, BA 81 Univ of LA Verne; MS 84 Univ of LA Verne; SLP, Los Angeles County Off of Educ, **SLP**

Swanson, Mrs Cynthia Louise 703 Edgemoor Road, Wilmington, DE 19809, (302) 764-7075, BS 83 Edinboro Univ of PA; MA 84 Edinboro Univ of PA; **SLP**

Swanson, Eleanor 1849 Portland, St Paul, MN 55104, (612) 348-6006, MS 53 Univ of IL - Urbana; SLP, Minneapolis Pub Schs, **SLP**

Swanson, Mrs Elizabeth Carver 1862 Teak Court, Henderson, NV 89015, (702) 736-5011, BS 84 Univ of WI - Eau Claire; MA 85 Univ of WI - Eau Claire; **SLP**

Swanson, Mrs Gineta Gann 965 Camino Anasazi, Santa Fe, NM 87501, (505) 438-0591, MS 83 OK St Univ; 88–Sp-Lang Path, InSpeech Inc, **SLP**

Swanson, Mrs Glenna 7102 South Plate Canyon Dr, Littleton, CO 80123, (303) 986-0680, BS 73 Northwestern Univ; MA 74 Northwestern Univ; Sp-Lang Path, SW Pediatric Habilitation Ctr, **SLP**

Swanson, Judith Danz Speech & Hearing Associates, 499 South Warren Street, Syracuse, NY 13202, (315) 471-2186, BS 65 Syracuse Univ; MS 68 Syracuse Univ; Sp-Lang Path, Private Practice, **SLP**

Swanson, Mrs Karen L 3408 Mock Orange Court S, Salem, OR 97302, (503) 363-1288, BA 65 Pacific Lutheran Univ; MS 71 Western OR St Coll; **SLP**

Swanson, Mrs Kay L 5133 Braun Street, Arvada, CO 80002, (303) 231-2467, BA 80 Univ of Northern CO; MA 82 Univ of Northern CO; Sp-Lang Path, Jefferson Co Pub Sch, **SLP**

Swanson, Leslie Helen 1485 Gatewood Avenue, Palatine, IL 60067, (312) 991-5143, BS 79 Northern IL Univ - De Kalb; MA 80 Northern IL Univ - De Kalb; SLP, Self Employed, **SLP**

Swanson, Leslie K 24032 North 40 Avenue, Glendale, AZ 85310, (602) 866-5958, BS 73 AZ St Univ; MS 79 AZ St Univ; SLP, Deer Valley USD, **SLP**

Swanson, Lori 5765 Heritage Hill Drive, Alexandria, VA 22310, (301) 981-4920, BA 72 Univ of TN - Knoxville; MA 73 Univ of TN - Knoxville; 88–Chief of Aud, Andrews Air Force Base, **A**

Swanson, Lori Ann Purdue University, 312 Young Graduate House, West Lafayette, IN 47906, (317) 494-3806, BS 80 Univ of WI - River Falls; MS 82 Univ of WI - Madison; Sp/Lang Path, Anoka-Hennepin Indep Sd #11, **SLP**

Swanson, Marie E 437 Rensvold Boulevard, Moorhead, MN 56560, (218) 236-2286, BS 67 Minot St Univ; MS 68 Minot St Univ; 70–Cl Superv/Asst Prof, Moorhead St U, **SLP**

Swanson, Mrs Martha B 44 Dalewood Road, Newington, CT 06111, (203) 584-7804, BA 77 Univ of CT; MS 80 Southern CT St Univ; SLP, Bristol Public Schools, **SLP**

Swanson, Nancy F 14720 Cardigan Square, Centreville, VA 22020-1818, (304) 599-5959, BS 78 WV Univ; MS 79 WV Univ; Audiologist, **A**

Swanson, Sally A 321 North Howard, Moscow, ID 83843, (605) 697-7617, BS 75 Univ of MI - Ann Arbor; MS 78 Univ of WA; Sp-Lang Path, Cen Co Home Hlth Serv, **SLP**

Swanson, Mrs Sharon Kay 602 South Belknap, Sugar Land, TX 77478-3210, (713) 498-8110, BA 79 CA St Univ - Northridge; MA 81 CA St Univ - Northridge; **SLP**

Swanson, Mrs Shirley Phelps Box 142 Rt 518, Hopewell, NJ 08525, (609) 466-2962, BS 51 SUNY - Coll at Geneseo; MA 87 Trenton St Coll; **SLP**

Swanson, Mrs Sonia C 991 Harvard Court, Highland Park, IL 60035, MS 78 Northeastern IL Univ; MA 84 Roosevelt Univ; Sp-Lang Path, District 37 Avoca Schools, **SLP**

Swanson, Stephanie Lu 53 Avondale Park, Rochester, NY 14620, (716) 257-5050, BS 83 Univ of AZ; MA 86 SUNY - Coll at Geneseo; **SLP**

Swanson, Susan Denise 605 Old U S Hwy 70 East, Black Mountain, NC 28711, (704) 669-7546, MS 81 Univ of WY; BS 77 SUNY - Coll at Geneseo; **A**

Swanson, Susan Marie Boys Town National Institute, 555 North 30th Street, Omaha, NE 68131, (402) 498-6557, 83–Sp-Lang Path, Boys Town Institute, **SLP**

Swanson, Teri 7971 Playmor Terrace, San Diego, CA 92122, (619) 691-5536, BA 69; MA 72 San Diego St Univ; SLP, Sweetwater Un Hs Dist, **SLP**

Swanson, Mrs Tracy L A 637 Albrook Drive, Allen, TX 75002-3013, (312) 742-3264, BS 77 IL St Univ - Normal; MS 78 IL St Univ - Normal; **A**

Swanson, Virginia Lee 2828 North Bristol #18, Santa Ana, CA 92706, (714) 633-7400, MA 85 San Diego St Univ; 88–Sp-Lang Path, Annette Levy & Assoc, **SLP**

Swanstrom, Gail J ENT Associates, 512 East Main Street, Hillsboro, OR 97123, (503) 648-8971, BA 70 Univ of CA - Irvine; BA 78 Humboldt St Univ; MS 82 Portland St Univ; Aud, ENT Assoc, **A**

Swany, Mrs Nancy B 633 Mackay Drive, Richmond Hill, GA 31324, (912) 727-2965, BA 74 Winthrop Coll; MA 76 Univ of TN - Knoxville; Slp, Bryan County Schools, **SLP**

Swapsy, Anita L 2901 South King Drive #509, Chicago, IL 60616, (312) 758-4520, BA 76 Southern IL Univ-Edwardsvill; MS 77 Southern IL Univ-Edwardsvill; Sp-Lang Path, Brookwood Sch Dist #167, **SLP**

Sward, Janet L 732 West Feemster, Visalia, CA 93277, (209) 625-6793, BA 72 CA St Univ - Fresno; MS 73 Univ of WY; Sp-Lang Path, Visalia USD, **SLP**

Swarthout, Shelly Jo 81 Whetstone Drive, Horsham, PA 19044, (215) 674-3091, BS 83 PA St Univ - Univ Park; MA 85 Temple Univ-Tyler Sch of Art; **SLP**

Swarts, Kevin Richard S-6801 Woodland Drive, Hamburg, NY 14075, (716) 878-7370, BS 72 SUNY - Coll at Geneseo; MS 74 Gallaudet Coll; Supvr Aud Svcs, Chldns Hosp Buffalo NY, **A**

Swartz, Anita L 8360 Calico Drive, Bozeman, MT 59715, (407) 586-0112, BS 69 Northeast MO St Univ; MA 69 Northeast MO St Univ; Sp-Lang Path, Private Practice, **SLP**

Swartz, Mrs Barbara Brewer PFC 1 Box 935, APO New York, NY 09292, (904) 678-8531, BA 76 Univ of MS; MS 78 Univ Southern MS-Hattiesburg; **A**

Swartz, Dr Bradford L 315 East May Street, Mount Pleasant, MI 48858, (517) 774-3471, BS 75 Central MI Univ; MA 76 Central MI Univ; PH 88 (Sp Science) MI St Univ; 80–Asst Prof, Ctrl MI U, **SLP ACE**

Swartz, Mrs Burnetta Flagg 600 Spruce Street, Lansdale, PA 19446, (215) 855-0975, BS 69 PA St Univ - Univ Park; MA 74 Trenton St Coll; Sp-Lang Path, Montgomery County Indepen Unit, **SLP**

Swartz, Mrs Carol C 7295 South Jefferson Road, Shreve, OH 44676, (216) 567-2837, BS 58 Kent St Univ; Sp-Lang Path, Triway Local Sch, **SLP**

Swartz, Mrs Judith L 4235-181 Porte DE Palmos, San Diego, CA 92122, BA 73 Queens Coll; MA 75 Hofstra Univ; Sp-Lang Path, Private Practice, **SLP**

Swartz, Kristin Kay 128 West Frack Street, Frackville, PA 17931, (717) 874-4228, MS 88 Bloomsburg Univ of PA; 88–Sp-Lang Path, InSpeech Inc

Swartz, Leslie A 150 Somerset Lane, Bolingbrook, IL 60439, (815) 467-2800, BS 78 IL St Univ - Normal; MS 80 Univ of AZ; Sp-Lang Path, Regional Educ Service Agency, **SLP**

Swartz, Mrs Linda Kay 7402 Wesboro Road, Louisville, KY 40222, (502) 454-8284, BA 69 CUNY - Queens Coll; MA 71 Montclair St Coll; SLP, Jefferson Co Bd of Ed Ky, **SLP**

Swartz, Susan R 2915 Tewksbury, Troy, MI 48098, (313) 858-1921, BA 68 Univ of IL - Urbana; MS 69 NY Univ; Sp-Lang Path, Oakland Sch ISD, **SLP**

Swartzlander, Paula M 963 South State Road 446, Bloomington, IN 47401, (812) 331-8712, MA 87 IN Univ - Bloomington; 88–Sp-Lang Path, Richland-Bean Blossom Sch Corp, **SLP**

Swast, Mrs Amy L Rd 7 Box 265, Kittanning, PA 16201, (412) 548-8020, BS 78 Clarion Univ of PA; MS 81 Indiana Univ of PA; Sp-Lang Path, Inter Ut #28, **SLP**

Swatek, Linda Kay 3433 Woodview Drive, Lafayette, CA 94549, (415) 828-4360, BA 62 Carlow Coll; MS 82 San Francisco St Univ; Sp-Lang Path, San Ramon Valley USD, **SLP**

Swayman, Debbie Meyers 9417 N W 46th Street, Sunrise, FL 33321, (305) 742-0326, BS 77 SUNY - Coll at Buffalo; MS 87 Nova Univ

Swearingen, Mrs Lisa McDonald 4200 W Memorial Road, Suite 107, Oklahoma City, OK 73120, (405) 755-4327, BS 82 OK St Univ; MS 84 Univ of OK - OK City; Aud, Okla Hearing Ctr, **A**

Swearingin, Marilyn K 307 Northmoor Drive, Jerseyville, IL 62052, (618) 498-5761, BS 76 Western IL Univ; MA 77 Western IL Univ; Sp-Lang Path, Caihoun District 40, **SLP**

Sweat, Linda Logan 199 Kenner Avenue #B, Nashville, TN 37205, (615) 320-5353, BA 81 Auburn Univ - Auburn; MA 83 Univ of FL; Sp-Lang Path, Bill Wilkerson Hrng & Sp Cen, **SLP**

Sweatt, Beverly Leverda 812 Countrywood Drive, Franklin, TN 37064, (615) 320-5353, BS 80 Univ of TN - Knoxville; MA 82 Univ of TN - Knoxville; Sp/Lang Path, Prof Hlth Servs, **SLP**

Sweatt, Mrs M Lynn 15627 Big Trail, San Antonio, TX 78232, (512) 496-8044, BS 73 TX Tech Univ; MS 74 TX Tech Univ; **SLP**

Sweda, Mrs Mary T 200 Adams Avenue, Second Floor - Headstart, Scranton, PA 18503, (717) 963-6633, **SLP**

Swedburg, Julie Siggelkow 2410 Calihan Avenue, Bemidji, MN 56601-4169, (218) 694-6528, BA 85 Univ of MN - Duluth; MS 86 Univ of WI - Eau Claire; 88–Sp-Lang Path, Bemidji Reg Interdist Council

Sweede, Mrs June W 10142 Dowling Road, Bowling Green, OH 43402, (419) 833-6771, BA 57 Bowling Green St Univ; ME 76 Univ of Toledo; Sp-Lang Path, Lake Local Sch

Sweeney, Mrs Anne Marie 106 Quaker Street, Northbridge, MA 01534, (508) 839-5484, BA 79 Assumption Coll; MS 84 Worcester St Coll; 84–Sp-Lang Path, Grafton Pub Schs, **SLP**

Sweeney, Colette M 4012 N W 5th Street, Rochester, MN 55901, (507) 289-8029, BA 75 Coll of Saint Teresa; MS 77 Saint Cloud St Univ; Sp-Lang Path, Rocheste Pub Sch, **SLP**

Sweeney, Hansine Schumacher Family Hospital & Nursing Home, 730 South Calhoun Road, Brookfield, WI 53005, (414) 937-2326, **SLP**

Sweeney, Judith Lorraine 143 Knollwood Drive, Wallingford, CT 06492, (203) 237-7835, BA 81 IN Univ - Bloomington; MA 83 IN Univ - Bloomington; 85–Sp-Lang Path, Easter Seals Rehab Ctr of Central Connecticut, **SLP**

Sweeney, Mrs Karin Alice 1574 North Cherry, Galesburg, IL 61401-1821, (309) 343-1481, MS 82 Univ of WI - Milwaukee; BS 80 Univ of WI - Milwaukee; BA 78 Marquette Univ; Sp-Lang Path, St Francis Chldrns Ctr, **SLP**

Sweeney, Lynn A 1600 Canterbury Trail #H, Mount Pleasant, MI 48858, (517) 774-7304, BS 78 Central MI Univ; MA 79 Central MI Univ; Sp/Lang Path, Midland Hosp Center, **SLP ACE**

Sweeney, Marion K 648 Roosevelt Avenue, Springfield, MA 01118, (413) 736-8173, BA 37 Elms Coll; MA 42 Emerson Coll; Prof Emerita, Coll of Our Lady of the Elms, **SLP LM**

Sweeney, Martha H 1201 Doregan Court, Lutherville, MD 21093, (301) 243-3800, BA 80 Loyola Coll; MS 81 Loyola Coll; Sp-Lang Path, **SLP**

Sweeney, Mrs Mary G P O Box 62, Zeigler, IL 62999, BS 33 IA St Univ; **A LM**

Sweeney, Mary M 221 Greystone Lane #20, Rochester, NY 14618, (716) 275-2991, BA 76 Univ of Rochester; MS 78 Purdue Univ - West Lafayette; Sp-Lang Path, U of Rochester, **SLP**

Sweeney, Maureen Ann 5350 North Lotus Avenue, Chicago, IL 60630, (312) 935-1301, BS 80 Northwestern Univ; MA 82 Northwestern Univ; Sp-Lang Path, Private Practice, **SLP**

Sweeney, Patrice Moore 7 Vine Street, Brattleboro, VT 05301, (802) 254-3748, BA 77 Univ of CT; MA 85 Univ of MA - Amherst; 88–Sp-Lang Path, Windham Southeast Supvr Union, **SLP**

Sweeney, Dr Ronald J VA Medical Center (126), Tomah, WI 54660, (608) 372-3971, BA 71 Univ of Denver; MA 72 Univ of Denver; ED 83 (NS) Loyola Univ of Chicago; Chief Aud/Sp-Path, VA Med Cen, **SLP**

Sweeney, Mrs Sandra Haire 9211-B Williams Boulevard, Albany, GA 31705, BS 82 Univ of GA; MS 84 Vanderbilt Univ; Aud, Western Memorial Regional Hosp, **A**

Sweeney, Warren A 41 Hamilton Avenue, Staten Island, NY 10301, **SLP**

Sweeny, Mrs Shirley Y 50 Shore Road, Mount Sinai, NY 11766, (516) 474-4752, BA 65 ID St Univ; ME 67 Western OR St Coll; **SLP**

Sweeny, Veronica A 639 Central Avenue, Dunkirk, NY 14048, (716) 992-3610, BS 79 Northeastern Univ; MS 81 SUNY - Coll at Fredonia; Speech-Language Pathologist, Eden Central Schools, **SLP**

Sweet, Mrs Nancy 3309 Kenneth Drive, Palo Alto, CA 94303, (415) 493-2887, BS 68 Univ of OR; MA 87 San Jose St Univ; 88–Sp-Lang Path, Mid Peninsula Sp & Lang Cl, **SLP**

Sweet, Thomas R 3489 Emerald Drive, White Bear Lake, MN 55110, (612) 623-5163, BA 65 Univ of Northern IA; MA 66 Univ of Northern IA; SLP, Minnesota Dept Health, **SLP**

Sweeting, Dr Patricia M 42 Beiden Avenue, Dobbs Ferry, NY 10522, (212) 584-7679, BA 56 Coll of New Rochelle; MA 73 Columbia Univ Teachers Coll; PH 79 (Sp-Lang Path) 2162; 88–Asst Prof, Teachers Coll-Columbia U, **SLP**

Sweetman, Rebecca J 3530 Smuggler Circle, Boulder, CO 80303, (303) 492-5375, BA 67 Univ of Northern CO; MA 75 Univ of CO - Boulder; Instr/Cl Dir, U of CO, **SLP**

Sweetman, Dr Richard H 4500 19th Street, #617 Countryside Village, Boulder, CO 80302, (303) 492-3040, BA 61 Univ of CO - Boulder; MA 62 Northwestern Univ; PH 68 (Aud) Northwestern Univ; 76–Professor, U of CO-Boulder, **A**

Sweetow, Dr Robert W 1234 Divisadero, San Francisco, CA 94115, (415) 921-7658, BA 70 Univ of IA; MA 72 Univ of Southern CA; PH 77 (Aud) Northwestern Univ; Dir of Aud & Res, San Francisco Hrng & Sp Cen, **A**

Swegle, M Valentin 3329 Loreto Drive, San Ramon, CA 94583, (415) 552-3771, BA 75 Univ of WA; MS 85 Univ of NM; 86–Sp-Lang Path, InSpeech Inc, **SLP**

Sweitzer, Dr Richard S Speech And Hearing Center, Childrens Hospital, 1600 7th Avenue South, Birmingham, AL 35233, (205) 939-9789, BA 62 Univ of IA; MA 64 Univ of IA; ED 73 (NS) Boston Univ; Dir, Chldn's Hosp of AL, **A**

Swen, Pamela Michelle 9349 Jornada Lane #7, Atascadero, CA 93422, (805) 541-3061, BA 82 Point Loma Nazarene Coll; MS 86 San Francisco St Univ; Sp-Lang Path, Pam Suess & Assoc, **SLP**

Swengel, Kristen E 1800 North Hills Road, Apt 223, York, PA 17402, (717) 755-1646, BS 86 Bloomsburg Univ of PA; MS 87 Bloomsburg Univ of PA; **SLP**

Swensen, W Dean 648 North 450 East, Orem, UT 84057, (801) 225-8463, BS 65 Brigham Young Univ; OM 70 Brigham Young Univ; Tchr Leader, Provo City Schs, **SLP**

Swenson, Mrs Catherine A 602 2nd Street North, Thompson, ND 58278, (701) 780-2447, BA 77 Univ of ND; MS 83 Univ of ND; Ped Sp-Lang Path, U of ND Med Cen Rehab Hosp, **SLP**

Swenson, David Wayne Idaho Elks Rehab Hospital, P O Box 1100, Boise, ID 83701, (208) 343-2583, BS 80 Univ of UT; MS 82 Univ of UT; Audiologist, Audiology Associates, **A**

Swenson, Donna E 25218 Lawton Avenue, Loma Linda, CA 92354, (714) 658-2171, BS 80 Walla Walla Coll; MS 82 Loma Linda Univ - Riverside; SLP, Hemet USD, **SLP**

Swenson, Katharine Freeburg 22415 132nd Street S E, Monroe, WA 98272, (206) 364-0300, BA 70 Univ of WA; OM 72 Univ of WA; **SLP**

Swenson, Rita L 1147 East 25th Street, Idaho Falls, ID 83401, **SLP**

Swenson, Virginia Ann 187 Arthur Moore Drive, Lake Asbury, FL 32043, (904) 282-1981, SLP, **SLP**

Swentkowski, Stanley M 1033 Lynn Street, Clarksdale, MS 38614, (601) 627-5247, BA 69 Alliance Coll; OM 75 Univ of MS; Superv-Lan-Sp-Hrng Path, Coahoma Co Sch-Clarksdale Ms, **SLP**

Swenton, Mrs Gail P 106 Melinda Lane, Bristol, CT 06010, (203) 589-7297, MS 77 Southern CT St Univ; Sp-Lang Path, Wheeler Cl, **SLP**

Swenty, Dr Vinita W Psc Box 999, APO Miami, FL 34002, BS 65 Purdue Univ - West Lafayette; MA 73 Univ of Houston - Univ Park; ED 78 (NS) Univ of Houston - Univ Park; Prin, Dodds-Panama Region, **SLP**

Swerdlow, Mrs Judith 46 Greenleigh Drive, Sewell, NJ 08080, (609) 227-6216, BA 76 Adelphi Univ; MA 78 Trenton St Coll; Sp-Lang Path, Winslow Twsp Bd of Ed, **SLP**

Swerdlow, Leonard S 514 12th Street, Eureka, CA 95501, **SLP**

Swerzenski, Mrs Davi-Ann Hunter 1006 Autumnwood Circle, Apex, NC 27502, (919) 832-8301, BA 79 Our Lady Lake Univ-San Anton; MA 81 Our Lady Lake Univ-San Anton; Sp-Lang Path, Rehab Svcs of Wake County, **SLP**

Swetkovich, Sherri Alicia 8202 Oak Knoll Drive, Roseville, CA 95678, (916) 791-2255, BA 85 Abilene Christian Univ; MA 87 Univ of the Pacific; **SLP**

Swett, Carol Lesher 101 Bahama Court, San Ramon, CA 94583, (818) 889-4004, OB 79 Indiana Univ of PA; MA 85 CA St Univ - Los Angeles; **SLP**

Swick, Mrs Joan B R R 2 Box 54, Casey, IL 62420, (217) 932-4660, BS 58 IN St Univ - Terre Haute; MS 64 IN St Univ - Terre Haute; Sp-Lang Path, Casey Comm Sch, **SLP**

Swidler, Arleen G Hopkins House #415, 602 Washington Square S, Philadelphia, PA 19106, (215) 238-2315, BS 67 PA St Univ - Univ Park; ME 68 Boston Univ; SLP, Sch Dist of Phila, **SLP**

Swiecki, Tamara Ann 246 Darwin, Westland, MI 48185-4504, MA 84 Eastern MI Univ; 87–Dir of Sp-Lang Path, Special Tree Ltd, **SLP**

Swierc, Mrs Regina Marie 122 Stonehenge Terrace, Clark, NJ 07066, BS 73 Univ of CT; MA 81 Montclair St Coll; Sp-Lang Path, South Plainfield Board of Educ, **SLP**

Swiercinsky, Mrs Carol A 25310 Starling Drive, San Antonio, TX 78255, (512) 696-7441, BA 61 Our Lady Lake Univ-San Anton; MA 76 Our Lady Lake Univ-San Anton; Sp-Lang Path, Northside ISD, **SLP**

Swift, Dr Carol Sch Of Human & Educational Ser, Oakland University, Rochester, MI 48063, (313) 377-4164, BA 67 Southern Methodist Univ; MA 68 Southern Methodist Univ; PH 78 (NS) Univ of AZ; Assoc Prof Ed, Oakland Univ, **SLP**

Swift, Carol A 5981 Arapaho Road #401, Dallas, TX 75248, (214) 235-4593, BA 73 Southern IL Univ-Edwardsvill; MS 75 Southern IL Univ-Edwardsvill; Tchr, Richardson ISD, **SLP**

Swift, Mrs Dawn Elizabeth 3730 Marseille Drive, Owensboro, KY 42303, (502) 683-2609, BS 84 Brescia Coll; MA 85 Eastern KY Univ; Sp-Lang Path, Wendell Foster Center, **SLP**

Swift, Mrs Estelle W 1108 Garfield Street, Madison, WI 53705, (608) 262-3951, MA 69 Northwestern Univ; Sp-Lang Path, Univ of Wisconsin, **SLP**

Swift, JoAnn Arlene 106 Wingate, Lee's Summit, MO 64063, (816) 525-1780, BS 75 Central MO St Univ; MS 78 Central MO St Univ; 76–Sp-Lang Path, Lee's Summit R-7 Sch Dist, **SLP**

Swift, Mrs Karen F 502 N E 7th Street, Ankeny, IA 50021, (515) 244-8173, BA 81 Bethel Coll; MA 82 Northeast MO St Univ; SLP, Heartland AEA, **SLP**

Swift, Kaye Armstrong P O Box 809, Clyde, NC 28721, (704) 452-1447, BS 77 Auburn Univ - Auburn; MS 80 Univ of AL- Tuscaloosa; Sp-Lang Path, Haywood Co Home Hlth Care, **SLP**

Swift, Margo I 212 Westwind Drive, Alton, IL 62002-2779, (309) 344-2141, BS 76 Western IL Univ; MA 77 Western IL Univ; Galesburg Mental Hlth Cen, **SLP**

Swift, Mrs Patricia McCollum 5150 Amesterdam Court, Lilburn, GA 30247-5197, (404) 921-7994, **SLP**

Swift, Phil I 502 N E 7th Street, Ankeny, IA 50021, (515) 270-9030, BS 81; MA 82; Sp/Lang Path, Heartland AEA II, **SLP**

Swift, Renee Jane 3012 Mohawk #1, Burlington, IA 52601, (319) 753-3386, MA 83 Northeast MO St Univ; BS 82 Northeast MO St Univ; Sp-Lang Path, Burlington Med Ctr, **SLP**

Swift, Roger W 508 Park Avenue, Greensboro, NC 27405, (919) 375-7570, BA 77 Univ of NC - Greensboro; MA 79 Univ of NC - Greensboro; 82–Sp-Lang Path/Aud, Dev Eval Cen-Nc Dept Hum Res, **SLP A**

Swift-Billings, Mrs Mary 305 East Shamrock Lane, Blue Springs, MO 64015, (913) 362-7518, MS 82 Central MO St Univ; BA 79 687A; BA 79 Univ of MO - KS City; 85–Sp-Lang Path, Deborah King MA & Assoc Inc, **SLP**

Swigart, Dr Elca Reading Hospital & Medical Ctr, Speech And Hearing Center, 6th And Spruce Streets, Reading, PA 19603, (215) 378-6694, BS Mount Union Coll; MA OH St Univ; PH 72 (NS) OH St Univ; Director, Reading Hosp & Med Cen, **A**

Swigert, Nancy B 2401 Regency Road Ste 204, Lexington, KY 40503, (606) 277-1949, BA 75 Centre Coll of KY; MA 77 Univ of TN - Knoxville; 80–Dir, Swigert & Associates Inc, **SLP ACE**

Swim, Mrs Debra Ann R R 1 Box 274, Fortville, IN 46040, (317) 485-6454, BA 79 Ball St Univ; MA 82 Ball St Univ; Sp-Lang Path, Hancock-S Madison Jnt Serv, **SLP**

Swindell, Carol S 807 Jefferson Avenue, Memphis, TN 38105, (412) 624-0425, BS 77 Edinboro Univ of PA; MA 81 Univ of Pittsburgh - Pittsburgh; PH 86 (NS) Univ of Pittsburgh - Pittsburgh; Asst Prof, Memphis State U, **SLP**

Swindell, Harriette Juanice 4202 Mahogany Run S E, Winter Haven, FL 33880, (305) 645-5800, MS 87 FL St Univ

Swindell, Peggy Jo Route 1 Box 107, Winchester, IN 47394, (317) 857-2554, BS 76 Ball St Univ; MA 77 Ball St Univ; Sp-Lang Path, Randolph Central Sch Corp, **SLP**

Swindle, Katherine Lucille 5813 Southall Road, Birmingham, AL 35213, (205) 595-1792, BS 84 Univ of Montevallo; MS 86 Univ of Montevallo; 87–Sp-Lang Path, Physicians Phys Ther Svc, **SLP**

Swinehart, Therese M 7332 North Van Ness Blvd, Fresno, CA 93711, (209) 432-2710, BA 76 Creighton Univ; MS 80 Univ of MI - Ann Arbor; **SLP**

Swing, Mrs Melissa Dawn 5230 Wheaton Drive, Fort Collins, CO 80525, (303) 229-9876, BA 84 CA St Univ - Northridge; MA 86 CA St Univ - Northridge; **SLP**

Swingle, Mrs Lynn H 206 Hobson Drive, Hockessin, DE 19707, (301) 651-2750, BS 66 Purdue Univ - West Lafayette; MS 68 Purdue Univ - West Lafayette; 86–Sp-Lang Path, Red Clay Consol Sch Dist, **SLP**

Swinney, Martha Brown 1055 Camino DE Chavez Pl, Bosque Farms, NM 87068, (505) 865-9611, BA 82 NM St Univ; MA 84 Memphis St Univ; Sp-Lang Path, Los Lunas Hosp & Training Sch, **SLP**

Swinny, Dr Frances R 317 Lamont, San Antonio, TX 78209, (512) 736-8580, BS 48 Univ of TX - Austin; ME 51 Univ of TX - Austin; PH 80 (Oral Perf of Lit & Linguistics) Univ of TX - Austin; Prof/Sp & Drama Dept, Trinity U, **SLP**

Swinson, Linda Jean 429 Moseley Drive #B, Charlottesville, VA 22903-4304, (804) 293-7368, ME 83 Univ of VA - Charlottesville; Aud, Wagner Hearing Aid Serv, **A**

Swirbul, Therese Jennie 8686 Coffman And Pico Road, Pico Rivera, CA 90660, (213) 924-9581, BA 85 Whittier Coll; MA 87 Whittier Coll; 88–Sp-Lang Path, College Hosp

Swisher, Alisa Rose 2804 Themis Apartment #2, Cape Girardeau, MO 63701, (314) 335-3795, MA 88 Southwest MO St Univ; 88–Sp-Lang Path, InSpeech Inc

Swisher, Dr Linda P Dept Speech & Hearing Science, University Of Arizona, Tucson, AZ 85721, (602) 621-7069, BA 62 OH St Univ; MA 63 Stanford Univ; PH 66 (NS) McGill Univ - Quebec; Assoc Prof, U of AZ, **SLP A F**

Swisher, Mrs Lynn Crabtree 1607 Strader Drive, Lexington, KY 40505, (606) 252-0658, MS 88 Univ of KY

Swisher, Pamela Ann 1006 Valley Road, Charleston, WV 25302, (304) 348-7776, BS 73 PA St Univ - Univ Park; MS 82 PA St Univ - Univ Park; 87–Sp-Lang Path, Kanawha County Schs, **SLP**

Swisher, Mrs Rosemarie Aileen HHC 3-64 Armor, APO New York, NY 09702, 011 49 97216 2754, BS 77 WV Univ; MS 83 Syracuse Univ; 87–Sp-Lang Path, US Army 24 Medac APO 09033, **SLP**

Swisher, Timothy A 97th General Hospital, Box 17, APO New York, NY 09757, BS 70 Indiana Univ of PA; MA 71 Western IL Univ; 87–Aud & Hrng Cons, US Army-Frankfurt Army Reg Med Ctr, **A**

Swisher, Dr Wayne Everett 420 Franklin Avenue, Grand Forks, ND 58201, (701) 775-7798, BS 66 CO St Univ; MS 67 CO St Univ; PH 74 (NS) Univ of WI - Madison; 86–Prof Sp/Lang Path, Univ of North Dakota, **SLP**

Swiss Rossi, Ellen Ann 1601 Ocean Parkway #2-G, Brooklyn, NY 11223, (718) 854-3737, BS 85 PA St Univ - Univ Park; MS 88 CUNY - Brooklyn Coll

Switzer, Emilia C 1810 North Roosevelt Avenue, Altadena, CA 91001, (818) 791-8323, BA 79 CA St Univ - Long Beach; MA 81 CA St Univ - Long Beach; Consult Sp-Lang Path, Private Practice, **SLP**

Switzer, Janet Lynne 1312 North Frances Avenue, Fullerton, CA 92631, (714) 738-5182, BA 83 CA St Univ - Fullerton; MS 85 Univ of Redlands; **SLP**

Switzer, Mrs Kathryn Beck 1015 Division, Charleston, IL 61920-2616, (217) 258-2568, BS 85 Baylor Univ; MS 86 Baylor Univ; 87–Sp-Lang Path, Sarah Bush Lincoln Health Ctr, **SLP**

Swoboda, Mrs Cecilia F 621 Jefferson Avenue, New Orleans, LA 70115, (504) 895-7094, BA 74 Univ of MD - College Park; MA 79 Hofstra Univ; SLP, Touro Hospital, **SLP**

Swoboda, Harvey J, Jr 19 Rambo Road, Red Lion, PA 17356, (301) 628-7330, **SLP**

Swonder, Linda K 114 Long Street, North Vernon, IN 47265, (812) 346-1529, BA 81 IN Univ - Bloomington; OM 82 IN Univ - Bloomington; 88–Sp-Lang Path, Jackson Co Schneck Mem Hosp, **SLP**

Swope, Dr Suzanne 8201 Shadowridge Drive, Fairfax Station, VA 22039, (617) 578-8530, BS 63 OH St Univ; MA 64 OH St Univ; ED 74 (NS) Boston Univ; Prfessor, Emerson Coll, **SLP**

Sword, Mrs Paula Ann 174 South Main, Terryville, CT 06786, (203) 879-0081, BS 79 IL St Univ - Normal; ME 81 Univ of NC - Greensboro; 84–Sp-Lang Path, Wolcott Bd of Ed, **SLP**

Sword, Valerie Ann 1223 Crescent Drive, Elizabeth City, NC 27909, (919) 338-4044, SLP, Albemarle Sp & Hrng Ctr, **SLP**

Syden, Mrs Sheree J Speech Lang & Hearing Rehab Pa, 1897 Palm Beach Lakes Blvd, Suite 222, West Palm Beach, FL 33409, (305) 471-3371, BA 76 FL Atlantic Univ; MA 77 Hofstra Univ; Admins/SLP, Sheree Syden Sp/Lang/Hrng Rehb, **SLP**

Syfert, Grace Privette Atlanta Rehabilitation Institute Incorporated, 5667 Peachtree-Dunwoody Road NE, Atlanta, GA 30342, (404) 252-5325, BS 68 Winthrop Coll; ME 71 Univ of VA - Charlottesville; Dir/Admin, Atl Rehab Inst Inc, **SLP ACE**

Syfert, Gretchen Adams Arlington Hearing Center, 3260 Wilson Boulevard, Arlington, VA 22201, (703) 525-1898, BS 67 Univ of ND; MA 68 MI St Univ; Aud, **A**

Sykes, Barbara T 307 Lamont, San Antonio, TX 78209, BA 70 Southern Methodist Univ; MA 78 Trinity Univ; MS 71 Vanderbilt Univ; **SLP**

Sykes, Debra L P O Box 38, East Glacier Park, MT 59434, (406) 338-6136, BS 76 Univ of MT; MS 79 Univ of MT; Aud, Private Contractor, **SLP A**

Sykes, Gaile Ala Wai Plaza, 500 University Avenue #911, Honolulu, HI 96826, BA 59 George Washington Univ; Tchr, McKinley Hs Prog Hrng Impaired, **SLP**

Sykes, Georgia Gail 1209 Towering Oaks, Jacksonville, AR 72076, (501) 985-6449, MS 86 TX Christian Univ; **SLP**

Sykes, Kim M 1010 Carondelet Drive Suite 224, Kansas City, MO 64114, (816) 942-7200, BS 83 KS St Univ; MA 85 KS St Univ; 87–Aud/Supvr, Old Westport Med Assoc,Inc, **A**

Sykes, Meredeth K 1393 N W 122nd Terrace, Pembroke Pines, FL 33026-3823, (305) 431-6454, **SLP**

Sykes, Susan P 47 Alleghany Road, Hampton, VA 23661, (804) 723-6892, BS 72 OK St Univ; MS 73 Univ of OK Medical Center; Sp-Lang Path, Newport News PS, **SLP**

Sylla, Mary Beth 2575 South Calhoun Road, Apartment 108, New Berlin, WI 53151-2754, (608) 483-2111, BA 82 Univ of WI - Eau Claire; MS 82 Coll of Saint Teresa; SLP, Waukesha Public Schools, **SLP**

Sylvan, Susan K 7 North Drive, Simsbury, CT 06070, **SLP**

Sylvester, Stephen F 13245 Glenhill Road, Silver Spring, MD 20904, (202) 254-4617, BA 72 Catholic Univ of America; MA 75 Catholic Univ of America; OD 85 (Law) George Washington Univ; 86–Attorney, VA Bd of Veterans Appeals, **SLP A**

Sylwester, John H 424 Oxford Street, Winnipeg, MB, Canada R3M 3J8, (204) 786-7841, BA 69 WA St Univ; MA 71 OR St Univ; Aud, Chld Guidance Cl, **A**

Syme, Michele F 11 Yantacaw Place, Nutley, NJ 07110, (201) 667-2065, BA 75 Montclair St Coll; MA 79 Montclair St Coll; 87–Sp-Lang Path, Lyndhurst Bd of Educ, **SLP**

Symington, Mrs Debbie Lynn 1602 Chittam, Euless, TX 76039, (817) 283-1583, BS 82 Baylor Univ; MS 83 Baylor Univ; Sp-Lang Path, Hurst-Euless-Bedford Sch Dist, **SLP**

Symington, Linda Bullock 32 Nassau Avenue, West Babylon, NY 11704, (516) 669-6514, BS 83 SUNY - Coll at Geneseo; MS 85 Columbia Univ Teachers Coll; 86–Aud, Pilgrim Psychiatric Ctr, **A**

Symon, Mrs Carol H 4512 Birchman Avenue, Fort Worth, TX 76107, (817) 336-8611, BS 71 Purdue Univ - West Lafayette; MS 72 Purdue Univ - West Lafayette; Dir, Child Study Cen, **SLP**

Symonaitis, Katherine M 1580 N W 90th Street, Des Moines, IA 50322, (515) 270-9030, BA 68 Augustana Coll; MS 70 Univ of WY; Sp-Lang Path, Heartland AEA, **SLP**

Symuleski, Joseph Stephen An 337 Lands End Apts, Laurel Road, Lindenwold, NJ 08021, (609) 861-2164, BS 81 East Stroudsburg Univ of PA; MS 82 Bloomsburg Univ of PA; Sp-Lang Path, Woodbine Dev Cen, **SLP**

Synakowski, Melanie C 231 Slocombe Avenue, Marcellus, NY 13108, (315) 673-2188, BS 81 Nazareth Coll of Rochester; MS 85 Nazareth Coll of Rochester; **SLP**

Synstelien, Mary Joan 3430 25th Avenue, Marion, IA 52302, (319) 398-2467, MS 84 Moorhead St Univ; Sp-Lang Path, Grant Wood AEA, **SLP**

Sysak, Mrs Marian Ernsberger Rural Delivery 5, 10 Markham Court, Hockessin, DE 19707, (302) 239-0661, BA 66 Univ of Toledo; MA 81 West Chester Univ of PA; Sp-Lang Path, Self Employed, **SLP**

Sysko, Linda M W 4438 Yanich, Troy, MI 48098, (313) 528-1539, BS 68 MI St Univ; ME 75 Wayne St Univ; Sp/Lang Path, Home Hlth Care Inc, **SLP**

Sytsma, Wendy Ham 19799 East Flora Place, Aurora, CO 80013, BS 78 Purdue Univ - West Lafayette; MS 80 Purdue Univ - West Lafayette; 87–Aud, VA Med Ctr, **A**

Szablicki, Mrs Joanne Cotroneo 32 Pomona Place, Buffalo, NY 14210, (716) 826-3877, BA 74 SUNY - Center at Buffalo; MS 80 SUNY - Coll at Buffalo; SLP, The Cen for Handicapped Chldn, **SLP**

Szabo, Mrs Donna 50-A Spruce Street, Elmwood Park, NJ 07407, (201) 926-1193, BA 81 Kean Coll of NJ; MA 82 Kean Coll of NJ; Aud, Bruce Str Sch F/T Deaf, **A**

Szabo, Gladys T 20 Milrose Lane, Monsey, NY 10952, (914) 634-4648, BS 56 Univ of WI - Madison; MS 73 CUNY - Hunter Coll; Coord Sp & Hrng Dept, Rockland Co Cen Phys Hndcpd, **SLP ACE**

Szafran, Mrs Karen M 8178 Old Sunridge Drive, Manlius, NY 13104, (716) 834-6549, BS 73 SUNY - Coll at Buffalo; MS 76 SUNY - Coll at Buffalo; Sp-Lang Path, Williamsville Ctrl Sch Dist, **SLP**

Szafran, Teri Lea 87 Schooner Lane, Shalimar, FL 32579, (904) 862-5622, BA 84 Univ of KS; MA 86 Univ of KS; Sp-Lang Path, Sch Dist of Okaloosa County, **SLP**

Szal, Mrs Regina M 16415 Colorado Avenue #408, Paramount, CA 90723, (213) 531-9423, BA 73 Case Western Reserve Univ; MA 74 MI St Univ; Aud, Private Practice, **A**

Szaller, Mrs Charlene N 25214 Deerfield Drive, North Olmsted, OH 44070, (216) 777-3961, BS 77 OH Univ - Athens; MA 79 Cleveland St Univ; Sp-Lang Path, Hospice Prog Lutheran Med Cen, **SLP**

Szari, Janice D 4407 Howard, Youngstown, OH 44512, **SLP**

Szczeck, Jeanne Larkin 2508 River Hills Drive, Burnsville, MN 55337, (612) 895-9325, BA 76 Univ of MN - Duluth; MA 77 Univ of WI - Eau Claire; Parent Child Instructor, Bloomington Sch Dist, **SLP**

Szczypka-Gay, Mrs Rene Marie 44 Dennison Drive, Glendale Heights, IL 60139, (312) 665-6200, BS 83 Northern IL Univ - De Kalb; MS 85 IL St Univ - Normal; Aud, Wheaton Medical Clinic, **A**

Szekely, Mrs Shelley Rosen 13609 Cherrydale Drive, Rockville, MD 20850-3637, (301) 598-8955, BA 72 Univ of MD - College Park; MS 73 Loyola Coll; Sp/Lang Path, Private Practice, **SLP**

Szekeres, Shirley F 415 Locust Street, Pittsburgh, PA 15218, (412) 521-9000, MA 67 SUNY - Center at Albany; PH 88 (Communications Disorders) Univ of Pittsburgh - Pittsburgh; Dir of Sp-Lang Path Dept, The Rehab Inst of Pittsburgh, **SLP**

Szewczyk, Catherine J 140 Oakville Drive, Pittsburgh, PA 15220, (513) 293-1588, **SLP**

Szewczyk, Susan Kay 505 Cherry S E #106, Grand Rapids, MI 49503, (616) 242-0427, BA 81 MI St Univ; MA 84 Wayne St Univ; **SLP**

Sziraki, Donna 2967 Fort Park, Lincoln Park, MI 48146, (313) 383-5195, BS 85 Central MI Univ; MA 87 Wayne St Univ; **SLP**

Szuba, Sandra W 1 Seaborne Drive, Pasadena, MD 21122, (301) 757-7007, BS 75 Towson St Univ; MS 77 Loyola Coll; Sp-Lang Path, Anne Arundel Co Sch, **SLP**

Szubeczak, Leslie A 15258 Travis, Southgate, MI 48195, (419) 471-4175, MA 81 Eastern MI Univ; BA 80 MI St Univ; 82–Sp-Lang Path, Toledo Hosp, **SLP ACE**

Szumlas, Mrs Janet J P O Box 577, North Bend, WA 98045, (206) 888-3678, BA 64 Sioux Falls Coll; MA 66 Northern IL Univ - De Kalb; Sp-Lang Path, St Joseph Hospital, **SLP**

Szumowski, Edward J, Jr Western Mich Hearing Services, 26 Sheldon S E, Suite 204, Grand Rapids, MI 49503, (616) 456-1441, BA 72 Univ of MI - Ann Arbor; MA 78 Wayne St Univ; Aud, Western MI Hrng Serv, **A**

Szykulski, Theresa Mary 1000 East 78th Street, Apartment #18, Richfield, MN 55423-4561, (612) 866-8506, BS 82 Univ of MN - Minneap-St Paul; MS 86 Mankato St Univ; 85–Sp-Lang Path, Bloomington PS ISD #271, **SLP**

Szymanski, Deborah A 990 Cressman Road, Rd 1, Schwenksville, PA 19473, BS 80 Indiana Univ of PA; MS 83 Indiana Univ of PA; 83–Sp-Lang Path, Montgomery Co Inter Unit, **SLP**

Szymczak, Constance Geonnotti 2547 Plumleaf Lane, Toledo, OH 43614, (419) 471-5680, BS 79 West Chester Univ of PA; MA 81 Univ of SC - Columbia; 86–Mgr-Neur, The Toledo Hospital, **A**

Szymoniak, Elaine Eisfelder 2116 44th Street, Des Moines, IA 50310, (515) 279-3115, BS 41 Univ of WI - Madison; MS 77 IA St Univ; **SLP LM**

Szymula, Mrs Annette 99 Jesson Parkway, Lockport, NY 14094, (716) 433-0714, BS 71 Nazareth Coll of Rochester; MA 74 SUNY - Center at Buffalo; Office Manager, Norbert J Szymula MD Pc, **SLP**

Szynski, Michael John 12415 Timber Ridge Drive, Kenosha, WI 53142, BS 85 Ball St Univ; MA 87 Ball St Univ; **A**

Szypulski, Edmund S 2144 Forest Lakes Blvd, Charleston, SC 29414, (803) 766-1515, MA 75 Univ of SD - Vermillion; OM 85 Univ of SD - Vermillion; Sp-Lang Path, Private Practice, **SLP A**

Szypulski, Mrs Theresha A 2144 Forest Lakes Blvd, Charleston, SC 29407, BA 70 Univ of SD - Vermillion; MA 78 Univ of SD - Vermillion; Sp-Lang Path, Charleston County Schools, **SLP**

T

Taarud, Nancy M Lynchville Park Road, Goffstown, NH 03045, (603) 524-8552, BS 80 Moorhead St Univ; MS 81 Saint Cloud St Univ; Sp-Lang Path, Private Practice, **SLP**

Tabakman, Shelly D 59 North Street, Katonah, NY 10536, (914) 232-7191, BA 74 CUNY - Brooklyn Coll; MS 76 CUNY - Brooklyn Coll; Aud, V M Dunn MD, **A**

Tabbut, Christina Stengel 306 West Upsal Street, Philadelphia, PA 19119, (215) 849-5181, BS 81 PA St Univ - Univ Park; MA 85 Temple Univ-Tyler Sch of Art; Sp-Lang Path, Delaware Co Memorial Hosp, **SLP**

Taber, Mrs Linda E 50-A Bates Street, Honolulu, HI 96817, (808) 533-6122, BS 78 Univ of HI - Manoa; MS 79 Univ of HI - Manoa; Sp-Lang Path, Private Practice, **SLP**

Taber, Mrs Marcia L 397 Beaver Lake Road, Tallahassee, FL 32312, (904) 488-3364, BS 78 FL St Univ; MS 79 FL St Univ; SLP, Leon Co Sch/Private Practice, **SLP**

Tabili-Kilmer, Mrs Julie Anne 2731 West Elm Road, Franklin, WI 53132, (414) 697-2113, BS 84 Univ of WI - Whitewater; MS 85 Univ of WI - Whitewater; **SLP**

Tabin, Mrs Barbara Russo 8649 Vista Del Boca Drive, Boca Raton, FL 33433, (305) 479-0945, SLP, Palm Beach Schl Dstr, **SLP**

Tabler, Tana Lynn 1608 Beacon Ridge Rd #721, Charlotte, NC 28210-8961, (704) 376-1342, MS 81 FL St Univ; Sp-Lang Path, Charlotte Sp & Hearing Clinic, **SLP**

Tables, Sanford A 13940 S W 109 Street, Miami, FL 33186, (305) 221-0284, **SLP**

Tabor, Mrs Carolyn K 120 North Mills Road, Ventura, CA 93003, (805) 525-1581, BS 80 Univ of HI - Manoa; MS 84 Univ of HI - Manoa; 85–Sp-Lang Path, Santa Paula Sch Dist, **SLP**

Tabor, Linda Kolwyck 239 Hermitage Place, Jackson, TN 38301, **SLP**

Tabor, Mrs Marie A 1838 Batten Hollow Road, Vienna, VA 22180, (703) 448-1704, BA 69 Boston Coll; MA 71 OH St Univ; Sp-Lang Path, Fairfax County Public Schools, **SLP**

Tabshey, Christine 8335 North 46th Street, Omaha, NE 68152, (402) 393-8910, BA 75 Univ of NE - Lincoln; MA 77 Univ of NE - Lincoln; Aud, ENT Assoc, **A**

Tace, Mrs Heather J 800 Adrian Drive, Virginia Beach, VA 23452, (804) 463-1688, BS 65 SUNY - Coll at Geneseo; MS 68 SUNY - Coll at Buffalo

Tackes, Mrs Linda Braun 820 Woodbine Circle, Lake Zurich, IL 60047, (312) 438-6591, BA 81 Univ of WI - Eau Claire; MS 83 Univ of WI - Madison; Sp-Lang Path, Clearbrook Ctr, **SLP**

Tackett, Annette Rene 9959 Adleta #421, Dallas, TX 75243, (214) 349-9136, BS 85 TX Tech Univ; MS 87 TX Tech Univ

Tackett, Mrs Deborah Berry P O Box 1542, Cleveland, MS 38732, (601) 843-4222, BS 83 Delta St Univ; MS 85 Univ Southern MS-Hattiesburg; **SLP**

Tackett, Katherine Holland 1121 Sara Cove #4, Cordova, TN 38018, (901) 757-0924, BS 82 AR St Univ; MA 84 Memphis St Univ; 85–Aud, Shea Clinic-Hrng Svcs Memphis, **A**

Taddeo, Dolores A 15 Satinwood Road, Bayville, NY 11709, (516) 628-8239, BA 83 Hofstra Univ; MS 87 Adelphi Univ; **SLP**

Tade, Mrs Wilma Jean 3705 Arborlawn Drive, Fort Worth, TX 76109, (817) 921-7620, BS 45 Eastern IL Univ; MS 49 IN St Univ - Evansville; MA 72 TX Christian Univ; Sp-Lang Path, Texas Christian U, **SLP**

Taden, Mrs Claudia E Department Of Communication Disorders, St Johns Hospital, 333 North F Street, Oxnard, CA 93030, (805) 988-2757, BS 64 Univ of IA; MS 65 Bradley Univ; 78–Dir-Sp-Lang Path, St John's Hospital, **SLP**

Taenaka, Patrice H 909 South Ledoux Road #5, Los Angeles, CA 90035, (213) 756-9114, BA 76 Univ of CA - Los Angeles; MA 84 CA St Univ - Northridge; 80–Sp-Lang Path, Los Angeles USD, **SLP**

Tafeen, Mrs Janet 31 Roundtree Drive, Melville, NY 11747, (516) 491-7182, BA 78 Long Island U - CW Post Ctr; MA 82 Long Island U - CW Post Ctr; Sp-Lang Path, North Merrick Elem Sch, **SLP**

Taff, Mrs Janet H 6200 Carriagehouse Lane, Charlotte, NC 28226, (704) 364-1543, BA 78 Univ of MD - College Park; MA 79 Univ of MD - College Park; Aud, **A**

Taffin, Leslie M 8395 Dynasty Drive, Boca Raton, FL 33433, BA 77 Univ of FL; MA 79 Univ of Miami; **SLP**

Taffner, Nancy L Fairmount Childrens Center, P O Box 69, Belle Isle Road, Solvay, NY 13209, BA 78 SUNY - Coll at Plattsburgh; MA 81 OK St Univ; Sp-Lang Path, Fairmount Chldns Cen, **SLP**

Taft, Lavonne Joyette 5436 Tandem Lane, El Sobrante, CA 94803, (415) 537-4211, BA 75 CA St Univ - Northridge; MA 79 Univ of Cincinnati; 84–Aud, Hayward Hearing Aid Ctr Inc, **A**

Taft, Patricia Michele 40 S W 12th Street, Suite A-102, Ocala, FL 32671, (904) 351-3977, MS 81 Univ of South FL; MS 84 Univ of FL; Sp-Lang Path/ Aud, Dr Christopher E Bald, Otolyng, **SLP A**

Taft, Sandra M 17 Flower Road, Sandia Park, NM 87047, (505) 884-3820, BS 79 Northern AZ Univ; MS 82 Univ of NM; 82–Aud, Pueb Coun Sp&Hrng Prog, **A**

Taggart, Mrs Leslie A 226 Foxwood Court, Jacksonville, NC 28540, (919) 763-1308, BA 83 San Diego St Univ; MA 87 CA St Univ - Long Beach; 88–Aud, Hrg & Sp Svc Inc

Taggart, Rebecca Sue 2658 Roxbury Road, Evansville, IN 47715-6527, (812) 479-1411, BS 82 IN Univ - Bloomington; OM 84 IN Univ - Bloomington; Supvr of Speech Pathology, The Rehabilitation Center, **SLP**

Taggart-Ross, Mrs Linda P O Box 88428, Steilacoom, WA 98388, (206) 581-3458, BA 76 WA St Univ; MS 79 Univ of WA; Sp-Lang Path/Aud, Steilacoom Sch Dist, **SLP A**

Taglia, Camille R 1022 South Menard Avenue, Chicago, IL 60644, (312) 261-6527, BS 62 Marquette Univ; BS 70 Marquette Univ; SLP, Chicago Board of Education, **SLP**

Taguchi, Mrs Estrelleta N 1661 Hale Loke Street, Hilo, HI 96720, (808) 935-9079, BS 63 Univ of OR; 73–Sp-Lang Path, CA-Hi Elks Major Proj Inc, **SLP ACE**

Taigman, Myra T 3931 Kamden Way, Las Vegas, NV 89119, (702) 733-3041, BA 73 CUNY - City College; MA 74 CUNY - City College; 88–Pres, Hearing Specialists of Nevada, **A**

Taigman, Susan 853 North Larrabee Street, West Hollywood, CA 90069, (213) 657-3678, BA 75 CUNY - Brooklyn Coll; MA 76 Univ of Denver; OM 83 CA St Univ - Dominguez Hills; 86–Gen Mgr, M Latter Inc, **A**

Taipale, Mrs Cynthia Jean 3007 Fort Worth Trail, Austin, TX 78748, (512) 476-7111, BA 81 MI St Univ; MS 85 Univ of IL - Urbana; Sp-Lang Path, St David's Comm Hosp, **SLP**

Tait, Dr Charles A Speech And Hearing Sciences, University Of Michigan, 1111 East Catherine Street, Ann Arbor, MI 48109, (313) 747-2495, BS 57 Wayne St Univ; ME 61 Wayne St Univ; PH 65 (NS) Stanford Univ; Associate Professor, University of Michigan, **SLP A**

Tait, Lorinda J 2010 Edwin Place, Lansing, MI 48911, (517) 374-4097, BA 70 MI St Univ; MA 72 MI St Univ; SLP, Lansing Schools, **SLP**

Tait, Nancy A 3679 Woodlake Drive S W, Bonita Springs, FL 33923, (813) 947-6730, BS 59 TX Woman's Univ; MA 76 Univ of KS; Sp-Lang Path, Lee Count School District, **SLP**

Takacs, Mrs Candace E Helen Sherman Hook Center, 2610 Philadelphia Drive, Dayton, OH 45405, (513) 276-6833, BS 78 Purdue Univ - West Lafayette; MS 80 Purdue Univ - West Lafayette; 85–Sp/Lang Path, Montgomery Cty Board of Mr, **SLP**

Takacs, Mrs Patricia Ann 744 Cedarwood Drive, Pittsburgh, PA 15235, (412) 793-4614, BS 79 SUNY - Coll at Fredonia; ME 84 Univ of NC - Greensboro; 88–Dir Adult Day & Personal Care, Regency Hall Nursing Home, **SLP**

Takagi, Mrs June K 8580 Graton Road, Sebastopol, CA 95472, (707) 545-0213, BA 80 Int'l Christian Univ - PR; MA 82 OH Univ - Athens; Sp-Lang Path, Agency for Infant Development, **SLP**

Takagi, Dr Yasuaki 8636 Arlington Boulevard, Fairfax, VA 22031, (703) 560-9700, MD 57 (NS); Private Practice

Takahashi, Mrs Candace L 719 9th Avenue, San Mateo, CA 94402, (415) 856-0732, BS 73 Univ of HI - Manoa; MA 75 Univ of CA - Santa Barbara; 75–Sp-Lang Path, Palo Alto USD, **SLP**

Takahashi, Janis L 15562 Quiet Oak Drive, Chino, CA 91709, (714) 597-1374, BA 79 CA St Univ - Fullerton; MA 82 CA St Univ - Fullerton; SLP, Ontario-Montclair Sch Dist, **SLP**

Takeda, Dr Keiichi 1-11-2-704, Sakasedai Takarazuka, Hyogo Prefecture, Takarazuka, Japan, BA 61 Asbury Coll; MA 62 Univ of Pittsburgh - Pittsburgh; MD 75 (NS) Keio Med Sch - Tokyo, Japan; 75–Prof/Dept of Commun Dis, Osaka Univ of Educ

Takekawa, Kristine Montgomery 678-C Kihapai Street, Kailua, HI 96734-3721, (808) 732-1853, MS 86 Univ of HI - Manoa; 88–Aud, HI Dept of Health, **A**

Takemoto, Charlotte 707 Hausten Street #D, Honolulu, HI 96826, (808) 423-2477, BA 72 Humboldt St Univ; MA 74 Humboldt St Univ; Sp-Lang Path, Hi Dept of Ed-Cen Dist Offi, **SLP**

Takeshita, Mrs Marolyn K 2200 Quitman, Denver, CO 80212, (303) 237-1379, BA 71 Univ of Denver; MA 72 Univ of Denver; SLP, Jefferson County Public Schs, **SLP**

Takeshita, Ruby Tsugie 3626 Courtney Way, Torrance, CA 90505, (213) 673-4660, BA 70 CA St Univ - Northridge; MA 86 CA St Univ - Northridge; **SLP**

Taketa, Janice Hanley 4705 48th Street N W, Washington, DC 20016, (202) 244-0819, Sp-Lang Path, Ridley & Fill Assoc, **SLP**

Takeuchi, Janice Sueko 1312 Lucile Avenue, Los Angeles, CA 90026, (213) 666-0647, BA 83 Univ of Southern CA; MA 86 CA St Univ - Long Beach; 86–Sp-Lang Path, Los Angeles USD

Takumi, Mona S 528 Kamoku Street, Honolulu, HI 96826, MS; **A**

Talamante, Patricia P 2436 East Fairmont Drive, Tempe, AZ 85281, (602) 835-3636, BA 62 WA St Univ; MS 79 AZ St Univ; Dir of Sp-Lang Path Svcs, Desert Samaritan Hosp, **SLP**

Talanian, Valerie Lee 655 Pleasant Street #6, Weymouth, MA 02190, (617) 848-6466, BS 81 Univ of MA - Amherst; MS 83 Boston Univ; **SLP**

Talbert, Linda B 15301 S E Highway 224, Clackamas, OR 97015, **SLP**

Talbert-Sterne, Cindy G 1201 West Buena Vista Road, Evansville, IN 47710, (812) 429-0700, BS 77 Southern IL Univ -Carbondale; MS 79 Southern IL Univ -Carbondale; 85–Sp-Lang Path, Holiday Speech & Lang Ctr, **SLP**

Talbot, Mrs Barbara G 3818 Woodbine Street, Chevy Chase, MD 20015, (301) 559-3956, BA 66 Catholic Univ of America; MA 78 Catholic Univ of America; Sp-Lang Path, Pg Co Bd of Ed, **SLP**

Talbot, Catherine 10 Florence Drive, Mystic, CT 06355, (203) 486-2629, BA 66 Coll of Wooster; MA 67 OH Univ - Athens; 78–Sp-Lang Path, U of Connecticut, **SLP**

Talbot, Elizabeth Parker P O Box 146, Hollister, CA 95024, (408) 637-5393, BA 82 Univ of CA - Santa Barbara; MA 84 Northwestern Univ; SLP, San Benito County Office of Ed, **SLP**

Talbot, Gwendolyn Sp Path Consultant Serv Inc, 8222 Wycliffe Court, Manassas, VA 22110, (703) 368-7357, BA 69 Univ of AZ; MA 71 Univ of AZ; Pres/Sp-Lang Path, Sp Path Conslt Serv, **SLP**

Talbott, Mrs Carolyn B Audiology Associates, 2222 NW Lovejoy Suite 607, Portland, OR 97210, (543) 227-5109, BA 62 Univ of CA - Berkeley; MA 64 Univ of WA; Aud, Aud Assoc, **A ACE**

Talbott, Dr Richard E University Of Georgia, 570 Aderhold Hall, Athens, GA 30602, (404) 542-1685, BS 64 WV Univ; MS 66 WV Univ; PH 73 (NS) Univ of OK Medical Center; Assoc Prof & Head, U of GA, **A F**

Talbott, Mrs Sally A 11533 Seafan Court, Indianapolis, IN 46236, (317) 823-4461, OM 76 Univ of WA; Aud, Indianapolis Pub Schs, **A**

Talbot-Yablon, Ruth J 3451 Harold Street, Oceanside, NY 11572, BA 69 CUNY - Queens Coll; ME 70 PA St Univ - Univ Park; Sp & Hrng Resource Tchr, Speech Services Ut-Bd of Ed, **SLP**

Talboy, Mrs Lori W 3554 South Crosspoint, Boise, ID 83706-5594, (208) 336-2016, BA 74 Creighton Univ; MS 75 Southern IL Univ -Carbondale; SLP, Boise Public Schools, **SLP**

Talburt, Mrs Valerie S 206 Euclid Avenue #407, Long Beach, CA 90803, (213) 674-7050, BS 82 Baylor Univ; MA 84 Memphis St Univ; 87–Sp-Lang Path, Daniel Freeman Hospital, **SLP**

Talerico, Frank B Margate Hearing Center, 5170 Coconut Creek Parkway, Margate, FL 33063, (305) 972-0524, BA 75 Baldwin-Wallace Coll; MA 76 Univ of Akron; ED 88 (Early Childhood Ed) Nova Univ; Aud, Margate Hearing Center, **A**

Taliaferro, Mrs Sharon P O Box 772781, Steamboat Springs, CO 80477, BA 64 Univ of Northern CO; MA 76 Univ of Northern CO; Sp-Lang Path, NW Co Bd of Coop Servs, **SLP**

Tallarico Cutter, Tina 730 Oakwood Trail, Fort Worth, TX 76112, (817) 457-6099, **SLP**

Tallent, Joy R 6100 Westchester Park #L-4, College Park, MD 20740, (301) 474-5112, BA 49 Wichita St Univ; MA 52 Univ of IL - Urbana; **SLP**

Talley, Mrs Anita M Route 2 Box 253A, Eddyville, KY 42038, (502) 825-6030, BA 82 Univ of KY; MS 83 Univ of KY; Sp-Lang Path, Hopkins County Schools, **SLP**

Talley, Frank James 918 Church Road, Forest City, NC 28043, (704) 287-2211, BS 74 Appalachian St Univ; MA 80 Appalachian St Univ; Sp-Lang Path, McDowell Dist Hlth Dept, **SLP**

Talley, Dr James N 2506 Tyron Road, Durham, NC 27705, (919) 286-0411, BS 61 East TN St Univ; MA 65 Univ of IL - Urbana; PH 70 (NS) Univ of IL - Urbana; Aud, Durham VA Med Cen, **A**

Talley, Mrs Mary Ellen 8227 Ashworth Avenue North, Seattle, WA 98103, (206) 839-0904, BA 75 Univ of WA; OM 77 Univ of WA; SLP, Fed Way Sch Dist, **SLP**

Talley, Ron Claire P O Box 3671, Boone, NC 28607, (704) 733-4532, BA 72 Univ of NC - Chapel Hill; MS 79 Univ of NC - Chapel Hill; SLP, Avery County Schs, **SLP**

Talley, Susan Harris 6511 West Higgins, Chicago, IL 60656, (312) 485-0216, BA 71 Elmhurst Coll; MS 82 IL St Univ - Normal; Sp-Lang Path, La Grange Dist #102, **SLP ACE**

Tallman, Travis M 18 Indiana Road, Somerset, NJ 08873, (201) 549-5580, BS 70 Towson St Univ; MS 72 PA St Univ - Univ Park; Dir Sp-Lang Path, Cp Assoc of Middlesex Co, **SLP**

Tallman, Valerie L Veterans Administration Medical Center, 2401 West Main, Marion, IL 62959, (618) 997-5311, BS 81 Southern IL Univ -Carbondale; MS 84 Southern IL Univ -Carbondale; 84–Sp-Lang Path, VA Medical Center, **SLP**

Tallon, Valerie McDonald 122 Tamwood Lane, Elgin, SC 29045, (803) 788-5420, BA 83 Columbia Coll; OM 84 Univ of SC - Columbia; Sp-Lang Path, Joseph Keels Ele Schl, **SLP**

Talmadge, Mrs Ann Rannazzi 38 Augusta Drive, Wayne, NJ 07470, (201) 239-9010, BA 79 William Paterson Coll; MS 83 William Paterson Coll; 80–Sp-Lang Path, Verona Bd of Ed, **SLP ACE**

Talmadge-Sessions, Susan Victoria 210 East 15th Street #62, Tuscaloosa, AL 35401, (205) 795-1395, MA 88 Univ of AL- Tuscaloosa

Talmage, Christine Devers Box 497-A, Kennebunkport, ME 04046, (207) 985-3137, BS 77 Univ of NH; MS 82 Univ of NH; 87–Sp-Lang Path, Private Practice, **SLP**

Talon, Mrs Pamela H 3714 Durham Court, Bloomfield Hills, MI 48013-1979, BA 78 MI St Univ; MA 79 Eastern MI Univ; SLP, Saratoga Hosp, **SLP**

Tamai, Laverne Mieko 45-088 Namoku Street, Kaneohe, HI 96744, BS 83 Univ of HI - Manoa; MS 85 Univ of HI - Manoa; 86–Sp-Lang Path, Dept of Educ, **SLP**

Tamari, Dr Pauline L 12 Pond View Drive, Syosset, NY 11791, (516) 921-5205, BA 65 CUNY - Queens Coll; MA 69 Univ of IA; ED 78 (NS); Prog Dir, Suffolk Child Devel Ctr, **SLP**

Tamashiro, Howard K 1040 South King Street, Suite 307, Honolulu, HI 96701, (808) 538-3922, BA 73 Univ of Northern CO; MA 74 Univ of Northern CO; Aud, Equip Corp, **A**

Tamashiro, Lynette S 98-761 Lealil Street, Aiea, HI 96701, (808) 486-0148, BA 73 Univ of Northern CO; MA 74 Univ of Northern CO; Sp-Lang Path, State Dept of Hlth, **SLP**

Tamayo, Eliana Isabel 87-30 Justice Avenue #7-D, Elmhurst, NY 11373, (212) 932-6620, BS 78 0500; MA 86 NY Univ; 86–Sp-Lang Path, Sydenham Nghbrhd Fam Ctr

Tamayo, Mrs Irene H 17411 Port Marnock Drive, Poway, CA 92064, (619) 487-2348, BS 79 Univ of HI - Manoa; MS 81 Univ of HI - Manoa; Aud, Communication Disorders Clinic, **A**

Tamblyn, Anne M 1311 Honeysuckle Road, Apartment A, Dothan, AL 36301, (205) 793-5771, BS 83 Auburn Univ - Auburn; OM 88 Auburn Univ - Auburn; 88–Sp-Lang Path, Steensland Ctr for Sp Path

Tambo, Mrs Josephine 100 Pine Hill Road, Chelmsford, MA 01824, (617) 256-5044, BA 56 MI St Univ; Sp-Lang Path, Private Practice, **SLP**

Tammone, Karen Lee 3131 Hayes Road #816, Houston, TX 77082, (713) 465-1572, BS 83 CO St Univ; MS 85 CO St Univ; **SLP**

Tan, Barbara Box 259, Edinboro, PA 16412, (814) 724-1440, BA 62 Western MI Univ; MS 69 IL St Univ - Normal; Sp-Lang Path, Private Practice, **SLP**

Tan, Grace M Y 3304 Heatherfield Drive, Hacienda Heights, CA 91745, (818) 330-8750, BA 69 Univ of Redlands; MA 70 Univ of Redlands; Aud, LA Co Super Sch, **SLP**

Tanabe, Karen Jo 13062 Cypress Street #19, Garden Grove, CA 92643, (213) 217-0427, BS 83 IL St Univ - Normal; MA 86 CA St Univ - Fullerton; **SLP**

Tanaka, Cathleen 38660 Lexington Street, Apartment 568, Fremont, CA 94536, (209) 478-2918, BA 86 San Diego St Univ; MA 87 Univ of the Pacific; **SLP**

Tanaka, Mrs Marsha U R R 1 Box 485-J, Kula, HI 96790, (808) 244-4223, BS 74 Western OR St Coll; ME 75 Western OR St Coll; Sp-Lang Path, Dept Ed-St O Mi, **SLP**

Tanaka, Mieko 1622 11th Street, Wichita Falls, TX 76301, (817) 322-6953, MS 86 Univ of TX - Dallas; 86–Aud, Head & Neck Surgical Assoc, **A**

Tanaka, Mrs Wanette Y 98-1952 Hoala Street, Aiea, HI 96701, (808) 455-2885, BS 73 Univ of HI - Manoa; MS 75 Univ of WA; Sp-Lang Path, Dept of Educ, **SLP**

Tanaka-Cameron, Audrey Takaoka 7348 South Coles Avenue, Chicago, IL 60649, (312) 942-8011, BS 80 Roosevelt Univ; MS 86 Rush Univ

Tanchak, Theresa L 2 F Holly Court, Harrisonburg, VA 22801, (703) 433-3255, BA 81 SUNY - Coll at Cortland; MS 86 James Madison Univ; 86–Sp-Lang Path, Woodrow Wilson Rehab Ctr, **SLP**

Tancredi, Mrs Joan L 15515 Sunset Boulevard, Apartment 216, Pacific Palisades, CA 90272, (213) 674-7050, BS 53 Univ of WI - Madison; MA 73 CA St Univ - Los Angeles; Prog Coord Nepathw Center, Daniel Freeman Mem Hosp, **SLP**

Tancredi, Sandra A 78 Oakwood Avenue, Providence, RI 02909, **SLP**

Tandarich, Mrs Charon B H 309 Yale Avenue, Broomall, PA 19008, (215) 539-8550, BA 73 Univ of MD - College Park; MA 75 Case Western Reserve Univ; Sp-Lang Path, Montgomery County Int Unit 23, **SLP ACE**

Tande, Dennis O 4965 Gilkeson Road, Waunakee, WI 53597-9506, (608) 249-6415, BA 73 Univ of IA; MS 74 Univ of WI - Madison; Sp-Lang Path, Madison Metro School District, **SLP**

Tandler, Joan Mary 22 Lake Avenue, High Bridge, NJ 08829, (201) 540-5202, BS 69 Miami Univ - Oxford; MS 73 Rutgers St Univ - Camdem; 83–Sp-Lang Path, Morristown Memorial Hosp, **SLP**

Tandy, Sharon G 3901 Lafayette Drive N E, Apartment 74, Albuquerque, NM 87107, (919) 638-4389, BA 77 Univ of FL; MA 79 Univ of TN - Knoxville; **SLP**

Tanenbaum, Mrs Sheila T 7433 Asman Avenue, Canoga Park, CA 91307, (805) 251-2901, BA 66 MI St Univ; MA 75 CA St Univ - Los Angeles; SLP, L A Co Supt Sch, **SLP**

Tanenhaus, Mrs Joan Beris 5 Tameling Road, East Rockaway, NY 11518, (516) 887-2814, BA 59 Univ of MI - Ann Arbor; MA 69 CUNY - Hunter Coll; Sp-Lang Path & Aud, Private Practice, **SLP A ACE**

Taney, Bernadette M 9 Genessee Street #4, Camillus, NY 13031-1121, BA 80 Marywood Coll; MS 84 Syracuse Univ; Sp-Lang Path, St Camillus Health Rehab Cen, **SLP**

Tangeman, Gretchen 36 Mainview Court, Randallstown, MD 21133, (301) 363-2758, BA 65 Miami Univ - Oxford; MA 69 Western MI Univ; 75–Dir, Leo Kanner Sp & Hrng Cen, **SLP**

Tani, Dr Allen H Associated Healthfocus-LA, 7516 Picardy Avenue, Suite B, Baton Rouge, LA 70808, (504) 766-6113, BA 66 Adams St Coll; MA 67 Adams St Coll; PH 70 (NS) OH Univ - Athens; Admin, Associated Healthfocus Inc, **SLP A**

Tani, Mrs Janis Nakanishi 1103 Winding Oak Drive, Chula Vista, CA 92010, (619) 482-1048, **SLP**

Taniguchi, Lori M 6931 East Princeton, Tucson, AZ 85710, (602) 747-4909, BS 75 Kent St Univ; MA 77 Kent St Univ; Sp-Lang Path, Tucson USD #1, **SLP**

Tanihana, Jami Hatsumi 16748 Tribune Street, Granada Hills, CA 91344, (818) 894-4588, BA 81 CA St Univ - Northridge; MA 83 CA St Univ - Northridge; **A**

Tanja, Mrs Virginia Kathleen 641 Thorpe Street, Auburn, AL 36830, (205) 821-6595, BS 67 Auburn Univ - Auburn; OM 86 Auburn Univ - Auburn; **A**

Tank, Joell I 5665 Lakepoint System, Johnston, IA 50131, **SLP**

Tanklefsky, Mrs Gay Sherman 289 Elm Street #66A, Medford, MA 02155, (617) 745-9300, **SLP**

Tannahill, Dr J Curtis Dept Speech Path & Audiology, Illinois State University, 204 Fairchild Hall, Normal, IL 61761, (309) 438-8641, BS 62 Univ of NE - Lincoln; MA 63 Univ of NE - Lincoln; PH 71 (NS) Univ of KS; Dir Sp & Hrng Cl, Il St U, **A**

Tannenbaum, Linda Joy 81 Westwood Court, Old Bridge, NJ 08857, (201) 679-0768, MS 80 CUNY - Brooklyn Coll; Sp-Lang Path, New York City Board of Educ, **SLP**

Tannenbaum, Madeline F 280 Burrage Court, Cheshire, CT 06410, (203) 272-8022, BA 74 SUNY - Center at Buffalo; MA 75 Case Western Reserve Univ; Aud, Julian Henley MD, **A**

Tannenbaum, Melissa Ann 46 Sharon Street, San Francisco, CA 94114, (415) 282-2551, BA 82 San Francisco St Univ; MS 85 San Francisco St Univ; **A**

Tannenbaum, Michelle S 4733 Prince Street, Downers Grove, IL 60515, (312) 960-5047, BS 78 Northern IL Univ - De Kalb; MA 80 Northern IL Univ - De Kalb; Sp-Lang Path, Naperville Schools, **SLP**

Tannenbaum, Sandra 105B Spring Woods Lake Pt, Columbia, SC 29223, (803) 782-0470, BA 67 CUNY - Hunter Coll; ME 73 Univ of SC - Columbia; Sp-Lang Path, Richland Co Sch Dist 2, **SLP**

Tanner, Amgela Maria Route 2 Box 800, Orangeburg, SC 29115, (803) 531-4874, BA 85 SC St Coll; MA 87 SC St Coll

Tanner, Barry Jon 3913 Calle Abril, San Clemente, CA 92672, (714) 496-1215, MA 74 CA St Univ - Long Beach; BA 64 CA St Univ - Long Beach; Sp-Lang Path, Capistrano USD, **SLP**

Tanner, Mrs Carol Jw 35 Old Still Road, Columbia, SC 29223, (803) 776-4000, BS 74 Univ of VA - Charlottesville; OM 75 Univ of SC - Columbia; 80–Sp-Lang Path, Dorn VA Med Cen, **SLP**

Tanner, Dr Dennis C Speech & Hearing Cons Serv Inc, 3320 South Gillenwater Dr, Flagstaff, AZ 86001, (602) 779-2489, BS 71 ID St Univ; MS 73 ID St Univ; PH 76 (NS) MI St Univ; 76–Assoc Prof, Northern AZ U, **SLP**

Tanner, Mrs Donna W 3911 South 3250 East, Salt Lake City, UT 84124, (801) 582-5534, BA 50 Brigham Young Univ; MS 51 Univ of UT; Sp-Lang Path, The Children's Center, **SLP A**

Tannock, Joy Ann 70 Steere Farm Road, Harrisville, RI 02830, (401) 294-4581, BS 82 Worcester St Coll; MS 87 Worcester St Coll

Tansey, Mrs Janet H 348 Park Lane, Lake Bluff, IL 60044, (312) 234-4215, BA 48 Coll of New Rochelle; MA 52 Univ of CO - Boulder; Retired, Spec Ed Dist of Lake Co, **SLP**

Tantillo, Mary W 60 Newkirk Road, Yonkers, NY 10710, BA 74 CUNY - Queens Coll; MA 76 CUNY - Queens Coll; Sp-Lang Path, Pelham Sch Dist, **SLP ACE**

Tapajna, Marilyn R Kent 4 Danube Way, Olympia Fields, IL 60461, (312) 481-3367, BS 73 Purdue Univ - West Lafayette; ME 78 IN Univ - Bloomington; 84–Sp-Lang Path, Ctr for Communication Disordrs Ltd, **SLP ACE**

Tapia, Mrs Mary Esteve 11469 Glenda Drive, Baton Rouge, LA 70815, (504) 275-4448, BA 81 Nicholls St Univ; OM 82 LA St Univ - N O Medical Ctr; Sp-Lang Path, East Baton Rouge Parish Sch Bd, **SLP**

Tapley, Lori Ann 136 Washington Street, Brewer, ME 04412, (207) 989-2249, BA 83 Univ of ME - Orono; MS 85 Northeastern Univ; Sp-Lang Path, Griffiths-Larrabee Inc, **SLP**

Tapp, Mrs Susan R 21630 Stanstead, Northville, MI 48167, (313) 553-8054, BA 73 Univ of OK - Norman; MS 74 Univ of OK Medical Center; **SLP**

Tapp-Gallegos, Mrs Jennifer Gisele 1318½ Bennett Avenue, Long Beach, CA 90804, (213) 985-0148, BA 85 Chapman Coll; MA 87 Whittier Coll; 88–Sp-Lang Path, Casa Colina Rehab Ctr So Bay, **SLP**

Tarantine, Deborah Pauline 1200 Saxonburg Boulevard, Glenshaw, PA 15116, (713) 847-3109, BA 84 Univ of Houston - Univ Park; MA 86 Univ of Houston - Univ Park; **SLP**

Taras, Mrs Ellen Epstein 29668 Strawberry Hill Dr, Agoura Hills, CA 91301, (818) 889-5790, BA 73 CA St Univ - Northridge; MA 74 CA St Univ - Northridge; Learning Handicapped Tchr, Los Angeles USD, **SLP**

Tarasick, Arlene L 701 Spring Street, Michigan City, IN 46360-3440, BS 66 IN Univ - Bloomington; OM 74 IN Univ - Bloomington; OD 83 (NS) IN Univ - Bloomington; Principal, MI Cty Area Sch, **SLP**

Taratoot, Mrs Deborah L 4960 Willeo Ridge Court, Marietta, GA 30067, (404) 992-1333, BS 69 Univ of FL; MA 70 Univ of MI - Ann Arbor; **SLP**

Tarbox, Mrs Gail Manin 205 Forest Street, North Andover, MA 01845, BS 76 Univ of MA - Amherst; MS 79 Boston Univ; Aud, ENT Cen, **A**

Tardanico, Jamie McBride 1375 Half Moon Road, Cheshire, CT 06410, (203) 238-7328, BA 80 SUNY - Coll at Cortland; MA 81 Bowling Green St Univ; MA 84 Bowling Green St Univ; Sp-Lang Path, Private Practice, **SLP**

Tardelli, Maureen M 11 Chester Avenue, Medford, MA 02155, (617) 726-2763, BA 64 Univ of CT; ME 71 Boston Univ; Assoc Dir/Sp-Lang Path, Mass Gen Hosp, **SLP**

Tardif, Joan Marie 427 N Tioga Street, Ithaca, NY 14850, (607) 272-5891, BS 81 Ithaca Coll; MS 87 Ithaca Coll

Tardiff, Catherine Carre 3511 Shepherd Street, Chevy Chase, MD 20815, (703) 360-8000, BS 70 Emerson Coll; ME 75 Northeastern Univ; SLP, Mt Vernon Hosp, **SLP**

Tardy, Mrs Kathryn K 2730 Country Club Blvd, Sugar Land, TX 77478, (713) 242-3690, BS 60 TX Woman's Univ; **SLP**

Targovnik, Nan Sudran 44 Sagamore Avenue, North Edison, NJ 08820, (201) 549-7265, BA 79 SUNY - Center at Buffalo; MA 82 Univ of CT; Aud, Center for Sp & Hring Sci, **A**

Tarkanian, Dr Lois 2905 Justice Lane, Las Vegas, NV 89107, (702) 870-2700, BA 55; MA 64; PH 79 (NS); Ed/Dir, Sound Foundation, **SLP A**

Tarlow, Gail I 25246 58th Avenue, Flushing, NY 11362-2114, BS 74 Univ of GA; ME 75 Univ of GA; Sp-Lang Path, Northern Westchester Ctr For Sp Dis, **SLP**

Tarlton, Mrs Tina S 301 McCall Drive, Forest City, NC 28043, (704) 245-5230, BA 79 Univ of TN - Knoxville; MA 81 Univ of TN - Knoxville; Aud, Rutherford/McDowell Co Sch, **A**

Tarman, Mrs Mary T 121 Chandler, Elmhurst, IL 60126, (312) 834-7620, BA 76 Elmhurst Coll; MA 78 Northwestern Univ; Sp-Lang Path, **SLP**

Tarnawski, Julia K T 9737 Wheatland, Sunland, CA 91040, **SLP**

Tarnoff, Terri Lynne 930 Westbourne Drive #302, West Hollywood, CA 90069, (213) 273-8480, BA 80 Temple Univ; MA 83 San Diego St Univ; Sp-Lang Path, Irwin Lehrhoff and Associates, **SLP**

Tarnow, Janet Elaine 324-D Pasadena Avenue, South Pasadena, CA 91030, (818) 405-1177, BA 81 CA St Univ - Los Angeles; MA 84 CA St Univ - Los Angeles; Sp-Lang Path, Frostig Center of Educ Therapy, **SLP**

Tarnpoll, Judith M 50 Ridgefield Avenue #320, Bridgeport, CT 06610, (203) 334-2467, BA 64 Rutgers St Univ - Newark; MA 66 Columbia Univ Teachers Coll; Aud, Private Practice, **SLP A**

Taromino, Mrs Jane Lee G 52 Archer Road, Rochester, NY 14624, (716) 889-1728, BS 77 SUNY - Coll at Geneseo; MA 81 SUNY - Coll at Geneseo; 79–Sp-Lang Path, BOCES #2, **SLP**

Tarpley, Jewel D 5101 Russett Road, Rockville, MD 20853, BS 78 Towson St Univ; MS 81 Tulane Univ; Cl SLP, Walter Reed Army Med Ctr, **SLP**

Tarr, Debi Lynne 1507 Glenwood Avenue, Fort Wayne, IN 46805, (219) 234-3136, BS 84 Ball St Univ; MS 85 Ball St Univ; **SLP**

Tarr, Dena M Route 4 Box 63-B, Reed City, MI 49677, (616) 832-5277, MA 86 Central MI Univ; 86–Sp-Lang Path, Mecosta-Osceola Intermed Sch Dist, **SLP**

Tartarka, Margery A P O Box 5839, Santa Fe, NM 87502-5839, (505) 984-1850, **SLP**

Tartter, Dr Vivien Rothman Psychology Department, CUNY, New York, NY 10031, (212) 535-2735, BA 73 Brown Univ; MA 75 Brown Univ; PH 77 (Psychology) Brown Univ; 88–Assoc Prof, City Coll-CUNY

Tarulli, Nancy Jo 24 Donnelly Drive, Dover, MA 02030, (508) 785-9832, BS 66 Kent St Univ; MA 69 Kent St Univ; Sp-Lang Path, Medway PS, **SLP**

Tarumoto, Elsie K 94-1135 Mo'Olelo Street, Waipahu, HI 96797, (808) 455-5986, BS 78 Univ of HI - Manoa; MS 79 Univ of HI - Manoa; Sp-Lang Path, Children with Spec Health Needs, **SLP**

Tarushka, Mrs Linda L 32 Harbor Street #3, Salem, MA 01970, (617) 396-9250, OB 84 Salem St Coll; MS 87 Northeastern Univ; 87–Sp-Lang Path, Lawrence Mem Hosp of Medford, **SLP**

Tarver, Carolyn Williams 5701 East Shirley Lane, Apartment 1002, Montgomery, AL 36117-1946, (404) 283-3140, BS 78 AL A & M Univ; MA 79 OH St Univ; Sp-Lang Path, Elbert Co Pub Sch, **SLP**

Tarver, Margaret Miller 5111 Maulding Pass, Austin, TX 78749, (512) 892-3968, BS 73 SUNY - Center at Albany; MA 74 Hofstra Univ; **SLP**

Tarzia, Mrs Eileen Rose 7 Glenn Lane, Vernon, CT 06066, (203) 872-1625, BS 80 Univ of MA - Amherst; MS 82 PA St Univ - Univ Park; Sp-Lang Path, East Hartford Pub Sch, **SLP**

Tasca, Martha Flynn 116 Fosdyke Street, Providence, RI 02906, (617) 234-8120, BA 79 Univ of RI; ME 81 Northeastern Univ; SLP, Johnston Pub Sch, **SLP**

Tasch, Melissa B 204 West 78th Street #3B, New York, NY 10024, (212) 877-3169, BA 74 NY Univ; MA 76 NY Univ; 86–Sp-Lang Path, Private Practice, **SLP**

Tassini, Donna M 6382 E Seneca Turnpike, Jamesville, NY 13078, (315) 470-3196, BS 79 Syracuse Univ; MS 80 Syracuse Univ; Sp-Lang Path, N Syracuse Early Ed Prog, **SLP**

Tatar, Gloria V 114 Hiawatha, Clarendon Hills, IL 60514, (312) 789-3617, BS 73 Marquette Univ; MS 74 Marquette Univ; SLP, Glen Ellyn Pub Schs, **SLP**

Tatchell, Dr Renny Hemsley Dept Of Communication Disorder, Central Michigan Univ, Mount Pleasant, MI 48858, (517) 774-7291, PH 84 Univ of CT; Assoc Prof, Central MI U, **SLP ACE**

Tate, Constance Route 9 Box 385, Statesville, NC 28677, BA 76 Wake Forest Univ; ME 78 Univ of NC - Greensboro; Spec Serv Coord, Barium Sprng Fmly/Chld Dev Cen, **SLP**

Tate, David Michael 40 Franklin Street, New Haven, CT 06511, (203) 777-1829, BA 82 Univ of CT; MS 85 Southern CT St Univ; **SLP**

Tate, Mrs Deborah Kellum 155 Watertown Way, Fayetteville, GA 30214, (404) 460-9651, BA 83 Harding Univ; MS 85 Univ of MS; 88–Sp-Lang Path, Sp Svcs for Children, **SLP**

Tate, Judith A 1755 Newark Road, Zanesville, OH 43701-2629, BS 75 Bowling Green St Univ; MA 77 Bowling Green St Univ; Sp/Lang Path, Muskingum Co Bd of Ment Ret, **SLP**

Tate, Kathleen 197 Belford Avenue, Rutherford, NJ 07070, BA 75 Univ of OR; OM 77 Univ of MT; SLP, Evergreen Stroke Association, **SLP**

Tate, Rebecca C 3215-A Liberty Road, Hill AFB, UT 84056, (801) 773-6553, BS 73 Univ of AR - Fayetteville; MA 74 Memphis St Univ; Sp-Lang Path, Rocky Mtn Rehab Cen, **SLP**

Tate, Susan M 788 Victoria Circle East, Ormond Beach, FL 32074, (904) 441-7852, BA 79 Univ of FL; MA 81 Univ of FL; **SLP**

Tate, Virginia May 14930 Faust, Detroit, MI 48223, (313) 286-8400, BA 75 Univ of CA - Santa Barbara; MA 84 Eastern MI Univ; Sp-Lang Path, State of Michigan, **SLP**

Tatge, Barbara A Germantown Speech & Hearing Clinic, 2028 Exeter Road #2, Germantown, TN 38138-3922, (901) 756-4499, BA 80 Auburn Univ - Auburn; MA 81 Memphis St Univ; 84–Aud, Private Practice, **A**

Tatham, Ellen G 805-2310 W 2, Vancouver, BC, Canada V6K 2J1, **SLP**

Tatich, Denise Marie Rehabilitation Services Incorporated, PO Box 310, Binghamton, NY 13902, (607) 722-5308, BS 84 SUNY - Coll at Geneseo; MS 85 Coll of Saint Rose; 86–Sp-Lang Path, Rehab Svcs Inc, **SLP**

Tatman, Linda D 6468 North Broadway, Indianapolis, IN 46220, (317) 872-4051, BS 80 Miami Univ - Oxford; MA 81 Univ of IL - Urbana; Sp-Lang Path, Americana Healthcare, **SLP**

Tator, Diann V P O Box 223, Dulce, NM 87528, (505) 759-3277, BS 74 Eastern NM Univ; MS 75 Eastern NM Univ; Sp-Lang Path, Jicarilla Headstart Prog, **SLP**

Tatoul, Corinne M 2621 East 20th Street #8, Signal Hill, CA 90804, (213) 597-9866, BA 59 FL St Univ; MS 60 FL St Univ; Progress Administrator, Los Angeles Co Office of Educ, **SLP**

Tattershall, Dr Sandra Susan Language And Learning Center, 6421 Dixie Highway, Florence, KY 41042, (606) 525-1570, BA 62 Univ of KY; MA 74 Univ of Cincinnati; PH 76 (Sp Path & Linguistics) Univ of Cincinnati; Sp-Lang Path/Dir, Private Practice, **SLP**

Tatum, Linda Marie 1038 W Jefferson St #11, Orlando, FL 32805, (305) 422-2470, BA 81 Univ of Central FL; MS 84 Univ Southern MS-Hattiesburg; **SLP**

Tatum, Pamela E 11718 Spring Dale, San Antonio, TX 78249, (512) 654-1041, BS 82 IN St Univ - Terre Haute; MA 86 Univ of Houston - Univ Park; 87–Sp-Lang Path, North East ISD, **SLP**

Tatum, Tom L 635 East Utah, Fresno, CA 93710, (209) 227-1552, BA 79 CA St Univ - Fresno; BA 79 CA St Univ - Fresno; MA 81 CA St Univ - Fresno; Pres/Sp-Lang Path, Sunrise A Speech Path Corp, **SLP**

Taub, Barbara Susan 1866 Lynton Circle, Wellington, FL 33410, BA 72 CUNY - Lehman Coll; OM 82 Governors St Univ; 87–Sp-Lang Path, Palm Beach County Schs, **SLP**

Taub, Claire F 52 Van Syckel Lane, Wyckoff, NJ 07481, **A**

Taub, Linda B 1451 John Street, Fort Lee, NJ 07024, (201) 585-1797, BA 69 Elmira Coll; ME 74 Bloomsburg Univ of PA; **SLP**

Taube, Mrs Wanda Watts 14246 Tornelia Lane, West Palm Beach, FL 33414, (305) 833-2070, BS 78 FL St Univ; MA 81 Univ of TN - Knoxville; Sp-Lang Path, Palm Beach County School Board, **SLP**

Tauber, Rosalyn 125 Woodbine Avenue, Larchmont, NY 10538, (212) 439-6570, BS 51 Newark St Coll; MA 56 Columbia Univ Teachers Coll; Sp-Lang Path, Private Practice, **SLP**

Tauberer, Mrs Gale M 21 Jeremy Avenue, Plainview, NY 11803, (516) 666-6346, BA 71 Case Western Reserve Univ; MS 76 Columbia Univ Teachers Coll; Sp-Lang Path, Assoc for Children with Learning Disabi, **SLP**

Taubman, Jacqueline 44 Hicks Street #2, Brooklyn, NY 11201, (718) 852-3445, **SLP**

Taubman, Miriam 2041 Naudain Street, Philadelphia, PA 19146, 85–Sp-Lang Path, YALE Sch, **SLP**

Tauchen, Aileen N3648 Cloverland Road, Ladysmith, WI 54848, (715) 532-5533, BA 76 Univ of WI - Eau Claire; MS 77 Univ of WI - Eau Claire; SLP, Ladysmith Hawkins Sch Dist, **SLP**

Tauger, Susan M 29562 Rainbow Hill Road, Golden, CO 80401-9709, (303) 526-1649, **SLP**

Taulman, Mrs Cheryl Ann 2754 Hilltop Drive, Sun Prairie, WI 53590, (414) 386-2655, BS 66 Purdue Univ - Calumet; MS 84 Univ of WI - Whitewater; **SLP**

Taussig-Leibow, Mrs Lisa 2856 North Burling #4, Chicago, IL 60657, (312) 702-1864, BS 75 Bradley Univ; MA 76 IN Univ - Bloomington; 87–Aud, Univ of Chicago Med Ctr, **A**

Tavares, Patricia L 377 Fisher Road, Westport, MA 02747, BA 78 Bridgewater St Coll; MS 85 Northeastern Univ; Sp-Lang Path, Wareham School System, **SLP**

Tavenner, Mrs Laura Mae Route 1 Box 114, Rigby, ID 83442, (208) 754-0469, 78 Northwest Nazarene Coll; BS 80 ID St Univ; MS 82 ID St Univ; **SLP**

Taves-Ruenzel, Mary Elizabeth 2014 N 51st Street, Milwaukee, WI 53208, (215) 631-0928, BA 75 Valparaiso Univ; MS 85 Marquette Univ; 87–Sp-Lang Path, InSpeech Inc, **SLP**

Tavlin, Mrs Karen Hayden 2 Harvard Terrace, West Orange, NJ 07052, (914) 634-4648, BS 80 IN Univ - Bloomington; MA 82 IN Univ - Bloomington; Sp-Lang Path, Rockland Co Cen/Phys Hndcpd, **SLP**

Tavolacci, Gina Marie 94 South Hamilton Street, Apartment 5, Poughkeepsie, NY 12601, (914) 677-5021, **SLP**

Tavormina, Barbara L 5349 West Crain, Skokie, IL 60077, (312) 446-0353, BA 77 IN Univ - Bloomington; OM 78 IN Univ - Bloomington; Sp-Lang Path, Winnetka Pub Sch, **SLP**

Taxy, Mrs Gail S 1123 Wade, Highland Park, IL 60035, (312) 433-0715, BS 69 Northwestern Univ; MS 72 Univ of MI - Ann Arbor; Sp-Lang Path, Private Practice, **SLP**

Taylert, Barbara J 310 Westage @ The Harbor, Rochester, NY 14617, **SLP**

Taylor, Abigail B 8509 Harrington Road, Indianapolis, IN 46256-1523, (913) 682-3672, **SLP**

Taylor, Alice Ross 41 Clarkes Crossing, Fairport, NY 14450, (716) 377-4660, BS 49 Univ of IL - Urbana; MS 77 Nazareth Coll of Rochester; Sp-Lang Path, BOCES Monroe Co, **SLP**

Taylor, Alicia 708 McKinley, Miami, OK 74354, BA 72 OK St Univ; MA 75 OK St Univ; Sp/Lang Path, Commerce Schs, **SLP**

Taylor, Alta Lou 3124 Alameda Street, Pasadena, CA 91107, (818) 449-5635, MA 69; 67–Sp-Lang Path, Villa Esperanza Sch, **SLP**

Taylor, Andrewena 1552 Kinnard Drive, Franklin, TN 37064, BA 73 Birmingham-Southern Coll; MS 75 Vanderbilt Univ; Case Manager, State of Tennessee, **SLP**

Taylor, Mrs Angela Audrey 2275 Gray Highway #L-16, Macon, GA 31211, (912) 825-3132, MA 83 Univ of SD - Vermillion; Sp-Lang Path, Mid GA Coop Educ Service Agcy, **SLP**

Taylor, Anita Kay 4906 66 Street #B, Lubbock, TX 79414, (806) 747-2641, BA 77 Harding Univ; MS 83 Univ of AR - Fayetteville; Sp/Lang Path, Lubbock ISD, **SLP**

Taylor, Ann L 21 Dorothy Drive, Plymouth, MA 02360, (617) 992-4756, BA 78 Loyola Coll; MS 79 Loyola Coll; Early Intervention Coord, Kennedy-Donovan Center, **SLP**

Taylor, April Jean P O Box 2753, Santa Maria, CA 93455, (805) 736-2371, BA 72 CA St Univ - Fresno; MA 74 CA St Univ - Long Beach; SLP, Lompoc USD, **SLP**

Taylor, Barbara Ann 1600 Pullen Road #7A, Tallahassee, FL 32303, (904) 656-4800, BS 86 FL St Univ; MS 87 FL St Univ

Taylor, Barbara Berry 510 Winstead Road, Greenville, NC 27834, (919) 756-2176, BS 80 WV Univ; MA 81 Marshall Univ; Sp/Lang Path, Private Practice, **SLP**

Taylor, Barbara Jean Five Village West Court, Apartment 302, Washington, MO 63090, (314) 239-7547, BS 86 Saint Louis Univ; MA 87 Saint Louis Univ; 88–Sp-Lang Path, Franklin County Coop

Taylor, Belinda Michelle 7752 South Winchester, Chicago, IL 60620, (312) 890-8366, BS 80 Western IL Univ; MA 83 Western MI Univ; **SLP**

Taylor, Beth P O Box 85, Hadley, MA 01035, (413) 737-7368, BS 77 SUNY - Coll at Utica-Rome; MA 81 Univ of MA - Amherst; Augmentative Comm Prog Coord, West MA Sp & Lang Serv Assoc, **SLP**

Taylor, Beth Nanette Nichols 270 Concord Drive, Casselberry, FL 32707, (407) 831-8034, BS 81 Edinboro Univ of PA; MA 86 Univ of Central FL; 82–Sp-Lang Path, Orange County Schs, **SLP**

Taylor, Bonnie Ellen 914 East Cochise Drive, Phoenix, AZ 85020, (602) 255-1181, BA 71 Univ of MI - Ann Arbor; MS 73 Univ of MI - Ann Arbor; MS 86 AZ St Univ; 87–Aud, Arizona Dept of Hlth Svcs, **A**

Taylor, Mrs Brenda K 627 Deer Acres Drive, Goldsboro, NC 27530-9238, (919) 734-2592, **SLP**

Taylor, Carmen Lisa HHC 299th Spt Bn, APO New York, NY 09137, 49-07161-33656, BA 86 Columbia Coll; MS 87 Univ of AL- Tuscaloosa; 88–Aud, **A**

Taylor, Carole A 4140 Fair Avenue #2, Studio City, CA 91604, **SLP**

Taylor, Carole J 7950 Seward Avenue, Cincinnati, OH 45231, (513) 729-4706, BS 73 Univ of TN - Knoxville; MA 76 Univ of TN - Knoxville; Sp-Lang Path, Talk to Me, **SLP**

Taylor, Carolyn F 101 Cameron Drive, Spartanburg, SC 29302, (803) 585-0322, BA 60 Univ of AR - Fayetteville; Sp-Lang Path, Charles Lea Center, **SLP**

Taylor, Catherine Rose 1360 Fraser Drive, Fayetteville, NC 28303, (919) 868-9459, OB 84 Univ of Toledo; MS 85 Univ of NC - Chapel Hill; Aud, Southeastern Sp & Hrng Servs, **A**

Taylor, Charles R 1216 Stuart Avenue S W, Decatur, AL 35601, (205) 534-2033, BS 71 Univ of Northern AL; MA 73 Univ of AL- Tuscaloosa; Aud, Huntsville Hrng Ser Inc, **A**

Taylor, Charles Reid 109 Atlantic Street, Jersey City, NJ 07304, BA 75 Jersey City St Coll; MA 77 Seton Hall Univ; Sp-Lang Path, Jersey City State College, **SLP**

Taylor, Mrs Cheryl Davidson 1119 Springfield Road, Union, NJ 07305, (201) 688-5150, BS 78 Univ of TX - Austin; MS 81 Univ of TX - Dallas; 88–Aud, Siemens Hearing Instruments, **A**

Taylor, Mrs Cynthia Lee 601 West Renner Road #222, Richardson, TX 75080, (214) 699-1095, BS 80 WV Univ; MS 83 Baylor Univ; Speech Language Pathologist, Lampasas ISD, **SLP**

Taylor, Dana R 7100 Louisiana N E #3206, Albuquerque, NM 87109, (505) 828-2028, MS 69 East TX St Univ - Commerce; Sp-Lang Path, Bernalillo Pub Sch, **SLP**

Taylor, Mrs Deborah S 14 Admas Road, Framingham, MA 01701, (617) 879-0752, SLP, **SLP**

Taylor, Deborah Susan 105 Eastview Drive, New Concord, OH 43762, (614) 826-7440, BS 84 Miami Univ - Oxford; MS 85 Miami Univ - Oxford; **SLP**

Taylor, Mrs Denise Catherine 7860 Boone Drive, Baton Rouge, LA 70808-6720, (504) 388-5356, BA 80 Western KY Univ; MS 81 Western KY Univ; Cl Superv, LA St U Sp/Hrng Cl, **SLP**

Taylor, Denise D Communication Therapy, Rt 1 Box 10, Farmerville, LA 71241, (318) 368-8142, BA 77 LA Tech Univ; MA 82 LA Tech Univ; Sp-Lang Path, Private Practice, **SLP**

Taylor, Denise Susan 130 Tara Drive, Roslyn, NY 11576, (516) 789-7342, BA 79 George Washington Univ; MA 81 Northwestern Univ; 86–Director of Sp-Lang Path, Brunswick Hosp Ctr Inc, **SLP**

Taylor, Diane I P 5537 South Atlanta Place, Tulsa, OK 74105-7214, (918) 245-5911, BS 68 Northeastern OK St Univ; MA 70 Univ of Tulsa; Superv Sp Lang Serv, OK Dhs Hissom Mem Cen, **SLP**

Taylor, Diane M 86-28 90th Street, Woodhaven, NY 11421, (212) 241-6153, BA 77 CUNY - Queens Coll; MA 79 CUNY - Hunter Coll; Aud, Mt Sinai Med Ctr, **A**

Taylor, Mrs Diane M 36055 Turpin Way, Fremont, CA 94536, (415) 792-0740, BS 78 UT St Univ; MS 81 UT St Univ; **SLP**

Taylor, Mrs Donna J 827 Moraine Drive, Lincoln, NE 68510, (402) 483-1115, BS 69 Univ of NE - Lincoln; MA 70 Univ of NE - Lincoln; Aud, Lincoln ENT Assoc, **A**

Taylor, Mrs Donna Lynn 2522 Camelot Court #144, Hollywood, FL 33026, (305) 435-1014, BS 79 Univ of IA; MA 81 Univ of IA; Aud, Hearx Ltd, **A**

Taylor, Donna M 2705 Folsom Avenue, Leavenworth, KS 66048, (919) 867-9203, BS 71 Univ of Science & Arts of OK; MS 76 Phillips Univ; **SLP**

Taylor, Ella Pat 95 Highpoint Drive, Gulf Breeze, FL 32561, (904) 432-6121, BA 49 LA St Univ - Baton Rouge; MA 76 LA St Univ - Baton Rouge; 78–Sp-Lang Path, Escambia Sch Dist, **SLP ACE**

Taylor, Mrs Esther Ruth Route 3 Box 17-B, Hope Mills, NC 28348, (919) 483-4037, BS 79 East Carolina Univ; MS 83 East Carolina Univ; SLP, Cumberland County Schools, **SLP**

Taylor, Evelyn J 354 Root Road, Modesto, CA 95351, (209) 571-6600, BA 77 CA St Univ - Stanislaus; MA 79 CA St Univ - Stanislaus; SLP, Stanislaus Co Schs, **SLP**

Taylor, Geraldine P O Box 1816, Fernley, NV 89408, (702) 789-1820, BS 75 Univ of NV - Reno; MS 81 Univ of NV - Reno; Sp-Lang Path, Associated Sp-Lang Path, **SLP**

Taylor, Harriet B Route 1 Box 711-P, Accokeek, MD 20607, (301) 283-3345, BA 54 Wayne St Univ - Sch of Med; MA 71 Univ of MD - College Park; Instr, Charles Cty Comm Coll, **SLP**

Taylor, Hazel E 2108 Bermuda Hills, Spring Valley, Columbia, SC 29223, **SLP**

Taylor, Mrs Honora Agnus 9401 South Forest, Chicago, IL 60619, (312) 264-6259, BS 59 Northern IL Univ - De Kalb; OM 87 Governors St Univ; 67–Sp-Lang Path, Chicago Bd of Educ

Taylor, Mrs Irma S Northwestern State University, Box 4133, Natchitoches, LA 71497, (318) 352-6193, BA 38 FL Southern Coll; MA 43 Univ of WI - Madison; **SLP LM**

Taylor, Mrs Jane E 4307 Saxonbury Way, Charlotte, NC 28213, (812) 376-6851, **SLP**

Taylor, Mrs Jeanne M Rt 4, 33 Dogwood Circle, Mechanicsville, MD 20659, (301) 862-2174, BA 74 George Washington Univ; MA 75 George Washington Univ; Sp/Lang Path, Green Holly Sch, **SLP**

Taylor, Joanne 2921 Foxcroft Drive, Tallahassee, FL 32308, **SLP**

Taylor, Dr Joyce S 90 Eastmoor, East Alton, IL 62024, (618) 692-3662, BS 60 Bradley Univ; MA 64 Bradley Univ; PH 69 (NS) Univ of MO - Columbia; Chmn, Southern Illinois University, **SLP**

Taylor, Dr Judy Ann 39 East 12th Street #808, New York, NY 10003, (212) 254-2331, BS 69 NY Univ; MA 70 NY Univ; DD 80 NY Univ; **SLP**

Taylor, Kathleen Helen 188 Shoshone Street #1, Buffalo, NY 14214, (716) 887-8063, BA 83 SUNY - Center at Buffalo; MA 85 SUNY - Center at Buffalo; **SLP**

Taylor, Mrs Kathleen Jeffrey 427 South Ninth Street, Chesterton, IN 46304, (219) 962-5751, BS 77 Purdue Univ - West Lafayette; MS 81 Northern IL Univ - De Kalb; 88–Sp-Lang Path, Cerebral Palsy of NW IN, **SLP**

Taylor, Mrs Kathleen Manuel 24 First Street, Mt Pearl, NF, Canada A1N 1X8, (709) 364-3402, BA 81 Memorial Univ - Newfoundland; MS 84 Dalhousie Univ - Nova Scotia; 86–Sp-Lang Path, Avalon Consolidated School Board, **SLP**

Taylor, Kathryn 1805 Mercury Drive, Garland, TX 75040, (214) 276-6357, BS 79 Southwest TX St Univ; MS 81 Minot St Univ; **SLP**

Taylor, Kathryn Bushman 625 Vallejo Villas, Los Angeles, CA 90042, (213) 464-3174, BA 73 CA Poly St Univ-San Luis Obi; MA 82 CA St Univ - Northridge; SLP, Los Angeles USD, **SLP**

Taylor, Dr Kenya S 1909 Pebblewood Drive, Arlington, TX 76006, (817) 921-7620, BA 73 Baylor Univ; MA 74 Baylor Univ; ED 85 (Counseling) Univ of TN - Knoxville; 88–Aud, Texas Christian Univ, **SLP A**

Taylor, Mrs Kerri Pool P O Box 1212, Friendswood, TX 77546, (808) 261-3234, **SLP**

Taylor, Mrs Kristine A 388 Main Street, Tonawanda, NY 14150, (716) 773-9100, BS 76 SUNY - Coll at Buffalo; MS 80 SUNY - Coll at Buffalo; SLP, Grand Island Sch Dist, **SLP**

Taylor, Mrs Lauren B 1187 Lawndale Road, Kenwood, CA 95452, (707) 528-5240, BA 69 Univ of CA - Los Angeles; MA 73 San Francisco St Univ; Sp-Lang Path, Santa Rosa City Schools, **SLP**

Taylor, Mrs Lilia Hinojo 1111 Eagle Drive #10, Denton, TX 76201, (817) 336-8611, BS 83 Univ of North TX; MS 86 Univ of North TX; 87–Sp-Lang Path, Child Study Ctr, **SLP**

Taylor, Linda Gayle 3739 Greenleaf Circle #205, Kalamazoo, MI 49008, (616) 674-8091, BA 66 Western MI Univ; MA 75 Western MI Univ; Sp-Lang Path, Van Buren Inter Sch Dist, **SLP**

Taylor, Linda J B 25 Burlington Road, Harwinton, CT 06791, **SLP**

Taylor, Mrs Lori Brosius 2113 Sir Lockesley Drive, Miamisburg, OH 45342, (513) 461-3000, BS 84 Miami Univ - Oxford; MS 85 Miami Univ - Oxford; **SLP**

Taylor, Lorraine Route 1 Box 77, Elora, TN 37328, (205) 539-6080, BS 85 AL A & M Univ; MS 86 AL A & M Univ

Taylor, Lynda Kay St Vincents Hospital, 1762 French Hill Road, Yorktown Heights, NY 10598, (212) 790-8678, **SLP ACE**

Taylor, Marcia H 312 King Richard Court, Jacksonville, NC 28540, (919) 451-2575, MA 76 Univ of IL - Champaign; 83–Sp-Lang Path, Camp Lejeune Dependent Schs, **SLP**

Taylor, Dr Margaret F 990 Sierra Madre Boulevard, San Marino, CA 91108, (818) 795-4454, BA Univ of MI - Ann Arbor; MA Univ of Southern CA; PH (Sp Path) Univ of Southern CA; **SLP LM**

Taylor, Mrs Margaret M 2519 Greenleaf Avenue, Wilmette, IL 60091, (312) 256-4699, BS 75 Northwestern Univ; MA 77 Northwestern Univ; Retired, Sch Dist 65, **SLP**

Taylor, Marilyn J 843-A Fairdale Road, Salina, KS 67401-8430, (913) 827-0301, BA 54 Ottawa Univ; MS 57 Univ of KS; Coord/Sp-Lang-Hrng Serv, Cent Kan Coop In Ed, **SLP**

Taylor, Mary Ann 2301 Waltham, Troy, MI 48098, (313) 258-3780, BA 83 MI St Univ; MA 86 Wayne St Univ; 88–Sp-Lang Path, William Beaumont Hosp, **SLP**

Taylor, Melissa C 321 Woodbury, Ponca City, OK 74601, (405) 762-4003, BS 84 OK St Univ; MA 86 OK St Univ; 86–Sp-Lang Path, Tonkawa PS, **SLP**

Taylor, Mildred S 7140 Talisman Lane, Columbia, MD 21045, **SLP**

Taylor, Mrs Myra Jane 8152 21st Street, Westminster, CA 92683, BA 33 Univ of Southern CA; MA 34 Univ of Southern CA; **A LM**

Taylor, Mrs Nancy Jane 1315 Shillington, Caty, TX 77450, (713) 578-5253, BS 67 Southwest TX St Univ; MS 69 Univ of North TX; Resource Teacher, **SLP ACE**

Taylor, Nancy L P O Box 361, East Winthrop, ME 04343, (207) 395-4553, BS 80 UT St Univ; MS 86 UT St Univ; 88–Sp-Lang Path, Mid State UCP, **SLP**

Taylor, Nancy Ruth Vizcaya Apt 5-H, 6101 34 Street West, Bradenton, FL 34210, (813) 756-3411, BS 62 CUNY - City College; MA 69 NY Univ; MA 83 Pace U -NY City; SLP, **SLP**

Taylor, Orlando L Howard University, Box 65, Washington, DC 20059, (202) 636-6711, BS 57 Hampton Univ; MA 60 IN Univ - Bloomington; PH 66 (NS) Univ of MI - Ann Arbor; Prof of Communications Science, Howard University, **SLP F**

Taylor, Mrs Pamela Beane 7650 County Road 65, Foley, AL 36535-9802, (205) 949-7794, BS 80 Auburn Univ - Auburn; MS 84 Univ of South AL; Sp-Lang Path, Baldwin Co Bd of Ed, **SLP**

Taylor, Pamela Hoffman 1609 Fenley Drive, Lebanon, IN 46052-1482, (317) 924-3251, **SLP**

Taylor, Mrs Patricia Ann 8918 River Road, Richmond, VA 23229, (804) 740-8244, **SLP**

Taylor, Patricia S 3350 Delmonte Blvd #A-6, Marina, CA 93933, (408) 649-1951, BA 73 Northwestern St Univ; MA 74 Northwestern St Univ; 84–Sp-Lang Path, Monterey Penn USD, **SLP**

Taylor, Paula N 500 Napa Valley #914, Little Rock, AR 72211, (501) 370-1830, OB 76 AR St Univ; OM 77 AR St Univ; SLP, AR Childrens Hosp, **SLP**

Taylor, Phyllis Ann P O Box 723821, Atlanta, GA 30339-0821, **SLP**

Taylor, Phyllis Arlene 1613 Camellia Drive, Elizabeth City, NC 27909, (919) 335-4305, BS 83 Univ of NC - Greensboro; MA 85 Hampton Univ; 85–Sp-Lang Path, Elizabeth City-Pasquotank Sch, **SLP**

Taylor, Phyllis B 745 West Palm, Reedley, CA 93654, **SLP**

Taylor, Rebecca Rae 3312 Central, Memphis, TN 38111, (901) 525-2682, BS 81 Purdue Univ - West Lafayette; MS 83 Purdue Univ - West Lafayette; 85–Aud, Memphis State Univ, **A**

Taylor, Renee R 117 West Rochester Apt 24, Ottumwa, IA 52501, (515) 682-8591, BS 86 Northeast MO St Univ; MA 87 Northeast MO St Univ; 87–Sp-Lang Path, Southern Prairie AEA

Taylor, Roxie G 118 Country Acres Road, Greenwood, SC 29646, (803) 223-4862, BA 76 St Andrews Presbyterian Coll; MA 79 Univ of TN - Knoxville; Sp-Lang Path, St Nicholas Sp & Hrng Cen, **SLP**

Taylor, Mrs Sandra Smith 2079 Royal Farms Drive #10, Salt Lake City, UT 84121, (801) 565-7100, BS 86 Brigham Young Univ; MA 87 Brigham Young Univ; **SLP**

Taylor, Sarah Oakley 3 Conver Drive, Saratoga Springs, NY 12866, (518) 587-3664, BA 78 Coll of Wooster; MA 79 Bowling Green St Univ; MA 83 Bowling Green St Univ; 87–Supvr of Sp-Lang Path, Sunnyview Hosp, **SLP**

Taylor, Mrs Sherri S 6713 Limestone, Houston, TX 77092, (713) 522-1051, BS 75 Univ of Central AR; MS 78 Univ of AR - Little Rock; Sp-Lang Path, Chldns Cen for Dev Ther, **SLP**

Taylor, Mrs Shirley Clarkston 608 Monnette Street, Pineville, LA 71360, (318) 487-5472, BA 84 Grambling St Univ; MA 87 LA Tech Univ; **SLP**

Taylor, Tamara Dawn 2307D Queen Street, Winston-Salem, NC 27103, (919) 777-0024, BA 82 Univ of NC - Chapel Hill; MS 84 Univ of NC - Chapel Hill; SLP, Davie County Schools, **SLP**

Taylor, Mrs Terri M 23472 Via Codorniz, Trabuco Canyon, CA 92679, (213) 598-7725, BA 83 CA St Univ - Long Beach; MA 85 CA St Univ - Long Beach; Audiologist, Private Practice, **A**

Taylor, Trudy A 154-A DE Sales Avenue, Mobile, AL 36607, (205) 473-8831, BA 75 Univ of South AL; MA 77 Univ of AL- Tuscaloosa; Sp-Lang Path, Mobile Co Pub Sch, **SLP**

Taylor-Walker, Ophelia 4722 41th Street N E, Tacoma, WA 98422, (206) 593-6814, BA 73 FL A & M Univ; MA 78 Univ of IA; Sp-Lang Path, Tacoma Pub Sch, **SLP**

Taymans, Dr Loretta M 14 West Cold Spring Lane, Apartment 813, Baltimore, MD 21210, (301) 243-3800, BA 56 Catholic Univ of America; MA 60 Catholic Univ of America; PH 76 (Sp Path) Northwestern Univ; Coord of Cl Serv, Hrng & Sp Agcy of Metro Balto, **SLP**

Tayrien, Mrs Lucille E 249 Beauregard Drive, Conroe, TX 77302, (409) 273-1782, BA 55 Univ of OK - Norman; 83–Sp-Lang Path, Curaflex Health Svcs, **SLP**

Tchaconas, Maria 233 East Wacker Drive, Apartment 3709, Chicago, IL 60601-5115, (312) 565-0786, BA 76 Baptist Bible Coll; MA 79 Northwestern Univ; Sp/Lang Path, Dist 45 Villa Park Il, **SLP**

Tea, Mrs Janice S 1128 North 300 East, Centerville, UT 84014, (801) 298-0481, MS 88 Univ of UT; Sp-Lang Path, Primary Children's Med Ctr

Teachman, Sandra E 16441 3rd S W, Seattle, WA 98166, (206) 242-6213, MA 88 Western WA Univ

Teachworth, Jill P 1441 Mill Race, Rochester, MI 48064-2089, (313) 651-2578, BA 71 CUNY - City College; MS 72 Columbia Univ Teachers Coll; MA 82 Oakland Univ; SLP, Utica Comm Schs, **SLP**

Teague, Mrs Cheryl C 905 North Columbus Street, West Liberty, IA 52776, (319) 627-4385, BA 68 Univ of OK - Norman; MS 69 CO St Univ; Sp-Lang Path, Grant Wood AEA, **SLP**

Teague, Laura Jo 1411 Audubon Avenue, Baton Rouge, LA 70806, (504) 343-2454, BA 75 LA St Univ - Baton Rouge; MA 78 LA St Univ - Baton Rouge; Sp-Lang Path, W Baton Rouge Parish Sch Bd, **SLP**

Teague, Mrs Melissa Carol 230 Silver Lake Road #F-11, Church Hill, TN 37642, (615) 246-4600, BA 84 East TN St Univ; OM 86 Univ of TN - Knoxville; Sp-Lang Path, Mountain Region Sp & Hrng Ctr, **SLP**

Teague, Rebecca Lynn 87 Whitfield Drive, Jackson, TN 38305, (901) 989-4611, BA 57 David Lipscomb Coll; MS 59 Vanderbilt Univ; ME 85 Memphis St Univ; 87–Sp-Lang Path, Pro Health Svc, **SLP**

Tear, Mrs Diane Louise 260 Morgan Street, Oberlin, OH 44074, (216) 775-1458, BA 82 OH St Univ; MA 86 Cleveland St Univ; Sp-Lang Path, Elyria City Schs, **SLP**

Tear, Susanne 7825 Northwest Skyline Blvd, Portland, OR 97229, (413) 592-4616, BA 72 Bucknell Univ; MA 81 Univ of MA - Amherst; Sp/Lang Path, Pioneer Devel Ctr, **SLP**

Teare, Sharon Wood 1312 North 52 Street, Omaha, NE 68132, (402) 346-2088, BS 74 SUNY - Coll at Buffalo; MS 76 SUNY - Center at Albany; Sp-Lang Path, Omaha Pub Sch, **SLP**

Teas-Hester, Dr Elizabeth A Teas NPI UCLA Center For Health Sci, 760 Westwood Plaza C8-692, Los Angeles, CA 90024-1759, (213) 825-0164, OB 55 Univ of KS; MA 76 Univ of CO - Boulder; PH 83 (NS) Univ of CO - Boulder; 85–Sp-Lang Path, Npi Univ of California at L A, **SLP**

Teas-Trudeau, Elizabeth C 170 Bartlett Street, Portsmouth, NH 03801, (603) 742-2676, BA 83 Univ of FL; MA 86 Univ of FL; Sp-Lang Path, Hillhaven Inc, **SLP**

Tebb, Michael Royal 8255 Buena Vista Road, Independence, OR 97351, (503) 838-2307, MA 70 San Jose St Univ; BA 68 Central WA Univ; 80–Pres & Sp-Lang Path, Cascade Sp & Hrng Cl PC, **SLP**

Tebbe, Bonnie C 7473 Rupert, Richmond Heights, MO 63117, (314) 658-2939, BA 69 Hanover Coll; MA 74 IN Univ - Bloomington; Clinic Coordinator, St Louis U/Dept Commun Dis, **SLP ACE**

Tebbetts, Ranier Barbara Box 379, Groton, MA 01472, (617) 448-6606, BS 77 Northeastern Univ; MS 83 Syracuse Univ; Sp-Lang Path, N Middlesex Reg Sch Dist, **SLP**

Tebinka, Jean A Audiology & Speech Pathology, Handicapped And Crippled Children's Unit, DC General Hospital, 19th & Massachusetts Avenue SE, Washington, DC 20003, (202) 675-7324, BS 71 Marquette Univ; MA 72 Bowling Green St Univ; Aud, Washington Dc Dept of Hum Serv, **A**

Tebow, Mrs Laura S 5109 Cheviot Road, Greensboro, NC 27405, (919) 288-3726, BA 77 Univ of NC - Greensboro; ME 81 Univ of NC - Greensboro; Sp-Lang Path, Greensboro Pub Sch, **SLP**

Tecca, Dr John E Constance Brown Hrng & Sp Ctr, 1521 Gull Road, Kalamazoo, MI 49001, (616) 343-2601, BS 76 WV Univ; MA 78 Memphis St Univ; PH 82 (Aud) Purdue Univ - West Lafayette; 84–Coord Aud Serv, Constance Brown Hrng/Sp Cen, **A**

Techler, Melinda Reily 9209 Seminok Blvd #122, Seminole, FL 34642, (813) 393-9790, **SLP**

Techler-Crowe, Helen 13702-B Utt, Tustin, CA 92680, (714) 634-5426, BA 73 Univ of South FL; MS 79 Univ of South FL; 83–Aud, Univ of Calif Med Ctr, **A**

Tedeschi, Jaye 1520 Eisenhower Drive, Apartment 234, Boulder, CO 80303, (303) 442-4650, MA 88 Univ of CO - Boulder

Tedesco, Brenda Elizabeth 41 Raff Avenue, Mineola, NY 11501, (516) 746-5789, BA 84 Adelphi Univ; MS 85 Adelphi Univ; **SLP**

Tedesco, Mrs Joni L 33047 Myrna Court, Livonia, MI 48154, (313) 557-3650, BA 78 Univ of MI - Ann Arbor; MA 80 CA St Univ - Los Angeles; Aud, Rontal, Rontal & Jacob, **A**

Tedesco, Mrs Karlyne A 6786 East Kettle Avenue, Englewood, CO 80112, (303) 753-9984, BA 67 Univ of Northern CO; MA 69 Univ of Northern CO; Sp-Lang Path, Cherry Creek Sch Dist, **SLP**

Teegardin, Kelly S 908 May Place, Fort Wayne, IN 46825, (219) 425-3053, BS 84 Purdue Univ - West Lafayette; MS 85 Purdue Univ - West Lafayette; **SLP**

Teekell, Mrs Joyce D 8809 Skyline Boulevard, Oakland, CA 94611, (415) 685-3533, BA 71 Univ of CA - Santa Barbara; MA 72 Univ of the Pacific; Sp-Lang Path, Mt Diablo USD, **SLP**

Teele, Mrs Miriam R 345 Chester Street #4, Glendale, CA 91203, (818) 240-7844, BS 84 Loma Linda Univ - Riverside; MA 85 CA St Univ - Los Angeles; **A**

Teeple, Gail 9 Ellen Heath Drive, Matawan, NJ 07747, (201) 750-3200, BA 62 Trenton St Coll; ME 66 Rutgers St Univ -N Brunswick; Sp-Lang Path, Woodbridge Board of Education, **SLP**

Teeter, Lee Harvill Route 1 Box 167, Tillar, AR 71670, (501) 392-2212, BS 84 Univ of AR - Little Rock; ME 87 Univ of Central AR; 88–Sp-Lang Path, Private Practice, **SLP**

Tefft, Donita R 220-A Roswell Avenue, Long Beach, CA 90803, (213) 940-7687, BS 80 OK St Univ; MA 82 OK St Univ; 88–Sp-Lang Path, Rancho Los Amigos Med Ctr, **SLP**

Tegeler, Robert Victor 102 South Main Street, Sioux Center, IA 51250, (712) 722-4374, BA 57 Univ of Northern IA; MA 65 Univ of Northern IA; 75–Dir Spec Educ, AEA 4, **SLP**

Tegfeldt, Joyce Ellen 307 N E Skipanon Drive, Warrenton, OR 97146, (503) 325-2862, Sp-Lang Path, Clatsop Education Service Dist, **SLP**

Tegtmeier, Diana Armbruster 4350 East Cherokee Road, Space 1, Stockton, CA 95205, (209) 468-6210, BA 61 Univ of the Pacific; MA 62 Univ of the Pacific; Sp-Lang Path, San Joaquin Gen Hosp, **SLP**

Tegtmeier, Mrs Mary E Teds Box D-1044, 2065 Half Day Road, Deerfield, IL 60015, (312) 940-9388, BS 78 Univ of WI - Stevens Point; MS 80 Univ of WI - Eau Claire; Sp-Lang Path, Excellcare Rehabilitation, **SLP**

Teich, Cathleen Box 770846, Eagle River, AK 99577, (907) 272-0586, BS 77 Univ of North TX; MS 82 East TX St Univ - Commerce; Sp-Lang Path, AK Treatment Ctr, **SLP**

Teich, Laurie 6 Lawterdale Circle, Asheville, NC 28804, (704) 251-6091, MS 73 Univ of SC - Columbia; Coord/Sp-Lang Path, Div of Health Svcs, **SLP**

Teich, Mrs Linda B Gill And Levinson Md Pc, 52 Beach Road, Fairfield, CT 06430, (203) 255-7424, BS 74 Boston Univ; MS 76 Columbia Univ Teachers Coll; 76–Aud, Gill and Levinson MD Pc, **A**

Teicher, Stephanie Hope 1012 Arcadia Avenue #8, Arcadia, CA 91006, (818) 445-4441, BS 84 SUNY - Coll at Fredonia; MA 86 Univ of CA - Santa Barbara; SLP, A Brown & Assoc, **SLP**

Teichert, Mrs Kathleen M 10958 Rock Island Road, Jacksonville, FL 32217, (904) 262-3048, MS 79 Auburn Univ - Auburn; BS 78 Auburn Univ - Auburn; **SLP**

Teig, Mary J 1400 Smokey Wood Drive, Apartment 602, Pittsburgh, PA 15218, **SLP**

Teigland, Dr Arne D Speech And Hearing Clinic, Moorhead State University, Moorhead, MN 56560, (218) 236-2286, BA 65 Moorhead St Univ; MA 68 Univ of WA; PH 76 (NS) Univ of WA; Dept Chair/Prof, Moorhead St U, **A**

Teitelbaum, Hedy 105 Popula Boulevard, Wappingers Falls, NY 12590, (914) 343-2424, BA 79 CUNY - Brooklyn Coll; MS 80 PA St Univ - Univ Park; Sp-Lang Path, Rehabilitation Programs Inc, **SLP**

Teitelbaum, Mrs Meryl A H 20 Waterford Drive, Wheately Heights, NY 11798, (212) 767-1593, BA 78 CUNY - Queens Coll; MA 79 Hofstra Univ; **SLP**

Teitelbaum, Mrs Susan Jane 9542 Netherway Drive, Huntington Beach, CA 92646, (714) 962-3663, BS 69 OH St Univ; MA 72 CUNY - Queens Coll; 84–Aud, Private Practice, **A**

Teitelreis-Sorenson, Judy 12104 Vienna Drive N E, Albuquerque, NM 87111, (505) 841-5135, BS 72 CUNY - Brooklyn Coll; MA 75 CUNY - Brooklyn Coll; Sp-Lang Path, Carrie Tingley Hosp, **SLP**

Teitscheid, Mrs Lorraine Quintero 200 Placerado Avenue, Auburn, CA 95603, BA 77 CA St Univ - Fullerton; MA 83 CA St Univ - Fresno; Sp-Lang Path, The Norma Bork Associates, **SLP**

Tek, Susan Downey 3920 King Drive, Brandon, FL 33511, (813) 654-1801, BA 81 Univ of MI - Ann Arbor; OM 86 Univ of SC - Columbia

Tekieli, Dr Mary E P O Box 187, 100 Idlewyle Lane, Fairmont, WV 26554, (304) 293-4241, **SLP F**

Telage, Dr Kal M Dept Speech Path & Audiology, New 310, Ithaca College, Ithaca, NY 14850, (607) 274-3248, BA 62 Univ of CT; MA 64 Univ of CT; PH 72 (NS) OH Univ - Athens; Assoc Prof, Ithaca College, **SLP**

Teleck, Verna Margaret 11790 S W Baker Street, Beaverton, OR 97005, (503) 649-0456, BS 56 Western OR St Coll; ME 59 Univ of OR; Sp/Lang Path, Beaverton Sch Dist #48, **SLP**

Telega, Mildred C 354 Hookstown Grade Road, Clinton, PA 15108, (412) 264-2288, BS 75 CA Univ of PA; ME 76 CA Univ of PA; Aug Comm Consult, Adaptive Commun Syst Inc, **SLP**

Telesmanic, Mrs Joanne C 6048 North Durant, Fresno, CA 93711, (209) 439-9190, BA 76 CA St Univ - Stanislaus; MA 78 CA St Univ - Stanislaus; Sp-Lang Path, Private Practice, **SLP**

Telesmanic, Dr Luciano P 6048 North Durant, Fresno, CA 93711, (209) 439-9190, BA 74 CA St Univ - Stanislaus; MA 76 CA St Univ - Stanislaus; ED 87 (Educational Management) Univ of LA Verne; Educational Consult, Fresno County Dept of Educ, **SLP**

Telian, Mrs Nancy Alemian 107 Lowe Avenue, Stoughton, MA 02072, (617) 341-2022, BA 76 Univ of CT; MS 78 Boston Univ; 86–Sp-Lang Path, Judith Wisnia & Associates, **SLP**

Tell, Mrs Elaine F 27355 Wellington, Franklin Village, MI 48025, (313) 966-3613, BA 73 CUNY - Queens Coll; MA 75 Wayne St Univ; 87–Coord/Sp-Lang Path, Grace Hosp, **SLP**

Telleen, Mrs Christine 701 Laurelwood Drive, San Mateo, CA 94403, (415) 666-5101, BA 69 Carleton Coll; MA 71 Northwestern Univ; MA 76 San Francisco St Univ; Aud, U of California, **A**

Telleen, Pamela Sue 4053 Dupont Avenue South, Minneapolis, MN 55409, (612) 627-3080, SLP, Minneapolis Public Schools, **SLP**

Telting, Diderika Marie 21 Steeplechase, Norman, OK 73072-2818, (405) 636-7434, BA 78 Univ of OK - Norman; MS 81 Univ of OK Medical Center; **SLP**

Telzak, Carol S 70 Riverside Drive #3E, New York, NY 10024, (212) 362-2097, BA 73 SUNY - Center at Buffalo; MA 75 SUNY - Center at Buffalo; 88–Sp-Lang Path, New York Hosp, **SLP**

Temin, Donna R 1264 Burnett Road, Huntingdon Valley, PA 19006, MS; **SLP**

Temin, Michael B 1264 Burnett Road, Huntingdon Valley, PA 19006, (215) 947-6939, BS 71 East Carolina Univ; ME 73 Northeastern Univ; Sp-Lang Path, Sch Dist of Phila, **SLP**

Tempalski, Karen 129 Frederick Drive, Ambridge, PA 15003, (412) 266-8640, MA 77 Edinboro Univ of PA; Sp-Lang Path, Allegheny Intermediate Unit, **SLP**

Tempel, Edward O 1234 Benjamin Holt Drive, Stockton, CA 95207, (209) 477-0478, BA 50 Univ of the Pacific; MA 62 Univ of the Pacific; Supvr Clinic, Univ of Pacific, **SLP**

Temple, Keryn Judith 3121 No Sheridan Rd #1414, Chicago, IL 60657, (312) 975-7053, BS 82 IL St Univ - Normal; MS 84 IL St Univ - Normal; Sp-Lang Path, Proviso Area for Exceptional Children, **SLP**

Temple, Linda Anne Apartment 308, 1781 Cherry Hill Road, Peterborough, ON, Canada K9K 1Y4, (705) 748-2221, BA 85 Minot St Univ; MS 86 Minot St Univ; 88–Sp-Lang Path, Five Counties Children's Centre, **SLP**

Temple, Vicki L 4411 Bank Drive #2, La Crosse, WI 54601, (608) 788-1271, BS 81 Univ of WI - Madison; MS 83 Univ of WI - Madison; Sp-Lang Path, Sch Dist of La Crosse, **SLP**

Templeman, Janette E 6032 Caprock Court #1906, El Paso, TX 79912, (915) 833-3917, BS 82 Eastern NM Univ; MS 85 TX Tech Univ; Sp-Lang Path, InSpeech Inc, **SLP**

Templeman, Mary A 632 S W 299th Street, Federal Way, WA 98023-3557, (206) 841-8744, BA 78 Univ of WA; OM 79 Univ of WA; SLP, Puyallup School District, **SLP**

Templet, Mrs Lisa Crochet 3604 Highway 70, Pierre Part, LA 70339, (504) 252-9824, BA 83 Nicholls St Univ; MS 85 Univ of Southwestern LA; 88–Sp-Lang Path, Ascension Parish Sch Bd, **SLP**

Templeton, Mrs Karla Mitchell 7210 Hosbrook Road, Madeira, OH 45243, BA 83 IN Univ - Bloomington; MA 84 IN Univ - Bloomington; Sp-Lang Path, Hamilton County Office of Educ, **SLP**

Templeton, Lillian Richeson 925 Alvarado Terrace, Walla Walla, WA 99362, (509) 525-3320, BA 65 Coll of Wooster; MA 66 MI St Univ; Sp-Lang Path, St Mary Med Cen, **SLP**

Templeton, Lynda Kay 1830 South Norwood, Independence, MO 64052, (816) 833-3433, MS 76 Central MO St Univ; Sp-Lang Path, Independence Sch Sys, **SLP**

Templin, Jessica Leigh Route 1 Box 428, Manson, WA 98831, (509) 687-3682, MA 88 Western WA Univ

Templin, Marilyn Susan 3146 Bennett, Wichita, KS 67217, (316) 942-4431, BA 83 Wichita St Univ; MA 87 Wichita St Univ; **SLP**

Templin, Dr Mildred C 521 5th Street S E, Minneapolis, MN 55414, (612) 331-5452, BA 36 Univ of WI - Madison; MA 37 Univ of WI - Madison; PH 47 (Child Psychology) Univ of MN - Minneap-St Paul; Prof Emerita, Univ of Minnesota, **SLP F H LM**

Tencza-Pinsonneault, Judith L 6205 36th Avenue East, Palmetto, FL 34221, (813) 729-2233, BS 80 Wayne St Univ - Sch of Med; MA 79 Wayne St Univ - Sch of Med; Sp-Lang Path, Manatee Co Schs, **SLP**

Tendler, Irene Oxford Heights, Tipton #9 Johnston Road, Albany, NY 12203, (518) 462-7187, BS 73 SUNY - Center at Albany; MS 74 SUNY - Center at Albany; Sp-Lang Path, Albany City School District, **SLP**

Tenenbaum, Mrs Joie K 5720 Reinhardt Drive, Fairway, KS 66205, BA 48 Univ of MO - Columbia; MA 70 Univ of KS; SLP, Ks Cty Mo Sch Dist, **SLP**

Tenenberg, Mrs Thelma K 1884 Clemens Road, Oakland, CA 94602, (415) 682-8000, BA 53 Roosevelt Univ; MA 65 San Francisco St Univ; Program Specialist, Mount Diablo USD, **SLP**

Tenenholtz, Elisabet Saudi Arabian Airlines, Cc 654, P O Box 167, Jeddah, Saudi Arabia 21231, OB 67 0181; OM 68 0180; MA 72 Northwestern Univ; 88–Sp-Lang Path, Juffali Help Ctr, **SLP**

Tennessen, Marilyn K 990 Southview Drive, Hastings, MN 55033, (612) 437-6111, BA 71 Univ of WI - Eau Claire; MS 74 Univ of WI - Eau Claire; Sp-Lang Path, Hastings Sch Dist #200, **SLP**

Tenney, Scott Charles 4412 Chestnut, P O Box 62, Cortland, IL 60112-9999, (312) 297-1022, BS 77 Southern IL Univ -Carbondale; MS 82 Southern IL Univ -Carbondale

Tennison, Mrs Shirley W 21 Highridge Road, Mount Kisco, NY 10549, (914) 241-2268, BS 65 MS Univ for Women; MA 66 OH Univ - Athens; Supvr/Instr, Tchrs Coll Columbia Univ, **SLP ACE**

Tennyson, Patricia J 231 West Cattle Call Drive, Apt 5, Brawley, CA 92227, (619) 344-8455, SLP, Imperial Co Ofc of Ed, **SLP**

Tenty, Linda Anderson 3828 Canterbury Court #GA, Richton Park, IL 60471, (312) 747-1801, OB 87 Governors St Univ; OM 87 Governors St Univ; 88–Sp-Lang Path, S Metro Assoc, **SLP**

Teodoro, Mrs Sally Ann 1125 East Utopia Road, Phoenix, AZ 85024, (602) 866-0147, BA 80 Brigham Young Univ; OM 81 Brigham Young Univ; Aud, Phoenix Chldrns Hosp, **A**

Teodoro, Stephen F 1125 East Utopia Road, Phoenix, AZ 85024, (602) 866-0147, BS 80 Brigham Young Univ; OM 81 Brigham Young Univ; Aud, Metro Hearing Svcs, **A**

Teodosio, Gail Elizabeth 36093 Cherry Street, Newark, CA 94560, (415) 796-0969, BA 82 San Jose St Univ; MA 87 San Jose St Univ; 85–Sp-Lang Path, Fremont USD

Teoman, Patricia Lynne 1401 S Harbor Boulevard, Apartment 4-J, La Habra, CA 90631, BA 84 Univ of MD - College Park; MS 86 PA St Univ - Univ Park

Tepe, Mrs Krista Lynn 1058 Webber Road, Loveland, OH 45140, (513) 742-2200, BS 82 Miami Univ - Oxford; MS 83 Miami Univ - Oxford; Sp-Lang Path, Hamilton Co Office of Ed, **SLP**

Tepper, Arthur S Danbury Hospital, 24 Hospital Avenue, Danbury, CT 06810, (203) 797-7504, BS 77 SUNY - Coll at Brockport; MA 78 Montclair St Coll; Aud, Danbury Hospital, **A**

Tepper, Mrs Carol M 65 Marvin Avenue, Rockville Centre, NY 11570, (516) 678-1395, BA 75 SUNY - Coll at Geneseo; MS 76 Ithaca Coll; **SLP**

Tepperberg, Mrs Iris Zimmerman 951 S W 133rd Terrace, Davie, FL 33325, MS 80 Univ of South FL; SLP, Broward Co Schs, **SLP**

Tepperman, Linda S 145 Commack Road, Commack, NY 11725, (516) 499-5360, BA 74 CUNY - Queens Coll; MA 76 Hofstra Univ; Sp-Lang Path/Dir, Commack Cen for Sp & Hrng Dis, **SLP ACE**

Terango, Dr Larry P O Box 457, Richmond, KY 40475, (606) 273-5000, BA 50 Kent St Univ; MA 52 Kent St Univ; PH 66 (Sp-Lang Path/Aud) Case Western Reserve Univ; **SLP A F**

Terasaki, Dr Diana Lynn 157 Seascape, Port Lavaca, TX 77979, (512) 552-5800, BA 74 Univ of Houston - Univ Park; MA 75 Univ of Houston - Univ Park; ED 80 (NS) Univ of Houston - Univ Park; Sp-Lang Path, Port Lavaca Clin Assoc, **SLP ACE**

Terbush, Connie Jean 2944 St Jude Drive, Drayton Plains, MI 48020, (313) 674-3760, MA 88 Eastern MI Univ

Terek-Ball, Linda M Route 1 Box 39-A, Talcott, WV 24981, (304) 466-3250, BS 76 Edinboro Univ of PA; MS 82 Radford Univ; Sp-Lang Path, Summers Co Sch, **SLP**

Tereshinski, Mrs Michele Renee 722 Montrose, Kalamazoo, MI 49008, (616) 427-7961, BS 82 Western MI Univ; MA 84 Western MI Univ; SLP, Van Buren Intermed School Dist, **SLP**

Tereshko-Ewart, Katherine Joan 165 Pierpont Street, Rochester, NY 14613, (716) 458-9409, BS 80 SUNY - Coll at Geneseo; MS 85 Nazareth Coll of Rochester; 88–Sp-Lang Path, Rochester City Sch Dist, **SLP**

Teresi, Pamela S 2612 Wildwood Drive, Haughton, LA 71037, (318) 949-3783, BA 78 Univ of NE - Lincoln; MA 80 Univ of NE - Lincoln; Sp-Lang Path, Bossier Parish Sch Bd, **SLP**

Ter Haar, Mrs Sandra S 3081 Locke S W, Grandville, MI 49418, (616) 677-3741, BS 79 Minot St Univ; MS 80 Minot St Univ; Sp-Lang Path, Holland Area Child Development, **SLP**

Terleski-Katz, Lynn R 1416 52nd Street, Sacramento, CA 95819-4121, (916) 736-2082, BS 76 East Stroudsburg Univ of PA; MS 80 AZ St Univ; 85–Sp-Lang Path/Neurodev Ther, Private Practice, **SLP**

Terr, Dr Arthur L 115 Old Shorthills Road, Apartment 564, West Orange, NJ 07052, (201) 736-3547, BA 48 Lebanon Valley Coll; MS 54 Syracuse Univ; ED 62 (NS) Columbia Univ Teachers Coll; Prof, Kean Coll, **SLP A**

Terran, Eileen M P O Box 1500, Santa Monica, CA 90406, (213) 394-8233, BA 68 Univ of MO - Columbia; MA 73 Univ of MO - Columbia; MA 85 Univ of CA - Los Angeles; **SLP**

Terrano, Cathy A R 15 Meroke Trail, Port Jefferson, NY 11777, MA 75 Hofstra Univ; Sp-Lang Path, Volz & Amato, **SLP**

Terranova, Susan Ann 30 Woodward Avenue, Buffalo, NY 14214, (716) 835-6009, BA 83 SUNY - Center at Buffalo; MS 84 2939; **A**

Terregino, Sr Antoinette 189 Brunswick Street, Jersey City, NJ 07302, (201) 596-3929, BS 49 Newark St Coll; MS 65 Fordham Univ; Sp-Lang Path, Mount Carmel Guild, **SLP**

Terrell, Dr Brenda Y School Of Speech Pathology And Audiology, Kent State University, Kent, OH 44242, (216) 672-2672, BS 72 Univ of TN - Knoxville; MA 73 Memphis St Univ; PH 83 (Communication Disorders) Univ of Pittsburgh - Pittsburgh; 88–Assoc Prof, Kent State Univ, **SLP**

Terrell, Joanne M 11146 Vance Jackson Road, Apartment 4005, San Antonio, TX 78230-2563, (512) 647-2100, BA 78 Our Lady Lake Univ-San Anton; MA 80 Our Lady Lake Univ-San Anton; Early Childhood Tchr, Northside ISD, **SLP**

Terrell, Dr Sandra L 5640 Cando Drive, Fort Worth, TX 76134, (817) 565-2262, BA 73 Univ of Pittsburgh - Pittsburgh; MA 74 Univ of Pittsburgh - Pittsburgh; PH 78 (Effects of Culture on Language) Univ of Pittsburgh - Pittsburgh; 79–Prof, Univ of No Texas-Div Comm Dis, **SLP ACE**

Terrero, Irene Aparatado 80616, Caracas, Venezuela 108, BA 72 George Washington Univ; MA 74 Northwestern Univ; OD 83 (NS); Dir of Sp & Lang Prog, Ministerio De Educ - Venezuela

Terrigno, Georgina B Rural Delivery 2, Peddlers Hill Road, Monroe, NY 10950, **SLP**

Terrill, Mrs Karen L 11650 North Annette Avenue, Mequon, WI 53092, (414) 242-3200, BA 77 Augustana Coll; MS 79 Univ of WI - Madison; 79–Sp-Lang Path, Mequon-Thiensville Sch Dist, **SLP**

Terrill, Mona C 638 East Teakwood Court, Highlands Ranch, CO 80126, (303) 861-3561, BS 76 CO St Univ; MS 78 Univ of AZ; 86–Sp-Lang Path, Kaiser Permanente, **SLP**

Terrill, Mrs Sally B 900 Orange Street, Chico, CA 95926, (916) 345-4500, BA 72 CA St Univ - Fresno; MA 73 Univ of the Pacific; SLP, Butte County Supntndnt Schools, **SLP**

Terrio, Dr Leelen M 2300 Lincoln Road #126, Hattiesburg, MS 39401, (601) 266-5224, BA 70 Nicholls St Univ; MS 74 Univ Southern MS-Hattiesburg; PH 82 (NS) FL St Univ; Asst Prof, U of Sn MS, **A**

Territo, Dr Jacqueline M 302 Field Club Ridge, Pittsburgh, PA 15238, (412) 963-1532, BS 69 Edinboro Univ of PA; ME 76 Duquesne Univ; PH 88 (Educ Curric & Superv) Univ of Pittsburgh - Pittsburgh; 83–Sp-Lang Path, Pittsburgh PS, **SLP**

Terrizzi, Dr Adrienne M 61 Pondview Drive, Amherst, MA 01002, (413) 594-2761, BA 63 Rutger's St Univ - Douglas Coll; MA 67 Seton Hall Univ; ED 87 (Higher Education) Univ of MA - Amherst; 78–Assoc Prof, Elms College, **SLP**

Terry, Anne C 111 Muirfield Court, Durham, NC 27712, (919) 575-7529, **SLP**

Terry, Barbara Graham 2011 Springdale Drive, Columbus, GA 31906, (404) 571-1090, BA 66 Southern Methodist Univ; ME 75 Trinity Univ; MA 67 Northwestern Univ; Aud, Rehab Serv of Columbus, **A**

Terry, Mrs Carole A 127 North 34th Street, Apartment 16-D, Richmond, IN 47374, (317) 935-2093, BS 61 IL St Univ - Normal; MA 79 Ball St Univ; 84–Sp-Lang Path, Reid Memorial Hospital, **SLP**

Terry, Mrs Diana B 3514 Shoreside Drive, Garland, TX 75043, (214) 240-7937, **SLP**

Terry, Joanna Lynn 229 Glenbrook Drive, New Braunfels, TX 78130, (512) 625-1674, **SLP**

Terry, Mrs Judith D 215 Shadowood Lane, Peachtree City, GA 30269, (404) 631-3265, BS 68 Univ of TX - El Paso; OM 70 Southern Methodist Univ; 82–Sp-Lang Path, Fayette Co Pub Sch Syst, **SLP**

Terry, Laura V 7117 Bobtail Drive, Shreveport, LA 71129, (318) 742-4210, BS 68 TX Woman's Univ; MA 76 LA Tech Univ; Sp/Lang Path, Bossier Parish Schs, **SLP**

Terry, Nancy Thomesn 1215 North Roosevelt, Wichita, KS 67208, (316) 689-9310, BA 81 Wichita St Univ; MA 83 Wichita St Univ; Aud, Wichita Cl, **A**

Terry, Susan E Broadwater Hearing Care, 4199 34th Street South, Suite C-101, St Petersburg, FL 33711, (813) 866-9365, BS 80 FL St Univ; MS 81 FL St Univ; 88–Aud, Private Practice, **A ACE**

Terry, Wayne S 1820 Barrs Street, Suite 322, Jacksonville, FL 32204, (904) 384-8088, BA 69 SUNY - Center at Buffalo; MA 72 SUNY - Center at Buffalo; 86–Aud, Dr Michael Lopez, **A**

Terway, Joanne August Lane #5-A, Flying Hills, Reading, PA 19607, (215) 777-7615, BS 60 Bloomsburg Univ of PA; MS 77 Bloomsburg Univ of PA; Sp/Lang Path, Reading Rehab Hosp, **SLP**

Teryek, Jo Anne E 359 Elvin Street, Staten Island, NY 10314, (718) 698-4153, BA 78 Saint Johns Univ - Staten Is; MA 81 Kean Coll of NJ; SLP, NYC Bd of Ed Speech Svc Unit, **SLP**

Teryl, Katherine J 94 Bramhill Court, East Amherst, NY 14051, (716) 837-2441, BS 83 SUNY - Center at Buffalo; MA 85 SUNY - Center at Buffalo; 85–Sp-Lang Path, Lang Dev Prog, **SLP**

Teselle, Nancy Eleanor 3287 Arizona Street, Oakland, CA 94602, (415) 531-5289, MS 87 San Francisco St Univ; 87–Sp-Lang Path, Richmond USD, **SLP**

Teske, Katherine 5837 Hithergreen Drive, Dayton, OH 45429, **SLP**

Tessandori, Mrs Joann S 1917 Stratford Drive, Owensboro, KY 42301, (502) 926-3030, BA 71 Univ of TX - El Paso; MS 76 Murray St Univ; Sp/Lang Path, Private Practice, **SLP**

Tessier, Mrs Amy B PO Box 87, Holden, MA 01520, (508) 832-5365, BA 73 Univ of MA - Amherst; MA 75 Univ of MA - Amherst; Pres, Hearing Care Delivered Inc, **SLP A**

Tessier, Maria Grazia 598 Moreland Avenue Apartment #1, Atlanta, GA 30307, (404) 377-1084, MA 88 Northwestern Univ; 88–Sp-Lang Path, The Davison Sch Inc

Testa, Carol Sue 193 Hickory Corner Road, Milford, NJ 08848, (201) 996-4751, BA 78 Montclair St Coll; MA 79 Ball St Univ; Aud, **A**

Testa, Donna Lee 122 Newbury Street, Framingham, MA 01701, (508) 872-5661, BS 84 Univ of MA - Amherst; MS 86 Northeastern Univ; 88–Aud, Otolaryngological Associates, **A**

Testa-Mack, Rosemary L 126 Cimarand Drive, Williamsville, NY 14221, (716) 688-2599, BS 79 SUNY - Coll at Buffalo; MS 81 SUNY - Coll at Buffalo; 79–Sp/Lang Path, Buffalo Publ Sch, **SLP**

Testut, Dr Eldred W Ithaca College, Dept Of Speech Path & Aud, Ithaca, NY 14850, (607) 274-3727, BA 68 SUNY - Coll at Cortland; MS 69 Univ of OK Medical Center; PH 80 (NS) Univ of OK Medical Center; Asst Prof of Aud, Ithaca College, **A**

Testut, Mrs Gay L 873 Taughannock Boulevard, Ithaca, NY 14850, BA 71 Abilene Christian Univ; MS 73 Univ of OK - OK City; **SLP**

Tetenman, Mrs Catherine Murray 75 Sunderland Drive, Auburn, ME 04210, (207) 783-0155, BA 72 Univ of ME - Orono; MS 83 Univ of NH; Sp-Lang Path, Lewiston Sch Dept, **SLP**

Teter, Constance Keenum 1700-A Utica Square, Suite 174, Tulsa, OK 74114, (918) 493-8498, BA 70 Wichita St Univ; MA 71 Wichita St Univ; Coord Sp-Path Serv, Cty of Faith Med and Res Cen, **SLP ACE**

Teter, Darrel Lee 6850 East Hampden Avenue, Denver, CO 80224, (303) 758-3415, BA 60; MA 61 Univ of Denver; PH 69 (NS) Univ of Denver; Pres, Private Practice, **SLP**

Teter, Mrs Mary G 85 Dunning Avenue, Webster, NY 14580, (716) 872-1770, BS 67 Bloomsburg Univ of PA; MA 68 OH Univ - Athens; Sp-Lang Path, Webster Ctrl Sch Dist, **SLP**

Teter, Mrs Wendy Beth 15 Honeysuckle Lane, Swedesboro, NJ 08085, (609) 769-0144, MA 84 Trenton St Coll; Sp-Lang Path, Woodstown-Pilesgrove Sch Dist, **SLP**

Tetlie, Rebecca Rice 1218 North Victoria Street, St Paul, MN 55117, (218) 487-3694, BA 80 Concordia Coll - Moorhead; MA 85 Univ of MN - Minneap-St Paul; **SLP**

Tetnowski, John A 3166 Stonecastle Road, Orlando, FL 32822, (305) 275-2328, **SLP**

Tett, Pamela G 12522 Blackstone Court, Houston, TX 77077, (713) 493-4438, BS 65 CO St Univ; MA 66 Univ of Houston - Univ Park; **SLP**

Tettemore, Barbara Lynn 11601 Suburnas Way, Santa Ana, CA 92705, (714) 821-3620, BA 71 Southern CA Coll; MA 79 CA St Univ - Fullerton; **SLP**

Tettinger, Mrs Kathryn Elaine 23 Kimberly Court, Sparta, NJ 07871, (201) 729-7851, **SLP**

Tetz, Mrs Shelley Marie/Rand 129 Cascade Street, Elgin, SC 29045, (803) 788-2383, BA 83 Univ of VT; MA 84 Western MI Univ; 88–Sp-Lang Path, New Medico Head Injury System, **SLP**

Tetzeli, Marta Christina 855 8OTH Street Apt #4, Miami Beach, FL 33141, (305) 861-9068, BA 85 Univ of CA - Santa Barbara; MS 87 Washington Univ

Teuber, Ann M 46 Ferncroft Road, Waban, MA 02168, (617) 527-0965, BS 74 Worcester St Coll; MS 77 Boston Univ; **SLP**

Teubl, Richard Joseph 4015 Kirtland Road, Willoughby, OH 44094, (216) 454-9461, BA 77 John Carroll Univ; MA 83 Cleveland St Univ; MA 87 Cleveland St Univ

Teubner, Mrs Cathy Briscoe 1310 Swifts Highway Unit H-103, Jefferson City, MO 65109, (314) 636-2720, OB 85 Univ of MO - Columbia; MA 87 Saint Louis Univ; **SLP**

Teubner-Rhodes, Mrs Louise 5 Orchard Road, Towson, MD 21204, (301) 823-4243, BA 75 Univ of MD - College Park; MA 77 Univ of KS; Sp-Lang Path, Private Practice, **SLP**

Tew, Mrs Lisa E H 2103 Monteray Court, Blacksburg, VA 24060, (703) 953-1402, BS 78 Purdue Univ - West Lafayette; MS 80 Purdue Univ - West Lafayette; Sp/Lang Path, **SLP**

Tew, Roy E 1303 N W 31st Street, Gainesville, FL 32605, PH (NS); **A LM**

Texada, Kristin E Southwest Human Development, 1366 East Thomas Road #100, Phoenix, AZ 85014-5739, (602) 997-8392, BS 76 Univ of NE - Omaha; MA 78 Univ of NE - Omaha; Dir Dine Cen, SW Human Dev, **SLP**

Textor, Mrs Catherine Tedder 700 Roberts Avenue, Apartment 202A, Lumberton, NC 28358, (919) 646-3524, MS 86 East Carolina Univ; 87–Sp-Lang Path, Dillon County Schs, **SLP**

Thachara, Babu Punan 94-29 Lefferts Boulevard, Richmond Hill, NY 11419, (718) 805-0250, BS 74 Univ of Mysore - India; MS 76 Univ of Mysore - India; PH 82 (Aud/Sp & Hrng) Univ of Mysore - India; 84–Sp-Lang Path/Aud, Bernard Fineson Developmental Ctr, **SLP A**

Thacker, Lynda JoAnne 724 Coral Ridge Circle, Rodeo, CA 94572, (415) 222-2161, BA 72 San Diego St Univ; MA 80 San Diego St Univ; Sp-Lang Path, Richmond USD, **SLP ACE**

Thacker, Mrs Susan Jane 11135-83 Avenue #509, Edmonton, AB, Canada T6G 2C6, BA 83 Western WA Univ; MA 85 Western WA Univ; **A**

Thacker, Mrs Teresa Ann R R 1 Box 142, Mc Lean, IL 61754, (309) 874-3242, BS 81 Eastern IL Univ; MS 82 IL St Univ - Normal; **SLP**

Thaden, Marilyn Joyce Box 21, Broadus, MT 59317, MS 72 Univ of MN - Minneap-St Paul; 88–Sp-Lang Path, Tri-County Spec Educ Co-op, **SLP ACE**

Thal, Dr Donna J 402 Brighton Avenue, Cardiff By Sea, CA 92007, (619) 534-2891, BA 68 CUNY - Brooklyn Coll; MS 71 CUNY - Brooklyn Coll; PH 78 (NS) CUNY - Grad Sch & Univ Cntr; 88–Asst Research Psych, Univ of California-San Diego, **SLP**

Thaler, Mrs Theresa K 8045 Hillrise Court, Elridge, MD 21227, (301) 796-7033, BA 80 Loyola Coll; MS 81 Loyola Coll; Sp-Lang Path, MD Sch for the Deaf, **SLP**

Thambooswamy, Leela 106 Van Wagner Road #1F, Poughkeepsie, NY 12603, **A**

Thames, Mrs Anita McNeece 1304 32nd Street, Laurel, MS 39440, (601) 426-6116, BS 75 Univ Southern MS-Hattiesburg; MS 81 Univ Southern MS-Hattiesburg; Sp-Lang Path, Laurel Sp-Lang-Hrng Center, **SLP**

Thamm, Mrs Merikaye Mitchell P O Box 520996, Big Lake, AK 99652, (907) 745-4822, BA 83 Eastern WA Univ; MS 84 Eastern WA Univ; 84–Sp-Lang Path, Matanuska-Susitna Sch Dist, **SLP**

Tharp, Patricia G 1410 East Glenoaks, Glendale, CA 91206, (213) 567-8871, MS 72 Univ of OK Medical Center; SLP, Los Angeles USD, **SLP**

Tharp, Paula L 1912 Parkwood, Olathe, KS 66062, **SLP**

Tharp, Roger L 15959 Leclaire, Oak Forest, IL 60452, BS 80 IL St Univ - Normal; MA 81 Western IL Univ; Aud, Oakforest Hosp, **A**

Tharpe, Anne M 1114 19th Avenue South, Nashville, TN 37212, (615) 320-5353, BS 79 Univ of AZ; MS 80 Vanderbilt Univ; Aud, Bill Wilkerson Hrng & Spch Cen, **A**

Thatcher, Deven M 110 Gilchrist, Punta Gorda, FL 33950, (813) 639-4071, BS 70 Univ of OK - Norman; MA 72 Univ of OK - Norman; **SLP**

Thau, Sandra Cohn 80 Prairie Avenue, Newton, MA 02166, (617) 536-7255, BA 76 Northwestern Univ; MA 77 Northwestern Univ; Dir, Emerson College, **SLP**

Thaxton, Loree D 412 East Goywood, Houston, TX 77079, BS; **LM**

Thayer, Dr Jean T 9439 Hickory View Place, Gaithersburg, MD 20879, (301) 424-5200, BA 59 Northwestern Univ; MA 75 Univ of CO - Boulder; PH 82 (NS) Univ of CO - Boulder; 87–Dir of Early Childhood Dev, Treatment & Learning Centers, **SLP**

Thayer, Mary Lape P O Box 167, West Hurley, NY 12491, (914) 338-9414, BS 75 SUNY - Center at Albany; MS 84 Coll of Saint Rose; Sp-Lang Path, NY State, **SLP**

Theadore, Mrs Geraldine Liguori Little Brook Road, Westerly, RI 02891, (401) 322-7875, BA 75 Univ of RI; MS 87 Univ of RI; 87–Sp-Lang Path, Bradley Hosp, **SLP**

Theander, Estelle J 56 Airmount Avenue, Ramsey, NJ 07446, (201) 327-3644, BA 49 Montclair St Coll; MA 54 Montclair St Coll; MA 69 Columbia Univ Teachers Coll; Sp-Lang Path, Bd of Ed, **SLP ACE**

Theard, Marie-Paule 4451 McClure Avenue, Gurnee, IL 60031, (312) 367-8000, BS 84 Marquette Univ; MS 87 Univ of WI - Milwaukee; 88–Sp-Lang Path, Hawthorn Sch Dist, **SLP**

Thebarge, Thomas N 3326 Ladoga Avenue, Long Beach, CA 90808, (213) 426-6522, BS 49 Univ of MN - Duluth; MA 51 Univ of CO - Boulder; Sp-Lang Path, Long Beach USD, **SLP**

Thebo, Mrs Jane L Hearing Associates Inc, 2700 Hospital Drive, Suite 320, North Kansas City, MO 64116, (816) 421-6262, BA 71 Univ of MO - KS City; MA 72 Univ of KS; Aud/Vice Pres, Hrng Assoc Inc, **A**

Theil, Carol Eastman 4246 Hertford Lane, Dublin, OH 43017, (614) 766-0753, BA 77 Allegheny Coll; MA 79 NY Univ; Sp-Lang Path, Delaware Sp & Hrng Ctr, **SLP**

Theimer, Lisa R 1875 West Seventh Avenue, Apartment 111, Vancouver, BC, Canada V6J159, (604) 584-2827, BS 82 McGill Univ - Quebec; MA 86 Univ of Pittsburgh - Pittsburgh; 87–Sp-Lang Path, B C Elks Aud Rehab Ctr

Theis, Mrs Denice K 20895 Coventry Drive, Brookfield, WI 53005, (414) 784-7294, BS 74 Univ of NE - Omaha; MS 75 Univ of NE - Omaha; **SLP**

Theis, Marsha Ann 210 Interwood Drive, Glencoe, MN 55336, (612) 864-4866, BA 68 Univ of MN - Minneap-St Paul; MA 70 Univ of MN - Minneap-St Paul; Sp-Lang Path, Hopkins Sch Dist #270, **SLP**

Theis, Mary Deany 1226 North Cedar, Hastings, NE 68901, (402) 463-4521, BA 80 Univ of NE - Lincoln; MS 82 Univ of NE - Lincoln; Coord of Sp-Lang Path, Mary Lanning Memorial Hosp, **SLP**

Theisen, Jane Elizabeth 105 Old Mill Pond #6, Grand Ledge, MI 48837, (517) 627-1384, BS 84 Western MI Univ; MA 85 Western MI Univ; **SLP**

Theiss, Kristen Jean 2215 Washington Avenue, Apartment 202, Silver Spring, MD 20910, (301) 495-0926, MA 84 Kent St Univ; Sp-Lang Path, Montg Co PS, **SLP**

Thelander, Mary J 95 Inglewood Drive, Toronto, ON, Canada M4T 1H7, (416) 965-6211, BS 71 Northwestern Univ; MS 72 Univ of MI - Ann Arbor; **SLP**

Thelen, Michael K 100 West Lawrence Street, Suite 106, Appleton, WI 54911, (414) 731-9611, BS 73 Univ of WI - Stevens Point; MS 79 Univ of WI - Oshkosh; Aud, Private Practice, **A**

Thelen, Patricia A 4763 East Plata Del Sol Drive, Las Vegas, NV 89121, (702) 486-5223, BS 74 Central MO St Univ; MS 86 Univ of WY; 87–Sp-Lang Path, State of Nevada-Health Div, **SLP**

Thelin, James W University Of Missouri, ENT MA314 Hsc, Columbia, MO 65212, (314) 882-8173, BA 68 Rice Univ; MA 73 Univ of IA; PH 80 (NS) Univ of IA; Chf Aud, Div of Otol/U of Mo Sch of Med, **A**

Thelin, Sara J 810 Yale, Columbia, MO 65203, (314) 474-9459, BA 68 CA St Univ - Los Angeles; MA 70 Univ of IA; 84–Sp-Lang Path, Missouri Dept of Health, **SLP**

Themides, Michelle Anne 4609 Birdie Court, Virginia Beach, VA 23462, (804) 497-5667, BS James Madison Univ; MS 86 James Madison Univ; 86–Sp-Lang Path, VA Bch Cty Sch Sys, **SLP**

Theo, Kathleen Johnson 32 Hurlbutt Road, Gales Ferry, CT 06335, (203) 464-7977, BA 76 Allegheny Coll; MS 78 Adelphi Univ; Sp/Lang Path, **SLP**

Theros, Jean A 704 Collier Road N W, Atlanta, GA 30318, (404) 233-5332, BS 74 Northwestern Univ; MA 75 Northwestern Univ; **SLP**

Therriault, Teresa Marie 3045 125th Avenue N E, Bellevue, WA 98005, (213) 273-8480, BS 83 Univ of WA; MS 85 Univ of AZ; **SLP**

Therrien, Kathleen Rose Route 3 Box 262-A, Mechanicsville, MD 20659, (301) 884-5033, **SLP**

Therrien, Mrs Sheila B 3 Langley Lane, Andover, MA 01810, (617) 681-9062, BA 69 Boston Coll; ME 70 Boston Univ; Sp-Lang Path, The Sp & Lang Ctr, **SLP**

Theurer, John J 215 Halsey Avenue, Jericho, NY 11753, (718) 470-8920, BA 56 Syracuse Univ; MS 65 Adelphi Univ; Chief/Aud, Lng Isl Jewsh-Hillside Med Cen, **A**

Theys, Debi A D 4432 Westmont, Ventura, CA 93003, (805) 644-0332, BA 75 CA St Univ - Chico; MA 76 CA St Univ - Chico; SLP, Moorpark USD, **SLP**

Theys, Mrs Leslie Ann 2365 Granville Road, West Bend, WI 53095, (414) 675-6784, BS 86 Univ of WI - Stevens Point; MS 87 Marquette Univ; 88–Sp-Lang Path, ABC Kids Care, **SLP**

Thibaudeau-Meyers, Camille 1460 37th Avenue, Kenosha, WI 53142, BS 71 Univ of WI - Milwaukee; MS 74 Univ of WI - Milwaukee; SLP, Kenosha USD #1, **SLP**

Thibedeau, Mrs Susan B 1851 Heritage Lane, New Brighton, MN 55112, (612) 422-5234, BA 67 Univ of IA; MA 70 Western MI Univ; Sp-Lang Path, Early Childhood Anoka-Henn 11, **SLP**

Thibodeau, Mrs Linda Mesloh Department Of Speech Communication, University Of Texas At Austin, Austin, TX 78715-1089, (512) 471-3841, BA 75 Univ of TX - Austin; MA 77 Univ of TX - Austin; PH 86 (Sp & Hrng Science) Univ of MN - Minneap-St Paul; 86–Asst Prof, Univ of Texas, **SLP A**

Thibodeaux, Carol Ann 254 Ridgewood Street, Lafayette, LA 70506, (318) 234-8083, MS 84 Univ of Southwestern LA; Sp-Lang Path, Private Practice, **SLP**

Thibodeaux, Darline Marie 254 Ridgewood Street, Lafayette, LA 70506, (318) 236-6800, BA 81 Univ of Southwestern LA; MS 87 Univ of Southwestern LA

Thibodeaux, Mrs Regina Cecile 1007 West St Mary Boulevard, Lafayette, LA 70506, (318) 981-3434, BA 81 Univ of Southwestern LA; MS 82 Lamar Univ; 87–Clin Supvr, Univ of Southwest LA, **SLP**

Thiebaut, Jeanine Marie RFD 3 Cushman Road, Amherst, MA 01002, (413) 548-9269, MA 83 Univ of MA - Amherst; 87–Sp-Lang Path, Amherst-Pelham PS, **SLP**

Thiel, Jeanne M 1412 East 54th Place, Chicago, IL 60615, **SLP**

Thiel, Sharon K 3629 Kevington, Eugene, OR 97405, (505) 334-9505, BS 80; MS 82; Sp-Lang Path, Albuquerque Public Schools, **SLP**

Thielemeir, Margaret Ann 2915 Harbor View Drive, Corona Del Mar, CA 92625, (714) 644-2910, BA 74 Univ of CA - Santa Barbara; MA 81 Univ of MN - Minneap-St Paul; Aud, **A**

Thielen, Joann C 1613 Littlejohn Circle #1, Council Bluffs, IA 51501, (515) 582-3382, BA 75 Univ of Northern IA; MA 76 Univ of Northern IA; SLP, Northern Trails AEA, **SLP**

Thieme, Amy 1005 Zinnia Street, Golden, CO 80401, (303) 674-3329, BA 72 Southeast MO St Univ; MS 74 Eastern IL Univ; R-1 Sch Dist Jeff Co Colo, **SLP**

Thiemkey, Mrs Roberta 9363 Riverside Drive, St Louis, MI 48880, (517) 681-5912, BS 76 Northeast MO St Univ; MA 77 Northeast MO St Univ; Consult/Sp-Lang Path, Schnepp Health Care Center, **SLP**

Thies, Mrs Harriet Fleischer 2223 Golden Meadow Drive, Duarte, CA 91010, (818) 357-6676, BA 63 CUNY - Brooklyn Coll; MA 71 CA St Univ - Los Angeles; Tchr, L A Co Supt of Schs, **SLP**

Thies, Dr Terry L 2223 Golden Meadow Drive, Duarte, CA 91010, (818) 960-3802, BS 64 Univ of IA; MA 70 CA St Univ - Los Angeles; PH 82 (NS) Univ of Southern CA; Assistant Principal, Los Angeles County Off of Educ, **SLP A**

Thiesen, Lauren Joy 408 Shabbona Drive, Park Forest, IL 60466, (312) 747-2329, BS 76 IL St Univ - Normal; MS 77 IL St Univ - Normal; **SLP**

Thietje, Mrs Joanne G 1535 West Linden Avenue, Fremont, NE 68025, (402) 727-3020, BS 64 Univ of NE - Omaha; MA 70 Univ of NE - Lincoln; Sp-Lang Path, Fremont Pub Sch, **SLP**

Thigpen, Mrs Carol Evangeline 19 Begonia Court, Jackson, MS 39206, (601) 956-5361, BS 77 Jackson St Univ; MS 86 Univ of MS; 79–Sp-Lang Path, Jackson PS, **SLP**

Thigpen, Mrs Mary Catherine 1005 Capri Court, Crestview, FL 32536, (904) 682-5153, BA 77 Univ of FL; MS 78 FL St Univ; Sp-Lang Path, Okaloosa County Sch Bd, **SLP**

Thigpen, Mrs Sheron S Route 4 Box 244, Waynesboro, GA 30830, (404) 554-9839, BS 87 Univ of GA; ME 87 Univ of GA; **SLP**

Thile, Dr Edmund L 3990 Old Town Avenue, Suite 102C, San Diego, CA 92110, (619) 265-6477, BA 53 San Diego St Univ; MA 55 Univ of Southern CA; PH 67 (NS) Univ of Southern CA; Prof, San Diego St U-Dept Commun Dis, **SLP**

Thinglum, Dr Harold J Oak Forest Hospital Speech, 15900 South Cicero Avenue, Oak Forest, IL 60452, (312) 687-7200, BA 71 Northern MI Univ; MA 72 Northern MI Univ; PH 78 (NS) Univ of IL - Urbana; Dir of Lang Sp & Hrng, Oak Forest Hosp, **SLP**

Thingvold, Jacqueline Williams Rural Route 1, Muscoda, WI 53573, (507) 454-2930, MS 80 Univ of WI - Whitewater; 86–Asst Prof Sp-Lang Path, Coll of St Teresa, **SLP**

Thios, Mrs Barbara M 461 Stublyn Road, Granville, OH 43023, (614) 587-6774, BS 67 WV Univ; ME 71 Univ of VA - Charlottesville; Instructor, Denison Univ, **SLP**

Thistlethwaite, Nancy L HC 79 Box 4223, Chugiak, AK 99567, (907) 688-3723, BA 75 Univ of FL; MS 77 Univ of OR; 86–Sp-Lang Path, Providence Hosp Rehab Ctr, **SLP**

Thole, Mrs Kim Price 1297 Birmingham Street, St Paul, MN 55106, (612) 780-9155, BA 81 Univ of MO - KS City; MS 83 Central MO St Univ; Sp-Lang Path, Coon Rapids Med Ctr, **SLP**

Thoma, Joan A 30 Grande Vista Drive, Novato, CA 94947, (415) 561-5267, BS Univ of Pittsburgh - Pittsburgh; MS Univ of Pittsburgh - Pittsburgh; Aud, Letterman Army Med Cen, **A ACE**

Thoma, Nancy Lynn 17275 S W Blanton, Aloha, OR 97007, (503) 648-1126, MA 84 Univ of Northern CO; Sp-Lang Path, Hillsboro Elem Sch, **SLP**

Thoma, Pamela Susan 2411 Solutaris #D-1, Cincinnati, OH 45206, (513) 732-9200, BS 83 Miami Univ - Oxford; MA 84 Miami Univ - Oxford; 87–Supvr, Southwest Ohio Dev Ctr, **SLP**

Thoman, Connie Lyn 2520 Nason Avenue, El Cerrito, CA 94530, (415) 456-9680, BA 83 Univ of Toledo; MS 85 Univ of MI - Ann Arbor; Sp-Lang Path, Kentfield Rehab Hosp, **SLP**

Thomas, Mrs Alice F 5715 Charlie Chan, San Antonio, TX 78240, (512) 680-0430, BS 80 Northwest MO St Univ; MS 81 Northwest MO St Univ; Sp/Lang Path, Northside ISD, **SLP**

Thomas, Angella Hough 5600 Molly's Place Court, Charlotte, NC 28212, (704) 535-4458, BA 80 Univ of SC - Columbia; MA 82 SC St Coll; SLP, Rockhill P S

Thomas, Mrs Ann Bosse 4819 West 64th Street, Prairie Village, KS 66208, (913) 384-6428, BS 80 LA St Univ - Baton Rouge; MA 81 LA St Univ - Baton Rouge; 85–Sp-Lang Path, Private Practice, **SLP**

Thomas, Ann Christine 5308 Abingdon Place, Austin, TX 78723-3117, (512) 471-3841, OB 75 Southwestern Univ; MA 85 Univ of TX - Austin; Sp-Lang Path, Univ of Texas at Austin, **SLP**

Thomas, Barbara Ann 2929 S Boston Court, Tulsa, OK 74114, (918) 747-2593, BA 78 Northeastern OK St Univ; MA 82 OK St Univ; 88–Sp-Lang Path, Owasso PS, **SLP**

Thomas, Barbara Cassidy 4212 Highview Drive, San Mateo, CA 94403, (415) 349-7434, BS 77 CO St Univ; MS 80 Portland St Univ; Sp-Lang Path, Assoc Lrng Lang Specialist, **SLP**

Thomas, Barbara E 1818 Riggs Place N W #109, Washington, DC 20009, (202) 462-6999, BA 76 Temple Univ; MS 87 Univ of the DC

Thomas, Barbara Ellen 1401-A Lochner Road, Baltimore, MD 21239, BA 70 Towson St Univ; MS 83 Towson St Univ; Sp/Lang Path, U of MD/Dept Neurology, **SLP**

Thomas, Beth Fullerton Arlington Hospital Pm&R Dept, 1701 North George Mason Dr, Arlington, VA 22205, (703) 558-6507, BA 76 Catholic Univ of America; MA 78 Catholic Univ of America; Sp-Lang Path, Arlington Hosp, **SLP**

Thomas, Bettie McLawhorn Route 2 Box 117, Zionville, NC 28698, (919) 246-7175, BS 74 Appalachian St Univ; MA 78 Appalachian St Univ; Sp-Lang Path, Ashe County Board of Education, **SLP**

Thomas, Mrs Billie J 2939 Eckert Road Route 9, Lexington, OH 44904, (419) 884-1792, BA 72 Marshall Univ; MA 73 Marshall Univ; 87–Sp-Lang Path, Highland Local Schs, **SLP**

Thomas, Bruce M 641 Bowen Street, Dayton, OH 45410-2422, **A**

Thomas, Mrs Carol L 364 Quarry Brook Drive, South Windsor, CT 06074, (203) 644-6334, BA 64 Univ of KY; MA 67 Univ of KY; ME 72 Univ of Louisville; Sp-Lang Path, Hartford Board of Education, **SLP A**

Thomas, Mrs Carolyn Denise 869 Woodford Avenue, Youngstown, OH 44511, (216) 726-8855, BA 75 Kent St Univ; MA 76 Kent St Univ; SLP, Youngstown Hrng & Sp Cen, **SLP**

Thomas, Carolyn Marie 5381 Big Tyler Rd #102, Charleston, WV 25313, (304) 776-8237, OB 83 Indiana Univ of PA; ME 85 Univ of VA - Charlottesville; **A**

Thomas, Celeste 5770 East Warren #308-C, Denver, CO 80222, (303) 690-1155, BS 77 Northwestern Univ; MA 79 Univ of Denver; Sp-Lang Path, Aurora Public Schools, **SLP**

Thomas, Cheryl Ann 12 Highland Circle, Hadley, MA 01035, (413) 549-5119, BS 83 Univ of MA - Amherst; MA 85 Univ of MA - Amherst; 85–Sp-Lang Path, Monson Developmental Center, **SLP**

Thomas, Mrs Claudell F 2634 Whippoorwill Lane, Enid, OK 73703, (405) 234-3734, BA 61 Phillips Univ; OM 64 Univ of OK Medical Center; Dir, Comm Sp & Hrng Cen, **SLP**

Thomas, Mrs Cleopatra Word 2692 Dusk Drive, San Diego, CA 92139, (619) 483-0690, **A**

Thomas, Mrs Connie S 67 Fawn Lake Forest, Hawley, PA 18428, (717) 698-5647, BS 69 IN St Univ - Terre Haute; MS 70 IN St Univ - Terre Haute; Dir-Rehab & Soc Svcs, Julia Ribaudo Home, **SLP**

Thomas, Constance Ann 1430 South First, Springfield, IL 62704, (217) 544-4459, BS 83 IL St Univ - Normal; MS 84 IL St Univ - Normal; 84–Sp-Lang Path, Springfield Sch Dist #186, **SLP**

Thomas, Mrs Corinne Adele 304 Masterson Pass #142, Austin, TX 78753, (512) 452-3028, MA 84 Brigham Young Univ; Sp-Lang Path, Austin ISD, **SLP**

Thomas, Curtis Gerald 96 East 900 North, Price, UT 84501, (801) 637-9255, BS 81 UT St Univ; OM 82 Brigham Young Univ; Chief of Aud, Castleview ENT Clinic, **A**

Thomas, Cynthia 7425 Armstrong Place #C11, San Diego, CA 92111, (619) 576-5837, BA 79 San Diego St Univ; MS 80 Univ of MI - Ann Arbor; **SLP**

Thomas, Mrs Cynthia Stager 4802 Rolling Meadows Lane, Signal Mountain, TN 37377, BS 77 Appalachian St Univ; ME 80 Univ of NC - Greensboro; 88–Sp-Lang Path, Associated Children's Therapies, **SLP**

Thomas, Deborah P O Box 187, Hoyt, KS 66440, (913) 986-6129, BS 73 Univ of KS; MS 74 Central MO St Univ; SLP, Holton Spec Ed Coop, **SLP**

Thomas, Mrs Debra Elizabeth 19272 Echo Pass Road, Trabuco Canyon, CA 92679, (714) 551-2301, BA 77 CA St Univ - Long Beach; MA 81 CA St Univ - Long Beach; Sp-Lang Path, Irvine USD, **SLP**

Thomas, Mrs Debra F 401 Beverly Island, Pontiac, MI 48054, (313) 828-6003, BS 78 Bowling Green St Univ; MA 79 MI St Univ; Sp-Lang Path, Wm Beaumont Hosp-Troy, **SLP**

Thomas, Mrs Dolores Adams 882 Kings Post Road, Rockledge, FL 32955, (407) 632-4491, BA 84 Univ of Central FL; MA 85 Univ of Central FL; 85–Sp-Lang Path, Brevard Co Sch Bd, **SLP**

Thomas, Donna Terry 1334 Craigmont, El Cajon, CA 92019-3108, (318) 742-2715, BA 85 LA St Univ - Shreveport; OM 86 LA St Univ - N O Medical Ctr; **SLP**

Thomas, Doreen M 418 Meadow Street #D-14, Agawam, MA 01001, (413) 789-1642, MS 79 Northwestern Univ; Chief Sp-Lang Path, Healthwin Hospital, **SLP**

Thomas, Mrs Elizabeth 3206 Casey Key Road, Nokomis, FL 34275, (813) 966-2338, BA 76 Duke Univ; MA 80 IN Univ - Bloomington; Cl Path, National Sp Hrng Servs, **SLP**

Thomas, Elizabeth Ruth 4308 Feldspar Court, Union City, CA 94587, (415) 636-1752, BA 81 CA St Univ - Hayward; MS 84 San Francisco St Univ; 85–Sp-Lang Path, Oakland USD, **SLP**

Thomas, Ellen Diane 1907 Yacht Enchantress, Newport Beach, CA 92660, (714) 644-9196, BS 77 Southwest MO St Univ; MS 79 Central MO St Univ; Sp-Lang Path, Irvine School District, **SLP**

Thomas, Faytrene Noyes 318 West 24th, Pine Bluff, AR 71601, (501) 536-7900, BS 79 Univ of AR - Pine Bluff; MS 86 Univ of Central AR; SLP, Pine Bluff School System, **SLP**

Thomas, Georgeanne Marie 526 Adler Drive, Montgomery, AL 36116, (205) 834-7221, MS 84 Univ of Montevallo; Audiologist, Montgomery Otolaryncology, **A**

Thomas, Mrs Gretchen Ann 3769 Harvard Acres, Cincinnati, OH 45227, (573) 742-2200, BS 78 Miami Univ - Oxford; MS 81 Miami Univ - Oxford; Sp/Lang Path, Hamilton Co Office Ed, **SLP**

Thomas, Inge Hinrichs PO Box 49142, Atlanta, GA 30359, (404) 321-6111, BS 77 Univ of Montevallo; MS 79 Univ of OK - OK City; PH 88 (Comm Disorders Lang) Univ of OK - OK City; 88–Sp-Lang Path, VA Med Ctr, **SLP**

Thomas, Jack E Speech Language Pathology, Mayo Clinic #E8A, Rochester, MN 55905, (507) 284-3112, BS 74 Univ of OR; MS 82 Portland St Univ; Sp-Lang Path, Mayo Clinic, **SLP**

Thomas, Jane D 1489 Massey Road, Memphis, TN 38119, (901) 683-8530, BS 70 Auburn Univ - Auburn; MS 72 Univ of AL- Tuscaloosa; **SLP**

Thomas, Janet E 392 Central Park West, New York, NY 10025, (212) 579-5440, BA 71 Barat Coll; MS 73 Columbia Univ Teachers Coll; Sp-Lang Path, Lincoln Hosp Cerc C-2, **SLP**

Thomas, Jayne F 5624-D Kingsgate Place, Charlotte, NC 28226, (803) 283-8547, BA 62 Winthrop Coll; MA 74 Winthrop Coll; MS 76 Winthrop Coll; SLP, Total Care Inc, **SLP**

Thomas, Mrs Jean Feddersen 500 Emmet Street, University Gardens H-9, Charlottesville, VA 22903, (804) 924-2050, BS 80 Bradley Univ; MS 84 Vanderbilt Univ; Aud, Univ of VA Med Center, **A**

Thomas, Mrs Jean Marie 121 Cedar Street, West Union, IA 52175, (319) 245-1480, **SLP**

Thomas, Mrs Jill E P O Box 643, Wampsville, NY 13163, (315) 363-3159, BS 73 SUNY - Coll at Fredonia; MS 78 Syracuse Univ; Sp-Lang Path, **SLP**

Thomas, Judith Allyn 6422 Amber Court, Mason, OH 45040, (513) 244-3109, BS 71 Saint Mary's Dominican Coll; MA 77 Univ of Cincinnati; Sp-Lang Path, Private Practice, **SLP**

Thomas, Julia Mae 700 Montgomery, Lee's Summit, MO 64063-3632, (816) 363-4606, BS 82 Central MO St Univ; MS 84 Central MO St Univ; Sp-Lang Path, Sherwood Center, **SLP**

Thomas, Mrs Karen L 4515 Whiteford Lane, Fort Wayne, IN 46816, (219) 447-1110, BS 79 Purdue Univ - West Lafayette; MS 81 Purdue Univ - West Lafayette; 88–Sp-Lang Path, Private Practice, **SLP**

Thomas, Kathleen Ann 76 Wellington Road, East Brunswick, NJ 08816, (201) 321-7765, BA 83 Rutger's St Univ - Douglas Coll; MA 84 Northwestern Univ; Sp-Lang Path, John F Kennedy Med Ctr, **SLP**

Thomas, Mrs Kathleen Palmer 86 Marlborough Street, Boston, MA 02116, (617) 424-8625, BA 72 Univ of TX - Austin; MA 74 LA St Univ - Baton Rouge; Supvr, InSpeech Inc, **SLP**

Thomas, Mrs Kathryn C 143 Thornwood Drive, Marlton, NJ 08053, BA 77 Asbury Coll; MA 79 Montclair St Coll; Sp-Lang Path, St John of God Comm Svcs, **SLP**

Thomas, Kathy Wright 5926 Penrose, Dallas, TX 75206, BS 82 Univ of North TX; MS 85 Univ of North TX; **SLP**

Thomas, Kenneth E P O Box 473, FPO Seattle, WA 98764, BA 72 Brigham Young Univ; MS 78 UT St Univ; 80–Sp-Lang Path, DoD Dep Sch, **SLP**

Thomas, Dr Kenneth P 506 East Cheves Street, Florence, SC 29501, BS 70 Univ of SC - Columbia; OM 75 Univ of SC - Columbia; PH 82 (NS); Aud, Private Practice, **A**

Thomas, Kimberly Roxanne Iowa Methodist Medical Center, 1200 Pleasant Street, Speech Path & Aud Dept, Des Moines, IA 50309, (515) 283-6344, BS 82 IA St Univ; MA 84 Univ of IA; Sp-Lang Path, Iowa Methodist Med Ctr, **SLP**

Thomas, Kirsten Lynn 515 Buford Drive East, Mobile, AL 36608, (205) 343-5177, MS 88 Univ of South AL

Thomas, Kristi Harbage 1208 Meadowwood Drive, Kinston, NC 28501, (919) 523-8071, BS 72 KS St Univ; MA 76 Kent St Univ; Aud, Lenoir Co Sch, **A**

Thomas, Mrs Laura O 3030 West Sacramento Avenue, Chico, CA 95926, (916) 891-0415, BS 67 CO St Univ; MA 70 CA St Univ - Chico; Supvr Sp-Lang Path, Butte Co Ofc of Educ, **SLP**

Thomas, Laurie Bunten 7021 Edwina Avenue, Albuquerque, NM 87110, (505) 884-8157, MS 86 Univ of NM; 87–Sp-Lang Path, Albuquerque PS, **SLP**

Thomas, Laurie J 153 Glenside Avenue, Linwood, NJ 08221, (609) 927-1916, BS 78 WV Univ; MS 79 WV Univ; 84–Sp-Lang Path, Winchell Sch, **SLP**

Thomas, Linda Kay 3100 Russell Way Lane, Winston-Salem, NC 27127, (919) 748-3103, BS 79 East Carolina Univ; MA 80 Univ of TN - Knoxville; Aud, N C Baptist Hospital, **A**

Thomas, Lori L 303 74th Street Court N W, Bradenton, FL 33529, (813) 792-6611, MS 81 Univ of South FL; Sp/Lang Path, L W Blake Memorial Hospital, **SLP**

Thomas, Mrs Margaret F 70 Eat Water Street, Toms River, NJ 08753, (201) 270-5269, BS 72 Trenton St Coll; MA 77 Trenton St Coll; Aud, Auditory Consulting, **A**

Thomas, Marjorie Dimeo Rd 2 Box 124 F-1, Corning, NY 14830, (607) 524-6761, BS 72 SUNY - Center at Albany; MS 76 Ithaca Coll; 72–Sp-Lang Path, Corning-Painted Post Sch Dist, **SLP**

Thomas, Mary Ann 561 Canyon Court, Connersville, IN 47331, (313) 625-4900, BS 69 Ball St Univ; MA 75 Ball St Univ; Sp-Lang Path, Educational Consultants Serv, **SLP**

Thomas, Mary Ann Soebbing 1 Cliff Park Circle, Ithaca, NY 14850, (607) 898-5853, BS 79 Ithaca Coll; MS 85 Ithaca Coll; 88–Sp-Lang Path, Spec Children's Ctr, **SLP**

Thomas, Mrs Mary Jacobs 4239 Ladoga Avenue, Lakewood, CA 90713, (213) 669-2137, BA 79 CA St Univ - Long Beach; MA 85 CA St Univ - Long Beach; Aud, Pacific Hearing Services, **A**

Thomas, Patricia B 10455 West Fremont Place, Littleton, CO 80127, (303) 235-4255, BS 59 Univ of OK - Norman; **SLP**

Thomas, Mrs Patricia B 5310 Elmridge Circle, Excelsior, MN 55331, (612) 474-0227, BA 62 Coll of New Rochelle; MA 64 Columbia Univ Teachers Coll; **SLP**

Thomas, Mrs Phyllis S 108 6th Street, Garden City, NY 11040, (516) 628-3210, BA 63 OH Univ - Athens; MA 75 Hofstra Univ; 77–Sp-Lang Path, Locust Valley Sch Dist, **SLP**

Thomas, Mrs Randolph S P O Box 404, Tennille, GA 31089, (912) 552-7679, BS 69 Univ of GA; ME 70 Univ of GA; **SLP**

Thomas, Rebecca Nurre 1108 Panhandle, Denton, TX 76201, (817) 565-9220, BS 84 Univ of North TX; MS 86 Univ of North TX; **SLP**

Thomas, Regina R 1349 Constitution Avenue N E, Washington, DC 20002, (202) 328-1550, BA 72; MA 74 George Washington Univ; Supvr-Comm, Georgetown Univ-Forest Haven, **SLP**

Thomas, Robert E 7 Ritenour Drive, St John, MO 63114, (314) 428-4859, BA 66 Western MI Univ; MS 88 Southern IL Univ-Edwardsvill

Thomas, Mrs Robin G School Street Box 660 R R#1, Kennebunkport, ME 04046, (207) 967-5154, BA 76 Univ of ME - Orono; MS 77 Ithaca Coll; Sp-Lang Path Consult, Sweetser-Chldns Home, **SLP**

Thomas, Steven Michael 8115 31st Avenue N E, Seattle, WA 98115, (206) 455-4042, BA 62 Univ of WA; MA 68 Univ of WA; Dir Sp/Lang Hrng Serv, Group Hlth Coop, **SLP**

Thomas, Susan Clark 310 Ross Road, Suite 3-F, Columbia, SC 29223, (803) 796-8024, BA 84 Univ of NC - Chapel Hill; MA 86 Univ of TN - Knoxville; 86–Dir of Sp-Lang Path, Manor Healthcare, **SLP**

Thomas, Susan K 5272 South Lewis Suite 35, Tulsa, OK 74105, BS 70 Univ of Tulsa; MA 71 Univ of Tulsa; Sp-Lang Path, Communication Services, **SLP**

Thomas, Susan Kay 3796 San Francisco Drive, Destrehan, LA 70047, (504) 764-8164, BS Univ Southern MS-Hattiesburg; MS 86 Univ Southern MS-Hattiesburg; **SLP**

Thomas, Susan Ridenhour 427 Rieck Road #137, Tyler, TX 75703, (214) 597-5067, BS 84 Univ of TX - Austin; MS 86 Lamar Univ; 88–Sp-Lang Path, Texas Dept of MHMR, **SLP**

Thomas, Mrs Sylvia S 15 Indian Head Road, Riverside, CT 06878, (203) 637-3458, BA 54 SUNY - Center at Albany; MA 55 Univ of IA; **SLP A**

Thomas, Mrs Terri Lynn 3513 Willow Lake Lane, Enid, OK 73703, (405) 234-2154, BS 84 Southern IL Univ-Edwardsvill; MS 85 Southern IL Univ-Edwardsvill; **SLP**

Thomas, Terry A 3700-B Wiley Avenue, East Ridge, TN 37412, (615) 877-8463, BA 76 Auburn Univ - Auburn; MS 78 Auburn Univ - Auburn; Sp-Lang Path, Chattanooga Pub Schs, **SLP**

Thomas, Timothy Michael 3312 Gatcombe Place, Raleigh, NC 27604, (919) 790-2500, BS 74 Northeast MO St Univ; MS 76 Northeast MO St Univ; 88–Sp-Lang Path, Wake County PS, **SLP**

Thomas, Mrs Tina Gaffney 4928 Caspian Court, Orlando, FL 32811, (305) 351-0675, BA 82 Auburn Univ - Auburn; MS 84 Univ of South FL; Aud, Clifford B Dubbin MD, **A**

Thomas, Tonda Lee Columbus Hearing Impaired Program, 1455 Huy Road, Columbus, OH 43224, (614) 365-5977, BS 75 OH St Univ; MA 76 OH St Univ; MA 83 OH St Univ; **A**

Thomas, William G Associated Hearing Services, 4002 Barrett Drive, Suite 101, Raleigh, NC 27609, (919) 783-8751, BS 57 Appalachian St Univ; MA 61 Washington Univ; PH 68 (NS) Univ of FL; Private Practice, Associated Hearing Services, **A F**

Thomas-Kersting, Corinne A 4142 N E Royal Court, Portland, OR 97232, (503) 231-0779, BS 80 Portland St Univ; MS 82 Portland St Univ; Sp/Lang Path, Portland Pub Sch, **SLP**

Thomas-Kincaid, Lauren 505 North Division #6, Ann Arbor, MI 48104, (313) 572-3565, BA 79 Oberlin Coll; MS 81 Boston Univ; 87–Sp-Lang Path, St Joseph Mercy Hosp, **SLP**

Thomason, Bonnie Carol B 17731 Tristania Place, San Diego, CA 92127-0814, (619) 485-7676, BA 77 Univ of Redlands; MS 80 Univ of Redlands; Sp-Lang Path, Private Practice, **SLP**

Thomason, Karen Patricia 1333 Coates Bluff Drive, Apartment 1035, Shreveport, LA 71104, (318) 869-3736, BA 84 LA Tech Univ; MA 85 LA Tech Univ; 88–Sp-Lang Path, Schumpert Medical Center, **SLP**

Thomason, Laura Stephenson 103 Pettingill Place, Southern Pines, NC 28387-6822, (919) 295-2342, **A**

Thomason, Mrs Nancy Loomis 1556 Perkins Street, Morehead, KY 40351, (606) 784-5792, MS 84 Univ of KY; SLP, Rowan Co Board of Education, **SLP**

Thomason, Mrs Pauline Claire 403 West Frederick Street, Anderson, SC 29621, (803) 231-0555, BS 81 Edinboro Univ of PA; MS 84 Indiana Univ of PA; Sp-Lang Path, Anderson Sch Dist 5, **SLP**

Thomas-Pender, Lori Jean 2408 Burnette Drive, Greensboro, NC 27406, (919) 495-1322, BS 83 Appalachian St Univ; ME 84 Univ of NC - Greensboro; **SLP**

Thomassee, Sharon M 217 Mimosa Place, Lafayette, LA 70506, **SLP**

Thomasset, Mrs Lindley G 344 Main Street, Suite 205, Mount Kisco, NY 10549, (914) 234-9032, BA 68 Bennington Coll; MS 83 Univ of VT; Sp-Lang Path, Private Practice, **SLP**

Thomasson, Mrs Alice Wilson 3621 Robin Circle, Birmingham, AL 35243, (205) 991-7048, BS 79 Auburn Univ - Auburn; MA 82 LA Tech Univ; 87–Sp-Lang Path, Private Practice, **SLP**

Thomasson, Mrs Elizabeth 9786 Dogwood Avenue, Palm Beach Gardens, FL 33410, (407) 622-9454, BS 69 LA St Univ - Baton Rouge; MA 71 Univ of TN - Knoxville; Aud, Rc Ifft MD, **A**

Thomasson, Jana R'Dean 4120 Prairie Avenue #232, Amarillo, TX 79109-6066, (806) 353-4652, BS 83 West TX St Univ; MS 87 Baylor Univ; 87–Sp-Lang Path, Amarillo ISD

Thomas-Stonell, Nancy L 61 Tudor Glen Crescent, Scarborough, ON, Canada M1C 2S3, (416) 424-3835, BS 76 Univ of Toronto - Ontario; OM 78 Univ of Toronto - Ontario; 85–Sp/Lang Path, Hugh MacMillan Med Ctr, **SLP**

Thomas-Will, Marjorie Bryant 9494 Jones Avenue, Durham, CA 95938, (916) 896-5380, SLP, Chico Co Hosp, **SLP**

Thomley, Nancy B 13 Lateer Drive, Normal, IL 61761, (309) 438-8643, BS 52 IL St Univ - Normal; ME 68 IL St Univ - Normal; Asst Prof, Il St U, **SLP**

Thompson, Angela M 10312 Way Avenue, Cleveland, OH 44105, (216) 641-0459, BS 85 OH Univ - Athens; MA 87 OH Univ - Athens; 87–Sp-Lang Path, Cleveland Hearing & Speech Ctr, **SLP**

Thompson, Angela M S 800 Ben Allen Road, Nashville, TN 37216-2698, (615) 262-6159, BA 77 Univ of KY; MS 79 Vanderbilt Univ; Regional Director/Sp-Hrng Serv, State of Tennessee, **A**

Thompson, Mrs Ann Diamond 8221 N W 49th Court, Coral Springs, FL 33067, (305) 755-6404, BS 72 Ithaca Coll; MS 73 Columbia Univ Teachers Coll; Sp-Lang Path, Jonas Pediatrics, **SLP ACE**

Thompson, Ann Marian 1522 Steffen Court #11, Fort Wright, KY 41011, (606) 341-1100, BS 85 Western KY Univ; MS 87 Vanderbilt Univ; 87–Aud, Head & Neck Surgery Assoc, **A**

Thompson, Annette L 15775 SE Kaslin Way, Milwaukie, OR 97267, (503) 655-2898, BA 75 Western WA Univ; MA 76 Western WA Univ; 87–Sp-Lang Path, Portland Ctr for Hrng & Sp, **SLP**

Thompson, Mrs Barbara 2313 Berwyn Road, Chalfonte, Wilmington, DE 19810, (302) 651-6057, BS 53 Saint Louis Univ; MS 58 Northwestern Univ; 73–Sp-Lang Path, Alfred I duPont Institute, **SLP**

Thompson, Mrs Barbara K 606 West High, Toledo, IA 52342, (515) 484-3803, MA 78 Univ of Northern IA; SLP, AEA 7, **SLP**

Thompson, Beverly B 9709 Water Oak Drive, Fairfax, VA 22031, (415) 685-5338, BA 71 Univ of FL; MA 72 Univ of FL; Aud, Treatment & Learning Centers, **A**

Thompson, Beverly B Route 1 Box 119, Lyons, GA 30436, (912) 526-8391, BS 74 Univ of GA; ME 75 Univ of GA; Sp/Lang Path, Toombs County School Systems, **SLP**

Thompson, Bonnie Baker 1819 Indiana, Peoria, IL 61603, (309) 692-8110

Thompson, Branita L 3415 Linden Avenue #210, Long Beach, CA 90807, (213) 426-0733, BA 79 Univ of NC - Chapel Hill; ME 86 GA St Univ; 86–Sp-Lang Path, Los Angeles USD, **SLP**

Thompson, Mrs Caprice M 2 Westwood Drive, Lawrence, KS 66044-4560, (913) 842-1931, BS 75 Univ of KS; MA 77 Univ of KS; Sp-Lang Path, USD #497, **SLP**

Thompson, Dr Carl L Audiology & Speech Path Service, VA Medical Center #629, 1601 Perdido Street, New Orleans, LA 70146, (504) 589-5566, BA 54 Baylor Univ; MA 57 Baylor Univ; PH 65 (NS) Univ of FL; 87–Sp-Lang Path, VA Med Cen-New Orleans LA, **A**

Thompson, Carol A 216 Alexander, Memphis, TN 38111, (901) 458-6291, BS 72 MS Univ for Women; MA 73 Memphis St Univ; Sp-Lang Path, Christian Psychol Cen, **SLP**

Thompson, Carol M 1435 Kinghorn, Pocatello, ID 83201, (208) 236-6000, BS 75 Worcester St Coll; MS 77 ID St Univ; Sp-Lang Path/Aud, Idaho Dept Health & Welfare, **SLP**

Thompson, Catherine Anderson 13709 S E Gladstone Street, Portland, OR 97236, (503) 255-4673, BS 74 OR St Univ; Sp-Lang Path, Reynolds Sch Dist, **SLP**

Thompson, Catherine Phelps 520 Sullivan Road, Statesville, NC 28677, (704) 873-9481, BA 70 Univ of NC - Greensboro; MA 87 Appalachian St Univ; **SLP**

Thompson, Mrs Christine M 2765 North Prospect, Colorado Springs, CO 80907, (719) 598-2566, BS 74 Western MI Univ; MA 80 CA St Univ - Long Beach; 80–Sp-Lang Path, Academy Sch Dist #20, **SLP**

Thompson, Christy L 3598 South 2300 East #B, Salt Lake City, UT 84109, (801) 581-3506, BA 77 Brigham Young Univ; OM 78 Brigham Young Univ; Clinical Spervisor, University of Utah, **SLP**

Thompson, Mrs Claire R 1831 South Norfolk, Westchester, IL 60153, (312) 279-4820, BA 74 Elmhurst Coll; MS 78 Governors St Univ; Sp-Lang Path, East Dupage Special Educ Dist, **SLP**

Thompson, Connie Annette P O Box 3696 Upb, Las Cruces, NM 88003, (505) 522-6816, MA 88 NM St Univ

Thompson, Cynthia A 5134 Timber Crest Drive, New Orleans, LA 70131, (504) 899-3505, BA 75 Univ of New Orleans; OM 79 LA St Univ - N O Medical Ctr; SLP, Orleans Parish Sch Bd, **SLP**

Thompson, Dr Cynthia Kay Department Of Speech, 335 Dauer Hall, University Of Florida, Gainesville, FL 32611, (904) 392-2041, BS 75 Univ of OR; MS 76 Univ of OR; PH 83 (NS) Univ of KS; Assoc Prof, U of FL, **SLP**

Thompson, Cynthia L PSC4 Box 17299 Apo, San Francisco, CA 96408-0006, (904) 725-4646, SLP, Dept of Defense, **SLP**

Thompson, Cynthia Susanne 228 Woodlawn Avenue, Richmond, IN 47374, (317) 935-2582, Sp-Lang Path/ Preschool, Wayne Co Assoc for Ret Citizen, **SLP**

Thompson, Dale R 1364 Starshine, Thousand Oaks, CA 91360-6203, (317) 529-0900, BS 70 Ball St Univ; MA 74 Ball St Univ; **SLP**

Thompson, Dr David J Chief Audiology Section (126), Dorn Veterans Hospital, Columbia, SC 29201, (803) 776-4000, BA 67 Brescia Coll; MS 69 Marquette Univ; PH 72 (Aud) Univ of WI - Madison; 83–Ch Aud Section, Dorn Veterans Hosp, **A**

Thompson, David Wayne 25 Pershing Avenue, Jamestown, NY 14701, (716) 458-3215, BS 81 Slippery Rock Univ of PA; MA 86 Edinboro Univ of PA; 87–Sp-Lang Path, WCA Hosp, **SLP**

Thompson, Mrs Deborah J 3789 C R 39, Auburn, IN 46706, (219) 925-5611, BS 72 IN St Univ - Terre Haute; MS 75 IN St Univ - Terre Haute; Sp-Lang Path, Dekalb Ctrl USD, **SLP**

Thompson, Dena Fletcher 6210 Wishing Well, Houston, TX 77088, (713) 896-9569, BA 81 Sam Houston St Univ; MA 83 Univ of Houston - Univ Park; 83–Sp/Lang Path, Mem Hosp Southwest, **SLP**

Thompson, Mrs Diana Outman 85 North 2nd Street, Allegany, NY 14706, (513) 492-4565, BS 82 SUNY - Coll at Geneseo; MA 83 Bowling Green St Univ; SLP, Putnam County Board of Educ, **SLP**

Thompson, Mrs Diane C 1611 East Calhoun Street, Seattle, WA 98112, (206) 467-4678, BA 61 Smith Coll; MS 77 Univ of WA; 88–Proj Coord, Fred Hutchinson Cancer Research Ctr, **A**

Thompson, Donald L 1001 East Magdalena Drive, Tempe, AZ 85283, (602) 973-0852, BA 59 Univ of Northern IA; MA 66 Univ of Northern IA; Private Practice, **SLP**

Thompson, Mrs Donna Marie 495 San Juan Street, Santa Rosa, CA 95409, (707) 538-0551, BA 83 CA St Univ - Chico; MA 85 Univ of CA - Santa Barbara; 87–Sp-Lang Path, Santa Rosa Sp & Lang Svcs Inc, **SLP**

Thompson, Mrs Donna Tercasio 112 Sycamore Circle, Stony Brook, NY 11790-3168, (516) 467-6010, BA 81 Hofstra Univ; MA 83 Hofstra Univ; Sp-Lang Path, Connetquot CSD, **SLP**

Thompson, Edward E 2310 Arrowhead Drive, McComb, MS 39648, (601) 249-3254, BS 68 Univ Southern MS-Hattiesburg; MS 69 Univ Southern MS-Hattiesburg; Aud, Private Practice, **A**

Thompson, Mrs Eloise Burn 33 Trinity Street, Newton, NJ 07860, (201) 383-1731, BA 62 Hood Coll; MA 64 Syracuse Univ; Director Speech Department, Fredon Township School, **SLP ACE**

Thompson, Eloise Shepherd 2608 West 166th Place, Torrance, CA 90504, (213) 437-2851, BA 78 Univ of the Pacific; MA 79 Univ of the Pacific; 88–Assoc Dir, LB USD, **SLP**

Thompson, Dr Gary 7531 41st Avenue N E, Seattle, WA 98115, (206) 545-2531, BA 53 Univ of IA; MA 55 Univ of IA; PH 67 (NS) Univ of MN - Minneap-St Paul; Prof, U of WA, **A**

Thompson, Genelle Huddleston Rt 23 Box 218, Terre Haute, IN 47802, (812) 898-2486, BS 81 IN St Univ - Terre Haute; MS 82 IN St Univ - Terre Haute; 83–Asst Dir of Sp-Lang Path, Union Hospital Inc, **SLP**

Thompson, Geraldine Gray 1435 Kenwood Road, Santa Barbara, CA 93109, (805) 963-4331, BA 49 Univ of CA - Santa Barbara; SLP, Santa Barbara Sch Dist, **SLP**

Thompson, Heather Immer 5640 West Judy Court, Visalia, CA 93277, (209) 625-6500, BA 82 Humboldt St Univ; OM Humboldt St Univ; **SLP**

Thompson, Heather Lee 12626 Blanco Road #2201, San Antonio, TX 78216, **SLP**

Thompson, James W Audiology & Hearing Aid Center, 306-1/2 Holton Avenue, Yakima, WA 98902, (509) 248-0933, BS 68 Brigham Young Univ; MS 69 Brigham Young Univ; Private Practice, **A**

Thompson, Janee S P O Box 3104, Auburn, CA 95604, (916) 885-7689, BS 64 Southern IL Univ -Carbondale; **SLP**

Thompson, Mrs Janet S 16 Yellowbrick Drive, Stillwater, OK 74074, (405) 624-8605, BS 67 Purdue Univ - West Lafayette; MA 69 MI St Univ; Aud, Private Practice, **A**

Thompson, Janice Ann 702 Euclid Avenue #4, Des Moines, IA 50313, (515) 244-8152, BS 77 Northern IL Univ - De Kalb; MA 83 Univ of IA; **A**

Thompson, Mrs Jeri L 121 Sandra Circle, Drew, MS 38737, (601) 745-2564, BS 77 Delta St Univ; MS 78 MS Univ for Women; SLP, Drew Public Schools, **SLP**

Thompson, Dr Jesse J 13282 Cedar Street, Westminster, CA 92683, (714) 893-4238, BA 41 Santa Barbara State Coll; OM 47 Univ of Southern CA; PH 57 (Sp Path) Univ of Southern CA; 79–Stress Management Consult, Private Practice, **SLP F LM**

Thompson, Jo Anne 535 Townsend Avenue, New Haven, CT 06512, (203) 787-0086, BS 64 Univ of NE - Lincoln; MA 66 Bradley Univ; Sp-Lang Path, James M Dowaliby MD Pc, **SLP**

Thompson, Mrs Josephine Dragan 38201 Bloomfield Drive, Livonia, MI 48154, (313) 421-0548, BS 76 Purdue Univ - West Lafayette; MS 78 Purdue Univ - West Lafayette; Sp-Lang Path, Sp-Lang Path Assocs, **SLP**

Thompson, Judith J 212 Hampton Trace Lane, Columbia, SC 29209, (803) 783-3185, BS 70 Marquette Univ; ME 76 Univ of Louisville; **SLP**

Thompson, Julie Kay N 85 W 17948 Ann Avenue #6, Menomonee Falls, WI 53051, (414) 255-9303, BA 83 Univ of WI - Eau Claire; MS 85 Univ of WI - Madison; **SLP**

Thompson, Karen M 1241 North Grant Road, Carroll, IA 51401, (712) 792-3102, BS 72 Univ of ND; MS 74 Univ of ND; Sp-Lang Path, **SLP**

Thompson, Kathleen 5915 Greendale Place #107, Johnston, IA 50131, **SLP**

Thompson, Kathleen 8233 Clear Brook Drive, Raleigh, NC 27615, BA 80 Univ of Pittsburgh - Pittsburgh; MA 82 Univ of Cincinnati; 87–Sp-Lang Path, InSpeech Inc, **SLP**

Thompson, Mrs Kathleen G 4506 Chateau Drive, Albany, GA 31707, (912) 431-1232, OB 74 Univ of GA; ME 75 Univ of GA; ES 87 Univ of GA; 88–Asst Dir of Spec Educ, Dougherty Co Sch Syst, **SLP**

Thompson, Lea M 650 Warburton Avenue #4-E, Yonkers, NY 10701, **SLP**

Thompson, Leesa C 837 Terrace Place, Peekskill, NY 10566, **SLP**

Thompson, Leigh Anne 701 Victory Terrace, Morganton, NC 28655-5702, **SLP**

Thompson, Mrs Linda Conley 8334 Saylynn Lane, Houston, TX 77075, (713) 527-7247, 75 East Carolina Univ; 81–Sp-Lang Path, Texas Souther Univ, **SLP**

Thompson, Linda D 913 South McClelland St, Santa Maria, CA 93454, BA 78 CA St Univ - Fresno; MA 80 CA St Univ - Fresno; Sp-Lang Path, Coastal Sp & Lang Gr/Orcutt USD, **SLP**

Thompson, Mrs Linda M R R 2 Box 50A, Omaha, IL 62871, (618) 378-3212, BS 76 Murray St Univ; MS 79 Southern IL Univ -Carbondale; Sp-Lang Path, Norris City-Omaha Grade Sch, **SLP**

Thompson, Lisa Mele 420 Cambridge Street, Fredericksburg, VA 22405, (703) 373-7458, **SLP**

Thompson, Mrs Lori Kaye 18259 Westover Drive, South Bend, IN 46637, (219) 271-0258, BA 84 Augustana Coll; MA 85 Western MI Univ; **SLP**

Thompson, Lori Rae 6158 Laurel Drive, Florence, KY 41042, (606) 594-4450, BS 83 IN St Univ - Terre Haute; MA 85 IN Univ - Bloomington; 88–Sp-Lang Path, Redwood Sch, **SLP**

Thompson, Mrs Lurline Glover 702 Archers Lane, Columbia, SC 29212, (803) 771-4591, BA 72 SC St Coll; MA 76 SC St Coll; Sp/Lang Path, Floyd Co Head Start

Thompson, Lynn Christine 4625 West Evington Way #1A, Indianapolis, IN 46254, MS 88 IL St Univ - Normal

Thompson, Mrs Margaret R Route 4 Box 584, Marshall, TX 75670, (214) 935-5420, OB 72 Southern Methodist Univ; MA 73 Univ of Denver; Sp-Lang Path, Mem Hosp, **SLP**

Thompson, Mrs Marie H 443 Coldstream Drive, Columbia, SC 29210-9781, (803) 734-4620, ME 71 Univ of SC - Columbia; **A**

Thompson, Mrs Mary C 173 Neal Street, Farmington, AR 72730, (501)267-3309, BA 77 Univ of AR - Fayetteville; MA 79 Univ of AR - Fayetteville; 88–Sp-Lang Path, Farmington PS, **SLP**

Thompson, Mary-Ellen RR #3, Stirling, ON, Canada K0K 3E0, (416) 586-8280, BS 81; MS 83 McGill Univ - Quebec; OM 85 Univ of Toronto - Ontario; 86–Research, Mt Sinai Hosp Research Institute, **SLP**

Thompson, Mrs Mary K 139 Behan, Natchitoches, LA 71457-3903, (318) 352-9076, MA 77 Northwestern St Univ; Sp-Lang Path, Private Practice, **SLP**

Thompson, Mary Krystowski R R 1 Box 35, North Liberty, IA 52317, (319) 626-3053, BS 73 Kent St Univ; MA 74 Kent St Univ; **SLP**

Thompson, Michele Dupay 34 Winterset Lane, Marlton, NJ 08053, (609) 596-2396, BS 82 WV Univ; MA 86 Trenton St Coll; Sp-Lang Path, Consultant for LARC Sch, **SLP**

Thompson, Mrs Mindy S 3335 Elliott Boulevard, Oceanside, NY 11572, BA 77 CUNY - Queens Coll; MA 79 Hofstra Univ; 83–Sp-Lang Path, Nassau Co BOCES, **SLP**

Thompson, Molly Kathleen S 4410 17th Street, Lubbock, TX 79416-5702, (806) 797-2115, BS 83 Univ of IA; MS 85 Minot St Univ; Sp-Lang Path, InSpeech Inc, **SLP**

Thompson, Nancy Ann 1001 East 77th Street #24, Richfield, MN 55423, (612) 227-8471, BS 79 Univ of WI - Madison; MS 81 Univ of WI - Madison; 83–Sp-Lang Path, St Paul Rehabilitation Center, **SLP**

Thompson, Mrs Nancy B 414 Hunters Trail, Greenville, SC 29615, (803) 244-0443, BA 75 Winthrop Coll; MS 77 Winthrop Coll; Sp-Lang Path, Sch Dist of Greenville Co, **SLP**

Thompson, Nancy Diane 2495 Schultz Road, Moscow, ID 83843, (208) 882-3279, BS 74 ND St Univ; MS 78 Moorhead St Univ; 86–Sp-Lang Path, Washington State Univ, **SLP**

Thompson, Nancy J 2314 North Burke Drive, Arlington Heights, IL 60004, (312) 965-4780, BS 67 Univ of IL - Urbana; MA 68 Univ of IL - Urbana; Sp-Lang Path, E Me Dist 63, **SLP**

Thompson, Nella C College Of St Teresa, Winona, MN 55987-5186, (507) 454-2930, BS 72 Miami Univ - Oxford; MS 74 Miami Univ - Oxford; MS 77 UT St Univ; Asst Prof, Coll of Saint Teresa, **SLP A**

Thompson, Owinda Moss 3493 Sacramento Street, San Francisco, CA 94118, (415) 921-6171, MS 79 Univ of the Pacific; Educational Therapist, Private Practice

Thompson, Pamela A P O Box 9787, Attn Speech Pathologist, Savannah, GA 31412, (912) 356-6227, BS 81 Univ of GA; ME 82 Univ of GA; 87–Dir Sp-Lang Path, Candler General Hosp, **SLP**

Thompson, Patricia Lynne 2248 San Anseline #2, Long Beach, CA 90815, (213) 515-3084, BA 79 CA St Univ - Long Beach; MA 81 CA St Univ - Long Beach; SLP, Los Angeles USD, **SLP**

Thompson, Patricia R 2204 Quinton Road, Silver Spring, MD 20910, (202) 727-2618, **A**

Thompson, Patryce F Army Audiology & Speech Clinic, Walter Reed Army Med Cen, Washington, DC 20307-5001, (202) 576-1677, BA 52 Univ of AL- Tuscaloosa; MA 70 Catholic Univ of America; **SLP ACE**

Thompson, Mrs Paula Marie 1931 Mediterranean Road, West Palm Beach, FL 33406, (305) 765-6744, BA 81 Univ of FL; MA 83 Univ of FL; 85–Aud, Sch Bd of Broward County, **A**

Thompson, Dr Robert C Childrens Medical Center, 5300 East Skelly Drive, Tulsa, OK 74135, (918) 664-6600, BS 57 Univ of WI - Milwaukee; MS 61 Univ of WI - Madison; PH 68 (NS) Univ of OK Medical Center; Dir SLP & Aud, Chldns Med Cen, **SLP A**

Thompson, Rosemary Munday 5717 W Wilshire Boulevard, Oklahoma City, OK 73132, (405) 721-3669, BS 71 Central St Univ; ME 87 Central St Univ

Thompson, Mrs Ruth Anne 47 Bell Road, Asheville, NC 28805, (704) 255-0675, BA 64 Univ of NC - Greensboro; ME 68 Univ of NC - Greensboro; Aud, Buncombe Co Sch, **A**

Thompson, Mrs Sandra Maria 664 Wilkinson Road, Macedon, NY 14502-8814, (315) 986-3507, BS 76 SUNY - Coll at Geneseo; MS 82 Nazareth Coll of Rochester; Sp-Lang Path, Newark Cen Sch, **SLP**

Thompson, Sarah G 4157 Reiland Lane, Shoreview, MN 55126, (612) 633-8150, BA 71 Elmira Coll; MA 74 Univ of MN - Minneap-St Paul; Sp-Lang Path, Roseville Area Sch 623, **SLP**

Thompson, Mrs Sarah S 2155 Geary Drive, Santa Rosa, CA 95404, (707) 528-4321, BA 70 Univ of MI - Ann Arbor; MS 71 Univ of MI - Ann Arbor; 88–Sp-Lang Path, Agency for Infant Development, **SLP**

Thompson, Sheryl Kesey 1609 West Main Street, Cottage Grove, OR 97424, (503) 942-1070, BA 83 Univ of OR; MA 85 Univ of OR; **SLP**

Thompson, Susan K 64 Highland Avenue, Arlington, MA 02174, (617) 254-3800, BA 80 Allegheny Coll; MA 81 SUNY - Coll at Geneseo; 88–Asst Dir for Sp-Lang Path, Kennedy Mem Hosp for Children, **SLP**

Thompson, Mrs Tamela Sue 1022 Lake Grove Avenue, Grand Rapids, MI 49506, (616) 242-0483, MA 81 OH St Univ; BS 79 Miami Univ - Oxford; Sp-Lang Path, Mary Free Bed Hosp & Rehab Cen, **SLP**

Thompson, Mrs Traudl Cheshire Hospital, Court Street, Keene, NH 03431, (603) 352-4111, OB 45; OB 52; MA 55 Case Western Reserve Univ; Sp/Lang Path, Cheshire Hosp, **SLP LM**

Thompson, Viki Lee 11 Washington Lane, Clifton Park, NY 12065, (518) 442-5385, BS 84 Coll of Saint Rose; MS 85 Coll of Saint Rose; **SLP**

Thompson, Virginia 5753 Otter View Trail, White Bear Lake, MN 55110, (612) 879-2249, SLP, Ebenezer Corp, **SLP**

Thompson, Mrs Virginia Leonard 47051 Iverson Point Road, Point Arena, CA 95468, BA 41 Univ of CA - Berkeley; MA 59 Univ of San Francisco; **SLP LM**

Thompson, Virginia M 5335 Rosita Way, Santa Rosa, CA 95409, (707) 539-9788, BS 73 Pacific Union Coll; MS 74 Loma Linda Univ - Riverside; Sp-Lang Path/Consultant, Private Practice, **SLP**

Thompson, Vivienne F 2647 North Van Dorn Street #103, Alexandria, VA 22302, (703) 379-7263, BS 79 OH Wesleyan Univ; MS 82 Columbia Univ Teachers Coll; 86–Sp-Lang Path, Alexandria Head Start, **SLP**

Thompson, Mrs Wendy Wade 2518 Back Bay Loop, Costa Mesa, CA 92627, (714) 631-7783, BS 84 Northern AZ Univ; MA 86 Northwestern Univ; 86–Sp-Lang Path, Newport Lang Sp & Aud Inc, **SLP**

Thompson-Heerlein, Judith A 171 East Lothrop Street, Beverly, MA 01915, (508) 922-1870, BA 77 Univ of RI; MS 79 PA St Univ - Univ Park; 84–Sp-Lang Path, Adult-Ped/Sp-Hrng-Lang Assoc, **SLP**

Thomsen, Mrs Susan M 1701 Edgewood Drive, Palo Alto, CA 94303, (415) 964-7555, BS 67 Northwestern Univ; MS 68 Univ of MI - Ann Arbor; Sp-Lang Path, Mountain View Sch Dist, **SLP ACE**

Thomsen, Susan W 209 5th Avenue, Camanche, IA 52730, (319) 242-6454, BS 69 Univ of IA; MS 70 Univ of IA; 84–Sp-Lang Path, Mississippi Bend AEA, **SLP**

Thomson, Caroline E 6219 Gaywind Drive, Charlotte, NC 28226, (704) 362-2925, MS; **SLP**

Thomson, Mrs Cynthia M P O Box 383, Adamsville, RI 02801-0383, (401) 423-0260, BA 71 Southeastern MA Univ; MS 76 Univ of RI; Sp/Lang Path, Dartmouth Pub Schs, **SLP**

Thomson, Janet L R 4130 42nd Avenue N E, Seattle, WA 98105, (206) 771-0665, BA 71 Univ of WA; OM 78 Univ of WA; Sp-Lang Path, Edmonds School District, **SLP**

Thomson, Jean E 30621 Open Circle, Temecula, CA 92390, (714) 676-9448, BA 71 Univ of WI - Madison; MS 75 Univ of WI - Madison; **SLP**

Thomson, Kathleen Stephenson P O Box 614, Silver City, NM 88062, (505) 538-2032, BS 79 Northern AZ Univ; MS 82 Northern AZ Univ; Sp/Lang Path, Silver Consolidated Schs, **SLP**

Thomson, Madora W 333 Adelphi Street, Brooklyn, NY 11238, (718) 789-0044, MA 88 NY Univ; Sp-Lang Path, Herbert G Birch Early Chld Ctr

Thomson, Mrs Vickie Rae 2431 Senator Drive, Louisville, CO 80027, (303) 441-0437, BA 76 Univ of Northern CO; MA 79 Univ of Northern CO; 86–Dir-Neurodiagnostic Lab, Memorial Hosp, **A**

Thordarson, Kathleen Wells 14932 Grant Creek Road, Arlington, WA 98223, (206) 653-0630, BA 75 Univ of WA; OM 76 Univ of WA; Sp-Lang Path, Marysville Sch Dist #25, **SLP**

Thorell, Mrs Mary C 1412 Independence Drive, Slidell, LA 70458, (504) 649-5026, BS 67 Marquette Univ; MA 70 Univ of AZ; **SLP**

Thoresen, Linda Rose 6907 Halifax River Drive, Apartment 102, Tampa, FL 33617, (813) 986-1287, BA 81 Univ of FL; MS 83 Vanderbilt Univ; 84–Sp-Lang Path, Hillsborough Cty Schs, **SLP**

Thorgesen, Constance L 7368 Tennessee Drive, Clarendon Hills, IL 60514, (312) 896-0522, MA 87 Northern IL Univ - De Kalb; 88–Aud, Arthur H Katz MD, **A**

Thorkelsson, Anne E 608 Avila Avenue, Winnipeg, MB, Canada R3T 3A4, BA 72; OB 75; MA 80 Univ of ND; Sp-Lang Path, Winnipeg Sch Div #1, **SLP**

Thorn, Nancy Fae 1200 South Oneida Street, Apartment 8-203, Denver, CO 80224, (303) 861-6800, BA 81 Univ of CO - Boulder; MA 83 Univ of Denver; Sp-Lang Path, Childrens Hosp, **SLP**

Thornbery, Carrie H 3506 Newland Road, Baltimore, MD 21218, (301) 243-3800, BS 66 East TN St Univ; ME 68 Emory Univ; Sp-Lang Path, Hrng & Sp Agcy Metro Balt Inc, **SLP**

Thornbrue, Sue Ann 513 Mohawk, Pauls Valley, OK 73075-3638, (405) 238-6401, BS 80 OK St Univ; MA 82 OK St Univ; Sp-Lang Path, Pauls Valley State School, **SLP**

Thornburg, Mrs Dianne Ghent 113 South Hazelton, Wheaton, IL 60187, (312) 968-2589, BA 79 Elmhurst Coll; MA 81 Northern IL Univ - De Kalb; SLP, Darien Sch Dist #61, **SLP**

Thornburg, Mrs Judith D 2804 West Purdue Road, Muncie, IN 47304, (317) 285-8173, BA 56 Depauw Univ; MA 64 Ball St Univ; 77–Assistant Professor, Ball State University, **SLP**

Thorne, Sr Ann Theresa Star Route 3 HC #63, Box 6, Lebanon, NH 03766, (603) 448-4322, BA 76 Catholic Univ of America; MA 82 Fairfield Univ; MS 86 Nazareth Coll of Rochester; **SLP**

Thorne, Dr B Clyde 200 East 74th Street #14A, New York, NY 10021, BA 52 CUNY - Brooklyn Coll; MA 54 CUNY - Brooklyn Coll; PH 69 (NS) Univ of Pittsburgh - Pittsburgh; **SLP A**

Thorne, Catherine 1579 Sunflower Drive, Missoula, MT 59802, (406) 549-1321, BA 71 Univ of MT; MA 73 Univ of MT; SLP, Missoula Sch Dist #1, **SLP**

Thorne, Roger Paul 5698 Cathedral Drive, Saginaw, MI 48603, (517) 790-1234, **SLP**

Thornhill, Mrs Fabian G 3418 Churchill Road, Raleigh, NC 27607, (919) 787-7171, BA 77 Univ of NC - Chapel Hill; MS 79 Univ of AL- Tuscaloosa; Aud, Raleigh ENT Head-Neck Surgery, **A**

Thornton, Dr Aaron R Audiology Department, Mass Eye And Eye Infirmary, 243 Charles Street, Boston, MA 02114, (617) 573-3266, BA 66 Univ of Northern IA; MA 68 Univ of Northern IA; PH 75 (Aud) Univ of IA; Dir Aud, MA Eye & Ear Inf, **SLP A**

Thornton, Cathy M 220 Tacoma Avenue South, Apartment 903, Tacoma, WA 98402-2510, BS 73 ID St Univ; MS 75 ID St Univ; 87–Owner, Neurotrauma Med Legal Research, **SLP**

Thornton, Mrs Cheryl G 839 East 300 North, Orem, UT 84057, (801) 224-6530, BS 78 Univ of UT; MS 80 Univ of UT; Sp-Lang Path, Provo Sch Dist, **SLP**

Thornton, Christine 1023 Pawnee Drive, Elizabethtown, KY 42701, (502) 769-6630, BA 69 Univ of KY; ME 72 Univ of KY; Sp-Lang Path, Ireland Army Hosp, **SLP ACE**

Thornton, Mrs Karen Himdmarsh P O Box 281, Sinclair, WY 82334, (307) 328-9234, BS 72 Univ of WY; MS 85 Univ of WY; **SLP**

Thornton, Mrs Kathy Lee 5935 Wayne Avenue #2, Philadelphia, PA 19144, (215) 662-3240, BA 77 Bucknell Univ; MS 79 PA St Univ - Univ Park; Sp/Lang Path, Hospital of the U of Penn, **SLP**

Thornton, Kimberly Wilson 1016 Seahawk Drive, Ponte Vedra Beach, FL 32082, (904) 285-8565, BS 85 TX Tech Univ; MA 87 Our Lady Lake Univ-San Anton; 88–Sp-Lang Path, InSpeech Inc, **SLP**

Thornton, Mrs Mary Beth 966 Sixth Lane, Vero Beach, FL 32962, (407) 589-4140, BA 79 MI St Univ; MA 80 Western MI Univ; Sp-Lang Path, Indian River County Schools, **SLP**

Thornton, Mary Susan 223 East Washington Street, Quincy, FL 32351, (904) 627-3100, BS 83 Univ of GA; ME 85 Univ of GA; Aud, Audiology Assoc of North FL, **A**

Thornton, Robin E 20616 N E 7th Court, North Miami Beach, FL 33179, (305) 923-7862, BA 74 Univ of FL; MS 76 FL St Univ; SLP, Broward Sch Bd, **SLP**

Thorpe, Kellee Ann 4330 North Grandview #910, Odessa, TX 79762, (915) 366-2223, BS 80 Univ of North TX; MS 82 Univ of North TX; **SLP ACE**

Thorpe, Mary O 871 Faulkwood Court, Sarasota, FL 34232-2549, (813) 377-3611, **A**

Thorsen, Claire B R R 1 Box 183, Casey, IL 62420, (217) 581-2712, BS 69 Eastern IL Univ; MS 73 Eastern IL Univ; 88–Supvr-Comm Hndcpd Prog, Covered & Bridge Spec Educ, **SLP**

Thorson, Gwen 314 Midway Avenue, Proctor, MN 55810, (218) 723-4150, BA 73 Univ of MN - Duluth; MA 74 Univ of MN - Duluth; SLP, ISD 709, **SLP**

Thorson, Mrs Janice 448 Grove Street, Oradell, NJ 07649, (201) 265-6780, BA 75 Montclair St Coll; MA 77 Montclair St Coll; Sp-Lang Path Special Ed Tchr, Early Childhood Center, **SLP**

Thorson, Janice H 373 Laredo Drive, Birmingham, AL 35226, (205) 322-1919, BA 69 Univ of AL- Tuscaloosa; MA 74 Univ of AL- Tuscaloosa; Sp-Lang Path, Birmingham Board of Education, **SLP**

Thorson, Kathryn A 1450 Larch Lane, Plymouth, MN 55441, (612) 546-1942, BS 84 Univ of WI - Madison; MA 86 Northwestern Univ; Aud, **A**

Thorstad, Mrs Janice Lee 1911 North Glagler Drive, West Palm Beach, FL 33407-6113, MS 73 Columbia Univ Teachers Coll; Sp-Path, Private Practice, **SLP**

Thorum, Dr Arden R Dept Of Speech Communication, California State Univ, 800 North State College Dr, Fullerton, CA 92634, (714) 773-3617, BA 67 CA St Univ - Los Angeles; MA 69 CA St Univ - Fullerton; PH 73 (NS) Univ of UT; Prof Communicative Dis, Calif St U, **SLP**

Thrall, Anne Marie 8555 Framewood Drive, Newburgh, IN 47630, (812) 853-5697, BS 80 IN St Univ - Terre Haute; MS 82 IN St Univ - Terre Haute; **SLP**

Thran, Kelly Sue 3407 S E 53rd Avenue, Portland, OR 97206-2978, (503) 771-8115, BA 84 Pacific Univ; 86–Sp-Lang Path, Good Shepherd Lutheran Home, **SLP**

Thrash, Mrs Paula Genice 2900-D Silver Spur Circle, Bryan, TX 77801, (409) 822-7568, BS 85 Baylor Univ; MS 86 Baylor Univ; 86–Sp-Lang Path, Brenham Independent Sch Dist, **SLP**

Thrasher, Gerald D BS 77 Univ of Montevallo; MS 78 Univ of Montevallo; **SLP**

Threats, Travis Terrence 740 South Cuyler Avenue, Oak Park, IL 60304, (312) 239-2191, BS 82 KS St Univ; MA 84 Univ of IL - Urbana; **SLP**

Threewits, Marla C R R 1 Box 201, Union City, IN 47390, (513) 548-4915, BS 77 IN Univ - Bloomington; MA 78 IN Univ - Bloomington; Pupil Pers Dir, Darke Co Offi of Ed, **SLP**

Thresher, Mrs Jill C 209 Wildcat Lane, Chapel Hill, NC 27514, (919) 967-1418, BA 77 Univ of FL; MA 79 Univ of MA - Amherst; Sp-Lang Path, Private Practice, **SLP**

Throckmorton, Verl John AI Workers Hlth Safety & Comp, 4th Floor Donsdale Place, 10709 Jasper Avenue, Edmonton, AB, Canada T8N 3X3, BA 64 Univ of UT; MS 72 ID St Univ; Co-Ord Occup Hrng Conserv, Alberta Worker Hlth, **A**

Thrope, Denise Weisblatt Sinai Hospital Of Baltimore, Audiology Section, Belvedere At Greenspring Avenue, Baltimore, MD 21215, (301) 578-5602, BA 77 Univ of MI - Ann Arbor; MS 80 Boston Univ; 85–Aud, Sinai Hosp of Balt, **A**

Thrope, Susan Dee 3 Orange Street #1, Newburyport, MA 01950, (617) 281-2878, BS 74 Northeastern Univ; MS 85 Univ of NH; **SLP**

Thul, Mrs Nancy Ann 304 West Main Box 1143, Washburn, ND 58577, (701) 857-4410, BS 83 Moorhead St Univ; MS 84 Minot St Univ; **SLP**

Thuman, Pamela R 2415 Espanola Northeast, Apartment B, Albuquerque, NM 87110, (505) 883-8421, BA 81 Univ of NM; MS 83 Univ of NM; 83–Sp-Lang Path, Albuquerque Pub Sch, **SLP**

Thunder, Thomas D Thunder Hearing & Noise Assoc Ltd, 520 North Hicks Road, Suite 110, Palatine, IL 60067, (312) 359-1068, BS 74 Northern IL Univ - De Kalb; MA 76 Northern IL Univ - De Kalb; Aud, Private Practice, **A**

Thunselle, Mary Lou Douglas County Hospital, 111 17th Avenue East, Alexandria, MN 56308, (612) 762-1511, BS 72 Moorhead St Univ; MS 80 Saint Cloud St Univ; Sp/Lang Path, Douglas Co Hosp, **SLP**

Thureau, Mrs Lani C 1605 Shipley Road, Wilmington, DE 19803, (302) 478-1740, BA 70 Univ of Miami; MA 79 Kent St Univ; 86–Sp-Lang Path, The Pilot Sch Inc, **SLP**

Thurman, Mrs Hattie Tingle 353 Hayward Mill Road, Concord, MA 01742, (617) 369-9500, BS 70 Purdue Univ - West Lafayette; ME 82 Northeastern Univ; Sp-Lang Path, Concord Pub Sch, **SLP**

Thurman, James E University Of Central Arkansas, Box 5096, Conway, AR 72032, (501) 450-3176, ED 79 (NS) Univ of Northern CO; Chmn/Assoc Prof, Univ of Central Arkansas, **SLP**

Thurman, Rita D 3948 Browning Place, Raleigh, NC 27609, (919) 783-5060, BS 76 UT St Univ; MS 77 UT St Univ; Sp-Lang Path, Private Practice, **SLP**

Thurman, Mrs Susan H 300 West Brown Street, Glasgow, KY 42141, (502) 651-6155, BA 71 Univ of FL; ME 72 Univ of FL; Sp-Lang Path, Private Practice, **SLP**

Thurman, Dr Wayne L 238 El Caminito, Carmel Valley, CA 93924, (408) 659-2378, BS 48 Southeast MO St Univ; MA 49 Univ of IA; PH 53 (NS) Purdue Univ - West Lafayette; Ch-Prof Dept SLP &Aud Retired, En IL U Ret, **SLP F LM**

Thursby, Mrs Janet R 4750 S W 22nd Place, Ocala, FL 32674, (904) 351-7225, BA 69 SUNY - Coll at New Paltz; MA 76 Univ of FL; Sp-Lang Path, Munroe Reg Med Cen, **SLP ACE**

Thurston, Mrs Kathryn 4008 Oleander Avenue, Fort Pierce, FL 33482, (305) 461-1002, MS 88 Nova Univ; 88–SLP, St Lucie County Schs

Thurston, Kenneth I Rural Delivery 1, Tully, NY 13159, (315) 488-0941, BS 70 SUNY - Coll at Geneseo; MA 73 Western MI Univ; Spec Ed Superv, Onon Madison BOCES, **SLP**

Thurston, Laural B 620 Long Hill Road, Gillette, NJ 07933, (201) 647-2055, BS 81 Kean Coll of NJ; MA 84 Kean Coll of NJ; 88–Sp-Lang Path, Comm Sp & Lang Svcs, **SLP**

Thurston, Mrs Susan Kay 4945 Cornell Avenue, Downers Grove, IL 60515, (312) 852-5586, BA 71 Augustana Coll; OM 87 Governors St Univ

Tibbetts, Susan H S 8526 Midas Court, Annandale, VA 22003, (703) 323-1744, BA 70 OH Univ - Athens; MA 75 Catholic Univ of America; Sp-Lang Path, Franklin Co Pub Sch, **SLP**

Tibbits, Dr Donald F Speech And Hearing Clinic, Central Missouri St Univ, Warrensburg, MO 64093, (816) 429-4993, BS 64 Univ of AR - Fayetteville; MS 68 Univ of AR - Fayetteville; PH 73 (Sp-Lang Path) Univ of MO - Columbia; 80–Sp-Lang Path, Ctrl MO St U, **SLP**

Tibbits, James D Rt 5 Box 268, Stillwell, OK 74960, (918) 696-6161, BA 75 Northeastern OK St Univ; MA 76 Univ of AR - Fayetteville; Sp-Lang Path, Wn AR Couns & Guid Cen, **SLP**

Tiburzi, James R R 1 Box 295, Staunton, IL 62088, (217) 835-2518, BS 73 Southern IL Univ-Edwardsvill; MS 76 Southern IL Univ-Edwardsvill; Sp-Lang Path, Gillespie Comm Ut Dist #7, **SLP**

Tice, Dr Robert E 2801 Bell Street, Sacramento, CA 95821, (916) 454-6601, BA 58 CA St Univ - Sacramento; MA 64 CA St Univ - Sacramento; PH 68 (NS) Univ of WA; Professor Audiology, Cal State Univ-Sacramento, **SLP A**

Ticich, Margaret M 2440 North Koa Drive, Rialto, CA 92376, (714) 887-2335, BA 78 Carroll Coll; MA 82 CA St Univ - Long Beach; Childhood Aphasia/Sp-Lang Path, San Bernardino Scottish Rite I, **SLP**

Tidik, Amy Valentine 157 Valley View Drive, Pismo Beach, CA 93449, (314) 878-4845, BA 76 San Diego St Univ; MA 79 Saint Louis Univ; Ch Sp & Lang Path, Good Shepherd Sch for Chldn, **SLP**

Tidwell, Melanie Hall 18700 S W Farmington #28, Aloha, OR 97007, (801) 374-9236, BA 84 Brigham Young Univ; OM 85 Brigham Young Univ; **SLP**

Tieche, Mrs Connie L S 11717 Douglas Street, Yucaipa, CA 92399, (714) 797-9681, BS 71 Pacific Union Coll; MS 76 Univ of Redlands; Sp-Lang Path, Nishikawa and Associates, **SLP**

Tiedemann, Jayne Novotny 1719 Colvin Avenue, St Paul, MN 55116, (612) 895-7304, BS 85 Univ of WI - Whitewater; MS 86 Univ of WI - Whitewater; Sp-Lang Path, ISD 191, **SLP**

Tiedemann, Mrs Susan B 296 Maple Street, Kearny, NJ 07032, (201) 955-5000, BA 78 Rutger's St Univ - Douglas Coll; MA 83 Montclair St Coll; 78–Sp-Lang Path, Kearny Bd of Ed, **SLP**

Tiegerman, Dr Ellenmorri 4 Grace Court North, Great Neck, NY 11021, (516) 773-4065, OM 78; MS 75 CUNY - Brooklyn Coll; PH 79 (NS) CUNY - Brooklyn Coll; Associate Professor, Adelphi University, **SLP**

Tiemann, Mrs Brenda Lynn 348 Quinby Road, Rochester, NY 14623, (716) 232-2310, MS; 88–Sp-Lang Path, Rochester City Sch Dist, **SLP**

Tiemann, Joann L 1009 Woodlake Village Dr, St Louis, MO 63141-6062, (314) 469-7437, BA 56 Elmhurst Coll; MA 59 Syracuse Univ; 84–Dir, Spec Sch Dist St Louis Co, **SLP**

Tiemann, Lynn Kay 1321 41st Place, Marion, IA 52302, (319) 373-0404, BA 80 Univ of Northern IA; MA 82 Univ of Northern IA; Sp-Lang Path, Grant Wood AEA, **SLP**

Tier, Eleanor Patricia 40 Bernard Drive, Tinton Falls, NJ 07753, (201) 922-1787, BA 82 William Paterson Coll; MS 85 Columbia Univ Teachers Coll; Sp-Lang Path, Private Practice, **SLP**

Tieri, Mrs Lynnee Luckett 1333 Jean Avenue, Redlands, CA 92374, (714) 781-1718, BS 75 Loma Linda Univ - Riverside; MS 77 Loma Linda Univ - Riverside; SLP, Jurupa USD, **SLP**

Tiernan, Mrs Sue Frick 1250 South Grandview, Dubuque, IA 52001, (319) 583-2808, BA 83 Univ of Northern IA; MA 87 Univ of Northern IA; 87–Sp-Lang Path, Keystone AEA, **SLP**

Tierney, Elizabeth 3635 Scott Drive, Troy, MI 48084, (313) 293-5100, BS 77 Central MI Univ; MA 78 MI St Univ; SLP, Fraser Pub Sch, **SLP**

Tierney, Martin Eugene 693 Arbor Drive, Westminster, MD 21157, (301) 848-6980, BA 80 Loyola Coll; MS 81 Loyola Coll; Sp-Lang Path, Carroll County Board of Educ, **SLP**

Tierney, Terry J 46 Allyn Street, Holyoke, MA 01040, (203) 668-7301, BS 79; MA 81; SLP, Suffield Pub Sch, **SLP**

Tiesi, Sharon Reich 9042 Meadow Oaks Drive, Allison Park, PA 15101, BS 77 Clarion Univ of PA; MA 78 Univ of Pittsburgh - Pittsburgh; Aud, Eye and Ear Hosp, **A**

Tieszen, Mrs Marion V 109 Grant Drive, Warrensburg, MO 64093, (816) 747-6725, BS 33 Northern St Coll; MS 65 Central MO St Univ; Consultant, Health Tech, **SLP LM**

Tietje, Mrs Betty Ann 5860 Highplace Drive, San Diego, CA 92120, (619) 449-0343, BS 66 Univ of WI - Madison; MA 85 San Diego St Univ; 88–Sp-Lang Path, Santee Sch Dist, **SLP**

Tietjens, Mrs Mary Ann 4708 King Bird Lane, St Louis, MO 63128, (314) 569-8233, BS 73 Saint Louis Univ; MA 74 Saint Louis Univ; Area Coord, St Louis Co Spec Sch Dist, **SLP**

Tievsky, Mrs Sharon L 7000 Endicott Court, Bethesda, MD 20817, (301) 229-3191, BA 72 Univ of Rochester; MA 74 George Washington Univ; **SLP**

Tiff, Richard Jefferson Rehab Center, Gaffney Drive, Watertown, NY 13601, BA 67 Bowling Green St Univ; MA 69 CA St Univ - Los Angeles; Sp-Lang Path, Jefferson Rehab Center, **SLP**

Tiffany, Mrs Sheila Ann 6 Howard Trail, Fredericksburg, VA 22401, (703) 371-7200, BA 70 Mary Washington Coll; MA 71 Univ of FL; Sp-Lang Path, Private Practice, **SLP**

Tiger, Ruth W 814 North Cushman, Tacoma, WA 98403, (206) 272-2087, BA 75 Univ of OR; MA 78 Univ of Denver; **SLP**

Tight, Mrs Jane T Altos Speech Lang & Lrng Ctr, 960 North San Antonio Road, Suite 170, Los Altos, CA 94022, (415) 948-3383, BA 76 Univ of Redlands; MS 77 Univ of Redlands; Dir, Altos Sp-Lang Lrng Cen, **SLP**

Tikofsky, Mrs Rita 6909 West Greenbrook Court, Milwaukee, WI 53223, (414) 355-5678, BS 53 Univ of Pittsburgh - Pittsburgh; MS 54 Univ of Pittsburgh - Pittsburgh; Sp-Lang Path, Private Practice, **SLP**

Tikofsky, Dr Ronald S 6909 West Greenbrook Ct, Milwaukee, WI 53223, (414) 257-6068, BA 52 CUNY - Brooklyn Coll; MA 53 CUNY - Brooklyn Coll; PH 57 (NS) Univ of UT; Prof of Radiology, Medical Col of Wisconsin, **SLP F**

Tilden-Browning, Mrs Stacy Ann 16960 S E Stanhelma Drive, Gladstone, OR 97027-1227, (503) 280-6322, BA 81 Pacific Univ; MS 85 Portland St Univ; **SLP**

Tilford, Michelle Renee 751 Runyan Drive, Apartment 813, Chattanooga, TN 37405, (615) 875-6089, BA 83 Univ of TN - Knoxville; MA 85 Univ of TN - Knoxville; 87–Sp-Lang Path, Chattanooga-Hamilton Co Sp & Hrng Ctr, **SLP**

Till, Dr James A Veterans Admin Med Center 126, 5901 East 7th Street, Long Beach, CA 90822, (213) 494-5415, BA 69 Univ of WA; MA 71 Univ of WA; PH 76 (NS) Univ of IA; Sp-Lang Path, VA Medical Center, **SLP**

Till, Jill Kane 3210 Arlington Avenue, Bronx, NY 10463, (212) 652-9790, BS 76 SUNY - Center at Albany; MS 78 Rutger's St Univ - Douglas Coll; SLP, UCP of NYC, **SLP**

Till, Kathleen Kiddon 7603 Woodland West, Houston, TX 77040, (713) 491-7100, BS 77 Kent St Univ; MA 79 Kent St Univ; Sp-Lang Path, Fort Bend ISD, **SLP**

Tiller, Mrs Charlene T 4400 Old Gee Road, Hopewell, VA 23860, (804) 458-8551, BS 68 East Carolina Univ; ME 72 East Carolina Univ; Sp/Lang Path, Hopewell Pub Schs, **SLP**

Tiller, Denise Marie 1630 Weiland Lane #6, Appleton, WI 54914, (414) 739-6021, BS 83 Univ of WI - Madison; MS 85 Univ of WI - Madison; **SLP**

Tiller, Gary Robert 999 E Baseline Road #3122, Tempe, AZ 85283, (602) 220-6176, BS 79 Univ of AZ; MA 83 Humboldt St Univ; 87–Sp-Lang Path, AZ State Hosp, **SLP**

Tiller, Rebecca N 102 Warmstone Path, Peachtree City, GA 30269, (404) 487-7650, ME 87 West GA Coll; 88–Sp-Lang Path, Oak Grove Elem, **SLP**

Tillery, Elizabeth Thompson 7060 Barcelona Boulevard, Macon, GA 31206, (912) 929-7899, BS 80 Ball St Univ; MA 81 Ball St Univ; Aud, Houston Co Bd of Educ, **A**

Tillett-Ferguson, Sandra 1223 Holly Avenue, Columbus, OH 43212, (614) 475-0564, BA 74 OH St Univ; MA 76 OH St Univ; Sp-Lang Path, Franklin County Bd MR/DD, **SLP**

Tilley, Mrs Connie Holland Route 3 Box 121, Pilot Mountain, NC 27041, (919) 368-2641, BS 83 Univ of NC - Greensboro; ME 85 Univ of NC - Greensboro; Sp-Lang Path, Surry County Sch Sys, **SLP**

Tillia, Pamela Ruth H 9 Madison Avenue, Lancaster, NY 14086, (716) 674-6300, BA 79 Baldwin-Wallace Coll; MA 81 SUNY - Center at Buffalo; **SLP**

Tillman, Mrs Marianne B 1439 Fawnbrook Court, Lilburn, GA 30247, (404) 483-4410, BA 70 Paterson St Coll; MS 71 Univ of MS; Sp-Lang Path, C J Hicks Elem Sch, **SLP**

Tillman, Patricia A 4314 Rockhill Road, Kansas City, MO 64110, (913) 588-5937, BA 84 Univ of Northern IA; MA 87 Univ of IA; Aud, Univ Ks Med Ctr, **A**

Tillman, Dr Tom W Northwestern University, SPC Bldg Room 204, Evanston, IL 60201, (312) 492-7023, BA 54; MA 55; PH 59; Prof Aud/Assoc Dean Sch Speech, Northwestern University, **A F**

Tillotson, Barbara L 503 Anderson Street, Manhattan Beach, CA 90266, (213) 372-9153, BS 71 Univ of MN - Minneap-St Paul; MA 78 Whittier Coll; SLP, LA Co Supt Sch, **SLP**

Tillquist, Candace Sheley 3815 Howard Avenue, White Bear Lake, MN 55110, (612) 653-0227, BA 77 Univ of CO - Boulder; MA 81 Univ of CO - Boulder; 88–Aud, ENT Pro Assoc, **A**

Timberlake, Mary J P O Box 749, Mount Carmel, IL 62863, (618) 445-2430, BS 75 Eastern IL Univ; MS 76 Eastern IL Univ; Sp-Lang Path, Mt Vernon City Schs, **SLP**

Timby, Mrs Marsha M 7500 San Felipe, Suite 460, Houston, TX 77057, MS 74 Southern Methodist Univ; 78–Sp-Lang Path, Sp & Lang Remed Ctr Inc, **SLP**

Timer, Mrs Loretta Ann 8917 Fleming Road, Fowlerville, MI 48836, (517) 223-8064, BS 77 Eastern MI Univ; MA 78 Eastern MI Univ; Sp/Lang Path, Livingston ISD, **SLP**

Timke, Margot Supervisor Audiology, Crippled Children's Service, 19th & Mass Aves S E, Washington, DC 20003, (202) 675-7324, BS 61 Northwestern Univ; ME 64 Univ of VA - Charlottesville; 68–Aud, DC Govt, **SLP A**

Timko, Andrew F Bucks Co Iu-22, Cross Keys Bldg, Routes 611 & 311, Doylestown, PA 18901, (215) 348-2940, BS 57 CA Univ of PA; ME 62 Temple Univ; 67–Superv, Lang & Sp Prog, Bucks Co Inter Unit, **SLP**

Timko, James Robert 1522 S Montgomery Street, De Land, FL 32720, (904) 736-9148, BS 84 OH Univ - Athens; MA 86 Univ of FL; Aud, North Florida Hearing Services, **A**

Timler, Geralyn R 12 Baton Rouge, Irvine, CA 92714, (714) 857-5092, BA 82 Univ of WI - Eau Claire; MS 84 Univ of WI - Madison; **SLP**

Timlin, Janice Hollenback 3 Nikhil Ct, Claymont, DE 19703, (215) 622-6087, BA 82 Temple Univ-Tyler Sch of Art; MA 86 Temple Univ-Tyler Sch of Art; **SLP**

Timlin, Mrs Katherine Love 8 Farrington Lane, Palm Coast, FL 32037, (904) 445-3991, BA 73 MT St Univ; OM 76 Univ of MT; Sp-Lang Path, Easter Seal Soc Volusia Cnty, **SLP**

Timmins, Garth Joseph 1950 8-1/2 Street S E #E, Rochester, MN 55904, (507) 289-1524, BS 80 UT St Univ; MS 82 ID St Univ; **A**

Timmis, Thomas W New Trier High School, 3013 Il Road, Wilmette, IL 60091, BS 54 Eastern IL Univ; MS 59 Univ of IL - Urbana; Dir of Pers, New Trier H S, **SLP**

Timmons, Barbara 10333 Oak Tunnel Road, Grass Valley, CA 95945, (916) 265-6256, **SLP**

Timmons, Mrs Lori Tocash 41 Euclid Avenue, Columbus, OH 43201, (614) 369-3650, BA 85 OH St Univ; MA 87 OH St Univ

Timmons, Mae 213 Old Chatham Road, Brewster, MA 02631, (508) 896-6563, MS 81 Boston Univ; 88–Sp-Lang Path, Harwich PS Sys, **SLP**

Timmons, Mary Catherine 8000 Rio Vista, Waco, TX 76712, (817) 776-0326, BA 82 TX Tech Univ; MA 88 Univ of TX - Austin; 86–Sp-Lang Path, Private Practice, **SLP**

Timmons, Dr Roy J Speech And Hearing Center, University Of The Pacific, Stockton, CA 95211, (209) 946-2381, BA 60 Univ of Northern IA; MA 63 Univ of KS; PH 66 (Sp Path) Univ of KS; 70–Prof, U of the Pacific, **SLP**

Timofey, Mrs Robin Marlene 73-10 173rd Street, Fresh Meadows, NY 11366, (718) 969-8196, BA 79 CUNY - Queens Coll; MA 81 NY Univ; SLP, NYC Bd of Ed/Sp Ser Vt, **SLP**

Timpone, Lauren Alissa 11401 9th Street North, Apartment 615, St Petersburg, FL 33716-2311, (813) 870-3560, BA 85 Hofstra Univ; MA 86 Hofstra Univ; **A**

Tinagero, Elizabeth 23 Wheatley Avenue, East Williston, NY 11596, (212) 899-8800, BA 77 CUNY - Queens Coll; MA 80 Hofstra Univ; Sp-Lang Path, Lexington Hrng & Sp Cen, **SLP**

Tindall, Reed B 229 West Seattle Street, Shelton, WA 98584, (206) 748-8681, BA 63 Western WA Univ; OM 70 Univ of WA; SLP, Chehalis School District 302, **SLP**

Tindel, Mrs Marilyn B 1646 Summit, Cardiff By Sea, CA 92007, (619) 943-1547, BA 64 Univ of CA - Riverside; MA 80 San Diego St Univ; Sp-Lang Path, San Diego USD, **SLP**

Tindell, Marsha Eloise 6770 N La Canada, Tucson, AZ 85704, BS 82 Univ of AZ; MS 83 Univ of AZ; **SLP**

Tinetti, Mrs Susan Marie 23658 Valley Starr, Novi, MI 48050, (313) 288-2370, **SLP**

Tingle, Meredith Kastner 518 Mount Vernon Drive, Wilson, NC 27893, (919) 291-5603, BA 71 SUNY - Coll at Plattsburgh; MA 72 OH Univ - Athens; Sp-Lang Path, Wilson County Schools, **SLP**

Tingum, Paulette Ann 336 Eastern Avenue, Grafton, ND 58237, (701) 352-2140, BA 83 Univ of ND; MS 84 Univ of ND; Sp-Lang Path, Grafton State Sch, **SLP**

Tinker, Mrs Agnes Z 35 Highland Drive, Yardley, PA 19067, (215) 493-6976, BS 62 Univ of Pittsburgh - Pittsburgh; MS 64 Univ of Pittsburgh - Pittsburgh; Sp-Lang Path, Mercer County Special Services, **SLP**

Tinker, Christine Bolen 708 Alexander Circle N W, Calgary, AB, Canada T2M 4B6, (306) 882-2633, **SLP**

Tinley, Gordon F 1128 Laura Street, Jacksonville, FL 32206, (904) 355-3404, BS 70 Maryville Coll; MA 73 Univ of TN - Knoxville; Chief Aud, Sp & Hrng Cen, **A**

Tinsley, Glen, Jr 1003 Laura, La Marque, TX 77568, (713) 337-1529, BS 66 Lamar Univ; MA 69 Central MI Univ; Quality Assurance Coordinator, Mc Ree Ford Inc, **SLP**

Tinsley, Judyth A 1934 Calvert Street N W, Washington, DC 20009, (202) 265-7335, BS 72 Morgan St Univ; MA 74 Kean Coll of NJ; Exec Dir, Wash Hrng & Sp Soc

Tinsley, Kerri D 1929 Denniston Avenue S W, Roanoke, VA 24015, (703) 344-2306, BS 84 James Madison Univ; MS 85 James Madison Univ; Sp-Lang Path, Roanoke City Schools, **SLP**

Tinsley, Sara S 2708 Sunnybrook, Jonesboro, AR 72401-9006, (501) 932-6799, OB 78 AR St Univ; OM 79 AR St Univ; 88–Sp/Lang Path, Cottage of Hope, **SLP**

Tinsley, Shelley 8412 Duncan South, Seattle, WA 98118, (206) 725-4149, BS 82 Univ of WA; MS 85 Univ of WA; 85–Sp-Lang Path, Highline Sch Dist #401, **SLP**

Tinsley-Teague, Mrs Louanne 201 Honeysuckle Lane, Cary, NC 27511, (919) 755-6485, BA 77 CA St Univ - Chico; MA CA St Univ - Fresno; **SLP**

Tintera-Jacobs, Karen A 432 65th Street, Westmont, IL 60559, (312) 826-3600, BS 75 Southern IL Univ -Carbondale; MS 79 Southern IL Univ -Carbondale; 79–Sp-Lang Path, Chicago Board of Education, **SLP**

Tintle, Mrs Patricia Ann 15110 Banner Lava Cap Road, Nevada City, CA 95959, (916) 265-9126, BA 82 CA St Univ - Sacramento; 87–Sp-Lang Path, Sierra Nevada Mem Hosp, **SLP**

Tipper, Raymond 110-20 71st Road, Forest Hills, NY 11375, (516) 543-5100, BA 75 CUNY - Queens Coll; MS 76 Adelphi Univ; Director/Clinical Services, UCP, **SLP**

Tippett, Mrs Cynthia Martino 4228 Sandcastle Lane, Olney, MD 20832, (301) 570-9024, BA 77 Univ of MD - College Park; MA 78 Western MI Univ; Sp-Lang Path, Prince Georges County Bd of Ed, **SLP**

Tippett, Donna Clark 38 Laurence Brooke Road, Baltimore, MD 21228, MA 84 Univ of MD - College Park; Sp-Lang Path, Good Samaritan Hosp, **SLP**

Tippett, Sally DeWitt 2919 West Kingston Court, Peoria, IL 61604, (309) 672-6510, BS 59 Northwestern Univ; MA 63 Stanford Univ; Sp-Lang Path, Peoria Pub Sch, **SLP**

Tipps, Mrs Deborah L 2920 Sycamore School Road #133, Fort Worth, TX 76133, (817) 346-8247, BS 74 TX Tech Univ; MS 75 TX Tech Univ; Sp-Lang Path, Private Practice, **SLP ACE**

Tipton, Carol B Carol B Tipton & Associates, 1901 Medi Park, Suite 1054, Amarillo, TX 79106, (806) 352-4721, BA 69 Southern Methodist Univ; MA 71 West TX St Univ; Sp-Lang Path, Private Practice, **SLP**

Tipton, Mrs Cindy H 3420 Cherry Tree Lane, Erlanger, KY 41018-1207, (606) 723-2465, BS 78 Eastern KY Univ; MA 81 Eastern KY Univ; Sp/Lang Path, Nazareth Home Health Agency, **SLP**

Tipton, Debra Rizek RR 1 Box 94, Munden, KS 66959, (913) 987-5362, BS 80 KS St Univ; MA 82 KS St Univ; Sp/Lang Path, Learning Coop of N Ctrl Ks, **SLP**

Tirello, Elaine C 6 Ziff Lane, Princeton Junction, NJ 08550, (609) 799-0238, BA 69 Kean Coll of NJ; MA 72 Trenton St Coll; Sp-Lang Path, Mercer Co Spec Svcs Sch Dist, **SLP ACE**

Tirnauer, Sandra S 8715 Garfield Street, Bethesda, MD 20817, (301) 897-8100, BS 55 Miami Univ - Oxford; MS 57 PA St Univ - Univ Park; 83–Dir, Rehabilitation Services Inc, **SLP**

Tirolo-Zaleski, Mrs Barbara 1 Stark Terrace, Boylston, MA 01505, **SLP**

Tirpak, Mrs Paula LaBute 532-B Alabama Avenue, Salisbury, MD 21801, (301) 632-1155, BS 84 CA Univ of PA; MS 86 CA Univ of PA; 88–Sp-Lang Path, Worcester Bd of Educ, **SLP**

Tischler, Mrs Joan Marie Rd 1 Box 208, Canadensis, PA 18325, (717) 595-3009, BS 81 East Stroudsburg Univ of PA; MA 83 Montclair St Coll; Sp-Lang Path, Wayne City Memorial Hosp, **SLP ACE**

Tisenchek, Mrs Cathryn Anne 107 Johnson, Cohoes, NY 12047, (518) 273-4911, BS 74 SUNY - Coll at Geneseo; MS 78 Coll of Saint Rose

Tishman, Mrs Shelley L 305 East 86th Street #8JW, New York, NY 10028, (212) 860-5383, BA 72 Hofstra Univ; MS 74 Columbia Univ Teachers Coll; Sp-Lang Path, Private Practice, **SLP**

Tisler, Mrs Susan Jone 10839 Mansfield Road, Cucamonga, CA 91730, (714) 788-7142, BA 81 CA St Univ - Fullerton; MS 85 Chapman Coll; SLP, Riverside USD, **SLP**

Tissiere, Michele 38 Saceamento Street, Cambridge, MA 02138, (617) 232-8390, BS 80 SUNY - Coll at Geneseo; MS 82 CO St Univ; Sp-Lang Path, Jude Baker Guidance Center, **SLP**

Tissot, Mrs Kathleen L R R Highway 92, Brooklyn, WI 53521, (608) 455-8451, BS 82 Univ of IL - Urbana; MA 83 Northern IL Univ - De Kalb; Sp-Lang Path, Rural Wisconsin Hosp Cooperative, **SLP ACE**

Tisthammer, Ladon A 715 Aspen, Cherokee, IA 51012, **SLP**

Tittel-Zuchowski, Karen 43 Hansen Drive, Edison, NJ 08820, (201) 668-8461, SLP, Bernards Township P S, **SLP**

Titze, Ingo R University Of Iowa, 127 A SHC, Iowa City, IA 52242, (319) 335-8732, BS 63 Univ of UT; MS 65 Univ of UT; PH 72 (NS) Brigham Young Univ; Prof, U of Iowa

Tivenan, Karen A PO Box 693, Hauppauge, NY 11788, (516) 724-5477, BA 85 SUNY - Coll at Plattsburgh; MS 86 Clarion Univ of PA; 87–Aud, Hearing & Speech Assoc Inc, **A**

Tjomsland, Lily Clara 407 West 25th Street, Sioux Falls, SD 57105, MS; **SLP LM**

Tkacs, Donna L 137 Brighton Avenue, Perth Amboy, NJ 08861, (201) 442-0228, BA 84 Kean Coll of NJ; MS 87 Northeastern Univ; 87–Aud, Dr F Catalfumo

Toal, Carmen S 932 Stonetrail Drive, Plano, TX 75023, (214) 424-5633, BS 76 Marquette Univ; MS 77 Southern Methodist Univ; Sp/Lang Path, Plano ISD, **SLP**

Toar, Janet W 14 Degel Reuven Street #8, Kfar Ganim, Petach Tekvah, Israel 49402, BA 75 Temple Univ-Tyler Sch of Art; MA 77 Temple Univ-Tyler Sch of Art; SLP, Ministry of Education, **SLP**

Toback, Frieda 6 Fiesta Court, Patchogue, NY 11772, (516) 434-5200, BA 69 CUNY - Hunter Coll; MA 80 CUNY - Queens Coll; Aud, Pilgrim Psychiatric Center, **A ACE**

Tobe, Mrs Judy Gail 4323 Camden Avenue, Dallas, TX 75206, (214) 826-9175, BS 82; MA 84 SUNY - Center at Buffalo; 84–Sp-Lang Path, Humana Hosp Med City Dallas, **SLP**

Tober, Mrs Allison Beth 67-33 150th Street, Flushing, NY 11367, (718) 428-7507, BS 83 Ithaca Coll; MS 86 Adelphi Univ; **SLP**

Tober, Mrs Barbara N 20324 Bassett Street, Canoga Park, CA 91306, (818) 997-2395, BA 64 Univ of CA - Los Angeles; MA 81 CA St Univ - Northridge; SLP, Los Angeles USD, **SLP**

Tobey, Dr Emily A Dept Of Communication Disorder, 1900 Gravier, New Orleans, LA 70112, (504) 568-4348, BA 73 NM St Univ; OM 76 LA St Univ - N O Medical Ctr; PH 81 (Sp Science) CUNY - Grad Sch & Univ Cntr; 86–Assoc Prof, LA St U Med Cen, **SLP F**

Tobias, Celeste V 55 Central Street, Woodstock, VT 05091, (802) 457-1213, BA 83 SUNY - Center at Buffalo; MS 86 Univ of VT; **SLP**

Tobias, Dr Jerry V Submarine Medical Research Lab, Box 900 Navsubase Nlon, Groton, CT 06349, (203) 449-3201, OM 83 Univ of OK - Norman; MA 54 Univ of IA; PH 59 (Psychoacoustics) Case Western Reserve Univ; 82–Head-Submarine Sys Div, US Navy, **F**

Tobias, Mrs Kathleen C 771 Lewiston Court, Sunnyvale, CA 94087, (415) 967-5541, BS 57 Univ of MN - Duluth; MA 65 Univ of MN - Minneap-St Paul; Sp-Lang Path, Whisman Sch Dist, **SLP**

Tobias, Marian Rosenthal 5786 Santa Ana Valley Road, Hollister, CA 95023, (408) 637-5393, BA 75 Stanford Univ; MS 78 San Francisco St Univ; Sp-Lang Path, San Benito Co Office of Ed, **SLP**

Tobias-Roach, Lisa c/o Boys Town National Institute, 555 North 30th Street, Omaha, NE 68131, (402) 449-6666, BA 78 San Diego St Univ; MS 81 Univ of Redlands; 85–Sp-Lang Path, Boys Town National Institute, **SLP**

Tobin, Annette R 7523 18th N E, Seattle, WA 98115, MS 69 Univ of WA; SLP, Seattle School District 1, **SLP**

Tobin, Bonnie L 23014 Ostronic Drive, Woodland Hills, CA 91367-6144, (818) 713-8242, **SLP**

Tobin, Mrs Deborrah Johnston Saint Francis Medical Center, Audiology Department, 4401 Penn Avenue Suite 1200, Pittsburgh, PA 15201, (412) 622-4488, BA 79 Univ of Pittsburgh - Pittsburgh; MA 81 Univ of Pittsburgh - Pittsburgh; 87–Chief of Aud, St Francis Med Ctr, **A**

Tobin, Mrs Deirdre Mary 112 Ralph Avenue, Babylon, NY 11702, (516) 667-6000, BA 84 Adelphi Univ; MS 85 Adelphi Univ; **SLP**

Tobin, Mrs Denise A 171 Woodward Avenue, Fond Du Lac, WI 54935, (414) 929-2890, BS 77 Univ of WI - Oshkosh; MA 78 Univ of WI - Oshkosh; Sp/Lang Path, Fond Du Lac Sch Dist, **SLP**

Tobin, Dr Henry 10662 Faulkner Ridge Circle, Columbia, MD 21044, (301) 477-1800, BA 56 CUNY - Brooklyn Coll; MA 62 CUNY - Brooklyn Coll; PH 68 (NS) Purdue Univ - West Lafayette; Aud, VA Medical Center, **SLP A**

Tobin, Mrs Janet P 109 Pleasant Street, Box 453, North Kingstown, RI 02852, (401) 277-5485, BS 67 Univ of VT; MS 68 Univ of NE - Omaha; Asst Dir, R I Hosp Hrng & Sp Cen, **SLP**

Tobin, Mrs Sherry Yolles 3733 Font Hill Drive, Ellicott City, MD 21043, (301) 498-5040, BA 74 Univ of MD - College Park; MA 76 Catholic Univ of America; Sp-Lang Path, Howard Co Bd of Ed, **SLP**

Tobin, Mrs Sylvia Magura Saudia Hearing Aids, PO Box 3460-81190, 3301 Menaul NE, Albuquerque, NM 87107, (505) 889-9100, MS 84 Univ of NM; MS 74 Univ of NV - Las Vegas; BA 71 Univ of KY; Aud, Sandia Hrng Aids, **A**

Tobin, William D 109 Pleasant Street, North Kingstown, RI 02852, (401) 294-4665, BA 64 Creighton Univ; MS 68 Univ of NE - Omaha; Private Practice, **SLP ACE**

Tobisman, Karen Bleier 251 Bellino Drive, Pacific Palisades, CA 90272, (213) 450-1649, BA 61 1939; MA 69 Univ of Southern CA; **SLP**

Tobochnik, Andrea Moll 412 Stuart Avenue, Kalamazoo, MI 49007, (212) 852-3220, BA 79 Clark Univ; MS 83 Columbia Univ Teachers Coll; Sp-Lang Path, Hrng & Sp Ctr Constance Brown, **SLP ACE**

Tobolowsky, Judith W 13325 Purple Sage, Dallas, TX 75240, (214) 239-9404, BA 70 Adelphi Univ; ME 71 Boston Univ; **SLP**

Tockert, Sr M 3600 Broadway, Great Bend, KS 67530, (316) 792-1232, BS; **SLP LM**

Toczylowski, Corinne A 8 Hemlock Street, Dupont, PA 18641, (717) 287-9680, BS 74 Bloomsburg Univ of PA; ME 75 Bloomsburg Univ of PA; SLP, Luzerne Intermediate Unit 18, **SLP**

Toczylowski, Darlene M 9219 Shields, 2nd Floor, Brookfield, IL 60513, (312) 850-7573, BA 78 Saint Xavier Coll; MA 79 Univ of IL - Urbana; Sp Ed-SLP, St Xavier College, **SLP**

Todd, Bonnie E 46 W 615 Dolly Lane, Big Rock, IL 60511, (312) 556-3031, BS 72 Northern IL Univ - De Kalb; MA 73 Northern IL Univ - De Kalb; **SLP**

Todd, Mrs Deborah S 6312 Stilwell, Plano, TX 75023, (214) 330-5253, BA 78 TX Tech Univ; MA 81 Univ of North TX; 81–Sp-Lang Path, Dallas ISD, **SLP**

Todd, Eleanor F 2208 Cabrillo Circle, Lodi, CA 95240, (209) 368-2056, BA 35 Univ of Redlands; ME 73 Univ of the Pacific; Consult - Deaf Infants, Private Practice, **LM**

Todd, Leann Pilkenton 2506 Teton Circle, Wichita, KS 67215-1504, BA 83 Wichita St Univ; MA 85 Wichita St Univ; 85–Sp-Lang Path, Sg County Coop, **SLP**

Todd, Linda I 2339 Kilborne Drive, Charlotte, NC 28205, (704) 343-6400, BS 73 East Carolina Univ; MS 76 East Carolina Univ; 79–Sp-Lang Path, Charlotte-Mecklenburg Schs, **SLP**

Todd, Mrs Margaret Florance 8302 Hot Springs Drive, Houston, TX 77095, (713) 926-0853, BS 80 Univ of TX - Austin; MA 82 Univ of Houston - Univ Park; SLP, Cypress ISD, **SLP**

Todd, Mrs Margit Juul 1844 Palisades Drive, Carlsbad, CA 92008, (619) 729-1496, MA 73 Univ of Southern CA; SLP, Los Angeles USD, **SLP**

Todd, Mrs Maureen F 7770 Ivygate Lane, Cincinnati, OH 45242, (513) 984-8922, BA 73 Univ of ME - Orono; MS 74 Ithaca Coll; **SLP**

Todd, Nancy A 1020 Sassafras Lane, Niles, MI 49120, (616) 684-0222, BS 65 Marquette Univ; MA 87 Western MI Univ; 87–Sp-Lang Path, Buchanan Comm Schs, **SLP**

Todd, Pamela R 112 Mackey Avenue, Butler, PA 16001, (412) 776-1581, BS 69 CA Univ of PA; ME 74 CA Univ of PA; 84–Sp-Lang Path, Seneca Valley Sch Dist, **SLP**

Todd, Susan M P O Box 506, Hammond, LA 70401, (504) 567-3111, BS 79 Murray St Univ; MS 83 Murray St Univ; Sp/Lang Path, Priv Pract, **SLP**

Todebush, Martha J 265 Garcia Avenue, San Leandro, CA 94577, (415) 635-6003, BS 76 CA St Univ - Hayward; MA 79 CA St Univ - Fresno; 79–Aud, **A**

Todtfeld, Mrs Michele Brenda 14404 N W 67th Street, Parkville, MO 64152, (913) 621-6255, BA 80 CUNY - Brooklyn Coll; MS 81 Columbia Univ Teachers Coll; SLP, Wyandotte Co Comp Sp Ed Coop, **SLP**

Toennies, Mrs Joanne Elizabeth 2497 Hillpoint Drive, McFarland, WI 53558, (608) 838-8745, MS 84 Univ of WI - Whitewater; Sp-Lang Path, Middleton Sch Dist, **SLP**

Toennies, Mrs Teresa Kanrhoff P O Box 312, Rural Delivery 1, New Baden, IL 62265, (618) 465-0105, MS 85 Southern IL Univ-Edwardsvill; BS 83 Southern IL Univ-Edwardsvill; **SLP**

Toepel, Gail A HC 61 Box 1325, Cle Elum, WA 98922, (509) 674-4527, BS 74 Wayne St Univ; MA 77 Wayne St Univ; 88–Aud, Mt View Hrng & Sp Ctr, **A**

Toerper, Mrs Billie Jean 499 Hunting Park Lane, York, PA 17402, (717) 755-5192, MA 75 Univ of Pittsburgh - Pittsburgh; **SLP**

Togami, Joan Allbright 110 East 10th Avenue, Belton, TX 76503, (817) 756-4447, BS 84 Baylor Univ; MS 85 Baylor Univ; 88–Sp-Lang Path, Scott & White Hosp, **SLP**

Tognan, Mrs Denise M 136 Roosevelt Street, Oceanside, NY 11572, (516) 825-8800, BA 75 Adelphi Univ; MA 76 Adelphi Univ; Aud, Franklin General Hospital, **A**

Togno, Mrs Lucille P 7 College Road, Netcong, NJ 07857, (201) 538-0339, BA 72 Montclair St Coll; MA 78 Montclair St Coll; 72–Sp-Lang Path, Morris Plains Bd of Ed, **SLP**

Tokarz, Mrs Jeanne G P O Box 546, St Michaels, MD 21663, (301) 745-5433, BA 39 Saint Joseph's Coll; Sp-Lang Path, Talbot Co Hm Hlth Agcy, **SLP**

Tokay, Mrs Carol B Smith-Garrison Road, Newmarket, NH 03857, (603) 778-0503, BA 68 Central MI Univ; MA 72 Univ of MA - Amherst; Sp-Lang Path, Exeter Sch Dist, **SLP**

Tokay, Dr F Harry Smith-Garrison Road, Newmarket, NH 03857, (603) 749-2444, BS 60 Saint Cloud St Univ; MA 62 MI St Univ; PH 67 (NS) MI St Univ; Aud, Atlantic ENT Pro Assoc, **A**

Tokishi, Walter H 410 Kahiki Street, Kahului Maui, HI 96732, (808) 877-7944, BS 62 Emporia St Univ, MS 70 Univ of OR; 79–Sp-Lang Path, Private Practice, **SLP**

Tokita, Mrs Shayne Horita 4427 UPA Road, Koloa, HI 96756, (808) 245-6983, BS 73 Univ of HI - Manoa; MS 74 Univ of HI - Manoa; Cen Dir, Er Sl So-Hawaii Inc, **SLP**

Tokoly, Mrs Alice A P 311 Black Oak Drive, Michigan City, IN 46360, (219) 879-2411, MA 79 Ball St Univ; SLP, MI Cty Area Schs, **SLP**

Tokosch, Ann Frances 110 Severn Way, Arnold, MD 21012, (301) 757-2440, BA 82 Univ of MD - College Park; MA 84 Univ of MD - College Park; Sp-Lang Path, Anne Arundel Public Schools, **SLP**

Tokusato, Mona A 1825 Anapuni Street #302, Honolulu, HI 96822, (808) 946-8443, BS 84 Univ of HI - Manoa; MS 86 Univ of HI - Manoa

Tolbert, Alfred J 1309 East Lincoln Highway, Coatesville, PA 19320, (215) 384-9211, BA 72 Wayne St Univ; MA 84 Trenton St Coll; 88–Pres, Quality Rehabilitation Svcs Inc, **SLP**

Tolbert, Brenda Rodgers 11861 Cato Drive, Florissant, MO 63033-6901, (314) 837-6664, **A**

Toleman, Cynthia F 30 Maple Leaf Circle, Penfield, NY 14526, **SLP**

Toler, Joyce Marie 202 J Saxony Place, Fayetteville, NC 28304, MS 80 East Carolina Univ; Sp-Lang Path, Dev Evaluation Center, **SLP**

Tolin, Mrs Paula Rupert 3281 Farber Road S E, Magnolia, OH 44643, BS 79 Kent St Univ; MA 79 Kent St Univ; Sp-Lang Path, Sandy Valley Local Sch Syst, **SLP**

Toll, Mrs Donna Marie 126 Strathmore Road, Havertown, PA 19083, (215) 891-2212, Sp-Lang Path, Elwyn Inst, **SLP**

Tolland-Lavey, Mrs Therese Maria 3319 Drummond, Toledo, OH 43606, BA 79 Univ of Toledo; MA 85 Eastern MI Univ; **SLP**

Tollefson, Brenda Kay 40 West 78th #304, Richfield, MN 55423, (612) 866-7957, BS 85 Mankato St Univ; MS 87 Mankato St Univ; 87–Sp-Lang Path, InSpeech Inc, **SLP**

Tollefson, Mrs Christine Hirahara 6717 Hillglen Way, Fair Oaks, CA 95628, (916) 961-5267, BA 71 CA Lutheran Coll; MS 83 San Francisco St Univ; 87–Sp-Lang Path, Burger Physical Therap & Rehab Agency Inc, **SLP**

Tollefson, Lori Ann 1201 Office Park Road #811, West Des Moines, IA 50265, (515) 224-0979, BS 86 Univ of IA; MS 88 Univ of IA

Tolley, Carolyn J Audiometric Services Inc, 2718 Hollandale, Suite 200, Dallas, TX 75234, (214) 521-1261, BS 75 Univ of AR - Fayetteville; MS 79 Southern Methodist Univ; Aud, Audiometric Sers Inc, **A**

Tolley, Patricia Banks 14 Wayne Drive, Poughkeepsie, NY 12601, (919) 851-7159, BS 83 Appalachian St Univ; MS 86 East TN St Univ; 88–Sp-Lang Path, Hudsen-Valley Sp Ctr, **SLP**

Tolley-Hindman, Mrs Christine Elaine 1216 40th Street West, Bradenton, FL 34205, (813) 747-4773, BA 81 Indiana Univ of PA; MS 83 WV Univ; Sp-Lang Path, Manatee County School System, **SLP**

Tolliver, Beverly Diane 11168 Roxbury, Detroit, MI 48224, BS 75 MI St Univ; MS 75 Miles Coll; MA 76 Wayne St Univ; Teacher, Detroit Bd of Ed, **SLP**

Tolliver, Janey K 8625 Nubbin Ridge Road, Knoxville, TN 37923, (615) 690-8961, BS 81 Univ of TN - Knoxville; MA 82 Univ of TN - Knoxville; Sp-Lang Path, East Tennessee Childrens Rehab, **SLP**

Tollos, Sandra Katherine 173 Quebec Avenue, Toronto, ON, Canada M6P 2T9, (416) 964-9595, BA 83 MI St Univ; MA 84 MI St Univ; Audiologist, The Canadian Hearing Society, **A**

Tolson, Maureen Bowes 31 Ellis Road, Southbridge, MA 01550, (617) 792-8500, BS 79 Univ of NH; MS 82 CO St Univ; Sp/Lang Path, Hahnemann Hospital, **SLP**

Tom, Cynthia Marie 604 Avery Avenue, Syracuse, NY 13204, (315) 425-4477, **SLP**

Tom, Kenneth Dept Of Sp Path & Aud, Speech And Hearing Center, Univ Of Iowa, Iowa City, IA 52242, MA 87 San Diego St Univ; **SLP**

Tom, Mrs Rosemarie N 204 Kingsman, Converse, TX 78109, (808) 423-2477, BS 73 Univ of HI - Manoa; MS 75 Univ of IL - Urbana; Sp-Lang Path, Dept of Ed, **SLP**

Tomaino, Deborah Walsh 624 Irving Place, Long Branch, NJ 07740, (201) 244-3100, BA 76 Kean Coll of NJ; MA 77 Kean Coll of NJ; 85–Dir/Sp-Lang Path, Garden State Rehab Hosp, **SLP**

Tomala, Mary P 38242 Briarwood Place, Wayne, MI 48184, (313) 729-3548, BS 68 Eastern MI Univ; MA 70 Eastern MI Univ; **SLP**

Tomalski, Suzanne F 236 Fredrick Drive, Athens, GA 30607, (404) 549-9319, BA 77 Loyola Coll; MS 80 Loyola Coll; ES 83 Univ of GA; Sp/Lang Path, Athens Gen Hosp, **SLP**

Toman, Mrs Barbara Kessler 14939 Rodstock Drive, Houston, TX 77062, (713) 488-7221, **SLP**

Tomanelli, Angie Marie 7516 Fair Avenue, Sun Valley, CA 91352, (818) 503-9826, BS 81 FL St Univ; MS 83 FL St Univ; Sp-Lang Path, New Sch for Child Development, **SLP**

Tomanovich, Sandra 210 Fairgate Street, Rochester, NY 14606, MS 68 SUNY - Coll at Geneseo; OM 84 SUNY - Coll at Brockport; SLP, City Sch Dist Rochester, **SLP**

Tomasic, Mrs Dorothy Ann 6113 Haverford Avenue, Indianapolis, IN 46220, (317) 843-0120, BS 84 Purdue Univ - West Lafayette; MA 85 Memphis St Univ; 88–Sp-Lang Path, The Ctr for Neuro Rehab, **SLP**

Tomassetti, Carole W P O Box 60671, Longmeadow, MA 01106, (413) 781-9100, BA 66 Univ of MA - Amherst; MA 68 Univ of MA - Amherst; OM 84 Western New England Coll; Director Sp-Hrng-Lang Center, Mercy Hospital, **A**

Tomassini, Daisy Suite 2, San Patricip Plaza Pcc, San Juan, PR 00920, MS; **SLP**

Tomasso, Mrs Jean Anne 901 Weiland Road, Rochester, NY 14626, (716) 225-6167, BS 76 SUNY - Coll at Geneseo; MS 81 Nazareth Coll of Rochester; Sp-Lang Path, **SLP**

Tomaszewski, Elaine M Box 35 Princess Point Road, Yarmouth, ME 04096, (207) 729-5577, BS 74 Univ of ME - Farmington; MS 79 SUNY - Coll at Buffalo; Sp-Lang Path, Brunswick School Dept, **SLP**

Tomblin, J Bruce Wendell Johnson Sp & Hrng Ctr, University Of Iowa, Iowa City, IA 52242, (319) 335-8745, BA 66 Univ of LA Verne; MA 67 Univ of Redlands; PH 70 (NS) Univ of WI - Madison; Prof, Univ of Iowa, **SLP F**

Tomchak, Mrs Ann Marie 2871 Graham Road #2, Stow, OH 44224, (216) 673-4514, BS 87 Kent St Univ; MA 87 Kent St Univ; 87–Sp-Lang Path, Field Local Sch Sys, **SLP**

Tomchik, Peggy Frances 23 Creekfield Drive, Sumter, SC 29154-4607, (803) 648-8344, MS 85 Univ of South FL; **SLP**

Tomei, Mrs Robin A 8933 Milton Morris Drive, Charlotte, NC 28212, (704) 343-6410, BS 83 East Carolina Univ; MA 87 Appalachian St Univ; 88–Sp-Lang Path, Charlotte-Mecklenburg Schs, **SLP**

Tomes, Mrs Ines A 5121 McCoy Road, Oxford, OH 45056, (513) 867-5960, BS 80 Univ of Cincinnati; MA 83 Univ of Cincinnati; 84–Sp-Lang Path, Butler Co Bd of MR/DD, **SLP**

Tomes, Lucrezia A 3555 North 1st Avenue #H-4, Tucson, AZ 85719, (402) 472-2068, BA 73 Coe Coll; MA 76 Univ of IA; University of Arizona, **SLP**

Tomiello, Mrs Marilyn R 465 Bell Street, Chagrin Falls, OH 44022, (216) 247-5024, BS 67 Kent St Univ; MA 69 Kent St Univ; 88–Asst Admin-Phys Med/Rehab Svcs, Lake Hosp System Inc, **SLP**

Tominac, Cheryl Ann 4332 West Oraibi Drive, Glendale, AZ 85308, BA 79 MI St Univ; MS 81 AZ St Univ; Sp-Lang Path, Deer Valley USD, **SLP**

Tomita, Mrs Bessie S 5985 Brace Road, Loomis, CA 95650, (916) 454-8291, BA 72 CA St Univ - Sacramento; MA 74 CA St Univ - Sacramento; SLP, Sacramento Cty USD, **SLP**

Tomkiewicz, Carol C Rd 1 Box 120, Sugarloaf, PA 18249, (717) 824-9742, BS 78 Bloomsburg Univ of PA; MS 79 Bloomsburg Univ of PA; Co-Dir, Wilkes-Barre Sp & Lang Cl, **SLP**

Tomko, Mrs Rosemary 2845 West Monroe Street, Bethel Park, PA 15102, (412) 622-4484, BS 74 Univ of Pittsburgh - Pittsburgh; MA 76 Univ of Pittsburgh - Pittsburgh; Sp-Lang Path, St Francis Medical Center, **SLP**

Tomko, Mrs Sharon Ann 1213 Tillicum Drive, Worthington, OH 43085, (419) 522-1214, BA 81 OH St Univ; MA 82 OH St Univ; SLP, Private Practice, **SLP**

Tomlin, Kathryn J 82 Unami Trail, Chalfont, PA 18914, (215) 822-5992, BS 78 PA St Univ - Univ Park; MS 80 Columbia Univ Teachers Coll; 84–Sp-Lang Path, Doylestown Hosp Rehab Ctr, **SLP**

Tomlinson, Mrs Cameron V 348 Bay Avenue, Huntington Bay, NY 11743, (516) 423-1499, ME 74 Univ of VA - Charlottesville

Tomlinson, Mrs Joan Hough 203 Felicity Street, Bay St Louis, MS 39520, (601) 467-2957, BA 50 Northwestern St Univ; ME 61 Northwestern St Univ; Sp-Lang Path, Bay St Louis Sch Dist, **SLP**

Tomlinson, Kristine Diegel 344-1/2 Meeting House Lane, Narberth, PA 19072, (215) 427-5469, BS 83 Trenton St Coll; MA 86 Hahneman Medical Coll; Audiologist, St Christophers Hospital, **A**

Tomlinson, Peggy Kosters 10343 Birkemeyer Drive, Cincinnati, OH 45242, (513) 984-2188, BS 71 Univ of IA; MA 72 Univ of IA

Tomlinson, Theresa Fay 2360 Thompson Bridge Road, Apartment G-4, Gainesville, GA 30501, (404) 532-8314, BS 86 Univ of GA; ME 87 Univ of GA; 87–Sp-Lang Path, Hall County Sch Sys

Tomoeda, Cheryl K Dept Of Speech & Hearing Sciences, Univ Of Arizona, Tucson, AZ 85721, (602) 629-9760, BS 80 Univ of HI - Manoa; MS 82 Univ of AZ; Res Asst/Sp-Lang Path, University of Arizona, **SLP**

Tomory, Raymond Julius 1961 Norene Street, Anchorage, AK 99508, (907) 272-5325, MA 85 KS St Univ; Sp-Lang Path, Anchorage Sch Dist, **SLP**

Tomosada, Ann Hatsumi 1923-G Fern Street, Honolulu, HI 96826, (808) 947-1884, BS 79 Univ of HI - Manoa; MA 83 Univ of KS; Sp-Lang Path, Dept of Ed, **SLP**

Tompkins, Mrs Charlene H 2630 Van Dam NE, Belmont, MI 49306, (616) 456-4207, BA 74 MI St Univ; MA 75 MI St Univ; SLP, Grand Rapids Public Schools, **SLP**

Tompkins, Dr Connie A 703 Woodland Drive, Pittsburgh, PA 15238, (412) 624-2311, BS 75 IL St Univ - Normal; MS 77 IL St Univ - Normal; PH 84 (NS) Univ of WA; Asst Prof-Comm Disorders, Univ of Pittsburgh, **SLP**

Tompkins, Mary M 504 Douglas, Elkhorn, NE 68022, (402) 721-7710, BS 71 Univ of NE - Omaha; MS 73 Univ of NE - Omaha; ES 85 Univ of NE - Omaha; 86–Dir-Spec Educ, Ed Ser Ut #2, **SLP**

Tompkins, Susan Morgan 12714 Miriam Lane, Houston, TX 77071, (713) 792-4744, BS 80 Univ of VA - Charlottesville; ME 82 Univ of VA - Charlottesville; Aud, U of TX Med Sch, **A**

Tomtishen, Mrs Louise F Rd 1 Box 17, Ringtown, PA 17967, (215) 799-4111, BS 77 Bloomsburg Univ of PA; MS 78 Bloomsburg Univ of PA; **SLP**

Tondra, Mrs Janice K 3737 Croydon Drive N W, Canton, OH 44718, (216) 493-7717, BA 73 Univ of Akron; MA 74 Kent St Univ; **SLP**

Toner, Katherine Young 1575 Sacramento #8, San Francisco, CA 94109, (415) 346-5874, BA 82 San Francisco St Univ; MS 84 San Francisco St Univ; Sp-Lang Path, California-Hawaii Elks Major Project Inc, **SLP**

Toner, Dr Mary A 862 North 10th, Laramie, WY 82070, (307) 766-6426, BS 76 Univ of WY; MS 78 Univ of WY; PH 85 (NS) Univ of OK Medical Center; Sp-Lang Path, U of WY, **SLP**

Toner, Susan M 75 Williams Street #B, Rutland, VT 05701, (802) 773-1919, MA 76 SUNY - Center at Buffalo; Sp-Lang Path, Rutland Cty Pub Schs, **SLP**

Toner, Mrs Tommie C 2045 Bermuda Hills Road, Columbia, SC 29204-6706, (803) 788-3792, BA 63 FL St Univ; ME 74 Univ of TN - Chattanooga; Elem Couns, Richland Sch Dist One, **SLP**

Tonetti, Mrs Suzanne Marie 14 Westview Avenue #700, Tuckahoe, NY 10707, (914) 961-3678, BS 84 James Madison Univ; ME 87 Univ of VA - Charlottesville

Tonge, Mrs Michele Stolar 16 Langton Lane, Newtown Square, PA 19073, (215) 356-2119, BA 79 Univ of MD - College Park; MA 81 Temple Univ-Tyler Sch of Art; **SLP**

Tongen, John L Professional Hearing Center, 925 West Villard, Dickinson, ND 58601, (701) 227-4403, BS 78 ND St Univ; MS 80 Minot St Univ; Dir, Private Practice, **A**

Tongier, Joan C Route 1 Box 140-D, Altamont, KS 67330, BS 70 Emporia St Univ; MA 76 Univ of Northern CO; Sp-Lang Path, Sek Spec Ed Coop USD #250, **SLP**

Tonini, Mrs Kathleen Burnett 3315 Nanz Avenue, Louisville, KY 40207, (502) 454-8205, BS 80 Eastern KY Univ; ME 82 Eastern KY Univ; Sp-Lang Path, Jefferson County Board of Educ, **SLP**

Tonini, Mrs Kathleen M 2 Whitecloud, Irvine, CA 92714, BA 76 Univ of Southern CA; MA 80 CA St Univ - Fullerton; Sp-Lang Path, **SLP**

Tonini, Ross E 110 North 8th Street #2, Allentown, PA 18101, (215) 434-1975, BS 81 Univ of AZ; MS 83 Univ of AZ; 86–Sp-Lang Path, RT Enterprises, **SLP**

Tonkin-Stickler, Marilyn J 12 Boud Avenue, Farmingdale, NJ 07727, (201) 591-1750, BS 77 Indiana Univ of PA; MA 81 Trenton St Coll; Sp-Lang Path, Children's Psych Cen, **SLP**

Tonkovich, John D Speech-Language Pathology Dept, Rehabilitation Institute, 261 Mack Boulevard, Detroit, MI 48201, (313) 745-9721, BA 72 Univ of MI - Ann Arbor; MS 73 Univ of MI - Ann Arbor; PH 78 (Sp/Hrng Sci) Univ of TN - Knoxville; 80–Dir/Sp-Lang Path, Rehabilitation Inst, **SLP A ACE**

Tonkovich, Mary J H 8295 Garnet Street, Juneau, AK 99801, (907) 789-2514, BA 68 MT St Univ; MA 75 WA St Univ; Reading Resource Teacher, Cty & Bor/Juneau Sch Dist, **SLP**

Tonkovich, Susana M 9878 Coledale Court, Union Lake, MI 48085, (313) 344-8415, MA 73 Eastern MI Univ; Sp-Lang Path, Northville Public Schools, **SLP**

Tonn, Martin 1115 12th Street South, Moorhead, MN 56560, (218) 233-3657, BA 49 Univ of IA; MA 50 Univ of IA; PH 64 (NS) Univ of IA; **SLP LM**

Tonokawa, Lisa Lynn 1962 North Allen Avenue, Altadena, CA 91001, (213) 483-9930, BA 81 Humboldt St Univ; MS 83 CO St Univ; 88–Coord, Otologic Med Group Inc, **A**

Tonsager, Mary L 1890 Helena Road North, Oakdale, MN 55119, (612) 520-5614, BA 77 Augsburg Coll; MA 81 MI St Univ; 88–Sp-Lang Path, ISD #622, **SLP**

Tooker, Patricia Ann 1406 Cherrywood Square, San Jose, CA 95117, (408) 923-1845, BA 60 San Jose St Univ; MA 72 San Jose St Univ; MA 81 Univ of Santa Clara; SLP, Berryessa Un Sch Dist, **SLP**

Tookey, Mrs Carol 1033 Rafael Street North, Salem, OR 97303, (503) 399-3163, BA 57 Linfield Coll; MS 76 Western OR St Coll; Sp/Lang Path, Salem Sch Dist, **SLP**

Toolajian, Mrs Anne Scala 633 Roosevelt Street, Westfield, NJ 07090, (201) 654-0098, BA 81 George Washington Univ; MA 83 George Washington Univ; Sp-Lang Path, Private Practice, **SLP**

Toole, Dolores M 1613 North Logan, Danville, IL 61832, (217) 431-8156, BA 64 Southern IL Univ -Carbondale; MS 81 Southern IL Univ-Edwardsvill; Aud, Central Assoc for Spec Ed, **A ACE**

Toole, Janet M 211 Burton Street, Grayslake, IL 60030-1409, (312) 578-3759, BA 73 CA St Univ - Los Angeles; MA 75 CA St Univ - Los Angeles; MA 86 Northwestern Univ; Audiology Supervisor, VA Medical Center, **A**

Tooley, Brenda J 111 Willow Road #17, Ruidoso, NM 88345, (505) 247-0371, BS 71 Univ of IL - Urbana; MA 71 Univ of IL - Urbana; SLP, All Indiana Pueblo Council, **SLP**

Toombs, Margaret S 242 Taranto Lane, Houston, TX 77015, (713) 455-3795, BA 76 Univ of Houston - Univ Park; MS 79 Univ of TX - Houston; Dir, Private Practice, **SLP ACE**

Toomer, Catherine Ann 7918 Sycamore, New Orleans, LA 70118, (504) 891-4072, **SLP**

Toomey, Mrs Carol S 2901 Gerard Avenue, Sinking Spring, PA 19608, (215) 670-0648, BA 69 Coll Misericordia; ME 71 Bloomsburg Univ of PA; Sp-Lang Path, Berks Co Intermediate Unit, **SLP**

Toomey, Mrs Marilyn Mantifel 7545 Graves Road, Cincinnati, OH 45243, (513) 369-4000, BS 64 Kent St Univ; MA 67 Case Western Reserve Univ; Sp-Lang Path, Cincinnati Pub Sch, **SLP**

Toomey, Dr Mary Fran St Michaels College, Winooski, VT 05404, (802) 655-2000, MA 63 Univ of CT; MA 79 Univ of VT; PH 80 (NS) Univ of VT; Dir Spec Ed Prog, St Michaels Coll, **SLP**

Toomey, Wendy J P O Box 584, Chico, CA 95927, (916) 741-6231, BA 78 CA St Univ - Chico; MA 80 CA St Univ - Chico; SLP, Yuba Co Sch, **SLP**

Toomey-Brigham, Rosemary 1106 North Bailey Road, Coatesville, PA 19320, (215) 384-7711, SLP, VA, **SLP**

Toonen, Mrs Margaret S 14014 White Birch Road, Minnetonka, MN 55343, (612) 544-2908, MA 76 Saint Louis Univ; Sp-Lang Path, Hennepin Technical Institute, **SLP**

Toor, Mrs Jane H 2152 Meadow Hills Court, Columbus, OH 43228, (614) 272-2924, BS 77 Purdue Univ - West Lafayette; MA 78 Ball St Univ; **SLP**

Toovy, Michael L 7432 Gazette Avenue, Canoga Park, CA 91306-2712, (213) 936-3411, **SLP**

Topa, Carole B 10804 Vernon, Huntington Woods, MI 48070, (313) 333-7435, BS 61 Univ of Detroit; MA 67 Eastern MI Univ; 86–Sp-Lang Path, Pontiac Bd of Educ, **SLP**

Topa, Mrs Christine Breen 25 Orchard Street, Warren, PA 16365, (800) 331-8840, **SLP**

Topalian, Tracy Ann 2926 Gregory Street, Madison, WI 53711, (608) 244-2411, BS 78 Univ of WI - Madison; MS 82 Univ of WI - Madison; SLP, Mendota Ment Health I, **SLP**

Tope, Dolores M 9604 Waterline Drive, Burke, VA 22015, (703) 455-1843, OM 87 AZ St Univ; 88–Sp-Lang Path, Comm Rehab Svcs PC

Topel, Ellyn 1725 Overland Trail, Deerfield, IL 60015, (312) 945-5980, MA 88 Northwestern Univ

Topf, A Bridget 111 North 49th Street #N-4, Philadelphia, PA 19139-2718, (215) 922-1188, BA 68 Clarke Coll; MA 78 Univ of SD - Vermillion; SLP, **SLP**

Topkin, Susan 903 Maple Lane, East Meadow, NY 11554, BA 74 SUNY - Center at Buffalo; MA 75 Hofstra Univ; Sp-Lang Path, Private Practice, **SLP**

Topp, Karen S 3071 Shamrock Place, Nanaimo, BC, Canada V9T 2Z6, (604) 755-7611, OB 76 Univ of Manitoba - Winnipeg; MA 79 Univ of ND; 87–Sp/Lang Path, Nanaimo Reg Gen Hosp, **SLP**

Topper, Diane Marie 736 Benton Court, Elmhurst, IL 60126, (312) 620-4433, BS 82 IL St Univ - Normal; MS 84 IL St Univ - Normal; **SLP**

Topper, Mrs Maureen Gallagher 30 Arden Lane, Bethlehem, PA 18015, BS 77 Villanova Univ; MS 79 Columbia Univ Teachers Coll; **SLP**

Topper, Nancy B 251-06 71st Road, Little Neck, NY 11426, (212) 470-2741, BA 78 CUNY - Queens Coll; MA 80 Hofstra Univ; Sp/Lang Path, Lng Insl Jewish-Hilside Med Ce, **SLP**

Toppin, Cynthia J 409 West 7th Street, Hastings, MN 55033, (612) 227-8471, BA 74 Univ of MN - Minneap-St Paul; MA 76 Univ of MN - Minneap-St Paul; 87–VP-Rehab Therapies, SPRC, **SLP**

Topping, Gary E 3212 Cranberry, Wichita, KS 67226-5174, (316) 689-3289, BA 71 Adams St Coll; MA 71 Adams St Coll; OD 77 (NS) Univ of CO - Boulder; 84–Dir of Aud Cl Serv, Wichita State U, **A**

Torabi, Mrs Elaine E Rural Route 1, Comfrey, MN 56019, (507) 877-2355, BA 64 Mankato St Univ; **SLP**

Toren, Linda R 835 Mix Avenue #309, Hamden, CT 06514, (203) 239-5865, BS 59 Purdue Univ - West Lafayette; MS 65 Stanford Univ; SLP, North Haven Pub Sch, **SLP**

Torf, Mrs Donna R 2210 Ash Lane, Northbrook, IL 60062, (312) 498-1147, BS 77 Loyola Univ of Chicago; MA 80 Northwestern Univ; Sp-Lang Path, **SLP**

Torfin, Deanna Janine 9510 Congdon Boulevard, Duluth, MN 55804, (218) 727-0900, MA 83 Univ of MN - Duluth; Sp-Lang Path, Polinsky Medical Rehabil Ctr, **SLP**

Torgerson, Mrs Elaine B 900 25th Street N W, Minot, ND 58701, (701) 727-6140, BS 68 Univ of ND; MS 72 Univ of ND; Sp-Lang Path, Souris Valley Spec Ed Ut, **SLP**

Torgerson, Dr John K Minot State University, 500 University Avenue West, Minot, ND 58701, BA 64 Moorhead St Univ; MS 66 Purdue Univ - West Lafayette; PH 75 (Sp-Lang Path) Wayne St Univ; 80–Prof, Minot State Univ, **SLP**

Torgerson, Judith Martha The Hear Center, 305 15th Avenue East, Seattle, WA 98112, (206) 322-0011, BA 80 Moorhead St Univ; MA 85 Western WA Univ; Aud, The Hear Center, **A**

Torgerson, Nancy Ann 1973 North Woodward Avenue, Bloomfield Hills, MI 48013, (313) 644-5197, MS 88 Univ of MI - Ann Arbor; 88–Sp-Lang Path, Oakwood Hosp

Torkelsen, Mrs Darla J 2020 South 360th E304, Federal Way, WA 98003, (206) 874-8514, BS 86 Loma Linda Univ - Riverside; MS 87 Loma Linda Univ - Riverside; Sp-Lang Path, Associated Home Health Care

Torkos, Gina Pretti 919 Smokey Wood Drive, Pittsburgh, PA 15218, (412) 622-4359, BS 82 Indiana Univ of PA; MA 85 Univ of Pittsburgh - Pittsburgh; 86–Chief Sp-Lang Path Rehab, St Francis Med Ctr, **SLP**

Torline, Mrs Lori L 11405 Howard Street, Whittier, CA 90601, (213) 695-0311, BA 77 Wichita St Univ; MA 78 Wichita St Univ; Sp-Lang Path, Los Angeles County Office Educ, **SLP**

Tormey, Kimberly A 394 Crawford St, New Shrewsbury, NJ 07724, (201) 747-0128, **SLP**

Tornblom, David H 523 Lamp Post Lane, Camp Hill, PA 17011, (717) 787-2271, BA 53 Waynesburg Coll; MS 64 Univ of UT; Pub Hlth Aud, PA Dept of Hlth, **SLP A ACE**

Torney, Catherine 1202 North Holden Road, Greensboro, NC 27410, (916) 852-6319, MA 74 Univ of IA; **SLP**

Toro, Bridget H 7410 Authon Drive, Dallas, TX 75248, (214) 960-1196, BS 73 Univ of MO - Columbia; MS 74 Southern IL Univ -Carbondale; **SLP**

Toro, Jaime Irizarry Box 40623, Minillas Station, San Juan, PR 00940, (809) 726-3695, MS 71 Univ of PR - Rio Piedras

Toro, Margaret Ross 34 Whitten Street, Dorchester, MA 02122, BS 73 SUNY - Center at Buffalo; MA 76 SUNY - Center at Buffalo; Adjunct Clinical Instructor, Boston U, **A**

Torp, Marilyn 116 Holway Drive, Santa Cruz, CA 95065, (408) 429-3805, BA 75 CA St Univ - Sacramento; MA 81 San Jose St Univ; Sp/Lang Path, Santa Cruz City Sch, **SLP**

Torpey, Dr Mary Clare C 4141 East Avenue, Rochester, NY 14618, (716) 381-3490, BA 52 Nazareth Coll of Rochester; MA 59 Nazareth Coll of Rochester; ED 68 (Sp Path & Aud) Boston Univ; 63–Prof, Nazareth Coll of Rochester, **SLP**

Torrans, Dr Anne Communication Department, Louisiana State University, One University Circle, Shreveport, LA 71115, (318) 797-5315, BA 55 Northwestern St Univ; MA 59 LA St Univ - Baton Rouge; PH 72 (NS) MI St Univ; 79–Prof, Commun Dept Lsu Shreveport, **SLP**

Torrence, Mrs Penny P 19832 Bazzellton Place, Gaithersburg, MD 20879, (301) 963-4957, MS 84 Bloomsburg Univ of PA; Sp-Lang Path, Mont Co Pub Schs, **SLP**

Torres, Mrs Dorothy V 113 Rugosa Drive, Folsom, CA 95630, (916) 733-3040, BA 76 San Jose St Univ; MA 78 CA St Univ - Sacramento; 85–Sp-Lang Path, Sutter General Hospital, **SLP ACE**

Torres, Mrs Irene Gilbert 737 E 9th Street, Brooklyn, NY 11230, (718) 434-2902, BA 73 CUNY - Brooklyn Coll; MS 78 CUNY - Brooklyn Coll; **SLP**

Torres, Mrs Jan Marie 107 St Anthony Street, Raceland, LA 70394, (504) 447-8181, **SLP**

Torres, Mrs Kristen Kay 1750 Martina Avenue #B, Torrance, CA 90501, (213) 618-0381, BA 84 Univ of NM; MA 86 CA St Univ - Northridge; 86–Sp-Lang Path, Mem Med Ctr, **SLP**

Torres, Nelida Bo Los Llanos, HC-01 Box 3415, Coamo, PR 00640-9713, (809) 825-5378, MS 88 Univ of PR - San Juan

Torres, Nellie Cond Camino Real, Apartment B-304, Guaynabo, PR 00657, (809) 783-6407, **SLP**

Torres, Mrs Terri F Route 1, Buhler, KS 67522, (316) 663-2671, BA 75 Wichita St Univ; MS 77 Wichita St Univ; 81–Sp-Lang Path, Early Educ Ctr, **SLP**

Torrey, Elizabeth Farrell 128 Pearl Street, Cambridge, MA 02139, (617) 354-7850, MS 81 Emerson Coll; Sp-Lang Path, University Hospital, **SLP**

Torrey, Mrs T Zoann Route 2 Box 57A, Satanta, KS 67870, (316) 649-2612, BS 73 Central MO St Univ; MS 74 Central MO St Univ; Sp-Lang Path, Uhigh Plains Ed Coop, **SLP**

Torry, Mrs Jane 314 Longridge Road, Elgin, IL 60120, **SLP**

Tortolani, Beth C 3 Westgate Boulevard, Plandome, NY 11030, (516) 338-4204, BA 65 PA St Univ - Univ Park; MA 76 Wichita St Univ; Research Coor & Curric Spec, Norht Shore Univ Hosp Pre-Sch, **SLP**

Tortorice, Pamela Jane 860 Cherry Valley Drive, Apartment 308-A, Vernon Hills, IL 60061, (312) 578-3759, BS 73 Marquette Univ; ME 79 CA Univ of PA; 85–Sp-Lang Path, VA Medical Center, **SLP**

Tortorich, Consuela 25 Nottingham Lane, Pine Bluff, AR 71603, (501) 535-5719, MS 86 Univ of AR - Little Rock; Aud, Pine Bluff ENT Clinic, **A**

Torvinen, Lisa C 11365 Albarar Path, Inver Grove Heights, MN 55075-7644, (612) 566-1814, MA 82 Univ of MN - Duluth; Sp-Lang Path, Northside Ther Serv, **SLP**

Toscano, Jacqueline Maria 309 5th Street, East Northport, NY 11731, (516) 368-2820, BA 80 SUNY - Coll at Cortland; MS 85 San Francisco St Univ; **SLP**

Toston-Edwards, Mrs Anna James 24 Magnolia Drive, Monroe, LA 71203, (318) 396-6300, BA 79 Northeast LA Univ; MA 83 LA Tech Univ; Sp-Lang Path, G B Cooley Hosp for Dev Disab, **SLP**

Toth, Jean L 3 Presque Isle Street, Fort Fairfield, ME 04742, (207) 476-5721, BS 77 Boston Univ; MA 81 Univ of MA - Amherst; 82–Aud, Farooki & Prasanna Otol Assoc, **A**

Toth, Mrs Kathleen M 164 East Gull Lake Drive, Augusta, MI 49012-9712, BS 82 Western MI Univ; MA 84 Wayne St Univ; **SLP**

Toth, Susan A W 26 Harmony Circle Court, Missoula, MT 59802, (406) 243-4131, BS 72 CO St Univ; MA 74 Univ of IA; 87–Aud, Univ of Montana, **SLP A**

Totten, Carol Orrin 940 Lester Avenue, Reno, NV 89502, (702) 463-2205, BA 71 Univ of NV - Reno; MS 85 Univ of NV - Reno; **SLP**

Totten, Holly Lynne 704 Coxwell Avenue, Toronto, ON, Canada M4C 3B9, (416) 469-6256, BS 78 Ball St Univ; MA 80 Ball St Univ; 88–Aud, Toronto East Gen Hosp, **A**

Totter, Dr Joseph J 1044 Bret Cove Court, San Jose, CA 95120, (408) 947-6618, BS 72 SUNY - Coll at Geneseo; MS 74 SUNY - Coll at Buffalo; PH 79 (Sp Path) SUNY - Center at Buffalo; 80–Sp-Lang Path, Santa Clara Co Offi of Ed, **SLP**

Tottle, Edward L 2993 Yorkway, Baltimore, MD 21222, PH (NS); **SLP**

Toubbeh, Dr Jamil I 1500 Harvard Drive N E, Albuquerque, NM 87106, (505) 766-1232, BA 54 Millikin Univ; MA 56 Univ of IL - Urbana; PH 65 (Sp Path/Aud) Univ of Denver; Dep Dir/Sensory Dis Prog, Indian Hlth Serv Phs Dhhs, **SLP F**

Toueg, Mrs Renee Eichler 239 East 79th Street, New York, NY 10021, (212) 744-1204, BA 61 CUNY - Brooklyn Coll; MS 63 PA St Univ - Univ Park; Adj Lect, Hunter College, **SLP**

Tourne, Patrice M Box PPP 282, Saipan, Mariana Islands 96950, (670) 322-9956, BA 85 Humboldt St Univ; MA 88 Univ of MT; 88–Aud, Comm of N Mariana Islands

Toussaint-Krutz, Mrs Lois C 3138 South Spruce, Mesa, AZ 85210, (602) 820-1780, BS 77 Eastern IL Univ; BS 77 Eastern IL Univ; MS 79 Purdue Univ - West Lafayette; 86–Sp/Lang Path, Private Practice, **SLP**

Toutain, Beverly Ambrosic 203 Stonewall Lane, Brewster, NY 10509, (914) 278-7259, BA 72 Rosary Coll; MS 75 Univ of IL - Urbana; **SLP**

Toward, Mrs Mary Margaret 16700 Washington Square, Apartment J, Fraser, MI 48026, (313) 792-3357, BS 80 Lamar Univ; MS 82 Lamar Univ; 86–Sp-Lang Path, The Child's Place, **SLP**

Towell, Marianne D Audiological Consultant, P O Box 1146, Biloxi, MS 39533, (601) 392-9506, BA 72 Univ of South AL; MS 74 Univ Southern MS-Hattiesburg; Aud, Private Practice, **A**

Tower, Mrs Nancy Ruth 8024 Geneva Street, Woodridge, IL 60517, (312) 985-8155, BA 81 Valparaiso Univ; MA 82 Edinboro Univ of PA; 88–Sp-Lang Path, Private Practice, **SLP**

Towers, Mrs Catherine Speech & Language Consultants, 1824 Blanding Boulevard, Jacksonville, FL 32210, (904) 388-8756, BA 66 Converse Coll; ME 68 Univ of VA - Charlottesville; 79–Sp-Lang Path, Private Practice, **SLP ACE**

Towey, Michael P Rural Free Delivery 3, Belfast, ME 04915, (207) 236-8381, BS 74 Univ of ME - Farmington; MA 75 Univ of ME - Orono; Dir-Sp & Hrng Dept, Waldo County Gen Hosp, **SLP**

Towle, Patricia M 5791 Southwest 74th Terr, Apartment 27, South Miami, FL 33143, (305) 387-4852, MS 87 WV Univ; 87–Aud, Univ of Miami Sch of Med, **A**

Towler, Mary Johnson 4701 Desmond Beach, Port Huron, MI 48060, OB 74 Univ of NH; BA 74 Univ of NH; MA 79 CUNY - Lehman Coll; 88–Sp/Lang Path, Nicolaysen Cen-Escondido Un Sh, **SLP**

Towler, Patience K 146 West 40th Avenue, Vancouver, BC, Canada V5Y 2RZ, (604) 736-9844, MS 68 Univ of MI - Ann Arbor; Sp-Lnag Path, Cty of Vancouver Hlth Dept, **SLP**

Town, Margaret J 381 Northwest 112, Seattle, WA 98177, (206) 475-6770, BA 63 Univ of MT; MA 68 Univ of MT; SLP, Tacoma Pub Sch, **SLP**

Towne, Dr Carol 1420 Locust Street-29AB, Philadelphia, PA 19102, (215) 985-0716, BA 50 Lawrence Univ; MA 51 Univ of WI - Madison; PH 61 (NS) Univ of WI - Madison; Retired, St Christophers Hosp Children, **SLP**

Towne, Judith Ann 5864 Ramona Drive, Greendale, WI 53129, **SLP**

Towne, Dr Roger L Southwest Missouri State Univ, Dept Commun Disorders, Springfield, MO 65804, (417) 836-5368, MA 72 Univ of MT; PH 85 (Comm Disorders & Sciences) Southern IL Univ -Carbondale; Asst Prof, SW MO St Univ, **SLP**

Towner, MaryJane E 15030 S W 104th Street, Apartment 2023, Miami, FL 33196, (305) 385-8954, BS 56 Northwestern Univ; MS 70 Long Island U - CW Post Ctr; Instructor, Florida Jr College, **SLP**

Townes, Valerie A 51 Hunters Hill Circle, Amherst, MA 01002, (413) 863-9311, BA 74 Univ of MA - Amherst; MA 79 Univ of MA - Amherst; 86–Sp-Lang Path, Gill-Montague Reg Sch Dist, **SLP**

Towns, Barbara Schulte St Joseph Mercy Hospital, 900 Woodward Avenue, Pontiac, MI 48053, (313) 858-3111, MA 85 Wayne St Univ; **SLP**

Townsend, Ann E D 27 West Avenue, Seekonk, MA 02771, (508) 336-2217, BS 72 Ithaca Coll; MS 73 Syracuse Univ; Sp/Lang Path, Attleboro PS, **SLP**

Townsend, Mrs Beatrice Kay 3902 Calle Andalucia, San Clemente, CA 92672, (714) 894-7311, BA 81 CA St Univ - Long Beach; MA 84 CA St Univ - Long Beach; SLP, Westminster School District, **SLP**

Townsend, Beverly J 2611 Boyd Road, Columbus, MS 39701, (601) 327-4145, BA 76 Univ of MS; MS 77 MS Univ for Women; **SLP**

Townsend, Mrs Deborah J 615 Normandie Blvd, Bowling Green, OH 43402, (419) 354-3963, BA 77 Bowling Green St Univ; MA 78 Bowling Green St Univ; 88–Aud, The Toledo Hosp, **A**

Townsend, Jean M 803 South Duncan, Marion, IL 62959, (618) 993-3198, BS 70 Northern IL Univ - De Kalb; MS 79 IL St Univ - Normal; Aud, School for Hearing Impaired, **A**

Townsend, Mrs Joan Adams 1001 South 450th East, Orem, UT 84058, (801) 227-8700, OM 87 Brigham Young Univ; 87–Sp-Lang Path, Alpine Sch Dist, **SLP**

Townsend, Mrs Joyce A 3118 Mason Way, Modesto, CA 95355, (209) 521-8544, BA 70 CA St Univ - Stanislaus; MA 75 CA St Univ - Stanislaus; Sp-Lang Path, Modesto City Sch, **SLP**

Townsend, Laura Anna 8054 Matterhorn Lane, Apartment D-130, Crown Point, IN 46307, (219) 736-6924, BS 83 IN St Univ - Terre Haute; MS 87 IN St Univ - Terre Haute; **SLP**

Townsend, Mrs Lisa M 11751 Stonegate Lane, Columbia, MD 21044-4300, (904) 255-2494, BA 79 Univ of FL; MA 81 Northwestern Univ; SLP, School Board of Volusia County, **SLP**

Townsend, Mrs Lorrie Blackmon 14537 Donald Drive, Austin, TX 78728, (512) 926-4701, BS 82 Univ of TX - Austin; 84–Sp-Lang Path, Austin ISD, **SLP**

Townsend, Mrs Lynne Hylton 7 Gulf Road, Derry, NH 03038, (603) 432-6869, BS 81 Northeastern Univ; MA 83 OH Univ - Athens; 88–Sp-Lang Path, Hampstead NH Sch Dist, **SLP**

Townsend, Nancy M 101 Larchwood Drive, Cambridge, MA 02138, (617) 536-7255, BA 50 Univ of Saint Andrews - Scotland; MA 68 Columbia Univ Teachers Coll; 78–Cl Staff Superv/Instr, Emerson Coll, **SLP ACE**

Townsend, Thomas H 321 Exeter Road, Devon, PA 19333, BA 66 Oberlin Coll; MS 69 Purdue Univ - West Lafayette; PH 71 (NS) Purdue Univ - West Lafayette; Prof, Phila Coll of Pharmacy & Sci, **A**

Towsley, Mary Frances 8 Wadsworth Street, Geneseo, NY 14454, (716) 475-6837, BS 86 SUNY - Coll at Geneseo; MA 87 SUNY - Coll at Geneseo; 87–Aud, NTID, **F**

Toyama, Susan G 5055 North Kilbourn, Chicago, IL 60630, (312) 282-4271, BS 79 Univ of IL - Urbana; MS 80 Univ of IL - Urbana; SLP, Divsn Services Crippled Childn, **SLP**

Toye, Andrea Rae 19728 Alida, Cerritos, CA 90701, (213) 494-5415, BA 82 CA St Univ - Fullerton; MS 85 Chapman Coll; **SLP**

Toyne, Mrs Julie Ann 3472 North Cramer, Milwaukee, WI 53211-2815, (414) 962-9997, BA 80 KS St Univ; MA 82 KS St Univ; Sp-Lang Path, Curative Rehabil Workshop, **SLP**

Toyzer-Ronis, Lee-Ellen Neurotology Unit, Surburban Hospital, 8600 Old Georgetown Road, Bethesda, MD 20814, (301) 530-3165, BA 80 George Washington Univ; MS 82 Vanderbilt Univ; 87–Aud, Suburban Hosp, **A**

Tozer, Cynthia S 223 Cassatt Road, Berwyn, PA 19312, (215) 647-0673, BS 66 PA St Univ - Univ Park; MA 80 West Chester Univ of PA; Consultant, Private Practice, **SLP**

Traba, Vickie M 857 South Oak Street #1, Ukiah, CA 95482, (707) 468-5193, BA 74 CA St Univ - Sacramento; MA 80 CA St Univ - Los Angeles; Sp-Lang Path, Susan Pollesel Speech Path Inc, **SLP**

Traboulsi, Mrs Margaret Ann Foothills Hospital, Dept Of Audiology, 1403-29 St N W, Calgary, AB, Canada T2N 2T9, (403) 270-1358, OB 78 Dalhousie Univ - Nova Scotia; BS 77 Dalhousie Univ - Nova Scotia; MS 80 Dalhousie Univ - Nova Scotia; Aud, Foothills Hosp, **A**

Trace, Melissa M 27 High Point Ridge, Franklin, TN 37064, **SLP**

Tracer, Gale E 4912 Corkwood, Irvine, CA 92715, (714) 667-3397, BA 68 Univ of CA - Los Angeles; MA 76 CA St Univ - Los Angeles; Instr/Sp-Lang Path, Rancho Santiago College, **SLP**

Tracey, Mrs Susan A 11090 Winding Brook Lane, Indianapolis, IN 46280, (317) 848-7409, BA 63 IN Univ - Bloomington; OM 69 IN Univ - Bloomington; Sp-Lang Path, **SLP**

Trachtenberg, Carol Ann 160 West End Avenue #2J, New York, NY 10023, BS 69 Univ of Bridgeport; MS 78 Columbia Univ Teachers Coll; Sp-Lang Path, NYC Bd of Ed, **SLP**

Trachtenberg, Nina S 6507 Markstown Drive, Tampa, FL 33617, (813) 988-3124, MS 88 Univ of South FL; 87–Sp-Lang Path, Bay Area Rehab Inc, **SLP**

Trachtenberg, Renee B 844 Crestview Avenue, North Woodmere, NY 11581, (516) 486-7711, BA 74 Adelphi Univ; MS 77 Adelphi Univ; Teacher of the Deaf, Nassau BOCES, **SLP**

Trachtenberg, William P O Box 300, Jenkintown, PA 19046, (715) 289-0504, BA 61 Temple Univ-Tyler Sch of Art; MA 63 Temple Univ-Tyler Sch of Art; SLP, Private Practice, **SLP**

Trachtenberg-Zutty, Marilyn R 50 Alpine Way, Huntington Station, NY 11746, (516) 673-3253, BA 75 Adelphi Univ; MA 79 Montclair St Coll; Sp-Lang Path, BOCES of Nassau Co, **SLP**

Trachtman, Mrs Michelle R 1998 Gainsborough Drive N E, Atlanta, GA 30341-1016, (404) 457-7963, BA 79 Hofstra Univ; MA 81 Northwestern Univ; SLP, Woodhill Medical Center, **SLP**

Trackman, Phyllis 309 North Essex Avenue, Margate, NJ 08402, (609) 822-2391, BA 66 William Paterson Coll; MA 78 Fairleigh Dickinson U-Ruther; MA 80 Trenton St Coll; Sp/Lang Path, Margate Bd of Ed, **SLP**

Tracy, Ellen D P O Box 745, Morongo Valley, CA 92256, **SLP**

Tracy, Dr John M, III 525 Orchard Drive, Monmouth, OR 97361, (503) 370-5486, BA 71 Whittier Coll; MS 74 Western OR St Coll; PH 83 (NS) Univ of OR; Supvr-Sp & Lang Path, Salem Hosp, **SLP**

Tracy, Mrs Julie F 3239 North Kenmore Unit 6, Chicago, IL 60657, (312) 908-8035, MA 83 Northwestern Univ; Sp-Lang Path, Northwestern Memorial Hospital, **SLP**

Tracy, Mrs Karen A 59 Chapin Parkway, Buffalo, NY 14209, MS 77 SUNY - Coll at Buffalo; **SLP**

Tracy, Kathleen McQuade Drewville Road, Brewster, NY 10509, (914) 279-6765, ME 81 SUNY - Coll at Fredonia; SLP, Nn Westcherter/Putnam BOCES, **SLP**

Tracy, Marilyn Louise 49 Oceanic Lane, Lake Havasu City, AZ 86403, (602) 855-6296, BS 55 Univ of UT; MA 60 Univ of UT; Sp-Lang Path, Private Practice, **SLP**

Tracy, Patricia J 631 North Kansas, Edwardsville, IL 62025, **SLP**

Tracy, Mrs Rebecca T 81 Governors Harbour, Hilton Head Island, SC 29928, (803) 681-6023, BS 74 Marshall Univ; ME 79 GA St Univ; Sp-Lang Path, Gibbes-Savage Assoc, **SLP**

Tracy, Mrs Susan Graben 3715 Poplar Road, Flossmoor, IL 60422, (312) 798-2080, BS 77 IL St Univ - Normal; MS 80 Southern IL Univ -Carbondale; Sp/Lang Path, South Metro Assoc, **SLP**

Trader, Miriam P 500 Overbrook Road, Baltimore, MD 21212, **SLP**

Traeder, Mrs Maxine D Route 1 Box 376, Ashland, WI 54806, (715) 682-8169, BA 53 Marquette Univ; Sp-Lang Path, Ashland Public Schools, **SLP**

Traficanti, Judy Phelan Rd 2 Box 194, Accord, NY 12404, (914) 626-3533, BA 78 SUNY - Coll at New Paltz; MS 86 SUNY - Coll at New Paltz; Sp-Lang Path, Childrens Annex In Kingston, **SLP**

Trafton, Judith Anne 2621 Wells Avenue, Raleigh, NC 27608, (919) 781-8318, BA 71 Univ of NC - Chapel Hill; MS 82 Univ of NC - Chapel Hill; Sp-Lang Path, Wake County Schools, **SLP**

Tragesser, Mrs Dorothy L 12679 Terrie Drive, North Huntingdon, PA 15642, (412) 864-0820, BS 70 Clarion Univ of PA; MA 73 Univ of Pittsburgh - Pittsburgh; Sp-Lang Path, Michael Gerard Rehab, **SLP**

Tragitt, Leslie Ann 801 Sierra Vista Way #28, Yreka, CA 96097, BS 75 OR St Univ; MS 84 Western OR St Coll; MS 86 Vanderbilt Univ; **SLP**

Tragler, Mrs Janice L 172 Main Street, Topsham, ME 04086, (207) 443-3341, BA 72 IA St Univ; MA 74 Western MI Univ; Sp/Lang Path, Pinetree Soc for Crpled Inc, **SLP**

Trahan, Mrs Carol A 5421 Superior Drive Suite B, Baton Rouge, LA 70816, (504) 292-4138, BS 80 1979; MS 81 1979; Dir, Abilities for Sp & L, **SLP**

Trahan, Henry P 2817 Johnston Street, Lafayette, LA 70503, (318) 235-6601, BA 74 Univ of Southwestern LA; OM 77 LA St Univ - N O Medical Ctr; Dir of Clin Svcs, ACI Hrng Ctr, **A**

Trahan, Sally A 307 Meecham Road, Petaluma, CA 94952, (415) 472-4110, BS 77 San Francisco St Univ; MS 79 San Francisco St Univ; Sp-Lang Path, Marin Co Office of Education, **SLP**

Trahan, Sherry E 24205 Welsh Road, Gaithersburg, MD 20879-9539, Sp-Lang Path, Private Practice, **SLP**

Trahan, Mrs Suzanne Karol 2245 College Drive #125, Baton Rouge, LA 70808, (504) 769-8160, BS 84 Kent St Univ; MA 86 Univ of IL - Urbana; 88–Aud, LA Sch for the Deaf, **A**

Trahey, Patricia Ann 11649 Glenview Drive, Orland Park, IL 60462, BS 81 IL St Univ - Normal; OM 86 Governors St Univ; **SLP**

Trail, Wayne D Route 1 Box 13, Basehor, KS 66007, BS 44 Wichita St Univ; **SLP LM**

Trainer, Mrs Rosa Lee 18906 North Golden Hawk Trail, Jupiter, FL 33458, (407) 747-1623, BS 78 Purdue Univ - West Lafayette; MS 80 Purdue Univ - West Lafayette; Sp-Lang Path, Private Practice, **SLP**

Trainor, Ana M 258 John Street, South Amboy, NJ 08879, (201) 721-3652, BS 82 Trenton St Coll; MS 84 Rutgers St Univ -N Brunswick; SLP, St Joseph's Hosp & Med Ctr, **SLP**

Trainor, Mary T 1025 Hancock Street #10-C, Quincy, MA 02169, (617) 573-3266, BS 81 Coll of Saint Rose; MS 83 Syracuse Univ; 87–Aud, MA Eye & Ear Infirmary, **A**

Trambert, Robyn E 37 Country Club Lane, Springfield, NJ 07081, (201) 792-8106, BA 79 Rutger's St Univ - Douglas Coll; MS 81 PA St Univ - Univ Park; 87–Supvr of Sp-Lang Path Dept, St Mary Hosp, **SLP ACE**

Tramel, Mrs Karen Ray 4795 Riveredge Cove, Lithonia, GA 30058, (404) 292-7272, BS 74 MS Univ for Women; MS 76 MS Univ for Women; **SLP**

Tramel, Mrs Kim Smith 1502 Green Mountain Drive, Apartment 177-R, Little Rock, AR 72211-1724, (501) 223-7558, **SLP**

Trammel, Rebecca J RR2 Box 63, Effingham, IL 62401, (217) 868-5302, BS 76 Southern IL Univ -Carbondale; MS 86 Eastern IL Univ; 86–Sp-Lang Path, Effingham Comm Unit #40, **SLP**

Trammell, Mrs Cynthia V Fulton County Schools, 580 College Street, Hapeville, GA 30354, (404) 763-0580, BA 75 Univ of MS; MS 76 FL St Univ; Consult Sp-Lang Path, Fulton Co Sch, **SLP**

Tramposch, Helga Kay 487 Chalfonte Avenue, Grosse Pointe Farms, MI 48236, **SLP**

Transue, Vicki E 117 East 5th, Goodland, KS 67735, **SLP**

Trantham, Carla Ann 1564 South Tucson Street, Aurora, CO 80012, (303) 755-5836, MA 68 Univ of Denver; BS 67 Northwestern Univ; Sp-Lang Path, Private Practice, **SLP**

Trantum, Dennis 135 East Emmett Street, Battle Creek, MI 49017, (616) 965-3206, BA 73 Western MI Univ; MA 75 Western MI Univ; Aud, Southwestern MI Rehab Hosp, **A**

Tranzillo, Katherine 847 Ridge Road, Lansing, NY 14882, (607) 533-4596, BS 81 SUNY - Coll at Buffalo; MS 84 Ithaca Coll; **SLP**

Traser, Mrs Erin McKee 6833 Spring Brook Road, Rockford, IL 61111-6701, (815) 338-7411, BS 84 Western IL Univ; MA 85 Western IL Univ; Sp-Lang Path, Spec Educ Dist McHenry County, **SLP**

Trask, Julie G 9 Olde Orchard Lane, Greenville, SC 29615, BA 68 Univ of NE - Lincoln; MA 69 Univ of NE - Lincoln; Sp-Lang Path, Greenville Co Sch Dist, **SLP**

Tratter, Deborah Suzanne 297 Buckner, Cleveland, OH 44123-1511, (216) 951-7272, **SLP**

Trattner, Naoma H 8105 N W 117th Street, Oklahoma City, OK 73132, (405) 722-3597, BA 38 Southeastern OK St Univ; ME 62 Univ of OK - Norman; **SLP LM**

Trauba, Jane A Hearing Aid Center, 444 Estudillo Avenue, San Leandro, CA 94577, (415) 483-5422, MS 82 Univ of UT; BA 79 Humboldt St Univ; Aud, Jeanette Von Khaelssberg, **A**

Trauber, Mrs Rochelle 264 East Broadway, New York, NY 10002, (212) 254-0967, BA 72 CUNY - City College; MA 73 NY Univ; Sp-Lang Path, Hosp for Jt Diseases, **SLP**

Trauernicht, Maxine J 1111 East Roosevelt Avenue, Nampa, ID 83651, (208) 466-9255, BA 63 Northwest Nazarene Coll; MS 74 ID St Univ; SLP, ID State Sch & Hosp, **SLP**

Trauger, Mrs Vicki C 2027 Cloverdale Road, Bethlehem, PA 18018-1442, (215) 861-8232, MS 85 Rutgers St Univ -N Brunswick; **SLP**

Traul-Anderson, Gail N 924 Riverside Drive SE, St Cloud, MN 56304, (612) 252-0857, BS 63 Univ of MN - Minneap-St Paul; MA 64 OH St Univ; **SLP A**

Traut, Mrs Edith M 7031 Cedar Street, Wauwatosa, WI 53213, (414) 447-2208, BS 79 Northwestern Univ; MA 81 Northwestern Univ; Sp/Lang Path, St Joseph's Hosp, **SLP**

Trautmann, Julie Beth 10863 East Beverly Drive, Whittier, CA 90601, (213) 695-6586, MA 88 Whittier Coll

Travers, Barbara Walker 5812 Winegrove Court, Rockville, MD 20855, (301) 258-0791, BS 72 Purdue Univ - West Lafayette; MS 73 PA St Univ - Univ Park; **SLP**

Travers, Capt Denise M 1319 St Andrews, San Antonio, TX 78248, (512) 652-5320, BA 74 Regis Coll; MS 77 Southern CT St Univ; Capt, USAF, **SLP**

Travers, Joan Marie 48 East Pacemont, Columbus, OH 43202, (614) 263-4968, BS 83 OH St Univ; MA 85 OH St Univ; SLP, Aasp, **SLP**

Travers, Nancy 101 Ralph Avenue, North Bellmore, NY 11710, (212) 650-6153, MA 86 CUNY - Queens Coll; **SLP**

Travis, Elizabeth B Higgins 2502 Mohawk Drive, Bowling Green, KY 42101, (502) 781-2254, BA 64 Morehead St Univ; OM 65 Morehead St Univ; MS 81 Western KY Univ; Sp/Lang Path, Bowling Green Inde Sch, **SLP**

Travis, Miriam Louise 34th General Hospital EFMS, APO New York, NY 09178-5000, BS 80 KS St Univ; MA 85 Wichita St Univ; 88–Sp-Lang Path, US Army, **SLP**

Travis, Dr Norma C 3111 Moss Point Drive, Baton Rouge, LA 70808, (504) 388-2545, BS 59 LA St Univ - Baton Rouge; MA 72 LA St Univ - Baton Rouge; PH 81 (Sp Path) LA St Univ - Baton Rouge; Coord of Cl Serv/Superv, LA St U, **SLP**

Travis, Teresa L 749 West Brookforest Drive, Peoria, IL 61615, (309) 688-8467, BS 79 Bradley Univ; MS 80 Bradley Univ; 88–Sp/Lang Path, Comm Action Agency-Head Start, **SLP**

Traweek, Dr Suzanne Calvert 2502 Briarhill, Ruston, LA 71270, (318) 257-4764, BS 59 MS Univ for Women; MS 74 MS Univ for Women; PH 79 (NS) Wichita St Univ; Asst Prof, Louisiana Tech U, **SLP ACE**

Traynor, Dr Robert M Dept Of Communicative Disorder, Colorado State University, Fort Collins, CO 80523, (303) 491-6981, BA 72 Univ of Northern CO; MA 73 Univ of Northern CO; ED 75 (NS) Univ of Northern CO; 82–Assoc Prof-Aud, Co St Univ/Dept of Comm Dis, **A**

Traynor-Duda, Hilary c/o Maj Francis Duda, 30th Field Hospital, APO New York, NY 09034, (496) 381-3577, BS 75 FL St Univ; MS 77 SC St Coll; Sp-Lang Path, Private Practice, **SLP**

Treacy, Margaret M 409-A Wakefield Drive, Charlotte, NC 28209, (704) 338-4430, BS 74 East Carolina Univ; MA 75 OH Univ - Athens; Dir of Sp-Lang Path, Charlotte Rehab Hosp, **SLP**

Treadwell, Mrs Pamela K Brevard School Board, 1450 Martin Boulevard, Merritt Island, FL 32952, (305) 631-1911, BS 72 Univ of ND; MS 74 Univ of ND; Coord Commun Dis Prog, Brevard Co Sch Dist, **SLP**

Treanor, Dr Ruth D 3579 Fiske Terrace, Silver Spring, MD 20906, (301) 598-8131, BA 41 Hiram Coll; MS 47 Univ of MI - Ann Arbor; ED 70 (NS) American Univ; SLP, Private Practice, **SLP**

Treb, William E 8361 Doolittle Road, Minequa, WI 54548, MS 71 Univ of WI - Stevens Point; Aud, **A**

Trebay, Dana Victoria 947 26th Place N E, Auburn, WA 98002, (206) 735-1487, BS 83 Univ of OR; MS 85 Univ of UT; 85–Aud, Group Health Coop, **A**

Treccani, Barbara Biro 17713 Larkspur, Homewood, IL 60430, (312) 210-2878, OB 84 Governors St Univ; OM 87 Governors St Univ; **SLP**

Trecek, Mrs Jeanette S 32 Yellow Brick Road, Wayne, NJ 07470, BA 64 Baylor Univ; MA 66 Univ of IA; Sp-Lang Path, Wayne Bd of Ed, **SLP**

Trecroce, Mrs Marie Suzanne 1128 Potter's Wheel Cres, Oakville, ON, Canada L6M 1J2, (416) 847-2698, BA 77 McGill Univ - Quebec; MS 80 McGill Univ - Quebec; 86–Sp-Lang Path, Oakville-Trafalgar Memorial Hosp, **SLP**

Tredinnick, Amy Marie 24 Scotland Street, Ansonia, CT 06401, (203) 754-5141, OB 84 SUNY - Center at Buffalo; 87–Sp-Lang Path, Easter Seal Rehab Ctr of Greater Waterbury, **SLP**

Trees, Anne T 10014 White Bluff Road, Apartment 104, Savannah, GA 31406, (912) 356-6634, BS 81 Univ of GA; ME 82 Univ of GA; 88–Sp-Lang Path, Candler General Hosp, **SLP**

Trees, Debra E 31 South Main Avenue, Albany, NY 12208, (518) 454-1375, BS 77 Coll of Saint Rose; MS 84 Syracuse Univ; Aud, St Peter's Hosp, **A**

Treese, Mrs Carol K Box 6021, Blue Jay, CA 92317, (714) 337-2485, BS 62 Kent St Univ; MA 68 CA St Univ - Los Angeles; SLP, Rim of World Sch, **SLP**

Treiber, Diane Marie 22 Patricia Lane, Syosset, NY 11791, (516) 921-4753, BS 84 Ithaca Coll; MS 85 Adelphi Univ; **SLP**

Treiber, Patricia M 17 High View Drive, High Bridge, NJ 08829, (201) 522-2215, BS 70 Marquette Univ; MA 71 Temple Univ-Tyler Sch of Art; Ch Sp-Lang Path, Overlook Hosp, **SLP**

Trela, Mrs Margaret F 137 San Juan, Los Alamos, NM 87544, (505) 662-5281, BA 58 Univ of VA - Charlottesville; MA 62 Stanford Univ; Sp-Lang Path, Los Alamos Pub Sch, **SLP**

Tremaglio, Barbara McLaughlin 893 Highland Avenue, Waterbury, CT 06708, (203) 754-5141, BS 81 Southern CT St Univ; MS 84 PA St Univ - Univ Park; 87–Sp-Lang Path, Easter Seal Rehab Cen of Wbury, **SLP**

Tremain, Mrs Debbie Hobbs 8338 Rose Lane, Wichita, KS 67207, (316) 682-9354, MA 88 Wichita St Univ; 88–Sp-Lang Path, Wichita PS

Tremaine, Deborah Angela 11 Kresswood Drive, Rochester, NY 14624, (716) 594-0372, MS 79 Nazareth Coll of Rochester; Sp-Lang Path, Private Practice, **SLP**

Treman, Terri Ann St Elizabeth Medical Center, 601 Edwin C Moses Blvd, Dayton, OH 45408, (513) 229-6081, BS 82 Miami Univ - Oxford; MA 83 Miami Univ - Oxford; Sp-Lang Path, St Eliz Med Cen/Rehab Ut, **SLP**

Trembacki, Mrs Debra J 937 Lehigh Circle, Naperville, IL 60565, (312) 961-9743, BS 80 Univ of IL - Urbana; MS 81 Univ of IL - Urbana; Sp-Lang Path, Kendall Co Spec Ed Coop, **SLP**

Trembath, Leigh Hartigan 208 South 12th Street, Clear Lake, IA 50428, (515) 357-6125, BS 79 Univ of IA; MA 82 Northwestern Univ; Aud, Northern Trails AEA, **A**

Trembath, Stuart G 208 South 12th Street, Clear Lake, IA 50428, (515) 357-6125, BA 79 MI St Univ; MA 81 Northwestern Univ; Aud, Northern Trails AEA, **A**

Tremblay, Michelle A 1105 West 11th Avenue, Anchorage, AK 99507-1103, (907) 278-5560, BA 79 Gonzaga Univ; MS 82 Portland St Univ; SLP, Anchorage Sch Dist, **SLP**

Tremel, Nancy A Upper Island Health Unit, 1729 Comox Avenue, Comox, BC, Canada V9N 3Z8, (604) 334-1254, BA 75 Univ of IA; MA 76 Univ of IA; Aud, Bc Ministry of Hlth, **A**

Trenkle, Margaret Mary 325 Westshire Road, 2nd Floor, Baltimore, MD 21229, (301) 788-2185, **SLP**

Trent, Deirdre R 429 O Street N W, Washington, DC 20001, (202) 673-7002, BS 70 OH Univ - Athens; MS 72 Univ of Pittsburgh - Pittsburgh; PH 86 (NS) Howard Univ; 84–Coord Sp-Lang & Aud, Dept of Human Svcs, **SLP**

Trent, Mrs Janice Diane 930 Lincoln Avenue, West Chester, PA 19380, (215) 696-8800, BS 76 Hampton Univ; ME 84 Northeastern Univ; 84–Aud, Chester County ENT Group Ltd, **A**

Trentacoste, Lori Ann 32 Cathedral Avenue Apartment 3F, Hempstead, NY 11550, (516) 565-9667, BS 85 SUNY - Coll at Fredonia; MA 87 SUNY - Center at Buffalo; Aud, Island Better Hearing Inc, **A**

Treon, Dr Martin Avery Communication Disorders Prog, University Of South Dakota, Vermillion, SD 57069-2390, (605) 677-6203, BS 59 Univ of MN - Minneap-St Paul; MA 61 Stanford Univ; PH 67 (NS) Univ of CA - Los Angeles; **SLP**

Trepasso, Mrs Carolyn S 327 I Avenue, Coronado, CA 92118, (619) 522-8932, BA 75 Univ of San Diego; MA 79 Univ of the Pacific; Sp-Lang Path, Coronado USD, **SLP**

Tresnak, Rosemarie 4539 Kingscup Court, Ellicott City, MD 21043, (301) 997-6482, BS 76 Bloomsburg Univ of PA; MS 77 Bloomsburg Univ of PA; Sp-Lang Path, Mt Vernon Hosp, **SLP**

Treston, Elizabeth Margaret 37 Wyoming Avenue, Long Beach, NY 11561, (516) 432-2617, BA 83 Hofstra Univ; MA 85 Hofstra Univ; **SLP**

Treuhaft, Mrs Eleanor Cohen 33 Knollwood Drive, Cherry Hill, NJ 08002, (609) 667-3303, BA 49 CUNY - Brooklyn Coll; MA 51 Univ of IA; Sp-Lang Path, Cherry Hill Bd of Ed, **SLP**

Trevennen, Mrs Betsy B 16302 Duchess Lane, Huntington Beach, CA 92647, (213) 862-0715, BA 71 CA St Univ - Long Beach; MA 74 CA St Univ - Long Beach; Sp-Lang Path, Los Angeles Cnty Ofc of Educ, **SLP**

Trevino, Mrs Carmen Hernandez 6608 Sprucewood Lane, Apt 1211, Arlington, TX 76017, (817) 478-6941, BS 84 Univ of North TX; MS 86 Univ of North TX; 88–Sp-Lang Path, Arlington ISD, **SLP**

Trevithick, Karen Refvem 943 Laguna Avenue, Burlingame, CA 94010, (209) 385-8404, BA 80 Univ of CA - Santa Barbara; MS 82 Western OR St Coll; Sp-Lang Path, Jefferson Elem Sch, **SLP**

Tribbett, Beth Waite 2801 Walmsley Circle, Lake Orion, MI 48035, (313) 464-4814, BS 83 Purdue Univ - West Lafayette; MA 86 Wayne St Univ; **A**

Tribble, Renee 3731 Deer Forest Drive, Memphis, TN 38115, Senior Product Analyst, Methodist Health Systems, **SLP**

Tribby, Sandra Roark 1215 Pine #A, Lebanon, MO 65536, (314) 346-5651, BS 85 Northeast MO St Univ; MA 86 Northeast MO St Univ; **SLP**

Triebert, Raymond F 1248 Farmington Avenue, Apartment 12A, West Hartford, CT 06107, (203) 727-1315, MS 50 Butler Univ; MA 55 Columbia Univ Teachers Coll; Aud, Amer Sch for the Deaf, **A**

Trier, Kelly Lynn Rural Route 1, Agency, IA 52530, (515) 937-5464, BS 84 Northeast MO St Univ; MA 85 Northeast MO St Univ; 85–Sp-Lang Path, Southern Prairie AEA, **SLP**

Trigg, Kimberly Jane 305 South Water Avenue, Philadelphia, MS 39350, (601) 656-1870, BS 86 Univ Southern MS-Hattiesburg; MS 86 Univ Southern MS-Hattiesburg

Triller, Maureen E 4014 Les Cherbourg Lane, Florissant, MO 63034, (314) 837-0754, OB 83 Saint Louis Univ; OM 85 Saint Louis Univ; **SLP**

Trilling, Terry G 11 Schermerhorn Street, Brooklyn Heights, NY 11201, (212) 624-2796, BA 62 CUNY - Hunter Coll; MA 64 NY Univ; 86–Assoc Prof, Kingsborough Community College, **SLP**

Trimboli, Barbara H 1428 Cole Avenue, Elkins, WV 26241, (304) 636-4560, BS 72 WV Univ; MS 75 WV Univ; Sp-Lang Path, Randolph Co Sch, **SLP**

Trimm, Mary Margaret 12 Hilltop Boulevard, Canfield, OH 44406, (216) 372-4599, **SLP**

Trimmer, Mrs Lisa Ann 7973 Lost Tree Drive, Boardman, OH 44512, (216) 758-0516, BS 74 Univ of PA; MA 79 Univ of PA; 87–Intern, Potential Dev Ctr

Trinch, Mrs Paula Jean 2111 Tanglewood Drive, Waldorf, MD 20601, BS 84 Clarion Univ of PA; MS 85 Clarion Univ of PA; **SLP**

Trinchero, Jennifer D 465 Capital Street #D, Oakland, CA 94610, (415) 465-9995, BS 85 CA St Univ - Hayward; MS 87 CA St Univ - Hayward; **SLP**

Tringale, Mrs Kathlene M 66 Cobb Lane, Scituate, MA 02066, (617) 471-8180, BA 71 Bridgewater St Coll; MS 74 Southern CT St Univ; SLP, Quincy Publ Sch, **SLP**

Tringham, Karen Sue K 512 Carmella, Arroyo Grande, CA 93420, (415) 427-1839, BA 77 CA St Univ - Fullerton; MA 81 CA St Univ - Fresno; Sp/Lang Path, **SLP A**

Trinwith, Gail E 204 Acorn Court, Schaumburg, IL 60193, (312) 742-3264, OB 79 Univ of WI - Whitewater; MS 80 Univ of WI - Whitewater; Commun Dis Dept Head, Jayne Shover Er Sl Rehab Cen, **SLP**

Triolo, Dennis J P O Box 22165, Agana, GU 96921, BS 74 Univ of OR; MS 83 Univ of UT; Aud, Dept Pub Hlth & Social Servs, **A**

Triplett, Mrs Julienne Kay Route 4 Box 75, Cheney, WA 99004, (509) 235-6691, BS 64 ID St Univ; MA 66 Univ of HI - Manoa; SLP, Cheney Pub Schs Dist 360, **SLP**

Triplett, Mrs Marilyn Jean 1745 Ewald S E, Salem, OR 97302, (503) 967-8822, BS 73 OR Coll of Education; MS 76 OR Coll of Education; 84–Sp-Lang Path, Educ Eval Ctr, **SLP**

Tripp, Jeanette Lois Armory Road, RFD #3, Milford, NH 03055, (603) 673-3616, BA 82 CA St Univ - Chico; MS 88 CA St Univ - Sacramento

Tripp, Karen Anne 4345 Raleigh #303, Alexandria, VA 22304, (202) 877-1440, MS 84 ID St Univ; 87–Sp-Lang Path, Natl Rehab Hosp, **SLP**

Trippe, Stuart J 7 Church Lane Suite 16, Baltimore, MD 21208, (301) 484-8383, BA 71 Univ of MD - College Park; MS 73 Loyola Coll; 87–Pres, Sp Rehab Assoc Inc, **SLP**

Trippel, Mrs Monique Cherie 133 Vickroy, Crown Point, IN 46307, (219) 662-1864, BA 82 IN Univ - Bloomington; MA 83 IN Univ - Bloomington; Sp-Lang Path, NW In Spec Ed Coop, **SLP**

Triscik, Bette 4642 Pinto River Court, San Jose, CA 95136, (408) 723-8924, BA 76 San Jose St Univ; MA 83 San Jose St Univ; Sp-Lang Path, San Jose USD, **SLP**

Trisdale, Miriam Edel 8 Maple Ridge Road, Seabrook, NH 03874, (603) 929-0553, BA 74 Suffolk Univ; ME 81 Northeastern Univ; Sp-Lang Path, Beverly Hospital, **SLP**

Trisolini, Margaret Mountjoy 19 North May Avenue, Athens, OH 45701, (614) 593-7204, BS 69 OH Univ - Athens; MA 75 OH Univ - Athens; Sp-Lang Path, Sp Lang Path Services, **SLP**

Tritsch, Mrs Martha M 675 J E George Boulevard, Omaha, NE 68132, (402) 976-7152, BS 73 Univ of NE - Lincoln; MA 74 Univ of NE - Lincoln; 86–Sp-Lang Path, Omaha PS, **SLP**

Tritschler, Helen L 1473 S Ponce DE Leon Avenue N, Atlanta, GA 30307, **SLP**

Tritz, Lois Catherine 3210 Blakely, Eau Claire, WI 54701, (715) 877-2411, BS 82 Univ of WI - Stevens Point; MS 84 Univ of WI - Stevens Point; Sp-Lang Path, Rehabilitation Assoc, **SLP**

Trivelpiece, Mrs Ruth Moskowitz Box 154, Medical College Of Virginia Hospital, Richmond, VA 23298, (804) 786-9318, BA 75 PA St Univ - Univ Park; ME 80 Univ of VA - Charlottesville; 88–Clinic Coord, MCV Hosp, **SLP**

Trochinski, Mrs Barbara A 510 East Tilson Street, West Salem, WI 54669, (608) 786-2467, BS 73 Univ of WI - Eau Claire; MS 74 Univ of WI - Eau Claire; Sp/Lang Path, Lacrosse Pub Sch, **SLP**

Trochlil, Margaret A 1011 Mound Avenue, South Charleston, WV 25309, (304) 345-8522, BS 85 WV Univ; MS 87 PA St Univ - Univ Park; 87–Aud, Aud & Hrng Aid Services Inc, **A**

Trocki, Edith M 167 Central Street, South Weymouth, MA 02190, (617) 335-7568, BA 80 Bridgewater St Coll; MS 82 Emerson Coll; Sp-Lang Path, Sp-Lang-Hrng Assoc, **SLP**

Trocki, Mona R 631 A Tilton Road, Northfield, NJ 08225, (609) 645-3055, MA Hahneman Medical Coll; 88–Aud Dir, Better Hearing Inc, **A**

Troesch, Peter J 421 College Avenue, Lincoln, IL 62656, (217) 735-2361, BS 65 IL St Univ - Normal; MA 67 Univ of IL - Urbana; Coord Sp-Lang Path/Aud Serv, Lincoln Dev Cen, **A**

Troester, Judith Hill 114 East 36th Street, Erie, PA 16504, (814) 870-6000, BS 80 Murray St Univ; MS 86 Southern IL Univ -Carbondale; 87–Aud, Hamot Med Ctr/Comm Rehab Spec, **A**

Trogdon, Mrs Laura Harris 633 Sunset Avenue, Asheboro, NC 27203, (919) 431-1027, BA 82 Univ of NC - Chapel Hill; MS 83 Univ of NC - Chapel Hill; Sp-Lang Path, Private Practice, **SLP**

Troia, Mrs Barbara Lynn 9359 Jones, Omaha, NE 68114, (402) 399-9120, **A**

Troio, Debra A Exeter West Condominiums, Kingston Rd Bldg 37 #8, Exeter, NH 03833, (603) 964-5501, BA 81 Anna Maria Coll; MS 88 Worcester St Coll

Trom, Michael Gene 4073 Beard Avenue North, Robbinsdale, MN 55422, (612) 535-6279, BA 80 Univ of MN - Minneap-St Paul; BS 81 Univ of MN - Minneap-St Paul; MA 86 Univ of MN - Minneap-St Paul; **SLP**

Trombetta, JeanMarie 1154 Hammond Avenue, Utica, NY 13501, (315) 736-0176, BS 81 SUNY - Coll at Geneseo; MS 82 Syracuse Univ; 85–Sp-Lang Path, Harts Hill Sch, **SLP**

Trombetta, Marla Handmaker 1456 Chippewa Trail, Wheeling, IL 60090, (312) 506-9254, BS 80 Northern IL Univ - De Kalb; MA 81 Northern IL Univ - De Kalb; 87–Aud, Otolarngology Med & Surg Assoc, **A**

Trombley, Jayne S 503 Campbell, Kalamazoo, MI 49007, (616) 685-5823, BA 77 Univ of CT; MA 78 Western MI Univ; SLP, Plainwell Comm Sch, **SLP**

Trombly, Janine Marie 54 Rutgers Street Apartment #1, Rochester, NY 14607, (716) 328-7340, BA 84 Univ of Rochester; MA 87 SUNY - Coll at Geneseo; 87–Sp-Lang Path, Assoc For Retarded Citizens

Trombly, Dr Thelma 938 South Kihei Road #612, Kihei, HI 96753, (808) 879-6434, BA 32; MA 33 Univ of MO - Columbia; PH 58 (Sp Path) Univ of MO - Columbia; Prof Emeritus, U of MO, **SLP F LM**

Tromburg, Mrs Ruth Ann 17734 East Colgate Place, Aurora, CO 80013, (303) 986-4587, **SLP**

Tromm, Kathleen Barry 206 6th Street, Beach Haven, NJ 08008, (609) 492-2185, BA 80 Rutger's St Univ - Douglas Coll; MS 85 Rutgers St Univ -N Brunswick; Sp-Lang Path, Long Beach Island Bd of Educ, **SLP**

Trommald, Mrs Dagne A Middlesex School, Concord, MA 01742, (201) 689-1222, BS 62 Boston Univ; MA 81 Montclair St Coll; Director/Head Teacher, The Childrens Meetinghouse, **A**

Trommer-Thaul, Mrs Nancy E 300 West 55th Street #5H, New York, NY 10019, (212) 439-3388, BS 76 Ithaca Coll; MS 78 Columbia Univ Teachers Coll; Sp-Lang Path, Lenox Hill Hospital, **SLP ACE**

Trompeter, Joyce L 5915 North Cedarcrest Ct, Apartment 809, Peoria, IL 61615, (309) 673-2341, BS 76 Bradley Univ; MS 77 Bradley Univ; Sp-Lang Path, Spec Ed Assn of Peoria Co, **SLP**

Troncho, Mrs Sue A 157 Arleta Drive, Downsview, ON, Canada M3L 2M3, (416) 633-5427, BS 79 Western KY Univ; ME 80 Univ of NC - Greensboro; Sp-Lang Path, Hamilton Bd of Educ, **SLP**

Trondsen, Mrs Lisa Anderson 2616 Escobar Way, Sacramento, CA 95827, (916) 985-0112, BA 80 CA St Univ - Sacramento; MA 83 CA St Univ - Sacramento; Sp/Lang Path, Norman Bork Assoc, **SLP**

Trone, Jill Phillips 140 South Hall #4, Virginia, IL 62691, (217) 544-6464, BS 82 Western IL Univ; MA 83 Western IL Univ; Sp-Lang Path, St Johns Hosp, **SLP**

Tronolone, Veronica 7108 Stockton Drive, Knoxville, TN 37909, (615) 584-4646, **SLP**

Troop, Mrs Pamela Bushart 5521 Nordica N E, Albuquerque, NM 87111, (505) 247-4224, BS 81 Baylor Univ; MS 82 Baylor Univ; Sp-Lang Path, Albuquerque, Hrng & Sp Cen, **SLP**

Troquato, Mrs Aileen Murphy 955 Catkin Court, San Jose, CA 95128, (408) 292-7482, BA 84 San Jose St Univ; MA 86 San Jose St Univ; 86–Sp-Lang Path, Santa Clara USD

Trost-Cardamone, Dr Judith E Dept Communicative Disorders, California St University, 18111 Nordhoff Street, Northridge, CA 91330, (312) 726-8220, BS 62 Northwestern Univ; MA 63 Northwestern Univ; PH 70 Northwestern Univ; Associate Professor, CA State U, **SLP F ACE**

Trostler, Nancy J County Hearing & Balance Inc, 464 Ocean Avenue, New London, CT 06320, (203) 443-6944, BA 75 Univ of Denver; MS 79 Univ of Redlands; 83–Aud, Co Hrng/Balnc, **A**

Trost-Steffen, Catherine Agronomy Dept Ag Science N, University Of Kentucky, c/o Kenneth Steffen, Lexington, KY 40546-0091, (608) 231-2601, BS 74 Univ of IL - Urbana; MA 77 Univ of IL - Urbana; **SLP**

Trotta-Boehler, Lynda L 42 Harding Avenue, Roslyn Heights, NY 11577, (516) 621-0806, BA 74 Hofstra Univ; MA 75 Hofstra Univ; Sp-Lang Path, Roslyn Pub Sch, **SLP**

Trotter, Alan Norman Rt 11 Box 470-K, Morganton, NC 28655, (704) 264-0566, MS 85 Univ Southern MS-Hattiesburg; SLP, Communi Care Inc, **SLP**

Trotter, Dr Alice Child 109 Defender Street, Lexington Park, MD 20653, MA 76 Pepperdine Univ - Los Angele; MA 83 San Diego St Univ; PH 87 (Comm Dis & Sci) Southern IL Univ -Carbondale; Sp-Lang Path, **SLP**

Trotter, Jessie Nesmith 13415 Reid Circle, Fort Washington, MD 20744, (703) 371-1211, **SLP**

Trotter, Paul James 439 North 50th Street, Milwaukee, WI 53208, BS 76 Marquette Univ; MS 77 Marquette Univ; Sp/Lang Path, Glendale-River Hills Sch Dist, **SLP**

Trotter, Dr William D 6404 West Wells Street, Wauwatosa, WI 53213, (414) 258-4269, BA 49 Queens Univ - Ontario; MA 51 Univ of IA; PH 53 (Sp Path) Univ of IA; 87–Prof Emeritus, Marquette Univ, **SLP LM**

Trotti, Melinda Ellen H 7 Peach Tree Lane, Madison, MS 39110, (601) 956-2744, BS 80 Univ Southern MS-Hattiesburg; MS 81 Univ Southern MS-Hattiesburg; Sp-Lang Path, Dogwood Sch Sp/Lang Imp Chldn, **SLP**

Trouba, Mrs Susan Sievers 296 Howe Avenue #F, Sacramento, CA 95825, (916) 736-3399, BS 85 Univ of NE - Lincoln; MA 87 Univ of CA - Santa Barbara; Aud, Sacramento ENT, **A**

Trouillier, Doreen Theresa 4062 Iroquois Street, New Orleans, LA 70126, (504) 947-3580, BS 80 Saint Mary's Dominican Coll; ME 85 Southeastern LA Univ

Trounson, Marilynn B 446 Theresa Lane, Sierra Madre, CA 91024, **SLP**

Trout, Elaine Addy 609 Alvarado N E, Albuquerque, NM 87108, (505) 255-2458, BS 76 Howard Payne Univ; MS 86 Univ of TX - El Paso; **SLP**

Trout, Mrs Janet L R R 14 Box 250, Haywood Farms, Brazil, IN 47834, (812) 448-2675, BS 74 IN St Univ - Terre Haute; MS 75 IN St Univ - Terre Haute; MS 77 IN St Univ - Terre Haute; Sp-Lang Path, Clay Co Hosp, **SLP**

Trout, Mrs Kimberly L 7133 Stone Mountain Rd S W, Roanoke, VA 24018, (703) 989-5033, BS 83 Edinboro Univ of PA; MA 84 Edinboro Univ of PA

Trout, Mrs Madonna N 105 North Bosart Avenue, Indianapolis, IN 46201, (317) 353-5429, BA 71 IN Univ - Bloomington; MA 72 IN Univ - Bloomington; 72–Sp-Lang Path, Comm Hosp of Inpls Inc, **SLP**

Trout, Dr Susan Struve 1200 North Nash Street, Apartment 261, Arlington, VA 22209, (202) 797-5522, BS 58 Ball St Univ; MA 60 Stanford Univ; PH 73 (Learning Disabilities) Northwestern Univ; 86–Exec Dir, Washington Cen for Att Healing, **SLP**

Trowbridge, Mrs Deborah A 396 Watson Street, Akron, OH 44305, (216) 794-0308, BS 79 PA St Univ - Univ Park; MA 81 Kent St Univ; Sp-Lang Path, Stow City Schools, **SLP**

Trowe, Pamela J 310 East 19th Street, Costa Mesa, CA 92627, (714) 645-4174, BA 72 CA St Univ - Long Beach; MA 74 CA St Univ - Long Beach; Super, Bernard Landes Phd, **SLP**

Trow-Steinman, Joyce 316 Atlantic Avenue, Massapequa, NY 11762, **SLP**

Troxell, Christine 8214 158th Street West, Taylor Ridge, IL 61284, (309) 798-2894, BS 78 Univ of WI - Oshkosh; MS 81 Univ of WI - Oshkosh; 81–Aud, Aud Consult, **A**

Troxell, Jay Lowell Route 1 Box 81, Landis Road, Hagerstown, MD 21740, **SLP**

Troxell, Mrs Lucinda B 449 West Middle Street, Hanover, PA 17331, (717) 624-4616, BS 73 Indiana Univ of PA; MS 78 Towson St Univ; Sp-Lang Path, Lincoln Interm Unit #12, **SLP**

Troxell-Klosterman, Julia Lynne 3606 Utica Drive, Dayton, OH 45439, (513) 866-4347, Sp-Lang Path, Miamisburg City Schs, **SLP**

Troxler, Mrs Terry Fink 5201 Timer Haven Lane, New Orleans, LA 70114, (504) 391-0985, BS 79 LA St Univ - Baton Rouge; OM 80 LA St Univ - N O Medical Ctr; Sp/Lang Path, Jefferson Parish Pub Sch Syst, **SLP**

Troy, Shirley Loretta 375 South Randolph Street, Apartment 802, Brea, CA 92621, (818) 969-2467, BA 80 Whittier Coll; MA 83 Whittier Coll; 88–Sp-Lang Path, Azusa USD, **SLP**

Troyert, Mrs Stephanie Stewart 1631 East Lark, Springfield, MO 65804, (816) 276-4023, BS 83 KS St Univ; MA 85 Whittier Coll; SLP, Research Med Cntr, **SLP**

Truan, Linda M 9605 Arden Street, Livonia, MI 48150, (313) 422-0438, BS 74 Central MI Univ; MA 76 Central MI Univ; Tchr, Wayne County Intermed Sch Dist, **SLP**

Trubey, Cindy Joy 10 Candlewick Court, Newcastle, DE 19720-3924, (217) 987-6155, BA 81 Valparaiso Univ; MS 83 Univ of IL - Urbana; **SLP**

Trucchi, Sharon A 28 Kilmer Avenue, Taunton, MA 02780, (508) 678-8336, BA 84 Bridgewater St Coll; MS 87 Northeastern Univ; 88–Aud, Azhar Q Mustafa MD

Trucco, Mrs Corinne R 815 Sturgeon Eddy Road, Wausau, WI 54401, MA 82 Univ of WI - Stevens Point; **SLP**

Trudeau, Gerard A 1606 Landquist Drive, Encinitas, CA 92024-4755, (619) 753-8355, BA 60 Central MI Univ; MA 65 Central MI Univ; MA 79 CA St Univ - Chico; Sp-Lang Path, San Diego USD, **SLP**

Trudeau, Mrs Linda A 2158 Cranford Road, Columbus, OH 43221, (614) 457-7464, BS 74 PA St Univ - Univ Park; MA 79 OH St Univ; 88–Aud, Ohio State Univ Sp/Hrng Cl, **A**

Trudeau, Dr Michael D Division Of Speech & Hearing Science, 324 Derby Hall, Columbus, OH 43210, (614) 422-8207, BA 72 OH St Univ; MA 80 OH St Univ; PH 82 (NS) OH St Univ; Asst Prof, OH St U-Sp & Hrng Sci, **SLP**

Trudelle, Terie M 372 Beacon Street #6, Somerville, MA 02143, (617) 576-2360, BA 82 CA St Univ - Northridge; MA 84 CA St Univ - Northridge; Sp-Lang Path, Perkins School for Blind, **SLP**

Truehart, Lisa A HCR 61 Box 178, West Plains, MO 65775, (417) 764-3441, BS 75 Bloomsburg Univ of PA; MS 81 Bloomsburg Univ of PA; Owner / Dir, Private Practice, **SLP**

Trueman, Mrs Janet Katherine 26832 Salinas Lane, Mission Viejo, CA 92691, (714) 667-3397, BA 65 Univ of CA - Los Angeles; MS 82 CA St Univ - Fullerton; SLP, Orange Coast College, **SLP**

Truesdale, Mrs Susanne Poulette 13 Birch Lane, Scotia, NY 12302, (518) 399-7970, BS 85 Coll of Saint Rose; MS 86 Coll of Saint Rose; 87–Sp-Lang Path, Schalmont Central Sch Dist, **SLP**

Truesdell, Paula Jean 4875 Linden Road #126, Freeport, IL 61109, (307) 864-2147, BA 82 Univ of Northern CO; MA 84 Univ of Northern CO; Sp-Lang Path, Gottsche Rehab Cen, **SLP**

Truett, Carol Pierce P O Box 125, Wellton, AZ 85356, (602) 782-2561, BS 75 Eastern IL Univ; MS 83 Northern AZ Univ; Sp-Lang Path, Yuma Dist #1, **SLP**

Truitt, Lisa E Box 123, New Gretna, NJ 08224, (609) 652-7000, BS 78 Stockton St Coll; MA 81 Montclair St Coll; 85–Supvr Sp-Lang Path, Betty Facharach Rehab Hosp, **SLP**

Trujillo, Denise E 2719 Oak Bluff, San Antonio, TX 78230, (512) 493-8327, BS 77 Univ of TX - Dallas; MS 79 Univ of TX - Dallas; **SLP**

Trujillo-Sanchez, Mrs Cynthia D Star Route Box 4B #82, Mesilla Park, NM 88047, (505) 526-3341, BA 80 NM St Univ; MA 84 NM St Univ; Sp-Lang Path, Las Cruces Public Schools, **SLP**

Trullinger, Dr Richard W Aud & Speech Path SVC (126), V A Medical Center, 4801 Linwood Blvd, Kansas City, MO 64128, (816) 861-4700, BS 72 Portland St Univ; MS 74 Portland St Univ; PH 80 (NS) Univ of OK Medical Center; 88–Sp-Lang Path, VA Medical Center, **SLP**

Trumbo, Charles R 1717 Homewood Boulevard, Apartment 255, Delray Beach, FL 33445, (407) 272-0831, BA 36 Transylvania Univ; MA 48 Univ of KY; **LM**

Trumbo, Mrs Michelle Keenan 261 28th Street, San Francisco, CA 94131, (415) 282-4883, BA 82 Univ of CA - Santa Barbara; MA 84 Chapman Coll; 84–Sp-Lang Path, Belmont Sch Dist, **SLP**

Trumbower, Mrs Eva Beth 2417 Beachview, Columbia, MO 65203, (314) 445-5541, BA 71 Univ of MO - Columbia; MS 72 Central MO St Univ; **SLP**

Trumbull, Lois King 5919 North 3rd Street, Arlington, VA 22203, (703) 528-6212, BA 71 Syracuse Univ; MA 76 Catholic Univ of America; MA 86 Catholic Univ of America; **SLP**

Trump, Stephanie Ann 3858-B Fox Chase Drive, Dover, PA 17315, (717) 767-6941, BS 83 PA St Univ - Univ Park; MS 85 PA St Univ - Univ Park; Dir Sp-Lang Path, Rehab Hosp of York, **SLP**

Trumpy, Carol Jean 191 Hickory Hollow Place, Antioch, TN 37013, (658) 885-5232, BA 85 Central MI Univ; MA 86 Central MI Univ; 88–Sp-Lang Path, Hillsboro Rehab Ctr, **SLP**

Trunk, Dr Joseph 1968 White Star Drive, Diamond Bar, CA 91765, (714) 861-8053, BA 73 CA St Univ - Los Angeles; MA 74 CA St Univ - Los Angeles; PH 79 (NS) Univ of the Pacific; Aud, Private Practice, **A**

Trunzo, Mary Jane 8501 East Sage Drive, Scottsdale, AZ 85253, (602) 946-6534, BA 72 Univ of Pittsburgh - Pittsburgh; MA 80 Wichita St Univ; Clinic Director, Arizona Inst for Com Disorders, **SLP ACE**

Trupe, Elizabeth Hillis Dir Speech-Language Pathology, Medical Rehab Ctr Of Md, 9512 Harford Road, Baltimore, MD 21234, (301) 661-7400, BA 81 George Washington Univ; MA 82 George Washington Univ; Director/Sp-Lang Path, Med Rehab Ctr of MD, **SLP**

Truschel, Mrs Mary Joan 103 Atterbury Road, Monroeville, PA 15146, (412) 856-5750, BS 65 Carlow Coll; MS 67 Univ of OK - Norman; Sp-Lang Path, Private Practice, **SLP**

Truse, Susan Shellar 1950 Osage Lane, Santa Fe, NM 87501, (505) 982-0038, MS 70 Univ of WI - Madison; BA 67 Saint Xavier Coll; Sp-Lang Path, Santa Fe Pub Sch, **SLP**

Truss, Marion Elida 517 North Hullen, Metairie, LA 70001, (504) 834-2654, BS 76 Univ of New Orleans; MA 77 Eastern KY Univ; OM 85 LA St Univ - N O Medical Ctr; Aud, Oschner Clinic, **A**

Trussell, Susan Elaine 8806 Wooded Glen Road, Louisville, KY 40220, (502) 491-7186, MS 88 Univ of Louisville; 88–Sp-Lang Path, InSpeech Inc

Trusso, Joseph Phillip 336 LaBarbera Lane, Jamestown, NY 14701, (716) 483-4408, BS 81 SUNY - Coll at Fredonia; MS 82 SUNY - Coll at Fredonia; 82–Sp-Lang Path, Jamestown Bd of Ed, **SLP**

Trutna, Phyllis 3110 Downhill Drive, Colorado Springs, CO 80918, **SLP**

Trutner, Mrs Patricia L 133 Cambon Avenue, St James, NY 11780, (516) 673-1672, BA 79 Adelphi Univ; MA 82 Hofstra Univ; Sp-Lang Path, Anne E Gordon Assoc, **SLP**

Truxler, Joan E 26 Banks Hill Place, Ridgefield, CT 06877, (203) 438-5562, BA 72 CA St Univ - Fresno; MA 73 San Jose St Univ; Sp-Lang Path, Private Practice, **SLP**

Tryba, Mary Jo 348 Foster Drive, Apartment E, Willimantic, CT 06226, (203) 423-8401, BS 84 Univ of WI - Whitewater; MS 87 Univ of WI - Madison

Trybus-Worniak, Mrs Paula M 17252 Summit Drive, Northville, MI 48167, (313) 347-0363, BS 75 Central MI Univ; MA 77 Central MI Univ; **SLP**

Trychel, Marc Robert 1127 Edgewater Drive, Orlando, FL 32804, (305) 843-8028, BS 83 Univ of Central FL; MS 85 FL St Univ; 85–VP, Oto-Audiological Hearing Service, **A ACE**

Trygg, Larry D 3627 35th, Spokane, WA 99203, (509) 299-3131, BA 71 Eastern WA Univ; MS 72 Eastern WA Univ; Sp-Lang Path, Lakeland Village, **SLP**

Tryggvason, Lilyanna Zmijak 72 Delong Drive, Gloucester, ON, Canada K1J 7E1, (613) 744-5731, BS 78 Univ of Toronto - Ontario; OB 79 Univ of Western Ontario; MA 82 Wichita St Univ; Sp-Lang Path, Carleton Bd of Educ, **SLP**

Tryon, Ruth E K P O Box 307, Eaton, CO 80615, (303) 454-3618, BA 72 Univ of LA Verne; MA 73 Univ of Northern CO; Sp-Lang Path, Weld BOCES, **SLP**

Trzcinski, Marie G 4158 Rahn Road, Apt 20, Eagan, MN 55122, (612) 454-1527, MA 73 Eastern MI Univ; **SLP**

Tsandikos, George Michael 98 Bowers Street, Lowell, MA 01854, (617) 459-6144, OB 54 New England Cons of Music; OM 58 New England Cons of Music; ME 62 Boston Univ; Admin of Spec Ed, Lowell Pub Sch, **SLP**

Tsappis, Anthony Stockton Hearing & Speech Ctr, Quail Lakes Office Plaza, 4623 Quail Lakes Drive, Stockton, CA 95207, (409) 951-6491, BA 73 CA St Univ - Sacramento; 74 CA St Univ - Sacramento; PH 87 (Psychoacoustics) Columbia Pacific Univ; 77–Aud, Private Practice, **A**

Tschaepe, Mrs Lois Miskovich 200 Blair Drive, Normal, IL 61761, (309) 452-4473, BS 71 Eastern IL Univ; MS 84 IL St Univ - Normal; Aud, Thomas C Ocheltree, **A**

Tschanz, Mrs Dina Marie 418 West Madison Street, Eau Claire, WI 54703, (715) 833-0048, BA 84 Univ of WI - Eau Claire; MS 85 Univ of WI - Eau Claire; SLP, Keystone AEA 1, **SLP**

Tschiderer, Mrs Patricia Archila 325 Darthmouth Avenue, Apartment E5, Swarthmore, PA 19081, (302) 651-6052, BS 82 WV Univ; MS 83 WV Univ; Sp-Lang Path, Alfred I Dupond Institute, **SLP**

Tse, Dr Sou-Mee 7 Cumber Avenue, Scarborough, ON, Canada M1E 1S7, (416) 281-7306, MA 76 Univ of MN - Minneap-St Paul; MS 83 Univ of British Columbia; PH 82 (Child Language) Univ of British Columbia; 86–Aud, Centenary Hosp, **A**

Tseng, Bi-Hwa 314 22nd Avenue, San Francisco, CA 94121, (415) 921-7658, OB 82 Nat'l Taiwan Normal Univ; MS 85 Univ of WI - Madison; 85–Aud, San Francisco Hrng & Sp Cntr, **A**

Tsugawa, Lance 5845 S W Arrowwood Lane, Portland, OR 97225, MS 75 Portland St Univ; Sp-Lang Path, Kaiser-Permanente, **SLP**

Tsujimoto-Cho, Gail Miyuki 7001 Blake Street, El Cerrito, CA 94530, (415) 233-6698, BA 83 San Francisco St Univ; MS 85 San Francisco St Univ; 85–Spec Educ Tchr, Richmond USD, **SLP**

Tsumpes, Mrs Cynthia Sue 29610 Heather Court, Agoura Hills, CA 91301, (213) 785-2911, **SLP**

Tucci, Mrs Judith P 150 Wendover Avenue, Kenmore, NY 14223, (716) 838-5815, BS 75 SUNY - Coll at Brockport; MS 81 SUNY - Coll at Buffalo; Sp-Lang Path, Buffalo Bd of Ed, **SLP**

Tuch, Mrs Claire H 300 Edwards Street, Roslyn Heights, NY 11577, (516) 484-5396, BS 50 Adelphi Univ; MA 53; Sp/Lang Path, Private Practice, **SLP LM**

Tuch, Doris P 4105 North 48th Avenue, Hollywood, FL 33021, (305) 987-0103, BA 72 CUNY - Brooklyn Coll; MS 77 CUNY - Brooklyn Coll; SLP, Broward Sch Bd, **SLP**

Tuchband, Mrs Daren 12 West Palmer Avenue, Nanuet, NY 10954, (914) 942-2700, BA 73 SUNY - Coll at New Paltz; MA 75 CUNY - Queens Coll; 86–Sp-Lang Path, North Rockland Centr Sch Dist, **SLP**

Tuchman-Rosen, Shari Marlene 444 East 86th Street #33C, New York, NY 10028, (212) 787-7070, **SLP**

Tuchscherer, Maria 2724 Sinton Avenue, Regina, SK, Canada S4S 1K1, (306) 586-4429, BA 73 Univ of Regina -Saskatchewan; MS 75 Minot St Univ; 87–Sp-Lang Path, Regina Child & Youth Services, **SLP**

Tuck, April E 1115 Burnley Road, Charlotte, NC 28210, (704) 552-0543, BS 78 Ithaca Coll; MS 80 Univ of WI - Madison; 87–Sp-Lang Path, Doylestown Hosp, **SLP**

Tuck, Robin Elizabeth 6530 Country Oaks Circle, Apartment 37, Memphis, TN 38115-5269, (901) 761-1500, BA 83 Univ of NC - Chapel Hill; MS 85 Univ of NC - Chapel Hill; 85–Aud, Colonial Hearing Eval Ctr, **A**

Tuck, Tara J 65 Berkeley Street, Reading, MA 01867, (617) 498-9269, BS 69 Lesley Coll; MS 76 Boston Univ; Sp-Lang Path, Cambridge Public Schools, **SLP**

Tucker, Abigail D 425 Lindbergh Dr #A2, Atlanta, GA 30305, (404) 266-9915, BA 76 Eckerd Coll; MS 88 GA St Univ; 88–Sp-Lang Path, Atlanta PS

Tucker, Mrs Alison Marsh 1044 Camino La Costa #1047, Austin, TX 78752, (512) 926-4112, BS 82 Univ of GA; ME 84 Univ of GA; Sp-Lang Path, Austin ISD, **SLP**

Tucker, Barb A 20324 Perkins Avenue, Torrance, CA 90503, BA 71 CA St Univ - Long Beach; MA 73 CA St Univ - Long Beach; Prog Spec, Off of LA Co Supt of Schs, **SLP**

Tucker, Barbara G 2639 Wyman Road, Winston-Salem, NC 27106, (919) 727-2442, MA 76 Appalachian St Univ; 88–Sp-Lang Path, Forsyth Central Public Health, **SLP**

Tucker, Mrs Barbara L 2701 Coronado Drive, Fullerton, CA 92635, (818) 443-6181, BA 66 Univ of CA - Santa Barbara; MA 68 Univ of CA - Santa Barbara; SLP, Los Angeles Cnty Supt Schools, **SLP**

Tucker, Mrs Beverly J 1360 Nottingham Drive, Casper, WY 82609, (307) 234-5903, BA 58 Univ of MT; Sp-Lang Path, Natrona County Sch Dist No 1, **SLP**

Tucker, Mrs Connie Montgomery 4040 South Ledbetter, Dallas, TX 75236, (214) 494-8348, BS 75 East TX St Univ - Commerce; MS 76 Southern Methodist Univ; Sp-Lang Path, Garland ISD, **SLP**

Tucker, Dawn D 7031 Flint Hill Road, Owings Mills, MD 20736, (301) 257-3083, BS 74 Univ of MD - College Park; MS 77 Towson St Univ; 81–Consult, Private Practice, **SLP**

Tucker, Deborah Ann 2529C West Jerome, Chicago, IL 60645, BS 78 Univ of IL - Urbana; OM 86 Governors St Univ; 86–Sp-Lang Path, Chicago PS, **SLP**

Tucker, Mrs Debra Bales 7342 Winnington Circle, Charlotte, NC 28226, (704) 364-6252, BS 78 Eastern MI Univ; MA 79 Eastern MI Univ; 84–SLP, Charlotte-Mecklenberg Schools, **SLP**

Tucker, Denise Anne Dept Of Otolaryngology, Univ Of VA Medical Center, P O Box 430, Charlottesville, VA 22908, (804) 924-2050, BS 79 Brigham Young Univ; OM 81 Brigham Young Univ; Audiologist, University of Virginia, **A**

Tucker, Mrs E Raylene 6737 Riviera Drive, Fort Worth, TX 76180, (817) 294-8408, BA 70 Bethany Nazarene Coll; MS 83 TX Christian Univ; Sp-Lang Path, Overton Sp & Lang Cen, **SLP**

Tucker, Frances M 3518 Vaughn, Knoxville, TN 37920, BA 66 Univ of CA - Santa Barbara; MA 68 San Francisco St Univ; 88–Sp-Lang Path, Univ Of TN-Knoxville, **SLP**

Tucker, Mrs Janice K Rd 1 Box 416-K, Seven Valleys, PA 17360-9801, (717) 428-1405, BS 78 Ashland Coll; MS 80 Loyola Coll; Sp-Lang Path, Private Practice, **SLP**

Tucker, Jayma Lee 5 Rolling Acres R R 5, Jacksonville, IL 62650, (217) 245-2111, BS 82 Eastern IL Univ; MS 83 Eastern IL Univ; 88–SLP, IL Mental Hlth Dev Disabilities, **SLP**

Tucker, Linda K 11291 Bristolwood, St Louis, MO 63126-3204, (314) 569-8235, BS 71 Western IL Univ; MS 73 Central MO St Univ; Area Coord, Spec Sch Dist of St Louis Co, **SLP**

Tucker, Mrs Linda M 14 Kensington Place, East Orange, NJ 07017, (201) 456-5347, BA 78 Cleveland St Univ; MS 79 TN St Univ; Sp-Lang Path, Univ of Med & Dentistry of Nj, **SLP ACE**

Tucker, Mrs Marsha B 7001 Meadowbrook Drive, Fort Worth, TX 76112, (817) 654-1106, BA 72 Univ of Redlands; MA 74 San Jose St Univ; SLP, Arlington ISD, **SLP**

Tucker, Melody A Watson Clinic, 1600 Lakeland Hills Blvd, Lakeland, FL 33805, (813) 680-7195, MS 80 Univ of South FL; Chief of Aud, Watson Clinic, **A**

Tucker, Mrs Nancy J C 11404 South Talman, Chicago, IL 60655, (312) 361-2121, BS 79 Northern IL Univ - De Kalb; MA 80 Northern IL Univ - De Kalb; Sp-Lang Path, Sertoma Cen/Commun Dis, **SLP**

Tucker, Mrs Nancy M RFD 2 Box 237-A, Randolph, VT 05060, (802) 728-3113, BA 73 Univ of CT; ME 75 Northeastern Univ; Aud, Private Practice, **A**

Tucker, Pamela J 1408 Spruce Street, Chico, CA 95926, (916) 342-7243, MA 88 CA St Univ - Chico

Tucker, Mrs Phoebe Simons 45 Honey Bee Lane, Huntington, CT 06484, (203) 929-6455, **SLP**

Tucker, Mrs Ruth Strong P O Box 5219, Birmingham, AL 35207, (205) 322-1460, MA 73 Univ of AL- Tuscaloosa; OM 83 Univ of AL-Birmingham; ED 88 (Ed Leadership) Univ of AL-Birmingham; 79–Tchr Coord, Birmingham Pub Sch Syst, **SLP**

Tucker, Mrs Sharon Lynn Route 3 Box 299, Luray, VA 22835, (703) 743-7633, ME 88 James Madison Univ; 88–Sp-Lang Path, Page County Sch Bd

Tucker, Mrs Susan L 120 Trafalgar Place, Longwood, FL 32779, (407) 779-6880, BA 66 FL St Univ; MS 67 FL St Univ; SLP, Seminole County School Board, **SLP**

Tucker, Thomas W 22 Brighton Street #1, Charlestown, MA 02129, (617) 424-4685, BA 76 Emerson Coll; ME 79 Northeastern Univ; Aud, Boston City Hosp, **A**

Tucker, Wendy Weiss 511 Alden Avenue, Westfield, NJ 07090, (201) 321-7063, BA 79 Univ of MD - College Park; MA 81 Montclair St Coll; Sp-Lang Path, JFK Medical Cen Sp-Hrng Dept, **SLP**

Tuder, Peggy Jean 25645 Longview Place, Hayward, CA 94541, BA 57 San Jose St Univ; MA 63 CA St Univ - Fresno; Palo Alto USD, **SLP A**

Tudor, Mrs Gail M 19 Locksley Lane, Brewer, ME 04412, (207) 862-3830, BA 72 Univ of ME - Orono; MA 73 Univ of ME - Orono; Sp-Lang Path, Maine Sch Admin Dist #22, **SLP**

Tudor, Patricia Lynn 613 Royal Crest Avenue, Nashville, TN 37214, (615) 865-2373, BA Butler Univ; MA Western MI Univ; SLP, TN Christian Medical Center, **SLP**

Tuecke, Susan K 5310 Terminal Drive, McFarland, WI 53558, (319) 245-1480, BS 79 Univ of IA; MS 80 Univ of IA; Sp-Lang Path, Verona Community Sch, **SLP**

Tufano, Mrs Sally 468 Salmon Creek Road, Brockport, NY 14420, (716) 325-4560, OM 83 SUNY - Coll at Brockport; BS 72 SUNY - Coll at Geneseo; MA 75 SUNY - Coll at Brockport; Dir of Pupil Pers, Rochester City Sch Dist, **SLP**

Tufte, Lori Jean 2034 15th Street, Eau Claire, WI 54703, (715) 834-8094, BS 80 ND St Univ; MS 86 Univ of WI - Eau Claire; 88–Sp-Lang Path, Eau Claire Area Sch Dist, **SLP**

Tufts, Devon C 26206 Valley Point Lane, Newhall, CA 91321, (805) 252-8444, BS 69 Brigham Young Univ; BS 70 Brigham Young Univ; ED 84 Pepperdine Univ - Los Angele; Asst Prin, Los Angeles Co Offi of Ed, **SLP**

Tufts, Dr La Rene C 3248 Tulip Lane, Stevens Point, WI 54481, (715) 346-4511, BA 50 Univ of WA; MA 58 Univ of WA; PH 83 (NS) IN Univ - Bloomington; 87 Assoc Dean, U WI-Sch of Commun Dis, **SLP A**

Tuite-Taffe, Anne Marie 1841 West 105th Street, Chicago, IL 60643, (312) 997-3648, BS 83 Western IL Univ; MA 84 Western IL Univ; **SLP**

Tukey, Laura Kapp 844 22nd Street, Santa Monica, CA 90403, (213) 828-1703, BA 78 OH Wesleyan Univ; MA 80 Univ of IL - Urbana; SLP, LA Co Supt Sch, **SLP**

Tukey, Sharyn Ann Hale 20 Chapel Street, Augusta, ME 04330, (207) 289-3311, BS 74 Univ of ME - Farmington; MA 80 Univ of ME - Orono; Sp-Lang Path, ME-Div of Maternal & Chld Hlth, **SLP**

Tulak, John M 6055 Boxer Drive, Bethel Park, PA 15102, BS 71 Clarion Univ of PA; ME 77 Clarion Univ of PA; Sp-Lang Path, Volusia County Schools, **SLP**

Tulak, Joseph, Jr P O Box 492, Daytona Beach, FL 32015, (904) 258-5471, BS 77 Clarion Univ of PA; ME 80 Clarion Univ of PA; Sp-Lang Path, Volusia County School Board, **SLP**

Tuller, Mrs Brenda Rems 5 Spradley Lane, Middletown, NJ 07748, (201) 826-3360, BA 69 Kean Coll of NJ; MA 84 Kean Coll of NJ; 79–SLP, Perth Amboy Bd of Educ, **SLP**

Tuller, Karen Burke 4522 Teas, Bellaire, TX 77401, (713) 785-6760, MA 85 Univ of Houston - Univ Park; **SLP**

Tuller, Linda Golden 5111 Glen Ridge #A25, San Antonio, TX 78229, (512) 434-6711, BS 75 TX Tech Univ; MS 76 Univ of North TX; Superv, Our Lady of the Lake U, **SLP**

Tullier, Mrs Amy Lynn 13341 Ott Lane, Gonzales, LA 70737, (504) 644-2865, BS 81 LA St Univ - Baton Rouge; MA 86 LA St Univ - Baton Rouge; 81–Sp-Lang Path, Ascension Parish Sch Bd, **SLP**

Tullos, Dr Daniel C Box 751 Station A, Searcy, AR 72143, (501) 268-6161, BA 73 Harding Univ; OM 74 Univ of MS; PH 88 (Communication Disorders) PA St Univ - Univ Park; 79–Sp-Lang Path, Harding University, **SLP**

Tully, Joanne B 346 Woodcock Lane, Feasterville, PA 19047, (215) 456-2900, BA 80 Temple Univ; MA 83 Temple Univ; Coord Sp&Aud Servs, Phila Geriatric Cen, **SLP A**

Tully, Mrs Miriam 355 South Main Street, Old Town, ME 04468, (207) 827-8077, BA 81 Univ of ME - Orono; MA 84 Univ of ME - Orono; 88–Sp-Lang Path, Union 90 Milford, **SLP**

Tuma, Mrs Aleta Dean 608 East Clark Boulevard, Murfreesboro, TN 37130, (615) 893-4618, BS 65 Univ of TN - Knoxville; MS 66 Vanderbilt Univ; Aud, ENT Office Dr Robert Tuma, **A**

Tuma, Elizabeth Rose 6466 Camino Viviente, Goleta, CA 93117, (805) 964-5626, BA 81 St Mary's Coll of CA; MS 84 San Francisco St Univ; **SLP**

Tumolo, Mrs Judith A 5597 Day Drive, Milford, OH 45150, (513) 791-7949, BS 68 Millersville Univ of PA; MA 73 Rutgers St Univ -N Brunswick; Sp-Lang Path, Sycamore Comm Schs, **SLP**

Tumpowsky, Audrey F K 25 Colony Road, Westport, CT 06880, (203) 854-4000, BA 63 CUNY - Brooklyn Coll; MS 67 CUNY - Brooklyn Coll; Sp-Lang Path, Norwalk Bd of Ed, **SLP**

Tuneski, Mrs Jean Pepin Naval Hospital, Audiology Division, Box 600, Groton, CT 06349, (203) 449-3870, **A**

Tunick, Phyllis 89-15 Parsons Boulevard, Apartment 7F, Jamaica, NY 11432, (212) 658-2680, BA 54 Columbia Univ Teachers Coll; MA 61 CUNY - Hunter Coll; Sp-Lang Path, Bd of Ed Sp Serv Ut, **SLP**

Tunin, Mrs Carolyn S 5100 West 300 South, Crawfordsville, IN 47933, (317) 362-2650, BA 59 IN Univ - Bloomington; MA 64 IN Univ - Bloomington; Sp-Lang Path, Crawfordsville Comm Sch Corp, **SLP**

Tunnell, John S 5850 North Star Road, Ferndale, WA 98248, (206) 384-8922, BA 69 Univ of WA; OM 74 Univ of WA; Aud, Private Practice, **A**

Tunney, Kathleen M 6 Elm Street, Assonet, MA 02702, (617) 823-5327, MS 83 Univ of RI; **SLP**

Tunney, Pamela Ann 1966 Inwood Road, Dallas, TX 75235, (214) 783-3039, BS 82 Saint Louis Univ; MA 83 Univ of Northern CO; Aud, Callier Cen, **A**

Tunningley, Georgiann 9135 Rolston Road, Gaines, MI 48436, (313) 735-4940, MS; **SLP**

Tunningley, Richard M 9135 Rolston Road, Gaines, MI 48436, (313) 735-4940, **SLP**

Tunstall, Christine M Speech Pathology Services, 1848 North Garey Avenue, Pomona, CA 91767, (714) 865-0114, BA 78 Univ of MI - Ann Arbor; MS 80 Univ of MI - Ann Arbor; Sp-Lang Path, Private Practice, **SLP**

Tunteri, Diane Shaffer Shaffer Hearing & Speech Ctr, 2625 Laurel, Beaumont, TX 77702, (409) 835-2791, BS 80 Lamar Univ; MS 82 Lamar Univ; Admin/Owner, Shaffer Hrng/Sp Cen, **A**

Tuohy, John L 12821 West Playfield Drive, Crestwood, IL 60445, MA 67 De Paul Univ; SLP, Evergreen Park School Dist 124, **SLP**

Tuohy-Eagan, Mrs Geralyn 17 Cumberland Road, West Hartford, CT 06119, (203) 232-7301, BA 78 Univ of CT; MS 81 Southern CT St Univ; 85–Sp-Lang Path, Hartford PS Sys, **SLP**

Tuomala, Mrs Kathleen A Longleaf Medical Ctr, Audiology Of The Sandhills, 1902-F N Sandhills Blvd, Aberdeen, NC 28315, (919) 692-6422, BA 73 Elmira Coll; MA 76 Kent St Univ; Aud, Audiology of the Sandhills, **A**

Tuomi, Dr Seppo K 10 Alexandra Avenue, Craighall 2196, Johannesburg, South Africa, BA 66 8140; MA 67 8140; PH 72 (Cleft Palate Sp) Northwestern Univ; 80–Sp-Lang Path, Private Practice, **SLP**

Tuozzolo, Jacquilin Ann 3 Patrician Terrace, Mays Landing, NJ 08330, (609) 646-9321, BA 67 Montclair St Coll; MA 84 Trenton St Coll; Sp-Lang Path, Egg Harbor Twp Board of Educ, **SLP**

Tupler, Ruth I 6570 S W 47th Court, Fort Lauderdale, FL 33314, (305) 583-0801, BA 54 CUNY - Queens Coll; Office Mgr, Austin Tupler Trucking Inc

Tupper, Mrs Billie Jo 2039 Hewitt Drive, Billings, MT 59102, BA 56 Univ of Southwestern LA; MA 65 Univ of SD - Vermillion; Sp-Lang Path, Billings Sch Dist 2, **SLP**

Turbeville, Dr Joseph B, Jr 11122 Sabine Valley Drive, Little Rock, AR 72212, (501) 224-6910, BS 69 Univ of Central AR; MA 71 Memphis St Univ; PH 74 (NS) Vanderbilt Univ; Aud, Private Practice, **A**

Turchin, Mrs Beverly K 1808 Altozano Drive, El Cajon, CA 92020, (619) 562-1808, BA 71 Rutger's St Univ - Douglas Coll; MS 73 Rutgers St Univ -N Brunswick; Sp-Lang Path, Private Practice, **SLP**

Turcich, Mrs Maryellen Lawlor P O Box 1076, Corrales, NM 87048, (505) 256-0507, BS 76 Western IL Univ; MA 77 Western IL Univ; Sp-Lang Path, Albequerque Pub Sch Syst, **SLP**

Turck, Sr Stephanie St Elizabeth Medical Center, 2100 Madison Avenue, Granite City, IL 62040, (618) 798-3133, BA 75 Fontbonne Coll; MS 81 Fontbonne Coll; SLP, St Eliz Med Cen, **SLP**

Turco, Tambria Marie 70 Trillium Court, Madison, WI 53719, (608) 263-8412, BA 82 Univ of CA - Santa Barbara; MS 85 Univ of WI - Madison; 88–Dir/Sp-Lang Path, Univ of WI Hosp Clnc, **SLP**

Turcotte, Mrs Mary Leclair 2411 Lexington Street, Steilacoom, WA 98388, (206) 582-0865, **SLP**

Tureen, Dr Phyllis 544 Mohawk Road East, West Hempstead, NY 11552, (212) 998-5265, BA 50 CUNY - Brooklyn Coll; MA 54 CUNY - Brooklyn Coll; PH 68 (Sp Path) NY Univ; 63–Assoc Prof & Program Director, New York U, **SLP**

Turek, Kathleen 5000 Town Center #2102, Southfield, MI 48075, **SLP**

Turek, Monica D 3437 Lovers Lane #B, Dallas, TX 75225, (214) 361-8408, BA 74 Southern Methodist Univ; MS 76 Southern Methodist Univ; Sp-Lang Path, Highland Park ISD, **SLP**

Turek, Sandra L 5336 East Kings Avenue, Scottsdale, AZ 85254, (602) 222-6412, BS 73 AZ St Univ; MS 78 AZ St Univ; Aud, VA Med Cen, **A**

Tures, Cathleen Roberta 14642 Rosemary Avenue, Moreno Valley, CA 92388, (714) 793-2631, BA 81 CA St Univ - Long Beach; MA 85 CA St Univ - Long Beach; **A**

Turetsky, Karen 12 Sandys Road, Andover, NJ 07821, **SLP**

Turgeon, Michelle 418-1/2 Carnation, Corona Del Mar, CA 92625, (714) 760-3406, BA 69 Univ of Santa Clara; MA 73 Univ of Southern CA; Sp-Lang Path, Newport-Mesa USD, **SLP**

Turgeonn, Mrs Kelly S 4038 Bell Grande Drive, Valrico, FL 33594, (813) 251-7744, BS 80 Auburn Univ - Auburn; MA 82 Memphis St Univ; SLP, Tampa General Hosp, **SLP**

Turgiss, Susan Marie 18 Briar Lane, Westwood, MA 02090, (617) 762-5288, BA 75 Bridgewater St Coll; ME 81 Northeastern Univ; 87–Sp-Lang Path, North River Collaborative, **SLP**

Turk, Helen 22 Creekside Road, Willowdale, ON, Canada M2M 2R6, (416) 431-8155, MA 88 Univ of MI - Ann Arbor

Turk, Mrs Jane E 98-51 64th Avenue, Rego Park, NY 11374, (718) 459-1008, BA 79 CUNY - Queens Coll; MA 84 CUNY - Queens Coll; 88–Sp-Lang Path, VTA Mgmt Svcs Inc, **SLP**

Turk, Rebecca S 1724 Morgan, Parsons, KS 67357-4344, **A**

Turkel, Nancy Beth 1101 Pine Heights Drive N E, Atlanta, GA 30324, (904) 266-9567, BA 84 Tulane Univ; MA 86 Univ of FL; SLP, Fulton Co Bd of Ed, **SLP**

Turkiew, Mrs Rachel A 11 Edward Street, Bethpage, NY 11714, (516) 681-8858, BA 74 CUNY - Brooklyn Coll; MS 78 CUNY - Brooklyn Coll; Sp-Lang Path, Private Practice, **SLP**

Turkin, Anita Beth 6986 Old Brentford Road, Alexandria, VA 22310, (301) 899-3033, BA 68 Univ of MI - Ann Arbor; ME 72 Wayne St Univ; Sp-Lang Path, Prince Geo Co Bd of Ed, **SLP**

Turkstra, Lyn Siobhan 190 Sorauren Avenue, Toronto, ON, Canada M6R 2E9, (416) 848-7286, BA 81; OB 85; MA 87 SUNY - Center at Buffalo; 87–Sp-Lang Path, The Mississauga Hosp

Turley, William A 609 Old Farm Lane, State College, PA 16803, (814) 237-3267, BS 66 Bloomsburg Univ of PA; BS 66 Bloomsburg Univ of PA; ME 70 Bloomsburg Univ of PA; Aud, Private Practice, **A**

Turley-Shuck, Jeanne C Speech-Language Pathology Serv PA, The Prevention & Treatment Center, 4501 East North Street Ext, Taylors, SC 29687, (803) 292-5154, BS 75 Univ of TN - Knoxville; MS 80 Univ of SC - Columbia; Pres/Dir, Sp Lang Path Serv, **SLP ACE**

Turnbaugh-McCormick, Karen Robin 4550 47th Street West, Apartment #609, Bradenton, FL 34210, (813) 794-3126, BA 76 Univ of VT; MS 77 Univ of VT; PH (Experimental Psychology) Univ of VT; 87–Sp-Lang Path, Sarasota County PS, **SLP**

Turnbull, Karen Koester 5732 Harding, Barryton, MI 49305, (517) 382-7027, BS 76 Central MI Univ; MA 83 Central MI Univ; Sp-Lang Path, Mt Pleasant Sch, **SLP**

Turnbull, Kathleen R 3722 Highland Avenue, Drexel Hill, PA 19026, (419) 423-0957, BS 76 Western MI Univ; MA 77 Central MI Univ; Sp-Lang Path, Crozer Chester Med Ctr, **SLP**

Turnbull, Laura Hammond 9133 Carlton Cricle, Knoxville, TN 37922, (615) 691-4428, BS 81 East TN St Univ; MA 86 Univ of TN - Knoxville; **A**

Turnbull-Norton, Carol A 3892 Trailwood, Okemos, MI 48864, BS 76 Western KY Univ; MA 78 Western KY Univ; **SLP**

Turner, Aina 661-A Prescott Avenue, Monterey, CA 93940, (408) 647-9545, BA 78 Univ of CA - Los Angeles; MA 82 CA St Univ - Northridge; Sp-Lang Path, Alisal Sch Dist, **SLP**

Turner, Mrs Ann M 2505 Devri Court, Mountain View, CA 94043, (415) 856-4744, MS 80 IL St Univ - Normal; Sp-Lang Path, Newark USD, **SLP**

Turner, Beverly Ann 2709 A Laclede Station Rd, St Louis, MO 63143, (314) 647-6808, BA 84 Univ of MS; MS 86 Univ of MS; 86–Aud, Washington Univ Sch of Med, **A**

Turner, Brenda A 94 Love Lane, Hartford, CT 06112, BA 78 Case Western Reserve Univ; MS 80 Bradley Univ; SLP, New Britain Bd of Ed, **SLP**

Turner, Mrs Carla Dawn 1332 West Meadowbrook Circle, Springfield, MO 65807, (314) 351-4395, BA 84 Ouachita Baptist Univ; MA 86 Saint Louis Univ; **SLP**

Turner, Carolyn T 232 Walnut Lane, Slingerlands, NY 12159, (518) 452-0654, BA 81 MI St Univ; MA 82 George Washington Univ; Sp-Lang Path, Private Practice, **SLP**

Turner, Charlcie H Audiology & Speech Path (126), VA Medical Center, Mountain Home, TN 37684, (615) 926-1171, BS 69 East TN St Univ; MS 70 Vanderbilt Univ; Aud, VA Medical Center, **A**

Turner, Charles R 700 South Bois D Arc, Tyler, TX 75701, (214) 597-8886, BA 69 Abilene Christian Univ; MA 73 Our Lady Lake Univ-San Anton; MS 77 Univ of TX - Austin; Ther/Couns, Turner Couns Stress & Pain Cen

Turner, Mrs Cheryl R 2405 Sunrise Court, Green Bay, WI 54301, (414) 465-8593, BA 77 MI St Univ; MA 78 MI St Univ; Sp-Lang Path, Green Bay Area Pub Sch, **SLP**

Turner, Dr Chris W Syracuse University, 805 South Crouse Street, Syracuse, NY 13244, (315) 443-9647, BA 73 Univ of WI - Madison; MA 79 Univ of MN - Minneap-St Paul; PH 82 (NS) Univ of MN - Minneap-St Paul; 83–Assoc Prof, Syracuse Univ, **A**

Turner, Claire Jean 10650 Weymouth Street #203, Bethesda, MD 20814, (301) 493-4124, BA 67 Univ of MD - College Park; MA 76 Stanford Univ; MA 68; Sp-Lang Path, Mont Co Pub Sch, **SLP**

Turner, Mrs Deborah Lynn 2321 Blue Hill, Chesterfield, MO 63017-7363, (314) 434-2753, **SLP**

Turner, Mrs Elizabeth Grimes 2846 Fairlane Drive S E, Atlanta, GA 30354, (404) 681-0251, BA 73 Trinity Univ; MS 79 Emory Univ; Special Education Specialist, Tea Division-Services F/T Deaf, **SLP**

Turner, Ernie W 265 North Cleveland Avenue, Orange, CA 92668, (714) 558-2666, BA 67 Eastern NM Univ; MS 69 UT St Univ; Vice President, Hearing & Sp Assoc Inc, **A**

Turner, Greg S 219 North Main Street, Deerfield, WI 53531, (608) 764-5139, BS 83 Western MI Univ; MS 86 Univ of WI - Madison; Proj Asst, State of Wisconsin, **SLP**

Turner, Jamie Galloway 4770 North Peachtree Road, Atlanta, GA 30338, (404) 393-7089, BS 76 IN Univ - Bloomington; MA 77 IN Univ - Bloomington; 78–Aud, GA Retardation Ctr, **A**

Turner, Dr Janet E 6639 West Dodge Place, Milwaukee, WI 53220, (414) 472-5204, BS 75 Indiana Univ of PA; MS 76 Syracuse Univ; PH 87 (Sp Communication) Univ of PA; Asst Prof, Univ of Wisconsin Whitewater, **SLP**

Turner, Janet Lois 35-2088 Pembina Highway, Winnipeg, MB, Canada R3T 2G8, (204) 256-4301, MS 85 Univ of ND; 85–Sp-Lang Path, St Amant Centre Inc, **SLP**

Turner, Mrs Jayne A 4477 Aragon Drive, San Diego, CA 92115-1716, (619) 286-7263, BS 75 Univ of UT; MS 77 Univ of UT; Sp/Lang Path, Assoc of Retarded Ctzns, **SLP ACE**

Turner, Mrs Jayne S 4040 East Piedmont Drive, Space 278, Highland, CA 92346, MS; **LM**

Turner, Mrs Joann R 3147 Avenue A, Council Bluffs, IA 51501, (402) 551-9908, BA 72 Univ of WY; MS 78 Univ of NE - Omaha; **SLP**

Turner, Julie L 85 Francis Street #3, Brookline, MA 02146, (617) 889-2523, BA 80 Temple Univ-Tyler Sch of Art; MS 85 Emerson Coll; SLP, Till Inc, **SLP**

Turner, Karel Lee 30 Park Avenue 9-C, New York, NY 10016, (212) 725-9422, BS 69 Ithaca Coll; MS 70 Ithaca Coll; OD 87 (Law) Yeshiva Univ; 87–Attorney, Jackson/Lewis/Schnitzler/Krupman, **A**

Turner, Laureen Theresa 2157 Patterson Street #3, Eugene, OR 97405, (503) 686-3591, BA 81 McGill Univ - Quebec; MS 84 Univ of South FL; 87–Clin Supvr, Univ of Oregon, **SLP**

Turner, Linda S 260 El Dorado Boulevard, Apartment 804, Webster, TX 77598, **SLP**

Turner, Lois Susan 916 54th Street, Brooklyn, NY 11219, (718) 317-3639, BS 76 CUNY - Hunter Coll; MS 86 Columbia Univ Teachers Coll; 87–Aud, Sea View Hosp & Home, **A**

Turner, Mrs Martha Morse 40 Ledgelawn Drive, Little Rock, AR 72212, (501) 776-0691, MS 83 Univ of AR - Little Rock; Sp-Lang Path, Pediatric Physical Therapy Clin, **SLP**

Turner, Martha P 164 Maple Avenue, Northport, NY 11768, (516) 261-5584, BS 44 Columbia Univ Teachers Coll; MA 49 Columbia Univ Teachers Coll; **SLP A LM**

Turner, Mary H U 1826 Ridgeover Place, Jackson, MS 39211, (601) 981-2611, BA 74 Millsaps Coll; MS 78 Univ of MS; Dir Dept Communication Disord, MS Methodist Rehabil Center, **SLP**

Turner, Mrs Nancy Aduddell 5541 1st Place, Lubbock, TX 79416, (806) 793-8257, BS 72 TX Tech Univ; MS 73 TX Tech Univ; Sp-Lang Path, Lubbock Pub Sch, **SLP**

Turner, Nancy N 405 High Court, Gladstone, OR 97027, (503) 255-1841, BS 76 ID St Univ; MS 77 ID St Univ; SLP, Multnomah Esd, **SLP**

Turner, Mrs Nancy Wilson 208 Roger Webster, Williamsburg, VA 23185, (804) 564-3372, BS 71 WV Univ; MS 73 WV Univ; SLP, Williamsburg James City County, **SLP**

Turner, Mrs Patricia Jo 219 North Main Street, Deerfield, WI 53531, (414) 699-2511, BS 82 Western MI Univ; MA 83 Western MI Univ; Sp-Lang Path, Johnson Creek School District, **SLP**

Turner, Patsy Ann 2125 Robinhood Drive, Miamisburg, OH 45342-2037, (513) 833-2181, BS 79 Northwest MO St Univ; MS 87 Miami Univ - Oxford

Turner, Paula Marie 4516 Barnett Road, Apt#2053, Wichita Falls, TX 76310, (817) 851-2143, BA 83 Univ of FL; MS 85 Univ of South FL; Aud, United States Air Force, **A**

Turner, Mrs Rebecca Goodwin Rt 4 Box 156, Stillwater, OK 74074, (405) 282-6484, BS 80 OK St Univ; MA 82 OK St Univ; Sp/Lang Path, Scottish Childhood Lang Clinic, **SLP**

Turner, Regina Q 3507 Halliday, St Louis, MO 63118, (918) 743-3268, BS 54 Central MO St Univ; MS 76 Univ of MO - Saint Louis; **SLP**

Turner, Richard W, Jr P O Box 20041, Birmingham, AL 35216, (205) 823-9387, BA 73 Auburn Univ - Auburn; MS 87 Univ of Montevallo; 88–Sp-Lang Path, InSpeech Inc, **SLP**

Turner, Dr Robert Graham 533 Panassus, Room U-494, UCSF, San Francisco, CA 94143, (415) 476-2928, BS 67 FL St Univ; MS 68 FL St Univ; PH 75 (Aud/Hrng Science) Univ of FL; 87–Dir-Aud & Sp Clinic/Assoc Prof, Univ of California-SF, **A**

Turner, Sherry B 30 South Ridge Road, Niantic, CT 06357, (203) 444-0931, BS 76 Univ of RI; MS 80 Southern CT St Univ; Owner/Pres, Private Practice, **SLP**

Turner, Mrs Sue Beth 179 Forest Place, Buffalo Grove, IL 60089, (312) 441-9300, BS 77 Univ of IL - Urbana; MS 78 Univ of IL - Urbana; Sp-Lang Path, The Cove School, **SLP**

Turner, Vicki Lynn Rt Box 775-8, Nixa, MO 65714, (417) 725-4644, BS 83 Southwest MO St Univ; MA 85 Southwest MO St Univ; **SLP**

Turocy, Lynn M 106 Timber Ridge, Madison, AL 35758, **SLP**

Turowski, Marjorie Roth 106 Delwood Drive, Morganton, NC 28655, (704) 433-2850, BS 71 Western IL Univ; MA 73 NM St Univ; Dir of Commun Serv, Western Carolina Cen, **SLP A**

Turpin, Linda L 1155 Briarhurst Drive, St Louis, MO 63021, BS 76 Fontbonne Coll; MS 78 Washington Univ; Audiologist, Hearing Associates of St Louis, **A**

Turpin, Mrs Pamela Lynn Box 26, Puxico, MO 63960, (314) 323-4296, BS 80 Southeast MO St Univ; MA 82 Southeast MO St Univ; K-12 Sp-Lang Path, Puxico R8 Sch Dist, **SLP**

Turpin, Mrs Renee E 1809 East Brosdway, Enid, OK 73701, (405) 237-6801, BA 59 Univ of MO - KS City; MA 60 Univ of MO - KS City; SLP, Enid Pub Schls, **SLP**

Turton, Mrs Carla Catherine 491 Rankin Boulevard, Windsor, ON, Canada N9B 2R6, (519) 258-6658, MA 85 Wayne St Univ; **SLP**

Turton, Dr Lawrence J Rd 2 Box 371, Indiana, PA 15701, (412) 357-2451, BA 62 John Carroll Univ; MA 64 Case Western Reserve Univ; PH 66 (Sp Path/Aud) Univ of KS; Professor, Indiana Univ of Pennsylvania, **SLP**

Tusa, Lynn R 7853 Wynnefield Drive, South Glens Falls, NY 12803, (518) 793-7721, BA 74 SUNY - Coll at Plattsburgh; MA 75 OH Univ - Athens; Aud, Southern Adirondack Educ Ctr, **A**

Tushkowski, Mrs Renae 612 Vilas Street, Onalaska, WI 54650, (414) 845-2371, BA 76 Univ of WI - Eau Claire; MS 77 Univ of WI - Eau Claire; SLP, Cesa 7 Seymour Sch Dist, **SLP**

Tusinski, Mrs Marcia R 421 South Van Ness Avenue, Unit 50, Los Angeles, CA 90020, (213) 384-4290, BS 69 Ithaca Coll; MA 75 CA St Univ - Los Angeles; Sp-Lang Path, Private Practice, **SLP**

Tusten, James D 3212 W 21st Place, Lawrence, KS 66046, (913) 843-8479, OB 84 Univ of KS; MA 87 Univ of KS; 87–Aud, Marston Hrng Ctr, **A**

Tuten, Laurie Elizabeth 3010 Northwood Drive #1004, Winston-Salem, NC 27106, (919) 723-1474, BS 84 Univ of NC - Greensboro; ME 85 Univ of NC - Greensboro; 87–Sp-Lang Path, SPEECHCENTER, **SLP**

Tutt, Marilyn Louise 57 Forest Avenue #1409, Hamilton, ON, Canada L8N 1X3, (416) 525-1910, BA 72 Univ of Cincinnati; MA 79 Univ of Cincinnati; 80–Aud, Charlton Aud Cl, **A**

Tutterrow, Mrs Susan Lynn 3260 Running Cedar Drive, Marietta, GA 30062-1363, (404) 578-9281, ME 77 Univ of NC - Greensboro; 84–Sp-Lang Path, Adaptive Learning Ctr, **SLP**

Tuttle, Doreen 1 Meadow Lane, Brewster, NY 10509, **SLP**

Tuttle, Dr Gerald A Department Of Public Health, 150 Tremont Street, Boston, MA 02111, PH 69 (NS) Univ of Pittsburgh - Pittsburgh; 88–Dir-Div Chldrn Spec Hlth Needs, MA Dept of Public Health, **SLP**

Tuttle, JoAnn 2077 Center Avenue #15-C, Fort Lee, NJ 07024, (914) 356-4100, BA 76 Univ of NE - Omaha; MS 79 William Paterson Coll; OM 86 SUNY - Coll at New Paltz; Sp-Lang Path, E Rampo Sch Dist, **SLP ACE**

Tuttle, Karen M 114 South Russell, Ames, IA 50010, (515) 232-1729, MA 73 Univ of NE - Lincoln; BA 72 Univ of Northern CO; 87–Sp-Lang Path, Heartland AEA II, **SLP**

Tveit, Holly L 8538 Delco Avenue, Canoga Park, CA 91306, (818) 718-8131, BA 78 Univ of CA - Santa Barbara; MA 80 CA St Univ - Northridge; Sp-Lang Path, LA USD, **SLP**

Twachtman, Diane D 332 Ash Swamp Road, Glastonbury, CT 06033, (203) 236-1919, BA 65 Univ of CT; MA 68 Univ of CT; 85–Coord-Commun Dis Prog, CREC-Day Treatment Service, **SLP**

Tweed, Rebecca Jean 226-F River Bend Drive, Altamonte Springs, FL 32714, (612) 739-0464, BS 79 Univ of MN - Minneap-St Paul; MA 82 Univ of WI - River Falls; Sp-Lang Path, Rehab Spec Inc, **SLP**

Tweed, Theodore S Dept Communicative Disorders, University Of Wisconsin, 1975 Willow Drive, Madison, WI 53706, (608) 262-3951, BA 55 Luther Coll; MA 60 Univ of IA; Cl Instr, U of WI, **A**

Tweedie, Dr David 324 North Fairfax Street, Alexandria, VA 22314, (703) 684-7079, BS 64 Univ of TN - Knoxville; MA 66 NY Univ; ED 73 (NS) Univ of GA; **SLP A**

Tweedie, Gary L 16-A Bond Street South, Dundas, ON, Canada L9H 3H1, (416) 521-2100, MA 88 SUNY - Center at Buffalo

Tweedy, Julia K 11150 4th Street North, Apartment 2816, St Petersburg, FL 33716, (813) 892-4141, BS 85 FL St Univ; MS 86 FL St Univ; 87–Sp-Lang Path, All Chldn Hosp, **SLP**

Twichell, Dr Doris Y 6926 N Orange Grove Circle, Tucson, AZ 85704, PH (NS); **SLP LM**

Twisselman, Mrs Karen Marie 1441 Linwood Drive, Salinas, CA 93906, (408) 443-3741, BA 80 Univ of Redlands; MS 82 San Francisco St Univ; **SLP**

Twitchell, Dr Mary C Dept Of Comm Sciences & Dis, Radford University, Radford, VA 24142, (703) 831-5453, BA 61 Univ of SD - Vermillion; MA 65 Univ of SD - Vermillion; PH 85 (Sp-Lang Path) MI St Univ; 86–Assoc Prof, Radford Univ, **SLP ACE**

Twomey, David L 1023 South Fleishel, Tyler, TX 75701, (214) 592-8374, BA 77 Univ of MD - College Park; MA 78 Univ of MD - College Park; Aud, Audiology Assoc of East Tx, **A**

Twomey, Karen Wilson 52 Saranac Street, Littleton, NH 03561, (603) 444-0322, BS Univ of NH; Boston Univ; **SLP**

Twomey, Mary Ellen 603 5th Avenue, New Hyde Park, NY 11040, (212) 498-2500, MS 82 Adelphi Univ; Sp-Lang Path, Little Village School, **SLP**

Twyman, Mrs Carol L 893 West Wooster, Bowling Green, OH 43402, (419) 352-2777, BS 78 Bowling Green St Univ; MA 80 Bowling Green St Univ; Sp-Lang Path, S L H Inc, **SLP**

Tyahla, Linda Gross 11981 Sarthe Drive, Maryland Heights, MO 63043, (314) 521-1501, BS 85 Radford Univ; MA 87 Saint Louis Univ; 87–Sp-Lang Path, Spec Sch Dist of St Louis Co, **SLP**

Tyczkowski, Mrs Barbara 523 East Carriage Drive, Glastonbury, CT 06033, (203) 633-5611, BA 79 Univ of CT; MA 81 Univ of CT; Sp-Lang Path, Private Practice, **SLP**

Tye-Murray, Dr Nancy University Hospital, Dept Of Otolarngology, Iowa City, IA 52242, (319) 356-3969, PH 84 (NS) Univ of IA; Aud, Univ/Iowa Hospitalls, **A**

Tygard, Elizabeth 80-W 2260 Sunderland Road, Winston-Salem, NC 27103, (919) 768-8095, BS 84 PA St Univ - Univ Park; MS 88 Univ of NC - Chapel Hill; 88–Aud, Forsyth Head & Neck Assoc

Tykol, Judy Mauterer 5715 Crow Lane, San Jose, CA 95123, (408) 227-3690, BS 73 LA St Univ - Baton Rouge; MA 76 LA St Univ - Baton Rouge; Sp-Lang Path, Oak Grove Sch Dist, **SLP**

Tyler, Ann A Department Of Speech Pathology & Audiology, SUNY Cortland, PO Box 2000, Cortland, NY 13045, (607) 756-5423, BS 75 Univ of NH; MS 78 Syracuse Univ; PH 88 (NS) Syracuse Univ; Prof, SUNY Coll at Cortland, **SLP**

Tyler, Audrey S 1250 S Pennsylvania Avenue, Apartment 1, Winter Park, FL 32789, **SLP**

Tyler, Elizabeth Randolph Mill Street Apartment, Apartment I-2, Athens, OH 45701, (616) 424-5750, BS 74 Southern IL Univ-Edwardsvill; MA 75 Saint Louis Univ; Doct Stud, OH U, **SLP**

Tyler, Mrs Jacqueline 11924 Continental Drive, St Louis, MO 63138, (314) 388-8000, BS 77 OK St Univ; MA 79 Univ of Tulsa; SLP, The Bellefontaine Hab Ctr, **SLP**

Tyler, James I Harmony Woods, 105 Melodie Drive, Newark, DE 19713, BA 77 Temple Univ-Tyler Sch of Art; MA 79 Temple Univ-Tyler Sch of Art; Aud, Med Cen of DE, **A**

Tyler, Jane F 9490 Valley Oak Way, Salinas, CA 93907, (408) 755-6446, BS 71 Emerson Coll; MA 74 NY Univ; MS 77 Univ of NM; Sp-Lang Path, Monterey Co Offi Ed, **SLP**

Tyler, Mrs Jeanne R 17 Court Street, Stamford, CT 06902, (203) 869-1685, BS 65 Emerson Coll; ME 68 PA St Univ - Univ Park; Sp-Lang Path, Greenwich Bd of Ed, **SLP**

Tyler, Mrs Lorraine D 1 Westchester Drive, Georgetown, DE 19947, (302) 856-7364, BA 71 Rosemont Coll; ME 73 Univ of VA - Charlottesville; 88–Sp-Lang Path, Easter Seal Rehab Ctr, **SLP**

Tyler, Melanie 7667 Callaghan Road Suite 315, San Antonio, TX 78229, (512) 340-6666, BS 80 Southern Methodist Univ; MS 81 Univ of WI - Stevens Point; Sp-Lang Path, Private Practice, **SLP**

Tyler, Dr Richard S Department Of Otolaryngolgy, Univ Of Iowa Hospital, Iowa City, IA 52242, (319) 356-2471, BS 74 Univ of Western Ontario; MS 75 Univ of Western Ontario; PH 78 (Psychoacoustics) Univ of IA; Prof & Dir of Aud, U of IA, **A**

Tyler, Sheila Marie 1652 Mapleleaf Court, Encinitas, CA 92024, (619) 436-0208, BS 81 Univ of ND; MS 83 Minot St Univ; **SLP**

Tyler, Tammie Rose 2106 Baker, Vicksburg, MS 39180, (502) 762-2457, MS 88 Murray St Univ

Tyll, Terry W 5430 Baltimore Drive #51, La Mesa, CA 92042, MA 77 San Diego St Univ; District Aud, San Diego City Schs, **A**

Tynan, Mary P 123 Vassar, San Antonio, TX 78212, (512) 696-1910, BA 74 Our Lady Lake Univ-San Anton; MA 75 Our Lady Lake Univ-San Anton; 75–Sp-Lang Path, Stx Chldn Hab Cen, **SLP**

Tynon, Mrs Debra J R R 1 Box 140, Moran, KS 66755, (316) 496-2587, BA 81 Wichita St Univ; MA 82 Wichita St Univ; Sp-Lang Path, Anw Spec Ed Coop 603, **SLP**

Tyree, Jean M 2011A North Halsted, Chicago, IL 60614, (312) 440-0929, BS 80 IL St Univ - Normal; MS 82 IL St Univ - Normal; Sp-Lang Path, PAEC, **SLP**

Tyrrell, Denise K 734 Prescott Place, Paramus, NJ 07652, (201) 967-4040, MS 77; Senior Clinical Supervisor, Bergen Pines County Hospital, **SLP**

Tyrrell-Jones, Louise M 5 West Colorado Avenue, Beach Haven, NJ 08008, (609) 652-7000, BA 71 Univ of RI; MS 72 Univ of RI; Dir of SLP & Aud, Betty Bacharach Rehab Hosp, **SLP**

Tysklind, Mrs Elizabeth S 6047 Crittenden Avenue, Indianapolis, IN 46220, (317) 871-2270, BS 79 IN Univ - Bloomington; MA 80 Ball St Univ; Aud, St Vincent Hosp, **A**

Tysklind, John Michael 3100 Vine, West Des Moines, IA 50265, (515) 274-4493, BS 81 Purdue Univ - West Lafayette; MS 83 Purdue Univ - West Lafayette; Aud, Iowa Head & Neck Assoc, **A**

Tyson, Mrs Joanne G 90 Joanie Lane, North Tonawanda, NY 14120, (716) 837-5238, BS 66 SUNY - Coll at Buffalo; MS 68 SUNY - Coll at Buffalo; Sp-Lang Path, Lang Dev Prog, **SLP**

Tyszka, Dr Frederic A The Sheboygan Clinic, 2414 Kohler Memorial Drive, Sheboygan, WI 53081, (414) 457-4461, BS 64 Univ of WI - Milwaukee; MS 66 Purdue Univ - West Lafayette; PH 68 (Aud) Purdue Univ - West Lafayette; Aud, Sheboygan Cl, **A**

Tytko, Cynthia A 527 Main Street, Oneida, NY 13421, (315) 363-5800, BS 70 SUNY - Coll at Geneseo; MA 71 Western MI Univ; Sp-Lang Path, Oneida City School District, **SLP**

Tytler, Mrs Carol Laureen 9 Stevenson Street, Cortland, NY 13045, (607) 753-7338, BA 81 SUNY - Coll at Plattsburgh; MA 83 Western MI Univ; 85–Sp-Lang Path/Consult, Private Practice, **SLP**

Tzanetopoulos, Karen Nelson 1745 Washington Avenue, Wilmette, IL 60091-2420, (312) 908-3689, BA 84 Univ of MI - Ann Arbor; MS 85 Univ of MI - Ann Arbor; **SLP**

Tzanis, Mrs Evmorfia Fotiou 1884 Pelham Parkway South, Bronx, NY 10461, (212) 584-9000, BA 78 CUNY - Lehman Coll; MA 80 NY Univ; 80–Aud, Bronx VA Med Ctr, **A**

U

Uberuaga, Phillip J P O Box 5545, Tucson, AZ 85703, (602) 628-5427, BA 63 ID St Univ; MA 68 Univ of AZ; 68–Audiologist, Arizona State Sch Deaf & Blind, **A**

Uchmanowicz, Mary Kay 45 Sylvia Road, Medford, MA 02155-4503, (617) 396-9051, **A**

Ucok, Mrs Marilyn Finch 37 Redrock Lane, Pomona, CA 91766-4912, (818) 917-3403, BA 74 Holy Names Coll; MS 76 CA St Univ - Northridge; 79–Asst Prin, Los Angeles Co Ofc of Educ, **SLP**

Udell, Mrs Deborah Brown 801 Society Hill, Cherry Hill, NJ 08003, (609) 424-7489, BA 73 PA St Univ - Univ Park; MA 77 Temple Univ-Tyler Sch of Art; SLP, Phila P S, **SLP**

Udell, Mrs Mary Lou 2385 Roscomare Road, Unit E-15, Los Angeles, CA 90077, (213) 472-0305, BA 81 CA St Univ - Northridge; MA 83 CA St Univ - Northridge; SLP, Valley Hospital Medical Center, **SLP**

Udell, Mrs Ruthe W 51 Birchwood Avenue, West Orange, NJ 07052, (201) 731-3600, BA 70 Montclair St Coll; MA 71 Montclair St Coll; Dir Sp & Aud, Kessler Inst for Rehab, **SLP ACE**

Uding, Ann M 1514 Swallow Drive, St Louis, MO 63144, (314) 878-3314, BS 76 Southeast MO St Univ; ME 81 Southeast MO St Univ; 83–Sp-Lang Path, St Louis Co Sp Sch Dist, **SLP**

Udwin, Mrs Lisa Home 355 Dublin Drive, Cardiff, CA 92007, (619) 747-6933, BS 77 Univ of MA - Amherst; MA 81 San Diego St Univ; Sp-Lang Path, Sharp Cabrillo Hospital, **SLP**

Udziela, Joan Nelke 7375 Overbrook Drive, St Louis, MO 63121, (314) 521-7811, BS 76 Univ of MO - Columbia; MS 77 Fontbonne Coll; **SLP**

Uehara, Mrs Ginny Sueko 1504-F Palo Avenue, Honolulu, HI 96816, (808) 531-7498, BS 79 Univ of HI - Manoa; MS 81 Univ of HI - Manoa; Sp-Lang Path, Dept of Ed St of Hawaii, **SLP**

Uffenheimer, Janis Blindman 1700 Madison, 1st Floor, Evanston, IL 60202-2038, (312) 367-4300, BA 76 Univ of MN - Minneap-St Paul; ME 78 Univ of WI - Madison; 79–Aud, Lake McHenry Reg Prog, **A**

Ufford, Amanda F 147 Honness Lane, Ithaca, NY 14850, (607) 273-8719, BA 66 Univ of Keele - England; MS 79 Ithaca Coll; 87–Sp-Lang Path, Spec Chldn Ctr, **SLP**

Uglem, Mrs Linda R H W 6111 Cth S, Onalaska, WI 54650, (608) 783-5528, BS 66 IN Univ - Bloomington; MS 71 Purdue Univ - West Lafayette; Sp/Lang Path, Holmen Scvhool District, **SLP**

Ugrin, Jerome G 1174 Bierly Road #68, Portsmouth, OH 45662, (614) 354-3026, BA 68 Univ of Northern CO; MA 72 Univ of Northern CO; Scioto Mem Hosp, **A**

Uhl, Jennifer Anne 110-B Somers-Point Road, Mays Landing, NJ 08330, BA 81 Loyola Coll; MS 82 Loyola Coll; Sp-Lang Path, Helmbold Ed Ctr, **SLP**

Uhl, Lizette M P O Box 731, Knoxville, IA 50138, (515) 828-6021, BA 79 Montclair St Coll; MA 80 George Washington Univ; Audiologist, Verterns Admin Medical Center, **A**

Uhl, Sandra McFall 9884 Zig Zag Road, Cincinnati, OH 45242, (513) 529-4432, BS 70 Miami Univ - Oxford; MA 71 Univ of IL - Urbana; Cl Coord, Miami U, **SLP**

Uhler, Mrs Karen Haugsjaa Box 64, 14 McCann Mill Road, Pottersville, NJ 07979, (201) 722-1500, BA 69 MT St Univ; MA 72 Western MI Univ; SLP, Bridgewater-Raritan Sch, **SLP**

Uhler, Sarah Bussier 1501 1st Street S E, Minot, ND 58701, (701) 852-2465, BS 85 Moorhead St Univ; MS 86 Minot St Univ; Sp-Lang Path, Souris Valley Special Services, **SLP**

Uhlman, Mrs Lorraine L 522 Airway Avenue, Lewiston, ID 83501, (208) 743-4240, BA 69 Eastern WA Univ; MS 72 Eastern WA Univ; Sp-Lang Path, Lewiston Public Schools, **SLP**

Uhlrich, Mrs Clara L W 8615 Hawthorne, Raytown, MO 64138, (816) 358-5433, BS 74 Pittsburg St Univ; MA 77 Univ of KS; **SLP**

Ujhelyi, Mary P 1678 East Swan Circle, Brentwood, MO 63144, BA 71 Fontbonne Coll; MS 81 Fontbonne Coll; SLP, Sp Sch Dist-St Louis Co, **SLP**

Ujiki, Nenon L M 521 Stratford Place, Chicago, IL 60657, (312) 477-1088, MS 68 Northwestern Univ; Sp-Lang Path, **SLP ACE**

Uken, Dennis Lee 620 East Plumb Lane, Suite 120, Reno, NV 89502, (702) 825-6006, BA 69 SD St Univ; MA 71 Univ of AZ; Aud, Reno Hearing Center, **A**

Ulbright, Deborah T P O Box 34, Geneseo, NY 14454, (607) 659-7185, BS 82 SUNY - Coll at Geneseo; MS 85 Ithaca Coll; **SLP**

Ulery, Beverly Ann 1944 McBain Avenue, San Jose, CA 95125, (408) 377-7988, **SLP**

Ulery, Norma Jean 5925 Mac Corkle Avenue S W, Apartment B, St Albans, WV 25177, (304) 766-6281, BA 81 Univ of Pittsburgh - Pittsburgh; MA 83 Univ of Pittsburgh - Pittsburgh; 87–Sp-Lang Path, Kanawha Co Bd of Educ, **SLP**

Ulfsdottir, Thora Saeunn Haaleitisbraut 107 108, Reykjavik, Iceland, OB 81 0500; MS 85 Univ of AL-Tuscaloosa; 88–Sp-Lang Path, The City Hosp, **SLP**

Ulius, Mrs Marilyn 510 East 86th Street, New York, NY 10028, Audiologist, Imc Audiology Services, **A**

Ulizio, Deborah Lynne 4111 Stonecliffe Drive, Monroeville, PA 15146, (216) 444-6693, BS 84 PA St Univ - Univ Park; MA 86 Univ of Pittsburgh - Pittsburgh; **A**

Ullberg, Mrs Renee Gould 4105 River Birch Road, Fort Worth, TX 76137, (817) 847-0007, BS 85 Northwestern Univ; MS 87 Univ of TX - Dallas; **SLP**

Ullman, Ann P 1545 Fay Road, Loveland, OH 45140, (513) 575-3646, BS 74 Miami Univ - Oxford; MS 77 Miami Univ - Oxford; Sp-Lang Path, Clermont Co Spec Ed Twsp Cen, **SLP**

Ullman, Merle Charmian 119 Alta Vista Way, Daly City, CA 94014, (415) 584-3593, SLP, San Francisco USD, **SLP**

Ullrich, Diane Rita 2013-A Woodburn Road, Waukesha, WI 53188, (414) 781-3030, BS 55 Marquette Univ; MS 65 Marquette Univ; Sp-Lang Path, Sch Dist of Elmbrook, **SLP**

Ullrich, Kenneth Albert Eye & Ear Clinic Of Wenatchee, P O Box 3027, Wenatchee, WA 98801, (506) 662-7143, MS 72 TX Tech Univ; Aud, Eye & Ear Clinic Inc, **A**

Ulman, Stephen G R R 2 Box 244A, Fort Fairfield, ME 04742, **SLP**

Ulmer, Julie Annette R R #3 Box 7, Hawarden, IA 51023, (712) 722-4374, BS 79 SD St Univ; MA 83 Univ of IA; **SLP**

Ulmer, Mrs Sue C 3427 North Hunter, Stockton, CA 95204, (209) 462-6262, BA 83 Univ of the Pacific; MA 84 Univ of the Pacific; Sp-Lang Path, Stockton USD, **SLP**

Ulmer, Mrs Susan Judith 1715 Chadwick Drive, Richmond, VA 23229, (804) 282-7068, BS 83 James Madison Univ; ME 85 James Madison Univ; **A**

Ulreich, Patty L 6332 Ohio Street, Kent, OH 44240, (216) 678-6561, BS 84 Bowling Green St Univ; MA 85 Bowling Green St Univ; Sp-Lang Path, Edwin Shaw Hosp, **SLP**

Ulrich, Colby Kendro 9733 North Lake Drive #1, Milwaukee, WI 53217, (414) 377-6103, BS 84 Univ of WI - Madison; MS 86 Marquette Univ

Ulrich, Kathleen M 4262 Kiem Road, Lisle, IL 60532, (312) 960-9346, BS 75 Northern IL Univ - De Kalb; MA 76 Northern IL Univ - De Kalb; Aud, Otol Head & Neck Surg Ltd, **A**

Ulrich, Mrs Margaret Littell Route 3 Box 413, Dayton, TN 37321, (615) 775-0603, BA 67 Southern Coll of S D A; ME 79 James Madison Univ; Aud, Rhea Co Schs, **A**

Ulrich, Mrs Miriam N 3587 S Leisure World Blvd, Silver Spring, MD 20906, (301) 598-7826, BS 30 Northwestern Univ; MA 60 Univ of MD - College Park; **SLP LM**

Ulrich, Paul D 3960 South Spruce, Denver, CO 80237, (303) 428-3511, BA 67 Baker Univ; MA 73 Wichita St Univ; SLP, Adams Co Dist 50 Pub Sch, **SLP**

Ulrich, Mrs Rhonda Bay 943 North 10th Street, Reading, PA 19604, (215) 775-8334, BS 82 Bloomsburg Univ of PA; MS 83 Bloomsburg Univ of PA; Sp-Lang Path, Reading Rehab Hosp, **SLP**

Ulrich, Sandra R 41 Partridge Hollow, Gales Ferry, CT 06335, (203) 486-2629, BS 59 PA St Univ - Univ Park; MA 71 Univ of CT; Dir Sp & Hrng Cl, University of Connecticut, **SLP F ACE**

Ulrich, Sara Lynn 3569 Old Brandon Road, Apt #33, Pearl, MS 39208, (601) 939-8640, BS 82 Delta St Univ; MS 84 Univ Southern MS-Hattiesburg; Sp-Lang Path, Hudspeth Ret Ctr, **SLP**

Ulrich, Vicki K Rural Route 2, Baldwin, KS 66006, **SLP**

Ulrichny, Cathy L Rd 5 Box 67, Choctaw Trail, Oak Ridge, NJ 07438, (201) 729-3107, BA 72 Montclair St Coll; MA 73 Montclair St Coll; SLP, Sparta Board of Education, **SLP**

Ultsch, Mrs Susan Lannert 403 Shoreline Highway, Mill Valley, CA 94941, (415) 282-2551, BA 83 CA St Univ - Sacramento; MS 87 San Francisco St Univ; Sp-Lang Path, St Luke's Hosp

Umano, Helen V 6 Kristy Drive, Beacon, NY 12508, (212) 430-5598, BA 54 CUNY - Hunter Coll; MA 70 CUNY - Hunter Coll; Sp-Lang Path, Albert Einstein Coll Med, **SLP**

Umansky-Sokol, Debra 1 Brewery Square #319, New Haven, CT 06513, (203) 384-8681, BA 78 Adelphi Univ; MA 79 Case Western Reserve Univ; Sp-Lang Path, Rehab Assoc of Ct, **SLP**

Umatum, Michael W 8811 Ruggles Street, Omaha, NE 68134, (712) 322-7354, BS 73 Univ of NE - Omaha; MS 75 Univ of NE - Omaha; Sp-Lang Path, Loess Hills AEA-13, **SLP**

Umberger, Dr Forrest Glen 630 Clifton Road N E, Atlanta, GA 30307, (404) 651-2310, BS 64 Univ of UT; MS 66 Univ of UT; PH 71 (NS) Univ of IL - Urbana; Coor Commun Dis, Georgia State U, **SLP**

Umble, Dr Roy H 403 Marilyn Avenue, Goshen, IN 46526, (219) 533-6598, BA 35 Goshen Coll; MA 38 Northwestern Univ; PH 49 (Sp Path) Northwestern Univ; **LM**

Umbro, Mrs Maria G Woodbine Developmental Ctr, DE Hirsch Avenue, Woodbine, NJ 08270, (609) 861-2164, MS 72 Boston Univ

Umen, Ilene A 4660 Kester Avenue #213, Sherman Oaks, CA 91403, (805) 658-8161, BA 75 SUNY - Coll at Buffalo; MA 77 Univ of CA - Santa Barbara; SLP, Private Practice, **SLP**

Umfleet, Mrs Katherine 1107 West Braddock Street, Tampa, FL 33603, MS 77 Univ of South FL; Aud, **A**

Umfress, Janel A 1924 35th Place NW, Washington, DC 20007, (202) 333-3992, BA 83 Univ of CA - Santa Barbara; MS 85 Univ of Redlands; 88–Sp-Lang Path, Private Practice, **SLP**

Umphlett, Marianne Parsons 1700-D Backbay Court, Charlotte, NC 28212, (704) 338-4430, BS 85 Appalachian St Univ; MS 86 Univ of SC - Columbia; Sp-Lang Path, Charlotte Rehab Hosp, **SLP**

Umstead, Mrs Monica Marie 2382 East Rock Road, Perkasie, PA 18944, (215) 297-8113, BS 80 Kutztown Univ of PA; MA 84 Trenton St Coll; 81–Sp-Lang Path, Pleasant Manor Inc, **SLP**

Umstead, Rebecca Skacel 1 Hillview Drive, Baltimore, MD 21228, BA 78 Franklin & Marshall Coll; MS 81 Purdue Univ - West Lafayette; 86–Sp/Lang Path, PG County Health Dept Cheverly, **SLP**

Undem, April Lee 2120 N Pacific Avenue #53, Santa Cruz, CA 95060, (408) 973-9933, BA 85 San Jose St Univ; MA 87 San Jose St Univ

Underdahl, Charles W 9215 Oak Valley Drive, De Soto, KS 66018, (913) 585-1771, BS 67 Mankato St Univ; MS 71 Univ of OR; 83–Sp-Lang Path, Therapy Assoc Limited, **SLP**

Underhill, Mrs Marianne S 510 South 18th, Coeur d'Alene, ID 83814, (208) 667-2837, BS 79 Univ of NE - Lincoln; MA 80 Univ of NE - Lincoln; 83–Sp-Lang Path, Joint Sch Dist 391, **SLP**

Underhill, Mrs Nancy A D 195 Topeg Drive, Severna Park, MD 21146, (301) 766-3390, BA 67 Rutgers St Univ - Newark; MA 76 Seton Hall Univ; Sp/Lang Path, Anne Arundel Bd of Ed, **SLP**

Underwood, Analeen J 705 Maple Lane, Oak Grove, MO 64075, (913) 448-3127, BS 76 Central MO St Univ; MS 78 Central MO St Univ; Sp-Lang Path, Lone Jack Sch Dist, **SLP**

Underwood, Mrs Debra Drumwright 2605 Stone Hollow Drive, Bedford, TX 76021, (817) 267-1280, BS 81 Baylor Univ; MS 82 Baylor Univ; Sp-Lang Path, Arlington ISD, **SLP**

Underwood, Linda L P O Box 1378, Rose Haven Unit, Thomasville, GA 31792, (912) 228-2239, BA 74 Emory Univ; MS 76 FL St Univ; SLP, St of GA/Dept Human Resource, **SLP**

Underwood, Mark A 2406 Swift, Richland, WA 99352, (907) 442-3472, BA 81 Central WA Univ; MA 85 WA St Univ; 88–Sp-Lang Path, Northwest Arctic Borough Sch Dist, **SLP**

Underwood, Patricia A 6011 N W 63rd, Suite A, Oklahoma City, OK 73132, (405) 843-1823, BS 74 OK St Univ; MA 76 Saint Louis Univ; Sp-Lang Path, Speech Pathology, **SLP**

Underwood, Paul S Aural Rehabilitation Center, 602 Jodi Drive, Hammond, LA 70401, (504) 345-3402, BA 74 Univ of AL- Tuscaloosa; MS 76 Troy St Univ - Montgomery; MS 76 Univ of Montevallo; Owner, Underwood Hearing Products, **A**

Ungar, Christophe David 2041 Euclid #9, Santa Monica, CA 90405, (213) 452-0544, BA 76 Humboldt St Univ; MA 85 CA St Univ - Los Angeles; 85–Sp-Lang Path, Glendale USD, **SLP**

Ungar, Mrs Elizabeth R 14444 Summerfield Road, University Heights, OH 44118, (216) 231-8787, BS 82 Ithaca Coll; MA 83 Case Western Reserve Univ; Sp-Lang Path, Cleveland Hearing & Sp Ctr, **SLP**

Ungemach, Deborah 3050 Coleridge Road, Cleveland Heights, OH 44118, (216) 951-5551, BA 78 Univ of Central FL; MA 80 Kent St Univ; Sp-Lang Path, Health Hill Hospital, **SLP**

Unger, Mrs Dorothy M 188 Highwood Avenue, Tenafly, NJ 07670, (201) 569-5061, BA 43 Emerson Coll; MA 48 Emerson Coll; ME 53 NY Univ; Dir Sp/Lang Path, Sp/Lang Therapy, **SLP LM**

Unger, Lori R 4 Commonwealth Court #7-D, Brighton, MA 02135, (617) 277-3982, BS 80 Ithaca Coll; ME 82 Northeastern Univ; SLP, The Neuro Cen Forest Manor, **SLP**

Unger, Sharon Joy 140-10 Jewel Avenue, Flushing, NY 11367, (718) 544-1834, MS 88 CUNY - Brooklyn Coll

Ungerleider, Deborah S New England Medical Center Hospital, 750 Washington Street, Speech & Hearing Department, Box 823, Boston, MA 02111, (617) 956-5300, BA 79 SUNY - Center at Buffalo; MA 80 SUNY - Center at Buffalo; 85–Aud, New England Medical Center, **A**

Ungricht, Susannah 267 East 500 North #62, Provo, UT 84601, (801) 374-5558, MS 88 Brigham Young Univ

Union, Mrs Roberta 4 Old English Road, Worcester, MA 01609, (617) 345-0172, BS 74 Worcester St Coll; MA 79 Univ of MA - Amherst; Sp-Lang Path, Private Practice, **SLP**

Unke, Alberta B 920 Falmouth Road, Victoria, BC, Canada V8X 3A3, (604) 382-6187, BA 71 Univ of Manitoba - Winnipeg; MS 73 Minot St Univ; **SLP**

Unke, Paul J 920 Falmouth Road, Victoria, BC, Canada V8X 3A3, (604) 592-1923, BS 72 Minot St Univ; MS 73 Minot St Univ; Sp-Lang Path, Greater Victoria Sch Dist #61, **SLP**

Unruh, Mrs Jane Barrick P O Box 266721, Houston, TX 77207-6721, (409) 763-2373, **SLP**

Unruh, Perry Wallace 1104 N Clouds Rest Drive, Diamond Bar, CA 91765, (808) 917-0515, BA 82 CA St Univ - Fullerton; MS 85 Univ of Redlands; Aud, Unruh Associates, **A**

Unsworth, Mrs Barbara L 11943 Ottawa Place, Chino, CA 91710, (714) 628-8613, BS 75 2559; MA 82 CA St Univ - Los Angeles; SLP, San Bernardino County Schools, **SLP**

Unterman, Dr Rosalie M 65 Goller Place, Staten Island, NY 10314, (718) 983-7599, BA 68 CUNY - Brooklyn Coll; MS 70 CUNY - Brooklyn Coll; PH 76 (NS) NY Univ; Sp-Lang Path, Private Practice, **SLP**

Unterseher, Marilyn 2924 Snelling Avenue North, Apartment 205, Roseville, MN 55113, (612) 781-6571, BS 83 Univ of MN - Minneap-St Paul; MS 85 Mankato St Univ; **SLP**

Untz, Sr Jeanne D'Arc 400 North Bluff, Clinton, IA 52732, (319) 242-4070, BS 73 Northern IL Univ - De Kalb; MS 74 Marquette Univ; Asst Dir, Mt St Clare Coll, **SLP**

Unverdorben, Marion Holly Hill Apts #21, Oxford, MS 38655, (601) 234-1476, MS 87 0840; 87–Aud, N MS Retardation Ctr, **A**

Uonelli, Mrs Elaine Martin 2879 Vermont Avenue, Perry, OH 44081, (216) 352-2300, BS 63 Kent St Univ; Sp-Lang Path, Painesville Twsp Sch Syst, **SLP**

Upchurch, Mrs Angela G C 151 Central Avenue, Los Gatos, CA 95030, (415) 793-1141, MA 76 San Jose St Univ; Prin, Fremont USD, **SLP**

Upchurch, Mrs Carla Blakley 14131 Prestonwood First Dr, Houston, TX 77070, (713) 469-0850, BS 76 Stephen F Austin St Univ; MS 77 Univ of North TX; Sp/Lang Path, Cypress Fairbanks ISD, **SLP**

Upchurch, Naida S Speech And Hearing Services, Murdoch Center, Butner, NC 27509, (919) 575-7529, BS 75 PA St Univ - Univ Park; MS 78 PA St Univ - Univ Park; 78–Aud, Murdoch Center, **A**

Upchurch, Mrs Pamela H 15 Springdale Road, Carrollton, GA 30117, (404) 832-6314, ME 87 West GA Coll

Upchurch, Tamara A Lantern Lane Elementary, 3323 Mission Valley Drive, Missouri City, TX 77459, (713) 437-1988, BA 72 Northwestern St Univ; MA 73 Northwestern St Univ; Sp-Lang Path, Ft Bend ISD, **SLP**

Updike, Mrs Suzanne Scott 3472 Oyster Bay Avenue, Davis, CA 95616-5606, (916) 753-9019, BA 73 Univ of CA - Los Angeles; BA 73 Univ of CA - Los Angeles; MA 79 CA St Univ - Fresno; Sp/Lang Path, Yolo Co Sch, **SLP**

Uppinghouse, Karen Marie West 2516 Lacrosse, Spokane, WA 99205, BA 79 Eastern WA Univ; MS 84 Eastern WA Univ; **SLP**

Upshaw, Helen P 3211 Country Walk Drive, Powder Springs, GA 30073, (404) 942-2443, **SLP**

Uptmor, Eileen M 2988 Warm Springs Road, Cottage, Glen Ellen, CA 95442-9704, (707) 938-9224, BA 84 CA St Univ - Chico; MA 87 Univ of the Pacific; SLP, Sonoma Dev Ctr, **SLP**

Upton, Mrs Beth M 2671 East Ridgewood Circle, Zanesville, OH 43701-1611, (614) 454-5453, BS 77 Bowling Green St Univ; MA 80 Bowling Green St Univ; Mgr-Dept SLP and Aud, Good Samaritan Medical Center, **SLP ACE**

Upton, Jane Duncan 1379 N Carolina N E, Washington, DC 20002, (504) 766-6113, OM 85 LA St Univ - N O Medical Ctr; **SLP**

Upton, Mrs Patricia S 3242 Parkhill Drive, Cincinnati, OH 45248, (513) 931-5441, BS 67 Univ of Cincinnati; MA 80 Univ of Cincinnati; Tchr, Green Hills-Forest Pk Sch, **SLP**

Uranga, Jimena B 2930 Day Avenue #106, Miami, FL 33133-5261, (305) 944-8378, BA 85 Univ of Denver; MA 87 Univ of FL; **A**

Urban, Dr Beth J Childrens Hearing & Speech Center, 111 Michigan Avenue NW, Washington, DC 20010, (202) 745-5600, BA 58 AZ St Univ; MA 63 Univ of MD - College Park; PH 68 (NS) Univ of MD - College Park; 85–Dir of Aud Svcs, Childrens Hosp Nat Medical Cen, **A**

Urbanc, Rebecca A 510 Jenkran Street #4, Morrison, IL 61270, **SLP**

Urbanczyk, Amanda Elizabeth 5907 Eckhert #404, San Antonio, TX 78240, (512) 342-0729, MS 88 Southwest TX St Univ

Urbanek, Mrs Elaine Diak 69 Frances Lane, Chicago Heights, IL 60411, (312) 754-4680, BA 73 Coll of Saint Francis; MA 74 Univ of IL - Urbana; **SLP**

Urbanski, Janice Dempster 139 Willow Lane, Scotia, NY 12302, (518) 374-6617, BS 81 SUNY - Coll at Geneseo; MS 82 Ithaca Coll; Sp-Lang Path, Burnt Hills Ballston Lake Ctrl, **SLP**

Urban-Wessinger, Cheryl 86 Duanesburg Road, Schenectady, NY 12306, (518) 482-3331, **SLP**

Urbina, Mariana Consuelo 220 Pelham Road #5C, New Rochelle, NY 10802, (212) 579-5693, MS 80 Columbia Univ Teachers Coll; Aud, New York Med Coll-Lincoln Aff, **SLP A ACE**

Urbistondo, Vincente J Nueva Street #1662, Santurce, PR 00909, (809) 781-3055, BS 83 Univ of PR - Rio Piedras; MS 87 Univ of PR - San Juan; Aud, Audifonos Audio Centro

Urborg, Anita M 701 West Indiana, Urbana, IL 61801, (217) 356-9176, MS 84 Univ of IL - Urbana; Sp-Lang Path, Dev Services Center, **SLP**

Urcuioli, Nancy Jean 65 Woodbridge Avenue, Chicopee, MA 01022, BS 81 Univ of NH; MA 85 Univ of CT; **A**

Uren, Julie A 445 Sullivan Lane #102, Sparks, NV 89431, (702) 789-3268, BS 86 Univ of NV - Reno; MS 87 Univ of NV - Reno

Uribe, Judy 1708 East Teague, Fresno, CA 93710, (209) 221-8272, BA 74 CA St Univ - Fresno; MA 76 CA St Univ - Fresno; 88–Sp-Lang Path, Fresno USD, **SLP**

Urig, Debbie 2623 Via Caballero, Del Norte, Santa Fe, NM 87505, (505) 471-8339, BA 76 Univ of Northern CO; MS 78 Univ of NM; Sp-Lang Path, **SLP**

Urioste, Karen J 47 Oak Street, Westport, CT 06880, (203) 384-8681, BS 67 Bucknell Univ; MS 79 James Madison Univ; Sp-Lang Path, Private Practice, **SLP**

Urreiztieta, Mrs Melissa Ann 1101 East Hedrick Drive, Tucson, AZ 85719, (602) 622-7857, BS 83 Univ of AZ; MS 85 Northern AZ Univ; 86–Sp-Lang Path, Tucson USD #1, **SLP**

Urrutia, Deborah Jean 95 East Bellaire, Fresno, CA 93704, (209) 233-8404, **SLP**

Ursel, David 2020 River Reach Drive, Apt #160, Naples, FL 33942, (813) 643-4680, BA 85 Univ of FL; ME 87 Univ of FL; 87–Sp-Lang Path, Collier County PS, **SLP**

Urso, Mrs Patricia A 33 Gilbert Place, West Orange, NJ 07052, (201) 736-3864, BA 64 Montclair St Coll; MA 69 Montclair St Coll; Sp/Lang Path, Montclair Bd of Ed, **SLP**

Uruski, Kathleen A 641 Morningside, Topeka, KS 66604, **A**

Uryase, Deborah 887 Hanover Street, Meriden, CT 06450, (203) 284-2880, MA 76 Univ of Chicago; MA 85 Univ of CT; PH 88 (Sp-Lang Path) Univ of CT; 87–Sp-Lang Path, The Gaylord Hosp, **SLP**

Uschold, Mrs Claudia Joan 111 London Road, Webster, NY 14580, (716) 266-3239, 88–Sp-Lang Path, Webster Central Sch Dist, **SLP**

Uschold, Mrs Kathie H 1104 Dorset Drive, West Chester, PA 19382, (215) 793-1805, BS 63 SUNY - Coll at Geneseo; MA 67 SUNY - Center at Buffalo; Educational Consultant, Tatnall Preschool, **SLP**

Usdan, Mrs Linda K 1475 Eastridge, Memphis, TN 38119, (901) 754-0567, BA 67 Tulane Univ; MS 69 Tulane Univ; **SLP**

Ushycky, Irene 14 Ridgevale Drive, Toronto, ON, Canada M6A 1K8, (416) 598-6100, OM 76 Univ of Toronto - Ontario; 77–Sp-Lang Path, The Hosp for Sick Children, **SLP**

Usiondek-Benjamin, Mrs Anne Marie Route 3 Box 264, Cambridge, MD 21613, (301) 228-4950, BA 76 Loyola Coll; MS 79 Loyola Coll; Sp-Lang Path, Dorchester County Pub Schools, **SLP**

Usner, Jean M 26896 Summerdale Drive, Southfield, MI 48034, (313) 356-6386, MA 86 Eastern MI Univ

Usrey, Mrs Ruth S 108 Wisteria Circle, Haughton, LA 71037, BS 70 Northwestern St Univ; MA 81 Northwestern St Univ; Sp-Lang Path, Webster Parish Sch Bd, **SLP**

Usrey, Tamara Lynn 4601 Brentwood Avenue #B, Independence, MO 64055, (816) 478-4040, BS 84 Univ of NE - Lincoln; MS 86 CO St Univ; **A**

Ussery, Loyd E 183 Sunset Drive, North Little Rock, AR 72118-2764, (501) 562-9310, Jones Volvo, **A**

Ustik, Gary 96 North Crescent Drive, Hermitage, PA 16148, (412) 347-0853, BS 80 Clarion St Coll; MS 84 Clarion Univ of PA; Asst Prof of SLP & Aud, Clarion Univ of PA, **SLP ACE**

Utain, Sharon Beth 1276 Mettler Road, Huntingdon Valley, PA 19006, (215) 539-8550, BS 84 PA St Univ - Univ Park; MA 86 Temple Univ; 87–Sp-Lang Path, M C Intermediate Unit, **SLP**

Uth, Deedra J S 3264 Chalfant Road, Shaker Heights, OH 44120, (216) 751-9794, BS 76 Ithaca Coll; MS 78 Emory Univ; Sp-Lang Path, Private Practice, **SLP**

Uthus, Megg Ann Searing Route, Sidney, MT 59270, (701) 839-7731, **A**

Utrup, Mary E P O Box 700, Tijeras, NM 87059, **SLP**

Utsumi, Mrs Patricia Jan 25542 Soto Road #9, Hayward, CA 94544, (415) 784-2000, BS 76 CA St Univ - Hayward; MS 79 San Francisco St Univ; Sp-Lang Path, Hayward USD, **SLP**

Utt, Dr Harold A, Jr Dept Of Com Dis, Uniov Of Central Florida, Orlando, FL 32816, (305) 275-2121, Asst Prof, U of Cewntral FL, **A**

Uttech, Shawn Lee 5017 Sundstein Road, Eagle River, WI 54521, (715) 362-7676, BA 71 San Diego St Univ; MA 72 Univ of WI - Milwaukee; SLP, Rhinelander School District, **SLP**

Utter, Julia 5412 Winthrop, Indianapolis, IN 46220, (317) 736-3399, BA 74 IN Univ - Bloomington; MA 84 Butler Univ; 87–Sp-Lang Path, Johnson County Mem Hosp, **SLP**

Uvodic, Kathleen T 5235 Glen Ridge #2308, San Antonio, TX 78229, (312) 352-1513, BS 74 Univ of IL - Urbana; MS 75 Univ of IL - Urbana; Sp-Lang Path, Lombard Pub Sch Dist 44, **SLP**

Uyehara-Isono, June M Audiological Cons & Serv, 1380 Lusitana, Suite 209, Honolulu, HI 96813, (808) 524-1432, BS 74 Univ of HI - Manoa; MS 77 Purdue Univ - West Lafayette; Aud, Aud Consult & Serv, **A**

Uyenoyama, Mrs Jayne Hayden 19 Ocean View Avenue, Cotuit, MA 02635, (508) 548-0411, BA 62 Univ of MA - Amherst; ME 64 Boston Univ; Sp-Lang Path, Vistng Nurse Assn, **SLP**

Uyesaka, Mrs Linda S L 24 Lalita Lane, Santa Barbara, CA 93105, (805) 682-3641, BA 72 San Diego St Univ; MA 74 San Diego St Univ; **SLP**

Uzdawinis, Dianne C 2745 Tramway Circle N E, Albuquerque, NM 87122, (505) 299-7870, BA 74 SUNY - Center at Buffalo; MA 76 SUNY - Center at Buffalo; Sp-Lang Path, InSpeech Inc, **SLP**

Uznis, Judith C 23901 Fordson, Dearborn, MI 48124, (313) 494-5727, BA 69 Central MI Univ; MA 76 Wayne St Univ; SLP, Chldn Hosp of MI, **SLP**

V

Vaccariello, Mrs Carol M 723 Trotter Lane, Berea, OH 44017, (216) 243-0076, BA 59 Baldwin-Wallace Coll; MA 61 OH Univ - Athens; Sp-Lang Path, Private Practice, **SLP**

Vaccaro, Nancy Louise 404 Windjammer Circle, Chula Vista, CA 92010, (619) 274-1191, BS 76 San Diego St Univ; MS 83 Chapman Coll; **SLP**

Vacek, Mrs Kathleen D 917 Aster Avenue, Newark, DE 19711, (302) 731-0575, BS 77 Purdue Univ - West Lafayette; MS 79 Purdue Univ - West Lafayette; 82–Sp-Lang Path, Private Practice, **SLP**

Vacel, Marilyn 6270 Greenwood Parway #505, Sagamore Hills, OH 44067, (216) 662-7455, BS 74 Kent St Univ; MA 76 Cleveland St Univ; Sp-Lang Path, Maple Heights City Schools, **SLP**

Vachal, Melody Ann 411 2nd Avenue N E, St Cloud, MN 56304, (612) 259-4414, BA 85 Univ of ND; MS 86 Univ of ND; 88–Sp-Lang Path, St Cloud Pub Schools, **SLP**

Vadakin, Cheryl Ann 68-A Marginal, Boston, MA 02128, (617) 561-3177, BS 85 Bowling Green St Univ; MS 86 Lamar Univ; **SLP**

Vadopalas, Mrs Patricia J 829 Northampton, Palo Alto, CA 94303, (408) 286-3807, BA 53 San Jose St Univ; MA 75 San Jose St Univ; Sp-Lang Path, Franklin-McKinley Sch Dist, **SLP**

Vahcic-Pierce, Barbara J 1999 Berger Avenue, Stow, OH 44224, (216) 688-6468, **SLP**

Vahling, Theresa Ann 1400-5 West Calhoun, Macomb, IL 61455, (309) 833-2871, BS 85 Eastern IL Univ; MS 86 Eastern IL Univ; 87–Sp-Lang Path, Macomb District #185, **SLP**

Vai, Donna G 11171 N W 39th Court, Coral Springs, FL 33065, (618) 277-0976, BS 74 Southern IL Univ -Carbondale; MS 76 Southern IL Univ -Carbondale; **SLP**

Vail, Mrs Beth H 9 Elysian Drive, Andover, MA 01810, (805) 957-4633, BA 54 Univ of MI - Ann Arbor; ME 68 Univ of Cincinnati; Sp-Lang Path & Aud Coord, Dracut Pub Sch, **SLP**

Vail, Florence Cameron 1511 Catalpa Street, Goldsboro, NC 27530, (919) 559-5371, BA 75 Univ of MD - College Park; MA 81 Univ of CO - Boulder; Clinic Mgr, Caswell Center, **SLP ACE**

Vail, Mrs Pamela Arnold 3555 Mark Twain Circle, Bethlehem, PA 18017, BS 74 Millersville Univ of PA; MA 76 Bucknell Univ; MS 79 Bloomsburg Univ of PA; Sp-Lang Path, Phillipsburg Pub Sch, **SLP**

Vaillancourt, Mrs Nyola R 1081 Lowell Road, Groton, MA 01450, (617) 251-4981, BS 62 Boston Univ; ME 65 Boston Univ; Sp-Lang Path, Chelmsford Sch Dept, **SLP**

Vaillancourt, Patricia Marie 25 Russell Street, Hull, MA 02045, (617) 925-3784, BS 84 Univ of MA - Amherst; MA 86 MI St Univ; **A**

Vair, Lauri R 1061 Deleone Drive, Kent, OH 44240, (216) 678-9064, BS 83 Kent St Univ; MA 83 Kent St Univ; PH (Special Education) Kent St Univ; 87–Sp-Lang Path, Stow Learning Center, **SLP**

Vajen, Mrs Mary Jane 1030 Woodlane Drive N E, Lancaster, OH 43130, (614) 687-8150, BS 78 Bowling Green St Univ; MA 80 OH Univ - Athens; **SLP**

Vakos, Toni L Oakland Hearing Service, 3324 Webster Street, Oakland, CA 94609, (415) 525-7145, BA 74 Univ of WI - Madison; MA 76 Univ of WA; Aud, Temporary Audiologic Services, **A**

Valaitis, Carol S 4691 Cardamon Lane, Rockford, IL 61111, **SLP**

Valarezo, Mrs Toni Thompson 1300 West 6th Street, Suite 1, San Pedro, CA 90732, (213) 831-8449, BS 80 Univ of WY; MS 83 Univ of WY; Aud, Audio-Diagnostics, **A**

Valbracht, Janice R 50 Parklane, Clinton, IL 61727, **SLP**

Valcarenghi, Tina 4419 Van Nuys Boulevard, Suite #205, Sherman Oaks, CA 91403, (818) 905-0243, BA 74 Loma Linda Univ - Riverside; MS 79 Loma Linda Univ - Riverside; Pres, Therapeutic Consult Serv, **SLP**

Valdes, Diane Theresa 64-61 84th Place, Middle Village, NY 11379, (212) 268-6280, BA 79 CUNY - Queens Coll; MA 83 CUNY - Queens Coll; Sp-Lang Path, The Summit Schl Inc, **SLP**

Valdez, Alfred J 5600 Domingo N E, Albuquerque, NM 87108, (505) 268-4592, OB 72 Univ of NM; MS 74 Univ of NM; Project Director, Albuquerque Area Ind Hlth Bd, **SLP**

Valdez, Dwight R 3609 Redondo Drive, Lafayette, IN 47905, (317) 494-3789, BS 80 Andrews Univ; MA 82 MI St Univ; Tchr, Purdue Univ, **A**

Valdez, Mrs Elizabeth S 2509 Highmont, Garland, TX 75041, (214) 271-8280, BA 82 Oral Roberts Univ; MS 87 Univ of TX - Dallas

Valdez, Geneva Nellie 895 Carriage Drive, Solvang, CA 93463, (805) 688-9846, BA 84 Univ of CA - Santa Barbara; MA 86 Univ of CA - Santa Barbara; SLP, Lompoc USD, **SLP**

Valenta, Kathleen Orr Inter-Communication Services/Ear Lab, 12-04 Saddle River Road, Fair Lawn, NJ 07410, (201) 796-3131, BA 66 Rutger's St Univ - Douglas Coll; MS 71 William Paterson Coll; 85–Owner, Inter-Communication Services/Ear Lab, **SLP A**

Valente, Elizabeth Helen 43 Georgia Street, Valley Stream, NY 11580, BA 84 CUNY - Queens Coll; MA 86 CUNY - Queens Coll; 87–Aud, Brooklyn VA Med Ctr, **A**

Valente, Michael Dept Of Otolaryngology, WA Univ School Of Medicine, 517 South Eucid Street, St Louis, MO 63110, BS 71 Adelphi Univ; MS 73 Adelphi Univ; PH 75 (NS) Univ of IL - Urbana; Aud, WA Univ Sch of Medicine, **A**

Valentik, Kathleen 367 Pelham Road, Philadelphia, PA 19119, (215) 549-4208, BS 69 Central MO St Univ; MA 74 Temple Univ; Dir Sp/Lang Path, Commun Rehab Inc, **SLP**

Valentine, Mrs Barbara J 15432 Canary, Grand Haven, MI 49417, (616) 725-7100, BA 77 Central MI Univ; MA 79 Central MI Univ; 79–Sp-Lang Path, Muskegon Pub Sch, **SLP**

Valentine, Mrs Courtney H 2404 Montebello Terrace, Baltimore, MD 21214, (301) 426-7128, BS 41 Morgan St Univ; MA 55 NY Univ; **SLP LM**

Valentine, Cynthia Birdsall 395 Pequot Avenue #2, New London, CT 06320, (203) 447-0301, BA 79 Coll of William & Mary; ME 85 Univ of VA - Charlottesville; 86–Sp-Lang Path, Seaside Ctr, **SLP**

Valentine, Mrs Melinda S 12832 Noel Road #1029, Dallas, TX 75230, (214) 358-5261, BS 76 OK St Univ; MS 77 Southern Methodist Univ; 82–Sp-Lang Path, Dallas Easter Seal Soc, **SLP**

Valentine, Susan Mairne 22 Brookmont Drive, Malvern, PA 19355, (215) 964-3000, MS 86 Rutgers St Univ - Newark; **SLP**

Valentino, Patricia A 29 Krystal Drive, Somers, NY 10589, BS 64 Emerson Coll; MA 68 Columbia Univ Teachers Coll; Placement Officer, NYC Bd of Ed-Spec Services Ut, **SLP**

Valent-Matsick, Mrs Nancy Lee Passer Road Box 242B, Coopersburg, PA 18036, (215) 282-2128, BS 77 WV Univ; MS 81 Clarion Univ of PA; Sp-Lang Path, Private Practice, **SLP**

Valenza, Beth 2773 Windswept Drive #305, Lantana, FL 32462, (407) 642-0059, BA 78 Loyola Coll; MS 80 Loyola Coll; Sp-Lang Path, Palm Beach Co PS, **SLP**

Valenza, Gary R Mednet, 18599 Lakeshore Boulevard, Cleveland, OH 44119, (216) 383-5913, BA 71 IN Univ - Bloomington; MA 77 Cleveland St Univ; Head Aud Serv, Mednet, **A**

Valeo-Gahn, Joanne 19 Virginia Avenue, Poughkeepsie, NY 12601, (914) 473-2124, BA 73 SUNY - Coll at Oneonta; MA 77 Hofstra Univ; Program Coordinator, Punman Assoc Retarded Chldn, **SLP**

Valerio, Dr Michael W VA Medical Center, Audiology (126), 800 Irving Avenue, Syracuse, NY 13210, (315) 476-7461, BA 66 SUNY - Coll at Geneseo; MA 68 SUNY - Coll at Geneseo; PH 79 (NS) Syracuse Univ; Aud, VA, **A**

Valero, Greg Martin 5335 Robinwood Road, Bonita, CA 92002, (619) 425-9600, BA San Diego St Univ; MA 85 San Diego St Univ; **SLP**

Valite-Andersen, Arlinda E 1641 Hakuaina Place, Honolulu, HI 96819, (808) 696-3531, BS 74 Eastern MI Univ; MA 75 Eastern MI Univ; Spec Educ Tchr, Dept of Educ, **SLP**

Valji, Susanna K 6341 Hartley Drive, La Jolla, CA 92037, (415) 826-2605, BA 78 Harvard Univ; MA 80 Northwestern Univ; **SLP**

Vallandingham, Dr Richard R 11111 West 59th Terrace, Shawnee, KS 66203, (913) 268-4101, BS 75 OK St Univ; MA 77 Univ of Tulsa; PH 82 (Rehab & Counseling) Univ of AZ; Aud, Aud/Couns Serv, **A**

Valle, Kathleen T 5350 Driftwood Court, Lisle, IL 60532, (312) 964-9420, BA 63 Saint Mary-of-the-Woods Coll; MA 66 IN Univ - Bloomington; Sp-Lang Path, Comm Ut Sch Dist 202, **SLP**

Valles, Luciano, Jr 515 South Sugar Road #20, Edinburg, TX 78539, (512) 381-3587, MS 83 TX Christian Univ; Asst Prof, Pan American Univ, **SLP**

Valletutti, Dr Peter James 2500 West North Avenue, Baltimore, MD 21216, (301) 383-7421, BA 51 CUNY - Brooklyn Coll; MA 54 CUNY - Brooklyn Coll; ED 66 (NS) Columbia Univ Teachers Coll; Chairperson/Dept Special Educ, Coppin State College, **SLP**

Vallier, Dr Fred J 2700 Pierce Avenue, Ames, IA 50010, (515) 294-5572, BA 59 Univ of the Pacific; MA 61 Univ of the Pacific; PH 77 (Sp-Lang Path) Univ of CO - Boulder; Sp-Lang Path, Iowa State University, **SLP**

Vallino, Dr Linda D The Children's Hospital-Boston, Department Otolaryngology & Communication Disorders, Boston, MA 02115, (617) 735-6467, BS 77 PA St Univ - Univ Park; MA 80 Univ of Pittsburgh - Pittsburgh; PH 87 (Sp-Lang Path/Aud) Univ of Pittsburgh - Pittsburgh; 88–Sp-Lang Path/Aud, The Children's Hosp-Boston, **SLP A**

Vallon, Jerome M 150 Overlook Avenue, Peekskill, NY 10566, (914) 245-6129, BA 51 Long Island U - Brooklyn Ctr; MA 52 NY Univ; Supvr-Spec Educ, Lakeland Sch, **SLP F**

Valot, Linda S 146 Birch Bend, Coventry, CT 06238, (203) 742-6174, BS 83 Bowling Green St Univ; MA 87 Kent St Univ; **SLP**

Valvezan, Rose N 209-39 23rd Avenue #4C, Bayside, NY 11360, (718) 224-0699, BA 79 NY Univ; MS 82 Adelphi Univ; Aud, Long Island Jewish Hosp, **A**

Vamos, Kathleen Marie 24289 Reservation Line, Curtice, OH 43412, (419) 885-1444, BS 82 Marquette Univ; MS 83 Case Western Reserve Univ; 88–Sp-Lang Path, The Toledo Hosp, **SLP**

Vanagas-Cote, Susan A P O Box 564, Porcupine, ON, Canada P0N 1C0, (705) 235-3985, BS 79 Northern MI Univ; MA 82 Univ of MN - Minneap-St Paul; Sp/Lang Path, Northern Speech-Lang Services, **SLP**

Van Aman, Mrs Debra E 246 Churchill Street, Northfield, IL 60093-3220, (312) 441-6507, BA 78 IN Univ - Bloomington; ME 79 IN Univ - Bloomington; Sp-Lang Path, Winnetka Sch Dist #36, **SLP**

Van Amburgh, Ruth C Box 29, Wallkill, NY 12589, **SLP**

Van Atta, Mrs Deborah W 493 Belvedere Street, San Francisco, CA 94117, (415) 759-0620, MS 87 San Francisco St Univ; 87–Sp-Lang Path, InSpeech Inc, **SLP**

Van Bebber, Sally J 1215 North Edison, Stockton, CA 95203, MS 63 Univ of OR; Tchr, Tracy Elem Sch Dist, **SLP**

Van Beek, Mrs Cynthia A 2915 Lynwood Drive, Billings, MT 59102, (406) 252-3927, BA 76 Univ of MI - Ann Arbor; MA 83 Central MI Univ; Sp-Lang Path, Billings Sch Dist #2, **SLP**

Van Bemmel, Charlotte 10 Danbury Court, Suffern, NY 10901-8026, (914) 638-1606, BS 73 Mercy Coll; MS 75 William Paterson Coll; Sp-Lang Path, ARC Adlt Day Treatment Cen, **SLP**

Van Buren, Annette Duckert 29 West 370 Grove Avenue, West Chicago, IL 60185, (312) 980-0726, BS 85 Univ of WI - Milwaukee; MS 86 Marquette Univ; **SLP**

Van Buren, Cynthia A 2051 West Lakeview Drive, Provo, UT 84604, (801) 225-1409, BS 80 Brigham Young Univ; MS 81 Brigham Young Univ; Sp-Lang Path, Pediatric Therap Servcs, **SLP**

Van Buskirk, Karen Lynn 3249-L Arrowhead Circle, Fairfax, VA 22030, (202) 745-5600, BS 83 Elmira Coll; MS 85 Boston Univ; 88–Sp-Lang Path, Children's Hosp Natl Med Ctr, **SLP**

Vancaeseele-Pontieri, Mrs Martha L P O Box 168, Bayport, NY 11705, (516) 244-2281, BA 73 SUNY - Coll at Plattsburgh; MS 78 Hofstra Univ; SLP, Connetquot Central Schools, **SLP**

Van Campen, Luann Elizabeth 11422 Lakeshore Drive East, Carmel, IN 46032, (317) 846-9262, BS 84 Miami Univ - Oxford; MS 86 Purdue Univ - West Lafayette; 86

Vance, Anne D 201 Amberwood Drive, Jamestown, NC 27282, (919) 378-9105, BA 71 Univ of NC - Greensboro; ME 72 Univ of NC - Greensboro; SLP, Greensboro City Schs, **SLP**

Vance, Bette Mae 6107 Galleon Way, Tampa, FL 33615, (813) 872-4530, BS 54 IN Univ - Bloomington; MS 57 IN Univ - Bloomington; Sp/Lang Path, Hillsborough Co Sch Syst, **SLP ACE**

Vance, Cynthia L 412 Red River Trail #2040, Irving, TX 75063, (214) 751-1700, BS 80 LA St Univ - Baton Rouge; MA 84 LA St Univ - Baton Rouge; 87–Sp-Lang Path, Bruel & Kjaer Instruments Inc, **SLP**

Vance, Henrietta Vernell 517 West 9th, Pine Bluff, AR 71601, (301) 628-5111, BS 78 Univ of AR - Pine Bluff; OM 85 Univ of Central AR; **SLP**

Vance, Margaret Pojman 13931 Oak Brook Drive #102, North Royalton, OH 44133, (216) 237-2604, BS 77 John Carroll Univ; MA 79 Kent St Univ; Sp-Lang Path, Nordonia City Sch Sys, **SLP**

Vance, Michelle Chamberlai 1301 Shelton Manor #B, Lehi, UT 84043, (801) 768-4353, BS 85 Univ of UT; OM 86 Brigham Young Univ; **SLP**

Vance, Mrs Rebecca Butler 5755 East River Road #119, Tucson, AZ 85715, (602) 887-5500, BA 81 Univ of AZ; MS 83 Univ of AZ; Sp-Lang Path, Amphitheatre School District, **SLP**

Vancey, Mrs Gail Richerson 5004 West Franklin Street, Richmond, VA 23226, (804) 924-8242, BA 73 Univ of AL-Tuscaloosa; MS 74 Marquette Univ; Sp-Lang Path, Medical College Virginia, **SLP**

Van Cleave, Mary L 9807 North Lamplighter Ln, Mequon, WI 53092, BS 71 Univ of WI - Madison; MS 72 Univ of WI - Madison; Audiologist, Private Practice, **A**

Van Coppenolle, Mrs Sylvia S 3409 Hackberry, Brownsville, TX 78521, (512) 546-3101, BS 78 Univ of TX - Austin; MA 81 Univ of TX - Austin; Sp-Lang Path, Brownsville ISD, **SLP**

Vancura, Mrs Rebecca Rose 1725 Van Buren Circle, Whitehall, PA 18052, (215) 799-4239, BS 82 PA St Univ - Univ Park; MS 83 Ithaca Coll; Pro Assoc, InSpeech Inc, **SLP**

Vandam, Mrs Vicki A M 1212 South Heron Street, Sebring Hills, FL 33870, (813) 382-1121, BS 79 Central MI Univ; MA 81 Central MI Univ; Sp-Lang Path, Highlands Co Sch Dist, **SLP**

Vandament, Mrs Vickie Sue 201 Gemini, Osborne, KS 67473, (913) 346-2657, BS 80 Fort Hays St Univ; MS 81 Fort Hays St Univ; SLP, Smith Co Pub Sch

Van De Boe, Caryl Ann 50 Ellers Drive, Chatham, NJ 07928, (201) 635-1508, BS 76 West Chester St Coll; OM 81 Hahneman Medical Coll; Aud, Ctr for Commun Dis, **A**

Vandecar, Mrs Susan E W 7708 24th Avenue West, Bradenton, FL 33529, (813) 955-8197, BS 75 Univ of IA; MA 77 Univ of NE - Lincoln; SLP, Sarasota County Schools, **SLP**

Vandeguchte, Dr Marten Dept Communication Arts & Sci, Calvin College, Grand Rapids, MI 49506, (616) 957-6284, BA 53 Calvin Coll; ME 54 Wayne St Univ; PH 69 (Sp Path) MI St Univ; Prof, Calvin Coll, **SLP**

Van Deinse, Steven Dale 4630 Tamarack Blvd #A9, Columbus, OH 43229, (614) 251-3740, BS 84 Univ of AZ; MA 86 Univ of IL - Urbana; SLP, St Anthony Med Cntr, **SLP**

Van Demark, Dr Ann A Special Tree Incorporated, 39010 Wabash, Romulus, MI 48197, (313) 942-1760, BA 59 Univ of NE - Omaha; MA 62 Univ of IA; PH 64 (Sp-Lang Path) IN Univ - Bloomington; 88–Dir, SpecialTree Inc, **SLP**

Van Demark, Dr D R Department Of Otolaryngology, University Hospital, Iowa City, IA 52242, (319) 356-2293, BA 58 Hiram Coll; MA 62 Univ of IA; PH 62 (NS) Univ of IA; Prof & Coord Cleft Palate Cl, Dept of Otol U Hosp, **SLP F**

Van Den Heuvel, Denise M 1208 7th Street, Stevens Point, WI 54481, (715) 341-2993, **SLP**

Van Den Hoven, Mrs Monica Heffernan 1166 Windermere Road, Windsor, ON, Canada N8Y 3E6, (519) 252-7281, MA 87 Wayne St Univ; **SLP**

VanDerBeek, Mrs Marcia Baird 1032 Washington Avenue, Old Tappan, NJ 07675, (201) 664-7717, BA 68 Elmira Coll; ME 70 Univ of VA - Charlottesville; Sp-Lang Path, Private Practice, **SLP**

Vanderbeek, Valerie Lanoa 3306 North Ohara Drive, Macon, GA 31206, (912) 788-5013, BS 76 FL St Univ; BS 81 FL St Univ; MS 84 FL St Univ; Aud, Middle Georgia Reg Ed Serv Agy, **A**

Vanderbrook, Mrs Lisa Pirrone 153 Jenell Drive, Grand Island, NY 14072, (716) 837-2441, BS 77 SUNY - Coll at Fredonia; MS 86 Western OR St Coll; 86–Sp-Lang Path, Lang Dev Prog of W NY, **SLP**

Van Der Heide, Mrs Joan Manze 401 N E 37th Street, Boca Raton, FL 33431, (305) 583-7383, BS 77 Ithaca Coll; MS 88 Nova Univ; 87–Sp-Lang Path, Pediatric Therapy Associates

Van Der Heiden, Edward William 2807 South Main Street, Burlington, IA 52601, (319) 753-3551, BS 73 Univ of WI - Oshkosh; MS 75 Univ of WI - Stevens Point; Dir Aud & Neuro Vestibular Labs, Burlington Med Cen, **A**

Vanderheiden, Dr Gregg C Trace Research And Dev Center, University Of Wisconsin, 1500 Highland Avenue, Madison, WI 53705, (608) 262-6966, BS 72 Univ of WI - Madison; MS 74 Univ of WI - Madison; PH 84 (Technology in Comm Rehab & Child Dev) Univ of WI - Madison; Director, University of Wisconsin

Vanderheyden, Denise 75 Fidler Green Road, London, ON, Canada N6H 4S8, (519) 432-2257, BS 84 Univ of Western Ontario; OM 86 Univ of Western Ontario

Vanderhoff, Joan H 2959 Mt Curve, Altadena, CA 91001, (818) 397-5458, BS 70 SUNY - Coll at Geneseo; MS 71 SUNY - Coll at Geneseo; 82–Sp-Lang Path, Huntington Mem Hosp, **SLP**

Van De Riet, Mrs Mary Margaret 740 Wickerleigh Terrace, Fenton, MO 63026, (314) 343-1210, BA 72 Fontbonne Coll; MA 73 Saint Louis Univ; **SLP**

Vander Laan, Carolin H 6 Fordham Road, West Newton, MA 02165, BA 60 Univ of Denver; MA 64 Univ of Denver; 77–Sp/Lang Path, Norwood Pub Sch, **SLP**

Vanderlip, Mrs Nancy A 4443 East 58th Place, Tulsa, OK 74135, (918) 299-4411, BA 75 Univ of MO - Columbia; MA 76 Wichita St Univ; Sp-Lang Path, Jenks Public Schools, **SLP**

Vanderpan, Lisa Calkins P O Box 116, Bridger, MT 59014-0116, (406) 662-3922, BS 81 WA St Univ; MS 85 Eastern WA Univ; Sp-Lang Path, Big Country Educational Coop, **SLP**

Vander-Ploeg, James 422 West G Street, Battle Ground, WA 98604, (406) 296-2131, BS 74 Western MI Univ; MA 75 Western MI Univ; Sp-Lang Path, Lincoln Co High School, **SLP ACE**

Vanderster, Diane S 2350 Broadway #1233, New York, NY 10024-3202, (914) 592-7555, BS 78 Emerson Coll; MS 80 Columbia Univ Teachers Coll; Sp-Lang Path, Blythedale Chld Hosp, **SLP**

Vander Veen, Mrs Daphnne Moore 8502 Saratoga Way, Stockton, CA 95209, (707) 257-8622, BA 82 CA St Univ - Stanislaus; MA 84 CA St Univ - Stanislaus; **SLP**

Vander Veen, Mrs Eileen E 684 Marylane Drive, Holland, MI 49423, (616) 335-3043, BS 76 Miami Univ - Oxford; MA 79 Bowling Green St Univ; Sp-Lang Path, W Ottawa Pub Sch, **SLP**

Van Derveer, Mrs Rita H Holiday Harbour #130-B, Canandaigua, NY 14424, (716) 357-3645, BA 48 Elms Coll; ME 51; MA 64 Coll of Saint Rose; Sp/Lang Path, Wayne Finger Lakes Bd Coop Ser, **SLP**

Vander Velde, Deborah L 2203 Parker-Baits, Ann Arbor, MI 48109-2082, (313) 764-4057, MS 88 Univ of MI - Ann Arbor

Van Der Ven, Dorothy S 8036 Indian Hill Road, Manlius, NY 13104, **SLP**

Vandervliet, Cornelia R 90 Warren Street #2-A, Nutley, NJ 07110, (201) 533-5786, BA 73 Montclair St Coll; MA 74 Montclair St Coll; 78–Aud, St Barnabas Med Cen, **A**

Van Der Voort, Mrs Denise Boyle 4027 Calavo Drive, La Mesa, CA 92041, (619) 697-7448, BS 76 Univ of NH; MA 78 Memphis St Univ; **SLP**

Vandervoort, Mrs Nicole Leman 2043-C North Halsted, Chicago, IL 60614, (312) 266-8133, BA 63; MA 65 Univ of Montreal - Quebec; Sp-Lang Path, SHV Corp, **SLP**

Vanderwaerden, Theresa Rose 11302 Alger, Warren, MI 48093, (313) 494-9721, BA 82 MI St Univ; MA 84 MI St Univ; Sp-Lang Path, Rehabilitation Institute, **SLP**

van Deusen, Diana Jean 3305 Irving Avenue South, Minneapolis, MN 55408, (612) 624-3322, BS 79 Univ of IA; MA 82 Univ of IA; Aud, Univ of Minnesota, **A**

Van Deusen, Elaine 108 Foote Street, Barrington, RI 02806, (401) 245-0602, BS 77 Emerson Coll; MS 79 Boston Univ; Sp-Lang Path, Private Practice, **SLP**

Vandeusen, Jamie S 5012 Waterford Road, Clarkston, MI 48016, (313) 627-4981, BS 76 Eastern MI Univ; MA 77 Central MI Univ; 83–Sp/Lang Path, Brandon Pub Sch, **SLP**

Vandevander, Gary M Greenbrier Aud & Hrng Aid Serv, P O Box 808, Lewisburg, WV 24901, (304) 647-5115, BS 69 WV Univ; MS 70 WV Univ; Aud, Greenbrier Aud & Hrng Aid Serv, **A**

Van De Water, Sandra M Colorado Otolaryngology PC, 601 East Hampden #390, Englewood, CO 80110, (303) 788-6377, BA 72 SUNY - Coll at Potsdam; MS 75 Syracuse Univ; Aud, Colorado Otolaryngology PC, **A**

Van Diggelen-Cooper, Kathleen Route 1 Box 511H, Fontana, WI 53125, (414) 275-5166, BA 78 Northeastern IL Univ; MS 82 Univ of WI - Whitewater; SLP, Spec Ed Dist of McHenry Co, **SLP**

Van Doorn-Conard, Elizabeth 105 East Alabama Street, Abbeville, AL 36310, (205) 793-4788, MA 74 Univ of AL-Tuscaloosa; Aud, Warren Rollins MD Pa, **A**

Van Doren, Cynthia Johanna 7211 Garland Avenue, Takoma Park, MD 20912, (301) 493-8342, BA 82 Pacific Union Coll; MA 86 Univ of MD - College Park; 87–Sp-Lang Path, Montgomery Co PS, **SLP**

Vandrew, Mrs Karen Singiser 104 E Simpson Street, Mechanicsburg, PA 17055, (717) 691-3700, BS 83 Bloomsburg Univ of PA; MS 84 Bloomsburg Univ of PA; Director, Mechanicsburg Rehab, **SLP**

Van Drie, Mary L 164 Katherine NE, Grand Rapids, MI 49505-2674, (616) 942-1660, BS 76 Central MI Univ; MA 78 MI St Univ; 87–Aud, Comprehensive Audiological Svcs, **A**

Van Driel, Margaret Anne 23 4th Street N E, Washington, DC 20002, (703) 323-4000, BA 69 Clarke Coll; MA 77 Catholic Univ of America; 86–Sp-Lang Path, Communicare Hrng & Sp Assoc, **SLP**

Van Duivenbode, Laurie Ann 85 South Lima # C, Sierra Madre, CA 91024, (818) 355-2642, BA 84 Univ of CA - Santa Barbara; MA 86 CA St Univ - Los Angeles; **A**

Van Dusen, C Raymond Plantation Apartment 6-C, 2105 Howell Branch Road, Miatland, FL 32751, (904) 622-1811, BA 31 IN Univ - Bloomington; MA 32 Univ of MI - Ann Arbor; OD 37 (Sp-Lang Path) Univ of MI - Ann Arbor; Sp-Lang Path, Mid-Florida Physical Therapy, **SLP F LM**

Vandy, S Ermon C 7975 Riggs Road #1, Adelphi, MD 20783, (301) 445-2516, BA 70 Hendrix Coll; OM 75 Cumberland Coll of Health Sciences - Australia; 87–Sp-Lang Path, Montgomery County PS, **SLP ACE**

Van Dyke, Elizabeth Anne Porter Hospital, 2525 South Downing, Denver, CO 80210, (303) 778-5645, BS 72 CO St Univ; MS 74 CO St Univ; Aud, Porter Hosp, **SLP A**

Van Dyke, Mrs Laura Beth 12736 Auburn Avenue, Palos Heights, IL 60463, (312) 687-0900, OB 84 Governors St Univ; OM 87 Governors St Univ; 87–Sp-Lang Path, SW Cook Co Coop for Spec Educ, **SLP**

Van Dyke, Linda M 9440 East Girard #5, Denver, CO 80231, BA 76 Univ of NE - Lincoln; MA 77 Univ of Northern CO; Aud, Arapahoe Hearing Assoc Inc, **A**

Van Dyken, Mrs Eleanore 88 Jog Hill Road, Trumbull, CT 06611, MS 76 Southern CT St Univ; SLP, Town of Fairfield, **SLP**

Van Dyne, Mrs Barbara Jean 238 Camille Avenue, Alamo, CA 94507, (415) 944-0153, BS 70 OK St Univ; MA 71 KS St Univ; 86–Dir, East Bay Sp & Lang Assoc, **SLP**

Van Eman, Janis B 425 Woburn Street #47, Lexington, MA 02173, (617) 523-6050, MA 75 Univ of AR - Fayetteville; **SLP**

Van Engen, Mrs Mary L Route 1 Box 73-A, Sioux Center, IA 51250, (712) 476-5888, BA 71 Univ of IA; MA 75 Univ of IA; SLP, AEA 4, **SLP**

Van Ess, Lisa M 3500 S 74 #C-6, Fort Smith, AR 72903, (501) 452-1786, BS 86 Univ of AR - Fayetteville; MS 87 Univ of AR - Fayetteville; 87–Sp-Lang Path, Ft Smith Rehab Hosp, **SLP**

Vanessen, Susan S 7301 N W Beaver Drive #14, Johnston, IA 50131, (800) 362-2720, BS 73 Northeast MO St Univ; MA 74 Northeast MO St Univ; SLP, AEA #11, **SLP**

Van Evra, Mrs Cathleen Maria 1-43 27th Street, Fair Lawn, NJ 07410, (201) 522-2283, BA 82 OH St Univ; MA 84 OH St Univ; 87–Aud, Overlook Hosp, **A**

Van Fleet, Mrs Kathleen Brennan 5111 West Cambridge Drive, McHenry, IL 60050, (312) 546-5200, BS 79 IL St Univ - Normal; MS 81 IL St Univ - Normal; 81–Sp-Lang Path, Round Lake Area Sch 116, **SLP**

Vanfossen, Linda 2700 Reynolds Road #911, Winston-Salem, NC 27106, (919) 768-3361, BA 77 Auburn Univ - Auburn; MS 79 Auburn Univ - Auburn; Aud, Salem ENT Assoc, **A**

Van Fossen, Lucinda Twitchell 24346 Parkside Drive East, Laguna Niguel, CA 92677, (714) 730-7333, BS 77 Auburn Univ - Auburn; MS 84 Auburn Univ - Auburn; **SLP**

Vanfrank, Mrs Leslie Cohan 52 Carolin Road, Upper Montclair, NJ 07043, BA 64; MA 70 Columbia Univ Teachers Coll; Sp-Lang Path, Jefferson Sch, **SLP A**

Van Gend, Patricia Lynn 5706 Fairwood Drive #20, Salt Lake City, UT 84118, (801) 375-3014, OM 86 Brigham Young Univ; **SLP**

Van Genderen, Joanne 214 Wren Street, Scotia, NY 12302, (518) 346-6044, BA 78 SUNY - Coll at Plattsburgh; MS 84 Coll of Saint Rose; Sp-Lang Path, Schalmnont School District, **SLP**

Van Giesen, Marjorie Fleck 3916 Linden Avenue, Fort Worth, TX 76107, (817) 870-1393, BS 70 Emerson Coll; OM 71 Tulane Univ; SLP, Assoc In Sp Path Ionc, **SLP**

Vanginderen-Wakeley, Ingrid 2 Fir Drive, Danbury, CT 06811, (203) 775-4700, BA 78 Marist Coll; MS 82 Boston Univ; 87–Sp/Lang Path, Datahr Inc, **SLP**

Van Gorder-La Porta, Joanne M 6605 74th Street, Middle Village, NY 11379, (212) 750-6787, MA 85 SUNY - Center at Buffalo; Supvr of Aud, Goldwater Memorial Hosp, **A**

Vangroesbeck, Mrs Patrice L 5 New Searles Road, Nashua, NH 03062, BA 68 Plymouth St Coll; ME 81 Northeastern Univ; Sp-Lang Path, Nashua Sch Dept, **SLP**

Van Groningen, Mrs Grace 516 Barringham Lane, Modesto, CA 95350, (209) 529-8462, BA 76 CA St Univ - Stanislaus; MA 79 CA St Univ - Stanislaus; 79–Sp-Lang Path, Modesto City Schs, **SLP**

Van Haalen, Teresa G 1484 Gemini, Houston, TX 77058, (713) 420-5706, BS 69 OR St Univ; MA 73 NM St Univ; 88–Asst Prin, Goose Crk Consol Ind Sch Dist, **SLP ACE**

Van Hagey, Mrs Connie W 27373W Lakeview Drive N, Wauconda, IL 60084, (217) 526-5082, BS 68 Univ of IL - Urbana; MA 70 Univ of IL - Urbana; Sp-Lang Path, Private Practice, **SLP**

Van Ham, Mrs Diane 849 Darlington Lane, Crystal Lake, IL 60014, (815) 455-1465, BS 76 Bradley Univ; MS 77 Bradley Univ; Sp-Lang Path, Spec Educ Dist of Mc Henry Co, **SLP**

Van Hecke, Deborah P Box 250 Cluster 11, Hyde Park Estates, Santa Fe, NM 87505, (505) 988-3719, BA 75 Univ of NC - Chapel Hill; MA 79 LA St Univ - Baton Rouge; Sp-Lang Path, Martha Hardwick Sp & Lang Assoc, **SLP**

Van Heertum, Mrs Ellen E 3 Pletcher Place, Morristown, NJ 07960, (201) 584-1200, BA 63 Newark St Coll; MA 66 Newark St Coll; 78–Sp-Lang Path, Roxbury Bd of Ed, **SLP**

Van Hemert, Margaret 452 Westmont Court, Bonita, CA 92002, (619) 479-7171, BA 72 San Diego St Univ; MA 77 San Diego St Univ; Spec Ed Tchr-Commun Hndcpd, Chula Vista Cty Sch Dist, **SLP**

Van Himbergen, Lori M 523 Pine Street #210, Sheboygan Falls, WI 53085, (414) 467-8669, BS 85 Univ of WI - Stevens Point; MS 87 Univ of WI - Stevens Point; 87–Sp-Lang Path, Plymouth Joint Sch Dist, **SLP**

Vanhoenacker, Christine 33 Northumberland Road, Pittsfield, MA 01201, (413) 442-0934, BA 67 Emmanuel Coll; MS 72 Univ of VT; Sp-Lang Path, Private Practice, **SLP**

Van Hoesen-Closs, Mrs Jane 4328 Pasadena Court, Sarasota, FL 33583, (813) 922-1050, BS 70 Purdue Univ - West Lafayette; MA 75 Kent St Univ; Sp-Lang Path, Sarasota County Schools, **SLP**

Van Horn, Billy J 5549 S E Pine Street, Portland, OR 97215, ME; **SLP**

Van Horn, Mrs Janis C 4018 Summersworth Run, Fort Wayne, IN 46804, (219) 425-7463, BS 77 IN Univ - Bloomington; MA 78 IN Univ - Bloomington; Sp-Lang Path, Ft Wayne Comm Sch, **SLP**

Van Horn, Mrs Judith E 914 Rose Avenue, Piedmont, CA 94611, (415) 537-1832, MA 73 San Francisco St Univ; BA 66 Univ of the Pacific; SLP, Castro Valley USD, **SLP**

Van Horn, Mrs Linda Marie 1384 North Wedgewood, Upland, CA 91786, (714) 624-9041, MA 82 CA St Univ - Los Angeles; 86–Tchr, Claremont USD, **SLP**

Van Horn, Robert H 914 Rose Avenue, Piedmont, CA 94611, (415) 889-5064, BA 65 Univ of the Pacific; MA 73 San Francisco St Univ; Sp/Lang Path, Private Practice, **SLP**

Van Horne, Mrs Lisa J 715 North 130th, Apartment A-403, Seattle, WA 98133, (206) 363-7618, BA 85 Luther Coll; MS 87 CO St Univ

Van Hout, Mary Ellen Hawthorne Beach, Rural 2 Box 245, Westfield, NY 14787, (716) 664-7212, BS 73 Clarion Univ of PA; ME 77 Clarion Univ of PA; SLP, Mary Ellen Van Hout, **SLP**

Vanhouten, Mrs Eleanor F 28 Arbolado, La Selva Beach, CA 95076, (408) 684-1861, BA 53 9687; MA 72 9687; Sp/Lang Path, Franklin-McKinley Sd, **SLP**

Van Huss, Margaret C 600 Chestnut Avenue, Waynesboro, VA 22980, (703) 949-7017, **SLP**

Vanier-Garcia, Jeannine M 1400 South Yale, Santa Maria, CA 93454, (805) 922-0334, BA 75 Loyola Marymount Univ; MA 79 CA St Univ - Northridge; SLP, Santa Barbara County Schools, **SLP**

Vanis, Patty Joan 2611 27th Street Apt 1-19, Great Bend, KS 67530, (316) 793-9579, BS 84 Kearney St Coll; MS 86 Kearney St Coll; **SLP**

Van Kessel, Joan Marie 839 Big Buck Circle, Winter Springs, FL 32708, (305) 699-9035, BS 82 Stephen F Austin St Univ; MS 85 Univ of TX - Dallas; **SLP**

Van Kleeck, Dr Anne E Dept Of Speech Communication, University Of Texas, Austin, TX 78712, (512) 471-4119, BA 73 SUNY - Center at Buffalo; MS 74 Columbia Univ Teachers Coll; PH 78 (NS) Univ of WA; Dir-Prog in Comm Sci & Disorders, U of TX/Austin, **SLP**

Vankleeck, Mrs Marilyn M 9002 Sharpview, Houston, TX 77036, (713) 776-2162, BS 73 TX Christian Univ; MS 79 Baylor Coll of Medicine; 82–Aud, Drs Warshaw Weycer and Weber, **A**

Vankooten, Linda K 5035 Pillar Creek S E, Kentwood, MI 49508, (616) 698-0530, BA 86 MI St Univ; MA 87 MI St Univ

Van Lancker, Dr Diana Roupas Department Of Neuroscience, University Of North Dakota, 1919 Elm Street North, Fargo, ND 58102, (701) 293-4101, BS 62 Univ of WI - Madison; MA 66 Univ of Chicago; PH 75 (NS) Brown Univ; 88–Assoc Prof, Univ of North Dakota

VanLier, Rebecca Lansing 2310 Highland Avenue, Charlottesville, VA 22903, (804) 293-5332, BS 84 James Madison Univ; MS 85 James Madison Univ; 86–Sp-Lang Path, Albemarle Co PS, **SLP**

Vanlierop, Henry G Speech & Language Path Serv, P O Box 853, Jamestown, NM 87347, (505) 488-5535, BA 72 CA St Univ - Long Beach; MA 76 CA St Univ - Long Beach; Sp-Lang Path, Private Practice, **SLP**

Van Liew, Mrs Felisa Villarin 1018 Kensington Avenue, Plainfield, NJ 07060, (201) 881-6006, MA 88 Kean Coll of NJ

Van Loozen, Dorothy Cox 3018 Townbluff, Plano, TX 75075, (214) 867-8778, **SLP**

Van Luven, Elizabeth 8528 East Virginia Avenue, Scottsdale, AZ 85257, PH (NS); **SLP A LM**

Van Meter, Adelia M University Of Michigan Medical Center, Department PM&R Speech/Language Pathology, Ann Arbor, MI 48109-0050, (313) 936-7080, BA 79 Univ of MI - Ann Arbor; MS 82 Univ of MI - Ann Arbor; Sp-Lang Path, Univ of MI Med Ctr, **SLP**

Van Meter, Mrs Cynthia Louise 7005 Glendora, El Paso, TX 79912, (915) 799-1010, BA 73 Univ of TX - El Paso; MA 83 Univ of TX - El Paso; 73–Sp-Lang Path, El Paso PS

Van Meter, Mrs Ellen Mary 69-20 213th Street, Bayside, NY 11364, (718) 423-7951, BS 82 SUNY - Coll at Oneonta; MS 85 Adelphi Univ; 85–Sp-Lang Path, Sch for Lang & Comm Development, **SLP**

Vann, Brenda J 2426 North 73rd Place, Kansas City, KS 66109, (816) 921-2488, BS 70 Univ of KS; MA 72 Univ of KS; Sp/Lang Path, Kansas City Pub Sch, **SLP**

Vann, Mrs Charlotte Hopkins 18 Springhill West, Greenbrier, AR 72058, (501) 679-3121, BS 80 Univ of Central AR; MS 87 Univ of Central AR

Vann, Peter D 6510 Old Coach Court, Alexandria, VA 22310, (703) 550-8538, BA 67 Univ of MT; ME 70 Univ of VA - Charlottesville; SLP, Pg Co Bd of Ed, **SLP**

Vann, Mrs Vicki Jo Rd 1 Box 86, Hollsopple, PA 15935, (814) 535-8531, MS 83 Indiana Univ of PA; 83–Sp-Lang Path, City County Clinic, **SLP**

Van Natta, Mrs Madeleine Aura Beth 1801 Avalon, Colleyville, TX 76034, (817) 283-3191, BA 80 Depauw Univ; ME 83 Southwest TX St Univ; Sp-Lang Path, N Cent Texas Rehab Agency, **SLP**

Vannerson, Mrs Judy R 1630 Enfinger Road, Pace, FL 32570, (904) 994-8203, BA 71 Murray St Univ; MS 72 Murray St Univ; SLP, Escambia Co Sch Dist, **SLP**

Van Nest, Devona S Easter Seal Society, P O Box 115, 510 Penn Street, Huntingdon, PA 16652, (814) 643-5724, BS 76 Bloomsburg Univ of PA; MS 77 Bloomsburg Univ of PA; 77–Sp-Lang Path, Er Sl So of Huntingdon Co, **SLP**

Van Nevel, Anita Marie 1720 Kenmar, Manhattan, KS 66502, (913) 632-3176, BA 81 Western MI Univ; MA 83 Western MI Univ; Sp-Lang Path, Twin Lakes Ed Coop, **SLP**

VanNostrand, Mrs Toni DeTraglia A-109 Grange Hall Road, Rural Delivery 4, Moravia, NY 13118, (315) 784-5460, BS 81 SUNY - Coll at Geneseo; MA 86 SUNY - Coll at Geneseo; 86–Sp-Lang Path, E John Gavras Cntr, **SLP**

Vannote, Mrs Michele G 1045 Broadway, Fargo, ND 58102, (701) 241-4961, OM 74 Univ of ND; MS 70 Univ of ND; 85–Pricipal, Fargo PS, **SLP**

Vanover, Cheryl Annette 4508 Landside Drive #2, Louisville, KY 40220, (502) 584-9781, BS 85 Murray St Univ; MS 87 Murray St Univ; 87–Sp-Lang Path, Easter Seal Hearing & Sp Ctr, **SLP**

Van Overbeke, Mrs Nancy Phillips 4641 40th Street South, St Cloud, MN 56301, (612) 251-6343, BS 77 Saint Cloud St Univ; MS 81 Saint Cloud St Univ; Sp-Lang Path, Dist #742 St Cloud Commun Sch, **SLP**

Van Patten, Christine K 150 Howell Circle #328, Greenville, SC 29615, (803) 292-7032, BA 72 MI St Univ; MA 73 MI St Univ; 88–Sp-Lang Path, Sch Dist of Greenville Co, **SLP**

Van Patten, Peggy Louise 2763 Pine Street, Napa, CA 94558, (707) 544-7822, BA 74 Univ of CA - Berkeley; MS 82 Univ of WA; Aud, Robert C Bruner MD, **A**

Van Reenen, Mrs Janie Lee S 3992 Gunnin Road, Norcross, GA 30092, (404) 447-9657, BS 71 LA St Univ - Baton Rouge; ME 84 GA St Univ; Sp-Lang Path, Private Practice

Van Riper, Dr Charles 3821 West Milham, Kalamazoo, MI 49001, (616) 323-1353, BA 26 1939; MA 30 Univ of MI - Ann Arbor; PH 34 (NS) Univ of IA; **SLP F H LM**

Van Riper, Mrs Lori Ann c/o Univ Of MI Hospital, 1500 E Medical Ctr Drive, Tc-1904, Ann Arbor, MI 48109-0312, (313) 936-8013, BA 83 MI St Univ; MS 85 Univ of MI - Ann Arbor; 87–Aud, Univ of Michigan Hosp, **A**

Van Rooyen, Mrs Jennifer Marie P O Box 462, Coquille, OR 97423, BS 83 Univ of OR; MS 86 Univ of OR; 83–Sp-Lang Path, Coos County Educ Svc Dist, **SLP**

Van Slyke, Mrs Patricia A 42W143 Empire Road, St Charles, IL 60174-9530, (312) 369-0575, BS 73 IL St Univ - Normal; MS 75 IL St Univ - Normal; Dir, Sp-Lang Hrng Cl, **SLP ACE**

Van Son, Dr L George Ithaca College, School Health Sciences & Human Performance, Ithaca, NY 14850, (607) 274-3248, BS 61 Boston Univ; ME 62 Boston Univ; ED 68 (NS) Boston Univ; Assoc Prof, Ithaca College, **SLP**

Vanston, Marylynn A 1600 Garrett Road, Apartment K305, Upper Darby, PA 19082, (215) 623-4994, BA 83 Univ of Pittsburgh - Pittsburgh; MS 85 PA St Univ - Univ Park; Aud, Hahnemann Univ Hosp, **A**

Vanta, K Sandra 2065 Wyandotte Avenue, Lakewood, OH 44107, (216) 421-8960, BS 70 OH St Univ; MA 77 Kent St Univ; Sp-Lang Path, Cleveland Pub Sch, **SLP**

Van Tasell, Dr Dianne J 2121 Folwell Avenue, St Paul, MN 55108, (612) 624-3322, BA 70 Coe Coll; MA 72 Univ of IA; PH 78 (Aud) Northwestern Univ; 88–Prof, U of MN, **F**

Van Tatenhove, Gail M 8322 Tangelo Tree Drive, Orlando, FL 32819, (305) 291-7469, BA 76 Univ of WI - Eau Claire; MS 77 Univ of WI - Eau Claire; MS 77 Univ of WI - Eau Claire; Sp-Lang Path, Prentke Romich Co, **SLP**

Van Thorre, Mrs Candace B 5251 Humboldt Avenue South, Minneapolis, MN 55419, (612) 827-3685, BS 73 Mankato St Univ; MA 75 Mankato St Univ; Sp-Lang Path, Mpls Pub Sch-Sp Sch Dist #1, **SLP**

Van Tine, Ruth H 1515 7th Avenue #307, Greeley, CO 80631, (303) 352-3320, BA 34 Univ of Northern CO; MA 49 Univ of Denver; **SLP LM**

Vant Land, Mrs Julie Lynn 946 West 220th Street #105, Torrance, CA 90501, (213) 439-6864, BA 83 Calvin Coll; MA 84 MI St Univ; 86–Sp-Lang Path, LA USD, **SLP**

Vantrease, Mrs Carma Morrow 6645 Ridge Rock Lane, Knoxville, TN 37909-2769, **SLP**

Van Tuyl, Mrs Mildred Thoeny 11 Friends Road, Setauket, NY 11733, BS 81 Univ of AZ; MA 83 Univ of CT; Sp-Lang Path, Volz/Amato Sp-Lang Path, **SLP**

Vanvliet, Dennis 1432 Old River Road, Fullerton, CA 92631, (714) 544-6043, BS 73 Univ of CA - Irvine; MA 76 CA St Univ - Fullerton; Dir of Aud, Newport Lang & Auditory Center, **A ACE**

Van Vliet, Louise 3743 Riggs Road, Oxford, OH 45056, (513) 529-2322, BS 68 OH St Univ; MA 71 OH St Univ; PH 74 (NS) OH St Univ; Miami U, **SLP A**

Van Vooren, Mrs Margaret S 400 5th Street, Manhattan Beach, CA 90266, (213) 540-7676, BS 53 Northwestern Univ; MA 78 CA St Univ - Long Beach; Aud, Independent Contractor, **A ACE**

Van Voy, Karen Guilford 10155 Fallen Leaf Court, Ventura, CA 93004, (805) 659-2735, BS 84 AZ St Univ; MA 86 Univ of CA - Santa Barbara; 86–Sp-Lang Path, Carpinteria USD, **SLP**

Van Wagner, Karen 168 Harbor Lane, Massapequa Park, NY 11762, (516) 798-0990, BS 85 Ithaca Coll; MS 86 Adelphi Univ; **SLP**

Vanwagoner, Richard S 187 E 200 N, Lehi, UT 84043, (801) 268-4141, BS 69 Brigham Young Univ; MS 70 Brigham Young Univ; Owner, Mountain West Hrng Cen, **A**

Van Wallenburgh, Mrs Mary Campbell 3621 Lodge Haven Drive, Gainesville, GA 30506, BS 57 OK Coll for Women; ME 86 GA St Univ; 87–Sp-Lang Path, Forsyth County PS

Vanwey, Linda W 6 Melanie Lane, Gales Ferry, CT 06335, (203) 464-2650, BA 74 Univ of CT; MA 76 Univ of CT; **SLP**

Van Winkle, Cynthia G 15 Turner Drive, Mount Vernon, IL 62864, (618) 985-3138, BS 74 Saint Louis Univ; MA 79 Memphis St Univ; Sp-Lang Path, Good Samaritan Hosp, **SLP**

Van Winkle, David L ASP-126, Veterans Administration Medical Center, 4100 West Third Street, Dayton, OH 45428, (513) 268-6511, BA 66 KS St Univ; MA 75 Univ of KS; PH 81 (Aud & Sp Path) Univ of KS; 88–Chief Aud & SLP, VA Medical Center, **A**

Van Wyck, Nancy 4162 East Ridgewood Avenue, Las Vegas, NV 89120, (702) 369-7853, MS 72 Univ of South FL; Sp-Lang Path, Desert Springs Hosp, **SLP**

Vanzandt, Mrs Joan C Rt 2 Box 35, Oak Grove, MO 64075, (816) 625-3383, BS 60 Northeastern OK St Univ; 88–Sp-Lang Path, Rainbow Ctr for Commun Dis, **SLP**

Vanzant, Mrs Nancy P 503 North 7th Street, Ponca City, OK 74601, (405) 765-8073, BS 74 Kent St Univ; MS 75 Univ of AZ; 84–Sp-Lang Path, Sp/Path Assoc of North Cen OK, **SLP**

Vanzino, Mrs Laura M 507 Leawood Avenue, Toms River, NJ 08753, (201) 244-7684, MA 81 Trenton St Coll; SLP, Stafford Township Bd of Educ, **SLP**

Vara, Mrs Eileen A W Coastal Bend Sp & Lang Assoc, Neurological Clinic Bldg, 3006 South Alameda, Corpus Christi, TX 78404, (512) 888-7020, BA 75 Our Lady Lake Univ-San Anton; MA 76 Our Lady Lake Univ-San Anton; Sp-Lang Path, Coastal Bend Sp/Lang Assoc, **SLP**

Varadi, Mrs Carol Anne 6 Southbury Drive, Columbia, SC 29209, (803) 783-6885, BS 78 Miami Univ - Oxford; ME 84 Old Dominion Univ; Sp-Lang Path, Private Practice, **SLP ACE**

Varadi, Rhea C 65-38 Booth Street, Rego Park, NY 11374, (212) 620-6306, BA 76 Hofstra Univ; MS 79 Columbia Univ Teachers Coll; Aud, VA Outpatient Cl, **A**

Varavvas, Mrs Denise M 2752 Cleveland Avenue N W, Canton, OH 44709, (216) 452-1201, BS 78 Miami Univ - Oxford; MS 80 Kent St Univ; Aud, Denise M Varavvas MA Aud, **A**

Vardiman, Karen 13410 Larkhaven Drive, Moreno Valley, CA 92388, (714) 653-5447, BS 78 Univ of MO - Columbia; MA 85 CA St Univ - Los Angeles; Sp-Lang Path, Private Practice, **SLP**

Vardsveen, Dorothy J 49 Southgate Road, Franklin, MA 02038, (617) 335-0191, BS 78 Minot St Univ; MA 79 Minot St Univ; **A**

Varelman, Dian W Route 3 Box 636, Wichita Falls, TX 76308, (817) 720-3055, BA 69 Memphis St Univ; MA 70 Memphis St Univ; Sp-Lang Path, Wichita Falls ISD, **SLP**

Varga, Mrs Tamara Elaine 2205 Northwest 22nd Street, Oklahoma City, OK 73107, (405) 272-5522, BS 86 Univ of OK - OK City; MS 88 Univ of OK - OK City

Vargas, Mrs Leslie Kahn 86-A 3rd Place, Brooklyn, NY 11231, (212) 834-1863, BS 67 Emerson Coll; MA 69 NY Univ; MA 84 Columbia Univ Teachers Coll; 68–SLP, NYC Bd Ed Sp Serv Dist 20, **SLP**

Vargo, Dr Steven William 102 West Chocolate Avenue, Hershey, PA 17033, (717) 533-7350, BS 54 IN St Univ - Terre Haute; MS 57 Purdue Univ - West Lafayette; PH 65 (NS) IN Univ - Bloomington; Owner/Aud, Audiology/Hearing Aid Service, **A**

Vargoshe, Mrs Barbara J 149 Millville Avenue, Naugatuck, CT 06770, (203) 723-4421, BA 73 Univ of CT; MS 74 Southern CT St Univ; SLP, Naugatuck Bd of Ed, **SLP**

Vargulich-Sinkuc, Valerie 728 South State Line Road, Masury, OH 44438, (216) 448-8393, BS 79 IN Univ - Bloomington; MS 81 OH Univ - Athens; 88–Sp-Lang Path, Easter Seals Society, **SLP**

Varjian, Doris 13 Wield Court, Park Ridge, NJ 07656, (201) 573-0742, BA 69 Montclair St Coll; MA 70 Seton Hall Univ; **SLP**

Varnado, Mrs Mollie Denise Route 1 Box 158, Iota, LA 70543, (318) 824-3038, BS 81 LA St Univ - Baton Rouge; MA 85 LA St Univ - Baton Rouge; 88–Sp-Lang Path, Acadia Parish School Board, **SLP**

Varnedoe, Danielle Reed Univ S Carolina Sp-Hrng Center, 1601 St Julian Place, Columbia, SC 29204, (803) 777-2614, BA 76 Univ of Akron; MA 79 Univ of Akron; Instructor, University of South Carolina, **SLP**

Varner, Mrs Harriet K 911 North Colonial Court, Indian Harbor Beach, FL 32937, (305) 773-3235, BA 41 PA St Univ - Univ Park; ME 55 PA St Univ - Univ Park; Sp-Lang Path, **SLP LM**

Varner, Mrs Pamela Hogge 3562 Dumosa Way, Beale AFB, CA 95903, (916) 788-0326, BA 81 NM St Univ; MA 83 NM St Univ; 86–Sp-Lang Path, Goldsworthy & Johnston Sp & Lang Path, **SLP**

Varney, Mrs Carol Ann 125 West Carpenter #4, Springfield, IL 62702, (217) 544-6464, BS 83 Northern IL Univ - De Kalb; MA 84 Northern IL Univ - De Kalb; **SLP**

Varney, Mrs Ruth P 546 Hillcrest Drive, Bowling Green, OH 43402, (419) 352-7656, BA 47 OH St Univ; BS 47 OH St Univ; MA 51 OH St Univ; Supervisor Teachers, Bowling Green State University, **SLP**

Varnon, Mrs Suzanne M 10407 Chesterton, Dallas, TX 75238, (214) 226-3922, BA 70 Baylor Univ; MS 76 Univ of North TX; Sp-Lang Path, Garland ISD, **SLP**

Varro, Emily Mauzy 62 Valley View Road, High Bridge, NJ 08829, (201) 822-3880, BS 79 Kutztown Univ of PA; MA 85 Montclair St Coll; **SLP**

Vasconcellos, Cynthia Jean 314 El Capitan, Manteca, CA 95336, (209) 948-7196, BA 86 CA St Univ - Stanislaus; MA 88 CA St Univ - Stanislaus; 88–Sp-Lang Path, Stockton Dev Ctr

Vasilauskas, Mrs Cherylyn Joy 419 Christopher, Holland, MI 49424, (616) 392-5141, BS 86 Central MI Univ; MA 87 Western MI Univ; 87–Sp-Lang Path, Holland Comm Hosp, **SLP**

Vasiloff, Richard M 37445 Fountain Park Circle, Apartment 450, Westland, MI 48185, BS 73 Central MI Univ; MS 75 Univ of Montevallo; Dept Analyst, Ment Health License& Accred, **SLP**

Vasilos, Stephanie 72 Cottage Park Road, Winthrop, MA 02152-2907, (401) 725-5798, Sp-Lang Path, Judith Wisinia & Assoc, **SLP**

Vasquez, Rachel 147-28 72nd Road #3-E, Flushing, NY 11367, (718) 793-0151, BA 78 CUNY - Queens Coll; MA 81 CUNY - Queens Coll; Aud, Private Practice, **A**

Vasquez, Therese Janine 2156 S 8th Avenue, Yuma, AZ 85364, (602) 343-1290, BS 83 Northern AZ Univ; MS 85 Northern AZ Univ; **SLP**

Vass, William K 10419 Lee Drive, Eden Prairie, MN 55344, (612) 941-6401, MS 78 WV Univ; National Sales Mngr, Danavox Inc, **A**

Vassallo, Lawrence A 127 Williamsburg Way, Mount Laurel, NJ 08054, (215) 735-0205, BS 61 SUNY - Coll at Buffalo; MS 62 PA St Univ - Univ Park; Dir of Trng/Data Proc Sng Mgr, Hrng Conserv Noise Ctrl Inc, **A**

Vasseur-Kwech, Virginia Marie 2112 Jonquil Avenue, Mc Allen, TX 78501, (512) 686-3669, BA 83 Univ of MN - Duluth; MA 84 Memphis St Univ; **A**

Vassilaros, Mrs Maria Athena 3 Edith Place, Pittsburgh, PA 15213, (412) 682-4143, BS 84 Miami Univ - Oxford; MA 85 Kent St Univ; **SLP**

Vassiliades, Diane G 1524 N W 109th Terrace, Coral Springs, FL 33065, (305) 752-1752, BA 68 Hofstra Univ; MA 73 Columbia Univ Teachers Coll; **SLP**

Vasta, Nicoletta M 61 Evans Street, Medford, MA 02155-4115, (617) 935-5050, BA 85 Bridgewater St Coll; MS 87 Northeastern Univ; SLP, New England Rehab Hosp, **SLP**

Vasterling, Margaret M 2128 North Booth, Milwaukee, WI 53212, (414) 259-3071, BS 61 Univ Southern MS-Hattiesburg; MS 62 Univ Southern MS-Hattiesburg; SLP, Curative Rehab Ctr, **SLP**

Vatz, Claire Santagati 884 Lovingston Drive, Pittsburgh, PA 15216, (412) 343-9391, BA 75 Adelphi Univ; MA 76 Univ of Pittsburgh - Pittsburgh; Director of Sp-Lang Path, Claire Santagati Vatz Ma Ccc, **SLP**

Vaubel, Ann W Route 3 Box 168, Mapleton, MN 56065, (507) 625-1811, BS 72 Univ of MN - Minneap-St Paul; MA 76 Univ of MN - Minneap-St Paul; 88–Aud, Dist 77 Mankato PS, **A**

Vaudin, Andrea #2 3025 Birch Street, Vancouver, BC, Canada V6H 2T8, (604) 589-4436, BA 79 Univ of Victoria - Bc; MS 82 Purdue Univ - Calumet; 88–Sp-Lang Path, North Delta Sch Dist, **SLP**

Vaughan, Mrs Donna Duewall 1953 Lakeview Drive, Madisonville, KY 42431, (502) 825-6036, BA 78 Univ of MS; MS 83 Western KY Univ; 82–Sp/Lang Path, Hopkins Cty Sch Sys, **SLP**

Vaughan, Dorothy H c/o Susan Baldwin, 1108 Indian Prairie Loop, Victor, MT 59875, BS 66 Vanderbilt Univ; MS 71 Vanderbilt Univ; 79–Sp-Lang Path, **SLP**

Vaughan, Mrs Jenni Anderson 5483-C Country Side Drive, Winston-Salem, NC 27105, (919) 744-0669, BS 86 Univ of AR - Fayetteville; MS 87 Univ of AR - Medical Sci; **SLP**

Vaughan, Linda Decker 5719 Glengate Lane, Cincinnati, OH 45212, (513) 531-2131, BA 63 Univ of Cincinnati; MA 82 Univ of Cincinnati; Sp-Lang Path, Hamilton Co Bd of Ed, **SLP**

Vaughan, Martha S 29011 Crags Drive, Agoura, CA 91301, (213) 419-2526, BS 74 Emerson Coll; MA 78 CA St Univ - Los Angeles; SLP, Los Angeles Co Supt of Sch, **SLP**

Vaughan, Dr Robin H 11346 Mt View Avenue #C, Loma Linda, CA 92354, (714) 796-9136, BS 76 Brigham Young Univ; OM 77 Brigham Young Univ; PH 87 (Allied Health Science) Columbia Pacific Univ; Aud, Private Practice, **A**

Vaughn, Cheryl R 2704 Arnold Drive, Marshalltown, IA 50158, (515) 753-4223, BA 73 Univ of Northern IA; MA 74 Univ of Northern IA; Sp-Lang Path, Iowa Vet Home, **SLP A**

Vaughn, Denise Lynn 3313 Harvest, Cibolo, TX 78108, (512) 620-6713, BS 86 Southwest TX St Univ; MS 88 Southwest TX St Univ; 88–Sp-Lang Path, InSpeech Inc

Vaughn, Dr Gwenyth R 2050-A Montreat Parkway, Birmingham, AL 35216, (205) 939-2163, BA 39 Univ of Denver; MA 42 Univ of Denver; PH 59 (Communication Methodology) Univ of Denver; 67–Chief Aud-SLP, VA, **SLP A F LM ACE**

Vaughn, Judith Campsie 3931 Hill Terrace, Jacksonville, FL 32211, (513) 559-4341, BS 75 Univ of MA - Amherst; MS 77 Rutger's St Univ - Douglas Coll; Sp/Lang Path, Cincinnati Childrens Hospital, **SLP**

Vaughn, Mrs Linda Robinson 1805 Hampton Drive, Harvey, LA 70058, (504) 361-7745, BS 71 Jackson St Univ; ME 80 Univ of MS; MS 80 Univ of MS; SLP, Jefferson Parish Schools, **SLP**

Vaughn, Maureen G 6407 Londonderry Drive, Gary, IL 60013, **SLP**

Vaughn, Mrs Suzanne Lee 3845 Saddle Rock Road, Colorado Springs, CO 80918, (719) 260-0092, BS 71 IN Univ - Bloomington; MS 72 Univ of IL - Urbana; Sp-Lang Path, El Paso Co Sch Dist #11, **SLP**

Vaughn, Mrs Teresa R 601 Ridgeview Drive #2, Frankfort, KY 40601-1426, (502) 695-5584, BS 82 Eastern KY Univ; MA 87 Eastern KY Univ; 82–Sp-Lang Path, Franklin Co PS, **SLP**

Vaughn, Tracey Jane P O Box 1303, Rhinelander, WI 54501, (715) 284-5028, BA 80 Univ of WI - Eau Claire; MS 81 Univ of WI - Eau Claire; SLP, Tomah Rehab Cen, **SLP**

Vaughn-Cooke, Dr Ana F 1501 Hamilton Street N W, Washington, DC 20011, (202) 727-2637, MS 76 Georgetown Univ; BA 70 Univ of MD - College Park; PH 76 (NS) Georgetown Univ; Assoc Prof, Udc, **SLP**

Vaught, Cheryl Sue 709 Brown, Liberty, MO 64068, (816) 781-1001, BS 83 Central MO St Univ; MS 84 Central MO St Univ; Aud, Hearing Specialists Inc, **A**

Vaught, Samuel F 534 South Lumina Avenue, Box 7815, Wrightsville Beach, NC 28480, (919) 343-7218, BA 80 Univ of NC - Chapel Hill; MS 82 Univ of NC - Chapel Hill; 85–Aud, New Hanover Mem Hosp, **A**

Vaughters, Donna Mosher 5981 South Lima Street, Englewood, CO 80111, (303) 693-0260, BS 58 IL St Univ - Normal; MS 67 IL St Univ - Normal; LD Tchr, Cherry Crk Sch Dist, **SLP**

Vaupen, Pearl 5005 Collins Avenue #708, Miami Beach, FL 33140, (305) 864-1573, BA 81 Univ of FL; OM 84 Emory Univ; Sp-Lang Path, Jackson Mem Hosp, **SLP**

Vaurio, Kathryn P 100 Elm Avenue, Swarthmore, PA 19081, (215) 543-6183, BA 35 OH Northern Univ; MS 42 Purdue Univ - West Lafayette; Sp-Lang Path, Private Practice, **SLP LM ACE**

Vause, Mark Wayne 12101 Peconic, Boise, ID 83709, (208) 338-3655, BS 73 UT St Univ; MS 75 UT St Univ; 75–Aud, Boise PS

Vause-Stapleton, Nancy 92-1141 Makamai Loop, Ewa Beach, HI 96707, (808) 672-3790, BS 75 East TX St Univ - Commerce; MA 77 Memphis St Univ; Audiologist - Asst Chief, Tripler Army Med Center, **A**

Vautier, Pamela D 5651 Briehtwood Lane, Mobile, AL 36608, BA 76 Auburn Univ - Auburn; OM 77 Auburn Univ - Auburn; 86–Aud, Dauphin W Eye Ear Nose & Throat Spec, **A**

Vavra, Mrs Alicia O R 16447 Parksley Drive, Houston, TX 77059, (713) 488-2249, BS 74 Univ of Houston - Univ Park; MA 76 Univ of Houston - Univ Park; **SLP**

Vayianos, Marissa C 330 Penns Way, Basking Ridge, NJ 07920, (201) 580-9362, BS 78 Elmira Coll; MA 80 Case Western Reserve Univ; Sp-Lang Path, Morristown Memorial Hosp, **SLP**

Vazquez, Rosa I Hato Rey Plaza #4-M, Hato Rey, PR 00918, (809) 751-5110, BA 55 Univ of PR - Rio Piedras; BA 61 Univ of PR - Rio Piedras; MA 67 (NS) Columbia Univ Teachers Coll; Assoc Prof, U of PR Med Sci Campus, **SLP**

Vazquez, Mrs Terry Linda 3007 N Black Canyon #33-B, Phoenix, AZ 85015, (602) 257-2800, BS 72 Southern IL Univ -Carbondale; MS 85 Governors St Univ; 87–Sp-Lang Path, Creighton Sch Dist, **SLP**

Veale, Mrs Tina K 8496 Windcrest Drive, West Chester, OH 45069-3486, BA 79 Miami Univ - Oxford; MA 80 Miami Univ - Oxford; Sp-Lang Path, Private Practice, **SLP**

Veatch, Dr John W 4708 64th Avenue West, Tacoma, WA 98466, (206) 564-8251, OB 51 WA St Univ; BA 46 WA St Univ; ED 70 (NS) Univ of ID; Private Practice, **SLP**

Veazey, Deborah Paschall Route #1, Puryear, TN 38251, (901) 498-8955, BS 77 Murray St Univ; MS 85 Murray St Univ; **SLP**

Veazy, Mrs Julia Woodard 12751 South Carpenter, Calumet Park, IL 60643, (312) 758-1410, BS 79 IL St Univ - Normal; OM 86 Governors St Univ

Vecchi, Melody Curphy 5324 East 114th Place, Thornton, CO 80233, (303) 452-8841, BS 75 CO St Univ; MA 76 Univ of Denver; 77–Sp-Lang Path, Adams Co Dist 12-Pub Sch, **SLP**

Vecchio, Mrs Deborah Strange P O Box 2272, Muskogee, OK 74402, (918) 682-6641, MA 74 Univ of Tulsa; 76–SLP, Oklahoma Sch for the Blind, **SLP**

Vecchio, Joan A L 18 Erie Street, Staten Island, NY 10309, (212) 596-5742, BA 69 CUNY - Brooklyn Coll; MS 72 CUNY - Brooklyn Coll; SLP, Citywide Speech Unit, **SLP**

Vecchio, Mrs Kathy Ann 98 Bassie Drive, Zelienople, PA 16063, (412) 728-7000, BS 83 0500; MS 84 CA Univ of PA; 87–Sp-Lang Path, The Medical Center of Beaver, **SLP**

Vedaa, Karen Ostlund 1944 Loma Vista, Pasadena, CA 91104, (818) 797-6985, BA 76 CA St Univ - Los Angeles; MA 86 Whittier Coll; 78–Sp-Lang Path, LA USD

Veder, Dr Robert A 14940 Penitencia Creek Rd, San Jose, CA 95132, (415) 881-3233, BA 61 San Jose St Univ; MA 64 Univ of WA; PH 66 (NS) Univ of WA; 71–Prog Dir, Cal St U-Hayward, **A ACE**

Vega, Allene C L W Blake Memorial Hospital, 2020 59th Street West, P O Box 25004, Bradenton, FL 33506, (813) 798-6220, MA 69 Univ of South FL; Dir-Sp-Lang Path, L W Blake Memorial Hospital, **SLP**

Vega-Barachowitz, Carmen Dolores 64 Blomerth Street, Malden, MA 02148, (617) 324-3637, BS 78 FL St Univ; MS 79 FL St Univ; Sp-Lang Path, Visiting Nurse Assoc of Boston, **SLP**

Vegter, Candace H Gillette Children's Hospital, University Avenue, St Paul, MN 55101, (612) 291-2848, BS 73 Univ of WI - Madison; MA 74 Univ of IA; Sp-Lang Path, Gillette Chldrn's Hosp, **SLP**

Vehr, Jeffrey Paul 7358 Perry Street, Cincinnati, OH 45231, (513) 729-4375, MA 88 Univ of Cincinnati

Vein, Mrs Paula Canarick 6050 Johnston Road, Slingerlands, NY 12159, (518) 489-2681, BS 78 SUNY - Center at Albany; MS 80 SUNY - Coll at Fredonia; Sp-Lang Path, Vna of Albany, **SLP**

Veis, Sharon L Northwestern Univ Medical Sch, 303 East Chicago Avenue, Ward 3-140, Chicago, IL 60611, (312) 908-8035, BS 81 Northwestern Univ; MA 83 Northwestern Univ; 83–Sp-Lang Path, Northwestern Univ, **SLP ACE**

Veitch, Mrs Genevieve 3607 South Florence, Tulsa, OK 74105, (918) 742-1582, BA 74 Univ of OK - Norman; MA 76 Univ of Tulsa; **SLP**

Veith, Karalee Colleen 91-D Harmony Hill Road, Albany, NY 12203-3222, (518) 674-2881, MA 85 SUNY - Coll at Fredonia; **SLP**

Veith, Mary C 3306 99th N E, Bellevue, WA 98004, (503) 567-8121, BA 79 WA St Univ; MA 81 WA St Univ; SLP, Edmonds School District, **SLP**

Vekovius, Mrs Gay Tate 210 Linden, Shreveport, LA 71104, (318) 227-5156, BA 65 Vanderbilt Univ; MS 66 Vanderbilt Univ; Assistant Professor, LA St U Med Cen, **A ACE**

Velasquez, Mrs Stacy Goodrich 405 Burnell Circle, Waco, TX 76712, (817) 562-2821, BS 83 Baylor Univ; MS 84 Baylor Univ; 85–Sp-Lang Path/Aud, Mexia State Sch, **SLP A**

Velde, Therese Marie 918 Simpson Street, Evanston, IL 60201, (312) 492-3165, BS 74 Univ of AZ; MS 76 Univ of AZ; OM 77 Univ of AZ; Northwestern U, **A**

Velez, Dora 4343 Baring Avenue, East Chicago, IN 46312, (219) 397-1917, BS 77 Purdue Univ - West Lafayette; MA 78 Ball St Univ; 86–Sp-Lang Path, St Anthony's Med Ctr, **SLP**

Velez-Davila, Wanda Damaris Ext Betances, #24A Bo Algarrobo, Vega Baja, PR 00763, (809) 780-2890, BS 85 Univ of PR - San Juan; MS 87 Univ of PR - San Juan; 88–Sp-Lang Path, Dept of Educ of PR at FL

Veligdan, Mrs Marietta Scuro 6 Stephanie Lane, Manorville, NY 11949, (516) 878-6098, BA 73 Univ of Pittsburgh - Pittsburgh; MA 75 Univ of Pittsburgh - Pittsburgh; Consult/Sp-Lang Path, Private Practice, **SLP**

Vella, Barbara 180 South Middleneck Road, Apartment 3-P, Great Neck, NY 11021, BA 74 CUNY - Queens Coll; MA 78 CUNY - Hunter Coll; 79–Sp-Lang Path, NYC Bd Ed Sp Serv Ut, **SLP**

Vella, Mrs Jo Ann Benfatta 5281 Crossbridge Drive, West Chester, OH 45069, **SLP**

Velleman, Dr Shelley Lynne 10 Morning Star Drive, Hadley, MA 01035, (413) 781-9100, MA 85 Univ of MA - Amherst; MA 78 Univ of WI - Madison; PH 83 (Linguistics (Child Lang)) Univ of TX - Austin; 88–Sp-Lang Path, Mercy Hosp Sp Hrng & Lang Ctr, **SLP**

Veloon, Paulette A 2921 Fish Hatchery Road, Apartment 206, Madison, WI 53713, (608) 873-7257, BS 77 Univ of WI - Madison; MS 79 Univ of WI - Stevens Point; SLP, Stoughton Area Schools, **SLP**

Velte-Jones, Phyllis C 6519 Shenandoah Drive, Sykesville, MD 21784, (301) 243-3800, BA 75 Loyola Coll; MS 76 Loyola Coll; Sp-Lang Path, Hrng & Sp Agcy of Metro Balt, **SLP**

Veltman, Anne Marie 4320 Mink, Casper, WY 82604, (307) 577-0253, **SLP**

Veltman, Mrs Sharon A 1270 Belmont Avenue, Schenectady, NY 12308, (518) 382-4519, BS 77 SUNY - Coll at Fredonia; MS 80 Coll of Saint Rose; Sp-Lang Path, Sunnyview Rehab Hosp, **SLP**

Venable, Gail P 156 Diamond Street, San Francisco, CA 94114, (415) 664-4646, BA 68 Occidental Coll; MS 74 McGill Univ - Quebec; Sp-Lang Path, Scottish Rite I-Chldhd Aphasia, **SLP**

Venable, Mrs Marsha Butler 1992 Hoods Creek Drive, New Bern, NC 28560, (919) 638-6845, BS 75 East Carolina Univ; MS 76 East Carolina Univ; SLP, Jefferson Par Sch, **SLP**

Venegoni, Mary L 400 Wilcox Street, Joliet, IL 60435, (815) 467-2261, BS 79 Western IL Univ; MA 80 Western IL Univ; Sp-Lang Path, Grundy Co Spec Ed Coop, **SLP**

Venegoni, Mary Margaret 113 Gillman Street, Washington, IL 61571, (309) 444-3497, BS 82 Marquette Univ; MA 84 Univ of IA; Sp-Lang Path, Creve Coeur Sch Dist 76, **SLP**

Venema, Theodore H 340 Mill Road #502, Etobicoke, ON, Canada M9C 1Y8, (416) 621-0685, MA 88 Western WA Univ; 87–Aud, The Canadian Hearing Society, **A**

Vener, Sharon 4348 Park Corona, Calabasas, CA 91302, **SLP**

Veness, Deborah Miracle 2500 Wigwam Road, Aliquippa, PA 15001, (412) 375-1588, BS 84 Indiana Univ of PA; MS 85 WV Univ; 88–Aud, Beaver Valley Interm Unit #27, **A**

Venezia, Robert 13 Kenyon Street, Providence, RI 02903, (401) 456-9330, BA 76 Univ of RI; MS 80 Univ of RI; Sp/Lang Path, Providence Spec Ed Dept, **SLP**

Veneziano, Mrs Charlotte 7 Fairwater Avenue, Massapequa, NY 11758, MA 73 Hofstra Univ; Teacher, Nassau County BOCES, **SLP**

Venezuela-Estavillo, Gladys Yadira 6451 Yarmouth Avenue, Reseda, CA 91335, (818) 996-3615, BS 78 Univ of PR - Rio Piedras; MS 80 Univ of PR - San Juan; 86–Sp-Lang Path, LA USD, **SLP**

Veniar, Dr Florence A 2254 Pine Grove Court, Ann Arbor, MI 48103, BA 43; MA 44 Columbia Univ Teachers Coll; PH 48 (NS) Columbia Univ Teachers Coll; Retired, Rutgers Univ, **A**

Venkatagiri, Dr Horabail Iowa State University, 210 Pearson Hall, Ames, IA 50011, (515) 294-6476, MS 69 Univ of Mysore - India; PH 77 (NS) Bowling Green St Univ; Assoc Prof, Iowa State U, **SLP**

Venkatesh, Mrs Sreedevi 13 Birch Lake Drive, Sherman, IL 62684, (217) 735-2361, BS 74; MS 76; Aud/SLP, Lincoln Dev Cen, **SLP A**

Venne, Dona P 15125 Farmington Road, Livonia, MI 48154, (313) 523-9366, BS 50 SUNY - Coll at Buffalo; MA 59 Eastern MI Univ; Sp-Lang Path, Livonia Pub Schs, **SLP**

Vento, Mrs Barbara A 250 Redoak Drive, Pittsburgh, PA 15239, (412) 828-1300, BA 74 Duquesne Univ; MS 77 Univ of Pittsburgh - Pittsburgh; Aud, Harmarville Rehab Cen, **A**

Ventola, Mrs Ellen M 365 Bloomfield Avenue Apartment 7A, Verona, NJ 07044, (201) 884-2030, BA 81 Montclair St Coll; MA 84 Montclair St Coll; 86–Sp-Lang Path, The Calais Sch, **SLP**

Ventry, Nona 155 West 91st Street, New York, NY 10024, (718) 830-1015, BS 64 NY Univ; MA 65 NY Univ; 65–Aud, Mt Sinai Hosp Serv City Hosp Elm, **A**

Ventuleth, Mrs Shannon M 1015 North Iowa Street, Fallbrook, CA 92028, (619) 740-2431, BA 75 Univ of the Pacific; Sp-Lang Path, Escondido Union Sch Dist

Ventura, Dr F Paul 2801 S E 122nd, Portland, OR 97236, (503) 761-1506, BA 48 IN St Univ - Terre Haute; MA 51 Northwestern Univ; PH 68 (Doctor of Philosophy) Univ of OR; Dir, Industrial Hearing Svc, **SLP A**

Ventura, Lisa Marie 445 Wood Street, New Bedford, MA 02745, (603) 646-5978, BS 85 Northeastern Univ; MS 86 Syracuse Univ; 87–Sp-Lang Path, Dartmouth-Hitchcock Med Ctr, **SLP**

Venturini, Mrs Susan Parkin 18 Lawrence Avenue, Warwick, RI 02888, (401) 467-5043, BA 77 Univ of RI; MS 79 Emerson Coll; 79–Sp-Lang Path, North Providence Schs, **SLP**

Venus, Dr Carol A O E Teague VA Medical Center, Audiology & Sp-Path (126), 1901 South 1st Street, Temple, TX 76504, (817) 778-4811, BS 73 Loyola Univ of Chicago; MA 75 Vanderbilt Univ; PH 83 (Commnication Disorders) Northwestern Univ; Coord Sp-Lang Path, Olin E Teague VA Med Ctr, **SLP ACE**

Veraldi, Mrs Janet J 242 Roscommon Place, Mc Murray, PA 15317, (412) 941-4746, BS 73 CA Univ of PA; ME 76 CA Univ of PA; SLP, Allegheny Intermediate Unit #3, **SLP**

Verbeck, Margaret Mary 411 Allenhurst Avenue, Ridgway, PA 15853, (814) 776-6531, BS 85 PA St Univ - Univ Park; MS 87 PA St Univ - Univ Park

Verble, Mrs Suzanne D 1505 Thrush Terrace, St Louis, MO 63144, (606) 269-6848, MS 88 Univ of KY

Verburg, Mrs Virginia L 3007 Edgewood, Sugar Land, TX 77479, (713) 232-4041, BA 70 Univ of Houston - Univ Park; MA 71 Univ of Houston - Univ Park; Ed Diagn, Lamar Cisd, **SLP**

Vercellone, Donna Cheryl 10107 Tramonte, St Louis, MO 63137, BS 78 Fontbonne Coll; MS 78 Fontbonne Coll; Sp-Lang Path, St Joseph Hospital, **SLP**

Verchot, Lucinda K 2018 Nelson Street S E, Decatur, AL 35601, **SLP**

Vercoe, Donna M 3320 Alsace Court, Mequon, WI 53092, BS 84 Univ of WI - Madison; MS 85 Univ of WI - Eau Claire; **SLP**

Vercruysse, Mrs Robin Ehrlich 1215 Pasteur Drive, Lancaster, CA 93535, (805) 942-1115, MA 80 Northeast MO St Univ; **SLP**

Verdecchia, Julie Marie 7808 East Lake Road, Erie, PA 16511, (814) 453-5602, BS 80 Indiana Univ of PA; MS 82 Vanderbilt Univ; 82–Sp-Lang Path, Lake Erie Inst of Rehab, **SLP**

Verderosa, Janet Noia 450-20 Atlantic Avenue #2B, East Rockaway, NY 11518, (516) 887-7679, BA 85 CUNY - Queens Coll; MA 87 CUNY - Queens Coll; **SLP**

Verdi, Janet Rosemarie 1225 Glenmere Street, West Covina, CA 91790, (714) 591-2653, BA 79 Univ of LA Verne; MS 83 Univ of LA Verne; Sp-Lang Path, China USD, **SLP**

Verdolini-Marston, Mrs Katherine Tuller 3022 Watson, St Louis, MO 63139, BS 75 IN Univ - Bloomington; OM 78; MA 82 IN Univ - Bloomington; 88–Sp-Lang Path, Wash U, **SLP**

Veremko, Gregory Steven 25 Pleasantview Drive, Dalton, MA 01226, (413) 655-8035, **SLP**

Veremko, Karen Eissmann 25 Pleasantview Drive, Dalton, MA 01226, (413) 743-5202, **SLP**

Veres, Sally Ard 2001 Dundee Road, Rockville, MD 20850, (301) 762-0632, BS 59 Univ of Houston - Univ Park; MA 67 Univ of Houston - Univ Park; **SLP**

Vergales, Phylis Ellen 12213 Poplar Forest Drive, Richmond, VA 23233, (804) 353-9780, BS 82 Bradley Univ; ME 84 Univ of VA - Charlottesville; Aud, Maico Hrng Aid Service Inc, **A**

Ver Hoef, Anne L 1675 Sitka Street #303, Anchorage, AK 99501, (907) 272-0586, BS 83 Univ of MN - Minneap-St Paul; MA 85 Univ of IA; **SLP**

Verhoef, Mrs Joan Fernandes 221 Ferguson Avenue, Newport News, VA 23601-4001, (314) 865-3333, BS 80 Bradley Univ; MA 81 Northern IL Univ - De Kalb; Aud, **A**

Ver Hoef, Niel Audiology Associates Pc, 2584-A Hubbell Avenue, Des Moines, IA 50317-6102, (515) 243-1283, BA 56 Univ of Northern IA; MS 61 Southern IL Univ -Carbondale; Aud, Aud Assoc Pc, **SLP A**

Verkest, Suzanne Bernice Dartmouth Hitchcock Med Cen, Department Of Audiology, 2 Maynard Street, Hanover, NH 03756, (603) 646-8125, BA 82 Wayne St Univ - Sch of Med; MA 84 Wayne St Univ - Sch of Med; 84–Aud, Dartmouth-Hitchcock Med Cen, **A**

Verkuilen, Mrs Kathleen Kimmel 5733 Restal Street, Madison, WI 53711, (608) 882-4606, BS 75 Univ of WI - Milwaukee; MS 76 Univ of WI - Milwaukee; Sp-Lang Path, Evansville Community Sch Dist, **SLP**

Verlo, Ellen Pringnitz Otologic Medical Services, 2440 Towncrest Drive, Iowa City, IA 52240, (319) 337-6879, BA 82 Univ of IA; MA 85 Northern IL Univ - De Kalb; Aud, Otologic Medical Services, **A**

Vermeulen, Rosalyn A 67 Beaconsfield Avenue, London, ON, Canada N6C 1B6, (519) 672-3729, BS 75 SUNY - Coll at Buffalo; MS 80 SUNY - Coll at Fredonia; Sp-Lang Path, Bd of Educ City of London, **SLP**

Vernamonti, Mrs Jane M O Ironstone Medical Bldg B, 120 Stokes Road, Medford, NJ 08055, (609) 654-6775, BA 75 Rutger's St Univ - Douglas Coll; MA 76 Trenton St Coll; Sp/Lang Path, Private Practice, **SLP**

Vernau, Lesley Anne 1605 White Cloud Court, Winter Springs, FL 32708, (305) 365-8815, MA 88 Univ of Central FL

Verner, Monica Marasco 16 Miller Heights, Middletown, NY 10940, (914) 342-2950, MA 85 Western MI Univ; **SLP**

Vernetti, Robert James 1722 Lasalle, Belleville, IL 62221, (618) 256-7545, BS 74 Southern IL Univ-Edwardsvill; MS 82 Southern IL Univ-Edwardsvill; Chief of Aud, USAF Med Ctr Scott/SGHSE, **A**

Vernon, Mrs Estelle R 10504 Stable Lane, Potomac, MD 20854, (301) 299-3259, BS 71 Syracuse Univ; MA 74 Temple Univ; Aud, **A**

Vernon, Mrs Jean C 1004 Yardley Road, Morrisville, PA 19067, (215) 295-2028, BA 35 Depauw Univ; MA 41 Northwestern Univ; **LM**

Vernon, Mary Lou 5605 Hempstead Road, Madison, WI 53711, (608) 262-3951, BA Mundelein Coll; MA Northwestern Univ; 84–Clin Instr, Univ of WI, **SLP**

Vernon, Mrs Sharon L 1916 Arboro Place, Louisville, KY 40220, (502) 491-1141, BS 70 Indiana Univ of PA; MS 74 Univ of SC - Columbia; Sp-Lang Path, New Albany Floyd Cnty Schools, **SLP**

Vertes, Dr Dianne Dept Of Communication Sciences, Case Western Reserve Univ, Cleveland, OH 44106, (409) 761-2711, BA 67 MI St Univ; MA 68 MI St Univ; PH 76 (NS) Univ of TN - Knoxville; Asst Prof, Case Western Reserve Univ, **A**

Vertrees, Mrs Nancy Marie 11915 Barkman, Creve Coeur, MO 63141, (314) 994-1600, MS 87 Fontbonne Coll; 87–Sp-Lang Path, UCP Assoc of Greater St Louis Inc, **A**

Vertz, Steven P PO Box 1059, Thomasville, GA 31799-1059, (912) 439-7061, BS 82 Abilene Christian Univ; MS 86 Univ of MS; 88–Sp-Lang Path, Southwest GA Easter Rehab Ctr, **SLP**

Vescovich, Margaret A 331 Franklin Avenue, Cheltenham, PA 19012, (215) 842-6595, BA 77 Ramapo Coll of NJ; MS 80 PA St Univ - Univ Park; Sp-Lang Path, Med Coll of PA, **SLP**

Vesel, Mary A 879 N W 84th Drive, Coral Springs, FL 33071, (407) 495-3070, BS 73 Trenton St Coll; MS 77 William Paterson Coll; Sp-Lang Path, Pinecrest Rehab Hosp, **SLP**

Vesely, Donna M 36 Montraver Drive, Monessen, PA 15062, (412) 394-5815, BS 58 CA Univ of PA; ME 71 CA Univ of PA; 70–Sp/Lang Path, Allegheny Inter Ut, **SLP**

Vesely, Jean Cenaida 208 First Street South #2, Newton, IA 50208, (515) 964-2550, BA 81 Univ of IA; MA 85 Univ of IA; **SLP**

Vesely, Mrs Lorenza 3245 Fairmount Avenue, Bronx, NY 10465, (212) 824-6787, BA 77 CUNY - Lehman Coll; MS 78 Adelphi Univ; **SLP**

Vesper, Julie Anne 105 Quail Run Drive, Athens, GA 30606, (404) 542-4598, BS 81 Univ of MI - Ann Arbor; MS 83 Univ of MI - Ann Arbor; 86–Aud, University of Georgia, **A**

Vessels, Tina Helena 2552 East Alameda #45, Denver, CO 80209, (303) 778-6790, BA 82 Univ of CO - Boulder; MA 84 Univ of CO - Boulder; **SLP**

Vessna Drosdick, Danielle 5620 North Keystone, Chicago, IL 60646, (312) 583-4036, BA 77 Loyola Univ of Chicago; MS 79 Georgetown Univ; MA 82 Northwestern Univ; Sp-Lang Path, Chicago Bd of Educ Dist 3, **SLP**

Vest, Denise L 6605 Clayton Avenue #412, St Louis, MO 63139, (314) 647-3079, MA 88 Saint Louis Univ; 88–Sp-Lang Path, Neurorehab Ctrs of St Louis

Vest, Mrs Joyce C 1111 Hermitage Drive, Florence, AL 35630, (205) 766-3234, BA 72 Southwest MO St Univ; MA 82 Southwest MO St Univ; **SLP**

Vestal, Kelli Bell St Francis Hospital, Physical Medicine, 6161 South Yale Avenue, Tulsa, OK 74136, (918) 494-1474, BA 69 Olivet Coll; MA 72 IN Univ - Bloomington; 79–Cord of SLP & Aud, St Francis Hosp, **SLP**

Vestri, Jean Barnhart 353 Kyle Drive, Coppell, TX 75019, (214) 879-6178, MS 87 Univ of South FL; 87–Sp-Lang Path, Children's Med Ctr of Dallas, **SLP**

Vetere, Mrs Mary T Rd 6 Box 279, Indiana, PA 15701, (412) 357-0768, BS 73 Indiana Univ of PA; MA 76 Ball St Univ; 85–Sp-Lang Path, Private Practice, **SLP**

Vetrano, Elaine M 37 Maple Avenue, Bellport, NY 11713-2010, (516) 585-0100, BA 79 SUNY - Coll at Potsdam; MS 80 Ithaca Coll; Aud Coord, Assoc for Help of Ret Chld Inc, **A**

Vetter, Dolores Kluppel Dept Communicative Disorders, University Of Wisconsin, 1975 Willow Drive, Madison, WI 53706, (608) 262-3951, BA 57 Univ of CA - Los Angeles; MA 59 Univ of CA - Los Angeles; PH 62 (Psychology) Univ of CA - Los Angeles; Prof, U of WI-Madison

Vetter, Virginia 1332 West Avenue #J-4, Lancaster, CA 93534, (805) 945-1429, BS 82 WA St Univ; MS 87 Univ of WA; **SLP**

Vetter-Powell, Mrs Julie 3283 Davies Street, Green Bay, WI 54311, (414) 845-2371, BS 81 Univ of WI - Stevens Point; MA 83 Central MI Univ; Sp-Lang Path, Luxemburg-Casco Sch Dist, **SLP**

Veydt, Nicole 5 Wabash Avenue, Morgan, PA 15064, (412) 221-6805, BS 84 CA Univ of PA; MA 86 OH Univ - Athens; **SLP**

Veys, Mrs Susan Boden 5991 Parkchester Place, Dayton, OH 45459, (312) 386-4015, BS 79 Univ of IL - Urbana; MS 80 Univ of IL - Urbana; Sp-Lang Path, Centerville City Schools, **SLP**

Via, Mrs Pamela Rae 17 Ashley Drive, Newburgh, NY 12550, MA 70 Marshall Univ; 87–Sp-Lang Path, Newburgh DLC, **SLP**

Viafore, Mrs Joyce S Box 351, West Main Street, North Canaan, CT 06018, (413) 443-3531, BS 78 Univ of MA - Amherst; MA 80 Univ of MA - Amherst; Sp/Lang Path, Berkshire Rehab Cen, **SLP**

Viall, Mrs Anne Gallacher 8499 Monticello Drive, West Chester, OH 45069, (513) 868-2000, BA 74 Boston Coll; MA 76 OH St Univ; Sp-Lang Path, Hamilton Cty Sch Dist, **SLP**

Viamari-Williamson, Gina L 2089 N W 86th Way, Coral Springs, FL 33071, (305) 755-2875, BS 76 Univ of MA - Amherst; ME 78 Univ of VA - Charlottesville; SLP, Sp Path Inc, **SLP**

Viamontes, Mrs Karen Marie 75 Second Street Southwest, Britt, IA 50423, BA 80 NM St Univ; MA 83 NM St Univ; **SLP**

Vian, Emily K 4348 Valley Avenue, Pleasanton, CA 94566, (415) 426-4290, BA 80 CA St Univ - Northridge; MA 82 CA St Univ - Northridge; Sp/Lang Path, Pleasanton USD, **SLP**

Vian, Linda P O Box 1144, Laguna Beach, CA 92652-1144, (714) 494-6510, **SLP**

Viani, Lynn Marie 17 5th Avenue Apt#46, Pelham, NY 10803, (718) 520-7358, BA 79 Iona Coll; MA 82 CUNY - Queens Coll; 82–Sp/Lang Path, Westchester Except Chldn Sch, **SLP**

Vicars, Lee Ann Rural Route 4, Carbondale, IL 62901, (618) 833-5161, BS 61 Univ of Central AR; MS 63 Southern IL Univ -Carbondale; Training Coordinator, Anna Mental Health & Dev Ctr, **SLP**

Vice, Mrs Janna Hilliard RR 7 Box 502, Bloomington, IL 61701, (309) 827-3979, BS 80 Univ of IL - Urbana; MS 81 Univ of IL - Urbana; Bloomington Public Schools, **SLP**

Vicino, Mrs Jeroma L 2 South 551 River Oaks Dr, Warrenville, IL 60555, (312) 393-6446, BS 82 Northern IL Univ - De Kalb; MA 84 Northern IL Univ - De Kalb; Sp-Lang Path, School District 89, **SLP**

Vick, Mrs Marianne U 14015 West Virginia Drive, Lakewood, CO 80228, (303) 421-6945, BA 77 Univ of CO - Boulder; MA 79 Univ of CO - Boulder; SLP, Jefferson Co Pub Sch, **SLP**

Vicker, Beverly Anne 133 Lexington Road, Bloomington, IN 47401, (812) 855-6508, BS 67 Univ of WI - Madison; MS 68 Univ of WI - Madison; Sp/Lang Path, IN U-Inst for the Study of Dev Dis, **SLP ACE**

Vickerman, Katherine 121 Ricelan Drive, Simpsonville, SC 29681, (803) 297-8088, MA 78 Univ of SD - Vermillion; **SLP**

Vickers, William E 2640 Delany Road #201, Waukegan, IL 60087, (312) 336-3100, MA 52 Northwestern Univ, Retired, **SLP LM**

Vickery, Mrs Lori A 190 Holly Lane, Athens, GA 30606, (404) 543-5146, BS 85 Univ of GA; MS 87 Univ of HI - Manoa

Vicknair, Rose Marie Messers Mobile Manor #31, Pearl River, LA 70452, (504) 863-3772, BS 81 Univ Southern MS-Hattiesburg; MS 83 Univ Southern MS-Hattiesburg; 86–Sp-Lang Path, Picayune School System, **SLP**

VickRoy, Mrs Mille 6161 East Oak Street, Tucson, AZ 85711, (602) 790-1601, BS 41 Black Hills St Coll; MA 68 Univ of AZ; Retired, Private Practice, **SLP LM**

Victor, Mrs Constance P 116 Rogers Road, Furlong, PA 18925, (215) 794-8584, BA 62 CUNY - Queens Coll; MS 64 FL St Univ; Sp-Lang Path, Private Practice, **SLP**

Victor, Henry P 679 Davis Drive, Suite 105, New Market, ON, Canada L3Y 5G8, (416) 895-1422, BS 74 Kent St Univ; MA 75 Kent St Univ; Aud, York Audiology Service, **A**

Victor, Judith A 9180 Lakeside Avenue, Angola, NY 14006, (716) 532-5522, BS 70 SUNY - Coll at Buffalo; MS 75 SUNY - Center at Buffalo; Sp-Path-Audiology Coord, Jn Adam Dev Disordrs Serv Off, **SLP**

Victor, Mrs Lois Ann 400 Fox Crest Court, Terre Haute, IN 46803, (812) 877-2071, BA 75 Bowling Green St Univ; MA 81 Bowling Green St Univ; Sp/Lang Path, **SLP**

Victor, Mrs Shelley J 4230 N W 107th Avenue, Coral Springs, FL 33065, (305) 475-7075, BA 73 SUNY - Center at Stony Brook; MA 78 Univ of Miami; 87–Sp-Lang Path, Nova Univ, **SLP ACE**

Victor-Beale, Margaret C 78 Satchell Boulevard, West Hill, ON, Canada M1C 3B4, BA 71 Univ of Akron; MA 73 Kent St Univ; **SLP**

Victoria, Kristen Jean Mount Vernon Drive #43D, Vernon, CT 06066, (203) 871-9294, MA 87 Univ of CT; 87–Sp-Lang Path, Enfield PS, **SLP**

Vidal, Nancy Stella 94-04 66th Avenue, Rego Park, NY 11374, (212) 960-2888, BS 80 CUNY - City College; MA 87 CUNY - Hunter Coll; Sp-Lang Path, Montefiore/NC Bronx Hosp, **SLP**

Videlock, Dr Joyce L Saint Christopher's Hospital For Children, 2603 North 5th Street, Philadelphia, PA 19133, (215) 427-5590, BS 71 Ithaca Coll; MA 76 Univ of Pittsburgh - Pittsburgh; PH 79 (Sp Path) Univ of Pittsburgh - Pittsburgh; 87–Mgr-Psych Svcs, Philadelphia Early Childhood Evaluation Ctr, **SLP**

Vidolin, Faith Friedland 575 New Dover Road, Iselin, NJ 08830, (201) 388-2493, BA 84 Kean Coll of NJ; MA 85 Kean Coll of NJ; 86–Sp-Lang Path, Monroe Twsp Bd of Educ, **SLP**

Vidrine-Bralley, Jean C 1720 Essex Road, Charlottesville, VA 22901, (804) 295-8472, BS 69 Univ of Southwestern LA; ME 76 Univ of VA - Charlottesville; **SLP**

Viedrah, Beverly G 15938 Addison Court, Southfield, MI 48075, (313) 258-1090, BS 56 Wayne St Univ; ME 62 Wayne St Univ; Super/Diagn Servs, William Beaumont Hosp, **SLP**

Viehweg, Elizabeth R 19350 Azure Road, Deephaven, MN 55391, (612) 473-9643, BS 79 Univ of TX - Austin; MS 82 Northwestern Univ; 88–Sp-Lang Path, Courage Ctr, **SLP**

Viehweg, Dr Steven H Dept Of Comm Disorders Umc 10, Utah State University, Logan, UT 84322-1000, (801) 750-1387, BS 63 UT St Univ; MS 65 UT St Univ; PH 68 (NS) Northwestern Univ; Assoc Prof, Utah St Univ, **A**

Vieira, Mrs Rhonda Honora 1041 Raymond Road, Hanford, CA 93230, (209) 584-1441, MA 84 CA St Univ - Fresno; SLP, Kings Co Supt of Schs, **SLP**

Vielgut, Mrs Kathleen Marie 4259 North 104th Street Apartment #5, Milwaukee, WI 53222, (414) 961-4174, BS 86 Marquette Univ; MS 87 Marquette Univ; 87–Sp-Lang Path, Columbia Hosp

Vienna, Barbara Hoefner 255 Arcadia Parkway, Rochester, NY 14612, (716) 663-7394, **SLP**

Vierima, Carol A 333 West Superior, Duluth, MN 55802, (218) 722-0775, BA 77 Univ of SD - Vermillion; MA 77 Univ of SD - Vermillion; Owner, Advantage Hearing Ctr, **A**

Vierling, Mrs Evelyn Annette W 927 Napoli Drive, St Louis, MO 63021, (314) 768-3037, BS 79 Southeast MO St Univ; MS 81 Fontbonne Coll; Sp-Lang Path, Deaconess Hosp, **SLP**

Viers, Mrs Davenda Allen 5136 West Timbervue Court, Peoria, IL 61615, **SLP**

Viers, Mrs Joellen Robertson 636 Ashley Avenue, Woodland, CA 95695, (916) 661-6145, BS 61 OH St Univ; MA 85 Humboldt St Univ; 88–Sp-Lang Path, Coastal Assess & Therapy Svcs

Vig, Sheri Eder 1748 Newcastle Drive, Jenison, MI 49428, (616) 457-1877, BA 83 MI St Univ; MA 84 MI St Univ; Sp-Lang Path, Jenison PS, **SLP**

Vigdor-Peck, Lisa 2723 Ordway Street N W #5, Washington, DC 20008, BS 80 Syracuse Univ; MA 82 IN Univ - Bloomington; 83–Sp-Lang Path, Montgomery Co Pub Sch, **SLP**

Viger, Mrs Wendy W 225 Silver Maple, Mandeville, LA 70448, (504) 626-3770, BS 76 LA St Univ - Baton Rouge; MS 77 Univ of AL- Tuscaloosa; SLP, Educational Associates of S E, **SLP**

Viggiano, Christine 2432 South Camac Street, Philadelphia, PA 19148, (609) 881-8678, BA 80 Temple Univ; MA 82 Temple Univ; Sp/Lang Path, UCP Ctr of Gloucester Salem Co, **SLP**

Vigil, Elizabeth Tuttle 714 Cardinal Street, Colorado Springs, CO 80911, (303) 423-4878, BA 75 Univ of Northern CO; MA 78; **SLP**

Vigil, Marie Elizabeth 2012 Calle DE Suenos, Las Cruces, NM 88001, (505) 523-5884, BA 80 NM St Univ; MA 83 NM St Univ; 88–Sp-Lang Path, Las Cruces PS, **SLP**

Vigilante, Carla 2536 Yorkstown #209, Houston, TX 77056, **SLP**

Viglietta, Sarah Marie 137 Olivia Drive, Rochester, NY 14626, (716) 225-1914, BA 84 SUNY - Center at Buffalo; MA 86 SUNY - Center at Buffalo; **A**

Viguerie, Susan Mouton 709 South Ryan, Lake Charles, LA 70601, (318) 433-1775, MS 84 Univ of Southwestern LA; 88–Sp-Lang Path, St Patrick Sp & Hrng Ctr, **SLP**

Vilardi, Mrs Mary Ann Miller 185 Roberts Street, Holbrook, NY 11791, (516) 543-5100, BA 83 SUNY - Coll at New Paltz; MS 86 CUNY - Hunter Coll; **SLP**

Vilda, Rebecca R 1220 Village Road #4, Iowa City, IA 52240, (319) 356-0445, BS 71 Univ of NE - Lincoln; MA 72 Univ of NE - Lincoln; 84–SLP, U of IA Hosp & Clinics, **SLP**

Vilensons, Mrs Virginia 3165 Wasteside Circle, Las Vegas, NV 89117-2055, (702) 363-9379, BS 70 Univ of IA; MA 71 Univ of IA; Sp-Lang Path, **SLP**

Vilker-Krause, Mrs Nancy K 331 S Kools Street #7, Appleton, WI 54914, (414) 749-9191, BS 85 Univ of WI - Madison; MS 87 Univ of WI - Madison; Sp-Lang Path, Menasha School District

Villani, Christine 6 Strawberry Hill Road, Milford, CT 06460, (203) 637-1440, BS 77 Mercy Coll; MA 78 Hofstra Univ; MA 85 New Sch for Social Research; Sp-Lang Path, Greenwich Bd of Ed, **SLP**

Villano, Dorothy Marie 17 Marwood Lane, Yonkers, NY 10701, (212) 860-7800, BA 71 CUNY - Hunter Coll; MA 81 NY Univ; SLP, Flower Hosp Dev Disabl Cl, **SLP**

Villarreal, Jesse J 5104 Crestway Drive, Austin, TX 78731, (512) 454-8075, BA 35 Univ of TX - Austin; MA 37 Univ of TX - Austin; PH 47 Northwestern Univ; **SLP F LM**

Villella, Gina M 4031 Emerald Lane #B, Bowie, MD 20716, (301) 297-7810, BS 80 Clarion Univ of PA; MS 81 Clarion Univ of PA; Sp-Lang Path, Prince Georges Public School, **SLP**

Villemaire, Judy A 105 Leclair Street, Winooski, VT 05404, (607) 272-8879, BS 86 SUNY - Coll at Plattsburgh; MS 87 Ithaca Coll; **SLP**

Villere, Kathleen C 18185 Lakeview Lane, Monument, CO 80132, (719) 630-5200, BA 77 Univ of WI - Eau Claire; MA 78 Univ of Northern CO; Sp/Lang Path, Penrose Hosp, **SLP**

Villwock, Mrs Martha M 1725 Winding Drive, North Wales, PA 19454, (215) 699-1966, BA 74 TX Woman's Univ; MS 80 TX Woman's Univ; Sp-Lang Path, Private Practice, **SLP**

Vilmos, Mrs Madeleine 8 Scarsdale Farm Road, Scarsdale, NY 10583, (914) 472-1911, BA 59 CUNY - Hunter Coll; MS 60 Syracuse Univ; Sp-Lang Path, St Cabrini Nurs Home, **SLP**

Vince, Mrs Virginia Jackson HC 69 Box 750, St Francisville, LA 70775, (504) 635-6579, BS 78 LA St Univ - Baton Rouge; MA 83 LA St Univ - Baton Rouge; Sp-Lang Path, Feliciana Forensic Facility, **SLP**

Vincent, Amy Elizabeth 1069 Mount Royal #1-A, Kalamazoo, MI 49009, (616) 375-3908, 88 Western MI Univ

Vincent, Mrs April 2624 Verano, Modesto, CA 95355, (209) 521-2609, BA 78 Brigham Young Univ; OM 79 Brigham Young Univ; **SLP**

Vincent, Mrs Carol A 1122 Lynnwood, Carthage, TX 75633, (214) 693-2410, BS 65 Stephen F Austin St Univ; MA 69 Stephen F Austin St Univ; Sp/Lang Path, Carthage ISD, **SLP**

Vincent, Mrs Linda J 2425 Benton, Granite City, IL 62040, (314) 645-8510, BA 74 Southern IL Univ-Edwardsvill; MS 75 Southern IL Univ-Edwardsvill; Dir of Rehab, Deaconess Hosp, **SLP**

Vincent, Lisa Ellen 1524 San Rocco Circle, Stockton, CA 95207, (209) 944-4486, BA 82 Univ of the Pacific; MS 84 Univ of TX - Dallas; SLP, Stockton USD, **SLP**

Vincent, Patricia J Pee Dee Speech & Hearing Ctr, P O Box 804, 153 North Baroody Street, Florence, SC 29503, (803) 662-7802, BS 58 East TN St Univ; MA 68 East TN St Univ; Exec Dir, Pee Dee Sp & Hrng Cen, **SLP**

Vincent, Tambra Russom 41 Hemlock, Altus, OK 73521, (405) 482-5944, BA 81 San Diego St Univ; MA 83 San Diego St Univ; Sp-Lang Path, Charleston Co Sch, **SLP**

Vincent, Vernon Lee 820 Alberta Avenue, Santa Barbara, CA 93101, (805) 966-7344, BA 84 Univ of CA - Santa Barbara; MS 86 Univ of CA - Santa Barbara; **A**

Vincent, Vicki Lynn East 3282 Highway 106, Union, WA 98592, (206) 898-3376, BA Eastern WA Univ; MS 85 Eastern WA Univ; SLP, Educational Services Dist #123, **SLP**

Vine, Deborah Louise 232 Florence Avenue, Willowdale, ON, Canada M2N 1G6, (416) 451-1710, BS 80 Univ of Western Ontario; OM 84 Univ of Western Ontario; **SLP**

Vines, Mrs Shannan Hinrichs 15955 S W Bull Mountain Rd, Tigard, OR 97224, (503) 228-6479, BA 82 UT St Univ; MS 84 Boston Univ; Sp-Lang Path, Portland Ctr Hring & Speech, **SLP**

Vinograd, Margaretha Miller Glenwood Estates, Saranac Lake, NY 12983, (518) 891-5802, BA 71 SUNY - Center at Stony Brook; MA 76 SUNY - Center at Buffalo; 84–Coordinator Speech & Hearing, Sunmount Developmental Center, **SLP**

Vinopal, Mary C 700 Salem Drive #315, Hoffman Estates, IL 60194, (312) 742-1040, BS 78 Eastern IL Univ; MS 79 Eastern IL Univ; Sp-Lang Path, Elgin Men Hlth Cen, **SLP**

Vinski, Mrs Cathy B 326 Libourel Road, South Plainfield, NJ 07080, (201) 754-4620, BS 80 Clarion Univ of PA; MA 81 Kent St Univ; Sp/Lang Path, S Plainfield Bd of Ed, **SLP**

Vinson, Mrs Betty P 1128 N W 36th Street, Gainesville, FL 32605, (904) 376-7533, BA 75 Emory Univ; OM 76 Emory Univ; Clin Super, U of FL, **SLP**

Vinson, Mrs Jennifer Herndon 1720 Ward Avenue, Huntsville, AL 35801, (205) 859-7368, BS 79 AL A & M Univ; MS 81 Radford Univ; Assist Dir/Cl Supvr, Alabama A & M University, **SLP ACE**

Vinson, Mrs Lynette Hanke Rt 2 Box 137-D, Odessa, MO 64076, (816) 229-3869, BS 80 Central MO St Univ; MS 83 Central MO St Univ; Sp-Lang Path, Rainbow Ctr for Cd, **SLP**

Vinton, Ava M 710 Wedgewood, Cortez, CO 81321, (303) 565-6666, BA 78 MI St Univ; MA 80 Western MI Univ; 88–Sp-Lang Path, Southwest Memorial Hosp, **SLP**

Vinyard, Mrs Allison J R R 6, Roxanne #92, Carbondale, IL 62901, (618) 549-6480, MS 88 Southern IL Univ -Carbondale

Violick-Boole, Kathryn 19 Ledgetree Road, Medfield, MA 02052, (617) 359-2324, BS 78 Univ of NH; MS 79 Columbia Univ Teachers Coll; Sp-Lang Path, Spaulding Rehab Hosp, **SLP**

Vircks, Bruce E Wolfe Clinic Pc, 309 East Church Street, Marshalltown, IA 50158, (515) 752-1565, BS 77 Univ of WI - Madison; MS 81 Univ of WI - Madison; Aud, Wolfe Clinic Pc, **A**

Virzi, Jerome I 23 Redfern Drive, Churchville, NY 14428, (712) 293-1586, BS 70 Univ of MA - Amherst; MS 75 SUNY - Coll at Geneseo; SLP, Spencerport Cen Sch, **SLP**

Visconti, Mrs Colleen Fitzgerald 801 Cooper Landing Road Apartment A411, Cherry Hill, NJ 08002, (609) 482-5943, BA 86 Case Western Reserve Univ; MS 88 PA St Univ - Univ Park; 88–Sp-Lang Path, Ken-Crest Services

Visconti, Joann Rose Marie 1211 Sandburg Place, Newark, DE 19702, (302) 733-1010, BS 82 Seton Hall Univ; MA 84 OH St Univ; Sp-Lang Path, Med Ctr of DE, **SLP**

Visencio, Louis H 1685 Heritage Trail, Camarillo, CA 93010, MA 75; 82–Sp-Lang Path, Camarillo State Hosp, **SLP**

Visnick, Mrs Joyce Dragash 7715 Falstaff Road, Mc Lean, VA 22102, (703) 821-1394, BA 67 MI St Univ; MA 68 Wayne St Univ; **SLP**

Visoky, Mrs Anita M 4979 South Barton Road, Lyndhurst, OH 44124, (216) 382-7700, BA 75 Cleveland St Univ; MA 76 Cleveland St Univ; 76–Sp/Lang Path, S Euclid-Lyndhurst Sch, **SLP**

Visser-Dumont, Leslie Jean 1757 Sitka Avenue, Simi Valley, CA 93063, (805) 522-6942, MA 87 CA St Univ - Northridge; 88–Aud, Kaiser Permanente Med Group, **A**

Vissering, Christine Denise Box 281, Hopewell, NJ 08525, (609) 466-3165, BA 72 SUNY - Center at Stony Brook; ME 78 Trenton St Coll; Sp-Lang Path, New Hanover Township School, **SLP**

Visto, Mrs Jane Ackerman Route 1 Box 21, Guelph, ND 58447, (605) 622-7716, BS 84 Northern St Coll; MS 87 Moorhead St Univ; 88–Dir of Sp-Lang Path, Northern State

Viswanath, Nagalapura S Stuttering Center, Baylor College Of Medicine, 6501 Fannin Street, Houston, TX 77030, (718) 799-6331, BS 67 All India Inst of Sp & Hrng; MS 72 All India Inst of Sp & Hrng; PH 86 (Sp Science & Sp Path) CUNY - Grad Sch & Univ Cntr; 86–Post-Doctoral Fellow, Stuttering Ctr/Baylor Coll, **SLP**

Vitagliano, Mary Louise 7758 #10 New Providence Dr, Falls Church, VA 22042, (301) 299-6714, BS 81 Radford Univ; MS 83 Radford Univ; **A**

Vitaglione, Mrs Joanne S 33 Fort Hill Road, Yonkers, NY 10710, (914) 337-3500, BA 75 CUNY - Lehman Coll; MA 77 CUNY - Lehman Coll; 80–Dir, Private Practice, **SLP ACE**

Vitale, Mrs Joyce D 8 Tinker Lane, Greenwich, CT 06830, (203) 869-8613, BA 65 Temple Univ; MA 67 Temple Univ; 88–Sp-Lang Path, Greenwich PS, **SLP**

Vitali, Gary John Eastern Ky Speech & Hrng Clinic, 2101 Nicholasville Road, Suite 104, Lexington, KY 40503, (606) 277-0491, BS 74 SUNY - Coll at Fredonia; MA 80 Marshall Univ; Dir of SLP Serv, Eastern KY Sp & Hrng Cln, **SLP**

Vitali, Marie Elizabeth Rt 4 Box 209, Versailles, KY 40383, (606) 873-5004, BS 78 SUNY - Coll at Geneseo; MA 83 Eastern KY Univ; SLP, Sp Therapy Assoc, **SLP**

Vito, Mrs Lia Uustal 17 Nardone Road, Needham, MA 02192, (617) 444-6197, BA 71 SUNY - Center at Albany; ME 79 Northeastern Univ; **SLP**

Vitone, Sherry Fundoots 215 South Mantua Street, Kent, OH 44240, (216) 425-8474, BS 78 Indiana Univ of PA; MA 85 Kent St Univ

Vitori, Mrs Laurie J 879 Crestwood Drive, North Huntingdon, PA 15642, (412) 864-5727, MA 83 Kent St Univ; 78–Sp-Lang Path, Struthers City Schools, **SLP**

Vitrano, Mrs Jennifer Duff 1020 Bayridge Terrace, Gaithersburg, MD 20878, (301) 330-9222, BS 81 Andrews Univ; MA 83 Eastern KY Univ; Sp-Lang Path, Treatment Centers, **SLP**

Vitt, Mrs Melissa Engelsmann 6016 Chalet Court #5220, Dallas, TX 75205, (214) 644-2076, BA 84 Denison Univ; MA 86 Saint Louis Univ

Vitulli, Deborah 1475 S W 53rd Street, Corvallis, OR 97333, (503) 753-0585, ME 87 Western OR St Coll

Vivaldi, Ann M Urb El Rosario 3 #36, Yauco, PR 00768, (809) 856-1171, **SLP**

Viviano, Ann K 2017 East Van Buren #7, Colorado Springs, CO 80909, (303) 630-5200, BS 75 CO St Univ; MA 82 Univ of Northern CO; 86–Sp-Lang Path, Penrose Hosp, **SLP**

Viviano, Cheryl S 359 Cold Spring Road, Syosset, NY 11791-1805, **SLP**

Viviano, Mrs Karen Elizabeth 13 Ridgelawn Court, Florissant, MO 63031, (314) 837-3662, MA 87 Saint Louis Univ; 87–Sp-Lang Path, Sisters of St Mary's Rehab Inst

Vivrette, Deanne 509 South Melton Drive, Jonesboro, AR 72401, (501) 935-5004, OM 86 AR St Univ

Vledder, Gayle Lynn 1765 Winchester Drive, Muskegon, MI 49441, (616) 866-2888, BS 80 Western MI Univ; MA 82 Western MI Univ; SLP, Northview Public Schools, **SLP**

Vockroth, Mrs Rebecca Dessauer 416 South Pierce Street, New Orleans, LA 70119, (504) 830-4424, BA 75 LA St Univ - Baton Rouge; OM 77 LA St Univ - N O Medical Ctr; Sp-Lang Path, Jefferson Parish Sch Bd, **SLP**

Voda, Jerrilyn A 1008 West 20th Place, Chicago, IL 60608, (312) 908-2556, BS 70 De Paul Univ; MS 71 Southern IL Univ -Carbondale; 79–Sp-Lnag Path, Rehab I of Chicago, **SLP ACE**

Vodev, Michelle C 2810 North Powers Drive, Apartment 60, Orlando, FL 32818, (305) 297-3776, BS 72 OH Univ - Athens; ME 74 Clarion Univ of PA; Sp-Lang Path, Magnolia School, **SLP**

Vodicka, Diana Mary 819 Dueno Court, Manitowoc, WI 54220, (414) 684-3138, BA 74 Coll of Notre Dame of MD; MS 86 Univ of WI - Stevens Point; 87–Sp-Lang Path, Holy Family Med Ctr, **SLP**

Voegeli, Mrs Beth Carson 549 Summit Avenue, Monticello, WI 53570, (608) 938-4194, BS 82 Univ of WI - Oshkosh; MS 84 Univ of WI - Stevens Point; 87–Sp-Lang Path, Monticello Sch Dist, **SLP**

Voeks, Dr Susan K P O Box 37, Nelsonville, WI 54458, (715) 341-9361, BS 71 Univ of WI - Stevens Point; MS 72 Univ of WI - Stevens Point; PH 84 (NS) Univ of IA; Sp/Lang Path, Private Practice, **SLP**

Voelker, Diane J Ross Hearing Center, 6111 Harrison Street, 311 Merrillville Center, Merrillville, IN 46410, (219) 980-6030, BS 75 Univ of WI - Oshkosh; MS 78 Univ of WI - Madison; Owner, Ross Hrng Cen, **A**

Voelker, Mrs Evelyn G 3716 Covert Road, Pontiac, MI 48054, (313) 673-7518, BS 46 Eastern MI Univ; MS 60 Univ of MI - Ann Arbor; **SLP A LM**

Voelpel, Mrs Judith Ann 19 Prince Street, Baldwin, NY 11510, (516) 825-9131, **SLP**

Voge, Mrs Margaret Lennertz 2531 East Richards Place, Tucson, AZ 85716, (602) 327-3712, BA 79 CA St Univ - Long Beach; MA 81 CA St Univ - Long Beach; Sp-Lang Path, Tucson USD, **SLP**

Vogel, Mrs Carolyn Sue 7890 Mulberry Street, Maineville, OH 45039, (513) 867-2473, OB 80 Miami Univ - Oxford; MS 81 Miami Univ - Oxford; Sp-Lang Path, Fort Hamilton Hughes Hosp, **SLP**

Vogel, Dr Deanie Speech Pathology Department, VA Hospital, 7400 Merton Minter Blvd, San Antonio, TX 78284, (512) 694-5209, BA 69 Univ of MO - KS City; MA 71 Univ of KS; PH 81 (Sp Path) Univ of KS; Sp-Lang Path, VA Hosp, **SLP ACE**

Vogel, Debra G 38 Windham Way, Englishtown, NJ 07726, (201) 536-7465, BA 76 CUNY - Brooklyn Coll; MS 80 Adelphi Univ; Sp-Lang Path, Bd of Ed Sp Servs Ut, **SLP**

Vogel, Donald Allen 439 16th Street, Brooklyn, NY 11215, (718) 604-5354, BA 75 Adelphi Univ; MS 77 Adelphi Univ; 85–Aud, Kingsbrook Jewish Med Ctr, **A**

Vogel, Karen L 104 Meadow Drive, Gretna, NE 68028, (402) 332-3341, BS 72 Northern IL Univ - De Kalb; MA 74 Northern IL Univ - De Kalb; Sp-Lang Path, Gretna Public Schools, **SLP ACE**

Vogel, Laura B 8415 Geyser Avenue, Northridge, CA 91324, (805) 482-1964, BA CUNY - Brooklyn Coll; MA CUNY - Brooklyn Coll; Sp-Lang Path, Pleasant Valley Sch Dist, **SLP**

Vogel, Mrs Lorilyn King 2932 Taylor Avenue, Ogden, UT 84403, (801) 479-8030, BS 83 Brigham Young Univ; OM 85 Brigham Young Univ; Sp-Lang Path, Weber Co Sch Dist, **SLP**

Vogel, Mrs Nancy Wind 11 Acorn Street #3, Cambridge, MA 02139, (617) 491-0600, BS 83 SUNY - Coll at Oneonta; MS 85 Emerson Coll; 88–Sp-Lang Path, Cambridge-Somerville Interv Prog, **SLP**

Vogelhuber, Barbara Wickson 119 Tree Crest Circle, The Woodlands, TX 77381, BA 76 OH St Univ; MA 78 OH St Univ; Aud, **A**

Vogelman, Mrs Lura H 620 Overbrook Road, Baltimore, MD 21212, (301) 377-9405, BA 69 Towson St Univ; MS 87 Loyola Coll; **SLP**

Vogelsang, Ellen Speech & Language Clinic, 111 N Last Chance Gulch, Suite 4C, Helena, MT 59601, (406) 449-2736, BA 77 Univ of MT; MA 79 Univ of Northern CO; Sp-Lang Path, Speech & Language Clinic, **SLP**

Vogelsang, Dr Mary Ann Trombetta Route 2 Box 538-M, Cape Girardeau, MO 63701, (314) 651-2488, BA 61 West Liberty St Coll; MA 62 OH St Univ; PH 76 (NS) OH St Univ; 62–Prof of Sp, S E MO St U, **SLP**

Vogelsang, Dr Robert W Department Of Speech, Portland State University, P O Box 751, Portland, OR 97207, (503) 464-3531, BA 53 Univ of CA - Santa Barbara; MA 58 WA St Univ; ED 65 (Curriculum & Instruct/Communication) WA St Univ; 70–Prof, Portland State Univ, **SLP**

Vogelson, Douglas O 408 9th Avenue, Charles City, IA 50616, (515) 394-2162, BS 73 Univ of WI - Whitewater; MS 75 Univ of WI - Stevens Point; Aud, Keystone AEA, **A**

Vogelstein, Mrs Ilene C 3700 Breton Way, Baltimore, MD 21208, (301) 653-0909, BS 74 Coll of Notre Dame of MD; MA 75 Loyola Coll; 88–Sp-Lang Path, Madeline Fox Assoc Inc, **SLP**

Vogen, Barbra Dickinson 950 Office Park Road, Suite 333, West Des Moines, IA 50265, (515) 224-0979, BS 72 Univ of WI - River Falls; MS 73 Southern IL Univ -Carbondale; Sp-Lang Path, Central Rehabilitation, **SLP**

Vogen, Dr Clifford Stin 4513 99th Street, Urbandale, IA 50322, (515) 438-2600, BS 64 Northern IL Univ - De Kalb; MA 66 Northern IL Univ - De Kalb; PH 74 (NS) Southern IL Univ -Carbondale; Treat Serv Dir, Woodward State Hosp Sch, **SLP A**

Voges, Kathryn Biles 502 Grant Place, Corpus Christi, TX 78411, (512) 884-2903, BS 76 Univ of TX - Austin; MA 82 Univ of TX - Austin; Aud, Ear Nose & Throat Assoc, **A**

Vogl, Beate R 324 Overdale Road, Pittsburgh, PA 15221, **SLP**

Vogl, Mrs Laura Anne 222 Ridgewood Drive, Syracuse, NY 13206-2458, (315) 437-6925, BA 81 SUNY - Coll at Cortland; MA 83 SUNY - Center at Buffalo; Sp-Lang Path, Syracuse City Sch Dist, **SLP**

Vogler-Ryan, Sasha 8505 Langtree Lane, Raleigh, NC 27612, (919) 846-2684, MS 80 Univ of NC - Chapel Hill; Dept Hd/SLP, Rehab Cen Hndcpd, **SLP**

Vogt, Mrs Anne Christine P O Box 818, Estes Park, CO 80517-0818, (303) 586-8607, BA 79 Univ of MI - Ann Arbor; MS 81 Univ of MI - Ann Arbor; Sp/Lang Path Tchr, Jefferson Parish Sch, **SLP**

Vogt, Mrs Donna Crinklaw 600 Country Club Road, Newport News, VA 23606, (804) 596-3049, BS 76 TX Christian Univ; MS 77 TX Christian Univ; Instr, Christopher Newport Coll, **SLP**

Vogt, Dr Eugenia F 8907 Odessa Avenue, Sepulveda, CA 91343, BA 45 Keuk Coll; MA 47 SUNY - Center at Albany; PH 73 (Commun Disord) Univ of Southern CA; Sp-Lang Path, LA Co Ofc of Educ, **SLP**

Vogt, Dr Gayle H 502 Riviera Court, Fullerton, CA 92635, (714) 992-0830, MA 72 Montclair St Coll; PH 85 (NS) Claremont Graduate Sch; Lecturer, CA State Fullerton, **SLP**

Vogt, Mrs Kathleen Casey 328 Metz Street, Erie, PA 16508, (814) 455-4150, BS 80 SUNY - Coll at Fredonia; MA 81 Bowling Green St Univ; Sp-Lang Path, Dr Gertrude A Barber Center, **SLP**

Voiers, William D Dynastat Inc, 2704 Rio Grande Suite 4, Austin, TX 78705, (512) 476-4797, BA 48; OM 49 Univ of TX - Austin; PH 52 (Psychology) Univ of TX - Austin; Pres/Dir Res, Dynastat Inc

Voita, Cathy Lynn 35755 Terrace Court, Farmington Hills, MI 48331, (313) 478-8734, BS 83 Western MI Univ; MS 85 Univ of MI - Ann Arbor; St Joseph Mercy Hosp, **SLP**

Voitier, Mrs Vicki Langston P O Box 938, Opelousas, LA 70570, (318) 948-8211, BA 69 LA St Univ - Baton Rouge; MA 71 LA St Univ - Baton Rouge; Sp-Lang Path, St Landry Parish School Board, **SLP**

Vojnovic, Olga 2940 Northway, Windsor, ON, Canada N93 4E9, (519) 969-2179, MA 88 Wayne St Univ

Vokes, Jimmie Ann 351 Thunderbird #16, El Paso, TX 79912, (915) 584-3403, BA 75 Univ of TX - El Paso; MS 86 Univ of TX - El Paso; 88–Assistive Devices Coord, Educ Svc Ctr

Volin, Dr Robert A 330 Alpine Drive, Peekskill, NY 10566, (212) 960-6084, BA 67 CUNY - Queens Coll; MA 74 CUNY - City College; PH 83 (Agrammatism) CUNY - Grad Sch & Univ Cntr; Assoc Dir-Sp-Lang Path, Lehman Coll, **SLP**

Volk, Barbara Berger 5806 Schade Drive, Midland, MI 48640-2598, (517) 835-5518, BS 73 Purdue Univ - West Lafayette; MA 82 Central MI Univ; 73–SLP, Midland Pub Sch, **SLP**

Volkert, Kristin Kay 13670 Valley View Road, #108, Eden Prairie, MN 55344, (612) 588-0811, BA 84 Univ of WI - Eau Claire; MS 87 Marquette Univ; 88–Sp-Lang Path, Courage Ctr

Volkland, Mrs Effie E Rural Route 3, Rolling Meadows, Nevada, MO 64772, (417) 667-3224, BS 69 Univ of KS; MA 70 Univ of KS; ED 79 (NS) Pittsburg St Univ; Sp-Lang Path, Nevada R5 Sch Dist, **SLP LM**

Volkman, Mrs Therese Marie 4061 Charleston Road, Matteson, IL 60443, (312) 496-3330, BS 82 IL St Univ - Normal; OM 85 Governors St Univ

Volland, Mrs Bonnie L 17071 Dolphin Drive, North Redington Beach, FL 33708, (813) 397-1431, BS 75 Univ of WI - Milwaukee; MS 76 Marquette Univ; **SLP**

Vollertsen, Cathleen M 850 Congdon Avenue #12, Elgin, IL 60120-2570, BS 78 IL St Univ - Normal; MS 80 IL St Univ - Normal; Sp/Lang Path, Commun Ut Sch Dist #300, **SLP**

Volles, Bianca Lauro 25 Stewart Place #712, Mount Kisco, NY 10549, (914) 277-4344, BA 80 Univ of CT; MS 82 Southern CT St Univ; Sp/Lang Path, Somers Ctrl Sch Dist, **SLP**

Vollmer, Mrs Deborah Kay 2807 North 49th Avenue, Omaha, NE 68104, (402) 331-6954, MS 79 Univ of NE - Omaha; SLP, Ralston Public Schools, **SLP**

Vollmer, Sandra Marie 5306 East Courtney Avenue, Castle Rock, CO 80104, (303) 688-9510, BS 82 TX Christian Univ; MA 84 Univ of Denver; Sp-Lang Path, Douglas Co Pub Sch, **SLP**

Volpe, Mrs Ann Lechner 115 Prairie #1, Highwood, IL 60040, (312) 256-0211, BS 76 IL St Univ - Normal; MS 78 IL St Univ - Normal; Sp-Lang Path, Wilmette Public School 39, **SLP**

Volpe, Kathleen A 9519 55th Street Court W, Tacoma, WA 98467, (206) 593-2068, OM 75 Univ of WA; BA 69 WA St Univ; SLP, Tacoma Sch Dist, **SLP**

Voltz, Mrs Kathy Ingram 1621 Alaca Place, Tuscaloosa, AL 35401, (205) 553-4550, BS 74 Auburn Univ - Auburn; OM 75 Auburn Univ - Auburn; Sp-Lang Path, Partlow State Sch & Hosp, **SLP**

Volz, Dr Helen Breon Rd 1 Box 459A, Centre Hall, PA 16828, (814) 234-6760, BS 58 PA St Univ - Univ Park; MS 65 PA St Univ - Univ Park; PH 75 (NS) PA St Univ - Univ Park; 88–Sp-Lang Path, Centre Community Hosp, **SLP ACE**

Volz, Pamela Rosen 139 Cypress Drive, Pittsburgh, PA 15241, (412) 622-4484, MA 83 Univ of IL - Urbana; Sp-Lang Path, St Francis Hospital, **SLP**

Vom Eigen, Beth Ann 711 Cooney Road, Caledonia, NY 14423, (716) 275-2992, BA 69 WV Wesleyan Coll; ME 74 Univ of Louisville; Asst Prof, Sp-Lang Path, **ACE**

Von Achen, Mrs Deborah Goldman 5792 Middlecoff Drive, Huntington Beach, CA 92649, (714) 840-6747, BA 76 CA St Univ - Fullerton; MS 77 Southern Methodist Univ; Sp-Lang Path, Easter Seals Living Skill Prog, **SLP**

Von Almen, Peggy G 729 Pleasantdale Crossing, Doraville, GA 30340, (404) 963-6713, BS 71 AR St Univ; ES 88 UT St Univ; 88–Aud, Gwinnett County PS, **SLP A ACE**

Vonasek, Denise Wamre 12355 Oak Park Boulevard NE #214, Blaine, MN 55434, (612) 754-0103, BS 86 ND St Univ; MA 87 Univ of MN - Duluth; 88–Sp-Lang Path, Cambridge-Isanti ISD #911, **SLP**

Von Bargen, Dawn Marie Kingswood Gardens, 218 Fulton Street #1 B, Farmingdale, NY 11735, (516) 454-0991, BS 84 Elmira Coll; MA 85 Bowling Green St Univ; **A**

Von Berg, Mrs Sarah J 35 Palermo Drive, Oroville, CA 95966, (916) 534-4241, BA 73 CA St Univ - Chico; MA 74 CA St Univ - Chico; SLP, Butte County Supt Schools, **SLP**

Von Boeck, Evonne Pusan American School, Apo, San Francisco, CA 96259-0005, BS 76 AZ St Univ; Sp-Lang Path, Dept of Defense Depend Sch, **SLP**

Von Cloedt, Dr Carol Denise 3715 Port Royale Lane, Phoenix, AZ 85023, (602) 279-2580, BA 72 Southeast MO St Univ; MA 73 Southeast MO St Univ; PH 81 (NS) Southern IL Univ -Carbondale; Owner/, Private Practice, **SLP**

Von Deck, Mrs Karin A 5245 Spring Run Avenue, Orlando, FL 32819, (407) 291-7501, BS 59 Fitchburg St Coll; MS 63 Boston Univ; Sp-Lang Path, Orange Co PS, **SLP**

Vonderhaar, Mrs Joan Mary 105 East Milligan Street, Fort Recovery, OH 45846, (419) 375-2781, BS 70 Ball St Univ; MA 78 Bowling Green St Univ; Sp-Lang Path, Darke Co Boe

Vonder Heide, Patricia Hall 124 Fuller Road, Hinsdale, IL 60521, (312) 789-1263, BS 77 Univ of IL - Urbana; MS 78 Univ of IL - Urbana; SLP, Tames, **SLP**

Von Drach, Dr Robert B Cross Keys Bldg, Routes 611 & 313, Doylestown, PA 18901, BA 54 Bloomsburg Univ of PA; ME 56 Temple Univ-Tyler Sch of Art; ED (NS) Temple Univ-Tyler Sch of Art; Asst Dir/Spec Ed, Bucks Co Inter Unit 22, **SLP F**

Von Ehrenkrook, Cathy 431 North Linden, Itasca, IL 60143, (312) 438-6378, **SLP**

von Hermann, Jean O 983 33rd Street, Richmond, CA 94804, (415) 236-9314, MA 70 San Francisco St Univ; **SLP LM**

Von Holten, Mrs Lori Jean 1620 Bruner Street, Rockford, IL 61103-4413, (815) 962-2316, BS 75 Western IL Univ; MS 76 IL St Univ - Normal; 87–Sp-Lang Path, Barbara Olson Sch of Hope, **SLP**

Von Leden, Dr Hans V 10921 Wilshire Boulevard, Los Angeles, CA 90024, (213) 208-3100, MD 41 (NS) Loyola Univ of Chicago; Private Practice, **F LM**

Vonnegut, Susan H 1695 2nd Street #401, Highland Park, IL 60035, (312) 256-5918, BA 69 Univ of WA; MA 77 CA St Univ - Long Beach; ME 86 Nat'l Coll of Ed - Evanston; 88–Sp-Lang Path, Wilmette Sch Dist #39, **SLP ACE**

Von Rembow, Deborah L 703 Elizabeth Street, Easton, MD 21601, (301) 225-4190, BA 71 American Univ; MA 73 Vanderbilt Univ; Resource Dev Spec, Govt Ofc for Children/Youth, **A**

Von Roos, Ingetraud 17255 Loggers Road North, Los Gatos, CA 95030, MA 75 MI St Univ; 88–Sp-Lang Path, Dominican Hosp, **SLP**

von Wolfseck, Dr Janie Wester 25 Gloria Lane, St Peters, MO 63376, (314) 889-1407, BS 63 Southeast MO St Univ; MA 72 Saint Louis Univ; PH 84 (Educ Focus-Spec Ed-Sp/Path) Saint Louis Univ; Chairperson, Fontbonne College, **SLP**

Voorakkara, Mrs Seeta Mylai 2400 Dante Avenue, Vineland, NJ 08360, (609) 696-6496, BA 58; MA 66 Temple Univ; SLP, Vineland Dev Cen, **SLP**

Voorhees, Mrs Gretchen M 411 Harrison Avenue, Westfield, NJ 07090, (201) 233-4286, BA 59 PA St Univ - Univ Park; MS 62 PA St Univ - Univ Park; SLP, South Plainfield Board of Educ, **SLP**

Vorbroker, Mrs Jane Annette 117 Billups Drive, Lawrenceburg, IN 47025, (812) 537-5940, **SLP**

Vorce, Mrs Deborah Jean 2505 E Allen, Howell, MI 48843, (517) 887-3059, BS 84 Northern MI Univ; MA 87 MI St Univ; 88–Sp-Lang Path, Lansing Sch Dist

Vorce, Eleanor R 2 Tudor City Place 12C So, New York, NY 10017, (212) 697-3818, MS; **A LM**

Vorce, Pamela P 2022 Edgewood Drive, Palo Alto, CA 94303, (415) 424-1189, BA 64 Univ of MO - KS City; MA 68 San Diego St Univ; MA 68 San Diego St Univ; Sp-Lang Path, Peninsula Chldn Ctr, **SLP**

Vornheder-Allendorf, Valerie Ann 2366 Victor Street, Cincinnati, OH 45219, (513) 661-2905, BS 73 Univ of Cincinnati; MA 78 Univ of Cincinnati; Aud, Private Practice, **A**

Voroba, Dr Barry Voroba Technologies Associates, 14853 Deveau Place, Minnetonka, MN 55345, (612) 935-8443, BA 67 CUNY - Brooklyn Coll; MS 70 CUNY - Brooklyn Coll; PH 73 (NS) CUNY - Grad Sch & Univ Cntr; President, Voroba Technologies Associates, **A**

Voroba, Jane S 218 Bedford Street #3-B, Stamford, CT 06901, (203) 327-2146, BA 79 Univ of CT; MS 81 Southern CT St Univ; Sp-Lang Path, Greenwich Ct Bd of Ed, **SLP**

Vortherms, Mrs Kimberly A 3936 Snug Harbor Drive, Virginia Beach, VA 23456, (804) 471-6164, BA 80 Univ of Northern IA; MA 81 Univ of Northern IA; **SLP**

Vorwerk, Susan J R 518 Buckley Court, University Park, IL 60466, (312) 534-6887, BS 60 Kent St Univ; ME 68 IN Univ - Bloomington; Sp-Lang Path, Crete-Monee Sch Dist 201-U, **SLP**

Vosburg, Mrs Elyse Hoytt 125 Cabro Courte, Novato, CA 94947, (415) 892-5903, BA 76 Univ of CA - Santa Barbara; MA 81 CA St Univ - Los Angeles; 88–Sp-Lang Path, Marin Co Ofc of Educ, **SLP**

Vosburgh, Mrs Gloria S 510 East Evy Lane, Arlington Heights, IL 60004, (312) 824-8044, BS 73 IL St Univ - Normal; MA 74 Ball St Univ; Sp-Lang Path, Elgin U-46 School District, **SLP**

Vosel, Sherrie Ruth P O Box 1008, Cedar Hill, TX 75104, (214) 291-2652, MS 81 Univ of South AL; 87–Reg Sls Rep, Nicloet Audiodiagnostics, **A**

Voss, Barbara T 555 Roddy Road #8-A, Salem, IL 62881, (618) 548-3172, BS 86 Eastern IL Univ; MS 87 Eastern IL Univ; Sp-Lang Path, Kaskaskia Special Educ Dist, **SLP**

Voss, Carla Jo 4310 Gayle Drive, Woodstock, IL 60098, (815) 338-8883, BS 81 Univ of WI - Madison; MS 83 Univ of WI - Madison; Sp/Lang Path, Dist 200 Woodstock Il, **SLP**

Voss, John H The Duluth Clinic Ltd, 400 East 3rd Street, Duluth, MN 55805, (218) 722-8364, BS 72 Mankato St Univ; ME 81 Univ of MN - Duluth; Aud, The Duluth Cl, Ltd, **A**

Voss, Mrs Lee Ann Box 782, Clarksville, IA 50619, (319) 273-8200, BA 72 Univ of Northern IA; MA 73 Univ of Northern IA; Sp-Lang Path, Ed Agcy 7, **SLP**

Voss, Mrs Marsha K 11257 War Cloud, El Paso, TX 79936, BA 71 Fort Hays St Univ; MS 74 KS St Univ; Sp/Lang Path, Beaumont Army Military Hosp, **SLP**

Voss-Schwartz, Kathleen N71 W27065 Meadowood Lane, Sussex, WI 53089, (414) 246-4323, BA 74 Univ of WI - Eau Claire; MS 78 Univ of WI - Milwaukee; 79–Sp-Lang Path, Hamilton Sch Dist, **SLP**

Vosu, Lorraine Wander The Audiology Centre Incorporated, 1333 Shepard Avenue East Suite 246, North York, ON, Canada M2J 1V1, (416) 498-4151, BS 74 SUNY - Coll at Brockport; MA 75 MI St Univ; Aud, Private Practice, **A**

Votaw, Mrs Lynn Kresheck 254 West Schreyer Place, Columbus, OH 43214, (614) 421-3818, BS 84 Miami Univ - Oxford; MS 85 Miami Univ - Oxford; Sp-Lang Path, Affiliated Aud & Sp Pathology, **SLP**

Votral, Karen Ann Forest Hills #2A, Rd 6 Box 2, Lewistown, PA 17044, (717) 242-7342, BS 84 Indiana Univ of PA; MS 86 James Madison Univ; 88–Sp-Lang Path, Lewistown Hosp, **SLP ACE**

Vottero, Lynn Maroney 2706 Bellwood Avenue, Columbus, OH 43209, (614) 263-5151, BA 80 Univ of Toledo; MA 82 Univ of TN - Knoxville; Sp-Lang Path, Columbus Speech-Hearing Center, **SLP**

Vourakis, Andrea L 3200 Hillsdale Drive, Visalia, CA 93291, MS

Vowell, Mrs Mary B 4200 Inwood Lane, Colleyville, TX 76034, (817) 498-3341, BA 68 Univ of AR - Fayetteville; MS 80 Univ of AR - Little Rock; Sp-Lang Path, Lewisville Public Schools, **SLP**

Vowels, Eleanor E 7718 Jaffrey Road, Fort Washington, MD 20744, **SLP**

Voyer, Carolyn R Folk 1536 East Mineral Avenue, Littleton, CO 80122, (303) 798-6232, BA 70 Univ of TX - El Paso; MA 71 Univ of TX - El Paso; 79–Sp-Lang Path, Littleton Sch Dist #6, **SLP**

Vrablic, Eleanor M 41 Edgewater Place, Edgewater, NJ 07020, **SLP**

Vrablik, Mrs Charlotte 149 Shenandoah Drive, Fairbanks, AK 99712, (907) 452-5771, BA 69 MT St Agnes Coll; ME 70 Loyola Coll; **SLP**

Vracin, Elizabeth 1680 La Loma Road, Pasadena, CA 91105, **SLP**

Vranizan, James M, Jr 104 N W Delaware, Bend, OR 97701, (503) 382-4321, BS 86 Portland St Univ; SLP, Nancy Ricker - Pp, **SLP**

Vrchota, Elizabeth A St Paul Rehabilitation Center, 319 Eagle Street, St Paul, MN 55102, (612) 227-8471, BS 74 Univ of MN - Minneap-St Paul; MS 75 Univ of WI - Madison; Aud, St Paul Rehab Cen, **A**

Vreeland, Dr Joella Box 1204, Mattituck, NY 11952, PH (NS); Retired, **SLP A**

Vreeland, Richard S 97 Via Arcerolo, Monterey, CA 93940, (408) 755-6431, BA 52 San Francisco St Univ; 57–Aud, Monterey County Office of Educ, **SLP A**

Vroman-Cooper, Carolyn R P O Box 352, Rancho Mirage, CA 92270, (619) 340-4566, BA 74 CA St Univ - Sacramento; MA 75 CA St Univ - Sacramento; 77–Aud, Desert ENT Med Group, **A**

Vruwink, Debra Lynn 278 North Seymour Street, Apartment J-206, Fond Du Lac, WI 54935, (414) 922-6206, BS 85 Univ of WI - Madison; MS 87 Univ of WI - Stevens Point; 88–Sp-Lang Path, Fond du Lac Sch Dist, **SLP**

Vuchetich, Julie Ann 104-1/2 Douglas Street #9, Princeton, WV 24740, (304) 487-1551, BA 84 Univ of WI - Eau Claire; MS 85 Univ of WI - Eau Claire; 87–Sp-Lang Path, Mercer County Schs, **SLP**

Vujanovic-Browne, Mrs Bosiljka Bessie 641 Walnut Court, Des Plaines, IL 60016, (312) 455-4060, **SLP**

Vukas, Cynthia 3000 Swallow Hill Road, Apartment 414, Pittsburgh, PA 15220, (412) 394-5815, BS 82 Indiana Univ of PA; MS 83 Indiana Univ of PA; 86–Sp-Lang Path, Allegheny Intermediate Unit, **SLP**

Vulanich, Mrs Nova Nicolette 1208 Fawn Court, Loveland, OH 45140, (513) 575-9845, OB 74 Kent St Univ; MA 75 Kent St Univ; 86–Sp-Lang Path, Cincinnati Sp & Hearing Ctr, **SLP**

Vulcano, Mrs Sally A M 15001 North 49th Way, Scottsdale, AZ 85254, (602) 952-0062, BS 78 Southern IL Univ -Carbondale; MA 79 Saint Louis Univ; Sp/Lang Path, Scottsdale Pub Schs, **SLP**

Vuolo, Mrs Janelle M 6/29 Church Street, Rockhampton, Queensland, Australia 4700, BA 79 Univ of Northern CO; MA 81 Univ of Northern CO; 88–Sp-Lang Path, Rockhampton Base Hosp, **SLP**

W

Waas, Karen D Waters 10650 S W 77th Court, Miami, FL 33156, (305) 667-5397, BA 79 Univ of Miami; MA 80 Univ of Miami; **SLP**

Wacaster, Mrs Pamela Vollmer 3207 Independence, Fort Smith, AR 72903, (501) 474-7059, OB 77 Univ of AR - Fayetteville; MS 83 Univ of AR - Fayetteville; Sp-Lang Path, Van Buren Pub Sch, **SLP**

Wachman, Cheryl Thomson 2 Indian Point Drive, New Ulm, MN 56073, (507) 354-1701, BA 77 Univ of MN - Minneap-St Paul; MS 78 Saint Cloud St Univ; Sp-Lang Path, GFW-ISD #735, **SLP**

Wachowiak, Mrs Joanne Elizabeth 135-A Chadd Road, Newark, DE 19711, BA 78 Univ of CT; MS 81 Southern CT St Univ; Sp/Lang Path, DE Autistic Prog, **SLP**

Wachowiak, Nancy Kubasek Rural Free Delivery, 34 Lamprey Lane, Durham, NH 03824, BA 79 Univ of CT; MS 81 Southern CT St Univ; Sp-Lang Path, Sav #53 Proj Tell, **SLP**

Wachs, Diane Kaufman 1010 Kater Street, Philadelphia, PA 19147, (215) 928-0341, BS 83 PA St Univ - Univ Park; MA 85 Temple Univ-Tyler Sch of Art; **SLP**

Wachs, Katharine Box 765, MacKenzie, BC, Canada V0J 2C0, (604) 997-6340, BS 75; OM 81 Univ of Western Ontario; Sp/Lang Path, Sch Dist #57, **SLP**

Wachtel, Mrs Clara Jacobs 892 Westview Drive, Boulder, CO 80303, (303) 441-0437, BS 64 PA St Univ - Univ Park; MA 65 Northwestern Univ; Sp-Path Senior Staff, Boulder Mem Hosp, **SLP**

Wachtel, Mrs Eve Tyroler 7 Everit Avenue, Hewlett, NY 11557, (516) 562-4600, BA 79 Univ of RI; MA 82 Univ of MD - College Park; Sp-Lang Path, North Shore Univ Hosp, **SLP**

Wachtel, Jayne Miller Carle Clinic, 602 University Avenue, Urbana, IL 61801, (215) 337-3130, BS 79 IL St Univ - Normal; MA 81 Univ of IL - Urbana; Sp-Lang Path, Carle Cl Assoc, **SLP ACE**

Wachtell, Marlene A 22 Smart Road, Acton, MA 01720, (617) 779-2821, BA 69 CUNY - City College; MS 74 Boston Univ; Sp/Lang Path, Town of Bolton-Emerson Sch, **SLP**

Wachtor, Carol T 17333 Brookhurst Street, Apartment E-1, Fountain Valley, CA 92708, (714) 963-6084, BS 75 IL St Univ - Normal; MA 76 IL St Univ - Normal; Sp-Lang Path, Garden Grove USD, **SLP**

Wack, Stephanie Ann 317 Chesterfield #206, Maumee, OH 43537-3812, (419) 893-8340, **SLP**

Wacker, Jean A 460 Academy Street, Madison, GA 30650, (404) 342-3475, BS 71 OH Univ - Athens; MA 72 OH Univ - Athens; 88–Sp-Lang Path, Morgan Co PS, **SLP**

Wacker-Mundy, Dr Roberta L Rd#1, Box 137, West Chazy, NY 12992, (518) 564-2170, BA 75 Capital Univ; MS 77 Purdue Univ - West Lafayette; PH 83 (Communication Disorders) PA St Univ - Univ Park; Assistant Professor, SUNY-College at Plattsburgh, **SLP**

Wacks, Mrs Joyce S 230 Glen Hills Drive, Cranston, RI 02920, (401) 946-4913, BS 72 Northeastern Univ; MA 73 Northwestern Univ; Sp-Lang Path, Providence Sch Dept, **SLP**

Wada, Celeste 7401 Asman Avenue, Canoga Park, CA 91307, (818) 997-2357, BS 53 Univ of CA - Los Angeles; MA 80 CA St Univ - Northridge; SLP, LA USD, **SLP**

Wada, Margaret K 1042 17th Avenue, Honolulu, HI 96816, (808) 847-2565, BS 67 Univ of HI - Manoa; MS 69 Univ of HI - Manoa; 72–Sp-Lang Path, State of HI-Dept of Hlth, **SLP**

Wadas, David A 29 Alpine Drive, P O Box 3192, Scranton, PA 18505-0192, (717) 344-7271, BS 69; MS 79 Bloomsburg Univ of PA; Aud, Hrng Aid Cen, **A**

Waddell, Jill 5217 Penrith Avenue #G, Durham, NC 27713-1722, **SLP**

Waddell, Mrs Judith S 114 Crestview Drive, Union, SC 29379, (803) 427-5624, BA 70 Trenton St Coll; MA 72 Univ of MD - College Park; Aud, Union Co Sch, **SLP A**

Waddell, Mrs Patricia Lewis 609 Hadley Court, Wilmington, NC 28405, (919) 762-1744, BS 75 NC A & T St Univ; ME 80 NC Central Univ; Sp-Lang Path, Dev Eval Cen, **SLP**

Wadden, Mrs Rosemary S 159 Frederick Court, Los Altos, CA 94022, (415) 949-1223, BA 67 Univ of MD - College Park; MA 72 George Washington Univ; **SLP**

Waddle, Mrs Janis Kay 14 Mohican Circle, Shawnee, OK 74801, (405) 273-8395, BA 65 Southern IL Univ -Carbondale; MS 74 Univ of NE - Omaha

Waddoups, Dr Milo O 2206 Knob Creek Road, Johnson City, TN 37604, (615) 929-4272, BS 67 Univ of UT; MA 71 Univ of UT; PH 81 (Sp-Lang Path) Univ of IA; Sp-Lang Path, East Tennessee State Universit, **SLP**

Wade, Barbara J 2705 Sycamore Street, Alexandria, VA 22305, (703) 683-5434, BS 78 IN Univ - Bloomington; OM 80 IN Univ - Bloomington; Sp-Lang Path, Private Practice, **SLP**

Wade, Betsy M 7210 Creveling, St Louis, MO 63130, (314) 726-2223, BA 72 Baylor Univ; OM 74 Emory Univ; Aud/Sp-Lang Path, St Joseph Hosp, **SLP A**

Wade, Mrs Cami Lynn 1910 Barak #17, Bryan, TX 77802, (409) 776-0101, BS 84 Lamar Univ; MS 85 Lamar Univ; Aud, Otolaryngology & Assoc, **A**

Wade, Curtis Nelson 2015 Garnet Avenue Suite 110, San Diego, CA 92109, (619) 581-2364, BS 77 Univ of CA - Santa Barbara; MS 80 Univ of TX - Dallas; 87–SLP, Nicolet Audiodiagnostics

Wade, Mrs Dorothy Dodge 12 Grasshopper Lane, Acton, MA 01720, (617) 635-0906, BA 71 Northeastern Univ; ME 72 Northeastern Univ; 72–Sp-Lang Path, Hudson PS, **SLP**

Wade, Elizabeth Parnell 229 Danby Road, Columbia, SC 29212, (803) 254-2495, BS 74 Univ of SC - Columbia; MA 76 Univ of SC - Columbia; Aud, Midland ENT Clinic, **A**

Wade, Mrs Elizabeth Ruth 1985 University Circle, Las Vegas, NV 89119, (702) 799-5650, BA 45 Waynesburg Coll; MS 54 Univ of Pittsburgh - Pittsburgh; PH 63 (Aud/Sp Path) Univ of WI - Madison; Sp-Lang Path, Clark Co Sch Dist, **SLP**

Wade, Dr G Michael Wade Institute, 9 Doris Avenue, Lancaster, NY 14086, BS 61 SUNY - Coll at Buffalo; MS 64 SUNY - Coll at Buffalo; OD 76 (NS) 2965; Dir, Wade I, **SLP**

Wade, Helen K Pc Werth Ltd, Audiology House, 45 Nightingale Lane, London, England SW12 8SU, BS 74 OH Univ - Athens; MA 76 OH Univ - Athens; Mgr Aud Servs, P C Werth, Ltd, **A**

Wade, Helen Sherman 15250 Ventura Blvd Suite 1015, Sherman Oaks, CA 91403, (818) 986-4114, BA 77; MA 75 CA St Univ - Northridge; Sp-Lang Path, Private Practice, **SLP**

Wade, Mrs Jacqueline Anne 3006 Kent Drive, Carbondale, IL 62901, (618) 549-7784, MS 88 Southern IL Univ -Carbondale; 88–Sp-Lang Path, Tri-County Special Educ Dist

Wade, Janice 1067-C Greta Lane, Centerville, OH 45458, (513) 435-8227, **SLP**

Wade, Mrs Leslie H 2002 Cottage Way, Vista, CA 92083, BA 80 Univ of the Pacific; MA 82 Univ of the Pacific; 86–Sp-Lang Path, Tri-City Med Ctr, **SLP**

Wade, Mary A R R 3 Box 26, Wamego, KS 66547, (913) 456-7317, MA 86 KS St Univ; 87–Instr, Kansas St Univ Sp and Hearing Ctr, **A**

Wade, Mrs Nancy M 1503 Spencer, Monroe, LA 71201, (318) 388-3601, BA 72 LA St Univ - Baton Rouge; MA 74 LA St Univ - Baton Rouge; Aud, Drs Taliaferro & Mickey, **A**

Wade, Patricia M 620 North Sweetzer #3, Los Angeles, CA 90048, (818) 846-7121, BA 75 Antioch Coll; MS 80 Univ of OR; Sp/Lang Path, Burbank USD, **SLP**

Wade, Rebecca Sue 2733 Avenue K, Fort Madison, IA 52627, (319) 372-8474, BA 80 CA St Univ - Fresno; MA 84 CA St Univ - Fresno; Aud, Great River AEA 16, **A**

Wade, Mrs Roxanne Marie 1409 West 32nd Street, Topeka, KS 66611, (913) 625-8442, BA 83 Fort Hays St Univ; MS 87 Fort Hays St Univ

Wade, Susan Jean 14469 East 1st Drive, Apt C-11, Aurora, CO 80011, (303) 360-8857, BA 76 Graceland Coll; MA 85 Central MI Univ; **SLP**

Wade-Kellar, Martha E 25913 Largo Court, Damascus, MD 20872, (703) 491-6060, BA 76 Univ of MD - College Park; MA 78 Catholic Univ of America; **SLP**

Wadle, Cherie L 1508 Boyd, Green Bay, WI 54301, (414) 468-1161, BA 77 Univ of Northern IA; MS 78 Univ of WI - Stevens Point; 79–Sp-Lang Path, Curative Rehab Ctr, **SLP**

Wadle, Kella Lynn 1805 West Fourth Avenue, Indianola, IA 50125, (515) 961-8191, OB 83 Northeast MO St Univ; MA 84 Northeast MO St Univ; Sp-Lang Path, Heartland AEA 11, **SLP**

Wadle, Mrs Sharon Lee 318 South 4th Street, De Kalb, IL 60115, (815) 895-2045, BA 64 Augustana Coll; MA 83 Northern IL Univ - De Kalb; 87–Sp-Lang Path/Instr, N IL Univ, **SLP**

Wadlinger, Mrs Carolyn M 1023 Rancho Road, Roswell, NM 88201, (505) 623-8319, BA 71 Temple Univ-Tyler Sch of Art; MA 73 Temple Univ-Tyler Sch of Art; Sp-Lang Path, SE Nm Sp & Hearing Clinic, **SLP**

Wadman, Patrick N 260 Hermosa, Bakersfield, CA 93305, (805) 327-3311, MS 84 Univ of Redlands

Wadsworth, Margaret Marie 5800 Steubenville Pike, Mc Kees Rocks, PA 15136, (412) 787-0590, BS 85 PA St Univ - Univ Park; MS 87 PA St Univ - Univ Park; 88–Sp-Lang Path, Harmarville Rehab Center Inc, **SLP**

Wadsworth, Pamela Joyce 5512 South Fresno, Fort Smith, AR 72903, (501) 632-5100, BA 75 Henderson St Univ; MS 83 Univ of AR - Fayetteville; SLP, Alma Pub Sch, **SLP**

Wadsworth, Dr Steven D 5184 North Del Mar, Fresno, CA 93704, (209) 294-2423, BS 62 UT St Univ; MS 63 UT St Univ; ED 72 (Communicative Disorders Hrng Handicapped) Brigham Young Univ; Prof of Comm Disord, CA St U-Fresno, **SLP**

Wage, Kathryn J 1189 East Brandywine, Fresno, CA 93710, (209) 222-6573, BA 72 CA St Univ - Fresno; MA 73 CA St Univ - Fresno; Asst Supt/Instr, Diagn Sch/Neurly Hndcpd Chldrn, **SLP**

Wagener, Dr John W VA Medical Center, Pensacola Outpatient Clinic, 312 Kenmore Road, Pensacola, FL 32503, (904) 479-6626, BA 65 Johns Hopkins Univ; MS 68 Lehigh Univ; PH 72 (Experimental Psychology) Lehigh Univ; 86–Coord Aud, VA Med Ctr, **A**

Wagenheim, Evonne Vaksman 672 Sproul Road, Bryn Mawr, PA 19010, (215) 527-7580, BA 77 Beaver Coll; MA 83 Temple Univ; **SLP**

Wagenknecht, Mrs Amy S 234 Jackson Street, Williamston, MI 48895, (517) 394-5100, BA 79 MI St Univ; MA 80 MI St Univ; Sp-Lang Path, Commun Serv for Dev Disabl, **SLP**

Wager, Glenda G 202-1221A West Haven Drive, Edson, AB, Canada T0E 0P0, **SLP**

Wagers, Mrs Gloria S 41332 Sequoia Lane, Hemet, CA 92343, (714) 925-1265, BS 60 Saint Louis Univ; MA 70 CA St Univ - Long Beach; SLP, Riverside Co Supt Sch, **SLP**

Wages, Dianne Bass Route 3 Box 94, Dublin, GA 31021, (912) 272-7494, OB 72 Univ of GA; ME 84 Columbus Coll; **SLP**

Waggener, Lloyd Denton 4240 Blue Ridge Boulevard Suite 434, Kansas City, MO 64133, (816) 358-7177, BS 77 Central MO St Univ; MS 85 Central MO St Univ; 84–Dir Aud/Hearing Aid Dept, Head & Neck Group, **A**

Waggoner, Mrs Barbara Joyce P O Box 24665, Fort Worth, TX 76124-1665, **SLP**

Waggoner, Edna Mae 307 North Singingwood #24, Orange, CA 92669, (213) 690-2340, MA 83 CA St Univ - Long Beach; Sp-Lang Path, LA Habra City Sch Dist, **SLP**

Waggoner, Mrs Nancy E 1012 Fairview Avenue, Prattville, AL 36067, (205) 293-7804, OB 65 OH Univ - Athens; MS 75 Miami Univ - Oxford; 77–Sp-Lang Path, Maxwell AFB Elem Sch, **SLP**

Waggoner, Peggy Perry 5527 Central, Kansas City, MO 64113, (913) 588-5937, BS 80 Univ of KS; MA 82 Wichita St Univ; 87–Clin Instr, Univ of KS Med Ctr, **SLP**

Wagman, Mrs Michele A 2611 North King Way, Claremont, CA 91711, (804) 353-1211, BA 75 SUNY - Center at Buffalo; MA 77 CUNY - Hunter Coll; Sp-Lang Path, Private Practice, **SLP**

Wagman, Mrs Rhoda K 17 Crommelin Court, East Brunswick, NJ 08816, (201) 297-5057, BS 49 Newark St Coll; MA 66 Newark St Coll; Supvr, Kean Coll of New Jersey, **SLP**

Wagner, Mrs Amelia A 4 Caroline Drive, Bennington, VT 05201, (802) 447-0414, BA 70 Univ of VT; MA 71 Wichita St Univ; 86–Sp-Lang Path, Southwest VT Union, **SLP**

Wagner, Aylene P 1013 Overbrook Road, Wilmington, DE 19807, (302) 655-1754, BA 61 Carson-Newman Coll; MA 64 Northwestern Univ; Sp-Lang Path, Pvt Practict/DE Prog for Deaf/Bl, **SLP ACE**

Wagner, Barry Thomas 800 North Smith Road Apartment X26, Bloomington, IN 47401, (812) 336-9484, BS 81 Ball St Univ; MS 84 Univ of WY; Sp-Lang Path, Bloomington Hosp, **SLP**

Wagner, Brenda R 307 Pebble Brook, Clinton, MS 39056, (601) 924-3533, BS 70 MS Univ for Women; OM 73 Univ of MS; SLP, Pearl Separate Mun Sch Dist, **SLP**

Wagner, Bruce Robert Route 1 Box 286, Crozet, VA 22932, (703) 886-6831, BA 78 5579; ME 82 James Madison Univ; Aud, Private Practice, **A**

Wagner, Charles Richard 1312 Hillcrest Drive, Frederick, MD 21701, (304) 263-0811, BA 81 Northeastern Univ; MS 83 Towson St Univ; Audiologist, VA Administration, **A**

Wagner, Charlotte 915 Terraine Avenue, Long Beach, CA 90804, (213) 498-1130, BA 37 Univ of WA; MA 41 Univ of WA; **SLP LM**

Wagner, Claudia M 21 Ann Road, Long Valley, NJ 07853, (201) 852-1953, BA 73 OH St Univ; ME 74 Bloomsburg Univ of PA; Sp-Lang Path, Long Valley Sp & Lang Cl, **SLP**

Wagner, Mrs Danette P 25225 118th Avenue S E, Kent, WA 98031, (206) 859-7513, BA 84 WA St Univ; MA 86 WA St Univ; 86–Aud

Wagner, Dawn M 7707 North Sheridan Road, Apartment 3-P, Chicago, IL 60626, (312) 508-9843, MA 88 Northwestern Univ

Wagner, Deanna Junell 911 East 15th St, Winfield, KS 67156, (316) 221-1200, BA 84 Northeastern OK St Univ; MA 87 OK St Univ; 87–Sp-Lang Path, Winfield State Hosp & Training Ctr, **SLP**

Wagner, Mrs Diana 18636 Walkers Choice Road, #3, Gaithersburg, MD 20879, (301) 490-1376, BA 84 MI St Univ; MA 86 MI St Univ; 88–Aud, Hearing Laboratory

Wagner, Elaine C R R 1 Box 413, Windfall Road, Olean, NY 14760, (716) 373-8888, BA 70 SUNY - Center at Buffalo; MA 72 SUNY - Center at Buffalo; Sp/Lang Path, Speech Pathology Serv, **SLP**

Wagner, Gwyneth Megan 3012 Miles Road, Burtonsville, MD 20866, (301) 464-6701, BA 81 Univ of MD - College Park; MA 83 Northwestern Univ; Aud, Bowie Hearing Ctr, **A**

Wagner, Mrs Irene Kay 3908 Clinton Avenue, Des Moines, IA 50310-4137, (515) 283-6344, BS 74 KS St Univ; MA 81 KS St Univ; Aud, IA Methodist Med Ctr, **A**

Wagner, Janet Resta 103 Terrace Street, Vicksburg, MS 39180, (601) 636-2847, BA 83 Univ of MS; MS 87 Univ of MS; **SLP**

Wagner, Mrs Joan Wasinger P O Box 4332, Lincoln, NE 68504-0332, (402) 471-2071, BA 75 Wichita St Univ; MA 76 Marshall Univ; Supervisor/Instructor, University of Nebraska Lincoln, **SLP**

Wagner, Joanne L 7061 North Mason Avenue, Chicago, IL 60616, BS 74 Stephen F Austin St Univ; MA 85 Northwestern Univ; **SLP**

Wagner, Jody Lynn 7698 Old Telegraph Road, Severn, MD 21144, (301) 969-3048, BA 83 Univ of MD - Baltimore CO; MS 88 Loyola Coll

Wagner, Joe Herman 3123 A Michigan, St Louis, MO 63118, (314) 644-7930, MA 87 Saint Louis Univ; **SLP**

Wagner, Kathleen Sparks P O Box 15, Westover, PA 16692, (814) 247-8499, BS 77 Indiana Univ of PA; MS 85 Indiana Univ of PA; Sp-Lang Path, Ebansburg Ctr, **SLP**

Wagner, Laura A 6252 Coleman, Dearborn, MI 48126, (313) 649-3755, BA 75 Univ of MI - Ann Arbor; MA 77 Wayne St Univ; Sp-Lang Path, Sp-Lang Rehab Serv, **SLP**

Wagner, Linda Carroll P O Box 11275, Albuquerque, NM 87192-0275, (505) 296-6207, BA 85 Univ of NM; MS 87 Univ of NM; 87–Aud, Albuquerque PS, **A**

Wagner, Marita L 114 West Allens Lane, Philadelphia, PA 19119, (215) 247-4034, BA 71 Mount Holyoke Coll; MA 73 Northwestern Univ; Sp/Lang Path, Sch Dist of Phila, **SLP**

Wagner, Mrs Mary C 1714 Westminster Way, Annapolis, MD 21405, BA 74 Marymount Coll; MS 77 Columbia Univ Teachers Coll; Sp-Lang Path, Private Practice, **SLP**

Wagner, Michele Louise 702 Barnhill Drive, Riley A-56, Indianapolis, IN 46223, (317) 253-9443, BS 82 Purdue Univ - West Lafayette; MA 84 Univ of IA; Aud, Indiana Univ Med Ctr, **A**

Wagner, Monica Palmieri 421 Queens Avenue, Massapequa, NY 11758, (516) 799-3631, BA 77 SUNY - Coll at Cortland; MA 79 CUNY - Queens Coll; Sp-Lang Path, Private Practice, **SLP**

Wagner, Mrs Nancy G 3534 Meadowridge, Howell, MI 48843, (313) 353-0310, BA 77 Univ of MI - Ann Arbor; MS 78 Univ of MI - Ann Arbor; Sp-Lang Path, Sp-Lang Rehab Serv, **SLP**

Wagner, Susan Adele 2058 Swans Neck Way, Reston, VA 22091, (703) 691-4063, MS 83 James Madison Univ; 85–Co-Dir/Sp-Lang Path, Communication Rehabilitation Services PC, **SLP ACE**

Wagner, Mrs Susan K 9511 Browns Mill Road, Greencastle, PA 17225, (717) 263-9281, BS 74 Indiana Univ of PA; MS 75 Indiana Univ of PA; 87–Sp-Lang Path, Chambersburg Area Sch Dist, **SLP**

Wagner, Susan Kay 6770 West 19th Place #205, Lakewood, CO 80214, (303) 659-4820, BA 82 Fort Lewis Coll; MA 86 Univ of CO - Boulder; SLP, Brighton School District, **SLP**

Wagner, Sylvia Clymer MEU Box 20, FPO Seattle, WA 98762-3300, 045-786-0788, 69 Syracuse Univ; MS 76 Syracuse Univ; Sp-Lang Path, Private Practice, **SLP**

Wagner, Valerie A 1530 Parker Avenue, Regina, SK, Canada S4S 4R8, (319) 399-6700, BA 73; MS 76; Sp-Lang Path, Saskatchewan Dept of Health, **SLP**

Wagner-Hill, Geraldine 456 Summit Avenue, Oradell, NJ 07649, (201) 385-8581, BA 67 Glassboro St Coll; MS 79 William Paterson Coll; 85–Sp-Lang Path, Bergenfield Pub Schs, **SLP**

Wagner-Otol, Cynthia A 3520 Northcliffe Road, Cleveland Heights, OH 44118, (219) 932-5976, BS 77 Purdue Univ - West Lafayette; MS 79 Purdue Univ - West Lafayette; **A**

Wagster, Mrs Cindy M 48 Windfield Cove, Jackson, TN 38305, (901) 668-6653, BS 79 Univ of TN - Knoxville; MA 81 Memphis St Univ; Sp/Lang Path, Jackson-Madison Co Gen Hosp, **SLP**

Wagster, Lora Octavia 380 South Moore, Piggott, AR 72454, (314) 688-2161, BS 82 AR St Univ; OM 85 AR St Univ; **SLP**

Waguespack, Glenn M 1118 Runningbrook Drive, Shreveport, LA 71118, (318) 226-1510, BA 67 Univ of Southwestern LA; MS 69 Purdue Univ - West Lafayette; 77–Aud, Private Practice, **A**

Waguespack, Mrs Mary K 2601 Hyman Place, New Orleans, LA 70114, (504) 392-7322, BS 74 Nicholls St Univ; OM 75 LA St Univ - N O Medical Ctr; 88–Sp-Lang Path, Jefferson Parish Sch Bd, **SLP**

Waguespack, Mrs Yvette R 728 26th Street, Laurel, MS 39440, (504) 876-3799, BA 79 Nicholls St Univ; OM 80 LA St Univ - N O Medical Ctr; SLP, Terrebonne Parish Sch Bd, **SLP**

Wahl, Lisa Hinze 5806 Crabapple Lane, Madison, WI 53711, (608) 271-1609, BS 80 Univ of WI - Madison; BS 81 Univ of WI - Madison; MS 84 Univ of WI - Madison; **SLP**

Wahl, Nancy M 5729 Sheffield, Riverside, CA 92506, MS 76 IN St Univ - Terre Haute; Sp/Lang Path, Riveside Comm Hosp, **SLP**

Wahl, Roger V R R 5 Box 17C, Council Bluffs, IA 51501, **SLP**

Wahl, Theresa Clark Route 2 Box 506, Lanesville, IN 47136, (812) 738-1985, BA 73 Brescia Coll; MA 75 Univ of KY; Sp-Lang Path, Private Practice, **SLP**

Wahlquist, Mrs Tracey Noelruchti 11117 Xylon Avenue North, Champlin, MN 55316, (612) 781-6571, **SLP**

Wahlstrom, Diane J c/o Medtronic, MST 266, 7000 Central Avenue, Fridley, MN 55432, BA 73 CA St Univ - Stanislaus; MA 76 Univ of MN - Duluth; Superv Cl Serv, Medtronic-Holland, **SLP**

Wahlton, Raymond E WI Dept Of Public Instruction, P O Box 7841, Madison, WI 53707, (608) 266-3890, BS 51 Univ of IL - Urbana; MS 54 Univ of IL - Urbana; Aud, WI Dept Pub Instr, **SLP A**

Wahoske, Patricia A Speech-Language Pathology Dept, Hennepin County Med Center, 701 Park Avenue South, Minneapolis, MN 55415, (612) 347-8550, BS 72 Univ of MN - Minneap-St Paul; MA 75 Univ of MN - Minneap-St Paul; 74–Sp-Lang Path Director, Hennepin County Medical Center, **SLP**

Wain, Tobey D 8 Fort Drive, Old Westbury, NY 11568, **A**

Waine, Zillah Bernidine P O Box 11987, Main Post Office, Edmonton, AB, Canada T5J 0J0, (403) 471-2262, BS 83 Univ of Alberta - Alberta; MA 84 Western IL Univ; 84–Sp-Lang Path, Glenrose Rehab Hosp, **SLP**

Wainer, Marilyn F 109 Bentley Drive, Mount Laurel, NJ 08054, (201) 835-5167, BA 66 William Paterson Coll; MA 69 William Paterson Coll; **SLP LM**

Wainer-Levi, Audrey L 42 Mill Road Extension, Woodcliff, NJ 07675, (201) 391-6737, BA 76 NY Univ; MS 77 NY Univ; SLP, Bergen County Spec Serv, **SLP**

Wainright, Mrs R LaNell 41724 S E 66th, Snoqualmie, WA 98065, (206) 888-3522, BS 80 Brigham Young Univ; OM 81 Brigham Young Univ; Sp-Lang Path, Private Practice, **SLP**

Wainright, Rebecca S 289 Wild Heron Road, St Simons Island, GA 31522, (912) 638-4314, BS 75 Ball St Univ; ME 78 Univ of GA; Sp-Lang Path, Glynn Co Sch Syst, **SLP**

Waintraub, Mrs Charnie Lynn 1542 Victoria Road, Teaneck, NJ 07666, (201) 836-5709, BS 80 CUNY - Brooklyn Coll; MS 82 CUNY - Brooklyn Coll; 85–Sp-Lang Path, Comm Disorder Ctr, **SLP**

Wainwright, Patricia Colby 5633 South 106th Street, Hales Corners, WI 53130, (414) 425-3755, BA 61 Carthage Coll; MS 87 Univ of WI - Milwaukee; 88–Sp-Lang Path, Lutheran Social Svcs, **SLP**

Waisman, Mrs Georgette B 3444 Laurelvale Drive, Studio City, CA 91604, BA 82 4108; BS 71 Boston Univ; MS 72 Univ of MI - Ann Arbor; 72–Sp-Lang Path, LA Co Supt of Sch, **SLP**

Waiss, Sharon L 7111 Cheshire Court, Alexandria, VA 22307, (703) 780-9466, BA 57 Univ of WA; SLP, Fairfax Co Pub Schs, **SLP**

Waissman, Rachael 5739 Mackerel Street, El Paso, TX 79924, (915) 778-4209

Waite, Beth A 3242 Sutherland Avenue, Indianapolis, IN 46205, (317) 924-3251, BS 84 Ball St Univ; MA 85 Ball St Univ; 85–Sp-Lang Path, Crossroads Rehab Ctr, **SLP**

Waite, Joanne Metzger 800 Magnolia Drive, Waukesha, WI 53188, (414) 679-1177, BA 76 Univ of WI - Eau Claire; MS 77 Univ of WI - Eau Claire; SLP, New Berlin Pub Schs, **SLP**

Waites, Mrs Danette Rene 1264 Brandl Drive, Marietta, GA 30060, (404) 436-0806, BA 80 Harding Univ; OM 82 GA St Univ; Cobb Co Schl Systm, **SLP**

Waitkus, Mrs Nancy A 106 River Street, Fair Haven, VT 05743, MS 72 Univ of VT; Sp-Lang Path, Addison Rutland Supervis Union, **SLP**

Wakefield, Mrs Lucille Atkinson 3 Waverly Drive, Hummelstown, PA 17036, (717) 566-6685, BA 81 Univ of Richmond; MA 83 Temple Univ; 84–Dir Sp Dept, Easter Seal Soc of Lebanon Co, **SLP ACE**

Wakefield, Maureen Pohn 125 Victoria Place, Sterling, VA 22170, (703) 481-4242, BA 83 PA St Univ - Univ Park; MA 85 George Washington Univ; 88–Sp-Lang Path, Fairfax Co Hlth Dept, **SLP**

Wakeley, Donna Adele 1 Holly Lane #8, Tonawanda, NY 14150-2854, (716) 693-0133, BS 85 SUNY - Coll at Fredonia; MS 86 SUNY - Coll at Fredonia; SLP, De Graff Hosp, **SLP**

Walbridge, Carol Box 5094, APO New York, NY 09179-5376, MS; **SLP**

Walbridge, Elizabeth Koestner 908 West Waveland #1-E, Chicago, IL 60613, (312) 971-0840, **SLP**

Walcek, Ann Marie 16866 Kingsbury Street, Apartment 215, Granada Hills, CA 91344, (213) 651-4651, BA 85 CA St Univ - Northridge; MA 87 CA St Univ - Northridge; 87–Aud, Doctor Freed, **A**

Walcher, Helen R 2055 Arlington, Las Cruces, NM 88001, MS; **SLP A LM**

Walchko, Jack C 11204 Veranda Court, Perico Island, Bradenton, FL 34209, (813) 792-2876, PH (NS); Aud, **A ACE**

Walck, Carol Ann 2733 Washington Street, Allentown, PA 18104, (215) 391-1111, BS 77 Indiana Univ of PA; MS 86 Bloomsburg Univ of PA; Sp-Lang Path, Carbon-Lehigh Intermediate Unit #21, **SLP**

Walczak, Necia B 13543 North Cedarburg Road, Mequon, WI 53092, (414) 675-2366, BS 74 Univ of WI - River Falls; MS 78 Univ of WI - Whitewater; 88–Sp-Lang Path, Rehabilitation Associates, **SLP**

Wald, Janice M M 10 Balcom Drive, East Aurora, NY 14052, (716) 655-0836, BS 72 SUNY - Coll at Brockport; MS 73 SUNY - Coll at Buffalo; Sp-Lang Path, Erie-Chataugua-Cattaraugus BOCES, **SLP**

Wald, Mrs Karen Pick 49 Meadowbrook Road, Chatham, NJ 07928, (201) 701-0286, BS 82 Syracuse Univ; MS 83 Columbia Univ Teachers Coll; Sp-Lang Path, Private Practice, **SLP**

Wald, Lisa Tuchman 134 Rowayton Woods Drive, Norwalk, CT 06854, (203) 866-5682, **SLP**

Wald, Mrs Pamela M 133 West Avenue, Darien, CT 06820, (203) 655-7097, BA 67 Simmons Coll; MS 71 Emerson Coll; 81–Sp-Lang Path, Darien Bd of Ed, **SLP**

Waldbillig-Gunn, Mrs Jamee 3309 Mackinaw Street, Saginaw, MI 48602, (517) 776-8307, BS 78 Central MI Univ; MA 81 Central MI Univ; Sp-Lang Path, St Marys Hosp, **SLP**

Walden, Mrs Bethany Lee 21327 Bassett Avenue, Port Charlotte, FL 33952, (813) 629-4112, MS 83 Univ of South FL; Aud, Audiological Associates, **A**

Walden, Dr Brian E 2116 Dexter Avenue #101, Silver Spring, MD 20902, (202) 576-4062, BA 67 San Diego St Univ; MS 69 Purdue Univ - West Lafayette; PH 71 (NS) Purdue Univ - West Lafayette; Dir of Research/Aud, Walter Reed Army Med Cen, **A F**

Walden, Ernest E, Jr University Of Florida, Department Of Comm Dis, Box J-174 JHMHC, Gainesville, FL 32610, (904) 395-0174, BS 75 East TN St Univ; MA 77 East TN St Univ; Asst Prof, Univ of FL, **A**

Walden, Mary Elizabeth 250 North Anderson Street, Morganton, NC 28655, (704) 433-3651, BS 84 Appalachian St Univ; MS 85 East Carolina Univ; **SLP**

Walder, Mrs Louise E 1303 Westbrook Drive, Mahomet, IL 61853, (309) 438-8455, BA 79 Univ of Northern IA; MA 81 Univ of IL - Urbana; Sp-Lang Path, Illinois State University, **SLP**

Waldkirch, Therese M 867 St Francis Road, De Pere, WI 54115, (414) 336-4172, BA 74 Coll of Saint Teresa; MS 81 Univ of WI - Stevens Point; Sp-Lang Path, Green Bay PS, **SLP**

Waldman, Deborah Scannell 27 Priscilla Avenue, Norfolk, MA 02056, (508) 856-3996, BA 79 Univ of MD - College Park; MS 81 Boston Univ; 88–Aud, Univ of Mass Med Ctr, **A**

Waldman, Lois Jean 798 President Street, Apartment 4R, Brooklyn, NY 11215, BA 80 SUNY - Center at Buffalo; MA 82 SUNY - Center at Buffalo; Sp-Lang Path, Visiting Therapy Associates, **SLP**

Waldman, Mrs Sandra M Freilich 8 Madison Lane 1E, Carle Place, NY 11514, (516) 746-7423, BA 80 Hofstra Univ; MA 81 Hofstra Univ; Sp-Lang Path, Levittown Pub Sch, **SLP**

Waldman, Susan E P O Box 859, Barnstable, MA 02630, (508) 778-6222, BS 73 Northeastern Univ; MA 76 Trenton St Coll; Sp/Lang Path, Cape Cod Collaborative, **SLP**

Waldman, Wanda S 1101-C Wright Street, Dodge City, KS 67801, (316) 225-5177, BA 78 Wichita St Univ; MA 79 Wichita St Univ; Sp-Lang Path, Arrowhead West, Inc, **SLP**

Waldmann, Frederick Northeast Hearing Aid Service, 170 37th Avenue North, St Petersburg, FL 33704, (813) 822-2132, BS 63 Upsala Coll; MA 66 Seton Hall Univ; Aud, Northeast Hearing Aid Service, **A**

Waldo, Mrs Judith M 1785 Oak Grove Avenue, San Marino, CA 91108, (818) 446-0131, BA 74 Univ of CA - Los Angeles; MA 80 CA St Univ - Los Angeles; Sp/Lang Path, Arcadia USD, **SLP**

Waldo, Lois J 2429 S E Gemini, Topeka, KS 66605, (913) 354-8232, BS 73 KS St Univ; MA 74 KS St Univ; **SLP**

Waldo, Mrs Lois Jean 367 Whispering Pines #1951, Estes Park, CO 80517, (303) 586-3470, BA 49 Western MI Univ; MA 66 MI St Univ; Retired, Ingham Inter Sch Dist, **SLP**

Waldo-Barr, Kelly 764 East 7th Street, Chico, CA 95928, (916) 894-3296, BA 84 CA St Univ - Chico; MA 86 CA St Univ - Chico; **SLP**

Waldon, Mrs Gloria B 2102 Rownd Street, Cedar Falls, IA 50613, (319) 266-6308, BA 65 Univ of Northern IA; MA 66 Univ of Northern IA; Retired, AEA 7, **SLP**

Waldorf, Mrs Pamela Crowder 6227 Ethan Place, Boise, ID 83704, (208) 378-0525, BA 81 CA St Univ - Long Beach; MA 84 CA St Univ - Long Beach; **SLP**

Waldron, Mrs Claire M 826 Tom's Creek Road, Blacksburg, VA 24060, (703) 381-5453, OB 71 Univ of MO - Columbia; MA 72 Univ of MO - Columbia; 88–SLP, Radford Univ, **SLP**

Waldron, Dr Daryle Lee 718 London Drive, Charleston, SC 29412, (803) 795-5936, BA 49 Univ of CA - Santa Barbara; MA 50 Univ of Southern CA; PH 60 (NS) Stanford Univ; Retired, Dept of Otol Med U of Sc, **A LM**

Waldron, Mrs Lynn Angevine RD 4 Box 4233, Newton, NJ 07860-9421, (201) 729-3557, BS 77 Indiana Univ of PA; MS 79 Vanderbilt Univ; 87–Aud, Private Practice, **A**

Waldron, Maybette Z 120 High Meadow Road, Southport, CT 06490, (203) 259-4551, BS 70 Univ of Bridgeport; MS 72 Southern CT St Univ; Sp-Lang Path, Wilton Bd Educ, **SLP**

Waldron, Sally J 1145 Commodore Street, Clearwater, FL 33515, (813) 442-1171, MS 79 Univ of South FL; SLP, Gulfcoast Cen/Pinellas Co Sch, **SLP**

Waldrop, Teresa Anne 1110 Rickenbacker, Tullahoma, TN 37388, (615) 454-1021, BS 81 Auburn Univ - Auburn; MS 83 Univ of Montevallo; Sp-Lang Path, Elk Valley Home Health Care, **SLP**

Walence, Mrs Barbara Kester 1099 Virginia Drive, Alden, NY 14004, (716) 937-3462, BS 80 Purdue Univ - West Lafayette; MA 82 OH Univ - Athens; **SLP**

Walence, William W 1099 Virginia Drive, Alden, NY 14004, (716) 937-3462, BA 72 Kent St Univ; MA 74 Kent St Univ; Admin, Southtowns Primary Care Ctr Inc, **A**

Walerstein, Mrs Joan I S 1340 N W 97th Avenue, Plantation, FL 33322, (305) 475-1745, BA 72 SUNY - Coll at Cortland; ME 75 Univ of Miami; 79–Sp-Lang Path, Sp/Lang Consult of West Broward, **SLP ACE**

Wales, Mrs R Joella 4970 Avila Way, Buena Park, CA 90621, (714) 521-7699, BA 82 CA St Univ - Fullerton; MA 84 Whittier Coll; Sp-Lang Path, Norwalk School District, **SLP**

Walet, Mrs Marla Ann 1001 East Dale #115, New Iberia, LA 70560, (318) 364-4075, BS 83 Univ of Southwestern LA; MA 86 Univ of Southwestern LA; 87–Sp-Lang Path, Iberia Parish Sch Bd, **SLP**

Walfish, Eleanor R Wilmot Circle #43, Scarsdale, NY 10583, **SLP**

Walford, Janet L 10116 Hefner Village Terrace, Oklahoma City, OK 73162, (405) 631-0137, BS 86 OK Christian Coll; MS 88 Univ of OK Medical Center; Sp-Lang Path, Med Sp Path Aud Assoc

Walhood, Mrs Mary-Kate G 1540 Lee Drive, Clarksdale, MS 38614, (601) 627-5247, BS 78 Delta St Univ; MS 80 Univ of MS; Sp-Lang Path, Clarksdale Sp & Hrng Cen, **SLP**

Waligora, Mrs Jane F 904 Westwood Drive, Herkimer, NY 13350, (315) 724-5101, BS 71 IN Univ - Bloomington; OM 72 IN Univ - Bloomington; Aud/Director, Childrens Hospital/Rehab Ctr, **A**

Walk, Jeanne B 10 Pat's Place, Metairie, LA 70001, BS 77 LA St Univ - Baton Rouge; OM 79 LA St Univ - N O Medical Ctr; Sp-Lang Path, Jefferson Parish Schools, **SLP**

Walker, Alice Irene 5281 M Street, Sacramento, CA 95819, (916) 823-7532, **SLP**

Walker, Ann B 1232 Cheyenne Drive, Richardson, TX 75080, **SLP**

Walker, Beverly S 1325 McBride Lane, Hayward, CA 94544, (415) 785-1361, MS 78 FL St Univ; 88–Sp/Lang Path, Hayward USD, **SLP**

Walker, Bobbie Lonsford 5863 Braesheather, Houston, TX 77096, (713) 541-4933, BS 64 Univ of Houston - Univ Park; Director, Maford Center, **SLP**

Walker, Brenda Dodson 14217 East 37th, Tulsa, OK 74134, (918) 366-4421, BS 75 AR St Univ; MS 76 AR St Univ; Sp-Lang Path, Bixby PS, **SLP**

Walker, Carol Ann 502 Baylor Road, Glen Burnie, MD 21061, (301) 766-8049, MS 87 Loyola Coll

Walker, Carolyn P O Box 363, Zebulon, GA 30295, (404) 567-8097, BS 74 Ithaca Coll; ME 84 GA St Univ; Sp-Lang Path, Pike Co Pub Sch, **SLP**

Walker, Mrs Cathleen Marie Swift Route 2 Box 372, Roseboro, NC 28382, (314) 364-0279, BS 84 Southeast MO St Univ; MA 87 Southeast MO St Univ; 87–Sp-Lang Path, LOGOS Inc, **SLP**

Walker, Mrs Cherie Burge 1205 Jeb Stuart Street, Tupelo, MS 38801, (601) 842-1891, BS 82 Univ of MS; MS 84 Univ of MS; Sp-Lang Path, Regional Rehabilitation Center, **SLP**

Walker, Mrs Cheron Glaze 14800 Private Drive, East Cleveland, OH 44112, (216) 761-6100, MA 81 Univ of Cincinnati; 81–Sp-Lang Path, Cuy Co Bd of Ment Ret, **SLP**

Walker, Christine 2260 E University Drive, Apartment 17-F, Auburn, AL 36830, (205) 826-5545, BA 71 FL St Univ; MS 72 FL St Univ; 86–Sp-Lang Path, Auburn Univ Sp & Hrng Cl, **SLP**

Walker, Dr Christophr Niles Truesdail Speech Center, University Of Redlands, Redlands, CA 92373, (714) 793-2121, BA 70 CA Lutheran Coll; MA 73 CA St Univ - Northridge; PH 81 (Sp Path) Univ of IA; Athletic Dir, University of Redlands, **SLP**

Walker, Clara E P O Box 36, Marietta, OK 73448, BS; **SLP LM**

Walker, Mrs Connie K 4134 Potomac Street, Abilene, TX 79605, (915) 692-1633, BS 79 TX Woman's Univ; MA 81 TX Woman's Univ; 87–Sp-Lang Path, Hendrick Med Ctr, **SLP**

Walker, Cori L S 686 Knox Road, Strafford, PA 19087, (215) 254-0424, BS 78 SUNY - Coll at New Paltz; MA 81 Temple Univ; Aud, Private Practice, **A**

Walker, Danya 519 Oxford St E Apt #2, London, ON, Canada N5Y 3H8, (519) 439-3271, BS 78 Univ of Toronto - Ontario; MS 83 Univ of British Columbia; **SLP**

Walker, David A Ayers Medical Plaza, 720 S W 2nd Avenue Ste 200, Gainesville, FL 32601, (904) 338-1166, BA 80 Univ of AL- Tuscaloosa; MS 82 Univ of AL- Tuscaloosa; Aud, Private Practice, **A**

Walker, Fred L 3330 South 11th Place #2, Sheboygan, WI 53081, (608) 233-2245, BS 76 Marquette Univ; MS 80 Marquette Univ; Sp-Lang Path, St Nicholas Hosp/ENT Cl, **SLP**

Walker, Mrs Gail M R R 1 Box 147, Byron, MN 55920, (507) 775-2596, BA 69 Univ of CA - Santa Barbara; OM 71 Univ of WA; **SLP**

Walker, Glynda Marie 200-B Betty Street, Wheeling, WV 26003, (304) 242-1390, BS 62 Southern IL Univ -Carbondale; MA 68 OH St Univ; 62–Dir Sp-Lang Path, Easter Seal Rehab Ctr, **SLP**

Walker, Mrs Helen S 116 Curtis Avenue, Maxwell Hill, Beckley, WV 25801, (304) 252-7355, BS 64 WV Univ; MS 71 WV Univ; 64–Sp-Lang Path, Raleigh Co Bd of Ed, **SLP**

Walker, Mrs Jacque D 2208 Beau Monde, Pine Bluff, AR 71603, (501) 535-3002, BA 59 Univ of AR - Fayetteville; MA 75 Univ of AR - Fayetteville; Sp-Lang Path, Pine Bluff ENT Cl, **SLP ACE**

Walker, James Anthony 6330 Lake Apopka Place, San Diego, CA 92119, (619) 697-8408, MS 88 Howard Univ

Walker, Mrs Jane A P O Box 907094, Gainesville, GA 30501, (404) 534-5141, BS 80 Western Carolina Univ; ME 81 Western Carolina Univ; Sp-Lang Path, NE Georgia Sp Ctr, **SLP**

Walker, Jane M 2760 Macby Avenue, Marietta, GA 30066-3620, (404) 977-2232, **SLP**

Walker, Mrs Janice L 1301 2nd Avenue, P O Box 1415, Zillah, WA 98953, (509) 829-5545, BA 77 WA St Univ; MA 80 WA St Univ; SLP, Sunnyside School District, **SLP**

Walker, Janice R 111 Washington Avenue, Hawthorne, NJ 07506, (201) 595-2208, BA 73 Univ of MA - Amherst; MA 75 Univ of MA - Amherst; Aud, Wm Patterson Col, **A**

Walker, Jena W 601 East 15th Street, Austin, TX 78626, (512) 480-1993, MS 85 Univ of TX - Dallas; Sp-Lang Path, Brackenridge Hosp, **SLP**

Walker, Jerry O P O Box 299, Grayson, LA 71435, (318) 640-0754, BA 59 Northwestern St Univ; MA 68 LA Tech Univ; 86–Sp-Lang Path, Pinecrest State Sch, **SLP**

Walker, Joan Peirce 5-20 Strawberry Bank Road, Nashua, NH 03062, (617) 649-6071, BS 69 CO St Univ, MA 70 Univ of Northern CO; Sp/Lang Path, Tyngsboro Pub Schs, **SLP**

Walker, Joanne M 35 Roosevelt Street, Babylon, NY 11702, (516) 543-5100, BA 85 SUNY - Center at Stony Brook; MS 86 Adelphi Univ; **SLP**

Walker, Johnnie C 1908 Carriage House Lane, Camden, SC 29020-2018, (803) 432-8416, BS 70 Univ of GA; ME Univ of SC - Columbia; 88–Sp-Lang Path, Kershaw Co Schs, **SLP**

Walker, Joyce Witzler 3296 Bellefonte Drive, Lexington, KY 40502, (606) 278-3126, BS 62 Kent St Univ; ME 67 Kent St Univ; Instr/Superv, Univ of Kentucky, **SLP**

Walker, Mrs Judith K 790 Oakhaven Drive, Roswell, GA 30075, (404) 998-2296, BS 66 Univ of NE - Lincoln; MA 75 CA St Univ - Fullerton; 87–Sp-Lang Path, Fulton Co Schs, **SLP**

Walker, Mrs Julia C 5529 Hickory Ridge, Bossier City, LA 71111, (318) 742-5308, MA 87 LA Tech Univ; **SLP**

Walker, Julie A 11324 Windmill Place, Oklahoma City, OK 73162, BS 78 KS St Univ; MS 80 CO St Univ; Sp-Lang Path, Oklahoma City Public Schools, **SLP**

Walker, Karen Elaine 657 24th #45, Santa Cruz, CA 95062, (408) 476-9568, BA 81 CA St Univ - Hayward; MA 83 Univ of San Francisco; Sp-Lang Path, Eldercare Conv Hospital, **SLP**

Walker, Karen Woodford 511 Dogwood Circle View, Pigeon Forge, TN 37863, (615) 453-7521, BS 65 CO St Univ; MS 66 Univ of WI - Madison; Sp-Lang Path, Douglas-Cherokee Knox Hd Start, **SLP**

Walker, Kathryn 1851 East South Mountain, Phoenix, AZ 85040, (602) 838-3688, **SLP**

Walker, Kimberley M 3 Lexington Road, Bordentown, NJ 08505, (609) 298-9215, BS 76 Trenton St Coll; MA 77 Trenton St Coll; **SLP**

Walker, Mrs Linda A 658 East Stottler Place, Chandler, AZ 85225, (602) 496-4720, BS 86 Univ of Southern CO; OM 87 AZ St Univ; 87–Sp-Lang Path, Kyrene Sch Dist

Walker, Mrs Linda Mathis 802 Comer Avenue, Eufaula, AL 36027, (205) 687-9647, BS 85 Auburn Univ - Auburn; OM 87 Auburn Univ - Auburn; **SLP**

Walker, Mrs Lisa Carol 3301 Rivercrest Drive #304, Melbourne, FL 32935, (305) 242-1469, BS 83 Western KY Univ; MS 84 Western KY Univ

Walker, Lois Alice 1100 West Chester Pike, Apartment E-9, West Chester, PA 19382, (215) 891-2380, BA 71 Rutger's St Univ - Douglas Coll; MS 72 PA St Univ - Univ Park; 88–Unit Mgr-Sp & Hrng, Elwyn Inc, **A**

Walker, Lola Deane 8707 East Fort Foote Terr, Fort Washington, MD 20744, (301) 839-9243, BA 80 Univ of MD - College Park; MS 86 Univ of the DC; **SLP**

Walker, Lynn A 10108 Chickadee Lane, Adelphi, MD 20783, (301) 439-5355, BA 80 Univ of MD - College Park; MS 82 Univ of MI - Ann Arbor; Sp/Lang Path, Montgomery County PS, **SLP**

Walker, Margaret E 301 20th Avenue #2, San Francisco, CA 94121, MA; **SLP**

Walker, Mrs Marianna Morris Route 1 Box 396-M, Bethel, NC 27812, (919) 825-0531, BS 79 East Carolina Univ; MS 82 East Carolina Univ; 88–Clin Instr, East Carolina Univ, **SLP**

Walker, Mary Elizabeth 251 Pearl Street, Newton, MA 02158, (617) 935-5050, Sp-Lang Path, New England Rehabilitatn Hosp, **SLP**

Walker, Mrs Mary Jo 902 West Lynwood Street, Phoenix, AZ 85007, (602) 234-3366, BS 73 OH St Univ; MS 78 AZ St Univ; Sp/Lang Path, Osborn Sch Dist #8, **SLP**

Walker, Maude J 770 Columbia Road N W, Washington, DC 20001, (202) 265-1126, BS Univ of the DC; MA 77 Univ of the DC; SLP, Dc Public Schools Special Educ, **SLP LM**

Walker, Maura Anne 725 Old County Road, Apartment N, Belmont, CA 94002, (415) 696-4300, OB 82 Univ of MO - Columbia; MA 84 Univ of KS; Sp-Lang Path, Mills Peninsula Hosp, **SLP**

Walker, Michael T 5765 Carranza Drive, Salt Lake City, UT 84118, (801) 967-9548, BS 80 Brigham Young Univ; OM 81 Brigham Young Univ; Aud, Intermountain Health Care, **A**

Walker, Michael W Toledo Clinic, Audiology Dept, 4235 Secor Road, Toledo, OH 43623, (419) 473-3561, BS 70 Purdue Univ - West Lafayette; MS 72 Purdue Univ - West Lafayette; Aud, Dept Head, Toledo Cl, **A**

Walker, Mrs Pamela Hoover 11904 Swallow Drive, Austin, TX 78750, (512) 444-4835, BS 79 Univ of TX - Austin; MA 82 Univ of Houston - Univ Park; SLP, Health Care Rehab Ctr, **SLP**

Walker, Pamela M 11291 South Sandy Creek Dr, Sandy, UT 84070, (801) 350-4689, BA 79 SUNY - Coll at Potsdam; MS 81 Ithaca Coll; Aud, Holy Cross Hospital, **A**

Walker, Patricia A Tkaczuk 50 Reed Street #6, Rockland, MA 02370, (617) 638-7370, BA 80 Southeast MO St Univ; BS 80 Southeast MO St Univ; MA 83 Memphis St Univ; Sp-Lang Path, Private Practice, **SLP**

Walker, Penelope Rice 2148 Eastwood Drive, Fort Collins, CO 80525, (303) 482-5712, BS 78 Elmira Coll; MS 82 Ithaca Coll; Sp-Lang Path, **SLP**

Walker, Phyllis Jinette 5312 Mays Drive, Jacksonville, FL 32209, (904) 765-2465

Walker, Randy Wayne 110 Anne Street, Beckley, WV 25801, (304) 574-2901, **A**

Walker, Rhonda Kim 2216 N Denton Road #D-3, Dothan, AL 36303, (205) 774-5132, BS 82 Univ of Montevallo; MS 85 Univ of Montevallo; **SLP**

Walker, Dr Richard W Harding University, Searcy, AR 72143, (501) 268-3180, BA 50 Harding Univ; ME 51 LA St Univ - Baton Rouge; PH 61 (NS) LA St Univ - Baton Rouge; Cl Dir, Harding U

Walker, Mrs Roberta A 15314 Bonita Springs Drive, Houston, TX 77083, (817) 980-6899, BS 76 Wayne St Univ; MA 78 Wayne St Univ; **SLP**

Walker, Sandra Gail 110 Barrett Road, Calhoun, GA 30701, (404) 382-0680, BS 79 Ball St Univ; ME 83 Columbus Coll; Sp-Lang Path, Bartow County Schools, **SLP**

Walker, Mrs Sandra Reese 3525 Esteva Place, Gainesville, GA 30506, (404) 532-7711, BS 79 Appalachian St Univ; ME 81 Univ of GA; ME 84 Univ of GA; Sp-Lang Path, Gainesville City Schools, **SLP**

Walker, Mrs Sherry McDaniel 4408 Turnberry Court, Douglasville, GA 30135, (404) 942-5330, BS 76 Univ of GA; ME 85 GA St Univ; 82–Sp-Lang Path, Cobb County Public Schools, **SLP**

Walker, Sherry Wilson Quarters 36-B, Francis E Warren AFB, WY 82001, (307) 632-0364, MS 87 Univ of WY

Walker, Susan M 3931 Round Hill Drive, Chesterfield, VA 23832, (804) 276-9434, BS 79 Univ of VA - Charlottesville; MA 81 Univ of TN - Knoxville; Sp-Lang Path, Richmond Pub Schs, **SLP**

Walker, Teresa Phillips 3417 Candy Drive, Hopkinsville, KY 42240, (502) 439-1927, BS 83 Murray St Univ; MS 84 Murray St Univ; 85–Sp-Lang Path, Ft Campbell Sch Sys, **SLP**

Walker, Thomas Lee 543 Bryant Street, Palo Alto, CA 94301, Director of Audiology, Industrial Health Inc, **A**

Walker, Mrs Virginia Ann 4760 West Forest Peak, Marietta, GA 30066, BA 82 Univ of NC - Greensboro; ME 83 Univ of NC - Greensboro; Sp-Lang Path, Cobb County Schs, **SLP**

Walker, Dr Virginia G 3220 Robinhood Road, Tallahassee, FL 32312, (904) 644-2238, BA 64 Longwood Coll; ME 65 Univ of VA - Charlottesville; PH 79 (NS) FL St Univ; Assoc Prof, FL St U, **SLP**

Walker-Casey, Amy Beth 15096 S W 104th Street, Apartment 1107, Miami, FL 33196, (305) 385-7985, BS 83 SUNY - Coll at Buffalo; MS 86 Univ of VT; **SLP**

Walkey, Mrs Joan E 50 Cedar Street, Duxbury, MA 02332, (617) 934-5588, BA 82 Bridgewater St Coll; MA 87 Bridgewater St Coll; **SLP**

Walkley, Dawn Dodder 307 West 35th Street #310, Steger, IL 60475-2024, (312) 957-7100, BS 84 Central MI Univ; MA 85 Central MI Univ; 86–Sp-Lang Path, S Metro Assoc Commun Dev Prog, **SLP**

Walko, Amy Clark 3607 N Seeley #3, Chicago, IL 60618, (312) 702-6687, BS 83 Univ of IL - Urbana; MS 86 Univ of WA; **SLP**

Walkup, Tami K 3815 Watkins Lane, Eugene, OR 97405, (503) 686-3591, BS 83 Univ of OR; MS 86 Univ of OR; **SLP**

Wall, Mrs Ann M Brabston Route 1 Box 92, Grove Hill, AL 36451, (205) 275-3390, BS 80 Univ Southern MS-Hattiesburg; MS 81 Univ Southern MS-Hattiesburg; 88–Sp/Lang Path, Thomasville City Schs, **SLP**

Wall, Mrs Brenda 8104 Backlash Court, Springfield, VA 22153, (703) 534-7712, BS 65 WV Univ; ME 66 Univ of VA - Charlottesville; SLP, Fairfax Co Pub Sch, **SLP**

Wall, Christine Joyce 200 Walnut Street, Pocomoke City, MD 21851, (301) 957-0990, BS 85 Towson St Univ; MS 87 Towson St Univ; 87–Sp-Lang Path, Somerset Co Bd of Educ

Wall, David John 3216 Victory Palm Drive, Edgewater, FL 32032-6512, (904) 734-3320, BA 77 Univ of Central FL; MA 83 Wayne St Univ; Sp-Lang Path, West Volusia Memorial Hosp, **SLP**

Wall, Mrs Debra J Box 246, Montezuma, KS 67867, (316) 855-3343, BA 73 Univ of KS; MS 74 KS St Univ; Sp-Lang Path, SW Ks Area Coop Dist, **SLP**

Wall, Jane C 33 Chestnut Street, Malden, MA 02148, (617) 298-7900, BS 51 Univ of NH; MA 70 Temple Univ; Sp-Lang Path, Mattapan Hosp, **SLP**

Wall, Mrs Janet Myrick 2630 Weymouth Road, Winston-Salem, NC 27103, (919) 765-6846, BS 76 Old Dominion Univ, ME 80 Univ of VA - Charlottesville; Sp-Lang Path, Winston-Salem Forsyth Co Sch, **SLP**

Wall, Kathleen 3703 Adams Drive, Wheaton, MD 20902, (703) 536-1666, BA 75 Univ of MD - College Park; MS 77 Towson St Univ; Aud, Arlington/Fairfax Hrng & Sp Ctr, **A**

Wall, Kathleen B 26 South M Street, Lake Worth, FL 33460, BS 53 Fordham Univ; MA 55 Columbia Univ Teachers Coll; **SLP A**

Wall, Kathryn Ellen 8440 Lafayette Way, Wilsonville, OR 97070, (503) 588-5330, BS 82 Western OR St Coll; MS 84 Western OR St Coll; 85–Sp-Lang Path, Marion Educ Svc Dist, **SLP**

Wall, Mrs Kelly Jo 1770 South Rock Road #604, Wichita, KS 67207-5176, (316) 684-6649, BA 84 Wichita St Univ; MA 85 Wichita St Univ; 88–Sp-Lang Path, Cowley Co Spec Svcs Coop Dist #465, **SLP**

Wall, Dr Lida Gayl Division Of Speech/Hearing Science, Ohio State University, 154 North Oval Drive, Columbus, OH 43210, (614) 292-8207, BA 61 Univ of Northern CO; MS 73 Univ of WY; PH 79 (NS) OH St Univ; Associate Professor, Ohio State University, **A**

Wall, Mrs Martha M 231 Monmouth Way, Clifton Park, NY 12065, (518) 355-2390, BS 86 SUNY - Coll at Plattsburgh; MS 87 Ithaca Coll; SLP, Schenectady Assn for Rc, **SLP**

Wall, Mrs Mary Elizabeth 2711 Grants Lake Blvd #124, Sugar Land, TX 77479, (713) 790-8634, BS 74 TX Tech Univ; MA 83 San Diego St Univ; 86–Sp-Lang Path, Alief ISD, **SLP**

Wall, Mary Ellen 44 Dunham Place, St Charles, IL 60174, (312) 420-6335, BA 82 Elmhurst Coll; MA 83 Northern IL Univ - De Kalb; Sp-Lang Path, Naperville Sch Dist #203, **SLP**

Wall, Dr Meryl Johnson 134 Garden Street, Roslyn Heights, NY 11577, (516) 294-8700, MS 64 Purdue Univ - West Lafayette; PH 77 (NS) CUNY - Grad Sch & Univ Cntr; 77–Assoc Prof, Adelphi U, **SLP**

Wall, Shellee D Route 6 Box 147-B #1, Peartree Village, Poplar Bluff, MO 63901, (314) 785-0101, BS 85 Murray St Univ; MS 87 Murray St Univ

Wall, Susan Mary 10740 Shedron Way, Lombard, IL 60148, (312) 916-0120, BS 82 IL St Univ - Normal; MS 79 Governors St Univ; SLP, Sch Dist #135 Orland Park II, **SLP**

Wallace, Beth E 2901 Rosedale, Dallas, TX 75205, (214) 373-7625, BS 83 LA St Univ - Baton Rouge; MS 84 LA St Univ - N O Medical Ctr; Sp-Lang Path, Prof Sp & Hrng Serv, **SLP**

Wallace, Dr Bill L Communication Sci & Dis Dept, Towson State University, Baltimore, MD 21204, (301) 321-3097, BS 57 Central MI Univ; MS 62 Central MI Univ; PH 66 (NS) OH St Univ; 68–Chmn, Towson State Univ, **SLP A**

Wallace, Brenda Reimer 3107 Indiana N E, Albuquerque, NM 87110, (505) 764-2000, BA 76 MI St Univ; MS 84 Univ of NM; 84–Sp-Lang Path, Albuquerque PS, **SLP**

Wallace, Mrs Brenda Sue 46 Sunset Drive, Bronston, KY 42518, (606) 678-5229, BS 74 Murray St Univ; MA 84 Eastern KY Univ; Sp-Lang Path, Pulaski Co Board of Ed, **SLP**

Wallace, Christine Morgan 201 Cedarcroft Road, Baltimore, MD 21212, (301) 532-7809, BS 72 Purdue Univ - West Lafayette; MS 74 Purdue Univ - West Lafayette; Consultant Sp-Lang Path, Madeline Fox Associates, **SLP**

Wallace, Dr Cynthia A 3745 East Nichols Avenue, P O Box 2336, Littleton, CO 80161, (303) 771-3990, MA 71 Univ of Denver; PH 88 (School Administration) Univ of Denver; Prin, Beacon Country Day Sch, **SLP**

Wallace, Mrs Dana D 1800 Long Drive, Richmond, TX 77469, (713) 342-3939, BA 73 Univ of Houston - Univ Park; MA 76 Our Lady Lake Univ-San Anton; 87–Sp-Lang Path, Living Waters Christian Sch, **SLP**

Wallace, Mrs Debora Hamilton 400 Cross Lake Dr, Fuquay-Varina, NC 27526, (919) 552-8276, BA 79 NC St Univ at Raleigh; ME 84 NC Central Univ; Sp-Lang Path, North Carolina Public Schools, **SLP**

Wallace, Debra S 18 Beechwood Lane, Glastonbury, CT 06073, (203) 633-9281, BS 74 Northwestern Univ; MA 75 Northwestern Univ; Sp-Lang Path, Private Practice, **SLP**

Wallace, Diane 900 Tepic, El Paso, TX 79912, (915) 581-3181, BA 83 Univ of TX - El Paso; MS 87 Univ of TX - El Paso; **SLP**

Wallace, Donald E Luzerne Intermediate Unit, 368 Tioga Avenue, Kingston, PA 18704, (717) 655-8509, MS 62 Univ of Scranton; Supervisor Special Education, Luzerne Intermediate Unit, **SLP**

Wallace, Dr Doris Davis , Anabel, MO 63431, (816) 699-2365, BS 37 Northeast MO St Univ; MA 45 Univ of MO - Columbia; PH 64 (Sp Path Stuttering) NY Univ; 72–Retired, **SLP LM**

Wallace, Mrs Dorothy A 415 Wayne, Salina, KS 67401, (913) 827-0301, BA 69 KS St Univ; MA 71 KS St Univ; Sp-Lang Path, Central Kans Coop In Ed, **SLP**

Wallace, Dyanne E 296 Grist Mill Lane, Lawrenceville, GA 30245, (404) 995-5327, BS 78 Univ of GA; ME 79 Univ of GA; 86–Sp-Lang Path, Bailey Sp & Lang Svcs, **SLP**

Wallace, Elizabeth M 2017 East Ocean Boulevard, Balboa, CA 92661, (714) 673-8955, BA 56 Univ of WA; MA 66 San Francisco St Univ; Retired, **F**

Wallace, Dr Gloriajean L Michigan State University, Dept Aud & Speech Sciences, 378 Comm Arts & Sci Bldg, East Lansing, MI 48824, BS 74 Miami Univ - Oxford; MA 76 Univ of CO - Boulder; PH 81 (NS) Northwestern Univ; Assistant Professor, Michigan State University, **SLP ACE**

Wallace, Mrs Jane Lambert 1808 Haynes Street, Clarksville, TN 37040, BS 76 Austin Peay St Univ; MS 78 Murray St Univ; SLP, Private Practice, **SLP**

Wallace, Kathleen Louise Boys Town National Inst, 555 No 30th St, Omaha, NE 68131, (402) 449-6668, BS 84 Univ of WI - Madison; MS 86 Univ of WI - Madison; Aud, Boys Town Nat'l Institute, **A**

Wallace, Kathleen P Route 3 Box 354, Brighton, TN 38011, (901) 476-7148, BS 80 Univ of TN - Martin; MA 82 Memphis St Univ; Sp/Lang Path, Tipton Co Dept of Pub Instr, **SLP**

Wallace, Laurie Link 25 Corinthian Road, Somerville, MA 02144, (617) 629-2729, BS 79 PA St Univ - Univ Park; MS 81 PA St Univ - Univ Park; Sp-Lang Path, Kennedy Mem Hosp for Chldn, **SLP**

Wallace, Linda Mary 30 Corbett Avenue, Dedham, MA 02026, (412) 421-6543, BS 85 Univ of MA - Amherst; MA 86 Univ of Pittsburgh - Pittsburgh; **A**

Wallace, Mrs Lori Ann/Borth 1 Carnelian, Irvine, CA 92714, (714) 552-5171, BA 82 CA St Univ - Long Beach; MA 85 Univ of CA - Santa Barbara; Sp-Lang Path, Irvine USD, **SLP**

Wallace, Mrs Marion M 8115 Amelia Drive, El Cajon, CA 92021, BA San Diego St Univ; MA 77 San Diego St Univ; SLP, Ramona USD, **SLP**

Wallace, Mrs Mary Louise 4686 Talbot Drive, Boulder, CO 80303, (303) 499-7677, BA 79 SUNY - Coll at Plattsburgh; MA 83 Univ of CO - Boulder; Sp/Lang Path, Peter Ramig Phd & Assoc, **SLP**

Wallace, Mrs Maureen Porter 191 West Burton Mesa Blvd, Lompoc, CA 93436, (805) 735-3396, BA 80 Univ of CA - Santa Barbara; MA 81 Univ of Northern CO; Aud, Dr Michel, **A**

Wallace, Mrs Neta Jane 624 North 13th, Apt N, Garden City, KS 67846, (316) 277-6583, **SLP**

Wallace, Patty Nesom 4317 South Baldwin #107, Fort Worth, TX 76115-1202, (915) 643-5610, BS 84 Baylor Univ; MS 86 Univ of OK - OK City; **SLP**

Wallace, Rita Baker 1533 Applewood Road, Baton Rouge, LA 70808, **SLP**

Wallace, Sarah A 117 Georgia Street, Lafayette, LA 70501, (318) 365-2341, BA 74 Univ of Southwestern LA; MA 75 Univ of Denver; Sp-Lang Path, Iberia Parish Sch Bo, **SLP**

Wallace, Sharon Kitina P O Box 554, Wallace, NC 28466, (919) 755-4845, BS 81 East Carolina Univ; MS 83 Univ of NC - Chapel Hill; **A**

Wallace, Sherry L 10223 Melrose, Overland Park, KS 66214, (913) 676-2444, BS 70 Univ of KS; MA 72 Univ of KS; 77–Sp-Lang Path, Private Practice, **SLP**

Wallace, Mrs Susan E 2959 Whispering Pines, Canfield, OH 44406, (216) 743-1151, BA 76 Temple Univ; MA 78 Temple Univ; Aud, Youngstown Bd of Ed, **A**

Wallace, Susan Mervin 1924 Alcoa Highway, Knoxville, TN 37920, (615) 544-9030, BA 65 Univ of VT; MA 76 Univ of TN - Knoxville; 76–Dir Sp-Hrng Ser, U of TN Hosp-Birth Defects Ctr, **SLP**

Wallace, Susan Shreffler 2664 Travis Drive, Wheelersburg, OH 45694, (614) 353-7774, **SLP**

Wallace, Suzanne Stacey 3240 Jupiter Road, Las Cruces, NM 88001, (505) 522-2226, OB 62 Univ of FL; OM 71 Univ of FL; 88–Sp-Lang Path, Las Cruces PS, **SLP**

Wallace, Mrs Teri Ann 4421 N E 3rd Street, Ocala, FL 32671, (904) 694-7289, **SLP**

Wallace, Thomas Claude 1051 South Main, Orem, UT 84057, (801) 225-3847, BA 67 Walla Walla Coll; MS 70 Western OR St Coll; 88–Predoctoral Psychology Intern, Timpanogos Mental Health Center, **SLP**

Wallace, Mrs Vicki Rush 121 East High Street, Kingwood, WV 26537, (304) 329-2129, BS 80 WV Univ; MS 81 WV Univ; Aud, Preston Co Bd of Ed, **A**

Wallace-Bates, Mrs Victoria Rose 3700 South Poplar, Casper, WY 82601, (307) 234-5619, BS 83 Univ of WY; MS 85 Univ of WY; **SLP**

Wallach, Dr Geraldine 4627 Roxbury Road, Corona Del Mar, CA 92625, (714) 760-9762, BA 68 Long Island U - Brooklyn Ctr; MA 69 NY Univ; PH 77 (NS) CUNY - Grad Sch & Univ Cntr; **SLP**

Wallach, Richard W 917 Pacific Street, Monterey, CA 93940, (408) 373-1209, BS 75 SUNY - Coll at Brockport; MS 81 Univ of MI - Ann Arbor; Exec Dir, Rehab Providers, **SLP**

Wallach-Delucia, Wendy 913-3 Wesley Avenue, Oak Park, IL 60304, (312) 567-5650, BA 83 Pace U -NY City; MS 85 Univ of VT; 86–Aud, Mercy Hosp & Med Ctr, **A**

Wallack, Wendy C 500-273B Peconic Street, Ronkonkoma, NY 11779, (516) 981-0814, BS 78 SUNY - Center at Albany; MA 79 Hofstra Univ; 84–Sp-Lang Path, Brentwood Pub Sch, **SLP ACE**

Wallander, Mrs Karen S 714 South Willow Road, Evansville, IN 47714, (812) 477-6109, BS 62 Univ of WI - Madison; MS 65 Univ of WI - Madison; SLP, Evansvile-Vanderburg Sch Coop, **SLP**

Wallber, M Josara National Tech Inst For Deaf, One Lomb Memorial Drive, 60-3135, Rochester, NY 14623, (716) 475-6294, BS 75 CO St Univ; MS 80 ID St Univ; Asst Prof/Rehab Aud, NTID, **A**

Walle, Eugene L 4609 Morgan Drive, Chevy Chase, MD 20815, (301) 799-3400, BA 50 Central MI Univ; MA 52 Univ of MI - Ann Arbor; **SLP A**

Wallen, Joyce A Univ Of Kentucky Medical Cen, Neurosen Disorders Rm N-1, 800 Rose Street, Lexington, KY 40536, (606) 233-5472, BA 71 Berea Coll; ME 75 Univ of Louisville; Aud, Univ of Kentucky Medical Cen, **A**

Wallenberg, Ellis A, III 178-25th Avenue, San Francisco, CA 94121, (415) 221-6260, BA 66 Glenville St Coll; MS 68 WV Univ; 85–VP of Mktg, Environmental Hlth Assoc, **SLP A**

Wallenius, Wesley A 2 Temi Road, West Peabody, MA 01960, (617) 535-1053, BA 37 Dartmouth Coll; ME 50 Boston Univ; **SLP LM**

Waller, Sharon Denny P O Box 831, Aromas, CA 95004, MA 86 San Jose St Univ; **SLP**

Waller-Lee, Mrs Rhonda Jean 1304 Jacob Drive, Yardley, PA 19067, (215) 860-6636, BA 77 Rutger's St Univ - Douglas Coll; MA 81 CUNY - Hunter Coll; SLP, Trenton Board of Education, **SLP**

Walley, Joy Brandt 4436 Swiss Stone Lane East, Apartment 2-A, Ypsilanti, MI 48197, (215) 631-9300, BA 83 Univ of MI - Ann Arbor; MS 85 Univ of MI - Ann Arbor; **SLP**

Walley, Mary L 1305 South Seaman, Eastland, TX 76448, (214) 569-2466, BS 70 East TX St Univ - Commerce; MS 75 East TX St Univ - Commerce; Sp-Lang Path, East End Educ Coop, **SLP**

Wallin, Mrs Ann Berstein 1424 East 85th Street, Brooklyn, NY 11236, (718) 780-5186, BA 82 CUNY - Brooklyn Coll; MS 84 CUNY - Brooklyn Coll; **A**

Wallin, Mrs Francine A 7504 Germane Trail, Apple Valley, MN 55124, (612) 432-1140, BA 66 Syracuse Univ; MA 68 OH Univ - Athens; MS 72 Canisius Coll; **SLP**

Wallis, Mrs Barbara A Route 1 Box 845, Louisa, KY 41230, (606) 638-9054, BA 69 Marshall Univ; MA 72 Marshall Univ; Sp-Lang Path, Private Practice, **SLP**

Wallis, Donna Lynn 3423 Oak Shadow Lane, Montgomery, AL 36116, (205) 281-6327, OM 84 Auburn Univ - Auburn; 84–Aud, Bruce F Holding MD, **A**

Wallis, Julie Ann 118 Rockland Dr, West Lafayette, IN 47906, (317) 643-3571, BS 81 Central MO St Univ; MS 83 Central MO St Univ; Sp-Lang Path, Hd State Sch Severe Hndcpd, **SLP**

Wallis, Mrs Karene Jones Head-Neck Specialty Group, 200 Route 16, Somersworth, NH 03878, (603) 749-2749, BS 81 Univ of NH; MS 84 Gallaudet Coll; 87–Aud, Head & Neck Speciality Group, **A**

Wallis, Mrs Kathryn D 272 2nd Avenue S E, New Brighton, MN 55112, (612) 347-8550, BA 77 Univ of ND; MS 81 Univ of WI - Madison; Sp-Lang Path, Hennepin Co Med Ctr, **SLP**

Walls, Mrs Brenda K 2112 Malvern Hill Drive, Austin, TX 78745, (512) 472-4240, BA 78 Marshall Univ; MA 79 Marshall Univ; Sp-Lang Path, Austin ISD, **SLP**

Walls, Mrs Carol S 6009 North State Street, Oklahoma City, OK 73122, (405) 949-3280, BS 62 Austin Coll; MA 79 Ball St Univ; Sp-Lang Path, Baptist Medical Center, **SLP**

Walls, Mrs Nancy F 346 Hotchkiss Road, Orange, CT 06477, BS 70 Emerson Coll; MS 72 Southern CT St Univ; Sp-Lang Path, Private Practice, **SLP**

Walls, Wilma Margarita 916 Ash Street, St Charles, IL 60174, (312) 859-1616, BS 80 Bradley Univ; MS 84 Bradley Univ; **A**

Wallschlaeger, Anne Marie 7718 West Howard Avenue #3, Milwaukee, WI 53220, (414) 321-5835, BA 84 Univ of WI - Eau Claire; MS 85 Univ of WI - Eau Claire; SLP, Milwaukee Ps, **SLP**

Walmsley, Dixie Maas 2100 47th S W, Seattle, WA 98116, (206) 326-7330, BA 62 Univ of WA; MA 64 Univ of WA; 87–Sp-Lang Path, Private Practice, **SLP**

Walmsley, Mrs Sandra D 2320 West Calle Iglesia, Mesa, AZ 85202, (602) 248-7503, BS 78 AZ St Univ; MS 80 AZ St Univ; Sp-Lang Path, Private Practice, **SLP**

Walner, Mrs Joan C 2609 Graphic Place, Plano, TX 75075, (214) 233-8471, BA 69 Univ of North TX; MS 73 Southern Methodist Univ; Sp/Lang Path, Pediatric Comm Dis Cl, **SLP**

Walpole, Elizabeth 620-D Sutton Apartment, Collingswood, NJ 08107, (609) 858-6860, BA 44 Univ of Cincinnati; MA 46 Case Western Reserve Univ; Sp-Lang Path, Private Practice, **SLP LM**

Walpool, Thomas W 9-11 Medical Court, 811 Pendleton Street, Greenville, SC 29601, (803) 235-9689, BS 59 East TN St Univ; MA 60 Univ of AL- Tuscaloosa; Exec Dir, Sp/Hrng/Lrng Cen Inc, **SLP**

Walrath, Mrs Pamela D 40 Pine Knoll Drive, Rochester, NY 14624, (716) 461-2800, BS 71 SUNY - Coll at Geneseo; MS 72 SUNY - Coll at Geneseo; Sp-Lang Path/Aud Prog Coord, Monroe Developmental Cen, **SLP**

Walser, Paula S 224 North Street, North Fond Du Lac, WI 54935, (414) 233-CESA, BS 80 Univ of WI - Oshkosh; MS 82 Univ of WI - Oshkosh; Sp/Lang Path, CES 6, **SLP**

Walseth, Mrs Wanda Colleen 709 South 9th Street, Moorhead, MN 56560, (218) 354-2300, BS 73 Moorhead St Univ; MS 79 Moorhead St Univ; SLP, Barnesville Public Schools, **SLP**

Walsh, Mrs Bobbie Jean Lee 1480 Muretic Lane, Cottonwood, AZ 86326, (602) 634-3965, BS 78 Northern AZ Univ; MS 81 Northern AZ Univ; Sp-Lang Path, Oak Creek Cottonwood Sch Dist, **SLP**

Walsh, Carol R 462 Greg Drive, Lilburn, GA 30247, (404) 320-4700, BA 68 MI St Univ; OM 71 IN Univ - Bloomington; 86–Aud, Children's Med Svcs, **A**

Walsh, Cindy Therese 1781 Spyglass Drive, #195, Austin, TX 78746, (512) 454-4731, SLP, Austin State School, **SLP**

Walsh, Daniel J Communication Clinic, P O Box 193, Spring Lake, MI 49456, (616) 842-9536, BS 60 Western MI Univ; Dir, Commun Cl, **SLP**

Walsh, Donna Wright 3989 Rowena Drive, Philadelphia, PA 19114, (215) 945-1730, BS 81 Bloomsburg Univ of PA; MS 86 PA St Univ - Univ Park; 86–Sp-Lang Path, Easter Seal Society, **SLP**

Walsh, Mrs Dorothy W 3 Smithfield Road, Whippany, NJ 07981, (201) 887-0632, BA 33 Rutger's St Univ - Douglas Coll; MA 64 Kean Coll of NJ; **SLP LM**

Walsh, Mrs Elizabeth 3 Hearthstone Drive, Simsbury, CT 06070, (203) 658-0451, BA 57 Emerson Coll; MS 79 Southern CT St Univ; **SLP**

Walsh, Mrs Gail P 14108 Canterbury Lane, Rockville, MD 20853, BA 74 Univ of VA - Charlottesville; ME 77 Univ of VA - Charlottesville; Sp-Lang Path, Mont Co Pub Sch, **SLP**

Walsh, Gail Shearer 6716 Curtis Way, Florence, KY 41042, (606) 781-3333, BA 79 Univ of KY; MS 82 Miami Univ - Oxford; Sp-Lang Path, Fort Thomas Indepen Schools, **SLP**

Walsh, Mrs Georgia Lou 2231 Laguna Court, Point Pleasant, NJ 08742, (201) 899-6534, BA 72 Marshall Univ; MA 80 Seton Hall Univ; 72–Sp-Lang Path, Toms River Board of Education

Walsh, Mrs Helen Alice 2339 Oxford Avenue, Cardiff, CA 92007, (619) 755-8000, MA 83 San Diego St Univ; **SLP**

Walsh, Jeanne M Children's Medical Center Of Dallas, Speech Pathology And Audiology Department, 1935 Motor Street, Dallas, TX 75235, (214) 879-6178, BA 76 MI St Univ; MA 79 Central MI Univ; 85–Sp-Lang Path, Childrens Med Ctr, **SLP**

Walsh, Mrs Joann M 1529 North 117th Street, Wauwatosa, WI 53226, (414) 354-9494, BA 70 Univ of WI - Eau Claire; MS 71 Univ of WI - Eau Claire; 77–Sp-Lang Path, Brown Deer Pub Sch, **SLP**

Walsh, Karen C 15606 Dove Meadow, San Antonio, TX 78248, (512) 493-2647, BS 65 Clarion Univ of PA; MS 68 PA St Univ - Univ Park; **SLP**

Walsh, Kate 28 Endora Drive, Baldwinsville, NY 13027-1208, (315) 451-2161, BA 72 Catholic Univ of America; ME 74 Univ of Pittsburgh - Pittsburgh; MS 80 Syracuse Univ; Sp-Lang Path, Baldwinsville Central Schools, **SLP**

Walsh, Katherine 3130 Walnut Road, Norman, OK 73072, (405) 321-4048, BS 73 Univ of OK - Norman; MA 75 Univ of OK - Norman; 75–Cl Dir/Sp-Lang Path, OK St Hlth Dept, **SLP ACE**

Walsh, Keith P 3 Johnson Road, Saranac Lake, NY 12983, (518) 561-2000, BA 74 SUNY - Coll at Plattsburgh; MA 81 SUNY - Coll at Plattsburgh; Aud, Cvph Medcen, **A**

Walsh, Kimberly K 1427 N Nash Street #22, Arlington, VA 22209, (703) 527-4525, BS 82 IL St Univ - Normal; MA 83 Western MI Univ; **SLP**

Walsh, Mrs Linda H 14 Sand Hill Road, Charlestown, RI 02813, BA 70 3672; MS 75 Univ of RI; 75–Sp-Lang Path, Chariho Sch Dist, **SLP**

Walsh, Lois G 36 Birch Lake Drive, Sherman, IL 62684, (217) 496-2021, BS 72 Southern IL Univ -Carbondale; MA 73 Univ of IL - Urbana; Sp-Lang Path, Sangamon Area Special Ed Dist, **SLP**

Walsh, Mary J 3102 Pleasant Court, Tallahassee, FL 32303, **SLP**

Walsh, Mary Justina Route 1 Box 525, Stateline Road, Beloit, WI 53511, (608) 676-2223, **SLP**

Walsh, Maureen A 1508 Second Avenue #6, New York, NY 10021, (212) 535-6694, BA 77 Univ of CA - Santa Barbara; MA 79 Univ of Denver; Private Practice, **SLP**

Walsh, Michael J VA Medical Center, 150 South Huntington Avenue, Jamaica Plain, MA 02130, (617) 232-9500, BA 69 Suffolk Univ; ME 71 Northeastern Univ; Sp/Lang Path & Cl Superv, VA, **SLP**

Walsh, Moira F 30 Brantwood Road, Arlington, MA 02174, MS 75 Boston Univ; Sp-Lang Path, Winthrop Public Schools, **SLP**

Walsh, Patricia 46 Fairfield Road, Yonkers, NY 10705, (914) 963-9210, BA 73 Saint John's Univ - Jamaica; ME 75 Univ of VA - Charlottesville; Instrictor/Clinical Super, Queens College of CUNY, **SLP**

Walsh, Dr Patricia S 3626 East Hiawatha, Okemos, MI 48864, (517) 355-8420, BA 59 Oberlin Coll; MA 62 IN Univ - Bloomington; PH 66 (Aud/Sp Sciences) MI St Univ; Asst to Provost, Michigan St U, **SLP**

Walsh, Mrs Robin McDonough 5 Ruland Road, Selden, NY 11784, (516) 281-3020, BS 81 Coll of Saint Rose; MS 82 Adelphi Univ; Sp-Lang Path, Sachem Central School District, **SLP**

Walsh, Susan M N 9539 Northwest 2nd Place, Coral Springs, FL 33071, (305) 755-3956, BA 78 Univ of MI - Ann Arbor; MA 81 Univ of CO - Boulder; Sp-Lang Path, Broward County Public SCHOOLS8, **SLP**

Walsh, Mrs Susan Weston 51 Devonshire Drive, Salisbury, MD 21801, (301) 546-1046, BS 65 Western IL Univ; MS 73 Old Dominion Univ; Sp-Lang Path, Private Practice, **SLP**

Walsh, Mrs Vanya Su 3536 Hungnam Place, Tarawa Terrace, NC 28543, (617) 324-8000, BS 82 Saint Louis Univ; MS 85 Univ of HI - Manoa; SLP, Malden Public Schools, **SLP**

Walsh, Mrs Vickie Clark 12617 Randolph Street, Crown Point, IN 46307, (219) 736-2210, BA 81 IN Univ - Bloomington; MS 82 IN St Univ - Terre Haute; Sp-Lang Path, Porter County Special Ed Coop, **SLP**

Walski, Mrs Roberta B 11730 Barranca Road, Camarillo, CA 93010, (805) 482-6544, BA 76 CA St Univ - Los Angeles; MA 77 CA St Univ - Los Angeles; Administrator, Burnwall Clinic, **SLP**

Walston, Theodora Flint 18BLUE Bonnet Drive, Los Lunas, NM 87031, (505) 865-5692, BS 54 Indiana Univ of PA; ME 63 PA St Univ - Univ Park; Sp/Lang Path, Los Lunos Schs, **SLP**

Walstrom, Mrs Rosemary E 504 North 11th Street, Marysville, KS 66508, (913) 562-3641, BS 74 Univ of NE - Lincoln; MA 77 Univ of NE - Lincoln; Sp-Lang Path, USD 364, **SLP**

Walter, Arlan E Cheyenne Hearing Clinic, 5320 Education Drive, Cheyenne, WY 82009, (307) 635-0435, BS 71 CO St Univ; MS 73 CO St Univ; Aud, Cheyenne Hearing Cl, **A**

Walter, Barbara J 325 Mc Clellan Boulevard, Davenport, IA 52803, (309) 762-5112, BA 74 Univ of IA; MA 75 Univ of IA; Editor, Linguisystems, **SLP**

Walter, Mrs Charlotte 1107 North Randall, Elk City, OK 73644, (405) 225-0951, BS 68 OK St Univ; MS 71 UT St Univ; **SLP**

Walter, Denise L 13319 Lamel, North Edwards, CA 93523, (619) 769-4305, BA 84 Univ of CA - Santa Barbara; MS 86 UT St Univ; Sp-Lang Path, Fillmore PS, **SLP**

Walter, Janet P R R 1 Box 490, 215 West South Street, Rossville, IN 46065, (317) 457-8273, BS 79 Purdue Univ - West Lafayette; MS 82 Purdue Univ - West Lafayette; 88–Sp-Lang Path, St Elizabeth Hosp, **SLP**

Walter, Mrs Jody L M 1418 Cedar Street, Alexandria, MN 56308, (612) 762-5463, MS 88 Saint Cloud St Univ; 87–Sp-Lang Path, Alexandria Sch Dist #206

Walter, Judith Marie 167 Diamond Street, New Haven, CT 06515, (215) 783-6010, BS 86 Bloomsburg Univ of PA; MS 87 Bloomsburg Univ of PA; **SLP**

Walter, Judy K 2361 Delaware Drive, St Charles, MO 63303, (918) 683-3040, BA 70 Univ of MO - KS City; MA 71 Univ of KS; Sp-Lang Path/Prescriptive Tchr, Reg Ed Serv Cen, **SLP**

Walter, Lisa Marie 1312 West Sitka, Tampa, FL 33604, (813) 251-7760, BA 81 Univ of FL; MS 82 FL St Univ; Sp-Lang Path, Tampa General Rehab Cen, **SLP**

Walter, Nancy Jane 9939 Rio San Diego Drive, #52, San Diego, CA 92108, (619) 283-7803, OM 85 Brigham Young Univ; Sp-Lang Path, Nebo School District, **SLP**

Walter, Mrs Rita N 315 Thistle Lane, Lake Zurich, IL 60047, (312) 438-4958, BS 73 Northwestern Univ; MA 77 Northern IL Univ - De Kalb; **SLP**

Walter, Mrs Susan Gail R R 5 Box 21-A, Seymour, IN 47274, (812) 523-3020, **SLP**

Walter, Teri A 1044 Cypress Point, Mansfield, TX 76063, (817) 274-5581, BA 76 McMurry Coll; MS 74 AZ St Univ; Sp-Lang Path, Arlington Mem Hosp, **SLP**

Walters, Mrs Florence M 1431 Stonebridge Circle, Lansdale, PA 19446, (215) 275-4151, BS 70 PA St Univ - Univ Park; MS 80 PA St Univ - Univ Park; Aud, ENT Assoc Cn Mont Co, **A ACE**

Walters, James E 222 North Pine, Vermillion, SD 57069, (607) 677-5381, BA 56 Univ of SD - Vermillion; MA 63 Univ of SD - Vermillion; Academic Advg/Testing Ctr, U of SD, **SLP**

Walters, John C 8660 S W 15th Street, Pembroke Pines, FL 33025, (305) 595-3175, **SLP**

Walters, Joyce 726 52nd Avenue North, St Petersburg, FL 33703, (813) 541-3521, BA 65 IN Univ - Bloomington; MA 76 Ball St Univ; ED 86 (Lang-Learning Disabilities) Univ of South FL; 82–Sp-Lang Path, Pinellas Co Sch, **SLP**

Walters, Mrs Judith Raucci 1000 East Brookdale, La Habra, CA 90631, (213) 691-8746, BS 70 Southern CT St Univ; MS 72 Syracuse Univ; Program Spec, Whittier Area Coop Spec Ed Prg, **SLP**

Walters, Mrs Karen L 4125 Sherel Lane, Cincinnati, OH 45209, (513) 871-6080, BS 76 Univ of Cincinnati; MA 78 Univ of Cincinnati; Sp-Lang Path, The Springer Sch, **SLP**

Walters, Lynn Perkins 5762 38th Street, Lubbock, TX 79407, (806) 792-6135, BA 83 TX Tech Univ; MS 85 TX Tech Univ; **SLP**

Walters, Martha Ann 804 North Everts, Fort Stockton, TX 79735, (915) 336-3651, MS 85 Univ of North TX; **SLP**

Walters, Mary Ann 255 Oakwood Drive, Lancaster, TX 75146-2821, (214) 227-4334, BS 78 Univ of North TX; MS 81 Univ of North TX; SLP, Visiting Nurse Assn of Texas, **SLP**

Walters, Melissa J 823 Carman Drive, Wyomissing, PA 19610, **SLP**

Walters, Noreen Marie 26400 Mallard Avenue, Euclid, OH 44132, BA 83 Cleveland St Univ; MA 85 Cleveland St Univ; SLP, Ashtabula County Soc for Hndcp, **SLP**

Walters, Dr Roger John 5711 Ridgedale Road, Baltimore, MD 21209, (301) 466-4711, BA 67 CUNY - Hunter Coll; MS 68 Univ of MI - Ann Arbor; OD 82 (NS) Johns Hopkins Univ; 88–Aud/Sp-Lang Path, Private Practice, **SLP A**

Walters, Sylvia Y 633 East 24 Street, Brooklyn, NY 11210, (212) 636-4573, BA 74 CUNY - Brooklyn Coll; MS 77 CUNY - Brooklyn Coll; 74–Preprimary Dept Super, St Francis De Sales Sch Deaf, **SLP**

Walters, Wellington P O Box 16, Wittensville, KY 41274, (606) 789-1440, BA 74 Marshall Univ; MA 76 Marshall Univ; Sp-Lang Path, Carl D Perkins Comp Rehab Ctr, **SLP ACE**

Walters, William B 102 Finch Court, La Place, LA 70068, (504) 652-4310, BA 76 Univ of Southwestern LA; OM 78 LA St Univ - N O Medical Ctr; Aud, Private Practice, **A**

Walters-Page, Linda 4540 Sandringham Drive, Columbus, OH 43220, (614) 261-4940, MA 83 OH St Univ; Sp-Lang Path, Neurological Rehabilitatn Ctr, **SLP**

Walter-Stephan, M Patricia 9428 Baymeadows Road, Suite 122, Jacksonville, FL 32256, (904) 730-7121, BS 80 Ithaca Coll; MS 82 Univ of NC - Chapel Hill; Sp-Lang Path, Private Practice, **SLP**

Walther, Bonnie J 9927 Southport, Houston, TX 77089, (713) 941-3943, BS 72 LA St Univ - Baton Rouge; MS 74 Lamar Univ; **SLP**

Walther, Mrs Kathleen O'Donnell 18 Morrislea Court, Baltimore, MD 21234, (301) 747-7710, BS 74 Towson St Univ; MS 75 PA St Univ - Univ Park; Sp-Lang Path, Baltimore County Pub Sch, **SLP**

Walton, Anne 8315 Mobud, Houston, TX 77036, (713) 774-9495, BS 83 TX Christian Univ; MA 87 Univ of Houston - Univ Park; **SLP**

Walton, Betty Reed 297 Colony Road, Newport News, VA 23602, (804) 723-3330, MA 83 Hampton Univ; BA 79 Univ of NC - Greensboro; **SLP**

Walton, Mrs J Andrea 823 First Street East, Scott City, MO 63780, (314) 334-5209, BS 75 AR St Univ; MS 76 AR St Univ; Sp-Lang Path, Mo Crpld Chldrns Serv, **SLP**

Walton, Dr Joseph Paul Strong Memorial Hospital, Audiology Department-Box 629, 601 Elmwood Avenue, Rochester, NY 14642, (716) 275-4852, BA 77 Univ of FL; MA 82 Univ of FL; PH 84 (Aud/Hrng Science) Univ of FL; Asst Prof of Otolaryngology, Univ of Rochester Med Ctr, **A**

Walton, Mrs Julie H Dept Communicative Disorders, University Of Mississippi, University, MS 38677, (601) 232-7271, BA 60 Univ of MS; MA 62 Univ of MS; OM 74 Univ of MS; Asst Prof, U of MS, **SLP**

Walton, Michael W 4141 N Braeswood #28, Houston, TX 77025, (713) 791-4298, MS 79 Lamar Univ; 86–Sp-Lang Path, TX Childrens Hosp, **SLP**

Walton, Patricia A 225 West 400 North, Logan, UT 84321, (801) 563-3866, BS 77 CO St Univ; MA 78 Univ of Northern CO; Sp-Lang Path, Cache County Sch Dist, **SLP**

Walton, Rosemary Rice 2600 Secota Drive, Hampton, VA 23661, (804) 723-1200, BA 62 Brown Univ; MA 64 Univ of MI - Ann Arbor; MA 84 Hampton Univ; 88–Sp-Lang Path, Peninsula Therapy Center, **SLP**

Walton, Ruth T 4085 Vanda Lane, Fairfax, VA 22031, (202) 994-7360, BA 60 Greensboro Coll; MA 75 George Washington Univ; Aud, GW U-Sp-Hrng Cen, **A**

Waltrip, Mrs LoAnne 24570 New Haven Drive, Murrieta, CA 92362, (714) 534-1041, BS 80 CA St Univ - Fullerton; MA 84 CA St Univ - Fullerton; Sp-Lang Path, **SLP**

Waltrip, Susan Grose 437 Dolphin Place, Corpus Christi, TX 78411, (512) 855-6290, **A ACE**

Waltz, Mary F 1950 Bellglade Terrace, Cincinnati, OH 45238, (513) 661-4327, BS 70 OH St Univ; MA 82 Univ of Cincinnati; 82–Sp-Lang Path, Cincinnati Cen for Improv Comm, **SLP ACE**

Waltzman, Dava L One Fall Ridge Road, Weston, CT 06883, BS 61 Univ of WI - Madison; MA 85 CUNY - Hunter Coll; Sp/Lang Path, Hunter Coll of CUNY, **SLP ACE**

Waltzman, Dr Susan Beth 333 East 30th Street #2J, New York, NY 10016, (212) 561-3564, BA 66 Univ of WI - Madison; MA 68 Columbia Univ Teachers Coll; PH 74 (NS) CUNY - Grad Sch & Univ Cntr; Dir, Hrng & Sp Serv, NYU-Bellevue Med Cen, **A**

Walvoord, Barbara B 818 E High Point Terrace, Peoria, IL 61614, (309) 676-1212, BA 62 Northwestern Univ; MA 64 Northwestern Univ; 85–Sp-Lang Path, Sp & Lang Rehab Svcs, **SLP ACE**

Walz, Mrs Laurie Peterson 2927 Crystal Boulevard # A, Inverness, FL 32652, (904) 344-0292, BS 83 Kearney St Coll; MS 87 Saint Cloud St Univ; **SLP**

Walz, Michelle Marian 1341 West Lake Cowdry, Alexandria, MN 56308, (612) 762-2141, BS 84 Moorhead St Univ; MS 86 Moorhead St Univ

Walzer, Jacalyn F 14 Sumter Road, Monsey, NY 10952, (914) 634-4648, OB 72 Univ of Miami; MS 73 PA St Univ - Univ Park; 85–Sp-Lang Path, Rockland Co Ctr for the Hndcpd, **SLP**

Wambaugh, Julie Lynn 329 Connell Avenue, Missoula, MT 59801, (406) 243-5637, BS 78 Indiana Univ of PA; MS 82 PA St Univ - Univ Park; PH 88 (NS) PA St Univ - Univ Park; 88–Asst Prof, Univ of Montana, **SLP**

Wambold, Mrs Constance Anne 208 Bull Street, Savannah, GA 31401, (912) 651-7161, BA 75 Molloy Coll; MS 79 Towson St Univ; 86–Sp-Lang Path, Savannah-Chatham Co Bd of Educ, **SLP**

Wambsgans, Sal J 2005 Arnold Street, Waveland, MS 39576, (601) 863-6617, BA 78 Univ Southern MS-Hattiesburg; MS 80 Univ Southern MS-Hattiesburg; Aud, Hearing & Balance Cen, **A**

Wan, Mrs Charisse Louie 229 Obsidian Way, Hercules, CA 94547, (415) 799-7874, BA 77 San Francisco St Univ; MA 78 Univ of IA; Sp-Lang Path, Vallejo County USD, **SLP**

Wanamaker, Abby 352 North Croft Avenue, Los Angeles, CA 90048, (213) 653-9759, MA 70 Univ of Southern CA; OM 78 Univ of CA - Los Angeles; SLP, Lincoln Ctr for Sp Path, **SLP ACE**

Wancket, Sari M 841 Roanoke Drive, Springfield, IL 62702, (217) 525-8593, OB 74 Univ of MI - Ann Arbor; MS 75 Univ of MI - Ann Arbor; 88–Sp-Lang Path, Il Easter Seals, **SLP**

Wanderman, Hope B 935 North Halifax #405, Daytona Beach, FL 32018, (904) 255-8750, MA 70 Univ of South FL; **SLP**

Wandland, Mrs Cynthia L R R 1 Box 173, Claypool, IN 46510, (312) 566-2272, BA 73 Saint Xavier Coll; MS 74 IL St Univ - Normal; SLP, Home Health Care, **SLP**

Wang, Dr Chester 1358 Highland Oaks Drive, Arcadia, CA 91006, (818) 577-7367, MA 69 Pepperdine Univ - Los Angele; MA 76 Pepperdine Univ - Los Angele; PH 79 (NS) Pepperdine Univ - Los Angele; Director Commun Dis, Huntington Mem Hosp, **SLP**

Wang, Hueiyao Sophia 1243 Beacon Street #7-D, Brookline, MA 02146, (617) 277-2975, BS 79 Nat'l Tawian Univ - Taipei, Tawian; MS 81 Nat'l Tawian Univ - Taipei, Tawian; MS 87 Columbia Univ Teachers Coll; **A**

Wang, Mrs Norene K P O Box 11231, Honolulu, HI 96828, (808) 522-3348, BS 69 Univ of HI - Manoa; MA 70 OH Univ - Athens; Aud, Straub Cl & Hosp Inc, **A**

Wanger, Cynthia K 1321 Tanglewood Drive, P O Box 444, Gwynedd, PA 19436-0444, (215) 368-5290, BA 74 Temple Univ-Tyler Sch of Art; MA 76 Temple Univ-Tyler Sch of Art; Audiologist, Intercounty Aud & Hrng Aid Cen, **A**

Wangerin, Kathleen Ann 1747 South 73rd Street, West Allis, WI 53214, (414) 649-6400, BS 74 Northern MI Univ; MA 77 Northern MI Univ; Sp-Lang Path, St Luke's Hosp-Milwaukee, **SLP**

Wanke, Mrs Janis Ann 637 East Upperline, La Grange, TX 78945, (918) 968-6927, MA 84 LA Tech Univ; Sp-Lang Path, InSpeech Inc, **SLP**

Wankoff, Mrs Lorain S 64-37 Alderton Street, Rego Park, NY 11374, (212) 459-3542, BA 69 CUNY - Queens Coll; MA 72 CUNY - Queens Coll; **SLP**

Wanner, Nancy Weakley 1011 Atlantic Drive, Stafford, VA 22554, (703) 659-2143, BS 84 Univ of VA - Charlottesville; ME 86 Univ of VA - Charlottesville; 86–Sp-Lang Path, Stafford County Public Schools, **SLP**

Wantuch, Debra J 47-48 196th Street, Flushing, NY 11358, MS 78 Columbia Univ Teachers Coll; 85–Dir Aud, St Lukes/Roosevelt Hospital, **A ACE**

Ward, Alicia Ann 4800 Highway 7, Apartment 301, St Louis Park, MN 55416, (612) 924-9365, BA 84 Univ of SD - Vermillion; MA 85 Univ of SD - Vermillion; Sp-Lang Path, Achievement Rehab Corp, **SLP**

Ward, Allan R 1103 South Summit #B-11, Newcastle, WY 82701-2969, (307) 766-6426

Ward, Mrs Annette Fulton 10037 South Lakewood, Tulsa, OK 74137, (918) 664-6600, ME 83 Central St Univ; Sp-Lang Path, Chldrns Med Ctr, **SLP**

Ward, Barbara Leilani 417 Hertford Court, Maumee, OH 43537, (419) 666-1120, OB 85 Univ of Toledo; MS 86 Bowling Green St Univ; 86–Sp-Lang Path, Penta County Voc Schs, **SLP**

Ward, Betty Jane 104 Rue Des Meurons, Winnipeg, MB, Canada R2H 2M3, (204) 237-2131, BA 70; MA 72; Dir Communication Disorders, St Boniface Gen Hosp, **SLP**

Ward, Mrs Carol K 611 Shore Road, Cape Elizabeth, ME 04107, BS 66 Carlow Coll; MA 67 Western MI Univ; 80–Sp-Lang Path, S Portland Sch, **SLP**

Ward, Catherine 131 Melrose Avenue, Ormond Beach, FL 32074, **SLP**

Ward, Dianne Gottlieb 3303 Judy Lynn Drive, Arlington, TX 76014, (817) 460-4191, BS 79 Baylor Univ; MS 80 Baylor Univ; Sp/Lang Path, Arlington ISD, **SLP**

Ward, Mrs Dolores M 9620 Windermere Turn, Fort Washington, MD 20744, (301) 839-0295, BS 62 Univ of the DC; MS 63 Gallaudet Coll; MS 63 Gallaudet Coll; **SLP A LM**

Ward, Dr Doyle G 510 Franklin Drive, San Marcos, TX 78666, (512) 245-2157, BA 56 Harding Univ; MA 58 Univ of IL - Urbana; PH 66 (NS) Univ of MO - Columbia; Prof Commun Dis, Southwest TX St U, **SLP**

Ward, Mrs Elisabeth 2112 Velez Drive, San Pedro, CA 90732, (213) 547-9383, BA 71 CA St Univ - Northridge; MA 75 CA St Univ - Northridge; **SLP**

Ward, Ellen W 4840 East Missouri Avenue, Denver, CO 80222-3244, (303) 756-6333, BA 74 Loretto Heights Coll; MA 81 Univ of Denver; Aud, **A**

Ward, Mrs Evelyn L 5 Hewitt Avenue, Bronxville, NY 10708, (914) 337-6026, BA 50 Marymount Coll; OM 52 Yale Univ; **SLP**

Ward, Gary L 3321 Greenwich Drive, Fairfield, OH 45014, (513) 559-6800, BA 69 Olivet Nazarene Coll; MA 75 Univ of Cincinnati; 80–Sp/Lang Path, Cincinnati Chdns Hosp, **SLP**

Ward, Mrs Judith H 604 Chatham Court, Neenah, WI 54956, (414) 722-2452, BS 66 Univ of WI - Madison; MS 67 Univ of WI - Madison; Sp-Lang Path, Menasha Jt Sch Dist, **SLP**

Ward, Mrs Kathleen 84 Palmer Avenue, Tenafly, NJ 07670, (201) 569-0880, MA 68 Trenton St Coll; Sp-Lang Path, Private Practice, **SLP**

Ward, Mrs Kelly A 306 East Main Street #1, Morehead, KY 40351, (606) 784-9688, **SLP**

Ward, Mrs Leslie G 1228 Cypress Drive, Richardson, TX 75080, (214) 699-9363

Ward, Lethe Finks 1242 South Stanley Avenue, Los Angeles, CA 90019, (213) 936-5491, BA 82 CA St Univ - Northridge; MA 84 Univ of Denver; 84–Sp-Lang Path, LA USD, **SLP**

Ward, Lisa P 14274 Lindendale Road, Dale City, VA 22193, (703) 670-7856, BS 75 Radford Univ; MS 81 James Madison Univ; 84–Sp-Lang Path, Fairfax Co PS, **SLP**

Ward, Louise M Dept Audiology & Speech Path, Memphis State University, 807 Jefferson Avenue, Memphis, TN 38105, (901) 525-2682, BS 50 Auburn Univ - Auburn; MA 51 Univ of AL- Tuscaloosa; Assoc Prof, Memphis St U, **SLP F LM**

Ward, Mrs Louise W 39 Hampshire Road, Reading, MA 01867, (617) 944-1907, OB 72 Southern Methodist Univ; MS 73 Southern Methodist Univ; Sp-Lang Path, Reading Pub Sch, **SLP**

Ward, Mrs Marcia C 4525 Real Del Sur, Las Cruces, NM 88001, (505) 522-2316, BA 70 NM St Univ; MA 72 NM St Univ; Sp-Lang Path, **SLP**

Ward, Mrs Martha Z 1821 North Racine Street, Appleton, WI 54911, (414) 733-9256, BS 62 Purdue Univ - West Lafayette; MS 63 Univ of WI - Madison; Sp-Lang Path, Appleton Area PS, **SLP**

Ward, Mary Frances 305 South 4th Street, Princeton, MN 55371, (612) 348-3562, BA 76 Univ of Northern IA; MA 77 Univ of Northern IA; Sp-Lang Path, Focus Homes Inc, **SLP**

Ward, Melanie Denise Regency Plaza #A-4, Route 9 Box 59, Russellville, AL 35653, (205) 345-2578, BS 85 Univ of AL- Tuscaloosa; MS 86 Univ of AL- Tuscaloosa; **SLP**

Ward, Nancy Lynn 4 Gary Court, Holmdel, NJ 07733, (201) 997-6464, BA 85 Univ of MD - College Park; MA 87 OH St Univ; 87–Aud, James P Murphy MD, **A**

Ward, Natalie E 1170 Massachusetts Avenue, Cambridge, MA 02138, BA 67 Univ of WI - Madison; MS 73 Emerson Coll; Sp-Lang Path, Boston Public Schools, **SLP**

Ward, Patricia A 1336 Greenwillow Lane, Townhouse 6-B, Glenview, IL 60025, (312) 880-3430, BA 81 Mundelein Coll; MS 82 Marquette Univ; 87–Sp-Lang Path, Children Memorial Hospital, **SLP**

Ward, Robert M 305 South Main, McAlester, OK 74501, (918) 426-4742, BA 76 Univ of OK - Norman; MS 78 Univ of OK Medical Center; Aud, McAlester Aud & Hrng Aid Cen, **A**

Ward, Sue Ellen 1317 Oakleigh N W, Grand Rapids, MI 49504, (616) 676-8932, BA 63 Western MI Univ; MA 68 Western MI Univ; Sp/Lang Path, Forest Hills PS, **SLP**

Ward, Mrs Susan M 1315 Albright Drive, Yardley, PA 19067, BS 75 Bloomsburg Univ of PA; MS 77 PA St Univ - Univ Park; **SLP**

Ward, Susan Schimmel 147 Bayberry Trail, Kitty Hawk, NC 27949, (919) 261-4126, BA 78 MI St Univ; MA 79 MI St Univ; Sp-Lang Path, Dare County Schs, **SLP**

Ward, Suzan Lynette 405 Brairwood, Yukon, OK 73099, (405) 354-4347, BS 81 OK St Univ; MS 83 Univ of OK Medical Center; Sp-Lang Path, Private Practice, **SLP**

Ward, Mrs Teresa Anne P O Box 1204, Corbin, KY 40701, (606) 864-2208, BS 82 Eastern KY Univ; ME 83 Eastern KY Univ; Sp-Lang Path, Seton Home Health Agency, **SLP**

Ward, Thomas G 2112 Wilmington Drive, Midland, MI 48640, (517) 835-9567, BA 55 MI St Univ; ME 61 Wayne St Univ; Dir of Spec Ed, Meridan Pub Sch, **SLP**

Ward, Virginia Gleason Street, Westborough, MA 01581, **SLP**

Ward, Dr W Dixon Hearing Research Lab, 2630 University S E, Minneapolis, MN 55414, (612) 627-4694, BS 44 SD Sch of Mines & Tech; PH 53 (NS) Harvard Univ; Prof, U of MN, **F**

Wardell, Ferman N Olin E Teague VA Center, Audiology Program (126), Temple, TX 76502, (817) 778-4811, BS 74 Univ of TX - Austin; MA 76 Univ of TX - Austin; Aud, Olin E Teague VA Cen, **A**

Warden, Mrs Mary Diane 12381 Arrowhead Street #37, Stanton, CA 90680, (714) 530-6116, BA 81 CA St Univ - Long Beach; MA 84 CA St Univ - Long Beach; 84–Sp-Lang Path, Providence Sp & Hearing Ctr, **SLP**

Warden, Rebecca M 1401 South Driscoll #307, Appleton, WI 54914, (414) 739-8469, **SLP**

Ward-Gravely, Mrs Valenta G #5 Severance Circle, Suite 701, Cleveland Heights, OH 44118, (216) 249-7177, BA 75 Cleveland St Univ; MA 77 Cleveland St Univ; 87–Dir-Aud, DIVA Assoc Lang Sp & Hrng Spec, **SLP A**

Ward Isbey, Mrs Julie A 1777 Holly Springs Road, Marietta, GA 30062-9244, (404) 980-9869, BS 80 IN Univ - Bloomington; OM 82 IN Univ - Bloomington; Acct Exec, Integon, **SLP**

Wardlaw, Francis G 716 Fern Street, Nampa, ID 83651, (208) 465-2700, BA 56 Northwest Nazarene Coll; MA 60 Univ of Denver; 69–Aud/Sp-Lang Path, Sch Dist #131 Nampa Id, **SLP A**

Wardner, Mrs Monique C 2810 Easy Street, Ann Arbor, MI 48104, (313) 764-8440, MA 84 SUNY - Center at Buffalo; BA 82 Univ of MI - Ann Arbor; Clinical Coor, Univ of MI, **A**

Wardrip-Fruin, Carolyn Dept Communication Disorders, California State Univ, Long Beach, CA 90840, (213) 498-4583, BA 62 Univ of Redlands; MA 76 Stanford Univ; PH 80 (NS) Stanford Univ; Assoc Prof, CA St Univ-Comm Dis, **SLP**

Wardrop, Cheryl M 15 Sterling Place, Glen Rock, NJ 07452, (201) 652-3068, BS 69 Boston Univ; MS 80 Montclair St Coll; 87–Sp-Lang Path, Dr E Shulman PhD & Assoc, **SLP**

Ware, Debra Davis 13 Byron Close, Laguna Niguel, CA 92677, (714) 643-8255, BA 78 Univ of CA - Irvine; MA 82 CA St Univ - Fullerton; 88–Dir, Laguna Niguel Sp/Lang Ctr, **SLP**

Ware, Donna P 15 Larkspur Drive, Latham, NY 12110, (518) 783-0098, BS 74 SUNY - Center at Albany; ME 75 Bloomsburg Univ of PA; Sp-Lang Path, Private Practice, **SLP**

Ware, Janice G P O Box 343, Rayne, LA 70578, BA 78 Univ of Southwestern LA; OM 80 LA St Univ - N O Medical Ctr; **SLP**

Ware, Justine M PO Box 89, Benedicta, ME 04733, (203) 365-4648, BS 79 Northeastern Univ; MA 82 Univ of KS; Aud, Otolaryngology Assoc, **A**

Ware, Kathryn J 445 North Hayden Bay Drive, Portland, OR 97217, (503) 280-4403, BA 75 LA Tech Univ; MS 77 Univ of TX - Arlington; Sp-Lang Path, Emanuel Rehabilitation Center, **SLP ACE**

Ware, Mrs Monica Combs 709 Terry Drive, Winchester, KY 40391, (606) 744-4983, BA 82 Univ of KY; MS 86 Univ of KY; 87–Sp-Lang Path, Lynn B Shearon Sp-Lang Svcs, **SLP**

Ware, Myra Jo 3234 South Keaton Avenue, Tyler, TX 75701, (214) 595-6767, BS 77 Southern IL Univ -Carbondale; ME 85 Stephen F Austin St Univ; 88–Sp-Lang Path, Tru Care Rehab Svcs Inc, **SLP**

Ware, Mrs Victoria Topp 115 Hilary Place, Cary, NC 27511, (919) 782-4184, BA 82 Univ of FL; MA 84 MI St Univ; 85–Sp-Lang Path, Assoc Healthfocus Inc, **SLP**

Ware, Mrs Virginia A 9040 N E 195th Street, Bothell, WA 98011, (816) 364-1501, BS 72 Purdue Univ - West Lafayette; MS 76 IN St Univ - Terre Haute; 87–Sp-Lang Path, Providence Hosp Childrens Ctr, **SLP**

Warfel, M Kay 209 Garth Road #6-H, Scarsdale, NY 10583, (212) 653-0835, BS 76 PA St Univ - Univ Park; ME 79 Univ of OR; OM 86 Iona Coll; Sp/Lang Path, NYC Bd of Ed, **SLP**

Wargo, Susan Shaw R R 1 Box 522, Hinesburg, VT 05461-9704, (802) 453-3673, BA 70 Ottawa Univ; MS 74 Bank Street Coll of Educ; MS 83 Univ of VT; Sp-Lang Path, Eee Anesu New Haven Vt, **SLP**

Warhit, Mrs Ilissa Carol 5400 Fieldston Road #11-C, Riverdale, NY 10471, (212) 548-5715, MA 86 CUNY - Queens Coll; 86–SLP, Burke Rehab Ctr, **SLP**

Waring, Mrs Carolyn H 1 Summit Ridge Drive, Vicksburg, MS 39180, (601) 636-4733, BA 72 Univ of TX - El Paso; MA 73 Univ of TX - El Paso; Sp-Lang Path, Warren County Public Schools, **SLP**

Waring, Mrs Margaret L 125 Orchard Hills, Boyertown, PA 19512, (215) 779-7111, BS 61 Northwestern Univ; MA 78 West Chester Univ of PA; Sp-Lang Path, Berks Co Intermediate Unit, **SLP**

Wark, Dr David J Memphis Speech & Hearing Ctr, 807 Jefferson, Memphis, TN 38105, (901) 525-2682, BA 65 Univ of AL- Tuscaloosa; MA 67 Univ of AL- Tuscaloosa; PH 71 (NS) IN Univ - Bloomington; Coord of Grad Studies, Memphis St U, **A**

Wark, Nancy H 5587 Murray Road Suite 201, Memphis, TN 38119, (901) 763-3858, MA 69 IN Univ - Bloomington; Sp-Lang Path, Nancy H Wark & Associates, **SLP**

Warlick, Joann 2714 N E 35th Avenue, Portland, OR 97212, (503) 636-4551, MS 83 Portland St Univ; Sp-Lang Path, Lake Oswego Sch Dist, **SLP**

Warman, Mrs Donna Sue 101 White Oak Court, Ashland, KY 41101, (606) 836-5143, BS 79 WV Univ; ME 83 Univ of VA - Charlottesville; Aud, **A**

Warman, Wendy B 234 Monroe Street, Dunedin, FL 34698, (813) 733-6326, MS 74 Univ of South FL; Owner/Dir, Dunedin Sp & Hrng Cen, **SLP ACE**

Warne, Mrs Deborah Ann R R 1 P O Box 46, Mankato, KS 66956, (913) 378-3008, MA 84 KS St Univ; 84–Sp-Lang Path, Beloit Spec Educ Cooperative, **SLP**

Warner, Brian D 114 Woodcliff Circle, Pineville, LA 71360, (318) 442-9707, BA 73 LA Tech Univ; MA 74 LA Tech Univ; 87–Dir, Center for Speech Pathology, **SLP**

Warner, Candis M 3904 Pine Glade Drive, Portage, MI 49002, (616) 383-0963, MS 70 Western MI Univ; Instructor, Wn MI U, **SLP**

Warner, Mrs Cheryl Busing 10234 Indian Princess Road, Jacksonville, FL 32257, (904) 390-1143, BS 79 TX Christian Univ; MS 80 TX Christian Univ; Sp-Lang Path, Baptist Med Ctr, **SLP**

Warner, Dianne Elizabeth Kennedy-Donovan Center, Early Intervention, 42 Washington Street 2nd Floor, Fairhaven, MA 02719, BS 85 Boston Univ; MS 86 Boston Univ; 86–Sp-Lang Path, Kennedy-Donovan Ctr, **SLP**

Warner, Mrs Janet K Grant Grove, Kings Canyon Natl Park, CA 93633, (209) 338-2511, BA 60 Phillips Univ; MA 70 CA St Univ - Sacramento; Program Spec, Kings Canyon USD, **SLP**

Warner, Janice Holmes 3104 Ulster Avenue, Greensboro, NC 27406, (919) 621-6490, BS 80 PA St Univ - Univ Park; MA 84 Univ of Pittsburgh - Pittsburgh; Aud, Central NC Sch for the Deaf, **A**

Warner, Joan Ellen 95 Star Lake Road, Bloomingdale, NJ 07403, (201) 697-3185, BA 80 William Paterson Coll; MS 83 William Paterson Coll; 82–Sp-Lang Path Hndcped Preschool, West Milford Board of Educ, **SLP**

Warner, Joann Marie 1400 East Newport Rd, Rothsville, PA 17543, (717) 627-1649, BS 81 Indiana Univ of PA; MA 85 Univ of Northern CO; SLP, Lancaster Lebinin Nter Unit 13, **SLP**

Warner, Joy C 2336 Forest, Denver, CO 80207, (303) 329-8959, ME 77 Univ of NC - Chapel Hill; **SLP**

Warner, Karen Simpson 5313 Hickory Hill Drive, Lynchburg, VA 24503, (804) 384-6306, **SLP**

Warner, Mrs Kathleen F 2 Douglas Road, Freehold, NJ 07728, (201) 780-2433, BA 75 Montclair St Coll; MA 78 Trenton St Coll; Sp/Lang Path, Indepedent Child Study Teams, **SLP**

Warner, Kathleen Jane 177 South 67th Street, Milwaukee, WI 53214, (414) 747-4423, BS 79; MS 80 Marquette Univ; Dir of Admin, WI Air Natl Guard, **SLP**

Warner, Kathleen Wright 10415 Cueva Del Oso N E, Albuquerque, NM 87111, (505) 262-7261, MS 87 CO St Univ; **A**

Warner, Kimberley Racheal I-302 Chateau-on-The-Lake Apts, Unit #30602, Pacific Highway South, Federal Way, WA 98003, (206) 456-7312, BA 80 CUNY - Brooklyn Coll; MA 86 CUNY - Hunter Coll; Sp-Lang Path, St Peter Hosp, **SLP**

Warner, Klaran Wyn P O Box 148, South Strafford, VT 05070, (802) 765-4586, BA 65 Univ of MI - Ann Arbor; MS 68 Syracuse Univ; Sp-Lang Path, Overton Speech-Language Center, **SLP**

Warner, Mark Richard 95 Star Lake Road, Bloomingdale, NJ 07403, (212) 584-9000, BA 81 William Paterson Coll; MS 83 William Paterson Coll; Aud, Bronx VA Med Cen, **A**

Warner, Mary Ellen 109 Laurel Avenue, Wilmington, DE 19809, (302) 792-2179, BS 78 East Carolina Univ; MS 79 PA St Univ - Univ Park; Sp-Lang Path, Alfred I Dupont Institute, **SLP**

Warner, Patricia 1250 Chateaugay Lane, Indianapolis, IN 46217, (317) 264-1452, MA 77 Saint Louis Univ; **SLP**

Warner, Robert C 6315 Lahring Road, Holly, MI 48442, (313) 634-4441, BA 56 Wichita St Univ; MS 64 Vanderbilt Univ; SLP, Holly Area Sch, **SLP**

Warner, Mrs Susan P Speech & Language Therapy Serv, 236 East 9th Street, Traverse City, MI 49684, (616) 947-6060, BA 66 Univ of IA; MA 68 Univ of IA; Sp-Lang Path, Speech & Language Therapy Serv, **SLP**

Warner, Therese Marie 171 Linwood Avenue #5D, Buffalo, NY 14209, (716) 837-2441, BS 80 SUNY - Coll at Buffalo; MS 86 SUNY - Coll at Buffalo; 88–Sp-Lang Path, Lang Dev Prog of W NY, **SLP**

Warnke, Mrs Ann Marie 16123 Indus Drive, Woodbridge, VA 22191-4334, (703) 680-7152, **SLP**

Warnke, Eileen Regina 297 Castlebar Road, Rochester, NY 14610, (716) 244-4433, BA 84 SUNY - Coll at Cortland; MS 87 Syracuse Univ; **A**

Warns, Deborah S 119 East Erie Road, Temperance, MI 48182, (313) 847-6736, OB 77 Univ of Toledo; BA 77 Univ of Toledo; MA 81 Eastern MI Univ; Sp-Lang Path, Bedford Pub Sch, **SLP**

Waronker, Mrs Sue Ann 3335 Muirfield Place, Lima, OH 45805, (419) 991-7532, BS 70 OH St Univ; OM 72 Emory Univ; Sp-Lang Path, Hosp, **SLP**

Warp, Mrs Sherry L D 1991 Camino A Los Cerros, Menlo Park, CA 94025, (415) 321-7053, BA 70 Western WA Univ; MA 76 San Diego St Univ; 88–Prog Spec, Santa Clara Co Office of Educ, **SLP**

Warren, Angela Dawn 5000 Ridgewood Road #1106, Jackson, MS 39211, (601) 956-3109, BA 85 Univ of MS; MS 87 Univ of MS; **SLP**

Warren, Barbara Crownover 359 East Hildebrand, San Antonio, TX 78212, (512) 828-5583, BS 75 Southwest TX St Univ; ME 76 Southwest TX St Univ; Director of Speech Pathology, Olmos Sp Lang & Lrng Clinic, **SLP**

Warren, Mrs Berniece B One Oceans West Boulevard, Apartment A-1204, Daytona Beach Shores, FL 32018, (904) 756-2942, **SLP LM**

Warren, Mrs Bliss Hemric P O Box 3371, Boone, NC 28607, (704) 264-4854, BS 85 Appalachian St Univ; MA 86 Appalachian St Univ; 88–Sp-Lang Path, Private Practice, **SLP**

Warren, Chuck Nathan 1093 Garlock Avenue South, Salem, OR 97302, (503) 399-3300, BS 72 Western OR St Coll; MS 80 Western OR St Coll; Sp-Lang Path, Salem Pub Sch Salem or, **SLP**

Warren, Mrs Deborah L 14401 Danes Circle, Huntington Beach, CA 92647, (714) 381-1180, BA 78 Chapman Coll; MS 80 Chapman Coll; Sp-Lang Path, San Bernardino City USD, **SLP**

Warren, Dr Donald William Dental Research Center, Bldg #7450, University Of North Carolina, Chapel Hill, NC 27514, (919) 966-5240, MS 61 Univ of PA; DD 59 Univ of NC - Chapel Hill; PH 63 (NS) Univ of PA; Prof & Dir, Univ of NC, **F**

Warren, Mrs Francine Marcia 304 6th Street #1, Brooklyn, NY 11215, (212) 875-0578, BA 79 SUNY - Center at Buffalo; MS 83 CUNY - Brooklyn Coll; SLP, NYC Bd Ed-Sp/Serv Un, **SLP**

Warren, Geralynn F P O Box 223, Sioux Falls, SD 57101, (605) 338-5633, BS 78 Univ of SD - Vermillion; MA 80 Univ of SD - Vermillion; SLP, Sioux Falls Sch Dist, **SLP**

Warren, Glenda Gale 19835 Haynes Street, Woodland Hills, CA 91367, (818) 784-4137, SLP, Self Employed, **SLP**

Warren, Dr Irene B 261 Dallam Road, Newark, DE 19711, PH 75 (NS) Univ of WA; **SLP**

Warren, Mrs Jane Anne 2158 Granite Drive, Walla Walla, WA 99362, (509) 525-2238, BS 71 OR St Univ; MS 75 Western OR St Coll; **SLP**

Warren, Joanne K 7180 S W 27th Court, Beaverton, OR 97005, (503) 299-2141, BS 70 De Paul Univ; MA 71 Northwestern Univ; SLP Super, St Vincent Hosp & Med Cen, **SLP**

Warren, Mrs Katherine 10221 Binter Lane, Wichita, KS 67212, (316) 722-1996, BA 75 Wichita St Univ; MA 76 Wichita St Univ; Sp-Lang Path, Private Practice, **SLP**

Warren, Kechia Virginia 11010 Southview, Houston, TX 77047, (713) 734-0151, BS 86 Univ of TX - Austin; MA 88 Hampton Univ; 88–Sp-Lang Path, Baylor Coll of Med

Warren, Kimberly Ann Saint Clair Medical Center, 222 Medical Circle, Morehead, KY 40351, (606) 784-6661, BA 84 MI St Univ; MA 85 MI St Univ; 88–Sp-Lang Path, St Claire Med Ctr, **A**

Warren, Linda S 9615 Scotch Haven Drive, Vienna, VA 22180, **SLP**

Warren, Mrs Margaret R Saint Vincent Health Center, 232 West 25th Street, Erie, PA 16544, (814) 452-5654, BS 80 WV Univ; MA 84 Kent St Univ; Aud, St Vincent Health Center, **A**

Warren, Mrs Margaret V 1815 Franklin, Enumclaw, WA 98022, (206) 825-2588, BS 62 Univ of MN - Minneap-St Paul; Sp-Lang Path, Enumclaw Sch Dist, **SLP**

Warren, Maribeth B 6141 Burgandy, Shreveport, LA 71105, (318) 227-5156, BS 55 Northwestern Univ; MA 73 LA Tech Univ; Cl Instr, LA St U Med Cen-Shreveport, **SLP**

Warren, Dr Marilyn Park The Childrens Hospital, Hearing & Speech Division, 300 Longwood Avenue, Boston, MA 02115, (617) 735-6476, BA 70 Middlebury Coll; MA 72 Univ of MA - Amherst; PH 76 (NS) Wichita St Univ; Coord Aud Serv, Chldn Hosp, **A**

Warren, Mrs Mary Kay 125 Ivy Lane, Hewitt, TX 76643, (817) 778-6785, MS 81 Baylor Univ; BS 80 Baylor Univ; Dir/SLP, Bell Co Rehab Cen, **SLP**

Warren, Mary L 6100 South Leix Road, Mayville, MI 48744, **SLP**

Warren, Mrs Nancy H 7227 George Burns, San Antonio, TX 78240, (512) 654-1041, BS 71 Southwest TX St Univ; MA 77 Our Lady Lake Univ-San Anton; Sp-Lang Path, Northeast ISD, **SLP**

Warren, Pamela G 215 Congress, Hot Springs, AR 71901-2677, (501) 624-7111, BA 69 Hendrix Coll; OM 71 Southern Methodist Univ; 77–Sp-Lang Path, Comm Counsl Svcs Inc, **SLP**

Warren, Dr Reg Lawrence Director Ctr For Comm Disorder, Braintree Hospital, 250 Pond Street, Braintree, MA 02184, (617) 848-5353, BS 69 Saint Louis Univ; MA 71 Saint Louis Univ; PH 75 Univ of KS; 88–Sr VP Clin Svcs, Braintree Hosp, **SLP**

Warren, Dr Richard M Psychology Department, University Of Wisconsin, Milwaukee, WI 53201, (414) 229-5328, BS 46 CUNY - City College; PH 51 (NS) NY Univ; Distinguished Prof, U WI Milwaukee

Warren, Roxanne Williams 1093 Garlock Avenue South, Salem, OR 97302, (503) 623-5539, BS 81 Western OR St Coll; MS 82 Western OR St Coll; Sp-Lang Path, Polk Co Ed Serv Dist, **SLP**

Warren, Sally C 610 High Street, Honesdale, PA 18431, (717) 253-1300, BS 74 Bloomsburg Univ of PA; ME 75 Bloomsburg Univ of PA; 85–Sp-Lang Path, Wayne County Memorial Hospital, **SLP**

Warren, Dr Steven Forest Box 328, Peabody At Vanderbilt, Nashville, TN 37203, (615) 322-8277, BS 74 Univ of KS; MA 75 Univ of KS; PH 77 (NS) Univ of KS; 82–Assoc Prof of Spec Educ & Psych, Vanderbilt Univ

Warren, Mrs Susan B 4312 Wallace Circle, Tampa, FL 33611-3438, (813) 837-6239, BS 77 Univ of FL; MS 79 FL St Univ; Sp-Lang Path, Seminole Heights Elem, **SLP**

Warren, Mrs Tracey Lynne 230 Sorrel Trail, Keller, TX 76248, (817) 431-9529, MS 88 Univ of North TX

Warren, Dr Virginia G 2124 Thorley Road, Palos Verdes Estates, CA 90274, (213) 985-4207, BA 60 Marymount Univ; MA 65 Univ of Southern CA; PH 72 (NS) Univ of Southern CA; Assoc Dean, CA St U-Long Beach, **A**

Warren, Yolanda Collean 403 Real Road #26, Bakersfield, CA 93309, (805) 398-3600, MS 88 Univ of AR - Little Rock; 88–Sp-Lang Path, Kern County Supt of Schs

Warren-Manning, Mrs Debby Anne Mile Post 0 71, Mabee Mines Road, Washougal, WA 98671, (206) 837-3853, BS 83 Univ of NE - Lincoln; MS 85 Univ of NE - Lincoln

Warrick, Mrs Debra Mattern 1001 West 18th Avenue, Spokane, WA 99203, (509) 455-3747, BA 82 Central WA Univ; MS 85 Eastern WA Univ; **SLP**

Warrick, Edward J B 4607 Dallas Place, Marlow Heights, MD 20748, (301) 899-3205, BA 73 William Paterson Coll; MS 75 Howard Univ; **SLP**

Warr-Leeper, Dr Genese Ann Department Of Communicative Disorders, Elborn College, University Of Western Ontario, London, ON, Canada N6G 1H1, (519) 661-2001, BS 69 Univ of OK - Norman; MS 71 Univ of OK Medical Center; PH 76 (Sp-Lang Path) Univ of OK Medical Center; 78–Professor, U of Western Ontario, **SLP**

Warshaw, Mrs Elyse W 1509 Rachel Lane, Buffalo Grove, IL 60089, (312) 506-1250, BS 77 Univ of IL - Urbana; MS 78 Univ of IL - Urbana; Sp-Lang Path, Highwood-Highland Park Sch Dist #111, **SLP**

Warshawsky, Mrs Adrienne E 700 Bellefonte Street, Pittsburgh, PA 15232, (412) 682-7503, BS 55 Northwestern Univ; Sp-Lang Path, Private Practice, **SLP**

Warshawsky, Linda M 6532 North Albany, Chicago, IL 60645, (312) 472-6688, BS 81 Northwestern Univ; MA 82 Northwestern Univ; Sp-Lang Path, Chicago Bd of Ed, **SLP**

Warsing, Suzanne Miller P O Box 234, Forestdale, MA 02644, (617) 548-7300, SLP, Falmouth Pub Schls, **SLP**

Warthaw, Lavonne 1232 Ridgepointe Drive, Indianapolis, IN 46234, **SLP**

Waryas, Dr Carol Lynn 2202 Garden Stream Court, Houston, TX 77062, (713) 792-4500, BA 68 Univ of MI - Ann Arbor; MA 69 OH Univ - Athens; PH 74 (NS) Univ of KS; Assoc Dir for Cl Serv, U of TX Hlth Sci Cen-Houston, **SLP F**

Waryas, Dr Paul Allen 2202 Garden Stream Court, Houston, TX 77062, (713) 749-4553, BA 68 Univ of MI - Ann Arbor; MA 69 OH Univ - Athens; PH 74 (Sp & Hrng Science) Univ of KS; Assoc Prof, U of Houston, **A**

Wascom, Mrs Lorrianne 204 Ragan Street, Ruston, LA 71270, (318) 255-3690, BA 78 Nicholls St Univ; MA 82 LA Tech Univ; MA 86 LA Tech Univ; 86–Sp-Lang Path/Aud, Green Clinic, **SLP A ACE**

Wasdin, Mrs Alice J 513 Knollwood Drive, Bremen, GA 30110, (404) 537-4739, BS 59 Univ of AL- Tuscaloosa; MA 72 Memphis St Univ; 85–Sp-Lang Path, Haralson Co Dev Dis Council, **SLP**

Washa, Laura K 5623 Kenny Drive, West Bend, WI 53095, MS; **LM**

Washam, Rita A 2532 North Blanchard, Davenport, IA 52804-1083, **SLP**

Washburn, Amy D 333 East Ontario Street, Apartment 3509-B, Chicago, IL 60611-3035, (312) 908-6134, BS 80 Northwestern Univ; MS 82 Purdue Univ - West Lafayette; Aud, Rehab I of Chicago, **A**

Washburn, Linda J R R 1 Box 1397, Greene, ME 04236, **SLP**

Washburn, Mrs Rosemary C 3176 Bryson Avenue, Boise, ID 83704, (208) 888-6701, BA 77 Eastern WA Univ; MS 80 Eastern WA Univ; Sp-Lang Path, Joint Sch Dist #2, **SLP**

Washchuk, Mrs Carol Keeler 24975 Van Horn Road, Flat Rock, MI 48134, (906) 228-5173, MA 73 Western MI Univ; Consultant, Private Practice, **SLP**

Washer, Constance 200 West 79th Street #3-T, New York, NY 10024, (212) 580-3231, MA 75 NY Univ; SLP, NYC Bd of Ed, **SLP**

Washer, Mrs Sandra 305 West Bergen Court, Fox Point, WI 53217, (414) 351-0722, BS 74 Univ of ND; MS 75 Univ of ND; Private Practice, **SLP**

Washington, Mrs Darlene Williams 313 Manor Drive, Oxford, MS 38655, (601) 252-1768, BA 80 Univ of MS; MA 82 Univ of TX - Austin; 88–Sp-Lang Path, Holly Springs City Schs, **SLP**

Washington, Dr Dora S 1351 Rockdale Drive, Jackson, MS 39213, (601) 968-2244, MA 57 Northwestern Univ; MA 72 IN Univ - Bloomington; PH 74 (Sp Lang Path) IN Univ - Bloomington; 86–Asst VP Academic Affairs, Jackson Ms US, **SLP**

Washington, Dorothy M 17-546 West 13th Avenue, Vancouver, BC, Canada V5Z 1V7, (604) 876-5282, BA 26 Univ of British Columbia; MA 53 Case Western Reserve Univ; **SLP LM**

Washington, Eileen C 1809 East Northern Parkway, Baltimore, MD 21239, (301) 433-4081, MS; **SLP**

Washington, Mrs Elaine Shackelfor 17806 Lassen Street #306, Northridge, CA 91325, (818) 772-6722, MS 87 Univ of MI - Ann Arbor; 87–Sp-Lang Path, Burnwall Clinic

Washington, Mrs Evelyn Douglas 4401 West 11th Street, Little Rock, AR 72204, (501) 778-1111, MS 84 Univ of AR - Little Rock; BA 54 Dillard Univ; Sp-Lang Path, Benton Services Center, **SLP**

Washington, Hazel Delois 1525 Winchester Avenue, Columbia, SC 29203, (803) 754-8189, MA 78 SC St Coll

Washington, Julie Ann 541 South Ashley #1, Ann Arbor, MI 48103, (313) 764-8440, BA 82 Spelman Coll; MS 84 Univ of MI - Ann Arbor; **SLP**

Washington, Sherry Gladys 416 East 13th Street #6, New York, NY 10009, (212) 340-6027, BS 83 Univ of WA; MA 87 Univ of MA - Amherst; **SLP**

Wasileski, Mrs Anita Arthur 25 Pine Avenue, Elysburg, PA 17824, (717) 672-2940, BS 76 Bloomsburg Univ of PA; MS 77 Bloomsburg Univ of PA; Sp-Lang Path, **SLP**

Wasilewski, Mrs Nancy A Route 3 Box 282, Ravenwood Circle, Piedmont, SC 29673, (803) 235-9689, BA 81 Purdue Univ - West Lafayette; MS 82 Purdue Univ - West Lafayette; 88–SLP, Sp Hrng & Learning Ctr, **SLP**

Wasilk, Barbara Miksch 800 West Rand Road #A403, Arlington Heights, IL 60004, (312) 632-1092, MA 87 Univ of IL - Urbana; 87–Sp-Lang Path, Therapeutic Systems, **SLP**

Waskom, Sheryl B 408 Ben Oaks Drive East, Severna Park, MD 21146, **SLP**

Wason, Kim Goudreau 933 Shiloh Court, Joliet, IL 60436, (815) 729-0453, MS 83 Rush Univ; Aud, Dupage Easter Seals Trtmnt Ctr, **A**

Wasser, Deborah S 106 Riversedge Drive, Little Silver, NJ 07739, (201) 747-2115, BA 72 Oberlin Coll; MA 74 Case Western Reserve Univ; **SLP**

Wasser, Mrs Janis K 7517 Red Cravat Court, Columbia, MD 21046, (301) 455-0820, BA 69 Temple Univ; MA 71 Temple Univ; Sp-Lang Path, Baltimore Co Pub Sch, **SLP**

Wasser, Wendy S 326 Cochran Place, Valley Stream, NY 11580, (212) 470-2741, BA 78 SUNY - Center at Buffalo; MA 80 OH St Univ; Sp-Lang Path, L Island Jewish/Hillside Med C, **SLP**

Wasserman, Mrs Barbara K 111 Livingston Avenue, Pittsfield, MA 01201, (413) 442-5201, BA 76 Univ of AL- Tuscaloosa; MS 77 Univ of AL- Tuscaloosa; Sp-Lang Path, Pittsfield Bd of Ed, **SLP**

Wasserman, Debra B 225 South Tropical Trail, Apartment 607, Merritt Island, FL 32952, (404) 329-5520, BS 80 Ithaca Coll; MA 81 Western MI Univ; SLP, Emory U, **SLP**

Wasserman, Helene Debra 2055 West Jarvis Avenue, Apartment 205, Chicago, IL 60645, (312) 262-8449, BA 79 Univ of MO - Columbia; MA 86 Northwestern Univ; 87–Sp-Lang Path, Northwestern Univ, **SLP**

Wasserman, Helene R 70 Colgate Road, Great Neck, NY 11023, (516) 773-3225, BA 76 CUNY - Queens Coll; MS 77 Columbia Univ Teachers Coll; SLP, Private Practice, **SLP**

Wasserman, Mrs Nancy H 169 Garfield Place, Brooklyn, NY 11215, (212) 499-5453, BS 66 Kent St Univ; MS 71 Columbia Univ Teachers Coll; Sp-Lang Path, Private Practice, **SLP**

Wasserman, Sandra A F 116 Church Street, Ashland, OR 97520, (503) 773-7717, BA 73 Univ of CA - Santa Barbara; OM 76 Univ of CA - Santa Barbara; MA 79 San Diego St Univ; SLP, Private Practice, **SLP**

Wasserman, Sara Ethel 1500 Rustie Drive, Bldg 83 Apartment 4, Ocean, NJ 07712, (201) 870-1261, BS 82 Trenton St Coll; MA 85 Montclair St Coll; **SLP**

Wasserman-Gwirtzman, Sarina 80 Park Avenue #6-J, New York, NY 10016, (212) 697-7157, BA 66 CUNY - Hunter Coll; MA 70 CUNY - Hunter Coll; 66–Coord/ Sp-Lang Trainer, Citywide Sp Unit Div of Spec Educ, **SLP**

Wasserstein, Mrs Sharon H 54 Sunrise Terrace, Staten Island, NY 10304, (718) 816-5179, BA 71 CUNY - Brooklyn Coll; MS 82 CUNY - Brooklyn Coll; Sp-Lang Path, Private Practice, **SLP**

Wassner, Paula Levy 47 Branch Avenue, Freeport, NY 11520, (212) 579-5425, BA 64 MI St Univ; MA 67 NY Univ; Sp-Lang Path, Lincoln Med & Ment Hlth Cen, **SLP**

Wasson, Mrs Alison Hasley 16 O'Donnell Court, Little Rock, AR 72205, (501) 225-1318, BS 85 Henderson St Univ; MS 87 Univ of AR - Medical Sci; 87–Sp-Lang Path, Little Rock Sch Dist, **SLP**

Wasson, Mrs Charlotte R R 4 Box 197, Effingham, IL 62401, BS 71 Eastern IL Univ; MS 72 Eastern IL Univ; Supervisor Instr, Eastern Illinois University, **SLP**

Wasson, Dr H Waldo 2311 Jackson Avenue, Joplin, MO 64801, (417) 781-2311, BS 39 Northeast MO St Univ; MA 47 Univ of MO - Columbia; PH 60 (NS) LA St Univ - Baton Rouge; Owner/Dir, Private Practice, **SLP A**

Wasson, Mary Ann Box 625, Sanibol, FL 33957, (813) 472-5373, BA 55 Univ of AR - Fayetteville; MA 75 Univ of AR - Fayetteville; **SLP**

Wasson, Miriam I 1706 Park Street, Houston, TX 77019, (713) 523-3633, BA 81 Tulane Univ; MA 85 Univ of Houston - Univ Park; Parent-Inf Advisr & Mainstream, Houston Schl for Df Chldrn, **SLP**

Wasson, Patricia M 104 Cherokee, San Antonio, TX 78232, (512) 271-7611, BA 57 Our Lady Lake Univ-San Anton; MA 74 Our Lady Lake Univ-San Anton; Consult, Ed Serv Cen Region 20, **SLP**

Wasson, Shari Angela 18404 Vincennes #7, Northridge, CA 91325, (818) 886-7033, MA 88 CA St Univ - Northridge; 88–Sp-Lang Path, Northridge Hosp Med Ctr

Wassum, Gregory P 2239 Ridgewood Drive, Lynchburg, VA 24503, (804) 384-2804, BA 79 Marshall Univ; MA 80 Marshall Univ; Sp-Lang Path, Cen VA Speech and Hearing Ctr, **SLP**

Wassum, Mrs Susan E K 2239 Ridgewood Drive, Lynchburg, VA 24503, BA 79 Marshall Univ; MA 80 Marshall Univ; Sp-Lang Path, Amherst Co Sch Sys, **SLP**

Wasylkewycz, Marta Lydia 2300 Aquila Avenue North, Golden Valley, MN 55427, (612) 591-0833, MS 85 Univ of ND; Speech/Language Pathologist, School District #279, **SLP**

Watamori, Toshiko S Metro Inst Of Gerontology, 35-2 Sakaecho, Itabashiku, Tokyo, Japan 173, BS 66; MA 71 Univ of WA; OD 82 (NS); Research Assoc, Tokyo Metro I of Gerontology

Watanabe, Noriko C 1453 South San Joaquin St, Stockton, CA 95206, (209) 473-5468, BA 78 Univ of the Pacific; MA 79 Univ of the Pacific; Spec Day Class Tchr, John R Williams/Lincoln USD, **SLP**

Waterbury, Olga A P O Box 43406, Austin, TX 78745, BS 40 TX A & I Univ; ME 51 Southwest TX St Univ; **SLP A**

Waterfall, Mrs Lorraine M 1600 Higgins Street, Newberry, SC 29108, (803) 276-1890, BA 61 Converse Coll; OM 78 Univ of SC - Columbia; SLP, Newberry Co Pub Schs, **SLP**

Waterman, Mrs Deborah S 303 Quail Drive, Eldersburg, MD 21784, (301) 655-2236, BA 76 Univ of MI - Ann Arbor; MA 77 Eastern MI Univ; Sp/Lang Path, Carroll Co Bd of Ed, **SLP**

Waterman, Jo Ellen Abbott 4795 Yarrow Place, Colorado Springs, CO 80917, (303) 596-3035, **SLP**

Waterman, Leann K 1905 Wooddea Apt 8, Flint, MI 48507, (313) 732-2160, BA 81 MI St Univ; MA 82 MI St Univ; 82–Sp-Lang Path, McLaren Gen Hosp, **SLP**

Waterman, Sarah Margaret 2516 Vartikian, Clovis, CA 93612, (209) 323-1308, BA 79 CA St Univ - Fresno; MA 82 CA St Univ - Fresno; Sp-Lang Path, State of CA, **SLP**

Waters, Betty Jean Department Communicative Disorders, Northern Illinois Univ, De Kalb, IL 60115, (815) 753-1893, MA 59 Case Western Reserve Univ; Superv, Nn IL Univ, **SLP A**

Waters, Mrs Chris T 13300 S W 101st Street, Miami, FL 33186, (305) 385-3636, MA 76 Univ of Miami; Sp-Lang Path, Private Practice, **SLP ACE**

Waters, Ellen K 1021 S Prospect St #F, Hartville, OH 44632, (216) 877-6320, BA 81 Univ of Akron; MA 87 Univ of Akron; **SLP**

Waters, Ellen Kay R R #1 Box 267, Payson, IL 62360, BS 72 Western IL Univ; MA 78 Western IL Univ; **SLP**

Waters, Gary D Route 1 Box 253-A, Opelika, AL 36801, (404) 568-0286, BS 76 Auburn Univ - Auburn; OM 79 Auburn Univ - Auburn; Asst Admin Sp-Lang Path, Columbus Sp-Lang Cen, **SLP**

Waters, Mrs Helen V 306 Ulster Street, Syracuse, NY 13204, (315) 473-4806, BS 76 Syracuse Univ; MS 77 Syracuse Univ; Aud Superv, Upst Med Cen-Commun Dis Ut, **A ACE**

Waters, Jana Michelle 12001 Belcher Road #B-25, Largo, FL 33543, (305) 898-0551, BA 79 FL St Univ; MS 80 FL St Univ; Sp-Lang Path, InSpeech Inc, **SLP**

Waters, Jeannette Leigh 5276 Wyoming N E #D-9, Albuquerque, NM 87111, (505) 345-7994, **SLP**

Waters, Dr Jerry E Department Of Psychology, Maryville College, Maryville, TN 37801, (615) 982-6412, BA 57 Maryville Coll; MA 60 Univ of KY; PH 64 (NS) Univ of KY; Chmn/Dept Behavior Scis, Maryville Coll, **A**

Waters, Judith A 300 Ridgewood Road, Linthicum, MD 21090, (301) 766-3390, BS 79 Towson St Univ; MS 81 Towson St Univ; 81–Sp-Lang Path, Anne Arundel Co Bd of Ed, **SLP**

Waters, Mrs Kathleen 103 Bradford Park Road, Baden, PA 15005, (412) 869-9393, BS 69 Carlow Coll; MA 73 Univ of Pittsburgh - Pittsburgh; Sp-Lang Path, Pittsburgh Bd of Ed, **SLP**

Waters, Mrs Kathleen H Heard School, 414 Lee Blvd, Savannah, GA 31405, (912) 355-3802, BA 67 Emory Univ; OM 80 LA St Univ - N O Medical Ctr; Sp-Lang Path, Savanna-Chatham Bd of Educ, **SLP**

Waters, Kimberly Jane 7255 Wilby Street, Apartment 28, Norfolk, VA 23505, (804) 440-2945, 88–Sp-Lang Path, Newport News PS, **SLP**

Waters, Larry D Texas St Hearing & Speech Inc, P O Box 90909, Houston, TX 77290, (713) 444-3877, MA 76 Univ of Northern CO; Admin/Pres, Texas State Hring & Speech Inc, **A**

Waters, Lori Kristina 25915 Vicar Way, El Toro, CA 92630, (714) 558-5871, **SLP**

Waters, Mrs Lynn M R 2356 Mission Hills Dr S E, Grand Rapids, MI 49506, (616) 956-0042, BA 75 MI St Univ; MA 77 MI St Univ; **A**

Waters, Melanie B 216 Berwyn Drive West #48, Mobile, AL 36608, (205) 342-4544, BS 81 Univ of South AL; OM 86 Auburn Univ - Auburn; **SLP**

Waters, Mrs Nancy Kay 708 White, Canton, MO 63435, (314) 288-5671, BS 76 Northeast MO St Univ; MA 75 Northeast MO St Univ; Sp-Lang Path, Canton Sch Dist R-V, **SLP**

Waters, Mrs Nancy Suzanne Rt 4 Box 266, Camden, TN 38320, (901) 584-6111, BS 81 Murray St Univ; MS 86 Murray St Univ; 81–Sp-Lang Path, Benton County Bd of Educ, **SLP**

Waters, Patricia A 7-9 Elmwood #7, Maynard, MA 01754, (617) 897-4615, BA 84 IN Univ - Bloomington; OM 85 IN Univ - Bloomington; Sp-Lang Path, **SLP**

Waters, Sandra Cristo P O Box 90909, Houston, TX 77090, (713) 444-3877, Vice President, Texas State Hearing & Speech, **A**

Waters, Mrs Saundra C 11906 McLeod's Lane, Houston, TX 77024, (713) 785-4605, BS 63 CO St Univ; MS 66 CO St Univ; 88–Sp-Lang Path, The Education Clinic, **SLP**

Waters, Susan 765 Oak Avenue, Westfield, NJ 07090, (201) 233-6411, BA 81 Rutger's St Univ - Douglas Coll; MS 82 Rutger's St Univ - Douglas Coll; Sp-Lang Path, St Barnabas Med Cen, **SLP**

Waterstone, Mrs Judith B 9347 Rubio, Sepulveda, CA 91343, (818) 988-5993, OB 67 Univ of MI - Ann Arbor; MA 68 Northwestern Univ; Sp-Lang Path, Tarzana Speech & Language Ctr, **SLP**

Waterstone, Stuart I 9347 Rubio, Sepulveda, CA 91343, (818) 960-3802, MA 69; OD 75 (NS); SLP, Los Angeles Cnty Supt Schools, **SLP**

Waterwall, Jeannit Elain 8506 Rockline, San Antonio, TX 78251, (512) 684-2373, BA 84 Our Lady Lake Univ-San Anton; MA 86 Our Lady Lake Univ-San Anton; 86–Sp-Lang Path, NISD, **SLP**

Wathen, Mrs Patricia Durbin 1726 Sherwood Forest Drive, Miamisburg, OH 45342, (513) 434-0562, BS 78 Eastern KY Univ; MA 85 Univ of Cincinnati

Watkin, Dr Kenneth L Biomedical Engineering, McGill University, 3775 University Street, Montreal, PQ, Canada H3A 2B4, (514) 630-4863, BA 66 Univ of Puget Sound; MA 69 Univ of WA; PH 71 (NS) Univ of WA; 87–Assoc Prof, McGill Univ

Watkin, Patrice S P O Box 216, Washingtonville, OH 44490, ME 78 Univ of VA - Charlottesville; BA 76 Mary Washington Coll; Sp-Lang Path, Youngstown Hrng & Sp Cen, **SLP**

Watkins, Alice Lee 823-33rd Avenue E #D, Seattle, WA 98112, (206) 324-7505, BA 81 Univ of OR; MS 83 Boston Univ; 85–Sp-Lang Path, VA Mason Clinic, **SLP ACE**

Watkins, Bonnie B 903 Larson Drive, Zumbrota, MN 55992, (507) 732-7611, BA 76 Bradley Univ; MS 77 Bradley Univ; SLP, Wasioja Area Sp Ed Coop, **SLP**

Watkins, Dr Carolyn W 2301 Henry Clower Boulevard, Snellville, GA 30278, (404) 979-2027, BS 70 Kent St Univ; MA 72 Kent St Univ; ED 87 (Educ/Sp Path) Univ of GA; Private Practice, **SLP**

Watkins, Christine L 1408 Thaddeus Cove, Austin, TX 78746-6322, (512) 328-5113, BA 72 Univ of TN - Knoxville; MA 74 Univ of TN - Knoxville; **SLP**

Watkins, Donna L 5 Bauer Place, Westport, CT 06880, (203) 661-8500, BA 77 Hofstra Univ; MA 79 Hofstra Univ; Sp/Lang Path, Greenwich Pub Sch, **SLP**

Watkins, Mrs Guinevere Ann 2200 Garfias Drive, Pasadena, CA 91104, (213) 625-4183, BA 67 CA St Univ - Los Angeles; MA 81 CA St Univ - Los Angeles; 88–Sp-Lang Path, Los Angeles USD, **SLP**

Watkins, Karen J 4200 Seabury Q233, Wichita Falls, TX 76308, (817) 322-0771, BA 75 TX Tech Univ; MA 79 Univ of North TX; Aud, The Wichita Falls Clinic, **A**

Watkins, Mrs Kay F 8345 Greenwood Circle, Lenexa, KS 66215, (913) 492-3044, BA 76 Samford Univ; MS 79 Univ of AL- Tuscaloosa; Sp-Lang Path, E Cen Ks Coop In Ed, **SLP**

Watkins, Mrs Leah B 31 Canterbury Woods Street, Glens Falls, NY 12801-1416, (518) 761-0157, BS 78 Bradley Univ; MA 80 Univ of MA - Amherst; Hd Dept of Sp & Lang Path, St Josephs Hosp, **SLP ACE**

Watkins, Lydia Steiner 2514 Kimberly Drive, Garland, TX 75040, (214) 484-0033, BS 81 Univ Southern MS-Hattiesburg; MS 83 Univ Southern MS-Hattiesburg; Sp-Lang Path, Trinity Easter Seals Soc, **SLP**

Watkins, Marla K c/o Pine Lane School, 6475 East Ponderosa Drive, Parker, CO 80134, (303) 841-0202, BS 77 CO St Univ; MS 79 CO St Univ; Sp-Lang Path, Douglas Co Sch Dist Re 1, **SLP**

Watkins, Paula 5 Colony Square Apartment, Dothan, AL 36301, (205) 794-1483, BS 82 Auburn Univ - Auburn; OM 83 Auburn Univ - Auburn; Sp-Lang Path, Dothan City Sch System, **SLP**

Watkins, Richard B 216 Way Station Trail, Knoxville, TN 37922, (314) 631-7800, BA 62 Saint Ambrose Coll; MA 79 Saint Louis Univ; Regional Manager, Pahlberg Inc 84, **A**

Watkins, Ronnie L 2100 Falling Creek Road, Silver Spring, MD 20904, (202) 724-4662, BS 77 Hampton Univ; MS 79 PA St Univ - Univ Park; SLP, Dist Columbia Pub Sch, **SLP**

Watkins, Thomas M 310 Greene Street, Augusta, GA 30901, (404) 722-8899, BA 74 Metropolitan St Coll; MA 75 Univ of Northern CO; Owner, Watkins Hrng Ctr, **A**

Watkis, Deborah J 1832 Metzerott Road #305, Adelphi, MD 20783, (301) 445-4979, BA 76 Howard Univ; MS 79 Howard Univ; 79–Sp-Lang Path, Watkis of Columbia PS Dist, **SLP**

Watman, Lizabeth M 1633 Thomas Court, Flossmoor, IL 60422, (312) 798-3720, BS 73 Eastern IL Univ; MS 74 Eastern IL Univ; SLP, Homewood School District #153, **SLP**

Watnick, Myra L 87 Macarthur Road, Trumbull, CT 06611, (203) 384-8681, BA 65 CUNY - Brooklyn Coll; MS 67 Southern CT St Univ; Dir, Rehab Assoc of Ct, **SLP**

Watroba, Cheryl Ann 2124 Hermosa Avenue #1, Hermosa Beach, CA 90254-2857, (213) 374-3578, BS 85 Eastern IL Univ; MS 86 Eastern IL Univ; 88–Sp-Lang Path, Paramount USD, **SLP**

Watrous, Mrs Betty S Sandie Medical Park, Bldg 3, 1101 Medica Arts N E, Albuquerque, NM 87102, (505) 424-3425, BS 70 Univ of TN - Knoxville; MS 72 Vanderbilt Univ; Aud, Private Practice, **SLP A ACE**

Watrous, Marie-Beth 47 Deforest Drive, North Branford, CT 06471, (203) 527-3139, BA 85 Assumption Coll; MA 88 Southern CT St Univ; 88–Sp-Lang Path, Hartford Bd of Educ

Watson, Ben C University Of Texas, Callier Center, 1966 Inwood Road, Dallas, TX 75235, (214) 783-3105, BA 77 George Washington Univ; MA 79 Univ of CT; PH 83 (NS) Univ of CT; Assistant Professor, University of Texas, **SLP**

Watson, Mrs Betty H P O Box 1221, Whiteville, NC 28472, (919) 642-3028, BA 71 Univ of NC - Greensboro; MS 76 Univ of NC - Chapel Hill; **SLP**

Watson, Dr Betty U Dept Of Speech & Hearing Sci, Indiana University, Bloomington, IN 47405, (812) 335-0710, BA 63 Univ of WI - Madison; PH 70 (NS) Washington Univ; Psychol, IN U

Watson, Bruce W P O Box 97, Gilbertsville, PA 19525, (215) 562-3816, BA 78 Temple Univ; ME 80 Clarion Univ of PA; Sp-Lang Path, Berks Co Inter Ut, **SLP**

Watson, Mrs Caroline 4413 Nancy Drive, Crystal Lake, IL 60014, (815) 455-6126, MS 70 Univ of WI - Madison; MA 71 Univ of WI - Madison; Sp-Lang Path, Crystal Lake Sch Dist #47, **SLP**

Watson, Charles Schoff Dept Of Speech & Hearing Sci, Indiana University, Bloomington, IN 47405, (812) 335-4156, BA 58 IN Univ - Bloomington; PH 63 (NS) IN Univ - Bloomington; Professor Dept Sp-Hrng Science, Indiana University

Watson, Mrs Cheryl Ann 5250 Williams Drive, Paris, TX 75460, (214) 737-3605, BS 81 Univ of North TX; MS 82 Univ of North TX; Sp-Lang Path, St Joseph's Hosp & Hlth Ctr, **SLP**

Watson, Cheryl Ann Route 3 Box 153, Brownsville, TN 38012, (901) 664-5538, BA 84 Univ of TN - Knoxville; MA 86 Univ of TN - Knoxville; **A**

Watson, Mrs Christine Bagalonis PO Box 2727, Roseville, CA 95746, (408) 977-4557, BS 82 PA St Univ - Univ Park; MS 84 PA St Univ - Univ Park; Sp-Lang Path, Meadowbrook Ranch-Sacramento, **SLP**

Watson, Donna Ann Felicita School, 980 North Ash, Escondido, CA 92027, BA 78 Univ of Southern CA; MA 82 CA St Univ - Northridge; Tchr, Escondido USD, **SLP**

Watson, Dorothy H 6611 Memphis Street, New Orleans, LA 70124, BA 76 Univ of Central FL; MS 77 Auburn Univ - Auburn; Sp/Lang Path, Private Practice, **SLP**

Watson, Emily Strauss 680 West 204th Street, New York, NY 10034, (201) 327-1159, BA 68 CUNY - City College; MA 69 Columbia Univ Teachers Coll; Sp-Lang Path, Ramsey Pub Sch, **SLP**

Watson, Jennie Sexton 5 Sedley Place, Durham, NC 27705, **SLP**

Watson, Dr Jennifer Barber 2915 Hilltop Drive, Euless, TX 76039, (817) 921-7620, BS 76 Northern AZ Univ; MA 79 Northwestern Univ; PH 81 (NS) Northwestern Univ; Assoc Prof, TX Christian U, **SLP ACE**

Watson, Mrs Jennifer Becker Route 3 Box 164 B, Brantley, AL 36009, (205) 527-3604, BS 83 Univ of Montevallo; ME 86 West GA Coll; Sp-Lang Path, Covington Co PS, **SLP**

Watson, Judy M 4065 Scotch Pine Drive, Colorado Springs, CO 80920, (719) 520-2230, BS 68 Northern IL Univ - De Kalb; MS 78 IL St Univ - Normal; Sp/Lang Path, El Paso Co Sch Dist 11, **SLP**

Watson, Karen Savage P O Box 421, Green Mountain Falls, CO 80819, (303) 684-9646, BA 71 Univ of FL; MS 72 Univ of South FL; Sp-Lang Path, Colorado Springs Sch Dist #11, **SLP**

Watson, Kay E P 2300 Mecca, Austin, TX 78733, **SLP**

Watson, Mrs Lea Donovan Auditory Verbal Commun Ctr, 1 Gardner Terrace, Gloucester, MA 01930, (617) 281-3293, BA 74 Univ of VT; MS 76 Emerson Coll; Sp-Lang Path, Auditory Verbal Commun Ctr, **SLP**

Watson, Linda Ann 706 South Edisto Drive, Apt Q, Florence, SC 29501, (803) 669-8891, BA 81 Marshall Univ; MS 82 WV Univ; 86–Neurorehab Prog Dir, Health South Rehab Center, **SLP ACE**

Watson, Linda D 6945 South Chappel #3-D, Chicago, IL 60649, (312) 925-1896, BA 77 Augustana Coll; MA 78 Western MI Univ; Sp-Lang Path, Chicago Pub Schs, **SLP**

Watson, Louise Gooch 4514 145th Avenue S E, Bellevue, WA 98006, (206) 641-0766, BA 75 Univ of WA; MA 77 Univ of WA; SLP, Bellevue Pub Sch, **SLP**

Watson, Mrs Luann M 2008 Parker Circle, Norfolk, NE 68701, (402) 371-6243, BS 82 Univ of NE - Lincoln; MS 84 Univ of NE - Lincoln; Sp-Lang Path, Norfolk Public Schools, **SLP**

Watson, Mrs Margaret Anne P O Box 101, Aubrey, TX 76227, (817) 365-9568, MS 83; 83–Sp-Lang Path, Private Practice, **SLP**

Watson, Marie May Moore Halle Room 441, Central Michigan, Mount Pleasant, MI 48859, (517) 774-3472, BA 79 Univ of WI - Stevens Point; MS 81 Univ of WI - Eau Claire; Assistant Professor, Central Michigan University, **SLP**

Watson, Mavis M 3406 Spangler Road, Cleveland Heights, OH 44112, (216) 623-1037, BS 74 Northwestern Univ; MA 75 Univ of Pittsburgh - Pittsburgh; Sp-Lang Pathcruiter, Visting Nurse Assoc, **SLP**

Watson, Michael Lyon 3272 300th Avenue West, Apartment B-104, Oak Harbor, WA 98277, (206) 679-5800, BA 84 Eastern WA Univ; MS 86 Eastern WA Univ; **SLP**

Watson, Mrs Micheleen M 1801 Eutaw Place, Baltimore, MD 21217, (301) 396-7227, BA 65 George Washington Univ; MS 80 Johns Hopkins Univ; 75–Sp-Lang Path, Baltimore City Schools, **SLP**

Watson, Mrs Patricia O 6 Edgewood Court, Decatur, IL 62522, (217) 424-3210, BS 71 Purdue Univ - West Lafayette; MS 72 Purdue Univ - West Lafayette; Sp-Lang Path, Macon-Piatt Special Education, **SLP**

Watson, Patti A 1324 G5 Holgate Drive, Ballwin, MO 63021, (314) 525-1948, MS 81 Central MO St Univ; BS 80 Univ of MO - Columbia; Sp-Lang Path, St Anthonys Medical Center, **SLP**

Watson, Paula Renee 9034 Westheimer Suite 101, Houston, TX 77063, (713) 781-2439, BS 85 Auburn Univ - Auburn; OM 86 Auburn Univ - Auburn; 86–Aud, Rosewood Aud & Hrng Aid Disp, **A**

Watson, Mrs Penny Camp Route 7 Box 59, Mayfield, KY 42066, (502) 345-2225, OB 85 Hardin-Simmons Univ; MS 87 Murray St Univ

Watson, Peter J University Of Arizona, Dept Of Speech And Hearing, Tucson, AZ 85721, (602) 621-7072, OB 74 Univ of IA; OM 80 Univ of AZ; MS 83 Univ of AZ; Research Assistant III, University of Arizona, **SLP**

Watson, Mrs Phyllis B 198 Camellia, Luling, LA 70070, (504) 785-0056, BA 73 Nicholls St Univ; MA 78 Tulane Univ; 88–Sp-Lang Path, Jefferson Parish Sch Bd, **SLP**

Watson, Mrs Sandra M 115 Northwind Trail, Fayetteville, GA 30214, (404) 460-3560, BS 73 Univ of GA; ME 74 Univ of GA; 88–Asst Prin, Fayette County Board of Educ, **SLP**

Watson, Sue B 2210 Cline Street, Tallahassee, FL 32312, (904) 488-5266, BA 68 CUNY - Hunter Coll; MA 71 Univ of KY; Sp-Lang Path, Leon Co Sch Bd, **SLP**

Watson, Mrs Tammy Dahlberg 18994 Avenue 300, Exeter, CA 93221, (209) 592-2157, MA 84 Humboldt St Univ; Sp-Lang Path, Shurson Hearing & Sp Ctr, **SLP**

Watson, Vivian L 7922 South Princeton, Chicago, IL 60620, (312) 723-5364, BS 75 Univ of IL - Urbana; MA 76 Memphis St Univ; SLP, Chicago Bd of Ed, **SLP**

Watson-Dodd, Mrs Brenda Lee 12588 East Pike, Cambridge, OH 43725, (614) 432-3395, MA 85 OH Univ - Athens; Aud, Private Practice, **A**

Watson-Florence, Winifred T 1310 Berkshire, Stow, OH 44224, (216) 375-7884, MS 71 Wichita St Univ; Assoc Prof, Univ of Akron, **SLP**

Watson-Holcomb, Judy 5425 Haverhill Drive, Dublin, OH 43017, (614) 792-1973, BS 76 Purdue Univ - West Lafayette; MA 77 OH St Univ; Self Employed, **SLP**

Watson-Zavodny, Mrs Barbara Ann 130 Westchester Dr, Amherst, OH 44001, (216) 988-2284, BS 76 Bowling Green St Univ; MA 84 Cleveland St Univ; 85–Sp-Lang Path, Private Practice, **SLP**

Watt, Cydney Harrington 1205 Leopard Street, Philadelphia, PA 19125, (215) 945-7200, BA 79 San Francisco St Univ; MA 80 Univ of the Pacific; 86–Suprv/Sp-Lang Path, Easter Seal Society, **SLP ACE**

Watt, Mrs Linda S c/o Kent Board Of Education, 321 North Depeyster Street, Kent, OH 44240, (216) 673-6515, BS 71 Bowling Green St Univ; MA 73 Kent St Univ; Sp-Lang Path, Kent Pub Sch, **SLP**

Watt, Rhonda J P O Box 104, Medina, TN 38355, (901) 422-4005, BS 81 Murray St Univ; MS 82 Murray St Univ; Sp-Lang Path, West Tenn Hrng & Sp, **SLP**

Watt, Susan J 716 Lasalle, Collinsville, IL 62234, BS 85 Southern IL Univ-Edwardsvill; MS 86 Southern IL Univ-Edwardsvill; 88–Sp-Lang Path, Illinois Ctr for Autism, **SLP**

Watters, Mrs Amany 939 Lake Christina Way S E, Calgary, AB, Canada T2J 2R2, (403) 278-2894, BS 79 Univ of Calgary - Alberta; MS 81 Univ of Toronto - Ontario; 81–Sp-Lang Path, Alberta Children's Hosp, **SLP**

Watters, Jack Allan 1187 Hidden Ridge Road, Toledo, OH 43615, (419) 475-3373, BS 52 Ball St Univ; MS 53 IN Univ - Bloomington; **SLP**

Watters, Mrs Mary Jo 5121 South David Street, Casper, WY 82601, (307) 237-9571, BA 73 Univ of Northern CO; ME 78 Clarion Univ of PA; Sp-Lang Path, Natrona Co Sch Dist #1, **SLP**

Watters, Sandra M 2217 Looscan, Houston, TX 77019, (713) 521-2690, BA 68 TX Tech Univ; MA 70 Southern Methodist Univ; **SLP**

Watterson, Mrs Kathye H 10255 Sutters Mill Lane, Reno, NV 89506, (307) 742-8217, BS 78 Univ of WY; MS 80 Univ of WY; **SLP**

Watterson, Dr Thomas L 10255 Sutters Mill Lane, Reno, NV 89506, (307) 766-6426, BS 71 Saint Louis Univ; MA 72 Saint Louis Univ; PH 76 (NS) Univ of OK Medical Center; Assoc Prof, U of NV, **SLP**

Watts, Ann K 11083 Corona Road, Cincinnati, OH 45240, (513) 825-5808, BA 56 Univ of DE; MA 60 Temple Univ-Tyler Sch of Art; Sp-Lang Path, Private Practice, **SLP**

Watts, Donna K 1816 S W 114th, Seattle, WA 98146, (206) 361-1736, BS 80 Univ of WA; OM 82 Univ of WA; Aud, NW Sp & Hrng Cen, **A**

Watts, Marvetta 4521 Granada Boulevard, Apartment 208, Warrensville Heights, OH 44128, (216) 581-8343, MA 88 Cleveland St Univ

Watts, Mrs Mary Clifford 49 Lake Avenue, Greenwich, CT 06830, (203) 869-0177, BA 68 Northeastern Univ; OM 70 Univ of MI - Ann Arbor; MS 83 Columbia Univ Teachers Coll; Audiologist, Associates of Otolaryngology, **A**

Watts, Mrs Michele L 140 Golden Pheasant, Slidell, LA 70461, (504) 847-1679, BS 76 Indiana Univ of PA; MS 81 Central MO St Univ; Aud, **A**

Watts, Mrs Michelle Therese 6563 Nod Hill Road, #21, Salt Lake City, UT 84121, (801) 565-7426, BS 84 Brigham Young Univ; MA 85 Brigham Young Univ; **SLP**

Watts, Mrs Rebecca C 808 South 25th Street, Terre Haute, IN 47803, (812) 232-1467, BS 78 IN St Univ - Terre Haute; MS 79 IN St Univ - Terre Haute; Sp-Lang Path, Paris Sch Dist #95, **SLP**

Watts, Rosalie Eiler 5956 Pinerock Place, Columbus, OH 43229, (614) 471-4007, BS 65 Univ of MN - Minneap-St Paul; MA 70 Univ of MN - Minneap-St Paul; Sp/Lang Path, Gahanna-Jefferson Schs, **SLP**

Watts, Vivian G c/o Southall, 4500 Portsmouth Boulevard, Chesapeake, VA 23321, MS; **LM**

Waugh, Janet Elaine 528 Myrtle Street, Milton, PA 17847, (717) 742-3635, BS 86 Bloomsburg Univ of PA; MS 87 Bloomsburg Univ of PA; **SLP**

Waugh, Marilyn M 411 S W Greenwood, Topeka, KS 66606, (913) 235-6122, BS 74 KS St Univ; MA 75 KS St Univ; **SLP**

Waugh, Patricia F 19309 34th Drive S E, Bothell, WA 98012, (206) 543-3134, BS 71 CO St Univ; MS 73 Univ of WA; Sp-Lang Path, U of WA Hosp, **SLP**

Wauthier, Kelly L 14 Starr Road, Aliquippa, PA 15001, (216) 424-9561, BS 78 Indiana Univ of PA; MS 80 Indiana Univ of PA; Sp-Lang Path, Columbiana Cty Bd of Ed, **SLP ACE**

Wavrek, Dorothy J 321 Exeter Road, Devon, PA 19333, BA 77 MI St Univ; MA 78 Central MI Univ; Aud, Temple Univ Health Sci Ctr, **A**

Wavrin, Nancy Ellen 1230 North Mesa Drive #167, Mesa, AZ 85201, (602) 345-2011, BA 86 Univ of ND; MS 87 Univ of ND; 88–Sp-Lang Path, Arizona Speech Pathology, **SLP**

Wawrykow, Margaret Jean 418 Tanquay Court, Kanata, ON, Canada K2L 3W9, (613) 592-3641, BA 73 Univ of Manitoba - Winnipeg; OB 74 Univ of Manitoba - Winnipeg; MS 84 Univ of ND; **SLP**

Wawrzyniak, Mary Theresa 846 Sacandaga Road, Scotia, NY 12302, (518) 399-2140, BS 82 Syracuse Univ; MS 85 Coll of Saint Rose; 85–Sp-Lang Path, Newmeadow Preschool, **SLP**

Wax, LCDR James P Naval Hospital, Hearing Conservation Division, Bremerton, WA 98312-1898, (206) 478-9560, BA 72 Univ of TX - El Paso; MA 73 Univ of Tulsa; Aud, U S Navy, **A**

Waxman, Ilene A 75 Kaye Vue Drive #2H, Hamden, CT 06514, (203) 274-5411, BA 71 CUNY - Queens Coll; MA 73 Hofstra Univ; OM 83 Univ of CT; SLP, Watertown Bd of Ed, **SLP**

Waxman, Mrs Jeanne H 45-A Appian Way, South San Francisco, CA 94080, (415) 991-6679, BS 79 CA St Univ - Hayward; MS 81 Phillips Univ; Sp-Lang Path, Independent Contractor, **SLP**

Way, Sheila A 15 Banfield Lane, Bloomfield, CT 06002, (203) 722-8635, **SLP**

Waybright, Mrs Cheryl J 1865 Mason Dixon Road, Gettysburg, PA 17325, (717) 334-8904, BS 76 Bloomsburg Univ of PA; MS 77 Bloomsburg Univ of PA; **SLP**

Wayburn, Mrs Laura P 26668 Franklin Pointe Dr, Southfield, MI 48034, (313) 358-3623, BS 71 Univ of MI - Ann Arbor; MA 72 Wayne St Univ; **SLP**

Waychoff, Mrs Tracy Tucker 1506 Sheffield Road, Oklahoma City, OK 73120, (405) 755-4327, BS 84 OK St Univ; MS 86 Univ of OK Medical Center; 86–Aud, Oklahoma Hearing Ctr, **A**

Wayne, Hollie D 1028 Rota Drive, Apo, San Francisco, CA 96334, (209) 358-7940, BS 78 Minot St Univ; MS 79 Minot St Univ; Sp-Lang Path, Private Practice, **SLP**

Wayne, Karen B 6 Hillside Drive, Fairfield, NJ 07006, (201) 575-5814, BA 76 Rutger's St Univ - Douglas Coll; MS 78 Rutgers St Univ -N Brunswick; **SLP**

Wayne, Lori Jo 401 Ide Street #C, Arroyo Grande, CA 93420-3442, (805) 543-7732, Sp-Lang Path, Private Practice, **SLP**

Wayner, Dr Donna Shpikula Hearing Rehabilitation Center, Albany Medical Center Hosp, New Scotland Avenue, Albany, NY 12208, (518) 785-6905, BA 61 Clarke Coll; MA 62 Northwestern Univ; PH 79 (Communications) Rensselaer Polytech Inst; Dir, Albany Med Cen Hosp, **A**

Wayson, Suzanne W 21 Trojan Horse Drive, Phoenix, MD 21131, (301) 444-5000, BS 75 Loyola Coll; MS 76 Loyola Coll; Superv Sp Serv, Maryland Sch for the Blind, **SLP**

Wayt, Paula M 465 Royal Oak Circle, Sebring, OH 44672, (216) 938-9504, BS 68 Capital Univ; MA 71 Kent St Univ; SLP, Salem Pub Schls, **SLP**

Waytashek, Tammy A 4011 Alabama Street, San Diego, CA 92104, (619) 296-9135, MA 87 San Diego St Univ; 88–Sp-Lang Path, Brenda Mann-Mercy Hosp, **SLP**

Wayte, Penelope H 2226 California Street, San Francisco, CA 94115, (415) 338-1001, BA 64 Univ of CA - Berkeley; MA 66 San Francisco St Univ; Sp-Lang Path, Private Practice, **SLP**

Wayte, Dr Rosemary F 825 N E 14th Street, Oklahoma City, OK 73104, BS 62 Northwestern Univ; MS 64 Univ of OK - OK City; PH 71 (NS) Univ of OK - OK City; Assistant Professor, University of Oklahoma, **SLP**

Wealton, Kate A 1008 South 30th Street, Milwaukee, WI 53215, (414) 554-6772, BS 78 Univ of WI - Madison; MS 79 Univ of WI - Stevens Point; Sp-Lang Path, Curative Rehab Ctr, **SLP**

Wean, Dennis F 631 Vine Court, Apopka, FL 32703, **A**

Weatherbee, Donald Scott 14 Green Street, Topsham, ME 04086, (207) 778-3501, BS 61 Boston Univ; ME 62 Boston Univ; Asst Prof In Spec Ed, Un Maine/Farmington, **SLP**

Weatherby, Lynn A Nicolet Instrument Corp, 5225-4 Verona Road, Madison, WI 53711, (608) 271-3333, BS 74 OH Univ - Athens; MA 76 OH Univ - Athens; PH 86 (Aud) Univ of WI - Madison; Product Manager, Nicolet Instruments, **A**

Weatherholt, Steven D 339 Marianna Drive, New Albany, IN 47150, (317) 285-6913, BA 74 IN Univ - Bloomington; MA 77 IN Univ - Bloomington; **SLP A**

Weatherill, Joy M 578 New Britain Road, Doylestown, PA 18901, MS 81 OH Univ - Athens; 84–Sp-Lang Path, Easter Seal Society, **SLP**

Weatherley-White, Dr R C A Plastic Surgery Clinic, 1578 Humboldt Street, Denver, CO 80218, (303) 830-7200, MA 53; MD 58 (NS) Harvard Univ; Chief of Surgery, Plastic Surgery Cl

Weatherly, Mrs Ann D 9014 South Gary, Tulsa, OK 74137, (918) 493-7048, BS 70 OK St Univ; MA 71 Univ of Tulsa; Sp-Lang Path, Assoc Speech & Lang Services, **SLP**

Weathers, Mrs Cynthia Wade P O Box 272, Mount Olive, MS 39119, (601) 765-4457, BS 77 MS Univ for Women; MS 78 MS Univ for Women; Sp-Lang Path/Psychometrist, Covington County Schs, **SLP**

Weathers, Debra Louise 509 Eleventh Street, Davis, CA 95616, (916) 756-1324, BA 85 CA St Univ - Sacramento; MS 87 CA St Univ - Sacramento

Weathers, Kathryn Saxon 14888 Clovercrest Drive, Huntsville, AL 35803, (205) 880-1644, BS 80 Auburn Univ - Auburn; OM 82 Auburn Univ - Auburn; **SLP**

Weathers, Patricia Reed Charleston Sp & Hrng Ctr, 30 Lockwood Drive, Charleston, SC 29401, (803) 577-5410, BS 80 Clarion Univ of PA; OM 83 Univ of SC - Columbia; Aud, Charleston Speech/Hearing Ctr, **A**

Weathersbee, Patricia A 155 Farm Hill Circle, Roswell, GA 30075, (404) 751-2642, BS 80 Univ of TX - Dallas; MS 82 Univ of TX - Dallas; 86–Sp-Lang Path, North Fulton Reg Hosp, **SLP**

Weatherton, Dr Maurice Allen 14106 Ridgewood Drive, Little Rock, AR 72211, (501) 569-3155, BA 61 Henderson St Univ; MA 65 Univ of AL- Tuscaloosa; PH 70 (NS) Univ of KS; Prof, Univ of Ark, **SLP A**

Weatherwax, Leslie Roberta 8115 Morningside Drive, Loomis, CA 95650, (707) 965-2026, **SLP**

Weaver, Amanda S P O Box 594, Norris, TN 37828, **SLP**

Weaver, Brenda K 13611 Scarlet Oak Drive, Little Rock, AR 72211, (501) 329-6851, BS 82 Univ of AR - Little Rock; MS 85 Univ of AR - Little Rock; SLP, Conway Human Dev Cent, **SLP**

Weaver, Carol Nan 24953 Paseo DE Valencia #14C, Laguna Hills, CA 92653, (714) 581-2800, BA 62 Stanford Univ; MS 87 CA St Univ - Sacramento; 88–Asst Dir, Newport Speech-Lang-Aud Ctr, **SLP**

Weaver, Mrs Catherine 103 Woodbine, Wilmette, IL 60091, (312) 251-1513, BS 71 Saint Louis Univ; MA 72 Univ of IL - Urbana; **SLP**

Weaver, Mrs Debra Joy 7349 West Boulevard Unit D, Youngstown, OH 44512, (216) 758-5071, BS 82 Kent St Univ; MS 84 Clarion Univ of PA; 87–Sp-Lang Path, St Elizabeth Hosp Med Ctr, **SLP**

Weaver, Dora C 18838 Watson Avenue, Cerritos, CA 90701, (213) 602-6000, BA 74 CA St Univ - Long Beach; MA 77 CA St Univ - Long Beach; Sp-Lang Path, Paramount USD, **SLP**

Weaver, Dr Ella H 215 East 68th Street #17S, New York, NY 10021, BA 32 Carnegie-Mellon Univ; MA 33 Univ of MI - Ann Arbor; PH 49 (NS) Northwestern Univ; **SLP LM**

Weaver, Mrs Emilie Jo 107 Country Hills, Terry, MS 39170, (601) 372-3838, BS 85 Univ of South AL; MS 87 Univ Southern MS-Hattiesburg; Sp-Lang Path, Hinds Co PS, **SLP**

Weaver, Frank P O Box 533, 1200 William Street, Buffalo, NY 14240, (416) 434-3532, **A**

Weaver, Gayle M 424 Waupelani Drive #M-32, State College, PA 16801, (717) 237-6368, BS 86 Bloomsburg Univ of PA; MS 87 Bloomsburg Univ of PA; 87–Sp-Lang Path, S G Rehab Agency Inc, **SLP**

Weaver, Janet Kathleen 4200 Two Lakes Avenue, Norman, OK 73072, BA 71 Univ of OK - Norman; MS 86 Univ of OK Medical Center; **SLP**

Weaver, Mrs Jennifer Ann 411 Clearwater Drive, Champaign, IL 61821, (217) 351-1243, Aud, Christie Clinic, **A**

Weaver, Mrs Jill M 468 Avila Circle N E, St Petersburg, FL 33703, (813) 522-5053, BS 80 Central MI Univ; MA 81 Central MI Univ; Sp-Lang Path, InSpeech Inc, **SLP**

Weaver, Dr John B 207 West Vermont, Urbana, IL 61801, (217) 351-3841, BS 56 Univ of IL - Urbana; MA 58 Univ of IL - Urbana; PH 70 (NS) Univ of IL - Urbana; 70–Dir Spec Educ, Champaign Commun Sch, **SLP**

Weaver, Mrs Joyce Holland 11719 West 54th Street, Shawnee, KS 66203, (913) 621-5155, BS 60 Phillips Univ; MA 83 Univ of KS; Sp-Lang Path, Kansas City Kansas PS, **SLP**

Weaver, Mrs Julia Cartrette Route 2 Box 56, Chadbourn, NC 28431, (919) 654-5790, **SLP**

Weaver, Kathryn Lois 2140 Lynch Drive, Las Cruces, NM 88001, (505) 522-2292, BS 78 NM St Univ; MA 84 NM St Univ; **SLP**

Weaver, Laura O P O Box 31, Coffee Springs, AL 36318, (205) 588-3937, BS 83 Univ of Montevallo; MS 84 Univ of Montevallo; Sp-Lang Path, Geneva Co Bd of Ed, **SLP**

Weaver, Leslie F 7140 Cypress Cove Road, Jacksonville, FL 32244, (904) 390-2074, BA 68 Univ of OR; MS 74 Univ of HI - Manoa; 87–Coord/Prog Compliance, Duval Co Sch Bd, **SLP**

Weaver, Marietta B 5105 Lucille, Fort Worth, TX 76117, BS 74 Univ of North TX; MS 75 Univ of North TX; SLP, Ft Worth ISD, **SLP**

Weaver, Nancy J Box 352, Accomac, VA 23301, (804) 787-7394, BA 73 Coll of William & Mary; ME 78 Univ of VA - Charlottesville; 88–SLP, Northampton County Schs, **SLP**

Weaver, Phoebe C 1923 General Jackson, Baton Rouge, LA 70810, (504) 261-2730, BA 67 Univ of Southwestern LA; MS 74 Bradley Univ; PH 88 (Sp Path Stuttering) LA St Univ - Baton Rouge; Consult, Greenwell Springs Hosp, **SLP**

Weaver, Mrs Rebecca O Harding University, Box 885, Searcy, AR 72143, (501) 268-6161, BA 73 Harding Univ; OM 74 Univ of MS; 84–Asst Prof, Harding U, **SLP**

Weaver, Dr Ross Maughan 1395 North Cherry Lane, Provo, UT 84604, BS 50 UT St Univ; MS 51 UT St Univ; PH 70 (NS) Univ of OK Medical Center; Aud, Utah State Training School, **SLP A**

Weaver, Mrs Sarah A 5400 South 37th Street, Lincoln, NE 68516, (402) 475-1081, BA 66 Wichita St Univ; MA 75 Wichita St Univ; Sp-Lang Path, Lincoln Pub Schs, **SLP**

Weaver, Stephen Craig 844 West Pampa, Mesa, AZ 85202-8226, (602) 833-6539, BA 69 Willamette Univ; MS 75 AZ St Univ; Sp-Lang Path, Mesa Public Schools, **SLP**

Weaver, Vickie Denise 9220 Shady Bend Lane, Knoxville, TN 37922, (615) 974-6702, BS 83 East TN St Univ; MA 85 Univ of TN - Knoxville; 88–Sp-Lang Path, Ped Lang Clinic-Univ of Tenn, **SLP**

Weaver, Violet Lorraine 2315 McKendree Church Road, Kevil, KY 42053, (502) 488-3077, Sp-Lang Path, Murray State University, **SLP**

Weaver, Mrs Virginia Leigh P O Box 1212, Live Oak, FL 32060-1212, (904) 973-4081, BA 86 Univ of Central FL; MA 87 Univ of Central FL; 87–Sp-Lang Path, Madison Co Schl Dstr

Webb, Bonnie Wootten Route 5 Box 155, Jackson, GA 30233, (404) 761-2745, BA 70 North GA Coll; MS 74 FL St Univ; Comptr Ctr Coord, PACT-GA Assoc Retarded Citizens, **SLP**

Webb, Mrs Catherine Sparacino P O Box 458, Narrows, VA 24124, (703) 726-7264, MA 73 Marshall Univ; Sp-Lang Path, Bluefield Community Hosp, **SLP**

Webb, Christophr A 305 Virginia Street, Marietta, OH 45750, (614) 374-2047, **SLP**

Webb, Dina-Marie 6935 Waterwood Court, Colorado Springs, CO 80918, (719) 593-2246, BA 82 Univ of Northern CO; MA 83 Univ of Northern CO; 88–Sp-Lang Path, Private Practice, **SLP**

Webb, Edward W 270 Crowell Street, Hempstead, NY 11550, (516) 483-8498, BA 67 Adelphi Univ; MS 68 Adelphi Univ; Dir Comm Dis Prog, Nassau Co Dept Hlth, **SLP**

Webb, Elaine W 122 Bethany Drive, Mc Murray, PA 15317, (412) 941-8155, BS 75 OR St Univ; MS 77 Univ of Pittsburgh - Pittsburgh; **A**

Webb, Gary W 4375 Confederate Point Road #22F, Jacksonville, FL 32210, (904) 845-4471, BA 72 Univ of FL; BS 76 FL St Univ; MS 78 FL St Univ; Aud, Nassau Co Sch Bd, **A**

Webb, Mrs Jane C 1333 Windsor Spring Court, Kirkwood, MO 63122, (314) 966-6491, BS 65 IL St Univ - Normal; MS 69 Southern IL Univ-Edwardsvill; Sp-Lang Path, Sp Sch Dist of St Louis Co, **SLP ACE**

Webb, Jane C 305 Virginia Street, Marietta, OH 45750, (614) 374-2047, BA 76 Univ of Pittsburgh - Pittsburgh; BA 76 Univ of Pittsburgh - Pittsburgh; MA 78 Univ of Pittsburgh - Pittsburgh; **A**

Webb, Mrs Janet E S 4949 S E 39th Street, Ocala, FL 32671-8573, (813) 541-1765, BA 76 Univ of FL; ME 77 Univ of FL; **SLP**

Webb, Mrs Jeanette C 1615 Big Horn Drive, Houston, TX 77090, (713) 792-4500, BS 61 East TN St Univ; MA 66 Univ of TN - Knoxville; Sp-Lang Path, U of TX Spc Shi, **SLP**

Webb, Mrs Jennifer Jill 4710 N W 18th Place, Gainesville, FL 32601, (904) 373-5080, **SLP**

Webb, Karen B 16 East 98th Street #2-B, New York, NY 10029, (212) 860-2094, BS 64 UT St Univ; MS 65 UT St Univ; Clinical Supvr, New York League for the Hard of Hearing, **SLP**

Webb, Mrs Katherine 2145 Pond View Court, Reston, VA 22091-3812, (703) 860-2493, BA 72 Temple Univ; MA 74 Northwestern Univ; **SLP**

Webb, Kelly Darleen 10 Vairo Boulevard, Box 404, State College, PA 16803, (814) 238-7020, BS 84 PA St Univ - Univ Park; MS 86 PA St Univ - Univ Park; 88–Clin Educ Coord, Nittany Valley Rehab Hosp, **SLP**

Webb, Kent L Audiological Services, Box 114, Red Oak, IA 51566, (712) 623-4802, BS 74 Northwest MO St Univ; MA 78 Univ of KS; Pres, Aud Servs, **A**

Webb, Dr Kevin C Speech & Hearing Clinic, Lima Memorial Hospital, 1001 Bellefontaine Avenue, Lima, OH 45804, (419) 226-5070, BS 78 Miami Univ - Oxford; MA 79 Bowling Green St Univ; PH 82 (Aud) Bowling Green St Univ; Director Sp & Hrng Clinic, Lima Mem Hosp, **A**

Webb, Kimberly Lynn 1534 Hayes Street #1, San Francisco, CA 94117, (415) 885-0331, BS 83 Univ of WY; MS 85 Univ of WY; **A**

Webb, Dr Loren L Dept Speech Path & Audiology, Western Washington Univ, Bellingham, WA 98225, (206) 676-3881, BS 51 Univ of CA - Berkeley; MA 58 Univ of Redlands; PH 68 (NS) Univ of WA; 88–Sp-Lang Path, Western Wash U, **A**

Webb, Marie J Eastern North Carolina School, For The Deaf, P O Box 2768, Wilson, NC 27894-2768, (919) 237-2450, BS 79 Bloomsburg Univ of PA; MS 80 FL St Univ; 88–Aud, Eastern NC Sch for the Deaf, **A**

Webb, Mrs Mary Susan 1695 East County Road D #211, Maplewood, MN 55109, (612) 439-5160, BA 82 Coll of Saint Teresa; MA 84 Univ of MN - Minneap-St Paul; Sp-Lang Path, Stillwater ISD 834, **SLP**

Webb, Michael O Sierra Hearing Center, 1989 South Frontage Road, Sierra Vista, AZ 85635, (602) 458-3383, BS 75 Univ of AZ; MS 77 Univ of AZ; Owner/Aud, Sierra Hearing Center, **A**

Webb, Mrs Michele E 1079 Timberwood Trls Drive, Florissant, MO 63031, (314) 838-1051, BA 71 MO Valley Coll; MA 75 Saint Louis Univ; Sp-Lang Path, Christian Hospital, **SLP**

Webb, Patricia H 205 Crofton Lane, Knoxville, TN 37922, (615) 974-6702, BA 74 Univ of FL; ME 75 Univ of FL; 87–Assoc Dir-Ped Lang Clin, Univ of Tenn-Knoxville, **SLP**

Webb, Ronald J P O Box 6961, Florence, SC 29502, (803) 669-8891, BA 79 Western KY Univ; MS 80 Western KY Univ; Sp-Lang Path, HealthSouth Rehab Ctr, **SLP**

Webb, Tina Daughtridg Route 4 Box 298, Rocky Mount, NC 27801, (919) 442-9926, BS 84 East Carolina Univ; MS 85 East Carolina Univ; **SLP**

Webb, Tina Renee 7059 West Boulevard #241, Boardman, OH 44512, (216) 726-8855, BA 81 Univ of South FL; MA 85 Case Western Reserve Univ; **A**

Webb, Dr Wanda G 5608 Hillview Drive, Brentwood, TN 37027, (615) 322-0100, BS 70 Middle TN St Univ; MS 71 Eastern IL Univ; PH 79 (NS) Vanderbilt Univ; Asst Prof, Vanderbilt University, **SLP**

Webb, Wendy Stewart 2080 Hermway Heights Place, Mount Vernon, WA 98273, (206) 445-4303, BA 82 Western WA Univ; MA 84 Western WA Univ; **A**

Webber, Mrs Ava L 219 West Wall, Fort Scott, KS 66701, (316) 223-1726, BS 53 Fort Hays St Univ; MA 59 Univ of Denver; Sp-Lang Path, Private Practice, **SLP LM**

Webber, Mrs Diane Ruotolo 1000 Hudson Street #301, Hoboken, NJ 07030, (201) 731-3600, MS 83 Columbia Univ Teachers Coll; SLP, Kessler Institute for Rehab, **SLP**

Webber, Mrs MaryKate E 96 Calumet Avenue, Worcester, MA 01606, (508) 443-9971, BS 79 Nazareth Coll of Rochester; ME 81 Nazareth Coll of Rochester; 86–Sp-Lang Path, Sudbury PS, **SLP**

Webber, Patricia Jane 3709 Madera, Columbia, MO 65203, (314) 882-1571, BS 82 Univ of MO - Columbia; OM 83 Univ of MO - Columbia; 83–Aud, U Hosp & Cl, **A ACE**

Webber, Paula R 815 West J Street #3, Forest City, IA 50436, (515) 582-3382, BA 85 Grinnell Coll; MA 87 Univ of IA; 87–Sp-Lang Path, Northern Trails AEA, **SLP**

Webber, Sharon Green 101 Don Drive, Greenville, SC 29607, (803) 242-0899, BS 80 Univ of GA; MS 81 Univ of SC - Columbia; President, The Compendium Corp, **SLP**

Webber, Susan Ann 44 Dufferin Avenue, St John, NB, Canada E2K 2T8, (506) 648-6741, BA 80 Univ of New Brunswick - Nb; OM 84 Univ of Western Ontario; **SLP**

Weber, Alison Leah 311 Elfinwild Road, Allison Park, PA 15101, (412) 486-2223, BA 82 Univ of Pittsburgh - Pittsburgh; MA 84 OH Univ - Athens; Aud, Pittsburgh Hr/Sp & Deaf Ser, **A**

Weber, Mrs Ann Drake 5846 Louisville Street, New Orleans, LA 70124, (504) 482-2315, **SLP**

Weber, Barbara S 175 Mill Pond Road #312, Hamden, CT 06514, (203) 248-5441, BS 79 Univ of WI - Madison; MS 79 Univ of WI - Madison; Sp-Lang Path, Private Practice, **SLP**

Weber, Bonita L 95 Butternut Street, Elmwood, WI 54740, **SLP**

Weber, Dr Bruce Arthur Ctr For Speech & Hearing Dis, Duke Univ Medical Center, Box 3887, Durham, NC 27710, (919) 684-3859, BA 59 Concordia Coll - Moorhead; MS 61 PA St Univ - Univ Park; PH 66 (NS) Univ of IL - Urbana; Aud, Duke U Med Cen, **A F**

Weber, Christine Maria Aus Dept Purdue University, Heavilon Hall, West Lafayette, IN 47907, (317) 742-6392, BS 81 Portland St Univ; MS 85 Purdue Univ - West Lafayette

Weber, Connie H 125 Mimosa Drive, Decatur, GA 30030, (404) 377-0221, BS 73 Moorhead St Univ; ME 76 GA St Univ; Dir, Sp Path Serv, **SLP**

Weber, Denise A 116 Alvina, Louisville, KY 40214, (502) 454-8261, MA 76 IN Univ - Bloomington; BA 75 Bellarmine Coll; Sp-Lang Path, Jefferson Co Pub Sch, **SLP**

Weber, Donna M 28 Heckle Street, Wellesley Hills, MA 02181, (617) 237-2278, BA 68 Simmons Coll; ME 70 Boston Univ; Sp-Lang Path, Private Practice, **SLP**

Weber, Elaine Dorothy 1847 Lincoln Avenue, Pittsburgh, PA 15235, (412) 828-1300, BA 82 Duquesne Univ; MA 85 Kent St Univ; **SLP**

Weber, Mrs Eleanor H 150 Forest Street, Montclair, NJ 07042, (201) 744-4289, **SLP A**

Weber, Ellen Schmoyer 2481 N E Coachman Road #403, Clearwater, FL 34625, BS 75 Kutztown Univ of PA; MS 82 Univ of South FL; SLP, Pinellas Co Sch Dist, **SLP**

Weber, Ethel Lynn c/o Weinroth, 19 East 88th Street #3B, New York, NY 10028, (212) 920-5445, BS 60 Boston Univ; MA 73 NY Univ; Aud, Montefiore Med Cen, **SLP A ACE**

Weber, Evan A F 1104 Magnolia Road, Teaneck, NJ 07666, (201) 836-6563, BS 75 SUNY - Center at Albany; MA 78 CUNY - Hunter Coll; 88–Clin Supvr, Private Practice, **SLP**

Weber, Frank Jacob, III 3711 Gay Road, Erie, PA 16510, (814) 868-0831, BA 84 Allegheny Coll; MA 86 Edinboro Univ of PA; 88–Sp-Lang Path, InSpeech Inc, **SLP**

Weber, Harold J 1926 Leyden, Denver, CO 80220, (303) 333-6681, BS 51 Univ of MO - Columbia; MA 52 Univ of MO - Columbia; 88–Pres, Colorado Hearing Systems Inc, **A**

Weber, Dr Jack L 76 Southwood Street, Oshawa, ON, Canada L1G 6L7, (416) 968-7877, BA 58 Univ of IA; MA 60 Univ of IA; PH 67 (Phonology) SUNY - Center at Buffalo; Sp-Lang Path, The Geneva Centre, **SLP**

Weber, Mrs Janet Martin 2014 Vanderbilt Court, Naperville, IL 60565, (412) 833-2471, BA 76 Univ of Cincinnati; MS 78 Univ of NC - Chapel Hill; Instr, Coll of Dupage, **SLP**

Weber, Jean A P O Box 67, Urbana, IL 61801, (217) 384-8406, MS 88 Univ of IL - Urbana

Weber, Jennifer E North Colorado ENT/Audiology Associates, 2528 16th Street, Greeley, CO 80631, (303) 356-4646, BS 78 CO St Univ; MS 80 CO St Univ; 80–Aud, N Colorado ENT/Aud Associates, **A**

Weber, Karee Lynn 8970 Dixie Highway, Clarkston, MI 48016, (313) 625-7270, BS 76 Eastern MI Univ; MA 80 Central MI Univ; Supervisor Sp-Lang Path, Education & Therapy Associates

Weber, Mrs Karen Wichelns Box 5361, Taos, NM 87571, (505) 758-8523, MS 77 Univ of NM; 82–Sp-Lang Path, Taos Municipal Schools, **SLP**

Weber, Larry Dwayne 381A Ogden City Mall, Ogden, UT 84401, (801) 627-3001, BA 64 Univ of Northern CO; MS 65 CO St Univ; Aud, Self Employed, **A**

Weber, Laura Gail 9405 Burt Street #20, Omaha, NE 68114, (402) 397-5606, BS 85 Univ of NE - Lincoln; MS 86 Univ of NE - Lincoln; **SLP**

Weber, Lisa Maria 6 Emerald Place, Somerset, NJ 08873, (201) 356-3569, BA 79 MI St Univ; MS 80 Columbia Univ Teachers Coll; Sp-Lang Path, NY League for Early Lrng Inc, **SLP**

Weber, Margaret Meister 141 Joralemon Street #5-C, Brooklyn, NY 11201, (718) 858-9648, MA 88 Univ of MA - Amherst; 88–Aud, Staten Island Aud Services

Weber, Marianne 1250 South Brookhurst, Apartment 2077, Anaheim, CA 92804, (213) 960-3802, BS 71 Fordham Univ; MS 74 Adelphi Univ; SLP, **SLP**

Weber, Mrs Mary Amelia 1508 Adam Road, Virginia Beach, VA 23455, (804) 583-0151, BA 44 Univ of TX - Austin; ME 50 Univ of TX - Austin; 66–Sp-Lang Path, Norfolk PS, **SLP LM**

Weber, Nancy C 191 Harbor View Court, Ventura, CA 93003, (805) 658-0242, BA 73 Towson St Univ; MS 77 James Madison Univ; Sp-Lang Path, CA-Hi Elks Major Proj Inc, **SLP ACE**

Weber, Renee M A Sr 1 Box 57, Pennsylvania Street, Paisley, FL 32767, (904) 738-1112, BS 72 IN Univ - Bloomington; OM 72 IN Univ - Bloomington; SLP, Volusia Co Sch Bd, **SLP**

Weber, Mrs Rosemary Feichtner 2665 Cathy Anne Drive, High Ridge, MO 63049, (314) 942-2565, BA 80 Purdue Univ - West Lafayette; MS 83 Purdue Univ - West Lafayette; Sp-Lang Path, Special Services Co-Op, **SLP**

Weber, Mrs Sandra S 13300 West Courtland Avenue, Brookfield, WI 53005, (414) 783-4266, MS 70 Marquette Univ; Sp-Lang Path, Milwaukee Pub Sch, **SLP**

Weber, Sharon Reiser 3 Sunflower Court, Edison, NJ 08820, (201) 668-6863, **SLP**

Weber, Dr Susan 2381 Carter Avenue, St Paul, MN 55108, (612) 729-4001, BA 67 San Francisco St Univ; MA 68 Northwestern Univ; PH 82 (NS) Univ of MN - Minneap-St Paul; Dir, Northstar Audiology Ltd, **A**

Weber, Mrs Susan Stuckey 9905 Mandeville Circle, Austin, TX 78750, (512) 250-5416, BS 77 Baylor Univ; ME 82 Southwest TX St Univ; SLP, Round Rock ISD, **SLP**

Weber, Theresa M P O Box 153, Springfield, SD 57062, (605) 369-2282, BA 77 9416; MA 78 Univ of SD - Vermillion; Sp-Lang Path, Bon Homme School Dist 4-2, **SLP**

Weber, Vaughan 750 Colony Circle, Pittsburgh, PA 15243, (412) 531-6892, BS 52 Univ of Pittsburgh - Pittsburgh; MS 54 PA St Univ - Univ Park; **SLP**

Weberling, Janet L 1521 Winterbury Lane, Darien, IL 60559, (312) 910-3284, BA 74 Saint Louis Univ; MS 75 Saint Louis Univ; **SLP**

Weber-Olsen, Dr Marcia M 280 West Tenaya, Fresno, CA 93704, (209) 225-3000, BA 72 San Jose St Univ; MA 73 Univ of KS; PH 78 (NS) Univ of KS; 88–Sp-Lang Path, Valley Childrens Hosp, **SLP**

Weber-Pagel, Vivian 2203 Evergreen Court, Plover, WI 54467, (715) 346-2273, BS 70 Univ of WI - Stevens Point; MS 71 Univ of WI - Stevens Point; 72–Sp-Lang Path, Stevens Point Bd of Ed, **SLP**

Weberpal, Molly 1830 Preble Avenue, Green Bay, WI 54302-2937, (414) 498-0635, BS 82 Univ of WI - Whitewater; MS 83 Univ of WI - Whitewater; Sp-Lang Path, Green Bay Area Public Schools, **SLP**

Webster, Ann H G 630 Oakhurst, Clarksdale, MS 38614, (601) 627-9681, BA 73 Univ of MS; OM 75 Univ of MS; Sp-Lang Path/Superv, Clarksdale Mun Sep Sch Dist, **SLP**

Webster, Beverly Nielsen 7907 John Adams Court, Apt 20, Annandale, VA 22003, (703) 938-5060, BS 84 Univ of VA - Charlottesville; MS 86 Vanderbilt Univ; 88–Aud, Vienna-Fairfax Hearing & Sp Ctr, **A**

Webster, Brendan O Ctr For Speech And Language, 851 Fremont Avenue #99, Los Altos, CA 94022-5602, (415) 948-7189, BA 70 San Jose St Univ; MA 72 San Jose St Univ; **SLP**

Webster, Cheryl Ann 187 Cottage Street, Woonsocket, RI 02895, (401) 769-9720, BA 74 SUNY - Coll at Cortland; MS 79 Ithaca Coll; Consult/Sp-Lang Path, Ri Assn/Retard Citizens, **SLP**

Webster, Cheryl Irene Post Office Box 622, 402 Washington Avenue, Woodbine, NJ 08270, (609) 861-5350, BA 77 Montclair St Coll; MA 80 Trenton St Coll

Webster, Dr Elizabeth J 2649 Crossgate Trail, Montgomery, AL 36117-2403, (205) 271-2564, OB 50 OH Univ - Athens; MA 51 Univ of AL- Tuscaloosa; PH 61 (NS) Columbia Univ Teachers Coll; Professor, Memphis State University, **SLP F**

Webster, John C Donovan Farm, Chestertown, NY 12817, (518) 494-4442, BA 41 Univ of IA; MA 43 Univ of IA; PH 53 (NS) Univ of IA; Nsf-Cnrs Exchange Scientist, Inst Phonetique Univ Provence, **F LM**

Webster, Kathy L 9218 King's Cross, San Antonio, TX 78250, (512) 647-8268, BS 80 Southwest TX St Univ; MA 81 Memphis St Univ; Sp-Lang Path, Jimmy Elrod Elem, **SLP**

Webster, Leslie H 2431 Northrup Drive, Tucker, GA 30084, (713) 387-6690, BA 71 Hobart-William Smith Coll; ME 75 SUNY - Center at Buffalo; OM 77 Emory Univ; **SLP**

Webster, Mrs Lynda F D 7510 Andiron Circle, Houston, TX 77041, (713) 937-7646, BS 74 Univ of TX - Austin; ME 75 Southwest TX St Univ; **SLP**

Webster, Mrs Mary McEvoy Elliot Hospital, Rehabilitation Medicine, 955 Auburn Street, Manchester, NH 03102, (603) 669-5300, BS 78 Univ of VA - Charlottesville; ME 80 Univ of VA - Charlottesville; SLP, Nashua Memorial Hospital, **SLP**

Webster, Dr Michael 14644 93rd Avenue, Edmonton, AB, Canada T5R 5G6, (403) 428-5886, BS 65 Southern IL Univ -Carbondale; MS 66 Southern IL Univ -Carbondale; PH 68 (Sp-Lang Path) Southern IL Univ -Carbondale; Pres, Canadian Communication Consult, **SLP F**

Webster, Nancy Sullivan P O Box 2250, Murphys, CA 95247, (209) 736-4662, **SLP**

Webster, Olive M 151 North Chestnut Street, Kent, OH 44240, (216) 743-1168, BS 53 Bowling Green St Univ; MA 76 Univ of Cincinnati; Dir of Commun & Soc Serv, Easter Seal Society, **SLP**

Webster, Patricia Marie 233 Parkside Avenue #A, Buffalo, NY 14214, (716) 439-6169, BS 82 SUNY - Coll at Buffalo; MS 83 SUNY - Coll at Buffalo; 88–Sp-Lang Path, Children's Hosp of Buffalo, **SLP**

Webster, Dr Penelope E Rural Route 1 Box 26, Canterbury, NH 03224, (603) 862-2110, BS 76 Northeastern Univ; MA 77 SUNY - Coll at Geneseo; ED 84 (NS) Boston Univ; Asst Prof, The University of New Ham, **SLP**

Webster, Richard V 15038 Wedgeworth, Hacienda Heights, CA 91745, (818) 333-1980, BS 57 Brigham Young Univ; Sp-Lang Path, Hacienda Lapuente Sch Dist, **SLP**

Webster, Mrs Teri Ellen P O Box 1107, Pittsboro, NC 27312, (919) 774-4634, BA 83 Univ of NC - Chapel Hill; MS 85 Univ of NC - Chapel Hill; Sp-Lang Path, Lee County Schs, **SLP**

Webster, Theda E 3106 El Dorado Lane, Hays, KS 67601, (913) 625-3257, BS 69 Phillips Univ; MS 73 Phillips Univ; 88–Exec Dir, Early Childhood Dev Ctr, **SLP**

Wechsler, Louise A 10981 Rose Avenue #9, Los Angeles, CA 90034, (213) 935-5272, BA 70 Univ of CA - Los Angeles; MA 73 CA St Univ - Northridge; SLP, LA Cty Unif Sch Dist, **SLP**

Wechsler, Mrs Rivi P O Box 1394, Bryn Mawr, PA 19010, (215) 296-6861, BA 65 Temple Univ; MA 82 West Chester Univ of PA; Sp-Lang Path, Devereux Foundation, **SLP**

Wechsler, Robert M 11550 S W 21st Court, Davie, FL 33325, (305) 962-4466, BS 67 Univ of AL- Tuscaloosa; MA 69 Univ of AL- Tuscaloosa; Aud, South Broward Hearing Diag Cen, **A**

Wecker, Mrs Susan A 5344 Woodland Avenue, Western Springs, IL 60558, (312) 246-1404, BS 78 Northern IL Univ - De Kalb; MS 80 Univ of IL - Urbana; Sp-Lang Path, Private Practice, **SLP**

Wedding, Kellye Ann 420 Redding Road #710, Lexington, KY 40502, (606) 271-0061, BS 84 Murray St Univ; MS 86 Murray St Univ; Sp-Lang Path, Franklin Co PS, **SLP**

Wedding, Mrs Sarah Beth 6039 Laurel Trail, Henderson, KY 42420, BS 83 Brescia Coll; MA 84 Univ of TN - Knoxville; Aud, Thomas Logan MD, **A**

Weddington, Gail L 8666 South Shepherd Road Apartment 14, Shepherd, MI 48883, (517) 774-3726, BA 80 Wayne St Univ; MA 81 Western MI Univ; MA 86 OH Univ - Athens; 88–Aud, Central Michigan Univ, **SLP A ACE**

Weddington, Dr Gloria T 16700 Oak View Circle, Morgan Hill, CA 95037, PH (NS) OH St Univ; Professor, San Jose State University, **SLP**

Weddle, Mrs Ginger Rock 257 Heatherton Way, Winston-Salem, NC 27104, (918) 250-1905, BA 74 Univ of OK - Norman; MS 76 Univ of OK Medical Center; **SLP**

Wedmore, Mrs Suellen 285 South Street, Rockport, MA 01966, (617) 546-7460, BA 65 Univ of MA - Amherst; MA 79 Northeastern Univ; Sp-Lang Path, Rockport Pub Sch, **SLP**

Wedzikowski, Mrs Rita Elizabeth 3106 Whispering Drive S, Largo, FL 34641, (813) 527-7175, BS 82 Eastern KY Univ; MA 83 Eastern KY Univ; 84–Sp-Lang Path, Pinellas Co Sch Bd, **SLP**

Weed, Sara Marie P O Box 813, APO New York, NY 09164-5000, BA 64 Fairmont St Coll; MA 65 OH St Univ; OD 83 (NS) Western St Univ Coll of Law; SLP, S Bay Un Sch Dist, **SLP**

Weed, Suzanne G 1055 9th Avenue, Suite A-1, Longview, WA 98632, (206) 636-4420, BA 68 Univ of OR; MA 69 Univ of OR; Sp-Lang Path, Suzanne G Weed Ma Ccc Sp, **SLP**

Weeker, Gail 197 Vista Del Monte, Los Gatos, CA 95032, (408) 353-4664, BA 78 San Jose St Univ; MA 79 San Jose St Univ; 82–Sp-Lang Path, Private Practice, **SLP**

Weekes, Mrs Barbara Blain 10333 Paris Drive, Whittier, CA 90604, (213) 693-0771, BA 69 CA Baptist Coll; MA 84 Whittier Coll; 88–Supvr/Instr, Whittier Coll, **SLP**

Weeks, Mrs Debra Kaye 1402 Mitts Drive, Tupelo, MS 38801, (601) 844-8888, BS 76 Univ Southern MS-Hattiesburg; MA 82 Memphis St Univ, Sp-Lang Path/Teacher Hrng Impd, Tupelo Sp-Lang-Hearing Clinic, **SLP**

Weeks, Joyce Marie 630 Sixth Street, Southfield, MI 48076, (313) 245-1317, BA 82 MI St Univ; MA 84 Eastern MI Univ; **SLP**

Weeks, Julia A 254 West Woodland, Ferndale, MI 48220, (313) 967-3001, BA 51 Grinnell Coll; MA 52 Northwestern Univ; 67–Sp-Lang Path, Oak Park School District, **SLP**

Weeks, Karen S Fire Road 11, Lancaster, MA 01523, (617) 534-6233, BS 75 Worcester St Coll; ME 79 Northeastern Univ; Sp/Lang Path, Fllac Collaborative, **SLP**

Weeks, Lucy E 628 North Treat Avenue, Tucson, AZ 85716, BA 74 Whittier Coll; MS 78 Univ of AZ; Sp-Lang Path, Tucson USD #1, **SLP**

Weeks, Mark S 628 East John #2, Carson City, NV 89706, (801) 489-6056, OM 82 Brigham Young Univ; Aud, Hearing Care of Carson City, **A**

Weeks, Mary S 144 Concord Avenue, Belmont, MA 02178, BS 78 Univ of NH; ME 81 Northeastern Univ; **SLP**

Weeks, Patricia Sue 5730 Libby Road N E, Olympia, WA 98506, (206) 829-1111, BA 75 Western WA Univ; MA 77 Western WA Univ; SLP, Dsh Ddd Ranier State School, **SLP**

Weeks, Mrs Paula B 1640 Maple Drive #61, Chula Vista, CA 92011, (619) 427-9978, MA 84 San Diego St Univ; Sp-Lang Path, Logan Heights Family Health Ctr, **SLP**

Weeks, Robert Alan 6818 Missouri Drive, Vancouver, WA 98664-1271, (206) 696-3945, BS 83 OR St Univ; MA 84 WA St Univ; **SLP**

Weeks, Sally J Bain 301 Chapel Lane, Midland, MI 48640, (517) 636-7011, BA 72 MI St Univ; MA 74 MI St Univ; **SLP**

Weeks, Sharon A 16 Rheola Street, Perth, West Australia, Australia 6005, BA 71 Univ of MT; MS 75 CO St Univ; Aud, Pub Hlth Dept of Wn Australia, **A**

Weems, Alisa Karen 2810 Malone Drive, Panama City, FL 32405, (904) 769-1511, MS 84 FL St Univ; 85–Sp-Lang Path, Bay Med Ctr, **SLP**

Weems, Althea A 1001 West Henry, Mount Pleasant, IA 52641, (319) 385-9005, BS 78 Univ of WI - Madison; MS 80 Univ of WI - Madison; Aud, Great River AEA 16, **A**

Weems, Dr Linda J Northern Arizona University, P O Box 15045, Flagstaff, AZ 86011, (602) 523-7432, BS 85 Univ of OK Medical Center; MS 74 Eastern NM Univ; PH 76 (NS) Univ of OK Medical Center; Asst Professor, Northern Arizona Univ, **SLP**

Weers, Werdna E 1116 S E 2nd Street, Willmar, MN 56201, (612) 235-3096, BS 57 Saint Cloud St Univ; MA 66 Univ of MN - Minneap-St Paul; **SLP LM**

Weesner, David Russell 148 Crest Avenue #3, Revere, MA 02151, (617) 421-5984, BA 85 Univ of FL; MA 87 Univ of FL; 88–Aud, Harvard Comm Health Plan, **A**

Weg, Mrs Susan T 32 Herrick Drive, Lawrence, NY 11559, (516) 239-2241, BA 77 CUNY - Brooklyn Coll; MA 79 CUNY - Queens Coll; 86–Sp-Lang Path, Private Practice, **SLP**

Wegen, Keely Jo 603 California Avenue, Deer Lodge, MT 59722, (406) 846-2268, MS 87 Saint Cloud St Univ; 87–Sp-Lang Path, Deer Lodge Elem Sch Dist #1

Wegener, John G Cincinnati Speech & Hearing Ct, 3021 Vernon Place, Cincinnati, OH 45219, (513) 221-0527, BS 64 Univ of WI - Madison; MA 66 IN Univ - Bloomington; Asst Dir/Coord Sp-Lang Serv, Cincinnati Sp&Hrng Cen, **SLP**

Weger, Frank Randy 2002 College South East, Grand Rapids, MI 49507, (616) 247-1947, BS 73 Purdue Univ - West Lafayette; MA 74 Western MI Univ; SLP, Grand Rapids Pub Sch, **SLP**

Wegienka-Vokal, Mrs Susan C 5733 Kaufman, Dearborn Heights, MI 48125, (313) 928-0462, BA 73 MI St Univ; MA 74 Wayne St Univ; Sp-Lang Path, Allen Park Pub Sch, **SLP**

Wegmann, Monica E 340 Fairway Drive, New Orleans, LA 70124, (504) 488-0155, BS 77 LA St Univ - Baton Rouge; OM 78 LA St Univ - N O Medical Ctr; SLP, Jefferson Parish School Board, **SLP**

Wegner, Jane R 3017 Harvard Road, Lawrence, KS 66044, (816) 582-2040, BS 70 Central MI Univ; MA 71 Central MI Univ; Sp/Lang Path, Private Practice, **SLP**

Wegner, Mrs Mary A Bosinski 4261 South Wayside, Saginaw, MI 48603, MS 75 Central MI Univ; Sp-Lang Path, Buena Vista Pub Schs, **SLP**

Wegner, Mrs Sara R Rural Route 2, Kemptville, ON, Canada K0G 1J0, (613) 820-1820, BA 72 IN Univ - Bloomington; MA 73 IN Univ - Bloomington; Sp-Lang Path, Carleton Board of Ed, **SLP**

Wegrzyn, Mrs Brenda J C 2640 Commercial Avenue, South Chicago Heights, IL 60411, (312) 755-1147, BS 84 IL St Univ - Normal; MS 87 IL St Univ - Normal

Wegrzynek, Lynn Ann 900 Macbeth Drive #1, Monroeville, PA 15146, (412) 372-1783, BS 75 Carlow Coll; ME 79 Indiana Univ of PA; 75–Sp-Lang Path, Allegheny Intermediate Unit, **SLP**

We Hara, Constance Sada 174 Kona Lane, Long Beach, CA 90805, (213) 922-7682, BA 81 Univ of CA - Santa Barbara; MS 85 San Francisco St Univ; Sp-Lang Path, Rancho Los Amigos Med Ctr, **SLP**

Wehmeyer, Mrs Jan Blair 10203 N Mac Arthur #302, Irving, TX 75063, (214) 506-8481, BS 84 Univ of AR - Fayetteville; MS 86 Univ of TX - Dallas; 86–Sp-Lang Path, Irving ISD, **SLP**

Wehnert, Jay L 2214 Pelham Avenue, Baltimore, MD 21213, (301) 243-3800, BA 78 Loyola Coll; MS 79 Loyola Coll; Sp-Lang Path, The Hrng & Sp Agcy, **SLP ACE**

Wehr, Mrs Diana R R R 2 Box 4, Sigourney, IA 52591-9701, (515) 622-3680, BA 75 Creighton Univ; MS 78 Univ of NE - Omaha; Sp-Lang Path, Private Practice, **SLP**

Wehrle, Anne Patricia 642 Jackson Avenue, West Paterson, NJ 07424, (201) 523-7282, BA 70 William Paterson Coll; MS 72 William Paterson Coll; 70–Sp-Lang Path, West Paterson Bd of Educ

Wehrle, Ellen L 1102-B South Maple, Oak Park, IL 60304, (312) 848-3015, BA 68 Coll of Wooster; MA 74 Case Western Reserve Univ; Sp-Lang Path, InSpeech Inc, **SLP**

Weichel, Kimberly Suzanne c/o Audiological And Hearing Aid Services, 501 Howard Avenue Bldg D, Altoona, PA 16601, (814) 946-0721, BS 84 Clarion Univ of PA; MS 85 Clarion Univ of PA; 86–Aud, Aud/Hrng Aid Svcs Inc, **A**

Weidenfeld, Susan H 830 Dorncliff Lane, Buffalo Grove, IL 60089, (312) 541-8048, BS 73 OH Univ - Athens; MA 74 Northwestern Univ; **SLP**

Weidenfeller, Geraldine 3 Banor Drive, Somerville, NJ 08876, (201) 359-8462, BS 54 Newark St Coll; MA 62 NY Univ; Sp-Lang Path, Private Practice, **SLP**

Weidman, Maja B 6635 Century Avenue, Middleton, WI 53562, MS; **SLP**

Weidner, Julie Lynne 35 Wood Street Apartment 113, Lewiston, ME 04240, (207) 782-1680, BS 82 Univ of SD - Vermillion; MA 84 Univ of SD - Vermillion; 84–Sp-Lang Path, Griffiths-Larrabee Inc, **SLP**

Weidner, Dr William E 1248 Cottonwood Circle, Auburn, AL 36830, (205) 826-5545, BS 49 Bowling Green St Univ; MS 52 Bowling Green St Univ; PH 71 (NS) Case Western Reserve Univ; Prof/Dept Head Commun Dis, Auburn U, **SLP F**

Weigel, Rebecca S 36 Annie Lou Drive, Hamilton, OH 45013, **SLP**

Weiger, Dr Myra L 38 Bedford Terrace, Irvington, NJ 07111, (201) 527-2175, BA 56 Montclair St Coll; MA 67 Kean Coll of NJ; ED 77 (NS) Rutgers St Univ -N Brunswick; Dept Chmn, Kean College of Nj

Weiglin, Mrs Jeanne T 421 Seville Way, San Mateo, CA 94402, (415) 573-9726, BA 63 Univ of OK - Norman; ME 67 Duquesne Univ; **SLP**

Weikel, Mrs Marilyn Lucy 340 Rockwell Road, Jackson, TN 38305, (901) 686-0840, BS 74 Brescia Coll; MS 78 East TN St Univ; 86–Sp-Lang Path, Polk-Clark Elementary, **SLP**

Weikel, Mrs Stephanie Suzette 627 Ames Place, Williamsport, PA 17701, (717) 323-8441, BS 79 Bloomsburg Univ of PA; MS 80 Bloomsburg Univ of PA; SLP, Blast Iu 17, **SLP**

Weikert, Mrs Barbara 302 Frances Street, Teaneck, NJ 07666, (201) 977-2435, BA 69 Elmira Coll; MA 70 Columbia Univ Teachers Coll; Superv Sp & Hrng, St Joseph's Hosp & Med Cen, **SLP**

Weil, Mrs Bette J 10 West Lane, Madison, NJ 07940, (201) 966-2843, BA 56 CUNY - Queens Coll; MA 81 Kean Coll of NJ; Sp-Lang Path, Speech Language Associates, **SLP ACE**

Weil, Elizabeth R 3508 North Paulina, Chicago, IL 60657, (312) 908-6134, MA 84 Northwestern Univ; 87–Sp-Lang Path, Rehab Inst of Chicago, **SLP**

Weil, Emily Jean 121 South Washington St #3, Genoa, IL 60135, (815) 338-7411, BA 81 Valparaiso Univ; MA 85 Northern IL Univ - De Kalb; **SLP**

Weil, Mrs Jerilyn Blatt 2066 Brighton Way, Merrick, NY 11566, (516) 379-7470, **SLP**

Weil, Mrs Miriam S 575 Laurent Road, Hillsborough, CA 94010, (415) 348-0992, BS 58 Univ of UT; MA 65 Univ of CA - Los Angeles; Sp-Lang Path, Hillsborough Cty Sch Dist, **SLP**

Weil, Patricia Messina 1241 Country Place, Redlands, CA 92374, (714) 639-4990, BS 81 Univ of AZ; MS 83 Univ of AZ; Aud/Aural Rehab Spec, Loma Linda Surgery Medical Group, **A**

Weil, Mrs Sara Magence 1390 Somerset Gate, Teaneck, NJ 07666, (201) 692-3917, BA 76 CUNY - Hunter Coll; MA 77 CUNY - City College; 85–Aud, Metro Aud, **A**

Weil, Stacy Rachelle 12202 Braxfield Court Apartment 13, Rockville, MD 20852, (301) 424-5200, BA 85 Univ of MD - College Park; MA 87 George Washington Univ; 87–Sp-Lang Path, Treatment & Learning Center, **SLP**

Weiland, Ellen B 1820 North Blossom Drive, Appleton, WI 54914, BS 74 Marquette Univ; MS 75 Marquette Univ; 86–Sp-Lang Path, Appleton Area Sch Dist, **SLP**

Weiland, Linda E 4211 Lincoln Swing #34, Ames, IA 50010, (515) 239-4480, BS 81 Univ of WI - Madison; MA 86 Univ of Denver; Aud, Mc Farland Clinic, **A**

Weiland, Susan Huber 3101 Toledo Avenue South, Minneapolis, MN 55416, (612) 559-3535, BA 75 Univ of MN - Minneap-St Paul; BA 75 Univ of MN - Minneap-St Paul; MA 77 Wayne St Univ - Sch of Med; 86–Aud, Hennepin Tech Inst Dist 287, **A**

Weiler, Charles W 20 Briggs Street, Wollaston, MA 02170, (617) 479-5345, BA 70 Boston Coll; ME 74 Northeastern Univ; OD 87 (Ed-Admin) Bridgewater St Coll; Sp-Lang Path, Qunicy Pub Sch, **SLP**

Weiler, Dr Nancy A Eastern Illinois University, Clinical Services Bldg, 7th & Hayes, Charleston, IL 61920, (217) 581-2712, BS 63 Univ of WI - Milwaukee; MS 66 Purdue Univ - West Lafayette; PH 76 (NS) Univ of IL - Urbana; Dir-Hrng Servs, Eastern IL U, **SLP A**

Weiler, Pamela A 425 Audubon Road, Apt 2-A, Danville, VA 24540, (804) 797-2553, BS 77 James Madison Univ; MS 87 James Madison Univ; 88–Sp-Lang Path, Danville Sp & Hrng Ctr, **SLP**

Weil-Lefkovith, Patricia 43 Ivy Road, Malden, MA 02148, (617) 683-4000, **A**

Weimer, Mary Margaret 99 Foster Street, New Haven, CT 06511, (203) 734-0783, **SLP**

Weinberg, Bernd 4950 North Apache Hills Tr, Tucson, AZ 85715, (602) 299-5286, BS 61 SUNY - Coll at Fredonia; MA 63 IN Univ - Bloomington; PH 65 (NS) IN Univ - Bloomington; Dir-Inst Rel, Research Corp Tech Inc, **SLP F**

Weinberg, Mrs Cheryl F 6913 Asher, Metairie, LA 70003, (504) 527-0303, BS 66 MS Univ for Women; MA 67 OH Univ - Athens; Sp-Lang Path, Orleans Parish Sch Bd, **SLP**

Weinberg, Donna L 150 Overlook Avenue, Apartment 3A, Hackensack, NJ 07601, (201) 343-3245, BA 78 Hofstra Univ; MA 80 NY Univ; Sp-Lang Path, Private Practice, **SLP**

Weinberg, Mrs Leslie R 11 Carefree Lane, Suffern, NY 10901, (914) 356-4100, BA 74 CUNY - Queens Coll; MA 76 CUNY - Lehman Coll; Sp-Lang Path, E Ramapo Cen Sch Dist, **SLP**

Weinberg, Mrs Marcia L 5324 Plains Drive, Lake Worth, FL 33463, (407) 439-4349, BS 71 Northeastern Univ; ME 72 Northeastern Univ; OM 75 Northeastern Univ; Sp-Lang Path, Sch Bd of Palm Beach Co, **SLP**

Weinberg, Marion J 77 Montvale Road, Newton Center, MA 02159, (617) 357-6000, BS 75 Miami Univ - Oxford; MA 79 Kent St Univ; Sp-Lang Superv, Act for Boston Comm Dev Hd Str, **SLP**

Weinberg, Mrs Marjorie F 2 Central Drive, Kings Point, NY 11024, (516) 466-5667, BA 56 Univ of MI - Ann Arbor; MS 60 Adelphi Univ; **SLP**

Weinberg, Norma Pasekoff 82 Hayes Road, Centerville, MA 02632, (508) 771-0164, BS 63 OH St Univ; MS 69 Emerson Coll; Sp-Lang Path, Corporate Comm, **SLP**

Weinberg, Mrs Randi Beth 34 Orchard Street, Blackstone, MA 01504, (617) 883-6232, BS 81 Univ of MA - Amherst; MA 83 Northeast MO St Univ; **SLP**

Weinberg, Susan Oppenheim 272 South 2nd Street, Philadelphia, PA 19106, (215) 928-1477, BA 64 Univ of PA; MA 66 Temple Univ

Weinberg, Mrs Sylvia Z 80 Steeplechase Drive, Marlboro, NJ 07746, (212) 447-0124, BA 71 CUNY - Brooklyn Coll; MS 81 Columbia Univ Teachers Coll; Sp-Lang Path, Community Dist 23 Bd of Educ, **SLP**

Weinberger, Mrs Giti Schachner 1745 58th Street, Brooklyn, NY 11204, (212) 232-6894, BA 75 CUNY - Brooklyn Coll; MS 82 CUNY - Brooklyn Coll; Sp-Lang Path, Giti Weinberger, **SLP**

Weinberger, Hadasa 23 Blueberry Hill Road, Monsey, NY 10952-1948, **SLP**

Weiner, Adeline E 17 Homestead Lane, Roosevelt, NJ 08555, (609) 448-2358, BA 65 Rutger's St Univ - Douglas Coll; MS 69 Rutgers St Univ -N Brunswick; **SLP LM**

Weiner, Mrs Barbara R 3562 South Poplar, Denver, CO 80237, (303) 693-0611, BA 67 1075; MA 75 Univ of CO - Boulder; Sp/Lang Path, Cherry Creek School District, **SLP**

Weiner, Carole May 31 Cantebury Drive, Athens, OH 45701, (614) 594-3539, MA 65 Univ of MA - Amherst; OM 63 CUNY - Brooklyn Coll; **SLP**

Weiner, Carolyn Ausberger 6739 North 16th Place, Phoenix, AZ 85016, (602) 277-7348, BA 67 Univ of MO - KS City; MA 70 Univ of IA; Pres, Syndactics, **SLP**

Weiner, Ellen S 2020 N E 163rd Street, Suite 209, North Miami Beach, FL 33162, (305) 949-1624, BS 76 Boston Univ; MA 79 Univ of Miami; Sp-Lang Path, Private Practice, **SLP**

Weiner, Frederick F 190 Sandy Ridge Road, State College, PA 16803, (814) 863-2012, BA 68 Wayne St Univ; MA 69 Wayne St Univ; PH 71 (Sp Path) Wayne St Univ; Assoc Prof, PA St U at U Park, **SLP**

Weiner, Dr Honore I 1011 Main Street, Concord, MA 01742, (617) 369-9500, BS 68 Emerson Coll; MS 70 Emerson Coll; ED 81 (Special Education) Boston Coll; 74–Prog Coord, Case Collaborative, **SLP**

Weiner, Jean C 153 West 82 Street, New York, NY 10024, **SLP**

Weiner, Mrs Johanna G 104 Bennington Drive, East Windsor, NJ 08520, (609) 448-6333, BA 57 CUNY - Brooklyn Coll; MA 65 CUNY - Brooklyn Coll; 87–Sp/Lang Path, Burlington Co Comm Action Prog Head Start, **SLP ACE**

Weiner, Judith A 26 Dorchester Road, Buffalo, NY 14222, (716) 886-4488, BA 72 SUNY - Center at Buffalo; MA 75 SUNY - Center at Buffalo; Aud, Hearing Evaluation Service, **A**

Weiner, Mrs Judith Kahn Achievement Resource Assoc Inc, 3140 Warbler Place, Highland Park, IL 60035, (312) 432-3410, BS 63 Univ of WI - Madison; MA 64 Northwestern Univ; Sp-Lang Path, Achievement Resource Assoc Inc, **SLP**

Weiner, Mrs Regina I P 91 Patton Drive, Yonkers, NY 10710, (914) 793-1703, MA 69 Pace U -NY City; MA 70 NY Univ; 70–Sp-Lang Path, NYC Citywide Sp Svc Unit, **SLP**

Weiner, Dr Ruth H 540 North Neville, Pittsburgh, PA 15213, (412) 381-0600, BS 36 Northwestern Univ; MS 60 Univ of Pittsburgh - Pittsburgh; PH 63 (NS) Univ of Pittsburgh - Pittsburgh; **SLP LM**

Weiner-Kahn, Mrs Sheila B 2293 Calle Conejera, Palm Springs, CA 92262, BA 75 San Diego St Univ; MS 82 Univ of Redlands; Sp-Lang Path, Desert Hospital, **SLP**

Weiner-Kaplow, Dawn F 6364 Musket Court, Bensalem, PA 19020, (215) 750-0563, BA 81 Univ of IL - Urbana; MS 83 Univ of WI - Madison; Sp/Lang Path, Cora Services In Philadelphia, **SLP**

Weinfeld, Brenda 1145 Barry #106, Brentwood, CA 90049, (213) 820-9270, BS 83 Univ of TX - Austin; MS 85 Univ of TX - Dallas; 88–Aud, Childrens Hosp of LA, **SLP A**

Weingart, Lori 5129 Foxon Road, Virginia Beach, VA 23464, (804) 474-2245, BS 77 Univ of WI - River Falls; MS 78 Univ of WI - River Falls; Aud, **A**

Weingarten, Barbara McNurney 3473 Fisher Place, Carmel, CA 93923, (408) 624-0801, BS 62 Emerson Coll; MS 65 Emerson Coll; 70–Sp-Lang Path, Carmel USD, **SLP**

Weingartner, Susan C 2604 Blackridge Avenue, Penn Hills, PA 15235, (412) 854-0507, BS 84 Northwestern Univ; MS 86 Univ of MI - Ann Arbor; **SLP**

Weingast, Mrs Beatrice M 145 Main Street, Ridgefield, CT 06877, (203) 438-5895, BA 44 CUNY - Brooklyn Coll; MA 66 Seton Hall Univ; SLP, Danbury Bd of Ed, **SLP**

Weingram, Mrs Florence N 1619 Sheridan Road, West Lafayette, IN 47906, (317) 463-1502, BA 56 CUNY - Brooklyn Coll; MS 59 PA St Univ - Univ Park; SLP, Indiana Veterans Home, **SLP ACE**

Weinheimer, Bernice Cecelia 5493 Trastevere Road, Clay, NY 13041-8930, (315) 425-4565, BS 82 Nazareth Coll of Rochester; MS 83 Radford Univ; **SLP**

Weinheimer, Sr LaVerne C 6505 Market Street, Youngstown, OH 44512, (216) 792-7636, BS 1955; MA 70 Seton Hall Univ; 70–Dir of Aud, Youngstown Hrng & Sp Cen, **SLP A**

Weinhouse, Dr Iris 114 Bedford Road, Hillsdale, NJ 07642, (201) 664-5195, BA 57 CUNY - Brooklyn Coll; MA 62 CUNY - Brooklyn Coll; PH 73 (Sp Path) CUNY - Brooklyn Coll; Dir Speech Clinic, Rockland Comm Coll, **SLP**

Weinman, Janice 10578 White Fir Court, Cupertino, CA 95014, (408) 923-1950, BS 64 Boston Univ; MA 71 San Jose St Univ; SLP, Berryessa Un Sch Dist, **SLP**

Weinreich, Mrs Patricia C 6982 Webster Road, Orchard Park, NY 14127, (716) 686-3219, BS 59 SUNY - Coll at Buffalo; MS 65 SUNY - Coll at Buffalo; Sp-Lang Path, Lancaster Ctrl Sch, **SLP**

Weinrib, Mrs Holly Jaci 445 Broadway #3-E, Hastings on Hudson, NY 10706, (914) 478-2165, BA 79 Dominican Coll of Blauvelt; MA 82 CUNY - Lehman Coll; SLP, Lakeland School District, **SLP**

Weinrich, Mrs Barbara D 1605 Gage Drive, Middletown, OH 45042, (513) 424-7711, BS 68 Miami Univ - Oxford; MA 73 Univ of Cincinnati; 75–Sp-Lang Path, Private Practice, **SLP**

Weinsaft, Mrs Gudrun Stehr Rt 2 Box 276, Rogersville, MO 65742, (417) 882-7501, BS 65 Northwestern Univ; MS 83 Southwest MO St Univ; 87–Dir, Bellwether Institute, **SLP**

Weinstein, Dr Barbara E 10 West 15th Street #9N, New York, NY 10011, (212) 960-8017, BA 75 SUNY - Coll at Buffalo; MA 76 Case Western Reserve Univ; PH 80 (Aud) 2162; 87–Assoc Prof of Aud, Lehman Coll-CUNY, **A**

Weinstein, Dayna S Boston Hearing Assoc Inc, O Emerson Suite 2C, Boston, MA 02114, (617) 523-0281, **A**

Weinstein, Mrs Emily A M 958 Lydia Place, Baldwin, NY 11510, (516) 678-1200, BS 74 SUNY - Center at Albany; MS 77 Adelphi Univ; Sp-Lang Path, Oceanside Pub Sch, **SLP**

Weinstein, Ilene G 18765 Braemore Road, Northridge, CA 91326, (818) 366-9410, BA 72 Univ of Pittsburgh - Pittsburgh; MA 74 Northwestern Univ; Sp-Lang Path, Burbank USD, **SLP**

Weinstein, Jeri 157 East 18th Street #6A, New York, NY 10003, (212) 420-2760, BS 77 Boston Univ; MS 78 Columbia Univ Teachers Coll; 88–Sp-Lang Path, Beth Israel Med Ctr, **SLP**

Weinstein, Marlene 2281 S W 15th Street #142, Deerfield Beach, FL 33441, (305) 937-1432, BA 79 CUNY - Queens Coll; MS 81 CUNY - Brooklyn Coll; SLP, Janet Sandler and Assoc, **SLP**

Weinstein, Philip 8210 Arrowhead Road, Baltimore, MD 21208, (301) 655-4234, BS 52 Bloomsburg Univ of PA; 84–Sp-Lang Path, Private Practice, **SLP**

Weinstein, Mrs Rena R K 18808 Briars Court, Olney, MD 20832, (301) 570-0322, BA 76 SUNY - Center at Buffalo; MA 77 NY Univ; 87–Sp-Lang Path, Howard County PS, **SLP**

Weinstein, Mrs Sherrie 6503 North Military Trail, Apartment 3100, Boca Raton, FL 33496, BA 75 Univ of MD - College Park; MS 76 PA St Univ - Univ Park; Sp-Lang Path, **SLP**

Weinstein, Mrs Susan Rydell 1529 East Oak Forest Spur Drive, St Louis, MO 63146, (314) 993-0406, OB 85 Univ of MO - Columbia; MA 87 Saint Louis Univ; **SLP**

Weinstein, Mrs Suzanne M 16501 Limerick Lane, Minnetonka, MN 55345, (612) 933-9343, BS 68 Univ of MN - Minneap-St Paul; MA 70 Univ of MN - Minneap-St Paul; Sp-Lang Path, Hopkins Sch Dist, **SLP**

Weinstein, Mrs Virginia Kopf 1359 Stanley Terrace, Elizabeth, NJ 07208, (201) 352-8789, BA 76 Long Island U - CW Post Ctr; MA 78 Seton Hall Univ; Sp-Lang Path, Elizabeth Bd of Ed, **SLP**

Weinstock, Holly H 209 Howard Avenue #2, Passaic, NJ 07055, (201) 773-3464, BS 84 Emerson Coll; MS 87 William Paterson Coll; 87–Sp-Lang Path, Miriam S Marzell, **SLP**

Weinstock, Susan E 1841 East Oak Knoll Circle, Fort Lauderdale, FL 33324, (305) 475-8350, BA 75 Tulane Univ; OM 77 LA St Univ - N O Medical Ctr; Sp-Lang Path, Hearing & Spch Cen of Florida, **SLP**

Weintraub, Suzanne 3797 Fallon Circle, San Diego, CA 92130, (619) 589-4108, BS 79 Univ of AZ; MS 81 Univ of AZ; Sp-Lang Path, Grossmont District Hospital, **SLP ACE**

Weintraub, Wendy S 6913 Bonnie Ridge Drive, Apartment T-2, Baltimore, MD 21209, (301) 486-1419, BA 85 OH St Univ; MA 87 Northwestern Univ; **SLP**

Weintrob, Sharon 306 Head House Court, Wayne, PA 19087, (215) 524-5000, BS 64 Univ of WI - Madison; Sp-Lang Path, Chester Co Iu #24, **SLP ACE**

Weir, Beth 2111 Refset Drive #22, Janesville, WI 53545, (608) 757-2386, MS 88 Univ of WI - Madison; 88–Sp-Lang Path, Janesville Sch Dist

Weir, Clara B 127 Whitney Street, Hartford, CT 06105, MA 32 Columbia Univ Teachers Coll; **SLP LM**

Weir, Jacqueline M 227 Oak Street, Binghamton, NY 13905, (607) 798-7117, BA 75 SUNY - Center at Buffalo; MA 77 Ball St Univ; 81–Sp-Lang Path, Hndcpd Chldn Assoc, **SLP**

Weir, Linda D Santa Fe Center For Audiology, 1454 St Francis, Santa Fe, NM 87501, (505) 988-9818, BA 72 Univ of TX - El Paso; MA 73 Univ of North TX; Aud Co Owner, Santa Fe Cen for Audiology, **A**

Weir, Lynn Hoffman 4513 North 35th Place, Phoenix, AZ 85018, (602) 957-3654, BA 72 Occidental Coll; MA 74 Northwestern Univ; Sr Acct, McGladrey & Pullen, **SLP**

Weir, Mitzi Hancock Route 7 Box 1002, Tyler, TX 75707, (214) 566-5885, BS 83 Murray St Univ; MS 83 Murray St Univ; **SLP**

Weirather, Dr Randy R Dept Of Communication Sciences, And Disorders, University Of Montana, Missoula, MT 59812, PH 76 (NS); Assoc Prof, Univ of MT, **SLP**

Weirich, Patricia Suzanne 1365 Cove Avenue, Lakewood, OH 44107, (216) 362-6450, MA 79 Cleveland St Univ; Sp-Lang Path, Cuyahoga Board of Ment Retardn, **SLP**

Weis, Carole Marie 4216 Kathleen Lane, Oak Lawn, IL 60453, (312) 385-2450, **SLP**

Weis, Mary Dvorak 9911 Kramer Drive, Sandy, UT 84092, (801) 565-7432, BS 78 UT St Univ; MS 80 UT St Univ

Weis, Patricia A 2354 W University Dr, Apt 2122, Mesa, AZ 85201, (601) 224-5970, BS 84 ND St Univ; MS 86 ID St Univ; 86–Aud, Southwest Audiology Inc, **A**

Weisbein, Mrs Wanda 44 Columbine Circle, Newtown, PA 18940, (215) 757-0227, BS 72 OH Univ - Athens; MA 75 Trenton St Coll; 72–Sp/Lang Path, Bucks Cty I U 22, **SLP**

Weisberg, Dr Doris F 145 East 92nd Street, New York, NY 10128, (212) 831-6539, BS 58 Univ of WI - Madison; MS 65 Columbia Univ Teachers Coll; PH 70 (NS) 2162; Assoc Prof-Chair Sp Dept, Cty Coll-Cuny, **SLP**

Weisberg, Mrs Jennifer Dale 40 Willow Gate Rise, Holliston, MA 01746, (617) 587-2121, **SLP**

Weisberg, Mrs Roberta 1 Nelson Road, Monsey, NY 10952, (914) 356-2975, BS 66 CUNY - Queens Coll; MS 72 CUNY - Brooklyn Coll; **SLP**

Weisbrod, Barbara M 1187 Fuhrman Road, Cincinnati, OH 45215, (513) 498-2131, BS 78 Univ of Cincinnati; MA 79 Miami Univ - Oxford; SLP, Sidney Cty Sch, **SLP**

Weisbrod, Mrs Kathleen Granahan West 611 23rd, Spokane, WA 99203, (509) 455-3287, BS 79 Univ of WI - Madison; MS 81 Univ of WI - Milwaukee; SLP, Sacred Heart Medical Center, **SLP**

Weise, Mrs Mary T 6319 104th Avenue, Clear Lake, MN 55319, (612) 743-2854, BS 63 Univ of MN - Minneap-St Paul; MS 71 Saint Cloud St Univ; Cl Dir, St Cloud St U, **SLP**

Weise, Susan L 27 Bourndale Road North, Manhasset, NY 11030, (516) 627-1355, BA 75 OH Wesleyan Univ; MA 77 Hofstra Univ

Weise, Timothy G 9106 Manchester, Grosse Ile, MI 48138, (313) 458-3385, BS 73 Eastern MI Univ; MA 77 Eastern MI Univ; Dir Sp-Lang Path, Garden Cty Hosp, **SLP ACE**

Weisel, Mrs Christine 685 Jasmine Place N W, Issaquah, WA 98027, (206) 391-2377, BA 74 WA St Univ; MA 81 CA St Univ - Long Beach; SLP, Los Alamitos USD, **SLP**

Weisel, Joyce Carol 6055 Harwood Avenue, Oakland, CA 94618, (415) 653-5143, MS 87 CA St Univ - Hayward; 88–Sp-Lang Path, Albany USD

Weisenburger, Carolyn M 12300 30th Avenue North, Plymouth, MN 55441, (612) 920 6377, BS 75 IL St Univ - Normal; MS 77 IL St Univ - Normal; Sp/Lang Path, Groves Lrng Cen, **SLP**

Weiser, Ellen B 30263 Regent Road, Wickliff, OH 44092, (216) 321-8787, BA 73 CUNY - Lehman Coll; MA 74 NY Univ; 88–Sp-Lang Path, Cleveland Hrng & Sp Ctr, **SLP**

Weiser, Michael Lawrence Central Kansas ENT Associates, 909 East Wayne, Salina, KS 67401, BA 76 Fort Hays St Univ; MA 78 Wichita St Univ; Aud, J E Cossette, M D P A, **A**

Weiser, Mrs Randi E 401 East 86th Street, New York, NY 10028, (212) 722-2304, BA 77 CUNY - Brooklyn Coll; MS 78 Columbia Univ Teachers Coll; 86–Sp-Lang Path, New York Communication Ctr, **SLP**

Weishan, Mrs Deborah A 1111 Crown Point Road West, Signal Mountain, TN 37377, MA 77 Western MI Univ; Audiologist, Chattanooga Speech/Hearing Ctr, **A**

Weisiger, Bradford, Jr Speech Pathology 126 Cvamc, 3200 Vine Street, Cincinnati, OH 45220, (513) 861-3100, BA 72 Univ of NC - Chapel Hill; MS 74 Univ of NC - Chapel Hill; **SLP**

Weisinger, Wendell Lynne 25 Harley Street 1st Floor, Dorchester, MA 02124, (617) 247-5467, BA 73 CUNY - Brooklyn Coll; MS 74 Univ of WI - Madison; Sp-Lang Path, Boston University Hospital, **SLP**

Weiskopf, Mrs Dianne E 961 Avon Crest Boulevard, Schenectady, NY 12309, BA 71 Case Western Reserve Univ; MS 72 Univ of MI - Ann Arbor; SLP, Wildwood Sch, **SLP**

Weiskopf, Mrs Donna T 920 Park Drive, Flossmoor, IL 60422, (312) 798-6227, BS 65 OH St Univ; MA 66 OH St Univ; **SLP**

Weiskotten, June S Box 21 Brookside Avenue, Morrisonville, NY 12962, (518) 563-8345, **SLP**

Weisleder, Mrs Jenny N 5249 40th Avenue NE Apartment 201, Seattle, WA 98105, (206) 525-1987, BA 84; MA 87 Univ of AZ; 88–Aud, Children's Hosp & Med Ctr

Weisman, Audrey T Speech & Language Associates, 5 Walnut Avenue, Stoughton, MA 02072, (617) 344-6502, BA 72 Univ of MA - Amherst; MA 73 Eastern MI Univ; Sp-Lang Path, Sp/Lang Assoc, **SLP**

Weisman, Linda J 10770 S W 131 Avenue, Miami, FL 33186, (305) 325-0470, MS 77 Univ of South FL; 81–Chief Sp-Lang Path, Er Sl So of Dade Co Inc, **SLP**

Weismer, Susan Ellis Department Of Communicative Disorders, 1975 Willow Drive, Madison, WI 53706, (608) 262-3951, BA 75 IN Univ - Bloomington; MA 76 IN Univ - Bloomington; PH 81 (NS) IN Univ - Bloomington; Asst Prof, University of Wisconsin, **SLP**

Weiss, Mrs Aileen A 4431 Ivy Hall Drive, Columbia, SC 29206, (803) 782-1772, BA 51 CUNY - Brooklyn Coll; MS 53 Purdue Univ - West Lafayette; Sp-Lang Path, Fort Jackson Dep Sch, **SLP**

Weiss, Dr Amy L Department Speech Pathology & Audiology, University Of Iowa, WJSHC, Iowa City, IA 52242, (319) 335-8731, BA 74 SUNY - Center at Buffalo; MA 76 Univ of IL - Urbana; PH 83 (NS) Purdue Univ - West Lafayette; Asst Prof, Univ of Iowa, **SLP**

Weiss, Dr Arthur I 4431 Ivy Hall Drive, Columbia, SC 29206, (803) 777-2824, BS 50 Pacific Univ; MA 52 Univ of NM; PH 54 (NS) Purdue Univ - West Lafayette; Prof, U of SC/Coll Ed, **SLP F LM**

Weiss, Barbara 9 Albion Road, Montreal, PQ, Canada H3X 3L8, (514) 934-8028, BS 77 McGill Univ - Quebec; MS 79 McGill Univ - Quebec; Aud, Montreal Gen Hosp, **A**

Weiss, Betty G 7415 Richards Road, Melrose Park, PA 19126, (215) 288-2102, BA 60 CUNY - Queens Coll; MS 62 Univ of Pittsburgh - Pittsburgh; Aud, ENT Consult Pc, **SLP A**

Weiss, Carol Ann 2630 Grunewald, Blue Island, IL 60406, (312) 481-6741, BA 78 Saint Mary's Coll; MA 84 Northern IL Univ - De Kalb; 88–Sp-Lang Path, South Metropolitan Assoc, **SLP**

Weiss, Mrs Carol Arenson Longwood Crossing, Lawrence, NY 11516, (516) 239-1917, **SLP**

Weiss, Cathryn Claudia 126 Helm Way, Downingtown, PA 19335, (215) 383-3862, BS 67 Bowling Green St Univ; MA 84 West Chester Univ of PA; 79–Sp-Lang Path, Chester Co Inter Unit, **SLP**

Weiss, Claudia J 192 Mt Vernon Road, Snyder, NY 14226, (716) 898-3217, BS 65 SUNY - Coll at Buffalo; MS 67 SUNY - Coll at Buffalo; Sp-Lnag Path, Erie County Medical Center, **SLP ACE**

Weiss, Dr Curtis E 324 Dungeness Meadows, Sequim, WA 98382, (206) 683-6194, BS 58 Dickinson St Coll; ME 62 Univ of OR; PH 68 (NS) Univ of MO - Columbia; Sp-Lang Path, Private Practice, **SLP**

Weiss, Mrs Deborah Edelstein 20 Trenor Drive, New Rochelle, NY 10804, (914) 235-2597, BA 72 CUNY - City College; MA 75 CUNY - Hunter Coll; SLP, Private Practice, **SLP**

Weiss, Mrs Deborah L 8 Eliot Drive, Lake Grove, NY 11755, (516) 585-5356, BA 73 Hofstra Univ; MA 75 Hofstra Univ; Sp-Lang Path, BOCES, **SLP**

Weiss, Deborah M 43 Mansfield Apartment, South Eagleville Road, Storrs, CT 06268, (203) 524-2462, BS 74 NY Univ; MA 78; SLP, Univ of Connecticut, **SLP**

Weiss, Donna M 1219 O Avenue Place NE #4, Cedar Rapids, IA 52402, (319) 365-6469, BS 84 Univ of WI - Stevens Point; MS 87 ID St Univ; 88–Aud, St Luke's Hosp, **A**

Weiss, Gail E 196-70 69th Avenue, Fresh Meadows, NY 11365, (212) 454-4940, BS 78 Syracuse Univ; MA 82 NY Univ; SLP, Gail Weiss, **SLP**

Weiss, Mrs Iris Fisher 8 Forrest Road, Randolph, NJ 07869, (201) 895-9331, BA 79 CUNY - Brooklyn Coll; MS 81 CUNY - Brooklyn Coll; **SLP**

Weiss, Mrs Judith Bellin 2106 East Wellington Road, Newtown, PA 18940, (215) 321-0727, BS 79 Kent St Univ; MA 79 Kent St Univ; Sp-Lang Path, Wilmette Jr High, **SLP**

Weiss, Judy Reva 421 East 81st Street #3RE, New York, NY 10028, (212) 360-5600, BA 76 CUNY - City College; MS 81 Columbia Univ Teachers Coll; **SLP**

Weiss, Mrs Karen Kaplan 2366 Stepping Stone Way, Colorado Springs, CO 80904, (303) 389-0475, MA 85 Univ of CO - Boulder

Weiss, Kathleen M 3852 10th Avenue South, Minneapolis, MN 55407-2624, (612) 348-8412, BS 75 Univ of WI - Madison; MS 77 Gallaudet Coll; Aud, Minneapolis Pub Schs, **A**

Weiss, Mrs Laurie K 252 Aspen Lane, Highland Park, IL 60035, (312) 433-6252, BA 64 Univ of MI - Ann Arbor; MS 65 Univ of MI - Ann Arbor; 71–Sp-Lang Path, Private Practice, **SLP**

Weiss, Mrs Lori Joyce 7360 116th Street, Flushing, MI 48433, (313) 639-7921, **SLP**

Weiss, Mrs Marion I 2977 Charlotte Drive, Merrick, NY 11566, BA 66 CUNY - Brooklyn Coll; MA 70 CUNY - Brooklyn Coll; OM 83 Hofstra Univ; SLP, NYC Bd of Education, **SLP**

Weiss, Mrs Mary Margaret 26 Normandy Drive, Northport, NY 11768, (516) 549-4900, BS 76 Marquette Univ; MA 77 Tulane Univ; Teacher Coordinator, BOCES III, **SLP**

Weiss, Dr Michael S Dept Communicative Disorders, West Chester University, West Chester, PA 19383, (215) 436-3403, BA 64 Long Island U - Brooklyn Ctr; MS 68 Purdue Univ - West Lafayette; PH 70 (NS) Purdue Univ - West Lafayette; Prof, West Chester University

Weiss, Mina 36203 Delaire Landing Road, Philadelphia, PA 19114, (215) 745-3287, BA 83 Temple Univ; MA 86 Temple Univ; **SLP A**

Weiss, Nancy Waring 110 Malverne Avenue, Malverne, NY 11565, (718) 780-1598, MS 84 Boston Univ; Sp-Lang Path, Long Island College Hospital, **SLP**

Weiss, Mrs Naomi R 30 Brook Drive, Milltown, NJ 08850, (201) 246-0417, BA 68 CUNY - City College; MA 69 Columbia Univ Teachers Coll; Sp/Lang Path, Elizabeth Molinari Defusco, **SLP**

Weiss, Phyllis Windwer 1363 Millwood Lane, Merrick, NY 11566, (212) 683-6970

Weiss, Rebecca L 1272 East 9th Street, Brooklyn, NY 11230, **SLP**

Weiss, Dr Rita S 801 Euclid Avenue, Boulder, CO 80302, (303) 492-8727, BS 45 Simmons Coll; MA 57 Univ of CO - Boulder; PH 67 (NS) Univ of CO - Boulder; Prof Emerita, U of CO-Boulder, **SLP**

Weiss, Samuel c/o P O Box 12067, Jerusalem, Israel 91120, BA 73 CUNY - City College; MA 74 CUNY - City College; Aud, Hadassah Hospital, **A**

Weiss, Mrs Shifra Lipshitz 1245 South Bedford Drive, Los Angeles, CA 90035-1014, (212) 220-8596, MA 69 Columbia Univ Teachers Coll; **SLP**

Weiss, Susan Eileen 18350 Hatteras Street #236, Tarzana, CA 91356-1668, (818) 997-2357, MA 84 Whittier Coll; Sp-Lang Path, LA City Schools, **SLP**

Weissberg- Smith, Amy Jo 733 West Canterbury Street, Apartment A, St Louis, MO 63132, (314) 968-4710, BS 84 Eastern IL Univ; MA 86 Northern IL Univ - De Kalb; 88–Aud, St Louis Hearing-Sp Ctr, **A**

Weissbrot, Sharon D 4555 Henry Hudson Parkway, Riverdale, NY 10471, (212) 543-1076, BA 74 CUNY - City College; MA 76 CUNY - City College; 79–Sp-Lang Path, NYC Bd of Ed-Sp Sers Ut, **SLP**

Weisslender, Mrs Diane P 21 Portland Street, New Haven, CT 06513, (203) 468-9667, BS 80 SUNY - Coll at Geneseo; MA 82 SUNY - Coll at Geneseo; Sp-Lang Path, Easter Seals Rehab Ctr, **SLP ACE**

Weissman, Mrs Cynthia C 764 Applegate Lane, Rosemont, PA 19010, (215) 527-8938, BA 76 Boston Coll; ME 80 Northeastern Univ; 85–Sp-Lang Path, Private Practice, **SLP**

Weissman, Linda L 24 South Park Place, Longmeadow, MA 01106, (413) 567-9139, BA 74 Hofstra Univ; MA 76 Univ of MA - Amherst; Sp-Lang Path, Ludlow Pub Sch, **SLP**

Weissman, Rita R 21 Benenson Drive, Cos Cob, CT 06807, (203) 869-4381, BA 78 CA St Univ - Long Beach; MA 81 CA St Univ - Northridge; **SLP**

Weissman, Mrs Ronee F 517 Almena Avenue, Ardsley, NY 10502, (914) 693-4289, BA 73 CUNY - Queens Coll; MA 78 CUNY - Queens Coll; Sp-Lang Path, Visiting Ther Assoc, **SLP**

Weissman, Sandra E 241 Lexington Street, Apartment 11-1C, Woburn, MA 01801, **SLP**

Weisz, Nancy Schatz 9109 Brierly Road, Chevy Chase, MD 20815, BA 76 Wesleyan Univ; MA 78 Northwestern Univ; 83–Sp/Lang Path, Private Practice, **SLP**

Weitenhagen, Janet Johnson 241 56th Street, Des Moines, IA 50312, (515) 274-6560, BS 81 Northeast MO St Univ; MA 84 Northeast MO St Univ; Ctr Manager, Des Moines Hrng & Sp Ctr, **SLP**

Weiter, Pamela Leigh 7021 A Green Tee Court, St Louis, MO 63129, (314) 846-6231, BS 83 Fontbonne Coll; MS 84 3216; Sp-Lang Path, Windsor Sch C-1, **SLP**

Weithman, Mrs Jodi Simmonds 2392 Sandstrom Drive, Worthington, OH 43085, (614) 761-3478, MA 82 OH St Univ; **SLP**

Weitman, Mrs Sheryl T 4517 Netherwood Drive, Tampa, FL 33624, (813) 968-6356, BA 76 Univ of Pittsburgh - Pittsburgh; MA 78 Univ of Pittsburgh - Pittsburgh; **A**

Weitz, Mrs Cynthia 3708 Calvend Lane, Kensington, MD 20895, BS 69 Cornell Univ; MA 73 George Washington Univ; 84–Sp-Lang Path, Montgomery Co MD PS, **SLP ACE**

Weitz, Mrs Geraldine Greenfield 5 Rosewood Court, Somerset, NJ 08873, (201) 846-7783, BA 67 SUNY - Center at Buffalo; MA 71 Montclair St Coll; 80–Sp-Lang Path, Franklin Township PS, **SLP**

Weitz, Julia M Dept Of Comm Disorders, Bloomsburg University, Bloomsburg, PA 17815, (717) 389-4436, MS; **SLP**

Weitz, Karen A Rd #3 Box 15J, Rhinebeck, NY 12572, (914) 876-4404, BS 85 Long Island U - CW Post Ctr; MS 87 WV Univ

Weitzenkorn, Mrs Patricia G 0040 Tanager Drive, Glenwood Springs, CO 81601, (303) 945-5444, BA 79 Univ of FL; MA 81 Univ of FL; 88–Sp/Lang Path, Hearing & Speech Associates, **SLP**

Weitzman, Dr Nancy Fried 20 Seward Lane, Stony Brook, NY 11790, (516) 751-2517, BS 64 NY Univ; MA 66 NY Univ; PH 83 SUNY - Center at Stony Brook; **SLP A**

Weitzmann, Erica E 336 West 95th Street #62, New York, NY 10025, (212) 584-9000, BA 84 SUNY - Coll at New Paltz; MS 85 Columbia Univ Teachers Coll; 86–Aud, VA Med Ctr, **A**

Weitzner, Maxine 212 West 22nd Street, New York, NY 10011, (212) 242-0464, MA 84 NY Univ; Sp-Lang Path, League Sch, **SLP**

Weitzner-Lin, Dr Barbara 171 Wellingwood Drive, East Amherst, NY 14051, (716) 878-5316, BA 73 SUNY - Center at Buffalo; MS 74 Columbia Univ Teachers Coll; PH 81 (NS) SUNY - Center at Buffalo; Prof, State Coll at Buffalo, **SLP**

Weix, Mrs Donna Jean Route 2 Box 210, Elk Mound, WI 54739-9532, (715) 879-5546, BA 83 Univ of WI - Eau Claire; OM 84 Univ of WI - River Falls; 87–Sp-Lang Path, Altoona Sch Dist, **SLP**

Welborn, Mrs Helen Giese 5537 Valhalla Drive, Carmichael, CA 95608, (916) 483-4608, BA 49 Univ of MI - Ann Arbor; MA 50 Northwestern Univ; Sp-Lang-Hrng Spec, San Juan USD, **SLP**

Welch, Mrs Alison Keene 2370 North Aspen, Hanford, CA 93230, (209) 584-1266, BS 79 Univ of NE - Lincoln; MA 81 Univ of NE - Lincoln; Sp/Lang Path, Sierra Speech & Hearing, **SLP**

Welch, Mrs Ann H 1435 East Crestwood, Memphis, TN 38119, (901) 386-0550, BA 57 Univ of MS; MA 74 Memphis St Univ; MA 74 Memphis St Univ; Sp-Lang Path, Memphis City Schs, **SLP**

Welch, Cara Suzette 120 East Beauregard, San Angelo, TX 76903, (915) 658-1511, BS 85 TX Tech Univ; MS 87 Univ of TX - Dallas; 87–Aud, Angelo Cl Assoc, **A**

Welch, Carolyn Louise 2108 Lansdown Drive, Carrollton, TX 75007, (214) 416-5555, BS 73 Univ of Central AR; MS 86 East TX St Univ - Commerce; 86–Sp-Lang Path, North Central Texas Rehab Agency, **SLP**

Welch, Catherine 20 Woolworth Street, Longmeadow, MA 01106, BA 56 Coll of William & Mary; ME 58 Boston Univ; OM 78 Boston Univ; **SLP**

Welch, Connie Renee Route 7 Box 365, Lebanon, MO 65536, (417) 588-4275, MS 83 Univ of MO - Columbia; 86–Sp-Lang Path, Pro Sp-Lang Svc of the Ozarks, **SLP**

Welch, Deborah Greengold 2113 North Sheffield, Chicago, IL 60614, (312) 975-4080, BA 72 Hofstra Univ; MA 74 Trenton St Coll; SLP, Welch Consulting, **SLP**

Welch, Mrs Denise Suzanne 17007 N E 136th Place, Redmond, WA 98053, (415) 935-7820, BS 81 CA St Univ - Hayward; MS 83 San Francisco St Univ; 87–Aud, The Hear Ctr, **A**

Welch, Donal M 1519 Rollin Street #B, South Pasadena, CA 91030, MA 87 Univ of CA - Santa Barbara

Welch, Elizabeth 5967 Arden Place, Baton Rouge, LA 70806, (504) 343-4232, Sp-Lang Path, Baton Rouge Sp-Hrng Foundation, **SLP**

Welch, Gary R 129 South 26th Street Ct, Blue Springs, MO 64015, (816) 228-7530, BS 76 Central MO St Univ; MS 78 Central MO St Univ; 85–Sp-Lang Path, Midwest Rehabilitation Ctr, **SLP**

Welch, Kathy W 230 Elizabeth Street, Wetumpka, AL 36092, (205) 288-0240, BS 70 Auburn Univ - Auburn; MA 72 Auburn Univ - Auburn; SLP, Ctrl Al Rehab Cen, **SLP**

Welch, Dr Lin Speech And Hearing Clinic, Central Missouri St Univ, Warrensburg, MO 64093, (816) 429-4606, BS 48 West TX St Univ; MA 49 Baylor Univ; PH 60 (NS) Univ of MO - Columbia; Chmn-SLP/Aud Dept, Central Missouri State Univ, **SLP F**

Welch, Nina J F 17451 Ojai Lane, Huntington Beach, CA 92647, (213) 225-6187, BA 77 CA St Univ - Long Beach; MA 79 CA St Univ - Long Beach; MA 83 CA St Univ - Los Angeles; Admin Asst, St Dept of Ed Diag Sch, **SLP**

Welch, Patricia Dare 1755 Michigan Street, Algonac, MI 48001-1323, (313) 765-8817, BS 73 Wayne St Univ; MA 76 Wayne St Univ; Sp-Lang Path, East China Sch, **SLP**

Welch, Mrs Sheila Swentzel 104 Simpson Drive, Huntington, WV 25705, BA 76 Marshall Univ; MA 77 Marshall Univ; SLP, Cabell Bd of Ed, **SLP**

Welchans, Bonita C 6704 Rexford Way, Bakersfield, CA 93309, BS 72 Northern IL Univ - De Kalb; MA 74 Northern IL Univ - De Kalb; SLP, Norland Speech Pathology, **SLP**

Weldele, Dr Frank J Pure Tone Hearing Center, Garden Square Plaza, 3622 Belmont Avenue, Youngstown, OH 44505, (216) 759-3593, BS 69 Bowling Green St Univ; MA 73 Kent St Univ; PH 77 (NS) Kent St Univ; Asst Executive Director, St Elizabeth Hospital Med Cen, **A**

Welge, Elizabeth H 1030 Entrada Road, Sacramento, CA 95864, (916) 482-7275, **SLP**

Welk, Mrs Genevieve 2905 South 4th Avenue, Sioux Falls, SD 57105, (605) 335-1468, BS 73 Creighton Univ; MA 75 SD St Univ; **SLP**

Welk, Mrs Joyce M 2609 Termini Drive, Muscatine, IA 52761, (319) 263-8476, BS 64 Univ of IA; MA 75 Univ of IA; Sp-Lang Path, Mississippi Bend AEA, **SLP**

Welker, Mrs Ann M Scottsdale Public Schools, 2519 East Carmel Avenue, Mesa, AZ 85204, (602) 898-3633, BA 79 Augustana Coll; MS 82 AR St Univ; 81–SLP, Scottsdale USD, **SLP**

Welker, Vivian A 9708 Greenmeadow Circle, Glen Allen, VA 23060, (804) 230-1388, BA 78 Univ of MD - College Park; MS 80 Old Dominion Univ; 81–Sp-Lang Path, VA Med Cen, **SLP**

Welland, Richard Joseph 1191 Olympus Avenue, Peterborough, ON, Canada K9H 6V8, (705) 743-2121, OM 80 Univ of Toronto - Ontario

Wellen, Mary J 811 Oakland Boulevard, Cambridge, OH 43725, (614) 432-7838, **SLP**

Weller, Patricia Blaisdell 167 Tumblebrook Drive, South Windsor, CT 06074, (203) 242-4431, BS 75 Univ of NH; MA 78 Univ of CT; 87–Admin, Mt Sinai Hosp Rehab Ctr, **SLP**

Weller, Dr Rosemary D Dept Communication Arts, Gallaudet University, 800 Florida Avenue N E, Washington, DC 20002, (202) 651-5616, BA 59 Saint Mary's Coll; MA 62 Catholic Univ of America; PH 84 (Special Education) Univ of MD - College Park; 85–Professor of Communicatn Arts, Gallaudet Univ, **SLP**

Weller, Susan Elizabeth 1173 Keeler Avenue, Berkeley, CA 94708, (415) 783-0216, 73 Univ of CA - Berkeley; MS 83 CA St Univ - Hayward; **SLP**

Welling, Ronda S East 2845 St James Avenue, Hayden Lake, ID 83835, (208) 664-8241, BA 69 Univ of WA; MS 75 Eastern WA Univ; Sp-Lang Path, Sch Dist #271 Coeur D'Alene, **SLP**

Welling, Mrs Rosalee Buhler Route 1 South Main Street, Warrensburg, MO 64093, (816) 747-6335, BS 58 Central MO St Univ; MS 87 Central MO St Univ; 87–Sp-Lang Path, Children's Therapy Ctr, **SLP**

Welliver, Mrs Susan Marie P O Box 06, Westminster, MD 21157, (301) 848-3125, **SLP**

Wellman, Beth Cox 6350 North Park Avenue, Indianapolis, IN 46220, (317) 259-0143, BS 75 Eastern IL Univ; MS 76 Eastern IL Univ; Sp-Lang Path, **SLP**

Wellman, Mrs Karen M 5365 J Knollwood Pkwy Ct, Hazelwood, MO 63042, (304) 523-1695, MA 86 Marshall Univ; **SLP**

Wellman, Linda Pyle 1058 Holz, Cincinnati, OH 45230-3661, (513) 232-0209, BS 84 Univ of Cincinnati; MA 86 Univ of Cincinnati; 86–Sp-Lang Path, Hamilton Co Ofc of Educ, **SLP**

Wellman, Robin Lynn 4380 Northridge Drive, Traverse City, MI 49684, (616) 941-0422, MA 84 Central MI Univ; 88–Aud, MI Hrng Aid Co Audio Svcs Inc, **A**

Wellmes, Debora 383 East Sycamore, Columbus, OH 43206, (614) 457-1548, BA 79 OH St Univ; MA 81 OH St Univ; 86–Sp-Lang Path, Affiliated Aud & Sp Path, **SLP**

Wells, Mrs Althea Boston 902 Vickers Avenue, Durham, NC 27701-3145, (216) 574-8000, BS 77 Hampton Univ; MA 80 Cleveland St Univ; SLP, Cleveland Pub Sch, **SLP**

Wells, Barbara 10411 South Drive #523, Houston, TX 77099, (713) 561-5006, MS; **SLP**

Wells, Mrs Barbara K 720 54th Avenue East, Tuscaloosa, AL 35404, (205) 652-9314, BS 71 Central MI Univ; MA 73 Univ of AL- Tuscaloosa; 87–Sp-Lang Path, Sumter County Bd of Educ, **SLP**

Wells, Betsy G 1604 Dalmatia Drive, San Pedro, CA 90732, BA 59 Pomona Coll; MA 86 CA St Univ - Long Beach

Wells, Carolyn R 2619 Success Road, Houston, TX 77068, (713) 440-3785, BA 70 Univ of Houston - Univ Park; MA 71 Univ of Houston - Univ Park; **SLP**

Wells, Dr Charlotte G 938 South Kihei Road #612, Kihei Maui, HI 96753, (808) 879-6434, OB 31 Univ of NE - Lincoln; MA 38 Univ of WI - Madison; PH 41 (NS) Univ of WI - Madison; **SLP F H LM**

Wells, Mrs Cheryl D 7905 Joreen, Fort Worth, TX 76180, (817) 387-3831, BS 76 Southwest TX St Univ; ME 77 Southwest TX St Univ; 86–Dir of Habilitative Therapies, TX Dept of Ment Hlth & Ret, **SLP**

Wells, Mrs Cindia Kinney 509 North Washington St, Ypsilanti, MI 48197, (313) 483-4941, MA 84 Eastern MI Univ; Sp-Lang Path, Livingston Sch Dist, **SLP**

Wells, David Bryan 836 Jefferson Place, Shreveport, LA 71104, (318) 221-8411, BA 80 Univ of Southwestern LA; MA 86 LA Tech Univ; Sp-Lang Path, Overton Brooks VA Med Ctr, **SLP**

Wells, Mrs Deanna Rea 8225 Peach Tree Lane, Wichita, KS 67207, (316) 689-8549, MA 88 Wichita St Univ

Wells, Donna Arnett 1004 Panferio Drive, Pensacola Beach, FL 32561, (904) 932-0016, BA 77 Univ of KY; OM 79 Auburn Univ - Auburn; Sp-Lang Path, Gulf Brze Phys Ther & Rehab Svcs, **SLP ACE**

Wells, Donna S 4016 Knoll Top Court, Carmichael, CA 95608-2173, (916) 454-8354, BS 79 CA St Univ - Hayward; MA 83 CA St Univ - Sacramento; Aud, Sacramento City USD, **A**

Wells, Mrs Edith Estrella 50 Budd Avenue, Pemberton, NJ 08068, (609) 894-2805, BA 67 Boston Univ; MS 69 Rutgers St Univ - Newark; Sp-Lang Path, Burlington Co Pub Hlth Nurs As, **SLP**

Wells, Mrs Elaine F 1844 San Miguel Drive, Suite 108, Walnut Creek, CA 94596, (415) 933-6152, BA 61 CA St Univ - Fullerton; MA 72 San Francisco St Univ; Sp-Lang Path, Private Practice, **SLP**

Wells, Jean A 818 North Florence Street, Burbank, CA 91505, (818) 840-0478, MA 76 Univ of Tulsa; BS 73 Phillips Univ; Dir, Commun Enrichment Cen, **SLP**

Wells, Jo Ann 21 Lonie Young Court, Baptist Village, Dothan, AL 36303, (205) 671-1707, BA 56 Samford Univ; ME 84 Columbus Coll; 88–Sp-Lang Path, Dothan City Schs, **SLP**

Wells, Mrs Judy Haselwood 6 Westover Place, Greenville, SC 29615, (803) 233-1652, BA 61 Columbia Coll; ME 64 Emory Univ; Sp-Lang Path, Greenville Co Sch Dist, **SLP**

Wells, Julia Ann 820 N Street, Fortuna, CA 95540, (707) 725-5063, BS 67 Univ of MI - Ann Arbor; MA 85 Humboldt St Univ; 87–Aquired Brain Inj/LD Spec, CA Comm Colleges Foundation, **SLP**

Wells, Karon 180 East 21st Street, Apartment #E1, Costa Mesa, CA 92627, (714) 957-5147, **SLP**

Wells, Mrs Kathryn Elizabeth 9474 Highland Avenue, Cincinnati, OH 45242, (513) 791-5456, BS 84 Miami Univ - Oxford; MS 85 Miami Univ - Oxford; **SLP**

Wells, Laura Jean 4883 Roswell Road N E #D3, Atlanta, GA 30342, (404) 252-6559, ME 74 Univ of GA; Sp-Lang Path, Private Practice, **SLP**

Wells, Lauraine Lorinda 1614 North Forgeus, Tucson, AZ 85716, (602) 795-6041, BS 83 Univ of IA; MS 85 Univ of AZ; **A**

Wells, Mrs Linda Dianne 14 Sequoia Drive, Troy, IL 62294, (618) 667-2271, BS 68 MS Univ for Women; MS 71 MS Univ for Women; **SLP**

Wells, Mrs Lori Romeo 7 Alva Drive, Latham, NY 12110, (518) 456-9066, MS 85 Coll of Saint Rose

Wells, Mrs Randi S 6315 Mill Point Circle, Dallas, TX 75248, (214) 250-3975, BS 73 Ithaca Coll; MS 74 Ithaca Coll; **SLP**

Wells, Mrs Rebecca Brenner 1817 McKee, Wichita, KS 67203, (316) 833-2515, MA 87 Wichita St Univ

Wells, Robin A 10999 Gillette Street, Overland Park, KS 66210, (913) 642-6200, BS 67 Central MO St Univ; MS 72 Central MO St Univ; Sp-Lang Path, Shawnee Mission Sch Dist, **SLP**

Wells, Mrs Sara Jane 800 South Suncrest, Hillsboro, MO 63050, (314) 789-3525, BS 71 Southeast MO St Univ; ME 80 Southeast MO St Univ; Sp-Lang Path, Hillsboro R-3 Sch, **SLP**

Wells-Friedman, Margaret 5230 39th Avenue North, St Petersburg, FL 33709, (813) 522-1114, MS 86 Univ of South FL; 88–Sp-Lang Path, All Children's Hosp, **SLP**

Wells-Walberg, Judith Christine 146 South 14th Street, San Jose, CA 95112, (408) 983-2164, OB 68 OH Univ - Athens; MA 87 San Jose St Univ; 85–Sp-Lang Path, Santa Clara USD, **SLP**

Wells-Weekly, Barbara J Dept Speech Path & Audiology, Western Washington Univ, Bellingham, WA 98225, (206) 676-3881, MS 75 East Carolina Univ; BS 72 East Carolina Univ; Dir Extern Prog, W WA U, **SLP ACE**

Welp, Gregory K 2709 Balboa Drive, Dubuque, IA 52001, (319) 588-0538, BA 70; MA 73 Univ of IA; SLP, Keystone AEA, **SLP**

Welp, Mrs Marjorie Monnin 2019 New Linden, Newport, KY 41071, (606) 261-1037, BS 84 Univ of Cincinnati; MA 87 OH St Univ; **SLP**

Welsch, Mrs Mary Ruth 4745 Oxbow Place, Boise, ID 83704, (208) 465-2700, BS 81 AZ St Univ; MS 84 Univ of OR; **SLP**

Welscher, Carmen A R 2 Box 139F, La Crescent, MN 55947, (608) 526-9080, BS 72 Minot St Univ; MS 77 Minot St Univ; Sp-Lang Path, Holmen WI Area Sch Dist, **SLP**

Welsh, Cathy Ann 425 West Surf Street, Apt 817, Chicago, IL 60657, (312) 975-3000, BS 83 Clarion Univ of PA; MS 84 Miami Univ - Oxford; Sp-Lang Path, St Josephs Hosp, **SLP**

Welsh, Mrs Darlene Fay 208 West Main Street, P O Box 816, Sheffield, PA 16347, (814) 723-5500, BS 76 Clarion Univ of PA; ME 77 Clarion Univ of PA; Sp-Lang Path, PA Warren St Hosp, **SLP**

Welsh, Donna Jean 15 Cooke Place, Cedar Knolls, NJ 07927, (201) 299-0166, BA 82 William Paterson Coll; MA 86 CUNY - Hunter Coll; **SLP**

Welsh, James J, Jr Holland Hearing Center, 601 Michigan Avenue, Suite 101, Holland, MI 49423, (616) 396-0440, BS 69 Western MI Univ; MA 70 Western MI Univ; 85–Aud/Dir, Holland Hrng Cen, **A**

Welsh, Mrs Janice Marie W 9132 West 250 South, La Porte, IN 46350, (219) 785-4352, BS 76 Clarion Univ of PA; ME 80 Clarion Univ of PA; Sp-Lang Path, Laporte Comm Sch Corp, **SLP**

Welsh, Mrs Joan Benner 3453 North Lake Drive, Milwaukee, WI 53211, (414) 962-4647, BA 61 Univ of Pittsburgh - Pittsburgh; MA 82 Univ of WI - Milwaukee; MS 65 Univ of Pittsburgh - Pittsburgh; **SLP**

Welsh, John W 26709 Herring Road, Greenwood, MO 64034-9804, MS; **SLP**

Welsh, John Woodford 3739 Garfield Avenue South, Minneapolis, MN 55409, (612) 827-3578, MA 83 Univ of MN - Minneap-St Paul; **SLP**

Welsh, Kim R 648 Syracuse Street, Colorado Springs, CO 80911, (719) 391-1338, BA 85 Univ of Northern CO; MA 86 Univ of Northern CO; 88–Aud, Cascade Ear Clinic

Welsh, Loren Patricia 619 McKinley, Klamath Falls, OR 97601, (503) 883-3621, BS 80 Univ of OR; MS 84 Western OR St Coll; Sp-Lang Path, Klamath Sp & Hrng Ctr, **SLP**

Welsh, Loretta A 3301 A Street, Philadelphia, PA 19134, (215) 634-5927, BS 64 Trinity Coll; ME 71 Univ of NC - Greensboro; Sp-Lang Path, Sch Dist of Phila, **SLP**

Welsh, Mrs Pamela S Rd 4 Box 500, Troutville, VA 24175-9221, BS 65 Bloomsburg Univ of PA; MA 68 Gallaudet Coll; SLP, Roanoke City Schools, **SLP**

Welsh, Richard J Route 6 Box 394, Sanford, NC 27330, (919) 776-3633, BA 75 Rutgers St Univ -N Brunswick; MS 80 Univ of NC - Chapel Hill; Sp-Lang Path, Fort Bragg Schs, **SLP**

Welsh, Terry D 4153 West Lane Avenue, Phoenix, AZ 85051, (602) 977-7281, BA 63 ID St Univ; MA 83 Northern AZ Univ; Sp-Lang Path, Dysart Sch Dist, **SLP**

Welt, Mrs Andrea Brodie 25 Shadowlawn Drive, Livingston, NJ 07039, (201) 992-8512, BS 74 Univ of MD - College Park; MA 75 MI St Univ; **SLP**

Welte, Renee 11001 S W 11th Place, Davie, FL 33324, (305) 476-1266, BS 68 Northland Coll; BS 81 FL St Univ; MS 83 FL St Univ; Sp-Lang Path, Dade Co Pub Sch, **SLP**

Welter, Julie Ann 500 West Rand Road, Apt B-404, Arlington Height, IL 60004, (312) 398-3210, BS 83 IL St Univ - Normal; MS 84 IL St Univ - Normal; 88–Sp-Lang Path, NSSEO-Parent-Infant Educ Prog, **SLP**

Welton, Karen Ann 19 Rudder Lane, Latham, NY 12110, (518) 766-3888, BS 78 SUNY - Center at Albany; MS 83 Coll of Saint Rose; Sp-Lang Path, East Greenbush Central Schools, **SLP**

Welwood, Deborah S 15 Stratton Brook Road, Box 141, Weatogue, CT 06089, (203) 566-6098, BS 73 Univ of CT; MA 79 3668; **SLP**

Wemmers, Mrs Sally W 7 Cottenwood Court, Hockessin, DE 19707, (302) 239-9698, BA 65 Wayne St Univ; MA 66 Univ of WI - Madison; **SLP**

Wempe, Mary Ruth 1001 Locust Street, Denver, CO 80220, (303) 333-2976, BS 80 Northern IL Univ - De Kalb; MA 82 Northern IL Univ - De Kalb; 87–Sp-Lang Path, Spalding Rehabilitation Hosp, **SLP**

Wenbourne, Deborah Pierce 15745 Zeigler Court, Ramona, CA 92065, (619) 749-1631, **SLP**

Wende, Richard A 1800 5th Street N W, Great Falls, MT 59404, (406) 791-2270, BS 64 Univ of WI - Madison; MS 69 Eastern Montana Coll; 88–Sp-Lang Path, Sch Dist #1 Great Falls Sch, **SLP**

Wendel, Mrs Karen M S 424 Havasu, Tooele, UT 84074, (801) 522-2259, BS 74 Univ of MD - College Park; MS 76 Towson St Univ; **SLP**

Wendell, Mary V 2630 Ridgecrest Avenue, Orange Park, FL 32073, BA 71 OH St Univ; MA 74 Univ of Cincinnati; **SLP**

Wender, Marilyn 418 East 77th Street #3-G, New York, NY 10021, (718) 990-3832, BA 65 George Washington Univ; MA 66 Northwestern Univ; Chief-Hearing & Speech, Queens Hosp Cen, **SLP ACE**

Wenderoth, Mrs Martha Cofer 712 Dakota S E, Albuquerque, NM 87108, (505) 255-7451, BS 75 Univ of NM; MS 83 Univ of NM; 87–Sp-Lang Path, Alb PS, **SLP**

Wendling, Mrs Donna L Reading Rehab Hospital, Box 250 Morgantown Road, Reading, PA 19607, (215) 777-7615, BS 83 Bloomsburg Univ of PA; MS 84 Bloomsburg Univ of PA; 84–Sp-Lang Path, Reading Rehab Hosp, **SLP**

Wendroff, Mrs Marta Gay 747 Dorian Road, Westfield, NJ 07090, BA 60 Univ of PR - Rio Piedras; MA 82 Kean Coll of NJ; Aud, David B Garmise MD, **A**

Wendrow, Sylvia D 818-1/2 E Hunt, Adrian, MI 49221, (517) 263-8931, BA 59 Univ of MI - Ann Arbor; MS 63 Univ of MI - Ann Arbor; 59–Sp-Lang Path, Lenawee Inter Sch Dist, **SLP**

Wendschlag, Mrs Sandra Jean 877 West Fremont Avenue Suite I-4, Sunnyvale, CA 94087, (408) 773-9933, BA 84 San Jose St Univ; MA 86 San Jose St Univ; 86–Aud, Golden State Aud Assoc Inc, **A**

Wendt, Mrs Deborah Cook 1160 Rambling Road, Simi Valley, CA 93065, (818) 908-8676, BA 73 Univ of CT; MS 75 Univ of WI - Stevens Point; 83–Sp-Lang Path, Valley Hosp Med Cen, **SLP**

Wendt, Katherine Lynn 4713 78th Place S W, Mukilteo, WA 98275, (206) 353-5839, BA 85 WA St Univ; MA 86 WA St Univ; **SLP**

Wendt-Harris, Barbara Lynn 2201 Pioneer Road, Evanston, IL 60201, (312) 883-7136, BA 77 SUNY - Coll at New Paltz; ME 79 Univ of VA - Charlottesville; 81–Aud, Il Masonic Med Cen, **A ACE**

Wener, Dr Deena Louise 883 Converse Street, Longmeadow, MA 01106, (413) 567-3839, BA 73 Univ of VT; MS 74 Univ of VT; PH 83 (NS) Univ of MA - Amherst; 87–Asst Prof, Southern CT St Univ, **SLP**

Wenger, Mrs Linda Bernhardt 125 Bagley Road, Southbury, CT 06488, BA 80 Univ of CT; MS 82 Southern CT St Univ; Sp-Lang Path, Waterbury Pub Schs, **SLP**

Wengert, Mary E 2617 Crestway, Utica, NY 13501, **SLP**

Wenick, Susan Fern 1708 East Lancaster Avenue, Suite 140, Paoli, PA 19301, (215) 698-1737, BA 81 Temple Univ; MA 83 Temple Univ; Aud, ENT Assoc, **A**

Wenner, Susan Kay 801 King Street, Lancaster, OH 43130, (614) 654-3690, BS 76 Bowling Green St Univ; MA 78 Bowling Green St Univ; Sp-Lang Path, Lancaster Cty Sch, **SLP**

Wennersten, Linda Kugler 11842 North 68th Street, Scottsdale, AZ 85254, (602) 948-4264, MA; 87–Sp-Lang Path, Paradise Valley Sch Dist, **SLP**

Wensman, Debra K 6534 Olympia Street, Golden Valley, MN 55427, (612) 593-1965, BS 75 Moorhead St Univ; MS 77 Moorhead St Univ; Sp-Lang Path, Courage Ctr, **SLP**

Wenters, Melissa Ilene Valley Audiology, 2322 Bacon Street Suite 1, Concord, CA 94520, (415) 676-8101, BS 79 Univ of CA - Santa Barbara; MS 82 Syracuse Univ; Aud, Valley Audiology, **A**

Wentland, Mrs Kathleen Anne 71 Camner Avenue, Lancaster, NY 14086, BS 81 SUNY - Coll at Buffalo; MA 83 SUNY - Center at Buffalo; SLP Asst, Erie Co Med Cen, **SLP**

Wentland, Marilynn F 227 Holley Drive, Apartment 209, Bowling Green, OH 43402, (419) 372-2515, BS 68 Univ of WI - Stevens Point; OM 73 Univ of MS; Asst Prof, Bowling Green St U, **SLP**

Wentland, Mrs Phyllis W 5818 Old Dominion, Columbus, GA 31909, (404) 545-5520, BS 69 East TN St Univ; MA 73 Memphis St Univ; OD 77 (NS) Univ of MS; Dir of Special Education, Ft Benning Sch, **SLP**

Wentland, Dr Thomas J Department Of Developmental Studies, Columbus College, Columbus, GA 31993, (404) 568-2196, BS 56 Northern IL Univ - De Kalb; MS 65 Univ of WI - Madison; PH 70 (NS) Univ of WI - Madison; Prof & Ch, Columbus Coll, **SLP**

Wentz, Linda Diane 345 East Portage Trail, Cuyahoga Falls, OH 44221, (216) 762-5425, BA 83 Univ of Akron; MA 84; Sp-Lang Path, Blick Clinic Devlpmntl Disabil, **SLP**

Wenz, Mrs Mary Antkowiak 53 Washington Avenue, Coxsackie, NY 12051, (518) 438-8785, BS 86 SUNY - Coll at Fredonia; MS 87 SUNY - Coll at Fredonia

Wenzlaff, Alice L 1536 Marquette, Naperville, IL 60565, (312) 420-6540, MS 79 Univ of OR; **SLP**

Weppler, Mrs Cynthia Levelle Rd 1 Box 16, Point Breeze Drive, Bethany, WV 26032, (304) 737-2063, BA 77 West Liberty St Coll; MS 79 WV Univ; Sp-Lang Path, Brooke County Board of Educ, **SLP**

Werbela, Mrs Madelyn Beth 2599 Elmwood Avenue, Rochester, NY 14618, (716) 245-5688, BS 77 SUNY - Coll at Brockport; MA 80 Univ of IA; Coord Commun Dept, ARC Childrens Serv, **SLP**

Werbowetzki, Cynthia Lynn 1528 Holland Avenue, Norfolk, VA 23509, (804) 623-7112, BS 80 Northern IL Univ - De Kalb; MA 81 Northern IL Univ - De Kalb; Sp-Lang Path, Rehab Ins of VA, **SLP**

Wermuth, Barbara C 95 Daytona Avenue, Webster, NY 14580, (716) 377-4660, BS 68 SUNY - Coll at Fredonia; MS 70 SUNY - Coll at Geneseo; Sp-Lang Path, Monroe Co BOCES #1, **SLP**

Wermuth, Nancy B 4781 Springfield Drive, Dunwoody, GA 30338, (404) 396-4991, BS 78 IN Univ - Bloomington; OM 79 IN Univ - Bloomington; Sp-Lang Path, Private Practice, **SLP**

Wernecke, Candace 16527 Hannah Drive, San Leandro, CA 94578, (415) 276-0254, BA 70 San Francisco St Univ; MA 72 San Francisco St Univ; SLP, Alameda Co Offi of Ed, **SLP**

Werner, Mrs Anita B 4321 East Beryl Lane, Phoenix, AZ 85028, (602) 996-2525, BS 74 AZ St Univ; MS 79 Southern Methodist Univ; Sp-Lang Path, Private Practice, **SLP**

Werner, Connie L 935 West Oak Street, Fort Collins, CO 80521, (303) 490-3212, BA 75 FL St Univ; MA 76 Univ of IL - Urbana; Sp-Lang Path, Poudre R-1 Sch Dist, **SLP ACE**

Werner, Mrs Ellen O Box 12, Sandwich, IL 60548, (312) 552-7771, BA 61 Saint John's Univ - Jamaica; MA 68 CUNY - Hunter Coll; Pres, Janelle Publications, **SLP**

Werner, James Lee RR1 Box 11 Site 6, Corner Brook, NF, Canada A2H 2N2, (709) 634-1869, OM 84 Brigham Young Univ; 77–Aud Dept Head, Western Mem Reg Hosp, **A**

Werner, Mrs Lorna S 4204 Center Pointe Lane, Sarasota, FL 34233, (813) 377-1866, BS 40 Northwestern Univ; MA 43 Northwestern Univ; **SLP LM**

Werner, Dr Marlin S 1292 Waianuenue Avenue, Hilo, HI 96720, (808) 961-6631, BA 50 Univ of MO - Columbia; MS 57 Johns Hopkins Univ; PH 66 (Sp & Hrng Science) OH St Univ; Aud/Sp-Lang Path, Private Practice, **SLP A**

Werner, Mary Kathryn 1401 North Powhatan Street, Arlington, VA 22205, (703) 754-7181, BS 78 WV Univ; MS 79 WV Univ; Sp-Lang Path, Prince William Co Pub Sch, **SLP**

Werner, Renee A 2840 Monte Cresta Way, San Jose, CA 95132, (408) 923-1800, BA 85 San Jose St Univ; MA 87 San Jose St Univ

Werner, Mrs Susan Angela 17 Branchwood Drive, Schaumburg, IL 60193, (312) 980-6700, BA 82 Elmhurst Coll; MA 84 Northern IL Univ - De Kalb; 84–Sp-Lang Path, Community Consolidated Sch Dist, **SLP**

Wernersbach, Mrs Margaret Baker Northern Kentucky Easter Seal Center, 212 Levassor Avenue, Covington, KY 41014, (606) 491-1171, BA 71; MS 80 Univ of Louisville; 87–Exec Dir, N KY Easter Seal Center, **SLP**

Wernikoff, Mrs Esta Ross 10228 Sardis Oaks Road, Charlotte, NC 28226, (704) 845-2299, BS 80 Ithaca Coll; MS 81 SUNY - Coll at Buffalo; SLP, Montgomery Co Intermediate Ut, **SLP**

Wernikoff, Nancy Kasdon 42 Somerset Drive, Woodcliff Lake, NJ 07675, (201) 391-8376, BA 62 NY Univ; MS 69 CUNY - Queens Coll; 69–Sp-Lang Path, Private Practice, **SLP ACE**

Wert, Kimberlee 3955 Walnut Wood Way, Uniontown, OH 44685, (216) 875-3347, BA 76 Univ of Akron; MA 78 Univ of Akron; Sp-Lang Path, Stark Co Bd Ment Ret/Dev Disab, **SLP**

Werth, Kathryn J P O Box 918, Omak, WA 98841-0918, (509) 826-3123, BS 60 Ithaca Coll; MA 65 Univ of Denver; **SLP**

Wertley, Kathleen M 501 North Bethlehem Park, Apartment 14-C, Ambler, PA 19002, (215) 539-8550, BA 69 Temple Univ-Tyler Sch of Art; MA 71 Temple Univ-Tyler Sch of Art; SLP, Mont Cty Inter Ut #23, **SLP**

Werts, Jeanne L 6206 Jeremy Circle, Salt Lake City, UT 84121, (801) 278-6507, **SLP**

Wertz, Mrs Florence C 700 Arbogast Road, St Paul, MN 55126, (612) 484-3708, BA 44 Augustana Coll; **SLP LM**

Wertz, Jean B Rd 2 Box 294, Johnstown, PA 15904, **SLP**

Wertz, Larry Ray 960 Camino Parocela, Palm Springs, CA 92262, 87, **SLP**

Wertz, Mrs Mildred B 1015 Indian Creek Road, Chesapeake, VA 23322, (804) 421-9261, BS 37 Southeast MO St Univ; MA 45 Univ of MO - Columbia; Prog Dir Sp-Lang Path, **SLP LM**

Wertz, Dr Robert T Department Of Speech Pathology, VA Hospital, 150 Muir Road, Martinez, CA 94553, (415) 228-6800, BA 59 CA St Univ - Long Beach; MA 64 Stanford Univ; PH 67 (NS) Stanford Univ; Ch Aud & SLP, VA, **SLP F**

Werve, Kathryn Symons 6907 52nd Avenue, Kenosha, WI 53142, (414) 656-6270, BS 71 Univ of WI - Madison; MS 75 Univ of WI - Milwaukee; SLP, Kenosha USD, **SLP**

Werven, Gerald Wayne 1216 South Higland Acres Road, Bismarck, ND 58501, (701) 222-4541, BA 83 Univ of ND; MS 85 Univ of ND; 86–Sp-Lang Path, Rehab Ctr, **SLP**

Wesemann, Theresa Ann 417 Bethel Drive #2N, Joliet, IL 60435, (815) 725-2194, BS 84 IL St Univ - Normal; MS 85 IL St Univ - Normal; **SLP**

Weskerna, Gail B 2733 5th Street, Peru, IL 61354, (815) 223-3982, BS 75 Western IL Univ; MA 76 Western IL Univ; Sp-Lang Path Preschool, Peru Pub Sch-Roosevelt Sch, **SLP**

Wesle, Cheryl L S P O Box 147, Calmar, IA 52132, (319) 422-5678, BS 74 Univ of WI - River Falls; MS 79 Univ of WI - River Falls; 84–Sp-Lang Path, Keystone AEA, **SLP**

Wesley, Carol Lorraine 1242 Colfax Drive, Richardson, TX 75080, (214) 783-3060, BS 76 Univ of VA - Charlottesville; MS 85 Univ of TX - Dallas; 88–Sp-Lang Path, UTD-Callier Ctr, **SLP**

Wesley, Mrs Lynette Ann P O Box 99, Snyder, OK 73566-0099, (601) 649-6391, **SLP**

Weslosky, Therese P 5877 Patterson, Troy, MI 48098, (313) 879-9518, BA 76 Univ of MI - Ann Arbor; MA 79 Wayne St Univ; Sp/Lang Path, Medi-Sp Serv Inc, **SLP**

Wesner, Mrs Barbara P 351 Kennard Street, Johnstown, PA 15906, (814) 472-5770, BS 78 CA Univ of PA; ME 81 Indiana Univ of PA; SLP, Intermediate Unit 08, **SLP**

Wesolowski, Mrs Anita M 2702 Bravado Drive, Rancho Cordova, CA 95670, (916) 366-6284, BS 79 Northern AZ Univ; MS 81 ID St Univ; Sp-Lang Path, **SLP**

Wesolowski, Mrs Beverly Denson 1301 Fairfax, North Tonawanda, NY 14120, (716) 625-8795, BS 77 SUNY - Coll at Buffalo; MS 81 SUNY - Coll at Buffalo; SLP, Orleans-Niagara BOCES, **SLP**

Wessel, Mrs Brenda 400 West King Street #400, Carson City, NV 89701, (702) 883-3119, BA 75 San Diego St Univ; MA 77 San Diego St Univ; SLP, Washoe Co Sch Dist, **SLP**

Wessell, Mrs Margery H 4650 Shavano Woods, San Antonio, TX 78249-1842, (512) 492-0823, BS 62 Case Western Reserve Univ; MA 64 CUNY - Queens Coll; Sp-Lang Path, San Antonio ISD, **SLP ACE**

Wesson, Mrs Bette C 4759 East Van Bruen, Las Vegas, NV 89110-1537, (702) 486-5223, BA 67 Univ of AZ; MA 70 Univ of AZ; Sp-Lang Path, Spec Chlrns Cl, **SLP**

Wesson, Kathleen B 6720 Waverly Place, Little Rock, AR 72207, (501) 686-5140, BA 68 Univ of AR - Fayetteville; MA 69 Southern Methodist Univ; Sp-Lang Path/Instr, Univ of Arkansas for Med Sci, **SLP ACE**

West, Alisa Rich 1437 Regency Court, Fort Collins, CO 80526, (303) 225-0508, BA 80 Univ of CO - Boulder; MA 83 Univ of MT; Sp-Lang Path, Capital Area Sp Ctr, **SLP**

West, Annette Rose 4478 Via Marina #P-94, Marina Del Rey, CA 90292, (213) 301-2032, BA 82 Univ of Southern CA; MA 86 CA St Univ - Los Angeles

West, Carol A Mass Eye And Ear Infirmary, 243 Charles Street, Boston, MA 02114, BA 74 Univ of HI - Manoa; MA 76 Univ of IA; Audiologist, Mass Eye and Ear Infirmary, **A**

West, Daniel Welch 814A Allison Gardens, Columbia, TN 38401, (615) 388-3646, MA 87 TN St Univ; 86–Aud, Middle Tennessee Hrng Aid Ctr, **A**

West, Mrs Deborah Route 2 Box 660, Sardis, MS 38666, (601) 627-5247, BA 83 Univ of MS; MS 85 Univ of MS; Aud, No MS ENT Surgical Cl, **A**

West, Debra A H 3103 Algoa Road, Jefferson City, MO 65101, **SLP**

West, Edwin Andre 2400 13th Street #1, Ashland, KY 41101, (606) 329-1329, BS 82 Andrews Univ; MA 85 Univ of Pittsburgh - Pittsburgh; **A**

West, Gayla Beth 1800 Briar Run, Benbrook, TX 76126, (817) 249-0352, BS 85 TX Christian Univ; MA 87 TX Woman's Univ

West, Mrs Geraldine 570 Road N, Redwood Valley, CA 95470, (707) 485-7730, BA 72 Humboldt St Univ; MA 73 Humboldt St Univ; Sp-Lang Path, Mendocino Co Sch, **SLP**

West, Harland J 104 Seymour Street, Fredonia, NY 14063, MS 69 SUNY - Coll at Geneseo; Coordinator Sp & Hrng, Gowanda Psychiatric Ctr, **SLP ACE**

West, Hazel Hill Colonial Vista, 657 Okanogan Avenue #234, Wenatchee, WA 98801, (415) 364-5417, BS 32 Univ of WA; MA 62 San Francisco St Univ; **LM**

West, Judy 710 Jackson Avenue, Oxford, MS 38655, (601) 234-1417, BA 71 Univ of MS; MS 76 Univ of MS; Pres, W Phoenix Sp/Lang Rehab Inc, **SLP**

West, Kathleen Loftus 63 Walnut Street, Belmont, MA 02178, (617) 254-3800, BS 75 Worcester St Coll; MA 76 SUNY - Coll at Geneseo; Aud, Chldn's Hosp, **A**

West, Lane 445 West Nees Avenue #227, Fresno, CA 93711, (209) 229-9600, OB 84 Hardin-Simmons Univ; MA 87 San Jose St Univ; **A**

West, Mrs Laurel Lynne 1438 Weatherby, St Louis, MO 63146, (314) 426-9581, BS 81 Southern IL Univ-Edwardsvill; MS 82 Southern IL Univ-Edwardsvill; **SLP**

West, Mrs Margy Theresa 8131 Hillcrest Lane, Tinley Park, IL 60477, (815) 485-6197, BS 78 IL St Univ - Normal; OM 83 Governors St Univ; **SLP**

West, Mary 406 Oxford Road, East Lansing, MI 48823, SLP, Lansing Pub Schs, **SLP**

West, Michael H c/o San Juan Hrng Center, 2713 East 20th Suite D, Farmington, NM 87401, (505) 325-7474, BA 72 William Carey Coll; MS 76 Univ Southern MS-Hattiesburg; Aud, San Juan Hrng Ctr, **A**

West, Mrs Nancy Lee 1405 Coral Drive, Laguna Beach, CA 92651, (714) 494-0469, BS 55 Slippery Rock Univ of PA; ME 66 Whittier Coll; SLP, Newport Mesa USD, **SLP**

West, Mrs Nora J 10 Oak Court, Allegan, MI 49010, (616) 694-9904, BS 79 Western MI Univ; MA 80 Western MI Univ; SLP, Otsego Public Schools, **SLP**

West, Mrs Patricia K 63 Karen Drive, Mahwah, NJ 07430, BA 54 Rutger's St Univ - Douglas Coll; MA 73 Temple Univ-Tyler Sch of Art; **SLP**

West, Ronda Shackelford 12514 Miriam Lane, Houston, TX 77071, (713) 498-8110, BS 78 Baylor Univ; MS 79 Baylor Univ; 81–Sp-Lang Path, Alief ISD, **SLP**

West, Suzanne Marie 19920 Buckhaven Lane, Saratoga, CA 95070, (408) 867-5863, BS 84 Abilene Christian Univ; MS 86 Univ of TX - Dallas; 87–Sp-Lang Path, Lee Francia MA & Assoc, **SLP**

West, Dr Terri Louise 2294 Bigelow Avenue, Simi Valley, CA 93065, (805) 581-9665, BS 71 Kent St Univ; MA 72 Kent St Univ; PH 83 (NS) Univ of CO - Boulder; **SLP**

West, Vicky Nowell 7451 Cessna, Corpus Christi, TX 78412, (512) 993-3166, BS 84 Southwest TX St Univ; ME 85 Southwest TX St Univ; Sp-Lang Path, Rehab Hosp of S TX, **SLP**

West, Dr W Barry 1324 Nelson Avenue Suite A, Modesto, CA 95350, (209) 522-7999, BA 63 Univ of Northern CO; MS 66 CO St Univ; PH 71 (NS) Stanford Univ; Dispensing Audiologist, Private Practice, **SLP A**

Westbay, Erin Christine 3256 Winton Road South, P-35, Rochester, NY 14623, (716) 546-5554, BA 83 SUNY - Coll at Plattsburgh; MA 85 SUNY - Coll at Plattsburgh; 88–Sp-Lang Path, Monroe Dev Ctr BOCES, **SLP**

Westbrook, Cathryn J Dept Of Speech Communication, Oregon State University, Shepard Hall, Corvallis, OR 97331, (503) 754-2461, BA 73 Univ of OR; MS 77 Western OR St Coll; Sp-Lang Path, Oregon State University, **SLP**

Westbrook, Janice B 6114 Waterway Drive, Garland, TX 75043, (214) 490-8701, BS 79 Univ of TX - Dallas; ME 81 Southwest TX St Univ; Sp-Lang Path, Dallas ISD, **SLP**

Westbrook, Linda A N 4400 Overlook Road, Birmingham, AL 35222, (205) 591-8936, BS 69 Univ Southern MS-Hattiesburg; MA 70 Univ of AL- Tuscaloosa; Sp-Lang Path, Private Practice, **SLP**

Westbrook, Mrs Mary K 2546 Oak Valley Drive, Vienna, VA 22180, (703) 369-0300, BS 74 Bowling Green St Univ; MA 77 Kent St Univ; Aud, Private Practice, **A**

Westby, Dr Carol E Programs For Children, 2600 Marble N E, Albuquerque, NM 87106, (505) 843-2950, BA 65 Geneva Coll; MA 68 Univ of IA; PH 71 (NS) Univ of IA; Sp-Lang Path, Programs for Chldn, **SLP ACE**

Westcott, Joanne M 9 Walton Drive, Sewell, NJ 08080, (609) 589-4965, BA 77 Loyola Coll; MS 78 Loyola Coll; Sp-Lang Path, St John of God Community Serv, **SLP**

Westcott, Mrs Judy Girdwood 2 Roosevelt Avenue, Binghamton, NY 13901, **SLP**

Wester, Derin C 820 2nd Avenue, Salt Lake City, UT 84103, OM 79 Brigham Young Univ; Aud, UT St Hlth Dept, **A**

Wester, Linda 15919 Wolf Creek, San Antonio, TX 78232, (817) 923-6706, MA 70 Our Lady Lake Univ-San Anton; **SLP**

Westerback, Ann Kathryn 7743 West 157th Street, Apple Valley, MN 55124, (612) 920-4595, BA 83 Univ of WI - Eau Claire; MS 85 Univ of WY; 86–Aud, Minneapolis ENT PA, **A**

Westerbeck, Sandra L 1486 Wittekind Terrace, Cincinnati, OH 45224, (513) 369-2474, BS 81 Univ of Cincinnati; MA 83 Univ of Cincinnati; Sp/Lang Path, Christ Hosp, **SLP**

Westerhold, Mrs Rosalie P Midlands Community Hospital, 11111 South 84th Street, Papillion, NE 68046, (402) 593-3753, BA 73 Univ of NE - Lincoln; MA 74 Univ of NE - Lincoln; 79–Aud, Midlands Comm Hosp, **A**

Westerholt, Laurel Ann 435 Otter Creek Court, Atlanta, GA 30328, **SLP**

Westerhouse, Janice June 712 West 27th Street, Wilmington, DE 19802, (302) 656-2521, BS 62 Purdue Univ - West Lafayette; MA 68 IN Univ - Bloomington; Sp-Lang Path, De Curatve Wrksp/Opd Rehab Cen, **SLP ACE**

Wester-Snyder, Ruth E 3050 Beauclerc Road, Jacksonville, FL 32217, BS 78 FL St Univ; MS 79 FL St Univ; Dir SLP, Healthsouth Rehab Corp, **SLP**

Westfall, Mary F 2404 Hillmont Drive, Murfreesboro, TN 37130, (615) 890-3927, BS 69 Middle TN St Univ; ME 72 Univ of VA - Charlottesville; **SLP**

Westfall, Michele Janine 1300 South Parker Road, Unit 204, Denver, CO 80231, (303) 671-8344, BS 76 CO St Univ; MA 81 Univ of Denver; SLP, **SLP**

Westfall, Patricia D Route 1 Box C, Glenville, WV 26351, (304) 853-2523, BS 75 Edinboro Univ of PA; MS 78 WV Univ; Sp-Lang Path, Braxton Co Bd of Ed, **SLP**

Westfall, Mrs Wendelyn Lori 25 Arrowhead #66, Algonquin, IL 60102, (312) 658-7466, BS 79 IL St Univ - Normal; MS 81 IL St Univ - Normal; Sp-Lang Path, Spec Educ Dist of McHenry Co, **SLP**

Westfall-Cox, Mrs Tammy L 216 Wadsworth Avenue, Avon, NY 14414, (716) 226-3833, MA 87 SUNY - Coll at Geneseo; 88–Sp-Lang Path, Monroe Co BOCES #1

Westheim, Mrs Adrienne Rd 2 Remington Rd Box NV36, East Stroudsburg, PA 18301, BS 78 SUNY - Center at Albany; MS 80 Columbia Univ Teachers Coll; Sp-Lang Path, **SLP ACE**

Westin, Jane C 7555 Parkview Road, Greendale, WI 53129, (414) 878-3717, BA 60 Ripon Coll; MS 74 Marquette Univ; Sp-Lang Path, Racine Co-Hndcpd Chldn Bd, **SLP**

Westlake, Dr Harold Rd 7 Box 8, Wellsboro, PA 16901, (717) 724-5132, MS 32; PH 38 (NS) Univ of MI - Ann Arbor; **SLP F H LM**

Westlake, Mrs 0ONNA Fridy 2072 Chelsea Lane, State College, PA 16801, (814) 234-6915, BS 82 East Stroudsburg Univ of PA; MA 87 West Chester Univ of PA; 88–Sp-Lang Path, SG Rehab Inc, **SLP**

Westle, Mrs Robin S D 68 Lexington Drive, Groton on Hudson, NY 10520, (914) 271-3056, BA 76 SUNY - Center at Buffalo; MS 78 Columbia Univ Teachers Coll; Sp-Lang Path, Private Practice, **SLP**

Westlund, Janet A 2030 Lehigh Street Suite 111, Easton, PA 18042, (215) 253-0287, BS 78 Univ of NH; MS 80 PA St Univ - Univ Park; Aud, Private Practice, **A**

Westmaas, Loralee Hamstra 1312 Chester Road, Lansing, MI 48912, (517) 655-1205, BA 81 MI St Univ; MA 83 MI St Univ; **SLP**

Westman, Charlene Ann 8211 S W 72nd Avenue, Apartment 118, Miami, FL 33143, (305) 547-6660, BA 85 Univ of FL; MA 87 Univ of FL; 88–Sp-Lang Path, Univ of Miami, **SLP**

Westman, Martha J Rural Route 1, Center City, MN 55012, (612) 464-8080, BS 64 Univ of WI - Madison; MA 66 Stanford Univ; SLP, North Branch School Dist 138, **SLP**

Westmoreland, Mrs Deborah E 2658 East Fox Street, Mesa, AZ 85213, (602) 827-0470, BS 72 CO St Univ; MS 74 CO St Univ; Sp-Lang Path, Valley Lutheran Hosp, **SLP**

Westmoreland, Mary M American River Hosp-Eskaton, Speech Pathology Dept, 4747 Engle Road, Carmichael, CA 95608, (916) 486-2049, MA 75 CA St Univ - Sacramento; Chief SLP, Eskaton American River Hosp, **SLP**

Weston, Dr Alan J Cleveland Chiropractic, 590 North Vermont, Los Angeles, CA 90004, (213) 660-6166, BA 63 Univ of AL- Tuscaloosa; MA 65 Univ of AL- Tuscaloosa; PH 69 (NS) Univ of KS; Professor, Univ of Wisconsin-Milwaukee, **SLP F**

Weston, Audrey 6517 Tottenham Road, Madison, WI 53711-4013, (402) 488-9192, BS 68 Univ of NE - Lincoln; MA 74 Univ of NE - Lincoln; Project Assistant, University of Wisconsin, **SLP**

Weston, Debra Cantey 2101 Lakeview Drive, Apartment 115, Ypsilanti, MI 48198, BA 82 Univ of SC - Columbia; MA 85 SC St Coll; **SLP**

Weston, DiAnne P 657 Jackson, Denver, CO 80206-4544, (303) 329-9710, BS 70 TX Christian Univ; MS 75 TX Christian Univ; 84–Sp-Lang Path, Spalding Rehab Hosp, **SLP**

Weston, Mrs Genecile Watts 11761 Inverness Circle, West Palm Beach, FL 33414, (407) 793-0683, BA 75 Univ of MS; OM 76 Univ of MS; **SLP**

Weston, Mrs Lisa Marie 335 Cliff View Court, Reno, NV 89523, (702) 789-0341, OM 84 Univ of NV - Reno; **SLP**

Weston, Mrs Lucinda C 2642 East Beverly Road, Shorewood, WI 53211, (414) 332-3527, BA 73 Univ of WI - Milwaukee; MA 75 Univ of WI - Milwaukee; SLP, Private Practice, **SLP**

Weston, Maria V 2740 North Racine, 2nd Floor Front, Chicago, IL 60614, BS 84 Western KY Univ; MS 86 Vanderbilt Univ; **SLP**

Weston, Mrs Marsha Lyn 181 South Sycamore Avenue #202, Los Angeles, CA 90036, (213) 931-0919, BA 63 Univ of AL- Tuscaloosa; MA 64 Univ of AL- Tuscaloosa; **A**

Weston, Stephanie 123 Georgina #7, Santa Monica, CA 90402, (213) 533-2743, MA 84 CA St Univ - Los Angeles; Aud, Harbor-UCLA Medical Center, **A**

Westra, Mrs Mary Oettinger 3435 Van Buren Street, Hudsonville, MI 49426, BA 77 Bucknell Univ; MA 82 Western MI Univ; Sp-Lang Path, Holland Comm Hosp, **SLP**

Westra, Susan E 454 Mount Curve Boulevard, St Paul, MN 55105, BA 73 Univ of MN - Minneap-St Paul; MA 83 Univ of MN - Minneap-St Paul; 81–Sp-Lang Path, St Paul PS, **SLP**

Westrich, Abby Jane 536 Melrose Place, South Orange, NJ 07079, (201) 783-4000, BA 63; MA 72; Sp/Lang Path, Montclair Bd of Ed, **SLP**

Westrup, Mrs Linda L 202 Whitehall Road, Camden, NC 27921, (919) 335-2705, BS 72 Purdue Univ - West Lafayette; MA 76 Northwestern Univ; Sp-Lang Path, **SLP**

Wetherald, Mrs Carol A 281 Shoreham Drive, Rochester, NY 14618, (716) 338-2810, BA 64 Oberlin Coll; MA 76 SUNY - Coll at Geneseo; Aud, Rochester Otol Group, Pc, **A**

Wetherbee Taggart, Mrs Maureen A 194 West Godfrey Avenue, Philadelphia, PA 19120, (215) 549-7569, BA 82 Case Western Reserve Univ; MA 83 Case Western Reserve Univ; Sp/Lang Path Dept Hd, Elwyn Inc, **SLP**

Wetherby, Dr Amy M Florida State University, Communication Disorders, Rrc 107, Tallahassee, FL 32306, (904) 644-2238, BA 77 SUNY - Center at Buffalo; PH 82 (Sp & Hrng Science) Univ of CA - San Francisco; 83–Assoc Prof, FL St U, **SLP**

Wethered, Dr Chris E 1011 West Holland Avenue, Nampa, ID 83651, (208) 466-9633, BS 72 ID St Univ; MS 76 ID St Univ; ED 83 (Special Education) Memphis St Univ; Sp-Lang Path, Joint Sch Dist #2, **SLP**

Wetterhahn, Marilyn J 2 Don Mills Court, Rockville, MD 20850, BA 67 CUNY - Queens Coll; MS 69 CUNY - Queens Coll; Sp-Lang Path, Rockville Nursing Home, **SLP**

Wetz, Cynthia Walsh 2801 West Broadway, L-4, Columbia, MO 65203, (314) 446-0506, BS 78 Univ of IA; MA 79 Univ of IA; Sp-Lang Path, **SLP**

Wetzel, Barbara 3303 Wooside Terrace #2, Altoona, WI 54720, **SLP**

Wetzel, Mrs Dawn Elizabeth 8725 Springmill Road, Indianapolis, IN 46260, (317) 353-5429, BS 83 IN Univ - Bloomington; MA 86 IN Univ - Bloomington; **SLP**

Wever, Mrs Jane R 23 Montague Circle, Winchester, VA 22601, (703) 662-3888, BS 74 Radford Univ; MS 83 James Madison Univ; Coord Sp-Lang Path Prog, Frederick Co Pu Sch, **SLP**

Wevrick, Mrs Patricia J 281 Crestview Road, Ottawa, ON, Canada K1H 5G4, (613) 737-2372, BS 56 Ball St Univ; MA 58 Univ of IL - Urbana; Sp-Lang Path, Childrens Hosp of Eastern Ont, **SLP**

Wexelblatt, Michael A Southern Indiana ENT, 1655 Gladstone Avenue, Suite E, Columbus, IN 47201, (812) 376-3071, BA 70 Hofstra Univ; MA 77 IN Univ - Bloomington; Aud, S In ENT Inc, **A**

Wexler, Mrs Donna Youkilis 13824 Southwest 108 Court, Miami, FL 33176, (305) 255-1028, BA 69 IN Univ - Bloomington; MA 70 Univ of Cincinnati; Sp-Lang Path/Intensive Sp Prog, Dade Co Bd of Ed, **SLP**

Wexler, Mrs Helen 737 Camino Lakes Circle, Boca Raton, FL 33486, (305) 392-4652, BS 70 Emerson Coll; ME 71 Boston Univ; Private Practice, **SLP**

Wexler, Mrs Hilary P 6142 Beachway Drive, Falls Church, VA 22041, (703) 671-6595, MA 76 George Washington Univ; Sp-Lang Path, Private Practice, **SLP**

Wexler, Dr Karin B 5 Roble Road, Suffern, NY 10901, (914) 354-7323, MA 71 Columbia Univ Teachers Coll; OM 77 Columbia Univ Teachers Coll; PH 78 (NS) Columbia Univ Teachers Coll; Sp-Lang Path, Private Practice, **SLP**

Wexler, Kathryn F 5258 Dijon Drive, Baton Rouge, LA 70809, (504) 769-1090, BA 72 Univ of MI - Ann Arbor; MS 74 Tulane Univ; Aud, ENT Medical Center, **A**

Wexler, Leslie Ann 141-59 72nd Crescent, Flushing, NY 11367, (212) 904-2677, MA 87 CUNY - Queens Coll; 87–Aud, Albert Einstein Coll of Med, **A**

Wexler, Melanie Ellen 164 Helen Street, Binghamton, NY 13905-3438, (607) 798-7117, BA 74 Univ of Akron; MA 76 Univ of Akron; Aud, Hndcpd Chldn's Assoc of Sn NY, **A**

Wexler, Robin 516 Cheryl Drive, Iselin, NJ 08830, BA 80 Rutger's St Univ - Douglas Coll; MS 83 Rutgers St Univ - Newark; 88–Sp-Lang Path, Volunteers of America-Early Learning Ctr, **SLP**

Wexler, Sharon B 1475 Hidden Hills Parkway, Stone Mountain, GA 30088, (404) 469-3943, BS 72 OH St Univ; OM 74 Emory Univ; Sp-Lang Path, Private Practice, **SLP**

Wexler, Mrs Sharon P Lincourt Hrng Aid & Aud Servs, 501 South Lincoln Avenue, Clearwater, FL 33516, (813) 461-6993, BS 68 McGill Univ - Quebec; MS 70 McGill Univ - Quebec; Aud, Lincourt Hrng & Aud Serv, **A**

Wey, Mary Jane 208 Hoodridge Drive, Pittsburgh, PA 15234, (412) 531-2445, BS 80 Towson St Univ; MS 81 Loyola Coll; Sp/Lang Path, Private Practice, **SLP**

Weyand, Natalie Ann 436 Canisteo Street, P O Box 94, Hornell, NY 14843, (607) 324-2495, BS 54 SUNY - Coll at Geneseo; ME 63 PA St Univ - Univ Park; 58–Sp/Lang Path, Hornell City Sch Dist, **SLP**

Weybright, Glenn D 7810 S W Calaveras Court, Beaverton, OR 97007, (503) 227-0671, BS 71 Portland St Univ; MS 74 Portland St Univ; Sp-Lang Path, Private Practice, **SLP**

Weyenberg, Debra J 313 West River Road, Oscoda, MI 48750, (806) 885-2313, BS 79 Univ of WI - Oshkosh; MS 81 Univ of WI - Madison; 86–Sp-Lang Path, Private Practice, **SLP**

Weyforth, Mara K 10524 Farley, Overland Park, KS 66212, (816) 373-4415, BA 62 Washington Univ; MS 81 Central MO St Univ; Coord of Sp-Lang Path, Truman Med Cen East, **SLP**

Weyhmuller, Mrs Arlene Mehl 16 Colgate Road, Somers Point, NJ 08244, (609) 399-5611, BA 72 Adelphi Univ; MA 79 Trenton St Coll; Sp-Lang Path, Ocean Ciy Bd of Ed, **SLP**

Weyland, Christina Seaborg MPC, 1801 N Senate Blvd, Suite 540, Indianapolis, IN 46202, (317) 929-5630, BS 75 IN Univ - Bloomington; MA 76 IN Univ - Bloomington; Aud, Methodist Hospital of Indiana, **A**

Wezalis-Webber, Kathleen Mary 27838 Whirlaway Trail, Evergreen, CO 80439-6425, (303) 674-9664, **SLP**

Whalen, Judith M West Road #G47 Box 5, Pleasant Valley, NY 12569, (914) 635-1514, SLP, Wassaic Dev Cntr, **SLP**

Whalen, Sr M Clare E 520 Plainfield, Joliet, IL 60435, (815) 727-3686, MA 55 Marquette Univ; 87, Private Practice, **SLP**

Whalen, Rosemary 5330 San Mateo N E, Bldg F Apartment 86, Albuquerque, NM 87109, BA 75 Univ of WI - Milwaukee; BA 80 Univ of WI - Milwaukee; MA 82 Univ of WI - Milwaukee; Sp/Lang Path, Roswell ISD, **SLP**

Whalen, Mrs Sherry L 101 Tudor, Barrington, IL 60010, (312) 255-6350, BA 70 MI St Univ; MA 79 Western MI Univ; Sp-Lang Path, NW Sub Spec Ed Org, **SLP**

Whaley, Celeste Patton 7908 Wilnoty Drive, Knoxville, TN 37931, (615) 562-8377, **SLP**

Whaley, Patricia 804 West Windsor, Phoenix, AZ 85007, (602) 265-2996, BA 64 Univ of GA; ME 66 Univ of GA; **SLP F**

Whalley, Michelle V 29 Hollister Street, Pittsfield, MA 01201, **SLP**

Whan, Mrs Mary Q 555 North 30th Street, Omaha, NE 68131, (402) 498-6665, BS 84 Marquette Univ; MA 87 Univ of IA; Aud, Boys Town Natl Ins, **A**

Whang, Lisa Ann 2825 Poelua Street, Honolulu, HI 96822, BS 83 Univ of HI - Manoa; MS 85 Univ of HI - Manoa; **SLP**

Wharam, Kate PO Box 84242, Fairbanks, AK 99708, (907) 479-3029, BA 81 Univ of MI - Ann Arbor; MS 85 Univ of WA; 88-Sp-Lang Path, Yukon-Koyukuk Sch Dist, **SLP**

Wharton, Jeanne Ann 1059 Beaconsfield, Grosse Pointe Park, MI 48230, (313) 876-3280, BS 85 Central MI Univ; MA 87 Central MI Univ; 88–Aud, Henry Ford Hosp, **A**

Whatley, Mrs Jean Scott 6719 Crestland Avenue, Dallas, TX 75252, (214) 248-3330, BA 77 Univ of NC - Greensboro; ME 78 Univ of NC - Greensboro; Sp-Lang Path, Plano ISD, **SLP**

Whatley, Mrs Vivian 422 Pinelea Road, Griffin, GA 30223, (404) 228-0262, BS 79 FL St Univ; MS 80 FL St Univ; 83–Parent Adv for Hrng Impr, Georgia Pines, **SLP**

Whatoff, Angela Brooke 3974 North Story Road, Apartment 933-B, Irving, TX 75038, (214) 358-8337, MS 86 Univ of OK Medical Center; 87–Sp-Lang Path, Dallas Rehab Inst, **SLP**

Whealon, Mrs Margaret McAdams 2796 Cedar Wood Place, Thousand Oaks, CA 91360, (805) 492-4938, BA 74 CA St Univ - Northridge; MA 76 CA St Univ - Northridge; SLP, Pleasant Valley Sch Dist, **SLP**

Whearty, Kathryn Annelle 3100 North Lake Shore Drive, Apt 211, Chicago, IL 60657, (312) 528-9347, BA 83 Univ of MI - Ann Arbor; MA 84 MI St Univ; Aud, Dr Jack Clemis, **A**

Wheat, Mrs Ann Chiles 228 Perth Drive, Dublin, OH 43017, (614) 761-2950, BS 80 Miami Univ - Oxford; MA 86 Univ of TX - Austin; Aud, Columbus Sp & Hrng Ctr-Columbu, **A**

Wheatley, Regina L 100 Arrowhead Court, Apartment A-8, Phillipsburg, NJ 08865, (201) 788-6424, BS 83 East Stroudsburg Univ of PA; MS 84 Bloomsburg Univ of PA; 87–Aud, Hunterdon Med Ctr, **A**

Wheaton, Karen S 1730 Hazelwood Avenue, Elmira, NY 14905, (607) 734-3911, BS 72 SUNY - Center at Albany; MA 76 SUNY - Coll at Geneseo; Assoc Prof of Speech/Hearing, Elmira Coll, **SLP**

Wheaton, Ronald E 1730 Hazelwood Avenue, Elmira, NY 14905, (607) 936-3704, BS 70 SUNY - Coll at Geneseo; MA 75 SUNY - Coll at Geneseo; Sp-Lang Path, Corning City Sch Dist, **SLP**

Wheelden, Julie Atwood Director, Speech-Language Pathology Dept, Massachusetts General Hosp, Boston, MA 02114, (617) 726-2762, BA Univ of MA - Amherst; ME 67 Boston Univ; 73–Dir, MA Gen Hosp, **SLP F**

Wheeler, Barbara Ann Primary Children's Medical Center, 320 Twelfth Avenue, Salt Lake City, UT 84103, (801) 521-1221, OM 86 Univ of MO - Columbia; 88–Sp-Lang Path, Primary Children's Med Ctr, **SLP**

Wheeler, Barbara Eleanor 1700 S W Blandenship Road, Apartment B-2, West Linn, OR 97068, (503) 271-3616, BS 77 Univ of OR; MS 82 Univ of OR; Sp-Lang Path, Douglas Co Ed Serv Dist, **SLP**

Wheeler, Mrs Betty K 1043 Waterford, Dallas, TX 75218, (214) 231-6301, BS 59 Univ of TX - Austin; MA 76 Southern Methodist Univ; Sp-Lang Path, Region 10 Ed Serv Cen, **SLP**

Wheeler, Mrs Carolyn S 309 Glenwood Avenue, Haddonfield, NJ 08033, (609) 783-3321, BS 71 Indiana Univ of PA; MA 79 Trenton St Coll; Sp-Lang Path, Stratford Board of Education, **SLP**

Wheeler, Catherine 126 Gereenhill Trail South, Trophy Club, TX 76262, (817) 430-4159, BA 67 Southern Methodist Univ; MS 69 Univ of OK Medical Center; **SLP**

Wheeler, Dale C N8 W30620 Broken Bow Trail, Waukesha, WI 53188, **SLP A**

Wheeler, Mrs Diane G 23 Langdon Terrace, Bronxville, NY 10708, (914) 337-9332, BA 73 Catholic Univ of America; MS 76 Columbia Univ Teachers Coll; Private Practice, **SLP**

Wheeler, Mrs Grete M Box 273, Agency, IA 52530, (515) 937-5313, BA 50; MA 57 Univ of IA; 74–Sp-Lang Path, Ottumwa Regional Health Ctr, **SLP LM**

Wheeler, Jan B Kerrick 12903 Springdale Village, Creve Coeur, MO 63146, (314) 878-6680, **A**

Wheeler, Janie S 1425 West Busch Blvd, Tampa, FL 33612, (813) 933-3477, BS 73 IN St Univ - Terre Haute; MS 76 IN St Univ - Terre Haute; SLP, Private Practice, **SLP**

Wheeler, Karen Marie Route 2, Box 2770, Hartsburg, MO 65039, (314) 443-2511, BA 79 Univ of MO - Columbia; MA 80 Univ of MO - Columbia; Sp-Lang Path, Harry S Truman Mem VA Hospital, **SLP**

Wheeler, Kathy M 6061 DE Zavala Road #1610, San Antonio, TX 78249, (512) 299-5500, BS 76 Univ of MA - Amherst; MS 78 Southern CT St Univ; 87–Sp-Lang Path, San Antonio ISD, **SLP ACE**

Wheeler, L Darrell Audiology/Sp Path Serv (126), VA Medical Center, 1515 West Pleasant Street, Knoxville, IA 50138, (515) 828-5007, BS 70 Northeast MO St Univ; MA 71 Northeast MO St Univ; Chief, Aud/Sp Path Ser, **SLP**

Wheeler, Linda Marie 4235 Ruskin Street, Houston, TX 77005-3550, (713) 667-0616, BA 80 Univ of MO - KS City; MS 85 Washington Univ

Wheeler, Mrs Lisa B 20 Mattern Road, Preston, CT 06360-8614, (203) 886-2787, MS 88 Southern CT St Univ

Wheeler, Mrs Nancy R 10 Crestwood Drive, Gulfport, MS 39503, (601) 865-4692, BA 53 Univ of MS; MS 66 Univ Southern MS-Hattiesburg; 88–Sp-Lang Path, Gulfport Mun Sep Sch Dist, **SLP**

Wheeler, Mrs Sara Lee T 13433 Featherstone Drive, St Louis, MO 63131, (314) 645-8510, BS 75 Fontbonne Coll; MA 79 Saint Louis Univ; Director Aud/SLP, Deaconess Hosp, **SLP ACE**

Wheeler, Sherwood 309 Glenwood Avenue, Haddonfield, NJ 08033, (609) 854-5844, BA Alderson-Broaddus Coll; MA 74 Kean Coll of NJ; Audiologist, H A McKee & Associates, **A**

Wheeler, Mrs Wendy Polsky 2017-A Woodriver Drive, Carbondale, IL 62901, (618) 549-4442, BS 81 Univ of MO - Columbia; MS 85 Southern IL Univ -Carbondale; Exec Dir, Archway Inc, **SLP**

Wheeling, Sandra Kay 9115 Marigold, Boise, ID 83714, (208) 454-0445, BS 80 ID St Univ; MS 82 ID St Univ; Sp-Lang Path, Canyon School District, **SLP**

Wheelock, Sandra Kaye 402-K Banana Cay Drive, South Daytona, FL 32019, (904) 767-2332, MA 81 Bowling Green St Univ; **SLP**

Whelan, Catherine 767 East Boulder Creek Lane, Fresno, CA 93710-1238, (209) 441-3328, BA 80 Pomona Coll; MA 82 Northwestern Univ; **SLP**

Whelan, Connie R Psychology-Speech Path Assoc, 1505 Strong Avenue, Greenwood, MS 38930, (601) 453-5066, BA 74 Sam Houston St Univ; MS 77 Univ Southern MS-Hattiesburg; Sp-Lang Path, Private Practice, **SLP**

Whelan, Mrs Debra J 5914 Shamrock Lane, Hubertus, WI 53033, (414) 628-2472, BS 78 Univ of WI - Stevens Point; MS 79 Univ of WI - Stevens Point; Sp-Lang Path, Mequon-Thiensville Sch Dist, **SLP**

Whelan, Donna D 124 Payne Whitney Lane, Manhasset, NY 11030, (516) 627-2567, BA 74 Univ of Dayton; MS 76 Adelphi Univ; SLP, Mill Neck Manor Sch for Deaf, **SLP**

Whelan, Mrs Janice M 1117 Gannon Drive, Plano, TX 75023, (214) 423-3146, BS 73 TX Tech Univ; MS 76 TX Tech Univ; SLP, Plano ISD, **SLP**

Whelan, Maureen Santos 206 South Mountain, Monrovia, CA 91016, (714) 623-5251, BA 75 Whittier Coll; MA 81 CA St Univ - Northridge; Sp-Lang Path, Pomona USD, **SLP**

Whelihan, Ann T 141 May Street #F, Addison, IL 60101, (312) 543-9644, BA 50 Rockford Coll; MA 61 Univ of WI - Madison; Sp-Lang Path-Lrng Dis Teacher, Elmhurst Pub Schs #205, **SLP**

Wheltle, Marian D 4619 Oakview Court, Ellicott City, MD 21043, (301) 730-8909, BA 76 Loyola Coll; MS 78 Loyola Coll; Sp-Lang Path, Hrng & Sp Agency, **SLP**

Wherley, Mrs Barbara 2462-0 Pleasant Way, Thousand Oaks, CA 91360, (805) 379-5226, BA 77 Marshall Univ; MA 78 Marshall Univ; Sp/Lang Path, **SLP**

Wherry, James Allen, Jr 365 McKinley Avenue, Washington, PA 15301, (412) 394-5815, BS 79 CA Univ of PA; ME 81 CA Univ of PA; SLP, Western Center

Whetstone, Clarence E, Jr Rd 4 Box 421, Bedford, PA 15522, (814) 623-1390, BS 54 Mansfield Univ of PA; ME 61 PA St Univ - Univ Park; Sp-Lang Path, Appalachia Iu 08, **SLP**

Whibbs, Rosemary 2120 Tronjo Road, Pensacola, FL 32503, **SLP**

Whichard, Mrs Susan P Lewis-Gale Clinic, 1802 Braeburn Drive, Salem, VA 24153, (703) 772-3430, BS 76 East TN St Univ; MS 82 Radford Univ; Aud, Lewis-Gale Clinic, **A ACE**

Whicker, Sheri Leigh 6368 Bethania-Tob Road, Tobaccoville, NC 27050, (704) 264-0566, BS 85 Appalachian St Univ; MS 86 East Carolina Univ; 87–Sp-Lang Path, Communi-Care Inc, **SLP**

Whidden, Rose 869 11th Street, Manhattan Beach, CA 90266, (213) 372-4345, BA 48 AR St Univ; MA 58 Univ of AL- Tuscaloosa; Sp-Lang Path, Manhattan Beach Cty Schs, **SLP**

Whinnery, Sheridan Elizabeth 2576 Millcreek Drive #156, Sacramento, CA 95833, (916) 985-0112, BS 85 CA St Univ - Sacramento; MS 87 San Francisco St Univ; **SLP**

Whippen, Leslie A Woodard, Hearing Aid Centers, 4217 University Avenue, Des Moines, IA 50311, (515) 255-2300, BS 76 UT St Univ; MS 77 UT St Univ; Aud, Woodard Hearing Aid & Sp Cen, **A**

Whipple, Linda Leigh Speech And Hearing Department, St Joseph's Hospital, 555 East Market Street, Elmira, NY 14902, (607) 733-6541, BS 81 Bloomsburg Univ of PA; MS 82 Bloomsburg Univ of PA; Sp-Lang Path, St Josephs Hosp, **SLP**

Whirledge, Rosemary A 8429 Shiredale Lane, Charlotte, NC 28212, (704) 596-6515, BA 73 OH St Univ; MA 76 IN Univ - Bloomington; SLP, Charlotte-Mecklenburg Sch, **SLP**

Whirt, Mrs Celeste A 5900 Suncreek Drive, Lake Oswego, OR 97035, (503) 639-9617, BS 78 WV Univ; MS 79 Paterson St Coll; Sp-Lang Path, St Vincent's Med Ctr, **SLP**

Whisler, Mrs Lanna J P O Box 635, Tipton, MO 65081, (816) 433-2213, BS 84 Northeast MO St Univ; MA 85 Northeast MO St Univ; 85–Sp-Lang Path, Tipton Ps, **SLP**

Whisonant, Brenda L 29 Round Hill Drive, Radford, VA 24141, (703) 639-0048, BA 63 Furman Univ; MS 82 Radford Univ; Sp-Lang Path, Sp Pathology Serv, **SLP**

Whitaker, Joanna R R 13043 Espinheira Drive, Cerritos, CA 90701, (213) 924-5306, BA 65 Loma Linda Univ - Riverside; MA 71 Univ of Southern CA; **SLP**

Whitaker, John M 2908 E Great Smokey Court, Thousand Oaks, CA 91362, (805) 379-9226, BA 77 WA St Univ; MA 78 WA St Univ; Sp-Lang Path, **SLP ACE**

Whitaker, Mrs Mary Mouer Campus Box 8116, Speech Pathology & Audiology, Idaho State University, Pocatello, ID 83209, (208) 236-3495, BS 84 Univ of UT; MS 86 Univ of AZ; Aud, Idaho State University, **A**

Whitaker, Mrs Nancy O 2511 Firstenberger Road, Marion, OH 43302, (614) 383-2513, BS 66 OH St Univ; MA 70 OH Univ - Athens; Sp-Lang Path, Marion Therapy Center, **SLP**

Whitaker, Oreno Faye 7222 Bellerive Drive #1503, Houston, TX 77036-1503, (919) 485-5145, BS 83 East Carolina Univ; OM 84 Univ of SC - Columbia; Sp-Lang Path, Southeastern Speech-Hearing, **SLP**

Whitaker, Pamela 2107 Canal Drive, Wilson, NC 27893, (919) 291-4029, BA 71 Southern Methodist Univ; MS 73 Emory Univ; **SLP**

Whitaker, Rebecca Schupbach 7458 South Fairfax Court, Littleton, CO 80122, (303) 694-3512, BA 78 Ottawa Univ; MA 81 Univ of CO - Boulder; Sp-Lang Path, Cherry Creek Schs, **SLP**

Whitaker, Stephanie 2819 Tell Street, Tell City, IN 47586, (812) 547-5541, BS 74 Brescia Coll; MS 78 IN St Univ - Terre Haute; 78–Sp-Lang Path, Dubois-Spencer-Perry, **SLP**

Whitaker, Susan E 2005 Court Street, Suite N, Redding, CA 96001, (916) 244-3260, BA 74 Whittier Coll; MA 76 San Diego St Univ; Sp/Lang Path, Susan E Whitaker Ma Ccc Sp, **SLP**

Whitaker, Mrs Susan M F 21 Jean Road, Arlington, MA 02174, (617) 862-7323, BA 68 Heidelberg Coll; MS 78 Emerson Coll; Sp-Lang Path Cl Supervisor, Cotting Sch, **SLP**

Whitaker, Tamara Ann 7440 Waterfront Drive #202, Indianapolis, IN 46214, (317) 745-5451, BS 85 Purdue Univ - West Lafayette; MS 87 Purdue Univ - West Lafayette; 88–Sp-Lang Path, InSpeech Inc

Whitby-Norman, Mrs Debra Marie 132 Wooden Carriage Drive, Hockessin, DE 19707, (302) 239-3661, BS 81 West Chester Univ of PA; MS 83 Boston Univ; Sp-Lang Path, Unified Cerebral Palsy, **SLP**

Whitcher, Mrs Abigail B 5965 Gladden Drive, Indianapolis, IN 46220, BS 60 Univ of WI - Madison; MS 73 Butler Univ; SLP, Indianapolis Pub Sch, **SLP**

Whitcomb, Curtis Joe 2103 Westgate Drive, Boise, ID 83704, (208) 343-2583, BS 78 Univ of OR; MS 82 ID St Univ; 85–Aud, Rehab Assoc Inc-Hearing & Sp Ctr, **A**

Whitcomb, Mrs Dale P 7914 Rocoso Lane, Carlsbad, CA 92009, (619) 753-1879, BA 72 Univ of CA - Santa Barbara; MA 74 San Diego St Univ; SLP, Carlsbad USD, **SLP**

Whitcomb, Rebecca Beukelman 2103 Westgate Drive, Boise, ID 83704, (208) 343-2583, BS 75 Univ of OR; MS 82 ID St Univ; 85–Sp-Lang Path, Rehab Assoc Inc-Hearing & Speech Ctr, **SLP**

White, Mrs Anita Moon 583 Unadilla Street, Shreveport, LA 71106, (318) 861-3464, BS 85 Univ of AR - Little Rock; MS 87 Vanderbilt Univ; **SLP**

White, Anne C 12422 Wethersfield, San Antonio, TX 78216, (512) 226-8982, BA 80 WV Univ; MS 81 WV Univ; Aud, Walter Bain Otol, **A**

White, Mrs Anne Elaine 2666 East Elmwood Street, Mesa, AZ 85203, BA 75 Univ of Akron; MS 76 AZ St Univ; SLP, Mesa Pubsch, **SLP**

White, Mrs Anne La Fave 10593 U S 31, Williamsburg, MI 49690, (616) 941-7070, BA 80 MI St Univ; MA 82 Central MI Univ; Sp-Lang Path, Northwest Michigan Human Serv, **SLP**

White, Barbara S 17 Boxwood Court, Poughkeepsie, NY 12601, (914) 877-6821, BA 74 CUNY - Queens Coll; MA 75 Long Island U - CW Post Ctr; Sp-Lang Path & Aud Prog Coord, Wassaic Dev Cen, **SLP**

White, Barbara Shultz 2600 Kelp Street, Oxnard, CA 93035, (805) 984-3591, ME 83 Univ of VA - Charlottesville; Aud, **A**

White, Barbara W 714 North Powers, Taylorville, IL 62568, (217) 824-9675, MS 74 Eastern IL Univ; BS 73 Eastern IL Univ; Sp-Lang Path, Christian Co Dev Cen, **SLP**

White, Mrs Betty Stallings 27 Walker Avenue, Morristown, NJ 07960, (201) 539-2030, BA 74 Univ of NC - Greensboro; ME 79 Univ of VA - Charlottesville; Sp/Lang Path/Consult, Private Practice, **SLP**

White, Blaik J 2140 East Sanos Drive, Tempe, AZ 85282, (602) 833-6220, BS 74 UT St Univ; MS 75 UT St Univ; SLP, Mesa Public Schools, **SLP**

White, Blanche B 706 Bragg Drive, Tallahassee, FL 32304, (904) 575-7684, **SLP**

White, Bridget K Box 572, 425 E 25th Street, New York, NY 10010, MS 88 CUNY - Hunter Coll

White, Carol Marie 214 North San Jose Street, Mesa, AZ 85201, (602) 835-7114, BS 77 Univ of ND; MS 87 Northern AZ Univ; **SLP**

White, Carol Rowene 1117 Arizona Avenue, Ames, IA 50010, (515) 432-6345, BS 81 IA St Univ; MA 83 Northeast MO St Univ; Sp-Lang Path, Heartland AEA, **SLP**

White, Mrs Carolyn Holmes 5509 Ursuline Drive, Alexandria, LA 71301, (318) 448-4165, BA 77 Univ of Southwestern LA; MA 81 Northwestern St Univ; SLP, Rapides School System, **SLP**

White, Mrs Carolyn Martin 414 Jolee Street, Richardson, TX 75080, (214) 669-3553, BS 82 Baylor Univ; MA 85 TX Woman's Univ; Sp-Lang Path, Richardson ISD, **SLP**

White, Cheryl A Lakeville Hospital, Lakeville, MA 02346, (617) 947-1231, BA 75; MA 78; Sp/Lang Path Dept Head, Lakeville Hosp Rehab Cen, **SLP**

White, Cheryl Jouret 818 Monumnet Road, Ponca City, OK 74604, (405) 762-7561

White, Christine 340 Foxboro Court, San Ramon, CA 94583, (415) 447-9500, BA 61 San Jose St Univ; SLP, Livermore Valley Unif Sch Dist, **SLP**

White, Mrs Cynthia J 157 Belle Grove, La Place, LA 70068, (504) 652-1925, BS 73 LA St Univ - Baton Rouge; OM 78 LA St Univ - N O Medical Ctr; Sp-Lang Path, St John Parish Schools, **SLP**

White, Daniel Raymond P O Box 371, Jamestown, TN 38556, (615) 879-8447, BS 79 East TN St Univ; MS 84 East TN St Univ; SLP, Fentress County Schools, **SLP**

White, Daniel Steven Bush Road, Clymer, NY 14724, (716) 355-9918, BS 86 SUNY - Coll at Fredonia; MS 87 SUNY - Coll at Fredonia

White, David L 346 West Mansion Avenue, Chico, CA 95926, (916) 895-4496, BA 42 Univ of CA - Santa Barbara; MS 58 Univ of Southern CA; Lecturer, CA State Univ, **SLP LM**

White, Mrs Deborah P 1639 Woodvale Drive, Charleston, WV 25314, BS 78 WV Univ; MS 79 WV Univ; **SLP**

White, Mrs Deborah Williams 3979 Springleaf Drive, Stone Mountain, GA 30083, (404) 299-7765, MS 84 Governors St Univ; Sp-Lang Path, Gwinnett Co Bd of Educ, **SLP**

White, Debra Lee 7915 South Pennsylvania Ct, Littleton, CO 80122, (303) 797-3929, BS 80 Central MO St Univ; MA 81 Univ of Northern CO; 86–Aud, Listen Acoupedic Ctr, **A**

White, Donna S 24631 Kipling, Oak Park, MI 48237, **SLP**

White, Mrs Dorenda T 2600 Rockybrook Road, Opelika, AL 36801, (205) 745-5966, BS 76 Auburn Univ - Auburn; MS 78 Auburn Univ - Auburn; **SLP**

White, Dr Doris Lee 2101 Mackenzie Drive, Columbus, OH 43220, (614) 365-5230, BA 48 OH St Univ; MA 55 Columbia Univ Teachers Coll; PH 75 (NS) OH St Univ; Superv, Columbus Pub Sch, **SLP A**

White, Dorothy J 70-9 Kirkland Street, Cambridge, MA 02138, (617) 491-1751, BS 64 Univ of IA; MS 73 Southern CT St Univ; Sp-Lang Path, Private Practice, **SLP**

White, E Rebecca 8830 Dollyhyde Road, Union Bridge, MD 21791, (301) 469-0228, BS 77 Auburn Univ - Auburn; MS 78 Univ of MS; 87–Sp/Lang Path, Ivymount Sch, **SLP**

White, Elease 2852 Booker Washington, Jackson, MS 39213, BS 72 Jackson St Univ; MS 76 Univ of IL - Urbana; SLP, Tougalon Cll

White, Mrs Elizabeth Jo 609 Robby Road, Burleson, TX 76028, (817) 335-2583, BS 82 Andrews Univ; MA 83 MI St Univ; Aud, Jack Jones Aud & Hrng Aid Ctr, **A**

White, Emily J 343 Sayre Drive, Princeton, NJ 08540, (609) 924-0534, BA 63 Smith Coll; MA 74 Temple Univ; Dir, Penta Hrng Care, **A ACE**

White, Ethel B Rural Free Delivery 6, Butler, PA 16001, BS; **SLP LM**

White, Gail Jean 1009 Rue DE La Banque West, Apartment G, Creve Coeur, MO 63141-5116, (314) 946-6546, **SLP**

White, Gayl A 10202 Cantertrot, Humble, TX 77338, (713) 446-0371, BS 59 Univ of Houston - Univ Park; MA 69 Univ of Houston - Univ Park; Sp-Lang Path, Private Practice, **SLP ACE**

White, Dr Harvey 86 Henry Street, Merrick, NY 11566, (516) 560-5507, BS 50 NY Univ; MS 57 SUNY - Coll at New Paltz; PH 63 (NS) NY Univ; Prof/Chmn, Hofstra U, **SLP**

White, Mrs Helen A B 88 Stonewood Court, Hickory, NC 28602, (704) 464-1257, BS 72 Appalachian St Univ; MA 73 Appalachian St Univ; ES 84 Appalachian St Univ; 73–Sp-Lang Path, Catawba Co Sch, **SLP**

White, Mrs Helen J 5133 North Old Highway #13, Springfield, MO 65803, ME 69 Drury Coll; 70–Consultant, US Med Center for Fed Prisonrs, **SLP**

White, Holly Meier 19 Rockaway Terrace, Mountain Lakes, NJ 07046-2012, (201) 316-8379, MA 87 OH Univ - Athens; 88–Sp-Lang Path, Lake Drive Sch for Hrng Impaired, **SLP**

White, Ingrid H W 1844 Malden Street, San Diego, CA 92109, (619) 239-1355, MS 78 San Diego St Univ; 86–Sp-Lang Path, Achievement Ctr for Lang Sp & Hearing, **SLP**

White, Mrs Irene F 17105 Laburnum Court, Rockville, MD 20855, (301) 253-5101, BS 68 Ithaca Coll; MS 70 Ithaca Coll; Sp-Lang Path, Mont Co Pub Sch, **SLP**

White, James Clyde, III 603 Goldleaf Drive, Goldsboro, NC 27530-0243, (919) 731-3620, BS 84 Western Carolina Univ; MA 86 Western Carolina Univ; **SLP**

White, Mrs Jane A RD 1 Box 12-A, Jones Road, Remsen, NY 13438, (315) 831-3797, BS 73 SUNY - Center at Albany; MS 77 SUNY - Center at Albany; Sp-Lang Path, Remsen Central Schools, **SLP**

White, Mrs Janet Ann R R 1 Box 211, Plainview, NE 68769, (402) 582-3672, BS 70 Univ of NE - Lincoln; MA 72 Univ of NE - Lincoln; Sp-Lang Path, Ed Ser Ut #8, **SLP**

White, Janet Dea P O Box 298, 30 North Walnut Street, Chillicothe, OH 45601, (614) 773-2679, OB 83 OH St Univ; BA 82 OH St Univ; MA 85 OH St Univ; Sp-Lang Path, S Cen Ohio Speech & Hrng Cen, **SLP**

White, Janie Lynee 800 East Washington Street, Apartment 208, Colton, CA 92324, (714) 350-7300, BS 86 Loma Linda Univ - Riverside; MS 86 Loma Linda Univ - Riverside; **SLP**

White, Janis Bryant 20981 Coastview Lane, Huntington Beach, CA 92648, (714) 730-7314, BA 70 CA St Univ - Sacramento; ME 76 Rivier Coll; MA 83 Northern IL Univ - De Kalb; Sp-Lang Path, Tustin USD, **SLP**

White, Mrs Jennifer W 6198 Northampton Drive, Bartlett, TN 38134, (901) 682-3730, BS 76 Appalachian St Univ; MS 82 Radford Univ; 88–Prog Dir/Head Injury Rehab Svcs, The Rehab Group Inc, **SLP**

White, Jessie G 4902 Euclid, East Chicago, IN 46312, (219) 949-4000, BA Univ of Pittsburgh - Pittsburgh; MS Univ of Pittsburgh - Pittsburgh; Associate Director, Gary Community Mental Hlth Cen, **SLP**

White, Joanne Elizabeth 2843 Marshall Street, Falls Church, VA 22042, (202) 832-4400, BS 78 Radford Univ; MA 81 Marshall Univ; Sp-Lang Path, The Hospital for Sick Children, **SLP**

White, Johanna M 26 Westpoint Terrace, West Hartford, CT 06107, (203) 486-2629, BA 80 Univ of CT; MS 82 Boston Univ; Clin Supvr-Sp-Lang Path, Univ of Connecticut, **SLP**

White, Mrs Judith Lee Judith L White & Associates, 8187 Inverness Ridge Road, Potomac, MD 20854, (301) 299-8418, BA 62 George Washington Univ; MA 74 Univ of MD - College Park; PH 88 (Psycho-Social Aspects of Deaf) Walden Univ - Minneapolis; 81–Dir/Sp-Lang Path, Judith L White & Assoc, **SLP ACE**

White, Dr Kathleen 8613 Trumbull Avenue, Skokie, IL 60076, (312) 633-2169, BA 72 Univ of Pittsburgh - Pittsburgh; MS 74 PA St Univ - Univ Park; PH 84 (NS) Northwestern Univ; Sp-Lang Path, VA, **SLP**

White, Cms Kathleen Sheryll 20401 S W 84th Avenue, Miami, FL 33189, (305) 253-9565, BA 78 SUNY - Coll at Cortland; OM 83 Governors St Univ; **SLP**

White, Kristen Mattson 17609 185th Avenue N E, Woodinville, WA 98072, (206) 259-5068, BA 80 Univ of Redlands; MS 82 Univ of Redlands; Sp-Lang Path, Pacific Hearing & Sp Svcs, **SLP**

White, Laurel M D Box 2134, Zweibruchen, Germany, BA 73 CA St Univ - Long Beach; MA 78 CA St Univ - Long Beach; Sp-Lang Path, Dept of Defense Dependents Sch, **SLP**

White, Leta D 2403 Yosemite, Lawrence, KS 66046-3564, BA 57 Wichita St Univ; **SLP**

White, Linda R 13528 Copper Bed Road, Herndon, VA 22071, ED 85 (NS) Vanderbilt Univ; **SLP**

White, Mrs Lisa Annette 603 Goldleaf Drive, Goldsboro, NC 27530-8867, (919) 731-3559, BS 84 Western Carolina Univ; MA 86 Western Carolina Univ; **SLP**

White, Lisa Pace 16 Echo Lane East, Fairhope, AL 36532, (205) 928-6124, BS 84 Univ of South AL; MS 86 Univ of South AL; 84–Sp-Lang Path, Baldwin Co Bd of Educ, **SLP**

White, Liza C 4233 Towhee Drive, Calabasas, CA 91302, (818) 888-0636, BA 68 Univ of CA - Los Angeles; MA 79 CA St Univ - Northridge; Sp-Lang Path, Private Practice, **SLP**

White, Lois D 7736 Alden Way, Fridley, MN 55432, (612) 476-3145, BA 57 Berea Coll; MA 71 Univ of MN - Minneap-St Paul; Sp-Lang Path, ISD 284 Wayzata, **SLP**

White, Mrs Lora Lee 1575 Anderson Lane, Buffalo Grove, IL 60089, (312) 882-2501, BS 74 Univ of WI - Stevens Point; MA 86 Northern IL Univ - De Kalb; **SLP**

White, Mrs Lynda McCall 8129 Oldmill Road, Pewee Valley, KY 40056, (502) 241-5606, BA 78 IN Univ - Bloomington; MS 82 Univ of Louisville; Sp-Lang Path, Pub Sch, **SLP**

White, Mrs Lynne M 3601 Bue Street, Norfolk, VA 23513, (518) 829-7303, BS 85 Univ of Akron; MA 87 Univ of Akron

White, Marcella Leigh H 1508 Cedar Lane, Ponca City, OK 74604, (405) 723-4582, BS 78 Phillips Univ; MS 82 Phillips Univ; Sp/Lang Path, Red Rock Pub Sch, **SLP ACE**

White, Margaret C Route 4 Box 588, Elizabeth City, NC 27909, (919) 335-0831, BS 72 East Carolina Univ; MA 80 Hampton Univ; 88–Dir, Camden County Sch Sys, **SLP**

White, Margaret J 140 Wood Road, Los Gatos, CA 95030, (408) 354-3793, MA 54 4637; **SLP LM**

White, Margaret R Rt 1 Box 93, Star Prairie, WI 54026, (715) 247-3311, BA 79 Univ of WI - Eau Claire; MS 80 Univ of WI - Eau Claire; Sp-Lang Path, Sch Dist-Somerset, **SLP**

White, Marshall K 1666 Elliott Avenue, Ashland, KY 41101, BA 56 Univ of KY; ME 58 Univ of KY; Sp-Lang Path, Ashland Cty Schs, **SLP**

White, Mary Anne 4208 Smithdeal Avenue, Richmond, VA 23225, (804) 231-0934, BS 79 Radford Univ; OM 81 Auburn Univ - Auburn; Sp-Lang Path, Crater Dist Program, **SLP**

White, Mrs Mary H 208 Mason Croft, Sumter, SC 29150, (803) 773-1893, BA 70 Columbia Coll; ME 73 Univ of SC - Columbia; 88–Sp-Lang Path, Sumter Sch Dist 17, **SLP**

White, Mrs Mary Hawkins 902 North Brandywine Lane, Corona, CA 91720, BA 78 CA St Univ - Long Beach; MA 80 CA St Univ - Long Beach; **SLP**

White, Mary Layden P O Box 1225, Telluride, CO 81435, (214) 373-3988, BS 72 Univ of TX - Austin; ME 74 Southwest TX St Univ; Sp-Lang Path, Private Practice, **SLP**

White, Melinda 1106 Bon Air Drive, Augusta, GA 30907, (404) 737-7533, BS 86 Univ of GA; ME 87 Univ of GA

White, Mrs Myrna Goff 121 Avenida #23, Pensacola, FL 32561, (904) 934-3810, BS 75 OH Univ - Athens; MA 77 Bowling Green St Univ; Sp/Lang Path, Escambia Co Sch Bd, **SLP**

White, Nancy C 1127 Holly Drive, Sioux Falls, SD 57105, (605) 332-8947, BS 66 Univ of MN - Minneap-St Paul; MA 68 Univ of MN - Minneap-St Paul; **SLP**

White, Nancy J 23556 Los Grandes, Laguna Hills, CA 92653, (714) 859-6807, BA 76 Univ of WI - Eau Claire; MS 77 Univ of WI - Eau Claire; SLP, Irvine USD, **SLP**

White, Nancy J 5949 Anna Lee, Hudson, OH 44236, (216) 650-4152, BS 76 SUNY - Coll at Geneseo; MA 77 SUNY - Coll at Geneseo; Aud, **A**

White, Nina G P O Box 5051, Shreveport, LA 71105, **SLP**

White, Mrs Patricia Fincher 306 Buena Vista Place, Memphis, TN 38112, (901) 726-1618, BA 80 LA Tech Univ; MA 83 Memphis St Univ; Sp-Lang Path, Methodist Hosp, **SLP**

White, Renee Spies 1194 West 30th Street #9, Los Angeles, CA 90007

White, Richard A 2228 Kensington Road, Salina, KS 67401, (913) 823-7263, BS 74 Emporia St Univ; MS 76 Fort Hays St Univ; MA 79 Univ of SD - Vermillion; Audiologist, Central Kansas Coop In Educ, **A**

White, Mrs Robin Renae Route 2 Box 205, Grand Rivers, KY 42045, (502) 444-2850, BS 84 Murray St Univ; MS 88 Murray St Univ; 87–Sp-Lang Path, Dr Laurie Ballew Inc

White, Mrs Sandra F 86 Henry Street, Merrick, NY 11566, (516) 378-3900, BA 76 Hofstra Univ; MA 77 Hofstra Univ; SLP, Merrick Un Free Sch Dist, **SLP**

White, Sandra S 3728 Gladney Drive, Chamblee, GA 30341, **SLP**

White, Sherry Elizabeth 4091 Briarforest Road West, Jacksonville, FL 32211, BS 70 FL St Univ; MS 71 FL St Univ; SLP, Duval Co Sch Bd, **SLP**

White, Mrs Sherry M Rural Route 3, Carlyle, IL 62231, (618) 594-3997, BS 74 Eastern IL Univ; MS 75 Eastern IL Univ; 88–Sp-Lang Path, Kaskaskia Spec Educ Dist #801, **SLP**

White, Dr Steven C ASHA, 10801 Rockville Pike, Rockville, MD 20852, (301) 897-5700, BS 66 Ithaca Coll; MS 69 Ithaca Coll; PH 74 (Aud) Wayne St Univ - Sch of Med; Dir Reimbursemen Policy Div, ASHA, **A ACE**

White, Mrs Susan G 1637 Waff Road, Virginia Beach, VA 23464, (804) 479-4547, BS 73 Univ of VA - Charlottesville; ME 74 Univ of VA - Charlottesville; 82–Sp/Lang Path, VA Beach Pub Sch, **SLP**

White, Susan J 55 Meadow Park, Bexley, OH 43209, (614) 252-2521, BA 68 Miami Univ - Oxford; MA 70 OH St Univ; Sp-Lang Path, Comm Hlth & Nursing Ser, **SLP**

White, Mrs Susan M L 605 West High Street, Edwardsville, IL 62025, (618) 635-8230, BS 76 IL St Univ - Normal; MS 77 IL St Univ - Normal; Sp-Lang Path, Staunton Co Dist #6, **SLP ACE**

White, Susan Marie P O Box 823-7, 348 East Lincoln Way, Coburg, OR 97401, (503) 343-2428, MS 87 Univ of OR; 87–Sp-Lang Path, Bethel Sch Dist #52

White, Therese B 3245 Richmond Avenue, Shoreview, MN 55126, (612) 559-3535, BS 78 Univ of WI - River Falls; MS 80 Univ of WI - River Falls; Aud, ISD 287 Henn Tech Ctr, **A**

White, Thomas P Buffalo Otologic Group, 897 Delaware Avenue, Buffalo, NY 14209, (716) 883-6800, BS 66 IN Univ - Bloomington; MA 67 IN Univ - Bloomington; 67–Asst Prof, Univ at Buffalo, **A**

White, Valorie Parker Boys Town National Institute, Audiology Dept, 555 North 30th Street, Omaha, NE 68131, (402) 449-6535, BS 74 SD St Univ; MA 76 Univ of NE - Lincoln; Aud, Boys Town National Institute, **A**

White, Vivian Dianne Route 3 Box 306, Highway 76, Springfield, TN 37172, (615) 384-4657, BS 85 Western KY Univ; MS 86 Western KY Univ; SLP, Upper Cumberland Hr/Sp/L Ctr, **SLP**

Whitebread, Bonnie P Rural Delivery 2, Sugarloaf, PA 18249, (717) 788-2394, BS 75 PA St Univ - Univ Park; MS 79 Bloomsburg Univ of PA; 88, Dr Geeta Krishnan MD, **A**

Whitebread, Debora Kay 431 North Bunker Hill, Tucson, AZ 85748, (602) 722-2040, BS 82 Univ of AZ; MS 84 Univ of AZ; 85–Sp-Lang Path, Carondelet Health Svcs, **SLP**

White-Chambers, Marcia J 5236 Kensington, Wichita, KS 67208, (316) 686-2404, BA 82 Fort Hays St Univ; MA 85 Wichita St Univ; **SLP**

Whitefield, Mrs Sylvia H 317 Willow Bough, Old Hickory, TN 37138, BA 59 David Lipscomb Coll; ME 79 Middle TN St Univ; Sp-Lang Path, Metro-Davidson Co Pub Schools, **SLP**

Whitehair, Mrs Patricia M 1903 Berue Drive, Coatesville, PA 19320, (215) 358-6615, BS 72 West Chester Univ of PA; MS 76 West Chester Univ of PA; 75–Coord/Sp & Lang Dept, Elwyn, **SLP**

Whitehead, Mrs Brenda Humphrey 12 Colonial Drive, Fairport, NY 14450, (716) 475-6260, BS 73 SUNY - Coll at Geneseo; MA 74 Western MI Univ; Sp-Lang Path, NTID, **SLP**

Whitehead, Mrs Charlotte Jones County Junior Coll, Ellisville, MS 39437, (601) 477-3622, BA 69; MS 71 Univ Southern MS-Hattiesburg; Teacher of Mathematics, Jones County Junior College, **SLP**

Whitehead, Jean M 3761 Plumb Street, Houston, TX 77005, (713) 795-7492, BA 68 David Lipscomb Coll; MA 71 LA St Univ - Baton Rouge; Sp-Lang Path, VA Med Cen, **SLP A**

Whitehead, Kathleen 644 DE Soto Lane, Indian Harbor Beach, FL 32937, (407) 773-2818, MS 75 Univ of South FL; Sp-Lang Path, Sch Bd of Brevard Co, **SLP**

Whitehead, Lisa M 42639 Northville Place Dr, Apt 809-A, Northville, MI 48167, (313) 347-1026, BA 85 Univ of MI - Ann Arbor; MS 87 Univ of MI - Ann Arbor; **SLP**

Whitehead, Dr Robert L Dept Of Communication Research, Ntl Tech Inst For The Deaf, 1 Lomb Mem Dr P O Box 9887, Rochester, NY 14623, (716) 475-6457, BS 65 Brigham Young Univ; MS 66 Brigham Young Univ; PH 70 (Communication Disorders) Univ of OK Medical Center; 74–Chmn-Dept of Commun Res, NTID, **SLP F**

Whitehead-Blen, Margaret L Rodgers Forge Elementary, Dumbarton Rd At Regester, Baltimore, MD 21212, (301) 472-4444, **SLP**

Whitehill, Tara Loraine A8 Rodrigues Court, 350 Victoria Road, Pokfulam, Hong Kong, BA 79 Oberlin Coll; MS 83 Columbia Univ Teachers Coll; 88–Lecturer/Practicum Supvr, Univ of Hong Kong, **SLP**

Whitehurse, Lisa J 107 South Austin, Butler, MO 64730, (816) 679-4931, BS 84 Central MO St Univ; MS 86 Central MO St Univ; 88–Sp-Lang Path, Nevada Habilitation Ctr, **SLP**

Whitehurst, Mrs Cynthia Stefanov 6321 Parkman Place, Cincinnati, OH 45213, (513) 731-8647, BA 82 OH St Univ; MA 87 Univ of TX - Austin; 86–Aud, Hearing & Balance Laboratory, **A**

Whitehurst, Jeanette L 113 Martinsborough Road, Greenville, NC 27834, **SLP**

Whitelaw, Gail Moira 178 Oakland Park Avenue, Columbus, OH 43214, (614) 268-5041, BS 81 Bowling Green St Univ; MA 83 MI St Univ; Aud, Ohio State University, **A ACE**

Whitely, Mrs Carolyn Chambers 544 River Road, Coldwater, MI 49036, (616) 467-9745, BS 79 Central MI Univ; MA 84 Western MI Univ; Sp-Lang Path, St Joseph Co Intermed Sch Dist, **SLP**

Whitely, Mrs Sherri Ranee P O Box 1293, Chilhowie, VA 24319, (703) 669-6331, BS 80 WV Univ; MS 81 Syracuse Univ; Sp-Lang Path, Bristol Sp & Hrng Ctr, **SLP**

Whiteman, Mrs Judy C P O Box 593, Ringgold, LA 71068, (318) 894-9483, BS 73 LA Tech Univ; MA 79 LA Tech Univ; 87–Sp-Lang Path, Evergreen Developmental Center, **SLP**

Whiteman, Leah Duncan 3923 Rampart, Boise, ID 83704, (208) 336-1360, BS 74 ID St Univ; MS 76 ID St Univ; SLP, Boise Sch Dist, **SLP**

Whiteman, Sheryl Foust 125 Steamboat Lane, Apartment 7, Ballwin, MO 63011, (314) 256-7275, BA 84 IN Univ - Bloomington; MA 86 IN Univ - Bloomington; **A**

White-Martin, Mrs Bonnie 905 North 59th Street, Elm Grove, WI 53122, (414) 384-2000, BS 79 Bowling Green St Univ; MS 81 Purdue Univ - West Lafayette; Sp/Lang Path, Zablocki VA Med Ctr, **SLP**

Whitener, Marilyn Klopper 626 Lakeview Road, Lake St Louis, MO 63367, (618) 398-7500, BS 78 Eastern IL Univ; MS 79 Eastern IL Univ

Whites, Margery M 1530 East Hwy 23, Apartment 204, St Cloud, MN 56304, (612) 255-2092, BA 74 SD St Univ; MA 81 Univ of SD - Vermillion; PH 88 (Sp-Lang Path/Child Lang) Univ of KS; 88–Asst Prof, St Cloud State Univ, **SLP**

Whitesell, Mrs Denise Jean 1662 Brookdale Road #13, Naperville, IL 60540, (312) 717-7054, MA 88 Univ of IA; 88–Sp-Lang Path, Aurora East PS

Whiteside, Mrs Emily Luttrell 2734 Barbara Avenue, Columbus, GA 31907, (404) 324-5661, BS 77 Auburn Univ - Auburn; ME 83 Columbus Coll; Sp-Lang Path, Muscogee Co Sch Dist, **SLP**

Whiteside, Dr Janet 1828 Valencia Place, Pekin, IL 61554, (309) 672-6340, BA 73 Augustana Coll; MA 75 Vanderbilt Univ; PH 83 (Philosophy) IN Univ - Bloomington; 87–Sp-Lang Path, UCP, **SLP**

Whitesides, Margie Karen 46 Cross Club Drive, Greenville, SC 29607, (803) 288-7774, BA 82 Winthrop Coll; MA 85 Univ of SC - Columbia; 88–Sp-Lang Path, Spartanburg Dist 5, **SLP**

Whiteway, Mrs Deborah Hare P O Box 1077, Warsaw, VA 22572, (804) 529-7406, BS 76 Univ of VA - Charlottesville; ME 77 Univ of VA - Charlottesville; Sp-Lang Path, Mid Peninsula/No Neck Comm Svcs Bd, **SLP**

Whitfield, Belva W 7004 Dellwood Road N E, Albuquerque, NM 87110, (505) 345-8531, BS 51 Hardin-Simmons Univ; MS 71 Univ of NM; 76–Sp-Lang Path, Albuquerque Public Schools, **SLP**

Whitfield, Donna E 6 Ridge Road #1A, Congers, NY 10920, (914) 268-7166, MA 84 Seton Hall Univ; Sp-Lang Path, Ramapo Cen Sch District, **SLP**

Whitfield, Mrs Elizabeth Anne P O Box 781, Jay, FL 32565, (904) 488-2819, MS 84 FL St Univ; Sp-Lang Path, Santa Rosa Co Schs, **SLP**

Whitfield, Jennifer B 4710 Sealand Lane, Nashville, TN 37220, **SLP**

Whitfield, Marie L P O Box 1496, Harlan, KY 40831, (606) 573-1523, BA 71 Univ of KY; MA 72 Univ of KY; **SLP**

Whitham, Joyce Merrie 920 Amherst Street #18, Buffalo, NY 14216, (716) 834-9200, BS 85 SUNY - Coll at Fredonia; MA 87 SUNY - Center at Buffalo; 88–Aud, VA Med Ctr, **A**

Whitham, Mrs Nancy Cox 90 Portsmouth Court, Holland, PA 18966, (215) 596-9125, BS 76 WV Univ; MS 77 WV Univ; 85–Aud, Chldrns Hosp of Phila, **A**

Whiting, Cheryl A 407 East 213rd Street, Carson, CA 90745, (213) 835-3642, BS 72 Southern IL Univ -Carbondale; MA 76 CA St Univ - Long Beach; Sp-Lang Path, Los Angeles USD, **SLP**

Whiting, Mrs Nell E 501 North Colorado, Gunnison, CO 81230, (303) 641-0251, BA 49 Univ of WI - Madison; MA 71 Western St Coll of CO; 81–Consult/Asst, Intermountain Sp/Hrng, **SLP**

Whitlatch, Mary Ellen 1211-C Lake Shore Drive, Columbus, OH 43204-3638, (614) 491-9296, BA 81 OH St Univ; MA 83 OH St Univ; MA 83 OH St Univ; SLP, Franklin Co Dept of Ed, **SLP**

Whitley, Mrs Brenda P Whitley & Associates Inc, PO Box 5067, Hudson, FL 34674, (813) 856-4597, MS 75 Univ of South FL; Dir of Rehab Serv, Private Practice, **SLP ACE**

Whitley, Mrs Jennifer W 183 Fairmont Circle, Danville, VA 24541-5210, (804) 799-3724, BS 80 East TN St Univ; MS 82 East TN St Univ; Sp-Lang Path, The Memorial Hosp, **SLP**

Whitley, Kenneth P 307 Inglewood Drive, Morganton, NC 28655, (704) 433-2873, BS 75 Appalachian St Univ; MA 77 Appalachian St Univ; Director-Aug Comm Resource Ctr, Western Carolina Ctr, **SLP**

Whitley, Mrs Ruth S 105 Buckingham Way, Taylors, SC 29687, (803) 268-0655, BA 77 Univ of NC - Greensboro; ME 76 Univ of NC - Greensboro; Sp/Lang Path, Private Practice, **SLP**

Whitley, Mrs Wendy Sue 2020 East 5th Street, Ontario, CA 91764, (714) 983-0042, BA 80 Univ of Redlands; MS 82 Univ of Redlands; Sp-Lang-Hrng Spec, San Bernardino Co Sch, **SLP**

Whitlock, Beverly H 900 Baltimore Road, Rockville, MD 20851, (301) 330-0300, BA 52 IN Univ - Bloomington; MA 55 Univ of MD - College Park; Dir, Head Injury Svcs, **SLP A F ACE**

Whitlock, Mrs Kathleen Staggs 851 Old Chapin Road, Lexington, SC 29072, (803) 359-7270, BS 70 WV Univ; MS 81 Univ of SC - Columbia; Sp-Lang Path, Lexington Sch Dist One, **SLP**

Whitlock, Maureen Maslowski 27 Arnold Terrace, Marblehead, MA 01945, (508) 745-9000, BA 77 Boston Coll; MA 78 Bowling Green St Univ; 86–Dir-Comm Dis, Shaughnessy-Kaplan Rehab Hosp, **SLP**

Whitlow, Mrs Holly J 1505 Via Arco, Palos Verdes Estates, CA 90274-2056, (213) 533-2743, BA 65; MA 66; Chief Sp-Lang Path, Harbor Gen UCLA Med Cen, **SLP**

Whitlow, Lucinda A 402 Converse, Lancaster, SC 29720-3863, (803) 286-0070, MA 87 Univ of Tulsa; **SLP**

Whitlow, Dr Roy E 1505 Via Arco, Palos Verdes Estates, CA 90274-2056, (213) 378-8679, BA 67; MA 69; PH 80 (NS); Dir, California Speech Pathologists, **SLP**

Whitman, Mrs Adrienne 3728 Springdell Avenue, Randallstown, MD 21133, BA 57 Univ of MD - College Park; MA 67 Univ of MD - College Park; Sp-Lang Path, Balto Co Bd Ed, **SLP**

Whitman, Allister C 72 Barrow Street #5-P, New York, NY 10014, (212) 427-2749, BS 47 Boston Univ; MA 60 Columbia Univ Teachers Coll; MA 80 Pace U -NY City; Superv, NYC Bd of Ed, **SLP**

Whitman, Gail L 8720 Elk Street, Highlands Ranch, CO 80126-2403, (303) 688-3675, BS 73 Minot St Univ; MS 74 Minot St Univ; Chld Find Coord, Douglas Co Sch, **SLP**

Whitman, Jo-Ann C M 573 Brook Street, Framingham, MA 01701, (617) 877-7823, BS 78 Northeastern Univ; ME 80 Northeastern Univ; Aud Suprv, W E Fernald State Sch, **A**

Whitman, Mrs Margherita 7830 Lexington Avenue, Philadelphia, PA 19152, (215) 331-4464, BS 76 West Chester Univ of PA; MS 78 Trenton St Coll; SLP, Cora Services, **SLP**

Whitman, Sandra L W P O Box 187, Choudrant, LA 71227, **SLP**

Whitman Reynolds, Kathleen Kelly 219 South 14th Street, Lewisburg, PA 17837, (301) 224-7152, BA 79 Loyola Coll; MS 80 Loyola Coll; 86–Sp-Lang Path, Private Practice, **SLP**

Whitman-Tims, Iowana 3160 Hyde Park Place, Pensacola, FL 32503, (904) 434-5926, BS 72 AL A & M Univ; MS 74 Purdue Univ - West Lafayette; Sp/Lang Path, Escambia Co Schools, **SLP**

Whitmore, Melodia Kay 20326 Cohasset Street #1, Canoga Park, CA 91306, (818) 702-8948, BS 80 Southern IL Univ -Carbondale; MS 82 Univ of MO - Columbia; **SLP**

Whitney, Mrs Billie B 1377 East Melrose, Westlake, OH 44145, (216) 282-4683, OB 64 Univ of GA; MA 65 Univ of TN - Knoxville; 84–Dir/Sp-Lang Path, Lorain Comm Hosp, **SLP**

Whitney, Mrs Carolyn J 108 West 5th Avenue, Ritzville, WA 99169, (509) 659-0232, BA 69 Univ of WA; BA 73 Univ of WA; OM 74 Univ of WA; Resource Tchr Dir Spec Ed, Ritzville Sch Dist, **SLP**

Whitney, Cynthia Walker 261 Main Street, Apartment A, Nashua, NH 03060, (603) 424-6211, BA 83 MI St Univ; MA 84 MI St Univ; 88–Sp-Lang Path, SE Reg Educ Svc Ctr Inc, **SLP**

Whitney, Elizabeth Jane 184 Brig Court, Half Moon Bay, CA 94019, (415) 726-0750, BA 79 Univ of CA - Santa Barbara; MA 81 Univ of WA; 88–Aud, San Mateo Hearing Ctr, **A**

Whitney, Dr Janet L VA Medical Center 126, 1201 NW 16th Street, Miami, FL 33125, (305) 324-3148, BA 62 Northwestern Univ; MA 70 Case Western Reserve Univ; PH 88 (Sp-Lang Path) Univ of Pittsburgh - Pittsburgh; 88–Sp-Lang Path/Coord, VA Med Ctr, **SLP**

Whitney, Joan C 8641 Geren Road, Silver Spring, MD 20901, (301) 565-4383, MA 88 Univ of MD - College Park

Whitney, M Cerinda 701 Whispering Pine Road, Little Rock, AR 72210, (501) 758-6560, BS 81 Univ of AR - Little Rock; MS 83 Univ of AR - Little Rock; 85–Aud, NLR ENT Clinic, **A**

Whitney, Valerie K 231 South Gore, Webster Groves, MO 63119, (314) 962-4378, BS 73 Univ of MO - Columbia; MA 74 Univ of MO - Columbia; Sp-Lang Path, Spec School District, **SLP**

Whitsell, Mrs Patricia L 1342 South Kimbrough, Springfield, MO 65807, (417) 836-3767, MS 77 Southern IL Univ-Edwardsvill; Director Speech & Hearing, Cox Medical Centers, **SLP**

Whitson, Cynthia Ann Route 2 Box 59, Rudy, AR 72952, (501) 632-3537, BS 86 Univ of Central AR; MS 87 Univ of Central AR; 87–Sp-Lang Path, Bost Human Dev Svcs

Whitson, Edward T, Jr Piedmont ENT Da, 701 Arlington Avenue, Greenville, SC 29601, (803) 233-6881, BS 64 East TN St Univ; MS 68 Vanderbilt Univ; Aud, Piedmont ENT Pa, **A**

Whitson, Sally H 10404 West Sheridan Avenue, Milwaukee, WI 53225, (414) 352-3100, BS 77 Univ of WI - Oshkosh; MS 79 Univ of WI - Oshkosh; Aud, Milwaukee Med Cl S C, **A**

Whitt, Mrs Becky M Focus on Hearing, 2250 North Road, Snellville, GA 30278, (404) 972-4327, BA 75 Univ of AL- Tuscaloosa; MS 80 Univ of AR - Little Rock; Owner, Focus On Hearing, **SLP**

Whittacre, Mrs Pamela Jo 22 Hardwood Street, Cumberland, MD 21502, (304) 788-3881, BS 77 Indiana Univ of PA; MS 79 WV Univ; Sp-Lang Path, Mineral County Bd of Education, **SLP**

Whittaker, Mrs Debroah G P O Box 39, Quincy, CA 95971, (916) 283-3375, BA 75 Humboldt St Univ; MA 77 Humboldt St Univ; Sp-Lang Path, Plumas USD, **SLP**

Whittaker, Janice Sepe C-31 Glen Hollow Drive, Holtsville, NY 11742, (516) 475-1785, BA 84 Montclair St Coll; MS 86 Adelphi Univ

Whittaker, Robbie H 11569 Baylor Drive, Baton Rouge, LA 70816, (504) 927-6130, BS 80 LA St Univ - Baton Rouge; MA 82 LA St Univ - Baton Rouge; Sp-Lang Path, E Baton Rouge Parish Sch Bd, **SLP**

Whitted, Joyce Elaine 2813 Kendallwood Parkway #6, Gladstone, MO 64119, (816) 453-5050, BS 80 Central MO St Univ; MS 85 Central MO St Univ; N KS City Sch Dis, **SLP**

Whittemore, Cynthia 1242 Hathaway, Lakewood, OH 44107, (216) 221-3768, BS 84 Saint Louis Univ; MA 86 Case Western Reserve Univ; 86–Sp-Lang Path, Cleveland Metropolitan Hosp, **SLP**

Whittemore, Karen E 30209 Barwell Road, Farmington Hills, MI 48018, (313) 477-3630, BS 57 SUNY - Coll at Geneseo; MS 64 Purdue Univ - West Lafayette; 88–Sp-Lang Path, Carlin Unlimited, **SLP**

Whitten, Carol Ann 1502 N E 205th Avenue, Troutdale, OR 97060, (503) 255-1841, BS 83 Portland St Univ; Sp-Lang Path, Multnomah Educ Service Dist, **SLP**

Whitten, David A R R 2 Box 37, Oakland City, IN 47660, (812) 425-3561, BS 62 IN St Univ - Terre Haute; MS 68 IN St Univ - Terre Haute; 88–Sp-Lang Path, Visiting Nurse Assoc, **SLP**

Whitten, Debra A 3 Blaisdell Terrace, Ipswich, MA 01938, (617) 922-8920, BA 79 CA St Univ - Fresno; 87–Prog Coord, Morgan Memorial Goodwill Inst, **SLP**

Whitten, Ida E 5821 Gullstrand, San Diego, CA 92122, MA 34 Univ of NE - Lincoln; **SLP LM**

Whitten, Pam J #2 Seminole, West Plains, MO 65775, (417) 257-9111, BS 81 AR St Univ; MS 82 Univ of AR - Little Rock; Sp-Lang Path, Ozarks Med Ctr, **SLP**

Whitten, Terrie Ann 9014 Bouquet Road, Lake Worth, FL 33467, (407) 964-5247, BA 81 Univ of ME - Orono; MA 83 Univ of ME - Orono; Sp/Lang Path, Sch Bd of Palm Beach Co, **SLP**

Whittie, Lisa Carolyn 2329 Sherwood Lane, Havre de Grace, MD 21078, (301) 391-3940, BA 81 Univ of MD - College Park; MA 85 Univ of MD - College Park; 85–Sp-Lang Path, Balt Co PS, **SLP**

Whittinghill, Mrs E Jane 849 Edgehill Road, Glenside, PA 19038, (215) 887-4754, BA 76 Middlebury Coll; MA 78 Univ of Denver; **SLP**

Whittington, Mrs Barbara Coleridge 1200 South Harbor City Boulevard, Melbourne, FL 32901, (407) 724-4991, BS 71 FL St Univ; MS 72 FL St Univ; Sp-Lang Path, Melbourne Speech Clinic, **SLP ACE**

Whittington, Diane M 105 Aron, Lafayette, LA 70503, (318) 981-2084, BA 73 Univ of Southwestern LA; MA 74 Bowling Green St Univ; 86–Sp-Lang Path, Univ of Southwestern LA Dept of Communicative Disorders, **SLP**

Whittington, Kathryn E 625 Zamora Avenue, Coral Gables, FL 33134, BA 74 Univ of NC - Chapel Hill; MS 77 Univ of NC - Chapel Hill; OM 82 FL Int'l Univ; Sp-Lang Path and Aud, VA, **SLP A ACE**

Whittington, Mrs Mitzi J 8710 Galena Drive, El Paso, TX 79904-2561, (915) 751-2993, BA 77 Univ of MS; OM 78 Univ of MS; 88–Sp-Lang Path, Region XIX Educ Svc Ctr, **SLP**

Whittle, J Kathryn 119 Oakhart Drive, Glendora, CA 91740, (818) 335-3009, BA 72 Univ of Redlands; MA 75 CA St Univ - Los Angeles; 88–Instr, Calif State Univ-Fullerton, **SLP**

Whitton, Mrs Janna Gordon 2238 Fort Point Drive, Gold River, CA 95670, (916) 638-1724, BA 79 TX Tech Univ; MA 80 Univ of North TX; SLP, Eds, **SLP**

Whitton, Laura Ballantyne 254 Arlen Drive, Rohnert Park, CA 94928, (707) 795-4020, BA 77 Brigham Young Univ; OM 80 Brigham Young Univ; **SLP**

Whitton, Leon K 1207 Sunset Drive, Enid, OK 73703, (405) 237-6801, MA 57 Wichita St Univ; 74–Sp-Lang Path, I Dist #57 Enid PS, **SLP**

Whittredge, Dorothy K 1301 North West, Wichita, KS 67203, (316) 945-5245, BA 79 Wichita St Univ; MA 85 Wichita St Univ; **A**

Wholey, Mrs Marilyn K 3342 Montlake Drive, Rockford, IL 61111, (815) 633-6442, BS 71 Nazareth Coll of Rochester; MS 72 Syracuse Univ; Sp/Lang Path, Children's Dev Ctr, **SLP**

Whytlaw, Elizabeth E 315 East 8th, Apt 5, Northfield, MN 55057, (507) 645-6292, BA 76 Saint Olaf Coll; MS 79 Phillips Univ; SLP, Dept of Hlth & Welfare, **SLP**

Wiatrek, Susan Long 306 Graham Road, Kenedy, TX 78119, (512) 655-0691, BS 81 Southwest TX St Univ; ME 82 Southwest TX St Univ; Sp-Lang Path, Northeast ISD, **SLP**

Wiberg, Wendy A 5 Bellvista Road #6, Brookline, MA 02146, (617) 787-3390, BS 78 Univ of MA - Amherst; MA 80 NY Univ; Sp-Lang Path, Greenery Nursing Hm, **SLP**

Wiblin, Judith B 1073 South Hague Avenue, Columbus, OH 43204, (614) 451-6418, BS 69 Central St Univ; MA 78 OH St Univ; Asst Prin, Franklin Co Bd MR/DD, **SLP**

Wichman, Angela M 1320 South Conway #4, Marshall, MO 65340, (816) 761-3223, BS 83 Kearney St Coll; MS 84 Kearney St Coll; SLP, Med Ctr of Independence, **SLP**

Wichman, Rachel L 4105 Whitman Avenue North, Apartment 2, Seattle, WA 98103, (206) 632-7191, BA 71 Boston Univ; MS 75 Southern CT St Univ; OM 85 Smith Coll; 87–Sp-Lang Path, Sherwood Lvng Ctr, **SLP**

Wick, Carol Ann 1247 Garden Circle, Wyoming, OH 45215, (513) 761-0375, BS 74 Miami Univ - Oxford; MS 78 Miami Univ - Oxford; 74–Sp/Lang Path, Mt Healthy Cty Sch Bd of Ed, **SLP**

Wick, Diane J 3327 12th Avenue, Anoka, MN 55303, (612) 421-3906, BS 76 Univ of WI - River Falls; MA 79 Univ of MN - Duluth; SLP, Anoka-Hennepin Sch Dist, **SLP**

Wick, Eleanor A 105 North Highland Avenue, Bala-Cynwyd, PA 19004, (215) 664-7839, BA 69 Univ of Charleston; MA 72 Wichita St Univ; Pres, Sp Ther Inc, **SLP**

Wick, Erika 166 Central Park Road, Plainview, NY 11803, (516) 931-6622, BA 74 Univ of RI; MA 76 NY Univ; Sp/Lang Path, Wick and Penzi, **SLP**

Wick, Mrs Jacquelyn Lande 712 South 6th Street, St Charles, IL 60174, (312) 844-4534, BS 64 Univ of MN - Minneap-St Paul; MA 78 Northern IL Univ - De Kalb; Sp-Lang Path, School District 129, **SLP**

Wick, Laura Mary Baron 853 #B East Lynwood, San Bernardino, CA 92404, MS; **SLP LM**

Wick, Sharon L 444 Walnut Lane, Apple Valley, MN 55124, **SLP**

Wicka, Mrs Donna K 6801 North Pointe Drive, Troy, MI 48098, (313) 689-6000, BS 64 Western MI Univ; MA 69 Wayne St Univ; Sp-Lang Path, Troy Sch Dist, **SLP**

Wicka, Dr James R 430 Lovell Street, Worcester, MA 01602, (617) 791-6305, MA 68; ED 77 (Aud) Columbia Univ Teachers Coll; Dir of Sp-Lang Path, Haelen Medical Center, **SLP A**

Wickens, Alice R Wanda Rest Home, Bradford, VT 05033, PH (NS); **LM**

Wicker, Ellen R 1400 Dufossat, New Orleans, LA 70115, (504) 897-6349, BA 74 Univ of Pittsburgh - Pittsburgh; MA 75 Case Western Reserve Univ; Sp-Path, Jefferson Parish Bd of Ed, **SLP**

Wicker, Sharon 3025 Lake Avenue, Cheverly, MD 20785, (202) 722-5860, BS 83 James Madison Univ; MS 85 Gallaudet Coll; Audiologist, Gallaudet College, **A**

Wickersham, Mrs Jill Horrow 253 S Main Street, Sharon, MA 02067, **SLP**

Wickham, Mrs Claudia A 208 Westbury Park Road, Watertown, CT 06795, (203) 274-1400, BS 75 Trenton St Coll; MA 77 CUNY - City College; Supervisor, Dept Pf Mental Retardation, **SLP**

Wickman, Mrs Katherine 1979 May Court, Pleasant Hill, CA 94523, (415) 820-6815, BA 74 Univ of CA - Santa Barbara; MS 76 Univ of AZ; Sp-Lang Path, San Ramon Valley USD, **SLP**

Wickstrom-Kane, Susan Kay Laurel Crest Manor, Loretto Road Box 360, Ebensburg, PA 15931, (814) 472-8100, MA 83 Univ of Pittsburgh - Pittsburgh; Sp-Lang Path/Research Coord, Crossroads Speech-Hearing Inc, **SLP**

Wiczer, Ellen S 4915 Glenwood Hills Dr N E, Albuquerque, NM 87111, (505) 296-4496, BA 74 Carleton Coll; MS 81 Univ of NM; Sp/Lang Path, Sp & Lang Svcs, **SLP**

Widan, Margot 83 Winchester Street #6, Brookline, MA 02146, (617) 254-3800, BS 78; MS 82 Boston Univ; Sp/Lang Path, Kennedy Meorial Hospital, **SLP**

Widder, Carol Ash 622 East Maple, Fayetteville, AR 72701, (501) 521-7507, MS 87 Univ of WI - Madison; 88–Spec Educ Tchr, Fayetteville Pub Sch, **SLP**

Widdowson, H Douglas Allen Audiology & Hearing Inst, Allentown Medical Center, 401 North 17th St Ste 101, Allentown, PA 18104, (215) 439-1196, BS 75 Bloomsburg Univ of PA; ME 76 Bloomsburg Univ of PA; Owner/Aud, Allen Audiology & Hearing Inst, **A**

Widen, Dr Judith E Mailman Ctr For Child Develop, University Of Miami, P O Box 016820, Miami, FL 33101, (305) 547-5937, BA 69 WA St Univ; MS 74 Portland St Univ; PH 82 (Sp & Hrng Sciences) Univ of WA; 83–Dir of Sp & Hrng, U of Miami, **A ACE**

Widener, Dr Anna H 132 So Ribaut Road, Beaufort, SC 29902, (803) 524-7920, BA 71 George Washington Univ; MS 73 Purdue Univ - West Lafayette; PH 75 (NS) Purdue Univ - West Lafayette; Aud, Private Practice, **A ACE**

Widenhouse, Betty Lynn Route 1 Box 541, Boone, NC 28607, (704) 264-5987, BS 81 Appalachian St Univ; MA 86 Appalachian St Univ; 88–Sp-Lang Path, Communi-Care, **SLP**

Widi, Mrs Maureen Y 5115 Pennsbury Drive, Tampa, FL 33624, (813) 249-2939, BS 76 Univ of WI - Whitewater; MS 77 Univ of WI - Stevens Point; Aud, Hillsborough Cty Sch Syst, **A**

Widin, Dr Gregory P 3M Center, Bldg 270-4S-11, St Paul, MN 55144, (612) 736-6708, OB 74 Kenyon Coll; PH 79 (Experimental Psychology) Univ of MN - Minneap-St Paul; Hearing Research Supvr, 3M

Widlitz, Pamela 54 Westchester Heights, Milford, NH 03055, (603) 672-3504, BA 77 George Washington Univ; MA 79 Univ of CO - Boulder; Aud, **A**

Widofsky, Mrs Maureen Epton 9 Kingswood Way, Manalapan, NJ 07726, (201) 446-5998, BA 77 Hofstra Univ; MA 79 Hofstra Univ; Sp-Lang Path, Private Practice, **SLP**

Wiebler, Ladona Cunningham 5024 Chesterfield Cove, Mapleton, IL 61547-9735, (309) 697-1298, **SLP**

Wieczner, Loretta Levin 70 Ridge Avenue, Newton Center, MA 02159, (617) 899-0620, BS 73 Univ of WI - Madison; MS 74 Univ of WI - Madison; Primary Language Class Teacher, Weston Pub Sch, **SLP**

Wieczorek, Gregory F 1204 Givens Road, Manhattan, KS 66502, BA 71 John Carroll Univ; MA 73 Cleveland St Univ; Chief, Audiology Services, Irwin Army Hospital, **A**

Wieczorek, Judy C 4440 Laguna #307, Boulder, CO 80303, (303) 447-1010, BS 79 Univ of NE - Omaha; MS 81 Univ of NE - Omaha; Sp-Lang Path, Boulder Valley Sch Dist, **SLP**

Wiede, Margaret R 6357 Thomas Corners Road, West Valley, NY 14171, (716) 592-9805, BS 79 Ithaca Coll; MA 81 OH Univ - Athens; Sp-Lang Path, League for the Hndcpd Inc, **SLP**

Wiedel, Mrs Ida M Personally & Professional Speakg, 6225 Brookside Boulevard, Kansas City, MO 64113, (816) 444-8540, MA 72 Western MI Univ; Sp-Lang Path, Private Practice, **SLP**

Wiedermann, Faigie F 1924 East 24th Street, Brooklyn, NY 11229, (718) 376-2161, BA 75 CUNY - Brooklyn Coll; MS 79 CUNY - Brooklyn Coll; Sp-Lang Path, Private Practice, **SLP**

Wiedmer, Beatrix E 8009 Brooklyn Avenue NE, Seattle, WA 98115, (206) 485-0498, BA 76 Univ of CA - Berkeley; MS 83 Univ of WA; 80–Sp-Lang Path, Northshore Sch Dist #417, **SLP**

Wiegand, Mrs Judith F 5 School Street, Salem, MA 01970, (617) 878-7100, BA 62 Syracuse Univ; ME 69 PA St Univ - Univ Park; Sp-Lang Path, Communication Rehab Spec Inc, **SLP**

Wiegand, Kristy A Surgical Clinic, 429 South 6th Street, Vincennes, IN 47591, (812) 882-3280, BS 78 Ball St Univ; MS 80 IN St Univ - Terre Haute; Aud, Surgical Clinic of Vincennes, **A**

Wiegel, Mrs Terry Breeze 730 Valley Street, Dayton, OH 45404, (513) 222-5597, BS 79 Miami Univ - Oxford; MS 80 Miami Univ - Oxford; Sp-Lang Path, Dayton Hrng/Sp Cen, **SLP**

Wiegel, Valerie Frangos 665 Boston Post Road, Sudbury, MA 01776, (617) 532-0303, **SLP**

Wiegert, Katherine Mary 6917 Colonial Woods #9, St Louis, MO 63129, (314) 487-9080, MS 83 Fontbonne Coll; 83–Sp-Lang Path, Spec Sch Dist of St Louis Co, **SLP**

Wieland, Jerome W 743 North Elm, Cresco, IA 52136, (319) 547-4834, BA 78 Univ of Northern IA; MA 80 Univ of Northern IA; SLP, Keystone AEA, **SLP**

Wieland, Sue M 706 East 2nd Street, Cresco, IA 52136, (319) 547-4834, BA 79 Univ of Northern IA; MA 80 Univ of Northern IA; 80–Sp-Lang Path, Keystone AEA, **SLP**

Wieler, Constance 78 Garfield Street, Garden City, NY 11530, **SLP**

Wiemann, Mrs Janet M 800 North Anton Street, Marshfield, WI 54449, (715) 255-8655, BS 75 Univ of WI - Oshkosh; MS 79 Univ of WI - Stevens Point; Sp-Lang Path, Loyal Pub Sch, **SLP**

Wiemers, Mrs Pat Ann 221 East Ormonde Road, Arroyo Grande, CA 93420, BA 62 Univ of CA - Santa Barbara; MA 68 CA Poly St Univ-San Luis Obi; 68–Sp-Lang Path, Co Superintendent of Schs, **SLP**

Wiemeyer, Mrs Sandra Lynn 960 East Bonita Avenue, Apartment 130, Pomona, CA 91767, (714) 593-7521, MA 83 Univ of CA - Santa Barbara; Clin Dir, Casa Colina Rehab Hospital, **SLP**

Wiener, Debra A 330 East 85th Street, New York, NY 10028, (212) 340-6027, BS 79 Northwestern Univ; MA 81 Univ of MN - Minneap-St Paul; Sp-Lang Path, Rusk I of Rehab Med, **SLP**

Wiener, Diane F L 7 Steeplechase Drive, Marlboro, NJ 07746, (201) 308-9577, BS 73 CUNY - Brooklyn Coll; MS 76 CUNY - Brooklyn Coll; SLP, New York City Board of Educ, **SLP**

Wiener, Mrs Elana Sue 2105 43rd Street SE, Grand Rapids, MI 49508, (616) 455-9780, BS 83 Univ of Cincinnati; MA 86 Cleveland St Univ; 88–Sp-Lang Path, Jenison PS, **SLP**

Wiener, Iris F 7150 Rockford Street, Portage, MI 49002, (616) 323-9523, BS 85 Western MI Univ; MA 86 Western MI Univ

Wiener, Mrs Marlene W 365 Constitution Circle, North Brunswick, NJ 08902, (201) 499-5632, BA 70 Jersey City St Coll; MA 79 Kean Coll of NJ; 70–Aud, Woodbridge Dev Ctr, **A**

Wiener-Maran, P 211-65 23rd Avenue, Apt 6-H, Bayside, NY 11360, (718) 224-7358, BA 76 CUNY - Hunter Coll; MS 77 Adelphi Univ; Exec Dir, Therapies Unlimited, **SLP**

Wienke, Susan Allyson 221 North Cross Street, Sycamore, IL 60178, (815) 895-6265, MA 87; 87–Sp-Lang Path, Genoa-Kingston Dist #424

Wierdo, Patricia L 37 N 23rd Street, Kenilworth, NJ 07033, (201) 766-7766, BA 82 Kean Coll of NJ; MA 83 Kean Coll of NJ; Sp-Lang Path, Private Practice, **SLP**

Wiers, Mrs Kathleen A 203 Scout Way, Depere, WI 54115, BA 69 Creighton Univ; MS 70 Purdue Univ - West Lafayette; **A**

Wiersema, Gregory N 567 South Park Avenue, Fond Du Lac, WI 54935, (414) 929-1224, BS 74 Univ of WI - Oshkosh; MS 77 Univ of WI - Oshkosh; 77–Aud, St Agnes Hospital, **A**

Wiese, Enid 142 Trent Road, Penn Wynne, PA 19151, **SLP**

Wiese, Mrs Marie Altmeyer 9639 Shipwright Drive, Burke, VA 22015, (703) 978-0113, BA 70 Fontbonne Coll; MS 84 SUNY - Coll at Buffalo; Sp-Lang Path, Fairfax Co Pub Schs, **SLP**

Wiese, Mrs Sally Bush 5173 South Laredo Way, Aurora, CO 80015, (303) 796-0109, **SLP**

Wiesenborn, Mrs Gloria K 1501 Spur Street, Alvin, TX 77511, (409) 935-3031, BS 54 Washington Univ; MA 70 Univ of Houston - Univ Park; SLP, La Marque ISD, **SLP**

Wiesner, Civia Renne 1821 East 5th Street #11, Long Beach, CA 90802, (213) 435-3042, BA 80 CA St Univ - Long Beach; MA 83 CA St Univ - Long Beach; SLP, Los Angeles USD, **SLP**

Wiesner, Eric C 1416 Creek Pointe, Farmington, NY 14425, (716) 924-4717, BA 79 SUNY - Center at Buffalo; MA 81 Long Island U - CW Post Ctr; 88–Sp-Lang Path, Monroe Dev Cen/BOCES II, **SLP**

Wiesner, Gaye B 86 Elson Street, Staten Island, NY 10314, (718) 761-6921, BA 73 CUNY - Brooklyn Coll; MS 75 CUNY - Brooklyn Coll; Sp-Lang Path, NYC Bd of Educ, **SLP**

Wiesner-Sims, Myra 206 South Plainville Avenue, Plainville, KS 67663, (913) 434-7295, BA 81 Fort Hays St Univ; MS 83 Fort Hays St Univ; Sp-Lang Path, N Ctrl Ks Spec Ed Coop, **SLP**

Wigall, Mrs Loleata D 296 Lowell Street, Lawrence, MA 01841, (617) 662-7499, BA 72 Univ of Redlands; MS 74 Bradley Univ; Dir of Aud, Atlantic Aud Assn, **A**

Wigent, Michael Robert 528 35-1/2 Road, Palisades, CO 81526, (303) 243-5236, BS 71 Western MI Univ; MS 72 Univ of RI; Sp-Lang Path, Mesa Co Valley Sch Dist #51, **SLP**

Wigent, Mrs Sue A Route 3 P O Box 39-Wa, Ligonier, IN 46767, (219) 894-3418, BS 63 Purdue Univ - West Lafayette; MA 67 Ball St Univ; SLP, Noble Co Trng Cen, **SLP**

Wiggins, Mrs Frances A 115 West Ann, New Braunfels, TX 78130, (512) 625-9514, BS 77 Southwest TX St Univ; ME 78 Southwest TX St Univ; Tchr, Comal ISD, **SLP**

Wiggins, M Eugene 11632 Stewart Lane #101, Silver Spring, MD 20904, (202) 727-2608, BS 63 Hampton Univ; MS 69 Univ of MI - Ann Arbor; Sp-Lang Path, U of the DC, **SLP**

Wiggins, Mrs Patsy J 529 Oak Street, Chattanooga, TN 37403, MS 65 Auburn Univ - Auburn; SLP, Chattanooga Speech Center, **SLP**

Wiggins, Mrs Sheri Freeman 9018 Theysen, Houston, TX 77080, (713) 461-3103, BS 84 Univ of OK - OK City; MS 86 Univ of North TX; 87–Sp-Lang Path, InSpeech Inc, **SLP**

Wigginton, Virginia M 4200 Norma Avenue, Arden Hills, MN 55112, (612) 626-3457, BS 66 Univ of TN - Knoxville; MA 77 Univ of MN - Minneap-St Paul; Sp-Lang Path, Chldn Rehab Cen-U of MN Hosp, **SLP**

Wiggle, Linda Lee 21286 Danbury, Trenton, MI 48183, (313) 246-1077, MA 85 Eastern MI Univ; SLP, Wyandotte Ps, **SLP**

Wight, Mrs Carol Ann 221 Park Street, Williamstown, MA 01267, (413) 458-3376, BS 63 SUNY - Center at Buffalo; MA 64 Univ of WI - Madison; Sp-Lang Path, Williamstown Pub Sch, **SLP**

Wight, Darlene V Gracelane College, Lamoni, IA 50140, MA Univ of KS; **SLP**

Wight, Karen M 2241 Yewell's Landing Nort, H Apt B, Owensboro, KY 42303, (502) 683-4250, BA 79 Univ of FL; MS 80 FL St Univ; 86–Sp/Lang Path, Private Practice, **SLP**

Wight, Mrs Marallyn M Rural Route 1, 307 West Franklin, Clinton, MI 49236, (517) 456-4694, BA 43 Univ of MI - Ann Arbor; MA 44 Univ of MI - Ann Arbor; 55–Retired, Lenawee Inter Sch Dist, **SLP LM**

Wigim, Elizabeth Ann 1756 Sherry Lane #33, Santa Ana, CA 92701, (714) 639-4990, BA 81 Univ of Redlands; MA 83 Univ of IA; Sp-Lang Path, Providence Sp & Hrng Ctr, **SLP**

Wiginton, Mrs Julie Solow 15231 Haley Drive, Choctaw, OK 73020, (405) 390-8585, MA 86 Univ of Science & Arts of OK; **SLP**

Wigton-Feetham, Mrs Lauri E 2750 Kern Avenue, San Jose, CA 95121, (408) 998-6030, BA 82 San Jose St Univ; **SLP**

Wiig, Dr Elisabeth H 7101 Lake Powell Drive, Arlington, TX 76016, (817) 478-5946, BS 56; MA 60 Case Western Reserve Univ; PH 67 (NS) Case Western Reserve Univ; Author, Private Practice, **SLP A F**

Wika, Carol L 5844 West Bernice Avenue, Chicago, IL 60634, (312) 272-5652, BA 76 Mundelein Coll; MA 78 Northwestern Univ; Sp-Lang Path, Northbrook Sch Dist, **SLP**

Wiksell, Carla Maria 113 Evergreen Ct Apt A, Bardstown, KY 40004, (502) 348-1302, BS 84 Murray St Univ; MA 85 Univ of TN - Knoxville; 86–Sp-Lang Path, Bardstown City Schs Sys, **SLP**

Wikstrom, Pia Rd #1 Parker Road Box 46, Lockwood, NY 14859, (607) 589-6444, BA 77 Hofstra Univ; MA 78 Hofstra Univ; **SLP**

Wilansky, Mrs Judith A P 2425 Knobhill Drive, North Bellmore, NY 11710, MA 76 CUNY - Queens Coll; 84–Sp-Lang Path, Hewlett-Woodmere Ufsd, **SLP**

Wilber, Kelly K 1137 Hawkins Grad House, West Lafayette, IN 47906, (317) 495-1655, BS 85 Purdue Univ - West Lafayette; MS 87 Purdue Univ - West Lafayette

Wilber, Dr Laura Ann 422 Skokie Boulevard, Wilmette, IL 60091, (312) 491-2470, BS 55 Univ Southern MS-Hattiesburg; MS 58 Gallaudet Coll; PH 64 (Aud) Northwestern Univ; 78–Prof of Aud, Nwnu, **SLP A F**

Wilbert, Dr Karen M 165 Fletcher Road, Ponchatoula, LA 70454, (504) 549-2214, BS 74 LA St Univ - Baton Rouge; OM 75 LA St Univ - N O Medical Ctr; PH 87 (Sp & Hrng Science) Univ Southern MS-Hattiesburg; 88–Coord of Cl Svcs, New Medico Rehab Ctr, **SLP**

Wilbourn, Mrs Carmen R Route 2 Box 417, Pullman, WA 99163, (509) 332-3581, BS 76 WA St Univ; MA 78 WA St Univ; Pullman Pub Schls, **SLP**

Wilbourn, Mrs Carolyn Springer 721 Brightridge Drive, Bridgeport, WV 26330, (304) 624-3254, BS 64 WV Univ; MS 65 WV Univ; Sp-Lang Path, Harrison Co Bd of Ed, **SLP**

Wilbur, Mrs Amelia O 3070 Eden Court, Medford, OR 97504, BS 68 UT St Univ; MA 69 UT St Univ; **SLP**

Wilbur, Anita A 7 Pheasant Ridge Circle, Henderson, NV 89014, (702) 451-0014, BS 77 Univ of SD - Vermillion; MA 78 Univ of SD - Vermillion; Sp-Lang Path/Sp Ed Tchr, Clark Co Sch Dist, **SLP**

Wilburn, Mrs Duana Charles 7406 Autumn Bent Way, Crestwood, KY 40014, (513) 385-0321, BS 76 Eastern KY Univ; MA 81 OH Univ - Athens; 86–Sp-Lang Path, Private Practice, **SLP**

Wilburn, Michael Alan 629 North Brainard, La Grange Park, IL 60525, (312) 687-0900, BS 77 Western IL Univ; MA 80 Western WA Univ; Sp-Lang Path, SW Cook Co Coop Assn Spec Ed, **SLP**

Wilcomb, Jennifer L 4541 Antique Lane, Raleigh, NC 27604, (919) 850-9246, **SLP**

Wilcott, Mrs Kathleen Marie 91 Cherry Street, (Upstairs), West Orange, NJ 07052, MA 83 Univ of Houston - Univ Park; Sp-Lang Path, **SLP**

Wilcox, Mrs Aneita R R 1 Box 26, Wakonda, SD 57073, (605) 267-2644, BS 73 Univ of SD - Vermillion; MA 74 Univ of SD - Vermillion; Coord Sp-Lang Path Svc, Southeast Area Coop, **SLP**

Wilcox, Aneita W D Route 2 Box 178-A, Jonesboro, TN 37659, (615) 753-3216, MA 69 East TN St Univ; SLP, Kingspoint City Schools, **SLP**

Wilcox, Dr Colleen Bridget Superintendent NSSED, 760 Red Oak Lane, Highland Park, IL 60035, (312) 831-5100, BS 71 Univ of IA; MS 74 Univ of AZ; PH 86 (NS) Univ of Southern CA; Supt, Northern Suburban Spec Educ Dist, **SLP**

Wilcox, Mrs Dana Lefler Route 2 Box 392, Greenbrier, AR 72058, (501) 679-2112, **SLP**

Wilcox, Edna B 1220 Northwood Road #2301, Seal Beach, CA 90740, MS; **SLP LM**

Wilcox, Mrs Jeri Milner HCR 32 Box 119OX 119, Fort Pierre, SD 57532, BA 77 Univ of SD - Vermillion; MA 78 Univ of SD - Vermillion; SLP, Stanley Co Sch Dist 57-1, **SLP**

Wilcox, Juli 519 West Riverside Drive, Yankton, SD 57078, (402) 254-3947, BS 67 SD St Univ; MA 68 Univ of SD - Vermillion; Dir Spec Ed/Sp-Lang Path, Hartington Pub Sch, **SLP**

Wilcox, Dr Kim Speech - Language - Hearing Science & Disorders, University Of Kansas, 2101 Haworth Hall, Lawrence, KS 66045, (913) 864-4690, BA 76 MI St Univ; MS 78 Purdue Univ - West Lafayette; PH 80 (NS) Purdue Univ - West Lafayette; Assoc Prof, U of KS, **SLP**

Wilcox, Laura Lynn 1345 Victoria Drive #D, Fullerton, CA 92631, BS 85 OH Univ - Athens; MA 87 OH Univ - Athens; **SLP**

Wilcox, Mrs Linda A 4657 Selkirk, Fremont, CA 94538, (415) 657-2350, BS 73 CA St Univ - Hayward; MA 76 San Jose St Univ; SLP, Fremont USD, **SLP**

Wilcox, Lynn H 1413 7th Street, Aurora, NE 68818, (402) 463-2848, BS 67 OK St Univ; MS 78 Phillips Univ; SLP, Educational Service Unit 9, **SLP**

Wilcox, Dr M Jeanne Speech And Hearing Clinic, Kent State University, Kent, OH 44242, (216) 672-2672, BA 74 KS St Univ; MA 76 Memphis St Univ; PH 79 (NS) Memphis St Univ; Associate Professor, Kent State University, **SLP**

Wilcox, Patricia Sue 2240 27th Avenue Court, Greeley, CO 80631, (330) 339-5360, OM 85 Fort Hays St Univ; **SLP**

Wilcox, Paulette M 1940 Pleasant Meadows, Portage, IN 46368, (219) 763-2087, BS 75 IN Univ - Bloomington; OM 76 IN Univ - Bloomington; **SLP**

Wilcox, Mrs Rebecca Ann 1350 Whispering Pine Road, Little Rock, AR 72210, (501) 821-4536, BS 83 Univ of Central AR; MS 86 Univ of Central AR

Wilcox, Sharon K Sharon Wilcox Speech Pathology, 3757 State Street, Suite 207, Santa Barbara, CA 93105, BA 74 Univ of Redlands; MS 76 Univ of Redlands; Sp/Lang Path, Private Practice, **SLP**

Wilcox, Mrs Susan Scott 653 Fallow Court, Gahanna, OH 43230, (614) 462-3270, BS 77 Bowling Green St Univ; MS 83 Miami Univ - Oxford; SLP, Groveport Madison Schs, **SLP**

Wilcox, Vonda L 640 13th Street N E, Mason City, IA 50401, (515) 423-8371, BS 72 Minot St Univ; MS 73 Minot St Univ; SLP, Northern Trails AEA, **SLP**

Wilcoxen, Dr Anne Glover 224 Eighth Street, Manhattan Beach, CA 90266, BS 66 Univ of OK - Norman; MA 69 George Washington Univ; PH 84 (Educ Psych) Univ of CA - Los Angeles; Lecturer, UCLA, **SLP**

Wilde, Dr Graham L 4126 Birchtree Drive, Martinez, GA 30907, (404) 868-8560, BS 72 Central MO St Univ; MS 64 Central MO St Univ; Aud, US Army, **A**

Wilde, Mrs Jana R 1390 Appomattox Trail, Carol Stream, IL 60188, (312) 377-4863, BA 80 Coll of Saint Francis; MS 81 Univ of IL - Urbana; Sp-Lang Path, Marianjoy Rehab Hosp, **SLP**

Wilde, Lorin F 48 Chestnut Street, Stoneham, MA 02180, (617) 876-6819, **A**

Wilde, Mrs Nancy Jo R Speech & Hearing Centre, PO Box 186, Wembley, West Australia, Australia 6014, BA 70 Univ of Detroit; MA 72 Wayne St Univ; Aud, Speech and Hearing Centre, **A**

Wilde, Dr Ronald A Curtin University Of Technology, Department Speech & Hearing SCI, GPO Box U 1987, Perth, West Australia, Australia 6001, BA 62 Univ of CO - Boulder; MA 68 Wayne St Univ; PH 77 (NS) Wayne St Univ; 83–Lecturer, Curtin Univ of Tech, **A**

Wilder, Dr Carol N Hemlock Hill Road, R R 4 Box 16, Pound Ridge, NY 10576, (212) 678-3415, OM 51 Univ of MI - Ann Arbor; MS 67 Columbia Univ Teachers Coll; PH 72 Columbia Univ Teachers Coll; Cl Assoc/Adj Assoc Prof, Tchrs Coll-Columbia U, **SLP**

Wilder, Carolyn S 12403 Alexander Cornell Dr, Fairfax, VA 22033, BA 69 Mary Washington Coll; MA 74 Our Lady Lake Univ-San Anton; 87–Sp-Lang Path, Fairfax County PS, **SLP**

Wilder, Mrs June Harris 2980 Sandstone Trail N W, Marietta, GA 30064, (404) 980-1744, BS 82 Univ of GA; ME 83 Univ of GA; Sp-Lang Path, Easter Seal, **SLP**

Wilder, Kathryn V 345 Linda Lane, West Palm Beach, FL 33405, BS 75 East Carolina Univ; MS 79 Univ of NC - Chapel Hill; Aud, ENT Assoc Inc, **A**

Wilder, Mrs Martha J Route 4 Box 394, Saluda, SC 29138, (803) 445-7800, BS 75 Western Carolina Univ; MA 79 Western Carolina Univ; Sp/Lang Path, Private Practice, **SLP**

Wilder, Mrs Mary K 4014 East 36th Avenue, Spokane, WA 99223, (509) 448-2180, BS 73 Southern IL Univ -Carbondale; MS 74 Univ of OK Medical Center; Aud, Edward L Treyve, M D, **A**

Wilder, Pauline L 1203 Big Rock Loop, Los Alamos, NM 87544, (505) 662-7768, BS 69 Phillips Univ; MA 71 Univ of Denver; 87–Sp-Lang Path, Private Practice, **SLP**

Wilder, Mrs Suzanne Marie 1344 Wild Rose Lane, Neenah, WI 54956, (414) 727-4989, BS 83 Univ of WI - Whitewater; MS 84 Univ of WI - Whitewater; 85–Sp-Lang Path, Central Wisconsin Rehab Assoc, **SLP**

Wildgen, Mrs Patricia Long 2036 Crestdale Drive, Stow, OH 44224, (216) 688-9549, BS 66 Dickinson Coll; MA 85 Kent St Univ; 88–Sp-Lang Path, Akron PS, **SLP**

Wildhagen, Dwayne L c/o Rocky Mountain Ear Inst, 4701 East 9th Avenue, Denver, CO 80220, (813) 293-8998, BS 74 CO St Univ; MA 75 Univ of Northern CO; Aud, Rocky Mountain Ear Institute, **A**

Wildman, Mrs Myra 9 Ramsgate Drive, St Louis, MO 63132, (314) 993-5797, BS 57 Washington Univ; MS 80 Washington Univ; **SLP**

Wildman, Susan L 52 Williamsburg Road, Evanston, IL 60203, BS 71 Ball St Univ; MA 74 Ball St Univ; MA 82 LA Verne Coll; Sp-Lang Path, Wildman Sp & Lang Ctr, **SLP**

Wilds, Daena Cheryl Huntertown Road, Versailles, KY 40383, (606) 873-3005, BA 83 Univ of TN - Knoxville; MS 85 Univ of Louisville; 86–Aud, Lexington Hearing and Sp Ctr, **A**

Wildt, Mrs Cathleen Frances 5517 North Bay Ridge, Whitefish Bay, WI 53217, (414) 225-8130, BS 82 Marquette Univ; MS 84 Marquette Univ; Supvr-SLP Dept, Saint Mary Hospital, **SLP**

Wilensky, Diane S Ear Nose & Throat Department, LSU Medical Center, 1542 Tulane Avenue, New Orleans, LA 70112, (504) 568-4785, BS 71; MS 73 Tulane Univ; Asst Prof, L S U Med Cen, **SLP**

Wiles, Dr Lora H 101 Broadview Court, Columbia, MO 65201, (314) 474-1580, BA 83 Univ of MO - KS City; MA 86 Univ of KS; PH 88 (Aud) Univ of KS; **A**

Wiley, Kay D 11542 Janette Lane, Garden Grove, CA 92640, (714) 530-5227, BS 74 CO St Univ; MS 76 CO St Univ; 86–Sp-Lang Path, Newport Lang Sp & Aud Ctr Inc, **SLP ACE**

Wiley, Mrs Linda Chisholm 8633 East Davies Avenue, Englewood, CO 80112, (303) 794-6225, BS 80 CO St Univ; MS 82 CO St Univ; SLP, Littleton Pub Schools 6, **SLP**

Wiley, Martha V 3930 Madison SE, Portland, OR 97214, (503) 236-9466, MS 88 Univ of OR; 88, Child Dev & Rehab Ctr

Wiley, Pam W 10 Tappan Court, Orinda, CA 94563, (415) 254-9073, BS 73 Univ of Southern CA; MS 75 Univ of WI - Madison; **A**

Wiley, Terry L Dept Communicative Disorders, Univ Of WI Goodnight Hall, 1975 Willow Drive, Madison, WI 53706, (608) 262-3951, BA 65 Univ of Northern IA; MS 68 CO St Univ; PH 72 (NS) Univ of IA; Prof, Commun Dis U of WI Madison, **A F**

Wiley-Shreffler, Yvonne Kay Route 1 Box 670, Grottoes, VA 24441-9521, (703) 249-3000, MA 86 Edinboro Univ of PA; 86–Sp-Lang Path, InSpeech Inc, **SLP**

Wilger, Terese Marie 1111 South 8th Street #A, Manitowoc, WI 54220-5309, (414) 683-4090, BS 84 Marquette Univ; MS 85 Marquette Univ; 85–Sp-Lang Path, Manitowoc Co Hndcpd Chldn Educ Prog, **SLP**

Wilhelm, Dr Charles L Box 432, Hays, KS 67601, (913) 628-5366, BS 65 Univ of KS; MS 67 Univ of KS; PH 70 (NS) Univ of KS; Dir/Commun Dis, Ft Hays State University, **SLP**

Wilhelm, Katherine Loridas 11 Carlton Club Drive, Piscataway, NJ 08854, (201) 968-9170, BS 83 Northern MI Univ; MA 86 Eastern MI Univ; **SLP**

Wilhelm, Mrs Sammie Sexton Box 432, Hays, KS 67601, (913) 628-5366, BA 68 Univ of KS; MA 72 Univ of KS; Supen Inst In Commun Clinic, Fort Hays State Universtiy, **SLP**

Wilhite, Mrs Diane R 1733 Lindy Drive, Lansing, MI 48917-9734, (517) 353-8780, BA 76; MA 79 Cleveland St Univ; Clinicaal Spec, MI St U, **SLP**

Wilhite, Irvin P O Box 23495, Baton Rouge, LA 70893, (504) 343-4232, BA 66 Tulane Univ; MA 73 LA St Univ - Baton Rouge; Sp-Lang Path /Aud, Ctr for Sp-Hrng-Lrng Dis, **SLP A**

Wilke, Mrs Debra D Route 20 Box 311, San Antonio, TX 78218, BS 78 Southwest TX St Univ; ME 79 Southwest TX St Univ; **SLP**

Wilke, Debra J 4582 Jonathan Lane N W, Cedar Rapids, IA 52405, (319) 390-3568, BA 79 Univ of Northern IA; MA 80 Univ of Northern IA; Sp-Lang Path, Grant Wood AEA, **SLP**

Wilke, Rosalie A 30 Santa Anita, Edwardsville, IL 62025, (314) 868-5330, MS 78 Southern IL Univ -Carbondale; SLP, **SLP**

Wilke, Mrs Sara Bachmann 609 Spruce, North Platte, NE 69101, (308) 534-1616, BS 85 Univ of NE - Lincoln; MS 86 Univ of NE - Lincoln; 88–Sp-Lang Path, Educ Service Unit #16, **SLP**

Wilke, Star Wood 1627 Green River Drive, Schaumburg, IL 60194-4510, (312) 628-2550, BS 67 Culver-Stockton Coll; MA 69 Univ of MO - Columbia; SLP, Bd of Ed Sch Dist #4, **SLP**

Wilkens, Connie Marie 1106 West 17th Street, Hutchinson, KS 67501, (316) 663-7178, BS 79 Fort Hays St Univ; MS 81 Fort Hays St Univ; 81–Sp-Lang Path, Reno County Educ Coop Dist #610

Wilkens, Jeannette 31-85 Crescent Street #315, Long Island, NY 11106, (212) 920-5894, BA 73 Long Island U - Brooklyn Ctr; MS 75 Columbia Univ Teachers Coll; ME 85 Columbia Univ Teachers Coll; Chief Sp-Lang Path & Hrng, Beth Abraham Hosp, **SLP**

Wilkerson, Mrs Dorian Lee 1785 Lisa Drive #12, Indiana, PA 15701, (412) 357-2454, BS 77 Hampton Univ; MS 78 Indiana Univ of PA; PH 88 (Sp Path) Howard Univ; 86–Asst Prof, Indiana Univ of PA, **SLP**

Wilkerson, Janet Ellen 1324 Essex Way Unit #1, San Jose, CA 95117, (408) 866-8552, BA 80 San Jose St Univ; MA 85 San Jose St Univ; 86–Sp-Lang Path, San Jose USD, **SLP**

Wilkerson, Mrs Jill K 17410 Marda Avenue, Yorba Linda, CA 92686, BA 78 Univ of SD - Vermillion; MS 80 AZ St Univ; 86–Sp-Lang Path, Casa Colina Hosp, **SLP**

Wilkerson, Kenneth Dwayne 725 West 17th Lane, Portales, NM 88130, (505) 356-5574, BS 81 Eastern NM Univ; MS 83 Eastern NM Univ; Sp-Lang Path, Portales Pub Sch, **SLP**

Wilkerson, Linda 9605 West 103rd St Terrace, Overland Park, KS 66212, **A**

Wilkerson, Mary Ann Route 2 Box 520-4, Scottsburg, IN 47170, (812) 948-5758, BA 70 Bellarmine Coll; ME 72 Univ of Louisville; SLP, Floyd Co Consolidated Sch Dist, **SLP**

Wilkerson, Michele L 2908 Cunnington Lane, Kettering, OH 45420, BS 85 Miami Univ - Oxford; MS 86 Miami Univ - Oxford; **SLP**

Wilkes, Mrs Deborah Egly 2002 Merrimac Trail, Garland, TX 75043, (214) 840-0822, BS 76 TX Tech Univ; MS 77 Univ of North TX; Sp-Lang Path, **SLP**

Wilkes, Elizabeth Reid 1784 Jameston Drive, Charlotte, NC 28209, (704) 376-1377, BA 84 Univ of SC - Columbia; OM 86 Univ of SC - Columbia; 87–Sp-Lang Path, LOGOS, **SLP**

Wilkes, Mrs Pamela Taylor 18 Old Pond Way, Columbia, SC 29212-5312, (803) 781-3686, BA 74 Columbia Coll; MS 76 Univ of SC - Columbia; 87–Sp-Lang Path, Private Practice, **SLP ACE**

Wilkes-Travers, Judith 520 Winding Way, Warminster, PA 18974, BA 76 West Chester Univ of PA; MS 78 Trenton St Coll; **SLP**

Wilkey, Mrs Marjorie C 9256 South Richmond Avenue, Evergreen Park, IL 60642, (312) 422-3462, BS 77 Western IL Univ; MA 78 Univ of IL - Urbana; Sp-Lang Path, Private Practice Consult, **SLP**

Wilkie, Mary Ellen 920-F South Dahlia, Denver, CO 80222, (303) 758-5152, BA 78 Univ of ND; MS 79 Minot St Univ; OD 84 (NS) Univ of ND; Association Attorney, Koransky Friedman & Cohen, **A**

Wilkie, Pamela C 38 Kensington Place, Brighton, England BN1 4EL, BA 57 Univ of Cambridge - England; OM 64 Univ of Cambridge - England; MA 81 George Washington Univ; Sp-Lang Path, Montgomery Co Pub Sch, **SLP**

Wilkins, Alice Maxine 173 Alabama Avenue, Hempstead, NY 11550, (516) 489-5490, BS 79 Saint John's Univ - Jamaica; MS 82 Adelphi Univ; 88–Sp-Lang Path, New York Foundling Hosp, **SLP**

Wilkins, Mrs Angela R 7427 Harbour Pt, Indianapolis, IN 46240, (317) 251-4563, BS 86 Ball St Univ; MA 88 Ball St Univ; 88–Aud, The Ear Institute Inc

Wilkins, Carol Marlene 56 Country Lane, London, ON, Canada N5Y 2H5, (519) 667-6558, BA 70 Univ of Western Ontario; MA 72 Univ of Western Ontario; OM 83 Univ of Western Ontario; 88–Sp-Lang Path, Victoria Hosp Corp, **SLP**

Wilkins, Mrs Deborah M 227 Rochester Road, Mobile, AL 36608, (205) 344-6514, BA 76 Univ of AL- Tuscaloosa; MA 81 LA St Univ - Baton Rouge; Sp-Lang Path, Private Practice, **SLP**

Wilkins, Elizabeth Kathleen 3500 Earlmont, Clovis, NM 88101, BS 84 Eastern NM Univ; MS 86 Eastern NM Univ; 87–Sp-Lang Path, Southeastern NM Sp & Hrng Clinic, **SLP**

Wilkins, Mrs Georgiann 4260 Braganza Avenue, Miami, FL 33133, (305) 661-1318, BS 71 G Peabody Coll-Vanderbilt U; MA 72 Univ of Houston - Univ Park; Sp-Lang Path, **SLP**

Wilkins, Lucinda M 23324 106th Avene S E, Kent, WA 98031, BA 79 WA St Univ; MA 81 WA St Univ; Sp-Lang Path, **SLP**

Wilkins, Mary Kathleen 266 East Carmel Drive, Mobile, AL 36608, **A**

Wilkins, Raymond A 306 Leveland Lane, Modesto, CA 95350, **SLP A**

Wilkins, Mrs Rita Ann 5515 Los Robles, La Verne, CA 91750, (818) 446-0131, BA 76 Univ of CA - Los Angeles; MA 80 CA St Univ - Northridge; Sp-Lang Path, Arcadia USD, **SLP ACE**

Wilkins, Sandra M Regional Guidance Center, 620 South 3rd, McAlester, OK 74501, (918) 423-1267, BS 66 Univ of KS; MS 71 Univ of OK Medical Center; Sp-Lang Path, Regional Guid Cen, **SLP**

Wilkinson, Mrs Carol R P O Box 711, Zuni, NM 87327, (505) 782-4441, BS 69 Bowling Green St Univ; MS 84 Eastern NM Univ; **SLP**

Wilkinson, Mrs Cheryl Shipman 1824 Park Lane Drive, Edmond, OK 73034, (405) 340-1416, BA 83 Univ of OK - Norman; MS 85 Univ of OK Medical Center; SLP, Speech and Hearing Associates, **SLP**

Wilkinson, Dianne Lynn 5528 Southdirle Drive #B, St Louis, MO 63129-6133, (712) 322-7354, **A**

Wilkinson, Dominique 503 Towne House Village, Hauppauge, NY 11788, (516) 673-1624, BS 76 Syracuse Univ; MS 77 Columbia Univ Teachers Coll; Sp-Lang Path, South Huntington Sch, **SLP**

Wilkinson, Mrs Esther Ruth 12620 West Atlantic Avenue, Lakewood, CO 80228, (303) 985-0610, BA 37 Dakota Wesleyan Univ; MA 38 Univ of Denver; **SLP LM**

Wilkinson, Glenna S N 112 Keeler Drive, Ridgefield, CT 06877, (203) 790-7613, BS 71 Northeast MO St Univ; MA 73 Northeast MO St Univ; Sp-Lang Path, Ridgefield Ct Sch Sys, **SLP**

Wilkinson, Jane Raub 124 Lee Ann Court, Bowling Green, KY 42101-9739, (502) 843-3296, BS 59 IN Univ - Bloomington; MS 83 Western KY Univ; Instructor/ Clinic Supervisor, Wn KY U, **SLP**

Wilkinson, Mrs Jean M 835 Linden Hall Road, Chattanooga, TN 37415, (615) 877-9458, BS 54 East TN St Univ; MA 59 G Peabody Coll-Vanderbilt U; Sp-Lang Path, Walker County Board of Educ, **SLP A**

Wilkinson, Mrs Margaret M 3 Jumping Brook Drive, Neptune, NJ 07753, (201) 528-6400, BA 71 Kean Coll of NJ; MA 75 Montclair St Coll; 71–Sp/Lang Path, Brielle/Sp Lake Hgts Bd of Ed, **SLP**

Wilkinson, Melissa K 625 Piney Branch #204, Virginia Beach, VA 23451, (919) 929-0929, MS 88 Univ of NC - Chapel Hill

Wilkinson, Mrs Pamela Meinders 10407 Windsor View Drive, Potomac, MD 20854, (301) 279-8592, BS 65 OH St Univ; OM 77 LA St Univ - N O Medical Ctr; Sp-Lang Path, Montgomery County Pub Schools, **SLP**

Wilkinson, Dr Robert J 3004 Grandin Road S W, Roanoke, VA 24018, (703) 774-5513, BA 62 Montclair St Coll; MA 67 Montclair St Coll; ED 70 (Sp-Lang Path) Univ of VA - Charlottesville; Sp-Lang Path, Private Practice, **SLP**

Wilkinson, Sue A C Route 4 Box 33, Brahman Road, Kingston, TN 37763, BA 73 Univ of Pittsburgh - Pittsburgh; MA 75 Univ of TN - Knoxville; Sp/Lang Path, Roane Co Sch Syst, **SLP**

Wilkinson-Sherman, Mrs Lucretia G Route 2 Box 17, Carrington, ND 58421, (701) 252-4100, BS 84 Northeast MO St Univ; MA 85 Northeast MO St Univ; 86–Sp-Lang Path, Sp & Hrng Svcs Inc, **SLP**

Wilkoff, Dr Joan B 1814 Tuscola, Flint, MI 48503, (313) 767-7337, BA 72 Univ of MI - Ann Arbor; MA 74 Wayne St Univ; DD 85 (Doctor of Dental Medicine) Temple Univ; **A**

Wilkoff, Mrs Margaret A 3416 Hilton Woods Drive, Columbus, GA 31906, (404) 561-4066, BS 72 Auburn Univ - Auburn; OM 76 Auburn Univ - Auburn; Exec Dir, Sp Ther Center, Pc, **SLP ACE**

Wilks, Mrs Gina Guillera 5828 Cedar Creek, Baton Rouge, LA 70817, (504) 295-3476, BS 82 LA St Univ - Baton Rouge; MA 85 LA St Univ - Baton Rouge; SLP, East Ascension Schl Bd, **SLP**

Wilks, Stuart R 290 Central Avenue, Lawrence, NY 11559, (516) 236-6400, BA 71 Hofstra Univ; MA 72 Hofstra Univ; President, Wilks Hearing Center Inc, **A**

Will, Darryl J 5464 Stein Court, Dublin, OH 43017, (614) 267-0570, BA 75 OH St Univ; MA 77 OH St Univ; Aud, Riverside Hrng Serv Inc, **A**

Will, David Albert 2408 West College Avenue, Visalia, CA 93277, (209) 734-9036, BS 61 Northern AZ Univ; MA 64 Northern AZ Univ; MS 65 CO St Univ; SLP, Private Practice, **SLP**

Will, Toni Iten 730 Alta Vista Road, Mill Valley, CA 94941, (415) 666-5101, **A**

Will, Virginia Laurence 307 Worth Street, Box 515, Dallas, NC 28034, (704) 922-3312, MA 86 Univ of TN - Knoxville; **SLP**

Willaman, Kathryn E 808 1st Avenue, Altoona, PA 16602, (814) 942-6629, BS 72 Miami Univ - Oxford; MA 81 Memphis St Univ; Sp-Lang Path, InSpeech Inc, **SLP ACE**

Willand-Adams, Jennifer 4773 Galaxie Avenue, Eagan, MN 55122, (612) 456-0026, BS 76 Univ of UT; MS 78 Univ of UT; Sp-Lang Path, ISD 622, **SLP**

Willard, Dr Cheralyn Tiffany P O Box 3737, Rancho Santa Fe, CA 92067, (619) 756-9654, BA 85 Univ of CA - Santa Barbara; MA 72 Univ of CA - Santa Barbara; PH 74 (NS) Univ of CA - Santa Barbara; Private Practice, **SLP**

Willard, Mrs Helen Nelson 1509 Primrose Lane, Cary, NC 27511, (919) 469-0913, OB 73 Univ of Miami; ME 88 NC Central Univ; 79–Sp-Lang Path, Wake Cty PS Sys, **SLP**

Willard, Mrs Marilyn Ness 424 Banner Avenue, Winston-Salem, NC 27127, (919) 723-7837, BS 72 SUNY - Center at Albany; MS 77 Coll of Saint Rose; Sp-Lang Path, Stokes Co Bd of Educ, **SLP**

Willard, Sandra M 60 Via Di Roma Walk, Long Beach, CA 90803, **SLP**

Willard, Mrs Sandra Shy 401 Winding Way, Shelbyville, KY 40065, (502) 633-0934, BA 84 Univ of KY; MS 87 Univ of Louisville; **SLP**

Willbrand, Dr Mary L 1201 Behavioral Science, University Of Utah, Salt Lake City, UT 84112, (801) 581-6725, BS 58 Univ of MO - Columbia; MA 69 Univ of MO - Columbia; PH 72 (NS) Univ of MO - Columbia; Prof, Univ of Utah, **SLP**

Willcox, Joyce 5789 Mulberry Ridge, Camarillo, CA 93010, (805) 987-1727, BS 67 Univ of TX - Austin; MA 70 Univ of TX - Austin; SLP, Private Practice, **SLP**

Willcox-Bein, Katherine 31 Westbourne Terrace, Brookline, MA 02146, (617) 745-9000, BA 82 Univ of CA - Los Angeles; MS 85 Northeastern Univ; **SLP**

Willeford, Dr Jack Allen 1200 East Stuart Street, Apartment 51, Fort Collins, CO 80525, (303) 491-6981, BA 51 Univ of Denver; PH 60 (NS) Northwestern Univ; Prof of Aud, Co St U, **A F LM**

Willems, Caroline C 3388 Pheasant Ridge S E, Grand Rapids, MI 49508, (616) 245-7210, MA 87 Western MI Univ

Willems, Mrs Sherry G 7504 Third Avenue, Kenosha, WI 53140, (414) 658-3389, BA 68 Saint Xavier Coll; MA 76 OH St Univ; Sp-Lang Path, Kenosha Memorial Hospital, **SLP**

Willen, Mrs Michelle Martin 645 Castle Boulevard, Akron, OH 44313, (216) 454-9461, BS Kent St Univ; MA 86 Kent St Univ; **SLP**

Willenborg, Janet Ann 788 Woodlyn Drive So, Cincinnati, OH 45230, (513) 732-3226, BS 71 Saint Louis Univ; MS 72 Purdue Univ - West Lafayette; Consult-Superv Sp/Lang Serv, Clermont Co Offi Ed, **SLP**

Willenborg, Mrs Kimberly M 302 Eden, Effingham, IL 62401, (217) 347-7761, BS 79 IN St Univ - Terre Haute; MS 81 IN St Univ - Terre Haute; Sp-Lang Path, Effingham Comm Unit #40, **SLP**

Willens, Diane 25495 Wareham, Huntington Woods, MI 48070, (313) 399-3586, BA 70; MA 74 Wayne St Univ; **SLP**

Willensky, Andi R 5535 Balboa Boulevard Suite 205, Encino, CA 91316, (818) 905-2700, BS 74 Syracuse Univ; MA 76 CA St Univ - Los Angeles; Sp-Lang Path, Private Practice, **SLP**

Willer, Mrs Phyllis Lorene 205 Elm Road, Hartford, SD 57033, (605) 528-3938, BA 72 Univ of SD - Vermillion; MA 74 Univ of IA; **SLP**

Willer-Urfer, Janene 1117 4 1/2 Street N W #5, Rochester, MN 55901, (507) 280-6421, BA 71 Univ of Northern IA; MA 72 Univ of Northern IA; 88–Sp-Lang Path, InSpeech Inc, **SLP**

Willett, Mrs Donna K 1833 218th Place N E, Redmond, WA 98053, (206) 868-4385, BA 70 Univ of WA; OM 72 Univ of WA; **SLP**

Willett, Mrs Irma Ramos 611 Merlin, Laredo, TX 78041, (512) 723-5898, BA 79 Univ of TX - Austin; MA 84 Univ of TX - Austin; Sp-Lang Path, Laredo ISD, **SLP**

Willett, Mrs Karen Mikesell 412 Salt Springs Road, Fayetteville, NY 13066, (315) 652-1300, MS 87 Syracuse Univ

Willett, Maryanne M R R 1 Box 415, Rome, NY 13440, (315) 336-2300, BS 74 SUNY - Center at Albany; MS 79 Syracuse Univ; Aud, Rome Dev Cen, **A**

Willhoit, Marilyn J 2051 Wheeler Lane, Route 76, Switzerland, FL 32259, (904) 737-2702, BA 68 Trenton St Coll; MA 70 Univ of CT; Dir-Mktg Sls, K&A Medical, **A**

Williams, Alice I 312 Clover Lane, Louisville, KY 40207, (502) 562-3395, BS 79 Eastern KY Univ; MS 80 Univ of Louisville; Clinical Supervisor, Univ of Louisville, **SLP ACE**

Williams, Amelia K 3874 Willis Road #11, Columbus, GA 31906, (404) 882-1411, BA 74 Auburn Univ - Auburn; OM 76 Auburn Univ - Auburn; Chief Audiology Department, West Georgia Medical Center, **A**

Williams, Mrs Amy Patricia General Delivery, Gilboa, WV 26671, (304) 872-6572, BA 84 Thiel Coll; MA 86 Edinboro Univ of PA; **SLP**

Williams, Angela Kay 8104 Chipplegate Drive, Richmond, VA 23227, (804) 262-4908, MA 88 Hampton Univ; 88–Sp-Lang Path, Richmond PS

Williams, Anita L 1271 Westmont Place, Pomona, CA 91766, (312) 769-5310, BS 78 WV Univ; MS 80 WV Univ; **SLP**

Williams, Dr Ann Marie 110 Bedford Avenue, Rockaway Point, NY 11697, (212) 988-9500, BA 61 CUNY - Hunter Coll; MA 64 Univ of IL - Urbana; PH 79 (Reading) 9995; Assoc Exec Dir, Kennedy Child Study Cen, **SLP**

Williams, Barbara H 2405 Rdius Drive, Sanford, NC 27330, (919) 774-3225, BA 74 Meredith Coll; MS 80 East TN St Univ; Sp-Lang Path, Natl Sp & Hrng Servs, **SLP**

Williams, Capt Barbara Jean Hearing Conservation Center, U S A Meddac, Fort Hood, TX 76544-5063, (817) 287-5504, BS 73 Univ of HI - Manoa; MA 76 Rice Univ; MA 82 OH Univ - Athens; Chief-Hrng Conservation, USA MEDDAC, **A ACE**

Williams, Becky A 1222 East 30th Street, Tulsa, OK 74114, (918) 438-4166, BS 68 OK St Univ; MA 70 OK St Univ; 88–Sp-Lang Path, Meadowbrook of Tulsa, **SLP**

Williams, Betsy M P O Box 340, Rural Hall, NC 27045-0340, (919) 969-2755, BA 75 NC St Univ at Raleigh; ME 81 Univ of NC - Greensboro; 85–Sp-Lang Path, Forsyth Co Health Dept, **SLP**

Williams, Betty Mae 1208 Bob Wallace Avenue S E, Huntsville, AL 35801, (309) 254-3360, MA 83 Talladega Coll; Sp-Lang Path, Lakeshore Rehabilitation Ctr, **SLP**

Williams, Mrs Beverly Renee 406 Dogwood Lane, Princeton, KY 42445, (502) 365-5150, **SLP**

Williams, Brenda Haas 218 Chandler Road, Chadds Ford, PA 19317, (215) 388-6053, BS 72 Bloomsburg Univ of PA; ME 73 Bloomsburg Univ of PA; 87–Sp-Lang Path Consult, Chester Co IU #24, **SLP**

Williams, Mrs Carol Troffer 320 73rd Street S W, Everett, WA 98203, (206) 259-5066, BA 57 Univ of WA; MA 59 Univ of WA; Owner/Aud, Pacific Hrng & Sp Serv, **SLP A**

Williams, Mrs Caroline Miller Box 451, Pleasanton, TX 78064, (512) 569-2643, BS 50 Southwest TX St Univ; MA 51 Southwest TX St Univ; **SLP LM**

Williams, Mrs Cathy J 637 South Spinningwheel Ln, Bloomfield Hills, MI 48013, (313) 577-3337, BA 75 MI St Univ; MA 76 MI St Univ; 88–Lecturer-Clin Supvr, Wayne State Univ, **SLP**

Williams, Charles 3046 Ladera, San Bernardino, CA 92405, (714) 829-5641, BA 59 Univ of Redlands; MS 71 Univ of Redlands; Sp-Lang Path, Southn Calif Permanente Med Gr, **SLP**

Williams, Cheryl Ann 313 South Maple, Oak Park, IL 60302, (312) 570-5204, BA 83 Augustana Coll; MA 85 Northeast MO St Univ; **SLP**

Williams, Clare W 19B Walnut Street, Palmer, MA 01069, (413) 534-2508, BA 81 Univ of FL; MA 85 Univ of FL; Aud, Holyoke Speecxh & Hring Ctr, **A**

Williams, Mrs Colleen Houston 5900 Riverdale Road #K-8, College Park, GA 30349, (404) 996-5752, BA 82 Univ of AL- Tuscaloosa; MS 83 Univ of AL- Tuscaloosa; **SLP**

Williams, Cynthia Kathleen 6603-A Bilberry Drive, Gloucester, ON, Canada K1C 4N5, (613) 737-2768, MS 87 Univ of VT; Childrens Hosp of Eastern On

Williams, Danna Duncan 9240 Shady Mill Lane, Knoxville, TN 37922, (615) 693-7908, BA 84 Univ of TN - Knoxville; MA 86 Univ of TN - Knoxville; 88–Aud, Hearing Conservation Assoc, **A**

Williams, Dr David K 21 Timothy Drive, Minot, ND 58701, PH 73 (NS) Univ of MO - Columbia; Chmn Dept Commun Dis, Minot State Coll, **SLP**

Williams, Dean E Speech And Hearing Center, University Of Iowa, Iowa City, IA 52240, (319) 335-8754, BA 47 Univ of IA; MA 49 Univ of IA; PH 52 (Psych-Sp Path) Univ of IA; Prof Emeritus, Univ of IO, **SLP F**

Williams, Mrs Deborah A 2319 Howard Road S W, Roanoke, VA 24015, (703) 982-3691, BS 79 James Madison Univ; MS 81 PA St Univ - Univ Park; Sp/Lang Path, Rehab Servs, **SLP**

Williams, Mrs Deborah Hopkins 9179 Trelawney Court, Cincinnati, OH 45251, (513) 742-1500, BS 86 Miami Univ - Oxford; MS 87 Miami Univ - Oxford

Williams, Debra A B 211 Foggy Bottom Drive, Carrollton, GA 30117, (404) 834-1868, BS 75 West GA Coll; ME 77 GA St Univ; 84–Sp-Lang Path, Carrollton City Sch System, **SLP**

Williams, Debra Bailey 3319 W Gladys Street, Chicago, IL 60624, (312) 826-3600, SLP, Chic Bd of Ed, **SLP**

Williams, Debra Elizabeth MCHR-Dept Oto-HNS, 825 Fairfax Avenue, Norfolk, VA 23507, (804) 446-5934, BS 81 Old Dominion Univ; MS 84 Old Dominion Univ; 87–Aud, MCHR-Dept Oto-HNS, **A**

Williams, Mrs Debra S 8511 S W 52nd Place, Gainesville, FL 32608, (904) 377-6529, BA 76 Univ of FL; MS 78 FL St Univ; **SLP**

Williams, Denise Ann 503 Victory Trail, Morganton, NC 28655, (704) 264-0566, BS 84 Appalachian St Univ; MS 85 East Carolina Univ; 86–Admin Supvr, Communi-Care Inc, **SLP**

Williams, Maj Dennis L 5705 Bear Creek Circle, Fayetteville, NC 28304, (919) 423-2263, BS 71 CO St Univ; MS 77 CO St Univ; Aud, US Army, **A ACE**

Williams, Mrs Diana Lynn 24151 Creekside Drive, Newhall, CA 91321, (805) 259-1660, MA 84 CA St Univ - Los Angeles; Sp-Lang Path, Newhall Sch Dist, **SLP**

Williams, Diane L 3405 Longview Avenue #18, Bloomington, IN 47401, (812) 335-6251, BS 76 Auburn Univ - Auburn; MA 78 Univ of TN - Knoxville; 87–Sp/Lang Path, Indiana Univ, **SLP**

Williams, Diane Ruley 1333 Ocean Avenue, Del Mar, CA 92014, (619) 594-6774, BA 66 Univ of KY; MA 67 Northwestern Univ; Asst Prof Coord of Aud Serv, Commun Cl San Diego St U, **A**

Williams, Donna L 710 Fairington View Drive, St Louis, MO 63129, **A**

Williams, Mrs Donna L 51 Long Ridge Road, Terre Haute, IN 47802-4743, BS 72; MS 73 IN St Univ - Terre Haute; Sp/Lang Path, Vigo Co Sch Corp, **SLP**

Williams, Mrs Dorothy J 558 Russell Road, De Kalb, IL 60115, (815) 756-6986, BA 43 Univ of Pittsburgh - Pittsburgh; MS 49 Univ of IA; Retired, Dekalb Comm Sch Dist 428, **SLP**

Williams, Dorythea C 1113 Irwin, Fresno, CA 93706, PH (NS); **SLP**

Williams, Elizabeth Marie 139 37th Avenue N W, Rochester, MN 55901, (507) 732-7611, OB 78 Univ of MN - Duluth; MS 86 Univ of WI - River Falls; **SLP**

Williams, Elsie Monterey 4 Cameron Court #H, Baltimore, MD 21236, (301) 922-2610, BS 54 Hampton Univ; Sp/Lang Path, Bd of Ed of Balt Co, **SLP**

Williams, Fern Elizabeth 291-B Newman Avenue, Harrisonburg, VA 22801, (703) 433-6534, BS 76 James Madison Univ; MS 86 James Madison Univ; **SLP**

Williams, Frances G Hotel Wilkes, North Wilkesboro, NC 28659, MS; **LM**

Williams, Gail A 12 Midship Lane, Patchogue, NY 11772-3411, (516) 758-7917, BA 76 New York Univ; MS 78 New York Univ; 87–Sp-Lang Path, South Co Central Sch Dist, **SLP**

Williams, Genice Nix 303 Fairmont Drive, Greenville, SC 29605, (803) 232-2494, BA 78 SC St Coll; MA 79 Univ of SC - Columbia; Aud, Sch Dis of Greenville Co, **A**

Williams, Geralyn Huzicka 1497 Burroak Drive, Cincinnati, OH 45230, (513) 221-4243, **SLP**

Williams, Gerilyn A 216 South 2-1/2 Street, Nederland, TX 77627, (409) 838-1485, BS 76 Lamar Univ; MS 78 Lamar Univ; Sp-Lang Path, Beaumont St Ctr for Human Dev, **SLP**

Williams, Gina M 524 El Camino Real #20, Burlingame, CA 94010, (415) 579-4400, BA 80 Holy Names Coll; MA 82 CA St Univ - Stanislaus; SLP, Russell Bede School, **SLP**

Williams, Mrs Grace O 5341 Thayer Drive, Raleigh, NC 27612, (919) 787-5109, BA 65 MT St Agnes Coll; ME 68 Univ of GA; Sp-Lang Path, Wake Co Pub Sch, **SLP**

Williams, Mrs Gretchen S 3351 Stoney Point Road, Grand Island, NY 14072, (716) 625-7281, BS 58 SUNY - Coll at Geneseo; Sp-Lang Path, Starpoint Cen Sch, **SLP**

Williams, Dr Harold N Nat Inc, 212 West California, El Paso, TX 79902, (915) 532-4765, BS 47 Bradley Univ; MS 49 Bradley Univ; ED 57 (NS) Bradley Univ; 80–Sp-Lang Path, Nat Inc, **SLP A**

Williams, Mrs Harriet Lee Route 7 Box 195, Lenoir City, TN 37771, (615) 986-2009, BA 75 Univ of TN - Knoxville; MA 77 Univ of TN - Knoxville; 77–Sp-Lang Path, Lenoir City Schs

Williams, Helen Hargadon 13908 Mathews Drive, Woodbridge, VA 22191, (703) 356-2833, 87–Sp-Lang Path, Sp & L Ctr of N VA, **SLP**

Williams, Dr J David 558 Russell Road, De Kalb, IL 60115, (815) 756-6986, BA 47 Univ of IA; MA 48 Univ of IA; PH 54 (Sp Path) Univ of IA; Professor Communicative Dis, Northern Illinois University, **SLP LM**

Williams, Mrs Jan Wallace 1959 Westfield Drive, Mount Sterling, KY 40353-8115, (606) 784-6661, BA 75 Univ of KY; MS 78 Univ of KY; Sp-Lang Path, St Claire Med Cen, **SLP**

Williams, Mrs Jane C 102 Mimosa Hills Drive, Morganton, NC 28655, (704) 433-2967, BA 49 Duke Univ; ME 65 Univ of NC - Chapel Hill; Assoc Prof Ed Dept, Lenoir-Rhyne Coll

Williams, Mrs Janice S Route 5 Box 161, Marianna, FL 32446, (904) 352-4204, BS 74 FL St Univ; MS 75 FL St Univ; Sp-Lang Path, Jackson Co Sch Bd, **SLP**

Williams, Mrs Janis Marie 1687 Rosebud Court, Wheaton, IL 60187, (312) 682-2055, BS 77 IL St Univ - Normal; MS 79 IL St Univ - Normal; 79–Sp-Lang Path, DuPage/West Cook Spec Educ Reg, **SLP**

Williams, Jennifer Anne 594 Channing Avenue, Palo Alto, CA 94301, (415) 327-2549, BS 82 Univ of WI - Madison; MS 86 Univ of North TX; 88–Sp-Lang Path, Peninsula Children's Ctr, **SLP**

Williams, Jennifer Derexa 5505 Clover Rise Lane, Norcross, GA 30093, (404) 925-7891

Williams, Mrs Jennifer Ellen P O Box 89, Grahamsville, NY 12740, (914) 985-7305, BA 81 SUNY - Coll at Cortland; MS 86 SUNY - Coll at New Paltz; **SLP**

Williams, Jerry O 1300 Wallace Boulevard, Amarillo, TX 79106, (806) 359-7681, BS 55 West TX St Univ; ME 57 West TX St Univ; Sp-Lang Path, Aisd/Reg Ed Prog for Deaf, **SLP**

Williams, Mrs Jill Koehler 209 North Gay Street, Mount Vernon, OH 43050, (614) 397-3853, BS 76 Capital Univ; MA 78 OH St Univ; SLP, Heinzerling Dev Cen, **SLP**

Williams, Jo Ellen 13503 Bartlett Street, Rockville, MD 20853, (301) 897-5700, BS 80 Univ of SC - Columbia; OM 83 Univ of SC - Columbia; 87–Mgr Aud Tech Asst Sec, ASHA, **A**

Williams, Jodi L 1411 Penrose, Olathe, KS 66062, (913) 829-5432, 85 KS St Univ; MA 87 KS St Univ; 87–Sp-Lang Path, USD #368 Paola, **SLP**

Williams, John Elliott 123 Alpine Road, Middlesboro, KY 40965-1406, (606) 248-8716, BS 74 Purdue Univ - West Lafayette; MA 83 Eastern KY Univ; SLP, Bell County Board of Education, **SLP**

Williams, Judy K Department Of Communicative Disorders, University Of New Mexico, 901 Vassar NE, Albuquerque, NM 87131, (505) 277-4453, BS 70 OK St Univ; MA 71 Northwestern Univ; Instr/Superv, U of NM, **SLP**

Williams, Julianna W 548 Inglewood Place, Macon, GA 31204, (912) 474-9440, ME 70 Univ of GA; SLP, Bibb Co Sch Syst, **SLP**

Williams, Kadyn Ochs Aud Consultants Of Atlanta Inc, 2550WINDY Hill Road #305A, Marietta, GA 30067, (404) 953-2223, BS 75 Univ of GA; ME 76 Univ of GA; Aud/Owner, Aud Consult of Atlanta Inc, **A**

Williams, Karen A 18185 Tabony Lane, Livingston, LA 70754, (504) 698-3818, BS 74 TX Tech Univ; MS 80 Central St Univ; 87–Sp/Lang Path, East Baton Rouge Par Sch Bd, **SLP**

Williams, Mrs Karen D 1203 Northlake Drive, Sanford, FL 32773, (407) 323-4946, BS 80 Univ of North TX; MS 81 Univ of North TX; **SLP**

Williams, Katharine Twin Lakes Village, Route 4 Box 5000, Rathdrum, ID 83858, (208) 687-1885, BA 78 Eastern WA Univ; MS 80 Univ of HI - Manoa; **SLP**

Williams, Kathleen 320 South Woodale, Decatur, IL 62522, (217) 877-8121, BS 83 Eastern IL Univ; MS 84 Eastern IL Univ

Williams, Kathleen A 776 Powder Springs Street, Smyrna, GA 30080, (404) 233-5332, BS 71 Univ of IL - Urbana; MA 72 Univ of IA; Sp-Lang Path, Atlanta Sp Sch, **SLP ACE**

Williams, Kathleen Joy 95 North Michigan #2, Pasadena, CA 91106-1816, (818) 577-9785, BA 83 CA St Univ - Northridge; MA 85 CA St Univ - Northridge; **SLP**

Williams, Kathryn D 856 Calle Vallarta, San Clemente, CA 92672, (714) 498-8909, BA 73 Univ of Redlands; MS 74 Univ of Redlands; Sp-Lang Path, Santa Ana USD, **SLP**

Williams, Kathy Linette 5316 Kansas Avenue N W, Washington, DC 20011, (202) 882-8539, MA 88 Univ of the DC

Williams, Mrs Katrina Belton Route 3 Box 379, Jackson, MS 39213, (601) 982-1437, BS 79 Univ Southern MS-Hattiesburg; MS 84 Univ Southern MS-Hattiesburg; 87–CL Supvr, Jackson State Univ, **SLP**

Williams, Mrs Kim Marie 3112 Cedar Lane, Bemidji, MN 56601, (218) 751-6622, BS 80 Univ of ND; MS 81 Univ of ND; 86–SLP, Bemidji Reg Interdistrict Council, **SLP**

Williams, Mrs Kimberly Ann 88 North Hamilton Street, Doylestown, PA 18901, (215) 340-0530, BS 84 Bloomsburg Univ of PA; MS 85 Bloomsburg Univ of PA; 86–Sp-Lang Path, Mont Co Inter Unit #23, **SLP**

Williams, Mrs Kimberly Perry 5011 N W 179th Terrace, Miami, FL 33055, (305) 620-4056, BA 78 Univ of FL; MS 80 FL St Univ; SLP, Professional Rehabil Assoc, **SLP**

Williams, Laura Lynn 2224 Norman Lane, Pueblo, CO 81005, (303) 574-1607, **SLP**

Williams, Lisa S 1030 Balfour Street, Midland, MI 48640, (517) 631-4331, OB 78 Univ of Miami; ME 80 GA St Univ; 88–Sp-Lang Path, Private Practice, **SLP**

Williams, Lori Anne 11729 Silvergate Drive, Dublin, CA 94568, (415) 682-8000, BA 83 San Francisco St Univ; MS 85 San Francisco St Univ; 85–Sp-Lang Path, Mt Diablo USD, **SLP**

Williams, Lori Lynn 100 Sea View Street, P O Box 703, Chatham, MA 02633, (304) 295-7357, BA 84 Marshall Univ; MA 86 Marshall Univ; **SLP**

Williams, Louise Ann 306 East Main Street, Smithville, TN 37166, (615) 597-4494, BS 83 Univ of GA; ME 84 Univ of GA; Sp-Lang Path, Professional Health Services, **SLP**

Williams, Mrs Luann M P O Box 262, Chester, NY 10918, (914) 469-7610, BA 77 Northern St Coll; MS 79 Phillips Univ; 88–Sp-Lang Path, Audiology and Speech Assoc, **SLP**

Williams, Mrs Lynn Dell 8902 Highland Avenue S W, Tacoma, WA 98499, (206) 588-0585, MS 88 Eastern WA Univ

Williams, Lynn L 1545 Downington, Salt Lake City, UT 84105, (801) 484-9848, BS 61 Univ of UT; MS 79 Univ of UT; Sp-Lang Path, Granite Sch Dist, **SLP**

Williams, Marcia J 716 Hemlock, Pocatello, ID 83201, (208) 678-9451, BS 83 ID St Univ; MS 85 ID St Univ; **SLP**

Williams, Mrs Margarette 3402 West 36th, Pine Bluff, AR 71603, (501) 879-3390, BA 74 Univ of AR - Pine Bluff; MS 79 9110; **SLP**

Williams, Mrs Marilyn G P O Box 304, Brenham, TX 77833, (409) 836-4511, BA 77 Sam Houston St Univ; ME 78 Southwest TX St Univ; **SLP**

Williams, Martha 2107 Kemp, Wichita Falls, TX 76309, (817) 322-8604, BS 70 Univ of North TX; MS 72 Univ of North TX; Cl Dir, Private Practice, **SLP**

Williams, Mrs Martha Skerrett 947 Nottingham Road, High Point, NC 27260, (919) 379-4120, ME 77 Univ of NC - Greensboro; 88–Sp-Lang Path, Moses H Cone Mem Hosp, **SLP**

Williams, Mary Catherine 3013 Dogwood Drive, Louisville, KY 40220, (502) 451-9750, MS 86 Univ of Louisville; 87–Sp-Lang Path, InSpeech Inc, **SLP ACE**

Williams, Mary Elizabeth 8200 Kroll Way #313, Bakersfield, CA 93311, (805) 327-3311, BA 80 Univ of OK - Norman; MS 83 Univ of OK - OK City; 83–Sp-Lang Path, Bakersfield City Sch Dist, **SLP**

Williams, Mary H 25331 68th Avenue South, Kent, WA 98032, BS 30 Univ of WA; **LM**

Williams, Mary Kay 6588 Sullivan Trail, Wind Gap, PA 18091, (215) 778-2544, BS 78 PA St Univ - Univ Park; MA 85 West Chester Univ of PA; 87–Sp-Lang Path, The Allentown Hosp, **SLP**

Williams, Mary Kim 1016 Pelham Street, Williamsburg, KY 40769, (606) 549-0145, BS 82 Univ of TN - Chattanooga; MA 84 Univ of TN - Knoxville; Sp-Lang Path, Williamsburg Schs, **SLP**

Williams, Merrilee M P O Box 2582, Avon, CO 81620, (303) 949-1110, BS 73 SUNY - Center at Albany; MA 75 Univ of CT; 81–Sp-Lang Path, Private Practice, **SLP**

Williams, Michael K 18931 Loretto Lane, Country Club Hills, IL 60477, (312) 798-4486, BS 62 IL St Univ - Normal; MA 73 Governors St Univ; Sp-Lang Path, Bloom Hs Dist #206, **SLP**

Williams, Mrs Michelle Kummerer RD #8271, Sinking Spring, PA 19608, (717) 272-7611, MS 81 Bloomsburg Univ of PA; Sp/Lang Path, Good Samaritan Hospital, **SLP**

Williams, Myra Jann Spence 1072 Birchwood Drive, Orange Park, FL 32065, (904) 272-8150, BS 76 Univ of GA; ME 80 Univ of GA; Sp-Lang Path, Clay Co Bd of Ed, **SLP**

Williams, Nancy 32 Woodcrest Avenue, Ithaca, NY 14850, (309) 454-2803, **SLP**

Williams, Mrs Nancy Ellen 201 Jefferson Avenue, Muscle Shoals, AL 35660, (205) 381-1324, BA 81 Univ of MS; MS 85 Univ of MS; **SLP**

Williams, Nancy H 2469 North Country Club, Tucson, AZ 85716, (602) 325-3540, BS 75 Purdue Univ - West Lafayette; MS 76 Auburn Univ - Auburn; Sp-Lang Path, Private Practice, **SLP**

Williams, Nancy Lynne 6750 Wilber Circle, Richmond, VA 23228, (804) 262-1262, BS 82 James Madison Univ; MS 87 James Madison Univ; Sp-Lang Path, Communi-Care Inc

Williams, Neta C 4634 Belfast Drive, Columbus, OH 43227, (614) 861-0983, MS 69; **SLP**

Williams, Mrs Nina C 12041 Captains Landing, North Palm Beach, FL 33408, (305) 622-7660, OB 64 Univ of FL; ME 65 Univ of FL; Sp-Lang Path, Palm Beach Co Sch Bd, **SLP**

Williams, Mrs Noreen Marie 134 Glasgow, Stockton, CA 95210, (209) 944-4486, BA 83 Univ of the Pacific; MA 84 Univ of the Pacific; SLP, Stockton USD, **SLP**

Williams, Patricia J 647 West Escalon, Fresno, CA 93704, (209) 441-3328, BA 66 Univ of IA; MA 68 Univ of IA; Sp-Lang Path, Fresno USD, **SLP**

Williams, Paula Sue P c/o Russell Williams, 10027 Nadina Drive, Huntsville, AL 35805, **SLP**

Williams, Dr Peggy S American Sp-Lang-Hearing Assn, 10801 Rockville Pike, Rockville, MD 20852, (301) 897-5700, BS 63 WV Univ; MS 64 WV Univ; PH 76 (Aud) Univ of WA; Deputy Executive Director, ASHA - National Office, **SLP A**

Williams, Penny Sue 3314 Felton Street, San Diego, CA 92104, (619) 588-3053, BA 72 CA St Univ - Northridge; MA 87 San Diego St Univ; **SLP**

Williams, Phyllis Cashen ENT Clinic, 1919 Lathrop Street #42, Fairbanks, AK 99701, (907) 456-7767, BA 71 Gonzaga Univ; MA 74 Univ of Northern CO; Aud, ENT Clinic, **A**

Williams, Rebecca Ann 103 Intermond Heights Road, Baxter, KY 40806, (606) 573-4330, BS 84 Eastern KY Univ; MA 85 Eastern KY Univ; **SLP**

Williams, Rita J 7817 Skylake, Fort Worth, TX 76179, **SLP**

Williams, Rita Murphy c/o Murphy, 15 Clark Court, Brookline, MA 02146, (617) 254-3800, BA 78 McGill Univ - Quebec; MS 82 Emerson Coll; 88–Sp-Lang Path, Kennedy Mem Hosp for Children, **SLP**

Williams, Dr Robert D 2 Raynan Drive, Ottumwa, IA 52501, (515) 682-8591, BS 68 Northeast MO St Univ; MA 68 Northeast MO St Univ; PH 80 (NS) Univ of KS; **SLP A**

Williams, Dr Robert G, Jr Speech And Hearing Center, Western Illinois Univ, Macomb, IL 61455, (309) 298-1649, BA 59 Marietta Coll; MA 62 OH Univ - Athens; PH 69 (NS) OH Univ - Athens; Associate Professor Audiology, Western Illinois University, **A**

Williams, Robert Harold 7152 Birchwood Drive, Mount Morris, MI 48458, (313) 767-5750, BA 55 MI St Univ; MA 60 MI St Univ; Aud, Flint Bd of Ed, **SLP A**

Williams, Robert L Rd 4 Box 4219, East Stroudsburg, PA 18301, (717) 421-2879, BS 50 East Stroudsburg Univ of PA; MA 57 Columbia Univ Teachers Coll; Hearing Conservation Consult, Private Practice, **A**

Williams, Mrs Roberta N 600 Sager, Danville, IL 61832, (217) 443-5665, BS 72 Purdue Univ - West Lafayette; MS 73 Purdue Univ - West Lafayette; 88–Aud, RJ Hearing Ltd, **A**

Williams, Robin Kaye 509 West James Street #4, Lancaster, PA 17603, (717) 293-1457, BS 85 Bloomsburg Univ of PA; MS 86 Bloomsburg Univ of PA; 86–Sp-Lang Path, Lancaster-Lebanon Intermed Unit 13, **SLP**

Williams, Mrs Ruth T P O Box 94, Halifax, NC 27839, (919) 445-3525, BS 72 East Carolina Univ; MS 77 East Carolina Univ; Sp-Lang Path, Halifax Co Bd of Ed, **SLP**

Williams, Sandra Fay 2225-H Kilborne Drive, Charlotte, NC 28205, (704) 892-3321, BA 81 Univ of SC - Columbia; MS 83 Univ of NC - Chapel Hill; SLP, Charlotte Mecklenburg Schools, **SLP**

Williams, Mrs Sara Sparkman 30 Camp Lane, Carrollton, GA 30117, (404) 834-5220, BS 80 MS Univ for Women; MS 81 Univ of AL- Tuscaloosa; Sp-Lang Path, **SLP**

Williams, Dr Sarah E 645 18th Avenue N E, St Petersburg, FL 33704, (813) 894-1586, MS 77 Univ of South FL; PH 80 (Sp-Lang Path) Northwestern Univ; Sp-Lang Path, Bay Pines Med Ctr, **SLP**

Williams, Seleria Jean 7276 East Caprice Drive, Baton Rouge, LA 70811, (504) 292-2682, BA 78 Southern Univ - Baton Rouge; MA 85 LA St Univ - Baton Rouge; 87–Sp-Lang Path, Maternal & Child Therapy Ctr, **SLP**

Williams, Mrs Sharon Louise 1635 Fir Meadow Court, Ferndale, WA 98248, (206) 384-9260, BA 75 Western WA Univ; MA 77 Western WA Univ; SLP, Ferndale Sch Dist, **SLP**

Williams, Mrs Shawn Markey 505 East 36th #6, Stillwater, OK 74074, (405) 377-3869, MA 88 OK St Univ

Williams, Sheila Carol 11468 Orchard Lane, Reston, VA 22090, (703) 437-3196, BS 78 Bowling Green St Univ; MA 79 Ball St Univ; 88–Sp-Lang Path, Ivymount Sch, **SLP**

Williams, Mrs Sheila Chase 641 Geranium Place, Oxnard, CA 93030, (805) 485-3115, BA 77 CA St Univ - Chico; MA 79 CA St Univ - Chico; SLP, Rio Sch Dist, **SLP**

Williams, Mrs Shelley Plath 302 West 26th, Sioux Falls, SD 57105-2901, BA 79 Univ of Denver; MA 82 Univ of WA; SLP, Sioux Falls School District, **SLP**

Williams, Mrs Sheryl Guda 4960 Lockwig Trail, Florissant, MO 63033, (314) 741-9694, Audiologist, Cardinal Glennon Memorial Hosp, **A**

Williams, Mrs Sonja Dean Route 1, Arbyrd, MO 63821, (314) 757-6200, **SLP**

Williams, Susan Berger 123 Alpine Road, Middlesboro, KY 40965, (606) 248-8716, BS 74 Purdue Univ - West Lafayette; MA 83 Eastern KY Univ; Sp-Lang Path, Bell Co Bd of Ed, **SLP**

Williams, Susan E 60 Arlene Avenue, Youngstown, OH 44512, (216) 758-2144, **SLP**

Williams, Susan G 4218 Jennie, Amarillo, TX 79106, (806) 352-0872, BS 78 Southwest TX St Univ; ME 79 Southwest TX St Univ; Sp-Lang Path, Amarillo ISD, **SLP**

Williams, Mrs Susan L K 810 Mann Road, Bartow, FL 33830, (813) 533-0456, MS 76 Univ of South FL; Sp/Lang Path, Polk Co Sch Bd, **SLP**

Williams, Mrs Susan M 1611 Todd Trail, College Station, TX 77840, BA 71 Univ of NC - Greensboro; MS 75 1816; **SLP**

Williams, Mrs Susan S 4128 North Stevens, Tacoma, WA 98407, (206) 858-6131, BA 68 WA St Univ; MS 69 Central WA Univ; SLP, Penisula Sch Dist #401, **SLP**

Williams, Mrs Susan Thomas 803 Stephen Court, Friendswood, TX 77546, (713) 996-7525, BS 78 Southern Methodist Univ; MS 84 UT St Univ; **A**

Williams, Thelma F 4206 Green Ivy Circle, Martinez, GA 30907-1619, (404) 790-2101, BS 65 FL A & M Univ; MA 77 SC St Coll; Sp-Lang Path, Gracewood St Sch & Hosp, **SLP**

Williams, Thema Johnson 507 Oak Crest Lane, Wallingford, PA 19086, (212) 566-7405, **SLP**

Williams, Theresa Aleise 5166 Lazy Oaks, Drive, Winter Park, FL 32792, (305) 671-2358, BS 83 Univ of DE; MA 86 Univ of Central FL; **SLP**

Williams, Dr Thomas F 2114 Moncrieff Street, Augusta, GA 30906, (404) 790-2101, BA 73 Univ of FL; MS 74 FL St Univ; PH 81 (NS) FL St Univ; Aud, Gracewood State School & Hosp, **A**

Williams, Mrs Thomasyne Hill 1025 South Beach Street, Apt #43, Daytona Beach, FL 32014, (904) 258-1635, BS 83 Univ of Montevallo; MS 87 Univ of Montevallo; 88–Sp-Lang Path, Volusia Co Sch Dist, **SLP**

Williams, Tina B 823 Loxford Terrace, Silver Spring, MD 20901, (301) 681-8403, BS 75 Syracuse Univ; MA 76 NY Univ; Sp-Lang Path, Bay Area Rehab Cen, **SLP**

Williams, Mrs Vanessa P 4866 Terrace Green Trace, Stone Mountain, GA 30088, (404) 792-9310, BS 77 Morris Brown Coll; MS 81 Univ of SC - Columbia; 88–Sp-Lang Path, DeKalb Co Sch Sys, **SLP**

Williams, Victoria L 9 Evans Drive, Simsbury, CT 06070, (203) 658-2658, BS 75 TX Christian Univ; MS 85 TX Christian Univ; **SLP**

Williams, Mrs Wanda S 3275 Ardmore, Memphis, TN 38127, (901) 358-6209, BA 83 MS Valley St Univ; MA 86 Western Carolina Univ

Williams, Waukita 432 North Denver, Kansas City, MO 64123, **SLP**

Williams, Dr William G 482 East 300 South, St George, UT 84770, (801) 628-1944, BA 57 Brigham Young Univ; MA 58 Brigham Young Univ; PH 62 (NS) Purdue Univ - West Lafayette; Retired, Dixie Hearing & Sp Cen, **SLP A LM**

Williams, Dr William Norman 214 S W 40th Street, Gainesville, FL 32607, (904) 392-4370, BA 63 FL St Univ; MS 64 FL St Univ; PH 69 (NS) Univ of FL; Assoc Prof, U of FL-Coll of Dentistry

Williams-Beintema, Teresa Marie P O Box 2137, Cody, WY 82414, (307) 587-4163, BS 82 Univ of WY; MS 85 Univ of WY; **SLP**

Williams-Butler, MaryAnn 44 Kinsley Road, Acton, MA 01720, (508) 635-0512, BS 79 Univ of MA - Amherst; MA 83 San Diego St Univ; 84–Sp-Lang Path, Hahnemann Rehab Cen, **SLP**

Williams-Garrow, Lynne R R 2 Box 221, Harrison, ME 04040, (413) 245-3132, BS 68 Indiana Univ of PA; MA 72 Univ of IL - Urbana; Sp-Lang Path, Hartford Er Sl So Rehab Cen, **SLP**

Williamson, Capt Angela Starr Wilford Hall USAF Medical Cen, Whmc/Sghsos, Lackland AFB, TX 78236, (512) 670-5421, BS 81 OK St Univ; MA 83 Univ of TX - Austin; Aud, US Air Force, **A ACE**

Williamson, Mrs Dale Anne 205 N E Orchard #B, Lee's Summit, MO 64063, (816) 921-2488, Aud, Kansas City School District, **A**

Williamson, Mrs Darlene S 3112 Trenholm Drive, Oakton, VA 22124, (703) 620-2445, BS 70 Purdue Univ - West Lafayette; MA 73 Univ of IL - Urbana; SLP, Commonwealth Hospital, **SLP**

Williamson, Denise Duncan 2122 Cleveland Avenue, Roseville, MN 55113, (612) 698-8349, MS 85 Univ of WI - River Falls; **SLP**

Williamson, Devyn Hogan 436 Winter Park Lane, Colorado Springs, CO 80919-2130, (405) 364-6364, BA 77 Univ of OK - Norman; MS 86 Univ of OK Medical Center; 88–Sp-Lang Path, Co Springs Dist #11 Schs, **SLP**

Williamson, Donna E 1 Evergreen Avenue, Rutland, VT 05701, (802) 247-5757, BA 81 Univ of VT; MS 82 Univ of VT; Sp-Lang Path, Rutland NE Superv Un, **SLP**

Williamson, Mrs Gail E Wing & Wheeler MD PA, Hearing Center, 899 NE Second Avenue, Delray Beach, FL 33444, (407) 278-2515, BS 79 Kent St Univ; MA 84 Kent St Univ; Chief Aud, Wing & Wheeler MD PA Hrng Ctr, **A**

Williamson, Juanita Transversal 2 #112-30, Apartment 701-A, Bogota, Colombia, (212) 860-7800, MS 84 Columbia Univ Teachers Coll; SLP, Private Practice, **SLP**

Williamson, Mrs Karen S 3110 Dunaway Drive, Albany, GA 31707, BS 80 FL St Univ; MS 81 FL St Univ; Sp-Lang Path, Dougherty Co Sch, **SLP**

Williamson, Kathleen Teresa 16 Merriam Road, North Oxford, MA 01537, (617) 365-4531, BS 80 Worcester St Coll; MS 82 Univ of RI; Sp-Lang Path, Clinton Hosp, **SLP**

Williamson, Kelly S 1017 Cynthia Crescent, Anniston, AL 36201, (205) 236-7023, BA 81 Univ of AL- Tuscaloosa; MS 87 Emerson Coll; 88–Sp-Lang Path, Cleburne County Bd of Educ, **SLP**

Williamson, Linda Lee 6954 Park Ridge Drive, Madison, WI 53719, (608) 267-6174, BS 69 Miami Univ - Oxford; MS 70 Univ of WI - Milwaukee; 72–Sp-Lang Path, Meriter Hosp-Madison Gen, **SLP**

Williamson, Mary 4111 Druid Hill #1, Memphis, TN 38128, (901) 388-6861, BS 72 Memphis St Univ; MA 76 Memphis St Univ; Sp-Lang Path, Memphis City Schs, **SLP**

Williamson, Mrs Nancy Alphin P O Box 14, Kenansville, NC 28349, (919) 296-0221, **SLP**

Williamson, Mrs Patricia McHale 2009 North Harding Street, Albany, GA 31701, (912) 439-7061, BS 80 PA St Univ - Univ Park; MS 82 PA St Univ - Univ Park; Chf Sp-Lang Path, SW GA Easter Seal Rehab Cen, **SLP**

Williamson, Mrs Rebecca Kinney PO Box 456, Iron River, WI 54847, (715) 372-4128, BA 74 Augustana Coll; MA 75 Univ of IL - Urbana; 88–Sp-Lang Path, InSpeech Inc, **SLP**

Williamson, Mrs Sharon L H 10431 El Dorado Way, Los Alamitos, CA 90720, (714) 536-7567, BA 63 Rocky Mountain Coll; MA 78 CA St Univ - Long Beach; Sp-Lang Path, Huntington Beach Cty Sch Dist, **SLP**

Williamson, Sherie M 1015 Pennsylvania N E, Albuquerque, NM 87110, (515) 268-2643, BS 76 Wichita St Univ; MA 81 Northeast MO St Univ; Sp-Lang Path, Albuquerque Public Schools, **SLP**

Williamson, Mrs Sue Ellen 417 Batesville Road, Greer, SC 29650, (803) 877-0931, BA 65 Lynchburg Coll; MA 67 IN Univ - Bloomington; Sp-Lang Path/Resource Cnsultnt, Grnv Co Sch Dist, **SLP ACE**

Williamson-Jenkins, Mrs Susan D 5185 Kimbark Woods Drive, Memphis, TN 38134, (901) 522-5199, BS 78 Memphis St Univ; MA 80 Memphis St Univ; Sp-Lang Path, Baptist Memorial Hosp, **SLP**

Williams-Rice, Mrs Teresa F 915 Gay Avenue, St Louis, MO 63130-2737, (314) 725-1278, BS 75 Saint Louis Univ; MA 77 Saint Louis Univ; Sp-Lang Path, Deaconess Hospital, **SLP**

Williamsson, Helene A 3323 Kings Highway #3F, Brooklyn, NY 11234, (718) 692-3178, MA 85 NY Univ; Sp-Lang Path, Private Practice, **SLP**

Williford, Christine Anne 2011 Headland Avenue, Dothan, AL 36303, (205) 793-5771, OM 87 Auburn Univ - Auburn

Willig, Sharon 4242 Eastwest Highway, Apartment 303, Chevy Chase, MD 20815, (202) 625-7891, BS 63 Univ of GA; MA 71 Univ of MD - College Park; Sp-Lang Path, Georgetown U Chld Dev Cen, **SLP**

Willig-Denise, Nancy E 424 Pinewood, Piqua, OH 45356, (513) 773-4321, BS 79 Purdue Univ - West Lafayette; MA 80 Ball St Univ; Sp/Lang Path, Piqua Cty Schs, **SLP**

Willing, Janice E 11835 Walmort Road, Galt, CA 95632, **SLP**

Willing, Mrs Mavis A 610 Western Star Place, Danville, CA 94526, (512) 837-5557, BS 70 Univ of NE - Lincoln; MS 74 Univ of NE - Omaha; 88–Sp-Lang Path, Livermore USD, **SLP**

Willinger, Mrs Rebecca L 621 North Broadview Lane, Andover, KS 67002, (316) 262-8271, BA 83 Fort Hays St Univ; MS 84 Fort Hays St Univ; 88–Sp-Lang Path, Institute of Logopedics, **SLP**

Willingham, Christina Maria 818 Spring, Arlington, TX 76012, (817) 882-2045, BS 85 Univ of TX - Austin; MA 87 Univ of TX - Austin; **SLP**

Willingham, Mrs Marjorie K 3653 Newcastle Creek Drive, Jacksonville, FL 32211, (904) 389-2230, BS 73 Kent St Univ; MA 74 Kent St Univ; SLP, Duval Co Sch Bd, **SLP**

Willingham, Mrs Rebecca S Route 1, Byromville, GA 31007, (912) 433-4770, BS 70 Auburn Univ - Auburn; ME 71 Univ of GA; SLP Consult, Dept of Human Resources, **SLP**

Willis, Mrs Deborah L P O Box 1328, Logan, WV 25601-1328, (304) 752-4180, BA 75 Marshall Univ; MA 76 Marshall Univ; Sp-Lang Path, Logan Co Bd of Ed, **SLP**

Willis, Mrs Diane Kay 105 12th Avenue West, Redfield, SD 57469, (605) 472-0562, BS 83 Univ of SD - Vermillion; MA 84 Univ of SD - Vermillion; Sp-Lang Path, North Central Spec Serv Coop, **SLP**

Willis, Diane Louise 6911 West 52nd Place #1-B, Mission, KS 66202, BA 82 Southwest MO St Univ; MA 85 Central MO St Univ; **A**

Willis, Mrs Dora W 3811 Flintwood Lane, Opelika, AL 36801-7613, (205) 745-0137, BS 76 Northeastern Univ; MS 81 San Francisco St Univ; Clin Supvr, Auburn Univ, **A**

Willis, Mrs Joyce Thomas 4555 Walton Creek Road, Cincinnati, OH 45243, (513) 232-4302, BA 58 Univ of Akron; MS 61 Univ of Pittsburgh - Pittsburgh; Aud, Richard B Fleming MD Inc, **A**

Willis, Lisa Jean PO Box 210, Derby, UT 05829, (802) 766-8092, BA 83 Univ of VT; MS 84 Univ of VT; Sp-Lang Path, Orleans Essex N Supervisory Union, **SLP**

Willis, M Anthony 1618 Brome Circle, Lee's Summit, MO 64063, BS 79 Univ of Tulsa; MS 81 Central MO St Univ; Sp-Lang Path, Mo Crpld Chldn Serv, **SLP**

Willis, Mary Ann 3612 West Warwick, Peoria, IL 61615-2551, (309) 672-6585, BS 82 Bradley Univ; MS 84 FL St Univ; 86–Sp-Lang Path, Peoria PS Dist 150, **SLP**

Willis, Mary Stoveken 1058 Shaker Road, Westfield, MA 01085, (413) 568-9357, BA 68 Trenton St Coll; ME 70 PA St Univ - Univ Park; Sp-Lang Path, Westfield PS, **SLP**

Willis, Mrs Michelle S 1618 Brome Circle, Lee's Summit, MO 64063, BS 73 Univ of MD - College Park; MS 75 Washington Univ; 86–Sp-Lang Path, Private Practice, **SLP**

Willis, Mina P 3600-B Foxridge Apartment, Blacksburg, VA 24060, (919) 683-6470, BS 68 Longwood Coll; ME 78 NC Central Univ; MA 84 NC Central Univ; Doctoral, Nc Ctrl Univ, **SLP**

Willis, Pamela Ruth 4920 Winters Chapel Road, Apartment I-5, Doraville, GA 30360, (404) 921-2400, BS 78 Univ of VA - Charlottesville; ME 80 Univ of VA - Charlottesville; Sp-Lang Path, Gwinnett County Schools, **SLP**

Willis, Patricia Speech And Language Resources, 225 Regency Court Suite 200, Waukesha, WI 53186, (414) 796-0760, BS 71 Univ of WI - Madison; MS 74 Univ of WI - Whitewater; Dir, Speech & Language Resources Inc, **SLP**

Willis, Mrs Toni M 601 West Michigan Avenue, Marshall, MI 49068, (616) 781-5379, BA 83 MI St Univ; MA 87 Western MI Univ; **SLP**

Willis, Tracy Lynn 7600 West 63rd Street Apartment 204, Overland Park, KS 66202, (816) 932-3262, BS 84 KS St Univ; MA 85 KS St Univ; 86–Sp-Lang Path, St Luke's Hosp, **SLP**

Willis, Tyra Jean 554 South Dorchester, Anaheim, CA 92805, (714) 828-8660, BA 71 Univ of NV - Reno; OM 77 Brigham Young Univ; SLP, Cypress ISD, **SLP**

Willis, Yvonne Ingram 6283 Holly Park, Memphis, TN 38115, (901) 575-7158, BA 76 Memphis St Univ; MA 78 Memphis St Univ; Sp-Lang Path, Reg Med Cen, **SLP**

Willis-Henry, Olivia Marie P O Box 80282, San Diego, CA 92138, (619) 589-0867, BA 77 Columbia Union Coll; MA 78 OH St Univ; OM 83 Temple Univ-Tyler Sch of Art; Aud-Sp-Lang Path, Christiana Aud Assoc Inc, **A**

Willis-Simek, Mrs Teresa 2420 Algodones Northeast, Albuquerque, NM 87112, (505) 275-1316, **SLP**

Williston, James 65 Oak Ridge Lane, Bridgewater, MA 02324, (508) 697-7085, BA 62 Boston Univ; ME 65 Boston Univ; 75–Sp Lang Path, Attleboro Sch Dept, **SLP**

Willitts, Rebecca L 1202 West Northwood Street, Greensboro, NC 27408, (919) 299-3911, BS 84 Saint Lawrence Univ; ME 87 Univ of NC - Greensboro; 87–Sp-Lang Path, Private Practice, **SLP**

Willkom, Bonnie S 7712 Wissota Drive, Chippewa Falls, WI 54729, (715) 836-4186, BA 65 Univ of WI - Eau Claire; MS 71 Univ of WI - Eau Claire; Sp-Lang Path, U of Wisconsin Eau Claire, **SLP**

Willmeng, Jane A 2211 Pioneer, St Joseph, MI 49085, **SLP**

Willock, Tracy Lynn 3920 Miners Court, Placerville, CA 95667, (916) 626-9438, BA 81 CA St Univ - Sacramento; MA 84 CA St Univ - Sacramento; El Dorado Co Ofc of Ed, **SLP**

Willoughby, Carol D 12389 N W Kearney, Portland, OR 97229, (503) 280-5860, BS 65 OR Coll of Education; ME 69 OR St Univ; 74–Sp-Lang Path/Aud, Portland PS, **SLP A**

Willoughby, Paul J 12389 N W Kearney, Portland, OR 97229, (503) 228-9497, BS 66 Portland St Univ; MS 70 OR Coll of Education; 71–Aud & Administration, Portland Ear Nose & Throat Cl, **A**

Wills, Edward C 5953 Deerfield Drive, Alexandria, LA 71301, (318) 640-0754, BA 71 Southern Univ - Baton Rouge; MA 74 Northwestern St Univ; Sp-Lang Path, Pinecrest St Sch, **A**

Wills, Edward J 26909 Russell Road, Bay Village, OH 44140, (216) 362-2000, BA 69 Denison Univ; MA 75 Case Western Reserve Univ; 78–Aud, Kaiser Permanente Health Plan Inc, **A**

Wills, Jonnie Charlyne 630 West Pope Road, Apartment 46, St Augustine, FL 32084, (904) 824-1654, BA 84 Univ of FL; MA 86 Univ of FL; 86–Aud, Florida Sch for Deaf & Blind, **A**

Wills, Richard W 5139 Mapleridge Road, Kalamazoo, MI 49008-3532, **SLP**

Willson, Becky Lynn 3092 S Oakland Forest Dr, Apt 1803, Oakland Park, FL 33309, (305) 739-6269, BS 84 IL St Univ - Normal; MS 85 IL St Univ - Normal; 85–Sp-Lang Path, Sch Bd of Broward Co, **SLP**

Willson, Mrs Jane C Box 240, Skippack, PA 19474, (215) 495-7654, BA 74 Case Western Reserve Univ; MA 75 Kent St Univ; Sp-Lang Path, Montgomery County Intermed Unit, **SLP**

Willson, Karen D 42 Strathmore Road #34, Brighton, MA 02146, (617) 735-6482, BA 78 SUNY - Center at Buffalo; MA 80 SUNY - Center at Buffalo; Aud, The Children's Hosp, **A**

Willson, Marcia G 816 Haynes Street, Denton, TX 76201-4072, (817) 382-7532, BS 79 Univ of North TX; MS 81 Univ of North TX; Sp-Lang Path, Denton St Sch-Hab Ther, **SLP**

Willson, Stephanie Ann 722 Grand Avenue Apt B, St Paul, MN 55105, (612) 227-5429, BA 86 Univ of WI - Eau Claire; MS 87 Univ of WI - Eau Claire; 88–Dir of Sp-Lang Path, ELR Systems Inc

Wilmes, Robin Thate R R 2 Box 170, Pilot Grove, MO 65276-9103, (816) 834-4415, BS 77 Northwest MO St Univ; MS 80 Northwest MO St Univ; SLP, Cooper Co R V Sch Dist, **SLP**

Wilmette, Valeria 925 Highland Avenue, Joliet, IL 60435, (815) 740-3196, BS 56 IL St Univ - Normal; MS 65 Univ of IL - Chicago; Sp/Lang Path, Joliet Pub Sch, **SLP**

Wilms, Herbert R 5608 Park Place, Minneapolis, MN 55424, **SLP**

Wilner, Lynda Katz 3905 Esgarth Way, Owings Mills, MD 21117, (301) 356-5666, BA 75 Univ of MD - College Park; MS 76 Univ of MI - Ann Arbor; Sp-Lang Path, Private Practice, **SLP**

Wilner, Susan Scott 10 Garfield Lane East, Andover, MA 01810, (617) 475-3806, **SLP**

Wilsens, Paul C Munson Medical Center, 6th & Madison, Traverse City, MI 49684, (616) 922-9455, BS 80 Univ of WI - Whitewater; MA 81 Western MI Univ; Aud, Munson Med Cen, **A**

Wilsey, Mrs Mary Martha 25 North Parsonage Street, Rhinebeck, NY 12572, (914) 229-8967, MS 84 Coll of Saint Rose; BS 80 SUNY - Coll at Geneseo; Speech-Language Pathologist, St Francis Hospital, **SLP**

Wilson, Allan J, III P O Box 121, Lunenburg, MA 01462, (617) 582-6232, BA 62 Univ of MA - Amherst; ME 84 Fitchburg St Coll; MA 67 Univ of MA - Amherst; Sp-Lang Path, Winchendon PS, **SLP**

Wilson, Barbara Ann 52 Greenwood Park, Pittsford, NY 14534, (716) 586-1950, BS 85 SUNY - Coll at Geneseo; ME 87 Univ of VA - Charlottesville; 88–Sp-Lang Path, Rochester Sch for the Deaf, **SLP**

Wilson, Dr Barbara C North Shore University Hospital, Center For Neuropsychological Services, 400 Community Drive, Manhasset, NY 11030, (516) 562-3054, PH 64 (Psychology (Neuropsych)) NY Univ; 72–Dir-Neuropsychology, North Shore Univ Hospital

Wilson, Mrs Beth Minick Psc Box 5159, APO New York, NY 09109, **SLP**

Wilson, Beverley L 16 Maynard Street, West Newton, MA 02165, MS; **SLP LM**

Wilson, Mrs Brenda W Afkn, Box 24, Apo, San Francisco, CA 96301, BS 76 Southern IL Univ -Carbondale; MS 76 Auburn Univ - Auburn; 87–Sp-Lang Path, Dept of the Army, **SLP ACE**

Wilson, Mrs Carole W1716 Mortensen Road, Rt 1 Box 34-W, Brooklyn, WI 53521, (608) 835-3161, BS 68 Univ of MI - Ann Arbor; MA 70 Marshall Univ; Sp-Lang Path, Oregon School District, **SLP**

Wilson, Mrs Carolyn C 4317 Willow Way Road, Fort Worth, TX 76133, (817) 293-6033, BS 74 TX Christian Univ; MS 75 TX Christian Univ; Sp-Lang Path, Crowley ISD, **SLP**

Wilson, Carolyn M 6700 Cottage Hill Road, Box 186, Mobile, AL 36695, (205) 460-6327, BS 76 MS Univ for Women; MS 82 Univ Southern MS-Hattiesburg; 88–Sp-Lang Path, Univ of South Alabama, **SLP**

Wilson, Mrs Catherine Ann 3636 S Jefferson, St Louis, MO 63118, (314) 772-6855, BA 74 Univ of OR; MA 76 Univ of MT; 87–Sp-Lang Path, Salvation Army Hope Ctr, **SLP**

Wilson, Cathy L 14131 Sandy Point Lane, Houston, TX 77066, (713) 893-9405, BS 76 Univ of North TX; MS 79 Univ of North TX; Sp/Lang Path, Peggy Wyatt-Engman Inc, **SLP**

Wilson, Mrs Cathy Sue 2306 S W 13th Street, Apartment 410, Gainesville, FL 32608, (904) 335-0758, BS 83 IA St Univ; MA 85 Univ of IA; 88–Sp-Lang Path, Alachua County Schs, **SLP**

Wilson, Cheri A 924 5th Avenue S #1, Fargo, ND 58103, (701) 280-0094, MS 88 Moorhead St Univ

Wilson, Christine M 435 East 26th Street, San Angelo, TX 76903, (915) 949-9535, BS 75 Northern MI Univ; MA 79 WA St Univ; 86–Sp-Lang Path, West Texas Rehab Ctr, **SLP ACE**

Wilson, Mrs Colleen Collins 40515 Chapel Way #48, Fremont, CA 94538, (415) 490-7315, BA 85 CA St Univ - Sacramento; MA 86 Univ of the Pacific; **SLP**

Wilson, Connie S 1481 Center Street Ext, Apartment 1208, Mount Pleasant, SC 29464, (803) 577-5410, BS 83 James Madison Univ; ME 87 Univ of NC - Greensboro; SLP, Charleston Sp & Hrng Ctr, **SLP**

Wilson, Mrs Courtenay Martindale 14964 Manor Ridge Drive, Chesterfield, MO 63017, (214) 492-2621, BS 77 Ball St Univ; MA 78 Ball St Univ; Sp-Lang Path, Psychologist & Educators Inc, **SLP**

Wilson, Dr D Kenneth 6310 Pelican Creek Crossin, St Petersburg, FL 33707, (813) 381-4058, BA 39 Western MI Univ; MS 47 Purdue Univ - West Lafayette; PH 50 (NS) Purdue Univ - West Lafayette; 79–Professor Emeritus, SUNY Center at Buffalo, **SLP A F LM**

Wilson, Mrs Debbie Jan 4619 Inspiration Drive S E, Albuquerque, NM 87108, (505) 266-0252, BS 79 Southwest TX St Univ; ME 80 Southwest TX St Univ; **SLP**

Wilson, Deborah A 10444 Melrose Drive, North Huntingdon, PA 15642, (412) 864-0230, MS 86 CA Univ of PA; 86–Sp-Lang Path, Mary Jo Truschel PC, **SLP**

Wilson, Deborah Suzanne 1114 19th Avenue South, Nashville, TN 37212, (615) 320-5353, BA 81 Western KY Univ; MA 83 Univ of TN - Knoxville; Aud, Billwilkerson Hearing Ctr, **A**

Wilson, Mrs Diane S 6050 Alpine Court, Rapid City, SD 57702, (605) 343-8500, BA 68; MA 70 Univ of IA; Sp-Lang Path, Black Hills Rehab Hospital, **SLP**

Wilson, Donald M 453 Helm Avenue, Clovis, CA 93612-0714, (209) 439-2304, BA 39 Western WA Univ; MA 48 Univ of Southern CA; PH 50 (NS) Univ of Southern CA; **SLP LM**

Wilson, Donna Dene 191 Webster Road, Grand Junction, CO 81503, (303) 245-2100, BS 82 Univ of NH; MA 84 Temple Univ; 87–Sp-Lang Path, Private Practice, **SLP**

Wilson, Mrs Donna Piercy 4527 Southern Parkway, Louisville, KY 40214, (502) 543-7252, **SLP**

Wilson, Elaine D 11503 February Circle #102, Silver Spring, MD 20904, (301) 622-3139, BS 77 Ithaca Coll; MS 78 Syracuse Univ; 87–Aud, The Hearing Center, **A**

Wilson, Elizabeth 4811 Washington Avenue, Gulfport, MS 39501, MS; **SLP LM**

Wilson, Elizabeth Jane 19448 Misty Lane, Strongsville, OH 44136, BS 72 OH St Univ; MA 73 Cleveland St Univ; 88–Sp-Lang Path, Brunswick Bd Educ, **SLP**

Wilson, Ellaine 4201 Saxon #D, Metairie, LA 70002, (504) 888-3316, OB 70 FL St Univ; MS 72 FL St Univ; Jefferson Sp and Lang Center, **SLP**

Wilson, Elma V 2562 Henderson Road, Lake Odessa, MI 48849, (616) 374-8073, BS 79 Western MI Univ; MA 81 Western MI Univ; **SLP**

Wilson, Mrs Evelyn L 11451 Purple Beech Drive, Reston, VA 22091, (703) 281-6143, BS 64 PA St Univ - Univ Park; ME 70 CUNY - City College; MS 74 Columbia Univ Teachers Coll; Sp-Lang Path, Fairfax Cty Pub Sch, **SLP**

Wilson, Mrs Frances P 6310 Pelican Creek Crossin, St Petersburg, FL 33707, (813) 381-4058, BA 33 Univ of IL - Urbana; MA 42 Univ of IL - Urbana; **A LM**

Wilson, Dr Frank B Dept Of Speech Pathology, University Of Alberta, Faculty Of Rehab Medicine, Edmonton, AB, Canada T6G 0T2, (403) 432-5990, BS 50 Bowling Green St Univ; PH 56 (NS) Northwestern Univ; Prof, U of Alberta, **SLP A F**

Wilson, Gail B 12 Marion Court, Pomona, NY 10970, (914) 577-6590, BS 80 Mercy Coll; MA 85 Montclair St Coll; 88–Sp-Lang Path, East Ramapo Central Sch Dist, **SLP**

Wilson, Gail Karen 1081 Rio Grande, Pasadena, CA 91104, (817) 526-9506, BS 80 Hardin-Simmons Univ; MA 82 Univ of TN - Knoxville; Sp-Lang Path, LA Co Ofc of Educ, **SLP**

Wilson, Geraldine Rockwell Hearing Services, 760 Market Street #307, San Francisco, CA 94102, (415) 397-4944, BS 62 Edinboro Univ of PA; MA 63 Stanford Univ; Aud/Sp-Lang Path, Private Practice, **SLP A**

Wilson, Greg A 52 Walhalla Road, Columbus, OH 43202, (614) 263-7497, OB 80 Univ of Toledo; BA 80 Univ of Toledo; MA 81 Bowling Green St Univ; Aud, St of Oh/Columbus Dev Cen, **A**

Wilson, Gregory Scott 1421 Ramsgate Lane #A, Lynchburg, VA 24501, (916) 648-8457, BS 85 CA St Univ - Sacramento; MS 87 CA St Univ - Sacramento; **A**

Wilson, Gwendolyn D South Carolina State College, 300 College Street NE, PO Box 1804, Orangeburg, SC 29117, (803) 536-8590, BA 67 SC St Coll; MS 73 Columbia Univ Teachers Coll; ME 87 Columbia Univ Teachers Coll; 82–Asst Prof of Aud, Sc State Coll, **A**

Wilson, Mrs Heidi Bergmuelle 14004 Walnut Creek Road, Midlothian, VA 23113-4810, (804) 796-5638, BA 80 Rutger's St Univ - Douglas Coll; MS 84 James Madison Univ; **SLP**

Wilson, Mrs Helen B F 3100 Monticello Boulevard, Cleveland Heights, OH 44118, (216) 371-1331, BA 49 Bishop Coll; ME 51 Bishop Coll; Sp/Lang Path, Cleveland Bd of Ed, **SLP**

Wilson, Dr Howard Franklin Speech And Hearing Program, Lamar University, P O Box 10076, Beaumont, TX 77710, (409) 880-8170, BS 71 FL St Univ; MS 72 FL St Univ; PH 80 (Sp Path) OH Univ - Athens; Assoc Prof, Lamar University, **SLP**

Wilson, Mrs I Nell Audio Recovery Inc, 3400 N W 56th Street, Oklahoma City, OK 73112, (405) 949-1906, BA 80 Univ of MS; MA 81 Memphis St Univ; 87–Aud, Otologic Med Clinic, **A**

Wilson, Illa R 17142 East Crestline Place, Aurora, CO 80015, (303) 690-8639, **SLP**

Wilson, Dr James R 113 Fairview Drive, Warrensburg, MO 64093, (816) 429-4916, BS 64 Univ of MO - Columbia; MA 65 Univ of MO - Columbia; PH 75 (NS) Univ of Denver; Coordinator of Clinical Serv, Central Missouri State U, **SLP**

Wilson, Mrs Jane C 1321 Farrington Road, Philadelphia, PA 19151, (215) 877-1075, BS 82 East Stroudsburg Univ of PA; MA 87 Trenton St Coll; 84–Sp-Lang Path, Haverford Township Sch Dist, **SLP**

Wilson, Janell A 7151 Bronson S E, Ada, MI 49301, (616) 676-3395, BS 81 Ferris St Coll; MA 86 Central MI Univ; 87–SLP, Forest Hills PS, **SLP**

Wilson, Janice A 1800 Augusta Suite 150, Houston, TX 77057, (713) 947-7987, BA 75 Univ of Houston - Univ Park; MS 78 Univ of TX - Houston; 85–Sp-Lang Path, Private Practice, **SLP**

Wilson, Jaye Stansbury Route 1 Box 293, Pilot Mountain, NC 27041, (919) 386-8211, BS 76 OK St Univ; MA 79 OK St Univ; SLP, Surry Co Pub Sch Sys, **SLP**

Wilson, Mrs Joan Powers 1601 Morris Avenue, Norfolk, VA 23509, (804) 623-0526, MS 82 FL St Univ; Coordinator of Audiology, Ear Nose & Throat Ltd, **A**

Wilson, Joanne E 910 Stern Lane, Oxnard, CA 93030, (805) 984-3922, BA 72 Univ of CA - Santa Barbara; MA 74 Univ of Southern CA; Sp-Lang Path, Rio Sch Dist, **SLP**

Wilson, Jodi L 2735 Lyle Street, Sarasota, FL 33577, **SLP**

Wilson, Mrs Josephine F 4228 North Walnut Grove, Rosemead, CA 91770, (213) 681-4641, BA 59 Univ of AZ; MA 60 Stanford Univ; Exec Dir, Hear Center, **A**

Wilson, Mrs Judith H 113 Fairview Drive, Warrensburg, MO 64093, (816) 747-8446, BS 66 Univ of MO - Columbia; MA 67 Univ of MO - Columbia; Sp-Lang Path, Private Practice, **SLP**

Wilson, Mrs Julie A Ponotoc County Health Dept, Guidance Department, 1630 East Beverly, Ada, OK 74820, (405) 332-2016, BA 71 Univ of OK - Norman; MA 73 IN Univ - Bloomington; Sp-Lang Path, St Dept of Hlth, **SLP**

Wilson, Julie Viola 18 Palomino Drive, Kanata, ON, Canada K2M 1L9, BS 82 Univ of Western Ontario; OM 84 Univ of Western Ontario; 88–Sp-Lang Path, Ottawa Children's Treat Ctr, **SLP**

Wilson, Karen Ashton 1309 Deerwood Drive, Eagan, MN 55123-1427, (612) 681-0631, BS 61 Univ of MN - Minneap-St Paul; MS 80 Univ of WI - River Falls; Spec Ed Superv, Burnsville Pub Sch, **SLP**

Wilson, Karen Lee 4201 Gann Store Road, Hixson, TN 37343, (615) 483-4203, BA 72 Univ of MI - Ann Arbor; MS 73 Univ of MI - Ann Arbor; 88–Sp-Lang Path, Private Practice, **SLP**

Wilson, Karen P 2404 Sandler N E, Albuquerque, NM 87112, (505) 344-1375, BA 76 Univ of NM; MS 78 Univ of NM; Sp-Lang Path, Albuquerque Pub Sch, **SLP ACE**

Wilson, Katheryn 200 Grand Boulevard, Abilene, KS 67410, (913) 263-7046, BA 70 Fort Hays St Univ; MS 71 Fort Hays St Univ; Sp/Lang Path, USD #305 Central KS Cooperative in Educ, **SLP**

Wilson, Mrs Kathryn 220 East Pennsylvania, Ottumwa, IA 52501, (515) 682-8591, BA 80 Univ of Northern IA; MA 82 Univ of Northern IA; Sp-Lang Path, Southern Prairie AEA, **SLP**

Wilson, Dr Kent J 12415 East Gold Dust Drive, Tucson, AZ 85749, (602) 621-7064, BS 64 Bradley Univ; MA 65 Bradley Univ; PH 74 (Speech Pathology) Univ of MI - Ann Arbor; 87–Asst Dir/Sp-Lang Clin, Univ of Arizona, **SLP A**

Wilson, Kenyon D Northern Trails Area Ed Agency, Box M, Clear Lake, IA 50428, (515) 357-6125, BA 64 Univ of Northern IA; MA 67 Univ of Northern IA; Supvr of Hearing Conservation-Educ Dept, Northern Trls AEA, **SLP**

Wilson, Kim Elizabeth 40 Dowsett Avenue #B, Honolulu, HI 96817, (808) 531-3511, MS 84 Univ of WA; 87–Mgr-Comm Disorders Dept, Rehab Hosp of the Pacific, **SLP ACE**

Wilson, Mrs Laura McNutt 2843 Paces Ferry Road West, Orange Park, FL 32073, (904) 269-4490, BS 74 AR St Univ; MS 76 Univ of North TX; Aud, Ron Rish MD, **A ACE**

Wilson, Leane Michele 3566 Ely Lake Drive, Eveleth, MN 55734, (218) 741 4772, BA 83 Univ of ND; MS 85 Univ of ND; 85–Sp-Lang Path, VA PS ISD #706, **SLP**

Wilson, Lee Otolaryngology & Head/Neck Sur, Central Medical Bldg, Suite 600, St Paul, MN 55104, (612) 645-0691, BS 59 SUNY - Coll at Fredonia; MS 61 PA St Univ - Univ Park; Aud, Otol & Hd & Neck Surg, **A**

Wilson, Lillian F 626 First Avenue, Berwyn, PA 19312, BS 54 Washington Univ; MS 56 Washington Univ; Superv/Prog & Serv for Hrng Im, De Co Inter Unit 25, **SLP**

Wilson, Linda A 1938 Kendall Avenue, Madison, WI 53705, (608) 238-6105, BA 80 Univ of WI - Eau Claire; MS 81 Marquette Univ; 82–Sp-Lang Path, Restorative Care Assoc Inc, **SLP**

Wilson, Linda F 569 Bayview Drive, Longboat Key, FL 34228, (813) 371-2484, BA 71 Dickinson Coll; MS 86 Univ of TX - Dallas; 88–Sp-Lang Path, Sarasota Co PS, **SLP**

Wilson, Dr Linda M 3424 North Utah, Oklahoma City, OK 73112, (405) 272-5545, Assistant Director, Oklahoma City Schools, **SLP**

Wilson, Mrs Linda S 2012 Hillcrest Road, Mobile, AL 36695, (205) 633-0241, BS 66 Bowling Green St Univ; MA 71 Northern IL Univ - De Kalb; Sp-Lang Path, Mobile Co Sch SW Reg Sch, **SLP**

Wilson, Linda S 3362 Marina Way, Spring Hill, FL 34606, (904) 683-5500, BA 76 Univ of FL; ME 78 Univ of FL; Owner/Sp-Lang Path, Commun Rehab Serv, **SLP**

Wilson, Mrs Lisa McCall 158 Londonderry Lane, Getzville, NY 14068, (716) 837-2441, BS 78 Baylor Univ; MA 80 TX Woman's Univ; SLP, Language Dev Programs of NY, **SLP**

Wilson, Mrs Luana S 7784 Pearl Road, Middleburg Heights, OH 44130, (216) 237-8800, OB 63 OH Univ - Athens; MA 64 OH Univ - Athens; Sp-Lang Path, North Royalton Cty Schools, **SLP**

Wilson, Margaret B 3280 Oak Court, Delmont, CA 94002-1340, (415) 469-1398, **SLP**

Wilson, Dr Margo E 8735 Adams Lane, Lexington, KY 40515, (606) 257-3390, BS 66 Univ of NE - Lincoln; MA 68 Univ of NE - Lincoln; PH 78 (Sp Path & Aud) Univ of KS; Sp-Lang Path, Univ of Kentucky Med Ctr, **SLP**

Wilson, Marilyn K 124 West Central Avenue, Winter Haven, FL 33880, (813) 299-7188, BS 74 LA St Univ - Baton Rouge; OM 75 LA St Univ - N O Medical Ctr; Aud, Cen Hearing Clin Inc, **A**

Wilson, Marsha L 7618 Farmgate Way, Citrus Heights, CA 95610, (916) 363-7323, BA 70 CA St Univ - Sacramento; MA 72 CA St Univ - Sacramento; Prog Spec-Spec Ed, Folsom Cordova USD, **SLP**

Wilson, Mary A 6333 Windswept Lane #16, Houston, TX 77057, (713) 782-3150, BA 85 Auburn Univ - Auburn; OM 87 Auburn Univ - Auburn; 88–Aud, Baylor Coll of Medicine

Wilson, Mrs Mary Amanda 4307 Overlook Road, Birmingham, AL 35222, (205) 591-0528, BS 75 FL St Univ; MS 86 Univ of Montevallo

Wilson, Mrs Mary Ann D 102 Tanglewood Place, Parkersburg, WV 26101, (304) 428-8139, BS 77 WV Univ; MS 78 WV Univ; **SLP**

Wilson, Mary Anne 833 Westcott Street, Syracuse, NY 13210, (315) 472-1263, BA 79 SUNY - Coll at Cortland; MS 82 Syracuse Univ; Aud, OCM BOCES, **A**

Wilson, Mary K 1713 Camina Placer, Farmington, NM 87401, (505) 327-6625, BS 72 Eastern NM Univ; MS 74 Eastern NM Univ; Sp-Lang Path, Aztec Mun Sch, **SLP**

Wilson, Mary Lois 8605 Clover Lane, Urbandale, IA 50322, (404) 938-6436, BA 28 Grinnell Coll; MA 45 Univ of IA; **SLP LM**

Wilson, Mary Pat 12412 Mt Pleasant Drive, Laurel, MD 20708, (202) 651-5328, BA 71 Catholic Univ of America; MS 74 Gallaudet Coll; Aud/Aud Habilitationist, Gallaudet Coll, **A**

Wilson, Dr Mary Sweig Laureate Learning Systems, Inc, 110 East Spring Street, Winooski, VT 05404, (802) 862-7355, BA 62 Smith Coll; MA 65 Emerson Coll; PH 68 (NS) Northwestern Univ; 82–Pres, Laureate Learning Systems Inc, **SLP F**

Wilson, Mrs Mary Z 3713 Greenbrier Road, Ashland, KY 41101, (614) 532-2905, BA 74 Univ of KY; MA 77 Marshall Univ; Sp-Lang Path, Russell ISD, **SLP**

Wilson, Michael J P O Box 15513, Seattle, WA 98115-0513, (206) 543-5230, BA 71 Wabash Coll; OM 75 IN Univ - Bloomington; MA 80 NM St Univ; 86–Aud, Otol Dept Univ of WA, **A**

Wilson, Dr Michele Drisko 2 Sunburst, Irvine, CA 92715-3607, (714) 854-3700, BA 68 Northwestern Univ; MA 71 Univ of KS; PH 78 (Aud) Vanderbilt Univ; Hrng & Sp Consult, Private Practice, **A**

Wilson, Mrs Minnie B P O Box 292, Rockaway, NJ 07866, (201) 361-6594, BS 71 SUNY - Center at Buffalo; BA 71 SUNY - Center at Buffalo; MA 76 SUNY - Center at Buffalo; Sp-Lang Path, PS 188 at JH 120, **SLP**

Wilson, Nancy 35 Osborne Street, Lynn, MA 01905, (617) 595-2845, BA 80 Boston Coll; MS 83 Boston Univ; 86–Sp-Lang Path, Newburyport PS, **SLP**

Wilson, Nancy A 821 S Williams #B505, Westmont, IL 60559, (312) 964-1273, BA 76 Univ of MI - Ann Arbor; MS 77 Univ of MI Ann Arbor; 87 Aud, Private Practice, **A**

Wilson, Nancy M 975 Easton Place, Dallas, TX 75218, (214) 943-2005, BS 63 Midwestern St Univ; MA 64 TX Woman's Univ; **SLP**

Wilson, Patricia A 2728 Francis, St Joseph, MO 64501, (816) 232-1446, BA 72 Univ of SD - Vermillion; MA 80 Univ of SD - Vermillion; Sp-Lang Path, State of Missouri, **SLP**

Wilson, Mrs Paula E B 10901 N Federal Blvd, Denver, CO 80234, (303) 466-6797, BS 71 CO St Univ; MA 75 Univ of Denver; **SLP**

Wilson, Mrs Paula S P O Box 485, Sterling, VA 22170, (703) 391-0480, BA 69 NM St Univ; MA 70 NM St Univ; **A**

Wilson, Phillip L Callier Cen For Comm Disorders, 1966 Inwood Road, Dallas, TX 75235, (214) 783-3000, BA 72 Southern Methodist Univ; MS 79 Univ of TX - Dallas; Aud, Callier Cen for Commun Dis, **A**

Wilson, Ramon L Route 1 Box 124, Carmel By Sea, CA 93923, BA 60 San Francisco St Univ; MA 61 San Francisco St Univ; Sp-Lang Path, Salinas City Sch Dist, **SLP**

Wilson, Mrs Rebecca A 8137 West Laurel Drive #F, Littleton, CO 80123, (303) 861-6800, MS 78 Central MO St Univ; Sp-Lang Path, Childrens Hosp Denver, **SLP**

Wilson, Dr Richard Hayes Audiology 126, VA Medical Center, 5901 East 7th Street, Long Beach, CA 90822, (213) 494-5414, BS 64 East TN St Univ; MS 65 Vanderbilt Univ; PH 70 (Aud) Northwestern Univ; Chief/Aud Sec, VA Med Ctr, **A**

Wilson, Robert Lynn 122 McClure Street, Gonzales, TX 78629, (512) 672-7561, BS 63 Henderson St Univ; ME 70 Southwest TX St Univ; 86–Dir, Childrens Diagnostic Cen, **SLP**

Wilson, Roberta Anne 939 Roanoke Avenue, Hillside, NJ 07205, (201) 558-3001, **SLP**

Wilson, Mrs Sabrina Fowler 7410 Sunlight Lane, Houston, TX 77095-1427, (713) 469-0351, BA 78 SC St Coll; MA 81 Univ of Cincinnati; Sp-Lang Path, Cypress Fairbanks ISD, **SLP**

Wilson, Sharon A Route 2 Box 77, San Marcos, TX 78666, (512) 396-8500, BS 81 Southwest TX St Univ; ME 82 Southwest TX St Univ; SLP, Brown Sch/San Marcos Treat Cen, **SLP**

Wilson, Mrs Sharon L P O Box 632, Rison, AR 71655, (501) 325-7293, BA 79 Univ of AR - Little Rock; MS 81 Univ of AR - Medical Sci; Sp-Lang Path, Private Practice, **SLP**

Wilson, Mrs Sherrie Lynn 24261 Via Aquara, Laguna Niguel, CA 92766, (312) 934-8299, MS 84 Bloomsburg Univ of PA; Sp-Lang Path, Newport Lang Sp Aud Center, **SLP**

Wilson, Susan B 70 Junco Court, Three Bridges, NJ 08887, (212) 439-3385, BA 82 Fairleigh Dickinson U-Madisn; MA 86 Hofstra Univ; 86–Aud, Lenox Hill Hosp, **A**

Wilson, Susan Marie 562 Kenmore Avenue, Buffalo, NY 14216, (716) 835-6145, BS 79 SUNY - Coll at Fredonia; ME 80 Clarion Univ of PA; Sp-Lang Path, Buffalo Bd of Ed, **SLP**

Wilson, Mrs Susan S 391 West Salisbury Street, P O Box 949, Pittsboro, NC 27312, (919) 542-5854, BS 81 Northwestern Univ; ME 82 Univ of NC - Greensboro; SLP, Chatham Co Schs, **SLP**

Wilson, Mrs Suzan Gayle 3001 South Jackson, San Angelo, TX 77690, (915) 949-9535, BS 78 Southwest TX St Univ; ME 79 Southwest TX St Univ; Sp-Lang Path, West Texas Rehabilitation Cen, **SLP**

Wilson, Suzanne Michelle 26241 Lakeshore Blvd #2054, Euclid, OH 44132, (216) 844-7660, BA 84 Abilene Christian Univ; MA 87 Case Western Reserve Univ; 86–Research Asst, Case Western Reserve Univ, **SLP**

Wilson, Mrs Suzanne Sinclair 1605 E Capitol Avenue, Bismarck, ND 58501, (701) 258-6556, MS 87 Minot St Univ

Wilson, Teresa E 1060 Aaron Road, North Brunswick, NJ 08902, **SLP**

Wilson, Terri K Rural Route 3 Box 58, Thompsonville, IL 62890, (618) 242-4600, BS 78 Eastern IL Univ; MS 79 Eastern IL Univ; 84–SLP, Good Samaritan Reg Health Ctr, **SLP**

Wilson, Terrie H 1553 Laureldale Drive, Raleigh, NC 27609-3572, (919) 790-2500, BA 76 Columbia Coll; OM 78 Univ of SC - Columbia; 85–Sp-Lang Path, Wake Co PS Sys, **SLP**

Wilson, Theresa Marie 1505 East 96th Street, Brooklyn, NY 11236, (212) 596-5742, BA 78 Hofstra Univ; MA 80 Hofstra Univ; SLP, Sp Ser U/NYC Bd of Ed, **SLP**

Wilson, Mrs Theresa S 55 Candlewood Drive, Yonkers, NY 10710, (914) 963-4567, BA 76 CUNY - Lehman Coll; MA 79 CUNY - Lehman Coll; SLP, Yonkers Public Schools, **SLP**

Wilson, V Denice 4204 Lankford, Springdale, AR 72764, (501) 575-4509, MS 86 Univ of AR - Fayetteville; **SLP**

Wilson, Vicki A 54 Webster Street, Hyde Park, MA 02136, (508) 824-5881, MS 85 Northeastern Univ; 86–Aud, Commonwealth of Massachusetts, **A**

Wilson, Dr Wesley R Dept Of Speech & Hearing Sci, (Jg-15), University Of Washington, Seattle, WA 98195, (206) 543-7966, BA 58 Univ of Redlands; MA 60 Univ of Redlands; PH 69 (Aud) Univ of WA; Professor, University of Washington, **SLP A F**

Wilson, Dr Willa Campbell Coll Ofallied Medical Sciences, Rehab Department, P O Box 10219 King Saud U, Riyadh, Saudi Arabia 11433, (803) 536-8176, BA 70 SC St Coll; MA 72 Univ of IL - Urbana; PH 75 (NS) Univ of IL - Urbana; Assoc Prof, Sc St Coll, **SLP**

Wilson, William Arthur 1406 West Walworth Street, Whitewater, WI 53190, (608) 255-5011, BA 70 Univ of WI - Madison; MS 86 Univ of WI - Whitewater

Wilson, William C 8839 Nebraska, Livonia, MI 48150, (313) 876-3289, BA 57 MI St Univ; MA 75 Wayne St Univ; Aud, Ford Hosp, **A ACE**

Wilson, Mrs Yvonne H 229 San Saba, Richwood Clute, TX 77531, (409) 265-6822, BS 72 TX Tech Univ; MS 73 TX Tech Univ; **SLP**

Wilson-Coleman, Mrs Phyllis Marie 16318 Hemitage, Markham, IL 60426, (312) 339-5788, Speech/Language/Pathologist, S Metro Assn Lo Incidence Hdcp, **SLP**

Wilsonn, Mrs Maria Johnson 49 Seminary Avenue, Binghamton, NY 13905, (607) 722-5308, BS 82 SUNY - Coll at Geneseo; MS 84 Ithaca Coll; Sp-Lang Path, Rehabilitation Services Inc, **SLP**

Wilson-Russell, Mrs Wendy 5 Roland Avenue, East Norwalk, CT 06855, (203) 762-8526, BS 80 Northeastern Univ; MS 81 Ithaca Coll; Sp/Lang Path, CES, **SLP**

Wilson-Vazquez, Mrs Kathleen G Veteran's Administration Medical Center, 1201 NW 16th Street, Miami, FL 33125, (305) 324-3148, BS 81 WV Univ; MS 82 FL St Univ; 88–Sp-Lang Path, VA Med Ctr, **SLP ACE**

Wilson-Ward, Kathleen 398 Argonne Drive, Kenmore, NY 14217, (716) 834-7200, BS 72 SUNY - Center at Buffalo; MS 73 Ithaca Coll; 86–Aud, NE Comm Achievement Ctr, **A**

Wilt, Dr Sonya M 262 Leech Road, Greenville, PA 16125, (412) 588-7700, BA 59 Muskingum Coll; MA 62 Univ of Pittsburgh - Pittsburgh; PH 75 (NS) Univ of Pittsburgh - Pittsburgh; Professor of Communication, Thiel College, **SLP**

Wiltcher, Cynthia G Route 1 Box 64, Moselle, MS 39459, (601) 428-1564, **SLP**

Wilton, Mrs Mary Martiny 3132 Pleasant Grove N E, Grand Rapids, MI 49505, (616) 363-4116, BS 82 Central MI Univ; MA 83 MI Tech Univ; **SLP**

Wiltsie, Dawn M 165 Kenville Road, Cheektowaga, NY 14215, BS 85 SUNY - Coll at Geneseo; MS 86 SUNY - Coll at Buffalo; 88–Sp-Lang Path, Buffalo Hrng & Sp Ctr, **SLP**

Wiltz, Muriel R P O Box 750186, New Orleans, LA 70175, (504) 897-0386, BA 50 Xavier Univ of LA; MS 57 Syracuse Univ; **SLP**

Wiman, Vicki L Tallahassee Ear Nose & Throat, 1401 Centerville Road, Suite 506, Tallahassee, FL 32308, (904) 877-0101, BS 73 Murray St Univ; MS 74 Vanderbilt Univ; 86–Aud, Tallahassee ENT, **A**

Wimberly, Annette C 2514 34th Avenue, Meridian, MS 39301, (601) 483-8121, BS 72 Univ Southern MS-Hattiesburg; MS 77 Univ Southern MS-Hattiesburg; 80–Dir, Meridian Sp & Hrng Cen, **SLP**

Wimberly, Sally Pettit P O Box 805, Presque Isle, ME 04769, (207) 455-4308, BS 75 Vanderbilt Univ; MS 77 Vanderbilt Univ; **SLP**

Wimmer, Vega H Moored Hearing Aid Service, 2311 F Stadium Boulevard, Ann Arbor, MI 48104, (313) 663-2915, BS 57 Northwestern Univ; OM 70 Wayne St Univ - Sch of Med; **SLP A**

Wimmer-Kuehl, Lonna G 7727 Benson, Overland Park, KS 66204, (816) 781-1600, BA 73 Univ of MO - KS City; MS 74 Central MO St Univ; Dir Sp & Hrng, Clay Co Hlth Cen, **SLP ACE**

Win, Susan M 6805 Mayfield Road, Suite 1401, Mayfield Heights, OH 44124, (216) 449-3567, MA 88 Case Western Reserve Univ

Winarski, Mrs Betty Ellen 222 Chittenden Road, Clifton, NJ 07013, (201) 239-5590, BA 64 Montclair St Coll; MA 67 Columbia Univ Teachers Coll; Sp-Lang Path, Verona Bd of Ed, **SLP ACE**

Winarsky, Sharon E 80 Crystal Avenue, West Orange, NJ 07052, (201) 533-5786, BA 72 Rutger's St Univ - Douglas Coll; ME 73 Northeastern Univ; Superv of SLP, St Barnabas Med Cen, **SLP ACE**

Winchell, George Corwin 2812 North Bryant, Portland, OR 97217, (503) 289 8751, MS 82 Portland St Univ, **A**

Winchester, Mrs Carol G 117 Dorado Avenue, Sewell, NJ 08080, (609) 582-6234, BA 77 Saint Mary's Coll; MS 79 Bradley Univ; SLP, Private Practice, **SLP**

Winchester, Cynthia P 4847 Pinedale Boulevard, Lumberton, NC 28358, (919) 738-7195, BS 82 East Carolina Univ; MS 84 East Carolina Univ; Director of Audiology, Southeastern General Hospital, **A**

Winchester, Madonna R R R 2 Box 358, Leeson Drive, New Castle, IN 47362, **LM**

Winder, Mrs Anette Schettino 8845 Stonebrook Lane, Columbia, MD 21046, (301) 964-8483, BA 77 Univ of MD - College Park; MS 79 Loyola Coll; Sp/Lang Path, Howard County Board of Educ, **SLP**

Winder, Deidre Ann 21388 S W Martinazzi Avenue, Tualatin, OR 97062, BA 79 Portland St Univ

Winder, Surline A 418 Franklin, Wapello, IA 52653, BS; **SLP LM**

Windhager, Julie Claire Dallas Easter Seal Society, 5701 Maple Avenue, Dallas, TX 75235, (214) 358-5261, BS 84 TX Christian Univ; MS 86 Vanderbilt Univ; 87–Sp-Lang Path, Dallas ESSC, **SLP**

Windham, Laurabeth 1054 East Seminole, Springfield, MO 65807, (417) 836-5368, BS 49 Southwest MO St Univ; MA 52 Univ of OK - Norman; Instr/Super, SW Mo St U, **SLP**

Windhausen, Perrian B 10302 Xavier Court, Westminster, CO 80030, (303) 466-2141, BA 82 Univ of OK - Norman; MA 84 Univ of CO - Boulder; **SLP**

Windle, Jill V 726 Diamond Leaf, Houston, TX 77079-3702, (713) 523-3633, BS 76 Univ of AR - Fayetteville; MA 77 Univ of AR - Fayetteville; Sp-Lang Path, Private Practice, **SLP**

Windman, Mrs Gail G 1617 North Fraser Drive, Mesa, AZ 85203, (319) 582-5088, BS 69 Univ of IA; MA 71 Univ of IA; **SLP**

Windmill, Dr Ian M Department Of Surgery, University Of Louisville, 129 East Broadway, Louisville, KY 40292, (502) 588-5274, BS 78 FL St Univ; MS 79 FL St Univ; PH 83 (Aud) FL St Univ; Asst Prof of Surg (Aud), U of Louisville, **A**

Windmill, Sue McDonnell 1002 Golden Maple Cove, Louisville, KY 40223, (502) 244-2779, BA 74 Univ of KY; MS 85 Univ of Louisville; 88–Sp-Lang Path, Frazier Rehab Ctr, **A**

Windom, Mrs Catherine C 254 Suffolk Road, Mobile, AL 36608, (205) 666-0901, BA 71 Univ of AL- Tuscaloosa; MA 73 Univ of AL- Tuscaloosa; 88–Sp-Lang Path, Mobile Co PS, **SLP**

Windsor, Jennifer Ann Dept-Audiology/Speech Sciences, Heavilon Hall, Purdue University, West Lafayette, IN 47907, (317) 494-3785, OB 81 Cumberland Coll of Health Sciences - Australia; MS 86 Purdue Univ - West Lafayette; 88–Grad Staff, Purdue Univ

Windsor, Shelley Box 763, Columbia Falls, MT 59912, (406) 752-0101, BA CA St Univ - Chico; MA 86 CA St Univ - Chico; 87–Sp-Lang Path, Evergreen Sch Dist #50, **SLP**

Windsor, Shirley M 230 South Hillcrest, Ada, OK 74820, (405) 332-8000, BS 73 Phillips Univ; MS 75 Phillips Univ; Sp-Lang Path, E Cen Ok St U, **SLP**

Wine, Mrs Ann Dogan 6718 Greenbark Drive, Memphis, TN 38115, (901) 522-6593, BA 79 Univ of MS; MA 81 Memphis St Univ; Sp-Lang Path, Baptist Memorial Hospital, **SLP**

Winegar, Rebecca Westra 912 Roseland, Kalamazoo, MI 49001, (215) 783-6010, **SLP**

Wineinger, Cynthia J 6236 East Coral Circle, Anaheim Hills, CA 92807, (714) 639-4990, BS 77 Northwestern Univ; MS 80 Univ of Redlands; Sp-Lang Path, Providence Sp & Hrng Cen, **SLP**

Wineman, Ellen Frey 608 Crum Creek Road, Wallingford, PA 19086, BA 71 George Washington Univ; MA 86 West Chester Univ of PA; **SLP**

Winer, Charlene Ava 2 Minuteman Road, Sharon, MA 02067, (617) 784-1935, BA 73 Univ of Toledo; MA 85 Univ of Pittsburgh - Pittsburgh; **SLP**

Winer, Mrs Heidi Eileen 1209 Camino Oro, Farmington, NM 87401, (505) 326-0928, BS 80 Univ of OR; MS 83 Western OR St Coll; SLP, Farmimgton Ps, **SLP**

Winer, Dr Marc E 6 Norfolk Avenue, Swampscott, MA 01907-1805, (617) 389-7950, BA 70 Salem St Coll; BS 73 Emerson Coll; ED 82 (NS) Boston Univ; Sp-Lang Path, Everett Public Schools, **SLP**

Winer-McWilliam, Yona 11690 Northwest 27 Court, Plantation, FL 33323-1827, (305) 556-0121, BA 74 CUNY - Queens Coll; MA 77 Univ of Miami; **SLP**

Winfrey, Joan Margaret 1627 South Jefferson Davis Parkway, New Orleans, LA 70125, MA 84 LA St Univ - Baton Rouge; BA 82 Univ of Southwestern LA; Sp-Lang Path, Children's Hosp, **SLP**

Wing, Christine 600 River Ridge, River Falls, WI 54022, (715) 425-9604, BS 72 Univ of WI - Madison; MS 73 Univ of VT; 88–Sp-Lang Path, Special Children Ctr, **SLP**

Wing, Dr Clara S 10631 Weymouth Street #203, Bethesda, MD 20814, (301) 384-4816, MA 66 American Univ; MA 72 Univ of MD - College Park; PH 78 (Sp-Lang Path) Univ of MD - College Park; Sp-Lang Path, Mont Co MD Pub Sch, **SLP**

Wing, Joy Chow 524 Inglewood, Vicksburg, MS 39180, (601) 638-7467, BA 77 Univ of MS; MS 80 Univ of MS; Sp-Lang Path, Vicksburg Warren Sch Dist, **SLP**

Wingard, Gary Lee 416 Smith Drive, Colby, KS 67701, (913) 462-6789, BA 60 Northwestern OK St Univ; MS 75 Fort Hays St Univ; 88–Sp-Lang Path, USD #315, **SLP**

Wingate, Cicely J Route 2 Box 102, Pullman, WA 99163, BA 67 Univ of WA; MA 69 Univ of WA; **SLP**

Wingate, Mrs Judith Maige 1515 N E 12th Terrace, Gainesville, FL 32601, (904) 378-0104, BA 76 Baptist Coll at Charleston; MS 83 Univ of South FL; 88–Sp-Lang Path, Michelle Jensen PhD, **SLP ACE**

Winger, Mrs Anita Marie 1007 Arlene Court #13, Bloomington, IL 61701, BS 85 IL St Univ - Normal; MS 87 IL St Univ - Normal; Sp-Lang Path, Hammitt Sch-The Baby Fold

Winger, Mrs Joan B 5126 Kay Lane, Sebring, FL 33872, (813) 382-1121, BS 71 PA St Univ - Univ Park; MS 74 Indiana Univ of PA; Sp-Lang Path, Highlands Co Sch, **SLP**

Winger, Joan M 7473 Pelican Drive, West Chester, OH 45069, (513) 867-2473, BS 73 Univ of WI - Oshkosh; MS 75 AZ St Univ; 84–Superv of Sp-Lang Path, Ft Hamilton Hughes Hosp, **SLP**

Winger, Dr Roger K 269 Rose Avenue, Marion, OH 43302, (614) 383-2513, BS 64 Ashland Coll; MA 66 OH St Univ; PH 69 (Aud) OH St Univ; Dir/Aud, Marion Ther Cen Inc, **A**

Wingfield, Jane Susan 1821 N W 82nd #405, Lawton, OK 73505, (405) 353-0334, BS 85 Univ of OK - OK City; ME 87 Central St Univ

Winik, Mrs Michelle Lester 12007 Garrison Forest Road, Owings Mills, MD 21117, (301) 396-1357, **SLP**

Winitz, Dr Harris University Of Missouri, 5216 Rockhill Road, Kansas City, MO 64110, (816) 276-2261, BA 54 Univ of VT; MA 56 Univ of IA; PH 59 (NS) Univ of IA; Prof, U of MO - Kansas Cty, **SLP F**

Winkel, Julie Ann 5175 Skylite, Utica, MI 48087, (313) 749-5131, BS 85 Central MI Univ; MA 87 Central MI Univ; Sp-Lang Path, Chippewa Valley PS, **SLP**

Winkleman, Mrs Dorothy E R R 2 Box 39, Sioux Falls, SD 57103, (605) 336-9277, BA 78 Northeast MO St Univ; MS 79 Northeast MO St Univ; Sp-Lang Path, Luverne Public Schools 670, **SLP**

Winkler, Cynthia Ann 26165 Sanz #D, Mission Viejo, CA 92691-2835, (505) 662-4087, BA 81 NM St Univ; MA 83 NM St Univ; SLP, Mesa Public Schs, **SLP**

Winkler, Mrs Erika C 835 North Rock Boulevard, Sparks, NV 89431, (702) 355-7722, BS 80 Univ of NV - Reno; MS 83 Univ of NV - Reno; Sp-Lang Path, Robison House Assoc, **SLP**

Winkler, Jeanne L 400 South Hamilton #2, Hillsboro, IL 62049-1437, (217) 532-6489, BS 79 Eastern IL Univ; MS 80 Southern IL Univ-Edwardsvill; Sp-Lang Path, Hillsboro Comm Sch Dist #3, **SLP**

Winkler, Karen Jean 134 Barkley Park #137, Fredericksburg, VA 22401, (313) 284-6068, BS 85 Eastern MI Univ; MA 86 Eastern MI Univ; **SLP**

Winkler, Lisa Ellen 705 B East 45th Street, Austin, TX 78751, (512) 451-6539, **SLP**

Winkler, Lois Jeanne 7918 Jones-Maltsberger, Apartment C-1, San Antonio, TX 78246, (512) 828-5534, BS 83 Bowling Green St Univ; MA 85 Bowling Green St Univ; **SLP**

Winkler, Mrs Marcia B 24 Doyle Road, Oakdale, CT 06370, (203) 443-3210, OM 83 SC St Coll; MS 76 CUNY - Brooklyn Coll; BA 70 CUNY - Queens Coll; Sp-Lang Path, Waterford Publ Sch, **SLP**

Winkler, Mindy R 3346 N E Alameda, Portland, OR 97212-1802, (503) 241-1811, BA 73 Univ of VT; MS 74 Univ of VT; SLP, Children's Program PC, **SLP**

Winkler, Dr Sheila J P O Box 641, Pittsburgh, PA 15230, (412) 566-2680, MS 70 Univ of Pittsburgh - Pittsburgh; PH 82 (Sp-Lang Path) Univ of Pittsburgh - Pittsburgh; 75–Sp-Lang Path, Private Practice, **SLP ACE**

Winkler, Suzanne J 442 Bambrick Street, Oceanside, NY 11572, (516) 536-7239, BA 84 SUNY - Center at Buffalo; MS 86 Adelphi Univ; **SLP**

Winkler, Wanda Joy 1932 Brynell Drive, Lexington, KY 40505, (606) 268-2843, BA 80 Univ of KY; MS 81 Univ of AL- Tuscaloosa; Aud, Comm for Hndcpd Chldrn, **A**

Winkowski, Teresa Banta P O Box 3031, San Pedro, CA 90731-0221, (213) 430-9624, **SLP**

Winn, Barbara B 15411 Valley Bend, Houston, TX 77068, (713) 583-1483, **SLP**

Winn, Conrad 432 North Prospect Avenue, Redondo Beach, CA 90277, (213) 540-2927, BS 70 Univ of CA - Riverside; MA 83 CA St Univ - Stanislaus; Sp-Lang Path, Private Practice, **SLP**

Winn, Patricia Elizabeth 212 Roosevelt Avenue, Northfield, NJ 08225, (609) 345-5191, BS 84 Stockton St Coll; MS 86 Univ of MI - Ann Arbor; **SLP**

Winn, Sandra Lee 20 Lori Lane, The Crossings Apts, West Carrollton, OH 45449, (513) 229-6081, **SLP**

Winn, Mrs Victoria L 1422 Queens Court Road, Peoria, IL 61614, (309) 671-2927, BS 71 Bradley Univ; MS 73 Bradley Univ; Sp/Lang Path, I of Phys Medic & Rehab, **SLP**

Winne, Deborah Ann 280 Washington Avenue, Kingston, NY 12401, (914) 338-8686, BS 78 SUNY - Coll at New Paltz; ME 84 Coll of Saint Rose; Sp-Lang Path, Edward L Aleo Phd & Associates, **SLP**

Winneg, Beth C 33 Union Square, Randolph, MA 02368, (617) 580-7360, BS 71 Emerson Coll; MS 72 Adelphi Univ; Sp-Lang Path, Brockton Pub Sch, **SLP**

Winner, Lori Ann 870 Main Street #2, Follansbee, WV 26037, (304) 748-8188, BS 85 WV Univ; MS 87 WV Univ; **SLP**

Winner, Mrs Michelle Garcia 635 South Woodlawn, Bloomington, IN 47401, (812) 335-6508, BA 82 Univ of CA - Santa Barbara; MA 85 IN Univ - Bloomington; Sp-Lang Path, Dev Trng Ctr, **SLP**

Winnett, Sharon Lee R R 1 Box 132, Hillsboro, IL 62049, (217) 532-2305, MS 84 Southern IL Univ-Edwardsvill; 86–Sp-Lang Path/Dir, Hillsboro CO D#3, **SLP**

Winney, Mrs Vernell 2241 Freeland Way, Dallas, TX 75228, (214) 381-1114, BS 76 Lamar Univ; MS 77 Lamar Univ; SLP, Dallas ISD, **SLP**

Winnik, Mrs Florence R 719 Washington Street, P O Box 384, Leonardtown, MD 20650, (301) 475-2975, BS 63 Univ of WI - Madison; MS 66 Univ of WI - Madison; Dir SLP, St Mary's Co Hlth Dept, **SLP ACE**

Winning, Mrs Maude I 28206 East Crown Point, Troutdale, OR 97060, (714) 520-5849, BA 68 CA St Univ - Fullerton; MA 74 CA St Univ - Fullerton; **SLP**

Winningham, Mrs Anthia K Box 130, Bradford, AR 72020, (501) 344-2707, BS 74 AR St Univ; MS 76 AR St Univ; Sp-Lang Path, Bradford Sch Dist, **SLP**

Winokur, Mrs Irene Synnott 93 Sunnyside Drive, Yonkers, NY 10705, (914) 376-3760, OB 75 CUNY - Lehman Coll; MA 82 CUNY - Lehman Coll; 79–Sp-Lang Path/Aud, NY City Bd of Educ, **SLP A**

Winship, Patricia Ann 22 Court Street, Apartment 4, Cortland, NY 13045, (607) 753-9631, BS 77 Ithaca Coll; MS 78 Bradley Univ; **SLP**

Winslow, Mrs Cynthia C Route 3 Box 451, Tappahannock, VA 22560, (804) 443-5301, BS 72 Appalachian St Univ; MA 74 Appalachian St Univ; 77–Sp-Lang Path, Essex County Public Schools, **SLP**

Winslow, Lydia J 831 North Highlands Drive, Hollywood, FL 33021, (305) 537-1323, BS 69 NY Univ; MA 74 CUNY - City College; Sp-Lang Path, Lydia Winslow MA & Assoc, **SLP**

Winson, Barbara 21 Cliffside Trail, Denville, NJ 07834, (201) 663-0520, BA 71 Bloomfield Coll; MA 74 Montclair St Coll; Sp-Lang Path, Jefferson Township Board of Ed, **SLP**

Winstead, Faye R 387 Olinda Drive, Brea, CA 92621, MS; **SLP**

Winstead, Mrs Nancy Hickling 2813 St Cloud Oaks Drive, Valrico, FL 33594, (919) 591-7204, BS 80 Ithaca Coll; MS 82 PA St Univ - Univ Park; Sp-Lang Path, Hillsboro Co Schls, **SLP**

Winstead, Renee Cannady 1021 Old Forge Road, Rocky Mount, NC 27804, (919) 937-8434, BS 77 East Carolina Univ; ME 78 Univ of NC - Greensboro; 88–Sp-Lang Path, Nash Co Schs, **SLP**

Winstead, Timothy Gene 182 Braelinn Court, Peachtree City, GA 30269, (404) 251-2925, BS 82 Univ of GA; ME 84 Univ of GA; Aud, Ahhas Hearing and Speech, **A**

Winston, Jon A 404 Vicksburg Court, Norman, OK 73071, **A**

Winston, Mrs Julia Stern 8404 Ensley Place, Leawood, KS 66206, (913) 642-2870, BS 73 Univ of FL; ME 75 Univ of GA; Admin, Aphasia-Sp Rehab Cen, **SLP**

Winston, Kim S Route 5 Box 196, Muskogee, OK 74401, (918) 683-0321, BA 64 FL St Univ; OM 66 Univ of OK Medical Center; 76–Sp Ser Superv, Muskagee Guid Cen/Hlth Dept, **SLP**

Winston, Dr Michael E 1200 Medical Towers, Little Rock, AR 72205, (501) 227-5050, BA 64 Northeastern OK St Univ; MA 66 Univ of KS; PH 74 (Aud) Univ of KS; 66–Dir of Aud, The ENT Clinic PA, **A**

Winston, Mrs Susan M 7851 Midday Lane, Alexandria, VA 22306, BA 68 Univ of San Francisco; MA 74 CA St Univ - Sacramento; **SLP**

Winter, Florian Davos 7000 Riverboat Way, Sacramento, CA 95831, (916) 395-6231, BA 81 CA St Univ - Sacramento; MS 85 San Francisco St Univ; 85–Sp-Lang Path, CarePoint Home Health Agency, **SLP**

Winter, Mrs Margaret E 22960 Garzota Drive, Valencia, CA 91355, (805) 296-6125, Aud, Audiology Inc, **A**

Winter, Marta Patricia Box 1189, Vicenza Elem School, APO New York, NY 09221, MA 79 Univ of TX - El Paso; 87–Sp-Lang Path, Federal Government, **SLP**

Winter, Miriam J 230 Ashley Drive, Rochester, NY 14620, (716) 473-1320, BA 58 CUNY - Brooklyn Coll; MA 60 CUNY - Brooklyn Coll

Winter, Nelda H 24410 Crenshaw Boulevard, Apartment 126, Torrance, CA 90505-5305, **SLP**

Winter, Mrs Susan K 2540 West Dunwood Road, Milwaukee, WI 53209, (414) 242-2400, BS 79 Univ of WI - Madison; MS 80 Univ of WI - Milwaukee; 86–Sp-Lang Path, Mequon-Thiensville PS, **SLP**

Winter, Yvonne P O Box 563, Redwood Valley, CA 95470, (707) 485-8681, BA 69; MA 73 Univ of IA; Sp-Lang Path, Willits USD, **SLP**

Wintercorn, Dr Eleanor S 9112 Cherbourg Drive, Potomac, MD 20854, (202) 745-8270, BA 56 Rockford Coll; MS 58 Univ of WI - Madison; PH 70 (Aud) Univ of MD - College Park; 80–Chief Aud & Sp-Path, VA Medical Center, **SLP A**

Winterling, Mrs Sharon Louise 7607 Windy Ridge, Baltimore, MD 21236, (301) 254-6413, BA 83 Loyola Coll; MS 84 Loyola Coll; Sp-Lang Path, Baltimore County Pub Schools, **SLP**

Wintermantel, Patricia 3 Mountain Avenue, Scranton, PA 18505, **SLP**

Wintermeyer, Dana B 206 Ralston Road, Richmond, VA 23229, (804) 288-5980, **SLP**

Winterrose, Mrs Maureen Rae 555 East Thornhill Drive, Apartment 103, Carol Stream, IL 60188-3103, (312) 462-4220, BA 84 Valparaiso Univ; MA 85 Western MI Univ; 85–Sp-Lang Path, Marianjoy Rehab Ctr, **SLP**

Winters, Debra A 203 Harris Drive, Sewell, NJ 08080, (609) 424-9084, BA 77 Rutger's St Univ - Douglas Coll; MA 78 Wayne St Univ - Sch of Med; Aud, Atrium Hrng & Sp Cen Inc, **A**

Winters, Mrs Emilia Ann 23 Ridgway Street, Mount Holly, NJ 08060-1437, BA 64 Montclair St Coll; MA 67 Paterson St Coll; Sp-Lang Path, Pemberton Twsp Bd of Ed, **SLP**

Winters, Mrs Rachelle 3777 Independence Avenue, Apartment 7L, Bronx, NY 10463, (212) 601-3698, BS 76 Rutger's St Univ - Douglas Coll; MS 78 Columbia Univ Teachers Coll; Sp-Lang Path, Private Practice, **SLP**

Winters-D'Amboise, Cynthia Lou 13 Guilder Place, Ballston Lake, NY 12019, (518) 371-6000, MS 81 Coll of Saint Rose; Sp-Lang Path, Shenendehowa Central Sch Dist, **SLP**

Wintersteen, Mrs Jane Noonan PO Box 695, Belvedere, CA 94920, (415) 387-0478, MA 83 MI St Univ; Sp-Lang Path, Private Practice, **SLP**

Wintersteen, Mrs Marylee Darlene 22711 Spatswood Lane, Katy, TX 77449, (713) 391-1113, **SLP**

Winthrop, Sandra J 3159 South Gilpin, Englewood, CO 80110, (303) 758-3415, BS 78 CO St Univ; MS 80 Univ of OK Medical Center; Aud, Darrel L Teter Phd & Assoc, **A**

Winthrop, Mrs Susan S 8060 S W Willowmere Drive, Portland, OR 97225, (503) 280-5729, BS 69 Univ of MN - Minneap-St Paul; MS 70 Univ of OR; Prog Coord, Regional Outreach Motor Svcs, **SLP**

Winton-Holland, Alice 442 South Paddock, Pontiac, MI 48053, (313) 664-2951, **A**

Wintringer, Mrs Cynthia L H 34 Lyrae Drive, Getzville, NY 14068, (716) 837-2441, BA 79 SUNY - Coll at Buffalo; MA 81 SUNY - Center at Buffalo; Sp-Lang Path, Lang Dev Prog of W NY, **SLP**

Winzelberg, Jody Stanford Univ Medical Center, Audiology Clinic R135, Stanford, CA 94305, (414) 497-6818, BA 78 CUNY - Queens Coll; MA 80 Univ of Denver; Aud, Stanford University, **A ACE**

Winzenried, Barbara B 811 Maydoll Drive, Kenton, OH 43326, (513) 599-5195, BA 57 OH St Univ; MA 75 Bowling Green St Univ; Sp-Lang Path, Logan Co Sch, **SLP**

Wipperling, Kathryn M 8931 York Road South, Bloomington, MN 55431, (612) 835-3399, BS 75 Minot St Univ; MS 79 Minot St Univ; Sp-Lang Path, Minnetonka School District, **SLP**

Wires, Karen N 9945 Ridgeline Drive, Gaithersburg, MD 20879, (301) 279-8490, ME 82 Loyola Coll; MA 69 Western MI Univ; Spec Educ Tchr, Montgomery Co Pub Sch, **SLP**

Wirt, Elizabeth C 5022 Hemlock, Irvine, CA 92715, (714) 534-1041, BS 59 Coll of Charleston; ME 60 Emory Univ; 88–Dir of SLP, Orangegrove Rehab Hosp, **SLP**

Wirt, Linda Sanford 1395 Farmdale Road, Mendota Heights, MN 55118, (612) 871-8665, BA 74 OH Univ - Athens; MA 75 Wayne St Univ; Coordinator of Sp/Lang Serv, Park Nicollet Med Cen, **SLP**

Wirtel, Sally K 11225 Fawnhaven Drive, St Louis, MO 63126, (314) 534-2273, BS 84 Southwest MO St Univ; MA 86 Saint Louis Univ; Sp-Lang Path, Childhaven, **SLP**

Wirth, Abigail J RFD 2 Box 247, St Johnsbury, VT 05819, (802) 748-5340, BA 80 CUNY - Queens Coll; MA 82 CUNY - Queens Coll; Adjunct Asst Prof, St Johns Univ, **SLP**

Wirth, David B 2857 Sunshine Circle, Fairfield, CA 94533, (707) 428-8736, BS 71 Univ of NE - Lincoln; MA 74 Univ of NE - Lincoln; 76–Aud, USAF, **A ACE**

Wirth, Mary Ruth 24747 Mound Road, Joliet, IL 60436, (815) 467-2800, BS 71 Western IL Univ; MA 72 Western IL Univ; Early Childhood Sp-Lang Path, Southern Will County Coop, **SLP**

Wirth, Richard W 5 East Fifth Street, Huntington Station, NY 11746, (516) 665-1900, BA 76 Hofstra Univ; MA 78 Hofstra Univ; Sp-Lang Path, BOCES, **SLP**

Wirzburger, Mrs Donna Ramos 1069 Westgate Street, New Bedford, MA 02745, (508) 778-6222, BA 82 Bridgewater St Coll; MS 84 Boston Univ; 86–Sp-Lang Path, Cape Cod Collaborative, **SLP**

Wisan, Arlene I 525 Ocean Parkway #3G, Brooklyn, NY 11218, (212) 990-6480, BA 68 CUNY - Brooklyn Coll; MA 70 CUNY - Queens Coll; Instructor, St Johns University, **SLP**

Wischner, George J 6280-301 Greenwood Parkway, Northfield, OH 44067, (216) 687-2543, BA 38 CUNY - Brooklyn Coll; MA 41 Univ of IA; PH 47 (NS) Univ of IA; Prof Emeritus, Cleveland St U, **SLP F LM**

Wischner, Mary Ellen 6280-301 Greenwood Parkway, Sagamore Hills, OH 44067, (216) 922-7445, BA Marshall Univ; MA Western MI Univ; 73–Sp-Lang Path, Private Practice, **SLP**

Wischner, Mrs Sary K Board Of Education, Havermere Bldg, Greenwich, CT 06830, (203) 531-9287, BA 45 Southern CA Coll; MA 46 Southern CA Coll; SLP, **SLP**

Wischow, Karen J 1394 East Monterey Drive, Boise, ID 83706-5077, (208) 338-3655, BS 77 ND St Univ; MS 82 Univ of ND; Sp/Lang Path, Boise Cty ISD, **SLP ACE**

Wiscombe, Cheryl Kay 724 West 1720 North #311, Provo, UT 84604, (801) 373-7850, BS 82; OM 83 Brigham Young Univ; 85–Aud, Utah Valley Reg Med Ctr, **A**

Wise, Birte H 7410-F Parkridge Blvd, San Diego, CA 92120, (619) 287-4382, OB 64 Statsseminariet PA Emdrupborg - Copenhagen, Denmark; MA 86 CA St Univ - Fullerton; 87–Sp-Lang Path, Grossmont Hosp, **SLP**

Wise, Cynthia 12 Blackwood B-8, Boston, MA 02115, (617) 732-5601, BS 86 Boston Univ; MS 87 Boston Univ; 88–SLP, Brigham & Warren's Hosp

Wise, Deborah L 837 Mansfield Ct, Schaumburg, IL 60194, (312) 885-6762, BA 79 MI St Univ; BA 80 MI St Univ; MA 82 Northwestern Univ; Sp-Lang Path, Dist 54, **SLP**

Wise, Donna Jean 35 Fern Street #2, Bangor, ME 04401, (207) 945-7365, BA 84 Univ of MD - College Park; MS 86 Towson St Univ; **A**

Wise, Mrs Dorothea Ann 760 Ridgecrest Road, Akron, OH 44303, (216) 434-1661, BS 69 Kent St Univ; MA 79 Kent St Univ; Sp-Lang Path, Akron Bd of Ed, **SLP**

Wise, Ida Dawn 7 Lake Street #7-0, White Plains, NY 10603, (914) 592-7555, MS 82 Columbia Univ Teachers Coll; 84–Aud, Blythedale Childrens Hospital, **A**

Wise, James A 11609 West 100th, Overland Park, KS 66214-2424, **A**

Wise, Janet L 3621 Los Alamos, Sacramento, CA 95825, (916) 922-3022, BA 74 CA St Univ - Sacramento; MA 76 CA St Univ - Sacramento; Sp-Lang Path, San Juan USD, **SLP**

Wise, Kay Louise 4909 Flint Drive, Bethesda, MD 20816-1747, (301) 424-6765, BA 83 Univ of MD - College Park; MA 86 George Washington Univ; 86–Aud, ENT Medical Group of Wash, **A**

Wise, Linda G 405 Tecumseh Street, Clinton, MI 49236-9510, (517) 456-7983, BA 75 Univ of MI - Ann Arbor; MS 76 Univ of MI - Ann Arbor; Sp/Lang Path, Lenawee Inter Sch, **SLP**

Wise, Patricia H 2395 East Co Road 36, Tiffin, OH 44883, (419) 447-9811, BA 59 MI St Univ; MS 63 MI St Univ; 67–Sp-Lang Path, The Betty Jane Rehab Ctr, **SLP**

Wise, Ruth S 8326 Lages Lane, Baltimore, MD 21207, (301) 768-3727, BS 73 Towson St Univ; MS 74 Towson St Univ; Sp-Lang Path, Anne Arundel Pub Schs, **SLP**

Wisely, Mrs Joanne M M 118 Deepdale Road, Wayne, PA 19087, (215) 688-7609, BA 73 Temple Univ; MA 76 West Chester Univ of PA; Sp/Lang Path, Private Practice, **SLP**

Wiseman, Mrs Peggy G 2504 Waterway Boulevard, Isle of Palms, SC 29451, (803) 886-6868, BA 59 Vanderbilt Univ; MS 60 Vanderbilt Univ; Aud, Charleston Sp & Hrng Cen, **A**

Wise-Siegel, Barbara Lynne 25 Harcourt Street, Greenville, SC 29601, (803) 233-2218, BA 77 Univ of TN - Knoxville; MA 79 Memphis St Univ; 87–Sp/Lang Path, Ctr for Dev Pediatrics, **SLP**

Wishkoski, Linda Slentz 7348 Keen Way North, Seattle, WA 98103, (206) 522-5978, BA 79 Univ of WA; OM 81 Univ of WA; SLP, Providence Hosp, **SLP**

Wishnick, Wendy R 12 Alvord Street, Oakhurst, NJ 07755, (201) 776-4495, BS 76 Univ of NH; MA 78 Kean Coll of NJ; 87–Aud, Jersey Shore Aud Ctr, **A**

Wisinski, Diane J 1518 West 45th Street, Erie, PA 16509, (814) 455-6711, BS 76 PA St Univ - Univ Park; MA 77 Edinboro Univ of PA; Sp/Lang Path, Hamot Medical Center, **SLP**

Wisinski, Mrs Judith 23W612 Woodworth Place, Roselle, IL 60172, (312) 529-1883, BA 69 Coll of Saint Francis; MA 71 Univ of IA; Sp/Lang Path, Roselle Sch Dist #12, **SLP**

Wisker, Mrs Nancy Ferree R R 1 Box 67, New Ross, IN 47968, (317) 723-1395, BS 79 Purdue Univ - West Lafayette; MA 82 IN Univ - Bloomington; **A ACE**

Wiskirchen, Mrs M Beth 5852 Crabapple Lane, Johnston, IA 50131, (515) 242-7714, BA 76 Univ of MO - Columbia; MA 77 Univ of MO - Columbia; Sp-Lang Path, Des Moines Indep Com Sch Dist, **SLP**

Wisnia, Judith F 20 Surrey Road, Winchester, MA 01890, (617) 272-4740, BS 66 Emerson Coll; Dir, Private Practice, **SLP**

Wisniewski, Mrs June Irene 767 Keith Lane, West Islip, NY 11795, (516) 422-3244, MS 86 Adelphi Univ; **SLP**

Wisnowski, Janine R 173 Wallace Street, Freeport, NY 11520, (516) 868-2336, BA 76 Hofstra Univ; MA 77 Hofstra Univ; **SLP**

Wiss, Mrs Deborah Crantz 7695 East Windrose Drive, Scottsdale, AZ 85260, (602) 991-3722, BA 77 MI St Univ; MA 78 MI St Univ; **SLP**

Wiss, Debra Ann 3602 NE Independence, Lee's Summit, MO 64064, (816) 525-9739, BS 83 Central MO St Univ; MS 86 Central MO St Univ; 88–Aud, Timbre Hrng & Sp Ctr, **A**

Wissel, Mrs Mary C 2310 North Elmwood, Peoria, IL 61604, (309) 672-6561, OB 55 IL St Univ - Normal; MA 66 Bradley Univ; Sp-Lang Path, Peoria Pub Sch, **SLP**

Wissner, Gail M 888 8th Avenue #314, New York, NY 10019, **SLP**

Wisutskie, April J C RFD 1 Box 3350, Poland Spring, ME 04274, (207) 998-2171, BA 75 Univ of CT; MS 78 Univ of OK Medical Center; Sp-Lang Path, Bureau of Ment Retard, **SLP**

Witczak, Kathryn Page 4304 Nutmeg Lane, Lisle, IL 60532-1117, (312) 653-7600, BS 79 Purdue Univ - West Lafayette; MS 81 Purdue Univ - West Lafayette; Sp-Lang Path, Marianjoy Rehab Hosp, **SLP**

Witecki, Cindy Ann 2545 North 9th Street, Kalamazoo, MI 49009, (616) 674-8091, MA 83 Western MI Univ; Sp-Lang Path, Van Buren Inter Sch Dist, **SLP**

Witek, Mrs Melanie McLean 2130 Teton Parkway, Algonquin, IL 60102, BS 82 Northwestern Univ; MA 83 Univ of IL - Urbana; 87–Sp-Lang Path, Comm Consolidated Sch Dist 15, **SLP**

Witham, James Todd 127 Wesleyan Way, Macon, GA 31210, (912) 825-3132, BS 84 Ball St Univ; MA 86 Ball St Univ; 85–Sp-Lang Path, Middle GA Reg Educ Svc, **SLP**

Witham, Richard F Southbury Training School, Box 66, Southbury, CT 06488, (203) 264-8231, BS 55 Gordon Coll; MS 75 Southern CT St Univ; Supervisor Sp-Hrng Clinicians, Southbury Training School, **SLP**

Witherell, Mrs Julie Korb 306 West Dean Avenue, Nonona, WI 53716, (618) 241-7589, MS 80 Univ of WI - Eau Claire; Sp-Lang Path, Jefferson Pub Schs, **SLP**

Withers, Mrs Lisa D 10147 Sassafras Woods Ct, Burke, VA 22015, (703) 250-8035, **SLP**

Withers, Mrs Mary T 6690 S W Parkwest Lane, Portland, OR 97225, MS 79 Portland St Univ; Sp-Lang Path, Portland State U, **SLP**

Witherspoon, Ann R Route 3 Box 220A, Durham, NC 27713, (919) 544-6288, **SLP**

Withowski, Mrs Barbara Therese 917 South 8th Avenue #1, La Grange, IL 60525-6924, (316) 431-7275, BS 83 Western IL Univ; MA 84 Western IL Univ

Witkin, Dr Belle Ruth 201 Union Avenue S E, SPC #132, Renton, WA 98056, (206) 271-1721, BA 39 Univ of Puget Sound; MA 51 Univ of WA; PH 62 (NS) Univ of WA; Consult, Witkin Associates, **SLP LM**

Witkin, Bonnie Joyce 1502 1/2 Lawrence, Eugene, OR 97401, (503) 344-3070, BA 83 Univ of CO - Boulder; MA 86 Univ of Denver; **SLP**

Witkind, Mark J 94-12 241st Street 2nd Fl, Floral Park, NY 11001, (516) 825-8800, BA 80 Univ of Miami; MS 82 Columbia Univ Teachers Coll; ME 86 Columbia Univ Teachers Coll; 87–Sp-Lang Path, Franklin Gen Hosp, **SLP ACE**

Witkowski, Mrs Jane B 850 Westbrooke Parkway, Waukesha, WI 53186, (414) 645-8600, BS 76 Univ of WI - Milwaukee; MS 77 Univ of WI - Milwaukee; Sp-Lang Path, Milwaukee Pub Sch, **SLP**

Witkowski, Paula Marie 338 East Adams, Kirkwood, MO 63122, MS 85 Fontbonne Coll; Sp-Lang Path, Northwest School District, **SLP**

Witlen, Sharon F 2 Richbell Road, White Plains, NY 10605, (914) 428-9329, BS 73 Syracuse Univ; MS 74 Univ of MI - Ann Arbor; Sp-Lang Path, Private Practice, **SLP**

Witman, Jamie Auxt Audiology & Speech Path (126), 112 Williams Circle, Williamsport, MD 21795, (301) 223-7447, BS 80 James Madison Univ; MS 81 WV Univ; 85–Sp-Lang Path, Private Practice, **SLP**

Witmer, Julie Deanne 2338 West Lindner #19, Mesa, AZ 85202, (602) 898-2953, BS 83 Univ of IA; MA 85 Univ of IA; 85–Sp-Lang Path, Mesa PS, **SLP**

Witmer, Lila A 2517 Dunks Ferry Road, #K-101, Bensalem, PA 19020, (215) 750-4062, BS 77 Bloomsburg Univ of PA; MS 78 Bloomsburg Univ of PA; SLP, The Woods Sch, **SLP**

Witsberger, Mrs Kathleen Ann 12916 N Cresap Street S W, Apartment 15, Cumberland, MD 21502, (301) 729-6026, MS 87 WV Univ; 88–Sp-Lang Path, Bd of Educ of Allegany Co

Witt, Anne M 247 South 9th Street, Burlington, IA 52601, BA 76 Univ of IA; MA 78 Univ of IA; 83–Sp-Lang Path, AEA #16, **SLP**

Witt, Bradley Kevin 25740 Rosebay Court, Moreno Valley, CA 92388, (714) 898-0968, BS 81 Brigham Young Univ; MA 83 Northwestern Univ; Aud, Pacific Aud, **A**

Witt, Eleanor B 2700 South Marion Circle, Denver, CO 80210, MS

Witt, Mrs Holly Burrell 3126 Mayfair, Carrollton, TX 75007, (214) 991-6383, BS 81 Univ of North TX; MS 82 Univ of North TX; 86–Sp-Lang Path/, Pediatric Therapy Assoc, **SLP**

Witt, Mrs Linda H 395 Persimmon Drive, St Charles, IL 60174, (312) 859-6872, BS 70 Purdue Univ - West Lafayette; MS 72 Washington Univ; Aud, Dreyer Med Clin, **A**

Witte, Kassie 2 Lords Highway, Weston, CT 06883, (212) 549-8700, BS 73 Adelphi Univ; MA 74 Adelphi Univ; Dir/Commun Dept, Hebrew Hm/Aged-Riverdale, **SLP A ACE**

Witte, Mrs Linda W Route 1 Box 190-A, Vandalia, MO 63382, (314) 594-2731, BS 77 Univ of MO - Columbia; MA 78 Univ of MO - Columbia; 80–Sp-Lang Path, Van-Far R-I Sch Vandalia Mo, **SLP**

Witte, Mrs Nancy R 4425 Crestlane, Hudsonville, MI 49426, (616) 457-4406, BS 77 Central MI Univ; MA 79 Central MI Univ; Sp-Lang Path, Hudsonville Pub Sch Sys, **SLP**

Wittenbach, Martha Green 3425 East English #106, Wichita, KS 67218, (316) 688-2730, BA 67 Wichita St Univ; MA 75 Wichita St Univ; Sp/Lang Path, Ruperto Mendlones MD, **SLP**

Wittenberg, Sherrie L 126 Whitmarsh Avenue, Worcester, MA 01606, (508) 481-1015, BS 77 SUNY - Center at Albany; MS 79 CUNY - Brooklyn Coll; 87–Sp-Lang Path, New England Ctr for Autism, **SLP**

Wittenstrom, Barbara B 4N034 Thornapple, St Charles, IL 60174, (312) 377-5005, BA 58 Univ of IA; **SLP**

Witter, Barbara H 306 Feronia Way, Rutherford, NJ 07070, (212) 828-9000, BA 71 Montclair St Coll; MS 76 Columbia Univ Teachers Coll; Aud, St Josephs Sch for the Deaf, **A**

Witter, Dr H L Rt 2 Box 333B, Liberty, IN 47353, (317) 458-6315, BS 65 Ball St Univ; MS 68 Purdue Univ - West Lafayette; PH 70 (NS) Purdue Univ - West Lafayette; 86–Owner, Private Practice, **A**

Witter, Mary Barbara 1066 Belvedere, Slidell, LA 70458, (504) 646-1148, BS 77 James Madison Univ; MA 79 LA St Univ - Baton Rouge; Sp-Lang Path, St Tammany Sch Bd, **SLP**

Wittkop, Peggy Ann 322 Jonquil, Eugene, OR 97404, (503) 689-1887, BA 66 Univ of Portland; MS 86 Univ of OR; **SLP**

Wittkopp, Jane E 1646 East High Street, Mount Pleasant, MI 48858, (517) 773-7921, BA 69 MI St Univ; MA 70 MI St Univ; Sp-Lang Path, Mount Pleasant Regional Center, **SLP**

Witt-Lajeunesse, Alane Kay 418 25th Street South, Lethbridge, AB, Canada T1J 3P3, (403) 320-5798, BA 76 Univ of MI - Ann Arbor; MS 77 Univ of MI - Ann Arbor; Sp-Lang Path, Private Practice, **SLP**

Wittle, Mrs Christine 7-H Phlox Circle, Owings Mills, MD 21117, (301) 356-6350, BS 86 East Stroudsburg Univ of PA; MS 88 Loyola Coll; 88–Sp-Lang Path, Baltimore City PS

Wittler, Mrs Maureen A 115 West 10th Street, Dover, OH 44622, (216) 343-6160, BS 70 Ball St Univ; MS 77 Saint Francis Coll; MA 79 OH Univ - Athens; Sp-Lang Path, Claymont City Schools, **SLP**

Wittler, Thomas P 115 West 10th Street, Dover, OH 44622, (216) 343-6160, BS 73 Indiana Univ of PA; MA 78 OH Univ - Athens; Consultant Sp-Lang Path, Eco Serrc, **SLP**

Wittman, Mrs Holly Diane 1284 Seventh Street, Hermosa Beach, CA 90254, (412) 232-7773, BA 82 IN Univ - Bloomington; OM 83 IN Univ - Bloomington; Sp-Lang Path, D T Watson Rehabilitation Hosp, **SLP**

Wittpenn, Denise Taneyhill 4 Old Field Lane, Mount Sinai, NY 11766, (516) 331-2118, BA 77 Loyola Coll; MS 78 Loyola Coll; Sp-Lang Path, **SLP**

Witwicky-Esden, Mrs Laila Anne 21337 Town Lakes Drive, Boca Raton, FL 33486, (315) 476-7441, MS 82 Nazareth Coll of Rochester; **SLP**

Witzel, Dr Mary Anne Speech Department, Hospital For Sick Children, 555 University Avenue, Toronto, ON, Canada M5G 1X8, (416) 598-6100, BA 71 Univ of Western Ontario; MS 74 Univ of Pittsburgh - Pittsburgh; PH 81 (NS) Univ of Pittsburgh - Pittsburgh; Dir Sp-Lang Path, The Hosp for Sick Childr, **SLP ACE**

Wizig, Mrs Carol Ann 11514 Ashcroft, Houston, TX 77035, (713) 791-4298, BS 70 Univ of TX - Austin; MA 72 OH St Univ; Sp-Lang Path, TX Childrens Hosp, **SLP**

Wladkowski, Mrs Elizabeth 184 Boston Street, Middleton, MA 01949, BS 76 Univ of MA - Amherst; MA 78 SUNY - Coll at Geneseo; 86–Sp-Lang Path, Lynn PS, **SLP**

Wladyka, Kateri Zook 646 Stumpville Road, Jefferson, OH 44047, (216) 743-1168, BA 70 Cleveland St Univ; MA 75 Cleveland St Univ; SLP, Easter Seal Soc, **SLP**

Wnek, Mary E P O Box 1768, Plant City, FL 34289-1768, (813) 754-6639, MS 87 Univ of South FL; **SLP**

Wnoroski, Christine Ellen 3939 Golden Wood Way, Uniontown, OH 44685, (216) 896-0870, MS 84 Kent St Univ; 78–Sp-Lang Path, Akron PS, **SLP**

Wnuk, Elizabeth Ann 4011 Neosho, St Louis, MO 63116, (618) 234-6876, BS 86 Saint Louis Univ; MA 88 Saint Louis Univ

Wobig, Terrence R Box 152, Minnesota City, MN 55959, (507) 454-1279, MA 72 Univ of IA; Sp-Lang Path, ISD, **SLP**

Wobosel, Carolyn Mary 1232 Wilson Drive, Eau Claire, WI 54703, (414) 494-6931, BA 85 Univ of WI - Eau Claire; MS 86 Univ of WI - Eau Claire; 88–Sp-Lang Path, Sch Dist of Alma Ctr, **SLP**

Wobst, Mrs Judy L Rhodes 18 Oxbow Creek Lane, Laguna Hills, CA 92653, (714) 997-6201, BS 76 Bowling Green St Univ; MA 79 Univ of Northern CO; Sdc Ch Pre-Schl Tchr, Orange USD, **SLP**

Woehr, Donna Yancy Manor Care Sharpview, 7505 Bellerive, Houston, TX 77036, (713) 774-9611, BS 75 Univ of North TX; MS 77 Univ of North TX; Sp/Lang Path Director, Manor Care Sharpview Nurs Ctr, **SLP**

Woerl, Dr Mary L 279 Kimberley Avenue, Asheville, NC 28804, (704) 252-0413, BS 44; MA 62 Univ of Notre Dame; PH 73 (NS) OH St Univ; **SLP LM**

Woerner, Wendy Lou 1329 Pitkin Avenue #8, Glenwood Springs, CO 81601-4159, (303) 945-9815, MS 87 CO St Univ; **A**

Woese, Jane Diane 471 St Patrick's Square #2, Thunder Bay, ON, Canada P7B 1G5, (807) 343-2407, OB 85 Univ of MN - Duluth; MS 86 Univ of WI - Eau Claire; 87–Sp-Lang Path, St Joseph's General Hosp

Woeste, Carol Ferris 3748 Frontenac Avenue, Cincinnati, OH 45236, (513) 271-2313, BS 81 Miami Univ - Oxford; MS 82 Miami Univ - Oxford; Sp-Lang Path, Hamltn Co Bd/Ment Ret & Dev Di, **SLP**

Wofford, Mrs Cynthia Holmberg Route 3 Box 764-5, Alma, AR 72921, (501) 997-1363, BS 83 Univ of AR - Fayetteville; MS 85 Univ of AR - Fayetteville; Sp-Lang Path, Mulberry Public Schools, **SLP**

Wofford, Dr Martha J 7639 Cambridge, Houston, TX 77054, (713) 795-7492, BS 67 Univ of TX - Austin; MA 69 Univ of TX - Austin; PH 77 (Aud) Univ of TX - Austin; Ch-Aud/Sp-Lang Path, VA Med Cen, **A**

Woge, Edward George 2 Glenwood Avenue, Lancaster, PA 17602, (717) 291-6275, BA 74 Edinboro Univ of PA; MS 82 PA St Univ - Univ Park; **SLP**

Wogrin, Mrs Lois B C A Wogrin, 121 Aubinwood Road, Amherst, MA 01002, (413) 253-2606, BA 70 Univ of MA - Amherst; MA 72 Univ of MA - Amherst; Sp-Lang Path, Chicopee Public Schools, **SLP**

Wohl, Mrs Laura M 1700 Northwest Avenue, Minot, ND 58701, (701) 839-8779, BA 78 Creighton Univ; MS 80 ID St Univ; 80–Dir, Private Practice, **SLP**

Wohlert, Amy B 1110 Church, Apt #1W, Evanston, IL 60201, (312) 864-8603, OB 78 Univ of NM; MS 80 Univ of NM; 86, Northwestern Univ, **SLP**

Wohlforth, Bettina Anne 7 Keller Lane, Westport, CT 06880, (203) 863-3240, BA 82 Adelphi Univ; MS 83 Adelphi Univ; Aud, Greenwich Hosp Hrng & Sp, **A**

Wohlrab, Lisa Marie 401 Albany Lane, Vernon Hills, IL 60061-1704, (312) 367-4565, BS 85 IL St Univ - Normal; MS 87 IL St Univ - Normal

Woicekowski, Laura 76 Jefferson Street, Metuchen, NJ 08840, (201) 549-1572, MA 87 Kean Coll of NJ

Woidtke, Cathy Rae W 1726 South 35th Street, Grand Forks, ND 58201, (701) 746-8056, BS 75 Univ of ND; MS 80 Univ of ND; SLP, Grand Forks Pub Sch, **SLP**

Woit, Ellen M 11389 Martin Street N W, Coon Rapids, MN 55433, (612) 434-9525, BS 76 Saint Cloud St Univ; MA 78 CA St Univ - Long Beach; Sp-Lang Path, ISD #15, **SLP**

Woiwode, Mrs Jo Anne Tazewell-Mason Special Ed Asso, 15 South Capitol Street, Pekin, IL 61554, BS 72 IL St Univ - Normal; MS 73 IL St Univ - Normal; Coord Sp/Lang Serv, Tazewell-Mason Spec Ed Assoc, **SLP**

Wojcik, Dorthy L 111 Colonial Hill Drive, Wallingford, CT 06492, (203) 828-6581, Southern CT St Univ; MS; Sp-Lang Path, Berlin Bd of Educ, **SLP**

Wojcik, Jodi K 1785 Coyote Court, Vista, CA 92083, **A**

Wojcik, Monica M G 7500 NW 5th Street, Suite 116, Plantation, FL 33317, (305) 583-7383, BA 74 Univ of ME - Orono; MA 76 Univ of Miami; 83–Sp-Lang Path, Pedia Ther Asoc, **SLP**

Wojcik, Steven A 1907 South 58th Avenue, Apt 2, Cicero, IL 60650, (312) 354-6929, BS 74 Southern IL Univ -Carbondale; MS 81 Southern IL Univ -Carbondale; SLP, Helping Hnd Rehab Cen, **SLP**

Wojcik-Davidson, Diane J 232 Walnut Street, Johnstown, PA 15901, (814) 535-5508, MS 83 WV Univ; Aud, Easter Seal Society, **A**

Wojtalewicz, Donna R 647 South Boulevard Apartment 2, Oak Park, IL 60302, (312) 848-3817, MS 87 Univ of WI - Stevens Point; Sp-Lang Path, River Grove Sch Dist 85½, **SLP**

Wolcott, Joanne M P O Box 421, 4 Myrtle Avenue, Hammondsport, NY 14840, (607) 776-7651, BS 74 SUNY - Coll at Geneseo; MA 79 SUNY - Coll at Geneseo; 81–Sp-Lang Path, Steuben Co Infirmary, **SLP**

Wolcott, Mrs Patricia M 1408 99th Street N W, Bradenton, FL 34209-9730, (813) 792-3949, MS 69 Univ of Cincinnati; Sp-Lang Path, Manatee County Schools, **SLP**

Wolcott, Mrs Rose C 916 Colonial Road, Franklin Lakes, NJ 07417, (201) 337-7784, BA 68 William Paterson Coll; MA 69 William Paterson Coll; Sp-Lang Path, Franklin Lakes Bd of Ed, **SLP ACE**

Wolczyk, Vicki R 600 Williamsburg Drive, Franklin, TN 37064, (615) 790-8015, BA 74 Univ of KY; MA 75 Univ of KY; Sp-Lang Path, Private Practice, **SLP**

Wold, Dr Donald C 38 Pine Manor Drive, Little Rock, AR 72207, (501) 569-3278, BA 55 Univ of WI - Madison; MA 57 Univ of WI - Madison; PH 68 (Theoretical Nuclear Physics) IN Univ - Bloomington; Chrprsn Dept of Physics & Astr, University of Arkansas

Wold, Dr James H 4300 15th Street, Gulfport, MS 39501, (601) 864-9292, MA 70 Univ of South FL; PH 74 (Sp & Hrng Science) Univ Southern MS-Hattiesburg; Sp-Lang Path/Aud, Private Practice, **SLP A**

Wolf, Mrs Adrienne Ollendorf 377 North Broadway #623, Yonkers, NY 10701, (914) 528-1354, BA 79 CUNY - Lehman Coll; MA 81 CUNY - Queens Coll; Sp-Lang Path, Lakeland Ctrl Sch Dist, **SLP**

Wolf, Ann Marie 736 West Ottawa, Lansing, MI 48915, (502) 456-3011, BA 80; MS 84 Univ of Louisville

Wolf, Mrs Barbara 199 Collins Road, Waban, MA 02168, (617) 965-4333, BA 65 MI St Univ; MA 66 MI St Univ; Adjunct Clin Instuctor, Boston Univ, **A**

Wolf, Beth Ann 1570 Eustis Street, #305, St Paul, MN 55108, (612) 636-3650, BS 84 Moorhead St Univ; MS 85 Moorhead St Univ; 88–Sp-Lang Path, Mounds View Sch Dist, **SLP**

Wolf, Carol K 2030 Falling Brook, Maryland Heights, MO 63043, (314) 542-9019, BS 66 Univ of IL - Urbana; MA 67 Univ of IL - Urbana; Sp-Lang Path, Spec Sch Dist-St Louis Co, **SLP**

Wolf, Clifford A 2037 Temblethurst Blvd, South Euclid, OH 44121, BA 73 OH Univ - Athens; MA 76 Case Western Reserve Univ; OM 85 Case Western Reserve Univ; 87–Dir-Ocu Hlh Pre-Adm Tes Sp Hrn, W G Nord Comm Mental Health Ctr, **SLP**

Wolf, Davidah St Michaels Hospital, 30 Bond Street, Toronto, ON, Canada M5B 1W8, (416) 864-5282, BA 67 CUNY - City College; MA 74 CUNY - Hunter Coll; Chief Aud, St Michaels Hosp, **A**

Wolf, Deborah L 186 Liberty Avenue, Norristown, PA 19403, (215) 539-8550, BS 72 Edinboro Univ of PA; MA 76 Temple Univ-Tyler Sch of Art; Sp-Lang Path, Montgomery County Intermed Unit, **SLP**

Wolf, Mrs Debra Zobel 1965 S W 81st Terrace, Davie, FL 33324, (305) 390-0799, BA 78 IN Univ - Bloomington; MS 79 IN St Univ - Terre Haute; Sp-Lang Path, Broward County Schs, **SLP**

Wolf, Diane S 5 Via Latigo, Rancho Santa Margarita, CA 92688, (714) 771-5276, BA 73 Univ of Northern CO; MA 74 Univ of Northern CO; 87–Sp-Lang Path, Winways Transitional Living Ctr, **SLP**

Wolf, Mrs Jean Marr 919 14th Street, Bismarck, ND 58501, (701) 663-7514, BS 72 Minot St Univ; MS 77 Minot St Univ; Mandan Pub Sch, **SLP**

Wolf, John M 43 Sunset Trail, Fairport, NY 14450, (315) 331-1700, BS 72 SUNY - Coll at Geneseo; MS 73 SUNY - Coll at Geneseo; Sp-Path & Aud Prog Coord, Newark Dev Disabil Svc Ofc, **SLP**

Wolf, Judith A 2411 Corriea Way, Fremont, CA 94539, (415) 657-5589, BS 62 Bloomsburg Univ of PA; MA 66 Temple Univ; **SLP**

Wolf, Mrs Karen B 14322 Ford Road, Madison, OH 44057, (216) 256-8483, BS 73 Univ of MD - College Park; MA 75 Case Western Reserve Univ; Superv Sp-Lang Path, E Shore Reg Resource Cen, **SLP**

Wolf, Dr Kenneth E 17350 Bronte Place, Granada Hills, CA 91344, (213) 603-4835, BA 70 Univ of CA - Santa Barbara; MA 72 Univ of CA - Santa Barbara; PH 77 (Aud) Univ of WI - Madison; Ch of Aud & Asst Prof Otolaryn, King/Drew Medical Center, **A ACE**

Wolf, Martha E 840B Forest Avenue, Evanston, IL 60202, (312) 480-8940, BS 79 Northwestern Univ; MA 80 Northwestern Univ; 87–Mgr-SLP Svcs, Timbre Hearing & Sp Ctrs, **SLP**

Wolf, Mary Ann 1140 Dartmouth Terrace, Inverness, FL 32652, (904) 726-2632, BA 83 Univ of FL; MA 85 Univ of FL; 85–Sp-Lang Path, Citrus County School Board, **SLP**

Wolf, Mary Faith 160 Wintersett Place, Winterville, GA 30683, (404) 742-8305, BA 85 Univ of Pittsburgh - Pittsburgh; MA 87 Univ of Pittsburgh - Pittsburgh; 88–Sp-Lang Path, Madison County Bd of Ed, **SLP**

Wolf, Dr Patricia L Speech And Language Institute, 3300 Webster #301, Oakland, CA 94609, (415) 834-6642, BA 70 Hofstra Univ; MA 75 Hofstra Univ; PH 76 (Sp-Lang Path) Edison Univ; Dir, Sp & Lang I, **SLP ACE**

Wolf, Mrs Phyllis B 312 Fawn Meadows Drive, Ballwin, MO 63011, BS 55 Univ of Pittsburgh - Pittsburgh; MS 57 Univ of Pittsburgh - Pittsburgh; Sp-Lang Path, Spec Sch Dist, **SLP ACE**

Wolf, Mrs Robin Hill 31 Lotus Street, Cedarhurst, NY 11516, (516) 569-3930, BA 71 CUNY - Queens Coll; MS 72 OH Univ - Athens; Audiologist-SLP, Private Practice, **A**

Wolf, Tracy Ellen 9 Abrams Place, Lynbrook, NY 11563, (516) 593-4280, MS 87 Univ of North TX

Wolfarth, Dr Donald L Dept Of Commun & Theatre Arts, University Of Wisconsin, 105 Garfield Avenue, Eau Claire, WI 54701, (715) 836-3153, BA 50 Hamline Univ; MA 53 Univ of MN - Minneap-St Paul; PH 59 (NS) Univ of MN - Minneap-St Paul; Prof/Sp Commun, U of WI

Wolfe, Anita R 131 Winslow Terrace, Glen Rock, NJ 07452, (201) 444-7149, BA 73 Paterson St Coll; MA 77 Montclair St Coll; Private Practice, **SLP**

Wolfe, Basil N, Jr 7324 Dawn Place, Mentor, OH 44060, (216) 289-0112, BS 64 Univ of TN - Knoxville; MA 71 Memphis St Univ; 71–Pres, Midwest Aud Inc, **A**

Wolfe, Cheryl L 131 McDowell Street, PO Box 15343, Asheville, NC 28813, (704) 252-6671, BA 78 Univ of NC - Greensboro; ME 79 Western Carolina Univ; Owner/Administrator, Asheville Cen for Commun Disor, **SLP**

Wolfe, Mrs Cynthia S 301 Tall Grass Drive, Lawrence, KS 66044, (913) 585-1107, BS 70 Univ of KS; MS 71 Univ of KS; Sp-Lang Path, Desoto Pub Sch, **SLP**

Wolfe, Cynthia S 508 18th Street, Huntington Beach, CA 92648, (760) 026-1747, BA 74 OH St Univ; MS 76 ID St Univ; SLP, Visiting Nurse Association, **SLP**

Wolfe, Donald L 1512 South Riegel Court, Spokane, WA 99212, (509) 534-7207, BA 66 Univ of Tulsa; MA 68 Univ of Tulsa; Owner, Hearing Conservation Consult, **A**

Wolfe, G Richard 9 Carmelita Court, Reisterstown, MD 21136, (301) 922-6880, BS 51 Clarion Univ of PA; ME 55 PA St Univ - Univ Park; **SLP**

Wolfe, Gwendolyn Talley 5504 East Sunset Road, Knoxville, TN 37914, (615) 525-4219, BA 65 FL St Univ; MA 66 Univ of TN - Knoxville; Assoc Director Sp-Lang Serv, Utk Aud Sp Path, **SLP**

Wolfe, Helen Stein 130 New Mark Esplanade, Rockville, MD 20850, (301) 279-4990, BA 66 Univ of MD - College Park; MA 70 Univ of MD - College Park; 88–Sp-Lang Path, Mont Co Pub Sch, **SLP**

Wolfe, Mrs Julie Atkins 108 Marylee, Hewitt, TX 76643-3731, (817) 754-9667, BS 83 Baylor Univ; MS 84 Baylor Univ; 85–Sp-Lang Path, InSpeech Inc, **SLP**

Wolfe, Mrs Karen M 64 Falcon Road, Livingston, NJ 07039, (201) 992-7574, BA 57 Newark St Coll; MA 63 Newark St Coll; Sp-Lang Path, Inglemoor Nursing Home, **SLP**

Wolfe, Mrs Kristina Marie 128 Madison Boulevard, Terre Haute, IN 47803, (812) 234-1955, MS 79 IN St Univ - Terre Haute; Sp-Lang Path, Vigo County School Corporation, **SLP**

Wolfe, Mrs Mary Ann E 1592 Oak Valley Dr, Fairfield, OH 45014, (513) 829-4685, BS 72 Miami Univ - Oxford; MA 77 Miami Univ - Oxford; SLP, Hamilton Co Office of Ed, **SLP**

Wolfe, Robert D, Jr Audiometric Associates, 1940 North 13th Street, Reading, PA 19604, (215) 929-3538, BS 74 James Madison Univ; ME 78 James Madison Univ; Aud, Audiometic Associates, **A**

Wolfe, Mrs Ruth V 1067 Village Drive, Hauppauge, NY 11788, (516) 361-4885, BS 80 SUNY - Coll at Fredonia; MA 82 OH Univ - Athens; Sp/Lang Path, Island Therapies, **SLP**

Wolfe, Mrs Sue Pearl Georgia Retardation Center, 4770 North Peachtree Road, Atlanta, GA 30338, BA 72; MA 74 CUNY - Brooklyn Coll; Sp-Lang Path, Georgia Retardation Cen, **SLP**

Wolfe, Susan G 10753 Wellerwoods Drive, Cincinnati, OH 45242, (513) 742-1500, BS 73 OH St Univ; MA 76 Univ of Cincinnati; Sp-Lang Path, Hamilton Co Bd Mr/Dd, **SLP**

Wolfe, Mrs Tracey Diane Therapeutic Learning Center, 32625 West Seven Mile, Suites 2 And 12, Livonia, MI 48152, (313) 474-1040, MS 84 Boston Univ; BA 82 MI St Univ; Owner and Dir, Therapeutic Learning Ctr, **SLP**

Wolfe, Victoria E 1566 Essex Road, Columbus, OH 43221, (614) 481-7904, BA 79 Boston Coll; MA 80 George Washington Univ; Sp-Lang Path, Private Practice, **SLP**

Wolfe, Dr Virginia S 2231 Long Wood Drive, Auburn, AL 36830, (205) 271-9410, BS 59 OH St Univ; MA 65 OH St Univ; PH 68 (NS) OH St Univ; Sp-Lang Path, Auburn University-Montgomery, **SLP F**

Wolfe, Vivian V 20247 Baltar Street, Canoga Park, CA 91306, (213) 997-2664, BA 65 Univ of ND; MA 69 CA St Univ - Northridge; **SLP**

Wolfenden, Mrs Deborah P RR 4 Box 4325, Freeport, ME 04032, (207) 874-1065, BA 73 Univ of Miami; ME 75 Univ of Miami; Exec Dir, NE Hrng & Sp Cen, **SLP**

Wolfer, Joseph Edward 40 North Grand Avenue, Fort Thomas, KY 41075, (606) 781-4900, BS 76 Univ of Cincinnati; MA 78 Univ of Cincinnati; **A**

Wolff, Adele M 2640 Bronholly Drive, Hollywood, CA 90068, (213) 462-8738, BA 76 Univ of Southern CA; MA 78 Whittier Coll; SLP, Los Alamitos USD, **SLP**

Wolff, Cissy 1203 4th Avenue, Salt Lake City, UT 84103, (801) 355-3841, BA 79 Univ of CA - Santa Barbara; MS 82 UT St Univ; Sp/Lang Path, Jordan School Dist, **SLP**

Wolff, Donald A 1376 6th Avenue, San Francisco, CA 94122, (415) 665-8344, BS 58 NY Univ; MA 70 Univ of Southern CA; 73–Aud, Comm Sp Lang Hrng Svcs, **A**

Wolff, Ellen S 69 Moran Avenue, Princeton, NJ 08542, (609) 683-8414, BA 73 Case Western Reserve Univ; MA 76 George Washington Univ; 82–Aud, The Medical Ctr at Princeton, **A**

Wolff, Mrs Karen Mitchell C2 Clairmont Court, Portland, ME 04103, (207) 874-0906, BS 83 Worcester St Coll; MA 85 CUNY - Hunter Coll; 88–Aud, Wilner-Greene Associates, **A**

Wolff, Lauri Joy 11 Alpine Road, Everett, MA 02149, (617) 389-7950, SLP, Everett Public Schools, **SLP**

Wolff, Mrs Linda Louise 40212 Hacienda Court, Fremont, CA 94539, (415) 797-9999, BA 75 SUNY - Center at Buffalo; MA 76 SUNY - Center at Buffalo; Aud, Private Practice, **A ACE**

Wolff, Sue Ostrow 212 Heathcliff Place, Winston-Salem, NC 27104, (919) 723-3571, BS 59 Syracuse Univ; MS 61 PA St Univ - Univ Park; 85–Sp-Lang Path, Child Guidance Ctr, **SLP**

Wolff, Suzanne Gits 301 Fall Creek Drive, Richardson, TX 75080, (214) 238-1651, BS 81 Marquette Univ; MA 85 Univ of TX - Austin; 88–Sp-Lang Path, Children's Med Ctr, **SLP**

Wolffer, Elaine A E 103 Jeffrey Drive, North Tonawanda, NY 14120, (716) 686-2462, BA 59 SUNY - Coll at Buffalo; MA 80 SUNY - Coll at Buffalo; Sp-Lang Path, Depew Sch Dist, **SLP**

Wolfgang, Mrs Lorelei D 5520 35th Avenue S, Minneapolis, MN 55417, (612) 431-8210, BS 78 Univ of MO - Columbia; MA 79 Univ of MO - Columbia; 88–Sp-Lang Path, ISD 196, **SLP**

Wolfley, Mary Elizabeth 4307 North Newhall Street, Shorewood, WI 53211, (414) 351-0450, BS 76 Marquette Univ; MS 77 Marquette Univ; Coord/Sp & Hrng Dept, WI Soc for Brain Injur Chldn, **SLP**

Wolfman-Wasserman, Mrs Wendy Jill 2404 Ohio Avenue, Apartment 7, Cincinnati, OH 45219, BS 84 Univ of WI - Madison; MS 85 Marquette Univ; SLP, Cincinnati Public School, **SLP**

Wolf-Moore, Carol Ann 352 Ridgecrest Avenue, Los Alamos, NM 87544, (505) 852-4244, BS 78 Univ of KS; MA 80 Univ of KS; 85–Sp-Lang Path, Santa Maria El Mirador, **SLP**

Wolfolk, William Bell Wayne State University, 503 Manoogian Hall, Detroit, MI 48202, (313) 577-3337, BS 71 Eastern MI Univ; MA 71 Eastern MI Univ; 87–Lecturer/Cl Supvr, Wayne State Univ, **SLP**

Wolford, Mrs Ellen Wolff 451 Harmony Drive, Wheeling, IL 60090, (312) 459-3474, BS 73 Univ of MD - College Park; MA 75 George Washington Univ; 87–Coord of Aud Svcs, Excellcare Inc, **A**

Wolford, Robert David, Jr Rt 7, 127 George Anderson Drive, Hillsborough, NC 27278, (919) 684-3859, MS Univ of NC - Chapel Hill; 85–Aud, Duke Univ Med Ctr, **A**

Wolfram, Walter A 12401 Venice Place, Silver Spring, MD 20904, (301) 622-0967, PH (NS)

Wolf-Schein, Dr Enid Gordon 1703 Andros Isle J-2, Coconut Creek, FL 33066, (305) 978-1368, BS 68 Temple Univ; ME 58 Temple Univ; ED 56 (NS) Boston Univ; Res Sci/Psycholinguist, Nysi/Res Dev Dis, **SLP**

Wolfson, Mrs Amy S 195 Independence Avenue, Apartment 141, Quincy, MA 02169, BS 81 Univ of MA - Amherst; MS 82 Univ of NC - Chapel Hill; Sp/Lang Path, S Shore Ed Collabor, **SLP**

Wolfson, Wendy Ruth 82 Wolcott Street, Medford, MA 02155, (617) 395-6680, MS 86 Northeastern Univ; **SLP**

Wolgat, Mrs Loretta 3118 Crazy Horse Drive, Simi Valley, CA 93063, (805) 527-1958, BA 76 CA St Univ - Northridge; MA 80 CA St Univ - Northridge; **SLP**

Wolgemuth, Lt Keith Stohman 114-A Avenida Las Brisas, Oceanside, CA 92056, (619) 725-4418, MA 84 Memphis St Univ; Aud, US Navy Naval Hosp, **A**

Wolinsky, Steven Wayne 8119 North Keeler, Skokie, IL 60076, (312) 685-9202, BS 72 Northern IL Univ - De Kalb; MA 74 Northern IL Univ - De Kalb; Dir, NW Audio-Vestibular Labs, **A**

Wolk, Lesley Dept Of Communication Sciences, 805 South Crouse Avenue, Syracuse, NY 13210, (315) 423-4121, BA 77 0500; MA 82 0500; Graduate Assistant, Syracuse University, **SLP**

Wolk, Phillis R 58 Graymoor Lane, Olympia Fields, IL 60461, (301) 484-7026, BS 71 Univ of TX - Austin; MA 73 Univ of TN - Knoxville; Sp-Lang Path, Private Practice, **SLP**

Wolkober, Martina M 3723 West Forest Home Avenue, Milwaukee, WI 53215, (414) 241-4240, BA 78 Mundelein Coll; MS 80 Marquette Univ; Dir Sp-Lang Path, Rehabilitation Associates, **SLP**

Wolkoff, Elaine S 93 Wedgewood Drive, P O Box 3066, Waterbury, CT 06705, (203) 754-1279, BS 72 Univ of Pittsburgh - Pittsburgh; MS 75 Univ of Pittsburgh - Pittsburgh; Sp-Lang Path, Private Practice, **SLP ACE**

Wolkowicz, Marilyn Heller 4664 North Andrews Avenue, Fort Lauderdale, FL 33309, BA 75 Towson St Univ; MS 78 Towson St Univ; **SLP**

Wolkowski, Robert Donald 4312 Montalvo Street, San Diego, CA 92107, (619) 438-3467, BA 78 San Diego St Univ; MA 81 San Diego St Univ; Sp-Lang Path, CA Sp Path Inc, **SLP**

Wollak, Barbara Ackermann 2225 Orkla Drive, Minneapolis, MN 55427, **SLP**

Wollenweber, Robert William 1580 East 3900 South Suite 210, Salt Lake City, UT 84124, (801) 277-8339, BA 80 Univ of CA - Santa Barbara; MS 83 UT St Univ; 87–Aud/Owner, Wasatch Sp & Hrng Ctr, **A**

Woller-Mummolo, Lauren 35 Ellen Road, Stoneham, MA 02180, (617) 438-5999, ME 82 Northeastern Univ; Sp-Lang Path, Boston Pub Sch, **SLP**

Wollerson, Beulah B R 3811 Brenda, Alexandria, LA 71301, (318) 445-2132, BA 56 Northwestern St Univ; MA 61 LA St Univ - Baton Rouge; SLP, Rapides Parish Sch Bd, **SLP**

Wolley, Jane K C 521 Fillmore Street, Herndon, VA 22070, (209) 441-3377, **SLP**

Wollin, Mrs Joan 10 Byrne Lane, Tenafly, NJ 07670, (201) 871-1672, BS 68 Emerson Coll; MA 71 CUNY - Hunter Coll; Sp-Lang Path, Tenafly Bd of Ed, **SLP**

Wollins, Dr Sally 1076-13 Lancaster Blvd, Mechanicsburg, PA 17055, (717) 787-2020, BA 53 Univ of Akron; MA 66 Univ of Akron; PH 73 (Aud) Univ of Pittsburgh - Pittsburgh; 88–Chief-Cleft Palate/Plastic Surg Prog, Commonwealth of PA-Dept of Health, **A**

Wollman, Irving L 2077 Butlersbridge Court, Cincinnati, OH 45244-2604, (513) 732-8223, BA 74 OH Univ - Athens; MA 78 OH Univ - Athens; Sp/Lang Path, Childrens Hosp Med Cen, **SLP**

Wollmann, Mrs Etta Marie 1409 Wellesley N E, Albuquerque, NM 87106, (505) 255-9091, MS 85 Univ of NM; 85–Sp-Lang Path, Albuquerque PS, **SLP**

Wollmuth, Wayne Robert 503 Sourdough, Buffalo, WY 82834, (307) 684-9328, BS 74 Univ of ND; MS 78 ID St Univ; Sp-Lang Path, Johnson Co Schl Dist, **SLP**

Wollner, Barbara A 385B Lexington Court, Pewaukee, WI 53072, (414) 542-8036, BS 76 Univ of WI - Stevens Point; MS 77 Univ of WI - Whitewater; Sp-Lang Path, Lutheran Social Services, **SLP**

Woloshen, D 2218 Chickering Lane, Nashville, TN 37215, BA 71 Univ of MA - Boston; ME 73 Boston Univ; Sp-Lang Path, **SLP**

Woloshin, Mrs Ronna Siegel 1607 Portsmith Lane, Arlington Heights, IL 60004, (312) 492-7974, BS 78 Northwestern Univ; MA 80 Northwestern Univ; Sp-Lang Path, Commun Consol Sch Dist #65, **SLP**

Wolosiansky, Sara Elizabeth 4644 Mars Road, Uniontown, OH 44685, (216) 434-5101, BS 81 Univ of Cincinnati; MA 83 Univ of Cincinnati; Sp-Lang Path, Private Practice, **SLP**

Wolosiansky, Walter B 4644 Mars Road, Uniontown, OH 44685, (216) 454-5101, **A**

Wolsch, Mrs Lois C 19 Homestead Avenue, Danbury, CT 06810, (203) 744-7232, BA 47 Univ of MI - Ann Arbor; MA 51 Univ of MI - Ann Arbor; Sp-Lang Path, Danbury Public Schools, **SLP**

Wolsch, Dr Robert A 19 Homestead Avenue, Danbury, CT 06810, (203) 744-7232, BA 49 NY Univ; MA 54 Columbia Univ Teachers Coll; ED 69 (NS) Columbia Univ Teachers Coll; Professor, Western Connecticut State Univ, **SLP**

Wolski, Dr William 1291 Arrowwood Lane, Grand Blanc, MI 48439, (313) 694-4258, BA 52 Univ of MI - Ann Arbor; MA 53 Univ of MI - Ann Arbor; PH 62 (NS) Univ of MI - Ann Arbor; Sp-Lang Path, Flint Bd of Ed, **SLP**

Wolslager, Jacqueline M 13214 Rockside Road, Garfield Heights, OH 44125, (216) 521-5050, Sp/Pathologist, Soc for Crippled Children, **SLP**

Wolst, Denise Kertsmar Rd 2 Box 427C, Hellertown, PA 18055, (215) 776-8480, BS 80 East Stroudsburg Univ of PA; MA 82 West Chester Univ of PA; Sp-Lang Path, Healtheast-1, **SLP**

Wolsten, Mrs Ava R S 630 Mountain Drive, South Orange, NJ 07079, BA 77 Montclair St Coll; MA 80 Seton Hall Univ; **SLP**

Wolstenholm, Jeanne L 187 Mill Road, Hampton, NH 03842, (603) 778-7772, BS 77 Univ of MA - Amherst; ME 79 Northeastern Univ; Sp-Lang Path, Exeter Pub Schs, **SLP**

Wolters, Brenda 1321 West Clarewood, Peoria, IL 61614, BA 60 Univ of IA; MA 72 Univ of CO - Boulder; 68–Sp/Lang Path, Pekin Pub Schs #108, **SLP**

Wolters, Mrs Cheryl Cartee Michael Reese Hospital, David T Siegel Institute, 3033 S Cottage Grove Avenue, Chicago, IL 60616, (312) 791-5487, BS 81 Baylor Univ; MS 83 Univ of TX - Dallas; 83–Aud, Michael Reese Hosp & Med Ctr, **A**

Wolthausen, Julie Pollock 15008 Southeast 51st, Bellevue, WA 98006, (206) 392-0700, BA 63 Univ of WA; MS 86 Univ of WA

Woltzen, Mrs Carol Ann R R 1 Box 94, Canistota, SD 57012, (605) 297-3773, BS 74 Northern St Coll; MA 82 Univ of SD - Vermillion; **SLP**

Wolvek, Dr Joseph 509 Southeast 3rd Street, Ankeny, IA 50021-3211, (515) 281-3294, MS 54 Univ of OR; OD 63 Univ of Northern IA; PH 73 (NS) IA St Univ; Ed Consult, IA St Dept of Pub Instr, **SLP A**

Womack, Audrey Faye 1823-D Fairfax Road, Greensboro, NC 27407, (919) 258-6599, **SLP**

Womack, Mrs Bethel Hissom P O Box 641, Knoxville, TN 37901, (615) 579-2474, BS 68 Univ of TN - Knoxville; OM 81 Univ of TN - Knoxville; MA 84 Univ of TN - Knoxville; 86–Sp-Lang Path, Tennessee Sch for the Deaf, **SLP**

Womack, Mrs Judy 201 Willowbrook, Hot Springs, AR 71913, (501) 623-5451, BS 75 Phillips Univ; MS 76 Vanderbilt Univ; Sp-Lang Path, St Joseph's Reg Health Ctr, **SLP**

Womack, Karen H 46-A Hill Road, Louisville, KY 40204, (502) 451-4600, BA 78 Marshall Univ; MA 79 Marshall Univ; Sp-Lang Path, Private Practice, **SLP**

Womack, Mrs Marylynn Hill 36855 Nicholas Street, Walker, LA 70726, (504) 766-1272, BS 74 FL St Univ; MS 75 FL St Univ; SLP, E Baton Rouge Parish Sch Bd, **SLP**

Womack, Patricia Gracewood State School & Hosp, Unit 4, Gracewood, GA 30812, (404) 790-2547, BA 71 Converse Coll; ME 72 Univ of SC - Columbia; Sp-Lang Path, Grace Wood St Sch & Hosp, **SLP**

Womack, Patty Kay 500 East Locust #B, Harrisburg, IL 62946, (618) 252-0030, MS 87 Eastern IL Univ

Womble, Mrs Amygayle Law 170 Penmoken Park, Lexington, KY 40503, (606) 271-3780, BA 83 Univ of NC - Chapel Hill; MS 84 Univ of NC - Chapel Hill; **SLP**

Wommack, Mrs Betty B 2179 Northlake Parkway, Suite 21, Tucker, GA 30084, BS 60 SUNY - Center at Buffalo; ME 69 Emory Univ; Sp-Lang Path, Atlanta Metro Sp Ctr, **SLP**

Wommer, Marcy K 35 Wallingford Road, Brighton, MA 02135, (617) 254-3227, MS 88 Northeastern Univ

Won, Terilyn Yukie 3758-A Manini Way, Honolulu, HI 96816, (808) 536-6993, BS 84 Univ of HI - Manoa; MA 86 OH Univ - Athens; **A**

Wonder, Coralie M 88 Headland Drive, Rancho Palos Verdes, CA 90274, BA 61 CA St Univ - Long Beach; MA 75 Whittier Coll; SLP, LA Co Supt of Sch, **SLP**

Wong, Anna 13386 Jarman Place, San Diego, CA 92130, (619) 481-5431, MA; Sp-Lang Path, Private Practice, **SLP**

Wong, Corinne M 340-16th Avenue, San Francisco, CA 94118, (415) 221-1920, BA 85 San Francisco St Univ; MS 88 San Francisco St Univ; 87–Sp-Lang Path, ACCESS Sp & Lang

Wong, Mrs Gloria Jackel Chicago Hearing Society, 10 West Jackson Boulevard, 2nd Floor, Chicago, IL 60604, (312) 939-6888, BA 80 Cleveland St Univ; MA 82 Cleveland St Univ; 86–Dir of Aud, Chicago Hearing Society, **A**

Wong, Helen Fung-Ying 430 Massachusetts Drive, #310, Stephenville, NF, Canada A2N 3C2, (709) 643-5111, BS 82 Acadia Univ - Nova Scotia; MS 87 Dalhousie Univ - Nova Scotia; 87–Sp-Lang Path, Sir Thomas Roddick Hosp

Wong, Lorraine Jean 1207 South Edith Avenue #1, Alhambra, CA 91803, (818) 576-5518, MA 83 San Jose St Univ; SLP, Miller & Standel, **SLP**

Wong, Lynette 266 Mather Street, Oakland, CA 94611, (415) 548-0180, BS 77 Univ of HI - Manoa; MS 79 Univ of HI - Manoa; 85–Sp-Lang Path, Sp-Lang Ctr Children's Hosp, **SLP**

Wong, Mrs Marleen N 2455 S W Timberline Drive, Portland, OR 97225, MA 73 Univ of OR; Sp-Lang Path, Portland Public Schools, **SLP**

Wong, Mrs Shirley A 372 Dollimore Road, Encinitas, CA 92024, BA 74 CA St Univ - Los Angeles; MA 77 CA St Univ - Los Angeles; 79–Sp-Lang Path, Chino USD, **SLP**

Wong, Mrs Susan A Fong 965 Via Enrico, San Lorenzo, CA 94580, (415) 783-2936, CA St Univ - Hayward; Sp-Lang Path, Hayward USD, **SLP**

Wong, Trudy T 95-116 Paikauhale Place, Mililani Town, HI 96789, (808) 423-2477, BS 77 Univ of HI - Manoa; MS 79 Univ of HI - Manoa; Sp-Lang Path, Dept of Ed Ctrl Dist, **SLP**

Wong, Mrs Virginia Young 1580 Frambuesa Dr, San Luis Obispo, CA 93401, (805) 543-6319, MA 84 CA St Univ - Fresno; **SLP**

Wong-Chin, Karen 15822 Cavendish Drive, Houston, TX 77059-4613, (713) 332-2411, BS 77 SUNY - Coll at Fredonia; MA 79 CUNY - City College; Sp-Lang Path, Clear Creek Indep School Dist, **SLP**

Wong-Trufanoff, Lonnie A Rd 3 Box 29-D, Highland, NY 12528, (914) 431-8801, BA 78 CUNY - Queens Coll; MA 80 SUNY - Coll at Geneseo; Sp-Lang Path, St Francis Hospital, **SLP**

Woociker, Mrs Jo Ann 4202 Prairie View Dr South, Sarasota, FL 34232, (813) 371-2878, BA 82 Auburn Univ - Montgomery; MS 85 Auburn Univ - Auburn; **SLP**

Wood, Dr Ann Stace 5709 Wayside, Cincinnati, OH 45230, (513) 281-6700, BA 62 Miami Univ - Oxford; MA 68 Univ of Cincinnati; PH 78 (NS) Univ of Cincinnati; Sp-Lang Path, Private Practice, **SLP**

Wood, Barbara G 5 Westwood Road, Santa Cruz, CA 95060, (408) 426-3686, BS 67 San Jose St Univ; **SLP**

Wood, Carolyn A P O Box 762, Laramie, WY 82070, (307) 745-7348, BS 72 Univ of WY; MS 73 Univ of WY; Educational Resource Spec, Albany Co School District #1, **SLP**

Wood, Christina 2023 Spanish Drive, St Louis, MO 63144, (314) 962-9229, BS 68 Jersey City St Coll; MS 70 Washington Univ; Aud, City Hosp #1 St Louis, **A**

Wood, Clarence A 440 NE C Street Apartment A, College Place, WA 99324, (509) 529-5005, BA 61 Loma Linda Univ - Riverside; MA 64 Univ of Denver; 88–Sp-Lang Path, Educational Service Dist 123, **SLP**

Wood, Cynthia C 1504 Branchwood Terrace, Gambrills, MD 21054, (301) 761-7196, BS 75 Frostburg St Coll; MA 79 Univ of MD - College Park; Sp-Lang Path, Anne Arundel Co Pub Sch, **SLP**

Wood, Mrs Cynthia C 16228 Culbert Road, Pascagoula, MS 39567, (601) 588-6001, BS 79 Univ of South AL; MS 81 Univ of South AL; 88–Sp-Lang Path, Jackson County Sch Dist, **SLP**

Wood, Mrs Dana Carrillo Route 2 Box 2193, Hermiston, OR 97838, (503) 276-6616, BA 80 Eastern WA Univ; MS 81 Eastern WA Univ; **SLP**

Wood, Debra Sue 1216 Colorado, Texarkana, TX 75503, (501) 774-9691, **SLP**

Wood, Mrs Diane C 316 Golf Club Lane, Mayfield, KY 42066, (502) 247-4392, BS 70 Murray St Univ; MS 71 Murray St Univ; OM 81 Murray St Univ; Sp-Lang Path, Mayfield ISD, **SLP**

Wood, Donald L 180 South Lake Avenue, Suite 420, Pasadena, CA 91101, (818) 792-8859, BA 72 Univ of Southern CA; MA 80 CA St Univ - Los Angeles; Owner, Private Practice, **SLP**

Wood, Mrs Dorothy H 4647 South Lake Drive, Cudahy, WI 53110, (414) 224-7349, BS 63 Marquette Univ; MS 68 Marquette Univ; Sp-Lang Path, Marquette U, **SLP**

Wood, Drucilla 218 High Street, Reading, MA 01867, (617) 396-9250, BA 73 Saint Lawrence Univ; MA 77 Univ of MA - Amherst; Coord Sp/Lang Path, Lawrence Memorial Hospital, **SLP**

Wood, Elaine Bay 2300 Cherokee Road, Janesville, WI 53545, (608) 754-2201, BS 62 Univ of WI - Madison; Sp-Lang Path, Janesville, **SLP**

Wood, Mrs Elizabeth 14119 North Suddley Castle, Houston, TX 77095, (713) 463-7265, BA 73 Univ of Southwestern LA; MS 75 Univ of Southwestern LA; Sp-Lang Path, Cypress-Fairbanks ISD, **SLP**

Wood, Elizabeth Ann 2902 Octavia Street, San Francisco, CA 94123, (415) 931-9479, BA San Diego St Univ; MA 86 San Diego St Univ

Wood, Gerald S Route 2 Box 88, Prince Frederick, MD 20678, (301) 535-2708, MS 72 Univ of MD - College Park; SLP, District Columbia Pub Schools, **SLP**

Wood, Mrs Gillian Christine 1201 145 Sandy Court, Saskatoon, SK, Canada S7K 6P7, (306) 934-7218, MA 87 Minot St Univ; 88–Dept Dir-Comm Disorders, Parkridge Centre

Wood, Dr James Fowle 215 East Watauga Avenue, Johnson City, TN 37601, (615) 929-9101, MD (NS) Univ of TN - Knoxville

Wood, Dr James Martin University Of Nebraska, Omaha, NE 68182, (402) 554-2201, BS 57 Univ of UT; MS 60 Univ of UT; PH 66 (NS) Univ of UT; Prof, U of Nebraska-Omaha, **SLP**

Wood, Mrs Jan M 46930 West Belmont, Firebaugh, CA 93622, (209) 364-6409, BA 79 Univ of the Pacific; MA 80 Univ of the Pacific; Sp-Lang Path, Dos Palos Jt Un Elem Sch Dist, **SLP**

Wood, Jewel A S Route 2 Box 244, California, MD 20619, (301) 863-7495, BS 73 WV Univ; MS 74 WV Univ; Sp-Lang Path, St Mary's County Public School, **SLP**

Wood, Julie Ann 1640 N W Rolling Hill Drive, Beaverton, OR 97006, (503) 643-2142, ME 83 Western OR St Coll; 87–Sp-Lang Path, Visiting Nurse's Association, **SLP**

Wood, Karen Hughes 41262 Erma Avenue, Fremont, CA 94538, (415) 659-6321, BA 77 1954; MA 79 Cleveland St Univ; Dir, Sun Coast Hosp, **SLP ACE**

Wood, Mrs Karen P English Village Apartment, Peter Hall #10, Newark, DE 19711, (302) 654-4327, BA 80 Univ of MD - College Park; ME 82 Univ of VA - Charlottesville; 84–Aud, Otol Consultants PA, **A**

Wood, Dr Kenneth Scott 1941 Potter Street, Eugene, OR 97405, (503) 686-2578, BS 35 OR St Univ; MA 38 Univ of MI - Ann Arbor; PH 46 (Sp & Clinical Psych) Univ of Southern CA; 42–Prof Emeritus, Univ of Oregon, **SLP A F LM**

Wood, Laurel B R 2223 Harvard Court, Visalia, CA 93277, (301) 687-1704, BA 71 CA St Univ - Long Beach; MA 75 CA St Univ - Long Beach; Sp/Lang Path, Balt Co Schs, **SLP**

Wood, Mrs Linda Thompson 59 Pebble Beach Boulevard, Naples, FL 33962, (813) 643-2700, BA 64 Univ of GA; ME 66 Univ of GA; Except Ed Facilitator, Collier Co Pub Sch, **SLP**

Wood, Lisa Ann 1081 Ambleside Drive #209, Ottawa, ON, Canada K2B 8C8, (613) 828-5376, BS 83 Purdue Univ - West Lafayette; MA 85 Memphis St Univ; 86–Sp-Lang Path, Chldn's Hosp of Eastern Ontario, **SLP**

Wood, Mrs Lori B RFD 1 Box 1420, Raccoon Hill Road, Salisbury, NH 03268, (603) 648-2603, BA 78 Univ of MT; MA 80 Memphis St Univ; 86–Sp-Lang Path, Merrimack Valley Schs, **SLP**

Wood, Mrs Lynn A 486 Parkside Drive, Carol Stream, IL 60188, (216) 678-5480, BA 81 Univ of Akron; MA 83 Univ of Akron; Audiologist, Hattie Larlham Foundation, **A**

Wood, Lynn Rodney 208 Montwood Court, Franklin, TN 37064, (615) 320-5353, BS 76 VA Commonwealth Univ; MA 79 NM St Univ; 88–Sp-Lang Path, Bill Wilkerson Hrng & Sp Ctr, **SLP**

Wood, Margaret 3900 Farmview Drive, Glenshaw, PA 15116, BS 67 Syracuse Univ; MS 68 Syracuse Univ; Sp/Lang Path, Allegheny Inter Unit, **SLP**

Wood, Margaret Louise Route 9 Box 91-F, Santa Fe, NM 87505, (505) 988-7239, BA 75 Hastings Coll; MS 87 Univ of NM; 88–Sp-Lang Path, Santa Fe PS

Wood, Marian Sharp 607 McRae Street #I-4, Waynesboro, MS 39367, (601) 368-1570, BS 85 MS Univ for Women; MS 86 Univ Southern MS-Hattiesburg; Sp-Lang Path, InSpeech Inc, **SLP**

Wood, Maria K P O Box 1176, Tomball, TX 77375-1176, BS 73 Univ of TX - Austin; MA 75 Univ of Houston - Univ Park; SLP, Spring Branch ISD, **SLP**

Wood, Mrs Martha S 2055 Tammarack Drive, Long Lake, MN 55356, (612) 933-9343, BS 65 Brenau Coll; MS 80 Univ of WI - River Falls; SLP, Hopkins Sch Dist 270, **SLP**

Wood, Mary Ann Duggan P O Box 1061, Barrow, AK 99723, (907) 852-5600, BA 76 Western WA Univ; MA 79 Western WA Univ; 88–Aud, North Slope Borough Hlth Dept, **A**

Wood, Mrs Mary C Box 396, Salem, MO 65560, (314) 729-3953, BS 68 Univ of MO - Columbia; MS 87 Central MO St Univ; 86–Sp-Lang Path, Exceptional Child Educ Co-op, **SLP**

Wood, Mary Ellen 400 91st Street, Daly City, CA 94015, **SLP**

Wood, Mrs Mary Helen 2305 Santiago Way #A, Stockton, CA 95209, (209) 473-7192, MA 40 Univ of IA; **SLP LM**

Wood, Dr Mary Lovey Austin Speech Lang & Lrng Clinic, 3724 Jefferson, Suite 101, Austin, TX 78731, (512) 459-0515, BA 64 Univ of TX - Austin; MA 66 Univ of TX - Austin; PH 76 (Sp-Lang Path) Univ of TX - Austin; Dir/SLP, Austin Sp Lang & Lrng Cl, **SLP F ACE**

Wood, Dr Mildred H 1825 Iowa Street, Cedar Falls, IA 50613, (319) 266-4453, MA 60 Univ of Northern IA; ES 62 Univ of Northern IA; ED 70 (Special Educ) IN Univ - Bloomington; **SLP LM**

Wood, Pamela Joyce 30 Ashland Street, Malden, MA 02148, (617) 324-3611, MS 85 Northeastern Univ; **SLP**

Wood, Mrs Pamela R 1775 West Saint Mary's Road #211, Tucson, AZ 85745, (602) 792-2044, BS 80 Towson St Univ; MS 82 Univ of AZ; 82–Aud, St Mary's ENT Assoc, **A**

Wood, Patricia F 1130 Woodmont Road, Anniston, AL 36201, (205) 831-5236, BS 74 Univ of Montevallo; MA 75 Univ of AL- Tuscaloosa; Sp-Lang Path, Private Practice, **SLP**

Wood, Patsy Ruth H 422 Peach Tree Street, Johnson City, TN 37601, (615) 623-0929, BS 74 East TN St Univ; MA 75 East TN St Univ; 87–Sp-Lang Path, Communi-Care Inc, **SLP**

Wood, Mrs Paulette J 8004 College Drive, Des Moines, IA 50322, (515) 283-6344, BA 65 Univ of Northern IA; MS 66 Purdue Univ - West Lafayette; 77–SLP, IA Methodist Med Cen, **SLP**

Wood, Penny Marie 1305 Virginia Avenue, Lakewood, OH 44107, (216) 261-4848, BA 81 Cleveland St Univ; MA 83 Cleveland St Univ; 85–Aud, Cleveland Ear Nose and Throat, **A**

Wood, Mrs Rachel S 30 W 265 Ridgewood Court, Warrenville, IL 60555, (312) 393-2391, BA 73 Western MI Univ; MS 74 IN Univ - Bloomington; Sp-Lang Path, Pediatric Sp & Lang Therapy, **SLP**

Wood, Rebecca E 324 Hamilton Road, Marquette Heights, IL 61554, (309) 685-0887, BS 75 Northern IL Univ - De Kalb; MA 76 Northern IL Univ - De Kalb; 86–Ofc Mgr, Beltone Hearing Aid Ctr, **A**

Wood, Mrs Rebecca H Box 33 Kelli Cove, Batesville, AR 72501, (501) 698-1529, BA 71 Hendrix Coll; MA 74 Univ of AR - Fayetteville; Sp-Lang Path, Batesville Therapy Services, **SLP**

Wood, Mrs Rebecca Marsh 1419 West Magnolia, San Antonio, TX 78201, (512) 680-0430, BS 78 Southwest TX St Univ; ME 79 Southwest TX St Univ; 85–Dept Chmn Spec Educ, Northside ISD, **SLP**

Wood, Mrs Suzanne Bess 438 N W 35th, Oklahoma City, OK 73118, (405) 525-2717, MS 85 Univ of OK Medical Center; Sp-Lang Path, Private Practice, **SLP**

Wood, Teresa Kay 81 Stoneledge Drive, Maumelle, AR 72118, (501) 490-2000, **SLP**

Wood, Terry Donovan 2369 Hidden Lake Drive, Palm Harbor, FL 33563, MA 72 Cleveland St Univ; Sp-Lang Path, Pinellas County Board of Educ, **SLP**

Wood, Timothy John 57 Senechal Drive, Somerset, MA 02725, (617) 672-9054, BA 84 Southern CT St Univ; MA 86 Univ of MA - Amherst; **SLP**

Wood, Tina Marie 4401 West Woodway Drive, Muncie, IN 47304, (317) 286-8004, BA 84 Ball St Univ; MA 85 Ball St Univ; Sp-Lang Path, Ball Memorial Hosp, **SLP**

Wood, Virginia Dixon J-174 Jhmhc, Gainesville, FL 32610, (904) 392-2636, BS 76 OH St Univ; MA 78 Univ of FL; SLP/Craniofacial Cl Coord, Univ of FL, **SLP**

Wood, Dr W Scott 6817 Circlecreek Drive, Pinellas Park, FL 34665, (813) 398-9395, BS 69 Maryville Coll; MA 71 Univ of TN - Knoxville; PH 81 (Hrng and Sp Sciences) Univ of TN - Knoxville; Aud, VA Med Cen, **A**

Wood, Mrs Zira A 18444 Clifftop Way, Malibu, CA 90265, (213) 454-6042, BA 65 Univ of CA - Los Angeles; MA 71 Univ of Southern CA; Sp/Lang Path, Priv Pract, **SLP**

Woodall, Mrs Laura Jean 120 Country Place, Stockbridge, GA 30281, (404) 957-6601, BA 81 Columbus Coll; ME 84 Columbus Coll; Sp-Lang Path, Henry County Bd of Education, **SLP**

Woodall, Martha Pickett P O Box 15853, Hattiesburg, MS 39401, (601) 582-7454, BS 69 Univ Southern MS-Hattiesburg; MS 70 Univ Southern MS-Hattiesburg; Sp-Lang Path, Voc & Hlth Serv Inc, **SLP ACE**

Woodall, Rosemary Vivian 1020 Waverly Street, Palo Alto, CA 94301, (415) 327-5494, MA 85 San Jose St Univ; **SLP**

Woodard, Mrs Beatrice E P O Box 248, Waxhaw, NC 28173-0248, (704) 843-6065, BA 73 Univ of ME - Orono; MS 75 Southern CT St Univ; Resource Teacher, Summer Institute - Linguistics, **SLP**

Woodard, Lottie 1337 Rimpau Boulevard, Los Angeles, CA 90019, MS 76; **SLP**

Woodard, Mrs Nancy Deann 9128 Peppertree Circle, Wichita, KS 67226, (316) 524-3181, MA 85 Wichita St Univ; SLP, USD 259, **SLP**

Woodbury, Keith 11 Maple Lawn Drive, RFD 3, Monson, MA 01057, (413) 323-6311, BS 76 SUNY - Coll at Geneseo; MA 77 SUNY - Coll at Geneseo; Dir of Sp & Hrng Serv, Belchertown St Sch, **SLP**

Woodcock, Linda W Speech & Language Services, 915 B Willowbrook Drive SE, Huntsville, AL 35802, (205) 882-0136, BS 58 Auburn Univ - Auburn; MS 60 Tulane Univ; 88–Sp-Lang Path, Private Practice, **SLP ACE**

Woodcox, Sharon Christine 65 Burgess Avenue, Toronto, ON, Canada M4E 1W9, (416) 492-3908, BA 83 MI St Univ; MA 84 MI St Univ; **A**

Woodfill, Marcia Jo Columbus Hearing Impaired Prgm, 1455 Huy Road, Columbus, OH 43224, (614) 451-2258, BS 75 Bowling Green St Univ; MA 82 OH St Univ; Aud, Columbus Bd of Ed, **A**

Woodfin, Linda Norris Ball Memorial Hospital, 2401 University Avenue, Muncie, IN 47303, (317) 747-4258, BA 65 LA St Univ - Baton Rouge; MS 74 Univ of TN - Knoxville; Clin Supervisor Sp-Lang Path, Ball Memorial Hospital, **SLP**

Woodfin, Shelia T 1405 Travis Heights Blvd, Austin, TX 78704, (512) 478-9131, BS 73 Univ of MO - Columbia; MA 74 Memphis St Univ; 88–Sp-Lang Path, Live Oak Ctr for Comm Dis, **SLP**

Woodford, Alice M Route 1, Potsdam, NY 13676, BS 67 SUNY - Coll at Buffalo; MS 71 SUNY - Coll at Geneseo; Consultant, Private Practice, **SLP**

Woodford, Dr Charles M West Virginia University, 805 Allen Hall, P O Box 6122, Morgantown, WV 26506, (304) 293-4241, BS 68 SUNY - Coll at Geneseo; MS 69 SUNY - Coll at Geneseo; PH 74 (Aud) Syracuse Univ; Prof, W VA U, **SLP A**

Woodford, Lee Lucas 2450 Simeon Court, Charlottesville, VA 22901, (804) 924-7107, BS 77 Radford Univ; MS 79 Marshall Univ; Sp-Lang Path, Univ of Virginia, **SLP**

Woodgate, Mrs Lisa J 2321 Melonie Trail, New Smyrna Beach, FL 32069, (904) 427-8416, BS 84 Southwest MO St Univ; MA 86 Southwest MO St Univ; SLP, InSpeech Inc, **SLP ACE**

Woodhams, Julia V 3456 Burbank Drive, Ann Arbor, MI 48105, (313) 662-6341, BS 78 Central MI Univ; MA 81 Eastern MI Univ; Sp-Lang Path, Our Lady of Providence, **SLP**

Woodhead, James S 32438 Celeste Court, Union City, CA 94538, BA 67 San Jose St Univ; MA 69 San Jose St Univ; SLP, Newark USD, **SLP**

Woodhouse, Toby 1335 Bounty Way, Laguna Beach, CA 92651, Syracuse Univ; 69 Univ of WI - Madison; **SLP**

Woodhull, Mrs Susan Z 1561 Burgundy Court, Elkhart, IN 46514, (219) 262-1471, BS 72 Ball St Univ; MA 75 Western MI Univ; **SLP**

Woodie, Sally Kay 40 Donovan Court, Merrimack, NH 03054, (603) 429-1769, BS 82 Ashland Coll; MA 83 OH St Univ; 87–Aud, Manchester ENT, **A**

Woodin, Mrs Devnet Trinkle P O Box 613, Lake George, NY 12845, (518) 434-4103, **SLP**

Woodley, Tricia Evans 349 West 31st Avenue, San Mateo, CA 94403, (415) 921-7658, BA 69 Univ of the Pacific; MA 72 San Diego St Univ; Sp-Lang Path, Sf Hrng & Sp Cen, **SLP**

Woodman, Patricia Anne 6635 S Staples #1334, Corpus Christi, TX 78413, (512) 853-9977, BA 82 Univ of WI - Stevens Point; MA 87 Univ of WI - Stevens Point; **SLP**

Woodmansee, Regina Gail 2020 Cheyenne #151, Modesto, CA 95356, (415) 228-6800, BA 85 CA St Univ - Chico; MA 87 CA St Univ - Chico

Woodruff, Mrs Rebecca Clifton 301 Woodards Ford Road, Chesapeake, VA 23320, (804) 482-3819, BS 85 Old Dominion Univ; ME 87 Old Dominion Univ

Woodruff, Susan A 372 H Street, Salt Lake City, UT 84103, (801) 278-2607, BS 58 Univ of UT; MS 73 Univ of UT; SLP, Granite Sch Dist, **SLP**

Woods, Dr C Lee Klamath Speech & Hearing Ctr, 1415 Esplanade, Klamath Falls, OR 97601, (503) 883-3621, BA 64 Culver-Stockton Coll; MA 67 Univ of IA; PH 69 (Sp-Lang Path) Univ of IA; Dir Sp-Lang Path, Klamath Sp and Hrng Cen, **SLP**

Woods, Mrs Carolyn J 2810 Shetland Drive, Winston-Salem, NC 27107, (919) 788-2826, BS 73 Appalachian St Univ; MA 74 Appalachian St Univ; Sp/Lang Path, Winston Salem/Forsyth Co Sch, **SLP**

Woods, Carrie Lynn 4900 Nichols Road #708, Bay City, TX 77414, (409) 245-6318, BS 81 Central St Univ; ME 82 Central St Univ; 87–Sp-Lang Path, Matagorda County Educ Svcs, **SLP**

Woods, Catherine 1585 Ridge Avenue #211, Evanston, IL 60201, (312) 864-6343, MS 49 Northwestern Univ; **SLP A LM**

Woods, Charline Joan 4524 Vista Del Monte #3, Sherman Oaks, CA 91403, (818) 997-2357, BA 78 CA St Univ - Northridge; MA 81 CA St Univ - Northridge; Sp/Lang Path, Los Angeles USD, **SLP**

Woods, Donald G 109 Joost Avenue, San Francisco, CA 94131, (415) 499-5807, BA 58 Univ of WA; MA 63 San Francisco St Univ; SLP, Marin Co Office of Ed, **SLP**

Woods, Mrs Donna J 1673 North 17th, Coos Bay, OR 97420, (503) 267-3104, BS 75 Univ of OR; Sp-Lang Path, Coos Bay School District, **SLP**

Woods, Mrs Elissa Bennack 3209 Conestoga Drive, Plano, TX 75074, (214) 231-4639, BS 81 Univ of North TX; MS 83 Univ of OK Medical Center; Sp-Lang Path, Richardson Speech & Language Clinic, **SLP**

Woods, Mrs Gay Ann J 1122 Maple Street, Klamath Falls, OR 97601, (503) 883-4745, BA 65 Univ of Denver; MA 67 Univ of IA; Sp-Lang Path, Klamath Falls Sch Dist, **SLP**

Woods, Jacqueline Ann 4212 Allendorf Drive #G-28, Cincinnati, OH 45209-1541, (513) 271-4318, BS 84 Univ of Cincinnati; MA 86 Univ of Cincinnati; 86–Sp-Lang Path, Cincinnati PS, **SLP**

Woods, Mrs Josephine 1950 Gardenia Street, Sykesville, MD 21784, (301) 795-5585, BS 74 Univ of MD - College Park; MA 76 Univ of MD - College Park; Sp-Lang Path, Carroll County Board of Educ, **SLP**

Woods, Mrs Laura Johnson P O Box 5226, Destin, FL 32541, (904) 243-8741, BS 85 Auburn Univ - Auburn; OM 86 Auburn Univ - Auburn; **SLP**

Woods, Leslie K 456 East 3335 South #14, Salt Lake City, UT 84115, (801) 565-7530, BA 74 Eastern WA Univ; MS 78 Eastern WA Univ; 81–Sp-Lang Path, Jordan Sch Dist, **SLP**

Woods, Sr M Lucy 2551 West 8th Street, Erie, PA 16505, (814) 838-1966, BS 42 Villa Maria Coll; ME 58 Duquesne Univ; **SLP LM**

Woods, Mrs Margaret Y 4440 Livingston Avenue, Dallas, TX 75205, (214) 358-5261, BA 52 Southern Methodist Univ; MA 69 Southern Methodist Univ; 69–Sp-Lang Path, Dallas Easter Seal Soc Fr Chil, **SLP**

Woods, Martha S 2175 Turk Road, Doylestown, PA 18901, (215) 348-9257, BS 64 Bloomsburg Univ of PA; MA 81 Trenton St Coll; Sp-Lang Path, Bucks County Independent Unit, **SLP**

Woods, Mary Ellen M 178 Whitman Avenue, West Hartford, CT 06107, (413) 781-9100, BA 83 Univ of CT; MA 85 Univ of CT; **SLP**

Woods, Richard T 916 Highland Terrace, Atlanta, GA 30306, (404) 979-8242, BS 72 Univ of TN - Knoxville; MA 74 Univ of TN - Knoxville; Reg Sales Mgr, 3-M Otolgic Products, **A**

Woods, Dr Robert W 143 Elmer Street, Westfield, NJ 07090, (201) 232-2900, BS 62 SUNY - Coll at Geneseo; MS 65 Purdue Univ - West Lafayette; PH 69 (NS) Purdue Univ - West Lafayette; Dir of Aud Prog & Serv, Speech & Hearing Associates, **A**

Woods, Roland E 909 East Pine Avenue, Olympia, WA 98506, BA 46 Univ of WA; **SLP LM**

Woods, Mrs Sarah N Route 1 Box 85-B, Lauderdale, MS 39335, (601) 483-0681, BS 70 Univ Southern MS-Hattiesburg; MS 72 MS Univ for Women; Sp-Lang Path, Meridian Pub Sch, **SLP**

Woods, Sheila P 9425 Shore Road, Brooklyn, NY 11209, (718) 330-1842, BA 50 Coll of New Rochelle; MA 54 Columbia Univ Teachers Coll; Assistant Director, New York City Board of Educ, **SLP**

Woods, Mrs Shirley L R 3115 Cherry Road N E, Washington, DC 20018, (202) 832-3472, BS 84 Univ of the DC; MS 87 Univ of the DC; 87–Sp-Lang Path, Comm Skills Consultants Inc, **SLP**

Wood-Sauer, Elizabeth Grace 361 Village Walk Circle, Spencerport, NY 14559, (716) 271-6423, BS 77 Nazareth Coll of Rochester; MS 80 Nazareth Coll of Rochester; Sp-Lang Path, UCP, **SLP**

Woods-Groves, Mrs Mary L 2304 Fairfax Road, South Charleston, WV 25303, (304) 345-6821, BS 78 WV Univ; MS 80 WV Univ; **A**

Woods-Viens, Mrs Elaine 260 Old Colchester Tpke, East Haddam, CT 06423, (203) 342-3131, BA 78 Univ of CT; MS 81 Southern CT St Univ; Sp-Lang Path, Portland Pub Sch, **SLP**

Woodward, Mrs Eleanor S P O Box 818, Experiment Station Road, Quincy, FL 32351, (904) 627-9651, OB 58 FL St Univ; MS 75 FL St Univ; Aud, Gadsen County School Board

Woodward, Mrs Laura D 802 Signal Ridge Place, Rockwall, TX 75087, (214) 328-9985, BA 80 IN Univ - Bloomington; OM 81 IN Univ - Bloomington; 82–Sp-Lang Path, Dallas ISD, **SLP**

Woodward, Lily L 125 Pine Valley, Huntsville, TX 77340, (409) 295-9495, BS 53 Univ Southern MS-Hattiesburg; MA 55 Univ Southern MS-Hattiesburg; **SLP**

Woodward, Sandra H Nicolet Instrument Corp, Audiodiagnostics Division, P O Box 7010, Madison, WI 53707, (608) 271-3333, BA 74 SUNY - Coll at Potsdam; MS 75 Ithaca Coll; Aud, Nicolet Instrument Corporation, **A ACE**

Woodweu, Linda P 2912 California #1, San Francisco, CA 94115, (415) 922-1998, BA 77 Univ of CO - Boulder; MS 79 IL St Univ - Normal; Sp-Lang Path, InSpeech Inc, **SLP**

Woodworth, Lorna G 561 Elizabeth Street, Oneida, NY 13421, **SLP**

Woodworth, Mrs Ruth MacCallum 28 Pettigrove Crescent, Fredericton, NB, Canada E3A 5P3, (506) 453-2472, BS 83 Univ of New Brunswick - Nb; MS 85 IL St Univ - Normal; 87–Sp-Lang Path, Dept of Health & Comm Services

Woody, Nancy Jean 1424 Kanawha Boulevard E, Apartment 23, Charleston, WV 25301, (304) 346-5109, BA 83 Univ of TN - Knoxville; MA 85 Univ of TN - Knoxville; Aud, Aud & Hrng Aid Srvcs Inc, **A**

Woofter, Herbert R Dept Of Communication Arts, Gallaudet University, 800 Florida Avenue N E, Washington, DC 20002, (202) 651-5420, BS 51 Northwestern Univ; MA 54 OH St Univ; Assoc Prof, Gallaudet Univ, **SLP**

Wool, Sharon Lee 102-G Community Drive, Shillington, PA 19607, (215) 378-6694, BS 85 Bloomsburg Univ of PA; MS 86 Bloomsburg Univ of PA; Sp-Lang Path, Reading Hospital & Medical Ctr, **SLP**

Woolbert, Kathi L 110 West Dawson Drive, Bridgeton, NJ 08302, (760) 455-3131, MA 88 Trenton St Coll

Woolbright, Wendy Lamont 174 Reservoir Avenue, Middletown, RI 02840, (401) 683-3570, BS 74 Kent St Univ; MA 79 Univ of Houston - Univ Park; Sp-Lang Path, Newport Co Reg Spec Ed Prog, **SLP**

Woolcock, Mrs Wendy Jane Rural Delivery 1, Box 115, Orangeville, PA 17859, (717) 966-0914, BS 81 Bloomsburg Univ of PA; MS 82 Bloomsburg Univ of PA; Sp-Lang Path, Cen Susquehanna Inter Unit #16, **SLP**

Woolcott, Mrs Sandra Butz 398 Vincent Place, Elgin, IL 60123, (312) 888-5185, BS 63 Northern IL Univ - De Kalb; MS 76 IL St Univ - Normal; Sp-Lang Path, Sch Dist U-46 Elgin Il, **SLP**

Wooldridge, Elaine L Speech & Language Consultants, 1824 Blanding Boulevard, Jacksonville, FL 32210, (904) 388-8756, MA 73 Univ of AR - Fayetteville; 79–Sp-Lang Path, Sp & Lang Consultants, **SLP ACE**

Wooldridge, Joyce M 4041 Crawford Avenue, Louisville, KY 40218, (502) 588-4459, BS 79 Murray St Univ; MS 81 Murray St Univ; Sp-Lang Path, Kentucky Comm for Hndcpd Chil, **SLP**

Woolet, Deborah J 2905 Pitkin Drive, Arlington, TX 76006-2043, (214) 255-2151, BS 78 Purdue Univ - West Lafayette; MS 79 Univ of North TX; Sp-Lang Path, Irving ISD, **SLP**

Wooley, Mrs Helen G 1301 Uila Street, Honolulu, HI 96818, (808) 695-9678, BA 65 MI St Univ; MA 67 Temple Univ; Sp-Lang Path, Dept of Ed Leeward Oahu, **SLP**

Wooley, Margaret E P O Box 706, Greenwood, NS, Canada B0P 1N0, (902) 678-8522, BA 77 Univ of Regina -Saskatchewan; OM 80 Univ of Western Ontario; 85–Sp-Lang Path, Kings County Dist School Board, **SLP**

Woolf, Dr Carole L 242 Dolphin Cove Court, Del Mar, CA 92014, (619) 481-0999, BA 73 Univ of Redlands; MS 74 Univ of Redlands; PH 83 (Learning Disabilities) Northwestern Univ; 85–Lecturer, San Diego State University, **SLP**

Woolf, Dr Gerald Dept Communication Sci & Dis, Montclair State College, Upper Montclair, NJ 07043, (201) 893-4227, BS 47 CUNY - City College; MS 50 Univ of Pittsburgh - Pittsburgh; PH 59 (NS) NY Univ; Prof, Montclair St Coll, **SLP**

Woolf, Rita F 4208 Manhattan Avenue, Brooklyn, NY 11224, (718) 236-3344, **SLP**

Woolf, Mrs Selma C 7521 Slade Avenue, Baltimore, MD 21208, (301) 356-0775, BA 52 CUNY - Hunter Coll; MA 54 CUNY - Hunter Coll; MS 76 Loyola Coll; Sp-Lang Path, Baltimore Ct Bd of Ed, **SLP**

Woolfolk, Mrs Elizabeth Carrow 11315 Smithdale Road, Houston, TX 77024, (713) 465-5467, BA 49 Our Lady Lake Univ-San Anton; ME 51 Univ of TX - Austin; PH 55 (NS) Northwestern Univ; **SLP F**

Woolie, Mrs Brenda Allen 16942 Culpepper Avenue, Baton Rouge, LA 70817, (504) 768-2838, MA 71 LA St Univ - Baton Rouge; SLP, Family Christian Academy, **SLP**

Woolley, Alice V 18529 Lyn Court, Homewood, IL 60430, (312) 798-4030, BS 56 Purdue Univ - West Lafayette; MA 59 Northwestern Univ; Sp-Lang Path, Private Practice, **SLP**

Woolley, Linda P 2545 S W 175th, Aloha, OR 97006, **SLP**

Woolley, Margaret L 212 Norcross Drive #48-C, Knoxville, TN 37923, (615) 544-3609, BS 73 Univ of TN - Knoxville; MA 77 Univ of TN - Knoxville; Sp/Lang Path, Knox County Schs, **SLP**

Woolley, Melissa O'Farrell 1519 Todd Street, Mountain View, CA 94040-2933, (415) 262-2100, BA 84 Univ of CA - Santa Barbara; MA 86 CA St Univ - Fresno; **SLP**

Wooten, Angela Lathem 457 Hidden Oaks, Elgin, TX 78621, (512) 458-3357, MS 77 Univ of North TX; Aud, Austin ENT Clinic, **A**

Wooten, Diana Styles 204 Castlegate Drive, Morganton, NC 28655-3621, (704) 437-1711, BS 75 Appalachian St Univ; MA 76 Appalachian St Univ; **SLP**

Wooten, Kathryn Wilkerson Route 9 Box 346, Albany, GA 31705, (912) 776-8605, BS 81 Univ of GA; ME 82 Univ of GA; Sp-Lang Path, Worth Co Bd of Ed, **SLP**

Wooten, Dr Philip Gary 1717 Robindale Road, Richmond, VA 23235, (804) 230-1402

Wootton, Joan W 33 South Martin Road, Janesville, WI 53545, (608) 756-8315, BA 50 Rockford Coll; MA 53 Northwestern Univ; 79–Sp-Lang Path, Janesville School District, **SLP A**

Wopata, Mrs Jeri Degraff 7908 North Park, Kansas City, MO 64118, (816) 932-3262, BS 80 IA St Univ; MA 82 Univ of KS; Sp-Lang Path, St Lukes Hosp Sp & Hrng Dept, **SLP**

Woppert, Mrs Diane L 910 North 60th Street, Milwaukee, WI 53213, (414) 476-3840, BS 80 Univ of WI - Milwaukee; MS 82 Univ of WI - Milwaukee; Sp/Lang Path, Milwaukee Pub Schs, **SLP**

Worachek, Jo A 286 Longwood Cove, Ridgeland, MS 39157, (601) 362-4471, BA 74 Univ of WI - Eau Claire; MS 77 Univ of WI - Stevens Point; Sp/Lang Path, VA Med Cen, **SLP**

Worachek-Jarocki, Mary 5926 North 37th Street, Milwaukee, WI 53209, (414) 475-8252, BA 83 Univ of WI - Eau Claire; MS 85 Univ of WI - Eau Claire; SLP, St Lukes Hospital, **SLP**

Worcester, Carol S 27910 Ridgecove Court, Rancho Palos Verdes, CA 90274, (213) 542-6608, BS 64 Northwestern Univ; BA 65 Northwestern Univ; ME 77 Loyola Marymount Univ; Princ, LA Co Office of Ed, **SLP**

Worde, Alfred B Cisd, 17111 G Drive North, Marshall, MI 49068, (616) 781-5141, BS 55 Western MI Univ; MA 61 Western MI Univ; Dir Spec Ed, Calhoun Inter Sch Dist, **SLP**

Worden, Diane C 8780 Glen Ferry Drive, Alpharetta, GA 30201, (404) 642-7236, BA 66 Jersey City St Coll; MS 80 William Paterson Coll; 88–Sp-Lang Path, Private Practice, **SLP**

Worden, Edwina Marie 15767 Tuscola Road #6, Apple Valley, CA 92307, (619) 247-2683, BA 82 Univ of the Pacific; MA 83 Univ of the Pacific; SLP, Apple Valley School District, **SLP**

Worgul, Jeffrey W 464 Ocean Avenue, New London, CT 06320, (203) 443-6944, BS 75 PA St Univ - Univ Park; MS 76 PA St Univ - Univ Park; Dir of Cl Serv, Co Hrng and Balance Inc, **A**

Work, Rhonda S 3323 Lakeshore Drive East, Tallahassee, FL 32312, (904) 487-2840, BS 55 Northwestern Univ; MA 68 Univ of FL; 75–Prog Spec Sp-Lang Path, FL Dept of Ed, **SLP F ACE**

Workinger, Dr Marilyn Seif Marshfield Clinic, 1000 North Oak Avenue, Marshfield, WI 54449, (715) 387-5128, BA 67 Univ of WI - Madison; MS 68 Univ of WI - Madison; PH 86 (Communicative Dis) Univ of WI - Madison; 79–Sp-Lang Path, Marshfield Clinic, **SLP**

Workman, Carol D 10 North Shore Drive, Seaford, DE 19973, (302) 629-9796, BA 75 Towson St Univ; MA 77 Univ of MD - College Park; Sp-Lang Path, Seaford Sch Dist, **SLP**

Workman, Oliver A 3500 University Blvd #3512, Jacksonville, FL 32211, **SLP**

Workmeister, Ann M 2245 Southorn Road, Baltimore, MD 21220, (301) 668-3236, BS 77 Towson St Univ; MS 79 Towson St Univ; Sp/Lang Path, Baltimore Co Pub Sch, **SLP**

Worley, Mrs Martha Lundy 1410 Rotherwood Drive, Johnson City, TN 37601, (615) 929-7453, **SLP**

Wormeli, Dale K 7422 Crawford Drive, North Delta, BC, Canada V4C 6X6, (604) 594-2750, **A**

Wormus, Catherine Ann 1627 Kenwood Lane, Olathe, KS 66062, (913) 888-4249, BS 83 KS St Univ; MA 85 Univ of KS; **SLP**

Wormus, Robert C 12510 South Hoxie Avenue, Norwalk, CA 90650, (213) 807-6511, BA 64 CA St Univ - Los Angeles; MA 65 CA St Univ - Los Angeles; Dir/Coord, So CA Permanente Med Gp, **A**

Worob, Mrs Phyllis Sacks 5716 Highland Hills Drive, Austin, TX 78731, (512) 454-8451, BS 77 Univ of TX - Austin; MS 79 Univ of North TX; Aud, **A**

Worrall, Mrs Christena 730 Woodside Avenue, Ripon, WI 54971, (414) 748-7531, BA 70 Univ of WI - Eau Claire; MS 72 Univ of WI - Madison; Sp-Lang Path, Oshkosh Public Schools, **SLP**

Worrell, Patricia A 708 Gretna Court, Winter Springs, FL 32708, (305) 695-4429, BA 82 Univ of Central FL; MA 86 Univ of Central FL; **SLP**

Worsek, Mrs Lisa David 1311 Linden, Highland Park, IL 60035, (312) 824-1136, BS 76 Univ of IL - Urbana; MS 77 Univ of IL - Urbana; **SLP**

Worsley, Mrs Martha W 101 Bristol Court, Victoria, TX 77904, (512) 576-3131, BA 62 Baylor Univ; ME 81 Univ of Houston - Victoria; Sp-Lang Path, Victoria Reg Dy Sch, **SLP**

Worster, Mrs Peggy A 562 Pearwood Court, Grand Junction, CO 81504, (303) 434-7262, MS 88 Northern AZ Univ

Worth, Catherine A Louelace Medical Center, Audiology Department, 5400 Gibson Boulevard S E, Albuquerque, NM 87108, (505) 262-7261, BA 74 Univ of Northern CO; MS 77 CO St Univ; Aud, Lovelace Med Cen, **A**

Worth, Janet C 178 Granville Street, Newark, OH 43055, **SLP**

Worth, Dr Loanne L 29W 381 Emerald Green Dr E, Warrenville, IL 60555, MS 70 Univ of MO - Columbia; ME 79 Northern IL Univ - De Kalb; Spec Ed Coord, Sased

Worth, Shannon Hulick Box 576 Rd 1, Gardiner, NY 12525, (914) 255-1537, BS 83 Trenton St Coll; MS 85 SUNY - Coll at New Paltz; **SLP**

Wortham, Mrs Bille Sintek Good Samaritan Hospital, Dept Of Audiology, 1040 N W 22nd Avenue, Portland, OR 97210, (503) 229-7860, BS 81 Univ of WY; MS 83 Univ of WY; Aud, Good Samaritan Hosp, **A**

Worthing, Donna Robichaud 8864 Warming Spring, Baldwinsville, NY 13027, (315) 455-7591, BS 81 Univ of ME - Farmington; MS 86 Syracuse Univ; 88–Sp-Lang Path, Schneier Comm Unit of Enable, **SLP**

Worthington, Colleen Kirley 9122 Bradford Road, Silver Spring, MD 20901, (202) 832-4400, BA 79 Univ of MD - College Park; MS 80 Loyola Coll; Cl Suprv, Howard U, **SLP**

Worthington, Dr Don W Boys Town Institute, 555 North 30th Street, Omaha, NE 68131, (402) 498-6526, BS 62 UT St Univ; MS 64 UT St Univ; PH 69 (Aud) Northwestern Univ; Aud, Boys Town Nat Instit, **A F**

Worthington, Mrs Jeannette 12917 South Arapaho, Olathe, KS 66062, (816) 932-3833, BS 76 Univ of KS; MS 77 Southern Methodist Univ; Sp-Lang Path, St Lukes Hospital, **SLP**

Worthley, Dr William J 3100 14th Street S W, #21, Minot, ND 58701, (503) 645-2958, MA 62 Univ of San Francisco; MS 68 Univ of OR; PH 70 (NS) Univ of OR; Adj Prof of SLP, Self Employed, **SLP**

Wortley, John S P O Box 325, Tarrytown, NY 10591, PH (NS); **SLP**

Wortman-Lowe, Linda 305 Inglewood Drive, Morganton, NC 28655-3656, (704) 433-2667, MA 77 Appalachian St Univ; Sp-Lang Path, Family Inf & Presch Prog, **SLP ACE**

Wortsman, Susan E 68 Rockledge Road #1-C, Hartsdale, NY 10530, (212) 241-6153, BA 74 CUNY - City College; MA 76 CUNY - City College; 78–Coord Aud, Mt Sinai Med Cen Comm Disorders Ctr, **A**

Woss, Mrs Debra Podvia Rd 3 Box 186D, Belle Vernon, PA 15012, (412) 439-1444, BS 81 CA Univ of PA; ME 82 CA Univ of PA; SLP, Sg Rehab Agcy Inc, **SLP**

Wothe, Carole A 8241 Hudson Drive, San Diego, CA 92119, (619) 469-9732, BA 66 Univ of Denver; MA 67 Univ of Denver; Sp/Lang Path, Co of San Diego Dept of Health Svcs, **SLP**

Wotus, Maryann 452 Garfield Avenue, Bridgeport, CT 06606, (203) 762-8526, BA 81 Univ of CT; MS 85 PA St Univ - Univ Park; **SLP**

Wouters, Mrs Jenny K 821 Vanceburg Drive, Indianapolis, IN 46241, (317) 241-7170, BA 75 Univ of TN - Knoxville; MS 77 FL St Univ; 86–Sp-Lang Path, MSD of Wayne Township, **SLP**

Woytowych, William 343 Clarke Avenue #6, Westmount, PQ, Canada H3Z 2E7, (514) 933-0349, OM 88 McGill Univ - Quebec

Woznak, Mrs Diana L 8661 Dunbar Lane, Brecksville, OH 44141, (216) 526-6169, BS 75 Bowling Green St Univ; MA 79 Univ of Akron; Sp-Lang Path, Parma City Schools, **SLP**

Wozniak, Linda A 5508 Cabot Place, Halifax, NS, Canada B3K 2J7, BA 79 SUNY - Center at Buffalo; MA 81 SUNY - Center at Buffalo; Sp-Lang Path, Nova Scotia Hearing & Sp Clin, **SLP**

Wozniak, Lorraine 9204 Wildwood Drive, Highland, IN 46322, (219) 933-2464, BS 74 Ball St Univ; MA 78 Ball St Univ; MA 81 Ball St Univ; Sp-Lang Path, Sch City of Hammond, **A**

Wozniak, Susan Marie 7 Spann Street, Buffalo, NY 14206, (716) 823-9658, MA 88 SUNY - Center at Buffalo

Wozny, Susan M 320 Ellen Place, Paramus, NJ 07652, (718) 317-3687, BA 83 Rutger's St Univ - Douglas Coll; MS 84 Rutgers St Univ -N Brunswick; Supvr Sp-Lang Path, Sea View Hospital and Home, **SLP**

Wozobski, Bette Schlanger 3927 South Florence Place, Tulsa, OK 74105, (918) 494-2093, BA 70 Univ of WI - Madison; MA 73 Univ of Tulsa; OM 76 Univ of Tulsa; Sp-Lang Path, St Francis Hosp, **SLP**

Wragg, Frances Rebecca 819 Miramar, Berkeley, CA 94707, (415) 836-8222, **SLP**

Wragge, Marcia Steinkruger 14439 Weir Circle, Millard, NE 68137, (402) 291-1297, BS 84 Kearney St Coll; MS 85 Univ of NE - Omaha; Sp-Lang Path, Bellevue PS, **SLP**

Wrasse, Kenneth W, Jr P O Box 9, San Carlos, CA 94070, **SLP**

Wray, Dr Denise F 412 Victoria Park Drive, Tallmadge, OH 44278, (216) 375-7883, BA 75 Univ of Akron; MA 77 Univ of Akron; PH 85 (NS) Univ of Akron; Assistant Professor, U of Akron, **SLP**

Wray, Doris Q 13309 Dove Street, Silver Spring, MD 20904, (301) 762-0635, BS 73 Howard Univ; MA 76 MI St Univ; Sp-Lang Path, Mongy Co Pub Sch, **SLP ACE**

Wray, Elinor C 156 Ocean Street, Narrabeen, New South Wales, Australia 2101, **SLP LM**

Wray, John Anthony 143 1/2 Moffatt Street #4, St Catharines, ON, Canada L2P 2L7, (705) 764-1320, BA 85 Univ of Western Ontario; MA 87 SUNY - Coll at Geneseo; **SLP**

Wreaks, Annette Catherine 408 West Portola Avenue, Los Altos, CA 94022, (415) 522-2600, BA 83 CA St Univ - Chico; MS 86 San Francisco St Univ; **SLP**

Wrege, Gail Lynn 2800 West Genesee, Saginaw, MI 48602, (517) 776-0200, BA 73 MI St Univ; MA 87 MI St Univ; 88–Sp-Lang Path, Saginaw PS

Wren, Susan Ann 1922 Hartel Avenue, Apartment 2, Philadelphia, PA 19111, (215) 643-3220, BS 83 Marywood Coll; MS 85 Bloomsburg Univ of PA; 88–Sp-Lang Path, Diane Morgan & Assoc, **SLP**

Wren, Mrs Thelma I 7536 35th N E, Seattle, WA 98115, (206) 522-2372, BA 68 Univ of WA; OM 71 Univ of WA; Retired, Lake Wash Sch Dist #414, **SLP**

Wrenn, Mary 2925-A Dwight Way, Berkeley, CA 94720, (415) 549-2467, MS 88 San Francisco St Univ; 88–Sp-Lang Path, Alameda Co Office of Educ

Wrens, Brenda M 1110 Bishop, Benton Harbor, MI 49022, (616) 927-1755, BA 84 MI St Univ; MA 85 MI St Univ; **SLP**

Wrich, Mrs Mary Jacquelyn 460 North Orlando Circle, Mesa, AZ 85205, (605) 832-9106, BA 77 Univ of NM; MS 79 Univ of NM; **SLP**

Wright, Adrienne 4838 East Harvard Lane, Denver, CO 80222, (303) 861-6800, BA 62 Univ of the Pacific; MA 64 Stanford Univ; Coord-Aud & Hrng-Impaired Svcs, The Children's Hosp, **A**

Wright, Mrs Anita Beth P O Box 296, Maxwell, NM 87728-0296, (505) 375-2464, BS 80 Univ of Tulsa; MA 83 Univ of Tulsa; 86–Sp-Lang Path, High Plains Regional Center, **SLP**

Wright, Anita L 2456 63rd Avenue S E, Mercer Island, WA 98040, (206) 545-2529, BA 68 Univ of WA; MS 78 Eastern WA Univ; Sp-Lang Path, U of WA, **SLP**

Wright, Ann G 14740 Maine Cove Terrace, Gaithersburg, MD 20878, (301) 251-1497, MS 75 Univ of NC - Chapel Hill; SLP, Fairfax Co Pub Sch, **SLP**

Wright, Mrs Anne T 13811 Crown Bluff, San Antonio, TX 78216, (512) 496-3783, BA 73 TX Tech Univ; MA 74 Our Lady Lake Univ-San Anton; Sp-Lang Path Consult, Skyview Living Cen-San Antonio, **SLP**

Wright, Mrs Betty Johnson 1941 Naylor Road S E #8, Washington, DC 20020, (202) 889-3254, Sp-Lang Path, Dc General Hospital, **SLP**

Wright, Mrs Betty T 28 Yellow Brick Road, Stillwater, OK 74074, (405) 372-1979, BS 65 IA St Univ; BS 81 OK St Univ; MA 83 OK St Univ; Sp-Lang Path, Payne Co Cuidance Clinic, **SLP**

Wright, Betty Tindel 404 Lutie Drive, Valrico, FL 33594, (813) 685-3585, MS 86 Univ of South FL; SLP, Hillsborough Cty Sch Sys, **SLP**

Wright, Mrs Beverly Brown 5890 Washington Boulevard, Indianapolis, IN 46220, BS 77 Vanderbilt Univ; MS 81 Vanderbilt Univ; **SLP**

Wright, Bonnie C 2908 Dunsinane Court, Raleigh, NC 27604, (919) 876-8787, BA 67 Wake Forest Univ; MS 78 Univ of NC - Chapel Hill; **SLP**

Wright, Mrs Carla Gasper 416 West 6th, Hays, KS 67601, (913) 628-2195, BS 84 KS St Univ; MS 87 Fort Hays St Univ; 88–Sp-Lang Path, North KS Educ Svc Ctr

Wright, Caroline 3220 Buckhorn Drive, Lexington, KY 40515, (606) 273-2050, BS 81 Eastern KY Univ; BS 84 Eastern KY Univ; MA 85 Eastern KY Univ; **SLP**

Wright, Cherry 2100 Friendly Drive #3014, Arlington, TX 76011, (214) 262-5545, BS 69 TX Tech Univ; MS 70 TX Tech Univ; Principal, Grand Prairie Ind Sch Dist, **SLP**

Wright, Cheryl A 16 Chesapeake Road, Holbrook, MA 02343, (617) 587-2121, BS 84 Boston Univ; MS 85 Boston Univ; **SLP**

Wright, Mrs China Allen 6737 Brentwood Stair Road #116, Fort Worth, TX 76112, (817) 429-2059, BS 77 Univ of North TX; MS 76 Univ of North TX; 88–Dir, Meadowbrook Hrng & Sp Ctr, **A**

Wright, Mrs Cynthia C 2162 East Laver Street, Sandy, UT 84092, (801) 565-7498, BS 75 AZ St Univ; MS 77 AZ St Univ; Sp-Lang Path, Jordan Sch Dist, **SLP**

Wright, Cynthia J 208 Cherry Hills Drive, Aiken, SC 29801, (803) 648-2364, BS 72 FL A & M Univ; MS 73 FL St Univ; Sp-Lang Path, Aiken Co Sch Dist, **SLP**

Wright, Cynthia L 412 Pebble Way #249, Arlington, TX 76006, (214) 579-0542, BS 77 Baylor Univ; MS 78 Baylor Univ; 88–Sp-Lang Path, Irving ISD, **SLP**

Wright, Debbie A 1420 South Montebello, Olathe, KS 66062-5707, (316) 776-2142, BS 78 Wichita St Univ; MA 80 Wichita St Univ; Sp/Lang Path, Spring Hill Sch Dist #230, **SLP**

Wright, Denise 70-33 65th Street, Glendale, NY 11385, (718) 456-2970, BA 85 Marymount Coll; MS 87 CUNY - Brooklyn Coll

Wright, Mrs E Devery 8748 Twelve Oaks Lane, Montgomery, AL 36116, (205) 272-3590, BA 77 Auburn Univ - Auburn; MS 78 Univ Southern MS-Hattiesburg; Sp-Lang Path, Madison Park Hope Cen, **SLP**

Wright, Elizabeth O 13 Via Palma, Laguna Niguel, CA 92677, (714) 828-7017, BA 74 CA St Univ - Long Beach; MA 80 CA St Univ - Long Beach; 77–Sp-Lang Path, Savanna Sch Dist, **SLP**

Wright, Ferne E 11927 W Appleton Avenue 9 #2, Milwaukee, WI 53224, BS; **SLP LM**

Wright, Geri C 1111 East Lynn, Seattle, WA 98102, (206) 461-7839, BA 70 Univ of FL; MS 72 Univ of South FL; SLP, Private Practice, **SLP**

Wright, Dr H N St Univ New York Hlth Sci Ctr, Dept Of Otolaryngology, 766 Irving Avenue, Syracuse, NY 13210, (315) 473-5573, BA 50 Grinnell Coll; MA 53 IN Univ - Bloomington; PH 58 (NS) Northwestern Univ; Associate Professor, St Univ New York Hlth Sci Ctr, **SLP A F**

Wright, Hope Vandegrift P O Box 565, Rustburg, VA 24588, (606) 436-2112, MA 85 Univ of TN - Knoxville; BS 82 James Madison Univ; Sp-Lang Path, Appalachain Regional Hosp, **SLP**

Wright, Janet C 93 Lessing Road, West Orange, NJ 07052, (201) 731-1879, BA 73 George Washington Univ; MA 74 NY Univ; SLP, UCP of N Jersey, **SLP**

Wright, Joanne M 911 Notre Dame Avenue, Concord, CA 94518, (415) 685-2747, BS 77 Pacific Union Coll; MS 79 Univ of Redlands; Reg Nurse, Kaiser Walnut Creek Hosp, **SLP**

Wright, Joanne Santoro 106 Harbourview Drive, Massapequa, NY 11758, BA 75 CUNY - Brooklyn Coll; MS 78 CUNY - Brooklyn Coll; **SLP**

Wright, Joyce E 2907 Woodmere Drive, Dallas, TX 75233, BA 61 Phillips Univ; MA 70 TX Christian Univ; SLP, Fort Worth ISD, **SLP**

Wright, Mrs Joyce H 1315 Cecelia Court, San Luis Obispo, CA 93401, (805) 541-1315, BA 65 San Diego St Univ; MA 68 San Diego St Univ; Assoc Prof Speech & Commun, California Polytechnic St Univ, **SLP**

Wright, Judith A 85 Wampum Road, Narragansett, RI 02882, (401) 847-2100, BA 72 Univ of RI; MS 75 Univ of RI; Sp-Lang Path, Newport Pub Sch, **SLP**

Wright, Mrs Judy Merrilyn 910 Aura Drive, Rockford, IL 61108, (815) 966-3184, BA 67 CA St Univ - Sacramento; MS 83 Northern IL Univ - De Kalb; Sp-Lang Path, Rockford PS, **SLP**

Wright, Mrs Julia Ann P O Box 1598, Gainesville, GA 30503, (504) 536-2222, BS 82 Univ of Central AR; MS 85 AR St Univ; 87–Sp-Lang Path, Hall County Sch Dist, **SLP**

Wright, Karen A P 7318 Shadywood Drive, Austin, TX 78745, (512) 440-5300, BS 74 Univ of TX - Austin; MA 78 Univ of TX - Austin; Aud, TX Sch for the Deaf, **A**

Wright, Karen Jo 203 Hancock Street #B, Beaufort, SC 29902, (803) 522-1302, BA 80 Columbia Coll; MS 81 Univ of SC - Columbia; 88–Sp/Lang Path, Private Practice, **SLP**

Wright, Mrs Kathleen T 3860 Wisteria, Seal Beach, CA 90740, (213) 865-1257, BA 77 San Diego St Univ; MA 81 CA St Univ - Los Angeles; SLP, ABC USD, **SLP**

Wright, Kelli Harris 3722 Seton Hall Drive, Decatur, GA 30034, (404) 297-7460, BS 80 TN St Univ; MA 81 Kent St Univ; Instructional Spec, Dekalb Co Sch System, **SLP**

Wright, Dr Kenneth L 1849 South Chinowth, Visalia, CA 93277, (209) 733-9433, MA 63 CA St Univ - Fresno; PH 73 (NS); **SLP**

Wright, Dr Laura F 13900 West Burleigh Road, Brookfield, WI 53005, (414) 781-7326, BA 26 Coll of Saint Teresa; MA 47 Marquette Univ; PH 52 (Sp Path & Therapy) Univ of WI - Madison; **SLP F LM**

Wright, Lelia C 1531 Hackett Avenue, Long Beach, CA 90815, (213) 436-9931, BS 51 Northwestern Univ; MA 77 CA St Univ - Long Beach; 88–Retired, Long Beach USD, **SLP**

Wright, Linda Dunn 329 East Haven Drive, Birmingham, AL 35215, (205) 854-9715, SLP, Physicians Physical Therapy S, **SLP**

Wright, Linda Fay 315 North Marshall, Burlington, IA 52601, (319) 753-6561, OB 71 Central MO St Univ; MS 72 Central MO St Univ; Sp-Lang Path, Great River AEA #16, **SLP**

Wright, Mrs Lisa Kay 1191 Gypsy Hill Road, Lancaster, PA 17602, (717) 569-7331, BA 80 Allegheny Coll; MS 85 Univ of NC - Chapel Hill; **SLP**

Wright, Lois M 339 Allendale Place, Flint, MI 48504, (313) 767-5750, BS 51 Bowling Green St Univ; MA 71 MI St Univ; Dept Head-Educ, Mott Childrens Health Ctr, **SLP**

Wright, Mrs Loretta L 7356 Gardner Road, Ripley, OH 45167, (513) 378-6118, BA 69 Asbury Coll; MA 75 Univ of Cincinnati; SLP, Brown Cty Bd of Ed, **SLP**

Wright, Lorna L 567 Verano Avenue, Sonoma, CA 95476, (707) 938-6472, BA 71 San Francisco St Univ; MA 75 San Francisco St Univ; SLP, Sonoma St Hosp & Dev Cen, **A**

Wright, Margaret Schmid 32304 Arlington, Birmingham, MI 48009, (313) 858-3111, BA Univ of MI - Ann Arbor; MS 86 Univ of MI - Ann Arbor; **SLP**

Wright, Maria Pavnica 903 Robert Street, Ruston, LA 71270, (318) 251-0146, BS 85 Univ of IA; MS 86 FL St Univ; **SLP**

Wright, Mrs Marianna Brogan 625 Old Towne Lane, Alabaster, AL 35007-9191, (205) 226-8116, ME 84 Univ of GA; Sp-Lang Path, Lakeshore Rehab Svcs, **SLP ACE**

Wright, Mary B 6404 Locke Avenue, Fort Worth, TX 76116, (817) 626-0321, BS 76 TX Christian Univ; MS 77 Southern Methodist Univ; SLP, Fort Worth ISD, **SLP**

Wright, Mrs Mary Beth Ebling 3041 Millsboro Road, Mansfield, OH 44903, (419) 524-6882, BS 83 Purdue Univ - West Lafayette; MA 85 Purdue Univ - West Lafayette; Aud, Martin Hearing Aid Service, **A**

Wright, Mrs Mary Catherine 300 Greenwood Avenue, Apartment C-11, Clarksville, TN 37040-3787, (615) 552-8057, BS 83 Ball St Univ; MA 85 Ball St Univ; 86–Sp-Lang Path, Clarksville-Mont Co Sch Sys, **SLP**

Wright, Monica L 115 Coral Drive, Safety Harbor, FL 34695, (813) 848-5244, BA 79 Univ of MD - College Park; MS 81 FL St Univ; 82–Coord Cl Sers, All Children's Hosp, **SLP**

Wright, Nancy J P O Box 70, Guthrie, OK 73044, (405) 282-6484, BS 78 OK St Univ; MA 81 OK St Univ; Sp-Lang Path, Guthrie Scot Rite Childhood La, **SLP**

Wright, Nancy Losaplo 42 Cat Path, Gilford, NH 03246, (603) 524-8444, BS 75 Univ of NH; MS 81 Univ of NH; Sp-Lang Path, Lakes Reg Early Inter Prog, **SLP**

Wright, Pamela Mabel 3630 Thomason Avenue, El Paso, TX 79904, (915) 565-2943, BA 84 Univ of TX - El Paso; MS 85 Univ of TX - El Paso; 86–Sp-Lang Path, Life Mgmt Ctr, **SLP**

Wright, Mrs Pamela N 9413 Danese Lane S E, Huntsville, AL 35803, (205) 353-6442, BS 75 Auburn Univ - Auburn; MS 77 Univ of AL- Tuscaloosa; 78–Sp-Lang Path, Morgan Co Bd of Ed, **SLP**

Wright, Mrs Patricia Boyd 1306 Cox Avenue, R R 1306, High Point, NC 27263, BS 84 East Carolina Univ; MS 85 East Carolina Univ; **SLP**

Wright, Patricia Kay 8896 East 30 1/2 Mile Road, Cadillac, MI 49601, (616) 846-1441, BS 82 Central MI Univ; MA 83 Western MI Univ; Sp-Lang Path, Gary L Nederveld & Associates, **SLP**

Wright, Revilla 840 Highland Avenue, Piedmont, CA 94611, (415) 548-0180, BA 45 Univ of CA - Berkeley; MA 47 Harvard Univ; Dir-Speech Lang Ctr, Chldn's Hosp Med Cen-N Ca, **SLP**

Wright, Richard D Audiology Associates, 3228 Shrine Road, Brunswick, GA 31520, (912) 267-1569, BS 68 FL St Univ; MS 69 FL St Univ; Aud, Audiology Associates, **A**

Wright, Sandra M 206 North L Street, Salt Lake City, UT 84103, BS 72 Univ of ND; MA 76 Northern MI Univ; Sp-Lang Path, Holy Cross Hosp, **SLP**

Wright, Sandra R Route 3 Box 1438, Appling, GA 30802, (404) 541-0945, BA 67 Western WA Univ; MA 70 KS St Univ; ME 80 Univ of Southern CA; Director Ed/Meetings, Amer College of Hlth Care Adm, **SLP**

Wright, Sandra Sue R R 1 Box 454, Parker City, IN 47368, (317) 288-4796, BS 79 Ball St Univ; MA 83 Ball St Univ; **SLP**

Wright, Sherrilyn R R 25 Box 252, Terre Haute, IN 47802, (812) 234-1898, BS 73 IN St Univ - Terre Haute; MS 74 IN St Univ - Terre Haute; **SLP**

Wright, Mrs Susan C 325 Burd Street, Pennington, NJ 08534, (201) 782-2314, MA 76 Trenton St Coll; SLP, Flemington Raritan Bd of Ed, **SLP**

Wright, Susan Meredith 409 North Blvd, Apt #2, Richmond, VA 23220, (804) 358-3985, BS 84 James Madison Univ; MA 86 Univ of CT; 88–Aud, Balance & Ear Ctr, **A**

Wright, Sylvia P 1319 East Cozy, Springfield, MO 65804, (417) 866-7803, MA 88 Southwest MO St Univ

Wright, Mrs Varla Jane 8529 North 33rd Drive, Phoenix, AZ 85021, (602) 973-2237, BS 64 UT St Univ; MS 85 Northern AZ Univ; Sp-Lang Path, Phoenix Elementary School Dist, **SLP**

Wright, Victoria H West Kentucky Easter Seal Ctr, 2229 Mildred Street, Paducah, KY 42001, (502) 444-9687, BS 69 MS Univ for Women; MS 70 MS Univ for Women; Dir-Sp-Lang Dept, West Kentucky Easter Seal Soc, **SLP**

Wright, Virginia A Box 304, Aschaffenburg American School, APO New York, NY 09162-0005, MA 69 Univ of KS; 81–Sp-Lang Path, Dod Dependents Schools, **SLP**

Wright, Virginia Thompson Warmister General Hospital, 225 Newtown Road, Warminster, PA 18974, (215) 662-2784, BS 81 MS Univ for Women; MA 83 Univ of TN - Knoxville; Aud, Warminster General Hospital, **A**

Wright-Edwards, Clark F 10323 West Coggins Drive, Sun City, AZ 85351, (602) 933-0143, BA 60 David Lipscomb Coll; MA 63 G Peabody Coll-Vanderbilt U; Owner, Aud Hrng Serv, **A**

Wright-Gard, Wanda K 1029 South Gretchen, Chanute, KS 66720, (316) 431-3770, BS 83 Fort Hays St Univ; MS 84 Fort Hays St Univ; Proj Dir Comm Hndcpd Res Prg, Anw Special Education Coop, **SLP**

Wright-Morrison, Amelia 126 Belmont Drive, Unit #24, London, ON, Canada N6J 4W1, (519) 434-7351, BS 80 Univ of Western Ontario; OM 82 Univ of Western Ontario; Sp/Lang Path, Thames V Chldn Cen, **SLP**

Wristen, Mrs Martha A 3355 Bee Cave Road #503, Austin, TX 78746, (512) 327-2083, ME 83 Southwest TX St Univ; Sp-Lang Path, Private Practice, **SLP**

Writsel, Mrs Leila V 2401 Riverview Drive, Mount Washington, KY 40047, (502) 538-6806, BS 71 Murray St Univ; MS 72 Murray St Univ; Sp-Lang Path, Spencer Co PS, **SLP ACE**

Wrobel, Mrs Mary Jamison 7184 Glenwood Lane, Hanover Park, IL 60103, (312) 885-6776, OB 76 IL Coll; MA 80 Western IL Univ; Sp/Lang Path, Comm Consolidated Sch Dist 54, **SLP**

Wrobel, Maureen M 1361 Post Oak Road, Lexington, KY 40502, (606) 272-3496, BA 64 Univ of MI - Ann Arbor; ME 76 Univ of KY; Prog Admin, Excepticon-Lexington Campus, **SLP**

Wroblewski, Anna Clare 4912 N Diversey Blvd, Whitefish Bay, WI 53217-2044, (608) 241-9543, BS 84 Univ of WI - Milwaukee; MS 86 Univ of WI - Madison; **A**

Wroblewski, Mrs Sandra Miller 541 N Waiola, La Grange Park, IL 60525, (312) 352-7364, BA 80 Univ of IA; MA 82 Univ of IA; Sp-Lang Path, School District 181/LADSE, **SLP**

Wrona, Mrs Sandra B S 127 Dover Drive, West Seneca, NY 14224, (716) 825-1011, BS 75 SUNY - Coll at Buffalo; MS 79 SUNY - Coll at Buffalo; Sp-Lang Path, Buffalo Board of Education, **SLP**

Wronski, Karen Louise H 81 East Main Street, Apalachin, NY 13732, (607) 625-4585, BS 79 Univ of WI - River Falls; MS 81 Southern Methodist Univ; SLP, St Paul Pub Sch, **SLP**

Wrotniewski, Elizabeth Ann Winding Wood #60, 4-B Bordentown Avenue, Sayreville, NJ 08872, (201) 390-5059, BA 83 Montclair St Coll; MA 85 Univ of FL; 86–Aud, Robert Wood Johnson Rehab Inst, **A**

Wrubel, Shulamith 2942 West 5th Street #2J, Brooklyn, NY 11224, (212) 372-1464, BA 75 CUNY - Brooklyn Coll; MS 77 CUNY - Brooklyn Coll; 82–Ch Sp-Lang Path, Hebrew I for Deaf & Excep Chld, **SLP**

Wruck, Dr Kurt 11035 87th Street, Kenosha, WI 53142, (414) 656-2209, PH 73 (NS) Bowling Green St Univ; Sp-Lang Path-Superv, Kenosha Mem Hosp, **SLP**

Wu, Janice K 449 Main Street, Shoemakersville, PA 19555, (215) 562-6108, BS 80 Bloomsburg Univ of PA; MS 81 Bloomsburg Univ of PA; **A**

Wu, Jorie T Chang Gung Memorial Hospital, Craniofacial Center, 199 Tung-Hwa N Rd 12th Fl, Taipei, Taiwan 10591, (716) 837-7235, MA 84 SUNY - Center at Buffalo; 84–Sp-Lang Path, Chang Gung Memorial Hosp, **SLP**

Wuebben, Renee L 460 West Rahn Road, Dayton, OH 45429, (513) 434-4404, BA 79 Cedarville Coll; MA 87 Univ of Cincinnati; 87–Sp-Lang Path, Dayton PS, **SLP**

Wuenstel, Mrs Peggy Sue 3710 South 34th Street, Greenfield, WI 53221, (414) 383-9925, BS 80 Marquette Univ; MS 82 Marquette Univ; Sp-Lang Path, Cen for Blind & Vis Imp Child, **SLP**

Wuestman, Cathryn 3 Fairfields Lane, Huntington Station, NY 11746, (516) 924-0008, **SLP**

Wuhl, Mrs Gail K 769 Harristown Road, Glen Rock, NJ 07452, (201) 444-9393, BA 67 2256; MA 69 Columbia Univ Teachers Coll; ED 85 (NS) Bank Street Coll of Educ; Sp-Lang Path, Janet Krebs Commun Ther Center, **SLP**

Wujcik, April Doehrel 2105 S Manor Drive, Erie, PA 16505, (814) 870-6000, BS 81 Clarion Univ of PA; MA 85 Kent St Univ; 88–Chief Aud, Hamot Med Ctr, **A**

Wujek, Christine Marie 406 Hickory Ridge #1D, Glenwood, IL 60425, (312) 957-7100, BA 86 Univ of WI - Eau Claire; MS 87 Univ of WI - Eau Claire; 87–Sp-Lang Path, South Metropolitan Assoc, **SLP**

Wulf, Ellen M 159 Fields Rock Road, Southport, CT 06490, (203) 255-8388, BA 75 Univ of CT; MA 77 Univ of CT; 77–Sp-Lang Path, Fairfield Public Schools, **SLP**

Wulf, Mrs Jan Morgan 3948 Rutgers Lane, Northbrook, IL 60062, (312) 480-0988, BS 71 IN Univ - Bloomington; OM 72 IN Univ - Bloomington; 88–Sp-Lang Path, Chicago PS, **SLP**

Wulfeck, Dr Beverly B 4755 Alta Rica Drive, La Mesa, CA 92041, (619) 447-0679, BA 69 Univ of CA - Santa Barbara; MA 71 Univ of CA - Santa Barbara; PH 87 (Psychology) Univ of CA - San Diego; 88–Asst Prof, Dept of Pediatrics/Univ of CA, **SLP**

Wulff, Cynthia J 4125 Drexel Drive, Binghamton, NY 13903, MA 71 Univ of FL; MS 84 Univ of Scranton; SLP, Broome Developmental Services, **SLP**

Wulkan, Jamie B Dept Comm Dis, 113 Rrc, Florida State University, Tallahassee, FL 32306-2007, **SLP**

Wunder, Mrs Vicki Charna 1021 West 69th Terrace, Kansas City, MO 64113, (816) 373-3131, BS 77 Northwest MO St Univ; MS 83 Northwest MO St Univ; Sp-Lang Path, Blue Springs R-IV Sch Dist, **SLP**

Wunderlich-Croft, Mrs Gabriele 1231 Astra Avenue, Oshawa, ON, Canada L1K 1H3, (416) 576-6150, BA 76 Queens Univ - Ontario; OM 78 Univ of Toronto - Ontario; Sp-Lang Path, Durham Reg R Cath Sep Sch Bd, **SLP**

Wunderly, Mrs Joan Lacki 207 Elrose Drive, Pittsburgh, PA 15237, (412) 471-4700, BA 75 Univ of Pittsburgh - Pittsburgh; MS 77 Univ of Pittsburgh - Pittsburgh; MS 83 Robert Morris Coll; **SLP**

Wundrow, Larry W 943 Stephens, Missoula, MT 59801, (406) 721-7414, BS 75 Univ of WI - Stevens Point; MS 76 Univ of WI - Stevens Point; **A**

Wunrow, Jean R 1610 North Palmetto Avenue, Marshfield, WI 54449, (715) 384-4909, BA 77 Coll of Saint Teresa; MS 79 Univ of WI - Madison; Sp-Lang Path, Marshfield Pub Schs, **SLP**

Wunschel, Karen L 1901 Clinch Avenue, Knoxville, TN 37916, (615) 971-1349, BA 85 Univ of TN - Knoxville; MA 87 Univ of TN - Knoxville; 87–Sp-Lang Path, Fort Sanders Regional Med Ctr, **SLP**

Wuorio, Mrs Judith Kaplan 2822 S W Carolina, Portland, OR 97201-1094, (503) 644-0510, MA 86 Univ of Denver; 88–Sp-Lang Path, Neurocare, **SLP**

Wu-Ramley, Mrs Grace Fei Min 122 Kathi Street, Redlands, CA 92373, (714) 798-3990, BS 85 Andrews Univ; MS 87 Univ of Redlands; 87–Sp-Lang Path, Bowden & Darringer Rehab Assoc, **SLP**

Wurfel, Mrs Karen K 44159 Gingham Avenue, Lancaster, CA 93535, (805) 948-4661, BA 71 Univ of AZ; MA 72 Univ of AZ; Sp-Lang Path, Lancaster Sch Dist, **SLP**

Wurgler, Lynn Renae Box 986, Watford City, ND 58854, (701) 842-4642, BS 86 Minot St Univ; MS 87 Minot St Univ

Wurl, Mrs Charlotte Box 20431, Wickenburg, AZ 85358, (602) 684-7423, BA 42 Univ of IA; MA 47 Univ of IA; **SLP**

Wurl, Holly L General Delivery, Charlo, MT 59824, (406) 745-2971, BA 73 Univ of MT; MS 76 Univ of MT; Sp-Lang Path, Missoula Rural Area Spec Serv Coop, **SLP**

Wurl, Melinda L 535 Mary Street East #5, Whitby, ON, Canada L1N 2R2, (416) 576-8711, BS 77 ND St Univ; MA 80 Univ of Denver; Sp/Lang Path, Oshawa General Hosp, **SLP**

Wurth, Charles W 8411 Peppertree, Wichita, KS 67226, (316) 262-4206, BA 50 Wichita St Univ; Sp-Lang Path, Mid America Health Center Inc, **SLP**

Wurth, Mary R 8411 Pepper Tree, Wichita, KS 67226, (316) 262-4206, BA 50 Wichita St Univ; Sp-Lang Path, **SLP**

Wurtman, Betty Grace P O Box 446, Princeton, KY 42445, (502) 365-6753, BS 78 Murray St Univ; MS 80 Murray St Univ; Sp-Lang Path, Lyon Co Bd of Ed, **SLP**

Wurtz, Judy R 930 Mona Brook Road, Muskegon, MI 49441, (312) 754-1989, BA 78 MI St Univ; MA 79 Western MI Univ; Sp/Lang Path, Chicago Heights Sch Dist, **SLP**

Wurtzel, Mrs Terese M 1000 West Madison, Ann Arbor, MI 48103, (517) 787-2800, BS 75 Central MI Univ; MS 77 Univ of MI - Ann Arbor; **SLP**

Wuschke, Joanne Box 661, Dover, MA 02030, (617) 697-1200, BS Boston Univ; ME Boston Univ; Asst Prof, Bridgewater State Coll, **SLP**

Wuth, James F 1201 116th N E, Suite 12, Bellevue, WA 98004, (206) 455-5596, BS 76 Univ of WA; OM 78 Univ of WA; Aud, Aud Assoc Inc, **A**

Wyandt, Katherine M 532 Forrer Avenue #D, Dayton, OH 45419, (513) 854-4832, BS 86 Miami Univ - Oxford; MS 87 Miami Univ - Oxford; **SLP**

Wyant, Cathy R 347 Oak Road, Oil City, PA 16301, (814) 437-7000, ME Clarion Univ of PA; Sp-Lang Path, Franklin Regional Med Cntr, **SLP ACE**

Wyant, Shawn Lee 305 Iowa Avenue, Decorah, IA 52101, (319) 382-2870, BS 81 Univ of WY; MS 83 Univ of WY; Aud, Keystone AEA, **A**

Wyant, Mrs Teresa Jane 203 Henry Place Sunny Hills, Orion, IL 61273, (319) 359-1371, BA 82 Augustana Coll; MA 83 Univ of Northern CO; Sp-Lang Path, Mississippi Bend AEA, **SLP**

Wyatt, Mrs Carla M N 2025 Dorset Lane, Modesto, CA 95355, (209) 576-4155, BA 76 CA St Univ - Fresno; MA 78 CA St Univ - Fresno; Sp-Lang Path, Modesto City Schools, **SLP**

Wyatt, Mrs Carolyn Anderson Audiology Department, The Washington Clinic Chartered, 5401 Western Avenue NW, Washington, DC 20015, (202) 244-9270, BA 65 George Washington Univ; MA 67 Univ of MD - College Park; 75–Aud, The Washington Clinic Chartered, **A**

Wyatt, Mrs Eldean Lines 116 West North Avenue, Belton, MO 64012, (816) 331-0264, BS 59 Central MO St Univ; MS 63 Central MO St Univ; **SLP LM**

Wyatt, Mrs Elizabeth Caroll 404 Willow Drive, Piedmont, SC 29673, (803) 233-6881, BS 82 WV Univ; MS 83 WV Univ; 85–Aud, Piedmont ENT Pa, **A**

Wyatt, Gertrud L 50 Grove Street #5512, Wellesley, MA 02181, PH (NS); **SLP LM**

Wyatt, Gwendolynn 540 East Van Dorn Avenue, Holly Springs, MS 38635, (601) 252-1768, BS 69 MS Univ for Women; MA 71 Univ of FL; **SLP A**

Wyatt, Mrs Linda Chatalian 8034 Ash Valley Drive, Spring, TX 77379-3422, (713) 367-2035, BA 74 Boston Coll; MS 75 Syracuse Univ; Sp-Lang Path, Sp & L Services, **SLP**

Wyatt, Linda M 1009 North Belmont, Arlington Heights, IL 60004, (312) 577-0745, BS 76 IL St Univ - Normal; MS 77 IL St Univ - Normal; Coord Aud Serv, Lutheran Gen Hosp, **A**

Wyatt, Martha R 1947 Edinburgh Terrace, Atlanta, GA 30307, **SLP**

Wyatt, Nancy Lucile 8054 Woodsboro Avenue, Anaheim Hills, CA 92807-2508, (714) 947-6693, BS 76 CA Poly St Univ-San Luis Obi; MA 83 Whittier Coll; 83–Sp-Lang Path, Chino USD, **SLP**

Wyatt, Teresa 7032 North Donatello Place, Tucson, AZ 85741, (602) 325-3671, BS 73 Univ of NE - Lincoln; MA 75 Univ of NE - Lincoln; 88–Therapy Svcs Prog Admin, AZ Dept of Hlth Serv, **A**

Wyatt, Toya A P O Box 619, North Amherst, MA 01059, (413) 256-1046, BS 80 Northwestern Univ; MA 81 Northwestern Univ; Clin Supvr/Lecturer, U of Massachusetts, **SLP**

Wyatt-Engman, Mrs Margaret F 4420 FM 1960 West #203, Houston, TX 77068, (713) 893-9405, BA 66 Tulane Univ; MS 69 Tulane Univ; Director, Private Practice, **SLP**

Wycech, Gertrude Howell 1505 Huntington, Grosse Pointe, MI 48236, (313) 977-6800, MA 82 Wayne St Univ; Sp-Lang Path, Warren Consol Sch, **SLP**

Wyckoff, Mrs Candice G 1920 Syringa, Pocatello, ID 83201, (208) 234-0120, BS 71 Bowling Green St Univ; MS 79 ID St Univ; Sp-Lang Path, Schl Dist #25, **SLP**

Wyeno, Gary L Foote & Beck Otolaryngology, 2115 North Kansas, Hastings, NE 68901, (402) 463-2431, BA 72 Univ of Northern CO; MA 73 Univ of Northern CO; Director of Audiology, Foote & Beck Otolaryngology, **A**

Wygoda, Barbara R 335 Victory Boulevard, New Rochelle, NY 10804, BA 70 Adelphi Univ; ME 71 Northeastern Univ; 79–Sp-Lang Path, Eastchester PS, **SLP**

Wygodny, Julie Kaplan 915 Dempster #2W, Evanston, IL 60201, (314) 362-7495, BA 78 Hofstra Univ; MS 80 Washington Univ; Aud, Otologic Professional Assoc, **A**

Wyhuske, Claire M 1808 Briggs Street, Stevens Point, WI 54481, (715) 346-4520, BS 74 Univ of WI - Stevens Point; MS 75 Univ of WI - Stevens Point; Clinical Asst Prof, Univ of WI Stevens Point, **SLP**

Wykhuis, Mrs Nicole Nesselroad Route 2 Cardinal Lane, Oostburg, WI 53070, (414) 459-3886, BS 77 Northeast MO St Univ; MA 78 Northeast MO St Univ; Sp-Lang Path, Lightfoot School, **SLP**

Wykis, Mrs Joan K 3409 Richmond, Mattoon, IL 61938, (217) 235-5446, BS 75 Eastern IL Univ; MS 76 Eastern IL Univ; Sp/Lang Path, Commun Ut-Il, **SLP**

Wylde, Mrs Barbara J 48 Elmthorpe Avenue, Toronto, ON, Canada M5P 2L7, (416) 482-1389, BA 71; OM 73; 88–SLP, Private Practice, **SLP**

Wylde, Dr Margaret A 428 North Lamar Boulevard, Oxford, MS 38655, (601) 234-0158, BA 72 Northern IL Univ - De Kalb; MS 72 Univ of OK Medical Center; PH 76 (Aud) Univ of OK Medical Center; 85–Director Living Systems, Inst Technology Development, **A**

Wyler, Mrs Michele R RD 4, Pottstown, PA 19464, (215) 469-0103, BS 79 East Stroudsburg Univ of PA; MA 83 West Chester Univ of PA; Sp-Lang Path, Montgomery Co Inter Unit, **SLP**

Wylie, Mrs Mary Theresa 631 N Terrace Avenue, Mount Vernon, NY 10552, (914) 699-7150, BS 82 Marywood Coll; MS 83 Ithaca Coll; SLP, St Agnes Hosp Chldrns Unit, **SLP**

Wylonis, Norraine C 180 High Street #24, Portland, ME 04101, (207) 761-5829, BA 75; MS 76 Columbia Univ Teachers Coll; 87–Sp-Lang Path, Maine Med Ctr, **SLP**

Wyman, Mrs Beverly Ann 590 Avocado Crest Road, La Habra Heights, CA 90631, (213) 944-6178, BA 80 Univ of LA Verne; MS 82 Univ of LA Verne; SLP, Norwak-La Mirada Sch Dist, **SLP**

Wyman, Kristina Kaye 2665 Franklin #1307, Mesquite, TX 75150, (214) 286-7300, MS 78 Univ of TX - Dallas; 88–Tchr, Dallas ISD, **SLP**

Wyman, Marion Resha 4138 Nakoma Road, Madison, WI 53711, (608) 257-6713, BA 70 Univ of MI - Ann Arbor; MA 71 Western MI Univ; Sp-Lang Path, Vn-Ser, **SLP**

Wyman, Renee Marie 65 Sympatica Crescent #605, Brantford, ON, Canada N3P 1M7, (519) 756-5368, BA 85 MI St Univ; MA 86 Western MI Univ; **SLP**

Wyman, Mrs Shirley V 816 West Plains, Clovis, NM 88101, (505) 762-3781, BS 68 Eastern NM Univ; MS 69 Eastern NM Univ; 69–Sp-Lang Path, Clovis Sch, **SLP**

Wymer, Wanda J P O Box 172, Hillsboro, WV 24946, (304) 653-4221, BS 73 WV Univ; MS 77 WV Univ; 75–Sp-Lang Path, Pocahontas Co Bd of Ed, **SLP**

Wynens, Maria Szczepanski 1298 Nalley Circle, Decatur, GA 30033, BS 84 Univ of GA; MS 86 Univ of GA; 87–Aud, R L Steenerson MD, **A**

Wynn, Barbara J 2218 Liberty Road, Stow, OH 44224, (216) 297-2778, BS 81 Kent St Univ; MA 81 Kent St Univ; Sp-Lang Path, Robinson Mem Hosp, **SLP**

Wynn-Dancy, Margaret L 1501 Hadley Court, Virginia Beach, VA 23456, (703) 820-0612, BS 63 Hampton Univ; MS 64 MI St Univ; MA 78 Univ of MI - Ann Arbor; **SLP**

Wynne, Michael K University Of Montana, Department Of Communication, Sciences And Disorders, Missoula, MT 59812, (406) 243-4131, BA 76 Whitman Coll; MA 79 Univ of MT; PH 88 (Aud) Univ of WA; Asst Prof, U of Montana, **SLP A ACE**

Wynter, Cecile A 15311 Ensenada, Houston, TX 77083-5032, (713) 933-5130, BA 75 CUNY - City College; MA 77 CUNY - City College; Sp-Lang Path, Milestones Child Develpmnt Ctr, **SLP**

Wyse, Marilyn A Virginia Mason Clinic G1-Sp, 1100 9th Avenue, Seattle, WA 98111-0900, (206) 223-6618, BA 72 Univ of WA; MS 74 Univ of WA; Sp-Lang Path, Virginia Mason Clinic, **SLP ACE**

Wyse, Thomas J, Jr 1231 Laurel Hill Drive, West Homestead, PA 15120, (412) 665-4985, BS 73 Indiana Univ of PA; MA 76 Univ of Pittsburgh - Pittsburgh; SLP, Pittsburgh Pub Sch Iu 2, **SLP**

Wyskiel, Mrs Debra MacKenzie 42 Pettit Drive, Meriden, CT 06450, (203) 238-1811, BA 80 Univ of CT; MA 82 Univ of CT; **SLP**

Wysocki, Mona Judith P O Box 286, 7299 Collins Street, Whitney Point, NY 13862, (607) 692-4289, BS 82 UT St Univ; ME 85 Univ of VA - Charlottesville; Sp-Lang Path, Private Practice, **SLP**

Wysocki, Rene Noel 5448 Tilly Mill Road, Dunwoody, GA 30338, (404) 547-8603, BS 84 Auburn Univ - Auburn; MS 86 Vanderbilt Univ; **A**

Wysuph, Mrs Pamela A 3310 Monument, Round Rock, TX 78664, (515) 244-6214, BA 76 Univ of NE - Lincoln; MS 77 Univ of NE - Omaha; Sp-Lang Path, Austin ISD, **SLP**

Wytrwal, Mrs Sandra Johnson 1596 Douglas Avenue, North Providence, RI 02904, (401) 253-4000, BA 76 Univ of RI; MS 78 Univ of RI; Sp/Lang Path, Bristol Publ Schs, **SLP**

X

Xanos, Mrs Janet Lynn 600 Old Street Road #E-203, Trevose, PA 19047, (609) 893-1400, BA 74 Syracuse Univ; MS 78 Syracuse Univ; Sp-Lang Path, Pemberton Sch Dist, **SLP**

Xenakis, Andrew G 10533 Dorchester, Westchester, IL 60153, (312) 562-3971, BS 79 Eastern IL Univ; MS 80 Eastern IL Univ; MS 85 Northern IL Univ - De Kalb; Sp-Lang Path, Chicago Bd of Ed, **SLP**

Xofillis, Athanasios Ostrovou 7, Thessaloniki, Greece 54453, (303) 199-9344, MS 87 Eastern IL Univ; **SLP**

Y

Yacavone, Carol Ann 10069 East Blue Lake Drive, Mecosta, MI 49332, (616) 972-7649, BS 74 Central MI Univ; MA 83 Central MI Univ; SLP, Mecosta Independent Sch Dist, **SLP**

Yacks, Dr C Thomas 1550 Eight Mile Road, Cincinnati, OH 45255, (513) 474-2499, BS 71 Univ of Cincinnati; MA 75 Univ of Cincinnati; PH 78 (NS) Univ of Cincinnati; Dir, Anderson Hrng & Sp Serv, **A**

Yacks, Colin Paul 7527 Lawyer Road, Cincinnati, OH 45244, **SLP A**

Yacullo, Dr William S Governors State University, Div Of Communication Dis, College Of Health Prof, University Park, IL 60466, (312) 534-5000, BS 74 Elmhurst Coll; MA 76 Northwestern Univ; PH 82 (NS) Univ of IA; 84–Univ Prof, Governors State U, **A**

Yadach, Kathleen Young 1990 Ypres Boulevard, Windsor, ON, Canada N8W 1S8, (519) 977-8123, MA 18 2120; Sp-Lang Path, Windsor Western Hospital, **SLP**

Yaffe, Linda S 2506 Stone Mill Road, Baltimore, MD 21208, (301) 323-1100, BS 75 Towson St Univ; MS 76 Towson St Univ; Private Practice, **A**

Yaffee, Nadine L 19590 Clinton Road, Jackson, CA 95642, (209) 223-1341, BA 78 San Jose St Univ; MA 80 Univ of the Pacific; Sp/Lang Path, Calaveras Co Offi Ed, **SLP**

Yaffe-Oziel, Susan 6 Owens Court, Rockville, MD 20850, (202) 994-7366, BS 76 Emerson Coll; OM 78 Emory Univ; Aud, George Wash Univ, **A**

Yager, Mrs Karen M 205-02 26th Street, Bayside, NY 11360, (718) 428-7507, BA 78 Long Island U - CW Post Ctr; MA 83 Adelphi Univ

Yagerman, Mrs Laurie Cooper 74 Miles Avenue, Albertson, NY 11507, (516) 746-5145, BA 77 CUNY - Brooklyn Coll; MA 78 Hofstra Univ; Sp-Lang Path, Laurie Cooper Yagerman, **SLP**

Yaghoubian, Mrs Emily B 1207 Selkirk Lane, Indianapolis, IN 46260, (317) 927-2212, BA 71 Northwestern St Univ; MA 72 Memphis St Univ; Sp-Lang Path, Winona RehabCare, **SLP**

Yaghoubian, Mrs Karen 1548 Granville #1, Los Angeles, CA 90025, (213) 428-1232, BA 76 CA St Univ - Northridge; MA 79 CA St Univ - Northridge; Sp-Lang Path, Long Beach USD, **SLP**

Yagi-Doi, Mrs Lori Ann Misa 8215 San Pablo Way, Stockton, CA 95209, (209) 477-8054, MA 85 Univ of the Pacific; 87–SLP, Castro Valley USD, **SLP**

Yahle, Patricia A 3014 North 75th Street, Milwaukee, WI 53210, (414) 449-2422, BS 71 Marquette Univ; MS 72 Marquette Univ; Sp-Lang Path, Milwaukee Pub Schs, **SLP**

Yahne, Elizabeth Jean 125 Ripley Blvd, Alpena, MI 49707, (517) 354-8162, BA 81 Univ of MI - Ann Arbor; MA 84 Eastern MI Univ; Sp-Lang Path, Self Employed, **SLP**

Yairi, Dr Ehud University Of Illinois, Department Of Speech & Hearing Science, 901 South 6th Street, Champaign, IL 61820, (217) 244-2547, BA 65 Tel Aviv Univ - Israel; MA 68 Univ of IA; PH 70 (Sp Path/Aud) Univ of IA; 77–Prof, U of IL, **SLP F ACE**

Yakaitis, Sr Kathleen J 3908 West 65th Street, Chicago, IL 60629, (312) 735-7118, BA 78 Mundelein Coll; MA 80 IN Univ - Bloomington; Sp-Lang Path, St Bede School, **SLP**

Yakel, Elizabeth 10840 North 52nd Street, Scottsdale, AZ 85254, (602) 991-1209, BS 71 Univ of WY; MS 74 Univ of WY; Sp-Lang Path, St Josephs Hosp, **SLP**

Yakir, Leslie C 3118 Natchez Avenue, Cleveland, OH 44109-4741, **A**

Yakupzack, Mrs Edwina M 109 Windham Drive, Houma, LA 70360, (504) 851-1550, BA 61 Nicholls St Univ; MA 72 Tulane Univ; Coord Chld Srch Spec Serv, Terrebonne Parish School Board, **SLP A**

Yale, Mrs Barbara 501 North High Street, Belleville, IL 62220, (618) 235-8083, BS 73 Southern IL Univ-Edwardsvill; MS 79 Southern IL Univ-Edwardsvill; Pres/Aud, Aud Consultations Inc, **A**

Yalowitz, Jan A 4527 191st Avenue SE, Issaquah, WA 98027, (206) 455-6077, BS 76 IL St Univ - Normal; MS 79 Southern IL Univ -Carbondale; Sp-Lang Path, Bellevue Sch Dist, **SLP**

Yama, Mrs Lauri M P O Box 1714, Lihue Kauai, HI 96766, (808) 245-4383, BS 78 Univ of HI - Manoa; MS 80 Univ of HI - Manoa; SLP, St of HI Dept of Ed Sp-Hrng Pa, **SLP**

Yamamoto, Mrs Gayle Y 119 Kai Nana Place, Kula, HI 96790, (808) 877-7890, BS 78 Univ of HI - Manoa; MS 80 Univ of HI - Manoa; Sp-Lang Path, Dept of Ed, **SLP**

Yamamoto, Irene Chieko 94-101 Palai Place, Waipahu, HI 96797, (808) 689-0075, BS 81 Univ of HI - Manoa; MS 83 Univ of HI - Manoa; SLP, Dept of Ed, **SLP**

Yamamoto, Mrs Satoko Fukada 480 Lincoln Circle #5, Millbrae, CA 94030, (415) 692-2538, OB 83 Yokohama Nat'l Univ; MS 87 Univ of NC - Chapel Hill; 87–Sp-Lang Path, Hillhaven Oakridge Conv Hosp

Yamasaki, Tim 14829 East Los Robles Avenue, Hacienda Heights, CA 91745, **A**

Yamauchi, Elinor H 157 Hoaloha Street, Hilo, HI 96720, (808) 961-7538, BA 75 Western WA Univ; MA 77 Western WA Univ; SLP, State of Hawaii-Dept of Educ, **SLP**

Yamauchi, Mrs Elinor Kim 2923 Vista Creek Drive, San Jose, CA 95133, (408) 735-6122, BA 82 CA St Univ - Fresno; MA 83 Univ of the Pacific; Sp-Lang Path, Fremont Union Hsd/Sunnyvale Sd, **SLP**

Yamauchi, Lori Lei 226 North Kuakini Street, Honolulu, HI 96817, (808) 531-3511, BS 84 Univ of HI - Manoa; MS 86 Univ of HI - Manoa; 87–Sp-Lang Path, Rehab Hosp of the Pacific, **SLP**

Yamazaki, Mrs Nancy K 2949 Military Avenue, Los Angeles, CA 90064, BA 69 Univ of Southern CA; MA 71 CA St Univ - Los Angeles; **SLP**

Yanagisawa, Erin Merle 1070 East Elgin Avenue, Salt Lake City, UT 84106, (801) 484-8272, BA 80 Univ of CO - Boulder; MS 85 Univ of UT; 84–Sp-Lang Path, Jordan Sch Dist, **SLP**

Yanagisawa, Kay 25 Hickory Road, Woodbridge, CT 06525, (203) 397-1620, MS 88 Southern CT St Univ

Yancey, Mrs Connie Sue Waldrop 7515 Saybrook Trail, Jonesboro, GA 30236, (404) 478-6090, BS 78 Baylor Univ; MS 79 Baylor Univ; SLP, Private Practice, **SLP**

Yancho, Dee Ann Munson Medical Center, 6th And Madison Street, Traverse City, MI 49684, (616) 922-9455, BS 82 Western MI Univ; MA 85 Western MI Univ; Aud, Munson Med Ctr, **A**

Yanchus, Elizabeth 2834 Harford Road, Fallston, MD 21047, MS; **SLP LM**

Yanco, Elissa Berg 4 Parker Road, Winchester, MA 01890, **SLP**

Yandell, Sara J Woodlake Country Club, 196-Cove, Vass, NC 28394, (919) 295-7927, BS 63 Kent St Univ; MA 68 Case Western Reserve Univ; Sp-Lang Path, Moore Regional Hospital, **SLP**

Yanero, Diane Everly Rt 3 Box 284-F, Old Morgan Ridge Road, Fairmont, WV 26554, (304) 367-1928, BS 75 WV Univ; MS 77 WV Univ; Sp-Lang Path, Marion Co Pub Sch Syst, **SLP**

Yaney, Karen K 410 North Raynor, Apt 3 E, Joliet, IL 60435, (815) 723-5048, BS 76 Northern IL Univ - De Kalb; MS 77 IL St Univ - Normal; Sp-Lang Path, Ada S McKinley, **SLP**

Yang, Hsu-Chun 19415 28 Avenue N E #C, Seattle, WA 98155, (206) 789-7029, MA 82 Univ of MN - Minneap-St Paul

Yanick, Dr Paul P O Box 549, Hamlin, PA 18427, (215) 862-3475, PH (NS); Hearing & Tinnitus Help Assoc, **A**

Yanke, Robert B Route 1 Box 66-A, Brooker, FL 32622, (904) 376-1611, BS 71 FL St Univ; MS 72 FL St Univ; Aud, VA Med Ctr, **A**

Yanklowitz, Mrs Sandra L 15 Stone Ridge Lane, Basking Ridge, NJ 07920, (201) 647-6922, BA 71 Rutger's St Univ - Douglas Coll; MA 74 Montclair St Coll; **SLP**

Yankovich, Carol Elaine 104 Granada Drive, Edinboro, PA 16412, (814) 474-2671, BS 67 Edinboro Univ of PA; ME 69 Edinboro Univ of PA; MA 81 (NS) Edinboro Univ of PA; Sp-Lang Path, NW Tri Co Inter Unit #5, **SLP**

Yankwitt, Mrs Suzanne Eisdorfer 1231 McFadden Drive, East Northport, NY 11731, (516) 543-5100, BA 63 CUNY - Brooklyn Coll; MA 69 CUNY - Brooklyn Coll; Sp-Lnag Path, Untd Cp Assoc of Grtr Sufolk, **SLP**

Yanoti, Mrs Diana T 22 Palmer Drive, Sayville, NY 11782, (516) 567-4073, BS 82 SUNY - Coll at Buffalo; MA 85 Hofstra Univ; **SLP**

Yantis, Mrs Elna M 1434 N W 204th Place, Seattle, WA 98177, (206) 670-7212, BA 53 Univ of WA; Prog Mgr/Sp & Hrng Ser, Edmonds Sch Dist #15, **SLP**

Yantis, Dr Phillip A Dept Of Speech & Hearing Sci, University Of Washington, 4101 N E 15th Street, Seattle, WA 98195, (206) 545-7400, BA 50 Univ of WA; MA 52 Univ of MI - Ann Arbor; PH 55 (NS) Univ of MI - Ann Arbor; Prof/Assoc Chmn, U of WA, **A F H**

Yanz, Dr Jerry L St Paul Hearing Clinic Inc, 280 North Smith, Suite 701, St Paul, MN 55102, (612) 227-0824, BA 71 Stanford Univ; MA 76 Univ of IA; PH 80 (Aud) Univ of IA; 85–Dir of Aud, St Paul Hrng Clinic Inc, **A**

Yanz, Michele F 2849 38th Avenue South, Minneapolis, MN 55406, (612) 729-1525, BA 72 Stanford Univ; MA 74 Univ of IA; Sp-Lang Path, Mpls Chldns Med Cen, **SLP**

Yao, Mrs Chie Cheng 8201 River Run, Northampton, MA 01060, (413) 585-5981, BS 82 Univ of OR; MA 85 Univ of OR; 88–Sp-Lang Path, Valley Rehabilitation Inc, **SLP**

Yap, Mrs Lynn Z 637 Parkhurst, Campbell, CA 95008, (408) 378-0473, BS 73 Bradley Univ; MS 75 SUNY - Center at Albany; 88–Sp-Lang Path, Bird & Kern, **SLP**

Yarboro, Mrs Kay D Route 2, Feather Ridge Farm, Lawndale, NC 28090, (704) 482-4416, BS 74 Appalachian St Univ; MA 75 Appalachian St Univ; **SLP**

Yarbrough, Carla 304 Housatonic Avenue, Stratford, CT 06497, **SLP**

Yarbrough, Mrs Donna Lavoy 1306 Rolling Hills South, Graham, TX 76046, (817) 549-8518, BA 83 Abilene Christian Univ; MA 87 Abilene Christian Univ

Yarbrough, Elizabeth 319 Ponderosa Trail, Eastaboga, AL 36260, (205) 237-6284, BS 65 Auburn Univ - Auburn; MS 74 Univ of Montevallo; Sp-Lang Path, Private Practice, **SLP**

Yarbrough, Rebecca Wilkes 68 Tiffany Lane, Warner Robins, GA 31093, (912) 922-7042, BA 78 Auburn Univ - Auburn; OM 79 Auburn Univ - Auburn; **A**

Yarkin, Reesa G 180 Baldwin Avenue, Framingham, MA 01701, (617) 456-3371, BA 66 OH St Univ; ME 67 Boston Univ; Sp-Lang Path, Harvard Pub Schs, **SLP**

Yarnell, Mrs Mary D 91 Meadowbrook Drive, Martinsburg, WV 25401, (304) 267-3500, BS 62 Marquette Univ; MS 66 Univ of WI - Milwaukee; 84–Coord of Related Serv, Berkeley Co Pub Sch, **SLP**

Yarrow, Joseph P O Box 890, Amherst, NS, Canada B4H 4E1, (902) 423-7354, BA 82 SUNY - Center at Buffalo; MA 84 SUNY - Center at Buffalo; 84–Sp-Lang Path, Nova Scotia Hrng & Sp Clin, **SLP**

Yarzebinski, Mrs Sally G 3337 Creekside Drive, Anchorage, AK 99504, (907) 337-2618, BS 77 Bloomsburg Univ of PA; MS 78 Bloomsburg Univ of PA; Sp-Lang Path, Anchorage Sch Dist, **SLP**

Yassi, Rosa Sara 1013 West Main Street, Lansdale, PA 19446, (215) 272-1160, BS 73 Temple Univ-Tyler Sch of Art; MA 75 Temple Univ-Tyler Sch of Art; SLP, Vna/Hhs of Montgomery County, **SLP**

Yastrov, Carol L 1501 E Palmyra Avenue, Orange, CA 92666, (714) 447-7735, MS 75 Univ of IL - Urbana; Teacher of Hndcp Class, Fullerton School District, **SLP**

Yates, Albert E Dept Speech Path & Audiology, California Univ Of Pa, California, PA 15419, (412) 938-4175, BS 60 CA Univ of PA; MA 62 WV Univ; 64–Chairman Dept of SLP/Aud, CA Univ of Pa, **SLP**

Yates, Brenda Faye 204 Bethel Street, Morganton, NC 28655, (704) 433-2754, BS 82 Appalachian St Univ; MA 85 Appalachian St Univ; Sp-Lang Path, Western Carolina Cntr, **SLP**

Yates, Mrs Carrie Norris 5432 Winthrop, Indianapolis, IN 46220, (317) 259-1449, BS 81 Stephen F Austin St Univ; MS 84 Univ of TX - Dallas; **SLP**

Yates, Dorisann 20433 Balfour #4, Harper Woods, MI 48223, (313) 881-2726, BA 85 MI St Univ; MA 87 Eastern MI Univ

Yates, Dr James T 117 Polihale Place, Honolulu, HI 96825, (808) 948-8279, BA 65 TX Tech Univ; MS 66 TX Tech Univ; PH 69 (NS) Univ of Denver; Prof & Chairman SLP/Aud, Univ of Hawaii Sch of Medicine, **A F**

Yates, Mrs Joan Diane 1626 North Prospect Avenue, Apartment 2303, Milwaukee, WI 53202-2443, (207) 773-2916, SLP, Private Practice, **SLP**

Yates, Dr Joann Ruth 6208 Tobruk Court, Long Beach, CA 90803, (213) 597-4265, BA 52 Univ of IL - Urbana; MA 61 CUNY - Hunter Coll; PH 71 (NS) Univ of Southern CA; Prof Commn Dis, Calif St Univ/Long Beach, **SLP F**

Yates, Mrs Judith Ann L 228 Fairview Drive, Lower Burrell, PA 15068, (412) 845-7348, BS 75 PA St Univ - Univ Park; ME 81 Indiana Univ of PA; SLP, Arin Independent Unit 28, **SLP**

Yates, Mrs Marilyn Anne 5855 97th Circle North, Pinellas Park, FL 34666, MS 79 Univ of South FL; 79–Sp-Lang Path, Sch Bd Pinellas County, **SLP**

Yates, Mrs Patricia Kay P O Box 125, Ulster Park, NY 12487, (914) 331-4300, BS 81 Univ of MO - Columbia; MA 85 Saint Louis Univ; Sp-Lang Path, Ulster Assoc for Ret Citizens, **SLP**

Yates, Phil P Good Samaritan Hospital, P O Box 1247, 407 14th Avenue S E, Puyallup, WA 98371, (206) 848-6661, BA 67 Univ of MT; MA 72 Univ of WA; SLP, Good Samaritan Hospital, **SLP**

Yates, Rebecca R 10016 Robin Hill, Dallas, TX 75238, (214) 340-7414, BA 72 Southern Methodist Univ; MS 73 Southern Methodist Univ; PH 87 (Sp Path) Univ of OK - OK City; **SLP**

Yates-Bennett, Mrs Sharon Michelle 216 Eureka Avenue, Lodi, CA 95240, (209) 369-7411, BA 80 Humboldt St Univ; MA 82 Humboldt St Univ; SLP, Linden USD, **SLP**

Yatogo, Mrs Julie Namie 6997 Pomaikai Street, Kapaa, HI 96746, (808) 245-4383, BS 82 Univ of HI - Manoa; MS 83 Univ of HI - Manoa; Sp-Lang Path, St of Hawaii DOE Kauai Dist, **SLP**

Yatrakis, Mrs Denise H 1 Wedgewood Way, Scotch Plains, NJ 07076, (201) 561-1359, BA 71 Georgian Court Coll; MA 74 Seton Hall Univ; Sp-Lang Path, Private Practice, **SLP**

Yauch, Lisa Diane P O Box 535, Sandwich, MA 02563-7575, (617) 947-9295, MS 87 Univ of MI - Ann Arbor; **SLP**

Yeager, Mrs Deborah Janice 19 East Colmar Circle, Margate, NJ 08402, (609) 465-2721, BS 78 Stockton St Coll; MA 80 Temple Univ; Sp-Lang Path, Cape May Co Sch Spec Serv, **SLP**

Yeager, Mrs Rhoni A 4910 Stuart Drive, Orcutt, CA 93455, (805) 937-6131, BA 75 CA St Univ - Long Beach; MA 79 CA St Univ - Long Beach; SLP, Orcutt USD, **SLP**

Yeager, Mrs Sandra D 5624 Knollwood Road, Bethesda, MD 20816, (301) 320-3951, BA 71 Univ of MD - College Park; MA 72 Univ of MD - College Park; **SLP**

Yeager-Williamson, Mrs Elizabeth Annette 1628 Hunters Branch Road, Antioch, TN 37013-3859, (615) 834-9621, BA 82 Univ of TN - Knoxville; MA 83 Univ of TN - Knoxville; Marketing Rep, Cumberland A Hosp for Chldrn, **SLP**

Yeakle, Mrs Jeanne Kelly 4725 Ocean Pines, Berlin, MD 21811, (302) 641-6517, MS 85 Loyola Coll; **SLP**

Yeamans, Carolyn J PO Box 6692, Richmond, VA 23230, (804) 254-6174, BS 74 Univ of VA - Charlottesville; ME 75 Univ of VA - Charlottesville; Sp-Lang Path, Sheltering Arms Rehab Hosp, **SLP ACE**

Yeamans, Elizabeth Louise 60-6 Hopeman West Apts, Hopeman Parkway, Waynesboro, VA 22980, (703) 885-9715, BA 80 VA Polytechnic Inst St Univ; ME 85 Univ of VA - Charlottesville; **SLP**

Yeaney, Mrs Barbara Bayless 4365 Holiday Drive, Erie, PA 16506, (814) 453-7661, BS 75 PA St Univ - Univ Park; MA 83 Edinboro Univ of PA; Sp-Lang Path, Gertrude A Barber Cen, **SLP**

Yearick, Mrs Ileen H 47 Market Street, Tamaqua, PA 18252, (717) 668-1885, BA 69 Catawba Coll; MA 72 Univ of Cincinnati; SLP, Easter Seal Society, **SLP**

Yeats, Susan Elizabeth 88 Cobb Street, Springfield, MA 01119-1022, (915) 692-8104, BS 80 OK Christian Coll; MA 86 Abilene Christian Univ; **SLP**

Yeatts, Rebecca Diane 1791 East Hampton, Tucson, AZ 85719, (602) 325-4402, BS 78 Univ of UT; MS 81 Univ of UT; Sp-Lang Path, Private Practice, **SLP**

Yeckley, Mrs Rebecca King 1155 North 9th Street, Colton, CA 92324, (714) 370-2561, MS 87 Univ of Redlands; **SLP**

Yedor, Katherine 26116 Geraldine Lane, Barrington, IL 60010, (312) 578-3759, BS 81 Bradley Univ; MA 82 Northwestern Univ; Supvr Sp-Lang Path, VA Med Cen-N Chicago, **SLP**

Yee, Curtis W 4945 Morella Avenue, North Hollywood, CA 91607, (213) 625-4183, BA 70 San Francisco St Univ; MA 71 San Francisco St Univ; OM 76 CA St Univ - Los Angeles; Aud, L A USD, **A ACE**

Yee, Patricia Anne 3275 Mountain Drive, Fremont, CA 94555, (415) 791-3450, MS 85 CA St Univ - Hayward; BS 83 CA St Univ - Hayward; 87–Sp-Lang Path, Washington Hosp, **SLP**

Yelich, Ann Marie 2400 North Braeswood #212, Houston, TX 77030, (713) 791-7010, BS 76 Univ of TX - Austin; MS 78 Baylor Coll of Medicine; Aud, Baylor Coll of Med, **A**

Yellin, Jill P 835 Milford Mill Road, Baltimore, MD 21208, BS 76 Towson St Univ; MS 77 Loyola Coll; Sp-Lang Path, Baltimore County Pub Schools, **SLP**

Yellin, M Wende Univ Of Texas Southwestern Medical Center, Dept Of Otolaryngology, 5323 Harry Hines, Dallas, TX 75235, (214) 688-4757, BS 76 Univ of TX - Austin; MS 81 Univ of TX - Dallas; Faculty Associate/Audiologist, Univ of Texas Health Sci Cen, **A**

Yelton, Donna E 7460 East 48th Street South, Apartment 54-105, Tulsa, OK 74145, (918) 663-6340, Sp-Lang Path, Broken Arrow Pub Schs, **SLP**

Yelvington, Cinda K 4808 North Locust, North Little Rock, AR 72116, (501) 758-3212, BA 75 Univ of AR - Monticello; MS 78 Univ of AR - Medical Sci; Sp-Lang Path, Southwestern Institute, **SLP**

Yeni-Komshian, Dr Grace H University Of Maryland, Dept Of Hrng And Sp Sci, College Park, MD 20742, (301) 454-6910, BA 57 Am Univ of Beirut - Lebanon; MS 61 Cornell Univ; PH 65 (Psychology) McGill Univ - Quebec; 85–Professor, U of MD

Yerger, Josephine C 1602 Overbrook Drive, Box 474, Gwynedd Valley, PA 19437, (215) 699-8022, BA 48 Univ of PA; MA 53 Temple Univ; Sp-Lang Path, Private Practice, **SLP**

Yerkes, Nancy Frances 266 Wolcott Avenue, Rochester, NY 14606, (716) 271-0761, MA 84 SUNY - Coll at Geneseo; 84–Sp-Lang Path, Mary Cariola Chldn Ctr, **SLP**

Yess, Mrs Denise A 21 Ledgewood Drive, Cohasset, MA 02025, (617) 383-6115, BS 70 Marquette Univ; MS 80 Boston Univ; 80–Sp-Lang Path, Cohasset Pub Sch, **SLP**

Yett, Judith Amend 11713 Rimrock Canyon Drive, Charlotte, NC 28226, (704) 541-8939, ME 74 Univ of FL; 87–Sp-Lang Path, Mercy Hosp, **SLP**

Yetter, Mrs Carol Johnson 1773 Talawa Court, North East, Salem, OR 97303, (503) 279-8510, BS 65 Univ of OR; OM 84 Western OR St Coll; 87–Aud, Oregon Health Sciences Univ, **A ACE**

Yetter, Mary Jean 204 Dove Creek, Mc Kinney, TX 75069, (214) 480-8034, BA 80 OH St Univ; MA 82 MI St Univ; Admin of Sp-Lang Path, Comm Rehab Svcs Inc, **SLP**

Yetzer, Mrs Marjorie S 1380 Center Lane Drive, Ashland, OH 44805, (419) 289-0000, BS 67 Ashland Coll; MA 69 Kent St Univ; SLP, Ashland Co Bd of Ed, **SLP**

Yeutter, Mrs Dale T 715 Glenside Road, Millville, NJ 08332, (609) 653-8652, BA 75 Montclair St Coll; MA 76 Montclair St Coll; Sp-Lang Path, Egg Harbor Twsp Bd of Ed, **SLP**

Yevick, Mrs Susan P 1536 Blue Course Drive, State College, PA 16801, BA 78 CA St Univ - Fresno; MA 79 CA St Univ - Fresno; **SLP**

Yevin, Barbara Ann 492 Bristol Drive, Carol Stream, IL 60188, (312) 690-2563, BS 73 Eastern IL Univ; MS 78 IL St Univ - Normal; Sp/Lang Path, Suburban Sp/Lang Hrng Assn, **SLP**

Yezierski, Denise M P O Box 573, Rocky Point, NY 11778, (516) 929-3833, BS 73 Radford Univ; MS 75 Univ of NC - Chapel Hill; 87–Coord of Sp-Lang Svcs, Preschooler's Pl for Learning, **SLP**

Yiannakis, Linda Carol 780 Merrow Road, Coventry, CT 06238, (203) 742-8116, BA 75 Univ of CT; MS 82 Univ of South FL; Sp-Lang Path/Clin Coord, **SLP**

Yick, Marilyn Jean 14018 Teaneck Terrace, Gaithersburg, MD 20878, (301) 840-7136, BA 81 George Washington Univ; MA 83 George Washington Univ; 86–Sp-Lang Path, Montgomery County PS, **SLP**

Yim, Janice Lee 3059 Maigret Street, Honolulu, HI 96816, (808) 531-3511, OB 71 Univ of HI - Manoa; MS 82 Univ of HI - Manoa; 85–Sp-Lang Path, Rehab Hosp of the Pacific, **SLP**

Ying, Elizabeth 6 Campbell Street, Amityville, NY 11701, **SLP**

Yinger, Mrs Kathleen 106-2 Tangley Road, Minot Afb, Minot, ND 58704, (701) 727-9576, BA 81 Univ of Northern CO; MS 85 Syracuse Univ; **A**

Yingling, Mary Alice N 2526 Highwood Lane, Cincinnati, OH 45239, (513) 931-6252, BA 80 Marshall Univ; MA 81 Marshall Univ; **SLP**

Yingst, Kathleen E 1036 North Lupine, Lompoc, CA 93436, (805) 922-0334, BA 81 Univ of the Pacific; MA 82 Univ of the Pacific; Sp-Lang Path, Santa Barbara Co Schs, **SLP**

Yinnon, Mrs Maya c/o H Yinnon, Fibronics MTM, Industrial Park, Haifa, Israel 31905, BS 80 Emerson Coll; MS 82 Emerson Coll; 83–Sp-Lang Path, Rambam Med Ctr, **SLP**

Ylvisaker, Mark S 1171 Van Antwerp Road, Schenectady, NY 12309, (412) 521-9000, BA 67 Concordia Coll - Moorhead; OM 68 Univ of Pittsburgh - Pittsburgh; MA 77 Univ of Pittsburgh - Pittsburgh; Director Sp-Lang Path, Rehab Institute of Pittsburgh, **SLP**

Ylvisaker, Velma S 1893 Shore Drive South, Apartment 209, St Petersburg, FL 33707, MS; **LM**

Yoas, Mrs Christine Begthel 48566 Harvest Drive, Plymouth, MI 48170, (313) 572-5112, MS 83 Univ of MI - Ann Arbor; 84–Aud, McAuley Clinic Corporation, **A**

Yoch, Lynne Krings 2570 Dianne Street, North St Paul, MN 55109-5117, (612) 779-0438, BS 81 Univ of MN - Minneap-St Paul; MS 82 IN St Univ - Terre Haute; 87–Sp-Lang Path, ISD #199, **SLP**

Yochim, Jill Elizabeth 462 Chestnut Neck Road, Port Republic, NJ 08241, (609) 345-5191, BS 77 2689; MA 85 Temple Univ-Tyler Sch of Art; **SLP**

Yockey, Kenton L 8712 114th Street Court SW, Tacoma, WA 98498, (206) 967-6496, MA 68 Univ of WA; 86–Sp-Lang Path, Madigan Army Med Cen, **SLP**

Yocom, Bonnie S 2881 Waterfield, Sparks, NV 89431, (702) 356-2990, BS 82 Univ of NV - Reno; MS 85 Univ of NV - Reno; 85–Sp-Lang Path, NY Comm Svcs, **SLP**

Yoder, David E Chair Med Allied Health Prof, Medical School Wing E, CB #7120, Univ Of NC At Chapel Hill, Chapel Hill, NC 27599-7120, (919) 966-2343, BA 54 Goshen Coll; MA 55 Northwestern Univ; PH 65 (NS) Univ of KS; 86–Chmn & Prof, Univ of NC at Chapel Hill, **SLP F**

Yoder, Dr Paul Jorden Peabody Box 154, Vanderbilt University, Nashville, TN 37203, (615) 322-8150, BS 78 LA St Univ - Baton Rouge; ME 79 G Peabody Coll-Vanderbilt U; PH 85 (Special Education) Univ of NC - Chapel Hill; 87–Res Asst Prof, Vanderbilt Univ

Yoder, Suzanne Ross 108 Beechwood Road, Louisville, KY 40207, (502) 584-4870, BA 79 OH St Univ; MA 81 IN Univ - Bloomington; Aud, S Eric Bergman MD, **A**

Yokaitis-Skutnik, Judith Ann 2235 Overlook Road #301, Cleveland, OH 44106, (216) 721-3942, BS 79 Univ of Scranton; MS 81 PA St Univ - Univ Park; **SLP**

Yoklic, Carol 9480 Princeton Square Blvd, South #1513, Jacksonville, FL 32216, (904) 399-6953, BA 77 Marshall Univ; MA 78 Marshall Univ; Sp-Lang Path, Memorial Reg Rehab Ctr, **SLP**

Yonclas, Dianne Goodnough 1816 Atlantis Place, Tallahassee, FL 32303, (904) 385-5983, BA 85 FL St Univ; MA 86 FL St Univ; 87–Sp-Lang Path, Dick Howser Center for UCP, **SLP**

Yoneshige, Yvonne S 34 Walcott Street, Stow, MA 01775, (617) 523-7900, BA 78 Cornell Univ; MA 80 Northwestern Univ; **A**

Yonick, Tracey A 2916 West Crockett, Seattle, WA 98199, (201) 522-2283, BS 76 Northwestern Univ; MS 78 Univ of WI - Madison; **SLP**

Yonovitz, Dr A 12841 Jones Road, Suite 101, Houston, TX 77070, (713) 469-7811, Assoc Prof, Univ of TX

York, Eleanor H 1607 Ruhland Avenue, Manhattan Beach, CA 90266, **SLP**

York, Jane Ellen 9219 Wenonga Road, Leawood, KS 66206, (913) 621-5155, BS 72 Univ of NE - Lincoln; MS 80 Central MO St Univ; Sp-Lang Path, USD 500, **SLP**

York, Mrs Jane Marie 2045 Prentiss Drive #D-201, Downers Grove, IL 60516, (312) 422-6200, BA 84 Valparaiso Univ; MS 86 Rush Univ; 88–Sp-Lang Path, Little Company of Mary Hosp, **SLP**

York, Julie A 4009 Washington Street, Westmont, IL 60559, (312) 354-5544, BS 80 Univ of IL - Urbana; MS 81 Univ of IL - Urbana; Sp-Lang Path, La Grange School District 102, **SLP**

York, Mrs Kate G 58 Shetland Lane, Willingboro, NJ 08046, (609) 871-1636, BA 65 Hampton Univ; MS 79 Rutger's St Univ - Douglas Coll; Exec Dir / Ed Dir, Githens Cen for Phys Hndcpd, **SLP**

Yorkston, Dr Kathryn M Dept Of Rehab Medicine Rj-30, University Of Washington, Seattle, WA 98105, (206) 543-3134, BS 70 Stanford Univ; MA 72 Univ of OR; PH 75 (NS) Univ of OR; Sp-Lang Path, University of Washington, **SLP**

Yoshiba-Medeiros, Christine Michle 4105 West 183rd Street, Torrance, CA 90504, (213) 602-6920, BS 74 Univ of HI - Manoa; MS 75 Univ of KS; MA 84 Whittier Coll; **SLP**

Yoshikawa, Courtney Smith 4905 Windbrooke Court, Virginia Beach, VA 23462, (804) 468-3140, **SLP**

Yoshinaga-Itano, Dr Christine 1995 Dartmouth Avenue, Boulder, CO 80303, (303) 871-3649, BA 72 Univ of Southern CA; MA 74 Northwestern Univ; PH 83 (Aud & Hrng Impairment) Northwestern Univ; Asst Prof, Univ of CO, **A**

Yoss, Dr Kathe A 920 7th Avenue S W, Rochester, MN 55902, (507) 285-8745, OB 51 Northwestern Univ; MA 70 FL St Univ; PH 72 (NS) FL St Univ; 73–Sup Sp-Lang & Prsch Hndcp Serv, Rochester Pub Sch Dept Spec Ed, **SLP F**

Yosses, Barbara A 2005 Mount Veron, Toledo, OH 43607, (419) 241-6219, MA 78 Eastern MI Univ; 85–Exec Dir, Toledo Hrng & Sp Ctr, **SLP**

Yost, Mrs Janet C 2837 East Overlook Road, Cleveland, OH 44118, (216) 321-2268, BA 53 Wellesley Coll; MA 72 Case Western Reserve Univ; Sp/Lang Path, Voice-Sp-Lang Consult, **SLP**

Yost, Dr William A Parmly Hearing Institute, Loyola University, 6525 North Sheridan, Chicago, IL 60626, (312) 508-2710, BS 66 CO Coll; PH 70 (NS) IN Univ - Bloomington; Dir & Prof, Psychol & Otol, Loyola U

Youatt, Amy Elizabeth 11425 West Gates, Romeo, MI 48065, (313) 752-2525, BS 83 Hope Coll; OM 86 Univ of SC - Columbia; **A**

Youdovin, Mrs Susan Schaalman 520 Sandy Hook Road, Treasure Island, FL 33706, (813) 367-6010, BA 64 Univ of WI - Madison; MA 66 De Paul Univ; Sp-Lang Path, Ssy Assoc, **SLP**

Youell, Mrs Janice D 11019 South Quebec Place, Tulsa, OK 74137, MS; **SLP**

Youmans, Albert Thomas 223 South Jefferson St, Lewisburg, WV 24901, (304) 645-1260, MA 85 Western MI Univ; SLP, Greenbrier Co Schools, **SLP**

Youmans, Patricia L 30 Sweetbriar Lane, Spartanburg, SC 29301, BA 64 Univ Southern MS-Hattiesburg; MS 65 Univ Southern MS-Hattiesburg; Sp-Lang Path, Spartanburg County Sch Dist 7, **SLP**

Younce, Mrs Susan Lynn 316 Columbia Avenue, Merced, CA 95340-0913, (209) 383-5920, BS 84 Eastern IL Univ; MS 85 Eastern IL Univ; **SLP**

Young, Abram O 75 East 250 North, St George, UT 84770, **SLP**

Young, Mrs Amy Bonnell 808 High Street, Worthington, OH 43085, (614) 846-6046, BS 77 Miami Univ - Oxford; MA 78 OH St Univ; Sp-Path/Myofunctional Ther, Private Practice, **SLP**

Young, Mrs Anamaria Bravo 993 North Holliston Avenue, Pasadena, CA 91104, (818) 398-8055, BA 85 CA St Univ - Long Beach; MA 87 CA St Univ - Long Beach

Young, Mrs Angela Marie 5206 Overlook Drive NE, Albuquerque, NM 87111, (505) 292-6528, ME 83 Columbus Coll; 83–Sp-Lang Path, Albuquerque Public Schools, **SLP**

Young, Ann M 420 1/2 S Baxter, Holyoke, CO 80734, (303) 774-6152, BS 79 Univ of WI - Stevens Point; MS 83 Univ of WI - Stevens Point; 88–Sp-Lang Path, Northeast Colorado BOCES, **SLP**

Young, Anne E 32 Nutmeg Ridge, Ridgefield, CT 06877, **SLP**

Young, Mrs Barbara Allen 250 Valle Vista Avenue, Monrovia, CA 91016, (213) 337-1820, BA 84 CA St Univ - Fullerton; MA 86 CA St Univ - Fullerton; **SLP**

Young, Bonnie Thorson 1003 Old Harrods Creek Rd, Anchorage, KY 40223, (502) 588-5320, BS 75 Univ of ND; MA 76 Univ of Northern IA; Sp-Lang Path, Private Practice, **SLP**

Young, Mrs Carol M 3840 Lyndell Street, Pittsburgh, PA 15234, (412) 521-9000, BA 73 Univ of CT; MA 76 OH Univ - Athens; 78–Sp/Lang Path, The Rehab Inst of Pittsburgh, **SLP**

Young, Carolyn E 5714 Arbor Vitae Place, Madison, WI 53705, (608) 252-8219, BA 67 San Diego St Univ; MA 76 San Diego St Univ; Aud, Dean Medical Center, **A**

Young, Carolyn Virginia 710 Beaver Road, Glenview, IL 60025, (312) 413-1495, BS 63 Purdue Univ - West Lafayette; MA 67 Northwestern Univ; Aud, Il Inst for Dev Dis, **SLP A**

Young, Casey Freeman P O Box 335, Celina, TN 38551, (615) 243-3310, BS 76 Middle TN St Univ; MA 82 Univ of TN - Knoxville; Sp/Lang Path, Clay Co Bd of Ed, **SLP**

Young, Catherine Rd 1 Box 97, Shermans Dale, PA 17090, (717) 582-4093, BA 75 Univ of CO - Boulder; MA 78 Univ of Northern CO; Dr Raymond J Wiss, **A**

Young, Cynthia H P O Box 304, Troy, AL 36081, (305) 793-6510, **SLP**

Young, Mrs Debbie Marsh 3813 Pendleton, Irving, TX 75062, (817) 882-2045, BS 85 Abilene Christian Univ; MS 86 Univ of TX - Dallas; **SLP**

Young, Mrs Deborah Dennis P O Box 467, Drumright, OK 74030, (918) 352-3234, BS 83 OK St Univ; MA 85 OK St Univ; 86–Sp-Lang Path, Cushing PS/Spec Svcs, **SLP**

Young, Deborah Melton 10330 Summer Creek Drive, Alpharetta, GA 30201, (404) 998-0368, BA 77 Furman Univ; MS 80 Emory Univ; Sp-Lang Path, Fulton Co Bd of Ed, **SLP**

Young, Denise M 55459 Monroe, Rochester, MI 48063, (313) 939-2290, BA 77 MI St Univ; MA 78 MI St Univ; Sp-Lang Path, MacOmb ISD, **SLP**

Young, Dr Edna Carter P O Box 629, 601 Elmwood Avenue, Rochester, NY 14642, (814) 863-3118, BS 68 Univ of TN - Knoxville; MA 70 Univ of TN - Knoxville; PH 85 PA St Univ - Univ Park; Asst Prof of Surg/Otol, Univ Rochester Medical Center, **SLP**

Young, Elizabeth 66 Sentry Lane, Merrimack, NH 03054, (603) 622-3623, BS 71 Ithaca Coll; MS 72 Syracuse Univ; Aud, ENT Specialists of So NH, **A**

Young, Elizabeth 1419 James Avenue, Rockford, IL 61107, (815) 966-3141, BS 79 Northern IL Univ - De Kalb; MA 81 Northern IL Univ - De Kalb; SLP, Rockford Bd of Ed, **SLP**

Young, Dr Elizabeth Bell 8104 West Beach Drive N W, Washington, DC 20012, (202) 723-4541, BA 48 NC Central Univ; MA 50 NC Central Univ; PH 59 (Sp Science and Sp Path & Aud) OH St Univ; Consultant, Office of Education, **SLP A F**

Young, Elizabeth Greene 392 Massachusetts Avenue, Trenton, NJ 08629, (609) 298-2500, BA 72 Rutger's St Univ - Douglas Coll; MA 76 Trenton St Coll; Sp-Lang Path, Johnstone Trng/Res Cen Nj, **SLP**

Young, Fay Elizabeth 61 Butler Road, West Harrow, Middx HA1 4DS, London, England NW3 3HY, MA 85 CA St Univ - Hayward; 85–Lecturer, Central Sch of Speech & Drama, **SLP**

Young, Heidi J 3 Charles Street, Apartment 2, Beverly, MA 01915, (716) 662-3349, BS 80 SUNY - Coll at Geneseo; MS 81 Ithaca Coll; Teacher of the Deaf, Beverly School for the Deaf, **A**

Young, Dr In Min 3209 Patricia Circle, Norristown, PA 19401, (215) 275-3179, MS 66; MD 48 (NS); Prof of Otolarynology, Thomas Jefferson U

Young, Mrs Jacqueline S 656 La Viveza Court, Santa Fe, NM 87501, BA 60 George Washington Univ; MA 63 San Francisco St Univ; **SLP LM**

Young, Janet L 7141 Cresheim Road, Philadelphia, PA 19119, BA 74 Temple Univ; MA 76 Temple Univ; 88–SLP, Sch Dist of Phla, **SLP**

Young, Mrs Janet Sue 19 Seminole Avenue, Lake Hiawatha, NJ 07034, (201) 672-7979, BA 80 William Paterson Coll; MA 84 Montclair St Coll; 82–Sp-Lang Path, Essex Co Educ Svcs Comm

Young, Mrs Janice J North 4918 Northwood Drive, Spokane, WA 99212, (509) 928-2352, BA 73 Whitworth Coll; MS 83 Eastern WA Univ; Sp-Lang Path, Sp-Path of Spokane, **SLP**

Young, Mrs Jeanette S 977 Campbellton Road, North Augusta, SC 29841, MA 64 Univ of TN - Knoxville; 87–Sp-Lang Path, Med Coll of GA Hosp, **SLP**

Young, Jeanne Hickey 822 Grand Avenue, Rochester, NY 14609, (716) 482-3212, BS 79 Nazareth Coll of Rochester; MS 82 Syracuse Univ; Sp-Lang Path, City Sch Dist, **SLP**

Young, Judy D Route 122, Glover, VT 05839, (802) 525-3115, BA 74 Lyndon St Coll; MS 81 Univ of VT; Sp-Lang Path, Orleans SW Super, **SLP**

Young, Judy Sue P O Box 7344, Dallas, TX 75209, (214) 783-3023, BS 69 Stephen F Austin St Univ; MA 70 Stephen F Austin St Univ; **SLP**

Young, Mrs Karen L 2114 Oak Peak, San Antonio, TX 78259, BA 64 Univ of OK - Norman; MA 77 CA St Univ - Long Beach; Sp-Lang Path, Northside Indep School Dist, **SLP**

Young, Karen Lyman 308 Cedar Brook Lane, Sandusky, OH 44870, BA 64 IN Univ - Bloomington; MA 66 IN Univ - Bloomington; **SLP**

Young, Karen S 16635 Shore Line Drive, Brookfield, WI 53005, (414) 781-1154, BS 63 Eastern IL Univ; MS 66 Univ of IL - Urbana; 88–Sp-Lang Path, St Luke's Med Ctr, **SLP**

Young, Karen W Route 20 Box 1688, Lexington, NC 27292, (704) 744-5706, **SLP**

Young, Mrs Kathleen Prout Haddonfield Sp & Hrng Ctr, 130 North Haddon Avenue, Haddonfield, NJ 08033, (609) 428-5618, BS 71 Ithaca Coll; MS 72 Ithaca Coll; Dir-Aud, Haddonfield Sp&Hrng Cen, **SLP A ACE**

Young, Kathryn Benton 9872 Hidden Drive, Highland, UT 84003, (801) 565-7446, BA 77 Univ of CA - Santa Barbara; MS 80 UT St Univ; 82–Sp-Lang Path, Jordan Sch Dist, **SLP ACE**

Young, Mrs Kathy Jean 1337 Raleigh Way, Lawrenceville, GA 30243, (404) 373-7288, **SLP**

Young, Dr Lamar L, Jr Shelby Hearing Clinic, P O Box 2503, Shelby, NC 28150, (317) 871-2270, BA 64 Wake Forest Univ; ME 69 Univ of VA - Charlottesville; PH 73 (NS) Northwestern Univ; Audiologist, Shelby Hearing Clinic, **A**

Young, Mrs Laura Carroll 4561 Dartmouth Drive, Sacramento, CA 95841, (916) 489-3296, BA 82 San Francisco St Univ; MS 84 Univ of OR; 86–Sp-Lang Path, Rehab Health Services, **SLP**

Young, Lind S 3222 Caroline Drive, East Petersburg, PA 17520, (717) 291-8295, BS 74 PA St Univ - Univ Park; MS 77 Indiana Univ of PA; 80–Dir Speech Pathology, St Joseph Hosp, **SLP**

Young, Linda L 831 Delray Street, Philadelphia, PA 19116, BA 72 Allegheny Coll; MA 76 Temple Univ; Tchr, School Dist of Philadelphia, **SLP**

Young, Linda L 506 Fern Street, New Orleans, LA 70118, (504) 866-8362, BA 81 Saint Mary's Dominican Coll; OM 87 LA St Univ - N O Medical Ctr; **SLP**

Young, Lisa Gay 4018 Beechwood, Norman, OK 73072, (405) 364-8065

Young, Lisa J 4977 Clinchstone, Memphis, TN 38128, (901) 373-5438, BA 86 LA Tech Univ; MA 87 Memphis St Univ; 88–Sp-Lang Path, Communi-Care Inc

Young, Lisa Trautwein 1101 Central Towers, Creighton University, Omaha, NE 68178, (402) 296-3361, BS 82 Eastern KY Univ; MS 87 Western KY Univ; 88–Sp-Lang Path, Plattsmouth Comm Schs, **F**

Young, Lore R 6416 Friars Road #215, San Diego, CA 92108-1022, (619) 221-6868, MA 81 CA St Univ - Sacramento; Sp-Lang Path, Private Practice, **SLP**

Young, Lori Ann 1449 Chelsea Avenue, Palatine, IL 60067, (312) 991-3552, BS 81 IL St Univ - Normal; MS 83 IL St Univ - Normal; SLP, Community Unit Schl Dstr #220, **SLP**

Young, Lorie Vaughn 1730 Saddlewood Drive, Fort Mill, SC 29715, (803) 323-2244, BS 82 Winthrop Coll; MS 84 Winthrop Coll; 87–Sp-Lang Path, Winthrop Coll

Young, Lynne T 16 Van Cortland Drive, Pittsford, NY 14534, (716) 385-2858, BA 70 OH Wesleyan Univ; ME 72 Boston Univ; 85–Sp-Lang Path, West Irondequoit Sch Dist, **SLP**

Young, Mariellen 166 Wildwood Drive, Calverton, NY 11933, (516) 369-1253, BA 77 Saint John's Univ - Jamaica; MA 78 NY Univ; Sp-Lang Path, Ctrl Suffolk Hosp, **SLP**

Young, Mrs Mariette A 340 Chestnut Street, West Newton, MA 02158, (617) 964-0950, BA 68 Boston Univ; ME 70 Boston Univ; Sp-Lang Path, Judith Wisnia & Assoc, **SLP**

Young, Marilyn J 3126 West Walnut Street, Johnson City, TN 37601, (615) 246-8155, BS 75 East TN St Univ; MA 77 East TN St Univ; Aud, Private Practice, **A**

Young, Mrs Marilyn Jane 4967 Sr 29, Sidney, OH 45365, (513) 498-4565, BA 60 OH Univ - Athens; MA 85 Univ of Cincinnati; **SLP**

Young, Dr Martin A 1021 Porter Lane, Normal, IL 61761, (309) 438-8643, BA 52 Univ of IA; MA 58 Univ of IA; PH 60 (NS) Univ of IA; Dept Chair, IL St Univ, **F**

Young, Mary B HC 61 Box 73, Etna, NH 03750, (802) 295-9363, BA 54 Loma Linda Univ - Riverside; MA 67 Case Western Reserve Univ; Sp-Lang Path, Veterans Administration, **SLP**

Young, Mary B 4701 South Snoqualmie Street, Seattle, WA 98118, (206) 324-8200, BA 76 IN Univ - Bloomington; MA 81 IN Univ - Bloomington; 86–Dir Sp-Lang Path, Greenery Rehabilitation Ctr, **SLP**

Young, Mary G S W Michigan Rehab Hospital, 183 West Street, Battle Creek, MI 49017, (616) 965-3206, BA 47 Albion Coll; MA 73 Western MI Univ; Sp-Lang Path, S W Mi Rehab Hosp, **SLP**

Young, Mrs Mary Kathryn 144 Sycamore Drive, Pittsburgh, PA 15237, (412) 486-2125, BS 80 Indiana Univ of PA; MA 85 Univ of Pittsburgh - Pittsburgh; Sp-Lang Path, Pittsurgh Mt Oliver Inter Unit, **SLP**

Young, Mrs Mary Sullivan 2533 Eagle, Ponca City, OK 74601, (405) 762-6366, **SLP**

Young, Maxine L 520 North Lansdowne Avenue, Drexel Hill, PA 19026, (215) 353-4138, BS 76 Carlow Coll; MS 78 Hahneman Medical Coll; Chief Aud Sp/Lang Path, Neuro-Otology Group, **SLP A**

Young, Michele A 43-60 Douglaston Parkway Apartment 317, Douglaston, NY 11363, (718) 423-9242, BS 78 SUNY - Center at Buffalo; MS 82 Univ of WI - Madison; Sp-Lang Path, Private Practice, **SLP**

Young, Mrs Michelle 1283 Kingsmead Crescent, Oakville, ON, Canada L6H 2K5, (416) 598-6558, BA 78 MI St Univ; MA 79 MI St Univ; Aud, Private Practice, **A**

Young, Mrs Nanci Cheryll 3945 Millbrook Street, San Angelo, TX 76904, (915) 942-6767, BS 83 Southeast MO St Univ; MA 85 Southeast MO St Univ; Sp-Lang Path, San Angelo ISD, **SLP**

Young, Dr Neil M Aud Sp Path Branch Otlg Ser, U S Naval Hospital, Portsmouth, VA 23708, (804) 398-7910, BS 60 Univ of VA - Charlottesville; ME 63 Univ of VA - Charlottesville; ED 75 (NS) Univ of VA - Charlottesville; 79–Head-Aud/SLP Branch, US Naval Hosp, **A**

Young, Dr Norton Bruce 77 Greenridge Court, Lake Oswego, OR 97034, (503) 225-8356, BS 50 Univ of WA; MA 53 Univ of WA; PH 57 (NS) Purdue Univ - West Lafayette; Prof Aud-Ch Aud, Crpld Chdrns Div or Hlth Sci U, **SLP A F**

Young, Mrs Pamela Jayne 1065 South Third, Albion, NE 68620, (402) 395-6647, BA 82 Fort Hays St Univ; MS 83 Fort Hays St Univ; Sp-Lang Path, Albion PS, **SLP**

Young, Mrs Pamela MacPherson 6520 Gaslight Lane North, Mobile, AL 36695, (205) 660-0507, BS 79 Univ of Montevallo; MS 80 Univ of Montevallo; **SLP**

Young, Patricia J 2880 Andover Avenue, Carlsbad, CA 92008, (619) 434-4850, BA 76 CA St Univ - Chico; MA 81 CA St Univ - Long Beach; Director Sp-Lang Path, Speech Pathology Services, **SLP**

Young, Mrs Paula Elaine 726 Oakhill Road, Texarkana, TX 75503, (214) 832-7043, BS 79 Henderson St Univ; MS 83 East TX St Univ - Commerce; SLP, Texarkana Arkansas Pub Schools, **SLP**

Young, Mrs Revonda W 250 St Johns Street, Arden, NC 28704, (704) 684-2502, BS 81 East TN St Univ; OM 83 Western Carolina Univ; Sp-Lang Path, Private Practice, **SLP**

Young, Richard J 4025 Farm Woods Lane, Hampstead, MD 21074, (301) 833-6830, BS 76 Towson St Univ; MS 77 Towson St Univ; MA 82 Johns Hopkins Univ; Aud, Balt Co Hlth Dept, **A**

Young, Richard N Valley Ear Nose And Throat, 3316 4th Street, Lewiston, ID 83501, (208) 746-0193, BS 68 UT St Univ; MA 70 Univ of NM; Audiologist, Private Practice, **A**

Young, Risa 150 West End Avenue #20G, New York, NY 10023, (914) 285-7294, BA 85 SUNY - Center at Binghamton; MS 87 Columbia Univ Teachers Coll; Sp-Lang Path, Westchester Co Med Cntr, **SLP**

Young, Mrs Sabrina Corey 25432 Santa Barbara Street, Moreno Valley, CA 92387, (714) 788-7366, 85–Sp-Lang Path, Riverside USD, **SLP**

Young, Sandra 1005 Ralston, Corpus Christi, TX 78404, (512) 853-9977, BA 74 Univ of MO - Columbia; MA 75 Univ of MO - Columbia; Dir of Sp Therapy Serv, Ada Wilson Hosp, **SLP**

Young, Sarah Baldwin 315 S Valley Forge Road A1, Devon, PA 19333, (215) 688-0334, MA 68 Columbia Univ Teachers Coll; 88–Dir, American English

Young, Mrs Susan Lisa 95 Pierpont Place, Staten Island, NY 10314-5946, (212) 683-6978, BA 80 CUNY - Brooklyn Coll; MS 83 CUNY - Brooklyn Coll; Sp-Lang Path, New York City Board of Educ, **SLP**

Young, Mrs Susan Marie 13309 Thomasville Circle, Apartment D, Tampa, FL 33617, (813) 985-9756, BS 83 Bradley Univ; MS 85 Vanderbilt Univ; Sp-Lang Path, Univ Comm Hosp, **SLP**

Young, Mrs Susanne H 3065 Windsor Place, Boca Raton, FL 33434, (407) 997-6171, BA 70 Rutger's St Univ - Douglas Coll; ME 72 Boston Univ; Sp-Lang Path, Private Practice, **SLP**

Young, Theresa Ann Box 188 CHRB, Saipan, Mariana Islands 96950, 67 322-9256, BA 80 Univ of Western Ontario; OM 85 Univ of Western Ontario; 86–Sp-Lang Path, CNMI PS Sys, **SLP**

Young, William L, Jr 1510 Addison Street, Philadelphia, PA 19146, **SLP**

Youngblood, Mrs Brenda K 1000 Lockhart, Plano, TX 75023, (214) 517-6482, BS 77 Baylor Univ; MS 80 Univ of TX - Dallas; 80–Sp-Lang Path, Richardson ISD, **SLP**

Youngblood, Deborah S P O Box 547, Green Mountain Falls, CO 80819-0547, (405) 233-0842, BS 76 OK St Univ; MA 78 OK St Univ; Chief/Sp-Lang Path & Audiology, Private Practice, **SLP**

Youngblood, Mrs Janet P 9706 South 235th E Avenue, Broken Arrow, OK 74014, (918) 496-1833, BS 74 Univ Southern MS-Hattiesburg; MS 75 Univ Southern MS-Hattiesburg; 88–Dir Sp-Lang Path, Muskogee Regional Med Ctr, **SLP**

Youngblood, Karen W 206 Pine Forest Lane, Wake Village, TX 75501, (214) 838-4879, BA 73 Sam Houston St Univ; MA 75 Univ of AL- Tuscaloosa; Sp/Lang Path, Texarkana ISD, **SLP**

Youngblood, Mae 214 Highland Avenue, Troy, AL 36081, **SLP**

Youngdale, Paula Lynn 1304 West Medicine Lake Drive #317, Plymouth, MN 55441, (612) 829-5376, BA 83 CA St Univ - Long Beach; MS 86 Univ of WI - Oshkosh

Youngelson, Vicki M 5197 Weatherwood Trace, Marietta, GA 30067, (404) 992-5000, BS 70 Boston Univ; MS 72 Emerson Coll; Sp-Lang Path, Private Practice, **SLP**

Youngman, Julie Anne Rd #2 Box 259, Dundee, NY 14837, (716) 674-6300, MA 87 SUNY - Center at Buffalo; **SLP**

Youngman, Patricia Kay c/o Good Samaritan Hospital CCR2, 407 14th Avenue SE, Puyallup, WA 98372, (206) 841-3859, MS 84 ID St Univ; BA 80 Northwest Nazarene Coll; Prog Mgr, Good Samaritan Hospital, **SLP**

Youngsma, Mrs Debra Schutt 5838 Hilltop Drive, Middleville, MI 49333, (616) 795-9793, BA 82 Calvin Coll; MA 84 MI St Univ; Aud, Drs Burton & Henry PC, **A**

Younkin, Elizabeth Marie 221 North Portage Path #8, Akron, OH 44303, (216) 867-9367, BS 82 Univ of WI - Whitewater; MS 84 Univ of WI - Whitewater; Sp-Lang Path, Manchester PS, **SLP**

Yount, Mrs Carol L 6235 Cresthaven Drive, La Mesa, CA 92041, (619) 464-2162, BA 69 Univ of WA; MA 75 San Diego St Univ; Sp-Lang Path, Adult & Child Speech & Lang Svcs, **SLP**

Yount, Margery Cameron P O Box 472, Statesville, NC 28677, (919) 642-5168, BA 84 Univ of NC - Chapel Hill; MS 87 Univ of NC - Chapel Hill; Aud, Columbus Co School System

Yourno, Jacquelyn Mary 16 Northcrest Drive, Clifton Park, NY 12065, (518) 489-8336, BA 85 SUNY - Coll at Cortland; MA 87 Coll of Saint Rose; **SLP**

Yourtz, Susan B 38 Rock Harbor Lane, Foster City, CA 94404, BA 63 Univ of IA; MA 64 Stanford Univ; 70–Sp-Lang Path, San Mateo County Office Educ, **SLP**

Youse, Mrs Lillian A 99 Northcrest Acres, Lebanon, PA 17042, BS 46 Elizabethtown Coll; ME 57 Temple Univ-Tyler Sch of Art; **SLP LM**

Yovetich, Sally Ann 158 Tarbart Terrace, London, ON, Canada N6H 3B2, (519) 451-1990, MS; 80–Sp-Lang Path, London Bd of Educ, **SLP**

Yovetich, Dr William S 158 Tarbart Terrace, London, ON, Canada N6H 3B2, (519) 661-2001, PH 85 (Cognitive Psychology) Univ of Western Ontario; 71–Asst Prof, Univ of Western Ontario, **SLP**

Yrchik-Shoemaker, Mrs Debra A 136 Briarwood Drive, Wakefield, RI 02879, (401) 783-1502, BS 76 Emerson Coll; MA 79 Univ of CA - Santa Barbara; 86–Sp-Lang Path, Cumberland Sch Dept, **SLP**

Yudkovitz, Dr Elaine 56 7th Avenue, New York, NY 10011, (212) 989-3689, MA 63 Columbia Univ Teachers Coll; OM 81 CUNY - Hunter Coll; PH 75 (NS) Columbia Univ Teachers Coll; Private Practice, **SLP**

Yudson, Mrs Kay C 611 South 25th Street, Arlington, VA 22202, (703) 684-8799, BA 72 CUNY - Brooklyn Coll; MS 76 CUNY - Brooklyn Coll; Sp-Lang Path, Comm Enrichment Services, **SLP**

Yuen, Mrs Eileen Dee 5 Canterbury Court, Marlton, NJ 08053, (609) 985-8541, MS 85 Univ of TX - Dallas; 87–Sp-Lang Path, Voorhees Township PS, **SLP**

Yukitomo, Mrs April S 761 Kapulena Lp, Honolulu, HI 96825-1011, (808) 396-7718, BS 73 Univ of HI - Manoa; MS 75 Univ of IL - Urbana; SLP, Dept Ed St of Hi, **SLP**

Yulich, Mrs Gail M 23465 Redding Circle, Salinas, CA 93908, (408) 757-4774, BA 71 Univ of the Pacific; MA 72 Univ of the Pacific; SLP, Monterey Co Offi of Ed, **SLP**

Yuncker, Kathy Annette 2421 Broadway, Mount Vernon, IL 62864-9, (618) 835-2206, MA 85 Ball St Univ; **A**

Yunker, Rosalind J 3 Shlomo Zemach, Yafe Nof, Jerusalem, Israel 96183, **SLP**

Yurchick, Rosann M 4452 N Winchester, 1st Floor, Chicago, IL 60640, (412) 845-8807, BA 84 Duquesne Univ; MA 86 Northwestern Univ; 86–Sp-Lang Path, Comm Consolidated Sch Dist #62, **SLP**

Yust, Valerie R Natl Tech Inst For The Deaf, Rit, 1 Lomb Memorial Drive, Rochester, NY 14623, (716) 475-6474, BS 71 Coll of Saint Francis; MS 73 Gallaudet Coll; Aud, NTID, **A**

Z

Zabawski, Charlene J 508 Elmside Boulevard, Madison, WI 53704, **SLP**

Zabel, Helen E R R 2 Box 50, Delmar, IA 52037, (319) 652-5621, MA 73 Univ of WI - Eau Claire; BS 69 Univ of WI - LA Crosse; SLP, MS Bend AEA #9, **SLP**

Zabinski, Mrs Denise A 640 North 2nd Street, Apollo, PA 15613, (412) 478-3042, BS 76 Edinboro Univ of PA; ME 78 Clarion Univ of PA; Sp/Lang Path, UCP W PA Inc, **SLP**

Zaborny, Anne M 210 North Main Street, Rear #1, Wilkes-Barre, PA 18702, (717) 824-9742, BS 74 Bloomsburg Univ of PA; ME 76 Bloomsburg Univ of PA; Co-Dir, Wilkes-Barre Sp & Lang Cl Inc, **SLP**

Zabriskie, Mrs Carol J K 401 Sunnybrook Lane, West Chester, PA 19382, (215) 436-4892, BS 73 SUNY - Coll at Fredonia; MA 76 Trenton St Coll; Sp-Lang Path, Private Practice, **SLP**

Zachar, Mrs Rosalie Theresa 4521 S W 25th Terrace, Fort Lauderdale, FL 33312, BS 48 Univ of WI - Madison; MS 71 Univ of South FL; **SLP LM**

Zachariah, Anne 94-29 Lefferts Boulevard, Richmond Hill, New York, NY 11419, (212) 464-7500, MS 80; SLP, Bernard Fineson Develpmntl Ctr, **SLP**

Zachariah, Dee M 734 Grandview Avenue, Martinez, CA 94553, (415) 685-4202, BA 68 Univ of OK - Norman; MS 70 Washington Univ; Tchr of Deaf/Hoh, Mt Diablo USD, **SLP**

Zachary, Mrs Ronda Kay 965 Villa Circle, Haughton, LA 71037, (318) 746-0137, BA 79 LA Tech Univ; OM 83 LA St Univ - N O Medical Ctr; SLP, Severe Language Disordered, **SLP**

Zacher, Catherine 3677 Thacher Road, Ojai, CA 93023, (805) 646-4860, BA 71 Univ of CA - Los Angeles; MA 76 CA St Univ - Northridge; SLP, Ojai USD, **SLP**

Zachman, Linda V 2401 27th Street, Moline, IL 61265, (309) 762-5112, BA 71 Northern IL Univ - De Kalb; MA 73 Northern IL Univ - De Kalb; Ch Exec Officer, LinguiSystems Inc, **SLP**

Zachman, Dr Thomas A 608 35th Avenue, Moline, IL 61265, (309) 762-1964, BA 59 Saint Cloud St Univ; MA 62 OH St Univ; PH 68 (NS) Univ of OK - Norman; Aud, Audiology Consultants, **A**

Zackey, Julie Engstrom 521 Andrea Doria Avenue, Sierra Vista, AZ 85635, (602) 458-6822, **SLP**

Zackin, Mrs Roselyn F Stonybrook Road, Middlebury, CT 06762, (203) 758-9512, BS 56 Syracuse Univ; MA 61 Univ of CT; Sp-Lang Path, Bethany Community Sch, **SLP**

Zador, Jane Burton 1504 Den Jean Drive, Warren, OH 44483-4314, (216) 638-5060, **SLP**

Zaengle, Mrs Janice Marie 47 Martindale Court, Clifton Park, NY 12065, (518) 383-3079, BA 82 Loyola Coll; MS 84 UT St Univ; Sp-Lang Path, Cerebral Palsy Center for the Disabled, **SLP**

Zafar, Kausar Humayon 1319 Emerald Green Blvd, Houston, TX 77094-3010, (713) 493-2494, MA 86 Wichita St Univ; 88–Sp-Lang Path, The Briarwood Sch, **SLP**

Zaffke, Linda O P O Box 198, Maribel, WI 54227, (414) 432-9261, BS 75 Univ of WI - Stevens Point; MS 76 Univ of WI - Stevens Point; Audiologist, E & E Associates, **A**

Zagajeski, Ellen Louise 9 Hemlock Drive, Natick, MA 01760, (617) 651-1990, BS 69 Wagner Coll; MS 82 WV Univ; Aud, City of Waltham Public Schools, **A**

Zagar, Linda Louise P O Box 293, Barnard, VT 05031, (802) 457-1213, BA 75 Univ of Stirling - Scotland; MA 82 Univ of MD - College Park; 85–Sp-Lang Path, Windsor Central Supervisory Un, **SLP**

Zagarella, Michael J Hear-Say Communication Disorders Spec, 109 Tavern Road, Martinsburg, WV 25401, (304) 267-8220, BS 68 SUNY - Coll at Geneseo; MA 69 Syracuse Univ; Aud, Hear-Say Commun Dis Spec, **A**

Zaggy, Mary Ann 7028 Stanford Avenue, St Louis, MO 63130, (314) 362-1443, Washington University, **SLP**

Zagier, Barbara 610 Clark Street, Linden, NJ 07036, (201) 862-3004, **SLP**

Zagurski, Kim Marie 15715 Farnam Street, Omaha, NE 68118, (402) 333-3495, BS 86 Univ of NE - Omaha; MS 87 Univ of NE - Omaha; 87–Sp-Lang Path, Omaha PS, **SLP**

Zagzebski, Mrs Mary Jean 8340 Duluth Street, Golden Valley, MN 55427, (612) 545-5645, BA 84 Univ of WI - Eau Claire; MS 85 Univ of WI - Eau Claire; **SLP**

Zahareas, Mrs Maria D 1015 South Mitchell, Arlington Heights, IL 60005, BS 64 Northwestern Univ; 64–Sp-Lang Path, Chicago Bd of Ed, **SLP**

Zahn, Marsha L 2708 N W 61st Street, Oklahoma City, OK 73112, (405) 840-2023, BS 66 Univ of OK - Norman; ME 78 Central St Univ; SLP, Private Practice, **SLP**

Zahner, Julianne R 3946A Redwood, Independence, MO 64055, (816) 478-4040, MA 88 Univ of IA; 88–Aud, Timbre Hearing & Sp Ctr

Zahner, Marie L 5300 Gulf Drive #406, Holmes Beach, FL 33509, (813) 953-2090, BA 77 Univ of FL; MS 78 FL St Univ; SLP, Sarasota Co Sch Bd, **SLP**

Zaichek, Mrs Randi Kay 11162 East 196th Street, Noblesville, IN 46060, (317) 274-8868, BS 63 IN Univ - Bloomington; MA 70 0105; Sp-Lang Path, Indiana Univ Sch of Medicine, **SLP**

Zaido, Patricia Hourihan 101 Lowell Street, Reading, MA 01867, (508) 741-6290, BA 61 Marymount Coll; ME 62 Boston Univ; Prof, Salem State College, **SLP**

Zajac, David J 313 Salk Hall, University Of Pittsburgh, Pittsburgh, PA 15261, (412) 648-8996, BS 78 Univ of Pittsburgh - Pittsburgh; MA 82 Univ of Pittsburgh - Pittsburgh; 85–Sp-Lang Path, Cleft Palate-Craniofacial Ctr, **SLP ACE**

Zajac, Patricia Barone 79-21 69th Road, Middle Village, NY 11379, (718) 296-1187, BA 77 CUNY - Queens Coll; MA 79 CUNY - Queens Coll; 87–Coord Sp-Lang Path, Lexington Hrng Sp Ctr, **SLP**

Zajac, Mrs Sandra S Box 23, Hailey, ID 83333, (208) 788-4752, BS 74 Northern IL Univ - De Kalb; MA 75 Northern IL Univ - De Kalb; SLP, Blaine Co Sch Dist 61, **SLP ACE**

Zakalik, Mrs Francene Zeplain 172 Forest Drive, Hillsdale, NJ 07642, (201) 666-1865, BS 71 Univ of IA; MA 72 Univ of IA, **SLP**

Zakar, Linda M Rural Delivery 2, 102 Carrage Lane, Clarks Summit, PA 18411, (717) 587-5101, BS 71 PA St Univ - Univ Park; MS 72 PA St Univ - Univ Park; Speech and Language Associates, **SLP**

Zakim, Shelley Pevner 10 Palm Court, Edison, NJ 08820, (201) 769-4233, BS 79 Boston Univ; MS 81 Columbia Univ Teachers Coll; Sp-Lang Path, Winston Prep Sch, **SLP**

Zakon, Mrs Susan 459 Old Connecticut Path, Wayland, MA 01778, (617) 443-9971, BS 57 Boston Univ; ME 75 Boston Univ; Sp-Lang Path, Sudbury Pub Sch, **SLP ACE**

Zaksek, Mrs Lorraine 48972 Woodway Drive, Plymouth, MI 48170, (313) 459-7030, BA 71 FL St Univ; MS 72 FL St Univ; SLP, Oakwood Hosp Canton Cen, **SLP**

Zalenski, Mrs Jane Reck 800 Allegheny River Blvd, 2nd Floor, Oakmont, PA 15139, (412) 856-9250, MS 83 Syracuse Univ; Case Coordinator, Transact Health Systems, **SLP**

Zaleski, Susan Marie 1912 Green Mountain Drive, Apartment 344A, Little Rock, AR 72212, (501) 374-3361, BS 83 Univ of Central AR; MS 85 Univ of Central AR; 87–Sp-Lang Path, Little Rock PS, **SLP**

Zalewski, Karen S 3854 Fort Street #18, Trenton, MI 48183, (313) 285-2047, BA 83 Western MI Univ; MA 84 Western MI Univ; SLP, Coummunity School District, **SLP**

Zallinger, Martha 38 Kilsyth Road, Brookline, MA 02146, (617) 734-9669, BS 68 Univ of MI - Ann Arbor; MS 77 Boston Univ; Sp-Lang Path, Waltham Public Schools, **SLP**

Zamadics, Cathy Louise 675 Woodale #147, Baton Rouge, LA 70806, (504) 924-5419, BS 84 Central St Univ; MA 86 LA St Univ - Baton Rouge; 88–Aud, Baton Rouge Sp and Hrng Found, **A**

Zambas, Chris S 2 Estate Drive, Hampton, VA 23666, (804) 380-3692, BA 70 Hampton Univ; MS 71 PA St Univ - Univ Park; Manager of Aud, Newport News Shipbuilding, **A**

Zamboldi, Mary D 850 Woodcrest Turn, Dover, DE 19901, (302) 734-4125, BS 81 Clarion Univ of PA; MS 82 Clarion Univ of PA; Sp-Lang Path, Kent-Sussex Presch Diag Center, **SLP**

Zambotti, Cynthia Lynn 308 Jacob Street, Kittanning, PA 16201, (412) 545-6209, MS 84 Indiana Univ of PA; 84–Sp-Lang Path, Moniteau Sch Dist, **SLP**

Zambuto, Mrs Julie Ellis 1898 Jackson Avenue, Seaford, NY 11783, (212) 860-4102, BA 79 SUNY - Coll at Oneonta; MA 82 CUNY - Hunter Coll; Sp-Lang Path, Private Practice, **SLP**

Zaminer, Marie M 159 Tiernan Avenue, Warwick, RI 02886, (401) 732-2632, BS 78 Auburn Univ - Auburn; MS 79 Auburn Univ - Auburn; 88–Sp-Lang Path, Woonsocket Dept of Educ, **A**

Zamora, Mrs Barbara L 513 Parkshore Drive, Shorewood, IL 60435, (815) 725-0053, MS 81 Northern IL Univ - De Kalb; 86–Sp-Lang Path, Private Practice, **SLP**

Zamora, Lourdez Dianna 4675 Oakwood #407, Odessa, TX 79761, (915) 332-8244, BA 84 Grand Canyon Coll; MA 86 Grand Canyon Coll

Zamore, Mrs Ellen R 7 Laurel Street, Garden City, NY 11530, (516) 742-2953, BA 59 Skidmore Coll; MA 61 Columbia Univ Teachers Coll; 75–Adj Assoc Prof of Commun, Nassau Commun Coll, **SLP**

Zampini, Mrs Nancy Diane 5610 West Redfield Road, Glendale, AZ 85306, (602) 866-5140, BS 84 Northern AZ Univ; MS 85 Northern AZ Univ; 86–Sp-Lang Path, Washington Sch Dist, **SLP**

Zamzow, Fran G 536 Windrift Drive, Belleville, IL 62221, (618) 233-9034, BS 79 Phillips Univ; MS 81 Phillips Univ; **SLP**

Zand, Dr Charlene Rooth 2098 Yorktown Drive, Ann Arbor, MI 48105, (313) 769-6410, BS 51 Northwestern Univ; MA 56 CUNY - City College; PH 82 (NS) Univ of MI - Ann Arbor; Consult SLP, Private Practice, **SLP**

Zander, Mrs Janet Sue 643 Illinois Road, Wilmette, IL 60091, (312) 998-5045, BA 64 Central MI Univ; OM 82 Governors St Univ; Sp-Lang Path, Glenview Sch Dist 34, **SLP**

Zane, Ellen Marcia 70 Lazell Street, Hingham, MA 02043, (617) 770-3082, BA 73 George Washington Univ; MA 75 Catholic Univ of America; 87–Assoc Dir, Quincy City Hosp, **SLP**

Zane, Jonna D 5944 Kalanianaole Highway, Honolulu, HI 96821, (808) 948-8279, BS 72; MS 74 Univ of HI - Manoa; **SLP**

Zane, Kim O'Hay 630 Concord Circle, Ewing, NJ 08618, (609) 466-0400, BS 78 Trenton St Coll; MA 82 Trenton St Coll; Sp-Lang Path, No Princeton Dev Ctr, **SLP**

Zanello, Mrs Costandina A 16 Violet Avenue, Mineola, NY 11501, (516) 560-5656, BA 77 SUNY - Coll at Cortland; MA 78 NY Univ; Cl Superv Instr, Hofstra U, **SLP**

Zaner, Dr Annette R 75 Bank Street, New York, NY 10014, (201) 596-3966, BA 49 CUNY - Queens Coll; MA 50 Univ of WI - Madison; PH 74 (Educational Psychology) NY Univ; 73–Dir Commun Dis, Mt Carmel Guild, **SLP A F**

Zanfordino, Joseph Peter 185 Oak Street #F, Binghamton, NY 13905, (607) 272-8990, BA 73 CUNY - Lehman Coll; MA 79 SUNY - Coll at Geneseo; 88–Sp-Lang Path, Spec Children's Ctr, **SLP**

Zangari, Carole P O Box 253, 504 Jewett Street, Battle Ground, IN 47920, (317) 494-7330, BA Univ of Pittsburgh - Pittsburgh; ME Trenton St Coll; Research Fellow, Prudue Univ, **SLP**

Zangel, Mrs Barbara B 1014 Mira Vista Drive, Huntsville, AL 35802, (205) 881-8289, BS 68 Univ Southern MS-Hattiesburg; MS 69 Univ Southern MS-Hattiesburg; Aud, State Crippled Children's Svc, **A**

Zangrando, Mary Zoe 15516 Sunset Boulevard, Pac Palisades, CA 90272, (213) 483-9930, BA 83 Loyola Marymount Univ; MA 86 CA St Univ - Northridge; **A**

Zangrilli, Donna M 711 Stevens Street, Utica, NY 13502, (315) 896-2654, BS 76 SUNY - Coll at Fredonia; ME 79 Univ of VA - Charlottesville; Sp-Lang Path, UCP of Greater Utica Area, **SLP**

Zangwill, Estelle R 109 Oak Park Place, Pittsburgh, PA 15243, (412) 531-0126, BS 50 Univ of Pittsburgh - Pittsburgh; MS 63 Univ of Pittsburgh - Pittsburgh; **SLP**

Zante, Mrs Sylvia M 626 Marigold Court, Fremont, CA 94538, (415) 657-2350, **SLP**

Zapala, David A 2822 Stoneway Lane #608, Memphis, TN 38128, (901) 525-2682, BA 80 CA St Univ - Fullerton; MS 83 UT St Univ; Aud, Memphis Sp & Hrng Ctr, **A**

Zapp, Mrs Marlene U 1001 Hilton Street, Aiken, SC 29801, (803) 648-0618, BA 72 CUNY - Queens Coll; MS 73 Univ of IL - Urbana; Sp-Lang Path, Private Practice, **SLP**

Zara, Carol V 17-49 166th Street, Whitestone, NY 11357, BA 85 Marymount Coll; MA 86 Northwestern Univ; 87–Sp-Lang Path, NY League for the Hard of Hrng, **SLP**

Zarajczyk, Mrs Deborah R 1515 Carmen Avenue, Holly Hill, FL 32017, (904) 255-4568, BA 73 SUNY - Coll at Brockport; MA 79 Univ of FL; Dir SLP & Aud, Er SI So/Volusia & Flagler Co, **A ACE**

Zarate, Nora Route 2 Box 9, Bellevue, TX 76228, (817) 928-2454, BS 77 Univ of North TX; MS 80 TX Christian Univ; 84–Sp-Lang Path, Sp Path Svcs of N TX, **SLP**

Zaremba, Mrs Diana T 57 Soundview Avenue, Oyster Bay, NY 11771, BA 80 OH Wesleyan Univ; MS 81 Miami Univ - Oxford; Sp-Lang Path, Maryhaven Therapeutic Presch, **SLP**

Zaremba, Mrs Natalie B 11 Linder Terrace, Newton, MA 02158, (617) 757-2756, BA 66 Colby Coll; ME 70 Boston Univ; 83–Sp-Lang Path, MA Er SI So, **SLP**

Zaretsky, Mrs Marcia P 5 Douglas Drive, Hillsdale, NJ 07642, BA 77 Hofstra Univ; MA 79 Hofstra Univ; **SLP**

Zarich, Mrs Karen L 951 Timber Trace, Brownsburg, IN 46112, (317) 852-2305, BS 73 IN Univ - Bloomington; MA 75 IN Univ - Bloomington; **SLP**

Zarider, Mrs Shirley Fox 5805 Windknoll Court, Cincinnati, OH 45243, (531) 561-6020, MS 84 Univ of Cincinnati; Sp-Lang Path, Indian Hill Schs, **SLP**

Zarnoch, Janet M St Francis Hospital, 25 McWilliams Place, Jersey City, NJ 07302, (201) 795-7156, MA 76 Univ of Denver; 83–Sp-Lang Path, St Francis Hosp, **A**

Zarth, Virginia Bonde 7601 Knox Avenue South, Apartment 308, Richfield, MN 55423, (612) 789-8575, BA 77 Augsburg Coll; MS 84 Saint Cloud St Univ; SLP, New York City Board of Educ, **SLP**

Zarwell, Lillian H 403 Fillmore Street, Clarksville, AR 72830, (501) 754-6614, BA 34 Univ of AR - Fayetteville; MA 59 Univ of AR - Fayetteville; **SLP LM**

Zaslow, Elinor L 10802 Lockridge Drive, Silver Spring, MD 20901, (301) 593-1821, BA 45 Univ of MN - Minneap-St Paul; **SLP**

Zastrow, Sharon Jean 3522 Walnut Street, Apartment C, Port Huron, MI 48060, (313) 982-0166, BA 84 MI St Univ; MA 85 MI St Univ; **A**

Zatwarnicki, Leslie 25 Poplar Avenue, Stony Brook, NY 11790, (516) 724-3626, **SLP**

Zatz, Anita F 2166 N W 37th Avenue, Coconut Creek, FL 33066, (305) 971-8827, BS 65 Syracuse Univ; MA 68 SUNY - Center at Buffalo; 82–Sp-Lang Path, N Broward Med Cen, **SLP**

Zaval, Janet K 150 Standish Road, Needham, MA 02192, (617) 782-3426, BA 75 Univ of MA - Amherst; MS 77 Syracuse Univ; Dir/Sp-Lang Path, Sp-Lang Therapy Serv, **SLP**

Zavala, Anna Bellott 3640 S Sepulveda #2-329, Los Angeles, CA 90034, (213) 836-3794, MA 86 CA St Univ - Los Angeles; **SLP**

Zavalkoff, Mrs Barbara H 5766 Westluke, Cote St Luc, PQ, Canada H4W 2N7, (514) 937-8411, BS 72 McGill Univ - Quebec; MS 74 McGill Univ - Quebec; Aud, Montreal Childrens Hospital, **A**

Zavalydriga, Mrs Susan Faler 2038 Lovers Lane, Shreveport, LA 71105, (318) 222-5317, BA 78 LA Tech Univ; MA 79 LA Tech Univ; 83–Sp-Lang Path, Caddo Parish Sch Bd, **SLP**

Zaversnik, Mrs Phyllis Robinson 9040 Cherry Creek Drive South #D, Denver, CO 80231, BA 62 Univ of Denver; MA 64 Univ of Denver; **SLP**

Zawacki, Mrs Julie D 1010 Marvin Street, Milan, MI 48160, (313) 994-8111, BS 76 Eastern MI Univ; MA 77 Eastern MI Univ; Sp-Lang Path, High Pt Washtenaw Ctr ISD, **SLP**

Zawadzki, Louise I 54 Burnside Avenue, Jeffersonville, PA 19403, (215) 277-0660, BS 74 Western IL Univ; MA 76 Univ of IA; **SLP**

Zazula, Mrs Elise Hoch 144-05 70th Road, Kew Gardens, NY 11367, (212) 261-0452, BA 63 CUNY - Hunter Coll; MA 67 CUNY - Hunter Coll; Sp-Lang Path, Private Practice, **SLP**

Zbieg, Mrs Mary Elizabeth 910 Treasure Lake, Du Bois, PA 15801, (814) 375-9100, BS 82 Edinboro Univ of PA; MA 83 Edinboro Univ of PA; Sp-Lang Path, InSpeech Inc, **SLP**

Zdenek, Mrs Constance 752 Harrell Street, Rock Hill, SC 29730, (803) 548-4677, BA 72 Winthrop Coll; MS 73 Winthrop Coll; Sp-Lang Path, Fort Mill School District 4, **SLP**

Zeagler, Mrs Clare Wells 7407 Whistlestop Drive, Austin, TX 78749, (512) 288-4191, BS 75 TX Tech Univ; MS 85 Univ of North TX; Sp-Lang Path, Private Practice, **SLP**

Zeaser, MaryLee 12148 Sadler Lane, Bowie, MD 20715, (301) 262-4594, MS 88 Loyola Coll; 88–Sp-Lang Path, Prince Georges Co PS

Zebro, Mrs Susan M M 169 Halston Parkway, East Amherst, NY 14051, (716) 688-5931, BA 72 SUNY - Coll at Plattsburgh; MS 76 SUNY - Coll at Buffalo; **SLP**

Zebrowski, Dr Patricia Finnerty 157 Glenn Drive, Iowa City, IA 52245, (319) 335-8735, BS 77 SUNY - Coll at Geneseo; MS 81 Syracuse Univ; PH 87 (Sp Path) Syracuse Univ; 88–Asst Prof, Univ of IA, **SLP**

Zech, Mrs Karen Pappas 34259 Macdonald, Sterling Heights, MI 48077, (313) 939-2290, BA 79 MI St Univ; MA 80 Central MI Univ; Sp-Lang Path, MacOmb ISD, **SLP**

Zeches, Jane Teresa 809 Nob Hill North #D, Seattle, WA 98109, (206) 632-0174, MS 84 ID St Univ; SLP, **SLP**

Zedler, Dr Empress Box 465, Luling, TX 78648, (512) 875-2259, BA 28 Univ of TX - Austin; MA 48 Univ of TX - Austin; PH 51 (NS) Univ of TX - Austin; Consult Psychol Sp-Lang Path, Private Practice, **SLP F LM**

Zeese, Mrs Dina Smith 890 North Lexington Street, Arlington, VA 22205, (301) 567-4877, BS 76 SUNY - Coll at Buffalo; MS 77 SUNY - Coll at Buffalo; Sp-Lang Path, Prince Georges County Bd of Ed, **SLP**

Zefo, Anna Marie 1921 Humboldt Avenue, Davis, CA 95616, (707) 422-3200, BA 83 CA St Univ - Sacramento; MA 84 Univ of the Pacific; Sp-Lang Path, Fairfield Suisun USD, **SLP**

Zegar, Marcia A 7712 Derksen Hill Road S E, Salem, OR 97301, (503) 399-3104, BS 76 Ball St Univ; MA 79 Univ of IL - Urbana; Prog Ass Sp/Lang Path, Salem Pub Sch, **SLP**

Zegarski-Isley, Elizabeth 1400 3rd Street, Manhattan Beach, CA 90266, (213) 625-6000, BA 79 San Diego St Univ; MA 85 CA St Univ - Los Angeles; **SLP**

Zegen, Mrs Joyce P O Box 6072, Incline Village, NV 89450, (702) 831-4395, BS 71 Northwestern Univ; MA 72 Northwestern Univ; **SLP**

Zehel, Dr Zoe Audiology & Speech Path Serv, Wilkes-Barre VA Med Center, 1111 East End Boulevard, Wilkes-Barre, PA 18711, (717) 824-3521, OB 64 CA Univ of PA; MS 67 WV Univ; PH 74 (NS) Univ of MD - College Park; Sp-Lang Path, Wilkes-Barre VA Med Cen, **SLP**

Zehm, Lucia Adrignola 1922 Donahue Drive, El Cajon, CA 92019, (619) 296-8344, BA 79; MS 81; Sp-Lang Path, **SLP**

Zehnder, Mrs Barbara Pajak 154 Cassia Drive, Clairton, PA 15025, (412) 653-7046, MA 83 Univ of Pittsburgh - Pittsburgh

Zehner, Cynthia Louise Rd #1 Box 159-A, New Ringgold, PA 17960, (717) 386-4073, BS 85 Bloomsburg Univ of PA; MS 86 Bloomsburg Univ of PA

Zehrer, Mary Battaglia 8 East Riverside, Melrose, MN 56352, (612) 256-4224, OB 80 Univ of MN - Duluth; MA 81 Univ of MN - Duluth; SLP, ISD #740 Melrose MN, **SLP**

Zehrt, Pamela Bartz R R 1 Box 226Z, Solon, IA 52333, (319) 337-6879, BS 81 Univ of WI - Stevens Point; MS 83 Univ of WI - Madison; Aud, Otologic Med Serv, **A**

Zeidner, Mrs Joan D 2034 Arch Street #P, Walden Walk, Philadelphia, PA 19103, (215) 952-8620, BA 50 Rutger's St Univ - Douglas Coll; MA 74 Temple Univ; Sp-Lang Path, Sch Dist of Phil Pa, **SLP**

Zeigler, Dana Joy 1737 Belle, Topeka, KS 66604, (913) 272-4060, SLP, Capper Fndt, **SLP**

Zeigler, James Alan ENT Surgical Group, Medical Arts Bldg, 35 W Linden Street Ste 320, Wilkes-Barre, PA 18702, (717) 826-6892, BS 81 Indiana Univ of PA; MS 84 PA St Univ - Univ Park; Aud, ENT Surgical Gp, **A**

Zeigler, John Trawick Lake County Hearing Clinic, Corner New Highway 441, Route 19, Tavares, FL 32778, (904) 343-4488, MA 73 Bowling Green St Univ; 78–Dir/Aud/Owner, Lake County Hrng & Sp Clinic, **A**

Zeigler, Laura B 949 Churchill Lane, Newport News, VA 23602, (804) 877-0278, BS 79 Radford Univ; MS 83 Radford Univ; Sp-Lang Path, Hampton City Schools, **SLP**

Zeigler-Waddell, Nancy E 11917 Indian Trail, Hales Corners, WI 53130, (414) 425-4807, BS 83 Univ of WI - Madison; MS 85 Marquette Univ; **SLP**

Zeihen, Mrs Connie Zaqzebski 904 Brown Street, Wausau, WI 54401, (715) 845-7150, **SLP**

Zeine, Dr Lina Western Washington University, Speech Path & Audiology, Parks Hall, Bellingham, WA 98225, (206) 676-3881, BA 69; MA 72 Univ of CO - Boulder; PH 84 (NS) Univ of KS; Assistant Professor, Western WA U, **SLP**

Zeisler, Carolyn 1278 Pacific Beach Drive, #7, San Diego, CA 92109, (619) 745-7000, BA 79 Stanford Univ; MA 86 San Diego St Univ; 85–Tchr, Escondido Union Sch Dist

Zeisloft-Falbey, Barbara C 1280 Ulupalakua, Kailua, HI 96734, (808) 842-8383, BS 69 MI St Univ; MS 71 Purdue Univ - West Lafayette; 86–Sp-Lang Path, Kamehameha Elem Sch, **SLP**

Zeit, Mrs Janice J 8312 S Tuckaway Shores Dr, Franklin, WI 53132, (414) 425-6040, BS 57 Univ of WI - Milwaukee; MS 76 Univ of WI - Whitewater; 88–Sp-Lang Path, Oak Creek-Franklin Sch Dist #1, **SLP**

Zeitler, Mrs Jill Richey 18W090 14th Street, Villa Park, IL 60181, (312) 916-0894, BS 79 Univ of IL - Urbana; MA 81 Northern IL Univ - De Kalb; Sp-Lang Path, Arl Heights Pub Sch Dist 25, **SLP**

Zeitlin, Debra J Box 497, Piermont, NY 10968, (914) 365-0372, BA 77 SUNY - Center at Buffalo; MA 79 NY Univ; Sp/Lang Path, Helen Hayes Hosp, **SLP**

Zeitlin, Rosalyn R c/o L Parker, 300 North State #4727, Chicago, IL 60610, MS; **LM**

Zeitlin, Mrs Virginia Riordan 1237 Ostrander Avenue, La Grange, IL 60525, (312) 579-3330, BS 81 Western IL Univ; MA 82 Western IL Univ; Sp-Lang Path, Cicero Sch Dist 99, **SLP ACE**

Zeitoun, Lisa Horowitz 246 Bronxville Road, Bronxville, NY 10708, (212) 519-4836, BA 78 CUNY - Lehman Coll; MS 80 Columbia Univ Teachers Coll; 84–Aud, Montefiore Hosp Affiliation, **A**

Zelasko, Mrs Mary C 2731 North Dayton, Chicago, IL 60614, (312) 883-9601, BA 76 Loyola Univ of Chicago; MS 80 Governors St Univ; Sp-Lang Path, Southern Schools, **SLP**

Zeldner, Michele J 454 Center Street, Collingswood, NJ 08108, (609) 858-0813, BS 73 Kent St Univ; MA 74 Case Western Reserve Univ; Sp-Lang Path, Haddon Township Bd of Educ, **SLP**

Zeleznik, Linda M Rd 1 Box 60-A, Salt Point, NY 12578, (914) 452-8000, BA 72 Coll of Saint Rose; MA 74 Coll of Saint Rose; Sp-Lang Path, Hudson River Psychi Cen, **SLP**

Zelgart-Evans, Jane K 4387 Wilson, Rolling Meadows, IL 60008, **SLP**

Zelinsky, Pamela S Rd 2 Box 568, Barto, PA 19504, (215) 631-9300, BS 80 Bloomsburg Univ of PA; MS 81 Bloomsburg Univ of PA; Mgr-Training & Continuing Educ, InSpeech Inc, **SLP ACE**

Zell, Abby B Box 95, Terre Hill, PA 17581, (717) 393-0425, BS 81 Univ of VA - Charlottesville; MS 83 PA St Univ - Univ Park; Sp-Lang Path, Lancaster Co Er SI Rehab Cen, **SLP**

Zeller, Mrs Carolyn S 36 Stilt Street, New Orleans, LA 70124, (504) 282-2464, BS 69 LA St Univ - Baton Rouge; OM 75 LA St Univ - N O Medical Ctr; 71–Sp-Lang Path, Jefferson Parish Sch Bd, **SLP**

Zeller, Dr Robin K 2 Meadowood Drive, Jericho, NY 11753, (516) 433-2373, BA 75 CUNY - Queens Coll; MA 77 CUNY - Queens Coll; PH 87 (Sp & Hrng Sciences Aud) CUNY - Grad Sch & Univ Cntr; 88–Asst Prof of Aud, Marymount Manhattan Coll, **A**

Zellhoefer, Paul 325 Winnebago Drive, Lake Winnebago, MO 64034, MS 78 Univ of NE - Omaha; Sp-Lang Path, Rainbow Mental Health Unit, **SLP**

Zellhoefer, Robin L T 325 Winnebago Drive, Lake Winnebago, MO 64034, (816) 942-7695, BS 76 Northwest MO St Univ; MS 78 Univ of NE - Omaha; **SLP**

Zellhofer, Carol M 10303-J Malcolm Circle, Cockeysville, MD 21030, (301) 772-0990, BS 79 Towson St Univ; MA 81 OH Univ - Athens; Sp-Lang Path, Prince George's Co Health Dept, **SLP**

Zellmer, Mary K Route 2 Box 235-D, Falls Creek, WI 54742, (715) 286-2236, BS 80 Univ of WI - Stevens Point; MS 81 Univ of WI - River Falls; Sp-Lang Path, Augusta Sch Dist, **SLP**

Zelman, Betty M 170 Avenida Majorca, Laguna Hills, CA 92653-4148, (714) 859-1304, BA 59 Univ of Redlands; MS 64 Loma Linda Univ - Loma Linda; **SLP LM**

Zelman, Dr Elizabeth 7222 Dartmouth, University City, MO 63130, (314) 679-7732, MA 66 Univ of MO - Columbia; MS 82 Southern IL Univ-Edwardsvill; PH 74 (NS) Univ of MI - Ann Arbor; Sp-Lang Path, Spec Sch Dist-St Louis Co, **SLP**

Zelski, Robert F K Atlanta Hearing Aid Service, 533 Peachtree Street N E, Atlanta, GA 30308, (404) 874-2893, BS 67 Univ of PA; OM 73 Emory Univ; Vp/Gen Mgr, Hearing Services Div, **A ACE**

Zeltmann, Mrs Frances Kay 1208 South Pecos, Brownfield, TX 79316, (806) 637-4282, BA 83 TX Tech Univ; MA 84 TX Woman's Univ; 88–Sp-Lang Path, Brownfield ISD Colonial Heights Elem, **SLP**

Zelvis, Dorothy Aphrodite 4021 Dryden, North Olmsted, OH 44070, (216) 529-4201, BA 69 Cleveland St Univ; MA 79 Cleveland St Univ; Sp-Lang Path, Lakewood Bd of Ed, **SLP**

Zeman, Richard D 12450 Sunnyglen Drive, Moorpark, CA 93021, (805) 583-6215, BA 73 SUNY - Center at Buffalo; MA 81 CA St Univ - Los Angeles; Aud, Simi Hills Hearing Ctr, **A**

Zeman, Mrs Tina Marie 5914 Greendale Place, Apt 108, Johnston, IA 50131, (515) 278-8340, BS 86 Northeast MO St Univ; MA 87 Northeast MO St Univ; AEA 11, **SLP**

Zemel, Jamie I 888A Corbett Avenue, San Francisco, CA 94131, (415) 922-9514, MS 87 San Francisco St Univ

Zemlin, Eileen 1519 West Park Avenue, Champaign, IL 61821, (217) 359-3416, BS 52 Univ of MN - Minneap-St Paul; ME 54 PA St Univ - Univ Park; **SLP**

Zemlin, Willard R 1519 West Park Avenue, Champaign, IL 61821, (217) 333-2230, BS 58 Univ of MN - Minneap-St Paul; MS 60 Univ of MN - Minneap-St Paul; PH 62 (NS) Univ of MN - Minneap-St Paul; Professor Emeritus, **F**

Zemmol, Mrs Caroline S 4962 Whispering Pine Lane, Bloomfield Hills, MI 48013, (313) 858-1918, BA 65 Wayne St Univ; ME 66 Wayne St Univ; Consult, Oakland Sch Sp & Hrng Cl, **SLP**

Zemper, F Anne 822 North Haddow Street, Arlington Heights, IL 60004, (312) 398-1188, BS 61 Western MI Univ; MS 86 Marquette Univ; **SLP**

Zencheck, Mrs Robin Fader RFD 10 Box 106, Teakettle Spout Road, Mahopac, NY 10541, (914) 832-6611, BA 76 CUNY - Queens Coll; MA 77 Hofstra Univ; Aud, Westchester Dev Cen, **A**

Zengel, Mrs Beverly J 1415 12th Avenue, Menomonie, WI 54751, (715) 235-0611, BS 64 Univ of MN - Duluth; MS 79 Univ of WI - Eau Claire; SLP, School Dist of Menomonie Area, **SLP**

Zenner, Dr Anthony A Zenner And Zenner Pa, Anderson Elementary School, Cross City, FL 32628, (813) 821-5746, BA 66 Univ of WI - Eau Claire; MA 67 Univ of TN - Knoxville; PH 71 (NS) Syracuse Univ; Sp-Lang Path, Zenner & Zenner Pa, **SLP**

Zenner, Mrs Natalie Argyris 108 Church Street, Fair Haven, NJ 07704, (201) 530-2425, BA 74 CUNY - City College; MA 77 CUNY - City College; 88–Sp-Lang Path, Riverview Med Ctr, **SLP**

Zenner, Sandra B Zenner And Zenner Pa, Anderson Elementary School, Cross City, FL 32628, (813) 821-5746, BA 70 Univ of WI - Eau Claire; MS 72 Univ of WI - Eau Claire; Asst Adm, Zenner & Zenner Pa, **SLP**

Zeno, Mrs Sara Hodge 3110 Rodney Parham, Little Rock, AR 72212, (501) 376-0377, BA 76 Univ of AR - Little Rock; OM 77 Univ of MS; 86–Sp-Lang Path, Ark Spec Educ Resource Ctr, **SLP ACE**

Zenon, Wendy Ann 3262 Florence Blvd, Omaha, NE 68110, (402) 453-8990, BS 83 Univ of NE - Lincoln; MS 85 Univ of NE - Lincoln; SLP, Omaha Public Schools, **SLP**

Zenorini, Brenda 2074 Bentwood Court, Arbor Pointe Apartment, Wilmington, DE 19804, (302) 998-7474, BA 79 Univ of DE; MA 82 Univ of Pittsburgh - Pittsburgh; Sp-Lang Path, Delaware Curative Workshop, **SLP**

Zentmeyer, Rebecca Beale 15746 Scrimshaw Drive, Tampa, FL 33624, (813) 886-4247, SLP, Temple Terrace Elementary Sch, **SLP**

Zentz, Bonnie Wisenauer 3025 Lavender Avenue, Baltimore, MD 21234, (301) 661-2400, BS 76 Towson St Univ; MS 77 Loyola Coll; Sp-Lang Path, Baltimore County Board of Educ, **SLP**

Zentz, Cynthia Klobuka 28 Freeport Street #D, Pittsburgh, PA 15223, (412) 366-3471, BS 82 PA St Univ - Univ Park; MS 84 PA St Univ - Univ Park; Aud, Metropolitan ENT Assoc, **A**

Zenz, Michael E ENT Audiology, Naval Hospital, Great Lakes, IL 60088, (312) 688-4533, BA 69 MI St Univ; MA 70 MI St Univ; Aud, US Govt, **A ACE**

Zepecki, Mrs Carol A H 17371 Lakeview Drive, Morgan Hill, CA 95037, (408) 779-5278, MA 71 Montclair St Coll; MA 85 San Jose St Univ; 88–Curriculum Coord, Morgan Hill Sch Dist, **SLP**

Zepeda, Isabel Castillo 7335 Lansbury, San Antonio, TX 78250, (512) 734-5770, BA 84 Our Lady Lake Univ-San Anton; MA 86 Our Lady Lake Univ-San Anton; **SLP**

Zerbst, Ellen S 2904 South 13th Street #2, Arlington, VA 22204, (703) 827-0980, BS 78 James Madison Univ; MA 79 Bowling Green St Univ; 87–Dir, Sp & Lang Services of McLean, **SLP**

Zerden, Stephanie 2 Mulberry Bluff Drive, Savannah, GA 31406, (912) 355-4602, BS 71 Emerson Coll; MS 72 Univ of NC - Chapel Hill; Sp-Lang Path, Savannah Sp & Hrng Cen, **SLP**

Zerebny, Roman 5822 Pathfinder Road, Rockford, IL 61109, (815) 229-2880, BA 72 Northern IL Univ - De Kalb; MA 74 Northern IL Univ - De Kalb; Aud, Nwn Il Assoc, **A**

Zerfas, Kimberly Jo 441 East Taro Lane, Phoenix, AZ 85024, (602) 375-0390, BA 83 Univ of Northern CO; MA 85 Univ of Northern CO; **SLP**

Zerfas, Mrs Terri Bumpas Route 2 Box 12-V, Rockwall, TX 75087, (214) 722-4667, BS 72 TX Tech Univ; MS 74 TX Tech Univ; Sp-Lang Path, Rockwall Independent Sch Dist, **SLP**

Zerlin, Dr Stanley Dept Of Audiology & Speech Sci, Purdue University, Heavilon Hall, West Lafayette, IN 47907, (317) 494-3804, BS 51 CUNY - City College; MA 53 Columbia Univ Teachers Coll; PH 59 (NS) Case Western Reserve Univ; Assoc Prof, Purdue University

Zervas, Mrs Rachel Hyman 1021 South 46th Street, Philadelphia, PA 19143, (215) 248-6877, BA 74 Colby Coll; MA 78 Temple Univ-Tyler Sch of Art; 87–SLP, North West Ctr, **SLP**

Zessin, Linda K 719 North Thomas, Oakland, NE 68045, **SLP**

Zetter-Kunze, Nola 2455 Lilac Lane, Fargo, ND 58102, (701) 234-5119, BS 73 ND St Univ; MS 75 Western OR St Coll; Sp-Lang Path, St Lukes Hospitals, **SLP**

Zey, Mrs Joyce Colleen 3904 S E Skylark Court, Topeka, KS 66605, BS 73 KS St Univ; MA 74 KS St Univ; SLP, Visiting Nurse Association, **SLP**

Zich, Cynthia Ann 4917 Melinda Court, Rockville, MD 20853, (301) 460-5286, MS 88 WV Univ

Zick, Mrs Autumn W 5415 Lincoln Avenue, St Joseph, MI 49085, (616) 473-2600, BA 76 MI St Univ; MA 77 Central MI Univ; Sp-Lang Path, Blossomland Learning Ctr, **SLP**

Zickar-Stranieri, Mrs Susan Elaine Waterside Gardens, 205 Schindler Dr Bldg 11, Brick, NJ 08723, (201) 240-2121, BA 81 Univ of Pittsburgh - Pittsburgh; MA 83 Kent St Univ; Sp-Lang Path, Early Intervention Program Inc, **SLP ACE**

Zidel, Mrs Marsha Rubin 221 Wynne Lane, Penn Valley, PA 19072, (215) 664-3097, MA 71 George Washington Univ; 88–Sp/Lang Path, Girard Coll, **SLP**

Ziebarth, Brenda Earlene 1209 Englewood, Royal Oak, MI 48073, (313) 542-3910, BS 84 Western MI Univ; MA 85 Central MI Univ; 85–Sp-Lang Path, Hazel Park Comm Schs, **SLP**

Ziebell, Andrea Powers 1012 Metro Circle, Palo Alto, CA 94303, (415) 493-5328, BA 83 San Jose St Univ; MA 87 San Jose St Univ; **SLP**

Zieber, David Alan P O Box 17104, Montgomery, AL 36117, (205) 567-8471, BA 81 Univ of CA - Santa Barbara; MS 84 Univ of Montevallo; Aud, J S Tarwater Dev Center, **A**

Ziegler, Brenda K 1669 Tiburon Court, Thousand Oaks, CA 91360, **A**

Ziegler, Jane E Rubin 3740 East Pima, Tucson, AZ 85716, (602) 881-0249, BA 84 Univ of SD - Vermillion; MA 86 Univ of MN - Duluth; 88–Sp-Lang Path, Arizona St Sch for the Deaf & the Blind, **SLP**

Ziegler, Mally Heaton 38W023 Heatherfield E Dr, Elgin, IL 60123, (312) 529-5670, BA 79 Elmhurst Coll; MS 81 Univ of WI - Milwaukee; Sp-Lang Path, Schl Assn for Spec Ed, **SLP**

Ziegler, Mrs Marilyn N R R 2 Box A19, Columbia, IL 62236, (618) 281-5707, BS 69 Ball St Univ; MA 78 Saint Louis Univ; **SLP**

Ziegler, Mrs Phyliss M 2311 13th Street, Monroe, WI 53566, (608) 328-9175, BA 75 Univ of WI - Eau Claire; MS 76 Univ of WI - Eau Claire; SLP, Sch Dist of Monroe, **SLP**

Ziegler, Teresa Schulze Route 2 Box 244 Ab, Clarksville, AR 72830, (501) 754-2893, BA 81 Ouachita Baptist Univ; MS 86 Univ of Central AR; 81–Sp-Lang Path, Clarksville PS, **SLP**

Ziegler, Willard D, Jr 303 North George Street, Hanover, PA 17331, (717) 783-6913, BS 59 Bloomsburg Univ of PA; ME 64 PA St Univ - Univ Park; Spec Ed Advisor, PA Dept of Ed, **SLP**

Ziegler-Blau, Mrs Carol 69-09 108th Street #412, Forest Hills, NY 11375, (718) 544-2289, BA 82 Univ of RI; MA 84 NY Univ; 87–Sp-Lang Path, St Mary's Hosp for Children, **SLP**

Zieha, Ellen E 2701 Navajo Pass-Arrowhead, Maple Glen, PA 19002, (816) 531-1200, BA 77 OH St Univ; MA 79 Saint Louis Univ; Sp-Lang Path, Vna, **SLP**

Zielinski, Ronald J 601 Tawas Street, East Tawas, MI 48730, BA 68; MA 77 Wayne St Univ; SLP, Private Practice, **SLP**

Ziemba, Mrs Michele Bidic 607 Guildford Rd, Cherry Hill, NJ 08003, (609) 424-8773, BA 79 Rutger's St Univ - Douglas Coll; MA 82 Trenton St Coll; Sp-Lang Path, Haddon Heights PS, **SLP**

Zieminski, Marianne 994 George Urban Boulevard, Apartment 4, Cheektowaga, NY 14225, (716) 626-9127, BS 82 SUNY - Coll at Buffalo; MS 85 SUNY - Coll at Buffalo; 88–Sp-Lang Path, West Seneca Central Sch Sys, **SLP**

Zieno, Janet H 33 Birch Lane, Fairport, NY 14450, (716) 271-0680, BA 72 SUNY - Coll at Oneonta; MA 77 SUNY - Coll at Geneseo; Aud, Hrng/Sp Cen of Rochester, **A**

Zientara, Mrs Betty K 8111 West Waterford Avenue, Milwaukee, WI 53220, (414) 259-1414, BS 76 Marquette Univ; MS 77 Marquette Univ; Asst Super/Sp-Lang Path, Curative Rehab Cen, **SLP**

Ziering, Deborah Jo 444 East 58th Street #2-A, New York, NY 10022, (212) 371-1413, BA 84 CUNY - Queens Coll; MA 86 NY Univ; **SLP**

Ziesel, Theresa Ann 4146 Zane Avenue North, Robbinsdale, MN 55422, (612) 535-5415, BS 80 Univ of NE - Omaha; MS 83 Saint Cloud St Univ; 87–Sp-Lang Path, Wayzata PS, **SLP**

Ziko, Connie Allen 534 Laurel Hill Road, Norwich, CT 06360, (203) 887-0816, BA 80 Univ of ME - Orono; MS 85 Univ of NH; 87–Sp-Lang Path, Windham PS, **SLP**

Zilber, Sharon Lisa 3210 Shelburne Road, #B2, Baltimore, MD 21208, (301) 328-5947, BA 83 Univ of MD - College Park; MS 85 Towson St Univ; Audiologist, Univ of MD Hospital, **A**

Zilch, Marsha L South 5176 Lake Shore Road, Hamburg, NY 14075, MA 67; **SLP**

Ziller, Georgia J 4107 N E 59th Street, Kansas City, MO 64119, (816) 453-7630, BS 73 Central MO St Univ; MS 74 Central MO St Univ; Sp-Lang Path, Research Med Cen, **SLP**

Zilowey, Stacey A 725 East Fox Hills Drive, Bloomfield Hills, MI 48013, (313) 333-7896, BA 78 Univ of MI - Ann Arbor; MA 80 Wayne St Univ; Sp-Lang Path, Nurse Home Hlth Svcs, **SLP**

Ziltz, Mrs Mary Termine 228 Regent Road, Harrisburg, PA 17112, (717) 657-7621, BA 77 Southern CT St Univ; MS 83 Southern CT St Univ; 86–Sp-Lang Path, Early Intervention Prog Inc, **SLP**

Ziman, Susan M 7204 Denberg Road, Baltimore, MD 21209, **SLP**

Zimbler, Mrs Enid B 975 Memorial Drive #609, Cambridge, MA 02138, MS

Zimdars, Mrs Judith Ann 4948 Edgewater Drive, Mound, MN 55364, (612) 533-2246, BS 76 IA St Univ; MA 80 Univ of IA; Sp-Lang Path, ISD 279, **SLP**

Zimmer, Barbara J 1331 Bolling Avenue, Norfolk, VA 23508, (804) 423-0525, BA 63 Rutger's St Univ - Douglas Coll; ME 64 Boston Univ; **SLP**

Zimmer, Catherine H 5567 North Diversey Blvd, Milwaukee, WI 53217, (414) 964-5269, BA 32 1183; MA 39 Northwestern Univ; **SLP F LM**

Zimmer, Millie Resweber 202 Bayou Bend Road, New Iberia, LA 70560, (318) 365-5910, BA 76 Univ of Southwestern LA; MS 87 Univ of Southwestern LA; 85–Dir/Sp-Lang Path, Rehab Assoc, **SLP**

Zimmer, Wendy A 7 Cleveland Road, Marblehead, MA 01945, (617) 631-6528, BA 73 Univ of MI - Ann Arbor; MA 75 Northwestern Univ; SLP, Private Practice, **SLP**

Zimmer-Jeger, Ronie 135-20 78th Road, Flushing, NY 11367, (718) 380-7682, MA 86 CUNY - Queens Coll

Zimmer-Lucas, Mary Elizabeth 121 1/2 N Wabash, Glendora, CA 91740, (818) 962-4011, BA 81 Univ of CA - Santa Barbara; MA 85 CA St Univ - Long Beach; **SLP**

Zimmerman, Mrs Barbara Kriedman 9917 Bluegrass Road, Potomac, MD 20854, (301) 299-2204, BA 64 Hofstra Univ; MA 65 NY Univ; Sp-Lang Path, Private Practice, **SLP**

Zimmerman, Dr Barbara R 21 Clear View Lane, Benton, LA 71006, (318) 227-5156, BS 54 Bowling Green St Univ; MA 62 Wayne St Univ; PH 68 (NS) OH Univ - Athens; Assoc Prof/Coord Cl Ser, LSU-Med Center, **SLP A**

Zimmerman, Beverly N 1503 Yale Drive, Ruston, LA 71270, (318) 255-8713, BA 49 Univ of FL; MA 73 LA Tech Univ; Asst Prof, LA Tech U, **SLP ACE**

Zimmerman, Carla Marie 2300 West San Angelo #1117, Gilbert, AZ 85234, (602) 833-3252, BA 84 Univ of SD - Vermillion; OM 85 AZ St Univ; 86–Sp-Lang Path, Mesa PS, **SLP**

Zimmerman, Mrs Carolyn W 14024 West 69th Street, Shawnee Mission, KS 66216, (913) 621-5155, BS 61 IL St Univ - Normal; ME 64 Southern IL Univ -Carbondale; Sp-Lang Path, Kansas Cty Pub Sch Dist #500, **SLP**

Zimmerman, Diane Power Davis Joint Unified School District, 1207 Sycamore Lane, Davis, CA 95616, (916) 757-5460, BA 72 Univ of CA - Davis; MA 75 Univ of the Pacific; 86–Elem Prin, Davis Joint USD, **SLP**

Zimmerman, Donna S 7808 Vista Del Arroyo N E, Albuquerque, NM 87109, (505) 888-4033, BS 75 Univ of NM; Sp/Lang Path, Albuquerque Pub Sch, **SLP**

Zimmerman, Harry R 1455 Wofford Drive, Las Cruces, NM 88001, (505) 526-4131, BA 62 IN Univ - Bloomington; MA 76 NM St Univ; 79–Owner, Private Practice, **A**

Zimmerman, Mrs Hilary Deborah 41 Carman Avenue, Cedarhurst, NY 11516-1904, (212) 544-3152, BA 80 Hofstra Univ; MA 82 Hofstra Univ; SLP, NYC Bd of Ed, **SLP**

Zimmerman, Jane S 235 Prospect Street, Leominster, MA 01453, **SLP**

Zimmerman, Janiece C 219 North Sage #1-D, Kalamazoo, MI 49007, (616) 673-5431, BS 63 Western MI Univ; MA 73 Western MI Univ; Sp/Lang Path, Allegan Publ Schs, **SLP**

Zimmerman, Mrs Jeanne L Kent General Hospital, 640 South State Street, Dover, DE 19901, (302) 734-4700, BS 73 Clarion Univ of PA; MS 76 Towson St Univ; 88–Sp-Lang Path, Kent Gen Hosp, **SLP**

Zimmerman, Joseph B 1530 Bellevue Way SE Suite B, Bellevue, WA 98004, (206) 454-1420, BA 64 Western WA Univ; ME 68 Western WA Univ; Owner, Bellevue Sp Clinic, **SLP**

Zimmerman, Judith Holloway 1455 Wofford Drive, Las Cruces, NM 88001, (505) 522-6444, BA 64 Univ of Redlands; MA 75 NM St Univ; Sp-Lang Path, Las Cruces Pub Sch, **SLP**

Zimmerman, Lauri Michele 1529 Hillside Drive, Cherry Hill, NJ 08003, (215) 339-4275, BA 83 Temple Univ; MA 85 Temple Univ; 87–Sp-Lang Path, St Agnes Med Ctr, **SLP**

Zimmerman, Mrs Lesta Lee 3405 South 126th Street, Omaha, NE 68144, (402) 334-2245, OB 77 Univ of NE - Lincoln; MA 80 Univ of NE - Lincoln; Sp-Lang Path, Yutan PS, **SLP**

Zimmerman, Mrs Loreen Landino Sertoma Center, 7330 College Drive, Palos Heights, IL 60463, (312) 361-2121, MA 85 Northern IL Univ - De Kalb; BS 83 Northern IL Univ - De Kalb; 85–Aud, Sertoma Ctr for Comm Dis, **A**

Zimmerman, Rae 5941 Pine Vista S E, Kentwood, MI 49508, (616) 455-5900, BA 73 MI St Univ; MA 79 MI St Univ; 87–Sp-Lang Path, Sojourners Trans Living Ctr, **SLP**

Zimmerman, Reila 17 Hoskier Road, South Orange, NJ 07079, (201) 763-7865, **SLP**

Zimmerman, Rita H 832 Ruskin, Edwardsville, IL 62025, (314) 569-8234, BA 70 Southern IL Univ-Edwardsvill; MS 79 Southern IL Univ-Edwardsvill; 87–Coord-Sp-Lang Path, Spec Sch Dist of St Louis Co, **SLP**

Zimmerman, Dr Robert Lee 10050 Pineledge Drive West, Clarence, NY 14031, BA 66 West Liberty St Coll; MS 69 5841; PH 77 (NS) Southern IL Univ -Carbondale; Chmn/Audiology-Spch Patholoigy, Veterans Admn Medical Center, **SLP A**

Zimmerman, Mrs Sandra J 740 Regency, Hurst, TX 76054, (817) 283-3191, BA 80 Valparaiso Univ; MS 83 TX Christian Univ; Sp-Lang Path, Mid Cities Sp & Hrng Clinic, **SLP**

Zimmerman, Susan Rural Route 2, Beloit, KS 67420, (913) 439-6665, BS 50 Emporia St Univ; MA 59 Univ of Denver; **SLP LM**

Zimmerman, Mrs Susan F Route 4 Box 322D, Manhattan, KS 66502, (913) 539-0301, BA 71 Univ of AZ; MA 73 KS St Univ; 88–Sp-Lang Path, USD 383, **SLP**

Zimmerman, Susan Mary 826 Fairmont Avenue, Madison, WI 53714, (608) 263-3141, BS 83 Univ of WI - Eau Claire; OM 86 Univ of WI - River Falls; 88–Research Spec, Waisman Early Childhood Prog, **SLP**

Zimmerman, Dr Terrance S Division Of Public Health, PO Box 637, Dover, DE 19903, (302) 736-4767, BS 73 Clarion Univ of PA; MS 76 Towson St Univ; PH 87 (Human Development) Univ of MD - Baltimore CO; 87–Prog Dir Sp-Lang Path, Delaware Div of Public Health, **SLP**

Zimmermann, Mrs Kelly J 3329 West Birchwood Avenue, Milwaukee, WI 53221, (414) 264-2535, MS 88 Univ of WI - Milwaukee; 88–Sp-Lang Path, Milwaukee PS

Zimmermann, Mrs Margo Townsend 1391 Broadway #A-12, Hewlett, NY 11557, (516) 569-7675, BS 83 Ithaca Coll; MS 85 Syracuse Univ; Sp-Lang Path, Syracuse City Schools, **SLP**

Zimmerman-Phillips, Susan R University Of Michigan Hospital, 1505 Tarbman Center, Department Of Otolaryngology, 1500 East Medical Center Drive, Ann Arbor, MI 48109-0312, (313) 936-8013, MS 86 Univ of WI - Stevens Point; Aud, Univ of MI Hospitals, **A**

Zinberg, Dr Mildred F 1071 Denton Avenue, New Hyde Park, NY 11040, (212) 631-6284, BA 48 Univ of WI - Madison; MS 50 Univ of Pittsburgh - Pittsburgh; PH 69 (Sp) CUNY - Grad Sch & Univ Cntr; Dr/Prof, Queensbor Commun Coll-CUNY, **SLP**

Zindel, Betsy Jane 9 White Birch Drive, Morris Plains, NJ 07950, (201) 539-5636, **SLP ACE**

Zindel, Elaine M 614 Meadow Lane, Oreland, PA 19075, **SLP**

Zinder, Mrs Christine Theriault 108 Park Lane, Ithaca, NY 14850, (607) 273-0742, BA 72 Coll of Mount Saint Vincent; MS 74 CO St Univ; **A**

Zingeser, Louise B 1715 Luzerne Avenue, Silver Spring, MD 20910-1510, (301) 585-3745, BA 79 Univ of OR; **SLP**

Zingg, Cynthia Callan 48 Country Lane, Hamilton, NJ 08690, (609) 396-5444, BA 69 Rutger's St Univ - Douglas Coll; MA 80 Trenton St Coll; Sp-Lang Path, Sr Georgine Lrng Cen, **SLP**

Zingg, Mrs Kathleen Hanrahan 1170 Center Street, Middleboro, MA 02346, (203) 859-0005, BS 80 Ithaca Coll; MS 82 Ithaca Coll; Sp-Lang Path, Morton Hosp Sp Dept, **SLP ACE**

Zink, Mrs Barbara A 2208 Tiffany Drive, Schaumburg, IL 60194, (312) 981-3670, BS 68 Northern IL Univ - De Kalb; MA 69 Univ of IL - Urbana; Aud, Elk Grove Hearing Center, **A**

Zink, G David 14371 Country Hills Drive, Brighton, CO 80601, (604) 387-1051, BA 60 Univ of Northern CO; MA 64 Univ of Northern CO; 88–Aud, Private Practice, **A**

Zinkowski, Debra Ann 1766-B 6th Place Northwest, Birmingham, AL 35215, (205) 854-4898, BS 82 Univ of NV - Reno; MS 85 Univ of NV - Reno; **SLP**

Zinn, Mrs Joan S 8406 Jefferson Street, Paramount, CA 90723, (213) 861-2891, BA 73 Whittier Coll; MA 75 Whittier Coll; Sp-Lang Path, Los Angeles Cnty Supt Schools, **SLP**

Zinna, Mario Anthony, Jr 7356 Radiant Circle, Orlando, FL 32810, (407) 299-0927, BS 81 Indiana Univ of PA; MS 83 James Madison Univ; Dir of Sp/Aud, Sea Pines Rehab Hosp, **SLP ACE**

Zinner, Elliott M 23249 South Woodland Road, Shaker Heights, OH 44122, PH (NS); **SLP**

Zinter, Mrs Irine Denis 122 Hiview Terrace, West Seneca, NY 14224, (716) 674-7856, BS 50 SUNY - Coll at Buffalo; MA 55 Case Western Reserve Univ; Sp-Lang Path, W Seneca Cen Sch, **SLP**

Ziol, Mrs Elaine J 2040 Marston Lane, Flossmoor, IL 60422, (312) 799-0562, MS 85 Governors St Univ; Sp-Lang Path, CARES, **SLP**

Ziolkowski, Lori J 1712 Washtenaw, Ypsilanti, MI 48197, (313) 295-5027, MA 78 MI St Univ; SLP, People's Comm Hosp Authority, **SLP**

Zionts, Mrs Laurie B 168 Penhurst Drive, Pittsburgh, PA 15235, (412) 823-7317, BA 77 Rutger's St Univ - Douglas Coll; MS 79 Hahneman Medical Coll; Sp-Lang Path/Aud, Private Practice, **SLP A**

Zipp, Judy Ann 17822 Beach Boulevard, Suite 325, Huntington Beach, CA 92647, (714) 842-2596, BA 80 CA St Univ - Long Beach; MA 88 CA St Univ - Long Beach; 88–Aud, Dr Castanon

Zipursky, Mrs Myrna A 173 West 22nd, Vancouver, BC, Canada V5Y 2G5, (604) 875-0872, BA 71 Univ of Manitoba - Winnipeg; OM 76 Univ of Toronto - Ontario; 88–Sp-Lang Path, Surrey Sch Bd, **SLP**

Zirbel, Jennifer Joan 1016 West Burnsville Pky, Apt 353, Burnsville, MN 55337-2357, (612) 890-0420, BS 78 Mankato St Univ; MS 83 Mankato St Univ; Sp-Lang Path, Dakota County Sp Serv Dist 917, **SLP**

Zirkelbach, Dr Thelma K 4907 Dumfries, Houston, TX 77096, (713) 777-6107, BS 57 Univ of TX - Austin; MA 70 Univ of Houston - Univ Park; ED 83 (NS) Univ of Houston - Univ Park; Dir, Assoc Sp-Lang Serv, **SLP**

Zirkin-Dagan, Sharon 118 Ford Road, Woodbridge, CT 06525, (203) 397-0558, SLP, Ansonia Bd of Ed, **SLP**

Zirkle, Mary Lynn 815 Sudbury Road, Atlanta, GA 30328, BA 75 Hollins Coll; MS 77 Emory Univ; **SLP**

Zirlen, Mrs Adrienne 147 Exeter Road, Hamden, CT 06518, (203) 281-4410, BS 60 Boston Univ; MS 74 Southern CT St Univ; Sp-Lang Path, Zirlen-Zirlen, **SLP**

Zirlen, David Michael 27 Trolley Crossing Lane, Middletown, CT 06457, (203) 635-6818, BS 84 Ithaca Coll; MS 87 Southern CT St Univ; 88–Dir Sp-Lang Path, Forestville Health & Rehab Ctr, **SLP**

Zirlin, Rachel Meisler 32 Winding Way West, Morrisville, PA 19067, (215) 752-8829, BA 79 Gordon Coll; MS 82 Columbia Univ Teachers Coll; Sp/Lang Path, Self Employed, **SLP**

Zisblatt, Mrs Sharon Wieder 1000 Ocean Parkway #5J, Brooklyn, NY 11230, (718) 253-6308, BA 81 CUNY - Queens Coll; MA 83 CUNY - Queens Coll; Sp-Lang Path, Bd of Ed, **SLP**

Zisk-Rosner, Lori B 131 Bennett Road, Teaneck, NJ 07666, (201) 837-8574, BS 75 Syracuse Univ; MS 77 Syracuse Univ; Sp-Lang Path, Private Practice, **SLP**

Zita, Jan 232 Mandel Drive, Southington, CT 06489, (203) 621-4613, BS 83 Central CT St Univ; MS 87 Southern CT St Univ

Zitalone, Mrs Kathleen Harder 406 Broad Street, Butler, PA 16001, (412) 445-3680, BS 77 Clarion Univ of PA; ME 81 Clarion Univ of PA; Sp-Lang Path, Karns City Area Sch Dist, **SLP**

Zitman, Mrs Diana Victoria 10266 Plum Tree Lane, Cupertino, CA 95014-1840, **SLP**

Zito, Roberta Kolstein 213 Ledden Terrace, South Plainfield, NJ 07080, (201) 593-6534, BS 80 Trenton St Coll; MA 83 Montclair St Coll; SLP, Glen Ridge Bd of Ed, **SLP**

Zittere, Judy Oakley 6853 Edgefield Lane, Orlando, FL 32822, (904) 395-1505, BA 78 Univ of FL; MA 85 Univ of FL; **SLP**

Zitzer, Ellyn R 117 Redlands Road, West Roxbury, MA 02132, (617) 735-6487, BS 71 Univ of WI - Madison; MA 74 Univ of WA; Aud, Boston Children's Hospital, **A**

Zitzer, Robert 796 Juniper Walk #A, Goleta, CA 93117, (805) 968-3978, BA 70 Southern IL Univ -Carbondale; MS 79 Univ of WI - Milwaukee; Sp-Lang Path, Santa Barbara Sch Dist, **SLP**

Zizz, Carol A Audiology-126, Veterans Administration Medical Center, 5901 East Seventh Street, Long Beach, CA 90822, (213) 494-5414, BS 84 Univ of AZ; MS 86 Univ of AZ; 87–Research Asst, VA Med Ctr, **A**

Zizzo, Robert 1648 N Arlington Place, Milwaukee, WI 53202, (414) 645-6271, BS 61 Univ of WI - Milwaukee; MS 66 Univ of WI - Milwaukee; 64–Sp-Lang Path, Public Schools, **SLP**

Zlotnick, Mrs Michele M 25 High Oaks Court, Huntington, NY 11743, (516) 351-8456, MA 85 Hofstra Univ; Sp-Lang Path, St Charles Hospital, **SLP**

Zlotnick, Phyllis H 624 Queen Anne Road, Teaneck, NJ 07666, (201) 836-4707, BA 74 SUNY - Center at Stony Brook; MA 76 CUNY - City College; Consult-Aud, **A**

Zlotnick, Rosemarie 17 Redwood Drive, Penfield, NY 14526, (716) 377-0527, BA 74 Univ of Denver; MA 75 Univ of Denver; **SLP**

Zlydaszek, Mrs Susan L 301 Marshall Road, North Brunswick, NJ 08902, (201) 321-6800, BA 65 Newark St Coll; MA 68 Newark St Coll; Sp-Lang Path, Roosevelt Hosp, **SLP**

Zoback, Mark S 520 Old Stafford Road, Tolland, CT 06084, (203) 456-3261, BA 75 CUNY - Brooklyn Coll; BA 75 CUNY - Brooklyn Coll; MS 77 CUNY - Brooklyn Coll; 88–Dir-Early Childhood Prog, Eastconn Reg Ed Ser Cen, **SLP**

Zodrow, Nancy S P O Box 356, Olympia, WA 98507-3775, (206) 456-8281, BA 74 Eastern WA Univ; MS 75 Eastern WA Univ; 86–Sp-Lang Path, Olympia Sch Dist, **SLP**

Zoellner, Ann M 1612 Chamberlain Avenue S E, Grand Rapids, MI 49506-4559, **SLP**

Zofcin, Michael Francis 305 East 197th Street, Euclid, OH 44119, (216) 761-6100, BA 79 OH St Univ; MA 81 OH St Univ; Sp-Lang Path, Cuyahoga Co Bd of M R, **SLP**

Zola, Mrs Pamela Dale 8727 Donahue Road, Batavia, NY 14020, (716) 344-2340, BS 80 SUNY - Coll at Buffalo; MA 81 George Washington Univ; Sp-Lang Path, Livingston Wy Arc Chldn Serv, **SLP**

Zola, Stefani 8471 Highton Court, Cincinnati, OH 45236, (513) 791-1235, BS 77 Northwestern Univ; MA 79 Univ of Cincinnati; Sp-Lang Path, Private Practice, **SLP**

Zolintakis, Linda 757 Redmaple Road, Salt Lake City, UT 84106, BS 73 Univ of UT; MS 75 Univ of UT; Sp-Lang Path, Jordan Sch Dist, **SLP**

Zoller, Mrs Mary N 9625 East Soutport Road, Indianapolis, IN 46259, (317) 862-5872, BS 71 Murray St Univ; MS 74 Murray St Univ; 80–Sp-Lang Path, Indianapolis Pub Sch, **SLP**

Zoller, Mrs Valerie Ann 418 Sedgewick Court, Virginia Beach, VA 23454, MA 83 Univ of SD - Vermillion

Zoller, Vicki A 57-D Troy Drive, Springfield, NJ 07081, (201) 547-3037, BS 68 Ithaca Coll; MA 69 Seton Hall Univ; 77–Sp-Lang Path, Moore Lab Sch/Jersey Cty St C, **SLP**

Zoltak, Mrs Ruth S 217-A Wildcat Road, Franklin, NJ 07416, (201) 697-1700, BA 69 Kean Coll of NJ; MA 74 Montclair St Coll; Tchr, W Milford Twnshp Pub Schs, **SLP**

Zoltowski, Mrs Elyse Malins 1225 West 1st Street, Elmria, NY 14905, (607) 734-5304, MS 76 Syracuse Univ; Sp-Lang Path, St Josephs Hospital, **SLP**

Zombar, Catherine Roll 7021 S W 10th Street, Pembroke Pines, FL 33023, (305) 739-6233, BA 77 Univ of FL; MA 79 Univ of FL; 80–Supervisor/Sp-Lang Path, Bertrand J Reese MS & Assoc Inc, **SLP ACE**

Zombeck, Mrs Suzanne M 8-A Osborne Street, Rochester, NH 03867, (603) 332-9399, BS 83 Univ of NH; MS 87 Univ of NH; 87–Sp-Lang Path, New Medico Highwatch Rehab Fac, **SLP**

Zoochi, Lawrence Michael Hearing Impaired Program, James Ward School, 2701 South Shields Avenue, Chicago, IL 60616, (312) 567-8661, BA 79 Univ of IL - Urbana; MA 82 Western IL Univ; 83–Aud, Chicago Pub Sch, **A**

Zopfi, Mrs Sarah D 180 Tashua Road, Trumbull, CT 06611, BA 78 Loyola Coll; MS 79 Loyola Coll; 83–Sp-Lang Path, Eagle Hill School, **SLP**

Zordell, John K 270 Robson Drive, Kamloops, BC, Canada V2E 1W1, (604) 376-5745, BA 73 Univ of IA; MA 77 Central MI Univ; Sp-Lang Path, Sch Dist #24 (Kamloops), **SLP**

Zorich, Mrs Donna June Indiana Audiology, 925 Philadelphia Street, Indiana, PA 15701, (412) 349-6462, BA 74 Humboldt St Univ; MS 76 Univ of OR; 88–Aud/Owner, Indiana Audiology, **A**

Zorthian, Anna L Touro Infirmary, Speech Pathology, 1401 Foucher Street, New Orleans, LA 70115, (504) 897-8563, BA 73 Lake Forest Coll; MS 78 Tulane Univ; Sp-Lang Path, Touro Infirmary, **SLP ACE**

Zoss, Donald C 1 Belmont Avenue North, Plattsburgh, NY 12901, (518) 564-2170, BS 59 SUNY - Coll at Geneseo; MS 63 SUNY - Coll at Geneseo; 81–Dir of Speech Ctr, St U Coll of Arts & Sci SUNY, **SLP**

Zouck, Elizabeth 4052 South 685 East #D, Salt Lake City, UT 84107, (801) 269-1648, BA 70 Univ of NC - Chapel Hill; MS 79 Univ of NC - Chapel Hill; **SLP**

Zozom-Guiheen, Mrs Arlene 813 Furlong Drive, Libertyville, IL 60048, (312) 367-4120, BA 75 Rutger's St Univ - Douglas Coll; MA 77 NY Univ; Sp-Lang Path, Oak Grove Sch, **SLP**

Zozulak, Helen Eva 2910 Evergreen Way, Ellicott City, MD 21043, (301) 461-2354, BA 79 Towson St Univ; MS 81 Towson St Univ; Sp-Lang Path, Commun Health Care Assoc, **SLP**

Zraick, Richard Isaac 8902 North 17th Drive, Phoenix, AZ 85021-4316, (602) 997-8571, BA 84 Univ of AZ; MS 87 Univ of AZ; 88–Sp-Lang Path, AZ Inst of Physical Med

Zuback, Jacqueline Robin 34 Hudson Terrace, Edgewater, NJ 07020, (212) 526-1000, SLP, VA Med Ctr St Albans, **SLP**

Zubick, Dr Howard H Speech And Hearing Division, Brigham & Womens Hospital, 75 Francis Street, Boston, MA 02115, (617) 732-5601, BS 64 Emerson Coll; MS 65 Univ of WI - Madison; PH 69 (NS) MI St Univ; Ch of Sp & Hrng Div, Brigham & Womens Hosp, **SLP A**

Zubrick, Dr Stephen R 5A Riverside Road, Fremantle, West Australia, Australia 6158, MS 73 Univ of MI - Ann Arbor; MA 78 Univ of MI - Ann Arbor; PH 79 (Psychology) Univ of MI - Ann Arbor; 79–Asst Prin-Clin Psych, Hlth Dept/Wn Australia, **SLP A**

Zuck, Mrs Roberta Draper 6632 South Buffalo Drive, Littleton, CO 80120, (303) 798-3108, BA 42 OH Wesleyan Univ; MA 70 Univ of Denver; Sp/Lang Path, Denver Pub Sch, **SLP**

Zucker, Barbara Loren 5440 Mayfield Road, Lyndhurst, OH 44124, (216) 352-8993, BS 84 Miami Univ - Oxford; MA 86 Kent St Univ; 86–Sp-Lang Path, Kerr-Brumbaugh Ctr for Rehab, **SLP**

Zucker, Carolyn M 246 Tavistock Avenue, Los Angeles, CA 90049, BA 65 Univ of CA - Los Angeles; MA 78 CA St Univ - Northridge; **SLP**

Zucker, Joan 18-75 Corporal Kennedy St, Bayside, NY 11360, **SLP**

Zucker, Karen D 436 Woodland Road, Highland Park, IL 60035, BS 74 Boston Univ; MS 76 Washington Univ; Consult, Private Practice, **A**

Zucker, Laura Sue 510 Sheridan #308, Evanston, IL 60202, (312) 336-3100, BS 83 Univ of WI - Madison; MA 84 Northwestern Univ; Sp-Lang Path, Niles Township High Schs, **SLP**

Zucker, Mrs Susan Robins 65 White Oak Drive, South Orange, NJ 07079, (201) 763-8877, BS 63 Univ of MI - Ann Arbor; MA 64 Syracuse Univ; **SLP**

Zucker-Krantz, Mrs Jerri 550 Thompson Boulevard, Buffalo Grove, IL 60089, BS 74 Univ of IL - Urbana; MA 75 Northwestern Univ; Sp-Lang Path, Private Practice, **SLP**

Zuckerman, Carol L 23738 Ingomar Street, West Hills, CA 91304, (818) 702-0763, BA 77 CA St Univ - Northridge; MA 80 CA St Univ - Northridge; Sp-Lang Path, Sepulveda VA Med Ctr, **SLP**

Zuckerman, Heidi L J 1390 East 19th Street, Brooklyn, NY 11230, (718) 998-0567, BA 76 CUNY - Brooklyn Coll; MS 79 CUNY - Brooklyn Coll; Sp/Lang Path, Private Practice, **SLP**

Zuckerman, Susan A 124 Hastings Avenue, Croton on Hudson, NY 10520, (914) 245-6697, BA 73 SUNY - Coll at Cortland; MA 77 CUNY - City College; Sp-Lang Path, Yorktown Cen Sch Dist, **SLP**

Zuckerman-Simon, Mrs Holly 546 Lasalle Court North, Buffalo Grove, IL 60089-1043, (312) 362-3120, BS 80 Northern IL Univ - De Kalb; MS 82 IL St Univ - Normal; Sp-Lang Path, Libertyville Pub Sch Dist 70, **SLP**

Zuehlsdorff, Kathleen Marie 3 Therrian Avenue, Saco, ME 04072, (603) 433-4015, BS 83 Univ of Northern CO; MS 85 Portland St Univ; 86–Mgr: Sp-Lang Path Dept, Portsmouth Reg Hosp, **SLP**

Zuena, Mrs Paulette B 10 Glen Meadow Road, Andover, MA 01810, (617) 470-1505, BA 74 Univ of RI; MS 76 Univ of South FL; Sp-Lang Path, Choate-Symmes Health Services, **SLP**

Zuga, Donna J 1255 Millers Landing, Cortland, OH 44410, (216) 372-2200, BS 73 OH St Univ; MA 74 Kent St Univ; Superv, Trumbull Co Bd of Ed, **SLP**

Zuk, Mrs Cynthia Anne 1600 Woodburn Road, Rural Route 1, Bimbrook, ON, Canada L0R 1CO, (416) 521-2100, BA 83 Brock Univ - Ontario; MA 86 SUNY - Center at Buffalo; 88–Sp-Lang Path, Chedoke-Mc Master Hosp, **SLP**

Zukoff, Pricilla J 23 Rockwood Circle, Bedford, TX 76021, (817) 545-3319, BS 77 CUNY - Brooklyn Coll; MS 79 Univ of WI - Milwaukee; Sp-Lang Path, Private Practice, **SLP**

Zukosky, Carol Anne 7902 Marks Street, Tampa, FL 33603, (813) 848-6451, MS 84 Univ of South FL; Sp-Lang Path, Pasco County, **SLP**

Zukowski, Glenna J 1192 Woodglen, Ypsilanti, MI 48198, (313) 481-0153, BS 79 Eastern MI Univ; MA 81 Eastern MI Univ; Sp-Lang Path, Willow Run Public Schools, **SLP**

Zuleski, Kathleen Elizabeth 501 Magnolia Street #107, South Pasadena, CA 91030, (818) 595-2297, BA 84 CA St Univ - Los Angeles; MA 86 CA St Univ - Los Angeles; 86–Sp-Lang Path, Los Angeles Dept of Educ, **SLP**

Zulewski, Richard 1132 Hellerman Street, Philadelphia, PA 19111, (215) 342-7660, BA 81 Duquesne Univ; MA 84 Temple Univ; 84–Sp-Lang Path, Cora Services, **SLP**

Zulli, Bonnie Hughes Rd 2 Simeon Road, Riverhead, NY 11901, (516) 929-8500, BS 78 SUNY - Coll at New Paltz; MS 86 Adelphi Univ; Sp-Lang Path, Shoreham Wading River Schl Dst

Zulofsky, Debra R Communication Resources, P O Box 10201, Portland, ME 04104, (207) 774-4440, BS 75 Boston Univ; ME 77 Northeastern Univ; Dir, Commun Res, **SLP ACE**

Zumbach, Kathy 708 38th Street, West Des Moines, IA 50265, (515) 225-0491, BS 72 IA St Univ; MA 75 Univ of IA; **SLP**

Zummo, Samuel R 5316 Grandview Drive, Milton, WI 53563-9420, BS 68; MS 72; OM 78; Director of Spec Education, Milton Area Sch Dist, **SLP**

Zuniga, Mrs Deborah Ann 1119 Lovera, San Antonio, TX 78201, (512) 532-9610, BS 86 Southwest TX St Univ; MS 87 Southwest TX St Univ; 88–Sp-Lang Path, TX Dept of MHMR

Zuniga, Monica 27 Whiton Avenue, Hingham, MA 02043, (617) 848-5353, BS 85 Bridgewater St Coll; MS 87 Columbia Univ Teachers Coll; **SLP**

Zunz, Gail C 37 Victoria Street, West Somerville, MA 02144, (617) 397-7252, BS 74 Ithaca Coll; MA 77 Univ of Denver; Sp-Lang Path, Malden Pub Schs, **SLP**

Zupan, Diane Marie 1808 North 42nd, Seattle, WA 98103, (206) 633-2123, BA 82 Univ of WA; MS 84 Univ of WA; **SLP ACE**

Zupan, Mrs Kathleen Lynn 5411 South Sherman Street, Littleton, CO 80121, (303) 762-9660, BS 79 Univ of WI - Milwaukee; MS 80 Univ of WI - Milwaukee; Sp-Path, Aurora Pub Sch, **SLP**

Zurales, Sue Kaminski 1351 South Lombard Avenue, Lombard, IL 60148-4618, (312) 310-0220, BS 81 Northern IL Univ - De Kalb; MA 83 Northern IL Univ - De Kalb; Aud, Mobilear Inc, **A**

Zurav, Mrs Frances S 1 Archbridge Lane, Springfield, NJ 07081, (201) 376-4355, BS 51 Syracuse Univ; MA 66 Newark St Coll; 66–Sp-Lang Path, Plainfield Bd of Ed, **SLP**

Zuraw, Edward Paul 2514 Warwick Court, Bay City, MI 48706, BS 60; MA 63 Central MI Univ; Sp-Lang Path, Carrollton Pub Sch, **SLP**

Zurenda, Joseph J 29 Wickman, Williamsville, NY 14221, (716) 834-9200, BA 72 Manhattan Coll; MA 77 CUNY - City College; **SLP**

Zurich, Mrs Sue A M 9 Berry Lane, Randolph, NJ 07869, BS 76 Ithaca Coll; MS 78 Rutgers St Univ -N Brunswick; Sp-Lang Path, State of New Jersey, **SLP**

Zurif, Dr Francoise L Speech & Language Center, 30 Tremont Street, Duxbury, MA 02332, (617) 934-0340, PH 84 (Psychology) Univ of Geneva - Switzerland; 85–Sp-Lang Path, Private Practice, **SLP**

Zurlinden, Mrs Patricia M 7885 Jolain Drive, Cincinnati, OH 45242, (513) 742-2200, BA 75 Cleveland St Univ; MA 76 Cleveland St Univ; Sp-Lang Path, Hamilton Co Office of Ed, **SLP**

Zurl-O'Day, Mrs Linda Mary 12 Beechwood Court, San Rafael, CA 94901, (415) 485-1912, MS 88 San Francisco St Univ; 88–Sp-Lang Path, Novato USD

Zurn, Michelle 1124 Wolf Street, Syracuse, NY 13208, (315) 253-6283, BS 77 SUNY - Coll at Fredonia; MS 82 Syracuse Univ; 85–Sp-Lang Path, Cayuga Co, **SLP**

Zurovski, Janet M L 1581 Redfield Court, San Jose, CA 95121, (408) 264-3803, BA 75 San Jose St Univ; MA 79 San Jose St Univ; Aud, West Vly Hrng Imp Cent, **A**

Zvejnieks, Mrs Anita Z 26912 Westwood Lane, Olmsted Township, OH 44138, (216) 574-8512, BA 75 Cleveland St Univ; MA 78 Cleveland St Univ; Sp-Lang Path, Cleveland Bd of Ed, **SLP**

Zwang, Fran S S 9 Pinewood Drive, Commack, NY 11725, **SLP**

Zwanziger, Mrs Dianne K 358 Rockhurst Court, Fairfield, CA 94533, (707) 426-2881, BS 70 Miami Univ - Oxford; MS 72 Purdue Univ - West Lafayette; **SLP ACE**

Zwaska, Janet Marie 5526 Englewood Drive, Madison, WI 53705, (608) 238-6152, BA 84 Univ of WI - Eau Claire; 87–Sp-Lang Path, M J Therapy Svcs, **SLP**

Zweben, Diane Mildred 62 Arlington Road, Devon, PA 19333, (215) 750-4001, BA 62 Jersey City St Coll; OM 85 Hahneman Medical Coll; 86–Sp-Lang Path, Beechwood Ctr for Head Injured, **SLP ACE**

Zweiban, Mrs Mira R 711 Essington Lane, Buffalo Grove, IL 60089, (312) 537-7455, BA 78 Univ of ND; MA 80 Univ of IL - Urbana; Admin Lang Rehab Pgm, Quality Hlth Care Ctrs Inc, **SLP**

Zweier, Jill Buttwinick Veterans Administration Medical Center, West Los Angeles (W126), Wilshire & Sawtelle Boulevard, Los Angeles, CA 90073, (213) 824-3100, BA 83 CA St Univ - Northridge; MA 85 CA St Univ - Northridge; 85–Sp-Lang Path, West LA VA Med Ctr, **SLP**

Zwick, Lynn K 1341 East 3rd Street, Brooklyn, NY 11230, (212) 998-1366, BA 77 CUNY - Brooklyn Coll; MS 79 CUNY - Brooklyn Coll; **SLP**

Zwier, Janet 602 Iowa Avenue S W, Orange City, IA 51041, (712) 737-3795, BS 72 KS St Univ; MA 73 KS St Univ; SLP, AEA 4, **SLP**

Zwierz, Judith Wolski 13024 South 71st Street, Palos Heights, IL 60463, (312) 687-7200, BA 79 Saint Xavier Coll; OM 82 Governors St Univ; Sp-Lang Path, Oak Forest Hosp, **SLP**

Zwink, Elizabeth Louise 33 Arthur Drive, Albany, NY 12208, (518) 732-7266, BS 82 Coll of Saint Rose; ME 84 Coll of Saint Rose; Sp-Lang Path, Rens-Col-Greene Counties BOCES, **SLP**

Zwir, Rosalie R 64 Linden Road, Barrington, RI 02806, **A**

Zwislocki, Dr Jozef J Institute For Sensory Research, Syracuse University, Syracuse, NY 13244, (315) 443-4164, OD 48 (Acoustics) Federal Inst of Tech - Zurich, Switzerland; 57–Prof, Syracuse U, **F**

Zwitman, Dr Daniel H 3556 Via Dolce, Marina Del Rey, CA 90292, (213) 208-6000, OB 64 Univ of Miami; MA 66 Western MI Univ; PH 70 (Sp Path & Aud) Univ of Pittsburgh - Pittsburgh; Private Practice, **SLP A**

Zwolan, Teresa A 320 West Illinois #2308, Chicago, IL 60610, (404) 971-6089, BS 83 Purdue Univ - West Lafayette; MA 85 Northwestern Univ; 88–Aud, Children's Mem Hosp, **A**

Zykorie, Bonnie E 6116 Rockwell Court, Burke, VA 22015, BS 66 Emerson Coll; MS 75 Univ of the DC; **SLP**

Zylla-Jones, Elizabeth M 5703 Alvarado, Houston, TX 77035, (713) 522-1051, BA 80 Univ of the Pacific; MS 82 Purdue Univ - West Lafayette; Sp/Lang Path, Childs Center for Dev Therapy, **SLP**

Zyrkowski, Mrs Nancy J Memorial Hospital, 615 North Michigan Street, South Bend, IN 46601, (219) 284-7953, BS 67 Marquette Univ; MA 68 De Paul Univ; Director Neuro Rehabilitation, Memorial Hospital South Bend, **SLP**

Zyskowski, Gladys Sophia 112 Wetzel Road, Pittsburgh, PA 15209, (412) 766-6615, BA 63 Carlow Coll; Sp Lang Cl, Allegheny Intermed Unit, **SLP**

GEOGRAPHICAL LIST OF MEMBERS

ALABAMA

Abbeville
Van Doorn-Conard, Elizabeth **(A)**

Alabaster
Boswell, Mrs Deborah Byrd **(SLP)**
Harris, Mrs Jodi Kennedy
Wright, Mrs Marianna Brogan **(SLP)**

Albertville
Calhoun, Mrs Cindy C **(SLP)**
Hamm-Sickles, Mrs Sharon K **(SLP)**
Iwankovitsch, Mrs Janet Jefferson **(SLP)**

Alexander City
Queen, Elizabeth Ann **(SLP)**
Smith, Sharon L **(SLP)**

Andalusia
Picking, Mrs Caroline Cumbie **(SLP A)**

Anniston
Babb, Mrs Elizabeth **(SLP)**
Diaz-Torres, Mrs Bonnie **(SLP)**
Kelley, Mrs Donna P **(SLP)**
Nevala, Betty Hill **(A)**
Ringer, Mrs Kayleen Mulford **(A)**
Rose, Carol Maj **(SLP)**
Rousey, Mrs Juliet S **(SLP)**
Williamson, Kelly S **(SLP)**
Wood, Patricia F **(SLP)**

Athens
Adams, H Gregory **(A)**
Sims, Mrs Laura Whitman **(SLP)**

Atmore
Jenkins, Terrilynn Faye **(SLP)**

Auburn
Baird, Dr Samera M **(SLP)**
Burns, Janet Zickfield **(SLP)**
Clark-Lewis, Sandra **(A)**
Cosgrove, Mrs Sheree H **(SLP)**
Couch, Mrs Gibbs Daniel **(SLP)**
Darling, Dr Rieko Marie **(A)**
Diebold, Dr Martin H **(SLP)**
Ferris-Reid, Gwen **(SLP)**
Finney, Virginia P **(SLP)**
Grant, Ann M **(SLP)**
Griffin, Mrs Margaret Ann **(SLP)**
Hargis, Mrs Janet V **(SLP)**
Hopkins, Mrs Ethel M **(A)**
Johnson, Victor Ross **(A)**
Miller-Wood, Deborah J **(SLP)**
Moore, Mary Virginia M **(SLP)**
Moran, Dr Michael J **(SLP)**
Payne, Robin L
Pindzola, Dr Rebekah Hand **(SLP)**
Ramsey, Mrs Pamela Davis **(SLP)**
Sayers, Mrs Leigh Camp **(SLP)**
Smith, Dr Curtis R **(SLP A)**
Tanja, Mrs Virginia Kathleen **(A)**
Walker, Christine **(SLP)**
Weidner, Dr William E **(SLP)**
Wolfe, Dr Virginia S **(SLP)**

Bellwood
Baker, Mrs Rita T **(SLP)**

Bessemer
Adams, Rita Lynn **(SLP)**
Bryant, Beverly J **(A)**

Birmingham
Adams, June B **(SLP)**
Alpiner, Dr Jerome G **(A)**
Anderson, Mrs Vicki Driver **(SLP)**
Arnold, Mrs Lynn C **(SLP A)**
Beckworth, Ralph M **(A)**
Bergren, Rebecca **(SLP)**
Betros, Cecil G, Jr **(SLP)**
Booker, Patricia E **(SLP)**
Borton, Mary Kealey **(SLP)**
Borton, Dr Thomas E, III **(A)**
Brown, Dr Loretta G **(SLP)**
Bryan, Debbie A **(SLP)**
Burke, Catherine Anne **(SLP)**
Caldwell, Mary A
Carmichael, Carol L **(A)**
Caudle, Mrs Teresa Harrison **(A)**
Chamblee, Mrs Barbara Fowler **(SLP)**
Churchill, Mrs Faye M **(SLP A)**
Clark, Lynnette **(A)**
Coley, Mrs Sherrill Quinn **(A)**
Crawford, Mary Schmalz **(SLP)**
Cunningham, Monyette W **(SLP)**
Cutchen, Mrs Judy Lee
Dagenais, Dr Paul A **(SLP)**
Dahle, Dr Arthur J **(SLP A)**
Davidson, Mrs Lanita Whitten
Dawkins, Patricia Harper
Dunivant, Mrs Janis H **(SLP)**
Durham, Mrs Kimberly Raybuck
Elkins, Dorothy B **(SLP)**
Enger, Nancy Christine **(SLP)**
Faucett, Mrs Ramona Aldridge **(SLP)**
Fendley, Frances M **(SLP)**
Fisher, Jeanne Hebert **(SLP)**
Flege, Dr James Emil
Fletcher, Dr Samuel G **(SLP A)**
Foster, Holly Krueger **(SLP)**
Freind, Mrs Deborah B **(A)**
Furio, Ellen D
Gant, Fiona Robertson **(SLP)**
Gilchrist, Mrs Shirley B **(SLP)**
Goldman, Dr Ronald **(SLP)**
Gray, Dorothy Davis **(SLP)**
Guerdat, Beverly Lambert **(SLP)**
Gullatt, Pamela E **(SLP)**
Hagood, Mrs Nancy P **(SLP)**
Hanvey, Sharon B **(SLP)**
Harrington, Shirley J **(SLP)**
Hays, Sylvia Samples **(A)**
Hemm, Dr Margaret E M **(SLP)**
Henderson, Rebecca W **(SLP)**
Hilyer, Mrs Tamela Hale **(SLP)**
Holifield, Mary M **(A)**
Hudson, Mrs Alane B **(A)**
Jackson, Dr Rosemary H **(SLP)**
Josof, Mrs Wadia Bolus **(SLP)**
Kanelos, Frank T **(SLP)**
Kauffman, Mary Jane **(SLP)**
King, Marie L **(SLP)**
Knapp, Brenda Kelly **(SLP)**
La Coste, Patricia A **(A)**
Lavender, Mrs Barbara Comstock **(SLP)**
Lessley, Elizabeth J
Lewis, Nancy Delaney **(SLP)**
Lott, Carol Lusco **(SLP)**
Luks, Susan Beall **(A)**
Mann, Mrs Judith G **(SLP)**
Marbury, Mrs Sharon Jeffcoat **(SLP)**
Marino, Gina Patricia **(SLP)**
Marshall, Nancy B **(SLP A)**
Mason-Clendaniel, Charlene Magaki **(SLP)**
Mayer, Mrs Theresa K **(SLP)**
McClintock, Mrs Ferne E **(SLP)**
McCollister, Mrs Faye Perry **(A)**
Moore, Mrs Joy Reed **(SLP)**
Moore, Mrs Susan Williams **(SLP)**
Morawetz, Mary Jean **(SLP)**
Murray, Mrs Gina Whatley **(SLP)**
Naccari, Angela Pumilia **(A)**
Nichols, Cynthia Gay **(SLP)**
Nolen, Bonnie Lynn **(A)**
O'Dell, Mrs Elizabeth Ward **(SLP)**
Ozley, Mrs Carleen F **(SLP)**
Price, Sandra Wayne **(SLP)**
Prince, Linda Price **(SLP)**
Putman, Donna Manning **(SLP)**
Reeves, Cintealia Paige **(SLP)**
Rentschler, Nancy S **(SLP)**
Richardson, Mrs Melissa Ann **(A)**
Riley, John Scott **(A)**
Roach, Dr Robert E **(A)**
Robertson, Patricia Rita **(A)**
Robinson, Leslie K **(SLP)**
Ross, Teresa Annette **(SLP)**
Rust-Miron, Mrs Jana Elizabeth **(SLP)**
Sahlie, Elizabeth **(SLP)**
Savasten, Patricia T **(SLP)**
Serota, Mrs Cynthia J **(SLP)**
Snell, Helen P **(SLP)**
Springfield, Mrs Amy P **(SLP)**
Summers, Mrs Janet T **(SLP)**
Sweitzer, Dr Richard S **(A)**
Swindle, Katherine Lucille **(SLP)**
Thomasson, Mrs Alice Wilson **(SLP)**
Thorson, Janice H **(SLP)**
Tucker, Mrs Ruth Strong **(SLP)**
Turner, Richard W, Jr **(SLP)**
Vaughn, Dr Gwenyth R **(SLP A)**
Westbrook, Linda A N **(SLP)**
Wilson, Mrs Mary Amanda
Wright, Linda Dunn **(SLP)**
Zinkowski, Debra Ann **(SLP)**

Brantley
Watson, Mrs Jennifer Becker **(SLP)**

Brundidge
Jones, Beverly Katrina **(SLP)**

Chatom
Montgomery, Dianne Dickey **(SLP)**

Clanton
Burlingame, Tammy L

Coffee Springs
Weaver, Laura O **(SLP)**

Columbiana
Ford, Joseph Edward **(A)**

Cropwell
Goodman, Peggy B **(SLP)**

Cullman
Canada, Mrs Conna **(A)**
Coffman, Mrs Angela Weston **(SLP)**
Cornett, Lynn H **(SLP)**

Dadeville
Britt, Mrs Colleen D **(SLP)**
Munson, Karen Slavens **(SLP)**

Daphne
Hosmer, Mrs Teri Lynn Johnson **(SLP)**
Murphy, Jan Marie **(SLP)**
Rodriguez, Pamela Hoffman **(SLP)**

Dauphin Island
Horn, Linda Diane **(SLP)**

Decatur
Boyd, Ronald D **(SLP)**
Burmester, Mrs Barbara Bridges **(SLP)**
Campbell, Mrs Margaret Anne **(SLP)**
Chalmers, Elizabeth **(SLP)**
Rowell, Mrs Tommye S **(SLP)**
Slack, Mrs Martha P **(SLP)**
Taylor, Charles R **(A)**
Verchot, Lucinda K **(SLP)**

Dothan
Arieux, Mrs Donna P **(SLP)**
Bell, Mrs Martha Groenendyk **(SLP)**
Clearman, Patsy Thomas **(SLP)**
Langford, Dr Ted L
Lawrence, Kimberly Ann **(SLP)**
Messer-Smith, Mrs Patricia D **(SLP)**
Peterman, Cheryl Stewart **(SLP)**
Schilder, Theresa D **(SLP)**
Steensland, Dianne D **(SLP)**
Tamblyn, Anne M
Walker, Rhonda Kim **(SLP)**
Watkins, Paula **(SLP)**
Wells, Jo Ann **(SLP)**
Williford, Christine Anne

Eastaboga
Yarbrough, Elizabeth **(SLP)**

Eufaula
Odom, Mrs Amelia M **(SLP)**
Walker, Mrs Linda Mathis **(SLP)**

Fairfield
Paxton, Anita T **(A)**

Fairhope
Barr, Mrs Audrey L C **(SLP)**
Broughton, Mrs Carol Kittrell **(SLP)**
Evans, Mrs Marilyn G **(SLP)**
Harmon, Electa M M **(SLP)**
Harmon, Harvey S **(SLP)**
Nason, Mrs Janet F **(SLP)**
White, Lisa Pace **(SLP)**

Fayette
Finley, Laurene T **(SLP)**

Fitzpatrick
Pickett, Mrs Gloria Oakes **(A)**

Florence
Baird, Mrs Beverly **(SLP)**
Burch, Donna **(SLP)**
Cocke, Carol B **(SLP)**
Maxwell, Mrs Rosalou S **(SLP)**
Novelli, Patsy Grissom **(A)**
Osborn, Mrs Diana Dickens **(SLP)**
Vest, Mrs Joyce C **(SLP)**

Foley
Taylor, Mrs Pamela Beane **(SLP)**

Fort Payne
Bowen, Deborah Trent
Green, Mrs Jeanie K **(SLP)**

Fort Rucker
Barson, Mrs Gay Lynn Flanders **(SLP)**
Nelson, William R **(A)**

Gadsden
Auerbach, Robin E **(A)**
Cusimano, Barbara Walker **(SLP)**
Hawkins, Mary F **(SLP)**
Newhoff, Dr Marilyn **(SLP)**

Gardendale
Cornelius, Donna Bean

Geneva
Helms, Mrs Donna Strickland **(SLP)**

Grove Hill
Wall, Mrs Ann M Brabston **(SLP)**

Gurley
Richardson, Joyce C **(SLP A)**

Haleyville
McDaniel, Mrs Diane F **(SLP)**

Hamilton
Barton, Marion Elizabeth

Harpersville
Johnston, Judy Franke **(SLP)**

Harvest
Bates, Mrs Ann Lloyd **(SLP)**
James, Mrs Sarah H **(SLP)**

Helena
Adams, Carroll M **(SLP)**
Adams, Dr Larry **(SLP)**
Barton, Mrs Vicki Parrish **(SLP)**
Crosby, Paula Critz
Harris, Mrs Pamela Seamon **(SLP)**
Rowe, Mrs Tammy De Boer **(A)**

Homewood
Baumgartner, Carolyn **(SLP)**
Phillips, Daniel E **(SLP)**

Hoover
Medlock, Sophia Anderton **(A)**
Miller, Judith C **(SLP)**
Patterson, Margaret J **(SLP)**

Hueytown
Parker, Mrs Mary Semrick **(SLP)**

Huntsville
Baker, Deborah E **(A)**
Barnes, Gertha Roberts **(SLP)**
Bernstein, Dr Joyce Edens **(SLP)**
Cady, Dr Barbara B **(SLP)**
Chvatal, Mrs Sarah Curtis **(SLP)**
Coffield, Phyllis Reel **(SLP)**
Fouts, Mrs Christine Mey **(SLP)**
Gaut, Katherine Carol **(SLP)**
Goltz, Nancy Carol **(SLP)**
Hall, Kim J **(SLP)**
Herrington, Mrs Dominique E Parish **(SLP)**
Holman, Mrs Eugenia Turner **(A)**
Humphrey, Mrs Anita
Johnson, Flora Renee
Lassiter, Josephine J **(SLP)**
Lehman, Mrs Donna Brooks **(SLP)**
Lehmann, Martha G R **(SLP)**
Mahone, Mrs Melissa McDonald **(SLP)**
McKinley, Anne C **(SLP)**
Miller, Nancy Joan **(SLP)**
Modlin, Mrs Marika G **(SLP)**
Moffet, Bethann
Murphree, George D, Jr **(A)**
Pennington, Mrs Gloria T **(SLP)**
Pierce, Mrs Roberta B **(SLP)**
Pruitt, Chris W **(A)**
Sharp, Mrs Deborah C **(SLP)**
Vinson, Mrs Jennifer Herndon **(SLP)**
Weathers, Kathryn Saxon **(SLP)**
Williams, Betty Mae **(SLP)**
Williams, Paula Sue P **(SLP)**
Woodcock, Linda W **(SLP)**
Wright, Mrs Pamela N **(SLP)**
Zangel, Mrs Barbara B **(A)**

Irvington
Blackard, Mrs Cornelia Nelms **(SLP)**

Jackson
Bridges, Mrs Dickie L **(SLP)**

Jacksonville
Roundtree-Newell, Janice **(SLP)**

Jasper
Briscoe-Hamilton, Patricia Lynn **(A)**
Simmons, Bettie B **(A)**

Lanett
Jackson, Mrs Jody Mayo **(A)**

Leeds
Adamson, Cathy **(A)**
Bell, Mrs Margaret L **(SLP)**
Borland, Laurie James **(SLP)**
Harrison, Tamara Davis **(SLP)**

Lowdesboro
McPherson, Mrs Lillian Lother **(SLP)**

Maddison
Lyons, Joy Lynn **(SLP)**

Madison
Biller, Maysoon Ibrahim **(SLP)**
Bunyard, Mrs Susan M G **(SLP)**
Jenkins, Mrs Melissa Kaye **(SLP)**
Nickey, Mrs Lynn M **(SLP)**
Turocy, Lynn M **(SLP)**

Marion Junction
Norton, Mrs Patricia R **(SLP)**

Maxwell AFB
Carter, Linda C F **(SLP)**

McCalla
Howton, Mrs Charlotte Powell **(SLP)**

Millbrook
Knight, Mrs Janice Knapp **(SLP)**

Mobile
Aldes, Maureen E **(SLP)**
Allen, Mrs Elizabeth Carter **(SLP)**
Atchison, Mrs Shirley A **(SLP)**
Austin, Lisa L **(SLP)**
Backes, Jeanne M **(SLP)**
Bell, Mrs Lynda G **(SLP)**
Botts, Lucia Marian **(A)**
Calogrides, Cynthia **(SLP)**
Cash, Rebecca A **(SLP)**
Cook, Theresa M **(SLP)**
Corley, Mrs Terry N **(SLP)**
Crary, Margaret A **(SLP A)**
Crenshaw, Fredda W **(SLP)**
Crowley, Mrs Grett Doneen **(SLP A)**
Deavours, Mrs Ross S **(A)**
Dorsey, Pamela Harrington **(SLP)**
Dranka, Mrs Sydney S **(SLP)**
Edwards, Laura J
Evans, Dr William Bryce **(SLP)**
Fitch, Dr James L **(SLP A)**
George, Mrs Melba E **(SLP)**
Gilbert, Sharon Lee
Hammock, Mrs Sandra W **(SLP)**
Hardaway, Mary Beth **(SLP)**
Hassell, Mrs Mary Cynthia **(SLP)**
Hearon, Mrs Betty C **(SLP)**
Hendrich, Betty G **(SLP)**
Hollon, Nancy B **(SLP)**
Holston, Joseph T **(A)**
Hood, Dr Stephen B **(SLP)**
Howse, Sandra F **(SLP)**
Huffman, Mrs Judith Bartels **(A)**
Johnson, Mrs Hettie P **(SLP)**
Jones, Nadine J **(SLP)**
Kotis, Christine Kelly **(SLP)**
Lattof, Mrs Marian T **(SLP)**
Lester, Leigh Ann
McDill, Dr Jim D **(A)**
Mitchell, Mrs Amy Burns **(SLP)**
Montgomery, Mrs Brenda Lynette **(SLP)**
Moseley, Mrs Susan M **(SLP)**
Newman, Connie Meyer **(SLP)**
Ogden, Patricia **(SLP)**
O'Hanlon, Mrs Angela M **(SLP)**
Perez, Mrs Randa A **(SLP)**
Rothaar, Thomas S **(SLP)**
Sellers, Dr Daniel E **(A)**
Sisk, E Diane **(SLP)**
Swan, Mrs Cynthia S **(SLP)**
Taylor, Trudy A **(SLP)**
Thomas, Kirsten Lynn
Vautier, Pamela D **(A)**
Waters, Melanie B **(SLP)**
Wilkins, Mrs Deborah M **(SLP)**
Wilkins, Mary Kathleen **(A)**
Wilson, Carolyn M **(SLP)**
Wilson, Mrs Linda S **(SLP)**
Windom, Mrs Catherine C **(SLP)**
Young, Mrs Pamela MacPherson **(SLP)**

Monroeville
Dozier, Betsy L **(SLP)**

Montevallo
Gibbs, Dr Denise P **(SLP)**
Gibbs, Steven D **(A)**
Meline, Nannette C **(A)**
Meline, Dr Timothy J **(SLP)**
Smith, Dr Wendell F **(SLP)**

Montgomery
Anderson, Laura Jean **(A)**
Belcher, Mrs Suzanne W **(SLP)**
Bess, Mrs Christine **(SLP)**
Brooks, Donna Kay **(SLP)**
Brown, Mrs Shirley W **(SLP)**
Caviness, Mrs Rebecca Parker **(A)**
Clark, Mrs Barbara S **(SLP)**
Cornell, Dr Richard A **(A)**
Cover, Mrs Suzanne Britt **(A)**
Davis, Melinda M **(A)**
Dennis, Mrs Laura Godbold
Faircloth, Mrs Betty Y **(SLP)**
Harmon, Hollie Ward **(SLP)**
Horner, Mrs Nettie K **(SLP)**
Johnston, Donna Lynn **(SLP)**
Laakman, Mrs Mary J **(SLP)**
Lammon, Mrs Kay L **(SLP)**
May, Mrs Betty Ann **(A)**
McGowin, Katherine Brown **(SLP)**
McGraw, Mrs Sandra A **(SLP)**
Morris, Mrs Sandra R **(A)**
Patton, Mrs Patricia A **(A)**
Posta, Elizabeth Anderson **(SLP)**
Pugh, Sallie Jeanette **(SLP)**
Richards, Darlene Marie **(SLP)**
Savage, David H **(SLP)**
Shook, Mrs Anita Mobley **(SLP)**
Shows, Dennis L **(SLP)**
Smiley, Rosemary **(SLP)**
Spivey, Mrs Kay W **(SLP)**
Tarver, Carolyn Williams **(SLP)**
Thomas, Georgeanne Marie **(A)**
Wallis, Donna Lynn **(A)**
Webster, Dr Elizabeth J **(SLP)**
Wright, Mrs E Devery **(SLP)**
Zieber, David Alan **(A)**

Mountain Brook
Ciamarra, Cheryl Ringuette **(SLP)**

Muscle Shoals
Beck, Joan Karen **(SLP)**
Williams, Mrs Nancy Ellen **(SLP)**

Northport
Bogardus, Ann Olson **(SLP)**
Charlton, Judith S **(A)**
Daffron, Margaret D **(SLP)**
Earley, Kenneth W **(SLP)**
Frederick, Mrs Roan K **(SLP)**
Graves, Laurel Nelson **(SLP)**
Hass, Mrs Margaret Slough **(SLP)**
Hindman, Mrs Sandra McGee **(A)**
Mansfield, Mrs Lynne N **(SLP)**
Sears, Loie P **(SLP)**

Odenville
Horton, Mrs Ellen Cowart **(SLP)**

Opelika
Crews, Richelle Webster **(SLP)**
Haynes, Maureen D **(SLP)**
Haynes, William O **(SLP)**
Middleton, Renee Annette **(A)**
Phillips, Mrs Sally M **(SLP)**
Rubio, Mrs Linda P **(SLP)**
Stearns, Mrs Cynthia Sims **(A)**
Waters, Gary D **(SLP)**
White, Mrs Dorenda T **(SLP)**
Willis, Mrs Dora W **(A)**

Ozark
Pryby, Mrs Helen Nessmith
Sherrard, Mrs Kyla C **(SLP)**

Pelham
Carroll, Mark Randolph **(A)**
Goossens', Dr Carol A **(SLP)**
Kent, Thomas P, Jr **(A)**
McFeeters, Donna S **(A)**

Phenix City
Bush, Patricia Mullin **(SLP)**
Nolin, Martha J **(SLP)**
Perdue, Mrs Annette P **(SLP)**

Pike Road
Knox, Mrs Jane Hastings **(SLP)**

Pinson
Blodgett, Lori Ruth **(SLP)**
Smith, Rebecca Dawn

Pleasant Grove
Lowry, James Keith **(A)**

Prattville
Coleman, Victoria Linder **(SLP)**
Comer, Mrs Judith W **(SLP)**
Fox, Dr Robert L **(SLP A)**
Fox, Sharon A **(SLP)**
Waggoner, Mrs Nancy E **(SLP)**

Ralph
Carver, Betty B **(SLP)**

Russellville
Ward, Melanie Denise **(SLP)**

Saraland
Reeves, Lisa Ann **(A)**

Satsuma
Knight, Doris Lee **(SLP)**

Scottsboro
Prickett, John M **(SLP)**

Selma
Newton, Mrs Lori J **(SLP)**

Semmes
Camilleri, Kathryn C **(SLP)**

Sheffield
Gresham, Richard Lee **(A)**
Smallwood, Anita E

Shorter
Hooks, Myra A **(A)**

Spanish Fort
Kissel, Ellen Elizabeth **(SLP)**
McDowell-Fleming, Martha M **(SLP)**

Sylacauga
Stover, Susan Eugena

Talladega
Hill, Mrs Mary B **(SLP)**
Overbey, William F **(A)**
Shackelford, Mrs Kathleen J **(SLP)**
Stiff, Janet Maria **(SLP)**

Theodore
Forman, Mrs Vernell S **(SLP)**
Garcia, Robert Gene **(A)**
Mertz-Garcia, Sara J **(SLP)**

Troy
Ingram, Rebecca Vinson **(SLP)**
Young, Cynthia H **(SLP)**
Youngblood, Mae **(SLP)**

Trussville
Crowley, Paula Wilson **(SLP)**
Peters, Mrs Cathy W **(SLP)**

Tuscaloosa
Bird, Mrs Linda Gray **(SLP)**
Brackett, Katherine **(A)**
Bradford, Pamela Walker **(SLP)**
Brockway, Nancy L
Brooks, Rebecca P **(A)**
Burch, Teresa S **(A)**
Burdick, Dr Jeanne H **(SLP)**
Burgess, Barbara B **(SLP)**
Byrd, Kathryn **(SLP)**
Charlton, Steve R **(A)**
Cooper, Mrs Crystal S **(SLP)**
Cooper, Dr Eugene B **(SLP)**
Culton, Dr Gerald Lee **(SLP)**
Curry, E Thayer **(SLP A)**
Dickard, Mrs Elizabeth Bentley **(SLP)**
Horne, Nancy L **(SLP)**
Johnson, Dr T Earle **(A)**
McCrary, Debra S **(SLP)**
McQueen, Karen Connor **(SLP)**
Nye, Denita Scott **(SLP)**
Pike, Lisa T **(SLP)**
Poole, Mrs Pamela B **(A)**
Robbins, Maxine G **(A)**
Rosen, Mrs Ella Zittrer **(SLP)**

Schmitt, Dr John F **(SLP)**
Schmitt, Lane S **(SLP)**
Sheeley, Dr Eugene C **(A)**
Talmadge-Sessions, Susan Victoria
Voltz, Mrs Kathy Ingram **(SLP)**
Wells, Mrs Barbara K **(SLP)**

Vestavia Hills
Horton, Sherri H **(SLP)**

Waverly
Jones, Mrs Patricia A **(A)**

Wetumpka
Hannah, Dr Joan B **(SLP)**
Hannah, Dr Joseph E **(A)**
Welch, Kathy W **(SLP)**

Winfield
McCullough, Mrs Eleanor B **(SLP)**

Woodland
McCord, Jill Stewart **(SLP)**

ALASKA

Anchorage
Agi, Mrs Esta-Dara **(SLP)**
Aufrecht, Joan B
Bowles, Marion D **(SLP)**
Brewer, Kelly Scannell **(SLP)**
Brueggemann, David J **(A)**
Canterbury, Dr David Richard **(A)**
Coe, Carolyn M **(SLP)**
Creegan, Elizabeth **(SLP)**
Duthie, Jill K **(SLP)**
Erb, Mrs Linda V **(A)**
Foley, Celia **(SLP)**
Garner, Betty **(A)**
Green, Laurie **(SLP)**
Griffo, Margaret K **(SLP)**
Hartke, Susanne **(SLP)**
Holmes, Mrs Pamela K **(SLP)**
Horne, Mrs Martine Elizabeth **(SLP)**
Hubbard, Nancy Ehle **(SLP)**
Hughes, Eileen Karen **(SLP)**
Kautzman, Laura Katherine **(SLP)**
Levesque, Ute D **(A)**
Libby, Mrs Christina Aldea **(SLP)**
Loutrel, Barbara H **(SLP)**
McBride, Gilda Chauvin **(SLP)**
McCarty, Thomas A **(A)**
McKinnis, Mrs Sandra K **(SLP)**
Miner, Kathleen **(SLP)**
Normandeau, Ann Renee **(SLP)**
Olsen, Lylis E **(A)**
Otwell, Freda Williams **(SLP)**
Powers, Jeri L **(A)**
Roberson, Mrs Carolyn J **(SLP)**
Roberts, Cathryn L **(SLP)**
Ross, Brenda K **(SLP)**
Roulo, Rosemary A **(SLP)**
Schilling, Marcia M **(SLP)**
Strutzel, Karla K **(SLP)**
Tomory, Raymond Julius **(SLP)**
Tremblay, Michelle A **(SLP)**
Ver Hoef, Anne L **(SLP)**
Yarzebinski, Mrs Sally G **(SLP)**

Angoon
Lane, Scott Robert **(SLP)**

Auke Bay
Blair, Mrs Kim M **(SLP)**
Gustine, Mrs Dixie A **(SLP)**

Barrow
Alexander, Mrs Twylla B **(SLP)**
Christianson, Mrs Pamela Paguia
Wood, Mary Ann Duggan **(A)**

Bethel
Lopez, M B **(A)**

Big Lake
Thamm, Mrs Merikaye Mitchell **(SLP)**

Chugiak
Sexton, Joyce Forrester **(SLP A)**
Thistlethwaite, Nancy L **(SLP)**

Clam Gulch
Martin, Mrs Karen Marie **(A)**

Eagle River
Anderson, Roy Bruce **(A)**
Goldstein, Joan Eagle **(SLP)**
Grinstead, Dr Geraldine LaCourt **(A)**
Marzonie-Devine, Monica **(SLP)**
Olmstead, Mrs Patricia J **(SLP)**
Poage, Mrs Diane Louise **(SLP)**
Stoebner, Mrs Ronda Palmer **(SLP)**
Teich, Cathleen **(SLP)**

Elmendorf AFB
Campbell, John C **(A)**

Fairbanks
Berrie, Mrs Elaine B **(SLP)**
Blockcolsky, Valeda N **(SLP)**
Cleworth, Mrs Janice E **(SLP)**
Dauenhauer, Sandra G **(SLP)**
Ferguson, Monica L **(SLP)**
Finstad, Linette Arloine **(SLP)**
Gish, Keith D **(A)**
Guinn, Suzanne Y **(SLP)**
Hall, Mrs Susan Larkins **(SLP)**
Kennedy, Susan Liff **(A)**
Pippin, Kerry Rae **(SLP)**
Rongstad, William Alver **(A)**
Vrablik, Mrs Charlotte **(SLP)**
Wharam, Kate **(SLP)**
Williams, Phyllis Cashen **(A)**

Fort Wainwright
Mitchell, Mrs Patricia D **(SLP)**

Girdwood
Le Levier, Suzanne Marie **(A)**

Homer
Hartigan, Mrs Nancy J **(SLP)**

Juneau
Bergeron, Laura **(SLP)**
Betit, Suzanne L **(A)**
Hatt, Shawn Terese
Murphy, Janice S **(SLP)**
Sanders, Mrs Rachel Johnson **(SLP)**
Tonkovich, Mary J H **(SLP)**

Ketchikan
Chandler, Cecelia M **(SLP)**
Packet, Linda L **(SLP)**
Schuerger, Karen Stafford **(SLP)**

Kodiak
Holzshu, Nancy Lee **(SLP)**

Kotzebue
Driscoll, Janene M **(SLP)**

Metlakatla
Ross, Dona R **(SLP)**

Nome
Arin, Merle Allan **(SLP)**
Lemaster, Mrs Beverly Joan **(A)**
Roy, Linda McCarty **(SLP)**

North Pole
Benshoof, Mrs Geraldine **(SLP)**
Cannon, Charlotte Perala **(SLP)**
Nelson, Mrs Patricia M **(SLP)**

Sitka
Bunting, Susan **(A)**
Morse, Stephen D **(SLP)**

Soldotna
Beeson, Mrs Cheryl A **(SLP)**
Burman, Barbara E **(SLP)**
Marsh, Diana M **(SLP)**
Powers, Mrs Bonnie R **(SLP)**
Springer-Hann, Patricia **(SLP)**

Valdez
Devens, Dr John S **(SLP A)**

Wasilla
Altman, Dr Mickey D **(SLP)**
Bikulcs, Lucy **(SLP)**
McNeese-Elliott, Linda **(SLP)**
Stein, Mrs Gary Bonita

ARIZONA

Apache Junction
Burke, Mrs Sharon Lynn **(SLP)**
Deans, Mary Frances **(SLP)**

Chandler
Andrews, Mrs Nancy A Lunde **(SLP)**
Baxter-Saari, Deborah **(A)**
Bishoff, Tracey Jeanne **(A)**
Bossuyt, Colette M **(SLP)**
Brown, Mrs Lenora Harden **(SLP)**
Casanova, Mrs Christine Digges **(SLP)**
Demars, Virginia Ella **(SLP)**
Gabriel, Mrs Roxanne Marie **(SLP)**
Hawkins, Mrs Carol J **(A)**
Heim, Clareen **(SLP)**
Holen, Deborah **(SLP)**
Horewitch, Mrs Laurie Lentz **(SLP)**
Kenna, Peggy T **(SLP)**
Meador, Mrs Jeanette D **(SLP)**
Measeles-Allen, Larwin Michele **(SLP)**
Pearson, Mrs Lisa M **(SLP)**
Seale, Linda Ruth **(A)**
Spaulding, Laura C **(SLP)**
Walker, Mrs Linda A

Chinle
Adams, Terri Ruth **(SLP)**

Clarkdale
Bliss, Beverly B **(SLP)**

Coolidge
Flenner, Carolyn Ferrell **(SLP)**

Cottonwood
Walsh, Mrs Bobbie Jean Lee **(SLP)**

Flagstaff
Gartland, Dr Margaret-Ann D **(SLP)**
Graham, Mrs Edith Elizabeth **(SLP)**
Gross, Gail Y **(SLP)**
Jacobs, Ellen L **(SLP)**
Jensen, Mrs Marilyn **(SLP)**
Koudelka, Garry Anthony **(SLP)**
Lamb, Wendy Meredith **(SLP)**
Mahosky, Katherine Passmore **(SLP)**
Martin, Mrs Susan C **(SLP)**
Nye, Dr Chad **(SLP)**
Palcich, William Joseph **(SLP)**
Reid, Karyn A **(SLP)**
Rotert, Teresa Marie **(SLP)**
Stubblefield, Dr James H **(SLP A)**
Tanner, Dr Dennis C **(SLP)**
Weems, Dr Linda J **(SLP)**

Fort Huachuca
Couey, Mrs Catherine W **(SLP)**

Fountain Hills
Card, Georgia Therese **(SLP)**

Ganado
Kennedy, Darlene A **(SLP)**

Gilbert
Ahlman, Mrs Pamela S **(SLP)**
Dees, Sharon E
Harding, Kim Jared **(SLP)**
Howard, Mrs Jackie A **(SLP)**
Kenney, Kathryn W **(SLP)**
Martin, Carol F **(SLP)**
Nelson, Cheryl Dee **(SLP)**
Pfeiffer, Mary P **(SLP)**
Slapper, Mrs Beth W **(SLP)**
Zimmerman, Carla Marie **(SLP)**

Glendale
Ackerman, Mrs Sonia Sperry **(SLP)**
Blewett, Mrs Jana L **(SLP)**
Buckler, Mrs Jennifer Margaret
Butler, Dr Myrtice R **(SLP)**
Camponovo, Mrs Trudie G **(SLP)**
Colyar, Terry C **(SLP)**
Coze, Elizabeth Alexandra **(SLP)**
Daniels, Mrs Kathy Colene **(SLP)**
Dobbins, Edward Anthony **(A)**
Dutton, Mrs Susan Marie **(SLP)**
Elliott, Christine **(SLP)**
Geldin, Irving H **(SLP)**
Gray, Mrs Susan Robinson **(SLP)**
Hoffman, Cindy Sue **(SLP)**
Jacobs, Donald W **(SLP)**
Julien, Mrs Judith Rae **(SLP)**
Labrozzi, Karen M **(SLP)**
Lepkowski, Mary Ellen Burns **(SLP)**
Maes-Serazio, Audrey Susan **(SLP)**
McCarthy, Mrs Constance **(SLP)**
Pearsall, Mrs Debra Ann **(SLP)**
Pourkaveh, Faith Alison **(SLP)**
Ryan, Mrs Patricia M **(SLP)**
Shoop, Deborah H **(SLP)**
Swanson, Leslie K **(SLP)**
Tominac, Cheryl Ann **(SLP)**
Zampini, Mrs Nancy Diane **(SLP)**

Green Valley
Rosenfeld, Laura S **(SLP)**

Holbrook
Scorse, Denise **(SLP)**

Kayenta
Alexander, Jan Wrather

Kingman
Collett, Holly Marjorie **(SLP)**
DeWeese, Mrs Barbara P **(SLP)**
Foster, Stephen C **(SLP)**
Jacobelli-Glass, Lucia Jo **(SLP)**

Lake Havasu City
McDonald, Barbara Jean **(SLP)**
Reeves, Toni Ann
Rosinski, Mrs Patrice Ann **(SLP)**
Tracy, Marilyn Louise **(SLP)**

Laveen
Royse, Catherine L **(SLP)**

Maricopa
Ormson, Mary Frances **(A)**

Mesa
Anderson, Daryrene
Bissinger, Kathy M **(A)**
Bloyer, Cynthia J **(A)**
Bonitati, Mrs Carolyn L **(SLP)**
Boragina, Annette
Brown, Mrs Mary E **(A)**
Byerly, Mary Ann **(SLP)**
Byrnes, Nona Jane **(SLP)**
Carter, Randall Harrison **(SLP)**
Carter, Mrs Rita Gail **(A)**
Caywood, Janet L **(SLP)**
Chery, Pamela L **(SLP)**
Comerchero, Sherry R **(SLP)**
Connell, Sheila M **(A)**
Cummard, Mrs Kathryn Anne **(SLP)**
Dormady, Elizabeth P **(SLP)**
Downing, Mrs Karla Deane **(SLP)**
Ehret, Mrs Patricia M **(A)**
Ely, Monica **(SLP)**
Farrand, Tad **(A)**
Forst, Mary Canon **(SLP)**
Frye, Mrs Linda Jambor **(SLP)**
Hellman, Laurie Jean **(SLP)**
Hevezi, Rose Ann **(SLP)**
Hines, Mrs Lisa Marie **(SLP)**
Jaffa, Mrs Helen S **(SLP)**
Jensen, Marian Mahfood **(A)**
Jensen, Mrs Nancy L **(A)**
Jensen, Robert J **(A)**

Kinney, Brenda L **(SLP)**
Lear, Dorothy Ann **(SLP)**
Loui, Calvin M **(A)**
Merritt, Mrs Susan J **(SLP)**
Migaki, Karen Jo **(A)**
Moore, Gregory Robert **(A)**
Morse, Anita Wooten **(SLP)**
Oltmann, Mrs Donna Sandquist **(SLP)**
Peters, Mrs Becky S **(SLP)**
Pezzelle, Mrs Sheryl Sue **(SLP)**
Pfrang, Mrs Cynthia L **(SLP)**
Powell, Colette Suzanne **(SLP)**
Proctor, Mrs Linda McCormick **(SLP)**
Ringdahl, Marian M **(A)**
Rumack, Mrs Nancy Berg **(SLP)**
Russell, Rebecca R **(SLP)**
Schall-Woodley, Dr Joann **(SLP)**
Scharber, Robert J **(A)**
Sheehan, Mary T **(SLP)**
Smith, Mrs Sherry Stewart **(A)**
Street-Speck, Mrs Diane M **(SLP)**
Sumner, Mrs Pamela J **(SLP)**
Toussaint-Krutz, Mrs Lois C **(SLP)**
Walmsley, Mrs Sandra D **(SLP)**
Wavrin, Nancy Ellen **(SLP)**
Weaver, Stephen Craig **(SLP)**
Weis, Patricia A **(A)**
Welker, Mrs Ann M **(SLP)**
Westmoreland, Mrs Deborah E **(SLP)**
White, Mrs Anne Elaine **(SLP)**
White, Carol Marie **(SLP)**
Windman, Mrs Gail G **(SLP)**
Witmer, Julie Deanne **(SLP)**
Wrich, Mrs Mary Jacquelyn **(SLP)**

Oracle
Huntington, Kathleen M **(SLP)**

Page
Lehn, Mrs Ann Marie **(SLP)**

Paradise Valley
Gerber, Mrs Marilyn S **(SLP)**
Kelley, Laura N **(A)**
Norman-Murch, Dr Trudi N **(SLP)**
Posner, Mrs Ellen S **(SLP)**

Patagonia
Fulcomer, Mrs Lauren Russell **(SLP)**

Peoria
Armour, Lucinda G **(SLP)**
Benge, Mrs Mary Riley **(SLP)**
Coughlin, Mrs Bonita G **(SLP)**
Olson, Mrs Laurel **(A)**
Plamondon, Emily Ann **(SLP)**
Plamondon, Keith Allen **(A)**
Sapp, Mrs Sally Sue **(SLP)**
Sedlacek, Virginia **(A)**
Siegelman, Steven M **(SLP)**

Phoenix
Adams, Lisa Ann **(SLP)**
Allen, Mrs Mary Kay DeBoer **(SLP)**
Anderson, Mrs Christina Susanne **(SLP)**
Anderson, Mrs LaVae M Hoffman **(SLP)**
Andriacchi, Catherine **(SLP)**
Balko, Karla Ann **(A)**
Benson, Mrs Mary Elizabeth **(SLP)**
Black, Margaret A **(SLP)**
Black, Mrs Muriel K **(SLP)**
Blair, Julie Ann **(SLP)**
Bloeser, Mrs Rubye H **(SLP)**
Borgeas, Mrs Serita B **(SLP)**
Brevoort, Sarah Hines **(SLP)**
Budrzysky, Julie Ann **(SLP)**
Burk, Mrs Cindy **(SLP)**
Burke, Nancy M **(SLP)**
Cantrill, Craig E **(SLP)**
Cantrill, Mrs Vicki C **(SLP)**
Carr, Cynthia D **(SLP)**
Cattey, Tommy J **(A)**
Chandler, Elizabeth Frances **(SLP)**
Charlesworth, Barbara S **(SLP)**
Chiapello, Dennis Albert **(SLP)**
Clark, Jeanne Paquette **(SLP)**
Clark, Mrs Karen Whipple **(SLP)**
Clarke, Mrs Donna M **(SLP)**
Clasgens, Mrs Pamela Sue **(A)**
Clees, Patricia B **(A)**
Colby, Mrs Eileen R **(SLP)**
Cooler, Sarah J **(SLP)**
Coope, Mrs Beverly Ray **(SLP)**
Cooper, Larry M **(SLP)**
Crowley, Kathleen Moynahan **(SLP)**
Cummins, Christine Ellen **(A)**
Cutsinger, Linda K **(SLP)**
Dahl, Cecilia W **(SLP)**
Dashefsky, Mrs Randy L **(SLP)**
Davids, Mrs Francine Elissa **(SLP)**
Davis, Mrs Kathleen Duffy **(SLP)**
Dean, Janet Therese **(SLP)**
Deangelis, Deborah Ann **(SLP)**
Derrick, Betty K **(A)**
Dillon, Debra Dawn **(SLP)**
Distin, Viki Linneman **(A)**
Dodge, Mrs Diane DiMaio **(SLP)**
Drake, Gloria S **(SLP)**
Duffy-Gillespie, Janet **(SLP)**
Edelberg, Mrs Ann Rita **(SLP)**
Elliott, Norma H **(SLP)**
Engle, Linda A **(SLP)**
Ensign, Patricia Moats
Fairbank, Mrs Carlene Marie **(SLP)**
Fairfax, Mrs Lyn M **(SLP)**
Farrell, Cynthia Fangman **(SLP)**
Fitz, Mrs Mary L **(SLP)**
Fitzgerald, Mrs Karen Ann **(SLP)**
Fitzgerald, Margaret Marie **(SLP)**
Flitner, Laurene Lukas **(SLP)**
Folsom, Laura Clark **(SLP)**
Frazer, Mrs Joan M **(SLP)**
Geclewicz, Mirla **(SLP)**
Getz, Phyllis **(SLP)**
Giordano, Mrs Lorraine A **(SLP)**
Goering, Mrs Danielle M **(A)**
Grady, Barbara J **(SLP)**
Guzman, Charles R **(SLP)**
Habgood, Karen Lynne **(SLP)**
Hackett, Mrs Anita C **(SLP)**
Hall, Dr Allen Sanders **(SLP)**
Haney, Patricia **(A)**
Harris, Mrs Amy B **(SLP)**
Hassett, Kelly Marie **(SLP)**
Hayes, Mrs Debra H **(SLP)**
Hill, Mrs Betsy P **(SLP)**
Hill, Mrs Sandra L **(SLP)**
Hixson-Robles, Cynthia **(A)**
Holtzapple, Pat Ann **(SLP)**
Hubschman, Dr Eva W **(SLP)**
Hurlbert, Linda L **(SLP)**
Jarvis, Mrs Kelly Michele **(SLP)**
Johnson, Geraldine **(SLP)**
Jolley, Ray Garth **(A)**
Jones, Mrs Amy J **(A)**
Jones, Mrs Cynthia Winham **(A)**
Jones, Mrs Dinah R **(SLP)**
Katz, Jodi Robin **(SLP)**
Keene, Mrs Lisa C **(SLP)**
Kendall, Deborah Anne **(SLP)**
Kohl, Mrs Evelyn P **(SLP)**
Kordek, Dolores A **(A)**
Krieski, Sandra Nan **(SLP)**
Kronberg, Linda Ann **(SLP)**
Kundin, Mrs K R **(SLP)**
Kurn, Mrs Barbara A **(SLP)**
Laikko, Terry McGrath **(SLP)**
Larson, Steven Kenneth
Law, Patricia L **(SLP)**
Lei, Linnea **(SLP)**
Linam, Virginia L **(A)**
Loudenslagel, Jean F **(SLP)**
Loudenslagel, Mark W **(SLP)**
Lukas, Julie S **(A)**
Lyons, Teresa S **(SLP)**
Martin, Margaret **(SLP)**
Marton, Karen D **(A)**
Mayfield, Bonnie L **(SLP)**
McClanahan, Deana Sue
McGary-Fynmore, Susan **(SLP)**
McIntosh, Margaret Swanson **(SLP)**
McKee, Mrs Joan Tolley **(SLP)**
McMillan, Don Fraizer **(A)**
Meschnark, Nancy Newell **(SLP)**
Meyer, Judith Pollack **(SLP)**
Mikkelsen, Debra Kay **(SLP)**
Miller, Mrs Kathryn A **(SLP)**
Miller, Kathryn A **(SLP)**
Miller, Suzanne D **(SLP)**
Miller, Suzanne Marie **(SLP)**
Moeller, Sharon A **(SLP)**
Mollison, Karen Kelly **(SLP)**
Morton, Mrs Cheryl Myers
Movitz, Linda **(A)**
Mullica, Karyn L **(SLP)**
Nagle, Mary Carlin **(SLP)**
Nelson, Mrs Barbara Mills **(SLP)**
Noonan, Mrs Krista Weinhold **(SLP)**
North, Mrs Kay Smith **(SLP A)**
Novy, Fred John **(A)**
Ober, Mrs Gail Silber **(SLP)**
O'Keefe-La Pratt, Nancy J **(SLP)**
Ouellette, Donna I **(A)**
Pappas, Ranae Tone **(SLP)**
Pellini, Mrs Jo Ann **(SLP)**
Perfect, Mrs Joni Boysen **(SLP)**
Pike, Gayle Lancaster **(SLP)**
Pohlman, Mrs Virginia Bregar **(SLP)**
Prather, Dr Elizabeth M **(SLP)**
Prather, Dr William F **(A)**
Quintana, Mrs Marilyn Miller **(SLP)**
Rasmussen, Catherine Ann **(SLP)**
Ray, Georgine Haines **(A)**
Raymond, Susan Benjamin **(SLP)**
Readhead, Donna Geralyn **(SLP)**
Reese, Gaylen L **(A)**
Romano, Mary Anne McMahon **(SLP)**
Rosen-Rudin, Robin Amy **(SLP)**
Rothberg, Susan Lori
Ruby, Trena G **(A)**
Runbeck, Mrs Robyn Goddard **(SLP)**
Runge, Cheryl A **(A)**
Runyon, Mrs Jill Lynn **(SLP)**
Ruzicka, Mrs Tamyra L
Sabo, Michael P **(A)**
Sarginger, Kathryn Steinbach **(SLP)**
Schaefer, Mrs Patricia **(SLP)**
Schlappi, Mrs Carole Rayline **(SLP)**
Schrader, Patricia F **(SLP)**
Schultz, Cynthia Lynn **(SLP)**
Schuster, Carolyn Susan **(SLP)**
Schwartz, Mrs Shawnee K **(SLP)**
Seiler, Susan **(A)**
Shannon, Mrs Michelle Renee **(SLP)**
Sheehy, Bruce Frank **(A)**
Shultz, Mrs Diane Carol **(A)**
Sloan, Debra Peacock **(SLP)**
Sotelo, Mrs Judith Connolly **(SLP)**
Squier, Sheryl Lynn **(SLP)**
Staab, Dr Wayne J **(A)**
Staffan, Kristin Ann
Stultz, Pamela Ann **(SLP)**
Sundstrom, Pat K **(SLP)**
Taylor, Bonnie Ellen **(A)**
Teodoro, Mrs Sally Ann **(A)**
Teodoro, Stephen F **(A)**
Texada, Kristin E **(SLP)**
Vazquez, Mrs Terry Linda **(SLP)**
Von Cloedt, Dr Carol Denise **(SLP)**
Walker, Kathryn **(SLP)**
Walker, Mrs Mary Jo **(SLP)**
Weiner, Carolyn Ausberger **(SLP)**
Weir, Lynn Hoffman **(SLP)**
Welsh, Terry D **(SLP)**
Werner, Mrs Anita B **(SLP)**
Whaley, Patricia **(SLP)**
Wright, Mrs Varla Jane **(SLP)**
Zerfas, Kimberly Jo **(SLP)**
Zraick, Richard Isaac

Pinetop
Gray, Mrs Wanda L **(SLP)**
Martin, Mrs Bobette Susanne **(A)**

Prescott
Crain, Rene A **(SLP)**
Foss, Cynthia **(SLP)**
Guile-Lange, Laurie M **(SLP)**
Holmes, David A **(A)**
Moses, Dr Elbert R, Jr **(SLP)**
Robbins, Colleen **(SLP)**

Prescott Valley
Brooks, Leonard L **(SLP A)**

Safford
Schade, Mrs Paula M **(SLP)**

San Manuel
Stager, Mrs Sharlene M **(SLP)**

Scottsdale
Amenson, Mrs Gail Arlene **(SLP)**
Andersen, Beverly H **(SLP A)**
Ball, Barbara Anne **(SLP)**
Bassett, Michele **(A)**
Bates, Dr Kathie Berles **(SLP)**
Beichel, Mrs Pamela Lory **(SLP)**
Bernstein, Lois M **(SLP)**
Brenner, Mrs Ann C **(SLP)**
Broner, Judy **(SLP)**
Bryant, Mrs Karen Theresa **(SLP)**
Burkett, Argyra Marie **(A)**
Bush, Mrs Catherine W **(SLP)**
Calvin, Mrs Sarah Ellis **(SLP)**
Carsch, Mrs Deborah Brown **(SLP)**
Cevette, Dr Michael J **(A)**
Chapman, Maureen Ann
Conley, Patricia Tautfest **(SLP)**
Cooper, Mrs Linda C **(SLP)**
Cosgrove, Dawn Michele **(SLP)**
Crew, Mrs Deanna H **(SLP)**
Currier, Mrs Laura Chesler **(SLP)**
Day, Dana Louise **(A)**
Drye, Cynthia A
Frame, Rebecca L **(SLP)**
Friedman, Mrs Ruth F **(SLP)**
Gnotta, Lillian S **(SLP A)**
Goldstein, Jill E K **(SLP)**
Gotsch, Mrs Linda Joyce
Graham, Lisa Fletcher **(SLP)**
Harper, Sandra Ann **(A)**
Heob, William G **(A)**
Herbst, Nancy Suzanne **(SLP)**
Hoole, Caroline E **(SLP)**
Kafer, Joan Desrochers **(A)**
Kurth, Cathy E **(A)**
Larson, Janet Inga **(SLP)**
Linovitz, Maeva P **(SLP)**
Martin, Joanne C **(SLP)**
Matheson, Linda A **(SLP)**
Maynor, Joyce Lynn **(SLP)**
Mazursky, Mrs Marcie Alpert **(SLP)**
McGuire, Jane E **(SLP)**
Miller, Terri Lynne **(SLP)**
Mills, Susan J **(SLP)**
Mongoven, Mary Elizabeth **(SLP)**
Nagy, Mrs Denise E **(SLP)**
Nedberg, Patricia J **(SLP)**
Neidlinger, Mrs Susan C **(SLP)**
Nelson, Joan **(SLP)**
Nicklawsky, Lisa Mary **(SLP)**
Noble, Mrs Lynn
Norwood, Elena D **(SLP)**
Novak, Constance W **(SLP)**
Okun, Mrs Sue Kneler **(SLP)**
Perry, Maureen Mooney **(SLP)**
Petersen, Mrs P Diane **(SLP)**
Peterson, Catherine H **(SLP)**
Peterson, Mrs Kathleen Evans **(A)**
Pristo, Ellen **(SLP)**
Rosher, Ellen M **(SLP)**
Row, Sandra M **(SLP)**
Savage, N Leslie **(SLP)**

Seplow, Mrs Marilyn K **(SLP)**
Shaw, Mrs Karen A **(SLP)**
Shepherd, Janet C **(SLP)**
Simpson, Mrs Vickie Myers **(SLP)**
Snyder, Mrs Francesca Engler **(SLP)**
Soli, Sydney Jane **(SLP)**
Spadafore, Mary Jo **(SLP)**
Sroda, Mrs Mary Ellen **(SLP)**
Stockman, Lavonne S **(SLP)**
Trunzo, Mary Jane **(SLP)**
Turek, Sandra L **(A)**
Van Luven, Elizabeth **(SLP A)**
Vulcano, Mrs Sally A M **(SLP)**
Wennersten, Linda Kugler **(SLP)**
Wiss, Mrs Deborah Crantz **(SLP)**
Yakel, Elizabeth **(SLP)**

Sedona
Jobe, Brenda **(A)**

Sierra Vista
Webb, Michael O **(A)**
Zackey, Julie Engstrom **(SLP)**

Sun City
Casebier, Dr Gabrielle **(SLP)**
Farrell, Kathleen Faye **(SLP)**
Lovering, Dr Larry J **(A)**
Runion, Dr Howard L **(SLP)**
Shotwell, Mrs Jeannette **(SLP)**
Wright-Edwards, Clark F **(A)**

Sun City West
Schaetzel, Mrs Anne Nottingham **(SLP)**

Sun Lakes
Patton, Mrs Eleanor Miller **(SLP)**

Tempe
Albright, Mrs Joy S **(SLP)**
Bacon, Dr Sid P
Balser, Elnora M **(SLP A)**
Belus, Gail Seiler **(SLP A)**
Blohm, Mrs Elizabeth J
Borman, Deborah Lynn **(SLP)**
Bostrom, Debra Withers **(SLP)**
Bourbouse, Janet M **(SLP)**
Brown, Jean C **(SLP)**
Call, Wendy M W **(SLP)**
Case, Dr James L **(SLP)**
Cedar, Ingrid Kristina **(A)**
Cheslik, Paula C **(SLP)**
Chouard, Jeanne Campbell **(SLP)**
Chubrich, Robert **(SLP)**
Chubrich, Mrs Ronda C **(SLP)**
Click, Marilyn J **(SLP)**
Cluff, Dr Gordon L **(SLP A)**
Colleran, Eileen Marie **(A)**
Compton, Mrs Gladys B **(A)**
Cordova-Voron, Mrs Cecilia
Cronin, Denise Lynn **(SLP)**
Dudley, Mrs Susan M **(SLP)**
Everts, Kathryn W **(SLP)**
Fausett, Mrs Linda R **(SLP)**
Fontes, Daniel **(SLP)**
Fontes, Kristine C **(SLP)**
Gitlis, Karyn R **(SLP)**
Hart, Merilyn Kay **(SLP)**
Hueffner, Debra Sue **(A)**
Johnson, Kathleen R **(SLP)**
Kelley, Mrs Anita Jaime **(SLP)**
LaPointe, Dr Leonard Lyell **(SLP)**
Loring, Mrs Julie K **(SLP)**
McBride, David Lawrence **(A)**
Mintz, Sandra Lee **(A)**
Moore, Kathleen A **(SLP)**
Mowrer, Dr Donald **(SLP)**
Parady, Susan K **(SLP)**
Pihl, Karen L **(SLP)**
Riding, Mrs Nancy Campbell **(A)**
Schaffer, Susan Renee **(SLP)**
Sharp, Mrs Sheryl Fursteneau **(SLP)**
Simon, Charlann S **(SLP)**
Solan, John Raymond **(A)**
Stein, Sharon Bengel **(SLP)**
Sunday, Deborah Lynne **(SLP)**
Talamante, Patricia P **(SLP)**
Thompson, Donald L **(SLP)**
Tiller, Gary Robert **(SLP)**
White, Blaik J **(SLP)**

Temple
Hawker, Marilyn Evans **(SLP)**

Tuba City
Johnson, Therese Ann **(SLP)**
Long, Susan Michele **(SLP)**
O'Connor, Ann Monsor **(SLP)**

Tubac
Hansen, Karen V **(SLP)**

Tucson
Aitken, Mrs Karen B **(SLP)**
Alfonso, Rosa Maria **(SLP)**
Altman, Mary Ellen **(SLP)**
Anderson, Ruth M **(SLP)**
Arthur, Susan Ann **(SLP)**
Avolio, Mrs Wendy F **(SLP)**
Bailey, Mary Ellen **(SLP)**
Baker, Karen Lee **(SLP)**
Barney, Riley J **(A)**
Barsky, Mrs Shari Lisa **(SLP)**
Bayles, Dr Kathryn A **(SLP)**
Beeson, Pelagie M **(SLP)**
Belk, Dr Judith B **(SLP A)**
Bellissima, Mary Ann L **(A)**
Berkin, Alissa M **(SLP)**
Blackmon, Shirley Renee **(SLP)**
Boone, Dr Daniel R **(SLP)**
Borga, Gerri Beth **(SLP)**
Branham, Charlotte Bandi **(SLP)**
Broom, Donna Raye **(SLP)**
Butler, Kevin William **(SLP)**
Campbell, Mrs Marcia **(SLP)**
Caryl, Carol A **(SLP)**
Cassidy, Mrs Renee Marcia **(SLP)**
Cheek, Ellen Berry **(A)**
Cheeseman-Foulk, Sara **(SLP)**
Childers, Dr Robert L **(A)**
Chuzi, Ken Martin **(SLP)**
Coppola, Lisa **(SLP)**
Curlee, Dr Richard F **(SLP)**
Davis, Mrs Betty J **(A)**
DeFeo, Anthony B **(SLP)**
Demetras, Dr Martha Jo-Ann **(SLP)**
Dengler, Judith **(SLP)**
Dilworth, Robin Powers **(SLP)**
Dunton, Mrs Sheryl Widen **(SLP)**
Edwards, Brian W **(SLP)**
Eilat, Mrs Rosie N **(SLP)**
Ellingsen, Mary Elizabeth **(SLP)**
Esckelson, Dorothy A **(SLP)**
Evans, Mrs Brenda E **(SLP)**
Faux, Cassandra **(SLP)**
Felix, Barbara G **(SLP)**
Findlow, Julie Gail **(SLP)**
Fitzsimmons, Lori K **(A)**
Formentini, Mrs Bonnie J **(SLP)**
Frevert, Corine T **(SLP)**
Frichtl, Mrs Joan Marie **(SLP)**
Friend, Mrs Carolyn Jean
Fulton, Dr Calvin W **(SLP A)**
Garcia, Graciela G **(SLP)**
Gasch, Mrs Janis Wolfe **(A)**
Gentry, Mrs Tina Marie **(SLP)**
Gertzulin, Rona S **(SLP)**
Gibb, Nancy Jo **(SLP)**
Gilabert, Nancy Rehn **(SLP)**
Gilliland, Eleanor Lauri **(SLP)**
Girardot, Karen D **(SLP)**
Glattke, Jean B **(SLP)**
Glattke, Dr Theodore J **(A)**
Goldberg, David H **(SLP)**
Goldman, Bernice Ellen **(A)**
Goodman, Debra L
Gordon-Siken, Donna
Gould, Judy **(SLP)**
Harris, Gail A **(SLP)**
Harrison, Wayne L **(SLP)**
Hawley-Gunckel, Janet **(SLP)**
Healey, Dr William C **(SLP)**
Heerboth, Jill K **(SLP)**
Hendrickson, Mrs Barbara Ann **(SLP)**
Hendrickson-Pfeil, Sharon **(SLP)**
Hernandez, Aleida M **(SLP)**
Herrboldt, Sydney O **(A)**
Hickey, Cynthia Spier **(SLP)**
Hill, Emmeline Kunde **(A)**
Hixon, Thomas J **(SLP)**
Hodgson, Dr William R **(A)**
Hoit, Dr Jeannette **(SLP)**
Holguin, Mrs Roxanna Ramirez **(SLP)**
Hopkins, Sharon Kay **(A)**
Horensten, Mrs Judith Greene **(SLP)**
Hosbjor, Lila **(SLP)**
Hosford-Dunn, Dr Holly L **(A)**
Howard, Sherril R **(SLP)**
Hunter, Mollie Annand **(SLP)**
Hurley-Vangerud, Mrs Heather **(SLP)**
Jacobs, Margaret A **(A)**
Jett, Ellen E **(A)**
Johnson, Mrs Anita Faye **(SLP)**
Johnson, Janice L **(SLP)**
Johnson, Karen H **(SLP)**
Johnson, M K Maddie **(SLP)**
Jones, Ann Katherine **(SLP)**
Jurkowitz, Mrs Chaya B **(SLP)**
Karibian, Dana **(A)**
Kelly, Mrs Carole R **(SLP)**
Kitzman, George H **(A)**
Krause, Eloise M **(SLP)**
Kriendler, John C **(SLP)**
Kristiansen, Mrs Mary Ann **(SLP)**
Kujawa, Sharon Guilds **(A)**
Kurick-McAnally, Mrs Linda **(SLP)**
Lamden, Mrs Frances F **(SLP)**
Lasseter, Mrs Susanne Wilkinson **(SLP)**
Libera, Mrs Jan A **(SLP)**
Little, Sharon F **(SLP A)**
Maguire-Bradley, Sheila Ann **(SLP)**
Maj, Barbara J **(SLP)**
Martin, Michele Hurst **(SLP)**
Martinez, Mrs Catherine Chreitzber **(SLP)**
Mather, Ronnie K **(A)**
Matkin, Dr Noel D **(A)**
Maxwell, Joellen **(SLP)**
McGrath, Mrs Kathe E K **(SLP)**
McGuire, Laurie D **(SLP)**
McLeod, Dr H Lee **(A)**
Melvin, Mrs Patricia W **(SLP)**
Miller, Mrs Jeannine Antoinnett **(SLP)**
Moncur, Dr John P **(SLP A)**
Mong, Tracy Irene **(SLP)**
Morris, Jacqueline **(SLP)**
Mosier, Laura F **(SLP)**
Mukherjee, Mrs Sarah W **(SLP)**
Murray, Mrs Elvira Lalli **(SLP)**
Nagel, Dr Robert F **(SLP A)**
Nation, Dr James E **(SLP)**
Ostlund, Nancy **(SLP)**
Oyler, Anne L **(A)**
Oyler, Robert F **(SLP A)**
Park, William B
Patick, Madelyne K **(SLP)**
Perez, Frank Joseph **(SLP)**
Person, J Brayton **(SLP A)**
Pipes, Marilyn Anne **(SLP)**
Plante, Elena Margaret **(SLP)**
Primeau, Richard L **(A)**
Psaltis, Mrs Cynthia Doyen **(SLP)**
Quigley, Dr Stephen P
Rabeau, Nancy Christine **(SLP)**
Rees, Marjorie Addie **(SLP)**
Reichman, Julie **(A)**
Rochlin, Gail D **(A)**
Rogers, Beth Ann **(SLP)**
Sabin, George Alfred **(SLP)**
Scanlan, Margaret
Schafer, David J **(SLP)**
Schrader, Margaret A **(SLP)**
Semrad, Sherry Noel
Shearer, Cynthia Ann **(SLP)**
Shelby, Theresa M **(SLP)**
Shelton, Dr Ralph L, Jr **(SLP)**
Simons, Janice L **(SLP)**
Slauson, Thomas Jay **(SLP)**
Smith, Christine Ann **(SLP)**
Smith-Eusebio, Mrs Falicia E **(SLP)**
Sokal, Mrs Rhoda H R **(SLP)**
Solomon, Mrs Nancy Pearl **(SLP)**
Spears, Mrs Iris E **(A)**
Stefanski-Brown, Margaret Bridget **(A)**
Stein, Mrs Sandra Jean **(SLP)**
Strautman, Susan **(SLP)**
Sukoneck, Lenore L **(SLP)**
Super, Sarah Lorraine **(A)**
Swisher, Dr Linda P **(SLP A)**
Taniguchi, Lori M **(SLP)**
Tindell, Marsha Eloise **(SLP)**
Tomes, Lucrezia A **(SLP)**
Tomoeda, Cheryl K **(SLP)**
Twichell, Dr Doris Y **(SLP)**
Uberuaga, Phillip J **(A)**
Urreiztieta, Mrs Melissa Ann **(SLP)**
Vance, Mrs Rebecca Butler **(SLP)**
VickRoy, Mrs Mille **(SLP)**
Voge, Mrs Margaret Lennertz **(SLP)**
Watson, Peter J **(SLP)**
Weeks, Lucy E **(SLP)**
Weinberg, Bernd **(SLP)**
Wells, Lauraine Lorinda **(A)**
Whitebread, Debora Kay **(SLP)**
Williams, Nancy H **(SLP)**
Wilson, Dr Kent J **(SLP A)**
Wood, Mrs Pamela R **(A)**
Wyatt, Teresa **(A)**
Yeatts, Rebecca Diane **(SLP)**
Ziegler, Jane E Rubin **(SLP)**

Wellton
Truett, Carol Pierce **(SLP)**

Wickenburg
Wurl, Mrs Charlotte **(SLP)**

Window Rock
Brutz, Mrs Loretta R **(SLP)**

Yuma
Broadhead, Mrs Sandra Lee
Defranco, Sharon A **(SLP)**
Dockins, Mrs Sharon F **(SLP)**
Madison, Lawanda D
Pohlman, Janie Lynn **(SLP)**
Popeck, Mrs Gay Lounsberry **(SLP)**
Vasquez, Therese Janine **(SLP)**

ARKANSAS

Alexander
Pickett, Larry R **(SLP)**
Sanford, Mildred M **(A)**

Alma
Wofford, Mrs Cynthia Holmberg **(SLP)**

Arkadelphia
Anderson, Dr Martha W **(SLP A)**
Crawley, Mrs Linda Pendleton **(SLP)**
Huckabee, Mrs Kimberly Ann **(SLP)**
Lisemby, Doris M **(SLP)**
McDonald, R Hilton **(SLP)**
Price, Mrs Dee Ann **(A)**

Ash Flat
Rabon, John Davis **(SLP)**

Ashdown
Gray, Mrs Ann Y **(SLP)**

Augusta
Branscum, Mrs Dixie C **(SLP)**

Austin
Pryor, Mrs Dana Richmond **(SLP)**

Batesville
Bruce, Kaye S
Dover, Mrs Pamela Reynolds
McElmurry, Mrs Susan P **(SLP)**
Wood, Mrs Rebecca H **(SLP)**

Bella Vista
Smith, Mrs Ruth E **(SLP)**

Benton
Caldwell, Mrs Credonna L
Durham, Glenda Dawn **(SLP)**
Eddington, Mrs Judith Anne **(SLP)**
Grimes, Mrs Karin Dale **(SLP)**
Hawkins, Mrs Diana Durham **(SLP)**
Hill, Vanessa Ruth **(SLP)**
Holland, Ange N **(SLP)**
Northern, Mrs Sandra W **(SLP)**
Rainwater-Ross, Janet **(SLP)**
Richey, Mrs Lisa C **(A)**
Snowden, Mrs Patricia Burke **(SLP)**

Bentonville
Sandlin, Vicki L **(SLP)**

Bigelow
Cooley, Sara Ann **(SLP)**

Blytheville
Keller, Dana Renee
Kleiman, Mrs Kay Seaton
Little, Tom Anthony, III **(SLP)**
Lynch, Kelly J
Myers, Mrs Tracy D **(SLP)**
Patterson, Mrs Molly G **(SLP)**

Blytheville AFB
Matthews, Kathleen McGinnis **(SLP)**

Booneville
Evans, Marcia Ann **(SLP)**

Bradford
Winningham, Mrs Anthia K **(SLP)**

Brookland
Murphy, Mrs Susan Phillips **(SLP)**

Cabot
Brooks, Mrs Bonnie H **(SLP)**
Kelley, Rhonda **(SLP)**
Miranda, Carla Yvette **(SLP)**

Carway
Case, Linda G D **(SLP)**

Cave City
Cruthis, Mrs Quinta Lockhart **(SLP)**

Clarksville
Harrison, Mrs Melinda A **(SLP)**
Kemp, John Patrick **(SLP)**
Zarwell, Lillian H **(SLP)**
Ziegler, Teresa Schulze **(SLP)**

Cleveland
Harris, Cristi O'Neal

Concord
O'Brien, Mrs Kathryn S **(SLP)**

Conway
Eubanks, Lillie Sharon **(SLP)**
Fusilier, Betty B **(SLP)**
Graham, Linda Ruth **(SLP)**
Hickey, Mrs Susan Bell **(SLP)**
Johnson, Cynthia L **(SLP)**
Jones, Lisa Kaye **(SLP)**
Logan, Dr Robert **(SLP A)**
McDaniel, Kathy Johnson **(SLP)**
McNiece, Dr Elaine M **(SLP)**
Moss, Susan A **(SLP)**
Nichols, Mrs Elizabeth Gillingham **(SLP)**
Poole, Mrs Marilyn R **(SLP)**
Powell, Mrs Vanessa Koonce **(SLP)**
Ross, Dr Frona S **(SLP)**
Ross, Mrs Sharon Elser **(SLP)**
Simon, Clara Rose **(SLP)**
Thurman, James E **(SLP)**

Crosett
Nutt, Margaret Elizabeth

Danville
Eitenmiller, Anna Marie **(A)**

Dardanelle
Choate, Rosmyr L, Jr **(SLP)**
Jackson, Charline B **(SLP)**

De Queen
Sikes, Mrs Kelly Dowdle **(SLP)**

Dermott
Hawkins, Margaret C **(SLP)**

El Dorado
Bennett, Mrs Angela Shaddock **(SLP)**
Davidson, James V **(A)**
Hammond, Mrs Debra Calaway **(SLP)**
Jones, Dr Carolane **(SLP)**
Morgan, Mrs Carol Wasson **(SLP)**
Post, Mrs Kathy Milner **(SLP)**

Eudora
Nelson, Janet L **(SLP)**

Farmington
Thompson, Mrs Mary C **(SLP)**

Fayetteville
Aslin, Larry W **(SLP)**
Aslin, Mary E **(SLP)**
Bersinger, Don D **(SLP A)**
Bourne, Jenny **(SLP)**
Bruns, Janet M M **(SLP)**
Caldarera, Mrs Dana M **(SLP)**
Calvert, Mrs Brenda Plourde **(SLP)**
Childers, Mrs Blake Brasel **(SLP)**
Dow, Mrs Beverly J **(SLP)**
Glenn, Marietta G **(SLP)**
Griffin, Suzanne A **(SLP)**
Hamilton, Mrs Treva K **(SLP)**
Hampton, Alice W **(SLP)**
Hays, Elizabeth D **(SLP)**
James, Linda L **(SLP)**
Jones, Mrs Martha Leigh
Jones, Mrs Sondra Carson **(SLP)**
Linam, Ruth **(SLP)**
McKenzie, Mrs Margaret
Norbash, Mrs Sherrie L **(A)**
Paas, Deborah T
Park, Martha G **(SLP)**
Raiford, Dr Carolyn Ann **(A)**
Roberts, Mrs Karen F **(SLP)**
Shadden, Dr Barbara B **(SLP)**
Widder, Carol Ash **(SLP)**

Forrest City
Fisher, Teriann **(A)**
Hill, Mrs Mary P **(SLP)**
Nimocks, Mrs Carla Morehead **(SLP)**
Phillips, Brenda Beck **(SLP)**

Fort Smith
Carner, Mrs Teresa Jo **(SLP)**
Cummings, Betty J **(SLP)**
Eady, Mrs Lady Martin **(SLP)**
Eoff, Elizabeth Haaser **(SLP)**
Harper, Mrs Carol P **(A)**
Kerbow, Kendra L **(SLP)**
Mason, Mrs Sydney Brooks **(SLP)**
Meeks, Lisa Rene **(SLP)**
Merrell, Mrs Laquita Southall **(SLP)**
Mueller, Phoebe S **(SLP)**
Ramey, Mrs Rita C Gray **(SLP)**
Slack, Mrs Carol Dianne **(A)**
Spradlin, Mrs Kelly T
Van Ess, Lisa M **(SLP)**
Wacaster, Mrs Pamela Vollmer **(SLP)**
Wadsworth, Pamela Joyce **(SLP)**

Fox
Barton, Kay Humphreys **(SLP)**

Garfield
Lee, Patricia Clark **(SLP)**

Gentry
Droho, Mary

Green Forest
Dillard, Elizabeth Marie **(SLP)**

Greenbrier
Vann, Mrs Charlotte Hopkins
Wilcox, Mrs Dana Lefler **(SLP)**

Greenwood
Davidson, Sharee Graddy **(SLP)**
Holloway, Micki W **(SLP)**

Hamburg
Smith, Michael Keith **(SLP)**

Hampton
Raney, Melissa Lynne **(A)**

Harrisburg
Byrd, Mrs Gwendolyn Everhart **(SLP)**
Kempf, Mrs Connie Lynn **(SLP)**
Noe, Elizabeth Ann **(SLP)**

Harrison
Fast, Mrs Patricia L **(SLP)**
Hudson, Amy Jo **(SLP)**
Hudson, Nancy T **(SLP)**
Melton, Ray E **(A)**

Hasty
Dunlap, Mrs D'Lorah Reddell **(SLP)**

Heber Springs
Gehle, Mrs Phyllis D **(SLP)**
Goff, Mrs Gail S **(SLP)**
Krug, Karen A **(SLP)**

Hope
Franks, Dr Christine H **(SLP A)**
Roe, Susan G **(SLP)**

Hot Springs
James, Kellye A **(SLP)**
Kennedy, Alicia Quinn **(SLP)**
Palmer, Clarence **(A)**
Palmer, Lee D **(SLP)**
Warren, Pamela G **(SLP)**
Womack, Mrs Judy **(SLP)**

Hot Springs Village
Pearson, Mrs Diana Johnson **(SLP)**

Jacksonville
Evans, Vicky Sue **(SLP)**
Schultz, Mrs Mary Lee C **(SLP)**
Starkey, Mrs Aleecia A **(SLP)**
Sykes, Georgia Gail **(SLP)**

Jonesboro
Burrow, Mrs Pamela Lee **(SLP)**
Frey, Marilyn Maclk **(SLP)**
Greenwald, Carol A **(SLP)**
Herndon, Dr George Y **(SLP)**
Leblanc, Jane H **(SLP A)**
McQuay, Sue M
Neeley, Richard A **(SLP)**
Prince, Jane B **(A)**
Roberson, Joan Lee **(SLP)**
Tinsley, Sara S **(SLP)**
Vivrette, Deanne

Lakeview
Burks, Dan A **(SLP)**

Little Rock
Allen, Christy Denise **(SLP)**
Alman, Martha Hirsch **(SLP)**
Bacon, Linda A M **(A)**
Baker, Lorie H **(SLP)**
Barlund, Mrs Sarah L **(SLP)**
Batie, Ramona L **(SLP)**
Beggs, Fred R **(A)**
Bellairs-Salemi, Mrs Luanna Lee **(SLP)**
Belveal, Mrs Sally Squires **(A)**
Bennett, Tammy Warren **(SLP)**
Berry, Virginia S **(A)**
Bracy, Mrs Connie Lynn **(SLP)**
Bradley, Leslie Ann **(A)**
Brannen, Kimberly Jean
Brosh, Mrs Lee Ann **(SLP)**
Butler, Patricia Ann **(SLP)**
Causey, Susan Jean **(SLP)**
Cherepski, Mary Ann **(SLP)**
Crumpler, Linda S **(SLP)**
Dancer, Dr Jesse E **(A)**
Dixon, Cynthia Anderson **(SLP)**
Drummond, Dr Sakina S **(SLP)**
Dunn, Mrs Nancy Susan **(SLP)**
Eaton, Sarah Butler **(SLP)**
Fleming, Deodis D **(SLP)**
Ford, Mrs Cindy C **(SLP)**
Frazier, Mrs Kate Erwin **(A)**
Frith, Mrs Charlotte **(SLP)**
Gentry, Betholyn R **(SLP)**
George, Gail S **(SLP)**
Graham, Sharon S **(A)**
Grever, Karl H **(A)**
Griffin, Kyle Mark **(SLP)**
Hampton, Mrs Karen H **(SLP)**
Harding, Marcia A **(SLP)**
Heard, Dr Kenneth W **(A)**
Hedges, Ann Mahon **(A)**
Henson, Mrs Mary Dian **(SLP)**
Highley, Patricia Ann **(A)**
Hillis, Mrs Aimee C **(SLP)**
Hoffman, Janice Kathryn **(SLP)**
Huff, Lou Ann Gioannini **(A)**
Hutton, Mrs Terri J **(SLP)**
Johnson, Mrs Susan King **(SLP)**
Josephson, Glenda M **(SLP)**
Karpe, Mrs Donna N **(SLP)**
Karpe, Larry M **(SLP A)**
Keiser, Dr Janet Hope **(A)**
Kirkland, Mrs Julie Ann **(SLP)**
Kizewski-Hill, Cynthia Maria **(A)**
Lewis, Carolyn Jean **(SLP)**
Lorenzo, Jackie C **(SLP)**
Losey, Jana P **(SLP)**
Martin, Patti F **(A)**
McElduff, Mary Kathleen **(SLP)**
McElrath, Mrs Lesli Overbey **(SLP)**
McMurtrey, Mrs Lisa G
McQueen, Ann B **(SLP)**
Montague, Dr James C, Jr **(SLP)**
Morse, Mrs Rachel Cates **(SLP)**
Nellum-Davis, Dr Priscilla **(SLP)**
Othold, Becky Jean
Park, Mrs Victoria L **(SLP)**
Pearsall, Valerie **(SLP)**
Petruk, Mrs Marilyn Harris **(SLP)**
Pine, Dr Shirley J **(SLP)**
Reynolds, Diana Lynn **(SLP)**
Rippy, Mrs Janice Gail **(SLP)**
Roberts, Mrs Kathleen B **(SLP)**
Romesburg, Jocelyn **(SLP)**
Rorie, Beverly Lewis
Rowe, Mrs Marjean S **(SLP)**
Rudd, Amy Key **(A)**
Rudolph, Deborah A **(SLP)**
Russell, Mrs Susan Scanlan **(SLP)**
Rutenberg, Mrs Judith B **(SLP)**
Ryan, Stephenie Pickering **(SLP)**
Sample, Mrs Mary Henderson **(SLP)**
Schaub, Mrs Lisa J **(SLP)**
Sims, Sue E **(SLP)**
Smith, Randall W **(SLP)**
Steelman, Mrs Mary L **(SLP)**
Taylor, Paula N **(SLP)**
Tramel, Mrs Kim Smith **(SLP)**
Turbeville, Dr Joseph B, Jr **(A)**
Turner, Mrs Martha Morse **(SLP)**
Washington, Mrs Evelyn Douglas **(SLP)**
Wasson, Mrs Alison Hasley **(SLP)**
Weatherton, Dr Maurice Allen **(SLP A)**
Weaver, Brenda K **(SLP)**
Wesson, Kathleen B **(SLP)**
Whitney, M Cerinda **(A)**
Wilcox, Mrs Rebecca Ann
Winston, Dr Michael E **(A)**
Wold, Dr Donald C

Zaleski, Susan Marie **(SLP)**
Zeno, Mrs Sara Hodge **(SLP)**

Lonoke
Bennett, Caroline T **(SLP)**
Henderson, Cathy Crow **(A)**

Lonsdale
Lewis, Mrs Mary Jane **(SLP)**

Mabelvale
Forbus, Mrs Sandra Sue **(SLP)**
Shearon, Mrs Nancy P **(SLP)**

Magnolia
Boaz, Mrs Paula H **(SLP)**
Groves, Marilyn E **(SLP)**

Malvern
Corley, Cecelia Elizabeth **(SLP)**
Erwin, Paul Michael **(SLP)**

Marion
Mayton, Mrs Pamela Sue **(SLP)**

Maumelle
Cox, Mrs Michelle Elizabeth **(SLP)**
Craig, Sherry Annette **(SLP)**
Hutson, Grover Henry **(A)**
Price, Mrs Juneanne Downs **(SLP)**
Russell, Mrs Glennae Anderson **(SLP)**
Rye, Carol V **(A)**
Wood, Teresa Kay **(SLP)**

McGehee
Gober, Mrs Paula J **(SLP)**

Melbourne
Jones, Mrs Elizabeth Dillin **(SLP)**

Mena
Deweese, Thomas E **(SLP)**
Lee, Ann S **(SLP)**
Ryburn, Mrs Charlotte Ferguson **(SLP)**

Morrilton
Hutchison, Mary Judith **(SLP)**

Mount View
Landrum, Mrs Anne T **(SLP)**

Mountain Home
Baker, Deborah Prince **(A)**
Barrows-Butler, Mrs Dorothy
Kent, Mrs Wanda Z **(SLP)**
Skrine, Mrs Rebecca A **(SLP)**

Nashville
Bell, Alicia A A **(SLP)**
Rowland, Rebecca R **(SLP)**

Newark
Flynn, Paula L I **(SLP)**

Newport
Montgomery, Mrs Janet K **(SLP)**

North Little Rock
Adkisson, Carol D **(SLP)**
Banks, Mrs Rhonda E **(SLP)**
Bingham, Mrs Marcia Roles **(SLP)**
Burl, Nola T **(SLP)**
Carr, Mrs Rebecca Ritchie **(SLP)**
Douglas, Mrs Kristiann **(A)**
Garnes, Mrs Willye M **(SLP A)**
Henderson, Mrs Nancy Biery **(SLP)**
Herrod, Robin McMahon **(SLP)**
Hettler, Mrs Elizabeth A **(SLP)**
Hildebrand, Dr Beverly H **(SLP)**
Holleran, Laine Mayer **(A)**
Hostler, Mrs Sandra Bradford **(SLP)**
Kiley, Kathy **(SLP)**
Krueger, Kathleen M **(SLP)**
Masters, Mrs Janis M
McKelvey-Burbage, June **(SLP)**
Parker, Mrs Glenda Chambers **(SLP)**
Pattison, Darcy S **(A)**
Rippy, James V **(A)**
Sowell, Mrs Barbara Fitzpatrck **(SLP)**
Sowell, Thomas William **(SLP)**

Ussery, Loyd E **(A)**
Yelvington, Cinda K **(SLP)**

Osceola
Richmond, Mrs Donna Porterfield

Ozark
Abbott, Thomas M **(SLP)**
Armstrong, Mrs Donna C **(SLP)**

Paragould
Camp, Kathy Vaughn **(SLP)**
Moore, Linda L **(SLP)**

Paris
Layes, Mrs Holly R Davis

Piggott
Wagster, Lora Octavia **(SLP)**

Pine Bluff
Bell, Mrs Sandra Sue **(SLP)**
Cockrum, Mrs Emily S **(SLP)**
Grimmett, Sharon G
Hamilton, Mrs Vikki Thompson
Jumper, Mrs Martha Melinda **(A)**
Moore, Rowene Caley **(SLP)**
Simmering, Brenda D **(SLP)**
Thomas, Faytrene Noyes **(SLP)**
Tortorich, Consuela **(A)**
Vance, Henrietta Vernell **(SLP)**
Walker, Mrs Jacque D **(SLP)**
Williams, Mrs Margarette **(SLP)**

Pocahontas
Couch, Teri C **(SLP)**
Jarrett, Catherine DeClerk **(SLP)**

Prescott
Barfield, Judy T **(SLP)**

Rector
Crancer, Michele **(SLP)**

Rison
Stewart, Carolyn Rose **(SLP)**
Wilson, Mrs Sharon L **(SLP)**

Rogers
Krish, Geneva A **(A)**
McGrail, Louis J **(A)**
Melton, Mrs Mary E **(SLP)**
Parenti, Mrs Margaret An **(SLP)**

Rudy
Whitson, Cynthia Ann

Russellville
Gardner, Mrs Mary Ellen **(SLP)**
Price, Margaret Mary **(SLP)**
Silkensen, Mary P **(SLP)**

Searcy
Biggs, Gail R **(SLP)**
Devan, Mrs Sheila Ann **(SLP)**
Jackson, Mary Ann **(SLP)**
Noble, Dennis R **(A)**
Stewart, Mrs Pamula Faye **(SLP)**
Tullos, Dr Daniel C **(SLP)**
Walker, Dr Richard W
Weaver, Mrs Rebecca O **(SLP)**

Sheridan
Horton, Mrs Betty A **(A)**

Sherwood
Patterson, Nancy Elaine **(SLP)**

Springdale
Buchanan, Mrs Susan H **(SLP)**
Edgmon, Donna M **(SLP)**
Pertile, Traci Lee **(A)**
Slaton, Mrs Teresa A **(SLP)**
Wilson, V Denice **(SLP)**

State University
Justen, Mary Sandra **(SLP)**
Neeley, Mrs Phyllis Miles **(SLP)**
Neumeyer, Jerry W **(SLP)**
Perez, Dr Emilio **(SLP)**

Stuttgart
Grabbe, Laura Leigh **(SLP)**
McGraw, Wilmer Tracy
Simpson, Carolyn S **(SLP)**

Taylor
Perry, Linda Gail **(SLP)**

Texarkana
Beck, Mrs Judith A **(SLP)**
Burdine, Mrs Judy Crisp

Tillar
Teeter, Lee Harvill **(SLP)**

Walnut Ridge
Reeves, Mrs Sheri Kaye **(SLP)**

Warren
Durmon, Mrs Laura Helen **(SLP)**

West Helena
Chesser, Beverly J **(A)**
Deitz, Laura F **(SLP)**
Reyna, Karen Ann **(SLP)**

West Memphis
Hood, Tamara Andrea

Wynne
Easley, Mrs Cynthia Renee **(SLP)**
Horton, Mrs Janice A **(SLP)**

CALIFORNIA

Agoura
Berry, Mrs Betsy L S **(SLP)**
Epstein-Roberts, Mrs Sharon L **(A)**
Gallenberg-Zieve, Felice R **(SLP)**
Hardeman, Christine **(SLP)**
Hardeman, Gary T **(SLP)**
Meisel, Janice B **(SLP)**
Nelson, Carol A **(SLP)**
Vaughan, Martha S **(SLP)**

Agoura Hills
Arons, Mrs Lauri Jill **(SLP)**
Breines, Gail L **(SLP)**
Comer, Mrs Patricia Fabiola **(SLP)**
Dzombar, Mrs Diane G **(SLP)**
Kulik, Mrs Linda **(SLP)**
O'Neal, Elaine **(SLP)**
Parlen, Mrs Marilyn J **(SLP)**
Stearn, Mrs Diane M **(SLP)**
Taras, Mrs Ellen Epstein **(SLP)**
Tsumpes, Mrs Cynthia Sue **(SLP)**

Alameda
Bay, Carolyn Amelia **(SLP)**
Bochner, Laurie Flamm **(SLP)**
Collins, Patricia J **(SLP)**
De Benedetto, Jane R **(SLP)**
Hachiya, Janet Schoen **(SLP)**
Hempstead, Megan **(SLP)**
Jackson, Linda Lee **(SLP)**
Kramer, Lisa **(SLP)**
Laurence, Marianna Louise **(SLP)**
Lefler, Mary Anne **(SLP)**
MacPherson, Mary A **(SLP)**
Matthews, Leslie Kandee **(SLP)**
Pennefeather, Ann **(SLP)**
Scott, Wallace G **(SLP)**
Smith, Mae Ann Levine **(SLP)**

Alamo
Mahon, Christine Shannon **(A)**
Porter, Dora Thea **(SLP A)**
Van Dyne, Mrs Barbara Jean **(SLP)**

Albany
Bonney, Susan D **(SLP)**
Salisbury, Mrs Dawn **(SLP)**
Schumacher, Marilyn E **(SLP)**

Alhambra
Bosso, Yu-Wen Shih **(A)**
Ghadialy, Fatema Beguwala **(A)**
Hunte, Frances **(SLP)**

Low, Elaine Yee Ling **(SLP)**
McGuire, Marion
Miller, Mrs Antoinette Marie **(A)**
Rivas, Monica
Wong, Lorraine Jean **(SLP)**

Alpine
Franklin, Marcia Reiss **(SLP)**

Alta Loma
Jones, Gary Lee **(A)**
Jones, Lisa Petersen **(A)**
Kay, Vicki D **(SLP)**
Logerfo, Catherine **(SLP)**

Altadena
Alexander-Stone, Elise **(SLP)**
Clingmon, Ilene C **(SLP)**
Duhon, Mrs Rosalind Williams **(SLP)**
Egge, Victoria Dreis **(SLP)**
Harris, Mrs Pamela Elizabeth
Houston, Robin G **(SLP)**
Johnson, Mrs Dovie Jean **(SLP)**
Mabie-DeRuyter, Ann Moninne **(A)**
Nakasone, Dr Hirotaka
Novell, Kathleen McGann **(SLP)**
O'Donnell, Connie C **(SLP)**
Sinclair, Dr John Stephen **(A)**
Sisskin, Vivian D **(SLP)**
Switzer, Emilia C **(SLP)**
Tonokawa, Lisa Lynn **(A)**
Vanderhoff, Joan H **(SLP)**

Anaheim
Ackerman, Mrs Randa R **(SLP)**
Ballmer, Mrs Irene Mary **(SLP)**
Bell, Brenda Lynn
Bossier, Mrs Ida J **(SLP)**
Bulloch, Mrs Kathleen L **(SLP)**
Chambers, Mrs Carole Schaffer **(SLP)**
Coates, Kathleen M **(A)**
Curfman, Mrs Susan Margaret **(SLP)**
Farley, Shauna L **(SLP)**
Fielder, Kay L G **(SLP)**
Foster, Debra K **(SLP)**
Gahre, Teri Lea **(SLP)**
Gilbert, Mrs Mary Ann M **(A)**
Glisson-Heffel, Denise L **(SLP)**
Goslin, Mrs Betty **(SLP)**
Greening, Naomi Karen **(SLP)**
Hayes, Victoria S **(SLP)**
Jahr, Mrs Katherine Layton **(SLP)**
Kelley, Mrs Kathleen Janice **(SLP)**
Kramer, Mrs Pamela M **(SLP)**
Kupris, Joseph J **(SLP)**
Larson, Jamie A **(SLP)**
Lippincott, Charles V **(SLP)**
McLean, Darlene **(SLP)**
Ornstein, Mrs Mary A **(SLP)**
Ozsvath, Nancy Lynn **(SLP)**
Parker, Judith A **(SLP)**
Pisakov, Mrs Nesta **(SLP)**
Price, Lynda McCann
Redden, William J **(SLP)**
Renck, Gene B **(A)**
Riley, Elizabeth **(SLP)**
Roberts, Mrs Sharon L **(SLP)**
Rogers, Mrs Margaret Denise
Schein-Sokolow, Adrian **(SLP)**
Shragg, Judith Metchik **(SLP)**
Sinclair, Beverly J **(SLP)**
Studebaker, Barbara Ann **(SLP)**
Weber, Marianne **(SLP)**
Willis, Tyra Jean **(SLP)**

Anaheim Hills
Barrett, Jean Lorene **(SLP)**
Becker, Mary R **(SLP)**
Bowman, Katie Monty **(SLP)**
Cepinko, Barbara H **(SLP)**
Mooney, Mrs Janice Griffin **(SLP)**
Moore-Brown, Barbara Joann **(SLP)**
Wineinger, Cynthia J **(SLP)**
Wyatt, Nancy Lucile **(SLP)**

Anderson
Griffin, Mrs Ruth Goesele **(SLP)**

Angwin
Emde, Mrs Jennifer **(SLP)**

Antioch
Baumgartner, Mrs Holly Fisher **(SLP)**
Ferrante, Mrs Marian E **(SLP)**
Hewitt, Joan Tillman **(SLP)**
Madura-Carroll, Karin **(SLP)**
McBride, Karen L **(SLP)**

APO San Francisco
Ahlgren, Mrs Marianne Collins **(A)**
Backlar, Annette Warren **(SLP)**
Campbell, Deborah L **(SLP)**
Dembeck, Pamela Mary **(SLP)**
Gurley, Susan A **(SLP)**
Jordan, Craig Eugene **(A)**
Litvinas, Carol J **(A)**
Mason, Marcia L **(SLP)**
Mullen, Joan M **(SLP)**
Smith, Mrs Ellen D **(SLP)**

Apple Valley
Mainess, Karen Joanne **(SLP)**
Worden, Edwina Marie **(SLP)**

Applegate
Hilton, Judith Ann **(SLP)**

Aptos
Hertel, Christina **(SLP)**
Hughes, Kathleen **(SLP)**
Kesterson, Suzanne B **(SLP)**
Murphy, Mrs Carol L **(SLP)**
Robin, Lois L **(SLP)**

Arcadia
Addicks, Connie S **(SLP)**
Barnes, Mrs Suzanne M **(SLP)**
Bennett, Daphne N **(SLP)**
Briggs, Dr Margaret H **(SLP)**
Brown, Alexandra **(SLP)**
Callaham, Marilyn Llewellyn **(SLP)**
Clark, Mrs Pearl Mary **(SLP)**
Dickinson, Mrs Cheryl L **(SLP)**
Eldredge, Mrs Patricia Devers **(SLP)**
Gottschalk-Grafman, Carole **(A)**
Gundrum, Gladys R **(SLP)**
Lake, Teresa Manlove **(A)**
Larner, Mrs Carolynn **(SLP)**
Nelson, John Patrick **(A)**
Palfrey, Cheryl C **(A)**
Platte-Worth, Mrs Susan Marie **(SLP)**
Shahak, Antoinette E **(SLP)**
Swanson, Christine B **(SLP)**
Teicher, Stephanie Hope **(SLP)**
Wang, Dr Chester **(SLP)**

Arcata
Dutra, Mrs Leslie R **(SLP)**
Gaasch, Isabel F **(SLP)**
Langlois, Dr Aimee **(SLP A)**
Long, Dr Steven H **(SLP)**
Mattison, Roger W **(A)**
Ranton, Debra Beth **(SLP)**

Arnold
Doenges, Donna Ada **(SLP)**

Aromas
Waller, Sharon Denny **(SLP)**

Arroyo Grande
Christensen, Mrs Susan S **(SLP)**
Cumley, Gary D **(SLP)**
Mahnke, Nancy C **(SLP)**
Tringham, Karen Sue K **(SLP A)**
Wayne, Lori Jo **(SLP)**
Wiemers, Mrs Pat Ann **(SLP)**

Artesia
Kampen, Karen Lynn **(SLP)**

Atascadero
Garrett, Bobbie Lee **(A)**
Rucci-Zimmer, Susan **(SLP)**
Steinke, Mrs Clella J **(SLP)**
Swen, Pamela Michelle **(SLP)**

Atherton
Jackson, Mrs Ruth M **(SLP)**
MacKenzie, Janet Hanbery **(SLP)**
Rattner, Dr Bonnie G **(SLP)**

Atwater
Beatty, Beth Marinne **(SLP)**
Mires, Joann M **(SLP)**
Reierson-Griffith, Karen J **(SLP)**
Sparkman, James L **(SLP)**
Suit, Kimberly A **(SLP)**

Auburn
Fitzpatrick-McKenzie, Susan Wills **(SLP)**
Krizman, Mrs Debora Johnson **(SLP)**
Lavoie, Mary E **(A)**
Levesque, Mrs Cynthia Hyatt **(SLP)**
Lloyd, Susan **(SLP A)**
Piette, Mrs Jean Ross **(SLP)**
Roy, Melody Bakos **(SLP)**
Teitscheid, Mrs Lorraine Quintero **(SLP)**
Thompson, Janee S **(SLP)**

Augoura Hills
Burt, Mrs Cheryl D **(SLP)**

Azusa
Euler, Catherine **(SLP)**

Bakersfield
Andersen, Douglas E **(A)**
Anderson, Jan P **(SLP)**
Anderson, William O **(SLP)**
Arbeit, Holley S **(SLP)**
Ashley, Mark J **(SLP)**
Ashley, Susan M **(SLP)**
Barrett, Julia Jeanne **(SLP)**
Beckham-Woodward, Mrs Paula L **(SLP)**
Bermejo, Dr Juan J **(A)**
Bermejo, Mrs Kathy Fletcher **(SLP)**
Bickett, Jeanne Lanovara **(SLP)**
Brandt, David A **(SLP)**
Braun, Mrs June E B **(SLP)**
Burroughs, Dr Glenn R **(SLP)**
Chavis, Mrs Marlene Cecilia
Deifel, Gayle R **(SLP)**
Del Val, Erica **(SLP)**
Dooley, Mrs Laurie Jeanne P **(SLP)**
Driver, Joyce Eileen **(SLP)**
Dukes-Mc Mahan, Sandra E **(SLP)**
Elieff, Linda M **(SLP)**
Ellis, Charles C **(SLP)**
Faulk, Jennifer Perkins **(SLP)**
Fitch, Jon M **(SLP A)**
Fonssagrives, Dianne **(SLP)**
Gallagher-Hornback, Julie G **(SLP)**
Garrett, Mrs Judith P **(SLP)**
Greenlee, Gloria M D **(SLP)**
Harness, Mrs Denise E **(SLP)**
Henry, Thomas E **(SLP)**
Jacobson, Mrs Robin Lynn **(SLP)**
Johnson, Mrs Dorothy E **(SLP)**
Justice, Ann L **(SLP)**
Keeter, Dr Larry G **(SLP)**
Krych, David K **(SLP)**
Lemieux, Janice M **(SLP)**
Livingston, Gregory Merrill **(SLP)**
Lotspeich, Nancy Ruonavaara
Lynch, Anna M **(SLP)**
Mahoney, M Elaine **(SLP)**
Manidok, Renee Ann **(A)**
May, Patricia **(SLP)**
Meyer, Mrs Madeline D **(SLP)**
Meyers, Edward Frederick **(SLP)**
Morrison, Mrs Helen M **(SLP A)**
Newquist, Mrs Cathy Robinson **(SLP)**
Norland, Betty M **(SLP)**
Oakes, Deborah K **(SLP)**
O'Hara, Mrs Diane A **(SLP)**
Olson, Joni L **(SLP)**
O'Rourke, Maureen Rose **(SLP)**
Otting-Blaine, Julia A **(SLP)**
Patton, Beverly Elaine **(SLP)**
Perkins, Scott Tucker **(SLP)**
Peterson, Ann Marie **(SLP)**
Phillips, Edgar W **(SLP A)**
Pierucci, Dr Rita A **(SLP)**
Plake, Terri L **(SLP)**
Roope, Mrs Jane E **(SLP)**
Secor, Julianna Louise **(SLP)**
Short, Gaylord R **(A)**
Skelton, Mrs Kathy Carter **(SLP)**
Skelton, Steven L **(SLP)**
Stewart, Mrs La Tricia Pritchard **(SLP)**
Wadman, Patrick N
Warren, Yolanda Collean
Welchans, Bonita C **(SLP)**
Williams, Mary Elizabeth **(SLP)**

Balboa
Bailey, Elizabeth
Buesking, Susan M **(SLP)**
Schnack, Lori Rae **(SLP)**
Wallace, Elizabeth M

Balboa Island
Davis, Doreen **(SLP)**
Gaunt, Susan M **(SLP)**
Keys, Mrs Tracy L **(SLP)**

Baldwin Park
Dyer, Mrs Helen A

Banning
Little, Kathy L **(SLP)**

Barstow
Long, Elaine K **(SLP)**
Meek, Mrs Denise Patricia R **(SLP)**

Bayside
Bank, Mrs Robin M **(SLP)**
Cole, Mrs Barbara Dolf **(SLP)**

Beale AFB
Varner, Mrs Pamela Hogge **(SLP)**

Beaumont
Hill-Brown, Mrs Carolyn J **(SLP)**

Bell Canyon
Cosaro, Mrs Janet A **(SLP)**

Bellflower
Gong-Guy, Ellen **(SLP)**

Belmont
Beuttler, Deborah B **(SLP)**
Dixon, Melinda S **(SLP)**
Kriesel, Mrs Leslie J **(SLP)**
Oeser, Julie Ann **(SLP)**
Rubin, Martha Chickering **(SLP)**
Solomon-Rice, Patti L **(SLP)**
Walker, Maura Anne **(SLP)**

Belvedere
Wintersteen, Mrs Jane Noonan **(SLP)**

Ben Lomond
Forbes, Carolin K **(SLP)**
Miles, John C **(A)**

Benicia
Barone, Mrs Deborah Sue **(SLP)**
Chalmers, Mrs Joyce S **(SLP)**
Cramer, Mrs Judy C **(SLP)**
Dirks, Thomas Jay **(SLP)**
Mills, Mary E **(SLP)**
O'Brien, Nancy L **(SLP)**
Schermerhorn, Carol Costa **(SLP)**

Berkeley
Agin, Dr Rhoda Leah **(SLP)**
Apple, Linda G
Baker, Catherine S **(SLP)**
Begen-Peltz, Linda Gail **(A)**
Bilecki, Mary Ann Schiffer **(A)**
Bluma, Susan Marie
Bowen, Carol Marie **(A)**
Brodersen, Shelach H **(SLP)**
Burkard, Amy Brown
Chomak, Joan E **(SLP)**
Clopper, Dr Donald L **(SLP)**
Davis, Sharon M **(SLP)**
Freundlich, Susan Gale **(A)**
Greenfield, Susan L R **(SLP)**
Greenlee, Dr Mary Ellen (Mel)
Gribben, Dana Jo **(SLP)**
Han, Dr Margaret **(SLP)**
Hunt-Berg, Mary **(SLP)**
Jacobs, Mary Kane **(SLP)**
Jacobs-White, Leona M **(SLP)**
Kaiser, Holly W **(SLP)**
Kessler, Dorcas **(A)**
Kirchner, Dr Diane M **(SLP)**
Kroll, William J **(SLP)**
Larvick, Jenny C **(SLP)**
Liles, Patricia A **(SLP)**
Ludden, Sarah Margaret **(A)**
Lyon, Jonathan Victor **(SLP)**
May, Ann R **(SLP)**
Mitchell, Terry **(A)**
Mussen, Dr Ethel F **(SLP A)**
Rosen, Cynthia D **(SLP)**
Ross, Dr Florence **(SLP)**
Sax, Eva Helene **(SLP)**
Scarborough, Sheri Lynn **(SLP)**
Weller, Susan Elizabeth **(SLP)**
Wragg, Frances Rebecca **(SLP)**
Wrenn, Mary

Beverly Hills
Braslau, Cynthia Gay **(SLP)**
Charnov, Mrs Ellen Klinenberg **(SLP)**
Glass, Dr Lillian **(SLP)**
Goldberg, Tova R **(SLP)**
Heffernan, H Patricia **(A)**
Kaufman-Katz, Valerie F **(SLP)**
Krissman, Mrs Rosalynn **(SLP)**
Roesch, Pauline Jean **(SLP)**
Schoenfeld, Debra **(SLP)**
Schulman, Linda S **(SLP)**
Simpson, Joanne C **(SLP)**
Smith, Dr Bettye W **(SLP A)**

Big Sur
Smith, Doris J **(SLP)**

Blue Jay
Treese, Mrs Carol K **(SLP)**

Bodega Bay
Fulton, Mrs Helen L **(SLP A)**
Illsley, Sylvia Jasso **(SLP)**

Bonita
Day, Charles E **(SLP)**
Griggs, April S **(SLP)**
Valero, Greg Martin **(SLP)**
Van Hemert, Margaret **(SLP)**

Boulder Creek
Graham, Harriet J **(SLP)**
Heyl, Donna Shanley **(SLP)**

Brawley
Asamen, Julie Kimiko **(SLP)**
Hajos, Mrs Anita B **(SLP)**
Tennyson, Patricia J **(SLP)**

Brea
Abrassart, Mrs Joanne Y **(SLP)**
Abrassart, Richard A **(SLP)**
Allard, Laura Ann **(A)**
Barger, Mary Jane **(SLP)**
Brown, George D **(SLP)**
Lichman, Mrs Jeanne M **(SLP)**
Mansur, Cs Wade A **(SLP)**
McCormick, Mrs Suzanne **(SLP)**
Rapp, Deborah E **(SLP)**
Rasmussen, Marjorie R **(SLP)**
Troy, Shirley Loretta **(SLP)**
Winstead, Faye R **(SLP)**

Brentwood
Weinfeld, Brenda **(SLP A)**

Brisbane
Halling, Mrs Shirley Ann **(SLP)**

Buellton
Mann, Mrs Donna J **(SLP)**

Buena Park
Blakeney, Mrs Rachel Joan **(SLP)**
Blauert, Mrs Gladys Gleason **(SLP)**
Landoe, Jurine **(SLP)**
Law, Mrs Sibylla M **(SLP)**
Madding, Carolyn **(SLP)**
Schunk, Marlene Joanne **(SLP)**
Shackelford, Allen El **(SLP)**
Wales, Mrs R Joella **(SLP)**

Burbank
Atkisson, Beth **(SLP)**
Baba, Ann Harumi
Donaldson, Mrs Donalyn B **(SLP)**
Edler, Elaine I **(SLP)**
Forquer, Brian Durand **(A)**
Gasson, Linda Dominguez **(SLP)**
Kesselring, Christina Leigh **(SLP)**
Low, Mrs Annie Chui **(SLP)**
Luger, Linda Suzanne **(SLP)**
Maund, Gay **(A)**
McIntosh-Skupen, Mrs Nancy Linden **(SLP)**
Shapero, Sheldon O **(SLP)**
Wells, Jean A **(SLP)**

Burlingame
Andersen, Jacqueline Barsoom **(SLP)**
Anderson, Daniel G **(SLP)**
Breakey, Margaret R **(A)**
Dotterweich, Mrs Margaret Faith **(SLP)**
Herman, Mrs Mary M **(SLP)**
Larson, Mrs Rita F **(SLP)**
Pestrong, V Monica **(SLP)**
Ratto, Mrs Lorene Lynne **(A)**
Sullivan, Judy M **(SLP)**
Trevithick, Karen Refvem **(SLP)**
Williams, Gina M **(SLP)**

Burney
Condry, Mrs Sherrill R **(SLP)**
Downs, Mrs Paula **(SLP)**

Calabasas
Currie-Crowell, Joanne
Durham, Mary Ellen **(SLP)**
Dwight, Mrs Maria T Campat **(SLP)**
Kysar, Carol B **(SLP)**
Vener, Sharon **(SLP)**
White, Liza C **(SLP)**

Calimesa
Achord, Mrs Sara H **(SLP)**
Schier, Mrs Dianne W **(SLP)**

Calistoga
Brown, Barbara **(SLP)**
Burnham, Nora Eileen **(SLP)**

Camarillo
Aitken, Mrs Sheryl Hooper
Blatt, Clayton L **(A)**
Blatt, Mrs Pamela Ptacek **(SLP)**
Brandt, Dr Grace Emery **(SLP)**
Cherno-Matievich, Mrs Joan **(SLP)**
Drogin, Mrs Brodea M **(SLP)**
Fletcher, Elisabeth Cheryl **(SLP)**
Graff, Shirlee H **(SLP)**
Groom, Mrs Barbara Bogdanoff **(SLP)**
Harrell, Mrs Ruth Ann **(SLP)**
Johnson, Jean T **(SLP)**
Kamino, Mrs Maureen Kay **(SLP)**
Koenigsberger, Mrs Bobbie Ariz **(SLP)**
Lee, Mrs Kathleen Collier **(SLP)**
Marion, Mrs Laurel J **(A)**
Marion, Michael W **(A)**
McDaniel, Mrs Mary Therese **(SLP)**
Moen, Gayl L **(SLP)**
Noonan, Catherine L **(SLP)**
Santora, Paula S **(SLP)**
Smith, Mrs Eleanor Colby **(SLP)**
Smith, Renee J **(SLP)**
Visencio, Louis H **(SLP)**
Walski, Mrs Roberta B **(SLP)**
Willcox, Joyce **(SLP)**

Cambria
Crujido, Mrs Lisa Payne **(SLP)**
Saphier, Marlene **(SLP)**

Campbell
Beckett, Mrs Lyda B **(SLP)**
Blake, Susan Emily
Hardt, Mrs Carol A **(SLP)**
Kearney, Margaret Mary
Kenyon, Kirsten M **(SLP)**
Labourdette, Janet Marie **(SLP)**
Leeman, Mrs Martha Wahl **(SLP)**
Lind, Terrie Lee **(SLP)**
Loeffler, Susanne M **(SLP)**
Mahaffie, Mrs Catherine Jean **(A)**
Maier, Valerie Judith
Sinatra, Kathleen S **(SLP)**
Stephens, Robert William **(SLP)**
Yap, Mrs Lynn Z **(SLP)**

Canoga Park
Burns, Mrs Joyce Shahan **(SLP)**
Cooper, Marsha M **(SLP)**
Flores, Grace A **(SLP)**
Gaulbon, Mrs Lenore B **(SLP)**
Glassman-Lee, Mrs Eileen M **(SLP)**
Guzel, Shakeh N **(SLP)**
Held, Mrs Stephena D **(SLP)**
Jones, Mrs Sheryl K **(SLP)**
Reeve, Dr Rolland Ralph **(SLP)**
Samuels, Barbara A **(SLP)**
Seid, Jill B **(SLP)**
Tanenbaum, Mrs Sheila T **(SLP)**
Tober, Mrs Barbara N **(SLP)**
Toovy, Michael L **(SLP)**
Tveit, Holly L **(SLP)**
Wada, Celeste **(SLP)**
Whitmore, Melodia Kay **(SLP)**
Wolfe, Vivian V **(SLP)**

Canyon Country
Chatterton, Bruce Kerr **(A)**
De La Cruz, Mrs Maritza Lucia **(SLP)**
Drinkwine, Janie **(SLP)**
Edwards-De La Vega, Maureen A **(SLP)**
French-Watts, Mrs Geraldine Anne **(SLP)**
Gatti-Smith, Mrs Filomena **(SLP)**
Hall, Jeffrey Lynn
Mullen, Linda Lee **(SLP)**
Napoli, Mrs Janet Alviani **(SLP)**

Canyon Lake
McEntire, Beverly Lynn **(SLP)**
Schreiner-Stotz, Mrs Dee Ann **(SLP)**
Stotz, William Albert **(A)**

Capistrano Beach
Damon, Mrs Kristine E **(SLP)**
Dermody, Mrs Joan A **(SLP)**

Capitola
Davis, Mrs Margaret W **(A)**

Cardiff
Domenie, Deborah Conard **(SLP)**
Kobernick, Deena Bornstein **(SLP)**
Merin, Diane S **(SLP)**
Salomon, Amy G **(SLP)**
Udwin, Mrs Lisa Home **(SLP)**
Walsh, Mrs Helen Alice **(SLP)**

Cardiff By Sea
Klinger, Mrs Susan Ames **(SLP)**
Thal, Dr Donna J **(SLP)**
Tindel, Mrs Marilyn B **(SLP)**

Carlsbad
Anderson, Mrs Leslie Giles **(SLP)**
Anderson, Randy L **(SLP)**
Birrenkott, Mrs Jan Marianne
Cates, Mrs Susan Mary **(SLP)**
Choy, Sharon Rose **(SLP)**
Croshier, Barbara B **(SLP)**
Dediminicantanio, Susan Paige
Diamond, Barbara S **(SLP)**
Egbert, Dr James H **(SLP)**
Garland-Jacobs, Nancy **(SLP)**
Hart, Terrill L **(SLP)**
Hewitt, Joan Glaser **(A)**
Hobson, Lisa Brewer **(SLP)**
Hofman, Mrs Eliza Kubota **(SLP)**
Johnson, Pearl E **(SLP)**
Koeneke-Varley, Meridith Ann **(SLP)**
Korek, Pamela Jean **(SLP)**
Kratze, Alexa Romain **(SLP)**
L'Esperance, Mrs Merry L **(SLP)**
Lockwood, Belva **(SLP)**
Miller, Mrs Marianne Flowers **(SLP)**
Moore, Sandra Lynne **(SLP)**
Mosele, Mardelle B **(SLP)**
Mueller, Kathleen J **(SLP)**
Murphy, Janice E **(SLP)**
Ryan, Karen Maria **(SLP)**
Saunders, Mrs Nedra J **(SLP)**
Todd, Mrs Margit Juul **(SLP)**
Whitcomb, Mrs Dale P **(SLP)**
Young, Patricia J **(SLP)**

Carmel
Anderle, Mrs Dawn Dershem **(SLP)**
Dalkey, Sharon Lee **(SLP)**
Danielson, Mrs Nenita P **(SLP)**
Hahn, Dr Elise S **(SLP)**
Hixon, Nancy M **(SLP)**
Ryan, Remy Karen **(SLP)**
Sanford, Mark Joseph **(A)**
Weingarten, Barbara McNurney **(SLP)**

Carmel By Sea
Wilson, Ramon L **(SLP)**

Carmel Valley
Thurman, Dr Wayne L **(SLP)**

Carmichael
Bass, Mrs Robbie A **(SLP)**
Beermann, Martha L L **(SLP)**
Bennett, Mrs Donna Faye **(SLP)**
Briggs, Milton M **(SLP)**
Chapple, Persis M **(SLP)**
Edwards, Mrs Suzanne T **(SLP)**
Ference, Terry **(SLP)**
Imada, Dr Dixie H **(A)**
Kamholz, Pamela Kay **(SLP)**
Kilian, Mrs Marianne M **(SLP)**
Kramer, Mrs Patricia Roberts **(SLP)**
Kreeger, Sandra F **(A)**
Mart, Mrs Margaret J **(SLP)**
Minella, Trina C **(SLP)**
Pine-Brandwein, Mrs Shefra T **(SLP)**
Reynolds, Mrs Judith T **(SLP)**
Schaefer-Norris, Christine **(SLP)**
Spector, Mrs Sima **(SLP)**
Studebaker, Diane Joy **(SLP)**
Welborn, Mrs Helen Giese **(SLP)**
Wells, Donna S **(A)**
Westmoreland, Mary M **(SLP)**

Carnelian Bay
Jurey, Ruth A **(SLP)**
Sonnenberg, Esther A **(SLP)**

Carpinteria
Hopkins-Acos, Mrs Patty **(SLP)**
O'Dell-Doiron, Mary Catherine **(SLP)**
Schiemann, Mrs Winifred W **(SLP)**
Smith, Katherine Virginia **(SLP)**

Carson
Whiting, Cheryl A **(SLP)**

Castro Valley
Devane, Margaret Edwards **(A)**
Franzwa, Agnes B **(SLP)**
Helwig, Mrs Mary M K **(A)**
Holland, William H **(A)**
Hyde, Mrs Eileen T **(SLP)**
Kent, Helen
McDonald, Mrs Vesta Betonte **(A)**
Palmer, Mrs Barbara Weisburd **(SLP)**

Cathedral City
Hensler, Eileen Hansen **(A)**

Ceres
Cabral, Claudia Jean **(SLP)**
Crouch, Georgia E **(SLP)**
Platt, Dr James H **(SLP)**

Cerritos
Henderson, Dr Barbara C **(A)**
Lew, Linda **(SLP)**
Martinet, Lenore A **(SLP)**
Rau, Charlene E **(SLP)**
Sanft, Mrs Suzanne B **(SLP)**
Toye, Andrea Rae **(SLP)**
Weaver, Dora C **(SLP)**
Whitaker, Joanna R R **(SLP)**

Chatsworth
Allen, Jacqueline F **(SLP)**
Cujino, Joan E **(SLP)**
Gastel-Pendarvis, Mrs Cristina **(SLP)**
Leeds-Horwitz, Susan B **(SLP)**
Loeb, Elise **(SLP)**
Martin, Sharil **(SLP)**
Satuloff, Mrs Marilyn B **(SLP)**

Cherry Valley
Baxter, Mrs Sandra D **(SLP)**

Chico
Abell, Mrs Jean C **(SLP)**
Barr, Mark Edward **(SLP)**
Birtcil, Mrs Susan Alice **(SLP)**
Blackmon, Dr Robert C **(A)**
Boles, Mrs Joy Liebman
Brasseur, Dr Judith A **(SLP)**
Cain, Mrs Jean Beauloc
Callahan, Robert Ross **(SLP)**
Clark, Marilyn Louise **(SLP)**
Craig, Michelle S **(SLP)**
Eckalbar, Mrs Anne Marie **(SLP)**
Glendinning, Shawn Patrice
Golden, Mrs Diane W **(SLP)**
Hall, Robert E **(SLP)**
Hall, Stacy Alma
Hassenstab-Brines, Mrs Catherine Marie **(SLP)**
Henneberry, Tamara Thompson **(SLP)**
Henry, Sherri Ann
Iseyama, Dee Ann **(SLP)**
Jimenez, Dr Beatrice C **(SLP)**
Johnston, Cheryl Ann **(SLP)**
Knight, Carolyn L **(SLP)**
Kreul, Dr E James **(SLP A)**
Leeson-Forner, Linda **(SLP)**
Lydon, Kathleen Ann **(SLP)**
McCaffrey, Dr Patrick K **(SLP)**
McGettrick, Peggy **(SLP)**
Miller, Mrs Nancy E **(SLP)**
Nissan, Kathleen B **(SLP)**
Palmer, Diane Carol **(SLP)**
Peart, Mrs Trixine Ratliff **(SLP)**
Pittman, Mrs Laura M **(SLP)**
Pulliam, Bonnie L **(SLP)**
Ray, Mrs Gayle C **(SLP)**
Roseberry, Celeste Arleen **(SLP)**
Shrum, Dr William F **(SLP)**
Slocum, Grace Ellen **(SLP)**
Sorenson, Brenda Ranee **(SLP)**
Stanton, Kay **(SLP)**
Starmer, Dr Garrett L **(SLP)**
Stutz, Sue Ann **(SLP)**
Terrill, Mrs Sally B **(SLP)**
Thomas, Mrs Laura O **(SLP)**
Toomey, Wendy J **(SLP)**
Tucker, Pamela J
Waldo-Barr, Kelly **(SLP)**
White, David L **(SLP)**

Chino
Craig, Mrs Emily D **(SLP)**
Dunhoff, Mrs Tess P **(SLP)**

Edgerton, Katharine M **(SLP)**
Jones, Mrs Marietta R **(SLP)**
Langridge, Mrs Diane R **(SLP)**
Lowell, Mrs Elizabeth L **(SLP)**
McMurtry, Mrs Janice Marshall **(SLP)**
Rowley, Carla Jean **(SLP)**
Spears, Mrs Dale Anne **(SLP A)**
Takahashi, Janis L **(SLP)**
Unsworth, Mrs Barbara L **(SLP)**

Chino Hills
Aine, Mrs Lavera F **(SLP)**
Balzer, Lorie A **(SLP)**
Hulme, Nancy A Slater **(SLP)**
Pasqualetto, Morgan **(SLP)**
Pike, Debbie Lynn **(SLP)**

Chula Vista
Bell, Mrs Patricia Gail **(SLP)**
Brown, Mrs Laurie McPhillips **(SLP)**
Chapman, Mrs Verna Jean **(SLP)**
Dashiell, Mrs Judith G **(SLP)**
Dixon, Carmen C **(SLP)**
English, Kristina Marie **(A)**
Harrison, Mrs Wendy Cox **(SLP)**
Laird, Mrs Beverly K **(SLP)**
Lockhart, Charles R **(SLP)**
Myers, Mrs Gladys I **(SLP)**
Sloane, Mrs Jeanine **(A)**
Tani, Mrs Janis Nakanishi **(SLP)**
Vaccaro, Nancy Louise **(SLP)**
Weeks, Mrs Paula B **(SLP)**

Citrus Heights
Findley, Mrs Suzy Streamer **(SLP)**
Jenkins, Mary A **(SLP)**
Phelan, Anna M **(SLP)**
Silkwood, Valerie Gail **(SLP)**
Staal, Donna J **(SLP)**
Wilson, Marsha L **(SLP)**

Claremont
Backus, Dr Ollie L **(SLP)**
Bailey, Mrs Linda K **(SLP)**
Bartholome, Kim Marie **(A)**
Burton, Pamela Y **(SLP)**
Case, Mrs Sally H **(SLP)**
Durall, Dr Maurice J **(SLP)**
Eisenberg, Richard **(SLP)**
Gould, Mrs Marsha L **(SLP)**
Graefe, Mrs Joan W **(SLP)**
Higgins, Dr Mary K **(SLP A)**
Higgins, Paul H **(A)**
Jolly, Mrs Faith **(SLP A)**
Kurland, Linda Sue **(SLP)**
Lott, Kay Ritchie **(SLP)**
Lucas, Gary Allen **(SLP)**
Oglesby, Barbara B **(SLP)**
Owen, Laurie Moeller **(SLP)**
Poole, Joann Neu **(SLP)**
Ragland, Donald Elliott **(SLP)**
Ribbler, Mrs Nancy S **(SLP)**
Schery, Teris Kim **(SLP)**
Selden, Kathleen E **(SLP)**
Shebesta, Mrs Jann K **(SLP)**
Wagman, Mrs Michele A **(SLP)**

Clayton
Dwyer, Cynthia A **(SLP)**
Meuel, Ann S **(SLP)**
Parish, Susan P **(SLP)**

Clovis
Adolph, Mrs Melinda Rae **(SLP)**
Bennett, Mrs Diane E H **(SLP)**
Carter, Mrs Diane Louise **(SLP)**
Foristiere, Melonie Y **(SLP)**
Morrisseau, Mrs Charlene R **(SLP)**
Pimentel, Elizabeth Anne **(SLP)**
Pomaville, Mrs Frances Marian **(SLP)**
Reynolds, Robert B, Jr **(A)**
Rogers, Mrs Cheryl W **(SLP)**
Sandoval-Pugh, Cheryl Ann **(SLP)**
Schuett, Mrs Carmen Bernice **(SLP)**
Sutherland, Mrs Lindsey Martin

Waterman, Sarah Margaret **(SLP)**
Wilson, Donald M **(SLP)**

Coarsegold
Foushee, David R **(SLP)**
Rothchild, Fred H **(SLP)**
Rothchild, Mrs Rita R **(SLP)**
Sherick-Bennett, Dana **(SLP)**

Cobb
La Rue, Janet Ruth **(SLP)**

Colma
Chalmers, Crystal L
O'Connor-Putman, Maureen **(SLP)**

Colton
Brown, Mrs Vivian J **(SLP)**
Fletcher, Mrs Sharon K L **(SLP)**
Godinez-Chan, Noreen Sycip **(SLP)**
Gustafson, Mrs Sharon Elaine
Moore, Marguerite **(SLP)**
Nishikawa, Lynne K **(SLP)**
White, Janie Lynee **(SLP)**
Yeckley, Mrs Rebecca King **(SLP)**

Columbia
Duffy, Mrs Janice E **(SLP)**

Concord
Ahonen, Michele A **(SLP)**
Benjamin, Ruth **(SLP)**
Bernstein-Ellis, Ellen Gay **(SLP)**
Cole, Carole Stimac **(SLP)**
Danforth, Patricia Martin **(SLP)**
Erickson, Mrs Nancy A B **(SLP)**
Esparza, Cami Lurita
Fulford, Mrs Julie O **(A)**
Gardner, Mrs Farrell T **(SLP)**
Gherzi, Barbara M **(SLP)**
Giles, Gerald L **(SLP)**
Grier, Mrs Tose Foote **(SLP)**
Hendrickson, Joseph G, Jr **(SLP)**
Kitchell, Dr Pat S **(SLP)**
Koan, Phyllis A **(SLP)**
Lake, Janet E **(SLP)**
Levy, Mrs Karen Brannigan **(SLP)**
Liniger, Harriet W **(SLP)**
McKissick, Kelly A **(SLP)**
Medsker, Susan A
Miller, Earl Lewis **(SLP A)**
Okanes, Mrs Barbara Marcus **(SLP)**
Sahley, Tony L
Schott, Mrs Kim S **(SLP)**
Shearer, Robert R **(SLP)**
Shubitowski, Yvonne Densie **(SLP)**
Wenters, Melissa Ilene **(A)**
Wright, Joanne M **(SLP)**

Corona
Amundson, Jill Katherine **(SLP)**
Barnes, Phyllis Julie **(SLP)**
Blatchley-Hibbard, Mary Lynn **(SLP)**
Buckley, Mary Maria **(SLP)**
Delahoyde, Mrs Charlene B **(SLP)**
Eagans, Karen K **(SLP)**
Lish, Mrs Jane Gesler **(SLP)**
McCleary, Diana S **(SLP)**
Pollock, Pattie L **(A)**
Powell, Laura Marie **(SLP)**
Reilly, Marilyn E **(A)**
White, Mrs Mary Hawkins **(SLP)**

Corona Del Mar
Aznavoorian, Karen Lea **(SLP)**
Berry, Patricia **(SLP)**
Kopecky, Adele **(SLP)**
Kroll, Paulette **(SLP)**
Thielemeir, Margaret Ann **(A)**
Turgeon, Michelle **(SLP)**
Wallach, Dr Geraldine **(SLP)**

Coronado
Graves, Laury Sanor **(SLP)**
Greathouse, Susan Renee **(SLP)**
Ninneman, Mrs Margaret Sue **(SLP)**

Sullivan, Mrs Mildred Alison **(SLP)**
Trepasso, Mrs Carolyn S **(SLP)**

Corte Madera
Desmond, Deborah Jean **(A)**
Fowler, Kathleen S **(SLP)**
Loring, Diane **(SLP)**
Martin, Karin Kligfield **(SLP)**
Super, Margaret S **(SLP)**

Costa Mesa
Arnesen, Carol B **(SLP)**
Brigham Do, Fleda M **(SLP)**
Dobkin, Mark S **(A)**
Dorf, Gary R **(A)**
Erickson, Constance Farran **(SLP)**
Garcia, Guadalupe **(A)**
Gilmore, Sheila Elizabeth **(SLP)**
Goud, Ramesh M **(SLP)**
Goud, Mrs Ranjan R **(SLP)**
Hansen, Mark H **(SLP)**
Hollingsworth, Mrs Carolyn D **(SLP)**
Kisner, Rita P **(SLP)**
Letostak, Jody Terry **(SLP)**
Lukins, Margaret Roblee **(SLP)**
McClanahan, Mrs Anne R
Medeles, Sandra Silva **(SLP)**
Melgares, Nancy **(SLP)**
Raimondis, Nina M **(SLP)**
Rausch, Mrs Kathleen S **(SLP)**
Smith, Glenn L **(SLP)**
Spear, Barbara H **(SLP)**
Supal, Connie Alane
Thompson, Mrs Wendy Wade **(SLP)**
Trowe, Pamela J **(SLP)**
Wells, Karon **(SLP)**

Covina
Borghi, Mrs Mary Jo **(SLP)**
Borghi, Dr Robert W **(SLP)**
Grisham, Robert C **(A)**
Hurley, Robert Lee, Jr **(SLP)**
Kistler, Blaze W **(A)**
Morris, Mary Ann **(SLP)**
Nagami, Pamela S **(SLP)**
Peart, Mrs Joan T **(SLP)**
Pitzer, Mrs Carol Woodruff **(A)**
Roberts, Mrs Leticia A **(SLP)**

Crescent City
Beatty-Hanko, Maya P **(SLP)**
Standring, Lorene Carver **(SLP)**

Crestline
Keller, Sharon Pillsbury **(SLP)**
Rashok, Katherine

Cromberg
Digby, Matthew J **(SLP)**

Cucamonga
Schlessinger, Amy Joan **(SLP)**
Tisler, Mrs Susan Jone **(SLP)**

Culver City
Allen, Mrs Lauri Marie **(SLP)**
Balber, Bethel **(SLP)**
Basner, Anne M **(A)**
Basner, Barry **(SLP)**
Cowan, Beth Ann **(SLP)**
Epport, Karen Lynn **(SLP)**
Hayes, Mrs Joanne G **(SLP)**
Horn, Stuart A **(A)**
Kutcher, Evelyn Gong **(A)**
McCladdie, Michelle R **(A)**
Medall, Lisa Zee **(SLP)**
Milner, Mrs Joyce Browning **(SLP)**
Osgood, Eleanor **(SLP)**
Richie, Dr Dolores J **(SLP)**
Saxman, Rosalie G **(A)**
Sheridan, Mrs Amelia P **(SLP)**
Shlaes, Toni E **(SLP)**

Cupertino
Biemer, Carole Ann **(SLP)**
Borengasser, Sara Lynn **(SLP)**

Cross, Mrs Gloria J **(SLP)**
Langdon, Dr Henriette W **(SLP)**
Melhus, Marina L **(SLP)**
Peterson, Susan Kathryn
Reading, Patricia **(SLP)**
Speed, Marilynn E **(SLP)**
Weinman, Janice **(SLP)**
Zitman, Mrs Diana Victoria **(SLP)**

Cyn Country
Essary, Mrs Rebecca Z **(SLP)**

Cypress
Arguijo, Edward **(SLP)**
Arguijo, Mrs Rebecca Lou **(SLP)**
Banchi, Charlotte A
Flohr, Mrs Pamela Lampshire
Furst, Mrs Dorothy J **(SLP)**
Gilmore, Willis C **(SLP)**
Harpole, Susan Lois
Kelley, Pamela J **(SLP)**
Lux, Cecelia Marie **(SLP)**
Rogers-Leimbach, Mrs Julie Ann **(SLP)**
Rose, Mrs Corie H **(SLP)**
Shapiro, Dr Irving **(A)**
Shotwell, Sue Christense
Stephenson, Cathy Lynne **(SLP)**

Daly City
Buzolich, Dr Marilyn J **(SLP)**
Draper, Patricia Louise
Ghio, Adele Ann **(SLP)**
Stone, Mrs Mary Pearsall **(SLP)**
Ullman, Merle Charmian **(SLP)**
Wood, Mary Ellen **(SLP)**

Dana Point
Abramson, Maria L K **(A)**
Becker, Catherine **(SLP)**
Brown, Mrs Susan Mathews **(SLP)**
Countryman, Darlene M
Frazee, Mrs Cynthia M **(SLP)**
McCool, Mrs Linda Jean **(SLP)**
Sanders, Stephen Jeffrey **(A)**

Danville
Bloom, Mrs Deborah B **(SLP)**
Bordogna, Marianne **(SLP)**
Brown-Myers, Stephanie **(SLP)**
Campbell, Mrs Patricia A **(SLP)**
Clark, Mrs Amy R G **(SLP)**
Daddio, Mary McLellan **(SLP)**
Davis, Edward T **(SLP)**
Eberline, Linda Jean **(SLP)**
Englehardt, Mrs Alyce C **(SLP)**
Laporte, Lynn M **(SLP)**
Mazzella-Gordon, Mrs Carmella **(SLP)**
Riley, Dr Russell V **(SLP)**
Robbins, Christine **(SLP)**
Ryan, Joelyn V **(SLP)**
Sakata, Mrs Karen Shigezumi **(SLP)**
Schatz, Nancy Troxel **(SLP)**
Steinhauser, Mrs Michal Urban **(SLP)**
Willing, Mrs Mavis A **(SLP)**

Davis
Ayer, Edith Annette **(SLP)**
Baecker, Frederick W **(SLP)**
Baecker, Phyllis J **(SLP)**
Borchers, Mrs Alice D **(SLP)**
Brodie, Maureen Nakazawa **(SLP)**
Burns, Mrs Danielle S **(SLP)**
Charley, Mrs Linda Kay **(SLP)**
Cliff, Mrs Susie Elaine **(SLP)**
Diamond, Laura A **(SLP)**
Grant, Mrs Theresa Terry **(SLP A)**
Greenhill, Ann Hirsh **(SLP)**
Hasek, Nancy Jane **(SLP)**
Hodell, Susan F **(A)**
Larssen, Karen **(SLP)**
Lewis, Mary F **(SLP)**
Louderback, Frances Mae **(SLP)**
Moore, Mrs Edra Lurae **(SLP)**
Nelson, Joanna Boettcher
Oldenburg, Lynda S **(SLP)**

Pollnow, Rita K **(SLP)**
Posner, Elizabeth H **(SLP)**
Reutter, Susan L **(SLP)**
Rivers, Jill **(SLP)**
Updike, Mrs Suzanne Scott **(SLP)**
Weathers, Debra Louise
Zefo, Anna Marie **(SLP)**
Zimmerman, Diane Power **(SLP)**

Del Mar
Deetz, Mrs Janis Lee **(SLP)**
Deftos, Mrs Linda H **(SLP)**
Fruehling, Beverly H **(SLP)**
Goerlitz, Cynthia Jo **(SLP)**
Kiel, Mrs Julia J **(SLP)**
Scheinberg, Dr Judith C **(A)**
Williams, Diane Ruley **(A)**
Woolf, Dr Carole L **(SLP)**

Delmont
Wilson, Margaret B **(SLP)**

Denair
Gauger-Crownover, Terry K **(SLP)**

Descanso
Perdomo, Celia F **(SLP)**

Desert Hot Springs
Dixon, Karen Sue **(SLP)**
Gorman, Stephen J **(SLP)**

Diamond Bar
Adolf, Kathryn A **(SLP)**
Chenoweth, Mrs Marybeth Keith **(SLP)**
Deasy, Mrs Laurie Noriega **(SLP)**
Goldblatt, Mary Anne **(SLP)**
Lawrie, Patricia Marie S **(SLP)**
Linehan, Mrs Cynthia Konow **(SLP)**
Nagey, Caroline **(SLP)**
Sclar, Judith **(SLP)**
Trunk, Dr Joseph **(A)**
Unruh, Perry Wallace **(A)**

Diamond Springs
English, Mrs Susan T **(SLP)**

Dinuba
Cochran, Ione M **(SLP)**
Gregory, Mrs Judith M **(SLP)**

Downey
Allen, Mark Eugene **(SLP)**
Bauer, Dr Cherie **(SLP)**
Cavanagh, John M **(A)**
Cross, Janet Ann **(SLP)**
DeRuyter, Dr Frank **(SLP)**
Hasler, Lorrie Marie **(SLP)**
Huff, Donna Todd **(SLP)**
Naranjo, Lucina A **(SLP)**
Pasta, Albert Stephen **(SLP)**
Popejoy, Maurice E **(A)**

Duarte
Dye, Mrs Linda McLean **(A)**
Thies, Mrs Harriet Fleischer **(SLP)**
Thies, Dr Terry L **(SLP A)**

Dublin
Hanna-Kraus, Mrs Linda Susan **(A)**
Moore, Mrs Betty E **(SLP)**
Moultrie, Mary Ann Taylor **(SLP)**
Staehle, Mrs Gayle Hornbeck **(SLP)**
Williams, Lori Anne **(SLP)**

Durham
Boone, Mrs Linda Ann **(SLP)**
Thomas-Will, Marjorie Bryant **(SLP)**

East Highland
Carper, Kelly Anne

East Palo Alto
Jackson, Patricia A **(SLP)**

El Cajon
Biggerstaff, Michele Ann **(SLP)**
Chinn, Andrea **(SLP)**
Cowen, Mrs Roberta Polgar **(SLP)**
Ehrlich, Cynthia L **(SLP)**
Hicks, Gayle E **(A)**
Hoeptner, Mrs Deborah Miller **(SLP)**
Hohn-Hizal, Mrs Diane Carol
Kitson, Mrs Laura G J **(SLP)**
Le Resche, Mrs Marilyn M **(SLP)**
Lewis, Mrs Shirley M **(SLP)**
Marino, Mrs Catherine **(SLP)**
McArthur, Cindy Biss **(SLP)**
McMahon, Kelley Kay **(SLP)**
Meyer, Marcia Ann **(SLP)**
Prebys, Paul T **(SLP)**
Rasmussen Noble, Shelly Rae **(SLP)**
Redding, Mrs Marguerite S **(A)**
Sablove, Audrey B **(SLP)**
Sandlin, Dr Robert E **(SLP A)**
Stephenson, Mrs Eleanor Alice **(SLP)**
Stowers, Richard A **(SLP)**
Stowers, Shirley Richard **(SLP)**
Susca, Mary Alice Schiff **(SLP)**
Susca, Michael **(SLP)**
Thomas, Donna Terry **(SLP)**
Turchin, Mrs Beverly K **(SLP)**
Wallace, Mrs Marion M **(SLP)**
Zehm, Lucia Adrignola **(SLP)**

El Centro
Berryman, Erika Linette **(SLP)**
Hubbard, Mrs Gail L **(A)**
Parker, Carmen K **(SLP)**

El Cerrito
Furst, Mrs Alice Coopersmith **(SLP)**
Gott, Mrs Sylvia Rulff **(SLP)**
Hylander, Diana Jo **(SLP)**
Panush, Robert Marc **(SLP)**
Rose, Carolyn Estelle **(SLP)**
Soneda, Mrs Rosaline Ong **(SLP)**
Thoman, Connie Lyn **(SLP)**
Tsujimoto-Cho, Gail Miyuki **(SLP)**

El Dorado Hills
Healey-Dame, Mary **(SLP)**
Helm, Alexis **(SLP)**

El Granada
Benson, Darcy E **(A)**
Edgren, Mrs Dawn S **(SLP)**
Ryan, Mrs Lori A **(SLP)**

El Monte
Hoglin, Mrs Sherrie **(A)**
Pomes, Mrs Leticia Flores

El Segundo
Kihara, Jane J **(SLP)**
Lanphere, Teresa **(SLP)**
Peterson, Mrs Linda Moyer **(SLP)**

El Sobrante
Jakubowitz, Melissa D **(SLP)**
McCullough, Mrs Peggy Crooks **(SLP)**
Taft, Lavonne Joyette **(A)**

El Toro
Avne, Mrs Laura **(SLP)**
Bates, Fredra D **(SLP)**
Cates, Mrs Cheryl A **(SLP)**
Day, Karen Loly **(SLP)**
Duggleby, Mrs Eileen H **(SLP)**
Estep, Mrs Janet M **(SLP)**
Gardiner, Maureen M **(A)**
Glasser-Woolf, Mrs Dorie Ann **(SLP)**
Holtzclaw, Mrs Lisa I S **(SLP)**
Hull, Barbara B **(SLP)**
Jackson, Mrs Lee Ann **(SLP)**
Konopisos, Mrs Melinda J **(SLP)**
McIntyre, Judith R **(SLP)**
Preston, Mrs Gwenn E **(SLP)**
Rosenthal, Michael J **(SLP)**
Shiffman-Sacks, Susan Lee **(A)**
Sullivan, Mrs Helen A **(SLP)**
Waters, Lori Kristina **(SLP)**

Eldridge
Noha, Martha H **(A)**

Elk Grove
Allison, Geraldine **(SLP)**
Cagle, Daphne **(SLP)**
Haskins, Sherry E **(SLP)**
Merritt, Cynthia Smith **(A)**
Perez, Elisa **(SLP)**
Pierson, Mrs Robin M M **(SLP)**
Sargisson, Lisa J **(SLP)**
Smith, Mrs Diane E O **(SLP)**

Elverta
Smith-Lehmann, Rebecca **(SLP)**

Emeryville
Leininger, Gail Lynn **(A)**

Encinitas
Berg, Joyce Kennedy **(SLP)**
Bondesson, Mrs Kelly Froning **(SLP)**
Boyarsky, Marcia J **(SLP)**
Casenave, Mrs Deeann Mari **(SLP)**
Chatfield, Mrs Janet Leutel **(SLP)**
Detweiler, Lynda G **(SLP)**
Devon-Frank, Mrs Gloria **(A)**
Edsall, Deborah Gail **(SLP)**
Edwards, Linda M **(SLP)**
Elam, David Scott **(SLP)**
Elam, Nancy Revelli **(SLP)**
Gavin, Linda V **(SLP)**
Hawkins, Cassandra Ann
Ill, Mrs Karen A **(SLP)**
Johns, Mrs Julie O'Donovan **(A)**
Llewellyn, Deborah Daniels **(SLP)**
MacHin, Mrs Karen Louise **(SLP)**
MacNeil-Brint, Kathleen M
Martin, Mrs Lisa King **(SLP)**
May, Mary E
Mills, Jane Burrington **(SLP)**
Riedler, Valerie L **(SLP)**
Schwartz, Teresa M **(SLP)**
Sims, Mrs Nancy Monroe **(SLP)**
Smith, Kathleen McCullum **(SLP)**
Trudeau, Gerard A **(SLP)**
Tyler, Sheila Marie **(SLP)**
Wong, Mrs Shirley A **(SLP)**

Encino
Aroesty, Mrs Fern **(SLP)**
Dubrovner, Mrs Shulamith **(SLP)**
Ferdows, Nazanin **(SLP)**
Freeman, Dr Ben **(SLP)**
Gerson, Barbara Beer **(SLP)**
Glick, Donna Rochelle **(A)**
Hestrin, Mrs Marcia K **(SLP)**
Hoisch, Mrs Ruth Pomeranz **(SLP)**
Knox, Nancy Shapiro **(SLP)**
Kreitzman, Jackie L **(SLP)**
Lew, Beverly **(A)**
Lopata, Leslie Faden **(SLP)**
Meckler, Marlys **(SLP)**
Oppenheim, Mrs Debra L **(SLP)**
Piner, Bruce D **(A)**
Poster, Mrs Roberta F **(SLP)**
Robin, Peggy T J **(SLP)**
Rome, Mrs Deborah K **(SLP)**
Rothman, Mrs Ruth S **(SLP)**
Schlosser, Mrs Barbara F **(SLP)**
Sedlik, Mrs Bernice M **(SLP)**
Shrira, Lois R **(SLP)**
Sniderman, Mrs Shirley G **(SLP)**
Steinberg, Mrs Ethel M **(SLP)**
Willensky, Andi R **(SLP)**

Escalon
Moss, Mary M **(SLP)**

Escondido
Bell, Pamela **(SLP)**
Bova, Lisa Gross **(SLP)**
Check, Christine Ann **(SLP)**
Daniel, Mrs Nina MacAulay **(SLP)**
Edwards, Mrs Elena G **(SLP)**
Grasberger, Jan E **(SLP)**
Hanson, Lyle Duane **(SLP)**
Hicks, Charlotte Visniski **(SLP)**
Illich, David Michael **(A)**
Kirpalani, Mrs Pamela Tadlock **(SLP)**
Lang, Dr Adrianne **(SLP)**
Noronha, Mrs Barbara Louise **(SLP)**
Schumacher, Janis Lynn **(SLP)**
Skutshek, Mrs Denise Lynne **(SLP)**
Watson, Donna Ann **(SLP)**

Eureka
Elliott, Mrs Ovieda Perra **(SLP)**
Freudiger-Grantham, Trish
Hunt, Mrs Janeth Nash **(SLP)**
Meek, Stephanie **(SLP)**
Murray, Dennis Paul **(SLP)**
Osredkar, Mark M **(SLP)**
Paulus, Janet Eileen **(SLP)**
Phoenix, Mary Lydon **(SLP)**
Swerdlow, Leonard S **(SLP)**

Exeter
Brenner, Clyde J **(SLP)**
Linik, Frank Joseph **(A)**
Watson, Mrs Tammy Dahlberg **(SLP)**

Fair Oaks
Anderson, Betty D **(SLP)**
Anuber, Susan Elizabeth **(SLP)**
Bowling, Dr Evelyn B **(SLP)**
Dae, Donna **(SLP)**
James, Mrs Kay Robbins **(SLP)**
Tollefson, Mrs Christine Hirahara **(SLP)**

Fairfax
Bauer, Mrs Lynn G **(SLP)**
Ross, Cindy A **(A)**

Fairfield
Bogart, Lynn M **(SLP)**
Bunselmeier, Karen Baxter **(SLP)**
Davis, Mrs Emily H **(SLP)**
Esposto-Franklin, Lesa **(SLP)**
Griffin, Beverly J **(A)**
Huddleston, Lynne A **(SLP)**
Kudszus, Ursula R **(SLP)**
Lawrence, Dr Frank R **(SLP)**
Plummer, Dr Bonnie A **(SLP)**
Puskas, Rene R **(SLP)**
Wirth, David B **(A)**
Zwanziger, Mrs Dianne K **(SLP)**

Fallbrook
Ventuleth, Mrs Shannon M

Felton
Petrovich-Larwood, Lou Yvonne

Ferndale
Baumgartner, Mrs Dawn M **(SLP)**

Fieldbrook
Meyer, Mary F **(SLP)**

Fillmore
Caldwell, Nancy A
Stafford-Litton, Bonnie Jean **(SLP)**

Firebaugh
Wood, Mrs Jan M **(SLP)**

Folsom
Baker, Carla Jean **(SLP)**
Bryant, Stephanie **(A)**
Eubank, P Gail **(SLP)**
McElroy, Nancy T **(SLP)**
Rawiszer, Steven J **(A)**
Rivard, Mrs Joan M **(SLP)**
Torres, Mrs Dorothy V **(SLP)**

Fontana
Juliano, Mrs Ethel D **(SLP)**
Maly, Mrs Debra Rhein **(SLP)**

Fort Bragg
Malnati, Cheryl
Menken, Dr Gregory E **(SLP)**
Neuwald, Kathleen Marie **(SLP)**
Patterson-Waters, Jann **(SLP)**

Fort Ord
Lane, Linda Carolyn **(SLP)**
Pardon, Donna M **(A)**

Fortuna
Howard, Mrs Renee L **(SLP)**
Johnson, Cynthia Clark **(SLP)**
Wells, Julia Ann **(SLP)**

Foster City
Chandler, Emily D **(SLP)**
Christiansen, Kay **(SLP)**
Deruy, Debora G **(SLP)**
Golden, Maureen Theresa **(SLP)**
Kasprisin, Dr Arlene **(SLP)**
McCollough, Yvonne D **(SLP)**
Mower, Laura D **(SLP)**
Pex, Carol M **(SLP)**
Rooney, Robin Theresa **(SLP)**
Yourtz, Susan B **(SLP)**

Fountain Valley
Barwick, Steven A **(A)**
Caforio, Mrs Judith Mae-England **(SLP)**
Forsythe, Mrs Linda A **(SLP)**
French, Mrs Wendolyn Houghton **(SLP)**
Joseph, Mrs Ida M G **(SLP)**
Knipprath, Mrs Cathleen H **(SLP)**
Lange, Barbara L **(SLP)**
Lehman, Jean S
Leveque, Mrs Grace
McNeill, Mrs Mannon B **(SLP)**
Mendenhall, Patricia Ann **(SLP)**
Mills, Donna S **(SLP)**
Montgomery, Dr Judith K **(SLP)**
Nimmo, Mrs Regina E **(SLP)**
Stephens Brown, Mrs Sally Willis **(SLP)**
Wachtor, Carol T **(SLP)**

Fowler
Cholakian, Cathy M **(SLP)**

FPO San Francisco
Pearson, Mrs Mary G **(SLP)**

Freestone
Rossman, Robin A **(SLP)**

Fremont
Ball, Arnetha **(SLP)**
Berzin, Audrey E **(SLP)**
Bolig, Loyola Leveroni **(A)**
Coles, Pamela L W **(A)**
Dugoni, Marianne C **(SLP)**
Garland, Cynthia A **(A)**
Hasson-Perakis, Karin Elise **(SLP)**
Jones, Mrs Karen P **(SLP)**
Kane, Janet T **(SLP)**
Lacey, Christine **(SLP)**
Lacosse, Mrs Brenda J S **(A)**
Laudenslager, Mrs Wanda Lee **(SLP)**
Mikulich, Danielle M **(A)**
Miller-Gordon, Deborah
Nelson, Mrs Michele **(SLP)**
Oza, Kalindi Uttam **(A)**
Perlewitz, Jo Ann **(SLP)**
Polsky, Marla R **(SLP)**
Rothaug, Mrs Wendy Wallach
Salzmann, Mrs Mary Anne **(SLP)**
Schmidt, Mrs Ann W **(A)**
Tanaka, Cathleen **(SLP)**
Taylor, Mrs Diane M **(SLP)**
Wilcox, Mrs Linda A **(SLP)**
Wilson, Mrs Colleen Collins **(SLP)**
Wolf, Judith A **(SLP)**
Wolff, Mrs Linda Louise **(A)**
Wood, Karen Hughes **(SLP)**
Yee, Patricia Anne **(SLP)**
Zante, Mrs Sylvia M **(SLP)**

Fresno
Abell, Mrs Jacqueline **(SLP)**
Allen, Mrs Elizabeth **(SLP)**
Amend, Mrs Gaylee M **(SLP)**
Arnst, Dr Dennis James **(A)**
Baker, Christopher **(SLP)**
Bernthal, Mrs Gail **(A)**
Blizard, Dorothy E **(SLP)**
Borofka, Debbie Marie **(SLP)**
Bryant, Jonathan D **(A)**
Buck, Sandra L **(SLP)**
Bunting, Mrs Janet Lanfranco **(SLP)**
Capelli, Robin Maria **(SLP)**
Chadwick, Jean M **(SLP)**
Chavira, Mrs Diane Noel **(SLP)**
Clark, Ione A **(SLP)**
Conae, Francine D **(SLP)**
Cottingham, Linda M **(SLP)**
Curry-Carter, Mrs Elena Maria **(SLP)**
De Laveaga, Mrs Sharon Ruth **(SLP)**
Donovan, Lori M
Duvall, Michelle P **(SLP)**
Eng, Marlene **(SLP)**
Eversole, Laura Marie **(SLP)**
Graves, Mrs Patricia Lynn
Gregg, Ann English **(SLP)**
Hanoian-De St Jeor, Mrs Sharon **(SLP)**
Heath, Shirley T **(SLP)**
Hegde, Dr M N **(SLP)**
Horsley, Beverly Jean M **(SLP)**
Huschle, Mary Patricia **(SLP)**
Jern, Mrs Lori E **(SLP)**
Johnson, Pamela Lynn **(SLP)**
Kelly, Dr Ben R **(A)**
King, Jody Lynette **(SLP)**
Krikorian, Mrs Lynn A **(A)**
Larson, Mrs Susan J **(SLP)**
Lauria, Joanne **(SLP)**
Long, Mrs Beverly E **(SLP)**
Lowe, Mrs Linnea Katherine **(SLP)**
Martin, Shena Wileman **(A)**
Massie, Sherin L T **(SLP)**
Mayeda, M Melinda Gaminde **(SLP)**
McMain, Deanna G **(A)**
McManaway, Emily Paula **(SLP)**
Mecham, Steven G **(A)**
Miller-Arnst, Charlene **(SLP)**
Miyamoto, Kay D **(SLP)**
Moats, Barbara H **(SLP)**
Murvay, Terri Elizabeth **(SLP)**
O'Brien, Mrs Lorraine K **(SLP)**
Olsen, Dr Clifford C **(A)**
Olson, Kimberly Kaye **(SLP)**
Osumi, Joy Lynne **(SLP)**
Parker, Dr Ron M **(A)**
Penza, Allison M **(SLP)**
Perl, Sarah Miriam **(SLP)**
Pinkerton, Susan Joy **(A)**
Powers, Mrs Myrna G **(SLP)**
Reichert, Judith A **(SLP)**
Reither, Mrs Linda P **(SLP A)**
Richesin, Kathy Nash **(A)**
Rittore, Carol B **(SLP)**
Roberts, Dr Stephen D **(A)**
Rollins, Mrs Teresa A **(SLP)**
Rowe, Mrs Karen A **(SLP)**
Sa, Theresa Rene **(SLP)**
Sacks, Stephen W **(SLP)**
Samuelian, Mrs Charlene J **(SLP)**
Schneider, Mrs Sandra V **(SLP)**
Schneiderman, Dr Carl Royce **(SLP)**
Scott, Mrs Kathleen Ann **(SLP)**
Shanks, Dr Susan **(SLP)**
Shipley, Dr Kenneth G **(SLP)**
Shumway, Erma J **(SLP)**
Smith, Mrs Janet Novella **(SLP)**
Speechly, Marla D **(SLP)**
Stines, Elizabeth A **(SLP)**
Stoddard, Jeanne Hagen **(SLP)**
Swinehart, Therese M **(SLP)**
Tatum, Tom L **(SLP)**
Telesmanic, Mrs Joanne C **(SLP)**
Telesmanic, Dr Luciano P **(SLP)**
Uribe, Judy **(SLP)**
Urrutia, Deborah Jean **(SLP)**
Wadsworth, Dr Steven D **(SLP)**
Wage, Kathryn J **(SLP)**
Weber-Olsen, Dr Marcia M **(SLP)**
West, Lane **(A)**
Whelan, Catherine **(SLP)**
Williams, Dorythea C **(SLP)**
Williams, Patricia J **(SLP)**

Fullerton
Brooks, Jacqueline Marie
Buckley, Mary E **(SLP)**
Bueermann, Donald William **(A)**
Chisum, Mrs Linda H **(SLP)**
Collins, Joan Pratt **(SLP)**
Corfariu, Mrs Manuela
Crane, Phyllis Taillon **(SLP)**
Crary, Delores F **(SLP)**
Dalton, Kathleen B **(SLP)**
Davis, Dr Michael J **(A)**
Grossman, Melvin R **(SLP)**
Hatcher, Caro C **(SLP)**
Heer, Pamela L **(SLP)**
Kitselman, Dr Kurt **(SLP)**
Lamberth, Mrs Ellen McGuirk **(SLP)**
Li, Dr Edith C **(SLP)**
Maenaga, Linda A
Marshall, Paulette A **(SLP)**
McLean, Kathleen Ann **(SLP)**
Merritt, Joanna Z **(SLP)**
Mondello, Linda Jean **(SLP)**
Nelson, Dr Max **(SLP A)**
Pellino, Phyllis Ann **(SLP)**
Pippert, Mrs Linda K **(SLP)**
Riggs, Mrs Kristy **(SLP)**
Sherman, Cynthia Jean **(A)**
Smitheran, Judith R **(SLP)**
Switzer, Janet Lynne **(SLP)**
Thorum, Dr Arden R **(SLP)**
Tucker, Mrs Barbara L **(SLP)**
Vanvliet, Dennis **(A)**
Vogt, Dr Gayle H **(SLP)**
Wilcox, Laura Lynn **(SLP)**

Galt
Willing, Janice E **(SLP)**

Garberville
Richardson, Wanda Arlene **(SLP)**

Garden Grove
Alters, Mrs Laura Lynn **(SLP)**
Archer, Mrs Jane B **(SLP)**
Barnes, Nancy Jean G **(SLP)**
Chiaromonte, Leatrice Auzenne **(SLP)**
Cragin, Mrs Karen Ann **(SLP)**
Crain, Mrs Cherie L **(SLP)**
Dietrich, Mrs Virginia Joyce **(SLP)**
Dutton, Donald E, Jr **(SLP)**
Etchepare, Teresa Lu **(SLP)**
Hernandez, Mrs Stephanie Day **(SLP)**
Jasman, Daniel Robert **(SLP)**
Letto, Claire **(SLP)**
Metz, Dr Michael J **(A)**
Rampey, Robin Sue
Rogers, Robert Kimsey **(A)**
Scherer, Dr Nancy J **(SLP)**
Sloniger, Diann Marie **(SLP)**
Smith, Mrs Karen Iati
Stockton, Nancy Miller **(SLP)**
Tanabe, Karen Jo **(SLP)**
Wiley, Kay D **(SLP)**

Garden Valley
Delongchamp, Mrs Kerri Joanne

Gardena
Blake, Susan L **(A)**
Fong, Craig Daniel **(A)**
Minson, Adrienne Ann

Gilroy
Carr, Sherrean Marie **(SLP)**
Ewing, Janice R **(SLP)**
O'Dea-Dooley, Kathleen **(SLP)**
Smith, Thomas D **(SLP)**

Glen Ellen
Goldstein, Patricia B **(SLP)**
Shandler, Phyllis **(SLP)**
Uptmor, Eileen M **(SLP)**

Glendale
Baghdassarian, Mrs Kathleen **(A)**
Czuzak, Mrs Alicia Mitter **(A)**
Dumaux, William E **(A)**
Elliott, Alicia **(SLP)**
Ferguson, Patricia Ann **(SLP)**
Frederick, Mrs Lois K **(SLP)**
Greig, Rhonda Banke **(SLP)**
Lamorey, Suzanne Grace **(A)**
Lewellen, Sherri Ann **(A)**
Lichtman, Andrea R **(SLP)**
Lowe, Raymond L **(SLP)**
Mamey, Joan F **(SLP)**
McKinney, Dr Virginia
McQuirk, Susan Jean
Michel, Linda Beth **(SLP)**
Obando, Nancy Moreno **(SLP)**
Olsen, Mrs Betty **(SLP)**
Orloff, Wendy L **(SLP)**
Simek, Sheryl L **(SLP)**
Teele, Mrs Miriam R **(A)**
Tharp, Patricia G **(SLP)**

Glendora
Anglin, Colleen Sue **(SLP)**
Atkisson, Nancy L **(SLP)**
Belak-Plenger, Barbara J **(SLP)**
Bonavich, Mrs Louise F **(SLP)**
Burggraaf, Cynthia Lieberg **(SLP)**
Dayne, Mrs Margaret N **(SLP)**
Kunze, Mrs Barbara Lou **(SLP)**
Miller, Mrs Nanette Malicki **(SLP)**
Pioli, Elizabeth **(SLP)**
Whittle, J Kathryn **(SLP)**
Zimmer-Lucas, Mary Elizabeth **(SLP)**

Gold River
Bergounous, Paulette M **(SLP)**
Dellasanta, Mrs Marcia L **(SLP)**
Edmiston, Karen P **(SLP)**
Poteet, Carol Elaine **(SLP)**
Whitton, Mrs Janna Gordon **(SLP)**

Goleta
Bhardwaj, Mrs Kathern A **(SLP)**
Garfinkel, Janine Boggs **(A)**
Gauvain, Joyce Eileen **(SLP)**
Gelberg, Bernice F **(SLP)**
King, Annabelle Joyce
Murphy, Mrs Lisa A **(SLP)**
Myles-Zitzer, Catherine A **(SLP)**
Pelland, Mrs Carmen M **(SLP)**
Tuma, Elizabeth Rose **(SLP)**
Zitzer, Robert **(SLP)**

Granada Hills
Arnold, Marcia L **(SLP)**
Bergman, Wendy O **(SLP)**
Cate, Carol Paulson **(SLP)**
Cook, Sally J **(SLP)**
Cornelius, Cathleen Adele **(SLP)**
Dankowski, Margaret Mary **(SLP)**
Gardner, Dr Julie O **(SLP)**
Geller, Ann Harding **(SLP)**
Harrington, Donna B **(SLP)**
Hogg, Jamie Marie
Honowitz, Stacey Rae **(SLP)**
Judkowitz, Mrs Joyce Palefsky **(SLP)**
Lisak, Mrs Myriam Tobon
Luter, Dr James G, Jr **(SLP)**
Mabel, Suzanne S **(A)**
Middleton, Lorraine D
Pehde, Mrs Harriet L **(SLP)**
Pleskus, Mrs Judy Lynn **(SLP)**
Rolls, Denise Patricia **(SLP)**
Tanihana, Jami Hatsumi **(A)**
Walcek, Ann Marie **(A)**
Wolf, Dr Kenneth E **(A)**

Grand Terrace
Scriven, Mrs Louise M **(SLP)**

Granite Bay
Haugh, Mrs Elise B **(SLP)**
King-Streit, Mrs Suzanne **(SLP)**

Grass Valley
Boss, Peggy Hawbecker **(SLP)**
Coley, Karen E **(A)**
Culhane, Karen D **(SLP)**
Levan, Dee A **(SLP)**
Lovestedt, Lucille K **(SLP)**
Nat, Mrs Melinda Fisk **(SLP)**
Timmons, Barbara **(SLP)**

Greenbrae
Cuttie, Vallarie Smith **(A)**
Luxenberg, Jan **(A)**
Sammis, Mrs Suzanne M **(SLP)**

Grover City
Erickson, Mrs Ellen A **(SLP)**

Hacienda Heights
Aguilera-Posen, Judith Diana **(SLP)**
Applebaum, Mrs Nikki A R **(SLP)**
Becker, Susan Nancy **(A)**
Herrera, Evelyn Catherine **(SLP)**
Majernik, Mrs Sylvia R **(A)**
Sue-O'Brien, Mrs Debora C **(SLP)**
Tan, Grace M Y **(SLP)**
Webster, Richard V **(SLP)**
Yamasaki, Tim **(A)**

Half Moon Bay
Baker, Dr Rochelle A **(SLP)**
Chambers, Patricia L **(SLP)**
Fox, M Elisa Lamb **(SLP)**
Whitney, Elizabeth Jane **(A)**

Hanford
Berg-Mattos, Wendy Marie **(SLP)**
Penn, Mrs Erta V **(SLP)**
Vieira, Mrs Rhonda Honora **(SLP)**
Welch, Mrs Alison Keene **(SLP)**

Harbor City
Fujimoto, June Mitsunaga **(SLP)**
Nozaki, Joanne M **(SLP)**
Orsten, Marguerite M **(SLP)**
Roush, Mrs Betty Michie **(SLP)**

Hawaiian Gardens
Bohleen-Ferguson, Ellen Elizabeth **(SLP)**

Hayward
Bercovitz, Karin R **(SLP)**
Bohntinsky, Mrs Dorothy J **(SLP)**
Ehrlich, Beth L **(A)**
Ho, Mrs Esther M **(SLP)**
Johnson, Charita B **(SLP)**
Kriege, Mari S **(SLP)**
Martin, Maureen McHugh
Masterman, Mrs Sandra J
Mayo, Kathleen Tina **(SLP)**
Roberts, Mrs Lynn **(SLP)**
Rosenthal, Dr William Sidney **(SLP)**
Schumacher, Dawn M
Slack, Patti Jo
Solomon, James R **(SLP)**
Tuder, Peggy Jean **(SLP A)**
Utsumi, Mrs Patricia Jan **(SLP)**
Walker, Beverly S **(SLP)**

Healdsburg
Crabtree, Chris Tina **(SLP)**
Hammer, Larry D **(SLP)**

Heber
Apodaca, Anna Rose

Hemet
Arcidiacono, Nina A **(SLP)**
Dalzell, Mrs Mary Ellen **(SLP)**
Jenkins, Mrs Helen Michelle **(SLP)**
Landes, Mrs Eileen Schaefer **(SLP)**
Porter-Cope, Judith L **(SLP)**
Ruybal, Alfredo E **(SLP)**
Wagers, Mrs Gloria S **(SLP)**

Hercules
Brady, Mrs Patricia A **(SLP)**
Wan, Mrs Charisse Louie **(SLP)**

Hermosa Beach
Boochever, Mrs Kathleen R **(SLP)**
Contieri-Pease, Mrs Carol F **(A)**
Demore, Janice Elaine **(SLP)**
Jackson, Catherine A **(SLP)**
Jones, Kathleen H **(SLP)**
Larson-Tuttle, Claudine Sandra **(A)**
Lewis, Janet E **(SLP)**
Myers, Roxanne Elizabeth **(SLP)**
Nugent, Therese M
Watroba, Cheryl Ann **(SLP)**
Wittman, Mrs Holly Diane **(SLP)**

Hesperia
Holmskog, Sevia Lynne **(SLP)**

Hidden Hills
Cooper, Dr Donna J **(SLP)**
Siegel, Marcia G **(SLP)**

Highland
Bachman, Mary Elizabeth **(SLP)**
Brossia, Mrs Martha Burrell
Harwood, Mrs Monica Anne **(SLP)**
Krause, Linda S **(SLP)**
Law, Debra L T **(SLP)**
Turner, Mrs Jayne S

Hillsborough
Buchwald, Mrs Janet S **(SLP)**
Erpen, AnnaMarie **(SLP)**
Fletcher, Dorothy L **(SLP)**
Luongo, Rhonda Ruth **(SLP)**
Weil, Mrs Miriam S **(SLP)**

Hilmar
Pace, Carlynn Marie **(SLP)**
Ramsey, Mrs Mary Lindsay **(SLP)**

Hollister
Belt, Dr Donald A **(SLP A)**
Morejohn, Nikki Lynn **(SLP)**
Rocco, Pamela Jean **(SLP)**
Talbot, Elizabeth Parker **(SLP)**
Tobias, Marian Rosenthal **(SLP)**

Hollywood
Brisbane, Glenda **(A)**
Davison, Michelle M **(SLP)**
Moss, Margaret Lynn **(SLP)**
Wolff, Adele M **(SLP)**

Hollywood Hills
Noffsinger, Dr P Douglas **(A)**

Huntington
Hart, Lauana J **(SLP)**

Huntington Beach
Bivens, Kathleen McCarty **(SLP)**
Blair, Mrs Jo Ann **(SLP)**
Boggs, Teresa Ann **(SLP)**
Bradley, Emilie S **(SLP)**
Briggs, Mrs Joanne S **(SLP)**
Brown, Marianne Kathryn **(SLP)**
Buchanan, Mrs Christine Mary **(SLP)**
Carter-Jackson, Cynthia A **(SLP)**
Chen, Rose Jenman **(SLP)**
Cochran, Mrs Evelyn C **(SLP)**
Cook, Nicholas J **(SLP)**
Creighton, Mrs Barbara B **(SLP)**
Currey, Lindsay A **(SLP)**
Deutsch, Shirley M L **(SLP)**
Diaz, Karen L **(SLP)**
Earlabaugh, Mrs Susanne **(SLP)**
Ehring, Dana Sue **(SLP)**
England, Kathie Elizabeth **(SLP)**
Ganulin, Mrs Karen Johnson **(SLP)**
Generous, Christine Leigh **(SLP)**
Goldberg-Stoter, Mrs Gail **(SLP)**
Gonsalves, Jan M **(SLP)**
Graves, Mrs Sharon R **(SLP)**
Green, Barbara Jean **(SLP)**
Guarnera, Mrs Susan E **(SLP)**
Guinn, Gail A **(SLP)**
Haunreiter, Mrs Rose Kathleen **(SLP)**
Hawk, Dr Elizabeth **(SLP)**
Hole, Karen Lynn **(SLP)**
Inamasu, Laura T **(SLP)**
Jackson, Kenneth J **(SLP)**
Jacobs, Mrs Nancy **(SLP)**
Jarvis, Mrs Elizabeth Wolz **(SLP)**
Jeffers, Donna P **(SLP)**
Johnson, Mrs Leeda G **(SLP)**
Kahn, Dr Nancy T **(SLP)**
Kaplan, Donald E **(SLP A)**
Kincaid, Vicki S Y **(SLP)**
Kohut, Carrie Ann **(A)**
Larkin, Patricia G **(SLP)**
Levy, Sheila Z **(SLP)**
Luth, Mrs Tracy R **(SLP)**
Mayer, Mrs Sharon Peach **(SLP)**
Miller, Joseph William **(SLP)**
Nichols, Mrs Brenda Jean **(SLP)**
Ordonez, Mrs Joan F **(SLP)**
Pearl, Bonnie P **(SLP)**
Quinn, Rhonda Rougelot **(SLP)**
Roland, Margaret G **(SLP)**
Sasano, Lynn A **(SLP)**
Schutte, Mrs Kris Dykstra
Schwartz, Lorene M **(SLP)**
Sheeks, Debra Sue **(SLP)**
Sinclair, Mrs Paula **(SLP)**
Sterkel, Mrs Mary J K **(SLP)**
Teitelbaum, Mrs Susan Jane **(A)**
Trevennen, Mrs Betsy B **(SLP)**
Von Achen, Mrs Deborah Goldman **(SLP)**
Warren, Mrs Deborah L **(SLP)**
Welch, Nina J F **(SLP)**
White, Janis Bryant **(SLP)**
Wolfe, Cynthia S **(SLP)**
Zipp, Judy Ann

Huntington Harbor
Selker-Adams, Judith M **(SLP)**

Idyllwild
Drolet, Cynthia J **(SLP)**
Latham, Mrs Nancy J **(SLP)**
Meyer, Neil N **(SLP)**

Imperial Beach
Richards, Jacqueline J **(A)**

Indian Wells
Barkemeyer, Maudene Wheeler **(SLP)**

Indio
Burson, Susan L
Fedrick, Pary K **(SLP)**

Inglewood
Brayton-Gerratt, Shaun **(SLP)**
Cawby, Jerry L **(SLP)**
Crumpler, Mrs Gloria T **(SLP)**
Hiersemann, Ruth L **(SLP)**
King, Joan **(SLP)**
Law-Till, Cindy B **(SLP)**
Levy, Joanne Schnee **(SLP)**
Mooney, Patricia V **(SLP)**

Irvine
Black, Mrs Natalye S **(SLP)**
Bochynski, Cathy K **(SLP)**
Bordok, Barbara Coons **(SLP)**
Brisbois, Susan G **(SLP)**
Busby, Robert A **(SLP)**
Butler, Mrs Rebecca **(SLP)**
Causino, Maryanne **(SLP)**
Chasin, Mrs Rachel L **(A)**
Cox, Ronald S **(SLP)**
Crews, Linda Johnston
Daily, Linda Jennings **(A)**
Dashiell, Sallie E **(SLP)**
Erickson, Cathy Suzan **(SLP)**
Evans, Laura F **(SLP)**
Fibel, Yvette J **(SLP)**
Fielder, Mrs Susan B **(SLP)**
Fujikawa, Dr Sharon E **(A)**
Gilmer, Mrs Mary Grace **(SLP)**
Gogolin, Marilyn T **(SLP)**
Gold, Mrs Lynn Dickson **(SLP)**
Goldstein, Mrs Beverly Ruth **(SLP)**
Gorback-Lopez, Nadzia Marie **(SLP)**
Hatzkilson, Mrs Jennifer A
Herring, Phyllis W **(SLP)**
Hill, Mrs Linda C **(SLP)**
Hilling, Mrs Christina A **(SLP)**
Hogan, Dolores A **(SLP)**
Hundley, Lucinda G **(SLP)**
Jackson-Colando, Patricia **(SLP)**
Keenan, Mrs Judy E **(SLP)**
Levine, Susan B **(SLP)**
Nielsen, Jan K P **(SLP)**
Novegrod, Mrs Marcia Kessert **(SLP)**
Parsons, Mrs Jennifer G **(SLP)**
Pellico, Mrs Janice Barbara **(SLP)**
Petersen, Christine Kay **(SLP)**
Pickett, Donna L **(SLP)**
Plass, Mrs Beverly Goodrich **(SLP)**
Rapp, Mrs Kathleen Wilks **(SLP)**
Rothwell, Karen R **(A)**
Schrenzel, Jane R **(A)**
Schroeder, Mrs Brenda Brownlee **(SLP)**
Sebby-Hornbruch, Mrs Ingrid **(SLP)**
Sheldon, Mrs Alexis H **(SLP)**
Singleton, Mrs Mary Susan **(A)**
Spiegel, Lisa Michelle **(SLP)**
Stetson, Mrs Roxanne E **(SLP)**
Still, Mrs Linda L **(SLP)**
Timler, Geralyn R **(SLP)**
Tonini, Mrs Kathleen M **(SLP)**
Tracer, Gale E **(SLP)**
Wallace, Mrs Lori Ann/Borth **(SLP)**
Wilson, Dr Michele Drisko **(A)**
Wirt, Elizabeth C **(SLP)**

Isla Vista
Mitsunaga, Faye F

Jackson
Kee, Linda M **(SLP)**
Yaffee, Nadine L **(SLP)**

Jamul
Harrelson, Michael **(SLP)**

Jamulpur
Montgomery, Mrs Kathryn D **(SLP)**

Janesville
Steele, Michele Shelly

Joshua Tree
Kirchmann, Olivia Augustina **(SLP)**
Maurer, Anne Berg **(SLP)**
Mitz, Mary E **(SLP)**

Kensington
Carman, Carol K **(A)**
Hartmann, Barbara Sheehy **(SLP)**
Silver, Jane **(SLP)**
Simrin, Shelley **(SLP)**

Kentfield
Dimeglio, Angela **(SLP)**
Goudy-Andrew, Sandra **(SLP)**
Hamilton, Mrs Dorothy T **(A)**
Rayman, Naomi Sinai **(SLP)**

Kenwood
Taylor, Mrs Lauren B **(SLP)**

Kings Beach
Seymour, Mrs Bonnie Lee **(SLP)**

Kings Canyon Natl Park
Warner, Mrs Janet K **(SLP)**

Kingsburg
Cole, Terrilynn **(SLP)**

La Canada
Balisy, Mrs Diane Elizabeth **(SLP)**
Brady, Bonnie B **(SLP)**
Brown, Melba V **(A)**

Chaplin, Mrs Beverly Fagen **(A)**
Cryder, Ellen Gail **(SLP)**
Drake, Mrs Patricia A **(SLP)**
Foley, Mary Josp **(SLP)**
Hoskins, Dr Richard A **(SLP)**
Knerl, Mary K **(SLP)**
Ogden, Helen Vaughan **(SLP)**
Senne, Allen John **(A)**
Senne, Mrs Catherine Ann **(A)**
Stein, Mrs Marilyn L **(SLP)**

La Costa
Goodman, Joan Lee **(SLP)**

La Crescenta
Bollier, Betty J **(SLP)**
King, Kathleen **(A)**
Linane, Mrs Valerie Ann **(SLP)**
Martin, Leslie Schroeder
Mudd, Sherri G **(SLP)**
Riner-Costantino, Patricia Collleen **(SLP)**

La Habra
Attaway, Mrs Judith Marie **(A)**
Bailey, Peggy L **(SLP)**
Burgess, Mrs Vicky L **(SLP)**
James, Susan Kathleen **(SLP)**
Lloyd, Mrs Rose M **(SLP)**
Menzel, Mrs Rita H **(SLP)**
Moore, Marti **(SLP)**
Teoman, Patricia Lynne
Walters, Mrs Judith Raucci **(SLP)**

La Habra Heights
Wyman, Mrs Beverly Ann **(SLP)**

La Honda
Chwalek, Maryann C **(SLP)**

La Jolla
Barclay, Mrs Pamela Harford **(SLP)**
Bastian, Jalinda A **(SLP)**
Brown, Rhea Strauss **(SLP)**
Bulley, Kathleen Ann **(A)**
Chandler, Mrs Mary Kay W **(SLP)**
Chien, Mrs Patricia Anne **(SLP)**
Clarke, Susan M **(SLP)**
Cohen, Ivan J **(A)**
Dodge-Sipan, Patricia **(SLP)**
Fischer, Mrs Marlowe W **(SLP)**
Foster, Holly Anne **(SLP)**
Gee, Erin M **(A)**
Hageman, Mrs Ruth A **(SLP)**
Halliwell, Nancy **(SLP)**
Harden, Dr Sheila H **(SLP)**
Hurd, Joyce A E **(SLP)**
Isenberg, Mrs Leslie Z **(SLP)**
King, Dr Susan H **(SLP)**
Kozin, Linda P **(SLP)**
Leisz, Jacquelin **(SLP)**
Marinkovich, Gayle E **(SLP)**
Poiset, Melissa L **(SLP)**
Rafkin, David **(SLP)**
Salo, Ladonna **(SLP)**
Sample, Pamela A **(A)**
Slovin, Susan Colvin **(SLP)**
Valji, Susanna K **(SLP)**

La Mesa
Augustine, Mrs Suzanne Renee **(SLP)**
Austerlitz, Mrs Francine S **(SLP)**
Baird, Patricia M **(A)**
Bleigh, Mrs Marjorie Eady **(SLP)**
Blitz-Noel, Elyse **(SLP)**
Boncher, JoAnne B **(SLP)**
Clark, Mrs Sara H **(A)**
Curwen, Mrs Vicki E
Dustin, Carla J **(SLP)**
Ghio, Mrs Carol Bennett **(SLP)**
Goldberg, Mrs Dianne **(SLP)**
Gupta, Mrs Anne Pottinger **(SLP)**
Hansen, Corine S **(SLP)**
Hoffer, Kathleen R **(SLP)**
Kesling, Randy Ann Marshall **(SLP)**
Kitson, Nancy Carolan **(SLP)**
Leduc, Mrs Sandra S **(SLP)**
Lindsey, Deanne Michelle **(SLP)**
McWilliams, Linda Leverenz
Merritt, Audree Huhn **(SLP)**
Morgan, Ann M **(SLP)**
Nobiensky, Wynne **(SLP)**
Porras-Bagingito, Tina L
Richardson, Marcelle R **(SLP)**
Schrock, Patricia Bradley **(SLP)**
Schroeder, Linda L **(A)**
Stengel, Mark L **(SLP)**
Storton, Deborah S **(SLP)**
Tyll, Terry W **(A)**
Van Der Voort, Mrs Denise Boyle **(SLP)**
Wulfeck, Dr Beverly B **(SLP)**
Yount, Mrs Carol L **(SLP)**

La Mirada
Beck, Michael David **(SLP)**
Deluca-Braccio, Virginia A **(SLP)**
Lambright, Barbara L **(A)**
McQueen, Mrs Carol B **(SLP)**
Provo, Deborah K **(SLP)**
Shanebeck, Mrs Camilla Diane

La Palma
Gulland, Melinda **(SLP)**
Imizu-Iwanaga, Darlene **(SLP)**
Lipe, Lisa Ann **(A)**
Mast, Barbara D **(SLP)**
Rutherford, Dr Karen M **(A)**

La Puente
Jones, Lenora L **(SLP)**

La Quinta
Bowman, Mrs Sylvia Ann **(SLP)**

La Selva Beach
Dunn, Lawrence E **(SLP)**
Vanhouten, Mrs Eleanor F **(SLP)**

La Verne
Bakhit, Lily Mary **(SLP)**
Klein, Dr M Diane **(SLP)**
Kraushar, Saundra Ann **(SLP)**
Little, Cassandra A **(SLP)**
Smith, Mrs Pamela Z **(SLP)**
Steinwinter, Sheryl S B **(SLP)**
Wilkins, Mrs Rita Ann **(SLP)**

Lafayette
Banker-Trotter, Anne **(SLP)**
Biasatti-Croak, Lynne **(SLP)**
Dobkin, Gloria A **(SLP)**
Hughes, Joanne M **(SLP)**
Levine, Mrs Cynthia S **(SLP)**
Malin, Susan S **(SLP)**
Melmed, Dr Paul J **(SLP)**
Newhart, Mrs Patricia Hassan **(SLP)**
Phillips, Mrs Loretta A **(SLP)**
Pickton, Mrs Alice Monosmith **(SLP)**
Rubins, Mrs Sue G **(SLP)**
Sears, Cathy L **(SLP)**
Sulprizio, Sandra L **(SLP)**
Swatek, Linda Kay **(SLP)**

Laguna Beach
Deyoung, Linda S **(SLP A)**
Hupp, Randall **(SLP)**
Jelinek, Mrs Judith E M **(SLP)**
Kolberg, Mrs Carolyn K **(SLP)**
Nelsen, Mrs Lynn E **(SLP)**
Oliveri, Geraldine **(SLP)**
Pendleton, Jewel A **(SLP)**
Perrault, Sara Jeanne **(SLP)**
Vian, Linda **(SLP)**
West, Mrs Nancy Lee **(SLP)**
Woodhouse, Toby **(SLP)**

Laguna Hills
Bourassa, Diane **(SLP)**
Brenner, Michelle Gowen **(SLP)**
Broida, Dr Helen **(SLP)**
Chin, Amy K **(SLP)**
Cline, Janna M **(A)**
Daly, Cynthia **(SLP)**
Erkel, Karen L **(SLP)**
Goodman, Mrs Sharlene **(SLP)**
Karpati, Janet M Knutson **(SLP)**
Katsuyama, Laurel H **(SLP)**
Larson, Mrs Thalia W **(SLP)**
Lee, Caroline M
Lynn, Karen Lee **(SLP)**
Mahoney, Mrs Barbara Katherine **(SLP)**
McJenkin, Mrs Dorothy F **(SLP)**
Puntil, Jo A **(SLP)**
Streicher, John Paul **(SLP)**
Weaver, Carol Nan **(SLP)**
White, Nancy J **(SLP)**
Wobst, Mrs Judy L Rhodes **(SLP)**
Zelman, Betty M **(SLP)**

Laguna Niguel
Block, Marie K **(SLP)**
Bollingmo, Susan Spivak **(SLP)**
Carley, Linda L M **(SLP)**
Daniels, Mary Rose Turley **(SLP)**
Davis, Rose Marie **(SLP)**
Delfosse, Mrs Anne L **(SLP)**
Delfosse, Michael L **(SLP)**
Flair, Mrs Erin M **(SLP)**
Ghan, Mary **(SLP)**
Greene, Margaret **(SLP)**
Hollenbeck, Mrs Judy E **(SLP)**
Jones, Donna L **(A)**
Kansas-Zahn, Mrs Kathleen Marie **(SLP)**
Krater, Mary K **(SLP)**
Lagourgue, Helen F **(SLP)**
Lagourgue, John R
Lipsett, Robert K **(SLP)**
Livesay, Laurel Y **(SLP)**
Martinez, Shari L **(SLP)**
Milburn, Mrs Rosemary L **(SLP)**
Miles, Mrs Janet A **(SLP)**
Schwallie, Mrs Lora L
Schwartz, Dr Edith M **(SLP A)**
Stewart, Mrs Sharon S **(SLP)**
Van Fossen, Lucinda Twitchell **(SLP)**
Ware, Debra Davis **(SLP)**
Wilson, Mrs Sherrie Lynn **(SLP)**
Wright, Elizabeth O **(SLP)**

Lake San Marcos
Manucia, Dr Charles F **(SLP)**

Lakeport
Hage-Brodnansky, Becky

Lakewood
Albosta, Karen **(SLP)**
Arismendi, Mrs Cheryl A **(SLP)**
Brine, Mrs Lou Ann **(SLP)**
Crosby, Mrs Brenda Weiland **(SLP)**
Curel, Julia Akimi **(SLP)**
Fagan, Leslie Lorraine **(SLP)**
Fee, Mrs Christine Diane **(SLP)**
Frankeberger, Robert D **(SLP)**
Hawkins, Elizabeth Rae **(A)**
Langsam, Susan Klaif **(SLP)**
Levinson, Shelly K **(SLP)**
McInally, Mrs Lynn Torigoe **(SLP)**
Mills, Dawna Mitchell **(A)**
Nathan, Debra E **(SLP)**
Oltman, Mrs Barbara Jean **(SLP)**
Rogers, Mrs Rebecca A **(SLP)**
Thomas, Mrs Mary Jacobs **(A)**

Lamesa
Frank, Sherry Southers **(SLP)**

Lancaster
Courtney, Thomas W **(SLP)**
Heidt, Sheryl Lee **(SLP)**
Kew, Joyce Margaret **(SLP)**
Knutson, Mrs Leah Joy **(SLP)**
McMillan, Jeanette Lum
McPherson, Larry T **(A)**
Schneider, Dr Elaine Fogel **(SLP)**
Stephenson, Heather Lucile
Vercruysse, Mrs Robin Ehrlich **(SLP)**
Vetter, Virginia **(SLP)**
Wurfel, Mrs Karen K **(SLP)**

Larkspur
Lococo, Jomar K **(SLP)**
Reilly, Mrs Katherine **(A)**

Lebec
Evans-McDowell, Mrs Judy K **(SLP)**

Lemon Grove
Beyer, Willena A **(A)**

Lemoore
Breen, Mrs Jennifer Gates **(SLP)**
Callaghan, Mrs Wendy M **(SLP)**
Mohr, Cheryl Kay **(SLP)**

Leona Valley
Eisbrener-Hester, Patricia Anne **(SLP)**

Leucadia
Casey, Victoria L **(SLP)**
Hightower, Caroline J **(SLP)**
Johnson, Kathryn A **(SLP)**

Linden
Datwyler, Bonita Brooks **(SLP)**

Little River
Brownson, Mariam Allen **(A)**

Livermore
Chace, Carmel Joan **(SLP)**
Dickerson, Dr Mary V Dearstone **(SLP)**
Eaton, Mrs Joyce P **(SLP)**
Gary, Mrs Caroline Jean **(SLP)**
Howard, Deborah K
Hoyle, Marsha **(SLP)**
Massey, Holly Joyce **(SLP)**
McGowan, Mrs Laurie Hendricks **(SLP)**
Meyer, Susan Marie **(SLP)**
Otting, Victoria Louise **(SLP)**
Stimatz-Elchesen, Marcia **(SLP A)**

Livingston
Moore, Mrs Judith A **(SLP)**

Lodi
Armstrong, Elizabeth Gale **(A)**
Christy, Mrs Janis Lynn **(SLP)**
Dickey, Mrs Lynette Case **(SLP)**
Diroll, Mrs Debbie J **(SLP)**
Edwards, Mrs Jacque J **(A)**
Field, Terri Lynne **(SLP)**
Graber, Gail Rust **(A)**
Hazen, Mrs Nancy White **(SLP)**
Hodgson, Margaret Murphy **(SLP)**
Maclel, Karen J **(SLP)**
McCoy, Dr Carolyn **(SLP A)**
Navone, Michelle L **(SLP)**
Nishizaki, Mrs Debra J **(SLP)**
Schock, Mrs Diane M **(SLP)**
Snyder, Mrs Annemarie Luginbuhl **(SLP)**
Sorenson, Dr Fay D **(A)**
Todd, Eleanor F
Yates-Bennett, Mrs Sharon Michelle **(SLP)**

Loma Linda
Baer, Juli Ann **(SLP)**
Barnard, Dr Logan W **(SLP)**
Erich, Mrs Kristen Lea **(SLP)**
Khoo, Mrs Keiko I **(A)**
Lawson, Janet Lee **(SLP)**
Lowry, Kathleen Mary **(SLP)**
Moon, Marjorie M **(SLP)**
Moore, Mrs Penny Louise W **(SLP)**
Racosky, Janice D **(SLP)**
Ratcliff, Ann E **(SLP)**
Rawson, Craig Allen **(A)**
Richards, Melonie Sauceda **(SLP)**
Roach, Robert A **(SLP)**
Robinson, Mrs Susan Mulder
Swenson, Donna E **(SLP)**
Vaughan, Dr Robin H **(A)**

Lomita
Berman, Ira Isaac **(SLP)**

Brown, Marsha A **(SLP)**
Moretti, Margaret E **(A)**
Nelson, Linda Lee **(A)**
Schafer, Stuart **(A)**

Lompoc

Arneson, James **(SLP A)**
Beebe, Margaret W **(SLP)**
Cross, Mrs Laura S **(SLP)**
Cruickshank, Teresa Lee **(SLP)**
Graves, Risa Hershman **(SLP)**
McReynolds, Barbara L **(SLP)**
O'Neill, Patricia Ilene **(SLP)**
Palmer, Marjorie M **(SLP)**
Runyon, Mrs Phyllis J **(SLP)**
Sankey, Carole J **(SLP)**
Wallace, Mrs Maureen Porter **(A)**
Yingst, Kathleen E **(SLP)**

Lone Pine

Echelbarger, Clara Dee **(SLP)**

Long Beach

Agranowitz, Aleen C **(SLP)**
Agranowitz, Sara **(SLP)**
Applbaum, Robyn Sue **(SLP)**
Aten, Dr James L **(SLP)**
Bangar, Diane M **(SLP)**
Barkell, Nancy Leigh **(SLP)**
Basil, Sherwin A **(SLP A)**
Beattie, Randall C **(A)**
Beber, Mrs Pamela Sue **(SLP)**
Bowden, Mrs Debra J **(SLP)**
Boyd, Mrs Sylvia Sturz **(SLP)**
Brannon, Mrs Laurie **(SLP)**
Brown, C Rebecca
Burt, Mrs Frances Corine **(SLP)**
Burton, Wendy Elizabeth **(SLP)**
Cecil, Mrs Elizabeth Ann **(SLP)**
Christensen, Mary V **(SLP)**
Cook, Barbara L **(SLP)**
Cooper, Dr June M **(SLP)**
Covert, Kathleen Gillin **(SLP)**
Craven, Dr Duane C **(SLP)**
Curtis, Mrs Gale H **(SLP)**
Dale, Elizabeth **(A)**
Davis, Traci Karlene **(SLP)**
Dewey, Susan Jean **(SLP)**
Dunbar, Mrs Fern S **(SLP)**
Duncan, Susan Louise
Epstein, Carolyn W **(SLP)**
Erratt, John David **(A)**
Eugenio-Nahina, Lianne G **(SLP)**
Faridani, Mrs Samina Ramzan **(SLP)**
Farman, Jill Pellerin **(SLP)**
Fidler, David B **(SLP)**
Forney, Jack L **(SLP A)**
Fowler, Cynthia G **(A)**
Franke, Lauren K **(SLP)**
Fugleberg, Ruth Ann **(A)**
Gallant, Maureen Victoria **(SLP)**
Garry, Mrs Elizabeth Philbrick **(SLP)**
Gasaway, Jane **(SLP)**
Geller Vogeli, Mrs Sherry R **(SLP)**
Gerlach, Mrs Kirsty E **(A)**
Gower-Alba, Mrs Lynne Ellen **(SLP)**
Hall, Maureen Bridget **(SLP)**
Hoekstra, Belinda **(SLP)**
Horner, Patricia **(SLP)**
Howe, Mrs Robin Lynne **(SLP)**
Huffman, Dr Elna S **(SLP)**
Isaacs, Elizabeth Ellen **(SLP)**
Jackson, Janancy S
Jeffery, Jill Coleen **(SLP)**
Johnson, Susan L **(SLP)**
Kaber, Dinneen L **(SLP)**
Kaplan, Susan K **(A)**
Kastagir, Penelope A **(SLP)**
Kidd, Joyce E **(SLP)**
Kisich, Esther S **(SLP)**
Klemin, Mrs Lisa Maria **(SLP)**
Knowles, Brooke O **(SLP)**
Kolmodin, Sally J **(A)**
Landes, Dr Bernard A **(SLP A)**
Lauless, Sandra L **(SLP)**
Lawson, Audrey C **(SLP)**
Lex, Mrs Sandra B **(SLP)**
Litton, Mrs Alene L **(SLP)**
Loganbill, Dr G Bruce
Marshall, Mrs Susan L **(SLP)**
Mazzocco, Diane M **(SLP)**
Merrill, Mrs Sharon Mares **(SLP)**
Mikami, Charlene Mieko **(A)**
Miller, Laura Dean **(A)**
Miniaci, Karen J **(SLP)**
Montague, Jean L **(SLP)**
Montgomery, Mrs Maureen Maguire **(SLP)**
Munzer, Mrs Susan W **(SLP)**
Noble, Marilyn L **(A)**
Oberle, Kristina Lynn **(SLP)**
Oliva, Constance **(SLP)**
Parker, Kristine J **(SLP)**
Partridge, Lyman M **(SLP)**
Pearson, Lynn R **(SLP)**
Pepitone, Celeste C **(SLP)**
Perkins, Denise Kay **(SLP)**
Perttula, Betty S **(SLP)**
Preece, Dr John P **(A)**
Rainey, Barbara J Trost **(SLP)**
Robinson-Murphy, Jennifer **(SLP)**
Rosen, Roberta A **(SLP)**
Ryan, Barbara V **(SLP)**
Ryan, Bruce P **(SLP)**
Sanderson, Tanya B **(SLP)**
Sandler, Eileen B **(SLP)**
Shanks, Janet E **(A)**
Sheridan, Susan M **(SLP)**
Shinn, Dr Joyce A **(SLP)**
Simpson, Anne E **(SLP)**
Simpson, Mrs Marianne **(SLP)**
Smith, Reginald Robin **(SLP)**
Sollecito, Kathy Jeanne **(SLP)**
Speirs, Dr James A **(SLP)**
Spokane, Frances G **(SLP)**
Stephan, Mrs Jean M **(SLP)**
Stiles, Mrs Sharon Kubacki **(SLP)**
Stuller, Mrs Arlene **(SLP)**
Svigals, Dolores J **(SLP)**
Talburt, Mrs Valerie S **(SLP)**
Tapp-Gallegos, Mrs Jennifer Gisele **(SLP)**
Tefft, Donita R **(SLP)**
Thebarge, Thomas N **(SLP)**
Thompson, Branita L **(SLP)**
Thompson, Patricia Lynne **(SLP)**
Till, Dr James A **(SLP)**
Wagner, Charlotte **(SLP)**
Wardrip-Fruin, Carolyn **(SLP)**
We Hara, Constance Sada **(SLP)**
Wiesner, Civia Renne **(SLP)**
Willard, Sandra M **(SLP)**
Wilson, Dr Richard Hayes **(A)**
Wright, Lelia C **(SLP)**
Yates, Dr Joann Ruth **(SLP)**
Zizz, Carol A **(A)**

Loomis

Conrad, Brenda K
Kinstler, Dr Donald B **(SLP A)**
Nolan, Barbara L **(SLP)**
Nolan, Steven C **(A)**
Tomita, Mrs Bessie S **(SLP)**
Weatherwax, Leslie Roberta **(SLP)**

Los Alamitos

Conway, Mrs Nancy A **(SLP)**
Curran, Nancy Voegeli **(SLP)**
Deutsch, Dr Steven E **(SLP)**
Dorsey, Cynthia Ann **(SLP)**
Kleiman, Larry I **(SLP)**
Korzeniowski, Mrs Roxanne F **(SLP)**
Mallory, Jocelyn Elaine **(SLP)**
Phelps, Mrs Elizabeth Waller **(SLP)**
Radaich, Susan J **(SLP)**
Reed, Andrea Brown **(A)**
Snyder, Dr Lynn Sebestyen **(SLP)**
Williamson, Mrs Sharon L H **(SLP)**

Los Altos

Bates, Bette B **(A)**
Baxter, Jane H **(A)**
Breslow, Karen Ann **(SLP)**
Gesell, Carol Grace **(SLP)**
Giudici, Mrs Henrietta Helen **(SLP)**
Hon, Mrs Christine Voye **(SLP)**
Jordan, Connie L **(A)**
Krebs, Mrs Barbara Ballard **(SLP)**
Lathrop, Jennifer Fargo **(A)**
Mannos, Mrs Ronnie S **(SLP)**
Martindale, Mrs Eleanor N **(SLP)**
O'Connor, M Catherine **(SLP)**
Parker, Jayne H **(SLP)**
Ratner, Mrs Ellen J **(SLP)**
Tight, Mrs Jane T **(SLP)**
Wadden, Mrs Rosemary S **(SLP)**
Webster, Brendan O **(SLP)**
Wreaks, Annette Catherine **(SLP)**

Los Altos Hills

Barrager, Dr Diane Copeland **(A)**
Bate, Mrs Christine Porter **(SLP)**
Henderson, Juliet M **(SLP)**

Los Angeles

Abshez, Mrs Wendy Ann **(SLP)**
Ackerman, Carol A **(SLP)**
Alcan, Christine Lynn **(SLP)**
Allsman, Catherine **(A)**
Antone, Deborah C **(SLP)**
Apper, Cheryl Wenkart **(SLP)**
Ash, Carol Diane **(A)**
Bader, Mrs Shellie Sue **(SLP)**
Baral, Mrs Sydell **(SLP)**
Bargelt, Hal James **(SLP)**
Barkan, Merle Beth **(SLP)**
Barkan, Vicki Lee **(SLP)**
Barrett, Betty A **(SLP)**
Baumwohl, Dana **(A)**
Beaufait, Kathleen B **(SLP)**
Bell, Karen J **(SLP A)**
Ben-Moshe, Mrs Felice **(SLP)**
Bennett, Carissa D **(A)**
Berkey, David A **(A)**
Bernstein, Mrs Diane Elizabeth **(SLP)**
Berry, Cheryl Denise **(SLP)**
Betsworth, Mrs Anne Hogue **(A)**
Bias-Scott, Mary Ellen **(SLP)**
Biegun, Deborah Lee **(SLP)**
Blank, Marcia Smith **(A)**
Bloch, Sharon Ruth/Cohen **(SLP)**
Bosko, Carmela Sansone **(SLP)**
Bower, Mrs Deborah R **(A)**
Bowers, Marilyn Darcel
Bradfield, Patricia Annette **(SLP)**
Bravos, Christine **(SLP)**
Brenner, Eve H **(SLP)**
Brough, Nancy Carroll **(SLP)**
Brown, Elizabeth A H **(SLP)**
Burnette, Jacqueline Tiongson **(SLP)**
Carlson, Terry E **(SLP)**
Carmen, Richard E **(A)**
Chavez-Law, Mrs Rita **(SLP)**
Christensen, Dr Arden H **(SLP)**
Christopher, Mrs Dana E **(SLP)**
Clark-Thomas, Mrs Eleanor M **(SLP A)**
Cohen, Dr Melvin S **(SLP)**
Coleman, John R **(A)**
Colman, Joan C B **(SLP)**
Cone-Wesson, Dr Barbara K **(A)**
Conrad, Susan J **(A)**
Cook, Timothy G **(A)**
Cooper, Dr Donald Stewart
Cooper, Mrs Marcia Hartung **(SLP)**
Cooper, Dr Morton **(SLP)**
Cort, Mrs Vianne K
Cravens-Matheson, Mrs Catherine **(SLP)**
Cummings, Marjorie D **(SLP)**
Cutler, Ellen S **(SLP)**
Dabney, Marsha Jo
Davidoff, Marsha N **(SLP)**
Day-Register, Mrs Patricia **(SLP)**
Delacy, Hester S **(SLP)**
Dersh, Laurie M **(A)**
Diament, Mrs Cynthia J **(SLP)**
Diamond, Linda Feldsott **(SLP)**
Dirks, Dr Donald D **(SLP A)**
Domb, Mrs Anik **(A)**
Douglass, Mrs Lois W **(SLP)**
Douglass, Dr Robert L **(SLP)**
Dubno, Dr Judy R **(A)**
Dupuy, Cheryl Bozik **(SLP)**
Ecung, Mrs Debra Ford **(SLP)**
Eisenberg, Laurie S **(A)**
Elvenstar, McRandon **(SLP)**
Englert, Frances Watson **(A)**
Epstein, Mrs Cheryl S **(A)**
Erman, Andrew Allen **(SLP)**
Feinberg, Louise S **(SLP)**
Feinberg, Regina R K **(SLP)**
Finkelstein, Naomi G **(SLP)**
Fisher, Helen F **(SLP)**
Flint-Greenberg, Sara **(SLP)**
Fox, Mrs Cydney M **(A)**
Francis, Nancy Spencer **(SLP)**
Freed, Cheryl S **(SLP)**
Freeman, Mrs Gertrude Anne **(SLP)**
Furman, Paul B **(A)**
Gamson, Mrs Joan J **(SLP)**
Gardner, Ingrid Jacqueline **(SLP)**
Gendelman, Mrs Evelyn G **(SLP)**
Gerratt, Bruce R **(SLP)**
Gerry, Lorna **(SLP)**
Getlin, Jules P **(SLP)**
Goodhill, Dr Victor
Gottlieb-Karp, Beverly N **(SLP)**
Gray, Dr Susan Gillen **(SLP)**
Greenberg, Donna C **(A)**
Greene, Mrs Soloris J **(SLP)**
Greenwald, Judy B **(SLP)**
Grimes, Mrs Marybess V **(SLP)**
Grossbard, Rebecca J **(SLP)**
Gunderson, Marsha L
Guzzardo, Sr Margaret **(SLP)**
Hanawalt, Katharine L **(SLP)**
Hanson, Dr David G
Harris, Audrey Axelrod **(SLP)**
Harris, Marjorie R **(A)**
Hasselberger, Warren William **(A)**
Heatley, Thomas W **(SLP)**
Hensel-Cohen, Sharon **(SLP)**
Herbert, Esther L **(SLP)**
Hill, Barbara Goodman **(SLP)**
Hill, George E, Jr **(A)**
Hirsch, Rheta R F **(SLP)**
Hobbs, Julia Ann **(SLP)**
Holle, Jean Louise **(SLP)**
Hopper, Bruce F **(SLP)**
Hopson, Mrs Karen Leslie **(SLP)**
Horowitz, Mrs Ruth Rappaport **(SLP)**
Hoversten, Gloria H **(A)**
Howell, Tina Marie **(SLP)**
Hubbard-Wiley, Pamela S **(SLP)**
Huotari, Mrs Janice Lynn **(SLP)**
Hyde Phd, Charlene J **(SLP)**
Ikuta, Michele J **(A)**
Ingram, Mrs Catherine **(SLP)**
Izumi, Mutsumi I **(SLP)**
Jackson, Dr Judith M **(SLP)**
Jackson, Mrs Maland Bunton **(SLP)**
Jacobson, Cheryl F **(SLP)**
Jespersen, Rhonda M
Johnson, Dr Alice L **(SLP)**
Jones, Joan Harris **(SLP)**
Jones, Patricia A **(SLP)**
Kandel, Mrs Jodi Murayama **(SLP)**
Kaplan, Judith G **(SLP)**
Karsh, Mrs Diane M **(SLP)**
Katz, Mrs Jean Yager **(SLP)**
Katz, Dr Richard C **(SLP)**
Keaster, Jacqueline **(A)**
Keirn, Susan Green **(SLP)**
Kempler, Dr Daniel **(SLP)**
Kenworthy, Diane **(A)**

Kirkland, Jean Clennon **(SLP)**
Knorr, Geralynn Snyder **(SLP)**
Kohler, Susan **(SLP)**
Kollender, Mrs Rona P **(SLP)**
Koven, Marvin V **(SLP)**
Ladefoged, Dr Peter N
Lahti, Dr Ganea P **(SLP)**
Lake, Mrs Ethel P **(SLP)**
Lambert, Mrs Beatrice Baker **(SLP)**
Lavine, Mrs Janice Helene **(A)**
Lehrhoff, Dr Irwin **(SLP)**
LeVine, Mrs Ricki **(SLP)**
Longerich, Dr Mary C **(SLP)**
Lovus, Dr Yvonne A **(SLP)**
Lowell, Edgar Lafayette
Lowell, Mrs Marilyn Olsen **(SLP A)**
Luis, Deborah N **(SLP)**
Lyons, Leslie Ann **(SLP)**
Marlis, Jane A L **(SLP)**
Marr, Molly Kay **(SLP)**
Martinez, Charles D **(A)**
Marx, Francis N **(SLP)**
Mason, Richard D **(SLP)**
Masters, Vera E **(SLP)**
Masuda, Ann **(A)**
Matheny, Dr Patricia A **(SLP A)**
Matsuda, Dr Maryon M **(SLP)**
Mauner, Gail Ann **(SLP)**
Maybruck, Dr Iris L **(SLP)**
McCoy, Nancy Ellen **(A)**
McDonald, Crystal Lynne **(SLP)**
McDowell, Cheryl L **(SLP)**
McFarland, Dr William H **(A)**
McGinnis, Amy R **(SLP)**
McKeon, Gerald Joseph **(SLP)**
Miller, Dr Charles James **(SLP)**
Miller, Mrs Sue F **(SLP)**
Mines, Sondra **(SLP)**
Mireles, Mrs Laura Ann **(SLP)**
Mitchell, Cecile A **(A)**
Monk, Barbara P **(SLP)**
Moore, Mrs Susan B **(SLP)**
Moreno, Cynthia E **(SLP)**
Morgan, Dr Donald E **(A)**
Moy, Susan **(SLP)**
Nassau-Taxon, Christy Ann **(SLP)**
Nassberg, Joan **(A)**
Netherland, Sherry **(A)**
Nielsen, Dr Donald W
Nolin, Mrs Traci E F
O'Connor, Jean-Ann Nelson **(SLP)**
O'Connor, Lisa C **(SLP)**
Off, C Elizabeth
Otto, Steven R **(A)**
Ou-Young, Lai-Shyang Melody **(SLP)**
Owens, Catherine Elaine **(SLP)**
Parker, Lucy L **(SLP)**
Perkins, Dr William H **(SLP)**
Peters, Mrs Kathleen M **(SLP)**
Peterson, Dr Miles E **(A)**
Picheny, Barbara M **(SLP)**
Pitre, Derek Jerome **(SLP)**
Polichar, Donna J **(SLP)**
Pomeranz, Shira Tolwin **(SLP)**
Porcella, Nancy Weldon **(SLP)**
Procopi, Nickolas **(SLP)**
Pruitt-Shough, Mrs Ann L **(SLP)**
Purcell, Sherry L **(SLP)**
Rauss, Laura C **(SLP)**
Rawson, Mark L **(SLP)**
Reisbaum, Margaret L **(SLP)**
Richardson, Mrs Natalie **(SLP)**
Robman, Jolie D **(A)**
Roper, Linda Joyce **(SLP)**
Rose, Karen **(SLP)**
Rosenthal, Judee Anne **(SLP)**
Roston, Amanda R **(SLP)**
Roth, Cicely Anne **(SLP)**
Rundberg, Elizabeth Ann **(SLP)**
Sacks, Linda Nancy **(SLP)**
Salick, Mrs Gloria **(SLP)**
Salisbury, Jean T **(A)**
Salkowitz, Bobbe Banks **(SLP)**
Savich, Dr Patricia A **(SLP)**
Schaap, Mrs Joni Martin **(SLP)**
Schaefer, Amy Beth **(A)**
Schall, Mrs Wendy Rosenthal **(SLP)**
Schramm, Britta J **(SLP)**
Sedat, Nancy A **(SLP)**
Seraydarian, Fredi Diamond **(SLP)**
Sharp, Dr Florence A **(SLP)**
Shoji, Leslie Shawn **(A)**
Shreiber, Mrs Ida F **(SLP)**
Sikov, Mrs Elaine Linda **(SLP)**
Silverman, Rita C **(SLP)**
Sininger, Dr Yvonne S **(A)**
Sklar, Dr Maurice **(SLP A)**
Slavin, Laverne A **(SLP)**
Smith, Connie J **(SLP)**
Smith, Veronica Nadine **(SLP)**
Smoller, Mrs Henny Perlmutter **(SLP)**
Snelgrove, Kathy A **(SLP)**
Soo Hoo, Marianne **(A)**
Spaner, Vicki Joanne **(SLP)**
Steckler, Jane F **(A)**
Sullivan, Jean A **(A)**
Summitt, Diana Lynn **(SLP)**
Swann, Maria T **(SLP)**
Taenaka, Patrice H **(SLP)**
Takeuchi, Janice Sueko
Taylor, Kathryn Bushman **(SLP)**
Teas-Hester, Dr Elizabeth A Teas **(SLP)**
Tusinski, Mrs Marcia R **(SLP)**
Udell, Mrs Mary Lou **(SLP)**
Von Leden, Dr Hans V
Wade, Patricia M **(SLP)**
Wanamaker, Abby **(SLP)**
Ward, Lethe Finks **(SLP)**
Wechsler, Louise A **(SLP)**
Weiss, Mrs Shifra Lipshitz **(SLP)**
Weston, Dr Alan J **(SLP)**
Weston, Mrs Marsha Lyn **(A)**
White, Renee Spies
Woodard, Lottie **(SLP)**
Yaghoubian, Mrs Karen **(SLP)**
Yamazaki, Mrs Nancy K **(SLP)**
Zavala, Anna Bellott **(SLP)**
Zucker, Carolyn M **(SLP)**
Zweier, Jill Buttwinick **(SLP)**

Los Banos
Amabile, Mrs Michelle Rico **(SLP)**

Los Gatos
Bergman, Kathleen S **(SLP)**
Berwald, Rosemary Rhines **(SLP)**
Choyce, John C **(SLP A)**
Hack, Mrs Zarita C **(A)**
Holder, Gregory Marc **(A)**
Kern, Carolyn A **(SLP)**
Lynn, Diana **(SLP)**
Miller, Geraldine **(A)**
Redmon, Melinda A **(A)**
Stockton, Martha **(SLP)**
Upchurch, Mrs Angela G C **(SLP)**
Von Roos, Ingetraud **(SLP)**
Weeker, Gail **(SLP)**
White, Margaret J **(SLP)**

Los Molinos
Steffen, Colette M **(SLP)**

Los Osos
Johnston, Michael Mary/Tiema **(SLP)**
Olson, Linda B **(SLP)**

Lotus Beach
McGinty, Mrs Barbara Peloquin **(SLP)**

Loyalton
Ludwig, Mrs Marsha S **(SLP)**

Mad River
Campain, Robert F **(SLP)**

Madera
Frazier, Sally L **(SLP)**
Leach, Mrs Linda R **(SLP)**
Morvay, Torrey Lee **(SLP)**
Sandness, Dr Donald L **(SLP)**

Magalia
Hostettler, Mrs Carmelita Ann **(SLP)**
Stimson, Linda C **(SLP)**

Malibu
Anderson, Mrs Susanne R **(SLP)**
Baumeister, Marilyn E **(SLP)**
Breault, Leslie M **(SLP)**
Hartenbaum, Mrs Susan G **(SLP)**
McAllister, Judith Boyden **(SLP)**
McCloud, Elizabeth **(SLP A)**
Stone, Beth V **(SLP)**
Wood, Mrs Zira A **(SLP)**

Mammoth Lakes
Morvay, Ruth McConnell **(SLP)**

Manhattan Beach
Basik, Carleen P **(A)**
Bluhm, Mrs Sharon B
Condit, Linda Christine
Hobbs, Lynne W **(SLP)**
Kohl, Mrs Cecilia M **(SLP)**
Lovelace, Lynne C **(SLP)**
Mandelbaum, Mrs Nancy J **(SLP)**
Popelka, Jean Sladek **(SLP)**
Tillotson, Barbara L **(SLP)**
Van Vooren, Mrs Margaret S **(A)**
Whidden, Rose **(SLP)**
Wilcoxen, Dr Anne Glover **(SLP)**
York, Eleanor H **(SLP)**
Zegarski-Isley, Elizabeth **(SLP)**

Manteca
Galli, Anthony P **(SLP)**
Natteford, Mary S **(SLP)**
Parker, Bruce David **(SLP)**
Vasconcellos, Cynthia Jean

Marina
Ellis, Mary Lucena **(SLP)**
Kelly, Jacqueline Lou **(SLP)**
McPherson, Hal C **(A)**
Rexroth, Donna Louise
Savage, Linda Amalia **(SLP)**
Taylor, Patricia S **(SLP)**

Marina Del Rey
Berg, Roberta J **(A)**
Borning-Cordova, Katherine Ellan **(SLP)**
D'Asaro, Dr Lois N **(SLP)**
Dawkins, Avis Wheeler **(SLP)**
Fallenstein, Sherry L **(SLP)**
Florence, Diane P **(SLP)**
Fromwiller, Sharon E **(SLP)**
McDermott, Patrick J **(SLP)**
Newman, Ann **(SLP)**
West, Annette Rose
Zwitman, Dr Daniel H **(SLP A)**

Mariposa
Gerken, Mrs Shelly Lynn **(SLP)**
Neal, Mrs Marjorie Solliday **(SLP)**

Martinez
Bern, Martha Graham **(SLP)**
Contastin, Francoise M **(SLP)**
Divenyi, Dr Pierre L
Getman, Laura Whipple **(SLP)**
Gillilan, Patricia A **(A)**
Hempel, Mrs Nancy J C **(SLP)**
Humphrey, Jane Ellen **(A)**
Kneale, Mrs Patricia Susan **(SLP)**
Preciado-Lumsden, Mrs Eva Maria
Quinn, Katherine C **(SLP)**
Romolino, Diane Duk **(SLP)**
Silverstein, Roberta J **(SLP)**
Wertz, Dr Robert T **(SLP)**
Zachariah, Dee M **(SLP)**

Marysville
Kelley, Leslie L
Lind, Richard C **(A)**

Mather AFB
Jenkins, Susan Leonard **(SLP)**
Lattig, Marcia Jo **(SLP)**

McArthur
Soares-Brown, Camille Pauline **(SLP)**

McClellan AFB
Schulz, Capt Theresa Yarber **(A)**

McKinleyville
Forbes, Kevin C **(SLP)**

Mendocino
Daggett, Mrs Helen C **(SLP)**
Stofle, Mrs Patricia Tewksbury **(SLP)**

Menlo Park
Boscamp, Patricia Ann **(SLP)**
Buschini, Gail M **(SLP)**
Cessaris, Ann Clarke **(SLP)**
Davis, Connee S **(SLP)**
Fung, Debra McDevitt **(SLP)**
Harris-Ryan, Margaret **(SLP)**
Hayes, Deborah Dawn **(SLP)**
Hecker, Dr Michael H L
Holeman, Lois J **(SLP)**
Lamb, Stanford H **(SLP A)**
Levy, Mrs Hillary Brook **(SLP)**
Metcalfe, Dr Jean V **(SLP)**
Nashban-Murphy, Mrs Janell P **(SLP)**
O'Connor, Maureen M **(SLP)**
Pollock, Mrs Norma Haegg **(SLP)**
Sattui, Melanie Anne **(SLP)**
Schnugg, Jill Taylor **(SLP)**
Seefeldt, Mrs Ellen Homann **(SLP)**
Stone, Mrs Sueann **(SLP)**
Warp, Mrs Sherry L D **(SLP)**

Merced
Allen, Mrs Elizabeth Alice
Carlsgaard, Rowena Mazzei **(SLP)**
Chenoweth, Robin **(SLP)**
Cook, Mrs Christine A **(SLP)**
Hamill, Mrs Pamela L P **(SLP)**
Karastathas, Mrs Susan E C **(SLP)**
Powell, Mrs Edna M M **(SLP)**
Ramirez, Aurora Parreno
Rowley, Melody **(SLP)**
Schemanske, Judith A **(SLP)**
Schuddeboom-Kelley, Mrs Joan **(SLP)**
Sortini, Dr Adam J **(SLP A)**
Stephenson, Ruthanne B
Younce, Mrs Susan Lynn **(SLP)**

Meridian
Becker, Stephanie **(A)**

Middletown
Beaudet, Rudy R **(SLP)**

Mill Valley
Buell-Chittenden, Mrs Claudia **(SLP)**
Eber, Francine L **(SLP)**
Gill, Joanne **(SLP)**
Kendrick, Mrs Clara A Yourman **(SLP)**
McCloskey, Deborah Burns **(SLP)**
Regalado-Robb, Mrs Sharon F **(SLP)**
Ultsch, Mrs Susan Lannert
Will, Toni Iten **(A)**

Millbrae
Anderson, Lloyd C **(SLP)**
England, Christina Ann **(SLP)**
Malekos, Karen Marie **(SLP)**
Ogawa, Mrs Diana K **(SLP)**
Yamamoto, Mrs Satoko Fukada

Milpitas
Chinn, Roxanne M **(SLP)**
Churich, Mrs Jan M **(SLP)**
Murdock, Dr Betty Jane **(SLP)**
Roberts, Dr Jan Avent **(SLP)**

Mira Loma
McGuire, Mrs Wendy Lynn **(SLP)**

Mission Viejo
Bennett, Mrs Susan N **(SLP)**
Bethke, Mrs Darla H **(SLP)**
Blinn, James F **(SLP)**
Crawford, Cynthia L **(SLP)**
Deliema, Mrs Kathy Ledeen **(SLP)**
Drazinski, Lynn Ann **(SLP)**
Duchon, Mrs Rebecca Ann **(SLP)**
Fash, Mrs Deborah S **(SLP)**
Fowler, Kymry Hart **(SLP)**
Jones, Howard C **(A)**
Jones, Mary Lou Herceg **(A)**
Litz, Stacy L **(SLP)**
Medina, Mrs Sherri Larson **(SLP)**
Penno, Catherine **(SLP)**
Pohlot, Mrs Nancy Elizabeth **(SLP)**
Puckett, Mrs Linda J **(SLP)**
Rigler, Mrs Caryl R **(SLP)**
Roe, Rochelle Williams **(A)**
Roy, Susan Holly **(SLP)**
Silver, Nancy Reguly **(SLP)**
Smyth, Thomas C **(SLP A)**
Starkey, Mrs Cynthia Lynn **(SLP)**
Trueman, Mrs Janet Katherine **(SLP)**
Winkler, Cynthia Ann **(SLP)**

Modesto
Adams, Bonnie Stalians **(SLP)**
Allen, Mildred **(SLP)**
Banghart-Bragg, Mrs Denise Helen **(SLP)**
Barnett, Mrs Lorrie Colleen **(SLP)**
Conley, Paul W
Cooley, Leslie Lynne **(SLP)**
Davis, Janice A **(SLP)**
Earp, Christine Joan **(SLP)**
Ewin, Mrs Carol I **(SLP)**
Fisher, Susan M **(SLP)**
Ford, Mrs Tresa Ann **(SLP)**
Fosnaught, Lynn M **(SLP)**
Gerber, Karen Elaine
Hansen, Lenore Anne **(SLP)**
Honey, Patricia **(SLP)**
Huff, Mrs Carolyn Ditman **(SLP)**
Jones, Christine Ann **(SLP)**
Justice-Brown, Mrs Joan L **(SLP)**
Knepp, Cynthia Susanne **(SLP)**
Kuliberda, Theresa A **(SLP)**
Lee, Sharon J **(SLP)**
Lustri, Jessye J J **(SLP)**
Lux, Mrs Elizabeth Pluim **(SLP)**
McKinney, Mrs Beverly Sue **(SLP)**
Mello-Smither, Susan A **(SLP)**
Moran, Rosalyn Soares **(SLP)**
Murray, Elsaree D **(SLP)**
Norton, Dr Max C **(SLP)**
Ringsby, Mrs Sandra Lynn **(SLP)**
Rokaitis, Mrs Beth Lorraine **(SLP)**
Santos, Mrs Bonita B **(SLP)**
Savage, Sandra McEwen **(SLP)**
Smith, Kristy Lynne
Sparkman, Coleen Kelley **(SLP)**
Summers-Johnson, Wendy **(SLP)**
Taylor, Evelyn J **(SLP)**
Townsend, Mrs Joyce A **(SLP)**
Van Groningen, Mrs Grace **(SLP)**
Vincent, Mrs April **(SLP)**
West, Dr W Barry **(SLP A)**
Wilkins, Raymond A **(SLP A)**
Woodmansee, Regina Gail
Wyatt, Mrs Carla M N **(SLP)**

Monrovia
Bell, Barbara Anne **(A)**
McConnell, Diane **(SLP)**
Mustain, Vivian Burke **(SLP)**
Newman, Mrs Linda Vaughan **(A)**
Ritchey, Rebecca Anne **(A)**
Simmons-Carr, Mrs Stephanie **(SLP)**
Whelan, Maureen Santos **(SLP)**
Young, Mrs Barbara Allen **(SLP)**

Montara
Krabbenschmidt, Mrs Katie J **(SLP)**
Patterson, Janice E

Montclair
Newman, Sandra Lee **(SLP)**

Monte Sereno
Noehr, Mrs Bonnie B **(SLP)**

Montebello
Kelleher, Loleati A **(SLP)**
Pedigo, Lois Verjean **(SLP)**

Montecito
Eve, Irwin Leigh **(A)**
Eve, Salli Elena **(A)**
Mershon, Virginia R **(SLP)**

Monterey
Blackstone, Dr Sarah W **(SLP)**
Bruno, Mrs Janet S **(SLP)**
Dunbar, Barbara Jean **(A)**
Frederick, Anne A **(SLP)**
Gelaro, Mrs Glynnis Ann **(SLP)**
Harr, Mrs Karen J **(SLP)**
Henderson, Mari Koda
Hilaire, Francine J **(SLP)**
Hugar, Lily A **(A)**
Moore, Carol Linda **(SLP)**
Odom, Terria Lee **(SLP)**
Parsons, Helene Herzfeld **(SLP)**
Paul, Mrs Christine Drescher **(SLP)**
Sigars, Judith Regina **(SLP)**
Turner, Aina **(SLP)**
Vreeland, Richard S **(SLP A)**
Wallach, Richard W **(SLP)**

Monterey Park
Barbosa, Maureen McLean **(SLP)**
Chin, Dr May Elizabeth **(A)**
Ikeuye, Colleen Teruko **(SLP)**
Kohama, Mrs Kathleen Albertoni **(SLP)**
Miyamura, Kelly Hisae
Monnin, Dr Lorraine M **(SLP)**
Pirrone, Mrs Elisa Golley **(SLP)**

Montrose
Ellis, Joan B **(SLP)**
Schmidt, Richard J, Jr **(SLP)**

Moorpark
Benko, Mrs Kay Lynn **(A)**
Caputo, Karen L **(SLP)**
Nagai, Mrs Jeanette F **(SLP)**
Zeman, Richard D **(A)**

Moraga
Anderman, Barbara B **(SLP)**
Boltz, Irene M **(SLP)**
Cogswell, Cynthia Church **(SLP)**
Glynn, Linda M
Jacobs, Mrs Mary T **(SLP)**
Ludolph, Leslie Baker **(SLP)**
Nash, Shirley B **(SLP)**

Moreno Valley
Ch'iu, Julie M **(SLP)**
Leffler, Mrs Donna Marie **(SLP)**
Tures, Cathleen Roberta **(A)**
Vardiman, Karen **(SLP)**
Witt, Bradley Kevin **(A)**
Young, Mrs Sabrina Corey **(SLP)**

Morgan Hill
Armstead, Dr Kay A G **(SLP)**
Bayless, Mrs Barbara **(SLP)**
Coates, Mrs Nadine H **(SLP)**
Murdoch, Mrs Cynthia Watjen **(SLP)**
Weddington, Dr Gloria T **(SLP)**
Zepecki, Mrs Carol A H **(SLP)**

Morongo Valley
Tracy, Ellen D **(SLP)**

Morro Bay
Moss, Stephanie Ecker **(A)**

Mountain View
Benham, Deborah Marie **(SLP)**
Benning, Caryl M **(SLP)**
Bergen, Karen Koppel **(SLP)**
Greene, Sheri Robin **(SLP)**
Mangan, Debra Hashimoto **(A)**
Meyer, Mrs Amalie **(SLP)**
Miller, Cheryl U **(SLP)**
Norton, Claire Margaret
Rosen, Dr Linda M **(SLP)**
Stephens, Mark J **(SLP)**
Stewart, Deborah L **(A)**
Stewart, Mrs Helga J **(SLP)**
Stong, Mont Edward **(A)**
Turner, Mrs Ann M **(SLP)**
Woolley, Melissa O'Farrell **(SLP)**

Murphys
Webster, Nancy Sullivan **(SLP)**

Murrieta
Waltrip, Mrs LoAnne **(SLP)**

Napa
Allen, Mrs Catherine **(SLP)**
Athey, Joseph T **(A)**
Bork, Dr Norma K **(SLP)**
Caldwell, Keith C **(A)**
Corwin, Mrs Bonnie Layerle **(SLP)**
Jones, James L **(SLP)**
Keyes, Mrs Alison M **(SLP)**
Lalich, Margaret Myrtle **(SLP)**
Litz, Paulette J **(SLP)**
Loyborg, Troels V **(A)**
Martin, Denise Louise **(A)**
Misch, Mrs Diane L **(SLP)**
Rooney, Nancy **(SLP)**
Sonderman-Thompson, Mrs Judith Clar **(SLP)**
Van Patten, Peggy Louise **(A)**

Nevada City
Green, Dr Rosalind N **(SLP)**
Tintle, Mrs Patricia Ann **(SLP)**

Newark
Bryan, Catherine **(SLP)**
Kleczewska, Maria K **(SLP)**
Nakai, Anne I **(SLP)**
Postle, Mrs Cleo B **(SLP)**
Teodosio, Gail Elizabeth

Newbury Park
Broughton, Mrs Janette Marie **(SLP)**
Brown, Carol D **(SLP)**
Harris, Stannye Seay **(SLP)**

Newhall
Ambrose, Cheryl Lee **(SLP)**
Anderson, Beth Louise **(SLP)**
Calams, Timothy J **(A)**
Lavin, Marian **(SLP)**
Lindemann, Norma M V **(SLP)**
Neft, Mrs Beth Weinstock **(SLP)**
Pitre, Retha White **(SLP)**
Tufts, Devon C **(SLP)**
Williams, Mrs Diana Lynn **(SLP)**

Newport
Mango, Howard T **(A)**

Newport Beach
Barrett, Kathleen Krock **(SLP)**
Diamond, Mrs Beverly A **(SLP)**
Dobkin, Renee Cencel **(A)**
Eaton, Mrs Susan Ann **(SLP)**
Hein, Judith Ann **(SLP)**
Howle, Barbara K **(SLP)**
Killian, Bobbye N M **(SLP)**
Murphy, Shawn A **(SLP)**
Owsley, Robert Michael **(A)**
Schmitz, Dr Henry D **(A)**
Snyder, Deborah S **(SLP)**
Specterman, Paul **(SLP)**
Thomas, Ellen Diane **(SLP)**

Nipton
Lang, Roxanne M **(SLP)**

North Edwards
Walter, Denise L **(SLP)**

North Highlands
Orozco, Mrs Susan Elizabeth **(SLP)**

North Hollywood
Calder, Mrs Pat E **(SLP)**
Card, Mrs Helen W **(SLP)**
Demuniz, Karen Anne **(SLP)**
Dunn, Marianne **(SLP)**
Faermark, Jory **(SLP)**
Fogelson, Mrs Janie Karen
Fried, Dr Leonard **(SLP)**
Gilbertson, Jean Marie **(SLP)**
Horasanian, Dena **(SLP)**
Nalls, Joseph C, II **(SLP)**
O'Grady, Gwendolyn M **(A)**
Pierson, Mrs Jan Latta **(A)**
Romack, Carolee A **(SLP)**
Russell, Mrs Sandra L **(SLP)**
Shanin, Sandra J **(SLP)**
Yee, Curtis W **(A)**

North San Gabriel
Holdridge, Julie Ann **(SLP)**

Northridge
Blitz-Weisz, Mrs Sally **(SLP)**
Brix, Tina G **(SLP)**
Deroo-Wagman, Carolyn J **(SLP)**
Deutsch, Mrs Sylvie R **(SLP)**
Doyle, Mary M **(SLP)**
Drake, Mrs Marion E **(SLP)**
Eastes, Lorene Ellen **(SLP)**
Epstein, Mrs Cynthia S **(SLP)**
Haber, Mrs Rita Patnoi **(SLP)**
Heck, Bonnie June **(SLP)**
Jonas, Jill G **(SLP)**
Langer, Mrs Deana K **(A)**
Lazaros, Mrs Sandra L **(SLP)**
Luckey, Richard S, Sr **(A)**
Manna-Levin, Karen Lee
McCracken, Mrs Rosanne D **(SLP)**
Meyers, Esther K **(SLP)**
Piner, Mrs Andrea Winters **(SLP)**
Reid, Mrs Gloria Ann **(SLP)**
Reid, Jeffrey Bruce **(A)**
Reid, Dr Philip **(SLP A)**
Roussos, Dr Christine Strike **(SLP)**
Schnee, Mrs Karen Fern **(SLP)**
Smoot, Rikki J **(SLP)**
Staley, Mrs Barbara Kay **(SLP)**
Trost-Cardamone, Dr Judith E **(SLP)**
Vogel, Laura B **(SLP)**
Washington, Mrs Elaine Shackelfor
Wasson, Shari Angela
Weinstein, Ilene G **(SLP)**

Norwalk
Keating, Shirley M **(SLP)**
Kestler, Carla J **(SLP)**
Perkins, Richard Alan **(SLP)**
Rossa, Denise Marie **(A)**
Wormus, Robert C **(A)**

Novato
Ahern, Janis C **(SLP)**
Ewart, Joanne **(A)**
Juskowitz, Susan **(SLP)**
Key, Jan C **(SLP)**
Kneeter, Judith **(SLP)**
Leidy, Susan W **(SLP)**
Long, Dr Nancy V **(SLP)**
Mordecai, Dr Dennis R **(SLP)**
Nelson, Alexandra **(SLP)**
Piltch, Michelle Ann **(A)**
Raye, Mrs Janine Solkov **(SLP)**
Thoma, Joan A **(A)**
Vosburg, Mrs Elyse Hoytt **(SLP)**

Oak Hills
Marienthal, Pamela P **(SLP)**

Oak View
Nofrey, Mrs Linda R **(SLP)**

Oakdale
Jackson, Mary G **(SLP)**

Keefe, Mrs Linda Marie **(SLP)**

Oakhurst
Pesetski, Loretta S **(SLP)**

Oakland
Arvold, Joan P **(SLP)**
Behrens, Kathleen Ann **(SLP)**
Blanchard, Dr Sumner L **(SLP)**
Bradley, Gerri A **(SLP)**
Bronstein, Dr Arthur J **(SLP)**
Byrne, Polly **(A)**
Corwin, Jan R **(SLP)**
Crosby, Nancy P **(SLP)**
De Costa, Virginia Nell **(SLP)**
Eichhorn, Patricia R **(SLP)**
Elman, Roberta J **(SLP)**
Faltz, Amy E **(SLP)**
Fankhauser, Charles E **(A)**
Felton, Janet Lynn **(SLP)**
Fernandez, Mrs Diane Piva
Fox, Shelly **(SLP)**
Fulghum, Sandra Casner **(A)**
Hanau, Kathleen **(SLP)**
Harman, Marjorie G **(SLP)**
Harmon, Mrs Gloria W **(SLP)**
Harris, Mrs Veronica M **(SLP)**
Harvell, Mrs Priscilla Saffold **(SLP)**
Heidkamp, Mrs Sada G **(SLP)**
Higgins, Mrs Christine Pauletich **(SLP)**
Humphrey-Zika, Mrs Jean M **(SLP)**
Hutchinson, Joan F **(SLP)**
Jong, Nancy Tomi Hamai **(SLP)**
Kahan, Candace Wice **(SLP)**
Kaji, Mrs Agnes O **(SLP A)**
Keblusek, Sue J **(SLP)**
Kerr, Debra L **(SLP)**
Kreutzer, Mrs Robin Jeanine **(SLP)**
Lage, Ray V **(SLP A)**
Lee, Jane **(SLP)**
Levin, Patricia Ann **(SLP)**
Lintner, Mary Emily **(A)**
Loomos, Dimitra J **(A)**
Maffeo, Angela Marie
Mangiapane, Patricia Ann **(SLP)**
McAleese, Patricia Marie **(SLP)**
McGrath, Mrs Cynthia Lundgren **(SLP)**
Milton, Mary P **(SLP)**
Minkler, Donna Beth **(SLP)**
Morgan, Sherrill Davis **(SLP)**
Murphy, Carol A **(SLP)**
Noyes, Mrs MaryLou **(SLP)**
Pankow, Deanna K **(SLP)**
Parker, Maria Guttentag **(SLP)**
Peppard, Ann Baker **(SLP)**
Peterson, June M **(SLP)**
Polonsky, Ronnie Jane **(A)**
Roberts-Yuen, Sharon **(SLP)**
Rose, Lauraine Sara **(SLP)**
Russell, Diane B **(SLP)**
Salus, Dr Mary W **(SLP)**
Scalione, Patricia **(SLP)**
Schantz, Deborah Lyn **(SLP)**
Siepser, Mrs Zell A **(SLP)**
Smith, D Wayne **(SLP A)**
Starck, MaryJo **(SLP)**
Stone, Rebecca Jane-Boyd **(SLP)**
Surgers, Brenda J **(SLP)**
Teekell, Mrs Joyce D **(SLP)**
Tenenberg, Mrs Thelma K **(SLP)**
Teselle, Nancy Eleanor **(SLP)**
Trinchero, Jennifer D **(SLP)**
Vakos, Toni L **(A)**
Weisel, Joyce Carol
Wolf, Dr Patricia L **(SLP)**
Wong, Lynette **(SLP)**

Oakland Hills
Benedict, Mrs Paula Maria **(SLP)**

Ocean Hills
Brown, Mrs Lavergne B **(SLP)**
Davidson, Mrs Irene E **(SLP)**

Oceanside
Allen, Dr Emma M **(SLP)**
Hall, Gregory William **(A)**
Hutchinson, Mrs Valerie Jean **(SLP)**
Jackson, Linda S **(SLP)**
Lytle, Mrs Mary E A **(A)**
MacLellan, Maryanne **(SLP)**
Mattes, Dr Lawrence J **(SLP)**
Moskowitz, Vickie L A **(A)**
O'Lowney, Mrs Patricia M **(SLP)**
Parr, Enid A **(SLP)**
Ray, Judy C **(SLP)**
Rowe, Linda Jo **(A)**
Shinn, Mrs Susan **(SLP)**
Sloniker, Mrs Sheila J **(SLP)**
Stults, Karen Marie **(SLP)**
Wolgemuth, Lt Keith Stohman **(A)**

Ojai
Bisek, Thorice S **(SLP)**
Charters, Dr Nancy **(SLP)**
Cooper, Mrs Georgia T **(SLP)**
Dearinger, Patricia McCombs **(A)**
Dugan, Mrs Patricia J **(SLP)**
Manion, Kathleen H **(SLP)**
Merkley, Dr Frances A Giannino
Mortensen, Sydnee Jean B **(SLP)**
Osbakken, Bonnie Rochelle **(SLP)**
Zacher, Catherine **(SLP)**

Old Orcutt
Silbernagle, Mary Jo **(SLP)**

Olivenhain
Hagen, Dr Chris **(SLP)**
Hagen, Mrs Suzanne G **(SLP)**

Olympic Valley
Ganong, Mrs Janice E **(SLP)**

Ontario
Carrick, Valerie C **(SLP)**
Cavanaugh, Martin Joseph **(SLP)**
Fraser, Mrs Leslie T **(SLP)**
Fritz, Mrs Lori Snow **(SLP)**
Neeley, Lambert W **(SLP)**
Neeley, Mrs Velma L **(SLP)**
Seaton, Stewart S **(A)**
Whitley, Mrs Wendy Sue **(SLP)**

Orange
Adams, Mary M **(A)**
Andersen, Mrs Katherine Kiehn **(SLP)**
Bell, Mrs Cheryl J **(A)**
Bellinger, Joyce H **(SLP)**
Brady, Patricia Eileen **(SLP)**
Burnell, Christine Switzer **(SLP)**
Conan, Mrs Eileen T **(SLP)**
Countryman, Cora A **(SLP)**
Critelli, Gloria Ellen **(SLP)**
D'Antonio, Dr Linda L **(SLP)**
De Clark, Janet Louise **(SLP)**
Ensworth, Mrs Leisa Kathleen **(A)**
Eszlinger, Mrs Elizabeth Hall **(SLP)**
Harnack, Mrs Carol Susan **(SLP)**
Hiser, Nancy M **(SLP)**
Hoerauf, Pamela D **(SLP)**
Hoey, Mrs Nancy Louise **(SLP)**
Honda, Mrs Bedonna J **(SLP)**
Hostetter, Melanie S **(SLP)**
Inman, Dr Margaret A **(SLP)**
Klinkert, Mrs Laurie Jackson **(SLP)**
Knight, Mrs Patricia D **(SLP)**
Kuluris, Mrs Joan J M **(SLP)**
Kurtzer-Metter, Mrs Karen **(SLP)**
Lillywhite, Beth Ann **(A)**
Lofink, Joanne L T **(SLP)**
McPherson, David L **(SLP A)**
Momtaz, Mrs Anita Ruth **(SLP)**
Morris, Harry A **(SLP)**
Petrovich, Mrs Leslie Kirchoff **(SLP)**
Post, Lorena Ann **(SLP)**
Power, Mark **(SLP)**
Serafin, Mary M **(SLP)**
Smith, Becky Lee **(A)**
Turner, Ernie W **(A)**
Waggoner, Edna Mae **(SLP)**
Yastrov, Carol L **(SLP)**

Orangevale
Fish, Alice McGorman **(SLP)**
Immer, Valerie J **(SLP)**
Johnson, Sandra **(SLP)**
Kidd, Cynthia Louise **(SLP)**
Marty, Mrs Mary J **(SLP)**
O'Connell, Maureen Ann **(A)**
Phillips, Laura L **(SLP)**

Orcutt
Yeager, Mrs Rhoni A **(SLP)**

Orinda
Arellano, Mrs Joan Sheridan **(SLP)**
Bjork-Hilsinger, Cristine A **(SLP)**
Lojacono, Marie S **(SLP)**
McCabe, Deborah Ann
McClatchie, Mrs Adeline D **(A)**
Seelinger, Janet W **(SLP)**
Wiley, Pam W **(A)**

Oroville
Cosart, Mrs Anne Rattray **(SLP)**
King, Bonnie L **(SLP)**
Lane, Mrs Cathy Walker **(SLP)**
Neben, Mrs Susan J **(SLP)**
Salerno, Margaret Gilbreath **(SLP)**
Von Berg, Mrs Sarah J **(SLP)**

Oxnard
Davis, Alice-Jean **(SLP A)**
Maeno, Alice H **(SLP)**
Martin, Mrs Elizabeth **(A)**
Ortenberg, Celia Louise **(SLP)**
Patterson, Patti L **(SLP)**
Rydgig, Kathleen Ann **(SLP)**
Taden, Mrs Claudia E **(SLP)**
White, Barbara Shultz **(A)**
Williams, Mrs Sheila Chase **(SLP)**
Wilson, Joanne E **(SLP)**

Oxnard Shores
De La Vallee, Dolores Meola **(SLP)**

Pac Palisades
Zangrando, Mary Zoe **(A)**

Pacific Grove
Blum, Mrs Stephanie Shaw **(SLP)**
Britton, Jane Natalie
Gertzulin, Michele
Kalashian, Verjene Eileen
Lorenzen, Mrs Anna L **(SLP A)**
McFadden-Wittrock, Mrs Margaret C **(SLP)**
Montanez, Mrs Virginia F
Mowry, Richmond Bruce **(A)**
Mueh, Mrs Ferne H **(A)**
Pearce, Margaret C **(SLP)**
Pulliam, Louis L **(SLP)**

Pacific Palisades
Baehr, Bonnie **(A)**
Block, Wendy Jayne **(SLP)**
Doose, Alexis **(SLP)**
Garwood, Dr Victor P **(SLP A)**
Gray, Dr Burl B **(SLP)**
Hadler, Bette L **(SLP)**
Hannah, Dr Elaine P **(SLP)**
Hanson, Dr Wayne R **(SLP)**
Hoffeller, Jill Marie **(SLP)**
Leshin, Mrs Phyllis **(SLP)**
Marx, Barbara Ruth S **(SLP)**
Schibel, Mrs Linda Grossman **(SLP)**
Tancredi, Mrs Joan L **(SLP)**
Tobisman, Karen Bleier **(SLP)**

Pacifica
Lane, Dr Vera Wall **(SLP)**
Maher, Mary E **(SLP)**
Neeley, Cynthia H **(SLP)**
Raggio, Marcia Eve **(A)**
Raymond, Jennifer Carniglia **(SLP)**

Palm Desert
Schwartz, Mrs Arlene Susan **(SLP)**

Palm Springs
Bellows, Liz Nathan **(A)**
Borthick, William Arnold **(SLP)**
Burney, Phillip A **(A)**
Griswold, Frank Orr **(SLP)**
Huber, Dr Mary Wehe **(SLP)**
Jaffe, Emily G **(A)**
Kalfuss, Dr Helene A **(SLP)**
Kaufman, Mrs Marilyn J **(SLP)**
Oldknow, Wendy K
Shippee, Frank H **(SLP)**
Weiner-Kahn, Mrs Sheila B **(SLP)**
Wertz, Larry Ray **(SLP)**

Palmdale
Foster, Mrs Beverly Cunningham **(SLP)**
Hembd, Mrs Bonita M **(SLP)**
Hunt, Marline Elam **(SLP)**
Jackson, Mrs Judith Ann **(SLP)**
Johnson, Mrs Michelle McDonald **(SLP)**
Kall, Mrs Maralyn Bettina **(SLP)**
Leibner, Aimee Kyle **(SLP)**
Olson, Dolores M **(SLP)**

Palo Alto
Beadle, Dr Kathryn R **(SLP)**
Bucquet, Susan Reed **(SLP)**
Bush, Dr Marcia A
Buttrill, Judith C **(SLP)**
Cunningham, Judith Rees **(SLP)**
Dagenais, Donna Jo **(SLP)**
Forse, Mrs Kathleen H **(SLP)**
Franklin, Dr Barbara **(A)**
Gregory, Anna Vagin **(SLP)**
Grimm, Diann D **(SLP)**
Hautala, Kelly T **(SLP)**
Hearn, Stella B **(SLP)**
Hibbs, Melanie June **(SLP)**
Hochscheid, Mrs Sylvia F
Holland, Joan B **(SLP)**
Jelonek, Susan Jean
Kiesling, Elizabeth Heath **(SLP)**
Kirkes, Mrs Bette L **(SLP)**
Lake, Mrs Sandra J **(SLP)**
Lunger, Judith Gloria **(SLP)**
Norris, Dr Jane C **(A)**
Sackler-Feldblum, Cynthia **(SLP)**
Schuman, Mrs Linda L Steiner **(SLP)**
Silver, Marsha A **(SLP)**
Simon, Susan Markowitz **(SLP)**
Spatafore, Julie Lizanne **(SLP)**
Stolpa, Mrs Rebecca T **(SLP)**
Stoner, Susan Ballew
Sweet, Mrs Nancy **(SLP)**
Thomsen, Mrs Susan M **(SLP)**
Vadopalas, Mrs Patricia J **(SLP)**
Vorce, Pamela P **(SLP)**
Walker, Thomas Lee **(A)**
Williams, Jennifer Anne **(SLP)**
Woodall, Rosemary Vivian **(SLP)**
Ziebell, Andrea Powers **(SLP)**

Palo Cedro
Blakemore, Mrs Susan K **(SLP)**

Palos Verdes Estates
Block-Miller, Joyce A **(SLP)**
Borgeson, Kathleen Ann **(SLP)**
Firemark, Rosalyn **(A)**
Martinoff, Rosemary V **(SLP)**
Mennis, Mrs Selma Tres **(SLP)**
Montague, Melanie F
Opatrny, Gay **(A)**
Perens, Margaret **(SLP)**
Warren, Dr Virginia G **(A)**
Whitlow, Mrs Holly J **(SLP)**
Whitlow, Dr Roy E **(SLP)**

Palos Verdes Peninsula
Etheridge, Barbara B **(SLP)**
Lavan, Mrs Leah D A **(SLP)**
Magee, Helmtrud Maria **(SLP)**

Purinton, Laural Wolfe **(A)**

Panorama City

Frazer, Dr Gregory J **(A)**
Harrison, Daniel Paul **(SLP)**

Paradise

Gilbertson, Mrs Kim Annette **(SLP)**
Hanawalt, Mrs Ladonna R **(SLP)**
Lunak, Bridget F **(SLP)**
McWilliams, Bonnie L
Sievert, Rosalind June **(SLP)**

Paramount

Miller, Mrs Stacey Anderson
Porteous, Mrs Mary Jane **(SLP)**
Szal, Mrs Regina M **(A)**
Zinn, Mrs Joan S **(SLP)**

Pasadena

Anderson, Andrea Stockard **(SLP)**
Beck, Karla Luise **(SLP)**
Boyle, Katherine **(SLP)**
Brockway, Debra Elizabeth **(A)**
Caples-Price, Mrs Sherrie D **(A)**
Clayton, Sue K **(SLP)**
Corfield, Joan **(SLP)**
Cotter, Mrs Debora Joyce **(SLP)**
Davis, Gehl M **(SLP)**
Donley, Noreen Jean **(SLP)**
Douglas, Judith Ann
Dryden, Marianne T **(SLP)**
Eldridge, Linda Karen **(SLP)**
Furuya, Yoshio J **(A)**
Hoffman, Lori Ann **(SLP)**
Holt, Mrs Lynne Jacobsen **(SLP)**
Hoskins, Dr Barbara B **(SLP)**
Hudson, Martha Frances **(SLP)**
Jewett, Judith E
Kawaguchi, Jean Noriko **(SLP)**
Kaylor, Carol L **(SLP)**
Kent, Edythe K **(SLP)**
Knepflar, Dr Kenneth J **(SLP)**
Krische, Karen L **(SLP)**
Luster-Carpenter, Mary J **(SLP)**
Monahan, Gail P **(SLP)**
Moody, Mrs Candice A'Lora **(SLP)**
Moody, Carla Susann **(SLP)**
Moscarello, Mrs Kathleen C **(SLP)**
Orona, Mrs Kathryn Marie **(SLP)**
Perez, Mrs Josephine Rivas **(SLP)**
Randel, Dr Elizabeth G **(SLP)**
Revis-Fax, Mrs Andrea Michelle **(SLP)**
Salisbury, John A **(A)**
Shirk, Charles F **(SLP)**
Slater, Robyn L **(SLP)**
Smith, Vera D **(SLP)**
Steinkohl, Mrs Sari H **(SLP)**
Taylor, Alta Lou **(SLP)**
Vedaa, Karen Ostlund
Vracin, Elizabeth **(SLP)**
Watkins, Mrs Guinevere Ann **(SLP)**
Williams, Kathleen Joy **(SLP)**
Wilson, Gail Karen **(SLP)**
Wood, Donald L **(SLP)**
Young, Mrs Anamaria Bravo

Paso Robles

Bray, Mary Petrea **(SLP)**
Deppler-Smith, Dr Doreen D **(SLP)**
Gibbons-Legros, Libby L **(SLP)**

Patterson

Kelly, Mrs Nancy Sue

Pebble Beach

Foy, Mrs Linda P **(SLP)**
Masica, Martha Denise **(SLP)**
Ohanian, Dr Edward **(SLP)**

Perris

Higbee, Nancy L C **(SLP)**

Petaluma

Bachman, David M **(SLP)**
Bates-Stokes, Barbara A **(SLP)**
Bryant, Barbara A **(SLP)**
Collins, David E **(SLP)**
Gratto, MaryEthel **(SLP)**
Marth, Julie E **(A)**
Porcaro, Mrs Susan C C **(SLP)**
Stevick, Mrs Elaine M **(SLP)**
Trahan, Sally A **(SLP)**

Pico Rivera

Marker, Sheila R **(SLP)**
Mendoza, Sylvia Ann **(SLP)**
Swirbul, Therese Jennie

Piedmont

Cohen, Jane S **(SLP)**
Fakoury, Mrs Noura S **(SLP)**
Herman, Mrs Mary Gage **(SLP)**
Lindenstein, Margaret G **(SLP)**
Salter, Mrs Charlotte **(SLP)**
Van Horn, Mrs Judith E **(SLP)**
Van Horn, Robert H **(SLP)**
Wright, Revilla **(SLP)**

Pine Valley

Fichter, Mrs Dana S **(SLP)**

Pinole

Eskilson, Jane E **(SLP)**
Samuels-Rojo, Linda **(SLP)**

Pismo Beach

Gorski, Cynthia Frances **(SLP)**
Tidik, Amy Valentine **(SLP)**

Pittsburg

Gering, Douglas A **(SLP)**
Lieber, Mrs Starr Ehmke

Placentia

Beckett, Dr Ralph L **(SLP)**
Chang, Mrs Laura Gethard **(SLP)**
Dominguez, Mrs Suzanne Marie **(SLP)**
Flatley, Mrs Susanne Gerace **(SLP)**
Huggins, Janice L **(SLP)**
Jarusek, Mrs Sandra L **(SLP)**
Kosel, Denise A **(SLP)**
Pendergast, Mrs Carmela T **(SLP)**
Piper, Mrs Jocelyn Ann **(SLP)**
Rau, Mrs Dale Pruim **(SLP)**

Placerville

Randolph, Laddie A **(SLP)**
Willock, Tracy Lynn **(SLP)**

Playa Del Rey

Camp, Mrs Susan E **(SLP)**
Eisler, Nancy Ann **(SLP)**
Gelman, Irene S **(SLP)**
Johnson, Joy Clark **(SLP)**
Sher, Diane Davis **(SLP)**
Stratton, Elizabeth **(SLP)**

Pleasant Hill

Hauge, Mrs Robin Elizabeth **(SLP)**
Lawson, Kris A **(SLP)**
Manning, Mrs Mary C **(SLP)**
Paulson, Dana M **(SLP)**
Wickman, Mrs Katherine **(SLP)**

Pleasanton

Billheimer, Kenneth D **(A)**
Boos, Bette A **(SLP)**
Edmonds, Vivian Kaita **(SLP)**
Ekren-Cambra, Mrs Susan G **(SLP)**
Fischer, Meredith A **(SLP)**
Hovorka-White, Mrs Carolyn A **(SLP)**
Palin, Sue Johnston **(SLP)**
Ratto-Joy, Mrs Elsie M **(SLP)**
Rivier, Susan Hamilton **(SLP)**
Rodgers, Mrs Brigitte E **(SLP)**
Sabo, Mrs Karen King **(SLP)**
Sharp, Angela Helen **(SLP)**
Vian, Emily K **(SLP)**

Point Arena

Thompson, Mrs Virginia Leonard **(SLP)**

Pomona

Davis, Lisa Ann **(SLP)**
Donahue, Mrs Karen Lee **(SLP)**
Gammon, Sarah E **(SLP)**
Johnson, Cindy Marie **(SLP)**
Knip-Ness, Rebecca L **(SLP)**
Pearman, Sophia Lee **(SLP)**
Rodenbuecher, Nancy Marie **(SLP)**
Smith, Ann L **(SLP)**
Sonti, Lakshmi V **(A)**
Tunstall, Christine M **(SLP)**
Ucok, Mrs Marilyn Finch **(SLP)**
Wiemeyer, Mrs Sandra Lynn **(SLP)**
Williams, Anita L **(SLP)**

Port Hueneme

Case, Mrs Sandra L **(SLP)**
Crawford, John W **(SLP)**
Murphy, Blanche M **(SLP)**

Porterville

Apilado, Benjamin C **(A)**
Buckles, Theresa Ann **(SLP)**
Mills, Sherry Lisa **(SLP)**
Ramirez, Julie Ann
Si-Tayeb, Betty G **(SLP)**

Portola Valley

Bredt, Polly W **(SLP)**
Dowler, Mrs Sharon J M **(SLP)**
Gage, Mrs Ann W **(SLP)**
Rubinstein, Carrie M **(A)**
Squier, Mrs Judith R **(SLP)**

Poway

Butler, Stephanie Alice **(SLP)**
Cegavske, Beth
Fagan, Mary K **(SLP)**
Horning, Judith K **(A)**
Knight, Mrs Georgianne **(SLP)**
Miller, Linda S **(SLP)**
Minard, Mrs Charlotte **(SLP)**
Pollard, Stephanie Crum
Recchia, Mrs Audrey T **(SLP)**
Seitz, Dr Michael R **(SLP)**
Shamasko, Ellenor K **(SLP)**
Tamayo, Mrs Irene H **(A)**

Quartz Hill

Honeycutt, Theresa **(SLP)**

Quincy

Whittaker, Mrs Debroah G **(SLP)**

Ramona

Hughes, Nancy Lee **(SLP)**
Leslie, Mrs Christina **(SLP)**
Wenbourne, Deborah Pierce **(SLP)**

Rancho Cordova

Campa, Connie L **(A)**
Mattson, Laurinda R
Nyland, Mrs Christylee Kinkaid **(SLP)**
O'Neill, Mrs Laura Lee **(SLP)**
Wesolowski, Mrs Anita M **(SLP)**

Rancho Cucamonga

Allison, Jane Mathys **(A)**
Bridges, Annette K **(SLP)**
Kremer, Mrs Susan Elaine **(SLP)**
McCown, Mrs Barbara Lorraine **(SLP)**
Mory, Mrs Kimberly Dews **(SLP)**
Osgood, Everett Clark **(SLP)**
Ruiz, Victor G **(SLP)**

Rancho Mirage

Vroman-Cooper, Carolyn R **(A)**

Rancho Murieta

Obley-Kilborn, Nancy N **(SLP)**

Rancho Palos Verdes

Chickedantz, Lise A **(SLP)**
Davis, Janet B **(SLP)**
Hanley, Mrs Joan C **(SLP A)**
Hollander, Beverly M **(A)**
Jeans, Mrs Rowena Marie **(SLP)**
Koehler, Mrs Mary P **(SLP)**
Lentz, Mrs Barbara S **(A)**
McDowell, Mrs Angela P **(SLP)**
Moir, Jane Magennis **(SLP)**
Nagy, Mrs Regina L **(SLP)**
Rennick, Sydelle **(SLP)**
Wonder, Coralie M **(SLP)**
Worcester, Carol S **(SLP)**

Rancho Santa Fe

Willard, Dr Cheralyn Tiffany **(SLP)**

Rancho Santa Margarita

Garber, Karen Bentley **(SLP)**
Mues, Catlin **(SLP)**
Wolf, Diane S **(SLP)**

Red Bluff

Craig, Mrs Mary L **(SLP)**
Depuy, Mrs Mabel B **(SLP)**
Eicholtz, Glenn Everett **(SLP)**
Eicholtz, Helen J **(SLP)**
Pack, Nancy J **(SLP)**

Redding

Blankenship, Mrs Sally Warner **(SLP)**
Carr, Jacquelyn Carney **(SLP)**
Chenoweth, Wayne L **(SLP)**
Crean, Mrs Joanne Ziegler **(SLP)**
Dawes, Patricia Jann **(SLP)**
Deetz, Debbie M **(SLP)**
Herrmann, Mrs Martha Ann **(SLP)**
Hinson, Susan Ann **(SLP)**
Howells, Mrs Cindy Wells **(SLP)**
Howells, Rod Carlyle **(A)**
Knell-Berg, Caron Anne **(SLP)**
Peterson, Anne K **(SLP)**
Ramsdell, Rebecca Sue **(SLP)**
Simko, Rita McWilliams **(A)**
Whitaker, Susan E **(SLP)**

Redlands

Ackley, Diane D **(SLP)**
Anderson, James Russell **(A)**
Argon, Janet Lynn **(SLP)**
Arguello, Nancy Kathryn **(SLP)**
Backstrom, Melissa Katherine **(SLP)**
Baer, Dr William P **(SLP)**
Balthazor, Dr Ronald J **(A)**
Billings, Bradley L **(A)**
Bjorklund, Kristen B **(SLP)**
Bongers, Libewij F **(SLP)**
Booth, Judith A **(SLP)**
Braxton, Mrs Patricia Lynn **(SLP)**
Brezsny, Mrs Felice J **(SLP)**
Burgraff, Dr Roger I **(SLP)**
Chicouris, Cynthia Lynn **(SLP)**
Cozad, Mrs Betty Berry **(SLP)**
Cozad, Dr Robert L **(SLP A)**
Deal-Tackett, Laurie K **(SLP)**
Delange, Mrs Sonya B **(SLP)**
Demler, Mrs Mary McDermott
Ellis, Christina Ann **(SLP)**
Gale-Sadler, Cheri **(SLP)**
Harrison, Mrs Jean M **(SLP)**
Hendryx, Patricia Mary **(SLP)**
Hofferber, Mrs Kelly Ann **(A)**
Inkmann, Mrs Constance Marie **(SLP)**
Jacobs, Frederick Paul **(A)**
Katkov, George W **(SLP)**
King-Webb, Robin **(SLP)**
Kiyan, Beverly Ng **(A)**
Livoni, Mrs Linda E **(SLP)**
Mallory, Donna M **(A)**
Maskin, Mrs Lynn N **(SLP)**
McCabe, Marianne Michele
Mirau, Mrs Maureen M **(SLP)**
Mitchell, Edgar D **(SLP)**
Morgan, Marianne Marie **(SLP)**
Morrison, Judith A **(SLP)**
Odell, Mrs Teresa Gail **(SLP)**
Ouellette, Dr Eugene G **(SLP A)**
Parr, Mrs Kristy Sjogren
Perenchio, Mrs Jan **(SLP)**
Petty, Anne M **(SLP)**

Reid, Annie Kathleen **(SLP)**
Rider, Dr Larry P **(SLP)**
Rogan, Jane Elizabeth **(A)**
Rowley, Dr Rodney Ray **(A)**
Shannon, Janet Louise **(SLP)**
Stauble, Ann-Marie Elizabeth **(SLP)**
Stephens, Mrs Christey H **(SLP)**
Sturlaugson, Dr William R **(SLP)**
Sukowske-Miles, Mrs Pauline G **(SLP)**
Tieri, Mrs Lynnee Luckett **(SLP)**
Walker, Dr Christophr Niles **(SLP)**
Weil, Patricia Messina **(A)**
Wu-Ramley, Mrs Grace Fei Min **(SLP)**

Redondo Beach

Airola, Catherine E **(SLP)**
Burkholz, Robin Aimee **(SLP)**
Calkins, Lynnell Flynn **(SLP)**
Clark, Mrs Michele Mary **(SLP)**
Dawson, Mrs Theresa T **(SLP)**
Dietiker, Terri A **(A)**
Faigen, Janet **(SLP)**
Fearman, Eleanor G **(SLP)**
Feldman, Mrs Linda Morris **(SLP)**
Halsey, Mrs Karen C **(SLP)**
Heino, Pamela Sue **(SLP)**
Huguet, Michelle **(SLP)**
Jared, Mrs Laura Lee **(SLP)**
Kaatz, Kathryn J **(SLP)**
Koebsell, Katherine Allison **(A)**
Likavec, Judith Marie **(SLP)**
Lippes, Beth C **(SLP)**
Maben, Nancy E **(SLP)**
Martin, James P **(A)**
Montes, Michelle Marie **(SLP)**
Moore, Johanna Lee **(SLP)**
Powell, Mrs Celia K **(SLP)**
Reid, Mary Elizabeth **(SLP)**
Robinson, Alice Jean **(SLP)**
Snider, Judith L **(SLP)**
Winn, Conrad **(SLP)**

Redwood City

Chaney, Dr Carolyn **(SLP)**
Dewitt, Mrs Carolyn Dankowski
Duignan, Mrs Sue E **(SLP)**
Friedlander, Mrs Barbara N **(SLP)**
Fukuhara, Mrs Victoria Lai **(SLP)**
Haas, Dr Gustav F **(A)**
MacChello, Ronda M **(SLP)**
Murakami, Karen Ayako
Nelson-Barber, Dr Sharon S **(SLP)**
Schwartzbord, Carolyn **(SLP)**
Soby, Mrs Annette M **(SLP)**
Spuhler, Barbara **(SLP)**

Redwood Valley

Phelan, Mrs Shannon B **(SLP)**
West, Mrs Geraldine **(SLP)**
Winter, Yvonne **(SLP)**

Reedley

Belden-Pope, Mrs Lori **(SLP)**
Enns, Mrs Janet M **(SLP)**
Neufeld, Rebecca A **(SLP)**
Taylor, Phyllis B **(SLP)**

Rescue

Jones, Alyce W **(SLP)**

Reseda

Aller, Dr Sonia Konialian **(SLP)**
Bell, Mrs Joan L **(SLP)**
Comroe, Mrs Judith S **(SLP)**
Cooney, Mrs Kathryn Mack **(SLP)**
Elswick, Mrs Nadine B **(SLP)**
Giraldo, Consuelo Gloria **(SLP)**
Girvan, Stephanie **(A)**
Kaye, Roberta Loren **(SLP)**
Kohn, Mrs Sybil W **(SLP)**
Lemoine, Noma R **(SLP)**
Mack, Ronald Andrew **(SLP)**
Smith, Janice C **(SLP)**
Venezuela-Estavillo, Gladys Yadira **(SLP)**

Rialto

Bilderback, Mrs Linda Lyon **(SLP)**
Chenoy, Sohrab Y **(SLP)**
Olson, Mrs Terry Lee **(SLP)**
Snavely, Christophr R **(A)**
Ticich, Margaret M **(SLP)**

Richmond

Adsit, Paula S **(SLP)**
Aleman, Mrs Malisa D
Allen, Mrs Cynthia Marie **(SLP)**
Deegan, Marywin **(SLP)**
Izdebski, Dr Krzysztof **(SLP)**
McDowell, Betty M
Mizell, Dr Diann **(SLP)**
Rappaport, Michele Coy **(SLP)**
Rosenberg, Trudy Lorraine **(SLP)**
von Hermann, Jean O **(SLP)**

Ridgecrest

Sorbo, Joann E **(SLP)**

Rimforest

Pope, Carol L **(SLP)**

Rio del Mar

Marietti-Benito, Mrs Valerie Ann **(SLP)**

Riverbank

Simonton, Mrs Martha Rae **(SLP)**

Riverside

Anderson, Diana Best **(SLP A)**
Anderson, Georgiana **(SLP)**
Bockover, Mrs Donna Louise **(SLP)**
Boshart, Charlotte **(SLP)**
Bothwell-Blanchet, Mrs Kathleen A **(SLP)**
Bowers, Mrs Brenda R **(SLP)**
Bradley, Mrs Janet Cheryl **(SLP)**
Britt, Dr Eulalia Evelyn **(A)**
Butterfield, Mrs Lisa Bennett **(SLP)**
Christenson, Merilyn J **(SLP)**
Clem, Mrs Karen L **(SLP)**
Coachbuilder, Dr Deenaz P **(SLP)**
Cowart, Mrs Rosa Cash **(SLP)**
Diaz, Suzanne Gail **(SLP)**
Eberlein, Nancy J **(SLP)**
Elliot, Mrs Linda Pighini **(SLP)**
Feldman, Mrs Sharon A **(SLP)**
Fiedler-Fuhrman, Judith Lynn **(SLP)**
Forrest, Jeanine Chapman **(SLP)**
Hartman, Robert S **(SLP)**
Jeffries, Angela L **(SLP)**
Kaplan, Mrs Kathleen L
Kline, Catherine **(SLP)**
Lewis, Kristy A **(SLP)**
Lowry, Dr Jean **(SLP)**
Lozoya, Mrs Maria Uribe **(SLP)**
Malle, Mrs Joyce Marie **(SLP)**
Mathis, Brian Roger **(SLP)**
Minsker, Marilyn **(SLP)**
Morrow, Michelle Renee **(SLP)**
Nielsen, Mrs Barbara Jean **(SLP)**
Peacher, William G **(SLP)**
Plumer, Elizabeth H **(SLP)**
Pope, Mrs Monica M **(SLP)**
Roberts, Joan Elizabeth **(SLP)**
Rohr, Mrs Kari Vj
Sakover, Mrs Patricia E **(SLP)**
Schaefer, Linda Dell **(SLP)**
Stoever, Jean E **(SLP)**
Wahl, Nancy M **(SLP)**

Rocklin

Baker, Mrs Connie K **(A)**
Gabria, Ronald C **(SLP)**
Labudde, Mrs Dorothy E **(SLP)**
Morris, Mrs Lynn Mae **(SLP)**
Reedy, Debra Strawhun **(SLP)**
Sherman, Mrs Leann A **(SLP)**
Starch, Mrs Sandy Abolins **(SLP)**

Rodeo

Condevaux-Dahlberg, Annie **(SLP)**
Thacker, Lynda JoAnne **(SLP)**

Rohnert Park

Bagley, Christine Maria **(SLP)**
Burt, Mrs Phyllis J **(A)**
Dundas, Lisa A **(A)**
Lipp, Rhandee Gail **(SLP)**
Whitton, Laura Ballantyne **(SLP)**

Rolling Hills

Ryker, Angela M

Rosemead

Maldonado, Monica **(SLP)**
Wilson, Mrs Josephine F **(A)**

Roseville

Babiak, Mrs Joann U **(SLP)**
Behrens, Leilani **(SLP)**
Bjekich, Karen Hauber **(SLP)**
Burnstad, Evelyn G **(SLP)**
Daulton, Mrs Donna S **(SLP)**
Donlon, Mrs Roswitha Heinicke **(A)**
Files, Mrs Wendy Welch **(SLP)**
Hauck, Mrs Margaret K **(SLP)**
Hess, Linda Kurani **(SLP)**
Lechthaler, Denise Ann **(SLP)**
Rosoff-Foster, Mrs Beverly **(SLP)**
Smith, Mrs Lisa K **(SLP)**
Stillman, Nancy M **(SLP)**
Swetkovich, Sherri Alicia **(SLP)**
Watson, Mrs Christine Bagalonis **(SLP)**

Rowland Heights

Arnhold, Mrs Linda M **(SLP)**
Gomez, Donna Hotra **(SLP)**
Loggins, Janice Ellen **(A)**
Smith, Yolanda **(SLP)**
Sperling, Terri Bukaitz **(SLP)**

Running Springs

Hayes, Tyler S **(SLP)**
Jaffe-Karp, Alison **(SLP)**

Sacramento

Addicott, John P **(SLP)**
Addicott, Mrs Margaret A **(SLP)**
Alberts, Cecil D **(SLP A)**
Ambalong, Mrs Gaudencia **(SLP)**
Armstrong, Timothy Patrick **(A)**
Barbaria, Lynn **(SLP)**
Becker, Mrs Chris Nunn **(SLP)**
Becker, Mrs Rosalind
Bennitt, Barbara A **(A)**
Berger, Mrs Barbara B **(SLP)**
Birkenstock, Nora Karla/Holl **(A)**
Bonds-Baird, Joy **(SLP)**
Bonslett, Merrylee M **(A)**
Brixey, Nancy L **(A)**
Calvert, Dr Donald Raymond **(A)**
Chuchas, James G **(SLP)**
Colbert, Martha S **(SLP)**
Coleman, Dr Colette L **(SLP)**
Cottor, Mary Kappel **(SLP)**
Darlow, Mrs Mary S **(SLP)**
Davis, Christine Herrick **(SLP)**
DeLorenzo-Guinn, Mrs Therese **(SLP)**
DeRoss, Mrs Sandy S **(SLP)**
Dokimos, Elizabeth **(SLP)**
Druliner, Mrs Barbette Carol **(SLP)**
Duck, Gordon L **(SLP)**
Dyer, Mrs Linda King **(A)**
Fawx, Linda L **(SLP)**
Fetherston, Cynthia Powell **(A)**
Flessatti, Paula Mary **(SLP)**
Foley, Rochelle Lynn **(SLP)**
Fong, Raymond G **(SLP A)**
Fong, Valerie
Forrest, Mrs Andrea Swenson **(SLP)**
Fusilier, Freida M **(SLP)**
Germ, Mrs Jane Mary **(SLP)**
Gilmore, Dr Susan L **(SLP)**
Goldsworthy, Dr Candace L **(SLP)**
Goodrich, Susan Jean **(SLP)**
Grimm, Gretchen A **(A)**
Guis, Amy H **(SLP)**
Hallam, Jerold J **(SLP)**
Hancock, Mrs Jennifer Kretz **(SLP)**
Hansen, Mrs Lynn M **(SLP)**
Harris, Shelley **(SLP)**
Hartnett, Debra Scott **(SLP)**
Hoadley, Barbara Robertson **(SLP)**
Hoey, Cathy A **(SLP)**
Holub, Karen Dorothy **(SLP)**
Hubbell, Robert D **(SLP)**
Huff, Frances Ann **(A)**
Huff, Dr Steven Jay **(A)**
Johnson, Judy Lynn **(A)**
Johnson, Mrs Mary A
Jones, Morris Val **(SLP A)**
Keck, Deborah Ann **(A)**
Kelly, Kerry A **(SLP)**
Kiester, Vicki A **(A)**
Kukla, Janis Ann **(SLP)**
Kuratomi, Christine
Lee, Patricia Spears **(SLP)**
Leonard, Perry C **(SLP)**
Leonard, Dr Rebecca J **(SLP)**
Lerner, Judith L S **(SLP)**
Loest, Deborag Gaye
Lohman-Ruiz, Patricia S **(SLP)**
Lydon, Mary D **(SLP)**
Lystrup, Laura D **(SLP)**
Mayer, Dr Carole L **(A)**
McCartney, Dr James H **(A)**
McCarty-Leet, Patricia A **(SLP)**
McMurtry, Mrs Carol A W **(A)**
Melarkey, Barbara Alexina **(SLP)**
Miller, Madge B **(SLP)**
Morgan, Barbara M **(SLP)**
Morrell-Trussell, Carol Anne **(A)**
Morrison, Mrs Judith G H **(SLP)**
Morse, Mrs Lynn Allison **(SLP)**
Murphy, Jane W **(SLP)**
Murphy, Kinzie S **(SLP)**
Murphy, Lynn B **(SLP)**
Nielsen, Patricia P **(SLP)**
Nigro, Mrs Kerri F **(SLP)**
Norris, Mrs Marcia M **(SLP)**
Osborn, Joan H **(SLP)**
Osborn, Richard Joseph **(A)**
Payne, Lonnie Mark
Phelan, Charlene A **(SLP)**
Phelps, Mrs Pamela Bernadette **(A)**
Phillips, Janice Kay **(SLP)**
Piazza, Carol Ann **(SLP)**
Pickens, Susan Alexander **(SLP)**
Pierce, Mrs Edwina S G **(SLP)**
Potter, Susan Dale **(SLP)**
Powell, Deborah Renee **(A)**
Press, Mrs Judy Reed **(SLP)**
Pressley, Glenda Earline **(SLP)**
Ramirez-Krambs, Mrs Olga V **(SLP)**
Reed, Gail A **(SLP)**
Rees Phd, Dr Maryjane **(SLP)**
Robison, Myrna Kay **(SLP)**
Sanchez-Boyce, Michele L **(SLP)**
Schetter, Jacqui L **(A)**
Sheaffer, David Bryan **(A)**
Sheppard, Douglas R **(SLP)**
Simon, Julie Ann **(SLP)**
Simpson, Jeffrey M **(SLP)**
Smith, Susan Carol **(SLP)**
Spacagna, Robert A **(A)**
Stennett, Mrs Nadine E **(SLP)**
Stevens, Mrs Patricia Kathleen **(SLP)**
Stone, Robin Gayle
Strickler, Carol J
Sunderland, Mrs Linda G **(SLP)**
Terleski-Katz, Lynn R **(SLP)**
Tice, Dr Robert E **(SLP A)**
Trondsen, Mrs Lisa Anderson **(SLP)**
Trouba, Mrs Susan Sievers **(A)**
Walker, Alice Irene **(SLP)**
Welge, Elizabeth H **(SLP)**
Whinnery, Sheridan Elizabeth **(SLP)**
Winter, Florian Davos **(SLP)**
Wise, Janet L **(SLP)**
Young, Mrs Laura Carroll **(SLP)**

Salinas

Brooks, Francis D **(SLP A)**
Cofer, Mrs Sandra K **(SLP)**
Dillon, James Anthony **(SLP)**
Hansen-Emery, Dawn L **(SLP)**
Hart, Major Loren Stephen **(A)**
Howe, Catherine Louise **(SLP)**
Johnson, Mrs Janice F **(SLP)**
McGuire, Tamara Jane **(SLP)**
McIntyre, Mrs Mary Ann **(SLP)**
Scarr, Mrs Gail A **(SLP)**
Schatz, Susan A **(SLP A)**
Smith, Mark Allen **(SLP)**
Solow, Dr Lawrence **(A)**
Twisselman, Mrs Karen Marie **(SLP)**
Tyler, Jane F **(SLP)**
Yulich, Mrs Gail M **(SLP)**

Salona Beach

Ryan, Janis C **(A)**

San Anselmo

Cogen, Lynn C **(SLP)**
Dillon, Diane Lynn **(SLP)**
Halverson, Joan Marie **(SLP)**
Honig, Melissa Rogosin **(SLP)**
Jarvis, Carol A **(SLP)**
Kaul, Joan W **(SLP)**
Meyer, Joanne L **(SLP)**
Sheviakov, Mrs Carole K **(SLP)**

San Bernardino

Balthazor, Mrs Patricia N **(SLP)**
Burch, Nancy Louise
Burson, Laura **(SLP)**
Campbell, Evelyn C **(SLP)**
Cepeda, Mrs Bernice Teresa **(SLP)**
Chalfant, Gail Ann **(SLP)**
Clifton, Mrs Sharon Jo **(SLP)**
Craig, Mary Helen **(SLP)**
Crandall, Cynthia D **(SLP)**
Czvik, Mrs Patsy Smith **(SLP)**
Demetrion-Boatright, Helen **(SLP)**
Elliott, Margaret L **(SLP)**
Gardner-Cyr, Mrs Theresa Marie **(SLP)**
Gorham, William J **(SLP A)**
Lade, Mrs Debra Moseley **(SLP)**
Milner, Floyd Eugene **(A)**
Persell, Evelyn S **(SLP)**
Peterson, Donna M **(SLP)**
Reed, Mrs Betty Lou **(SLP)**
Salzman, Gilbert M **(SLP)**
Sitts, Joanne P B **(SLP)**
Wick, Laura Mary Baron **(SLP)**
Williams, Charles **(SLP)**

San Bruno

Blazek, Barbara Lynn **(A)**
Evans, Mrs Susan Lynn **(SLP)**
O'Leary, Lauren Jean **(SLP)**

San Carlos

Ahern, Ellen Louise **(SLP)**
Campbell, Virginia A **(SLP)**
Cassanego, Diane L P **(SLP)**
Goold-Caulfield, Jane Evelyn **(SLP)**
Henderson, Mrs Barbara A **(SLP)**
Holden, Mrs Kelley A **(A)**
Joy, Mrs Pamela Colston **(SLP)**
Kowalka, Linda H **(SLP)**
Najac, John W **(SLP)**
Nikodym, Deanna L **(SLP)**
Powell, Mrs Terren **(SLP)**
Powell-Todd, Gwendolyn **(SLP)**
Shaw, John D **(SLP)**
Wrasse, Kenneth W, Jr **(SLP)**

San Clemente

Allison, Regina M **(SLP)**
Bromm, Mary **(SLP)**
Douthett, Mary Beth **(SLP)**
Galyean, Barbara B **(SLP)**
Geller, Karla V S **(SLP)**
Hanaford, Mrs Laura Ann **(SLP)**
Hard, Vallori K **(SLP)**
Jenson, Gloria R **(SLP)**
Kugler, Karen J **(SLP)**
McDaniels, Karen E **(SLP)**
Prenovost, Annette Louise **(SLP)**
Richardson, Darlene Marie **(SLP)**
Schade, Mary Beth **(SLP)**
Schade, William A **(A)**
Tanner, Barry Jon **(SLP)**
Townsend, Mrs Beatrice Kay **(SLP)**
Williams, Kathryn D **(SLP)**

San Diego

Abrams, Annette
Adamo, Brian
Adams, Mrs Julia G **(SLP)**
Adler, Jacqueline **(A)**
Allen, Brenda May **(SLP)**
Allen, Elizabeth **(SLP)**
Allen, Mrs Elizabeth Bishop **(SLP)**
Altomare, Lynn Woods **(SLP)**
Anderson, Mrs Diane Carolan **(SLP)**
Arnn, Cheryl McDougall **(SLP)**
Atherton, Deanna J **(SLP)**
Badam, Kimberly K **(SLP)**
Barbieri-Welge, Rene L **(SLP)**
Barnes, Dr Gary J **(SLP)**
Barnett, Mrs Debra L **(SLP)**
Basser, Mrs Roberta Ilene **(SLP)**
Bellugi, Dr Ursula
Bennett, Dr Clayton L **(SLP)**
Berman, Judy S **(SLP A)**
Bernstein, Mrs Patricia E **(SLP)**
Best, Mrs Pamela O'Bryan
Betzig, Lynn Louise **(A)**
Bianco-Vasquez, Andrea Louise **(SLP)**
Billman, Mrs Kimberly Smith **(SLP)**
Bishop-St Clair, Mrs Cynthia M **(SLP)**
Black, Mrs Joyce Elizabeth **(SLP)**
Blackmer, Kathryn M **(SLP)**
Blake, Lynn Ann **(SLP)**
Blanck, Mrs Cathy Pryatel **(SLP)**
Bliler, Dr Robert L **(SLP)**
Blount, Mrs Shirley M **(SLP)**
Boehringer, Hans Walter **(SLP)**
Boehringer, Mrs Marilyn **(A)**
Bradshaw, Denise **(SLP)**
Brammer, Melanie Ann **(A)**
Branch, Mrs Carol **(A)**
Braverman, Mrs Sharon G **(SLP)**
Bronson, Kathryn Thelen
Brown, Anita Gibson **(SLP)**
Brown, Geraldine Harris **(SLP)**
Bushnell, Dale R
Byrd, Susan Marie **(A)**
Cabe, Donna J **(A)**
Cabello, Arturo **(SLP)**
Camenzuli, Dr Lorraine F **(SLP)**
Cannon-Kramer, Mrs Kathleen A **(SLP)**
Cate, Jeanne Beatrice **(SLP)**
Catterall, Mrs Kathleen A **(SLP)**
Catton, Mrs Barbara Anne
Cheng, Dr Li-Rong L **(SLP)**
Christensen, Dr Kathee Ann
Christensen, Michelle K **(SLP)**
Cicotte, Mrs Carol Alvord
Clark, Mrs Janice Burnett **(SLP)**
Clark, Linda Jean **(SLP)**
Clarke, Ronnie M **(A)**
Clerkson, Marion **(SLP)**
Clifton, Gina Anne **(SLP)**
Cohen, Mrs Penny Lynn **(SLP)**
Cole, Dr Robert C **(SLP)**
Cook, Mary Ann **(SLP)**
Cook, Sharon Lynne **(SLP)**
Coonce, Gayle S **(SLP)**
Currie, Sally Jo **(SLP)**
Davies, Darlene Gould **(SLP)**
Davis, Ann M **(SLP)**
Davis, Karlyn H **(SLP)**
Dickinson, Mrs Stella C **(SLP)**
Don, Eujania B **(SLP)**
Dowling, Claire J **(A)**
Doyle, Carol Anne **(SLP)**
Dukas, Marilyn D **(SLP)**
Dunaway, Claudia L **(SLP)**
Duncan, Teresa K **(SLP)**
Earnest, Dr Sue W **(SLP)**
Edwards, Barbara B **(SLP)**
Eshelman, Mrs Chris Winters **(SLP)**
Fisher, Mrs Joni Jane **(SLP)**
Flaherty, James Peter **(SLP)**
Fleming, Terrilyn E **(SLP)**
Frank, Ruby Ann **(SLP)**
Funkhouser, Kristen Dee **(A)**
Gardner-Reichley, Mrs Elizabeth **(SLP)**
Garrett, Mrs Sharon Ellen **(SLP)**
George, Louise Eddy **(A)**
Gevanthor, Peter Greene **(SLP)**
Gilden, Laurie Susanne **(SLP)**
Gimbel, Mrs Iris M **(SLP)**
Glasheen, Mrs Marie C **(SLP)**
Glines, Lisa Wasick **(SLP)**
Goldman, Stephen Norman **(SLP)**
Golub-Roberts, Mrs Amy B **(SLP)**
Gordon, Yvonne C **(SLP)**
Gowan-Baker, Mrs Daralee **(SLP)**
Gray, Carol Jeanne
Greene, Dr Nancy E **(SLP)**
Grote, Dr Carole Ann **(SLP)**
Hale, Mrs Maryjane Bialomizy **(SLP)**
Hammerton, Mrs Cynthia A **(SLP)**
Harding, Deborah B
Harris, Barbara Jane **(SLP)**
Hartman, Dr Paul W **(A)**
Hashimoto, Naomi **(SLP)**
Hein, Herbert R **(SLP)**
Hein, Joanne Gerstein **(SLP)**
Hiatt, Christine L
Hinshaw, Mary C M **(SLP)**
Hippert, Mrs Carol Lowrey **(A)**
Hoffelmeyer, Melissa Guss **(SLP)**
Hoke, Mrs Jody Lynn Hilles **(SLP)**
Holtz, Mrs Tami Anne **(SLP)**
Howard, Mrs Lauranne M **(SLP)**
Howell, Lynne M **(SLP)**
Huffer, Mrs Frances C **(A)**
Hurley, Mary M **(SLP)**
Imhoff, Timothy E **(SLP)**
Irvin, Merle J **(SLP)**
Jackson, Dr Colleen O **(A)**
Jalowayski, Mrs Irene R **(SLP)**
Jansen-Petersen, Jane E **(A)**
Johnson, Mrs Dorothy C **(SLP)**
Johnson, Dr Kenneth O **(SLP A)**
Johnston, Eloise R **(SLP)**
Jones, Dr Barry W
Kafoure, Dory Rigopoulos **(SLP)**
Kahn, Mrs Alison P **(A)**
Kalter, Eleanor R **(SLP)**
Kasanoff, Julie Lynn **(A)**
Kellerhouse, Sylvia Pittman **(SLP)**
Kessler-Heiberg, Mrs Heike A **(SLP)**
Kim, Erin Jamie **(A)**
Kirsch, Christine Lynn **(A)**
Kissh, H Laura **(SLP)**
Kohrs, Charlotte **(SLP)**
Kopp, Dr Harriet G **(A)**
Kramer, Dr Steven J **(A)**
Krebs, Dr Donald F **(A)**
Krupp, Rita S **(SLP)**
Kuhn, Beth Ann **(SLP)**
Kvaal, Jolene Teresa **(SLP)**
Langkabel, Terry Lynn **(SLP)**
Larkin, Carol D B **(SLP)**
Larson, Mark H **(SLP)**
Last, Stephanie **(SLP)**
Launer, Dr Patricia B **(SLP)**
Law, Deborah A **(A)**
Lewis, Mary Frances **(SLP)**
Lopes, Charlotte Marie **(SLP)**
Lorber, Nina P **(SLP)**
Lovely, Leslee Susan **(SLP)**
Ludwig, Gail Ann **(SLP)**
Ludwig, Janelle Lynne
MacLearie, Elizabeth **(SLP)**
Maher, Mrs Lynne Meyer **(SLP)**
Malchow-McCarty, Deborah Lee **(A)**
Mann, Brenda Pakier **(SLP)**
Marchette, Mrs Susan Nealon **(SLP)**
Marino, Anne Jean **(SLP)**
Martinez, Rita Teran
Mattison, Mindy Susan **(SLP)**
May, Suzanne **(SLP)**
McAlister, Shirley W **(SLP)**
McClendon, Mary Kay **(SLP)**
McCullough, Brenda Carol **(SLP)**
McGee, Mrs Laura Ferreira **(SLP)**
McGowan, Charlene Green **(SLP)**
McGrane, Mrs Susan Driver **(SLP)**
McManus, Margaret Theresa **(SLP)**
McMillen, Joanne Lynn
Merrick, Mrs Paula Lenocker **(SLP)**
Merrick, Roy L **(SLP)**
Merrick, Mrs Theadora Smith **(SLP)**
Michaletz, Mary Patricia **(SLP)**
Mickowski, Jois Ann **(SLP)**
Miller, Sara F **(SLP)**
Mitchell, Mrs Christine D
Monaghan-Maxson, Mrs Cindy M **(SLP)**
Monger-Massie, Mrs Tamara Jo **(SLP)**
Mooers, Janet E **(SLP)**
Mopper, Marjorie Ann **(SLP)**
Morgan, Yvonne **(SLP)**
Mornout, Mrs Claudia W **(SLP)**
Muncy, Dr M Jean **(SLP)**
Munoa, Marissa Hunt **(SLP)**
Murry, Dr Thomas **(SLP)**
Nakamura, Patricia Shigetomi **(SLP)**
Naliboff, Mrs Ellen C **(SLP)**
Natkin, Mrs Karen L **(SLP)**
Navratil, Shirley Ann **(A)**
Neubauer, Christine A
Nevitt, Susan G **(SLP)**
Nichols, Dr Alan C **(SLP)**
Nies, Linda Ann **(SLP)**
Nigro, Carolyn Griffith **(SLP)**
Novak, Robert E **(A)**
O'Hara, James J **(A)**
Olsson, Robert J **(A)**
Papuga, Susan Kathryn **(SLP)**
Pearson, Mrs Jane S **(SLP)**
Perry, Mrs Susan M **(A)**
Pfeifer, Mrs Christina Hunter **(SLP)**
Pichurko, Joann J **(SLP)**
Popp, Sharon Ad **(SLP)**
Rannard, Elizabeth Joan
Raymond, Susan J C **(SLP)**
Reed, Nancy J **(SLP)**
Rhodes, Diane I **(SLP)**
Rickon, Sandra **(SLP)**
Riedman, Dr Richard M **(SLP A)**
Rieker, Carole Sue **(A)**
Ring, Mrs Ngareta E **(SLP)**
Rissman, Mrs Marlene S **(SLP)**
Rivera, Enid M
Robinson, Mrs Leslie Susan **(SLP)**
Rosen, Perry Alan **(SLP)**
Rosenberg-Alpert, Mrs Beth **(SLP)**
Rosenfeld, Ronni J **(SLP)**
Rosenquist, Mrs Teresa Davis **(SLP)**
Rost, Mrs Mara L
Rothstein, Mrs Roberta Arlene **(SLP)**
Ruhm, Dr Howard B **(A)**
Ryan, Mrs Sandra Lee **(SLP)**
Sallee, Mrs Gayle A D **(SLP)**
Sanderson, Pamela M **(A)**
Satin, Terry L **(SLP)**
Schickler, Judy Sobel **(SLP)**
Schlosser, Dr Frances D **(SLP)**
Servetter, Miriam **(SLP)**
Shellenberger, Sharon L T **(SLP)**
Shipstead-Cox, Mrs Nancy Jean **(SLP)**
Shorn-Fletcher, Amy M **(SLP)**
Shurtleff, Mrs M'Liss Marler
Siblesz, Ana Maria **(SLP)**
Siegel, Constance **(SLP)**
Silverman, Laurie A **(SLP)**

Singh, Dr Sadanand
Sofen, Linda N
Stansell, Dr Barbara J **(SLP)**
Steckbeck, Mrs Pamela Meza **(SLP)**
Stecker, Kay E S **(A)**
Steffan, Karen Anne **(SLP)**
St Onge, Tracie Lee **(SLP)**
St Peters, Mary C **(SLP)**
Stringer, Jerrie S **(SLP)**
Strommer, Amy **(SLP)**
Sullivan, Mrs Elizabeth Mascolo **(SLP)**
Summers, Judith A **(SLP)**
Swanson, Teri **(SLP)**
Swartz, Mrs Judith L **(SLP)**
Thile, Dr Edmund L **(SLP)**
Thomas, Mrs Cleopatra Word **(A)**
Thomas, Cynthia **(SLP)**
Thomason, Bonnie Carol B **(SLP)**
Tietje, Mrs Betty Ann **(SLP)**
Turner, Mrs Jayne A **(SLP)**
Wade, Curtis Nelson
Walker, James Anthony
Walter, Nancy Jane **(SLP)**
Waytashek, Tammy A **(SLP)**
Weintraub, Suzanne **(SLP)**
White, Ingrid H W **(SLP)**
Whitten, Ida E **(SLP)**
Williams, Penny Sue **(SLP)**
Willis-Henry, Olivia Marie **(A)**
Wise, Birte H **(SLP)**
Wolkowski, Robert Donald **(SLP)**
Wong, Anna **(SLP)**
Wothe, Carole A **(SLP)**
Young, Lore R **(SLP)**
Zeisler, Carolyn

San Dimas

Adzovich, Mrs Nancy Lea **(A)**
Dunn, Mrs Jean B **(SLP)**
Erdos, Elaine M **(SLP)**
Fried, Marla G **(SLP)**
Ginther, Judith A **(SLP)**

San Fernando

Klein, Patty A **(A)**
Montaug-Martin, Linda J **(SLP)**

San Francisco

Ahonen, Judi Elizabeth **(SLP A)**
Almon, Mrs Grace M **(SLP)**
Arana, Margot A **(SLP)**
Bargman, Kathleen **(SLP)**
Barrett, Dr Lyman Stewart **(SLP A)**
Beilke, Richard Marshall **(SLP)**
Black, Peggy S **(SLP)**
Blumenthal, Reeva S
Bond, Flavia Michelle **(SLP)**
Breshike, Kevin John **(A)**
Brockman, Loreen Rita **(SLP)**
Buchwald, Gerald J
Buhr, Barbara Ann **(SLP)**
Burke, Sheila Burnett **(A)**
Callaghan, Carol A **(SLP)**
Campbell, Leslie M L **(SLP)**
Carr, Ann B **(SLP)**
Ceriotti, Mary Ann **(SLP)**
Chang, Robert K **(A)**
Charpentier, Cynthia A **(SLP)**
Clark, Mrs Teresa Marie **(A)**
Claus, Russell S **(SLP)**
Claus, Mrs Theresa A **(SLP)**
Clumeck, Dr Harold V **(SLP)**
Compton, Dr Arthur J
Connell, Jane S
Conover, Kathleen D **(SLP)**
Conry, Christine Patricia **(SLP)**
Converse, Marilyn V **(SLP)**
Corinblit, Barbara **(SLP)**
Cross, A Donald **(SLP)**
Croutch, Carl A **(A)**
Darby, John L
Defrantz, Dr Anita P **(SLP)**
Deppe, Janet A **(SLP)**
Dill, Ann Lawrence **(SLP)**
Doherty, Dr E Thomas
Drew, Nancy **(SLP A)**
Edelson, Martha **(SLP)**
Egan, Sylvia
Ehrlich, Mrs Ruth H **(SLP)**
Eng, Lawrence M **(A)**
Etkin, Reuma
Facer, M Christina **(SLP)**
Feinstein, Marjorie S **(SLP)**
Ferris, Virginia A **(A)**
Fertman-Wolff, Dr Joan C **(SLP)**
Fleming, Dr Carol A **(SLP)**
Flower, Dr Richard M **(SLP A)**
Flower, Mrs Wilda M **(SLP A)**
Flynn, Diane Marie **(SLP)**
Focht, Christofer
Foreman, Joyce Ellen **(SLP)**
Forrest, Shelley H **(SLP)**
Freeman, Patty L **(SLP)**
Freidenberg, Carol J **(SLP)**
Friedman, Janice Ruth **(SLP)**
Friedman, Jerome L **(A)**
Fuller, Susan T **(SLP)**
Furnish-Kollman, Mrs Jean **(SLP)**
Galant, Mrs Michelle N **(SLP)**
Gambert, Debby **(SLP)**
Garber, Gerry Beth **(SLP)**
Gardi, Dr John N **(A)**
Geile, Suzann M **(SLP)**
Gennai-Rizzi, Janet L **(SLP)**
Gilbert, Ellen W **(SLP)**
Goldberg, Dr Stanley A **(SLP)**
Golub, Shirley L **(SLP)**
Goodman, Mrs Naomi **(SLP)**
Gottsleben, Robert H **(SLP)**
Graham, Mrs Minnie S **(SLP)**
Grahamjones, Frances **(SLP)**
Green, Robert Baron **(A)**
Grekin, Terry Rosenblatt **(A)**
Grimes, Alison M **(A)**
Hairston, Anne Heinrich **(SLP)**
Hamilton, Mrs Elizabeth V **(A)**
Hanbery, John G **(SLP)**
Harris, Mason Derring **(A)**
Hartman, Mrs Melissa Kay **(SLP)**
Haspiel, Dr George S **(SLP A)**
Hefner, Pamela Sue
Hellinga, Jewel **(SLP)**
Henderson, Alicia Box **(SLP)**
Hendricks, Jennifer Lynn **(SLP)**
Hojem, Leslie Eileen **(A)**
Hopkins, Judith Anne **(SLP)**
Hue, Mrs Eva M **(SLP)**
Jason, Henry C, Jr **(SLP)**
Jones, Lucille W **(SLP)**
Jordan, Vesper Quarti **(SLP)**
Kalbfleisch, Kathleen E **(A)**
Kamaka, Mrs Anita Riebeling **(SLP)**
Kaplan, Joel J **(SLP)**
Kaufmann, Tiphanie J **(SLP)**
Keatinge, Connie **(SLP)**
Kennedy, Josephine **(SLP)**
King, Mrs Jillian Suzanne **(SLP)**
King, Karolyn Louise **(SLP)**
Kleid, Terry Lynne **(SLP)**
Kopay, Kathleen **(A)**
Kraemer, Maxine G **(SLP)**
Langman, Iris **(A)**
Loumbas, Dean George **(SLP)**
Lusk, Elise Bernadette **(SLP)**
Madory, Robert David **(A)**
Manning, Mary E **(SLP)**
Matonak, Kathy Elaine **(A)**
McClendon, Marian E **(SLP)**
McKeown, Maureen **(SLP)**
McMahon, Mrs Kelly Ann **(SLP)**
Meyerson, Dr Marion D **(SLP A)**
Michaels, Meredith G **(SLP)**
Michels, Mrs Sonia L H **(SLP)**
Miksak, Joseph A **(SLP)**
Miller, Meredith Lee **(SLP)**
Miller, Randi
Molyneaux, Dr Dorothy Munz **(SLP A)**
Moore, Charlotte Marie **(A)**
Moy, Marcia E H **(SLP)**
Mueller, Dr H Gustav **(A)**
Nau, Pamela R **(SLP)**
Nicholson, Mrs Nancy Gregory **(A)**
Nisbet, Mrs Jean Boling **(SLP)**
Novak-Szarek, Mrs Jean M **(SLP)**
Obermann, C Esco **(SLP)**
Oleary, Mrs Roberta M **(SLP)**
Owens, Prof Elmer **(SLP A)**
Palmer, Cheryl B **(SLP)**
Pearse-Storey, Mrs Marla A **(SLP)**
Pena, Elizabeth D **(SLP)**
Pengilly, Kathryn Ann
Pennington, Mrs Valerie Joan **(SLP)**
Peterson-Falzone, Dr Sally J **(SLP)**
Prinz, Dr Philip M **(SLP)**
Rachek, Patricia A **(SLP)**
Rademaker, Mrs Nancy M **(SLP)**
Reddell, Dr Rayford C **(A)**
Reed, Dr Charles G **(SLP)**
Reed, Mrs Jane M **(SLP)**
Richards, Dr Griffith G **(SLP)**
Rockman, Dr Barbara Karp **(SLP)**
Rodriguez, Dr Joyce M **(A)**
Rogers, Gail Karen **(SLP)**
Rolff, Susan B **(SLP)**
Rosenblatt, Mrs Erica W **(SLP)**
Rosson, Grace L **(SLP)**
Rotunno, Rosemarie **(A)**
Rowland, Elizabeth Jane **(SLP)**
Saber, Mrs Diana Powell **(SLP)**
Salamy, Dr Alan
Schmidt, Barbara M **(SLP)**
Schuler, Adriana L **(SLP)**
Schumacher, Walter C **(SLP)**
Schwartz, Anna S **(SLP)**
Seid, Phyllis H **(SLP)**
Shaber, A David **(SLP)**
Shapiro, Lori S
Shelton, Mrs Carole W **(A)**
Shinn, Wanda L **(SLP)**
Shipp, Dr Thomas **(SLP)**
Silverman, Lenore A **(SLP)**
Simon, Dr Helen J **(SLP A)**
Sisk, Michael V **(A)**
Slack, Mrs Mary Beth G **(A)**
Smith, Norma J **(SLP)**
Sopp, Nancy Ruth **(SLP)**
Sorenson, Mrs Danita D **(SLP)**
Spencer, Sara **(SLP)**
Stevenson, Sarah A H **(SLP)**
Strauss, Paul Karel **(SLP A)**
Sturiale, Mrs Madeleine M **(SLP)**
Sussman, Mrs Beryl M **(SLP)**
Sutton, Cheryl Anne **(SLP)**
Sweetow, Dr Robert W **(A)**
Tannenbaum, Melissa Ann **(A)**
Thompson, Cynthia L **(SLP)**
Thompson, Owinda Moss
Toner, Katherine Young **(SLP)**
Trumbo, Mrs Michelle Keenan **(SLP)**
Tseng, Bi-Hwa **(A)**
Turner, Dr Robert Graham **(A)**
Van Atta, Mrs Deborah W **(SLP)**
Venable, Gail P **(SLP)**
Von Boeck, Evonne **(SLP)**
Walker, Margaret E **(SLP)**
Wallenberg, Ellis A, III **(SLP A)**
Wayne, Hollie D **(SLP)**
Wayte, Penelope H **(SLP)**
Webb, Kimberly Lynn **(A)**
Wilson, Mrs Brenda W **(SLP)**
Wilson, Geraldine **(SLP A)**
Wolff, Donald A **(A)**
Wong, Corinne M
Wood, Elizabeth Ann
Woods, Donald G **(SLP)**
Woodweu, Linda P **(SLP)**
Zemel, Jamie I

San Gabriel

Copley, Mrs Marilyn J **(SLP)**
Cottier, Cynthia A **(SLP)**
Figueroa, Lorraine **(SLP)**
Gaman, Marthelma Catherine **(SLP)**
Hjelte, Mrs Phyllis P **(SLP)**
Hopkins, Gayle L **(SLP)**
Kappe, Mrs Terry Highstreet **(SLP)**
Lautz, John R, II **(A)**
Malakoff, Iris Mae **(SLP)**

San Jose

Allen, Mrs Lois N **(SLP)**
Antonucci, Mrs Lorraine D **(SLP)**
Arambula, Gustavo Guerrero **(SLP)**
Bauquier, Oliver W **(SLP)**
Bird, Marilyn R **(SLP)**
Breakey, Lisa K **(SLP)**
Brouwers, Simone Elisabeth **(SLP)**
Brown, Georgia C **(SLP)**
Buck, Mrs Beverly Douglas **(SLP)**
Burchfiel, Michele F **(SLP)**
Burgei, Thomas J **(SLP)**
Burns, Deborah H **(SLP)**
Butler, Lori Lee
Campbell, Carola R **(SLP)**
Capano, Dr Richard F **(A)**
Carpenter, Gaye H **(SLP)**
Castillo, Kathleen Ann **(SLP)**
Ceballos, Patricia Ann **(SLP)**
Chandler, Jill S **(SLP)**
Childress, Marian M S **(SLP)**
Christman, Mary Ann **(SLP)**
Crowe, Cheryl A **(SLP)**
Day, Mrs Susan M B **(SLP)**
Dickinson, Mrs Muriel E **(SLP)**
Didech, Marleen S **(SLP)**
Diederich, Nancy Ann **(SLP)**
Dietrich, Mrs Jill Molock **(SLP)**
Eccleston, Vincent **(SLP)**
Elash, Mrs Eletah Paula **(SLP)**
Elggren, Barbara Lorille
Enns, Mrs Joan Y **(SLP)**
Fadness, Mrs Aiko Ruth **(SLP)**
Fallico, Peter G **(SLP)**
Fariss, Mrs Marcia K **(A)**
Farmer, Dr Alvirda **(SLP)**
Felmus, Mrs Veta R **(SLP)**
Ferrito, Joseph R **(A)**
Fowler, Mrs Martha J **(SLP)**
Francia, Leonette J **(SLP)**
Galvan, Minerva M **(SLP)**
Gericke, Marian Baldacchino **(SLP)**
Gibson, Linda Lou **(SLP)**
Gitin, David L **(SLP)**
Gitin, Eileen B **(SLP)**
Good, Alison Mary **(SLP)**
Grossman, Mrs Linda S **(SLP)**
Grossman, Ronald A **(SLP)**
Grupp, Patricia B **(A)**
Gusdorf, Mrs Katherine V **(SLP)**
Harding, Mrs Mary Jane **(SLP)**
Henoch, Dr Miriam A **(A)**
Heydon, Linda Joy **(SLP)**
Hing, Julie Diana **(SLP)**
Hollibaugh, Mrs Jennifer Susan **(SLP)**
Homan, Deborah Ann **(A)**
Horrocks, Barbara L **(SLP)**
Iwamoto, Karen Chizuko **(SLP)**
Johnson, Mrs Marilyn Spears **(SLP)**
Jones, Mary Ellen Therese **(SLP)**
Judd, Rebecca Muhleka **(SLP)**
Keesling, Julie Tate **(A)**
Kiel, Carol Ann **(SLP)**
Kirkpatrick, Lorie Lyn **(SLP)**
Kovarik, Anne M **(SLP)**
Krumm, Laurence Charles **(SLP)**
Krupit, Mrs Felicia Mindy
Landis, Marcia H **(SLP)**
Laraway, Lee Ann **(SLP)**
Lindberg, Mrs Jodie Ann **(SLP)**
London, Mrs Sylvia Claire **(SLP)**
Looper, Callie A **(SLP)**

Lopopolo, Mrs Theresa J **(SLP)**
Louis-Dodson, Dr Patricia Jo **(SLP)**
Malavey, Mohan Rao **(A)**
Mazzeo, Larry Paul
McCarthy, Mrs Mary **(SLP)**
McCullough, Dr June Antablin **(A)**
McDermid, Mrs Susan Renee **(SLP)**
McInnes, Mrs Vera K
Meredith, Rebecca Lynn **(A)**
Michael, Liane E **(SLP)**
Mize, Christina Joyce **(SLP)**
Montgomery, Patricia B **(A)**
Montilla, Florence Mary G **(SLP)**
Moore, Dr Carmen E **(SLP)**
Moore, James E **(SLP)**
Morejohn, Linda Celeste **(SLP)**
Nellany, Kim Ann
Nichols-Klocke, M Sue **(SLP)**
Nightengale, Mary Finan **(SLP)**
Nishikawa, Mrs Dianne Haruye **(SLP)**
Nordheim, Mrs Lee T **(SLP)**
Notor, Nancy Schell **(A)**
Ostrowski, Audrey A **(SLP)**
Pearson, Mrs Patricia Hanrahan
Pinelli, Mrs Pamela Sears **(SLP)**
Potts, Maryann Wenner **(SLP)**
Rasmussen, Louise A **(SLP)**
Ray, Mrs Kristin Elaine **(SLP)**
Reinis, Belinda Jane **(SLP)**
Roach, Virginia A **(SLP)**
Roberts, Barbara Ann **(SLP)**
Rouse, Mrs Radyne P
Rowan, Mrs Cynthia Lee **(SLP)**
Savage, M Martha **(SLP)**
Schnabel, Mary Frances
Semans, Susan L **(SLP)**
Shank, Julie E **(SLP)**
Smith-Ray, Brenda J **(SLP)**
Snyder, Gayle P **(SLP)**
Snyder, Janet Kaye F **(A)**
Sousa, Veronica M **(SLP)**
Springer, Clare S **(SLP)**
Sterner, Teri Lee **(SLP)**
Stuart, Carole Levinson **(SLP)**
Tooker, Patricia Ann **(SLP)**
Totter, Dr Joseph J **(SLP)**
Triscik, Bette **(SLP)**
Troquato, Mrs Aileen Murphy
Tykol, Judy Mauterer **(SLP)**
Ulery, Beverly Ann **(SLP)**
Veder, Dr Robert A **(A)**
Wells-Walberg, Judith Christine **(SLP)**
Werner, Renee A
Wigton-Feetham, Mrs Lauri E **(SLP)**
Wilkerson, Janet Ellen **(SLP)**
Yamauchi, Mrs Elinor Kim **(SLP)**
Zurovski, Janet M L **(A)**

San Juan Capistrano

Bouck, Joanne King **(SLP)**
Brunell-Nelson, Mrs Sheyla Loren **(SLP)**
Ferris, Mrs Linda M **(SLP)**
Hart, Holly Dixon **(SLP)**
Johnson, Mrs Cynthia Kelley **(SLP)**

San Leandro

Barranti, Mary F **(SLP)**
Clark, Ann L **(SLP)**
Dvorsky, Mrs Isobel G **(SLP)**
Jove-D'Amato, Martha **(A)**
Killeen, Denise M **(SLP)**
Saunders, Mrs Deborah Lynn **(SLP)**
Todebush, Martha J **(A)**
Trauba, Jane A **(A)**
Wernecke, Candace **(SLP)**

San Lorenzo

Hill, Lyman M **(SLP)**
Wong, Mrs Susan A Fong **(SLP)**

San Luis Obispo

Bernhardt, Mrs Ann S **(SLP)**
Frady, Dr Lynn **(SLP)**
Genereux, Mrs Kay Swanson **(SLP)**
Johnstone, Patti Michele **(SLP)**
Kent, William C **(SLP)**
Lindamood, Patricia Conway **(SLP)**
Luckett, Catherine **(SLP)**
McElhinney, Dana **(SLP)**
McQuade, Rosalyn F **(SLP)**
Palmquist, Cheryl Louise **(SLP)**
Peters, Jane Marie **(SLP)**
Ramirez, Jennifer Thompson **(SLP)**
Scarry-Larkin, Marna Kathryn **(SLP)**
Sena, Nancy **(SLP)**
Shirar, Lynda C
Wong, Mrs Virginia Young **(SLP)**
Wright, Mrs Joyce H **(SLP)**

San Marcos

Burgeson, Marilee Burnett **(SLP)**
Campbell, Kay **(SLP)**
Lasswell, Mrs Carolyn Jean **(SLP)**
Pastore, Marc **(SLP)**

San Marino

Katz, Francine H **(SLP)**
Seligman, Darlene **(SLP)**
Smith, Patricia H **(SLP)**
Sutherland, LaVerne Deel **(SLP)**
Taylor, Dr Margaret F **(SLP)**
Waldo, Mrs Judith M **(SLP)**

San Mateo

Brekke, Jody Ann **(A)**
Calavano, Mrs Joycelyn R **(SLP A)**
Cohen, Mrs Carol Berman **(SLP)**
Field, Elizabeth McCracken **(SLP)**
Fowler, Mary M **(SLP)**
Frazzini, Mrs Karen A **(SLP)**
Golden, Ellen Nan
Jaye, Robin Lynne **(SLP)**
Klinger, Mrs Deborah S **(SLP)**
Krasow, Mrs Dyane Schrager **(SLP)**
Lampert, Jeffrey J **(A)**
Low, Patricia **(SLP)**
Macey, Mrs Esther B **(SLP)**
Matthes, Mrs Paula K **(SLP)**
McConnell, Nancy L **(SLP)**
Peck, Jillian B **(SLP)**
Price, Mrs Barbara J **(SLP)**
Rodriguez, Mrs Carroll Jane
Skinner, Elaine **(A)**
Stitt, Dr Clyde L **(SLP)**
Takahashi, Mrs Candace L **(SLP)**
Telleen, Mrs Christine **(A)**
Thomas, Barbara Cassidy **(SLP)**
Weiglin, Mrs Jeanne T **(SLP)**
Woodley, Tricia Evans **(SLP)**

San Pablo

Leverenz, A Florence **(SLP)**
Nordahl-Aldape, Carol A

San Pedro

Avriett, Mrs Paula Hayes
Canetti, Mrs Marianne **(SLP)**
Flaherty, Mrs Carol **(SLP)**
Kopilow, Ellen D **(SLP)**
Newcomb, Mrs Kathy A **(A)**
Rill, Kathryn Elizabeth **(SLP)**
Schott, Marcella K **(SLP)**
Valarezo, Mrs Toni Thompson **(A)**
Ward, Mrs Elisabeth **(SLP)**
Wells, Betsy G
Winkowski, Teresa Banta **(SLP)**

San Rafael

Bingea, Rebecca L **(A)**
Blum, Arthur M **(SLP)**
Bott, Mrs Diane E Z **(SLP)**
Bridgewater, Mrs Barbara Gilford **(SLP)**
Danjelic, Erica **(SLP)**
Engel, Mrs Karen **(SLP)**
Gordon, Mrs Sharon A **(SLP)**
Green, Maureen Raedy **(SLP)**
Jensen, Susan K **(SLP)**
Jones, Mrs Marny S **(SLP)**
Keenan, Laura Jean **(SLP)**
Kurtz, Paula Marie Zanker **(SLP)**
Lithgow, Joan Ann **(SLP)**
McGinnis, Maxine S **(A)**
Mery, Dr Barbara D **(SLP A)**
Rollin, Dr Walter J **(SLP)**
Zurl-O'Day, Mrs Linda Mary

San Ramon

Ashford, Mrs Pamela C **(SLP)**
Austin, Jill M **(SLP)**
Berris, Anastasia
Buckles, Krista M **(A)**
Hardy, Richard D **(SLP)**
Huff, Mrs Janet Lee **(SLP)**
Jansen, Cindy Larson **(SLP)**
Kaye, Jennifer E **(SLP)**
Man, Hilda **(SLP)**
Mullen, Ann Marie **(A)**
Nicholson-Barcal, Nancy K **(SLP)**
Petersdorf, Susan Hewitt **(SLP)**
Price, Roslyn R **(SLP)**
Swegle, M Valentin **(SLP)**
Swett, Carol Lesher **(SLP)**
White, Christine **(SLP)**

San Ysidro

Choy, Ines

Sanger

Adams, Mrs Janet Olive **(SLP)**
Craycroft, Jessica T **(A)**
Lee, Karen **(SLP)**

Santa Ana

Baker, Richard D **(SLP)**
Bermudez, Mrs Leona Brauns **(SLP)**
Bottorf, Lucinda E **(SLP)**
Colosimo, Mrs Ruth A G **(SLP)**
Conant, Janet Lynn **(A)**
Cone, Martha A **(SLP)**
Delorenzis, Anne M **(SLP)**
DeuPree, Dr Robert M
Edwards, Mrs Patricia S **(SLP)**
Ezra, Mrs Cheryl Diane **(SLP)**
Gavin, Mrs Nancy D **(SLP)**
Herscovitz, Toby Lois **(SLP)**
Jarvis, Ruthann Reis **(SLP)**
Jones-Brown, Mrs Robin Elane **(SLP)**
Kenworthy, Dr O T **(A)**
Kirsch, Laurie Jean **(SLP)**
Kogler, Clare **(SLP)**
Lawrence, Jan J **(SLP)**
Logue, Anne L **(SLP)**
Mandiola, Mrs Claudine Allamand **(SLP)**
Matthews, Mrs Judith L **(A)**
McMicken, Dr Betty Lou **(SLP)**
Meves, Mrs Julia Renee **(SLP)**
Moore, Dr Walter H, Jr **(SLP)**
Perez, Mrs Linda Maurine
Reid, Mrs Janell D **(A)**
Rogers, Stacy Leigh **(A)**
Roice, Mrs Susan E **(SLP)**
Saucier, Mrs Linda Jill **(SLP)**
Schulist, Carol
Sikorski, Lorna D **(SLP)**
Silverman, Mrs Nancy E **(SLP)**
Smith, Donna Marie **(A)**
Swanson, Virginia Lee **(SLP)**
Tettemore, Barbara Lynn **(SLP)**
Wigim, Elizabeth Ann **(SLP)**

Santa Barbara

Ament, Annemarie
Anderson, Ellen K **(SLP)**
Armstrong, Mrs Chandler Loomis **(SLP)**
Beaver, Elizabeth **(SLP)**
Berns, Donna B **(SLP)**
Burleigh, Sally **(SLP)**
Camarata, Dr Stephen M **(SLP)**
Cole, Susan Jeanette **(SLP)**
Cubert, Mrs Catherine L **(A)**
Czuleger, Mrs Collette Moulton **(SLP)**
Danhauer, Dr Jeffrey L **(A)**
Dean, Kathryn N **(SLP)**
Dibartolomeo, Dr Joseph R
Ellis, Maxine **(A)**
Gerber, Dr Sanford E **(SLP A)**
Gilchrist, Diane B **(SLP)**
Gillette, Barbara B **(SLP)**
Gostow, Terry Lynn **(SLP)**
Greenbaum, Rochelle I **(SLP)**
Gulje, Mrs Kathleen K **(SLP)**
Haines, Harold H **(SLP)**
Hanley, Dr Theodore D **(SLP)**
Hartzman, Deborah Dosick **(A)**
Hill, Edith M **(SLP)**
Hollander, Mrs Ruth E H **(SLP)**
Ingham, Dr Janis Costello **(SLP)**
Ingham, Dr Roger J
Ingram, Maria M **(SLP)**
Jackson, Roberta E **(SLP)**
Jackson, Theresa L **(SLP)**
Joachim, Mrs Pamela Christlieb **(SLP)**
Johnson, Mrs Christine Smith **(A)**
Keeney, Linda E **(SLP)**
Kirkpatrick, Mrs Diane Yvonne **(SLP)**
Kiselewich, Mrs Anne S **(SLP)**
Koegel, Lynn Kern **(SLP)**
Lewis, Mary Anne **(SLP)**
Lynaugh, Mae A **(SLP)**
Mamolen, Eleanor G **(SLP)**
Mannon, Janice Evelyn **(SLP)**
McGann, William Morris **(SLP)**
Mentis, Michelle **(SLP)**
Moskovitz, Laurie Jane **(SLP)**
Palmer, Carole C **(SLP)**
Prutting, Carol Ann **(SLP)**
Ratliff, Janis Lynn **(SLP)**
Riffle, Paige A **(SLP)**
Ronneberg, Mrs Gail V **(SLP)**
Stuman, Lillian Yvonne **(SLP)**
Thompson, Geraldine Gray **(SLP)**
Uyesaka, Mrs Linda S L **(SLP)**
Vincent, Vernon Lee **(A)**
Wilcox, Sharon K **(SLP)**

Santa Clara

Bruner, Mrs Marianne **(SLP)**
Carmack, Mrs Brooke Alene **(A)**
Hutchinson, Julie Irene **(SLP)**
Hutto, Brenda **(SLP)**
Johnston, Virginia J **(SLP)**
Maiani, Mrs Rhonda Jeannette **(SLP)**
Musko, Sally E S **(A)**
Orgera-Mandey, Rena A **(SLP)**
Osada, Diane G **(A)**
Spurlock, Shelley Lynn **(SLP)**
Stovall, Susan Marie **(SLP)**

Santa Cruz

Bell, Deborah A **(SLP)**
Beveridge, Susan Eileen **(SLP)**
Bowden, Pamela S **(SLP)**
Dragavon, Paul **(SLP)**
Ehritt, Donelle **(A)**
Eldridge, Sandra J **(SLP)**
Felton-Sheldon, Mrs Melody **(SLP)**
Fuller, Paula T **(SLP)**
Galt, Cynthia F **(SLP)**
Jackson, Jean Marie **(SLP)**
Kamian, Colette Alice **(SLP)**
Kinney-White, Dr Barbara A **(SLP)**
Krieger, Mrs Judith **(SLP)**
Lang, Dr Janna Smith **(A)**
Linzer, Deborah R **(SLP)**
Mathewson, Peggy A **(SLP)**
McIvers, Janice **(SLP)**
Morrison, Claire V **(A)**
Nahin, Melinda J **(SLP)**
Nakanishi, Laurel Ann **(SLP)**
Pierini, Sr M Paul Francis **(SLP)**
Rockoff, Carrie Ellen **(SLP)**
Stagnaro, Mrs Phyllis C **(SLP)**
Torp, Marilyn **(SLP)**
Undem, April Lee
Walker, Karen Elaine **(SLP)**
Wood, Barbara G **(SLP)**

Santa Maria
Bertoldi, Janet Thayer **(SLP)**
Crandall, James R **(SLP)**
Lara, Cynthia **(SLP)**
Leo, Victoria Ireland **(SLP)**
Mayfield, Norman K **(A)**
Scott, Karen M **(SLP A)**
Simon, Vicki Jean **(SLP)**
Taylor, April Jean **(SLP)**
Thompson, Linda D **(SLP)**
Vanier-Garcia, Jeannine M **(SLP)**

Santa Monica
Arnold, Peggy Lee **(SLP)**
Bensussen, Jane O **(SLP)**
Berman, Bonnie **(SLP)**
Blatt, Mrs Susan R **(SLP)**
Bost, Sheila P **(SLP)**
Brown, Mrs Helen E D **(SLP)**
Butler, Karen L **(SLP)**
D'Asaro, Dr Michael J **(SLP)**
Davidow, Mrs Diana Sue **(SLP)**
Di Santo, Susan M **(SLP)**
Francis, Catherine Moacanin **(SLP)**
Freiman, Susan **(SLP)**
Galin, Susan Joy **(SLP)**
Gilder-Sloane, Lorie E **(SLP)**
Griffith, Patricia M **(SLP)**
Haim, Saralyn Polon **(SLP)**
Heller, Naomi C **(SLP)**
Hellman, Mrs Hilary **(SLP)**
Hermann, Nancy T **(SLP)**
Jacobs, Dr Teri G **(SLP)**
Jessup, Georgia L **(SLP)**
Karz, Mrs Lynn Anita **(SLP)**
Katzman, Mrs Jeanne **(SLP)**
Kerns, Pamela A **(SLP)**
Kidd, Margaret L **(SLP)**
Kolda, Sr Felice Marie **(A)**
Kondra, Jeanne Smith **(SLP)**
Kurtzer, Denise Wynne **(SLP)**
Lansky, Pamela Stewart **(SLP)**
Lessac, Prof Arthur **(SLP)**
Likens, Barbara A
Lomonaco, Mrs Beatrice Joros **(SLP)**
Manassero, Robynn **(SLP)**
May, Dr Annette Anisman **(SLP)**
Milgrom, Patricia Mondro **(SLP)**
Miller, Robin P **(SLP)**
Milton, Sandra B **(SLP)**
Neumeier, Marianne **(SLP)**
Paulson, Mrs Janet Elizabeth **(SLP)**
Punt, Mrs Ruth B **(SLP)**
Ross, Harriet Pearlston **(SLP)**
Sharp, Deena S **(SLP)**
Sheehan, Vivian Mowat **(SLP)**
Stanley, Mrs Sue L **(SLP)**
Terran, Eileen M **(SLP)**
Tukey, Laura Kapp **(SLP)**
Ungar, Christophe David **(SLP)**
Weston, Stephanie **(A)**

Santa Paula
Banks, Mrs Carolyn G **(SLP)**
Linn, Dr George B **(SLP)**

Santa Rosa
Agee-Burton, Debra Lynn **(SLP)**
Anderson, Karen Alanna **(SLP)**
Bencivenga, Anthony J **(A)**
Casper, Judy R **(SLP)**
Conway, Mrs Jane Parker **(SLP)**
Davis, Dianne Lynn **(SLP)**
Flanary, Heather Molly **(SLP)**
Fletcher, Mrs Margaret I **(SLP A)**
Harris, Jeffrey Paul **(SLP)**
Hiatt, Anne Louise **(SLP)**
Huhn, Mrs Kathleen L **(SLP)**
Hutchinson, Barbara J **(SLP)**
Leaf, Antony **(SLP)**
Lehrer, Mrs Carol M **(SLP)**
Lord, Mrs Joan Cashin **(SLP)**
Marcopulos, E Gail **(A)**
Marincovich, Dr Peter J **(A)**
Mattern, Ann Louise **(SLP)**
McManus, Penny E
Oliver-Hurt, Susan Kay **(A)**
Rodman, Melissa
Ross, Mrs Deborah G **(SLP)**
Samples, Dianne L **(SLP)**
Samples, Dr John Mar **(SLP)**
Schwab, Ingrid Ursula **(SLP)**
Skillicorn, Patricia Lynn **(SLP)**
Slager, Sara **(SLP)**
Snavely, Jan Allyson **(SLP)**
Sorensen, Eugenia R **(A)**
Stemach, Gerald J **(SLP)**
Thompson, Mrs Donna Marie **(SLP)**
Thompson, Mrs Sarah S **(SLP)**
Thompson, Virginia M **(SLP)**

Santa Ynez
Boisen, Mrs Sandra K **(SLP)**
Porter, Wyne W **(SLP A)**

Santee
Amundsen, Joanne E **(SLP)**
Daniel, Mrs Julie Ann
Moroney, Donna Patrice **(A)**
Summy, Mrs Barbara Ann **(SLP)**

Saratoga
Boardman, Laura Jo **(SLP)**
Dinucci, Linda Miller **(SLP)**
Ehlers, Mrs Michele M **(SLP)**
Havard, Joan L **(A)**
Mastman, Mrs Ellen Sue **(A)**
Murphy, Beverly S **(A)**
Smith, Mrs Elizabeth Mary **(SLP)**
West, Suzanne Marie **(SLP)**

Saugus
Hartmann-Kott, Catherine Marie **(SLP)**
Koutstaal, Dr Cornelis W **(SLP A)**

Sausalito
O'Donnell, Mrs Cynthia **(SLP)**

Scotts Valley
Evans, Mrs Dianne Harvey **(SLP)**
Frandle, Kathy Jo **(SLP)**
MacLaren, Jeanne E **(SLP)**

Seal Beach
Carin, Sandy **(SLP)**
Chattler, Mrs Lisa Kalisher **(SLP)**
Donoghue, Kathleen Anne **(SLP)**
Dunan-Vittori, Leslie Richmond **(SLP)**
Himes, Mrs Barbara Endle **(A)**
Jax, Dr Vicki A **(SLP)**
Klein, Ellen S **(SLP)**
Klisanin, Mrs Joan **(SLP)**
McKeown, Mrs Milfred R **(SLP)**
Morrison, Margaret **(SLP)**
Palaski, Mrs Dorothy **(SLP)**
Wilcox, Edna B **(SLP)**
Wright, Mrs Kathleen T **(SLP)**

Seaside
Davis, Mrs Shirley C **(SLP)**
Saleh, Michele J **(SLP)**

Sebastopol
Agnello, Virginia L **(SLP)**
Bisbee, Julie Kathleen **(SLP)**
McGinty, Patricia Josephine **(SLP)**
Potts, Mrs Linda A N
Takagi, Mrs June K **(SLP)**

Selma
Katayama, Kerri Misao **(SLP)**
Neufer, Mrs Susan L **(SLP)**

Sepulveda
Becker, Mark M **(A)**
Birmingham, Mrs Ingrid B **(SLP)**
Boschma, Mrs Wendy R F **(SLP)**
Hurvitz, Joel A **(A)**
Kamber, Mrs Beverly F **(SLP)**
Nusser, Mrs Michele J **(SLP)**
Reeves, Mrs Marilyn Ziton
Vogt, Dr Eugenia F **(SLP)**
Waterstone, Mrs Judith B **(SLP)**
Waterstone, Stuart I **(SLP)**

Shasta
Casey, Moira H **(SLP)**

Sherman Oaks
Bennett-Briscoe, Edna A **(SLP)**
Bezonsky, Deborah A **(SLP)**
Bildner, Betty R **(SLP)**
Bizoza, Bonnie H **(SLP)**
Bloom, Lucy
Brainin, Mrs Blanche M **(SLP)**
Brock, Mrs Gaby **(SLP)**
Cohen, Siri Ilene **(SLP)**
Coulter, Jody Katt **(SLP)**
David, Lisa K **(SLP)**
Dickter, Mrs Farryl Suplin **(SLP)**
Eckberg MD, Dr Theodore J
Eskwitt, Dr Donna L **(A)**
Fils, Mrs Deborah J **(A)**
Giammarino, Denise Vega **(SLP)**
Goldman, Sheila Ochs **(SLP)**
Grant, Susan V **(SLP)**
Hull, Mrs Ruth Elmore **(SLP)**
Johnson, Dr E W **(A)**
Keer, Mrs Francine E **(SLP)**
Larson, Leslie A **(SLP)**
Leffler, Pamela **(SLP)**
Manzella, Dr Diane S **(SLP A)**
McKitrick, Edward F **(SLP)**
McNary, Doris
Melcon, Melinda A **(SLP)**
Miller, Susan Lynn **(SLP)**
Norris, Wendy Elaine **(SLP)**
Plaisance, Cynthia L **(SLP)**
Rabin-Posner, Mrs Debra Sue **(SLP)**
Rafkind, Mrs Shirley M **(SLP)**
Robbin, Barbara Lee **(SLP)**
Sabah, Mrs Debra Brim **(A)**
Salisbury, Joan L **(SLP)**
Schaeffer, Kathleen **(SLP A)**
Semow, Shirley P **(SLP)**
Seymour, Patricia Jean-Anne **(SLP)**
Umen, Ilene A **(SLP)**
Valcarenghi, Tina **(SLP)**
Wade, Helen Sherman **(SLP)**
Woods, Charline Joan **(SLP)**

Shingle Springs
Costello, Mrs Jean F O **(SLP)**
Kimzey, Mary Whitfield **(SLP)**
Storrs, Jack L **(SLP)**

Sierra Madre
Braff, Dr Reba G **(SLP)**
McClurg, Lisa B **(A)**
Sharp, Karen Link **(SLP)**
Trounson, Marilynn B **(SLP)**
Van Duivenbode, Laurie Ann **(A)**

Signal Hill
Edwards, Marilyn J **(SLP)**
Fortine, Yvonne Marie **(SLP)**
Grant, Felene F **(SLP)**
Huckaby, Geraldine **(SLP)**
Schiffmacher, Pamela W **(SLP)**
Tatoul, Corinne M **(SLP)**

Simi Valley
Battle, Marie Josephine **(SLP)**
Daitch, Wendy L **(SLP)**
Fiala, Louise Ann
Frank, Leslie H **(SLP)**
Hall, Dr Edward Pierce **(SLP A)**
Johnson, Mrs Denise Loy **(SLP)**
Kruse, Mrs Lisa Polino **(SLP)**
Lambden, Kristi Ann
Leslie, T Anne Harris **(SLP)**
Namson, Mrs Sandra Kohn **(SLP)**
Pizzano, Theresa Marie **(SLP)**
Ruditsky, Sherry Lynn **(SLP)**
Seldin, Lila Bergman **(SLP)**
Shaban, Helen **(A)**
Visser-Dumont, Leslie Jean **(A)**
Wendt, Mrs Deborah Cook **(SLP)**
West, Dr Terri Louise **(SLP)**
Wolgat, Mrs Loretta **(SLP)**

Solana Beach
Andre, Janice J **(SLP)**
George, Mrs Priscilla Hayfield **(A)**
Irwin, Mrs Dina Minish **(SLP)**
Johnson, Roxanna M **(SLP)**
MacKenzie-Laxague, Judy L **(SLP)**
Surch, Patricia Joyce **(SLP)**

Solvang
Franklin, Leslie Mason **(SLP)**
Grant, Mrs Deborah Lee **(SLP)**
Homyack, Mrs Elizabeth Baysa **(SLP)**
Valdez, Geneva Nellie **(SLP)**

Somis
Cartwright, Cathrine **(SLP)**

Sonoma
Cobb, Leslie Louise **(SLP)**
Lang, Mrs Linda J **(SLP)**
Marshall, Mrs Bonnie B **(SLP)**
Presley, Karen June **(SLP)**
Ruebush-Gonzales, Lynn N **(SLP)**
Southard, Susan D **(SLP)**
Southard, William Michael **(A)**
Spencer, Raymond E **(A)**
Wright, Lorna L **(A)**

Sonora
Dunbar, Jessica Ann
Haverstock, Mrs Linda C **(SLP)**
Paxton, Mrs Alice H **(SLP)**

Soquel
Kelly, Paula E **(SLP)**
Kessinger, Jacque L **(SLP)**
Kirkland, Wendy Rita **(SLP)**

South El Monte
Martinez, Catherine Rose **(SLP)**

South Gate
McGlothlin, Beth A

South Laguna
Holmer, Janice A **(SLP)**
Lukoff, Mrs Linda G **(SLP)**

South Lake Tahoe
Schaefer, Lynn A **(SLP)**
Swain, Mrs Robin H **(SLP)**

South Pasadena
Barrows, Jane Deringer
Borgatti, Mrs Juliana Zimmer **(SLP)**
Bright, Janice L **(SLP)**
Endo, Janet K **(A)**
Fishel, Anne Marlene **(SLP)**
Rohr, Mrs Elaine H **(SLP)**
Schwieder, Jane **(SLP)**
Scott, Rosemary **(SLP)**
Stratton, Constance Cutter **(SLP)**
Tarnow, Janet Elaine **(SLP)**
Welch, Donal M
Zuleski, Kathleen Elizabeth **(SLP)**

South San Francisco
Sack, Dr Leo P **(SLP)**
Waxman, Mrs Jeanne H **(SLP)**

South San Gabriel
Matsumoto, Mrs Lillian S **(SLP)**

Spreckels
Madsen, Betsy **(SLP)**

Spring Valley
Buteau, Mrs Carol Liddiard **(SLP)**
Farrell, Lesley A **(SLP)**
Heiser, Margaret **(SLP)**
Honea, Mrs Marilyn Jean **(SLP)**
Keating, Mrs Carol Ann **(SLP)**
Luse, Dr Eleanor M **(SLP)**

Nelson, Mrs Barbara L **(SLP)**
Nelson, Mrs Eudora P **(SLP)**
Nelson, Dr Robert G **(SLP A)**
Smith, Patricia E **(SLP)**

Squaw Valley

Sandness, Serena Marie **(SLP)**

St Helena

Bishop, Thomas Everett **(SLP)**
Green, Carol J **(SLP)**
Minifie, Mrs Ferne **(SLP)**

Stanford

Ciaranello, Mrs Nancy J R **(SLP A)**
Eisenson, Dr Jon **(SLP)**
Haggerty, Holly Susan
McBeath, Karen Haymond **(SLP)**
Winzelberg, Jody **(A)**

Stanton

Warden, Mrs Mary Diane **(SLP)**

Stinson Beach

Orton, Clodagh **(A)**

Stockton

Abbott, Mrs Christine Malone **(SLP)**
Adams, Mrs Nancy Engel **(SLP)**
Arsanis, David J **(SLP)**
Aspiras, Rose Angela
Beeson-Holmes, Melissa **(SLP)**
Brodie, Gail R **(SLP)**
Carlson, Bertha K **(SLP)**
Davis, Deborah **(SLP)**
Davis-Drake, Mrs Lisa J **(SLP)**
Doyle, Mrs Harriett E **(SLP)**
Eakes-Frush, Mrs Wendy E **(SLP)**
Flentge, Mrs Margaret Louise **(SLP)**
Fogle, Paul T **(SLP)**
Friedman, Lawrence J **(SLP)**
Gerlach, Janelle **(SLP)**
Hanyak, Robert E **(A)**
Heine, Marilyn K **(SLP)**
Hirota, Carol S **(SLP)**
Hue Gunawan, Marcia Denise **(SLP)**
Johnson, Thomas R **(SLP)**
Judson, Mrs Dee Anne Barker
Kidwell, Mrs Susan Marie **(SLP)**
Kroese, Judith M G **(SLP)**
Laverty-Reves, Robin M **(SLP)**
Nimtz, Mrs Janet Marie **(SLP)**
Okawachi, Pearl K **(SLP)**
Omiya, Grace Michiyo **(SLP)**
Ortize, Nancy M **(SLP)**
Otis, Lindsay Ann **(SLP)**
Otte, Mrs Catherine Ann **(SLP)**
Polk, Katherine Elaine **(SLP)**
Puich, Virginia L **(SLP)**
Rathhaus, Mrs Coralita **(SLP)**
Reed, Susanne **(SLP)**
Reed-Musto, Mrs Barbara
Royer, Patricia A **(SLP)**
Schmitt-Chan, Mrs Christine **(SLP)**
Serventi, Edwina R **(SLP)**
Skeels, Kathleen Fujinaka **(SLP)**
Smith, Denise Marie **(SLP)**
Smith, Simalee Carol **(SLP)**
Spencer, Mrs Nancy Bolton **(SLP)**
Standley, Mrs Christine A **(SLP)**
Tegtmeier, Diana Armbruster **(SLP)**
Tempel, Edward O **(SLP)**
Timmons, Dr Roy J **(SLP)**
Tsappis, Anthony **(A)**
Ulmer, Mrs Sue C **(SLP)**
Van Bebber, Sally J **(SLP)**
Vander Veen, Mrs Daphnne Moore **(SLP)**
Vincent, Lisa Ellen **(SLP)**
Watanabe, Noriko C **(SLP)**
Williams, Mrs Noreen Marie **(SLP)**
Wood, Mrs Mary Helen **(SLP)**
Yagi-Doi, Mrs Lori Ann Misa **(SLP)**

Studio City

Greenstate, Mrs Judith Willens **(SLP)**
Gutowicz, Barbara **(SLP)**
Levatter, Theodore D **(SLP)**
Lewis, Susan Myra
Ross, Gail **(SLP)**
Taylor, Carole A **(SLP)**
Waisman, Mrs Georgette B **(SLP)**

Summerland

McCall, Mrs Laurie Elizabeth **(SLP)**

Sun Valley

Abel, Joseph H, Jr **(SLP)**
Tomanelli, Angie Marie **(SLP)**

Sunland

Tarnawski, Julia K T **(SLP)**

Sunnyvale

Ball-Kimball, Pamela L **(A)**
Bautch-Daniels, Doreen A **(SLP)**
Cato, Patricia Elizabeth **(A)**
Christensen, Mrs Connie Kay
Clark, Marion B **(SLP)**
Doane, Michele E **(SLP)**
Goodreau, May Hoefling **(SLP)**
Graham, Mrs Laurie I **(SLP)**
Gray, Mrs Beverly K **(SLP)**
Hartz, Mrs Julie Diane **(A)**
Heller, Lisa Lethin **(SLP)**
Higgins, Janice Logg **(SLP)**
Kamitses, Kim L **(SLP)**
Kashinsky, Mrs Eileen D **(SLP)**
McEwen, Susan K **(SLP)**
Melamid, Juliet A **(SLP)**
Niizawa, Judy J **(SLP)**
Pettygrove, Laura Ann **(SLP)**
Plevin, Francine S **(SLP)**
Robinson, Gayle R **(SLP)**
Shatz, Mrs Phyllis Goldstein **(SLP)**
Steel, Mrs Kelly N **(SLP)**
Tobias, Mrs Kathleen C **(SLP)**
Wendschlag, Mrs Sandra Jean **(A)**

Sunset Beach

Culibrk, Janine **(SLP)**

Susanville

Fleckenstein, Mrs Julie Jeanette **(SLP)**

Sylmar

Baer-Forman, Mrs Mary Ann **(SLP)**
Casper, Marilyn E **(SLP)**
Cooper, Mrs Shirley A **(SLP)**
Polk, Teresa C **(SLP)**

Tarzana

Alpert, Fay Ellen **(SLP)**
Canter, Janet C C **(SLP)**
Feinberg, Evelyn Maj **(SLP)**
Gordon, Linda L **(SLP)**
Harris, Mrs Ruth L **(SLP)**
Haus, Gilda K **(SLP)**
Johnston, Laura Assante
Kissel, Robert J **(SLP)**
Norton, Norma Bain **(SLP A)**
Nyman, Mrs Peggy Graham **(SLP)**
Offsay, Mrs Pamela S **(SLP)**
Weiss, Susan Eileen **(SLP)**

Tehachapi

McPheeters, Deborah H **(SLP)**

Temecula

Johnson, Erin Michelle **(SLP)**
Mark, Kathy Jane **(SLP)**
Phelps, Mrs Cathen H **(SLP)**
Saline, Jerry W **(A)**
Thomson, Jean E **(SLP)**

Temple City

Benedict, Kathleen Whalen **(SLP)**
Canar, Nelly Teresa **(SLP)**
Cuffia, Mrs Deborah Anne **(SLP)**
Florensa, Montse **(SLP)**
Sporleder, Jeannie A **(SLP)**

Templeton

Porter, James F **(SLP)**

Thousand Oaks

Abrahams, Mrs Karen Joy **(SLP)**
Adriansen, Therese J **(SLP)**
Auer, Karla M **(SLP)**
Baker, Mrs Pattie W **(SLP)**
Bannon, Kelley Ann **(A)**
Broesamle, Mrs Katharine Sue **(SLP)**
Burns, Mrs Lisa Anne **(SLP)**
Carr, Mrs Camille Slavin **(SLP)**
Driggs, Phyllis T **(SLP)**
Frank, Arthur **(SLP)**
Hurst, Maria Antonietta **(SLP)**
Jarett, Mrs Irene G **(SLP)**
Kimes, Cheryl Jane **(SLP)**
Klein, Patricia K **(SLP)**
Lavorato, Dr Alfred S **(SLP)**
Lazerson-Ross, Mrs Susan Gail **(SLP)**
Long, Mrs Karen V **(SLP)**
Lynn, Mrs Corinne W **(SLP)**
Miech, Mrs Maureen Rose
Miraglia, Jean Ann M **(SLP)**
Shapiro, Mark J **(SLP)**
Sternberg, Mrs Joan Fuertes **(SLP)**
Thompson, Dale R **(SLP)**
Whealon, Mrs Margaret McAdams **(SLP)**
Wherley, Mrs Barbara **(SLP)**
Whitaker, John M **(SLP)**
Ziegler, Brenda K **(A)**

Three Rivers

Gurcinas, Birute J **(SLP)**

Toluca Lake

Barsook-Schwartz, Barbara **(A)**

Torrance

Anthony, Mrs Lea Love **(SLP)**
Auerbach, Sylvia S **(SLP)**
Bellevue, Mrs Dorothy I **(SLP)**
Boyce, Maureen A
Brunson, Nancy M **(SLP)**
Canales, Mrs Betty H **(SLP)**
Cook, Carolee B **(SLP)**
Crowley, Mrs Therese M **(SLP)**
Edgar, Mrs Nancy R **(A)**
Ginsberg, Esther B **(A)**
Head, Mrs Pamela G **(SLP)**
Hill, Mrs Karen L **(SLP)**
Hosier-Holt, Karen Leslie **(SLP)**
Iverson, Sharon A **(SLP)**
Joga, Mrs Regina Vilkas **(SLP)**
Johnston, Maureen M **(SLP)**
Kamdar, Aditi Vijay **(SLP)**
Kastner, Deborah Butler **(SLP)**
Kropf, Mrs T Janet **(SLP)**
Lanna-Farris, Karyn M **(SLP)**
Liles, Barbara H **(SLP)**
Long, Suzanne L **(SLP)**
Mangels, Barbara J **(SLP)**
McCoy, Michael J **(SLP)**
Parker, Dr William L **(A)**
Peirce, Mrs Terrilee **(SLP)**
Pfannenstiel, Mrs Karen Stinson **(SLP)**
Pumphrey, Mrs Debra Lehman **(SLP)**
Renge, Joyce Lynn **(SLP)**
Sahlberg, Richard A **(SLP)**
Savage, Roberta A **(SLP)**
Schenasi, Mrs Carol L **(SLP)**
Stansbury, Mrs Carol Lee **(SLP)**
Stauber, Shoshana **(SLP)**
Takeshita, Ruby Tsugie **(SLP)**
Thompson, Eloise Shepherd **(SLP)**
Torres, Mrs Kristen Kay **(SLP)**
Tucker, Barb A **(SLP)**
Vant Land, Mrs Julie Lynn **(SLP)**
Winter, Nelda H **(SLP)**
Yoshiba-Medeiros, Christine Michle **(SLP)**

Trabuco Canyon

Atkins, Mrs Carol J **(A)**
Taylor, Mrs Terri M **(A)**
Thomas, Mrs Debra Elizabeth **(SLP)**

Tracy

James, Cynthia Rae **(SLP)**
Mottershead, Janet Lee **(SLP)**

Tujunga

Foldvary, Sherry Lee **(SLP)**
Hill, Marilyn Taube **(SLP)**
Orth, Susan J **(SLP)**

Tulare

Beauchamp, James A **(A)**
McAdams, Mrs Lisa Rasenti
McBride, Mrs Lois A **(SLP)**

Turlock

Bacca, Glenda G **(SLP)**
Bamberg, Mrs Gail A **(SLP)**
Du Frane, Mrs Michele McKinnon **(SLP)**
Genzoli, Linda Qualle **(SLP)**
Lefevre, Mrs Cecily S **(A)**
McDearmon, Dr James R **(SLP)**
Pannier, Mrs Audrey Forster **(SLP)**
Parolini, Mrs Pauline F **(SLP)**
Sasaki, Mrs Elaine Kaoru

Tustin

Barnhart, Kimberly Marie **(SLP)**
Dobeck, Connie Sue **(SLP)**
Doyle, Louise Marie **(SLP)**
Grigsby, Cynthia L **(SLP)**
Kane, Sandra Bordner **(SLP)**
Reese, Katherine Thomas **(SLP)**
Richards, Douglas **(A)**
Ridder, Mrs Jane **(SLP)**
Riley, Dr Glyndon D **(SLP)**
Riley, Dr Jeanna N **(SLP)**
Rott, Mrs Betty Baker **(SLP)**
Rzepnick, Adrienne **(SLP)**
Techler-Crowe, Helen **(A)**

Twain Harte

McKee, Gill Grimsley **(SLP)**
Pogroszewski, Janis M

Ukiah

Andrus, Gary Wyatt **(A)**
Arnett, Patricia **(SLP)**
Chadd, Nancy L **(SLP)**
Larsen, Mrs Joyce F **(A)**
Mery-Rutledge, Mrs Renee Louise **(SLP)**
Pollesel, Susan S **(SLP)**
Traba, Vickie M **(SLP)**

Union City

Fiori, Carolyn E **(SLP)**
Mason, Mrs Kelly Ann **(SLP)**
Stevens, Mrs Joanne M **(SLP)**
Thomas, Elizabeth Ruth **(SLP)**
Woodhead, James S **(SLP)**

Upland

Bance-Davis, Mrs Angela Velma **(SLP)**
Berasi, Karen Marie **(SLP)**
Brinegar, Dr Kimberly Park **(SLP)**
Brittain, Mary Jean **(SLP)**
Eckel, Mrs Roberta H **(SLP)**
Elder, Frances J **(SLP)**
Fisher, Mrs Christine **(SLP)**
Gerety, Martha Blessey **(SLP)**
Goode, Lisa Lepore
Granger, Misty Leann **(SLP)**
Henderson, Carol L **(SLP)**
Ishimoto, Sharon Kiku **(SLP)**
Madkin, Mrs Mary E A **(SLP)**
Reed, Mrs Pamela Pickering **(SLP)**
Robinson, Michael E **(A)**
Schmidt, Mrs Sandra Jeanne **(SLP)**
Schneider, Dr Marie J **(SLP)**
Sortor, Kathryn E **(SLP)**
Stevenson, Hideko **(SLP)**
Van Horn, Mrs Linda Marie **(SLP)**

Vacaville

Allen, Mrs Claudia Koller **(SLP)**
Curtis, Mrs Christine **(SLP)**
Gilson, Eileen K **(SLP)**

Grimard, Dianne D **(SLP)**
Keiser, Mrs Diane **(SLP)**
Knight, Jody L **(SLP)**
Lewis, Debra Marie
Maul, Mrs Rosalie W **(SLP)**
Meyers, Jeanne C **(SLP)**
Mickelson, William D **(SLP)**
Naggi, Elaine J **(SLP)**
Phelps-Lindsay, Lucy **(SLP)**

Valencia

Aronson, Mrs Nola Clark **(A)**
Feinholz, Mrs Lori Adrienne **(SLP)**
Flickinger, Mrs Kimberly L **(SLP)**
Goldner, Mrs Debra L **(SLP)**
Legler, Mrs Lannie T **(SLP)**
Parmenter, Mrs Wendy I **(SLP)**
Stone-Gross, Dale Ellen **(SLP)**
Winter, Mrs Margaret E **(A)**

Vallejo

Beaton, Suzanne Kay **(SLP)**
Buck-Gordon, Susan **(SLP)**
Collins, Robert P **(SLP)**
Lytle, Pauline **(SLP)**
Melton, Mrs Sally A
Ray, Mrs Deidre Wright
Read, Mrs Laurie Smith **(SLP)**
Strickler, Mrs Ruth E **(SLP)**

Valley Center

Redding, Mrs Sandra Lea **(SLP)**

Van Nuys

Bargelt, Dr James Hager **(SLP)**
Cohen-Essig, Shary I **(SLP)**
Cozzi, Angela **(SLP)**
Cramer, Cathleen L **(SLP)**
Cutler, Mark Jay **(SLP)**
Enman, Mrs Sharon L **(SLP)**
Everett, Karen Herman **(SLP)**
Finkelstein, Mrs Lorraine Sheila **(SLP)**
Firestone, Dr Barbara A **(SLP)**
Frank, Dr Grace W **(SLP)**
Glucksman-Weiss, Vivian **(SLP)**
Goldojarb, Mrs Muriel F **(SLP)**
Grey, Dr Howard A **(SLP A)**
Gurnick, Ellen B **(SLP)**
Higgins, Thomas M **(A)**
Hirsch, Caryl **(SLP)**
Jenkins, David W **(A)**
Kunes, Ellen Blair **(A)**
Laris, Emily Joan **(SLP)**
Miller, Lori G **(SLP)**
Moskowitz, Mrs Sheila I F **(SLP)**
Peale, Janet L **(SLP)**
Prentice, Dr Abbie Shuford **(SLP)**
Reagan, William G **(SLP A)**
Sadigh-Behzadi, Mrs Marianne Morrisey **(SLP)**
Sadja-Thompson, Lynn **(SLP)**
Segal, Judy Marilyn **(SLP)**
Simon, Ellen Shapiro **(A)**
Smith, Terrie Lynn **(SLP)**

Vandenberg AFB

Brawner, Christine Marie **(SLP)**

Venice

Criswell, Martha S **(SLP)**
Karbelnig, Amy Bade **(SLP)**
Kopelow, Nancie Lynn **(SLP)**
Rudin, Steffi W **(A)**

Ventura

Aguirre, Guadalupe Maria **(SLP)**
Barnett, Carol L **(SLP)**
Bennett, Trudy B **(SLP)**
Blare, Lindy Elizabeth **(SLP)**
Bolson, Mrs Virginia A **(SLP)**
Borel, Denise A **(SLP)**
Bramer, Jean M **(SLP)**
Buffon, Katherine Prince **(SLP)**
Burkhart, Mrs Nancy Ellen **(SLP)**
Cataldo, Mary N **(SLP)**
Chase, Tara C **(SLP)**
Crawford, Sandra V **(SLP)**
Doane, Suzanne Catherine **(SLP)**
Edwards, Mrs Cathleen Pew **(SLP)**
Gomez, Mrs Beverly Hopper **(SLP)**
Greene, Bonnie M **(SLP)**
Ito, Arlene Karen **(SLP)**
Johnstone, Mrs Rhetta **(SLP)**
Leamy, Donald P **(A)**
Linton, Anita L **(SLP)**
Magnusson, Ronald L **(A)**
Marshall, Linda **(SLP)**
Murray, Maurice E **(SLP)**
Muth, Sharon S **(SLP)**
Pedersen, Judy Elizabeth **(SLP)**
Power, Paula A W **(SLP)**
Quintanilla, Jerilyn B **(SLP)**
Roberts, Elizabeth **(SLP)**
Saunders, Mrs Joyce E **(SLP)**
Shinder, Mrs Anne **(SLP)**
Slack, Mrs Kirsten Nielsen **(SLP)**
Sporn, Marcia W **(SLP)**
Stiles, Mrs Jean E **(SLP)**
Tabor, Mrs Carolyn K **(SLP)**
Theys, Debi A D **(SLP)**
Van Voy, Karen Guilford **(SLP)**
Weber, Nancy C **(SLP)**

Victorville

Girard, Mrs Brenda Lindquist **(SLP)**
Kelly, Lela M **(SLP)**

Villa Park

O'Malley, Mrs Carol E L **(SLP)**

Visalia

Aldrich, Richard S **(SLP)**
Calloway, Mrs Kristal Smith **(A)**
Chambers, Mrs Jane C **(SLP)**
Cruzen, Linda Louise **(SLP)**
Darling, Linda Joy **(SLP)**
Ditmanson, AnnaDell **(SLP)**
Grant, Andrea Elaine **(SLP)**
Hoffman, Mrs Robin Menge **(SLP)**
Hofstetter, Mrs Lynn P **(SLP)**
Johnson, Mrs Carole Fornell **(A)**
Kitaoka, Jennifer Yoshiko **(SLP)**
Krikorian, Marvel J **(SLP)**
McCabe, Ronald L **(SLP)**
Nickols, Mrs Linda S **(SLP)**
Schaeffer, Mindy I **(SLP)**
Shearon, Mrs Mary E **(SLP)**
Shurson, Tedd Dennis **(A)**
Sward, Janet L **(SLP)**
Thompson, Heather Immer **(SLP)**
Vourakis, Andrea L
Will, David Albert **(SLP)**
Wood, Laurel B R **(SLP)**
Wright, Dr Kenneth L **(SLP)**

Vista

Baumel, Mrs Deborah W **(SLP)**
Christianson, Mary Lou **(SLP)**
Grosse, Mrs Patricia Elizabeth **(SLP)**
Hagood, Brenda Britton **(SLP)**
Hoffman, Beth Gilbertson **(SLP)**
Johnson, Cynthia W **(A)**
Lesser, Karen Anne **(SLP)**
Rohrbacher, Mrs Susan H **(SLP)**
Singleton, Sandra L **(SLP)**
Wade, Mrs Leslie H **(SLP)**
Wojcik, Jodi K **(A)**

Walnut

Brown, Debra A **(SLP)**
Green, Steven Michael **(SLP)**
Jones, Mrs Theresa T **(SLP)**
Kipper-Hall, Mechele **(SLP)**
Kyker, Mrs Judy Catherine **(SLP)**
Navarro, Mrs Jacquelyn **(SLP)**
Noble, Mrs Deborah Lynn **(SLP)**
Piper, Mrs Lisa C S **(SLP)**
Rust, Roxanna Lou **(SLP)**

Walnut Creek

Austin, Mrs Jolynn Sanborn **(SLP)**
Burger, Mrs Linda H **(SLP)**
Callery, Ingrid Margot
Epstein, Mona R **(SLP)**
Furbacher, Ellen A **(SLP)**
Gilmartin, Eva Marie **(SLP)**
Hall, C Mike **(A)**
Hall, Mrs Malinda M **(SLP)**
Hodes, Mrs Cynthia Blair **(SLP)**
Holzhueter, Ann Marie **(SLP)**
Husby, Deborah Louise **(SLP)**
Kelley, Mrs Karin Wolverton **(SLP)**
LaVallee-Kennedy, Mrs Janet Mary **(SLP)**
Maj, Mrs Elizabeth **(SLP)**
Minardi, Mrs Lisa M **(SLP)**
Moreno, Melinda V **(SLP)**
Newman, Mrs Kristen Elizabeth **(SLP)**
Nyman, Darlene Patricia **(SLP)**
Outman, Richard R **(SLP)**
Peterson, Colleen O'Brien **(A)**
Rasmus, Dr Ward **(SLP)**
Rudman, Mrs Cynthia M **(SLP)**
Schuster, Mrs Bette **(SLP)**
Wells, Mrs Elaine F **(SLP)**

Waterford

Clover-Mallory, Mrs Jill **(SLP)**

Watsonville

Myers, Raymond Dan **(SLP)**

Weed

Sanders, Mrs Karen S **(SLP)**

West Covina

Alexander, Shirley J **(A)**
Bourgeois, Pamela Chevreaux **(SLP)**
Bridgman, Connie Marie **(SLP)**
Dabul, Dr Barbara L **(SLP)**
Devitt, Elizabeth Ann West **(SLP)**
McGregor, Mrs Theodora F **(SLP)**
Offstein, Lois **(SLP)**
Osacho, Jennifer Marie **(SLP)**
Smith, Mrs Frances A **(SLP)**
Verdi, Janet Rosemarie **(SLP)**

West Hills

Morgan, Mrs Karen S **(SLP)**
Zuckerman, Carol L **(SLP)**

West Hollywood

Dean, Jeffery Lynn **(A)**
Goubeaux, Jocelyn H **(A)**
Gumbiner, Tracy Ann **(SLP)**
Mahoney, Elaine Marie **(SLP)**
Mindes, Miriam Joane **(SLP)**
Taigman, Susan **(A)**
Tarnoff, Terri Lynne **(SLP)**

West Los Angeles

Ginsberg, Bernard L **(SLP A)**
Gomeztrejo, Patricia Elena **(SLP)**
Sabado, Mrs Diane Duclos **(SLP)**

Westchester

Ryal, Mary Kay **(SLP)**

Westlake Village

Borelli, Nancy R **(SLP)**
Copeland, Mrs Barbara R **(SLP)**
Herr, Mrs Beverly B **(SLP)**
Johnson, Sue Burns **(SLP)**
Mactague, Mrs Janet Mary **(SLP)**
McKnight, Deborah E
Murray, Mrs Patti Z **(SLP)**
Shriftman, Mrs Eileen C **(SLP)**

Westminster

Duffield-Hunthausen, Janice L **(A)**
Glance, Steven Eugene **(SLP)**
Horvath, Ellen M J **(SLP)**
McIsaac, Mrs Pamela Dianne
Perry-Wilock, Linda L **(SLP)**
Richey, Mrs Cheryl Merdgen **(SLP)**
Taylor, Mrs Myra Jane **(A)**
Thompson, Dr Jesse J **(SLP)**

Westport

Pettit, Alyse Edwards **(SLP)**

Whittier

Apel, Dr Kenn **(SLP)**
Burica, Cathleen Sue **(SLP)**
Carlyle, Irene Varcados **(SLP)**
Conner, Mrs Joanne Kathleen **(SLP)**
Delgado, Lupe L **(SLP)**
Drown, Mrs Carol M **(A)**
Harris, Lester L **(SLP)**
Henderson, Amy Kathleen **(SLP)**
Jennings-Reimer, Terry D **(SLP)**
Klein, Dr Edward S **(SLP)**
Lara, Anastasia M
Lewman, Mrs Lucie E **(SLP)**
Lund, Mrs Shanna J E **(SLP)**
Martens, Dale M **(SLP)**
Meydag, Mrs Vana L **(SLP)**
Novina, Joan **(SLP)**
Olden, Mrs Clara E **(SLP)**
Paquette, Mrs Michelle K **(SLP)**
Peel, Laurie Welsh **(SLP)**
Peirson, Mrs Lorelei **(SLP)**
Peter, Laurie Ann
Santo, Daniel J **(SLP)**
Schnell, Roxanne **(SLP)**
Torline, Mrs Lori L **(SLP)**
Trautmann, Julie Beth
Weekes, Mrs Barbara Blain **(SLP)**

Willits

Horowitz-Moilanen, Nancy **(SLP)**

Windsor

Frost, Don I **(SLP)**
Sowell, Mrs Janis Belkin **(SLP)**

Winton

Rohrer, Rosemary Elizabeth **(SLP)**

Woodland

Behrends, Bernadette Cotta
Gray, Mrs Carol Aimee **(SLP)**
Guillermo, Carmen R **(A)**
Huff, Mrs Marcia L **(SLP)**
Shipley, Jean E **(SLP)**
Viers, Mrs Joellen Robertson

Woodland Hills

Aptakin, Sammye Jean **(SLP)**
Brown, Karen D **(SLP)**
Calderon-Dworetzky, Dianne L **(SLP)**
Campbell, Diane **(SLP)**
Ceragioli, Mrs Joan D **(SLP)**
Cook, Connie S **(SLP)**
Forman, Ruth L **(SLP)**
Givner, Jodi **(SLP)**
Gould, Jody Anne **(SLP)**
Grover-Gaffney, Mary Corinne **(SLP)**
Harwin, Mrs Lisa S **(SLP)**
Kayl, Susan N **(SLP A)**
Lehrhoff, Terri L **(SLP)**
Lehrman, Karen E **(SLP)**
Leiman, Mrs Sheilla Irene **(SLP)**
Mautner, Mrs Diane S **(SLP)**
McCulloch, Mrs Joan Helene **(SLP)**
Milne, Charlynn J **(SLP)**
Mulick-Altuna, Dianne Jean **(SLP)**
Piasecki, Charlene P **(SLP)**
Priceman, Lorraine R **(SLP)**
Quinn, Mary K **(SLP)**
Rosenblatt, Mrs Judith M **(SLP)**
Schulkin, Mrs Florence P **(SLP)**
Shafton, Mrs Judith H **(SLP)**
Skopp, Elaine R **(SLP)**
Solomon, Mrs Greta N **(SLP)**
Soroky, Dr Doris L **(SLP)**
Tobin, Bonnie L **(SLP)**
Warren, Glenda Gale **(SLP)**

Woodside

Barker, Mrs Ruth A **(SLP)**
Scott, Dr Carl H **(SLP)**

Worthridge
Rothstein, Rabbi S **(SLP)**

Wrightwood
Bricca, Barry Steven **(A)**
Clements, Darlene C **(SLP)**

Yorba Linda
Bendroff, Mrs Ann Denise **(SLP)**
Bergert, Mrs Sandra G V **(SLP)**
Bonsangue, Nancy J **(SLP)**
Bretney, Louise E **(SLP)**
Cory, Thomas L **(SLP)**
Drost, Kathleen Anderson **(SLP)**
Ferrara, Linda Mizenko **(SLP)**
Garcia, Mrs M Erin O'Toole **(SLP)**
Harms, Mrs Karen Lee **(SLP)**
Horn, Mrs Gail Boedeker
Inouye, Mrs Karen Gail T **(SLP)**
Izumi, Mrs Marsha **(SLP)**
Kohlenberger, Lisa Karen **(SLP)**
Martin, Mrs Sara Lee M **(SLP)**
McCann, Mrs Ann H **(SLP)**
McDonald, Mrs Barbara A **(SLP)**
Napoli, Dennis M **(SLP)**
Profet, Sharon Beth **(SLP)**
Rendon, Anita S **(SLP)**
Robins, Mrs Laurie Galey **(SLP)**
Schneider, Michael D
Stone, Mrs Ann Marie **(SLP)**
Wilkerson, Mrs Jill K **(SLP)**

Yreka
Ellis, Marian Leigh **(SLP)**
Tragitt, Leslie Ann **(SLP)**

Yuba City
Alexander, Joan W H
Arnold, Kathy L **(SLP)**
Bock, Bonna Dee **(SLP)**
Brierly, Anne Carolyn **(SLP)**
Cummings-Ingram, Peggy Jean **(SLP)**
Dyrhsen, Mrs Judith C **(SLP)**
Jackson, Janice E **(SLP)**
Johnston, Gerry P **(SLP)**
Miller, Doris Jane **(SLP)**

Yucaipa
Baernstein, Mrs Denise Marie C **(SLP)**
McGann, David **(A)**
Mitson, Linda A **(SLP)**
Moran, Joyce A **(SLP)**
Rider, Mrs Janice Lynn **(SLP)**
Tieche, Mrs Connie L S **(SLP)**

Yucca Valley
Farris, Mrs Ruth B

Yucuipa
Millhouse-Smith, Mrs Susan A **(SLP)**

COLORADO

Alamosa
Jones, Judy K **(SLP)**
Katauskas, Linda Marie
McPherson, Lorrane Marie **(SLP)**
Merkley, Mary J **(A)**

Arvada
Agnes, Stephanie **(SLP)**
Burke-Daoust, Jeanette Eileen
Evans, Terrell Riley **(SLP)**
Fuller, Karlene C **(SLP)**
Gannon, Marlene M **(SLP)**
Gilmore, Dee A **(SLP)**
Herder, Julie Christy **(SLP)**
Hoffman, Mrs Jolene Slocum **(A)**
Hurt, Jerri Johnson **(SLP)**
Ireland, Nancy D **(SLP)**
Jones, Mrs Patricia Presnall **(SLP)**
Lentz, Mrs Terri Colleen **(SLP)**
McKenna, Sue M **(SLP)**
Melton, Suzanne Spears
Oligschlaeger, Mrs Elayne Joy **(SLP)**
Polk, Pamela M R **(SLP)**
Rodriguez, Terry J **(SLP)**
Siems, Mrs Deborah A **(SLP)**
Swanson, Mrs Kay L **(SLP)**

Aspen
Brubaker, B J **(SLP)**
Landis, Marjorie A **(SLP)**

Ault
Steg, Mrs Katherine **(SLP)**

Aurora
Baker, Jane Meier **(A)**
Bihr, Mrs Roxann P **(SLP)**
Braden, Marcia M **(SLP)**
Browne, Maureen Therese **(A)**
Burney, Ellen V **(SLP)**
Chambers, Patricia Rodney **(SLP)**
Connelly, Mrs Corliss Ann **(SLP)**
Cripe, Dr Antje E **(SLP)**
Csargo, Georganne Marie **(SLP)**
Dale, Mrs Sharon R **(SLP)**
Davis, Mrs Ronda L **(SLP)**
Dekas-Marafiote, Elizabeth **(SLP)**
Dey, Vanda Lee **(SLP)**
Dickey, Sarah K B **(SLP)**
Dienhart, Susan E **(SLP)**
Enix, Mrs Candice S **(SLP)**
Farina, Mary Kay **(SLP)**
Ferrer-Vinent, Susan T **(A)**
Gibbons, Mrs Carole Curtis **(SLP)**
Gibson, Susan A **(A)**
Goldstein, Dr Jerod **(A)**
Goldstein, Vicki Morris **(SLP)**
Gross, Michelle Leblanc **(A)**
Hall, Carolyn J **(SLP)**
Hall, Patricia Sanders **(SLP)**
Hasbargen, Jerene M **(SLP)**
Hasbrouck, Dr Jon M **(SLP)**
Hastings, Anne Cecile **(A)**
Haxby, Marsha F **(SLP)**
Hinckley, Penny F **(SLP)**
Huzzard-Trombly, Deborah **(SLP)**
Ingve, Kathleen Jane **(A)**
Inman, Mrs Denise Elaine **(SLP)**
Jones, Jo Ann P **(SLP)**
Klein, Dr Estelle E **(SLP)**
Kuhn, Lynn Erica **(SLP)**
Lardent, Jeanne P **(SLP)**
Leary, Kimberly Anne **(SLP)**
Ley, Mrs Kathleen Ann **(SLP)**
Loveless, Mrs Barbara Louise **(SLP)**
Lowry-Romero, Mary Frances **(SLP)**
Matyk, Mrs Karen A **(SLP)**
Mazeau, Zoe Ann **(SLP)**
Moynihan, E A **(SLP)**
Otness, Mrs Martha A M **(SLP)**
Palmer, 1Lt Richard Lee **(A)**
Parks, Virginia W **(SLP)**
Piche, Mrs Leslie Donelan **(SLP)**
Pitts, Janice K **(SLP)**
Pollack, Mrs Doreen M **(SLP A)**
Post, Gail-Susan F
Randle, Bonnie **(SLP)**
Redwine, Linda Simpson **(SLP A)**
Rodie, Mrs Sharon Marie **(SLP)**
Rollert, Linda Cooper **(SLP)**
Schachterle, Bruce D **(A)**
Schurr, Margaret S **(A)**
Schuster, Martha Lee **(SLP)**
Shores, Linda Sue
Shriver, Carla Jean **(SLP)**
Snelling, Theresa Marie **(SLP)**
Snipes, Mrs Ann Rae **(SLP)**
Stickney, Lycia Lauka **(SLP)**
Sytsma, Wendy Ham **(A)**
Trantham, Carla Ann **(SLP)**
Tromburg, Mrs Ruth Ann **(SLP)**
Wade, Susan Jean **(SLP)**
Wiese, Mrs Sally Bush **(SLP)**
Wilson, Illa R **(SLP)**

Avon
Bielmaier, Catherine Ann
Williams, Merrilee M **(SLP)**

Avondale
Pooler, Shannon Gill

Boulder
Beatty, Janet G
Bihum, Virginia C **(SLP)**
Blatchford, Katheryn Dean **(A)**
Brown, Arlene Stredler **(SLP)**
Bryan, Janie C **(SLP)**
Byrd, Faythe S **(SLP)**
Call, Timothy A **(SLP)**
Carter, Mrs Christine McGregor **(SLP)**
Cassel, Tami S **(SLP)**
Cory, Mrs Martha W **(SLP)**
Curran, Catherine Elizabeth **(SLP)**
Dean, Nadine Salacone **(SLP)**
Downey, Dr Doris Marie **(SLP)**
Driscoll, Julia Ann
Elling, Susan Mary **(SLP)**
Fischer, Mrs Anne W **(SLP)**
Fox, Mrs Nanci Goldsmidt **(SLP)**
Gang, Mrs Shirley J **(SLP)**
Gitterman, Dena **(SLP)**
Goetz, Sheila L **(SLP)**
Hahn, Wilma J **(SLP)**
Haywood, Marialys G **(SLP)**
Hedberg, Dr Natalie L **(SLP A)**
Hickey, Carla Yim **(SLP)**
Horii, Dr Yoshiyuki
Hyink, Mrs Pamela J **(SLP)**
Jackson, Judith Lynn **(SLP)**
Jacobson, Terry A **(SLP)**
Johnson, Georgiana **(SLP)**
Judkins, Mary Gold **(SLP)**
Kail, Sandra L **(SLP)**
Kalb, Marti B **(SLP)**
Keatley, Dr Mary A W **(SLP)**
King, Judy Bell **(SLP)**
Krug, Dr Richard F **(SLP A)**
Krug, Terri L **(SLP)**
Landry, Beth M **(SLP)**
Levine, Jodie L **(SLP)**
Linville, Dr Sharon S **(A)**
Mann, Andrea L **(SLP)**
Matthews, Cynthia A **(A)**
McGrane, Rhonda L **(SLP)**
Mecklenburg, Dr Dianne Jorgi **(SLP A)**
Miller, Karan K **(SLP)**
Miller, Patricia Kay **(SLP)**
Moore, Susan M **(SLP)**
Nunemaker, Kathy L **(SLP)**
Ochsner, Patricia Cady **(SLP)**
Papper, Margaret A **(SLP)**
Raforth, Donna F **(SLP)**
Ramig, Dr Lorraine Olson **(SLP)**
Ramig, Dr Peter R **(SLP)**
Ramsberger, Dr Gail **(SLP)**
Redstone, Fran **(SLP)**
Rende, Barbara **(SLP)**
Sackschewsky, Louise B **(SLP)**
Sementelli, Catherine Ann
Shallop, Dr Jon K **(SLP A)**
Shay, Donna M **(SLP)**
Smadbeck, Diana W **(SLP)**
Smathers, Jessica C **(SLP)**
Smith, Elizabeth Imle **(SLP)**
Snyder, Mrs Christine **(SLP)**
Stockman, Diane S
Strobridge, Mary Ann **(SLP A)**
Summers, Patricia **(SLP)**
Sweetman, Rebecca J **(SLP)**
Sweetman, Dr Richard H **(A)**
Tedeschi, Jaye
Wachtel, Mrs Clara Jacobs **(SLP)**
Wallace, Mrs Mary Louise **(SLP)**
Weiss, Dr Rita S **(SLP)**
Wieczorek, Judy C **(SLP)**
Yoshinaga-Itano, Dr Christine **(A)**

Breckenridge
Johnston, Sally L **(SLP)**

Brighton
Fudala, Dr Janet B **(SLP A)**
Zink, G David **(A)**

Broomfield
Dixon, Dr James D **(A)**
Ellison, Lisa A
Fagler, Mrs Patricia A **(SLP)**
Guberud, Jane Croce **(SLP)**
Nicholas, Mrs Leslie Denise **(SLP)**

Brush
Castrup, Mrs Jacqueline R **(SLP)**
Prascher, Elaine C **(SLP)**

Buena Vista
Evans, Robin Unger **(SLP)**
Miller, Donna **(SLP)**

Calhan
Matthews, Mrs Nancy Shubella **(SLP)**

Canon City
Cozzette, Rose M D **(SLP)**
Cranston, John E **(SLP A)**
Ertmer, David **(SLP)**

Cascade
Bosley, Mrs Elizabeth C **(SLP)**
Coman, J Michael, II **(SLP)**
Erickson, Pamela Kaye **(SLP)**
Koshak, Karen K **(SLP)**

Castle Rock
John, Anne Farquhar **(SLP)**
Johnson, Mrs Mary L T **(SLP)**
Look, Lois Neff **(A)**
Slevin, Mrs Barbara J **(SLP)**
Vollmer, Sandra Marie **(SLP)**

Clifton
Meyers, Judith A **(SLP)**

Colorado Springs
Allison, Mrs Carolyn Barth
Altman, Mrs Jill Cook **(SLP)**
Andersen, Mrs Pamela Mary S **(SLP)**
Anderson, Mrs Arlene K **(SLP)**
Arterbury, Mrs Tammy S **(SLP)**
Ashley-Smutko, Mrs Nan N **(SLP)**
Atlas, Deborah **(SLP)**
Bechtold, Patricia A **(SLP)**
Bellis, Mrs Teri James **(A)**
Biga, Judith M
Bjork, Jean Anne W **(SLP)**
Blythe, Mrs Debra Lorraine **(SLP)**
Bonin, Betsy Jean **(SLP)**
Brady, Deborah H **(SLP)**
Champlin, Jeanne M **(SLP)**
Cichowitz, Mrs Deborah J **(SLP)**
Cluxton, Kelly Jo **(SLP)**
Cowan, Mrs Dorothy R **(SLP)**
Crary, Suzan B **(SLP)**
Creekmore, Mrs Susan A **(SLP)**
Curry, Mrs Kerin Cunning **(SLP)**
Davidson, Kathryn Pohlit **(SLP)**
Davis-Pedrle, Mrs Denise **(SLP)**
Detwiler, Mrs Cathleen A **(SLP)**
Dickson, Mrs Lori Sue **(SLP)**
Difoggio, Jacy Doumas **(SLP)**
Dige, Janet L T **(SLP)**
Dolata, Mrs Cindi L **(SLP)**
Dueber, Mrs Sandee Horton **(A)**
Duncan, Dr Melba Hurd **(SLP)**
Everett, Mrs Siri Ann **(SLP)**
Faraguna, Mrs Debra L Smith **(SLP)**
Goodwin, Mrs Karen Rae **(SLP)**
Grace, Patricia **(SLP)**
Green, Mrs Patricia Ann **(SLP)**
Grimes, Ruth Katherine **(SLP)**
Hahn, Patricia M **(SLP)**
Harms, Gail N **(SLP)**
Hartlaub, Alice W **(SLP)**
Hennessy, Fran Rochelle **(SLP)**

Hoedl-Bayer, Mrs Denise M **(SLP)**
Horton, Penelope S **(SLP)**
Hulse, Christine Jo **(SLP)**
Hutchins, Jerilyn **(A)**
Jobe, Meredith A **(SLP)**
Jones, Mrs Lynette **(SLP)**
Judy, Joanna Michele **(SLP)**
Kessler, Mrs Monica Balsano **(SLP)**
Kesting, Mrs Lisa Mortimer **(SLP)**
Kibbe, Kathleen McGrann **(SLP)**
Komarow, Patricia W **(SLP)**
Korf, Mrs Patricia C **(SLP)**
Leaf, S Michael **(A)**
Leonard, Lisa Jean **(SLP)**
Lizzul, Lee Ann **(A)**
Malone, Susan M **(SLP)**
Martin, Susan K **(SLP)**
Martin-Boehs, Mrs Sally Sue **(SLP)**
Mathias, Mrs Dana **(A)**
May-Landes, Annette Lynn **(SLP)**
McClow-Kinsey, Sheila **(SLP)**
McDavid, Dorothy S **(SLP)**
McGlynn, Becky A **(A)**
McHugh, Dr Eugene Rice **(A)**
Meyers, Mrs Carol A **(A)**
Munson, Doris M **(SLP)**
Nichols, Cynthia Marie **(SLP)**
Parlet, Mrs Rebecca Jane **(SLP)**
Pattillo, Mrs Janis S **(SLP)**
Pennington, Dr R Corbin
Ross, Mrs Dana **(SLP)**
Roth, Nancy K **(SLP)**
Scheidhauer, Karen Elizabeth **(SLP)**
Sera-Budney, Kathryn K **(A)**
Short, Shirley Crandall **(SLP)**
Sieck, Mrs Sharon **(SLP)**
Slack, Lisa Cheryl **(SLP)**
Stohr, Kathleen M
Straka, Mrs Elizabeth M **(SLP)**
Streeter-Discenzo, Mrs Suzanne **(SLP)**
Sugimura, Cathryn Michiko
Thompson, Mrs Christine M **(SLP)**
Trutna, Phyllis **(SLP)**
Vaughn, Mrs Suzanne Lee **(SLP)**
Vigil, Elizabeth Tuttle **(SLP)**
Viviano, Ann K **(SLP)**
Waterman, Jo Ellen Abbott **(SLP)**
Watson, Judy M **(SLP)**
Webb, Dina-Marie **(SLP)**
Weiss, Mrs Karen Kaplan
Welsh, Kim R
Williamson, Devyn Hogan **(SLP)**

Commerce City
Reed, Agnes Faye **(SLP)**

Cortez
Marshall, Edwina Catherine
Vinton, Ava M **(SLP)**

Crawford
Reed, Mrs Wanda B **(SLP)**

Denver
Angstman, Mrs Jean Ward **(SLP)**
Bachrach, Annette M **(SLP)**
Baker, Kathy Sue **(A)**
Ball, Mary M **(A)**
Barilko, Margaret R **(SLP)**
Barrows, Susan Miller **(SLP)**
Bell, Tina A **(SLP)**
Bemski, Mrs Sandra L **(A)**
Bernard, Patricia Jane **(SLP)**
Birkle, Mrs Lydia S **(A)**
Blager, Dr Florence B **(SLP)**
Blando, Barbara Owens **(SLP)**
Bloom, Barbara J **(SLP)**
Bodenhemier, Dr Wayne G **(A)**
Boone, Mary J G **(SLP)**
Brewer, Mrs Gwendolyn Harland **(SLP)**
Brown, Debra J **(SLP)**
Burtness, Carol Diffenbaugh **(SLP)**
Butterly, Beth **(A)**
Cairella, Cynthia A **(SLP)**
Carey, Barbara L **(SLP)**
Carpenter, Mrs Barbara L **(SLP)**
Carrico, Mrs Denise Marie
Carrieri, Laura Jean **(SLP)**
Christensen, Sally A **(SLP)**
Clement, Mrs Ann Morrison **(SLP)**
Crennen, Cynthia L **(SLP)**
Dance, Dr Frank E X
Daniel, Linda L **(A)**
Danielson, Sarah J **(SLP)**
Denton, Sandra Sue **(A)**
Diehl, Mrs Adeline E **(SLP)**
Dinner, Dr M Bernice **(A)**
Dionigi, Cynthia Marie **(SLP)**
Dixon, Leeann Hanson **(SLP)**
Domko, Jo Anne Camp **(SLP)**
Donohoe, Robert W **(A)**
Dorn, Abigail M **(SLP)**
Downs, Mrs Marion P **(A)**
Dreith-Ratcliffe, Susan **(A)**
Eckert, Joan A **(SLP)**
Ehrlich, Carol H
Emerson-Anderson, Shari Lynne **(SLP)**
England, Mrs Rosemary B **(A)**
Erickson, Paula Lois **(SLP)**
Ernst, Mrs Marian M **(SLP A)**
Esch-Johnson, Mrs Geraldine Gerry **(SLP)**
Faingold, Mrs Sandra Pribble **(SLP)**
Felker, Donna Lea **(A)**
Fogg, Patricia Lettko **(SLP)**
Foster, Susan F **(SLP A)**
Fox, Eileen J **(A)**
Fox, Mary E **(SLP)**
Franklin, Dana Bendigkeit **(SLP)**
Freeland, Dr E Elaine **(SLP A)**
Gabbard, Sandra Abbott **(A)**
Galloway, Ann R **(SLP)**
Gerber, Judy A **(SLP)**
Glenn, Sharon Murphy **(SLP)**
Gould, Mrs Jeanne K **(SLP)**
Greb, Kathryn Diana **(SLP)**
Green, Nancy E **(SLP)**
Greene, Patricia D **(A)**
Grossman, Rhonda K **(SLP)**
Gruber, Janet L **(SLP)**
Gugenheim, Susan M **(SLP)**
Haddow, Judith A **(SLP)**
Haglund, Janet M **(SLP)**
Hall, Mrs Teresa Lynn **(SLP)**
Harding, Julie Ann **(SLP)**
Hartung, Barbara A **(SLP)**
Hayes, Dr Deborah **(A)**
Hayward, Mrs Deborah Carol **(SLP)**
Higgins, Patti A **(SLP)**
Holloway, Martha J **(SLP)**
Horan, Margaret **(SLP)**
Horton, Mrs Barbara L **(SLP)**
Householder, Julie A **(SLP)**
Howard, R Ann **(SLP)**
Hubbard, Jenita Lynn **(A)**
Hurst, Karen Diane **(SLP)**
Hutson, Debra Kay
Hynes, Patricia A **(SLP)**
Jaeger, Ellen Louise **(SLP)**
Jansen, John W **(A)**
Johnson, Mrs Janice R **(SLP)**
Johnson, Judith C **(SLP)**
Jones, Judith Burch **(SLP)**
Kagan, Laurie **(SLP)**
Kelley, Kathy A **(SLP)**
Kidd, Mrs Margaret R **(SLP)**
Killian, Dr Patricia **(SLP)**
Killius, Kristin Ann **(SLP)**
Kinder, Deborah L **(A)**
Kiyota, Linda K **(A)**
Kurtz, Joellen **(SLP)**
Lackner, Susan L **(SLP)**
Lake, Patricia **(SLP)**
Larson, Kristin
Lebold, Christine Laurie **(A)**
Le Brun, Mrs Karen Lee **(A)**
Lehmann-Epstein, Mrs Carolyn **(SLP)**
Levander, Jane M **(A)**
Levisohn, Ruth L **(SLP)**
Lowry, Mrs Laura D G **(SLP)**
Lozow, Mrs Karen Simmons **(SLP)**
Luellen, Betty Ruth **(SLP)**
Lukanic, Bill A
Luke-Gysin, Patricia A **(SLP)**
Lunde, Laura Katherine **(A)**
Maertens, Mrs Maria Hidalgo **(SLP)**
Mallory, Kathleen E **(SLP)**
Markin, Lori Ann **(SLP)**
Marshall-Siegel, Mrs Susan **(SLP)**
Martin, Lesa A **(A)**
McBride, Teresa Lyn **(SLP)**
McCabe, Carol Lee **(SLP)**
McCray, Jeri L **(SLP)**
Mercer, Louise B **(SLP)**
Methven, Dr Margaret P **(SLP)**
Mikami, Karen Akemi **(A)**
Minkler, Pearllynne **(SLP)**
Mundil, Donna B **(A)**
Murphy, Maureen A **(SLP)**
Myland, Jackie **(SLP)**
Newman, Wendy **(SLP)**
Northern, Dr Jerry L **(A)**
Nuanes, Ladean **(SLP)**
Obert, Allan Dale **(A)**
Papilla, Mrs Minerva Windham **(SLP)**
Parkes, Jo Anne S **(SLP)**
Pautler, Rosemary D **(SLP)**
Pike, Patricia A **(SLP)**
Prescott, Dr Thomas E **(SLP)**
Pruet, Mrs Mary Montera **(SLP)**
Reis, Kathy S **(SLP)**
Riley, Deborah Schwied **(SLP)**
Riordan, Mrs Jean E **(SLP)**
Roberts, Linda Sobel **(SLP)**
Robinson, Maureen C **(SLP)**
Romano, Tina Lisa **(A)**
Roth, Mrs Tammy Buss **(SLP)**
Salamy, Jacque **(SLP)**
Salo, Rhonda Lee **(SLP)**
Sanborn, Barbara A **(SLP)**
Santivasi, Jill G **(SLP)**
Schaefer, Susan Brown **(SLP)**
Scharfenaker, Sarah Koehne **(SLP)**
Scherer, Dr Ronald C
Schock, Pamela Lynn **(SLP)**
Seagren, Mrs Jill C **(A)**
Selinger, Dr Marilyn **(SLP)**
Simone, Danielle **(SLP)**
Sinopoli, Terese Adele **(A)**
Smiderski, Sarah J **(SLP)**
Smith, Catherine M **(SLP)**
Smith, Janet G **(SLP)**
Sorensen, Pamela M **(SLP)**
Speirs, Jan Carol **(SLP)**
Spencer, Jodene
Spohn-Grall, Kelly Jeanne **(SLP)**
Stannard, Margaret K **(SLP)**
Steighner, Richard Lee **(A)**
Stockdale, Marianne Elizabeth **(SLP)**
Swallow, Barbara **(SLP)**
Takeshita, Mrs Marolyn K **(SLP)**
Teter, Darrel Lee **(SLP)**
Thomas, Celeste **(SLP)**
Thorn, Nancy Fae **(SLP)**
Ulrich, Paul D **(SLP)**
Van Dyke, Elizabeth Anne **(SLP A)**
Van Dyke, Linda M **(A)**
Vessels, Tina Helena **(SLP)**
Ward, Ellen W **(A)**
Warner, Joy C **(SLP)**
Weatherley-White, Dr R C A
Weber, Harold J **(A)**
Weiner, Mrs Barbara R **(SLP)**
Wempe, Mary Ruth **(SLP)**
Westfall, Michele Janine **(SLP)**
Weston, DiAnne P **(SLP)**
Wildhagen, Dwayne L **(A)**
Wilkie, Mary Ellen **(A)**
Wilson, Mrs Paula E B **(SLP)**
Witt, Eleanor B
Wright, Adrienne **(A)**
Zaversnik, Mrs Phyllis Robinson **(SLP)**

Dolores
Anderson, Mrs Maxine Ulyate **(SLP)**

Dumont
Pals, Mrs Marjorie E **(SLP)**

Durango
Dorr-Hendry, Janis **(A)**
Hendry, Carl John **(A)**
Keen, Mrs Joyce M **(SLP)**
Monger, Mrs Marilyn M **(SLP)**

Eaton
Allsup-Armstrong, Peggy **(SLP)**
Kehl, Cynthia Ann
Tryon, Ruth E K **(SLP)**

Edgewater
Bowsher, Robert B **(SLP)**

Elbert
Ferrer, Patricia McGowan **(SLP)**

Englewood
Abrams, Deborah Shanok **(SLP)**
Alderson, Mrs Carol Vagge **(SLP)**
Angelo, Mary Ann **(A)**
Arthur, Gail Wimp **(SLP)**
Barrow, Jeannette Carr **(SLP)**
Beighley, Nancy Ruttenberg **(SLP)**
Beiter, Anne L **(SLP A)**
Bohlen, Holly Heiser **(A)**
Brimacombe, Judith A **(A)**
Carroll, Dr Anne W **(SLP A)**
Childs, Mrs Barbara L **(SLP)**
Dart, Cheryl Bennett **(SLP)**
Dietz, Mrs Judith **(SLP)**
Edwards, Judith Shoemaker **(SLP)**
Emlen, Mrs Mary K **(SLP)**
Ernst, Trudy Eileen **(A)**
Ferrigno, Sharon J **(SLP)**
Florick, Wendy M **(SLP)**
Friebus, Maxine B **(SLP)**
Fudge, Mrs Linda Marlene **(A)**
Goodwin, Dr Patricia E **(A)**
Hansen, Mrs Terrilou **(SLP)**
Johnson, Mary Lou Brecht **(SLP)**
Kaufman, Glenda F **(SLP)**
Kaufmann, Linda B **(SLP)**
Kirton, Mrs Susan J **(SLP)**
Knuter, Lynnette M **(SLP)**
Kottenstette, Claire M **(SLP)**
Laycob, Carol L
Leiser, Mrs Jane Bronstien **(SLP)**
Lemon, Phyllis D **(SLP)**
Levy, Mrs Robyn K **(SLP)**
Mathiasen, Antoinette Tucker **(SLP)**
Mehlmann, Mrs Marybeth Ames **(SLP)**
Miller, Connie Jean **(SLP)**
Monroe, Patricia A **(SLP)**
Morse, Mrs Julie A A **(A)**
Mulhern, Margaret Dianne **(SLP)**
Murray, Elwood **(SLP)**
Nathan, Mrs Linda L **(SLP)**
Owen, Cynthia B **(A)**
Panasci, Mrs Nancy E **(SLP)**
Pierini, Mrs Carolyn Kuhn **(SLP)**
Purswell, Jeralyn K **(SLP)**
Rich, Mrs Joan Pedersen **(SLP)**
Ringger, Joy M **(A)**
Rittenberg, Mrs Susan Vincent **(SLP)**
Searles, Linda M **(SLP)**
Staller, Dr Steven J **(A)**
Tedesco, Mrs Karlyne A **(SLP)**
Van De Water, Sandra M **(A)**
Vaughters, Donna Mosher **(SLP)**
Wiley, Mrs Linda Chisholm **(SLP)**
Winthrop, Sandra J **(A)**

Erie
Chadwick, Carol **(SLP)**

Estes Park
Alexander, Nancy J **(A)**
Connelly, Mrs Elva A **(SLP)**
Knudson, Mrs Wendy K **(A)**
Lindell, Helen Alma
Spector, Mrs Diane J **(SLP)**
Vogt, Mrs Anne Christine **(SLP)**
Waldo, Mrs Lois Jean **(SLP)**

Evans
Davies, Cheryl Delight **(SLP)**

Evergreen
Anderson, Cheryl C **(SLP)**
Caleffe-Schenck, Nancy S **(A)**
Clinton, Kathy Lunstrum **(SLP)**
Larsen, Mrs Donna A **(SLP)**
Leue, Debra Ann **(SLP)**
Miller, Margaret A **(SLP)**
Robertson, Darlene M **(SLP)**
Roth, Jill G G **(SLP)**
Wezalis-Webber, Kathleen Mary **(SLP)**

Flagler
Smith, Mrs Charlotte **(SLP)**

Florence
Sazama, Melissa D **(SLP)**

Fort Carson
Moisan, Patricia Lee **(A)**

Fort Collins
Abkarian, G G **(SLP)**
Ackley, Robert S **(A)**
Bennett, Steven R **(SLP)**
Blomberg, Mrs Barbara A **(SLP)**
Brown, Suzanne Logan **(SLP)**
Bruxvoort, Evelyn Jo **(SLP)**
Burleigh, Andrew J **(A)**
Burleigh, Mrs Joan M **(SLP A)**
Cantrell, Mrs Susan Kay
Chonzena-Clark, Lareen K **(SLP)**
Cunningham, Peter Douglas **(A)**
Dickson, Jean **(SLP)**
Duffy, Dr Marjorie Richards **(SLP)**
Edgerton, Judith P **(SLP)**
Enell, Mark William
Ferguson, Mrs Ellen F **(SLP)**
Foos, Rhonda Kaye **(SLP)**
Friedlieb, Victoria Josephine **(SLP)**
Garretson, Lisa Durey **(SLP)**
Haden, Nedah L **(SLP)**
Hall, Cora Belle **(SLP)**
Hull, Mary E **(SLP)**
Julian, Mrs R Marlene **(SLP)**
Krappes, Mrs Teresa Kathleen **(SLP)**
Lanza, Carol K
Larimore, Dr Howard W **(SLP)**
Larsen, Joan Ellen **(SLP)**
Leidholt, Kathleen W **(SLP)**
Lentz, Dr William Edwin **(A)**
McLean, Shelle Donn **(A)**
McNab, Teresa Marie
Miles, Marcia C **(SLP)**
Miller, Mrs Kimberly Inez **(A)**
Mulford, Mrs Terri R **(SLP)**
Ostergren, Daniel Eugene, Jr **(A)**
Pacior, Brenda E **(SLP)**
Paleski, Tanya Elizabeth **(SLP)**
Parker, Anne Whitney **(SLP)**
Pendley, Ann Louise **(SLP)**
Peters, Ellen B **(SLP)**
Rodel, Michael J **(A)**
Romine, Mark Laurence
Rupp, Susan K **(SLP)**
Schaack, Anita L
Scholer, Sally E **(A)**
Skinner, Barbarba K **(A)**
Soraci, Mrs Lynne L **(SLP)**
Starling, Mrs Julia Mary
Swing, Mrs Melissa Dawn **(SLP)**
Traynor, Dr Robert M **(A)**
Walker, Penelope Rice **(SLP)**
Werner, Connie L **(SLP)**
West, Alisa Rich **(SLP)**
Willeford, Dr Jack Allen **(A)**

Fort Morgan
Gertge, Lynn Marie **(SLP)**

Fraser
Knudsen, Lisa Anne

Frisco
Steeves, Sherri Lee **(SLP)**

Fruita
Krebs, Mrs Ann Winn

Glenwood Springs
Burke, Terry L **(A)**
Mincer, Shelia Rae **(SLP)**
Saathoff, Mrs Susan L S **(SLP)**
Weitzenkorn, Mrs Patricia G **(SLP)**
Woerner, Wendy Lou **(A)**

Golden
Adams, Kathryn L **(SLP)**
Arndt, Donna K Morehead **(SLP)**
Asher, Margaret **(SLP)**
Ekberg, Judith W **(SLP)**
Gordon, Mrs Garnet Michelle **(SLP)**
Kepler, Laura Jennings **(A)**
Livingston, Mary Brace **(SLP)**
Mack-Hess, Mrs Joalyn Dawn **(SLP)**
Manninen, Jean L M **(SLP)**
McClelland, Linda G **(SLP)**
Mehring, Martha Jane **(SLP)**
Ratkiewicz, Brenda J **(A)**
Seymour, Deborah T **(SLP)**
Silver, J Diane **(SLP)**
Stellini, Mrs Deborah A **(SLP)**
Streit, Mrs Ann Ralsten **(SLP)**
Tauger, Susan M **(SLP)**
Thieme, Amy **(SLP)**

Grand Junction
Browne, Kelly Dolores **(SLP)**
Carbone, Mrs Susan P **(SLP)**
Duffey, Mrs Christine Polito **(SLP)**
Hagan, Adrienne J **(SLP)**
Kasper, Mrs Andrea G **(SLP)**
Keener, Christine Bebee **(SLP)**
Knackendoffel, Mrs Becky S **(SLP)**
Kolano, S Kay Wiseman **(SLP)**
Martin Ochsner, Deborah Ann **(SLP)**
Mealler, Mrs Jo-An Murch **(A)**
Neilsen, Amy Marie **(SLP)**
Olson, Rosalind **(SLP)**
Patrick, Sandra Lynn **(SLP)**
Pearlstein, Ruth Conis **(SLP)**
Prevett, Mrs Donna K **(SLP)**
Rouse, Mrs Lucy W **(SLP)**
Russell, Belinda Brooks **(SLP)**
Succo, Peter Jay **(A)**
Wilson, Donna Dene **(SLP)**
Worster, Mrs Peggy A

Greeley
Bartels, Mrs Jane Lennon **(SLP)**
Bottenberg, Dr Donna J **(SLP)**
Carey, Sharon L **(SLP)**
Chase, Tamara K
Cleeland, Linda K **(A)**
Connett, Mrs Nancy R **(SLP)**
Deconde-Johnson, Dr Cheryl **(A)**
Fields, Mrs Jody Thompson **(SLP)**
Fletcher, Deborah G **(SLP)**
Frankwick, Rita
Geary, Arlene Kopperud **(SLP)**
Gregg, Dr Ellen Meyer **(SLP)**
Griffith, Mrs Dawn Robertson **(SLP)**
Griffith, Dr Francis A **(SLP)**
Hanks, Julie McShane **(SLP)**
Hoff, Mrs Elaine D **(SLP)**
Hull, Dr Raymond H **(SLP A)**
Ingrisano, Dr Dennis R S **(SLP)**
Lamp, Mrs Gayle **(SLP)**
Littke, Jean M **(SLP)**
Lundeen, Dr Dale J **(SLP)**
McNear, Claire Tyrrell **(SLP)**
Meinke, Mrs Deanna Kay **(A)**
Miccio, Adele Whiting **(SLP)**
Neece, M Maxine **(SLP)**
Shotland, Dr Lawrence **(A)**
Sullivan, Barbara A **(SLP)**
Van Tine, Ruth H **(SLP)**
Weber, Jennifer E **(A)**
Wilcox, Patricia Sue **(SLP)**

Green Mountain Falls
Watson, Karen Savage **(SLP)**
Youngblood, Deborah S **(SLP)**

Gunnison
Blair, Mrs Shirley L **(SLP)**
Bramble, Mrs Margaret W **(SLP)**
Davenport, Dr Richard W **(SLP)**
Whiting, Mrs Nell E **(SLP)**

Haxtun
Gartin, Donna M R

Highlands Ranch
Cooney-Eickelman, Margaret Peggy **(SLP)**
Jessiman, Sherril Daun **(A)**
McJunkin, Leslie D **(A)**
Smith, Mrs Linda Emrich **(SLP)**
Soderlind, Mrs Isabel M **(SLP)**
Terrill, Mona C **(SLP)**
Whitman, Gail L **(SLP)**

Holyoke
Young, Ann M **(SLP)**

Hotchkiss
Carlson, Kathleen Sue **(SLP)**

Iliff
Lueck, Mrs Margaret F **(SLP)**

Indian Hills
Diedrich, Joan Marie **(SLP)**

Keenesburg
Gustafson, Mrs Brigitte Josi **(SLP)**

La Salle
Delafuente, Jose R **(SLP)**

Lafayette
Acimovic, Mary Lou **(SLP)**
Biegner, Laura Marie **(SLP)**
Guenther, Mrs Claudia Park **(SLP)**
Heublein, Elizabeth **(SLP)**

Lakewood
Adams, Amy L **(SLP)**
Bladow, Catherine Mary **(SLP)**
Brockmeier, Laura L **(SLP)**
Carter, Nanette E **(SLP)**
Coomes, Barbara Lynn
Cooper, Mrs Avis P **(SLP)**
Dawson, Mrs Susan H **(SLP)**
Fujioka, Carol A **(SLP)**
Gessini, Lisa J **(SLP)**
Gonzalez, Mrs Robin Tapp **(SLP)**
Gray, Mrs Sheila Ruth **(SLP)**
Gwinner, Debra Atkinson **(A)**
Hafner, Mary Beth **(SLP)**
Hahn, Mrs Carole Kravec **(SLP)**
Hiltenbrand, Marion G **(SLP)**
Hurd, Mrs Mary E **(SLP)**
Hurst, Kathleen M **(SLP)**
Kannenberg, Patricia C **(SLP)**
Konrath, Mrs Eileen Finucane **(SLP)**
Kovach, Therese M **(SLP)**
Lauter, Karen **(SLP)**
Lightfoot, Mrs Pamela S E **(SLP)**
Martin, Jannette J **(SLP)**
Merten, Dr Karol Kay **(SLP)**
Milane, Lynne A **(SLP)**
Nissen, Mrs Janet Siddens **(SLP)**
Perchacz, Teresa J **(SLP)**
Peters, Colleen Kay **(SLP)**
Petiya, Nancy Philips **(SLP)**
Pitcher-Fisher, Donna **(A)**
Pittenger, Mrs Gail S **(SLP)**
Potter, Cilinda G **(SLP)**
Pred, Dr Lynne B **(SLP)**
Smith, Lana Sue **(SLP)**
Swafford, Katherine **(SLP)**
Vick, Mrs Marianne U **(SLP)**
Wagner, Susan Kay **(SLP)**
Wilkinson, Mrs Esther Ruth **(SLP)**

Lamar
Beverly, Robin C **(SLP)**
Francis, Mrs Victoria Tramontano **(SLP)**

Larkspur
Knafelc, Valerie **(SLP)**

Limon
Hellwig, Robin Kay

Littleton
Allison, Mrs Frances T **(SLP)**
Andre, Susan L **(SLP)**
Arnold, Mrs Claire L **(SLP)**
Bagnall, Mrs Tracy Ann **(A)**
Bane, Mary J **(SLP)**
Barber, Mrs Ronda Joyce **(SLP)**
Berkowitz, Marjorie B **(SLP)**
Bland, Mrs Cheryl Ready **(SLP)**
Brant, Paula Rae **(SLP)**
Byrd, Mrs Mary Delamar **(SLP)**
Casey, Pauline Eilert **(SLP)**
Chaffee, Kim A **(SLP)**
Chamberlain, Lisa Lynn **(SLP)**
Curry, Genevieve Marie **(SLP)**
Dahlberg, Cynthia A **(SLP)**
Dethmers, Anna Ayers
Diederich, Jane B **(SLP)**
Dougan, Janet E **(SLP)**
Eberly, Mrs Teresa Yengich **(SLP)**
Esslinger-Heger, Robin E **(SLP)**
Fischer, Mrs Kathleen **(SLP)**
Frazier, Mrs Jacqueline Bolders **(SLP)**
Fry, Mrs Elizabeth **(SLP A)**
Fung, Mrs Thelma N **(SLP)**
Garb, Mrs Hildreth R **(SLP)**
Gerkin, Katherine Pike **(A)**
Gordan, Mrs Wenda L **(SLP)**
Hoffman, I Brenda **(SLP)**
Holder, Elizabeth **(SLP)**
Holtz, Mrs Pamela E **(SLP)**
Howard, Sherry H **(SLP)**
Jaeger, Sharon Elizabeth **(SLP)**
Jillson-Cook, Kathryn Dayle **(SLP)**
Kenna, Mrs Marcia Jo
King, Betty A M **(SLP)**
Korona, Karen Joyce **(SLP)**
Lemme, Dr Margaret L **(SLP)**
Lilley, Mrs Patricia Reed
Loeffler, Susanne Ellen **(SLP)**
Maloney, Mrs Beth Ann **(SLP)**
McElhaney, Paula R S **(SLP)**
Miller, Mrs Susan Matteson **(A)**
Preshaw, Linda Sue **(SLP)**
Preslan, Mrs Jacque Schmidt **(SLP)**
Puckey, Roberta M **(SLP)**
Quirico, Dorothy **(SLP)**
Schlueter, Sandra S **(SLP)**
Shipley, Kathryn Hendrick **(SLP)**
Silverstein, Jan W **(SLP)**
Silvestain, Carol B **(SLP)**
Smith, Donna M **(SLP)**
Souther, Mrs Nancy S **(SLP)**
Stewart, Judy **(SLP)**
Strange, Beth Arlene **(SLP)**
Stuebe, Mrs Sara C **(SLP)**
Swanson, Mrs Glenna **(SLP)**
Thomas, Patricia B **(SLP)**
Voyer, Carolyn R Folk **(SLP)**
Wallace, Dr Cynthia A **(SLP)**
Whitaker, Rebecca Schupbach **(SLP)**
White, Debra Lee **(A)**
Wilson, Mrs Rebecca A **(SLP)**
Zuck, Mrs Roberta Draper **(SLP)**
Zupan, Mrs Kathleen Lynn **(SLP)**

Livermore
Mahoney, Melanie **(A)**

Longmont
Artigliere, Julia Marie **(SLP)**
Bledsoe, Mrs Irma M **(SLP)**
Borkowski, Mrs Linda L **(SLP)**
Friesenborg, Laurie Ann **(SLP)**
Lake, Mrs Susan E **(SLP)**
McFarling, Mrs Faith Ann **(SLP)**
McKinley, Mrs Susan H **(SLP A)**
Miller, Dr Nancy L **(SLP)**
Mohr, Mrs Barbara A **(SLP)**
Moler, Sandra T **(SLP)**
Peterson, Mrs Beverly H **(SLP)**
Roberts, Christina Lee **(SLP)**
Schmunk, Mrs Linda M **(A)**
Schuetze, Bronwyn L **(SLP)**
Snyder, Mrs Beverly Jo **(A)**
Soman, Bonnie L **(SLP)**
Specht, Mrs Sally R **(A)**
Stewart, Ellen W **(SLP)**

Louisville
Baum, Mrs Sherry Ann **(SLP)**
Grant, Patricia Jude **(SLP)**
Ross, Lori Louise **(SLP)**
Shearer, Paulette B **(SLP)**
Snead, Nancy A S **(SLP)**
Stadjuhar-Watson, Mrs Karen G **(SLP)**
Thomson, Mrs Vickie Rae **(A)**

Loveland
Barron, Mrs Nancy J **(SLP)**
Cox-Willms, Carol C **(A)**
Davis, Polly Welty **(SLP)**
Einertson, Mrs Janice Loraine **(SLP)**
Nussbaumer, Mrs Carol W **(SLP)**
Patterson, Mrs Janet R **(SLP)**

Lyons
Branum, Mrs Cynthia **(SLP)**
Nellist, Susan Gay **(SLP)**

Manitou Springs
Shapiro, Mrs Barbara B **(SLP)**

Montrose
Godsey-Neubert, Jamie Kathryn **(SLP)**
Herr, Mrs Leslie C **(SLP)**
Stevenson, R Jeneine **(SLP)**

Monument
Kiernan, Susan C **(SLP)**
Smoot, Mrs Karen Marty **(SLP)**
Villere, Kathleen C **(SLP)**

Morrison
Hornbecker, Mrs Renee **(SLP)**
Moore, Joanna M **(SLP)**
Smith, Randall D **(SLP)**

Nederland
Nelson, Diana L G **(SLP)**

Northglenn
Buckler, Mrs Georgiana S **(SLP)**
Burke, Mrs Kathleen McVicar **(A)**
Myers, Robin Lynn **(SLP)**

Oak Creek
Hunera, Darlene T **(SLP)**

Palisades
Carter, Cleo Irene **(SLP)**
Slosson, Cynthia Worth **(SLP)**
Wigent, Michael Robert **(SLP)**

Paonia
Petersen, Mrs Pam R **(A)**

Parker
Barker, Mrs Mary Jean **(A)**
Kirk, Nancy C **(SLP)**
Rehling, Mrs Jan D **(SLP)**
Stuart, Debra M **(SLP)**
Watkins, Marla K **(SLP)**

Pueblo
Adams, Eleanor **(SLP)**
Ballantyne, Margaret Morgan **(SLP)**
Barickman, Barbara L **(SLP)**
Clark, Mona M **(SLP)**
Combs, Diana Sue **(A)**
Daugherty, Dale E **(A)**
Flipping, Joette Leslie **(SLP)**
Garrett, Barbara R B **(A)**
Hall, Rachelle Reines **(SLP)**
Hof, Catherine **(SLP)**
Keleher, Elizabeth Lee
Kuntz, Patricia A **(SLP)**
Martinez, Cecilia A **(SLP)**
Nelson, Kristin K **(SLP)**
O'Leary, Dr Emmett L **(SLP)**
Schoenmakers, Steve Dell **(SLP)**
Smith, Mrs Nancy A **(SLP)**
Squires, Ty Warren **(A)**
Stouffer, John **(SLP)**
Strait, Mrs Rose **(SLP)**
Stringert, Terese Dunlavy **(SLP)**
Williams, Laura Lynn **(SLP)**

Rangely
Miller, Andrea Sue **(SLP)**

Rifle
Chesley, Mrs Mary Kay **(SLP)**

Rocky Ford
Maxwell, Mrs Patricia **(SLP)**

Salida
Meythaler, Mrs Gwendolyn J **(SLP)**

Sedalia
Fockler, Mrs Victoria Gene **(SLP)**
Gulley, Mrs Barbara Ann **(SLP)**

Springfield
Larson, Katherine O'Neil **(A)**

Steamboat Springs
Burke, John R **(SLP A)**
Johnston-Rowland, Mary F **(SLP)**
Matson, Denise Kay **(SLP)**
Pfeiffer, Debra A **(SLP)**
Taliaferro, Mrs Sharon **(SLP)**

Sterling
Brunkhardt, Melinda Sue
Mertens, Debra Sue **(SLP)**
Stern, Meryl J **(SLP)**

Telluride
White, Mary Layden **(SLP)**

Thornton
Jacobson, Dr Edward J **(SLP A)**
Lay, Karen Susan
Martinson, Mrs Elizabeth **(SLP)**
McKamy, Mrs Vicky L W **(SLP)**
Molinski, Mrs Kathleen A **(SLP)**
Omafray, Mary Jo **(SLP)**
Potter, Cyndy O **(A)**
Vecchi, Melody Curphy **(SLP)**

USAF Academy
Cargo, Elizabeth A **(A)**

Vail
Duffy, Theresa Marie
Logan, Mrs Susan Anderson **(SLP)**

Wellington
Mizushima, Margaret **(SLP)**

Westminster
Bailey, Mrs Jill Anne **(SLP)**
Cyphers, Mrs Nancy W **(A)**
Durnford, Mrs Susan Elaine **(SLP)**
Elgart-Light, Candace **(SLP)**
Hepner, Mrs Sharon Doane **(SLP)**
Mason, Mrs Sharon Lee **(SLP)**
Ogrodnick, Patricia Ann **(SLP)**
Osterkamp, Mrs Kaye A **(SLP)**
Sundberg, Mrs Darleen H **(SLP)**
Windhausen, Perrian B **(SLP)**

Wheat Ridge
Darrow, Will T **(SLP)**
Heppe, Jo Anne T **(SLP)**
Reid, Carol A **(A)**

Wheatridge
Gillis-Cooper, Paulette Karen **(SLP)**
Rankin, Kristin Lee **(A)**

Woodland Park
Lundstrom, Sheila L **(SLP)**
Ostop, Mrs Janet L **(SLP)**

CONNECTICUT

Abington
Peacock, Mrs Judy H **(SLP)**

Andover
Carroll, Mrs Elaine M **(A)**
Desmone, Linda Few **(SLP)**
Garosshen, Mrs Cynthia B **(SLP)**

Ansonia
Baughn, Cynthia E **(SLP)**
Loda, Robert A **(SLP)**
Tredinnick, Amy Marie **(SLP)**

Avon
Buff, Mrs Judith S **(SLP)**
Gloth, Joanne B **(SLP)**
Monte, Denise Anne **(A)**
Osbourn, B Neil **(SLP)**
Parker, Christine **(SLP)**
Richilson, Mary Jane **(SLP)**

Beacon Falls
Moritz, Susan Ann

Bethany
Kaye, Mrs Arlene D **(SLP)**
Murdock-Abell, Roberta Ann **(SLP)**
Orzechowski, John, Jr **(SLP)**
Orzechowski, Kathleen M **(SLP)**
Simon, Mrs Marilyn C **(SLP)**

Bethel
Antanaitis, Robert J **(SLP)**
Atkinson, Mrs Lavonne Lynne **(SLP)**
Baird, Mrs Barbara H
Ehrlickman, Gail S **(SLP)**
Evans, Mrs Denise S **(SLP)**
Jankowski, Janet Marie **(SLP)**
Lakatos, Mrs Catherine **(SLP)**
Muller, Beth L F **(SLP)**

Bethlehem
Jacaruso, Mrs Maryanne Chesko **(SLP)**
Loucks, Sr Yvonne Mary **(SLP)**

Bloomfield
Boyle, Dr Thomas **(A)**
Cornell, Mrs Marcia **(A)**
Donatelli, Deborah Ann **(SLP)**
Needham, Alan C **(A)**
Reitman, Gail S **(SLP)**
Rutstein, Irving T **(SLP)**
Sandler, Steven J **(SLP)**
Way, Sheila A **(SLP)**

Branford
Babey, Lois J **(SLP)**
Chipkin, Mrs Linda B **(SLP)**
Everson, Mrs Cheryl Ann **(SLP)**
Farat, Mrs Mary MacDonald **(A)**
Green, Dr David S **(SLP A)**
Law, Elaine M **(SLP)**
Mobeck, Mrs Jeanette G **(SLP)**
Morris, Margaret Fraser **(SLP)**
Ridarelli, Susan L **(SLP)**
Romano, Grace Mary **(SLP)**

Bridgeport
Burton, Annette A **(A)**
Caldwell, Carol A **(A)**
Cherry-Cruz, Mrs Teresa Ann **(SLP)**
Corrigan, Mrs Cynthia Marie **(SLP)**
Foreman, Tryphena Hyacinth **(SLP)**
Grady, Elizabeth **(SLP)**
Herrick, Carol **(SLP)**
Leddo, John J **(SLP A)**
Strohmeyer, Linda J **(SLP)**
Tarnpoll, Judith M **(SLP A)**
Wotus, Maryann **(SLP)**

Bristol
Conrod, Mrs Jo Ann Bisignano **(SLP)**
Cronin, Mrs Nadine Merrihew **(SLP)**
Freimuth, Cynthia Anne **(SLP)**
Jung, Marjorie D **(A)**
Kasmer, Mrs Shelia H **(SLP)**
Knight, Kimberly K **(A)**
Knoegel, Mrs Roberta G **(SLP)**
Malavenda, Anthony **(SLP)**
Reade, Mrs Robin L **(SLP)**
Stoots, Mrs Sheri L **(A)**
Swenton, Mrs Gail P **(SLP)**

Broad Brook
Deffley, Monica Ann **(SLP)**

Brookfield
Calmels, Mrs Anne Trautmann **(SLP)**
Fraistat, Judith B **(SLP)**
Kane, Linda A **(SLP)**
McAleer, Patricia Kathleen **(SLP)**
Siciliano, Mrs Linda G **(SLP)**
Spencer, Leigh C **(SLP)**

Brookfield Center
Halek, Kathleen A **(SLP)**

Burlington
D'Angelo-Carley, Mrs Kathleen **(SLP)**
Malkin, Cheryl Felmus **(SLP)**
Sullivan-Shepard, Karen Marie **(SLP)**

Canton
Duran, Vicki Holbrook **(SLP)**

Centerbrook
Leach, Clifford J **(SLP)**

Chaplin
Chuk, Ann E **(SLP)**

Cheshire
Bauman, Dr Natan **(A)**
Bookbinder, Julia Dwyer **(SLP)**
Breeze, Christine **(SLP)**
Callow, Mrs Mary M **(SLP)**
Capozzi-Lombard, Mrs Lisa Marie **(SLP)**
Carley, Marvin E **(SLP)**
Chaback, Mrs Laurey W **(SLP)**
Cirmo, Mrs Nancy L **(SLP)**
Coelho, Dr Carl A **(SLP)**
Connor, Catherine John **(SLP)**
Eterginio, Richard M **(SLP)**
Fay-Coelho, Elaine **(SLP)**
Fiss-Zeiger, Ann V **(SLP)**
Gelb, Mrs Carol S **(A)**
Golymbieski, Lisa **(SLP)**
Jackson, Caroline R **(SLP)**
Landis, Lydia J **(SLP)**
Leder, Dr Steven B **(SLP)**
Moscato-Biondino, Mrs Paula **(SLP)**
Pearce, Beth Anne **(SLP)**
Penna, Mrs Joan Urniezus **(SLP)**
Pinkerton, Mrs Hope Leeger **(SLP)**
Rozak, Mrs Deanna Podhorn **(SLP)**
Tannenbaum, Madeline F **(A)**
Tardanico, Jamie McBride **(SLP)**

Chester
Steigleder, Susan Mane **(SLP)**

Clinton
Bowen, Beverly A **(SLP)**
Gluck, Nancy A **(SLP)**

Colchester
Kendzior, Laurel R **(SLP)**
Mellen, Mrs Mary Ellen **(SLP)**
Neri, Lorraine M **(SLP)**
Sandberg, Deborah Tavalaro **(SLP)**

Colebrook
Banas, Mrs Adele S **(SLP)**

Collinsville
Saidel, Susan M R **(SLP)**

Columbia
Hokanson, Mrs Joanne Marie **(SLP)**

Cornwall
Austin, Janet H **(SLP)**

Cos Cob
Chen, Josephine **(SLP)**
Dillon, Lorie Houston **(SLP)**
Weissman, Rita R **(SLP)**

Coventry
Covell, Mrs Jane Scory **(SLP)**
Platz, Janet A **(SLP)**
Pryce, Jane Watson **(A)**
Valot, Linda S **(SLP)**
Yiannakis, Linda Carol **(SLP)**

Cromwell
McMahon, Mrs Ann Carney **(A)**

Danbury
Akeson, Marcia L **(SLP)**
Connell, Mrs 0ARY S **(SLP)**
Friedman, Rochelle Z **(SLP)**
Hoban, Mrs Ann Marie **(SLP)**
McCall, Colleen K **(SLP)**
Merrer, Mrs Christine M **(SLP)**
Powell, Mrs Lynne S **(SLP)**
Ralabate, Mrs Patricia Kelly **(SLP)**
Salata, Marie E **(SLP)**
Seifert, Janet L
Shortsleeve, Mary **(SLP)**
Smith, Janet L **(SLP)**
Starman, Christine Joy **(SLP)**
Strenkert, Dr Nancy T **(SLP)**
Tepper, Arthur S **(A)**
Vanginderen-Wakeley, Ingrid **(SLP)**
Wolsch, Mrs Lois C **(SLP)**
Wolsch, Dr Robert A **(SLP)**

Danielson
Haney, Mary R **(SLP A)**
Mondor, Mrs Blair Gauthier **(SLP)**

Darien
Anderson, Mrs Marilynne Anne **(SLP)**
Armstrong, Charlotte Butterfield **(SLP)**
Hughes, Mrs Patricia M **(SLP)**
Melough, Mrs Nancy S **(SLP)**
Rhyne, Mrs Tina M **(SLP)**
Wald, Mrs Pamela M **(SLP)**

Dayville
Galante-Plucenik, Mrs Michelle E **(SLP)**

Deep River
Merlini, Mary Elizabeth **(SLP)**
Mosca, Susan Roy **(SLP)**

Derby
McInerney, Louise M **(SLP)**

Durham
Boylin, Catherine **(SLP)**
Frost-Gaffey, Mrs Jill **(A)**
Mekrut-Suzio, Mrs Joy M **(SLP)**

East Haddam
Woods-Viens, Mrs Elaine **(SLP)**

East Hampton
Bisantz, Jane L **(SLP)**
Gaffney, Mary Susan **(SLP)**

East Hartford
Corcoran, Kathie A **(SLP)**
Owens, Aljean H **(SLP)**
Rondino, Joyce A **(SLP)**
Schoen, Mrs Mary Stephanie **(SLP)**
Shervanian, Anna Ethel **(SLP)**

East Haven
Augustine, Russell Albert **(SLP)**
Avallone, Mrs Margaret T **(SLP)**
De Paolo, Kathleen M **(SLP)**
Ingersoll, Mary J **(SLP)**
Massini, Paula A
Rybacki, Mary-Jean **(SLP)**

East Lyme
Legg, Mrs Bonnie Kay **(SLP)**

East Norwalk
Wilson-Russell, Mrs Wendy **(SLP)**

Easton
Giannone, Toni L **(SLP)**
Rosenberg, Jacqueline **(SLP)**

Ellington
Boylan, James E **(SLP)**
Bymers, Susan **(SLP)**
Jury, Mrs Vernice Liljenberg **(SLP)**
Metty, Debra I **(SLP)**

Enfield
Brion, Jennifer Smith **(SLP)**
Curtis, Hillary
Holeman, Deborah A **(SLP)**

Essex
Graff, Lynn L **(SLP)**

Fairfield
Bender, Mrs Wendy E A **(SLP)**
Campbell, Mrs Ruby P **(SLP)**
Clarke, Mrs Susan M **(A)**
Curran, Mrs Kathryn Lambros **(SLP)**
Faulkner, Mrs Evelyn R **(SLP)**
Gill, Dr Alan Jay
Goodman, Deborah J **(SLP)**
Hannafey, Christine A **(SLP)**
Hermele, Mrs Jean O **(SLP)**
Jacke, Patti Jean **(A)**
Jennings, Mrs Carole S **(SLP)**
Joy, Patricia E **(SLP)**
Karpinski, Lauren Barbara **(SLP)**
Landsman, Carol D **(SLP)**
Laurent, Deborah
McGrath, Kim Irene **(A)**
Offeney, Sharon L **(SLP)**
Pipenur, Denise R **(SLP)**
Polley, Mrs Mary Ann Key **(SLP)**
Redler, Sherry P **(SLP A)**
Russo, Arlyne E **(SLP)**
Schneider, Dorothy E **(SLP)**
Silverstein, Cheryl Rita **(A)**
Teich, Mrs Linda B **(A)**

Falls Village
McGuire, Mrs Carole L K **(SLP)**

Farmington
Butterfield, Mrs Ann Fickes **(SLP)**
Dobkin, Ceil K **(SLP)**
Groob, Mrs Lisa S **(SLP)**
Hayford, Donna S **(SLP)**
Jordan, Annemarie H **(SLP)**
Kane, Mrs Angela Marie **(SLP)**
Knudsen, Karen E **(SLP)**
Levine, Mrs Arlene Greneman **(SLP)**
Mulpeter, Virginia A **(SLP)**
Papp, Mrs Nancy E **(SLP)**
Rhodes, Linda T **(SLP)**
Schloss, Sharon Merker **(SLP)**
Stern, Cynthia Billian **(SLP)**

Forestville
Rosenblatt, Judith E **(SLP)**
Smythe, Linda T **(SLP)**

Gales Ferry
Jones, Mrs I Terry **(SLP)**
Schnur, Mrs Jane R **(SLP)**
Schnur, Dr Marvin R **(SLP)**
Theo, Kathleen Johnson **(SLP)**
Ulrich, Sandra R **(SLP)**
Vanwey, Linda W **(SLP)**

Glastonbury
Abrams, Mrs Ellen J **(SLP)**
Bacolini, Paula **(SLP)**
Bartlett, Susan E **(SLP)**
Edwards, Mrs Susan S **(SLP)**
Farrell, Jeanne Nicole **(A)**
Firestone, Mrs Lynn M **(A)**
Jamroga, Elizabeth **(SLP)**
Lukas, Margaret Kay **(SLP)**
May, Suzanne J **(SLP)**
Newman, Mrs Diana B **(SLP)**
Pearson, Mrs Karen L **(SLP)**
Powell, Lynn E **(SLP)**
Schwartzkroin, Gail M **(SLP)**
Twachtman, Diane D **(SLP)**
Tyczkowski, Mrs Barbara **(SLP)**
Wallace, Debra S **(SLP)**

Goshen
Herman, Evelyn M **(SLP)**

Granby
Barberino, Mrs Lorraine E **(SLP)**
Fahan, Linda MacKay **(SLP)**
Kelly, Mrs Claudia M **(SLP)**

Greenwich
Balmuth, Stacy Brucker **(A)**
Berk, Mrs Barbara B **(SLP)**
Goldschmid, Mrs Leslie S **(SLP)**
Henniges, Marian P **(A)**
Hiles, Mrs Mary O **(SLP)**
Skorney, Debra A **(A)**
Stillman, Gail Y **(SLP)**
Vitale, Mrs Joyce D **(SLP)**
Watts, Mrs Mary Clifford **(A)**
Wischner, Mrs Sary K **(SLP)**

Groton
Ahearn, Barbara Lynne **(SLP)**
Colgan, Karen Koudal **(SLP)**
Lefker, Madeleine Sherwood **(SLP)**
Marshall, Dr Lynne **(A)**
Tobias, Dr Jerry V
Tuneski, Mrs Jean Pepin **(A)**

Groton Long Point
Sergeant, Dr Russell L **(SLP)**

Guilford
Bulakites, Mrs Debra L **(SLP)**
Canny, Rickie Ann **(SLP)**
Granger, Mrs Eileen R **(SLP)**
Ketaineck, Mrs Francie E **(SLP)**
Lund, Mrs Carrol G **(SLP)**
Megargee, Mary Eigler **(SLP)**
Ricci, Paula Ann **(SLP)**
Rosenzweig, Luann B **(SLP)**
Sills, Mrs Margaret S **(SLP)**

Hamden
Bader, C Sarah **(SLP)**
Beaudette, Paula A **(SLP)**
Bergamini, Mrs Marcia Higney **(SLP)**
Bicknell, Mrs Gertrude L **(SLP)**
Bolton, Kathleen **(SLP)**
Bossenberry, Julie **(A)**
Cade, Elisabeth L
Casso, Thomas, Jr **(SLP)**
Cutler, Cheryl Ellen **(SLP)**
D'Alessio, Linda J **(A)**
Dardick, Leila R **(SLP)**
Donohue, Mrs Helen Shay **(SLP)**
Eldrich, Civia Reich **(SLP)**
Giffin, Frances E **(SLP)**
Goldberg, Donald R **(SLP)**
Gross, Carl David **(SLP)**
Held, Roberta J **(SLP)**
Herd, Mrs Carol H **(SLP)**
Highsmith, Mrs Deborah A **(SLP)**
Jamron, Susan Carol
King, Carolyn V **(SLP)**
Kopff-Schaefer, Helen L **(SLP)**
Kosowsky, Alice Puchalsky **(SLP)**
Levitan, Tamar K **(SLP)**
Matteo, Jo-Anne B **(SLP)**
Morton, Mrs Betty Jean **(SLP)**
Mowry, Lisa Jeannine **(SLP)**
Oltzik-Ladin, Mrs Barbara **(SLP)**
Paier, Susan Barbara **(A)**
Reich, Mrs Janet Riggan **(SLP)**
Saportin, Charlene T **(SLP)**
Smith, Nancy Jean **(SLP A)**
Toren, Linda R **(SLP)**
Waxman, Ilene A **(SLP)**
Weber, Barbara S **(SLP)**
Zirlen, Mrs Adrienne **(SLP)**

Hartford
Campbell, Kristen E **(SLP)**
Carroll, Jane E **(SLP)**
Cook, Sandra **(SLP)**
Cormier, Carolann Marie **(SLP)**
Lampe, Henrica C **(SLP)**
Melnick, Beth K **(SLP)**
Perez, Juan M **(SLP)**
Smith, Dr Norma D **(SLP)**
Turner, Brenda A **(SLP)**
Weir, Clara B **(SLP)**

Harwinton
Fields, Mrs Marjorie R
Taylor, Linda J B **(SLP)**

Hebron
Maio-Duffy, Maureen E **(SLP)**
Mogensen, Mrs Mary Beringer **(SLP)**

Higganum
Hewitt, Pamela Rose **(SLP)**
Nagler, Mrs Janie D **(SLP)**

Huntington
Breuer, Wanda R **(SLP)**
Giovanetti, Laura T **(SLP)**
Latino, Susan B **(SLP)**
Tucker, Mrs Phoebe Simons **(SLP)**

Jewett City
Lathrop, Mrs Debra C **(SLP)**

Kensington
Grant, Martha Zadrozny **(SLP)**
Polgroszek, Mrs Beverly B **(SLP)**

Kent
Kahrs, Sharon Girardey **(SLP)**

Killingworth
Hunsicker, Deborah Jane **(SLP)**

Lebanon
Horan-Senechal, Mary Catherine **(SLP)**

Ledyard
Hans, Jay C **(A)**
Hausmann, Joan B **(SLP)**
Jaworski, Sandra Ann
McLaughlin, Karen Neilan **(SLP)**
Sandman, Sharon Elizabeth **(SLP)**
St Rock, Kathleen A **(SLP)**

Litchfield
Meyer, Judith A **(SLP)**

Lyme
Delisa, Diana C **(A)**

Madison
Burdick, Mrs Edythe O **(SLP)**
Duques, Wendy Bowden **(SLP)**
Goodman, Mrs Mona B **(SLP)**
Gosin-Lynch, Barbara R **(SLP)**
Harrigan, Christine **(SLP)**
Keating, Maryann Pozycki **(SLP)**
McGlinchey, Kathleen S **(SLP)**
Ressler, Jane E **(SLP)**

Manchester
Donovan, Donna M **(SLP)**
Griffin, Eileen Leahy **(SLP)**
Laidig, Margaret Anne **(SLP)**
Maury, Cynthia Ann **(SLP)**
Mazur, Mrs Barbara P **(SLP)**
Moore, Mrs Lynda S **(SLP)**
Persico, Dena **(SLP)**

Robert, Alice C **(SLP)**
Stebbins, Willard P **(SLP)**

Mansfield
Bishop, Candace H **(SLP)**

Mansfield Center
Dunham, Janet L **(SLP)**
Maxon, Dr Antonia Brancia **(A)**
Randolph, Dr Karin M **(SLP)**
Randolph, Dr Kenneth J **(A)**

Mansfield Depot
McLaughlin, Donna C **(A)**

Marlborough
Duff, Lynn A Bampton **(SLP)**
Passacantando, Mrs Janice Elaine **(SLP)**

Meriden
Barillaro, Mrs Judith Ann **(SLP)**
Dominello, Anne Marie **(SLP)**
Dominello, Matthew C, Jr **(SLP)**
Durr, Mrs Karen Breininger **(SLP)**
Kumnick, Mrs Laurie C **(SLP)**
Morse, Diantha **(SLP A)**
Ostby, Karen J **(SLP)**
Przywara, Mrs Kathy I **(SLP)**
Rutt, Diane E
Sasso, Laraine M **(SLP)**
Uryase, Deborah **(SLP)**
Wyskiel, Mrs Debra MacKenzie **(SLP)**

Middlebury
Albanese, Susan Gillis **(SLP)**
Zackin, Mrs Roselyn F **(SLP)**

Middletown
Cragin, Mrs Elizabeth Papiro
Darrow, Mrs Mary Ann M **(SLP)**
Dunn, Avery E W **(SLP)**
Howard, Eleanor W **(SLP)**
Katten, Mrs Laurie **(SLP)**
Kiernan, Robert Leddy, Jr **(SLP)**
Lyman-McCann, Mrs Janet M **(SLP)**
McDermott, Mrs Rita P **(SLP)**
McIntyre, Rebecca J **(SLP)**
Moran, Catherine Ann **(SLP)**
Roeder, Mrs Sharon L **(SLP)**
Zirlen, David Michael **(SLP)**

Milford
Algiere, Elaine Catherine **(SLP)**
Brownsberger, Susan L **(SLP)**
Casey, Mrs Helen M **(SLP)**
Colliton, Kathleen Ann **(SLP)**
Cutler, Michelle J **(SLP)**
Dotson, Kimberley Wray **(A)**
Estabrook, Mrs Elizabeth T **(SLP)**
Kaufman, Mrs Carol M **(SLP)**
Kimberly, Pamela Silva **(SLP)**
Lippman, Mrs Leslie Gaye **(SLP)**
Lukas, Patricia A
McNamara, Kevin Michael **(SLP)**
McVay, Robyn **(SLP)**
Miller, Mrs Maureen A **(A)**
Mitaly, Mrs Barbara J **(SLP)**
Moretz, Mrs Linda P **(SLP)**
Mountzouris, Christine Farakos **(SLP)**
Murray, Mrs Leslie Tishler **(SLP)**
Newton, Mrs Kathryn K **(SLP)**
Silver, Mrs Roberta A Lotreck **(SLP)**
Villani, Christine **(SLP)**

Milldale
Lapierre, Rhonda Irion **(SLP)**

Moodus
English, Susan Hollister **(SLP)**

Mystic
Dyslin, Mrs Margery M **(SLP)**
Hanson-Schade, Kathleen M **(SLP)**
Maclone, Michael John **(A)**
Robertson, Margaret Alexandra **(SLP)**
Talbot, Catherine **(SLP)**

Naugatuck
Kirdzik, Constance B **(SLP)**
Klawiter, Mrs Pamela Sue **(SLP)**
Lapidge, Barbara L **(SLP)**
Vargoshe, Mrs Barbara J **(SLP)**

New Britain
Adams, Susan L **(SLP)**
Bingham, Donna G **(SLP)**
Cole, Mrs Irma J **(SLP)**
Friday, Mrs Kathleen MacElroy
Leibowitz, Mrs Martha Sue **(SLP)**
Lernihan, Andrea Joyce **(SLP)**
Mancino, Diane Marie **(SLP)**
Mostoller, Theresa Keating
O'Connell, Mrs Susan D **(SLP)**
Owen, Elizabeth A **(SLP)**
Pecora, Jolanta M **(A)**

New Canaan
Coleman, Mrs Diana Blachly **(SLP)**
Dinan, Mrs Shelley **(SLP)**
Dolan, Ann Goyda **(SLP)**
Dwenger, Mrs Sandra G **(SLP)**
Goldblatt, Mrs Judith A **(SLP)**
Gravel, Dr Judith S **(A)**
Karger, Vera V **(SLP)**
Keepnews, Susan B **(SLP)**
Squitieri, Elena **(SLP)**

New Fairfield
Jacobs, Mrs Arleen G **(SLP)**
Joram, Mary Fazzino **(SLP)**
Klages, Mrs Catherine **(SLP)**
Plevan, Mrs Janet C **(SLP)**

New Hartford
Charest, Mrs Linda R **(SLP)**
Deschenes-Desmond, Mrs Anita **(SLP)**

New Haven
Altro, Moira O'Neill **(SLP)**
Alfonso, Dr Peter J **(SLP)**
Bailey, Beryl Irene
Bloom, Andrea **(SLP)**
Brancato, Elizabeth Ann **(SLP)**
Bynum-Welfare, Mrs Harriett Lettitia **(SLP)**
Celotto, Janet **(SLP)**
Cole, Mrs Sarah **(SLP)**
Cooper, Dr Franklin S
Coppola, Valarie A **(SLP)**
Cozean, Mrs Jeanne Marie **(SLP)**
Ellis, H Sherrill
Engel, Alida **(SLP)**
Eule, Mrs Althea Marshall **(SLP)**
Evans, Brian J **(SLP)**
Fischer, Mary L **(SLP)**
Flynn, Barry James **(SLP)**
Gadsden-Lopez, Wanda Lenore
Glenn, Larry E **(SLP)**
Hindenlang, Jane E **(SLP)**
Holley, Dr Sandra C **(SLP)**
Honigman-Hellman, Mrs Sharon Ann
Horowitz, Hilda L **(SLP)**
Kelly, Jody Goggins **(SLP)**
Lipin, Bernard **(A)**
Loos-Cosgrove, Margaret Myriah **(SLP)**
Marans, Wendy Dalton **(SLP)**
Miller, Seth Bruce **(SLP)**
Morrow, Rose A **(SLP)**
Nicol, Mrs Lori Sue **(SLP)**
Rakfeldt, Mrs Kristi R **(SLP)**
Rini, Mrs Denise L **(SLP)**
Ruby, Josephine R **(SLP)**
Sansone, Dr Frank E, Jr **(SLP)**
Schiaroli, Kathryn Ada
Schwartz, Arlene Randy **(SLP)**
Selden, Mrs Deborah Holston **(SLP)**
Shachar-Hill, Susan Cogan **(SLP)**
Stoll, Bernard **(SLP)**
Story, Mrs Robin Seider **(SLP)**
Sussman, Anita Jones **(SLP)**
Tate, David Michael **(SLP)**
Thompson, Jo Anne **(SLP)**
Umansky-Sokol, Debra **(SLP)**
Walter, Judith Marie **(SLP)**
Weimer, Mary Margaret **(SLP)**
Weisslender, Mrs Diane P **(SLP)**

New London
D'Huy, Kathy Ann **(SLP)**
Maclone, Mrs Nancy E L **(SLP)**
Marven, Elaine Maria **(SLP)**
Trostler, Nancy J **(A)**
Valentine, Cynthia Birdsall **(SLP)**
Worgul, Jeffrey W **(A)**

New Milford
McGrath, Mrs Christine **(SLP)**
Natale, Janet Sue **(SLP)**
Pelliciari, Thomas A **(SLP)**
Purcell, Mrs Laura Kelley **(SLP)**

Newington
Anthony, Karen Jane **(SLP)**
Beveridge, Lynn Ruth **(SLP)**
Bonino, Joanne O **(SLP)**
Brown, Mrs Judith Ann **(SLP)**
Deranleau, Madeleine T **(SLP)**
Haddad, Layth Nadim **(SLP)**
Harvey, Mrs Maresa M **(SLP)**
Krutt, Susan Sidranksy **(A)**
McMillen, Malcolm E **(SLP)**
Paterno, Melissa Anne
Saunders, Zane G **(SLP)**
Schneider, Bonnie S **(A)**
Swanson, Mrs Martha B **(SLP)**

Newtown
Burak-Bertram, Virginia **(SLP)**
Gates, Mrs Karen S **(A)**
Keane, Mrs G Marie **(SLP)**

Niantic
Davis, Mrs Patricia A **(SLP)**
Doyle, Mrs Karen Crocker
Havens, Richard M **(A)**
Raymond, Mrs Debra Sue **(SLP)**
Turner, Sherry B **(SLP)**

Noank
Barron, David Pitt **(SLP A)**
Covin, Regina R **(SLP)**
Rathbun, Evelyn Kowalysyn **(SLP)**

Norfork
Baldwin, Virginia H **(SLP)**

North Branford
Calvo, Raymond J **(SLP)**
Golod, Mrs Camille Dedomenico **(SLP)**
Jauernig, Mrs Joan R **(SLP)**
Mirakian, Barbara Y **(SLP)**
Watrous, Marie-Beth

North Canaan
Viafore, Mrs Joyce S **(SLP)**

North Granby
Chiocca, Barbara J **(SLP)**

North Haven
Booker, Denise M **(SLP)**
De Poto, Mrs June M **(A)**
Gormley, Mrs Patricia Teggi **(SLP)**
Huttner, Mrs Sharon G **(SLP)**
Landino, Daniel **(SLP)**
Soriano, Deborah Ann **(SLP)**
Spose, Mrs Beth Ann **(SLP)**

North Stonington
Carlson, Mrs Elaine C **(A)**
Rich, Mrs Gay Dingman **(SLP)**

Northfield
Lynn, Mrs Elizabeth A **(SLP)**
Lynn, William M **(SLP)**

Northford
Kos-Flanagan, Mrs Stephanie Jo

Norwalk
Adair, Sharon **(SLP)**
Brooks, Roberta L **(SLP)**
Cascella, Paul W **(SLP)**
Copeland, Mrs Mary Hammond **(SLP)**
Cuttner, Nancy Kratzer **(SLP)**
Dell, Katherine **(SLP)**
Faugno, Joanne M **(SLP)**
Fors, Karen A **(SLP)**
Green-Tucknall, Margaret Ann
Gunnip, Debra **(SLP)**
Hartzer, Mrs Linda Egener **(SLP)**
Jeffery, Mrs Karin L **(SLP)**
Jones, Bronwen L **(A)**
Kaczmarek, Monica Carin **(SLP)**
Lettko, Mrs Carol Shearer **(SLP)**
Liljeqvist, Christine **(SLP)**
Ristau, Mrs Elizabeth S **(SLP)**
Sneider, Mrs Cecile D **(SLP)**
Strunin, Bonnie H **(SLP)**
Wald, Lisa Tuchman **(SLP)**

Norwich
Botchis, Mrs Gloria **(SLP)**
Combs, Mrs Deborah Jean
Davey, Mrs Terry Kay **(SLP)**
Etra, Joel L **(SLP)**
Gill, Mrs Cynthia Davis **(SLP)**
Heely, Mary Archibald **(SLP)**
Landry, Mrs Anne Ligocki **(SLP)**
Middel, Mrs Lori Ann **(SLP)**
Mussler, J James **(A)**
Schnip, Barbara S **(SLP)**
Starr, Mrs Lee Anne M **(SLP)**
Stockton, Karen D **(A)**
Ziko, Connie Allen **(SLP)**

Oakdale
Mellisy, Carolyn R **(SLP)**
Winkler, Mrs Marcia B **(SLP)**

Oakville
Kisatsky, Thomas J **(SLP A)**
Masayda, Barbara Lynn **(SLP)**

Old Greenwich
Lorenzut, Mrs Geraldine **(A)**
Schiff-Myers, Dr Naomi B **(SLP)**

Old Lyme
Danenberg, Mary A **(SLP)**
Phelan, Katherine A **(SLP)**
Schaaf, Mrs Jeanne Dolph **(SLP)**

Orange
Baumgarten, Mrs Rachel Bazant
Bell, Walter J **(SLP)**
McGowan, Margaret M **(SLP)**
Overchuk, Cynthia Lynne
Sinclair, Kathleen E **(SLP)**
Spiewak, Lauren N **(SLP)**
Walls, Mrs Nancy F **(SLP)**

Oxford
Bachyrycz, Mrs Jayne J **(SLP)**
Kostka, Mrs Candice E **(SLP)**
Lynn, Anne H **(A)**
Sokol, Mrs Mary G **(SLP)**

Pawcatuck
Hewson, Sara A **(SLP)**
O'Connor, Constance **(SLP)**

Plainfield
Marchesseault, Marie Ann **(SLP)**
Stephen, Mrs Patricia McShane **(SLP)**

Plainville
Reiss, Debra Elizabeth **(SLP)**

Plantsville
Burns, Janet Pasteris **(SLP)**
Lyon, Mrs Maureen C **(SLP)**

Pomfret Center
Danielson, Holly L **(SLP)**

Portland
Boske, Mrs Laurie J S **(SLP)**
Malecky, Susan M **(SLP)**

Spencer, Loretta B **(SLP)**

Preston
Wheeler, Mrs Lisa B

Prospect
Schain, Mrs Judith W **(SLP)**

Quaker Hill
Spence, Mrs Lee Ann M **(SLP)**

Quinebaug
Hebert, Michele A **(SLP)**
Krogul, Mrs Valerie A **(SLP)**

Redding Ridge
Nurin, Marabeth W **(SLP)**

Ridgefield
Bier, Barbara N **(SLP)**
Budweiser, Mrs Judith D **(SLP)**
Doidge, Mary C Bayer **(SLP)**
Dolan, Cormack J **(SLP)**
Edley, Carol D **(SLP)**
Falzone-Mangone, Maryellen **(SLP)**
Hackman, Mrs Lesley J **(SLP)**
Hudson, Tracy L **(SLP)**
Lodewick, Mrs Christine Lobeck **(SLP)**
Maneri, Mrs Marilyn S **(SLP)**
McDonald, Patricia Marie
Nayor, Mrs Rhoda A **(A)**
Peraino, Madonna Katherine **(SLP)**
Sturges, Mrs Patricia Mazza **(SLP)**
Truxler, Joan E **(SLP)**
Weingast, Mrs Beatrice M **(SLP)**
Wilkinson, Glenna S N **(SLP)**
Young, Anne E **(SLP)**

Riverside
Barshop-Molberger, Jill E **(SLP)**
Friedman, Mrs Ann D **(SLP)**
Thomas, Mrs Sylvia S **(SLP A)**

Riverton
Heasley, Frederick H **(SLP)**

Rockville
Doffek, Mrs Margaret A **(SLP)**
Gottier, Mrs Daryl-Lynne K **(SLP)**
Schoen-Rene, Mrs Patricia Anne **(SLP)**

Rocky Hill
Boyko, Robin K **(SLP)**
Delconte, Laurie Ann
Gash, Mrs Allyson D **(SLP)**
Janusko, Mrs Claudia Ripinski **(A)**
Kelly, Janet Anne **(SLP)**
Liss-Bronstein, Linda **(SLP)**
Radin, Mrs Hyla Beth **(SLP)**
Rischall, Mrs Cindy E **(SLP)**
Smiley, Ann M **(SLP)**

Rowayton
Rambusch, Mrs Nancy-Jo Geiger **(SLP)**

Salem
Bateman, Mrs Julie **(SLP)**
Kennedy, Mrs Marianne D **(SLP)**

Sandy Hook
Nelson, Mrs Patricia S **(SLP)**
Shanahan, Mrs Denise Kotyk **(SLP)**

Seymour
Doyle, Jane Seymour **(SLP)**
Hauburger, Janice Raineault **(SLP)**
Herne, Mrs Robin Mirante
Johns-Elmy, Mrs Lisa Anne
Rhodes, Rebecca Sue **(SLP)**

Shelton
Beck, Mrs Blanche F **(SLP)**
Goldstein, Mrs Francene C **(SLP)**
Lazarus, Mrs Barbara A **(SLP)**
Passaro, Mrs Nancy J **(SLP)**
Pennell, Connie R **(SLP)**
Sochrin, Mrs Phyllis L **(SLP A)**

Simsbury
Berke, Mrs Lisa A **(SLP)**
Coster, Mrs Judianne Longfield
Cote, Mrs Janet Marion **(SLP)**
Defrancesco, Mrs Joyce M **(SLP)**
Kerrigan, Mrs Janet B **(SLP)**
Lescher, Mrs Ellen B **(SLP)**
Mule, Lisa Nystrom **(SLP)**
Munroe, Susan Bessette **(SLP)**
Piehl, Mrs Ann G **(A)**
Salzberg, Beth Friedman
Sargent, Mrs Irene **(SLP)**
Sylvan, Susan K **(SLP)**
Walsh, Mrs Elizabeth **(SLP)**
Williams, Victoria L **(SLP)**

Somers
Butler, Barbara Ann **(SLP)**
Caravella, Mrs Yvonne L **(SLP)**

South Kent
Johnson, Adele S **(SLP)**

South Killingly
Gubernat, Laura A **(SLP)**

South Windsor
Chun, Raquel Ortiz **(SLP)**
De Rosa-Lukach, Patricia Ann **(SLP)**
Doherty, Karen
Eduardo, JoAnn L **(SLP)**
Eisenberg, Judith Faith **(SLP)**
Fanning, Mrs Lucretia **(SLP)**
Gore, Donna R **(SLP)**
Griffith, Mrs Gail S **(SLP)**
Heikoff, Raisa Ann
Hermes, Estelle L **(SLP)**
Jachym, Mrs Jane A **(SLP)**
Kerensky, Nancy A **(SLP)**
McKnerney, Lorraine **(SLP)**
Schneider, Mrs Sandra S **(SLP)**
Sloate, Mrs Meryl H **(SLP)**
Starr, Mrs Marilyn W **(SLP)**
Thomas, Mrs Carol L **(SLP A)**
Weller, Patricia Blaisdell **(SLP)**

Southbury
Alex, Cathleen A **(A)**
De Voe, Anne S **(SLP A)**
Dumoch, Mrs Amy M **(SLP)**
Hibbard, Mrs Marybeth Kemp **(SLP)**
Kippur, Mrs Mary Scharpf **(SLP)**
Lord, Kathleen M **(SLP)**
Olliver, Jodie Eileen **(SLP)**
Perriello, Elizabeth M **(SLP)**
Ramsey, Mrs Barbara A **(SLP)**
Wenger, Mrs Linda Bernhardt **(SLP)**
Witham, Richard F **(SLP)**

Southington
Carabetta, Mrs Denise Donovan **(SLP)**
Fors, Mrs Sarah Drake **(SLP)**
Glass, Mrs Lori Waldo **(SLP)**
Jesudowich, Mrs Barbara W **(SLP)**
Kania, Mrs Eileen S **(SLP)**
Lees, Andrew B **(SLP)**
Massucci, Ellen Marie **(SLP)**
Mattie, Mrs Linda Larosa **(SLP)**
Merriman, Ronda Gaita **(SLP)**
Niezgorski, Mrs Angela **(SLP)**
Rubano, Mrs Nancy G **(SLP)**
Schmittgens, Jane T **(SLP)**
Zita, Jan

Southport
Artemenko, Sherry Younger **(SLP)**
Messinger, Maris S **(SLP)**
Waldron, Maybette Z **(SLP)**
Wulf, Ellen M **(SLP)**

Stafford Springs
Fers, Mrs Therese **(SLP)**
McDuffee, Mrs Cynthia Delores **(A)**
Pallanck, Patricia Gregorio **(A)**

Stamford
Alberti, Deborah Ann **(SLP)**
Aronin, Meryl W **(SLP)**
Bailey, Pauline G **(A)**
Bollard, Dr Priscilla Eaves **(SLP A)**
Bush, Margaret S **(SLP)**
Callahan, Rosemary E **(SLP)**
Cariri, Benjamin A **(SLP)**
Cariri, Mrs Marilyn W **(SLP)**
Erichson, Mrs Elaine G **(SLP)**
Farber, Mrs Karen S **(SLP)**
Feder, Mrs Karen S **(SLP)**
Fillinger-Kraus, Francine **(SLP)**
Gordon, Mrs Adele B **(SLP)**
Greenman, Denise A **(SLP)**
Harris, Mrs Mary Helen **(SLP)**
Hornlein, Rita H **(SLP)**
Kalter, Mrs Carol Cepler **(SLP)**
Kanter, Mrs Carol S **(SLP)**
Kirschblum, Mrs Elyse K **(A)**
Kolbrenner, Mrs Susan G **(SLP)**
Lane, Mrs Lynne S **(SLP)**
Lipsitz, Mrs Margaret A **(SLP)**
MacKenzie, Vicki **(SLP)**
Means, Sharon H **(SLP)**
Nass, Mrs Susan Simpson **(SLP)**
Osta, Norma Kalil **(SLP)**
Perez, Mrs Aldana S **(SLP)**
Prabhudas, Jayne M **(SLP)**
Rakowitz, Mrs Julie C **(SLP)**
Roth, Mrs Harriet T **(SLP)**
Rothman, Mrs Gayle Hannah **(SLP)**
Sabia, Mrs Sharon A **(SLP)**
Seelig, Mrs Renee Cohen **(SLP)**
Sichel, Mrs Ronnie N **(SLP)**
Slaine, Mrs Joan Shearer **(SLP)**
Stark, Lois D **(SLP)**
Stein, Mrs Louise I **(SLP)**
Suchow, Linda Beth **(A)**
Tyler, Mrs Jeanne R **(SLP)**
Voroba, Jane S **(SLP)**

Stonington
Butterworth, Mrs Kathleen Marie **(SLP)**
Fort, Mary K **(SLP)**
Robinson, Mrs Janet E **(SLP)**

Storrs
Abramson, Dr Arthur S
Birkenruth, Mrs Honore H **(SLP)**
Cohen, Dr Marion F **(A)**
Demars, Sally S **(SLP)**
Duffy, Dr Robert J **(SLP)**
Giolas, Marilyn H **(A)**
Giolas, Dr Thomas G **(A)**
Goldberg, Dr Donald M **(SLP A)**
Hogan, Nicholas **(SLP)**
Jordan, Janet W **(SLP)**
Lerman, Dr Jay William **(SLP)**
Liles, Dr Betty Zoe **(SLP)**
Lynch, Onita C **(A)**
McLaughlin, Joseph G **(SLP)**
Oxman, Barbara Louise **(SLP)**
Paesani, Andrew, Jr **(SLP)**
Ross, Mrs Helen **(SLP)**
Ross, Dr Mark **(A)**
Stone, Mrs Maryalice **(SLP)**
Weiss, Deborah M **(SLP)**

Stratford
Beatty, Lizabeth Mary **(SLP)**
Bryant, Gretchen R **(SLP)**
Codeghini, Donna M **(SLP)**
Fein, Cathy Rochelle **(SLP)**
Glasow, Mrs Georgiana Quest **(SLP)**
Gold, Amy Joy **(SLP)**
Howard, Janice Ann **(A)**
Korth, Gail Dennison **(SLP)**
Meth, Phyllis R **(SLP)**
Owens, Katharine **(SLP)**
Yarbrough, Carla **(SLP)**

Suffield
Damon, Sheryl A **(SLP)**
Murdock, Mrs Susan A **(SLP)**
Shaffer-Bartley, Susan **(SLP)**

Terryville
Sword, Mrs Paula Ann **(SLP)**

Thomaston
Beccia-Blakeslee, Marisa Ann **(SLP)**
Fentress, Mrs Deborah P **(SLP)**
Hapken, Mrs Kim R **(SLP)**

Tolland
Avino, Mrs Gail J **(SLP)**
Garabedian, Mrs Nancy Anne **(SLP)**
Goldenberg, Nancy **(SLP)**
Horsfield, Mrs Lisa M C **(SLP)**
Zoback, Mark S **(SLP)**

Torrington
Conger, Sharon J **(SLP)**
Gibbs, Marilyn S **(SLP)**
Gonya, Linda Marie
Lloyd, Shelley Hornik **(SLP)**
MacCalous, Jean **(SLP)**
Pagano, Mrs Julie Anna **(SLP)**
Stearns, Mrs Phyllis Brusie **(A)**

Trumbull
Jositas, Mrs Susan M **(SLP)**
Kruzshak, Lauren L **(SLP)**
Rabine, Mrs Nina P **(SLP)**
Rader, Suzanne **(SLP)**
Schary, Mrs Varda Feinsilber **(A)**
Schumaker, Anita Drost **(SLP)**
Sullivan, Mrs E Barbara **(SLP)**
Van Dyken, Mrs Eleanore **(SLP)**
Watnick, Myra L **(SLP)**
Zopfi, Mrs Sarah D **(SLP)**

Unionville
Ashmont, Janice Gomez **(SLP)**
Baldwin, Mrs Barbara S **(SLP)**
Pickering, Mrs Mary Fletcher **(SLP)**

Vernon
Breslau, Susan R Z **(SLP)**
Johnson, Dr Marie Love **(SLP)**
Kessler, Myles A **(A)**
Paullo, Ronald D **(SLP)**
Riordan, Anne E **(A)**
Sexton, Mrs Valerie Anne **(SLP)**
Tarzia, Mrs Eileen Rose **(SLP)**
Victoria, Kristen Jean **(SLP)**

Voluntown
Pellinen, Mrs Sandra P **(SLP)**

Wallingford
Borsari, Mrs Carol Hintz **(SLP)**
Charette, Mrs Lori Wills **(A)**
Liska, Mrs Robin Susan **(SLP)**
Murray, Mrs Mary Scanlon **(SLP)**
Ruminski, Mrs Marion G **(SLP)**
Surowiecki, Mrs Patricia D **(SLP)**
Sweeney, Judith Lorraine **(SLP)**
Wojcik, Dorthy L **(SLP)**

Washington Depot
Biancardi Krukowski, Mrs Dawn **(SLP)**

Waterbury
Daniels, Karen Jeanne **(SLP)**
Essency, Nadine G **(SLP)**
Farrand, Julie Ann **(SLP)**
Fontano, Joan Alice **(SLP)**
Healey, Patricia **(SLP)**
Huerta, Dr Lynn Ellen **(A)**
Klipp, Abbie J **(SLP)**
Martin, Janice L **(SLP)**
McGrath, Susan R **(SLP)**
Rayel, Doreen Ann **(SLP)**
Ringenberg, Dr Carol Watson **(SLP)**
Sanford, Mrs Jill T **(SLP)**
Sember, Margaret D **(SLP)**
Sirois, Diane Patricia **(SLP)**
Tremaglio, Barbara McLaughlin **(SLP)**
Wolkoff, Elaine S **(SLP)**

Waterford
Bingaman, Mrs Donna Mitchell **(SLP)**

Dell'Angelo, Denise Dominique **(SLP)**
Downie, Mrs Ellen Mary **(SLP)**
Jones, Mrs Julie Lavezzoli **(SLP)**
Moss, Lynne R **(SLP)**
Nesdill, Mrs Judith Michele **(SLP)**
Rothman, Frederick **(SLP)**

Watertown
Cianciolo, Alison Grace **(SLP)**
Gagnon, Donna Marie **(SLP)**
Lagno, Joan A **(SLP)**
McCleary, Mrs Gail Vontobel **(SLP)**
Rubano, Mrs Bernedette **(SLP)**
Wickham, Mrs Claudia A **(SLP)**

Weatogue
Welwood, Deborah S **(SLP)**

West Gramby
Smith, Mrs Cynthia Griffin **(SLP)**

West Hartford
Abbott, Mrs Robin K **(SLP)**
Alfin, Marlene V **(SLP)**
Alfke-Norman, Dorothy C **(SLP)**
Auber, Patricia Anne **(SLP)**
Bard, Dr Barbara **(SLP)**
Breiter, Mrs Ronni F **(SLP)**
Burger, Mrs Teresa A **(SLP)**
Curylo, Caroline Patricia **(SLP)**
Falkowski, Sr Mary Felicia **(SLP)**
Forman, Mrs Joann Querner **(SLP)**
Gaines, Ellen Lynn
Gay, Mrs Joan M **(SLP)**
Geetter, Mrs Ava F **(SLP)**
Grasso, Susan G **(SLP)**
Hayes, Mrs Carol Benjamin **(SLP)**
Howe, Linda B **(SLP)**
Isakson, Mrs Carolyn Weiner **(SLP)**
Jardin, Mrs Irene M **(SLP)**
Jones, Dr Martha E **(SLP)**
Jordan, Mrs Sheryl A **(SLP)**
Kahoud, Mrs Judith L **(SLP)**
Kass-Levy, Maxanne **(SLP)**
Kessler, Maurine E **(A)**
La Russa, Mrs Karen M **(SLP)**
Layden, Doris L **(SLP)**
Lerman, Joanne Linda
Lewis, Mrs Janet S **(SLP)**
Mahaffey, Kevin Brooks
Marks, Mrs Elizabeth **(SLP)**
McGowan, Judith D **(SLP)**
Montano, Mrs Marleen Graf **(SLP)**
Mooradd, Mrs Theresa H **(SLP)**
Morgenstern, Nancy **(SLP)**
Poe, Mrs Esther F **(SLP)**
Przybycien, Mrs Julianne MacFadden **(SLP)**
Scott, Homer W **(SLP)**
Siegel, Elaine S **(SLP)**
Silverberg, Mary H **(SLP)**
Smiley, Kathy H **(SLP)**
Smith, Dr Rosalie H **(SLP)**
Triebert, Raymond F **(A)**
Tuohy-Eagan, Mrs Geralyn **(SLP)**
White, Johanna M **(SLP)**
Woods, Mary Ellen M **(SLP)**

West Haven
Biondi, Gina
Hawley, Connie Vie **(SLP)**
Kisner, Carol Helen **(A)**
Lucas-Cooley, Mrs Ann Marie **(SLP)**
Mazur, Carol L
Spitzer, Dr Jaclyn Barbara **(A)**

West Mystic
Beach, Cynthia M **(SLP)**

West Redding
Robinson, Mrs Myrna B **(SLP)**

West Simsbury
Carey, Linda R **(SLP)**
Hopfer, Mrs Adrienne P **(SLP)**
Innes, Mary R **(SLP)**
Johnson, Mrs Joanne Phelps **(SLP)**
Sharpless, Mrs Clair **(SLP)**

West Suffield
Fahrenholz, Kathryn A **(SLP)**
Gardner, Mrs Alice L **(SLP)**
Simison, Paul R **(A)**

West Willington
Paine, Pamela J **(A)**

Westbrook
Bock, Mrs Margaret Buckridge **(SLP)**

Weston
Attisani, Donna M **(SLP)**
Morris-Neufeld, Vonnie V **(SLP)**
Rajotte, Margaret **(SLP)**
Schwartz, Dr Nancy Z **(SLP)**
Sculnick, Mrs Gloria Nevard **(SLP)**
Seideman, Mrs Avonne P **(SLP)**
Waltzman, Dava L **(SLP)**
Witte, Kassie **(SLP A)**

Westport
Aron, Mrs Arlis **(SLP)**
Brooke, Donna **(SLP)**
Burigo, Janice R **(SLP)**
Duchan, Mrs Lynn S **(A)**
Gist, Kenneth T **(SLP)**
Goldberg, Betty L **(SLP)**
Goldschmidt, Mrs Catherine **(SLP)**
Harper, Dr Edith **(SLP)**
Levine, Judith G **(SLP)**
Lowes, Mrs Victoria Sue **(SLP)**
Luterman, Mrs Lillian B **(SLP)**
Tumpowsky, Audrey F K **(SLP)**
Urioste, Karen J **(SLP)**
Watkins, Donna L **(SLP)**
Wohlforth, Bettina Anne **(A)**

Westville
Holland, Richard Wayne **(SLP)**

Wethersfield
Batory, Mrs Nancy Anderson **(A)**
Cox, Deborah A **(SLP)**
Dumaine, Alan J **(A)**
Maliszewksi, Michelle Barbara **(SLP)**
Matos, Karen Ann **(SLP)**
Purdy, Mrs Mary Harlin **(SLP)**
Regan, Mary Margaret S **(A)**

Willimantic
Ashton, Lori Jean **(SLP)**
Costa, Carol A **(A)**
Horrocks, Mrs Pamela **(SLP)**
Merritt, Dr Donna D **(SLP)**
Richards, Deborah J **(SLP)**
Rollinson, Mrs Frances M **(SLP)**
Tryba, Mary Jo

Wilton
Aubrey, Mrs Joan A V **(SLP)**
Fieber, Deborah Osman **(SLP)**
Gould, Alan B **(SLP)**
Graham, Margaret S **(SLP)**
Jaffe, Mrs Sharon B **(SLP)**
Lopez, Sandra **(A)**
Minsky, Mrs Shelley W **(A)**
Nessel, Mrs Jo Ann M **(SLP)**
Overland, Mrs Lori L **(SLP)**
Smith, Mrs Shirley Mayo **(SLP)**

Windham Center
Gillcash, Mrs Judith Ann Sansone **(SLP)**

Windsor
Bentrup, Sarah Kickham **(SLP)**
Berta, Mrs Susan Lea **(SLP)**
Boysen, Dona Hudson **(SLP)**
Daves, Mrs Rita Rome **(SLP)**
Golbabai, Mrs Carolyn J **(SLP)**
Oliverio, Alexis Matko **(SLP)**
Reeves, Paula J

Winsted
Baker, Kathy L **(SLP)**
Corcoran, John Allen **(SLP)**

Wolcott
Coburn, Mrs Pamela Lee **(SLP)**
Groody, Mrs Maria **(SLP)**
Lewis, Susan K **(SLP)**

Woodbridge
Buffa, Phyllis M **(SLP)**
Burt, Mrs Linda R **(SLP)**
Gottlieb, Mrs Linda Haas **(SLP)**
Gregg, Mrs Jean Westerman **(SLP)**
Kapleau-Lebov, Mrs Nancy B **(SLP)**
Krevolin, Mrs Evelyn S **(SLP)**
Lerea, Dr Louis **(SLP A)**
Pleckaitis, Carolyn D **(SLP)**
Ravski, Barbara **(SLP)**
Yanagisawa, Kay
Zirkin-Dagan, Sharon **(SLP)**

Woodbury
Albert, Mrs Judith I **(SLP)**
Harris, Mrs Elizabeth H **(SLP)**

Woodstock
Laflamme, Joanne **(SLP)**

Woodstock Valley
Collins, Kevin P **(SLP)**

DELAWARE

Bear
Mann, Richard Clarke **(A)**

Bridgeville
Cera, Nancy M **(SLP)**

Claymont
Sabo, Denise R **(SLP)**
Timlin, Janice Hollenback **(SLP)**

Delaware
Fleming, Paul L **(SLP)**

Dover
Bilton, Regina R **(SLP)**
Brown, Linda L **(A)**
Chapman, Mrs Francine L **(SLP)**
Cooke, Patricia Ann **(SLP)**
Fisher, John C **(SLP A)**
Frick, Mrs Jill Tiedemann **(SLP)**
Holden, Mrs Helen Q **(SLP)**
Hutchison, Lynne Michele
Jones, Lisa Marie **(A)**
Jones, Mrs Merry M **(SLP)**
Kahl, W Bailey **(SLP A)**
Kupiec, Karen Jean **(A)**
Mardis, Mrs Emily J **(SLP)**
Patterson, Pamela J **(SLP A)**
Slentz, Patricia C **(SLP)**
Smith, Eric Lamont **(A)**
Suleski, Mrs Nancy L **(SLP)**
Zamboldi, Mary D **(SLP)**
Zimmerman, Mrs Jeanne L **(SLP)**
Zimmerman, Dr Terrance S **(SLP)**

Elsmere
Marks, Mrs Robin D **(SLP)**

Georgetown
Himes, Thomas Alan **(SLP)**
Tyler, Mrs Lorraine D **(SLP)**

Greenville
Landrey, Mrs Lynne Herring **(SLP)**

Hockessin
Clark, Nancy T **(SLP)**
Davis, Mrs Ann W **(SLP)**
Herrmann, Elizabeth **(SLP)**
Lenk-Roberts, Susan Colleen **(SLP A)**
Mineo, Dr Beth Ann **(SLP)**
Peck, Mrs Cynthia Reynolds **(SLP)**
Swingle, Mrs Lynn H **(SLP)**
Sysak, Mrs Marian Ernsberger **(SLP)**
Wemmers, Mrs Sally W **(SLP)**
Whitby-Norman, Mrs Debra Marie **(SLP)**

Lewes
Moellenbeck, Karen Ann **(SLP)**
Packman, Ellen R **(SLP)**

Middletown
Lantz, Eleanor Piazza **(SLP)**

Milford
Berry, Mrs Susan Lynn **(SLP)**
Sommerfield, Sandra Lee **(SLP)**

Millsboro
Coffman, Mary Beth **(SLP)**

New Castle
Bartlett, Jennifer L **(A)**
Byrnes, Mrs Arlene **(SLP)**
Jensen, Mrs Senta H **(SLP)**

Newark
Azzara, John P **(SLP)**
Azzara, Mrs Marie Randolph **(SLP)**
Barnett, Marsha S **(SLP)**
Courtright, Illene C **(SLP)**
Demond, Elizabeth Lambert **(SLP)**
Geib, Mrs Janet R **(SLP)**
Hammond, Mrs Patricia Ann **(SLP)**
Hill, Jo Anne K **(SLP)**
Klimowicz, Mrs Donna Hug **(SLP)**
Langsdorf, Anne M
Litchfield, Mrs Marilyn K **(SLP)**
Mandel, Jeri Lynn **(SLP)**
Marencin, Gary Joseph **(A)**
Markowitz, Michelle **(SLP)**
Maxwell, Pamela A **(SLP)**
McGregor, Sarah S **(SLP)**
Meadows, Mrs Polly E **(A)**
Meisel, Edith Schneider **(SLP)**
Mejia-Hershberger, Mrs Yvonne M **(SLP)**
Melton, Donna Hicks **(SLP)**
Moses, Mrs Andra A **(SLP)**
Muller, Mrs Carolyn Wheeler **(SLP)**
Nigro, Jill Lewis **(SLP)**
Novakoski, William E **(SLP)**
Owens, Mrs Sarah J **(SLP)**
Riley, Kathleen J **(A)**
Schantz, Elizabeth R **(SLP)**
Soper, Mrs Ellen A **(SLP)**
Spiegler-Gordon, Karin Ethel **(SLP)**
Stokes, Mary Hug **(SLP)**
Tyler, James I **(A)**
Vacek, Mrs Kathleen D **(SLP)**
Visconti, Joann Rose Marie **(SLP)**
Wachowiak, Mrs Joanne Elizabeth **(SLP)**
Warren, Dr Irene B **(SLP)**
Wood, Mrs Karen P **(A)**

Newcastle
Trubey, Cindy Joy **(SLP)**

Rehoboth Beach
Connolly, Mary Ann S **(A)**

Seaford
Laddbush-Lecompte, Mrs Diane M **(SLP)**
Parker, Mrs Cynthia Foxwell **(A)**
Workman, Carol D **(SLP)**

Smyrna
Reynolds, Mrs Eileen Kahl **(A)**

Wilmington
Badick, Martha **(SLP)**
Baker, Mrs Janet Ann **(SLP)**
Ball, Mrs Nancy J **(SLP)**
Baryla, Joanne **(SLP)**
Bouchard, Ellen **(SLP)**
Brown, Ruth Elizabeth **(A)**
Budovitch, Mrs Rona L **(SLP)**
Burstein, Susan A **(SLP)**
Burtch, Mrs Roberta F **(SLP)**
Conboy, Elizabeth A **(SLP)**
Costanzo, Marcia **(SLP)**
Danielson, Priscilla Mary **(SLP)**
Davidson, K Rochelle **(SLP)**
Eareckson, Jane B **(SLP)**
Ehrenkaufer, Louise Pauze **(SLP)**

Fallon, Gary E **(SLP)**
Finnigan, Cynthia S **(SLP)**
Fitzgerald, Carol Reese **(A)**
Giacoma, Beth Feeney **(SLP)**
Glazier, Marijane **(SLP)**
Goldstein, Mrs Amy Helene **(SLP)**
Gregore, Dale Rebhan **(SLP)**
Grumbacher, Mrs Suzanne W **(SLP)**
Hagen, Susan T **(SLP)**
Hertzfeld, Debra B **(SLP)**
Jankowski, Mrs Catherine Jane **(SLP)**
Kagel, Mrs Marion C **(SLP)**
Kerr, Mrs Marlys Mae **(SLP)**
Kirchner, Maryanne **(SLP)**
Kline, Kathy Kay **(SLP)**
Latocha, Mrs Diane C **(SLP)**
Lindsay, Ann M
Lofquist, Beverly Henke **(SLP)**
Mikola, Judy Marie **(SLP)**
Montanaro, Mrs Janet J **(SLP)**
Pehrson, Julie J **(A)**
Peltz, Beverly R **(SLP)**
Prasad, Mrs Kamala R **(SLP)**
Rapkin, Mrs Enid S **(SLP)**
Roberson, Mrs Judith E **(SLP)**
Rodriquez, Rebecca Angeli
Ronnei, Mrs Eleanor C **(A)**
Straitman, Nina P **(SLP)**
Swanson, Mrs Cynthia Louise **(SLP)**
Thompson, Mrs Barbara **(SLP)**
Thureau, Mrs Lani C **(SLP)**
Wagner, Aylene P **(SLP)**
Warner, Mary Ellen **(SLP)**
Westerhouse, Janice June **(SLP)**
Zenorini, Brenda **(SLP)**

Wyoming

Smith, Mrs Valerie Crawford **(SLP)**

DISTRICT OF COLUMBIA

Washington

Albinson, Mrs Sharon J **(SLP A)**
Alprin, Mrs Linda Ann **(SLP)**
Anderson, Annette McKenzie **(SLP)**
Arthur, Priscilla S **(A)**
Attorri, Judith Treadwell **(SLP)**
Babbs, Barbara S **(SLP)**
Bales, Joel D **(A)**
Bally, Scott J **(SLP)**
Baquet, Glenn M **(A)**
Barnes, Dr Norman S **(SLP)**
Barnwell, Dr Ysaye Maria **(SLP)**
Baron, Christine Rochelle **(SLP)**
Barry, Mary M **(A)**
Bassin, Mrs Beatrice Kellner **(SLP)**
Berlinsky, Dr Stanley L **(SLP)**
Berman, Mrs Carol P **(SLP A)**
Bernero, Dr Raymond J **(A)**
Bettigole, Donna Klein **(SLP)**
Bielski, Mrs Lee S **(SLP)**
Black, Lillian M **(SLP)**
Bost, Dianne M **(SLP)**
Boysen, Dr Allen E **(SLP)**
Braverman, Leonard **(SLP)**
Brewer, Diane M **(A)**
Britton, Barbara D **(SLP)**
Brock, Karen Elizabeth **(A)**
Brown, Marcia Linda **(SLP)**
Brown, Ralph Elton **(SLP)**
Brunner, Barbara Jarboe **(A)**
Bunting, Bonita M **(SLP)**
Capobianco, Maria Carrescia **(A)**
Carmon, Mrs Sharon Marie **(SLP)**
Carroll, Dawn Felice
Coleman, Mrs Marcella Bell **(SLP)**
Comer, Pamela J **(SLP)**
Compton, Cynthia L **(A)**
Conlon, Dr Sara E **(SLP)**
Coppel, Marcia E **(SLP)**
Cord, Mary T **(SLP A)**
Corliss, Mrs Edith L R
Daley, Dr William T **(SLP)**
Davis, Johnetta G **(SLP)**
Dexter, Mark Edward **(SLP)**
Dickman, Donna M **(SLP A)**
Drayton, Augusta P **(SLP)**
Egan, Dr James J **(SLP A)**
Eskew, Mrs Lorraine W **(SLP)**
Evans, Gail E **(SLP)**
Fabry, David Alan **(A)**
Favors, Dr Aaron **(SLP A)**
Favors, Vanessa Wilson **(SLP A)**
Feeley, John J, Jr **(SLP)**
Fiedler, Rosmarie **(SLP)**
Fischer, Dr Martin A **(SLP)**
Fogelstrom, Suzanne S **(SLP)**
Foster, Mrs Teresita Lourdes E M
Foster, Wesley A **(A)**
Freeman, Ena Gail **(SLP)**
Garrett, Debra M **(SLP)**
Geron, Lynda B **(SLP)**
Glazer, Shirley L **(SLP)**
Gould, Nancy **(SLP)**
Grady, Ellen Grace **(SLP)**
Green, Marcia H **(A)**
Greenley, Diane Carol **(SLP)**
Gurevich-Uvena, Joyce **(SLP)**
Haley, Eileen T **(SLP)**
Handy, Mrs Dianne Janette **(SLP)**
Harris, Mrs Elizabeth **(SLP)**
Harris, Marilyn Jill **(SLP)**
Helminski, Carole A **(SLP)**
Hilliard, Annette Walser **(SLP)**
Hillis, Dr James W **(SLP A)**
Honeygosky, Robert A **(SLP)**
Horowitz, Sabra
Hosty, Kathleen A **(SLP)**
Houle, Dr Gail Ruppert **(SLP)**
Hughes, Mary Catherine **(SLP)**
Hussey, Deborah Heath **(SLP)**
Jenkins, Mrs Lucille B
Johnson-Lawrence, Paula Faith **(A)**
Jons, Catherine Riedel **(A)**
Joyner, Jeanette **(SLP)**
Klacan, Ann Marie **(A)**
Kline, Marcia S **(SLP)**
Kress, Mary F **(SLP)**
Kuerbis, Tracy L **(A)**
LaCoss, Mrs Joan Harkin **(A)**
Lamm, Joanne Schwartz **(SLP)**
Leek, Dr Marjorie R **(A)**
Lindholm, Sylvia B **(SLP)**
Linebaugh, Dr Craig W **(SLP)**
Lotterman, Dr Stephen H **(A)**
MacNeil, Donna M **(A)**
Maddox, Chere
Madison-Land, Mrs Sharron R **(SLP)**
Mahshie, Dr James J **(SLP)**
Marshall, Stephanie Scott **(A)**
Martin, Laurel Campbell
Massey, April **(SLP)**
McCardle, Dr Peggy D **(SLP)**
McGee, Dr Donald I **(SLP)**
McKnight, Laura W **(SLP)**
McQueen, Jo Ella **(SLP)**
Melendy, Lorna K **(SLP)**
Miller, Eddie Jack **(A)**
Mitchener-Colston, Mrs Wanda K **(SLP)**
Monsen, Dr Randall B
Moore, Jean P **(A)**
Moss, Sharon Elizabeth **(SLP)**
Munsey, Mrs Bernice Wilson
Murray, Dr Sharon L **(SLP)**
Neale, Mrs Tawana M **(SLP)**
Ney, Elise **(A)**
Nichols, Ann Pryor **(SLP)**
Nichols, Maureen T **(SLP)**
Nuru, Dr Njeri **(A)**
Oliver, Mrs Jean G **(SLP)**
Oliver, Vincent T
Overton, Vivian F **(SLP A)**
Payne, Dr Kay T **(SLP)**
Payne-Johnson, Dr Joan C **(SLP)**
Pearlman, Dr Ronald C **(SLP A)**
Pickett, Dr James M
Pietranton, Arlene Arrigan **(SLP)**
Postove, Mrs Mary A **(A)**
Prosek Phd, Robert A
Queene, Lisa Annette **(SLP)**
Reagan, Mrs Deborah A **(SLP)**
Reed, Dr L Deno **(SLP A)**
Reveron, Dr Wilhelmina **(SLP)**
Revoile, Dr Sally G **(A)**
Richner, Mrs Susan Mayes **(SLP)**
Riecken, Frances B **(SLP)**
Roberts, Robbie Dethelia **(A)**
Robier, Therese Clarke **(A)**
Robinson, Tommie L **(SLP)**
Rosenberg, Jeanette **(SLP)**
Rosenman, Dr Patricia **(SLP)**
Rosenstein, Dr Joseph **(A)**
Russell, Cynthia A **(SLP)**
Schafer, Dr Judy D **(A)**
Schandl, Kathleen Marie **(SLP)**
Schenker, Roz **(A)**
Schmitt, Dr Philip J **(A)**
Schnack, Mrs Susan Guthrie **(A)**
Schnitzer, Ruth Ellen
Shekim, Dr Lana O **(SLP)**
Shervin, Mrs Cheri Jeannette **(A)**
Shipley-Brown, Frances Hawpe **(SLP)**
Shulman, Carole **(SLP)**
Silberman, Judith R **(SLP)**
Silverwood, Pamela **(SLP)**
Singer, Louis **(SLP)**
Smalls, Jacquelyn Elaine **(SLP)**
Soso, Verafran **(SLP)**
Stern, Zina G **(SLP)**
Stokes, Nona B **(A)**
Surr, Mrs Rauna K **(A)**
Taketa, Janice Hanley **(SLP)**
Taylor, Orlando L **(SLP)**
Tebinka, Jean A **(A)**
Thomas, Barbara E
Thomas, Regina R **(SLP)**
Thompson, Patryce F **(SLP)**
Timke, Margot **(SLP A)**
Tinsley, Judyth A
Trent, Deirdre R **(SLP)**
Umfress, Janel A **(SLP)**
Upton, Jane Duncan **(SLP)**
Urban, Dr Beth J **(A)**
Van Driel, Margaret Anne **(SLP)**
Vaughn-Cooke, Dr Ana F **(SLP)**
Vigdor-Peck, Lisa **(SLP)**
Walker, Maude J **(SLP)**
Weller, Dr Rosemary D **(SLP)**
Williams, Kathy Linette
Woods, Mrs Shirley L R **(SLP)**
Woofter, Herbert R **(SLP)**
Wright, Mrs Betty Johnson **(SLP)**
Wyatt, Mrs Carolyn Anderson **(A)**
Young, Dr Elizabeth Bell **(SLP A)**

FLORIDA

Alachua

Holmes, Dr Alice E **(A)**
Molyneux, Mrs Carol Snapp **(SLP)**

Altamonte Springs

Almon, Mrs Ledonna H **(SLP)**
Ballard, Paige Marten **(SLP)**
Bennett, Dr Gladys H **(SLP)**
Chari, Dr Nallan C A **(A)**
Crossmier, Mrs Judith Lynn **(SLP)**
Gurecki, Rebecca J **(SLP)**
Hardy, Cynthia L **(SLP)**
Harrigan, Deborah Conley **(SLP)**
Harvey, Charlotte M **(SLP)**
Henderson, Dana Paige **(A)**
Hiser, Kathy Ann **(A)**
Judge, Mrs Pamela Monroe **(SLP)**
Keeney, Janice Marie **(SLP)**
Kowalski, Gwen Laura **(SLP)**
Kowalski, Timothy P **(SLP)**
La Motte, Carolyn **(SLP)**
Nash, Deborah Jo **(SLP)**
Robinson, Deirdre
Russell, Mrs Vicki R **(SLP)**
Shultz, Karla Jean **(SLP)**
Skinner, Mrs Linda S **(SLP)**
Spires, Diantha K **(SLP)**
Tweed, Rebecca Jean **(SLP)**

APO Miami

Kerksiek, Charlotte **(SLP)**
Schwarz-Cordier, Mrs Jean Marie **(SLP)**
Swenty, Dr Vinita W **(SLP)**

Apollo Beach

Holdsworth, Mrs Leslie Plowman **(SLP)**
Shepherd, Dr David C **(A)**

Apopka

Fowle, Dawn Renee **(SLP)**
Gordon, Nancy M **(SLP)**
James-Trychel, Michele **(SLP A)**
Juskie, Mrs Dorothy Bartosh **(SLP)**
Wean, Dennis F **(A)**

Arcadia

Mizell, Marilyn Purvis **(SLP)**

Atlantic Beach

Brantley, Maxie C **(SLP)**
Brooks, Mrs Cecelia A **(SLP)**
Nusbaum-Hollenback, Mrs Janis **(SLP)**
Sidoff, Mrs Chris Ellen Alexis **(SLP)**

Auburndale

French, Mrs Lydia L **(SLP)**
Haack, Mrs Dean S **(SLP)**

Avon Park

Berger, Shirley L **(SLP)**
Heilig, Barbara McConihe **(SLP)**

Babson Park

Harr, Rhonda Ruth **(SLP)**

Barefoot Bay

Jackson, Bernard R **(SLP)**

Bartow

Smith, Virginia G **(SLP)**
Stidham, Mrs Patricia Joanne **(SLP)**
Williams, Mrs Susan L K **(SLP)**

Bay Pines

Abrams, Dr Harvey B **(A)**
Butler, Sheila Ann **(SLP A)**
Nelson, T Russell **(SLP)**

Belleair

Crockett, Lawrence O **(A)**
Haicken, Vivian G **(SLP)**

Belleair Beach

Edwards, Rosemary C **(SLP)**
Michels, Ida Ann **(SLP)**

Biscayne Park

Langhauser, Karen A **(SLP)**

Boca Raton

Anderson, Mrs Rebecca S **(A)**
Bargas, Lori R **(SLP)**
Capitena, Mrs Vickie Wallace **(SLP)**
Cohen, Mrs Joy B **(SLP)**
Cook, Mrs Linda G **(SLP)**
Cutler-Held, Dr Marcia **(SLP)**
Desousa, Rhonda Ann
Dorne, Dr William P **(SLP)**
Eisenberg, Mrs Marlene **(SLP)**
Engelhardt, Mrs Marian K **(SLP)**
Epstein, Mrs Ruth Elias **(SLP)**
Ezring, Mrs Barbara M **(SLP)**
Ferry, Nancy Ann **(SLP)**
Friedman, Mrs Joan A **(SLP)**
Furick, Mrs Paula K **(SLP)**
Garlick, Mrs Judith A **(SLP)**

Goodman, Deborah G **(SLP)**
Greenwald, Mrs Audrey B **(SLP)**
Greer, Ruth Ellen **(SLP)**
Hammesfahr, Judith Ann **(SLP)**
Hepner-Dion, Susan Meryl **(A)**
Heyer, Mrs Mary Haynie **(SLP)**
Isert, Mrs Deanna S
Jaffe, Dr Mata B **(SLP)**
Jordan, Mrs Angela Fox **(SLP)**
Kostis, Sandy Hughes **(SLP)**
Levy, Regina H **(SLP)**
Lipnack, Robin Lori **(SLP)**
Listokin, Sandra Arlene
Meisler, Beatrice R **(SLP A)**
Michelman, Margot **(SLP)**
Molt, Alexandra Rowland **(SLP)**
Molt, Dr Lawrence F **(SLP A)**
Morrissey, Kathleen M **(SLP)**
Murray, Shelly Arthur **(SLP)**
Ness, Michanne Alexis **(A)**
Oungst, Carmen Dee **(SLP)**
Putney, Mrs Jill Isler **(SLP)**
Rees, Mrs Muriel **(SLP)**
Scarpa, Gaye A **(SLP)**
Schosheim, Joanne Katz **(SLP)**
Schwartz, Robin N **(SLP A)**
Sharf, Dr Donald J
Sorkowitz, Melvin J **(A)**
Susskind, Mrs Cathy A **(SLP)**
Tabin, Mrs Barbara Russo **(SLP)**
Taffin, Leslie M **(SLP)**
Van Der Heide, Mrs Joan Manze
Weinstein, Mrs Sherrie **(SLP)**
Wexler, Mrs Helen **(SLP)**
Witwicky-Esden, Mrs Laila Anne **(SLP)**
Young, Mrs Susanne H **(SLP)**

Bokeelia
Ford, Carolyn S **(SLP)**
Sexton, Mrs Florence E **(SLP)**

Bonifay
Helms, Dr Beverly **(SLP)**

Bonita Springs
Barickman, Julia A **(SLP)**
Sheff, Martha I **(SLP)**
Tait, Nancy A **(SLP)**

Boynton Beach
Adamson, Benita McCarthy **(SLP)**
Gotlib, Kenneth S **(A)**
Judice, Kathy Theriot **(SLP)**
Martin, Anita C **(SLP)**
Myrick, Lisa Drummond
Rosenzweig, Meri Sue **(SLP)**
Shaw, Jill D **(SLP)**

Bradenton
Barnes, Beth L **(SLP)**
Becher, Diane L **(A)**
Caputa, Antoinette Marie
Cleary, Carol Sue **(SLP)**
Dardas Rn, Mrs Kathryn D **(SLP A)**
Davis, Diane Dorothy **(SLP)**
Deane-Watson, Edie Hope **(A)**
Edwards, Dorothy A **(SLP)**
Gregg-Chlebina, Jerilyn Kay **(SLP)**
Hardee, Mrs Shirley Jean **(SLP)**
Harrison, Mrs Anne **(A)**
Henslick, Katharine Haag **(SLP)**
Heyen, Donna Louise **(SLP)**
Higgins, Cheryl J **(SLP)**
Holub, Janet Marie **(SLP)**
Jemelka, Victor J **(SLP)**
Klein, Helen P G **(SLP A)**
Koshnick, Tami Rose **(SLP)**
Krival, Catherine R **(SLP)**
Livingston, Mrs Janetta P **(SLP)**
Mancusco, Catherine **(SLP)**
Martin, Sherrie **(SLP)**
Meissner, Mrs Deborah E **(SLP)**
Mulkern, Marie T **(SLP)**
Roller, Rena Paulette **(SLP)**

Schneiderman, Dr Jeffrey R **(SLP)**
Simpson, Mrs Joanne Medeiros **(SLP)**
Sterns, Gladys M **(SLP)**
Streu, Mrs Patricia Erickson **(SLP)**
Taylor, Nancy Ruth **(SLP)**
Thomas, Lori L **(SLP)**
Tolley-Hindman, Mrs Christine Elaine **(SLP)**
Turnbaugh-McCormick, Karen Robin **(SLP)**
Vandecar, Mrs Susan E W **(SLP)**
Vega, Allene C **(SLP)**
Walchko, Jack C **(A)**
Wolcott, Mrs Patricia M **(SLP)**

Brandon
Blackwell, Lisa Freeman **(A)**
Broussard, Mrs Mary Margaret **(SLP)**
Carr, Mrs Patricia Irene **(A)**
Graham, Mrs Sandra Jean **(SLP)**
Ingram, Dr Beth A **(SLP)**
Kaplan, Mrs Carol Beth **(SLP)**
Morgan, Mrs Denise L **(SLP)**
Robbins, Sharon Bowen **(SLP)**
Tek, Susan Downey

Brooker
Yanke, Robert B **(A)**

Brooksville
Cockin, Mrs Margaret A **(SLP)**
Conter, Joanne Born **(A)**

Cantonment
Miller, Mrs M Annette **(SLP)**

Cape Canaveral
Girdvainis, Cheryl Marie **(SLP)**
Kolsch, Angela M **(SLP)**

Cape Coral
Adams, John (Jack) H **(A)**
Brown, Janet Ann **(SLP)**
Burton-Tihen, Mrs Deborah L **(SLP)**
Coleman, Mrs Ann Marie **(SLP)**
Gale, John E **(SLP)**
Halstead-Elser, Mrs Sammie **(A)**
Holmes, Joseph John, Jr **(A)**
Schell, Mrs Kathy G **(SLP)**

Casselberry
Anastario, Patricia Kelley **(SLP)**
Hasan, Mrs Mary Jo
Kloiber, Margaret A **(SLP)**
O'Hara, Anne **(SLP)**
Osborn, Mrs Sandra R
Taylor, Beth Nanette Nichols **(SLP)**

Chiefland
Alexander, Jane E **(SLP)**

Chipley
Kirkland, Mrs Sheila Laney **(SLP)**

Clearwater
Abjanich, Patricia B **(SLP)**
Amspaugh, Gilbert D **(SLP)**
Anderson, Regina W **(SLP)**
Brown, Beverly P **(SLP)**
Caiaccio, Mrs Marjorie V **(SLP)**
Caste, Debra Fay
Chinnick, Phyllis S **(SLP)**
Cline, Mrs Joan A **(SLP)**
Farrington, Mitzi G **(SLP)**
Focaracci, Mrs Laura Weiss **(SLP)**
Garcia, Mrs Suzanne G **(SLP)**
Gaspelin, Mrs Shirley Mershon **(SLP)**
Gates, Valerie Ann **(SLP)**
Harrison, Melinda K **(A)**
Hosner, Rochelle G **(SLP)**
Hough, Mrs Karen S **(SLP)**
Locke, Shirley Walker **(SLP)**
McClary, Annette Edmonds **(SLP)**
McCusker, Ann **(SLP)**
McManamon, Donna W **(SLP)**
Miller, Mrs Elizabeth G **(SLP)**
Osborn, Courtney D **(A)**
Parrish, Shauna Lori **(SLP)**
Robinson, Kathryn A **(SLP)**

Saives, Christine Ann
Sauers, Mrs Judith F **(SLP)**
Schwartz, Mrs Sherry F
Schwartz, Mrs Susan **(SLP)**
Sloan, Mrs Helen Ann **(SLP)**
Waldron, Sally J **(SLP)**
Weber, Ellen Schmoyer **(SLP)**
Wexler, Mrs Sharon P **(A)**

Clearwater Beach
Arlt, Mrs Phyllis B **(SLP)**

Clermont
Abderrahman, Mrs Carole Jean **(SLP)**

Cocoa
Healey, Mrs Barbara N **(SLP)**

Cocoa Beach
Burke, Kathleen F **(SLP)**
Keane, Mrs Sandra O'Neill **(SLP)**

Coconut Creek
Berlin-Stern, Mrs Euna **(SLP)**
Cooley, Mrs Carol Durkin **(SLP)**
Jones, Mrs Fay Linda Schlimper **(SLP)**
Meizel, Ellen Stacey
Miric, Leigh Anne **(SLP)**
Mohardt, Karen Diane
Wolf-Schein, Dr Enid Gordon **(SLP)**
Zatz, Anita F **(SLP)**

Coconut Grove
Brooks, Jill **(SLP)**
Freeman, Eddi-Ann R **(SLP)**
Rodriguez, Judith T **(SLP)**
Shapiro, Mrs Joyce Reich **(SLP)**

Cooper City
Cavanagh, George J **(SLP)**
Farrell, Carol A **(SLP)**
Gellick, Mrs Ramona Rodery **(SLP)**
Golembieski, June Oster **(SLP)**
Reisinger, Mrs Joan H **(SLP)**

Coral Gables
Becker, Leonard V **(SLP A)**
Berkley, Rita K **(SLP)**
Bragman, Mrs Janet Strawgate **(SLP)**
Brian, Mrs Jody D **(SLP)**
Cummings, Mrs Jolie E **(SLP)**
Garland, Mrs June M **(SLP)**
Gathman, Mrs Jacqui D
Gould, Linda R **(A)**
Green, Dr Joni Grant **(SLP)**
Jenkins, Paula Kay **(SLP)**
Kelly, Mrs Bea B **(SLP)**
Shea, Dr William L **(SLP)**
Whittington, Kathryn E **(SLP A)**

Coral Springs
Adamowicz, Michael F **(A)**
Allen, Robin Janine **(SLP)**
Brooks, Mrs Andrea S **(A)**
Fischler, Mrs Barbara L **(SLP)**
Freedman, Mrs Deborah Meckler **(SLP)**
Garrett, Mrs Mary F **(SLP)**
Gober, Mrs Ruth H **(SLP)**
Goldstein, Gwenn S **(SLP)**
Goodman-Saia, Mrs Shari I **(SLP)**
Halper, Betty D **(SLP)**
Haverfield, Mrs Mary **(SLP)**
Hirschberg, Joyce G **(SLP)**
Hoffman, Mrs Kathy D **(SLP)**
Hurwitz, Morton William **(SLP)**
Kareff, Gary R **(A)**
Kogen-Scharf, Mrs Kim **(SLP)**
Krantz, Mrs Joan H **(SLP)**
Levine, Sharon W **(SLP)**
Nacht, Andrea B **(SLP)**
Oremland, Betty J **(A)**
Oxenhandler, Gail H **(SLP)**
Randel, Roberta Malat **(A)**
Robbins, Wendy M **(SLP)**
Robinson, Charlene **(SLP)**
Roffman, Mrs Carol A **(A)**

Rood, Mrs Leah Berman **(SLP)**
Rothberg, Suzanne G **(SLP)**
Russell, Marcus Randall **(A)**
Schwartz, Mrs Paula Carol
Skeegan, Mrs Joan M **(SLP)**
Thompson, Mrs Ann Diamond **(SLP)**
Vai, Donna G **(SLP)**
Vassiliades, Diane G **(SLP)**
Vesel, Mary A **(SLP)**
Viamari-Williamson, Gina L **(SLP)**
Victor, Mrs Shelley J **(SLP)**
Walsh, Susan M N **(SLP)**

Crawfordville
Holbrook, Mrs Johanna G **(SLP)**

Crestview
Freeman, Angela Whitehurst **(SLP)**
Harrison, Jean M **(SLP)**
Riley, Cynthia J **(SLP)**
Thigpen, Mrs Mary Catherine **(SLP)**

Cross City
Smith, Mrs Lydia H **(SLP)**
Zenner, Dr Anthony A **(SLP)**
Zenner, Sandra B **(SLP)**

Crystal River
Hickle, Mrs Polly Ann L **(SLP)**
Hubbard, Tana Witte **(SLP)**

Davie
Bautista, Christina Diane **(SLP)**
Daskin, Barbara J **(SLP)**
Elmore, Suzanne **(SLP)**
Gale, Mrs Stacy S **(SLP)**
Gorlin, Mrs Ruth Annette **(SLP)**
Gorlin, Todd Nelson **(A)**
Gundersen, Mrs Debra H **(A)**
Gundersen, Fredrik **(A)**
Higgins, Barbara F **(A)**
Markey, Mrs Shari Kligman **(A)**
Reisberg, Mrs Susan Scalise **(SLP)**
Tepperberg, Mrs Iris Zimmerman **(SLP)**
Wechsler, Robert M **(A)**
Welte, Renee **(SLP)**
Wolf, Mrs Debra Zobel **(SLP)**

Daytona Beach
Brock, Angela
Burgess-Hall, Mrs Nancy Dyer **(SLP)**
Day, Carol Sue **(SLP)**
Doyle, Mrs Joann L **(SLP)**
Greene, Janet D **(SLP)**
Missal, Mrs Donna M **(SLP)**
Sofiak, Nancy T **(A)**
Tulak, Joseph, Jr **(SLP)**
Wanderman, Hope B **(SLP)**
Williams, Mrs Thomasyne Hill **(SLP)**

Daytona Beach Shores
Warren, Mrs Berniece B **(SLP)**

De Land
Barbare, Diane E **(SLP)**
Bezdek, Kathleen Terese **(A)**
Harrington, Dr Don A
Klock, Mrs Lila **(SLP)**
Landau, Claudia **(SLP)**
Snedeker, Dr Leo W, Jr **(SLP A)**
Stewart, Marjorie M **(SLP)**
Timko, James Robert **(A)**

Deerfield Beach
Horowitz, Mrs Louise P **(SLP)**
Jonas, Dr Renai K **(SLP)**
Oare, Katherine Adele **(A)**
Paolini, Elizabeth Anne **(SLP)**
Weinstein, Marlene **(SLP)**

Delray Beach
Brecker, Rona Carol **(SLP)**
Cheskin, Mrs Adele **(SLP)**
Da Pra, Denise M **(SLP)**
Friedley, Mrs Sheridan Coale **(SLP)**
Harmon, Mrs Jacqueline Prince **(SLP)**
Hunt, Mrs Barbara S **(SLP)**

Johnson, Mrs Denise L **(SLP)**
Keyser, Beverly Ann
Klauk, Susan W **(SLP)**
McClain, Linda S **(SLP)**
Meltzer, Mrs Elaine F Gantman **(SLP)**
Nichols, Clare M **(SLP)**
Reese, Martha M **(SLP)**
Rothman, Mrs Ruth Agert **(SLP)**
Rutz, Terry A **(A)**
Seiler, Mrs Nancy E **(SLP)**
Simons, Doris Ilene **(SLP)**
Spence, Dr Nancy Long **(SLP)**
Trumbo, Charles R
Williamson, Mrs Gail E **(A)**

Deltona

Herod, Linda R **(SLP)**
Howden, Shaune B **(SLP)**
Johnson, John D, III **(A)**
McNiece, Mrs Judith Ann **(SLP)**

Destin

Woods, Mrs Laura Johnson **(SLP)**

Dunedin

Clobridge, Carol Ann **(A)**
Embrey, Janice K **(SLP)**
Karow, Mrs Colleen Marie **(SLP)**
Murphy, Conrad V **(SLP)**
Solomon, Charles **(A)**
Storey, Julia Lynn **(SLP)**
Warman, Wendy B **(SLP)**

East Palatka

Knisley, Marianne Murray **(SLP)**

Eaton Park

Malloy, Brenda Lane **(SLP)**

Edgewater

Wall, David John **(SLP)**

Englewood

Clines, Sharon Marie **(SLP)**
de Laubenfels, Prof Richard J **(SLP)**

Estero

Judge, Robert D **(SLP)**

Eustis

Amman, Debra A **(SLP)**
Birr, Sydney R **(SLP)**
Hale, Mrs Cathy P **(SLP)**
Harrison, Mrs Denise Sprouse **(SLP)**

Fern Park

Johnson, Mrs Lee Ann **(SLP)**
Smith, Mrs Patricia **(SLP)**

Fort Lauderdale

Aitken, Susan E **(SLP)**
Albritton, Thelma **(SLP)**
Behrman, Eileen Ann
Brimberry, Alexis C
Bruno, Mrs Patricia S **(SLP)**
Brunz, Mrs Janice J **(SLP)**
Campbell, Doris R **(SLP)**
Centini, Philippa G **(SLP)**
Champion, William N **(SLP)**
Ciely, Paula M **(A)**
Conway, Kathleen M **(SLP)**
Crane, Jane Pack **(SLP)**
Daes, Evelyn I
Dudley, Fay J C **(SLP)**
Falzarano, Mrs Alisa Lee **(A)**
Fischer, Michelle Anne
Friedel, Elane R **(A)**
James, Daniel H **(A)**
Kopp, Mrs Margaret B **(SLP)**
Krakower, Barbara J **(SLP)**
Leeds, Linda Nadelman **(SLP)**
Lonegan, Dr Charles **(SLP)**
Martin, Mrs Anne H **(SLP)**
Marto, Robert J **(SLP)**
Marx, Linda Carol **(SLP)**
Masarsky, Iris Abbe
McDonald, Alexis C **(SLP)**
McMillan, Susan B **(SLP)**
Mendelewicz, Mrs Dianne S **(SLP)**
Miller, MS3C Carole Ann **(SLP)**
Mills, Dr Jack R **(SLP A)**
Montanti, Dr John C **(SLP A)**
Nelson, Laurie Ellen **(A)**
Palmeri, Daniel J **(SLP)**
Rinehart, Gaye Michelle **(SLP)**
Rohrbach, Kay E **(SLP)**
Rollins-Bellows, Joan C **(SLP)**
Rowe, Nancy **(A)**
Ruymann, Mrs Marilyn Q **(SLP)**
Saul, Barbara J **(SLP)**
Scerri, Janice M L **(SLP)**
Selby, Elizabeth **(SLP)**
Siller, Mrs Evelyn Anne
Smith, Janet K **(SLP)**
Steelman, Carol R **(SLP)**
Stewart, Wren **(SLP)**
Tupler, Ruth I
Weinstock, Susan E **(SLP)**
Wolkowicz, Marilyn Heller **(SLP)**
Zachar, Mrs Rosalie Theresa **(SLP)**

Fort Myers

Davis, Mrs Judith J **(SLP)**
De Leon, Carmen M **(SLP)**
Dixon, Patricia Lynch **(SLP)**
Edington, Mrs Dian N **(SLP)**
Erwin, Betty J **(A)**
Grim, Mrs Elli **(SLP)**
Hawthorne, Mrs Maura Lynne **(A)**
Hayford, Dr Jane Morris **(SLP A)**
Hooper, Dr Robert Lane **(A)**
Karr, Lawana R **(SLP)**
Koste, Marilyn B **(SLP)**
Levy, Diane D **(SLP)**
Loughridge, Anne H **(SLP)**
Luna, Denise E **(SLP)**
Martina, Mark Charles **(A)**
Maxwell, Mrs Catherine T **(SLP)**
Naf, Mrs Jane H **(SLP)**
Nandur, Srinivaskumar Udyavar **(SLP A)**
Oden-Greenberg, Sandra E **(SLP)**
Padnuk, Andrew S **(SLP)**
Richardson, Deborah Young **(A)**
Roesch, Mrs Margaret Anne **(SLP)**
Sijan, Amy O **(SLP)**
Spevak, Ronald E **(SLP)**

Fort Myers Beach

Rdzanek, Irena R **(A)**

Fort Pierce

Becker, Alan M **(A)**
Orlando-Hayes, Carol **(SLP)**
Perry, Dr William D **(A)**
Spangler, Laurie Gail **(SLP)**
Thurston, Mrs Kathryn

Fort Walton Beach

Baker, Mrs Beth **(SLP)**
Cauley, Mrs Kathleen O'Neill **(SLP)**
Cavanah, Mrs Elizabeth **(SLP)**
Rivers, Susan W **(SLP)**
Ross, Rebecca Gould **(SLP)**
Sotile, Kathryn Marie **(SLP)**

Gainesville

Abbott, Dr Thomas B **(SLP)**
Andersen, Dr Helen G **(SLP)**
Barker, Constance J **(A)**
Bartlett, Mrs Cynthia Denise L **(SLP)**
Bevins, Carla McKenzie **(SLP)**
Bock, Mrs Martha R **(SLP)**
Boydstun, Mrs Sherry Bechard **(SLP)**
Brice, Alexander Emris
Brice, Caroline B **(SLP)**
Brinsko, Mrs Kit Evans **(SLP)**
Brown, Dr William S, Jr
Bzoch, Dr Kenneth R **(SLP A)**
Calkins, Dr Janice Lockhart **(SLP)**
Caranasos, Dr Constance **(SLP)**
Childers, Dr Donald G
Clements, Cheryl Marie **(SLP)**
Coomer-Rothman, GloryAnn M **(SLP)**
Crary, Dr Michael A **(SLP)**
Crawley, Brenda J
Crowley, Albert Brian **(A)**
Crowley, Margaret Stanton **(SLP)**
Cutler, Dr William H **(SLP A)**
Davidson, Mrs Linda Fox **(SLP)**
De Paz, Brunilda Gomzalez
Dillon, Ann Smith
Dyson, Dr Alice Tanner **(SLP)**
Faircloth, Barbara H **(SLP)**
Fink, Maxine E **(SLP)**
Formby, Dr Charles Craig **(A)**
Frostholm, Linda K **(SLP)**
Gerhardt, Dr Kenneth J **(A)**
Gerhardt, Mrs Melissa K **(SLP)**
Goldstein, Dr Lewis P **(SLP)**
Gomez, Malvy Carmen
Gonzalez-de Paz, Mrs Brunilda **(SLP)**
Gonzalez-Rothi, Dr Leslie J **(SLP)**
Gravel, Jane S **(SLP)**
Green, Mrs Rhonda M **(SLP)**
Haak, Dr Nancy Jeanne **(SLP)**
Hall, Mrs Gilda E F **(SLP)**
Hamilton, Mrs Nancy Chase **(A)**
Hammer, Dr Lowell Clarke **(SLP)**
Hicks, Dr Douglas M **(SLP)**
Hoffmann, Mrs Susan Kreis **(SLP)**
Hollien, Dr Harry
Hong-Wang, Mrs Marian Man-Hwei **(SLP)**
Irish, Mrs Patricia White **(A)**
Jensen, Dr Michelle W **(SLP)**
Jensen, Dr Paul J **(SLP)**
Kemker, Dr Francis Joseph **(A)**
Kim, Young Tae
Kricos, Dr Patricia **(A)**
Kristal-Bryant, Linda Gail **(SLP)**
Kwock, Dana S Y **(A)**
Lane, Angela Bollich **(SLP)**
Lazarus, Gloria J **(SLP)**
Leadon, Margaret Rose **(SLP)**
Lombardino, Linda Jean **(SLP)**
Mack, Linda **(SLP)**
Maher, Lynn M **(SLP)**
Mase, Dr Darrel J **(SLP)**
McCann, Beth **(SLP)**
McDilda, Dalzell G **(SLP)**
McIntosh, Mrs Jennifer Baur **(SLP)**
Meadows, Amanda L
Molden, Ivy Tutein **(A)**
Moore, Dr G Paul **(SLP)**
Morgese, Zoe L **(SLP)**
Murphy, Mrs Amy Waters **(A)**
Mutch, P Jane **(SLP)**
Niederkohr, Mrs Carolyn H **(SLP)**
Ochipa, Cynthia **(SLP)**
Page, Margaret R
Payne, Amy J **(SLP)**
Penner, Kandace A **(SLP)**
Phipps, Mrs Janet T **(SLP)**
Pierce, Mrs Lorraine M **(SLP)**
Post, Kathryn N **(A)**
Richard, Mrs Twana S **(SLP)**
Richtner, Ulla E M **(SLP)**
Ross, Cynthia Marie **(A)**
Rothman, Dr Howard B
Rutenberg, Mrs Kirsten V **(SLP)**
Sarkis, Joanna L **(A)**
Sarrett, Mrs Elizabeth G **(SLP)**
Schenck, Betty Jo **(SLP)**
Scroggie, Everett, Jr **(A)**
Shapiro, Susan L **(SLP)**
Shipp, Polly Moore **(A)**
Silverman, Dr S Richard **(A)**
Sloate, Mrs Carolyn Reid **(SLP)**
Sparks, Joseph D **(A)**
Stapell, Mrs Jamie Michele **(SLP)**
Stone, Mrs Peggy L **(SLP)**
Tew, Roy E **(A)**
Thompson, Dr Cynthia Kay **(SLP)**
Vinson, Mrs Betty P **(SLP)**
Walden, Ernest E, Jr **(A)**
Walker, David A **(A)**
Webb, Mrs Jennifer Jill **(SLP)**
Williams, Mrs Debra S **(SLP)**
Williams, Dr William Norman
Wilson, Mrs Cathy Sue **(SLP)**
Wingate, Mrs Judith Maige **(SLP)**
Wood, Virginia Dixon **(SLP)**

Golden Beach

Mongiello, Mrs Ann **(SLP)**

Green Cove Springs

Dooley, Mrs Judith R **(SLP)**

Greenwood

Clark, Ira B

Gulf Breeze

Allen, Mrs Linda Bronerwine **(A)**
Collier, Mrs Cheryl W **(A)**
Delisle, Shirley H **(SLP)**
Kahalley, Barbara Jean **(SLP)**
Kian, Mrs Martie A **(SLP)**
LaPorta, Rosemary A **(SLP)**
Steadham, Renee G **(A)**
Taylor, Ella Pat **(SLP)**

Gulfport

Cohen, Mrs Harriet B **(SLP)**
Costello, Dr Mary R **(SLP A)**

Haines City

Chaney, Mrs Sarah Lanier **(SLP)**

Hallandale

Beechler, Margaret Lydia **(SLP)**

Havana

Leinaar, Mrs Anne Rhodes **(SLP)**

Hawthorne

Eisen, Susan H **(SLP)**

Hernando

Donovan, Debra Ayleen **(SLP)**

Hialeah

Fernandez-Roque, Natalie **(A)**
Hullen, Mrs Virginia B **(SLP)**
Maisel, Vivian T **(SLP)**
Sueiro, Mrs Gladys V **(A)**

Holiday

Gladwin, Helen J **(A)**
Kalodoukas, Debra Economos **(SLP)**

Holly Hill

Sirk, Mrs Carolyn King **(SLP)**
Zarajczyk, Mrs Deborah R **(A)**

Hollywood

Brelinsky, Mrs Sandra Kaplan **(SLP)**
Bush, Marcia Frances **(SLP)**
Cantor, Mrs Hedia M D **(SLP)**
Chizner, Mrs Susan **(SLP)**
Ehrlich, Mrs June W **(SLP)**
Feingold, Robin E **(SLP)**
Fichtel, Mrs Dina Helene **(SLP)**
Goldberg, Mrs Sara Ann
Gorlin, Barbara Helene
Harrison, Mrs Patricia A **(SLP)**
Israel, Mrs Marian A **(SLP)**
Kurtz-Califf, Mrs Rebecca A **(SLP)**
Light, Mrs Leah Karen **(A)**
Newman, Barbara **(SLP)**
Rosenberg, Mrs Barbara C **(SLP)**
Ryll, Carolyn M **(SLP)**
Slapin, Mrs Anita E **(SLP)**
Sotiropoulos, Peter D **(A)**
Taylor, Mrs Donna Lynn **(A)**
Tuch, Doris P **(SLP)**
Winslow, Lydia J **(SLP)**

Holmes Beach

Barbe, Joann **(SLP)**
Di Orazio, Nicholas **(SLP)**
Dougherty, Mrs Dana Braswell **(SLP)**
Kurtz, Deborah Ann **(SLP)**

Lindemann, Patricia Ann **(SLP)**
Zahner, Marie L **(SLP)**

Homestead AFB
Brannon, Cindy Sue **(SLP)**

Hudson
Stemmerman, Mrs Anne Farley **(A)**
Whitley, Mrs Brenda P **(SLP)**

Indialantic
Berger, Charlene B **(SLP)**
Coleman, Mrs Linda G **(SLP)**
Reinecke, Mrs Joy G **(SLP)**

Indian Harbor Beach
Blauel, Susan B **(A)**
Varner, Mrs Harriet K **(SLP)**
Whitehead, Kathleen **(SLP)**

Indian Rocks Beach
Eisen-Siegel, Samantha **(SLP)**
Folden, Mrs Julie Sardinha **(SLP)**

Inverness
Algeo, Mark A **(SLP)**
Brumm, Robin Ann
Donovan, Mrs Beverly G **(SLP)**
Glandon, Mrs Margaret P **(SLP)**
Orlando, Ann-Marie
Regan, M Clare **(SLP)**
Smith, Audrey Lynn **(SLP)**
Walz, Mrs Laurie Peterson **(SLP)**
Wolf, Mary Ann **(SLP)**

Jacksonville
Abbott, Mrs Pamela P
Aberwald, Leslie Allison **(A)**
Allen, Mrs Susan G **(SLP)**
Allison, Mrs Cathi Pierce **(SLP)**
Aschliman, Mrs Teri L
Austin, Teresa Dawn **(SLP)**
Beckwith, Rosalind Lorraine **(SLP)**
Block, Mrs Beverly S **(SLP)**
Blumberg, Mrs L B **(SLP)**
Bungard, Mrs Elizabeth Ann **(SLP)**
Campos, Chris Timothy **(A)**
Carter, Eunice Trask **(SLP A)**
Chase, Mrs Julie Rhodes **(SLP)**
Chennault, Mrs Yanira Caparros **(SLP)**
Cherry, Mrs Barbara Waterman **(SLP)**
Cohen, Mrs Vicki C **(SLP)**
Crosby, Lisa T **(SLP)**
Cummings, Mrs Lori A **(A)**
Cummings, Robinson **(A)**
Deadrick, Mrs Dana Lynn **(A)**
Douberley, Joy L
Dunn, Mrs Lisa Baldwin **(SLP)**
Edwards, Mrs Anne Bruzzese **(SLP)**
Eilers, Mrs Gail M **(SLP)**
Franklin-Tillman, Vivian C **(SLP)**
Fuller, Mrs Susan H **(SLP)**
Gallagher, Mrs Debra L **(SLP)**
Geiger, Mrs Julia O **(SLP)**
Goggans, Shirley Dale **(SLP)**
Green, Mrs Nancy N **(A)**
Hadley, Mrs Shannon Wilder **(SLP)**
Hull, Mrs Mary O'Shea **(SLP)**
Kanter, Mrs Nancy E **(A)**
Kerley, Mrs Paula Wall **(SLP)**
Kesler, Sharon S **(SLP)**
Lawrence, Lois K **(SLP)**
League, Roslynn P **(SLP)**
Lee, Myra Amy **(SLP)**
Lightle, Mrs Susan Hall **(SLP)**
Lingenfelter-Proper, Lisa Marie **(SLP)**
Lingor, Mrs Gail J **(SLP)**
Lotowycz, Mrs Nancy Carol **(SLP)**
Mattimoe, Mrs Susan Gleespen **(SLP)**
McCray, Mrs Phyllis E **(SLP)**
McDearman, Mrs Terri Turner **(SLP)**
Memminger, Anna Belle **(SLP)**
Merritt, Mrs Dana M **(SLP)**
Moss, Mrs Amy Lee **(SLP)**
Norvid, Gail S
Ort, Ruth G **(SLP)**
Pagel, Mrs Janice Ruth **(SLP)**
Papale, Mrs Lynda P **(SLP)**
Peoples, Nancy Velma **(SLP)**
Poston, Mrs Allison Evans **(A)**
Potter, Deborah Shidler **(SLP)**
Powell, Mrs Gail C **(SLP)**
Reddick, Genevieve Nottingham **(SLP)**
Regan, Mrs Kathy Ossi **(SLP)**
Roberts, Sandra E **(SLP)**
Rose, Dr Darrell Eugene **(A)**
Russo, Sheila D **(SLP)**
Salitsky, Maureen E **(A)**
Schoenberg, Mrs Rena Dreskin **(SLP)**
Schuh, Mrs Mary Joanne **(A)**
Self, Mrs Jennifer Nass **(SLP)**
Shackelford, Mrs Helen Carolyn **(SLP)**
Singletary, Mrs Floris F **(SLP)**
Smith, Bettye H **(SLP)**
Smith, Dr Frances S **(SLP A)**
Snyder, Rosanne Marie **(SLP)**
Stewart, Adele **(SLP)**
Stringfellow, Mrs Verna W **(SLP)**
Sullivan, Glenda Moss **(SLP)**
Sutton, Mrs Kathleen Johns **(SLP)**
Teichert, Mrs Kathleen M **(SLP)**
Terry, Wayne S **(A)**
Tinley, Gordon F **(A)**
Towers, Mrs Catherine **(SLP)**
Vaughn, Judith Campsie **(SLP)**
Walker, Phyllis Jinette
Walter-Stephan, M Patricia **(SLP)**
Warner, Mrs Cheryl Busing **(SLP)**
Weaver, Leslie F **(SLP)**
Webb, Gary W **(A)**
Wester-Snyder, Ruth E **(SLP)**
White, Sherry Elizabeth **(SLP)**
Willingham, Mrs Marjorie K **(SLP)**
Wooldridge, Elaine L **(SLP)**
Workman, Oliver A **(SLP)**
Yoklic, Carol **(SLP)**

Jay
Evans, Shirley D **(SLP)**
Whitfield, Mrs Elizabeth Anne **(SLP)**

Jensen Beach
Dzikowski, Nancy Ann **(A)**
Fleming, Mrs Kimberly O'Hara **(SLP)**
Koch, Sarah Cooper **(SLP)**

Jupiter
Conner, Eleanor Sophia
Davis, Lois-Anne W **(SLP)**
Kitchings, Mrs Anne H **(SLP)**
Kitchings, Donald A **(SLP)**
Loeser, Mrs Nancy A **(SLP)**
Moore, Mrs Ilene S **(SLP)**
Snook, Robert Winson **(SLP)**
Trainer, Mrs Rosa Lee **(SLP)**

Key Biscayne
Lipman, Sharon H **(SLP)**
Musson, Nan Denise **(SLP)**
Rabassa-Thompson, Mrs Ana Maria **(SLP)**
Smith, Mary Ann **(SLP)**

Key West
Corbin, Elizabeth **(SLP)**
Freedman, Maurene M **(SLP)**
Goldner, Dr Beverly Boling **(SLP)**
Hartzell, Susan Rae **(SLP)**
Laskey-Kemnitz, Alisa J **(SLP)**

Keystone Heights
Sistrunk, Cathy Rawls **(SLP)**

Kissimmee
Allen, Wendy Leyfert **(SLP)**
Hervey, Mrs Terry O'Hair **(SLP)**
Hjelm, Jane D **(SLP)**

Lake Asbury
Swenson, Virginia Ann **(SLP)**

Lake City
Atwood, Elizabeth May **(SLP)**
Lord, Karen Sampson **(SLP)**
Powell, Jeannette H **(SLP)**
Seehorn, Mrs Terry E

Lake Mary
Bayly, Mrs Debra Ann **(SLP)**
Glantz, Michael J **(A)**
Piacentine, Mrs Marjorie Hipp **(SLP)**
Ragland, Mrs Rebecca Raye
Sackett, Karen M **(SLP)**
Steiniger, Mrs Peggy Carroll **(SLP)**

Lake Park
Pankey, Mrs Catherine Norwood **(SLP)**
Shore-Rushfeldt, Bette H **(SLP)**

Lake Vales
Johnson, Mrs Rebekah Jahna **(SLP)**

Lake Wales
Hall, Mrs Judith K **(SLP)**

Lake Worth
Crutcher, Deborah G **(SLP)**
Flory, William C **(SLP)**
Meadows, Cynthia Lynn **(A)**
Perez, Margaret Manley **(SLP)**
Spottiswood, Lydia Lynne **(A)**
Wall, Kathleen B **(SLP A)**
Weinberg, Mrs Marcia L **(SLP)**
Whitten, Terrie Ann **(SLP)**

Lakeland
Altman, Betsy Jean **(A)**
Blanchard, Mrs Diane Tooke **(SLP)**
Bodolay, Kerry Broussard **(SLP)**
Carswell, Sandra G **(SLP)**
Cary, Shelley R **(SLP)**
Copp, Mrs Martha Lamb **(A)**
Derx, Mrs Corinne Houlis **(SLP)**
Fendrick, Jennifer Elaine **(SLP)**
Golub, Latricia Daigle **(SLP)**
Gottsche, Linda L **(SLP)**
Grady, Mrs Lynn B **(SLP)**
Haskins, Mrs Janice H **(SLP)**
Haubner, Mrs Dorothy Bennett **(SLP)**
Hayes, Norma H **(SLP)**
Ittleman, Mark A **(SLP)**
Kruhm, Carolyn M **(SLP)**
Mansfield, Kelly Lyn **(SLP)**
Mercadante, Anthony J **(A)**
Moore, Mrs Ann Siman **(SLP)**
Pafunda, Mrs Katherine C **(A)**
Ratcliff, L Gay **(A)**
Reesor, Myrna Diane **(SLP)**
Rosegger, Mrs Leslie K **(A)**
Saari, Mrs Kay Ann W **(SLP)**
Seamens, John B **(SLP A)**
Tucker, Melody A **(A)**

Land O'Lakes
Cox, Linda Ruth **(A)**
Gardner, Daniel P **(A)**
Hierlmeier, Debra K **(SLP)**
Long, Mrs Marsha M Y **(SLP)**
Musalo, Sylvia C **(SLP)**

Lantana
Francis, Annjala **(SLP)**
Gough, Mrs Karen Frances **(SLP)**
Nichols, Mary Ploumis **(SLP)**
Valenza, Beth **(SLP)**

Largo
Anderson, Dr Elaine R **(SLP)**
Atkinson, Mrs Pamela M **(SLP)**
Blanchard, Deborah Jeanne **(SLP)**
Buck, Mrs Deborah Cockrell **(SLP)**
Butler, Nancy Elizabeth **(A)**
Carver, Mrs Phyllis W **(SLP)**
Gibbons, Mrs Marguerite F **(SLP)**
Gosche, Bruce Paul **(A)**
Goudie, Janice L **(SLP)**
Holstein, Diane Z **(A)**
Hutson, Mrs Patricia Fitzwillia **(SLP)**
Johanon, Rebecca R **(SLP)**
Kostakis, Cynthia **(SLP)**
Lashley, Clare Oliveri **(SLP)**
McFadden, Mrs Janice E **(A)**
Moss, Mrs Beverly A **(SLP)**
Oleksiuk, Adriana B **(SLP)**
Waters, Jana Michelle **(SLP)**
Wedzikowski, Mrs Rita Elizabeth **(SLP)**

Lauderhill
Gordon, Fran Widelitz **(SLP)**
Hershey, Beverly M **(SLP)**
Horowitz, Mrs Iris Friedman **(SLP)**
Juster, Mrs Suzanne F **(SLP)**
Maisenhalder, Laurie Evelyn **(SLP)**
Neil, Gilbert G **(SLP)**
Shapiro, Mrs Ruth Wagner **(SLP)**

Lecanto
Brown, Mrs Madeline G **(SLP)**
Dunn, Mrs Diana Bailey **(SLP)**

Leesburg
Burdick, Eve C **(SLP)**
Moat, Mrs Dorothy J **(A)**
Poulos, Thomas H **(A)**
Stroney, Mrs Mary Q **(SLP)**

Lehigh Acres
Favaro, Frank J **(A)**
Luttrell, Mrs Sherri Robin **(SLP)**

Lighthouse Point
Heise, Mrs Cynthia D **(A)**

Live Oak
Weaver, Mrs Virginia Leigh

Longboat Key
Klapman, Mrs Phyllis L **(SLP)**
Learned, Mrs Helen S **(SLP)**
Wilson, Linda F **(SLP)**

Longwood
Barnes, Janet C James **(A)**
Beckman, Debra S **(SLP)**
Coverman, Mrs Gail B **(SLP)**
Dorsey, Mrs Gillian C **(SLP)**
Gornto, Peggy D **(SLP)**
Keefer, Mrs Barbara L **(SLP)**
Lasris, Mrs Manette E **(SLP)**
McDowell, Thomas J **(SLP)**
Pensack, Irwin **(A)**
Roblee, Mrs Lorraine A **(SLP A)**
Tucker, Mrs Susan L **(SLP)**

Lutz
Brassard, Mrs Tracy Blevins **(SLP)**
Espy-Leroy, Roberta **(SLP)**
Fischer, Jayne M **(SLP)**
Freeman, William B **(A)**
Heath, Lynn C **(SLP)**
Heintz, Heather Reneee
Kinsinger, Susan I **(SLP)**
Lee, May L **(A)**
O'Brien, Ann Dorsey **(SLP)**
Sarginger, Maryrose Sharkey **(SLP)**
Saslow, Katherine **(A)**
Stefanakos, Karlene M **(SLP)**

Madeira Beach
Gray, Dr Eugene T **(SLP)**

Maitland
Buckman, Gerald F, Jr **(SLP)**
Buncher, Robert Martin **(A)**
Director, Larry **(SLP)**
Kazek, Mrs Ruth Elizabethk **(A)**
Kissel, Mrs Joan S
McNeill, Marguerite **(A)**
Medland, Julie **(SLP)**
Rubin, Cynthia B **(SLP)**
Stump, Mrs Lynn Ahrenbeck **(SLP)**

Marathon
Horn-Quarberg, Susan **(SLP)**

Margate
Lynn, Mrs Phyllis A **(SLP)**
McIntyre, Regina A **(SLP)**
Reese, Bertrand **(SLP)**
Rosso, Audrey P **(SLP)**
Talerico, Frank B **(A)**

Marianna
Lowe, Albert G, III **(SLP)**
Pruitt, Debra Michelle **(SLP)**
Williams, Mrs Janice S **(SLP)**

Mary Esther
Caravello, Cecelia LeAnn **(SLP)**

Melbourne
Campbell, Rosolyn C **(SLP)**
Carter, Tracy J
Chappotin, Laura Pierce **(A)**
Epstein, Mrs Joan Pless **(SLP)**
Faull, Mrs Rosann Wood **(A)**
Harpold, Mrs Karen Shumate **(SLP A)**
Harrison, Dr Janet Snyder **(SLP)**
Hering, Mrs Laurie Works **(SLP)**
Kurjack, Mrs Paula Reed **(SLP)**
Logsdon, John Paul **(SLP)**
Moore, Leslie Virginia **(SLP)**
Peters, Cindy L **(SLP)**
Pharo, William R **(A)**
Phillips, Janet Cheryl **(A)**
Plyler, Juliana Gibbs **(SLP)**
Rhodes, Mrs Janice Lynne **(SLP)**
Siter, Mrs Vicki Evans **(SLP)**
Stewart, Marianne **(SLP)**
Susmar, Ann E **(SLP)**
Walker, Mrs Lisa Carol
Whittington, Mrs Barbara Coleridge **(SLP)**

Melbourne Beach
Gelbert-Inbornone, Mrs Lisa **(SLP)**
Latta, Mary **(SLP)**
Porter, Elizabeth Mulligan **(SLP)**

Melrose
Neale-Tobener, Mrs Elisa **(SLP)**

Merritt Island
Bernstein, Mrs Rena S **(SLP)**
Morgan, Mrs Patsy Hardin **(SLP)**
Russo, Barbara P **(SLP)**
Treadwell, Mrs Pamela K **(SLP)**
Wasserman, Debra B **(SLP)**

Miami
Adam, Linda Peebles **(SLP)**
Adams, Lennon C, Jr **(A)**
Aiello, Margaret Guinan **(SLP)**
Applebaum, Fredrica **(SLP)**
Archer, Judith Ann
Barksdale, Mrs Linda M **(SLP)**
Batista, Mrs Lourdes **(SLP)**
Beaton, Mrs Lillian L **(SLP)**
Bender, Barbara Lynn **(SLP)**
Berger-Landau, Janice M **(SLP)**
Bergeson, Mary H P **(SLP)**
Bersson, Robin S **(SLP)**
Betancourt, Lisette M **(SLP)**
Binder, Margaret Dunn **(SLP)**
Bollinger, Dr Rick L **(SLP)**
Brashears, Margaret M **(SLP)**
Buchanan, Julia N **(SLP)**
Buldas, Nancy M **(SLP)**
Cabeza, Mrs Constance H L **(A)**
Canfield, Dr Norton **(A)**
Carlson, Dr Deborah Lynn **(A)**
Castellanos, Ana E **(SLP)**
Cetak, M J
Clarke, Pamela Yvonne **(SLP)**
Cochran, Cynthia E **(SLP)**
Connors, Janet Marie **(SLP)**
Corradini, Mrs Carol A **(SLP)**
Criswell, Wendy **(SLP)**
Dale, Dr Paulette **(SLP)**
Danse, Mrs Marian Burnett **(SLP)**
Danz, Dr Alan D **(A)**
Dawson, Clara Virginia **(SLP)**
De La Cruz, Mrs Omayda G
De La Paz, Alina **(SLP)**
Diamond, Linda **(SLP)**
Dickson, Dr David Ross **(SLP)**
Douglas, Bettye B **(SLP)**
Draizar, Dr Andrea **(SLP)**
Drucker, Mrs Judith C **(A)**
Dubosar, Mrs Stacey Meryl **(SLP)**
Eddins, Carolyn L **(SLP)**
Eifert, Anna Louise **(SLP)**
Eilers, Dr Rebecca E
Elliott, Wendy Lee **(SLP)**
Fein, Dr Louis I **(SLP)**
Fein, Rebecca B **(SLP)**
Felton, Joy E **(SLP)**
Ferguson, Betty T **(SLP)**
Figueroa, Rosario Annette **(SLP)**
Forcina, Debra L **(SLP)**
Gans, Dr Richard E **(A)**
Genet, Mrs Ellen F **(SLP)**
Giannoni, Rosa Esther **(SLP)**
Goldberg, Mrs Phyllis K **(SLP)**
Gonzalez, Mrs Julie Gonzalez **(SLP)**
Green, Mrs Nancy S **(SLP)**
Greenberg-Cordero, Barbara Alice **(A)**
Guerra, Maria Zoila
Gyant, Mrs Marie Goldson **(SLP)**
Hamrock, Marilyn Angela **(SLP)**
Harrison, Dr Robert J **(SLP A)**
Heffernan, John W **(A)**
Henretig, Max D **(SLP)**
Hernandez, Denise **(SLP)**
Hirsh, Mrs Vera Anne **(SLP)**
Hudson, Mrs Tinamarie Petrillo **(A)**
Hutchins, Deborah D **(SLP)**
Iglesias-Golden, Mrs Olga **(SLP)**
Johnson, Barbara F **(SLP)**
Kaplan, Robin Jacobs **(SLP)**
Karbowski, Laurie L **(A)**
Katzman, Mrs Shirley Rose **(SLP)**
Kay, Aimee **(A)**
Kemp, Dr James Charles **(SLP)**
Kinsora-Joseph, Mrs Peggy **(SLP)**
Korenvaes, Cynthia B **(SLP)**
Lane, Bette **(SLP)**
Langer, Dr Roy M **(SLP)**
Lavoie, Mrs Evelyn Fairchild **(SLP)**
Leon-Rodriguez, Mrs Maria E **(SLP)**
Leveen, Mrs Nancy C **(SLP)**
Lewis, Nancy E **(A)**
Light, Malcolm H, II **(A)**
Lipscomb, Mrs Gwendolyn **(SLP)**
Lundy, Donna S **(SLP)**
Malsin, Janie **(SLP)**
Mandell, Jacqueline Kramer **(SLP)**
Manners, Lori Sue **(SLP)**
Marcus, Mrs Geraldine **(SLP)**
Marks, Sharyn E **(SLP)**
Marlin, Mrs Elaine A **(SLP)**
McVoy, Esther Marie **(SLP)**
Mitrani, Mrs Laurie Cohen **(A)**
Nebel-Gould, Mrs Amy Sue **(SLP)**
Newbauer, Mrs Alisa J **(SLP)**
Nullman, Mrs Susan L **(SLP)**
Nunziata, Gale Margaret **(SLP)**
Olarte, Dr Gerardo **(SLP)**
Olarte, Mary P H **(SLP)**
O'Reilly, Ana Santos **(A)**
Parris, Rachel K **(SLP)**
Pascual, Lydia **(SLP)**
Pasternack, Karen Franco **(SLP)**
Pernick, Andrea Dale **(A)**
Pero, M Theresa **(A)**
Peters, Adrienne K **(SLP)**
Petty, Nancy A **(SLP)**
Pierce, Sondra Michelle **(SLP)**
Plager, Mrs Sara S **(SLP)**
Plumley, G Joyce **(SLP)**
Pollak, Mrs Renee **(SLP)**
Poms, Mrs Lillian R **(SLP)**
Rabin, Mrs Elizabeth Ahrenbeck **(A)**
Redd, Phillip M **(A)**
Reddin, Mrs Marcelle Cherry **(SLP)**
Reynolds, Dr Garnet L **(SLP)**
Richardson, Wendy J **(SLP)**
Richardson-Zizi, Mrs Pamela A **(SLP)**
Riley, Mrs Janet A H **(SLP)**
Roberts, Barbara Kubasta **(SLP)**
Rogatz, Linda B **(SLP)**
Rosenberg, Mrs Lillian R **(SLP)**
Rosenberg-Stein, Mrs Jan **(SLP)**
Rosenblatt, Mrs Ellen S **(SLP)**
Saul, Dr Richard S **(A)**
Schachner, Janet Smallberg **(SLP)**
Scherker, Mrs Dorothy Sholin **(SLP)**
Schwartz, Dr Melvin J **(SLP)**
Selesnick, Mrs Randy L **(SLP)**
Serrano, Maria A **(A)**
Sheckman, Iris Ettelman **(SLP)**
Shohet-Hamel, Francine L **(SLP)**
Shriner, Jane Nemec **(SLP)**
Silny, D Elaine **(SLP)**
Smith, Mrs Stacie Rubin **(SLP)**
Spector, Toby Rose **(A)**
Splitter, Marianne **(SLP)**
Steffens, Michele Leigh **(A)**
Stein, Mrs Leslie G **(SLP)**
Steinhart, Susan M **(SLP)**
Stone, Anita T **(SLP)**
Suarez, Mrs Mildred Martinez **(SLP)**
Tables, Sanford A **(SLP)**
Towner, MaryJane E **(SLP)**
Uranga, Jimena B **(A)**
Waas, Karen D Waters **(SLP)**
Walker-Casey, Amy Beth **(SLP)**
Waters, Mrs Chris T **(SLP)**
Weisman, Linda J **(SLP)**
Westman, Charlene Ann **(SLP)**
Wexler, Mrs Donna Youkilis **(SLP)**
White, Cms Kathleen Sheryll **(SLP)**
Whitney, Dr Janet L **(SLP)**
Widen, Dr Judith E **(A)**
Wilkins, Mrs Georgiann **(SLP)**
Williams, Mrs Kimberly Perry **(SLP)**
Wilson-Vazquez, Mrs Kathleen G **(SLP)**

Miami Beach
Gluck, Vivian F **(SLP)**
Goodwin, Mrs Selma Rabinovitz **(SLP A)**
Hanzman, Mrs Debi K **(SLP)**
Murphy, Marilyn Holm **(SLP)**
Stryker, Dr Stephanie **(SLP)**
Tetzeli, Marta Christina
Vaupen, Pearl **(SLP)**

Miami Lakes
Courtney, Joan Bedford **(SLP)**
Eliot, Mrs Joanne **(SLP)**
Fields, Mrs Susan E Gould **(A)**
Freiwald, Mrs Julianne Flick
Piccardo, Nancy J **(SLP)**
Ramsey, K Judith **(SLP)**

Miami Shores
Garrett, Mrs Ellen Gordon **(SLP)**
Kane, Susan Beverly **(SLP)**
Phillips, Mrs Kathleen **(SLP)**

Miami Springs
Burbey-Flingos, Mrs Jill **(SLP)**

Miatland
Van Dusen, C Raymond **(SLP)**

Middleburg
Overman, Mrs Virginia S **(A)**
Stanilonis, Daisy Nelson **(SLP)**

Mims
Kramer, Mrs Sharon Parker **(SLP)**

Miramar
Arechavaleta, Maria Teresa **(SLP)**
Dubin, Dennis C **(A)**
Panichella, Amy G **(SLP)**

Mount Dora
McAfee, Jacqulea S **(SLP)**
Miller, Mrs Irene W **(SLP)**

Mulberry
Roquemore, Leslie C **(SLP)**

Naples
Bentley, Mrs Peggy Weakland **(SLP)**
Erickson, Mrs Mary Earl **(SLP)**
Esber, Elizabeth C **(SLP)**
Foley, Michele Susan **(SLP)**
Goldman, Gail R **(SLP)**
Jacobs, Beverly Jean **(SLP)**
Ludlow, Ellen D **(SLP)**
Pittman, Mrs Mary Lou **(SLP)**
Russell, Mrs Leigh Ann **(A)**
Smith, Carolyn Jo **(SLP)**
Ursel, David **(SLP)**
Wood, Mrs Linda Thompson **(SLP)**

Neptune Beach
Cooper, Deborah Lynn
Hinton, Mrs Judy E **(SLP)**

New Port Richey
Beauclair, Lynette M **(SLP)**
Chancey, Mrs Ina M **(SLP)**
Dettman, Kim Annette **(SLP)**
Johansen, Connie Marie **(SLP)**
Metilly, Mrs Doric G **(SLP)**
Rothschild-Goldman, Mrs Lynn **(SLP)**

New Smyrna Beach
Green, Karen Denise **(SLP)**
Harvey, Kathleen **(SLP)**
Somers, Dr Janet M **(SLP)**
Woodgate, Mrs Lisa J **(SLP)**

Newberry
Rummel, Mrs Veronica Kadala

Niceville
Collins, Alicia J

Nokomis
Fitzgerald, Donna **(SLP)**
Leach, Mrs Judy S **(SLP)**
Thomas, Mrs Elizabeth **(SLP)**

North Bay Village
Blake, Mrs Jane G **(SLP)**

North Fort Myers
Carrasquillo, Mrs Ann Jabsen **(SLP)**
Conroy, Barbara B **(SLP)**
Lahaie, Dr Ralph V **(SLP)**

North Indiatlantic
Happ, J Yvonne **(SLP)**

North Lauderdale
Finnegan, Eileen Marquerite **(SLP)**
Frankel, Lynn E **(SLP)**
Pilelsky, Rhoda Gail **(SLP)**
Rosenberg, Mrs Sandra M

North Miami
Abecassis, Nancy F **(SLP)**
Bruno, Concetta **(SLP)**
Donalson, Valerie Ann **(SLP)**
Feldman, Irene R **(SLP)**
Pike, Vicki Jean
Schrager, Mrs Rhea H **(SLP)**
Slate, Suzanne I

North Miami Beach
Adler, Mrs Elaine T **(SLP)**
Altman, Mrs Stephanie R **(SLP)**
Bicky, Linda **(SLP)**
Center, Dr Benjamin **(SLP)**
Failla, Carl **(SLP)**
Ganz, Mrs Elinor C **(SLP)**
Glickstein, Laurel Chertow **(SLP)**
Goldenberg, Mrs Jean **(SLP)**
Jackerson, Cathy Briggs **(SLP)**
Kahn, Adrienne L **(SLP)**
Kates, Mrs Adele Dalinsky **(SLP)**
Klein, Carla L **(SLP)**

Mayer, Mrs Shelli Susan **(SLP)**
Perlstein, Marie Maffeo
Sattinger, Karen **(SLP)**
Thornton, Robin E **(SLP)**
Weiner, Ellen S **(SLP)**

North Palm Beach
Ciavarella, Carol **(SLP)**
Domb, Mrs Elona G **(A)**
Williams, Mrs Nina C **(SLP)**

North Port
Mraz, Norma Rivera **(A)**
Savell, Mrs Mildred S **(SLP)**
Smith, Thomas C **(SLP A)**

North Redington Beach
Volland, Mrs Bonnie L **(SLP)**

O'Brien
Moses, Mrs Nancy Johnson **(SLP)**

Oakland Park
Druckman, Mindy Lynn **(SLP)**
Dworkin, Valerie **(SLP)**
Lechtenberg, Mrs Cheryl Lynn **(A)**
Willson, Becky Lynn **(SLP)**

Ocala
Branson, Page Strickland **(SLP)**
Carl, Maureen Ellen **(SLP)**
Grubaugh, Karen J **(SLP)**
Hargrave, Mrs Jill Stewart **(SLP)**
Jones, Anne M **(SLP)**
Ludwig, Karen Lanice **(SLP)**
Metzger, Patricia R **(SLP)**
Mills, Joyce S **(SLP)**
Padgett, Mrs Carolynn J **(SLP)**
Phillips, Mrs Lorey House **(SLP)**
Pierce, Mrs Claudia Grooms **(SLP)**
Rigsby, Mrs Donna Brock **(SLP)**
Taft, Patricia Michele **(SLP A)**
Thursby, Mrs Janet R **(SLP)**
Wallace, Mrs Teri Ann **(SLP)**
Webb, Mrs Janet E S **(SLP)**

Odessa
Lavin, Kathryn D **(SLP)**

Okeechobee
Joselson, Dr Maurice Louis **(SLP)**
Kaufman, Mrs Diane Boehler **(SLP)**

Oklawaha
Miller, Mrs Dorothy S **(SLP)**

Opa-Locka
Johnson, Carla W **(SLP)**

Orange City
Dasso, Mrs Sandra Sandstrom **(SLP)**

Orange Park
Anderson, Mrs Therese Ann **(SLP)**
Benson, Mrs Nancy S **(SLP)**
Clarke, Debbie W **(SLP)**
Dipzinski, Christine Ann **(SLP)**
Green, Mrs Frances A **(SLP)**
Hugghins, Mrs Marcia L **(SLP)**
Jacquin, Mrs Diane Rubinski **(SLP)**
Kaswinkel, Mrs Patricia T **(SLP)**
Lucente, Mrs Laura Dykes **(SLP)**
Lucente, Warren R **(A)**
McKinney, Elizabeth Ann **(SLP)**
Muilenburg, Diane D **(A)**
Proctor, Roy E **(SLP)**
Sanders, Albert G, III **(A)**
Slayden, Mitzie Michele **(A)**
Wendell, Mary V **(SLP)**
Williams, Myra Jann Spence **(SLP)**
Wilson, Mrs Laura McNutt **(A)**

Orlando
Arias, Carmen M **(SLP)**
Ashley, Donna Debolt **(SLP)**
Berardino, John T **(A)**
Berger, Mrs Jeri Skolkin **(SLP)**
Brockman, Mrs Nancy A **(SLP)**
Byrd, Juliane Federico **(SLP)**
Caton, Ann **(SLP)**
Chambers, Carol J **(A)**
Clair, Mrs Margaret Goss **(SLP)**
Collins, Elizabeth A **(SLP)**
Collins, Mrs Jean Tallyn **(SLP)**
Cordero, Mrs M Suzanne **(SLP)**
Coward, Paula Joan **(A)**
Dahn, Barbara Gordon **(SLP)**
Dechant, Joseph Michael **(A)**
Flemming, Mrs Alison Hedden **(SLP)**
Flynn, Mrs Linda Denese **(SLP)**
Flynn, Patricia Aileen **(A)**
Franklin, Mrs Edith P **(SLP)**
Freeland, Susan M **(SLP)**
Gottsleben, Sheila Ann **(A)**
Graves, Mrs Linda Dawn P **(SLP)**
Hancock, Kelly Kathleen **(SLP)**
Hayduk, Roberta Jo **(A)**
Hemphill, Rhonda H **(SLP)**
Higley, Mrs Beulah S **(SLP)**
Hodges, Sue H **(SLP)**
Jensen, Denise A **(SLP)**
Johansen, Mrs Floye V **(SLP)**
Jones, Carmen Lynne **(SLP)**
Kennedy, Dr June Ford **(SLP A)**
Lefkov, Carol S **(SLP)**
Lemp, Janice Wright **(SLP)**
Lovegreen, Mrs Valerie Ann
Maggi-Thomas, Debra Jane **(SLP)**
Maher, Catherine A **(SLP)**
Marincov, Mrs Elizabeth Ellen **(SLP)**
Mattox, Helen M
McClung, Linda N **(SLP)**
McNamara, Mrs June Bilotta **(SLP)**
Miller, Lynn M **(SLP)**
Morilak, Deborah Jeanne **(SLP)**
Mowers, Mrs Karen Chesser **(SLP)**
Mullin, Dr Thomas A **(SLP A)**
Munson, Patricia Ann **(SLP)**
Nelson, C Van **(SLP)**
Nichols, Dean G **(SLP)**
Nichols, Murdayne A **(SLP)**
Olson, Mrs Mary S **(SLP)**
Osborne, Charles Arno **(SLP)**
Osborne, Jane A **(A)**
Parker, Hazel **(SLP)**
Pellosie, Mrs Elizabeth **(SLP)**
Peters, Mrs Anne Hains **(A)**
Petronio, Mrs Martha Jo **(SLP)**
Pickering, Mrs Joanna Hayes **(SLP)**
Redmond, Mrs Beatrice Myers **(A)**
Revoir, Katherine Elaine **(SLP)**
Rierson, Mrs Terrie Stanley **(SLP)**
Seal, Mrs Joy M **(SLP)**
Shirek, Mrs Paula G **(SLP)**
Stokes, Mrs Rosemary H
Tatum, Linda Marie **(SLP)**
Tetnowski, John A **(SLP)**
Thomas, Mrs Tina Gaffney **(A)**
Trychel, Marc Robert **(A)**
Utt, Dr Harold A, Jr **(A)**
Van Tatenhove, Gail M **(SLP)**
Vodev, Michelle C **(SLP)**
Von Deck, Mrs Karin A **(SLP)**
Zinna, Mario Anthony, Jr **(SLP)**
Zittere, Judy Oakley **(SLP)**

Ormond Beach
Belden, Christine Shanks **(SLP)**
Fink, Dr William H **(SLP)**
Hanson, Mrs Kathleen O **(SLP)**
Leorza, Mrs Susan C **(SLP)**
Marois, Denis A **(SLP)**
McMahon, Constance **(SLP)**
Ritter, Lynne M G **(A)**
Sheehan, Linda S **(SLP)**
Tate, Susan M **(SLP)**
Ward, Catherine **(SLP)**

Osprey
Peters, Dorothy M **(SLP)**

Oviedo
Clark, Mrs Janet Maurine
Hedrick, Dr Dona Lea **(SLP)**
Ingram, Dr David B **(SLP)**
Schmucker, Sheryl E **(SLP)**

Pace
De Vuyst, Mrs Anita Comfort **(SLP)**
Vannerson, Mrs Judy R **(SLP)**

Paisley
Weber, Renee M A **(SLP)**

Palatka
Clark, Joyce Fretz **(SLP)**
Richter, Ellen M **(SLP)**

Palm Bay
Aker, Dr Charles Randall **(SLP)**
Cowan-Oberbeck, Catherine **(A)**
Hermanowicz, Carol Jean **(SLP)**
Kinsey, Joanmarie Therese **(SLP)**
Lange, Mrs Nancy Slate **(SLP)**
Pegram, Nancy Metcalf **(SLP)**
Rushing, Susan Yvonne **(SLP)**

Palm Beach
Kelly, Mrs Kristina Larsen **(SLP)**
Olmstead, Mrs Mary J **(SLP)**
Rozelle, Anne M M **(SLP)**
Spencer, Nedra Elaine **(SLP)**

Palm Beach Gardens
Ancona, Beverly Wolfe **(SLP)**
Buttner, Patricia E **(SLP)**
Duhl, Mrs Sherrie J **(A)**
Kushner, Mrs Linda Ross **(SLP)**
Poterek, Theresa Marie
Schlanger, Dr Bernard B **(SLP)**
Schlanger, Mrs Phoebe H **(SLP)**
Stein, Mrs Helene F **(A)**
Thomasson, Mrs Elizabeth **(A)**

Palm Coast
Timlin, Mrs Katherine Love **(SLP)**

Palm Harbor
Alcorn, Stephen R **(SLP A)**
Bohling, Ellen Roslyn **(SLP)**
Fillmore, Rebecca Gail **(SLP)**
Glover, Mrs Toni A **(SLP)**
Hart, Ann Ross **(SLP)**
Kinde, Dr Stewart **(SLP A)**
Malone, Martha L **(SLP)**
Nikjeh, Mrs Deborah Adams **(SLP)**
Nowikowski, Kayte **(SLP)**
Rophie, Mrs Sharon Slaughter **(A)**
Sanborn, Mrs Pamela H **(SLP)**
Wood, Terry Donovan **(SLP)**

Palmetto
Bell, Fred E **(SLP)**
Hogan, Mrs Diane J **(SLP)**
McErlain, Eileen Margaret **(SLP)**
Tencza-Pinsonneault, Judith L **(SLP)**

Panama City
Benci, Mrs Dee Yvonne
Bohac, Mrs Carol A **(SLP)**
Davis, Diane A **(SLP)**
Drawbaugh, Lana Rae **(SLP)**
Hardy, Mrs Jocerlyn L **(SLP)**
Kennedy, Patricia A **(SLP)**
Loiry, Mrs Carol J **(SLP A)**
O'Gallagher, Elizabeth F **(A)**
Phillips, Janice Lynn **(SLP)**
Sewell, Mrs Jill N **(SLP)**
Siegel, Mrs Terri M **(A)**
Skinner, Mrs Betty R **(SLP)**
Staley, Anne **(SLP)**
Straub, Charles S **(A)**
Weems, Alisa Karen **(SLP)**

Panama City Beach
Sullivan, Carol R **(SLP)**
Sullivan, Dr James L **(A)**

Parkland
Alfonso, Mrs Jilana B **(SLP)**
Becker, Mrs Jill J **(SLP)**
Geller-O'Dwyer, Kathie **(SLP)**
Lack, Mrs Barbara S **(SLP A)**

Parrish
Morgan, Janet L **(SLP)**

Pembroke Lakes
Kevelson, Margery Gale **(SLP)**

Pembroke Pines
Burchyett, Shane Mulias **(SLP)**
Casale, Mrs Sandra Eskinzes **(SLP)**
Comiter, Mrs Marilyn T **(SLP)**
Esposito, Catherine **(SLP)**
Hale-Haniff, Mary **(SLP)**
Kishter, Mrs Helen H M **(SLP)**
Olicker, Mrs Charlene L **(SLP)**
Park, Michele A **(SLP)**
Pyers, Mrs Marilyn J
Roberts, Mrs Joanne S **(A)**
Stark, Mrs Irene Anstendig **(SLP)**
Sykes, Meredeth K **(SLP)**
Walters, John C **(SLP)**
Zombar, Catherine Roll **(SLP)**

Pensacola
Baggett, Julie Evan **(SLP)**
Baily, Mrs Linda B **(SLP)**
Beeman, Marsha L **(SLP)**
Behrends, William H, Jr **(A)**
Bruner, Mrs Barbara J **(SLP)**
Buckley, Mrs Vicki Annette **(SLP)**
Burns, William Joseph
Caldwell, Ethlyn D **(SLP)**
Cross, Mrs Sharon Thomas **(SLP)**
Cross, Mrs Sherrie Nesmith **(SLP)**
Dannheisser, Karen S **(A)**
De Stafney, Jan Elisabeth **(A)**
Duffy, Mrs Melita Tillery **(SLP)**
Eckert, Celeste F **(SLP)**
Goll, Mrs Margaret C **(SLP)**
Gowens, Pamela A R **(SLP)**
Gray, Molly Buckles **(A)**
Gridley, Mrs Katherine L **(SLP)**
Griffith, Jeffrey Samuel **(A)**
Hall, Jane Elizabeth
Haupt, Mrs Robin Terry **(A)**
Howard, Mrs Kay H **(SLP)**
Jones, J Paula **(SLP)**
Kahn, Janet S **(A)**
Kennedy, Linda E **(SLP)**
Lanphier, Melanie Ledyard **(SLP)**
Lozier, Dr Carol Whitcomb **(A)**
Nichols, Deborah H **(SLP)**
Overstreet, Paige Alise
Porch, Mrs Robyn Bailey **(SLP)**
Reeves, Mrs Marsha M **(SLP)**
Roberts, Gay W **(SLP)**
Robertson, Dr Ronald McDonald **(A)**
Robinson, Sheila Caleria **(A)**
Smead, Kathleen **(SLP)**
Wagener, Dr John W **(A)**
Whibbs, Rosemary **(SLP)**
White, Mrs Myrna Goff **(SLP)**
Whitman-Tims, Iowana **(SLP)**

Pensacola Beach
Gelfand, Mrs Dolores E **(SLP)**
Haney, Nancy Brannon **(SLP)**
Moss, Mrs Deborah C **(SLP)**
Oyama, Mrs Katherine Ann **(SLP)**
Wells, Donna Arnett **(SLP)**

Perry
Maxwell, Mrs Elizabeth D **(SLP)**

Pinellas Park
Counts, Lou H **(A)**
Fritz, Mrs Michelle I **(SLP)**
Kelly, Mrs Christine **(SLP)**
Sullivan, Burton H **(SLP)**
Wood, Dr W Scott **(A)**

Yates, Mrs Marilyn Anne **(SLP)**

Plant City
Falany, Mrs JoEllen H **(SLP)**
Wnek, Mary E **(SLP)**

Plantation
Adler, Ellen T **(SLP)**
Akar, Mrs Christine Hintz **(SLP)**
Arnold, Linda Jean **(SLP)**
Arroyo, Mrs Marian L **(SLP)**
Bianco, Carol **(SLP)**
De La Torre, Mrs Jodi Tice **(SLP)**
Foxman, Carol Ann **(SLP)**
Goldman, Diane M **(SLP)**
Heinrich, Jennifer Anne
Kahn, Mrs Andrea Port **(SLP)**
Karp, Mrs Roxanne L **(SLP)**
Kessler, Robin Ann **(A)**
Kluesing, Mrs Marsha A **(A)**
Lerner, Mrs Carol J **(SLP)**
Lowell, Judy Z **(SLP)**
Newman, Mrs Cindy Karesky **(SLP)**
Newman, Mrs Gail D **(SLP)**
O'Donnell, Grace B
Passman, Beth S **(SLP)**
Rahe, Frederick A **(A)**
Rey, Mrs Janice Whitehead **(SLP)**
Roberts, Cheri T **(SLP)**
Roth, Donald E **(SLP)**
Rudel, Debra L **(SLP)**
Saunders, Elizabeth O **(SLP)**
Shnider, Dr Arline **(A)**
Steinfeld, Mrs Marcia L **(SLP)**
Walerstein, Mrs Joan I S **(SLP)**
Winer-McWilliam, Yona **(SLP)**
Wojcik, Monica M G **(SLP)**

Plymouth
Fogarty, Cynthia Ann **(A)**

Pompano Beach
Breslow, Ellen N **(SLP)**
Burnett, Melodi Anne **(A)**
Casey-Wolff, Jeannette **(SLP)**
Cherof, Mrs Ruby C **(SLP)**
Diamond, Matthew **(SLP)**
Gabryel, Mrs Nini W **(SLP)**
Kerr, Mrs Cynthia Canipe **(SLP)**
Lieberman, Mrs Nancy K **(SLP)**
McCall, Patricia Lynn **(A)**
McConaughey, Lori A **(SLP)**
Pomerantz, Joan K **(SLP)**

Ponte Vedra Beach
Bell, Lisa Conover **(SLP)**
Chapa, Virginia Fiastro **(SLP)**
Crawford, Nancy P **(SLP)**
Knowles, Mary Susan **(SLP)**
Thornton, Kimberly Wilson **(SLP)**

Port Charlotte
Baisler, Perry E **(SLP)**
Beers, Mrs Ann Mackey **(SLP)**
Brown, Mrs Joan M **(SLP)**
Brown, Dr Robert A **(SLP)**
Chamberlain, Ruth I **(SLP)**
Dancek, Mrs Laura F P **(SLP)**
Draeger, Mrs Katherine Louise **(SLP)**
Holmes, Mrs Imogene L **(SLP)**
Muir, Katherine C Jones **(A)**
Stombaugh, Linda A **(SLP)**
Walden, Mrs Bethany Lee **(A)**

Port Orange
Hartman, Lisa D **(SLP)**
Miller, Vaughn P **(SLP)**
Palitz, Marsha E **(SLP)**
Sharkey, Laurie Ann **(SLP)**
Skowronsky, Susan A **(SLP)**

Port Richey
Balogh, Mrs Lucille M **(SLP)**
Kline, Constance Church **(SLP)**

Port St Lucie
Alfera, Mrs Valerie A **(SLP)**
Barno, Jeanne Ellen **(A)**
Carpenter, Michele D **(A)**
Ferch, Mrs Pamela A **(SLP)**
Hancock, Laura Ellen **(SLP)**
Magill, Shanda Barger **(SLP)**

Punta Gorda
Newby, Dr Hayes A **(SLP A)**
Stublen, Mrs Greta Pilson **(SLP)**
Thatcher, Deven M **(SLP)**

Quincy
Emery, Mrs Alice Ford
Penrod, Dr John P **(A)**
Thornton, Mary Susan **(A)**
Woodward, Mrs Eleanor S

Redington Beach
Millar, Stewart Wilson **(SLP A)**

Redington Shores
Miller, Claudia F **(SLP)**

Riverview
Sutherland, Alan C

Riviera Beach
Ernst, Barbara M **(SLP)**
Portera, Rosemary V **(SLP)**

Rockledge
Barr, Dr David F **(A)**
Holloway, Mrs Kathleen R **(SLP)**
Karlow, Carol Marie **(SLP)**
Thomas, Mrs Dolores Adams **(SLP)**

Rotonda West
Schaeffer, Remle Sue **(SLP)**

Royal Palm Beach
Pendleton, Suzanne McDavid **(SLP)**

Safety Harbor
Barton, Lori Jean **(SLP)**
Millns, Jennifer **(SLP)**
Olsen, Sue King **(SLP)**
Slaby, Mrs Robin Dale **(SLP)**
Wright, Monica L **(SLP)**

Sanford
Mercer, Ellen F **(A)**
Williams, Mrs Karen D **(SLP)**

Sanibel
Forster, Mrs Charlotte Fich **(SLP)**
Krival, Dr Molly P **(SLP)**
Wasson, Mary Ann **(SLP)**

Santa Rosa Beach
Linke, Charles E **(SLP A)**

Sarasota
Aronoff, Mrs Rebecca C **(SLP)**
Bennett, Leigh Holtby **(SLP)**
Berger, Mildred B **(SLP)**
Blaustein, June H **(SLP)**
Bowen, Katherine Ricchetti **(SLP)**
Brunner, Joseph L **(SLP)**
Burdette, Regina L **(SLP)**
Carmel, Norman Hirsch **(SLP A)**
Dinenna, Mrs Doreen S
Dolan, Lesley Pinel **(A)**
Dove, Hilary **(SLP)**
Eshelman, Mrs Mary P **(SLP A)**
Frawley, Janis R **(SLP)**
Gay, Mrs Helen S **(SLP)**
Godwin, Bernadette Augustine **(SLP)**
Gormley, Patricia Ryland
Haigh, Amy Lee **(SLP)**
Harrison, Patricia S **(SLP)**
Hotard, Mark Drake
Hudak, Mrs Deborah Wright **(A)**
Inbar, Mrs Betsy L **(SLP)**
Jones, Karin A **(SLP)**
Joseph, Phyllis Harris **(SLP)**
Knight, Dr Elmo L **(SLP A)**
Kraemer, Iris T **(SLP)**
Krassowski, Mrs Elaine Burke **(SLP)**
Lloyd-Jones, Mrs Rebecca Jo **(SLP)**
Morgan, Mrs Noel Garvin **(A)**
Oleen, Cornelia J **(SLP)**
Palmeri, Janine M **(A)**
Pedicini, Kathryn A **(SLP)**
Pickering, Mrs Joyce **(SLP)**
Rawlings, Diane Lynne **(SLP)**
Rogers-Brunner, Cindy L **(SLP)**
Rosenberg, Gail Gegg **(A)**
Rowe, Mrs Susan E B **(SLP)**
Rush, Mrs Juliann Finegan **(A)**
Schneider, Sandra L **(SLP)**
Simmons, Donna M **(A)**
Simons, Barbara H **(SLP)**
Stafford, Barbara S **(SLP)**
Thorpe, Mary O **(A)**
Van Hoesen-Closs, Mrs Jane **(SLP)**
Werner, Mrs Lorna S **(SLP)**
Wilson, Jodi L **(SLP)**
Woociker, Mrs Jo Ann **(SLP)**

Satellite Beach
Abrahamson, Debbie Lynn **(SLP)**
Ransom, Mrs Nina D **(SLP A)**
Rooks, Mrs Mary P **(SLP)**

Sebring
Ashley, Stephen J **(SLP)**
Chambliss, Mrs Colleen M **(SLP)**
Livingston, Andrea Dawn **(A)**
Puzel, Vicki Renken
Winger, Mrs Joan B **(SLP)**

Sebring Hills
Vandam, Mrs Vicki A M **(SLP)**

Seffner
Moran, Susan Schutz **(SLP)**

Seminole
Ekren, Wayne K **(SLP)**
Freeman, Mrs Nancy C **(SLP)**
Gillespie, Mrs M Beth **(SLP)**
Langhans, Dr Joseph J **(SLP)**
McKillop, Mrs Marcia Ann **(SLP)**
Miller, Pamela Moore **(SLP)**
Mokotoff, Mrs Barbara C **(A)**
Richman, Mrs Eileen K **(SLP)**
Speake, Mrs Jennifer Araj **(SLP)**
Sterensis, Mrs Barbara G **(SLP)**
Techler, Melinda Reily **(SLP)**

Shalimar
Cornell, Dr Rhonda Holmes **(SLP)**
Newsome, Cheryl Ann **(SLP)**
Szafran, Teri Lea **(SLP)**

Sopchoppy
Harriss, Judith C **(SLP)**

South Daytona
Prater, Laura Chappell **(A)**
Wheelock, Sandra Kaye **(SLP)**

South Miami
Lewis, Barbara Jean **(SLP)**
Simon, Cindy Ann **(A)**
Towle, Patricia M **(A)**

South Pasadena
Lorand, Mrs Marjorie J **(SLP)**

Spring Hill
Di Cristofalo, Mrs Karen Margaret **(SLP)**
Kania, Mrs Cathy S **(SLP)**
Noblin, Mrs Katherine Marie **(SLP)**
Schott, Deborah M **(SLP)**
Wilson, Linda S **(SLP)**

St Augustine
Hall, Vicki Lynn **(SLP)**
Kanofsky, Dorrie Lynne **(A)**
Long, Kai M **(SLP)**
Matsumoto, Judy Ann **(A)**
Parsons, Steven Taylor **(SLP)**
Prokes, Jerry E **(A)**
Stone, Mrs Karen Ann **(SLP)**
Wills, Jonnie Charlyne **(A)**

St Cloud
Cloud, Mrs Zletta K **(SLP A)**
Mungall, Teresa Kelly **(SLP)**

St Petersburg
Ahrndt, Gretchen Mary **(SLP)**
Ayers, Cathi Anne **(SLP)**
Barker, Daniel Edward **(A)**
Billings, Mrs Catherine A **(SLP)**
Boger, Janice Arlene **(A)**
Burgett, Sally A **(SLP)**
Burrows, Mrs Kimberly Ann
Chisholm, Mrs Katrina E **(A)**
Collins, Shelley Kay **(SLP)**
Cook, Jeannie Marie **(SLP)**
Davis, Emily H **(SLP)**
Davis, Mary Lynn **(SLP)**
Durkin, Teresa K **(SLP)**
Ebaugh, Mrs Elaine Dinst **(SLP)**
Eckhardt, Jenny L
Flacinski, Ann Frances **(SLP)**
Foster, Kathleen D **(SLP)**
Fularz-Sendker, Mrs Kathleen **(SLP)**
Fulton, Mrs Susan Ellison **(A)**
Gorski, Janice F **(SLP)**
Gray, Elizabeth Anne **(SLP)**
Herbert, Mrs Dale Frances **(SLP)**
Horton, Ann Smyth **(SLP)**
Hunsinger, Andrea S **(SLP)**
Jones, Carol Elise **(SLP)**
Langworthy, Jack Allen **(A)**
Lefevre, Margaret C **(SLP)**
Mason, Mrs Luane C **(SLP)**
McCulloch, Frances Harriet **(SLP)**
Mellon, Mrs Karen M Percy **(SLP)**
Meyer, Robert R **(A)**
Milliken, Joy J **(A)**
Misenhelder, Mrs Faye Cagle **(SLP)**
Montanari, Mrs Therese Marie **(SLP)**
Morris, Mary Clare **(SLP)**
Moss, Ellen N **(SLP)**
O'Gara, Susan Curran **(SLP)**
Paris, Melvin J **(SLP)**
Pendry, Dr Barry L **(SLP)**
Perrott, Karen Margaret **(SLP)**
Picantine, Jayna Lynn **(SLP)**
Rains, Jennifer Lee **(SLP)**
Reimer, Patricia Thompson **(SLP)**
Rossi, Carla Anne
Rowsey, Lisa Renae
Scurr, Deborah D **(SLP)**
Shelby, Ronald J **(SLP A)**
Sheppard, Susan Saynt **(SLP)**
Terry, Susan E **(A)**
Timpone, Lauren Alissa **(A)**
Tweedy, Julia K **(SLP)**
Waldmann, Frederick **(A)**
Walters, Joyce **(SLP)**
Weaver, Mrs Jill M **(SLP)**
Wells-Friedman, Margaret **(SLP)**
Williams, Dr Sarah E **(SLP)**
Wilson, Dr D Kenneth **(SLP A)**
Wilson, Mrs Frances P **(A)**
Ylvisaker, Velma S

St Petersburg Beach
Cane, Paula B **(SLP)**

Starke
Adams, Denise S **(SLP)**

Stuart
Edick, Mrs Lisa Irby **(SLP)**
Moore, Phyllis C **(SLP)**
Sawyer, Linda Delgado **(A)**

Summerfield
Hunter, Carolyn Jean

Summerland Key
Baker, Mrs Marjorie L **(SLP)**

Sun City
Roberts, Mrs Kathylene **(SLP)**

Sun City Center
Meissner, Mrs Nancy Fay **(SLP)**

Sunrise
Beck, Mrs Bonnie R **(SLP)**
Braverman, Mrs Meryl Spector **(SLP)**
Ehren, Dr Barbara J **(SLP)**
Ehren, Tom C **(SLP)**
Friedman, Gary **(A)**
Hess, Mrs Janell T **(SLP)**
Jones, Mrs Sara J **(SLP)**
Marmor, Mrs Francine Levy **(SLP)**
Mindell, Audrey Robin **(A)**
Reiff, Mrs Janice Roper **(SLP)**
Ronczkowski, Mrs Mary Ann **(SLP)**
Sheroff, Rita J **(SLP)**
Swayman, Debbie Meyers

Sunset Beach
Gerber, Beth Pressner **(SLP)**

Switzerland
Eye, Mrs Marcia P **(SLP)**
Willhoit, Marilyn J **(A)**

Tallahassee
Adams, Amy Kathryn **(SLP)**
Alford, Denise A **(SLP)**
Atkinson, Mrs Kimberly Harder **(SLP)**
Bachman, Mary L **(SLP)**
Bailey, Jean F **(SLP)**
Bailey, Larry Jerome **(SLP)**
Bauer, Steven **(SLP)**
Bechtold, Mrs Judith Alexander
Berry, Mrs Anna Whitley **(SLP)**
Bischoff, Deborah Cohen **(SLP)**
Blumsack, Dr Judith T **(A)**
Brisendine, Maria K **(A)**
Brosnan-Maddox, Susan **(SLP)**
Brown, Harriet Patricia **(SLP)**
Brown, Mrs Mary Ellen **(SLP)**
Clifton, Mrs Carrie Campbell
Cline, Mrs Lezlie H **(SLP)**
Collins, Virginia Rose **(A)**
Crawford, Mrs Gladys H **(SLP)**
Crawford, Lorri Couch **(SLP)**
Crowley, Donna J **(SLP)**
Davidson, Thomas Oferrell **(A)**
Disarno, Neil J **(A)**
Emanuel, Mrs Renee Miller **(SLP)**
Evans, Mrs Adeline L **(SLP)**
Franklin, Thomas Claiborne **(A)**
Goodwin, Mrs Rebecca Leach **(SLP)**
Graf, Mrs Ann Jones **(SLP)**
Grayson, Mrs Lori Savage **(SLP)**
Haas, Dr William H **(SLP A)**
Ham, Dr Richard E **(SLP)**
Hardiman, Mrs Carole M **(SLP)**
Harper, Mrs Gaye O **(SLP)**
Hatton, Nina E **(SLP)**
Headley, Mrs Carol McDaniel **(SLP)**
Holbrook, Dr Anthony **(SLP)**
Hudson, Delores Y **(SLP)**
Jimenez, Mary Rutledge **(SLP A)**
Johnson, Mrs Nancy J **(SLP)**
Johnson, Pamela C **(SLP)**
Katz, Debra Friedland **(SLP)**
Kessing, Elizabeth Ann **(SLP)**
Law, Mrs Marilyn Ayers **(SLP)**
Madsen, Sitka Ann **(SLP)**
Maxwell, Mrs Bess Sirmon **(SLP)**
May, Mrs Joan P **(SLP)**
McClung, Mrs Janice Wester **(SLP)**
McRae, Catherine L **(SLP)**
Miles, Linda F B **(SLP)**
Morgan-Landing, Kathleen Anne **(A)**
Morris, Dr Richard J **(SLP)**
Morrison, Mrs Carol Roberts **(SLP)**
Ogletree, Billy Townsend **(SLP)**
Ostendorf, Joseph C **(SLP)**
Payne, Dr John A
Pellegrino, Mrs Mary M **(SLP)**
Peyton, Katharine Taylor **(SLP)**
Pittman, Barbara Ann **(SLP)**
Pooser, Mrs Polly B **(SLP)**
Pope, Mrs Catherine Turner **(A)**
Rodriguez, Gary P **(A)**
Rose, John S **(SLP)**
Sande, Laninda Arisa
Scharein, Edna Ward **(SLP)**
Schendel, Laurel L **(SLP)**
Shelfer, Janet S **(A)**
Solberg, Larry C **(SLP)**
Stutzman, Mrs Anne Reidelberg **(A)**
Sumner, Mrs Nancy C **(SLP)**
Taber, Mrs Marcia L **(SLP)**
Taylor, Barbara Ann
Taylor, Joanne **(SLP)**
Walker, Dr Virginia G **(SLP)**
Walsh, Mary J **(SLP)**
Watson, Sue B **(SLP)**
Wetherby, Dr Amy M **(SLP)**
White, Blanche B **(SLP)**
Wiman, Vicki L **(A)**
Work, Rhonda S **(SLP)**
Wulkan, Jamie B **(SLP)**
Yonclas, Dianne Goodnough **(SLP)**

Tamarac
Carlson, Judith Marie **(SLP)**
Colton, Sophia S **(SLP)**
Moonen, Diane E **(A)**
Rubin, Sylvia **(SLP)**

Tampa
Ballagh, Brenda Johnson **(SLP)**
Barimo, Joseph Patrick **(SLP)**
Barth, Mrs Jeanne M **(SLP)**
Beckley, Linda S **(SLP)**
Berlinger, Susan M **(SLP)**
Bloch, Patricia J **(SLP)**
Boas, Beverly S **(SLP)**
Bonavico, Joni Cristine **(A)**
Booher, Kenneth **(A)**
Bosy, Anne Elizabeth **(A)**
Brand, Kathleen Ann **(SLP)**
Branham, Mrs Nancy G J **(SLP)**
Brinson, Joann
Cantor, Mrs Linda L **(SLP)**
Carlson, Rebekah L **(SLP)**
Case-Dehaven, Mrs Candace Ann **(SLP)**
Chase, Caren Ann **(SLP)**
Chilton, Mrs Shelley Kermeen **(SLP)**
Cline, Debbie Nilwon **(A)**
Cooperman, Susan N **(SLP)**
Corneau, Janette B **(SLP)**
Cox, Herbert A, III **(A)**
Crockett, Dr Karen E **(SLP)**
Davidson, Mrs Leah Adler **(SLP)**
Davis, Dr Julia M **(A)**
Davis, Mrs Pamela K **(SLP)**
Decker, Deborah Jean **(SLP A)**
Delotto, Antoinette **(SLP)**
Dickson, Maribeth
Diss, Mrs Nancy Muscato **(A)**
Dubrow, Janine Renee **(SLP)**
Eastman, Kimble Manley **(SLP)**
Edwards, Joyce A **(SLP)**
Evans, Sandra L **(SLP)**
Faulkner, Douglas H **(A)**
Fernandez, Mrs Carol L **(SLP)**
Fernandez, Lisa Ann **(A)**
Fones, Mrs Susan Plumb **(SLP)**
Forrestel, Mrs Kim H **(SLP)**
Frans, Mrs Noreen P **(A)**
Frost, Carol Ann **(SLP)**
Frueh, Dr Frank **(A)**
Garbrecht, Mrs Mary Ellen Ahern **(A)**
Gaskell, Alice Gail **(A)**
Genuardi, Sharon C **(SLP)**
Gilbert, Marcia Anne **(A)**
Gildar, Mrs Enid S **(SLP)**
Gordon, Pearl A **(SLP)**
Guilford, Dr Arthur **(SLP)**
Hargrave, Rose Kersey **(SLP)**
Higgins, Anne Weise **(SLP)**
Hildick, Dorothy Caccamo **(SLP)**
Hnath-Chisolm, Theresa E **(A)**
Hofmann, Betty Jane **(SLP)**
Holder, Mrs Suzanne Wooten **(A)**
Hollahan, Mrs Kelmie K **(SLP)**
Holliman, Dr Doreen G **(SLP)**
Howland, Denise Gayle **(SLP)**
Hunter, Patricia S **(SLP)**
Ingraham, Mrs Velda Chemise **(SLP)**
Ingram, Mrs Renee Morris **(SLP)**
Jablonski, Mrs Terry Anne **(SLP)**
Jackson, Mrs Valerie P **(SLP)**
Jones, Stacey Dawn
Kasan, E A Lee **(SLP)**
Kasan, Mrs Marilyn F **(SLP)**
Katz, Robin Beth **(SLP)**
Keller, Winifred Jean **(A)**
Kelly, Mrs Jackie Miller
Klingman, Kathy C **(SLP)**
Kuffel, Constance F **(SLP A)**
Kurtzrock, Dr George H **(SLP A)**
Labrake, Mrs Barbara A **(SLP)**
Lawson, Mrs Elisabeth M **(SLP)**
Lubert, Mrs Barbara D **(SLP)**
Mackay, Ann Catherine **(SLP)**
Madell-Charles, Mrs Nancy **(SLP)**
Malloy, Mrs Mylene Tamayo **(SLP)**
Manelli, Leslie Thedford **(SLP)**
Mattai, Susan Lentz **(SLP)**
McClowry, Dr Danny P **(SLP)**
McCormick, Michael John **(SLP)**
McDonald, Mrs Dawn Daganhardt **(SLP)**
Murphy, Mrs Alicia Ranon **(SLP)**
Nightingale, Mrs Lorie Marie **(SLP)**
O'Brien, Bennie Kay **(SLP)**
Ottinger, Mrs Mariann F **(SLP)**
Ownby, Mrs Jenifer C **(SLP)**
Pendry, Margaret M **(SLP)**
Pierce, Mrs Karen Dawn **(SLP)**
Piernick, Sherry Melinda **(A)**
Poklepovic, Mrs Michel Stewart **(A)**
Polka, Linda
Pomerantz, Harris I **(SLP A)**
Price, Jenny Brown **(SLP)**
Price, Margaret J **(SLP)**
Reice, Mrs Jeanne B **(A)**
Reidenbach, John **(SLP)**
Rice, Mrs Janet G **(SLP)**
Richardson, Dr Sylvia O **(SLP)**
Ricker, Lynn Marie **(A)**
Robinson, Evelyn B **(SLP)**
Roverts, Mrs Diana Lynn **(SLP)**
Ryals, Karen E **(SLP)**
Samson, Beth **(SLP)**
Saraceno, Mrs Maria Panico **(A)**
Scanio, Dr Tom S **(SLP)**
Scheuerle, Dr Jane F **(SLP)**
Seitz, Mrs Christine Schrock **(SLP)**
Shelton, Shirlene Matthews **(SLP)**
Shonbrun, Susan H **(SLP)**
Silliman, Elaine R **(SLP)**
Silverman, Henrietta C **(SLP)**
Sinsley, Mrs Debbie M **(SLP)**
Skiff, Pamela J **(SLP)**
Skinner, Mrs Holly Katherine **(A)**
Skotko, Mrs Janet Y **(SLP)**
Snyder, Maripat Pyatok **(SLP)**
Spruce, Wayne Vee **(SLP)**
Sternig, Pamela A **(SLP)**
Sullivan, Paula A **(SLP)**
Superfine, Donald M **(SLP)**
Thoresen, Linda Rose **(SLP)**
Trachtenberg, Nina S **(SLP)**
Umfleet, Mrs Katherine **(A)**
Vance, Bette Mae **(SLP)**
Walter, Lisa Marie **(SLP)**
Warren, Mrs Susan B **(SLP)**
Weitman, Mrs Sheryl T **(A)**
Wheeler, Janie S **(SLP)**
Widi, Mrs Maureen Y **(A)**
Young, Mrs Susan Marie **(SLP)**
Zentmeyer, Rebecca Beale **(SLP)**
Zukosky, Carol Anne **(SLP)**

Tarpon Springs
Du Mond, Glenna Colleen
Galant, Kimberly Rae **(SLP)**
Hill, Sharon Malure **(SLP)**
Payne, Joyce S **(SLP)**
Stieren, Angelika Janas **(A)**

Tavares
Donnelly, Mrs Judith A S **(SLP A)**
Zeigler, John Trawick **(A)**

Temple Terrace
Craig, Denise **(SLP)**
Haseman, Dr Elizabeth Owens **(SLP)**
Modahl, Mrs Jackie P **(SLP)**
Sanders, Bettina D **(A)**

Tequesta
Adler, Mrs Dianne L

Titusville
Hagerty, Mrs Lynette Reville

Treasure Island
Plumridge, Mrs Teri Salter **(SLP)**
Youdovin, Mrs Susan Schaalman **(SLP)**

Tyndall AFB
Miller, Nancy White **(A)**

Valrico
England, Lynne L **(SLP A)**
Foster, Tina L Sobel **(SLP)**
Franz, Mrs Janet L S **(SLP)**
Gardner, Mrs Deborah Bowen **(SLP)**
Riggs-Stites, Mrs Kathy Marie **(SLP)**
Turgeonn, Mrs Kelly S **(SLP)**
Winstead, Mrs Nancy Hickling **(SLP)**
Wright, Betty Tindel **(SLP)**

Venice
Boone, Shirley Reynolds **(SLP)**
Devlin, David Lawrence **(A)**
Devlin, Mrs Robin W **(A)**
Falk, Dr Joy W **(SLP)**
Gaunt, Mrs Barbara Brown **(A)**
King, Mrs Wilma G **(SLP)**
Stallings, Debra Marlene **(SLP)**

Vero Beach
Beneroski, Kimberly Jo **(SLP)**
Brown, Mrs Donna S **(SLP)**
Filosa, Alfred A **(A)**
Gangale, Debra Carmela **(SLP)**
Gregson, Jo Ann **(SLP)**
Hall, Mrs Martha Williams **(SLP)**
Horchler, Julia W **(SLP)**
Jones, Anna M
Lukomski, Mrs Joy Ellen **(SLP)**
Lukomski, Thomas Stephen **(SLP)**
McKee, Maribeth Caya **(SLP)**
O'Brien, Renee McMullen **(A)**
Rose, Heidi Fleck
Sauls, Lauri Ann **(A)**
Smith, Mrs Michele G **(SLP)**
Thornton, Mrs Mary Beth **(SLP)**

Virginia Gardens
Sawyer, Lori Elizabeth **(SLP)**

Wauchula
Galiano-Sanders, Mrs Roberta A **(SLP)**

Wellington
Brown, Mrs Kathy Taylor
Hayes, Dr Claude S **(A)**
Taub, Barbara Susan **(SLP)**

Wesley Chapel
Bruneau-Ritterman, Mrs Sharen **(A)**
Ritterman, Dr Stuart I **(SLP)**

West Melbourne
Day, Patsy W **(A)**

West Palm
Kerin, Alberta Rugh **(SLP)**

West Palm Beach
Albee, David C **(A)**

Berryman, Janice Lynn **(SLP)**
Blake, Lizanne P **(SLP)**
Bultemeyer, Christine Denise **(SLP)**
Coale, Sharon Ann **(SLP)**
Cohen, Mrs Elizabeth **(SLP)**
Deconna, Mrs Susan McCue **(SLP)**
Dobbert, Mrs Ruth Rohl **(SLP)**
Dreyfus-Landerman, Jamie D **(SLP)**
Epstein, Lynn Ellen **(SLP)**
Froehlin, Julia Mary **(SLP)**
Garrigus, Mrs Rosemary D **(SLP)**
Grant, Mel **(A)**
Grant, Mrs Wendy Levin **(SLP)**
Hartung, Mrs Mayra Teresita **(SLP)**
Hays, Debra Engelstein **(SLP)**
Hebert, Mrs Diane Marie
Hinish, Susan Gayle **(SLP)**
Israel, Dr Leonard **(SLP)**
Labrutto-Wilson, Janis D **(SLP)**
Lavallie, Patrick Dennis **(SLP)**
Loughran, Mrs Judith Tanner **(SLP)**
Lozano-Rodriguez, Jose Rafael **(SLP)**
Manning, Mrs Joan B **(SLP)**
Morgan, Susan **(SLP)**
Peyton, Mrs Bonnie Neukircher **(SLP)**
Phoebus, Maudie P **(SLP)**
Piersall, Mrs Marcia C **(SLP)**
Robinson, Elizabeth Prudence **(SLP)**
Rohm, Susan Marie **(A)**
Samuels, Ruth F **(A)**
Schultz, Moritz L **(A)**
Seligman, Daryl A **(SLP)**
Silverman, Sheryl **(SLP)**
Smith, Suzanne Marie **(SLP)**
Svarc-Hopkins, Joyce **(SLP)**
Syden, Mrs Sheree J **(SLP)**
Taube, Mrs Wanda Watts **(SLP)**
Thompson, Mrs Paula Marie **(A)**
Thorstad, Mrs Janice Lee **(SLP)**
Weston, Mrs Genecile Watts **(SLP)**
Wilder, Kathryn V **(A)**

Wilton Manors

Kenyon, Mrs Diana Lynn **(SLP)**
Oliver, Mrs Barbara J **(SLP)**

Windermere

Sullivan, Mrs Jacqueline Jones **(SLP)**

Winter Garden

Morgan, Ann F **(SLP)**

Winter Haven

Ancheta, Maria Celeste
Anderson, Mrs Sally B **(SLP)**
Barlow, Kevin Thomas **(A)**
Bunn, Thomas T **(A)**
Butler, Terrence Robert **(SLP)**
Chayt, Mrs Meryl B **(SLP)**
Comkowycz, Sharon M **(SLP)**
Dobson, Patricia T **(SLP)**
Dunn, Laura Anne **(SLP)**
Fry, Carolee **(SLP)**
Harper, Mrs Jo L **(SLP)**
Holmes, Mrs Cynthia Ken **(A)**
Johnson, Mrs Debra Brosseau **(SLP)**
Siner, Cheryl B **(SLP)**
Swindell, Harriette Juanice
Wilson, Marilyn K **(A)**

Winter Park

Adicks, Jennifer E
Baker, Elizabeth **(SLP)**
Becker, Carolyn A **(SLP)**
Busbee, Jane B **(SLP)**
Evans, Mrs Susan Ann Holmes **(SLP)**
Fegebank, Mrs Julie A **(A)**
Gitles, Toni **(A)**
Huskey, Mrs Sarah Farley **(A)**
King, Brian G **(A)**
Lyle, Dr Martha B **(SLP A)**
Marlowe, Judith A **(A)**
McClelland, Mrs Alison P **(SLP)**
Moroux, Danielle M **(SLP)**
Overley, Mrs Cheryl Morton **(SLP)**
Pohl, Mrs Joan K **(SLP)**
Rassmann, Diane L **(SLP)**
Ratusnik, Dr David L **(SLP)**
Rizner, Constance B **(SLP)**
Roberts, Mrs Patricia Jean S **(SLP)**
Roberts, Dr William H **(SLP A)**
Silvernail, Karen M **(SLP)**
Tyler, Audrey S **(SLP)**
Williams, Theresa Aleise **(SLP)**

Winter Springs

Bradbury, Rosanne B **(SLP)**
Butts, Catherine P **(SLP)**
Champ, Carmela L **(SLP)**
Eldridge, Mrs Darby B **(SLP)**
Furgason, Kristine Kaiser **(SLP)**
Gersen, Robin F **(SLP)**
Goldsmith, Carole B **(SLP)**
Moore, Mrs Janet Marie **(SLP)**
Phillips, Kathleen Morris **(SLP)**
Van Kessel, Joan Marie **(SLP)**
Vernau, Lesley Anne
Worrell, Patricia A **(SLP)**

Zephyrhills

Mason, Mrs Pamela M **(SLP)**

GEORGIA

Acworth

Berger-Reynolds, Mrs Lisa C **(SLP)**
Cain, Mrs Elizabeth Houseman **(SLP)**
Kenig, Mrs Janet A **(SLP)**

Albany

Bennett, Mrs Cynthia Wright **(SLP)**
Boyer, Barbara M **(SLP)**
Chaney, Joyce Marie **(SLP)**
Hancock, Mrs Lydia Ashton **(SLP)**
House, Donnita Ann **(SLP A)**
Lorber, Douglas Radman **(SLP A)**
Matthews, Lynn Hale **(SLP)**
Schorn-Bellows, Marilyn T **(A)**
Shell, Mrs Melanie Peacock **(SLP)**
Stone, Mrs Cynthia V
Sweeney, Mrs Sandra Haire **(A)**
Thompson, Mrs Kathleen G **(SLP)**
Williamson, Mrs Karen S **(SLP)**
Williamson, Mrs Patricia McHale **(SLP)**
Wooten, Kathryn Wilkerson **(SLP)**

Alpharetta

Browne, Mrs Mary Anne Turner **(SLP)**
De Corso, Jill Buelow **(SLP)**
Green, Mrs Cynthia Shealey **(SLP)**
House, Mrs Mary R **(SLP)**
Keough, Mrs Sharon Alexander **(SLP)**
Lieberman, Mrs Maura Elizabeth **(A)**
Malgeri, Roberta **(SLP)**
Orr, Lisa Ann **(SLP)**
Sisterhen, Mrs Christa C **(SLP)**
Sisterhen, Dr Daniel H **(SLP A)**
Worden, Diane C **(SLP)**
Young, Deborah Melton **(SLP)**

Americus

Daughtry, Mrs Susan Carreker **(SLP)**

Appling

Wright, Sandra R **(SLP)**

Arlington

Smith, Mrs Beverly B **(SLP)**

Athens

Adams, Deborah Lynn **(A)**
Andrews, Mrs Susan Beth **(SLP)**
Berryman, Joan D **(SLP)**
Blue, Dr Carl M **(SLP)**
Bogner, Mrs Phyllis M **(SLP)**
Bowman, Tamara Replogle **(SLP)**
Cary, Marilynn **(SLP)**
Curtis, Dr W Scott **(SLP)**
Dellaria, Nancy Broadhurst **(SLP)**
Duclos, Mrs Karen Meinert **(SLP)**
Froehlich, Mrs Deborah Sue **(SLP)**
Hardegree, Deborah Kay **(A)**
Hardin, Robin Barnes **(A)**
Harvey, Mrs Jane Hunt **(SLP)**
Jenkins, Mrs Shelley L **(SLP)**
Kahn, Ange **(SLP)**
Kools, Dr Joseph A **(SLP)**
Lauderdale, Linda F **(SLP)**
Laughton, Dr Joan **(SLP)**
McCarthy, Dr Patricia A **(A)**
McCoy, Dr Malcolm B **(A)**
Neal, Dr W Ray, Jr **(SLP A)**
Peach, Dr Richard K **(SLP)**
Risler, Susan Stinson **(SLP)**
Scarborough, Sarah Catherine **(SLP)**
Seaton, Jane B **(SLP A)**
Snyder, Florence H **(SLP)**
Steinkraus, Susan I
Street, Sherry Lynn **(SLP)**
Talbott, Dr Richard E **(A)**
Tomalski, Suzanne F **(SLP)**
Vesper, Julie Anne **(A)**
Vickery, Mrs Lori A

Atlanta

Abernathy, Donna Carol
Alexander, Mrs Marilyn K **(SLP)**
Alexander, Martha E **(SLP)**
Allen, Mrs Jane Law **(SLP)**
Anderson, Patricia A **(SLP)**
Atkins, Mrs Janet L **(SLP)**
Babcock, Shirley Joan **(SLP)**
Bailey, Mrs Suzanne B **(SLP)**
Baird, Mrs Virginia G **(SLP)**
Baltzell, David R **(A)**
Bates, Susan M V **(SLP)**
Beegle, Barbara B **(SLP)**
Binkow, Mrs Nancy H **(SLP)**
Blackstone, Lynn Gibbons **(SLP)**
Blalock, Dr Jane Wade **(SLP)**
Blane, Mrs Ann D **(SLP)**
Botstein, Laurie K **(SLP)**
Bourgeois, Debra Ann **(SLP)**
Branan, Georgiana **(SLP)**
Bridges, Jean Ellen **(SLP)**
Brokaw, Mrs Sonia P **(SLP)**
Brooks, Nondi Carol
Bucher, Doris A **(SLP)**
Buffington, Jenny Lin **(SLP)**
Burleson, Paula Deyon **(SLP)**
Bush, Katheryn B **(SLP)**
Busko, Mrs Sally C **(SLP)**
Byars, Susan W **(SLP)**
Calhoun, Janna K **(SLP)**
Callahan, Ruth A **(SLP)**
Cantwell, Marilyn M **(SLP)**
Cargill, Sharon A **(SLP)**
Carter, Camille Denise
Case, Elizabeth Fuller **(A)**
Cesari, Mrs Belinda Ann **(SLP)**
Chaiken, Rita Rosinek **(A)**
Clanton, Andrea Doris
Clegg, Stanley J **(A)**
Coakley, Mrs Mabel W **(SLP)**
Cobb, Justine C **(SLP)**
Coffie, Mrs Lucie Callaway **(A)**
Cohen, Mrs Melissa R **(A)**
Comerford, Michael A **(A)**
Conners, Marjory A **(SLP)**
Cook, Mrs Julie Alderman **(SLP)**
Crouse, Mrs Marjorie K **(SLP)**
Davison, Louise D **(SLP)**
Dinges, Dr Maureen McGarvey
Drost, Anne Scalise **(SLP)**
Elliott, Samuel B **(SLP)**
Enck, Mrs Carol A **(SLP)**
Erlinger, Karen S **(SLP)**
Eudaly, Mary J **(A)**
Ezzell, Debra Demaray **(SLP)**
Fletcher, Mrs Cornelia H **(SLP)**
Fowler, Marilynn **(SLP)**
Franco, Janis W **(SLP)**
Friedman, Rochelle **(SLP)**
Frist, Eve Judith **(SLP)**
Fudge, Suzanne V **(SLP)**
Georges, Jill B **(SLP)**
Glenz, Susan Marlyn **(SLP)**
Glicksberg, Susan P **(A)**
Graham, Dr James T **(A)**
Graham, Dr Louella W **(A)**
Graham-Pool, Leslee **(A)**
Greenberg, Marjorie W **(SLP)**
Hairston, Karen Jeannine **(SLP)**
Hamilton, Victoria Anne **(A)**
Hand, Julia W **(SLP A)**
Harnden, Pamela Sue **(SLP)**
Hawkins, Marianne S **(SLP)**
Henry, Evelyn Carol **(SLP)**
Hill, Mrs Winn Warner **(SLP)**
Hinman-Dudley, Mrs Narda F **(SLP)**
Hope, Donna **(SLP)**
Hoskins, Mrs Katherine Fleming **(A)**
Hullihan, Mrs Michelle Martina **(SLP)**
Jaques, Mrs Julie McGee **(SLP)**
Jensen, Dr Myltreda L **(SLP)**
Jones, Mamie J **(SLP)**
Joyce, Mrs Patricia Pamela **(SLP)**
Kaplan, Shelley A **(SLP)**
Kasriel, Mrs Ernestine **(SLP)**
Kaufman-Lennon, Andrea **(SLP)**
Klein, Mrs Ellen R **(SLP)**
Klingman-Palk, Paula C **(SLP)**
Kopel, Lydia Ann **(SLP)**
Lang, Susan K **(SLP)**
Lardner, Mrs Mary L **(SLP)**
Laseter, Carrell **(SLP)**
Lewis, Rosemary Brown **(SLP)**
Lisicia, Katherine Ann **(SLP)**
Long, Carla L
Lowe, Mrs Audrey D **(A)**
Lynn, Cindy F
Majeska, Jo Anne W **(SLP)**
Marshall, Dr Mary H **(SLP)**
Martin, Mrs Virginia Bruce **(SLP)**
Massey, Mrs Amy Reichard **(SLP)**
McCown, Marilyn C **(SLP)**
McDonald, Erin E **(SLP)**
McHale, Kathleen Patricia **(SLP)**
McSween, Mrs Nena Etheridge **(SLP)**
Meadows, Cynthia Kay **(A)**
Merkel, Amanda Schneider **(SLP)**
Milton, Octavia W
Monk, Dr Janice Walls **(SLP)**
Mullin, Vivian L S **(SLP)**
Myland, Debra Jay
Newlin, Rhonda T **(SLP)**
Parker, Tommie Corbett **(SLP)**
Parks, Mrs Mary Dean **(SLP)**
Parlato, Mrs Patricia L **(SLP)**
Pavlik, Loriann **(SLP)**
Payne-Blanton, Rebecca L **(SLP)**
Phelps, Mrs E Patrice **(SLP)**
Philp, Sandrya M **(SLP)**
Pinsky, Mrs Debra Chetlin **(SLP)**
Piroli, James Robert **(SLP)**
Poythress, Mrs Darla H **(SLP)**
Pressnell, Dr Lucille M **(SLP)**
Prine, Amy Pratt **(SLP)**
Reuben, Eileen R **(SLP)**
Rhodes, Catherine Anne **(SLP)**
Rickoff, Mrs Olga Feldman **(SLP)**
Ride, Kristen Jane **(SLP)**
Robinson, Lillian E **(SLP)**
Romski, Dr Maryann **(SLP)**
Ross, Francie **(SLP)**
Saunders, Mrs Anne Z **(A)**
Schroder, Mrs Karen K **(SLP)**
Seifarth, Mrs Victoria W **(SLP)**
Sharbaugh, Donna P **(SLP A)**
Sikes, Mrs Terri Eith
Smith, Mrs Susan P **(SLP)**
Sprinkle, Ruth S **(A)**
Stanek-Prats, Susan **(A)**
Steward, Dr Noreen **(SLP)**

Stewart, Mrs Suzanne Johnson **(SLP)**
Strahle, Jane C **(SLP)**
Sunshine, Betty **(SLP)**
Syfert, Grace Privette **(SLP)**
Taylor, Phyllis Ann **(SLP)**
Tessier, Maria Grazia
Theros, Jean A **(SLP)**
Thomas, Inge Hinrichs **(SLP)**
Trachtman, Mrs Michelle R **(SLP)**
Tritschler, Helen L **(SLP)**
Tucker, Abigail D
Turkel, Nancy Beth **(SLP)**
Turner, Mrs Elizabeth Grimes **(SLP)**
Turner, Jamie Galloway **(A)**
Umberger, Dr Forrest Glen **(SLP)**
Wells, Laura Jean **(SLP)**
Westerholt, Laurel Ann **(SLP)**
Wolfe, Mrs Sue Pearl **(SLP)**
Woods, Richard T **(A)**
Wyatt, Martha R **(SLP)**
Zelski, Robert F K **(A)**
Zirkle, Mary Lynn **(SLP)**

Augusta

Anderson, Kathleen C **(SLP)**
Anderson, Mary Kathryn **(SLP)**
Armstrong, Jane E **(SLP)**
Black, Linda S **(A)**
Bohannon, Edgar Robin **(A)**
Brathwaite, Mrs Charlotte Denise **(SLP)**
Brophy, Mrs Kathryn Kuykendall **(SLP)**
Clark, Sylvia Yvonne **(SLP)**
Darnell, Mrs Suzanne H **(SLP)**
De Chicchis, Dr Albert R **(A)**
Flanagin, Mrs Virginia W **(SLP)**
Garner, Mrs Gloria Donathan **(A)**
Gilbreath, Mrs Susan Hollowell **(SLP)**
Griffin, Mrs Fannie D **(SLP)**
Grubbs, Rosanne **(SLP)**
Halchishick, Janice Marie **(SLP)**
Kernaghan, Mrs Jean F **(SLP)**
Krakowiak, Mrs Marianne V **(SLP)**
Lane, Mrs Jerrie N **(SLP)**
Larson, Dr Vernon Dale **(A)**
Maund, Mrs Christie Young **(SLP)**
McClary, Barbara A **(SLP)**
Miller, Burnice D **(SLP)**
O'Connor, Thomas E **(A)**
Pigott, Janice F **(SLP)**
Pope, Zandra M **(A)**
Pursley, Martha Elaine **(SLP)**
Renie, Tamara Ann
Rogers, Mrs Mary Ann **(SLP)**
Sahaj, Erika Loring **(SLP)**
Skenes, Dr Linda Lilley **(SLP)**
Sleister, Cheryl A **(A)**
Stringer, William E **(SLP A)**
Watkins, Thomas M **(A)**
White, Melinda
Williams, Dr Thomas F **(A)**

Avondale Estates

Kropa, Jean J **(SLP)**

Bainbridge

Gibbs, Angela R
Parker, Mrs Margaret A **(SLP)**

Bishop

Dean, Mrs Manita B **(SLP)**

Blairsville

Colwell, Teresa B **(SLP)**
Sorth, Mrs Mary Emma **(SLP)**

Blythe

Fowler, Mrs Catherine **(SLP)**

Bogart

Mitchell, Mrs Lynn Farrell **(SLP)**

Bremen

Wasdin, Mrs Alice J **(SLP)**

Brunswick

Lennon, Dr E James **(SLP)**
Wright, Richard D **(A)**

Buford

Edwards, Mrs Dorothy S **(SLP)**
Spillane, Mrs Lisa Palazzolo **(SLP)**

Butler

Peavy, Angela McCall **(SLP)**

Byromville

Willingham, Mrs Rebecca S **(SLP)**

Cairo

Cooper, Mrs Mona R

Calhoun

Cannon, Mrs Karen Ann **(SLP)**
Walker, Sandra Gail **(SLP)**

Canton

Codwise, L Jody Mitchell **(SLP)**
Johnson, Charles S **(SLP)**

Carrollton

Meadows, Mary Beth M **(SLP)**
Meine, Cathy L **(SLP)**
Still, Mrs Deborah Beth **(SLP)**
Sullivan, Melissa Stagg
Upchurch, Mrs Pamela H
Williams, Debra A B **(SLP)**
Williams, Mrs Sara Sparkman **(SLP)**

Cave Spring

Hanson, Mary Elizabeth **(SLP)**
Keefer, C Helen

Chamblee

Sims, Leslie Ellen **(A)**
White, Sandra S **(SLP)**

Chula

Hudson, Mrs Cheerie Gentry **(SLP)**

Clarkesville

Allen, Ralph Charles **(SLP)**
Morgan, Mrs Michele Cole

Clarkston

Allen, Nancy R **(A)**
Stout, Mrs Tamara Worrell **(SLP)**

Cobbtown

Edenfield, Nikki Anita **(SLP)**

Cohutta

Allison, Lynn M **(SLP)**

College Park

Barksdale, Mrs Ethelyn Burton **(SLP)**
Jackson, Valerie White **(SLP)**
Williams, Mrs Colleen Houston **(SLP)**

Columbus

Betty, Charles Jones **(SLP)**
Broom, Mrs Stacey P **(SLP)**
Burrus, Mrs Jennifer Ann **(SLP)**
Cantrell, Mrs Judy Eileen **(SLP)**
Chappelle, Mrs Eva Ulrich **(SLP)**
Conner, Mrs Janis Nunnally **(SLP)**
Ford, Dr Susie C **(SLP)**
Fuller, Jennifer Kaye **(SLP)**
Grigsby, Diana Mizell **(SLP)**
Ingram, June M **(SLP)**
Johnson, Mrs Leslie M **(A)**
McCollum, Mrs Carolyn W **(SLP)**
Odom-Winn, Danni S **(SLP)**
Pate, Robyn Jo **(SLP)**
Perryman, Hugh Bryant **(SLP)**
Piskator, Mrs Tara Mullins
Slaughter, Robert L **(SLP)**
Smith, Mrs Sue McQuaig **(SLP)**
Speer, Mrs Rebecca Baker
Sutherland, Dr Dorothy F **(SLP)**
Terry, Barbara Graham **(A)**
Wentland, Mrs Phyllis W **(SLP)**
Wentland, Dr Thomas J **(SLP)**
Whiteside, Mrs Emily Luttrell **(SLP)**
Wilkoff, Mrs Margaret A **(SLP)**
Williams, Amelia K **(A)**

Conley

Hill-Latimer, Linda **(SLP)**

Conyers

Bryant-Sawyers, Carol Y **(SLP)**
Hooper, Mrs Iris R **(SLP)**
Nelson, Betty E **(SLP)**
Sorenson, Diane Lorene **(SLP)**

Coolidge

Kennedy, Kathy S

Cordele

Buford, Mrs Jennifer Perry **(SLP)**
Cayton, Mrs Georgianne M **(SLP)**

Cornelia

Cain, Debra Hubley **(SLP)**
Irvin, Mrs Elaine H **(SLP)**

Covington

Brown, Mrs Frances T **(SLP)**
Higgins, Mrs Teresa Nunn **(SLP)**

Crawford

Brubaker, Mrs Mary Booth

Cumming

McMillian, Susan McPherson **(SLP)**

Dacula

Edwards, Julia Ann **(SLP)**
Kenzel, Sherri Lynn **(SLP)**

Dahlonega

Dockery, David Ray **(SLP)**
Reed, Mrs Anne Free **(SLP)**

Dalton

Bacon, Hope H **(SLP)**
Riddle, Peggy Denise **(A)**

Decatur

Aleksa-Parr, Mrs Barbara **(SLP)**
Berman, Dr Marilyn S **(SLP)**
Bounds, Mrs Angelique Harrison **(SLP A)**
Boykin, Mrs Estelle V **(SLP)**
Canahl, Sue E Basore **(A)**
Cody, Shirley R **(SLP)**
Crook, Dalise Taylor **(SLP)**
Evans, Glenda Kay **(SLP)**
Ford, Mrs Sue Fillingim **(SLP)**
Fugate, Danna Lisa **(SLP)**
Garner, Margaret L **(SLP)**
Gilmore, Virginia Arbuckle **(SLP)**
Harney, Mrs Anne Paris **(SLP)**
Harris, Norma Jane **(SLP)**
Hilliard-Franks, Parthenia Evonne **(SLP)**
Hudson, Mrs Louise V **(SLP)**
Hutton, Dr Chas L, Jr **(SLP A)**
Kramer, Charles G **(SLP)**
Ludlow, Patricia A **(SLP)**
Morgan-Wasserman, Leslie L **(A)**
Newland, Stephanie Ann **(A)**
Perry, Mrs Connie Bone **(SLP)**
Roche, Mrs Luella **(SLP)**
Rogers, Mrs Linda Phifer **(SLP)**
Shaw, Anne E **(SLP)**
Stein, Mrs Cynthia Hall **(SLP)**
Weber, Connie H **(SLP)**
Wright, Kelli Harris **(SLP)**
Wynens, Maria Szczepanski **(A)**

Doraville

Harris, Linda Trammell **(SLP)**
Marx, Mrs Brenda Vest **(SLP)**
Owens, Alma D **(SLP)**
Reynolds, Deborah A **(SLP)**
Schaffer, Mrs Rochelle N **(SLP)**
Von Almen, Peggy G **(SLP A)**
Willis, Pamela Ruth **(SLP)**

Douglas

Dedmond, Cindy Lynn **(SLP)**

Douglasville

Cook, Irita Diane **(SLP)**
Gilman, Carol Lynn **(SLP)**
Kirkland, Mrs Susan Rice **(SLP)**
Kosater, Leigh Bowen **(SLP)**
Prince, Mrs Elizabeth Dent **(SLP)**
Walker, Mrs Sherry McDaniel **(SLP)**

Dublin

Belcher, Mrs Patricia Y **(SLP)**
Gordon, Martha Elizabeth **(SLP)**
Hall, Debra Lee **(A)**
Wages, Dianne Bass **(SLP)**

Duluth

Boettcher, Mrs Terry Latham **(SLP)**
Finnegan, Mrs Teri Lynn
Graham, Sandra Kay **(SLP)**
MacDonald, Elizabeth Anne **(A)**
McHugh, Mary Susan
Peterson, Nancy Mary **(SLP)**
Rietta, Mrs Katrina Hamilton **(SLP)**
Rodriguez, Mrs Joan E **(A)**
Smitherman, Mrs Arlene Palumbo **(SLP A)**
Sorrell, Mrs Angela Fisher **(SLP)**
Southerland, Mrs Patricia Elizabeth **(SLP)**

Dunwoody

Austin, Mrs Ellen L **(SLP)**
Bailey, Mrs Elizabeth P **(SLP)**
Bellaire, Karen J **(SLP)**
Cardwell, Mrs Janet Bush **(SLP)**
Harrah, Mrs Barbara Bente
Isbell, Lisa Angelyn **(A)**
Johnson, Mrs Jane C **(SLP)**
Jones, Mrs Cheri Benge **(SLP)**
Mainguy, Susan E **(SLP)**
McLemore, Mrs Sarah Lee **(SLP)**
Olthoff, Mary Jo **(SLP)**
Schaude, Mrs Bonnie A S **(SLP)**
Spigener, Laurie Toy **(SLP)**
Wermuth, Nancy B **(SLP)**
Wysocki, Rene Noel **(A)**

East Point

Bostick-Morgan, Oreather J **(SLP)**

Eastman

Ethridge, Brenda Revier **(SLP)**

Ellijay

Dorth, Donna Woodward **(SLP)**

Fairburn

Christy, Felicia Ann **(SLP)**

Fayetteville

Roberts, Mrs Roselyn C **(SLP)**
Tate, Mrs Deborah Kellum **(SLP)**
Watson, Mrs Sandra M **(SLP)**

Forsyth

Andrews, Janet Patricia **(A)**

Fort Benning

Stevens, Capt Marc J **(A)**

Fort Oglethorpe

Stephens, Louis M **(A)**

Fort Valley

Ballard, Mara L **(A)**
Butler, Mrs Roseann Walker **(SLP)**
Hatin, Mrs Darcy A **(SLP)**

Gainesville

Brady, Mrs Rebecca Mills **(SLP)**
David, Cleone F **(SLP)**
Miller, Mrs Teresa C **(SLP)**
Mundy, Mrs Alice Ann Edwards **(SLP)**
Neck, Wayne Walter **(SLP)**
Roesser, Mrs Sheryl L **(SLP)**
Smith, Dr Laura Ann **(SLP)**
Tomlinson, Theresa Fay
Van Wallenburgh, Mrs Mary Campbell
Walker, Mrs Jane A **(SLP)**
Walker, Mrs Sandra Reese **(SLP)**
Wright, Mrs Julia Ann **(SLP)**

Gracewood

Belcher, Marsha Davis **(SLP)**
Elmore, Ralph M **(SLP)**
Womack, Patricia **(SLP)**

Griffin
- Harris, Frances P **(SLP A)**
- Karam, Mrs Laurie Montgomery
- Martin, Mrs Sheryl Branan **(SLP)**
- Whatley, Mrs Vivian **(SLP)**

Guyton
- Stevens, Dr Linda B **(SLP)**

Hapeville
- Trammell, Mrs Cynthia V **(SLP)**

Hartwell
- Martin, Linda J **(SLP)**

Hephzibah
- Periman, Mrs Peggy Gish

Jackson
- Webb, Bonnie Wootten **(SLP)**

Jasper
- Gabriel, Mrs Chrystal A **(SLP)**

Jefferson
- Eisele, Dr Wendell A **(A)**
- Schwartz, Mrs Michelle L **(SLP)**

Jekyll Island
- McMillan, Mrs Olga Christina **(SLP)**

Jonesboro
- Feathers, Anne H **(SLP)**
- Hess, Mrs Carla Vehling **(SLP)**
- Nestor, Andrea Faye **(SLP)**
- Yancey, Mrs Connie Sue Waldrop **(SLP)**

Kennesaw
- Bancroft, Kathleen Stanton **(SLP)**
- Beasley, Cynthia Oslin **(SLP)**
- Bednarz, Maryann **(A)**
- Bunn, Deidra L **(SLP)**
- Eager-Kessel, Betsy L **(SLP)**
- Hoefer, Mrs Kathryn O **(SLP)**
- King-Debaun, Patricia **(SLP)**
- Murray-Johnson, Gwendolyn **(SLP)**
- Rhodes, Franklin E **(SLP)**
- Sebastian, Mrs Karen D **(SLP)**

Kingston
- Jones, Byron Lee **(SLP)**

La Grange
- Anderson, Mrs Kathleen Ann
- Gunter, Mrs Kathy Braden **(SLP)**
- Jordan, Eugenia **(SLP)**
- Malloy, Mrs Deborah Marlitt **(SLP)**

Lavonia
- Doll, Mrs Lea Daniel **(SLP)**

Lawrenceville
- Akerman, Judith L **(SLP)**
- Bailey, Beverly S **(SLP)**
- Brannen, Mrs Ann Marie **(SLP)**
- Crook, Margaret Blackwell **(SLP)**
- Davis, Regina Lynne **(A)**
- Elliott, Mrs Susan Kay **(SLP)**
- Fennell, Mrs Nena C H **(SLP)**
- Hilton, Larry W **(SLP)**
- Hosek, Mrs Paula Ann **(SLP)**
- Marshall, Sheri Caplan **(A)**
- Raymond, Mrs Carol A **(SLP)**
- Reed, Lisa Carriker **(SLP)**
- Simmons, Beth H **(SLP)**
- Stein, Andrea Vallen **(A)**
- Wallace, Dyanne E **(SLP)**
- Young, Mrs Kathy Jean **(SLP)**

Leesburg
- Arnold, Marcia M **(SLP)**
- McGhee, Connie D **(SLP)**

Lilburn
- Aronson, Joan Leach **(SLP)**
- Baron, Marla Balak **(A)**
- Fritz, Mrs Harriet Cannon **(SLP)**
- Frobose, Mrs Jane Scaglione **(SLP)**
- Judd, Mrs Catherine Whitehouse **(SLP)**
- Leet, Mrs Sandra P **(SLP)**
- Manning, Mrs Bonnie Krawczyk **(SLP)**
- Nuttall, Dawn M D **(SLP)**
- Swift, Mrs Patricia McCollum **(SLP)**
- Tillman, Mrs Marianne B **(SLP)**
- Walsh, Carol R **(A)**

Lindale
- Cox, Beth P **(SLP)**

Lithia Springs
- Pope, Gina Denise

Lithonia
- Gattis-McLendon, Mrs Patricia **(SLP)**
- Hilton, Mrs I Rose W **(SLP)**
- Hughart, Jiovanne N **(A)**
- Lafayette, Carol Jean **(SLP)**
- Lesley, Marie G **(SLP)**
- Nixon, Pamela H **(SLP)**
- Patton, Mrs Carolyn D **(SLP)**
- Peery, Mrs Peggy C **(SLP)**
- Pendergast, Mrs Terri Miller **(SLP)**
- Reeves, Mrs Rebecca K **(SLP)**
- Tramel, Mrs Karen Ray **(SLP)**

Lumpkin
- Henson, Claudia Carline **(SLP)**

Lyons
- Thompson, Beverly B **(SLP)**

Mableton
- Rackliffe, Roberta A **(SLP)**
- Snyder, Loretta S **(SLP)**

Macon
- Abbott, Mrs Phyllis Annette **(A)**
- Andrews, Robin S **(A)**
- Barber, Winde Jeanne **(SLP)**
- Bayme, Mrs Anne B **(SLP)**
- Bohn, Alexis Jane **(SLP)**
- Bragg, Mrs Virginia D **(SLP)**
- Cannon, Linda Carol **(SLP)**
- Grant, Mrs Saundra Bone **(SLP)**
- Harrell, Diane Ahola **(A)**
- Hatcher, Candace Ann **(SLP)**
- Hill, Dr Wathina Smith **(SLP A)**
- Johnson, Deloris R **(SLP)**
- Johnson, Julia **(A)**
- Labarge, Joann Mareen **(SLP)**
- Logan, Dr Richard Lanham **(SLP)**
- McKinnon, Frances Louise
- Milleman, Mrs Vicky B **(SLP)**
- Murphy, Patricia Daniels **(SLP)**
- Nackashi, Mrs Cynthia N **(SLP)**
- Peppard, Mrs Annette Rhoda **(A)**
- Pollard, Kenneth H **(A)**
- Ruffin, Mrs Patricia Dean **(SLP)**
- Scully-Burch, Julie Ann **(SLP)**
- Taylor, Mrs Angela Audrey **(SLP)**
- Tillery, Elizabeth Thompson **(A)**
- Vanderbeek, Valerie Lanoa **(A)**
- Williams, Julianna W **(SLP)**
- Witham, James Todd **(SLP)**

Madison
- Wacker, Jean A **(SLP)**

Manchester
- Evans, Randall P **(SLP)**
- Harman, Mrs Jill Brainerd **(SLP)**

Manetta
- Gierke, Mrs Suzanne V **(SLP)**

Marietta
- Adler, Dr Richard K **(SLP)**
- Albert, Mrs Lu-Anne M **(A)**
- Allen, Paula H Carpenter **(SLP)**
- Atkin, Leanne Lynn **(SLP)**
- Austin, Elizabeth **(SLP)**
- Barlow, Elizabeth K **(A)**
- Barrios, Martha E **(SLP)**
- Bering, Charles W **(SLP A)**
- Calhoun-Peters, Mrs Susan N **(SLP)**
- Campbell, Mrs Judith R **(SLP)**
- Carmichael, Joyce K **(SLP)**
- Carpenter, Mrs Patricia B **(SLP)**
- Casten, Leslie Ann **(SLP)**
- Chabon, Dr Shelly S **(SLP)**
- Christensen, Mrs Susan Hoster **(SLP)**
- Cobb, Pamela Patrice **(SLP)**
- Coddington, Robert K **(SLP)**
- Cohen, Mrs Minda J **(SLP)**
- Cress-Bush, Louise B **(SLP)**
- Dobos, Jennifer **(SLP)**
- Dorsey, Mrs E Peggy **(SLP)**
- Doyle, Beth Ann
- Duff, Dr Marigine M **(SLP)**
- Duncan, Carmen Alcyone **(SLP)**
- Eason, Mrs Barbara D **(SLP)**
- Emerson, Mrs Helen Wagner **(SLP)**
- Escott, Judith **(SLP)**
- Fink, Patricia L **(SLP)**
- Fisher, Mrs Maryjo Harlin **(SLP)**
- Foster, Linda D L **(SLP)**
- Frick, Lesa Renee **(A)**
- Fuller, Mrs Cynthia E **(SLP A)**
- Gerst, Joy B **(SLP)**
- Ginburg, Mrs Laurie Orkin **(SLP)**
- Goldstein, Celia Cohen **(SLP)**
- Haarbauer-Krupa, Mrs Juliet K **(SLP)**
- Hale, Mrs Wanda Richardson **(SLP)**
- Heflin, Kay Frances **(SLP)**
- Hess, Carole D **(SLP)**
- Holmes, Sandra S
- Howald, Mrs I Gayle **(SLP)**
- Howard, Mrs Mary Tolton **(A)**
- Jett, Madonna T **(SLP)**
- Kaminsky, Barbara M **(SLP)**
- Kassing, Jane M **(A)**
- Kendrick, Mrs Julie E **(SLP)**
- Kirkman, Judith A **(SLP)**
- Kviklys, Karen Anne **(SLP)**
- Larson, Mrs Sharon Kay **(SLP)**
- Laster, Mrs Cheryl Elizabeth **(SLP)**
- La Vine, Mrs Arlene K **(SLP)**
- Lawrence, Mrs Barbara Cullen **(SLP)**
- Lipscomb, Marsha Ann **(A)**
- Marks, Mrs Julie F **(SLP)**
- Marquis, Mrs Catherine Toney **(A)**
- Martin, Elaine G **(SLP)**
- McBee, Mrs Lucy Rush **(SLP)**
- McKee, Suzanne Wagnon **(SLP)**
- McLean, Mrs Elizabeth Ann
- Medved-Diangelo, Mrs Karen **(SLP)**
- Miller, Michele T **(SLP)**
- Mims, Sondra F K **(SLP)**
- Moskowitz, Susan Baer **(SLP)**
- Nutt, Mrs Lucille C **(SLP)**
- Omiecinski, Mrs Mary K **(A)**
- Otero, Jane Hanich **(SLP)**
- Perera, Patricia M **(SLP)**
- Pierce, Dr Bruce R **(SLP)**
- Plenge, Teresa F **(SLP)**
- Rose-Kroll, Mrs Deborah **(A)**
- Rydarowski, Mrs Lisa Neff **(SLP)**
- Shuler, Glenda D **(SLP)**
- Shuster, Mrs Nancy Lite **(A)**
- Silverman, Miriam Beth **(SLP)**
- Smolar, Aimee L **(SLP)**
- Solodar, Mrs Helena Stern **(SLP A)**
- Stasiak, Mrs Vicki W **(SLP)**
- Strader, Mrs Ann Teas **(SLP)**
- Strange, Karen W **(SLP)**
- Taratoot, Mrs Deborah L **(SLP)**
- Tutterrow, Mrs Susan Lynn **(SLP)**
- Waites, Mrs Danette Rene **(SLP)**
- Walker, Jane M **(SLP)**
- Walker, Mrs Virginia Ann **(SLP)**
- Ward Isbey, Mrs Julie A **(SLP)**
- Wilder, Mrs June Harris **(SLP)**
- Williams, Kadyn Ochs **(A)**
- Youngelson, Vicki M **(SLP)**

Martinez
- Ahlstrom, Jayne B **(A)**
- Cook, Mrs Kathy Elaine **(A)**
- Cranston, Cathi **(SLP)**
- Fox, Virginia R **(SLP)**
- Glover, Mrs Andrea K L **(SLP)**
- Larson, Patricia **(SLP)**
- Meehan, Mrs Carolyn Schindler
- Reed, Mrs Lynn J **(SLP)**
- Schroder, Thomas L **(A)**
- Stula, Mrs Trudy Jolene **(SLP)**
- Wilde, Dr Graham L **(A)**
- Williams, Thelma F **(SLP)**

Metter
- Lanier, Delores Spaid **(SLP)**

Milledgeville
- Bloodworth, Freida Dale **(SLP)**
- Childs, Mrs Lynne B **(SLP)**
- Pritchett, Mrs Joy W **(A)**

Monroe
- Bowers, Mrs Jane P **(SLP)**

Morrow
- Henegan, Sandra R **(A)**

Moultrie
- McCall, Kathryn J **(SLP)**
- Mercer, Mrs Elizabeth Lawson **(SLP)**
- Norman, Opal Jean **(SLP)**

Newnan
- McCloud, Mark Allen **(SLP)**
- Mooney, Mrs Diane K
- Steed, Susie F **(SLP)**

Nicholson
- Hulett, Kelly Cavadel **(SLP)**

Norcross
- Akridge, Mrs Jill J **(SLP)**
- Boruff, Mrs Susan Flynn **(SLP)**
- Feldman, Myrna G **(SLP)**
- Forkner, Mrs Vera C **(SLP)**
- Frank, Patricia R **(SLP)**
- Lindstrom, Mrs Sue A **(SLP)**
- Maio, Mrs Debra Dawkins **(SLP)**
- Marquis, Brenda Sue **(SLP)**
- Sticher, Jenny Lee **(SLP)**
- Van Reenen, Mrs Janie Lee S
- Williams, Jennifer Derexa

Oakwood
- Parker, Mrs Susan C **(SLP)**

Oxford
- McCanless, Mrs Carol S **(SLP)**

Peachtree City
- Dwight, Debra M **(SLP)**
- King, Mrs Iva L **(SLP)**
- Lodholz-Horton, Rita M **(SLP)**
- Marting, Ann McCay **(SLP)**
- Mascara, Mrs Eleanor S **(SLP)**
- Terry, Mrs Judith D **(SLP)**
- Tiller, Rebecca N **(SLP)**
- Winstead, Timothy Gene **(A)**

Pine Mountain
- Davis, Mrs Amy Paul **(SLP)**

Powder Springs
- Carter, Vicky L **(SLP)**
- Lozo, Deborah A **(SLP)**
- Upshaw, Helen P **(SLP)**

Quitman
- Roberts, Mrs Patricia Leigh **(SLP)**

Richmond Hill
- Allen, Mrs Margaret F **(SLP)**
- Swany, Mrs Nancy B **(SLP)**

Rincon
- Anderegg, Mrs Pamela P **(SLP)**

Ringgold
- Bowman, Jan M **(SLP)**
- Castleberry, Mrs Debra J **(SLP)**
- Frazee, Mrs Ellen Frances **(SLP)**
- Miller, Linda S **(SLP)**

Riverdale
- Alverson, Robin P **(A)**

Croft, Heather K **(SLP)**
Lashley, Mrs Rebecca E **(SLP)**
Laster, Mrs Jan Colwick **(SLP)**

Rome
Ayers, Mrs Susan Kay **(SLP)**
Corn, Pamela Leisa **(A)**
Fellows, Steven Arnold **(A)**
Grant, Cathryn B **(A)**
McGuire, Mrs Ann C **(SLP)**
Payne, James Sanford, Jr **(A)**
Samples, David M **(SLP)**
Sheeley, Mrs Elizabeth Ann **(SLP)**

Rossville
Allsup, Debra L **(A)**
Hosterman, Pamela Sue **(SLP)**

Roswell
Amis, Judith L **(SLP)**
Anderson, Mrs Kathleen **(SLP)**
Bogner, Mrs Frayne A **(SLP)**
Bohan-Shults, Mrs Jill **(SLP)**
Brown, Mrs Christine **(SLP)**
Brunson, Mrs Alance **(SLP)**
Conrad, Mrs Janet Bohling **(SLP)**
Cook, Mrs Nancy W
Dunn, Deborah A **(SLP)**
Farr, Mrs Rebecca Ray **(SLP)**
Gustin, Mrs Nancy Hess **(SLP)**
Hastings, Mrs Kathryn N **(SLP)**
Krantz, Mrs Susan Eileen **(SLP)**
Lipman, Mrs Heidi Rappaport **(SLP)**
Magid, Lee T **(SLP)**
McNabb, Mrs Kathy O **(SLP)**
Moulin, Dr Linda K **(SLP A)**
Porter, Mrs Claudia **(SLP)**
Routenberg, Linda P **(SLP)**
Storch-Joiner, Mrs Kimberly Yvonne **(A)**
Walker, Mrs Judith K **(SLP)**
Weathersbee, Patricia A **(SLP)**

Sandersville
Grabiak, Susan M **(SLP)**

Savannah
Beckley, Mrs Karen W **(SLP)**
Brackin, Cheryl A **(SLP)**
Brown, Lorena Ann **(SLP)**
Bruner, Mrs Diane Lynn **(SLP)**
Callaway, Mrs Mary Ann **(SLP)**
Cassidy, Maureen **(A)**
Chavez, Mrs Juli Ann Church **(SLP)**
Davis, Susan Edge **(SLP)**
Depue, Mrs Deborah Guidry **(SLP)**
Despain, Mrs Susan Christine **(A)**
Dickson, Mrs Dana Javo **(SLP)**
Eichholz, Mrs Susan Odrezin **(A)**
Etheridge, Carolynn R **(SLP)**
Fort, Mrs Elizabeth W **(SLP)**
Gatens, Barbara E **(A)**
Gates, Brenda J **(SLP)**
George, Mrs Netia Lillian **(SLP)**
Hay, Karla K **(SLP)**
Kuenzli, Timothy R **(SLP)**
Labrot, Mrs Marquerite Wilford **(A)**
Larrimore, Elizabeth F **(SLP)**
Lewis-Barnette, Helen Candice **(SLP)**
Meeks, Linda **(SLP)**
Miller, Martha Louise **(A)**
Millwood, Rebecca R **(SLP)**
Moeller, Mrs Debra Ann **(SLP)**
Myhre, Dr Steven J **(A)**
Parsons, Carla Ann **(SLP)**
Pellett, Faith Susan **(A)**
Pyle, Karla J **(A)**
Rundbaken, Sol **(SLP A)**
Smith, Linda Poppell **(SLP)**
Thompson, Pamela A **(SLP)**
Trees, Anne T **(SLP)**
Wambold, Mrs Constance Anne **(SLP)**
Waters, Mrs Kathleen H **(SLP)**
Zerden, Stephanie **(SLP)**

Shellville
Paul, Miriam Beth **(SLP)**

Smyrna
Forbes-Garner, Mrs Lynn **(SLP)**
Hornstein, Julie Lynn **(SLP)**
Sarris, Mrs Melanie L **(SLP)**
Williams, Kathleen A **(SLP)**

Snellville
Higgins, Patricia M **(SLP)**
Jones, Mrs Linda J
Rush, Mrs Mary B **(SLP)**
Watkins, Dr Carolyn W **(SLP)**
Whitt, Mrs Becky M **(SLP)**

St Marys
Gross-Barlow, Lucinda **(SLP)**
Medeiros, Myra Ann **(SLP)**

St Simons Island
Barrett, Mrs Sarah Davison **(SLP)**
Ivey, Dr Sara M **(SLP)**
Jopling, Bobbie Jean **(SLP)**
Rowell, Rebecca E **(SLP)**
Smead, Mrs Lucille J **(SLP)**
Wainright, Rebecca S **(SLP)**

Statesboro
Klick, Susan Lee **(SLP)**
Palfy, Susan Bieger **(SLP)**
Rushing, Robert O, Jr **(A)**
Silcox, Terry L **(A)**

Stockbridge
Woodall, Mrs Laura Jean **(SLP)**

Stone Mountain
Ahlstedt, Gayla Blythe **(SLP)**
Ambrose, Dr William Rufus **(A)**
Boutwell, Mrs Margaret **(SLP)**
Cosby, Sancha Sharon **(SLP)**
Dean, Mary A **(SLP)**
Fowler, Diane Tumlin **(SLP)**
Hartsell, Kimberly Gayle **(SLP)**
Hopper, Jenny D **(SLP)**
Ketchum, Mrs Linda Harrison **(SLP)**
Kosinski, Patricia Jean **(SLP)**
McCormick, Mrs Frances H **(SLP)**
McCullough, Mrs Pamela S **(SLP)**
McGough, Mrs Donna Woods **(A)**
McGregor, Kathleen J **(SLP)**
Newcomer, Mrs Jill Lyerla **(SLP)**
Phillips, Mrs Gwendolyn Hoff **(SLP)**
Rambow, Mary W **(SLP)**
Sherrill, Mrs Vonnie K **(SLP)**
Wexler, Sharon B **(SLP)**
White, Mrs Deborah Williams **(SLP)**
Williams, Mrs Vanessa P **(SLP)**

Summerville
Brown, Cheryl Annette **(SLP)**
Parker, Mary D **(SLP)**

Swainsboro
Palmer, Dr Julia Rountree **(SLP)**

Talmo
Brower, Diane M **(SLP)**

Tennille
Thomas, Mrs Randolph S **(SLP)**

Thomaston
Leonard, Sarah L M **(SLP)**

Thomasville
Cox, Mrs Betty T **(SLP)**
Davis, Mrs Ivey Jean **(SLP)**
Poss, David Robert
Underwood, Linda L **(SLP)**
Vertz, Steven P **(SLP)**

Tifton
Alt, Phillip J **(A)**
Branch, Judith B **(SLP)**
Dunn, Lisa H
Hathcock, Jacquelyn Rae **(SLP)**
Helton, John R **(SLP)**
Peirolo-Alt, Mrs Corine **(SLP)**
Roberts, Deborah Morris **(SLP)**

Toccoa
Crowe, Mrs Suzanne S **(SLP)**

Tucker
Bailey, Melinda Robin **(SLP)**
Bruce, Alice Thompson **(SLP)**
Coleman, Cynthia Lynn **(SLP)**
Hardy, Ruth Ann D **(SLP)**
Miller, Patricia Wheeler **(SLP)**
Rosenberg, Pamela H **(SLP)**
Slaff, Laurie Ann **(A)**
Webster, Leslie H **(SLP)**
Wommack, Mrs Betty B **(SLP)**

Tybee Island
Hosti, Bonnie S **(SLP)**

Union City
Acree, Laura **(SLP)**

Valdosta
Andrew, Diane **(SLP)**
Andrews, Alice E **(SLP)**
Consolini, Mrs Mary Therese **(A)**
Crowe, Dr Barbara J **(SLP)**
Deavours, Dr George M **(A)**
Dowling, Mrs Sue Y **(SLP A)**
Fountain, Mrs Sandra Elizabeth
Given, Mrs Patricia Lynn **(SLP)**
Griffin, Mrs Janice Hunter **(SLP)**
Hull, Robert A, Jr **(SLP)**
Neeley-Marshall, Vangie **(A)**
Pierdon, Laurie E **(SLP)**

Varnell
Kimbrough, Graham F **(SLP)**

Vienna
Davis, Jacqueline Denise

Villa Rica
Long, Mrs Cynthia Lynne **(SLP)**
Smith, Mrs Denise Elliott **(SLP)**

Waleska
Baggett, Donna D **(SLP)**

Warm Springs
Darby, Jon A **(SLP)**

Warner Robins
Bareither, Mrs Joan McCarthy **(SLP)**
Barnes, Mrs Helen H **(SLP)**
Clarke, Justine L **(SLP)**
Ethier, Mrs Laurel A **(SLP)**
Ethier, Mark E **(A)**
Hubbard, Kim Niemi **(SLP)**
Hunt, Mrs Norma M **(SLP)**
Jones, Mrs Vickie Kay Handley **(SLP)**
Lehman, Maj Jay W **(A)**
Pearson, Gwendolyn Marie **(SLP)**
Reaser, Mrs Ann R **(SLP)**
Yarbrough, Rebecca Wilkes **(A)**

Washington
Bowen, Mrs Judy W **(SLP)**

Watkinsville
Hatch, Judith E **(SLP)**

Waverly Hall
Boddie, Geraldine **(SLP)**

Waycross
Dukes, Mrs Luann Bashur **(SLP)**
Hankla, James W **(A)**
Herndon, Lolita Lorraine

Waynesboro
Thigpen, Mrs Sheron S **(SLP)**

West Point
Davenport, Florence E **(A)**

Winston
Carroll, Susan P **(SLP)**

Winterville
France, Betty Ann/Davis **(SLP)**
Gant, Mrs Leslie Osborne **(A)**
Wolf, Mary Faith **(SLP)**

Woodstock
Cantele, Mrs Susan Marie **(SLP)**
Cash, Wanda M **(SLP)**
Jacob, Lisa Anne **(A)**
Kononen, Mrs Patricia T **(SLP)**
Morrison, Mrs Linda A **(SLP)**
Murley, Mrs Laura Lynne **(SLP)**
Pufnock, Mrs Joyce Gatlin **(SLP)**
Rones, Mrs Cynthia Nothan **(SLP)**
Spears, Judy L **(A)**

Zebulon
Walker, Carolyn **(SLP)**

GUAM

Agana
Blaz, Margaret G **(SLP)**
Triolo, Dennis J **(A)**

Tamuning
Hanson, Mrs Lori Ann H **(SLP)**

HAWAII

Aiea
Amano, Mrs Sandra E **(SLP)**
Canubida, Mrs Carolyn E **(SLP)**
Chow-Hoy, Mrs Diane M S **(SLP)**
Fisher, Diane Marie **(SLP)**
Fukumoto, Paulette Tamie **(SLP)**
Goo, Shari Yuk Sum
Kido, Patricia F **(SLP)**
Lam, Mrs Winona Lau **(SLP)**
McGraw, Charlene S **(SLP)**
Mun, Coralee K **(SLP)**
Noh, Judy L **(SLP)**
Sato, Mrs Sharon K **(A)**
Sekine, Dennis T **(A)**
Sumida, Fay S M **(SLP)**
Tamashiro, Lynette S **(SLP)**
Tanaka, Mrs Wanette Y **(SLP)**

Captain Cook
Livingston, Mary Lou **(SLP)**
Reynolds, Bruce E **(SLP)**

Ewa Beach
Gregorio, Mrs Barbara Joan **(SLP)**
Gubenski, Mrs Mary Kaye Yeakle **(SLP)**
Vause-Stapleton, Nancy **(A)**

Hilo
Akama-Lapinta, Jean E **(SLP)**
Asato, Joanne Chiemi **(A)**
Dittmer, Judy **(SLP)**
Gale, Christine Annette **(SLP)**
Kanno, Dr Leila Okino
Kossick, Laurie Ann **(SLP)**
Martin, Steven Leroy **(SLP)**
Pruitt, Mrs Joy **(SLP)**
Suzuki, Gwen Mitsuko **(SLP)**
Taguchi, Mrs Estrelleta N **(SLP)**
Werner, Dr Marlin S **(SLP A)**
Yamauchi, Elinor H **(SLP)**

Honolulu
Abernethy, Pearl Mary **(SLP)**
Ansberry, Dr Merle **(A)**
Armstrong, Daryl Vesper **(SLP)**
Benjamin, Carolyn D **(SLP)**
Bielecki, Debra Shiro **(SLP)**
Billingsley, Mrs Marilyn M V **(SLP)**
Bishop, Mrs Sumie **(SLP)**
Chinen, Mrs Verna Mae Kn **(SLP)**
Ching, Shannon Y **(A)**
Chong, Sandra G H **(SLP)**
Chun, Darleen G **(SLP)**
Chun, Mrs Jan E Arakaki **(SLP)**

Clamp, Mrs Jana Poynor
Coronado, Marcia Chur **(SLP)**
Craven, Mrs Dorothy D **(SLP A)**
Davies, Dr Jeffrey W **(A)**
Dizon, Mary B **(SLP)**
Dufon, Margaret A **(SLP)**
Festerling, Jane S **(SLP)**
Fong, Cheryl Lou **(SLP)**
Geary, Mrs Joan C **(SLP)**
Gipe, Patricia Neal **(A)**
Gokan, Lynn Y
Grubb, Mrs Susan F **(SLP)**
Halevi, Dr Lynne Grossman **(SLP)**
Harada, Clark **(SLP)**
Higa, Mrs Doreen Yurie **(SLP)**
Hu, Mrs Lorna Kiyoko **(SLP)**
Ihara, Grace R **(SLP)**
Ip, Lai-Fan Renee **(SLP)**
Iwamoto, Valerie Iyeko **(SLP)**
Jerke, Thomas A **(SLP)**
Jones, Fay M **(SLP)**
Kam, Kellie W J **(SLP)**
Kau, Darlene M **(SLP A)**
Kauhane, Mrs Jere A **(SLP)**
Kelley, Susan P **(SLP)**
Kimata, Cheryl Lynn **(SLP)**
Kimoto, Kathleen Y **(SLP)**
Kobayashi, Lynn M
Krammer, Katherine **(SLP)**
Larkins, Deborah A **(A)**
Lee, Mrs Dee Ann H **(SLP)**
Lyon, Barbara J **(SLP)**
Maemori, Kathy Sadanaga **(SLP)**
Maki, Jerilyn Satomi
Marasovich, Mary Louise **(SLP)**
Mashima, Pauline Matsumoto **(SLP)**
Mashiyama, Dee K
Mason, Mrs Judith Asbury **(A)**
Masuda, Mrs Irene S **(SLP)**
Matsumoto, Mrs Haunani K **(SLP)**
Mayfield, Mrs Rhonda Moore **(SLP)**
Meyer, Mrs Lauren Rene **(SLP)**
Michael, Mrs Mary W
Mirafuentes, Noreen Nenita **(SLP)**
Moody, Donna Michelle **(SLP)**
Morisato, Teale Misae **(SLP)**
Moto, Eric Hiroshi **(SLP)**
Mow, Mrs Sally Mulder **(SLP)**
Muramaru, Mrs Ruth Y **(SLP)**
Nakasato, Mrs Jean M **(SLP)**
Nash, Cynthia Lynne **(A)**
Ng, Mildred Y B **(SLP)**
Ogawa, Mrs Toshiko O **(SLP)**
Okamura, Kay Emiko **(SLP)**
O'Leary, Mrs Geraldine **(SLP)**
Pang, Denise K **(SLP)**
Pang-Ching, Dr Glenn K **(A)**
Pearson, Mrs Christina Zavrotny **(SLP)**
Phillips, Dorothy C **(SLP)**
Pirone, Kim Cheryl **(SLP)**
Powell, Renee J **(SLP)**
Reed, Robbin C **(SLP)**
Richard, Dr Nancy B **(SLP)**
Robb, Dr Michael Paul **(SLP)**
Ruth, MaryLee **(A)**
Sakai, Grace M **(SLP)**
Sandefur, Mrs Dona Rae **(SLP)**
Schultz, Joanne M **(SLP)**
Shigemoto, Joan Hamatake **(SLP)**
Shotwell, Cherrie L **(SLP)**
Simmons, Johnny O **(SLP)**
Smith, Tracey S **(SLP)**
Spelman, Mrs Sylvia L K **(SLP)**
Stewart, Jean L **(A)**
Suematsu, Kikuyo **(SLP A)**
Suenaga, Patricia S Y **(SLP)**
Sykes, Gaile **(SLP)**
Taber, Mrs Linda E **(SLP)**
Takemoto, Charlotte **(SLP)**
Takumi, Mona S **(A)**
Tamashiro, Howard K **(A)**
Tokusato, Mona A
Tomosada, Ann Hatsumi **(SLP)**
Uehara, Mrs Ginny Sueko **(SLP)**
Uyehara-Isono, June M **(A)**
Valite-Andersen, Arlinda E **(SLP)**
Wada, Margaret K **(SLP)**
Wang, Mrs Norene K **(A)**
Whang, Lisa Ann **(SLP)**
Wilson, Kim Elizabeth **(SLP)**
Won, Terilyn Yukie **(A)**
Wooley, Mrs Helen G **(SLP)**
Yamauchi, Lori Lei **(SLP)**
Yates, Dr James T **(A)**
Yim, Janice Lee **(SLP)**
Yukitomo, Mrs April S **(SLP)**
Zane, Jonna D **(SLP)**

Kahului
Rejzer, Alexandra A **(SLP)**

Kahului Maui
Abe, Mrs Agnes O **(SLP)**
Tokishi, Walter H **(SLP)**

Kailua
Ban, Dr Paul K **(SLP)**
Camara, Mrs Ann Marie Heffron **(SLP)**
Campbell, Kathleen Haunani **(A)**
Eversmann, Mrs Jill Grant **(SLP)**
Failla, Peggy P **(A)**
Glamb, Mary D **(SLP)**
Hellreich, J Miriam **(SLP)**
Jensen, Mrs Joyce H **(SLP)**
Kimura, Mrs Kathleen C **(SLP)**
Looney-Burman, Patricia L **(SLP)**
Matsumoto, Ann S T **(SLP)**
Ranney, Mrs Elizabeth Anne **(SLP)**
Rausch, Shelia Marc-Aurel **(SLP)**
Roos-Marr, Ellen Juhl **(SLP)**
Singson, Maile Tanaka **(SLP)**
Survant, Mrs Maureen Connell **(SLP)**
Takekawa, Kristine Montgomery **(A)**
Zeisloft-Falbey, Barbara C **(SLP)**

Kailua Kona
Ashworth, Myra Y **(SLP)**
Gillam, Suzanne F **(A)**

Kalaheo
Harlacher, John C **(SLP)**

Kamuela
Ruddle, Eugenia Marie **(SLP)**

Kaneohe
Caballero-Somawang, Julieta **(SLP)**
Coons, Sandra La Verne **(SLP)**
Fushikoshi, Kellie Ann
Hadrick, Nancy Z **(SLP)**
Iwamoto, Vickie M **(SLP A)**
Lindsey, Deborah A **(A)**
Lum, Mrs Eydie Emi **(SLP)**
Matheson, Mrs Joan **(A)**
Matsunaga, Faye A T **(A)**
Mogi, Mrs Jonet Ahuna **(SLP)**
Muraoka, Mrs Eileen Kikue **(SLP)**
Nakayama, Mrs Pat **(SLP)**
Shiroma, Charlene E **(SLP)**
Tamai, Laverne Mieko **(SLP)**

Kapaa
Clark, Mrs Joan H **(SLP)**
Yatogo, Mrs Julie Namie **(SLP)**

Kapaa Kauai
Nishimitsu, Holly T **(SLP)**

Kaunakakai
Brito, Cynthia Kojima **(SLP)**

Kealakekua
Stewart, Lynne Tsuchida **(SLP)**

Kealakekua-Kona
Hata, Mrs Susan Sowa **(SLP)**

Kihei
Chapman, Mrs M Janet **(SLP A)**
Trombly, Dr Thelma **(SLP)**

Kihei Maui
Wells, Dr Charlotte G **(SLP)**

Koloa
Tokita, Mrs Shayne Horita **(SLP)**

Kula
Tanaka, Mrs Marsha U **(SLP)**
Yamamoto, Mrs Gayle Y **(SLP)**

Lahaina
Galloway-Curtis, Anne **(A)**

Laie
Anae, Mrs Annabel Porter **(A)**

Lihue Kauai
Yama, Mrs Lauri M **(SLP)**

Maui
Barnes-Shankel, Loretta Ann **(SLP)**

Mililani Town
Andres, Mrs Cecilia Basilio **(SLP)**
Bennett, Ana Aurora **(SLP)**
Doi, Mrs Betty S **(SLP)**
Matsumoto, Dale T
Matsuwaki, Mrs Beverly A **(SLP)**
Shintani, Janice S **(SLP)**
Wong, Trudy T **(SLP)**

Mountain View
Carey, Susan W **(SLP)**

Papaikou
Seaman, Constance **(SLP)**

Pearl City
Ho, Evelyn Z **(SLP)**
Kaminaga, Gail Naomi **(SLP)**
Kato, Wendy Yuriko **(SLP)**
Ohta, Debra Ann K **(SLP)**
Sato, Mrs Karen S K **(SLP)**

Punaluu Oahu
Bjornson, Mrs Jean N **(SLP)**

Wahiawa
Oshiro, Susan Ruth **(SLP)**
Suzuki, Deborah S **(A)**

Waialae Maui
Suson, Karen Anne **(SLP)**

Waianae
Pell, Florene **(SLP)**

Wailuku
Ikeda, Mrs Pamela F **(SLP)**
Miyamoto, Naomi H **(SLP)**

Waipahu
Arakaki, Gaye Keiko **(SLP)**
Demello, Mrs Corazon Nievera **(SLP)**
Manding, Mrs Glorilynn O
Tarumoto, Elsie K **(SLP)**
Yamamoto, Irene Chieko **(SLP)**

IDAHO

Blackfoot
Bevan, Mrs Debora Lee **(SLP)**
Dalton, Penny M Summers **(SLP)**

Blanchard
Saunders, Steven James **(SLP)**

Bliss
Bowler, Dr Ned W **(SLP)**

Boise
Adkins, Laurie Murray **(SLP)**
Allen, Carol S **(SLP)**
Belknap, Barbara A **(SLP)**
Blaesing, Martha E **(A)**
Butler, Linda Bartron **(SLP)**
Carpenter, Dr Jane M **(SLP)**
Collings, James Everett **(SLP)**
Collins, Judith W **(SLP)**
Drebin, Mrs Kathleen C **(A)**
Edwards, Dr Marcia Sue **(SLP)**
Gillette, Mrs Kamara Laree **(SLP)**
Hanson, Maxine R **(SLP)**
Hardy, Steven Dwight **(SLP)**
Hart, Karen A **(SLP)**
Hughes, Mrs Diane Hutchinson **(SLP)**
Hurley, Margaret Rose **(SLP)**
Jaeger, Karen S **(SLP)**
Jordan, Mrs Ethel S **(SLP A)**
Losasso, Sharon A **(SLP)**
Martin, Mrs Brenda K **(SLP)**
McElhinney, Gwynne **(SLP)**
McKain, Virginia Kraft **(SLP)**
Merris, Mrs Margaret **(SLP)**
Miller, Mary Margaret **(SLP)**
Moeller, Susan Jeannette **(SLP)**
Motley, Mrs Carla H **(SLP)**
Olsen, Cynthia Kathleen **(A)**
Peachey, Galen L **(SLP)**
Peterson, Perry Jo **(SLP)**
Purcell, Debra A **(SLP)**
Reese, Lynn Marie **(A)**
Rigg, M Leslie **(SLP)**
Roberts, Judith L **(SLP)**
Steiling, Mrs Margaret **(SLP)**
Steinauer, Judith A **(SLP)**
Strong, Rebecca Ann **(SLP)**
Sturmak, Michael J **(A)**
Swenson, David Wayne **(A)**
Talboy, Mrs Lori W **(SLP)**
Vause, Mark Wayne
Waldorf, Mrs Pamela Crowder **(SLP)**
Washburn, Mrs Rosemary C **(SLP)**
Welsch, Mrs Mary Ruth **(SLP)**
Wheeling, Sandra Kay **(SLP)**
Whitcomb, Curtis Joe **(A)**
Whitcomb, Rebecca Beukelman **(SLP)**
Whiteman, Leah Duncan **(SLP)**
Wischow, Karen J **(SLP)**

Burley
Reynolds, Mrs Jennifer Elaine **(SLP)**

Chubbuck
Crookston, Garr J **(A)**
Milbrandt, Mrs Mariette **(SLP)**

Coeur d'Alene
Hamilton, Lana H **(SLP)**
Merriman, Mrs Ruth Alice **(SLP)**
Riplinger, Patricia S **(SLP)**
Rossi, Louise F **(SLP)**
Stranger, Linda Paine **(SLP)**
Underhill, Mrs Marianne S **(SLP)**

Cottonwood
Allen, Mrs Carletta M **(SLP)**
Gwinn, Mrs Velma Rose

Eagle
Banks, Mrs Teresa M **(SLP)**
Boeder, Jess Seymour **(SLP)**

Eden
Maxwell, Jeannene **(SLP)**
Michener, Mary C J **(SLP)**
Mingo, Carla SJ **(SLP)**

Hailey
Bruhy, Sharon **(SLP)**
Zajac, Mrs Sandra S **(SLP)**

Hayden Lake
Welling, Ronda S **(SLP)**

Hope
Middleton, Mrs Janet M **(SLP)**

Ida Grove
Farnham, Todd A **(A)**

Idaho Falls
Dahlke, Joan M **(SLP)**
Hammond, Joann **(SLP)**
Harker, Mrs Eileen Orchard
Hogg, Mrs Debra F **(SLP)**
Horkley, Mrs Jeanette S

Hutterman, Lorraine G **(SLP)**
Kirchgasler, Claudia Roberts **(SLP)**
Kirn, June H **(SLP)**
Loomis, Janet Paider **(SLP)**
Marlette, Amy **(SLP)**
McCaffrey, Mrs Anne Randler **(SLP)**
McGee, Sandra R **(SLP)**
Mill, Dr Gerald P **(A)**
Nelson, Mrs Tammie Lou **(A)**
Olsen, Karel McSween **(SLP)**
Straka, Elizabeth A **(SLP)**
Swenson, Rita L **(SLP)**

Inkom
Huffman, Frances H **(SLP)**

Iona
Huntsman, Mrs Angela Abundis

Jerome
Harris, Mrs Nancy Lee **(SLP)**
Suter, Cherri A **(SLP)**

Kooskia
Brankey, Mrs Fern T **(SLP)**

Kuna
Carter, Marilyn J **(SLP)**

Lewiston
Anderson, Kathleen Caliendo **(SLP)**
Miller, Mrs Maxine Christa **(A)**
Norton, Jennifer Salka **(SLP)**
Uhlman, Mrs Lorraine L **(SLP)**
Young, Richard N **(A)**

McCall
Olde, Karen Leslie **(SLP)**
Robinson, Cindy L **(SLP)**

Meridian
Ray, Mrs Amy Sue **(SLP)**

Moscow
Bouillon, Mrs Rita Wetzstein **(SLP)**
Goff, Mrs Cindy Robinson **(SLP)**
Hall, Mrs Joyce E **(SLP A)**
Inglebret, Ella R **(SLP)**
Jones, Carla A **(SLP)**
Katz, Jean Becker **(SLP)**
Skelly, Mrs Alicia **(SLP)**
Swanson, Sally A **(SLP)**
Thompson, Nancy Diane **(SLP)**

Mountain Home
Ennis, Kimberly Ann **(SLP)**
Haney, Mrs Sheree J **(SLP)**
Hendrickson, Mrs Susan G **(SLP)**

Nampa
Boulette, Donna M **(A)**
Bowman, Rick G **(A)**
Deleo, Mrs Barbara Marie **(SLP)**
Owens, Dr Earl R **(SLP)**
Siedenstrang, Mrs Lynn Littleton
Trauernicht, Maxine J **(SLP)**
Wardlaw, Francis G **(SLP A)**
Wethered, Dr Chris E **(SLP)**

Orofino
Espinosa, Mrs Melinda A **(SLP)**

Osburn
Norris, Cathi D **(A)**

Pocatello
Bitton, Sidena Gardner **(SLP)**
Brockett, Jeff E **(A)**
Deputy, Dr Paul N **(SLP)**
Ferris, Linda L **(SLP)**
Gordon, Dr Kathleen Clegg **(SLP)**
Haffner-Spencer, Linda Jean **(SLP)**
Hutchinson, Dr John M **(SLP)**
Kline, Lorrie L S **(SLP)**
Longhurst, Dr Thomas M **(SLP)**
Malepeai, Brenda Bertsch **(SLP)**
Matkin, Mrs Susan Stewart **(SLP)**
Medley, Kennard E
Miller, Laura Blanco **(SLP)**
Moore, Betty Jean **(SLP)**
Musetti, Margaret C **(SLP)**
Nelson, Rachelle Louise
O'Donnell, Jody Sue **(SLP)**
Richards, Mrs Natalie Ann
Ross, Theresa L **(SLP)**
Schow, Ronald L **(A)**
Smedley, Dr Thayne C **(A)**
Smith, Jane Coe **(SLP)**
Smith, Stephany Myatt
Sorensen, Dr David N **(SLP)**
Springer, Mrs Leann Marie **(SLP)**
Stahlecker, Sue Schoenrock **(SLP)**
Thompson, Carol M **(SLP)**
Whitaker, Mrs Mary Mouer **(A)**
Williams, Marcia J **(SLP)**
Wyckoff, Mrs Candice G **(SLP)**

Post Falls
Gleesing, Mrs Cindy K **(SLP)**

Rathdrum
Williams, Katharine **(SLP)**

Rexburg
Godfrey, Mrs Sally C **(SLP)**
Hillier, David B **(SLP)**
Kerr, Mrs Caroline J **(A)**
Mortensen, Mrs Camille Heward **(SLP)**
Robinson, Mrs Kaloha Lloyd **(SLP)**

Rigby
Tavenner, Mrs Laura Mae **(SLP)**

Rupert
McKee, Sonna Cherie **(SLP)**
Miller, Marcia Lynne **(SLP)**

Salmon
Cook-Westfall, Deborah A **(SLP)**
Crowley, John Francis **(SLP)**

Sandpoint
Britton, Michelle A **(SLP)**
Carlson, Wendy Allen **(SLP)**
Gerth, Jean Louise **(SLP)**
Lund, Mrs Marion **(SLP)**
Rucklos, Kimberly Dawn **(SLP)**
Sleyster, Mrs Tina Shaffer **(SLP)**

Silverton
Adamson, Clark R **(SLP)**
Carpenter, Eileen M **(SLP)**

St Anthony
Bunnell, Mrs Maryann Riesland **(SLP)**
Dalin, Stephen Raymond **(SLP)**
Frugoli, Pamela Rae **(SLP)**

St Maries
Benda, Mrs Teresa Ann **(SLP)**

Troy
Engelhardt, Christine **(SLP)**

Twin Falls
Casabonne, Janet Houston **(SLP)**
Harville, Mrs Karen C **(SLP)**
Hesse, Audrey Lynn **(SLP)**
Langkopt, Linda Kay **(SLP)**
Lenkner, Melody A **(SLP)**
Lloyd, Jay C **(A)**
Nielsen, Elizabeth Ann
Standley, Mrs Cathie H **(SLP)**

Weiser
Huck, Barbara **(SLP)**

ILLINOIS

Adair
McCall, J Louise **(A)**

Addison
Anderson, Mrs Barbara B **(SLP)**
Conran, Mrs Kathleen S **(SLP)**
Hall, Kathleen E **(SLP)**
Whelihan, Ann T **(SLP)**

Albers
Dennison, Mrs Kelly Hamilton **(SLP)**

Algonquin
Aggen, Mrs Janet S **(SLP)**
Greco, Mrs Mary L **(SLP)**
Keen, Mrs Jeanmarie **(A)**
Nelmes, Dale A **(SLP)**
Reining, Penny **(SLP)**
Westfall, Mrs Wendelyn Lori **(SLP)**
Witek, Mrs Melanie McLean **(SLP)**

Alsip
Lopez-Chaney, Anna Marie **(SLP)**

Alton
Anderson, Cheryl L **(SLP)**
Gray, Mellaney **(SLP)**
Harman, Kathryn T **(SLP)**
Heppner, Nancee L **(SLP)**
Maag, Gregory J **(A)**
Martin, Diane C **(SLP)**
Murphy, Jerry B **(A)**
Pakosta, Judith Lynn **(SLP)**
Sherman, Janine Buehling **(SLP)**
Swift, Margo I **(SLP)**

Altona
Johnson, Mrs Christine L W **(SLP)**

Ancona
Cassady, Mrs Debbie D **(SLP)**

Anna
Ellison, Mrs Marcia F **(SLP)**
Pengress, Mrs Tanya Kay **(SLP)**
Rose, Pamela S **(SLP)**

Antioch
Crawford, Lynn J **(SLP)**
Denny, Marcia C **(SLP)**
Passarella, Mrs Rosanne G **(SLP)**

Arlington Height
Effa-Hill, Catherine Ann **(A)**
Froehlich, Mrs Paula Irene **(SLP)**
Holmes, Geraldine A **(SLP)**
Leonard-Pitts, Lori A **(SLP)**
Miller, Kathleen Grace **(SLP)**
Petro, Mrs Gail Lynn **(SLP)**
Shorey, Mrs Carrie Elizabeth **(SLP)**
Spells-Thompson, Mrs Vanessa R **(SLP)**
Stauber, Ronald C
Stephani, Mrs Lauren Fae **(SLP)**
Welter, Julie Ann **(SLP)**

Arlington Heights
Baker, Rita J **(SLP)**
Bieber, Catherine R **(SLP)**
Bonno-King, Carmelita M **(SLP)**
Breiding, Philip R **(SLP)**
Burnett, Mrs Judy C **(SLP)**
Cooper, Mrs Diana L B **(SLP)**
Danekas, Andrea Nicholas **(SLP)**
Drop, Mrs Judith Waterwash **(SLP)**
Eberhardt, Nancy B **(SLP)**
Elliott, Marian **(SLP)**
Faems, Mrs Debra H **(SLP)**
Goldberg, Lori E **(A)**
Graser, Nan Stutzman **(SLP)**
Haines, Sarah Elizabeth **(SLP)**
Herbst, Mrs Inger A **(SLP)**
Hill, Alice Baer **(A)**
Huebner, Mrs Debra S **(SLP)**
Jensen, Sherry E **(SLP)**
Kroupa, Molly J **(SLP)**
LeMaster, Sharon Lyn
Loftin, Rosemary B **(SLP)**
Mantilla, Mary W **(SLP)**
McClure, Lavonne K **(SLP)**
Metzger, Mrs Mary E **(SLP)**
Mito, Marion J **(SLP)**
Murphy, Mrs Barbara R **(A)**
Neidich, Jay S **(SLP)**
Neidich, Mrs Robin B **(SLP)**
Paxson, Mrs Carmel Dowd **(SLP)**
Powers-Richard, Vivian L **(SLP)**
Pulver, Maija G **(SLP)**
Resnik, Jane I **(SLP)**
Schlofner, Denise Barsella **(SLP)**
Scurry, Donna Jean **(SLP)**
Thompson, Nancy J **(SLP)**
Vosburgh, Mrs Gloria S **(SLP)**
Wasilk, Barbara Miksch **(SLP)**
Woloshin, Mrs Ronna Siegel **(SLP)**
Wyatt, Linda M **(A)**
Zahareas, Mrs Maria D **(SLP)**
Zemper, F Anne **(SLP)**

Ashkum
Rankin, Mrs Deena W **(SLP)**

Aurora
Callahan, Mrs Susan Finegan **(SLP)**
Carpenter, Nancy M **(SLP)**
Carson, Loretta S **(SLP)**
Fitzpatrick, Wilma L **(SLP)**
Hoover, Lisa **(SLP)**
Kline, Joann I **(SLP)**
Krantz, Susan Sanders **(SLP)**
Krieter, Mrs Mary Kathleen **(SLP)**
Leonard Allen, Patricia Ann **(SLP)**
McGinnis, Lisa M **(SLP)**
Miller, Charlene W **(SLP)**
Nordmeyer, Valerie Marie **(SLP)**
Radzimanowski, Kathryn Anne **(SLP)**
Russell, Mrs Charleen G **(SLP)**
Sibon, Brenda Dice **(SLP)**
Steele, Judith M **(SLP)**

Avon
Chatterton, Mrs Suzanne V **(SLP)**
Lock, Mrs Sally A **(SLP)**

Barlett
Hughes, Kara L

Barrington
Archer-Chmela, Mrs Kristin Marie
Hammes, Barbara Phillips **(SLP)**
Jaekel, Mrs Susan M **(SLP)**
Kitz, Janice H **(A)**
Luensman, Karen Butler **(SLP)**
Retzlaff, Wesley **(SLP)**
Whalen, Mrs Sherry L **(SLP)**
Yedor, Katherine **(SLP)**

Barrington Hills
Ellis, Mrs Lavonne **(SLP)**

Bartlett
Alt, Mrs Susan P **(SLP)**
Pastor, Mrs Lois **(SLP)**

Batavia
Braunsky, Mrs Susan B
Bromstrup-Garrity, Mrs Kathleen F **(SLP)**
Castellani, Mrs Laurelyn Mary **(SLP)**
Helfrecht, Mrs Paula Jean **(SLP)**
Hoffer, Kimberly Skarin **(SLP)**
Horbus, Mrs Marilyn **(SLP)**
Lewis-Hyde, Mrs Mary Lee
Manigold, Mrs Rebecca D **(SLP)**
Rohr, Mrs Linda J **(SLP)**
Samelson, Mrs Vicki Weiss **(SLP)**

Belleville
Beuckman, Sharon P **(SLP)**
Boyne, Sandra Olsson **(SLP)**
Brennan, Florence A **(SLP)**
Brennan, Frances M **(SLP)**
Calhoun, Melissa Hotto **(SLP)**
De Franco, Mrs Kathleen D **(SLP)**
Edris, Capt Robert W **(A)**
Gruneich, Mrs Mary Pacatte **(A)**
Gurr, Linda **(SLP)**
Hagan, Mrs Donna M **(SLP)**
Haman-Miller, Karen J **(SLP)**
Hamilton, Joyce **(SLP)**
Harres, Susan C **(SLP)**
Katzman, Mrs Sherry Hecht **(SLP)**
Kuhn, Mrs Margaret E **(SLP)**

Martin, Nancy S **(SLP)**
McLaughlin, Susan M **(SLP A)**
Miller, Cecilia C **(SLP)**
Nimmons, Mrs Ellen Marie **(SLP)**
Phillips, Gayle A **(SLP)**
Puhl, Janice Lee **(SLP)**
Rhein, Stephanie A **(SLP)**
Richards, Mrs Janice M **(SLP)**
Svec, Mrs Mary Arnold **(SLP A)**
Vernetti, Robert James **(A)**
Yale, Mrs Barbara **(A)**
Zamzow, Fran G **(SLP)**

Belvidere
Blascoe, Marcia O **(SLP)**
Hightower, Mrs Deborah Swank **(SLP)**
Liston, Lynn R **(A)**
Magill, Mrs Kathleen O'Grady **(SLP)**
Neil, Mrs Linda Sue **(SLP)**
Stenerson, Mrs Cynthia Hemmens **(SLP)**

Bensenville
Beiter, Dr Robert C **(A)**
Dettlaff, Krystina **(SLP)**

Benton
Doughty, Patricia Jo **(SLP)**

Berwyn
Baron, Fern A **(SLP)**
Cervenka, Mrs Linda Marie **(SLP)**
Hirschmann, Mary **(SLP)**
Merten, Mrs Joyce G **(SLP)**

Bethalto
Morrison, Mrs Patricia Walters **(SLP)**
Murbarger, Susan D M **(SLP)**

Big Rock
Todd, Bonnie E **(SLP)**

Bloomingdale
Angermeier, Dr Cynthia B **(SLP)**
Blaige, Judith Frances **(SLP)**
Chudik, Eileen M **(SLP)**
Sinnott, Mary A **(SLP)**

Bloomington
Blankenship, Sue A
Bowles, Mrs Patsy H **(SLP)**
Bowman, Linda Susan **(SLP)**
Burnett, Marsha K **(SLP)**
Burtis, Mrs Barbara D **(SLP)**
Cox, Mrs Kathleen M **(SLP)**
Dachauer, Mrs Joyce Susan **(SLP)**
Diemer, Barbara K **(SLP)**
Duffee, Mrs Penelope H **(SLP A)**
Eichenauer, Patricia Louise **(SLP)**
Evans, Mrs Donna S **(SLP)**
Moore, Maryevelyn R **(SLP)**
Prendergast, Susan G **(A)**
Schramm, Sara Ann **(SLP)**
Semanko, Gay E **(SLP)**
Sidak, Julie Ann **(A)**
Smoski, Dr Walter J **(A)**
Stevens, Mrs Nancy J H **(SLP)**
Vice, Mrs Janna Hilliard **(SLP)**
Winger, Mrs Anita Marie

Blue Island
Harting, Mrs Marlene A
Kane, Margaret Mary **(SLP)**
Weiss, Carol Ann **(SLP)**

Bolingbrook
Berg, Jeanette M **(A)**
Colletta, Marsha A **(SLP)**
Decarlo-Erickson, Mrs Ginny **(SLP)**
Felt, Mrs Catherine Renee **(SLP)**
Kloep, Karen Langenfeld **(A)**
Laszewski, Carol Lynn **(SLP)**
Meyer, Mrs Eileen R **(SLP)**
Meyer, Mrs Kay B **(SLP)**
Nielsen, Mrs Susan McGuckin **(SLP)**
Swartz, Leslie A **(SLP)**

Bourbonnais
Barber, Mrs Ellen J **(SLP)**
Bowman, Mrs Carol J **(SLP)**
Dattilo, Carol Langford **(SLP)**
Decker, David I **(SLP)**
Muchmore, Teresa Ann **(SLP)**
Shafland, Karen J **(SLP)**
Sublette-Sloan, Mrs Cynthia B **(SLP)**

Bradley
Croix, Mrs Patricia J **(A)**
Poen, Beth D **(SLP)**

Bridgeport
Rose, Deborah L **(SLP)**

Bridgeview
Coughlin, Mary Therese **(SLP)**
Kavouriaris, Kathleen Waldron **(SLP)**

Bristol
Petri, Pamela S **(SLP)**

Brookfield
Bombick, Dianne L **(SLP)**
Kral, Rhonda S **(SLP)**
Toczylowski, Darlene M **(SLP)**

Buffalo Grove
Avishar, Mrs Nancy J **(A)**
Behnken, Susan A **(SLP)**
Belasco, Mrs Carol W **(SLP)**
Bentley, Mrs Patricia K **(SLP)**
Breit, Mrs Miriam C **(SLP)**
Cohen, Mrs Nancy Fell **(SLP)**
Colick-Hapner, Edie R **(SLP)**
Downie, Mrs Linda K **(SLP)**
Eggert, Mrs Christine **(SLP)**
Galinsky, Mrs Franci M **(SLP)**
Gittelman-Nadeau, Mrs Debbie **(A)**
Jaffe, Mrs Nancy E R **(SLP)**
Kaplan, Mrs Ilene L **(SLP)**
Kirschner, Susan B **(SLP)**
Klein-Koonin, Mrs June E **(SLP)**
Lambert, Gerald T
Leibach, Ronna B **(SLP)**
Lovendahl, Crisler Magor **(SLP)**
MacIsaac, Diane M **(SLP)**
Meyers, Karen L **(SLP)**
Miller, Syndee F W **(SLP)**
Palella, Marietta C **(SLP)**
Robinson, Mrs Carol M **(SLP A)**
Rugg, Mrs Joanne D **(SLP)**
Schur, Mrs Karen G **(SLP)**
Sefcik, Mrs Jan B **(SLP)**
Segal, Mrs Renee R **(SLP)**
Shapiro, Dr Holly Rose **(SLP)**
Stern-Weisman, Phyllis **(A)**
Turner, Mrs Sue Beth **(SLP)**
Warshaw, Mrs Elyse W **(SLP)**
Weidenfeld, Susan H **(SLP)**
White, Mrs Lora Lee **(SLP)**
Zucker-Krantz, Mrs Jerri **(SLP)**
Zuckerman-Simon, Mrs Holly **(SLP)**
Zweiban, Mrs Mira R **(SLP)**

Burbank
Baker, Judith Ann
Garner, Mrs Marie A **(SLP)**
Greene, Maribeth **(SLP)**
Sabatini, Joyce A **(SLP)**

Burr Ridge
Eilers, Karen R **(SLP)**
Pikscher, Barbara A **(SLP)**
Salerno, Linda L **(SLP)**

Cairo
Browning, Janice L **(SLP)**

Calumet City
Clark, Lisa Michelle **(SLP)**
Davis, Dr Diane Vennessa **(SLP)**
Keever, Lyn G **(SLP)**
Muckian, Mrs Cathy A **(SLP)**

Calumet Park
Veazy, Mrs Julia Woodard

Cambridge
Morey, Mrs Ann Patrice **(SLP)**

Camp Point
Passley, Mrs Bonnie Jean **(A)**

Carbondale
Anderson, John O **(SLP)**
Blache, Dr Stephen E
Black, Katherine **(SLP)**
Booziotis, Kathy Kelly **(SLP)**
Brackett, Dr Isaac P **(SLP)**
Brewster, Cynthia Constance
Brutten, Dr Gene J **(SLP A)**
Corker, Mrs Susan Chase **(A)**
Craig, Dr Lillian M **(SLP A)**
Davie, Mrs Cynthia C S **(SLP)**
Deakin, Carol Stephens
Drew, Barbara Ann
Dunham, Elizabeth **(SLP)**
Friend, Connie Marie **(SLP)**
Garbutt, Dr Cameron W **(SLP)**
Gonzalez, Lori Stewart **(SLP)**
Hager, Mrs Nancy S **(SLP)**
Hashi, Michiko
Hoshiko, Dr Michael **(SLP)**
Kammlade, Mrs Helen S **(SLP)**
Leighty, Elizabeth G **(SLP)**
Masoner, Judith Collins
Mitchener, Karl K **(SLP)**
Mitchener, Mrs Marilyn H **(SLP)**
Newman, Mrs Sheree L
Reimbold, John **(A)**
Robb, Mrs Tommye L **(SLP)**
Robey, Dr Randall R **(SLP)**
Ruder, Dr Kenneth F **(SLP)**
Schultz, Dr Martin C **(A)**
Simpson, Richard Peerman **(SLP)**
Sinnott, Jan Morris **(SLP)**
Vicars, Lee Ann **(SLP)**
Vinyard, Mrs Allison J
Wade, Mrs Jacqueline Anne
Wheeler, Mrs Wendy Polsky **(SLP)**

Carlinville
Nolan, Mrs Laurie Jean **(SLP)**

Carlyle
Cardwell, Barbara Ann **(SLP)**
White, Mrs Sherry M **(SLP)**

Carmi
Broughton, Jill Glass **(SLP)**
Fritschle, Patricia **(SLP)**

Carol Stream
Furlano, Deborah Seubert **(SLP)**
Jones, Mrs Mary B **(SLP)**
McHenry, Eileen M
Mika, Mrs Ann Marie **(SLP)**
Schmeltzer, Marguerite **(SLP)**
Wilde, Mrs Jana R **(SLP)**
Winterrose, Mrs Maureen Rae **(SLP)**
Wood, Mrs Lynn A **(A)**
Yevin, Barbara Ann **(SLP)**

Carterville
Covey, Lee Ellen **(SLP)**
Ruder, Charlotte **(SLP A)**

Carthage
Nicholas, Rosalind H **(SLP)**

Cary
Bear, Mrs Annette Marie **(SLP)**
Darling, Angela Kay

Casey
Swick, Mrs Joan B **(SLP)**
Thorsen, Claire B **(SLP)**

Caseyville
Canty, Mrs Pamela Sue **(SLP)**

Catlin
Deck, John W **(SLP)**
Ingram, Mrs Linda Liggett

Centralia
Bodem, John Anthony **(A)**
Broughton, Jennifer Lee **(SLP)**
Bryan, Mrs Linda D **(SLP)**

Cerro Gordo
Strole, Mrs Christy O **(SLP)**

Champaign
Bennett, Laurie Floren **(A)**
Bilger, Robert C
Braden, Mrs Linda F **(SLP)**
Britten, Mrs Karin Elisabeth **(SLP)**
Brown, Michael Patrick **(A)**
Burwell, Mrs Donna **(SLP)**
Cartwright, Jenifer M **(SLP)**
Cetin, Patricia Davis **(SLP)**
Chambers, Dr Ron D **(A)**
Colwell, Andrea Thompson **(SLP)**
Dalene, Mrs L Juli **(SLP)**
Day, Mrs Marylou M **(SLP)**
De La Mar, Mrs Melody A **(SLP)**
Dowell, Bonita Lynne **(SLP)**
Eastin, Debra P **(SLP)**
Echols-Chambers, Lou **(A)**
Erickson, Dr Joan Good **(SLP A)**
Fifer, Dr Robert C **(A)**
Firszt, Mrs Jill Blair **(A)**
Forrest, Diana K **(SLP)**
Foss, Michelle Piper
Goller, Monica C **(A)**
Grant, Monica G **(A)**
Grater, Mrs Ruth D **(SLP)**
Greenwald, Carolyn R **(A)**
Hankinson, Anita J **(SLP)**
James, Mrs Jane G **(SLP)**
Johnson, Dr Cynthia J **(SLP)**
Kuehn, Dr David P
Laird, Mrs Kathryn A **(SLP)**
Lee, Sarah Britt **(SLP)**
Matthies, Dr Melanie L **(A)**
McKenzie, Terri A **(SLP)**
Metcalf, Mrs Kathleen Highland **(SLP)**
Mueller-Alms, Mrs Elizabeth A **(SLP)**
Neill, Michele Caroline **(SLP)**
Nichols, Mrs Shari A **(SLP)**
O'Neill, John J **(SLP A)**
Parker, Mrs Carol Louise **(A)**
Paxton, Kenneth Lowell **(SLP)**
Raso, Susan D **(SLP)**
Reed, Mrs Donna M **(SLP)**
Reeder, Ruth M **(A)**
Robertson, Kiz W
Roth, Judith A **(SLP)**
Rowan, Dr Lynne E **(SLP)**
Russell, Ann Faith **(A)**
Salinger, Roberta Lynn
Schmidt, Mrs Ellen D **(SLP)**
Schober-Peterson, Debra Lynn **(SLP)**
Seitzinger, Joanne R **(SLP)**
Siegle, Diane H **(SLP)**
Simpson, Robert Kennedy **(SLP)**
Weaver, Mrs Jennifer Ann **(A)**
Yairi, Dr Ehud **(SLP)**
Zemlin, Eileen **(SLP)**
Zemlin, Willard R

Charleston
Augustine, Dr Robert M **(SLP)**
Bumpus, Mrs Mary C **(SLP)**
Castle, Mrs Janell Dawn **(SLP)**
Chambers, Mrs Toni Furman **(SLP)**
Claeys, Polly E F **(SLP)**
Compton, Kathy S
Dell, Dr Carl W, Jr **(SLP)**
Dodson, Betty L **(SLP)**
Eason-Sons, Virginia Alberta **(SLP)**
Forrest, Jean Marie
Goble, Mrs Linda P **(SLP)**
Hall, Janet E **(SLP)**

Harper, Shelley D
Hay, Mrs Susan D **(SLP)**
Hollowell, Mrs Margaret **(SLP)**
Jacques, Dr Richard D **(SLP)**
King, Mrs Dona D **(SLP)**
Lovall, Susan Marie **(SLP)**
McKee, Mrs Gail **(SLP)**
Nilsen, Dr Jill F **(SLP)**
Paul, Mrs Pamela Dudley **(SLP)**
Richard, Dr Gail J **(SLP)**
Slattery, Margaret I
Snider, Eunice A **(SLP)**
Switzer, Mrs Kathryn Beck **(SLP)**
Weiler, Dr Nancy A **(SLP A)**

Chatham

Christ, Mrs Paula J **(SLP)**
Raycraft, Mrs Laura Beth **(SLP)**

Chester

Granger, Mardell Moeller

Chicago

Abrams, Mrs Wendy Chukerman **(SLP)**
Ackerman, Martha G **(SLP)**
Adamczak, Jeffrey E **(SLP)**
Alicea, Eileen E **(SLP)**
Allen, Kelly A **(SLP)**
Alpern, Jane A
Anderson, Dr Bernadette **(SLP)**
Anderson, Mrs Kathleen M **(SLP)**
Andrew, Lisa M **(SLP)**
Ankenbruck, Paula Jean **(SLP)**
Apel, Mrs Carolann D **(SLP)**
Armstrong, Catherine Ann **(SLP)**
Aron, Mrs Elizabeth Foreman **(SLP)**
Aufricht, Dr Hedda **(SLP A)**
Austin, Mrs Carolyn S **(SLP)**
Axelrod, Jennifer K **(SLP)**
Badofsky, Mrs Ellen Potischman **(SLP)**
Bady, Harold L **(SLP)**
Bailey, Dr Donn Fritz **(SLP)**
Baker, Mrs Ida Carter **(SLP)**
Barnes, Gwendolyn **(SLP)**
Baughman, Amy **(SLP)**
Baumgartner, Dr John M **(SLP)**
Bayley, Mrs Bonnie Z **(SLP)**
Baynard, Catherine Elizabeth
Beastrom, Susan Lynn **(SLP)**
Becker, Dr Nancy G **(SLP)**
Berger, Mrs Mary I **(SLP)**
Bernard, Kathryn Ann **(SLP)**
Berry, Debra Marie **(SLP)**
Berry, Mrs Kathleen M **(SLP)**
Beukema, Hermine **(SLP)**
Billington, Carla Jill **(SLP)**
Blanc, Julie Kay
Blayer, Nancy O **(SLP)**
Block, Evelyn S W **(SLP)**
Block, Mrs Frances K **(SLP)**
Bobrick, Mrs Jane A **(SLP)**
Bodolay, Deborah L **(SLP)**
Bondi, Terry M **(SLP)**
Bondy, Pamela S **(SLP)**
Bookshester, Dr Joyce C **(SLP)**
Bracey, Ann M **(SLP)**
Bradley, Kathy Cobbs **(A)**
Brady, Arnell A **(SLP)**
Brennan, Henry Patrick **(SLP)**
Brennan, Judy Ann **(SLP)**
Bresnock, Sr Catherine L **(SLP)**
Britt, Debbie Lynne **(SLP)**
Brodsky, Barbara
Brookner-Stein, Mrs Sheryl P **(SLP)**
Brown, B Evelyn **(A)**
Brown, Lisa C **(SLP)**
Brownlee, Lavinia Joyce **(SLP)**
Brownstein, R Dede **(A)**
Budney, Mrs Elizabeth Allison **(A)**
Budney, Seth Martin **(A)**
Burke-Peterson, Mary D **(A)**
Butcher, Dr Jaynee A **(A)**
Bycraft, Mrs Helen B **(SLP)**
Calabrese, Barbara J **(SLP)**
Canetta, Dr Robert **(SLP)**
Carroll, Denise Ann **(SLP)**
Chan, Susie **(SLP)**
Chisholm, Mary C **(A)**
Chrystal, Jean L
Chwierut, Barbara J **(SLP)**
Cilella-Meyer, Mrs Janet Mary **(SLP)**
Clarke, Mary A **(SLP)**
Clausen, Carol L **(SLP)**
Clements, Denise A **(SLP)**
Coghlan, Mrs Patricia M **(SLP)**
Colby, Janet Catherine **(A)**
Cole, Pamela Sue **(SLP)**
Conaway, Patrick Kelly **(A)**
Connelly, Gail J **(SLP)**
Conway, Peggy Ann **(SLP)**
Crane, Mary F **(SLP)**
Crotty, Dr Carol M **(SLP)**
Curley, Margaret M **(SLP)**
Czyzewski, Mrs Helen J **(SLP)**
Dalton, Mrs Donna Anne **(SLP)**
Dargan, Margaret A **(SLP)**
Dean-Myrda, Mrs Nancy E **(SLP)**
De Cesari, Rico **(SLP)**
Defoor-Hill, Lori A **(SLP)**
Dennis, Dr Kyle C **(A)**
Devine, Mary Ellen **(SLP)**
Dispensa, Mrs Kristine Mary **(SLP)**
Donahue, Dr Mavis L
Donner, Mrs Jean K **(SLP)**
Dorf, Debra S **(SLP)**
Downs, Mary Patricia **(SLP)**
Driscoll, Mark Stephen
Dritsas, Jane H **(A)**
Drower, Mrs Laura Anne **(SLP)**
Drudge, William Ralph **(SLP)**
Dubin, Erin Hope **(A)**
Dugan, Constance **(SLP)**
Duval, Chris L **(SLP)**
Dykema, Clarice B **(A)**
Eannace, Mrs Mary E **(SLP)**
Edelstein, Karen Feldman **(SLP)**
Einhorn, Rebecca Elizabeth
Elenbogen, Janet C **(SLP)**
Exelrod, Iris C **(SLP)**
Fabiszak, Dr Angie Jo **(SLP)**
Falkenberg, Inge **(SLP)**
Federhar, Lisa Joy **(SLP)**
Fedyniak, Lillian H **(SLP)**
Fisher, Ronna Labovitz **(A)**
Fitch, Mrs Adina Jarvinen **(SLP)**
Flaherty, Kathleen Anne **(A)**
Flarity, Jane A **(SLP)**
Fleming, Joanne **(SLP)**
Frade, Marilyn Frances **(SLP)**
Frazier, Mrs Herease **(SLP)**
Frenkiel, Leah **(SLP)**
Freund, Nancy Jo **(SLP)**
Friedlander, Renee S **(SLP)**
Friel, Eileen Marie
Gallagher, Helen F **(SLP)**
Garber, Mrs Debra Bell **(A)**
Gartenberg, Terri E **(SLP)**
Gary, Mrs Leiana Jae **(SLP)**
Gebelein, Mary Lynn **(A)**
Gentner, Debarra S **(SLP A)**
Geschwint, Jill Elizabeth **(SLP)**
Glass, Dr Rita M **(SLP)**
Glick, Mrs Susan S **(SLP)**
Goffman, Lisa Alice **(SLP)**
Goldwater, Mrs Joan Mullan **(SLP)**
Graber, Sarah Rachelle **(SLP)**
Gradassi, Renee A **(SLP)**
Gruger, Melissa M **(SLP)**
Gucwa, Judith Anne **(SLP)**
Gutstein, Mrs Carol F
Haber, Dr Lyn Roland **(SLP)**
Hadley, Debra L **(SLP)**
Hahn, Susan E **(SLP)**
Hairston, Kathryn **(SLP)**
Hall, James E **(SLP)**
Halper, Mrs Anita S **(SLP)**
Halvorson, Lori Ann **(A)**
Hamada, Cheryl L **(SLP)**
Hamel, Catherine Ross **(SLP)**
Hamilton, Kimberley Clarice **(SLP)**
Hammel, Diane Roberts **(A)**
Hanses, Sr Carmelia **(SLP)**
Harano, JoAnn N **(A)**
Harding, Janis Louise **(SLP)**
Harris, Jody Lee **(SLP)**
Harris-Schmidt, Dr Gail P **(SLP)**
Hartzog, Melody Althea **(SLP)**
Haydek, Cheryl Jean
Hayes, Mrs Cheryl Fouts **(SLP)**
Hecht, Mrs Mindy S **(SLP)**
Hedberg, Karen **(A)**
Hedman, Linda J **(A)**
Heinz, Carolyn Lake **(SLP)**
Hellen, Julia Kirwan **(SLP)**
Hill, Kathy D **(SLP)**
Hinson, Carl L **(SLP)**
Hoban, Mary Angela **(SLP)**
Hodge, Crystal Camille **(A)**
Holt, Mrs Virginia R **(A)**
Hopwood, Debbie Leigh **(SLP)**
Horsfall, Ruth M **(SLP)**
Hubner, Mary Ellen **(SLP)**
Huey-You, Dr Patricia **(SLP)**
Jacobs, Merle **(SLP)**
Jeglum, Mrs Marilynn J **(SLP)**
Jensen, Dr Thomas Wendell **(SLP)**
Jesse, Barbara Lynne **(A)**
Johnson, Sheryl R **(SLP)**
Judlo, Jodi **(SLP)**
Kasa, Felicia Marie **(SLP)**
Kastel, Joan H **(SLP)**
Kathrein, Paula C **(SLP)**
Katz, Nancy Suslick **(A)**
Kaufman, Mary E **(SLP)**
Kawell-Meskan, Mary E **(A)**
Kelleher, Mrs Tamara Jo **(SLP)**
Kelton, Debra D **(SLP)**
Kendall, Geralyn M
Kennedy, Margaret M **(SLP)**
King, Glynis Dawn **(SLP)**
Kirschner, Doris Ann **(SLP)**
Klafter, Carmem E **(SLP)**
Klaver, Mary Melissa **(A)**
Kobritz, Lauren Susan **(SLP)**
Kominsky, Mrs Perrie M **(SLP)**
Koonmen, Karin Elizabeth **(SLP)**
Kraus, Dr Nina J **(SLP)**
Krause, Dr SueEllen **(SLP)**
Krauss, Mrs Zehava **(SLP)**
Kukler, Linda B **(SLP)**
Laderta, Paul P **(SLP)**
Lapidus, Ghita A **(SLP)**
Larson, Nancy M
Lazarus, Cathy L **(SLP)**
Lazowski, Laura Elizabeth **(A)**
Leaks, Denise **(SLP)**
Le Duc, Judith A **(SLP)**
Lee, Corinne C **(SLP)**
Leonard, Mrs Kathleen M **(SLP)**
Levin, Betsy **(SLP)**
Levy, Laura Robin **(SLP)**
Lichtenberg, Dr Eva F
Lieberman, Gayle **(SLP)**
Lindaman, Sandra L **(SLP)**
Linkenheld, Debbie A **(SLP)**
Loggie, Bonnie Lee **(SLP)**
Long, Kathleen E **(SLP)**
Longinotti, Cheryl S **(A)**
Lucker, Nancy J **(SLP)**
Ludden, Sr Mary A **(SLP)**
Maddock, Mrs Janet Lyle **(SLP)**
Maddox, Carol M **(SLP)**
Mandell, Elizabeth Ann **(A)**
Marshall, Dr Rita K **(SLP)**
Mayberry, Dr Rachel I **(SLP)**
Mayfield, Dr Sandra A **(SLP)**
Mayster, Lynda W **(SLP)**
McCraven, Patricia Leslie **(SLP)**
McCurry, Jeanne K **(SLP)**
McEneaney, Joseph Peter **(SLP)**
McLaughlin-Wheat, Mrs Darlene L **(SLP)**
Mecklenburger, Jill E **(A)**
Melnick, Carol R **(SLP)**
Menard, Mrs Donna M **(SLP)**
Merrick, Kathleen **(SLP)**
Meyers, Francine G **(SLP)**
Miller, Barbara B **(SLP)**
Miller, Carole S **(SLP)**
Miller, Trudy K **(SLP)**
Moch, Mrs Corinne Sylvia
Mogil, Shelley I **(SLP)**
Monaco, H Cynthia **(A)**
Monhart, Charlotte Knaus **(SLP)**
Moore, Denis G **(A)**
Moore, Mrs Janet **(SLP)**
Moore, Mrs Terri **(A)**
Moseley, Juanita **(SLP)**
Murley, Judith Lynn **(SLP)**
Murphy, Catherine **(SLP)**
Murphy, Kathy S **(A)**
Murray, Allison Slaughter **(SLP)**
Nathanson, Dr Susan N **(SLP)**
Nelson, Susan H **(SLP)**
Neyhus, Dr Arthur I **(A)**
Niblack, Mrs Yolonda C
Nisivaco, Mrs Julie Caulfield **(SLP)**
Noell, Elizabeth **(SLP)**
Nofal, Mrs Charlotte **(SLP)**
Nolan, Judith Anne **(SLP)**
Nordstrom, Vereen Ann **(SLP)**
Norris, Paulette B **(SLP)**
Oakley, Judith L **(SLP)**
O'Brien, Mrs Ellen M **(SLP)**
O'Connor, Kathleen **(SLP)**
O'Donnell, Sheila **(SLP)**
Okonek, Ann Martha **(SLP)**
O'Leary, Mary Bridget **(SLP)**
Olofsson, Mrs Sheila Michaels **(A)**
Olson, Dr Don A **(SLP)**
O'Neill, Peter **(SLP)**
Ongley, Leena Marianna **(SLP A)**
Ostreicher, Harvey J **(SLP)**
Oswald, Sharon H
Otto, Karen D **(SLP)**
Padish, Gail R **(A)**
Pahle, William F **(SLP A)**
Pane, Kimberly M
Papillon, Nadjia Marie **(SLP)**
Pasko, Dr Stanley J **(SLP)**
Paustian, Glenn R **(SLP)**
Pearson, Mrs Karen **(A)**
Perkins, Dorothy Rose **(SLP)**
Perschon, Nancy **(SLP)**
Petras, Dru Anne **(A)**
Petru, Mrs Janis Ann M **(SLP)**
Phillips, Nevis C **(SLP)**
Pichler, Cindy Beth **(A)**
Pierce, Mrs Jill Walker **(SLP)**
Pimental, Dr Patricia Ann **(SLP)**
Pitcher, Cindy L **(SLP)**
Platt, Mrs Judy Lynn **(SLP)**
Plotkin, Dr William H **(SLP)**
Popowych, Daria Teresa **(A)**
Pott, Mrs Evanne M
Prince, Annette J **(SLP)**
Quinn, Barbara K **(SLP)**
Redmond, Kathleen J **(SLP)**
Reimer, Faith Forman **(SLP)**
Reppa, Cathleen Joan **(SLP)**
Reticker, Mrs Aleyda De Jesus **(SLP)**
Ricci, Carol Lisa **(A)**
Richter, Mrs Theresa Webber **(SLP)**
Rieger, Mrs Pearl H
Roche, Maryjo **(SLP)**
Roggatz, Karyn Joan **(A)**
Roll, Julia B **(SLP)**
Rollins, Laurel D **(SLP)**
Roninson, Olga Z **(SLP)**
Rooney, Lisa E **(SLP)**
Ross, Ilene Simon **(SLP)**

Roth, Mrs Judith S **(SLP A)**
Rouser, Mrs Holly Elaine **(SLP)**
Rusnak, Julianna **(SLP)**
Sadler, Mrs Dorothy O **(SLP)**
Saiki, Kenneth J
Sallas, Victoria Ann **(SLP)**
Sanchez, Mrs Linda **(SLP)**
Sandler, Mrs Marilyn **(SLP)**
Santucci, Michael Joseph **(A)**
Sasso, Anne Vickery **(SLP)**
Sayers, Patricia J **(SLP)**
Schuler, Janice M **(SLP)**
Schur, Mrs Lenora Singer **(SLP)**
Schust, Judith Ann **(SLP)**
Seiler, Elizabeth **(SLP)**
Selin, Mrs Ann Bulmash **(SLP)**
Sennett, William Fitzgerald
Sexton, Sandra Sue **(SLP)**
Shaffer, Dr Deborah J **(SLP)**
Shepherd, Suzanne C **(SLP)**
Shervanian, Chris C **(SLP)**
Shields-Cole, Mrs Sara L **(SLP)**
Shindler, Andrea Gellin **(SLP)**
Sieczko, Christine Krys **(SLP)**
Siegel, Ilene S **(SLP)**
Silver, Roberta **(SLP)**
Simon, Mrs Marguerite Feeley **(SLP)**
Smith, Mrs Esther Goldwasser **(SLP)**
Snyder, Kathleen Jean **(SLP)**
Spier, Susan Ann **(A)**
Spitz, Robin Leah **(SLP)**
Splawski-Roach, Jill L **(SLP)**
Stein, Dr Laszlo K **(A)**
Steingold, Gail H **(SLP)**
Steinhoff, Rin C **(A)**
Stenberg, Margaret L **(SLP)**
Stevens, Kathleen A **(SLP)**
Stillerman, Wendy **(SLP)**
Stone, Paula **(SLP)**
Stull, Mrs Sheila Ann
Sullivan, Dorothy S **(SLP)**
Summers, Sharon H **(SLP)**
Surace, Patricia **(SLP)**
Susser, Robin D **(SLP)**
Swapsy, Anita L **(SLP)**
Sweeney, Maureen Ann **(SLP)**
Taglia, Camille R **(SLP)**
Talley, Susan Harris **(SLP)**
Tanaka-Cameron, Audrey Takaoka
Taussig-Leibow, Mrs Lisa **(A)**
Taylor, Belinda Michelle **(SLP)**
Taylor, Mrs Honora Agnus
Tchaconas, Maria **(SLP)**
Temple, Keryn Judith **(SLP)**
Thiel, Jeanne M **(SLP)**
Toyama, Susan G **(SLP)**
Tracy, Mrs Julie F **(SLP)**
Tucker, Deborah Ann **(SLP)**
Tucker, Mrs Nancy J C **(SLP)**
Tuite-Taffe, Anne Marie **(SLP)**
Tyree, Jean M **(SLP)**
Ujiki, Nenon L M **(SLP)**
Vandervoort, Mrs Nicole Leman **(SLP)**
Veis, Sharon L **(SLP)**
Vessna Drosdick, Danielle **(SLP)**
Voda, Jerrilyn A **(SLP)**
Wagner, Dawn M
Wagner, Joanne L **(SLP)**
Walbridge, Elizabeth Koestner **(SLP)**
Walko, Amy Clark **(SLP)**
Warshawsky, Linda M **(SLP)**
Washburn, Amy D **(A)**
Wasserman, Helene Debra **(SLP)**
Watson, Linda D **(SLP)**
Watson, Vivian L **(SLP)**
Weil, Elizabeth R **(SLP)**
Welch, Deborah Greengold **(SLP)**
Welsh, Cathy Ann **(SLP)**
Weston, Maria V **(SLP)**
Whearty, Kathryn Annelle **(A)**
Wika, Carol L **(SLP)**
Williams, Debra Bailey **(SLP)**
Wolters, Mrs Cheryl Cartee **(A)**
Wong, Mrs Gloria Jackel **(A)**
Yakaitis, Sr Kathleen J **(SLP)**
Yost, Dr William A
Yurchick, Rosann M **(SLP)**
Zeitlin, Rosalyn R
Zelasko, Mrs Mary C **(SLP)**
Zoochi, Lawrence Michael **(A)**
Zwolan, Teresa A **(A)**

Chicago Heights

Maydew, Linda S **(A)**
Mina, Mrs Sheila D **(SLP)**
Morrin, Mrs Catherine Anne **(A)**
Murzyn, Mrs Barbara Klabunde **(SLP)**
Reif, Mrs Tamara Kay **(SLP)**
Urbanek, Mrs Elaine Diak **(SLP)**

Chicago Ridge

Hall-Ferchau, Theresa Margaret **(A)**
MacGregor, Mrs Charlene J **(SLP)**

Chillicothe

Dell, Mrs Lynn Ann **(SLP)**

Cicero

Wojcik, Steven A **(SLP)**

Cisne

Ray, Nancy J **(SLP)**

Clarendon Hills

Gardina-Wolfe, Anna M **(SLP)**
Hurley-Bularzik, Debra C **(SLP)**
Kingman, Mrs Janice L **(SLP)**
Moneka, Mrs Wynnette J **(A)**
Morlock, Julianne M **(SLP)**
O'Neal, Carol M **(SLP)**
Sullivan, Karen L **(SLP)**
Tatar, Gloria V **(SLP)**
Thorgesen, Constance L **(A)**

Clinton

O'Connor, Carol J **(SLP)**
Valbracht, Janice R **(SLP)**

Cobden

Saken, Toby J **(SLP)**

Collinsville

Holtzscher, George S **(A)**
Holtzscher, Judith M **(SLP)**
Justice, Mrs Frances L **(SLP)**
Moore, Melissa M **(A)**
Niman, Mrs Barbara A
Sanders, Mrs Lisa Carolyn **(SLP A)**
St Onge, Keith R **(SLP)**
Watt, Susan J **(SLP)**

Columbia

Fox, Lisa Latinette **(SLP)**
Stork, Mrs Kristine A **(SLP)**
Ziegler, Mrs Marilyn N **(SLP)**

Cortland

Tenney, Scott Charles

Country Club Hills

Bell, Delores C **(SLP)**
Chertok, Susan Gail **(SLP)**
Christ, Marlene N **(SLP)**
Foster, Sharon **(SLP)**
Williams, Michael K **(SLP)**

Creal Springs

Heidelbach, Cora **(SLP)**

Crestwood

Emery, Virginia Joanne **(SLP)**
Paolini, Barbara A **(SLP)**
Skarzynski, Mrs Shelly Elving **(SLP)**
Tuohy, John L **(SLP)**

Crete

Krizic, Lynn Soprych **(SLP)**
Schaller, Sheran M **(SLP)**

Crystal Lake

Beebe, Karen M **(SLP)**
Depalma, Mrs Janet **(A)**
Few, Linda J **(SLP A)**
Hoefer, Carol S **(SLP)**
Jakubec, Mrs Christine Smith **(A)**
Kehoe, Katherine M **(SLP)**
Kenney, Mary Kathryn **(SLP)**
McCullagh, Mrs Bette C **(SLP)**
Mitchell, Lora Porter **(SLP)**
Nanna, Mrs Patricia McGuire
Perz, Catherine **(SLP)**
Root, Mrs Linnea S **(SLP)**
Van Ham, Mrs Diane **(SLP)**
Watson, Mrs Caroline **(SLP)**

Cuba

Falk, Mrs Terese L **(SLP)**

Dahinda

Saline, Jocelyn Barnstead **(A)**

Danvers

Birky, Nanette Rummel **(SLP)**

Danville

Apodaca, Mrs Jane F **(SLP)**
Beck, Dr Ann R **(SLP)**
Brandy, Dr William T **(A)**
Edmonds, Mrs Kaye Louise **(SLP)**
Frankino, Ellen Connelly **(SLP)**
Frazier, Barbara **(SLP)**
Kelley, Mrs Leanne Brittany **(A)**
Killough, Mrs Candace L **(SLP)**
Leath, Laurie Jones **(A)**
Russell, Jan Elaine **(SLP)**
Toole, Dolores M **(A)**
Williams, Mrs Roberta N **(A)**

Darien

Barry, Mrs Mary Chiodo **(SLP)**
Behnke, Charles R **(A)**
Belcastro, Mary Elizabeth **(SLP)**
Heery, Mrs Anna R **(SLP)**
Kupensky, Sandra S **(SLP)**
Many, Mrs Marina Teglia **(SLP)**
Mueller, Jill Elizabeth **(SLP)**
Weberling, Janet L **(SLP)**

Davis

Spielman, Beth Ann

De Kalb

Andrews, Dr James R **(SLP)**
Bishop, Mrs Lilli Ann **(SLP)**
Blickhan, Janice P **(SLP)**
Brennan, Mary K **(SLP)**
Delorier, Joseph R **(A)**
Fisher, Dr Cletus G (Raydon) **(SLP A)**
Husa, Florence A **(SLP)**
Jackson, Melissa Foens **(SLP)**
Jackson, Dr Pamela L **(A)**
Kapper, Mrs Carol Sisler **(SLP)**
Kresheck, Dr Janet **(SLP)**
Lankford, James E **(A)**
Meyer, Robert G **(SLP)**
Sandridge, Dr Sharon A **(A)**
Seaver, Earl J **(SLP)**
Shearer, Dr William M **(SLP A)**
Slana, Audrey Ann
Slivinski, Ann L
Stephens, Dr Mary Irene **(SLP)**
Wadle, Mrs Sharon Lee **(SLP)**
Waters, Betty Jean **(SLP A)**
Williams, Mrs Dorothy J **(SLP)**
Williams, Dr J David **(SLP)**

De Soto

Keys, Wade Tyrone **(SLP)**

Decatur

Ankrom, Judith M **(SLP)**
Curlin, Elizabeth Kramer **(SLP)**
Ferracane, Mrs Barbara J **(SLP)**
Hills, Mrs Andrea Mary **(SLP)**
Honings, Mrs Barbara Entrican **(SLP)**
Klemens, James A **(A)**
Klemens, Mrs Miriam P **(SLP)**
Leiser, Mrs Ann Gail **(SLP)**
McVey, Richard K **(A)**
Pine, Rhoda Zucker **(SLP)**
Prince, Mrs Karen Janes **(SLP)**
Sly, Joanne Ruth **(SLP)**
Watson, Mrs Patricia O **(SLP)**
Williams, Kathleen

Deerfield

Edgeworth, Mrs Ann Blazek **(SLP)**
Hill, Cynthia L **(SLP)**
Horn, Mrs Deborah G **(SLP)**
Kanter, Mrs Ann B **(SLP)**
Lane, Mara H **(SLP)**
Loring, Mrs Arlene G **(SLP)**
Mangurten, Mrs Brucene B **(SLP)**
Pessis, Michelle G **(SLP)**
Pessis, Paul **(A)**
Roemer, Mrs Janet DeGrazia **(SLP)**
Romano, Mrs Lois J **(SLP)**
Schwanke, Mrs Janet L H **(SLP)**
Schwartz, Mrs Illeane Epstein **(SLP)**
Selgrad, Mrs Carol Cinnick **(SLP)**
Smolin, Louanne I **(SLP)**
Tegtmeier, Mrs Mary E **(SLP)**
Topel, Ellyn

Des Plaines

Baumbich, Brenda **(SLP)**
Briskey, Robert J **(SLP A)**
Burroughs, Mrs Peggy Ann **(SLP)**
Campbell, Catherine Edwards **(SLP)**
Conrick-Gaborek, Maryann **(A)**
Elkayam, Judith M **(A)**
Guenette-Wagner, Barbara **(A)**
Halpern, Barbara E **(SLP)**
Hart, Kathleen **(SLP)**
Kaetzel, Esther B **(SLP)**
Klor, Dr Barry **(SLP)**
Klor, Laura A **(SLP)**
Koszczuk, Georgette **(A)**
McAuliffe, Christine Matrice **(SLP)**
Mishler, Mrs Shelley Steel **(A)**
Rea, Sharon Patricia **(SLP)**
Rosedale, Mrs Judith B **(SLP)**
Shifrin, Susan **(SLP)**
Smith, Mary Beth **(SLP)**
Vujanovic-Browne, Mrs Bosiljka Bessie **(SLP)**

Dixon

Barber, James L **(SLP)**
Barber, Mrs Prudence S **(SLP A)**
Hiatt, Joann Marie **(A)**
Huffman, Mrs Jeanine Marie **(A)**
Kavanaugh, Mrs Kirsten P **(SLP)**
Lenkey, Laura E **(SLP)**
Mayer, Katherine K **(SLP)**
McBride, Glen Dale, Jr **(SLP)**
Metzger, Rolland
Pratt, Roger Sayers **(SLP)**
Stewart, Cheri L **(SLP)**

Dolton

Jackson, Lisa Gibson **(SLP)**
Mayerak, Dawn A **(SLP)**

Dongola

Miltenberger, Damaris S **(SLP)**
Miltenberger, Gerald E **(SLP A)**

Downers Grove

Batalia, Eugenia Rabias **(SLP)**
Bischof, Mrs Katharyn Worthingto **(SLP)**
Burnside, Patricia S **(SLP)**
Desai, Mrs Nivedita N **(SLP)**
Diestler, Mrs Kathryn E **(A)**
Dykas-Fierke, Cheryl M **(SLP)**
Gaul, Mrs Roxane Rosy **(SLP)**
Geen, Judy M **(SLP)**
Gleeson, Nancy J **(SLP)**
Holmes, Mrs Dorothy V **(SLP)**
Hoskins, Glee C **(SLP)**
Korsgard, Mrs Susan Victoria **(A)**
Kotula, Mrs Heather Bloecher **(SLP)**
Larson, Mrs Micki McGuire **(SLP)**

Meck-Eisenberg, Diane Marie **(SLP)**
Nojiri, Mrs Georgianne Hirota **(SLP)**
O'Reilly, Mrs Victoria Guerrieri **(A)**
Ori, Mrs Katherine P **(SLP)**
Podbelski, Mrs Susan Novak **(SLP)**
Schuler-Volger, Maria **(A)**
Shawron, Mrs Virginia Miller **(SLP)**
Simon, Bonita **(A)**
Stukas, Natalie Latoza **(A)**
Suesse, Karen S **(SLP)**
Tannenbaum, Michelle S **(SLP)**
Thurston, Mrs Susan Kay
York, Mrs Jane Marie **(SLP)**

Du Quoin
Olson, Mrs Donna K **(SLP)**
Rhoades, Mrs Jeanne C **(SLP)**

Dundee
Osth, Jodi A **(SLP)**
Smith, Deborah Lynn **(A)**

Dunlap
McCullough, Patricia J **(SLP)**
Phelps, Mrs Mary Anderson **(SLP)**
Reiser, Lawrence A **(A)**
Reiser, Mrs Trude M **(A)**

Durand
Broughton, Mrs Ann L **(A)**

Dwight
Neville, Mrs Lynn Bertino **(SLP)**

East Alton
Birmingham, Mrs Shirley **(SLP)**
Engelman, Mrs Dixie A **(SLP)**
Herndon, Mrs Claudia K **(SLP)**
Hotson, Peggy Flach **(SLP)**
Taylor, Dr Joyce S **(SLP)**

East Moline
Lytton, Beverly J **(SLP)**

East Peoria
Randle, Mrs Mary Ann **(SLP)**
Sedgwick, Linda S **(A)**

Edwardsville
Anderson, Mrs Dona C **(SLP)**
Becher, Mrs Nancy A **(SLP)**
Blair, Mrs Sara Beth **(SLP)**
Bullard, Mrs Irene W **(SLP)**
Clarkston, Mrs Jane Marshall **(SLP)**
Criswell-Baird, Mrs Barbara A **(SLP)**
Diak, Mrs Kathryn R **(SLP)**
Gardner, Mrs Paula J **(A)**
Harrison, Jean M **(SLP)**
Hoge, Dr Debra Reichert **(SLP)**
Joshu, Dan R **(A)**
Kostyshock, Linda Marie **(SLP)**
Lieblich, Dr Malcolm **(SLP)**
Luber, Lucille M **(SLP)**
Maag, O Eugene **(SLP A)**
Mozley, Audrey Marie **(SLP)**
Pinkley, Mrs Frances Clare **(SLP)**
Ray, Cathy Coldren **(SLP)**
Stack, Janet R **(SLP)**
Staten, Mrs Kathleen Ann **(SLP)**
Tracy, Patricia J **(SLP)**
White, Mrs Susan M L **(SLP)**
Wilke, Rosalie A **(SLP)**
Zimmerman, Rita H **(SLP)**

Effingham
Badders, Mrs Debra M **(SLP)**
Coen, Mrs Laura E **(SLP)**
Hartke, Mrs Susan K **(SLP)**
Potts, Mrs Ellen P H **(SLP)**
Trammel, Rebecca J **(SLP)**
Wasson, Mrs Charlotte **(SLP)**
Willenborg, Mrs Kimberly M **(SLP)**

Elburn
Fleming, Jami Ann **(SLP)**
Hucker, Mrs Patricia **(SLP)**
Lock, Robin B **(SLP)**

Eldorado
Bentley, Mrs Rebecca D **(SLP)**

Elgin
Bartz, Mrs Lynn O'Brien **(SLP)**
Becker, Mrs Myra M **(SLP)**
Clausen, Helen Kay **(SLP)**
Dunlop, Diane L **(SLP)**
Fiedler, Mrs Mary Byrne
Friebus, Mrs Cheryl A **(SLP)**
Hendricksen, Sandra Lee **(SLP)**
Hoeft, Mrs Elizabeth **(SLP)**
Kline, Margaret S **(SLP)**
Martini, Mrs Valerie Fitch **(A)**
Niggemann, Debra J
Olson, Carol Jean **(SLP)**
Olson, Saundra L **(SLP)**
Resener, Mrs Ann M **(SLP)**
Richards, Mrs Nancy C **(SLP)**
Rider, Mrs Molly Carlson **(SLP)**
Scrimshire, Linda B **(SLP)**
Steenhausen, Joan M **(SLP)**
Stewart, Joanne S **(SLP)**
Torry, Mrs Jane **(SLP)**
Vollertsen, Cathleen M **(SLP)**
Woolcott, Mrs Sandra Butz **(SLP)**
Ziegler, Mally Heaton **(SLP)**

Elk Grove
Anderson, Roger P **(SLP)**
Herman, Mrs Maria Luciani **(SLP)**

Elk Grove Village
Andriopoulos, Cheryl Lynn **(SLP)**
Braun, Lori A
Calderone, Susan C **(SLP)**
Jacobson, Tracy L
Killion, Mead C

Elmhurst
Baumgartner, Linda Strear **(SLP)**
Clark, Lamont L **(SLP)**
Fazzio, Mrs Elizabeth Merkel **(SLP)**
Frantz, Marilyn Kay
Gaetto, Anita M **(SLP)**
Gills, Ann C **(SLP)**
Goodban, Dr Marjorie T **(SLP)**
Goodman, Mrs Mary Rice **(SLP)**
Grobe, Loanne R **(SLP)**
Gruhlke, Mrs Susan Pruitt **(SLP)**
Heavey, Ann E **(SLP)**
Jerger, Margaret A **(SLP)**
Johnson, Mrs Debra Sue **(A)**
Koch, Catherine Marie **(SLP)**
Lepold, Mrs Lori Richter **(SLP)**
Massa, Mrs Georgiann K **(SLP)**
McGonigle, Mrs Patricia **(SLP)**
Methling, Mrs Catherine Camasto **(SLP)**
Milianti, Dr Franklin J **(SLP)**
Modlin, Diane M **(SLP)**
Reidy, Jeanne S **(SLP)**
Smith, Mrs Nancy B **(SLP)**
Tarman, Mrs Mary T **(SLP)**
Topper, Diane Marie **(SLP)**

Elmwood
McFall, Bonnie U **(SLP)**

Elmwood Park
De Julius, Bernadette Picardi **(SLP)**
Grubb, Mrs Lynn Marie **(SLP)**
Lovis, Mrs Emmy A **(SLP)**

Eureka
Moestue, Mrs Mary Jean **(SLP)**

Evanston
Albrecht, Judy R **(SLP)**
Anderson, Ellen L **(SLP)**
Aylesworth, Mrs Margaret R **(SLP)**
Blanning, Linda C **(SLP)**
Bolger, Beth-Lynn **(SLP)**
Brown, Gail F **(A)**
Brown, Mrs Kimberly Demary **(A)**
Burkland, Mrs Marjorie B **(SLP)**
Burns, Dr Martha S **(SLP)**
Canter, Dr Gerald J **(SLP A)**
Canter, Mrs Susan M **(SLP)**
Carmichael, Mrs Wendy A **(SLP)**
Cawley, Anna P **(SLP)**
Cheng, Joan Elizabeth **(SLP)**
Cohan, Joan Strandberg **(SLP)**
Dallos, Peter
Dancull, Denise Marie **(SLP)**
Drapekin, Mrs Susan Gail **(SLP)**
Duval, Nicole L **(SLP)**
Eggert, Gertrude H **(SLP)**
Elliott, Dr Charles R **(SLP)**
Elliott, Dr Lois Lawrence
Fiebig, Pamela J **(A)**
Fisher, Dr Hilda B **(SLP)**
Friend, Tressa J **(SLP)**
Garstecki, Dr Dean C **(SLP A)**
Goodman, Mrs Jane Y **(SLP)**
Gregory, Carolyn B **(SLP)**
Gregory, Dr Hugo H **(SLP)**
Hedlund, Larrain Ann
Hill, Mrs Diane G **(SLP)**
Hochberg, Dr Judith Golden
Hux, Karen Ann **(SLP)**
Jewett, Janet M **(SLP)**
Johnson, Doris Joan **(SLP)**
Katz, Susan J **(SLP)**
Kearns, Geralyn Harvey **(SLP)**
Keeley, Mrs Susanne Phillips **(SLP)**
Kobara-Mates, Mrs Mindy S **(SLP)**
Kobrin, Meryl
Kuhnsman, Liane M **(SLP)**
Lapping, Leslye **(SLP)**
Lehner, Leslie H **(SLP)**
Maas, Anne D **(SLP)**
Messerschmidt, Anita Borsdorf **(SLP)**
Meyer, Dr Toby **(SLP)**
Middleton, Mrs Susan H **(SLP)**
Molstad, Mary Anne **(SLP)**
Neils, Mrs Lynn Reimers **(SLP)**
Newby, Mrs Bonita Perkins **(SLP)**
Opie, Jane Maria **(A)**
Palmer, Catherine Vea **(A)**
Peters, Maryrita D **(SLP)**
Power, Mary S **(SLP)**
Reynolds, Ellen B
Rezabek, Mrs Barbara Campbell **(A)**
Ross, Deborah **(SLP)**
Rubinowitz, Linda **(SLP A)**
Russ, Mrs Diane Mendelsohn **(A)**
Rutherford, David R **(SLP)**
Sapir, Dr Shimon **(SLP)**
Sargent, Laura Elizabeth **(SLP)**
Savage, Mary Jo **(SLP)**
Seifer, Patricia J **(SLP)**
Shaffer, Mrs Paula P **(SLP)**
Shapiro, Mrs Marian C **(SLP)**
Shayne, Ava B **(SLP)**
Shields, Mrs Dianne T **(SLP)**
Sletteland, Hildegarde **(SLP)**
Smider, Wilma J E **(SLP)**
Smith, Dr Bruce L
Smith, Nancy L **(SLP)**
Smith, Dr Stephen J **(SLP)**
Steuben, Nancy R **(SLP)**
Stoddart, Mary B **(SLP)**
Tillman, Dr Tom W **(A)**
Uffenheimer, Janis Blindman **(A)**
Velde, Therese Marie **(A)**
Wendt-Harris, Barbara Lynn **(A)**
Wildman, Susan L **(SLP)**
Wohlert, Amy B **(SLP)**
Wolf, Martha E **(SLP)**
Woods, Catherine **(SLP A)**
Wygodny, Julie Kaplan **(A)**
Zucker, Laura Sue **(SLP)**

Evergreen Park
Alber, Denise Marie **(A)**
Barnard, Mrs Norma J **(SLP)**
Briggs, Noreen V **(SLP)**
Connelly, Diane Schwarz **(SLP)**
Doherty, Valerie A **(SLP)**
Getsinger, Ruth H **(SLP)**
Leshyn, Mrs Carolyn B **(SLP)**
Levin, Mrs Angela Fuoco **(SLP)**
McNamara, Sheila Marie
Muting, Elaine Kallas **(SLP)**
Salkas, Mrs Theresa Melican **(SLP)**
Schultz, Mrs Colleen Mary **(SLP)**
Wilkey, Mrs Marjorie C **(SLP)**

Fairbury
Hammer, Mrs Kay N **(SLP)**

Fairfield
Keele, Susan Laraine **(SLP)**

Fairview Heights
Brinkmann, Mrs Dawn Cross **(SLP)**
Buck, Caroline M **(A)**
Carey, Dr Ann Lee **(SLP A)**
Hughes, David G
Ott, Kimberly K **(A)**
Scott, James E **(A)**

Flora
Stevens, Robin Lynn **(SLP)**

Flossmoor
Anderson, Bettye E **(SLP)**
Bintz, Mrs Sally H **(SLP)**
Bochek, Dawn **(SLP)**
Greven, Mrs Carol Maloff **(SLP)**
Jacobson, Norma S **(SLP)**
Kaplan, Mrs Ellen W **(SLP)**
Mazza, Michael A **(SLP)**
Smith, Diana Ep
Tracy, Mrs Susan Graben **(SLP)**
Watman, Lizabeth M **(SLP)**
Weiskopf, Mrs Donna T **(SLP)**
Ziol, Mrs Elaine J **(SLP)**

Forest Park
Edgar, Julia D **(SLP)**
Kingsbury, Nancy **(SLP)**
Mullen, Georgine Frank **(SLP)**
Phillips, Nancy Marie **(SLP)**

Fox River Grove
Fister, Mrs Joy Wallace **(SLP)**
Karson-Bach, Mrs Lisa Ann **(SLP)**
Muenzenberger, Mrs Elizabeth **(A)**

Frankfort
Daniels, Kurt R **(SLP)**
Ingmire, Mrs Janet U **(SLP)**
Perkins, Mrs Jeanne P **(SLP A)**
Smith, William J

Franklin Grove
Nusbaum, Mrs Gloria Shoemaker **(SLP)**

Freeport
Myers, Margaret A **(SLP)**
Shriver, Rebecca L **(SLP)**
Truesdell, Paula Jean **(SLP)**

Fulton
Huisingh, Mrs Rosemary A **(SLP)**
Orman, M Jane **(SLP)**

Gages Lake
Maida, Lorraine Ann **(SLP)**

Galesburg
Carey, Sarah Jane **(A)**
Collins, Sonia G **(SLP)**
Sweeney, Mrs Karin Alice **(SLP)**

Gary
Vaughn, Maureen G **(SLP)**

Geneseo
Crane, Terrence L **(SLP)**
Dial, Bill Dean **(SLP)**
Robertson, Mrs Cheryl A K **(SLP)**

Geneva
Adams, Heidi Marie **(SLP)**
Brems, Stephen C **(A)**
Cleave, Doris C **(SLP)**
Dudzinski, Mrs Barbara Jean **(SLP)**

Hetzler, Mrs Marilyn J **(SLP)**
Hill, Mrs Mary E **(SLP)**
Malik, Joan M **(SLP)**
Nelson, Barbara H **(SLP)**
Skaar, Mary George **(SLP)**

Genoa
Weil, Emily Jean **(SLP)**

Georgetown
Galyen, Mrs Kathryn J **(SLP)**

Gilman
Stratton, June R **(SLP)**

Glen Carbon
Bahmani, Amy Frances
Bauer, Pamela Rae **(SLP)**
Colligan-Kovarik, Michelle K **(SLP)**
Parks, Mrs Kathleen Schneider **(SLP)**
Shultz, Cathleen M **(SLP)**

Glen Ellyn
Aach, Mrs Lori Fishman
Burba, Linda Ann R **(A)**
Dagley, Mrs Glenna M **(A)**
Gartlan, Kimberly A **(SLP)**
Gillespie, Mrs Janet Vandevelde
Haas, Mrs Joanne Ryan **(SLP)**
Hadley, Beth Eleanor **(SLP)**
Hibberd, Mrs Mary G **(SLP)**
Hull, Mrs Nancy D **(SLP)**
Linderman, Timothy D **(SLP)**
Lowery, Rita L **(SLP)**
Simon, Elaine B **(SLP)**

Glencoe
Alpert, Cynthia M **(SLP)**
Canel, Mrs Judith Forman
Graller, Mrs Lois C **(SLP)**
Hoenig, Mrs Ann S **(SLP A)**
Johnston, Charles E
Mack, Erminia D **(SLP)**
Miller, Nancy R **(SLP)**
Pasikov, Renee G **(SLP)**

Glendale Heights
Altersohn, Mrs Kathleen Ann **(SLP)**
Czaplewski, Mrs Cathleen Marie **(SLP)**
Eneberg-Farruggia, Karen G **(SLP)**
Malbon, Pamela **(SLP)**
Mealins, Amy **(SLP)**
Perry, Jana Timm **(A)**
Szczypka-Gay, Mrs Rene Marie **(A)**

Glenview
Arbanas, Marybeth **(SLP)**
Benedict, Ellen T **(A)**
Braverman, Devida Michelle **(SLP)**
Camastro, Mrs Theresa Seeber **(SLP)**
Connery, Patricia K **(A)**
Croasmun, Mrs Patricia A **(SLP)**
Demler, Jane W M **(SLP)**
Derman, Sheila K **(SLP)**
Donovan, Dorothy R **(SLP)**
Farrell, Mrs Patricia **(A)**
Froehling, Mrs Doreen Ann **(SLP)**
Gershenzon, Mrs Bonnie Esserman **(SLP)**
Graham, Marguerite **(SLP)**
Hill, David **(A)**
Jones, Mrs Marybeth D **(SLP)**
Knight, Mrs Helen Sullivan **(SLP)**
Knight, Paul D **(SLP)**
Levy, Lisa Jan **(SLP)**
Malina, Mrs Sheila **(SLP)**
Meyers, Martha M **(SLP)**
O'Dell, Mrs Nancy Smith **(SLP)**
O'Gara, Mary M **(SLP)**
Person, Joanne Tierney **(SLP)**
Pilcher, Mrs Ellen Elizabeth **(SLP)**
Rogal, Mrs Carol J **(SLP)**
Steinken, Terri L **(SLP)**
Ward, Patricia A **(SLP)**
Young, Carolyn Virginia **(SLP A)**

Glenwood
Fox-Gleason, Susan A **(SLP)**
Joseph, Mrs Vivian **(SLP)**
Sperti, Mrs Karen Nancy **(SLP)**
Wujek, Christine Marie **(SLP)**

Godfrey
Johnson, Sharon K **(SLP)**

Granite City
La Velle, Connie Marie **(SLP)**
Siegel-Grieves, Cheryl M **(A)**
Turck, Sr Stephanie **(SLP)**
Vincent, Mrs Linda J **(SLP)**

Grayslake
De Carlo, Mrs Susannah Mathis **(SLP)**
Dilallo, Mary D **(SLP)**
Reis, Mrs Michelle Ann **(SLP)**
Rejc, Cheryl S **(SLP)**
Toole, Janet M **(A)**

Great Lakes
Zenz, Michael E **(A)**

Greenville
Bayless, Becky Lynn **(SLP)**
Brewer, Mrs Karen M **(SLP)**

Gridley
Looney, Carol Ruch **(SLP)**

Gurnee
Anastasia, Mrs Stefanie Carol **(SLP)**
Jones, Sharen **(SLP)**
Theard, Marie-Paule **(SLP)**

Hampshire
Adham, Mrs Mary Lenschow **(A)**

Hanover Park
Ford, Mrs Constance Lynn **(SLP)**
Wrobel, Mrs Mary Jamison **(SLP)**

Harrisburg
Jerrels, Mrs Elaine Glynn **(SLP)**
Nelson, Linda C **(SLP)**
Speaks, Mrs Nancy Jo J **(SLP)**
Stearns, Terah Ann Martin **(SLP)**
Womack, Patty Kay

Harvard
Grieshop, Mrs Cheryl Graves **(SLP)**
Slater, Sandra Lee

Harwood Heights
Kohlin, Carol Marie **(A)**

Hawthorne Woods
Stauber, Mary Brudnicki **(SLP)**

Hazel Crest
Holden-Bryant, Diane **(A)**
Shepard, Janice Tucker **(SLP)**

Hennepin
Dean, Ronald J **(SLP)**
Justice, Natalie **(A)**

Herrin
Clanahan, Karen J **(SLP)**
Newcom, Robert D **(A)**
Saylor-Connell, Deborah Sue **(SLP)**

Hickory Hills
Czarnik, Karen A **(SLP)**
Luneckas, Mrs Ina Kristina **(SLP)**
Mackowiak, Diane Stec **(SLP)**
Rose, Patricia M **(SLP)**
Stewart, Corinne Kelly **(SLP)**

Highland
Bolton, Mrs Judith Murphy **(SLP)**
Randant, Mrs Barbara F **(SLP A)**

Highland Park
Brenner, Mrs Jan **(SLP)**
Brown-Grant, Mrs Elaine L **(SLP)**
Burstein, Caryn L S **(SLP)**
Cawn, Mrs Charleyne K **(SLP)**
Cosentine, Mrs Brenda H **(SLP A)**
Davies, Jacquelyn R D **(SLP)**
Doroff, Mrs Judi Anne **(SLP)**
Emmerman, Mrs Esther P **(SLP)**
Ferencz, Mrs Marla J **(SLP)**
Fish, Margaret Sidock **(SLP)**
Freedman-White, Laura B **(SLP)**
Hoffman, Mrs Randy A **(SLP)**
Holtzman, Mrs Naomi S **(A)**
Huseth, Nancy J **(SLP)**
Kabaker, Mrs Barbara S **(SLP)**
Katz, Mrs Debra R **(SLP)**
Lahm, Mary Elizabeth **(SLP)**
Lavin, Mrs Ellen **(SLP)**
Marcus, Mrs Beth Kraus **(SLP)**
Newman, Joanne Jacobs **(SLP)**
Novak, Ellen Sue **(SLP)**
Ordower, Elaine L **(SLP)**
Piper, Mrs Elizabeth **(SLP)**
Stein, Mrs Sharon P **(SLP)**
Streicker, Mrs Carol R **(SLP)**
Swanson, Mrs Sonia C **(SLP)**
Taxy, Mrs Gail S **(SLP)**
Vonnegut, Susan H **(SLP)**
Weiner, Mrs Judith Kahn **(SLP)**
Weiss, Mrs Laurie K **(SLP)**
Wilcox, Dr Colleen Bridget **(SLP)**
Worsek, Mrs Lisa David **(SLP)**
Zucker, Karen D **(A)**

Highwood
Volpe, Mrs Ann Lechner **(SLP)**

Hillsboro
Winkler, Jeanne L **(SLP)**
Winnett, Sharon Lee **(SLP)**

Hillside
Napolitano, Patricia Ann
Phillips, Carol Marie **(SLP)**
Rachlin, Holly Fiebert **(SLP)**
Smith, Mrs Susan Kalas **(A)**

Hines
Cook, Barbara S **(SLP)**
Graner, Darlene **(SLP)**
Mlcoch, Dr Anthony G **(SLP)**

Hinsdale
Burns, Mrs Rosealee L **(SLP)**
Davis, Deborah J **(SLP)**
Edens, Mrs Linda Ann **(SLP)**
Evans, Mary P **(A)**
Everette, Lisa Sandrolini **(SLP)**
Guild, Mrs Ann S **(SLP)**
Jackson, Mrs Adrianne **(SLP)**
Larose, Roger Walter
Meyer, Dr Dianne **(A)**
Newton, Pamela Kay **(SLP)**
Smith, Mrs Hilary C Y **(SLP)**
Socolofsky, Ginger K **(SLP)**
Spigos, Mrs Janet C **(SLP)**
Vonder Heide, Patricia Hall **(SLP)**

Hoffman Estates
Connelly, Robert J **(A)**
Darr, Christine **(SLP)**
Evans, Mrs Annette B **(SLP)**
Gudmundsen, Gail I **(A)**
Henriques, Mrs Jan Heymann **(A)**
Laferle, Kenneth R **(A)**
Leclercq, Mrs Julie P **(SLP)**
Lewallen, Barbara Hewitt **(A)**
Maguire, Mrs Lisa Carlson **(SLP)**
Martin, Elizabeth Pleune **(SLP)**
Orr, Cynthia Sue **(SLP)**
Patel, Mrs Sonal R **(SLP)**
Pidek, Catherine Monica **(SLP)**
Schneeberger, Jeanne **(A)**
Vinopal, Mary C **(SLP)**

Homewood
Bjella, Michele Angrisano **(SLP)**
Dolan, Mrs Laurie E **(SLP)**
Drucker, Gail S
Eisenbart, Karen S **(SLP)**
Frazek, Melanie **(SLP)**
Iverson, Mrs Mary W **(SLP)**
Karnell, Dr Michael Peter **(SLP)**
Lipuma, Cynthia L **(SLP)**
Nathan, Mrs Diane Z **(SLP)**
Ostarello, Denise R **(SLP)**
Palmer, Michele Tullier **(SLP)**
Searcy, Karyn Lewis **(SLP)**
Sheehy, Loretta M **(SLP)**
Treccani, Barbara Biro **(SLP)**
Woolley, Alice V **(SLP)**

Huntley
Kearns, Mrs Dacia L **(SLP)**
Miller, Cynthia Stewart **(SLP)**

Indian Creek
Olson, Mrs Sylvia E L **(SLP)**

Indian Head Park
Krcmar, Jean Gebhart **(SLP)**

Ingleside
Carsella, Mrs Janice R **(SLP)**

Inverness
Schrock, Kathleen C **(SLP)**

Island Lake
Farrell, Mrs Diana Jones **(SLP)**
Karson Gries, Allyson Sue **(SLP)**

Itasca
Dunn, Mrs Joann Hoffmann **(SLP)**
Von Ehrenkrook, Cathy **(SLP)**

Jacksonville
Carson, Mary Ellen **(A)**
Fetterer, Mrs Kimberly James **(SLP)**
Hill, Mrs Dolores Berry **(SLP)**
Hoard, Ann **(A)**
Silverio, Albert P **(A)**
Spangenberg, Sheryl L **(SLP)**
Tucker, Jayma Lee **(SLP)**

Jerseyville
Swearingin, Marilyn K **(SLP)**

Joliet
Bari-Bayci, Mrs Anna M **(SLP)**
Bates, Tempie M **(SLP)**
Brass, Mrs Edna M **(SLP)**
Chouinard, David R **(SLP)**
Connors Miller, Mrs M Chris **(SLP)**
Doszak, Arlene L **(SLP)**
Downey, Marlene G **(SLP)**
Kinsella, Colleen Therese
Liscic, Debra Schumann
Luthanen, Mrs Carol Jokisch **(SLP)**
Monahan-Tomasino, Christine **(SLP)**
Pauloski, Dr Barbara Roa
Riordan, Peg **(SLP)**
Scygiel, Sr M Dominica **(SLP)**
Smith, Patricia Ann **(SLP)**
Venegoni, Mary L **(SLP)**
Wason, Kim Goudreau **(A)**
Wesemann, Theresa Ann **(SLP)**
Whalen, Sr M Clare E **(SLP)**
Wilmette, Valeria **(SLP)**
Wirth, Mary Ruth **(SLP)**
Yaney, Karen K **(SLP)**

Justice
Prokes, Mrs Kim C **(SLP)**

Kankakee
Burgard, Theresa C **(SLP)**
Hildebrand, Susanne Y **(SLP)**
Hunnicutt, Darla Jo **(SLP)**
Kurzeja, Barbara A **(SLP)**
Mathews, Burma J **(SLP)**
McDermott, Therese M **(SLP)**
Milone, Marjorie **(SLP)**
Notton, Mrs Janet M **(SLP)**
Olsen, Dr Richard H **(A)**
Pierson, John R **(SLP)**
Schweigert, Mrs Ruth Annette **(SLP)**

Kansas
Hallock, Viola K

Kenilworth
Coughlin, Susan S **(SLP)**
Granum, Arline S **(SLP)**

Kewanee
Burns, Mrs Sharon **(SLP)**
Christiansen, Loretta M **(SLP)**

Kingston
Crouch, Mrs Starline R **(SLP)**

Kingston Mines
Dunn, Mrs Darlene T **(SLP)**

Knoxville
Gibbs, Mrs Cathy E **(SLP)**

La Grange
Bedore, Joan McGarry **(SLP)**
Clark, Susan M Kilgore **(SLP)**
Elliott, Jill Louise **(SLP)**
Graef, Mrs Felicia Harrington **(SLP)**
Hennessy, Betsy H **(SLP)**
Herman, Mrs Anne Hansen **(SLP)**
Hogan, Patricia Ellen **(SLP)**
Jarrick, Nancy A **(SLP)**
Jaskierski, Sheila P **(SLP)**
Kielp, Therese Anne **(A)**
Landis, Keith Duane **(SLP)**
McMahon, Mrs Helen M **(SLP)**
Moore, Janaan Schmuhl **(A)**
Petras, Mrs Gail E **(SLP)**
Schotland, Henrietta L **(SLP)**
Short, Mrs Mary Ann Marik **(SLP)**
Withowski, Mrs Barbara Therese
Zeitlin, Mrs Virginia Riordan **(SLP)**

La Grange Park
Baker-Buchalter, Mrs Darlene **(SLP)**
Blank, Candace Rose **(A)**
Dante, Joanne H **(SLP)**
Doyle-Kushner, Mrs Patricia **(SLP)**
Pudlo, Linda Mainiero **(SLP)**
Wilburn, Michael Alan **(SLP)**
Wroblewski, Mrs Sandra Miller **(SLP)**

La Salle
Bernardini, Deborah M **(SLP)**

Lake Barrington
Bocian, Mark A **(SLP)**
Sasala, John C **(A)**

Lake Bluff
Albrecht, Phyllis H **(SLP)**
Barry, Cheryl A **(SLP)**
Harms, Sherry S **(SLP)**
Hoenk, Megan O **(SLP)**
Schewitz, Mrs Sheila **(SLP)**
Tansey, Mrs Janet H **(SLP)**

Lake Forest
Arends, Mrs Jill Gallup **(SLP)**
Biety, Karen Ann **(SLP)**
Drumright, Judy D **(A)**
Eland, Mrs Marla H **(SLP)**
Hoover, Julia M **(SLP)**
Kohlmeyer, Anne M
Mulhern, Mrs Susan Taber **(SLP)**
Murphy, Mrs Linda F **(SLP)**
Nieds, Barbara G **(SLP A)**
Schugar, Linda R **(SLP)**

Lake Villa
Broy, Mrs Kathleen I **(SLP)**
Chilsen, Mrs Jody Marie **(A)**
Dahlke, Mrs Nanette Carlmark **(SLP)**

Lake Zurich
Alzos-Howe, Elaine I **(SLP)**
Avant, Mrs Susan L **(SLP)**
Gear, Mrs Ann V **(A)**
Givens, Kathleen A **(SLP)**
Napp, Mrs Ann P **(A)**
Nasca, Vincent P **(SLP)**
O'Leary, Jody B **(SLP)**
Poole, Julia Ann **(SLP)**
Qualiardi, Virginia Pangburn **(SLP)**
Tackes, Mrs Linda Braun **(SLP)**
Walter, Mrs Rita N **(SLP)**

Lansing
Fox, Kathryn M **(SLP)**
Hill, Mrs Karen S **(SLP)**
Kiester, Mrs Jeanette L **(SLP)**
Marquardt, Mrs Lillian A **(SLP)**
McIntyre, Claire Galloway **(SLP)**
Nyberg, Ruth M **(SLP)**

Leland
Schou, Mrs Linda Ann **(SLP)**

Lemont
Baker, Mrs Marletta A **(SLP)**
Crull, Mrs Sharon I D **(SLP)**
Hoffmann, Mrs Dale E **(SLP)**

Lena
Merchant, Mrs Cheryl Terese **(SLP)**

Libertyville
Albrecht, Mrs Elizabeth **(SLP)**
Chickey, Janet Hagan **(SLP)**
Dyer, Patricia Joan **(SLP)**
Kramer-Kohlbrenner, Mrs Claudia **(SLP)**
Lukens, Mrs Ann M **(SLP)**
Luplow, Catherine Ann **(SLP)**
Mandeltort, Susan G **(SLP)**
Manek, Mrs Doris J **(SLP)**
Remensnyder, Linda S **(A)**
Silvertrust, Joanne E **(SLP)**
Zozom-Guiheen, Mrs Arlene **(SLP)**

Lincoln
Borbely, Steven J **(SLP)**
Custis, Mrs Wendy Lu **(SLP)**
Knutilla, Cynthia Cooper **(SLP)**
Pollett, Pamela A L **(SLP)**
Troesch, Peter J **(A)**

Lincolnshire
Lucci, Mrs Bonnie D **(SLP)**

Lincolnwood
Belson, Mrs Muriel F **(SLP)**
Klodd, Dr David **(A)**
Korman, Arlene C **(SLP)**
Levin, Julie Anne **(SLP)**
Ostro, Mrs Gayle Patrice **(SLP)**
Pliskin, Mrs Doris K **(SLP)**
Ropek, Renee Marilyn **(SLP)**
Rukin, Sharon Faye **(SLP)**

Lindenhurst
Geary-Cook, Kathleen **(SLP)**

Lisle
Channon, Mrs Lisa Kerstin
Gron, Karen M **(SLP)**
Jelm, Judith Michels **(SLP)**
Kelly, Mrs Geralyn Helen **(SLP)**
Moore, Mrs Cindy S **(SLP)**
Popp, Stephanie L **(SLP)**
Ramakrishnan-Rothe, R K **(SLP)**
Reed, Mrs Alice N **(A)**
Samalot, Diana Isabel **(SLP)**
Schuman, Gayle **(SLP)**
Siefert, Michael J **(A)**
Spencer, Sarah Lynne **(SLP)**
Steury, Marlyn Ligner **(SLP)**
Ulrich, Kathleen M **(A)**
Valle, Kathleen T **(SLP)**
Witczak, Kathryn Page **(SLP)**

Litchfield
Harms, Christine **(SLP)**
Nelson, Mrs Stephanie Broom **(A)**

Lockport
Miller, Jane E **(SLP)**
Morrison, Michelle Kaleen **(SLP)**
Paskiet, Clare Ann **(SLP)**
Porter, Mrs Sandra P **(SLP)**

Lombard
Alberts, Mrs Alice S **(SLP)**
Bultas-Ryba, Mrs Karen Marie **(SLP)**
Cassin, Mrs Mary Padula **(SLP)**
Clery, Mrs Carolsue Harr **(SLP)**
Groenewold, Mrs Linda J **(SLP)**
Jenkins, Edna Margaret **(SLP A)**
Johnson, Mrs Catherine Carty **(SLP)**
King, Kathleen Anne **(SLP)**
McDonough, Mrs Mary Young **(A)**
McElroy, Mrs Anne-Marie C **(SLP)**
Murthy, Vasudha K **(A)**
Parratore, Mrs Christine Larsen **(SLP)**
Potanos, Mrs Jenny Fritsch **(SLP)**
Pulikowski, Mrs Gail Ponte **(SLP)**
Steinhauser, Elizabeth R **(SLP)**
Stover, Joanne Elizabeth **(A)**
Wall, Susan Mary **(SLP)**
Zurales, Sue Kaminski **(A)**

Long Grove
Gardner, Mrs Nancy Kriz **(SLP)**

Loves Park
Lehenbauer, B Ellen **(SLP)**

Lovington
Born, Lori Ann

Lyndon
Kelley, Edward L **(SLP)**

Lynn Center
Hills, Mrs Sherrill A Swanson **(SLP)**

Lynwood
Jakosh, Terri Lynn **(SLP)**
Kooy, Dr Linda Klesker **(SLP)**

Machesney Park
Burns, Mrs Debra J **(SLP)**
Jacobsen, Lee Ann G **(SLP)**

MacKinaw
Sommer, Mrs Deborah J **(SLP)**

Macomb
Boatz, Mrs Donna Sheryl **(A)**
Burrows, Dr Dennis Lee **(A)**
Burrows, Mrs Judith A **(SLP)**
Calderone, Mrs M Lynn **(A)**
Collins, Dr Carolyn S **(SLP)**
Francis, Dr William C **(SLP)**
Frankenberger, Dr Robert L **(SLP)**
Johlfs, Connie T **(SLP)**
Marx, Mrs Maureen G **(SLP)**
Passmore, Susan Whiteley **(SLP)**
Severinsen, Mrs Rosalie H **(SLP)**
Vahling, Theresa Ann **(SLP)**
Williams, Dr Robert G, Jr **(A)**

Mahomet
McCaughrin, Dr Wendy B **(SLP)**
Walder, Mrs Louise E **(SLP)**

Makanda
Hill, Mrs Susan Eileen **(SLP)**

Maltoon
Sandage, Michelle R **(A)**

Manteno
Brown, Mrs Anita J **(SLP)**
Glidden, Melissa B **(SLP)**

Mapleton
Wiebler, Ladona Cunningham **(SLP)**

Marengo
Sawallisch, Mrs Mary Beth

Marine
Kutz, Sheila L **(A)**
Ladd, Mrs Ruth A **(SLP)**

Marion
Drury-Young, Roberta F **(SLP)**
Tallman, Valerie L **(SLP)**
Townsend, Jean M **(A)**

Markham
Shannon, Donna Jo **(SLP)**
Wilson-Coleman, Mrs Phyllis Marie **(SLP)**

Marquette Heights
Wood, Rebecca E **(A)**

Marseilles
Gemberling, Dorothy E **(SLP)**

Mascoutah
Ostrom, Mrs Kay Ann F **(SLP)**

Mason City
Naylor-Shelabarger, Mrs Barbara Ann **(SLP)**

Matteson
Hawes, Mary Z **(SLP)**
Stachowicz, Karen Schultz **(A)**
Volkman, Mrs Therese Marie

Mattoon
Coffman, James M **(SLP)**
James, Sylvia E **(SLP)**
Milner, Mrs Lynnette Kay **(SLP)**
Wykis, Mrs Joan K **(SLP)**

Maywood
Anderson-Pelec, Karen Marie **(SLP)**
Harrold, Vickie M **(A)**
O'Brien, Mary E

Mc Lean
Hewitson, Mrs Deborah Hulbert **(SLP)**
Thacker, Mrs Teresa Ann **(SLP)**

McHenry
Boeldt, Elmer A **(SLP)**
Diedrich, Julie L **(SLP)**
Lawson, Mrs Cathy S **(SLP)**
Mowery, Charlane W **(SLP)**
Rossetti, Marybeth **(A)**
Stilling, Catherine M **(SLP)**
Van Fleet, Mrs Kathleen Brennan **(SLP)**

Melrose Park
Buhrke, Mrs Cheryl K **(SLP)**
Pryble-Dattalo, Susan M **(SLP)**
Puccio, Linda M

Merdota
Goy, Mrs Karen Miller **(SLP)**

Merrionette Park
Monahan, Judith A **(SLP)**

Metamora
Eckhardt, Mrs Lori **(SLP)**

Metropolis
Lunsford, Marla Dee **(SLP)**

Midlothian
Mittler, Thomas F **(SLP)**
Riedel, Mary Ellen **(SLP)**

Milan
Cero, Lianne Christine **(SLP)**

Milledgeville
Bergstrom, Mrs Larrabeth Fendler **(SLP)**

Millstadt
Aubuchon, Mrs Pamela R **(SLP)**
Kilhoffer, Royce L **(SLP)**

Milmine
Peterson, Linda B **(SLP A)**

Minooka
Casey, Suzanne J **(SLP)**
Raino-Hoglund, Mrs Kimberly **(SLP)**

Mokena
Foose, David B **(SLP)**
Ihrke, Mrs Ann G **(SLP)**
Maclejewski, Theresa Marie
Murskyj, Chrystyne L **(SLP)**
Rigoni, Mrs Karen E **(SLP)**

Moline
Barrett, Mark D **(SLP)**

Bielefeldt, John M **(SLP)**
Blagden, Carolyn M **(SLP)**
Brosius, Mrs Valerie Ann **(SLP)**
Castle, Terrina Marie **(SLP)**
Creen, Mrs Gloria F T **(SLP)**
Dondanville, Mrs Karen M **(SLP)**
Felstehausen-White, Susan L **(A)**
Hage, Mrs Luella R T **(SLP)**
Johnson, Debra Lois **(SLP)**
Kirkwood-Johnson, Mrs Karla **(SLP)**
Lind, Mary N **(SLP)**
Marten, Mrs Treasure A **(SLP)**
McDoniel, Margaret Burke **(A)**
Mueller, James Charles **(SLP)**
Ryder, Mrs Susan Klann **(SLP)**
Zachman, Linda V **(SLP)**
Zachman, Dr Thomas A **(A)**

Monee
Meyers-Hafner, Ellen Joan **(SLP)**

Monmouth
Ohlweiler, Sr Zita **(SLP)**

Montgomery
Hall, Nancy **(SLP)**

Morris
Bronk, Mrs Maxine M **(SLP)**
Crowder-Wile, Marilyn Theresa **(SLP)**
Gottlieb, Sheri Lee **(SLP)**
Mosey, Mrs Gail Patricia **(SLP)**
Sommers, Mrs Chandra D **(A)**

Morrison
Urbanc, Rebecca A **(SLP)**

Morton
Loscheider, Mary Jo **(SLP)**
Pollock, Gail Lynn **(A)**
Smith, Jane Anne **(SLP)**

Morton Grove
Amesquita, Mrs Rikki K **(SLP)**
Bucher, Mrs Irene R **(SLP)**
Davey, Mrs Karen M **(SLP)**
Goldman, Deborah S
Gurolnick, Mrs Joyce W **(SLP)**
Johnson, Mrs Jan Marsden **(SLP)**
Luecht, Kim L **(SLP)**
Pinkin-Troyk, Mrs Marianne **(A)**
Silverman, Mrs Barbara K **(SLP)**

Mounds
Russell, Kimberly K
Stout, Mrs Carol Elizabeth **(SLP)**

Mount Carmel
Newkirk, Mrs Alice B W **(SLP)**
Spruell, Mrs Sheri L **(SLP)**
Timberlake, Mary J **(SLP)**

Mount Morris
Erhart, Mrs Louise M **(SLP)**

Mount Prospect
Biegert, Mrs Janice L **(SLP)**
Davis, Catherine D **(SLP)**
Deranleau-Urban, Lisa Catherine
Ellwood, Marti Maloney **(SLP)**
Forgione, Angela M **(SLP)**
Frank, Lori Mitchell **(SLP)**
Klein, Marc I **(A)**
Lindelof, Laura **(SLP)**
Morreale, Carol Clifford **(A)**
Nichols, Marie A **(A)**
Rau, Mrs Elaine K **(SLP)**
Riddle, Rebecca Elaine **(SLP)**

Mount Vernon
Allen, Mrs Barbara Anne **(SLP)**
Burke, Mrs Elaine Brown **(A)**
Henderson, Lori J
Van Winkle, Cynthia G **(SLP)**
Yuncker, Kathy Annette **(A)**

Moweaqua
Gaines, Marilyn D **(SLP)**

Mulkeytown
Doerner, Mrs Sheila Mondino **(SLP)**
Sloan, Mrs Paula S **(SLP)**

Mundelein
Gauger, Mrs Jane E **(SLP)**
Haenze, Mrs Karen Crafford **(SLP)**
Jans-Kaplan, Mrs Gayle S **(SLP)**
Johnson, Mrs Michele F **(SLP)**
Kripal, Joni Peters **(A)**
Raz, Dr Israel **(A)**
Sagendorph, Mrs Lynn Legate **(SLP)**
Skowron, Christine **(SLP)**

Murphysboro
Brown, Marcia Jean **(SLP)**
Hungerford, Suzanne Mary **(SLP)**

Naperville
Bajusz, Mrs Goldie A **(SLP)**
Bazan, Mrs Theresa Caruso **(SLP)**
Bedell, Joy Anne **(SLP)**
Blank, Linda Rodgers **(SLP)**
Butera, Mrs Judith C **(A)**
Caffarella, Janice M **(A)**
Costigan, Linda D **(SLP)**
Durachta, Mrs Judith A **(SLP)**
Eades, Sheila N **(SLP)**
Ederer, Mrs Tami Duncan **(SLP)**
Feigh, Mrs Lori **(SLP)**
Fett, Cynthia Marie
Garlich, Mrs Deberah M **(SLP)**
Gonio-Colaluca, Mrs Lynn Ann **(SLP)**
Green, Diana L G **(SLP)**
Grissom, Mrs Susan E H **(SLP)**
Guttman, Dr Newman
Hammar, Mrs Carolann Corbit **(SLP)**
Hayes, Mrs Myra Lynn **(SLP)**
Henderson, Christine D **(SLP)**
Hilger, Sandra I **(SLP)**
Holden, Mary Ann
Jennings, Mrs Diana R
Johnson, Mrs Barbara Faye **(SLP)**
Keeler, Darlene D
Komes, Linda W **(SLP)**
Konrad-Wood, Patricia **(SLP)**
Kramer, Mrs Catharine Milligan **(SLP)**
Lamb, Donald P **(A)**
Lazerov, Florence Elise
Leccia, Jocelyn M A **(SLP)**
Lipman, Roberta B **(SLP)**
Mantel, Heather P **(SLP)**
McConaghy, Mrs Kathleen D **(A)**
O'Connor, Cathleen A **(A)**
Oker, Susan Lynn **(SLP)**
Olson, Lynn M **(SLP)**
Ormsby, Catherine Sarah **(SLP)**
O'Rourke, Mrs Margaret **(SLP)**
Palasz, Richard W **(A)**
Petrauskas, Mrs Geralyn M **(SLP)**
Plawecki, Mrs Lynne Myers **(SLP)**
Riegler, Mrs Marilyn G **(SLP)**
Robertson, Penny S **(SLP)**
Rooney, Mrs Bridget Knowles **(SLP)**
Roth, Mrs Christine L **(SLP)**
Russell, Elizabeth **(SLP)**
Sampat, Jyoti D **(A)**
Schachtschneider, Mrs Marietta Sobocinski **(SLP)**
Schiffler, Linda P **(A)**
Schoenberg, Barbara **(SLP)**
Schwartz, Dr Howard D **(SLP)**
Schwin, Evelyn Boyle **(A)**
Sihler, Mrs Patricia C **(SLP)**
Singer, Mrs Tina H **(SLP)**
Trembacki, Mrs Debra J **(SLP)**
Weber, Mrs Janet Martin **(SLP)**
Wenzlaff, Alice L **(SLP)**
Whitesell, Mrs Denise Jean

Neoga
Alexander, Mrs Rebecca Lynn

New Baden
Toennies, Mrs Teresa Kanrhoff **(SLP)**

New Lenox
Chalupa, Linda A **(SLP)**
Ghosh, Constance R **(SLP)**
Healy, Mrs Carolyn Schmitz **(SLP)**
Karneboge, Mrs Monica D **(SLP)**
Rendleman, Mrs Gail Anne **(SLP)**

New Milford
Kleinmeyer, Mrs Kathleen Joanne **(SLP)**

New Windsor
McGaughy, Sandra L **(SLP)**

Newman
McGee, Marylee N **(SLP)**

Normal
Anderson, Mrs Nancy A D **(SLP)**
Anderson, Patti W **(SLP)**
Bloomer, Dr H Harlan **(SLP)**
Bowman, Dr Clarence A **(SLP)**
Brickell, Mrs Nancy A **(SLP)**
Brunt, Dr Michael A **(A)**
Charles, Linda Kathryn **(SLP)**
Davidson, Keith C **(SLP)**
Howard, Dr Merle Ray **(SLP)**
Hufnagle, Dr Jon **(SLP)**
Hulit, Dr Lloyd M **(SLP)**
Hunt, Deanna Johnson **(SLP)**
Mahrt, Vickie Krause **(SLP)**
Monoson, Dr Patricia Komiss **(SLP)**
Pitcher, Mrs Deborah S **(A)**
Richards, Dr Doris M **(SLP A)**
Ricketts, Mrs Kristyn Jean **(SLP)**
Ritter, Dawn Ranee **(SLP)**
Spitz, Mrs Roberta E **(SLP)**
Steck, Mrs Mary Theresa **(SLP)**
Tannahill, Dr J Curtis **(A)**
Thomley, Nancy B **(SLP)**
Tschaepe, Mrs Lois Miskovich **(A)**
Young, Dr Martin A

Norridge
Schuster, Lauren K **(SLP)**
Skoulikaris, Sonya **(SLP)**

North Chicago
Kearns, Kevin P **(SLP)**

Northbrook
Alsaker, Nora V **(SLP)**
Avner, Ellen Rosenblatt **(SLP)**
Bendikas, Sylvia C **(SLP)**
Brown, Mrs Sandra E **(SLP)**
Brown-Sweeney, Sharon G **(SLP)**
Cariola, John W **(A)**
Chandler, Julie Scharff **(SLP)**
Chin, Linda Chang **(SLP)**
Comstock, Mrs Diane Reichert **(SLP)**
Cowin, Eileen Cotovsky **(SLP)**
Dahlstrand, Mrs Cheryl A **(SLP)**
Derrick, Kathryn G **(SLP)**
Feldman, Mrs Sheree Y **(SLP)**
Gottfred, Dr Catherine H **(SLP)**
Hagan, Marilyn L
Kaplan, Mrs Carrie Levine **(A)**
Kistenbroker, Mrs Valerie Spera **(SLP)**
Kohn-Lau, Annette M **(SLP)**
Lybolt, Dr John T **(SLP)**
Meltzer, Mrs Bonnie Rosett **(SLP)**
Meltzer, Mrs Jill B H **(A)**
Minick, Ellen G **(SLP)**
Neighbors, Mrs Victoria Ruth **(SLP)**
Noeth, Mrs Carolyn Frances **(SLP)**
Peterson, Linda A **(SLP)**
Rozen, Mrs Audrey L **(SLP)**
Schimel, Mrs Alison B **(SLP)**
Schneider, Susan B **(SLP)**
Schoen, Constance M **(SLP)**
Scolaro, Celeste P **(SLP)**
Shneider, Mrs Carole A **(SLP)**
Stoioff, Madonna M **(A)**
Torf, Mrs Donna R **(SLP)**
Wulf, Mrs Jan Morgan **(SLP)**

Northfield
Bidwill, Bettye J **(SLP)**
Paul, Mrs Cindy L **(SLP)**
Van Aman, Mrs Debra E **(SLP)**

Northlake
Koch, Mrs Victoria W **(SLP)**

O'Fallon
Chamblin, Diana Lynne **(SLP)**
Dillaplain, Jeanne L **(SLP)**
Fruehling, Mrs Janet Marlene **(SLP)**
Haney, Patricia L **(A)**
Hanko, Mrs Joyce M **(A)**
Schaefer, Mrs Mary K **(SLP)**

Oak Brook
Craig, Mrs Constance **(SLP)**
Kayner, Mrs Janet G **(SLP)**

Oak Forest
Bednarz, Therese F **(SLP)**
Birmingham, Debra A **(SLP)**
Dolk, Michaela L **(SLP)**
Dybala, Mrs Ellen Irene **(SLP)**
Fiala, Kathleen J
Hammer, Mrs Marcia Mary **(SLP)**
Placek, Susan Gale **(SLP)**
Tharp, Roger L **(A)**
Thinglum, Dr Harold J **(SLP)**

Oak Lawn
Alfirevic, Janine R **(SLP)**
Bielinski, Mrs Di Anne S **(SLP)**
Bohne, Michele Beth **(SLP)**
Bulka, Nancy Ann
Burklund, Lee Marie **(SLP)**
Cendejas, Deena L **(SLP)**
Chen, Diana N G **(A)**
Corcoran, Mrs Judith Allison **(SLP)**
Elsen, Julie Ann
Evans, Marion McTigue
Gaw, Mrs Sally A **(SLP)**
Klick, Mrs Pamela **(SLP)**
Kok, Mrs Jean H **(SLP)**
Maier, Kathleen M **(SLP)**
Miller, Mrs Kimberly Marie **(SLP)**
Prohaska, Mrs Denise I **(SLP)**
Stwora, Linda Swiatkowsk **(SLP)**
Weis, Carole Marie **(SLP)**

Oak Park
Aarts, Nancy Lee **(A)**
Abraham, Annabel S **(SLP)**
Agliata, Dana Ann **(SLP)**
Alper, Mrs Elaine G **(SLP)**
Anderson, Eunice **(SLP)**
Andrews, Mrs Rachel E **(SLP)**
Armstrong, Mrs Ann H **(SLP)**
Barber, Marian E **(SLP)**
Bell, Kathryn J **(SLP)**
Bligh, Mrs Sally B **(SLP)**
Bork, Debra A B **(SLP)**
Brann, Eileen **(SLP)**
Brenn-White, Bonnie M
Brown, Mrs Valerie Leon **(SLP)**
Byers, Mrs Suzanne K **(SLP)**
Carney, Mary S **(SLP)**
Carpenter, Mrs Margaret J **(SLP)**
Durham, Mrs Candace Kaye **(SLP)**
Farrelly, Mary Walsh **(SLP)**
Ferre, Dr Jeanane M **(A)**
Gamble, Mrs Mary Ellen **(SLP)**
Goodman, Elise Sue **(SLP)**
Goulding, William P **(SLP)**
Greenspan, Wendy Whalen **(SLP)**
Heimerle, Becki S **(SLP)**
Herendeen, Mrs Patricia **(SLP)**
Hughes, Vanessa
Kempster, Dr Gail B **(SLP)**
King, Mary T **(SLP)**
Kupperman, Phyllis P **(SLP)**
Kupperman, Susan J **(SLP)**
MacAuley, Kelly Ann **(A)**
MacWhirter-Holbrook, Carol A **(SLP)**

McAllister-Strong, Mrs Laurie Anne **(SLP)**
McCormick-Dunsmore, Virginia **(A)**
Merrick, Niki P **(SLP)**
Mitchell, Thomas R
Nickels, Janet K **(A)**
Osborne, Dr George S **(SLP A)**
Parker, Frances Jennings **(SLP)**
Pecora, Roberta L **(SLP)**
Pevsner, Janet H **(SLP)**
Peyser, Barbara Truax **(SLP)**
Pierson, Mrs Blair Alison **(SLP)**
Quane, Patricia G **(SLP)**
Rasley, Alexis Gray **(SLP)**
Rubin, Mrs Phyllis B **(SLP)**
Shugars, Mrs Lori Ann **(SLP)**
Smith, Dr Bonnie E **(SLP)**
Strong, Brian K **(SLP)**
Threats, Travis Terrence **(SLP)**
Wallach-Delucia, Wendy **(A)**
Wehrle, Ellen L **(SLP)**
Williams, Cheryl Ann **(SLP)**
Wojtalewicz, Donna R **(SLP)**

Oakbrook Terrace
Hubatch, Dr Leona M **(SLP)**

Oakland
Hanner, Mary Anne **(SLP)**

Odin
Hildreth, Sharon L **(SLP)**

Okawville
Sunnquist, Ellen Catherine **(SLP)**

Olney
Hartrich, Mrs Debra L **(SLP)**
Kesler, Mrs Lucy C **(SLP)**

Olympia Fields
Beemsterboer, Priscilla **(SLP)**
Gertler, Mrs Susan Joy **(A)**
Goodman, Mrs Edith Teper
Hoffman, Sheri R **(A)**
Johnson, Helen Gutmann **(SLP)**
Matlock, Renee H **(SLP)**
Ross, Mrs Francine C **(SLP)**
Russell, Susan Moore **(A)**
Smith, Mrs Joanne Parsons **(SLP)**
Tapajna, Marilyn R Kent **(SLP)**
Wolk, Phillis R **(SLP)**

Omaha
Thompson, Mrs Linda M **(SLP)**

Onarga
Hoy, Connie Lynn **(SLP)**

Orion
Lambert, Laura J **(SLP)**
Moon, Sharon E **(SLP)**
Wyant, Mrs Teresa Jane **(SLP)**

Orland Hills
Bilina, Faith B **(SLP)**
Kambic, Laura Esler **(SLP)**

Orland Park
Balsavich, Mrs Donna Marie **(SLP)**
Bandera, Elizabeth Ann **(SLP)**
Chilcutt, Virginia Wozniak **(SLP)**
Dosen, Mrs Laura Ann **(SLP)**
Fremarek, Mrs Carole M **(SLP)**
Johnson, Meredith A **(SLP)**
Jones, Elizabeth A
Lubinsky, Dr Jay **(SLP A)**
Maida-Cantone, Kathleen **(SLP)**
McDonough, Donna M **(SLP)**
Mirabella, Mrs Susan M **(SLP)**
Morrison, Kathleen A **(SLP)**
Presbitero, Mrs Michele Marie **(A)**
Stahl, Mrs Judith A **(SLP)**
Statkus, Donna Ahlert **(SLP)**
Trahey, Patricia Ann **(SLP)**

Ottawa
Butzen-Sheridan, Mrs Joanne M **(SLP)**
Caba, Mrs Mary W **(SLP)**
Feltes, Mrs Carol Urbanski **(SLP)**
Finley, Mrs Eleanor L **(SLP)**
Gayan, Lou Ann K **(SLP)**
Harte, Barbara A **(SLP)**
Kaiser, Holle Aungst **(A)**
Kirkpatrick, Mrs Julie M **(A)**
Meyer, Mrs Andrea M **(SLP)**
Mucci, Mrs Vicki Lee **(SLP)**
Scholz-Raben, Mrs Jane J **(SLP)**

Palatine
Beaudette, Mrs Kristine M **(SLP)**
Born, Rebecca A **(SLP)**
Brault, Judith C **(SLP)**
Diewald, Lisa Ann **(A)**
Gray, Barbara Johnson **(SLP)**
Hughes, Mrs Stacey B **(SLP)**
Iuorio, Mrs Barbara Baldwin
Nolan, Mrs Carol H **(SLP)**
Peters, Mrs Heidi Sawall **(SLP)**
Pollard, Michele M **(SLP)**
Reed, Dr Nancy Larkin **(SLP)**
Richter, Katherine **(SLP)**
Sanders, Aliceann C **(SLP)**
Sheehy, Judith M **(SLP)**
Shipman, Linda Marie **(SLP)**
Smiley, Mrs Deborah T **(SLP)**
Smith, Lisa Joan **(SLP)**
Swanson, Leslie Helen **(SLP)**
Thunder, Thomas D **(A)**
Young, Lori Ann **(SLP)**

Palos Heights
Adam, Mrs Kathryn L **(SLP)**
Bosack, Linda B **(A)**
Carney, Patricia Ann **(SLP)**
Kutlik, Mrs Roberta Emilie **(SLP)**
Lang, Mrs Judith Ann
Mahoney, Mrs C Michelle
Mattes, Nancy Ann **(SLP)**
Van Dyke, Mrs Laura Beth **(SLP)**
Zimmerman, Mrs Loreen Landino **(A)**
Zwierz, Judith Wolski **(SLP)**

Palos Hills
Bartusch, Mrs Mary Ann R **(SLP)**
Ihnat, Ruthanne Melfi **(SLP)**
Piechna, Linda Lee **(A)**

Palos Park
Andereck, Amy **(SLP)**
Binotti, Mrs Nancy Lea Wester **(SLP)**
Buchaniec, Mary Elisabeth **(SLP)**
Hackl, Mrs Margery B
Risinger, Lois Ann
Simpson, Dr Joann Margaret **(SLP)**

Pana
Amling, Mrs Frances Williamson **(SLP)**

Paris
David, Joan E **(SLP)**
Good, Mrs Elaine R **(SLP)**

Park Forest
Andres, Mrs Sandra A **(SLP)**
Ansai, Patricia Susan **(SLP)**
Arnold, Maretta J **(SLP)**
Cabanting, Erlinda **(SLP)**
Janota, Mrs Deloris A **(SLP)**
Lindmark, Janice Clare **(SLP)**
Perry, Mrs Pamela J **(SLP)**
Rogers, Alpha S **(SLP)**
Saunders-Culp, Mrs Karen T **(SLP)**
Shipley, Janet L **(SLP)**
Thiesen, Lauren Joy **(SLP)**

Park Ridge
Atanowsky, Orysia I **(SLP)**
Brandt, Lynne Marie **(SLP)**
Brooks, Sandra D **(SLP)**
Courtney, Anne Sheffield **(SLP)**
Harker, Darlene R **(SLP)**
Holloway, Suzanna K **(SLP)**
Kalas, Beth Hoffman **(A)**
Kiriluk, Ellaine A **(SLP)**
Kosinski, Mrs Diane T **(SLP)**
McGovern, Theresa L **(SLP)**
Michalowski, Mrs Alice J **(SLP)**
Shicotte, Cynthia Louise **(SLP)**

Patoka
Hopper, Anna L **(SLP)**

Pawnee
Clarizio, Mrs Katharine Rutherford **(SLP)**

Payson
Waters, Ellen Kay **(SLP)**

Pearl
Bess, Mrs Nanette Monygomery **(SLP)**

Peioria
John, Sunita

Pekin
Cassidy, Robert D **(SLP)**
Constable, Constance **(SLP)**
Emerson, Mrs Sharon S **(SLP)**
Heilman, Mrs Joanne Y **(SLP)**
Johnson, Mrs Lorraine Deutsch **(A)**
Rohren, Linda Michele **(SLP)**
Whiteside, Dr Janet **(SLP)**
Woiwode, Mrs Jo Anne **(SLP)**

Peoria
Aldrich, Mrs Mary K **(SLP)**
Aldrich, Dr William M **(A)**
Anderson, Lynn Froehling **(SLP)**
Anderson, Sue Ellen **(SLP)**
Andrejasich, Mrs Deirdre Kogan **(SLP)**
Bazil, Mrs Connie **(A)**
Brak, Mrs Sheila M **(SLP A)**
Brown, Elizabeth A **(SLP)**
Bullock, Gwynetta Y **(SLP)**
Carrara-O'Brien, Catherine Lynn **(SLP)**
Creager, Mrs Joan E **(SLP)**
Englert, Pamela K **(SLP)**
Ferguson, Mrs Elizabeth **(SLP)**
Giunta, Mrs Geralyn B **(SLP)**
Hansmann, Mrs Dawn Monchelle **(SLP)**
Hendricksen, Mrs Carol B **(SLP)**
Heslinga, Mrs Barbara A **(SLP)**
Huck, Jeanne E N **(SLP)**
Justice, Mrs Suzanne M **(SLP)**
Karr, David R **(SLP)**
Knight, Mrs Regina C **(SLP)**
Koller, Donald E **(SLP)**
Kwarta, Keri L
Lehmann, Mrs Billie Kay **(SLP)**
Leson, Mary A **(SLP)**
Lighter, Mrs Audrey Gail **(A)**
Lindberg, Mrs Patricia B **(SLP)**
Lindberg, Dr Robert F **(A)**
Mawhinney, Dr Clara K **(SLP)**
McAsey, Danila B **(SLP)**
McNamara, Mrs Tena Workman **(A)**
Meissner, Dr William August **(A)**
Moerman, Jane Francis **(SLP)**
Morris, Mrs Paula F **(SLP)**
Mullendore, Dr James M **(SLP A)**
Murphy, Mrs Connie J **(SLP)**
Nudo, Dr Lawrence A **(SLP A)**
Nunn, Mrs Carolyn M **(SLP)**
Ryan, Mrs Elizabeth MacKle **(SLP)**
Sanderson, Mrs Sandra A **(SLP)**
Seacrist, Anne M
Stafford, Mrs Evelyn S **(SLP)**
Stalling, Judith E **(SLP)**
Steinau, Stanley J **(SLP)**
Stelling, Martha D **(SLP)**
Stoner, Mrs Julia B **(SLP)**
Thompson, Bonnie Baker
Tippett, Sally DeWitt **(SLP)**
Travis, Teresa L **(SLP)**
Trompeter, Joyce L **(SLP)**
Viers, Mrs Davenda Allen **(SLP)**
Walvoord, Barbara B **(SLP)**
Willis, Mary Ann **(SLP)**
Winn, Mrs Victoria L **(SLP)**
Wissel, Mrs Mary C **(SLP)**
Wolters, Brenda **(SLP)**

Peoria Heights
Adams, Mrs Renee P S **(SLP)**
Lambert, Mrs Susan Therese **(SLP)**
Rupert, Mrs Catherine **(SLP)**

Peru
Weskerna, Gail B **(SLP)**

Petersburg
Spath, Kathy B **(SLP)**

Pittsfield
Little, Odette Kay **(SLP)**
Maher, Mrs Angela Maria **(SLP)**

Plainfield
Kovacik, Mrs Dawn R **(A)**

Polo
Bowlin, Tina M McLean **(SLP)**

Pontiac
Curry, Joan E **(SLP)**

Posen
Mikrut, Terry Agnes **(A)**

Prairie View
Kwiecinski, Bruce Gerard **(A)**

Preemption
Robb, Delores A

Princeton
Dahlen, Elizabeth **(SLP)**

Prospect Heights
Dean, Karen J **(A)**

Quincy
Harris, Willie V **(SLP)**
Obrock, Ellen L **(SLP)**
Siebers, Mrs Judith M K **(SLP)**

Rantoul
Sessoms, Mrs Melody Ann **(A)**

Richton Park
Baker, Jill Andrea
Bliss, Mrs Dorothy A **(SLP)**
Goode, Jay M **(A)**
Jones, Dr Mary E **(SLP)**
MacCracken, Ellen Louise **(SLP)**
Peterson, Susan B **(SLP)**
Reithal, Kathryn Frances **(SLP)**
Reynolds, Mrs Marylou F **(SLP)**
Tenty, Linda Anderson **(SLP)**

River Forest
Adducci, Helen Josephine **(A)**
Bray, Mrs Deborah Rea **(SLP)**
Handel, Mrs Janice A **(A)**
Holmes, Mrs Judith C **(SLP)**
Lecrone, Susan Kay **(SLP)**
O'Brien, Mary E **(SLP)**
Sheline, Linda M **(SLP)**

River Grove
Mahoney, Mrs Susan Ann **(SLP)**
Malnar, Debra D **(SLP)**

Riverside
Anderson, Jenifer Lyn
Kastenholz, Maribeth Ann **(SLP)**
McHatton, Mrs Laurene Hanlon **(SLP)**
Moser, Mrs Hannah S **(A)**

Riverwoods
Greene, Mrs Beverly Katz **(A)**
Haley, Judy **(SLP)**

Roanoke
Sauder, Frank D **(SLP)**

Robbins
Payne, Mrs Eva L T **(SLP)**

Rochelle
Chaplin, Mrs Beulah Mae **(SLP)**

Degolier, Mrs Elinor J **(SLP)**
McNamee, Melissa St George **(SLP)**

Rock City
Fischer, Natalie B **(SLP)**

Rock Falls
Krabbenhoeft, Cathy A

Rock Island
Coyner, Marilyn R **(SLP)**
Davis, Dr Donald C **(SLP)**
Faigen, Mrs Rogene M **(SLP)**
Frank, Mrs Patricia Ann **(A)**
Heinze, Mrs Barbara A **(SLP)**
Johnson, Mrs Karin L L **(SLP)**
Lange, Michael W **(SLP)**
Lemon, Pamela G **(SLP)**

Rockford
Berry, Dr Mildred F **(SLP)**
Butler, Mrs Debra Kay **(SLP)**
Christen, Mrs Marjorie Trainor **(SLP)**
Cicolello, Beverly **(SLP)**
Clayton, Lawrence G **(A)**
Cook, Mary S **(SLP)**
Debes, Phyllis R **(SLP)**
Dewey, Ellen Gano **(SLP)**
Diekelman, Mrs Suzanne M **(SLP)**
Doubek, Mrs Barbara A **(SLP)**
Foltz, Michael J **(A)**
Franzen, Kathleen A **(SLP)**
Gallant, Susan J **(SLP)**
Grusy, Ronald E **(SLP)**
Guedet, Mrs Ann F **(SLP)**
Harryman, Elizabeth **(SLP)**
Hartinger, Joel D **(A)**
Hartman, Melody Becker **(A)**
Hofflund, Violet Marian **(SLP A)**
Hoffman, Dr Jeanette A **(SLP)**
Knodle, Mrs Lauren M **(SLP)**
La Bella, Renee **(SLP)**
Miller, Leigh Ann **(A)**
Molitor, Guy Thomas **(A)**
O'Toole-Granberry, Mrs Cynthia O **(SLP)**
Pfau, Mrs Margaret Klym **(SLP)**
Rittmanic, Dr Paul A **(SLP A)**
Saichek, Susan Lynn **(SLP)**
Saint Blancard, Carol Ann
Schuster, Cheryl Jahn **(SLP)**
Seiler, Mrs Amy A **(SLP)**
Shaver, Robert S **(SLP)**
Smith, Mrs Sheila L **(SLP)**
Stevens, George H **(SLP)**
Sturtevant, Arlene Frances **(SLP)**
Sudderberg, Mrs Jane Marie **(SLP)**
Traser, Mrs Erin McKee **(SLP)**
Valaitis, Carol S **(SLP)**
Von Holten, Mrs Lori Jean **(SLP)**
Wholey, Mrs Marilyn K **(SLP)**
Wright, Mrs Judy Merrilyn **(SLP)**
Young, Elizabeth **(SLP)**
Zerebny, Roman **(A)**

Rockingford
Foecking, Ann Leslie **(SLP)**

Rockton
Herrick, Susan A **(SLP)**

Rolling Meadows
Appleby, Rena Beth
Hansel, Mrs Susan **(A)**
Ness, Vicki Lynn **(SLP)**
Zelgart-Evans, Jane K **(SLP)**

Roscoe
Brook, Mrs Jane J **(A)**
Spandet, Diane C **(SLP)**

Roselle
Labelle, Dr Joseph L **(SLP)**
Nash, Mrs Georgia E **(SLP)**
Wisinski, Mrs Judith **(SLP)**

Round Lake Beach
Glay, Mrs Karen Rynish **(A)**

Roxana
Stickels, Dorothy L V

Salem
Goostree, Mary Carol **(SLP)**
McLaughlin, Florence E **(SLP)**
Voss, Barbara T **(SLP)**

Sandwich
Werner, Mrs Ellen O **(SLP)**

Savoy
Dahlem, Mrs Laura Theil **(SLP)**

Schaumburg
Balogh, Mrs Trudy C **(SLP)**
Brown, Michael J **(SLP)**
Fairchild, Mrs Nancy J **(SLP)**
Hagan, Mrs Debra L **(SLP)**
Kucharski, Mrs Kimberlea Panuce **(SLP)**
Lande, Mrs Briana L N **(SLP)**
Larkin, Mrs Alecia Stafford **(SLP)**
Lauer, Marianne **(SLP)**
Lesniak, Mrs Donna Lynn **(SLP)**
Lewis, Peta Janice **(A)**
Norris, Mrs Diane L **(SLP)**
Pacer, Sally A **(SLP)**
Photos, Maria **(A)**
Rhodes, Mrs P Joyce **(SLP)**
Salemi, Joseph **(SLP)**
Smith, Marlene Therese
Stark, Mary Beth Van Osten **(SLP)**
Trinwith, Gail E **(SLP)**
Werner, Mrs Susan Angela **(SLP)**
Wilke, Star Wood **(SLP)**
Wise, Deborah L **(SLP)**
Zink, Mrs Barbara A **(A)**

Scott AFB
Prichard, Mrs Deborah Gray **(SLP)**

Seneca
Reardon, Mrs Nina A

Seymour
Difilippo, Mrs Suzanne D **(SLP)**

Shelbyville
Brownfield, Mrs Janet S **(SLP)**

Sherman
Heisler-Rapoff, Mrs Valerie A **(SLP)**
Peterman, Mrs Vicki Vaughn **(SLP)**
Venkatesh, Mrs Sreedevi **(SLP A)**
Walsh, Lois G **(SLP)**

Shorewood
Zamora, Mrs Barbara L **(SLP)**

Skokie
Baranchik, Debra H K **(SLP)**
Bass, Mrs Iris Goldberh **(SLP)**
Berman, Mrs Lois M **(SLP)**
Bertucci-Maratea, Susan **(SLP)**
Blumofe, Amy Wulf **(SLP)**
Cammarata, Mrs Ann M **(SLP)**
Camnitz, Amy S **(SLP)**
Cherney, Leora Reiff **(SLP)**
Corbett, Jodi G **(SLP)**
Doty, Maureen A **(A)**
Dvoret, Ken R **(A)**
Fine, Janis B **(SLP)**
Karlin, Andrea S **(A)**
Leeb, Mrs Sherry Samson **(SLP)**
Levy, Mrs Inez B **(SLP)**
Margolis, Norma C **(SLP)**
Meltzer, Mrs Evelyn S **(SLP)**
Reich, Tamara J **(SLP)**
Reiff, Sharyn Lachman **(SLP)**
Richman, Mrs Ann R **(SLP)**
Sherman, Susan L **(A)**
Stone, Mrs Harriet Cohen **(SLP)**
Tavormina, Barbara L **(SLP)**
White, Dr Kathleen **(SLP)**
Wolinsky, Steven Wayne **(A)**

Sleepy Hollow
Fendler, Mrs Marla Jacobson **(SLP)**

Sedlak, Mrs Ginnie Deangelis **(SLP)**

South Barrington
Barad, Mrs Dianne D **(SLP)**

South Chicago Heights
Wegrzyn, Mrs Brenda J C

South Holland
Buoscio, Ronald M **(SLP)**

Spring Grove
Eckardt, Judith Borchardt **(SLP)**

Spring Valley
Happ, Karen R **(SLP)**
Kozikowski, Mary A **(SLP)**

Springfield
Beveridge-Wavering, Mrs Agnes **(SLP)**
Bretz, Mrs Barbara A B **(SLP)**
Crain, Mrs Sheila F **(SLP)**
Cullen, Margaret **(SLP)**
Curtiss, James Willard **(SLP)**
Fisher, Dayna P
Glynn, Joni Lee **(SLP)**
Green, Evelyn M **(SLP)**
Green, Sharon H **(A)**
Hanisits, Christine Marie **(A)**
Johnson, Cynthia Ann **(SLP)**
Ketterer, Connie **(SLP)**
Koepke, Sandra Hann **(SLP)**
Lee, Virginia G **(SLP A)**
Long, Mrs Alice Jo **(SLP)**
Matthews, Kathleen Marie **(A)**
McDonald, Joan K **(SLP)**
Mlacnik, Mrs Victoria Sowinski **(SLP)**
Mosley, Mrs Eleanor R **(SLP)**
Mulholland, Elizabeth Lucille
Noska, Mrs La Vonne I **(SLP)**
Oliveri, Paula Jean **(SLP)**
Robinson, Mrs Kathleen L **(SLP)**
Roth, Mrs Julie Ann **(SLP)**
Strohmeyer, Karen Lynn
Swain, Dr Charles E, Jr **(SLP A)**
Thomas, Constance Ann **(SLP)**
Varney, Mrs Carol Ann **(SLP)**
Wancket, Sari M **(SLP)**

St Anne
Bachand, Mrs Patricia S **(SLP)**
Sutherland, Martin **(SLP)**

St Charles
Blahut, Donald C **(A)**
Blahut, Mrs Ingrid **(A)**
Buckham, Mrs Barbara A **(SLP)**
Bugh, Judith R **(SLP)**
Harnish, Janet A **(SLP)**
Kelso, Mrs Joanne P **(A)**
Mathers, Marilyn Sue **(SLP)**
Nicholson, Mrs Sandra **(SLP)**
Pelman, Kathleen Grace **(SLP)**
Reynolds, Mrs Catherine **(A)**
Smidt, Janet C **(SLP)**
Van Slyke, Mrs Patricia A **(SLP)**
Wall, Mary Ellen **(SLP)**
Walls, Wilma Margarita **(A)**
Wick, Mrs Jacquelyn Lande **(SLP)**
Witt, Mrs Linda H **(A)**
Wittenstrom, Barbara B **(SLP)**

St Joseph
Ball, Jennifer Leigh **(SLP)**

Staunton
Tiburzi, James **(SLP)**

Steger
Walkley, Dawn Dodder **(SLP)**

Sterling
Carpenter, Laurence John **(A)**
Henson, Mrs Evelyn Bruns **(SLP)**
Lew-Stolzoff, Angela A **(A)**
Martin, Mary Arney **(A)**
Peterson, Mrs Lynn J **(SLP)**

Stockton
Levan, Mrs Kathleen **(SLP)**

Streamwood
Bush, Janie P **(SLP)**
Doshier, Mrs Ronita Kay **(A)**
Rummelhart, Patricia D **(SLP)**
Stier, Mrs Carolyn Schaefer **(SLP)**

Streator
Beutke, Kenneth Paul **(SLP)**
Kreier, Kathi Sue
Richards, Mrs Julia Ficek **(SLP)**

Summit
Roza, Robert T **(SLP)**

Sumner
Cotterell, Mrs Kathy L **(SLP)**

Sycamore
Schairer, Mrs Loretta Martin **(SLP)**
Sinclair, Mrs Janet K **(SLP)**
Wienke, Susan Allyson

Taylor Ridge
Coon, Merriel C **(SLP)**
Troxell, Christine **(A)**

Taylorville
Akers, Edwin L **(SLP)**
Butler, Mrs Jill Cosby **(SLP)**
Emerson, Mary Michele **(SLP)**
White, Barbara W **(SLP)**

Thompsonville
Wilson, Terri K **(SLP)**

Tinley Park
Caputo, Susan Marie **(SLP)**
Chicvara, Joann M **(SLP)**
Dovantzis, Mrs Marylou Buckler **(A)**
Feldner-Pikula, Mrs Janeen M **(SLP)**
Gumz, Mrs Lynn M **(SLP)**
Murphy, Mrs Susan Lee **(SLP)**
Rapinchuk, Mrs Laurie E **(SLP)**
Rompala, David J **(SLP A)**
West, Mrs Margy Theresa **(SLP)**

Tremont
Brown, Mrs Carol T **(SLP)**

Troy
Mersinger, Sue Ann
Wells, Mrs Linda Dianne **(SLP)**

Tuscola
Best, Lorraine D **(SLP)**
Chaplin, Mrs Cathy M **(SLP)**

University Park
Conrad, Dr Carolyn Thera **(SLP)**
Goodman-Malamuth, Dr Leo, II **(SLP)**
Lowe, Dr John, III **(SLP)**
Vorwerk, Susan J R **(SLP)**
Yacullo, Dr William S **(A)**

Urbana
Ahart, Mrs Alice G **(SLP)**
Ascher, Christine Ann
Barry, Mrs Jane D **(SLP)**
Baszler, Stephanie Ann **(SLP)**
Black, Jennifer Marrer **(A)**
Des Jardins, Jane S **(SLP)**
Edwards, Linda Kathleen **(SLP)**
Evans, Mary Lee **(SLP)**
Goldacker, Frank E **(SLP)**
Griffiths, Scott Keith **(A)**
Hall, Janice **(SLP)**
Hall, Mrs Kelly Dailey **(SLP)**
Harris, Patricia A **(SLP)**
Hunt, Tracey L **(SLP)**
Iversen, Mrs Judith A **(A)**
Johnson, Frances L **(SLP)**
Kalinka, Mrs Marian Quinn
Kizer, Mrs Julia Bante **(SLP)**
Loftiss, Eugene W **(A)**
Miller, Mrs Joan S **(SLP)**
Miron, Mrs Helen K **(SLP)**

Murray, Nancy Ann **(SLP A)**
Novak, Denise Foss **(A)**
Osterling, Ann M **(SLP)**
Paden, Dr Elaine P **(SLP)**
Porter, Belinda J **(SLP)**
Salas-Provance, Marlene B **(SLP)**
Sanders, Dr Lois Joan **(SLP)**
Stack, Mrs Christine R **(SLP)**
Urborg, Anita M **(SLP)**
Wachtel, Jayne Miller **(SLP)**
Weaver, Dr John B **(SLP)**
Weber, Jean A

Vandalia
Boch, Mrs Caryl L **(SLP)**

Vernon Hills
Fine, Susan Kaplan **(A)**
Schrepfer-Mekemson, Sheryl **(SLP)**
Siedleck, Teri Moser **(SLP)**
Tortorice, Pamela Jane **(SLP)**
Wohlrab, Lisa Marie

Versailles
Staton, Mrs Deborah P **(SLP)**

Villa Grove
Knox, Ann Elizabeth **(SLP)**

Villa Park
Ashworth, Mrs Michelle A **(A)**
Brown, Michele G **(A)**
Celli, Anita M **(SLP)**
Farrimond, Mrs Glenda H
Lynch, Lauren L **(SLP)**
Mayworm, Sylvia L **(SLP)**
McInerney, Judy Peplowski **(SLP)**
Novak, Mrs Janet Eaton **(SLP)**
Srbeny, Joy Brown **(SLP)**
Zeitler, Mrs Jill Richey **(SLP)**

Virginia
Trone, Jill Phillips **(SLP)**

Walnut
Hansen, Nancy L B **(SLP)**

Warrenville
Finnegan, Mrs Carolyn Marie **(SLP)**
Marseille, Patricia A **(SLP)**
Vicino, Mrs Jeroma L **(SLP)**
Wood, Mrs Rachel S **(SLP)**
Worth, Dr Loanne L

Washington
Beard, Mrs Diane Y **(SLP)**
Dorward, Agnes K **(SLP)**
Venegoni, Mary Margaret **(SLP)**

Wauconda
Krimmel, Mrs Margaret W **(SLP)**
Kwit, Paula D **(SLP)**
Lapin, Mrs Monica Ann M **(SLP)**
Riordan, Patricia Martin **(SLP)**
Van Hagey, Mrs Connie W **(SLP)**

Waukegan
Beiriger, Mrs Antonia A **(SLP)**
Bickham, Carol M **(SLP)**
Borkman, Nancy L **(SLP)**
Brett, Richard J **(SLP)**
Hawkins, Mrs Mary E W **(SLP)**
Hewlett, Catherine Margaret **(SLP)**
Monnier, Wilnette E **(SLP)**
Morris, Mrs Karen Pawlowski **(A)**
Serdar, Mrs Marla Joy **(SLP)**
Vickers, William E **(SLP)**

Wayne
Reed, Mrs Nikki Doreen **(SLP)**

West Chicago
Frey, Rosemarie C **(SLP)**
Sorensen, Nancy E **(SLP)**
Van Buren, Annette Duckert **(SLP)**

West Dundee
Lane, Mrs Tracie L **(SLP)**
McCarthy, Mrs Monica Van Vleet **(SLP)**
McCoy, Barbara Isabel **(SLP)**

Westchester
Dugo, Susan M **(SLP)**
Fogg, Deborah A **(SLP)**
Foote, Mrs Carol Jean **(SLP)**
Hollowed, Barbara Lynn
Koehnemann, Donald F **(SLP)**
Lamich, Mrs Kathleen Horan **(SLP)**
Rollins, Mrs Kara M **(SLP)**
Thompson, Mrs Claire R **(SLP)**
Xenakis, Andrew G **(SLP)**

Western Springs
Anderson, Mrs Janice S **(A)**
Bacon, Mary J **(SLP)**
Benedek, Diane K **(A)**
Cumby, Polly B **(SLP)**
Denny, Mary L S **(SLP)**
Fleming, Mrs Susan K **(SLP)**
Frigo, Mrs Sylvia Alexandra **(SLP)**
Gemmell, Terrance G **(A)**
Houghton, Marion F **(SLP)**
Kane, Bridget R **(A)**
Leenheers, Mrs Karen Woerner **(SLP)**
Mahan, Dr Guy H **(SLP)**
Mayer, Carol A M **(SLP)**
O'Ryan-Fox, Irene R **(SLP)**
Stiemann-Brown, Mrs Kathleen T **(SLP)**
Wecker, Mrs Susan A **(SLP)**

Westmont
Bonet, Mrs Jeanne Spinoso **(SLP)**
Kish, Karen L **(SLP)**
Maxwell, Mrs Donna Hesslau **(SLP)**
Rogan, Susan Denise **(A)**
Schupbach, Joanne E **(SLP A)**
Tintera-Jacobs, Karen A **(SLP)**
Wilson, Nancy A **(A)**
York, Julie A **(SLP)**

Wheaton
Brown, Sue Ellen **(SLP)**
Cook, Mrs Katherine **(SLP)**
Costenero, Mrs Joan M **(SLP)**
Cummings, Mrs Laura **(SLP)**
Dalby, Mrs Pamela **(SLP)**
Figi-Murzyn, Mrs Denise Ann **(SLP)**
Goodman, Rebecca A **(SLP)**
Hasegawa, Mrs Joanne G **(SLP)**
Hawkins, Alicia Wylie **(SLP)**
Hutchins, Bradley **(SLP)**
Jordan, Marya T **(SLP)**
Kmetz, Julianne **(SLP)**
Laesch, Kelley Bowers **(SLP)**
Larkin, Mrs Patricia Jo **(SLP)**
Larowe, Mrs Barbara **(SLP)**
Lothers, Dr William T **(SLP)**
Lutz, Mrs Judith G **(SLP)**
Madeira, Mrs Shelley S **(SLP)**
Nold, Mrs Sally Smith **(SLP)**
Nystrom, Dr Clarence L **(SLP)**
Olson, Judith Buell
O'Rourke, Mrs Melanie Z **(SLP)**
Raack, Catherine Brown **(SLP)**
Roberts, Mrs Susan M **(SLP)**
Skarin, Dr Brenda Dudley **(SLP)**
Skow, Mrs Nancy Lee **(SLP)**
Thornburg, Mrs Dianne Ghent **(SLP)**
Williams, Mrs Janis Marie **(SLP)**

Wheeling
Baltowski, Marianne **(A)**
Burns, Mrs Bethany A **(SLP)**
Connell, Phil J **(SLP)**
Duling, Mrs Leah Obert **(SLP)**
Elliott-Blondin, Mrs Robin Ann
Eymann, Kristy A **(SLP)**
Fischman, Ilene Shapiro **(A)**
Hillner, Mrs Kathleen A **(SLP)**
Mihaly-Waldman, Janet Sue **(SLP)**
Trombetta, Marla Handmaker **(A)**
Wolford, Mrs Ellen Wolff **(A)**

White Hall
Surbeck, Kathryn Silvis **(SLP)**

Willow Springs
Ryan, Patrice M **(SLP)**

Willowbrook
Bergstrom, Sue A **(SLP)**
Dorgan, Mrs Barbara G **(SLP)**
Johnson, Mrs Margaret Mary **(SLP)**
Kilgren, Lori Ann **(SLP)**

Wilmette
Addy-Cantieri, Carol **(SLP)**
Braskamp, Frederick **(SLP)**
Brentan, Anne G **(SLP)**
Campbell, June Haerle **(SLP)**
Clark, Geraldine **(SLP)**
Decker, Mrs Joann A **(SLP)**
Desser, Mrs Linda **(SLP)**
Dunn-Engel, Dr Elaine **(SLP A)**
Fishman, Merle A **(A)**
Gideon, Mrs Sheila Sered **(SLP)**
Gold, Mrs Phyllis G **(SLP)**
Gomberg-Hirsch, Beth M **(SLP)**
Keer, Mrs Barbara D **(SLP)**
Logemann, Jerilyn Ann **(SLP)**
Lunz, Ellen D **(SLP)**
Malstrom, Linda K **(SLP)**
Okrent, Mrs Kathleen Mary **(A)**
Petersen, Mrs Donna V **(SLP)**
Potechin, Dr Gail Carol **(SLP)**
Rassi, Judith A **(A)**
Rom, Patricia **(SLP)**
Rosen, Arlene S **(SLP)**
Singerman, Mrs Susan H **(SLP)**
Taylor, Mrs Margaret M **(SLP)**
Timmis, Thomas W **(SLP)**
Tzanetopoulos, Karen Nelson **(SLP)**
Weaver, Mrs Catherine **(SLP)**
Wilber, Dr Laura Ann **(SLP A)**
Zander, Mrs Janet Sue **(SLP)**

Wilmington
Johnson, Constance Cowing **(SLP)**

Winfield
Anderson, Frances S **(SLP)**
Miller, Marta G **(SLP)**

Winnetka
Carey, Mrs Mary F **(SLP)**
Economou, Helen M **(SLP)**
Molinary, Dolores H **(SLP)**
Sugden, Mrs Frances B **(SLP)**

Winthrop Harbor
Clarke, Michael J **(SLP)**

Wood Dale
Gober, Carol A **(SLP)**

Wood River
Doughney, Mrs Sharon Perozzi

Woodridge
Ahrens, Jill Ann **(SLP)**
Baum, Lori Jean **(SLP)**
Collins, Teresa Kay **(SLP)**
Guyette, Thomas W **(SLP)**
Henry, Mary Geralyn **(SLP)**
Hughes-Fenchel, Carolyn P
Jastrzab, Joyce A **(SLP)**
Jenkins, Mrs Marija M **(A)**
Kalec, Ann Elizabeth **(SLP)**
Larose, Giselle Mary **(A)**
Logeman, Mrs Deborah J **(SLP)**
Manuell, Karen E Hassmer **(SLP)**
Molek, Mrs Christine Marie **(SLP)**
Sallmann, Nancy Ann **(SLP)**
Sullivan, Kathleen M **(SLP)**
Tower, Mrs Nancy Ruth **(SLP)**

Woodson
Malone, Terry P **(SLP)**

Woodstock
Donato, Elizabeth Ann **(A)**
Prichard, Carole J **(SLP)**
Raymond, John W **(SLP)**
Riner, Mrs Elaine Bottari **(SLP)**
Short, Mrs Judith H **(A)**
Voss, Carla Jo **(SLP)**

Worth
Stack, Frances M **(SLP)**

Yorkville
Lavin, Nancy J **(SLP)**

Zeigler
Sweeney, Mrs Mary G **(A)**

Zion
Ford, Donna Lynn **(SLP)**
Nelson-Lehman, Mrs Susan L **(SLP)**

INDIANA

Albany
Niner, David K **(SLP)**
Niner, Mrs Holly Lee **(SLP)**

Anderson
Bailey, Mrs Beth Ann **(SLP)**
Gale, Linda C K **(SLP)**
Gomer, Mrs Betty Jean **(SLP)**
Hare, Timothy R **(SLP)**
Hoover, Hal N **(A)**
Jack, Mrs Mary D **(SLP)**
Lakes, Mrs Dana L **(SLP)**
Lightfoot, Jean E **(SLP)**
Lynch, Beverly Jean **(A)**
Miller, Harriett Leggett **(SLP)**
Poffenbarger, Kathryn L **(SLP)**
Reed, Mrs Martha K **(SLP)**
Sheward, Lois Ellen W **(SLP)**

Arcadia
Stover, Gale Lynn **(SLP)**

Auburn
Thompson, Mrs Deborah J **(SLP)**

Bainbridge
Jackson, Mrs Martha F **(SLP)**

Battle Ground
Smith, Theresa A **(A)**
Zangari, Carole **(SLP)**

Bedford
Elliott, Phyllis R **(SLP)**
Pitman, Mrs Rosamond M

Bicknell
Phipps, Mrs Mary Elizabeth **(SLP)**

Bloomingdale
Pendleton, Mrs Juliene R **(SLP)**

Bloomington
Anderson, Jean L **(SLP)**
Andrews, Dr Moya L **(SLP)**
Bosin, Mrs Elizabeth W **(SLP)**
Cokely, Jeffrey A **(A)**
Cromer, Patricia A **(SLP)**
Crowe, Mrs Beth Ann **(SLP)**
Densmore, Ann E **(SLP)**
Devane, Gladys F **(SLP)**
Dinnsen, Daniel A
Duckett, Kathy **(SLP)**
Elbert, Dr Mary F **(SLP)**
Epstein, Dr Aubrey **(A)**
Espinoza-Varas, Blas
Garner, Mrs Carolyn Ball **(A)**
Garrison, James H **(SLP)**
Gelfer, Dr Marylou Pausewang **(SLP)**
Geltman, Carol Lynn **(A)**
Gierut, Dr Judith A **(SLP)**
Gospel, Mrs Mary Dragoo **(SLP)**
Gousha, Mrs Catherine **(SLP)**
Hall, Mrs Cathleen Thompson **(SLP)**
Harman, Mrs Deborah Rae **(SLP)**
Heller, Mrs Audrey B **(SLP)**
Hipskind, Dr Nicholas M **(A)**

Hultz-Sheriff, Mrs Georgia **(SLP)**
Humes, Dr Larry E **(A)**
Jones, Lynn M **(A)**
Kalhan, Mrs Behroze E **(SLP)**
Kewley-Port, Dr Diane
Marker, Margaret M **(SLP)**
McCrea, Dr Elizabeth S **(SLP)**
Mecca, Annamaria **(SLP)**
Milisen, Dr Robert L **(SLP)**
Naremore, Rita C
Riddle, Laura S **(SLP)**
Ritter, Dr E Gene **(SLP)**
Ryalls, Dr John Herman
Saltzman, Dorothy Jeanne
Shank, Dr Kennon H **(SLP)**
Shea, Patricia A **(A)**
Sterne, Susan L **(SLP A)**
Summers, Mrs Anne C **(SLP)**
Swartzlander, Paula M **(SLP)**
Vicker, Beverly Anne **(SLP)**
Wagner, Barry Thomas **(SLP)**
Watson, Dr Betty U
Watson, Charles Schoff
Williams, Diane L **(SLP)**
Winner, Mrs Michelle Garcia **(SLP)**

Bluffton
Johnson, Ellen Harshey **(SLP)**

Brazil
Reeve, Mrs Leighton M **(A)**
Trout, Mrs Janet L **(SLP)**

Brownsburg
Antony, Mrs Christine Holly **(SLP)**
Fifer, Mrs Sara Jane **(SLP)**
Snyder, Mrs Ruth **(SLP)**
Zarich, Mrs Karen L **(SLP)**

Cambridge City
Fain, Mrs Vicki C **(SLP)**
Hodowal, Mrs Deborah Anne C **(SLP)**

Carmel
Bryant, Mrs Barbara L **(SLP)**
Busard-Cates, Susan **(SLP)**
Campbell, Kathryn M **(A)**
Donahue, Diann F **(SLP)**
Gibstine, Mary A S **(SLP)**
Gilday, Mrs Sheila Q **(SLP)**
Hofeling, Christine Mary S **(SLP)**
Holbert, Mrs Susan M **(SLP)**
Josephson, Mrs Jane C **(SLP)**
Kainrath, Marilyn Joyce **(SLP)**
Kolodny, Dr Marvin R **(A)**
Lewis, Mrs Nancy J H **(SLP)**
McBeath-Benner, Susan **(SLP)**
Nix, Anita L **(SLP)**
Pakula, Cynthia Ann **(SLP)**
Quilligan, Donna H **(SLP)**
Rice, Mrs Marcia E **(SLP A)**
Shilling, Mrs Noel Sue **(SLP)**
Simmons, Mrs Deborah A **(A)**
Van Campen, Luann Elizabeth

Chandler
Mabis, Janet H **(SLP)**

Chesterton
Cobbs, Marlene H **(SLP)**
Holaway, Mrs Kathy Kubasiak
Nallenweg, Mrs Mary K **(SLP)**
Seibert, Mrs Pamela J **(SLP)**
Taylor, Mrs Kathleen Jeffrey **(SLP)**

Cicero
Bell, Ellen R **(SLP)**

Claypool
Wandland, Mrs Cynthia L **(SLP)**

Clinton
Barnes, Martha D **(SLP)**

Columbus
Beavers, Mrs Renee Marie **(SLP)**
Dillon, Mary Ellen **(A)**
Fleming, Mrs Patricia **(SLP)**
Glover, Mrs Karen A **(SLP)**
Henry, Mrs Deborah A **(SLP A)**
Hood, Valerie Hunsinger **(SLP)**
Ingmire, Susan M **(SLP)**
Kevitt, Christine **(SLP)**
King, Mrs Catherine Arthur **(SLP)**
Liddle, Mrs Lorene Swanson **(SLP)**
McDonald, Elaine Ketner **(A)**
Morone, Mrs Rebecca S **(SLP)**
Pence, Mrs Kimberly Lynne **(SLP)**
Sheehy, Mrs Kathleen **(SLP)**
Swank, Mrs Jo-Ann B **(SLP)**
Wexelblatt, Michael A **(A)**

Commiskey
Haney, Dr Russell **(SLP)**

Connersville
Newton, Karen R **(SLP A)**
Thomas, Mary Ann **(SLP)**

Crawfordsville
Bowes, Nancy Jane **(SLP)**
Tunin, Mrs Carolyn S **(SLP)**

Crown Point
Bartholomew, Karen Jane **(SLP)**
Bechthold, Mary Lee
Deloria, Anne Frances **(SLP)**
Mamrila, Mrs Suzanne **(SLP)**
Oglesby, Margo Ann **(SLP)**
Owens, Mrs Sandra Lee **(SLP)**
Proctor, Jaclin K **(A)**
Rieder, Katharine Ann **(SLP)**
Robbins, Deborah Cameron **(SLP)**
Stahr, Karen Coleman **(SLP)**
Townsend, Laura Anna **(SLP)**
Trippel, Mrs Monique Cherie **(SLP)**
Walsh, Mrs Vickie Clark **(SLP)**

Daleville
McManus, Deborah M **(SLP)**

Danville
Belcher, Jane Marie **(A)**
Catt, Mrs Mary J **(SLP)**
Pope, Mary Anne L **(A)**

Dugger
Edwards, Elsie M **(SLP)**
Palmer, Mrs Deborah Hill **(SLP)**

Dyer
Krol, Mrs Sheree Sarko **(A)**
MacKin, Susan C **(A)**
Nutley, Mrs Mandy Hubner **(SLP)**

East Chicago
Kokot, Mrs Nadyne T **(SLP)**
Velez, Dora **(SLP)**
White, Jessie G **(SLP)**

Elkhart
Blackwood, Mrs Toni W **(SLP)**
Breckenridge, Cora S **(SLP)**
Emerson, Mrs Sharon Kay **(SLP)**
Gildner, Christy L **(SLP)**
Healy, Mrs Sandra K **(SLP)**
Meagher, Mary Kane
Odlaug, Mrs Patricia B **(SLP)**
Price, Tobianne **(SLP)**
Rodgers, Dwight Carew **(SLP)**
Romine, Mrs Linda K P **(SLP)**
Russell, Mrs Suan **(SLP)**
Sharp, Mrs Cheryl S **(A)**
Woodhull, Mrs Susan Z **(SLP)**

Ellettsville
Huberty, Marsha L **(SLP)**
Price, Mary Beth McCreery **(SLP)**

Elnora
Etcheson, Mrs Barbara V **(SLP)**

Elwood
Garrison, Sherry Lynne **(A)**
Pettijohn, Mrs Kathy A **(SLP)**
Stanger, Jessica Ann **(SLP)**

Evansville
Balbach, Mrs Julia Jochum **(A)**
Donewald, Marian **(SLP)**
Gray, Mrs Susan Nuss **(SLP)**
Hawa, Elias M **(A)**
Heim, Karen M **(SLP)**
Herre, Debra L **(SLP)**
Jones, Edith T **(SLP)**
Kuhn, Joan Smith **(SLP)**
Lingo, Mrs Maryann S **(SLP)**
Martin, Terry M **(A)**
May, Susan J
Mayer, Mrs Carolyn M **(SLP)**
Miller, Mrs Margaret Bumgardner **(SLP)**
Pendley, Rosemary Verner **(SLP)**
Raibley, Ann B **(A)**
Robinson, Cheryl B **(SLP)**
Robinson, Mrs Lynn D **(A)**
Smith, Mrs Jamie Lynn **(SLP)**
Taggart, Rebecca Sue **(SLP)**
Talbert-Sterne, Cindy G **(SLP)**
Wallander, Mrs Karen S **(SLP)**

Fairland
McGown, Christine L **(SLP)**

Farmersburg
Pruiett, Mrs Mary Clift

Floyds Knobs
Boesing, Mrs Marguerite T Dague **(SLP)**
Krammes, Mrs Lynn H **(SLP)**

Fort Wayne
Amick, David K **(SLP)**
Atkins, Mrs Patricia Lynn **(SLP)**
Auburn, Dr Sandra K **(SLP)**
Barry, Mrs Martha L **(SLP)**
Bowen, Mrs Lynn Wehrenberg **(SLP)**
Carter, Edmund P **(A)**
Carter, Mark P
Clark, Mrs L Genie **(SLP)**
Clevenger, Mary F **(SLP)**
Collier, Pamela Lesak **(SLP)**
Collins, Mrs Junelle M **(SLP)**
Davis, Sue E Anderson **(SLP)**
Dean-Floridis, Dorothy **(SLP)**
Dix, Beth Ann
Doctor, Cynthia K **(SLP)**
Dubenion, Kimberly Rena **(A)**
Everett, Mrs Pamela Joyce **(SLP)**
Fairchild, Janice M **(SLP)**
Farny, Mrs Beth N S **(SLP)**
Federspiel, Marsha J **(SLP)**
Feichter, Jill Robbins **(SLP)**
Flynn, Dr Pauline T **(SLP)**
Ford, Mrs Rebecca L **(SLP)**
Foust, Robin Ann **(SLP)**
Funk, Lisa Kay **(SLP)**
German, Mrs Cathy McCracken
Gossman, Mrs Sandy Kay **(A)**
Green, Brenda M **(SLP)**
Gualdoni, Mrs Valerie Lynn
Henn, Mrs Teresa A **(SLP)**
Hess, Dr Lucille K **(SLP)**
Hill, Elizabeth Ann **(SLP)**
Hiltner, Mrs Rory Anne Musto **(SLP)**
Holman, Mrs Lynn S **(SLP)**
Ketcham, Julie F **(SLP)**
Kincaid, Laura Leanne **(SLP)**
Koehl, Dolores I **(SLP)**
Kornell, Mrs Tamara Ann **(A)**
Lewis, Mrs Nancy S **(A)**
Lowe, Dr R Gregory **(A)**
Maginn, Mary Margaret **(SLP)**
Markham, Amy Joyce **(A)**
Michalski, John A **(A)**
Millard, Mrs Rosemarie Lynn **(SLP)**
Moore, Rosalie Marie **(SLP)**
Mosshammer, Mrs Deborah E **(A)**
Neff, Mrs Marilyn Gennarelli **(SLP)**
Nitterauer, Richard A **(SLP)**
Offerle, Mrs Melanie Reszel **(A)**
Ottenweller, Mrs Laura Hagedorn **(SLP)**
Post-Hyndman, Patricia M **(A)**
Ranochak, Patricia **(SLP)**
Riggs, Mrs Sandra Fritz **(SLP)**
Rosenblatt, Enid S **(SLP)**
Rowe, Mrs Mary K **(SLP)**
Ruffolo, Mrs Linda P **(SLP)**
Rupp, Mrs Virginia H **(SLP)**
Schafer, Diane S **(SLP)**
Scheidt, Mrs Susan Vae **(SLP)**
Schmelz, Mrs Janice S K **(SLP)**
Schrimper, Mrs Patricia Beilhart **(SLP)**
Searer, Wilbur G **(SLP)**
Shepherd, Mrs Cynthia Skurner **(SLP)**
Shively, Larry E **(SLP)**
Skillicorn, Mrs Jane E **(SLP)**
Spillers, Nancy Sansom **(SLP)**
Summy, Cynthia K **(SLP)**
Tarr, Debi Lynne **(SLP)**
Teegardin, Kelly S **(SLP)**
Thomas, Mrs Karen L **(SLP)**
Van Horn, Mrs Janis C **(SLP)**

Fortville
Swim, Mrs Debra Ann **(SLP)**

Franklin
Bryan, Marjorie N **(SLP)**
Miller, Mrs Diane O **(SLP)**

Fremont
Crisman, Mrs Diane R **(SLP)**

Garrett
Miller, Mrs Kelly McFann **(SLP)**

Gary
Akins, Mrs Myra Jean C **(SLP)**
Besmark, Anna Marie **(SLP)**
Prewitt, Deborah F **(SLP)**

Goodland
Hedberg, Mrs Janet A **(SLP)**

Goshen
Bender, Ruth E **(A)**
Stack, Mrs Mary W **(SLP)**
Umble, Dr Roy H

Grabill
Roush, Mrs Mary Renee **(SLP)**

Granger
Andrews, Dianne G **(SLP)**
Bergstrand, Mrs Cynthia M **(SLP)**
Brown, Phyllis Franke **(SLP)**
Fisher, Dorothy **(SLP)**
Harmon, Mary Lou **(SLP)**
Heflick, Lamonte O **(SLP)**
Kujawski, Mrs Cindy D **(SLP)**
McVey, Kerry Lea
Papczynski, Mrs Janice L **(SLP)**

Greencastle
Kelly, Mrs Judith Cox **(SLP)**
MacPhail, Mrs Josephine Ruth **(SLP)**

Greenfield
Anderson, Carol A **(SLP)**
Cox, Mrs Karen L **(SLP)**
Hill, Mrs Baird McDonald **(SLP)**
Kindler, Mrs Barbara Hickey **(SLP)**
Meyerhoff, Mrs Linda M T **(SLP)**
Nixon, Margaret Foster **(SLP)**
Sturm, Mrs Mary. C G **(SLP)**

Greenville
Peak, Denise M **(SLP)**

Greenwood
Alley, James R **(SLP)**
Chatham, Barry Gene
Corbin, Mrs Kathleen K **(A)**
Freed, Sharron Eva **(SLP)**
Hewitt, Veronica G **(SLP)**
Konopka, Mrs Glenda B **(SLP)**
Lewark, Mrs Nancy Marie **(SLP)**

Lines, David L **(SLP)**
May, Janet E **(SLP)**
Powers, Mrs Diane B **(SLP)**
Sanders, Mrs Terri T **(SLP)**
Steeb, Carol L **(A)**

Griffith
Brush, Debra Irene **(SLP)**

Hammond
Geberin, Mrs Joanne White **(SLP)**
Hamlin, Mrs Juanita Rochelle **(SLP)**
Hudson, D Ann **(SLP)**
Nagdeman, Mrs Kathryn J **(SLP)**
Pallotto, Michele Louise **(SLP)**
Rompa, Kathleen Patricia **(A)**
Stanis, Mrs Elizabeth **(SLP)**

Harrodsburg
Olges, Kathleen N **(SLP)**

Hebron
Rice, Robyn R **(A)**

Highland
Gulledge, Kristine Joan **(SLP)**
Partyka, Cynthia Marie **(SLP A)**
Wozniak, Lorraine **(A)**

Hobart
Streit, Gloria Jane **(SLP)**

Hope
Hewitt, Mrs Danielle A **(A)**

Huntingburg
Clark, Mrs Nila M F **(SLP)**

Huntington
Leedy, Mrs Susan C **(SLP)**

Huron
Pruett, Mrs Ruby Toliver **(SLP)**

Indianapolis
Albright, Doris Ann **(SLP)**
Alcala, Mrs Sheri Kae **(SLP)**
Anderson, Charone B **(SLP)**
Armin, Mary Jo **(SLP)**
Armstrong, Sheri A **(A)**
Balmert, Donna M **(SLP)**
Bareither, Mrs Theresa M **(SLP)**
Behringer, Mrs Sandra M **(SLP)**
Berger, Elliott H
Blom, Dr Eric D **(SLP)**
Bollinger-McNall, Mrs Sondra Kay **(SLP)**
Bonham, Mrs Carlene Snider **(SLP)**
Bowman, Mrs Sally Ann **(SLP)**
Bowron, Mrs Dawn Ann **(A)**
Brantingham, Bruce F **(SLP)**
Braunagel, Becky J **(SLP)**
Breeden, Nancy D **(SLP)**
Bright, Florence D **(SLP)**
Buck, Julie Rene' **(SLP)**
Cameron, Mrs Carol B **(SLP)**
Camp, Mrs Cheryl Ann **(SLP)**
Carrigan, Mrs Norma L **(SLP)**
Casey-Harvey, Deborah G **(SLP)**
Chaplin, Robert G **(A)**
Charlebois, Linda Marie **(A)**
Chunn, Patricia C **(SLP)**
Cole, Roselyn R **(SLP)**
Cole-Crawford, Nancy **(SLP)**
Combs, Deadra Havens **(SLP)**
Combs, Mary Elizabeth **(SLP)**
Cornelia, Barbara Jane **(A)**
Correll, Judith T **(A)**
Coyne, Linda Borgmann **(SLP)**
Cronin, Diana Lynn **(SLP)**
Cullar, Ann
Curtis, Janet S **(SLP)**
Czerwinski, Mrs Charlene Stringer **(SLP)**
Danielson, Mrs Jan M **(SLP)**
Da Silva, Mrs Maria M P
Davis, Susan Elaine **(A)**
Dean, Carol Kaliebe **(SLP A)**
De Innocentes, Maryann Rose **(SLP A)**
Delaney, Mrs Laura Robbins **(SLP)**
Deutsch, Karen G **(SLP)**
Diener, Bethany L
Dilthey-Griggss, Mary Jean **(SLP)**
Drexler, Mrs Geraldine **(SLP)**
Driver, Lois L **(SLP)**
Dunn, Mrs Julia E T **(SLP)**
Dusckas, Sallie Jeanne **(SLP)**
Eberle, Rebecca Dawn **(SLP)**
Elftman, Mrs Elizabeth **(A)**
Engels, Mrs Tamara Lewis **(A)**
Farley, Mrs Debbie Reiff **(SLP)**
Faulkner, Christina Bender **(SLP)**
Fleenor, Mrs Diana Lynne **(SLP)**
Forbes, Mrs Janice M **(SLP)**
French, Mrs Julie Ann **(A)**
Fuller, Dr Carl W **(SLP A)**
Gadbury, Mrs Kathryn Miller **(SLP)**
Garrett, Mrs Deloris B **(SLP)**
Gebhardt, Dr Carol J **(A)**
Geddes, David Andrew **(A)**
Gray-Richardson, Laurel **(A)**
Greever, Glenna Sue **(SLP)**
Grove, Mrs Mary Jo R **(SLP)**
Hampton, Mrs Annie Winchester **(SLP)**
Hart, Mrs Virginia **(SLP)**
Hartz, Mrs Paula Ann **(SLP)**
Heck, Mrs Frances A **(SLP)**
Holzhausen, Mrs Julie Kay
Hornaday, Nila **(SLP)**
Jackson, Mrs Mari Ann Levandowsk **(SLP)**
Joest, Mrs Kathleen Fleming **(SLP)**
Johnson, Mrs Toni D **(SLP)**
Jones, Jeremy K **(A)**
Joyce, Mrs Natalie J **(SLP)**
Kelly, Michele Yvonne **(SLP)**
Kesner, Mrs Betsy Bannen **(SLP)**
Kessler, Kathy Sharon **(SLP A)**
Kienle, Marjorie L **(SLP)**
Kitch, Mrs Connie Joan S **(A)**
Klaus, S Elizabeth **(A)**
Knight, Mrs Shelly Kay **(A)**
Knotts, Jennifer L **(SLP)**
Koch, Elaina Sunas **(SLP)**
Kuhn, Mrs Elizabeth Ellen **(SLP)**
Kurtz, Janet Leigh **(SLP)**
Kyle, Amy Louise **(SLP)**
Lagler, Mrs Claudia A **(SLP)**
Lawrence, Mrs Cynthia Louise **(A)**
Levin, Stephanie Lynn **(A)**
Loser, Cindy P **(A)**
Lupton, Mrs Linda K **(A)**
Lybarger, Mrs Marceda W **(SLP)**
Lynn, Cheryl **(SLP)**
MacHinske, Kevin Arthur **(A)**
Maillet, Cassandra Joan **(A)**
Maultra, Alisa L **(A)**
May, Charlene M **(SLP)**
McGarvey, Susan Denise **(SLP)**
McNeill, Linda E **(SLP)**
Mesalam, Linda M **(SLP)**
Meyers, Carolyn Ann **(SLP)**
Monsey-Kavanaugh, JoAnn **(SLP)**
Moore, Denise Knisel **(SLP)**
Morrell, Mrs Ruth Ann **(SLP)**
Muldrow, Beverly Jo **(SLP)**
Munroe, Kathleen A **(SLP)**
Murphy, Margaret E **(SLP)**
Myres, Wendy A **(A)**
Ney, William I **(SLP)**
Noble, Nancy A **(SLP)**
Nordstrom, Patricia Torri **(A)**
O'Connor, Mrs Suzanne S **(A)**
Osberger, Dr Mary J **(A)**
Oser, Mrs Tamara S **(A)**
Payne, Melitta H **(SLP)**
Payne, Robert H **(A)**
Petrovic, Mrs Kathleen K **(SLP)**
Phillips, Lisa Kay **(SLP)**
Potter, Mrs Donna J **(SLP)**
Prather, Mrs Julia E C **(SLP)**
Pulley, Dawn A **(A)**
Raymond, Henry A **(A)**
Reinholt, Lisa Ann **(A)**
Reitz, Mrs Patricia Schrodt **(A)**
Renshaw, Julia J **(A)**
Robbins, Amy McConkey **(SLP)**
Roberts, Mary D **(SLP)**
Rockafellow, Susan S **(SLP)**
Ross, Susan K **(SLP)**
Roysdon, Valisa Jean **(A)**
Russel, Mrs Gina P **(SLP)**
Russel, Mark **(SLP)**
Sage, Annette Marie
Schipper, Mrs Catherine **(SLP)**
Schrager, Mrs Brenda D **(A)**
Schroeder, Mrs Ann Lawrence **(SLP)**
Secondino, Kathryn Susan **(SLP)**
Seiferth, Ellen Walk **(A)**
Shanks, Dr James C, Jr **(SLP)**
Siegel, Barbara G **(SLP)**
Smanda, Debra S **(SLP)**
Smith, Dr Kathryn J **(SLP)**
Sonday, Dr Francis L **(A)**
Speer, Mrs Jessica Christine **(A)**
Spenia, Lisa A **(SLP)**
Statland, Alexandra **(SLP)**
Steckler, Mrs Susan Elizabeth **(SLP)**
Steele, Lynne Jeck **(A)**
Steenbarger, Mrs Donna D **(SLP)**
Stehman, Helen E S **(SLP)**
Stumpf, Mrs Teresa Flahive **(SLP)**
Talbott, Mrs Sally A **(A)**
Tatman, Linda D **(SLP)**
Taylor, Abigail B **(SLP)**
Thompson, Lynn Christine
Tomasic, Mrs Dorothy Ann **(SLP)**
Tracey, Mrs Susan A **(SLP)**
Trout, Mrs Madonna N **(SLP)**
Tysklind, Mrs Elizabeth S **(A)**
Utter, Julia **(SLP)**
Wagner, Michele Louise **(A)**
Waite, Beth A **(SLP)**
Warner, Patricia **(SLP)**
Warthaw, Lavonne **(SLP)**
Wellman, Beth Cox **(SLP)**
Wetzel, Mrs Dawn Elizabeth **(SLP)**
Weyland, Christina Seaborg **(A)**
Whitaker, Tamara Ann
Whitcher, Mrs Abigail B **(SLP)**
Wilkins, Mrs Angela R
Wouters, Mrs Jenny K **(SLP)**
Wright, Mrs Beverly Brown **(SLP)**
Yaghoubian, Mrs Emily B **(SLP)**
Yates, Mrs Carrie Norris **(SLP)**
Zoller, Mrs Mary N **(SLP)**

Jasper
Lichlyter, Cynthia A
Schneider, Mrs Mary Jane **(SLP)**
Sternberg, Mrs Marsha L Smith **(SLP)**

Jeffersonville
Allen, Mrs Joan L **(A)**
Ballinger, Mrs Susan E **(SLP)**
Fresh, Mrs Jacqueline Finch **(SLP)**
Schipper, Mrs Beverly Lynn **(SLP)**
Stone, Mrs Susan B **(SLP)**

Kokomo
Grady, Mrs Linda D **(SLP)**
Huggins, Mrs Terri Sue **(SLP)**
Long, Gloria K **(SLP)**
Schlais, Mrs Susan Elaine **(SLP)**

La Porte
Anserello, Mrs Kathi Vogt **(SLP)**
Eklund, Mrs Michaeleen **(SLP)**
O'Dell, Evelyn S **(SLP)**
Osenga-Manolovits, Diana L **(A)**
Retseck, Mrs Kathleen Kuzydym **(SLP)**
Welsh, Mrs Janice Marie W **(SLP)**

Lafayette
Allen, George D
Bassett, Katherine Evans **(SLP)**
Binnie, Dr Carl A **(A)**
Bocko, Elizabeth Ann **(SLP)**
Bower, Mrs Julie Ann **(A)**
Brennan, Gayle C J **(SLP A)**
Caccavo, Dr Mary T **(A)**
Cecilsennett, Teresa Marie **(SLP)**
Cochran, Mrs Debra Jo **(SLP)**
Dunn, Kristin Kiekhaefer **(SLP)**
Frye, Dorothy A **(SLP)**
Fuller, Dr Donald Ray
Hill, Donna Brooks **(SLP)**
Hover-Parker, Teri Lynn **(SLP)**
Lewis, Debra Lyn **(SLP)**
McFerren, Druscilla Kaye **(SLP)**
Miller, Stephanie Mcllwain **(SLP)**
Mohler, Sally A **(SLP)**
Mulhaupt, Mrs Dorothy Ellen **(SLP)**
Murphy, Debora Sandquist **(SLP)**
Shields, Anne Ruppe **(A)**
Showalter, Robert G **(SLP A)**
Valdez, Dwight R **(A)**

Lanesville
Wahl, Theresa Clark **(SLP)**

Lawrenceburg
Devita, Ann Marisa **(SLP)**
Vorbroker, Mrs Jane Annette **(SLP)**

Lebanon
Schellenberg, Mrs Carol Faye **(A)**
Suggs, Shelly Jones **(SLP)**
Taylor, Pamela Hoffman **(SLP)**

Liberty
Witter, Dr H L **(A)**

Ligonier
Wigent, Mrs Sue A **(SLP)**

Logansport
Edgerly, Mrs Gayle A **(A)**
Lozier, Barbara L **(SLP A)**
Ruhl, Mrs Kelly Sue **(SLP)**

Madison
Gibson-Dossey, Sandra Jean **(SLP A)**
Sullivan, Joanna K **(SLP)**

Marion
Bachnivsky, Mrs Valentina H **(A)**
Blum, Mrs Dana J **(SLP)**
Huber, Mrs Linda K **(SLP)**
Johnson, Robert James **(A)**
Kraai, Mrs Rhonda V **(SLP)**
Lucas, Mrs Patricia J **(SLP)**
Morgan, Teresa Gail **(SLP)**

Martinsville
Dixon, Susan D **(SLP)**
Ruble, Marilou Gerhardt **(A)**
Salamander, Philip **(A)**

Merrillville
Backoff, Lori S
Heidtman, Cathryn I **(SLP)**
Sciackitano, Gwenn **(SLP)**
Shay, Mrs Margaret Irene **(SLP)**
Voelker, Diane J **(A)**

Metamora
Paras, Teresita A **(SLP)**

Michigan City
Argabright, Margaret L **(SLP)**
Bischof, Ellen Marie **(SLP)**
Eades, Kristin G **(A)**
Hahn, Carol Ann
Hathoot, Mary M **(A)**
Jensen, Dianna Leah **(SLP)**
Lee, Mrs Kathryn Lyness
Long, Nancy Michelle **(SLP)**
Martin, Nancy Jane **(SLP)**
Tarasick, Arlene L **(SLP)**
Tokoly, Mrs Alice A P **(SLP)**

Middletown
Shockley, Suzanne H **(SLP A)**

Milan
Davis, Mrs Lynne D **(SLP)**

Mishawaka
Barnett, Rebecca Sue **(SLP)**
Blanchard, Mrs Laurie J **(SLP)**
Davis, Kelley Marie **(SLP)**
Erlandson, Denise Burch
Hodges-Stillson, Cheryl L **(SLP)**
Hoerstman, Karen Lee **(A)**
Ihns, Mary J **(SLP)**
Lovett, Mrs Janet A **(SLP)**
Melda, Keith A **(A)**
Moon, Mrs Caryl **(SLP)**
Nelson, Mrs Cathy Ann
Phillips, Dena A **(SLP)**
Soderberg-Stefanek, Mrs Beth E **(SLP)**

Mitchell
Lee, Teresa Dawn S **(SLP)**

Monticello
Richardson, Mrs Connie D **(SLP)**

Mooresville
Buchanan, Sharon Elizabeth **(SLP)**
Hunteman, Kathy L H **(SLP)**

Morgantown
Olds, Mrs Leesa Kae **(SLP)**

Muncie
Artes, Dr Richard **(SLP)**
Beekman, Mrs Jane Kyhl **(SLP)**
Bode, Janet L **(SLP)**
Brown, Mrs Patricia A **(SLP)**
Clark, Donald I **(A)**
Corey, Mrs Suzanne Kincaid **(SLP)**
Edler, Mrs Marita **(SLP)**
Farling, Glenn T **(SLP)**
Halling, Dan C **(A)**
Hayes, Deborah A **(SLP)**
Heady, Mrs Linda Sue **(SLP)**
Hemeyer, Thomas F **(A)**
Hill, Mrs Carrie Kae **(SLP)**
Hoops, Mrs Helen W **(SLP)**
Hoops, Dr Richard A **(SLP A)**
Houk, Mrs Melanie L **(SLP)**
Kaufman, Mrs Joyce E **(SLP)**
Kolb, Jacqueline S **(SLP)**
Kramer, Dr William L **(SLP)**
Lemon-Updike, Dr Claudia D **(A)**
Lindell, Dr Gary A **(SLP)**
Lindell, Mrs Melinda J **(SLP)**
Martin, Dr Charles W **(SLP)**
Myers, Mrs Barbara L **(SLP)**
Powell, Thomas W **(SLP)**
Ratliff, Mrs Janet Hall **(SLP)**
Repp, Mrs Lora E E **(SLP)**
Ritz, Mrs Susan C **(SLP A)**
Shrack, Mrs Amy J **(A)**
Siebenaler, Ginia K
Stanley, Mrs Margaret D **(SLP)**
Thornburg, Mrs Judith D **(SLP)**
Wood, Tina Marie **(SLP)**
Woodfin, Linda Norris **(SLP)**

Munster
Ajdinovich, Mrs Suzanne P **(SLP)**
Bewley, Mrs Nancy A **(SLP)**
Cafmeyer, April M **(A)**
Glasgow, Kimberly Joanne **(SLP)**
Keil, Mrs Sharon G **(SLP)**
Kyriakides, Laura
Richardson, Sharon A **(A)**
Sufana, Mrs Karen Kicho **(SLP)**

New Albany
Attar, Vickie Lynne **(SLP)**
Baete, Mrs Phyllis Pharis **(A)**
Buchanan, Mrs Susanna W **(SLP)**
Duncan, Kimberly Ann **(A)**
Huber, Kimberly Ann **(SLP)**
Martin, Mrs Kristi Jean **(A)**
Oglesby, Carole S **(SLP)**
Weatherholt, Steven D **(SLP A)**

New Carlisle
Ford, Juilann Marie **(SLP)**

New Castle
Winchester, Madonna R

New Haven
Jones, Mrs Judith S **(SLP)**

New Ross
Wisker, Mrs Nancy Ferree **(A)**

Newburgh
Ahlbrand, Mrs Karen P **(SLP)**
Andis, Jennifer Jean **(SLP)**
Blackford, Mrs Connie L **(SLP)**
Brideweser, Mrs Darlene R **(SLP)**
Brooks, Mrs Jean Naeye **(SLP)**
Hartsaw, Mrs Lee Ann **(SLP)**
Miller, Jane P **(SLP)**
Stringfellow, Mrs Johannah Goodman **(SLP)**
Thrall, Anne Marie **(SLP)**

Noblesville
Burford, Ann Elaine **(SLP)**
Chalfin, Mrs Ellen M **(SLP)**
Hoefer, Sylvia Casper **(A)**
Land, Mrs Carol R **(SLP)**
Milburn, Mrs Lana Jo **(SLP)**
Schneider, Marsha Jolene **(SLP)**
Stitt, Mrs Cheryl Christine **(SLP)**
Zaichek, Mrs Randi Kay **(SLP)**

North Liberty
Anderson, Susan Marie

North Vernon
Dickerson, Linda L **(SLP)**
Knowlton, Mrs Janice Lynne **(SLP)**
Swonder, Linda K **(SLP)**

Oakland City
Whitten, David A **(SLP)**

Osceola
Spradlin, Sally J **(SLP)**

Otterbein
Baker, Helen L **(SLP)**

Parker City
Wright, Sandra Sue **(SLP)**

Pekin
Mason, Carolyn G **(SLP)**

Petersburg
Radcliff, Kendrea D'Lyn **(SLP)**

Pittsboro
Pamula-Murray, Mrs Karen **(SLP)**

Plainfield
Barlow, Karen S **(SLP)**
Deweese, Mrs Pamela D **(SLP)**
Fischer, Mrs Clare O **(SLP A)**
Jenkins, Tina Louise **(SLP)**
Naab, Mrs Jennifer Slagle **(SLP)**
Risley, Mrs Laura Dreiman **(A)**
Rudder, Nancy L **(A)**

Plymouth
Frey, Mrs Marsha **(SLP)**
Hunt, Mrs Jane Evelyn **(SLP)**

Portage
Anderson, Kenneth E **(SLP)**
Largura, Marjorie Jo **(SLP)**
Lehmann, Mrs Joanne Laatsch **(SLP)**
Wilcox, Paulette M **(SLP)**

Portland
Badders, Mrs Bonnie Barrett **(SLP)**
Johnsonbaugh, Mrs Susan H **(SLP)**
McMillan, Mrs Jeanne Kay **(SLP)**

Princeton
Goldberg, Mrs Sharon G **(SLP)**

Ramsey
Schmidt, Mrs Donna Gail

Rensselaer
Raff, Mrs Joan Warrick **(SLP)**

Richmond
Flint, V H **(SLP)**
Hertzog, Bonnie B **(SLP)**
Hull, Mrs Corrine F **(SLP)**
McDermott, Glenn W **(SLP)**
Regal, Darah J **(A)**
Regal, Jeffrey D **(A)**
Rodal, Mrs Jacquelyn Egger **(SLP)**
Terry, Mrs Carole A **(SLP)**
Thompson, Cynthia Susanne **(SLP)**

Rising Sun
Stowell, Mrs Virginia Harrel **(SLP)**

Rochester
Newcomer, Mrs Juleen S **(SLP)**
Smith, Dr Nancy W **(SLP)**
Stephen, Frances Leslie **(SLP)**

Rockville
Shaw, Carla Market **(SLP)**

Rossville
Walter, Janet P **(SLP)**

Schererville
Glover, John D **(SLP)**
Goldsberry, Mrs Gail Edelman **(A)**
Hoffman, Lauren P **(SLP)**
Legler, Mrs Danielle Michaelene **(SLP)**
Mecklenburg, Mrs Deborah V **(SLP)**

Scottsburg
Wilkerson, Mary Ann **(SLP)**

Sellersburg
Muncy, Mrs Denise B **(SLP)**

Selma
Carmichael, Mrs Jennifer J **(SLP)**

Seymour
Bywaters, Mrs Eleanor B **(SLP)**
Dominik, Lygia **(SLP)**
Ralph, Michael Ray
Walter, Mrs Susan Gail **(SLP)**

Shelbyville
McDaniel, Mrs Ann S **(SLP)**

South Bend
Blount, Dr Mary Ann Records **(SLP)**
Bodle, Mrs Carol Ann **(SLP)**
Brown, Heather L **(SLP)**
Burradell, Amy Lee
Clemons, Sara Jayne **(SLP)**
Cook, Michelle Ann **(SLP)**
Craig, Pamela J **(SLP)**
Craig, Dr Richard K **(A)**
Davis, Mrs Khris Mumby **(SLP)**
Donigan, Mary Kellagher **(A)**
Donigan, Rodney Craig **(A)**
Ekart, Sally Ann **(SLP)**
Engels, Laurie E **(SLP)**
Gennicks, Mrs Barbara A **(SLP)**
Goldstein, Fred **(SLP)**
Grover, Cynthia Denise **(SLP)**
Hanstra, Linda Lee **(SLP)**
Hay, Mary Alice **(SLP)**
Hooker, Polly Ann **(SLP)**
Horvath, Mrs Jana Lee M **(SLP)**
Jacobs, Dr Anita Isaacson **(SLP)**
Jarvis, Mrs Julie Ann **(SLP)**
Kallio, Pamela DeBoer **(SLP)**
Lake, Nancy A **(SLP)**
Lynch, Mrs Elizabeth J **(SLP)**
McKinley, Susanna C **(SLP)**
Moore, Charles Glenn **(SLP)**
Moore, Kem E **(A)**
Murphy, Mrs Linda J T **(A)**
Nathanson, Mrs Julie O'Connor **(SLP)**
Olson, Mrs Kathryn S **(SLP)**
Patterson, Mrs Julie Neeley **(SLP)**
Rakestraw, Rebecca C **(SLP)**
Ross, Jill B **(SLP)**
Self, Michele Lynn **(SLP)**
Shock, Charles A, Jr **(A)**
Star, Alice Jo **(SLP)**
Thompson, Mrs Lori Kaye **(SLP)**
Zyrkowski, Mrs Nancy J **(SLP)**

Speedway
Haug, Mrs Mary R **(SLP)**
Patterson, Mrs Kathryn K **(SLP)**

Springport
Kissick, Mrs Donann Hoopingarn **(SLP)**

Star City
Bucks, Mrs Patricia J **(SLP)**

Sullivan
Nichols, Mrs Marilyn Casey **(SLP)**

Sunman
Lauber, Mrs Vicky Sue N **(SLP)**
Norman, Peggy L **(SLP)**

Sweetser
McDonald, Mrs Mary Ann Lefavour **(SLP)**

Tell City
Whitaker, Stephanie **(SLP)**

Terre Haute
Albright, Mrs Susan Colson **(SLP)**
Allega, Nancy Louise **(SLP)**
Baer, Dr Sherwin H **(SLP A)**
Barker, Lynn D **(SLP)**
Baysinger, Mrs Kathleen S **(SLP)**
Begines, Mrs Terry Walker **(A)**
Brinza, Tamera Ann **(A)**
Brown, Mrs Kathleen R **(SLP)**
Buethe, Diane D **(SLP)**
Carpenter, Mrs Janice Grissom
Goodier, Mrs Brenda M **(SLP)**
Goodier, Jay A **(SLP)**
Hagness, Dr Don Edward **(A)**
Hambrecht, Dr Georgia **(SLP)**
Hansen, Lorraine Hendricks **(SLP)**
Heien, Marilyn J **(SLP)**
Kerins, Mrs Elynore P **(SLP)**
Lofland, Kristie Brown **(A)**
Luers, Ann E **(SLP)**
Lusco, Alene M S
Meeker, Joan B **(SLP)**
Melloh, Mrs Crispin Mary **(SLP)**
Oxendine, Karen Ellis **(SLP)**
Pittman, Mrs Susan K **(A)**
Quist, Dr Raymond W **(SLP)**
Randall, Rebecca Sue **(SLP)**
Rowe, Dr Margaret L **(SLP)**
Ruddock, Mrs Gay L **(SLP)**
Sapp, Mrs Helen D **(SLP)**
Thompson, Genelle Huddleston **(SLP)**
Victor, Mrs Lois Ann **(SLP)**
Watts, Mrs Rebecca C **(SLP)**
Williams, Mrs Donna L **(SLP)**
Wolfe, Mrs Kristina Marie **(SLP)**
Wright, Sherrilyn **(SLP)**

Tipton
Atchley, Pamela Sue **(SLP)**
Maynard, Mrs Conita S **(SLP)**

Union City
Threewits, Marla C **(SLP)**

Valparaiso
Anderson, Susan H **(SLP)**
Annen, Mrs Lonette Marie **(SLP)**
Carpenter, Neil E **(SLP)**
Daily, Mrs Mary S **(SLP)**
Dickey, Nancy **(A)**
Drew, Ruby Louise **(SLP)**
Dryer, Kathleen Mary **(SLP)**
Hayford, Cathy R **(SLP)**
Kapke, Christine Ruth
Kashani, Joanne S **(SLP)**
Kostrzeba, Susan Marie **(SLP)**
Little, Mrs Mary E **(SLP)**
McAfee, Mrs Patricia H **(SLP)**

Nantau, Judy L **(SLP)**
Paul, Roger D **(A)**
Pearson, Michele L **(SLP)**

Vevay
Ross, Mrs Rita Waltz **(SLP)**
Stephenson, Bonita K

Vincennes
Lankford, Mrs Isabelle S **(SLP)**
Piper, Mrs Rebecca Ann **(SLP)**
Spurrier, Mrs Jean M A **(SLP)**
Wiegand, Kristy A **(A)**

Warsaw
Elsbury, Christine Carol **(SLP)**
Lenke, Nancy E **(A)**
McCaman, Gary E **(A)**
Southwood, Mrs Jane W **(SLP)**

Washington
Rohweder, Deborah Lynn **(SLP)**

Waynetown
Selby, Mrs Karen J **(SLP)**

Wesport
Franke, Mrs Cindi **(SLP)**

West Lafayette
Ansel, Dr Beth Mindy **(SLP)**
Black, Mrs Judy K **(SLP)**
Blackwell, Pat B **(SLP)**
Boggess, Dr G Jean **(A)**
Bopanna, Dr Ballachanda Belliappa **(A)**
Brackney, Mrs Teresa Marie **(SLP)**
Brown, Mrs Barbara Lynn **(SLP)**
Buhler, Jill L **(SLP)**
Cassidy, Terrence J
Chan, Mrs Brenda Miu-Ying **(SLP)**
Clemons, Mrs Sue Ellen **(SLP)**
Cook, Mrs Madelyn K **(SLP)**
Dorn, Patricia Ann **(A)**
Downard, Mrs Carol Sue **(A)**
Fristoe, Dr MacAlyne **(SLP)**
Gleitman, Ronald
Goldstein, Dr David P **(A)**
Grim, Michael Allan
Hahne, Sharon K **(SLP)**
Hawkins, Mrs Joyce A **(A)**
Hession, Carol M **(A)**
Hickman, Mrs Karen M **(A)**
Irzyk, Barbara Kathleen **(SLP)**
Kangas, Kathleen A **(SLP)**
Keetay, Victoria **(A)**
Koschmann, Dawn Arleen **(A)**
Leonard, Jeanette S **(SLP A)**
Leonard, Dr Laurence B **(SLP)**
Lloyd, Dr Lyle L **(SLP A)**
Loeb, Mrs Diane Frome **(SLP)**
Loeding, Barbara L **(SLP)**
Long, Dr Glenis Raewyn
McFarland, David Harmon, II
McGregor, Karla Kay
Mills, Mrs Mary A **(SLP)**
Montgomery, James Wasson **(SLP)**
Moskal, Nancy **(A)**
Murphy, William P **(SLP)**
Noll, Dr J Douglas **(SLP)**
Ostroy, Zipora P **(SLP)**
Pennington, Penny P **(SLP)**
Piercy, Mrs Susan K **(SLP)**
Raghavendra, Parimala
Ringel, Dr Robert L **(SLP)**
Schmierer, Mrs Kimberly Marie **(A)**
Schwartz, Dr Richard G **(SLP)**
Shaffer, George **(SLP A)**
Shiffman, Mrs Elizabeth **(SLP)**
Smith, Anne
Solomon, Mrs Barbara S W **(SLP)**
Sommer, Anne Elizabeth **(A)**
SooHoo, Leo **(A)**
Stark, Dr Rachel E **(SLP)**
Steer, Dr Mack David **(SLP)**
Steer, Ruth K **(SLP)**
Stimley, Lisa L **(SLP)**
Stimley, Mark A **(SLP)**
Swanson, Lori Ann **(SLP)**
Wallis, Julie Ann **(SLP)**
Weber, Christine Maria
Weingram, Mrs Florence N **(SLP)**
Wilber, Kelly K
Windsor, Jennifer Ann
Zerlin, Dr Stanley

West Terre Haute
Milliren, Brenda F **(SLP)**

Wheatfield
Bradley, Margaret T **(SLP)**

Whiting
Mihalo, Mrs Deborah A **(SLP)**

Winchester
Swindell, Peggy Jo **(SLP)**

Woodburn
Burnett, Mrs Kathleen Smith **(SLP)**

Worthington
Powell, Mrs Teresa B **(SLP)**

Yorktown
Rennie, Mrs Kathleen A **(SLP)**

Zionsville
Harper, Mrs Nancy Neibert **(SLP A)**
Montgomery, Mrs Suzanne V **(SLP)**

IOWA

Adel
Holcomb, Tammi A
Lane-Hill, Carol A **(SLP)**
Pomper, Michael S **(SLP)**

Agency
Trier, Kelly Lynn **(SLP)**
Wheeler, Mrs Grete M **(SLP)**

Albion
Feltz, Mrs Kay Yvonne **(SLP)**

Algona
Adermann, Annette **(SLP)**
Kinne, Mrs L Kay **(A)**

Alton
Mueting, Mrs Karen H **(SLP)**

Altoona
Brown, Mrs Belinda R **(SLP)**
Gillon, Laura Ann **(SLP)**
Lohmeier, Jean A **(SLP)**

Ames
Albright, Shirley Mona **(A)**
Anderson, Mrs Nancy Bales **(SLP)**
Burke-Martin, Laura Ann **(A)**
Daley, Mrs Sue Ann Kenlee **(SLP)**
Doss-Schliesman, Mrs Patricia Marie **(SLP)**
Finn, Mrs Marilyn S **(SLP)**
Gunter, Dr Cheryl Darcel **(SLP)**
Hamilton, Kurt O **(SLP)**
Heady-Erickson, Mrs Barbara J **(SLP)**
Helland, Martha R **(SLP)**
Helms, William A **(A)**
Huntley-Kraus, Nancy Ann **(A)**
Kushner-Johnson, Mrs Miriam Leslie **(SLP)**
Lamkey, Mrs Becky Marie **(SLP)**
Link, Mrs Miriam Ruth
McCartan, Dr Kathleen **(SLP)**
Moen, Mrs Lucille A **(SLP)**
Schneider, Susan L **(SLP)**
Smith, Mrs Judith Ann
Tuttle, Karen M **(SLP)**
Vallier, Dr Fred J **(SLP)**
Venkatagiri, Dr Horabail **(SLP)**
Weiland, Linda E **(A)**
White, Carol Rowene **(SLP)**

Ankeny
Swift, Mrs Karen F **(SLP)**
Swift, Phil I **(SLP)**
Wolvek, Dr Joseph **(SLP A)**

Aplington
Rucksdashel, Mrs Sharon V **(SLP)**

Arthur
Oxendale, James **(SLP)**

Atlantic
Miller, Jill M E **(SLP)**
Spittler, Karen A **(SLP)**

Attumwa
Molek, Christine **(A)**

Audubon
Levis, Mrs Gayle Ann **(SLP)**
Olson, Douglas M **(A)**
Smith, Nancy L **(SLP)**

Baldwin
Cavanagh-Bruns, Cynthia **(SLP)**

Bennett
Goemaat, Jean A **(SLP)**

Bettendorf
Baldes, Robert A **(SLP)**
Bowles, Martha A **(SLP)**
Christensen, Mrs Janet Z **(SLP)**
Dryg, Lori Devore **(SLP)**
Eisenlauer, Mrs Ann L **(SLP)**
Ford, Dr Pamela S **(SLP)**
Foster-Hunter, Mrs Shirley A **(SLP)**
Halfman, Mrs Patricia J **(SLP)**
Hasken, Mrs Janet B **(SLP)**
Heaton, Constance **(SLP)**
Hildebrand, Lezlie A **(SLP)**
Huddleston, Ronald L **(SLP A)**
Jager, Lori L **(SLP)**
Krupke, David L **(SLP)**
Marttila, Joan D **(A)**
Moore, Donna K **(SLP)**
Morency, Claire D **(SLP)**
Morgan, Maria L **(SLP)**
Murray, Mrs Anne M **(SLP)**
Ordona, Heather Ann **(SLP)**
Pohlmann, Karen Trissel **(SLP)**
Sunderbruch, Roberta L **(SLP)**

Bloomfield
Rezai, Mrs Terry F **(SLP)**

Bondurant
Davis, Deborah **(SLP)**
Hood, Jack Richard **(SLP)**

Boone
Gunderson-Moses, Cynthea L **(A)**
Lucas, Jeanne Rossmiller **(SLP)**

Britt
Viamontes, Mrs Karen Marie **(SLP)**

Burlington
Kongable, Trisha Marie **(SLP)**
Krueger, Beverly M **(SLP)**
Minard, Edwin E, II **(A)**
Phillips, Sandra Lea **(A)**
Snowden, Bruce Oswald **(A)**
Strother, Terry Lee **(SLP)**
Swift, Renee Jane **(SLP)**
Van Der Heiden, Edward William **(A)**
Witt, Anne M **(SLP)**
Wright, Linda Fay **(SLP)**

Calmar
Wesle, Cheryl L S **(SLP)**

Camanche
Larsen, Leanne Shaff **(SLP)**
Thomsen, Susan W **(SLP)**

Carroll
Deshaw, Mrs Donna **(SLP)**
Rohlf, Jo Ann **(SLP)**
Simons, Monica Jean **(SLP)**
Stockbridge, Judith L **(SLP)**
Thompson, Karen M **(SLP)**

Cedar Falls
Beykirch, Dr Hugh L **(A)**
Boots, Mrs Myra Ruth **(SLP)**
Carver-Kagy, Deborah L **(SLP)**
Eblen, Roy E **(SLP)**
Fossum, Dr Ernest C **(SLP)**
Hageman, Dr Carlin F **(SLP)**
Harrington, Judith F **(SLP)**
Highnam, Dr Cliff L **(SLP)**
Highnam, Mrs Diane Bell **(SLP)**
Kelly, Mrs Dawn M **(SLP)**
Plakke, Dr Bruce L **(A)**
Pollock, Dr Karen E **(SLP)**
Potter, Lois S **(SLP)**
Relph, Mrs Theresa Lynne **(SLP)**
Romanin, Kay E B **(SLP)**
Schwartz, Dr Ralph J **(SLP A)**
Smaldino, Dr Joseph J **(A)**
Stubbe, Mrs Mary Bolgren **(SLP)**
Waldon, Mrs Gloria B **(SLP)**
Wood, Dr Mildred H **(SLP)**

Cedar Rapids
Aller, Kathleen L **(SLP)**
Anderson, Barbara H **(SLP)**
Boehne, Le Ann F **(SLP)**
Brackey, Mrs Pamela L S **(SLP)**
Brandenburg, Sara A **(SLP)**
Briggie, Ann M H **(SLP)**
Bryant, Mrs Jacqueline F **(SLP)**
Carlson, Claudia Ann **(SLP)**
Claflin, Donna L W **(SLP)**
Colton, Kathleen Cook **(SLP)**
Cowley, Debra **(A)**
Dahle, Alice L **(SLP)**
Edwards, Dr Dorothea B **(SLP)**
Erickson, Jean M **(SLP)**
Frana, Mrs Julie Dolan **(SLP)**
Gasway, Mrs Julie Gay/Hansen **(SLP)**
Kelly, Cheryl Mills **(SLP)**
Larson, Mrs Kristen Hansen **(SLP)**
Lynn, Susan G **(A)**
Mills, Debra Q **(SLP)**
Murphy, Margaret Kelley **(SLP)**
Nagel, Helen Moran **(SLP)**
Nicholson, Cynthia C **(SLP)**
Pate, Terri Lynn **(A)**
Petersen, Tracy Wesbrook **(SLP)**
Polehna, Mrs Priscilla **(SLP)**
Preisser, Debra A **(SLP)**
Romaniszak, Vivian Marie **(A)**
Schaubert, Mrs Lynn M **(A)**
Sebetka, Mrs Patricia M **(SLP)**
Steffensmeier, Anne E **(SLP)**
Weiss, Donna M **(A)**
Wilke, Debra J **(SLP)**

Centerville
Price, Peggy Gayle
Robinson, Raymond A, II **(SLP)**
Sidles, Mrs Sherry Elise **(SLP)**

Charles City
Johnson, Mrs Barbara Zintz **(SLP)**
Sharp, Carol Ann **(SLP)**
Vogelson, Douglas O **(A)**

Cherokee
Brodale, Mrs Vicky Ann **(SLP)**
Rhoads, Mrs Lynn T **(SLP)**
Tisthammer, Ladon A **(SLP)**

Clarinda
Finck, Carolyn D **(SLP)**
Honken, Mrs Connie Halverson **(SLP)**
Mellencamp, Sheila F **(SLP)**

Clarion
Hill, Mrs Connie S **(SLP)**

Clarksville
Voss, Mrs Lee Ann **(SLP)**

Clear Lake
Broghammer, Mrs Jane A **(A)**
Howitz, Michael J

Notestine, Patricia Eireen **(SLP)**
Scherber, Mrs Connie J **(SLP)**
Trembath, Leigh Hartigan **(A)**
Trembath, Stuart G **(A)**
Wilson, Kenyon D **(SLP)**

Clinton
Callen, John R **(SLP)**
Carter, Sherry J **(A)**
Dellit, Pamela M **(SLP)**
Dixson, JoAnne Alma **(SLP)**
Donnelly, Katherine M **(SLP)**
Narlock, Sr Marcella **(SLP)**
Untz, Sr Jeanne D'Arc **(SLP)**

Clive
Johannesen, Mrs Jane Lizette **(A)**
Rigler, Cheryl C **(SLP)**

Coralville
Bean, Carolyn **(SLP)**
Bebensee, Julia Gaudineer **(SLP)**
Brobeck, Teresa Carol **(SLP)**
Carpender-Robin, Debra K **(SLP)**
Clanfield, Kathleen Kiehl **(SLP)**
Fesenmeyer, Nancy **(SLP)**
Kelsay, Mrs Danielle Rubino **(A)**
Kiely, Michael A **(SLP)**
Kloberdanz, Jennie A
Kos, Sue Dusenbery **(SLP)**
Lowder, Kenneth L **(SLP A)**
McCracken, Wendy Margaret
Merry, Carol D **(SLP)**
Nelson, Jodi E

Council Bluffs
Armstrong, Mrs Marjorie K **(SLP)**
Baumert, Kathleen A **(SLP)**
Crouch, Mrs Diane Powell **(SLP)**
Farrell, Dr Dudley E **(A)**
Heiden, Sharon Denise **(A)**
Pekny, Marvin **(A)**
Pekny, Sharlene Clark **(A)**
Peton, Eileen D **(SLP)**
Smith, Jonette T **(SLP)**
Sullivan, Mrs Marsha Dawn **(SLP)**
Thielen, Joann C **(SLP)**
Turner, Mrs Joann R **(SLP)**
Wahl, Roger V **(SLP)**

Cresco
Wieland, Jerome W **(SLP)**
Wieland, Sue M **(SLP)**

Creston
Caputo, Valorie K **(A)**
Cross, Donald M **(SLP)**
Cross, Kathleen R **(SLP)**

Dallas Center
Smith-Fox, Lynn B **(SLP)**

Davenport
Barker, Mrs Ann M **(A)**
Bear, Ronald D **(SLP)**
Benjamin, Kathleen M **(SLP)**
Bernstein, Mrs Jo Ellen **(SLP)**
Blinkinsop, Paula H **(SLP)**
Bucher, Nancy A **(SLP)**
Crooks, Deborah Jo **(SLP)**
Hartman, Micheal C **(A)**
Hawkinson, Suzanne B **(SLP)**
Hollensbe, Mrs Deborah Aumann **(SLP)**
Huebner, Debbra K **(SLP)**
Ianni, Marilyn Annette **(SLP)**
Martin, Kellie Sue **(SLP)**
McGarry, Maureen Elizabeth **(SLP)**
McNeill, Linda D **(SLP)**
Meyer, Vicki L **(SLP)**
Peterson, Mrs Jane Long **(SLP)**
Regan, Mrs Mary M **(SLP)**
Samuelson, Virginia C **(SLP)**
Schieber, Cindy C **(SLP)**
Schillne, Sheryl Marie
Schmeltz, Leslie R **(A)**
Simonton, Mrs Kamala Joy **(SLP)**
Stephens, Dr Myrna Mannila **(SLP A)**
Walter, Barbara J **(SLP)**
Washam, Rita A **(SLP)**

Davis City
Boswell, Gary Lee **(A)**
Boswell, Mrs Nancy Jane **(SLP)**

De Witt
Sheldon, Mrs Dorothy L **(SLP)**

Decorah
Bril, Mrs Mary R **(SLP)**
Einck, Julie Mensing **(SLP)**
Juffer, Mary Jane **(SLP)**
Lubbert, Larry L **(SLP)**
McKee, Dorothy L **(SLP)**
Rowlette, Sandra M **(SLP)**
Wyant, Shawn Lee **(A)**

Delmar
Zabel, Helen E **(SLP)**

Denison
Eller, Connie **(SLP)**
Miller, John P **(SLP)**

Denver
Nelson, Joy I **(A)**

Des Moines
Alexander, Elizabeth Ann **(A)**
Anderson-Balch, Rhonda **(SLP)**
Augspurger, Mrs Jane Schmida **(SLP)**
Baird, Ann Elizabeth **(SLP)**
Bole, Mrs Patricia L **(SLP)**
Brown, Karen J **(SLP)**
Bunge, Mrs Cindy Whisler **(SLP)**
Calvin, Julie Marie **(SLP)**
Cheeseman, Nancy E K **(SLP)**
Cox, Susan E **(SLP)**
Cranberg, Mrs Norma A **(SLP)**
Davis, Debra Moon **(A)**
Davis, Lisa E **(SLP A)**
Deal, Dr Jon L **(SLP)**
Dobson, Mary **(SLP)**
Folkerts, Mrs Susan Miller **(SLP)**
Freilinger, Dr J Joseph **(SLP)**
Freshwaters, Karin Jean **(SLP)**
Gardner, Judith B **(SLP)**
Genz, Michael G **(A)**
Glazebrook, Mrs Evelyn N **(SLP)**
Griglione, Mrs Dolores Bertucco **(SLP)**
Gude, Stephen Sweeney **(SLP)**
Haberman, Mrs Gale Anne **(SLP)**
Herring, Mrs Rebecca Alleman **(SLP)**
Hobson, Sandra Gehling **(A)**
Horvath, Anthony **(A)**
Huff, Gary L **(SLP)**
Jenkinson, Phillip H **(SLP)**
Jepsen, Liane Marie **(SLP)**
Kayser, Dean J **(A)**
Kerst, Kathryn A **(A)**
Kiester, Jerry D **(A)**
Klungtvedt, Steven L **(A)**
Laville, Lisa J **(SLP)**
Lemke, Alison Easley **(SLP)**
Lovell, Sheryl Dee **(A)**
Lyons, Joy I **(SLP)**
McMurray, Christine Ann **(SLP)**
Mountsier, Mrs Deborah R **(A)**
Nebel, Mrs Barbara Lynn **(SLP)**
Nelson, DeeAnn B **(SLP)**
Newton, Mrs Sonna K **(SLP)**
Petersen, Eugenia Kay **(SLP)**
Pray, Mrs Rita S **(SLP)**
Ramsey, Sidney L **(A)**
Reams, Kenneth L **(SLP A)**
Reese, Mrs Sharon H **(SLP)**
Schmiechen, Susan Elizabeth **(A)**
Symonaitis, Katherine M **(SLP)**
Szymoniak, Elaine Eisfelder **(SLP)**
Thomas, Kimberly Roxanne **(SLP)**
Thompson, Janice Ann **(A)**
Ver Hoef, Niel **(SLP A)**
Wagner, Mrs Irene Kay **(A)**
Weitenhagen, Janet Johnson **(SLP)**
Whippen, Leslie A **(A)**
Wood, Mrs Paulette J **(SLP)**

Dubuque
Allen, Laurie A **(A)**
Bauchiero, Rosemary **(A)**
Bodnar, Andrew **(SLP)**
Burke, Mrs Elizabeth H F **(SLP)**
Coyle, Mrs Kathryn M **(SLP)**
Errthum, Joanne Starrett **(SLP)**
French, Mrs Barbara H **(SLP)**
Gard, Mrs Adeline Alderson **(SLP)**
Hattel, Mrs Susan Carson **(SLP)**
Johnson, Clayton R **(A)**
Kleppe, Kamela Joy **(SLP)**
Lepp, Daniel S **(SLP)**
McFarlane, Christine Mazurk **(SLP)**
Posch, Susan C **(SLP)**
Stockwell, Dean A **(A)**
Tiernan, Mrs Sue Frick **(SLP)**
Welp, Gregory K **(SLP)**

Early
Fredericks-Weber, Jeannette L F **(SLP)**

Eddyville
Lewman, Mrs Linda A **(SLP)**

Eldora
Bekemeier, Linda Grace **(SLP)**

Eldridge
Hawes, Kenneth C **(SLP)**

Elkader
Bronson, Peggy J **(SLP)**
McGaan, Mary Ellen
Shirley, Jeanette M **(SLP)**

Emmetsburg
Hersom, Roberta G **(SLP)**
Hill, Dianna Sue **(SLP)**

Fairfield
Dimmitt, Mrs Sandra C **(SLP)**
Emonin, Mrs Emily L **(SLP)**
Hinshaw, Judith A **(SLP)**

Fontanelle
Glassell, William L **(SLP)**

Forest City
Webber, Paula R **(SLP)**

Fort Dodge
Cochrane, Lorelei A **(SLP)**
Dreasler, Mrs Pauline F **(SLP)**
Jackson, Maureen Therese
Johnson, Roma Lee **(A)**
Maehl, Mrs Cheri P **(SLP)**
Maggio, Mrs Laura Lynn **(SLP)**
Salmon, Paul N **(A)**
Schlader, Susan Stuedemann **(SLP)**

Fort Madison
Brock, Mrs Linda J **(SLP)**
Pickford, Susan Kay **(A)**
Steflik, Gary L **(SLP)**
Wade, Rebecca Sue **(A)**

Gladbrook
Hildahl, Barbara B **(SLP)**

Glenwood
Brooks, Joyce McCurley **(SLP)**
Hensley, Jan L **(A)**
Johnson, Susan K **(SLP)**

Grinnell
Barber, Judith Louise **(SLP)**
Hiser, Mrs Velma B **(SLP)**

Guthrie Center
McCarty, Cynthia Ann **(SLP)**

Harlan
Haney, Sandra L **(SLP)**
Norris, Mrs Mary P **(SLP)**

Hartwick
Maschmann, Carolyn R **(SLP)**

Hawarden
Ulmer, Julie Annette **(SLP)**

Hubbard
Raney, Sandra Lee **(SLP)**

Hudson
Lindeman, Mrs Mary Ann **(SLP)**

Humboldt
Drevs, Lori Jane **(SLP)**
Nelson, Penny O **(SLP)**
Rhode, Kathy Lyn **(SLP)**

Ida Grove
Chase, Mrs Maribeth D **(SLP)**

Independence
Curphey, Mrs Kathleen Theresa **(SLP)**

Indianola
Boothe, Tamara Jan Adkins **(A)**
Gjerstad, Marlys Anderson **(SLP)**
Heideman, Barbara Smith **(SLP)**
Hoffa, Daniel C, Jr **(SLP)**
Hoffa, Esther K **(SLP)**
Larks, Mrs Sheri Moeckler **(A)**
Wadle, Kella Lynn **(SLP)**

Iowa City
Anderson, Charles V **(A)**
Barkmeier, Julie
Beisler, Jean Madsen **(SLP)**
Benishek, Mrs Lois Ann **(SLP)**
Bentler, Ruth A **(A)**
Bentley, Bruce O, Jr **(A)**
Betts, Dr Carl E **(SLP)**
Brady, Barbara Ann **(A)**
Brown, Dr Carolyn J **(SLP)**
Campbell, Kathleen C Murphey **(A)**
Cilek, Toni D **(SLP)**
Colson, Karen A **(SLP)**
Crump, Elizabeth S **(A)**
Dell'Aringa, Judith E **(SLP)**
Elfenbein, Dr Jill Libbie **(SLP A)**
Felling, Charles R **(SLP)**
Fix, Cynthia C **(SLP)**
Folkins, Dr John W
Fryauf-Bertschy, Holly **(A)**
Gebhardt, Tamara Jayne **(SLP)**
Getta, Mrs Jan P **(A)**
Gingerich, Mrs Peggy Joanne **(SLP)**
Goetz, Kathryn Lynn **(SLP)**
Greenwald, Daniel H **(A)**
Hall, Penelope K **(SLP)**
Hardy, Dr James C **(SLP)**
Hinton, Virginia A **(SLP)**
Hubbard, Mrs Rebecca Johnson **(SLP)**
Hubbard, William Conway **(SLP)**
Jones, David Lowry **(SLP)**
Jordan, Dr Herbert N **(A)**
Jordan, Dr Linda S **(SLP)**
Kahn, Dr Gerri **(A)**
Kallaus-Gay, Anne M **(SLP)**
Kaylor, Kristen A **(SLP)**
Keesee, Patricia D **(SLP)**
Kennedy, Margaret F **(SLP)**
Kirk, Mrs Karen Iler **(SLP)**
Knabe, Mrs Judith Milisen **(SLP)**
Knox, Dr Jeffrey A **(SLP)**
Kuk, Dr Francis Kok-Ming **(A)**
Lansing, Dr Charissa R **(SLP A)**
Le Peau, Nancy S **(SLP)**
Lorson, Ann W **(SLP)**
Lowder, Mary W **(A)**
Majerus, Anita
McMillin, Lois C **(SLP)**
Moll, Dr Kenneth L **(SLP)**
Moon, Dr Jerald B
Morris, Dr Hughlett L **(SLP)**
Niebuhr, Mrs Diane Dooley **(A)**
Nordquist, Carol L **(SLP)**
Parker, Barbara J **(SLP A)**

Pavlovic, Dr Chaslav V **(A)**
Perlman, Dr Adrienne L **(SLP)**
Petersen, Mrs Jacqueline **(SLP)**
Prieve, Beth Anne **(A)**
Records, Nancy L **(SLP)**
Retish, Mrs Esther S **(SLP)**
Robin, Dr Donald A **(SLP)**
Roegiers, Jane Michelle **(SLP)**
Rogers, Mrs Margaret A **(SLP)**
Schum, Dr Robert L
Seyfried, Deborah Ann **(A)**
Sherman, Dr Dorothy **(SLP)**
Show, Mrs Sandra Dickinson **(SLP)**
Simpson, Marcia S **(SLP)**
Small, Dr Arnold M
Smith, Prof Jeanne K **(SLP A)**
Spicknall, Mrs Diane D **(SLP)**
Spriestersbach, Mrs Bette **(SLP)**
Spriestersbach, D C **(SLP)**
Steele, Mrs Connie Elaine **(SLP)**
Titze, Ingo R
Tom, Kenneth **(SLP)**
Tomblin, J Bruce **(SLP)**
Tye-Murray, Dr Nancy **(A)**
Tyler, Dr Richard S **(A)**
Van Demark, Dr D R **(SLP)**
Verlo, Ellen Pringnitz **(A)**
Vilda, Rebecca R **(SLP)**
Weiss, Dr Amy L **(SLP)**
Williams, Dean E **(SLP)**
Zebrowski, Dr Patricia Finnerty **(SLP)**

Jefferson
Martino, Jane H **(SLP)**
Michels, Catherine Jean **(SLP)**
Rasmussen, Mrs Susan Gayle **(SLP)**

Johnston
Beck, Mrs Darlene Iverson **(SLP)**
Morris, Valerie Ann **(SLP)**
Tank, Joell I **(SLP)**
Thompson, Kathleen **(SLP)**
Vanessen, Susan S **(SLP)**
Wiskirchen, Mrs M Beth **(SLP)**
Zeman, Mrs Tina Marie **(SLP)**

Keokuk
Fyfe, Dorothy Grace **(A)**
Morgan, Mrs Kay Hutchinson **(SLP)**

Knoxville
Evans, Janet M S **(SLP)**
Graca, Mrs Lori E **(SLP)**
Lux, Lynn Louise **(SLP)**
Nesheim, Carolyn C **(A)**
Sayers, Elizabeth S **(SLP)**
Uhl, Lizette M **(A)**
Wheeler, L Darrell **(SLP)**

Lake City
Miller, Mrs Joan Mostoller **(SLP)**
Remsburg, Mrs Rebecca K **(SLP)**

Lamoni
Sinclair, Cynthia S **(SLP)**
Wight, Darlene V **(SLP)**

Laurens
Hopkins, Mrs Wendy B **(SLP)**

Le Claire
Leemans, Mrs Christine Marie **(SLP)**

Le Mars
Hanson, Connie D **(SLP)**
Laplante, Elaine N **(SLP)**

Lehigh
Larson, Debra A **(SLP)**

Lytton
Berkler, Carla S **(SLP)**

Manchester
Lafond, James Rolland **(SLP)**
Palmer, Mrs Anita Marie

Maquoketa
Koski, Kathleen M **(SLP)**
Snyder, Linda **(SLP)**

Marion
Aarni, John D
Cranny, Constance Joan **(SLP)**
Kent, Mrs Connie L **(SLP)**
Merrifield, Elizabeth **(SLP)**
Synstelien, Mary Joan **(SLP)**
Tiemann, Lynn Kay **(SLP)**

Marshalltown
Bennett-Porter, Sandra M **(SLP)**
Hollander, Janine Gail **(SLP)**
Hull, Mrs Christine Carter **(A)**
Jahnke, Katherine Anne **(A)**
Keiser, Nancy Jo **(SLP)**
Kimm, Gayle A **(SLP)**
Vaughn, Cheryl R **(SLP A)**
Vircks, Bruce E **(A)**

Mason City
Beshir, Mary **(SLP)**
Dockum, Gary D **(A)**
Dreyer, Sharon K **(SLP)**
Hanson, Mrs Shirley S **(SLP)**
Mastin, Bonnie Yegge **(SLP)**
Nielsen, Mrs Nancy **(SLP)**
Sarb, Mrs Eileen Ayres **(A)**
Simpson, Kenneth O **(SLP)**
Wilcox, Vonda L **(SLP)**

Milo
King, Franklin T **(SLP)**

Montrose
Senf, Linda K **(SLP)**

Mount Pleasant
Barker, Kenneth D **(SLP)**
Barker, Verla Lee **(SLP)**
Lindeen, Ruth N **(SLP)**
Roth, Mrs Janet E **(SLP)**
Weems, Althea A **(A)**

Mount Vernon
Clute, Jan Hayes **(SLP)**
Filkins, Emily **(SLP)**

Muscatine
Adkins, Bonnie Riepe **(SLP)**
Bridges, Mrs Susan K **(SLP)**
Clausen, Larry E **(SLP)**
Creasey, Kay W **(SLP)**
Kundel, Mrs Margaret N **(SLP)**
Mills, Mrs Mary L **(A)**
Quam, Mrs Colleen Ann **(SLP)**
Reeb, Paul R **(SLP)**
Welk, Mrs Joyce M **(SLP)**

Nevada
Hale, Nancy Tara
Parker, Barbara D **(SLP)**

Newton
Andrews, Mrs Pamela K **(SLP)**
Bell, Niki Sue **(SLP)**
Burke, Sherri S **(SLP)**
Gibbons, Peggy M **(SLP)**
McLaughlin, Wendy Irene **(A)**
Reinheimer, Rita K **(SLP)**
Vesely, Jean Cenaida **(SLP)**

North Liberty
Bingham, Dale S **(SLP)**
Maas, Mrs Lynne Bradbury **(SLP)**
McMellor, Gladys M **(SLP)**
Thompson, Mary Krystowski **(SLP)**

Oelwein
Jepsen, Debbie L **(SLP)**
Pasker, Julie Kay **(SLP)**
Stewart, Karen Moran **(A)**

Ogden
Reis, John W **(SLP)**

Orange City
Hansen, Dennis L **(A)**
Zwier, Janet **(SLP)**

Osage
Kloberdanz, Mrs Brenda K **(SLP)**

Oskaloosa
Asperheim, Kelly Lynn **(SLP)**
Hansen, Daniel L **(A)**

Ottumwa
Bonnell-Farmer, Mrs Cathy Ann **(SLP)**
Bramschreiber, Mrs Joy A **(SLP)**
Miller, Denise Renee **(A)**
Millsap, Mrs Lynn N **(SLP)**
Moore, Gregory K **(A)**
Nitzsche, Deborah S **(SLP)**
Taylor, Renee R
Williams, Dr Robert D **(SLP A)**
Wilson, Mrs Kathryn **(SLP)**

Panora
Meredith, Mrs Renita R **(SLP)**

Parkersburg
Neymeyer, Nancy R **(A)**

Pella
Jackson, Mrs Bonnie M V **(SLP)**
McMains, Lynn A **(SLP)**
Mozena-Fetty, Mrs Jane Nile **(SLP)**
Roush, Ted L **(SLP)**

Perry
Shelley, Mrs Erin E **(SLP)**

Pleasant Hill
Sherman-Proehl, Dr Laurabelle **(SLP)**

Pocahontas
Baier, Pamela Louise **(SLP)**

Primghar
Cole, Mrs Lynn Charlton **(SLP)**

Red Oak
Hartung, Colleen Dzingle **(SLP)**
Langland, Mrs Martha F **(SLP)**
Webb, Kent L **(A)**

Richland
Pacha, Sandra J **(SLP)**

Rock Valley
Jungemann, Susan Elaine

Rockwell City
Burt, Darla H **(SLP)**

Runnells
Brown, Dr Jerome D **(A)**

Sergeant Bluff
Harrold Webb, Mrs Mary Lynn **(SLP)**

Sheldon
Harts, Kenneth V **(SLP)**

Shenandoah
Broermann, Elaine S **(SLP)**
Erickson, Jill Peterson **(SLP)**

Sibley
Mehlbrech, Mrs Debra A G **(SLP)**

Sidney
Bateman, Mrs Sally F **(SLP)**

Sigourney
Wehr, Mrs Diana R **(SLP)**

Sioux Center
Ashelin, Cynthia A **(SLP)**
Biehl, Larry V **(SLP)**
Heidecker, Alan K **(A)**
Tegeler, Robert Victor **(SLP)**
Van Engen, Mrs Mary L **(SLP)**

Sioux City
Appletoft, Mrs Nancy C **(SLP A)**
Askeland, Mrs Susan R **(SLP)**
Bennett, Pama L **(SLP)**
Beran, Janine Ann **(SLP)**
Bloustine, Mrs Karen S **(SLP)**
Booth, Mrs Margaret L **(SLP)**
Daane, Tami Jo **(SLP)**
Dailey, Daniel J **(A)**
Deck, Mrs Janette H **(SLP)**
Dehaan-Hill, Julie Mae **(SLP)**
Ferris, James M **(SLP)**
Germann, Mrs Paula Jo S **(SLP)**
Grubel, Mrs Karen B **(SLP)**
Hauff, Latomah F **(SLP)**
Hendriks, Mary Cavanaugh **(SLP)**
Lamaster, Craig A **(SLP)**
Lamaster, Sandra K **(SLP)**
Langland, Julia Ann **(SLP)**
Lyle, Mrs Barbara A **(SLP)**
McLaughlin, Colette M
Momsen, Mrs Joy J **(SLP)**
Monson, Mark A **(SLP)**
Moulton, Byron Jess **(A)**
Munn, Cynthia Ann **(SLP)**
Nebuda, Marlene F **(SLP)**
Ownby, Robert L **(A)**
Plummer, Susan Lynn
Reiss, Evelyn P **(SLP)**
Shuminsky, Diane M **(SLP)**
Smith, Jaclyn D S **(SLP)**
Stump, Ann Howell **(SLP)**

Solon
Zehrt, Pamela Bartz **(A)**

Spencer
Harms, Mrs Cheryl Sue **(SLP)**
Howe, Katherine J **(SLP)**
Nelson, R David **(A)**
Poppe, Mrs Nancy I **(SLP)**
Rowland, Mrs Debra Spencer **(A)**
Rudkin, Jean M **(A)**

Spirit Lake
Davis, Mrs Jane B **(SLP)**

Stanton
Lundgren, Gerry H **(SLP)**
Nelson, Barbara A **(SLP)**
Peterson, Laurie Denning **(SLP)**

Storm Lake
Altringer, Kerry Mack **(SLP)**
Schons, Barbara R **(SLP)**

Tipton
Ford, Teresa Hobbs

Toledo
Christensen, Karen T **(SLP)**
Thompson, Mrs Barbara K **(SLP)**

Tripoli
Kerr, Kathie Reid **(SLP)**

Urbandale
Doggett, Mrs Andrea Jo Tyler **(SLP)**
Garner, Lynne Marie **(SLP)**
Kleber, Patricia E
Kurth, Donald D **(A)**
Vogen, Dr Clifford Stin **(SLP A)**
Wilson, Mary Lois **(SLP)**

Victor
Stiefel, Betty Jean **(SLP)**

Vinton
Ritchie, Bruce W **(SLP)**

Wapello
Winder, Surline A **(SLP)**

Waterloo
Anderson, Mrs Susan Elizabeth **(SLP)**
Bell, Mrs Alison C **(SLP)**
Blenderman, Phyllis Ruth **(SLP)**
Buzynski, Mrs Kathleen S **(SLP)**
Craven, Roberta L **(SLP)**
Ernster, Stanley M **(SLP)**
Evans, Julia C **(SLP)**
Fagre-Springer, Ann L **(SLP)**

Larson, Beth Ann
McGarvey, Margaret Zeis **(SLP)**
Murphy, Michele L **(SLP)**
Olson, Mrs Teri Daw **(SLP)**
Paulsen, Larae J **(SLP)**
Payne, Carey Meredith, III **(SLP)**
Pons, Kevin C **(A)**
Raecker, Shirley H **(SLP)**
Salkeld, Mrs Virginia L **(SLP)**
Schmitz, Julianne O **(SLP)**
Spaulding, Mrs Kay H **(SLP)**

Waukon
Grimes, Jan Elaine **(SLP)**
Montet, Thomas Herman **(SLP)**

Waverly
Larson-Fagre, Mrs Kristen M **(SLP)**
Sandor, Mrs Susan S **(SLP)**

Webster City
Campbell, Mrs Marian Fagin **(SLP)**
Ferguson, Cathleen **(SLP)**

West Branch
Picek, Mrs Mary Colleen **(SLP)**
Schnieders, Mrs Susan S **(SLP)**

West Des Moines
Boyd, Mrs Carole G **(SLP)**
Boyd, Thomas C **(A)**
Christensen, Barbara Michele **(SLP)**
Daly-Daysden, Julianne **(SLP)**
Fagg, Susan Gardner **(SLP)**
Forcucci, Angela K C **(SLP)**
Forcucci, Frank R **(SLP)**
Hillman, Sueann N **(SLP)**
Johnson, Richard W **(SLP)**
Martin, Amy Jane **(SLP)**
Price, Mrs Denise Faye **(SLP)**
Runner, Sandra J **(SLP)**
Schoen, Madelyn K **(SLP)**
Sederburg, Mrs Claudette N
Tollefson, Lori Ann
Tysklind, John Michael **(A)**
Vogen, Barbra Dickinson **(SLP)**
Zumbach, Kathy **(SLP)**

West Liberty
Teague, Mrs Cheryl C **(SLP)**

West Point
Sporkman-Link, Mrs Ann Grace **(SLP)**

West Union
Bishop, Lewis D **(SLP A)**
Carspecken, Ronald J **(SLP)**
Grafenberg, Janice E **(SLP)**
Thomas, Mrs Jean Marie **(SLP)**

Westside
McCampbell, Pamela M **(SLP)**

Wever
Drollinger, Jeanne M **(SLP)**

Wilton
Henning, Mrs Kay L **(SLP)**

Winterset
Bauer, Mrs Mary L **(SLP)**

Woodward
Marston, Mark Dewayne **(A)**

KANSAS

Abilene
Hilton, Mrs Judy L **(SLP)**
Wilson, Katheryn **(SLP)**

Altamont
McCoskey, Anita M **(SLP)**
Tongier, Joan C **(SLP)**

Andover
Willinger, Mrs Rebecca L **(SLP)**

Arkansas City
Campbell, Jane Siever **(A)**
Gilliland, Sharon B **(SLP)**
Hettrick, Mrs Chrystine M

Atchison
Lickhart, Candy Ann **(SLP)**

Auburn
Bird, Mrs Luann L **(SLP)**

Augusta
Constance, Jane **(SLP)**
Crawford, Mrs Deanna M **(SLP)**

Baldwin
Ulrich, Vicki K **(SLP)**

Basehor
Trail, Wayne D **(SLP)**

Belleville
Meyer, Eileen R **(SLP)**

Beloit
Andrews, Mrs Amy Correan **(SLP)**
Zimmerman, Susan **(SLP)**

Bonner Springs
Foley, Elaine H **(SLP)**

Bucyrus
Svoboda, Kathleen D **(SLP)**

Buhler
Heizelman, Mrs Jody Kay
Torres, Mrs Terri F **(SLP)**

Carbondale
Bourne, Mrs Lynne M **(SLP)**

Chanute
Wright-Gard, Wanda K **(SLP)**

Chapman
Pfannenstiel, Mrs Gloria L **(SLP)**

Clay Center
Bohnenblust, Brenda Diane **(SLP)**
McKee, Thomas L **(SLP)**
Meier, Mrs Susan M **(SLP)**

Coffeyville
Hogan, Toni Lea **(SLP)**

Colby
Wingard, Gary Lee **(SLP)**

Columbus
Richman, Mrs Nancy S **(SLP)**

Council Grove
Luce, Michael S **(SLP)**
Patrzykont-Horning, Patricia Jo **(SLP)**

De Soto
Underdahl, Charles W **(SLP)**

Derby
Black, Margaret J **(SLP)**
Brock, Mrs Sharon L **(SLP)**
Burnell, Mrs Marilyn K **(SLP)**
Hunter, Marilyn B **(SLP)**
Kallail, Dr Ken James **(SLP)**

Dighton
Campbell, Mrs Lisa M **(SLP)**

Dodge City
Herrmann, Mrs Colleen Robben **(SLP)**
Lehmkuhler, Mrs Elaine R **(SLP)**
Newell, Mrs Mary Jo Shapland **(SLP)**
Snyder, Cheryl Ann
Streit, Mrs Diane K **(SLP)**
Waldman, Wanda S **(SLP)**

Edgerton
Baird, Mrs Judy File **(SLP)**

El Dorado
Greenbank, Mrs Debbra A **(SLP)**
Karner, Mrs Karen Kay **(SLP)**
Keller, Mrs Sherry C **(SLP)**

Stoskopf, Mrs Sharon L **(SLP)**

Emporia
Baalman, Lee **(SLP)**
Davidson, Lloyd E **(SLP)**
Davis, Mrs Linda W **(SLP)**
Goodwin, Vicki **(SLP)**
Hadaway, Mrs Sharon Joy **(SLP)**

Eureka
Downing-Ball, Mrs Debbie J **(SLP)**

Fairway
Mitchell, Mary Wagner **(SLP)**
Tenenbaum, Mrs Joie K **(SLP)**

Fort Leavenworth
Sinclair, Mrs Joan B **(SLP)**

Fort Scott
Elliott, Mrs Patti Jo **(SLP)**
Webber, Mrs Ava L **(SLP)**

Fowler
Devine, Mrs Laura Elizabeth **(SLP)**

Galva
Larson, Rose Mary **(SLP)**

Garden City
Conroy, Mrs Sally Joan **(SLP)**
Hamlett, Mrs J Ann **(SLP)**
Hendricks, Kim Marie
Shook, Mrs Ellen Stephens **(SLP)**
Wallace, Mrs Neta Jane **(SLP)**

Geuda Springs
Hutchins, Betty J **(SLP)**

Girard
Boultinghouse, Mrs Sherry Arlene **(SLP)**

Goodland
Transue, Vicki E **(SLP)**

Great Bend
Cruse, Caroline M **(SLP)**
Donahue, Belita A **(SLP)**
Heinrich, Dixie A **(SLP)**
Magers, J L, Jr **(A)**
Magers, Mrs K Diane **(SLP)**
Tockert, Sr M **(SLP)**
Vanis, Patty Joan **(SLP)**

Halstead
Graham, KaAnn A **(SLP)**
Lathen, Jill E **(SLP)**

Harper
Fox, Gayla DiAnn

Hays
Bannister, Dr Marcia L **(SLP)**
Britten, Dr Frederick **(A)**
Byrne, Marie E **(SLP)**
Dome, Andrea Rene **(SLP)**
Dreiling, Mrs Sheryl L **(SLP)**
Herndon, Dr Geneva **(SLP)**
Knittel, June M **(A)**
Maddy, Mrs Julie Kay
Staab, Marla Schmidt **(SLP)**
Webster, Theda E **(SLP)**
Wilhelm, Dr Charles L **(SLP)**
Wilhelm, Mrs Sammie Sexton **(SLP)**
Wright, Mrs Carla Gasper

Healy
Jennison, Pamela Faye **(SLP)**

Herington
Haage, Constance L **(SLP)**

Hiawatha
Fleenor, Rebecca Ann **(SLP)**
Morrison, Rick Alan **(SLP)**

Hill City
Stark, Elizabeth A **(SLP)**

Holton
Esry, Mrs Linda J **(SLP)**

Hoyt
Thomas, Deborah **(SLP)**

Hutchinson
Adams, Mrs Esther Young
Coffey, Mrs Jill Renee **(SLP)**
Cuda, Mrs Rae A **(SLP)**
Gibson, Ruth B **(SLP)**
Hardin, Monte F **(A)**
Jensen, Jeffery Paul **(A)**
Lang, Micheal D **(SLP)**
Morgan, Mike David **(SLP)**
Ray, Mrs Susan Jordan **(SLP)**
Roberts, Mrs Linda D **(SLP)**
Swank, Mrs Linda K **(SLP)**
Wilkens, Connie Marie

Independence
Jackson, Jerry John
Kelly, Mrs Eloise Kathleen **(SLP)**
Mears, Mrs Treva J **(SLP)**

Iola
Arnott, Mary Ann **(SLP)**
Foster, Mrs Karrie Diane **(SLP)**
Larson, Mrs Stephanie Brock **(SLP)**

Junction City
Bruce, Mrs Dara A **(SLP)**
Flanagan, Dr Bruce C **(SLP)**
Gillum, Charles Jr Lindsey **(A)**
Heldstab, Mrs Peggy S **(SLP)**
Lake, Shirley K **(SLP)**

Kansas City
Bahrainwala, Lubaina E
Carpenter, Mary Ann **(SLP)**
Diedrich, William M **(SLP)**
Ferguson, Roxann **(A)**
Ferraro, Dr John A
Geier, Lisa Lyn **(A)**
Karlsen, Dr Elizabeth **(A)**
Keener, Sandy K **(A)**
Mayberry-Langston, Claudia L **(A)**
Mustain, Teresa B **(SLP)**
Norton, Dr Susan Joy **(A)**
Price, Sharon R **(SLP)**
Robinson, Joan Nancy **(SLP)**
Shubat, Sally Jo **(SLP)**
Snorgrass, Mrs Cheryl J **(SLP)**
Sostarich, Mary Elizabeth **(A)**
Stark, Diane Elizabeth **(SLP)**
Vann, Brenda J **(SLP)**

Kismet
McVey, Lola C **(SLP)**

Lawrence
Abegg, Mrs Michelle Lynn **(SLP)**
Bowline, Mrs Wilma L **(SLP)**
Brandt, Dr John F
Brandt, Dr Sara Dale **(SLP)**
Brinkley, Mary L **(SLP)**
Buhr, Joann Coleen **(SLP)**
Bunce, Dr Betty H **(SLP)**
Catts, Dr Hugh W
Chappell, Mrs Elizabeth Hamm **(SLP)**
Clark, Dr Frances L
Cockrell-Santee, Mrs Trena **(SLP)**
Dreiling, Mrs Alica Johnson **(SLP)**
Erdmann, Julie Lynn
Evans, Elizabeth Anne **(SLP)**
Gardiner-Morgan, Mrs Beverly **(SLP)**
Gatts, Julie J **(SLP)**
Gottlieb, Kathleen Ann **(SLP)**
Haack, Sharon L **(SLP)**
Hogan, Mrs Susan C **(A)**
Howard, Mrs Sydney W **(SLP)**
Johnson-Powell, Valerie K **(SLP)**
Kautsch, Mrs Elaine M **(SLP)**
Kelly, Donna J **(SLP)**
Ketter, Mrs Nancy R **(SLP)**
Langnau-Morris, Candace J **(SLP)**
Loushine, Patricia L **(A)**
Marston, Dr Larry E **(A)**

Maykulsky, Vicki W **(SLP)**
Michel, Dr John Frederich
Michel, Dr Lorraine I **(SLP)**
Morrison, Annette Yvonne **(SLP)**
Ott, Mrs Elizabeth Gayle **(SLP)**
Rice, Dr Mabel L **(SLP)**
Rohl, Mrs Nancy Dee **(SLP)**
Rose, Mrs Patricia Ann **(SLP)**
Saricks, Dr Margaret C Byrne **(SLP)**
Schiefelbusch, Dr Richard L **(SLP)**
Schulte, Edward J **(SLP)**
Still, Sheri Frances **(SLP)**
Thompson, Mrs Caprice M **(SLP)**
Tusten, James D **(A)**
Wegner, Jane R **(SLP)**
White, Leta D **(SLP)**
Wilcox, Dr Kim **(SLP)**
Wolfe, Mrs Cynthia S **(SLP)**

Leavenworth
Dickson-Loreti, Mrs Linda K **(SLP)**
Taylor, Donna M **(SLP)**

Leawood
Carter, Scott A **(A)**
Cheek, Mrs Diane Jones **(SLP)**
Corder, Mrs Barbara L **(SLP)**
Elliott, Mrs Cathy C **(SLP)**
McCluggage, Mrs Vicki Sue **(SLP)**
McGiffert, Mrs Maura Robinson **(SLP)**
Scheerer, Jennifer J **(SLP)**
Starks, Janet Marie **(SLP)**
Winston, Mrs Julia Stern **(SLP)**
York, Jane Ellen **(SLP)**

Lenexa
Atkinson, Mrs Lanoma **(A)**
Ballard, Mrs Kathleen Schwarz **(SLP)**
Bradfield, Mrs Karen S **(SLP)**
Browning, Dorothea J **(SLP)**
Cottone, Debra Ann **(A)**
Dopp, Shelley R **(SLP)**
Dziewior, Regina **(A)**
Fenley, Hannah L **(SLP)**
Haynes, Mrs Deborah Gordon
Howard, Elizabeth **(SLP)**
Jeffers, Sarah Jane **(SLP)**
Joens, Mrs Vicky De Witte **(SLP)**
Johnson, Mrs Barbara Jo **(SLP)**
Johnson, Kristin Matheson **(SLP)**
Mather, Diann **(SLP)**
Mulkey, Katherine Ann **(SLP)**
Pulvino, Patricia Jeanne **(SLP)**
Riordan, Ann R **(SLP)**
Runyan, Laura Kathleen **(A)**
Schottler, Laura D **(SLP)**
Seavertson, Dr John M **(A)**
Silberberg, Rhonda L **(SLP)**
Watkins, Mrs Kay F **(SLP)**

Liberal
Akey, Phyllis Irene **(A)**
Pennington, Gwendolyn **(SLP)**
Quiring, Lillian D **(SLP)**

Louisville
Jones, Alice Ott

Lyons
Beaver, Lora L **(SLP)**

Manhattan
Astrue, Carol Marie **(SLP)**
Bedrosian, Dr Janice L **(SLP)**
Cooper, Mrs Anna Wagg **(SLP)**
Goll, Annette Aerts **(SLP)**
Gray, Mrs Mary Ann D **(SLP)**
Gray, Dr Thomas F **(SLP A)**
Grubb, Mrs Betty F **(SLP)**
Hoag, Linda A **(SLP)**
Maatta, M'Elizabeth Ritchie **(A)**
Nelson, Peggy Bull **(A)**
Notestine, Mrs Patricia I **(SLP)**
Rainbolt, Harry R **(A)**
Rainbolt, Mrs Rosella T **(SLP)**
Reagan, Mrs Sharon S **(SLP)**
Riley, Mrs Peggy Jo **(SLP)**
Salva, Caroline Teresa **(SLP)**
Smit, Dr Ann B **(SLP)**
Smith, Anne Jaquette **(SLP)**
Van Nevel, Anita Marie **(SLP)**
Wieczorek, Gregory F **(A)**
Zimmerman, Mrs Susan F **(SLP)**

Mankato
Warne, Mrs Deborah Ann **(SLP)**

Marysville
Smith, Lauri Sue **(SLP)**
Walstrom, Mrs Rosemary E **(SLP)**

Mayfield
Gerberding, Mrs Karen E **(SLP)**

McCracken
Rogers, Mrs Sheryl Robinson **(SLP)**

McPherson
Franz, Celia Ann **(SLP A)**
Hunter, Mrs Caroline J **(SLP)**
Seymore, Mrs Charla Belle **(SLP)**

Meade
Goldsberry, Mrs Shirley W **(SLP)**
Kirkland, Erin E **(SLP)**

Mission
Cox, Sandy K **(A)**
Culbertson, Cheryl Ellen **(SLP)**
Hancock, Pamela K **(SLP)**
Ryding, Melanie C **(SLP)**
Schulte, Luanne **(SLP)**
Willis, Diane Louise **(A)**

Moline
Daniels, Katherine A **(SLP)**

Montezuma
Wall, Mrs Debra J **(SLP)**

Monument
Berry, Jana Marie **(SLP)**

Moran
Cole, Mrs Julie Spangler **(SLP)**
Tynon, Mrs Debra J **(SLP)**

Mound City
Hickman, Mrs Pamela Fay **(SLP)**

Mulvane
Allen, Rose L **(SLP A)**
Mason, Mrs Mickie Flora **(SLP)**
Meeker, Sidney A **(SLP)**
Meitl, Mrs Pamela A **(SLP)**
Rodd-Marks, Jane J **(SLP)**

Munden
Tipton, Debra Rizek **(SLP)**

Neodesha
Barry, Mrs Linda H **(SLP)**

Ness
Pfannenstiel, Michael C **(SLP)**

Newton
Anderson, Galen B **(SLP)**
Bonewitz, Mrs Karen S **(SLP)**
Bradbury, Steven H **(A)**
Clark, Mrs Carol Kopp **(SLP A)**

North Newton
Ellis, Mrs Ellen K **(SLP)**

Oakley
Rose, Mrs Opal L **(SLP)**

Olathe
Brewster, Elaine M **(SLP)**
Burns, Mrs Catherine Pelham
Burns Daniels, Mrs Debora A **(SLP)**
Byarlay, Mrs Diane Lynn **(SLP)**
Cicero, Carol Ann **(SLP)**
Cline, Mrs Roberta Mae **(SLP)**
Galbraith, Marla J **(SLP)**
Glankler, Kathleen C **(SLP)**
Goetzinger, Cornelius Peter **(A)**
Haeusler, Sheryl G **(SLP)**
Hettinger, Teresa Lynne
Knight, Colleen W **(SLP)**
Lenertz, Ann Schweitzer **(SLP)**
Mattson, Mrs Patty J **(SLP)**
Mercer, Mrs Lynn Weismiller **(SLP)**
Meyerowitz, Elizabeth Ann **(SLP)**
Newkirk, Mrs Carol Stelting **(SLP)**
Porter, Dr Thomas A **(A)**
Schaper, Mrs Nan D **(SLP)**
Schmidt, Mrs Melissa Ann
Skaggs, Mrs Kyle Grenda **(SLP)**
Smith, Mrs Elaine Ann **(SLP)**
Smyth, Troy **(SLP)**
Sullivan, Mrs Karen A **(SLP)**
Tharp, Paula L **(SLP)**
Williams, Jodi L **(SLP)**
Wormus, Catherine Ann **(SLP)**
Worthington, Mrs Jeannette **(SLP)**
Wright, Debbie A **(SLP)**

Osborne
Vandament, Mrs Vickie Sue

Ottawa
Bobbish, Mrs Ruth E **(SLP)**
Gaeddert, Mrs Connie L **(SLP)**

Overland Park
Alexander, Sharon Z **(SLP)**
Anderson, Mrs Robyn Lynette **(SLP)**
Baker, Sara Ann **(SLP)**
Barr, Mrs Rebecca Welch **(SLP)**
Bauman, Sheila M **(SLP)**
Becker, Katie Ann **(SLP)**
Bisang, Sharon J **(SLP)**
Booton, Barbara Lynne **(SLP)**
Brooks, Mary M **(SLP)**
Brown, Mrs Sandra A **(A)**
Bruhn, Mrs Margaret L **(SLP)**
Chapman, Mrs Kyle Anne **(A)**
Chinn, Mrs Deborah Lee **(SLP)**
Christison, Lori Sue **(SLP)**
Crain, Rebecca Andes **(SLP)**
Daniels, Cynthia Krug **(SLP)**
Dashiell, Mrs Pamela B **(SLP)**
Dethlefs, Mrs Kathleen **(SLP)**
Dethlefs, Richard D **(SLP)**
DiPasquale, Mrs Priscilla R **(SLP)**
Durley, Debra L **(SLP)**
Dyke, Carol Lee **(SLP)**
Embree, Michelle Cordes **(SLP)**
Ensminger, Rosanne M **(SLP)**
Ferraro, Mrs Jamie B **(SLP)**
Fitzgerald, Mrs Susan Swickard **(SLP)**
Franks, Harriet Tia **(SLP)**
Gahagan, Teresa Marie **(SLP)**
Gasser, Valerie Katz **(SLP)**
Gatlin, Kaye L **(SLP)**
Gerstner, Mrs Janet C **(SLP)**
Gordon, Mrs Betty J **(SLP)**
Haas, Celeste E **(SLP)**
Halpin, Mrs Kathy S W **(SLP)**
Hammer, Candice Ann **(SLP)**
Jordan, Corinne M **(SLP)**
Kerrigan, Patricia Leann
Krantz, Mrs Miriam L **(A)**
Kubin, Mrs Leigh Ann **(SLP)**
Lane, Marilyn J **(SLP)**
Leaf, Mrs Kim D **(SLP)**
Loeser, Gregory J **(SLP)**
McLain, Julie Ann **(SLP)**
McLennan, Roderick O, Jr **(A)**
Metzger, Mrs Mary L **(SLP)**
Mims, Mrs Lisa N
Morenz, Kim Renee **(SLP)**
Moster, Mrs Jean Ann MacGregor **(SLP)**
Mulligan, Laurie S **(SLP)**
Nelson, Beverly K **(SLP)**
O'Neil, Mrs Lynn Scroggs **(SLP)**
O'Renick, Pamela Sue **(SLP)**
Press, Mrs Joy A **(A)**
Press, Steven E **(A)**
Pyle, Marilyn W **(SLP)**
Reiz, Mrs Zelda L **(SLP)**
Schonbrun, Mrs Vita **(SLP)**
Smith, Mary C **(SLP)**
Steichen, Mary L **(SLP)**
Stone, Nicola F R **(SLP)**
Wallace, Sherry L **(SLP)**
Wells, Robin A **(SLP)**
Weyforth, Mara K **(SLP)**
Wilkerson, Linda **(A)**
Willis, Tracy Lynn **(SLP)**
Wimmer-Kuehl, Lonna G **(SLP)**
Wise, James A **(A)**

Oxford
Corn, Richard K

Paola
Lutz, Konnie Clarke **(SLP)**

Park City
Heck, Mrs Kendee Fawn

Parsons
Aistrup, Suzann **(SLP)**
Brady, Nancy Caroline **(SLP)**
Brinton, Dr Bonnie **(SLP)**
Coate, Melanie Lynn **(SLP)**
Etter, Rhonda R **(SLP)**
Flaton, Rebecca Lynn **(SLP)**
Fujiki, Dr Martin **(SLP)**
McLean, Dr James E **(SLP)**
McNay, Valerie J **(SLP)**
Messick, Anna M N **(SLP)**
O'Connor, Annette Marie **(SLP)**
Pound, Kathy Jo **(SLP)**
Pound, Rebecca Walker **(SLP)**
Reinthal, S Heidi **(A)**
Ritthaler, Christophr R **(SLP)**
Sack, Dr Sara H **(SLP)**
Simmons, Sheila **(SLP)**
Snyder-McLean, Dr Lee K
Turk, Rebecca S **(A)**

Pittsburg
Ensminger, Shelly Maxine **(SLP)**
Holt, Richard L **(SLP)**
Kilcher, Mary Frances **(SLP)**
Spry-Packard, Sheila M **(SLP)**

Plainville
Wiesner-Sims, Myra **(SLP)**

Prairie Village
Berlau, Mrs Marcia L **(SLP)**
Buchanan, Mrs Mary Anne **(SLP)**
Carrell, Mrs Marilyn F **(A)**
Carroll, Valeree S **(SLP)**
Ebeling, Ann E S **(SLP)**
Ensminger-Waldman, Mrs Lindi Ann **(SLP)**
Ford, Marty Suzanne **(SLP)**
Hoefer, Julie Ann **(SLP)**
Holbert, Heather Jayne **(SLP)**
Huston, Janet K **(SLP)**
Keels-Miller, Mrs Rita Ann **(SLP)**
Kendrick, Norma L **(SLP)**
Knox, Dr Albert W **(SLP A)**
Murphy, Mrs Glynis Barbosa **(A)**
Murray, Mrs Cheryl A **(SLP)**
Petigna, Lucrezia E **(SLP)**
Quirk-Stauch, Kathleen A **(SLP)**
Rubin, Arlene S **(A)**
Ryan, Cynthia Bird **(SLP)**
Sachs, Shirley A **(SLP)**
Siren, Kathleen Ann
Thomas, Mrs Ann Bosse **(SLP)**

Pratt
Barker, Mrs Ann C

Republic
Hurley-Sandell, Nancy Lee **(SLP)**

Riley
Neidenthal, Mrs Julie Schraeder **(SLP)**
Norris, Mrs Janice Sue **(SLP)**

Rose Hill
Gerber, Mrs Lynn Holland **(SLP)**
Perry, Cecyle K **(SLP)**

Sabetha
Kellenberger, Mrs Paula Hansen **(SLP)**

Salina
Duell, Mrs Margaret Green **(SLP)**
Edmands, Mrs Judith D **(SLP)**
Ewy, Jane Ann Davenport **(SLP)**
Hulstine, Margaret M **(SLP)**
McGinley, Mrs Mary R **(SLP)**
Modin, Mrs Nancy G **(SLP)**
Putnam, Christina Rena **(SLP)**
Putzier, Patrick Vincent **(A)**
Taylor, Marilyn J **(SLP)**
Wallace, Mrs Dorothy A **(SLP)**
Weiser, Michael Lawrence **(A)**
White, Richard A **(A)**

Satanta
Torrey, Mrs T Zoann **(SLP)**

Scott City
Faurot, Judy Carol **(SLP)**
Hess, Mrs Karen L **(SLP)**

Shawnee
Barforoush, Kathleen Bauman **(A)**
Bilyeu, Connie L **(SLP)**
De Haan, Mrs Shellee Cates **(SLP)**
Ethridge, Nancy L **(SLP)**
Foreman, Dalyn D **(SLP)**
Gartland, Sandy **(SLP)**
Grant, Evelyn Bergh **(SLP)**
Lawrence, Dr Donald L **(SLP A)**
L'Ecuyer, Mrs Rebecca Lee **(SLP)**
Phelps, Gail Z **(SLP)**
Schafer, Nancy Neilan **(SLP)**
Swain, Beth Carver **(SLP)**
Vallandingham, Dr Richard R **(A)**
Weaver, Mrs Joyce Holland **(SLP)**

Shawnee Mission
Breen, Katherine A **(SLP)**
Cherry, Mrs Peggy R **(SLP)**
Clore-Phillips, Sandra Kay **(SLP)**
Coleman, Mrs Jeanne F **(SLP)**
Condron, Mrs Ellen W **(SLP)**
Fish, Pamela S **(SLP A)**
Grant, Joan **(SLP)**
Hartley, Jack L **(SLP)**
King, Deborah A **(SLP)**
Lamb, Nancy L **(SLP)**
McDonald, Amelia A **(SLP)**
McReynolds, Dr Leija V **(SLP)**
Miller, Dr June B **(A)**
Moseley, Cathy **(SLP)**
Omer, Mrs Jane Lewis **(A)**
Powell, James E **(A)**
Powell, Janna Y **(SLP)**
Schwartz, Mrs Susan R **(SLP)**
Smith, Dr Kenneth E **(A)**
Zimmerman, Mrs Carolyn W **(SLP)**

Silver Lake
Lindstrom, Mrs Karen I **(SLP)**

South Haven
Strickland, Mrs Martha R **(SLP)**

Spring Hill
Acinger, Mrs Rhonda **(SLP)**

St Francis
Grace, Deborah Gorthy **(SLP)**

St Marys
Flannigan, William J **(SLP)**

Stilwell
Bingham, Mrs Lisa W **(SLP)**
Helton, Mrs Sally G **(SLP)**

Stockton
Haines, Marsha Bouchey **(SLP)**

Topeka
Baer, Mildred I **(SLP)**
Barber, Dr J Manford, III **(SLP A)**
Beardslee, Mary Lou L **(SLP)**
Berreth-Brazier, Lorraine Shelley **(SLP)**
Blasing, Mrs Carolyn Jo **(SLP)**
Bower, Dr Glenda Gay **(SLP)**
Bradford, Dr Larry J **(SLP A)**
Bruntzel, Melvin D **(SLP)**
Carr, Mrs Margaret Diane **(SLP)**
Colson, Connie J **(SLP)**
Dolezal, Pamela S **(SLP)**
Edmund, Mrs Elizabeth George
Fasulo, Elaine B **(SLP)**
Fisher, Mrs Patricia Trent **(SLP)**
Freund, Lise A **(SLP)**
Gentry, Mrs Joan Arrington **(SLP)**
George, William D, Jr **(SLP)**
Gober, Mrs Susan L **(SLP)**
Golos, Neila J **(SLP)**
Hall, Maura K M **(SLP)**
Hess, Teresa Holdren **(SLP)**
Hunter-Morehead, Cindy L **(SLP)**
Jacka, Mrs Janice Christine **(SLP)**
Johnson, Mrs Mary Ann **(SLP)**
Kenzy, Karol **(SLP)**
Krug, Karen E **(SLP)**
Lewis, Dr Jeffrey Ian **(SLP)**
McFarland, Brenda Kay **(SLP)**
Mize, Carole G **(SLP)**
Molineux, Barry R **(SLP)**
Oblander, Catherine Miller **(A)**
Poulton, Dr Karen T **(SLP)**
Reynolds, Deb S **(SLP)**
Ricke, Dianna M **(SLP)**
Rousey, Dr Carol H **(SLP)**
Rousey, Dr Clyde L **(SLP A)**
Rutherford, Gorin **(SLP)**
Shannon, Mrs Claudia J **(SLP)**
Simpson, Mike Alan **(SLP)**
Strand, Mrs Valerie Wilson **(SLP)**
Uruski, Kathleen A **(A)**
Wade, Mrs Roxanne Marie
Waldo, Lois J **(SLP)**
Waugh, Marilyn M **(SLP)**
Zeigler, Dana Joy **(SLP)**
Zey, Mrs Joyce Colleen **(SLP)**

Towanda
Pohlenz, Mrs Mary Lynn **(SLP)**

Valley Center
Jones, Winifred Brandt **(SLP)**
Snodgrass, R E **(SLP)**

Valley Falls
Schmidt, Mrs Janet K V **(SLP)**

Wakeeney
Deines, Rick Raymond **(A)**

Wamego
Boyd, Mrs Kimberly Ann **(SLP)**
Wade, Mary A **(A)**

Westwood
Bradley, Gary Kent

Wheaton
Kufahl, Mrs Susanne Suther **(SLP A)**

Whitewater
Henderson, Julie Hallenbeck **(SLP)**

Wichita
Alberts, Dr Ruby W
Arnold, Kay L **(SLP)**
Bailey, Mrs Anita S **(SLP)**
Barker, Mrs Susan Leigh **(SLP)**
Bates, Dana Marie **(SLP)**
Batson, Laura Guthrie **(A)**
Bayless, Elizabeth Marie **(SLP)**
Beasley, Mrs Mary J **(SLP)**
Bennett, Dorothy J **(SLP)**
Bennett-Kastor, Dr Tina L
Black, Dana B **(SLP)**
Blankenship, Mrs Terre Kay **(SLP)**
Bohn, Mrs Lilah M **(SLP)**
Bolin, Julianne C **(SLP)**
Boose, Martha Anne **(SLP)**
Branson, Renee D **(SLP)**
Brown, Sue Ann **(SLP)**
Browne, Marilyn K **(SLP)**
Burgess, Cynthia A **(SLP)**
Burk, Cathy Guinty **(SLP)**
Burk, Dr Kenneth W **(SLP)**
Cable, Jetta L **(SLP)**
Cary, Diane Alane **(SLP)**
Chambers, Dr Ronald Dean **(SLP)**
Champley, Mrs Jill Leslie **(SLP)**
Clark, Mary Ann B **(SLP)**
Clemons, Bobbie Jo **(SLP)**
Cole, Mrs Libbie Sisto
Cooper, Teresa Ann **(A)**
Crandall, Nancy M **(SLP)**
Cranford, Dr Jerry Lynn **(A)**
Debano-Burns, Dee Ann **(SLP)**
Dotson, Nancy J **(SLP)**
Draper, Dr David J **(SLP)**
Dyck, Kay Bartel **(SLP)**
Edwards, Dr Harold T
Faires, Dr Wesley L **(SLP)**
Fisher, Mrs Jean Marie
Fowler, Mrs Janet Sprecher **(SLP)**
Gazaway, Armen
Ginest, Mrs Joan H **(SLP)**
Girrens, Mrs Ellen Claire **(SLP)**
Givens, Teresa S **(SLP)**
Glenn, Mrs Almetta M **(SLP)**
Graham, Barbara Bennett **(SLP)**
Graham, Dr J Keith **(SLP)**
Gray, Mrs Kathryn O **(SLP)**
Gray, Terri S **(SLP)**
Greenwood, Becky Zirnstein
Groves, Mrs Deborah S **(SLP)**
Gurske-Hladik, Mrs Ellen **(SLP)**
Hageman, Mrs Cindy **(SLP)**
Hammar, Elaine G **(SLP)**
Hammond, Brian Reed **(A)**
Hanks, Joseph David **(SLP)**
Harr, Debra A **(SLP)**
Harris, Teresa S **(SLP)**
Henry, David F **(A)**
Hentzen, Mrs Cheryl W **(SLP)**
Herron, Victoria R **(SLP)**
Hilyard, Mrs Shelley W **(SLP)**
Hoch, Mrs Gail Lynn **(SLP)**
Hodson, Dr Barbara W **(SLP)**
Hoyt, Mrs Dianna K E **(SLP)**
Hubbard, Mrs Karen D **(SLP)**
Hyder, Elizabeth **(SLP)**
Irwin, Trudy Lorain **(SLP)**
Jared, Carol Beth **(A)**
Johnson, Jennifer A **(SLP)**
Johnson, Mrs Judy C
Kasten, Dr Roger N **(A)**
Kennalley, Mrs Teresa L **(A)**
King, Sheri-Lyn R **(SLP)**
Kirkpatrick, Anita G **(SLP)**
Kissick, Mrs Kara Miller **(SLP)**
Kleffner, Frank R **(SLP)**
Kneil, Dr Thomas R
Koerbel, Jane McCann **(SLP)**
Krumm, Mark Paul **(A)**
Ladnier, Carol A D **(SLP)**
Lampros, Nancy P **(SLP)**
Lee, Sheila R **(SLP)**
Levine, Elizabeth Fernandez **(SLP)**
Lies, Mrs Leigh A **(SLP)**
Long, Mrs Kari Sue **(SLP)**
Mabe, Denise M **(SLP)**
Mabee, Susan **(SLP)**
Mai, Mrs Deborah L **(SLP)**
Manion, Mary Beth **(SLP)**
Martin, Douglas R **(A)**
Matheson, Barbara Gail **(SLP A)**
Matsusaka, Eileen Kiyomi **(A)**
Mawdsley, Brenda **(SLP)**
McAtee, Mrs Linda Jo **(SLP)**
McCroskey, Dr Robert L **(SLP A)**
McMaster, Nancy R **(SLP)**
Menges, Joanna L **(SLP)**
Mills, Mrs Charlotte **(SLP)**
Moore, Dr Christopher Alden
Morphis, Gayle Thompson **(SLP)**
Neher, Mrs Winifred **(SLP)**
Nelson, Chelie Ann **(SLP)**
Northcutt, Jana L H **(SLP)**
Nyenhuis, Sharon K **(SLP)**
Overstake, Carol H **(SLP)**
Overstake, Dr Charles P **(SLP)**
Park, Kathleen Sarah **(SLP)**
Parmiter-Jacobs, Linda J **(A)**
Pasmore, Ronald R **(SLP)**
Phythian, Carla Andrews **(SLP)**
Pottorf, Mrs Molly **(SLP A)**
Pratt, Mrs Jeanne S **(SLP)**
Ralstin, Robert H **(SLP)**
Rapp, Mrs Amy L **(SLP)**
Reeves-Lamson, Sharon **(SLP)**
Rhatigan, Rebecca J
Robl, Mrs Janet T **(A)**
Rogers, Therese M **(SLP)**
Romereim, Beverly May **(A)**
San Martin-Edmunds, Mrs Mary P **(SLP)**
Sawyer, Mrs Judith Cooper **(SLP)**
Scherz, Julie W **(SLP)**
Schodorf, Dr Jean Kurtis **(SLP)**
Scudder, Dr Rosalind **(SLP)**
Self, Mrs Trisha Lynn **(SLP)**
Shea, Mrs Catherine Ann **(SLP)**
Shick, Karen Zamberlan
Simmons, Joanne **(SLP)**
Simpson, Joan Adele **(A)**
Songster, Mrs Pamela J
Spradling, Mrs Janabeth W **(SLP)**
Stephens, Jane M **(SLP)**
Strattman, Mrs Kathy H **(SLP)**
Stucky-Pirner, Angela Kay **(SLP)**
Templin, Marilyn Susan **(SLP)**
Terry, Nancy Thomesn **(A)**
Todd, Leann Pilkenton **(SLP)**
Topping, Gary E **(A)**
Tremain, Mrs Debbie Hobbs
Wall, Mrs Kelly Jo **(SLP)**
Warren, Mrs Katherine **(SLP)**
Wells, Mrs Deanna Rea
Wells, Mrs Rebecca Brenner
White-Chambers, Marcia J **(SLP)**
Whittredge, Dorothy K **(A)**
Wittenbach, Martha Green **(SLP)**
Woodard, Mrs Nancy Deann **(SLP)**
Wurth, Charles W **(SLP)**
Wurth, Mary R **(SLP)**

Winfield
Cooper, Victoria A **(SLP)**
Lay, Ruth Ann **(SLP)**
Wagner, Deanna Junell **(SLP)**

Yates Center
Herring, David H **(A)**

KENTUCKY

Alvaton
Patterson, Jeanne M **(SLP)**

Anchorage
Boden, Kimberly **(SLP)**
Stivers, Ann B **(SLP)**
Stoutt, Tyleen Roe **(SLP)**
Young, Bonnie Thorson **(SLP)**

Arlington
Hocker, Mrs Mary Helen **(SLP)**

Ashland
Bartram, Margaret Lynne **(SLP)**
Bowling, Mrs Karin Ann **(SLP)**
Crose, Elizabeth **(SLP)**
McKenzie, Kimberly Rhodes **(SLP)**

Reynolds, Judith L **(SLP)**
Sherwood, Dr Karen Heerse **(A)**
Strait, Mary Wells **(SLP)**
Warman, Mrs Donna Sue **(A)**
West, Edwin Andre **(A)**
White, Marshall K **(SLP)**
Wilson, Mrs Mary Z **(SLP)**

Auburn
Dorris, Mrs Tammy Fox **(SLP)**

Bardstown
Burgess, Stephanie Dawn **(SLP)**
Wiksell, Carla Maria **(SLP)**

Baxter
Williams, Rebecca Ann **(SLP)**

Beattyville
Perdue, Susan W **(SLP)**

Benton
Erwin, Mrs Ellen **(SLP)**
Sutherland, Dee Mills **(SLP A)**

Bowling Green
Bunch, Mrs Barbara Jean **(SLP)**
Buntzman, Louise B **(SLP)**
Congdon, Christina Margaret **(SLP)**
Cooke, Dr Stan S **(SLP)**
Dunlap, Kim E **(SLP)**
Fisher, Mrs Virginia E **(SLP)**
Hale, Mark Bates
Hill, Denzle L **(SLP)**
Kersting, Frank M **(SLP)**
Kielty, Pamela J **(SLP A)**
Laird, Mrs Emily W G **(SLP)**
Martis, Janet A **(A)**
Moore, Kathleen Claire **(SLP)**
Parsley, Debbie Barnett **(SLP)**
Raney, Judith Kellogg **(SLP)**
Shinn, Dr Roy E, Jr **(A)**
Simpson, Alice Young **(SLP)**
Smith, Mrs Anne Maven **(A)**
Travis, Elizabeth B Higgins **(SLP)**
Wilkinson, Jane Raub **(SLP)**

Brandenburg
Shellner, Mrs Jacqueline **(SLP)**

Bronston
Wallace, Mrs Brenda Sue **(SLP)**

Brooksville
Case, Sue Anne **(SLP)**

Burlington
Chaffee, Shon M **(A)**

Cadiz
Allen, Kerry L **(SLP)**
James, Mrs La Reeca Meador **(SLP)**
Myatt, Mrs Kelley Pipkin
Sheehan, Charlene Cox **(SLP)**

Calvert City
Nordloh, Mrs Sharon J **(SLP)**

Campbellsville
Haynes, Glenda Marie **(SLP)**

Columbia
Havens, Dr Dolores **(SLP)**
Hutchison, Linda A **(SLP)**

Corbin
Marlowe, Cynthia L **(SLP)**
Parulekar, Dr Leela S **(A)**
Ward, Mrs Teresa Anne **(SLP)**

Covington
Markiewicz, Lori Ann **(SLP)**
Riemer, Gayle P **(A)**
Snyder, Lee Z **(A)**
Wernersbach, Mrs Margaret Baker **(SLP)**

Crescent Springs
Air, Dr Dorothy H **(SLP)**

Crestwood
Farrow, Mrs Cheryl Coleman **(SLP)**

Liebman, Joyce Kay **(SLP)**
Wilburn, Mrs Duana Charles **(SLP)**

Crofton
Daniel, David Aubrey **(SLP)**
Daniel, Martha Hardin **(SLP)**
Summers, Jerry G **(SLP)**

Cunningham
McColgin, Leslie S **(SLP)**

Danville
Derringer, Ann R **(SLP)**
Dinielli, Marion L **(A)**
Ellis, Mrs Jane M S **(SLP)**
Hoover, Carla Therese **(A)**
Kleinert, Sheila B **(SLP)**
Mills, Thelma B **(A)**

Dawson Springs
Chappel, Mrs Jan Marie **(SLP)**
Nichols, Kathy Lynn **(SLP)**

Dexter
Coursey, Mrs Susan **(SLP)**

Eastwood
Bennett, Karen Isaacs **(SLP)**

Eddyville
Stewart, Janet C
Talley, Mrs Anita M **(SLP)**

Edgewood
Broeg, Charlotte Marie **(SLP)**

Elizabethtown
Beasley, Mrs Joyce Bramley **(SLP)**
Bohaning, Teresa Lynn **(SLP)**
Borders, Jennifer Carole **(A)**
Degraffenried, Dr Helen Lee **(SLP A)**
Lesher, Judith L **(SLP)**
Lukat, Rita K **(SLP)**
Thornton, Christine **(SLP)**

Elliottville
Doerrfeld, Karen Dlugosz **(SLP)**

Erlanger
Bernardo, Mrs Anita R **(SLP)**
Stuart, Keith **(SLP)**
Tipton, Mrs Cindy H **(SLP)**

Ermine
Danford, Daniel Ernest **(SLP)**
Simmons-Miles, Rhonda Z **(SLP)**

Flemingsburg
Kinder, Mrs Mary Beth **(SLP)**
Ross, Diane B **(SLP)**

Florence
Sipple-Wallace, Connie **(SLP)**
Tattershall, Dr Sandra Susan **(SLP)**
Thompson, Lori Rae **(SLP)**
Walsh, Gail Shearer **(SLP)**

Fort Campbell
Bogue, Dr John Phillip, Sr
Bond, Loretta A **(A)**

Fort Mitchell
Caufield, Laurie C **(SLP)**
Dickman, Jahnett L **(SLP)**
Durkin, Teresa M **(SLP)**

Fort Thomas
Clayton, Katherine J **(A)**
Gruenhagen, Carol Lynn **(A)**
Hines, Susan D **(SLP)**
Knauf, Mrs Marguerite **(SLP)**
Koopmans, Sherri Lynn **(SLP)**
Ogden, Dr Christine E **(SLP A)**
Slater, Mrs Glenda Richmond
Wolfer, Joseph Edward **(A)**

Fort Wright
Frickman, Mrs Gail Adkins **(SLP)**
Gilbert, Jane Marie **(A)**
Schnorbus, Ann Elizabeth **(SLP)**
Thompson, Ann Marian **(A)**

Frankfort
Brennan, Michelle R **(SLP)**
Edelstein, Mrs Holly G **(SLP)**
Herr, Sally Blanche **(SLP)**
Strode, Robin M **(SLP)**
Vaughn, Mrs Teresa R **(SLP)**

Franklin
Simmons, Mrs Mary E **(SLP)**

Georgetown
Mulholland, Mrs Julie B **(SLP)**
Sams, Mrs Helen V **(SLP)**
Smith, Stephanie Stewart **(SLP)**

Glasgow
Harper, Mrs Pandora Slinker **(SLP)**
Napier, Julie Denise **(SLP)**
Perkins, Geneva **(SLP)**
Simmons, Mrs Patricia C **(SLP)**
Thurman, Mrs Susan H **(SLP)**

Glensfork
Cranfill, Tamara B **(SLP)**

Goshen
Rash, Mrs Joni Louise **(SLP)**

Grand Rivers
White, Mrs Robin Renae

Hager
Arnett, Tammy Ann **(SLP)**

Hager Hill
Curtsinger, Barbara Gayle **(SLP)**

Hardinsburg
Moore, Mrs Janice L H **(SLP)**

Harlan
Goss, Rebecca Singleton **(SLP)**
Spear, Douglas James **(A)**
Whitfield, Marie L **(SLP)**

Harrodsburg
Rassiga, Malinda Ann **(SLP)**

Hartford
Hutchison, Mrs Leisa Smith **(SLP)**

Hazard
Combs, Barbara Sue **(SLP)**
Davis, Corieta J **(SLP)**
Fields, Dorothy J
Krumm, Kent M **(SLP)**

Henderson
Bethel, Mrs Patsy M **(A)**
Kramer, Lynne C **(A)**
Mathis, Mrs Kathy Chandler **(SLP)**
Stroud, Linda Payne **(SLP)**
Wedding, Mrs Sarah Beth **(A)**

Highland Heights
Johnson, Dr John P **(SLP)**

Hopkinsville
Bastin, Mrs Lana L **(SLP)**
Grable, Mrs Patty Cannon **(SLP)**
Ison, Mrs Pamela A **(A)**
McKenzie, Thelma M **(SLP)**
Middleton, Mrs Barbara M **(SLP)**
Pigage, Mrs Martha Jacqueline **(SLP)**
Smith, Mrs Caroline **(SLP)**
Walker, Teresa Phillips **(SLP)**

Independence
Howard, Barbara H **(SLP)**
Payne, Linda C **(SLP)**

Jamestown
Huckaby, Mrs Rose M **(SLP)**

Jeffersontown
Staggs, Mrs Susan F **(SLP)**

Kevil
Weaver, Violet Lorraine **(SLP)**

Lakeside Park
De Angelis, Cynthia Stone **(SLP)**

Lebanon
Gordon, Mrs Katherine Chism **(SLP)**
Hamilton, Jennifer

Lexington
Alford, Emily Cheryl **(SLP)**
Ash, Mrs Mary S **(SLP)**
Bader, Paula D **(SLP)**
Banton, Mrs Ann E **(SLP)**
Becht, Kelly Marie
Bell, Mrs Sandra A **(SLP)**
Bertram, Christie C **(SLP)**
Besten, Mrs Michelle Borror **(SLP)**
Bolling, Mrs Julie F **(SLP)**
Brennan, Mary Margaret **(SLP)**
Brush-Lorey, Patricia M **(SLP)**
Burchett, Julie Lynn
Byrd, M Rita **(SLP)**
Carroll, Jacqueline D **(SLP)**
Castle, Tracy Calpin **(SLP)**
Chamberlain, Mrs Catherine **(SLP)**
Colwell, Mrs Wanda Ward **(SLP)**
Coman, Mary Judson
Cook, Patsy Ruth **(SLP)**
Cooper, Pauline Anne **(SLP)**
Craig, Mrs Betty C **(SLP)**
Cripe, Mrs Kimberly A **(SLP)**
Culatta, Janet D **(SLP)**
Cutshall, Susan Kennedy **(SLP)**
Erl, Marjorie **(SLP)**
Fackler, Mrs Ann G **(SLP)**
Farrar, Mrs Deborah Schaefer **(SLP)**
Fleenor, Mrs Elizabeth Gloyeske **(SLP)**
Fleming, Lucy Ann **(SLP)**
Fox, Joseph P **(SLP)**
Graff, Mrs Victoria C **(SLP A)**
Gray, Mary S **(SLP)**
Green, Dr William W **(A)**
Greene-Vaughan, Betty **(SLP)**
Hagerman, Ellen C **(SLP)**
Hall, Susan **(SLP)**
Harwood, Teresa Carolyn **(SLP)**
Horn, Dr Donna G **(SLP)**
Hughes, Mary H **(SLP)**
Irwin, Dr John V **(SLP)**
Jones, Lou Ann **(A)**
Kleinert, Jane E O'Regan **(SLP)**
Knight, Terryl M **(SLP)**
Langley, Elizabeth McCoy **(SLP)**
Lawless, Kimberly H **(A)**
Lawson, Mrs Jane Withers **(SLP)**
Mabry, Lisa Rai **(SLP)**
Manning, Robert Dean **(A)**
Martin, Barbara Lynn **(SLP)**
Mason, Nancie C **(SLP)**
McDowell, Mary Louise **(SLP)**
Meilinger, Cynthia Smith **(SLP)**
Miller, Mrs Jean M A **(SLP)**
Monahan, Mrs Dana O **(SLP)**
Nabity, Mrs Regina M **(SLP)**
Nutter, Mrs Susan Botts **(SLP)**
Page, Dr Judith L **(SLP)**
Polk, Jane Midkiff
Porterfield, Wendy Sue **(SLP)**
Powell, Amy J **(A)**
Ragsdale, Elizabeth **(SLP)**
Reeves, Mrs Cindy W
Richardson, Mrs Virginia Ratliff **(SLP)**
Rutledge, Mrs Shelby Mullins **(SLP)**
Ryan, Mrs Alesia Houston **(SLP)**
Sandusky, Kathryn A **(A)**
Secrest, Mrs Mary Miller **(SLP)**
Shelton, Mrs Kathleen Mary **(SLP)**
Shook, Janelle B **(SLP)**
Sisson, Susan Lynn **(SLP)**
Sloan, Karla Ann **(SLP)**
Sloneker, Mrs Kathy R **(SLP)**
Soper, Donna Marie **(SLP)**
Southerland, Donna Jan **(SLP)**
Sparks, Mrs Sheldia Bishop **(SLP)**
Springate, Nancy Leigh **(SLP)**
Stacy, Ann Rhoten **(A)**
Stanley, Beverly A **(SLP A)**

Stephens, Gay **(SLP)**
Stewart, Sharon **(SLP)**
Stratton, Terry L **(SLP)**
Swigert, Nancy B **(SLP)**
Swisher, Mrs Lynn Crabtree
Trost-Steffen, Catherine **(SLP)**
Vitali, Gary John **(SLP)**
Walker, Joyce Witzler **(SLP)**
Wallen, Joyce A **(A)**
Wedding, Kellye Ann **(SLP)**
Wilson, Dr Margo E **(SLP)**
Winkler, Wanda Joy **(A)**
Womble, Mrs Amygayle Law **(SLP)**
Wright, Caroline **(SLP)**
Wrobel, Maureen M **(SLP)**

Louisa
Wallis, Mrs Barbara A **(SLP)**

Louisville
Abromaitis, Mrs Kay Marie **(SLP)**
Adornato, Viki Ann **(SLP)**
Ater, Judy A **(SLP)**
Baker, Janet L **(SLP)**
Barnett, Kathleen Ann
Baustien, Mrs Julie B **(SLP)**
Bechard, Mrs Maria Fotias **(SLP)**
Becker, Leslie A **(SLP)**
Bell, Ann Elizabeth **(SLP)**
Bellville, Judith Gail **(SLP)**
Binger, Mrs Annette T **(SLP)**
Bivins, Cynthia F **(SLP)**
Bland, Lauren Elaine **(SLP)**
Blodgett, Mrs Nancy H **(SLP)**
Bradley, Rose Oswald **(SLP)**
Breighner, Sr M Wilma **(SLP)**
Brown, Dr William J **(SLP A)**
Burtnett, Mrs Pamela L **(SLP)**
Burysek-Cherry, Mrs Denita J **(SLP)**
Calvert, Marianne Jordan **(SLP)**
Carden, Denise Gregson **(SLP)**
Carpenter, Susan S **(SLP)**
Cazden, Robert P
Chaudoin, Barbara Ann **(A)**
Clark, Mark E **(A)**
Clift, Mildred Ann **(SLP)**
Coan, Susan Lee **(SLP)**
Craven, Lisanne Simms **(SLP)**
Crowder, Joy Lynn **(SLP)**
Cunningham, Dr David Robert **(A)**
Dattilo, Mrs Joan L **(SLP)**
Dausman, Rebecca Carroll **(SLP)**
Davis, Sharon W **(SLP)**
Dermody, Rebecca Lynn
Donaldson, Mrs Cheryl W **(SLP)**
Draewell, Susan K **(SLP)**
Driskill, Susan W
Drury, Mrs JoLynn B **(SLP)**
Dunn, Mrs Donna S **(SLP A)**
Dunn, Thomas M **(A)**
Dyer, Barbara Jane **(A)**
Edlin, Mrs Vicki M **(SLP)**
Eisenmenger, Barbara A **(A)**
Emrich, Mrs Mary J **(SLP)**
Epstein, Mark S **(SLP)**
Farzi, Fred Edward
Flores, Marsha D **(A)**
Ford, Kathryn Lawson **(SLP)**
Fourman, Laura Ann
Fox, Susan M **(SLP)**
Frankrone, Sr M Dorothy **(SLP)**
Funk, Dr Harry E **(SLP)**
Galchick, Mrs Janis Milligan **(SLP)**
Garland, Priscilla **(SLP A)**
Geis, Rose Marie **(SLP)**
Gilda, Dr Barbara Baker **(SLP)**
Gorin, Mrs Mary B **(SLP)**
Gottschalk, Mrs Becky Rene **(SLP)**
Green, Mrs Patricia Mary
Gregory, Mrs Roberta A **(SLP)**
Grider, Mrs Elizabeth Callaway **(SLP)**
Hall, Rita Marie **(SLP)**
Hammer, Mary B **(SLP)**
Hancock, Mrs Melissa Dowse **(SLP)**
Hayden, Cecilia Marie **(A)**
Hepp, Cheryl L **(SLP)**
Herman, Mrs Terry S **(SLP)**
Higgins, Portia R **(SLP)**
Hoza, Sherry T **(SLP)**
Huffman, Mrs Myra Jean **(SLP)**
James, Marcy Ann **(SLP)**
Johnson, Margaret Anne **(A)**
Johnston, Sr Anna Mae
Jones, Deanna Suenette **(A)**
Just, Lynn B **(SLP)**
Kaelin, Charlotte **(SLP)**
Katz, James B **(A)**
Katzman, Dr Elizabeth A **(SLP)**
Keen, Mrs Peggy A **(SLP)**
Kieta, Mrs Mary Julie **(SLP)**
King, Michelle F **(A)**
Kirsch, Jane **(SLP)**
Knight, Jane Kiser **(SLP)**
Krebs, Mrs Mary B V **(SLP)**
Laemmle, Jane M **(SLP)**
Larson, Mrs Nancy S **(SLP)**
Lazich, Richard W **(A)**
Lockhart, Maureen Flannery **(A)**
Mabe, Joan Loeffler **(A)**
MacHtolff, Kim M **(SLP)**
Maier, Linda Carol **(SLP)**
Masden, Susan L **(SLP)**
McAllister, Mary Elizabeth **(SLP)**
McCall, Rosanne Bennion **(SLP)**
Montana, Amy L
Moriarty, Daniel Gerard **(A)**
Morris, Mrs Terry L **(SLP)**
Mudd, Mrs Mary Ann **(SLP)**
Myers, Mrs Gail S **(SLP)**
Newbery, Mrs Rosemary Motley **(A)**
Newett, Norma J **(SLP A)**
Newman, Mrs Jill Hess **(SLP)**
Niemann, Mrs Mary Kay **(SLP)**
Nitzken, Syl J, Jr **(SLP)**
Norfleet, Sheila G
Norris, Michael L **(A)**
Olin, Geraldine **(SLP)**
Panther, Mrs Kathy M **(SLP)**
Patterson, Dr Ramelle F **(SLP A)**
Paul, Christine **(A)**
Pearlman, Peter Michael **(A)**
Peebles, Mary Jane Delauter **(SLP)**
Perkins, Ann N G **(SLP)**
Persenaire, L Ann **(A)**
Pierce, Patricia D **(SLP)**
Pollom, Mrs Judy L **(SLP)**
Porter, Mary S **(SLP)**
Prendergast, Sandra Kay **(SLP)**
Proffitt, Kimberly G **(SLP)**
Purvis, Dr George O'Neill **(A)**
Rachford, Sharon L **(SLP)**
Ransaw, Mrs Anna K **(SLP)**
Reynolds, Lisa C **(SLP)**
Ridge, Mrs Holly Share **(SLP)**
Riordan, Barbara Baldwin **(SLP)**
Rivette-Smith, Mrs Patricia Walker **(SLP)**
Rouse, Mrs Carolyn B **(SLP)**
Rowlett, Mrs Karen L **(SLP)**
Russell, Mrs Luanne S **(SLP)**
Ryan, Mrs Elizabeth **(SLP)**
Sakaguchi, Mrs Linda M **(SLP)**
Saling, Reanna L **(SLP)**
Sanders, Mrs Sarah Mullaney **(SLP)**
Savage, Mrs Judy A **(SLP)**
Schmit, Pamela S **(SLP)**
Scott, Mrs Brenda Mueller **(SLP)**
Searcy, Deborah A **(SLP)**
Seligman, Mrs Lillian O **(SLP)**
Shouse, Sherry W **(SLP)**
Silverman, Dr Irving **(SLP A)**
Smith, Mrs Cynthia B **(SLP)**
Somer, Ellen S **(SLP)**
Spalding, Mrs Catherine Lucas **(SLP)**
Starr, Mrs Nancy S **(SLP)**
Steckol, Dr Karen Faye **(SLP)**
Stein, Dr Dorothy M **(A)**
Stenhouse, Sylvia T **(SLP)**
Stoltz, Mrs Terri Lynn **(SLP)**
Stone, Mrs Joan Marie **(SLP)**
Swartz, Mrs Linda Kay **(SLP)**
Tonini, Mrs Kathleen Burnett **(SLP)**
Trussell, Susan Elaine
Vanover, Cheryl Annette **(SLP)**
Vernon, Mrs Sharon L **(SLP)**
Weber, Denise A **(SLP)**
Williams, Alice I **(SLP)**
Williams, Mary Catherine **(SLP)**
Wilson, Mrs Donna Piercy **(SLP)**
Windmill, Dr Ian M **(A)**
Windmill, Sue McDonnell **(A)**
Womack, Karen H **(SLP)**
Wooldridge, Joyce M **(SLP)**
Yoder, Suzanne Ross **(A)**

Madisonville
Arnold, Laura Jean **(A)**
Badgett, Carol Elizabeth **(SLP)**
Beshear, Mrs Deborah Wood **(SLP)**
Boe, Debra J **(SLP)**
Edwards, Thomas Wayne **(SLP)**
France, Pamela Joyce **(SLP)**
Gover, Mrs Misha W **(SLP)**
Miner, Mrs Lista G R **(SLP)**
Morgan, Marian T **(A)**
Reasonover, Patricia Dianne **(A)**
Vaughan, Mrs Donna Duewall **(SLP)**

Manchester
Cornett, Mrs Lona Ghent **(SLP)**
Hughes, Lela J **(SLP)**
Sizemore, Ramona

Martin
Kissel, Sr Judith Ann **(SLP)**

Mayfield
Downing, Mrs Carolyn Butler **(SLP)**
Holloway, Mrs Shelia Allene **(SLP)**
Neely, Ann N N **(SLP)**
Watson, Mrs Penny Camp
Wood, Mrs Diane C **(SLP)**

Middlesboro
Flanigan, Steve George **(SLP)**
Williams, John Elliott **(SLP)**
Williams, Susan Berger **(SLP)**

Monticello
Botts-Penrod, Mrs Elizabeth **(SLP)**
Coffey, Elizabeth **(SLP)**
Miniard, Holly P **(SLP)**

Morehead
Thomason, Mrs Nancy Loomis **(SLP)**
Ward, Mrs Kelly A **(SLP)**
Warren, Kimberly Ann **(A)**

Morganfield
Brantley, Mrs Susan Lee **(SLP)**
Ebbeskotte, Karen A **(SLP)**
Harman, Deborah M **(SLP)**

Mount Olivet
Lally, Eleanore Coomes **(SLP)**

Mount Sterling
Gillaspie, Prudence Lynn **(SLP)**
Rice, Mrs Vicki Colliver **(SLP)**
Williams, Mrs Jan Wallace **(SLP)**

Mount Vernon
Gregory, Mrs Mary **(SLP)**

Mount Washington
Writsel, Mrs Leila V **(SLP)**

Munfordville
Anderson, Mrs Mary Lou **(SLP)**

Murray
Alexander, Mrs Eldonna Marie **(SLP)**
Blackford, Mrs Susan H **(SLP)**
Blodgett, Dr Elizabeth **(SLP)**
Chamberlain, Martha H **(SLP)**
Condon, Marilyn T **(A)**
Deem, Jodelle F **(SLP)**
Gradisher, Mrs Myra Summervill **(SLP)**
Hart, Mrs Sharon Blodgett
Hopkins, Dixie G **(SLP)**
Hornback, Mrs Marilyn A **(SLP)**
Kodman, Dr Frank, Jr **(SLP A)**
McCuiston, Patricia Robinson **(SLP)**
Miller, Dr Viola P **(SLP)**
Richardson, Cherie M **(SLP)**
Roberts, Mrs Wanda T **(SLP)**
Schempp, Mrs Nancy F **(SLP)**
Seargent, Mrs Janice W **(SLP)**
Severns, Mrs Jennifer Renee' **(SLP)**
Snell, Susan J **(A)**

Nancy
Sheets, Mrs Cheryl C **(SLP)**

Nerinx
Gutzwiller, Mary L **(A)**

New Castle
Bell, Mrs Jean L

New Hope
Fischer, Linda G **(SLP)**

Newport
Welp, Mrs Marjorie Monnin **(SLP)**

Nicholasville
Lach, Edythe T **(SLP)**

Owensboro
Ambrose, Mrs Bobbie Robertson **(SLP)**
Clark, Joan **(SLP)**
Cripps, Mrs Gina Nation **(SLP)**
Embry, Cynthia Anne
Etienne, Joseph E **(A)**
Gerteisen, Mrs Rita A **(A)**
Goodlett, Donna L **(SLP)**
Harrington, Mrs Hadley R **(SLP)**
Hein, Caroline Ann **(SLP)**
Holder, Hugh Scott **(SLP)**
Lee, Kathleen Kehoe **(SLP)**
Leonard, Mrs Melodie Kincaid
Litsey, Mrs Lisa Everhard **(SLP)**
McKown, Mrs Patricia D **(A)**
Mueller, Pam **(SLP)**
Naas, Dr James F **(SLP)**
Nall, Patricia Louise **(SLP)**
O'Bryan, Mrs Anne L **(SLP)**
Oldham, Mrs Elizabeth Belle **(SLP)**
Shown, Suzanne **(SLP)**
Swift, Mrs Dawn Elizabeth **(SLP)**
Tessandori, Mrs Joann S **(SLP)**
Wight, Karen M **(SLP)**

Owingsville
Roehrig, Sharon A **(SLP)**

Paducah
Amundson, Martin A **(A)**
Ballew, Dr Laurie Kay **(SLP)**
Borders, Mrs Mary Sue **(SLP)**
Chester, Mrs Enda Elaine **(SLP)**
Coughlin, Mrs Janel McKinney **(SLP)**
Cummings, Charlene D **(SLP)**
Fowler, Mrs Patricia Kay **(SLP)**
Gillespie, R David **(A)**
Griffin, Mrs Candice Burgess **(SLP)**
Gunn, Mrs Cynthia **(SLP)**
Hosford, Mrs Patti Miller **(SLP)**
Lang, Georgie Lee **(SLP)**
Luker, Edward E **(A)**
Nelson, Patricia E **(SLP)**
Ogden, Ruth A **(SLP)**
Simmons, Margaret E **(SLP)**
Spiceland, Joseph Cecil **(SLP)**
Wright, Victoria H **(SLP)**

Paintsville
Crigger, Mrs Kathryn H **(SLP)**
Mullins, Mrs Lynn D **(SLP)**

Park Hills
Becher, Donna K **(SLP)**
Hogan, Deborah S **(SLP)**

Pewee Valley
White, Mrs Lynda McCall **(SLP)**

Philpot
Gilbert, Ginger T **(SLP)**
Millay, Karyl Sue **(SLP)**

Pikeville
Furby, Robert Leon **(A)**

Prestonsburg
Fannin, Virginia L **(SLP)**
Reynolds, Sandra Gayle **(SLP)**

Princeton
Williams, Mrs Beverly Renee **(SLP)**
Wurtman, Betty Grace **(SLP)**

Printer
Dye, Mrs Gaye D **(SLP)**

Prospect
Dillingham, Mrs Nancy T **(SLP)**
Schoder, Mrs Debra J **(SLP)**

Radcliff
Coker, Mrs Jena Davis **(SLP)**
Purdy, Richard H **(A)**

Richmond
Baker, Mary Blank **(SLP)**
Coulter, Linda W **(SLP)**
Dapkus, Mrs Kathy Heil **(SLP)**
Eldot, Dr Howard L **(A)**
Erdmann, Mrs Michele **(SLP)**
Goldstein, Mrs Gail D **(SLP)**
Harris, Mrs Leta L **(SLP)**
Harris, Dr Lonnie G **(SLP)**
Kendrick, Kathryn Ann **(SLP)**
Mahanna-Boden, Susan **(SLP)**
Meckler, Mrs Deanna L **(A)**
Shearon, Lynn B **(SLP)**
Shelton, Ivy L **(SLP)**
Terango, Dr Larry **(SLP A)**

Rousseau
Holbrook, Wanda Kaye

Russell
Brown, Debra V
Fryling, Lori Jean **(SLP)**
Kupsky, Barbara L **(SLP)**
Lyman, Charlotte Kay **(A)**

Russell Springs
Grider, Mrs Joy Stephens
McKinley, Mrs Sheila Ison **(SLP)**

Russellville
Militana, Mrs Norma K S **(SLP)**

Shelbyville
Brammer, Mrs Brenda G **(SLP)**
Goss, Marilyn Mauck **(SLP)**
Willard, Mrs Sandra Shy **(SLP)**

Somerset
Durham, Kathleen V **(A)**
Flynn, Mrs Ronda Cain **(SLP)**
Kasica, Antoinette P **(SLP)**
Marcum, Debra L **(SLP)**
Noe, Lana C **(SLP)**
Peavie, Linda Fairchild **(SLP)**

Southgate
Dance, Joan L **(A)**

Summer Shade
Hammer, Mrs Shirley Jean **(SLP)**

Van Lear
Boswell, Teresa Clay **(SLP)**
Gregory, Charlotte Keane **(SLP)**

Versailles
Hundley, Claire L **(SLP)**
Knauss, Judith D S **(SLP)**
Leeper, Dr Linda H **(SLP)**
Vitali, Marie Elizabeth **(SLP)**
Wilds, Daena Cheryl **(A)**

Williamsburg
Greer, Mrs Lola B **(SLP)**
Williams, Mary Kim **(SLP)**

Wilmore
Chapman, Darwin Lee **(SLP)**

Winchester
Million, Dr Phillip C **(A)**
Ware, Mrs Monica Combs **(SLP)**

Wittensville
Walters, Wellington **(SLP)**

LOUISIANA

Abbeville
Degraauw, Mrs Claudette **(SLP)**
Ducote, Dianna Deshotels **(SLP)**

Abita Springs
Andries, Julie Gement **(SLP)**

Alexandria
Akridge, Jeanie Dupuy **(SLP)**
Brown, Carol Lynn **(SLP)**
Cataldie, Mary **(SLP)**
Colle, Mrs Josephine **(SLP)**
Daiy, Kelly Ann **(SLP)**
Hamilton, Nora L **(SLP)**
Jeanmard, Frances Lee **(SLP)**
Juneau, Cynthia Cheek **(SLP)**
Landry, Katherine Denise **(SLP)**
Masson, Mrs Ella Marie **(SLP)**
Mayeux, Deborah Anne M **(SLP)**
McDonald, Mrs Pamela Bonnette **(SLP)**
Mercer, Deena L **(SLP)**
Owens, Mrs Alice Risley **(SLP)**
Roberts, Terry Lynn **(A)**
Rozier, Mrs Judith Ann **(SLP)**
Seal, Mrs Nelda C **(SLP)**
White, Mrs Carolyn Holmes **(SLP)**
Wills, Edward C **(A)**
Wollerson, Beulah B R **(SLP)**

Amite
Mobley, Mrs Mary Morgan **(SLP)**

Arabi
Donnell, Mrs Betty A **(SLP)**
Doody, M Patricia **(SLP)**

Arnaudville
Mathews, Barbara Lucy **(SLP)**

Baker
McKann, Mrs Sallie M **(SLP)**

Bastrop
Cable, Mrs Virginia Evans **(SLP)**
Miller, Mrs Rhonda Rene **(SLP)**

Baton Rouge
Abshire-Jumonville, Mrs Wendy Marie **(A)**
Adcock, Aleta Millet **(SLP)**
Anderson, Marzene Elizabeth
Arnold, Mrs Julia L **(SLP)**
Babin, Mrs Sharon B **(SLP)**
Barbay, Judy Hammonds **(SLP)**
Barton, Dr James P **(SLP)**
Baucum, Kay **(SLP)**
Beard, Janice Holcomb **(SLP)**
Beridon, Brenda T **(SLP)**
Bird, Elisabeth Grace **(SLP)**
Blanco, Felicia
Blount, Hal Russell **(SLP)**
Brockhaus, Rebecca Watson **(SLP)**
Brzuszek, Melissa Gibb **(SLP)**
Buckingham, Dr Hugh W, Jr
Byers, Mrs Judith Braud **(SLP)**
Cage, Johnnye Annzanetta **(SLP)**
Campbell, Dr Lynda R **(SLP)**
Canon, Eleanor K **(SLP)**
Carey, Mrs Barbara Chicola **(SLP)**
Carville, Mrs Lynn B **(SLP)**
Casey, Beth M **(SLP)**
Civils, Mrs Carol Ann **(SLP)**
Collins, M Jane **(A)**
Cottrell, Dr Mary M **(SLP)**
Crary, Sharon Kay **(SLP)**
Damico, Dr Jack S **(SLP)**
Damico, Mrs Sandra K **(SLP)**
Daniloff, Raymond
Davidson, Gayle A **(SLP)**
Delaune, Mrs Pamela L **(SLP)**
Dickinson, Lynn M **(SLP)**
Ditty, Karen Markuson **(A)**
Dolan, Cynthia Jo **(SLP)**
Drumm, Marcelle Bergeron **(SLP)**
Ducombs, Sherry C **(A)**
Ducombs, Thomas V **(A)**
Dykes, Sandy Frank **(SLP)**
Dykes, Mrs Sharon H **(SLP)**
Earp, Rebecca J **(SLP)**
Eichler, Kaye B **(SLP)**
Eilts, Judith T **(SLP)**
Fairchild, Mrs Leslie P
Ferris, Lora M C **(SLP)**
Fisher, Mrs Francine Kaplan **(SLP A)**
Fletcher, Pat F **(SLP)**
Freeman, Clarence J **(A)**
Fuoto, Ellen M **(SLP)**
Garcia-Giese, Mrs Maria E **(SLP)**
Gavin, Jo Lynn **(SLP)**
Germany, Barbara T **(SLP)**
Gouvier, Rebecca Harrell **(SLP)**
Guidry, Annette Marie **(SLP)**
Guntrum, Dwana **(SLP)**
Hale, Dr Lester L **(SLP)**
Hall, Deanne Brenda **(A)**
Hall, Don Raymond **(SLP)**
Hamilton, Julie Barfield **(SLP)**
Hamilton, Marilyn A **(SLP)**
Hammatt, Mrs Nancy N **(SLP)**
Henderson, Mrs Patricia **(SLP)**
Hill, Brent W **(A)**
Hoffman, Paul R **(SLP)**
Hudson, Dr Amelia I **(SLP)**
Iturralde, Mrs Joy Harvey
Jetty, Dr Albert J **(SLP A)**
Johnson, Mrs Katherine Vaughn **(SLP)**
Johnston, Mrs Elizabeth **(SLP)**
Judice, Donna Felecia **(SLP)**
Kees, Maxwell G **(SLP A)**
Knecht, Mrs Gail B **(SLP)**
Lastrapes, Carolyn Hall **(SLP)**
Lauve, Jane F **(SLP)**
Le Blanc, Sherry A **(SLP)**
Lee, Mrs Barbara B **(A)**
Levert, Stephanie M **(SLP A)**
Lierman, Mrs Cynthia L **(SLP)**
Littman, Thomas A **(A)**
Loewy, Eva Susanna
Mangan, Dr James **(SLP A)**
Mangin, Nancy L **(SLP)**
Marshall, Dr George Matthews, Jr **(SLP)**
McCoy, Catherine Gordon
McKey, Frances D **(SLP)**
McKnight, Mrs Anne Elmore **(SLP A)**
McKnight, Mrs Kathleen N **(SLP)**
Means, Teresa Elizabeth **(SLP)**
Michaelson, Mrs Melanie C **(SLP)**
Miller, Jamie A
Mitchell, Dr Oscar, Jr **(SLP A)**
Monjure, Joann **(SLP)**
Moock, Mrs Judy N **(SLP)**
Moore, Marlyn D **(SLP A)**
Morgan, Gilda Fay
Norris, Dr Janet A **(SLP)**
Parker, Dr Frank P
Pennigton, Mrs Denise Amedee **(SLP)**
Pevey, Mrs Jo Rhea B **(SLP)**
Proctor, Nancy H **(SLP)**
Rappold, Patrick Wynn **(A)**
Richards, Pamela R **(SLP)**
Riely, Mrs Joann Edwards
Robertson, Mrs Helen **(SLP)**
Rockhold, Mrs Thayne Hamilton **(A)**
Rogers, Cathy Sue **(SLP)**
Safer, Deborah Griffin **(SLP)**
Sams, Mrs Lois Buchanan **(SLP)**
Schmidt, Janice O **(SLP)**
Schoen, Paula Hollins **(SLP)**
Sills, Marsha H **(SLP)**
Sims, Mrs Alice M **(SLP)**
Solanas, Elizabeth **(SLP)**
Sonnier, Eileen R **(SLP)**
Speeks, Emelda L **(SLP A)**
Stevenson, Dedra Michelle **(SLP)**
Sturkie, Mrs Bernice Barrett **(SLP)**
Suire, Mrs Lisa T **(SLP)**
Tani, Dr Allen H **(SLP A)**
Tapia, Mrs Mary Esteve **(SLP)**
Taylor, Mrs Denise Catherine **(SLP)**
Teague, Laura Jo **(SLP)**
Trahan, Mrs Carol A **(SLP)**
Trahan, Mrs Suzanne Karol **(A)**
Travis, Dr Norma C **(SLP)**
Wallace, Rita Baker **(SLP)**
Weaver, Phoebe C **(SLP)**
Welch, Elizabeth **(SLP)**
Wexler, Kathryn F **(A)**
Whittaker, Robbie H **(SLP)**
Wilhite, Irvin **(SLP A)**
Wilks, Mrs Gina Guillera **(SLP)**
Williams, Seleria Jean **(SLP)**
Woolie, Mrs Brenda Allen **(SLP)**
Zamadics, Cathy Louise **(A)**

Belle Chasse
Chauvin, Mrs Leslie Ann **(SLP)**

Benton
Zimmerman, Dr Barbara R **(SLP A)**

Berwick
Burchfield, Mrs Bella Parro **(SLP)**

Bogalusa
Briese, Mrs Anne D **(SLP)**
Pierce, Shonna Medell

Bossier City
Brown, Janet Barnett **(SLP)**
Collins, Mrs Dorla Durr **(SLP)**
Hill, Mrs Beth S **(SLP)**
Locke, Patricia **(SLP)**
Morgan, Jeanne Boose **(SLP)**
Phipps, Mrs Linda M **(SLP)**
Sprute, Debra Bengoa **(SLP)**
Walker, Mrs Julia C **(SLP)**

Boyce
Charrier, Sheila Crosby **(SLP)**

Breaux Bridge
Hobbs, Brenda Castille **(SLP)**
Romano, Alex T **(SLP)**
Romano, Mrs Jacqulyn **(SLP)**

Broussard
Fontenot, Mrs M Christy **(A)**

Bunkie
Ripley, Mrs Barbara Deville **(SLP)**

Calhoun
Bush, Mrs Lisa L **(SLP)**

Carencro
Barousse, Mrs Melanie S **(SLP)**
Parker, Mrs Kay Bruno **(SLP)**

Chalmette
Childress, Gloria G **(SLP)**
Clements, Charmaine **(SLP)**
Cooper, Mrs Sheilah Auderer **(SLP)**
Gremillion, Michelle Ann
Kelty, Mrs Pauline Cotaya **(SLP)**

Choudrant
Whitman, Sandra L W **(SLP)**

Church Point
Ousse, Anne M **(SLP)**

Covington
Boudreaux, Dr Jean Rose **(SLP)**
Desporte, Edward J **(A)**
Duke-Morvant, Deborah A **(SLP)**
Homer, Emily M **(SLP)**
Istre, Dr Clifton O, Jr **(SLP A)**
McInerney, Mrs Laurie Stehwien **(SLP)**
Parker, Catherine Spadaro **(SLP)**
Pounds, Mrs Gayle Montrevil **(SLP A)**
Robert, Jan M **(SLP)**
Stiegler, Mrs Lillian Nielsen **(SLP)**

Crowley
Bier, Margaret C **(SLP)**
Cunningham, Barbara C **(SLP)**

De Ridder
Bradley, Mrs Catherine **(SLP)**
Lestage, Rosemary B **(SLP)**

Destrehan
Clancy, Mrs Annemarie Bock **(SLP)**
Goitia, Mrs Lorena Desalvo **(SLP)**
Thomas, Susan Kay **(SLP)**

Duson
Desormeaux, Mrs Linda B

Ethel
Annison, Mrs Marguerite **(SLP)**
Blouin, Mrs Carolyn K **(SLP)**

Eunice
Chachere, Mrs Arlene Caillier **(SLP)**
Devillier, Mrs Wanda Normand **(SLP)**
Lacalle, Mrs Evelyn S **(SLP)**

Farmerville
Austin, Mrs Sue M **(SLP)**
Taylor, Denise D **(SLP)**

Folsom
Ducote, Dr Charlotte **(SLP)**
King, Gwen Sparkman **(SLP)**
Negrotto, Mrs Carol Anne **(SLP)**

Fort Polk
Baca, Capt Margaret Louise

Glynn
Mounger, Dorothy C **(SLP)**

Gonzales
Tullier, Mrs Amy Lynn **(SLP)**

Grambling
Jackson, Mrs Betty J J **(SLP)**

Gray
Prejean, Barbara A **(SLP)**

Grayson
Walker, Jerry O **(SLP)**

Gretna
Breaud, Mrs Jane Maness **(SLP)**
Brent, Mrs Elizabeth Rabalais **(SLP)**
Del Toro, Janice Feagin **(SLP)**
Hamilton, Mrs Nancy Welsh **(SLP)**
Lipchak, Andrea M **(SLP)**
Murphy, Mrs Donna Caswell **(SLP)**
Peat, Mrs Melinda Myhres **(A)**

Hammond
Bartels, Kathleen **(SLP A)**
Fajoni, Angela Crim **(SLP)**
Hughes, Mrs Kathleen Gilbert **(A)**
Lerner, Dr Brenda J **(SLP)**
Lomax, Mrs Teresa Ann **(SLP)**
Phares, Mrs Georgette Statham **(SLP)**
Robinson, John E **(SLP)**
Sroges, Cara Bianca **(SLP)**
Todd, Susan M **(SLP)**
Underwood, Paul S **(A)**

Harahan
Broussard, Robin Elizabeth **(SLP)**
Callia, Ramona Leydecker **(SLP)**
Deus, Julia B **(SLP)**
Duplantis, Myra B **(SLP)**
Guidry, Mrs Joan Pavur **(SLP)**
Kenney, Mrs Kerry Ann **(SLP)**
Lillich, Mrs Maureen Cronan **(SLP)**
Smyke, Anna T **(A)**

Harvey
Naseman, Suzanne Laborde **(SLP)**
Reynolds, Deborah L **(SLP)**
Scott, Mrs Atheria C **(SLP)**
Slater, Rebecca H **(SLP A)**
Vaughn, Mrs Linda Robinson **(SLP)**

Haughton
Jones, Linda H **(SLP)**
Teresi, Pamela S **(SLP)**
Usrey, Mrs Ruth S **(SLP)**
Zachary, Mrs Ronda Kay **(SLP)**

Houma
Allen, Mrs Sharon A **(SLP)**
Dagate, Robin Ann **(A)**
Ellender, Mrs Elizabeth **(SLP)**
Mire, Steve P **(SLP)**
Yakupzack, Mrs Edwina M **(SLP A)**

Iota
Hadaway, Mrs Mary Ann **(SLP)**
Varnado, Mrs Mollie Denise **(SLP)**

Jeanerette
Eldridge, Mrs Flavia H **(SLP)**

Jennings
Bourque-Ardoin, Deborah **(SLP)**
Carter, Mrs Regilyn W **(SLP)**
Hebert, Mrs Lynne R **(SLP)**
Marcantel, Kathleen Doherty **(SLP)**

Jonesboro
Oliver, Dr Paxton E **(SLP)**

Kenner
Anderson, Jill Marie **(A)**
Ariail, Alison Millet **(SLP)**
Cugin, Janet Melissa
Davis, Mrs Kay D **(SLP)**
Dodds, Holly Jo **(A)**
Hagstette, Sharon Murray **(SLP)**
Hebert, Mrs Lisa Anne **(SLP)**
Heuer, Deborah Joseph **(SLP)**
Jackson, Mrs Cynthia G **(SLP)**
Klibert, Mrs Elizabeth W **(SLP)**
McGee, Dr Annell **(SLP)**
Miciotto, Deanna P **(SLP)**
Mickleberry, Darlene Marie **(SLP)**
Smith, Mrs Dianne P **(A)**
Smith, Mrs Lisa W **(SLP)**
Soyez, Mrs Debbie D **(SLP)**

La Place
Coleman, Yvette St Martin **(SLP)**
Jones, Mrs Caroline Selig **(SLP)**
Neupert, Catherine Cangelosi **(SLP)**
Ocmond, Wilbert J, Jr **(SLP)**
Robottom, Mrs Natalie Claire **(SLP)**
Walters, William B **(A)**
White, Mrs Cynthia J **(SLP)**

Lacombe
Schaeffer, Mrs Lynne Guggenheim **(SLP)**

Lafayette
Arehole, Dr Shalini **(A)**
Audiffred, Martin J **(A)**
Augustine, Dr Lloyd E **(SLP)**
Badon, Linda Cain
Baker, Dr La Verne L **(SLP)**
Baxter, Dr Kelmer D **(SLP)**
Bennett, Cecile S **(SLP)**
Billeaud, Mrs Frances P **(SLP)**
Boulanger, Mrs Sue P **(SLP)**
Brooks, Mrs Lee Ann **(SLP)**
Cornyn, Aprel L F **(SLP)**
Coughlin, Bobette Marie **(SLP)**
Daigle, Theresa Kay
Davis, Margaret Alsworth **(SLP)**
Duhon, Mrs Andree S **(SLP)**
Foreman, Mrs Jan C **(SLP)**
Foret, Lois L **(SLP)**
Fruge, Karen Kay **(A)**
Godshall, Laurie C **(SLP)**
Gordon, Mary Jo **(SLP)**
Greenwood, Suzanne **(SLP)**
Guillory, Dr Jimmy John **(SLP A)**
Hammond, Mrs Rosemary Dupree **(SLP)**
Hanks, Felice A **(SLP)**
Hardesty, Dr Patricia E **(SLP A)**
Harris, Mrs Andrea Pappas **(SLP)**
Hebert, Mrs Marianne Lahaye **(SLP)**
Kane, Joan G **(SLP)**
Kiefer, Mrs Susan Deborah **(SLP)**
Laborde, Mrs Karen Dorsey **(SLP)**
Lacombe, Mrs Idell H **(SLP)**
Lacy, Mrs Aleyce Bluestein **(SLP)**
Landry, Mrs Laura Christman **(SLP)**
Lobdell, Mary Moseley **(SLP)**
Lock, Patricia Swinburne **(SLP)**
MacLeod, Mrs Cynthia Soforenko **(SLP)**
Meche, Peggy A **(SLP)**
Messonnier, Mrs Pamela G
Miller, Lisa Marie **(SLP)**
Moore, Mrs Sherri A **(SLP)**
Nugent, Mrs Lynn B
O'Pry, Mrs Judy **(SLP)**
Payne, Dr Peter D **(SLP A)**
Prejean, Mrs Sheila Duplechain **(SLP)**
Rainwater, Mrs Jenny Hook **(A)**
Rigo, Dr Thomas G **(A)**
Ruffin, Margaret A **(SLP)**
Sample, Mrs Walterine Britt
Sibille, Mrs Claudette B **(SLP)**
Stephens, Terirae **(SLP)**
Supler, Rebecca A **(SLP)**
Thibodeaux, Carol Ann **(SLP)**
Thibodeaux, Darline Marie
Thibodeaux, Mrs Regina Cecile **(SLP)**
Thomassee, Sharon M **(SLP)**
Trahan, Henry P **(A)**
Wallace, Sarah A **(SLP)**
Whittington, Diane M **(SLP)**

Lake Charles
Cagle, Mrs Lotus M **(SLP)**
Caldwell, Mrs Susan Aguzin **(SLP)**
Champagne, Jodie Richard **(SLP)**
Mize, Mrs Maura C **(SLP)**
Morris, Steven W **(A)**
Nileshwar, Ramgopal S **(A)**
Schrepfer, Mrs Betty P **(SLP)**
Smith, Mrs Valerie A **(SLP)**
Viguerie, Susan Mouton **(SLP)**

Lake Providence
Salemi, Kelly Joseph, Jr **(SLP)**

Larose
Doverspike, Cyd Triche **(SLP)**

Livingston
Williams, Karen A **(SLP)**

Lockport
Fletchinger, Sr M Therese **(A)**
Simpson, Mrs Mary P **(SLP)**

Luling
Hymel, Susan Cassagne
Lucky, Joan **(SLP)**
Watson, Mrs Phyllis B **(SLP)**

Mandeville
Bernard, Dorothy Jean **(SLP)**
Brown, Mrs Elizabeth **(SLP)**
Dempsey, Mrs Stacy P **(SLP)**
Farwell, Mrs Dorothy W **(SLP)**
Leyrer, Gina Raie **(SLP)**
Liuzza, Rosalie **(SLP)**
Perry, Karen Sue **(SLP)**
Rupard, Mrs Robyn Chandler **(SLP)**
Sins, Mrs Bonnie T **(SLP)**
Skinner, Mrs Dawn Viosca **(SLP)**
Strain, Mrs Donna Spiers **(SLP)**
Viger, Mrs Wendy W **(SLP)**

Mansfield
Calhoun, Marian Hope **(SLP)**
Jackson, Frances H **(SLP)**

Marrero
Bailey, Mrs Demetriel Poche **(SLP)**
Banks, Mrs Sandra Garrity **(SLP)**
Brown, Mrs Deborah Landry **(SLP)**
Hurley, Mrs Wanda L **(SLP)**
Mooney, Dorothy D **(SLP)**

Maurice
Aubin, Mrs Myra L
Christman, Mrs Sarah Slack **(SLP)**
Dugas, Mrs Anne B **(SLP)**
Harer, Carol J **(SLP)**
Skipton, Mrs Anne Broussard **(SLP)**

Meraux
Caplan, Bonnie Jean **(SLP)**

Metairie
Albrecht, Dana Sue
Allen, Dr Sylvia K **(A)**
Asaro, Danna Valdin **(SLP)**
Banajee, Mrs Meher Hormazd **(SLP)**
Barr, Dr Nona Lee **(SLP)**
Barranco, Jody **(SLP)**
Barron, Joan S **(SLP)**
Berins, Mrs Jane Z **(SLP)**
Billens-Ivory, Dr Susan **(SLP)**
Bode, Mary G **(SLP)**
Brumfield, Dr Shannon **(SLP)**
Buthman, Joanne **(SLP)**
Campo, Angene M **(SLP)**
Chaiklin, Dr Joseph B **(A)**
Corcoran, Susan Evans **(SLP)**
Creel, Lynn P **(A)**
Crews, Patricia Lynn **(A)**
Currie, Paula Sue **(SLP)**
de Brueys, Mrs Mary T **(SLP)**
Dyer, Anna J **(SLP)**
Edie, Mrs Patricia D **(SLP)**
Emrick, Mrs Nita P **(SLP)**
Ewing, Allison M **(SLP)**
Exnicios, Jill D **(SLP)**
Exnicios, Sharon Beth **(SLP)**
Finger, Sylvia S **(SLP)**
Gabler, Mary Jean **(SLP)**
Gardes, Christy G **(SLP)**
Glaser, Patricia R **(SLP)**
Glazer-Gordon, Dena Lee **(SLP)**
Gremillion, Grace P **(SLP)**
Griener, Tania D **(SLP)**
Guichard, Jeanne Marie **(SLP)**
Gulotta, Mrs Cynthia T **(A)**
Haar, Carolyn A **(SLP)**
Handy, Dr Pamela Lucy **(SLP)**
Hannan, Frances D **(SLP)**
Harbert-Joseph, Euna M **(SLP)**
Heine, Mrs Kymberly Smith **(SLP)**
Hess, Claire Louise **(A)**
Ivory, Dr Peter J **(A)**
Jenison, Virginia Williams **(A)**
Johnson-Welch, Mrs Judith S **(SLP)**
Judge, Mrs Annette Foreman **(SLP)**
Koniditsiotis, Dr Cornelia Y **(SLP)**
Laiche, Grace Marie
Lampard, Lucille Brinz **(SLP)**
Lang, Mrs Jane D **(SLP)**
Leidenheimer, Cathy L **(SLP)**
Lejeune, Sarah C **(SLP)**
Mayer, Mrs Mavis E **(SLP)**
Meade, Mrs Lynn T **(SLP)**
Muller, Mrs Windie Karen **(SLP)**
Murphy, Mrs Kathleen K **(SLP)**
Nagim, Mrs Denise H **(SLP)**
Paternostro, Mrs Jennifer F
Patterson, Mrs Sheila Ann B **(SLP)**
Piggott, Susan L **(SLP)**

Pollack, Peggy Blum **(A)**
Prucha, Mrs Kathleen Barnum **(SLP)**
Rebstock, Therese E **(SLP)**
Reynolds, Mrs Nancy B **(SLP)**
Richard, Mrs Mimi Barry **(SLP)**
Roppolo, Mrs Cynthia M **(SLP)**
Rufin, Virginia Dare **(SLP A)**
Russ, Lugene A **(SLP)**
Samuels, Paula M **(SLP)**
Semmes, Joan L **(SLP)**
Truss, Marion Elida **(A)**
Walk, Jeanne B **(SLP)**
Weinberg, Mrs Cheryl F **(SLP)**
Wilson, Ellaine **(SLP)**

Minden

Metzker, Mrs Peggy L **(SLP)**
Stull, Mrs Mary Young **(SLP)**

Monroe

Aitken, Mrs Paula Robertson **(SLP)**
Blackbourn, Jennifer W **(SLP)**
Bradford, Mrs Karen Ann **(SLP)**
Carmack, Dr Fairy **(SLP)**
Clark, Mrs Linda C **(SLP)**
Copeland, Lisa Kay **(SLP)**
Cunningham, Mrs Nancy M **(SLP)**
Fellows, Judy A **(SLP)**
Fudickar, Mrs Jane Z **(SLP)**
Gibson, Mrs Suzanne Strickland **(SLP)**
Haddad, Harriet Jane **(SLP)**
Huckleberry, Mrs Helen Carol B **(SLP)**
Irwin, Dr David L **(SLP)**
Jones, Sandra Tucker **(A)**
Miller, Leonard G **(SLP)**
Mullican, Willis L **(SLP)**
Pruett, Paula M **(SLP)**
Toston-Edwards, Mrs Anna James **(SLP)**
Wade, Mrs Nancy M **(A)**

Natalbany

Johnson, Terri K **(SLP)**

Natchitoches

Brown, Mrs Cynthia Roberson **(SLP)**
Horton, Mrs Virginia H **(SLP A)**
Matis, Dr Edward Eugene **(SLP A)**
Matis, Mary J **(SLP)**
Pippin, Mrs Jane B **(SLP)**
Taylor, Mrs Irma S **(SLP)**
Thompson, Mrs Mary K **(SLP)**

New Iberia

Barnewold, Mrs Melinda Magruder **(SLP)**
Burke, Mrs Alice W **(SLP)**
Dietlein, Mrs Dona Lopez **(SLP)**
Dougherty, Kathleen Mary **(SLP)**
Dugas, Jane Lassalle **(SLP)**
Hayes, Phebe Marie **(SLP)**
Marie, Mrs Georgia Breaux **(A)**
Walet, Mrs Marla Ann **(SLP)**
Zimmer, Millie Resweber **(SLP)**

New Orleans

Akins, Mrs Tanya M P **(SLP)**
Albright, Melissa De Shong **(A)**
Allen, Nell R **(SLP A)**
Alworth, Mrs Lois Anne **(SLP)**
Appleby, Mary Patricia **(SLP)**
Baker, Linda Veronica **(SLP)**
Bardon, Constance Lynn **(SLP)**
Batiste, Dierdra M **(SLP)**
Beale, Catherine **(SLP)**
Belding, Donna Lynn
Bendana, Frances B **(A)**
Benton, Steven Lamar **(A)**
Berlin, Dr Charles I **(SLP A)**
Bock, Julie M **(SLP)**
Bondy, Alice **(SLP)**
Bowen, Mrs Barbara M **(SLP)**
Boyle, Mrs Virginia Galvin **(A)**
Breen, Mrs Elise S **(SLP)**
Bristow, Diane C **(SLP)**
Brown, Judy H **(SLP)**
Broyard, Jennifer Bernadette **(SLP A)**
Bryant-Landry, Mrs Linda M **(SLP)**
Buchler, Mrs Deborah Tribou **(A)**
Burgess, Mrs Carla Dodd **(SLP)**
Burns, Regina Coeli **(SLP)**
Byers, Dr Vincent W **(A)**
Cocke, Mrs Carol B **(A)**
Courville, Adele R L **(SLP)**
Crabtree, Mrs Tammy Hudson **(A)**
Daniels, Stephanie Kay **(SLP)**
Davis, Beth A **(SLP)**
Davis, Dr Sylvia M **(SLP)**
De Kemel, Kathryn Patrice **(SLP)**
Dennis, Mary E **(SLP)**
Diament, Mrs Elise Trader **(SLP)**
Dopson, Deborah R **(SLP)**
Douglas, Jacqueline B **(SLP)**
Drichta, Dr Carl E **(SLP)**
Dunn, Tracey Michelle
Edmonson, Mrs Terry Lynn **(SLP)**
Farr, Lorraine E **(SLP A)**
Fertitta, Mrs Annette T **(SLP)**
Fischman, Diana L **(SLP)**
Fogleman, Mrs Jana Dunn **(SLP)**
Folse, Mrs Kathleen P **(SLP)**
Forstall, Janice M **(SLP)**
Fowler, Suzie **(SLP)**
Friedman, Mrs Susan B **(SLP)**
Gant, Deborah Elaine **(A)**
Gant, Linda R **(SLP)**
Gibian, Laura G **(SLP)**
Gibson, Mrs Christina Rogers
Gochnour, Mrs Elizabeth **(SLP)**
Gould, Susan Hosmer **(SLP)**
Grenier, Mrs Julienne Haro **(A)**
Guidry-Marks, Rose **(SLP)**
Guillory, Sandra F **(SLP)**
Haley, Evelyn C **(SLP)**
Hall, Melissa Wiegand **(A)**
Harlan, Mrs Cynthia A **(SLP)**
Harwell, Mrs Robin W **(SLP)**
Hoffman, Kitty Biven **(SLP)**
Hood, Dr Linda J **(A)**
Hood, Mrs Louise W **(SLP)**
Hughes, Mrs Jane S **(SLP)**
Irby, Mrs Rachel Ragsdale **(A)**
Jacobs, Linda W **(SLP)**
Javier, Nancy T **(SLP)**
Jernigan, Lesley Ray **(SLP)**
Johnson, Jana Lee **(SLP)**
Johnson, R C **(SLP)**
Jones, Dr M Carolyn **(SLP)**
Kelley, Dr Rhonda H **(SLP)**
Kenner, Patricia **(SLP)**
Kepper, Mrs Jo Nelle S **(SLP)**
Kimelman, Dr Mikael D Z **(SLP)**
King, Mrs Fannie E **(SLP)**
Kirkwood, Mrs Catherine Faust **(A)**
Kirtland, Mrs Margaret T **(SLP)**
Kobiernicki, Mrs Brenda Bwel **(SLP)**
Kruse, Caroline Gann **(A)**
La Bauve, Sonya M **(A)**
Laborde, Mrs Suzanne Mayer **(SLP)**
Lachmann, Teresa D **(SLP)**
Laguaite, Dr Jeannette **(SLP A)**
Leach, Mary S **(SLP)**
Lee, Lynne M **(SLP)**
Leonard, Loretta Ann **(SLP)**
Lykes, Aloma Reed **(SLP)**
Manzy, Y'Shua **(A)**
Marcel, Mrs Beth Marie **(SLP)**
Martin, Bonnie Marie **(SLP)**
Martin, Karen Maria **(A)**
McGhee, Wendy Gale **(SLP)**
McVay, Mary **(SLP)**
Meintel, Mary Kay **(SLP)**
Melcher, Dr Joe A **(A)**
Meunier, Kathy C **(SLP)**
Miller, Judith Ann **(SLP)**
Miller, Paul S **(SLP)**
Monteleone, Ila K **(SLP)**
Morehouse, Charles Robin **(A)**
Mounce, Deborah Downing **(SLP)**
Mowrey, Marinnette **(SLP)**
Myrick, Dean Kent **(SLP)**
Neu, Mrs Barbara J **(SLP)**
Nodurft, Judith B **(SLP)**
Norman, Michael C **(SLP)**
Orlesh, Mrs Dianne P **(SLP)**
Orth, Mrs Kay M **(SLP)**
Oswalt, Lisa H **(SLP)**
Pace, Mrs Melanie B **(SLP)**
Pailet, Mrs Janet Joseph **(SLP)**
Pappas, Frances O **(SLP)**
Patterson, Mrs Kathy Coleman **(SLP)**
Pfeifer, Dr Rosemary C **(SLP)**
Pincus, Mrs Clara F **(SLP)**
Pisa, Mrs Lisa G **(SLP)**
Pleasonton, Dr Anna **(SLP A)**
Porter, Dr Robert J, Jr
Prejean, Marsha J **(SLP)**
Ragan, Mrs Anita Louise **(SLP)**
Rampp, Dr Donald L **(SLP)**
Remsberg, Cheryl Ann **(SLP)**
Rich, Rose Rubel **(SLP)**
Richards, Mrs Carol Schmidt **(SLP A)**
Rose, Linda B **(A)**
Rosen, Dr Jack **(SLP A)**
Rubins, Mrs Merry Sumner **(SLP)**
Rusch, Mrs Catherine Rea **(SLP)**
Samuels, Mrs Carole **(SLP)**
Sarrat, Larry J **(SLP)**
Schroeder, Karen Elizabeth
Seidemann, Dr Michael F **(A)**
Shaiman, Dr Susan **(SLP)**
Simmons, Nina N **(SLP)**
Smith, Elliott Gregory **(A)**
Smith, Mrs Geraldine Jones **(SLP)**
Smith, Mrs Linda G **(SLP)**
Smith, Mrs Mary Brousseau **(SLP)**
Sogin, Ruth R **(SLP)**
Spencer, Mrs Maureen M **(SLP)**
Stassi, Dr Eugene J **(SLP)**
Steger, Nancy H **(SLP)**
Stewart, Myralyn A **(SLP)**
Strickland, Margaret J **(SLP)**
Swoboda, Mrs Cecilia F **(SLP)**
Thompson, Dr Carl L **(A)**
Thompson, Cynthia A **(SLP)**
Tobey, Dr Emily A **(SLP)**
Toomer, Catherine Ann **(SLP)**
Trouillier, Doreen Theresa
Troxler, Mrs Terry Fink **(SLP)**
Vockroth, Mrs Rebecca Dessauer **(SLP)**
Waguespack, Mrs Mary K **(SLP)**
Watson, Dorothy H **(SLP)**
Weber, Mrs Ann Drake **(SLP)**
Wegmann, Monica E **(SLP)**
Wicker, Ellen R **(SLP)**
Wilensky, Diane S **(SLP)**
Wiltz, Muriel R **(SLP)**
Winfrey, Joan Margaret **(SLP)**
Young, Linda L **(SLP)**
Zeller, Mrs Carolyn S **(SLP)**
Zorthian, Anna L **(SLP)**

Oakdale

McManus, Edna L **(SLP)**

Opelousas

Chevis, Mrs Mary Melanie
Christy, Dianne **(SLP)**
Dejean, Jeanne V **(SLP)**
Deranger, Mrs Cynthia A **(SLP)**
Guillory, Joseph A **(SLP A)**
Hess, Mrs Gay S **(SLP)**
Johnson, Mary R
Leblanc, Mrs Marie K **(SLP)**
Montgomery, Mrs Helena Cefalu **(SLP)**
Voitier, Mrs Vicki Langston **(SLP)**

Oscar

Songy, Cherie T **(SLP)**

Patterson

Felterman, Nancy J
Kornegay, Mrs Lisa Felterman **(SLP)**

Pearl River

Harris, Dr Marsha R **(SLP)**
Vicknair, Rose Marie **(SLP)**

Pierre Part

Templet, Mrs Lisa Crochet **(SLP)**

Pineville

Benedetti, Nancy L **(SLP)**
Coorpender, Linda M T **(SLP)**
Craig, Mrs Mary S **(SLP)**
Gass, Albert H, Jr **(A)**
Larvadain, Janice M **(SLP)**
McQuaig, Jean S **(SLP)**
Simpson, Carol A **(SLP)**
Taylor, Mrs Shirley Clarkston **(SLP)**
Warner, Brian D **(SLP)**

Pollock

Bonner, Mrs Jerri Lynn

Ponchatoula

McIntyre, Patricia M **(SLP)**
Wilbert, Dr Karen M **(SLP)**

Port Allen

Aguillard, Mary Christie **(SLP)**

Port Sulphur

Chauvin, Mrs Cathy Schroder **(SLP)**

Prairieville

Fleet, Audrey Ann **(SLP)**
Haydel, Tina H **(SLP)**
Rodgers, Mrs Theresa H **(SLP)**

Raceland

Chisholm, Mrs Rebecca Wise **(SLP)**
Gremillion, Mrs Suzanne B **(SLP)**
Torres, Mrs Jan Marie **(SLP)**

Rayne

Ware, Janice G **(SLP)**

Ringgold

Batchelor, Barbara M **(SLP)**
Whiteman, Mrs Judy C **(SLP)**

River Ridge

Brown, Mrs Karissa Taylor **(SLP)**
Gravois, Mrs Jean Breaux **(SLP)**
Risey, John A, Jr **(A)**

Ruston

Avallone, Sharon Rose **(SLP)**
Balloun, Lois Ann **(SLP)**
Dans, Dr Jimmie C **(SLP)**
Daugherty, Mrs Kathleen Gaydos **(SLP)**
Hall, Mrs Leah Adele **(SLP)**
Hammock, Mary E
Hipp, Donna Lynn **(SLP)**
Leake, Guy Dudley, Jr **(SLP A)**
Leake, Mrs Harriet B **(SLP)**
Meyer, Robert C **(A)**
Moore, Mrs Gladys B **(SLP)**
Rockett, Mrs Leda Watson **(SLP)**
Sheehan, Mrs Kimberly Jowers **(SLP)**
Sheeler, Betty Ward **(SLP)**
Traweek, Dr Suzanne Calvert **(SLP)**
Wascom, Mrs Lorrianne **(SLP A)**
Wright, Maria Pavnica **(SLP)**
Zimmerman, Beverly N **(SLP)**

Scott

Juckett, Mrs Lauri Woods **(A)**

Shreveport

Atkins, Mrs Elizabeth C **(SLP)**
Beck, Mrs Sherri Madden **(A)**
Blackwood, Mrs Sherry Lane **(SLP)**
Blow, Georgia W **(SLP A)**
Bolton, Mrs Debra Jean **(SLP)**
Bond, Beth B **(SLP)**
Box, Mrs Jane D **(SLP)**
Breland, Kristi J **(A)**
Bundrick, Mrs Judy S **(SLP)**
Butler, Mrs Mary A G **(SLP)**
Carmouche, Margaret A **(SLP)**
Carpenter, Dorothy Jan **(SLP)**

Carroll, Mrs Carolyn M **(SLP)**
Chance, Mrs Linda B **(SLP)**
Churchill, Santi Jane **(SLP)**
Clements, Mrs Gracie Thoman **(A)**
Crane, Susan Lake **(SLP)**
Critcher, Dr C Robert **(SLP)**
Eaves, Mrs Constance T **(SLP)**
Edwards, Mrs Diane M **(SLP)**
Elwinger, Dr Elyda S **(SLP)**
Evans, Mrs Becky Seidensticker **(SLP)**
Ferguson, Mrs Marie N **(SLP)**
Ferguson, Mrs Maxine Williams
Garner, Donna J **(SLP)**
Grussendorf, Betty P **(SLP)**
Harris, Mrs Jennifer W **(SLP)**
Harriss, Connie Clinton **(SLP)**
Herrin, Debra D **(SLP)**
Jameson, Shelby Denise
Johnson, Mrs Norma O **(SLP)**
Kiihnl, Linda L **(SLP)**
Lavelle, Renee Marie **(SLP)**
Leavell, Suanne M **(SLP)**
Lott, Rosalie **(SLP)**
Luck, Mrs Sheryl F R **(SLP)**
Martin, Mrs Cheryl Ann **(SLP)**
McDougald, Mrs Claire Conrad **(SLP)**
Mitchell, Clydie K **(SLP)**
Moch, Ozzie Ree **(SLP)**
Monk, Janis Smith **(SLP)**
Monroe, Mrs Cora M **(SLP)**
Morris, Belinda Denise **(SLP)**
Otto, Dr Walter C, Jr **(A)**
Pannbacker, Mary Dirickson **(SLP)**
Pendergrass, Merrie Gibson **(SLP)**
Poole, Mrs Anne P **(SLP)**
Prothro, Jana K **(SLP)**
Puett, Valerie King **(SLP)**
Randolph, Beverly **(SLP A)**
Reeves, Rebecca Fulghum **(SLP)**
Remmel, Dr Kerri Simpson **(SLP)**
Schuckers, Dr Gordon Howard **(SLP)**
Schuckers, Mrs Rita Carole **(SLP)**
Shefield, Cynthia N **(SLP)**
Slette, Renee Downs **(A)**
Stricklin, Mrs Delaine L **(SLP)**
Terry, Laura V **(SLP)**
Thomason, Karen Patricia **(SLP)**
Torrans, Dr Anne **(SLP)**
Vekovius, Mrs Gay Tate **(A)**
Waguespack, Glenn M **(A)**
Warren, Maribeth B **(SLP)**
Wells, David Bryan **(SLP)**
White, Mrs Anita Moon **(SLP)**
White, Nina G **(SLP)**
Zavalydriga, Mrs Susan Faler **(SLP)**

Slidell
Beeson, Joann Regina
Cocran, Cynthia Diane
Dixon, Marilyn Marie
Foley, Theresa Dawn **(SLP)**
Gagliardi, Mrs Beverly A **(A)**
Griffin, Cheryl B **(SLP)**
Henderson, Mrs Cathy G **(SLP)**
Lee, Diane M **(SLP)**
Lyle, Mrs Cheryl W **(SLP)**
McDonough, Dr Dayle Davis **(SLP)**
McLemore, Brenda Davis **(SLP)**
Needham, Thyria H **(SLP)**
Olroyd, Dr Marie Hiern **(SLP A)**
Payne, Mrs Virginia Anne **(SLP)**
Peffley, Mrs Mara S **(SLP)**
Reeves, Mrs Jerri Jo **(SLP)**
Schuber, Mrs Suzanne Perez **(A)**
Susslin, Margaret Ann **(SLP)**
Thorell, Mrs Mary C **(SLP)**
Watts, Mrs Michele L **(A)**
Witter, Mary Barbara **(SLP)**

St Amant
Le Blanc, Mrs Barbara M **(SLP)**

St Francisville
Allen, Mrs Teresa Grant **(SLP)**
Vince, Mrs Virginia Jackson **(SLP)**

St Martinville
Delhommer, Jan M **(A)**
Martin, Vicky Cecile **(SLP)**

St Rose
Dermody, Lynn Ann **(SLP)**

Stonwall
Butler, Mrs Kathy Jean **(SLP)**

Sunset
Corbello, Mrs Patricia B **(SLP)**

Thibodaux
Armstrong, Mary B **(SLP)**
Bodet, Glen P **(A)**
Bourgeois, Mrs Lynne L **(SLP)**
Knight, Dan P, Jr **(SLP)**
Nolen, Dr Jo Carol **(SLP)**
Simon, Mrs Bobbie L **(SLP)**
Simpson, William L, II **(A)**

Ville Platte
Boyne, Rita B **(SLP)**

Walker
Womack, Mrs Marylynn Hill **(SLP)**

Washington
Gomez, Charlotte Casto **(SLP)**

West Monroe
Fisher, Brenda F **(A)**
Fleming, Mrs Carolyn **(SLP)**
Gates, Rebecca H **(SLP)**
Irwin, Mrs Vickie Hammer **(SLP)**
Moore, Mrs Susan Rowe **(A)**
Naron, Clyde Allen **(SLP)**
Rogers, Kerrilyn Kaye **(SLP)**

Winnfield
Monk, Mrs Sharon P **(SLP)**

Winnsboro
Little, Charlotte **(SLP)**
Rhodes, Mrs Jean **(SLP)**

Zachary
McKenney, Mrs Ann Therese **(SLP)**
Samuel, Mrs Sheran L

MAINE

Acton
Steffens, Janet S **(SLP)**

Alfred
Andrews, Mrs Martha G **(A)**

Anson
Plourde, Lynn M **(SLP)**

Auburn
Bussiere, Mrs Deborah Joline **(A)**
Sinclair, Mrs Leona D **(SLP)**
Tetenman, Mrs Catherine Murray **(SLP)**

Augusta
Adams, Susan E **(A)**
Duncan, Richard A **(SLP)**
Larrabee, Holly A H **(SLP)**
Tukey, Sharyn Ann Hale **(SLP)**

Bangor
Ames, Janis G **(SLP)**
Backiel, Thomas C **(SLP)**
Cutting, Michael W **(A)**
Dean, James **(A)**
Emerson, Elizabeth W
Field, Mrs Elizabeth Ives **(SLP)**
Green, Mrs Mary Elizabeth **(SLP)**
Johansen, Mrs Nancy E **(SLP A)**
Kauffman, Mrs Laura Lee **(SLP)**
McElroy, Mrs Jo **(SLP)**
Mitchell, Mrs Marilyn P **(SLP)**
Olson, Mary Ellen **(SLP)**
Pease, Mrs Cathy Treer **(SLP)**
Pinette, Judy D **(SLP)**
Roscoe, Barbara Wais **(SLP)**
Specyal, Laura A **(SLP)**
Wise, Donna Jean **(A)**

Bath
Berman, Deborah A **(A)**
Ouellette, Marlene M **(SLP)**

Belfast
Curtis, Nathan Holbrook **(SLP)**
Towey, Michael P **(SLP)**

Benedicta
Ware, Justine M **(A)**

Biddeford
Butler, Mrs Maureen O'Neill

Blue Hills Falls
McKerns, Dorothy M **(SLP)**

Boothbay Harbor
Korwatch, Yvonne N **(SLP)**

Bowdoinham
Goddu, Mrs Kathleen A **(SLP)**
Guerette, Jean Ingram **(SLP)**
Guerette, Paul R **(SLP)**
Simmons, Deborah S **(SLP)**

Brewer
Fossa, Mrs Lorriann Prickett **(SLP)**
Spooner, Mrs Ellen L **(SLP)**
Tapley, Lori Ann **(SLP)**
Tudor, Mrs Gail M **(SLP)**

Brunswick
Carroll-Martini, Jean Frances **(SLP)**
Elsaesser, Susan **(A)**
Foley, Mrs Joyce J **(SLP)**
Kroc, Robin **(SLP)**
O'Donnell, Susan I **(A)**
Pyne, Katharine Dyer **(SLP)**

Camden
Bex, Mrs Margaret Ann **(SLP)**
Pelletier, Dr Louis P, Jr **(SLP)**

Cape Elizabeth
Hearns, Virginia M **(SLP)**
Lebel Curran, Mrs Jana M **(SLP)**
Levasseur, Mrs Mary T **(SLP)**
Saffer, Susan K **(SLP)**
Ward, Mrs Carol K **(SLP)**

Cape Neddick
Carey, Barbara Jocelyn **(SLP)**

Caribou
Bruce, Alton J, Jr **(SLP)**
Hosick, Heidi Ann **(A)**
Parente, Renee Freiman **(SLP)**

Casco
Ross, Clara Murch **(SLP)**

Cherryfield
Olday, Mrs Linda Jean **(SLP)**

Cornish
Shiland, Mrs Sybil B **(SLP)**

Costigan
La Riviere, Dr Conrad Louis **(A)**

Cumberland
Gillis, Patricia Sullivan
Spaulding, Mrs Rose Pesce **(A)**

Cumberland Center
Kotkas, Karen P **(SLP)**
Norton, Heidi Lynn

Damariscotta
Anderson, Christine **(SLP)**

Deer Isle
Hance, Mrs Ebba Carola **(SLP)**

Dexter
Breton, Janice G **(SLP)**

Dresden
Madore, Donna P

East Holden
Eichenlaub, Diane M **(SLP)**

East Millinocket
Loney, Helen E **(SLP)**

East Winthrop
Taylor, Nancy L **(SLP)**

Eliot
Cresta, Mrs Debra Roberts **(SLP)**
Romoser, Mrs Mechthild A **(SLP)**
Samson, Molly **(SLP)**
Sokol-Cass, Helene M **(SLP)**

Falmouth
Avallone, Paula **(SLP)**
Siegle, Peggy **(SLP)**
Siviski, Marsha T **(SLP)**

Farmington
Holmes, Richard Woodbury **(SLP)**
Mathers, Jolayne R **(SLP)**

Fort Fairfield
Briscoe, Anthony C **(SLP)**
Toth, Jean L **(A)**
Ulman, Stephen G **(SLP)**

Freeport
Fitzgerald, Susan Lochren **(SLP)**
Hudson, Mary S **(SLP)**
Kaczor, Kathy E **(SLP)**
Peterson, Mrs Eileen M **(A)**
Sleek, James Edward **(A)**
Wolfenden, Mrs Deborah P **(SLP)**

Gardiner
Griffiths, Heather **(SLP)**
Snow, Linda B **(A)**

Gorham
Boyko, Mrs Janice Carter **(SLP)**
Dabel, Mrs Debora Klein **(SLP)**
De Cotiis, Ellen H **(SLP)**
Hall, Mrs Linda C **(SLP)**

Greene
Washburn, Linda J **(SLP)**

Hampden
Hanson, Ronella V **(SLP)**
Heath, Jean L **(SLP)**
Hoar, Colleen J **(SLP)**

Harrison
Williams-Garrow, Lynne **(SLP)**

Houlton
Burleson, Paula L **(SLP)**
Mintz, Mrs Barbara W **(SLP)**

Hudson
Ellis, Joan J **(SLP)**

Kennebunk
Einsiedler, Mrs Stephanie L **(SLP)**
Hearn, Mrs Demetria Bilycia **(SLP)**
Henri, Dr Bernard P **(SLP)**
Joncas, Nancy Martin **(SLP)**

Kennebunkport
Owen, Geraldine **(SLP)**
Schlegel, Rita A **(SLP)**
Talmage, Christine Devers **(SLP)**
Thomas, Mrs Robin G **(SLP)**

Kittery
Kelly, Christine Delort **(A)**
Leonard, Colleen C **(A)**
Marsh, Mrs Carolynn K **(SLP)**

Lee
Sutter, Jane C **(A)**

Leeds
Mazzola, Lynda J **(SLP)**

Levant
Curtis, Mrs Kerry H **(SLP)**
Gwinn, Mrs Crystal Andrea **(SLP)**

Lewiston
Cote-Akerley, Stephanie **(SLP)**
Edgecomb, Pamela Ward **(SLP)**
Geller, Norman **(SLP)**
Hannah, Kevin Allen **(A)**
Peters, Maureen Ann **(SLP)**
Weidner, Julie Lynne **(SLP)**

Limington
Myers, Melissa P **(SLP)**

Lincolnville
Barbetta, Christine **(SLP)**
Kosmo, Helen L **(SLP)**

Lisbon Falls
Allen, Laurie E **(SLP)**

Loring AFB
Cole, Janice Kuioka **(SLP)**
Rutland, Mrs Kjaeren Aleece **(SLP)**

Madawaska
Castleberry, Charlotte J **(SLP)**

Mount Desert
Sanderson, Virginia S **(SLP)**

New Sharon
Lattz, Audrey L **(SLP)**

North Leeds
Rote, Ronda **(SLP)**

North Windham
Swander, Donald E **(SLP)**

Oakfield
Carter, Miriam Walker **(SLP)**

Oakland
Clark, Mrs Laurie Jane **(SLP)**
Dubois, Mrs Melinda Walsh **(SLP)**

Old Orchard Beach
Garland, Sharon Marie **(SLP)**

Old Town
Tully, Mrs Miriam **(SLP)**

Orland
Rosinski, Joyce E **(SLP)**

Orono
Camp, Mrs Polly N **(SLP)**
Carlson, Laurette L **(SLP)**
Dopheide, William R **(SLP)**
Kertoy, Marilyn K **(SLP)**
Miller, Lori Lynn **(SLP)**
Pettit, Dr John M **(SLP)**
Pickering, Dr Marisue **(SLP)**
Riley, Susan K P **(SLP)**

Orrington
Dufkin-Britt, Dawn A **(A)**
Gunn, Mrs Barbara J **(SLP)**
MacLeod, Mrs Kimberly S **(SLP)**

Oxford
Derry, Andrea Rebecca **(SLP)**
Gilliam, Pamela P **(SLP)**

Pittsfield
Gallagher, Mrs Helen S **(SLP)**

Poland Spring
Wisutskie, April J C **(SLP)**

Portland
Armstrong, W Jean **(SLP)**
Bachelder, Mrs Katherine **(SLP)**
Beagle, Mrs Linda D **(SLP)**
Catanzano, Annemarie **(SLP)**
Cheraso, Samuel C **(SLP A)**
Dionne, Carole S **(SLP)**
Fagan, Roger **(A)**
Greenblatt, Nancy L **(SLP)**
Heinrich, Ann **(SLP)**
Helms, Suzanne B **(SLP)**
Lalone, Dale T **(A)**
Lalone, Mrs Faye Bonnie **(A)**
Layne, Martha A **(A)**
Leland-Philbrook, Mrs Marilyn **(SLP)**
Maxsimic, Mrs Katherine **(SLP)**
Nielsen, Susan E **(SLP)**
Sacco, Lynne M **(A)**
Sparr, Mrs Sandra B **(SLP)**
Wolff, Mrs Karen Mitchell **(A)**
Wylonis, Norraine C **(SLP)**
Zulofsky, Debra R **(SLP)**

Presque Isle
Culp, Deidra Beth
Dwyer, Mrs Rosalie **(SLP)**
Wimberly, Sally Pettit **(SLP)**

Richmond
Coltharp, Mary Beth **(SLP)**

Saco
Caylor, John E **(A)**
Flores, Anita H H **(SLP)**
Roedner, Doris C
Sallis, Judith L P **(SLP)**
Zuehlsdorff, Kathleen Marie **(SLP)**

Sanford
Bisbee, Donna Joy **(SLP)**
Laflamme, Karen A **(SLP)**

Scarborough
Chase, Judith A **(SLP)**
Haley, Mrs Susan W **(SLP)**
Lever, Mrs Katharine Rando **(SLP)**

Sebago Lake
Goldberg, Joyce S **(SLP)**
Steeves, Nancy C **(A)**

Skowhegan
Gillis, Barbara **(SLP)**

Solon
Gray, Diane W **(SLP)**

South Berwick
Randall, Mrs Linda Mallick **(A)**

South Harpswell
Schaare-Denio, Regina **(SLP)**

South Paris
Collins, Virginia Betts **(SLP)**

South Portland
Baker, Mrs Arlene M **(SLP)**
Hillman, Kimberly Ann **(SLP)**
McOsker, Cynthia Crandall **(SLP)**
McOsker, Thomas Gerard **(SLP)**
Sexton, Barbara M **(SLP)**

Southwest Harbor
Ott, Jeanne Carolyn **(SLP)**

Thomaston
Fahy, Davene S **(SLP)**
Sobchuk, Lucille H **(SLP)**

Topsham
Cahill-Norton, Mrs Kelly **(SLP)**
Hodges, Jane
Marco, Catherine Mary **(SLP)**
Tragler, Mrs Janice L **(SLP)**
Weatherbee, Donald Scott **(SLP)**

Union
Birk, Janice Thompson **(SLP)**

Waterville
Baldwin, Anne L **(SLP)**
Fulling, Thomas M **(SLP)**
Olsen, Dr Bruce D **(SLP A)**
Pronovost, Dr Wilbert **(SLP A)**
Ratner, Mrs Roberta E **(SLP)**
Schwartzberg, Gary David **(A)**
Spence, Elizabeth Ann **(SLP)**
Stevens, Mrs Elaine R **(SLP)**

Wayne
Bornstein, Margaret Burn **(SLP)**

Weatherville
Sanagorski-Phillips, Mrs Susan Beth **(SLP)**

Wells
Caron, Mrs Susan Pagluica **(SLP)**

West Peru
Hazelton, Cathy A **(SLP)**

West Scarborough
Michaud, Mrs Janet Sullivan **(SLP)**

Westbrook
Dipple, Annette Lynn **(SLP)**

Windham
Hammond, Mark R **(SLP)**
Swander, Camille Grace **(SLP)**

Winslow
Giroux, Mrs Anne P **(A)**

Winterport
Pettit, Betty C **(SLP)**

Winthrop
Curtis, Dr Ann P **(SLP)**

Wiscasset
Garber, Mrs Betsy L **(SLP)**

Yarmouth
Hyde, Caroline C **(A)**
Koss, Mrs Anita Diamond **(SLP)**
Nangle, Martha Barry **(SLP)**
Tomaszewski, Elaine M **(SLP)**

York
Oates, Kim Victoria **(SLP)**
Parker, Mrs Janet Gallant **(SLP)**

MARIANA ISLANDS

Rota
Blodgett, Mary Jo **(SLP)**

Saipan
Blaisus, Jacqueline Treichler **(SLP)**
Brown, Sherry B **(A)**
Fraser, Leslie Ann **(SLP)**
Hammer, Carol Scheffner **(SLP)**
Smith, Carleen Wendt **(SLP)**
Tourne, Patrice M
Young, Theresa Ann **(SLP)**

MARYLAND

Aberdeen
Horst, Carol Jo W **(SLP)**
Phillabaum, Leeann Sue

Aberdeen Proving Ground
Ohlin, Doug W **(A)**

Abingdon
Bauer, Mrs Nancy S **(SLP)**
Brown, Mrs Deborah M **(SLP)**
Brown, Mrs Jacqueline Anita **(SLP)**
Ford, Mrs Robin Sommer **(SLP)**
Gotsch, Mrs Donna T **(SLP A)**
Kocher, Judith L **(SLP)**
Meinert, Mrs Lisa Pieger **(SLP)**
Rushing, Mrs Karen C **(SLP)**

Accident
Lander, Mrs Joyce I P **(SLP)**

Accokeek
Flanagan, Maureen Ann **(SLP)**
Taylor, Harriet B **(SLP)**

Adelphi
Dzime-Assison, Mrs Venita Gragg **(A)**
Gager, Patricia Nimeskern **(SLP)**
Jervay, Debra M **(SLP)**
Robinson, Joe Ann **(SLP)**
Shores, Mrs Ann Christine **(SLP)**
Vandy, S Ermon C **(SLP)**
Walker, Lynn A **(SLP)**
Watkis, Deborah J **(SLP)**

Andrews AFB
Gross, Leslie Ann **(SLP)**

Annapolis
Alexopulos, Janet Vitelozzi **(SLP)**
Beck, Edwin L **(A)**
Becker, Mrs Christine **(A)**
Brett, Rory C **(SLP)**
Campbell, Sylvia Marie **(SLP)**
Clark, Bonita L **(SLP)**
Crum-Sweely, Lori L **(SLP)**
Davis, Mrs Marie Talarico **(SLP)**
Drexler, Allan B **(SLP A)**
Drexler, Catherine **(SLP)**
Edward, Donna Marie
Flanders, William E **(A)**
Galetsky, Nancy G **(SLP)**
Goldsmith, Mrs Therese M **(SLP)**
Logan, Kimberly Denise **(A)**
Lombardo, Maureen F **(SLP)**
McCabe, Margaret K **(A)**
Nussbaum, Mrs Debra **(A)**
Ostrom, Mrs Sara W **(SLP)**
Remenick, Mrs Deedee **(SLP)**
Risher, Mrs Barbara E **(SLP)**
Robinson, Barbara B **(A)**
Sachs, Mrs Anne Quinn **(SLP A)**
Seckinger, M Suzanne Tomlinson **(SLP)**
Settele, Mrs Alison L Bradbury **(SLP)**
Silberman, Mrs Judith **(SLP)**
Stewart, Judy Laverne **(SLP)**
Wagner, Mrs Mary C **(SLP)**

Arbutus
Hixon, Mrs Cynthia Ellen **(SLP)**

Arnold
Aulbach, Melanie B **(SLP)**
Bond, Jennifer L **(SLP)**
Bruce, Christina **(SLP)**
Coover, Mrs Amy Cohen **(SLP)**
Glorioso, Mrs Lisa M **(SLP)**
Lee, Mrs Deborah Ann **(SLP)**
Magee, Mrs Rebecca D **(SLP)**
Newton, Margaret **(SLP)**
Tokosch, Ann Frances **(SLP)**

Ashton
Buckley, Mrs Emily Susan **(A)**

Baldwin
Leberknight, Jean C **(SLP)**
Rocchio, Catherine **(SLP)**

Baltimore
Abrams, Marjorie C **(SLP)**
Adams, Karen Mary **(SLP)**
Albright, Mrs Susan M **(SLP)**
Alterman, Merrill J **(A)**
Amos-King, Phyllis W **(SLP)**
Anderson, Carey Lynn **(SLP)**
Anshell, Susan Ellen **(A)**
Applestein, Mrs Shiela A **(SLP)**
Bailey, Mrs Kathryn C **(SLP)**
Baker, Correan M **(SLP)**
Barba, Caressa Maria
Bassich, Celia J **(SLP)**
Bauersfeld, Mrs Margaret M
Beetz, Ann L **(SLP)**
Beitsch, Mrs Estelle L **(SLP)**
Berman, Carol Bauer **(SLP)**
Berman, Judy B **(SLP)**
Bessel, Harriet W **(SLP)**
Bethke, Nancy Lanell **(SLP)**
Bevacqua, Yvette Lynn **(SLP)**
Biales, Mrs Cynthia Dipaola **(SLP)**
Bishop, Sandra G **(SLP)**
Blackman, Jasmin **(SLP)**

Blackstone, Sylvia Renee **(SLP)**
Bleile, Dr Kenneth Mitchell **(SLP)**
Blum, Mrs Wendy Beth **(SLP)**
Blumberg, Mrs Lisa Stein **(SLP)**
Bolton, Kathy C **(SLP)**
Bookstein, Mrs Ellen W **(A)**
Bounds, Dawn Leigh **(SLP)**
Brandner, Mrs Tamara Dee **(SLP)**
Breakey, Mrs Angela Raphael **(SLP)**
Briskin, Dr Ilene Hearn **(A)**
Brown, Eloise Furiga **(A)**
Burke, Margaret C **(A)**
Callahan-Smerdzinaki, Judith **(SLP)**
Caplan, Mrs Sharon Freeman **(SLP)**
Cassatt-James, Mrs Edith Lucinda **(SLP)**
Cawkwell, Mrs Elizabeth **(SLP)**
Chaffinch-Coyne, Janie Olivia **(A)**
Chapman, Mrs Diane H **(SLP)**
Chazen, Patricia B **(SLP)**
Chelminiak, Mrs Diane K **(SLP)**
Christie, Carol Schramm **(SLP)**
Chwang, Mrs Karen Malick **(SLP)**
Cicci, Dr Regina L **(SLP)**
Clasing, Anita T **(SLP)**
Clingerman, Mrs Judith Jump **(SLP)**
Conners, D Elizabeth **(SLP)**
Coons, Mrs Donna M **(SLP)**
Cooper, Mrs Iris P **(SLP)**
Coughlin, Mrs Sheryl Thomas **(SLP)**
Crowl-Gallagher, Renee **(SLP)**
Cummins, Mrs Melissa Grier **(SLP)**
Davis, Kelly J **(SLP)**
Davis, Mrs Marjorie Lee **(SLP)**
Davis, Mrs Naomi W **(SLP)**
Devlin, Judith C **(SLP)**
Dewey, Mrs Martha N **(SLP)**
Diaz-Plaja, Dr Ruth R **(SLP A)**
Diener, Dr Stuart **(SLP A)**
Diener, Mrs Wendy P **(SLP)**
Dobson, Robbie Ann **(SLP)**
Doyle, Deborah S **(A)**
Drayton, Mrs Peggy Cardwell **(SLP)**
DuChane, Ann Shaughnessy **(SLP)**
Eastman, Sheila J **(SLP)**
Efros, Paul L **(A)**
Eichelberger, Mrs Brenda Jones **(SLP)**
Endres, Arlene M
Eney, Mrs Stephanie **(A)**
Epstein, Gloria L **(SLP)**
Erskine, Mary Cara **(SLP A)**
Etzel, Carmel Dewaal **(SLP)**
Evans, John R **(SLP)**
Evers, Rev Robert T **(SLP)**
Ewing, Elizabeth R **(SLP)**
Favinger, Mrs Karen Britt **(SLP)**
Feinstein, Barry L **(SLP)**
Filbert, Mrs Susan W **(SLP)**
Firey, Trina Diane **(SLP)**
Fischer, Mrs Kayleen Lutts **(SLP)**
Florin, Suzanne **(A)**
Forget, Karen Aleen **(SLP)**
Fox, Mrs Madeline F **(SLP)**
Fox, Tina D **(SLP)**
Frankle, Bonnie C **(SLP)**
Fridman, Mrs Christine **(SLP)**
Gambone, Mrs Mary Lynn W **(SLP)**
Gerson, Deborah E **(SLP)**
Gimbel, Phyllis **(SLP)**
Gladstone, Robin A **(SLP)**
Gladstone, Dr Vic S **(A)**
Glasgow, Susan Haynes **(SLP)**
Glasner, Philip J **(SLP)**
Glick, Dr Alan H **(SLP)**
Glickman, Lisa Sue **(SLP)**
Goldberg, Mrs Rosalyn Berger **(A)**
Goldstein, Dr Moise H
Goodman, Mrs Mina Silesky **(SLP)**
Goodman-Schulman, Dr Roberta **(SLP)**
Grant, Dr Leslie Edwina **(SLP)**
Gray, Shareyfah Allyse
Green, Dr Lawanda **(SLP)**
Greenberg, Frederick **(SLP)**
Greenberg, Joan **(SLP)**
Greenhood, Johanna M **(SLP)**
Guyther, Robin E **(SLP)**
Haag, Mrs Joan S **(SLP)**
Haden, Ricole Hayley
Hallameyer, Mrs Claire M **(SLP)**
Hamburger, Mrs Ina **(SLP)**
Hammond, Hugh S, Jr **(SLP)**
Hanson, Ann V **(SLP)**
Hardy, Dr Miriam P **(SLP A)**
Harris, Mrs Elizabeth Wheeler **(SLP)**
Harrison, Bartel H **(SLP)**
Hart, Mrs Margart R **(SLP)**
Heinz, Dr John M
Hendricks, Mrs Rosemary **(SLP)**
Henninger, Mrs Debra R **(SLP)**
Hersey, Martha J **(SLP)**
Hersh, Michelle Zacharia **(SLP)**
Herzog, Harvey T **(SLP)**
Hession, Lucy Anne **(SLP)**
Holland, Mrs Ann Mitchell **(SLP)**
Horn, Mary Jo Donnelly **(SLP)**
Hoyt, Katherine Marie **(SLP)**
Hutton-Johnson, Mrs Iona Irene **(SLP)**
Inglis, Mrs Beverly Shank **(SLP)**
Isaacson, Rosalie **(SLP)**
Jinks, Andrew F **(SLP)**
Kaplan, Ronald Marc **(A)**
Kaplon, Mrs Marsha J **(SLP)**
Kappelman, Mrs Joan G **(SLP)**
Kasprzak, Carolyne Mary **(SLP)**
Katzenberger, Kathleen Anne **(SLP)**
Kelmenson, Florence **(SLP)**
Kennedy, Louise A **(SLP)**
Kenney, Mrs Teresa Plevyak **(SLP)**
Kerins, Marie R **(SLP)**
Keystone, Lori B
Kibby, Carol M **(A)**
Kidwell, Marcella Elizabeth **(SLP)**
Kiernan, Kim L **(SLP)**
Kirsh, Isidore M
Kobus, Mrs Anna H **(SLP)**
Kolman, Dr Ira H **(SLP A)**
Kotula, Carol A **(SLP)**
Kotula, Mrs Nora R **(SLP)**
Kramer, Mrs Carol W **(SLP)**
Kremer-Stern, Mrs Sharon L **(SLP)**
Kuntz, Mrs Marlene B **(SLP)**
Kuper, Mrs Eolin C **(SLP A)**
Landis, Patricia Ann **(SLP)**
Lando, Mrs Leah F **(SLP)**
Langlois, Jean Ann **(SLP)**
Lederer, Barbara Anne **(SLP)**
Lefton-Greif, Maureen A **(SLP)**
Lewis, Angela Utena **(SLP)**
Liberman, Thelma Wattenberg **(SLP)**
Liberto, Samuel **(SLP)**
Linden, Patricia L **(SLP)**
Litt, Bonnie **(SLP)**
Long, Mrs Martha S **(SLP A)**
Lynch, Mrs Gwendolyn **(SLP)**
MacHen, Mrs Nancy Knapp **(SLP)**
Maddox, Carol Maria **(SLP)**
Manlove, Sr Christine **(SLP)**
Marchetti, Patricia **(SLP)**
Markowski, Mrs Ruth Ann **(SLP)**
Mazurek, Mrs Susan McHugh **(SLP)**
McCune, Ellen Carol **(SLP)**
McGillick, Maureen C **(SLP)**
Meehan, Mrs Maria Gonzalez **(SLP)**
Mehring, Mrs Sheila Osman **(SLP)**
Messing, Barbara Pisano **(SLP)**
Miceli, Bernard Vincent **(SLP)**
Miiman, Susan **(SLP)**
Miller, Esther F **(A)**
Minarovic, Kathryn A **(SLP)**
Minghetti, Nancy J **(SLP)**
Moon-Luethke, Mrs Alison **(SLP)**
Morris, Colleen L
Morrow, Mrs Jean Levan **(SLP)**
Myers, Jane F **(SLP)**
Nichols, Mrs Kathleen M **(SLP)**
Nooney, Mary-Jo **(SLP)**
Novak, William Michael **(SLP)**
Nuckels, Patricia M **(SLP)**
Ogle, Mrs Mary E **(SLP)**
Oliver-Hoge, Mrs Patricia D **(SLP)**
Ourand, Mrs Patricia Regina **(SLP)**
Pachino, Judith L **(SLP)**
Padden, James Vincent **(SLP)**
Paige, Patricia Ann R **(SLP)**
Panitch, Adine R **(SLP)**
Parker, Diane Vanessa **(SLP)**
Paskowitz, Pamela A **(SLP)**
Patterson, Mrs Catherine Swift **(SLP)**
Pazornik, Sheri Robyn **(SLP)**
Perlmutter, Deborah Judith **(A)**
Peterson, Kathleen Q **(SLP)**
Pfeifer, Patricia Ann **(SLP)**
Phillips-Arthur, Sandra H **(SLP)**
Phoebus, Barbara M **(SLP)**
Pierce, Tina D **(SLP)**
Pillion, Dr Joseph Paul **(A)**
Pinerman, Eileen **(SLP)**
Poag, Linda J **(SLP)**
Posner, Mrs Annette Chester **(SLP)**
Pottash, Karen W **(SLP)**
Powell, Myrna T **(SLP)**
Preis-O'Brennan, Janet **(SLP)**
Reckord, Catherine Elizabeth **(SLP)**
Regler, Fred, Jr **(SLP)**
Rembe, Raymond R **(A)**
Resnick, Dr Steffi B **(A)**
Richmond, Jessica Jane **(SLP)**
Ridgley, Tami Michelle **(SLP)**
Riedner, Dr Erwin D **(A)**
Ries, Dr Julie E **(SLP)**
Ritgert, Barbara A **(SLP)**
Roebuck, Marsha Roberta **(SLP)**
Rombro, Nancy Block **(SLP)**
Romoser, Patricia R **(SLP)**
Roos, Sharon Williams **(A)**
Rosenbloom, Mrs Anita G **(SLP)**
Rosenfeld, Carol Dee **(SLP)**
Rossman, Mrs Katharine Crews **(SLP)**
Ryback-Cohen, Mrs Rachelle **(SLP)**
Saltysiak, Mrs Elaine B **(SLP)**
Sattem, Karen Ann **(SLP)**
Scales, Kim D **(SLP)**
Scharff, Laury Gold
Schauer, Mrs Paula C **(A)**
Schmalzer, Mrs Nancy **(SLP)**
Schnider, Mrs Evelyn H **(SLP)**
Schwartz, Roberta **(SLP)**
Searles, Mrs Carol L P **(SLP)**
Sheafor, Mrs Patricia F **(SLP)**
Shimizu, Dr Hiroshi **(A)**
Siffrin, Sandra L **(SLP)**
Skladany, Leah Ann **(SLP)**
Sklare, Daniel A **(A)**
Skrivan, Mary Anne **(SLP)**
Sloan, John M **(SLP)**
Smith, Catherine Patricia **(SLP)**
Sochaczewski, Mrs Ruth W **(SLP)**
Spector, Mrs Judith K **(SLP)**
Spencer, Dr Linda E **(SLP)**
Spliedt, William J **(SLP)**
Stein, Mrs Kathleen Noel **(SLP)**
Sterling, Debra G **(A)**
Sterling, Doris A **(SLP)**
Sterry, Mrs Merri Lynne **(SLP)**
Stevens, Bette J **(A)**
Stevenson, Susan Farr **(SLP)**
Stocksdale, Carla Portney **(SLP)**
Styer, Susan L **(SLP)**
Surell, Mrs Susan H **(SLP)**
Swanson, Brad Lauren **(SLP)**
Taymans, Dr Loretta M **(SLP)**
Thomas, Barbara Ellen **(SLP)**
Thornbery, Carrie H **(SLP)**
Thrope, Denise Weisblatt **(A)**
Tippett, Donna Clark **(SLP)**
Tottle, Edward L **(SLP)**
Trader, Miriam P **(SLP)**
Trenkle, Margaret Mary **(SLP)**
Trippe, Stuart J **(SLP)**
Trupe, Elizabeth Hillis **(SLP)**
Umstead, Rebecca Skacel **(SLP)**
Valentine, Mrs Courtney H **(SLP)**
Valletutti, Dr Peter James **(SLP)**
Vogelman, Mrs Lura H **(SLP)**
Vogelstein, Mrs Ilene C **(SLP)**
Wallace, Dr Bill L **(SLP A)**
Wallace, Christine Morgan **(SLP)**
Walters, Dr Roger John **(SLP A)**
Walther, Mrs Kathleen O'Donnell **(SLP)**
Washington, Eileen C **(SLP)**
Watson, Mrs Micheleen M **(SLP)**
Wehnert, Jay L **(SLP)**
Weinstein, Philip **(SLP)**
Weintraub, Wendy S **(SLP)**
Whitehead-Blen, Margaret L **(SLP)**
Williams, Elsie Monterey **(SLP)**
Winterling, Mrs Sharon Louise **(SLP)**
Wise, Ruth S **(SLP)**
Woolf, Mrs Selma C **(SLP)**
Workmeister, Ann M **(SLP)**
Yaffe, Linda S **(A)**
Yellin, Jill P **(SLP)**
Zentz, Bonnie Wisenauer **(SLP)**
Zilber, Sharon Lisa **(A)**
Ziman, Susan M **(SLP)**

Bel Air

Banick, Patricia L **(SLP)**
Beckelheimer, Alice F **(SLP)**
Belt, Charles William **(SLP)**
Boso-Suggs, Rhonda Lynn **(SLP)**
Bowers, Mary Ellen **(SLP)**
Ciampaglio, Mrs Susan N A **(SLP)**
Ciliax, Dr Donald R **(A)**
Deibert, Beverly Diane **(SLP)**
Donahue, Amy M **(A)**
Fisher, Frances F **(SLP)**
Gallagher, Mrs Beverly Jo **(SLP)**
Granger, Joyce Deany **(SLP)**
Harnden, Mrs Kathie Ann **(SLP)**
Kennedy, Mrs Marilyn A **(SLP)**
MacDonell, Mrs Ellen Mindy **(SLP)**
Mawhinney, Mrs Linda M **(SLP)**
Miller, Cynthia Lee **(SLP)**
Moffa, Mrs Barbara C **(SLP)**
Monk, William H **(A)**
Muir, Mrs Sue S **(SLP)**
Newberg, Michael R **(SLP)**
Noplock, Marie L **(SLP)**
O'Connell, Mrs Marybeth O **(SLP)**
Peters, Elaine Claire **(A)**
Popowych, Mrs Katherine **(SLP)**
Sonnichsen, Mrs Lucille B **(SLP)**

Belcamp

Benson, Donna Patricia **(SLP)**
Callaghan, Kathy Lynn **(SLP)**

Beltsville

Andrews, Valerie Elizabeth **(SLP)**
Anzelone, Deborah Kristen **(A)**
Coachman, Valerie Leah S **(SLP)**
Gomez, Donna Marie **(SLP)**
Henke, Mrs Deborah Barson **(SLP)**
Ludke, Judy Lavon **(A)**
Mellott, Kathleen Eccard **(A)**
Price, Dr Carol M **(SLP)**
Struntz, Brian Gerard **(SLP)**

Berlin

Baer, Karen Marie **(SLP)**
Cathell, Kathleen Wimmer **(SLP)**
Yeakle, Mrs Jeanne Kelly **(SLP)**

Berwyn Heights

Ahrens, Mrs Joan Ellen **(SLP)**

Bethesda

Anderson, Francis Martin **(SLP)**
Barwise, Kathryn T **(SLP)**
Berz, Mrs Sherry K **(SLP)**
Campbell, Nancy Jane **(SLP)**

Carr, Mary E **(SLP)**
Caruso, Dr Anthony J **(SLP)**
Chernikoff, Leslie R **(SLP)**
Cherow, Evelyn **(A)**
Coale, Mrs Sharon Smithey **(SLP)**
Coffman, Mrs Susan V **(SLP)**
Cooper, Dr Judith Ann **(SLP)**
Day, Dr Pat Spencer
Dingwall, William O
Eisenberg, Diane **(SLP)**
Feldman, Deborah G **(A)**
Ferketic, Michelle Mary **(SLP)**
Ferretti, Arlene V **(SLP)**
Ferry, Dr Peggy C
Fill, Michelle **(SLP)**
Fleischman, Mrs Stacy Brott **(SLP)**
Frable, Mrs Kimberly Demara **(A)**
Gans, Lynne Golubow **(SLP)**
Goldstein, Sandra D **(SLP)**
Goodman, Martha V **(SLP)**
Himler, Mrs Linda Edwards **(A)**
Hoskote, Vidya **(SLP)**
Johnson, Neal Blanchard
Kahn, Barbara **(SLP)**
Kefauver, Leslie F
Kushmeider, Susan Lynn **(SLP)**
Levine, Mrs Linda K **(SLP)**
Levine, Susan **(SLP)**
Levi-Shandler, Karen L **(SLP)**
Ludlow, Dr Christy L **(SLP)**
Ludtke, Beverly M **(SLP)**
Lynch, Mrs Gere C **(SLP)**
Mason, Pamela Ann **(A)**
McTernan, Mrs Carolyn L **(SLP)**
Meyerer, Mrs Margaret Lloyd **(SLP)**
Mrozowski-Starr, Mrs Marianne **(SLP)**
Naunton, Dr Ralph F **(A)**
Naylor, Dr Rex V **(SLP)**
Pines, Patricia L **(SLP)**
Polangin, Arlene K **(SLP)**
Pollack, Dr Helen A **(SLP)**
Racoosin, Mrs Suzanne D **(SLP)**
Raczynski, Mrs Sharon M **(SLP)**
Rankin, Julie H **(SLP)**
Ranney, Dr J Buckminster **(SLP A)**
Rhein, Ingeborg **(SLP)**
Ridley, Donna **(SLP)**
Ross, Lori Linwood **(SLP A)**
Sacks, Leslie S **(SLP)**
Sarnecky, Dr Ellen A **(A)**
Schulz, Geralyn Marie **(SLP)**
Sedory, Susan Elaine **(SLP)**
Semmes, Dr Marilyn Beverly **(SLP A)**
Shaw, Wendy H **(SLP)**
Spuehler, Dr H E
Stevens, Mrs Dorothy C **(SLP)**
Strohmaier, Alison A **(SLP)**
Strumpf, Sylvia G **(SLP)**
Tievsky, Mrs Sharon L **(SLP)**
Tirnauer, Sandra S **(SLP)**
Toyzer-Ronis, Lee-Ellen **(A)**
Turner, Claire Jean **(SLP)**
Wing, Dr Clara S **(SLP)**
Wise, Kay Louise **(A)**
Yeager, Mrs Sandra D **(SLP)**

Bladensburg
Singh, Dr Davinder **(SLP A)**

Bowie
Burns, Marcia Smith **(SLP)**
Cevasco, Rita Marie **(SLP)**
Elmore, LtCol John Howard **(A)**
Hurley-Forget, Mrs Patricia Anne **(SLP)**
James, Evelyn Louise
La Borwit, Dr Louis J **(SLP)**
Nelson, Beth V **(A)**
Parrucci, Mrs Regina Lucia **(SLP)**
Pestone, Robin Ross **(A)**
Stevenson, Virginia E
Villella, Gina M **(SLP)**
Zeaser, MaryLee

Brandywine
MacDonald, Mrs Theresa D **(A)**
Miles, Amy Fulton **(SLP)**

Brookeville
Sabin, Mrs Joanne M **(SLP)**

Bryans Road
Dillon, Mrs Donna Witerski **(SLP)**

Buckeystown
Hoyt, Mrs Linda **(SLP)**

Burtonsville
Alley, Lynda Laura **(A)**
Chandler, David W **(A)**
Ero, Lauren C **(A)**
Fogleman, Mrs Karen Hayes **(SLP)**
King-Grant, Mrs Caryl **(SLP)**
Wagner, Gwyneth Megan **(A)**

Butler
Clemmens, Mrs Jan M **(SLP)**

California
Wood, Jewel A S **(SLP)**

Cambridge
Marino-Tomey, Mrs Denise T **(SLP)**
Pender, F William **(SLP)**
Rivkin, Mrs Harriet B **(SLP)**
Usiondek-Benjamin, Mrs Anne Marie **(SLP)**

Capitol Heights
Mickelson, Mrs Faye E **(SLP A)**
Powers, Mrs Rita Jackson

Catonsville
Blasdel, Mary McKay **(SLP)**
Cohen, Susan Reincke **(SLP)**
Councill, Cheryl Anne **(SLP)**
Demorest, Dr Marilyn Elizabeth
Dorsey, Joseph Earl, Jr **(SLP)**
Melizzi, Mary A **(SLP)**
Rao, Mrs Martina M **(SLP)**
Rao, Dr Paul Richard **(SLP)**

Centerville
Baer, Elizabeth Cardwell **(SLP)**
Gregory, Mrs Marian Frances **(SLP)**
Kuhn, Mrs Kathleen Beskid **(SLP)**

Charlotte Hall
Bowling, Dr Lloyd S **(A)**

Chester
Aland, Mrs Caroline Holland **(A)**
Robinson, Richard Mark **(SLP)**

Chestertown
McSorley, Mrs Mary Kim **(SLP)**

Cheverly
Boudreaux, Mrs Ellen F **(SLP)**
Rilla, Mrs Donna C **(SLP)**
Surowicz, Christal Maria
Swailes, Winifred Louise **(SLP)**
Wicker, Sharon **(A)**

Chevy Chase
Anderman, Dr Bernard **(SLP A)**
Bates, Kimberly K **(SLP)**
Beck, Dr Lucille B **(A)**
Benitez, Mercedes J **(SLP)**
Causey, Dr G Donald **(SLP A)**
Connor, Adrienne G
Demb, Nancy L **(SLP)**
Epstien, Rhona G **(SLP)**
Friedman, Lisa Michele
Gaarder, Marie S **(SLP)**
Gaylin, Mrs Rita A **(SLP)**
Halstead, Margaret **(SLP)**
Hege, Mrs Gloria S **(SLP)**
Liebman, Mrs Roberta N **(SLP)**
O'Keeffe-Blue, Lisa Brooks **(SLP)**
Paul-Brown, Dr Diane **(SLP)**
Stein, Mrs Shirley P **(SLP A)**
Talbot, Mrs Barbara G **(SLP)**
Tardiff, Catherine Carre **(SLP)**
Walle, Eugene L **(SLP A)**
Weisz, Nancy Schatz **(SLP)**
Willig, Sharon **(SLP)**

Churchville
Peters, Dr Leslie J **(SLP A)**
Pierson, Capt Linda Davis **(A)**

Clarksburg
Lilly, Mrs Karen Bates **(SLP)**

Clarksville
Anderson, Mrs Elizabeth J **(SLP)**
Counts, Dr Alfred B **(SLP)**
Counts, Clarice R **(SLP)**

Clinton
Nance, Georgie C **(A)**
Rivers, Esther

Cockeysville
Jackson, Lauri Sleeth **(A)**
Shawver-Stearns, Heidi Ann **(SLP)**
Zellhofer, Carol M **(SLP)**

College Park
Bhathal, Inderjit Kaur **(SLP)**
Doudna, Dr Mark E **(A)**
Fitzgibbons, Dr Peter J **(A)**
Gordon-Salant, Dr Sandra M **(A)**
Graham, Geneva Louise **(SLP)**
Hool, Mrs Peggy Noroski **(SLP)**
McCall, Dr Gerald N **(SLP)**
Misback, Mrs Peggy S **(SLP)**
Penner, Dr Merrilynn J
Tallent, Joy R **(SLP)**
Yeni-Komshian, Dr Grace H

Columbia
Aisenberg, Sondra Lee **(SLP)**
Aliminosa, Donna **(SLP)**
Allen-Talley, Antoinette **(SLP)**
Baker, Mrs Laura L **(SLP)**
Binder, Mrs Marilyn R **(SLP)**
Breslow, Mrs Roberta K **(SLP)**
Brill, Mrs Barbara F **(SLP)**
Brown, Pamela I
Brown, Sue Anne **(SLP)**
Buchanan, Patricia K **(SLP)**
Carnahan, Cheryl F **(SLP)**
Chase, Mrs Carole J **(SLP)**
Cohen, Mrs Rita U **(SLP)**
Colegrove, Katherine A
Conner, Mrs Patricia Ann **(SLP)**
Copmann, Dr Kathryn S **(A)**
Coulter, Mrs Susan Green **(SLP)**
Cunningham, Dr Everlene Giles **(A)**
Diggs, Jayne Carithers **(SLP)**
Dinsmoor, Joyce H **(SLP)**
Dix, Cynthia A **(SLP)**
Downey, Amy Hottes **(SLP)**
Edwards, Mrs Jill Dejewski **(SLP)**
Erdman, Sue Ann **(A)**
Flanagan, Linda B **(SLP)**
Foote, Martha R **(SLP)**
Fuller, Linda Kay **(A)**
Glennen, Sharon **(SLP)**
Gold, Mrs Susan L **(SLP A)**
Grau, Arthur M **(SLP)**
Greyerbiehl, Dr Dianne H **(SLP)**
Haas, Joann **(SLP)**
Hall, Alberta W **(SLP A)**
Henry, Joan M **(SLP)**
Hester, Eva J **(SLP)**
Hoffmann, Mrs Ellen L **(SLP)**
James, Mrs Jacquelyn **(SLP)**
Jeffreys, Hanna Helane **(SLP)**
Johnson, Randolph Scott **(SLP)**
Koch, Mrs Deborah Georgian **(SLP)**
Kumin, Dr Libby B **(SLP)**
Matthews, Mary J K **(SLP)**
McCoy, Mrs Ellen D **(SLP)**
Meredith, Mrs Marti A **(SLP)**
Miller, Mrs Janice E **(SLP)**
Miller, Mary Alice **(A)**
Moore, Denise P **(SLP)**
Morin-Connolly, Gisele **(SLP)**
Moul, Maj Michael J **(A)**
Page, Leslie Ann **(A)**
Paige, Gretchen Marie **(A)**
Parker, Virginia W **(SLP A)**
Peterson, Mrs Colleen E Murphy **(SLP)**
Providence, Christophr Alan **(SLP)**
Raab, Katherine Anne
Rivers, Mrs Paula R **(SLP)**
Roberts, Marcy Diane **(SLP)**
Rosenberg, Margo H **(SLP)**
Rothenberg, Mrs Carol E **(SLP)**
Sarro, Mrs Victoria Anne **(SLP)**
Schiffer, Mrs Judith Mason **(SLP)**
Schoonover, Priscilla A **(SLP)**
Schwab, Constance **(SLP)**
Sedge, Dr Roy Kenneth **(A)**
Shamoo, Mrs Joan H **(SLP)**
Shriro, Dr Marjorie J **(SLP)**
Snope, Trudy L **(SLP)**
Soloff, Dr Hillary E **(SLP)**
Stalling, Paulette **(A)**
Sullivan, Holly Lynn **(SLP)**
Suter, Laura Jane **(SLP)**
Swanson, Allen F **(SLP)**
Taylor, Mildred S **(SLP)**
Tobin, Dr Henry **(SLP A)**
Townsend, Mrs Lisa M **(SLP)**
Wasser, Mrs Janis K **(SLP)**
Winder, Mrs Anette Schettino **(SLP)**

Crofton
Bulich, Brenda L **(SLP)**
Carey, Mrs Diane Turecamo **(SLP)**
Carr-Kraft, Linda Elaine **(A)**
Dillon, Lexa L **(SLP)**
Grigson, Mrs Sharon **(SLP)**
Hakala, Mrs Claudia G **(SLP)**
Kossman, Barbara A **(SLP)**
Luebkert, Mrs Frances R **(SLP A)**
Milone, Kate **(SLP)**
Resnick, Dr David M **(SLP A)**
Stern, Mrs Barbara K **(SLP)**

Crownsville
Barry, Pamela **(SLP)**
Kennington, Mrs Sabra Grant **(SLP)**
Roderick, Janice Mattei **(SLP)**

Cumberland
Fitzgerald, Michael G **(SLP)**
Nelson, Susan B **(SLP)**
Robb, Mrs Edith C **(SLP)**
Whittacre, Mrs Pamela Jo **(SLP)**
Witsberger, Mrs Kathleen Ann

Damascus
Blankinship, Mrs Mary C **(SLP)**
Cox, Leslie Woody **(SLP)**
Kurjan, Mrs Randy M **(SLP)**
Masters-Moore, Christine Aileen **(SLP)**
Sugrue, Mrs Joan Coughlan **(SLP)**
Wade-Kellar, Martha E **(SLP)**

Darlington
Horley, Mrs Mary B **(SLP)**

Darnestown
Gerber, Mrs Teresa Ellen **(SLP)**

Davidsonville
Brady, Judith W **(SLP)**

Delmar
Duerr, Mrs Leslie A **(A)**

Denton
Peksa, Paul E, Jr **(A)**
Peksa, Robin R **(A)**

Derwood
Boyd, Diane K **(A)**
Dalton, Marilyn G **(SLP)**
Kamara, Dr Carol Anne **(SLP A)**
Lillo, Mrs Margaret A **(A)**
Scarcella, Mrs Lori S **(SLP)**

Schofer, Mrs Joan W **(A)**

District Heights-Forestville
Cooper, Debra H **(A)**

Dunkirk
Millikin, Cynthia C **(SLP)**

Easton
McGuire, Cynthia L **(SLP)**
Morris, Mrs Barbara K **(SLP)**
Von Rembow, Deborah L **(A)**

Eden
Shively, Mrs Patricia D **(SLP)**

Edgewood
Perry, Mrs Natalie Colleen **(SLP)**
Schutt, Carol Jean **(SLP)**

Eldersburg
Benson, Donna M **(SLP)**
Waterman, Mrs Deborah S **(SLP)**

Elkridge
Antolick, Sharron Andeara **(SLP)**
Devlin, Susan M **(SLP)**

Elkton
Graser, Mrs Ann Derthick **(SLP)**
Reichenbach, Mrs Valerie C **(SLP)**
Steinemann, Mrs Lorri C **(SLP)**

Ellicott City
Banikiotes, Florence G **(SLP)**
Bishop, Libby K **(SLP)**
Collins, Carol L **(SLP)**
Curtis, Patricia Lou G **(SLP)**
Eikenberg, Mrs Mary Ann Sortore **(SLP)**
Geisler, Lisa O **(SLP)**
Haughey, Sr Kathleen **(SLP)**
Johnson, Mrs Bonnie J S **(SLP)**
Kellinger, Denise Litrenta **(SLP)**
Kinigopoulos, Mrs Helen Galinis
Laufer, Dr M Barbara **(A)**
Lazar, Mrs Sandra E **(SLP)**
Mancini, Frederic J **(A)**
Markotic, Klare K **(SLP)**
Martinez, Mrs Janet R **(SLP)**
McAuliffe, Mrs Shelley A **(SLP)**
McVey, Mrs Theresa A **(SLP)**
Resau, Christine **(SLP)**
Schoenbrodt-Myers, Mrs Lisa Ann **(SLP)**
Shannon, Dr Dorothy A **(SLP A)**
Tobin, Mrs Sherry Yolles **(SLP)**
Tresnak, Rosemarie **(SLP)**
Wheltle, Marian D **(SLP)**
Zozulak, Helen Eva **(SLP)**

Elridge
Thaler, Mrs Theresa K **(SLP)**

Fallston
Daddura, Mrs Rosalie E **(SLP)**
Gaines, Donnamarie Basta **(SLP)**
Johnston, Mrs Nancy N **(SLP)**
McCarthy, Valerie Baldwin
Yanchus, Elizabeth **(SLP)**

Federalsburg
Duda, Mrs Karen Borrello **(SLP)**

Ferndale
Dennis, Mrs Teresa Agnew **(SLP)**

Finksburg
Richards, Richard Mark **(SLP)**

Forest Hill
Borneman-Eckels, Dr Janice B **(SLP)**
Chellappa, Mariam
Heaps, Dana C **(SLP)**
Hensley, Carol Ann **(SLP)**
Schoenagel, Mrs Alyce Tomiko **(SLP)**

Forestville
Bowden, Brenda Jones **(SLP)**
Malilay, Marirose Martha **(SLP)**

Fort Howard
Eckenrode, Maribeth Vogel **(A)**
Koziol, L Steve **(SLP)**

Fort Meade
Anderson, Mrs Maureen **(SLP)**
Franklin, Susan Cheryl **(SLP)**
Notarianni, Julia **(SLP)**

Fort Washington
Durrette, Wanda G **(SLP)**
Engleking, Allen F **(SLP)**
Gadson, Pamela Jean **(SLP)**
Leighton, Terry True **(SLP)**
Locks, Francis M **(A)**
Trotter, Jessie Nesmith **(SLP)**
Vowels, Eleanor E **(SLP)**
Walker, Lola Deane **(SLP)**
Ward, Mrs Dolores M **(SLP A)**

Frederick
Bell, Julie Ann **(SLP)**
Birdsall, Marian P **(SLP)**
Boyer, Mrs Gail S **(SLP)**
Castle, Sandra **(A)**
Cherry, Jay D **(A)**
Cherry, Mrs Nancy C **(SLP)**
Copeland, Janet E **(SLP)**
Dorrell, Robert M **(SLP A)**
Duncan, Catherine B **(SLP)**
Fox, Mrs Donna Marie
Hedges, Cecelia H **(SLP)**
Hughes, Judy A G **(SLP)**
Jensen, Betty L **(A)**
Kent, Margaret S
Kritz, Kenneth W
Neumann, Grace Ellen **(SLP)**
Ryan, Mrs Sara Daly **(A)**
Sadownik, Sharyn M **(SLP)**
Wagner, Charles Richard **(A)**

Freeland
Landa, Dr Rebecca **(SLP)**
Miller, Mrs Barbara R **(SLP)**

Frostburg
Cockey, Mrs Elizabeth Ann **(SLP)**
Firestone, Pamela
Hanna, Mrs Theresa Marie **(SLP)**

Gaithersburg
Barber Kwolek, Mrs Cathleen M
Barwell, David R **(A)**
Bateman, Mrs Susan Blair **(SLP)**
Beverly-Ducker, Mrs Karen L **(A)**
Book, Susan Fields **(SLP)**
Bortnick, Mrs Rosalie M **(SLP)**
Bressler, Mrs Emily Gordon **(SLP)**
Carino, Mrs Mary H **(SLP)**
Casner, Mrs Mary Witham **(SLP)**
Copeland, Mrs Judith L **(SLP)**
Dennis, Elaine A **(SLP)**
Dorsey, Lisa Gainer **(SLP)**
Dublinske, Mrs Leslie H **(SLP)**
Dublinske, Dr Stan **(SLP)**
Feldman, Shirley Charney **(SLP)**
Frechette, Mrs Roberta S **(SLP)**
Gengel, Roy Werner **(A)**
George, Patricia R **(SLP)**
Gershman, Jennifer C **(SLP)**
Gillespie, Gerry G **(A)**
Golding, Gayla Siegal **(SLP)**
Goldman, Roberta L **(SLP)**
Goley, Irene Frances **(SLP)**
Goodwin, Karen K **(SLP)**
Grimes, Mrs Beth **(SLP)**
Gwyn, Susan E **(SLP)**
Hartman, Mrs Sandra Lee **(SLP)**
Healy, Maureen Elaine **(A)**
Howard, Mrs Myra N **(SLP)**
Kabatchnick, Ruth Karen **(SLP)**
Katz, Mrs Sally M **(SLP)**
Kendrick, Teresa Louise **(A)**
Klingler, Laura Rae **(A)**
Kruszewski, Christine **(SLP)**
Lowe, Mrs Fonda **(SLP)**
Martin, Mrs Janet B **(SLP)**
Miller, Ellen S **(SLP)**
Miller, Mrs Margery S **(SLP)**
Moody, Mary E **(SLP)**
Motto, Mrs Jane R **(SLP)**
Mulhern, Mrs Vickie **(SLP)**
O'Toole, Dr Thomas J **(SLP)**
Peller, Barbara F **(SLP)**
Pesti, Emily Conrad **(SLP)**
Pfeffer, Mrs Lynette S **(SLP)**
Postal, Mindy B **(SLP)**
Reinfrank-Dedo, Mrs Susan Ann **(A)**
Rosenberg, Mrs Nancy Anne **(SLP)**
Schramm, Mrs Teresa Natale **(SLP)**
Scott, Mrs Anne Marie
Shafer, Margaret Sorenson **(SLP)**
Shander, Mrs Sari G **(SLP)**
Sharer, Anita Marie **(A)**
Small, Judith L **(SLP)**
Stinson, Mrs Robin H **(A)**
Sutton, Valerie S **(A)**
Thayer, Dr Jean T **(SLP)**
Torrence, Mrs Penny P **(SLP)**
Trahan, Sherry E **(SLP)**
Vitrano, Mrs Jennifer Duff **(SLP)**
Wagner, Mrs Diana
Wires, Karen N **(SLP)**
Wright, Ann G **(SLP)**
Yick, Marilyn Jean **(SLP)**

Gambrills
Wood, Cynthia C **(SLP)**

Germantown
Bindert, CarolLynn **(SLP)**
Bjornsti, Patricia Hill **(A)**
Blomberg, Karen R **(SLP)**
Debelius, Sarah Costlow **(SLP)**
Engel-Sambrana, Mrs Patricia Jeanette **(SLP)**
Kiesow, Marion Sabrina **(SLP)**
Kovacevic, Mrs Jan D **(SLP)**
Miller, Cheryl J **(SLP)**

Glen Arm
Heckel, Mrs Donna M **(SLP)**
Mattingly, Marilyn T **(SLP)**
Rowe, Mrs Susan E **(SLP)**

Glen Burnie
Frank, Mrs Mary Elizabeth **(SLP)**
Gruen, Andrew Karl **(SLP)**
Gruen, Mrs Lynn S **(SLP)**
Longo, Karen Brode **(A)**
Nix, Tonya L **(SLP)**
Walker, Carol Ann

Glen Echo
Flaherty, M Kathleen **(SLP)**
Moore, M Patricia **(SLP)**

Glenelg
Smith, Romayne A **(SLP)**

Glenn Dale
Gary, Mrs Mary E **(SLP)**
Herring, Mrs Janice Pechter **(SLP)**

Glenwood
Humphrey-Lahayne, Joan **(SLP)**

Grantsville
Adams, Mrs Pamela Martin **(A)**

Greenbelt
Deal, Vicki R **(SLP)**
Haley, Ann M **(SLP)**
Hendrix, Jane H **(A)**
Kelley, Elisa Meredith **(SLP)**
Russell, Shari L **(SLP)**
Shevitz, Stephen D **(SLP)**

Hagerstown
Adams, R Kathleen **(A)**
Brennan, Mrs Elizabeth Long **(SLP)**
Conyers, Mrs Annette Wilson **(SLP)**
Day-Shockey, Mrs Diane **(A)**
Gloyer, Carol A **(SLP)**
Jicha, John James, III **(SLP)**
Kalin, George **(A)**
Kayser, Kathy Ann **(A)**
Kirchenbauer, Susan H **(SLP)**
McGuire, Karen A **(A)**
Merritt, Mrs Sarah Luanne **(A)**
Phares, Mrs Meredith M **(SLP)**
Sanford, Karl R **(SLP)**
Schukraft, Nancy V **(SLP)**
Troxell, Jay Lowell **(SLP)**

Hampstead
Holdt, Mrs Sarah J **(SLP)**
Suder, Mrs Nancy Higgs **(SLP)**
Young, Richard J **(A)**

Hanover
Barton, Deborah S **(SLP)**
McCauley-Fisher, Mrs Heather R **(SLP)**
O'Neill, Pamela Jean **(A)**

Havre de Grace
Cohen, Betsy Jane **(A)**
Whittie, Lisa Carolyn **(SLP)**

Hebron
Bartrug, Donna Briddell **(SLP)**

Hollywood
McGuffie, Mrs Alyce Lynne **(SLP)**

Huntingtown
Gibson, Mrs Patricia A **(SLP)**
Libertini, Nancy S **(SLP)**
Sasser, Mrs Mercedes P **(SLP)**

Hyattsville
Chisholm, Genie L **(SLP)**
Crawley, Mrs Lois Freeman **(SLP)**
D'Agostino, Christine L
Heck, Mrs Kathleen Denise **(SLP)**
Ifft, Linda Marie **(SLP)**
Kimbrough, Channing Michelle
McCreary, Dawn Evans **(SLP)**
Nelson, Elizabeth Ann **(SLP)**
Ottley, Melanie Dawn **(A)**
Roberts, Tamra Sarita **(A)**

Hydes
Fink, John J **(A)**

Jarrettsville
Compton, Judith G **(SLP)**

Jefferson
Morris, Mrs Amy Catherine

Jessup
Skrodzki, Mrs Cheryl T **(SLP)**

Joppa
Brockmeyer, Mrs Valerie Ann **(SLP)**
Cook, Mrs Barbara G **(SLP)**

Kensington
Goldberg, Mrs Lynette R **(SLP)**
Hart, Kathleen Gibson **(A)**
Hum, Mrs Carolyn C **(SLP)**
Hyde-Smith, Mrs Jennifer **(SLP)**
Lambert, Karen Marie **(SLP)**
Mason, Mrs Mary Golsen **(SLP)**
McDonough, Mrs Mary C **(SLP)**
Pyatak, Patricia Suzanne **(SLP)**
Racoosin, Mrs Lauren Schoenfeld **(A)**
Ratner, Dr Nan E Bernstein **(SLP)**
Schopmeyer, Betty B **(SLP)**
Stifel, Judith L **(A)**
Weitz, Mrs Cynthia **(SLP)**

Kingsville
Neville, Mrs Elizabeth **(SLP)**
Schulten, Mrs Margaret **(SLP)**

La Plata
Kondas, Lois Flavin **(SLP)**

La Vale
Clulee, Carol K **(SLP A)**
Freas, William Erdice, Jr **(SLP A)**

Ort, Marlee **(SLP)**

Landover

Crum, Robyn L **(A)**
Freeman, Mrs Evelyn Veney
Harlan, Mrs Nancy T **(SLP)**
Lebron-Ortiz, Maria G **(SLP)**
Stough, Mrs Susan Jane **(SLP)**

Lanham

Mack, Mrs Constance P Fearn **(SLP)**
Pontorno, Deborah Rewee **(SLP)**

Largo

Brockenborough, Mrs Ann Barrick **(SLP)**
Fisher-Minor, Gerri L **(SLP)**
Grant, Wanda Joyce **(SLP)**
Sayles, Adriane Hope **(SLP)**

Laurel

Arnoff, Mrs Judith B **(A)**
Dwyer, Mrs Aurion Louise **(A)**
Einolf, Michele M **(SLP)**
Elliott, Mrs Marsha K **(SLP)**
Fischetti, Mrs Jill Lorraine **(SLP)**
Gowin, Susan Ann Myers **(SLP)**
Marsicek, Jeanne Marie **(SLP)**
Miller, Mrs Bethany Wilson
O'Brien, Dr Maureen S **(SLP)**
Raymer, Anne Church **(SLP)**
Shaw-Holmes, Mrs Faith Suzanne **(SLP)**
Smallets, Sharon Marie **(A)**
Smetana, Wayne R **(A)**
Wilson, Mary Pat **(A)**

Leonardtown

Winnik, Mrs Florence R **(SLP)**

Lexington Park

Berger, Linda C **(SLP)**
Dove, Francine **(SLP)**
Elliott, Betty T **(SLP)**
Freed, Diane Joy **(SLP)**
Kent, Mrs Carrie E **(SLP)**
Olson-Silva, Mrs Sandra **(SLP)**
Smith, Jeanne A **(SLP)**
Trotter, Dr Alice Child **(SLP)**

Linthicum

McKenny, Mrs Irene F **(SLP)**
McKenny, M Joseph, Jr **(SLP)**
Waters, Judith A **(SLP)**

Linwood

Landy, Mrs Barbara Jo **(SLP)**

Lusby

Marsh, Mrs Michele Poynton **(SLP)**

Lutherville

Blumberg, Mrs Joan L **(A)**
Carberry, Patricia C **(SLP)**
Coughlin, Mrs Jane R **(SLP)**
Engnoth, Dr Gloria **(SLP)**
Harrison, Mrs Rosalind **(SLP)**
London, Mrs Denise Marie **(SLP)**
Marsh, Niki Pappas **(SLP)**
Martin, Katherine **(SLP)**
McDonald, Dr James M **(A)**
McDonald, Dr James M **(A)**
Nikoomanesh, Mrs Susan M Amini
Panzarella, Linda Theresa **(SLP)**
Papel, Mrs Leslie Bellah **(A)**
Saltsman, Robert H, Jr **(A)**
Seipp, William S **(SLP A)**
Sweeney, Martha H **(SLP)**

Marlow Heights

Datel, Tanya Marie **(A)**
Warrick, Edward J B **(SLP)**

Maugansville

Borland, Mrs Susan

Mechanicsville

Fowler, Susan E **(SLP)**
Taylor, Mrs Jeanne M **(SLP)**
Therrien, Kathleen Rose **(SLP)**

Middletown

Perich, Audrey Hare **(SLP)**

Millersville

Claybaugh, Gloria Petitclair **(SLP)**
Gallena, Mrs Sally K **(SLP)**
Iacarino, Judith E **(SLP)**
Kurek, Mrs Patricia A **(SLP)**

Mitchellville

Cuyjet, Carol L **(SLP)**

Monkton

Creticos, Ruth Morton **(SLP)**
Harris, Donald **(SLP)**
Martin, Mrs Carolyn C **(SLP)**

Mount Airy

Hutchins, Mrs Mary M **(SLP)**
Streett, Mrs Sharon S **(SLP)**

Mount Rainer

Pantano, Marilyn J **(SLP)**

Mount Rainier

Burrow, Cathy Lynn

New Carrollton

Miller, Wanda Louise **(SLP)**

New Windsor

Goettee, Mrs Marian S **(SLP)**

North Beach

Levy, Robin C W **(SLP)**

Oakland

Graybill, Mrs Joanne C
Graybill, Thomas J **(SLP)**

Olney

Andersen, Dr Catherine Finneran **(SLP A)**
Baker, Robert **(A)**
Brinker, Mrs Debra S
Coleman, Mrs Susan E **(A)**
Cullison, Bonita L **(SLP)**
Cygnarowicz, Mrs Teresa Marie **(A)**
Farmer, Mrs Wilma R **(SLP)**
Freedman, Amy Cushner **(SLP)**
Kramer, Mrs Bonnie S **(SLP)**
Miller, Joan
Natalo, Kelly D **(A)**
Rosenfeld, Mrs Diane S **(SLP)**
Stier, Arlene J **(SLP)**
Stinnett, Lisa Dawn **(SLP)**
Tippett, Mrs Cynthia Martino **(SLP)**
Weinstein, Mrs Rena R K **(SLP)**

Owings Mills

Abramowitz, Marvin R **(SLP)**
Adler, Mrs Janet Louis **(SLP)**
Alliker, Mrs Esta R **(SLP)**
Blaker, Mrs Sandra Weinberger **(SLP)**
Coddington, Colleen T **(A)**
Cohen, Eileen F **(SLP)**
Conner, Dr Thomas N **(SLP)**
Grant, Dr Susan R **(SLP)**
Greenwald, Jill R **(SLP)**
Hart, Mrs Sharon Elizabeth **(SLP)**
Hubert, Mrs Amy Bell **(SLP)**
Lubin, Joyce R **(SLP)**
McGarrell, Mrs Stephanie L
Misler, Mrs Donna T **(SLP)**
Neckrich, Jaclyn S **(SLP)**
Nevin, Nancy Patricia **(SLP)**
Principe, Sharon A **(SLP)**
Raphael, Mrs Rachel Aaron **(A)**
Roseman, Marcia L **(SLP)**
Rosenshein, Sandra **(SLP A)**
Scher, Mrs Stephanie B **(SLP)**
Shpritz, Mrs Ruth B **(SLP)**
Silverman, Mrs E Sara **(SLP)**
Slosberg, Marion G **(SLP)**
Tucker, Dawn D **(SLP)**
Wilner, Lynda Katz **(SLP)**
Winik, Mrs Michelle Lester **(SLP)**
Wittle, Mrs Christine

Parkville

Doyle, Dolores M **(SLP)**
Roese, Mrs Constance **(SLP)**

Pasadena

Brandenburger, Nancy **(SLP)**
Jabaay, Julie **(SLP)**
Leopold, Mrs Leslie Peterson **(SLP)**
Lyness, Elizabeth Susanne **(SLP)**
Ominsky, Mrs Karen Fults **(A)**
Szuba, Sandra W **(SLP)**

Patexent River

Conlon-Johnson, Mrs Ann **(SLP)**

Perry Hall

Girken, Mrs Karen C **(SLP)**
Godsey, Leslie Ann **(A)**
Kucera, Stephen Alan **(SLP)**
Suchowiecki, Jill Ann **(SLP)**

Phoenix

Gould, Mrs Cecelia A **(SLP)**
Kerr, Linda G T **(A)**
Smither, Donna Lauber **(SLP)**
Wayson, Suzanne W **(SLP)**

Pikesville

Eidelman, Mrs Jill Finkelstein **(SLP)**
Gardiner, Holly Jean **(SLP)**
Gilmore, Lloyd W **(SLP)**

Pocomoke City

Wall, Christine Joyce

Poolesville

Marsh, Sandra Evers **(SLP)**

Potomac

Abrams, Mrs Jane F **(SLP)**
Alexander, Rosanne Lessin **(SLP)**
Blane, Kathleen F **(A)**
Blumberg, Mrs Ina S **(SLP)**
Boris, Mrs Linda T **(SLP)**
Braunstein, Joan J **(SLP)**
Braunstein, Mrs M Sue **(SLP)**
Brick, Mrs Mara Green **(SLP)**
Brown, Earl J **(SLP A)**
Chi-Fishman, Mrs Gloria **(SLP)**
Chvotkin, Mrs Lynn Simmons **(SLP)**
Colodzin, Louise M **(A)**
Cox, Dr Bernard P **(A)**
Dobies, Mrs Sandra C **(SLP)**
Dorrow, Mrs Cecilia F **(SLP)**
Dougherty, Mrs Bonnie G **(SLP)**
Ellenbogen, Mrs Nancy Jo **(SLP)**
Ely, Mrs Nancy Meril **(A)**
Flatte-Hendel, Mrs Daryl F **(SLP)**
Fleming, Katherine J **(SLP)**
Glaser, Naomi B **(SLP)**
Goodman, Alice N **(SLP)**
Grimley, Mrs Judith L **(SLP)**
Hutkoff, Mrs Emily I **(SLP)**
Karl, Mrs Edith L **(SLP)**
Karr, Mrs Susan T **(SLP)**
Kirchner, Mrs Patricia Johnson **(SLP)**
LaNeve, Marion Yavener **(SLP)**
Lerner, Mrs Janet **(SLP)**
Levine, Mrs Judith D **(SLP)**
Lingwall, Dr James Bernard **(SLP)**
Lingwall, Maxine Campbell **(SLP)**
Mathrani, Jolanda W **(SLP)**
Mendelson, Gary L **(A)**
Menzin, Roberta Szalavetz **(SLP)**
Nepo, Mrs Hellaine Drucker **(SLP)**
Novak, Mrs Karen R J **(SLP)**
Oestreicher, Mrs Nancy K **(SLP)**
Patigalia, Mrs Barbara S **(SLP)**
Picard, Mrs Marianne T **(SLP)**
Pikus, Mrs Anita **(A)**
Rosenberg, Marylynn **(SLP)**
Roumel, Maria H **(SLP)**
Rubinoff, Mrs Laura A **(SLP)**
Saidel, Joan Fox **(SLP)**
Salwin, Mrs Nancy K **(SLP)**
Salzman, Lenore R **(SLP)**
Sandler, Ronna **(A)**
Schectman, Mrs Barbara L **(SLP)**
Scherr, Charlene K **(A)**
Schneider, Carol Ruth **(SLP)**
Schneider, Mrs Ilene F **(SLP)**
Siegel, Mrs Marjory Ellen Marks **(SLP)**
Silver, Clara M **(SLP)**
Skidmore, Mrs Sydney H **(SLP)**
Sonies, Dr Barbara C **(SLP)**
Vernon, Mrs Estelle R **(A)**
White, Mrs Judith Lee **(SLP)**
Wilkinson, Mrs Pamela Meinders **(SLP)**
Wintercorn, Dr Eleanor S **(SLP A)**
Zimmerman, Mrs Barbara Kriedman **(SLP)**

Prince Frederick

Paine, Mrs Wendy Luecker **(SLP)**
Wood, Gerald S **(SLP)**

Princess Anne

Haynes, Spencer H **(SLP)**

Queenstown

Butler, Mrs Sharon S **(SLP)**

Randallstown

Adams, Richard T **(SLP)**
Blank, Lillian Lurie **(SLP)**
Frazer, Mrs Deborah Seaman **(SLP)**
Goldstein, Mrs Barbara Feldman **(SLP)**
Grossman, Susan Leverah **(SLP)**
Harris, Howard I **(A)**
Johnson, Craig W **(A)**
Malin, Jerald A **(SLP A)**
Montgomery-Loy, Mrs Nancy L **(SLP)**
Pearl, Susan Z **(SLP)**
Pollock, Debra Kotelchuck **(SLP)**
Rabin, Susan L **(SLP)**
Tangeman, Gretchen **(SLP)**
Whitman, Mrs Adrienne **(SLP)**

Reisterstown

Bordenick, Roy M **(A)**
Goldman, Mrs Karon R **(SLP)**
Hornsby, Mrs Beth Ann **(SLP)**
Kaplan, Mrs Marsye W **(SLP)**
Le Donne, Diana Frances **(SLP)**
Miller, Mrs Linda O **(SLP)**
Resnik, Mrs Kathleen Collins **(SLP)**
Rowinsky, Mrs Wendy Sue **(SLP)**
Sarmir, Mrs Wendy L **(SLP)**
Scherr, Daun Willoughby **(SLP)**
Sherman, Roslyn S **(A)**
Wolfe, G Richard **(SLP)**

Relay

Moran-Grap, Mrs Lynn Marie **(SLP)**

Rising Sun

Kerns, Barbara J **(SLP)**
Marousek, Diane R **(SLP)**

Riva

Henline, Mrs Maureen **(SLP)**

Riverdale

Cook, Lynn E **(A)**

Rockville

Abrams, Susan M **(SLP)**
Anello, Mrs Elizabeth Lois **(SLP)**
Anglin, Mrs Michele Susan **(SLP)**
Baker, Karen P **(SLP)**
Berman, Mrs Jeri K **(SLP)**
Blasier, Mrs Marcia W **(SLP)**
Bouck, Janis K **(SLP)**
Cafritz, Donna M **(A)**
Carney, Mrs Sharon Sonnek
Cohen, Lucy L **(A)**
Cole, Dr Lorraine T **(SLP)**
Colen, Robin D **(SLP)**
Cornett, Dr Becky Sutherland **(SLP)**
Cowan, Bonnie Weinberg **(SLP)**
Curran-Zahra, Pamela E **(SLP)**
Dally, Mrs Anne E **(SLP)**
Dato, Dr Daniel P **(SLP)**
Diggs, Dr Charles C, Jr **(SLP)**

Emery, Mrs Susan S **(SLP)**
Fagan, Ellen C **(SLP)**
Feldman, Carin Bea **(SLP)**
Fleishman, Glenda C **(SLP)**
Forseter, Annette S **(A)**
Hankinson, Mrs Audrey L
Hart, Mandy Susan **(SLP)**
Havens, Mrs Laurie A **(SLP)**
Heller, Nancy **(SLP)**
Herer, Dr Gilbert R **(SLP A)**
Herson, Mrs Andrea **(SLP)**
Hilker, Patricia J **(SLP)**
Jacobs, Virginia V **(SLP)**
Johnston, Dr Frances J **(SLP)**
Kempner, Heidi N **(SLP)**
Kenton, Mrs Hedda S **(SLP)**
Kordell, Karen Ann **(A)**
Lake, Hope G
Lebowitz, Mrs Sandra S **(SLP)**
Levinson, Karen Beth **(SLP)**
Lourie, Bonita F L **(A)**
Malone, Margueritte S **(SLP)**
Malone, Dr Russell L **(SLP)**
Marks, Joan Marie **(A)**
Marks, Susan F **(SLP)**
Meisler, Mrs Barbara Altman **(SLP)**
Miller, Elizabeth Lonam **(SLP)**
Moe, Eunice W **(SLP)**
Moidel, Barbara **(SLP)**
Moriarty, Patricia L **(SLP)**
Peckarsky, Mrs Lori S **(SLP)**
Pellegrino, Joann McInnis **(SLP)**
Pelton, Marcia G **(SLP)**
Perlroth, Mrs Lynn Block **(A)**
Perreca, Mrs Dorothy **(SLP A)**
Pitarque, Patricia A **(SLP)**
Pons, Shayna Karas **(SLP)**
Proger, Laura Ellen **(A)**
Reeser, Mrs Judith P **(SLP)**
Regnell, Mrs Joan Roddy **(SLP)**
Richards, Grace Marcum **(A)**
Rosenfeld, Mrs Miriam Siegel **(SLP)**
Roth, Dr Froma P **(SLP)**
Schneiders, Marie H **(SLP)**
Scully, Martha S **(SLP)**
Seidman, Joyce H **(A)**
Shewan, Dr Cynthia M **(SLP)**
Singer, Beth Renee **(A)**
Spahr, Frederick T **(SLP)**
Stewart, Dr Billie Ackerman **(SLP)**
Striffler, Nancy S **(SLP)**
Szekely, Mrs Shelley Rosen **(SLP)**
Tarpley, Jewel D **(SLP)**
Travers, Barbara Walker **(SLP)**
Veres, Sally Ard **(SLP)**
Walsh, Mrs Gail P **(SLP)**
Weil, Stacy Rachelle **(SLP)**
Wetterhahn, Marilyn J **(SLP)**
White, Mrs Irene F **(SLP)**
White, Dr Steven C **(A)**
Whitlock, Beverly H **(SLP A)**
Williams, Jo Ellen **(A)**
Williams, Dr Peggy S **(SLP A)**
Wolfe, Helen Stein **(SLP)**
Yaffe-Oziel, Susan **(A)**
Zich, Cynthia Ann

Ruxton
Dearchs, Mrs Marianne Jackson **(SLP)**
Kubik, Dr Alexander W **(SLP A)**

Sabillasville
Phares, T Michael **(SLP)**

Salisbury
Anthenelli, Mrs Monica H **(SLP)**
Dalfonso, David L **(SLP)**
Gallivan, Paula C **(SLP)**
Glaze, Patricia Lynne
Hu, Mrs Florence Sun
MacAllister, Lance J **(SLP)**
Ollinger, Mrs Pamela L **(SLP)**
Scherr, Dr Robert **(SLP)**
Tirpak, Mrs Paula LaBute **(SLP)**
Walsh, Mrs Susan Weston **(SLP)**

Sandy Spring
Bonifant, Debra Croft **(SLP)**

Savage
Dellinger, David H **(A)**

Seabrook
Ferguson-Kinney, Mrs Gwendolyn C
Harman, Pamela M
Ridky, Dr Joseph R **(SLP)**

Severn
Boylan, Linda Carol **(A)**
Disanti, Mrs Catherine A **(A)**
Wagner, Jody Lynn

Severna Park
Basili, Dr Annanmaria **(SLP)**
Bowman, Brooks A **(SLP)**
Burkhart, Elizabeth Hohl **(SLP)**
Hutto, Charles L **(A)**
Irey, Linda **(SLP)**
Kraus, Mrs Kirsten Lacy **(SLP)**
Lynn, Mrs Cornelia Conrad **(SLP)**
Martini, Regina M **(SLP)**
Merrill, Pauline Reid **(SLP)**
Moeller, Mrs Leslie A **(SLP)**
Pallett, Stephen B **(A)**
Silverman, Mrs Fran L **(SLP)**
Styer, Mrs Brenda McAfee **(A)**
Underhill, Mrs Nancy A D **(SLP)**
Waskom, Sheryl B **(SLP)**

Silver Spring
Abrams, Mrs Kathleen M **(SLP)**
Acri, Jane B **(A)**
Anderson, Dr Noma B **(SLP)**
Anzelmo, Mrs Mary E **(SLP)**
Atack, Dr Rodney M **(A)**
Baker, Dr Donald J **(A)**
Balin, Mrs Betty W **(SLP)**
Barakat, Zeina Christine **(SLP)**
Barbour, Myra Maxwell **(SLP)**
Bass, Mrs Janice Heller **(SLP A)**
Beach, Rita Marie **(SLP)**
Beaman, Wynne B **(A)**
Beckford, Andrea Marcelle
Berman, Mrs Rita W **(SLP)**
Bialostozky, Franklin **(A)**
Blake, Mrs Donna M **(SLP)**
Bland, Linda Marie **(SLP)**
Bond, Marcia D **(SLP)**
Bove, Celeste F **(A)**
Bradley-Boggi, Mrs Jayne Anne **(SLP)**
Braithwaite, Beverley Ann
Breitler, Mrs Elaine K **(SLP)**
Brennan, Joan K **(SLP)**
Brooks, Lisa Colette **(SLP)**
Brozgal, Ruth **(SLP)**
Buckley, Regina **(SLP)**
Byers, Katherine Merchlinsk **(SLP)**
Byers, Mrs Patricia Ann **(SLP)**
Byrne-Hamilton, Mrs Karen Lyn **(SLP)**
Carter, Mrs Susan P **(SLP)**
Castner, Cheryl L **(SLP)**
Clausen, Roseanne P **(SLP)**
Cole, Patricia A **(SLP)**
Cornelius, Judith Marie **(SLP)**
Cowan, Dr Nancy S **(SLP)**
Crowley, Joanne M **(A)**
Dabbs, Terri Anne
Daniel, Marilyn J **(SLP)**
Del Polito, Dr Gene A **(A)**
De Pola, Mrs Adeline S **(SLP)**
Depola, John J **(SLP)**
Devlin, Lisa C **(A)**
Doris, Stacy A
Edmonds, Henriette **(SLP)**
Elkins, Dr Earleen **(A)**
Emme, Mrs Patricia C **(SLP)**
Evans, Christy Robin **(SLP)**
Farquhar, Mary S **(SLP)**
Finley, Deborah A **(SLP)**
Flack, Mrs Marilyn Neder **(A)**
Flinchum, Mary Brennan **(A)**
Forbes, Susan **(SLP)**
Fuso-de-Sevilla, Mrs Silvia **(SLP)**
Gaffigan, Mrs Hannah Clarke **(SLP)**
Gams-Ehrlich, Alma J **(SLP)**
Goldberg, Mrs Lynn Potashnick **(A)**
Greenfeld, Diane N **(SLP)**
Gritz, Mrs Janet M **(SLP)**
Gross, Johanna **(A)**
Hankinson, Mrs Arline L **(SLP)**
Hill, Elaine Maria **(SLP)**
Holden-Pitt, Lisa Denise
Hurst, Dr Charles G, Jr **(A)**
Ingersoll, Solveig H **(A)**
Inglisa-Vernetti, Mrs Marylou Joan
Israel, Dr Richard H **(SLP A)**
Iverson, Jeannine **(SLP)**
Jessen, Joanne K **(SLP A)**
Johnson, Mrs Barbara Powell **(SLP)**
Jones, Mrs Ann C **(SLP)**
Joseph, Mrs Sheryl S **(SLP)**
Jylkka, Margaret **(A)**
Kaplan, Dr Harriet F **(A)**
Kavanagh, Dr James F **(SLP)**
King, Mary L A **(SLP)**
Kinsella-Meier, MaryAnn **(A)**
Kryzer, Mrs Katherine **(SLP)**
Larkins, Dr Patricia Gail **(SLP)**
Lewis, Diane **(SLP)**
Lewis, Sharon Klich **(SLP)**
Light, Mrs Giselle Hope **(SLP)**
Loomis, Susan Roberta **(SLP)**
Lowery, Deborah Hodges **(A)**
Lynch, Constance E **(SLP)**
MacIver, Mrs Margaret L **(SLP)**
Marcot, Mrs Maryanne A **(SLP)**
Maslow, Lisa Abell
Mastroianni, Mary Ann P **(A)**
McGill, Barbara A **(SLP)**
Mechelis, Mrs Koula S K **(SLP)**
Mills, Dr Yvonne L **(SLP)**
Moore, Darlene Yvonne **(SLP)**
Moseley, Dr Mary June **(SLP)**
Muldoon-Donohue, Mrs Maureen **(SLP)**
Nash, Kimberly Rene **(SLP)**
Nelson-Drake, Janice K **(A)**
Norton, Darryl E **(SLP)**
Novakovich, Harriet V **(SLP)**
Oertli, Julene May **(SLP)**
Ortega-Hillyer, Nereida I **(SLP)**
Pafitis, Irene A **(A)**
Patrick, Susan B **(SLP)**
Peters-Johnson, Dr Cassandra **(SLP)**
Peterson, Mrs Mary B **(SLP)**
Redington, Mrs Mary O **(SLP)**
Reiner, Dr Barbara J **(SLP)**
Rensin, Mrs Katherine **(SLP)**
Reynolds, Anne T **(SLP)**
Rosenberg, Mrs Karen J **(SLP)**
Rosenthal, Susan Richards **(SLP)**
Rothberg, Mrs Caryl R **(SLP)**
Runnels-Contee, Cathy **(SLP)**
Schindler, Susan Kahalas **(SLP)**
Schroeder, Katherine Marie
Schuchman, Dr Gerald I **(A)**
Schultz, Jean S **(SLP)**
Schwartz, Mrs Gail S **(SLP)**
Schwartz, Marsha S **(A)**
Shapiro, Gail Andrea **(SLP)**
Sheridan, Catherine **(SLP)**
Simpkins, William T, Jr **(SLP)**
Spencer, Stephanie **(SLP)**
Stafford, Mrs Sally H **(SLP)**
Stern, Susan Bette **(SLP)**
Stewart, Mrs Carolyn H **(SLP)**
Suter, Dr Alice H **(A)**
Sylvester, Stephen F **(SLP A)**
Theiss, Kristen Jean **(SLP)**
Thompson, Patricia R **(A)**
Treanor, Dr Ruth D **(SLP)**
Ulrich, Mrs Miriam N **(SLP)**
Walden, Dr Brian E **(A)**
Watkins, Ronnie L **(SLP)**
Whitney, Joan C
Wiggins, M Eugene **(SLP)**
Williams, Tina B **(SLP)**
Wilson, Elaine D **(A)**
Wolfram, Walter A
Worthington, Colleen Kirley **(SLP)**
Wray, Doris Q **(SLP)**
Zaslow, Elinor L **(SLP)**
Zingeser, Louise B **(SLP)**

Smithsburg
Reynolds, Carol Suzanne **(SLP)**

Sparks
Buppert, Mary Blair **(SLP)**
Flood, Patricia Anne

St Leonard
Stanley, Mrs Susan Plaster **(SLP)**

St Michaels
Tokarz, Mrs Jeanne G **(SLP)**

Stevensville
Higgins, Mrs June Eden **(SLP)**
Lepczyk, Mrs Susan Guess **(SLP)**

Sudlersville
Rose, Mrs Bonnie Mae **(SLP)**

Sunderland
Fabiszak-Harrison, Mrs Michele K **(SLP)**

Swanton
Friend, Debra E **(SLP)**
Mauro, Darla M **(SLP)**

Sykesville
Albright, Mrs Linda M **(SLP)**
Ball, Mrs Theresa L **(SLP)**
Brimigion, Mrs Barbara Joan
Knipp, Anne **(SLP)**
Velte-Jones, Phyllis C **(SLP)**
Woods, Mrs Josephine **(SLP)**

Takoma Park
Alexander-Feasley, Mrs Margaret A **(SLP)**
Jacobs, Mrs Lucille Karas **(SLP)**
Leonard, Mrs Bernita Elin Z **(SLP)**
Levy, Sharon H **(SLP)**
Mason, Susan Reddan **(SLP)**
Murata, Hiroko **(SLP)**
Narsiah, Ravindra Enjaty **(SLP)**
Van Doren, Cynthia Johanna **(SLP)**

Temple Hills
Alexander-Whiting, Mrs Harriett **(SLP)**
Gee, Zilphia T **(SLP)**
Minus, Mrs Bertha D **(SLP)**

Timonium
Bacon, Mrs Mariana Goytisolo **(SLP)**
Brooks, Beverly Ann **(A)**
Cupples, Dr Willie P, Jr **(SLP)**
Herbert, Marybeth
Heyde, Mrs Wendy K **(SLP)**
Hitchcock, Virginia M **(SLP)**
Knox, Brenda Bonuccelli **(SLP)**
Kundrat, Donna M **(SLP)**
London, Cynthia J **(SLP)**
Makres-Polites, Olga D **(SLP)**
Norlin, Peter F **(SLP)**
Rysticken, Noreen Ann **(SLP)**
Schwartz-Reitzel, Dr Joyce **(SLP)**

Towson
Angle, Mrs Ann M **(SLP)**
Beauchamp, Mrs Terese D **(A)**
Bunker, Mrs Rosemary O **(SLP)**
Diaz, Maria-Hele
Elliott, Mrs Margaret Tampieri **(SLP)**
Ghitter, Dr Rosalyn **(SLP)**
Gordon, Mrs Edith Marie **(A)**
Heller, Mrs Judith A **(SLP)**
Kilburg, Dr Gail Donahue **(SLP)**
Larsen, Maren Lynn **(SLP)**

Lilly, Mrs Linda P **(SLP)**
Lynch, Mrs Carol Queen **(SLP)**
Seidel, Mrs Susan J **(A)**
Shrewsbury, Dr Margaret E **(SLP)**
Teubner-Rhodes, Mrs Louise **(SLP)**

Union Bridge
Mastalerz, Vickie R **(A)**
White, E Rebecca **(SLP)**

University Park
Brewer, Dr Carmen C **(A)**
Stone, Dr Maureen L **(SLP)**

Upper Marlboro
Carlson-Geer, Mrs Susan L **(A)**
Criss, Judith O **(SLP)**
Edelen, Kathleen Gail **(SLP)**
Edmonds, Celestina **(SLP)**
Ferralli, Sharon A **(SLP)**
Jones, Shirley A **(SLP)**
Mele-McCarthy, Joan A **(SLP)**
Moore, Evette Renee **(SLP)**
Pugh, Mrs Wilhelmina Scott **(SLP)**
Raab, Eileen W **(SLP)**
Reiter, Linda Jo **(A)**
Sales, Debra B **(SLP)**
Smith-Greene, Mrs Joyce **(SLP)**

Waldorf
Blake, Mrs Sandra Leona **(A)**
Clark, Donna C **(SLP)**
Davis, Barbara J **(SLP)**
Kline, Mrs Jamie Kay **(SLP)**
Mount, Mrs Amelia Willis **(A)**
Trinch, Mrs Paula Jean **(SLP)**

Walkersville
Ford, Mrs Alice B **(SLP)**
Ramirez, Cynthia Anne **(SLP)**

West River
Giannini, Coni J **(SLP)**

Westernport
Moran, Mrs Mary Ann **(SLP)**

Westminster
Alles, Catherine Dykstra **(A)**
Davidson, Barbara **(SLP)**
Katz, Mrs Iris L **(SLP)**
Mathias, Mrs Deborah Ann **(SLP)**
Tierney, Martin Eugene **(SLP)**
Welliver, Mrs Susan Marie **(SLP)**

Wheaton
Autry, Mrs Alice M **(SLP)**
Bennett, Lisa J W **(SLP)**
Busse, David J **(SLP)**
Busse, Mrs Mary S **(SLP)**
Epstein, Dr Stephen
Fischer, Alecia S **(SLP)**
Fontaine, Lisa M **(SLP)**
Herschfeld, Mrs Michele Waldman **(SLP)**
Kracov, Mrs Marion **(SLP)**
Rosenthal, Susan J **(SLP)**
Scheib, Donna S **(SLP)**
Wall, Kathleen **(A)**

White Hall
Demps, Mrs Karen Nelson **(SLP)**
McGraw, Mrs Paula Louise **(SLP)**

White Plains
Starkey, Mrs Marta I **(SLP)**

Williamsport
Witman, Jamie Auxt **(SLP)**

Woodbine
Murphy, Margaret A **(SLP)**

Woodstock
King, Mrs Margaret F **(SLP)**

MASSACHUSETTS

Abington
Kearney, Kathleen M
Somers, Mrs Andrea C **(SLP)**

Acton
Bergart, Mrs Marlene H **(SLP)**
Cohen, Susan **(SLP)**
Emer, Robin Burrows **(SLP)**
Gabay, Mrs Galina V **(SLP)**
Johnson, William Paul **(SLP)**
Lelchook, Alex K **(SLP)**
Pommers, Mrs Susan G **(SLP)**
Prosnitz, Gabrielle C **(SLP)**
Sayre, Mrs Vivien L **(SLP)**
Wachtell, Marlene A **(SLP)**
Wade, Mrs Dorothy Dodge **(SLP)**
Williams-Butler, MaryAnn **(SLP)**

Adams
Carmel, Norman R **(SLP)**

Agawam
Heyman, Beth Ann **(A)**
Perreault, Marilyn **(A)**
Thomas, Doreen M **(SLP)**

Allston
Adams, Patricia Agnes **(SLP)**
Anis, Helen **(SLP)**
Eisengart, Anne Edith **(SLP)**
Johnston, Jennifer **(SLP)**
Salzbank, Sharon L **(SLP)**
Schudrich, Brynna Joy **(SLP)**

Amesbury
Enos, Mrs Joann Hiehle **(SLP)**
Fletcher, Wendy J
O'Neil, Therese M **(SLP)**
Peyton, Eileen M **(SLP)**

Amherst
Arnold, Barbara J **(A)**
Balasubramanian, Dr Venugopal **(SLP)**
Baran, Dr Jane A **(SLP A)**
Bergman, Judith L **(SLP)**
Boscardin, Dr Mary Lynn **(SLP)**
Brush, Mrs Eleanor L **(SLP)**
Cann, Mrs Anne Garside **(SLP)**
Clower, Laura Ruth **(SLP)**
Conti, Mrs Judith R **(SLP)**
Cronen, Myrna P **(SLP)**
Davis, Dr G Albyn **(SLP)**
Estrany-Frau, Ingrid **(SLP)**
Falkowski, Marilyn K **(SLP)**
Freyman, Dr Richard L **(A)**
Garson, Blaine A **(SLP)**
Garvey, Judith P **(SLP)**
Hannahan, Mrs Lisa Barbara **(SLP)**
Harris, Jessica R **(SLP)**
Helfer, Karen S **(A)**
Hersh, Gene B **(SLP)**
Huntley, Ruth A **(SLP)**
Jenkins, Barbara Benda **(SLP)**
Jillson, Mrs Sheila Rose
Jubien, Ghislaine **(SLP)**
Levitt, Ellen **(SLP)**
Melrose, Dr Jay **(SLP A)**
Mullin, Mrs Sandra C **(SLP)**
Nerbonne, Dr G Patrick **(SLP)**
Nober, Dr E Harris **(SLP A)**
Nober, Dr Linda W **(SLP)**
Peirce, Dr Henry B, Jr **(SLP)**
Seymour, Dr Charlena Moten **(SLP)**
Seymour, Dr Harry N **(SLP)**
Terrizzi, Dr Adrienne M **(SLP)**
Thiebaut, Jeanine Marie **(SLP)**
Townes, Valerie A **(SLP)**
Wogrin, Mrs Lois B **(SLP)**

Andover
Block-Selwyn, Rochelle **(SLP)**
Bromberg, Mrs Elinor J **(SLP)**
Burton, Mrs Pearl B **(SLP)**
Gordon, Barbara J **(SLP)**
Johnston, Mrs Susan Yates **(SLP)**
Jolie, Kim R **(SLP)**
Krentcil, Bonnie **(SLP)**
Maietta, Dr Donald Francis **(SLP A)**
Miller, Mrs Robin Schelzi **(SLP)**
Rubin, Audrey S **(SLP)**
Ruderman, Mrs Ruth S **(SLP)**
Shapiro, Robert B **(SLP)**
Therrien, Mrs Sheila B **(SLP)**
Vail, Mrs Beth H **(SLP)**
Wilner, Susan Scott **(SLP)**
Zuena, Mrs Paulette B **(SLP)**

Arlington
Cummings, Mary A **(SLP)**
Dextraze, Kelly Mulrooney **(SLP)**
Dwyer, Sharon Patricia **(SLP)**
Farber, Marilyn E **(SLP)**
Gerstein, Leonore **(SLP)**
Giacone, Mrs Cheryl A **(SLP)**
Hargrave, Joan K **(SLP)**
Kelley, Elizabeth Anne **(SLP)**
Kelly, Ann Marie **(SLP)**
Levin, Wendy Gail **(SLP)**
Lincoln, Karen Lee **(A)**
Malone, Sr Patricia **(SLP)**
McEwen, Mrs Judy Laura **(SLP)**
Miller, Ellen R **(SLP)**
Mussa, Laraine **(SLP)**
Nicholas, Marjorie L **(SLP)**
Payton, Mrs Rebecca Z **(SLP)**
Reed, Charlotte
Samuels, Mrs Cynthia R **(SLP)**
Smith, Mrs Susan Vansant **(SLP)**
Thompson, Susan K **(SLP)**
Walsh, Moira F **(SLP)**
Whitaker, Mrs Susan M F **(SLP)**

Ashburnham
Murphy, Ann E **(SLP)**
Reid, Louise **(SLP)**

Ashby
Daigle, Mrs Teresa A **(SLP)**
Manney, Anne M **(A)**

Ashfield
Ferris, Jean B **(SLP)**
Pike, Harriet H **(A)**

Ashland
Barbera-Hanson, Cheriann **(SLP)**
Gilman, Sherri Lynne **(SLP)**

Assonet
Cooper, Judith K **(SLP)**
Loftus, Mrs Paula Megan **(SLP)**
Sullivan, Mrs Karen Schneider **(SLP)**
Tunney, Kathleen M **(SLP)**

Athol
Ambrozy, Dr Carol A **(SLP)**

Attleboro
Atwood, Iris Brastow
Quaglia, Mrs Margo Grace

Attleboro Falls
Cherecwich, Mrs Barbara J **(A)**

Auburn
Bialas, Susan Nallen **(SLP)**
Holden, Debra Lynn **(SLP)**
Lada-Butterworth, Joan E **(SLP)**
Lukaskiewicz, Janet **(A)**
Riley, Loy Dona **(SLP)**
Rucho, Patricia Ann **(SLP)**
Russell, David F **(SLP)**

Auburndale
Barbee, Mrs Mary Ann F **(SLP)**
Crimmins, Diana C **(SLP)**
Martin, Sandra Beth **(SLP)**
Read, Mrs M Margaret **(SLP A)**

Barnstable
Cullen, Patrick Edward **(SLP A)**
Sullivan, Margaret M **(SLP)**
Waldman, Susan E **(SLP)**

Barre
Howard, Barbara Morrison **(SLP)**

Barre Plains
Landry, Mrs Lisa D **(SLP)**

Bedford
Campbell, Mrs Jeanne P **(SLP)**
Dolan, Marie D
Felins, Mary Angela **(SLP)**
Heath, Linda M **(SLP)**
Howard, Craig L **(SLP)**
Mondello, Mrs Debra Ford **(SLP)**
Rabinowitz, Christine **(A)**
Sumner, Elizabeth **(SLP)**

Belchertown
Campbell, Cheryl A **(SLP)**
Hoag, Mrs Diane M **(SLP)**
Lambert, Mrs Carolyn **(SLP)**
Mercaitis, Dr Patricia A **(SLP)**
Scott, Laura M **(SLP)**

Bellingham
Albrigo, Angela Marie **(SLP)**

Belmont
Anderson, Elaine Rohde **(SLP)**
Banker, Dr Michele S **(SLP)**
Crawley, Kathryn **(SLP)**
Dalton, Maureen Lisbeth **(SLP)**
Derse, Christine Louise **(SLP)**
Eirich, Mrs Mary Sullivan **(SLP)**
Elias, Katherine M **(SLP)**
Fennell, Ann M **(SLP)**
Fishman, Mrs Sally W **(SLP)**
Kaplan, Jerome H **(SLP)**
McLean, Sharon Nellis **(SLP)**
Nissen, Sheryl E **(SLP)**
Rosowski, Mrs Jean Trelawny **(A)**
Sanders, R Richard **(SLP)**
Schadelbauer, Margaret J **(SLP)**
Segal, Dr Denise Erica **(SLP)**
Weeks, Mary S **(SLP)**
West, Kathleen Loftus **(A)**

Beverly
Bellevue, Beverly Walker **(SLP)**
Beswick, Jane D **(SLP)**
Chiusano, Roseann Atkin **(SLP)**
Connor, Jacqueline **(A)**
Conrad, Mrs Faith F **(SLP)**
Doring, Mrs Pamela Kodis **(SLP)**
Fernandes, Jean Keeffe **(SLP)**
Haight, Mrs Diane DaveKos **(SLP)**
Hamilton, Robert S, Jr **(SLP)**
Heller, Meryl A **(SLP)**
Kowalski, Kathryn R **(SLP)**
Letien, W Cary **(A)**
Levesque, Caren Ann **(SLP)**
McGovern, Dona M **(A)**
Merrill, Elizabeth Warner **(SLP)**
Peraino, Antoinette **(SLP)**
Schlein, Mrs Elizabeth Golden **(SLP)**
Sullivan, Kathleen K **(SLP)**
Thompson-Heerlein, Judith A **(SLP)**
Young, Heidi J **(A)**

Beverly Farms
Baker, Linda T **(SLP)**
Byrne, Lisa

Blackstone
Broderick-Backman, Mrs Katherine A **(SLP)**
Hendricks, Mrs Barbara Rodier **(SLP)**
Weinberg, Mrs Randi Beth **(SLP)**

Blandford
Caron, Alfred L **(SLP)**

Bolton
Janson, Diane B **(SLP)**

Bondsville
Sears, Valerie Ann

Boston
Arsenault, Joan Kelly **(SLP)**
Ashland, Jean E **(SLP)**
Bankson, Dr Nicholas Webb **(SLP)**
Bashir, Anthony **(SLP)**
Bean, Susan M **(A)**
Bennett, Dr Suzanne **(SLP)**
Blatt, Susan Lori **(SLP)**
Burkard, Robert F **(A)**
Cox, L Clarke **(A)**
Cumpata, Joellen Frere **(SLP)**
Damian, Judith Abriol **(SLP)**
Davis, Dr Robin L **(A)**
Drake, Karen Lynn **(SLP)**
Drummond, Martha E **(A)**
Dybka, Dr Michael E **(A)**
Ebersole, Amy K **(SLP)**
Eisenberg-Dorfman, Mrs Melody **(A)**
Ferullo, Dr Robert J **(SLP A)**
Florentine, Dr Mary
Frankoff, Denise J **(SLP)**
Freedman, Mrs Amy Curhan **(SLP)**
Gagliardi, David M **(A)**
Gavett, Elizabeth **(SLP)**
Germono, Dr Joseph Frederick **(SLP)**
Gold, Sharon J **(A)**
Hallahan, Thomas Jude **(A)**
Hellman, Rhona Phyllis
Helm-Estabrooks, Dr Nancy **(SLP)**
Karas, Irene D **(SLP)**
Katz, Cindy Miller **(SLP)**
Klein, Marie **(SLP)**
Koehnke, Dr Janet D **(A)**
Limtiaco, Theresa M G **(SLP)**
Locke, Dr John L **(SLP)**
Lorendo, Leah C **(SLP)**
Mason, Ruth **(SLP)**
Mastrandreas, Margaret **(SLP)**
McCormick, Kathleen Ann **(SLP)**
Miller, Dr Joanne L
Moll, Judith
Moneghan, Pamela Annette **(A)**
Monte, Karen L **(SLP)**
Morrison, Rhoda K **(A)**
Naeser, Dr Margaret A **(SLP)**
Norris, Michelle Marie **(SLP)**
Raffin Phd, Dr Michael J M **(A)**
Richardson, Mrs Elizabeth Bressler **(SLP)**
Ridgway, Alice Emily **(SLP)**
Romer, Susan O'Day **(SLP)**
Rosenblatt, Janet **(SLP)**
Rubin, Nan P **(SLP)**
Russo, Lorraine A **(A)**
Scavuzzo, Annebelle **(SLP)**
Shane, Dr Howard C **(SLP)**
Stangler, Sharon Lynn
Stewart, Deborah C **(A)**
Stitt, Barbara J **(SLP)**
Strand, Dr Kristine E **(SLP)**
Thomas, Mrs Kathleen Palmer **(SLP)**
Thornton, Dr Aaron R **(SLP A)**
Tuttle, Dr Gerald A **(SLP)**
Ungerleider, Deborah S **(A)**
Vadakin, Cheryl Ann **(SLP)**
Vallino, Dr Linda D **(SLP A)**
Warren, Dr Marilyn Park **(A)**
Weinstein, Dayna S **(A)**
West, Carol A **(A)**
Wheelden, Julie Atwood **(SLP)**
Wise, Cynthia
Zubick, Dr Howard H **(SLP A)**

Bourne
Chilson, Mrs Ruth F **(SLP)**
Donaldson, Anne Chalfin **(SLP)**

Boxborough
Barker, Elisabeth **(SLP)**
Meyers, Margaret Mae **(SLP)**

Boxford
Amidon, Mrs Joy W **(SLP)**
Haynes, Charles W **(SLP)**

Boylston
Donnelly, Nancy Carver **(SLP)**
Hochman, Ruth M **(SLP)**
Mitchell, Mrs Michelle Cullerton **(SLP)**
Tirolo-Zaleski, Mrs Barbara **(SLP)**

Bradford
De Roche, Jane Frances **(SLP)**
Hayes, Mrs Judith Anne **(SLP)**
Howland, Karole A

Braintree
Bloom, Harriet Debra **(SLP)**
Finnegan-Kelly, Janet E **(SLP)**
Gomes, Dr Barbara A **(SLP)**
Hurstak, Jane M **(SLP)**
La Dew, Lisa A **(SLP)**
Loverso, Dr Felice L **(SLP)**
Marcarelli, Karen H **(A)**
Nesbeda, Christina **(SLP)**
Pucillo, Mrs Joan M **(SLP)**
Sturm-Getchell, Joanne **(SLP)**
Warren, Dr Reg Lawrence **(SLP)**

Brant Rock
Graham, Mrs Joanne Louise **(SLP)**

Brewster
Green, Patricia W **(SLP)**
Stoia, Louis **(SLP A)**
Timmons, Mae **(SLP)**

Bridgewater
Homer, Judy R **(SLP)**
Kirby, Sr Alice M **(SLP)**
Popovics, Alice M **(SLP)**
Roza, Diane M **(SLP)**
Williston, James **(SLP)**

Brighton
Bess, Laura Ann **(SLP)**
Costello, John Michael **(SLP)**
Gross, Mrs Phyllis **(SLP)**
Kalotkin, Madoline **(SLP)**
Karas, Karen Joy **(A)**
Kennedy, Mary M **(SLP)**
Lannon, Mary Beth **(A)**
Lewis, Andrea Jill **(SLP)**
Loeb, Randi Chudnow
Lynch, Eileen Marie
Mahoney, Mary H **(SLP)**
Mark, Carol **(SLP)**
Markus, Theodore **(SLP)**
Perkins, Judy Marie **(SLP)**
Reynolds, Mary J **(SLP)**
Ronan, Mrs Gail A **(SLP)**
Rothenstein, Amy Jill **(SLP)**
Simons, Lynn **(SLP)**
Sperry, Elizabeth Ellen **(SLP)**
Stevens, Shelley L **(SLP)**
Unger, Lori R **(SLP)**
Willson, Karen D **(A)**
Wommer, Marcy K

Brimfield
Niemitz, Mrs Ann F **(SLP)**

Brockton
Brezner, Ellen L **(SLP)**
Bulgaris, Valerie A **(SLP)**
Carroll, Sara Beth **(SLP)**
Fruth, Janice K **(SLP)**
Hunyadi, Martha A **(SLP)**
Perry, Julie **(A)**
Rodriguez, Lisa Zimmerman **(SLP)**
Sullivan, Mrs Diane Riser **(SLP)**

Brookline
Adler, Carol R **(SLP)**
Arick, Judith T **(A)**
Avni, Nitza Movshovitch **(A)**
Berger, Jill Melodie **(SLP)**
Berliner, Ronna **(SLP)**
Birman, Marina **(A)**
Bonander, Lynn A **(SLP)**
Brenner, Sheila K **(SLP)**
Chaikin, Lauren B
Chasin, Judith G **(A)**
Cleveland, Sandra S **(A)**
Colton, Mrs Carolyn Mensh **(A)**
D'Artista, Diane F **(SLP)**
Ehrlich, Pauline **(SLP A)**
Fox, Mrs Lodiana E **(SLP)**
Goldenberg, Amy **(SLP)**
Goldstein, Marjorie J **(SLP)**
Gordon, Henrietta **(SLP)**
Green, Dr Meryl C **(SLP)**
Haas, Gretchen L **(SLP)**
Hanopole, Dr Martin S **(SLP A)**
Havens, Judith W **(SLP)**
Isaacson, Nancy Lynn **(SLP)**
Jones, Susan Lynne **(A)**
Kates, Leslie V **(SLP)**
Klaiman, Mrs Paula Gayle **(SLP)**
Laufer, Debora **(SLP)**
Lessem, Margot L
Levy, Carol B **(SLP)**
Lewis, Mrs Janice Rechnitz **(SLP)**
Lipschultz, Rochelle W **(SLP)**
Lubar, Phyllis **(SLP)**
Margolis, Lynn A **(A)**
Maxwell, Lesley Anne **(SLP)**
Menno, Kathleen Ann **(SLP)**
Menyuk, Prof Paula
Odessa, Susan Iris **(SLP)**
Proctor, Dr F Adele **(SLP)**
Ramirez, Irma Leticia **(SLP)**
Rees, Dr Norma S **(SLP A)**
Rubin, Julie K **(A)**
Schloff, Laurie **(SLP)**
Schwartz, Lynn Thomas **(A)**
Scobell, Lynnette **(SLP)**
Severson, Debra D **(A)**
Small, Dr Anita Ruth **(SLP)**
Sullivan, Kathleen Elizabeth **(SLP)**
Turner, Julie L **(SLP)**
Wang, Hueiyao Sophia **(A)**
Wiberg, Wendy A **(SLP)**
Widan, Margot **(SLP)**
Willcox-Bein, Katherine **(SLP)**
Williams, Rita Murphy **(SLP)**
Zallinger, Martha **(SLP)**

Burlington
Abbott, Cynthia D **(A)**
Cobb, Jane Emily **(SLP)**
Cohen, Nancy L **(A)**
Enders, Carolyn Diane
Howard, Marilyn R **(SLP)**
Rees, Deidre G **(SLP A)**

Byfield
Barry, Mrs Karen McNaught **(SLP)**

Cambridge
Arcus, Doreen M **(SLP)**
Bejoian, Linda C **(SLP)**
Besing, Joan M **(A)**
Bradford, Judith Ann **(SLP)**
Chen-Hall, Mrs I-Fan M **(SLP)**
Counter, S Allen **(A)**
Couts, Nancy **(SLP)**
Delhorne, Lorraine Anne
Dinapoli, Joseph M **(SLP)**
Epstein, Lisa Brazel **(SLP)**
Fayad, Donna M **(SLP)**
Garel, Susan Kathleen **(A)**
Gottlieb, Suzanne Del **(SLP)**
Grant, Kenneth Wayne
Haring, Karen Hardin **(SLP)**
Hirsch, Susan **(SLP)**
Hitschman, Mrs Hedwig **(SLP)**
Jacob, Loyal J **(SLP)**
Kleinman, Sandra Nan **(SLP)**
Mahoney, Dennis G **(SLP)**
Maurer, Charlo Jean
McGrath, Patricia M **(SLP)**
Midkiff-Borunda, Shelley S **(SLP)**
Rosenfield, Dr Irma B **(SLP)**
Stevens, Dr Merle **(SLP)**
Tissiere, Michele **(SLP)**
Torrey, Elizabeth Farrell **(SLP)**
Townsend, Nancy M **(SLP)**
Vogel, Mrs Nancy Wind **(SLP)**
Ward, Natalie E **(SLP)**
White, Dorothy J **(SLP)**
Zimbler, Mrs Enid B

Canton
Aronson, Anne Jody **(SLP)**
Clark, Marybeth G **(SLP)**
Goetze, Anne S **(SLP)**
Greenstein, Gayle Kaplan **(SLP)**
Hoffman, Martha-Sue **(SLP)**
Okun, Denise Riley **(SLP)**
Parker, Mrs Maria Elena **(SLP)**

Carlisle
Dimatteo, Pamela Kay **(SLP)**

Centerville
Alexander, Elizabeth W **(SLP)**
Battles, Kathy J **(SLP)**
Garreffi, Mrs Fern Feinberg **(SLP)**
Hosford, Joyce T **(SLP)**
McPhillips, M Regina **(A)**
Weinberg, Norma Pasekoff **(SLP)**

Charlemont
Golann, Adria J
Howatt, Sara L **(SLP)**

Charlestown
Cotter, Nancy Brennan
Tucker, Thomas W **(A)**

Charlton
Coderre, Mrs Tina R **(A)**
Dingle, Mrs Ann E **(SLP)**
Duff, Abigail C **(SLP)**
Gergich, Mrs Joyce Andrea **(SLP)**

Chatham
Colby, Mrs Jane Campion **(SLP)**
Williams, Lori Lynn **(SLP)**

Chelmsford
Babon, Mrs Wendy Diane **(SLP)**
Briand, Claire Marie **(SLP)**
Mayfield, Mrs Margaret Topian **(SLP)**
McGowan, Jean Marie **(A)**
Newman, Mrs Judith C **(SLP)**
Porter-Couto, Bonnie J **(SLP)**
Tambo, Mrs Josephine **(SLP)**

Chelsea
Curatolo, Jill Maloney **(SLP)**
O'Neil-Kayal, Jennifer Mary **(A)**

Chesterfield
D'Agostino, Eliza D **(SLP)**
Erb, Margaret Quinn **(SLP)**

Chestnut Hill
Adler, Eve **(A)**
Berlad, Tina Beth **(SLP)**
Catz, Mrs Judith C **(SLP)**
Dawson, Kathryn E **(SLP)**
Gray, Mrs Lillian W **(SLP)**
Krishnan, Ranjani
Levenson, Mrs Sondra H **(SLP)**
Linsky, Sharon E **(SLP)**
Malmad, Susan J **(SLP)**
Reinhardt, Susan E **(SLP)**
Sallet, Mrs Lauren Lazeroff **(SLP)**
Sauer, Margaret Lois **(SLP)**
Sonnenschein, Mrs Tamar G **(SLP)**
Stoia, Dr George **(SLP)**

Chicopee
Brault, Mrs Mary Ann Scavotto **(SLP)**
Burke, Lois E **(A)**
Deltoro, Mrs Karalynne Pope **(SLP)**
Hamel, Mrs Cecilia **(SLP)**
O'Malley, Marguerite Theresa **(SLP)**

Rickarby, Janet H **(SLP)**
Rosa, Janice Ann **(SLP)**
Starn, Cynthia Jo **(A)**
Urcuioli, Nancy Jean **(A)**

Clinton
Lee, Laurie
Martel, Susan Lynne **(SLP)**
Rauscher, Debra Lynn **(SLP)**
Strickland, Sherrill Moll **(SLP)**

Cohasset
Dunphy, Diana Gould **(SLP)**
Fradette-Sebell, Jeanne **(SLP)**
Johnston, Mrs Diane T G **(SLP)**
Lundgren, Kristine M **(SLP)**
Yess, Mrs Denise A **(SLP)**

Colrain
Abels, Mrs Jeanne **(SLP)**

Concord
Eisenhaure, Dorothy C **(SLP)**
Hekman, Mrs Carol Ann **(SLP)**
Mate, Cynthia A **(SLP)**
Morgan, Dr Alisa L R **(SLP)**
Shur, Mrs Iris B **(A)**
Thurman, Mrs Hattie Tingle **(SLP)**
Trommald, Mrs Dagne A **(A)**
Weiner, Dr Honore I **(SLP)**

Conway
Childs, Deborah H **(SLP)**

Cotuit
Conway, Marjorie J **(SLP)**
Fitton, Mrs Barbara Falese **(SLP)**
Uyenoyama, Mrs Jayne Hayden **(SLP)**

Cummaquid
Doll, Julie Burns **(SLP)**

Cummington
Arbib, Brenda Sullivan **(SLP)**
Steadman, Maryanne **(SLP)**

Dalton
Carmel, Mrs Barbara R **(SLP)**
Veremko, Gregory Steven **(SLP)**
Veremko, Karen Eissmann **(SLP)**

Danvers
Babbitt, Douglas A **(SLP)**
Barbaro, Anne L **(A)**
Coccoluto-Davidson, Donna M **(SLP)**
Leblanc, Denise Pendergast **(A)**
Middleton, Janet B **(SLP)**
Rowan, Karen A **(A)**

Dedham
Baye-Kaye, Lisa **(A)**
Bernstein, Sharon P **(SLP)**
Diamond, Shari R
Dixon, Carol H **(SLP)**
Galt, Sally Ann **(SLP)**
Kidd, Gerald D, Jr **(A)**
Lesinski, Mrs Kathleen Niven **(SLP)**
Mason, Christine **(A)**
Naughton, Marie A **(SLP)**
Niziak, Kathleen J **(SLP)**
Rossi, Mrs Bernice Liberatore **(SLP)**
Wallace, Linda Mary **(A)**

Deerfield
McHale, Jane Elizabeth **(SLP)**

Dennis
Peterson, Nancy E **(A)**

Dorchester
Ciambrone, Gary **(SLP)**
Ciambrone, Sarah W **(SLP)**
Dewey, Mrs Claire C **(SLP)**
Dubois, Mrs Ann Marie Jepsen **(SLP)**
Goldsmith, Tessa Ann **(SLP)**
Goode, Matthew Edward **(SLP)**
Griffin, Stephen J **(SLP)**
Toro, Margaret Ross **(A)**
Weisinger, Wendell Lynne **(SLP)**

Dover
Buus, Dr Soren
Tarulli, Nancy Jo **(SLP)**
Wuschke, Joanne **(SLP)**

Dracut
Czarnota, Annemarie **(A)**

Dudley
Grimes, Mrs Marian M **(SLP)**
Orsini, Mrs Barbara D **(SLP)**
Ruda, Linda C **(SLP)**

Duxbury
Domineau, Susanne Breen **(SLP)**
Jones, Janet P **(SLP)**
Kerr, Mrs Carol M **(SLP)**
Petrucelli, Lauren A **(SLP)**
Walkey, Mrs Joan E **(SLP)**
Zurif, Dr Francoise L **(SLP)**

East Boston
Perry, Cassandra Eve **(SLP)**
Stern, Evelyn Frances **(SLP)**

East Bridgewater
Rice-Fenstermaker, Mrs Claire **(SLP)**

East Dennis
Ellis, Suzanne **(SLP)**

East Freetown
Knight-McKenna, Mary T **(SLP)**

East Gloucester
Flynn, Linda F **(SLP)**

East Hampton
Albino, Susan G **(SLP)**

East Longmeadow
Bankoski, Susan Marie **(A)**
Berger, Cynthia D **(SLP)**
Entwistle, Mrs Nancy Vogenbergr **(SLP)**
Ferris, Mrs Holly E **(SLP)**
Harrison, Robert A **(SLP)**
Lekberg, Mrs Rebecca Stetson **(SLP)**
Parzivand, Harriet J **(SLP)**
Soforenko, Rhonda A **(SLP)**

East Taunton
Abel, Cullen D **(SLP)**
O'Brien, Mrs Mary Borsari **(SLP)**

East Walpole
Flaherty, Mrs Patricia E

East Weymouth
Clark, Patricia Marie **(SLP)**

Eastham
Gould, Mrs Rosario G **(A)**
Skoler, Mrs Charlotte **(A)**

Easthampton
Bernier-Gawle, Carol A **(SLP)**
Biladeau, Mrs Julie A **(SLP)**
Blackwood, Linda Carol **(SLP)**
Moreau, Mrs Maryellen Rooney **(SLP)**
Mortenson, Erin Kathleen **(SLP)**
Oleary, Mrs Joanne **(SLP)**

Easton
Augustyniak, Carol Ann **(SLP)**
Cribbs-Heenan, Lee Ann **(SLP)**
McGowan, Deborah Mirra **(SLP)**
Shepro, Wendy J **(SLP)**

Edgartown
Kelly, Susan White **(SLP)**

Everett
Anderson, Mrs Margaret Keating **(SLP)**
Puopolo, Edward C **(SLP)**
Spencer, Denise Bradshaw **(SLP)**
Wolff, Lauri Joy **(SLP)**

Fairhaven
Furtado, Stephen J **(SLP)**
Mello, Mrs Maureen Murphy **(SLP)**
Sciarappa, Jaryl Ann **(SLP)**

Warner, Dianne Elizabeth **(SLP)**

Fall River
Bigelow, Mrs Joanne Leduc **(SLP)**
Lucier, Penny J **(A)**

Falmouth
Caton, Nanette M
Erwin-Miller, Lisa N **(SLP)**
Florance, Kathleen **(SLP)**

Feeding Hills
Little, Noreen Hughes **(SLP)**

Fiskdale
Harrington, Mrs Kathleen H **(SLP)**

Fitchburg
Crawford, Suzanne F **(SLP)**
Dumas, Evelyn Sue **(A)**
Ehnstrom, Mrs Jane Anne **(A)**
Jakubosky, Mrs Ann Leblanc **(SLP)**

Florence
Carlson, Susan Mae **(SLP)**
Nadler, Amy **(SLP)**

Forestdale
Emery, Patricia A **(SLP)**
Warsing, Suzanne Miller **(SLP)**

Fort Devens
Owens, Gary W **(A)**

Foxboro
Capone, Mrs Lorraine Schulz **(SLP)**
Elliott, Charlene B **(SLP)**
Forgione, Mary-Anne **(SLP)**

Framingham
Apkon, Susan Debra **(SLP)**
Baskin, Roger B **(SLP)**
Beatch-Tilden, Susan C **(A)**
Boland, Sr M
Bromley, Maryellen
Conway, Mrs Rosemary Morse **(SLP)**
Cuneo, Margaret Elaine **(A)**
Feaver, Ann Tisdel **(SLP)**
Foley, Beth E **(SLP)**
Fournier, Denise Ann **(SLP)**
Fraher, Arlene L **(A)**
Gaither, Mrs Leslie L **(SLP)**
Hochstadt, Mrs Mindy S **(SLP)**
Kushinsky, Sharon L **(A)**
Lambert-Galtman, Mrs Pennie **(A)**
Miller, Sherri F **(SLP)**
Miller-Cook, Mrs Stephanie **(SLP)**
Pelc, Michael **(SLP A)**
Roditi, Mrs Denise Sher **(SLP)**
Safian, Marilyn **(SLP)**
Shapiro, Joyce A **(SLP)**
Steinkrauss, Mrs Barbara L **(SLP)**
Taylor, Mrs Deborah S **(SLP)**
Testa, Donna Lee **(A)**
Whitman, Jo-Ann C M **(A)**
Yarkin, Reesa G **(SLP)**

Franklin
Adams, Mrs Marla R **(SLP)**
Amoroso, Patricia **(SLP)**
Fitz-Patrick, Tijen Beker **(SLP)**
Vardsveen, Dorothy J **(A)**

Gardner
Heilman, Colette M **(SLP)**
Jordan, Mrs Terri Jolene **(SLP)**
Klash, Donna Marie **(SLP)**

Gilbertville
Gareau, Mrs Kim Marie **(SLP)**

Gloucester
Buchanan, Robert J **(A)**
Kane, Jane Lois
Lawless-Lane, Charlene Ann **(SLP)**
Phillips, Jean M **(SLP)**
Stevens, Anne Richardson **(SLP)**
Watson, Mrs Lea Donovan **(SLP)**

Grafton
El Khoury, Mrs Jo-Ellen Oleary **(SLP)**
Martin, Lynda M **(A)**

Granby
MacKenzie, Shirley R **(SLP)**

Great Barrington
Brewer, Ellen Jane **(SLP)**

Greenfield
Anderson, Laura O **(SLP)**
Bernier, Carla Ann **(SLP)**
Berson, Ellen M **(SLP)**
Hempel, Blanche V **(SLP)**
Hickey, William **(SLP)**
Morris, Norman W **(A)**

Groton
Siener, Mrs Mary Ellen **(SLP)**
Tebbetts, Ranier Barbara **(SLP)**
Vaillancourt, Mrs Nyola R **(SLP)**

Hadley
DiSalvo, Mrs Maureen Foster **(SLP)**
Taylor, Beth **(SLP)**
Thomas, Cheryl Ann **(SLP)**
Velleman, Dr Shelley Lynne **(SLP)**

Hamilton
Faust, Marlene A **(SLP)**

Hampden
Di Simoni, Rosemary **(SLP)**
Laflamme, Mrs Laurel L **(SLP)**

Hanover
Cunningham-Egan, Mrs Jacqueline **(SLP)**
Demakis, Marianne McDonald **(SLP)**
Doherty-Edlund, Barbara A **(SLP)**
Farrell, Marian E **(SLP)**
Pelissier, Mrs Paula Ann **(SLP)**
Somers, Louise Z **(SLP)**

Hanson
Spencer, Mrs Donna Kent **(A)**

Hardwick
Dykstra, Steven J **(SLP)**

Harvard
Brooks, Susan Katz **(SLP)**
Oliva, Deborah B **(SLP)**

Harwich
Sokoloff, Dr Martin A **(SLP)**

Hatfield
Mazurski, Phyllis A **(SLP)**

Haverhill
Gallivan, Kerin Mary **(A)**
Kern, Susan Wilson **(SLP)**
Silva, Susan C **(SLP)**

Haydenville
Eklof, Peter

Hingham
Broker, Carol A **(SLP)**
Dahill, Carol Ann **(SLP)**
Murphy, John F **(SLP)**
Perron, Gale L **(SLP)**
Rosseel, Lorraine **(SLP)**
Shea, Kathleen L **(A)**
Stenson, Mary Hartley **(SLP)**
Zane, Ellen Marcia **(SLP)**
Zuniga, Monica **(SLP)**

Holbrook
Donnelly, Regina C **(A)**
Jones, Elisa Saccardo **(SLP)**
Schwartz, Sandi **(SLP)**
Wright, Cheryl A **(SLP)**

Holden
Connolly, Mrs Loretta DeCrou **(SLP)**
Morocco, Katherine Creen **(SLP)**
Rezen, Dr Susan V **(A)**
Shapiro, Karen **(SLP)**
Skinner, Mrs Mary E **(SLP)**

Tessier, Mrs Amy B **(SLP A)**

Holliston
Ashe, Mrs Frances Marie **(SLP)**
Howe, Elizabeth Boehme **(SLP)**
Iversen, Thomas Richard
Sampson, Mrs Arlene F **(SLP A)**
Weisberg, Mrs Jennifer Dale **(SLP)**

Holyoke
Abdel-Wahab, Dr Aly Ezzat **(SLP)**
Conley, Lynne J
Devlin-De Lisle, Kathleen **(SLP)**
Ezzat, Mrs Esmat H **(SLP)**
Fradkin, David Lawrence **(A)**
Goren, Mrs Jenine G **(SLP)**
Howell, Marianne **(SLP)**
Judd, Mrs Diane F **(SLP)**
Lafontaine, Linda M **(SLP)**
Markt, Maureen F **(SLP)**
Tierney, Terry J **(SLP)**

Hopedale
Apicella, Mrs Susan Ellen **(SLP)**
Burberry, Jacqueline **(SLP)**
Miller, Mrs Cheryl Harding **(SLP)**

Hopkinton
Banik, Mrs Jan M **(SLP)**
Chenet, Patricia **(SLP)**
Fortin, Deborah A **(SLP)**
Jurado-Hilton, Antoinette **(SLP)**
McCowan, Leslie S **(A)**
Melvin, Mrs Julie Terese **(SLP)**

Hudson
Heerde, Sally M **(SLP)**
Role, Ellen B **(SLP)**

Hull
Cheney, Mrs Caron **(A)**
Vaillancourt, Patricia Marie **(A)**

Humarock
Riccardi, Linda M **(SLP)**

Huntington
Jordan, Richard O **(A)**

Hyannis
Bishop, Mrs Patricia Lee **(A)**
Bowser, Terri Louise **(SLP)**
Hayes, Mrs Elizabeth Connors **(SLP)**
Speirs, Louise Hope **(SLP)**

Hyde Park
Mason, Jane Marie **(SLP)**
McLaughlin, Barbara Ann **(SLP)**
Ruscito, Mary Ann **(SLP)**
Wilson, Vicki A **(A)**

Ipswich
Aurelio, Katherine Spiers **(SLP)**
Glennon, Kristine **(SLP)**
Larson-Schofield, Mrs September **(SLP)**
Whitten, Debra A **(SLP)**

Jamaica Plain
Borrero, Aixa **(SLP)**
Coderre, Maryann **(A)**
Courtney, Julia A **(SLP)**
Craig, Robin Lee **(A)**
Davis, Kathleen V **(SLP)**
McIntosh, Bonnie J **(SLP)**
Pierce, Mrs Thelma Hilton **(SLP)**
Price, Karen M **(SLP)**
Recchia, Jayne **(A)**
Robbins, Nancy V **(A)**
Sanderson, Robert G **(A)**
Sullivan, Mrs Martha M **(SLP)**
Walsh, Michael J **(SLP)**

Kingston
Gosselin, Mrs Lisa A **(SLP)**
Ingenito, Debra J

Lakeville
Spencer, Mrs Mary-Jo Ferreira **(SLP)**
Stewart, Carol C **(SLP)**

White, Cheryl A **(SLP)**

Lancaster
Weeks, Karen S **(SLP)**

Lawrence
Bateson, Mrs Cynthia Lee **(SLP)**
Broadbent, Josephine M **(SLP A)**
Hughes, Patricia M **(SLP)**
Karamourtopoulos, Donna Hollander **(SLP)**
Lynch, Kathleen E **(SLP)**
Skrabut, Diana H **(SLP)**
Wigall, Mrs Loleata D **(A)**

Ledminster
Jacques-Twichell, Mrs Kathy Ann

Lee
Bassen, Mrs Alice M **(A)**
Feinsod, Miriam G **(SLP)**

Leeds
Southwick, Renee E **(SLP)**

Leicester
Cooney, Cheryl Staruk **(SLP)**

Leominster
Caponi, Karen **(A)**
Donatelly, Mrs Maureen Crowley **(SLP)**
Fagan, Paula Louise **(A)**
Hume, Mrs Dayna Lisanne **(A)**
O'Connell-Goodfellow, Eileen Mary **(SLP)**
Reynolds, Patricia Ann **(A)**
Scarpino, Christiane Jane **(SLP)**
Schack-Hanson, Nancy **(SLP)**
Zimmerman, Jane S **(SLP)**

Leverett
Shinner, Deborah B **(A)**
Shinner, Glenn T **(A)**

Lexington
Black, Sandra M **(SLP)**
Di Russo, Mrs Irma B **(SLP)**
Ferrier, Linda J **(SLP)**
Frame, Mrs Suzanne Parizeau **(SLP)**
Frazer, Mrs Sylvia D **(SLP A)**
Goldstein, Phyllis R **(SLP)**
Haynes, Maria N **(SLP A)**
Johnson, Valerie J **(SLP)**
Kanter, Mrs Karen **(SLP)**
Leelman, Maryellen Alicia **(SLP)**
Liberman, Jane R B **(A)**
Luterman, David M **(A)**
O'Neil, Meghan Reardon **(SLP)**
Pace, Salvatore Anthony **(SLP)**
Pawliczek, Catherine **(SLP)**
Rubin-Haskell, Mrs Hinda P **(SLP)**
Rudy, Mrs Janice **(SLP)**
Strominger, Ann Z **(SLP)**
Van Eman, Janis B **(SLP)**

Littleton
Shenk, Amy L **(SLP)**

Longmeadow
Bailey, Dena A **(SLP)**
Beaulieu-Chalke, Mrs Norma J **(SLP)**
Breeding, Albert G **(A)**
Freedman, Mrs Sheryl Beth **(SLP)**
Gianelly, Mrs Cynthia C **(SLP)**
Kahan, Mrs Candace R **(SLP)**
Rothschild, Jane Lowenthal **(SLP)**
Rubin, Rona B **(SLP)**
Schneider, Megan Allen **(A)**
Seigel, Mrs Laurie B **(SLP)**
Stone, Mrs Hortense W **(SLP)**
Tomassetti, Carole W **(A)**
Weissman, Linda L **(SLP)**
Welch, Catherine **(SLP)**
Wener, Dr Deena Louise **(SLP)**

Lowell
Blake, Mrs Elaine B **(SLP)**
Boyd, Suzanne C **(SLP)**
Foote, Carolyn Elyse **(SLP)**
McCabe, Mrs Janice L **(SLP)**

Pershey, Monica Gordon **(SLP)**
Ross, Jo-Ann F **(SLP)**
Selger, Donna J **(A)**
Smith, Robinann S **(A)**
Tsandikos, George Michael **(SLP)**

Lunenburg
Brown, Suzanne Greening **(A)**
Hill, Diane Pagnotto **(SLP)**
McKenna, James C **(SLP)**
Stanley, Mrs Jane Tartre **(SLP)**
Storm, Mrs Pamela Adele **(SLP)**
Wilson, Allan J, III **(SLP)**

Lynn
Brown, Beth Ann **(SLP)**
Cutts, Elaine Valerie **(SLP)**
Myers, Laura J **(SLP)**
Wilson, Nancy **(SLP)**

Lynnfield
Barras, June M **(A)**
Bodek, Mrs Laurie J **(SLP)**
Dalton, Mrs Wilma K **(SLP)**

Malden
Cerullo, Mrs Jane K **(A)**
Chirichetti, Joann M **(SLP)**
Friedlander, Penney Helene **(SLP)**
Gosselin-Alfieri, Marcia **(SLP)**
Halpin, Dr Christopher Francis **(A)**
Klim, Dr Charles J **(SLP)**
Klim, Mrs Helen S **(SLP)**
Konnerth, Lynn A **(SLP)**
London, Louise A **(SLP)**
Mendes, Diane G **(SLP)**
San Martino, Mrs Alice Pauline **(SLP)**
Vega-Barachowitz, Carmen Dolores **(SLP)**
Wall, Jane C **(SLP)**
Weil-Lefkovith, Patricia **(A)**
Wood, Pamela Joyce **(SLP)**

Mansfield
Frank, Mrs Sharon D **(SLP)**
Gleason, Mrs Ellen C **(SLP)**
Mahan, Mrs Anne Marie **(SLP)**
Marks, Dr Maura G **(A)**
Martin, Mrs Rosalind Shope **(A)**
Sopko, Heidi G **(SLP)**

Marblehead
Arst, Linda B **(SLP)**
Becker, Mrs Marilyn H **(SLP)**
Goodwin, Diana J **(SLP)**
Gurman, Mrs Martha L **(SLP)**
Indresano, Susan L **(SLP)**
Isquith, Mrs Amy E **(SLP)**
Joseph, Janet M **(A)**
Main, Mary Ann **(SLP)**
Mazow, Mrs Maxine S **(SLP)**
Ogan, Susan S **(A)**
Parks, Linda Anne **(SLP)**
Rothbard, Mrs Elise L **(A)**
Rubin, Mrs Maxine S **(SLP A)**
Schrenko, Mrs Joanna C **(SLP)**
Whitlock, Maureen Maslowski **(SLP)**
Zimmer, Wendy A **(SLP)**

Marborough
Moffa, Carol Ludwig **(SLP)**

Marina Bay
Rivkind, Sheryl W **(A)**

Marlboro
Eisenhardt, Christine Marie **(SLP)**
Manning, Carol Ann **(A)**
Mastrogiacomo, Sharon Jean **(SLP)**
Sullivan, Wendy R **(SLP)**

Marshfield
Anderson, Joanne C **(A)**
Briggs, Dr Sandra Lee **(A)**
Brigham, Ellen Taer **(SLP)**
Corcoran, Mrs Maureen Patricia
Delisa, Mrs Sally T **(SLP)**
Maley, Susan P H **(SLP)**

Moore, Susan Beth **(SLP)**
Sampson-Lester, Alice M **(SLP)**

Marshfield Hills
Stewart, Gail P **(SLP)**

Mattapan
Leonard, Muriel J **(SLP)**

Mattapoisett
Campbell, Mrs Louise M **(SLP)**
Kattermann, Debora Ann **(SLP)**
Sager, Mrs Lois Gibbons **(SLP)**

Maynard
Bryant, Leslie A **(SLP)**
Dailey, Ann Madsen **(SLP)**
Waters, Patricia A **(SLP)**

Medfield
Mawhiney, Allan L **(SLP)**
McGillicuddy, Marjorie **(SLP)**
Nilson, Mrs Holly M **(SLP)**
Violick-Boole, Kathryn **(SLP)**

Medford
Ambrosi, Denise Maria **(SLP)**
Bartlett, Cynthia L **(SLP)**
Bennett, Mrs Jana C **(SLP)**
Champagne, Mrs Virginia Greeley **(SLP)**
Goldstein, Diann **(SLP)**
Gully, Ladonna Lea **(SLP)**
Howard, Joanne Catherine **(A)**
McFarland, Mrs Ann D **(SLP)**
Mizerak, Deborah Jean **(SLP)**
Mullen, Mrs Charlotte Houck **(A)**
O'Connell-Hanifan, Anne M **(SLP)**
Sieling, Mary Margaret **(SLP)**
Stromeyer, Katharina M
Tanklefsky, Mrs Gay Sherman **(SLP)**
Tardelli, Maureen M **(SLP)**
Uchmanowicz, Mary Kay **(A)**
Vasta, Nicoletta M **(SLP)**
Wolfson, Wendy Ruth **(SLP)**

Medway
Albertelli, Mrs Aprile Antosh **(SLP)**
Fleischer-Hill, Lisa Ann **(SLP)**
Komros-Hachenburg, Mrs Gail **(SLP)**
Myers, Kathleen Kub **(SLP)**
Rosoff, Nancy E **(A)**

Melrose
Aurelia, Joseph C **(SLP)**
Bagarella, Diane R **(SLP)**
Digrande, Adriana Jole **(SLP)**
Doyle, Kathleen Marie **(SLP)**
Henken, Bernard S **(SLP)**
Herrington, Mrs Patricia L **(SLP)**
Lyon, Katherine **(SLP)**
Merrill, Judith L **(SLP)**
Porter, Susan Swigart **(SLP)**
Primiano, Christine R **(SLP)**
Schweihs, Mrs Karen Mascolo **(SLP)**

Mendon
Costello, Jacalyn Rose **(SLP)**

Merrimac
Cosgrove, Yvonne Beth **(SLP)**

Methuen
Milewski, Diane Marie **(SLP)**

Middleboro
Baillargeon, Jocelyne G
Hartford, Renee S **(SLP)**
Kuhns, Evelyn Mae **(SLP)**
Zingg, Mrs Kathleen Hanrahan **(SLP)**

Middleton
Wladkowski, Mrs Elizabeth **(SLP)**

Milford
Bradley, Nancy Wilson **(SLP)**
Compagnone, Angela R **(SLP)**
Costigan, Sharon L
D'Agostino, Mrs Ann M **(SLP)**
Luchini, Ann **(A)**

Otlin, Mrs Jo-Ann F **(SLP)**
Pool, Grace Gismondi **(SLP)**
Redden, Mrs Joan R **(SLP)**
Redden, Dr Robert B **(A)**

Millbury
Pease, Mrs Leane E **(SLP)**

Millis
Micucci, Betsy C **(SLP)**

Milton
Barron, Cynthia Patricia **(SLP)**
Dunne, Lee Anne **(SLP)**
Feldmann, Mrs Madeline
Gagne, Adele Y **(SLP)**
Mahoney, Ruth Elizabeth **(SLP)**

Minot
MacKin, Mrs Anita Marion **(SLP)**

Monson
Ekstrom, Barbara I **(A)**
Matrow, Mrs Elizabeth **(SLP)**
Woodbury, Keith **(SLP)**

Montague
Keighley, Patricia **(SLP)**

Monument Beach
Kingman, Mrs Wendy S **(SLP)**
McMorrow, Mrs Dorothy Murray **(SLP)**

Nagog Woods
Morrison, Mrs Priscilla **(SLP)**

Nahant
Johnson-Liscio, Christine **(SLP)**

Natick
Chesnick, Dr Marie A **(SLP)**
Dziwulski, Mrs Margery Slosek **(SLP)**
Gerstman, Dr Hubert L **(SLP A)**
Gilmore, Robert Alan **(A)**
Harding, Katherine M **(A)**
Horowitz, Susan Goodman **(SLP)**
Hoyt, Margaret **(SLP)**
Owaroff, Carol R **(SLP)**
Ralen, Mrs Sally Rigelhaupt **(SLP)**
Seeto, Debra Ann **(SLP)**
Zagajeski, Ellen Louise **(A)**

Needham
Barresi, Barbara A **(SLP)**
Barry, Dorothy A **(SLP)**
Burt, Mrs Susan M **(SLP)**
Caplan, Frances A **(SLP)**
Dunsky, Mrs Patricia Lee **(SLP)**
Friedman, Dr Frances A **(A)**
Gershman, Mrs Linda P **(SLP)**
Hershberg, Karen Fran **(SLP)**
Kaufman-Mamon, Mrs Lauren Jan **(SLP)**
Kranefuss, Mrs Ellen Norton **(SLP)**
Landay, Sheila D H **(SLP)**
Maibor, Debra K **(SLP)**
Marcus, Sharon Lee **(SLP)**
Marshak, Mrs Elizabeth **(SLP)**
Needleman, Harriet L **(SLP)**
O'Hara, Jane M **(SLP)**
Podolsky, Vivian W **(SLP)**
Rabinovitz, Mrs Jane Ena **(SLP)**
Schneller, Mrs Wendy D **(SLP)**
Seiler, Roberta S **(SLP)**
Shapiro, Mrs Carole L **(SLP)**
Shubow, Gerri Feuer **(A)**
Smock, Mrs Nancy E **(SLP)**
Vito, Mrs Lia Uustal **(SLP)**
Zaval, Janet K **(SLP)**

Needham Heights
Haward, Cynthia P **(SLP)**
Roberts, Keyenna **(SLP)**

New Bedford
Barber, Sylvia E V **(SLP)**
Bejtlich, Mrs Janet Lynne **(SLP)**
Bernier, Mrs Cheryl E **(SLP)**
Ferreira, Beatriz M **(SLP)**
Jacobvitz, Lynda O **(SLP)**
Mahon, Mrs Florence L **(SLP)**
McCann, James Edward, Jr **(A)**
Nunez, Lilliam
Roussos, Catherine Athena
Ventura, Lisa Marie **(SLP)**
Wirzburger, Mrs Donna Ramos **(SLP)**

New Salem
Brown, Wendi Dempsey **(SLP)**

Newbury
Cooper, Debra Huther **(SLP)**
Petersen, Mary Lou **(SLP)**
Stavolone, Patricia A **(SLP)**

Newburyport
Anderson, Dierdre M **(A)**
Bagni, Martha J **(SLP)**
Thrope, Susan Dee **(SLP)**

Newton
Bedard, Janet Linda **(SLP)**
Ben-Azay, Marcie Lyn **(SLP)**
Berkowitz, Mrs Mozelle **(SLP)**
Chaiet, Lori **(SLP)**
Cook, Harriet Sacks **(SLP)**
Daniels-Miller, Dr Lenore **(SLP)**
Godine, Frances S **(SLP)**
Goldberg, Faye R **(SLP)**
Hattis, Mrs Beverly K **(SLP)**
Kelley, Kara Beth
Knapp, Cynthia **(SLP)**
Levin-Charns, Dr Judy **(SLP)**
Levy-Millen, Mrs Meta J **(SLP)**
Liebergott, Dr Jacqueline **(SLP)**
Loewenthal, Terri **(A)**
MacLean, Christina Marie **(SLP)**
Mittman, Mrs Ellen K **(SLP)**
Mosehauer, Anne Lally **(SLP)**
Oppenheimer, Barbara B **(SLP)**
Patton, Jennifer Sallman **(SLP)**
Richards, Roberta D **(SLP)**
Rosenfeld, Mrs Rene Gail **(SLP)**
Salzbank-Barron, Mrs Shelley **(SLP)**
Scheps, Amy Heller **(SLP)**
Semel, Dr Eleanor
Shulak, Cynthia B **(SLP)**
Sigel, Mrs Meryl L **(SLP)**
Thau, Sandra Cohn **(SLP)**
Walker, Mary Elizabeth **(SLP)**
Zaremba, Mrs Natalie B **(SLP)**

Newton Center
Becker Caplan, Laura **(SLP)**
Binus, Gale Z **(SLP)**
Brown, Mrs Betsy Shulkin **(SLP)**
Citron, Louise G **(A)**
Greenberg, Bonnie B **(SLP)**
Greenstein, Mrs Vicki **(A)**
Isserow, Mrs Rachelle Rosenberg **(SLP)**
Krupat, Barbara R **(SLP)**
Lopacki, Sandra R **(SLP)**
Marrinan, Eileen **(SLP)**
Masters, Eileen T **(SLP)**
Pollock, Mrs Marion C **(SLP)**
Ross, Suzanne L **(SLP)**
Weinberg, Marion J **(SLP)**
Wieczner, Loretta Levin **(SLP)**

Newton Corner
Rich, Mrs Lori A **(SLP)**
Rosenthal, Marjorie Hodes **(SLP)**

Newton Highlands
Finn, Dr Myrna W **(SLP)**
Seletsky, Mrs Marcia Gail **(SLP)**
Shugarts, Dawn Denise **(SLP)**

Newton Lower Falls
Granfield, Gretchen Lynn **(SLP)**
Mele, Maryteresa Colette **(SLP)**
Paver, Stacey Ann **(SLP)**

Newton Upper Falls
Michelow, Diane **(SLP)**
Shikiar, Karen A **(SLP)**

Newtonville
Brown, Jane A **(SLP)**
Cohen, Beth D **(SLP)**
Gross, Paula Herman **(SLP)**
Heiman, Sharon K **(SLP)**
Superior, Karen M **(SLP)**

Norfolk
Byrne, Mrs Debra D **(SLP)**
Waldman, Deborah Scannell **(A)**

North Abington
Geronimo, Mrs Kathy Murphy **(SLP)**
Katz, Susan L **(SLP)**

North Adams
Murray, Sandra R **(SLP)**

North Amherst
Wyatt, Toya A **(SLP)**

North Andover
Carlson, Mrs Mary Ginder **(SLP)**
Chambers, Constance **(SLP)**
Curran, Mrs Joan Donovan **(SLP)**
Dignam, Francis X **(SLP)**
George, Eleanor M **(SLP)**
Gray, Patricia A **(SLP)**
Gress, Carla Delassus **(SLP)**
Kunin-Phillips, Cathy **(SLP)**
Sadowski, Teresa Buckley **(SLP)**
Tarbox, Mrs Gail Manin **(A)**

North Attleboro
Austin, Paul W **(SLP A)**
Bailey, Kristi Anne **(SLP)**
Buchanan, Judith Sutherland **(SLP)**
Coblentz, Hope M **(SLP)**
Daugherty, Marybeth **(SLP)**
Kurtzer, Ellen A **(A)**
Manoogian, Mrs Judy L **(SLP)**

North Avington
Dodaro, Dr Robert Raymond **(SLP)**

North Billerica
Pusey, Mrs Kim Karla

North Chatham
Maxon, Carleen O **(SLP)**

North Chelmsford
Baker, Mrs Karen M **(SLP)**
Bezdeny, Barbara Drake **(SLP)**

North Dartmouth
Bihldorff, Mary F **(A)**
Raymon, Mrs Ruth R **(SLP)**
Sarmento, Nidia B **(SLP)**

North Easton
Denham, Patricia Gail **(SLP)**
McIntyre, Donna Kudzy **(SLP)**
Odabashian, Eileen **(SLP)**
Paul, Donald W **(A)**
Reams, Virginia F **(SLP)**

North Falmouth
Arectos, Linda A **(A)**
Ball, Susan R **(SLP)**

North Grafton
Casassa, Arlene J **(SLP)**

North Hampton
Murray, Carol A **(SLP)**

North Oxford
Dutra, Maria D F **(SLP)**
Goodwin, Jane Boutiette **(SLP)**
Williamson, Kathleen Teresa **(SLP)**

North Quincy
Knudson, Cherylanne **(SLP)**
Kobrin, Mrs Marjorie S **(A)**
Maloney, Anita Louise **(SLP)**

North Reading
Feeney-Grater, Pearl **(SLP)**

North Weymouth
Gaughan, Maureen E **(SLP)**
Hey, Mary L **(SLP)**

Northampton
Altman, Holly M **(A)**
Becker, Kathleen Marie **(SLP)**
Bickford, David L **(SLP)**
Bittel, Dr Peter J **(SLP)**
Duryee, Mrs Virginia **(SLP)**
Korza, Laurie Jane **(SLP)**
Meisner, John R **(A)**
Munson, Mrs Joy E **(SLP)**
Musante, Elizabeth Ann **(SLP)**
Shea, B David **(A)**
Singer, Janice L **(SLP)**
Snoek, Mrs Barbara B **(SLP)**
Yao, Mrs Chie Cheng **(SLP)**

Northboro
Coseo, Jane Melanie **(SLP)**
Dawe, Mary J **(SLP)**
Harris, Maureen A **(SLP)**
Simon, Joanne Miller **(SLP)**

Northbridge
Emond, Judith A **(SLP)**
King, Penney Reissis **(SLP)**
Kissell-Ariel, Veronica C **(SLP)**
Sweeney, Mrs Anne Marie **(SLP)**

Northfield
Reid, Mrs Dorothy F **(SLP)**

Norton
Daly, Mrs Barbara Balboni **(A)**
Friedman-Hanna, Karen Lynn **(SLP)**
Niedringhaus, Richard **(SLP)**
Price, Mrs Susan M **(SLP)**
Schmidt, Janet C **(SLP)**

Norwell
Conover, Elizabeth **(SLP A)**
Kearsley, Nancy Conlin **(SLP)**
O'Grady, Kathleen A **(SLP)**

Norwood
Brown, Donna Glaser **(SLP)**
Concannon, Julia Ann **(SLP)**
Douglass, Mrs Rebecca Floyd **(SLP)**
King, Danielle Coppes **(SLP)**
Krah, Mrs Kerrie Mc Manus **(SLP)**
Levine, Mrs Beth Shapiro **(A)**
Manchester, Ellen Morris **(SLP)**
O'Neil, Ellen Mary **(A)**
Rose-Jones, Kathleen A **(SLP)**
Russell, Dawn **(SLP)**
Shuster, Carol A **(SLP)**

Oxford
Bradford, Susan C **(SLP)**
Craig, Roberta May **(SLP)**
Harvey, Mrs Barbara C **(SLP)**
Harvey, Paul M **(A)**
Helpa, David P **(SLP A)**
Miller-Zuidema, Mrs Valerie Jean
Nystrom, Mrs Rita Visceto **(SLP)**

Palmer
Banigan, Dr Rae Loraine **(SLP)**
Williams, Clare W **(A)**

Paxton
Boria, Carolyn A **(SLP)**
Power, Dr Maryann H **(SLP)**

Peabody
Dancewicz, Susan Pulli **(SLP)**
Feinstein, Linda S
Freshman, Mrs Roberta Connolly **(SLP)**
Lapointe, Constance **(SLP)**
Makie, Patricia A **(SLP)**
Martin, Mrs Kathleen Sheehan **(SLP)**
McCready, Lynn R **(SLP)**
Nathanson, Mrs Karen L **(SLP)**
Quinlan, Karen Marie **(SLP)**
Rothman-Hazard, Mrs Loree Gay **(SLP)**

Sacco-Andree, Maryann **(SLP)**

Pelham
McClung, Emily Weiss **(SLP)**
Mis-Palley, Cindy **(SLP)**
Osbahr, Tracy C **(SLP)**
Servos, Mrs M Virginia **(SLP)**

Pembroke
Olsen, Pamela M **(SLP)**
Oppenheimer-Eidlin, Marsha **(SLP)**

Pepperell
Ryden, Mrs Karen Lawson **(SLP)**

Pittsfield
Brisimitzakis, Mrs Joan G **(SLP)**
Desnoyers, Anne M
Digaudio, Mrs Anna B **(SLP)**
Fritz, Mrs Wendy Anne **(SLP)**
Laragione, Mrs Evelyn Keeler **(SLP)**
Noonan, Mary Katherine **(SLP)**
O'Bert, Pamela A **(A)**
Porreca-Mansilla, Mrs Patricia L **(SLP)**
Vanhoenacker, Christine **(SLP)**
Wasserman, Mrs Barbara K **(SLP)**
Whalley, Michelle V **(SLP)**

Plainville
Hummel, Lauren J **(SLP)**

Plymouth
Borgia, Roberta L **(SLP)**
Candito, Carol Landers **(SLP)**
Cody, Mary M **(A)**
Draper-Parker, Linda Kaye **(SLP)**
McSharry, Edward J **(SLP)**
McSharry, Mrs Margaret Tassinari **(SLP)**
Mercure, Roland **(SLP)**
Taylor, Ann L **(SLP)**

Plympton
Hagan, Rebecca Wilcox **(SLP)**
Hansen, Dr Barin L **(SLP)**

Princeton
Green, Katie W **(SLP)**
Krouse, Maureen Casey **(SLP)**
Skrzypczak, Mrs Ann M **(SLP)**

Quincy
Alden, Carol L **(SLP)**
Briganti, Lisa Marie
Buffington, Kimberly Marie **(SLP)**
Clifford, Clare **(SLP)**
Conte, Beverly M **(SLP)**
Garabedian, Charlene B **(SLP)**
Lochner, Mrs Nancy Kaufman **(SLP)**
O'Hara, Nancy Lee **(A)**
O'Sullivan, Mary E **(SLP)**
Pitti, Mary John
Ridge, Ellen M **(SLP)**
Trainor, Mary T **(A)**
Wolfson, Mrs Amy S **(SLP)**

Randolph
Abdelahad, Linda L **(SLP)**
Fellman, Mrs Fern D **(SLP)**
Grolnic, Stephen S **(A)**
Hershfield, Kathy Seigel **(SLP)**
Lapon, Mrs Donna M **(SLP)**
McDonald, Sr Margaret M **(A)**
Parisi, Mrs Sharon A **(SLP)**
Rogers, Mrs Anastasia Maria **(SLP)**
Steinberg, Caren L **(SLP)**
Sullivan, Sr Declan **(A)**
Winneg, Beth C **(SLP)**

Raynham
Larkin, Elizabeth Anne **(A)**
Smith, Constance Cheryl **(SLP)**

Reading
Berndtson, Deborah L **(A)**
Briggs-Whittaker, Janice **(SLP)**
Cuthbertson, David Alan **(A)**
Donahue, Patrice Ann **(SLP)**
Dowling, Mrs Michelle Micciche **(SLP)**
Escher, Jane Murray **(SLP)**
Fitzpatrick, Patricia M **(SLP)**
Griffin, Pamela T
Grizzell, Mrs Barbara Schwinger **(SLP)**
Logsdon, Mrs Celia W **(A)**
Mayberry, Jill Marian **(SLP)**
Miles, Elizabeth **(SLP)**
Nemergut, Joy C **(SLP)**
Salter, Lorraine Zaisser **(SLP)**
Tuck, Tara J **(SLP)**
Ward, Mrs Louise W **(SLP)**
Wood, Drucilla **(SLP)**
Zaido, Patricia Hourihan **(SLP)**

Readville
Spears, Mrs Ann I **(SLP)**

Rehoboth
Hass, Mrs Rita L **(SLP)**

Revere
Brent, Susan A **(SLP)**
Federico, Rita Phyllis **(SLP)**
Hunt, John Robert
Menard, Mrs Karen Lynne **(SLP)**
Simmons, Judi I **(SLP)**
Weesner, David Russell **(A)**

Richmond
Hildreth, Mrs Katherine Morton **(SLP)**

Rochdale
Cashman, Debra A **(SLP)**

Rockland
LoSciuto, Mrs Ruth Ann **(SLP)**
Walker, Patricia A Tkaczuk **(SLP)**

Rockport
Chambers, C Lynn **(SLP)**
Dwinell, Mrs Maureen M **(SLP)**
Kaplan, Barbara F **(SLP)**
Wedmore, Mrs Suellen **(SLP)**

Roslindale
Atkins, Alice E **(SLP)**
Borg, Nancy E **(SLP)**
Finneran, Mary F **(SLP)**
Kent, Debora D **(SLP)**
Scheer, Paula **(SLP)**

Rowley
Bernier, Mrs Judith C **(SLP)**
Johnson, Alison A **(SLP)**
St Peter, Katherine A **(SLP)**

Salem
Aiello, Arlene R **(SLP)**
Breslouf, Lynne Diane **(SLP)**
Cudworth, Hilary F **(SLP)**
Dolan, Patricia Susan **(SLP)**
Felt, Suzanne R **(SLP)**
Grabowski, Kathleen S **(SLP)**
Harrison, Beverly J Hagen **(SLP)**
Hutchinson, Cynthia Baur **(SLP)**
Kemper, Dr Robert L **(SLP)**
Louisos-Kramer, Elaina **(SLP)**
Luongo, Patricia Marie **(SLP)**
Nalipinski, Mrs Paige McLarnon **(SLP)**
Papanicolaou, Irene **(SLP)**
Pincus-Clatterbuck, Laurie **(SLP)**
Sullivan, Jean L **(SLP)**
Tarushka, Mrs Linda L **(SLP)**
Wiegand, Mrs Judith F **(SLP)**

Salisbury
Juntunen, Janet K **(SLP)**

Sandwich
Mantenfel, Ellen McDonald **(SLP)**
Yauch, Lisa Diane **(SLP)**

Saugus
Gosselin, Patricia M **(A)**
Queen, Sheila M **(A)**

Scituate
Berry, Maureen M **(SLP)**
Flynn, Janis E **(SLP)**
Lavin-Arcand, Maureen **(SLP)**
Manning, Mrs Colleen M **(SLP)**
Norod, Mrs Carol N **(A)**
Tringale, Mrs Kathlene M **(SLP)**

Seekonk
Berson, Esther **(SLP)**
Caron, Mrs Debra Lynne **(SLP)**
Delude, Mrs Nancy L **(SLP)**
Rennick, Patricia Ann **(SLP)**
Townsend, Ann E D **(SLP)**

Sharon
Berman, Leslie W **(SLP)**
Bunting, Glenn W **(SLP)**
Clougherty, Mrs Melinda E **(SLP)**
Cochrane, Dr Rosalind McCrae **(SLP)**
Faye, Mrs Ruth A **(SLP)**
Fistel, Mrs Amy Rena **(A)**
Francer, Mrs Holly Jean **(SLP)**
Gale, Carrie G **(SLP)**
Granoff, Mrs Rosaline I **(SLP)**
Klecak, Lucinda B **(SLP)**
Koppel, Mrs Tina R **(SLP)**
Miller, Mrs Nancy J **(A)**
Milner, Dr Paul **(A)**
Schill, Dr Herman Allan **(A)**
Schweber, Mrs Susan Baer **(SLP)**
Seidman, Mrs Arleen B **(SLP)**
Semel, Donna R **(SLP)**
Wickersham, Mrs Jill Horrow **(SLP)**
Winer, Charlene Ava **(SLP)**

Shelburne Falls
Rice, Sally J

Sherborn
Goldsmith, Dr Sharon C **(SLP)**
Pitts, Dr Willis N, Jr **(SLP)**
Savery, Janice S **(SLP)**

Shrewsbury
Duffy, Denise M **(SLP)**
Feehily, Lynne Marie **(SLP)**
Finnerty, Joan S **(A)**
Flynn, Teresa F **(A)**
Friedman, Deborah Ann **(SLP)**
Gay, Susan Marie **(SLP)**
McCarthy, Mary Melissa **(SLP)**
McCormack, Susan M **(SLP)**
Struthers, Polly J **(SLP)**

Siasconset
Newman, Mrs Jody Vanderdonc **(SLP)**

Somerset
Bailey, Mrs Madeleine Marie L **(SLP)**
Denison, Peter B **(SLP)**
Sigal, Mrs Paula Ellen B **(SLP)**
Wood, Timothy John **(SLP)**

Somerville
Arzt, Aliza C P **(SLP)**
Balinskas, Carolyn
Bardsley, Ellen M **(SLP)**
Bluestone, Ruth **(SLP)**
Buianowski, Eileen M **(SLP)**
Casscles, Sheri
DiBenedetto, Donna J **(SLP)**
Flaherty, Robin Eileen **(SLP)**
Gyory, Mrs Sabina M **(SLP)**
Jumonville, Lynn Chisholm
Keenan, Mary Colleen
Livesay, Luanne L **(SLP)**
Moran, Marion C **(A)**
Rousse, Valerie M **(SLP)**
Trudelle, Terie M **(SLP)**
Wallace, Laurie Link **(SLP)**

South Ashburnham
Paquette, Mrs Sharon Ann Murray **(SLP)**

South Attleboro
Lyon, Deborah Lee **(A)**

South Boston
Kinas, Christophe N **(SLP)**

South Deerfield
Oeky, Deborah F **(SLP)**
Pfannebecker, Annette Eleanor **(SLP)**

South Easton
Abramson, Mrs Arlene F **(A)**
Buffman, Mrs Julie Kay **(SLP)**
Kone, Chris Jay **(SLP)**
Miller, Wayne D **(SLP A)**

South Hadley
Beauregard, Cynthia **(A)**
Bernier, Karen Marie **(SLP)**
Favro, Mary Alice **(SLP)**
Harris, Ann Sullivan **(SLP)**
Kershlis, Kimberley Ingrid
Landry, David D **(SLP)**
Paquin, Denise A **(SLP)**
Sierra, Mrs Lynne Marie **(SLP)**

South Hamilton
Hillman, Carol E **(SLP)**
Hillman, Dr Robert E **(SLP)**

South Hampton
Mathias, Mrs Daisy E **(SLP)**
McGrath, Mrs Maryann Cooney **(SLP)**

South Lancaster
Clark, Barbara J **(A)**

South Lawrence
Kowalkowski, Katharine **(SLP)**

South Natick
Rutberg, Barbara L **(SLP)**

South Weymouth
Chamberlain, Cheryl E **(SLP)**
Citron, Dr David, III **(A)**
Curran, Dr Michael F **(SLP)**
Grass, Catherine **(SLP)**
Kopp, Irene Rudzinski **(SLP)**
Moyer, Donna J **(A)**
Spinale, Marilyn R **(A)**
Trocki, Edith M **(SLP)**

Southborough
Berkowitz, Susan **(SLP)**
Goldberg, Robin **(SLP)**
Luloff, Arlyne K **(SLP)**
Snyder, Mrs Sue P **(A)**

Southbridge
Casaubon, Kathleen Katka **(SLP)**
Duke, Carla
Tolson, Maureen Bowes **(SLP)**

Southwick
Germaine, Lesley J **(SLP)**

Spencer
Amprimo-Beer, Mrs Arlene Mary **(SLP)**

Springfield
Conway, Mary Patricia **(SLP)**
Downie, Susan M **(SLP)**
Dudley, Mary Dipalma
Fidrych-Puzzo, Mrs Holly **(SLP)**
Gardner, Mrs Edna Gadsden **(SLP)**
Hebert, Edward C **(SLP)**
High, Jacklyn Joyce **(SLP)**
Karmelek, Eugene Joseph **(SLP)**
Mansolillo, Angela **(SLP)**
Monson, Mrs Susan K **(SLP)**
Murphy, Mrs Patricia Mary Paolino **(SLP)**
Pruyne, Karen Ziemba **(SLP)**
Pupulidy, Susan Ann **(SLP)**
Rhicard, Ellen **(SLP)**
Scofield, Michelle Renee **(A)**
Stagnitti, Charles D **(SLP)**
Stahelek, Mrs Linda M **(A)**
Stanton, Lisa Ann **(SLP)**
Sweeney, Marion K **(SLP)**
Yeats, Susan Elizabeth **(SLP)**

Sterling
Carlin, Kathleen C **(SLP)**

Sterling Junction
Percia, Valerie C **(SLP)**

Still River
Sanford, Catherine Izzi **(SLP)**

Stoneham
Bond, Christine M **(A)**
Cullen, Mrs Gail F **(SLP)**
Hill, Mrs Marcia Claudette **(SLP)**
Leahy, Mrs Deborah **(SLP)**
Sarmanian, Mrs Donna S **(SLP)**
Shiebler, Karen Merullo **(SLP)**
Sullivan, Mary Jane **(A)**
Wilde, Lorin F **(A)**
Woller-Mummolo, Lauren **(SLP)**

Stoughton
Becker-Olans, Mrs Jacquie Michelle **(SLP)**
Clark, Mark Charles **(SLP)**
Goldman, Mrs Mary Ann **(SLP)**
Raymond, Sandra L **(SLP)**
Rosenfield, Helaine W **(SLP)**
Siref, Judith E **(SLP)**
Smith, Mrs Linda Ellen **(A)**
Stickler, Nancy Sima **(A)**
Telian, Mrs Nancy Alemian **(SLP)**
Weisman, Audrey T **(SLP)**

Stow
Genereux, Jeanne C **(SLP)**
Lindner, Dr Laurie Gilden **(SLP)**
Yoneshige, Yvonne S **(A)**

Sturbridge
Clifford, Maureen Louise **(SLP)**
Destefano, Lori McNamara **(SLP)**
Grunthalt, Laura Lynn
Raskin-Holmes, Mrs Wendy Fae **(SLP)**
Reynolds, Marilyn Ostrowski **(A)**

Sudbury
Berkowitz, Mrs Laurie S **(SLP)**
Donahue, Ellen **(SLP)**
Feudo, Dr Peter, Jr **(SLP A)**
Rand, Marilyn A **(SLP)**
Wiegel, Valerie Frangos **(SLP)**

Sunderland
McQuade, MaryAlice **(SLP)**

Swampscott
Greenstein, Arlene T **(SLP)**
Mauceri, Patricia Murphy **(A)**
Moynihan, Judith B **(SLP)**
Mulroy, Mrs Esther D **(SLP)**
Nellhaus, Susan L **(SLP)**
Pressman, Mrs Karla S **(SLP)**
Schauben-Fuerst, Renna S **(SLP)**
Winer, Dr Marc E **(SLP)**

Swansea
Biancuzzo, Mrs Marjorie Beth **(SLP)**
Smith, Linda Hicks **(SLP)**

Taunton
Cains, Lynne G **(SLP)**
Cookerly, Karen Marie **(SLP)**
Henderson, Jennifer **(SLP)**
McLaughlin, Patricia **(SLP)**
Mukherjee, Constance S **(SLP)**
Sowle, Elizabeth Margaret **(SLP)**
Stumpf, Sandra E **(A)**
Trucchi, Sharon A

Tewksbury
Aglieco-McDonald, Mrs Susan M **(A)**
Green, Patti Lubowitz
Mango, Frances **(SLP)**
McDonough, Paula Sharkey **(SLP)**
Mitchell, Mrs Jane O'Connor **(SLP)**

Topsfield
Draper-Small, Lisa Monique **(SLP)**
Goldstein, Mrs Anne L **(SLP)**
Lunn, Mrs Joan Morgan **(SLP)**
McMullin, Mrs Carolyn R **(SLP)**

Turners Falls
Gore, Linda G **(SLP)**

Tyngsboro
Piscitelli, Mrs Maureen A M **(SLP)**

Upton
House, Cynthia Schultz **(SLP)**
Secrest, Molly **(SLP)**

Uxbridge
Hamelin, Mrs Paula Turpack **(SLP)**
Livingston, Laura A **(SLP)**

Waban
Arnold, Ruth Levine **(SLP)**
Eller-Miller, Eileen Faythe **(SLP)**
Henderson, Terry L **(SLP)**
Horowitz, Eva B **(SLP)**
Polishook, Mrs Robin Paige **(SLP)**
Savitsky, Mrs Sheila Krute **(SLP)**
Teuber, Ann M **(SLP)**
Wolf, Mrs Barbara **(A)**

Wakefield
Green, Robin W **(SLP)**

Walpole
Hanifin, Cynthia Quackenbus **(A)**
Herrmann, Dr Barbara Sprague **(A)**
Matthews, Mrs Bonnie G **(SLP)**

Waltham
Andre, Vicki Linn **(SLP)**
Archambault, Gayle M **(SLP)**
Bennett, Debra G **(SLP)**
Brown, Mrs Robyn A **(SLP)**
Buchanan, Dr Leo H **(A)**
Carlson, Charlotte E **(SLP)**
Casper, Mary Ellen **(A)**
Foster, Joan E **(SLP)**
Gaynor, Mary **(SLP)**
Gordon, Pamela J **(A)**
Leiboff, Francine R **(SLP)**
Mangipudi, Latha D **(A)**
Morgenstern, Doris A **(SLP)**
Morse, Elizabeth Desomery **(SLP)**
Peterson, Linda Ann **(SLP)**
Petrucci, Mary E **(SLP)**
Richards, Mrs Patricia Hartigan **(SLP)**
Ross, Michele Ilene **(SLP)**
Russo, Jo-Ann B **(SLP)**
Searle, Linda Lee

Waquoit
Lajoie, Claudette S **(SLP)**

Ware
Dunham, Judy-Ann Parker **(SLP A)**
Glime, Kathernie C **(SLP)**
Healey, Daniel K **(A)**

Wareham
Morrison, Sally **(SLP)**
Pizzolato, Gene W **(SLP)**

Warren
Flanagan, Linda N **(SLP)**

Watertown
Adams, Linda **(SLP)**
Bowz, Renee D **(SLP)**
Breazeale, Theresa Faye
Carlevale, Jean Karen **(SLP)**
Clifford, Mrs Martha Susan **(SLP)**
Crowder, Elaine Mayhall **(SLP)**
Daly, Eleanor Mary **(SLP)**
Di Luzio, Angela Maria **(SLP)**
Forst, Ellen G **(SLP)**
Fuess, Cynthia Jane **(SLP)**
Gramigna, Gary David **(SLP)**
Grieco, Jayne Fagan **(SLP)**
Irving, Susan Elizabeth **(SLP)**
Johnson, Lisa Ann **(SLP)**
Katz, Lisa Beth **(A)**
Kennedy, Grace M **(SLP)**
Kravitz, Ellen M **(SLP)**
MacDougall, Maryann Izzo **(SLP)**
Malitz-Katz, Mrs Karen L **(SLP)**
McGrath, Karen Marie **(SLP)**
Meisel, Ruth M **(SLP)**
Moore, Kate C **(SLP)**
Moore, Margaret Holland **(A)**
Morris, Alison Lee **(SLP)**
O'Neill-Baker, Mary Catherine **(SLP)**
Ricker, Margaret M
Rollins, Pamela Rosenthal **(SLP)**
Rosen, H Fabrien **(SLP)**
Salkaus, Joan T **(A)**
Sherman, Kathie J **(SLP)**

Wayland
Brant, Mrs Lynne M **(SLP)**
Elkin, Esther B **(A)**
Finn, Debra L **(SLP)**
Okoomian, Mrs Phyllis N **(SLP)**
Ouellette, Mrs Anita **(SLP)**
Zakon, Mrs Susan **(SLP)**

Webster
Aiken, Cynthia Lou **(SLP)**
Fournier, Steven R **(A)**
Messier, Mrs Susan Gail **(SLP)**

Wellesley
Albertson, Nancy **(SLP)**
Andersen, Carol L **(A)**
Cantor, Paul E **(SLP)**
Conti-Ramsden, Dr Gina Maria **(SLP)**
Densmore, Ann **(SLP A)**
Fishkin, Elyse Gustin **(SLP)**
Harvey, Pamela Lynn **(SLP)**
Kapp, Sharon W **(SLP)**
Miller, Gabrielle Judith **(SLP)**
Moore, Elizabeth **(A)**
Myerow, Barbara G **(A)**
Rosenberg, Terry C **(SLP)**
Rotman, Mrs Iris Kline **(SLP)**
Siegal, Mrs Dorothy R **(SLP)**
Stiernberg, Jeanne A **(SLP)**
Wyatt, Gertrud L **(SLP)**

Wellesley Hills
Dogon, Mrs Sally Sinaiko **(SLP)**
Weber, Donna M **(SLP)**

West Barnstable
Nevins, Mrs Arniel F **(SLP)**

West Boxford
Benas, Jacquelyn **(SLP)**

West Bridgewater
Henderson, Mrs Patricia Callahan **(A)**
Pike, Janet Marie **(SLP)**

West Chatham
Shaughnessy, Dale H **(SLP)**

West Falmouth
Blair, Cathleen Ann **(SLP)**

West Harwich
Langtry, Donna Martin **(SLP)**

West Hatfield
Davis, Janice M **(SLP)**

West Holyoke
Gorski, Mrs Kathleen Mary **(SLP)**

West Hyannisport
Arruda, Patricia A **(SLP)**

West Medford
Bloom, Diane L **(SLP)**
Friedl, Christina Ute

West Newburg
Smallcomb, Kathleen **(SLP)**

West Newbury
Carne, Maureen E **(SLP)**
Costa-Natario, Karen Lee **(SLP)**

West Newton
Bergstresser, Mrs Rene Marie **(SLP)**
Granberg, Paula L **(SLP)**
Graybeal, Dr Carolyn M **(SLP)**
Guthermann, Mrs Deborah M **(A)**
Lyons, Patricia Rose **(SLP)**
Noe, Mrs Beth J **(SLP)**
O'Leary, Virginia Marie **(SLP)**
Vander Laan, Carolin H **(SLP)**
Wilson, Beverley L **(SLP)**
Young, Mrs Mariette A **(SLP)**

West Peabody
Kelleher, Candice J **(SLP)**
Krinsky, Martin S **(SLP)**
Suber, Mrs Patricia A **(SLP)**
Wallenius, Wesley A **(SLP)**

West Quincy
Ruguleiski, Michelle Anne **(A)**

West Roxbury
Braun, Mrs Marianne L **(SLP)**
Casey, Margaret M **(A)**
Ferrara-Bowler, Mrs Kathleen Monique **(SLP)**
Feuer, Lois Rachel **(SLP)**
Newman, Lisa A **(SLP)**
Runfola, Rosanne M **(SLP)**
Zitzer, Ellyn R **(A)**

West Somerville
Zunz, Gail C **(SLP)**

West Springfield
Carroll, Mary L **(SLP)**
Dandy, Mrs Annemarie P **(SLP)**
Gillispie, Kathryn P **(A)**
St Pierre, Dianne Marie **(SLP)**

Westborough
Allen-Smith, Mrs Charlotte J
Burke, Mrs Leslie Croft **(SLP)**
Cole, Madeleine Burch **(SLP)**
Guiou, Debra Higgins **(SLP)**
Hnatiow, Gail Z **(SLP A)**
Kruse, Prof Richard W **(SLP)**
Lopatin, Rickey N **(SLP)**
Ward, Virginia **(SLP)**

Westfield
Adamovich, Dr Brenda L B **(SLP)**
Brach-Bonkowski, Mrs Valerie **(SLP)**
Chamberlain, Mrs Sandra L D **(SLP)**
Craig, Sarah Culver **(SLP)**
Flynn, Rosemary E **(SLP)**
Ireland, Nancy E **(SLP)**
Kenney, Karen Jean **(SLP)**
Miers-Lazas, Mrs Debby Rae **(A)**
Sibley, William C **(SLP)**
Stroetzel, Deborah L **(A)**
Willis, Mary Stoveken **(SLP)**

Westford
Chadwick, Donna M **(SLP)**
Faherty, Darlene N **(SLP)**
Hamalainen, Susan W **(SLP)**
Sirois, Doris Petrauskas **(SLP)**

Westminster
Remelius, Fae Ellen **(SLP)**

Weston
Ciampa, Elaine N **(SLP)**
Nussbaum, Rhoda Kahn **(SLP)**
Smart, Mrs Mary L **(SLP)**

Westport
Tavares, Patricia L **(SLP)**

Westwood
Atchue, Catherine Mary **(SLP)**
Bornstein, Byrna Arron **(SLP)**
Campagna, Barbara A **(SLP)**
Cohen, Mrs Diane H **(SLP A)**
Elk, Mrs Debby N **(SLP)**
Herren, Johanna **(SLP)**
Maxwell, Dr David L **(SLP)**
Maxwell, Sara Elizabeth **(SLP)**
Scollins, Beth Anne **(SLP)**
Shapiro, Jeanne Kantauskis **(SLP)**

Turgiss, Susan Marie **(SLP)**

Weymouth
Jones, Dena M **(SLP)**
Oteri, Stephen E **(SLP)**
Segelman, Sheera T **(SLP)**
Smith, Sarah Williston **(SLP)**
Talanian, Valerie Lee **(SLP)**

Whately
Blatt, Beverly Mara **(SLP)**
Ensslin, William R **(SLP)**
Haffey, Eileen F **(SLP)**

Whitinsville
Arbuckle, Priscilla **(SLP)**
Leone, Mrs Susan L **(SLP)**

Whitman
Averell, Lois H **(SLP A)**
Dorn, Lynne D **(SLP)**
Gould, Elaine Rose **(SLP)**
Laffy, Glenn Joseph **(SLP)**

Whittinsville
Daly, Deborah S **(A)**

Wilbraham
Ciocci, Sandra R **(SLP)**
Cook, Deborah C **(SLP)**
Kostek, Mary J **(SLP)**
Morris-Scharl, Barbara **(SLP)**
Quin, Paul E **(SLP)**
Shaw, Mrs Debra Young **(SLP)**

Williamsburg
Hankins, Ronald Joe **(SLP)**
Nicholls, Gloria H **(SLP)**
Restrepo, Maria Adelaida **(SLP)**

Williamstown
Derosier, Paula E S **(SLP)**
Wight, Mrs Carol Ann **(SLP)**

Winchester
Bzdula, Paula A **(SLP)**
Carlisle, Ellen W **(SLP A)**
Erdos, Mrs Caryl Ann **(SLP)**
Govostes, George J **(SLP)**
Grossbard, Mrs Marcia V **(SLP)**
Hines, Cathleen Ann **(SLP)**
Layte, Donna L **(SLP)**
McCabe, Margaret R **(SLP)**
Pavelle, Mrs Anne D P **(SLP)**
Slye, Tracy Rice **(SLP)**
Sullivan, Martha Anne **(SLP)**
Wisnia, Judith F **(SLP)**
Yanco, Elissa Berg **(SLP)**

Winthrop
Dempesy-Hart, Deborah **(A)**
Kushner, Laura **(SLP)**
Lewis, Mary C **(SLP)**
Papa, Elaine Marie **(SLP)**
Vasilos, Stephanie **(SLP)**

Woburn
Abele, Mary E P **(SLP)**
Berniger, Therese Marie **(SLP)**
Briggs, Kim Varoutsos
Burdulis, Miriam M **(SLP)**
Chin, Jeanie **(SLP)**
D'Addario, Mary Ann **(SLP)**
Fuller, Mrs Jan H **(SLP)**
Haring, Linda **(A)**
Hughes, Barbara S **(SLP)**
Kessaris, Mrs Claire Connolly **(SLP)**
Lefkowitz, Nancy G **(SLP)**
McCormack, Joan E **(A)**
O'Connor, Patricia Mary **(SLP)**
Pardo, Patricia A **(SLP)**
Schmidt, Valerie J **(SLP)**
Weissman, Sandra E **(SLP)**

Wollaston
Cody, Mary Teresa **(SLP)**
Weiler, Charles W **(SLP)**

Worcester
Bastardo, Mrs Susan Marie **(SLP)**
Blake, Patricia Celina **(SLP)**
Bove, Mrs Doreen Quiry **(SLP)**
Bove, Lydia Jean **(SLP)**
Capellari, Mrs Reva K **(A)**
Cohen, Dr Anna B **(SLP)**
Crosby, Janis L **(SLP)**
Cunningham, Mrs Linda G **(A)**
Dean, Marcia Southwell **(A)**
Freed, Mrs Helene P **(A)**
Granger, Mrs Diana Osik
Greenberg, Joyce M **(SLP)**
Hagstrom, Fran W **(SLP)**
Halligan, Colene Patricia
Hengen, Dr C Garth **(SLP A)**
Hertz, Robin L **(A)**
Horwitz, Susan B **(SLP)**
Jones, Kristina Marie
Kervick, Mrs Janice H A **(SLP)**
Kirby, Kathleen F **(A)**
Kurland, Mrs Carol L **(SLP)**
Larson, Linda Elizabeth **(SLP)**
Leddy, Karen A **(SLP)**
McCann, Carole J **(SLP)**
McGinn, Carey Elizabeth **(SLP)**
McGinn, Joan M **(SLP)**
McLaughlin, John F **(SLP)**
McLean-Muse, Dr Ann **(SLP)**
Murphy, Lynne Brackett **(SLP)**
O'Day, Marlene Jankowski **(SLP)**
Petty, Sr Alice G **(SLP)**
Rovezzi, Mrs Susan C **(A)**
Savitt, Mrs Amy E P **(A)**
Skillings, Linda J **(SLP)**
Slizeski, Kimberly Ann **(SLP)**
Sloane, Deborah S **(SLP)**
Smith, Mrs Susan L **(A)**
Soiles, Mrs Leslie Peterson **(A)**
Stein, Garie Morgonstem **(SLP)**
Union, Mrs Roberta **(SLP)**
Webber, Mrs MaryKate E **(SLP)**
Wicka, Dr James R **(SLP A)**
Wittenberg, Sherrie L **(SLP)**

Worthington
Fosnot, John D **(A)**
Gauger, Jaclyn **(A)**

Wrentham
Dubendris, Peter C **(SLP)**
Fraley, Mrs Marie R **(SLP)**

Yarmouth Port
McLean-Stead, Constance **(SLP)**
Stoia, John **(SLP A)**

MICHIGAN

Ada
Makuch, Mrs Denise Regina **(SLP)**
Robertson, Jane Ann **(SLP)**
Wilson, Janell A **(SLP)**

Addison
Fannin, Mrs Annette L **(SLP)**

Adrian
Hanks, Daniel A **(SLP)**
Henagan, Mrs Deanne C **(SLP)**
Lysaght, Mrs Mary Conn **(SLP)**
Nicola, Sharon F **(SLP)**
Scheuerman, Martha A **(SLP)**
Wendrow, Sylvia D **(SLP)**

Albion
Gilbert, Mrs Jo Ellen **(SLP)**
Longhurst, Lynn D **(SLP)**

Algonac
Shovan, Diane R **(SLP)**
Welch, Patricia Dare **(SLP)**

Allegan
Adams, Sally Lynne **(SLP)**
Hotchkiss, Dr John C **(SLP)**
West, Mrs Nora J **(SLP)**

Allen Park
Arkwright, Mrs Judy C **(SLP)**
Edwards, Mrs Beverly A **(SLP)**
Ford, Dr Ronald W **(SLP A)**
Johns, Patricia Lynn **(A)**
Peters, Dr Gilmour M **(SLP A)**
Salisbury, Mrs Lynda L **(SLP)**
Shirley, Dr Judith G **(SLP)**

Alma
Atkinson-Goward, Mrs Kathryn B **(SLP)**
McConkie, Mrs Karen E **(A)**
Scurfield, Mrs Jerri L

Alpena
Anderson, Dr Elwood G **(SLP)**
Boboltz-Kitchen, Janice K **(SLP)**
Kitchen, Dr Dale Western **(SLP A)**
LaCross, Kimberly A **(A)**
Yahne, Elizabeth Jean **(SLP)**

Alto
Parker, Vicki S **(SLP)**

Amasa
Saario, Mrs Laurie **(SLP)**

Anchorville
Brengman, Mrs Christine Janet **(A)**

Ann Arbor
Alley, Deborah Justice **(SLP)**
Al-Saadi, Karen S **(SLP)**
Backoff, Patricia M **(A)**
Baines, Kathleen Anderson **(SLP)**
Balmer, Irene W **(SLP)**
Bentrum, Sheila M **(SLP)**
Berger, Mary K **(SLP)**
Block, Margery E **(SLP)**
Boonin, Mrs Joan M **(SLP)**
Bowles, Pamela Elizabeth
Breier, Mrs Martha Helen **(SLP)**
Calder, Dr H B **(A)**
Callaway, Elizabeth **(SLP)**
Collins, Linda G **(SLP)**
Comstock-Reid, Ann K **(SLP)**
Coughlin, Joanne Perdzock **(A)**
Cox, Mrs Juanita Z **(SLP)**
Craig, Dr Holly K **(SLP)**
Crane, Robin Snedeker **(SLP)**
Daly, Dr David A **(SLP)**
Darian, Rosemary B **(SLP)**
Darnton, Sue Wilder **(SLP)**
Daugherty, Jamey A K **(A)**
deMink-LeDuc, Julaine Elizabeth **(SLP)**
Devine, Mrs Patricia B **(SLP)**
Dibble, Mrs Linda Crandall **(SLP)**
Driver, Mrs Lynn E **(SLP)**
Elaswad, Mary Beth **(SLP)**
England, Mrs Kathleen K **(SLP)**
Ensrud, Susan Karolyn **(SLP)**
Evans, Julia Lynne **(SLP)**
Fast, Carol Martha
Fell, Mrs Alice **(SLP)**
Fiegenbaum, Ilana Reiss **(SLP)**
Field, David G **(SLP)**
Finkbiner, Nina G **(SLP)**
Furlette, Deborah Sell **(SLP)**
Glazer, Diane Lynn **(A)**
Goode, Carolann **(SLP)**
Gorenflo, Dr Carole Wood **(SLP)**
Hall, Barbara **(SLP)**
Harrison, Barbara Lynn **(SLP)**
Henry, Dr Frances V **(SLP A)**
Herman, Elise K **(SLP)**
Higgins, John D **(A)**
Higman, Barbara J **(SLP)**
Hinckley, Jacqueline J
Hoffer, Dr Pamela C **(SLP)**
Hoodin, Dr Ronald Bruce **(SLP)**
Huber, Connie M **(SLP)**
Jarrell, Rita Coval **(SLP)**
Johnson, Mrs Letitia L **(SLP)**
Joyce, Patricia E **(A)**
Kileny, Dr Paul R **(A)**
Kluin, Karen J **(SLP)**
Koch, Larry John **(A)**
Koster, Marilyn H **(SLP)**
Landau, Cecelia Charest **(SLP)**
Langmore, Dr Susan L **(SLP)**
Larson, Sherri C **(SLP)**
Ledwon-Robinson, Elaine **(SLP)**
Lehman, Mark Edward **(SLP)**
Lewin, Jan S **(SLP)**
Limoges, Mrs Suzanne D **(SLP)**
Lowell, Sarah L
Maahs, Anne Marie **(SLP)**
Martin, Ann W **(SLP)**
Martin, Dr Daniel E **(SLP)**
Matz, Susan C **(SLP)**
McClure, Ramona Anne **(SLP)**
McConahy, Mrs Renee L **(SLP)**
McMartin, Heidi Therese **(SLP)**
McMillan, Mrs Pamella M **(A)**
Meador, Dr Helen Elisa
Melnyk, Lesia Anna
Milburn, Dr Braxton **(A)**
Mills, Dr Russell H **(SLP)**
Miltich, Dr Suzanne Hogan **(SLP)**
Morley, D E **(SLP)**
Morris, Sandra Ann **(SLP)**
Natoci, Mrs Karen Musselman **(SLP)**
O'Shaughnessey, Mrs Mary Susan **(A)**
Otto, Kay Anne S **(SLP)**
Oviatt, Carol C **(A)**
Oviatt, Dana L **(A)**
Peelle, Louise M **(SLP)**
Peters, James L **(SLP)**
Pozza, Carrie Anne **(SLP)**
Pulford, Laureen Rizzo **(SLP)**
Putz, Janine Lynette **(A)**
Roberts, Mrs Debra V **(SLP)**
Rogers, Ronald M **(A)**
Sansbury, Dr Russell J **(SLP)**
Saulles, Mrs Lisa Kanagur **(A)**
Schatz, Kenneth H **(SLP)**
Schultz, Mrs Jeanie Barry **(SLP)**
Schultz, Sara Joanne
Shapiro, Caryn L **(SLP)**
Shepard, Dr Neil T **(A)**
Siehl, Georgiana Pacini **(SLP)**
Silbergleit, Alice Klain **(SLP)**
Snead, Colleen **(A)**
Solon, Laurel Frassinell **(SLP)**
Spak, Constance **(A)**
Spalding, Jody L P **(SLP A)**
Stark-Nemon, Barbara A **(SLP)**
Stinson, Danita A **(SLP)**
Tait, Dr Charles A **(SLP A)**
Thomas-Kincaid, Lauren **(SLP)**
Vander Velde, Deborah L
Van Meter, Adelia M **(SLP)**
Van Riper, Mrs Lori Ann **(A)**
Veniar, Dr Florence A **(A)**
Wardner, Mrs Monique C **(A)**
Washington, Julie Ann **(SLP)**
Wimmer, Vega H **(SLP A)**
Woodhams, Julia V **(SLP)**
Wurtzel, Mrs Terese M **(SLP)**
Zand, Dr Charlene Rooth **(SLP)**
Zimmerman-Phillips, Susan R **(A)**

Atlanta
Russell, Mrs Mary Jo Burns **(SLP)**

Au Gres
Heinrich, Richard Allen **(SLP)**

Auburn Hills
Fields, Mrs Michelle **(SLP)**
Kilar, Carolyn Yandura **(SLP)**
Perry, Karen F **(SLP)**
Seidman, Kathryn Allison **(SLP)**
Sundt, Mrs Christi Morrow

Augusta
Eddy-Lasich, Mrs Mary Ellen **(A)**
Toth, Mrs Kathleen M **(SLP)**

Bad Axe
Lupinski, Michael Felix **(SLP)**

Barryton
Turnbull, Karen Koester **(SLP)**

Battle Creek
Blaising, Mrs Janice C **(SLP)**
Drikakis, Christine Ann **(SLP)**
Holub, Carl A **(SLP)**
Kracht, Colleen H **(A)**
Leaders, Mrs Linda **(SLP)**
Locke, William L **(SLP)**
Mumford, Albert **(SLP)**
Oman, Mrs Linda N **(SLP)**
Osborn, Laura W **(SLP)**
Shehabi, Mrs Pamela Lou **(SLP)**
Sims, Mrs Pamela M **(SLP)**
Sparks, Mrs Shirley N **(SLP)**
Trantum, Dennis **(A)**
Young, Mary G **(SLP)**

Bay City
Andrzejewski, Sally Ann **(SLP)**
Duffy, Mary Kate **(SLP)**
Emge, Mrs Judith Ann **(SLP)**
Goodell, Mrs Cynthia A **(SLP)**
Jalovaara, Rosemary A **(SLP)**
Neier, Mrs Kathryn R **(SLP)**
O'Brien, Mrs Carol Powell **(SLP)**
Zuraw, Edward Paul **(SLP)**

Belding
Granzo, Mrs Cheryl Marie **(SLP)**

Belleville
Henry, Robert J, Jr **(A)**
Kehn-Nichols, Judith Lynn **(SLP)**

Belmont
Konarska, Keith P **(SLP)**
Konarska, Kevin A **(SLP)**
Konarska, Laurie Hughes **(SLP)**
Tompkins, Mrs Charlene H **(SLP)**

Benton Harbor
Wrens, Brenda M **(SLP)**

Berkley
Candor-Kennedy, Peggy A **(SLP)**
Daniels, Paulette Gerard **(A)**
Finn, Karen Wimmer **(A)**
Silverstein, Mrs Lori Michele **(SLP)**
Stevens, Mrs Lizbeth **(SLP)**

Berrien Springs
Canaday, Mary Jo **(SLP A)**
Dutcher, Pamela S **(SLP)**
Grix-Kossakoski, Mrs Mary Whelan
Maki, Dr Jean E **(SLP)**
McNeil, Mrs Lystra E **(A)**

Big Rapids
Halpert, Helen V **(SLP)**
Kahn, Mrs Deborah Ann **(SLP)**
Storm, Mrs Florence R **(SLP)**

Birch Run
Potts, Rebecca Kay **(A)**

Birmingham
Bator, Mrs Cecilia J **(SLP)**
Bayleran, Mrs Ann Sarkis **(SLP)**
Beckwith, Mrs Barbara Ann **(SLP)**
Bell-Hiett, Cynthia J **(SLP)**
Borson, Carol Ann **(SLP)**
Brubaker, Susan Howell **(SLP)**
Bura, Marilyn B **(SLP)**
Cooper, Mrs Denise L **(SLP)**
Derkacz-Bolen, Mrs Mary Ann **(SLP)**
Dilgard, Susan S **(SLP)**
Dolan, Patricia Eades **(SLP)**
Donahue, Mrs Miriam L **(SLP)**
Ernst, Mrs Lorraine F **(SLP)**
Ewing, Susan A **(SLP)**
Farhat, Teri Rae **(SLP)**
Fenyes, Mrs Shelley R T **(SLP)**
Galper, Marcie R **(A)**
Garfield, Ilene F **(SLP)**
Green, Mrs Leslie R **(SLP)**
Harrington, Jo Ann **(SLP)**
Hemmerlein, Mrs Vicki Diane **(SLP)**
Hoban, Janet Louise **(SLP)**
Houser, Nancy E **(SLP)**
Hull, Mrs Joyce M **(SLP)**
Mathers, Dr Pamela L **(SLP)**
Mathews, Lynne L **(SLP)**
Mayhew, Nancy Craig **(SLP)**
McCarus, Carol H **(SLP)**
Morelli-Neddy, Mrs Aimee Beth **(SLP)**
Murphy, Mary J **(SLP)**
Nickles, Deborah L **(SLP)**
Nunn-Krieger, Barbara J **(SLP)**
O'Leary, Karen Schultz **(SLP)**
Orlandoni, Nancy J **(SLP)**
Potter, Mrs Susan W **(A)**
Robinson, Dr Dale Omar **(SLP A)**
Romanelli, Constance Ann
Rutkowski, Mrs Kristine Arlene **(SLP)**
Shell, Shirley J **(SLP)**
Sherbin, Mrs Lillian K **(SLP)**
Sidman, Helene Ruth **(SLP)**
Simpson, Dr Mark Louis **(SLP)**
Sloan, Annette Virginia **(SLP)**
Stephenson, Elizabeth Z **(SLP)**
Stephenson, William T **(SLP A)**
Stulberg, Ellen W **(SLP)**
Sviland, Carmen C **(SLP)**
Wright, Margaret Schmid **(SLP)**

Bloomfield Hills
Balay, Georgean **(A)**
Brandt-Guckes, Deborah **(SLP)**
Case, Carol Lynn **(SLP)**
Chucales, Katherine Anne **(SLP)**
Costin, Karen S **(SLP)**
Daines, Mrs Nancy C **(SLP)**
Eurich, Mrs Kathleen A **(SLP)**
Feiwell Ma, H Aubrey **(SLP)**
Henson, Ruth Annette **(SLP)**
Jaynes, Beverly Ann **(SLP)**
Kroell, Mrs Anne Carroll **(SLP)**
McIlrath, Mrs Pauline R **(SLP)**
Ramsey, Belinda R **(SLP)**
Schreck, Karen Tulin **(SLP)**
Shargel, George M
Shifman, Suzanne K **(A)**
Smiley, Helen Nutter **(SLP)**
Stoneman, Janice Green **(A)**
Talon, Mrs Pamela H **(SLP)**
Torgerson, Nancy Ann
Williams, Mrs Cathy J **(SLP)**
Zemmol, Mrs Caroline S **(SLP)**
Zilowey, Stacey A **(SLP)**

Boyne City
Shane, Carole J **(SLP)**

Brighton
Barlow, Kathleen G **(SLP)**
Crain, Sheri L **(SLP)**
Hollier, Mrs Anne S **(SLP)**
Mascow, Susan Zievers **(SLP)**
Sochocki, Mrs Rita Gail **(SLP)**

Brimley
Parish, Mrs Janine Diaz **(SLP)**

Buchanan
Pruitt, Mary Eliz **(SLP)**

Cadillac
Blackburn, Mrs Sharon L **(A)**
Hurni, Jill E **(SLP)**
Sayler, Julie Ann **(SLP)**
Wright, Patricia Kay **(SLP)**

Canton
Burgess, Mrs Anne D D **(SLP)**
Carter, Mrs Diana M **(SLP)**
Dawn-Kosteva, Laura Ann **(SLP)**
Dimusto, Mrs Lisa
Dirvonas, Mrs Deborah F **(SLP)**
Fine, Roslyn A **(SLP)**
Grey, Yona Leigh **(SLP)**
Harris, Marilyn Sue **(SLP)**
Lobelle, Donald E **(A)**
MacPherson, Colin A **(SLP)**
Rich, Mrs Janice Smithbauer **(A)**

Caro
Coats-Garrett, Mrs Paula C **(SLP)**
Daniels, Marjorie C **(SLP)**
Laeder, Ronald L **(SLP)**
Peter, Frederick F **(SLP)**
Shiffler, Therese Anstead **(SLP)**
Surabian, Julia Ann **(SLP)**

Cedarville
Sitz, Janet M B **(SLP)**

Charlevoix
Aiman, Eliece B **(SLP)**
Campbell, Mary Lee **(SLP)**
Mayhew, Preston W, II **(SLP)**

Charlotte
Jones, Julie Gail **(A)**

Chassell
Reed, Nancy L **(A)**
Scow, Mrs Cecilia H **(SLP)**

Chelsea
Andraska, Ann K **(SLP)**
Boshoven, Margaret M **(SLP)**
Denison, Marsha Figg **(SLP)**
Olson, Mrs Gail Lynn **(SLP)**
Robinson, Robin Lee **(SLP)**

Clare
FitzGerald, Ann E **(SLP)**
Patterson, Linda Jean **(SLP)**

Clarkston
Baker, Palma C **(SLP)**
Doty, Carolyn Ann **(SLP)**
Edmond, Mary Beth **(SLP)**
Fitton-Neville, Dr Roxie A **(A)**
Forster, Mrs Catherine C **(SLP)**
Harlton, Mrs Kathryn R **(SLP)**
Kirchgessner, Janice A P **(SLP)**
Vandeusen, Jamie S **(SLP)**
Weber, Karee Lynn

Clinton
Connors, Mrs Ronnie Marolf **(SLP)**
Wight, Mrs Marallyn M **(SLP)**
Wise, Linda G **(SLP)**

Clio
Farrell, Mrs Elizabeth **(SLP)**
Schultz, Norman R **(SLP)**

Coldwater
Fischer, Mrs Maureen R **(SLP)**
Gleason, Erland W **(SLP)**
Haas, Mrs Carol Ann **(SLP)**
Snyder, Mrs Louise M **(SLP)**
Whitely, Mrs Carolyn Chambers **(SLP)**

Coleman
Cashin, Mrs Joan L **(SLP)**

Coloma
Stader, Mrs Cynthia E

Comstock Park
Harpe, Janice N **(SLP)**

Dansville
Brandon, Judith K **(SLP)**

Davison
Higgerson, Michele M **(SLP)**

Dearborn
Andrews, D Karen **(SLP)**
Auffenberg, Mrs Nancy Ann Whatley **(SLP)**
Curran, Lynn M **(SLP)**
Dickson, Mrs Linda G Bradham **(A)**
Fink, Karen Smillie **(SLP)**
Gimpel, Mrs Colleen Marie **(SLP)**
Graham, Dr A Bruce **(A)**
Hoy, Carol Joan **(SLP)**
Kirk, Mary L **(SLP)**
McAdam, Carol C **(SLP)**
McAdam, Malcolm A **(A)**
McClung, Dr Betty Beranek **(SLP)**
Narkiewicz, Patricia Ann **(SLP)**
Novelli, Janine H **(SLP)**
Sarr, Mrs Jean Bills **(SLP)**
Sears, Richard B **(SLP)**
Stec, Mrs Jonelle Irene **(SLP)**
Uznis, Judith C **(SLP)**
Wagner, Laura A **(SLP)**

Dearborn Heights
Agemy, Evangeline **(SLP)**
Bonanno, Mrs Diane Hope **(SLP)**
Flowers, Arthur
Gorski, Mrs Therese Marie **(SLP)**
MacDonald, Shirley R **(SLP)**
Schroeder, Virginia Marie **(A)**
Wegienka-Vokal, Mrs Susan C **(SLP)**

Detroit
Adams, Clarinda T **(SLP)**
Allen-Peoples, Mrs Yvonne **(SLP)**
Bentzen, Ernestine **(SLP)**
Bliss, Lynn S **(SLP)**
Boyer, Kathryn K **(SLP)**
Boykin, Pamela T **(SLP)**
Covington, Dr Ann J **(SLP A)**
Covington, Sheryl J S **(SLP)**
Crawford, Mrs Valerie Y **(SLP)**
Denham, Linda **(A)**
Dibble, Lawrence M **(SLP A)**
Dickerson, Mrs Bertha M **(SLP)**
Dreyer, Dr Dorothy E **(SLP)**
Dzikowski, Richard John **(SLP)**
Eldis, Dr Frances E **(SLP A)**
Fleming, Dr Susan M **(SLP)**
Hadeed, Nabhan **(SLP)**
Hamlet, Dr Sandra Lee
Handel, Julie D **(A)**
Haney, Linda Kay **(SLP)**
Holste, Dr Herman M **(SLP)**
Hudson-Graham, Karen Marie
Hyter, Yvette Delaine **(SLP)**
Jacobson, Dr Gary P **(A)**
Johnson, Carolyn **(SLP)**
Jones, Mrs Roma B **(SLP)**
Kauffman, Dorothy Carlson
Kolarov, Margaret **(SLP)**
Krouse, Dr Carl W **(SLP A)**
Lacey, Elaine Marie
Leith, Dr William R **(SLP)**
Linander, Mrs Esther S **(SLP)**
Lindahl, Raymond F **(SLP)**
Luce, Roberta E **(SLP)**
Luster, Mrs Thelma B **(SLP)**
Massenberg, Angela Renee **(SLP)**
Matlock, Dr Mildred P **(SLP)**
Means, Paulette G **(SLP)**
Montgomery, Gay Ann **(SLP)**
Newman, Dr Craig W **(A)**
Polk, Mrs Gloria H **(SLP)**
Popielec, Eugene A **(SLP)**
Powell, Sheila L **(SLP)**
Rintelmann, Dr William F **(SLP A)**
Rucker, Lila **(A)**
Sbaschnig, Kristine V **(SLP)**
Scales, Phyllis Z **(SLP)**
Small, Mary Elizabeth
Starnes, Deborah Kaye **(A)**
Tate, Virginia May **(SLP)**
Tolliver, Beverly Diane **(SLP)**
Tonkovich, John D **(SLP A)**
Wolfolk, William Bell **(SLP)**

Dewitt
Stewart, Gregory D **(A)**

Dexter
Angelocci, Dr Angelo A **(SLP)**
Bertelsen, Mrs Beth Billman **(SLP)**

Dowagiac
Anderson, Roy K **(SLP)**

Drayton Plains
Terbush, Connie Jean

Dundee
Roe, Mrs Joan L **(SLP)**
Schultz, Laura Lee

East Grand Rapids
MacHiorlatti, Mrs Carol Oddo **(SLP)**
Scott, Mrs Anne C **(SLP)**

East Lansing
Alkistis, Charalambo
Beamon, Lehua L **(SLP)**
Bilkovsky-Johnson, Margie Renee **(SLP)**
Bridges, Sheila J **(SLP)**
Bruce, Mrs Elvy **(SLP)**
Bruno, Leonard **(A)**
Carr, Mrs Lisa A **(SLP)**
Carter, Roxanne Lanae
Casby, Dr Michael W **(SLP)**
Clugston, Deidra K W **(SLP)**
Davis, Charlotte A **(SLP)**
Deal, Dr Leo V **(SLP A)**
Eulenberg, Dr John Bryson
Fouts, Mrs Ann Pierce **(SLP)**
Frumkin, Neva **(SLP)**
Gaulden, Mrs Phyllis Kay B **(SLP)**
Gehl, Mrs Ellen Louise **(SLP)**
Gould-MacDonald, Carol L **(SLP)**
Hadjian, Dr Sophia **(SLP)**
Harding, Jeanne **(SLP)**
Herzog, Elizabeth Ellen **(A)**
Hooper, Arthur D **(SLP)**
Johnson, Mrs Kathleen Rose **(SLP)**
Kapur, Dr Y P **(A)**
Kortyka, Mrs Alice Ann **(A)**
LaPine, Dr Peter R **(SLP)**
Lesmez, Rebecca Mohn **(A)**
Lewis, Mrs Helga Lauretta **(A)**
Martin, Cheryl L **(SLP)**
Moore, Dr Ernest J
O'Leksy-Villarruel, Mrs Gail Anne
Palmer, Margaret L **(SLP)**
Pender, Mrs Evelyn H **(SLP)**
Redfearn, Mrs Deborah P **(SLP)**
Rintelmann, Mary J **(SLP)**
Sadasivan, Mangala Gowri **(SLP)**
Scott, Diane M **(A)**
Semela, Jacob J M Ne **(A)**
Smith, Dr Linda Lou **(A)**
Spieth, Martha L **(SLP)**
Stewart, Michael G **(A)**
Stockman, Ida Jones **(SLP)**
Wallace, Dr Gloriajean L **(SLP)**
West, Mary **(SLP)**

East Leroy
Jones, Frederick M **(A)**

East Tawas
Zielinski, Ronald J **(SLP)**

Eastport
Clark, Mrs Judith M **(SLP)**

Eaton Rapids
Hanthorne, Gloria D **(SLP)**
Kenyon, Mrs Julie Hudson **(SLP)**

Ecorse
Covington, Zenara Walthea **(SLP)**
Nelson, Sigfred A **(SLP)**

Elsie
Howe, Patricia Weston **(SLP)**

Escanaba
Rogero, Mrs Elaine A **(SLP)**

Essexville
Fox, Mrs Vernie R **(SLP)**

Farmington Hills
Afflerbaugh, Carol P **(SLP)**
Bahra, Mrs Joan A **(SLP)**
Baldwin, Mrs Anne C **(SLP)**
Beckerleg, Mrs Wendy **(SLP)**
Bielak, Mrs Elizabeth Ann **(SLP)**
Blugerman, Mrs Denise F **(SLP)**
Bryant, Antoinette **(SLP)**
Burtka, Mary Jo **(A)**
Cali, Thomas F **(SLP)**
Caverly, Patricia Jean **(A)**
Craine, Teri **(SLP)**
Cummins, Lori Gealer **(SLP)**
Dean, Karen Louise
Drozdowski, Mrs Emily C **(SLP)**
Duerr, Barbara Mikus **(A)**
Eick, Lisa Hill **(SLP)**
Ellis, Mrs Lori Klisman **(SLP)**
Falk, Dr Mervyn L **(SLP)**
Felsenfeld, Mark A **(SLP)**
Fenton-Jones, Jill **(SLP)**
Fineman-Singer, Mrs Sharon A **(SLP)**
Flevaris, Dr Carole A **(A)**
Gabe, Mrs Deborah Cogan **(SLP)**
Goff, Stephen William **(A)**
Goodman, Mrs Perri Marlene **(SLP)**
Greer, Mrs Deborah Corrine **(SLP)**
Gross, Elizabeth Ann **(SLP)**
Haberek, Theresa **(SLP)**
Harnisch, Mrs Diane L **(SLP)**
Henderson, Myrna **(SLP)**
Hobbins, Keith E **(SLP)**
Jahnke, Kathryn Ann **(SLP)**
Jenison-Hemmye, Susan **(SLP)**
Jeter, Mrs Christine M **(SLP)**
Kay, Mrs Janice Terry **(SLP)**
Kinsman, Mrs Georgene J **(SLP)**
Klegon, Ilene Z **(SLP)**
Klobucar, Mrs Cheryl L **(SLP)**
Klueger, Mrs Ruth Elizabeth **(SLP)**
Kulick, Kathleen Callan **(A)**
Lennon, Kim **(SLP)**
Levandowski, Mary Kaye
Lewsley, Mrs Sandra J **(SLP)**
Lieberman, Mrs Rochelle Rotblatt **(SLP)**
Lieberman, Mrs Susan G H **(SLP)**
Lipshaw, Mrs Lori Robin
Lubanski, Mrs Cathy Michele **(SLP)**
Mammoser, Lisa Marie **(SLP)**
McPherson, Neal I
Milstein, Rochelle Fern **(SLP)**
Mosier, Karen L **(SLP)**
Neuvirth, Debra Lynn **(SLP)**
Oleson, Susan H **(SLP)**
Palazzo, Mrs Jill Gannon **(SLP)**
Pall, Roberta Granke **(SLP)**
Pinkney, Mrs Ruth G **(SLP)**
Proteau, Dawn Agnes **(SLP)**
Riley, Anita Marcott **(SLP)**
Roeder, Kathleen Ventre **(SLP)**
Rogers, Amy H **(SLP)**
Royal, Verne G **(SLP)**
Sarpa, Mrs Nancy Needham **(SLP)**
Schloff, Sandra Joan **(SLP)**
Schneider, Paula Kathleen **(A)**
Schwartz Rostker, Mrs Jill **(SLP)**
Shultz, Mrs Sharon L **(SLP)**
Simons, Mrs Candace Rosenbaum **(SLP)**
Slowley, Jeanne I **(SLP)**
Smith, Harlie R **(A)**
Sowinski, Christine **(SLP)**
Stockwell, Dr Charles Warren
Voita, Cathy Lynn **(SLP)**
Whittemore, Karen E **(SLP)**

Fenton
Drake, Mrs Diana L **(SLP)**

Ferndale
Scheel, Joan M **(SLP)**
Weeks, Julia A **(SLP)**

Flat Rock
Washchuk, Mrs Carol Keeler **(SLP)**

Flint
Bas, Helen S **(SLP)**
Belford, Mrs Linda Morris **(SLP)**
Brooks, Mira J
Brown, Mrs Betty L **(A)**
Everitt, David Max **(A)**
Fronheiser, Glenn S **(A)**
Goddard, David E **(SLP)**
Hamann, Mrs Kathryn Louise **(A)**
Herrick, Jeryl Lynne **(SLP)**
Lonsway, John Alan **(A)**
Meyer, Becky Blodgett **(A)**
Parsons, Julie Marie
Poss, Mrs Edith S **(A)**
Rhodes, Cheryl D **(SLP A)**
Ritchie, Mrs Lynda C **(SLP)**
Stahl, John E **(SLP)**
Strahle, Marjorie James **(SLP)**
Waterman, Leann K **(SLP)**
Wilkoff, Dr Joan B **(A)**
Wright, Lois M **(SLP)**

Flushing
Boulter, Mrs Kathryn **(SLP)**
Carlsen, Mrs Vause S **(SLP)**
Purcell, Roberta L **(SLP)**
Rose, Margaret A **(SLP)**
Weiss, Mrs Lori Joyce **(SLP)**

Fountain
Gulembo-Plato, Mrs Terri Leah **(SLP)**

Fowlerville
Timer, Mrs Loretta Ann **(SLP)**

Frankfort
Steele, Mrs Sandra D **(A)**

Franklin
Gilbert, Shyrle I **(SLP)**
Hoyt, Michael B **(A)**
Sax, Mrs Mary R **(SLP)**
Schram, Judith R **(SLP)**
Silverman, Sandra D **(SLP)**

Franklin Village
Tell, Mrs Elaine F **(SLP)**

Fraser
Toward, Mrs Mary Margaret **(SLP)**

Fremont
Densmore, Cynthia George **(SLP)**
Panyard, Vickie Lynn **(A)**

Gaines
Tunningley, Georgiann **(SLP)**
Tunningley, Richard M **(SLP)**

Galesburg
Ellis, Mrs Nancy A **(SLP)**

Gaylord
Brooks, Penny McClard **(SLP)**
Coger, Patricia Johnson **(SLP)**
Karabacz, Mrs Nancy C **(SLP)**
Lamy, Mrs Lori Kay **(SLP)**
Rademacher, Mrs Ann D **(SLP)**
Slominski, Thomas J **(SLP)**

Gladstone
Aschbacher, Mrs Julie Agnes **(SLP)**
Dougherty, Leona Mae **(SLP)**
Featheringill, David Michael **(SLP)**
Hampton, Susan M **(SLP)**

Gladwin
Manninen, Mrs Debra Lynn **(SLP)**

Grand Blanc
Bouvier, Mrs Maryann Janet **(SLP)**
Flynn, Deanna Colleen **(SLP)**
Gentzel, Melora Jane
Lamson-Uhelski, Karen Dianne
Losinski, Mrs Jayne F **(SLP)**
Miller, Mrs Cynthia Cox **(SLP)**
Powell, Mrs Donna J **(SLP)**
Spence, Donna Joan
Wolski, Dr William **(SLP)**

Grand Haven
Bassett, Mrs Nancy L **(SLP)**
Johnson, Patricia Gasiciel **(SLP)**
Sjoberg-Anderson, Cynthia **(SLP)**
Valentine, Mrs Barbara J **(SLP)**

Grand Ledge
Graham, Jacqueline **(SLP)**
Hincher, Joanne Louise
Hoffman, Kathryn E **(A)**
Reath, Mrs Lisa Ann
Theisen, Jane Elizabeth **(SLP)**

Grand Rapids
Alexander, Kathleen **(SLP)**
Alsum, Mrs Terese Diane **(A)**
Ayala, Aurea Margarita **(SLP)**
Beachler, Cindy Robbins **(A)**
Befus, Mrs Barbara H **(SLP)**
Beyer, Kerry Lee **(SLP)**
Bonnema, Mrs Christine Monticello **(SLP)**
Brynelsen, Charles Allen **(SLP)**
Buth, Mrs Lisa L **(SLP)**
Buurma, Kathleen A **(SLP)**
Bylsma, Bruce Alan **(A)**
Carlson, Linda K **(SLP)**
Carlson, Norrene L **(SLP)**
Clabuesch, Rebecca P **(SLP)**
Coleman, Mrs Diane L **(SLP)**
Cragwall, Mrs Kathryn D **(SLP)**
Davis, Mrs Janet Van Orsdel **(SLP)**
Deboer, Jack A **(A)**
Denton, Rebecca Bennert **(SLP)**
Dietrich, Frances Harag **(SLP)**
Duisterhof, Julie K **(SLP)**
Eardley, Mary Dudek **(SLP)**
Ellison, Cynthia L **(A)**
Fausone, Beth Anne **(SLP)**
Gessner, Barbara Joy **(A)**
Gibson, Cinda Lou **(SLP)**
Haveman-Kruyf, Susan **(A)**
Jacobs, Mrs Karen Ann **(A)**
Johnson, Dr Kenneth R **(A)**
Jones, Mary Lynne **(SLP)**
Katerberg, Jane E **(SLP)**
Keeton, Mary F **(SLP)**
Keller, Barbara R **(SLP)**
Kurowski, Karen Susan **(A)**
Lang, Mrs Lori Jean **(A)**
Lanning, Jackie Christine
Ludwig, Denise A **(SLP)**
Maitland, Mrs Holly McKinley **(SLP)**
McBride, Laura A **(SLP)**
McCarthy, Diane L **(SLP)**
McLelland, Mrs Rosann Elizabeth
Mulford, Julie J **(SLP)**
Novak, Barbara A **(SLP)**
O'Connor, Anita M **(SLP)**
Ofield, Mrs Mary C **(SLP)**
Owens, Jerry Lee **(A)**
Raymonds-Sharp, Marianne **(SLP)**
Ricciardi, Mrs Geraldine Dunaway
Root, Susan D **(SLP)**
Rossio-Edwards, Mrs Patricia A **(SLP)**
Russo, Mrs Deborah Piehler **(SLP)**
Sass, Margaret M
Schreuder, Mary Sue **(A)**
Scogg, Mrs Renee Ann **(SLP)**
Silbar, Jean C **(SLP)**
Smith, Renee Lynne **(SLP)**
Stahl, Michael T **(A)**
Szewczyk, Susan Kay **(SLP)**
Szumowski, Edward J, Jr **(A)**
Thompson, Mrs Tamela Sue **(SLP)**
Vandeguchte, Dr Marten **(SLP)**
Van Drie, Mary L **(A)**
Ward, Sue Ellen **(SLP)**

Waters, Mrs Lynn M R **(A)**
Weger, Frank Randy **(SLP)**
Wiener, Mrs Elana Sue **(SLP)**
Willems, Caroline C
Wilton, Mrs Mary Martiny **(SLP)**
Zoellner, Ann M **(SLP)**

Grandville
Ter Haar, Mrs Sandra S **(SLP)**

Grass Lake
Reel, Kathryn Elizabeth **(SLP)**

Grayling
Bush, Gregory Alan **(SLP)**
Moss, Catherine **(SLP)**

Greenville
Borucki, Donna Kay **(SLP)**

Gregory
Clark, Michele Marie **(SLP)**

Grosse Ile
Loomer, Delores M **(SLP)**
Weise, Timothy G **(SLP)**

Grosse Pointe
Boykin, Lesley L **(SLP)**
De France, Mrs Nancy L R **(SLP)**
Evans, Roland S **(SLP)**
Jackson-Menaldi, Dr Maria Cristina
Johnston, Dr Robert G **(SLP)**
Rogers, Carolyn L **(SLP)**
Schutza, Mrs Patricia Frances **(SLP)**
Schwan, Mrs Sabina A **(A)**
Stemmelen, Maureen Therese **(SLP)**
Wycech, Gertrude Howell **(SLP)**

Grosse Pointe Farms
Burke, Mrs Mary Anne **(SLP)**
Leiphart, Janet R **(SLP)**
Mansfield, Mrs Carol S **(SLP)**
Smith, Mrs Barbara Varkoly **(SLP)**
Tramposch, Helga Kay **(SLP)**

Grosse Pointe Park
Liening, Maryellen Gleason **(SLP)**
Peters, Donna Lee **(SLP)**
Wharton, Jeanne Ann **(A)**

Grosse Pointe Pk
Craig, Mrs Peri M **(SLP)**
Evans-Batalucco, Georgianna **(SLP)**
Malis, Mrs Alexis Pervanis **(SLP)**
Scott, Mrs Christie Miller **(SLP)**
Sibley, Michele T **(SLP)**
Stuckey, Mrs Patricia A **(A)**

Grosse Pointe Woods
Cooper, Gary J **(SLP)**
Koester, Mrs Margaret M **(SLP)**
Monsour, Rosemary J **(SLP)**

Guam
Guiry, Sibyl D **(SLP)**

Haflett
Houser, Michele M **(SLP)**

Hamtramck
Stoll, Julie Bethea **(SLP)**

Hancock
Mannisto, Marilisa **(SLP)**

Harbor Springs
Leach, Mrs Susan M **(SLP)**
Scheerhorn, Mrs Cindy Dykstra **(SLP)**

Harper Woods
Edwards, Bruce M **(A)**
Gallagher, Lynn Marie **(SLP)**
Yates, Dorisann

Harrison
Kelke, Sandra A **(SLP)**

Harrisville
Jackson, Mrs Barbara J

Hartford
Kuehnle, Lisa G **(SLP)**

Hartland
Alterman, Mrs Maureen M **(SLP)**

Haslett
Alexander, Linda Lamison **(SLP)**
Alexander, Mrs Rise Barnett **(SLP)**
Carson, Kelly Marie **(SLP)**
Degennaro, Andrea T **(SLP)**
Flagg, Mrs Kelly Jo **(SLP)**
Lunsted, Carol Lappin **(SLP)**
Roberts, Rosemarie Stavros **(SLP)**

Hastings
Ainslie, Mrs Ann Ironside **(SLP)**
Huntley, Jill Allison **(SLP)**

Hemlock
Haveman, Jack A

Hillman
Scramlin, Mrs Cheryl D **(SLP)**

Hillsdale
Hayes, Robert **(SLP)**
Hepker, Mrs Sandra Jean **(A)**
Mallar, Mrs Mary M **(SLP)**
Myron, Susan J **(SLP)**
Shields, Mrs Karen F **(SLP)**

Holland
Beh-Arendshorst, Monica **(SLP)**
Fu, Mrs Mary Claire **(SLP)**
Gant-Johnston, Sheryl S **(SLP)**
Geiger, Mrs Gail A **(SLP)**
O'Rourke, Mrs Betty L **(SLP)**
Schripsema, Lois Elaine **(SLP)**
Vander Veen, Mrs Eileen E **(SLP)**
Vasilauskas, Mrs Cherylyn Joy **(SLP)**
Welsh, James J, Jr **(A)**

Holly
Hansz-Ax, Holly K **(SLP)**
Prechowski, Catherine Anne **(SLP)**
Warner, Robert C **(SLP)**

Holt
Cline, Jennifer Marie **(SLP)**

Houghton
Freedman, Linda Shepard **(SLP)**
Graham, Carol M **(SLP)**

Howell
Barnett, Constance **(SLP)**
Charron, Dechantal Marie **(SLP)**
Hairston, Valeri Lyn **(SLP)**
Schardein-Smith, Mrs Carolyn Lee **(SLP)**
Stankov, Mary Anne
Vorce, Mrs Deborah Jean
Wagner, Mrs Nancy G **(SLP)**

Hudsonville
Helmer, Mrs Penney Lynn **(SLP)**
Westra, Mrs Mary Oettinger **(SLP)**
Witte, Mrs Nancy R **(SLP)**

Huntington Woods
Brandt, Mrs Antoinette **(SLP)**
Frank, Mrs Mary A
Gordon, Charlene B **(A)**
Graef-Ferman, Denise B **(A)**
Kauffman-Mally, Mrs Helene **(SLP)**
Kujawski, Claudia Ezman **(SLP)**
McDonald, Mrs A Joan Ronan **(A)**
Mikon, Deena **(SLP)**
Morris, Mrs Cynthia G **(SLP)**
Potter, Suzanne **(SLP)**
Stiebel, Hart Henry **(SLP)**
Topa, Carole B **(SLP)**
Willens, Diane **(SLP)**

Ida
Campbell, Dr Mary E **(A)**

Inkster
Hanrahan, Donna E **(SLP)**

O'Rourke, CarolAnn **(A)**

Ionia
Hausserman, Julie L **(SLP)**

Iron Mountain
Holmes, Mrs Colleen J **(SLP)**
Jacobson, Paul Alan **(SLP)**

Ishpeming
Finney, John David **(A)**

Jackson
Baird, Mary P **(A)**
Berthiaume, Mrs Mary Ann **(SLP)**
Goyings, Mrs Joann S **(SLP)**
Hulbert-Wilson, Susan S **(SLP)**
Limmer, Kathleen **(A)**
Morris, Mrs Gail Marie **(SLP)**
Morrison, Mrs Sheila Kies **(SLP)**
Rehor, Linda S **(SLP)**
Reisdorf, Mrs Jean Marie **(SLP)**
Remsperger, Annette **(A)**
Stoner, Mrs Janet Lynn **(SLP)**

Jenison
Dehaus-Mattson, Mrs Mary Carol **(SLP)**
Vig, Sheri Eder **(SLP)**

Jerome
Saroli-Taylor, Mrs Diane Antoinette **(SLP)**

Kalamazoo
Allen, Mary Kay
Asciutto, Mrs Marium Al-Oboudi
Bate, Dr Harold L **(A)**
Bodtke, Mrs Liana Shreve **(SLP)**
Burton, Patricia H **(SLP)**
Cavanaugh-Doud, Crystal **(SLP)**
Clark, Dr Michael J **(SLP)**
Cox, Cynthia A **(SLP)**
Crumpton, Teresa B **(A)**
Davis, Alvin J **(SLP A)**
Deyoung, Bonnie Marie **(SLP)**
DeZwaan, Mrs Janet **(SLP)**
Dickerson, Mrs Janet L
Dingwall, Louise L **(SLP)**
Doscher-Thompson, Mrs Gail K **(SLP)**
Dowsett, Mrs Beth Ann **(SLP)**
Erickson, Dr Robert L **(SLP)**
Glista, Sandra O **(SLP)**
Kanna, Rhoda Mae **(SLP)**
Keeler, Andrew S
Kelley, Ronald W **(SLP)**
Kerr, Victoria A **(SLP)**
Kieft, Susan D **(A)**
Kovacs, Mrs Kathleen Ann **(SLP)**
Lager, Mrs Mary Jo **(SLP)**
Lawson, Gary D **(SLP A)**
Lohr, Dr Frances E **(SLP)**
Mathews, Gwendolyn Shereese
McBratnie, Barbara P **(SLP)**
McGlasson, Mrs Peggy Adele **(SLP)**
Mountjoy, Marjorie P
Phillips, Jane Marie **(A)**
Pollens, Robin Dovitz **(SLP)**
Polmateer-McKnight, Mrs Carol R **(SLP)**
Potter, David R **(A)**
Richards, Theodora Rinck **(SLP)**
Robinson, Frank B **(SLP)**
Robinson, Dr Jane E **(SLP)**
Roesler, Mary L **(A)**
Sacks, Cheryl L **(SLP)**
Seelig, Mrs Karen S **(SLP)**
Stromsta, Courtney **(SLP A)**
Taylor, Linda Gayle **(SLP)**
Tecca, Dr John E **(A)**
Tereshinski, Mrs Michele Renee **(SLP)**
Tobochnik, Andrea Moll **(SLP)**
Trombley, Jayne S **(SLP)**
Van Riper, Dr Charles **(SLP)**
Vincent, Amy Elizabeth
Wills, Richard W **(SLP)**
Winegar, Rebecca Westra **(SLP)**
Witecki, Cindy Ann **(SLP)**

Zimmerman, Janiece C **(SLP)**

Kawkawlin
Acker, Mrs Jane M **(SLP)**
Dauer, Theresa Mae **(SLP)**

Keego Harbor
Lubbers, Dr Donald E **(A)**

Kentwood
Blumer, Janet G **(SLP)**
Brady, Carolyn C
Dodge, Mrs Diane Wood **(SLP)**
Farnham, Mrs Susan L **(SLP)**
Freese, Paula Rae **(SLP)**
McCulley, Mrs Marilyn Joy **(SLP)**
Penning, Dr Marge S **(SLP)**
Phelps, Bridgit Helene
Schuler, Susan L **(SLP)**
Vankooten, Linda K
Zimmerman, Rae **(SLP)**

Kincheloe
Bosshart, Mrs Carole **(SLP)**
Montero, Mrs Gloria B **(SLP)**

Kingsford
Pickett, Len W **(SLP)**

L'Anse
Dougovito, Mrs Elaine B **(SLP)**

Laingsburg
Cribbs, Mrs Janet L **(SLP)**

Lake Odessa
Wilson, Elma V **(SLP)**

Lake Orion
Cote, Mary Particia **(A)**
Gibbens, Noreen Daly **(A)**
Ingram, James E **(SLP)**
Murphy, Lori Lillian **(SLP)**
Presnell, Eileen Kanczak **(SLP)**
Tribbett, Beth Waite **(A)**

Lambertville
Abood, Valerie L **(SLP)**
Holbrook, Mrs Susan Marie **(SLP)**

Lansing
Bates, Mrs Kim M **(SLP)**
Bolton-Hunt, Lisa Clark **(SLP)**
Bower, Wendy Anne **(SLP)**
Bryant, Susan McPhail **(A)**
Burns, Frank R **(A)**
Clift, Tamra Ann **(SLP)**
Crecine, Mrs Kathleen B **(SLP)**
Dimon, Mrs Elise Bolen **(A)**
Esch, Barbara E **(SLP)**
Foltner, Kathy A **(A)**
Gatesy, Nancy Matthews **(SLP)**
Johnson, William M **(A)**
Katt, David F **(SLP A)**
Kragt, Cynthia A **(SLP)**
Laprad, Debra C **(SLP)**
McKenna, Lori Kay **(SLP)**
Miller, Patricia M **(SLP)**
Murray, Rosemary M **(SLP)**
Neering, Diane Towns **(A)**
Nelson, Nancy B **(A)**
Pawluk, Michael Francis **(A)**
Piirainen, Paulette **(SLP)**
Poke, Mrs Lynn Washington **(SLP)**
Ripley, Bethann Weiss **(SLP)**
Rubendunst, Mrs Marilyn L **(SLP)**
Sanders, Jeannine Meyer **(SLP)**
Simpson, Dr Thomas Henry **(A)**
Sleight, Marsha A **(SLP)**
Stewart, Catherine Yeakle **(A)**
Tait, Lorinda J **(SLP)**
Westmaas, Loralee Hamstra **(SLP)**
Wilhite, Mrs Diane R **(SLP)**
Wolf, Ann Marie

Lapeer
Chadden, Marguerite **(SLP)**
Demko, Karen L **(SLP)**

Frazee, Mrs Cathy L **(SLP)**
Jacobs, Mrs Sharon R **(SLP)**
Kelly, Mrs Nancy G D **(SLP)**
Sexton, Mrs Susan M **(SLP)**

Lathrup Village
Mullen-Lynn, Patricia A **(SLP)**

Lexington
Brooks, Mrs Jacqueline E **(SLP)**
Mitchell, Megan Anne **(SLP)**

Lincoln Park
Rauch, Rita A **(SLP)**
Remus, Ruth **(SLP)**
Sziraki, Donna **(SLP)**

Linden
Ferguson, Mrs Cheryl Lynn **(SLP)**

Linwood
Learman, Lindsay McIntyre **(SLP)**

Livonia
Cangelosi, Natalie Joan **(SLP)**
Christian, Mrs Debra A **(SLP)**
Collins, Jacqueline **(SLP)**
Douglas, Barbara Jean **(A)**
Easterbrook, Marylou Harrington **(SLP)**
Enright-Stacey, Ellen H **(SLP)**
Faulkner, Karen Young **(SLP)**
Foley, Eileen Grace **(A)**
Hartman-Brockman, M Denise **(SLP)**
Igrisan, Lori J **(SLP)**
Keefe, Mary Jo **(SLP)**
Mitchell, John C, Jr **(SLP)**
Nagle, Janice Oja **(SLP)**
Nastas, Laurie S **(A)**
O'Brien, Mrs Valerie Lee **(SLP)**
Ploch, Janice Ann C **(SLP)**
Ponte, Mrs Colleen M **(SLP)**
Restum, Dr William H **(SLP)**
Riley, Leslie Denise **(SLP)**
Smith, Mrs Suzanne Ryder **(SLP)**
Tedesco, Mrs Joni L **(A)**
Thompson, Mrs Josephine Dragan **(SLP)**
Truan, Linda M **(SLP)**
Venne, Dona P **(SLP)**
Wilson, William C **(A)**
Wolfe, Mrs Tracey Diane **(SLP)**

Lowell
Kidder, Claude K **(SLP)**
Kidder, Mrs Roselyn J **(SLP)**

Ludington
Bergman, Nikki K
Flynn-Tinsley, Nancy Elaine **(SLP)**
Rice, Teresa Denese **(SLP)**

Madison Heights
Carney-Jankoviak, Cathy Marie **(SLP)**
Downing, Kenneth N **(SLP)**
Irla, Joni **(SLP)**
Lovsin, Carol **(SLP)**
Maness, Lisa Diana **(SLP)**
Stegeman, Susan

Mancelona
Miller, Heather Neary **(SLP)**

Manchester
Billetdeaux, Mrs Laura E **(SLP)**

Manistee
Russell, Cynthia Ramsey **(SLP)**

Manistique
Davis, Russell E **(SLP)**

Marcellus
Meyers, Lynn Denise **(SLP)**

Marquette
Bradtke, Farral J **(SLP)**
Bullock, Mary Beth **(SLP)**
Davis, Dr James **(A)**
Eaton, Janice Kay **(SLP)**
Eiben, Melissa M **(SLP)**
Emerick, Lon L **(SLP)**
Ford, Mrs Patricia H **(SLP)**
Friedman, Kathryn Klein
Goodman, Mrs Linda T **(SLP)**
Hartom, Jeannine Nappe **(SLP)**
Johnson, Mrs Mary B **(SLP)**
Knuff, Mrs La Vonne **(SLP)**
Larson, Mrs Mary K **(SLP)**
Lewis-Strong, Cheryl M **(SLP)**
McClellan, Sara Greer **(SLP)**
O'Donnell, Michael B **(A)**
Rapport, Karlyn I **(SLP)**
Sirovy, Mrs Karen Lynn **(SLP)**
Smith, Mrs Barbara Berglund **(SLP)**
Smith, Dr Peter B, Jr **(SLP)**

Marshall
Edwardson, Walter John **(SLP)**
Rosko, Mrs Sue A **(SLP)**
Willis, Mrs Toni M **(SLP)**
Worde, Alfred B **(SLP)**

Marysville
Adams, Mrs Deborah A **(SLP)**

Mason
Park, Marilyn L **(SLP)**
Rabidoux, Mrs Susan W **(SLP)**
Reckell, Mrs Barbara J **(SLP)**

Mass City
Morehouse, Mrs Julie J **(SLP)**

Mattawan
Byrne, Mary Lou C **(SLP)**

Maybee
Damico, Mrs Gem E **(SLP)**

Mayville
Warren, Mary L **(SLP)**

Mecosta
Yacavone, Carol Ann **(SLP)**

Melvin
Sheridan-Schell, Patricia Louise **(SLP)**

Melvindale
Allen, Angela Raphael **(SLP)**

Menominee
Arger, Mrs Janice L **(SLP)**

Merrill
Polzin, Franklin Dow **(SLP)**

Middleville
Youngsma, Mrs Debra Schutt **(A)**

Midland
Brennan, Anne E **(SLP)**
Brinkman, Mrs Rosemary Patricia **(SLP)**
Devries, Luanne K **(SLP)**
Dunn, Mrs Valerie Strzalka
Elliott, Mrs Cheryl Walker
Evans, Mrs Karen E **(SLP)**
Griffin, Theresa M **(SLP)**
Haggerty-Paolucci, Mrs Sharla J **(A)**
Haine, Mrs Geraldine **(SLP)**
Hampton, Julie Anne **(SLP)**
Jackson, Mrs Lorraine Mae
Leahy, Mrs Jane Dennis **(SLP)**
Lorden, Jill B **(A)**
Meyers, Mrs Barbara J **(SLP)**
Morgan, Terry A **(SLP)**
Parkhurst, Mrs Connie H **(A)**
Petrini, Mary E T **(SLP)**
Ringle-Bartels, Janet E **(SLP)**
Robert, Mrs Carolyn A **(SLP)**
Roe, Barbara W **(SLP)**
Rothman, Mrs Ann R **(SLP)**
Story, Mrs Tamara Beazell **(SLP)**
Volk, Barbara Berger **(SLP)**
Ward, Thomas G **(SLP)**
Weeks, Sally J Bain **(SLP)**
Williams, Lisa S **(SLP)**

Milan
Early, Elizabeth Ann **(SLP)**
Zawacki, Mrs Julie D **(SLP)**

Milford
Burke, Veronica A **(SLP)**
Heilman, Mrs Susan N **(SLP)**
Polan, Pam L **(SLP)**
Schmitz, Mrs Carol A W **(SLP)**
Stewart, Mary Jo G **(SLP)**

Monroe
Stanifer, Mary Jo **(SLP)**

Mount Clemens
Cadaret, Mrs Sally Joan **(SLP)**
Gryzenia, Mrs Sharon S **(SLP)**
Hansen, Kristen Maria **(SLP)**
Haxer, Marc J **(SLP)**
Hegler-Jackle, Cheri L **(SLP)**
Kaczor-Czech, Bonita Marie **(SLP)**
Kelke, Dr Carl A **(A)**
Lange, Terry Ann **(SLP)**
Mackey, Maureen Jane **(SLP)**
Mandel, Rae L K **(SLP)**
Miller, Sallie Annette **(SLP)**
Pandori, Joann **(SLP)**
Reed, Marlene J **(SLP)**
Snape, Cynthia A **(SLP)**

Mount Morris
Williams, Robert Harold **(SLP A)**

Mount Pleasant
Baker, Judith Diane **(A)**
Black, Mrs Nancy Strainic **(SLP)**
Brandell, Mary E **(SLP)**
Church, Dr Gerald T **(A)**
Coughlin, Suzanne Sobaski **(SLP)**
Faust, Geralyn Marie **(SLP)**
Fenlason, Catherine D **(SLP)**
Fisher, Valerie Jean **(SLP)**
Grasel, Theresa C **(SLP)**
Hughes, Diana L **(SLP)**
Huston, Leona M **(SLP)**
Hutchison, Donna M **(SLP)**
Kipfmueller, Dr Leo J **(SLP)**
Kopin, Sr Marie **(SLP)**
Lutz, Mrs Carolyn Louise **(SLP)**
Martineau, Deborah R **(SLP)**
McLauchlin, Dr Robert M **(SLP A)**
Nerbonne, Dr Michael A **(A)**
Poynor, Robert E **(SLP)**
Stanford, Linda Seestedt **(A)**
Swartz, Dr Bradford L **(SLP)**
Sweeney, Lynn A **(SLP)**
Tatchell, Dr Renny Hemsley **(SLP)**
Watson, Marie May **(SLP)**
Wittkopp, Jane E **(SLP)**

Munising
Schlicher, Karen S **(SLP)**

Muskegon
Andary, Diane Kelly **(SLP)**
Armstrong, Mrs Karen Marie **(SLP)**
Bancroft, Robert L **(SLP A)**
Egyed-Schultz, Glyce A **(A)**
Ellis, Susan Kay **(A)**
Frarey, Shawn Evans **(SLP)**
Geller, Nancy Josephine **(SLP)**
George, Linda Ann **(SLP)**
Gorbach, Penelope J **(SLP)**
Kane, Debra S **(SLP)**
Kolb, Maxine Angel **(SLP)**
Quarto, Nick J **(SLP)**
Reed, Penelope D **(SLP)**
Rogalla, Leonard T **(SLP)**
Shank, Sandra J
Sokoly, MD Judith Gootjes **(SLP)**
Vledder, Gayle Lynn **(SLP)**
Wurtz, Judy R **(SLP)**

New Baltimore
Fabian, Shari L **(SLP)**

New Boston
Niswonger, Donna L **(SLP)**

New Buffalo
Marshall, Luan F **(SLP)**
Mrozek, Nancy J **(SLP)**

New Era
Budzenski, Mrs Donna E B **(SLP)**

Newberry
Anderson, Mrs Caroline A **(SLP)**
Hermann, Gregory Paul **(SLP)**
Maki, Mrs Paula D **(SLP)**
Sischo, Luther W **(SLP)**

Niles
Henderson, Mrs Leslie Jones
Nelson, Dr Nickola W **(SLP)**
Todd, Nancy A **(SLP)**

North Muskegon
Clark, Mrs Dawn M **(SLP)**
Phelps, Laura Beth **(A)**

Northville
Barry, Marianne B **(SLP)**
Coleman, Lynne **(A)**
Crotteau, Mary Catherine **(SLP)**
Damron, Nancy Ann **(A)**
Dimambro, Mrs Laurie Anne
Gay, Mrs Yvonne Louise **(SLP)**
Grainer, Mrs Kathleen Shpiece **(SLP)**
Harmer, Mrs Sandra L **(SLP)**
Kelly, Mrs Chris-Anne **(SLP)**
Klinkhamer, Luci H **(SLP)**
Kochans, Joyce B **(SLP)**
Kroll, Susan Faye **(SLP)**
Krupic, Kathryn Lynn **(SLP)**
Lockwood, Elizabeth Loring
Mason, Molly Ann **(SLP)**
Perrine, Mrs Linda Rouhan **(SLP)**
Siman, Dr Robin K **(SLP)**
Simon, Candace A **(SLP)**
Stuart, Carolyn M **(SLP)**
Tapp, Mrs Susan R **(SLP)**
Trybus-Worniak, Mrs Paula M **(SLP)**
Whitehead, Lisa M **(SLP)**

Novi
Beaton, Mrs Susan L **(A)**
Conn, Mrs Julie W G **(SLP)**
Dunham, Dr Judy K
Gregory, Janis A **(SLP)**
Levinger, Bonnie Kwasman **(SLP)**
Pagano, Janice Ameen **(SLP)**
Quine, Doris Meacham **(SLP)**
Shevin-Finck, Eileen Carol **(A)**
Tinetti, Mrs Susan Marie **(SLP)**

Oak Park
Bazell, Cindy Lynn **(A)**
Blount, Sharon Alexis **(SLP)**
Hoze, Brenda Joyce **(SLP)**
Lasson, Sheryl R
Rothman, Mrs Ralle K **(SLP A)**
White, Donna S **(SLP)**

Okemos
Anderson, Gloria M **(SLP)**
Cooke, Dr Paul Alan **(SLP)**
Hatfield, Mrs Mary Lou **(SLP)**
Lepoire, Mrs Deborah J **(SLP)**
Leroi, Mrs Ellen S **(A)**
Loose, Dr Frances F
Murphy, Patricia **(SLP)**
Rosen, Gale Goodman **(SLP)**
Rysberg, Mrs Linda M **(SLP)**
Smith, Annette M **(SLP A)**
Smith, Nancy S **(SLP)**
Turnbull-Norton, Carol A **(SLP)**
Walsh, Dr Patricia S **(SLP)**

Orchard Lake
Bassin, Mrs Randee Levick **(SLP)**
Brukoff, Mrs Bonnie L **(SLP)**
Herman, Mrs Joyce **(SLP)**

Seitzman, Sheila D **(SLP)**
Selden, Beverly L **(SLP)**

Oscoda
Weyenberg, Debra J **(SLP)**

Otsego
Nebel, Cheryl Lehr **(SLP)**

Owosso
Lea, Mrs Sue Ellen **(SLP)**
Lincoln, Joyce Marie **(SLP)**
Parker, Hugh G **(SLP)**
Spencer, Mary E J **(SLP)**

Oxford
Gepner, Rebecca S **(SLP)**
Nauseda, Bonnie F **(A)**

Parchment
Mulford, Nicki M **(A)**

Paw Paw
Oas, Mrs Donna Billington **(SLP)**

Pentwater
Heidelberger, Tina E **(SLP)**

Perry
Schultz, Susan Schaner **(SLP)**

Petersburg
Kaires, Patti Lee **(A)**

Petoskey
Griffin, Michael W **(SLP)**
Koskus, Dr Michael W **(A)**
Sarosi, Mrs Nancy G P **(SLP)**

Pigeon
Brown, Carol Jean **(SLP)**

Pinckney
Langford, Mrs Ann L **(SLP)**

Plainwell
Goy, John Michael **(A)**

Pleasant Ridge
Archer, Susan E **(A)**
Chaput, Patricia Ann **(SLP)**

Plymouth
Beedle-Johnson, Debra Leah **(SLP)**
Cashin, Janice M **(A)**
Collop, Kathy Marie
Davies, Janet Barbara **(SLP)**
Dillon, Terese Marie **(SLP)**
Ferens, Mrs Donna J
Freels, Dale **(SLP A)**
Jetchick, Jeannie Marie **(SLP)**
Magnani, Nancy M **(SLP)**
Mallow, Pamela Ann **(SLP)**
Page, Dr Edwin R **(SLP)**
Schmidt, John H **(SLP)**
Souders, Kimberly Jenine **(SLP)**
Yoas, Mrs Christine Begthel **(A)**
Zaksek, Mrs Lorraine **(SLP)**

Pontiac
Blasingame, Mrs Kelly **(SLP)**
Duffy, Mrs Nancy Hagle **(SLP)**
Fontanive, Dr Lynn **(A)**
Frazier, Dr Larry A **(A)**
Knittel, Mary Ann Lyon **(A)**
Koonter, Martha M **(SLP)**
Munro, Betsy Craig **(SLP)**
Richard-Edwards, Deborah A **(A)**
Robertson, Mary Lu **(SLP)**
Thomas, Mrs Debra F **(SLP)**
Towns, Barbara Schulte **(SLP)**
Voelker, Mrs Evelyn G **(SLP A)**
Winton-Holland, Alice **(A)**

Port Huron
Buchanan, Denise M **(SLP)**
Currie, Kathleen M **(SLP)**
Koglin, Diane Campoli **(A)**
Prause, Mrs Jacqueline **(SLP)**
Spiess, Mrs Gwen H **(SLP)**

Towler, Mary Johnson **(SLP)**
Zastrow, Sharon Jean **(A)**

Portage
Brown, Mrs Logan L **(SLP)**
Cornelius-Randt, Mrs Tamara J **(SLP)**
Hillenbrand, Kathryn L **(SLP)**
Hurd, Mrs Kathy Ann **(SLP)**
Pierson, Joanne Marttila **(SLP)**
Pyke, Mrs Arlene May **(SLP)**
Saddler, Karen B **(SLP)**
Warner, Candis M **(SLP)**
Wiener, Iris F

Redford
Diacono, Lori Kay **(SLP)**
Fernandez-Soberal, Ana V **(SLP)**
Millard, Sidney Ann **(SLP)**

Reed City
Tarr, Dena M **(SLP)**

Reford
Piette, Sharon Louise **(SLP)**

Richland
Anderson, Patricia Anne **(SLP)**
Boersma, Mrs Susan K **(A)**
Hunt, Mrs Mary Ida **(SLP)**
Lavene, Mrs Phyllis L **(SLP)**

Riverview
Carlson, Connie C **(A)**
Chase, Christina Cheryl **(SLP)**

Rochester
Byle, Larry J **(A)**
Carpenter, Mrs Janice Lynn **(SLP)**
Cummings, Mrs Marlene Rayner **(SLP)**
Englehart, Mrs Catherine **(SLP)**
Even, Mrs Helen H **(SLP)**
Froeman, Dr Gerald G **(SLP)**
Joswiak, Laura Marie **(SLP)**
Krebs, Mary Ann P **(SLP)**
Manetta-Lawson, Margaret A **(SLP)**
Quinette, Karen Sue **(SLP)**
Sidor, Paula M **(SLP)**
Smith, Patricia S **(SLP)**
Stonestreet, Dr Ruth H **(SLP)**
Swift, Dr Carol **(SLP)**
Teachworth, Jill P **(SLP)**
Young, Denise M **(SLP)**

Rochester Hills
Burke, Mrs Christie Lynn **(SLP)**
Childs, Mrs Phyllis **(SLP A)**
Christina, Mrs Margaret **(SLP)**
Darcy-Campbell, Karen **(SLP)**
DeVreugd, Paul E **(SLP)**
Formanczyk, Karen M **(SLP)**
Frankovich, Mary Jo **(A)**
Greve, Mrs Nancy L J
Hartman, Mrs Jane D **(SLP)**
Lagrant, Margaret A **(SLP)**
Lindstrom, Mrs Kathryn S **(A)**
Shunk, Mrs Laurel Sue **(SLP)**
Simpson, Leslie A

Rockford
Gilewski, Mrs Suzanne Eardley
Hendricks, Betsy A **(SLP)**
Lisenbee, Catherine **(A)**
Mabie, Denise Ann **(SLP)**
Mayerik, Mrs Christine Annette **(SLP)**
Peterson-Combs, Mary E **(A)**
Romanow, Judith Lynn **(SLP)**

Romeo
Berlin, Donna Susan **(A)**
Kerrigan, Ann H **(SLP)**
Materna, Mary E **(SLP)**
Rose, Darryl R **(SLP)**
Youatt, Amy Elizabeth **(A)**

Romulus
Van Demark, Dr Ann A **(SLP)**

Roscommon
Eva, Michael L **(SLP)**
Murray, Jeanette E **(SLP)**

Roseville
Cosentino, Cathy A
McNelis, Mrs Linda Marie **(SLP)**
Prytula, Sandra Joanne **(A)**

Royal Oak
Allen, Doris Virginia
Beauregard, Barbara Ann **(SLP)**
Bolton, Maureen Talbot **(SLP)**
Chudej, Mrs Mary M **(SLP)**
Clarke, Stacey Lynn **(SLP)**
Crowe, Mrs Carol **(SLP)**
Deman, Jill Susan **(SLP)**
Duchene, Charlene A **(SLP)**
Fairchild, Janet M **(SLP)**
Finan, Colleen Marie **(A)**
Fouchey, Susan Kay **(SLP)**
Goff, Carole L **(SLP)**
Graham, Fatin A **(A)**
Grande, Mrs Anne Pinkerton **(SLP)**
Jacques, Jeanette Marie **(SLP)**
Jakubiak, Dawn Marie **(SLP)**
Jepsen, Mrs Maureen McGowan **(SLP)**
Kaufman, Nancy R **(SLP)**
Kiefer, Julie A **(SLP)**
Pianin, Alissa M **(A)**
Rhein, Alice Laster **(SLP)**
Rolnick, Dr Michael I **(SLP)**
Russell-Marquard, Erin Marie
Sheehan, Eileen Marie **(SLP)**
Swain, Joan Kasabach **(SLP)**
Ziebarth, Brenda Earlene **(SLP)**

Saginaw
Bell, Bert H **(SLP)**
Coone, Mrs Lori K **(SLP)**
Davey, Mrs Joan L **(SLP)**
Hare, Dr Gary **(A)**
Horny, Mrs Anita Louise **(SLP)**
Lutey, James Christophe **(SLP)**
Malone, Michael J **(A)**
Malott, Mrs Celeste Marie **(SLP)**
Mejeur, Mrs Judy L **(SLP)**
Mikolaski, Martha Ann **(A)**
Riedel, Mrs Barbara **(SLP)**
Schillio, Mrs Vivian Burness **(SLP)**
Smith, Mrs Michele Elizabeth **(SLP)**
Sommerville, Dr Suzanne **(A)**
Steih, Mrs Gail Marie **(SLP)**
Thorne, Roger Paul **(SLP)**
Waldbillig-Gunn, Mrs Jamee **(SLP)**
Wegner, Mrs Mary A Bosinski **(SLP)**
Wrege, Gail Lynn

Saline
Huelsberg, Susan R **(SLP)**
McClure, Pamela Sue **(SLP)**
Robinson, Kathleen **(SLP)**

Sandusky
Goddard, Deborah Crawford **(SLP)**

Sanford
Krauklis, Mrs Rita H **(SLP)**

Sault Sainte Marie
Henne, Joseph F **(A)**

Scotts
Hanley, Dr John M **(SLP)**
Hosken, Ann E **(SLP)**

Shaftsburg
Giebink, Lisa Kim **(SLP)**

Shepherd
Pufpaff, Marcia Ward **(SLP)**
Weddington, Gail L **(SLP A)**

South Lyon
Elick-Wolyniak, Mrs Katherine L **(SLP)**
Martin, Colleen Marie **(A)**

South Rockwood
Rillston, Mrs Mary J **(SLP)**

Southfield
Aaron, Sheryl A **(SLP)**
Adler, Dr Raphael **(SLP)**
Beckerman, Lynn P **(SLP)**
Bigham, Artan **(SLP)**
Braslaw, Mrs Michele D
Brown, Marcie V **(A)**
Carlson, Mrs Susan Ellen **(SLP)**
Chelst, Dr Tamy S **(SLP A)**
Clark, Mrs Raynell Brown **(SLP)**
Cook, Mrs Rita Spiller **(SLP)**
Coursen, Judith Denenberg **(A)**
Daitch-Dell, Suzanne Beth **(SLP)**
Edelstein, Esther K **(SLP)**
Fairbrother, Ellen J **(SLP)**
Finck, Mrs Jo Anne M **(A)**
Fishman, Arlene T
Goldsmith, Howard D **(SLP)**
Gutmann, Sharon Deborah **(SLP)**
Halpern, Barbara J **(SLP)**
Helman, Lori Dee **(SLP)**
Howard, Mrs Mary Ann **(SLP)**
Kanar, Fay Carol **(SLP)**
Klein, Leah Abigail **(A)**
Kligman, Mrs Audrey **(SLP)**
Leiser, Rosalind P **(A)**
Long, Helen J **(A)**
Mandell, Dr Theodore **(SLP)**
Marchildon, Claudia E **(SLP)**
Marcotte, Mrs Sally B **(A)**
Marcus, Mrs April Came **(SLP)**
Marlow, Mrs Lisa Burnett **(A)**
Merritt, Judith A **(SLP)**
Millman, Mrs Arlene **(SLP)**
Millstone, Eileen M **(SLP)**
Mobley, Mrs Patricia A **(SLP)**
Neumann, Brenda T **(SLP)**
Northway, Nancy Ann **(A)**
Novetsky, Paula Rosner **(A)**
Peterson, Rochelle C **(SLP)**
Rives, Cheryl R **(SLP)**
Rosen, Robert Gerald **(SLP)**
Salomon, Joanna L **(SLP)**
Seffinger, Debra **(SLP)**
Soffin, Bonnie S **(A)**
Sprague, Linda L **(A)**
Stein, Dr Leon **(A)**
Turek, Kathleen **(SLP)**
Usner, Jean M
Viedrah, Beverly G **(SLP)**
Wayburn, Mrs Laura P **(SLP)**
Weeks, Joyce Marie **(SLP)**

Southgate
Everett, Mrs Sue Thayer **(SLP)**
Szubeczak, Leslie A **(SLP)**

Spring Lake
Kauffman, Mrs Cynthia A **(SLP)**
McBeth, Mrs Gloria J **(SLP)**
Smits, Mrs Millicent **(SLP)**
Spyker, Margaret Mary **(SLP)**
Walsh, Daniel J **(SLP)**

St Charles
Kitchen, Mrs Linda L R **(SLP)**

St Clair
Beier, Pamela Marie **(A)**

St Clair Shores
Beich, Diane L **(SLP)**
Bloch, Mrs Nancy Masnado **(SLP)**
Burman, Mrs Brenda J **(SLP)**
Curtis, Ruth **(SLP)**
Duker, Gail S **(SLP)**
Fonville-Mitchell, Mrs Dianne Lyn **(SLP)**
Furest, Mrs Eileen Kerrigan **(SLP)**
Hausler, Walter E **(SLP)**
Pangori, Mrs Theresa Michele **(SLP)**
Pistono, Dr Kathleen Susan
Schmanski, Karen M **(SLP)**

Seitz, Mrs Gail Metta **(SLP)**
St Pierre, Karrie A **(SLP)**

St Ignace
Hawkins, Mrs Grace Morreale

St Johns
Drumwright, Mrs Cynthia Dodson **(A)**
Nemcik, Lawrence E **(SLP)**
Sandahl, Maureen Darin **(SLP)**
Schafer, Mrs Linda M **(SLP)**

St Joseph
Buckman, Mrs Gwenda P **(SLP)**
Franceschini, Thomas G **(SLP)**
Jonatzke, Mary Elizabeth
Kasewurm, Mrs Gyl Ann **(A)**
Miller, Mrs Renee S **(SLP)**
Powley, Carl E **(A)**
Reigle, Carol A **(SLP)**
Scharrer, Breena Lynn **(A)**
Smit, Beth G **(SLP)**
Willmeng, Jane A **(SLP)**
Zick, Mrs Autumn W **(SLP)**

St Louis
Cassidy-Goffnett, Mrs Mary Ellen **(SLP)**
Connaughton, Kathryn Bernice **(SLP)**
Thiemkey, Mrs Roberta **(SLP)**

Sterling Heights
Bugli, Mrs Terri Lynn **(SLP)**
Campion, Mrs Lori Ann **(SLP)**
Capoferi, Laurie Kyle **(SLP)**
Couchenour, Laurie Ann **(SLP)**
Delisle, Colleen Ann **(A)**
Fish, Mrs Marianne MacHala **(SLP)**
Gerbino, Thomas C **(A)**
Hennessey, Carolyn A **(SLP)**
Hogan-Henk, Christine J **(SLP)**
Kewak, Debra Lynn
Klump, Margaret A **(A)**
Krol, Mrs Mary Chambers **(SLP)**
Loman, Mrs Renee Coleen **(SLP)**
Mellis, Eugenia **(SLP)**
Mucci, Mrs Kathleen A **(SLP)**
Pape, Mrs Theresa Bender **(SLP)**
Pfalzgraf, Beth **(SLP)**
Segel, Cheri Buck **(SLP)**
Segel, Mitchell **(SLP)**
Steck, Mrs Rosemary A **(SLP)**
Zech, Mrs Karen Pappas **(SLP)**

Stevensville
Perry, Dennis Robert **(SLP)**
Perry, Mrs Donna Marie **(SLP)**
Spencer, Kathleen Mary **(SLP)**

Stockbridge
Bickerstaff, Mrs Jane Hanneman
Hickox, Sharon Kay **(A)**

Swartz Creek
Lake, Constance Ann **(SLP)**

Tawas City
Huck, Mrs Nancy E **(A)**

Taylor
Blair, Rebecca Lucille **(A)**
Charney, Elaine Ann **(SLP)**
Jaffe, Robert **(SLP)**
Korman, Darlene Marie **(SLP)**
Koschnitzke, Carol D **(SLP)**
Powell, Kathleen A **(SLP)**

Tecumseh
Da Silva, Mrs Virginia G **(SLP)**
Spillman, Denise Ann **(SLP)**

Temperance
Scheuerman, Sandi L **(SLP)**
Simon, Mrs Lisa McKay **(SLP)**
Warns, Deborah S **(SLP)**

Three Rivers
Kittredge, Deborah Luff **(SLP)**
Kleidon, Mrs Brenda K **(SLP)**

McLeod, Mrs Dara B **(SLP)**

Traverse City
Bearup, Patricia H **(SLP)**
Bevan, Dr Marlene A **(A)**
Braidwood, Lynne A **(SLP)**
Clyde, Mrs Connie Marie
Cope, Sharon Leah **(SLP)**
Friedlander, David Gerald, Jr **(SLP)**
Gleason, Carol Lyon **(SLP)**
Keyes, Carynne A **(SLP)**
Kinnish, Kathleen Monica **(SLP)**
Laird, Ralph F **(SLP)**
McPhee-Van Hevel, Judith A **(SLP)**
Monroe, Mrs Cindy M F **(SLP)**
Olney, Charlotte Anne
Parker, Mrs Suzanne H **(SLP)**
Smith, Norbert E **(A)**
Solomonson, Barbara Ann **(SLP)**
Spencer, Mrs Rena Elizabeth **(SLP)**
Warner, Mrs Susan P **(SLP)**
Wellman, Robin Lynn **(A)**
Wilsens, Paul C **(A)**
Yancho, Dee Ann **(A)**

Trenton
Arsenault, Michael Dennis **(A)**
Arsenault, Patricia Ann **(A)**
Fortuna-Roy, Mrs Patricia Kay **(SLP)**
Howey, Mrs Karla Buschle **(SLP)**
Korany, Mrs Dielynda Sue
Seal, Mrs Sharon B **(A)**
Wiggle, Linda Lee **(SLP)**
Zalewski, Karen S **(SLP)**

Troy
Athans, Olga **(SLP)**
Bakonyi, Susan Marie **(SLP)**
Bardsley, Mrs Karen L **(SLP)**
Bessell, Laura Anne **(SLP)**
Brady, Laura Loraine **(A)**
Brennan, Mrs Carol Resch **(SLP)**
Charchian, Martha M **(SLP)**
Cole, Dr Richard M
Coster, Mrs Judy L **(SLP)**
Davee, Veralyn T **(A)**
Dehem, Cynthia S **(SLP)**
Delong, Mrs Sally Ann **(A)**
Fike, Mrs Suzanne R **(SLP)**
Foster, Mrs Karen L **(SLP)**
Frank, Mrs Judith Lein **(SLP)**
Gray-Hoffman, Mrs Karen **(SLP)**
Hampton, Mrs Suzanne R **(SLP)**
Hodgdon, Mrs Linda Q **(SLP)**
Johnson, Mrs Mary Blaine **(SLP)**
Kahn, Mrs Denise J **(SLP)**
Kurtz, Mrs Connie JoAnn **(SLP)**
Miller, Catherine Ann
Palmer, Mrs Lorraine M **(SLP)**
Paul, Robert L **(A)**
Regan, Jeanette N **(SLP)**
Rizzo, Wendy Suzanne **(A)**
Runyan, Mrs Kathryn A **(SLP)**
Schlager, Mrs Sandra **(SLP)**
Schmitz, Mrs Judy C **(SLP)**
Stamos-Bushey, Elizabeth **(SLP)**
Sterling, Gail R **(A)**
Swartz, Susan R **(SLP)**
Sysko, Linda M W **(SLP)**
Taylor, Mary Ann **(SLP)**
Tierney, Elizabeth **(SLP)**
Weslosky, Therese P **(SLP)**
Wicka, Mrs Donna K **(SLP)**

Twining
Morgan, Michele M **(SLP)**

Union Lake
Deters, Mrs Christina Flynn **(SLP)**
Hengtgen, Sharon Wolfram **(SLP)**
Stempien, Mrs Theresa L **(SLP)**
Tonkovich, Susana M **(SLP)**

Utica
Fudold, Karen Marie

Hendricks, Mary L **(SLP)**
Knight, Karen F **(SLP)**
Megel, Mary J **(SLP)**
O'Hara, Daniel S **(A)**
Quinn, Mrs Joanne S **(SLP)**
Winkel, Julie Ann **(SLP)**

Vassar
Gast, Linda Sue **(SLP)**
Guthrie, Mrs Roxann A **(SLP)**
Merry-Aranyos, Mrs Elizabeth Jane

Vicksburg
Braat, Mrs Dortha Buchtel
Garvey, Lynelle Bailey

Walled Lake
Hug, Gerald August **(A)**

Warren
Bennefield, Mrs Susan Carol **(SLP)**
Caramagno, Mrs Leslie Marie **(SLP)**
Charron, Deanne M
Cook, Timothy Paul
Cortright, Mrs Joan E M **(SLP)**
Laraia, Karen Marie **(SLP)**
McCornack, Mrs Mariann W **(SLP)**
Molloy, Janet Lynn **(SLP)**
Santoro, Mary Anne **(A)**
Schlaman, Suzanne Marie
Vanderwaerden, Theresa Rose **(SLP)**

Washington
Baran, Judith M **(SLP)**
Koleda, Carolyn M **(SLP)**

Waterford
Norbury, Aaron William **(SLP)**

Wayland
Pittelkow, Lynne Hebert **(SLP)**

Wayne
Anderson, Robert H N **(SLP)**
Tomala, Mary P **(SLP)**

Webberville
Forbord, Mrs Janis L **(A)**

Wells
Barron, Mrs Sara Elizabeth **(SLP)**

West Bloomfield
Bank, Mrs Nancy **(SLP)**
Bloom, Dr Richard M **(SLP)**
Bouchard, Dr Kenneth R **(A)**
Debrincat, Mrs Geraldine **(SLP)**
Dedinas, Anthony S **(A)**
Engel, Mrs Helen L **(SLP)**
Fishkind-Faber, Mrs Toby G **(SLP)**
Freund, Mrs Judith Garber **(SLP)**
Fried, Mrs Janis E Sattler **(SLP)**
Garber, Sandra L **(SLP)**
Gillum, Dr Linda H **(SLP)**
Gonik, Andrea Shumaker **(SLP)**
Holcman, Mrs Janis F **(SLP)**
Horn, Mrs Julie Bloom **(SLP)**
Jacobs, Linda A **(SLP)**
Keramedjian, Lisa **(SLP)**
Kitain, Mrs Sonia S **(SLP)**
Klein, Cynthia F **(SLP)**
Krainen, Gordon **(SLP)**
Lax, Linda Sue **(SLP)**
Lipson, Mrs Joni Freed **(SLP)**
Lopatin, Nina S **(A)**
Meach, Mrs Barbara S **(SLP)**
Miller, Mrs Pamela Crowe **(SLP)**
Pesick, Paul I **(SLP)**
Ritter, Mrs Juliann V **(SLP)**
Root, Karen L **(A)**
Rosenthal, Mrs Laurie Shcolnek **(SLP)**
Salesin, Mrs Susan S **(SLP)**
Schwartz, Gail E **(SLP)**
Scott, Kathleen L **(SLP)**
Serrano-Flaisher, Mrs Enid **(SLP)**
Siegel, Mrs Heather B **(SLP)**

Westland
Bengel, Mrs Patricia Ellen **(SLP)**
Bixler, Ralph W **(SLP)**
Farran, Mary Zimmerman **(SLP)**
Gerlach, Mrs Maureen Kay **(SLP)**
Gomrick, Denise Elaine **(SLP)**
Gregory, Karen Sue **(SLP)**
Lohman, Mrs Tricia M
Ostrosky, Mrs Pamela Ann **(SLP)**
Samet, Julie B **(SLP)**
Shonce, Jan Doughty **(SLP)**
Swiecki, Tamara Ann **(SLP)**
Vasiloff, Richard M **(SLP)**

Westphalia
Peterson-Schroeder, Dr Janet M **(SLP)**

Whitehall
Dombrowski, Jane E O **(SLP)**

Williamsburg
Schnurr, Ruth Glesne **(SLP)**
White, Mrs Anne La Fave **(SLP)**

Williamston
Finelli, Alexandra **(SLP)**
Krino, Mrs Susan F **(SLP)**
Kuhn, Janeen G **(SLP)**
Minard, Nora Ann
Wagenknecht, Mrs Amy S **(SLP)**

Wixom
Deighton, Mrs Karen McQuade **(SLP)**
Lund, Mary Melissa **(SLP)**
Maziarz, Jennifer Lynn

Woodhaven
Pytel, Mrs Linda Lee-Kolasa **(SLP)**
Starll, Steven **(SLP)**

Wyoming
Cron, Mrs Marla Coulton **(SLP)**
Damore, Gina Marie
Dettloff, Mrs Julie Greenop **(SLP)**
Evans, Nancy K
Kraak, Christie L **(SLP)**
Middleton, Tammy Louise **(SLP)**
Potrykus, Rebecca A
Shumway, Sally Louise **(SLP)**

Ypsilanti
Barr, Lynn H **(SLP)**
Brown, Jennifer L **(SLP)**
Brown, Lauretha V
Clinton, Arlene M **(A)**
Crittendon, Anne Marie C
Davis, Mrs Sharon **(SLP)**
Erby, Rosalyn F **(SLP)**
Gabe, Dr Kathleen M **(A)**
Galli, Mrs Claudia S **(SLP)**
Galli, Danny, Jr **(SLP)**
Gitre, Mrs Carol Ann
Gitterman, Susan L **(A)**
Kenney, Katherine Mary **(SLP)**
Klein, Mrs Deanna Lynne **(SLP)**
Koski, Mrs Sandra Jennings **(SLP)**
Mosher, Robert A **(A)**
Norman, Laurie Ann **(SLP)**
Palmer, David E **(SLP)**
Quinn, Dr Kathleen S **(SLP A)**
Rupp, Dr Ralph R **(SLP A)**
Schall, Cheryl Castellana
Smith, K Roger **(A)**
Standish, Claire Ann **(A)**
Walley, Joy Brandt **(SLP)**
Wells, Mrs Cindia Kinney **(SLP)**
Weston, Debra Cantey **(SLP)**
Ziolkowski, Lori J **(SLP)**
Zukowski, Glenna J **(SLP)**

MINNESOTA

Albert Lea
Bryson, Elizabeth Ann **(SLP)**
Erickson, Mrs Bonnie Rae O **(SLP)**

Linn, Debra R

Alexandria
Forster, Mrs Cynthia Knoll **(SLP)**
Forster, Thomas Paul **(SLP)**
Lange, Ruth Anne **(SLP)**
Schurmann, Deborah Jean **(SLP)**
Thunselle, Mary Lou **(SLP)**
Walter, Mrs Jody L M
Walz, Michelle Marian

Andover
Custer, Kathryn K **(SLP)**
Holm, Ann Czajka **(SLP)**
Iserman, Blake F **(A)**
Iserman, Mrs Joan K **(SLP)**

Anoka
Krull, Mrs Alice M **(SLP)**
La Due, Mrs Cecilia M **(SLP)**
Larock, Mrs Beatrice B **(SLP)**
Parker, Mrs Beverly **(SLP)**
Wick, Diane J **(SLP)**

Apple Valley
Gleim, Mrs Eileen A **(SLP)**
Grissom, Mrs Susan J H **(SLP)**
Jensen, Mrs Debra Cyd **(SLP A)**
Poepping, Mrs Kathleen Marie **(SLP)**
Purdy, Mrs Dianne Ella
Soderlind, Ann Hittner **(SLP)**
Wallin, Mrs Francine A **(SLP)**
Westerback, Ann Kathryn **(A)**
Wick, Sharon L **(SLP)**

Appleton
Paulson, Margaret Rose **(SLP)**

Arden Hills
Berg, Mrs Cherie Jo **(SLP)**
Ferguson, Mrs Mary Elizabeth **(SLP)**
Kespohl, Beverly J **(SLP)**
Margolis, Janet C **(SLP)**
Meneghel, Susan L **(SLP)**
Wigginton, Virginia M **(SLP)**

Aurora
Krikelas, Mrs Alma Laurila **(SLP)**

Austin
Blaser, Joy O **(SLP)**
Gullickson, Joan Michelle **(SLP)**
Ollman, Jeffrey J **(SLP)**
Reese, Scott J **(SLP)**

Becker
Hartmann-Plath, Jane Susan **(SLP)**

Bemidji
Asper, Nancy Jo **(SLP)**
Fisher, Lee I **(SLP A)**
Geddes, Roger Charles **(SLP)**
Halcrow, Jeanette Van Camp **(SLP)**
Johansen, Anna Lee **(SLP)**
Oja, Gregory Lawton **(A)**
Olson, Mrs Joan Abrahamson **(SLP)**
Peterson, Deborah Ann **(SLP)**
Swedburg, Julie Siggelkow
Williams, Mrs Kim Marie **(SLP)**

Benson
Moorse, Mrs Deborah L **(SLP)**

Blaine
Baldwin, Ann M **(SLP)**
Heisterkamp, Jean Christiansen **(SLP)**
Vonasek, Denise Wamre **(SLP)**

Bloomington
Ambroe, Mary H **(SLP)**
Bartsh, Lorrie Lynette **(SLP)**
Becker, Mary T **(SLP)**
Berman, Julie Seibert **(SLP)**
Dileo, Mrs Elizabeth Kirby **(A)**
Engel, Michelle Lea **(SLP)**
Gault, Lynda M **(SLP)**
Johnson, Nancy Ellen **(SLP)**
Kaynatma, Martha Janecky **(SLP)**
Lindgren, John H **(SLP)**
Luke, Charlene M
Olson, Mary Christine **(SLP)**
Pehringer, James L **(A)**
Ryder, Joyce P **(SLP)**
Sayler, Sherri Lynn **(A)**
Schaub, Dr Janette M **(SLP)**
Strand-Janicek, Mrs Michele Darlene **(SLP)**
Wipperling, Kathryn M **(SLP)**

Blue Earth
Boos, Mrs Kay Turbett **(SLP)**
Gerdts, Marlin W **(SLP)**

Brainerd
Bartels, Charles E **(SLP)**

Britt
Jacklen, Kathleen Ann **(A)**

Brooklyn Center
Arnott, Mrs Lora Lynn **(SLP)**
Haugen, Kathleen **(SLP)**
Mathieu, Ardie E **(SLP)**

Brooklyn Park
Boever, Anne E **(SLP)**
Bradshaw, Clive Robert
Cleland, Sally B **(SLP)**
Deja, Patricia Ann **(SLP)**
Lanctot, Virginia L **(SLP)**
Neis, Kimberly Kae
Piette, Catherine Mary **(SLP)**
Strohfus, Brenda Kay **(SLP)**

Buffalo
Cassady, Bonnie Lee
Harnois, Karmen Hanson
Lindeman, Janet M **(A)**

Buhl
Kayfes, Mareve **(SLP)**

Burnsville
Appleby, Mrs Maribelle F **(SLP)**
Besser, Joyce A T **(SLP)**
Bluth, Yvonne F **(SLP)**
Counters, Thomas A **(A)**
Crock, Janet Lynn **(A)**
Fancher, Candis R **(SLP)**
Gallaher, Mrs Wendy J **(SLP)**
Graber, Mrs Adele A **(SLP)**
Hanson, Mrs Judith Lynn **(SLP)**
Kenefick, Kimberly Lindell **(SLP)**
Kothe, James Donald **(A)**
Kothe, Sylvia Lynn **(A)**
Peterson, Theodore L **(SLP)**
Reynolds, Dean E **(SLP)**
Segriff, Carla Helene **(A)**
Shelquist, Darleen M **(SLP)**
Stein, Mrs Cheryl Stern **(SLP)**
Swanhorst, Lisa Carole **(SLP)**
Szczeck, Jeanne Larkin **(SLP)**
Zirbel, Jennifer Joan **(SLP)**

Byron
Breneman, Alyce I **(A)**
Haselhorst, Mrs Susan Santema **(SLP)**
Walker, Mrs Gail M **(SLP)**

Cambridge
Slabaugh, Gerri K **(SLP)**

Cannon Falls
Sandquist, Mrs Mary Anne **(SLP)**

Canyon
See, Lavonne E **(SLP)**

Center City
Halbach, Rita Mary **(SLP)**
Westman, Martha J **(SLP)**

Centerville
Knockel, Mrs Brenda Renee **(SLP)**
Sullivan, Mrs Wendy Sue **(SLP)**

Champlin
Knourek, Marge Ann **(SLP)**
Wahlquist, Mrs Tracey Noelruchti **(SLP)**

Chanhassen
Brown, Mrs Diane Lynn **(A)**
Estrem, Theresa Serbus **(SLP)**
Peterson, Teri Kaminski **(SLP)**

Chaska
Kochenash, Mrs Susan D **(SLP)**
Schepers, Christine M **(SLP)**

Circle Pines
Penner, Dr Sharon Gail **(SLP)**

Clear Lake
Commers, Barbara Elaine **(SLP)**
Weise, Mrs Mary T **(SLP)**

Clearwater
Mork-Adix, Delores Arlene **(SLP)**

Cokato
Nelson, Howard D **(SLP)**

Columbia Heights
Paulson, Mrs Christine Ellen **(SLP)**

Comfrey
Torabi, Mrs Elaine E **(SLP)**

Coon Rapids
Adamski, Mrs Jeanette Johnson **(SLP)**
Albus, Marianne L **(SLP)**
Anderson, Ann L **(SLP)**
Belpedio, Katherine Elizabeth **(SLP)**
Lider, Barbara R **(SLP)**
Litecky, Mrs Rene Dubois **(SLP)**
Marquardt, Valerie Anne **(SLP)**
Mlinar, Theresa Patricia **(SLP)**
Pasek, Mrs Jill H
Reiners, Cheryl Joy **(SLP)**
Schee, Jon Erik **(A)**
Scheid, Sandra Lee **(SLP)**
Woit, Ellen M **(SLP)**

Corcoran
Arntson, Mrs Rachel M **(SLP)**
Carney, Mrs Jeanne Arnell **(SLP)**

Cottage Grove
Cory, Mrs Miriam E **(SLP)**
Love, Mrs Susan Odegaard
Rogers, Carla Jean **(SLP)**

Cotton
Maher, Roger Lee **(SLP)**

Crystal
Baldwin, Linda Mae **(SLP)**
Hagen, Mary E **(SLP)**

Deephaven
Viehweg, Elizabeth R **(SLP)**

Deerwood
Cousins, Mrs Gayle R **(A)**

Detroit Lakes
Heitmann, Mrs Marceda **(SLP)**
Lamb, Mrs Mary Londergan **(SLP)**
Shoemaker, Jeffrey R **(SLP)**

Dilworth
Lockrem, Mrs Tracey MaryEllen

Duluth
Allie, Kathleen Marie **(SLP)**
Betz, Susan E **(SLP)**
Bjorkman, Karen D **(SLP)**
Brungardt, Mrs Kristie Rae **(SLP)**
Burns, Gail Ann **(SLP)**
Burress, Bruce E **(A)**
Burress, Kathleen J **(SLP)**
Bussa, Denise Wetherille **(SLP)**
Everett, Mary K **(SLP)**
Friedman, Pacy **(SLP A)**
Gatlin, Tamara Anne **(SLP)**
Glynn, Christine Alice **(SLP)**
Goldfarb, Elizabeth Jane **(SLP)**
Gustafson, Mrs Kathy Ann Peterson **(SLP)**
Hanning, Luella M
Hatten, Dr John T **(SLP)**
Hawk, Dr Ash M **(SLP)**
Hougas, Wayne W **(A)**
John, Mrs Lynda Barker
Johnson, Cheryl Mae **(SLP)**
Johnson, Kathryn Ann-Hagen **(SLP)**
Johnson, Mrs Susan Hilburn
Jung, Mrs Cynthia Farkas **(A)**
Komarek, Rachel Ann **(SLP)**
Landin-Bohbot, Deborah Pears **(A)**
Levar, Lavonne **(SLP)**
Loven, Dr Faith C **(A)**
Melander, Laura B **(SLP)**
Miller, Judith A **(SLP)**
Mizuko, Dr Mark I **(SLP A)**
Newton, Patricia **(SLP)**
Pappas, Dr Nicholas James
Pierce, Robert F **(SLP)**
Polson, Mrs Kathryn E **(SLP)**
Renier, Michelle P
Rosenzweig, Betsy J **(SLP)**
Ryks, Joan Gilbertson
Sandness, Mrs Beret S **(SLP)**
Sazama, Carol Lee Repensky **(SLP)**
Spillers, Dr Cindy S **(SLP)**
Stauffer, Regis Jean **(SLP)**
Stromquist, Dagmar T **(SLP)**
Torfin, Deanna Janine **(SLP)**
Vierima, Carol A **(A)**
Voss, John H **(A)**

Dundas
Dierksen, Carol A **(SLP)**

Eagan
Barth, Tami Feland **(SLP)**
Bryant, Mrs Mary Kay **(SLP)**
Deans, Nancy C **(SLP)**
Galloway, Dawn Renee **(A)**
Hamilton, Laura Hinderer **(SLP)**
Heino, Jean Marie **(SLP)**
Lesiecki, William **(A)**
Maesaka, Michele Lynn **(SLP)**
McCool, Mrs Patti J **(SLP)**
Pearson, Mrs Marilyn M **(SLP)**
Roberts, Mrs Nancy Kaye **(SLP)**
Slanina-Orfei, Caroline Frances **(SLP)**
Snyder, Mrs Denise Nelson **(SLP)**
Trzcinski, Marie G **(SLP)**
Willand-Adams, Jennifer **(SLP)**
Wilson, Karen Ashton **(SLP)**

Eden Prairie
Anderson, Pamela J **(SLP)**
Branum, Mrs Anne Chandler **(SLP)**
Braun, Jeri Brynildson **(SLP)**
Des Lauriers, Dione Marie **(SLP)**
Eakle, Mrs Mary Jo **(SLP)**
Johnson, Mrs Bonnie F **(SLP)**
Korb, Mrs Loree Vivatson **(SLP)**
Marth, Mrs Suzanne S **(A)**
Okonek, Barbara J S **(A)**
Olson, Susan Hewitt **(SLP)**
Olson-Thomsen, Margaret **(SLP)**
Raskind, Linda Ann **(A)**
Satorhelyi, Mrs Donna Gail **(A)**
Vass, William K **(A)**
Volkert, Kristin Kay

Edina
Arenson, Mrs Diane K **(SLP)**
Bigham, Mrs Dona E **(SLP)**
Brown, Mrs Joan Moede **(SLP)**
Brown, Richard K **(A)**
Carlson, Carol H **(SLP)**
Davis, Mrs Ann M **(SLP)**
Doyle, Mrs Shirley S **(SLP)**
Doyle, Dr Timothy N **(A)**
Goergen, Sharon Ann **(SLP)**
Hagen, Kathryn J **(SLP)**
Kundel, Dr Karl J **(A)**
Laukka, Suzanne Mary **(SLP)**
Leibman, Joyce A **(SLP)**
Noonan, Mrs Mary Beth **(SLP)**

Stone, Charles R **(A)**

Elk River
Goetsch, Melinda K **(SLP)**
Haugen, Mrs Michelle Ann **(SLP)**
Marsh, Janice Ruth **(SLP)**

Esko
Johnson-Russell, Vickie **(SLP)**

Eveleth
Oliver, Kathryn Venaas **(SLP)**
Oliver, William C **(SLP)**
Wilson, Leane Michele **(SLP)**

Excelsior
Boo, Meredith L **(SLP)**
Hawley, Claudia D **(A)**
Mar, Margaret A **(SLP)**
Thomas, Mrs Patricia B **(SLP)**

Fairmont
Stein, Mrs Jacqueline A **(SLP)**

Faribault
Anderson, Samira B **(A)**
Bullock, Craig W **(SLP)**
Rice, Pat M **(A)**
Sommers, Nancy Henrikson **(SLP)**

Farmington
Otness, Shirley M **(SLP)**

Fergus Falls
Adams, Virginia S **(SLP)**
Gunderson, Gerald D **(SLP)**
Hoekstra, Lowell J **(SLP)**
Johnson, Judith Ann **(SLP)**
Johnson, Mrs Mary Kay
Matter, Dr Linda S **(SLP)**
Moen, Christine Spece **(SLP)**
Sanderson, Paul Daniel **(A)**

Fertile
Moore, Mrs Myrna Fladeland **(SLP)**

Fisher
Flaat, Kathryn Gay **(SLP)**

Forest Lake
Harris, Mrs Ann Mary
Koehler, Sheree Lynn **(SLP)**
Newman, Donald D **(SLP)**
Raarup, Beth Bellgowan **(SLP)**

Fridley
Bonine, Louann Marie **(SLP)**
Ekegren, Corinne A **(SLP)**
Gerdin, Mrs Meredith A **(SLP)**
Goran, Kristin A **(SLP)**
Sticha, Lee Ann **(SLP)**
Wahlstrom, Diane J **(SLP)**
White, Lois D **(SLP)**

Glencoe
Larsen, Janell Marie **(SLP)**
Theis, Marsha Ann **(SLP)**

Golden Valley
Aggen, Carol J **(SLP)**
Beck, William Gregory **(A)**
Berg, Kristi **(SLP)**
Ecklund, Sally Kay **(SLP)**
Frank, Marla T **(SLP)**
Lebow, Mrs Katherine **(SLP)**
Luker, Janice K **(SLP)**
Polikowsky, Ann Wennblom **(SLP)**
Raver, Mrs Cynthia Litman **(A)**
Wasylkewycz, Marta Lydia **(SLP)**
Wensman, Debra K **(SLP)**
Zagzebski, Mrs Mary Jean **(SLP)**

Gonvick
Nielsen, Kris T **(SLP)**

Grand Rapids
Bounds, Mrs Suzanne L **(SLP)**
Crea, Raymond John **(SLP)**
Lemahieu, Thomas William **(SLP)**
Sayward, Catherine

Granite Falls
Diebold, Rene **(SLP)**

Ham Lake
Glowacki, Mrs Connie Sangren

Hastings
Tennessen, Marilyn K **(SLP)**
Toppin, Cynthia J **(SLP)**

Hibbing
Daniels, Mrs Lynn Ann **(SLP)**

Hopkins
Allen, Sonia Rodriguez **(A)**
Bushey, Mrs Tahirih Rose
Fehst, Dr Christine **(SLP)**
Locker, Mrs Christine **(SLP)**
Olson, Cindy L **(A)**

Hugo
Gallagher, Diane Elmquist **(SLP)**

Hutchinson
Schulstad, Lorie Jean **(SLP)**

Inver Grove Heights
Carter, Jane Hicks **(SLP)**
Torvinen, Lisa C **(SLP)**

Kandiyohi
Depetro, William A **(SLP)**

La Crescent
Jones, Ernest I **(SLP A)**
Welscher, Carmen A **(SLP)**

Lake Elmo
Lay, Jacqueline **(SLP)**
Lorence, Karen Carr **(SLP)**
Nelson, Mrs Joy Kiersted **(SLP)**

Lake Park
Ronken, Mrs Donna M Ongalo **(SLP)**

Lakeland
Cunico, Lucille A **(SLP)**

Lakeville
Berberet, Mrs Susan Buss **(SLP)**
Grothe, Teresa Harrington **(SLP)**
Harris, MaryJane B **(SLP)**
Larsen, Mrs Kay **(SLP)**
McElmurry, John David **(A)**
Shiplett, Mrs Laura J **(A)**

Le Center
Schmidt, Catherine **(SLP)**

Lindstrom
OeltjenbrunsLindblad, Patricia Ann **(SLP)**

Litchfield
Johnson, Mrs Kimberly Ann **(SLP)**
Lewis, Mrs Judith Kay **(SLP)**
Nicholson, Sandra E **(SLP)**

Little Canada
Belf, Lee A **(A)**
Runa-Hencley, Mrs Cynthia **(SLP)**

Little Falls
Fox, James M **(SLP)**
Schoepf, Thomas J **(SLP)**

Long Lake
Boentgen, Mrs Rae **(SLP)**
Englund, Bette Visgar **(SLP)**
Ruprecht, Audrey J **(SLP)**
Wood, Mrs Martha S **(SLP)**

Madison
Brehmer, Ann Kathryn **(A)**

Mahtomedi
Johnson, Randall Kent **(SLP)**
Marion, Lori Marie **(A)**
Neff, Richard Wayne **(A)**

Mankato
Arndt, Mrs Kristine K **(SLP)**
Asthana, Mrs Pamela Sulochini
Baughn, Helen **(SLP)**
Birbeck, Dr Herbert E
Brooks, Dr Robert S **(SLP)**
Johnson, Karen Ann **(A)**
Mordue, Mrs Lavella Y **(SLP)**
Paquin, Roger Lyle **(SLP)**
Pedersen, Sharon L **(A)**
Poole, Ronald D **(A)**
Seppmann, Jody Lee **(SLP)**
Sheran, Christina Pietro **(SLP)**
Stevens, Susan M **(SLP)**

Mantorville
Pederson, Mrs Deborah A **(SLP)**

Maple Grove
Alvig, Kathleen **(SLP)**
Anderson, Coleen P **(SLP)**
Anderson, Vicki M **(SLP A)**
Bieber, Karen M **(SLP)**
Bonato, Mary M **(SLP)**
Gauthier, Mrs Gertrude **(SLP A)**
Irwin, Sandra Sue **(SLP)**
Kaldor, Mrs Cindy O **(SLP)**
Magsam, Loren A **(SLP)**
Maher, Mrs Elaine Dubois **(SLP)**
Marohn, Mrs Judith Riley **(SLP)**
Olson, Mrs Alice Jane **(SLP)**
Peel, Gretchen L **(SLP)**
Revling-Kreb, Roberta A **(SLP)**
Roth, Dr Carole R **(SLP)**

Mapleton
Nienow, Patricia M **(SLP)**
Vaubel, Ann W **(A)**

Maplewood
Ryberg, Wendy Sue **(SLP)**
Sommers, Tami Jo **(SLP)**
Webb, Mrs Mary Susan **(SLP)**

Marine St Croix
Lennes, Mrs Karna **(SLP)**

Marshall
Grong, Linda Stewart **(SLP A)**
Summers, Mrs Mary **(SLP)**

Melrose
Prax, Mary Louise **(SLP)**
Zehrer, Mary Battaglia **(SLP)**

Menahga
Holzworth, Mrs Annamae **(SLP)**

Mendota Heights
Carl, Mrs Suzanne C **(SLP)**
Fabian, Mrs Frances L **(SLP)**
Gollinger, Mrs Deirdre L
Nichols, Jill H **(SLP)**
Slobof, Maxine S **(SLP)**
Wirt, Linda Sanford **(SLP)**

Milan
Anderson, Shirley Mae **(A)**

Milrose
Nelson, Kimberly Wood **(SLP)**

Minneapolis
Adams, Mrs Ruth W **(SLP)**
Argetsinger, Elaine **(SLP)**
Balog, Katherine Marie
Barbatsis, D Lynne **(A)**
Barnes, Cherise Crozier **(SLP)**
Bathke, Robert E **(SLP)**
Berg, Janet Beth **(SLP)**
Berntsen, Jilayne Susan **(SLP)**
Biller, Ann Elizabeth **(SLP)**
Bol, Susan Hanson **(SLP)**
Brandt, Jane Ann **(SLP)**
Briesemeister, Mrs Karen Ruth **(SLP)**
Broen, Dr Patricia A **(SLP)**
Brookshire, Dr Robert H **(SLP)**
Brooks-James, Ossie **(SLP)**
Burdick, Eleanor W **(A)**
Carlstrom, Jane E **(A)**
Chandler-Rosenblatt, Cheryl Gay **(SLP)**
Cirrin, Dr Frank M **(SLP)**
Cohen, Mrs Lillian K **(SLP)**
Cooley, Mary Josephine **(SLP A)**
Cooper, Martha A **(SLP)**
Dahlquist, Lois H **(SLP)**
Dobran, Esther Mindy **(SLP)**
Doughman, Sheril L **(SLP)**
Dunn, Laurie Ann **(SLP)**
Engen, Mary Everson **(SLP)**
Evans, Barbara Liston **(SLP)**
Farr-Petterson, Abigail L **(SLP)**
Feinstein, Mrs Susan C **(A)**
Fenske, Kay Annette **(SLP)**
Freeman, Janet Gumprich **(SLP)**
Fried, Joy Michele **(SLP)**
Friedman, Barbara Jo **(A)**
Froehlich, Elizabeth O **(SLP)**
Garrison, Mrs Mary E M **(SLP)**
Gatten, Joy Marie **(SLP)**
Geiger, Mrs Kristen L **(SLP)**
Gorski, Sally Majetich **(SLP)**
Goulett, Diane M **(SLP)**
Gower, Kathy J G **(SLP)**
Grider, Robert B **(SLP)**
Gross, Gloria R **(A)**
Hafner, Mrs Teresa Dreyer **(SLP)**
Halverson, Mrs Lisa Anne **(SLP)**
Halvorson, Julia M **(SLP)**
Haroldson, Samuel K **(SLP)**
Hartman, J L **(A)**
Haug, Mrs Kathleen Liljemark **(SLP)**
Hawkins, Kristine J **(SLP)**
Hempe, Deidre Marie **(SLP)**
Henderson, Carol A **(SLP)**
Henrikson, Ernest H **(SLP)**
Herr, Laura Renee **(A)**
Hickey, Kathleen M **(A)**
Hildebrandt, Jane Kastner **(SLP)**
Hinderscheit, Linda R **(SLP)**
Hoistad, Mrs Kathleen Slick **(SLP)**
Horn, Mrs Jane H **(SLP A)**
Imhoff, Karen L **(SLP)**
Jaquith, Mrs Barbara A **(SLP)**
Johnson, David Warren **(A)**
Johnson, Iris E **(A)**
Johnson, Mrs Jody A **(SLP)**
Johnson, Michael G **(SLP)**
Johnson, Mrs Nancy Jean **(SLP)**
Karsh, Abbie Jean **(SLP)**
Kephart, Maggie B **(SLP)**
Kimball, Roberta R **(SLP)**
Klosterman, Julie A **(A)**
Knoblauch, Elizabeth Renee **(SLP)**
Knutson, Andrea J **(SLP)**
Kornov, James J **(SLP)**
Kosek, Steven **(SLP)**
Kozan, Anita L **(SLP)**
Krieger, Mrs Dorothy H **(SLP)**
La Luzerne, Dawn Marie **(SLP)**
Lassman, Dr Frank M **(SLP A)**
Laven, Frances J **(SLP)**
Leighton, Kellie Ann **(SLP)**
Lester, Karen Sue **(SLP)**
Linde, Diane Marie **(SLP)**
Lunda, Todd A **(A)**
Lynch, Teresa Ryan **(SLP)**
MacDonald, Catherine **(SLP)**
Maclosek, Rae Ann **(SLP)**
Maj, Jennifer Rea **(SLP)**
Manthie, Mrs Martha A **(SLP)**
Margolis, Dr Robert H **(A)**
Marrinan, Diane Margaret **(A)**
Marsala, Penelope D **(A)**
Marshall-Thoreen, Janet S **(SLP)**
Martin, Dr Richard R **(SLP)**
McCarty, Patricia A **(SLP)**
McDermott, Dr Richard P **(SLP)**
McLaughlin, Colleen Marie **(SLP)**
McMonigal, Lizabeth J **(SLP)**
Mickelson, Mrs Carol Mohan **(SLP)**
Molck-Ude, Roberta **(SLP)**
Montelibano, Michelle Burg **(SLP)**

Mueller, Rita J **(A)**
Nelson, Dr David A
Nelson, Mrs Kerri Rykal **(A)**
Nicholas, Linda Elmore **(SLP)**
Nispel, Cheri L **(SLP)**
Nitzke, Anne E **(SLP)**
Ojakangas, Catherine Lee **(SLP)**
Ouren, Mary J **(SLP)**
Oxman, Emily K **(SLP)**
Palmberg, Colleen Marie **(SLP)**
Pilcher, Beverly Michele **(SLP)**
Porrazzo, Shirley **(SLP)**
Preminger, Jill **(A)**
Prettner, Laurie K **(A)**
Ptak, Lori Avends **(SLP)**
Rankovic, Christine Marie **(A)**
Ratelle, Constance Briscoe **(SLP)**
Reece, Joann M **(SLP)**
Reece, Richard E **(SLP)**
Rogers, Donna B G **(SLP)**
Rosenblatt, Michael P **(A)**
Rowland, Mrs M Annette **(SLP)**
Rutherford, Berneice R **(SLP)**
Scheller, Mrs Lorrie Drake **(A)**
Schirber, Carol M **(A)**
Schloff, Mary J
Schnoebelen, Judy Shackman **(SLP)**
Schumacher, James Gregory **(SLP)**
Schwake, Mrs Eileen M **(SLP)**
Schwarzrock, Lorraine **(SLP)**
Scipior, Joan Marie **(SLP)**
Selb, Louise Kathryn **(SLP)**
Sellars, Carole A **(SLP)**
Seltz, Ann Eleanor **(A)**
Siegel, Dr Gerald M
Sigelman, Joye A **(A)**
Slater, Mary E **(A)**
Smayling, Mrs Lyda M **(SLP)**
Smolak, Lisa Hunter **(A)**
Sommerville, Patricia J **(SLP)**
Spates, Eleanor F
Starr, Dr Clark D **(SLP)**
Storti, Dr Susan **(SLP)**
Strait, Marcia M **(SLP)**
Strickland, Elizabeth Ann **(A)**
Struck, Richard E **(A)**
Sullivan, Michael Patrick **(SLP)**
Telleen, Pamela Sue **(SLP)**
Templin, Dr Mildred C **(SLP)**
van Deusen, Diana Jean **(A)**
Van Thorre, Mrs Candace B **(SLP)**
Wahoske, Patricia A **(SLP)**
Ward, Dr W Dixon
Weiland, Susan Huber **(A)**
Weiss, Kathleen M **(A)**
Welsh, John Woodford **(SLP)**
Wilms, Herbert R **(SLP)**
Wolfgang, Mrs Lorelei D **(SLP)**
Wollak, Barbara Ackermann **(SLP)**
Yanz, Michele F **(SLP)**

Minnesota City
Wobig, Terrence R **(SLP)**

Minnetonka
Bissonette, Mrs Linda L **(SLP)**
Bootsma, Jan Rasmusson **(SLP)**
Byrne, Sharon Fandrey **(SLP)**
DeMers, Mrs Gayle Hare **(SLP)**
Diachok, Kathleen M **(SLP)**
Dosen, Mrs Susan Gail **(SLP)**
Fuller, Janice S **(SLP)**
Gardner, Jacqui **(SLP)**
Hesselroth, Marcia L **(SLP)**
Kane, Joann S **(SLP)**
Levy, Mrs Mary A R **(SLP)**
Lovdahl, Ann S **(SLP)**
Magnusson, Dr Deanne L **(SLP)**
Marold, Jacqueline **(SLP)**
O'Brien, Mrs Kathleen Sue **(SLP)**
Patton, Mrs Kathryn M **(SLP)**
Raskin, Cynthia Landis **(SLP)**
Schur, Wendy Broker **(SLP)**
Toonen, Mrs Margaret S **(SLP)**
Voroba, Dr Barry **(A)**
Weinstein, Mrs Suzanne M **(SLP)**

Monticello
Crocker, Mrs Kathleen Ann
Holker, Nancy L **(A)**

Moorhead
Alm, Mrs Janice M **(SLP)**
Fortney, Molly Campbell **(A)**
Fridgen, Mrs Marvilyn Kay **(SLP)**
Gronhovd, Dr K Dale **(SLP)**
Hanson, Bruce Roy **(SLP)**
Hanson, Margaret Jean **(SLP)**
Holter, Barbara R **(SLP)**
Jons, Mrs Sarah M **(SLP)**
Kulla, Karen Kirsten
Magelky, Mrs Phyllis J **(SLP)**
McGillivray, Larae A **(SLP)**
Moyano, Mrs Anne M **(SLP)**
Schultz, Mrs Karen Marie **(SLP)**
Scott, Davis A **(SLP)**
Swanson, Marie E **(SLP)**
Teigland, Dr Arne D **(A)**
Tonn, Martin **(SLP)**
Walseth, Mrs Wanda Colleen **(SLP)**

Moose Lake
Lief, Rebecca L **(SLP)**

Morris
Stock, Sharon Nyquist **(SLP)**

Mound
Harnett, Betty W **(SLP)**
Zimdars, Mrs Judith Ann **(SLP)**

Mounds View
Enzenhauer, Mrs Sheila Barrett
Felsenfeld, Susan **(SLP)**
Matt, Mrs Doris E **(SLP)**

New Brighton
Flotten, Marcella S **(SLP)**
Frick, Mrs Lisa Faller **(SLP)**
Goepel, Judy T **(SLP)**
Schippits, Sandra Renee **(SLP)**
Thibedeau, Mrs Susan B **(SLP)**
Wallis, Mrs Kathryn D **(SLP)**

New Hope
Culhane, Colleen Ann **(SLP)**
Schumacher, Mary Martha **(SLP)**

New Richland
Bullock, Keith Eldon **(SLP)**
Hansen, James J **(SLP)**

New Ulm
Kuster, Judith Maginnis **(SLP)**
Peters, Debra N **(SLP)**
Schultz, Cynthia Bishop **(SLP)**
Wachman, Cheryl Thomson **(SLP)**

North Branch
Naggatz, Kay Lynn **(A)**

North Mankato
Hargrove, Dr Patricia Marie **(SLP)**
Mertesdorf, Donna H **(SLP)**

North Oaks
Muellerleile, Steve **(SLP)**
Murrans, Linda E **(A)**

North St Paul
Yoch, Lynne Krings **(SLP)**

Northfield
Amundson, Martha Z **(SLP)**
Day, Janice Eisma **(SLP)**
Draves, David William **(SLP)**
Gibbs, Mrs Inez G **(SLP)**
Noyes, Joanne Gislason **(SLP)**
Schnorr, John R **(SLP)**
Sorenson, Thomas A **(SLP)**
Whytlaw, Elizabeth E **(SLP)**

Northome
Kindred, Mrs Sheryl A **(SLP)**

Oakdale
Gergen, Ann Bauer **(SLP)**
Tonsager, Mary L **(SLP)**

Olden Valley
Peterson, Julie Lynn **(SLP)**

Osseo
Klitzke, Carol Ann **(SLP)**

Owatonna
Anderson, Mrs Karen Maxton **(SLP)**
Homuth, Anna K **(SLP)**
MacIntosh, Karen M **(SLP)**
Maki, Mrs Francyne A **(SLP)**

Park Rapids
Schellack, Carol B **(SLP)**

Pelican Rapids
Haugen, Stacy Jo

Pengilly
Eliason, Mrs Deborah T **(SLP)**

Pequot Lakes
Butcher, Mrs Barbara Kaufman **(SLP)**
Hoel, Richard L **(A)**

Perham
Schmitz, Mrs Nancy Wicker **(SLP)**

Pine City
Lange, Gail Larson **(SLP)**

Pipestone
Dalin, Galen E **(SLP)**

Plymouth
Anderson, Mrs Marlis E **(SLP)**
Baggett, Jewell M **(A)**
Biel, Mrs Joanne Ring **(SLP)**
Fox, Douglas E **(SLP)**
Fox, Mrs Susan E **(SLP)**
Francis, Mrs Carolyn J **(SLP)**
Goldetsky, Judy M **(SLP)**
Gray, Mrs Susan J B **(SLP)**
Grossman, Pearl G **(SLP A)**
Harmon, Mrs Lucia C **(SLP)**
Haug, Kirsten Marie **(SLP)**
Jensen, Julie Lynn **(SLP)**
Jude, Susan M **(SLP)**
Kornhauser, Debora S **(SLP)**
Lehman, Mrs Annie Laurie H **(SLP)**
Meester, Cindy Lee Dickinson **(SLP)**
Miller, Keri Ann **(SLP)**
Perlman, Eve S **(SLP)**
Polson, Cynthia Brown **(SLP)**
Rowland, Anne Bigelow **(SLP)**
Sandler, Mrs Judith A **(SLP)**
Skelly, Barbara Graves **(SLP)**
Skramstad, Mrs Mary K **(SLP)**
Thorson, Kathryn A **(A)**
Weisenburger, Carolyn M **(SLP)**
Youngdale, Paula Lynn

Princeton
Beattie, Mrs Rosanne Thubauvill **(SLP)**
Sabrowsky, Norman J **(SLP)**
Ward, Mary Frances **(SLP)**

Prior Lake
Funk, Carol Lee
Jacobson, Mrs Rebecca M **(SLP)**
Koblas, Linda Tutewohl **(A)**
Krueger, Sharon Lee **(SLP)**
Lenling, Camille M **(SLP)**

Proctor
Nordell, Christine Allen **(SLP)**
Thorson, Gwen **(SLP)**

Red Lake Falls
Erickson, Elizabeth **(SLP)**
Erickson, Keith D **(SLP)**

Red Wing
Boser, Jody G **(SLP)**
Halvorson, Alice Mae **(SLP)**
Hess, Wayne J **(SLP)**
Johnson, Mrs Pamela A **(SLP)**
Rauterkus, Mrs Mary Beth **(SLP)**

Redwood Falls
Nelson, R Elizabeth **(SLP)**

Richfield
Blum, Patricia L **(SLP)**
Bodensteiner, Carole Julia **(SLP)**
Goff, Jo Ellen Andersen **(SLP)**
Grey, Linnea R **(SLP)**
Johnson, Robin Christine **(SLP)**
McInroy, Mrs Cynthia Kay **(SLP)**
Rossman, Harry Richard **(A)**
Szykulski, Theresa Mary **(SLP)**
Thompson, Nancy Ann **(SLP)**
Tollefson, Brenda Kay **(SLP)**
Zarth, Virginia Bonde **(SLP)**

Robbinsdale
Haider, Donna M **(A)**
Hengst, Julie A **(SLP)**
Klein, Mrs Patricia L **(SLP)**
Krumm, John B **(SLP)**
Trom, Michael Gene **(SLP)**
Ziesel, Theresa Ann **(SLP)**

Rochester
Anderson, Mrs Ann Brown **(A)**
Aronson, Dr Arnold E **(SLP)**
Bauch, Chris D **(A)**
Darley, Dr Frederic L **(SLP)**
Dieter, Mrs Wendy Kay **(SLP)**
Dodge, Susan R **(SLP)**
Doenges, Mrs Karen Marie Stene **(SLP)**
Doty, Charles L **(SLP)**
Duffy, Dr Joseph R **(SLP)**
Eagen, Mrs Marla L Anderson **(SLP)**
Etzel, Mrs Tracy L
Franqui, Marisol **(A)**
Freeman, Douglas C **(A)**
Hayes, Harriet M **(SLP)**
Hedgecock, Dr Leroy D **(SLP A)**
Hill, Rowena Resnick **(SLP)**
Holt, Dennis Lavern **(SLP)**
Hunt, Mrs Barbara Ann
Kay, Melinda Harrison **(SLP)**
Keith, Robert Lee **(SLP)**
Kvols, Martha **(SLP)**
Nerison, Anne H **(SLP A)**
Olsen, Dr Wayne O **(A)**
Petersen, Daylene Patricia **(A)**
Peterson, Mrs Annamary **(A)**
Phillips, Lynn Bjork **(SLP)**
Robinette, Dr Martin S **(A)**
Rodwell, Mary C
Scardino, Virginia J **(SLP)**
Schaulis, Susan Ann **(SLP)**
Schreurs, Kevin K **(SLP A)**
Shaw, Rebecca E **(SLP)**
Stoeckel, Mrs Ruth B **(SLP)**
Sweeney, Colette M **(SLP)**
Thomas, Jack E **(SLP)**
Timmins, Garth Joseph **(A)**
Willer-Urfer, Janene **(SLP)**
Williams, Elizabeth Marie **(SLP)**
Yoss, Dr Kathe A **(SLP)**

Rosemount
Lund, Lori Ellen **(SLP)**

Roseville
Abbott, Mrs Laura Jean **(SLP)**
Bergauer, Judith H **(SLP)**
Harbison, Judith K **(SLP)**
Hinnerichs, Mrs Connie K **(SLP)**
Iwan, Susan Kelly **(SLP)**
Jacobs, Mrs Janet S **(SLP)**
Letcher-Glembo, Dr Lisa **(SLP)**
Paatalo-Nelson, Heidi E **(SLP)**
Stovall, Mrs Janice J **(SLP A)**

Sullivan, Darcy Nordquist **(SLP)**
Unterseher, Marilyn **(SLP)**
Williamson, Denise Duncan **(SLP)**

Saginaw
Sisson-Alness, Julia A **(SLP)**

Sandstone
Folkestad, Ann Elizabeth **(SLP)**

Sauk Rapids
Kuhl, Kathryn Trcka **(SLP)**
Peterson, Marty F **(A)**

Savage
Gustafson, Linda Houge **(SLP)**
Lyons, Mrs Charisse Diane **(SLP)**
Ness, Amber Cordahl **(SLP)**

Shakopee
Block, Joanne K **(SLP)**
Kirley, Mrs Mary S **(SLP)**

Shoreview
Buck, Jeanne L **(SLP)**
Dahlquist, Mrs Marcia E **(SLP)**
Hockett, Mrs Debra Cole **(SLP)**
McDaniels, Janis M **(SLP)**
McMahon, Margaret A **(SLP)**
Moller, Dr Karlind Theodore **(SLP)**
Monson, Mrs Loretta J **(SLP)**
Myers, Penelope S **(SLP)**
Shablow, Mrs Denise Conroy **(SLP)**
Thompson, Sarah G **(SLP)**
White, Therese B **(A)**

South St Paul
Biehn, Susan S **(SLP)**
Falkavage, Jean A **(A)**
Mazar, Linda Nylen
Reichle, Patti S A **(A)**

St Anthony
Kruger, Anita L **(SLP)**
Prekker, Janet Erren

St Charles
Reetz, Mrs Deborah K **(SLP)**

St Cloud
Blonigen, Mrs Julie A **(SLP)**
Busta, Mrs Julie I **(SLP)**
Carlson, Gerald A **(SLP)**
Ebert, Douglas Dwight **(SLP)**
Flakus, Theresea Marie **(SLP)**
Jacobson, Joan **(SLP A)**
Jensen, Cynthia A **(SLP)**
Kammermeier, Dr Martin A **(SLP)**
Kein, Joni Suzanne **(SLP)**
Kessler, Jodell Peterson **(SLP)**
Kloer, Cheryl N **(A)**
Larsen, Judith Persoon **(SLP)**
Larsen, Sveinar Y **(A)**
LaVoi, Dr Gerald W **(SLP)**
Munson, Leslie Jean **(SLP)**
Rolle, Mrs Jean T **(SLP)**
Schimnich, Kaye M **(SLP)**
Shirley, Mrs Maureen Kluegel **(SLP)**
Sokoloski, Danette K
Traul-Anderson, Gail N **(SLP A)**
Vachal, Melody Ann **(SLP)**
Van Overbeke, Mrs Nancy Phillips **(SLP)**
Whites, Margery M **(SLP)**

St Louis Park
Baumgarten, Deborah Susan **(SLP)**
Brown, Mrs Debra L **(SLP)**
Cartwright, Jane C **(A)**
Chargo, Steven J **(A)**
Cutler, Mrs Gayle Moyer **(SLP)**
Fox, Jennifer L **(A)**
Halter-Heifetz, Andrea
Harford, Dr Earl R **(A)**
Herrington-Hall, Barbara Lee **(SLP)**
Konikoff, Mrs Anita C **(A)**
Lefty, Dianne K **(SLP)**
Ruah, Catarina Korn **(A)**
Sievert, Amy Jo **(A)**
Ward, Alicia Ann **(SLP)**

St Paul
Adams, Judy K **(SLP)**
Armus, Sharon Roberta **(SLP)**
Baird, Deborah Gustafson **(SLP)**
Bearden-Rettger, Theresa Faye **(SLP)**
Berntsen, Harold R **(SLP)**
Bree, Loris G **(SLP)**
Brusegaard, Mrs Leann M **(SLP)**
Brust, Suzanne E **(SLP)**
Burce, Carrie Alma **(SLP)**
Busch, Cynthia R **(SLP)**
Canfield, Helen Jean **(SLP)**
Carlson, Beverly Kay **(SLP)**
Casselman, Sharon H **(SLP)**
Cheple, Mark A **(A)**
Christensen, Judith Eileen **(SLP)**
Clarke, Dr Christina **(A)**
Cox, Mrs Sharon O **(SLP)**
Crain, Thomas R
Dachtera, Linda Byrne **(SLP)**
Dauer, Kathleen E **(SLP)**
Derr, Ann C Nelson **(SLP)**
De Zelar, Lynne M **(A)**
Doroff-Johnson, Karen Lynn **(SLP)**
Drvota, Sandra I **(SLP)**
Dunn, Thomas F **(SLP)**
Durand, Paulette Ann
Emmerling-Knox, Mrs Lois
Fahnestock, Kristina Bergland **(SLP)**
Fax, Mrs Joanne Cantlon **(SLP)**
Fox, William J **(A)**
Freeman, Mrs Sheila Anne **(SLP)**
Garon, Bernard R **(SLP)**
Glaser, Mrs Rena H **(A)**
Goiffon, Joann C **(SLP)**
Greenfield, Donna G **(A)**
Harbers, Heidi M **(SLP)**
Harper, David E **(SLP)**
Harty, Particia E **(SLP)**
House, Kathleen M **(SLP)**
Humphrey, Brian D **(SLP)**
Imhoff, Susan H **(SLP)**
Johansen, Mrs Sheila Rae **(SLP)**
Johnson, Mrs Kara L **(SLP)**
Johnson, Karen Lee **(SLP)**
Johnson, Linda J **(SLP)**
Johnston, Kathleen L
Juntunen, Lynn **(SLP)**
Kestel, Lisa Marie **(SLP)**
Kiewel, Mrs Linda Lou **(SLP)**
Kinlaw, Sarah H B **(SLP)**
Kirby, Virginia M **(A)**
Kluz, Ellen L **(SLP)**
Kramer, Mrs Susan Elizabeth **(SLP)**
Lacher, Linda Lea **(SLP)**
Lewis, Mrs Nancy Shackman **(A)**
Mabbs, Linda Lu **(SLP)**
McCauley, Susanne Mary **(SLP)**
McDevitt, Mary A **(SLP)**
Oliveira, Dr Robert J
Olsen, Mrs Elizabeth Field **(SLP)**
Olson, David Ray **(SLP)**
Opsal, Cynthia R **(SLP)**
Park, Mary J **(SLP)**
Paulson, Joan Marie **(SLP)**
Paz, Christine Mary
Pearson, Judith E **(A)**
Peck, Anne Rouleau **(A)**
Pennino, John Arthur **(SLP)**
Plum, Sandra R **(SLP)**
Rankinen, Lynn M **(SLP)**
Romuld, Kathy Sue Kiewel **(SLP)**
Salmon, Rita A **(SLP)**
Schermer, Anita Dorn **(SLP)**
Schoenberg, Mrs Marlene C **(SLP)**
Scott, Lewis Henry, Jr **(SLP)**
Sexton, Janet D **(SLP)**
Sherry, Linda W **(SLP)**
Sineps, Mrs Diane Barber **(SLP)**
Slegman, Dorothy **(SLP)**
Smith, Patricia A **(SLP)**
Snyder, Mrs Jill Marie **(SLP)**
Soli, Dr Sigfrid D
Stoerzinger, Helen C **(A)**
Strom, Mary T **(SLP)**
Swanson, Eleanor **(SLP)**
Tetlie, Rebecca Rice **(SLP)**
Thole, Mrs Kim Price **(SLP)**
Tiedemann, Jayne Novotny **(SLP)**
Van Tasell, Dr Dianne J
Vegter, Candace H **(SLP)**
Vrchota, Elizabeth A **(A)**
Weber, Dr Susan **(A)**
Wertz, Mrs Florence C **(SLP)**
Westra, Susan E **(SLP)**
Widin, Dr Gregory P
Willson, Stephanie Ann
Wilson, Lee **(A)**
Wolf, Beth Ann **(SLP)**
Yanz, Dr Jerry L **(A)**

St Peter
Kallaus, Dan M **(A)**

Stacy
Moorman, Mrs Marilyn S **(SLP)**

Staples
Pipek, Merrie **(SLP)**
Scipkes, Pamela Elizabeth **(SLP)**

Stewartville
Stacy, Laurence W **(SLP)**

Stillwater
Banas, Mrs Debbie
Bauer, Mrs Laurie Marie **(SLP)**
Cannon, Linda Ann **(SLP)**
Herr, Patricia Mae E **(SLP)**
Niccum, Dr Nancy Ellen
Peters, Mrs Alice A **(SLP)**
Smith, Mrs Betty A **(SLP)**
Speaks, Dr Charles E

Thief River Falls
Enger, Janet K **(A)**

Tracy
Hicks, Naomi Jean

Vadnais Height
Bentley, Julie A **(SLP)**

Virginia
Bennetts, Mrs Genevieve Gillett **(SLP)**
Fridgen, Michael J **(A)**

Waconia
Gundlach, Marcia S **(SLP)**
Humphries, Mrs Patricia S **(SLP)**

Wadena
Johnson-Olsonk, Jeanne **(SLP)**

Wahkon
Heitschmidt, Larry Dean **(SLP)**

Waubun
LaVoy, Mrs Anita Kay **(SLP)**

Wayzata
Bailey, Mrs Annmarie Doyle **(SLP)**
Johnson, Dr Bonnie Diedrich **(SLP)**
Rigas, Lucinda Luhman

Wells
Schultz, Nancy Ruth **(SLP)**

West St Paul
Baldinger, Wendy R **(SLP)**
Hinke, Rebecca A **(SLP)**
Sershen, Elizabeth **(SLP)**
Stovall, Joan Cody **(SLP)**

White Bear Lake
Connelly, Jane Elizabeth **(A)**
Linnell, Dr Craig O **(A)**
MacKenzie, Barbara B **(A)**
Sweet, Thomas R **(SLP)**
Thompson, Virginia **(SLP)**
Tillquist, Candace Sheley **(A)**

Willmar
Johnson, Diane M **(SLP)**
Knoll, Cheryl L **(A)**
Mehmel, Mrs Norma J **(SLP)**
Ochsendorf, Mrs Karen L B **(SLP)**
Weers, Werdna E **(SLP)**

Willow River
Mikrot, Dee Ann Lynn

Windom
Gitter, Beatrice Joan
Peterson, Wayne Charles **(SLP)**

Winona
Briggs, Mrs Susan Anderson **(SLP)**
Ericksen, Todd D **(A)**
Fallenstein, Judith F **(SLP)**
Meska, Mrs Susan Boldon **(SLP)**
Thompson, Nella C **(SLP A)**

Woodbury
Hutt, Stephen Charles
Johnson, Dr Jeannette Seloover **(A)**
Kamrath, Mrs Gail C **(SLP)**
Koski, Ruby Vitalis **(SLP)**

Zumbrota
Watkins, Bonnie B **(SLP)**

MISSISSIPPI

Aberdeen
Camp, Mrs Nancy W **(SLP)**

Amory
Hall, Mrs Jan McKay **(SLP)**

Baldwyn
Bishop, Doris Lynn **(SLP)**

Bay St Louis
Benvenutti, Mrs Elizabeth **(SLP)**
Burns, William W **(SLP)**
Craig, Ava Brodie **(SLP)**
England, Dr Juliana E **(SLP)**
Lowe-Bell, Dr Sena E S **(SLP)**
Paul, Kelly S
Reinhart, Mrs Daren Deslatte **(SLP)**
Tomlinson, Mrs Joan Hough **(SLP)**

Belden
Price, Mrs Vickie H **(SLP)**

Biloxi
Balius, Mrs Andrea S **(SLP)**
Boehmer, Janet Nabozny **(SLP)**
Breeland, Mrs Nancy S **(SLP)**
Carraway, Mrs Bobbye A W **(SLP)**
Clarke, Gay Jean **(SLP)**
Hankins, Mrs Joan M **(SLP)**
Stanfield, Dr Gordon Lee **(A)**
Stoppenbach, Daniel T **(A)**
Towell, Marianne D **(A)**

Bonneville
Jumper, Mrs Eleshia Geno **(SLP)**

Brandon
Bullock, Mrs Charlene **(SLP)**
Chaudron, Donna Dellinger **(SLP)**
Leddy, Mrs Sharon F Wright **(SLP)**
May, Dr Jane V **(A)**
Mosley, Carol Ann **(SLP)**
Nesbit, Linda C **(SLP)**
North, Janice Carol

Brookhaven
Goodson, Ginger Lynette **(A)**
Ray, Beverly N **(SLP)**

Caledonia
Carrigan, Mrs Sharon **(SLP)**

Charleston
Groner, Cathy Sanders

Clarksdale
Belenchia-Huggins, Mrs Patricia Laura **(SLP)**
Burkes, Mrs Susan C **(SLP)**
Carroll, DeAnne **(A)**
Chamoun, Vivian Louise **(SLP)**
Cocke, Robin Page **(SLP)**
Gibson, Mrs Frances Lane **(SLP)**
Lavender, Mrs Celia Curcio **(SLP)**
Millis, Robert Guy **(SLP)**
Peacock, Ann C **(SLP)**
Swentkowski, Stanley M **(SLP)**
Walhood, Mrs Mary-Kate G **(SLP)**
Webster, Ann H G **(SLP)**

Cleveland
Brister, Mrs Gloria R **(SLP)**
Eley, Mrs Burnice Bailey **(SLP)**
Ouzts, Mrs Florence L **(SLP)**
Ouzts, Dr James W **(A)**
Tackett, Mrs Deborah Berry **(SLP)**

Clinton
Arnold, Dr Godfrey E
Depriest, June M
Greene, Martha Julia **(SLP)**
Holiman, Linda Hankins **(SLP)**
Johnson, Mrs Mary T Kremeyer **(SLP)**
Lu, Fang-Ling
McAlexander, Mary Lee **(A)**
Wagner, Brenda R **(SLP)**

Coldwater
Davis, Lisa D

Colombus AFB
Kovach, Pamela Gay **(SLP)**

Columbus
Akerman, Mrs Cynthia I **(SLP)**
Brown, Mrs Louise G **(SLP)**
Cattle, Sally F **(SLP)**
Dobbel-Brown, Mrs Andra L **(SLP)**
Fortenberry, Vivian Joyce **(SLP)**
Galloway, Camille C **(SLP)**
Golovin, Roselyn W **(SLP)**
Graves, Lynn Leonelli **(SLP)**
Hanners, Dr Barbara A **(A)**
Hanson, Mrs L Lynn **(SLP)**
Harmon, Mrs Michelle G **(SLP)**
Johnson, Mrs Susan N
Kerr, Linda M **(SLP)**
Leonard, Mrs Marilyn Greene **(SLP)**
Mitchell, Nancy A **(SLP)**
Revord, Marceia Joyce **(SLP)**
Townsend, Beverly J **(SLP)**

Corinth
McClamroch, Linda A **(SLP)**

Decatur
Boggan, Mrs Deborah A **(SLP)**

Drew
Thompson, Mrs Jeri L **(SLP)**

Ellisville
Whitehead, Mrs Charlotte **(SLP)**

Florence
Buller, Leisa Joy **(SLP)**

Flowood
Rush, Mrs Patricia A **(SLP A)**

Forest
Grice, Rita B **(SLP A)**

Gautier
Arnold, Mary Duncan **(A)**
Reeves, Ossie R **(SLP)**
Shaw, Mrs Marian Watts **(SLP)**

Goodman
Newton, Mrs Judy Prather **(SLP)**

Greenville
Lowe, Mrs Rebecca J **(SLP)**
Martin, Denise Marie **(SLP)**
McGregor, Mrs Crystal Higgins **(SLP)**
McRight, K Renee H **(SLP)**

Greenwood
Cook, Catherine **(SLP)**
Kimbrell, Steve Morris, Jr
Whelan, Connie R **(SLP)**

Grenada
Friday, Mrs Lisa T **(SLP)**
Garner, Mrs Mitzie A **(SLP)**
Garrick, Mrs Martha Tonos **(SLP)**
Gore, Mrs Darlene A **(SLP)**
Lawrence, Teresa Gail
Plunket, Jane M **(SLP)**

Gulfport
Ashe, Betty C **(SLP)**
Bailey, Mrs Martha Yvette **(SLP)**
Bise, Penny S **(SLP)**
Hanser, Mrs Gladys L **(SLP)**
Holcomb, Charlie McIlwain, Jr **(A)**
Layton, Mrs Carolyn D **(SLP)**
MacH, Mary Ann L **(SLP)**
Murphy, Joan F **(SLP)**
Powell, Ramona Kellie **(A)**
Price, Cynthia Lee **(SLP)**
Roberts, Mary Elizabeth **(SLP)**
Stokes, Martha A **(SLP)**
Wheeler, Mrs Nancy R **(SLP)**
Wilson, Elizabeth **(SLP)**
Wold, Dr James H **(SLP A)**

Hattiesburg
Alford, Mrs P Wynn **(A)**
Anderson, Mrs Lynn Lowe **(A)**
Boyer, Debra A **(A)**
Bradley, Dr Doris Parker **(SLP)**
Brown, Ann Thompson **(SLP)**
Buttross-Brinegar, Margaret **(SLP)**
Carlin, Dr Margaret F **(SLP A)**
Coleman, Mrs Patricia A **(SLP)**
Cornett, Mrs Daphne S **(SLP)**
Cox, Mrs Nancy L **(SLP)**
Dubard, Dr Etoile **(SLP A)**
Emrick, Sandra Catherine **(SLP)**
Farish, Olivia W **(SLP)**
Ferrell, Mrs Pamela M **(SLP)**
Keller, Dr Mildred G **(SLP A)**
Konefal, Dr Joanne **(SLP)**
Lang, Mrs Tammy T **(SLP)**
Lott, Mrs Linda M **(SLP)**
Magee, Mrs Linda B **(SLP)**
Martin, Maureen K **(SLP)**
Marx, Charles Gordon **(A)**
McClelland, Dr Keener D **(A)**
Mettler-Stephenson, Jean Marie **(SLP)**
Mullican, Megan McDaniel
Myers, Mrs Barbara Jean **(SLP)**
Myers, Mrs Betty B **(SLP)**
Myrick, Celia B **(SLP)**
New, Janie Cirlot **(SLP)**
Oshrin, Dr Stephen E **(A)**
Perry, Mrs Susan Saulters **(SLP)**
Read, Mrs C Renee Goodin
Rhodes, Lynne S **(SLP)**
Rhodes, Dr Robert C **(SLP)**
Saniga, Dr Richard D **(SLP)**
Sawyer, Mrs Diana I **(SLP)**
Schaub, Mrs Mary T **(SLP)**
Sellers, Mrs Kathryn Brabec **(A)**
Shute, Mary Julia **(SLP)**
Sofra, Mrs Brita Elina **(SLP)**
Speed, Peggy H **(SLP)**
Stevens, Sharon F **(SLP)**
Terrio, Dr Leelen M **(A)**
Woodall, Martha Pickett **(SLP)**

Hazlehurst
Daniels, Betty J **(SLP)**

Hernando
Bryant, Diane Marie S **(SLP)**

Holly Springs
Wyatt, Gwendolynn **(SLP A)**

Houston
Bowen, Brigitta P

Hurando
Buntin, Bonnie P **(SLP)**

Jackson
Bean, Melinda Joyce **(A)**
Berry, Sarah E **(SLP)**
Bradshaw, Janice F **(A)**
Callaway, Deborah **(SLP)**
Cannon, Carol L
Carruth, Letricia Louise **(SLP)**
Edwards, Mrs Lurie Ann **(SLP)**
Farmer, L Judson **(SLP A)**
Felker, Mrs Sharron S **(A)**
Ford, Karen Gay **(SLP)**
Gammel, Dr Charles L **(A)**
Griffith, Mrs Susan H **(SLP)**
Hall, Mrs Mary Ann Langford **(SLP)**
Hays, Mrs Lisa Michelle **(SLP)**
Hegwood, Mrs Merleen M **(SLP)**
Johnson, Mrs Cindy Jan **(A)**
Johnson, Margaret L **(SLP)**
Laskin, Mrs Rebecca D **(SLP)**
Linson, Mrs Linda Carol **(SLP)**
Lyon, Carolyn Kassel **(SLP)**
Malphurs, Dr Ojus, Jr **(SLP A)**
McGuffey, Mrs Annice Houston **(SLP)**
Morere, Karen L **(SLP)**
Morse, Diane M **(SLP)**
Mustain, Dr William D **(A)**
O'Leary, Georgia A **(SLP)**
Peck, Dr James E **(A)**
Pettit, Reba R **(SLP)**
Rasche, Laura Baggett **(SLP)**
Shields, Sarah E **(SLP)**
Sicard, Lisa Anne **(A)**
Sims, Dr Juanita L **(SLP)**
Slay, Matilda W **(SLP)**
Smith, Theresa A **(SLP)**
Thigpen, Mrs Carol Evangeline **(SLP)**
Turner, Mary H U **(SLP)**
Warren, Angela Dawn **(SLP)**
Washington, Dr Dora S **(SLP)**
White, Elease
Williams, Mrs Katrina Belton **(SLP)**

Kosciusko
McCoy, Mrs Patricia Helen **(SLP)**

Lauderdale
Woods, Mrs Sarah N **(SLP)**

Laurel
Allred, Mrs Penelope Graves
Coats, Mrs Sherry L **(SLP)**
Hall, Mrs Frances S **(SLP)**
Lomax, Brenda S **(SLP)**
Nowell, Kathy Jean **(SLP)**
Richert, Dr M Jeanne **(SLP)**
Thames, Mrs Anita McNeece **(SLP)**
Waguespack, Mrs Yvette R **(SLP)**

Leland
Fratesi, Regina Faye **(SLP)**

Lexington
Phillips, Mrs Kathy D **(SLP)**

Liberty
Dixon, Carol Zimmerman **(SLP)**

Long Beach
Cress, Pamela S **(SLP)**
Ganley, Dr Peter J **(SLP)**
Goshorn, Dr Edward L **(SLP A)**
Halterlein, Maria Bernadette

Louisville
Crawford, Mrs Beth **(SLP)**
Eaves, Emma L K **(SLP)**

Lucedale
Bauman-Waengler, Dr Jacqueline Ann **(SLP)**
Prill, Pamela Renae **(SLP)**

Lumberton
Kraft, Mrs Frances L **(SLP)**

Madison
Burns, Angele W **(SLP)**
Fairly, Mrs Pamela H **(SLP)**
Lamb, Mrs Lisa Guy **(SLP)**
Portera, Mrs Suzanne Haley **(SLP)**
Trotti, Melinda Ellen H **(SLP)**

Magee
Pudas, Marilynn A **(SLP)**

Magnolia
Price, Teresa Clark **(SLP)**

Marks
Scarbrough, Mrs Elizabeth **(SLP)**

McComb
Bates, Mrs Joyce W **(SLP)**
Jones, Anna L **(SLP)**
Lipscomb, Mary Winders **(SLP)**
Thompson, Edward E **(A)**

McCool
Kennedy, Glenda Lynette

Meridian
Covington, Mrs Kathy Lynn
Ferree, Mrs Ann J **(SLP)**
Gould, Trina A **(A)**
Hammack, Judy F **(A)**
McEntyre, Karen **(SLP)**
Mosley, Mrs Adrian Tureaud **(SLP)**
Nichols, Lucinda **(SLP)**
Norman, Mrs Kitzi Colbert **(SLP)**
Scott, Mrs Jacquelyn S **(SLP)**
Wimberly, Annette C **(SLP)**

Moselle
Wiltcher, Cynthia G **(SLP)**

Mount Olive
Johnston, Mrs Robin Lee **(SLP)**
Weathers, Mrs Cynthia Wade **(SLP)**

Natchez
Ayres, Mrs Ruth Young **(SLP)**
Easton, Mrs Celia Elaine **(SLP)**
Powers, Mrs Ruth M S **(SLP)**

Ocean Springs
Lucas-Alexander, Mrs Nancy **(SLP)**
McCool, Mrs Kathryn B **(SLP)**
Pittman, Jimmy D **(A)**

Okolona
Holloway, Cynthia Marie

Oxford
Atkinson, Connie G **(SLP)**
Bagwell, Cynthia L **(A)**
Bounds, Mrs Cynthia Green **(SLP)**
Chadwick, Julie Carr **(SLP)**
Cheek, Mrs Sharon G **(SLP)**
Colbert, Lisa Carol **(SLP)**
Corbin, Mrs Kim Caffey **(SLP)**
Hale, Mrs Sue T **(SLP)**
Holley, Mrs Jamie Sellers **(SLP)**
King, Janet Little **(SLP)**
Simmons, Katrina June **(SLP)**
Unverdorben, Marion **(A)**
Washington, Mrs Darlene Williams **(SLP)**
West, Judy **(SLP)**
Wylde, Dr Margaret A **(A)**

Pascagoula
Freeman, Mrs Jeanne S **(SLP)**
Lovorn, Mrs Vickey G **(SLP)**
O'Neil, Mrs Patricia M **(SLP)**
Rust, Mrs Lyann Louise **(SLP)**
Wood, Mrs Cynthia C **(SLP)**

Pass Christian
Kurbanick, Gloria **(SLP)**

Pearl
Ulrich, Sara Lynn **(SLP)**

Pelahatchie
Freeman, Cassie Lynn **(SLP)**

Petal
Cassatt-Hicks, Linda L **(SLP)**
McCrory, Mrs Barbara G **(SLP)**
Mulling, Mrs Sherry Lynne **(SLP)**

Philadelphia
Cole, Mrs Laura Stokes **(SLP)**
Trigg, Kimberly Jane

Picayune
Carver, Mrs Rachelle Lizette **(SLP)**
Hill, Mrs Joy H **(SLP)**
Keen, Mrs Janis Dyar **(SLP)**
Nunez, Mrs Kaysea Copeland **(A)**
Porter, Donna S **(SLP)**

Pontotoc
Hodge, Rickey F **(A)**
Jones, Linda G **(SLP)**
Odom, Mrs Joyce R **(SLP)**

Port Gibson
Massingill, Joyce L Lyle **(SLP)**

Purvis
Roseberry, Sherry Kay **(SLP)**

Quitman
Blackledge, Mrs Hilda A **(SLP A)**

Richton
Edwards, Mrs Claudette **(SLP)**

Ridgeland
Bryant, Maureen Ann **(SLP)**
Clay, Mrs Molly Quin **(SLP)**
Cobb, Mrs Julia Trainum **(A)**
Grantham, Leslie Alison **(SLP)**
Owen, Melanie Jean **(SLP)**
Parker-Bright, Mrs Kimberly D **(A)**
Stricker, Mrs Maureen Jones **(A)**
Worachek, Jo A **(SLP)**

Rolling Fork
Botts, Mrs Dawn Cultra **(SLP)**
Harris, Mrs Eloise Tenney
May, Mrs Helen C P **(SLP)**

Sanatorium
Barnes, Beverly Gaither **(SLP)**

Sardis
Shook, Janice Victoria
West, Mrs Deborah **(A)**

Senatobia
Skelton, Ann G **(SLP)**

Silver Creek
Hutchinson, Mrs Tracy King

Soso
Holifield, Mrs Deborah Wilson **(SLP)**

Starkville
Blackbourn, Mrs Betty N **(SLP A)**
Craig, Laurie Mandly **(SLP)**
Koenig, Mrs Brenda P **(SLP)**
Linton, Mrs Regina Dreher **(SLP)**
MacMillan, Kathleen W **(SLP)**

Sumrall
Cook, Mrs Pamela R **(SLP)**

Terry
Weaver, Mrs Emilie Jo **(SLP)**

Tupelo
Davis, Connie L **(SLP)**
Hines, Mrs Elaine L **(A)**
Johnson, Lennette Ruby
Jolly, Peggy R **(A)**
Slack, Mrs Rhonda Ivy **(SLP)**
Walker, Mrs Cherie Burge **(SLP)**
Weeks, Mrs Debra Kaye **(SLP)**

Tylertown
Stogner, Cindy Smith **(SLP)**

Union
Johnson, Mrs Denise H **(SLP)**

University
Bateman, Dr Hugh Elton **(SLP)**
Crowe, Dr Thomas A **(SLP)**
Hoops, Dr H Ray **(SLP)**
Jackson, Dr Patricia Daugherty **(A)**
Kellum, Dr Gloria Dodwell **(SLP)**
Masterson, Dr Julie J **(SLP)**
Nason, Mary Virginia **(SLP)**
Walton, Mrs Julie H **(SLP)**

Vicksburg
Cofrancesco, Mrs Deborah T **(SLP)**
George, Mrs Carol P **(SLP)**
Gerber, Mrs Christine Grace **(SLP)**
Kilgo, Deborah Cherie D **(SLP)**
Matthews, Mrs Shellie B **(SLP)**
Potter, Frances T **(SLP)**
Tyler, Tammie Rose
Wagner, Janet Resta **(SLP)**
Waring, Mrs Carolyn H **(SLP)**
Wing, Joy Chow **(SLP)**

Water Valley
McKenzie-Goodwin, Phyllis D **(SLP)**

Waveland
Lynch, Amy R **(SLP)**
Norton, Kathryn A J **(SLP)**
Wambsgans, Sal J **(A)**

Waynesboro
Britton, Shelia Ann Greene **(SLP)**
Wood, Marian Sharp **(SLP)**

West Point
Johnson, Susan Hurt **(SLP)**
O'Connor, Mrs Tommie Lou **(SLP)**

Whitfield
Power, Mrs Peggy J **(SLP)**

Yazoo City
Currie, Yolanda K **(SLP)**
Myers, Mrs Jean T **(SLP)**

MISSOURI

Affton
Griesenauer, Mrs Diane Marie **(SLP)**

Albany
Pile, Donna K Hughes **(SLP)**

Anabel
Wallace, Dr Doris Davis **(SLP)**

Arbyrd
Williams, Mrs Sonja Dean **(SLP)**

Arnold
Gault, Jennie **(SLP)**
Guess, Laurie Lee
McKeirnan, Mrs Karla K **(SLP)**
Prindiville, Rita Ann **(SLP)**

Ashland
Powell, Mrs Jeanne Marie **(SLP)**

Ava
Berger, Mrs Sue C **(SLP)**

Ballwin
Altepeter, Mrs Audrey E **(SLP)**
Andrich, Margo Louise **(SLP)**
Banford, Rhonda J **(SLP)**
Daugherty, Mrs Saundra H **(SLP)**
Fox, Mrs Carol L **(SLP)**
Guyer, Mrs Deborah Dalin **(SLP)**
Haislup, Linda J **(SLP)**
Jackson, Margaret Kathleen **(SLP)**
Jones, Carol **(A)**
Lindhorst, Suzanne L S **(SLP)**
Martin, Sandra H **(SLP)**
Mason, Dr David I **(A)**
Mason, Deborah B **(SLP)**
Meyer, Mrs Donna L **(SLP)**
Moore, Mrs Rebecca N **(SLP)**
Shay, Mrs Lynne Mason **(A)**
Watson, Patti A **(SLP)**
Whiteman, Sheryl Foust **(A)**
Wolf, Mrs Phyllis B **(SLP)**

Belton
Wyatt, Mrs Eldean Lines **(SLP)**

Bethany
Drew, Robert P **(SLP)**
Richert, Daniel R **(SLP A)**

Billings
Steinbaugh-Kristek, Jeanette Marie **(SLP)**

Blue Springs
Amick, Jeana M
Burbridge, Mrs Sherry L **(SLP)**
Duddridge, Mary Kathryn **(SLP)**
Gunderson, Mrs Teresa A W **(SLP)**
Henderson, Jana L **(SLP)**
Jones, Virginia Sue **(SLP)**
Kellison, Carol Sue **(SLP)**
Laskowski, Randy Paul **(A)**
Lee, Stephanie M
Porter, Linda I **(SLP)**
Sharp, Patricia Ann **(SLP)**
Swift-Billings, Mrs Mary **(SLP)**
Welch, Gary R **(SLP)**

Bolckow
Potter, Mrs Sallie J H **(SLP)**

Bolivar
Neill, Janet F **(SLP)**

Bonne Terre
Fischer, Allen L **(SLP)**

Boonville
Hinderer, Jeana **(SLP)**
Huff, Mrs Debra Sue **(SLP)**
Lenz, Mrs Susan Roberta **(SLP)**

Branson
Coats, Mrs Jo Anne J **(SLP)**

Brentwood
Blount, Mary Lucille **(SLP)**
Diekmann, Teri Lynn **(SLP)**
Messner, Karen Courtney **(SLP)**
Ujhelyi, Mary P **(SLP)**

Bridgeton
Carter, Tammy Lee **(SLP)**
Eppel, Mrs Jane Carol **(A)**
Hicks, Terry C **(SLP)**
Mayer, Mrs Judith H **(SLP)**
Roberts, Susan **(A)**

Butler
Whitehurse, Lisa J **(SLP)**

Camden Point
Percell, Lisa Michele **(SLP)**

Cameron
Fawkes, Mrs Suzanne A **(SLP)**

Canton
Waters, Mrs Nancy Kay **(SLP)**

Cape Girardeau
Austin, Mrs Sue Ann **(SLP)**
Brannock, Mrs Betty B **(SLP)**
Brown, Steven L **(A)**
Donnelly-Billmeyer, Mary L **(SLP)**
Eckelmann, Dorathy **(SLP)**
Hensley, Dr Leita Ballew **(SLP)**
Hoffmeister, Cheryln Kaye **(SLP)**
Hurt, Mrs Linda Marie **(A)**
Kelley, Patrick R
Kirn, Tamara Sue **(SLP)**
Le Page, Mrs Linda Theresa **(SLP)**
Long, Dr John B **(SLP A)**
McClanahan, Mrs Barbara A **(SLP)**
McLain, Mrs Judy Lynne **(SLP)**
Morgan, Mrs Donna Lynn R **(SLP)**
Rieman, Mrs Deirdre Ann **(SLP)**
Squibb, Kevin Dexter **(A)**
Swisher, Alisa Rose
Vogelsang, Dr Mary Ann Trombetta **(SLP)**

Carthage
Coffield, Eleanor **(SLP)**

Cedar Hill
Johanningmeier, Mrs Marcia Kemp **(SLP)**
Landers, Mrs Madie L **(SLP)**
Landers, Millard T

Centertown
Beyer, Norman L **(SLP A)**

Centralia
McClure-Beck, Jane A **(SLP)**

Charleston
Felker, Diana Lynn E **(SLP)**

Chesterfield
Bailey, Mrs Marie A **(SLP)**
Bartell, Carol W **(A)**
Bloomberg, Mrs Ruth M **(SLP)**
Blumenthal, Elizabeth Georgia **(SLP)**
Brown, Suzanne **(SLP)**
Buck, Christine Wahler **(SLP)**
Cohen, Mrs Kathy J **(A)**
Deckert, Mrs Linda Koehler **(SLP)**
Donohue, Sally Jo **(A)**
Dorney, Diane C **(A)**
Gustus, Mrs Christine Hilleary **(SLP)**
Hurt, Mrs Rhonda K **(SLP)**
Kiem, Tami Sue **(SLP)**
Krejci, Evelyn C **(SLP)**
Meyer, Mrs Barbara S **(SLP)**
Murphy, Mrs Nancy **(SLP)**
Murray, Mrs Kathleen A **(SLP)**
Olson, Mrs Linda Kay **(SLP)**
Ovca, Nancy H **(SLP)**
Parker, Mrs Susan M **(SLP)**
Peacock-Pearse, Mrs Mary E **(A)**
Pierce, Nancy Broo **(SLP A)**
Preuss, Mrs Kathleen M **(SLP)**
Robbins, Christine **(SLP)**
Stone, Barbara F **(SLP)**
Turner, Mrs Deborah Lynn **(SLP)**
Wilson, Mrs Courtenay Martindale **(SLP)**

Chillicothe
Dedrick, Marsha Lee **(SLP)**

Clayton
Huddart, M Susan F **(SLP)**
Johnston, Mrs Annette Plourde **(A)**
Marwit, Dr Karen L **(SLP)**
Schreiber, Dale L **(A)**
Spector, Lizabeth

Clinton
Christenson, Russell L **(SLP)**
Kimble-Smith, Carlotta **(SLP)**

Columbia
Amerman, Dr James D
Barker, Diane Shelton **(SLP)**
Bauer, Karen E **(A)**
Blanton, Mrs Mary Jacqueline **(SLP)**
Borts, Mary Wilcox **(SLP)**
Carleton, Linda Diane **(A)**
Cowherd, Mrs Ruth Karen **(SLP)**
Day, Linda Susan **(SLP)**
Dunn, Marilee G **(SLP)**
Earley, Marilyn H **(SLP)**
Ferguson, Mrs Jane W **(SLP)**
Forrester, Mrs Debora A **(SLP)**
Gillam, Dr Ronald B **(SLP)**
Ginsburg, Sharon Faubel **(SLP)**
Golden, Diane Cordry **(A)**
Harper, Mrs Judith S **(SLP)**
Hildebrand, Mrs Maurine H **(SLP)**

Hildebrand, Mrs Pamela Lea **(SLP)**
Hughley, Mrs Mary Michelle **(SLP)**
Johnston, Mrs Arlene M **(SLP)**
Karl, Mrs Belinda Louise **(SLP)**
Lamphear, Judith M **(SLP)**
Moore, Patti E **(SLP)**
Muckerman, Cynthia Bell **(SLP)**
Mullen, Sharon Fries **(SLP)**
Murphy, Mrs Janice E **(SLP)**
Myers-Schultz, Mrs Cheryl **(SLP)**
Parnell, Dr Martha M **(SLP)**
Patterson, Shirley Sue **(SLP)**
Polniak, Alan Martin **(A)**
Renner, Lisa A **(A)**
Richardson, Mrs Soundra Thomason
Riley, Mrs Lyanne **(SLP)**
Salvatore, Dr Anthony Paul **(SLP)**
Scroggs, Dana J **(SLP)**
Shariff, Kelly Bur **(SLP)**
Shumate-Houston, Mrs Stacie **(SLP)**
Silberg, Kathryn S **(SLP)**
Stephens, Mrs Jane B **(SLP A)**
Strawn, Mrs Charlotte R **(A)**
Thelin, James W **(A)**
Thelin, Sara J **(SLP)**
Trumbower, Mrs Eva Beth **(SLP)**
Webber, Patricia Jane **(A)**
Wetz, Cynthia Walsh **(SLP)**
Wiles, Dr Lora H **(A)**

Crestwood
Duckett, Mrs Barbara Ann T **(SLP)**
Newberry, Dr George W **(SLP)**

Creve Coeur
Bayer, Mrs Helen K **(SLP)**
Glovinsky, Mrs Eleanor B **(SLP)**
Keller, Mrs Susan L F **(SLP)**
Koncen, Ruth Kay **(SLP)**
Livingston, Cheryl **(SLP)**
McCann, Janet S **(SLP)**
McCartney, Mrs Jacqueline M **(SLP)**
McCarty, Mary Margaret **(SLP A)**
McGrath, Mrs Jeanne Z **(SLP)**
Preston, Mrs Janet Kowalsky **(A)**
Vertrees, Mrs Nancy Marie **(A)**
Wheeler, Jan B Kerrick **(A)**
White, Gail Jean **(SLP)**

Crystal City
Ganey, Mrs Dorothy Ann **(SLP)**

Cuba
Branson, Mrs Ann **(SLP)**

De Soto
Rumping, Mrs Jane Bles **(SLP)**

Defiance
Graves, Elaine E **(SLP)**

Des Peres
Cassin, Dr Roxanne Marie **(SLP)**
Drago, Mrs Jane Cooper **(SLP)**
Sander, Mrs Cindy Lee **(SLP)**
Sullivan, Mrs Audrey Tichacek **(SLP)**

Dexter
Lilley, Mrs Terri A C **(SLP)**

Eldon
Bond, Mrs Jennifer L **(SLP)**

Ellisville
Sumner, Jane E **(SLP)**

Eureka
Sindel, Mrs Lisa Lynn **(SLP)**

Excelsior Springs
King, Shelley L **(SLP)**
Rucker, Mrs Merrie Dee **(SLP)**
Siegel, Kim Stevens **(SLP)**

Fair Grove
Bacon, Mrs Karen Elizabeth **(SLP)**

Fairfax
Hunter, Mrs Janet L **(SLP)**

Farmington
Barnes, Mrs Charla Kaye **(SLP)**
Brown, Judith Ann **(SLP)**
Gray, Mrs Kelley Beth **(SLP)**
Sohn, Lucinda Anne **(SLP)**

Fenton
Bronnert, Lois Marie **(SLP)**
Kutz, Mrs Jane Ann Talmage **(SLP)**
McEntyre, Carol Mitchell **(SLP)**
Robison, Mrs Jan M **(SLP)**
Van De Riet, Mrs Mary Margaret **(SLP)**

Ferguson
Dixon, Rhoda Thomas **(SLP)**
Eldringhoff, Judy L **(SLP)**

Festus
Killoren, Mary Jo **(SLP)**

Florissant
Ackermann, Diane Lillian **(SLP)**
Ackermann, Lynne Marie
Brown, Mrs Claire E **(SLP)**
Carlberg, Mike Oscar **(SLP)**
Clancy, Ann Marie **(SLP)**
Clausen, Margaret A **(SLP)**
Coffey, Cynthia **(SLP)**
Cornwell, D Jeanne **(SLP)**
Elliott, Mrs Mary B **(SLP)**
Gambill, Mrs Kay L **(SLP)**
Grames, Lynn Marty **(SLP)**
Grindstaff, Mrs Barbara D **(SLP)**
Held, Donald Theodore **(SLP)**
Huneke, Mary J **(SLP)**
Jester, Mrs Deanna Kay **(SLP)**
Kocs, Diane S **(SLP)**
Neuner, Mrs Sharon A **(SLP)**
Niewoehner, Debra K **(A)**
Pike, Sheryl Kay **(SLP)**
Pinkowski, Jodi Lynne **(SLP A)**
Podleski, Jane P **(SLP)**
Scheibel, Mrs Mary C **(SLP)**
Schuster, Mrs Renee M **(SLP)**
Sisul, Leonard A **(SLP)**
Spina, Mrs Nancy Claire **(SLP)**
Streiler, Kathi **(SLP)**
Tolbert, Brenda Rodgers **(A)**
Triller, Maureen E **(SLP)**
Viviano, Mrs Karen Elizabeth
Webb, Mrs Michele E **(SLP)**
Williams, Mrs Sheryl Guda **(A)**

Forest City
Holstine, Mrs Mary Lucile **(SLP)**

Fort Leonard Wood
Larson, Arthur Francis **(A)**

Frontenac
Ragen, Lauren M **(A)**

Fulton
Bartholomy, Dr John M **(SLP)**
Bastean, Judith Ann P **(A)**

Gideon
Matson, Mrs Shari S **(SLP)**

Gladstone
Heisserer, Tina M **(SLP)**
Pace, Karmen Suzette **(SLP)**
Peterson, Jacqueline Kay **(SLP)**
Whitted, Joyce Elaine **(SLP)**

Glencoe
Chivetta, Antoninett **(SLP)**
Hendricks, Mrs Carolyn G **(SLP)**
Mercer, Mrs Linda Marie **(SLP)**

Glendale
Cady, Mrs Patricia Nash **(SLP)**
Fagan, Marcy M **(SLP)**
Ross, Mrs Rhonda E **(SLP)**

Grand Pass
Dierking, Mrs Patricia Elizabeth

Grandview
Blake, Marilu W **(SLP)**
Christensen, Mrs Diana M B **(SLP)**
Goodseal, Wilbur D **(SLP)**
Hemsath, Melissa Beth **(A)**

Greenfield
Dustman, Jami Lynne **(SLP)**

Greentop
Byrd, Mrs Lisa J **(SLP)**

Greenwood
Welsh, John W **(SLP)**

Hamilton
Alden, Judith Ann **(SLP)**
Chapman, Janet L

Hannibal
Lewis, Debra Karen **(SLP)**
Salter, Kathryn Meyer **(SLP)**
Shepherd, Carrie Lynn **(SLP)**

Hartsburg
Reznicek, Virginia L **(SLP)**
Wheeler, Karen Marie **(SLP)**

Harwood
Hazel, William O, II **(A)**

Hazelwood
Autrey, Theresa Lynn **(SLP)**
Bechtold, Janice M **(SLP)**
Becker, Helen Kay **(SLP)**
Bohannon, Donald Lee **(SLP)**
Bohannon, Mrs Melisa Wilcox **(SLP)**
Mareing, Robert J **(A)**
Wellman, Mrs Karen M **(SLP)**

Henley
Bultmann, Mrs Carole Sweeney **(SLP)**

High Ridge
Hall, Mrs Carol Jean **(SLP)**
Weber, Mrs Rosemary Feichtner **(SLP)**

Hillsboro
Wells, Mrs Sara Jane **(SLP)**

Hillsdale
Ross, Elva Ann **(SLP)**

Holts Summit
Brown, Donna U **(SLP)**

Houston
Hansen, Susan Marie **(SLP)**

Huggins
Lybyer, Mrs Mary J **(SLP)**

Iberia
Hopkins, Mrs Harriett F **(SLP)**

Imperial
Church, Mrs K L **(SLP)**
Otto, Mrs Peggie Ann **(SLP)**

Independence
Bartshe, Judy Diann **(SLP)**
Bennett, Mrs Floy L
Caccamo, Dr James M **(SLP)**
Chipman, Elizabeth Anne **(SLP)**
Foster, Marcia L **(SLP)**
Gimmarro, Patricia Lynora **(SLP)**
Griffall, John **(SLP)**
Magers, Mrs Claudia A **(SLP)**
Maloney, John B **(SLP)**
Mitchell, Willa May **(SLP)**
Morris, Mrs Cheryl A **(SLP)**
Mullies, Ronna McClanahan **(SLP)**
Readecker, Alece A **(A)**
Richards, Dorothy J **(SLP)**
Ruder, Larry Lee **(A)**
Shook, Sharon J **(SLP)**
Templeton, Lynda Kay **(SLP)**
Usrey, Tamara Lynn **(A)**
Zahner, Julianne R

Jackson
Ludwig, Dr Carol S K **(SLP)**
Schaefer, Shirley **(SLP)**

Jefferson City
Becker, Mrs Carolyn F **(SLP)**
Boechler, Julie A **(SLP)**
Doerhoff, Mrs Ruth Ann **(SLP)**
Doyne, Mrs Marcella P **(SLP)**
Ennis, Mrs Linda Jo **(SLP)**
Glascock, Mrs Mary Jane **(SLP)**
Goodding, Dr Patricia Jean **(SLP)**
Graham, Mrs Marsha G **(SLP)**
Hall, Julie T **(SLP)**
Hemphill, Mrs Sandra J **(SLP)**
Hilger, Mrs Manuela W **(SLP)**
Huhman, Evelyn Nilges **(SLP)**
Kuebler, Mrs Linda K **(SLP)**
Maclas, Lori Anne **(SLP)**
McCafferty, Mrs Mary A M **(SLP)**
Robuck, Mrs Sally J **(SLP)**
Siebert, Susan Marie
Teubner, Mrs Cathy Briscoe **(SLP)**
West, Debra A H **(SLP)**

Joplin
Arnold, Kelly Ann **(SLP)**
Barcus, Janet Sue **(SLP)**
Bohannon, Dorothy E
Coiner, Juanita L **(SLP)**
Cole, Mrs Donna I **(SLP)**
Gordon, Mrs Brenda Lee **(SLP)**
Grombka, Darlene P **(SLP)**
Hafner, Mrs Margaret S **(SLP)**
Lee, Linda L **(SLP)**
Leverett, Dr Ralph G **(SLP)**
Mullin, Cynthia M **(SLP)**
Peterson, Kimberly Jeanne
Smith, Judy G **(SLP)**
Sowder, Sharon C **(SLP)**
Stacy, Mrs Lisa Marie **(SLP)**
Wasson, Dr H Waldo **(SLP A)**

Kansas City
Allen, Mrs Evelyn Y **(SLP)**
Arndt, Patti L **(A)**
Arvin, Regina S B **(SLP)**
Bannister, Susan Marie **(SLP)**
Barco, Diana C **(SLP)**
Barron, Diana R **(SLP)**
Bayton-Langford, Angela Joann **(A)**
Bellassai, Mrs Kimberly Ann **(SLP)**
Bellerose, Betty **(SLP)**
Bennett, Mrs Virginia Gallup **(SLP)**
Brooks, Karen Bruns **(SLP)**
Brown, Sharon A **(SLP)**
Bullock-McConnell, Janna Lu **(SLP)**
Cain, James V **(A)**
Clark, Mrs Jacquelyn **(SLP)**
Cooper, Susan J **(A)**
Corbaley, John L, II **(SLP)**
Davis, DeMaris A **(SLP)**
Davis, Robert W **(SLP)**
Diaz, Elizabeth Ann **(SLP)**
Dolson, Mrs Kay Marie **(SLP)**
Easley, Kristin Mueller **(SLP)**
Engelmann, Mrs Linda A
Fishman, Sheryl L **(SLP)**
Fortune-Swartz, Mrs Lynn M **(SLP A)**
Frazier-Fuemmeler, Mrs Elizabeth Sophia **(SLP)**
Fuller, Mrs Candice T **(SLP)**
Gauer, Judith L **(SLP)**
Green, Suzanne K **(SLP)**
Grilo, Nanette Renee **(SLP)**
Hagerman, Evie J **(SLP)**
Hartung, Deedra L **(SLP)**
Hemphill, Mrs Maureen Kay **(SLP)**
Hourigan, Mrs Rebecca B **(SLP)**
Jacobsen, Dr Cynthia H **(SLP)**
Johnson, Sarah Jo **(A)**
Jouras, Nikki A **(SLP)**
Kloster-Doohan, Kristine Kay **(SLP)**
Laschkewitsch, John M **(SLP A)**

Licausi, Josephine **(SLP)**
Martin, Mrs Anita P **(SLP)**
Martucci, Mrs Julie S **(SLP)**
Maslin, Mrs Joyce L **(SLP)**
McGuire, Jane Ann **(SLP)**
McPartland, Mrs Tracy Stoecker **(SLP)**
Metzl, Dr Marilyn N **(SLP)**
Michalson, Mrs Cheryl Kay Burt **(SLP)**
Miller, John W **(A)**
Miller, Jonathan P **(A)**
Miller, M Katherine **(SLP)**
Mills, Sharyn Sapp **(SLP)**
Moore, Mrs Mary C **(SLP)**
Mos, Mrs Martha A **(SLP)**
Moses, Frances R **(SLP)**
Munkers, Mrs Linda Sue **(SLP)**
Newman, Sandra G **(SLP)**
Newton, Mrs Renee Pryor **(SLP)**
Noon, Gary C **(A)**
O'Brien, Mrs Alice Hargens **(SLP)**
O'Reagan, Margaret Mary **(SLP)**
Otsuka-Davis, Evelyn **(SLP)**
Parmely, Janet C **(A)**
Perkins, Shawna Ann **(A)**
Price, Susan Crain **(SLP)**
Ragan, Mrs Judith Logan **(SLP)**
Raycraft, Melissa Lee **(A)**
Reed, Sherry Y **(SLP)**
Renner, Mrs Sherlyn S **(SLP)**
Richards, Mrs Marilyn M **(SLP)**
Ritschl, Nancy V **(SLP)**
Robinson, Dr Donald L **(SLP)**
Salmon, Dr Shirley J **(SLP)**
Saturday-Rollet, Mrs Kelly Lynne **(SLP)**
Schaaf, Joan Annette **(A)**
Schutzel, Elizabeth A
Sheward, Douglas John **(SLP)**
Smiley, Nancy Marie **(SLP)**
Soisson, Margaret **(A)**
Solomon, Dr Linda Z **(SLP)**
Steen, Cynthia A **(A)**
Sterrett, Michael L **(A)**
Street, Brenda Brehob **(A)**
Stucky, Lynda R **(SLP)**
Sykes, Kim M **(A)**
Tillman, Patricia A **(A)**
Trullinger, Dr Richard W **(SLP)**
Waggener, Lloyd Denton **(A)**
Waggoner, Peggy Perry **(SLP)**
Wiedel, Mrs Ida M **(SLP)**
Williams, Waukita **(SLP)**
Winitz, Dr Harris **(SLP)**
Wopata, Mrs Jeri Degraff **(SLP)**
Wunder, Mrs Vicki Charna **(SLP)**
Ziller, Georgia J **(SLP)**

Kearney
Mans-Leary, Linda L **(SLP)**

Kennett
De Pew, Mrs Teresa J **(SLP)**
Niederkorn, Terry Lynn **(SLP)**
Pelts, Mrs Carol P **(SLP)**

Kirksville
Applegate, Dr John A **(SLP)**
Cochran, Dr Paula S **(SLP)**
Costello, Mrs Nancy L
Daniels, Sheila J **(SLP)**
Hall, Dr William F **(SLP)**
Hunt, Dr J Paul **(A)**
Jimenez, Patricia Gordon
Kline, Mary Barbara **(SLP)**
Maloney, Nina Belle **(SLP)**
McClanahan, Mrs Carolyn A **(SLP)**
McClelland, Dr William D **(SLP)**
McGuire, Dr Kenneth Martin **(SLP)**
Przybylski, Sandra M H **(SLP)**
Simpson, Mrs Diane Lynette **(SLP)**

Kirkwood
Anderson, Colleen **(SLP)**
Baker, Terry L **(SLP)**
Baumer, Mrs Judith E **(A)**
Brake, Kristy Lunt **(A)**
Brannon, Dr John B, Jr **(A)**
Childress, Mrs Margaret W **(SLP)**
Davis, Marilyn J **(SLP)**
Fagin, Kathleen Marie **(SLP)**
Keefe, Karen R **(SLP)**
Leeds, Sherry Ann **(SLP A)**
McHugh, Joan E M **(SLP)**
Polys, Christine Meyer **(SLP)**
Richardson, Kari Sandvig **(SLP)**
Simmons-Martin, Dr Audrey Ann **(A)**
Smeltzer, Mrs Joan E **(SLP)**
Webb, Mrs Jane C **(SLP)**
Witkowski, Paula Marie **(SLP)**

Ladue
Lumaghi, Nancy Dowd **(SLP)**

Lake St Louis
Sansted, Phyllis H **(SLP)**
Whitener, Marilyn Klopper

Lake Winnebago
Cole, Diane M **(A)**
Zellhoefer, Paul **(SLP)**
Zellhoefer, Robin L T **(SLP)**

Lancaster
Silvey, A Anne **(SLP)**

Lathrop
Coleman, Patricia A **(SLP)**

Lawson
Gardner, Diane Lynn **(SLP)**

Lebanon
Baughman, Jane Kirsten **(SLP)**
Hargrave, Mrs Elisabeth K **(SLP)**
Knowles, Russell D **(SLP)**
Tribby, Sandra Roark **(SLP)**
Welch, Connie Renee **(SLP)**

Lee's Summit
Blanchard, Shirley A **(SLP)**
Brown, Tonya Graham **(SLP)**
Cavanaugh, Cathleen Marie **(SLP)**
Ellis, Mrs Julia Reiman **(SLP)**
English, Mrs Lisa Suzanne **(SLP)**
Harris, Mrs Judith L **(SLP)**
Hogan, Claire Marie **(A)**
Marshall, Merri Lea **(SLP)**
Nelson, Colleen Ann **(SLP)**
Shrull, Sharla Sue **(SLP)**
Swift, JoAnn Arlene **(SLP)**
Thomas, Julia Mae **(SLP)**
Williamson, Mrs Dale Anne **(A)**
Willis, M Anthony **(SLP)**
Willis, Mrs Michelle S **(SLP)**
Wiss, Debra Ann **(A)**

Lee's Summitt
Grote, Mrs Beth Ann **(SLP)**
Gutekunst, Mrs Cheryl Lee **(SLP)**
Hanson, Joanne Alness **(SLP)**
Lawrence, Mrs Wanda Sue **(SLP)**
McKee, Mrs Dianne Kay **(SLP)**
Nichols, Mrs Lisa K
Pennington, Mrs Patricia Louise **(SLP)**

Lexington
Jenkins, Mrs Donna L **(SLP)**

Liberty
McNair, Mrs Kay M **(SLP)**
Russell, Jamie Sue **(SLP)**
Stefanini, Mrs Sally Butler **(SLP)**
Vaught, Cheryl Sue **(A)**

Linneus
Ledbetter, Mrs Jane Frances **(SLP)**

Lockwood
Kahre, Mrs Vina Maureen **(SLP)**

Lutesville
McFarland, Mrs Alice Anne

Manchester
Auton, Mrs Vicky A **(SLP)**
Barmeier, Janet M **(SLP)**
Biere, Julia Ann
Cooper, Mrs Mary C **(SLP)**
Cramer, Sue Rae **(SLP)**
Crawford, Mrs Cynthia L **(SLP)**
Crowe, Mary R **(SLP)**
Cuquet, Mrs Elizabeth Atkinson **(SLP)**
Fressola, Diane R **(SLP)**
Friesen, Ellen A **(SLP)**
Grueter, Mrs Claire Cuddy **(SLP)**
Hyatt, Bonnie D **(SLP)**
Le Grand, Carol Devine **(A)**
Luckett, Joan L **(A)**
McGinnis, Mrs Carol Boyle **(SLP)**

Maplewood
Schmid, Mrs Kathleen A **(SLP)**

Marceline
Ravens, Eleanor I **(SLP)**

Marshall
Franklin, Mrs Deborah R **(SLP)**
Hedderig, Charles Theodore **(SLP)**
Pippes, Mrs Mary Kay **(SLP)**
Wichman, Angela M **(SLP)**

Marshfield
De Priest, Donald Lee **(SLP)**

Marthasville
Long, Janice M **(SLP)**
Platenberg, Lynn **(SLP)**

Maryland Heights
Brown, Suzanne Redmond **(SLP)**
Davied, Leah Anne **(SLP)**
Dreyer, Marla Lynn **(SLP)**
Fishman, Robyn Lynn **(SLP)**
Gaylor, Mrs Minnie Jean **(SLP)**
Lanius, Julia K **(SLP)**
Meyer, Mrs Victoria **(SLP)**
Shaw, Linda **(SLP)**
Tyahla, Linda Gross **(SLP)**
Wolf, Carol K **(SLP)**

Maryville
Euler, Mrs Pamala D **(SLP)**
Maxwell, Sandra Rose **(SLP)**
Spire, Mrs Victoria Ann

Mexico
Hagan, Mrs Jacquelyn **(SLP)**
McDannold, Steven Bernard **(SLP)**

Moberly
Rutledge, Wynne Sutter **(SLP)**

Montgomery City
Hull, Mrs La Donne Buck **(SLP)**
O'Connor-Beringer, Mrs Patricia Anne **(A)**
Steffan, Sharon H **(SLP)**

Morehouse
Grant, Mary Thea **(SLP)**

Mount Vernon
Campbell, Mary Lucia **(SLP)**

Neosho
Kern, Mrs Sandra Paulson

Nevada
Coons, Ellen E **(SLP)**
Gobin, Donald D **(SLP)**
Volkland, Mrs Effie E **(SLP)**

New Madrid
Davis, Mrs Mary Kay **(SLP)**

Nixa
Carrington, Terri L **(SLP)**
Turner, Vicki Lynn **(SLP)**

North Kansas City
Dollison, Janet Lynn **(A)**
Suman, Mrs Mary Katherine
Thebo, Mrs Jane L **(A)**

Novinger
Miller, Terri Lynn **(SLP)**

O'Fallon
Anderson, Mrs Elizabeth S **(SLP)**
Kinder, Kathy Meyer **(SLP)**
Littleton, Mrs Katherine **(SLP)**
Lukos, Lizz **(SLP)**
Marion, Michelle Renee **(SLP)**

Oak Grove
Underwood, Analeen J **(SLP)**
Vanzandt, Mrs Joan C **(SLP)**

Oakville
Hoffman, Patricia Diane **(SLP)**
May, Regina Margaret **(SLP)**

Odessa
Caine, Joyce Barker
Mallette, Julie Lynn **(SLP)**
Smith, Mrs Sandra Kay **(SLP)**
Vinson, Mrs Lynette Hanke **(SLP)**

Olivette
Blank, Karen W **(SLP)**
Eldridge, Mrs Doris D **(SLP)**
Schoenfeld, Sidney L **(A)**

Oran
Anthony, Jackie Gail
Hamm, Mrs Victoria Lou **(SLP)**

Overland
Cohen, Kenneth D **(SLP)**
Kelley, Carolyn A **(SLP)**
Lally-Barton, Judy Ann **(SLP)**

Ozark
Martien, Brenda M **(SLP)**

Parkville
Sanderford, Patricia Murphy **(A)**
Todtfeld, Mrs Michele Brenda **(SLP)**

Patterson
Dildine, Mrs Mary Sue **(SLP)**

Perry
Fuqua, Stacy G **(SLP)**

Perryville
Edwards, Mrs Jane Elizabeth **(SLP)**
Renaud, Mrs Joyce Rita **(SLP)**

Pilot Grove
Wilmes, Robin Thate **(SLP)**

Pomona
Keeney, Mrs Sandra D **(SLP)**

Poplar Bluff
Keeling, James D **(SLP)**
Keeling, Leslie Thompson **(SLP)**
Morse, Mrs Nancy Elizabeth **(SLP)**
Rodgers, Patricia L **(SLP)**
Sagharichi, Mahmoud **(A)**
Wall, Shellee D

Portage Dessioux
McClelland, Mrs Brenda Kelly

Portageville
Delisle, Anita L **(SLP)**
Heydon-Wrather, Norma Jean **(SLP)**

Princeton
Finney, Brenda Jo **(SLP)**

Puxico
Turpin, Mrs Pamela Lynn **(SLP)**

Raytown
Bachmann, Glenda J **(SLP)**
Dalton, Beth Marie **(SLP)**
Dunning, Mrs Cheryl R **(SLP)**
Harms, Jana Ewart **(SLP)**
Henslee, Yvonne Annette
Kallstrom, Rolfe D **(SLP)**
Madison, Ted Keith **(A)**
Queen, Marlene S **(A)**

Uhlrich, Mrs Clara L W **(SLP)**

Republic
King, Mrs Patricia S **(SLP)**

Richmond Heights
Bradshaw, Mary H **(SLP)**
Sieger, Ann Parsons **(A)**
Tebbe, Bonnie C **(SLP)**

Rocheport
Allard, Dr Juan Bradley **(A)**
Blackburn, Mrs Susan Marjorie **(SLP)**

Rogersville
Weinsaft, Mrs Gudrun Stehr **(SLP)**

Rolla
Breeding, Marcia Keller **(SLP)**
Deardeuff, Mrs Linda **(SLP)**
Morris, Mrs Helen Anderson **(SLP)**
Schlemper, Mrs Kathie Laraine **(SLP)**
Sells, Mrs Susan Elizabeth **(SLP)**

Rosebud
Oltman, Mrs Shirley G **(SLP)**

Salem
Wood, Mrs Mary C **(SLP)**

Scott City
Kam, Ernie K **(SLP)**
Walton, Mrs J Andrea **(SLP)**

Sedalia
Bivens, Cheryl Jean **(SLP)**
Dust, Mrs Donita K **(SLP)**
Edwards, Susan J **(SLP)**
Harris, Maude M **(SLP)**
Horacek, Shirley M **(A)**
Opfer, Nanci B **(SLP)**

Shelbina
Greenwell, Mrs Alice R **(SLP)**

Sikeston
Ancell, Mrs Gale Skalsky **(SLP)**
Giles, Richard B **(SLP)**
Moll, Mrs Delores M **(SLP)**
Rubenacker, Kenneth W **(A)**
Smothers, Celeste

Springfield
Aasby, Mrs Susan McGuinn **(SLP)**
Acton, Shari Kay **(A)**
Andrews, Betsy Jean **(SLP)**
Angell, Steven N **(A)**
Arkebauer, Dr Herbert J **(SLP)**
Baker, Mrs Norma Jean **(SLP)**
Baker, Mrs Trudy Annette **(A)**
Brooker, Mrs Gayle E **(SLP)**
Burgess, Mrs Nancy Gallier **(SLP)**
Burgess, Dr Ruth Vassar **(SLP)**
Chapman, Mrs Janet Sidmon **(SLP)**
Cochran, Amy Lynn **(SLP)**
Coleman, Mrs Kathy L **(SLP)**
Deal, Dr Randolph E **(SLP)**
Denton, Mrs Carolyn Jo **(SLP)**
Devries, Donna A **(SLP)**
Egbert, Mrs Polly Young **(SLP)**
Frieda, Linda B **(SLP)**
Gallatin, Rhonda Lee **(A)**
Gaut, Mrs Snowdrop **(SLP)**
Gilbert, Martha Malone **(SLP)**
Gordon, Mrs Terri Lou **(SLP)**
Herron, Dr Edna R **(SLP)**
Hill, Mrs Debbie Robinson **(SLP)**
Hunter, Jenny Lynn
Kemper, Mrs Marilyn Ruth **(SLP)**
Kinloch, Dr Diane L **(SLP)**
Landess-Towne, Susan Carol **(SLP)**
Lewis, Debra A **(SLP)**
Lynch, Susan L T **(SLP)**
Madden, Mrs Shirley **(SLP)**
Martin, Kathleen Anne **(SLP)**
Means, Wanda R **(SLP)**
Meyers, Dr Harold W, Jr **(A)**
Monson, Donna L **(SLP)**
Oswalt, M Jill **(SLP)**
Page, Mrs Christy Ann **(SLP)**
Reed-Curbow, Mrs Linda **(A)**
Richter, Mrs Judy Kathryn **(SLP)**
Rush, Mrs Sandra L **(SLP)**
Schilling, Mrs Kristin Mary **(SLP)**
Shikany, Susan Dye **(SLP)**
Smith, Lori Denise **(SLP)**
Spicer, Harry S
Stephens, Nancy Jo **(SLP)**
Towne, Dr Roger L **(SLP)**
Troyert, Mrs Stephanie Stewart **(SLP)**
Turner, Mrs Carla Dawn **(SLP)**
White, Mrs Helen J **(SLP)**
Whitsell, Mrs Patricia L **(SLP)**
Windham, Laurabeth **(SLP)**
Wright, Sylvia P

St Ann
Gamache, Mary E **(SLP)**

St Charles
Barinotti, Mrs Margaret **(SLP)**
Borgmeyer, Ann P **(SLP)**
Borgsmiller, Paul T **(A)**
Boyd, Mrs Mary Jane **(SLP)**
Budnick, Bonnie M **(SLP)**
Engel, Mrs Suzanne Keppel **(SLP)**
Fischer, Mrs Debra Joy **(SLP)**
Gessert, Eugene Kelly
Hallemeier, Kit Maureen
Hotchkiss, Karen Vail **(SLP)**
Jeans, Karen K **(SLP)**
Ketcherside, Jane **(SLP)**
Meissner, Mrs Alice N **(SLP)**
Ortscheid, Mrs Cynthia Morris **(SLP)**
Pape, Mrs Sue M **(SLP)**
Peters, Regina C **(SLP)**
Phon, Gilbert **(A)**
Ponche, Mrs Diane K **(SLP)**
Saville, Mrs Sharon Drysdale **(SLP)**
Schneider, Mrs Deborah L **(SLP)**
Schultze, Dr Betty Robb **(SLP)**
Scott, Mrs Elizabeth **(A)**
Walter, Judy K **(SLP)**

St Genevieve
Grass, Mrs Dorcas E **(SLP)**
Stange, Wanda Jean

St James
Kinkead, Steven Dale **(SLP)**

St John
Thomas, Robert E

St Joseph
Cook, Annette Lajean **(A)**
Durkin, Mrs Barbara T **(SLP)**
Larson, Penny S **(SLP)**
Louderback, Mrs Kristen Wakelin **(SLP)**
Norton, Mrs Robin Kellogg **(SLP)**
Roesle, Sue A **(A)**
Wilson, Patricia A **(SLP)**

St Louis
Aaron, Roxanne Jennemann **(A)**
Akin, Wendla R W **(SLP)**
Andrus, Mrs Pamela Bergkamp **(SLP)**
Angle, Pamela Marie **(A)**
Askew, Wanda **(SLP)**
Backer-Conklin, Sue **(SLP)**
Bante, Alice J **(SLP)**
Barnkow, David Scott **(A)**
Bass, Mrs M Virginia **(SLP)**
Bauer, Monica Lynn **(SLP)**
Beachy, Mrs Teresa S **(SLP)**
Beard, Ellen Kay **(SLP)**
Bender, Mrs Jessica D **(SLP)**
Bene, Mrs Kay **(SLP)**
Bingley, Mrs Katherine **(SLP)**
Binzer, Susan M **(A)**
Blackshear, Mrs Angela Denise **(SLP)**
Bock, Lynn Annette **(SLP)**
Bolesta, Mary Melinda **(SLP)**
Boschen, Mrs Sara Lou **(SLP)**
Brading, Mrs Christine Ann **(SLP)**
Brandmeyer, Mrs Georgina Cagas **(SLP)**
Breckwoldt, Dr Gerhard H
Brennan, Dr Donald G **(SLP)**
Brennan, Martha K **(SLP)**
Brooks-Miller, Mrs Susan Lynne **(SLP)**
Buchanan, Sr Dorothea **(SLP)**
Buckler, Dr Joyce **(A)**
Bumbry, Linda Leanna **(SLP)**
Bushmann, Mrs Maureen Murphy **(SLP)**
Butler, Mrs Janice Good **(SLP)**
Cannon, Mrs Loretta Frances **(SLP)**
Carlbery, Carol Fitzgerald **(SLP)**
Carver, Dr William F **(A)**
Caul, Mrs Linda Doherty **(SLP)**
Christopher, Patricia A **(SLP)**
Conner, Dennis E **(A)**
Corr, Jill Ziegler **(A)**
Crites, Laura S **(SLP)**
Dasovich, Dr Mary O **(SLP)**
Davenport, Wanda A **(SLP)**
Davidson, Mrs Lisa Surber **(A)**
Davis, Deanna Sue P **(SLP)**
Davis, Jay P **(A)**
Davis, Mrs Joan Marie **(SLP)**
Day, David R **(SLP)**
Dicarlo-Kramer, Annette Marie **(SLP)**
Doerr, Cynthia J **(SLP)**
Duddy, Mrs Diane Freiert **(A)**
Eichacker, Niclole Elana
Eilermann, Denise Ann **(SLP)**
Engel, Tracy Lynn **(SLP)**
Enger, Mrs Joan Kathleen **(SLP)**
Ess, Jacqueline S **(SLP A)**
Everding, Mrs Vicki Love **(SLP)**
Flannery, Donna Kay **(SLP)**
Floyd, Dr Larry R **(SLP)**
Frankel, Jacqueline A **(SLP)**
Frerker, Mrs Victoria G **(SLP)**
Frieberger, Mrs Susan M **(A)**
Frye, Jeri Ann **(SLP)**
Fuller, Dr Dennis P **(SLP)**
Fust, Rita Jean **(SLP)**
Gaffney, Theresa
Geers, Dr Ann Elizabeth
Globokar, Andrea R **(SLP)**
Godar, Marilyn R **(SLP)**
Goldwasser, Mrs Marilyn K **(SLP)**
Goodman, Karen Totty **(SLP)**
Green, Ellen **(SLP)**
Greenberg-Waxman, Faith E **(SLP)**
Gunn, Kathleen **(SLP)**
Haasis, Mrs Mary A **(SLP)**
Handley-Thompson, Mrs Louisa B **(SLP)**
Hartman, Jacqueline S **(SLP A)**
Hartz, Mrs Kathryn S **(SLP)**
Hartzler, Sharon Busch **(SLP)**
Hayes, Sr Janet M **(SLP)**
Hecht, Kimberly Anne **(SLP)**
Heffner, Dr David J **(A)**
Helton, Beverly Gean **(SLP)**
Hirsh, Dr Ira J
Hollander, Jeanne B **(SLP)**
Houlihan, Patricia Ann **(SLP)**
Hubbard, Dr Dee Jay **(SLP)**
Huber, Mary Elizabeth **(SLP)**
Hull, Laura Kay **(A)**
Hutchison, Alice N **(SLP)**
Hynes, Ann Maureen **(SLP)**
Ingram, Mrs Glenda Christine **(SLP)**
Jahneke, Anna Maria **(SLP)**
Jay, Anne Octavia **(SLP)**
Jensen, Mrs Karen Hick **(SLP)**
Johnston, Linda S **(SLP)**
Juelich, Margaret Fritsch **(A)**
Kadas, Thelma E **(SLP)**
Katz-Weintraub, Sharon Elaine **(SLP)**
Kayser, Marianne Catherine **(SLP)**
Keidar, Anat **(SLP)**
Kelley, Arthur L **(SLP)**
Kelly, Mrs Martha K **(SLP)**
Kinsella, Debra A **(SLP)**
Komerous, Sharon Sahrmann **(SLP)**
Koprowski, Pamela A N **(A)**
Korte, Carol Lynn **(SLP)**
Kramer, Kathleen Laura **(SLP)**
Kramer, Sallie Phyliss **(SLP)**
Kuergeleis, Bonita Jean **(SLP)**
Lablance, Dr Gary R **(SLP)**
Lane, Dr Helen S
Lay, Dr Thomas N **(SLP)**
Leeker, Mrs Linda **(SLP)**
Lejeune, Joseph B **(SLP)**
Lenza, Mrs Aurora B **(SLP)**
Lenzen, Mrs Polly Metzger **(SLP)**
Levary, Mrs Esther Feldman **(SLP)**
Levine, David S **(SLP A)**
Levy, Alice Marie **(SLP)**
Lewis, Mrs Diane H **(SLP)**
Lieberman, Susan B **(SLP)**
Lisson, Mrs Jennifer Kaye **(SLP)**
Liuzza, Nancy Merlotti **(SLP)**
Lodholz, Mrs Dorleta Oetting **(SLP)**
Loehr, Lynda K B **(SLP)**
Lohse, Katherine A **(SLP)**
Longo, Mrs Janine Marie **(SLP)**
Loomis, Robert A **(A)**
Lorenzen, Susan R **(SLP)**
Louiselle, Theresa Lahood **(SLP)**
Luis, Maureen Elizabeth **(SLP)**
Mader, Mrs Marjorie A **(SLP)**
Malke, Mrs Tracy L **(SLP)**
Mannarelli, Julie A **(SLP)**
Mannion, Marianne Theresa **(SLP)**
Marmonti, Mrs Mary Kathleen **(SLP)**
Marrah, Sr Marita Anne **(SLP)**
Marshall, Susan A V **(A)**
Marzano, Lisa Ann **(SLP)**
Matthews, Dr Claire **(SLP)**
McCormick, Mrs Candace A **(SLP)**
McDonnell, Patricia Kim **(SLP)**
McFarland, Robert Taylor **(A)**
McGartland, Marilyn A **(SLP)**
McKenzie, Bonnie Sue **(SLP)**
McLaughlin, Patricia A **(A)**
Meister, Mrs Martha J **(A)**
Meredith, Grace **(SLP)**
Miller, Patricia D **(SLP)**
Mishler, Mrs Tracy Mehan **(A)**
Monet, Mrs Natalie S **(SLP)**
Moog, Mrs Jean S
Moore, Mrs Paula E **(SLP)**
Morgan, Kathleen Elizabeth **(SLP)**
Mueller, Mrs L Jeannie **(SLP)**
Mueth, Mrs Patricia F **(SLP)**
Murphy, Mrs Tracy Agne **(SLP)**
Nagle-Weible, Nancy Ann
Napoli, Janet H **(A)**
Nelson, Sharon Woodcock **(SLP)**
Nichols, Lynn Wagner **(SLP)**
Nollau, Mrs Michaela K **(SLP)**
Norton, Kathleen Marie **(SLP)**
Nowland, Margaret F **(SLP)**
Nussbaum, Mrs Susan Martin **(SLP)**
O'Leary, Mrs Barbara L **(SLP)**
Olree, Mrs Kathy S **(SLP)**
Owens, Susan M **(SLP)**
Padberg, Anne Montgomery **(A)**
Park, Kay D **(A)**
Parthasarathy, Dr Teralandur K **(A)**
Pascoe, Dr David P **(SLP A)**
Peak, Margaret F **(A)**
Pearson, Mrs Debra Ann
Peterein, Judy Lynne **(A)**
Peterson, Mrs Marshalita Sims **(SLP)**
Piccirilli, Mrs Mary Schmitt **(SLP)**
Pilson, Mrs Susan C M **(SLP)**
Polinsky, Mrs Debra Shapiro **(SLP)**
Popelka, Dr Gerald Raymond **(A)**
Portnoy, Mrs Mary Regina **(SLP)**
Portnoy, Robert A **(SLP)**
Praechter, Dawn Marie
Price, Kathleen Gerianne **(SLP)**

Pugh, Bradley Keith **(A)**
Quante, Cheryl L **(SLP)**
Rector, Mrs Susan Ann **(SLP)**
Reisch, Mrs Beryl Stanley **(SLP)**
Reynolds, Mary D **(A)**
Rice, Gale Borkowski **(SLP)**
Richardson, Mrs Kelli Taylor **(SLP)**
Riordan, Mrs Jeanine W **(SLP)**
Robertson, Eugene L, Jr **(SLP)**
Roth, Mrs Linda Louise **(SLP)**
Ruhlin, Amy Noggle **(SLP)**
Ruskey, Debra Ann **(SLP)**
Sandler, Mrs Louise Gilles **(SLP)**
Sandretto, Gary Charles **(SLP)**
Santagato, Mrs Jeannette M **(SLP)**
Santucci, Gayle M **(A)**
Schaeffer, Cheryl A **(SLP)**
Schinsky, Mrs Lorraine B **(SLP)**
Schmidt, Mrs Anita M **(SLP)**
Schuman, Leslie E **(SLP)**
Schutzenhofer, Tom **(SLP)**
Scott, Dr Lorel M **(SLP)**
Shasserre, Mrs Mary L **(SLP)**
Sherrod, Barbara W **(SLP)**
Shields, Lynne W **(SLP)**
Sieve, Patricia Ann **(SLP)**
Skelly-Hakanson, Dr Madge **(SLP)**
Skinner, Dr Margaret W **(A)**
Slein, Joan Strassner **(SLP)**
Smith, Constance **(SLP)**
Sparks, Mrs Laurie Newell **(A)**
Steffen, Mrs Paula S
Stein, Margo E **(SLP)**
Stensrud, Kathryn Jo **(SLP)**
Stephens, Suzann K **(SLP)**
Stern, Jeane **(SLP A)**
Stoker, Dr Richard Glen **(A)**
Stroble, Susan Michele **(A)**
Stroer, Mrs Barbara S **(A)**
Sullivan, Lori Chirnside **(SLP)**
Suter, Mrs Carole P **(SLP)**
Swanson, Barbara L **(SLP)**
Tiemann, Joann L **(SLP)**
Tietjens, Mrs Mary Ann **(SLP)**
Tucker, Linda K **(SLP)**
Turner, Beverly Ann **(A)**
Turner, Regina Q **(SLP)**
Turpin, Linda L **(A)**
Tyler, Mrs Jacqueline **(SLP)**
Uding, Ann M **(SLP)**
Udziela, Joan Nelke **(SLP)**
Valente, Michael **(A)**
Verble, Mrs Suzanne D
Vercellone, Donna Cheryl **(SLP)**
Verdolini-Marston, Mrs Katherine Tuller **(SLP)**
Vest, Denise L
Vierling, Mrs Evelyn Annette W **(SLP)**
Wade, Betsy M **(SLP A)**
Wagner, Joe Herman **(SLP)**
Weinstein, Mrs Susan Rydell **(SLP)**
Weissberg- Smith, Amy Jo **(A)**
Weiter, Pamela Leigh **(SLP)**
West, Mrs Laurel Lynne **(SLP)**
Wheeler, Mrs Sara Lee T **(SLP)**
Wiegert, Katherine Mary **(SLP)**
Wildman, Mrs Myra **(SLP)**
Wilkinson, Dianne Lynn **(A)**
Williams, Donna L **(A)**
Williams-Rice, Mrs Teresa F **(SLP)**
Wilson, Mrs Catherine Ann **(SLP)**
Wirtel, Sally K **(SLP)**
Wnuk, Elizabeth Ann
Wood, Christina **(A)**
Zaggy, Mary Ann **(SLP)**

St Peters
Bumb, Mrs Chrys C **(SLP)**
Davidson, Mrs Laura Krieger **(SLP)**
Dougherty, Mrs Cynthia Lee **(SLP)**
Droste, Mrs Janet M **(SLP)**
Dulle, Catherine **(SLP)**
Guntli, Mrs Janice A **(SLP)**
Hass, Pamela Kay **(SLP)**
Lamzik, Mrs Jean Marie **(SLP)**
Langlois, Mary Ane **(SLP)**
Madak, Terri Wilson **(SLP)**
Murphy, Julie A **(SLP)**
Roderick, Mrs Barbara A **(SLP)**
Shelley, Mrs Gina Lee **(SLP)**
von Wolfseck, Dr Janie Wester **(SLP)**

Sugar Creek
Salva, Lora Lei **(SLP)**

Sunrise Beach
Houston, Mrs Mary Agnes **(SLP)**

Tarkio
Beckman, Mrs Debra Sue **(SLP)**

Thayer
Humphreys, Anita B **(SLP)**

Tipton
Whisler, Mrs Lanna J **(SLP)**

Town & Country
Childs, Carol Ann **(SLP)**
Huskey, Dr Robert L **(SLP)**

Troy
Fitzgerald, Mrs Glenda Frances **(SLP)**

University City
Deitchman, Pamela Susan **(SLP)**
MacHefsky, Kathryn A **(SLP)**
Molloy, Sr R
Zelman, Dr Elizabeth **(SLP)**

Van Buren
Sulsen, Mrs Katherine Lee **(SLP)**

Vandalia
Witte, Mrs Linda W **(SLP)**

Warrensburg
Dejonge, Mrs Linda B **(SLP)**
Dejonge, Dr Robert R, Jr **(A)**
Harlan, Dr Carl L, Jr **(SLP)**
Kerr, Mrs Dee Schaefer **(SLP)**
Magyar, Karla J W **(SLP)**
Patterson, Dr Karen A **(SLP A)**
Pendarvis, 8167476713 I **(SLP)**
Schmidt, Dr Marilynn Jo **(SLP)**
Stengel-Wittke, Mrs Patricia Ann **(SLP)**
Tibbits, Dr Donald F **(SLP)**
Tieszen, Mrs Marion V **(SLP)**
Welch, Dr Lin **(SLP)**
Welling, Mrs Rosalee Buhler **(SLP)**
Wilson, Dr James R **(SLP)**
Wilson, Mrs Judith H **(SLP)**

Warson Woods
Brandenburg, Mrs Louise A **(SLP)**

Washington
Paasch, Kathryn Ann **(SLP)**
Taylor, Barbara Jean

Wasola
Adair, Mrs Victoria Lynne

Waynesville
Shortridge, Mrs Judith C **(SLP)**

Webb City
Miller, Ronald W **(A)**

Webster Groves
Clote, Mrs Cynthia Ann **(SLP)**
Fearon, Mrs Donna Maria **(SLP)**
Ford, Mrs Nanette J **(SLP)**
Gaeth, Janice Schaefer **(A)**
Hamlin, Jeanne F **(SLP)**
Kane, M Eileen **(SLP)**
Karzon, Dr Roanne K **(SLP A)**
McWhorter, Tina D **(A)**
Whitney, Valerie K **(SLP)**

West Plains
Hubbard, Mrs Cynthia Hatley **(SLP)**
Truehart, Lisa A **(SLP)**
Whitten, Pam J **(SLP)**

MONTANA

Absarokee
Reynolds, Mrs Rosemary **(SLP)**

Belgrade
Purdy, Daryl A **(SLP)**

Big Timber
Fjare, Cheri L **(SLP)**

Billings
Allen, Annalee A **(SLP)**
Bartsch, Mrs Nancy R A **(SLP)**
Bukowski, Gene W **(A)**
Caputo, Linda A **(SLP)**
Chisholm, Mrs Sally Ann Ruehr **(SLP)**
Foss, Kristy Layne **(A)**
Hammerquist, Teresa L **(SLP)**
Hauptman, Linda K **(SLP)**
Hladek, Glenn **(A)**
Hoagland, Tina Louise **(A)**
Hogan, Mrs Susan H **(SLP)**
Johnson, E Suzanne **(A)**
Kilzer, Jeanne Marie
Klatt, Mrs Sallyanne Eichler **(SLP)**
Martin, Margaret H **(SLP)**
Morse, Mrs Carol J **(SLP)**
O'Leary, Christine Marie **(SLP)**
Pitts, Mrs Christine **(SLP)**
Rehder, Douglas E **(SLP A)**
Rice, Mrs Nancy J M **(SLP)**
Schmidt, Mrs Danielle D **(SLP)**
Shue, Michelle Marie **(SLP)**
Tupper, Mrs Billie Jo **(SLP)**
Van Beek, Mrs Cynthia A **(SLP)**

Boulder
Coutts, Marylou **(SLP)**

Bozeman
Davis, Laura S **(A)**
Hawkinson, Susan **(SLP)**
Micken, Darrell J **(A)**
Micken, Lee E **(A)**
Olson, Mrs Valerie S **(SLP)**
Purkett, Joseph C **(SLP)**
Swartz, Anita L **(SLP)**

Bridger
Vanderpan, Lisa Calkins **(SLP)**

Broadus
Thaden, Marilyn Joyce **(SLP)**

Butte
Chiodini, Valerie J **(SLP)**
Ingalls, Patricia M **(A)**
McClafferty, Kathleen M **(SLP)**
Morris, Tom M **(SLP)**

Charlo
Wurl, Holly L **(SLP)**

Choteau
Schauer, Mrs Glenda M **(SLP)**

Civa
Beste, Ann Margaret **(SLP)**

Clancy
Bloxsom, Mrs Jan L **(SLP)**
Paulson, Mrs Lucy H **(SLP)**

Colstrip
Francis-Dinstel, Mrs Sharon **(SLP)**
Petersen, Mrs MaryJoan Donahue **(SLP)**

Columbia Falls
Cordier, Mrs Charlene L **(SLP)**
Heider, Mrs Katherine **(SLP)**
Windsor, Shelley **(SLP)**

Conrad
Gremaud, Janice M

Corvallis
Kenngott, Carolyn L **(SLP)**

Culbertson
Mason, Kristen Elizabeth **(SLP)**

Deer Lodge
Wegen, Keely Jo

Dillon
Strudthoff, Jean Marie **(SLP)**

East Glacier Park
Barnard, Laurie W **(A)**
Strobbe, Mrs Margaret Irene **(SLP)**
Sykes, Debra L **(SLP A)**

Fort Benton
Streit, Mrs Joanne M **(SLP)**

Fort Shaw
Roy, Beverly J **(SLP)**

Galata
Sisk, Mrs Lore A **(SLP)**

Glasgow
Schmidt, Richard P **(SLP A)**

Glendive
Burrows, Cashwell L **(SLP)**

Great Falls
Bock, Chuck E **(SLP)**
Borgreen, Julia A **(SLP)**
Bouman, Joan **(A)**
Brasch, Marilyn L **(SLP)**
Conklin, Caroline **(SLP)**
Deck, Christie Reichert **(SLP)**
Ellis, Elizebeth **(SLP)**
Farabaugh, Kathleen Siobhan **(SLP)**
Griffin, Jeffrey D **(A)**
Grosfield, Jane E **(SLP)**
Hansen, Rebecca L **(SLP)**
Lewis, Mrs Jean S **(SLP)**
Meech, Mrs Sandy Swank **(SLP)**
Norberg, Diane **(SLP)**
Nowak, Gwen F **(SLP)**
Paulauskis, Mrs Jana L **(SLP)**
Pence, John R **(SLP)**
Perry, Paul J **(A)**
Reeves, Martha **(SLP)**
Rintoul, Mrs Dorothy Blake **(SLP)**
Rue, Ken **(SLP)**
Wende, Richard A **(SLP)**

Hamilton
Athman, Teresa M **(SLP)**
Johnson, Rose Mary Davis **(SLP)**

Harlem
Bardanouve, Mrs Venus T **(SLP A)**

Havre
Combs, Margaret R **(SLP)**
Coons, Mrs Lynn Westlake **(SLP)**
Schiefer, Penelope B **(SLP)**

Helena
Bartz, Mrs Patricia R **(SLP)**
Caniglia, Christine Ann **(SLP)**
Clark, Barbara A **(SLP)**
Devoe, Merle F **(A)**
Devoe, Shirley J **(SLP)**
Grover, Christian **(A)**
Inseth, Bette J **(A)**
Johnson, Mrs Elizabeth Jackson **(SLP)**
McCain, Mrs Kathleen C **(SLP)**
McDonough, Mrs Ruth Ann Stergar **(SLP)**
Metropoulos, Theresa S **(SLP)**
Miller, Mary M **(SLP)**
Molineux, Mrs Mary F **(SLP)**
Pearson, Marilyn M **(SLP)**
Reagor, Terrylea M **(SLP)**
Vogelsang, Ellen **(SLP)**

Kalispell
Bailey, Leslie Ann **(SLP)**
Biedscheid, Melia Collette **(SLP A)**
Graff, Mary H **(SLP)**
Gray, Mrs Karen C **(SLP)**
Retzer, Mrs Chare N **(SLP)**

Laurel
Boyd, Carolyn J **(SLP)**

Libby
Burley, Mrs Rachel S **(SLP)**

Livingston
Drexler, Dr Hazel G **(SLP A)**

Lolo
Bobowiec, Mrs Mary Suzanne **(SLP)**

Miles City
Hamano, Pearl Y **(SLP)**
Harris, Lynn V **(SLP A)**
Love, James M **(SLP)**

Milltown
Hall, Susan Grasso **(SLP)**

Missoula
Ammons, Dr Robert B
Bain, Dr Barbara A **(SLP A)**
Boehmler, Dr Richard M **(SLP)**
Brooks, Mrs Julie Ann **(SLP)**
Chaney, Dr Robert B, Jr **(A)**
Connell, Nancy J **(SLP A)**
Curtis, James F **(A)**
Davison, Mrs Janet Clark **(SLP)**
Egeland, Carol S **(SLP)**
Fifer, Linda S **(SLP)**
Folsom, Loreen C **(SLP)**
Frantz, Joy Lee **(A)**
Frost, Jamie Ruffatto **(SLP)**
Green, Margaret **(SLP)**
Harris, Cynthia Bacon **(SLP)**
Harrison, Rosemary S **(SLP)**
Holder, Ronald Lee **(SLP)**
Johnson, Sara Jane **(A)**
Jordan-Trestik, Jill Marie **(A)**
Laforest, Mary Pat **(SLP A)**
Love, Kathleen Mary **(SLP)**
Lowe, Mrs Marsha S **(SLP)**
Lyndes, Dr Kellogg O **(SLP)**
Miller, Debra L **(SLP)**
Miller, Sheila Marie **(A)**
Moffatt, Rose Ann **(SLP A)**
Nagel-Niehl, Patricia **(SLP)**
Parker, Dr Charles D **(SLP A)**
Pederson, Alane Kay **(SLP)**
Reynolds, Mrs Beverly R **(SLP)**
Richardson, Sharon L **(SLP)**
Scott, Mrs Carol Virginia **(A)**
Sims, Kathleen Dawn **(SLP)**
Small, Jamie Ann **(A)**
Smith, Mrs Alice E **(SLP)**
Thorne, Catherine **(SLP)**
Toth, Susan A W **(SLP A)**
Wambaugh, Julie Lynn **(SLP)**
Weirather, Dr Randy R **(SLP)**
Wundrow, Larry W **(A)**
Wynne, Michael K **(SLP A)**

Plains
Booth, Denise S **(SLP)**
Booth, Thomas **(SLP)**

Polson
Merriman-Sorensen, Christine Ainsworth **(SLP)**

Red Lodge
Schenkein, Lisa C **(SLP)**

Ronan
Friedlander, Rhonda Lynn **(SLP)**

Sidney
Allmaras, Geri Anne **(SLP)**
Uthus, Megg Ann **(A)**

Stevensville
Schaffer, Mrs Elizabeth Willen **(SLP)**

Ulm
McCann, Kim L **(SLP)**

Victor
Baldwin, Susan **(SLP)**
Vaughan, Dorothy H **(SLP)**

Whitefish
Cooper, Christophr **(SLP)**
Law, Mrs Kathleen L **(SLP)**
Penzi, Lori M **(SLP)**
Solberg, E Jane **(SLP)**
Swanson, Ann Marie **(SLP)**

NEBRASKA

Adams
Storz, Mrs Debra McClung

Ainsworth
Kinzie, Coralene **(SLP)**

Albion
Haave, Mrs Amy Nore **(SLP)**
Young, Mrs Pamela Jayne **(SLP)**

Alliance
Bond, Karen S **(SLP)**
Foster, Mrs Penny Felix **(SLP)**
Kees, Mrs Mary A **(SLP)**

Ashland
Sanger, Dr Dixie D **(SLP)**

Auburn
Anthony, Gene M **(SLP)**
Jamison, William J **(A)**

Aurora
Farrand, Mrs Diane M **(SLP)**
Shively, Philip Thomas **(SLP)**
Wilcox, Lynn H **(SLP)**

Axtell
Poole, Mrs Jean O **(SLP)**

Beatrice
Blackwell, Joyce R **(SLP)**
Freed, Mrs Julienne Marie **(SLP)**
Jenson, Mrs Barbara Jean **(SLP)**

Bellevue
Anderson, Karen Gail **(SLP)**
Buglewicz, Mrs Ellen Theresa **(SLP)**
Marquard, Mrs Virginia K **(SLP)**
McMillion, Mrs Leslie Ann **(SLP)**
Powers, Cynthia Ann **(SLP)**
Stevens, Dr James H **(A)**

Blair
Korte, Solveig Sperati **(SLP)**
Reed, De Etta Marie **(SLP)**

Burr
Hammond, Mrs Teresa R **(SLP)**

Ceresco
Johnson, Mrs Glenda L

Chadron
Moody, Pauline F **(SLP)**
Peak, Cynthia E **(SLP)**
Schallenkamp, Dr Kay K **(SLP)**

Chappell
Kinoshita, Mrs Sheryl M **(SLP)**

Clay Center
Reichmuth, Sara **(SLP)**

Columbus
Behm, Mrs Julia A **(SLP)**
Herbolsheimer, Marla Luella **(SLP)**
Koenig, Mary A **(SLP)**
McDanniels, Nora Lee **(A)**
Phillips, Mrs Erva J **(SLP)**

Comstock
Hickman-Kamarad, Mrs Bonita M **(SLP)**

Cozad
Nelsen, Ann S
Strickland, Cynthia S **(SLP)**

Crete
Lothrop, Sondra Swartz **(SLP)**

Curtis
Garrison, Mrs Sheila Anne **(SLP)**

Decatur
Dunning, Georgann **(SLP)**

Dodge
Grabowski, Carola Mary **(SLP)**

Elgin
Gunderson, Duane Nils **(SLP)**

Elkhorn
Hurst, Breta **(SLP)**
MacKlem, Mrs Janet Sixel **(SLP)**
Starks, Mary Alice **(SLP)**
Tompkins, Mary M **(SLP)**

Ewing
Eppler-Kropp, Sheila R **(SLP)**

Fairbury
Mannschreck, Brenda S **(SLP)**
Prince, Mrs Joyce Ann **(SLP)**
Reams, Mrs Virginia K **(SLP)**

Firth
McConnell, Mrs Jill B **(SLP)**

Fremont
Essex, Mrs Wanda E **(SLP)**
Gildersleeve-Maffitt, Joanna Louise **(SLP)**
Jeter, Mrs Patti A **(SLP)**
Kierstead, James M **(SLP)**
McKnight, Evelyn Vinduska **(A)**
Thietje, Mrs Joanne G **(SLP)**

Funk
Larson, Mrs Mardell R **(SLP)**

Gering
Rutter, Vicki **(SLP)**
Steadman, Sharon K **(SLP)**

Gordon
Prust, Jeanette Hickey **(SLP)**

Gothenburg
Gengenbach, Mrs Muriel L **(SLP)**
Peterson, Paula Smead **(SLP)**

Grand Island
Anderson, Karen M **(SLP)**
Bixenmann, Mrs Carolyn Faulder **(SLP)**
Boggs, James R **(SLP)**
Duennerman, Mrs Wanda G **(SLP)**
Foss, Craig A **(A)**
Grimes, Nancy Jensen **(SLP)**
Haynes, LeEllen R **(SLP)**
Howard, Mrs Jeni L **(SLP)**
Kenyon, Karen K **(SLP)**
Kohtz, Mrs Jane K **(SLP)**
Sims, Vicki J D **(SLP)**
Smedra, Carol Ann **(SLP)**
Splattstoesser, Deanne J **(SLP)**

Gretna
Salser, Bobbie C **(SLP)**
Vogel, Karen L **(SLP)**

Hastings
Adam, Mrs Colleen **(A)**
Eigenberg, Sigrid R **(SLP)**
Holt, Mrs Laurie B **(A)**
Moss, Mrs Donna J **(SLP)**
Quinn, Mrs Margaret F **(A)**
Rater, Rae J **(SLP)**
Ross, Dr Irwin **(SLP)**
Smith, Rosemary B **(SLP A)**
Theis, Mary Deany **(SLP)**
Wyeno, Gary L **(A)**

Holdrege
Carlson, Mrs Margo Elaine **(SLP)**
Hild, Mrs Patricia J **(SLP)**

Kearney
Ahrendts, Dr Harold L **(SLP)**
Anderson, Cynthia A **(A)**
Barry, Mrs Jean Kaer **(SLP)**
Beatty, Mrs Gertrude D **(SLP)**
Beavers, Rosemarie Joyce
Cochran, Mrs Averil C C **(SLP)**
Cochran, Dr John R **(SLP)**
Eggert, Mrs Sandra J **(SLP)**
Emal, Kent Clayton **(SLP)**
Falconer, Mrs Kathryn O **(SLP)**
Koenig, Vera Lee C **(SLP)**
Larsen, Mrs Connie S **(SLP)**
Larson, Lillian C **(SLP)**
McCammond, Mrs Shirley Pease **(SLP)**
McConnell, Mrs Leisa Kay **(SLP)**
Morrow, Mrs Mary Jo McCune **(SLP)**
Mosig, Mrs Edna Alice Ramsey **(SLP)**
Mues, Dwana Urbom **(SLP)**
Rosenwinkel, Deborah A **(SLP A)**
Stevens, Mrs Marcy Lynne **(SLP)**

La Vista
Spencer, Mrs Terri Lynn **(SLP)**

Lexington
Egenberger, Sheila S **(SLP)**
Roberts, Mrs Maxine J **(SLP)**

Lincoln
Alberts, Carol Ann **(SLP A)**
Arrowsnith, Amy L
Baack, Kris L **(SLP)**
Beaty, Carol A **(SLP)**
Bennett, Mrs Debra K **(SLP)**
Bernthal, John E **(SLP A)**
Bessler, Mrs Ramona M **(SLP)**
Beukelman, Dr David R **(SLP)**
Bodine, Cathy Sue **(SLP)**
Boldt, Winifred F **(SLP)**
Boney, Stephen J **(A)**
Brazda-Witters, Jorja M **(SLP)**
Brown, Carol Anne **(SLP)**
Brunken, Mrs Cynthia Diane **(SLP)**
Burton, Ellen Howard **(A)**
Combs-Denavs, Debra K **(A)**
Davis, Mrs Abbe Denise
Decker, Dr T Newell **(A)**
Denton, David R **(SLP)**
Deshayes, Irvin L **(A)**
De Vries, Mrs Sherri Marie **(A)**
Doak, Kathryn M Fikse **(A)**
Dongilli, Paul A, Jr **(SLP)**
Durgin-Clinchard, Mrs Jean **(SLP)**
Ellis, Gayle J **(SLP)**
Ellis, Mrs Susan L **(SLP)**
Evasco, Mrs Kathleen M **(SLP)**
Franklin, Kate
Gaines, Mrs Sharon L **(SLP)**
Garrett, Kathryn L **(SLP)**
Gutkin, Mrs Barbara Arlene **(SLP)**
Hakel, Mark Edward **(SLP)**
Halpern, Mrs Marsha Lommel **(SLP A)**
Hamnett, David **(SLP)**
Harvey, Eileen F **(SLP)**
Healey, Dr E Charles **(SLP)**
Hiatt, Eloise Bonebright **(SLP)**
Honeycutt, Kathy V **(SLP)**
Howe, Dr Susan W **(A)**
Hutchison, Kathleen **(SLP)**
Jensen, Janet K **(SLP)**
Kennedy, Anne Aileen **(SLP)**
Konz, Ruth A **(SLP)**
Kurtenbach, Mrs Janet Ruth **(SLP)**
Kushner, Marcia R **(A)**
Lacy, Donna F **(SLP)**
Lehman, Kimberly Ann **(SLP)**
Leising, Mrs Kathleen P **(SLP)**
Lunsford, Mrs Deanna Roberts
Marvin, Dr Christine A **(SLP)**
Mattas, Maureen C **(SLP)**
McCulloch, Barbara J **(A)**
Meduna, Marian Kay **(A)**
Meyer, Denise K **(SLP)**
Mirenda, Dr Pat
Monson, Kay E **(SLP)**
Morehouse, Toni B **(SLP)**
Morris, Dr Mary Jane **(SLP)**

Morrison, Mrs Roberta Jane **(SLP)**
Morrow, Mrs Deanna R
Morton-Anderson, K Anne **(SLP)**
Nielsen, Carol Sue **(SLP)**
Perkins, Mrs Marlene M **(SLP)**
Pleskac, Mrs Claudia L **(A)**
Potthoff, Mrs Patricia Tagler **(SLP)**
Prochaska-Charf, Mrs Mary Jane **(SLP)**
Rauscher, Mrs Ann Wall **(SLP)**
Riggs, Mrs Shelli D
Rittgarn, Mrs Gwendolyn **(SLP)**
Rydell, Patrick J **(SLP)**
Sakurada, Faith A
Sand, Mrs Nancy L **(SLP)**
Schliesser, Barbara H **(SLP)**
Schliesser, Dr Herbert F **(SLP)**
Schreiber, Sue G **(SLP)**
Sheets, Mrs Loretta W **(SLP)**
Sherrill, Dr Donald D **(SLP)**
Smolek-Sharp, Mrs Joyce Ann
Sohler, Rhonda A
Stick, Dr Sheldon L **(SLP)**
Summers, Kristine J **(SLP)**
Taylor, Mrs Donna J **(A)**
Wagner, Mrs Joan Wasinger **(SLP)**
Weaver, Mrs Sarah A **(SLP)**

McCook
Ficke-Richtarik, Mrs Karen Lynne
Otto, Judith A **(SLP)**
Salyer, Mrs Karen S **(SLP)**

Millard
Wragge, Marcia Steinkruger **(SLP)**

Minden
Featherston, Mrs Virgianne **(SLP)**

Nebraska City
Andrews, Mrs Evalin W **(SLP)**

Niobrara
Calvillo, M Kimberly **(SLP)**

Norfolk
Eggleston, Mrs Georgena K **(SLP)**
Honke, Lawrence E **(A)**
Keeler, Mrs Linda W **(SLP)**
Mettler, Mrs Laura Lynn **(SLP)**
Stevens, Pamela Thomas
Watson, Mrs Luann M **(SLP)**

North Platte
Cooper, Mrs Kimberley **(SLP)**
Hergert, Mrs Doylene K **(SLP)**
Jasnoch-Fairchild, Debra **(A)**
Mendenhall, Kay **(SLP)**
Mohs, Mrs Margaret Jo K **(SLP)**
Mueller, Mrs Linda L F **(SLP)**
Schwartz, Mrs Judith M **(SLP)**
Stefka, Mrs Paulette Sue **(SLP)**
Wilke, Mrs Sara Bachmann **(SLP)**

Oakland
Zessin, Linda K **(SLP)**

Ogallala
Graff, Nancy J **(SLP)**
Meyer, Annalisa K **(SLP A)**

Omaha
Adams-Davis, Mrs Pamela M **(SLP)**
Alexander, Lynn Gunn **(SLP)**
Anton, Larry J **(A)**
Auslander, Martha Clifford **(A)**
Banks, Mrs Cheryl **(SLP)**
Barlow, Dr Steven Michael
Barton, Kathleen Ann **(SLP)**
Beauchaine, Kathryn A **(A)**
Berberich, Mary E **(SLP)**
Bernstein, Bonnie Lynn **(SLP)**
Beste, Patrick D **(SLP)**
Birch, Bruce J **(A)**
Bird, Mrs Ann Olsen
Brown, Colleen Kenny **(SLP)**
Camp, Marita J **(SLP)**
Caniglia, Dr Joseph A **(SLP)**
Carney, Dr Arlene E **(A)**
Carotta, Mrs Catherine Cronin **(SLP)**
Chadwell, Daniel L **(A)**
Chappell, Cheryl R **(SLP)**
Christensen, Dr John Eric **(SLP)**
Claassen, Mary **(SLP)**
Clark, Pamela S **(SLP)**
Clark, Mrs Sharon Mitchell **(SLP)**
Cleary, Mrs Anne M **(SLP)**
Coltrane, Connie Jo **(SLP)**
Cook, Mrs Phyllis Newell
Cordes, Mrs Claudia A **(SLP)**
Coufal, Kathy L **(SLP)**
Cunningham, Mrs Nancy **(SLP)**
Cyr, Dr David G **(A)**
Davidson, Sandra Bushey **(SLP)**
Davis, Carol Ann **(SLP)**
Dinsdale, Mrs Dawn L S **(A)**
Dunning, Dennis P **(SLP)**
Edwards, Joel Allen **(A)**
Edwards, Mrs Kathleen Marie **(SLP)**
Ekstrom, Anita M **(SLP)**
Engel, Lisa Gustin **(SLP)**
Evans, Kathy
Feigin, Judith G **(A)**
Fielder, Mrs Jeanne Holmberg **(SLP)**
Fitzmaurice, Kathleen Anne **(SLP)**
Frisbie, Kris A **(A)**
Froehlich, Mrs Judy A **(SLP)**
Gasnick, Mary Elizabeth **(SLP)**
Gdowski, Becky Sue **(SLP)**
Gibbs, Kathy L **(SLP)**
Gilbert, Mrs Kristy K **(SLP)**
Gogenola-Rothberg, Ann **(SLP)**
Gordon, Mrs Kathleen B **(SLP)**
Gorga, Dr Michael P **(A)**
Goscha, Mrs Rebecca J **(SLP)**
Gossman, Mary A **(A)**
Gottsch, Barbara Mayer **(SLP)**
Goudreau, Anne L **(A)**
Grachek, Mrs Doris Jeanne **(A)**
Grandy, Mrs Victoria V **(SLP)**
Gray, Katherine A **(SLP)**
Guinane, Mrs Kathleen Ann **(SLP)**
Hanks, Lori Kim P **(SLP)**
Hansen, Susan H **(SLP)**
Hansler, Mrs Barbara Jean **(SLP)**
Hawkes, Mrs Donna Marie **(SLP)**
Hayford, Margaret Louise **(SLP)**
Henningsen, Mrs Dorothy L **(SLP)**
Hevrdeys, Sylvia A **(SLP)**
Hicks, Ann Michelle **(SLP)**
Hixson, Dr Peter K **(SLP)**
Hoefer, Mary McCormick **(SLP)**
Hofmeister, Risa Kay **(SLP)**
Humlicek, Elizabeth Eledge **(SLP)**
Jensen, Mrs Valerie Carda **(SLP)**
Jesteadt, Dr Walt
Johannes, Susan Underwood **(SLP)**
Johnson, Bonnie Marshall **(SLP)**
Johnson, Deborah L **(SLP)**
Johnson, Sally Grace **(SLP)**
Kalberer, Ann Elizabeth **(A)**
Karlquist, Mrs Suzanne Winslow **(SLP)**
Keck, Mrs Patricia Joan **(SLP)**
Kelly, Mrs Jean A **(SLP)**
Kempster, Marjory I **(SLP)**
Kingkade, Sandra Kirchmann **(SLP)**
Kladde, Annette G **(SLP)**
Knauss, Mrs Genevieve M **(SLP)**
Knudsen, Mrs Jana L **(SLP)**
Kopun, Mrs Judy G **(A)**
Kreifels, Mary Margaret **(SLP)**
Kreis, Mrs Mary Katherine **(SLP)**
Krieger, Kim M **(SLP)**
Krohn, Mrs Myrna L **(SLP A)**
Kutler, Debra **(SLP)**
Kyros, Mrs Victoria H **(SLP)**
Laikko, Paul E **(SLP)**
Langenfeld, Kelene Kelly **(SLP)**
Larsen, Joni K **(SLP)**
Larson, Lori Beth **(SLP)**
Lauren, Maureen A **(SLP)**
Leach, Marilyn M **(SLP)**
Lewis, Dawna E **(A)**
Lillegard, Linda R **(SLP)**
Litz, Mrs Laurie Donelan **(SLP)**
Lorenz, Mrs Lori J
Lotz, Wendy Kay **(SLP)**
Low, Mrs Linda K M **(SLP)**
Loyd, Rebecca R **(SLP)**
Maher, Barbara Anne **(SLP)**
Mangus, Robin Elizabeth **(SLP)**
Mathy-Laikko, Pamela **(SLP)**
Matthiesen, Mrs Linda L **(SLP)**
McDaniel, Mrs Ruth H **(SLP)**
McDermott, Catherine Ann **(SLP)**
McDermott, Susan **(SLP)**
McGargill, Dr Roger L, Jr **(SLP A)**
McLeod, Joye L **(SLP)**
Merrill, Gloria S **(SLP)**
Meyer, Mrs Diane Lynn **(SLP)**
Miklas, Mary Kathleen **(SLP)**
Miles, Mrs Mary Suzanne **(SLP)**
Mlotek, Mrs Janet Ritter **(SLP)**
Moe, Janet M S **(SLP)**
Moeller, Mrs Mary P **(A)**
Molacek, Mrs Vicki Louise **(SLP)**
Monaco, Christine **(SLP)**
Morgan, Suzanne E **(SLP)**
Morrow, Patricia Ellen **(A)**
Mote, Mrs Nina S **(SLP)**
Muehling, Linda Schutz
Muller, Julie Anne **(SLP)**
Naple, Mrs Ann M **(SLP)**
Neary, Mary Elizabeth **(SLP)**
Neff, Dr Donna Lynn
Nelson, Mrs Evelyn Mae **(SLP)**
Nelson-Barlow, Nancy L **(A)**
Netsell, Ronald **(SLP)**
Nittrouer, Dr Susan N
Noodell, Marcy Anne **(SLP)**
Norris, Dr Thomas W **(SLP A)**
O'Connor, Deborah Ann **(SLP)**
Olson, Andrea B **(SLP)**
Parrish, Mrs Sheryl Bruns **(SLP)**
Peters, Jo E **(SLP)**
Philips, Dr Betty Jane **(SLP)**
Pitts, Dawna Gail **(SLP)**
Pollok, Mrs Janice J **(SLP)**
Potter-Manion, Ann M **(SLP)**
Pribyl, Julianne L **(SLP)**
Quinn, Michelle A **(SLP)**
Rachow, Roger L **(SLP)**
Ransom, Kathleen M **(SLP)**
Reed, Cynthia Ann **(SLP)**
Richter-McEathron, Virginia Strohmeyer **(SLP)**
Roberts, Dr Kenneth R **(SLP)**
Robinson, Dale H **(A)**
Roelfs, Mrs Donna S **(SLP)**
Ronci, Eileen Stanton **(SLP)**
Rook, Mrs Judith Ann Morrison **(SLP A)**
Schaefer, Linda K **(SLP)**
Schick, Dr Brenda S
Schicker, Mrs Patricia L **(SLP)**
Schulze, Theresa Wulff **(SLP)**
Seger, Dr Cheryl A D **(SLP)**
Sennett, Mrs Holly Ann **(SLP)**
Shannon, Robert V
Sheppard, Shirley Jean **(SLP)**
Sherrets, Mrs Trish Anne **(SLP)**
Sims, Leslie Leanne **(A)**
Slattery, Linda K **(SLP)**
Smith, Debra L **(A)**
Smith, Sharon K **(SLP)**
Snyder, Rebecca M **(SLP)**
Srb, Mrs Charlene J **(SLP)**
Stelmachowicz, Dr Patricia G **(A)**
Stimbert-Guck, Karen F **(SLP)**
Sullivan, Dr Patricia M
Svingen, Julianne P **(SLP)**
Swanson, Susan Marie **(SLP)**
Tabshey, Christine **(A)**
Teare, Sharon Wood **(SLP)**
Tobias-Roach, Lisa **(SLP)**
Tritsch, Mrs Martha M **(SLP)**
Troia, Mrs Barbara Lynn **(A)**
Umatum, Michael W **(SLP)**
Vollmer, Mrs Deborah Kay **(SLP)**
Wallace, Kathleen Louise **(A)**
Weber, Laura Gail **(SLP)**
Whan, Mrs Mary Q **(A)**
White, Valorie Parker **(A)**
Wood, Dr James Martin **(SLP)**
Worthington, Dr Don W **(A)**
Young, Lisa Trautwein
Zagurski, Kim Marie **(SLP)**
Zenon, Wendy Ann **(SLP)**
Zimmerman, Mrs Lesta Lee **(SLP)**

Orchard
Meyer, Kathy Sue Dean **(SLP)**

Ord
Galvan, Mrs Valerie Ann **(SLP)**

Papillion
Bargstadt, Mrs Grace H **(SLP)**
Himmelberg, Kebbelin Keith **(SLP)**
Levell, Mrs Marilyn M **(SLP)**
Renfro, Mrs Elizabeth M **(SLP)**
Westerhold, Mrs Rosalie P **(A)**

Peru
Harper, Mrs Judith W **(SLP)**

Pickrell
Goracke, Mrs Loretta M **(A)**

Plainview
White, Mrs Janet Ann **(SLP)**

Plymouth
Schroeder, Mrs Catherine **(SLP)**

Prague
Sloup, Patricia Lackovic **(SLP)**

Ralston
Jones, Sheila L N **(SLP)**

Ravenna
McInroy, Mrs Judy W **(SLP)**

Raymond
Crowe, Linda Kay **(SLP)**

Scottsbluff
Burke, Marlene W
Douglas, Martha J **(SLP)**
Svoboda, Mrs Cheryl L **(SLP)**
Svoboda, James S **(SLP)**

Seward
Gauthier, Rita Dresp **(SLP)**

Shickley
Straight, Jenise Schroeder **(SLP)**

Sidney
Nienhueser, Mrs Kathleen E **(SLP)**

South Sioux City
Grier, Mrs Marla S **(SLP)**
Kielhold, Mrs Nancy Louise **(SLP)**

Springfield
Shuck, Anna Marie **(SLP)**

Steele City
Marsh, Lucille T

Superior
Alexander, Anna S **(SLP)**

Syracuse
Hillman, Mrs Pamela R **(SLP)**
Palmer, Mrs Gail L **(SLP)**

Valparaiso
Masek, Mrs Carol M **(SLP)**
Ryan, John P **(SLP A)**

Wahoo
Hakel-Dailey, Mrs Lori J

Wakefield
Luhr, Mrs Vernae Ivone **(A)**
Schroeder, Mrs Catherine **(SLP)**

Walthill
Kruse, Mrs Sydney Lynne B **(SLP)**

Wausa
Eckstrom, Carol Ann **(SLP)**

West Point
Hotovy, Mrs Patricia E **(SLP)**

Wilber
Max, Mrs Becky Sue **(SLP)**

York
Burrell, Mrs Sandra Cozad **(SLP)**

NEVADA

Boulder City
Giltner, Elizabeth (Toni) T **(SLP)**

Carson City
Baker, Mrs Susan K **(SLP)**
Christiansen, Diana J **(SLP)**
Eberle-Brinson, Jane Anne **(SLP)**
Erickson, E Joy **(SLP)**
Jones, Mrs Ruth E **(SLP)**
Patterson, Mrs Barbara A **(SLP)**
Reeves, Mrs Rita **(SLP)**
Weeks, Mark S **(A)**
Wessel, Mrs Brenda **(SLP)**

Dayton
Devaney, Mrs Jane M **(SLP)**

Fallon
Anderson, Mrs Patricia M **(SLP)**

Fernley
Taylor, Geraldine **(SLP)**

Gardnerville
Keele, Judy Smith **(SLP)**

Henderson
Harpster-Kazen, Barbara Jean **(SLP)**
Lund, Josette V **(SLP)**
Mackey, Mrs Teresa Ann **(SLP)**
Swanson, Mrs Elizabeth Carver **(SLP)**
Wilbur, Anita A **(SLP)**

Incline Village
Steele, Mrs Nancy R **(A)**
Zegen, Mrs Joyce **(SLP)**

Lamoille
Grinsell, Mrs Valerie Ann **(SLP)**

Las Vegas
Anderson, David E **(A)**
Austin, Mrs Judith K **(SLP)**
Bady, Janet A **(SLP)**
Banis, Mrs Carolyn J **(SLP)**
Blackford, Michele A **(SLP)**
Blair, Greta B **(SLP)**
Bokelmann, Dorothy T **(SLP)**
Bunderson, Karin **(A)**
Callahan, Barbara Heinz **(SLP)**
Cardwell, Cindy L **(SLP)**
Carpi, Mary Wibbert **(A)**
Caruso, Mrs Nancy Sowka **(SLP)**
Casini, Mrs Louann Jo **(SLP)**
Cremen, Mrs Lynn K **(SLP)**
Cromwell, Kenalyn Morrow **(SLP)**
Curran, Mrs Jean L **(SLP)**
Devlin, Kim R **(SLP)**
Dinsmore, Cassandra Elizabeth **(SLP)**
Emmer, DeeAnn **(SLP)**
Gerbino-Redick, Mrs Sharlette **(SLP)**
Gertz, Mrs Jil Marie **(SLP)**
Glovinsky, Mrs Marilyn G **(SLP)**
Goings, Mrs Regina E **(SLP)**
Hansen-Jones, Karen L **(SLP)**
Hanson, Mrs Pamela Marie **(SLP)**
Harkson, Janet Snyder **(SLP)**
Harrington, Mrs Kathleen A **(SLP)**
Hughes, Mrs Wendy L **(SLP)**
Jolls, Gwen Marie **(SLP)**
Kalman, Janet **(SLP)**
Kaner, Mrs Debra **(SLP)**
Kearns-Crockett, Patricia M **(SLP)**
Krueger, Charles Kent **(SLP)**
Laub, Mrs Clarice C **(SLP)**
Lloyd, Mrs Susan R **(A)**
Lovell, Mary E **(SLP)**
Malmgren, Virginia A **(SLP)**
Maschgan, Marilyn G **(A)**
Maxam, Patricia D **(SLP)**
Mayfield, Mrs Francine A **(SLP)**
Mekus, Mrs Deborah Drake **(SLP)**
Miks, Mrs Marilyn G **(SLP)**
Moss, Pamela G **(SLP)**
Paulson, Mrs Shelley Baker **(SLP)**
Rew, Mrs Christy Jackson **(SLP)**
Romeo, Mrs Teri Louise **(SLP)**
Schwartz, Barbara R **(SLP)**
Stevens, Ellen B **(A)**
Sutton, Cynthia F **(SLP)**
Taigman, Myra T **(A)**
Tarkanian, Dr Lois **(SLP A)**
Thelen, Patricia A **(SLP)**
Van Wyck, Nancy **(SLP)**
Vilensons, Mrs Virginia **(SLP)**
Wade, Mrs Elizabeth Ruth **(SLP)**
Wesson, Mrs Bette C **(SLP)**

Reno
Andersen, Lucie C
Anderson, Dr Bernard A **(SLP)**
Benning, Mrs Lori Joan **(SLP)**
Bensen, Court M **(SLP)**
Biondo, Barbara J **(SLP)**
Brick-Goodman, Nancy G **(SLP)**
Coburn, Lisa Marie **(A)**
Colang, Cheryl M **(SLP)**
Cunningham-Wong, Patricia Ann **(A)**
Dixon, Michelle Marie **(SLP)**
Fitch, Mrs Lucy Ann **(SLP)**
Froslie, Lucille L **(SLP)**
Golberg, Mrs Leslie Levin **(SLP)**
Green, Mrs Kelly E **(A)**
Healy, Colleen Ellen **(SLP)**
Hobbs, Linda L **(SLP)**
Karlin, Torrey S **(SLP)**
Klotz, Susan Lisa **(SLP)**
Knauf, Mrs Loren W **(SLP)**
Knauf, Dr Vincent H **(SLP A)**
Kuhles, Nancy Lillian **(SLP)**
Levitt, Mrs Linda Ruth **(SLP)**
Liljeblad, Mrs Astrid **(SLP)**
Lyon, Dr Jon G **(SLP)**
Mathews, Mrs Cheri Rene **(SLP)**
McFarlane, Dr Stephen C **(SLP)**
Menicucci, Andrea Lynn
Mirch, Marie Brown **(SLP)**
Morris, Thomas W **(A)**
Murph, Laura B **(SLP)**
Navarro, Dr M Richard **(A)**
Richardson, Mrs Debra Lee **(SLP)**
Ross, Diane C **(SLP)**
Rue, Mrs Patricia A **(SLP)**
Sakelaris, Patricia G **(A)**
Shapiro, Mrs Janet R **(SLP)**
Shrigley-Parker, Mrs Sandra Jo **(SLP)**
Sommer, Sue A **(SLP)**
Stone, Terry A **(SLP)**
Totten, Carol Orrin **(SLP)**
Uken, Dennis Lee **(A)**
Watterson, Mrs Kathye H **(SLP)**
Watterson, Dr Thomas L **(SLP)**
Weston, Mrs Lisa Marie **(SLP)**

Silver Springs
Erickson, Susan D **(SLP)**

Sparks
Bohman, Mrs Renee J **(SLP)**
Keats-Rigby, Mrs Caren S **(SLP)**
Leavitt, Phillip A
Penny, Mrs Lynn B **(SLP)**
Spuhler, Linde M **(SLP)**
Uren, Julie A
Winkler, Mrs Erika C **(SLP)**
Yocom, Bonnie S **(SLP)**

Verdi
Clark, Mrs Cheryl **(SLP)**

NEW HAMPSHIRE

Andover
Mishcon, Victoria Louise **(SLP)**

Ashland
Nadeau, Gail Brenda **(SLP)**

Atkinson
Stewart, Mrs Catherine M **(SLP)**

Barnstead
Dodge, M Cynthia **(SLP)**

Barrington
O'Neil-McCabe, Mrs Jana **(SLP)**

Bedford
Bailey, Deborah Hinton **(SLP)**
Chabot, Theresa E **(SLP)**
Fossum, Carol A **(SLP)**
Freeman, Toby Ellen **(SLP)**
Glennan-Brethauer, Nancy **(SLP)**
Nachbar, Mrs Charlotte **(SLP)**

Berlin
Schaffmeyer, Mrs Mary Jeanne **(SLP)**

Bethlehem
Lister, Paul B **(SLP)**

Bow
Cote, Mrs Donna Jane **(SLP)**
Culbertson-Egan, Maurine A **(A)**

Bradford
St Pierre, Mrs Melissa **(SLP)**

Brookline
Morgan, Marlene S **(SLP)**

Canterbury
Webster, Dr Penelope E **(SLP)**

Center Harbor
Di Cecca, Charles Louis **(SLP)**
Dorval, Mrs Bertha Mae **(SLP)**

Center Ossipee
Fairchild, Linda Ann **(SLP)**

Chichester
Prickett, Mrs Anita Louise **(SLP)**

Claremont
Bowen, Kathryn H **(SLP)**
Gosselin, Mrs Lisa R **(A)**
Shidlovsky, Cathy M **(SLP)**

Concord
Cieliczka, David J **(A)**
Dennis, Susan Gay **(SLP)**
Dinan, Christine Anderson **(SLP)**
Hanrahan, Dr Linda L **(SLP)**
Hicks, Patricia Rogers **(SLP)**
Iarussi, Jane M **(SLP)**
Jillette, Mrs Janet D W **(SLP)**
Jobin, Mrs Barbara Ann **(SLP)**
Krasner, Sherri L **(SLP)**
Lauze, Susan Flanders **(SLP)**
Nadeau, Leon N **(A)**
Scranton, Mrs Judith Whitacre **(SLP)**
Sherman, Ann Cheryl **(SLP)**

Contoocook
Knox, Joanne Elles **(SLP)**

Conway
Browning, Marla Anne **(SLP)**
Fishman, Susan Paula **(SLP)**
Hawkins, Mrs Catherine M **(SLP)**

Danville
Hull, Mrs Eileen M **(SLP)**

Derry
Caplan, Mrs Elizabeth A **(SLP)**
Gillette, Debra H **(A)**
Pelunis, Jill Dee **(SLP)**
Robertshaw, Mrs Kristan Kulch **(SLP)**
Townsend, Mrs Lynne Hylton **(SLP)**

Dover
Baker, Martha Sue **(SLP)**
Bertsch-Hill, Paula **(SLP)**
Bloom, Joanne A **(SLP)**
Boggis, Ivy Marie **(SLP)**
Brandon, Andrew E **(A)**
Cavalieri, Elizabeth Huckins **(A)**
Deminoff, Anne Louise
Holak, Mrs Susan M **(SLP)**
Laverty, Barbara Ann **(SLP)**
Looker, Susan N **(SLP)**
McKone, Ann M **(SLP)**
Stram, Sarah T **(SLP)**

Dunbarton
Haywood, Emily Jo **(SLP)**

Durham
Hilliard, Clinton Thielens, Jr **(SLP)**
Issokson, Roberta G **(SLP)**
Machon, Marsha W **(SLP)**
Murray, Dr Frederick P **(SLP)**
Wachowiak, Nancy Kubasek **(SLP)**

East Derry
Stevenson, J Marie **(SLP)**

Eaton
Kelly, Joann Linda **(SLP)**

Etna
Aulis, Patricia S **(SLP)**
Young, Mary B **(SLP)**

Exeter
Berry, Robert A **(SLP A)**
Dunnan, Judith R **(SLP)**
Gram, Mrs Margaret **(SLP)**
Hiney, Mrs Debra Stanley **(SLP)**
Hughes-O'Sullivan, Jeanne M **(SLP)**
Kirsch, Mrs Martha Rose **(SLP)**
Prescott, Marian H **(SLP)**
Troio, Debra A

Georges Mills
Marrin, Joan **(SLP)**

Gilford
McKinster, Mrs Katherine **(SLP)**
Seed, Mrs Pamela F **(SLP)**
Wright, Nancy Losapio **(SLP)**

Goffstown
Taarud, Nancy M **(SLP)**

Greenfield
Johnson, Michael Dewees **(SLP)**
Rube, Jean R **(SLP)**

Greenland
Lippmeier, Linda Lee **(SLP)**
Rahilly-Coviello, Sandra J **(SLP)**

Hampstead
Plante, Theresa Clark **(SLP)**

Hampton
Dow, Mrs Marie L
Fowler, Diana Teague **(A)**
Mahler, Mrs Linda Marie
Wolstenholm, Jeanne L **(SLP)**

Hampton Falls
Scott, Mrs Ruth **(SLP)**

Hancock
Quinn, Janet M **(SLP)**

Hanover
Gollegly, Karen M **(A)**
Musiek, Dr Frank E **(A)**

Verkest, Suzanne Bernice **(A)**

Henniker
Glover, Mrs Margaret **(A)**

Hollis
Banks, Pamela Fallon **(SLP)**
Butler, Mrs Kim-Ellen Schombert **(SLP)**
Cegalis, Mrs Nancy Ritchie **(SLP)**

Hooksett
Babineau, Mary Kathleen **(SLP)**
Beaudette, Mrs Jane Irene **(SLP)**
Storm, Patricia Grady **(SLP)**

Jaffrey
Salvione, Lisa Angela **(SLP)**

Keene
Crain, Lydia H **(SLP)**
Fellendorf, George W
Gaylord, Donna J **(SLP)**
Hill, William Blaine **(A)**
Hutcherson, Leslie Elaine **(SLP)**
Keene, Risa G **(SLP)**
Loughrey, Susan Elizabeth **(SLP)**
Quinn, Bernadette Mary **(A)**
Schroeder, Susan Hill **(SLP)**
Thompson, Mrs Traudl **(SLP)**

Laconia
Abikoff, Laurence **(A)**
Belanger, Steven A **(SLP)**
Boyd, Lynda Ann
Eshelman, Mrs Sally L **(SLP)**
Evans, Anne Eliza **(A)**
Green-Barber, Lisa J **(SLP)**
Muse, Diane **(SLP)**
Reinhardt, Donna
Santostefano, Joyce A **(SLP)**
Shea, Mrs Judith Orrill **(SLP A)**

Lebanon
Bouchard, Mrs Anne B **(SLP)**
Thorne, Sr Ann Theresa **(SLP)**

Lee
Colombo, Mrs Christine E **(SLP)**

Littleton
Twomey, Karen Wilson **(SLP)**

Londonderry
Arcidiacono, Nancy **(SLP)**
Bever, Mrs Donna J **(SLP)**
Blake, Mrs Barbara A **(SLP)**
Girard, Andree **(A)**
Gratton, Deborah **(SLP)**
Hayes, Amy Schweigert **(SLP)**
Kandle, Virjean Camp **(SLP)**
Madigan, Mrs Anne McClave **(A)**
Piper, Mrs Teresa Kathryn **(SLP)**
Renza, Geraldine **(SLP)**

Manchester
Greenberg, Mrs Dawn Jennifer **(SLP)**
Hamlet, Elizabeth G **(SLP)**
Izen, Joan M **(SLP)**
Levine-Stern, Ilene **(A)**
McCormack, Jane Ellen **(SLP)**
McHugh, Lea M **(SLP)**
Paskevich, Jeanne B **(SLP)**
Ramsay, Carolyn M **(SLP)**
Scanlan, Mrs Crista C
Singer, Mrs Rivelle Feldman **(SLP)**
Skruck, Connie Belleville **(SLP)**
Stickney, Joyce Karen **(SLP)**
Webster, Mrs Mary McEvoy **(SLP)**

Mason
Abbott, Virginia Miller **(SLP)**

Meredith
Ryan, Constance M **(SLP)**

Meriden
Allen, Deborah W **(SLP)**

Merrimack
Brooks, Martha Wisly **(SLP)**
Herbert, Mrs Linda May **(SLP)**
Nadeau, Mrs Karen L G **(SLP)**
Schulze, Victoria Lynne **(SLP)**
Woodie, Sally Kay **(A)**
Young, Elizabeth **(A)**

Milford
Beldin, Annette Teresa **(SLP)**
Tripp, Jeanette Lois
Widlitz, Pamela **(A)**

Nashua
Becker, Leanne Marie **(SLP)**
Bradley, Marcia E F **(SLP)**
Brown, Cheryl Ann **(A)**
Cheshire, Mrs Anne M **(SLP)**
Chesterley, Victoria L **(SLP)**
Daniels, Charleen Mary **(SLP)**
Desaulniers, Renee Michelle **(SLP)**
Drury, Carolyn Ruth **(A)**
Finn, Mary Cecelia **(SLP)**
Foss, Cynthia Diane **(SLP)**
Holmberg, Sandra L **(SLP)**
Kirk, Rita A **(SLP)**
Manning, Cynthia Wheeler **(SLP)**
Martin, Mrs Bonnie S **(SLP)**
Masse-Arikian, Jody Lynne **(SLP)**
Moran, Carolann **(SLP)**
Myska, Mrs Carol B D **(SLP)**
Potter, Anne T M **(SLP)**
Roberts, Mrs Karen Aicher **(SLP)**
Rosen, Mrs Karen P **(SLP)**
Schulz, Nancy A **(SLP)**
Scott, Mrs Mary Anne S **(SLP)**
Skibinski, Stephanie J **(SLP)**
Smith, Barbara M **(SLP)**
Strollo, Janet Ann K **(SLP)**
Vangroesbeck, Mrs Patrice L **(SLP)**
Walker, Joan Peirce **(SLP)**
Whitney, Cynthia Walker **(SLP)**

New Boston
Austin, Mrs Jane E **(SLP)**
Dana, Diane Sniegoski **(SLP)**
Ruddock, Jane Levine **(SLP)**

New Ipswich
Kress, Linda Elizabeth

New London
Prohl, Mrs Maureen Foy **(SLP)**

Newfields
Griffin, Sharon Louise **(SLP)**

Newmarket
Mikami, Judith Hinds **(SLP)**
Tokay, Mrs Carol B **(SLP)**
Tokay, Dr F Harry **(A)**

North Conway
Cargill, Susannah Halpern **(SLP)**
McHugh, Mrs Maria Stella

North Hampton
Hoffmann, Kit A **(SLP)**
Marshall, Eileen Frances **(A)**
Martin-Nadeau, Kimberly **(SLP)**

Northwood
Cullinan, Denise Graziano **(SLP)**

Ossipee
Estes, Mrs Patricia T **(SLP)**

Oxford
Lahey, Dr Margaret M **(SLP A)**

Pelham
Sherman, Barbara C **(SLP)**

Peterborough
Holmes, Jane F **(SLP)**
Maguire, Mrs Katherine Cypher **(SLP)**
Pore, Sally G **(SLP)**
Salciccia, Cathy E **(SLP)**

Plainstow
Rosati, Juliann Marie **(SLP)**

Portsmouth
Bowes, Alice H S **(SLP)**
Donigian, Christine A **(A)**
Fiske, Dana R **(A)**
Goodman, Deborah Ann
Hutchison, Thomas L **(A)**
Lewis, Frederick, Jr **(SLP)**
Minot-Seabrook, Jill Michele **(SLP)**
Teas-Trudeau, Elizabeth C **(SLP)**

Raymond
Lister, Jocelyn **(SLP)**

Rochester
Carignan, Mrs Karen Linda **(SLP)**
Knight, Mrs Karen Jean/Bell **(SLP)**
Leman, Mrs Lori Berry **(SLP)**
Michel, Mrs Karen Elaine **(SLP)**
Mortimer, Mrs Jean A W **(SLP)**
Poulin, Cynthia Anne **(SLP)**
Zombeck, Mrs Suzanne M **(SLP)**

Rye
McPherson, Cynthia Keddy **(SLP)**

Salem
Bassett, Mrs Jane T **(SLP)**
Brockway, Mrs Mary Ann **(A)**
Capuano, Mrs Dale W **(SLP)**
Faller, Jean Marie **(SLP)**
Koocher, Aida Louise **(SLP)**
Lucas, Dr Karen Hawver **(SLP)**
Mitchell, Mrs Lisa Ann **(SLP)**
Niemeyer, Judith Mary **(SLP)**
Stewart, Irene E **(SLP)**

Salisbury
Wood, Mrs Lori B **(SLP)**

Sanbornton
Stoecklin, Mrs Judy L **(SLP)**

Seabrook
Trisdale, Miriam Edel **(SLP)**

Somersworth
Calculator, Mrs Jean M **(SLP)**
Calculator, Dr Stephen **(SLP)**
Cullinane, Mrs Ruth Ann **(SLP)**
O'Day, James Marshall **(A)**
Wallis, Mrs Karene Jones **(A)**

South Lyndeboro
Bonner, Sue J **(SLP)**

Stratham
Crosland-Real, Marybeth **(SLP)**
Lacroix, Dr Paul G **(A)**
Sexton, Mrs Jill D **(SLP)**

Tilton
Brown-Herman, Catherine **(SLP)**
Murray, Marie Elsie **(SLP)**

Walpole
Seelye, Dr Barbara J **(SLP)**

Warner
Skoglund, Mrs Dianne Boutwell **(SLP)**

Weare
Heckman, Maureen Weitzel **(SLP)**
Lassonde, Mrs Christena L **(SLP)**
Poulin, Linda Lee **(SLP)**

West Nottingham
Plante, Amy Solomon **(SLP)**

Wilton
Galica, Roxanne Lee **(SLP)**

Winchester
Bierman, Mrs Marie S **(SLP)**

Windham
Gumbel, Gail E S **(SLP)**

Wolfeboro
Antonak, Carol Christine **(SLP)**

NEW JERSEY

Aberdeen
Easton, Mrs Patricia Lee **(SLP)**
Gura, Mrs Gloria Antebi **(SLP)**
Pedinoff, Cara Susan **(SLP)**

Absecon
Connor, Mrs Kathleen S **(SLP)**
Helsabeck, Mary R **(SLP)**
Johnson, Diane L
Kates, Alison Dale **(A)**
Potkay, Raymond J **(SLP)**

Allamuchy
Freeborn, Mrs Carol Hunt **(SLP)**

Allendale
Alexander, Suzanne **(SLP)**
Hovey, Mrs Karen Kane **(SLP)**
Kaufman, Mrs Tobie Nan **(SLP)**
Piliero, Mrs Mildred H **(SLP)**
Sukernick, Gail Rubini **(SLP)**

Andover
Turetsky, Karen **(SLP)**

Annandale
Blaus, Mrs Jane Hamrick **(SLP)**
Delsack, Barbara Stern **(SLP)**
Rakay, Cynthia J **(SLP)**
Simmonds, Nancy G **(SLP)**
Stephan, Mrs Roberta J **(SLP)**

Asbury
Norton-Darr, Sally **(SLP)**

Asbury Park
Hoff, Susan L **(SLP)**

Atco
Graham, Mrs Nancy Dunn **(SLP)**
Molloy, Julia Sale

Atlantic City
Bannister, Stacy G
Hershenfis, Hilda A **(SLP)**
Kaloustian, Houri Khatcher **(SLP)**

Atlantic Highlands
Gelber, Mrs Susan S **(SLP)**

Audubon
Janowicz, Pamela J **(SLP)**
McGinley, Joan Marie **(SLP)**

Avenel
Kreitzman, Natalie Rae **(SLP)**
Lasky-Broecker, Brenda **(A)**

Baptistown
McKenna, Ellen Mary **(SLP)**

Barrington
Gibson, Barbara A **(SLP)**
Kennedy, Elizabeth **(A)**

Basking
Robertson-Soriano, Mrs Kristie **(SLP)**

Basking Ridge
Boland, Barbara A **(SLP)**
Cohen, Mrs Terri Haskins
Del Coro, Paula Sosulski **(SLP)**
Donohue, Mrs Susann Islami **(A)**
Faust, Mrs Ruth S **(SLP)**
Levy, Mrs Cynthia **(SLP)**
Malkin, Darcie Ellen **(SLP)**
Polignano, Mrs Maria L **(SLP)**
Salvo, Mrs Donna Arthur **(SLP)**
Vayianos, Marissa C **(SLP)**
Yanklowitz, Mrs Sandra L **(SLP)**

Bayonne
Burke, Margaret Noel **(A)**

Bayville
- Constanza, Mrs Kathleen M **(SLP)**
- Herring, Mrs Karen Kissane **(A)**
- Multari, Bruno D **(SLP)**

Beach Haven
- Tromm, Kathleen Barry **(SLP)**
- Tyrrell-Jones, Louise M **(SLP)**

Bedminster
- Gaines, Mrs Lynn Susan **(SLP)**
- Marvin, Joanne **(A)**

Belford
- Rella, Anthony Robert

Belle Mead
- Della Sala, Eugenia Valeria **(SLP)**
- Denekas, Mrs Susan W **(SLP)**
- Fenster, Mrs Joan G **(SLP)**
- Millman, Ilene K **(SLP)**
- Smithyman, Rosemary L **(SLP)**

Belleville
- Browne, Alan, Jr **(SLP)**
- Freda, Elizabeth L
- Latona, Madelaine J **(SLP)**
- McDonald, Mrs Nancy Chamberlain **(SLP)**
- Miterman, Gail Pamela **(SLP)**

Belmar
- Fox, Dr Daphne S **(A)**
- Keane, Dr Vincent E **(SLP)**
- McCorry, Mrs Suzanne B **(A)**
- Rath, Mrs Antoinette Petrillo **(SLP)**

Bergenfield
- Auerbach, Dr Lawrence **(SLP)**
- Carter, Leslie A **(SLP)**
- Cirelli, Richard A **(SLP)**
- Nemec, Elizabeth Kathryn **(A)**

Berkeley Heights
- Albamonte, Stefanie J **(SLP)**
- Ben'Ary, Adele N **(SLP)**
- Borack, Mrs Sheila **(SLP)**
- Burnett, Arlene E **(SLP)**
- Fisher, Mrs Gayll A **(SLP)**
- Lecomte, Dr Barbara V **(SLP)**
- Minogue-Byrne, Mrs Maureen **(SLP)**

Berlin
- D'Armi, Mrs Patricia Cipoletti **(SLP)**
- Poussart, Mrs Susan B **(SLP)**

Beverly
- Bogush, Laurie J **(SLP)**

Blackwood
- Drake, Mrs Janis S **(SLP)**
- Jenkins, Mrs Leslie A **(SLP)**
- Miers, Deanne Kaye
- Schaffer, Lori Foster **(SLP)**
- Stepkin, Richard L **(A)**

Blairstown
- Lacken, Vivienne E **(SLP)**
- Schneider, Grace E **(SLP)**

Bloomfield
- Adubato, Felicia A **(SLP)**
- Hilt, Gary D **(SLP A)**
- Jalonack, Mary Louise T **(SLP)**
- Lollos, Mrs Virginia Farese **(SLP)**
- Moseson, Susan Shedd **(SLP)**
- Porrino, Mrs Andrea Mittleman **(SLP)**

Bloomingdale
- Warner, Joan Ellen **(SLP)**
- Warner, Mark Richard **(A)**

Blue Anchor
- Foster, Cecelia **(SLP)**

Bogota
- Hinchman-Giuffre, Mrs Joanne **(SLP)**
- Schaffer-Cohen, Mrs Phyllis Beth **(A)**

Boonton
- Gervasio, Mrs Anita F **(A)**
- McCarthy, Mrs Jean Marie **(SLP)**

Bordentown
- Kelley-Smith, Mrs Susan **(SLP)**
- Mitchell, Linda Sue **(SLP)**
- Walker, Kimberley M **(SLP)**

Bound Brook
- Brady, Granville Y, Jr **(SLP A)**
- Calderone, Mrs Tancine W **(SLP)**

Bradley Beach
- Eyer, Mrs Deborah L **(SLP)**

Brick
- Brooks, David H **(SLP)**
- Hurst, Mrs June Manger **(SLP)**
- Levine, Terri **(SLP)**
- Rinehart, Phyllis M **(SLP)**
- Sager, Mrs Gwen Hahn **(SLP)**
- Zickar-Stranieri, Mrs Susan Elaine **(SLP)**

Bricktown
- Cleary, Denise Elizabeth **(SLP)**
- Ferguson, Hugh D **(A)**
- Ferrie, Adrienne C **(SLP)**
- Gibbons, H Elizabeth **(SLP)**
- Kearney, Ruth S **(SLP)**
- Kurmin, Kathi E **(A)**
- Markell, Debra L **(A)**
- Smith, Mrs Joanne Geraldine **(SLP)**

Bridgeton
- Bickings, Mrs Jayme J **(SLP)**
- Ingraldi, Cynthia Ann **(SLP)**
- Martelli, Lisa **(SLP)**
- Masters, Nancy E **(A)**
- Woolbert, Kathi L

Bridgewater
- Bevan, Ronnie E **(SLP)**
- Blake, Mrs Rhoda S **(SLP)**
- Carswell, Mrs Lynn E **(SLP)**
- Constad, Mrs Ann B **(SLP)**
- Eagar, Miriam O **(SLP)**
- Fink, Mrs Joan Ann
- Hansch, Debra Jean **(SLP)**
- Lubinsky, Natalie B **(SLP)**
- Murphy, Patricia A **(SLP)**
- Pescevich, Lucille M **(SLP)**

Browns Mills
- Boyea, Mrs Jill Ann **(SLP)**

Brunswick
- Riccobono, Mrs Pina Tosca

Budd Lake
- Artis, Mrs Carmen W **(SLP)**
- Botto, Michelle **(SLP)**
- De Luca, Renee Marie **(SLP)**

Burlington
- Burik, Christine E **(SLP)**
- Knoff, Mrs Shari Rohloff **(SLP)**
- Martin, Barbara H **(SLP)**
- Mastrocola, Mrs Phyllis A **(SLP)**
- Schiavone, Diane Adele **(SLP)**

Butler
- Bruno, Mrs Alexandra H **(SLP)**

Byram Township
- Ellicott, Mrs Barbara A **(SLP)**

Caldwell
- Arcell, Paul C **(SLP)**
- Goldsmith, Mrs Regina D **(SLP)**
- Harmony, Leslie Jean **(SLP)**
- Henry, Elaine M **(A)**
- Hill, Mrs Patricia Vazquez **(SLP)**
- Marcus, Sheryl **(SLP)**
- McGuire, Eileen J **(SLP)**
- Rinaldi, Donna M **(SLP)**

Califon
- Newsome, Linda A **(SLP)**
- Robison, Mrs Lynn Bruckner **(SLP)**

Camden
- Bey, Krista M **(SLP)**

Cape May Court House
- Meade, Edwina **(SLP)**
- Schellinger, Mrs Debra D **(SLP)**
- Smith, Elizabeth Helen **(SLP)**

Carteret
- Gliniecki, Mrs Karen L **(SLP)**
- Nigro, Louis J **(SLP)**

Cedar Grove
- Anthony, Mrs Marilyn H **(SLP)**
- Cheskin, Mrs Arlene C **(SLP)**
- Cohen, Mrs Sharon F **(A)**
- Gualtieri, Mrs Sherry Ann Alfano
- Kaufman, Renee C **(SLP)**
- Koch, Evanne N S **(SLP)**

Cedar Knolls
- Glus, Mrs Kathleen A **(SLP)**
- Welsh, Donna Jean **(SLP)**

Chatham
- Aitchison, Dr Carole J **(SLP)**
- Brack, Barbara Anne **(SLP)**
- Fleming, Mrs Geraldine **(SLP)**
- Goepfert, Mrs Laura Picetti **(SLP)**
- Knox, Alexandra Brittain **(SLP)**
- Lutolf, John J **(A)**
- Mink, Amy Sipes **(SLP)**
- Myers, Sally A **(SLP)**
- Shirley, Beth Ann **(SLP)**
- Smith, Carol A **(SLP)**
- Smith, Joann **(SLP)**
- Van De Boe, Caryl Ann **(A)**
- Wald, Mrs Karen Pick **(SLP)**

Chatham Township
- Auriemma, Mrs Donna M S **(SLP)**
- Ruvane, Anne B **(SLP)**

Cherry Hill
- Baskies, Susan Baer **(SLP)**
- Berman, Mrs Laura N **(A)**
- Boardman, Mrs Francine Presser **(SLP)**
- Bross, Mrs Caryn H **(A)**
- Cherkas, Mrs Anne Blumenthal
- Clark, Elizabeth **(SLP)**
- Cowper, Mrs Ellen Elizabeth **(SLP)**
- De Masi, Cheryl Drumheiser
- Dressler, Diane Peck **(SLP)**
- Dreyfuss, Elaine E **(SLP)**
- Eisenberg, Mrs Hope Sandra **(SLP)**
- Etish, Mrs Barbara Levin
- Feidt, Arlene S **(SLP)**
- Feldbaum, Jill M **(SLP)**
- Field, Dr William G
- Freedman, Mrs Roni S **(SLP)**
- Glazer, Mrs Jacqueline Gray **(SLP)**
- Goldhaber, Danna **(A)**
- Goldman, Amy S **(SLP)**
- Herman, Donna L **(SLP)**
- Hurwitz, Marcia Rogers **(SLP)**
- Ivans, William **(SLP)**
- Joseph, Linda Dorr **(SLP)**
- Kaufman-Plenn, Beth **(SLP)**
- Kellerman, Mrs Sandra Volusher **(SLP)**
- Kipnis, Mrs Joan E K **(A)**
- Korngold, Mrs Debra L **(SLP)**
- Kozlov, Enid M **(SLP)**
- Kushner-Rulnick, Rhonda L **(SLP)**
- Lightman, Mrs Karen Mandelkehr **(SLP)**
- Miller, Mrs Ann Rochelle **(SLP)**
- Orel, Sylvia P **(SLP)**
- Orichowskyj, Rose Marie **(SLP)**
- Pearl, Sharon K **(SLP)**
- Perlman, Mrs Cathy A
- Platt, Felice Ruth **(SLP)**
- Polonsky, Mrs Adrienne **(SLP)**
- Powell, Diane J **(SLP)**
- Rudolph, Donna Ellen **(SLP)**
- Shore, Mrs Karen M **(SLP)**
- Shubach, Nancy K **(SLP)**
- Simon, Mrs Ann H **(SLP)**
- Treuhaft, Mrs Eleanor Cohen **(SLP)**
- Udell, Mrs Deborah Brown **(SLP)**
- Visconti, Mrs Colleen Fitzgerald
- Ziemba, Mrs Michele Bidic **(SLP)**
- Zimmerman, Lauri Michele **(SLP)**

Chester
- Collins, Mrs Sally A **(SLP)**
- Levinn, Mrs Karen A **(SLP)**
- Martin, Mrs Barbara Jeanne **(A)**

Cinnaminson
- Arey, H Regina Smith **(SLP)**
- Bornstein, Pamela S **(SLP)**
- Girson, Mrs Norma R H **(SLP)**
- Kaplan, Carol M **(SLP)**

Clark
- Koebli, Mrs Judith Rose **(SLP)**
- Regan, Peggy Anne **(SLP)**
- Seavy, Judith L **(A)**
- Snyder, Mrs Linda Huber **(SLP)**
- Swierc, Mrs Regina Marie **(SLP)**

Clarksboro
- McCairns, Mrs Lillian O'Leary **(SLP)**

Clementon
- Bower, Robert D **(SLP)**
- De Narie, Mrs Mary Young **(SLP)**

Cliffside Park
- Kuehn, Marilyn K **(SLP)**
- Lawton, Joan S **(SLP)**

Clifton
- Abruzzese, Rosalie Mary **(SLP)**
- Carucci-Fenyar, Mrs Linda E **(SLP)**
- Cohen, Mrs Susan Wynn **(SLP)**
- Colligan, Mrs Helen Claire
- Fraulo, Marlene K **(SLP)**
- Fredericks, Catherine **(SLP)**
- Gotlieb, Mrs Talia F **(A)**
- Hain, Mrs Rosalind J **(SLP)**
- Hayes, Kathleen H **(SLP)**
- Lynch, Mrs Sharon A **(SLP)**
- Paccioretti, Mrs Lorraine A **(SLP)**
- Richvalsky, Stephanie
- Staron, Maryann **(SLP)**
- Sullivan, Mrs Lynn Stein **(SLP)**
- Winarski, Mrs Betty Ellen **(SLP)**

Closter
- Glick, Freda **(SLP)**
- Kligerman, Dr Anne Barbara **(A)**
- Mintz, Susan M **(SLP)**
- Sperber-Halprin, Marilyn S **(SLP)**
- Sprung, Mrs Mindy Parmett **(SLP)**

Collingswood
- Harker, Mrs Deborah Burns **(SLP)**
- Heuer, Dr Reinhardt **(SLP)**
- Johnson, Pamela L **(SLP)**
- Marcinkevich, Mrs Paula Ruth
- Walpole, Elizabeth **(SLP)**
- Zeldner, Michele J **(SLP)**

Colonia
- Murawski, Mrs Donna L **(SLP)**
- Partyka, Bernadette **(A)**

Colts Neck
- Britton, Joal H **(SLP)**
- Garito, Mrs Arlene Gold **(SLP)**
- Roth, Mrs Sue E **(SLP)**

Columbus
- Anghelone, Mrs Joyce G **(SLP)**

Convent
- Reuben, Gail D **(A)**

Cranbury
- O'Flaherty, Dr Kevin Paul **(A)**

Cranford
- Buonaguro, Dr Antonia J **(SLP)**
- Fanelli, Maria Elena **(SLP)**

Michaels, Mrs Lisa R **(SLP)**
Moura-Durkin, Yvonne **(SLP)**
Shapiro, Gertrude G **(SLP)**

Dayton
Dennehy, Mrs Jane G **(SLP)**
Hoos, Barbara L **(SLP A)**
Leibner, Fran Reiner **(SLP)**
Levine, Mrs Ronnie Elaine Freedman **(SLP)**
Portnoy, Mrs Mona Semel **(SLP)**

Delran
Brady, Mrs Nancylee Emerson
Steiner, Debra Marie **(SLP A)**

Demarest
Levenson, Jodi Lynn P **(SLP)**
Slaven, Margaret **(SLP)**

Denville
Ciurczak, Judith G **(SLP)**
Fiedel, Paula L **(SLP)**
Gallagher, Mrs Katherine **(SLP)**
Lunn, Ronald A **(SLP)**
Schumann, Nancy V **(SLP)**
Winson, Barbara **(SLP)**

Deptford
Hill, Mrs Joy Perlove **(SLP)**

Dover
Munson, Joan Mary **(A)**
Roseman, Marcia H **(SLP)**
Ryerson, Wayne Scott **(SLP)**
Sederholm, Steven Daniel **(A)**
Smolaga, Mrs Deborah Jean **(SLP)**

Dumont
Dewald, Patricia A **(SLP)**
Morgan, Sylvia **(A)**

East Brunswick
Cancro, Mrs Janice Hinsley
Dondes, Mrs Susan T **(A)**
Flieder, Mrs Sally Willner **(SLP)**
Flug, Mrs Gail **(SLP)**
Griepenburg, Mrs Susan Tanger **(SLP)**
Hall, Flavia Bernado **(SLP)**
Kapur, Mrs Revati D **(SLP)**
Katz, Mrs Gloria B **(SLP)**
Kelly, Ellen Maderski **(A)**
Kurland, Mrs Cecelia J **(SLP)**
Molinari-Defusco, Mrs Elizabeth **(SLP)**
Natalicchio, Stefanie
Nickel, George John, Jr
Oberweis, Susan P **(SLP)**
Pearl, Meredith E **(A)**
Peter, Mrs Marcia J R **(SLP)**
Robinson, Mrs Helaine Winakor **(A)**
Rudy, John Michael
Shulman, Dr Martin D **(SLP)**
Thomas, Kathleen Ann **(SLP)**
Wagman, Mrs Rhoda K **(SLP)**

East Hanover
Siu, Tai Ling Wong **(A)**
Smith, Mrs Gloria M **(SLP)**

East Orange
Snead, Linda J **(SLP)**
Tucker, Mrs Linda M **(SLP)**

East Windsor
Brandner, Susan Miller **(A)**
Cooper, Andrea S **(SLP)**
Ettman, Susan B S **(SLP)**
Gold, Mrs Susan J **(SLP)**
Johnson, Christine **(A)**
Matthes, Dr Elisa Fuchs **(SLP)**
McCarthy, Eileen M **(SLP)**
Miller, Mrs Barbara Kamm **(SLP)**
Newman, Suzanne M **(SLP)**
Ohanian, Rosemary C **(SLP)**
Potts, AnnMarie Desandre **(SLP)**
Richman, Linda G **(SLP)**
Weiner, Mrs Johanna G **(SLP)**

Eatontown
Greenfield, Mrs Deborah Goodman **(SLP)**
Slovin, Mrs Loretta R **(SLP)**

Edgewater
Vrablic, Eleanor M **(SLP)**
Zuback, Jacqueline Robin **(SLP)**

Edgewater Park
Fiore, Mrs Carol B **(SLP A)**

Edison
Batshaw, Marilyn Seidner **(A)**
Blumstein, Penny R **(SLP)**
Capezza, Lenora M B **(SLP)**
Cohen, Mrs Amy J **(SLP)**
Davis, Mrs Anita C **(SLP)**
Diament, Mrs Deborah S **(SLP)**
Dumas, Mrs Mary Teresa **(SLP)**
Ehrlich, Jonathan S **(SLP)**
Engel, Marcy Eileen **(SLP)**
Epstein, Mrs Helene Grande **(SLP)**
Gruenling, Carol Ann **(SLP)**
Guilder, Mrs Marcy Leitman **(SLP)**
Hoernlein, Theresa R **(SLP)**
Kline, Mrs Cindi M **(SLP)**
Krchnavek, Elizabeth Pfeiffer **(SLP)**
Mintz, Mrs Laura Brill
Needleman, Betty Unger **(A)**
Neuder, Cynthia I **(SLP)**
Peins, Dr Maryann **(SLP A)**
Reid-Malleck, Linda **(SLP)**
Reiss, Phyllis Hochberg **(SLP)**
Sisolak, Debra J **(SLP)**
Smith, Mrs Deborah Shontz **(A)**
Sperling, Heidi **(SLP)**
Spillman, Donna Ellen **(SLP)**
Tittel-Zuchowski, Karen **(SLP)**
Weber, Sharon Reiser **(SLP)**
Zakim, Shelley Pevner **(SLP)**

Egg Harbor
Hughes, Amy Jean **(SLP)**

Elizabeth
Anastasia, Antoinette Marie **(SLP)**
Canavan, Maria Rose **(A)**
Dee, Anita D **(SLP)**
Hoffman, Mrs Madelene **(SLP A)**
Kleinman, Marvin A **(A)**
Mandel, Mrs Susan Y **(SLP)**
McCall, Margaret Ann **(SLP)**
Salutsky, Rita Gale **(SLP)**
Weinstein, Mrs Virginia Kopf **(SLP)**

Elmer
Richards, Karen B **(SLP)**

Elmwood Park
Cusumano, Mrs Marilyn T **(SLP)**
Szabo, Mrs Donna **(A)**

Emerson
Cohen, Mrs Erica A **(SLP)**

Englewood
Cohen, Mrs Noemi F **(SLP)**
Danto, Dr Joseph **(A)**
Eftekhar, Mrs Barbara Lee **(SLP)**
Kornhaber, Arlene Cohen **(A)**
Masland, Mary W **(SLP)**
Strauss, Dr Raymond B **(SLP A)**

Englishtown
Chassin, Beryl **(A)**
Csatari, Marjorie Pizer
Henry, Mrs Patricia Bokan **(SLP)**
Hurewitz, Mrs Karen Ellyce **(SLP)**
Oconnor, Mrs Mary Gerilyn **(SLP)**
Vogel, Debra G **(SLP)**

Ewing
Guendler, Laverne Quadt **(SLP)**
Zane, Kim O'Hay **(SLP)**

Fair Haven
Bade, Marlane T **(SLP)**
Zenner, Mrs Natalie Argyris **(SLP)**

Fair Lawn
Becker, Mrs Irma Weiss **(SLP)**
Bray, Mrs Robin J **(A)**
Brunetti, Mrs Vicki Catherine **(SLP)**
Defrank, Lois Young **(SLP)**
Drucker, Sharon Stern **(SLP)**
Fenick, Blanca V **(A)**
Glaser, Mrs Sharon Naomi **(SLP)**
Heymann, Mrs Lois K **(SLP)**
Ianuzzi, Mrs Gayle S **(SLP)**
Jaffe, Norma S **(SLP)**
Kotek, Mrs Beth Schuldiner **(SLP)**
Lambert, Evalyn Feller **(SLP)**
Lukavich, Susan E **(SLP)**
Miller, Mrs Cindy B **(SLP)**
Moore, Mrs Lynn Savasta **(A)**
Nadel, Jill S **(SLP)**
Neuman, Faye J **(SLP)**
Rosenthal, Mrs Loren B **(SLP)**
Silverman, Shirley S **(SLP)**
Susser, Mrs Bonnie S **(SLP)**
Valenta, Kathleen Orr **(SLP A)**
Van Evra, Mrs Cathleen Maria **(A)**

Fairfield
Bachmann, Mrs Grace **(SLP)**
Wayne, Karen B **(SLP)**

Fanwood
Bassoul-Restivo, Regina **(SLP)**
Berry, Barbara Suzanne **(SLP)**
Farb, Mrs Gwene S **(SLP)**
Fisher, Mrs Roberta Helene

Far Hills
Gottlieb, Mrs Linda Lehrer **(SLP)**
McKirdy, Dr Laura Spielvogel **(SLP)**

Farmingdale
Bloom, Mrs Nancy L **(SLP)**
Tonkin-Stickler, Marilyn J **(SLP)**

Flanders
Baker, Kelly Taylor **(SLP)**
Meade, Mrs Margaret B **(SLP)**

Flemington
Applegate, Mrs Debra Ann **(SLP)**
Demarco, Mrs Ann W **(SLP)**
Florio, Mrs Amarilis **(SLP)**
Genovese, Mary Beth **(SLP)**
Hart, Mrs Deborah L C **(SLP)**
Leutholt, Mrs Barbara Dugger **(SLP)**
Neville, Margaret M **(SLP)**
Rossetti, Mrs Colleen Sneddon **(SLP)**

Florham Park
Bohan, Mrs Eileen Finnegan
Capano, Sharon A **(SLP)**
Carlson, Joan M **(SLP)**
De Angelis, Mrs Nadine W **(SLP)**
Picon, Edith J **(SLP)**
Price-Goldman, Mrs Wendi **(SLP)**
Rynar, Mrs Susan G **(SLP)**

Fords
Branderbit, Pamela Lynne **(A)**
Hochman, Mrs Roberta L **(SLP)**

Forked River
Grant, Karen Eileen **(SLP)**

Fort Lee
Aisner, Claudia Gail **(A)**
Fellerman, Nanc E **(SLP)**
Garfinkel, Carrie Lyn **(SLP)**
Gaynes, Mrs Andrea Sue **(SLP)**
Gettenberg, Mrs Phyllis C **(SLP)**
Glass, Jeffrey L **(SLP)**
Haber, Barbara **(SLP)**
Katsantonis, Joann V **(A)**
Kusher-Smith, Ilyse Beth **(SLP)**
Miller, Joan **(SLP)**
Perrotta, Brigitte
Rossman, Mrs Terri L **(SLP)**
Sandler, Janet L **(SLP)**
Semon, Diane Leiman **(SLP)**

Sigal, Beverly **(A)**
Taub, Linda B **(SLP)**
Tuttle, JoAnn **(SLP)**

Franklin
Baird, Mrs Bonnie Stuart **(SLP)**
Zoltak, Mrs Ruth S **(SLP)**

Franklin Lakes
Degeeter, Judith W **(SLP)**
Polizzi, Anne Maureen **(SLP)**
Roesler, Mrs Cynthia P **(SLP)**
Wolcott, Mrs Rose C **(SLP)**

Franklin Park
Broomer, Mrs Mona S **(SLP)**

Freehold
Cheifetz, Mrs Myrna Fox **(SLP)**
Cheslow, Martha Frimer **(SLP)**
DiSogra, Robert M **(A)**
Hellrigel, Diane Patricia
Hess, Mrs Carol P **(SLP)**
Kaplan, Mrs Tola E **(SLP)**
Lehrer, Stuart **(SLP)**
Pauker, Mrs Gail G **(SLP)**
Payton, Mrs Laurie A **(SLP)**
Peters, Brenda W **(SLP)**
Siegel, Mrs Julie Regina **(SLP)**
Strugatch, Mrs Mindy K **(SLP)**
Warner, Mrs Kathleen F **(SLP)**

Freehold Township
Heaps, Mrs Irene S **(SLP)**
Klein, Mrs Judy B **(SLP)**

Garfield
Marzitelli, Mrs Gail Russin **(SLP)**

Gillette
Geissel, Jean **(SLP)**
Pelszynski, Mrs Patricia A **(SLP)**
Thurston, Laural B **(SLP)**

Glassboro
Batten, Claudia P **(SLP)**

Glen Gardner
Belsante, Mrs Susan Zohn **(SLP)**
Kupets-Mannon, Deborah L **(SLP)**
Sailer, Mrs Sarah B **(SLP)**

Glen Ridge
Harris, Mrs Carolyn M **(SLP)**
Kwiatkoski, Mrs Janet E **(A)**

Glen Rock
Ermey, Mary Jean **(SLP)**
Freund, Mrs Anna Daube **(SLP)**
Gelfer, Carole E **(SLP)**
Selikowitz, Jeanne E **(SLP)**
Shulman, Dr Edward **(SLP A)**
Silvestri, Susan C **(SLP)**
Wardrop, Cheryl M **(SLP)**
Wolfe, Anita R **(SLP)**
Wuhl, Mrs Gail K **(SLP)**

Glendora
Pezzano, Garry Richard **(SLP)**

Glenwood
Del Grosso, Mrs Gail Anne

Green Brook
Stainken, Mrs Marie A O **(SLP)**

Grenloch
Shipley, Larry B **(A)**

Guttenberg
Kafkafi, Ilana **(SLP)**
Klein, Marilyn **(SLP)**

Hackensack
Axelrod, Mrs Lauren Sherri
Blackwell, Mrs Dabney Woolford **(SLP)**
Disher-Hobeika, Linda Marie **(SLP)**
Frontera, Patricia **(SLP)**
Gordon, Dr Ellen J **(SLP)**
Kase, Lynn C **(A)**

Kriney, Valerie Pinto **(A)**
Lippe, Mrs Shirel W **(SLP)**
Margolis, Leonard H **(SLP)**
Roberts, Mrs Deborah I **(SLP)**
Sperling, Andrew L **(A)**
Spiegel, Susan L **(SLP)**
Weinberg, Donna L **(SLP)**

Hackettstown
Buin, Susan M **(SLP)**
Massaro, Mrs Donna M **(SLP)**
McCurdy, Joanne Lee **(SLP)**
Ramage, Mrs Margaret McClure **(SLP)**
Strachn-Hunt, Josephine **(SLP)**

Haddon Heights
Porcelli, Mrs Janet J **(SLP)**
Sanders, Mrs Elizabeth M **(SLP)**

Haddonfield
Hering, Mrs Ruth E **(SLP)**
Jones, Mrs Alix N **(SLP)**
Jones, Mrs Patricia **(SLP)**
Levitt, Mrs Patricia Joseph **(SLP)**
Mastriano, Barbara P **(SLP)**
Metrione, Mrs Mary Ann L **(SLP)**
Pearce, Mrs Jeanne K **(A)**
Reel, Sharon Marie **(SLP)**
Rottenberg, Paula A **(SLP)**
Schultz, Adeline R **(SLP)**
Silver, Joy E **(SLP)**
Speakman, Dianne Melody **(SLP)**
Wheeler, Mrs Carolyn S **(SLP)**
Wheeler, Sherwood **(A)**
Young, Mrs Kathleen Prout **(SLP A)**

Hamburg
Plaza, Yvonne S

Hamilton
Molnar, Suzanne **(SLP)**
Sinclair-Weitzner, Leslie Victoria **(SLP)**
Zingg, Cynthia Callan **(SLP)**

Hamilton Square
Dono, Deborah Tobias **(SLP)**
Giardina, Candida **(SLP)**

Hampton
Cody, Kathleen Maloney **(SLP)**

Harrington Park
Kaliski, Myra S **(SLP)**
Seneca, Eileen Coyle **(SLP)**

Harrison
Cislo, Mrs Heidi M **(SLP)**

Hasbrouck Heights
Gaur, Mrs Cathryn Lea **(SLP)**
Lynch, Mrs Mary P **(SLP)**
Scalo, Marilyn **(SLP)**

Haskell
Howard-Porter, Mrs Sara **(SLP)**

Haven Beach
Jones, Dr William O **(SLP A)**

Haworth
Dyer, Ruth S **(SLP)**
Fass, Karen E F **(SLP)**
Horning, Mrs Ruth S **(SLP)**
Mittnight, Helen Hill **(SLP)**
Pistrang, Judith A **(SLP)**
Schreiber, Meryl A **(SLP)**

Hawthorne
Bergen, Mrs Geraldine Gibbia **(SLP)**
Conyers, Olivia Wallace **(A)**
Fairly, Rebecca Ann
Klink, Dr Marcia L **(SLP)**
Lanza, Elizabeth Hope **(A)**
Mahometa, Mrs Maryann Retkwa **(SLP)**
Sanders-Mascari, Mrs Aviva **(SLP)**
Strang-Wolf, Christina Mayer **(SLP)**
Walker, Janice R **(A)**

Hazlet
Finchler, Mrs Michele Salzberg **(SLP)**
Oberstein, Mrs Lori Andra **(SLP)**

High Bridge
Tandler, Joan Mary **(SLP)**
Treiber, Patricia M **(SLP)**
Varro, Emily Mauzy **(SLP)**

Highland Lakes
Roche, William J **(SLP)**

Highland Park
Aziza, Mrs Elana Flori **(SLP)**
Caterson-Marshall, Mary **(SLP)**
Cohn, Helene T **(SLP)**
Donatelle, Christine Ruth **(A)**
Firgau, Eileen Mary
Footerman, Mrs Gittel G **(SLP)**
Hoyt, Mrs Kathryn P **(A)**
Kaminetzky, Aviva L **(SLP)**
Nathan-Gruber, Mrs Ellen **(SLP)**
Ratiner, Sharon Paula **(SLP)**
Rosedale, Michelle **(SLP)**
Rosenberg, Terri Godlas **(SLP)**
Stott, Beverly Liddicote **(SLP)**

Highlands
Carlesimo, Mrs Patricia B **(SLP)**

Hillsborough
Dellibovi, Regina Marino
Fitzgerald, Mrs Nancy L **(SLP)**
O'Neill-Fox, Barbara J **(SLP)**
Ruggiero, Mrs Gina Marchese **(SLP)**

Hillsdale
Duggan, Mrs Marguerite Orlandi **(SLP)**
Harrison, Mrs Susan I **(SLP)**
Nagaraja, Girija **(SLP A)**
Ohtaka, Mrs Keiko H **(SLP)**
Pfeifer, Helen K **(SLP)**
Philip, Beverly Siegel **(SLP)**
Rosenstein, Mrs Beverly B **(SLP)**
Shenkler, Mrs Barbara Effron **(SLP)**
Weinhouse, Dr Iris **(SLP)**
Zakalik, Mrs Francene Zeplain **(SLP)**
Zaretsky, Mrs Marcia P **(SLP)**

Hillside
Barsky, Dr Lisa
Chipelo, Mrs Helena Maria **(SLP)**
Kaufman, Randi E **(SLP)**
Wilson, Roberta Anne **(SLP)**

Hoboken
Bryde, Regina L **(A)**
Dagle, Kathleen Minna **(SLP)**
Greenstein, Diane B **(SLP)**
Hallihan, Ellen Elizabeth **(SLP)**
Webber, Mrs Diane Ruotolo **(SLP)**

Holmdel
Bottari, Mrs Cynthia L **(SLP)**
Kotler, Mrs Sheila B **(SLP)**
Rauchwerk, Mrs Starling Mara **(SLP)**
Shapanka, Judith M **(SLP)**
Ward, Nancy Lynn **(A)**

Hopatcong
Hruby, Bernadette **(A)**

Hopewell
Ennis, Thomas G **(SLP)**
Lowe, Sandra Rae **(SLP)**
Swanson, Mrs Shirley Phelps **(SLP)**
Vissering, Christine Denise **(SLP)**

Howell
Alter, Mrs Susan White **(SLP)**
Ellner, Scott A **(SLP)**
Nadkarni, Mrs Kausalya Sunil **(SLP)**

Indian Mills
Jordan, Barbara May **(SLP)**

Interlaken
McBride, Lloyd A

Irvington
Weiger, Dr Myra L

Iselin
Clarke, Mrs Ellen V **(SLP)**
Shifrin, Rosalyn Davis **(SLP)**
Vidolin, Faith Friedland **(SLP)**
Wexler, Robin **(SLP)**

Jackson
Brown, Karen Elman **(SLP)**
Galvin, Mrs Julie Malzone **(SLP)**
Lukenda, Mrs Karen Bornheimer **(SLP)**
McLoughlin, Judy L **(SLP)**
Sarason, Linda A **(SLP)**

Jamesburg
Anastasio, Joan
Caputo-Giancola, Mary J **(SLP)**
Cox, Mrs Marielise Kress **(SLP)**
Heinz, Mrs Margaret M **(SLP)**
Perrine, Mrs Rita Kass **(SLP)**

Jersey City
Amabile, Mrs Lisa Boardman **(SLP)**
Bragen, Deborah E **(SLP)**
Brown, Rhomas Jacqueline **(SLP)**
Cassiday, Jacqueline Ann **(SLP)**
Cornelius, Suzanne **(SLP)**
Enderle, Elizabeth Elaine **(SLP)**
Freeman, Sondra G **(SLP)**
Goh, Annette Wen-Li **(SLP)**
Jackson, Terri Alexa **(A)**
Levine, Elizabeth **(A)**
Miskell, John J **(SLP)**
Parker, Mrs Caroline J **(SLP)**
Scholl, Dr Hannah H **(SLP)**
Scholl, Dr Harold M **(SLP A)**
Smith, Mrs Beth Ann **(SLP)**
Taylor, Charles Reid **(SLP)**
Terregino, Sr Antoinette **(SLP)**
Zarnoch, Janet M **(A)**

Kearny
Canaley, James R **(SLP)**
Cancro-Welling, Deborah Regina **(A)**
Lindorff, Mrs Vicki M **(SLP)**
Murphy, Mrs Cynthia R
Tiedemann, Mrs Susan B **(SLP)**

Keasbey
Pullen, Mrs Cynthia P

Kendall Park
Arnson, Cheryl Byer **(A)**
Brady, Patricia E O'Rourke **(SLP)**
Lobaina, Elizabeth Sarah **(SLP)**
Mehler, Mrs Beth M **(A)**

Kenilworth
Wierdo, Patricia L **(SLP)**

Kinnelon
Cooper, Mrs Eleanor A **(A)**
Jockel, Mrs Carol M **(SLP)**
LeBlanc, Valerie Foster **(SLP)**
Santana, Mery Luz H **(SLP)**
Shenker, Joan Buchman **(A)**

Lafayette
Heitzman, Mrs Linda J **(SLP)**

Lake Hiawatha
Young, Mrs Janet Sue

Lake Hopatcong
Sheppard, Dr Justine Joan **(SLP)**

Lake Parsippany
Kabath, Mrs Ellen **(A)**

Lakehurst
Colon, Joann Sposini **(SLP)**

Lakewood
Berman, Sondra P **(SLP)**
Brown, Mrs Therian N **(A)**
Diskind, Mrs Faiga **(SLP)**
Fink-Flam, Vivian C **(SLP)**

Freundlich, Ruth **(SLP)**
Henningson-Vanucci, Mrs Marjori A **(SLP)**
Hill-Albanowicz, Kerry Lee **(SLP)**
Ingberman, Jeanne Ellen
Sabo, Mrs Marilyn E **(SLP)**
Schonbrun, Les Edward **(SLP)**

Landing
Garroway, Mrs Anne Anderson **(A)**

Lanoka Harbor
Gotti, Margaret E **(SLP)**
Springsted, Mrs Kim Ann R **(SLP)**

Laurence Harbor
Phillips, Janice A **(SLP)**

Laurenceville
Pretsfelder, Loreen Horowitz **(SLP)**

Lavallette
Brockwell, Mrs Celeste Micchelli **(SLP)**
Buscema, Michele Marie **(SLP)**

Lawrence
Holmes, Mrs Anne S **(SLP)**

Lawrenceville
Cahill, Mrs Judy G **(A)**
Campos, Susan A **(SLP)**
Devaney, Janet Shaw **(SLP)**
Grieco, Mrs Nancy Boyd **(SLP)**
Hastings, Lisa **(SLP)**
Lamendola, Rita Gandelman
Lapin-Pastorella, Robin **(SLP)**
Livecchi, Patricia Rosato **(SLP)**
Lustig, Beth E **(SLP)**
Markoe, Ruth **(SLP)**
Maxwell, Camille M **(SLP)**
Puchalski, Maureen A **(A)**
Raymond, Mrs Maryann Perugino **(SLP)**
Redder, Alice T **(SLP)**
Schalick, Nadine H **(SLP)**
Schwartz, Mrs Harriett **(SLP)**
Seaman, Bruce D **(SLP)**
Sherman, Mrs Bernadette G **(SLP)**
Smith, Carol A **(SLP)**

Lebanon
Carmen, Mrs Elizabeth M **(SLP)**

Leonardo
Hopkins-Rossabi, Theresa Marie **(SLP)**

Leonia
Sokol, Mrs Betty Ann **(SLP)**

Lincoln Park
Klimovitch, Mrs Michele O **(SLP)**
Purdy, Barbara Elaine **(SLP)**
Sarrow, Mrs Anne M **(SLP)**
Scarpellino, Susan **(SLP)**
Somerville-Pedi, Rae Ann **(SLP)**

Lincroft
Gribin, Barbara A **(SLP)**
Rembisz, Linda S **(SLP)**
Sens-Azara, Mary Catherine **(SLP)**

Linden
Chiarello, Alice G **(SLP)**
Conder, Eileen
Zagier, Barbara **(SLP)**

Lindenwold
Martin, Dr Nadine **(SLP)**
Milliken, Deborah Lynne **(SLP)**
Symuleski, Joseph Stephen **(SLP)**

Linwood
Ablonczy-Popeson, Joanne **(SLP)**
Arabia, Janet C **(SLP)**
Cohen, Ronnie K **(SLP)**
Laverdure, Mrs Edythe S **(SLP)**
Maletto, Mrs Patricia M **(SLP)**
Schermerhorn-Grossman, Mrs Siobhan **(SLP)**
Siegel, Mrs Karen C **(A)**
Thomas, Laurie J **(SLP)**

Little Falls
Adler, Mrs Kathleen **(SLP)**
Frain, Avria Bultz **(SLP)**
Malinowski, Marylou **(SLP)**
Petronchak, Mrs Joann V **(SLP)**

Little Silver
Impey, Gillian M **(SLP)**
Menist, Mrs Cynthia R **(SLP)**
Relyea, Linda A **(SLP)**
Straus, Mrs Harriet D **(SLP)**
Wasser, Deborah S **(SLP)**

Livingston
Aber, William **(SLP A)**
Auslander-Chroman, Mrs Barbara **(SLP)**
Bukantz, Mrs Carol I **(A)**
Bylo, Marianne G **(SLP)**
Cooper, Allyn D **(SLP)**
Dollinger, Lillian S **(SLP)**
Fenichel, Mrs Rita B **(SLP)**
Gershwin, Mrs Laynie G **(SLP)**
Goldfaden, Mrs Debra Rhonda **(SLP)**
Graber, Mrs Barbara R **(SLP)**
Hornstein, Mrs Cynthia S **(SLP)**
Jager, Mrs Susan H **(SLP)**
Levitt, Dr Harry
Lichtman, Mrs Heather Novy **(SLP)**
Marzell, Miriam S **(SLP)**
Negrin, Jane D **(SLP)**
Pepe-Caffrey, Christine E
Schenkel, Lynne B **(SLP)**
Slavitt, Mrs Stephanie **(SLP)**
Spigel, Francine B **(SLP)**
Sugarman, Mrs June **(SLP)**
Welt, Mrs Andrea Brodie **(SLP)**
Wolfe, Mrs Karen M **(SLP)**

Lodi
Di Mauro, Judith A **(SLP)**
Natale, Christine Clarino **(SLP)**

Long Branch
Tomaino, Deborah Walsh **(SLP)**

Long Valley
Coble, Teresa Goldman **(SLP)**
Costantino, Evelyn Suib **(SLP)**
Donleavy, Mrs Mary Ella **(SLP)**
Hamer, Carol Schneck **(A)**
Ludwig, Mrs Alisa L **(SLP)**
O'Brien-Fallon, Mrs Maureen E **(SLP)**
Wagner, Claudia M **(SLP)**

Lyndhurst
Gettings, Sharon M **(SLP)**
Gordon, Mrs Jill Suzanne **(A)**

Madison
Draegert, Margaret E **(SLP)**
Migliore, Lawrence Edward
Richardson, Mrs Karen Hill **(A)**
Schessler, Mrs Carol J **(SLP)**
Shinder, Mrs Jane F **(SLP)**
Weil, Mrs Bette J **(SLP)**

Mahwah
Cirillo, Mrs Lisa A **(SLP)**
West, Mrs Patricia K **(SLP)**

Manalapan
Friedman, Mrs Rhonda L **(SLP)**
Holzberg, Melanie C **(A)**
Margolis, Natalie M **(SLP)**
Widofsky, Mrs Maureen Epton **(SLP)**

Manalapan Township
Horowitz, Mrs Tinece L **(SLP)**
Katzin, Betsy Sue **(A)**
Levine, Mrs Ruth **(SLP)**
Sandler, Mrs Judith G **(A)**

Manasquan
Anderson, Susan Ruth **(SLP)**

Mantua
Garrigan, Kathleen D **(SLP)**

Manville
Gangwer, Kathleen Gissoni
Pritchard, Annette D **(SLP)**

Maple Shade
Gross, Mrs Georgia H **(SLP)**
Levinson, Susan
Litz, Nancy F **(SLP)**
Ryan, Teresa Ann **(SLP)**
Surowitz, Ellen **(SLP A)**

Maplewood
Certner-Smith, Marilyn **(SLP)**
Kraemer, Mrs Nancy B **(SLP)**
Lainer, Harriet **(SLP)**
Meador, Kathryn A **(SLP)**
Mittleman, Penny S **(A)**
Neu, Mrs Patricia B **(SLP)**
Newman, Mrs Barbara K **(SLP)**
Okeke, Irene N **(A)**
Paolino, Mrs Camille Marie **(SLP)**
Pepe, Tara Lynn **(SLP)**
Rothschild, Patricia K **(SLP)**

Margate
Blum, Mrs Joanne Amodeo **(SLP)**
Trackman, Phyllis **(SLP)**
Yeager, Mrs Deborah Janice **(SLP)**

Marlboro
Alterman, Mrs Lorraine **(SLP)**
Derris, Sandy J **(SLP)**
Goldblatt, Ree Ellen Lewen **(SLP)**
Herschberg-Muntner, Mrs Nancy R **(SLP)**
Ionin, Mrs Joyce M **(SLP)**
Lucey-Sparacio, Patricia **(SLP)**
Sarill, Debra Beth **(SLP)**
Schaen, Nancy R F **(SLP)**
Weinberg, Mrs Sylvia Z **(SLP)**
Wiener, Diane F L **(SLP)**

Marlton
Catherwood, Kay P **(A)**
Chapman, Cathy A **(SLP)**
Glod, David J **(SLP)**
Glod, Mrs Linda M **(SLP)**
Goodman, Mrs Barbara Lynne **(SLP)**
Kaplan, Beth **(SLP)**
Kushner, Mrs Sandra Gerson **(SLP)**
Lewis, Mrs Arlene **(SLP)**
Olanoff, Rachel **(A)**
Porter-Kanel, Mrs Robin **(SLP)**
Ravin, Judith Barbara **(A)**
Russell, Mrs Andrea I P **(SLP)**
Siegel, Robert B **(A)**
Stomel, Mrs Andrea W **(SLP)**
Thomas, Mrs Kathryn C **(SLP)**
Thompson, Michele Dupay **(SLP)**
Yuen, Mrs Eileen Dee **(SLP)**

Marmora
Greenberg, Mrs Lauri I **(SLP)**

Martinsville
Musial-Slowey, Vera J **(SLP)**

Matawan
Bean, Jerrilyn Akins **(SLP)**
Beilis, Mrs Rosalie **(SLP)**
Elson, Nancy Beth **(A)**
Farry, Mrs Corliss C **(SLP)**
Frommer, Mrs Shelley Berg **(SLP)**
Kozlik, Ethel Weimer **(SLP)**
Kristoff, Mrs Barbara L **(SLP)**
Levinson, Mrs Teri Solomon **(SLP)**
Nehlsen, Kerri Savage **(SLP)**
Schwander, Teresa Jane **(A)**
Teeple, Gail **(SLP)**

Mauricetown
Hoffman, Mrs Jennifer Sue

Mays Landing
Morales, Joanne Lynn
Roeske, Christine Ann **(SLP)**
Tuozzolo, Jacquilin Ann **(SLP)**
Uhl, Jennifer Anne **(SLP)**

Maywood
Morris, Mrs Linda Beth **(SLP)**
Oratio, Dr Albert R **(SLP)**
Oratio, Mrs Suzanne Lange **(SLP)**

Medford
Appert, Mrs Alice M **(SLP)**
Germinario, Mrs Carol Flagg **(SLP)**
Kamish, Stacey Jean
Kuzio, Beverlee M
Smeraski, Joan Ellen
Vernamonti, Mrs Jane M O **(SLP)**

Medford Lakes
Garth, Shirley C **(SLP)**
Huggins, Sherry A **(SLP)**

Mendham
Barth, Craig T **(A)**
Reilly, Kathleen **(SLP)**

Mercerville
Greenberg, Mrs Marilyn B **(SLP)**
Steck, Cynthia Diane

Metuchen
Abrams, Mrs Rosalie Gelfand
Dombrowski, Mrs Deborah Mary **(SLP)**
Marcus, Mrs Sandra S **(SLP)**
Nielsen, Lucille T **(SLP)**
Santo Pietro, Dr Mary Jo Cook **(SLP)**
Woicekowski, Laura

Middlesex
Bird, Mrs Ann L **(SLP)**
Bittel, Cynthia S **(SLP)**

Middletown
Avrin, Mrs Lois Silver **(SLP)**
Eckert, Anne Marie **(A)**
Ghigliotti, Sarah J D **(SLP)**
Kalb, Mrs Madelyn G **(SLP)**
Klane, Bonnie E **(SLP)**
Lombardo, Frank C **(A)**
Lynch, Mrs Joann L V **(A)**
Tuller, Mrs Brenda Rems **(SLP)**

Midland Park
Burke, Mrs Catherine Anne
Cronan-Polhemus, Anne **(SLP)**

Milford
Kenyon, V Talley **(SLP)**
Klein, Mrs Carol A **(SLP)**
Reilly, Mrs Camille Acquaviva **(SLP)**
Testa, Carol Sue **(A)**

Millburn
Berko, Mrs Deborah R **(A)**
Malkin, Edward S **(SLP)**
Pfeffer, Ellen B **(A)**

Millington
Auld-Whalen, Mrs Linda A **(SLP)**
Rothstein, Mrs Carole Gray **(SLP)**

Milltown
Glazewski, Dr Barbara D **(SLP)**
Murray, Mrs Eloise P **(SLP)**
O'Rourke, Eileen P **(SLP)**
Pellichero, Mrs Patricia **(SLP)**
Weiss, Mrs Naomi R **(SLP)**

Millville
Yeutter, Mrs Dale T **(SLP)**

Monmouth Junction
D'Andrea, Gerald Arthur **(SLP A)**
Fellner, Evangeline Estever **(SLP)**
Lisbona, Bonnie Zients **(SLP)**
Moses, Dr Nelson **(SLP)**
Quinlan, Mrs Lorraine W **(SLP)**

Montclair
Caracciolo, Dr Gerard L **(SLP)**
Eisenstadt, Dr Arthur A **(SLP)**
Kadijevic, Vojislav **(A)**
Levy, Mrs Miriam S **(SLP)**
Schwolow, Rhoda Jacobs **(SLP)**
Smith, Mrs Helen K **(SLP)**
Stern, Doris Rapisardi **(A)**
Weber, Mrs Eleanor H **(SLP A)**

Montvale
Donovan, Mrs Noreen Catherine **(SLP)**
Gordon, Gloria G **(SLP)**

Montville
Henry, Mrs Mary Ann D **(SLP)**
Hoberman, Mrs Fran S **(SLP)**
Nadler, Mrs Susan L **(A)**

Moorestown
Condoluci, Mrs Patricia W **(SLP)**
Cummons, Gail Ann **(A)**
Groh, Margaret E **(SLP)**
Hansen, Mrs Mary Hedenberg **(SLP)**
Nanni-Zacher, Deborah **(SLP)**
Paul-Cohen, Rhona S **(SLP)**

Morganville
Chodos, Lynn E **(SLP)**
Dix, Mrs Cheryl Herman **(SLP)**
Gold, Mrs Andrea Just **(SLP)**
Johnson, Barbara Louise **(SLP)**
Kass, Mrs Carole L **(SLP)**

Morris Plains
Blumenfeld, Mrs Sandra Alswang **(SLP)**
Briant, June E **(SLP)**
Cook, Yvette Marie
Dikengil, Angela Tipton **(SLP)**
Florman, Mrs Ellen Holly **(SLP)**
Garrett, Mrs Lisa Anne **(SLP)**
Gohde, Mrs Sandra E **(SLP)**
Levine, Mrs Rose Beverly **(SLP)**
McDonough, MaryEllen **(SLP)**
Quinn, Linda B **(SLP)**
Roth, Mrs Lori L **(SLP)**
Zindel, Betsy Jane **(SLP)**

Morris Township
Gilbert, Mrs Carol R **(A)**
Lavigne, Mrs Benjie Panesh **(SLP)**

Morristown
Brigante, Marie **(SLP)**
Grossberg, Mrs Donna Sue **(SLP)**
Hammer, Mrs Ronnie W **(SLP)**
Judkowitz, Mrs Helen F **(SLP)**
Kamm, Dr Candace A **(A)**
Kassel- Petrocco, Mrs Janice **(SLP)**
Kertesz, Laurie Ann **(SLP)**
Levitt, Nina **(SLP)**
Ludington, Mrs Noreen Malone **(SLP)**
Ruhalter, Wendy Baer **(SLP)**
Smiley, Melinda E **(SLP)**
Van Heertum, Mrs Ellen E **(SLP)**
White, Mrs Betty Stallings **(SLP)**

Mount Arlington
MacArthur, Karen **(SLP)**
Schlosser, Wendy Lynn **(SLP)**

Mount Holly
Gates, Kathy Elaine **(A)**
Jansen, Kathleen M **(A)**
Kowalski, Mrs Joanne M
Moore, Lori J
Pajares, Toni Mancuso **(SLP)**
Samson, Sarla Wyn **(SLP)**
Squires, Mrs Gail Ann **(SLP)**
Winters, Mrs Emilia Ann **(SLP)**

Mount Laurel
Barkand, Dixie **(SLP)**
Busillo, Mrs Judith E **(SLP)**
Discount, Mrs Kathy Debra **(SLP)**
Fauser, Mrs Janice L S **(SLP)**
Hall-Olsen, Kathleen **(SLP)**
Holmes, Marian Frances **(SLP)**
McGuire, Mrs Madelyn T **(SLP)**
Mintz-Bitman, Sari **(SLP)**
Rella, Mrs Marguerite Sheridan **(SLP)**
Rock, Marian V **(SLP)**
Say, Mrs Frances P **(SLP)**

Simpson, Mrs Elizabeth Taylor **(SLP)**
Stow, Mrs Carol Jean **(SLP)**
Vassallo, Lawrence A **(A)**
Wainer, Marilyn F **(SLP)**

Mountain Lakes
Eisenberg, Sarita H **(SLP)**
McGranahan-Eiring, Sarah **(SLP)**
White, Holly Meier **(SLP)**

Mountainside
Fine, Paula S **(SLP A)**
Mishkin, Mrs Lois W **(SLP)**
Ricciardi, John G **(SLP)**

Mullica Hill
Harrick, Mrs Elma M **(SLP)**

Murray Hill
Curtis, Mrs Nancy Wildstein **(A)**
Heller, Mrs Pamela G **(SLP)**
Olive, Debra A **(SLP)**
Shapiro, Mrs Susan G **(SLP)**

Neptune
Burden, Cynthia J **(SLP)**
Wilkinson, Mrs Margaret M **(SLP)**

Neshanic Station
Friedman, Mrs Debbie A **(SLP)**

Netcong
Togno, Mrs Lucille P **(SLP)**

New Brunswick
Cotterell, Patricia A **(A)**
Hindes, Dr Sally K **(SLP)**
Kennedy, Dr Kathleen B **(SLP)**

New Gretna
Truitt, Lisa E **(SLP)**

New Milford
Cohn, Mrs Susan Greenberg **(SLP)**
Janso, Christine Maria **(SLP)**
Skvarla, AnneMarie **(SLP)**

New Providence
Davis, Helen S **(SLP)**
Huebner, Mrs Christie Elizabeth **(A)**
Messineo, Maryanne D **(A)**

New Shrewsbury
Tormey, Kimberly A **(SLP)**

New Vernon
Goldring, Mrs Sondra K **(SLP)**

Newark
Hourihan, Dr John P **(A)**
Johnson, Mrs Cheryl Bennett
Mercurio, Mary Ann R **(SLP A)**

Newton
Decker, Marie N **(SLP)**
Delaney, Mrs Kathleen Ann **(A)**
Feenstra, Mrs Catherine B **(SLP)**
Holla-Aschenbrenner, Anne Marie Elizabeth
Ostuni, Elizabeth **(SLP)**
Reisen, Patricia D **(A)**
Thompson, Mrs Eloise Burn **(SLP)**
Waldron, Mrs Lynn Angevine **(A)**

North Bergen
Dapuzzo, Theresa **(SLP)**
Rubin, Arlene Faye **(SLP)**
Stopol, Joy E **(SLP)**

North Brunswick
Barry, Mrs Carol B **(SLP)**
Clancy, Donnamae Fitz **(SLP)**
Finkelstein, Mrs Dianne Lynn **(SLP)**
Pavloff, Patricia E **(SLP)**
Schimmel, Mrs Ellen S **(SLP)**
Schneier, Mrs Dorothy B **(SLP)**
Slavik-Moreau, Mrs Debra A **(SLP)**
Snyder, Mrs Nancy Bredbenner **(SLP)**
Wiener, Mrs Marlene W **(A)**
Wilson, Teresa E **(SLP)**

Zlydaszek, Mrs Susan L **(SLP)**

North Caldwell
Oolie, Marjorie R **(SLP)**

North Edison
Armel, Sarah Douek **(SLP)**
Targovnik, Nan Sudran **(A)**

North Haledon
McCain, Mrs Permelia A **(SLP)**

North Plainfield
Benham, Jayne Ann **(SLP)**
Gelmetti, Lisa Winters **(SLP A)**
Parker, Mrs Lois M **(A)**

North Wildwood
Savarese, Sharon Jean **(SLP)**

Northfield
Gross, Mark Warren **(SLP)**
Schmincke, Janet Lee **(A)**
Trocki, Mona R **(A)**
Winn, Patricia Elizabeth **(SLP)**

Northvale
Rizzo, Crystal S **(SLP)**

Norwood
Avari, Dinci N **(SLP)**

Nutley
Bates, Elsie C **(SLP)**
Cortese, Emma E **(SLP)**
Gagen, Venisse Theresa **(SLP)**
McGovern-Lawler, Janine M **(SLP)**
Syme, Michele F **(SLP)**
Vandervliet, Cornelia R **(A)**

Oak Ridge
Burke, John J **(SLP)**
Evans-Wezel, Mrs Ann Marie **(SLP)**
Hollander, Deann Janine **(SLP)**
Ulrichny, Cathy L **(SLP)**

Oakhurst
Rothfuss, Martha J **(SLP)**
Sutor, Ann Crawford **(SLP)**
Wishnick, Wendy R **(A)**

Oakland
Codd, Dorothy S **(SLP)**
Kane, Mrs Susan B **(SLP)**
McDonough, Mrs Diane T **(SLP)**

Ocean
Helmsing, Theresa Ann **(A)**
Wasserman, Sara Ethel **(SLP)**

Ocean City
Dincher, Barbara Jean **(SLP)**
Fulton, Pamela Ann Mager **(SLP)**
Rudisill, Mrs Harlene C **(SLP)**

Ocean Gate
Rando, Carolyn E M **(SLP)**

Ocean View
Deuter, Carol Breckley **(SLP)**
Grecco, Russell **(A)**

Oceanport
Jaworski, Mrs Suzanne Marie **(A)**

Ogdensburg
Jacobitti, Carmela A **(SLP)**

Old Bridge
Betines, Mary Alice **(A)**
Bosner, Mrs Cynthia R **(SLP)**
Goldhecht, Debra W **(SLP)**
Ragovin, Lori E **(SLP)**
Tannenbaum, Linda Joy **(SLP)**

Old Tappan
VanDerBeek, Mrs Marcia Baird **(SLP)**

Oradell
Anderson, Carol Jane **(A)**
Delaney, Kathleen Anne **(SLP)**
Demott, Dr Lois E **(SLP)**

Duggan, Katherine MacFarlane **(A)**
Lynn, Mrs Mary Martha **(SLP)**
Thorson, Mrs Janice **(SLP)**
Wagner-Hill, Geraldine **(SLP)**

Palisades Park
Goldberg, Mary Jane **(SLP)**

Paramus
Block, Alyse Glaser **(SLP)**
Bores, Mrs Joyce Anne Costello **(SLP)**
Diamantes, Helen **(SLP)**
Friedman, Judith Pierce **(SLP)**
Heaps, Mrs Nancy I **(A)**
Malacrida, Mrs Joan K **(SLP)**
Maramaldi, Mrs Carolyn Roger **(SLP)**
Mikiewicz, Patricia Treacy **(SLP)**
Rubin, Mrs Harriet Levinson **(SLP)**
Spindler, Kristine **(SLP)**
Suarez, Janet Kalina **(SLP)**
Tyrrell, Denise K **(SLP)**
Wozny, Susan M **(SLP)**

Park Ridge
Varjian, Doris **(SLP)**

Parlin
Dembner, Mrs Elissa C **(SLP)**
D'Errico, Irene **(SLP)**
Engel, Mrs Jean Catherine **(SLP)**
Grabowski, Ann J **(SLP)**
McInnis, Ellen M **(SLP)**
Redwood-Pilgrim, Mrs Rosemary

Parsippany
Fried, Mrs Barbara R **(SLP)**
Grenker, Mrs Harriet A **(SLP)**
Hoffman, Mrs Christine **(A)**
Moog, Ellen Reiter **(SLP)**
Murray, Cheryl Anne **(A)**
Purn, Janet M **(A)**
Pyontek, Alaina May **(SLP)**
Reich, Mrs Janet E **(SLP)**
Rhoades, Mrs Lynn Margaret **(SLP)**
Slavin, Sandra H **(SLP)**

Passaic
Abreu, Rosa A **(A)**
Armstrong, Andrea F **(SLP)**
Monaloy, Gail E **(SLP)**
Pernikoff, Naomi Stilman
Reiss, Mrs Judith D **(SLP)**
Reuter-Donato, Cathleen Anne **(SLP)**
Roth, Mrs Francine Feder **(SLP)**
Simon, Mrs Toby Lazar **(SLP)**
Weinstock, Holly H **(SLP)**

Paterson
Mathis, Carla L
McArdle, Mrs Mary **(SLP)**
Perez, Daisy
Salvatore, Carol A **(SLP)**
Slutsky, Marsha Joan **(SLP)**

Pemberton
Wells, Mrs Edith Estrella **(SLP)**

Pennington
Naffziger, Diane J D **(SLP)**
Sternberg, Mrs Lois W **(SLP)**
Wright, Mrs Susan C **(SLP)**

Pennsauken
Burgin, Marilyn R **(SLP)**
Eddy, Debra S **(SLP)**
Kocher, Beth Karen **(SLP)**
Lee, Kathleen D **(SLP)**
Leven, Kathy Breese **(SLP A)**
Rine, Helen E **(SLP)**
Sims, Carole Latice **(SLP)**

Pequannock
Rudolph, Ann Elizabeth **(SLP)**

Perth Amboy
Herron, Margaret M **(SLP A)**
Schulz, Ronald E **(SLP)**
Tkacs, Donna L

Phillipsburg
Nash, Karen Erickson
Wheatley, Regina L **(A)**

Pine Beach
Bright, Robbie Yesilonis **(A)**

Pine Brook
Fenton, Mrs Jacqueline Koss **(SLP)**
McClurkin, Robert H **(SLP)**
Miller, Mrs Beverly L **(SLP)**

Pine Hill
Jeanes, Barbara Cree **(SLP)**

Piscataway
Berman, Rachel G **(SLP)**
Crespy, Marilyn Steinberg **(SLP)**
Garrigan, Verita M **(SLP)**
Powers, Dr Thomas A **(A)**
Rhein, Mrs Catherine T **(SLP)**
Wilhelm, Katherine Loridas **(SLP)**

Pitman
Buzash, Mrs Lola M **(SLP)**
Meeks, Mrs Constance Dove **(SLP)**

Pittstown
Campanile, Mrs Joyce Lynn **(A)**

Plainfield
Garrison, Mrs Patricia M **(SLP)**
Hall, Mrs Geraldine A **(SLP)**
Lucas, Annie Hall
Sherman, Ellen Sue **(SLP)**
Van Liew, Mrs Felisa Villarin

Plainsboro
Baum, Mrs Meryl **(SLP)**
Callery, Mrs Donna L S **(SLP)**
Fields, Yolanda Gail **(SLP)**
Galasso, Laura Ann **(A)**
Hye, Jane Linda **(SLP)**
Linder, Lori Renee **(SLP)**
Sacca, Janet S **(A)**
Schneider, Mrs Donna Segal **(A)**
Sinett, Eileen N **(SLP)**
Spiegel, Elisa L **(SLP)**

Pleasantville
Lees, Cheryl K **(SLP)**
Schwartz, Joyce K **(SLP)**

Point Pleasant
Akins, Joan M **(SLP)**
Burd, Laurie Lee
Colonno, Cynthia **(SLP)**
Roy, Patricia V **(SLP)**
Walsh, Mrs Georgia Lou

Pomona
Berry, Richard C **(SLP A)**
Hershman, Marsha Jo **(SLP)**

Pompton Lakes
Faucetta, Mrs Patricia Mary **(SLP)**
Hunziker, Mrs Cheryl Copeland **(SLP)**
Krantz, Mrs Joan Berkowitz **(SLP)**
Le, Tuyet Mai Thi **(SLP)**

Pompton Plains
Anderson, Angela **(SLP)**
Hohorst, Suzanne Marie **(A)**
Reinhardt, Lynn K K **(SLP)**

Port Reading
Coghlan, Mrs Catherine H **(SLP)**

Port Republic
Garrison, Maria R
Yochim, Jill Elizabeth **(SLP)**

Pottersville
Uhler, Mrs Karen Haugsjaa **(SLP)**

Princeton
Bolton, Mrs Margaret G **(SLP)**
Borden, Dr Gloria Jones **(SLP)**
Colburn, Dr Norma M **(SLP)**
Cook, Mrs Mildred B **(SLP)**

Dixon, Mrs Richard E **(SLP)**
Farzad, Mrs Shapar **(SLP)**
Gantwerk, Barbara F **(SLP)**
Gibb, Lisa C **(SLP)**
House, Arthur S
Jenson, Dr Pauline M **(SLP A)**
Ketay, Barbara Biggin **(SLP)**
Kimble, Carline S **(SLP)**
Metzger, Mrs Mary Jean B **(SLP)**
Oppenheim-Errera, Gabrielle
Pomplun, Mrs Beverlee J **(SLP)**
Sans, Mrs June Gordon **(A)**
Savage, Mrs Barbara A **(SLP)**
Shoemaker, Sheela **(SLP)**
Stein, Mrs Sandra J **(SLP)**
White, Emily J **(A)**
Wolff, Ellen S **(A)**

Princeton Junction
Binney, Mrs Janet Jarrell **(SLP)**
Ficca, Mrs Jo-Ann G **(SLP)**
Gross, Susan K **(SLP)**
Kuller, Mary Ehrlich **(A)**
Perry, Isabelle **(SLP)**
Tirello, Elaine C **(SLP)**

Quakertown
Murray-Hoff, Kelly Ann **(SLP)**

Rahway
Argentiere, Mrs Barbara Elaine
Jordan, Mrs Miriam **(SLP)**
Lobato, Mrs Cecelia B **(SLP)**

Ramsey
Connelly, Dr Patricia E **(A)**
James, Cynthia A **(SLP)**
Kenny, Mrs Elena F **(SLP)**
Lieberman-Altman, Denise Elayne **(SLP)**
Theander, Estelle J **(SLP)**

Randolph
Deming, Mrs Jeanne Marie **(SLP)**
Fogel, Deborah Jeanne **(A)**
Gudis, Sheila Chesnov **(SLP)**
Pearl, Mrs Ellen G **(SLP)**
Peitzer, Mrs Wendy Sarner **(SLP)**
Rose, Myrna F **(SLP)**
Weiss, Mrs Iris Fisher **(SLP)**
Zurich, Mrs Sue A M **(SLP)**

Red Bank
Keelen-D'Amore, Mrs Karen Ann
Litzelman-Scoles, Janne **(SLP)**
Smith, Mary Ellen **(SLP)**
Stack, Jean H **(SLP)**

Ridgefield
Dowling, Mrs Ernestine Noferi **(SLP)**

Ridgefield Park
Deierlein, Therese Marie **(A)**
Frimmer, Mrs Barbara **(SLP)**

Ridgewood
Archibald, Judith A **(SLP)**
Bornstein, Steven P W **(A)**
Brady, William P, Jr **(SLP)**
Capozzelli, Mary G **(A)**
Dubner, Mrs Harriet **(SLP)**
Gromack, Gary R **(A)**
Gropper, Mrs Nancy R **(SLP)**
Kennedy, Mrs Mary Zimmerman **(SLP)**
Krebs, Janet Misita **(SLP)**
Matthey, Mrs Doris S **(SLP)**
O'Donnell, Georgette **(SLP)**
Schnaittacher, Mrs Esther Kimberg **(SLP)**
Sheridan, Patricia A **(SLP)**

Ringoes
Higgins, Mrs Candie L **(SLP)**

Ringwood
Hsu, Dr Jennifer R

River Edge
Formica, Deborah N **(SLP)**
Lipman, Lori H **(SLP)**
McVeigh, Patricia Sutley **(SLP)**
Ohanyan, Regina E **(SLP)**
Spiniello, Therese M **(SLP)**

River Vale
Kaffee, Mrs Jacqueline **(SLP)**
Laden, Mrs Joan **(SLP)**
Price, Mrs Karen S **(SLP)**

Riverdale
Haug, Mrs Laura Ann **(SLP)**
Kallet, Mrs Adele M **(SLP)**
Russinko, Mrs Valerie Louise **(SLP)**

Riverside
Chiarello, Joseph P **(A)**
Fuoco-McCooley, Barbara **(SLP)**

Riverton
Carroll-Ranieri, Nancy E **(SLP)**

Robbinsville
Acton, Lynn M
Stern, Howard J **(A)**

Rochelle Park
Sibbald, Julie Monroe **(SLP)**

Rockaway
Ayres, Mrs Deborah Ann **(SLP)**
Blair, Mrs Lillian Kurtz **(SLP)**
Einhorn, Mrs Elinor S **(SLP)**
Flanick, Mrs Ann Gilligan **(SLP)**
Wilson, Mrs Minnie B **(SLP)**

Rockaway Township
Porcelan, Mindy Abrams **(SLP)**

Rocky Hill
Seither, Mary Regan **(SLP)**

Roebling
Staaf, Susan J **(SLP)**

Roosevelt
Weiner, Adeline E **(SLP)**

Roselle
Eisenberg, Susan Burde **(SLP)**

Roselle Park
Casper, Rosemarie Ann **(SLP)**

Rumson
Graber, Kathleen A **(SLP)**

Rutherford
Chopek, Dr Elena D **(SLP)**
Douglas, Laquita **(A)**
Simone, Mrs Carol A K **(SLP)**
Tate, Kathleen **(SLP)**
Witter, Barbara H **(A)**

Saddle Brook
Schwerin, Barbara Jean **(SLP)**
Seidman, Mrs Marlene Dymant **(SLP)**

Sayreville
Haber, Sandra K **(SLP)**
Wrotniewski, Elizabeth Ann **(A)**

Scotch Plains
Alberts, Mrs Novela Pinckney
Buccola, Mrs Susan Mary **(SLP)**
Buckley, John E **(SLP A)**
Ehrlich, Barbara O **(SLP)**
Kanfer, Ruthe T **(SLP)**
Kelner, Mrs Gail Siegel **(SLP)**
Rubin-Flukman, Ellen D **(SLP)**
Stewart, Mrs Catherine **(SLP)**
Yatrakis, Mrs Denise H **(SLP)**

Sea Bright
Schechter-Stein, Elaine **(SLP)**

Sea Girt
Ariff-Karrberg, Judy A **(A)**

Secaucus
Calvanico, Donna Marie
Levine, Marion **(SLP A)**
Shore, Linda Suzanne **(SLP)**

Sewell
Dorais, Mrs Brenda Marcus **(SLP A)**
Feuer, Tammy Ebeling **(SLP)**
Hawkins, Eloise Rainey **(A)**
Marano, Karen A **(SLP)**
O'Kane, Mrs Florence K **(A)**
Paternoster, Debra L G **(SLP)**
Swerdlow, Mrs Judith **(SLP)**
Westcott, Joanne M **(SLP)**
Winchester, Mrs Carol G **(SLP)**
Winters, Debra A **(A)**

Short Hills
Flax, Dr Judith Fivis **(SLP)**
Hermele, Mrs Lynn Freeman **(SLP)**
Kaffel, Joyce W **(SLP)**
Kuchon, Dr Patricia P **(SLP)**
Lippe, Sylvia P **(SLP)**
Paris, Deanne R **(A)**
Perl, Mrs Ilene E **(SLP)**
Phillips, Mrs Susan D **(SLP)**
Schmidt, Dr Jean W **(SLP)**
Schneider, Mrs Harriet Shapiro **(SLP)**

Shrewsbury
Behr, Tina **(SLP)**

Sicklerville
Bramblett, Dixon A **(A)**
Demby, Linda Ann
Hatala, Mrs Susan Davis **(SLP)**
Leipert, Mrs Nancy J **(SLP)**

Skillman
Enstrom, Dr Daly H **(SLP)**

Slanders
Cofoni, Mrs Diane Elizabeth **(SLP)**

Smithville
Abdelhak, Catherine Ann **(SLP)**
Maitland, Mrs Merryl G **(SLP)**

Somerdale
Gliva, Mrs Denise Panella **(SLP)**
Perica, Ellen G **(SLP)**
Petersen, Florence M **(A)**

Somers Point
Dougherty, Mrs Dorothy Marie **(SLP)**
Weyhmuller, Mrs Arlene Mehl **(SLP)**

Somerset
Firling, Mrs Janice D **(SLP)**
Gerlach-Pastor, Julie Ann **(SLP)**
Hersh, Julie Dawn **(SLP)**
Ingram-Colotti, Mrs Allison **(SLP)**
Lambiase, Barbara A **(SLP)**
Mesulam, Mrs Audrey S **(SLP)**
Nowalk, Barbara Covert **(SLP)**
Perretta, Mrs Rosemarie **(SLP)**
Tallman, Travis M **(SLP)**
Weber, Lisa Maria **(SLP)**
Weitz, Mrs Geraldine Greenfield **(SLP)**

Somerville
Albers, Mrs Carol **(A)**
Arshen, Mrs Joan R **(SLP)**
Atkins, Mary D **(SLP)**
Buzby, Janet R **(SLP)**
Cleary, Mary Ellen **(SLP)**
Ford, Mrs Diane Molitoris **(SLP)**
Hartner, Laura L **(SLP)**
Levinston, Mrs Donna H Adler **(SLP)**
Pollins, Mrs Judith L **(SLP)**
Scotti, Mark R **(SLP)**
Shovlin, Rose Ann **(A)**
Weidenfeller, Geraldine **(SLP)**

South Amboy
Baranowski, Maryanne V **(SLP)**
De Roche, Lisa Anne **(A)**
Gabriel, Catherine **(SLP)**
Murphy, Mrs Rita Ann **(SLP)**
Schonberger, Eve B **(SLP)**
Trainor, Ana M **(SLP)**

South Belmar
Bonhag-Hansen, Mrs Elizabeth **(SLP)**

South Hackensack
Kurman, Barbara L **(A)**

South Orange
Amato, Mrs Sylvia R **(SLP)**
Campbell, Susan P **(SLP)**
Kronman, Mrs Sharon M **(SLP)**
Pannullo, Theresa A **(SLP)**
Polow, Dr Nancy Gross **(SLP)**
Prather, Mrs Phyllis Crew **(SLP)**
Simon, Marilyn F **(SLP)**
Slevin, Mrs Elizabeth M **(SLP)**
Westrich, Abby Jane **(SLP)**
Wolsten, Mrs Ava R S **(SLP)**
Zimmerman, Reila **(SLP)**
Zucker, Mrs Susan Robins **(SLP)**

South Plainfield
La Verne, Mrs Dianne A **(SLP)**
Lepelstat, Anita R **(SLP)**
Vinski, Mrs Cathy B **(SLP)**
Zito, Roberta Kolstein **(SLP)**

South River
Le Blon, Deirdre H **(SLP)**
Malone, Mrs Jane Grace **(SLP)**
McMenimen, Annemary M **(SLP)**
Provenzano, Nora **(SLP)**

Sparta
Gallagher, Mrs Wanda F **(SLP A)**
Landrock, Rose-Marie **(SLP)**
Lohner, Mrs Denise M **(SLP)**
Tettinger, Mrs Kathryn Elaine **(SLP)**

Spotswood
Almog, Donna Raspa **(SLP)**
Leszczynski-Weber, Mrs Dorene Lisbeth **(SLP)**
Roy, Melissa Passaro **(SLP)**

Spring Lake
Nixon, M Colleen **(SLP)**

Springfield
Cincotta, Martha F **(SLP)**
Cohen, Mrs Shirley A **(SLP)**
Conway, Joan Marie
Drew, Carolyn Ann **(A)**
Manheimer, Mrs Sandra **(SLP)**
Siegel, Mrs Rona N **(SLP)**
Trambert, Robyn E **(SLP)**
Zoller, Vicki A **(SLP)**
Zurav, Mrs Frances S **(SLP)**

Stanhope
Davis, Mrs Dorinne S **(A)**
May, Mrs Mary **(SLP)**
Schwartz, Mrs Camilla M **(SLP)**

Stirling
Dickson, Jacqueline T **(SLP)**

Stockton
Hughes, Jacqueline Deets **(SLP)**

Succasunna
Braunstein, Mrs Pamela R **(SLP)**
Farber, Mrs Heidi F **(SLP)**
Kantor, Mrs Rita H **(SLP)**
Kojak, Mrs Dolores J **(SLP)**
Kraft, Mrs Susan E **(SLP)**
Luchs, Mrs Deana M **(SLP)**
Meissner, James H **(SLP)**
Sundar, Girija S **(A)**

Summerset
Heath, Judith Lynn **(SLP)**

Summit
Burnett, Mrs Sherilyn Powell **(SLP)**
Elzer, Judyth A A **(SLP)**
English, Mrs Roberta Kent
Herman, Leslie E **(A)**
Johnson, Dr Jane I **(A)**
Knight, Mrs Nancy F **(SLP)**

Lasser, Amy B **(SLP)**
Lederer, Mrs Barbara Freedman **(SLP)**
Liebman, Anita H **(SLP)**
Rafferty, Richard A **(A)**

Sussex
Boehm, Mrs Kathleen Ann W **(SLP)**

Swedesboro
Bombara, Tracy Anne **(SLP)**
Kernoschak, Jeanne Opeil **(SLP)**
Oldt, Lucy Altersitz **(SLP)**
Teter, Mrs Wendy Beth **(SLP)**

Tabernacle
Osman, Ruth Folkman **(SLP)**

Teaneck
Alper, Randi R **(A)**
Anderson, Mrs June Elizabeth **(SLP)**
Balaban, Dr Mae J **(SLP A)**
Boisselle, Mrs Dolores Crichlow **(A)**
Cohen, Martin **(SLP A)**
Cunningham, Clare F **(A)**
Edelstein, Mrs Jacqueline L **(SLP)**
Esral, Naomi T **(SLP)**
Goetz, Dr Norma J **(SLP)**
Gregg, Harriette **(SLP)**
Gross, Beth C **(SLP)**
Hiltzik, Linda K **(SLP)**
Kadison, Jerilyn G **(SLP)**
Kornbluth, Joanne Z **(SLP)**
Kricheff, Mrs Marjorie G **(SLP A)**
Lazar-Reskakis, Julie **(A)**
Marcucci, Carol Ann **(SLP)**
Margulies, M Lee **(A)**
Margulies, Dr Maris K **(SLP A)**
Neuman, Dr Arlene C **(A)**
Payne, Mrs Edna Koonce **(SLP)**
Rosenthal, Stephen M **(A)**
Salisch, Sandra L **(SLP)**
Schwarz, Diane **(SLP)**
Simon, Mrs Deborah Ann **(A)**
Solomon, Mrs Elaine W **(SLP)**
Waintraub, Mrs Charnie Lynn **(SLP)**
Weber, Evan A F **(SLP)**
Weikert, Mrs Barbara **(SLP)**
Weil, Mrs Sara Magence **(A)**
Zisk-Rosner, Lori B **(SLP)**
Zlotnick, Phyllis H **(A)**

Tenafly
Brown, Mrs Shirley R **(SLP)**
Dumeer, Betsy H **(SLP)**
Egert, Allison B **(SLP)**
Erlebacher, Mrs Marlene **(SLP)**
Gentry, Donna M **(A)**
Goldberger, Mrs Rhoda S
Grossman, Mrs Marcia **(SLP)**
Kosta, Dr Joan C **(SLP)**
Schwartz, Elisa F **(SLP)**
Unger, Mrs Dorothy M **(SLP)**
Ward, Mrs Kathleen **(SLP)**
Wollin, Mrs Joan **(SLP)**

Three Bridges
Sorge, Mrs Carol Nolan **(SLP)**
Wilson, Susan B **(A)**

Tinton Falls
Collazo, Nilda **(SLP)**
Kimberlin, Karen T **(SLP)**
Tier, Eleanor Patricia **(SLP)**

Titusville
Cannon, Mrs Claire Wynn **(SLP A)**
Hansen, Judith Ann **(SLP)**

Toms River
Belli, Mrs Sharon Catherine **(SLP)**
Brodkey, Mrs Estelle W **(SLP)**
Butensky, Mrs Jane E **(SLP)**
Cook, Jill Ann **(SLP)**
Fontanella, Mrs Renee Nancy **(A)**
Gertner, Alan B **(A)**
Liston, Mrs Joan F **(SLP)**
Malles, Dr Irwin Hal **(A)**
Molitores, Jan Marie **(SLP)**
Noroski, Mrs Susan E **(SLP)**
Poane, Mrs Lydia Luttrell **(SLP)**
Reisberg, Marni H **(SLP)**
Sarte, Mrs Pamela Lois **(SLP)**
Sickles, Robin E **(SLP)**
Thomas, Mrs Margaret F **(A)**
Vanzino, Mrs Laura M **(SLP)**

Totowa
D'Antonio, Mrs Cynthia Cinderella

Totowa Boro
Ashworth, Kathleen F

Towaco
Kaplan, Mrs Judith L **(SLP)**

Trenton
Andriot, Celeste F **(SLP)**
Bishop, Mrs Susan A **(SLP)**
Bruch, Mrs Rosemary B **(A)**
Carter, Michele C **(SLP)**
Cavalier, Lynn Ann **(SLP)**
Constance, Eugene J, Jr **(SLP)**
Didun, Lisa DeAngelo **(SLP)**
Di Meglio, Mrs Susan Anne **(SLP)**
Drukier, Dr Gale S **(A)**
Fischer, Mrs Nadine S U **(SLP)**
Flesher, Barbara L **(SLP)**
Hornyak, Andrew J **(SLP)**
Jarvis, Susan E **(SLP)**
Kamrad, Joseph F **(A)**
Katz, Mrs Sally L **(SLP)**
Ludwig, Cheryl L C **(SLP)**
Malkiewicz, Jane M **(A)**
McCarthy-O'Donnell, Mrs Lyn Ann **(SLP)**
McDowell, Elizabeth **(SLP)**
McMullen, Mary Chattin **(SLP)**
O'Brien, Dr Audrey **(SLP)**
Paul, Patricia Ann **(SLP)**
Redmerski, Mrs Christina Murdza **(SLP)**
Saponaro, Patricia P **(SLP)**
Stankus, Mrs Marlene L **(SLP)**
Young, Elizabeth Greene **(SLP)**

Tuckerton
Ray, John G **(A)**

Turnersville
Eskilson, Mrs Barbara C **(SLP)**
Sanginiti, Janette Christine **(SLP)**

Union
Blake, Dr Joan B **(SLP)**
Caha, Anne Margaret
Gens, Dr George W **(SLP)**
Heller, Dr Joyce C **(SLP)**
Hershon, Roberta Beth **(A)**
Kuzan, Mrs Kathleen Massotto **(SLP)**
Maskevich, Judith S **(SLP)**
Pachtman, Prof Ruth Solow **(SLP)**
Pona, Rosemary
Schneider, Nancy **(A)**
Schuhmacher, Mrs Anita Hood **(SLP)**
Slugaski, Mrs Nancy **(SLP)**
Sommerer, Claudia Villanova **(SLP)**
Taylor, Mrs Cheryl Davidson **(A)**

Union City
Douros, Mrs Maria John **(SLP)**

Upper Montclair
Aronson, Hannah U **(SLP)**
Attanasio, Joseph S **(SLP)**
Barden, Dr Elaine **(SLP)**
Kauffman, Ellen K **(SLP)**
Levey, Sandra K **(SLP)**
Lindenman, Dr Michael **(A)**
Lowenthal, Phyllis **(SLP)**
Mauney, Mrs Mardi J **(A)**
McKendall, Maureen D **(SLP)**
Payne, Pamela C **(SLP)**
Polledri, Mrs Diane M **(SLP)**
Seidler, Ann G **(SLP)**
Vanfrank, Mrs Leslie Cohan **(SLP A)**
Woolf, Dr Gerald **(SLP)**

Upper Saddle River
Germain, Ellen G **(SLP)**
Johnson, Judith A **(SLP)**
Lotierzo, Mrs Christine **(SLP)**

Ventnor
Campbell, Ann M **(SLP)**
Casel, Mrs Brenda H **(SLP A)**
Feder, Mrs Lee V **(A)**

Vernon
Smoly, Mrs Eleanor **(SLP)**
Stefkovich, Donna M **(SLP)**

Verona
Cohen, Lenore W **(SLP)**
Maher, Betty Jane **(SLP)**
Snogans, Mrs Kathryn Laborioso **(SLP)**
Ventola, Mrs Ellen M **(SLP)**

Vincentown
Lafferty, Roxane Kreger **(SLP)**
Paul, Linda L **(SLP)**

Vineland
Butler, Daniel J **(A)**
Crescenzo, Warren Lewis **(SLP)**
Engstrom-Bauman, Karen Joyce **(A)**
Glovsky, Leon **(SLP)**
Klinge, Donald J
Rhubart, Myla Ann **(SLP)**
Rosenwasser, Linda Tucker **(SLP)**
Voorakkara, Mrs Seeta Mylai **(SLP)**

Voorhees
Apple, Mrs Janice Kanter **(SLP)**
Blackman, Mrs Ruth Rose **(SLP)**
Cohen, Mrs Robin B **(SLP)**
Cracknell, Meredith E **(SLP)**
Edelstein, Mrs Leah L **(SLP)**
Feldman, Janet M **(SLP)**
Ganzman, Ilene P **(SLP)**
Gardner, Ellen M **(SLP)**
Gibson, Mrs Kathy W **(SLP)**
Israelsky, Mrs Roberta Schwartz **(SLP)**
Katz, Mrs Heidi Rathe **(SLP)**
Kitley, Mrs Deborah Sweeney **(SLP)**
Levin, Lynne S **(SLP)**
Pettijohn, Mrs Susan **(SLP)**
Protti-Patterson, Mrs Elizabeth **(A)**
Provenzale-Buono, Judith **(SLP)**
Romaniello, Mrs Diane **(SLP)**
Sieff, Dr Sherri L **(SLP)**
Steinberg, Randee C **(SLP)**
Steventon, Bonnie M **(SLP)**

Voorhees Township
Berlin, Faye M **(SLP)**

Waldwick
Gorski, Margaret M **(SLP)**
Gorski, Vincent J **(SLP)**
Kratchman, Robynne F **(SLP)**

Wanamassa
Heleotis Rn, Joni Lee **(SLP)**
Lawlor, Mrs Josephine Losito **(SLP)**

Wanaque
Mercer, Linda R **(SLP)**

Warren
Hampton, Tama Labreche **(SLP)**
Ruderman, Mrs Lois Grebelsky **(SLP)**
Shulman, Mrs Audrey **(SLP)**

Washington
Engborg, Rebecca J **(SLP)**

Washington Township
Cush, Gina **(SLP)**
Gonzenbach, Stephen A **(SLP A)**
Gregorio, Maryann R **(SLP)**
Nichols, Mrs Laura Rypkema **(SLP)**

Watchung
Hollander, Cynthia S **(SLP)**
Rusignola, Kathryn Sosnicky **(SLP)**
Salzberg, Mrs Arlene M **(SLP)**
Steckley, J Lynn **(SLP)**

Wayne
Bates, Mrs Diane E **(SLP)**
Bleicher, Patti P **(A)**
Buonpane, Sharyn L E **(SLP)**
Carroll, Mrs Susan C D **(SLP)**
Coppola, Michael J **(SLP)**
Fabiano, Mrs Susan Rosa **(SLP)**
Franzblau, Carol G **(SLP)**
Gelman, Mrs Nancy R **(SLP)**
Heimrich, Joan Ann **(SLP)**
Honeycutt, Mrs Phyllis Cole **(SLP)**
Hughes, Barbara E **(SLP)**
Jelinsky, Barbara M **(SLP)**
Kapura, Mrs Diane Kaczka **(SLP)**
Kraft, Arlene F **(SLP)**
Larranaga, Catherine A **(SLP)**
Liebowitz, Mrs Linda J **(A)**
Likman, Edward A **(SLP)**
Pomeranc, Mrs Carol R **(SLP)**
Reyna, Mrs Diane S **(SLP)**
Schwartz, Mona Serotta **(SLP)**
Schwarz, Mrs Sheryl Lynn **(SLP)**
Serwin, Gaynol N **(SLP)**
Solomon, Mrs Estelle W **(SLP)**
Stempler, Mrs Jacqueline Abbe **(SLP)**
Suozzi, Laura **(SLP)**
Talmadge, Mrs Ann Rannazzi **(SLP)**
Trecek, Mrs Jeanette S **(SLP)**

Wayside
Sprung, Susan C **(SLP)**

Weehawken
Czesak, Beth A **(SLP)**
Douros, Mrs Angie P

West Berlin
Peterson, Belinda F **(SLP)**

West Caldwell
Felix, Mrs Maureen A **(SLP)**

West Collingswood
Marks, Mrs Nancy R F **(SLP)**

West Deptford
Sanders, Mrs Irene M **(SLP)**

West Long Branch
Fields-Kuhn, Mrs Sandra **(A)**

West Milford
Einbinder, Monique Sheryl **(SLP)**
Ferraioli, Mrs Mary Anne Malone **(SLP)**
Piatek, A **(SLP)**
Rudolph, Mrs Patricia Marguerite **(SLP)**
Smith, Mrs Gregoria A **(SLP)**

West Orange
Bodner, Mrs Ellen F **(SLP)**
Cherchio, Noella A **(SLP)**
Cuccaro, Mrs Joann Valentine **(SLP)**
Eisnitz, Phyllis Scher **(SLP)**
Jacob, Barbara **(A)**
Kaslon, Karen W **(SLP)**
Kupferer, Albert F **(SLP)**
Pires, Mrs Helen Marshall
Pressman, Hilda T **(SLP)**
Prime, Karen Anne **(SLP)**
Rabner, Mrs Hilary Feig **(SLP)**
Roessler, Lisa Beth **(SLP)**
Schwarzbaum, Mrs Elisa M **(SLP)**
Smith, Mrs Christine Buscaino **(A)**
Spinrad, Myrna Z **(SLP)**
Stylman, Randi L **(SLP)**
Tavlin, Mrs Karen Hayden **(SLP)**
Terr, Dr Arthur L **(SLP A)**
Udell, Mrs Ruthe W **(SLP)**
Urso, Mrs Patricia A **(SLP)**
Wilcott, Mrs Kathleen Marie **(SLP)**
Winarsky, Sharon E **(SLP)**

Wright, Janet C **(SLP)**

West Paterson

Shoobs, Mrs Diane S Naiman **(SLP)**
Wehrle, Anne Patricia

West Trenton

Britton, Mrs Barbara L
Pope-Hartman, Florence **(SLP)**

Westfield

Alspector, Mrs Helen W **(SLP)**
Bartok, Mrs Susan V **(SLP)**
Blake, Dr Irwin H **(SLP)**
Breakstone, Mrs Beth Ellen **(SLP)**
Brewster, Maureen C **(SLP)**
Chien, Patricia S
Cohen, Elisha Beth
De Martino, Edna M R **(SLP)**
Diffley, Mary M **(SLP)**
Di Girolamo, Mrs Linda A **(A)**
Eisner, Eileen **(SLP)**
Essington, Marianne W **(SLP)**
Hammer, Debra Beth **(SLP)**
Hansen, Ellen Kathryn **(A)**
Harvey, Mrs Joan L **(SLP)**
Kandel, Ellen B **(SLP)**
Mihalker-Scrudato, Mrs Diane **(SLP)**
Navrotski, Darlette Sue **(SLP)**
Rothenberg, Meredith H **(A)**
Sherman, Mrs Lorene H **(SLP)**
Toolajian, Mrs Anne Scala **(SLP)**
Tucker, Wendy Weiss **(SLP)**
Voorhees, Mrs Gretchen M **(SLP)**
Waters, Susan **(SLP)**
Wendroff, Mrs Marta Gay **(A)**
Woods, Dr Robert W **(A)**

Westwood

Erickson, Mrs Alice Marie **(SLP)**

Wharton

Sleasman, Mrs Katherine **(SLP)**

Whippany

Walsh, Mrs Dorothy W **(SLP)**

White House Station

Mazzetta, Kay **(SLP)**
Parolie, Mrs Donna O **(SLP)**

White Meadow Lake

Gerber-Weshnak, Mrs Arlene G **(SLP)**

Whiting

Ciaccia-Woskey, Mrs Kathleen **(SLP)**

Williamstown

Fowler, Susan M **(SLP)**
Keely, Cynthia Meier **(SLP)**
Krady, Kimberly Ann **(A)**

Willingboro

Atwater, Tonja Fayette **(SLP)**
Cohen, Dr Alan H **(SLP)**
Gibbons, Mrs Ahtoi
Stockton, Charles R **(SLP)**
York, Mrs Kate G **(SLP)**

Winslow

Cohan, Donnajo A **(SLP)**
Dotoli, Geraldine A **(SLP)**

Winslow Township

Chapman, Mrs Beth Ellen **(SLP)**

Wood Ridge

Rohsler, Maria Susan **(SLP)**

Woodbine

Adams, Mrs Barbara M **(SLP)**
Umbro, Mrs Maria G
Webster, Cheryl Irene

Woodbridge

Blitzer, Mrs Sheree B **(SLP)**
Edelstein, Dr Beatrice D **(SLP)**
Gamm, Carrie Beth **(SLP)**
Lorenzen, Mrs Geraldine **(SLP)**
Lucov-Lenox, Mrs Jerilyn **(SLP)**
McEwen-Sosnovich, Dr Kathleen **(SLP)**

Woodbury

Frierson, Marsha **(SLP)**
Harper-Bundens, Constance **(SLP)**
Perry, Mrs Alberta H **(SLP)**

Woodcliff

Wainer-Levi, Audrey L **(SLP)**

Woodcliff Lake

Hall, Mrs Ann M M **(SLP)**
Schwarzwalder, Mrs Susan D **(SLP)**
Wernikoff, Nancy Kasdon **(SLP)**

Woodridge

Calamaras, Dr Peter **(SLP A)**
Smith, Mrs Joann Caiola **(SLP)**

Wyckoff

Cipolletti, Michael W **(SLP)**
Colgan, Linda T **(SLP)**
Delmonico, Mrs Terri A R **(SLP)**
Keeler, Dr Christine Siss **(SLP)**
McCarthy, Mrs Debra Porco **(SLP)**
McInerney, Maryrose Hannon **(A)**
Reinitz, Mrs Francine Lynn S **(SLP)**
Taub, Claire F **(A)**

Yardville

Gural-Toth, Virginia J **(A)**
Martin, Nancy Schoenhut **(SLP)**

NEW MEXICO

Alamogordo

Crotteau, Nancy R **(SLP)**
Doyle, Margaret Marie **(SLP)**
Hays, Mrs Barbara West **(SLP)**
Mays, Carla Marie **(SLP)**
Morrison, George S, Jr **(SLP A)**
Morrison, Susan Tinker **(SLP)**

Albuquerque

Albonico, Sharon Lee **(SLP)**
Anderson, Cara Wright **(SLP)**
Anderson, Susan Alice **(SLP)**
Angel, Mrs Amelia Ayala **(SLP)**
Applebaum, Merle S **(SLP)**
Ballantine, George Herbert **(SLP)**
Barnes, Judith E M **(SLP)**
Bartley, Cynthia Ann **(SLP)**
Beauparlant, Mrs Pamela Ann **(A)**
Belitz, Mrs Leslie **(SLP)**
Bivins, Mrs Linda M **(SLP)**
Bjornberg, Vianne Larson **(SLP)**
Bolton-Koppenhaver, Mrs Mary L **(SLP)**
Bond, Mrs Jean M **(SLP)**
Bosworth, Mary Ann **(SLP)**
Brown, Christina M **(SLP)**
Brown, Dr Jean B **(SLP A)**
Brown, Lauren Krimsky **(SLP)**
Brya, Mrs Catherine Anne **(SLP)**
Burnett, Ardyce Elaine **(SLP)**
Butt, Dolores S **(SLP)**
Callaghan, Sheelagh A **(SLP)**
Cameron, Kristine S **(SLP)**
Campbell, Ellen Jane **(SLP)**
Carl, Mrs Rada B **(SLP)**
Carlson, Mrs Judith Marie **(A)**
Casaus, Robin A **(SLP)**
Cervetti, Carma Call **(SLP)**
Chavez, Mrs Marian A **(SLP)**
Cherniak, Gary B **(SLP)**
Christensen, Carol S **(SLP)**
Christensen, Patricia **(SLP)**
Clark, Mrs Hollie- Quillayne **(SLP)**
Class, Lois Wunker
Coachman, Lin **(SLP)**
Cohenour-Sexson, Suzanne M **(SLP)**
Cone, Charlene Pease **(SLP)**
Costlow, Linda Ann
Creveling, Regina C **(SLP)**
Crown, Mrs Kathleen M **(SLP)**
Crum, Dr Michael A **(A)**
Denker, Nancy B **(SLP)**
Detorie, Deborah **(SLP)**
Dickerson, Mrs Debra Oakley **(SLP)**
Dixon, Nancee L **(SLP)**
Dolan, Mrs Julie Powell **(SLP)**
Doran, Paul James **(SLP)**
Dowler, Susan **(SLP)**
Drumm, Dr Denise A **(SLP)**
Dugas, Mrs Jean Klar **(A)**
Dupuis, Jo Ann **(SLP)**
Eichelberg, Debbie Sue
Elledge, Patti L **(SLP)**
Emery, James F **(A)**
Erickson, Mrs Laurie Aldrich **(A)**
Erickson, Mrs Terri Louise **(SLP)**
Fitzgerald, Mrs Ardell C B **(SLP)**
Foley, Veronica D **(A)**
Franks, Daniel Chris **(A)**
Frese, Donna Essington **(SLP)**
Gabioud, Barbara Harris **(SLP)**
Gallegos, Mrs Wendy J **(A)**
Garcia, Priscilla L **(SLP)**
Garihee, Laura V **(SLP)**
Gibel, Rosalind **(SLP)**
Gilbert, Ramona Jane **(A)**
Gillis, Victoria Joann **(SLP)**
Goldberg, Rhona J **(SLP)**
Gonzales, Victoria Christine **(SLP)**
Goodman, Janice K **(SLP)**
Gordon, Mrs Candace J **(SLP)**
Goss, Linda L **(SLP)**
Gossage, Nona Ann **(SLP)**
Grover, Marsha J **(SLP)**
Gryniuk, Ronda P **(SLP)**
Guenley, Kay F **(SLP)**
Guidice, Mrs Elaine J **(SLP)**
Gunn, Deritha C **(SLP)**
Haase, Kathryn S **(SLP)**
Hackney, Maxine L **(SLP)**
Harper, William Frederic, Jr **(SLP)**
Hattler, Dr Karl William **(A)**
Henkel-Silva, Amy Dodd
Herman, Mrs Lauren W **(SLP)**
Hess, Sharon A **(SLP)**
Hicks, Shannon K **(SLP)**
Hill-Rue, Mary Elizabeth **(SLP)**
Holland, Dr Lynn J **(SLP)**
Holpp, Mrs Maryan M **(SLP A)**
Homiak, Mrs Suzanne MacCallum **(SLP)**
Hood, Dr Richard B **(A)**
Hoodwin, Marcia L **(SLP)**
Hooper, Mary U **(SLP)**
Horan, Margaret **(SLP)**
Horness, Paula Gay **(SLP)**
Hough, Judith M **(SLP)**
Howard, Phyllis **(SLP)**
Hudson-Edwards, Allison **(SLP)**
Hunt, Mrs Mary N **(SLP)**
Hutchinson, Pamela A **(SLP)**
Irving, Deborah A **(SLP)**
Jackson, Joanne K **(SLP)**
Jackson, Margaret **(SLP)**
Jasinski, Andrew Joseph **(SLP)**
Jennings, Susan M **(SLP)**
Kane, Karen Hilary **(SLP)**
Kenney, Michael J **(SLP)**
Kerschen, Kim Elizabeth **(SLP)**
King, Christi Lee **(SLP)**
Klein, Selma Alperen **(SLP)**
Kocipak, Susan **(SLP)**
Krueger, Mrs Barbara A
Kubala, Virginia **(SLP)**
Kuhn, Michael Robert **(SLP)**
Lamb, Dr Lloyd E **(A)**
Larsen, Jule Anne **(SLP)**
Latham, Mrs Sandra **(A)**
Laurel, Marci K **(SLP)**
Lewis, Jan Summers **(A)**
Lewis, Nancy P **(SLP)**
Lilley, Pat Krchmar **(SLP)**
Lindberg, Paul William **(SLP)**
Linden, Sharon **(SLP)**
Long, Charles L **(SLP)**
Lough, Mrs Charlotte Benefield **(SLP)**
Loyd, Sharon K **(SLP)**
Lujan, Kathleen Wheeler **(A)**
Mager, Mrs Lisa Z
Maier, Mrs Deborah M **(SLP)**
Malach, Randi S **(SLP)**
Manchester, Mary Elizabeth **(SLP)**
Marquis, Marjorie A **(SLP)**
Marrero, Francenia **(SLP)**
Marshall, Elizabeth **(SLP)**
Martinez, Cecilia Monica **(A)**
Martinez, Shannon Kay **(SLP)**
Maulsby, Emily Potts **(A)**
Mayfield, Sheryl Melinda **(SLP)**
McCarney, Teresa D **(SLP)**
McClellan, Max E **(A)**
McClure, Mrs Janice K **(SLP)**
McGuckin, Cynthia Jean **(SLP)**
McMahon, Nancy B **(A)**
McMullen, Mrs Gayle Mohorcich **(A)**
McNown, Vicki P **(SLP)**
Meader, Nancy Kay **(SLP)**
Mehlhorn, Mrs Noelle R **(A)**
Merrill, Laurel J P **(SLP)**
Metarelis, Mrs Sharon Eilzabeth **(SLP)**
Meyers, Linda Suzanne **(SLP)**
Middleton, Lisa Annise **(SLP)**
Miller, Marilyn W **(SLP)**
Miller, Mrs Suzanne Slayback **(A)**
Molecke, Constance **(SLP)**
Monast, Shelia A **(SLP)**
Montgomery, Mrs Rose B **(SLP)**
Morrison, Mrs Vida R **(SLP)**
Moya, Mrs Manuela Helen **(SLP)**
Moyer, Mrs Joyle Wiederspan **(SLP)**
Myers, Mrs Nadynne A **(SLP)**
Myers, Virginia C **(SLP)**
Nichols, Wanada Lorraine **(A)**
Oliver, Cynthia **(SLP)**
Ormiston, Sharon Jean **(SLP)**
Orsak, Janice L **(SLP)**
Osbourn, Patricia S **(SLP)**
Pacini, Mrs Claudette A **(SLP)**
Palmer, Phyllis Mary **(SLP)**
Parker, Mrs Kathleen Diane **(SLP)**
Patterson, Janet L **(SLP)**
Paxton, Judith Lynn **(SLP)**
Payne, Lynette Smith **(SLP)**
Peercy, Martha W **(SLP)**
Pelsor, Jeanell Catherine **(A)**
Perrott, Emily H **(SLP)**
Peterson, Mrs Katherine Garity **(SLP)**
Petrov, Susan Ann **(SLP A)**
Peura, Robin Elayne **(SLP)**
Porch, Dr Bruce **(SLP)**
Porch, Meg **(SLP)**
Porec, John Paul **(SLP)**
Powell, Jane **(SLP)**
Prothero, Emily Diane **(SLP)**
Pugh, Gaylen S **(SLP)**
Rappaport, Dr Bruce Z **(A)**
Rathge, Mrs Karen Maureen **(SLP)**
Raymond, Charlean **(A)**
Remegio-Loges, Lorilee Mariko **(A)**
Richards, Sharol L **(SLP)**
Riensche, Dr Linda **(SLP)**
Righter, Mrs Amanda Kirman **(SLP)**
Rimbert, Mrs Susan Lynn **(SLP)**
Robinson, Jacqueline **(SLP)**
Rodriguez, Barbara Salazar **(SLP)**
Romero, Mrs Jeannie G **(SLP A)**
Ross-Brennan, Laurie **(SLP)**
Rotondi, Paula E **(A)**
Rouse, Geraldine Rodriguez **(SLP)**
Saltman, Norva G **(SLP)**
Schmitt, Mrs Joyce Beckey **(SLP)**
Schoenleber, Gloria Jean **(SLP)**
Shenuski, Doris Marie **(SLP)**
Shirkey, Dr Edward A **(SLP)**
Shoemaker-Scott, Debra **(SLP)**
Sisneros, Lisa Therese **(SLP)**

Slattery, Timothy Michael **(SLP)**
Smith, Lourie Elaine **(SLP)**
Smith, Margaret J **(SLP)**
Smith, Matthew W F **(A)**
Smith, Mrs Verna Elaine **(SLP)**
Snyder, Kristi S **(A)**
Soales, Madelyn G **(SLP)**
Spear, Susan Therese **(SLP)**
Stacy, Susan J **(SLP)**
Stafford, Lucinda K **(SLP)**
Stallcup, Thomas Allan **(A)**
Stefan, Loretta **(SLP)**
Steffens, April **(SLP)**
Steinpress, Rene J **(A)**
Stewart, Stacie Jo **(SLP)**
Stockbower, Martha L **(SLP)**
Stout, Yvette C **(SLP)**
Stremsterfer, Mrs Jerry McIlvaney **(SLP)**
Suber, Margaret C **(SLP)**
Tandy, Sharon G **(SLP)**
Taylor, Dana R **(SLP)**
Teitelreis-Sorenson, Judy **(SLP)**
Thomas, Laurie Bunten **(SLP)**
Thuman, Pamela R **(SLP)**
Tobin, Mrs Sylvia Magura **(A)**
Toubbeh, Dr Jamil I **(SLP)**
Troop, Mrs Pamela Bushart **(SLP)**
Trout, Elaine Addy **(SLP)**
Uzdawinis, Dianne C **(SLP)**
Valdez, Alfred J **(SLP)**
Wagner, Linda Carroll **(A)**
Wallace, Brenda Reimer **(SLP)**
Warner, Kathleen Wright **(A)**
Waters, Jeannette Leigh **(SLP)**
Watrous, Mrs Betty S **(SLP A)**
Wenderoth, Mrs Martha Cofer **(SLP)**
Westby, Dr Carol E **(SLP)**
Whalen, Rosemary **(SLP)**
Whitfield, Belva W **(SLP)**
Wiczer, Ellen S **(SLP)**
Williams, Judy K **(SLP)**
Williamson, Sherie M **(SLP)**
Willis-Simek, Mrs Teresa **(SLP)**
Wilson, Mrs Debbie Jan **(SLP)**
Wilson, Karen P **(SLP)**
Wollmann, Mrs Etta Marie **(SLP)**
Worth, Catherine A **(A)**
Young, Mrs Angela Marie **(SLP)**
Zimmerman, Donna S **(SLP)**

Alto
Holt, Mrs Margaret C **(SLP)**
Holt, William A, Jr **(SLP)**

Artesia
Beardemphl, Jessica W **(SLP)**
Johns, Leslie A **(SLP)**

Aztec
Atencio, Rebecca Leora **(SLP)**

Belen
Brook, Janet Vallese **(SLP)**
Harper, Mrs Diane Michel **(A)**

Bosque Farms
Swinney, Martha Brown **(SLP)**

Carlsbad
Bird, Joyce Elaine **(SLP)**
Dennis, Mrs Suzanne Garcia **(SLP)**
Denton, Mrs Elisabeth **(SLP)**
Stidworthy, Helen Lavora **(SLP)**

Cedar Crest
Carpenter, Mrs Judy D **(SLP)**
Palmquist, Mrs Pamela Louise **(SLP)**

Clovis
Burger, Lori Lee **(SLP)**
Clark, Mrs Deanna M **(SLP)**
Defoor, Mrs Joy C **(SLP)**
Goldbaum, Mrs Donna D **(A)**
Henderson, Mrs Linda McRae **(SLP)**
Mapes, Mrs Lonna K **(SLP)**
Osburn, Cynthia H **(SLP)**
Simnacher, L Sharon M **(SLP)**
Wilkins, Elizabeth Kathleen **(SLP)**
Wyman, Mrs Shirley V **(SLP)**

Corrales
Brummer, Mrs Candice L **(SLP)**
Clauser, Mrs Patricia S **(SLP)**
Eaton, Gail G **(SLP)**
Shafer, Joyce T **(SLP)**
Turcich, Mrs Maryellen Lawlor **(SLP)**

Deming
Andrews, Jonni Anne **(A)**
Lindsay, Thomas N **(SLP)**

Dixon
Maes, Daniel R **(SLP)**

Dulce
Fryman, M Jeanne **(SLP)**
Tator, Diann V **(SLP)**

Espanola
Hester, Melissa Driskell
McDonald, Lynn Price **(A)**
Montoya-Maestas, Mrs Mary K **(SLP)**

Farmington
Buyok, Gloria Mascarenas **(SLP)**
Buyok, Nancy Elizabeth **(SLP)**
Carlsen, Mrs Susan G S **(SLP A)**
Crispin, Bonnie Lynn **(SLP)**
Dynneson, Philip L **(A)**
Fagrelius, Maryann Bush **(SLP)**
Green-Dragony, Jo Allison **(SLP)**
Jacquez, Teddy M **(A)**
Kelly, Sarah T **(SLP)**
Letey, Abbie J **(A)**
Reinhardt, Mary A **(SLP)**
West, Michael H **(A)**
Wilson, Mary K **(SLP)**
Winer, Mrs Heidi Eileen **(SLP)**

Gallup
Aldrich, Donna Reed **(SLP)**
Beamsley, Virginia Bacon **(SLP)**
Hansen, Mary Kathleen

Grants
Sanchez, Mrs Mary E **(SLP)**

Hatch
Luchini, Mrs Lizabeth Torres **(SLP)**
Nesseth, Virginia Marie **(SLP)**

High Rolls
Burch, Mrs Gloria Haynes **(SLP)**

Hobbs
Erickson, Carol Vesta
Fahrlander, Daniel C, Jr **(A)**
Ricklefs, Sheila
Schend, Mary B **(SLP)**

Jamestown
Vanlierop, Henry G **(SLP)**

Kirtland
Hilley, Carol Gourley **(SLP)**

Las Cruces
Aguirre, Marguerite **(SLP)**
Baca, Maria Langereis **(SLP)**
Baker, Karen Ann **(SLP)**
Bowser, Barbara M **(SLP)**
Briggs, Mrs Beverly M **(SLP)**
Christie, Mrs Judith Ann **(SLP)**
Coon, Mrs Jeannie Rose
Dalton, Dr Leslie W, Jr **(SLP A)**
Dearholt, Janice Lange **(SLP)**
Diemer, Mrs Marlane J **(SLP)**
Farmer, Mrs Judith L **(SLP)**
Farmer, Dr Stephen S **(SLP)**
Feuerberg, Mrs Lydia E **(SLP)**
Fudge, Jerri **(SLP)**
Garrett, Dr Edgar Ray **(SLP)**
Genin, Grace-Ann **(SLP)**
Grijalva, Lillian Dolores **(SLP)**
Hain, Marsha K **(SLP)**
Hartman, Mrs Kerry McGoldrick **(A)**
Harvey, Mrs Jane Bibeau **(SLP)**
James, Vivian Kirkpatrick **(SLP)**
Lightfoot, Adrienne R **(SLP)**
Lombard-Brundage, Eileen **(SLP)**
Loncarich, Patricia A **(SLP)**
Marquez, Mrs Frima K **(SLP)**
McIntyre, Sue Ellen Glenda **(SLP)**
Mizar-Ortiz, Kathryn A **(SLP)**
Morales-Pena, Blanca M **(SLP)**
Moran, Veronica Carreras **(SLP)**
Rhoades, Inez B **(SLP)**
Salamon, Judy T **(SLP)**
Schoeppner, Mrs Carol T **(SLP)**
Schutz, Mrs Barbara J McLemore **(SLP)**
Stern, Elaine L **(SLP)**
Stuve, Mrs Carolyn S Manthei **(SLP)**
Stuve, Mark K **(SLP)**
Thompson, Connie Annette
Vigil, Marie Elizabeth **(SLP)**
Walcher, Helen R **(SLP A)**
Wallace, Suzanne Stacey **(SLP)**
Ward, Mrs Marcia C **(SLP)**
Weaver, Kathryn Lois **(SLP)**
Zimmerman, Harry R **(A)**
Zimmerman, Judith Holloway **(SLP)**

Las Vegas
Foreman, Paul Michael **(SLP)**
Hallsten, Roger D
Linzie, William Robert **(SLP)**
Lundergan, Mrs Mia Houk **(SLP)**
Schmitz, Sarah E **(SLP)**
Stevenson, Carol Ann **(SLP)**

Los Alamos
Anderson, Mrs Kathryn Larson **(SLP)**
Carroll, Janice Santogrossi **(SLP)**
Cook, Mrs Kathryn H **(SLP)**
Fazely, Mrs Mondra R **(SLP)**
Fife, Pamela B **(A)**
Knox, Susan C **(SLP)**
Laughlin, Mrs Yvonne O **(SLP)**
Martz, Mrs Cynthia S **(SLP)**
Smith, Elaine M **(SLP)**
Stewart, Elizabeth **(SLP)**
Trela, Mrs Margaret F **(SLP)**
Wilder, Pauline L **(SLP)**
Wolf-Moore, Carol Ann **(SLP)**

Los Lunas
Anderson, Mrs Rebecca D **(SLP)**
Ogas, Mrs Teresa O **(SLP)**
Stein, Deborah **(SLP)**
Walston, Theodora Flint **(SLP)**

Lovington
Ridenour, Mrs Melanie Bridgforth **(SLP)**

Maxwell
Wright, Mrs Anita Beth **(SLP)**

Mesilla Park
Trujillo-Sanchez, Mrs Cynthia D **(SLP)**

New Mexico
Glorig, Aram **(A)**

Placitas
Martin, Katherine Louise **(SLP)**

Portales
Ferguson, Mrs Shirley Gail **(SLP)**
Hill, Mrs Debra G **(SLP)**
Hopper, Dr G Robert **(SLP)**
King, Dr Henry L **(A)**
Shearer, Mrs Janet L
Wilkerson, Kenneth Dwayne **(SLP)**

Raton
Amen, Linde Ann
Stack, Mary F **(SLP)**

Rio Rancho
Barron, Peter Bedford **(SLP)**
Gonzales, Maria **(SLP)**
Hill, Helen H **(SLP)**
Murphy, Mrs Jolyn Luna **(SLP)**
Rost, Michele P **(SLP)**

Rociada
Berwick, Mary Jo **(SLP)**

Roswell
Bohon, Mrs Marian Vandenoven **(SLP)**
Campos, Debra Sue **(SLP)**
Chelius, Mrs Leah Marlene **(SLP)**
Chelius, Stephen Michael **(A)**
Dickinson, Barbara **(SLP)**
Driscoll-Morgan, Diane **(SLP)**
Ebara, Yukie **(A)**
Hemingway, Karen Louise **(SLP)**
Hernandez, Morene E **(SLP)**
Homschek-Grooms, Eileen **(SLP)**
Jordan, Kaye **(SLP)**
Madrid, Joe **(SLP)**
McClure, Mrs Susan D **(SLP)**
McCutcheon, Gloria K **(SLP)**
McLean, Robin Rae **(SLP)**
Neff, Scott R **(SLP)**
Robinson, Rhonda M
Wadlinger, Mrs Carolyn M **(SLP)**

Ruidoso
Rogalla, Susan A **(SLP)**
Tooley, Brenda J **(SLP)**

San Miguel
Geanious, Gregory Kevin **(SLP)**

San Ysidro
Gachupin, Rosalind **(SLP)**

Sandia Park
Dismuke, Ruth P **(SLP)**
Hopkins, Susan G **(A)**
Schwebach, Lee Ann **(SLP)**
Taft, Sandra M **(A)**

Santa Fe
Adams, Mrs Phyllis S **(SLP)**
Blakeley, Janet C **(SLP)**
Boyd, Jean **(SLP)**
Bright, Donna Marie **(A)**
Chumley, Audrey **(A)**
Clarke, Jane C **(SLP)**
Fields-Cohen, Mary T **(SLP)**
Fitch, Ruth Ann L **(SLP)**
Gamm, Mrs Penelope Ann **(SLP)**
Haecker, Ernest E **(A)**
Hamre, Susan Dean **(SLP)**
Hardwick, Martha Anne **(SLP)**
Jebb, Jeanne Frances **(SLP)**
Kaplan, Dr Michael A **(SLP)**
Kessler, Joan **(SLP)**
Lacey, Mrs Francis Karen **(SLP)**
Lilienthal, Jeanette Roberta **(SLP)**
Lujan, Erin Hayes **(SLP)**
Mellencamp, Virginia L **(SLP A)**
Neal, Vicki K **(SLP)**
O'Connor, Larry **(A)**
Owings, Dr Nathaniel **(SLP)**
Pirhofer, Lenore Anne **(SLP)**
Reese, Sheryl **(SLP)**
Roybal, Bernadette Trujillo **(SLP)**
Scheib, Rebecca L **(SLP)**
Stephens-Johnson, Pamela S **(SLP)**
Strimple, Kathleen **(SLP)**
Swanson, Mrs Gineta Gann **(SLP)**
Tartarka, Margery A **(SLP)**
Truse, Susan Shellar **(SLP)**
Urig, Debbie **(SLP)**
Van Hecke, Deborah P **(SLP)**
Weir, Linda D **(A)**
Wood, Margaret Louise
Young, Mrs Jacqueline S **(SLP)**

Santa Teresa
Bacchus, Mrs Cathy **(SLP)**
Brown, David Russell **(SLP)**
Card, Deborah L **(SLP)**

Shiprock
Gilchrist, Cheryl O **(SLP)**

Silver City
Brown, Russell Cooper **(SLP)**
Herzog, Eileen Gavin **(SLP)**
Noel, Mrs Kristine Karen **(SLP)**
Thomson, Kathleen Stephenson **(SLP)**

Taos
Weber, Mrs Karen Wichelns **(SLP)**

Tesuque
Clarke, Leanne Liden **(SLP)**

Tijeras
Bonner, Katherine Ann **(SLP)**
Jones, Judy Davidson **(SLP)**
Reel, Mrs Carla Jean **(SLP)**
Utrup, Mary E **(SLP)**

Truth or Consequences
Gillespie, Teri Evans **(SLP)**

Zuni
Bell, Jeannette **(SLP)**
Wilkinson, Mrs Carol R **(SLP)**

NEW YORK

Accord
Knowlton, Linda M M **(A)**
Traficanti, Judy Phelan **(SLP)**

Adams
Hudson, Mrs Laura Bachner **(SLP)**

Addison
Mitchell, Mrs Gail H **(SLP)**

Akron
Hilton, Mrs Debra Ellen **(SLP)**

Albany
Anslow, Barbara Ellen **(SLP)**
Banner, Barbara C **(SLP)**
Behrmann, Georgette E **(SLP)**
Biggio, Stacey Margaret
Blasting, Tami H **(SLP)**
Blessington, Therese Eileen **(A)**
Bloom, Dr Charleen Marie **(SLP)**
Bollin, Katherine M **(SLP)**
Boomsliter, Dr Paul C **(SLP)**
Burke, Kathleen Smith **(SLP)**
Carrigan-Peek, Mrs Mary Ann **(SLP)**
Clements, Sr Elizabeth **(SLP)**
Connor, Karla Kae **(SLP)**
Corcione, Mrs Sarah W **(SLP)**
Dodge, Mrs Susan Delong **(A)**
Dudek, Mrs Quincey Marie **(SLP)**
Edwards, Mrs Maura M **(SLP)**
Ferrandino, Regina Mary **(A)**
Ferraro, Judy **(SLP)**
Frantsov, Marilyn Casaceli **(A)**
Gesser-Winter, Mrs Janet S **(SLP)**
Hess, Mrs Mary Loughney **(SLP)**
Insalaco, Deborah Michelle **(SLP)**
Julien, Joan E **(SLP)**
Karcher-Hewitt, Mrs Sherry Lynne **(SLP)**
Keener, Lynn Diane **(SLP)**
Koblenz, Mrs Marta B R **(SLP)**
Labier, Francesca M **(SLP)**
La Posta Donohue, Mrs Constance A **(A)**
Le Mark, Mary Elizabeth **(SLP)**
Leto, Mrs Deborah Leonard **(SLP)**
Levine, Deborah Biskin **(SLP)**
Liebman, Aaron H **(A)**
Maguire, Mabel C **(SLP)**
Margulies, Vivian **(SLP A)**
Metzger, Janet Marie **(SLP)**
Mooney, Marilyn Decker **(SLP)**
Moore, Claudia Contess **(SLP)**
Morris, Mrs Renee Warshaw **(SLP)**
Mueller, Grace A **(SLP)**
Osterhout, Cheryl A **(SLP)**
Pickett, Maureen Duane
Raffo, Christine M **(A)**
Ravalli, Susan Linda **(SLP)**
Reed, Mrs Dora Ruskin **(SLP)**
Rheingold, Gail **(SLP)**
Roach, Mary Jane **(SLP)**
Rosen, Rebecca G **(SLP)**
Rosenthal, Mrs Carolyn M **(SLP)**
Ross, Dr M Gerlene **(SLP)**
Saleem-Brodsky, Laura Fern
Salmon, Kimberly Ann **(SLP)**
Schilp, Mrs Carol D **(SLP)**
Seidner, Roslyn F J **(SLP)**
Shetler, Susan K **(SLP)**
Spring, Karen A **(SLP)**
Stonefield, Ross **(SLP)**
Tendler, Irene **(SLP)**
Trees, Debra E **(A)**
Veith, Karalee Colleen **(SLP)**
Wayner, Dr Donna Shpikula **(A)**
Zwink, Elizabeth Louise **(SLP)**

Albertson
Kramer, Mrs Marilyn L **(SLP)**
Martin, Dr Edwin W **(SLP)**
Yagerman, Mrs Laurie Cooper **(SLP)**

Alden
Garas, Mrs Donna M
Kurpita, Barbara J **(A)**
Walence, Mrs Barbara Kester **(SLP)**
Walence, William W **(A)**

Allegany
Crouse, Mrs Mary Ellen **(SLP)**
Medinger, Sue Ellen **(SLP)**
Monachino, Sandra Bullock **(SLP)**
Montague, Barbara P **(SLP)**
Thompson, Mrs Diana Outman **(SLP)**

Altamont
Heller, Mrs Gaye G **(SLP)**

Amenia
Appleton, Rozanne S **(SLP)**

Amherst
Bala, Mrs Sandra M **(SLP)**
Colling, Mrs Maryellen D **(SLP)**
Cunningham, Virginia **(SLP)**
Donovan, Alice Estelle **(SLP)**
Joyce, Jerri Kaplan **(A)**
Lubinski, Dr Rosemary B **(SLP)**
Martin, Charyleen **(SLP)**
Redino, Michelle A **(SLP)**
Stecker, Dr Nancy A **(SLP A)**

Amity Harbor
Freshley, Nancy L **(SLP)**

Amityville
Dellapenna, Loren A
O'Reilly, Mrs Ann E **(SLP)**
Resnitzky, Lauren Cwenar **(SLP)**
Rifkind, Mrs Susan Huck **(SLP)**
Ying, Elizabeth **(SLP)**

Amsterdam
Filiberto, Mrs Lisa Ann **(SLP)**
Lasky-Case, Mrs Lynnemarie **(SLP)**
Miskinis, Mrs Angela Lalla
Piechnik-Briggs, Diane C **(SLP)**
Rutnik, Margaret Mary **(SLP)**
Schwartz, Mrs Ellen S **(SLP)**
Seward, Mrs Helen M **(SLP)**

Angola
Mazur, Carolyn **(SLP)**
Piccillo-Stokes, Mrs Lois D **(SLP)**
Victor, Judith A **(SLP)**

Apalachin
Johnson, Linda W **(SLP)**
Strack, Mrs Alison Kay **(SLP)**
Wronski, Karen Louise H **(SLP)**

APO New York
Abbott-Cason, Susan **(SLP)**
Aker, Mrs Adelyn Ramoni **(SLP)**
Allen, Maj John R **(SLP A)**
Allen, Mrs Sue Sharp **(SLP)**
Aspinall, Dr Kenneth B **(A)**
Ball, Laura J **(SLP)**
Beamer, Sharon L **(A)**
Becker, Beverly Adelaide **(SLP)**
Benedict, Mary K **(SLP)**
Bennett, Howard D **(SLP)**
Bergeron, Linda P **(SLP)**
Blessing, Mrs Elizabeth Armstrong
Budinger, Ann Calkins **(A)**
Bunzendahl, Vivianne Wilson **(SLP)**
Calbos, Eleni T **(SLP)**
Cambon, Marjorie Burwell **(SLP)**
Carlson, Mrs Teresa H **(SLP)**
Carter, June Marie **(SLP)**
Carter, Mrs Terry T **(SLP)**
Clay, Marcy Dumoch **(SLP)**
Clement, Maj Augustus T **(SLP)**
Cohen, Gail E **(SLP)**
Conway, Mrs Valerie Hilliard **(SLP)**
Courtney, Mrs E LaWanda **(SLP)**
Cousins, Mrs Becky R **(SLP)**
Cramer-Richards, Janet **(SLP)**
Crampton, Joann M **(SLP)**
Crettol, Elaine L T **(SLP)**
Crouse, Maureen Elizabeth **(SLP)**
Cruthirds-Meyers, Mrs Lynda Lee **(SLP)**
Cullop, Joann Robertson **(SLP)**
Cutright, Mrs Jayne F **(SLP)**
Dixon, Mrs Jennifer L
Donovan, Mrs Rachael Anne **(SLP)**
Egblomasse, Sonja Cosby **(SLP)**
Fagan, Mrs Pamela J **(SLP)**
Flanagan, Sheila Ann **(SLP)**
Friedman, Deborah Walker **(SLP)**
Frisard, Louise M **(SLP)**
Galbreath, Mrs Jan Kathryn
Garnett, Mrs Mary Jane **(A)**
Gilbert, Susan C **(SLP)**
Girdler, Donna M **(SLP)**
Goodman, Pamela F **(SLP)**
Gordon, Debra Ann Long **(SLP)**
Green, Billye Marie **(SLP)**
Hadley, Mrs Beverly B **(A)**
Haines, Constance Dee **(SLP)**
Hallmark, Mary Hulett **(A)**
Heath, Mrs Susan Neff **(SLP)**
Hepler, Dr Ernest L, Jr **(A)**
Hessler, Teresa Ann **(SLP)**
Hill, Merry G **(SLP)**
Hogan, Gerardine **(SLP)**
Holloman, Angela Law **(SLP)**
Horsfall, Dr Geoffrey H **(SLP A)**
Huet, Elizabeth M **(SLP)**
Hyland, Mrs Sandra Ann Colema **(SLP)**
Jablonski, Gregory Michael **(SLP)**
Jerome, Maj James J **(A)**
Jeske, Agnes N **(SLP)**
Jones, Mrs Pamela R L **(SLP)**
Jones, William B **(SLP)**
Knaack, Patricia **(SLP)**
Krause, Karlene Ann **(SLP)**
La Fleur, Mrs Michele B
Lane-Marko, Joanne **(SLP)**
Lange, Gail T **(SLP)**
Leary, Judith E **(SLP)**
Leboeuf, Mrs Julie D **(SLP)**
Livingston, Dana Lou **(SLP)**
Lloyd, Rachel **(SLP)**
Loovis, Dr Carl F **(A)**
Lovorn, Sallie Beraud **(A)**
Lynch, Dr Constance J **(SLP)**
MacDougall, Mrs Mary Donnelly **(SLP)**
Mattern, Patricia C **(A)**
McCarthy, Diane Elizabeth **(A)**
Metrogen-Prieto, Karen Lea
Mikkelsen, Marie E **(A)**
Miller, Mrs Josephine Schulze **(SLP)**
Mohr, Waynette F **(SLP)**
Moody, Donna K **(SLP)**
Morton, Mrs Karen Deann **(SLP)**
Murphy, Mrs Letitia Wicker **(SLP)**
Neihardt, Carol **(SLP)**
Niklaus, Phyllis Marie **(SLP)**
Noda, Ann **(SLP)**
Novak, Mrs Janet Lynn W **(SLP)**
O'Keeffe, Kathleen Noonan **(SLP)**
Osborne, Carmela Bari **(SLP)**
Overton, Elaine Cecilia
Pengelly, Michael H **(A)**
Peterson, Laura Ide **(SLP)**
Polakof, Isabel
Rettgers, Bonnie J **(A)**
Richards, Denise S **(SLP)**
Rinschler, Roger Jay **(SLP)**
Rolfe, Brenda Smith **(A)**
Ross, Vicki K **(SLP)**
Rush, Mrs Debra Shelton **(SLP)**
Sessions, Mrs Judith M **(SLP)**
Shipp, Mrs Susan S **(SLP)**
Sinclair, Mary Patrcia **(SLP)**
Smolin, Lori Kay
Sternsdorff, Donna Lee **(A)**
Stevens, Mrs Janetta Buchner **(SLP)**
Storm, Jill B **(SLP)**
Swartz, Mrs Barbara Brewer **(A)**
Swisher, Mrs Rosemarie Aileen **(SLP)**
Swisher, Timothy A **(A)**
Taylor, Carmen Lisa **(A)**
Travis, Miriam Louise **(SLP)**
Traynor-Duda, Hilary **(SLP)**
Walbridge, Carol **(SLP)**
Weed, Sara Marie **(SLP)**
Wilson, Mrs Beth Minick **(SLP)**
Winter, Marta Patricia **(SLP)**
Wright, Virginia A **(SLP)**

Ardsley
Goodman, Dr Allan C **(SLP A)**
Metsch, Susan Ellen
Parris, Mary **(SLP)**
Phillips, Martha A **(A)**
Rickler, Irwin **(SLP)**
Schuman, Lois J **(SLP)**
Weissman, Mrs Ronee F **(SLP)**

Armonk
Callaghan, Janet Turansky **(SLP)**
Cascardo, Mrs Debra **(A)**
Kaufman, Mrs Eleanor G **(SLP)**
Rosen, Adrienne Z **(SLP)**
Schwartz, Dr Judith Stockheim
Solomon, Mrs Sandra P **(A)**

Astoria
Brachfeld, Jill Robin **(SLP)**
Centeno, Jose Gregorio **(SLP)**
De Ciccio, Maria **(SLP)**
Fee, Anne Elizabeth **(SLP)**
Gale, Laura J **(SLP)**
Gardella, Teresa D'Angelo **(A)**
O'Connor, Anna **(SLP)**
Paul, Zoe Lillian **(SLP)**
Schillinger, Karen M **(SLP)**
Short, Julie A **(SLP)**

Atlantic Beach
Johnson, Alan L **(SLP)**
Rosen, Mrs Stacey Jill **(SLP)**

Auburn
Cleaver, Mrs Patricia Quigley **(SLP)**
Damalt, Mrs Nancy Lisano **(SLP)**
Graham, Marjorie K **(SLP)**
Leciejewski, Ruth Klonowski **(SLP)**
McCarthy, Mrs Mary E Payne **(SLP)**
Nodzo, Ellen B **(SLP)**
Sarofeen, Carole Bishop **(SLP)**
Sullivan, MaryBeth **(SLP)**

Ava
Quattrini, Debra Jacobson **(A)**
Rasmussen, Mrs Delia Graham **(SLP)**

Averill Park
Cioffi, Lisa M

Gallant, Dr Olivia A **(A)**
Murray, Susan E **(SLP)**

Avon
Martens-Pitts, Lucinda A **(SLP)**
Nugent, Margaret Jo **(SLP)**
Proper, Marcia Lee **(SLP)**
Westfall-Cox, Mrs Tammy L

Babylon
Cronk, Mrs Rebecca A
Fisher, Karen Elizabeth **(A)**
Johnson, Mrs Lucille Mary **(SLP)**
Lebel, Mrs Debra Karen **(SLP)**
Lefkowitz, Mrs Beverly B **(SLP)**
Linko-Bellavia, Mrs Susan Claire **(SLP)**
Sutter, Mrs Ann Marie **(SLP)**
Tobin, Mrs Deirdre Mary **(SLP)**
Walker, Joanne M **(SLP)**

Baiting Hollow
Peters, Judy Woodall **(SLP)**

Baldwin
Barnwell, Veronica Bernadette **(A)**
Barrere, Mrs Eleni **(SLP)**
Binderoff, Randy **(A)**
Cohen, Mrs Patricia A **(A)**
Hetzel, Trudy Gordon **(A)**
Hollander, Barbara E **(A)**
Kolpon, Mrs Suzanne W **(SLP)**
Morvay, Christine Marie
Nissenfeld-Sells, Mrs Lisa Rachel **(SLP)**
Plotnick, Charlotte B **(SLP)**
Satir, Mrs Roxana E
Summerhayes, Elizabeth **(SLP)**
Voelpel, Mrs Judith Ann **(SLP)**
Weinstein, Mrs Emily A M **(SLP)**

Baldwin Harbor
Ashinoff, Mrs Ellen Herbst **(SLP)**
Barrow, Mrs Meryl B **(SLP)**
Blau, Deborah A **(SLP)**
Karlan, Mrs Andrea **(SLP)**

Baldwinsville
Colligan, Mrs Margaret Raby
Gibbons, Janet M E **(SLP)**
Goodwin, Harry S **(SLP)**
Grimes, Mrs Linda L **(A)**
Kenney, Arthur Joseph **(SLP)**
Stimson, Mrs Linda D **(SLP)**
Walsh, Kate **(SLP)**
Worthing, Donna Robichaud **(SLP)**

Ballston Lake
Donigan, Margaret **(SLP)**
Hart, Mrs Linda Carol **(SLP)**
Horgan, Mary C **(SLP)**
Winters-D'Amboise, Cynthia Lou **(SLP)**

Ballston Spa
Brennan, Mrs Jacalyn M **(SLP)**
Decker, Mrs Synnove E **(SLP)**
Drosky, Mrs Ceil Dicerbo **(SLP)**
Hite-Hare, Mrs Susan C **(SLP)**
Howatt, Kelly Ann **(SLP)**
Kavanaugh, Diane E **(SLP)**
Morehouse, Margaret P **(SLP)**
Schwartz, Sandra Levine **(SLP)**
Shisler, Mrs Wendy S **(SLP)**

Barneveld
Gajewski, Mrs Mary C **(SLP)**
Mahanna, Mary Christine **(SLP)**

Batavia
Friedman, Mrs Kathleen Anne **(SLP)**
Puleo, Shirley Bragg **(SLP)**
Zola, Mrs Pamela Dale **(SLP)**

Bath
Colomaio, Robert James **(SLP)**
Gwinner, Mrs Nanette Hawks **(A)**
Jablonovsky, Melanie S **(SLP)**
Ormsby, Rose A G **(SLP)**
Rodrigues, Mrs Barbara **(SLP)**

Bay Shore
Fox, Mrs Nancy Lynn
Harrison, Rhonda L **(SLP)**
Horton-McGinley, Mrs Diane E **(SLP)**
Jordan, Rebecca Semenak **(A)**
Jorgensen, Debra Ann **(SLP)**
Maggio, Mrs Michele W **(SLP)**
Nappo, Cheryl Ann **(SLP)**
Patchen, Mrs Laura Gerardi **(SLP)**
Podesta, Mindy T **(SLP)**

Bayport
Fiore-Powell, Joanne P **(SLP)**
Vancaeseele-Pontieri, Mrs Martha L **(SLP)**

Bayside
Abrams, Scott David
Alimaras, Constance Siomkos **(SLP)**
Baval, Bonnie D **(SLP)**
Bayone Cook, Ilene **(SLP)**
Bianco, Ellenbeth **(SLP)**
Buckles, Patricia Kay
Burhans-Ross, Wendy Ann **(SLP)**
Cooperman, Estelle B **(SLP)**
Cortez, Richard A **(A)**
Dimarco, Mrs Carol Fruchtman **(SLP)**
Forman, Mrs Carol Fern **(SLP)**
Gillis, Dr Herbert R **(SLP)**
Gold, Mrs Mindy Rose **(SLP)**
Goldberg, Donna Lynn **(A)**
Griffer, Mona R **(SLP)**
Gura, Mrs Randi Paige
Haft, Debra Joy **(SLP)**
Heller-Ringer, Mrs Donna L **(SLP)**
Henaghen, Jill Ann **(SLP)**
Hendler-Lederer, Mrs Susan G **(SLP)**
Kelly, Maureen Theresa **(SLP)**
Klipper, Rhonda D **(SLP)**
Lipkind, Vicki L **(SLP)**
Mirandona, Mrs Kathleen B **(SLP)**
Nedbalsky, Anna M **(SLP)**
Peckins, Susan Tracey **(A)**
Pollack, Mrs Dorothy H **(SLP)**
Popowsky, Karen Rudnick **(SLP)**
Rath, Jessica Lynn **(SLP)**
Ratnofsky-Reiss, Selma Esther **(SLP)**
Reich, Rita Daum **(SLP A)**
Resnick, Mrs Sylvia **(SLP)**
Rochlen, Mrs Libby Beth **(SLP)**
Rosado, Mrs Maria L **(SLP)**
Rosenzweig, Lisa P **(SLP)**
Rotches, Meryl **(SLP)**
Rubin, Barbara R **(SLP)**
Ruhalter, Fern Gayle **(SLP)**
Schlisselberg, Dr Gloria F **(SLP)**
Schroeder, Mrs Tamara P **(SLP)**
Shapiro, Mrs Melissa Malis **(A)**
Shapiro, William H **(A)**
Shusterman, Mrs Joan S **(SLP)**
Smith, Deborah Ann **(SLP)**
Studley, Mrs Lisa Sharon **(A)**
Sturm, Andrea E **(SLP)**
Valvezan, Rose N **(A)**
Van Meter, Mrs Ellen Mary **(SLP)**
Wiener-Maran, P **(SLP)**
Yager, Mrs Karen M
Zucker, Joan **(SLP)**

Bayville
Herbst, Jean **(SLP)**
Taddeo, Dolores A **(SLP)**

Beacon
Demetros, Mrs Cheryl Irene **(SLP)**
Horan, Roseann F **(SLP)**
Krass, Jay J **(SLP)**
Kunkel, Mrs Amy Elizabeth **(SLP)**
Umano, Helen V **(SLP)**

Bedford
Hurwitz, Mrs Jane S **(SLP)**
Joffee-Meszaros, Mrs Janis A **(SLP)**
Ormond, Mary Frances **(SLP)**
Scheffler, Mrs Frances Vandenburg **(SLP)**

Bedford Hills
Glotzer, Patti Ann **(SLP)**
Gould, Mary Devaney **(SLP)**

Belle Harbor
Chapey, Dr Geraldine **(SLP)**
Dube, Mrs Nina K **(SLP)**
Stathis, Eileen **(SLP)**

Bellerose
Duffy, Mrs Gloria Beth **(SLP)**
Genna, Carolyn Marie
Gozdziewski, Mrs Terry Hausner **(SLP)**
Houlihan, Mrs Jane Cooke **(A)**
McCoy, Noreen Lynn **(SLP)**
Sternemann, Mrs Phyllis M **(SLP)**

Bellmore
Abes, Karen Susan **(SLP)**
Brown, Ellen R **(SLP)**
Goldstein, Marilyn K **(SLP)**
Kushner, Mrs Roslyn Schachter **(SLP A)**
Siperstein, Mira S **(SLP)**
Stember, Lynn G **(SLP)**
Stetson, Mrs Joan Ruth **(SLP)**

Bellport
Becerra, Mrs Candice **(SLP)**
Vetrano, Elaine M **(A)**

Bethpage
Bedard, Laurie Gay **(A)**
Burn, Mrs Lois Murphy **(SLP)**
Candiotte, Elayne **(SLP)**
Clarke, Kim Spina **(A)**
Daley, Mrs Elysse B **(SLP)**
Fontana, Dr Marie **(SLP)**
Krinsky, Ruth Tammi
Nimmo, Mrs Debra Ryan **(SLP)**
Rafenski, Janet G **(SLP)**
Turkiew, Mrs Rachel A **(SLP)**

Big Flats
Kotacska, Rosina M G **(SLP)**

Binghamton
Arnaboldi, Loren Joseph **(SLP)**
Carpenter, Kyle M **(A)**
Cashman, Marianne **(SLP)**
Colpoys, Brian P **(SLP)**
Duncan, Kathleen P **(SLP)**
Gitlitz, Shelia R **(SLP A)**
Haas, Mrs Catherine Ann **(SLP)**
Hamzik-Mills, Mrs Suzanne **(SLP)**
Lepre-Clark, Mrs Camille **(SLP)**
Lewis, Karla Clair **(A)**
Luckern, Marie P **(SLP)**
McKissick, Mrs Karen E Bernardo **(SLP)**
Meredith, Mrs Theresa **(SLP)**
Moran-Burton, Mrs Judith A **(SLP)**
Palombaro, Mary Mason **(SLP)**
Quain-Krukowski, Mrs Elizabeth J **(SLP)**
Rose, Mrs Emily S **(SLP)**
Rozen, Charlotte **(SLP)**
Schindelman, Maxine **(SLP)**
Sommer, Mrs Lillian S **(SLP)**
Spitz, Diane E **(SLP)**
Spring, Mrs Theresa M **(SLP)**
Stephanie, Sandra G **(A)**
Tatich, Denise Marie **(SLP)**
Weir, Jacqueline M **(SLP)**
Westcott, Mrs Judy Girdwood **(SLP)**
Wexler, Melanie Ellen **(A)**
Wilsonn, Mrs Maria Johnson **(SLP)**
Wulff, Cynthia J **(SLP)**
Zanfordino, Joseph Peter **(SLP)**

Blasdell
Fritz, Barbara A **(SLP)**

Bloomingburg
Schleser, Marilyn Melis **(SLP)**

Bloomington
Massimi, Mrs Theresa Shanley **(SLP)**

Blue Point
Kopf, Karen P **(SLP)**

Brentwood
Crane-Riley, Catherine **(SLP)**

Brewerton
Finkenstadt, Mrs Susan C **(SLP)**

Brewster
Deperno, Denise **(SLP)**
Gerlt, Elaine A **(SLP)**
Meyer, Mrs Karen A G **(SLP)**
Toutain, Beverly Ambrosic **(SLP)**
Tracy, Kathleen McQuade **(SLP)**
Tuttle, Doreen **(SLP)**

Briarcliff Manor
Hammond, Judith G **(SLP)**
Kraft, Dr Anita R **(SLP)**
Prouty, Sharon W **(SLP)**
Sankin, Susan J P **(SLP)**

Briarwood
Hasan, Zahida M
Mesa-Ariss, Mrs Maria E **(SLP)**
Schaeffer, Natalie G **(SLP)**

Brighton
Heimrath, Karen **(SLP)**

Brightwaters
Scifo, Marianne Conrad **(SLP)**

Brockport
Boatfield, Mary Elizabeth **(SLP)**
Bouwes, Nona G **(SLP)**
Gehringer, Mary Louise **(SLP)**
Tufano, Mrs Sally **(SLP)**

Brocton
Perez, Dr Dennis M **(SLP)**

Bronx
Baron, Barbara Schwartz **(SLP)**
Bartolotta, Mrs Theresa E **(SLP)**
Berenhaus, Sandra R **(A)**
Bieker, Rebecca R **(A)**
Borger, Mrs Michele Strauss **(SLP)**
Brown, Gail Ann **(SLP)**
Brown, Joan C **(SLP)**
Cantor, Susan Helene **(SLP)**
Cave, Cornelia **(SLP)**
Cirkiel-Naftel, Karen **(A)**
Cohen, Robert A **(A)**
Contento, Kathryn Ann **(SLP)**
Dolan, William B **(A)**
Felder, Lynda J **(SLP)**
Fenster, Susan Ann **(SLP)**
Fertig-Friedman, Beth L **(SLP)**
Golding-Kushner, Mrs Karen J **(SLP)**
Goldman, Lisa Mendes **(SLP)**
Goodman, Paula Jodi **(A)**
Goshit, Mrs M Yvonne **(SLP)**
Greene, Renee Y **(A)**
Group, Mrs Joyce Regenbogen **(SLP)**
Herman, Mrs Ilana H F **(SLP)**
Hoffman, Blair Lynne **(SLP)**
Hyams, Mrs Sheila S **(SLP)**
Jones, Dr Jacqueline
Kelleher, Thomas Peter **(SLP)**
Kishon-Rabin, Mrs Liat
Konig, Diana G **(SLP)**
Laporte, Patricia Lynn **(SLP)**
Lipsky, Mrs Sharon Braver **(SLP)**
London-Samuels, Mrs Shelley D **(SLP)**
Lunde, Mrs Florence K **(SLP)**
Luther, Mary C **(SLP)**
Marks-Hershey, Leslie A **(SLP)**
Martinez, Martha R **(SLP)**
Modell, Lisa Fern **(SLP)**
Nelson, Carol Ann **(SLP)**
Ortiz, Ivette
Perez, Nilsa Rubin **(SLP)**
Person, Dr Carolyn J **(SLP)**
Rahman, Sahara **(SLP)**
Riccio, Susan E **(SLP)**

Rivas, Jeanne **(SLP)**
Rivera, Velma L **(SLP)**
Ruben, Dr Robert J
Schroeder, Ellen K **(SLP)**
Scotti, Mrs Amy B **(SLP)**
Sender, Dina L **(SLP)**
Shprintzen, Dr Robert J **(SLP)**
Simon, Geraldine **(SLP)**
Stapells, Dr David Richard
Stern, Mrs Barbara J **(SLP)**
Stracci, Mary E **(SLP)**
Strawder, Veronica G **(SLP)**
Till, Jill Kane **(SLP)**
Tzanis, Mrs Evmorfia Fotiou **(A)**
Vesely, Mrs Lorenza **(SLP)**
Winters, Mrs Rachelle **(SLP)**

Bronxville

Colonna, Alexandria **(A)**
Donohue, Mrs Joelen M **(SLP)**
Hayden, Patricia A **(SLP)**
Manno, Lorane **(SLP)**
Puncar, Josephine Anselmo **(SLP)**
Rade, Susan J **(SLP)**
Rooney, Barbara Ann **(A)**
Sherretta, Mrs Carrie Hirschhorn **(SLP)**
Ward, Mrs Evelyn L **(SLP)**
Wheeler, Mrs Diane G **(SLP)**
Zeitoun, Lisa Horowitz **(A)**

Brookland

Silman, Dr Shlomo **(A)**

Brooklyn

Abott, Ellen Fran **(A)**
Adamousky, Dawn Julie
Adasko, Mrs Mary Hardy **(SLP)**
Adler, Beryl T **(SLP)**
Alexander, Valerie M
Alterbaum, Irene P **(SLP)**
Annunziata, Christine Russo **(A)**
Ansbacher, Mrs Riva Hankel **(SLP)**
Applebaum, Mrs Valerie K **(SLP)**
Atkins, Wendy F **(SLP)**
Aversano, Anthony Michael **(SLP)**
Babb, Maxine Althea **(SLP)**
Bader, Sheryl **(SLP)**
Baker, Ellen P B **(SLP)**
Baker, Lisa Ann **(SLP)**
Bakke, Matthew H
Baraz, Julie E **(SLP)**
Becker, Mrs Irene A **(SLP)**
Becker, Laurence R **(SLP)**
Benjamin, Francine H **(A)**
Bennett, Barbara A **(SLP)**
Bernholz-Balsam, Lisa H **(SLP A)**
Bernstein, Mrs Susan R **(SLP)**
Biscow, Gail M **(A)**
Blackman, Ellen D **(SLP)**
Blackman, Mrs Sylvia B
Bleakney, Mary E **(A)**
Bloodstein, Dr Oliver **(SLP)**
Blumstein, Linda H **(SLP)**
Bochbot, Mrs Deborah Robin **(SLP)**
Bonadies, Mrs Pamela Ryan **(SLP)**
Borinsky, Janet S **(SLP)**
Bowens, Sandra Felecia **(SLP)**
Bradley, Willie B **(SLP)**
Brafman, Alicia H L
Brandes-Meyerfeld, Mrs Holly
Brandt, Mela B **(SLP)**
Brody, Philip **(SLP A)**
Budgar, Laurie Beth **(SLP)**
Butler, Chana L **(SLP)**
Caracciolo, Laurie Ann
Carey, Vanessa Aliesa **(SLP)**
Carrubba, Mrs Roberta Linda **(SLP)**
Castellano, Joseph **(A)**
Champion, Tempii Bridgene **(SLP)**
Chapey, Dr Roberta **(SLP)**
Cherry, Dr Rochelle S **(SLP A)**
Christian, Kathryn Farnen **(SLP)**
Cooper, Kimberly Hanna **(SLP)**
Coulon, Ellen L **(SLP)**
Cymerman, Shmuel **(A)**
Dadon, Angela Russo **(SLP)**
Davis, Deidre Marie **(SLP)**
Davis, Michelle **(SLP)**
Dear, Mrs Rickly Neiman **(SLP)**
Decicco, Barbara A **(SLP)**
Deeb, Barbara M **(SLP)**
Delapenha, Sandra Elaine **(A)**
Depasquale, Maria C **(SLP)**
Digiovanni, Mrs Kathleen Marie **(A)**
Dreifus, Vicky Greenberg **(SLP)**
Drillings, Mrs Flora M **(SLP)**
Dwyer, Bridget M **(SLP)**
Egbert, William S **(A)**
Einhorn, Allan Jack **(A)**
Eisert, Susan Y
Engel, Heather Lee **(SLP)**
Epstein, Ellayne S **(SLP)**
Epstein, Harold **(SLP)**
Fain, Dorothy Marie **(SLP)**
Fay, Catherine **(SLP)**
Fein, Deborah L **(SLP)**
Fein, Shelley **(SLP)**
Ferree, Mrs Celine M C **(SLP)**
Firestein, Mrs Laura H **(SLP)**
Fisher-Medina, Julia Ann **(SLP)**
Forestieri, Grace
Foster, Nyli **(SLP)**
Frankel, Henny **(SLP)**
Friedman, Susan E **(SLP)**
Frischman, Anne Weiss **(SLP)**
Gallagher, Linda Ann **(SLP)**
Gallo, Mrs Diane I **(SLP)**
Gaudin, Diane Shearer **(SLP)**
Geller, Elaine Fleisher **(SLP)**
Gelzer-Hill, Brenda Eleanor **(SLP)**
Gingold, Iris N **(SLP)**
Girlando, Lucy M **(SLP)**
Giuliano, Mrs Lynne C **(SLP)**
Golden, Mrs Sharon R **(SLP)**
Goldman, Charles **(SLP)**
Goldman, Mrs Donna Sue **(SLP)**
Grant, Lauren **(SLP)**
Green, Cynthia **(SLP)**
Greenstein, Mrs Evelyn Beller **(SLP)**
Greenstein, Richard A **(SLP)**
Gross, Ilene **(A)**
Grosvenor, Mrs Kathleen P **(SLP)**
Grunblatt, Mrs Henna Baila R **(A)**
Guardo, Elaine R **(SLP)**
Gurland, Dr Gail **(SLP)**
Halberstam, Feigi Taub **(A)**
Harari-Raful, Michela S **(SLP)**
Hart, Mrs Janice Schreier **(A)**
Hauben, Mrs Esther C Grinblat **(A)**
Heinsen-Combs, Alexandra **(SLP)**
Hershey-Miller, Mrs Sadelle **(SLP)**
Hessing, Mark **(SLP)**
Himmel, Jacquelin **(SLP)**
Hoffstead, Veronica **(SLP)**
Huie, Mrs Nancy Eng **(SLP)**
Jacobson, Mrs Rose **(SLP)**
Jacobson, Susan Gail **(A)**
Jakubovics, Helena Alter **(SLP)**
Janow, Mrs Ethel W **(SLP)**
Jeffery, Carol
Jennings, Joan Mary
Jessamy, Linda E **(SLP)**
Johnson, Mrs Gertrude L **(SLP)**
Kahane, Denise H **(A)**
Kamalic, Linda J S **(SLP)**
Kaner, Richard P **(A)**
Kapassakis, Georgea **(SLP)**
Kaplan, Betty Marsha **(SLP)**
Kasdorf, Susan Cohen **(SLP)**
Katzen, Sheri H **(SLP)**
Kaye, Debra Naiztat **(SLP)**
Kelly, Robert **(SLP)**
Kiersh, Nancy E **(SLP)**
Kinsberg, Helene K
Klein, Phyllis **(SLP A)**
Klein, Shelia **(A)**
Klinsky, Shirley Dombrow **(SLP)**
Kohn, Mrs Debra Glass **(SLP)**
Koller, Jerry J **(SLP)**
Korkes, Nancy L **(SLP)**
La Bella, Georgianna Teresa
Labriola, Mrs Cheryl Hicklen **(SLP)**
Landman, Chana **(SLP)**
Laufer-Turk, Mrs Stella Claire **(A)**
Lefkowitz, Freya **(SLP)**
Lefkowitz, Laurie E **(SLP)**
Lehrman, Mrs Aliza **(SLP)**
Leibowitz, Mrs Jane S **(SLP)**
Levine Esq, Mrs Barbara Pearlman **(SLP)**
Lieberburg, Ellen H **(SLP)**
Littlefield, Mrs Catherine M **(SLP)**
Litwin, Zelda **(SLP)**
Lorowitz, Lori Michele **(SLP)**
Louick, Mrs Karen Kronheim **(SLP)**
Lurie, Bonnie **(A)**
Maida-Schmieder, Debora **(SLP)**
Malfitano, Amanda A
Manela, Mrs Temmy L **(SLP)**
Mann, Marcia P **(SLP)**
Manzo, Frances Marie **(SLP)**
Maranga, Gina **(SLP)**
Martin, Brett A **(A)**
Matthes, Dr Richard W **(A)**
McMillan, Aundria R **(SLP)**
Meade, William F **(SLP)**
Mehler, Mrs Esther **(SLP)**
Mendez-Kurtz, Lucy P **(A)**
Mermelstein-Epner, Lillie E **(SLP)**
Messinger, Sue A **(A)**
Meyers, Laura I **(SLP)**
Montag, Mrs Maxine S **(SLP)**
Morris, Mrs Susan Edberg **(SLP)**
Murry, Laura Silverberg **(SLP)**
Nahmias, Mrs Gail A
Nathanson, Janis K **(SLP)**
Neuschotz, Carmen Kowalski **(SLP)**
Offenbacher, Barbara Levine **(SLP)**
Olenick, Gail M **(SLP)**
Ostrovsky, Steven N **(SLP)**
Ovadia, Mrs Joanne **(SLP)**
Papoutsakis, Catherine Christine **(SLP)**
Parker, Marilyn F **(SLP)**
Pasternack, Barbara **(SLP)**
Pavona, John T **(SLP)**
Pearlstein, Meryl R **(SLP)**
Pekler, Mrs June M **(SLP)**
Pelowitz, Helene M **(SLP)**
Perl, Mrs Marlene Ruth
Piascik, Laura Catherine **(SLP)**
Pieras, Dr Guillermo J **(SLP)**
Pilewski, Mrs Denise Ellen **(SLP)**
Pinter, Naomi L **(SLP)**
Pinter, Shaindy **(SLP)**
Pivor, Nadine R **(SLP)**
Poll, Mrs Karen Richler **(SLP)**
Posner, Carol Lynn **(SLP)**
Pratt, Mrs Miriam Markowitz **(SLP)**
Press, Mrs Ivy L **(A)**
Qualley, Michael David **(A)**
Quiles-Contreras, Sara Yleana **(SLP)**
Raber, Mrs Maya Gerkina **(SLP)**
Raeder, Celia R **(SLP)**
Rain, Keirsten **(SLP)**
Reich, Denise Michele **(SLP)**
Reichlin, Holly **(SLP)**
Reinman, Miriam K **(SLP)**
Reisberg, Debra R **(SLP)**
Reisler, Laura M **(SLP)**
Reiter, Dr Levi A **(A)**
Riquelme, Luis F **(SLP)**
Rivkin, Gail R
Rodin, Dr Alan **(SLP)**
Rosen, Mrs Annie Rebecca **(SLP)**
Rosen, Shirley Rona **(SLP)**
Rosengarten, Robert E **(A)**
Rosengarten, Mrs Susan H **(A)**
Rosenstock, Mrs Arlene S **(SLP)**
Rothwax, Helen Frances **(SLP)**
Rubin, Mrs Helen Leser **(SLP)**
Rudnick, Sherry J **(SLP)**
Rupp, Shayne D Y **(SLP)**
Rush, Carol Schaffer **(SLP)**
Russell, Mary C **(SLP)**
Salih, Mrs Ursula Fulcher **(SLP)**
Santana, Altagracia A **(SLP)**
Santaniello, Jean L **(SLP)**
Santisi, Rosemarie **(SLP)**
Savad, Mrs Libby **(SLP)**
Schacter, Chedva **(SLP)**
Schiavone, Diane C **(SLP)**
Schiavone, James Robert **(SLP)**
Schwabe, Annette Marie **(SLP)**
Schwartz, Mrs Debra Goldzweig **(A)**
Schwartz, Linda Raskin **(SLP)**
Schwebel, Rochelle Feifer **(SLP)**
Segal, Mrs Beverly D **(SLP)**
Shapiro, Carrie Janine
Shulman, Marc A **(SLP)**
Silverman, Kathe F **(SLP)**
Simpson, Patricia J **(SLP)**
Slotnick, Phyllis Beth **(A)**
Solomon, Mona Schechter **(SLP)**
Somma, Christine A **(SLP)**
Spears, Mrs Amy Beth **(SLP)**
Stefankiewicz, Sabina P **(SLP)**
Stein, Cyndi J **(SLP)**
Stein, Debra J **(SLP)**
Steinberg, Mrs Randi Joy **(A)**
Stein-Meyers, Anita Robin **(A)**
Stok, Mrs Vivian Kallus **(SLP)**
Stromer, Dr Jeffrey M **(SLP)**
Styczynski, Celeste R **(SLP)**
Suede, Mrs Diane Randie **(SLP)**
Sullivan, Maria A **(SLP)**
Swiss Rossi, Ellen Ann
Taubman, Jacqueline **(SLP)**
Thomson, Madora W
Torres, Mrs Irene Gilbert **(SLP)**
Turner, Lois Susan **(A)**
Vargas, Mrs Leslie Kahn **(SLP)**
Vogel, Donald Allen **(A)**
Waldman, Lois Jean **(SLP)**
Wallin, Mrs Ann Berstein **(A)**
Walters, Sylvia Y **(SLP)**
Warren, Mrs Francine Marcia **(SLP)**
Wasserman, Mrs Nancy H **(SLP)**
Weber, Margaret Meister
Weinberger, Mrs Giti Schachner **(SLP)**
Weiss, Rebecca L **(SLP)**
Wiedermann, Faigie F **(SLP)**
Williamsson, Helene A **(SLP)**
Wilson, Theresa Marie **(SLP)**
Wisan, Arlene I **(SLP)**
Woods, Sheila P **(SLP)**
Woolf, Rita F **(SLP)**
Wrubel, Shulamith **(SLP)**
Zisblatt, Mrs Sharon Wieder **(SLP)**
Zuckerman, Heidi L J **(SLP)**
Zwick, Lynn K **(SLP)**

Brooklyn Heights

Leddy, Mark Hodge **(SLP)**
Righetti, Dennis **(SLP)**
Rosen, Penny A **(SLP)**
Trilling, Terry G **(SLP)**

Brookville

Grey, Mrs Laura S **(SLP)**

Brown

Soto, Mrs Betty A

Brownville

Callahan, Mrs Patricia **(SLP)**

Brunswick

Joyce-O'Toole, Patricia Edna **(SLP)**

Buchanan

Burke, Susan **(SLP)**

Buffalo

Arnold, Dr Sally A **(A)**

Arvedson, Dr Joan Carol **(SLP)**
Ash, Wendy Lynn **(SLP)**
Avella, Richard D **(SLP)**
Bacon, Marilee J **(SLP)**
Baskervill, Mrs Maxine A **(SLP)**
Baskervill, Dr Robert David **(SLP)**
Blair, Mrs Lisa Annette **(SLP)**
Boland, Lynne Marie **(SLP)**
Bonfante, Laurie Ann **(SLP)**
Bowen, Jeanie Gurney
Brummett, Mrs Theresa A **(SLP)**
Bugman, Laura Marie **(SLP)**
Campbell, Carol D **(SLP)**
Campbell, Dr Richard A
Carney, Kathleen M **(SLP)**
Connare, Lynn Puliafico **(SLP)**
Coover, Mauri J
Coscia, Mary Ellen **(SLP)**
Crabtree, Beverly Anne **(SLP)**
Croasdale, Helen Lee **(SLP)**
Deboth, Renee Marie
Deltuva, Mrs Janet M **(SLP)**
Douglas, Ann V **(SLP)**
Duchan, Dr Judith F **(SLP)**
Duguay, Dr Marshall J **(SLP)**
Dunwoodie, Rosemary T
Edbauer, Margaret M **(SLP)**
Freundschuh, Laurie Weber **(SLP)**
Gallagher, Dr Betty **(SLP)**
Gallagher, Jerry D **(SLP)**
Geelan, Mrs Susan Barber
Giess, Sallyann
Gold, Jennifer R **(SLP)**
Gorman, Barbara Marie **(SLP)**
Gratton, Michael Anne **(A)**
Green, Catherine C **(SLP)**
Gruttadauria, Salvatore A **(SLP)**
Gutheil, Kathryn R **(SLP)**
Hayes-Pugh, Christine Ann **(SLP)**
Henderson, Dr Donald
Hewitt, Lynne Elizabeth **(SLP)**
Higginbotham, D Jeffery **(SLP)**
Hill, Sandra E **(SLP)**
Hittle, Mrs Susan A **(A)**
Holley, Mrs Bessie L **(SLP)**
Houk, Ronald R **(SLP)**
Jarmolowski, Patricia Ann **(SLP)**
Jarvis, Susan Marie **(SLP)**
Johnson, Mrs Susan H **(SLP)**
Juliano, Mrs Janice Jerris **(SLP)**
Katz, Dr Jack **(SLP A)**
Kelly, Mrs Gloria J R **(SLP)**
Kirkham, Cherie Cooper **(SLP)**
Krengulec, Kathleen **(A)**
Kunz, Audrey J **(SLP)**
Kuttesch, Cynthia Rose **(SLP)**
Laspisa, Lisa A **(A)**
Leiper, Mrs Norah Mary **(SLP)**
Loonan, Diane Bourhis **(SLP)**
Lorber, Pamela Ann **(SLP)**
Luppino, Marilyn A **(SLP)**
Marple, Mrs Christine Anne **(SLP)**
Masters, M Gay **(SLP)**
Matricardi, Mrs Natalie L **(SLP)**
Mendola, Noreen G **(SLP)**
Mirabella, Joann **(SLP)**
Monagle, Cathy Moira **(SLP)**
Morris, Diane M **(SLP)**
Murphy, Dolores Marie **(SLP)**
Nold, Anna M
Page, Joseph M **(SLP A)**
Pfeiffer, Rebecca Rupley **(SLP)**
Pfohl, Ann Marie Catherine
Pollock, Mrs Pamela K **(SLP)**
Pomerantz, Bonnie K **(SLP)**
Ramm, Elaine **(SLP)**
Richmond, Dr Allen M **(SLP)**
Robinson, Janet A **(SLP)**
Rogers, Cheryl Ann **(SLP)**
Rogerson, Brenda S **(SLP)**
Rosica, Sebastian Joseph **(SLP A)**
Russell, Dr Nancy K **(SLP)**
Rychnowski, Sharon L **(SLP)**
Rycyna, Mrs Mary E **(SLP)**
Rzadkiewicz, Joan K **(SLP)**
Salerno-Reed, Mrs Marianne **(SLP)**
Salvi, Dr Richard J
Sanders, Dr Derek A **(SLP A)**
Schneider, Daniel C **(A)**
Sciarrino, Sr Maralynn **(SLP)**
Segal, Lesley E **(A)**
Seidenberg, Susan B **(SLP)**
Seitz, Sandra L
Shaughnessy, Mrs Margaret Ann **(A)**
Shaw, Barbara K **(SLP)**
Smith, Alice B **(SLP)**
Smith, Mrs Judith Michelle **(SLP)**
Smith, Michele L **(SLP)**
Solecki, Janet M **(A)**
Sonnenmeier, Rae M **(SLP)**
Spring-Whiddon, Diane Rita **(SLP)**
Stadelmaier, Ann Elizabeth **(A)**
Stathopoulos, Dr Elaine T **(SLP)**
Sussman, Dr Joan E **(SLP)**
Szablicki, Mrs Joanne Cotroneo **(SLP)**
Taylor, Kathleen Helen **(SLP)**
Terranova, Susan Ann **(A)**
Tracy, Mrs Karen A **(SLP)**
Warner, Therese Marie **(SLP)**
Weaver, Frank **(A)**
Webster, Patricia Marie **(SLP)**
Weiner, Judith A **(A)**
White, Thomas P **(A)**
Whitham, Joyce Merrie **(A)**
Wilson, Susan Marie **(SLP)**
Wozniak, Susan Marie

Burnt Hills
Jackowski, Mrs Linda A **(SLP)**

Burt
Goodling-Beals, Karen M **(SLP)**

Caledonia
Glucksman, Catherine Mary **(A)**
Vom Eigen, Beth Ann

Calverton
Young, Mariellen **(SLP)**

Cambridge
Bowens, Virginia Nmn **(SLP)**

Camillus
Easton, Mrs Sally Jo **(SLP)**
Kelman-Maziuk, Margot E **(SLP)**
Mack-Balitz, Mrs Aileen **(SLP)**
Taney, Bernadette M **(SLP)**

Campbell Hall
Nowak, Mrs Patricia L **(SLP)**

Canandaigua
Burley, Kathryn L **(SLP)**
Canfield, Karen Lyn **(SLP)**
Forster, Linda Bates
Kukol, Dr Robert J **(SLP)**
Metting, Mrs Pamela Jean **(A)**
Van Derveer, Mrs Rita H **(SLP)**

Canastota
Mutz, Laurie Fisher **(SLP)**

Canton
Bush, Mrs Yolanda R **(SLP)**
Erdige-Holz, Susan **(SLP)**
Krafft, Karen Marie **(SLP)**

Carle Place
Waldman, Mrs Sandra M Freilich **(SLP)**

Carmel
Bonerbo-Marino, Mrs Marie Louise **(A)**
Sorell, Jeannie M **(SLP)**

Cassadaga
Keyser, MaryAnn C **(SLP)**

Castleton
Hancock, Mrs Judith Hanson **(SLP)**
Rosenbaum, Mrs Kathleen Margaret **(SLP)**

Castleton on Hudson
Plumb, Norma Hansen **(SLP)**

Catskill
Franz, Cheri Nanette **(SLP)**

Cazenovia
Allway, Linda J L **(SLP)**
Paonessa-Loftus, Carole L **(SLP)**
Schmit, Mrs Sharon A **(SLP)**

Cedarhurst
Blaustein, Steven **(SLP)**
Brenner, Karen F **(SLP)**
Ganz, Mrs Sheryl Klein **(SLP)**
Hersh, Helen **(SLP)**
Hudesman, Jill Aber **(A)**
Kalina, Andrea F **(SLP)**
Mayerhoff, Caryn Sue **(A)**
Reich, Mrs Arliene E **(SLP)**
Wolf, Mrs Robin Hill **(A)**
Zimmerman, Mrs Hilary Deborah **(SLP)**

Center Brunswick
Geary, Mrs Patricia J **(SLP)**

Center Moriches
Kronman, Mrs Joan Safier **(SLP)**

Centereach
Cassar, Dorothy A **(SLP)**
Gomes, Mrs Suellen MacEdonia **(SLP)**
Lee, Geralyn Marie **(SLP)**
Liberman, George A **(SLP)**
Mandell, Mrs Roni K **(SLP)**

Centerport
Bivona, Mrs Theresa G **(SLP)**
Stevenson, Mrs Maureen Dempsey **(SLP)**

Central Valley
Jolly, Mrs Sharon C **(SLP A)**

Chappaqua
Klatsky, Mrs Iris Ann **(SLP)**
Lopez, Sharon Rosen **(SLP)**
Nir, Talma **(SLP)**
Sullivan, Theresa P **(SLP)**

Chateaugay
Cook, Mrs Brenda L **(A)**
Kenny, Maureen Elizabeth **(SLP)**

Chatham
Hill, Mrs Ruth E **(SLP)**

Cheektowaga
Acevedo, Mrs Ann M **(SLP)**
Blackmore, Denise A **(A)**
Cych, Susan Jeanette **(SLP)**
Gavacs, Nancy M **(SLP)**
Moll-Richmond, Mrs Deborah **(SLP)**
Rosenfeld, Mrs Cathy Ann **(SLP)**
Sanderson, Laurie B **(SLP)**
Slowinski, Deidre E **(SLP)**
Stachowiak, Linda Ann **(SLP)**
Wiltsie, Dawn M **(SLP)**
Zieminski, Marianne **(SLP)**

Chenango Fork
Martin, Leona Dee **(SLP)**
Slocum, Barbara B **(SLP)**

Chester
Morico, Patricia Helen **(SLP)**
Williams, Mrs Luann M **(SLP)**

Chestertown
Behrens, George R **(SLP)**
Boggia, Mrs Susan Bucalo **(A)**
Webster, John C

Chestnut Ridge
Cohen, Dianne E **(SLP)**
Kantor, Elaine B **(SLP)**
Mills, Mrs Janis Ellyn **(SLP)**

Chittenango
Goeler, Mrs Nettie Wagner **(SLP)**
Meyer, Mrs Jacqueline **(SLP)**

Churchville
Huffman, Mrs Nancy P **(SLP A)**
Penney, Christine Ann **(SLP)**
Podyma, Mrs Noreen Susan **(SLP)**
Schockow, Mrs Tammy Anne **(SLP)**
Virzi, Jerome I **(SLP)**

Cincinnatus
Denmeade, Patti Buell **(SLP)**

City Island
Dikeman, Karen Joyce **(SLP)**
Laskowski, Margaret M **(SLP)**

Clarence
Carter, Thomas J **(SLP)**
Gray, Alice Roll **(SLP)**
Herzog, Mrs Winifred P
Rosica, Lenore M **(SLP)**
Stachowski, Mrs Claudia C **(SLP)**
Zimmerman, Dr Robert Lee **(SLP A)**

Clarence Center
Ross, Mrs Nancy D **(SLP)**

Clay
Caiella, Mrs Josephine Shuman **(SLP)**
Massey, Cathey L A **(SLP)**
McDonald, Elizabeth **(SLP)**
Natale, Marianne Irene **(SLP)**
Powers-Rabideau, Debora L **(SLP)**
Riese, Mrs Diane Hinkley
Weinheimer, Bernice Cecelia **(SLP)**

Clifton Park
Bailey-Jones, Karen E **(SLP)**
Brayton, Dr Evelyn R **(SLP)**
Brescher, Sherri A **(SLP)**
Fitsik, Mrs Lauren B **(SLP)**
Iandoli, Dr Edward W **(SLP A)**
Jacobsen, Ellen D **(SLP)**
Jones, Dr Gary W **(SLP)**
Klein, Dale Ginny **(SLP)**
Millington, Mrs Kelly Ann **(SLP)**
Norsigian, Mrs Deirdre Doran **(A)**
Quan, Karyn Lynne **(SLP)**
Riggi, Mrs Cynthia L **(SLP)**
Rosage, Kristine B **(SLP)**
Ross, David Hugh
Smiley-Slocum, Mrs Kimberly Marie
Sumithra, Mrs Radha Simhadri **(A)**
Thompson, Viki Lee **(SLP)**
Wall, Mrs Martha M **(SLP)**
Yourno, Jacquelyn Mary **(SLP)**
Zaengle, Mrs Janice Marie **(SLP)**

Clifton Springs
Rogers, Cheryl Ann **(SLP)**

Clymer
White, Daniel Steven

Cobleskill
Lupatkin, Robin Mara **(A)**

Cohocton
Duclos, Deborah A **(SLP)**

Cohoes
Emerick, Mrs Nancy J **(SLP)**
Hassett, Maryclaire T **(SLP)**
Orsini, Terri Ann **(SLP)**
Tisenchek, Mrs Cathryn Anne

Cold Spring
Neuroth-Gimbrone, Cindy **(SLP)**

Cold Spring Harbor
Liebowitz, Mrs Maxine A
Mathews, Pamela J M **(SLP)**
O'Reilly, Mrs Sandra B **(SLP)**

Colden
Dilapo, Deborah Lagodna **(SLP)**

College Point
Reddan, Patricia M **(SLP)**

Colonie
Ryan-Rivers, Michelle M **(SLP)**

Commack
Best, Robin **(SLP)**
Blanco, Patricia M **(SLP)**
Elgort, Janice Dale **(SLP)**
Glatman, Mrs Ilene Sheryl **(SLP)**
Goldhagen, Gregg A
Klein-Hall, Karen J **(SLP)**
Kruger, Dr Barbara **(SLP A)**
Kruger, Dr Frederick M
Levine, Mrs Sandra Young **(SLP)**
Levy, Stephanie **(SLP)**
Morseon, Mrs Marlene Volpe **(SLP)**
Nafman, Cheryl Sacks **(SLP)**
Newman, Peggy H **(SLP)**
Pincus, Mrs Karen Bernstein **(SLP)**
Schleifer, Randi **(SLP)**
Tepperman, Linda S **(SLP)**
Zwang, Fran S S **(SLP)**

Conesus
Davis, Mrs Marie W **(SLP)**
Schreiner, Mrs Elaine Holbrook **(SLP)**
Stachowski, David E **(SLP)**

Congers
Whitfield, Donna E **(SLP)**

Conklin
Kaufman, Mrs Marjorie J **(SLP)**

Constable
Lane-Johnson, Mrs Catherine Ann **(SLP)**

Cooperstown
Doig, Lori C **(SLP)**
Grosshans, Stephanie Garben **(SLP)**

Copake
Jacoby, Dr Beatrice F **(SLP A)**

Copiaque
Pocoroba, Mrs Catherine Mary **(SLP)**

Coram
Bevans, Denise Dardaris **(SLP)**
Buchanan, Maureen J **(SLP)**
Davis, William A **(SLP)**
Farbstein, Mrs Resa **(SLP A)**
Krolikowski, David Milker **(SLP)**
Progebin-Graffe, Barbara L **(SLP)**
Strauss, Anne M **(SLP)**

Corfu
Lazik, Michael Jerome **(SLP)**

Corning
Barker, Dianne Lynne **(SLP)**
Rossettie, Kathleen Santilli **(SLP)**
Thomas, Marjorie Dimeo **(SLP)**

Cornwall
Borger, Mrs Linda A **(SLP)**
Dicarrado, Mrs Connie P **(SLP)**
Lewis, Mrs Roberta A **(SLP)**
Meccia, Nancy **(SLP)**

Cornwall on Hudson
Brooks, Wendell M **(SLP)**

Cortland
Billet, Jacqueline Maria **(SLP)**
Cecconi, Christine **(SLP)**
Courtney, Margie Lynn **(SLP)**
Green, Dr Kathleen W **(SLP A)**
Jackson, Mrs Rita H **(SLP)**
Louko, Linda J **(SLP)**
McMahon, Mrs Judith A
Moss, Mrs Barbara Castiglion **(SLP)**
Newton, Mrs Kimberly Kahler **(A)**
Overhiser, Mrs Sandra T **(SLP)**
Pelletier, Cathy A **(SLP)**
Pitcher, Mrs Mary M **(SLP)**
Pitcher, Michael Joseph **(A)**
Pudish-Holland, Mrs Elizabeth **(SLP)**
Ramer, Deborah S **(SLP)**
Tyler, Ann A **(SLP)**
Tytler, Mrs Carol Laureen **(SLP)**
Winship, Patricia Ann **(SLP)**

Coxsackie
Wenz, Mrs Mary Antkowiak

Cross River
Eggleston, Mrs Maryann D **(SLP)**
Klein, Barbara Greenstein **(SLP)**

Croton on Hudson
Aufrichtig, Sandra Joseph **(SLP)**
Coleman, Thomas D **(SLP)**
Custer, H Dean **(SLP)**
O'Rourke, Patricia Herrmann **(SLP)**
Pasierb, Meridith C **(SLP)**
Powers, Barbara Colbert **(SLP)**
Zuckerman, Susan A **(SLP)**

Cuyler
Saya, Mrs Nancy Cabana

Cypress Hills
Reyes, Jacqueline G **(SLP)**

Dalton
Latona, Patricia C **(SLP)**

Dansville
Akrin, Donna C **(SLP)**
Buck, Virginia R **(SLP)**
Day, Mrs Kim Martin
Delong, Mrs Lisa F **(SLP)**
Pape, Robin A **(A)**

De Witt
Benson, Mrs Nancy K **(SLP)**
Cohen, Carol G **(SLP)**
Halbert, Charlene Georgetti **(A)**
Schneider, Mrs Lianne P **(SLP)**

Deansboro
Seely, Kathleen W **(SLP)**

Deer Park
Amira, Carol J **(A)**
Katz, Roberta Ann **(SLP)**
Kesselman, Toby
Murphy, Kathleen M **(SLP)**

Delhi
Morales, Mrs Susan M **(SLP)**

Delmar
Cammisa, Elaine **(SLP)**
Carcich, Mariann **(SLP)**
Cassidy, Mrs Janet Marsala **(SLP)**
Conklin, Jane S **(SLP)**
Coplin, Mrs Robin S **(SLP)**
Eaton, Mrs Mary A **(SLP)**
Fleming, Barbara Hoyt **(SLP)**
Gottlieb, Mrs Eileen Haber **(SLP)**
Johnston, Kathleen Kennelly **(SLP)**
Kahn, Mrs Debra W **(SLP)**
Kuta, Mary D **(SLP)**
Norrix, James M **(SLP)**

Depew
Bartkowiak, Mrs Elaine P **(SLP)**
Cardwell, Elizabeth M **(SLP)**
Halbert, Mrs Carolyn Cohen **(SLP)**
Jones, Kathleen **(SLP)**
Kopra, Leonard F **(SLP)**
Streebel, Laurie Aileen **(SLP)**

Derby
Le Roy-Rojek, Mrs Patricia Marie **(SLP)**
Sonnenberg, Joseph P **(SLP)**

Dix Hills
Blumling, Mrs Rochelle Cullen **(SLP)**
Bogin, Esther **(SLP)**
Boniciolli, Lori Marie **(SLP)**
Buechler, Mrs Carolyn C **(SLP)**
Cohen, Mrs Ronnie D **(SLP)**
Davis, Carole A **(SLP)**
Ellenbogen, Judith Lichtiger **(SLP)**
Exelbert, Mrs Trudy L **(SLP A)**
Fischbein, Sylvia G **(SLP)**
Glantz, Lisa **(SLP)**
Kaufman, Carol C **(SLP)**
Levy, Debra Renee
Motola, Mrs Natalie G **(SLP)**
Rothlein, Laurie Goodman **(SLP)**
Sabia-Peters, Toni M **(SLP)**
Siegel, Helen Lillian **(SLP)**
Sommers, Rona S **(A)**
Stein, Mrs Judith E **(SLP)**
Strickler, Karen G **(SLP)**

Dobbs Ferry
Cumiskey, Sr Marian **(SLP)**
Fingerhood, Barbara **(SLP)**
Laczay, Mary Koltay **(SLP)**
Neeck, Catherine Elizabeth **(SLP)**
Samsky, Jay G **(SLP)**
Shulman, Marsha A
Sweeting, Dr Patricia M **(SLP)**

Douglaston
Crane, Mrs Bonnie F S **(SLP)**
Kassel, Karen Hochstein **(SLP)**
Kreinik, Mrs Andrea Dorice **(SLP)**
Martucci, Phyllis Joy **(SLP)**
Oken, Cheryl Lynn **(SLP)**
Rein, Mrs Sheila G **(SLP)**
Sitver-Kogut, Marsha **(SLP)**
Young, Michele A **(SLP)**

Dover Plains
Herbert, Mrs Diane Procopio **(A)**

Dryden
Bierbaum, Mrs Agnes M **(SLP)**

Dundee
Youngman, Julie Anne **(SLP)**

Dunkirk
Harms, Mrs Eileen Cole **(SLP)**
Kelley-Manzella, Mary Ann **(SLP)**
Manzella, Dr Robert A **(SLP)**
Sweeny, Veronica A **(SLP)**

East Amherst
Coleman, Maryann **(SLP)**
Hatcherson, Mrs Vivianne S **(SLP)**
Liemberger, Kathleen A **(SLP)**
Mahon, Mrs Donna Weckerle **(A)**
Nock, Mrs Janet Lynn **(SLP)**
Schory, Maria Emmi **(SLP)**
Teryl, Katherine J **(SLP)**
Weitzner-Lin, Dr Barbara **(SLP)**
Zebro, Mrs Susan M M **(SLP)**

East Aurora
Druelinger, Nancy Jean **(SLP)**
Herold, Joan C **(SLP)**
Lindstrom, Mrs Sandra Harris **(SLP)**
Piske, Kathleen L **(SLP)**
Smaldino, James M **(SLP)**
Stewart, Leslie **(A)**
Wald, Janice M M **(SLP)**

East Berne
Mulson, Terri Lee **(SLP)**
Reese, Mary Landry **(SLP)**

East Bloomfield
Havey, Michele Tousley **(SLP)**

East Greenbush
Brehm, Mrs Elaine **(SLP)**
Gaffney, Ellen P **(SLP)**
Gorman, Nancy Ann **(SLP)**
Hart, Susan K **(SLP)**
Kramerson, Mrs Sherri F **(SLP)**
Monkhouse, Dr Kay M **(SLP)**
Quenelle, C P **(A)**
Sardynski, Susan Q **(SLP)**
Secor, Virginia M **(SLP)**

East Hampton
Smith, Patricia Fennell **(SLP)**

East Hills
Bayer, Mrs Gail V **(SLP)**
Dessen, Mrs Mimi Lynne **(SLP)**
Gutenplan, Mrs Lori Mandel **(A)**
Halpern, Mrs Linda D **(SLP)**
Hersch, Hariet K **(SLP)**
Richards, Dr Alan M **(A)**

East Islip
Bailis, Barbara L **(SLP)**
Cartusciello, Rosemarie **(SLP)**
Curley, Kathleen Mary **(SLP)**
Nestler-Faccini, Mrs Heidi Marie **(SLP)**
Purver, Jessica A **(SLP)**

East Meadow
Abramson, Lois Michele **(SLP)**
Andrews-O'Hearn, Mrs Joanne **(SLP)**
Babas, Linda **(SLP)**
Berman, Beth D **(SLP)**
Berman, Mrs Dorothy M **(SLP)**
Celentano, Nancy A
Clayburn, Alisa Boykin **(SLP)**
Dluhos, Mrs Anna Patricia **(SLP)**
Finley, Adam Lewis
Francis, Shelley Lynn **(A)**
Friedman, Mrs Sandra M **(SLP)**
Goldman, Mrs Eileen R **(SLP)**
Kolker, Maura F **(SLP)**
Lambros, Georgette Koskovolis **(SLP)**
Meisel, Diane Leslie **(SLP)**
Mistretta, Anna **(SLP)**
Regina, Mrs Jane McNamara **(SLP)**
Riedl, Patricia L **(SLP)**
Snyder, Mrs Patricia D **(SLP)**
Stein, Mrs Barbara Tepper **(SLP)**
Strassberg, Mrs Miriam Anne
Topkin, Susan **(SLP)**

East Northport
Agresta, Mrs Lillian P **(SLP)**
Alberti, Mrs Gail G G **(SLP)**
Ambrosio, Mrs Susan Ellenis **(SLP)**
Amorillo, Thomas P **(SLP A)**
Austen, Stacey L **(SLP)**
Di Lillo, Michelle Anne **(SLP)**
Flood, Margaret A **(SLP)**
Guerriero, John A **(A)**
Halton, Elizabeth Frances **(SLP)**
Jacobson, Peggy F **(SLP)**
Kadin, Mrs Shelly M **(SLP)**
Karn, Mrs Regina-Jo **(SLP)**
Newton, Susan Mary **(SLP)**
Schildkraut, Mrs Roberta H **(SLP)**
Schwartz, Leslie **(SLP A)**
Toscano, Jacqueline Maria **(SLP)**
Yankwitt, Mrs Suzanne Eisdorfer **(SLP)**

East Norwick
Slattery, Mrs Linda Carole **(A)**

East Otto
Johnson, Karen A **(SLP)**

East Patchogue
Cooper, Mrs Janet M **(SLP)**
Korn, Jeffrey Michael **(SLP)**

East Patchoque
Simpson-Sears, Marion June **(SLP)**

East Pembrooke
Calnan, Jeanne Zellner **(SLP)**

East Quogue
Dawson, Mary Ridgeway **(SLP)**
Miller, Mrs Andrea Jeanne **(SLP)**

East Rochester
Alfieri, Linda M
Dunn, Joanne C **(SLP)**
Knigge-Dartt, Ann E **(SLP)**
Naukam, Mrs Beth King **(SLP)**
Paciulli-MacAluso, Mrs Loretta **(SLP)**
Rambo, Elizabeth J **(SLP)**

East Rockaway
Bloch, Joyce Katinka **(SLP)**
Broome, Mrs Maxine A B **(SLP)**
Chizzik, Stacey G **(SLP)**
Stein, Mrs Beth I **(SLP)**
Tanenhaus, Mrs Joan Beris **(SLP A)**

Verderosa, Janet Noia **(SLP)**

East Setauket

Beaton, Mrs Wendy Sue **(SLP)**
Gordon, Ann E **(SLP)**
Kearns, Barbara A **(A)**

East Syracuse

Allmayer-Beck, Rosemary **(SLP)**
Kelly, Ellen M **(SLP)**
Lavigne, Cheryl Ann

East Williston

Devaney, Eileen M **(SLP)**
Sokol, Ellen R **(SLP)**
Tinagero, Elizabeth **(SLP)**

Eastchester

Fenzel, Mrs Catherine Curtin
Forcello, Juliana C **(SLP)**
Konchan, Teresa Briguglio **(SLP)**
Longo-Silvestri, Joann **(SLP)**
Shimizu, Mrs Carol A **(SLP)**
Simpson, Mrs Emily F **(SLP A)**

Eden

Crowell, Tama S **(SLP)**

Eggertsville

Bauer, Mrs Carmille A **(SLP)**
Jadd, Mrs Ellen Barron **(SLP)**
Pasternak, Judith A **(SLP)**
Stone, Mrs Sharon Rala **(SLP)**

Elizaville

Gayton, Gidget K **(SLP)**

Ellenville

Logan, Lorri Backer **(SLP)**
Sloan, Rosemary Minogue **(SLP)**

Ellicottville

Robinson, Mrs Robin Maines **(SLP)**

Elmhurst

Candido, Mrs Anna Rodriguez
Chou, Michele Ann **(SLP)**
Del Vecchio, Ruth Bretan **(SLP)**
Dostal, Suzanne Marion **(SLP)**
Haas-Belash, Mrs Barbara **(SLP)**
Hennessey, Ann-Marie B **(A)**
Langot, Helene
O'Brien, Mary Rita **(SLP)**
Sirovatka, Anne Therese **(SLP)**
Tamayo, Eliana Isabel

Elmira

Ahearn, Mary E **(SLP)**
Brady, Mrs Margaret S **(SLP)**
Bullett, John J **(SLP)**
Bullett, Maryann Shelton **(A)**
Ciccariello, Mrs Mary P **(SLP)**
Cowan, Pamela R **(SLP)**
Dipetta, Mrs Mary Ann **(SLP)**
Giovannini-De Renzo, Sheila **(A)**
Holtgrewe, Phyllis P **(SLP)**
Ivanick, Mrs Jane E **(SLP)**
Katz, Jeffrey A **(A)**
Katz, Mrs Sheila E **(SLP)**
Mathieu, Lawrence H **(A)**
Miller, Erik G **(SLP)**
Paone, Charles A **(SLP)**
Peros-Paone, Mariann **(SLP)**
Price, Mary Jo **(SLP)**
Wheaton, Karen S **(SLP)**
Wheaton, Ronald E **(SLP)**
Whipple, Linda Leigh **(SLP)**

Elmira Heights

Hartman, Victoria A

Elmont

McGinnis, Diane S **(A)**
Stapleton, Eileen T **(SLP)**

Elmria

Zoltowski, Mrs Elyse Malins **(SLP)**

Elmsford

Happas, Diane **(SLP)**

Endicott

Constantz, Mrs Grace A **(SLP)**
Every, Donna J **(SLP)**
Gilfoyle, Mary Nicol **(SLP)**
Manzo, Barbara J **(SLP)**
Murphy, Anne Marie **(SLP)**
Rucker, Mrs Brenda M **(SLP)**
Skrobacz, Mrs Margaret Mary **(SLP)**

Endwell

Goldsmith, Marian **(A)**
Mattise, Mary Ellen **(SLP)**
Pochily, Mrs Barbara Mahone **(SLP)**
Redington-Gilroy, Mrs Eileen Marie **(SLP)**

Evans Mills

Snyder, Winona M **(SLP)**

Fabius

Godlewski-Wise, Karen Ann **(SLP)**

Fairport

Bergin, Mary P **(SLP)**
Byrne, Patricia A **(SLP)**
Carlson, Diane B **(SLP)**
Couch, Meredith Ellen **(SLP)**
Crane-McCall, Debra Ann **(SLP)**
Cushman, Melissa J **(A)**
Degraff, Mrs Sheila Norton **(SLP)**
Deyoung, Mrs Barbara J **(SLP)**
Donlin-Smith, Colleen M **(SLP)**
Druziak, Mrs JoAnn Murphy **(SLP)**
Earnst, Mrs Elizabeth Ann/Holpit **(SLP)**
Gallagher, Kathleen Hennessy **(SLP)**
Grady, Mrs Francine E **(SLP)**
Hope-Bly, Mrs Connie A **(SLP)**
Keller, Sarah E **(SLP)**
La Salle, Lori Jo **(SLP)**
Lynch-Bennett, Maureen E **(SLP)**
Marasco, Kendra L **(SLP A)**
Miller, Dr Thomas D **(SLP)**
Nardi, Mrs Deborah Jenene **(SLP)**
Newman, Mrs Susan Howe **(A)**
O'Brien, Mary Ann **(SLP)**
Organ, Dairlis Jane **(A)**
Rosedale, M Yvonne **(SLP)**
Salisbury, John R **(A)**
Scarpulla, Margaret Ciak **(SLP)**
Schindler-Wale, Barbara **(SLP)**
Schmidt, Mrs Diana Ferga
Scott, Mrs Kathleen Ann R **(SLP)**
Shadd, Nancy Griffin **(SLP)**
Smith, Mrs Camille St Hilaire **(SLP)**
Taylor, Alice Ross **(SLP)**
Whitehead, Mrs Brenda Humphrey **(SLP)**
Wolf, John M **(SLP)**
Zieno, Janet H **(A)**

Far Rockaway

Engelstein, Renee Nancy **(A)**
Gelfand, Mrs Shira G **(SLP)**
Klahr, Lynn R **(SLP)**
Maslow, Shari Debra **(SLP)**
Pfeiffer, Mrs Laya Alyssa **(SLP)**
Pollack, Sheri **(SLP)**
Shenker, Mrs Basi Krasnow

Farmingdale

Bedford, Mrs Leslie V **(SLP)**
Domingo, Robert A **(SLP)**
Flynn, Mary Anne **(SLP)**
Giminaro, Mrs Ruth F **(SLP)**
Macari, Marylou **(A)**
Mulcahy, Juli Panepinto **(SLP)**
Von Bargen, Dawn Marie **(A)**

Farmington

Askins, Mrs Judith C **(SLP)**
Reid, Mrs Sheryl Guest **(A)**
Wiesner, Eric C **(SLP)**

Farmingville

Coppola, Anthony **(SLP)**

Murch, Mrs Donna Nicole **(SLP)**
Shikowitz, Mrs Sheila Marilyn **(SLP)**

Fayetteville

Allen, Mrs Korie L **(SLP)**
Barber, Kathy L **(SLP)**
Coughlin, Dr William A **(SLP)**
Fishbein, Gail Sherman **(SLP)**
Hankin, Mrs Wendy F **(SLP)**
Kagan, Sara B **(A)**
Krawitz, Beverly G **(SLP)**
Kristall-Sclar, Anita Joy **(SLP)**
Marge, Dorothy K **(SLP)**
Marge, Dr Michael **(SLP)**
Saxman, Dr John H
Willett, Mrs Karen Mikesell

Ferdonia

Champlain, Mary Catherine

Feura Bush

Gloeckler, Karen I **(SLP)**

Fillmore

Cwiklinski, Mrs Karen A **(SLP)**

Fishkill

Alloy, Linda K **(SLP)**
Hess, Mrs Sandra Lynn **(SLP)**
Kjellson, Mrs Sylvia Yeaton **(A)**
O'Reilly-Rao, Christine **(A)**

Fleetwood

Stall, Robin C **(SLP)**

Fleischmanns

Cook, Mrs Elaine Harris **(SLP)**

Floral Park

Abramowitz, Judith Sarah **(SLP)**
Azzara, Alice C G **(SLP)**
Cohen, Harriet R **(SLP)**
Costa, Victoria M
Hernandez-Grein, Ana Lourdes **(SLP)**
Hesselblad, Janet Elizabeth **(A)**
Insler-Gross, Mrs Marilyn A **(SLP)**
Kay-Newman, Mrs Susan **(SLP)**
Lee, Wanda W **(SLP A)**
O'Neill, Patricia M **(SLP)**
Witkind, Mark J **(SLP)**

Flushing

Aruta, Donna Marian **(SLP)**
Avignone, Olympia **(SLP)**
Barr, Mrs Delores **(SLP)**
Berezow, Mrs Adeana Tova **(SLP)**
Bichler, Amy C **(SLP)**
Blumenfeld, Mrs Vera G **(SLP)**
Burger, Robin R **(A)**
Cirillo, Richard R **(SLP)**
Conca, Mrs Cindy R **(SLP)**
Creedon, Francine Locastro **(SLP)**
Daddiego, Randi S **(SLP)**
Daniels, Lisa G
Deutsch, Dr Lawrence **(A)**
Fader, Denise Robin **(SLP)**
Fishman, Glenn Sean
Forman, Mrs Shari G R **(SLP)**
Gavarin, Mindy L **(SLP)**
Gillman, Sherry F **(SLP)**
Goldman, Sara B **(SLP)**
Gray, Marnetta J **(SLP)**
Grossman, Wendy S **(SLP)**
Hamill, Mrs Victoria Reed **(A)**
Hertzberg, Herman **(A)**
Hopman, Mrs Phyllis **(SLP)**
Horkans, Sr Lelia Mary **(SLP)**
Hurtubise, Gabrielle Marie **(SLP)**
Jonay, Adrienne **(SLP)**
Katz, Carolyn **(SLP)**
Kennedy, Mrs Kathleen D **(SLP)**
Kirschner, Mrs Randi **(A)**
Klapholz, Renee **(SLP)**
Klinger, Dr Herbert N **(SLP)**
Kolatch, Mrs Francine R **(SLP)**
Kramer, Mrs Tamar Feder **(A)**
Landau, Mrs Sharon **(A)**
Leong, Kathleen Jayne **(SLP)**
Levinson, Elizabeth Arla **(SLP)**
Lukin, Susan S **(SLP)**
Lustbader, Wendy **(SLP)**
Marks, Dr Sidney **(SLP)**
Martin, Denise A **(SLP)**
McCarron, Jeanne Marie **(SLP)**
Mermelstein, Pamela B
Metrik, Lynn R **(SLP)**
Monane, Ellen
Montano, Joseph J **(A)**
Morse, Wendy Lynn **(SLP)**
Murray, Eugene Raymond **(SLP)**
Nat, Leba Y **(SLP)**
Nedelka, Anne M **(SLP)**
Oleaga-Labriola, Mrs Josephine **(SLP)**
Pasinkoff, Mrs Maureen M **(SLP)**
Perkins, Susan S **(SLP)**
Pernick, Mrs Dina Mae **(SLP)**
Pruzansky, Mrs Karen I **(SLP)**
Punzi, Lucille M **(SLP)**
Rollhaus, Mrs Gila **(A)**
Rosete, Mrs Louise **(SLP)**
Rutigliano, Cynthia J **(SLP)**
Salata, Linda T **(SLP)**
Sappol, Davida W **(SLP)**
Savitz, Deborah R
Schindler-Reich, Mrs Wendy **(SLP)**
Schoen, Rosanne Z **(SLP)**
Silverman, Judith **(SLP)**
Sokol, Heidi **(A)**
Somerstein, Esther Deborah **(SLP)**
Sorice, Mrs Diane Patricia **(SLP)**
Stark, Dr Joel **(SLP)**
Tarlow, Gail I **(SLP)**
Tober, Mrs Allison Beth **(SLP)**
Unger, Sharon Joy
Vasquez, Rachel **(A)**
Wantuch, Debra J **(A)**
Wexler, Leslie Ann **(A)**
Zimmer-Jeger, Ronie

Fly Creek

Barnowsky, Mrs Joyce C **(SLP)**

Fonda

Kovian, Theresa Maria **(SLP)**

Forest Hills

Adler, Vivian Kahn **(SLP)**
Ash-Bernstein, Melissa Hillary **(SLP)**
Auslander, Susanne **(SLP)**
Bader, Ellen K **(SLP)**
Beckoff, Esther Miller **(SLP)**
Berkman, Sheryl A **(SLP)**
Blatt, Arlene L **(SLP)**
Chin, Margaret Wai-Yee
Duksin, Sherry **(SLP)**
Ehrlich, Roberta Elise **(SLP)**
Fedge, Marilyn J **(A)**
Feitel, Mrs Rhonda Rochelle **(SLP)**
Frydenberg, Helen R **(SLP)**
Glanzman, Adina Rachel **(SLP)**
Gordon, Dr Toni Gold **(A)**
Hoch, Lynn R **(SLP)**
Hoffman, Denise
Horn, Sydney G **(A)**
Kahlenberg-Picciano, Trudi **(SLP)**
Kahn, Joan Herman **(SLP)**
Kane-Markowitz, Rochelle **(SLP)**
Leccese, Linda R **(SLP)**
Levinson, Janice Sue **(SLP)**
Longtin, Dr Susan E **(SLP)**
Lumpkin, Sindy Stickler **(SLP)**
Meisel, Mrs Sara M **(SLP)**
Nachmias, Pamela G **(SLP)**
Rosenbaum, Robert Lee **(SLP A)**
Rubin, Deborah **(SLP)**
Seiler, Mrs Sheri Elyse **(SLP)**
Skydell, Mrs Sandra S **(SLP)**
Solomon, Anita K **(SLP)**
Solomon, Loryn Maude **(SLP)**
Stephens, Cynthia **(SLP)**

Tipper, Raymond **(SLP)**
Ziegler-Blau, Mrs Carol **(SLP)**

Fort Edward
Hillman, Barbara J **(SLP)**

Fort Johnson
Gillis, Roberta Clark **(SLP)**

Fort Salonga
D'Aquisto, Maureen **(SLP)**
Schruntek, Dr Agnes M **(SLP)**

FPO New York
Brady, Litha K **(SLP)**
Crane, Mrs Patricia Anne **(SLP)**
Dupree, Laureen T **(A)**
Hartmann, Kathleen G **(A)**
Prystalski, Sharon M **(SLP)**
Sandhofer, Jean S **(SLP)**

Frankfort
Eisinger, Mrs Joanne Mary **(SLP)**
Fraser-Almeida, Sarah B **(SLP)**

Franklin
Haney, Lori Ann **(SLP)**

Franklin Square
Antonellis, Mrs Susan A **(A)**
Devane, Susan Mary **(SLP)**
Giles, Susan J **(SLP)**
Gross, Robin Ansel **(SLP)**
Klein, Mrs Mary Ann **(SLP)**

Fredonia
Borst, Mrs Noreen Nelson **(SLP)**
Burkowsky, Dr Mitchell R **(SLP)**
Hinton, Douglas K **(SLP A)**
McKenna, Mrs Beth Wheelock **(SLP)**
Nachtigall-Harley, Aline **(SLP)**
Nasca, Michele Jasinski **(SLP)**
Notte, Mrs Michele T **(SLP)**
Onufrak, Mrs Betty J **(SLP)**
Onufrak, Dr John A **(SLP)**
Schaffer, Dr Elliott J **(SLP A)**
Sedota, Anthony R **(SLP)**
West, Harland J **(SLP)**

Freeport
Fee-Olsen, Barbara Jean **(A)**
Goldstein, Pia Mindy **(SLP)**
Hanna, Mrs Rhonda Fran **(SLP)**
Newberger, Jeanne Ellen **(SLP)**
Rothblum, Mrs Alice G **(SLP)**
Schnipper, Philip D **(SLP)**
Shufer, Sylvia F **(SLP)**
Wassner, Paula Levy **(SLP)**
Wisnowski, Janine R **(SLP)**

Freeville
Saleh, Mrs Florence B **(SLP)**

Fresh Meadows
Abramovitz, Dr Rachelle S **(A)**
Adams, Elizabeth Mantione **(SLP)**
Berkowitz, Sherry Lee **(SLP)**
Branfman, Dorrise **(SLP)**
Carbone, Olga Cordero **(SLP)**
MacKin, Karen Marie **(SLP)**
MacLachlan, Dr Barbara Gayle **(SLP)**
McGuire, Carol A **(A)**
Mischell-Schnitzer, Alane Myra
Simon, Mrs Linda J **(SLP)**
Timofey, Mrs Robin Marlene **(SLP)**
Weiss, Gail E **(SLP)**

Frewsburg
Hall, Kathleen D **(SLP)**
Piede, Mrs June E W **(SLP)**
Piede, Robert M **(A)**
Rowley, Elaine M **(SLP)**

Fulton
Colby-Coveney, Mrs Marianne **(SLP)**
Koehler, Mrs Ann Malcolm **(SLP)**

Fultonham
Nahrwold, Mrs Marcia A **(SLP)**

Galway
Cancio, Mrs Jane Elizabeth **(SLP)**

Gansevoort
Becker, Mrs Mary Sheldon **(SLP)**
McCarthy, Mrs Linda Palin **(SLP)**

Garden City
Bonich, Diane Scarcelli **(SLP)**
Caddy, Charna B **(SLP)**
Maj, Mary B
Mascia, John **(A)**
Mortensen-Mascia, Nancy Ann **(A)**
Myers, Dr Florence L **(SLP)**
Pappas, Lisa Marie **(SLP)**
Radziewicz, Dr Christine **(SLP)**
Sullivan, Mrs Carol A **(SLP)**
Sullivan, Dr Roy F **(A)**
Thomas, Mrs Phyllis S **(SLP)**
Wieler, Constance **(SLP)**
Zamore, Mrs Ellen R **(SLP)**

Gardiner
Nadoolman, Joanna **(SLP)**
Pierson, Janet E **(SLP)**
Worth, Shannon Hulick **(SLP)**

Garnerville
Blattstein, Mrs Barbara M **(A)**

Geneseo
Book, Terrel D **(SLP)**
Conklin, John M **(SLP)**
Jones, Kathleen **(SLP)**
Marean, Prof Charles E **(SLP A)**
McKeown, Carol Petito **(SLP)**
Muck, Jane E **(SLP)**
Orlando, Nicholas A **(SLP)**
Owens, Robert E, Jr **(SLP)**
Pinhas, Dr Joan **(SLP)**
Restifo, Cheryl Ann **(SLP)**
Schiavetti, Dr Nicholas **(SLP A)**
Towsley, Mary Frances
Ulbright, Deborah T **(SLP)**

Germantown
Buhler, Mrs Rita G **(A)**

Gerry
Bedient, Laurie K White **(A)**

Getzville
Moonay, Ruth J
Wilson, Mrs Lisa McCall **(SLP)**
Wintringer, Mrs Cynthia L H **(SLP)**

Glen Cove
Cooperman, Dr Donna Klur **(SLP)**
Kvietok, Camilla Maria **(SLP)**
Lazar, Gloria Schertz **(SLP)**
Ruffen, Frederick **(A)**
Schreiber, Betsy C **(SLP)**

Glen Falls
Peca, Margaret B **(SLP)**

Glendale
Beckmann, Dr Dorothy A **(SLP)**
Beckmann, Frieda J **(SLP)**
Laul, Alfred Christopher **(SLP)**
Wright, Denise

Glenford
Lane, Mrs Joanne W **(SLP)**

Glenhead
Bilko, Mrs Sheila Monica **(SLP)**

Glenmont
Hoffman, Mrs Barbara Carey **(SLP)**

Glens Falls
Abrams, Peter C **(SLP)**
Bruce, Clifford E **(SLP)**
Calvert, Elizabeth Mary **(SLP)**
Clynes, Mrs Deborah Dewey **(SLP)**
Crall, Brenda M **(SLP)**
Gancher, Paul D **(A)**
Haanen, Donna H **(SLP)**

Luckenbaugh, Mrs Sharon Hughes **(SLP)**
O'Connor, Mrs Barbara Ann **(SLP)**
Paolicelli, Catherine A
Sellig, Sara G **(SLP)**
Watkins, Mrs Leah B **(SLP)**

Gloversville
Alric, Mrs Ellen M **(SLP)**
Rockwell, Sharon Sue **(SLP)**

Goldens Bridge
Malfer, Nancy Rose **(SLP)**

Goshen
Bochnovich, Elaine **(A)**
Herbert, Mrs Jeanne T **(SLP)**
Mathieu, Lori Elizabeth **(A)**

Gowanda
Paul, Mrs Barbara Weller **(SLP)**

Grahamsville
Greene, Abigail Martha **(SLP)**
Williams, Mrs Jennifer Ellen **(SLP)**

Grand Island
Couch, Marla Floy **(SLP)**
DeBole, S Mario **(SLP A)**
DeRose, Joseph **(SLP)**
Geldin, Alan M **(A)**
Grabiec, Mrs Barbara J **(SLP)**
Hess, Dr Donald A **(SLP)**
Kavanaugh, Mrs Michelle M **(SLP)**
Lavallee, Mrs Donna Marlin **(A)**
Peter, Tracy A **(SLP)**
Popiel, Rebecca L **(SLP)**
Purdy, Rosemary Mallor **(SLP A)**
Schiro, Mrs Suzanne Y **(SLP)**
Schultz, Janet Marie **(SLP)**
Vanderbrook, Mrs Lisa Pirrone **(SLP)**
Williams, Mrs Gretchen S **(SLP)**

Great Neck
Anderson, Marcia L **(A)**
Bogatch, Mrs Amy R **(SLP)**
Bosboom, Lisa Beth **(SLP)**
Dallal, Mrs Rhonda G **(SLP)**
Duboff, Mindy L **(A)**
Eneman, Laura Sue **(SLP)**
Finkelstein, Mrs Ellen **(A)**
Fischer, Alva S **(SLP)**
Gastwirth-Masone, Judy S **(A)**
Gildston, Dr Harold M **(SLP A)**
Gildston, Dr Phyllis S **(SLP A)**
Goldberg, Mrs Debra Lynn **(SLP)**
Goldberger, Mrs Joan F **(SLP)**
Gould, Hope Weinrod **(A)**
Halpern, Harvey **(SLP)**
Kasten-Feintuch, Dr Frances **(SLP)**
Kirsch, Ida **(SLP)**
Klein, Mrs Jill W **(SLP)**
Lasky, Mrs Helene **(SLP)**
Leavitt, Mrs Nancy J R **(SLP)**
Marcus, Mrs Rovena S **(SLP)**
Merwin, Alice K **(SLP)**
Milhauser, Lynn **(SLP)**
Modugno Okin, Paula **(SLP)**
Morton, Deanna R **(SLP)**
Mostel, Rebecca **(SLP)**
Nathanson, Susan **(SLP)**
Platt, Roberta S **(SLP)**
Raphael, Dr Lawrence J
Rock, Mrs Jo Ann L **(SLP)**
Rosenmeyer, Debra D **(A)**
Schiano, Ilene Lieberman **(SLP)**
Schwartz, Mrs Amy Bruckner **(SLP)**
Segal, Mrs Andrea Sue **(SLP)**
Segalowitz, Mrs Bernice S **(SLP)**
Sloane, Dr Neal A **(A)**
Sobelson, Mrs Marna G **(SLP)**
Solotoff, Mrs Barbara B **(SLP)**
Stone, Jeannine **(SLP)**
Tiegerman, Dr Ellenmorri **(SLP)**
Vella, Barbara **(SLP)**
Wasserman, Helene R **(SLP)**

Greenfield Center
Baldwin, Janice Louise **(SLP)**
Howard, Pamela **(SLP)**

Greenvale
Sheldon, Dr Neil **(SLP)**

Greenwich
Snyder, Carol Thurlow **(SLP)**

Greenwood Lake
Mollica-Butfilowski, Diane **(A)**

Groton
Allerton, Leslie Ruth
Pericozzi, Mrs Alice T L **(SLP)**

Groton on Hudson
Westle, Mrs Robin S D **(SLP)**

Guilderland
Del Rosso, Darlene Kay **(SLP)**
Downey, Jane Capria **(SLP)**
Falcone-Miller, Judith A **(SLP)**
Freedman, Janie B **(SLP)**
Gralow, Mrs Sheila M **(SLP)**
Moreland, Judith Pickett **(SLP)**

Hamburg
Cornell, Mrs MaryAnn **(SLP)**
Garvin-Lease, Mrs Carol A **(SLP)**
Gelbaugh, Mrs Carole L **(SLP)**
Gill, Lynn Ann **(SLP)**
Jaworek, Sherry Ann **(SLP)**
Kasprzyk, Mrs Sarah J **(SLP)**
Krawczyk, Rita A **(SLP)**
Mallette-Tschaepe, Judi **(SLP)**
McQuade, Mrs Veronica Balicki **(SLP)**
O'Connor, Mrs Linda Basile **(SLP)**
Swarts, Kevin Richard **(A)**
Zilch, Marsha L **(SLP)**

Hamilton
Cohen, Mrs Marjorie H **(A)**

Hammondsport
Wolcott, Joanne M **(SLP)**

Hampton Bays
Hoberman, Mrs Shirley E **(SLP A)**
Leaden, Lynn Wagner **(SLP)**
Ruffner, Mrs Michele A **(SLP)**

Hancock
Homer, Gene Wesley

Harriman
Ohnsman, Sharon Anne **(SLP)**
Sobel, Catherine Mary **(SLP)**

Harris
Fadden-Herron, Cynthia A **(A)**

Harrison
Bufi, Doreen Elizabeth **(SLP)**
Cianci, Ann Marie **(A)**
Decere, Mrs Genevieve **(SLP)**

Hartsdale
Gaines, Mrs Barbara Wayne **(SLP)**
Holas, Marlene Ann **(SLP)**
Hurd, Mrs Diane A **(SLP)**
Jacob, Sheryl R **(SLP)**
Kalik, Barbara G **(SLP)**
O'Hara-Taylor, Mrs Patricia A **(SLP)**
Quirolo, Mrs Josephine **(SLP)**
Radner, Susan Rebecca **(SLP)**
Raubicheck, Letitia E **(SLP)**
Stern, Lori Robbin **(A)**
Wortsman, Susan E **(A)**

Hartwick
Garrity, Linda Lee **(SLP)**

Hastings
Gualandi, Rhea Evelyn **(SLP)**

Hastings on Hudson
Blank, Mrs Meryl **(SLP)**
Frankel, Phyllis **(SLP)**
Weinrib, Mrs Holly Jaci **(SLP)**

Hauppauge
Carnesi, Karyn Ann
Ehrlich-Herzfeld, Sherry Beth **(SLP)**
Filaseta, Mrs Hope G **(SLP)**
Havel, Lynn A **(SLP)**
Kievman-Young, Mrs Lisa M **(SLP)**
Kreider, Mrs Gloria A **(SLP)**
Lenahan, Joan Frances **(SLP)**
Morgan, Mrs Gerry Gardner **(SLP)**
Poillon, Patricia **(SLP)**
Santalone, Marianne T **(SLP)**
Selden, Mrs Louise M **(SLP)**
Tivenan, Karen A **(A)**
Wilkinson, Dominique **(SLP)**
Wolfe, Mrs Ruth V **(SLP)**

Haverstraw
Huebner, Sheila

Hawthore
Conway, Mrs Eileen Lyons **(SLP)**

Hecksville
De Nicola, Mrs Barbara Catherine **(SLP)**

Hemlock
Di Carlo, Susan M **(SLP)**

Hempstead
Brantley, Denise S **(A)**
Cohn, Mrs R Phyllis **(SLP)**
Eskridge, Marlene **(SLP)**
Trentacoste, Lori Ann **(A)**
Webb, Edward W **(SLP)**
Wilkins, Alice Maxine **(SLP)**

Henrietta
Feeney, Tawn R **(SLP)**
Johnson, Mrs Elaine S **(SLP)**
O'Connor, Mrs Anne Elizabeth **(SLP)**
Storm, Henry W, Jr **(SLP)**

Herkimer
Raymonda, Mrs Barbara Jean **(SLP)**
Waligora, Mrs Jane F **(A)**

Hewlett
Addis, Dr Judith T
Epstein, Mrs Caron Shohet **(SLP)**
Ganz, Ilene S B **(SLP)**
Genn, Mrs Brenda D S **(SLP)**
Genn, Shari Joy **(SLP)**
Gettinger, Daniel P **(A)**
London, Janet S **(SLP)**
O'Anna, Lisa Anne **(SLP)**
Rosenblum, Mrs Michele **(A)**
Stechel, Barbara Gordon **(SLP)**
Wachtel, Mrs Eve Tyroler **(SLP)**
Zimmermann, Mrs Margo Townsend **(SLP)**

Hicksville
Britton, Karen Ann **(SLP)**
Crosby, Donna Jane **(A)**
Ericksen, Janet L **(SLP)**
Heidrich, Mrs Lorraine **(SLP)**
Larrick, Susan Marie **(SLP)**
Loechel, June E **(SLP)**
Moone, Marianne F **(SLP)**
Pecora, Mrs Grace A **(SLP)**
Schmitt, Lisa L **(SLP)**
Smedley, Elaine Ann
Sussman, Susan T **(SLP)**

High Falls
Elmore, Carolyn Grace **(SLP)**

Highland
Dorn, Kathleen Cecilia **(SLP)**
Frisina, Mrs Joann **(SLP)**
Giangrasso, Carol J **(SLP)**
Wong-Trufanoff, Lonnie A **(SLP)**

Highland Mills
Lewis, Mrs Kathy E **(SLP)**

Hillcrest
Maurer, Joan E **(SLP)**

Hillsdale
Farrere, Carol A **(SLP)**

Hilton
Eppeira, Mrs Kathleen Maurer **(SLP)**

Holbrook
Berg, Virginia K **(SLP)**
Fox, Wendy Sillick **(SLP)**
Keller, Cindy Melanie
Richards, Mrs Maureen M **(SLP)**
Ryan, Mrs Cecilia H **(SLP)**
Vilardi, Mrs Mary Ann Miller **(SLP)**

Holland Patent
Aubertine, Mrs Jane Sullivan **(SLP)**

Holley
Kinsey, Charles R **(SLP)**

Hollis
Auriemmo, Jane **(A)**

Hollis Hills
Minear, Dr David J **(SLP)**
Stein, Mrs Harlee A L **(SLP)**

Holmes
Kurland, Miriam B **(SLP)**

Holtsville
Colon, Mrs Marieclaud Ganthier **(SLP)**
Holland, Kathleen **(SLP)**
Levine, Carol A **(SLP)**
Marcum, Gladys Charlene **(SLP)**
Newman, Diana **(SLP)**
Whittaker, Janice Sepe

Homer
Priest, Mrs Linda Wadsworth **(SLP)**

Honeoye
Cochrane, Susan Mary **(SLP)**

Honeoye Falls
Bonanni, Christine Marie **(SLP)**
Bredes, Diane E **(SLP)**
Castle, Dr Diane Sklar **(A)**

Hoosick Falls
McMartin, Colleen M **(SLP)**

Hopewell Junction
DeMartino, Karen A **(SLP)**
Krider, Jane A **(SLP)**
Munger, Mrs Carol P **(SLP)**
Preuss, Jodie R **(SLP)**
Riedell, Gail M **(SLP)**

Hornell
Hooper, Mrs Patricia Hamelin
Weyand, Natalie Ann **(SLP)**

Horseheads
Ek, Bette J **(SLP)**
Jernigan, Mrs Anne L **(SLP)**
Mryglot, Kimberly Smith **(SLP)**
Scanlon, Dr Patrick J **(A)**

Howard Beach
Cohen, Lauren Stephanie
Corazza, Antoinette Mignano **(SLP)**
Gertner, Mrs Jody M **(SLP)**
Letzter, Carol B **(A)**
Maio, Carmela A **(SLP)**
Ripinsky, Sharon **(A)**

Hudson
Sacco, Deborah J **(SLP)**
Swagemakers, Kimberly Anne **(SLP)**

Huntington
Andrews, Diana L **(SLP)**
Bongiorno, Joseph A **(SLP)**
Daniels, Joyce Sak **(SLP)**
Deluca, Joseph A **(SLP)**
Dickson-Serenita, Kerrin **(SLP)**
Epstein, Mrs Elaine G **(SLP)**
Feldman, Amy B **(SLP)**
Gallagher, Meghan L **(SLP)**
Gardner, Dr Harvey J **(SLP A)**
Girolamo, Nanette **(SLP)**
Glassmann, Deanna M **(SLP)**
Harmon, Bernard **(A)**
Herzfeld, Mrs Melanie W **(A)**
Hinchliffe, Mrs Nancy **(SLP)**
Lauria, Toni Ann M
Leonard, Jacqueline F **(SLP)**
Lupoletti, Nina L **(SLP)**
Markel, Edith G **(SLP)**
O'Neill, Mrs Andrea Bonchonsky **(SLP)**
Perlin, Ilene Gail **(SLP)**
Peter, Judith Herz **(A)**
Quinoa, Joanne T **(SLP)**
Rohrecker, Allison Clare **(SLP)**
Sabanos, Mrs Debra Tiffany **(SLP)**
Schapiro, Mrs Dorris B **(SLP)**
Sedovsky, Donna Cheryl **(SLP)**
Shalley, Mrs Carol J **(SLP)**
Zlotnick, Mrs Michele M **(SLP)**

Huntington Bay
Tomlinson, Mrs Cameron V

Huntington Station
Adler, Mrs Nancy H **(SLP)**
Crespo, Patricia **(SLP)**
Doris, Marie J **(SLP)**
Eagen, William H **(SLP A)**
Friedman, Deborah K **(SLP)**
Gerofsky, Mrs Deborah Diton **(SLP)**
Riegel, Marsha Fay
Rock, Katherine Ann **(SLP)**
Sanginario-Victor, Mrs Jeanne Marie **(SLP)**
Schwartz, Mrs Pearl E **(SLP)**
Trachtenberg-Zutty, Marilyn R **(SLP)**
Wirth, Richard W **(SLP)**
Wuestman, Cathryn **(SLP)**

Hyde Park
Attanasio, Dr Frederick G **(SLP)**
Cohn, Laurie E **(SLP)**
Eckwall, Randy S **(SLP)**
Osika, Michele M **(SLP)**
Phillips, Kathleen C **(SLP)**
Rielle, Mrs Judith L **(SLP)**

Ilion
Marley, Melinda M **(SLP)**
May, Mrs Elizabeth **(SLP)**

Interlaken
Reitema, Gordon Harrison **(SLP)**

Inwood
Capobianco, Mrs Martha L

Irvington
Bloom, Ronald L **(SLP)**
Dworkis, Audrey Beth **(SLP)**
Ferraro, Judith Ann **(A)**
Penn, Dr Jacques P **(A)**
Silverman, Jane M **(SLP)**
Singerman-Berman, Beth M **(SLP)**

Island Park
Baxter, Lisa R
Davis, Mrs Virginia L **(SLP)**
Dworkis, Mrs Andrea P **(SLP)**
Jacobs, Mrs Lori **(SLP)**
Ruscio, Mrs Denise R **(SLP)**

Islip
Kazandjian, Marta S **(SLP)**

Islip Terrace
Nikodem, Caroline **(SLP)**

Ithaca
Allen, Barbara E **(SLP)**
Ash, Harry B **(SLP)**
Bartishevich, Karen Y **(SLP)**
Bates, Dawn **(SLP)**
Begley, Liz H **(SLP)**
Boettger, Mrs Lynn S **(SLP)**
Bowman, Alison Faith **(SLP)**
Broadwell, Mrs Josephine Ann **(SLP)**
Budney, Sheryl Edwards **(SLP)**
Carroll, Christine **(SLP)**
Cross, Dr Douglas E **(SLP)**
Emerson, Nancy **(SLP)**
Finnerty, Patricia Cubells **(A)**
Garrity, Mrs Julie Schor **(SLP)**
Gottfried, Sorel D **(SLP)**
Gravani, Eileen H **(SLP)**
Green, Jacqueline **(SLP)**
Hagerty, Eileen R **(SLP)**
Halfast, Laurie Ann **(SLP)**
Hill, Colleen C **(SLP)**
Katz-Brown, Mrs Barbara D **(SLP)**
Kriegisch, Patricia **(SLP)**
Lacy, Susan D **(SLP)**
McDonald, Marie G **(SLP)**
Parsons, Charlotte **(SLP)**
Petrash, Marian Elizabeth
Sanford, Marie **(SLP)**
Sargent, Kenneth John **(SLP)**
Schissel, Mrs Ann **(SLP)**
Schissel, Dr Richard J **(SLP)**
Schoenfelder, Gail L **(SLP)**
Schultz, Mrs Katherine Clark **(SLP)**
Simpson, Maryann S **(SLP)**
Snyder, Charles J, Jr **(SLP)**
Svitko, Dr Carol Schnippert **(A)**
Tardif, Joan Marie
Telage, Dr Kal M **(SLP)**
Testut, Dr Eldred W **(A)**
Testut, Mrs Gay L **(SLP)**
Thomas, Mary Ann Soebbing **(SLP)**
Ufford, Amanda F **(SLP)**
Van Son, Dr L George **(SLP)**
Williams, Nancy **(SLP)**
Zinder, Mrs Christine Theriault **(A)**

Jackson Heights
Bernard-Morris, Mrs Laura M **(A)**
Brevda, Mrs Shelley Newman **(SLP)**
Brevda, Yale **(A)**
Cudahy, Dr Edward A
Donovan, Kathleen E **(SLP)**
Forde, Mrs Doreen Fisher **(SLP)**
Hallock, Geraldine P **(SLP)**
Krotick, Mindy Gayle **(SLP)**
Radbel, Mrs Shelley Jacovsky **(SLP)**
Sancilio, Susan Lisa **(SLP)**
Satin, Sally J **(SLP)**

Jamaica
Avignone, John L **(SLP)**
Bell-Berti, Dr Fredericka
Boyle, Dr Mary **(SLP)**
Esposito, Josephine Rose **(SLP)**
Fennimore, Rosalind Longley **(SLP)**
Gang, Karen D **(A)**
Geffner, Dr Donna **(SLP A)**
Gifford, Mrs Catherine **(SLP)**
Gonzalez, Myrna Doris **(SLP)**
Inniss, Melissa Elvira **(A)**
Kamerman, Joan D **(SLP)**
Moore, Roslyn H **(SLP)**
Obrien, Dr Denise P **(SLP)**
Pisacano, Margaret S **(SLP)**
Rapkin-Berger, Mrs Ellen **(SLP)**
Tunick, Phyllis **(SLP)**

Jamaica Estates
Kurzman, Esther Rachel **(SLP)**
Rothman, Mrs Sandra W **(SLP)**
Stoff, Mrs Nancy L
Straus, Monica B W **(SLP)**

Jamestown
Bennett, Mary Slattery **(SLP)**
Favata, Philip J **(SLP)**
Hedin, Mrs Anne K **(A)**
Hopkins-Lorenc, Mrs Cynthia A **(SLP)**
Johnson, Mrs Sheryl L **(SLP)**
Pascatore, Linda Concetta **(SLP)**
Rone, Mrs Linda H **(SLP)**
Spear, Rebecca Felton **(SLP)**
Swanson, Bonnelynn M **(SLP)**
Thompson, David Wayne **(SLP)**

Trusso, Joseph Phillip **(SLP)**

Jamesville

O'Connell, Dr Pamelia F **(SLP)**
Tassini, Donna M **(SLP)**

Jericho

Frank, Susanne O **(SLP)**
Gelfand, Mrs Janice K **(SLP)**
Gelfand, Dr Stanley A **(SLP A)**
Goldblatt-Kass, Mrs Mindy Gayle **(SLP)**
Harrison, Mrs Norma K **(SLP)**
Hertz, Mrs Nina R **(SLP)**
Hirsch, Linda M **(SLP A)**
Kornet, Renee H **(SLP)**
Krasner, Mrs Gladys R **(SLP)**
Levine, Phylis **(SLP)**
Pearlman, Mrs Ilene G **(SLP)**
Pochtar, Mrs Linda S **(SLP)**
Rosenbaum, Mrs Elise Rosen **(SLP)**
Rosenbaum, Dr S Steve **(SLP A)**
Rosenberg, Robin **(SLP)**
Schneider, Mrs Linda R **(SLP)**
Shapiro, Elizabeth De Ritter **(SLP)**
Theurer, John J **(A)**
Zeller, Dr Robin K **(A)**

Johnson City

Fahrenbach, Mrs Patricia E **(SLP)**
Gregoire-Koba, Mrs Lucille S **(SLP)**
Mieczkowski, Susan Lynn **(SLP)**

Johnstown

Kovalovich, Andrew **(A)**
Lefebvre, Richard H **(SLP)**

Katonah

Fiebert, Janet Diaz
Tabakman, Shelly D **(A)**

Keene

Goodwin, Emily Apthorp **(SLP)**

Kenmore

Frascatore, Beth Bailey **(SLP)**
Golanka, Janet M **(SLP)**
Grantham, Mrs Regina B **(SLP)**
Lawrence-Dederich, Susan Michele **(SLP)**
O'Donnell, Patricia L **(SLP)**
Parker, Ann Orlando **(SLP)**
Renken, Susan Marie **(SLP)**
Rizzo, Anne Marie
Skeels, Susan F **(SLP)**
Tucci, Mrs Judith P **(SLP)**
Wilson-Ward, Kathleen **(A)**

Kennedy

Eckendorf, Pamela S **(SLP)**

Kew Gardens

Abrahamson, Marilyn Samberg
Bromberg, Mrs Betsy **(A)**
Garson-Selevan, Barbara
Greenwald, Anne L **(SLP)**
Kunreuther, Mrs Gene R **(SLP)**
Loewe, Elaine H **(A)**
Matz, Dr Rita B **(SLP)**
Morgenroth, Nancy L **(SLP)**
Rothschild, Mrs Linda Rothenstei **(SLP)**
Siva, Mrs Sue Ann **(SLP)**
Zazula, Mrs Elise Hoch **(SLP)**

Kiamesha Lake

Baidowsky, Pamela Michele **(A)**

Kings Park

Deutsch, Andrea Sachs **(A)**
Goldstein, Angelyn G **(SLP)**
Mastrocinque, Mrs Meryl **(SLP)**
Smith, Lynn Goldberg **(SLP)**

Kings Point

Weinberg, Mrs Marjorie F **(SLP)**

Kingston

Aleo, Dr Edward L **(SLP A)**
Caughey, Mary B **(SLP)**
Darrow, Mrs Marianne D **(SLP)**
Fletcher, Mrs Eileen **(SLP)**
Glass, Susan Ruth **(A)**
Kelly, Richard James **(SLP)**
Mannello, Deborah C **(SLP)**
Miller, Harriet R **(SLP)**
Parete, Rose Marie **(SLP)**
Redmond, Mary Catherine **(A)**
Winne, Deborah Ann **(SLP)**

Kirkwood

Fernandez, Paula Ann **(SLP)**

La Grangeville

Brown, Shelli L **(SLP)**
Grady, Mrs Joan G **(SLP)**

Lake Carmel

Dadabo, Michele Marie **(SLP)**
Smith, Dr Clarissa R **(A)**

Lake George

Schmiel, Mrs Katherine Elizabeth **(SLP)**
Silva, Mrs Michele R **(SLP)**
Woodin, Mrs Devnet Trinkle **(SLP)**

Lake Grove

Weiss, Mrs Deborah L **(SLP)**

Lake Lucerne

Fox, Mrs Maura D **(SLP)**
Matthews, Linda Jenkins **(SLP)**

Lake Ronkonkoma

Bloechle, Mrs Lisa M **(SLP)**
McArthur, Mrs Barbara Mattson **(A)**

Lake Success

Abrahams, Arlene G **(SLP)**

Lake View

Allison, Richard E **(SLP A)**
Blair, Mrs Carol Ann **(SLP)**
Garra, John **(SLP)**
Kumiega, Santina Mantione **(SLP)**

Lakewood

Moynihan, Donna B **(SLP)**

Lancaster

Ciepiela, Mrs Lisa Marie **(SLP)**
Drews, Mrs Christine Lutz **(SLP)**
Krajewski, Mrs Christine **(SLP)**
Tillia, Pamela Ruth H **(SLP)**
Wade, Dr G Michael **(SLP)**
Wentland, Mrs Kathleen Anne **(SLP)**

Lansing

Bruno, Mrs Janet Kay **(SLP)**
Stephens, John Charles **(A)**
Tranzillo, Katherine **(SLP)**

Larchmont

Bialo, Nancy Kaye **(SLP)**
Gaiser, Mrs Gail H
Gasthalter, Mrs Margery Atkins **(SLP)**
Haas, Mrs Margot A **(SLP)**
Kleinman, Madeline Karter **(SLP)**
Krenkel, Paula S **(SLP)**
Needham, Mrs Leslie F **(SLP)**
Tauber, Rosalyn **(SLP)**

Latham

Burgess, Sr Augusta Ann **(SLP)**
Coffey, Christine Beth **(SLP)**
Davidoff-Adelson, Mrs Rita C **(SLP)**
Devlin, Sr M **(SLP)**
Hammer, Susan F **(A)**
Hoffman, Mrs Sharon Leitgeb **(SLP)**
Marotta, Mrs Beth Karol **(SLP)**
Marra, Cynthia Keller **(SLP)**
Martenis, Mrs Barbara Jeanne **(SLP)**
Redfield, Susan Stewart **(SLP)**
Rowley, Mrs Anne Toolan **(SLP)**
Senick, Denise Ann
Siegel, Harlan C **(SLP)**
Siegel, Mary Ann **(SLP)**
Ware, Donna P **(SLP)**
Wells, Mrs Lori Romeo
Welton, Karen Ann **(SLP)**

Lawrence

Barr, Beth Kalman **(SLP)**
Bernstein, Dr Deena K **(SLP)**
Feibusch, Arlene W **(SLP)**
Miller, Dr Maurice H **(SLP A)**
Rosenberg, Michaelle **(A)**
Weg, Mrs Susan T **(SLP)**
Weiss, Mrs Carol Arenson **(SLP)**
Wilks, Stuart R **(A)**

Leicester

House, Dr Linda Infante **(SLP)**
House, Thomas Duane

Leroy

Barefoot, Sidney M **(SLP)**

Levittown

Ardito, Vito **(A)**
Braunstein, Carol S **(SLP)**
Devlin, Brigitte Margaret **(SLP)**
Esposito, Paul R **(A)**
Mulreany, Sue **(SLP)**
Raffoni, Mrs Theresa Beller **(SLP)**

Lewiston

Marineau, Robyn Lee

Liberty

Blakey, Barbara Hackett **(SLP)**
Harrison, Mrs Nancy Ann **(SLP)**
Stuart, Frank J **(SLP A)**

Lido Beach

Jankeloff, Lois **(SLP)**

Lindenhurst

Byrne, Suzanne M **(SLP)**
Hursala, Mrs Dafna
Kahler, Linda B **(SLP)**
Lucas, Linda J **(SLP)**
Medwetsky, Leslie Weigel **(SLP)**
Russini, Teri-Anne

Little Falls

Maricle, Carlton A **(A)**

Little Neck

Axelson, Mrs Audrey M **(SLP)**
Broffman, Dr Sylvia **(SLP)**
Katz, Herman G **(SLP)**
Kirsh, Risa **(SLP)**
Levy, Mrs Ellyn B **(SLP)**
Safir, Mrs Irene J **(A)**
Serpanos, Yula Cherpelis **(A)**
Topper, Nancy B **(SLP)**

Littleneck

Jordan, Mrs Karen Donna **(SLP)**

Liverpool

Boneberg, Joan Marie **(SLP)**
Carr, Nancy Goodman **(SLP)**
Clapper, Mrs Nanette Doran **(SLP)**
Costello, Colleen Austin
Dennison, Beth Ann **(SLP)**
Engfer, Christine Mary **(SLP)**
Folger, Mrs Roscha B **(SLP)**
Geller, Daniel **(A)**
Good, Amy L R **(SLP)**
Graham, Mrs Judith Miller
Habicht-Grundner, Mrs Marcy J **(SLP)**
McKinney, Mrs Lee Ann Scharbach **(SLP)**
Meday-Rozwod, Mrs Susan **(SLP)**
Palmer, Mrs Floris N **(SLP)**
Ramstad, Mrs Margaret R **(A)**
Robinson, Valerie **(A)**
Suffredini, Carol Roser **(SLP)**

Livonia

Blood, Marie Anne
Hawk, Mrs Cynthia Tabolt **(SLP)**

Lockport

Behnke, Kim L
Benoit, Mrs Jeannine Brayer
Cassidy, Mrs Karen S **(SLP)**
Ivey, Kathryn Teresa **(SLP)**
Kaminski, Mrs Sherri A **(SLP)**
Kozlowski, Barbara A **(SLP)**
Macaluso, James T **(A)**
Nerone, Mrs Michelle M **(SLP)**
Reardon, John J M **(SLP)**
Showalter, Maria R T **(SLP)**
Szymula, Mrs Annette **(SLP)**

Lockwood

Wikstrom, Pia **(SLP)**

Londonville

Mack Nair, Mrs Anne Elizabeth **(SLP)**

Long Beach

Alpern, Dr Carol Sober **(SLP)**
Colucci, Mrs Maryann M **(SLP)**
Forman-Franco, Bonnie S **(A)**
Gross, David I **(SLP)**
Guba, Barbara H **(SLP)**
Hittleman, Warren Lee **(SLP)**
Kooper, Rebecca F **(A)**
Lugo, Mabeline **(SLP)**
Mazor, Rosemarie **(A)**
Mendlik, David F **(A)**
Merenstein-Brooks, Mrs Debra Karen **(SLP)**
Miller, Mrs Jan K **(A)**
Neiman-Diamond, Abby B **(SLP)**
Pagano-Piacente, Geraldine **(SLP)**
Page, Kathleen E **(A)**
Phillips, Mrs Arlene **(SLP)**
Posner, Dr Judd E **(SLP A)**
Scaglione, Matthew Paul **(SLP)**
Smith, Laurie Ellen **(SLP)**
Treston, Elizabeth Margaret **(SLP)**

Long Island

Brown, Jack B **(SLP A)**
Cron, Deborah A **(SLP)**
Dunne, Mrs Judith Gordon **(A)**
Gelbwasser, Mrs Rhonda B **(SLP)**
Greenberg, Mrs Lorraine R **(SLP)**
Marquez, Tamara Elizabeth **(A)**
Masone, Patrick **(A)**
Pettas, Dr Mary **(SLP)**
Rahman, Mrs Persephone **(SLP)**
Wilkens, Jeannette **(SLP)**

Long Lake

Plumley, Jeffrey Lew **(A)**
Plumley, Mrs Vickie Lynn **(SLP)**

Loudonville

Brockman, Mrs Nancy A **(SLP A)**
Buss, Denise P **(SLP)**
Delisa, Lauren R **(SLP)**
D'Orazio, Paula C **(SLP)**
Ferguson, Robert N **(A)**

Lowville

Johnson, Mrs Elizabeth **(SLP)**

Luzerne

Bagan, Mary Ann **(SLP)**

Lynbrook

Baren, Mrs Robin Prince **(SLP)**
Bonomo, Dorothy Hughes **(A)**
Boshnack, Arlene B **(SLP)**
Goldbach, Mrs Eileen D **(SLP)**
Letizia, Mrs Marina Roberta **(SLP)**
McNally, Mrs Helen Strobel **(SLP)**
Schneider, Debra Ann **(SLP)**
Spund, Ellen H **(SLP)**
Wolf, Tracy Ellen

Lyons

Hogan, Cynthia Ann **(A)**
Maslyn, Mary Lisa **(SLP)**

Macedon

Bigler-Burke, Mrs Linda G **(SLP)**
Criss, Mrs Carol C
Roat, Mrs Shirley E Renner **(SLP)**
Salitan, Mrs Kathleen Joanne **(SLP A)**
Thompson, Mrs Sandra Maria **(SLP)**

Mahopac
Aufiero-Sanchez, Joanne **(SLP)**
Fariselli, Mrs Lucille K **(SLP)**
Mansourian, Anne Louise **(SLP)**
Zencheck, Mrs Robin Fader **(A)**

Mahopac Falls
Prevost, Mrs Susan **(SLP)**

Malone
Dupuis, Mrs Robin Deborah **(SLP)**
Langdon, Jo Ann Mills
Storrs, Sherrill Gonyea **(SLP)**

Malverne
Sorrentino, Gayle E **(SLP)**
Weiss, Nancy Waring **(SLP)**

Mamaroneck
Anchin, Mrs Ellen **(SLP)**
Canil, Amy Jean **(SLP)**
Cohen, Dr Frederick **(SLP A)**
Datino, Nancy Louise **(A)**
Goldberg, Sunny Yeddis **(SLP)**
Kressner, Mrs Debra F **(SLP)**
O'Shea, Mrs Julie B **(A)**
Schaenman, Helene K **(A)**

Manhasset
Anderson, Mrs Vera L **(A)**
Bermack, Dr Elaine **(SLP)**
Conlan, Maureen T **(SLP)**
Dunn, Kathleen Siobhan **(SLP)**
Fayache, Zina P **(SLP)**
Guttenberg, Mrs Hope Stall **(A)**
Henrickson, Janine Diane **(A)**
Lorenzo, Adrienne M **(A)**
Mandelker, Mrs Cheryl Z **(SLP)**
Marzouk, Mrs Sheila Warren **(A)**
Sears, Lillian Wright **(SLP)**
Weise, Susan L
Whelan, Donna D **(SLP)**
Wilson, Dr Barbara C

Manhattan
Cooper, Mrs Cindy Rosenberg **(SLP)**
Heller, Janet Sue N **(SLP)**

Manlius
Frumkin, Mrs Judith R **(SLP)**
Giraudi-Perry, Dr Diane **(A)**
Glatter, Mrs Marsha R **(SLP)**
Kells, Mrs Lynn D **(SLP)**
Lockwood, Sally **(SLP)**
Lord, Sherman G **(A)**
Panels, Mrs Floria G **(SLP)**
Ryan, Helen Rose **(SLP)**
Szafran, Mrs Karen M **(SLP)**
Van Der Ven, Dorothy S **(SLP)**

Manorville
Freudendorf, Karen V **(SLP)**
Rose, Leah Z **(SLP)**
Veligdan, Mrs Marietta Scuro **(SLP)**

Marcellus
Ladd, Mrs Sandra Jane **(SLP)**
Overmann, Susan M
Synakowski, Melanie C **(SLP)**

Marcy
Beha, Deborah Mary

Marilla
Beebe, Mrs Judith P **(SLP)**
Schabel, Mrs Diana Phyllis **(SLP)**

Maryland
Benedict, Dr William S **(SLP)**

Maspeth
Both, Linda Elise **(SLP)**
Brennan-Kania, Blanche Frances **(SLP)**
Sheppard, Sr Mary F **(SLP)**

Massapequa
Antignano, Mrs Karin **(SLP)**
Cumisky, Mrs Joan Gavitt **(SLP)**
Festa, Dorothy Colucci **(SLP)**
Gelbs, Linda Susan
Gill, Mrs Kim Ann **(SLP)**
Hogan, Robert T **(A)**
Howe, Mrs Camille **(SLP)**
Jiran, Marygrace **(SLP)**
Lee, Eileen J **(SLP)**
Majlinger, Kathleen A **(SLP)**
Peters, Mrs Janet A **(SLP)**
Ross, Mrs Nancy M **(SLP)**
Scigliano, Vikki S **(SLP)**
Trow-Steinman, Joyce **(SLP)**
Veneziano, Mrs Charlotte **(SLP)**
Wagner, Monica Palmieri **(SLP)**
Wright, Joanne Santoro **(SLP)**

Massapequa Park
Castagna, Mrs Christine Marie **(SLP)**
De Ninno, Joanne Patricia **(SLP)**
Domni, Suzanne Halise **(SLP)**
McMillen, Anne Purdy **(SLP A)**
Mosca-Heisig, Dawn **(SLP)**
Oleksiak, Colleen P **(A)**
Van Wagner, Karen **(SLP)**

Mattituck
Bales, Mrs Debra Nicosia **(SLP)**
Vreeland, Dr Joella **(SLP A)**

Maybrook
Datres, Glen Phillip **(A)**

Mayville
Saunders, Mrs Wilma W **(SLP)**

Mechanicville
D'Alberto, Cindy Jane **(SLP)**
Krasuski, Mrs Mary J A **(SLP)**

Meddletown
Sumner, Theresa J **(SLP)**

Medford
Angelo, Veronica Rose **(SLP)**
Bayley, Geraldine **(SLP)**
Maneri, Mrs Dina A **(SLP)**
Perlmutter, Robert Bennett **(SLP)**

Medina
Barber, Diana Linda **(SLP)**
McGaughey, Derrick L **(SLP)**

Melville
Capazzi, Amy November **(SLP)**
Christensen, Jean C **(SLP)**
Elbaum, Marjorie **(SLP)**
Flam, Madeline **(SLP)**
Friedman, Debra Heller **(SLP)**
Gavin, Beatrice **(SLP)**
Press, Mrs Linda Corrie **(SLP)**
Savage, Mrs Trudy H **(SLP)**
Shelley, Suzanne Rosenast **(SLP)**
Stone, Mrs Marilyn L **(A)**
Tafeen, Mrs Janet **(SLP)**

Menands
Berkun, Elaine Rose **(SLP)**
Skapik, Gail S **(SLP)**

Mendon
Jones, Mrs Anne Evans **(SLP)**

Merrick
Bezozo, Sheila G **(SLP)**
Bloom, Bryna Schoffel **(SLP)**
Borten, Mrs Norma T **(SLP)**
Braterman, Francine **(SLP)**
Dunn, David L **(SLP)**
Elliott, Franklyn **(SLP)**
Flum, Dr Leonard **(SLP A)**
Kostes-Fiorella, Ellen H **(SLP)**
Kranz, Karen A **(SLP)**
Kruh-Meyer, Nancy L **(A)**
Pine, Bernard **(SLP A)**
Portnoy, Mrs Frances W **(SLP)**
Quirk-McGloin, Mrs Jennifer Marie **(SLP)**
Roeder, Mrs Melissa Jane **(SLP)**
Rose, Mrs Rochelle Honig **(SLP)**
Roy, Susan Jane **(SLP)**
Rutt, Marjorie North **(SLP)**
Schultz, Mimi Dryce **(SLP)**
Singer, Mrs Mindy Z **(SLP)**
Weil, Mrs Jerilyn Blatt **(SLP)**
Weiss, Mrs Marion I **(SLP)**
Weiss, Phyllis Windwer
White, Dr Harvey **(SLP)**
White, Mrs Sandra F **(SLP)**

Mexico
Forbes, Gary Richard **(A)**
Geer, Mrs Patricia Gartung **(SLP)**

Middle Grove
Friedel, Dianne M **(SLP)**
St Pierre Hetz, Mrs Michelle Marie **(SLP)**

Middle Island
Barsky, Steven S **(SLP)**
Malerba, Louis **(SLP)**

Middle Village
Belozerco, Laura Gail
Paluszek, Suzanne F **(SLP)**
Rodriquez, Linda Iris **(SLP)**
Valdes, Diane Theresa **(SLP)**
Van Gorder-La Porta, Joanne M **(A)**
Zajac, Patricia Barone **(SLP)**

Middlesex
Stover, Mrs Joan L **(SLP)**

Middletown
Burke, Mary Eileen S **(SLP)**
Goodman-Bowden, Jenny Louise **(SLP)**
Knox, Barbara D **(SLP A)**
Myruski, Janet **(SLP)**
Newman, Mrs Judith H **(SLP)**
Plain, Maureen O **(SLP)**
Sherman, Debra Lynne **(A)**
Snyder, Rebecca Ann **(A)**
Sotelo, Kathy M **(SLP)**
Verner, Monica Marasco **(SLP)**

Milford
Bliss, Joanne M **(SLP)**

Mill Neck
Klotz, Marianne R **(SLP)**

Millbrook
Braga, Mrs Danielle B **(SLP)**
MacPeek, June Marie **(SLP)**
Masters, Susan Roberta **(A)**
Sudaka, Mrs Martha F **(SLP)**

Miller Place
Dreyfus, Mrs Barbara Aronow **(A)**
Mahoney, Theresa Ann **(SLP)**
McCartin-Clark, Marguerite **(SLP)**
Pappas, Chrissi **(SLP)**
Schierwagen, Mrs Karin Ann **(SLP)**

Millwood
Kovac, Lisa Barone **(SLP)**

Mineola
Bernacchio, Mrs Carmela Granata **(SLP)**
Frost, Miriam B **(SLP)**
Lufrano, Nancy **(SLP)**
Sabella, Darleen Sue **(SLP)**
Springer, Ira Steven **(A)**
Tedesco, Brenda Elizabeth **(SLP)**
Zanello, Mrs Costandina A **(SLP)**

Minoa
Sacco, Linda J **(SLP)**
Sullivan-Witmer, Deborah J **(SLP)**

Mohawk
Ball, Karen A **(SLP)**

Mohegan Lake
Kahn, Melanie Susan **(SLP)**
Schwaid-Antin, Sandra **(SLP)**

Monroe
Gannon, J Kevin **(SLP)**
Kanis, Mrs Karen Lee **(SLP)**
Lombardo, Mrs Rose Ann Schirripa
Meth, Mrs Margaret Ann **(SLP)**
Migdel, Mrs Meryl Marla **(SLP)**
Perlov, Betty **(SLP)**
Shirley, Mrs Ellen M **(SLP)**
Terrigno, Georgina B **(SLP)**

Monsey
Adler, Mrs Jean L **(SLP)**
Baron, Mrs Phyllis G **(SLP)**
Fromowitz, Mrs Betty S **(SLP)**
Gross, Mrs Harriette **(SLP)**
Heinrich, Mrs Sharon **(SLP)**
Kaplan, Max **(SLP)**
Konstam, Mrs Marilyn Leah **(SLP)**
Kuzmik, Susan D **(SLP)**
Levitin, Mrs Rochelle **(SLP)**
Lipsky, Adrianne **(SLP)**
Rubin, Sharon Tepfer
Steinberg, Mary D **(SLP)**
Szabo, Gladys T **(SLP)**
Walzer, Jacalyn F **(SLP)**
Weinberger, Hadasa **(SLP)**
Weisberg, Mrs Roberta **(SLP)**

Montauk
Proctor, Minnie B **(SLP)**

Monticello
Cohon, Mrs Robin Y **(SLP)**

Montour Falls
Deroche, Maija A **(SLP)**

Montrose
Robinson, Stephanie Elaine **(A)**
Servedio, Dominick **(A)**
Servedio, Mrs Kathleen **(SLP)**

Moravia
VanNostrand, Mrs Toni DeTraglia **(SLP)**

Morrisonville
Schnob, Carol A **(SLP)**
Stadnicki, Mrs Barbara A **(SLP)**
Weiskotten, June S **(SLP)**

Mount Kisco
Bisbano, Mrs Carol W **(SLP)**
Caspi, Mrs Judy H **(SLP)**
Cohen, Marsha S **(SLP)**
Cook, Lois B **(SLP)**
Frank, Mrs Marlene Sharon **(SLP)**
Kazer, Mrs Joan G **(SLP)**
Levin, Mrs Susan Schwartz **(SLP)**
Tennison, Mrs Shirley W **(SLP)**
Thomasset, Mrs Lindley G **(SLP)**
Volles, Bianca Lauro **(SLP)**

Mount Morris
Hoey, Mrs Crystal Thornton **(SLP)**
Sacco, Mrs Adrienne G **(A)**
Sacco, Pat Richard **(SLP)**

Mount Sinai
Amato, John J **(SLP)**
Rhoads-Leslie, Janet **(SLP)**
Sweeny, Mrs Shirley Y **(SLP)**
Wittpenn, Denise Taneyhill **(SLP)**

Mount Vernon
Alvarenga, Joyce E **(SLP)**
Baron, Helen **(A)**
Brubacher, Margaret **(A)**
Bryan, Mrs Cecelia Davidson **(SLP)**
Faust, Kathleen Louise **(SLP)**
Hazim, Karolyn **(SLP)**
Heslin, Susan B
Phillips, Marie **(SLP)**
Pine, Mrs Anne Danetz **(SLP)**
Wylie, Mrs Mary Theresa **(SLP)**

Mumford
Gullo, Mrs Mae Ann **(SLP)**

Muttontown
Cooper, Ellen D **(SLP)**
Morgenstern, Carol S **(SLP)**

Nanuet
Berman, Laura B **(SLP)**
Coccaro, Mrs Lynda R **(SLP)**
Cohen, Nathan M **(SLP)**
Luther, Mrs Laurie Lynn **(SLP)**
Marlow, Mrs Mollie Zaffos **(SLP)**
Petersen, Donna L **(SLP)**
Schwartz, Mrs Sally Yevette **(SLP)**
Shapiro, Arnold **(SLP)**
Sullivan, Karen E **(SLP)**
Tuchband, Mrs Daren **(SLP)**

Naples
Peete, Brenda Carol **(SLP)**

Nassau
Byers, Mrs Shirley D **(SLP)**
Noll, Paula Jodoin **(SLP)**

Nelliston
Kilpatrick, Janet I **(SLP)**

Nesconset
Bauman, Gary M **(SLP)**
Becker, Mrs Shari Brown
Hoffer, Sheila Ann **(SLP)**
Sullivan, Kathleen E **(SLP)**

New City
Barabell, Mrs Fran H **(SLP)**
Brenner, Mrs Arlene O **(SLP)**
Buro, Mrs Jeanne R **(SLP)**
Cantor, Mrs Gail B **(SLP)**
Deering, Rosemary M **(SLP)**
Domroe, Sandy W **(SLP)**
Fishman, Jane S **(SLP)**
Friedman, Elaine C **(SLP)**
Lieberman, Mrs Bobbi M **(SLP)**
Loavenbruck, Dr Angela M **(SLP A)**
Mandel, Mrs Ellen W **(SLP)**
Mandell, Mrs Sue-Ellen **(SLP)**
Peterson, Mrs Debby L **(SLP)**
Refkin, Ilene M **(SLP)**
Rigrodsky, Dr Seymour **(SLP)**
Ritter, Mrs Lynn E **(SLP)**
Schiano, Maria Angela **(SLP)**

New Hampton
Kowalik, Mrs Norene Davitt **(SLP)**

New Hartford
Bero, Judy A **(A)**
Ketkar, Dr Indira S **(SLP A)**
Rinehard, Jean M **(SLP)**

New Hempstead
Faska-Kahana, Eva S **(SLP A)**

New Hyde Park
Gehan, Mrs Karen K **(SLP)**
Jask, Barbara Ann **(SLP)**
Lange, Diana Louise **(SLP)**
Levy, Mrs Cara S **(SLP)**
Levy, Mrs Marcia K **(SLP)**
Mayer-Weinstock, Daniela **(SLP)**
Rubenstein, Dr Joyce **(SLP A)**
Schwartz, Mrs Estelle N **(SLP)**
Twomey, Mary Ellen **(SLP)**
Zinberg, Dr Mildred F **(SLP)**

New Paltz
Bender, Lisa J **(SLP)**
Benjamin, Helise I **(SLP)**
Bienvenue, Dr Gordon R **(A)**
Haas, Dr Adelaide Nacamu **(SLP)**
Houston, Mrs Ladonna **(SLP)**
Kelner, Morgan Martha **(SLP)**
Madoff, Gretchen G **(SLP)**

New Rochelle
Ackerman, Mindy W **(SLP)**
Alessandroni, Mrs Gale M **(SLP)**
Aptaker, Ruth **(SLP)**
Arrow, Mrs Donna K **(SLP)**
Bach, Mrs Barbara **(SLP)**
Bergman, Mrs Marla Darefsky **(SLP)**
Boczko, Mrs Faerella E **(SLP)**
Brewer, Mrs Sharon C **(SLP)**
Capri, Linda Susan
Chassen, Mrs Deborah **(SLP)**
Chinitz, Shari K **(SLP)**
Danwitz, Sr M Winifred **(SLP)**
Dicairano, Nancy Louise **(SLP)**
Fredner, Mrs Marian Swanson **(A)**
Gelb, Laura B **(SLP)**
Gettelfinger, Mary Beth **(SLP)**
Grey, Monica Willoughby **(SLP)**
Guterson, Mary **(SLP)**
Heller, Francie H **(SLP)**
Israel, Mrs Jaclyn Sue **(SLP)**
Kamer, Mrs Arlene R **(SLP)**
Kramer, Mrs Roberta J **(SLP)**
Lew, Mrs Rhoda M B **(SLP)**
Price, Karen Jo **(SLP)**
Samuels, Ellen M **(SLP)**
Serber, Rhonda L **(SLP)**
Simon, Gail Beth **(SLP)**
Sirlin, Dr Mindy Wertheimer **(A)**
Urbina, Mariana Consuelo **(SLP A)**
Weiss, Mrs Deborah Edelstein **(SLP)**
Wygoda, Barbara R **(SLP)**

New Windsor
Henderson, Mrs Diane L **(SLP)**
Quicksell, Mrs Joanne Scully **(SLP)**
Rizzuto, Frances Pauline **(SLP)**
Rosa-Reed, Clare M **(SLP)**

New York
Abeloff, Suzanne P **(SLP)**
Abraham, Dr Suzanne Stephanie
Abrams, Beth L **(SLP)**
Abrams, Suzanne Lori **(SLP)**
Adler, Robin Birnbaum **(SLP)**
Allen, Dr Elizabeth **(SLP)**
Alper, Dina Pachino **(SLP)**
Altman, Elaine K **(SLP)**
Appelbaum, Maris Joan **(A)**
Armbruster, Joan M **(A)**
Arshen, Beverly S **(SLP)**
Ashkinaze, Barbara **(A)**
Babb, Carol **(SLP)**
Baden, Phyllis M **(SLP)**
Baken, Dr Ronald J
Baker, Dr Elmer E, Jr **(SLP)**
Balick, Dr Sylvia G **(SLP)**
Barnett, Janie P **(A)**
Bartfeld, Leslie M **(A)**
Barzey, Mrs Beverly F **(SLP)**
Beckman, Sandra L **(SLP)**
Belkin, Dr Amy S **(SLP)**
Belmont, Suzanne Snipes **(A)**
Bennardo, Lois Mary **(A)**
Berg, Abbey L F **(A)**
Berkowitz, Dr Alice O **(SLP A)**
Berkowitz, Helene Rapp **(SLP)**
Bertaccini, Ruona M **(SLP)**
Berti, Martha Carol **(SLP)**
Birnbaum, Michele J **(SLP)**
Bleiberg, Dr Aaron H **(SLP)**
Bloch, Carole S **(SLP)**
Bloom, Dr Lois **(SLP)**
Blue, Samual, Jr **(SLP)**
Bohne, Susan K **(SLP)**
Boothroyd, Arthur **(A)**
Bosler, Mrs Jenine **(SLP)**
Brackett, Diane **(SLP)**
Braunfeld, Giselle H **(SLP)**
Brief, Mrs Caryl Alterbaum **(SLP)**
Brodnitz, Dr Friedrich S **(SLP)**
Brookner, Christine Labenski **(A)**
Buck, Dr Joyce F **(SLP)**
Budde, Mark J **(SLP)**
Budnick, Amy S **(A)**
Burgess, Paul D, Jr **(SLP A)**
Burns, Susan Walsh **(SLP)**
Canfield, Dr William H **(SLP A)**
Carozza, Linda S **(SLP)**
Cavallo, Dr Stephen A **(SLP)**
Cayne, Dr Patricia Denner **(SLP)**
Ceron, Mrs Mildred Viera **(SLP)**
Chawkin, Phyllis Thorne **(SLP A)**
Chobor, Karen Lynn **(SLP)**
Chute, Mrs Patricia Molinelli **(A)**
Chwat, Sam E **(SLP)**
Ciuberkis, Arunas Jonas **(SLP)**
Clateman, Mrs Joyce Z **(SLP)**
Cohen, Barbara A **(SLP)**
Cohen, Shelley Robin **(SLP)**
Connolly, Susan B **(SLP)**
Davidson, Marjorie E **(SLP)**
Davis, Anne Varner **(SLP)**
Davis, Mrs Karla Frost **(SLP)**
De Hirsch, Katrina **(SLP)**
Diamond, Susan S **(SLP)**
Dichter, Mrs Carol A **(SLP)**
Dickinson, Dr Sandra **(SLP)**
Disibio, Diane L **(SLP)**
Doob, Dr Dorothy **(SLP)**
Dowd, Dorothy Ann **(SLP)**
Doyle, Catherine **(SLP)**
Dreyfuss, Nancy Matis **(SLP)**
Dubin, Madeline S **(SLP)**
Duciaume, Patricia A **(SLP)**
Dungan, Dr Ellen Love **(SLP)**
Dupre, Michael Joseph **(SLP)**
Dvosin, Mrs Edna **(A)**
Dyckes-Berke, Diana M
Edelman, Dr Florence **(SLP A)**
Edvardsson, Kerstin B **(SLP)**
Edwards, Dr Jan **(SLP)**
Eilat, Mrs Laurie W
Eisen, Dr Audrey H **(SLP)**
Ellis, Martha Anne **(A)**
Engel, Ellen M **(A)**
Ettenger, Vicki S **(SLP)**
Fabricant, Phyllis L **(SLP)**
Falk, Arlene Sue **(SLP)**
Faskowitz, Michele B **(SLP)**
Fay, Dr Thomas H **(SLP A)**
Feldman, Dr Bernice K **(SLP)**
Feldman, Susan L **(SLP)**
Feldman, Wendy K **(SLP)**
Feltman, Arlene J Kessler **(SLP)**
Fenton, Dr Elaine Reiman **(SLP)**
Ferguson, Mrs Marian N **(SLP)**
Feuerman, Laurie **(SLP)**
Fine-Marker, Sandra Bea **(SLP)**
Finger, Mrs Myrna L **(SLP)**
Finkelstein, Susan Fay **(SLP)**
Fisher, Liliane E **(SLP)**
Fishman, Iris **(SLP)**
Flaxman, Sheila Belkin **(SLP A)**
Fleming, Michelle **(A)**
Flynn, Karen Anne **(SLP)**
Fowlkes, Dr Thomas Eugene **(A)**
Fox, Mrs Marion Rosenbaum **(SLP A)**
Fox, Pamela Debbie **(SLP)**
Freeman, Dr Sandra F **(SLP)**
French, Stephanie M **(SLP)**
Freund, Anne Gustafsson **(SLP)**
Frey, Barbara S **(SLP)**
Fried, Debra **(A)**
Friedman, Dr Lynne Rosen **(SLP)**
Friedman, Rachel A
Friedman, Shari Arleen **(SLP)**
Fries, Ellen Feinerman **(A)**
Friess, Susan Sara **(A)**
Furst, Mrs Rachel Tova **(SLP)**
Gardner, Rex **(SLP)**
Garshman, Terry Diane **(SLP)**
Gaynes, Vivien **(SLP)**
Gaynor, Colleen Edith **(SLP)**
Gelman-Kukin, Phyllis **(SLP)**
Gerber, Dr Sima D **(SLP)**
Giattino, Dr Jill Arion **(SLP)**
Gilson, Natalie Ellen **(SLP)**
Gilston, Mrs Nancy Siwoff
Ginsberg, Patricia Davis **(SLP)**
Gleimer, Ellen F **(SLP)**
Glenn, Cheryl R **(SLP)**
Glick, Miriam **(SLP)**
Goldblum, Amy Denise **(SLP)**
Goldfarb, Dr Robert M **(SLP)**
Goldfein, Susan K **(SLP)**
Goldman-Gluck, Heryl **(SLP)**
Goldstein, Dr Barbara A **(SLP A)**
Goldstein, Helena Deutsch **(SLP)**
Goldstein, Sheila H **(SLP)**
Golub, Dr Arnold J **(SLP)**
Gomolin, Railey Helen **(A)**
Good, Mrs Leatrice Faye **(SLP)**
Grandis, Mrs Joan Eisenson **(SLP)**
Granson, Marian Kaplan **(A)**
Greenfield, Mrs Sharon Jakubowicz **(SLP)**
Greenwald, Mrs Robin Cassel **(SLP)**
Groher, Dr Michael E **(SLP)**
Grossberg, Reva Hillary **(SLP)**
Grossman, Barbara Ellen **(A)**
Guarino, Christine **(SLP)**
Gura, Rhonda Beth **(SLP)**
Hacker, Lynne R **(SLP)**
Hafitz, Miriam J **(SLP)**
Hagen, Mrs Debra Knauer **(SLP)**
Hager, Caryn D
Hahner, Jeffrey C
Hailparn, Ellen L **(SLP)**
Hamberg, Mrs Mildred S **(SLP)**
Hanson, Donna M **(SLP)**
Harmon, Barbara G **(SLP)**
Harris, Mrs Barbara C **(SLP)**
Harris, Dr Katherine
Harris, Laura R **(SLP)**
Haskell, Dr John A **(SLP)**
Heiko, Mrs Phyllis L **(SLP)**
Heit, Mrs Barbara S **(SLP)**
Held, Mrs Judith M **(SLP)**
Hendel, Deborah **(SLP)**
Hennessy, Ruth F **(SLP)**
Hickerson, A M **(SLP A)**
Hill, Dr Nina M **(SLP)**
Himler, Mrs Barbara A **(SLP)**
Hirsch, Judith **(A)**
Hochberg, Dr Irving **(A)**
Holderbaum, Flora M **(A)**
Horowitz, Mrs Virginia **(SLP)**
Horowitz-Ranzi, Karen A **(SLP)**
Horwitz, Dr Betty L **(SLP)**
Houchin, Dr Thomas D **(SLP)**
Hoyo, Elaine **(A)**
Hunter, Mrs Elaine J **(SLP)**
Hyman, AnnJoan **(SLP)**
Indursky, Beatrice **(A)**
Jablon, Dr Ann D **(SLP)**
Jacobson, Susan M **(SLP)**
Jacoby, Randi Faith **(SLP)**
Jaffe, Brenda S
Jassem, Harriet Lois **(SLP)**
Jennings, Joan M **(SLP)**
Jones, Marilyn
Jordan, Star M **(SLP)**
Judge, Mrs Jean **(SLP)**
Jupiter, Dr Tina Z **(A)**
Kahgan, Arnold **(A)**
Kahn, Robin Sue **(SLP)**
Kann, Cheryl M **(SLP)**
Kaplan, Mrs Claire G **(SLP)**
Karle, Mrs Linda J **(SLP)**
Karpel-Freilich, Anne R **(SLP)**
Karpoff, Marilyn A **(SLP)**
Kasper, Helen Hall **(SLP)**
Kaufman, Dr Gale A **(SLP)**
Kenvin, Kathy Elyse **(A)**
Kerman-Lerner, Patricia **(SLP A)**
Kisiel, Dr Dennis L **(A)**
Kistenberg, Lisa B **(SLP)**
Klein, Dr Harriet B **(SLP)**
Klein, Michelle Gloria **(SLP)**
Kling, Irene Frances
Kollia, Haralambia
Kornberg, Michelle Caren **(SLP)**
Kove, Mrs Rose **(SLP)**
Kramer, Dr Marc B **(A)**
Kreeger, Deborah

Kretschmer, Dr Robert E
Kriegel, Ellen S **(SLP)**
Krishnaswamy, Latha **(SLP)**
Kuhl, Susan Lisa **(SLP)**
Lamm, Tina Senders **(SLP)**
Landau, Ellen Jill **(SLP)**
Lande, Anita **(SLP)**
Lazarus, Susan B **(A)**
Leader, Barbara J **(SLP)**
Leffel, Myra P **(SLP)**
Leiter, Everett R **(SLP)**
Leitner, Lisa Helen **(SLP)**
Lenz, Carol F **(SLP)**
Levy, Dr Constance Andrea **(SLP)**
Levy, Mrs Joan R **(SLP)**
Levy, Louise **(A)**
Levy, Mrs Rosalind R **(SLP)**
Liberman, Robin L L **(SLP)**
Lichtenstein, Sandra **(SLP)**
Linden, Neil J **(SLP)**
Lindley, Katherine E **(SLP)**
Lipsky, Walter **(SLP A)**
Litsky, Jay **(A)**
Liu, Margaret Eichel **(SLP)**
Loren, Blanche M **(SLP)**
MacKersie, Carol L **(A)**
MacKins, Cynthia Campos
MacQuilken, Christine Marie **(SLP)**
Madell, Dr Jane Reger **(SLP A)**
Madonia, Julie Anne **(SLP)**
Mahecha, Mrs Nancy R **(SLP)**
Mahler, Marla Cooper **(SLP)**
Makman, Judith M
Malanaphy, Kathleen A **(SLP)**
Malinoff, Dr Rochelle L **(A)**
Manly, Dr Carol Ann **(SLP)**
Manning, Judy Ellen **(SLP)**
Marchese, Dr Judith **(SLP)**
Margulies, Cecele **(SLP)**
Margulies, Mrs Selma K **(SLP)**
Marino, Mrs Corinne A **(SLP)**
Marks, Adrienne L **(A)**
Markwitz, Adele **(SLP A)**
Martinez-Pita, Mrs Rowena Lee **(SLP)**
Mason, Susan S **(SLP)**
Mates, Dr Barbara **(SLP)**
May, Judith S **(A)**
Mazor, Marvin **(SLP A)**
McGarr, Dr Nancy S **(SLP A)**
McLaughlin, Noreen A **(A)**
McTighe, Audrey R **(SLP)**
Mead, Brenda Cammon **(SLP)**
Melley, Clare **(SLP)**
Meltsner, Sheryl Eve **(SLP)**
Meyrowitz, Gail S **(SLP)**
Milch, Karole K **(SLP)**
Miller, Joan P
Miller, Sarah Ann **(A)**
Miller, Susan D **(SLP)**
Mittler, Amy **(SLP)**
Molly, Leda S **(SLP A)**
Moncarz-Attinson, Freda Deborah **(SLP)**
Monzon, Robert **(A)**
Morales, Amparo Elsa **(SLP)**
Morganstein, Shirley **(SLP)**
Morisco, Jacqueline **(SLP)**
Morrison, Dr Eleanor B **(SLP)**
Mueller, Theresa Pinsky **(SLP)**
Mulholland, Dr Ann M **(A)**
Murphy, Patricia Ann **(SLP)**
Murray, Sharon S **(SLP)**
Mysak, Dr Edward D **(SLP A)**
Nadell-Siegel, Ellen **(SLP)**
Namm, Rosanne Bishop **(SLP)**
Nemeth, George
Newman, Ann Birns **(A)**
Nieburgs, Dr Tamara R **(SLP)**
Nousak, Jo Manette K **(A)**
Oates, Margaret Ann **(A)**
Oberndorfer, Adrienne P **(SLP)**
Obler, Dr Loraine K
O'Malley, Dr Honor
Orion, Dr Gertrude **(SLP)**
Ornstein, Mrs Amy Fleisher **(SLP)**
Ornstein, Myrna **(SLP)**
Otto, Catherine **(SLP)**
Packness, Louise **(SLP)**
Papir, Wendy Hope **(SLP)**
Paris, Vasilikie Sophia **(SLP)**
Parkhurst, Dr Barbara G **(SLP)**
Peacher, Dr Georgiana M **(SLP)**
Peretsman, Debora Russo **(SLP)**
Perschetz, Babs H **(A)**
Phatate, Dr Darlynne Devenny **(SLP A)**
Phillips, Renee Jean **(SLP)**
Platt, Robin Dale
Plotnick, Cheryl H **(A)**
Pollack, Evelyn **(SLP)**
Poor, Nancy **(SLP)**
Powell, Paulette I **(A)**
Prager, Mrs Marlene Mitauer
Press, David **(SLP A)**
Putter, Phyllis S **(SLP)**
Rabinowitz, Marcia G **(A)**
Ramos, Rosalva A **(SLP)**
Randall, Yolaine G **(SLP)**
Rappaport, Margery F **(SLP)**
Raskin, Mrs Carol Wolitzky **(SLP)**
Rein, Mrs Susan Lee Cuba **(SLP)**
Reiss, Dorothy **(SLP A)**
Remillaro, Susan Marie
Rhodes, Alice E **(SLP)**
Richardson, Elton **(SLP)**
Riedel, Dr Karen L **(SLP)**
Ronson, Dr Irwin **(SLP)**
Rosaly, Maria DeLourdes **(SLP)**
Rosenberg, Joan M **(SLP)**
Rosenberg-Levi, Mrs Meta **(SLP)**
Rosenthal, Phyllis H **(A)**
Rosenthal, Robin Shari **(SLP)**
Rosenthal, Dr Ruth Dorothy **(SLP A)**
Rosenwasser, Marian **(SLP)**
Rosner, Sharon E **(A)**
Rossi, Edith A **(SLP)**
Rottersman, Judy E **(SLP)**
Rubin, Mrs Gail **(SLP)**
Rubin, Dr Martha Teichholtz **(A)**
Rubinstein, Julie A **(SLP)**
Rudin, Bonnie L **(SLP)**
Russo, Robert L **(A)**
Sacks, Pamela Enid **(SLP)**
Safran, Valerie **(SLP)**
Samuels, Devorah Yoshpe **(SLP)**
Sapora, Mrs Laurie M **(SLP)**
Sarno, Martha Taylor **(SLP)**
Sauber, Mrs Kitty F **(SLP)**
Scheinfeld, Debra B **(SLP)**
Schmelzer, Mindy Sue **(A)**
Schoepflin, Janet Reath **(A)**
Schon, Terry D **(A)**
Schor, Ronnie M **(SLP)**
Schorrman, Dorothy **(SLP)**
Schreter, Beatrice **(SLP)**
Schuler, Eileen **(SLP)**
Schultz, Deborah **(A)**
Schutzer, Barbara M **(SLP)**
Schwartz, Anita B **(SLP)**
Schwarzberg, Rona Sheryl **(SLP)**
Seekamp, Sandra J **(SLP)**
Seff, Jane **(SLP)**
Sforza, Suzanne **(SLP)**
Sherman, Deborah Murtaugh **(SLP)**
Shulman, Dr Brian B **(SLP)**
Shuster, Lia **(A)**
Sidtis, Dr John J
Silberman, Hilary Joy
Silver, Dr Marilyn B **(SLP A)**
Silverman, Dr Carol A **(A)**
Silverman, Mrs Eleanor T **(SLP)**
Silverman, Dr Sidney I
Slavin, Dianne C **(SLP)**
Slingerland, Barbara M **(SLP)**
Slotnick, Karen Rochelle **(SLP)**
Snyder, Paula M **(SLP)**
Sokol, Rose Taubenfeld **(SLP)**
Solomon, Beth I **(SLP)**
Spanier, Paul M **(SLP)**
Spierer, Lili **(SLP)**
Spitzer, Linda **(SLP)**
Spivak, Dr Lynn G **(A)**
Sputz, Carla Ann **(SLP)**
Staloff, Mrs Debbie C **(SLP)**
Steiner, Mrs Elissa Beth **(SLP)**
Stern, Adele Jones **(SLP)**
Stewart, Celia F **(SLP)**
Stocker, Mrs Beatrice **(SLP A)**
Stovall, Inger Benedikte **(SLP)**
Sullivan, Margaret Ann **(SLP)**
Surkis, Eleanor **(A)**
Sutcliffe, Natalie M **(SLP)**
Tartter, Dr Vivien Rothman
Tasch, Melissa B **(SLP)**
Taylor, Dr Judy Ann **(SLP)**
Telzak, Carol S **(SLP)**
Thomas, Janet E **(SLP)**
Thorne, Dr B Clyde **(SLP A)**
Tishman, Mrs Shelley L **(SLP)**
Toueg, Mrs Renee Eichler **(SLP)**
Trachtenberg, Carol Ann **(SLP)**
Trauber, Mrs Rochelle **(SLP)**
Trommer-Thaul, Mrs Nancy E **(SLP)**
Tuchman-Rosen, Shari Marlene **(SLP)**
Turner, Karel Lee **(A)**
Ulius, Mrs Marilyn **(A)**
Vanderster, Diane S **(SLP)**
Ventry, Nona **(A)**
Vorce, Eleanor R **(A)**
Walsh, Maureen A **(SLP)**
Waltzman, Dr Susan Beth **(A)**
Washer, Constance **(SLP)**
Washington, Sherry Gladys **(SLP)**
Wasserman-Gwirtzman, Sarina **(SLP)**
Watson, Emily Strauss **(SLP)**
Weaver, Dr Ella H **(SLP)**
Webb, Karen B **(SLP)**
Weber, Ethel Lynn **(SLP A)**
Weiner, Jean C **(SLP)**
Weinstein, Dr Barbara E **(A)**
Weinstein, Jeri **(SLP)**
Weisberg, Dr Doris F **(SLP)**
Weiser, Mrs Randi E **(SLP)**
Weiss, Judy Reva **(SLP)**
Weitzmann, Erica E **(A)**
Weitzner, Maxine **(SLP)**
Wender, Marilyn **(SLP)**
White, Bridget K
Whitman, Allister C **(SLP)**
Wiener, Debra A **(SLP)**
Wissner, Gail M **(SLP)**
Young, Risa **(SLP)**
Yudkovitz, Dr Elaine **(SLP)**
Zachariah, Anne **(SLP)**
Zaner, Dr Annette R **(SLP A)**
Ziering, Deborah Jo **(SLP)**

Newark
Aradine, Rebecca A
Cole, Mary Jo **(SLP)**
Gordon, Eric S **(SLP)**
Jackson, Mrs Bonnie Lee N **(SLP)**
Luss, Sandra L **(A)**
Segmond, Andrea M **(A)**
Stephens, Mrs Christine Bender **(SLP)**

Newark Valley
Breese, Kathleen Munroe

Newburgh
Cunningham, Mrs Elizabeth Anne **(SLP)**
Hales, Nancy Burch **(SLP)**
Jeffrey, Mrs Jennifer S **(SLP)**
Kapilow, Carin P **(SLP A)**
Via, Mrs Pamela Rae **(SLP)**

Niagara Falls
Godino, Nancy A **(SLP)**
Hamilton, Esther I **(SLP)**
Marillo, Mrs Marie J **(SLP)**
Mazur, Jill Gleason **(A)**
McKnight, Donna Rountree **(SLP)**
McNally, Mrs Lorraine **(SLP)**
O'Brien, Diane Lynn **(SLP)**
O'Toole, Mrs Dale L **(SLP)**
Smith, Paula Susan **(A)**

Niskayuna
Miller, Mary Frances Coniglio **(SLP)**

Nissequogue
Santoro, Mrs Judy S **(SLP)**

Niverville
Stegmann, Nina Valente **(SLP)**

North Babylon
Copithorne, Nancy Adelle
Illingworth, Barbara M **(SLP)**
Pickus, Mrs Francine S **(SLP)**
Scelfo, Rosemarie **(SLP)**
Sheiffele, Wendy Ann **(SLP)**
Soriano, Mrs Lynn Friedlande

North Bellmore
Breslau, Lewis B **(A)**
Brown, Mrs Debra Mines **(SLP)**
Dank, Seth **(A)**
Goldstein, Michele **(SLP)**
Heller, Mrs Wendy Jacobson **(SLP)**
Lupu, Susan Picker **(A)**
Proct, Mrs Marlene P **(SLP)**
Seaman, Victoria Ann **(SLP)**
Sussman, Karen A **(SLP)**
Travers, Nancy **(SLP)**
Wilansky, Mrs Judith A P **(SLP)**

North Buffalo
Pietrafesa, Christina Inez **(SLP)**

North Massapequa
Ellis, William R **(A)**
Muscasella, Carol Frances **(SLP)**
Sanders, Patricia Mary **(SLP)**

North Merrick
Burns, Patricia J Yurko **(SLP)**
Fitzgerald, Mrs Patricia De Koning **(SLP)**
Rose, Mrs Eileen A **(SLP)**
Sirota-Rosen, Lori **(SLP)**

North Syracuse
Grant, David Alan **(SLP)**
Stayer, Mrs Janet H **(A)**

North Tarrytown
Billharz, Constance **(SLP)**
Compton, Carol A **(SLP)**
Farrell, Cathleen P **(SLP)**
Loffredo, Lisa Catherine **(SLP)**
Rubin, Bonnie R **(A)**

North Tonawanda
Donlavage-Craft, Sandra L **(SLP)**
Duffy, Nancy Rose **(SLP)**
Galland, Elizabeth M **(SLP)**
Gawrys, Mrs Elaine E **(SLP)**
Jacobi, Mrs Mary Elizabeth **(SLP)**
Lang, Mrs Kathryn Samway **(SLP)**
Lebold-Ruska, Mrs Suzanne **(SLP)**
Lute, Virginia M **(SLP)**
Lynch, Mrs Margaret Mary D
Pisarek-Freatman, Susan **(SLP)**
Rizzo, Mrs Valerie Jp
Skomski, Diane Csizmar **(SLP)**
Smith, Mrs Margaret Girton **(SLP)**
Tyson, Mrs Joanne G **(SLP)**
Wesolowski, Mrs Beverly Denson **(SLP)**
Wolffer, Elaine A E **(SLP)**

North Valley Stream
Berkman, Mrs Laurel H **(SLP)**
Hirsch, Mrs Jodi Sanoff **(A)**
Simon, Mrs Joanne V **(SLP)**

North White Plains
Egan, Christina Marie **(SLP)**

North Woodmere
Drexler, Mrs Shelley **(SLP)**
Eiger, Jaclyn S **(SLP)**
Galimidi, Mrs Robin E **(SLP)**
Rockfield, Naomi M **(SLP)**
Seplowe, Mrs Robin Lori **(SLP)**
Shaller, Randy Lynn **(SLP)**
Trachtenberg, Renee B **(SLP)**

Northport
Crawford, Nancy C **(SLP)**
D'Onofrio-Zizzo, Mrs Denise M **(SLP)**
Grow, Mrs Maryann Milich **(A)**
Larsen, Mrs Debra Penzi **(SLP)**
Lemli, Jayne Abrams **(SLP)**
Lorber, Sharyn S
Morrison, Mrs Carolyn **(A)**
Norman, Mrs Carol Slingerland **(SLP)**
Poveromo, Judith A G **(SLP)**
Turner, Martha P **(SLP A)**
Weiss, Mrs Mary Margaret **(SLP)**

Northville
Begeal, Mrs Anne T **(SLP)**

Norwich
Horovitz, Linda J **(A)**

Norwood
Gibson, Mrs Carolyn B **(SLP)**
Hartman, Adrienne Smith **(A)**

Nunda
Payne, Mrs Linda **(SLP)**

Nyack
Clark, Dr Lynne W **(SLP)**
Harris, Mrs Meryl K **(SLP)**
Kalinoski, Laurie A **(SLP)**
Knoebel, Mrs Constance **(SLP)**
Schwartz, Caryl H **(SLP)**

Oakdale
Dyer, Mrs Georgia Ann **(SLP)**
Greenberg, Marsha Rhonda **(SLP)**
Hornstein, Prof Sara Carol **(SLP)**
Langella-Pristera, Mrs Lori Lynn **(SLP)**
Masten, Irving **(SLP)**

Oakland Gardens
Stechel, Sandra S **(SLP)**

Oceanside
Bernstein, Abby Lou **(A)**
Blinderman, Michael **(SLP)**
Carfagna, Mrs Freda **(SLP)**
Froehlich, Mrs Elaine Mary **(SLP)**
Gargano, Debra Ann **(A)**
Grossman, Heather Lynn
Hassid, Mrs Janis D A **(SLP)**
Hoffnung, Dr Audrey S **(SLP)**
Keller, Mrs Claire B **(SLP)**
King, Mrs Laurie R **(SLP)**
Kirshenbaum, Rachelle P **(SLP)**
Koenig, Mrs Ellen Gitter **(SLP)**
Malamud, Mrs Gloria S **(SLP)**
Marcus, Debbie Beth **(SLP)**
McCarthy, Mrs Kathleen Byrnes **(SLP)**
Principe, Donna L **(SLP)**
Riemma, Angela Z **(A)**
Stamm, Lenore K **(SLP)**
Steinholz, Mrs Bonnie Fern **(SLP)**
Talbot-Yablon, Ruth J **(SLP)**
Thompson, Mrs Mindy S **(SLP)**
Tognan, Mrs Denise M **(A)**
Winkler, Suzanne J **(SLP)**

Ogdensburg
Rimas, Mrs Ramune V **(SLP)**
Ritter, Dr Patricia **(SLP)**

Old Bethpage
Fields, Elyse J **(SLP)**
Jacobs, Arthur H **(SLP)**
Mandor, Sandra A **(SLP)**

Old Westbury
Kropf, Anne N **(SLP)**
Wain, Tobey D **(A)**

Olean
Bolles, Tamara S **(SLP)**
Butler-Rybicki, Anne E **(SLP)**
Groth, Pamela W **(SLP)**
Hilliard, Pamela J **(SLP)**
Simon, Mrs Michele B **(A)**
Simon, Pamela J **(SLP)**
Wagner, Elaine C **(SLP)**

Oneida
Peterson, Catherine E **(SLP)**
Tytko, Cynthia A **(SLP)**
Woodworth, Lorna G **(SLP)**

Oneonta
Batill, Anthony Scott **(A)**
Berman, Lynne Winter **(SLP)**
Hillis, Carolyn **(SLP)**
Kabat, Deborah G **(SLP)**
Palmer, Karen Joyce **(SLP)**
Rech, Karl H **(A)**
Rogers, Evelyn M **(SLP)**

Orangeburg
Contino, Karen Carmela **(SLP)**

Orchard Park
Battle, Dr Dolores **(SLP)**
Drainville, Mrs Teresa Prusak **(SLP)**
Kaminski, Mrs Susan Gold
Kurzawski, Bernadette Ann **(SLP)**
McCartney, Mary Eileen **(SLP)**
Monofo, Mary Ellen **(SLP)**
Weinreich, Mrs Patricia C **(SLP)**

Oriskany
Buehler, Sandra A R **(SLP)**

Ossining
Baumann, Mrs Patricia B **(SLP)**
Cohill, Kathleen A **(SLP)**
Constable, Catherine M **(SLP)**
Deland, Mrs Nancy E **(SLP)**
Jackson, Mrs Shirley W **(SLP)**
Jaffe, Mrs Amy Goldman **(A)**
Levine, Mrs Helene B **(SLP)**
Lucker, Dr Jay R **(SLP A)**
Miller, Phyllis Jane **(SLP)**
Moulton, Mrs Janet Elizabeth **(SLP)**
Petruzzi, Pia M **(SLP)**
Riordan, Mrs Karin Salline **(SLP)**

Oswego
Hoehman, Karen J
Knoerl, Annmarie
Moore, Mrs Marcia Czyewski **(SLP)**
Morman, Mrs Patricia C **(SLP)**
Smith, Mary E **(SLP)**

Otego
Brown, Mrs Suzanne Reid **(SLP)**

Owego
Burnett, Catherine Patricia **(SLP)**
Hilliker, Allison Marie **(SLP)**
Luckhurst, Mrs Joan A **(SLP)**
Luckhurst, John M **(A)**

Oyster Bay
Bard, Madeline **(SLP)**
Multer, Mrs Regina Hedberg
Zaremba, Mrs Diana T **(SLP)**

Ozone Park
De Luca, Kathleen **(SLP)**

Painted Post
Carr, Mrs Faith Casey **(SLP)**
Nelson, Mrs Mary F **(SLP)**
Schramm, Molly Jean
Stunson, Mrs Da Fayne R **(SLP)**

Palisades
Allen, Deidre J **(SLP)**
Bowen, Mary B **(SLP)**

Palmyra
Drake, Jack **(SLP A)**
Faas, Mary Elizabeth
Murray, Matthew Richard **(SLP)**

Patchogue
Dole, Barbara R **(A)**
Larsen, Robert E **(SLP)**
Rocco, Mrs Cynthia R **(SLP)**
Toback, Frieda **(A)**
Williams, Gail A **(SLP)**

Pattersonville
Kralovic, Mrs Susan Dora **(SLP)**
Paul-Evenden, Renee A **(SLP)**

Pavilion
Johns, Mrs Catherine Beatrice **(SLP)**

Pawling
Reilly, Mary C **(SLP)**

Pearl River
Chirico, Jo Ann T **(SLP)**
Schaible-McArdle, Helen F **(SLP)**

Peconic
Mehrman, Mrs Normajean **(SLP)**

Peekskill
Berger, Mrs Rochelle **(SLP)**
Brown, Mrs Karen J **(SLP)**
Clarke, Mrs Marianne McKenna
Conetta, Elizabeth Hannaberry **(SLP)**
Darragh, Mrs Staci Haines **(SLP)**
De Micco, Lisa Jane **(SLP)**
DiFilippo-Angelo, Renee E **(A)**
Goodman, Mrs Colette Claire **(SLP)**
Greco, Cynthia Micali **(SLP)**
Lane, Susan **(A)**
Levine, Rochelle **(A)**
Murphy, Mrs Nancy R **(SLP)**
Plucknett, Janet F **(SLP)**
Poggi, Karen J **(SLP)**
Thompson, Leesa C **(SLP)**
Vallon, Jerome M **(SLP)**
Volin, Dr Robert A **(SLP)**

Pelham
Viani, Lynn Marie **(SLP)**

Pelham Manor
Magnani, Mrs Bernadette **(SLP)**
Nappi, Claire A **(SLP)**

Penfield
Boxbaum, Allen H **(A)**
Boxbaum, Michele Cerio **(SLP)**
Jameson, Janet W **(SLP)**
Jameson, Scott G **(A)**
Parlet, Mrs Theresa Rita **(SLP)**
Robinson, Shelley Elizabeth **(SLP)**
Rocco, Mrs Marcia M **(SLP)**
Russell, Linda Kay **(SLP)**
San Filippo, Jane Wicks **(SLP)**
Senio, Mrs Judith E **(SLP)**
Toleman, Cynthia F **(SLP)**
Zlotnick, Rosemarie **(SLP)**

Perry
Paddock, Jody Lynne **(SLP)**
Shumway, Teresa J **(A)**
Sitler, Dr Ronald W **(A)**

Peru
Bilyeu, Mrs Katherine Michele **(SLP)**
Demers, Margaret Hoey
Derrick, Mrs Virginia J **(SLP)**

Phelps
Power, Mrs Lorraine Liput **(SLP)**

Philadelphia
Doherty, Dr Joseph W **(SLP A)**

Piermont
Strikowsky, Shari D **(SLP)**
Zeitlin, Debra J **(SLP)**

Piffard
Feuerstein, James F **(A)**

Pine Bush
Niebel, Susan K **(SLP)**

Pine City
Hannah, Virginia Ann **(SLP)**

Pittsford
Austin, Allen A **(SLP)**
Benedict, Lois Anne **(SLP)**
Bornstein, Mrs Carolyn S **(SLP)**
Cupini, Mrs Mariellen **(SLP)**
Flewelling, Mrs Barbara B **(SLP)**
Goldberg, Mrs Donna **(SLP)**
Gray, Ann D **(SLP)**
Loughery, James H **(SLP)**
Loughery, Jean M **(SLP)**
Marlow, Patricia A
McCabe, Mrs Mary Ann Jenkins **(SLP)**
Ormandy, Dr Roderick B **(SLP)**
Robins, Arlene G **(SLP)**
Silva, Deborah B **(SLP)**
Sima-Eichler, Elizabeth **(SLP)**
Spector, Mrs Susan Naimark **(SLP)**
Subtelny, Dr Joanne D **(SLP)**
Wilson, Barbara Ann **(SLP)**
Young, Lynne T **(SLP)**

Plainview
Albala, Brent M **(SLP)**
Bennett, Joel **(SLP)**
Bressi, Susan Ann **(A)**
Cantor-Apfel, Debra E **(SLP)**
Cohen, Mrs Roberta S **(A)**
Cole, Mrs Babette W **(SLP)**
Diener, Mrs Rhonda Ash **(SLP)**
Fishkin, Mrs Debbie S **(SLP)**
Goldberg, Mrs Linda M **(SLP)**
Goldstein, Leslie B
Grossman, Mrs Lynn Shapiro **(SLP)**
Kallem, Ellen **(SLP)**
Katz, Lori E **(SLP)**
Krostich, Mrs Linda Gordon **(SLP)**
Kukelka, Mrs Tina R **(SLP)**
Lapidus, Deborah Cohen **(SLP)**
Leibowitz, Hope **(SLP)**
Lisabeth, Mrs Susan Fern **(SLP)**
Miller, Maureen L **(SLP)**
Morvitz, Mrs Sandra Alperin **(SLP)**
Naftol-Levitch, Mrs Linda **(SLP)**
Rabinowitz, Allan Jay **(SLP)**
Rattiner, Rochele G **(SLP)**
Roschwalb, Adena **(SLP)**
Sloan, Ellen C **(A)**
Tauberer, Mrs Gale M **(SLP)**
Wick, Erika **(SLP)**

Plandome
Tortolani, Beth C **(SLP)**

Plattsburgh
Conners, Mrs Cindy L **(SLP)**
Dewey, Charlene M **(SLP)**
Domenico, Dr Raymond A **(SLP)**
Dufort, Mrs Mary Margaret **(SLP)**
Freeman, Hyman S **(SLP A)**
Giroux, Lucy A **(SLP)**
Kelsey, Nancy Dorothy **(SLP)**
Kyea, Mrs Gail G **(SLP)**
Lafontaine, Sandra D **(SLP)**
Quesal, Mrs Donna Livingston **(SLP)**
Quesal, Dr Robert W **(SLP)**
Seiden, Mrs Bucky Rogers
Zoss, Donald C **(SLP)**

Pleasant Valley
Angiulo-Pugnali, Jayne Ann **(SLP)**
Bower, Mrs Wendy Obourn **(SLP)**
Goddard, Karla Sargent **(A)**
Hayes, Sandra M **(SLP)**
Kehrli, Karen S **(SLP)**
Kenney, Mary E **(SLP)**
Maulucci, Fred V **(SLP)**

Russo, Maryhelen **(SLP)**
Whalen, Judith M **(SLP)**

Pleasantville
Brandt, Tina C **(SLP)**
Carnes, Robert C **(SLP)**
Engel-Rudolph, Robin **(A)**
Faughnan, Mrs Theresa Joanne **(A)**
Fay, Mrs Kathleen A **(SLP)**
Fitzpatrick, Deanne B **(A)**
Ganis, Mrs Rosemary T **(SLP)**
Jaffe, Denise A **(SLP)**
Marshall, Deborah Durst **(SLP)**
Nuytkens, Pamela Ann **(SLP)**

Poestenkill
Shepard, Shari Ann **(SLP)**

Point Lookout
Falabella, Mrs Linda Q **(SLP)**

Pomona
Baumann, Mrs Pamela Dunn **(SLP)**
Cohen, Ellyn M **(SLP)**
Fisher, Helene Rosman **(SLP)**
Greenberg, Stephanie Robin **(SLP)**
Halpern, Mrs Karen T **(A)**
Jackson, Mrs Karen Ehrlich **(SLP)**
Kaplan-Greenberg, Mrs Vicki **(A)**
Marber, Mrs Marilyn Seltzer **(SLP)**
Robinson, Rosanne Theresa **(SLP)**
Subrizi, Laurie Perry **(SLP)**
Wilson, Gail B **(SLP)**

Port Chester
Black, Mrs Marjorie Blass **(SLP)**
Kach, Stacey Rabin **(SLP)**
Kennard-MacKenzie, Kathy **(SLP)**
Keslinger, Annette S **(SLP)**

Port Jefferson
Carter, Joyce R **(SLP)**
Craig, Mrs Jenise Palermo **(SLP)**
Dooley, Lizbeth Jean **(SLP)**
Fox, Mrs Deborah A **(SLP)**
Halegoua, Perla P **(SLP)**
Jonas, Linda F **(SLP)**
Reggio-Seng, Donna Regina **(SLP)**
Shapiro, Lawrence S **(SLP)**
Terrano, Cathy A R **(SLP)**

Port Jefferson Station
Davis, Mrs Diane Marsh **(A)**
Gilroy, Mrs Maureen Anne **(SLP)**
Martinetti, John Alan **(SLP A)**
Metzendorf, Diane E **(SLP)**
Polzer, Mrs Kathleen R **(SLP)**
Rodemack, Mrs Kayleen Hawker **(SLP)**
Rowlett, Lisa Kathleen **(SLP)**

Port Washington
Bradley, Mrs Claire Ledden **(SLP)**
Davidson, Barbara Sara
Duffy, Dr John K **(SLP A)**
Englander, Mrs Harriet **(SLP)**
Friedman, Eileen Savage **(SLP)**
Karp, Mrs Adrienne **(A)**
Lee, Mrs Patricia B **(SLP)**
Parker, Dr Ellen **(SLP)**
Peck, Lois Robyn **(SLP)**
Rogovin, Karen Susan **(SLP)**
Sands, Dr Elaine S **(SLP)**
Smith, Betty M **(SLP)**
Smitheimer, Dr Luella Sude **(SLP)**

Potsdam
Evans-Welpe, Mrs Mary C **(SLP)**
Kemp, Pamela J **(SLP)**
Woodford, Alice M **(SLP)**

Poughkeepsie
Ansley, Mrs Ellen R **(SLP)**
Buhler, Helen C **(SLP)**
Gallagher, Mrs Donna P B **(SLP)**
Galleher, Jerrold L **(A)**
Glick, Mrs Bonnie Greenberg **(SLP)**
Griffin-Gomez, Rosemary **(SLP)**
Hecht, Susan Karnes **(SLP)**
Himelstein, Emily Zimmer **(SLP)**
Keenan, Nancy C **(SLP)**
Kricheff, Adele M **(SLP)**
Kricheff, Barry **(A)**
Lashway, Mrs Carolanne Polizzi **(SLP)**
Longa, Robin L **(A)**
Nassar, Kim Ann **(SLP)**
Ottaviani, Roberta M **(SLP)**
Procopio, Mrs Karen A Teeling **(SLP)**
Raichle, Ruth Ann **(SLP)**
Scalzi, Karen W **(SLP)**
Schwartz, Fmdr Elsie Newman **(SLP)**
Scott, Allan **(SLP)**
Seifert, Elizabeth Dean **(SLP)**
Tavolacci, Gina Marie **(SLP)**
Thambooswamy, Leela **(A)**
Tolley, Patricia Banks **(SLP)**
Valeo-Gahn, Joanne **(SLP)**
White, Barbara S **(SLP)**

Pound Ridge
Heath, Dr Richard G **(SLP)**
Johnson, Mrs Sara M **(SLP)**
Wilder, Dr Carol N **(SLP)**

Putnam Valley
Ammann, Mrs Susan **(SLP)**
Mello, Mrs Mary L **(SLP)**
Patrick, Mrs Theresa A **(SLP)**

Queens
Carmeli, Sara **(SLP)**
Goldner, Mrs Kathleen M **(SLP)**
Haber, Diane Sue **(SLP)**
Hofflin, Lois E **(SLP)**

Queens Village
Cutrone, Linda R **(SLP)**
Esposito, Geraldine Anne **(SLP)**
Horowitz, Dr Leola S **(SLP)**
Koffler, Lori H **(SLP)**
Lochansky, Sydney Beth **(SLP)**

Red Creek
Martin, Molly A **(SLP)**

Red Hook
Karr, Linda A **(SLP)**
Montpetit, Isabelle **(SLP)**
Richmond, Mrs Prudence **(SLP)**

Rego Park
Berliant, Yola **(SLP)**
Faine, Susan D **(SLP)**
Friedman, Meryl L **(SLP)**
Hanin, Laurie **(A)**
Henderson, Dorita **(SLP)**
Kalish, Phylis L **(SLP)**
Kane, Deborah A **(SLP)**
Kessler, Stewart C **(SLP)**
Lipner, Hildy S **(SLP)**
Loaiza-Suarez, Rosario Maria **(SLP)**
Marcovici, Mrs Selma Goldstein **(SLP)**
Resnick, Mrs Cynthia B **(SLP)**
Turk, Mrs Jane E **(SLP)**
Varadi, Rhea C **(A)**
Vidal, Nancy Stella **(SLP)**
Wankoff, Mrs Lorain S **(SLP)**

Remsen
White, Mrs Jane A **(SLP)**

Rensselaer
Fox, Mrs Janis A **(SLP)**
Maloy, Marianne C **(SLP)**
McBride, Marie Francesca **(SLP)**
Spencer, Mrs Maryann M **(SLP)**
Standarski, Susan M **(SLP)**

Rexford
Higgins, Mrs Judy Herold **(SLP)**

Rhinebeck
Brodsky, Geraldine **(SLP)**
Jeffreys, Maureen B **(SLP)**
Knupp, Laura L **(SLP)**
Natale, Mrs Patricia G **(SLP)**
Pittman, Cecilia L **(SLP)**
Weitz, Karen A
Wilsey, Mrs Mary Martha **(SLP)**

Richfield Spring
Armstrong, Mrs Marcia J **(SLP)**

Richmond Hill
Anson, Lynn T
Ashley, Betty Ann Marie **(SLP)**
Gambino, Mrs Karen **(SLP)**
Thachara, Babu Punan **(SLP A)**

Ridgewood
Lewandowski, Elaine Cecilia **(A)**
Limbacher, Rosemarie Barbara **(SLP)**
Petschauer, Mrs Rosemarie S **(A)**
Smith, Debra Ann **(SLP)**

Riverdale
Baker, Rachelle D S **(SLP)**
Balkin, Barbara Hollis **(SLP)**
Bell-Vollandt, Clarice Angela
Biskup, Charlotte Lou **(A)**
Blau, Andrea F **(SLP)**
Cohen, Mrs Elisa Susan **(SLP)**
De Santis, Brenda R **(SLP)**
Ferber-Lerner, Rosanne **(SLP)**
Gilmartin, Theresa **(SLP)**
Grosser, Mrs Abbe C **(SLP)**
Liss, Lorri P **(SLP)**
Lynn, Deborah J **(A)**
Orloff, Donna P **(SLP)**
Prusslin, Gail F **(SLP)**
Reisfeld, Mrs Lora Schachter **(SLP)**
Santore, Frances C **(SLP)**
Schneider, Mrs Elaine Dolgin **(SLP)**
Schneider, Dr Phillip A **(SLP)**
Soifer, Dr Lydia H **(SLP)**
Warhit, Mrs Ilissa Carol **(SLP)**
Weissbrot, Sharon D **(SLP)**

Riverhead
Larkin, Mrs Marilyn K **(A)**
Lutz, Ellen Ruth **(SLP)**
Zulli, Bonnie Hughes

Rochester
Adornato, Denise Marie **(SLP)**
Anderson, Catherine Howley **(SLP)**
Antinore, Deborah Ann **(SLP)**
Antonik, Susan P **(SLP)**
Ater, Mrs Jacquelyn **(SLP)**
Atherton, Nancy J **(SLP)**
Aucoin, Cheryl Lynne **(A)**
Begner, Mrs Patricia **(SLP)**
Bell, David J **(SLP)**
Bement, Linda Bryant **(A)**
Bennett, Mary S **(SLP)**
Bianco, Penny L **(SLP)**
Block, Dr Michael G **(A)**
Bobry, Mrs Doris R **(SLP)**
Bondurant, Lynn Swain **(SLP)**
Boyer, Regina U **(SLP)**
Bradley, Mrs Mary Catherine **(SLP)**
Braeges, Judy L **(SLP)**
Bricault, Melody **(A)**
Brown, Mary J S **(SLP)**
Brown, Dr Paula M **(SLP)**
Burgess, Mrs Eleanor H **(SLP)**
Bushman, Nancy Jeanne
Caccamise, Dr Frank C **(A)**
Camardo, Mrs Joan L **(SLP)**
Caputo-Schwarz, Carol A **(SLP)**
Carney, Kathleen Mary **(A)**
Castle, Dr William E **(SLP)**
Cavalier, Mrs Margaret Grady **(SLP)**
Clark, Catherine Celeste **(A)**
Clonan, Ann F **(SLP)**
Clymer, Mrs Beryl F **(SLP)**
Crandall, Dr Kathleen Eilers
Culleton, Ruth S **(SLP)**
Culp, Ann E
Dalzell, Larry E **(A)**
Dalzell, Mrs Sheila M **(A)**
De Clerck, Mrs Ingrid Gundersen **(SLP)**
De Filippo, Dr Carol L **(A)**
Demott, Anne **(A)**
De Silva-Elich, Elaine Theresa **(SLP)**
Dicesare, Jeanette M **(SLP)**
DiPaola, Phyllis A **(SLP)**
Diraimo, Laura Wisniewski **(SLP)**
Dischiav, Kristine Marie **(SLP)**
Dobkowski, Karen G **(SLP)**
Donahue, Jeanne E **(SLP)**
Drake, Mrs Lilianne Jacqueline **(SLP)**
Dumigan, Mrs Lorrie Anne **(SLP)**
Durant-Jones, Mrs Lisa Anne **(SLP)**
Durfee, Barbara Lee **(SLP)**
Eamon, Diane W **(SLP)**
Ebner, Mary Jo **(A)**
Ernst, Suzanne M **(A)**
Evans, Chris Hawrylak **(A)**
Fallat, Claudia J **(SLP)**
Feehan, Deborah Anne **(A)**
Fettinger, Maryfran Camelio **(A)**
Frankel, Mrs Sandra L **(SLP)**
Freitag, Martha Helen **(SLP)**
Frohlich, Mrs Laraine Anne **(SLP)**
Gambee, Mrs Veronica **(SLP)**
Gammons, Mrs Roberta Poslusny **(SLP)**
Geglia, Mary-Jo **(SLP)**
Gerlach, Mrs Melanie L
Giesow, Virginia Ellen **(SLP)**
Golder, Kyle A **(SLP)**
Goldhawk-Haag, Mrs Kelly S **(SLP)**
Goodwin, Mrs Jeanne M **(SLP)**
Gottermeier, Linda G F **(A)**
Gratzer, Mrs Susan H **(SLP)**
Graver, Constance Marie **(SLP)**
Graziano, Adrienne Lee
Greenfield, Mrs Ellen Braiman
Greer, Mrs Carol A **(A)**
Hanna, Susan Denise **(SLP)**
Hart, Stephen Thomas **(A)**
Hendrick, Mrs Nancy A M **(SLP)**
Hess, Sr Wanda J **(SLP A)**
Holtzman, Mrs Eleanor Benes **(SLP)**
Hooey, Kimberlee Ann **(SLP)**
Hopf, A Gidget **(SLP)**
Houde, Dr Robert A
Huber, Mrs Patricia Marie **(SLP)**
Hymes, Enid F **(SLP)**
Ivsan, Carol Falbo **(A)**
Jarema-Mongeau, Ann **(SLP)**
Jeffers, Stephanie **(SLP)**
Johnson, Dr Barbara Ann **(SLP)**
Johnson, Dr Donald D **(A)**
Johnston, Suzanne Flockhart **(SLP)**
Kelly, Jacquelyn F **(SLP)**
Kennedy, Judith L **(SLP)**
Kirkey, Karen P **(A)**
Kowba, Mrs Joyce B **(SLP)**
Kozelsky, Joseph D **(A)**
Kozlowski-Willmarth, Jean M **(SLP)**
Kriegel, Janice Manolopoul **(SLP)**
Kunken, Mrs Naomi S **(A)**
Kuzel, Christina M **(SLP)**
Lavriha, Nancy Anne **(SLP)**
Lengefeld, Joyce Mary **(SLP)**
Leventer, Dr Susan L **(SLP)**
Lockamyeir, Mrs Judith Ann **(SLP)**
MacKenzie, Douglas Joseph **(A)**
MacMullin, Keith A **(SLP)**
Manello, Mrs Ephros **(SLP)**
Mantione, Denise Ann **(SLP)**
Martinelli, Mrs Laureen J **(SLP)**
McAndrew, Joyce Kathryn **(SLP)**
McCarron, Maureen P **(SLP)**
McCarthy, Mrs Jean D **(SLP)**
McCrossen, Karen B **(SLP)**
McDermott, Patricia Lynn **(SLP)**
McDonald, Maureen **(A)**
McKenna, Patricia S **(SLP)**
McMullin, Kelly Kristine **(SLP)**
McNamara, John Joseph **(A)**

Merle, Kathleen S **(A)**
Metz, Dr Dale E **(SLP)**
Metz, Mrs Wendy Susan **(SLP)**
Miele, Ellen Bronson **(A)**
Molner, Janet Ann **(SLP)**
Moroni, Mrs Susan M H **(SLP)**
Moss, Mrs Cheryl Ann **(SLP)**
Motiwala, Tina S **(SLP)**
Mull, Rebecca J **(SLP)**
O'Connell, Mrs Mary Lou **(SLP)**
Oftedahl, Mrs Geraldine Ann **(SLP)**
O'Neill, Mrs Ellen R **(SLP)**
Palmer, Mrs Linda Oltman **(A)**
Papso, Catherine F
Parasnis, Dr Ila
Paris, John N **(SLP)**
Pariser, Karen G **(SLP)**
Petote, Cynthia Anne
Ponticello, Michelina Ann **(SLP)**
Prucy, Nancy Ann **(A)**
Pudup, Mrs Kathleen M **(SLP A)**
Quarfot, Laney Jean **(SLP)**
Rahn, Dawn Renee **(A)**
Regoord, Sally **(SLP)**
Reiff, Donald Gene **(SLP)**
Reiss, Mrs Kathleen A **(SLP)**
Rende, Mrs Sharon Sue **(A)**
Renner, Mrs Carol M **(SLP)**
Rentschler, Paula C **(SLP)**
Reynolds, Toni A **(A)**
Ricci, Mrs Rosanne Palermo **(SLP)**
Richmond, Deserie J **(SLP)**
Roberts, Laura Montgomery **(SLP)**
Rossborough, Meredith Morgan **(SLP)**
Rozestraten, Mrs Elizabeth D **(SLP)**
Ruflin, Joan Marie **(SLP)**
Sadick, Robert H **(SLP)**
Salamone, Lisa Gail
Samar, Dr Vince Joseph
Sanderson, Mrs Deborah Briggs **(A)**
Santangelo, Mrs Gretchen L **(SLP)**
Schultze, Laura J **(SLP)**
Schumacher, Edith Kathryn **(SLP)**
Sconfietti, Sandra C **(SLP)**
Scott, Lawrence C, Jr **(A)**
Sennett, Susan Jank
Shoen, Cathy Jo **(A)**
Shulman, Ellen L **(SLP)**
Silver, Jane Ellen **(SLP)**
Sims, Dr Donald George **(A)**
Smith, Jean McKernan **(SLP)**
Sorrentino, Mrs Marie R **(SLP)**
Spadoni, Kimberly Anne **(SLP)**
Sperling, Mrs Deborah Lea **(SLP)**
Stanzel, Laurel **(A)**
Steen, Mrs Lisa Ann **(SLP)**
Stinson, Dr Michael S
Stotz, Mrs Valorie **(SLP)**
Sudore, Mrs Deborah E **(SLP)**
Summa, Maureen E **(A)**
Swanson, Stephanie Lu **(SLP)**
Sweeney, Mary M **(SLP)**
Taromino, Mrs Jane Lee G **(SLP)**
Taylert, Barbara J **(SLP)**
Tereshko-Ewart, Katherine Joan **(SLP)**
Tiemann, Mrs Brenda Lynn **(SLP)**
Tomanovich, Sandra **(SLP)**
Tomasso, Mrs Jean Anne **(SLP)**
Torpey, Dr Mary Clare C **(SLP)**
Tremaine, Deborah Angela **(SLP)**
Trombly, Janine Marie
Vienna, Barbara Hoefner **(SLP)**
Viglietta, Sarah Marie **(A)**
Wallber, M Josara **(A)**
Walrath, Mrs Pamela D **(SLP)**
Walton, Dr Joseph Paul **(A)**
Warnke, Eileen Regina **(A)**
Werbela, Mrs Madelyn Beth **(SLP)**
Westbay, Erin Christine **(SLP)**
Wetherald, Mrs Carol A **(A)**
Whitehead, Dr Robert L **(SLP)**
Winter, Miriam J
Yerkes, Nancy Frances **(SLP)**
Young, Dr Edna Carter **(SLP)**
Young, Jeanne Hickey **(SLP)**
Yust, Valerie R **(A)**

Rock Hill
Druse, Mrs Jean Marie **(SLP)**
Dunitz, Anne Elizabeth **(SLP)**

Rockaway Park
Rogers, Jean A **(A)**

Rockaway Point
Fox, Janet **(A)**
Williams, Dr Ann Marie **(SLP)**

Rockville
Katzman, Mrs Karen B

Rockville Centre
Alagna, Mrs Pauline R **(SLP A)**
Cartusciello, Mrs Christine V **(SLP)**
Dellicarpini, Mrs Carla J **(SLP)**
Gilmartin, Ann **(SLP)**
Goldstein, Mrs Merle Ruth **(SLP)**
Goore, Mrs Deborah S **(SLP)**
Greene-Luba, Mrs Jill A **(SLP)**
Greenhall, Mrs Irene Leav **(SLP)**
Israel, Hollis B R **(SLP)**
Lederer, Barbra **(SLP)**
Leicht-LeBron, Rachelle **(SLP)**
Malone, Christina **(SLP)**
Max, Mrs Phyllis R **(SLP)**
Paderewski, Ilyse **(A)**
Quinn, Shirley B **(SLP)**
Richards, Jerome F **(SLP)**
Riolo, Mrs Eva Banham **(SLP)**
Rooney, Joan Franzese **(SLP)**
Rosen, Mrs Barbara L **(A)**
Ross, Mrs Margaret M **(SLP)**
Rothfeld, Diddy L **(SLP)**
Schmidt, Mrs Barbara Teresa **(SLP)**
Stegman, Robin Eckstein **(A)**
Tepper, Mrs Carol M **(SLP)**

Rocky Point
Ekstrom, Cathy Faeger **(SLP)**
Keller, Gary A **(SLP)**
McGeehan, Mrs Maryellen Gallagher **(SLP)**
Reilly-Sardegna, Gerri M **(SLP)**
Yezierski, Denise M **(SLP)**

Rome
Badolato, Sheryl Ann **(SLP)**
Beatty, Raymond L, Jr **(SLP)**
Frank, Mrs Karen E **(SLP)**
Fullagar, Ann Elise **(SLP)**
Howell, Ella M **(SLP)**
Mero, Mrs Janette Lee **(SLP)**
Middleby, Maria Theresa **(A)**
Millett, Karen J **(SLP)**
Mokry, Deborah L **(SLP)**
Morganti, Mrs Denise Ann Borek **(SLP)**
Oleski, Mrs Theresa Ann **(SLP)**
Schatz, Joan Ann **(SLP)**
Short, Cynthia Anne **(SLP)**
Sims, Patricia A **(SLP)**
Willett, Maryanne M **(A)**

Ronkonkoma
Menzies-O'Leary, Pamela Jeanne **(SLP)**
Ponticiello, Michelle Maria **(SLP)**
Reidlich, Mrs Carole E **(SLP)**
Rosengarten, Amy
Wallack, Wendy C **(SLP)**

Rosedale
Abruzzo, Lynette **(SLP)**
Scheinman, Brenda Robin **(SLP)**
Schraub, Stacy
Sheridan, Mrs Maria G **(SLP)**

Rosendale
Hasson-Axblad, Marcia A **(SLP)**
Jacquart, John E **(A)**
Miller, Ruth A **(SLP)**

Roslyn
Cohen, Rhoda T **(SLP)**
Feldman, Dr Ronald L **(SLP)**
Hantman, Mrs Lesli R **(SLP)**
Miller, Linda R **(SLP)**
Millman, Gladys **(SLP)**
Rosenberg, Marion W **(SLP)**
Rosenberg, Mrs Taube Shiffman **(SLP)**
Santoro, Mrs Elizabeth **(SLP)**
Setzen, Sheryl D **(SLP)**
Taylor, Denise Susan **(SLP)**

Roslyn Estates
Hananel, Robin J **(SLP)**
Hollander, Mrs Marilyn R **(SLP)**
Kachel, Robin B **(SLP)**
Seaman, Mrs Linda S **(SLP)**
Sterling, Mrs Tinette D **(SLP A)**

Roslyn Harbor
Casper, Muriel Klein **(SLP)**

Roslyn Heights
Barse, Mrs Elinor A S **(A)**
Callahan, Dr Joan B **(SLP A)**
Paticoff, Mrs Ellen Sara **(SLP)**
Rasin, Mrs Judy Warshaver **(A)**
Rosenthal, Mrs Lori Sternig **(A)**
Saravay, Mrs Elizabeth Schiller **(SLP)**
Schnabel, Corinne V **(SLP)**
Sigman, Myrna K **(SLP)**
Trotta-Boehler, Lynda L **(SLP)**
Tuch, Mrs Claire H **(SLP)**
Wall, Dr Meryl Johnson **(SLP)**

Roxbury
Giella, Mrs Patricia **(SLP)**

Rush
Reilly, Cathleen Reap **(SLP)**

Rushville
Blackwood, Christina Newgarden **(SLP)**
Rogers, Linda S **(SLP)**

Rye
Barton, Amy Veerhoff **(SLP)**
Gluck, Shelley S **(A)**
Kaufman, Rosalind E **(SLP)**
Newburger, Dr Doris S **(SLP)**
Reap, Anne Roussel **(A)**
Riso, Mrs Claire A **(SLP)**
Roth, Mrs Barbara Edeson **(SLP)**
Schlossberg, Mrs Pamela Mitchell **(SLP)**
Shotland, Mrs Rochelle C **(A)**

Rye Brook
Berkowitz, Mrs Nancy E **(SLP)**
Genova, Mrs Wanda K **(SLP)**
Goldberg, Rachelle K **(A)**
Potter, Ellen Mittelman **(SLP)**
Sherman, Dr Randi S **(A)**
Stokes, Christine Montelone **(SLP)**

Sag Harbor
Button, Mrs Arlys S **(SLP)**
Ruch, Shirley Ann **(SLP)**

Salt Point
Zeleznik, Linda M **(SLP)**

Samsonville
Fraser, Maryann **(SLP)**

Sanborn
Human, Mrs Carol A **(SLP)**

Sand Lake
Steinberg, Mrs Marcy Gail **(SLP)**

Sands Point
Kirschenbaum, Mrs Bonnie L **(SLP)**
Sirow, Dr Lynn W **(A)**

Saranac
Haley, Cynthia S **(SLP)**

Saranac Lake
Gardner, Robert H **(SLP)**
Reyell, Joan K **(SLP)**
Reyor, Lea J B **(SLP)**
Vinograd, Margaretha Miller **(SLP)**
Walsh, Keith P **(A)**

Saratoga Springs
Ambrosino, Mrs Barbara Marie **(SLP)**
Christy, Mary Ellen **(A)**
Dart, Dawn Marie **(SLP)**
Grassi, Mrs Susan Marie **(SLP)**
Metz, Mrs Pandora Frank **(SLP)**
Pelone, Carolyn R **(SLP)**
Rose, Mrs Carol Ann **(SLP)**
Taylor, Sarah Oakley **(SLP)**

Saugerties
Gershon, J Casey **(SLP)**
Hogan, Leigh A **(SLP)**
Naccarato-Gage, Mrs Susan Lyn **(SLP)**
Schneider, Helene Mary **(SLP)**

Sauquoit
Douglas-Fee, Elyse **(SLP)**

Sayville
Azzaretti, Anne **(SLP)**
Barrick, Mrs Wendy Laura **(SLP)**
Beechley, Mrs Rena Bryant **(SLP)**
Gatta, Mrs Janice E **(SLP)**
Masche, Patricia A **(SLP)**
Nepote, Mrs Karen A **(SLP)**
Scrima-Castelli, Mrs Lisa Marie **(SLP)**
Sealy, Lynn **(SLP)**
Yanoti, Mrs Diana T **(SLP)**

Scarborough
Gavin, Sharon K **(A)**

Scarsdale
Ahearn, Natalie D **(SLP)**
Bucci, Linda Ann **(SLP)**
Defendi, Christel C **(SLP)**
Doolan, Mrs Theresa A **(A)**
Doolittle, Dr Jacqueline Baxter **(SLP)**
Dowling, Leslie B **(SLP)**
Glickenhaus, Mrs Sarah Brody **(SLP)**
Goda, Dr Sidney **(SLP A)**
Henricks, Mrs Barbara D **(SLP)**
Kavarsky, Mrs Joan M **(SLP)**
Liebowitz, Mrs Roni S **(SLP)**
Lowenfels, Barbara B **(SLP)**
Mahoney, Carol Ann **(SLP)**
Malpica, Frida L **(A)**
Manchester, Karen Z **(SLP)**
Marcus, Ivy April **(SLP)**
Markoff, Maxine N **(A)**
Nagle, Maureen Elizabeth **(SLP)**
O'Connor-Hodgdon, Eileen M **(SLP)**
Pollack-Klein, Sandra R **(SLP)**
Pravda, Mrs Lynn F **(SLP)**
Roberts, Mrs Elise R **(SLP)**
Rogalski, Dr Lois A **(SLP)**
Scheinberg, Mrs Louise G **(SLP)**
Schiller, Dr Newton M **(SLP)**
Shatz, Mrs Karen S **(SLP A)**
Smith, Arlene R **(A)**
Spiegel, Mrs Donna R **(SLP)**
Vilmos, Mrs Madeleine **(SLP)**
Walfish, Eleanor R **(SLP)**
Warfel, M Kay **(SLP)**

Schaghticoke
Perry, Mrs Barbara Ann **(A)**

Schenectady
Abba, Mrs Deborah Graham **(SLP)**
Abreu, Katherine Oconnor **(SLP)**
Bianchi, Patricia **(A)**
Boehlert, Lenora Therese **(SLP)**
Brooks, Valerie L **(SLP)**
Comer, Cynthia J **(SLP)**
De Bonis, David A **(A)**
Garbowitz, Mrs Barbara H **(SLP)**
Gregory, Carrie Frances **(SLP)**
Haller, Timothy Leonard **(SLP)**
Hasko, Joanna Joan **(SLP)**
Hatch, Mrs Janet M **(SLP)**

Hodges, Kathleen **(SLP)**
Hoorwitz, Marion K **(SLP)**
Jensen, Mrs Linda Jeanne **(SLP)**
Johnson, Mrs Lori **(SLP)**
Kenna, Ellen Therese **(SLP)**
Keough, Susan Ann **(A)**
Knupp, Diane T **(SLP)**
Lanza, Mrs Elaine Rehgie **(SLP)**
Leder, Arthur Lawrence **(SLP)**
Liebman, Dr Jerome **(SLP A)**
Marchewka, Carol C **(SLP)**
Margagliotti-Money, Sandra **(SLP)**
McDonald, Nancy **(SLP)**
Oneill, Margaret M **(A)**
Porter, Dr Lois S **(A)**
Preisman, Mrs Barbara **(SLP)**
Rossmeisl, Mrs Kathryn L **(SLP)**
Shields, Mrs Michele K **(A)**
Urban-Wessinger, Cheryl **(SLP)**
Veltman, Mrs Sharon A **(SLP)**
Weiskopf, Mrs Dianne E **(SLP)**
Ylvisaker, Mark S **(SLP)**

Schuyler Falls
Hay, Mrs Veronica W **(SLP)**

Scotia
Auriemma, Joseph R **(SLP)**
Eoannou, Susan A **(SLP)**
Grabo, Mrs Diane E E **(SLP)**
Greer, Marion P **(SLP)**
Hainey-Flacke, Martha J **(SLP)**
Jicha, Sandra Lynn **(SLP)**
Lariviere, Mrs Lisa Ann **(A)**
Leonard, Lois L **(SLP)**
Lynn, Mrs Gerene **(SLP)**
MacIver, Nora L
Maksail, Tricia C **(SLP)**
McCloskey, Mrs Debra Vitello
Rafalak, Susan Laura **(SLP)**
Schilke, Mrs Margaret L **(SLP)**
Skibinski, Mrs Diane K **(SLP)**
Truesdale, Mrs Susanne Poulette **(SLP)**
Urbanski, Janice Dempster **(SLP)**
Van Genderen, Joanne **(SLP)**
Wawrzyniak, Mary Theresa **(SLP)**

Scottsville
Boggs, Margaret J **(SLP)**

Sea Cliff
Boehm, Mrs Marian B **(SLP)**
Desanti, Susan M **(SLP)**
Kearney, Anne Ferguson **(SLP)**

Seaford
Bradley, Mary Katherine **(A)**
Lynn, Mrs Gail G **(SLP)**
Meyer, Mrs Hope Bonnie
Sturtz, Robin E **(A)**
Zambuto, Mrs Julie Ellis **(SLP)**

Searingtown
Bravstein, Mrs Linda L B **(SLP)**
Goodman, Mrs Helene R **(A)**
Hollander, Jane G K **(SLP)**

Selden
Walsh, Mrs Robin McDonough **(SLP)**

Selkirk
Kelleher-Assael, Kathleen **(SLP)**

Seneca Falls
Bondi, Marcel M **(SLP)**
Hedler, Mrs Charlotte Ellen **(SLP)**
Loucks, Mrs Natalie Frappolli **(SLP)**
Morton, Kathleen Susan **(SLP)**

Setauket
Boren, Grace Daly **(SLP)**
Feldman, Eileen Weisen **(SLP)**
Jones, Mrs Dianne Delaney **(SLP)**
Kamil, Mrs Eileen B **(SLP)**
Kaspar, Mrs Susan M **(SLP)**
Keahon, Sonia M V **(SLP)**
Laufer, Dr Marsha Z **(SLP)**
Lee, Mrs Nancy B **(A)**
Van Tuyl, Mrs Mildred Thoeny **(SLP)**

Sherburne
Kurtz, Debra J **(SLP)**

Sheridan
Monacelli, Mrs Melanie Lynn **(SLP)**

Shokan
Benson, Mrs Pamela **(SLP)**

Shoreham
Albert, Susan **(SLP)**
Squires, Deborah Pershern **(SLP)**

Sidney
Ross, Karen Pontius **(SLP)**

Silver Creek
Ark, Mary P **(SLP)**
Metzger, Mrs Judy A **(SLP)**

Sinclairville
Carlson, Mrs Vicki Lynn **(SLP)**

Skaneateles
Borsh, Mrs Frances L **(SLP)**
Sommers, Lisa K **(SLP)**

Slingerlands
Dececco, Mrs E Patricia Becker **(SLP)**
Ryan, Mrs Lavonne B **(SLP)**
Turner, Carolyn T **(SLP)**
Vein, Mrs Paula Canarick **(SLP)**

Smallwood
Godlewski, Mrs Alyce T

Smithtown
Bruno, Mrs Lorraine Schultz **(SLP)**
Caruso, Mrs Judith Mona **(SLP)**
Ferraro, Mrs Lynn Marie **(SLP)**
Fischthal, Mrs Lorraine Buchman **(SLP)**
Furlong, Sheila N **(SLP)**
Gerson, Lauri D H **(SLP)**
Goldberg, Sheila C **(SLP)**
Hartmann, Lydia Avallone **(SLP)**
Hoffman, Janet S **(SLP)**
Hoffman, Mrs Mary Elaine **(SLP)**
Klingelhoefer, Paula H **(SLP)**
Kyrk, Rochelle Racanelli **(SLP)**
Levine, Judith **(SLP)**
Longo, Mrs Barbara L **(SLP)**
O'Bray, Lynnann Susan **(A)**
Post, Lonni T **(SLP)**
Sturm, Mrs Mindy Robin **(SLP)**

Snyder
Byrne, Maj Clyde D **(A)**
Gettys, Mrs Jill Marie **(SLP)**
Grantham, Mrs Charlotte L **(A)**
Greenman, Mrs Carol Sellers **(SLP)**
Hadyn-Hawkins, Nancy P **(SLP)**
Harris, Patricia L **(SLP)**
Jones, Carol A **(SLP)**
Kurzius, Colette E **(SLP)**
Lund, Dr Nancy J **(SLP)**
Pagliaroli, Mrs Michele Terese **(SLP)**
Palen, Sharon B **(SLP)**
Ritter, Dona H **(SLP)**
Stocking, Christina **(A)**
Weiss, Claudia J **(SLP)**

Sodus
Andela, Mrs Christine Rita **(SLP)**

Solvay
Marascalchi, Carole Anne **(SLP)**
Orzell, Lisa O
Parkes, Mrs Barbara Joan **(SLP)**
Taffner, Nancy L **(SLP)**

Somers
Hocker, Mrs Susan G **(SLP)**
Valentino, Patricia A **(SLP)**

Sound Beach
Martinetti, Mrs Helen Catherine **(SLP)**

South Bellmore
Goldstein, Amy R G **(SLP)**
Krebs, Mrs Kay D **(A)**

South Farmingdale
Molinelli, Clifford J, Jr **(SLP)**

South Glens Falls
Berube, Michele E **(SLP)**
Tusa, Lynn R **(A)**

South Hempstead
Molinelli-Spatz, Mrs Roseann Judy **(A)**
Rein, Mrs Lorraine C **(A)**

South Huntington
Dempsey, Dr James J **(A)**
Rigby, Denise Frances **(SLP)**

South Ozone Park
Cappellano, Joseph G **(SLP)**
Jones, Jean T **(SLP)**

South Salem
Gilinson, Mrs Pamela F **(SLP)**
Hickey, MaryEllen **(SLP)**
Lamanna, Mary Lyon **(SLP)**

Southampton
Jackson-Bruyn, Mrs Sherryl A **(SLP)**

Sparrow Bush
Bird, Raymond J **(SLP)**

Spencerport
Gendrou, Mrs Diane Marie **(SLP)**
Kwiatkowski, Mrs Susan Mack
Wood-Sauer, Elizabeth Grace **(SLP)**

Spring Valley
Adler, Julie A
Blau, Chava **(SLP)**
D'Aurio, Mrs Gale M **(SLP)**
Dworkin, Mona L S **(SLP)**
Feldman, Julie G **(A)**
Flynn, Mrs Barbara Barry **(SLP)**
Friedman, Mrs Carol **(SLP)**
Goldberg, Linda D **(SLP)**
Laker, Etta-Jo **(SLP)**
Mackey, Mrs Sandra M O **(SLP)**
Schwartz, Mrs Caren S **(SLP)**
Seedman, Mrs Jamie Chalfon **(SLP)**
Seery, Joyce Bowen **(SLP)**
Spector, Dr Cecile C **(SLP)**

Springville
Beyer, Mrs Elaine M **(SLP)**
Carr, Charlene A **(SLP)**
Heary, Mrs Lori J **(SLP)**
Krezmien-Grasso, Susan M **(SLP)**

St James
Corvini, Mrs Joann D **(SLP)**
D'Orazio, Mrs Helene Cecelia **(SLP)**
Higgins, Mrs Kathleen Kelley **(SLP)**
Lieberman, Beth Susan **(SLP)**
Phillips-Springer, Lisa Ann **(SLP)**
Trutner, Mrs Patricia L **(SLP)**

Staatsburg
Kelleher, Sheila H **(SLP)**

Stamford
Graham, Dr Victoria S **(SLP)**

Stanfordville
Brondel, Florence **(SLP)**
Kelly, Mrs Sondra I **(SLP)**
Lepore, Nancy P **(SLP)**
Shanley, Valerie J **(SLP)**

Stanley
Mayton, Mrs Linda Mary **(SLP)**

Staten Island
Adriatico, Terry **(A)**
Arnao, Susan Geri **(A)**
Bernstein, Mrs Phyllis Carol **(SLP)**
Blaine, Mrs Maryanne **(SLP)**
Brennan, Mrs Josephine **(SLP)**
Brill, Linda P **(SLP)**
Brown, Mrs Gail Berger
Cammarata, Jerry F **(SLP)**
Chaitkin, Barbara A **(SLP)**
Cooney, Mrs Marion K **(SLP)**
Coyle, Mrs Jane Cannon **(SLP)**
Criscione, Regina Barbieri **(A)**
Cruz, Mayra **(SLP)**
Currie, Cathleen Marie **(SLP)**
Davies, Judy E **(SLP)**
Deford, Sheila Andrea **(SLP)**
Dickstein, Lisa Zucker **(SLP)**
Di Meglio, Angela **(SLP)**
DiPalma, Felix M **(SLP)**
Diresta, Diane **(SLP)**
Dorfman, Jodi M **(SLP)**
Felsenstein, Dr Bernard
Flynn, Mrs Margaret **(SLP)**
Franks, Janice L **(SLP)**
Friedman-Wilson, Harriet **(A)**
Gambardella, Mrs Janet Gail **(SLP)**
Gams-Golub, Mrs Stephanie **(SLP)**
Giamboi, Lois E
Goldsman, Mrs Susanna Klein **(SLP)**
Goldstein, Robin Diane **(SLP)**
Guttsman, Mrs Claire **(SLP)**
Haimowitz, Audrey R **(SLP)**
Hanrahan, Joan Cirillo **(SLP)**
Hechtman, Dr Marvin **(A)**
Henry, Catherine **(A)**
Hill, Miriam **(SLP)**
Horowitz, Christine **(SLP)**
Hose, Mrs Marilyn K **(SLP)**
Kaplan, Mrs Marsha Helene **(SLP)**
Kubiak-Cherkaski, Lisa D **(SLP)**
Legrand, Roseanne **(SLP)**
Levinson, Steven M **(SLP)**
Lubin-Sulzman, Mrs Karen **(SLP)**
Maida, Michele S **(SLP)**
Marinello, Robert P **(SLP)**
Mazzaro, Mrs Patricia E **(SLP)**
Mazzucco, Mrs Sandra B **(SLP)**
McEvoy, Jane P **(SLP A)**
McGarry, Marian M **(A)**
Merrefield, Gayle Emery **(SLP)**
Messano, Mrs Risa Lamia **(SLP)**
Neuhaus, Anne Rachel **(SLP)**
Newman, Mrs Cora Sandra **(SLP)**
Norman, Natasha
Poleshuck, Deborah S **(SLP)**
Redden, Camille Josephine **(SLP)**
Rosano, Anne **(A)**
Rosen, Carol **(SLP)**
Rosenberg, Lynn **(SLP)**
Ross, Rhonda F **(SLP)**
Rothstein, Michael J
Rubinstein, Adrienne **(A)**
Schwartz, Rebecca Levine **(SLP)**
Seminara, Dr Gloria F **(SLP)**
Stoddard-Schneider, Mrs Mary **(SLP)**
Sweeney, Warren A **(SLP)**
Teryek, Jo Anne E **(SLP)**
Unterman, Dr Rosalie M **(SLP)**
Vecchio, Joan A L **(SLP)**
Wasserstein, Mrs Sharon H **(SLP)**
Wiesner, Gaye B **(SLP)**
Young, Mrs Susan Lisa **(SLP)**

Stewart Manor
Curry, Laura Ann **(SLP)**

Stillwater
Mason, Mrs Kathleen Marie **(SLP)**

Stittville
Borawski, Karen S **(A)**

Stone Ridge
Roosa, Kelly Ann **(SLP)**

Stony Brook
Brener, Dr Rosemary Young **(SLP)**
Burger, Hannah J **(SLP)**
Cohen, Mrs Terri Baltier **(SLP)**

Dworkin, Nadine Sheri **(SLP)**
Harver, Mrs Nancy Hall **(SLP)**
Lazarus, Susan Beth **(SLP)**
Leonard, Mrs Roberta Millrod **(SLP)**
Marinelli, Mrs Kathleen A **(SLP A)**
McCauliff, Mrs Claire A **(SLP)**
Thompson, Mrs Donna Tercasio **(SLP)**
Weitzman, Dr Nancy Fried **(SLP A)**
Zatwarnicki, Leslie **(SLP)**

Stony Point
Farkas, Beth H **(SLP)**
Genchur-Lukas, Janet Anne **(A)**
Lukas, Robert Alan **(A)**
Rose, Mrs Karen Marie **(SLP)**
Stedge, Mrs Patricia F **(SLP)**
Stein, Kathie L **(A)**

Stormville
Anzovino, Mrs Sharon Weber **(SLP)**
Dubois, Ann C **(SLP)**

Stuyvesant
Birdsell, Denise Lasnier **(SLP)**
Masella, Alice Karen **(SLP)**

Suffern
Dowling, Jean Marie **(SLP)**
Goodman, Joanne **(SLP)**
Greenfeld-Furman, Mrs Debra **(SLP)**
Hansen, Mark **(A)**
Julis, Thelma R **(SLP)**
Kaplan, Mrs Ellen D **(SLP)**
Mass, Mrs Hagit Pur **(SLP)**
Nicholas, Dr Jo Ann **(A)**
Van Bemmel, Charlotte **(SLP)**
Weinberg, Mrs Leslie R **(SLP)**
Wexler, Dr Karin B **(SLP)**

Swan Lake
Lacey, Susan F L **(SLP)**

Synder
Bainbridge, Mrs Patricia P **(SLP)**

Syosset
Blond, Mrs Marylouise Ann **(SLP)**
Galluzzo, Andrea **(SLP)**
Glick, Robin J **(SLP)**
Griffin, Mary Elizabeth **(SLP)**
Jeddah, Janet Z **(A)**
Kahne, Mrs Lenore B **(SLP)**
Kornberg, Stanley Saul
Lamendola, Paula Fueller **(A)**
Lannig, Mrs Joanne Wiegand **(SLP)**
Lederman, Mrs Donna G **(SLP)**
Levitan, Mrs Peggy **(SLP)**
Link, Mrs Linda R **(SLP)**
Malgeri, Mrs Suzanne Elizabeth **(SLP)**
McLeer, Mrs Una Lee **(SLP)**
Orlando, Rosanna Marie **(SLP)**
Plotkin, Mrs Donna B **(SLP)**
Podwall, Dr Arthur **(SLP A)**
Podwall, Marcia Sue **(SLP)**
Popper, Mrs Roberta Antell **(SLP)**
Powers-Jakimo, Benay **(SLP)**
Resnick, Mrs Fern Phillips **(SLP)**
Schoer, Felicia E **(SLP)**
Sperling, Mrs Ilene **(SLP)**
Tamari, Dr Pauline L **(SLP)**
Treiber, Diane Marie **(SLP)**
Viviano, Cheryl S **(SLP)**

Syracuse
Amster, Dr Walter W **(SLP)**
Anderson, Mrs Maureen J **(SLP)**
Bergman, Stephanie **(SLP)**
Bowe, Angela J **(SLP)**
Brown, Douglas G **(A)**
Brown, Kathleen H **(SLP)**
Burritt, Grace Aletha **(SLP)**
Butler, Dr Katharine Gorrell **(SLP)**
Byron, Michael K **(SLP)**
Casper, Dr Janina K **(SLP)**
Cereo, Carol A **(SLP)**
Chadwick, Marilyn A **(SLP)**
Challenger, Mrs Sandra S
Clark, David Paul **(SLP)**
Colton, Dr Raymond H
Conture, Dr Edward G **(SLP)**
Conture, Mrs Shelley Smith **(SLP)**
Cross, M Stephanie **(SLP)**
Deboer, Bonnie L **(SLP)**
Del Guidice, Mary D **(SLP)**
Deptula, Patrick M **(A)**
Diminuco, Frank G **(SLP)**
Donn, Jane E **(SLP)**
Driscoll, Patricia Montani **(SLP)**
Driscoll, Mrs Therese Ann **(SLP)**
Edwards, Dr Mary Louise
Elliott, Ann Driscoll **(SLP)**
Feldman, Dr Alan S **(SLP A)**
Floch, Margot Jean **(SLP)**
Frieder, Mrs Dalia **(SLP)**
Garbinski, Kimberly Ann **(SLP)**
Garrett, Mrs Joyce Ellen **(SLP)**
Grimes, Dr Charles T **(A)**
Hardy, Robin M **(SLP)**
Higgins, Maureen B
Holte, Lenore A **(A)**
Hurst, Nancy Ann **(A)**
Karp, Elaine Barbara **(SLP)**
Katko, Mrs Suzanne M
Kim, Munah
Kosoff, Tess O **(SLP)**
Koss, Lynn C R **(SLP)**
Lavine, Laura Beth **(SLP)**
Leitner-Lockwood, Judith C **(SLP)**
Levett, Mrs Colleen Ann
Lowther, Maria Anne **(SLP)**
Lyons, Susan Blake **(SLP)**
McGrath, Patricia L **(A)**
Milosky, Linda M **(SLP)**
Montes, Michelle L **(A)**
Newby, Mrs Kathleen K **(SLP)**
Nezelek, Karen Lee **(SLP)**
Nydam, Marion R **(SLP)**
Olender, Mrs Rosemary **(SLP)**
O'Malley, Mrs Colleen Corbett **(SLP)**
Pastore, Mrs Caterina Anne **(SLP)**
Puma, Michelle A **(SLP)**
Roberts, Mary C K **(SLP)**
Rohn, Cheri L **(SLP)**
Rothenberg, Dr Martin
Rothschild, Laurie **(SLP)**
Ryan-Hammon, Patricia Ann **(A)**
Scheibe, Peter H **(SLP)**
Schubert, Annegret **(SLP)**
Spaulding, Mary E **(SLP)**
Spillane, Eileen M **(SLP)**
Stevens, Mrs Joanne K **(SLP)**
Swanson, Judith Danz **(SLP)**
Tom, Cynthia Marie **(SLP)**
Turner, Dr Chris W **(A)**
Valerio, Dr Michael W **(A)**
Vogl, Mrs Laura Anne **(SLP)**
Waters, Mrs Helen V **(A)**
Wilson, Mary Anne **(A)**
Wolk, Lesley **(SLP)**
Wright, Dr H N **(SLP A)**
Zurn, Michelle **(SLP)**
Zwislocki, Dr Jozef J

Tanglewood Hills
Moore, Mrs Debra E **(SLP)**

Tarrytown
Christopher, Dr Judith L **(SLP)**
Gabel, Michele **(SLP)**
Lovecky, Drusilla Dulcy **(SLP)**
Miscioscia, Mrs Elizabeth S **(SLP)**
Pogue, Dr Elizabeth **(SLP)**
Smith, Debra Kay **(SLP)**
Stassen, Raymond A **(A)**
Strandberg, Mrs Roberta Harnois **(SLP)**
Wortley, John S **(SLP)**

Tomkins Cove
Dries, Margaret Burton **(SLP)**
Gruberger, Carole Ann **(SLP)**

Tonawanda
Anello, Denise Marie **(SLP)**
Balsavage-Fritzinger, Lynn **(SLP)**
Cohen, Helene Janis **(SLP)**
Davis, Mrs F Teresa Runzo **(SLP)**
Demarco, Mrs Kathy Clarkson
Dentino, Monica Dixon **(A)**
Fillmore, Mrs Jane M **(SLP)**
Gerovac, Mrs Michelle Marie **(SLP)**
Grieve, Mrs Susan M K **(SLP)**
Harper, Arleen R **(SLP)**
Lawson, Mrs Gail Marie Cook **(SLP)**
Locicero, Jeanne Marie
McLean, Mrs Nancy J **(SLP)**
Medler, Diane **(SLP)**
Messineo, Marc Joseph
Miles-Fahs, Margaret Ellen **(SLP)**
Nemmer, Mrs Ruthe L **(SLP)**
Pullman, Pamela K **(SLP)**
Roussi, Lisa Ann
Sapienza-Crowley, Mrs Patricia **(SLP)**
Steiger, Cynthia J **(SLP)**
Stewart, Mrs Barbara J **(A)**
Taylor, Mrs Kristine A **(SLP)**
Wakeley, Donna Adele **(SLP)**

Troy
Cannon, Audrey S **(SLP)**
Cassidy, Kathleen R **(SLP)**
Check-Tapler, Maureen Lynn **(SLP)**
Cioffi, Mrs Maribeth Matthews **(SLP)**
Clemente, Mrs Dorothy Anne **(SLP)**
Donovan, Mrs Carol M **(SLP)**
Gallagher, Lynn A **(SLP)**
Ives-Kline, Kathleen Mary **(SLP)**
Marble, Elaine Mary **(SLP)**
Rabe, Maureen R **(SLP)**

Tuckahoe
Harsch, Mrs Debra Gallo **(A)**
Houston, Mrs Colleen Dibble
Marvin, Lynda **(SLP)**
Tonetti, Mrs Suzanne Marie

Tully
Thurston, Kenneth I **(SLP)**

Tupper Lake
Comeau, Betty Lynn **(SLP)**

Tuxedo Park
Buckley, Mrs Maureen Cahill **(SLP)**

Ulster Park
Yates, Mrs Patricia Kay **(SLP)**

Union Springs
deRoos, Diane Elizabeth **(SLP)**

Uniondale
Harkin, Mrs Mary Friel

Upper Brookville
Siris, Teresa P **(SLP)**

Upper Nyack
Gould, Laura D **(SLP)**
Kittay, Mrs Judith L **(SLP)**

Upper Schnectady
Chrusciel, Judy Beth **(SLP)**

Upton
Frank, Phyllis R **(SLP)**

Utica
Balutis, Karen A **(SLP)**
Cardillo, Mrs Kathleena **(SLP)**
Daley, Linda A **(SLP)**
Della Cava, Andrea **(SLP)**
Freed, Dolores F **(SLP)**
McDonald, Kathleen A **(SLP)**
Pietrafesa, Barbara Jane **(SLP)**
Trombetta, JeanMarie **(SLP)**
Wengert, Mary E **(SLP)**
Zangrilli, Donna M **(SLP)**

Valatie
Deily, Dr Ann Beth S **(SLP)**

Valhalla
Checchi, Anne M **(SLP)**
Morriss, Mrs Judy M **(SLP)**

Valley Cottage
Bakst, Julie S **(SLP)**
Cohen, Mrs Karen Hope **(SLP)**
De Cola-Samoylo, Mrs Debi Patricia **(SLP)**
Goldin, Marci H
Jagoda, David R **(SLP)**
Kotorac, Rita Erlbaum **(SLP)**

Valley Falls
Messier-Grilli, Mrs Nancy Ann **(SLP)**

Valley Stream
Bentley, Carolyn Sullivan **(A)**
Blumstein, Vivian H **(SLP)**
Desola, Deborah M **(SLP)**
Inkles, Mrs Sharon M **(SLP)**
Jakimetz, Dr John R **(A)**
Kornsweig, Mrs Carole Linda **(SLP)**
Krauss, Jeffrey D **(A)**
Leventhal, Mark L **(SLP)**
McDermott, Sandra **(A)**
Ognibene, Rocco James **(SLP)**
Parisi, Frances Ellen
Raad, Mrs Mary Gorman **(A)**
Reynolds, Mrs Mary Patricia **(SLP)**
Sachs, Lori Weisberger **(SLP)**
Scherr, Pia Sadowsky **(A)**
Schmierer, Merri S **(A)**
Semper-Veith, Mrs Cynthia Ann **(SLP)**
Valente, Elizabeth Helen **(A)**
Wasser, Wendy S **(SLP)**

Vernon Center
Deal, Margaret Elizabeth **(SLP)**

Verona
Kelsey, Valerie B **(SLP)**

Vestal
Agnew, Sue Ann **(SLP)**
Baldovin, Mrs Jill **(SLP)**
Covey-McKeage, Mrs Jennifer Lu **(SLP)**
Docster, Mrs Lisa D **(A)**
Keegan, Mrs Melody Ann **(SLP)**

Victor
Brannen, Susan J **(A)**
Cecere, Mrs Debra Lynn **(SLP)**
Leitgeb, Mrs Diane D **(SLP)**
Messineo-Cowles, Jacqueline **(SLP)**

Voorheesville
Bogert, Penny Smith **(SLP)**
Cacace, Anthony T **(A)**
Leombruno, Joseph A **(SLP)**
Pfeil-McGlynn, Mrs Marsha A **(A)**

Wading River
Bender, Mrs Dianne C **(SLP)**
Perkins, Ellen U **(SLP)**
Pollack, Janet Lynn **(SLP)**

Walden
Carroad, Pamela **(SLP)**
Decker, Mrs Patricia Alice **(SLP)**

Wallkill
Aller, Mrs Virginia K **(SLP)**
Cornell, Mrs Pamela Pope **(SLP)**
La Moy, Juli R **(SLP)**
Liseski, LuAnn Davis
Van Amburgh, Ruth C **(SLP)**

Walton
Breese, Mrs Judith **(SLP)**
Munk, Mrs Marilyn W **(SLP)**

Walworth
Elwell, Mrs Mary Margaret **(SLP)**
Gibala, Janice Lynn **(SLP)**
Keller, Mrs Susan B **(SLP)**
Murray, Mrs Jane E **(SLP)**

Wampsville
Thomas, Mrs Jill E **(SLP)**

Wantagh
Abenis-Cintron, Anna M **(SLP)**
Baumann, Mary Ellen **(SLP)**
Carr, Mrs Ellen S **(SLP)**
Friedman, Mrs Francine Rosenzweig **(SLP)**
Hecker, Mrs Nancy Greenwald **(SLP)**
Herbert, Judith L **(SLP)**
Kleinman, Mrs Frances R **(SLP)**
Palleja, Mrs Mary M **(SLP)**
Partridge, Mrs Marcia
Simon, Mrs Dana Lee **(SLP)**
Soman, Mrs Bonnie Commander **(SLP)**

Wappingers Falls
Brooks Ma Ccc, Gerard B **(SLP)**
Burke, Mrs Patricia E **(SLP)**
Gahn, James N **(A)**
Price, Georgianna La Rocque **(SLP)**
Stempler-Bloom, Susan **(A)**
Teitelbaum, Hedy **(SLP)**

Warsaw
Lane, David M **(SLP)**
Serventi, Gail W **(SLP)**

Warwick
Burriss, Mrs Pamela W **(SLP)**
Isaacson, Mrs Susan B **(SLP)**
Rounds, Brenda Cook **(SLP)**
Schuman, Ronda Lynn **(A)**
Skow, Mrs Marie L **(SLP)**

Washingtonville
Canady, Mrs Pamela Cooper **(SLP)**
Feuer, Mrs Shari Lynn **(SLP)**

Waterford
Abelson, Mrs Lori Haskins **(SLP)**
Pawlick, Mrs Judy Ann **(SLP)**

Waterloo
Abraham, Mrs Melinda Sue **(SLP)**

Watertown
Curtin, Sr Rose **(SLP A)**
Kuhne, Sylvia Marie **(SLP)**
Powell, Emily H
Redmond, Mrs Janice Munday **(SLP)**
Tiff, Richard **(SLP)**

Watervliet
Busi, Susan Elizabeth **(SLP)**
Jojo, Susanne Marie **(SLP)**
Lilienthal, Andrea Elsita **(SLP)**
Sherman, Arleen Abzug **(SLP)**

Webster
Backman, Nancy S **(SLP)**
Brennan, Mrs Colleen Curcillo **(SLP)**
Dailey, Kimberly K **(SLP)**
Dell, Mrs Naomi R **(SLP)**
Goodsell, Mrs Kathleen C **(SLP)**
Hanley, Mrs Martha Travis **(SLP)**
Heaney, Nancy Curchin **(SLP)**
Kitz, Margaret D **(SLP)**
Kohler, Polly Wagner **(SLP)**
Levey, Mary Jean
Manscuk, Mrs Theresa C **(SLP)**
McAfee, Mrs Mary Cincotta **(SLP)**
Moosmann, Anne F **(SLP)**
Ricciardi, Karen M **(SLP)**
Swain, Elizabeth Ann
Teter, Mrs Mary G **(SLP)**
Uschold, Mrs Claudia Joan **(SLP)**
Wermuth, Barbara C **(SLP)**

Wellsville
Canfield, Dr Kenneth L **(SLP)**
Carlson, Elizabeth Ann **(SLP)**
McGowan, Marie E **(SLP)**

West Amherst
Duguay, Douglas M **(SLP)**

West Babylon
Aherne-Lang, M Theresa **(SLP)**
Cianci, Susan Williamson **(SLP)**
Harrington, Nancy Anne **(SLP)**
Leister, Cheryl M **(A)**
Sande, Caren D **(SLP)**
Slack, Mrs Linda J **(SLP)**
Symington, Linda Bullock **(A)**

West Chazy
Wacker-Mundy, Dr Roberta L **(SLP)**

West Falls
Gavin, Carol P **(SLP)**
Kearns, Timothy M **(SLP)**
Malone, Patricia A **(SLP)**

West Hempstead
Goldenback, Robin **(SLP)**
Keen, Gerald Lawrence **(SLP)**
Keller, Sheri Glass **(SLP)**
Phillips, Carol Halpert **(SLP)**
Pizzuti-Almazan, Annamaria **(SLP)**
Pressel, Gene **(SLP)**
Tureen, Dr Phyllis **(SLP)**

West Hurley
Lotito, Heather Tobias **(SLP)**
Thayer, Mary Lape **(SLP)**

West Islip
Bjorkfelt, Christine Marie **(SLP)**
Gottsch, Mrs Jean Ann Quigley
Hill, Carolyn M **(SLP)**
Kane, Ellen M **(SLP)**
Lapenna, Aimee M **(SLP)**
Multer, Mrs Patricia C **(SLP)**
Wisniewski, Mrs June Irene **(SLP)**

West Lawrence
Schwartz, Mrs Leanne Greenwald **(SLP)**

West Nyack
Bonagura-Grehl, Mrs Debra Rose **(SLP)**
Klapper, Mrs Deborah **(SLP)**
Pulliam, Diana E **(SLP)**
Simos, Karen S **(SLP)**

West Park
Churan, Cynthia S **(SLP)**

West Point
Bergner, Mrs Carla Muntz **(SLP)**
Singleton, Mrs Linda W **(SLP)**

West Sand Lake
Krohel, Mary Beth K **(SLP)**
Seeger, Cynthia S **(SLP)**

West Sayville
Schoepp, Mrs Donna J **(SLP)**

West Seneca
Boulange, Mrs Linda A **(SLP)**
Josefiak, William R **(SLP)**
Klas, Lisa Marie **(SLP)**
Moran, Patricia Elizabeth **(SLP)**
Sudlik, Susan Ruth **(SLP)**
Wrona, Mrs Sandra B S **(SLP)**
Zinter, Mrs Irine Denis **(SLP)**

West Valley
Wiede, Margaret R **(SLP)**

West Winifield
Goodier, Janet **(SLP)**
Huxtable, Susan J **(SLP)**

Westbury
Abdale, Mrs Edna K V **(SLP)**
Ackerman, Marjorie Cimmet **(SLP)**
Amsel, Mrs Lynn J **(A)**
Coreys, Mrs Esther **(SLP)**
D'Andrea, Linda **(SLP)**
Foronjy, Eileen M **(SLP)**
Horan, Maryanne Kathleen **(SLP)**
Lambert, Judith C **(A)**
O'Connor, Jeanne A Dunn **(SLP)**
Pobjecki, Donna Pauline **(SLP)**
Rosenberg, Edward S **(A)**
Rubin, Marsha J **(SLP)**
Santoro, Mrs Susan Foglia **(SLP)**
Schwartz, Laurie I **(SLP)**
Sheridan, Mrs Joanne M A **(SLP)**

Westernville
Dicarlo, Louis M **(SLP A)**

Westfield
Van Hout, Mary Ellen **(SLP)**

Westhampton Beach
Resnick, Mrs Robin Ellen **(SLP)**

Westtown
Stevens, Mrs Linda V **(SLP)**

Wheately Heights
Teitelbaum, Mrs Meryl A H **(SLP)**

Wheatfield
Olsen, Mrs Amy R **(SLP)**

Wheatley Heighs
Markowitz, Meryl Lynn

White Plains
Achiron, Mrs Michele R **(SLP)**
Anik, Mrs Margie Abrahamson **(SLP)**
Awerbuch-Schwartz, Felicity **(SLP)**
Blumenfeld, Amy Elizabeth
Chalfin-Rosenblum, Roberta **(A)**
Christian, Beverly A **(SLP)**
Crouse, Mrs Mary Ann B **(SLP)**
Deckinger, Mrs Gloria May **(SLP)**
Garrett, Mrs Susan Casey **(SLP)**
Goldstein, Susan L **(SLP)**
Goldstein-Schneider, Mrs Joy
Halvorson, Kathryn A **(SLP)**
Hampton, Dr Dennis C **(A)**
Harper, Mary K **(SLP)**
Haverson, Mrs Nancy Ellen **(SLP)**
Hersh, Myra G **(SLP)**
Jones, Lynette Susan **(A)**
Katz, Mrs Barbara Ruth **(SLP)**
Klein, Edward D **(SLP)**
Klein, Mrs Estelle R **(SLP)**
Mandel, Mrs Jill **(A)**
McArthur, Eileen Birchett **(SLP)**
Murray, Mary E **(SLP)**
O'Connell, Christine J D **(SLP)**
Pedro, Mrs Judite Vida **(SLP)**
Penn, Nancy E **(SLP)**
Risi, Mrs Laurie **(SLP)**
Rosenkranz, Diane F **(SLP)**
Schwartz, Mrs Deborah F **(SLP)**
Smith, Sonja M
Stein, Dr Cecile L **(SLP)**
Wise, Ida Dawn **(A)**
Witlen, Sharon F **(SLP)**

Whitesboro
Knepka, Mrs Cynthia W **(SLP)**
Pikul, Mrs Angela R **(SLP)**

Whitestone
Bernstein, Sheila H **(SLP)**
Evelyn, Karen **(SLP)**
Jarmel, Mrs Fredi M **(A)**
Kraat, Arlene **(SLP)**
Smith, Mrs Lynn Z
Zara, Carol V **(SLP)**

Whitney Point
Wysocki, Mona Judith **(SLP)**

Williamsville
Abbott, Mrs Susan Harvey **(SLP)**
Bleichfeld, Sharla R **(SLP)**
Brenner, Merle Joan **(SLP)**
Carroll-Kenna, Mrs Mary J **(SLP)**
Clabo, Mrs Pamela A **(SLP)**
Cooper, Mrs Diane Hirschbeck **(SLP)**
Dickson, Dr Stanley **(SLP A)**
Ditusa, Mrs Mildred M **(SLP)**
Dubin, Mrs Lillian O **(SLP A)**
Eichelberger, Mrs Barbara S **(SLP)**
Evans, Bonita M **(SLP)**
Graziano-Tiso, Mrs Susan **(SLP)**
Henderson, Terri Siegel **(A)**
Hintermeier, Ann L **(A)**
Holt, Linda A **(SLP)**
Koenigsberg, Linda R **(SLP)**
Kowalski, Mrs Joanne D **(SLP)**
Mann, Dr Mary B **(SLP)**
Misso, Mrs Anita S **(SLP)**
Perlow, Steven **(A)**
Perlow, Susan R **(SLP)**
Pitzonka, Linda J **(SLP)**
Pranikoff, Merle G
Rosen, Sherrill S **(SLP)**
Sawyer, Sarah A **(SLP)**
Sinclair, Mrs Jennifer Josik **(SLP)**
Slomovitz, Linda Faye **(SLP)**
Steur, Elizabeth **(A)**
Stuart, Diana M **(A)**
Testa-Mack, Rosemary L **(SLP)**
Zurenda, Joseph J **(SLP)**

Williston Park
Brody, John J **(A)**
Rogan, Ellen Walsh **(SLP)**

Windsor
Morrissey, Mrs Elizabeth C **(SLP)**

Wolcott
Sparnon, John R **(SLP)**

Woodbury
Levy, Mrs Barbara G **(A)**
Mendelsohn, Mrs Priscilla **(SLP)**
Sandler, Mrs Marcia G **(SLP)**
Sepe, Mrs Barbara C **(SLP)**

Woodhaven
Cram, Janet Ellen **(SLP)**
Schmidt, Elizabeth Anne **(SLP)**
Severance, Mrs Maria Dispenzier
Taylor, Diane M **(A)**

Woodmere
Bizoza, Stuart Lee **(SLP)**
Carp, Mrs Jane R **(SLP)**
Davis, Leslie Faye **(SLP)**
Eichler, Mrs Estelle Miller **(SLP)**
Gershwin, Mrs Dolores R **(SLP)**
Kaplan, Mrs Joan R **(SLP)**
Kaplowitz, Mrs Lotte T **(A)**
Karkowsky, Faith G **(SLP A)**
Monin, Stacey Schlaff **(SLP)**
Robbins, Dr Myra G **(SLP A)**
Rom, Mrs Anita Block **(SLP)**
Rotter, Dr Paul **(A)**
Schneider, Barbara Ann **(SLP)**
Shomberg, Mrs Jane Ellen **(SLP)**

Woodridge
Gagliardo, Mrs Jill Levy **(SLP)**

Woodsburgh
Arker, Dina **(SLP)**

Woodside
Barile, Veronica Maria **(SLP)**
Garvin-Cullen, Allison J **(SLP)**
Melcer, Martin P **(SLP)**
Riffkin, Constance B **(SLP)**
Rothstein, Lisa Ilene

Woodstock
Jamison, Gayle **(SLP)**

Worcester
Lewis, Kathryn Carroll **(SLP)**

Wurtsboro
Doyle, Carmela Christine **(SLP)**

Yonkers
Bengston, Susan D **(SLP)**
Birkmann, Mrs Mildred Harnett **(SLP)**
Conte, Rosemarie
Csicsay, Mrs Katalin M **(SLP)**
D'Amico, Josephine **(SLP)**
Davis, Mrs Pota J **(SLP)**
De Gomez, Elizabeth A M **(SLP)**
Digilio, Mrs Carolyn A **(SLP)**
Eckerle, Mrs Andrea Rauso **(SLP)**

Egan, Kathleen A **(SLP)**
Elkan, Mrs Mindy C R **(SLP)**
Farrell, Gina L **(SLP)**
Gross-Handler, Mrs Iris Beth **(SLP)**
Haughton, Norma E **(SLP)**
Hernandez, Paloma Izquierdo **(SLP)**
Ivankovic, Susan E L **(SLP)**
Josephson, Mrs Judith A **(SLP)**
Katz, Melanie W **(A)**
Levine, Irma L **(SLP)**
McCarthy, Mrs Bridget S **(SLP)**
Nemetz, Tobyann **(SLP)**
Nevers, Maxine Lorraine **(A)**
Plaut, Joyce Felice **(SLP)**
Sadarangani, Karin Lee
Seda, Mrs Susan Tavernia **(SLP)**
Tantillo, Mary W **(SLP)**
Thompson, Lea M **(SLP)**
Villano, Dorothy Marie **(SLP)**
Vitaglione, Mrs Joanne S **(SLP)**
Walsh, Patricia **(SLP)**
Weiner, Mrs Regina I P **(SLP)**
Wilson, Mrs Theresa S **(SLP)**
Winokur, Mrs Irene Synnott **(SLP A)**
Wolf, Mrs Adrienne Ollendorf **(SLP)**

Yorkshire
Hanney, Mrs Elizabeth A **(SLP)**

Yorktown Heights
Cohn, Gail Cartenuto **(SLP)**
Coppel, Miriam L **(A)**
Ehrenfreund, Joseph **(SLP)**
Finsmith, Nancy B **(SLP)**
Galeotti, Mrs Lorraine M **(A)**
Giordano, Mrs Ellen Angela **(SLP)**
Leslie, Mrs Susan P **(SLP)**
Rosenthal, Felice Marsha **(SLP)**
Schlosser, Joan E **(SLP)**
Schutzbank, Myrna P **(SLP)**
Seiden, Lea F **(SLP)**
Taylor, Lynda Kay **(SLP)**

Youngstown
Metke, Debra L **(SLP)**

NORTH CAROLINA

Aberdeen
MacMillan, Dana Lillian **(A)**
McLeod, Mrs Susan Seagroves **(SLP)**
Tuomala, Mrs Kathleen A **(A)**

Advance
May, Dr Jo Whitten **(SLP)**
Meader, Diane D **(SLP)**
Money, Merrie R **(SLP)**
Rhyne, Mrs Lauren Clarkson **(SLP)**
Steelman, Mrs Anna A **(SLP)**

Ahoskie
Brown, Dr Arthur **(SLP)**
Camper, Tina Karen **(SLP)**
Hobbs, Mrs Linda Harrell **(SLP A)**
Jackson, Patricia Carol **(SLP)**
Mileur, Mari C **(SLP)**

Albemarle
Patterson, Mrs Merry Watson

Almond
Duven, Mrs Channa Gae **(SLP)**

Andrews
Hall, Mrs Valerie Marie **(SLP)**

Apex
Blackley, Mrs Lynn G **(SLP)**
Faherty, Monica A **(SLP)**
Johnson, Gloria J **(SLP)**
Meiburg, Mrs Diane Sanderson **(SLP)**
Plymale, Mrs Judy D **(SLP A)**
Swerzenski, Mrs Davi-Ann Hunter **(SLP)**

Arden
Corn, Sharon K **(SLP)**

Parobek, Susan Elizabeth **(SLP)**
Scott, William C **(SLP)**
Young, Mrs Revonda W **(SLP)**

Asheboro
Brown, Jane L Wommack **(SLP)**
Garcia, Mrs Morrine Moody **(SLP)**
Gehlhausen, Pamela Sue **(SLP)**
Gilmer, Mrs Joanna Hudgins **(SLP)**
Trogdon, Mrs Laura Harris **(SLP)**

Asheville
Allen, Kimberlee M
Baker, Lynn S **(SLP)**
Barker, David James **(SLP)**
Barker, Mrs Francine P **(SLP)**
Bennett, Mrs Janet M **(SLP)**
Berger, Mrs Mary B **(SLP)**
Brackett, Vanessa **(SLP)**
Coppedge, Mrs Lynn F **(SLP)**
Cox-Andrews, Helen Kaye **(SLP)**
Craig, Dr Rebecca Sue **(SLP)**
Dover, Mrs Crystal C **(SLP)**
Earle, Cynthia B **(SLP A)**
Germano, Donna M **(SLP)**
Ghandour, Leila A **(SLP)**
Grant, Mrs Janet Minner **(A)**
Leblanc, Marcelle Catherine **(SLP)**
Litton, Mrs Ellen Freeman **(SLP)**
MacPherson, Dr Robert H **(SLP A)**
Martin, Le'Ann L **(SLP)**
Miller, Yolanda E **(SLP)**
Muffley, Mrs Charlotte **(SLP)**
Mulligan, Margo McKay **(SLP)**
Musselwhite, Dr Caroline R **(SLP)**
Neeriemer, William R **(SLP)**
Nichols, Teresa Jane
Parrish, Mary Anne **(SLP)**
Queen, Laurie Ann **(SLP)**
Rider, John Milton **(SLP)**
Robinson, Mrs Norma Lou **(SLP)**
Rose, Shannon E **(SLP)**
Schwandes, Jean K **(SLP)**
Shore, Gretchen Lubov **(SLP)**
Small, Stacy A **(SLP)**
Teich, Laurie **(SLP)**
Thompson, Mrs Ruth Anne **(A)**
Woerl, Dr Mary L **(SLP)**
Wolfe, Cheryl L **(SLP)**

Ayden
Nipple, Mrs Donna Alligood **(SLP)**
Smith, Mrs Martha L **(SLP)**

Bahama
Downs, Mrs Debra B **(SLP)**

Bailey
Pittman, Mrs Frankie L **(SLP)**

Banner Elk
Cody, Patsy Davis

Beaufort
Ferrell, Elizabeth Bowman **(SLP)**
Malone, Dr James Charles **(A)**

Belhaven
Smith, Roberta Leigh **(SLP)**

Belmont
Pope, Mrs Denise L **(SLP)**

Benson
Hampton, Virginia Feldick **(SLP)**
Jones, Andrea Andrews **(A)**

Bethel
Walker, Mrs Marianna Morris **(SLP)**

Black Mountain
Swanson, Susan Denise **(A)**

Blanch
Roberts, Marilyn Baugham **(SLP)**

Blowing Rock
Blust, Mrs Cynthia Boyd **(SLP)**
Loftin, Mrs Joni Grey **(SLP)**

Boone
Carpenter, Mrs Jessie Lou **(SLP)**
Culatta, Dr Richard A **(SLP)**
English, Joy **(SLP)**
Franklin, Bruce William **(A)**
Harris, Dr Timothy B **(SLP)**
Hockaday, Rebecca Carol **(SLP)**
Hubbard, Dr Kenneth A **(SLP)**
Hubbard, Mrs Lynn R **(SLP)**
Hutchinson, Edward C **(SLP)**
Kite, Robert H
Lieberman, Dr R Jane **(SLP)**
Mattox, Katrina Ann **(SLP)**
Meador, Joan **(SLP)**
Meador, Dr Millard M **(A)**
Michael, Ann **(SLP)**
Parker Chapman, Mrs Susan B **(SLP)**
Talley, Ron Claire **(SLP)**
Warren, Mrs Bliss Hemric **(SLP)**
Widenhouse, Betty Lynn **(SLP)**

Brevard
Johnson, Mrs Judith Callan **(A)**
Polmanteer, Mrs Kathryn N **(SLP)**

Bryson City
Pedersen, Mrs Elizabeth Dickson **(SLP)**

Burlington
Beaman, Kimberly Elaine **(SLP)**
Faucette, Mrs Janet E **(SLP)**
Joseph, Thomas S **(A)**
Loy, Mrs Carla Fogleman **(SLP)**
Manning, Mrs Susan Slack **(SLP)**
McCollum, Diane Elaine
Reinhartsen, Debra A **(SLP)**
Smith, Donna W **(SLP)**

Burnsville
Christon, Mrs Michele **(SLP)**
Holland, Judi A

Butner
Upchurch, Naida S **(A)**

Camden
Westrup, Mrs Linda L **(SLP)**

Camp Lejeune
Kasselmann, Mrs Amanda Bennett **(SLP)**

Candler
Simpson, Brenda Gail

Canton
Caldwell, Sherrie Delores

Carrboro
Gaitros, Mrs Sonita Sue **(SLP)**
Khan, Susan Antaki **(SLP)**
Schuele, Clare Melanie **(SLP)**

Cary
Bartoli-Izquierdo, Mrs Paula **(SLP)**
Cesnik, Mrs Sharon Doyle **(SLP)**
Chaney, Amy M **(SLP)**
Cox, Mrs Robbie Rice **(SLP)**
Devine, Nancy F **(SLP)**
Gouge, Mrs Cynthia G **(SLP)**
Gracie, Georgie C **(SLP)**
Jochem, Macie J **(SLP)**
Kaye, Helen Donaldson **(SLP)**
Koerner, Mrs Susanne L **(SLP)**
Matthews, Karen Bettina **(A)**
McNeillie, Mrs Lynn K **(SLP)**
Overly, Mrs Patricia Hargett **(SLP)**
Pachura, Mrs Cristie W **(SLP)**
Perry, Mrs Carolyn S **(SLP)**
Showers, Mrs Drusilla Ramsay **(SLP)**
Stone, Mary F **(SLP)**
Tinsley-Teague, Mrs Louanne **(SLP)**
Ware, Mrs Victoria Topp **(SLP)**
Willard, Mrs Helen Nelson **(SLP)**

Cashiers
Baker, Mrs Marcia T **(SLP)**

Castle Hayne
Jenkins, Carol **(SLP)**
Moore, Alan Gregg

Chadbourn
Bullock, Michele Koenig **(SLP)**
Weaver, Mrs Julia Cartrette **(SLP)**

Chapel Hill
Allred, Julia D **(SLP)**
Barrett-Ensby, Cherilyn **(SLP)**
Brown, Martha B **(SLP)**
Bruton, Debbie S **(A)**
Butler, Estella Denise **(SLP)**
Carroll, Mrs Anita Matthews **(A)**
Carter, Sara C **(SLP)**
Clifford, Virginia Varner **(SLP)**
Crais, Dr Elizabeth R **(SLP)**
Crissey, Joan Florence **(SLP)**
Dalston, Eileen T **(SLP)**
Dalston, Dr Rodger M **(SLP)**
Didow, Sharon M **(SLP)**
Fennimore, Pauline **(A)**
Gral, Elizabeth J **(SLP)**
Greeson, Mrs Patty Dorsett **(SLP)**
Groder, Raquel Strauss
Hall, Dr Joseph W **(A)**
Harrison, Melody F **(SLP)**
Haythorn, Dr Mark M **(A)**
Heller, James H **(SLP)**
Henderson, Mrs Pamela Jackson **(SLP)**
Kegg, Stephen Earl **(SLP)**
Knebel, Karlene **(SLP)**
Lesesne, Mrs Jean P **(SLP)**
Lineberger, Susan Todd **(SLP)**
Lubker, Dr Bobbie B **(SLP)**
Ludington, Harriet Jane R **(SLP)**
Mahaffey, Dr Robert B **(SLP)**
Martinkosky, Dr Stanley J **(SLP)**
Mason, Dr Robert M **(SLP)**
McCallum, James T, Jr **(A)**
McDonald-Bell, Connie R **(SLP)**
McGill, Mrs Haley P **(A)**
Mims, Sarah S **(SLP)**
Mount, Marianne **(SLP)**
Paxson, Traci Meadows
Peters, Robert W **(SLP A)**
Puffenberger, Beth Larue **(A)**
Repass, Mrs Grace S **(SLP)**
Ringwalt, Sharon S **(SLP)**
Roberts, Dr Joanne Erwick **(SLP A)**
Roush, Dr Jackson **(A)**
Roush, Patricia A **(A)**
Saleeby, Nancy C W **(SLP)**
Spencer, Nancy B **(SLP)**
Stewart, Andrew P **(A)**
Stitsinger, Gretchen **(SLP)**
Swank, Phyllis M **(SLP)**
Thresher, Mrs Jill C **(SLP)**
Warren, Dr Donald William
Yoder, David E **(SLP)**

Charlotte
Armstrong, Sharon Kay **(SLP)**
Arrington, Mrs Roberta Barker **(A)**
Badman, Arlene Luberoff **(SLP)**
Bartels, David D **(A)**
Bashor, Pamela H **(SLP)**
Beam, Mrs Mary P **(SLP)**
Bender, Mrs Kathleen O **(SLP)**
Berniard, Terry Peterson **(SLP)**
Beverly-Walker, Amy S **(SLP)**
Bible, Judith Anne **(A)**
Binford, Kimberly Sue **(SLP)**
Bingler, Mrs Julie Lentz **(SLP)**
Bivens, Cathy Ann **(SLP)**
Bledsoe, Mrs Vicki Lynn **(SLP)**
Bynum, Donald F **(A)**
Clontz, Mrs Connie Rae **(SLP A)**
Cole, Dorothy C **(SLP)**
Conrad, Marybeth S **(A)**
Cox, Edith Lynne **(A)**
Crosby, Cynthia Pamela **(SLP)**

Culler, Ted A **(SLP)**
Darr, Claudia E **(A)**
Davidson, Mrs Deborah S **(SLP)**
Denson, Anna Haines **(SLP)**
Domenico, Debbie Lee **(SLP)**
Dornbusch, Mrs Deborah Swartz **(SLP)**
Dowd, Kathryn R **(A)**
Doyle, Julieanne M **(SLP)**
Drum, Markel K **(SLP A)**
Erickson, Eleanor R **(SLP)**
Evans, Diane **(SLP)**
Faires, Joan W **(SLP)**
Fastenau, Julianna **(SLP)**
Fedor, Karen Hardin **(SLP)**
Felton, Mrs Louise Black **(SLP)**
Foushee, Mrs Deborah Dawson **(SLP)**
Gardner, Donna H **(SLP)**
Gissy, Marie Clare **(SLP)**
Goddard, Linda Renee **(SLP)**
Graham, Frank Richard, Jr **(SLP)**
Grese, Carolyn A **(SLP)**
Griffith, Elizabeth **(SLP)**
Groover, Mrs Nancy D **(SLP)**
Hannan-Merwin, Mrs Mary Frances **(SLP)**
Hanson, Donna M **(SLP)**
Heitman, Dr Frederick **(SLP)**
Helms, Deborah D **(A)**
Henderlite, Mrs Patricia B **(SLP)**
Henry, Bonnie S **(SLP)**
Highfill, Melanie K
Hill, Rosemary A **(SLP)**
Hood, Amelia Toland **(SLP)**
Howell, Mrs Alison Shoulars **(SLP)**
Hudson, Mrs Judith T **(SLP)**
Hunter, James L **(A)**
Jeffries, Judith Ann **(A)**
Johnstone, Mrs Carol M **(SLP)**
Kelly, Mrs Louise Ellen **(SLP)**
Kibler, Janice Marie **(SLP)**
Kidd, Danielle O **(A)**
Kirby, Kristy A **(SLP)**
Kirkland, James Wade **(A)**
Kirschner, Mrs Ellyn Goodman **(SLP)**
Kirschner, Neil L **(SLP)**
Klockenkemper, Barbara Anne **(SLP)**
Knott, Margaret R **(SLP)**
Kosuda, Mrs Maria A **(SLP)**
Kuhn, Marilynn Harvit **(SLP)**
Lancaster, Leslie Ann **(A)**
Langdon, Frances P **(SLP)**
Law, Mrs Lyana L S **(SLP A)**
Lay, Deborah Anne **(SLP)**
LeDoux, Leonelle M **(SLP)**
Leister, Mrs Catherine M **(SLP)**
Liljefors, Janet Lee **(SLP)**
Lockhart, Sarah K **(SLP)**
Logan, Robert A **(SLP)**
Lohsen, Brenda W **(SLP)**
Lucas, Mary Anne L **(SLP)**
Lybrand, Roberta H **(SLP)**
Mack, Janne Himes **(A)**
Mann, Karen Eileen **(SLP)**
May, Mrs Thomasena Glover **(SLP)**
McCorkel, Mrs Stephanie Lynn **(SLP)**
McLean, Linda B **(SLP)**
Miller, Victoria H **(A)**
Monroe, Cynthia E **(SLP)**
Montali, Phyllis M **(SLP)**
Nadler, Mrs Suzanne Smith **(SLP)**
Nelli, Jean Marie **(SLP)**
Ogden, Mrs Brenley A **(SLP)**
Olson, Anne Desmarais **(A)**
Olynick, Mrs Miriam Smoot **(A)**
Parker, Anna L **(SLP)**
Phipps, Mrs Pamela P **(SLP)**
Rabon, Mrs Donna Switzer **(SLP)**
Rasner, Mrs Janine Dee
Richter, Mrs Ellen Wilcox **(SLP)**
Roland, Nancy M L **(SLP)**
Ruane, Mrs Ruth Schalk **(SLP)**
Rutledge, Cynthia Lynn **(SLP)**
Shelton, Mrs Diane Welsh **(SLP)**
Siragusa, Mrs Susan Marie **(SLP)**
Smaston, Mrs Sharon **(SLP)**
Smith, Mrs Gina Lynne **(SLP)**
Smith, Sharon Elaine **(SLP)**
Snead, Sarah Ann
Snow, Mrs Katherine L **(SLP)**
Stiles, Cynthia L **(SLP)**
Strom, Mary Patrice **(SLP)**
Sullivan, Mrs Rosemary **(SLP)**
Tabler, Tana Lynn **(SLP)**
Taff, Mrs Janet H **(A)**
Taylor, Mrs Jane E **(SLP)**
Thomas, Angella Hough
Thomas, Jayne F **(SLP)**
Thomson, Caroline E **(SLP)**
Todd, Linda I **(SLP)**
Tomei, Mrs Robin A **(SLP)**
Treacy, Margaret M **(SLP)**
Tuck, April E **(SLP)**
Tucker, Mrs Debra Bales **(SLP)**
Umphlett, Marianne Parsons **(SLP)**
Wernikoff, Mrs Esta Ross **(SLP)**
Whirledge, Rosemary A **(SLP)**
Wilkes, Elizabeth Reid **(SLP)**
Williams, Sandra Fay **(SLP)**
Yett, Judith Amend **(SLP)**

Cherryville
Markland, Sandra Hill **(SLP)**

Clemmons
Dickey, Mrs Claire W **(SLP A)**
Evans, Karen Kathleen **(SLP)**
Harless, Mrs Vivian A **(SLP A)**
Nicholas, Marlee W **(SLP)**
Parra, Mrs Anne Sullivan **(SLP)**
Pittaway, Carmel I **(SLP)**

Clinton
Carroll, Kathy Lynn **(SLP)**
Hudson, Mrs Nellie H **(SLP)**

Clyde
Swift, Kaye Armstrong **(SLP)**

Columbus
Scott, Duncan R **(SLP A)**

Concord
Boger, Jennie L **(SLP)**
Carpenter, Susan Annette **(SLP)**
Fink, Joy Elizabeth
Foard, Mrs Donna S **(SLP)**
Linker, Mrs Barbara Jean **(SLP)**
Seaford, Nancy I **(SLP)**
Sellers, Clarence **(SLP A)**

Cullowhee
Alt, Patricia E **(SLP)**
Baxley, Mary Beth **(SLP)**
Bowers, Mrs Linda Sandusky **(SLP)**
Collins, Mrs Susan H **(SLP)**
Colville, Mrs Mary B **(SLP)**
Core, Nancy Reighley **(A)**
Loeffler, Dr Donald Lee **(SLP)**
Saddler, Mrs Yvonne N **(SLP)**
Shapiro, Dr David A **(SLP)**
Smith, Dr Michael Douglas **(SLP)**

Dallas
Nutter-Will, Mrs Debra Jean **(SLP)**
Will, Virginia Laurence **(SLP)**

Danbury
Ring, Mrs Karen Overby **(SLP)**

Davidson
Hampton, Mrs Louise P **(SLP)**

Deep Gap
Clark, Beverly Anne **(SLP)**
Dirr, Susan **(SLP)**

Drexel
Hollifield, Laura Jan **(SLP)**
Junkins,, Robert William, Jr **(SLP)**

Durham
Aarons, Marlene **(SLP)**
Abernathy, Susan Gower **(SLP)**
Baldwin, Mrs Rachel Anne **(SLP)**
Blumhagen-Gill, Anne L **(SLP)**
Casey, Karen Marie **(SLP)**
Chase, Mrs Karen Nailling **(SLP)**
Chase, Michele **(SLP)**
Clark, Jo-Anna P **(SLP)**
Clayton, Mrs Elizabeth Patterson **(SLP)**
Constable, Anne Parnell **(SLP)**
Crabb, Mrs Carol S **(SLP)**
Duskey, Mrs Janet East **(SLP)**
Fitzwilliam, Mrs Heather M **(SLP)**
Gage, Rhea Jacobson **(A)**
Gibson, Terrie Denise **(SLP)**
Hatch, Debora R **(A)**
Hawk, Del Lynn **(A)**
Hogenkamp, Margaret Angelina **(SLP)**
Holland, Mrs Luanne G **(SLP)**
Horner, Dr Jennifer **(SLP)**
Jackson, Sandra Michelle **(SLP)**
King, Burton B **(A)**
Knobeloch, Dr F X Calvin **(SLP A)**
Korman, Rebecca B **(SLP)**
Kunze, Dr Luvern H **(SLP)**
Lambright, Laura G **(A)**
Layton, Dr Thomas L **(SLP)**
Leach, Mrs Carol N **(SLP)**
Liberty, Dr Timothy D **(SLP)**
Lochman, Mrs Linda K Bauwens **(SLP)**
Logue, Mrs Barbara H **(SLP)**
Lucas, Minnie B **(SLP)**
Mack, Karolyn J **(SLP)**
Mangum, Mrs Susan B **(A)**
McMullen, Catherine Therese **(SLP)**
Mirrett, Penny L **(SLP)**
Paul, Dr Robert G **(A)**
Quick, Gloria G **(SLP)**
Riski, Dr John E **(SLP)**
Robinson, Michael T **(SLP)**
Rush, Mrs Elizabeth S **(SLP)**
Scharver, Mrs M Candice **(SLP)**
Shade, Mrs Teresa Ellis **(SLP)**
Simpson, Bessie C **(SLP)**
Stephans, Kathy Hurst **(SLP)**
Talley, Dr James N **(A)**
Terry, Anne C **(SLP)**
Waddell, Jill **(SLP)**
Watson, Jennie Sexton **(SLP)**
Weber, Dr Bruce Arthur **(A)**
Wells, Mrs Althea Boston **(SLP)**
Witherspoon, Ann R **(SLP)**

Eden
Eackles, Jay Donald **(A)**
Harrold, Mrs Starr S **(SLP)**

Elizabeth City
Caldwell, Helen M **(SLP)**
Green, Dr Lois W **(SLP)**
Hartman, Kathy L **(SLP)**
Lamorte, Mrs Frances B **(SLP)**
Sword, Valerie Ann **(SLP)**
Taylor, Phyllis Arlene **(SLP)**
White, Margaret C **(SLP)**

Elkin
Barrie-Blackley, Sandie **(SLP)**

Fayetteville
Addison, Tina Marie **(SLP)**
Anderson, Linda Christine **(SLP)**
Armstrong, Debra J **(SLP)**
Axtell, Sherri Lee **(SLP)**
Bergeron, Sena M **(A)**
Boutte-Chambers, Mrs Janice S **(SLP)**
Burrows, Evelyn H **(SLP)**
Carnes, Patricia B **(SLP)**
Carter, Mrs Cynthia Janelle **(SLP)**
Craycraft, Constance Taylor **(SLP)**
Danzeisen, Nancy B **(SLP)**
Dewar, Mrs Sally Rule **(SLP)**
Evans, Susan A **(A)**
Faulkner, Angela Hammond **(SLP)**
Fitzsimmons, Laurie Ann **(A)**
Garber, Mrs Tammy Brooks **(A)**
Gore, Dr Larry B **(A)**
Gottardi, Donna L **(SLP)**
Green, Brenda
Griffiths, Cecilia Marie **(SLP)**
Hardesty-Pittard, Mrs Judith L **(SLP)**
Hill, Desdy Joforeka **(SLP)**
Husted, Mrs Valerie Lynne **(SLP)**
Jenuwine, Karen Jean **(SLP)**
Kemerling, Julie Ann **(SLP)**
Little, Marilyn D **(SLP)**
Lowsky, Debra C **(SLP)**
Lubell, Patricia A **(SLP)**
Lukat, R Michael **(A)**
Mangum, Mrs Connie West **(SLP)**
Matzinger, Darcy **(SLP)**
Owens, Byron **(SLP A)**
Powers, Alice G **(SLP)**
Ralph, Dawn Marie **(SLP)**
Ricker, Stephanie Anne **(A)**
Rierson, Mrs Patricia Louise **(SLP)**
Shuler-Scott, Carolyn Anita **(SLP)**
Sibbett, Kathy Sheridan **(SLP)**
Sibley, Mrs Kathryn H **(SLP)**
Stephens, James F **(A)**
Stewart, Brenda Lou **(SLP)**
Taylor, Catherine Rose **(A)**
Toler, Joyce Marie **(SLP)**
Williams, Maj Dennis L **(A)**

Fletcher
Merrell, Mrs Mary Bishop **(SLP)**

Forest City
Talley, Frank James **(SLP)**
Tarlton, Mrs Tina S **(A)**

Fort Bragg
Beaver, Mrs Jennifer Bennett **(A)**

Fountain
Irvin, Howard Van **(SLP)**

Franklin
Bruton, Mrs Cynthia Lee **(SLP)**
Cabe, Patricia M **(SLP)**

Franklinton
Burrell-Griffin, Jane **(SLP)**
Gogarty-Gajan, Kathleen R **(SLP)**

Fremont
Corwin, Carole **(SLP)**

Fuquay-Varina
Lindsay, Mrs Nadean F **(SLP)**
Sorrels, Lynne Walker **(SLP)**
Wallace, Mrs Debora Hamilton **(SLP)**

Garner
Furlough, Cynthia L **(SLP)**
Hicks, Loretta A **(SLP)**
Irons, Susan K **(SLP)**
Johnson, Mrs Maryann Shields **(SLP)**
Maddry, Ellen Ann **(SLP)**
Patton, Mrs Laura Lee **(SLP)**

Gastonia
Ratliff, Dr Sandra Sue **(SLP A)**
Simpson, Jane L W **(A)**

Glade Valley
Caldwell, Mrs Katy E **(SLP)**

Goldsboro
Angelo, Victor M **(SLP)**
Butcher, Joanie Siverston **(SLP)**
Butler, Mrs Ida Canady
Daniels, Larose S **(SLP)**
Darden, Celia Parker **(SLP)**
Dennler, Mrs Debra J **(SLP)**
McCall, Gerard A **(SLP A)**
McCall, Mrs Nancy Demeter **(SLP)**
Pearson, Mrs Patricia C **(A)**
Rogers, Sheila Kathleen **(SLP)**
Rowe, Mrs Barbara Munnerlyn **(SLP)**

Snodgress, Kathleen L **(SLP)**
Stone, Dr Mary Ann **(SLP A)**
Taylor, Mrs Brenda K **(SLP)**
Vail, Florence Cameron **(SLP)**
White, James Clyde, III **(SLP)**
White, Mrs Lisa Annette **(SLP)**

Graham
Capps, Mrs Ruby Ann **(SLP)**
Coleman, Patsy Pierce **(SLP)**
Gray, Susan G
Stoehr, Roxanne Wright **(SLP)**

Greensboro
Alexander, Marcia L **(SLP)**
Ambro, Mrs Lilli Moore **(SLP)**
Amos, Mrs Bonnie W **(SLP)**
Avent, Fayma L H **(SLP)**
Ball, Mrs Joyce S **(SLP)**
Beasley, Mrs Jean L **(SLP A)**
Berlin, Melanie Ann **(A)**
Boner, Mrs Maureen Maney **(SLP)**
Bonner, Sheri Nelson **(SLP)**
Brown, Mrs Donna J R **(SLP)**
Browning, Tammy Kim
Burks, Cheryl Lynn **(SLP)**
Carroll, Mrs Deborah Elliott **(A)**
Carter, Anna Y P **(SLP)**
Causby, Ralph E **(A)**
Chappell, Pamela A **(SLP)**
Chastain, Mrs Alice Veach **(A)**
Cheshire, Mrs Margie G **(SLP)**
Clenseur, Mrs Jane MacLeod **(SLP)**
Clontz, Kimberly B
Compton, Mary V **(SLP)**
Cook, George R, Jr **(A)**
Cunningham, Mrs Judith Harber **(SLP)**
Davis, Sherri Allred **(A)**
Delagrange, Teryl N **(A)**
Dixon, Dr Richard F **(SLP A)**
Earle, Dr Floyd E **(SLP)**
Earle, Dr Patty A **(SLP)**
Edwards, Mrs Colette M **(SLP)**
Flinn, Mrs Mary Perkins **(SLP)**
Flynn, Perry F **(SLP)**
Foster, Wayne A **(SLP A)**
Froelich, Cathy Dianne **(SLP)**
Gayler, Rebecca R **(SLP)**
Gordon, Mrs Margaret O **(SLP)**
Graff, Cordelia Dahl **(SLP)**
Gravley, Patricia M **(SLP)**
Hawkes, Mrs Cynthia H **(SLP)**
Hay, Mrs Bonnie W **(SLP)**
Hornfelt, Lori M **(SLP)**
Hudson, Diane Lorraine **(SLP)**
Ingels, Ginger L
Jeffrey, Mrs Judith Lynn **(SLP)**
Jirsa, Dr Robert E **(A)**
Jobe, Mrs Ruth B H **(SLP)**
Jones, Karen E **(SLP)**
Jones, Ronda Diane
Jones, William Dixon **(A)**
Kerr, Mrs Miriam G **(SLP)**
Kingsley, Mrs Georgia F **(SLP)**
Koehler, Gwen Ensley **(SLP)**
Krikorian, Carol Ann **(SLP)**
Leland, Leslie Culbertson **(SLP)**
Lewandowski, Deborah Lynne **(A)**
Long, Karen Dene **(SLP)**
Lucente, Maria Frances **(SLP)**
McCraw, Virginia L **(SLP)**
McLaughlin, Diane Jean
McWilliams, Mrs Maren L **(SLP)**
Montefusco, Mrs Marta Baucom **(SLP A)**
Newton, Dr Mariana **(SLP)**
Pahel, Carey W **(A)**
Patterson, Mrs Linda Lee
Perkins, Mrs Charlotte **(SLP)**
Powers, Joyce S **(SLP)**
Prater, Dr Rex Joe **(SLP)**
Raleigh, Mrs Louise Ferguson **(SLP)**
Reynolds, Mrs Jerri Bolling **(SLP)**
Richardson, Claretta C **(SLP A)**
Robbins, Mrs Rosalyn J **(SLP)**
Robinson, Sarah Barham **(SLP)**
Robson, Mrs Nancy L **(SLP)**
Rodman, Mrs Martha Fitzsimmon
Salvin, Bernice Y **(SLP)**
Seaton, Kay P **(SLP)**
Sexton, Johnnie E **(A)**
Shepard, Linda J **(SLP)**
Sligh, Julie Elizabeth **(SLP)**
Smith, Jill Pierce **(SLP)**
Smith, Nancy Edwards
Southall, Julia M **(SLP)**
Strong, Dr Jacqueline C **(SLP)**
Swift, Roger W **(SLP A)**
Tebow, Mrs Laura S **(SLP)**
Thomas-Pender, Lori Jean **(SLP)**
Torney, Catherine **(SLP)**
Warner, Janice Holmes **(A)**
Willitts, Rebecca L **(SLP)**
Womack, Audrey Faye **(SLP)**

Greenville
Allen, Jo Ann **(SLP)**
Bengala, Mrs Deborah E **(SLP)**
Bremer, Mrs Barbara Waaland **(SLP)**
Davis, Jacquelyn Irene **(SLP)**
Demarco, Salvatore **(SLP)**
Dixon, Mrs Martha M **(SLP)**
Downes, Mrs Meta M **(SLP)**
Dupree, Tammy Richelle **(SLP)**
Flynt, Cynthia Roberts **(SLP)**
Fratzke, Melvin L **(SLP A)**
Gay, Helen Kemp **(SLP)**
Givens, Dr Gregg D **(A)**
Graham, Mrs Caryl A **(A)**
Grantham, Mary Linda **(SLP)**
Hale, Mrs Dianne Louise **(SLP)**
Hicks, Mrs Alison F **(SLP)**
Hough, Dr Monica S **(SLP)**
Hume, Dr William G **(A)**
Johnson, George William, III **(SLP A)**
Joyner, Rhonda H **(A)**
McCabe, Robert B **(SLP)**
McFall, Mrs Bonnie Lois **(SLP)**
Moore, Sharon L **(SLP)**
Muzzarelli, Robert A **(SLP A)**
Preston, Stuart R **(SLP)**
Royals, Mrs Waverlyn Jones **(SLP)**
Shine, Dr Richard E **(SLP)**
Speier, Nancy E **(SLP)**
Stevenson, Mrs Marina Lynch **(SLP)**
Taylor, Barbara Berry **(SLP)**
Whitehurst, Jeanette L **(SLP)**

Grimesland
Phillips, Mrs Paula Brady **(SLP)**

Halifax
Williams, Mrs Ruth T **(SLP)**

Hampstead
Rand, Mrs Diane J **(SLP)**

Harrisburg
Kramer, Mrs Julie Miller **(SLP)**
Marcum, Mrs Terry D **(SLP)**

Havelock
Piech, Mrs Sharon C **(SLP)**

Haw River
Pennington, Mrs Elisabeth Bulla **(SLP)**

Hazelwood
Franklin, Sara Scruggs **(SLP)**

Henderson
Cyrus, Sandra A **(SLP)**

Hendersonville
Caserio, Marcia B **(SLP)**
Hirshburg, Mrs Sandra Tanner **(SLP A)**
Jameson, Mrs Joyce Eileen **(SLP)**
Kenzik, Mark Anthony **(A)**
Perella, Karen D **(SLP)**

Hickory
Allred, Mrs Patricia Choate **(SLP)**
Brown, Donna M **(SLP)**
Cannupp, Mrs Kathryn E **(SLP)**
Fletcher, Gordon L **(A)**
Heater-Lohrman, Mrs Julie Ann **(A)**
Johnson, Mrs Patricia Rhyne
McVay, Maureen Elizabeth **(SLP)**
Miller, James R **(A)**
Neill, Rebecca Ann **(SLP)**
Smith, Judith A **(A)**
White, Mrs Helen A B **(SLP)**

High Point
Brewer, Mrs Mary L M **(SLP)**
Clegg, Mrs Tina Carter **(SLP)**
Duke, Kathryn **(SLP A)**
Fosnaugh, Steven W **(SLP)**
Hawk, Mrs Eloise B **(SLP)**
House, Jennifer A
Ike, Tami Lee **(A)**
Jay, Dr Robert E **(SLP A)**
Lawrence, Clara Jane **(SLP)**
Meyers, Carol A **(SLP)**
Pope, Mrs Patricia L **(SLP)**
Stirewalt, Tina Marie **(SLP)**
Stonestreet, Rebecca Vernon **(SLP A)**
Williams, Mrs Martha Skerrett **(SLP)**
Wright, Mrs Patricia Boyd **(SLP)**

Highlands
Koepp-Baker, Dr Herbert **(SLP)**

Hillsborough
Ballard, Mrs Dail Daly **(SLP)**
Cameron, Dr Thomas H **(A)**
Mines, Arthur B **(SLP A)**
Parker, Mrs Claire V **(SLP)**
Wolford, Robert David, Jr **(A)**

Holly Ridge
Daughtry, Dr Ginger H **(SLP)**

Hope Mills
Harris, Dr Cheryl **(SLP)**
Taylor, Mrs Esther Ruth **(SLP)**

Horse Shoe
Ashley, Mrs Melinda Varda **(SLP)**

Jacksonville
Amos, Mrs Opal Chavis **(SLP)**
Barham, Mrs Renay Painter **(SLP)**
Benfield, Kathy Jean **(A)**
Choate, Mrs Jane G T **(SLP)**
Taggart, Mrs Leslie A
Taylor, Marcia H **(SLP)**

Jamestown
Scott, Mrs Donna Jean **(SLP)**
Vance, Anne D **(SLP)**

Kannapolis
Austin, Mrs Patricia H **(SLP)**
Cooper, Amy Marie **(A)**
Edscorn, Jane F **(SLP)**
Paolino, Donna S **(A)**

Kenansville
Williamson, Mrs Nancy Alphin **(SLP)**

Kernersville
Eanes, Martha Robinson **(SLP)**
Jordan, Deborah P **(SLP)**

Kill Devil Hills
Rose, Denise Fisher **(SLP)**

King
Nelson, Mrs Hunter McCorkle **(SLP)**

Kinston
Adams, A Barbara **(SLP)**
Bain, Sue McDevett **(A)**
Berry, Mrs Maryann B **(SLP)**
Camp, Kelly MacLeod **(A)**
Collins, Dr Bill M **(SLP)**
Dooling, Jim **(A)**
Galambush, Nancy **(A)**
Glassman, Mrs Harriet C **(SLP)**
Glassman, Joel R **(SLP)**
Griffin, Mrs Wendy N
Lapas, Annette Kuzdenyi **(SLP)**
McCabe, Mary Ann **(SLP)**
Parker, Colette Albritton **(SLP)**
Scott, Mrs Pamela S **(SLP)**
Thomas, Kristi Harbage **(A)**

Kitty Hawk
Ward, Susan Schimmel **(SLP)**

Knightdale
Nichols, Elizabeth **(SLP)**

La Grange
Cobb, Mary Dawn **(SLP)**

Lake Waccamaw
Edens, Kelly A **(SLP)**

Lamberton
Smith, Linda Aldridge **(SLP)**

Laurel Park
Glassman, Connie K **(SLP)**

Laurinburg
Mason, Mrs Lynn M **(SLP)**

Lawndale
Yarboro, Mrs Kay D **(SLP)**

Leland
Blinson, Mrs Sharon Moore **(SLP)**

Lenoir
Hawn, Mrs Debra Greene **(SLP)**
Parmelee-Regittko, Mrs Luann Mary **(SLP)**

Lewisville
Blevins, Mrs Michelle Hampton **(SLP)**
Brown, Dr Catherine S **(SLP)**

Lexington
Fritts, Ann Caron **(SLP)**
Hendren, Mrs Jan Plyler **(SLP)**
Michaud-Patterson, Mrs M **(SLP)**
Shoaf, Mrs Betsy Barber **(SLP)**
Young, Karen W **(SLP)**

Lincolnton
Millwood, Mrs Dessa Hampton **(SLP)**
Packer, Karen Alane **(SLP)**
Smith, Mrs Judy Shaw **(SLP)**

Locust
Austin, Jeannine **(SLP)**

Louisburg
Sledge, Mrs Kim L **(SLP)**

Lumberton
Hammond, Doylena **(SLP)**
Moore, Stacy Jane **(SLP)**
Textor, Mrs Catherine Tedder **(SLP)**
Winchester, Cynthia P **(A)**

Manteo
Baum, Helen C **(SLP)**
Goforth, Mrs Lee S **(SLP)**

Marion
Donahue, Blevin M **(SLP)**
Stewart, Michelle **(SLP)**

Mars Hill
Fields, Mrs Kathryn Ann **(SLP)**
Scruggs, Susan Dianne **(SLP)**

Marshall
Ramsey, Gale Mayhew **(SLP)**

Marshville
Simpson, Mrs Elizabeth **(SLP)**

Matthews
Barbour, Mrs Elaine J **(SLP)**
Buffie, Mrs Sandra Merritt **(SLP)**
Campbell, Mrs Sharon T **(A)**
Escher, Mrs Constance **(SLP)**
Griffith, Mrs Avis B **(SLP)**

Hensley, Betty Harden **(SLP)**
Kopsch, Janet H **(SLP)**
Laverick, Mrs Charlotte Lorraine **(SLP)**
Powell, Mrs Sharon S **(SLP)**
Prevatte, Beverly Elizabeth **(SLP)**
Rockwell, Mrs Amy White **(SLP)**

McLeansville
McCready, Carolyn V **(SLP)**

Mebane
Champion, Cynthia Carter **(SLP)**
Everhart, Katherine **(SLP)**
Norwood, Phyllis Lloyd **(SLP)**

Mill Spring
Pennington, Mrs Sharon Alicia **(SLP)**

Millers Creek
Goodman, Gilbert B, Jr **(SLP)**

Moncure
Fowler, Carolyn Cameron **(SLP)**

Monroe
Dickerson, Janice V **(SLP)**
Eklund, Mrs Tami Hemby **(SLP)**
Hutaff, Mrs Susan East **(SLP)**
McWhorter, Susan Jane

Morehead City
Austin, Mrs Katharine Thorne **(A)**
Laroque, Mrs Roseann T **(SLP)**
Parker, Martha V **(SLP)**

Morganton
Bartholomew, Patrick Cary **(SLP)**
Bergl, Mrs Burkett K **(SLP A)**
Blades, Mrs Janet Hamby **(SLP)**
Brassell, Mrs Esther G **(SLP A)**
Callahan, Edith E Corley **(SLP)**
Clifford, Lucinda A **(SLP)**
Coffey, Geneva J **(SLP)**
Coffey, Thomas S **(A)**
Compton, Gayle Renee **(SLP)**
Ervin, Dr Jean C **(SLP)**
Fox-Helser, Debra E **(SLP)**
Rhame, Leland W **(A)**
Robbie, Marguerite Pryor **(SLP)**
Schlein, Charles M **(SLP)**
Schoeberle, Leesa Jones **(SLP)**
Showman, Rebecca N **(SLP)**
Singleton, Mary K L **(SLP)**
Thompson, Leigh Anne **(SLP)**
Trotter, Alan Norman **(SLP)**
Turowski, Marjorie Roth **(SLP A)**
Walden, Mary Elizabeth **(SLP)**
Whitley, Kenneth P **(SLP)**
Williams, Denise Ann **(SLP)**
Williams, Mrs Jane C
Wooten, Diana Styles **(SLP)**
Wortman-Lowe, Linda **(SLP)**
Yates, Brenda Faye **(SLP)**

Morrisville
Goodwin, Mrs Diana Kay **(SLP)**

Mount Airy
Brewington, Mrs Theresa K **(SLP)**
Cole, Emily M **(SLP)**
Dixon, Emily H **(SLP)**
Smith, Sandra Jean **(SLP)**

Mount Olive
Jernigan, Gina Merle **(SLP)**
Kephart, Beth Casey **(SLP)**
Sutton-Merritt, Mrs Rhonda Jean **(SLP)**

New Bern
Buchanan, Virginia **(SLP)**
Cleland, Mrs Michele Tripp **(A)**
Cowling-Reed, Dr Karen M **(SLP)**
Hall, Mrs Brenda Bullock **(SLP)**
Hall, Terry A **(A)**
Hunter, Deborah Chaney **(SLP)**
Junak, Shelly Ann **(SLP)**
Moffitt, Mrs Peggie Collins **(SLP)**
Perdue, Nancy E **(SLP)**
Venable, Mrs Marsha Butler **(SLP)**

Newport
Farmer, Marian Taylor **(SLP)**
Harrell-Mizerak, Roxanne M **(SLP)**
Simmons, Mrs Ruby Kelly **(SLP)**

North Wilkesboro
Absher, Mrs Fern S **(SLP)**
Goodman, Pamela Jean **(SLP)**
Pruitt, Mrs Lisa Hendrix **(SLP)**
Williams, Frances G

Oak Ridge
Peters, Melissa R **(SLP)**

Otto
Shephard, Mrs Cheryl Lynn **(SLP)**

Pfafftown
Peele, Vicki Noeth **(SLP)**

Pikeville
Costa, Vivian Camille **(SLP)**

Pilot Mountain
Tilley, Mrs Connie Holland **(SLP)**
Wilson, Jaye Stansbury **(SLP)**

Pinehurst
Allison, Mrs Scarlett M **(SLP)**
Offill, Mrs Elinor B **(SLP)**

Pineville
Elkins, Patricia Anne **(SLP)**

Pisgah Forest
Austin, Mrs Lynn Hogsed

Pittsboro
Erhardt, Sandra Dee
Gaines, Mrs Merle B **(SLP)**
Hooper, Dr Celia R **(SLP)**
Webster, Mrs Teri Ellen **(SLP)**
Wilson, Mrs Susan S **(SLP)**

Raleigh
Barker, Nancy Tripp **(SLP)**
Betancourt, Susan Wahl **(SLP)**
Branker, Mrs Cheryl R **(SLP)**
Breedlove, Vickey **(SLP)**
Brinkerhoff, Diane Sue **(SLP)**
Brogden, Mrs Sharon I W **(SLP)**
Brooks, Elizabeth Alicia **(SLP)**
Comer, Sally D **(SLP)**
Cooper, Marie D
Courter, Teresa Marie **(SLP)**
DeJoy, Dr Daniel A **(SLP)**
Denning, Mrs Susan Whitener **(SLP)**
Derrenbacher, Carol Cooke **(SLP)**
Eacho, Mrs Caroline Jones **(SLP)**
Elleman, Mrs Charlotte Ann **(SLP)**
Farrow, Mrs Judy Little **(SLP)**
Folsom, Sarah D **(SLP)**
Gerhard, Mrs Barbara Foreman **(SLP)**
Gibson, Lynda S **(SLP)**
Goulding, Virginia R **(SLP A)**
Hardin, Elisa M **(SLP)**
Harris, Mrs Elizabeth A **(SLP)**
Harris, Mrs Holly F **(SLP)**
Helfrich, Deborah A **(SLP)**
Henson, Mrs Pamela M **(SLP)**
Howard, Mrs Mary Lynn **(SLP)**
Isaacs, Gale Joann
James, Jan Lynnette **(SLP)**
Kaufmann, Mrs Arlene J **(SLP)**
Kramer, Heidi A **(SLP)**
Lansing, Jeanne Georgia **(A)**
Laughlin, Veronica **(SLP)**
Leake, Linda S **(SLP)**
Leslie, Mrs Cynthia M **(SLP)**
Lewis, Dr Harold Donell **(A)**
Little, Julie Arlen **(SLP)**
Matthews, Mrs Ann **(SLP)**
McCormick, Mrs Mary Helen **(SLP)**
McDougal, Cheryl M **(SLP)**
McMillan, Deborah Mosely **(SLP)**
Middendorf, Kathi Ann **(SLP)**
Mills, William David **(SLP)**
Moroge, Mrs Phyllis A **(SLP)**
Morros, Joy S **(A)**
Murray, Mrs Ninevah W **(SLP)**
Murray, Patricia Snow **(SLP)**
Musgrave, Teresa L W **(SLP)**
Nichols, Mrs Cynthia Dawson **(SLP)**
Nychka, Helen B **(SLP)**
O'Donnell, Constance Martello **(SLP)**
Oettinger, Tambrey C **(A)**
Oliver, Lisa Michele
Olson, Nancy Elizabeth **(SLP)**
Perrine, Anne W **(SLP)**
Player, Mrs Marian Gray **(SLP)**
Porter, Dr Patricia B **(SLP)**
Psalidas, Mrs Joyce Y **(SLP)**
Rogister, Stephanie **(SLP)**
Royall, Julia B **(SLP)**
Royster, Dr Julia Doswell **(SLP A)**
Schroeder, Marjorie A **(SLP)**
Simmons, Mrs Marie Vest **(SLP)**
Sorice-Clark, Mary Jo **(SLP)**
Strong, Mrs Nancy A B **(SLP)**
Sullivan, Danita Whitworth **(SLP A)**
Summer, Sheila Jones **(SLP)**
Thomas, Timothy Michael **(SLP)**
Thomas, William G **(A)**
Thompson, Kathleen **(SLP)**
Thornhill, Mrs Fabian G **(A)**
Thurman, Rita D **(SLP)**
Trafton, Judith Anne **(SLP)**
Vogler-Ryan, Sasha **(SLP)**
Wilcomb, Jennifer L **(SLP)**
Williams, Mrs Grace O **(SLP)**
Wilson, Terrie H **(SLP)**
Wright, Bonnie C **(SLP)**

Reidsville
Keeling, Sandra D **(A)**
McMichael, Mrs Shirley O **(SLP)**

Richfield
Poolos, Mrs Hazel P **(SLP)**

Roanoke Rapids
Brightman, William P **(SLP)**
Harp, Bonnie Wilson **(SLP)**

Rockwell
Odom, Tina A **(SLP)**

Rocky Mount
Batts, Kathryn P **(SLP)**
Boone, Susan Michelle **(SLP)**
Dailey, Mrs Vicki C **(SLP)**
Dameron, Mrs Hannah H **(A)**
Galvin, Mrs Michelle Kinley **(SLP)**
Hudson, William E **(A)**
Manning, Kathy Lynn **(SLP)**
Mize, David Lee **(A)**
Ohree, Mrs Nathlyn B **(SLP)**
Shampain, Lisa Plattner **(SLP)**
Webb, Tina Daughtridg **(SLP)**
Winstead, Renee Cannady **(SLP)**

Ronda
Allen, Charlotte Anne **(SLP)**

Roseboro
Walker, Mrs Cathleen Marie Swift **(SLP)**

Roxboro
Carroll, Kathryn B **(SLP)**

Ruffin
Herr, Emma Rose **(SLP)**

Rural Hall
Conner, Mrs Deborah Boyd **(SLP)**
Williams, Betsy M **(SLP)**

Rutherford College
Martinat, Mrs Martha G **(SLP)**

Rutherfordton
Davis, Jill S **(SLP)**
Lane, Susan Melinda **(SLP)**

Salisbury
Black, Mrs Cheryl Sexton **(SLP)**
Calderon, Mrs Judith Roman **(SLP)**
Chaplin, Mrs Ruth T **(SLP)**
Harless, Dr Edwin L **(A)**
Ketner, Mrs Holly C **(SLP)**
Leonard, Kimberly Sue **(SLP)**
Linhart, Julie G **(SLP)**
Moore, Mrs Sylvia Pope **(SLP)**
Mundy, Rosanna McGraw **(SLP)**
Murray-Peterson, Mrs Marilyn Ann **(SLP)**
Robertson, Mrs Cecilia Dianne **(SLP)**
Shannon, Jeanette Manning **(SLP)**

Sanford
Bins-Hattaway, Alice Taylor **(SLP)**
Carraway, Mrs Tonda Pierce **(A)**
Freeman, Francine Carmody **(SLP)**
Stevens, Mrs Sheila Rhodes
Welsh, Richard J **(SLP)**
Williams, Barbara H **(SLP)**

Seagrove
King, Mary Ella **(SLP)**

Shelby
Bagby, Mrs Jill Rebecca G **(SLP)**
Brown-Young, Kay M **(A)**
Eckstein, Karen Lind **(SLP)**
Harrill, Janet Leigh **(SLP)**
Kirby, Mrs Sherry Maddox **(SLP)**
Young, Dr Lamar L, Jr **(A)**

Smithfield
Robinson, Diane C **(SLP)**
Simpson, Mrs Sally Herman **(SLP)**

Southern Pines
Hartman, Katherine L
Jones, Terri Lee **(SLP)**
Thomason, Laura Stephenson **(A)**

Southmont
Pickett, Owena Alston **(SLP)**

Southport
Conrad, G Beth **(SLP)**

Spindale
Hamrick, Mrs Mara C **(SLP)**

Spruce Pine
Baldwin, Laurel R **(SLP)**
Baldwin, Steven J **(SLP)**

Statesville
Bullard, Lynn T **(SLP)**
Falter, Brenda G **(SLP)**
Foster, Mrs Patricia Y Brown **(SLP)**
Howard, Sharon J **(A)**
Parker, Dianne L **(SLP)**
Penland, Mrs Amy K **(SLP)**
Stephens, Ginger R **(SLP)**
Tate, Constance **(SLP)**
Thompson, Catherine Phelps **(SLP)**
Yount, Margery Cameron

Summerfield
Guthrie, Patricia A **(SLP)**
Isaacs, Linda D **(SLP)**
Steele, Mrs Elizabeth **(SLP)**

Swansboro
Gaines, Patricia J **(SLP)**

Sylva
Salyer, Gregory W **(A)**
Sumner, Florence Greis **(SLP)**

Tarawa Terrace
Walsh, Mrs Vanya Su **(SLP)**

Tarboro
Anderson, Elizabeth **(SLP)**
Chapman, Mrs Tina H **(SLP)**

Taylorsville
Hall, Mrs Martha Nadler **(SLP)**

Thomasville
Moore, Mrs Charlotte W **(SLP)**
Prevo, Mrs Cheryl Allen **(SLP)**
Scarboro, Mrs Kim Schirrman **(SLP)**

Tobaccoville
Sebastian, Judith Jackson **(SLP)**
Whicker, Sheri Leigh **(SLP)**

Todd
Sizer, Mary R A **(A)**

Trinity
Bair, Mrs Janice J **(SLP)**
Blair, Mrs Patricia M **(SLP)**
Shore, Mrs Jeanne B **(SLP)**

Troy
Haywood, Louise **(SLP)**

Union Grove
Herring, June J **(SLP A)**

Valdese
Kibler, Lucy Maud **(SLP)**

Vass
Yandell, Sara J **(SLP)**

Wadesboro
Martin, Mrs Patricia Arnold **(SLP)**

Wake Forest
Gordon, Mrs Anita Shaw **(SLP)**

Wallace
Wallace, Sharon Kitina **(A)**

Washington
Lang, Edmonia L
Murray, Mrs Jeanne McAmis **(SLP)**
Smithwick, Mrs Connie G **(SLP)**

Waxhaw
Eichenbaum, Roberta Wyffels
Woodard, Mrs Beatrice E **(SLP)**

Waynesville
Kelly, Delores L **(SLP)**
Loomis, Wilda Brown **(SLP)**

Weaverville
Hutchinson, Dianna Ball **(SLP)**
Riddle, Sherri Lynne **(SLP)**

Webster
Nicholson, Anne T **(SLP)**

Weddington
Brownell, Mrs Karen J L **(SLP)**
Karolak, Mrs Donna Lucia **(SLP)**

Whiteville
Beck, Mrs Beverly Atwood **(SLP)**
Ezzell, Lisa Gayle **(SLP)**
Watson, Mrs Betty H **(SLP)**

Whittier
Salyer, Betty Jean H **(SLP)**

Wilmington
Abernathy, Mrs Barbara M **(SLP)**
Allman, Mrs Jean Wheeler **(A)**
Bloomfield, Barbara C **(SLP)**
Brooks, Mrs Stephanie B **(SLP)**
Caulfield, Mrs Patricia **(SLP)**
Cooper, Mrs Kimberly Sturgis **(SLP)**
Costin, Gail **(SLP)**
Dressler, Richard A **(SLP)**
Felton, Karen Kent **(SLP)**
Feske, Mrs Susanne R **(SLP)**
Frasier-Lilley, Dixie L **(SLP A)**
Harbour, Anne Marie **(SLP)**
Keating, Lisa Beekman **(SLP)**
Maddock, Mary Laird **(A)**
Mayer, Mrs Melanie H **(SLP)**
Mintzes, Dr Susan S **(SLP)**
Motteler, Elizabeth **(SLP)**
Parker, Aimee Bennett **(A)**
Payton-Parr, Pamela **(SLP)**
Redfearn, Barbara **(SLP)**
Shoemaker, Barbara Knapp **(A)**
Smith, Mrs Susan Harris **(SLP)**
Stewart, Eleanor K **(SLP)**
Waddell, Mrs Patricia Lewis **(SLP)**

Wilson
Darling, Mrs Nancy H **(SLP)**
Smith, Mrs Jeanne Lynn **(SLP)**
Tingle, Meredith Kastner **(SLP)**
Webb, Marie J **(A)**
Whitaker, Pamela **(SLP)**

Winston-Salem
Adams, McKinnie D
Biggam, Mrs Lynn Lincoln **(SLP)**
Blalock, Philip D **(SLP)**
Blank, Janet Louise **(A)**
Block, Mrs Linda D **(A)**
Blumenthal, Ida L **(SLP)**
Blumke, Shelby Poindexter **(SLP)**
Butts, Mrs Deborah Banks
Cagle, Lonna Faye **(A)**
Calhoun, Sarah Ann **(SLP)**
Callahan, Mrs Barbara M **(SLP)**
Carlton, Janet C **(SLP)**
Demo-Anderson, Laura **(SLP)**
Di Cola, George A **(SLP)**
Faker, Mrs Elisa Colasanto **(SLP)**
Favruzzo, Barbara Shoffner **(SLP)**
Ferguson, Mrs Mary A M **(SLP)**
Hanna, Mrs Alexis W **(SLP)**
Harris, Mrs Dora Mae **(SLP)**
Haynie, Mrs Christine Buchholz **(SLP)**
Hite, Deborah Simpson **(SLP)**
Houfek, Katherine Ann **(SLP)**
Hunter, Margaret S **(SLP)**
Johnson, Mrs Susan Payne **(SLP)**
Karstaedt, Marcelle M **(A)**
Kennedy, Mrs Suzanne N **(SLP)**
Killam, Alma Ellis **(SLP)**
Magee, Sheryl Kinsey **(SLP)**
McCullough, Cheryl Ann **(SLP)**
McLaurin, Paul Andrew **(SLP)**
Meier, Irene Marie **(SLP)**
Meis, Mrs Marcia D **(A)**
Mikol, Mrs Page Norris
Mills, Carlon Scott **(A)**
Moore, Sherye Leigh **(SLP)**
Owen, Mrs Karen Whisenhunt **(SLP)**
Pace, Melissa J **(SLP)**
Pena, Mrs Cheryl Swaim
Pillsbury, David C **(A)**
Preslar, Joyce W **(SLP)**
Ramsey, Deborah J **(A)**
Rinehart, Monica Joy
Shamey, Lenore T **(SLP)**
Sheldon, Sandra M **(SLP)**
Soisson, Dianne C
Taylor, Tamara Dawn **(SLP)**
Thomas, Linda Kay **(A)**
Tucker, Barbara G **(SLP)**
Tuten, Laurie Elizabeth **(SLP)**
Tygard, Elizabeth
Vanfossen, Linda **(A)**
Vaughan, Mrs Jenni Anderson **(SLP)**
Wall, Mrs Janet Myrick **(SLP)**
Weddle, Mrs Ginger Rock **(SLP)**
Willard, Mrs Marilyn Ness **(SLP)**
Wolff, Sue Ostrow **(SLP)**
Woods, Mrs Carolyn J **(SLP)**

Winterville
Fagundus, Kay W **(A)**

Woodleaf
Bost, Mrs Katherine **(SLP)**

Wrightsville Beach
Vaught, Samuel F **(A)**

Yadkinville
Huffstetler, Mrs Donna Gail **(SLP)**
Repa, Donna Bromiel **(SLP)**

Zebulon
Hinson, Mrs Mary C **(SLP)**

Zionville
Thomas, Bettie McLawhorn **(SLP)**

Zirconia
Stierwalt, Mrs Debra D **(SLP)**

NORTH DAKOTA

Arnegard
Kellogg, Mrs Debra J **(SLP)**

Beach
Fahlstrom, Merrill S **(SLP)**

Bemidji
Grismer, Tamara J **(SLP)**

Berthold
Schaan, Mrs Linda L **(SLP)**

Beulah
Rubbelke, Mrs Cynthia M **(SLP)**

Bismarck
Arneson, Debra J **(A)**
Beatty, Sherry M **(SLP)**
Bowman, Susan E **(SLP)**
Bradford, Mrs Mary James **(SLP)**
Brossart, Carol Marie **(SLP)**
Condon, Mrs Shelley J **(SLP)**
Deboer, Debbie Diann
Dyk, Diane A **(SLP)**
Gronhovd, Lee D **(A)**
Gunderson, Fiona Walton **(SLP)**
Melby, Mrs Carol Rhoades **(SLP)**
Ness, Joe A **(A)**
Pedersen, Klaudia M **(SLP)**
Peschong, Elizabeth Johns **(SLP)**
Richins, Jon C **(A)**
Smyth, Jill Flynn **(SLP)**
Sullivan, Mary Ann **(SLP)**
Werven, Gerald Wayne **(SLP)**
Wilson, Mrs Suzanne Sinclair
Wolf, Mrs Jean Marr **(SLP)**

Bottineau
Kornkven, Colleen **(SLP)**

Burlington
Scurlock, Mrs Margaret L **(SLP)**

Carrington
Wilkinson-Sherman, Mrs Lucretia G **(SLP)**

Casselton
Gilbery, Mrs Josie Ann **(SLP)**

Center
Pilsner, Judith Ann **(SLP)**

Chaseley
Heintz, Laurene B **(SLP)**

Crosby
Ingebo, Mrs Mildred H **(SLP)**

Devils Lake
Haaland, Phil J **(SLP)**
Skiftun, Annette Breider **(A)**

Dickinson
Ault-Teeters, Ronna L **(SLP)**
Callahan, Mrs Kim Bauer **(A)**
Herauf, Mrs Jean L **(SLP)**
Hilden, Rhoda I **(SLP)**
King, Catherine H **(SLP)**
Kuske, Trudy Kay **(SLP)**
Nelson, Jill Annette **(SLP)**
Tongen, John L **(A)**

Douglas
Price, Mrs Maryjo Anna **(SLP)**

Fargo
Black, Virgil L **(SLP)**
Dekrey, Silvia **(SLP)**
DeMaio, Dr Louis J **(SLP)**
Dignan, Mrs C Louise **(SLP)**
Dufek-Swegarden, Barbara **(SLP)**
Flagtwet, Katherine Kania **(SLP)**
Friend, Helen H **(SLP)**
Hauff, Eileen K **(SLP)**
Hovden, Dawn L **(SLP)**
Johnson, Ronald D **(A)**
Jurgens-Haberlack, Mrs Cheryl Ann
Kahn, Helen J **(SLP)**
Krush, Mrs Gail Owan
McGuire, Marjorie S **(SLP)**
Miller, Deborah Ann **(SLP)**
Olson, Ardell E **(A)**
Olson, Paulette Marie D **(SLP)**
O'Relley, E Annette **(SLP)**
Petersen, Kate **(SLP)**
Simonson, Faith Hiney **(SLP)**
Smette, Mrs Alice Marie
Sullivan, Patricia C **(SLP)**
Van Lancker, Dr Diana Roupas
Vannote, Mrs Michele G **(SLP)**
Wilson, Cheri A
Zetter-Kunze, Nola **(SLP)**

Gackle
De Voll-Dahl, Tracy Lynn **(A)**

Grafton
Lotlikar, Swati M **(A)**
Ottoel, Chris Ann **(SLP)**
Tingum, Paulette Ann **(SLP)**

Grand Forks
Becker, Michelle Ann **(SLP)**
Biberdorf, Peggy Schorsch **(SLP)**
Bushfield, Dr Martee R **(SLP)**
Carlson, Mrs Barbara H **(SLP)**
Carriere, Diane Renee **(SLP)**
Davies, Laurel James **(A)**
Elbert, Mrs Dora L R **(SLP)**
Engel, Dr Dean C **(SLP)**
Fickenscher, Saundra R **(SLP)**
Fitzgerald, Mary C **(SLP)**
Frana, Nancy Ann **(SLP)**
Glick, Audrey M **(SLP)**
Goertel-Breen, Mrs Marilyn Joyce **(SLP)**
Groth, Lynn R **(SLP)**
Groth, Mrs Susan F **(SLP)**
Harris, Barbara Zine **(SLP)**
Hartwick, Nancy Ann **(SLP)**
Haug, Holly T **(SLP)**
Hess, Dr Carla W **(SLP A)**
Hollifield, S Gail **(SLP)**
Imes, Mary Ellen **(SLP)**
Johnson, Mrs Debra Ann **(SLP)**
McPhail, Fay Lois **(SLP)**
Mercer, Anne L **(SLP)**
Olson, Leila M **(SLP)**
O'Shea, Beverly M **(SLP)**
Peterson, Mrs Carole W **(SLP)**
Qvammen, Brian Dale **(A)**
Reynolds, Dr Brian W **(A)**
Ridl, Mrs Jane E O **(A)**
Sander, Mrs Diane Quam **(SLP)**
Schill, Mrs Mary Jo S **(SLP)**
Schubert, Dr George W **(SLP)**
Selland-Lichter, Sandra **(SLP)**
Steffen, Susan Rae **(SLP)**
Swisher, Dr Wayne Everett **(SLP)**
Woidtke, Cathy Rae W **(SLP)**

Granville
Loftesnes, Mrs Lucille M **(SLP)**

Guelph
Visto, Mrs Jane Ackerman

Hillsboro
Lee, Terry L **(SLP)**

Jamestown
Charlton, Georgina **(SLP)**
Coppin, Mrs Rachel Irene **(SLP)**
Cornforth, Mrs Marilyn Voth **(SLP)**
Helfenstein, Sheila Darlene **(SLP)**

Kleingartner, Michelle Stock **(A)**
Lochow, Carol A **(SLP)**
Murphy, Eileen M **(SLP)**

Lansford
Cunningham, Mrs Colette Adele

Lisbon
Krivarchka, Mrs Cheryl M **(SLP)**

Mandan
Gumeringer, Mrs Antonia Bullinger **(SLP)**
Hochhalter, Susan M **(SLP)**
Hollingsworth, Rebecca A **(SLP)**

Manuel
Hankey, Mrs Cynthia Mooibroek **(SLP)**

Mayville
Parker, Jo Ann M Roscoe **(SLP)**

McGregor
Santella-Johnson, Mary Elizabeth

Michigan
Lozeau, Mrs Colleen Doody **(SLP)**

Minot
Beale, Dr Cecilia R **(SLP)**
Birnbaum, Lisa V
Bostow, Vicki V W **(SLP)**
Bradley, Dr Scott T **(A)**
Burbach, Cathy Ann **(SLP)**
Carpenter, Mrs Barbara Kay **(SLP)**
Dean, Marla Rae **(SLP)**
Dorrell, Cheryl Ann **(SLP)**
Fitzmaurice, Karen M
Froelich, Thomas M **(A)**
Fylling, Colleen E **(SLP)**
Gefroh, Tracy Ann **(SLP)**
Gehl, Mrs Pamela L **(SLP)**
Gietzen, Deborah D **(SLP)**
Hance, Mrs Joan Ostlund **(SLP)**
Johnson, Faye Guttormson **(SLP)**
Kane, Jane F **(SLP)**
Kienzle, Mrs Nancy L **(SLP)**
Kincheloe, Dr John W **(SLP)**
Knapp, Gerald A **(A)**
Kukurudz, Kim Marie
Lunday, Dr Audrey Mostoller **(SLP)**
Lunstad, Mrs Penny E
MacDonald, Mrs Diane Newell **(A)**
Maupin, Dianne C **(SLP)**
Nelson, David G **(A)**
Nering, Gayle N **(SLP)**
Pochant, Marylou Boots **(SLP)**
Renfandt, Mrs Paula E **(SLP)**
Schettler, Mrs Jamie Rae **(SLP)**
Torgerson, Mrs Elaine B **(SLP)**
Torgerson, Dr John K **(SLP)**
Uhler, Sarah Bussier **(SLP)**
Williams, Dr David K **(SLP)**
Wohl, Mrs Laura M **(SLP)**
Worthley, Dr William J **(SLP)**
Yinger, Mrs Kathleen **(A)**

North Fargo
Krogh, Stanley O **(A)**

Oberon
Rushfeldt, Mrs Betty Jane **(SLP)**

Oriska
Owen, Mrs Barbara E **(SLP)**

Rugby
Neumann, Mrs Jacqueline Denise **(SLP)**

Stanley
Erickson, Mrs Kathryn G **(SLP)**

Tappen
Bodvig, Merrilee Jane **(SLP)**

Thompson
Carroll, Dr Jack Adien **(SLP A)**
Kalash, Mrs Sharon U **(SLP)**
Swenson, Mrs Catherine A **(SLP)**

Underwood
Machart, Victor Eugene **(SLP)**

Valley City
Anderson, Katherine Mary **(SLP)**

Velva
Linrud, Mrs Carlotta Jean

Wahpeton
Johnson, Richard M **(SLP)**
Pankratz, Lori Dee **(SLP)**

Washburn
Thul, Mrs Nancy Ann **(SLP)**

Watford City
Wurgler, Lynn Renae

West Fargo
Mittag, Lori Anderson **(SLP)**
Riedinger, Vicki Lynn **(SLP)**

Westhope
Neumann, Marie Olin **(SLP)**

Wildrose
Peterson, Mrs Ila C **(SLP)**

Williston
Gormally, Susan Ulness **(SLP)**
Koble, Carolyn A
Kyllo, Mrs Teresa Marie **(SLP)**
Ross, Mrs Joann Horner **(SLP)**

OHIO

Ada
Oliver, Mrs Kristina Weiskittle **(SLP)**
Peterson, Mrs Gail A H **(SLP)**

Akron
Adams, Debbie M **(SLP)**
Ameris, Mrs Kimberly Kay **(SLP)**
Bahas-Horattas, Mrs Karen Marie **(SLP)**
Baker, Audrey Vendeland **(SLP)**
Bartlebaugh, Susan C **(SLP)**
Besozzi, Ella June **(SLP)**
Blickle, Jennifer **(A)**
Blosser, Dr Jean L **(SLP)**
Bogdanoff, Mrs Eleanor L **(SLP)**
Boyd, Christina A **(SLP)**
Brayer, Mary Ann **(SLP)**
Casterline, Judy **(SLP)**
Castor, Devorah L **(A)**
Clarke, Mrs Gloria Lynn **(A)**
Considine, Kathleen A **(SLP)**
Conti, Donna Marie **(SLP)**
Cowen, Alexandra Lee **(SLP)**
Davis, Dr George D **(SLP A)**
Dedinsky, Karen **(SLP)**
Dohner, Mrs Nancy P **(SLP)**
Ellsworth, Mrs Kathleen Marie **(SLP)**
Ferrara, Kristine Louise
Franck, Mrs Ardath Amond **(SLP)**
Gibson, Jay Howard **(SLP A)**
Gibson, Mrs Mary **(SLP A)**
Glass, Sandra D
Greenblatt, Mrs Debra A **(SLP)**
Hall, Dr Donald E **(SLP)**
Hansson, Marta Jean **(A)**
Holland, Frances L **(SLP)**
Hudgins, Mrs Judith M **(SLP)**
Huggins, Sharon DeNise **(SLP)**
Hunter, Mrs Judith P **(SLP)**
Ireland, JoAnn Chirakos **(A)**
Joachim, Marilyn Jean **(SLP)**
Jones, Mrs Roseann D **(SLP)**
Katz, Dr Karyn Bobkoff **(SLP)**
Korosa, Mrs Luan Davidson **(SLP)**
Kreeger, Virginia Flechtner **(SLP)**
Lawrence, Dr Carol W **(SLP)**
Lesner, Dr Sharon A **(A)**
Little, Mrs Janet M **(SLP)**
Lynn, Dr James M **(A)**
Lynn, Mrs Karen Sue **(A)**
Malinsky, Ann Elizabeth **(SLP)**
McGuckin, Mrs Virginia Bader **(SLP)**
Metzger, Barbara Ann
Miller, Mrs Deborah W **(A)**
Mockbee, Mrs Jo Anne Valcho **(SLP)**
Newcomb, Sandra S **(A)**
Norin, Mrs Helene S R **(A)**
Osburn, Catherine **(SLP A)**
Pascu-Godwin, Victoria **(SLP)**
Peterson, Joan M **(SLP)**
Richman, Harriet U **(SLP)**
Samples, Sheila Carol **(A)**
Sawan, Denise M **(SLP)**
Segal, Mrs Teri B **(SLP)**
Seitz, Andrew Joseph, Jr **(A)**
Siloac, Dr Kenneth T **(SLP)**
Soberano, Mrs Carol A W **(SLP)**
Steinberger, Andrea R **(A)**
Stephenson, Lydia Jane **(SLP)**
Stevenson, Kristen K **(A)**
Sudler, William H **(SLP)**
Trowbridge, Mrs Deborah A **(SLP)**
Willen, Mrs Michelle Martin **(SLP)**
Wise, Mrs Dorothea Ann **(SLP)**
Younkin, Elizabeth Marie **(SLP)**

Albany
Martin, Mrs Barbara K **(SLP)**

Alliance
Abel, Debra B **(A)**
Glazier, Susan Thomas **(SLP)**
Lee, Robert E **(A)**
McConahy, Regina Ellen **(SLP)**

Amelia
Fangman, Mrs Margaret White **(SLP)**

Amherst
Burkhart, Nancy L **(A)**
Watson-Zavodny, Mrs Barbara Ann **(SLP)**

Amlin
Crook, Mrs Randi Richter

Anna
Berning, Mrs Alison Ruese **(SLP)**
Massey, Mrs Joan Benanzer **(SLP)**

Ashland
Cadley, Donald K **(SLP)**
McCanna, Donald **(SLP A)**
Mullenix, Mrs Betty G **(SLP)**
Yetzer, Mrs Marjorie S **(SLP)**

Ashtabula
Bottorf, Barrie O **(SLP)**
Hutchinson, Peggy Diane **(SLP)**

Athens
Bond, Dr Zinny I
Buckberry, Emily S **(SLP)**
Collins, Linda B **(SLP)**
Conover, Helen B **(SLP)**
Dean, Charles R **(SLP)**
Fokes, Joann
Fucci, Dr Donald J
Fucci, Mrs Joan Y **(SLP)**
Garber, Maryann **(SLP)**
Garber, Dr Norman B **(SLP)**
Girmatzion, Mrs Phyllis Jenkins
Hoffman, Cheryl P **(SLP)**
Isele, Ronald Woodward **(SLP A)**
Kalweit, Linda M **(A)**
McVey, Diane E **(A)**
Nance, Mrs Rita F Carpenter
Pickering, John Edmund, Jr **(SLP)**
Sakadales, M Susanne **(SLP)**
Seaton, Dr William H **(A)**
Spangler, Carol S **(SLP)**
Trisolini, Margaret Mountjoy **(SLP)**
Tyler, Elizabeth Randolph **(SLP)**
Weiner, Carole May **(SLP)**

Aurora
Firestone, Harvey B **(A)**
Hoffman, Mrs Florence Eaton **(SLP)**
Moody, Mrs Laurie J **(SLP)**

Avon Lake
Cramer, Mrs Sandra Kay **(A)**
Heun, Mrs Joanne M **(SLP)**
Hoy, Rebecca B **(SLP)**

Barberton
Jackson, Mrs Sue M **(A)**
McGill, Mrs Pamela C W **(SLP)**
Moomaw, Mrs Edna L **(SLP)**

Bay Village
Cady, Mrs Susan Lynn **(SLP)**
Dawson, Mrs Theresa Sheahen **(SLP)**
Joyce, Mrs Peggy M **(SLP)**
Karnuta, Maryann L **(A)**
Langhenry, Mrs Debra Dlouhy **(SLP)**
Laurence, Deanna Glaser **(SLP)**
Peterson, Mrs Elizabeth R **(SLP)**
Ramsayer, Mrs Carolyn B **(SLP)**
Striegl, Mrs Janet W **(SLP)**
Wills, Edward J **(A)**

Beachwood
Aster, Christine Pampush **(SLP)**
Barricklow, Susan R **(SLP)**
Baum, Mrs Ginette A **(SLP)**
Biel, Mrs Claire D **(SLP)**
Bir, Mrs Margaret F **(SLP)**
Doris, Fran N **(SLP)**
Leavitt, Jane Freiberg **(A)**
Polster, Mrs Cindy Miller **(SLP)**
Siegel, Cheryl Lester **(SLP)**
Sloan-Brown, Nancy **(SLP)**

Beaver Creek
Cole, Kimberlee **(SLP)**
Douville, Rosanne R **(SLP A)**
McDevitt, Marcella Gertrude **(A)**
Myers, Mrs Sara W **(SLP)**
Rhodehamel, Mrs Susan E **(SLP)**

Bedford
Lamb, Mrs Kathryn Marie **(SLP)**
McClain, Wendy L **(A)**
Prasen, Patricia A **(SLP)**
Sadler, Laura L **(A)**
Spremulli, Mary **(SLP)**

Bedford Heights
Beach, Mrs Mary Nisbet **(SLP)**
Russell, Mrs Cheryl Winchester **(SLP)**

Bellefontaine
Beach, Suzanne Lynn **(SLP)**
Dunn, Theresa Ann **(SLP)**
Oda, Mrs Susan Idell **(SLP)**

Bellevue
Griffith, Cheryl Ann **(SLP)**
Middleswarth, Mrs Karen L **(SLP)**
Raifsnider, Mrs Jacquie S

Berea
Grekco, Mrs Kathy **(SLP)**
Hines, Joanne L H **(SLP)**
Kramer, Mrs Carol Anne **(SLP)**
Madden, Dr Deirdre Peters **(SLP)**
Packwood, Gary L **(SLP)**
Regas-Yutzy, Mrs Mary A **(SLP)**
Vaccariello, Mrs Carol M **(SLP)**

Bexley
Lieberman, Mrs Shelley M **(SLP)**
White, Susan J **(SLP)**

Blacklick
Bernard, Carolyn Nicrosi **(SLP)**

Blue Ash
Murray, Donna Smith **(SLP)**

Boardman
Firestone, Mrs Denise Dickman **(SLP)**
Norman, Mrs Carol A **(SLP)**
Salata, Bonnie J **(SLP)**
Trimmer, Mrs Lisa Ann
Webb, Tina Renee **(A)**

Bolivar
Partridge, Kathleen Jones **(A)**
Petrella, Christine Ann **(SLP)**

Bowling Green
Baker, Susan Kay **(SLP)**
Burroughs, Dr Elizabeth Irene **(SLP)**
Cohen, Judith L **(SLP)**
Colcord, Mrs Donna Jo **(SLP)**
Colcord, Dr Roger D **(SLP)**
Cruz, Mrs Eneida Maldonado **(SLP)**
Dittman, Mrs Kim Elias **(SLP)**
Dusenbery, Luanne Kay **(SLP)**
Gay, Lynn
Greenberg, Dr Bonita R
Greenberg, Dr Herbert J **(A)**
Hyman, Dr Melvin **(SLP)**
Infante, Alicia Anne **(SLP)**
Jackson, Mrs Faith L **(SLP)**
Kurcz, Mrs Karen Brasie **(SLP)**
Marchitelli-Martin, Mrs Karen A **(SLP)**
Mize, Cathleen S **(SLP)**
Neidecker, Elizabeth **(SLP)**
Norris, Cynthia Ferguson **(SLP)**
Olscamp, Ruth P **(SLP)**
Perlmutter, Marilyn **(SLP)**
Petrosino, Dr Linda A **(SLP)**
Popplewell, Deatra Ann **(A)**
Scukanec, Gail Patricia **(SLP)**
Simmons, Mrs Diana Strauss **(A)**
Simmons, Dr Frederick **(A)**
Small, Dr Larry H **(A)**
Stokes, Dorothy W **(SLP)**
Sweede, Mrs June W
Townsend, Mrs Deborah J **(A)**
Twyman, Mrs Carol L **(SLP)**
Varney, Mrs Ruth P **(SLP)**
Wentland, Marilynn F **(SLP)**

Brecksville
Engler, Robin Janus **(SLP)**
Robertson, Mrs Lois A **(SLP)**
Rowsey, Linda Margaret **(A)**
Sopko, Mary Helen **(SLP)**
Woznak, Mrs Diana L **(SLP)**

Bristolville
Reinhart, Mrs Rae L **(SLP)**

Broadview Heights
Hallal, Joseph Daniel **(A)**
Hof, Mrs Lenore R **(SLP)**
Korczynski, Mrs Beth Ann **(SLP)**
Ottaway, Ruth **(SLP)**

Brook Park
Bobowicz, Mrs Karen Harper **(SLP)**
Jakischa, Mrs Katherine Pauer **(SLP)**
McDonnell, John J

Brookfield
Rubano, Dennis P **(SLP)**

Brooklyn
Bodrock-Raksi, Mrs Mary Katherine **(A)**

Brunswick
Henchey, Cara Elaine **(SLP)**
Lepi, Mrs Carol L **(A)**
Marchionda, Mrs Jeannie Anne **(A)**
Stiegle, Mrs Melissa Elkins **(SLP)**

Brunswick Hills
Lavely-Planisek, Debra Sue **(SLP)**

Bryan
Curtis, Glen W **(SLP)**
Nott, Mrs Jane Richards **(SLP)**

Cambridge
Nash, Oliver A **(SLP)**
Slater, Emma Lu **(A)**
Watson-Dodd, Mrs Brenda Lee **(A)**
Wellen, Mary J **(SLP)**

Campbell
Svagerko, James Michael **(A)**

Canal Fulton
Hall, William T **(A)**
Segers, Mrs Vicki Ann **(SLP)**

Canal Winchester
Harter, Mrs Rene Stiteler **(SLP)**
Maguire, Jeanette Porter **(SLP)**

Canfield
De Matteo, Mrs Annette P **(SLP)**
Kuchmaner, Mrs Lauri Dahman **(SLP)**
Pfahler, Mrs Lorene A **(SLP)**
Schneider, Mrs Mary Walters
Sick, Steven Wesley
Trimm, Mary Margaret **(SLP)**
Wallace, Mrs Susan E **(A)**

Canton
Allman, Mrs Jeannette **(SLP)**
Brubaker, Susan L **(SLP)**
DeFrance, Mrs Dorothy Wells **(SLP)**
Di Giantonio, Heidi A Hathaway- **(SLP)**
Everett, Darlene Welton **(A)**
Finefrock, Mrs Joan Forney **(SLP)**
Fitzmaurice, Peggy E **(SLP)**
Larke, Lynn Marie **(SLP)**
Neading, Mrs Diana Loechel **(SLP)**
Previtera, Mrs Susan Leaman **(SLP)**
Ragosin, Mrs Edria M **(SLP)**
Schnebelen, Cheryl H **(SLP)**
Seich, Diane Marie **(SLP)**
Sheil, Mrs Francine Fister **(A)**
Simpson, Victoria Lynn **(A)**
Sklar, Mrs Linda Ellen **(SLP)**
Tondra, Mrs Janice K **(SLP)**
Varavvas, Mrs Denise M **(A)**

Castalia
Smith, Jean D **(SLP)**

Centerville
Bethke, Mrs Dorothy P **(SLP)**
Davis, Denise Homes **(SLP)**
Dean, Charlene **(SLP)**
Donaldson, Linda Larson **(A)**
Estes-Waddell, Anna Gale **(SLP)**
Gregory, Bonnie R **(SLP)**
Lacon, Mrs Donna Lynn **(SLP)**
Merrill, Patricia N **(SLP)**
Minutilli, James Benjamin **(SLP)**
Peach, Mrs Cherylin J **(SLP)**
Pentenburg, Ellen Kay **(SLP)**
Reitz, Janet L S **(A)**
Sekely, Mrs Bonnie Ann **(SLP)**
Skeel, Mary L **(SLP)**
Wade, Janice **(SLP)**

Chagrin Falls
Anthony, Mrs Julie Virginia **(SLP)**
Belobradic-Joyce, Lynn Christine **(SLP)**
Brotman-Domoracki, Sandra R **(A)**
Cox, Mrs Barbara M **(SLP)**
Domoracki, Dr David **(A)**
Goodrich, Frances H **(SLP)**
Green, Mary R **(SLP)**
Hornstein, Jennifer Lee **(SLP)**
Lewis, Sally M **(A)**
O'Rourk, Catherine **(SLP)**
Schafer, Mrs Karen S **(SLP)**
Tomiello, Mrs Marilyn R **(SLP)**

Chardon
Loomis, Mrs Selene G **(SLP)**
Norton, Mrs Nan C **(SLP)**
Sombat, Margaret M **(SLP)**

Chesapeake
Campbell, Mrs Bambi Lynn **(SLP)**
Clark, Mrs Bonita P **(SLP)**

Chesterland
Gustetic, Stanley J, Jr **(A)**
Minick Starke, Heidi **(SLP)**
Oppenheim, Mrs Carol Maple **(SLP)**

Chillicothe
Barada, Mrs Patricia Beam **(SLP)**
Rizzo,, Dr Stephen R, Jr **(A)**
White, Janet Dea **(SLP)**

Cincinnati
Adams, Maryln Allen **(SLP)**
Agnello, Dr Joseph G **(SLP)**
Albanese, Santina D **(SLP)**
Anderson, Mrs Donna L **(SLP)**
Antunes-Smith, Katherine **(SLP)**
Armstrong, Suzanne Elaine **(SLP)**
Augsburger, Julie B **(SLP)**
Badanes, Mrs Amy L **(SLP)**
Baker, Marilyn Ruth **(SLP)**
Bakie, Bruce E **(SLP)**
Banks, Nora Jacqueline **(SLP)**
Baron, Billie Lynn **(SLP)**
Bauer, Meier H **(SLP)**
Bayliss, Mrs Kim I M **(SLP)**
Beatty, Janice K **(SLP)**
Bennett, Marilyn S **(SLP)**
Bishop, Mrs Elaine Legler **(SLP)**
Bonds, Elisabeth Via **(A)**
Bowling, Stephen Dale **(A)**
Bradley, Sarah E
Brass, Mrs Raye Simon **(SLP)**
Braverman, Kathleen M **(SLP)**
Bredemeier, Mrs Nancy Sorn **(SLP)**
Breen, Mrs Phyllis O **(SLP)**
Brennan, Mrs Mary Schindler **(SLP)**
Brickner-Hoath, Sheri **(SLP)**
Burgan, Mrs Rebecca Sieck **(SLP)**
Burns, Kathryn L
Buschbacher, Pamelazita Wilbur **(SLP)**
Byrnes, Mrs Cathy Hicks **(SLP)**
Castilla, Carla **(A)**
Chalfonte-Evans, Melinda **(SLP)**
Champlin, Lisa D **(SLP)**
Chaney, Mrs Jeanine Schmidt **(SLP)**
Christopherson, Sharon **(A)**
Chute, Wendy Wenker **(A)**
Clark, Dr John Greer **(SLP A)**
Clements, Mrs Linda W **(SLP)**
Coen-Cummings, Martha Carol **(SLP)**
Cohen, Mrs Judith Marks **(SLP)**
Cohen, Dr Ronald Lee **(A)**
Coleman, Julie Marie **(SLP)**
Collins, Sharon K **(SLP)**
Colussi, Jane Marie **(SLP)**
Cone, Sarah W **(SLP)**
Cook, Mrs Marcia L **(SLP)**
Cornuelle, Robert Keith
Coulter, Leanne McJunkin **(SLP)**
Cox, Billie P **(SLP)**
Creaghead, Dr Nancy Acra **(SLP)**
Daggett, Mary D **(A)**
Dapollonio, Joann **(SLP)**
Dean, Mrs Cheryl C **(SLP)**
Dean, Mrs Susan Ann **(A)**
Deane, Janis Hartsfield **(SLP)**
Dell'Aira, Angel L **(SLP)**
Demaree, Gina L **(SLP)**
De Rosa, Kimberly Marie **(SLP)**
Devine, Mrs Jeanne Canty **(A)**
Dewine, Laurie J **(A)**
Disney, Sarah Thompson **(SLP)**
Dobson, Deborah Ruth
Donnelly, Dr Carole D **(SLP)**
Donnelly, Kenneth G **(A)**
Donovan, Mrs Barbara Ann **(SLP)**
Duwell, Lisa Iacobucci **(SLP)**
Emerson, Melanie S **(SLP)**
Farrenkopf, Mrs Linda C **(SLP)**
Farrer, Susan M **(A)**
Fleming, Dorsey A **(A)**
Fluharty, Mrs Nancy Buono **(SLP)**
Freeman, Patricia A **(SLP)**
Games, Diane C **(SLP)**
Gardner, Carol B **(SLP)**
Garland, Mrs Lori Ann **(A)**
Gear, Mrs Susan Campbell **(A)**
Geiger, Judy A **(SLP)**
Givler, Mrs Susan Kay **(SLP)**
Goldberg, Mrs Hazel P **(SLP)**
Goldman, Dr Thomas M **(A)**
Gottlieb, Gayle Pauline **(SLP)**
Grant, Michelle L **(A)**
Grasha, Mrs Carol H **(SLP)**
Griffin, Margaret Macy **(SLP)**
Gross, Lynn F **(SLP)**
Guiliano, Teresa Stehlin **(A)**
Guttman, Mrs Marlene B **(SLP)**
Hadsell-Brickler, Linda Denise
Hamant, Mrs Karla Feuchter **(SLP)**
Hamilton, Jean Wetter **(A)**
Harris, Mrs Pamela Glynn **(SLP)**
Hedgebeth, Mrs Mary Helen **(SLP)**
Hedges, Janet **(SLP)**
Henke, Mrs Karen **(SLP)**
Hennings, Cheryl Marie
Hepfner, Mrs Sharon T **(SLP A)**
Hereth, Mrs Kay Carolyn **(SLP)**
Hill, Michael Lee **(A)**
Himes, Terri K **(SLP)**
Hoke, Mrs Sharon A **(A)**
Hollenkamp, Mrs Teresa A **(SLP)**
Hotelling, Elaine Gracelyn **(SLP)**
Huntress, Mrs Linda M **(SLP)**
Ireland, Mrs Peggy G **(SLP)**
Isaacs, Lois E **(A)**
Jacobs, Mrs Carol Donnelly
Jacobson, Mrs Ina B **(SLP)**
Johnson, Jill M **(SLP)**
Johnson, Jilonda L
Jones, Beverly **(SLP)**
Jones, Leslie E **(SLP)**
Jones, Mrs Lynn A **(SLP)**
Jump, Jill Ellen **(SLP)**
Justice, Kathryn P **(SLP)**
Kagy, Jane E **(SLP)**
Keith, Dr Robert W **(A)**
Keperling, Marcia Lynn **(SLP)**
Kercher, Robyn K **(SLP)**
Kessel, Marjorie Wasserman **(SLP)**
Kortekamp, Mrs Carol W **(SLP)**
Krapp, Dr Dwight E **(A)**
Kretschmer, Dr Laura W **(A)**
Kugelman, Sandra Marli **(SLP)**
Kummer, Ann W **(SLP)**
Lawson, Mrs Cynthia King **(SLP)**
Lawson, Jeanne Marie **(SLP)**
Lee, Dr Linda **(SLP)**
Lehmann, M Drue **(SLP)**
Leslie, Dr Carol Prahl **(SLP)**
Linz, Joseph R **(SLP)**
Lipp, Lori S **(A)**
Lipson, Mrs Marilyn E **(SLP)**
Long, Joann Verville **(SLP)**
Lorenz, Mary Grace **(SLP)**
Lowenthal, Mrs Laura Lee **(A)**
Luebbe, Judith M **(SLP)**
Luhn, Kathleen Krabacher **(A)**
Lukes-Miller, Mrs Barbara E **(SLP)**
Lupella, Dr Robert O **(SLP)**
Lustiber, Mrs Laurie A **(SLP)**
Mackey, Barbara Raymond **(A)**
Mahoney, Patricia **(SLP)**
Mahorney, Mrs Lori Jean **(SLP)**
Mantel, Pamela Marie **(SLP)**
Marsh, Mrs Janet H **(SLP)**
Martin, Amy Rose **(SLP)**
Mauch, Mrs Janice **(SLP)**
McAvoy, Kathleen Anne
McClanahan, Mrs Sharolyn A
McConnell, Patricia **(SLP)**
McConnell-Stephen, Patricia Lynn **(SLP)**
Meade, Kathleen N **(SLP)**
Mecklenborg, Mrs Janis Pohlman **(SLP)**
Meek, Mrs Sylvia D **(SLP)**
Metz, Mrs Carol Neuner **(SLP)**
Metzger, Dr Hope H **(A)**
Meyer, Mrs Deborah Scully **(SLP)**
Miller, Claire Kane **(SLP)**
Miller, J Michael **(SLP)**
Miller, Dr Nancy K **(SLP)**
Moccia, Diane T **(SLP)**

Moler, Robin Seltzer **(SLP)**
Moll, Mrs Mollie A M **(SLP)**
Monahan, Mrs Sarah McGinnis **(A)**
Moore, Mrs Linda R **(SLP)**
Morningstar, Janet C **(SLP)**
Mouk, Betty Jean **(SLP)**
Mount, Kathy Requarth **(SLP)**
Murphy, Tracey Dawn **(SLP)**
Mussman, Mrs Jill Marie **(A)**
Napier, Deborah L **(SLP)**
Neils, Dr Jean Rankin **(SLP)**
Nuck, Martha Ellen **(SLP)**
Oetzel, Mrs Judith Yohman **(SLP)**
O'Hearn, Victoria Moluse **(A)**
Owens, Shirley E **(A)**
Padgett, Karen L **(SLP)**
Paff, Patricia Lee **(SLP)**
Parker, Sharon Lynn
Perin, Mrs Trina Ann **(SLP)**
Pleasant, Kelly J **(SLP)**
Pohl, Mrs Anne M **(SLP)**
Porter, Betty J **(A)**
Porter, Elizabeth Ann White **(A)**
Prelock, Dr Patricia A **(SLP)**
Prendeville, Jo-Anne **(SLP)**
Prudhomme, Maria R **(SLP)**
Quinn, Ruth Marie **(SLP)**
Raykovics, Patricia Marie **(SLP)**
Reich, Susan B **(SLP)**
Relojo, Mrs Patricia Lira **(SLP)**
Rickert, Mary T **(SLP)**
Riley, Judi Carey **(SLP)**
Rohrbaugh, Mrs Christine Ann **(SLP)**
Ross, Amanda M **(SLP)**
Ross, Mrs Karen Young **(SLP)**
Rothstein, Mrs Lori J **(SLP)**
Rudge, Nancy Joan **(SLP)**
Rudolph, Mrs Carolyn R **(SLP)**
Ryan-Carpenter, Sheila M **(SLP)**
Sammis, Barbara G **(SLP)**
Sandore, Lisa M **(SLP)**
Sapinkopf, Mrs Ellen F **(SLP)**
Schalk-Russell, Dr Mary C **(SLP)**
Schellman, Mary Jeanne L **(SLP)**
Schleicher, Melaine Ann **(SLP)**
Schleifer, Nancy I **(SLP)**
Short, Deborah L **(A)**
Shuller, Janis C **(SLP)**
Simmons, Juanita Faye **(SLP)**
Singleton-Filio, Kimberly Faye **(SLP)**
Slavik, Mrs Cynthia Ann
Slone, Ann M **(SLP)**
Spence, Mrs Mary E **(SLP)**
Stankiewicz, Ann W **(SLP)**
Stein, Janet A **(A)**
Stein, Lindsay M **(A)**
Steinsapir, Carolyn Denise **(SLP)**
Stern, Lynn Davidow **(A)**
Stewart, Dianne B **(SLP)**
Stewart, Mrs Nancy L **(SLP)**
Stromberg, Eleanor M **(A)**
Sudman, Mrs Joanne A **(SLP)**
Sunderhaus, Mrs Erika Courlander **(SLP)**
Taylor, Carole J **(SLP)**
Thoma, Pamela Susan **(SLP)**
Thomas, Mrs Gretchen Ann **(SLP)**
Todd, Mrs Maureen F **(SLP)**
Tomlinson, Peggy Kosters
Toomey, Mrs Marilyn Mantifel **(SLP)**
Uhl, Sandra McFall **(SLP)**
Upton, Mrs Patricia S **(SLP)**
Vaughan, Linda Decker **(SLP)**
Vehr, Jeffrey Paul
Vornheder-Allendorf, Valerie Ann **(A)**
Walters, Mrs Karen L **(SLP)**
Waltz, Mary F **(SLP)**
Watts, Ann K **(SLP)**
Wegener, John G **(SLP)**
Weisbrod, Barbara M **(SLP)**
Weisiger, Bradford, Jr **(SLP)**
Wellman, Linda Pyle **(SLP)**
Wells, Mrs Kathryn Elizabeth **(SLP)**
Westerbeck, Sandra L **(SLP)**
Whitehurst, Mrs Cynthia Stefanov **(A)**
Willenborg, Janet Ann **(SLP)**
Williams, Mrs Deborah Hopkins
Williams, Geralyn Huzicka **(SLP)**
Willis, Mrs Joyce Thomas **(A)**
Woeste, Carol Ferris **(SLP)**
Wolfe, Susan G **(SLP)**
Wolfman-Wasserman, Mrs Wendy Jill **(SLP)**
Wollman, Irving L **(SLP)**
Wood, Dr Ann Stace **(SLP)**
Woods, Jacqueline Ann **(SLP)**
Yacks, Dr C Thomas **(A)**
Yacks, Colin Paul **(SLP A)**
Yingling, Mary Alice N **(SLP)**
Zarider, Mrs Shirley Fox **(SLP)**
Zola, Stefani **(SLP)**
Zurlinden, Mrs Patricia M **(SLP)**

Cleveland

Aram, Dr Dorothy W **(SLP)**
Beastrom, Mrs Diane Reynolds **(SLP)**
Booher, Sheryl Anne **(A)**
Braverman, Mrs Janet M **(SLP)**
Carothers, Patrice Orosz **(SLP)**
Chapman, Dr Kathy L **(SLP)**
Cohen, Gail Katz **(SLP)**
Collard, Mary E **(A)**
Cook, Dr Darrell R **(SLP)**
Dettman, Mary Jane **(SLP)**
Dutka, Debra A **(SLP)**
Embry, Loretta Hill
Engelberg, Dr Marvin W **(SLP A)**
Fendrich, Mrs Dale P **(A)**
Forsythe, Susan I **(SLP)**
Gall, Michaelann **(SLP)**
Gerling, Dr Irvin J **(A)**
Goldstein, Dr Beverly A **(A)**
Graham, Mrs Marian Vargo **(SLP)**
Greenwald, Mrs Glenna Griffin **(SLP)**
Gromek, Mrs Marilyn M **(SLP)**
Hadzima, Susan G **(A)**
Haight, Patti Lynn **(SLP)**
Hardin, Mary A **(SLP)**
Harkin, Brigid C **(SLP)**
Harwood, Angela Bartel **(SLP)**
Hoopingarner, Mrs Carla Elaine **(SLP)**
Horwitz-Danzinger, Mrs Helen **(SLP)**
Hoynacke, Mrs Bonnie **(SLP)**
Jirecek, Amy Louise **(SLP)**
Johnson, Janice M **(A)**
Johnson, Kathleen Therese **(SLP)**
Joseph, Cynthia Beth **(A)**
Kay, Mrs Lois F **(SLP)**
Kearns, Thomas J **(SLP)**
Kimbarow, Dr Michael L **(SLP)**
Kostura, Michelle Marie
Kruzer, Mrs A Tammy **(SLP)**
Kulway, Joann M **(A)**
Leon, Julian P **(SLP)**
Lubowicz, Patricia Barniak **(A)**
Marvis, Elenny Michelle **(SLP)**
McGinnis, Mrs Wanda M
Mole, Arlene F **(SLP)**
Morey, Kathryn R **(SLP)**
Murray, Murraileen **(SLP)**
Myers, Mrs Karen Beecher **(SLP)**
Nodar, Dr Richard H **(A)**
Pizzuti, Mary R **(SLP)**
Riley-Blazina, Mrs Roberta J **(SLP)**
Ripich, Dr Danielle N **(SLP)**
Rosenbaum, Mrs Mary R **(A)**
Ruble, Cynthia E **(SLP)**
Rynes, Dr Edward J **(SLP A)**
Sander, Prof Eric Kurt **(SLP)**
Sanek, Gregory Paul **(A)**
Satterfield, Cindy Lee **(SLP)**
Scheckel, Joanne C **(SLP)**
Schwartz, Dr Arthur H **(SLP)**
Sipp, Myrita Yvonne **(A)**
Sitler, Susan Elizabeth **(SLP)**
Spilar, Kathleen Therese **(A)**
Stansberry, Gloria Bisson **(SLP)**
Sudak, Mrs Diane R **(SLP)**
Suty, Dr Karen A **(A)**
Thompson, Angela M **(SLP)**
Tratter, Deborah Suzanne **(SLP)**
Valenza, Gary R **(A)**
Vertes, Dr Dianne **(A)**
Yakir, Leslie C **(A)**
Yokaitis-Skutnik, Judith Ann **(SLP)**
Yost, Mrs Janet C **(SLP)**

Cleveland Heights

Ballard, Melissa J **(SLP)**
Blount, Mrs Adella H **(SLP)**
Courtney, Deborah P **(SLP)**
Gemler, Marcia J **(SLP)**
Gilson, Abigail Ellen **(A)**
Hall, Mrs Ruth L G **(SLP)**
Hamila, Mrs Debra L **(A)**
Henderson, Kathryn Ann **(SLP)**
Heyer, Judith L **(SLP A)**
Ho, Margaret Lew **(SLP)**
Huxel, Mrs Linda Noyes **(SLP)**
Jones, Mrs Patricia Marie **(SLP)**
Lesniak, Dennis P **(A)**
Manuel, Bettina R **(SLP)**
McLaughlin, Joann Nancy **(SLP)**
Messerly, Dr Carol L **(SLP)**
Metz, Dr David Abraham **(A)**
Pitts, Mrs Geraldine Mae **(SLP)**
Pitts, William M **(SLP)**
Richards, Sarah Lee **(SLP)**
Routman, Frank Joseph **(SLP)**
Salzbrenner, Mrs Lynn G **(A)**
Sapharas, Barbara A **(SLP)**
Smith, Carolyn Dana **(SLP)**
Ungemach, Deborah **(SLP)**
Wagner-Otol, Cynthia A **(A)**
Ward-Gravely, Mrs Valenta G **(SLP A)**
Watson, Mavis M **(SLP)**
Wilson, Mrs Helen B F **(SLP)**

Clinton

Butler, Mrs Margaret Smith

Columbia Station

Carpenter, Mary **(SLP)**
Conaway, Jo Adele **(SLP)**
Meister, Mrs Beth A **(SLP)**

Columbiana

McQuilkin, Jean S **(SLP)**
Parsly, Mrs Cinthia Rae **(SLP)**
Smith, Mrs Linda **(SLP)**

Columbus

Aeder, Mrs Nancy G **(SLP)**
Allamanno, Mrs Judith Carole **(SLP)**
Anketell, Mary T **(SLP)**
Backus, Mrs Marcia L **(SLP)**
Badgley, Mrs Janelyn Voigt **(SLP A)**
Bakhshi, Christine Lowe **(SLP)**
Banchefsky, Mrs Debra Kirshner **(SLP)**
Barnes, Dr Janice B **(SLP)**
Bartlinski, Jonette Ann **(A)**
Bauer, Dr Harold R
Becher, Leitsa K **(SLP)**
Beckler, Deanne Mary **(SLP)**
Berkman, Linda S **(SLP)**
Bodnar, Bonnie M **(SLP)**
Bolan, Mrs Margaret Ellen **(SLP)**
Booth, Mary J Y **(SLP)**
Boring, Mrs Melinda Lee **(SLP)**
Bowersock, Mrs Lisa A
Boylan, Mary F **(SLP)**
Brown, Mrs Sandra L **(SLP)**
Canright, Lynnette Jo **(A)**
Chambers, Mrs Helen G **(SLP)**
Chapa, Mrs Mary Anne **(SLP)**
Coddington, Jane H **(SLP)**
Cola-Schuh, Ann L **(A)**
Cook, Mrs Patricia M **(SLP)**
Crawford, Jean Verleny **(SLP)**
Cummins, Mrs Diane M
Davis, Lauren A **(SLP)**
Deboard, Mrs Cheryl J **(SLP)**
Dendiu, Paula D **(A)**
Dietch, Ellen L **(SLP)**
Dillon, Eileen A **(SLP)**
Donohue, Joann S **(SLP)**
Drake, Marla Colleen **(SLP)**
Evans, Sherri Lynne
Feth, Dr Lawrence L
Finnell, Dee Ann **(SLP)**
Flinta, Mrs Andrea J
Florance, Dr Cheri L **(SLP)**
Fox, Robert A
Fraher, Mrs Karen Theresa **(SLP)**
Gafford, Mrs Susan M **(SLP)**
Gardner, Robin Frances **(SLP)**
Gerdeman, Bernice Smith **(SLP)**
Gillette, Yvonne **(SLP)**
Gleason, Dawn E **(A)**
Gokcen, Jeanne Holloway **(SLP)**
Griffiths, Jana Lee **(SLP)**
Hall, Brenda Bogart **(A)**
Harris, Julie Ann **(SLP)**
Hedges, Susan F **(SLP)**
Heller, Mrs Susan Goebel **(A)**
Heron, Mrs Marguerite **(SLP)**
Holland, Carla E **(SLP)**
Holsinger, Mrs Esther L **(SLP)**
Hruschak, Jean M **(SLP)**
Hubbard, Dr Patricia B **(SLP)**
Igel, Joyce Diane **(SLP)**
Irwin, Dr Ruth B **(SLP)**
Ivinskas, Ann E **(SLP)**
Jarrow, Dr Jane E **(SLP)**
Johnson, Mary Elizabeth
Johnson, Michael H **(SLP)**
Kauffman, Carol L **(SLP)**
Kaufman, Paula W
Keller, Dr Geraldine Bermay **(SLP A)**
Kent, Daphne H **(A)**
Kephart, Mary Lisa **(SLP)**
Kiefer, Patricia J **(SLP)**
King, Mrs Deborah Crow **(SLP)**
Kline, Paula Jo **(SLP)**
Klingensmith, Ruth E **(SLP)**
La Chance, Susan Carol **(A)**
La Fleur, Mrs Kathryn E **(SLP)**
LaRosa, Mrs Marianne Kuhar **(SLP)**
Lazer, Dianne Ellen **(SLP)**
Leemhuis, Jane E **(SLP)**
Limburg, Mrs Laura Anne **(SLP)**
Lindsey, Patricia B **(SLP)**
Long, Wanda Baltes **(SLP)**
Luebbe-Gearhart, Mrs Mary Lou **(A)**
Lundblad, Anne Marie **(SLP)**
Lyons, Sr M Justine **(SLP)**
MacDonald, Dr James D **(SLP)**
Manley, Anita Odell **(SLP)**
Manley, Rita O **(SLP)**
Marsh, Mary Beth **(SLP)**
McClure, Mrs Elisa Markle
McGarvey, Judith Lombardo **(SLP)**
Mearan, Judith U **(SLP)**
Melnick, Dr William **(A)**
Mirman, Anne M **(SLP)**
Muccio, Maria A E
Mumm, Myrna N **(SLP)**
Nelson, Dr Lauren K **(SLP)**
Nickles, Dr Aleki C **(SLP)**
Nilo, Dr Ernest R **(A)**
Niswander, Dr Paul S **(A)**
Northrup, Barbara K **(SLP)**
O'Leary, Ann H K **(SLP)**
Oyer, Dr Herbert J **(SLP A)**
Paolucci, Annita Louise **(SLP)**
Paul, Constance L **(A)**
Paxton, Kelli Lynne
Penn, Kathryn L **(SLP)**
Plummer, Sally Ann **(A)**
Rabidoux, Paula C **(SLP)**
Ratcliff-Fais, Mary Beth **(A)**
Ridenour, Ellen H **(SLP)**

Roberts, Dr Margaret Mills **(SLP)**
Rogers, Julianna C **(SLP)**
Roth, Mrs Mary Hawkins **(SLP)**
Rubin, Mrs Shellie G **(SLP)**
Schlanser, Mrs Theresa Dianne **(SLP)**
Schroeder-Oswalt, Ann **(SLP)**
Secord, Dr Wayne A **(SLP)**
Seliskar, Jeanne R **(SLP)**
Sells-Rabold, Mrs Denise E **(SLP)**
Sherry, Mrs Melinda Lewis **(SLP)**
Smith, Mrs Judy K
Smith, Mrs Lyna L **(SLP)**
Sohner, Linda L **(SLP)**
Soukup, Connie Marie **(SLP)**
Squier, Victoria J **(SLP)**
Starr, Sheryl Silver **(A)**
Steele, Eileen R **(SLP)**
Steinbuch, Mrs Debra Wolkoff **(SLP)**
Thomas, Tonda Lee **(A)**
Tillett-Ferguson, Sandra **(SLP)**
Timmons, Mrs Lori Tocash
Toor, Mrs Jane H **(SLP)**
Travers, Joan Marie **(SLP)**
Trudeau, Mrs Linda A **(A)**
Trudeau, Dr Michael D **(SLP)**
Van Deinse, Steven Dale **(SLP)**
Votaw, Mrs Lynn Kresheck **(SLP)**
Vottero, Lynn Maroney **(SLP)**
Wall, Dr Lida Gayl **(A)**
Walters-Page, Linda **(SLP)**
Watts, Rosalie Eiler **(SLP)**
Wellmes, Debora **(SLP)**
White, Dr Doris Lee **(SLP A)**
Whitelaw, Gail Moira **(A)**
Whitlatch, Mary Ellen **(SLP)**
Wiblin, Judith B **(SLP)**
Williams, Neta C **(SLP)**
Wilson, Greg A **(A)**
Wolfe, Victoria E **(SLP)**
Woodfill, Marcia Jo **(A)**

Convoy
Benya, Dr John, Jr **(SLP)**

Cortland
Zuga, Donna J **(SLP)**

Coshocton
Gelacek, Mrs Mimi Tobias **(SLP)**
Pike, Mrs Diane Jones **(SLP)**
Skuza, Karen Ann **(SLP)**

Curtice
Schlievert, Mary Ellen **(SLP)**
Vamos, Kathleen Marie **(SLP)**

Cuyahoga Falls
Barr, Mrs Jennifer Kay **(SLP)**
Bedell, Mrs Beverly Lynn **(SLP)**
Cistone, Mary Padula **(SLP)**
Cochran, Jane Doak **(SLP)**
Daddario, Mrs Cynthia Carol **(A)**
Deering, Mrs Kathleen Mary **(SLP)**
Edgar, Mrs Judith Ann **(SLP)**
Edgerly, Barbara **(SLP)**
Francis, Mrs Shelly **(SLP)**
Hazlett, Mrs Joan M
Herzler, Stephan Charles **(A)**
Klingler, Mrs Mona L **(A)**
Manning, Annette Louise **(SLP)**
Pollack, Dr Michael C **(A)**
Powers, Mrs Linda M **(A)**
Ryan, Mrs Caryl Thomas **(SLP)**
Sabol, Barbara Ann **(SLP)**
Skinner, Christina T **(SLP)**
Steinberg, Mrs Virginia **(SLP)**
Wentz, Linda Diane **(SLP)**

Dayton
Adams, Mrs Vickie L **(A)**
Ali, Mrs Angela Catherine **(SLP)**
Anderson, Mrs Ann N **(SLP)**
Arnovitz, Mrs Elaine S **(SLP)**
Austing, Elisa M **(A)**
Birk, Angela C **(SLP)**
Blair, Jolynn Hopkins **(A)**
Brill, Mrs Cynthia Lawson **(SLP)**
Bunni, Maureen Bridget **(SLP)**
Clement, Diane E **(A)**
Coleman, Mrs Heidi J **(SLP)**
Connell, Mrs Sharon Marie **(SLP)**
Coulles, Mrs Linda C **(SLP)**
Creager, Mrs Carol F **(SLP)**
Darata, Mrs Carrie E **(A)**
Deloach, Michelle Logensie
Doerpinghaus, Mary Jude **(SLP)**
Donahue, Phyllis A **(SLP)**
Edly, Linda Marie **(SLP)**
Ege, Diane D **(SLP)**
Ehrenpreis, Mrs Elaine R **(SLP)**
Glaser, Dr Robert G **(A)**
Haley, Donna Jean **(SLP)**
Hazen, Jayne L **(SLP)**
Johnson, Dr Charles **(SLP)**
Johnson, Susan Straute **(SLP)**
Jones, Mrs Judith J **(SLP)**
Joyner, Mrs Gayle Merrix **(SLP)**
Justus, Molly Ann **(A)**
LaFosse, Maryann **(A)**
Lane, Pamela Pruitt
Leiter, Mrs Ann Cheryl **(SLP)**
McGinnis, Mrs Landa J **(A)**
McGinnis, Linda Rieser **(A)**
Merker, Mrs Corina E **(A)**
Monachino, Mrs Julie Kay **(A)**
Patty-Schwab, Dixie R **(SLP)**
Pavlakos, Dr Chris M **(A)**
Roberts, Mrs Juanita Dundon **(SLP)**
Rudy, Jane Hunter **(A)**
Schmidt, Robert K **(SLP A)**
Schumacher, Gretchen Klopf **(SLP)**
Seifferth, Susan Kay **(SLP)**
Shupe, Dr Lewis K **(SLP)**
Silver, Mrs Susan A **(SLP)**
Sisk, Mrs Belinda Kathleen C **(SLP)**
Skinner, Patricia F **(SLP)**
Spinnato, Ann **(SLP)**
Stahl, Mrs Lisa Marie **(SLP)**
Stemple, Dr Joseph C **(SLP)**
Stitt, Signe Lynn **(SLP)**
Stobbs, Kathryn J **(SLP)**
Surber, Barbara Kaufman **(SLP)**
Takacs, Mrs Candace E **(SLP)**
Teske, Katherine **(SLP)**
Thomas, Bruce M **(A)**
Treman, Terri Ann **(SLP)**
Troxell-Klosterman, Julia Lynne **(SLP)**
Van Winkle, David L **(A)**
Veys, Mrs Susan Boden **(SLP)**
Wiegel, Mrs Terry Breeze **(SLP)**
Wuebben, Renee L **(SLP)**
Wyandt, Katherine M **(SLP)**

Defiance
Schroeder, Mrs Nancy H **(A)**

Delaware
Burns, Mrs Carol J **(A)**
Jenkins, Linda Jean **(SLP)**
King, Mrs Marjorie C **(SLP)**
Meyer, Phyllis R **(SLP)**
Naples, Mrs Christy G **(A)**
Naples, Guy M **(SLP A)**
Porterfield, Mrs Janet L **(SLP)**
Robbins, Mrs Janice Schwenk **(SLP)**
Stadler, Marie Alice **(SLP)**

Delta
Kanagy, David N **(SLP)**

Dover
Dugan, Nancy C **(A)**
Ross, Barbara Ann **(SLP)**
Wittler, Mrs Maureen A **(SLP)**
Wittler, Thomas P **(SLP)**

Dublin
Brown, Paula Christine **(SLP)**
Chester, Kathleen Arvidson **(SLP)**
Davis, Lynne A **(A)**
deBondt, Susan Maynard **(A)**
Dickerson, Jan Marie **(SLP)**
Edwards, Joyce M **(SLP)**
Goeke, Lorraine A **(SLP)**
Goodin, Mrs Gina Lea
Johanns, Mrs Cindy J **(A)**
Leach, Helen M **(SLP)**
Lecks-Chernett, Nancy **(A)**
Minekime, Karen Johnstone **(A)**
Quantz-Ratliff, Patricia **(SLP)**
Scalzone, Mrs Diane Boehler **(SLP)**
Shahbazpour, Mrs Karin-Lyn **(SLP)**
Theil, Carol Eastman **(SLP)**
Watson-Holcomb, Judy **(SLP)**
Wheat, Mrs Ann Chiles **(A)**
Will, Darryl J **(A)**

East Canton
Bushey, Philip A **(SLP)**

East Cleveland
Mims, Dr Howard A **(SLP)**
Walker, Mrs Cheron Glaze **(SLP)**

East Liverpool
Malcomson, David L **(SLP)**
Peshel, Mrs Cynthia A **(SLP)**

Eaton
Farmer, Mrs Paula Ann **(SLP)**

Elida
Purdy, Lori Ebling **(A)**

Elyria
Coffin, Mrs Jo Ann B **(A)**
Degirolamo, Dale A **(SLP)**
Delf, Debra Susan **(SLP)**
Hetsko, Richard James **(A)**
Jones, Marlene L **(SLP)**
Koch, Gerald C **(SLP)**
Rosenbaum, Cynthia L **(SLP)**
Smola, Kimberly Ann **(SLP)**

Englewood
Dean, Mrs Sheila A **(SLP)**
George, Jill Ann **(SLP)**
Graef, Mrs Barbara A **(SLP)**

Euclid
Ardys, Inore A
Bowman, Mrs Susan Cherry **(A)**
Brooks-King, Kimberly Diann
Finney, Dollye P
Harrold, Mrs Yvonne Rhodes **(SLP)**
Lebowitz, Mrs Trudy Eilbaum **(SLP)**
McMurray, Mrs Mary Erdani **(SLP)**
Simenc, Bridget Garin
Smith, Katherine Dunn **(SLP)**
Walters, Noreen Marie **(SLP)**
Wilson, Suzanne Michelle **(SLP)**
Zofcin, Michael Francis **(SLP)**

Fairborn
Cunningham, Rosemary A J **(A)**
Grant, Leslie M **(SLP)**
Hardee, Terry H **(SLP)**
Hudson, Mrs Susan B **(SLP)**

Fairfield
Borgemenke, Mrs Jana Kay **(SLP)**
Bowman, Melinda Vice **(SLP)**
Fisher, Mrs Patricia K **(SLP)**
Gortner, Rebecca Lynn **(SLP)**
Gross, Melvin K **(A)**
Guthrie, Denise Cornett **(SLP)**
Holzhauser-Peters, Leslie Susan **(SLP)**
Jacobs, Molly Ann **(SLP)**
Kahn, Dr Alice R **(SLP)**
King, Roger D **(SLP)**
McCracken, Mrs Patrice Marie **(SLP)**
Singer, Tina Marie **(SLP)**
Ward, Gary L **(SLP)**
Wolfe, Mrs Mary Ann E **(SLP)**

Fairview Park
Bringman, Norman A **(A)**
Grispino, Mrs Linda M **(SLP)**
Kolas, Christy **(SLP A)**
Sabino, Ann Marie **(SLP)**
Smith, Mrs Karen Weller **(A)**

Findlay
Bade, Mrs Joan Elaine **(SLP)**
Chiles, Joleen A
Haugh, Mrs Elizabeth **(A)**
Howell, Mrs Marsha Eidnier **(SLP)**
Mielke, Mrs Martha Mary **(SLP)**
Mitchell, Mrs Lillian R **(A)**
Schrock, Laura L **(SLP)**
Schultz, Mrs Marilyn C **(SLP)**

Forest Park
Daum, Katherine Kuhn

Fort Recovery
Staugler, Mrs Kathy M **(SLP)**
Vonderhaar, Mrs Joan Mary

Fremont
Gamble, Robert P **(A)**

Gahanna
Dronberger, Mrs Elizabeth Anne **(SLP)**
Dunn, Lisa Maria **(A)**
Gingerich, Mrs Rhonda Schoon **(SLP)**
Klute, Mrs Jacqueline Monk **(SLP)**
Lockett, Ann Victoria **(SLP)**
Progar-Borowy, Mrs Pamela J **(SLP)**
Shnider, Mrs Doris Fern **(A)**
Wilcox, Mrs Susan Scott **(SLP)**

Galena
Davidson, Stephanie Ann **(A)**

Gallipolis
Koch, Mrs Lisa McHugh **(A)**
MacKenzie, Charla Bodimer **(SLP)**

Garfield
Pelley, Mrs Karen S **(SLP)**

Garfield Heights
Burns, Mrs Julianne Zielaski **(SLP)**
Kukula, Jane M **(A)**
Wolslager, Jacqueline M **(SLP)**

Gates Mills
Dicioccio, Mrs Patricia B **(SLP)**
Garrison, Mrs Mary Jo F **(A)**
Murray, Dr Gail S **(A)**
Schreiber, Rebecca Cronin **(A)**

Genoa
Placko, Mrs Judith Ryan **(SLP)**

Germantown
Leppla, Mrs Patricia Lindenmuth **(SLP)**

Gibsonburg
Hiser, Mrs Luann W **(SLP)**

Girard
Baumblatt, Mrs Gladys R **(SLP)**
Cera, Mrs Roselyn M **(SLP)**
Gaylord, Mrs Sondra P **(SLP)**
Lesinski, Mrs Marilyn Feicht **(SLP)**

Goshen
Massett, Mrs Kathryn H **(SLP)**

Grafton
Prokop, Mrs Terry Hall **(SLP)**

Grand Rapids
Smith, Mrs Debra L **(SLP)**

Grandview Heights
Blott, Mrs Judith P **(SLP)**

Granville
Lechner, Barbara K **(SLP)**
Stypula, Mrs Roseann C **(SLP)**
Thios, Mrs Barbara M **(SLP)**

Greenville
Fulk, Melissa Anne **(SLP)**
Jessup, Rita Ann **(SLP)**
McElwain, Judy Ann M **(SLP)**
Munn, Kimberly Stump **(SLP)**
Paschall, Mrs Frances Gulley **(SLP)**
Poeppelman, Lisa Louise **(SLP)**

Grove City
Kelly, Linda Lee **(SLP)**
Kleinline, Lisa Jane **(A)**

Hamilton
Dailey, Kathleen **(SLP)**
Fike, Mrs Suzanne M
Haid, Mrs Sheila Ann **(SLP)**
Hubbard, Mrs Sally A **(A)**
Keating, Mrs Linda Susan **(SLP)**
Lerer, Pamela Batson **(SLP)**
Ott-Jones, Lori Kay **(SLP)**
Pigg, Mrs Sue Ann
Polson, Debra L **(SLP)**
Poston, Alison Kirschner **(SLP)**
Rogers, Mrs Susan E **(SLP)**
Ryan, Victoria Ganz **(SLP)**
Smith, Mrs Karen Beth **(SLP)**
Stone, Mrs Katrinka L **(SLP)**
Weigel, Rebecca S **(SLP)**

Harrison
Davis, Teresa Martinelli **(SLP)**
Noxsel, Mrs Jennifer Lee **(SLP)**

Hartville
Milligan, Mrs Mary Louise **(SLP)**
Waters, Ellen K **(SLP)**

Heath
Jones, Mrs Janice Lohman **(SLP)**

Highland Heights
D'Alessandro, JoAnn Marie
Di Mare, Mrs Mateja J **(A)**
MacKin, Christine Lynn **(SLP)**

Hilliard
Carroll, Mrs Inez B **(A)**
Mandelbaum, Tricia Ann **(A)**

Hillsboro
Blischak, Doreen M **(SLP)**
Bruckner, Kristy Sue **(SLP)**
Gilmore, Joy E M **(SLP)**
Kelly, Dr Dan H **(SLP)**
Lucas, Tana Roush **(SLP)**

Hinckley
May, Mrs Sarah Jane **(SLP)**

Hiram
Hollinger, Susan Anne **(SLP)**

Hockingport
Slater, Carol Ann **(SLP)**

Holland
Drake, Lisa Ann **(A)**
Gill, Terri L F **(SLP)**

Howard
Luna, Ann L W **(SLP)**

Hubbard
Bross, Mrs Maureen Patrick **(SLP)**
Snyder-Williams, Mrs Mary Ann **(SLP)**

Huber Heights
Brenneman, Mrs Mary A T **(A)**
Fisher, Mrs Pamela A **(SLP)**
Hawkes, Mrs Kirsten J **(SLP)**
McPhail, Paula A **(A)**
Rich, Rita Dushman **(SLP)**

Hudson
Dworkin, Mrs Doris R R **(SLP)**
Flanagan, Mrs Barbara M **(SLP)**
Hall, Mrs Katherine Marie **(SLP)**
Kilpatrick, Kathryn M **(SLP)**
Newton, Mrs Ingeborg B **(SLP)**
Stolle, Mrs Marcia Zieman **(SLP)**
White, Nancy J **(A)**

Huron
Beatty, Kathy V **(SLP)**
Carter, Margaret **(SLP)**
Fox, Frank Lynn, Jr **(A)**
Kozar, Nadia E **(SLP)**
Kuhn, Mrs Charleene L

Independence
Montague, Mrs Karen Alm **(SLP)**
Pretzloff, Mrs Lucia Kowalski

Jamestown
Brown, Mrs Sandra Stiles **(SLP)**

Jefferson
Wladyka, Kateri Zook **(SLP)**

Johnstown
Buck, Paula King **(A)**

Kent
Andreani, Bonita K **(SLP)**
Awan, Karen Judith **(SLP)**
Awan, Shaheen Nazir **(SLP)**
Bacon, Susanellen **(SLP)**
Berger, Kenneth W **(SLP A)**
Bloch, Gerald A **(A)**
Bose, Nancy DuBois **(SLP)**
Clark, Julie M
Cottrell, Gary T **(A)**
Derk-Gans, Dr Karen **(SLP)**
Downs, David W **(A)**
Favetta, Fred Joseph **(A)**
Flexer, Dr Carol S **(A)**
Gans, Dr Donald P **(A)**
Germani, Mary Jo **(SLP)**
Grogan, Susan Lynn **(SLP)**
Herrick, Mrs Margaret Hatton **(SLP)**
Kaltenborn, Arthur L, Jr **(SLP)**
Klich, Dr Richard John
Kouri, Theresa A **(SLP)**
McCall, Judith Ann **(A)**
McGuffin, Donaldine E **(SLP)**
McLoughlin, Mrs Patricia J **(SLP)**
Neiman, Dr Gary S **(SLP)**
Palen, Dr Chester **(SLP)**
Pierce, Mrs Christine W **(SLP)**
Pierce, Dr Robert S **(SLP)**
Place, Patti J **(SLP)**
Puskaric, Nada Jane **(SLP)**
Ryland, Mark Gordon **(A)**
Sleight, Dr Christine C **(SLP)**
Sommers, Dr Ronald K **(SLP A)**
Stagray, James Ronald **(A)**
Terrell, Dr Brenda Y **(SLP)**
Ulreich, Patty L **(SLP)**
Vair, Lauri R **(SLP)**
Vitone, Sherry Fundoots
Watt, Mrs Linda S **(SLP)**
Webster, Olive M **(SLP)**
Wilcox, Dr M Jeanne **(SLP)**

Kenton
Morris, Mrs Elizabeth **(SLP)**
Winzenried, Barbara B **(SLP)**

Kettering
Galbreath, Mrs Debbie Dodge **(SLP)**
Hagerty, Mary B **(SLP)**
Kiefaber, Mrs Victoria L **(SLP)**
Lolan, Thomas C **(A)**
McKenna, Mrs Marla **(SLP)**
Mishler, Pamela J **(A)**
Phillips, Suzanne K **(A)**
Reichard, Mrs Joan M **(SLP A)**
Wilkerson, Michele L **(SLP)**

Kinsman
Davis, Sherry Renee **(SLP)**

Kirtland
Lewis, Mrs Barbara M **(SLP)**

Lagrange
Burke, Mrs Linda M **(SLP)**

Lakemore
Huff, Mrs Sheryl Joy Serbin **(SLP)**

Lakewood
Breen, Melissa Anne **(SLP)**
Burhans, Mrs Denise Strickler **(A)**
Dahler, Mrs Mary F Z **(SLP)**
D'Amore, Donald D **(SLP)**
DiFilippo, Mrs Marla A **(SLP)**
Filipek, Kathleen Ready **(SLP)**
Forkosh, Ronna Heidi **(SLP)**
Kuhn, Deborah Jean **(SLP)**
Magdinec, Melanie **(SLP A)**
Malinak, Betty S **(SLP)**
Maresco, Kathy D **(SLP)**
McAndrew, Patricia Burke **(SLP)**
McSweeney, Aileen Marie
Monroe, William M **(SLP)**
Powers, Susan M **(SLP)**
Razum, Cheryl A **(SLP)**
Schulz, Mrs Mary E **(SLP)**
Smith, Mrs Regina Teresa **(SLP)**
Vanta, K Sandra **(SLP)**
Weirich, Patricia Suzanne **(SLP)**
Whittemore, Cynthia **(SLP)**
Wood, Penny Marie **(A)**

Lancaster
Bickley, Mrs Minda S **(SLP)**
Lewis, Douglas Augustus **(A)**
Miller, Mrs Tracey Anne **(SLP)**
Snider, Bonita J **(SLP)**
Vajen, Mrs Mary Jane **(SLP)**
Wenner, Susan Kay **(SLP)**

Lebanon
Barry, June D **(SLP)**
Hawke, Mrs Carol Ann **(SLP)**

Lexington
Thomas, Mrs Billie J **(SLP)**

Libson
Amick, Katherine Ann **(SLP)**

Lima
Appaya, Monjula N **(SLP)**
Baker, Jennifer Cox **(SLP)**
Field, Mrs Janice Lynn **(SLP)**
Guagenti, Virginia M **(SLP)**
Jones, Mrs Lyda B **(SLP)**
Nadler, Mrs Alexis Rauch **(A)**
Waronker, Mrs Sue Ann **(SLP)**
Webb, Dr Kevin C **(A)**

Little Hocking
Cline, Sue Ellen **(SLP)**

Lodi
Simmons, Mrs Sally D **(SLP)**

London
Patterson, Pamela J **(A)**
Pinkerton, Mrs Judith A **(SLP)**

Lorain
Mentch, Mace W **(SLP)**
Miller, Thomas W **(SLP)**

Louisville
Best, Karen P **(SLP)**

Loveland
Brom, Carole Ann **(SLP)**
Cesco, Penny Suzanne **(SLP)**
Deboer, Carolyn **(SLP)**
Foster, Mrs Michele Marie **(SLP)**
Holcomb, Barbara J **(SLP)**
Housel, Mrs Susan I **(SLP)**
Redmon-Trame, Mrs Billie **(SLP)**
Songer, Judy A **(SLP)**
Tepe, Mrs Krista Lynn **(SLP)**
Ullman, Ann P **(SLP)**
Vulanich, Mrs Nova Nicolette **(SLP)**

Lynchburg
Dean, Julia Ann **(SLP)**

Lyndhurst
Camiener, Mrs Michele Schwartz
Isaacs, Mrs Laura J P **(A)**
Merriman, Mrs Elizabeth **(A)**
Nyer, Mrs Rochelle Rubin **(SLP)**
Phoenix, Mrs Lynann V C **(SLP)**
Visoky, Mrs Anita M **(SLP)**
Zucker, Barbara Loren **(SLP)**

Madeira
Templeton, Mrs Karla Mitchell **(SLP)**

Madina
Hertrick, Kathy Lynn **(SLP)**

Madison
Lapish, Marisa Joy **(SLP)**
Wolf, Mrs Karen B **(SLP)**

Magnolia
Tolin, Mrs Paula Rupert **(SLP)**

Maineville
Hopkins, Jennifer Marie **(SLP)**
Johnson-Glaser, Mary Ann **(SLP)**
Krejmas, Mrs Jodee **(SLP)**
Palmer, Mrs Kim Kokus **(SLP)**
Vogel, Mrs Carolyn Sue **(SLP)**

Manchester
Stwarka, Mrs Jeanne Ann **(SLP)**

Mansfield
Boals, Mrs Carol Martini **(SLP)**
Braun, Mary Beth **(SLP)**
Broege, Barbara Heermeier **(A)**
Czuchna, Paul E **(SLP)**
Giles, Nanette A **(SLP)**
Gyurek, Deborah Lynn **(SLP)**
Hire, Mrs Janeen Mabee **(SLP)**
Huprich, Mrs Joann S S **(SLP)**
Jabre, Mrs Angele Debbane **(SLP)**
Kerg, Mrs Gail B **(A)**
Kinstle, Frances Lillian **(SLP)**
Kreinbihl, Mrs Beth A **(SLP)**
Lukach, Lynne M **(SLP)**
Murphy, Mrs Jan Hughes **(SLP)**
Nichols, Mrs Cynthia Zender **(SLP)**
Palmer, Mrs Susan A **(SLP)**
Sakellakis, Tessie Jean **(SLP)**
Signoracci, Christine Jeanette **(SLP)**
Steele, Mrs Dedra L **(SLP)**
Wright, Mrs Mary Beth Ebling **(A)**

Mantua
Braden, Mrs Pamela King **(SLP)**
Gharky, Mrs Marylou F **(SLP)**
Phillips, Mrs Martha Zarzour **(SLP)**

Maple Heights
De Roia, Mrs Marielaine Dicillo **(SLP)**
Kriynovich, Linda G **(SLP)**

Mariemont
Foxman, Mrs Leanne K **(SLP)**

Marietta
Behun, Elizabeth K
Elliott, Virginia **(SLP)**
Neal, Julie A **(A)**
Shimer, Mrs Linda L **(SLP)**
Webb, Christophr A **(SLP)**
Webb, Jane C **(A)**

Marion
Finnegan, Mrs Sarah Meffley **(SLP)**
Whitaker, Mrs Nancy O **(SLP)**
Winger, Dr Roger K **(A)**

Martin
Padley, Susan Kay **(SLP)**

Martins Ferry
Davies, Jenny Frances **(A)**
Domyan, Steve R **(A)**

Mason
Bailey, Jill M **(SLP)**
Davis, Mrs Lynn A **(SLP)**

Doben-Stevens, Mrs Monica Elaine **(SLP)**
Kurtz, Mrs Carla Ann **(A)**
Lahrmer, Mrs Jackie S
Nelcamp, Valerie Grace **(SLP)**
Potter, Elizabeth Walker **(SLP)**
Smith, Mrs Sherry Sue **(SLP)**
Thomas, Judith Allyn **(SLP)**

Massillon
Avers, Kenneth William **(SLP)**
Bussard, Mrs Susan Hill **(A)**
Deal, Jane E **(SLP)**
Dickerhoof, Richard Gary **(A)**
Gole, Mrs Lisa
Kirven, Laura Ann **(SLP)**
Oser, Carla Kay **(SLP)**
Paul, Beth **(SLP)**

Masury
Vargulich-Sinkuc, Valerie **(SLP)**

Maumee
Amadio, Phillip H **(SLP)**
Baessler, Jane K **(SLP)**
Eaton, Mrs Jennifer Ann **(SLP)**
Farrell, Mrs Martha Domitio
Harrison, Diann Micka **(A)**
Irmen, Antonia Sares **(SLP)**
McAllister, Mrs Linda Ruth **(SLP)**
Mullee, Cynthia Ann **(SLP)**
Phillips-Littrell, Mrs Mary Ann **(A)**
Wack, Stephanie Ann **(SLP)**
Ward, Barbara Leilani **(SLP)**

Mayfield Heights
Bailys, Wendy Susan **(SLP)**
Beremana, Mrs Pamela J **(SLP)**
Body, Carmen Renee **(SLP)**
Burman, Laurie E **(A)**
Jackson, Shelley L **(A)**
Nisenboom, Jean M **(SLP)**
Starp, Carolyn Gail **(SLP)**
Win, Susan M

McDonald
Entzi, Mrs Judith L

Medina
Binnie, Mrs Doreen **(SLP)**
Conrad, Mrs Barbara Jean **(SLP)**
Derga, Kathleen E **(SLP)**
Ginesi, Linda A M **(SLP)**
Greytak, Sharyn P **(SLP)**
Huefner, Deborah Petro **(SLP)**
Prakup, Barbara R **(SLP)**
Ruhlin, Mrs Susan U **(SLP)**
Stepp, Mrs Helen Elizabeth **(SLP)**

Mentor
Cappello, Mrs Domenica Vitale **(SLP)**
Cortelezzi, Mrs Deborah A **(SLP)**
Harrison, Kathleen M Odonnell **(SLP)**
Munson, Deborah **(SLP)**
Roman, Elfriede **(SLP)**
Sak, Carla A **(SLP)**
Scott, Mrs Jane R **(SLP)**
Srsen, Mrs Paula M **(SLP)**
Wolfe, Basil N, Jr **(A)**

Miamisburg
Holdsworth, Mrs Joy Lindsey **(SLP)**
Hopping, Louise A **(A)**
Maine, Mrs Candy R **(SLP)**
Noel, Penny Kay **(SLP)**
Perrine, Helen J **(A)**
Ricks, Mrs Barbara G **(SLP)**
Roth, Susan Peio
Taylor, Mrs Lori Brosius **(SLP)**
Turner, Patsy Ann
Wathen, Mrs Patricia Durbin

Middleburg Heights
Wilson, Mrs Luana S **(SLP)**

Middleport
Call, Janell **(SLP)**

Middletown
Campbell, Terri Lynn
Halsey, Mrs Judith Snyder **(SLP)**
Hill, Alan R **(SLP)**
Noble, Paula L **(A)**
Weinrich, Mrs Barbara D **(SLP)**

Milford
Dacey, Deborah A **(SLP)**
Garrett, Jill **(SLP)**
Klein, Mrs Barbara Jones
Tumolo, Mrs Judith A **(SLP)**

Millersburg
Pratt, Mrs Linda S **(SLP)**

Mineral Ridge
Cerni, Mrs Carol A **(SLP)**
Slipski, Mrs Geralyn Balchak **(A)**

Mingo Junction
Graves, Mrs Karen B **(A)**

Mogadore
Atha, Mrs Karen J B **(SLP)**
Shaffer, Lori J **(SLP)**

Monclova
Blair, Bruce Bennett **(SLP)**
Sechler, Mrs Linda **(SLP)**

Montgomery
Kreisle, Alice E **(A)**

Moreland Hills
Braun, Mrs Susan W

Mount St Joseph
Kemble, Sr Carita **(SLP)**

Mount Vernon
Fish, Mrs Brenda S **(SLP)**
Garver, Mrs Gladis G **(SLP)**
Hoar, Rochelle Anne **(SLP)**
Oelker, Colleen Sue **(SLP)**
Romas, Mrs Debra B **(SLP)**
Williams, Mrs Jill Koehler **(SLP)**

Munroe Falls
Chafin, Mrs Patricia A **(SLP)**
Fleming, Lorna J **(SLP)**
Jones, Mrs Cynthia Pinney **(SLP)**
Lettieri, Mrs Mary M **(SLP)**

Napoleon
Kottman, Yvette Fischbach **(SLP)**

Navarre
Moulos, Tammy Jean **(SLP)**

New Carlisle
Current, Mrs Jeanne Louise **(SLP)**
Susnik, Jackie L **(SLP)**

New Concord
Patterson, Robert E **(SLP)**
Taylor, Deborah Susan **(SLP)**

New Philadelphia
Sanders, Mrs Marla Watson
Smith, Ruth Joyce **(SLP)**

New Richmond
Kennedy, Mrs Janice D **(SLP)**

New Waterford
Lipp, Linda A **(SLP)**

Newark
Badger, Mrs Shelli M **(SLP)**
Blakely, Mrs Patricia Smith **(SLP)**
Lacko-Pries, Mrs Diane **(SLP)**
Matesich, Martha Anne **(SLP)**
McCrory, Mrs Elizabeth Flynn **(SLP)**
Worth, Janet C **(SLP)**

Newburg Heights
Bonko, Mrs Julie Anne

Newton Falls
Pliszka, Katherine Lynn **(SLP)**

Niles
Austin, Juanita T **(SLP)**
Coleman, Mattie B **(SLP)**
Pezzano, Mrs Diane B **(SLP)**

North Bend
Clark, Mrs Lynn **(SLP)**

North Canton
Besozzi, Thomas E **(SLP)**
Brumbaugh, Mrs Brenda J **(SLP)**
Defazio, Dr Jean Levin **(SLP)**
Doyle, Mrs Debora H **(SLP)**
Gluck, Mrs Dolores Wells **(SLP)**
Greenfelder, Mrs Debra Diane **(SLP)**
Hein, Karen L **(SLP)**
Kodama, Mrs Mildred Riley **(SLP)**
Lutz, Arlene Mae **(SLP)**
Pfeiffer, Mrs Bonnie McClellan **(SLP)**
Rowan, Mrs Lydia A **(A)**
Schwitzgebel, Rita A **(SLP)**
Steckel, Laura Ann

North Olmsted
Abahazi, Dr Dennis A **(SLP A)**
Barnes, Mary Z **(SLP)**
Colo, Denise Marie **(A)**
Dittrick, Ginger Lee **(SLP)**
Lyall, Lisa Ann **(SLP)**
Marks, Mary D **(SLP)**
O'Malley, Mrs Nancy S **(SLP)**
Szaller, Mrs Charlene N **(SLP)**
Zelvis, Dorothy Aphrodite **(SLP)**

North Ridgeville
Gustetic, Susan M **(SLP)**
Heston, Robert E **(A)**
Lenters-Hansen, Marjorie S **(SLP)**
Limbert-Lerch, Carol Sue

North Royalton
Cherpillod, Deborah Lee **(A)**
Clink, Mrs Pamela J **(SLP)**
Platt, Cindy Lyn **(A)**
Stibora, Debra Ann **(SLP)**
Vance, Margaret Pojman **(SLP)**

Northfield
Foley, Mrs Sheila M **(SLP)**
Wischner, George J **(SLP)**

Northfield Center
Shotwell, Mrs Rochelle **(SLP)**

Northwood
Lynch, Mrs Carol L **(SLP)**

Norwalk
Hegemier, Lisa Renee **(A)**
Koupal, Mrs Margaret Thomson
Riley, Mrs Cindra Lee **(SLP)**
Schmidt, Mrs Susan Todd **(SLP)**
Strayer, Lorna Schwab **(SLP)**

Novelty
Arkis, Peter N **(A)**
Batza, Dr Eugene M **(SLP A)**

Oberlin
Tear, Mrs Diane Louise **(SLP)**

Olmsted Falls
Ledinsky, Judith A **(SLP)**
Mossman, Mary M **(SLP)**
Sommer, Mrs Carol Galbany **(A)**

Olmsted Township
Zvejnieks, Mrs Anita Z **(SLP)**

Orange Village
Elmets, Laurie Melamed **(A)**
Engler, Shelley F **(SLP)**
Schwartz, Mrs Sharon Salzman **(SLP)**

Oregon
Bosse, Mrs Julie K **(SLP)**
Griebner, Mrs Sandra S **(SLP)**

Orrville
Butzer, Mrs Jan Renner **(SLP)**

Ottawa
Affholder, Thomas G **(SLP)**
Meyer, Mrs Sheila Rose **(A)**

Oxford
Angello, Martha J **(SLP)**
Brown, Vicki C **(SLP)**
Grandstaff, Harvey L **(SLP)**
Hutchinson, Mrs Dianne C **(SLP)**
Johnston, Dr Elizabeth **(SLP)**
Kelly, Laura J **(A)**
Kneier, Barbara Louise **(SLP)**
Malott, Paul James **(SLP)**
Marron, Kathleen Hutchinson **(A)**
Tomes, Mrs Ines A **(SLP)**
Van Vliet, Louise **(SLP A)**

Painesville
Adomaitis, Christine Marie **(SLP)**
Cratcha, Stanley G **(SLP)**
Levin, Molly **(SLP)**
Sheterom, Mrs Helen Ronke **(SLP)**
Snyderwine, Mrs Carol Hazlett **(A)**
Spence, Scott W **(A)**

Parma
Alesnik, Christina **(SLP)**
Bartoul, Millet J **(A)**
Carns, Carol Louise **(SLP)**
Crowl, Mrs Kathy W **(SLP)**
Mackall, Jane M **(A)**
Mueller, Nancy Bitto **(SLP)**
O'Brien, Mrs Marti Marianne **(SLP)**
Olsen, Randall R **(A)**
Smith, Mrs Agatha **(SLP)**
Smith, Mrs Janet Darchuk **(SLP)**

Parma Heights
Baranek, Thomas Paul **(A)**
Blanda, Denise J **(SLP)**
Danko, Mrs Angela N **(SLP)**
Fraser, Janet R **(A)**
Mester, Leslie J **(A)**
Neff, Sue Ann **(SLP)**

Pataskala
Kean, Mrs Sally Ann **(SLP)**
Mielnik, Mrs Lynn K **(SLP)**

Paulding
McGrath, Mrs Julia B **(SLP)**

Pepper Pike
Meeker, Susan Scott **(SLP)**

Perry
Uonelli, Mrs Elaine Martin **(SLP)**

Perrysburg
Bowlus, Janet Mae **(SLP)**
Kaderavek, Joan N **(SLP)**
Kindt, Jacqueline L **(SLP)**
Lakis, Mrs Karen Terhune **(SLP)**
Mauk, Mrs Cornelia L **(SLP)**
Moser, Georgia Jean **(SLP)**
Persiani, Mrs Nancy Hank **(SLP)**
Rastatter, Dr Michael P **(SLP)**
Ridge, Michelle Manyak **(SLP)**
Rittenhouse, Sharon S **(SLP)**
Spletzer-Cheetwood, Mrs Barbara **(SLP)**

Pickerington
Boyer, Pauline M **(A)**
Fiorelli, Maria Tirabasso **(SLP)**
Monnin, Mrs Jean A **(SLP)**

Piqua
McHone, Mrs Molly Miller **(SLP)**
Willig-Denise, Nancy E **(SLP)**

Poland
Banks, Mrs Frances M **(SLP)**
Hicken, Susan J **(SLP)**
Malone, Mrs Charleen Campbell **(SLP)**

Pomeroy
King, Mrs Cheryl Ann **(SLP)**

Portsmouth
Kraft, Kathryn Irene **(SLP)**
Lashley, Luann L **(SLP)**
Snyder, Elizabeth Ellen **(A)**
Stimpert, Kevin Alan **(SLP)**
Ugrin, Jerome G **(A)**

Powell
Hofbauer, Carol L **(SLP)**
Lazor, Mrs Judy L **(A)**

Proctorville
Mayo, Mrs Lizabethe **(SLP)**

Ravenna
Deeter, Arlyce K **(SLP)**
Harrison, Linda D **(A)**
Johnson, Janet L

Reminderville
Bodziony, Mrs Beverly Bucell **(SLP)**

Reynoldsburg
Amberg, Cheryl D **(SLP)**
Beachy, Mrs Jane Ellen **(SLP)**
Brosius, Michele **(SLP A)**
Cartwright, Barbara A **(SLP)**
Erhart, Diana Marie **(SLP)**
George, Jeanne Hegarty **(SLP)**
Greening, Marti Netler **(SLP)**
Martin, Orville W **(A)**
Martin, Mrs Susan J **(A)**
Rodriguez, Carol Shade **(SLP)**
Starkey, Mrs Martha Krisko **(SLP)**

Richfield
McCann, Mrs Lawrette Jane **(SLP)**

Richmond Heights
Bingle, Janice M **(A)**
Cercone, Judith A **(A)**
Daryoush, Mehrdad Samimi
Daubenspeck, Deborah **(SLP)**
Friedman, Ellen Noreen **(SLP)**
Johnston, Mrs Clarion E **(SLP)**
Koenig, Linda A **(SLP)**
Kowalczyk, Deborah Jean **(SLP)**

Ripley
Wright, Mrs Loretta L **(SLP)**

Rittman
Bauer, Mrs Cathy Lynn **(SLP)**

Rocky River
DeVito, Teresa **(SLP)**
Karnes, Mrs Dianne E **(SLP)**
McNeal, Kathryn Marie **(SLP)**
Otto, Mrs Lucia Marie **(SLP)**

Sagamore Hills
McDonald, Mrs L Christine **(SLP)**
Vacel, Marilyn **(SLP)**
Wischner, Mary Ellen **(SLP)**

Salem
Mansfield, Mrs Mary Lee **(SLP)**
McDevitt, Amy Michelle

Sandusky
Blaesing, Basille Evelyn **(SLP)**
Millott, Mrs Marian Schlicht **(SLP)**
Schlett, Carolyn Elizabeth **(SLP)**
Young, Karen Lyman **(SLP)**

Sebring
Wayt, Paula M **(SLP)**

Seven Mile
Rockwell, Mrs Jackie M **(SLP)**

Shadyside
Cook, Leslie Ann **(SLP)**

Shaker Heights
Anglin, Joyce Ann **(A)**
Bachner, Mrs Lisa Dawn **(SLP)**
Bass, Mrs Nancy F **(SLP)**
Brown, Mrs Marilyn K **(SLP)**
Colombo, Patricia M **(SLP)**
Dent, Dr Ruth I **(SLP)**
Dettelbach, Mrs Joan A **(SLP)**
Ekelman, Barbara Lee **(SLP)**
Elliott, Mrs Mary-Anne **(SLP)**
Glasson, Dr Chloe C **(SLP)**
Jackson, Eleanor J **(SLP)**
Kirby, Mrs Karen Berg **(SLP)**
Koblenz, Mrs Maxine **(SLP)**
Kramer, Laura K **(SLP)**
Lezak, Mrs Mary H W **(A)**
Lezak, Dr Raymond J **(SLP A)**
MacIntyre, Patricia G **(SLP)**
Maimbourg, Mrs Odette M **(SLP)**
McNamara, Mrs Gail Marie **(SLP)**
McWilliams, Carol S **(SLP)**
Rauch, Mrs Roberta J **(SLP)**
Ringler, Dr Norma M **(SLP)**
Root, Mrs Lynn E **(A)**
Rubins, Sherry R **(SLP)**
Super, Mrs Encie J **(SLP)**
Uth, Deedra J S **(SLP)**
Zinner, Elliott M **(SLP)**

Sheffield Lake
Crum, Marian

Sherwood
Jones, Mrs Anne Marie **(SLP)**

Shreve
Swartz, Mrs Carol C **(SLP)**

Sidney
Husemann, Mrs Diana A **(SLP)**
Jay, Mrs Ellen R R **(SLP)**
Kirsch, Theresa Ann **(SLP)**
Young, Mrs Marilyn Jane **(SLP)**

Silver Lake
Byerly, Susan Jane **(A)**

Solon
Austin, Mrs Barbara A **(SLP)**
Hirsch, Mrs Marilyn S **(SLP)**
Hoffman, Jeri L **(A)**
Kaczuk, Mrs Priscilla A **(SLP)**
Knox, Mrs Leona L **(SLP)**
Spence, Marcia Gillcrist **(SLP)**

South Euclid
Altman, Mrs Pamela Ruth **(SLP)**
Blauner, Mrs Betty Jo Bass **(SLP)**
Carlin, Judith Ann **(A)**
Dorfman, Cathy **(SLP)**
Ellis, Mrs Eva M **(SLP)**
Guzauskas, Ann Helen K **(A)**
Hall, Nancy Edna **(SLP)**
Johnson, Dr Alex F, Jr **(SLP)**
Kay, Mrs Nancy S **(SLP)**
Kliszczuk-Gilbert, Mrs Mary Ann **(SLP)**
Lang, Mrs Elizabeth
Lorell, Daryl M **(SLP)**
Martin, Margaret Allison **(SLP)**
Mills, Mrs Cheryl Renee **(SLP)**
O'Connor, Mrs Lisa M **(SLP)**
Rachek, Mrs Sally Anne **(A)**
Salomon, Mrs Bethany Chaitoff **(SLP)**
Segel, Mrs Holly Ann **(SLP)**
Segel, Philip Allen **(A)**
Stalter, Margaret L **(SLP)**
Stein, Dr Seline **(SLP)**
Wolf, Clifford A **(SLP)**

South Point
Mays, Nancy Miller **(SLP)**

South Russell
Owens, Mrs Leslie H **(SLP)**

Spring Valley
Dugan, Mrs Mary Pavilonis **(SLP)**
Kelchner, Lisa K N **(SLP)**
Rastetter, Mrs Marcelle T **(SLP)**
Sakada, Mrs Janet P **(SLP)**

Springdale
Kuvshinoff, Mrs Barbara Elizabeth **(SLP)**

Springfield
Clark, John D **(SLP)**
Clark, Sharon H **(SLP)**
Coon, Diana Lynne **(SLP)**
Crossley, Marilyn Rivkin **(SLP)**
Dickey, Mrs Sally R **(SLP)**
Eichelberger, Mrs Diane S **(SLP)**
Evans, Barbara A **(SLP)**
Flum, Mary Therese
Hiles, Marcia M **(SLP)**
Komendat, Karen Ann **(SLP)**
Leher, Mrs Phyllis M **(SLP)**
Lineberger, Robert D **(SLP)**
Payne-Stikes, Lynda Denise
Rachlin, Paul **(A)**
Schemmel, Mrs Phyllis J **(SLP)**
Smith, Rayma E **(SLP)**

St Clairsville
Davison, Mrs Linda Lesnick **(A)**
Martinelli, Mrs Ann U **(A)**
Ross, Linda Jane **(SLP)**

St Mary's
Dammeyer, Mrs Denise L

St Marys
Laird, Mrs Jane Ellen **(SLP)**

Steubenville
Baughman, Sherry L **(SLP)**
Coen, Donald P **(SLP)**
Gelety, Mrs Beverly L **(SLP)**

Stoutsville
Schafer, Susan Ashley **(A)**

Stow
Angell, Robin L **(SLP)**
Basom, Mrs Susan Marckese **(SLP)**
Chandler, Mrs Yolande V **(SLP)**
De Pompei, Galvin John **(SLP)**
De Pompei, Mrs Roberta F **(SLP A)**
Durig, Anthony **(A)**
Griffith, Dr Penny L **(SLP)**
Hargreaves, Joyce M **(A)**
Hazenfield, Mrs Susan L **(SLP)**
Jacobsen, Roxann K **(A)**
Kavulla, Patrick S **(SLP)**
Keller, Mrs Linda Takahata **(SLP)**
Kline, Karen K **(A)**
Kluge, Mrs Mary Beth **(A)**
Lorman, Janis S **(SLP A)**
Murray, Lisa Elizabeth **(SLP)**
Nens, Mrs Diane D **(A)**
Nunez, Loretta M **(SLP A)**
Patterson, Janet P **(SLP)**
Profant, Deborah Susan K **(SLP)**
Savage, Dr Hallie E **(SLP)**
Saxe, Mrs Kathryn S **(SLP)**
Silvidi, Alfred C **(SLP)**
Tomchak, Mrs Ann Marie **(SLP)**
Vahcic-Pierce, Barbara J **(SLP)**
Watson-Florence, Winifred T **(SLP)**
Wildgen, Mrs Patricia Long **(SLP)**
Wynn, Barbara J **(SLP)**

Streetsboro
Hamilton, Margaret J **(A)**

Strongsville
Allen, Constance **(SLP)**
Bradford, Sheryl Ann **(SLP)**
Busta-Kolick, Kathleen A **(SLP)**
Chamberlain, Lourdes Marie **(SLP)**
Hobe, Elizabeth A
Lash, Mrs Susan Bour **(A)**
Serabin, Margaret **(SLP)**
Wilson, Elizabeth Jane **(SLP)**

Suffield
Ewing, Mrs Susan E **(SLP)**

Sunbury
Crandall, Tracy Teal **(SLP)**

Sylvania
Bechtol, Linda S **(SLP)**
Benjamin, Dr Barbaranne J **(SLP)**
Cousino, Pamela H **(SLP)**
Dalack-Ellias, Laila Marie **(SLP)**
Darah, Mrs Linda Sue **(SLP)**
David, Deborah J **(SLP)**
Drudge, Mrs Mary K **(SLP)**
Helmke, Mrs Carla S **(SLP)**
Kantner, Elizabeth **(SLP)**
Keeler, Patricia Sue **(SLP)**
Klamut, Mrs Kathryn L **(SLP)**
Meier, Mrs Ann Lynn **(SLP)**
Moore, Mrs Christine E **(SLP)**
Pakosz, Elizabeth H **(SLP)**
Read, Allison L **(SLP)**
Rhodes, Mrs Jerilyn Deboer **(A)**
Ripple, James Michael **(SLP)**
Roberts, Mary Ann K **(SLP)**
Roche, Rosanne V **(SLP)**
Schellschmidt, Joyce **(SLP)**
Sheppard, Susan Elizabeth **(SLP)**

Tallmadge
Coleman, Lynne G **(SLP)**
Croskey, Cheryl S **(SLP)**
Flower, Susan Lynne **(SLP)**
Jackson, Patricia W **(SLP)**
Messick, Dr Cheryl K **(SLP)**
Millin, Jennybel M **(SLP)**
Millin, Dr Joseph P **(A)**
Wray, Dr Denise F **(SLP)**

The Plains
Ellis, Lee W **(SLP)**

Thurman
Jennewine-Mullins, Jewelyn L **(SLP)**

Tiffen
Coker, William B, Jr **(SLP)**

Tiffin
Baxter, Mrs Katherine R **(SLP)**
English, Constance Reser **(SLP)**
Eppley, Kerry Ward **(SLP)**
Kiesel, Lucinda J **(SLP)**
Meiring, Peggy L **(A)**
Reed, Linda L **(SLP)**
Schmidbauer, Lawrence M **(A)**
Stoneham, Mrs Martha Transue **(SLP)**
Wise, Patricia H **(SLP)**

Tipp City
Bowman, Judith K **(SLP)**

Tippecanoe
Bear, Mary C **(SLP)**

Toledo
Aring, Mrs Mary Root **(SLP)**
Bradford, Debra Bukwaz **(SLP)**
Copeland, Terrilyn Denise **(SLP)**
Cousino, Mrs Mary E **(SLP)**
Davis, Regina Lloyd **(SLP)**
De Fosse, Dr Carlton O **(SLP A)**
Dirando, Mrs Maria **(SLP)**
Downing, Mrs Jude M **(SLP)**
Drake, Laurie Ede **(A)**
Drucker, Lawrence J **(A)**
Dunn, Cecilia Ann
Euton, Ruth Marie **(SLP)**
Frissell, Mrs Diane **(SLP)**
Giddan, Mrs Jane Jaffe **(SLP)**
Gottfried, Linda L Wood **(SLP)**
Grimm, William A, III **(A)**
Grossmann-Morris, Mrs Therese M **(SLP)**
Heminger-Cowell, Mrs Laurie Jean **(A)**
Hill, Larry Jay **(SLP A)**
Hull, Mrs Johanna R **(SLP)**
Hunt, Mrs Aileen **(SLP)**
Hyman, Mrs Joy Anne K **(SLP)**
Johansen, Catherine Louise **(SLP)**
Kinker, Joyce R **(A)**
Krasniewski, Christine **(SLP)**
Krill, Mrs Mary Louise **(SLP)**

Lance, Karen Lloyd **(SLP)**
Lawrence, Mrs Francine M **(SLP)**
Liber, Teena J **(SLP)**
Lopez, Mrs Carolyn Calhoun **(SLP)**
Lopez, Elizabeth Swanson
Mansour-Shousher, Mrs Randa **(A)**
Marsrow-Jablonski, D'Orcie **(SLP)**
McGreevy, Patricia **(SLP)**
Metz, Mary A **(SLP)**
Metzger, Thomas G **(SLP)**
Okarski, Kim J **(A)**
Paul-Bramer, Lisa Ann **(SLP)**
Pawlas, Annette Arnone **(SLP)**
Pinheiro, Marilyn L **(A)**
Price, Barbara **(A)**
Riley, Daniel S **(A)**
Rowen, Jane F **(A)**
Schumacher, Mrs Kimberly Renee
Sciplin, Mrs Camille L **(SLP)**
Shalda, Susan L **(A)**
Smith, Mrs Colleen Kroswek **(A)**
Spang, Peter J **(SLP)**
Spiegel, Bernard B **(SLP)**
Spudie, Annette Ryerson **(A)**
Szymczak, Constance Geonnotti **(A)**
Tolland-Lavey, Mrs Therese Maria **(SLP)**
Walker, Michael W **(A)**
Watters, Jack Allan **(SLP)**
Yosses, Barbara A **(SLP)**

Trotwood
Holmes, Nancy Rae **(A)**
Sacher, Martin H **(SLP)**

Troy
Curtis, Sue Llewellyn **(SLP)**
Gillespie-Rieck, Mrs Eva Marie **(SLP)**
Hiland, Mrs Kristin J **(SLP)**
Isham, Lorie **(SLP)**

Twinsburg
Ricci-Braum, Diane **(SLP)**

Uniontown
Caswell, Mrs Susan Beth **(SLP)**
Inglis, Robert H, Jr **(A)**
Prince, Mrs Nada **(SLP)**
Wert, Kimberlee **(SLP)**
Wnoroski, Christine Ellen **(SLP)**
Wolosiansky, Sara Elizabeth **(SLP)**
Wolosiansky, Walter B **(A)**

University Heights
Bruening, Dr Robert A **(SLP)**
Fabian, Stephanie Lynne
Freedman, Mrs Judy D **(SLP)**
Holland, Leslie Spahr **(A)**
Johnson, Lamont S **(SLP)**
Kaufmann, Evelyn M **(SLP)**
Kwait-Cohen, Mrs Darcee
Levenson, Mrs Roberta M **(SLP)**
Meyer, Sandra Jilek **(SLP)**
Nilson, Mrs Mary S M **(SLP)**
Phillips, Gene B **(SLP)**
Richman, Mrs Kim S **(SLP)**
Ungar, Mrs Elizabeth R **(SLP)**

Upper Arlington
Martello-Shepard, Nadine J **(A)**

Upper Sandusky
Beeler, Mrs Charlene C **(SLP)**

Valley City
Hawkins, Edwina **(SLP)**

Vermillion
Burley, Dr Robert M **(A)**
Novak, Mrs Tranette M **(SLP)**

Vienna
Pilati, Mrs Eleanor M **(SLP)**

Wadsworth
Blanar, Mrs Carol Braman
Smith, Mrs Margo Schenck **(SLP)**

Waldo
Seitter, Mrs Rebecca **(SLP)**

Walton Hills
Goga, Mrs Judith J **(SLP)**
Klukan, Katherine Ann **(SLP)**

Warren
Bandy-Palmer, Elizabeth **(SLP)**
Cornicelli, Mildred H **(SLP)**
Economos, Dorian L **(A)**
England, Ellen F
Feldmann, M C **(SLP)**
Hughes, Mrs Kathy E H **(SLP)**
Ireland, Jerry V **(SLP)**
Jones, Grant W **(SLP)**
Love, Mrs Patricia Lehner
Manser, Joseph Stephen, III **(A)**
Newman, Mrs Geraldine Gerson **(SLP)**
Sabo, William Joseph **(SLP)**
Schiesser-Manser, Mrs Pamela Susan **(SLP)**
Sescourka, DeAnna M
Shields, Richard W **(SLP)**
Zador, Jane Burton **(SLP)**

Warrensville Heights
Brown, Vicki Lynn **(SLP)**
Watts, Marvetta

Washingtonville
Watkin, Patrice S **(SLP)**

Waterville
Beaton, Janice M C **(A)**
Riley, Kathryn S **(SLP)**
Rondinelli, Michelle L **(SLP A)**

Wauseon
Dominique, Patricia Ann **(SLP)**
Restivo, Mrs Susan Marold **(SLP)**

Waynesville
Rickey, Mrs Carol Edna **(SLP)**

Wellington
Henderson, Mrs Nancy C **(SLP)**

West Carrollton
Konzen, Dolores Anne Marie **(SLP)**
Suddath, Mrs Carol R Gordon **(SLP)**
Winn, Sandra Lee **(SLP)**

West Chester
Armstrong, Mrs Paula Johnston **(SLP)**
Bastin, Mrs Carol E **(SLP)**
Davis, Lynn C **(SLP)**
McGraw-House, Mrs Deborah **(SLP)**
Pankratz, Mrs Judy M **(SLP)**
Pritz-Mullin, Christina **(SLP)**
Veale, Mrs Tina K **(SLP)**
Vella, Mrs Jo Ann Benfatta **(SLP)**
Viall, Mrs Anne Gallacher **(SLP)**
Winger, Joan M **(SLP)**

West Worthington
Esparza, Mrs Deborah A **(SLP)**
Jackson, Mrs Mary Kathleen

Westerville
Bogner, Laura Ann **(SLP)**
Burkholder, Joann E **(SLP)**
Huffman, Dianna Lynne **(SLP)**
Lea, Joan Pickens **(SLP)**
Lehman, Tamra Lea **(SLP)**
Mangino, Patrick N **(A)**
Mansfield, Lynn A **(SLP)**
Nelson-Picrenpaugh, Mrs Susan Jane **(SLP)**
Pursglove, Janet T **(SLP)**
Rupert, Sandra **(SLP)**
Shepherd, Mrs Laurie Barr **(SLP)**
Simpkins, Mrs Bernadine **(SLP)**

Westlake
Bird, Mrs Carolyn T **(SLP A)**
Bird, Richard Albert **(A)**
Comstock, Judith K **(SLP)**
Damiano, Laura Marie **(A)**
Hohman, Mrs Beth Ann **(SLP)**
Holmes, Karol Ann **(SLP)**
Jacob, Fae Jean **(SLP)**
Kunicki, Mrs Elizabeth **(SLP)**
Laraway, Mrs Ginette Marie **(SLP)**
McCown, Mrs Jacqueline **(SLP)**
Murnen, Kathleen Sackman **(SLP)**
Orr, Mrs Katie C **(A)**
Perla, Mrs Christine **(SLP)**
Ruggiero, Mrs Judith Lynn **(SLP)**
Whitney, Mrs Billie B **(SLP)**

Wheelersburg
Bushong, Mrs Laurel Lynn **(SLP)**
Hollback, Jenni Kay **(SLP)**
Lindley, Mrs Connie Lou **(SLP)**
Shaw, Tonya J **(SLP)**
Wallace, Susan Shreffler **(SLP)**

Whitehouse
Gay, Mary Lee
Kelsey, Susan G **(SLP)**

Wickliff
Weiser, Ellen B **(SLP)**

Willard
Frederick, Patricia A **(SLP)**

Willoughby
Bencin, Maryann E **(A)**
Catullo, Stephen Joseph
Cymbal, Edith Wickli **(SLP)**
Del Calzo, Dr Primo V **(SLP)**
Fugate, Mrs Mae Elizabeth **(SLP)**
Gowman, Marilyn **(SLP)**
Halas, Mrs Christine **(SLP)**
Newman-Teubl, Mrs Margaret **(SLP)**
Teubl, Richard Joseph

Willowick
Destro, Diane R **(SLP)**

Wilmington
Black, Thomas S **(A)**
Buckley, Anne H **(SLP)**
Hein, Mrs Diane C **(SLP)**
Hubert, Mrs Donna A **(SLP)**
Myers, Mrs Donna L **(SLP)**
Ruse, Susan Dankovich **(SLP)**

Wintersville
Braley, Karen Kathleen

Wooster
Bender, Lisa H **(SLP A)**
Brock, Mrs Sharon F **(SLP)**
Bruno, J Joan **(SLP)**
Calderwood, Rebecca W **(SLP)**
Cunningham-Grant, Mrs Jean D S **(SLP)**
Higgins, Dr Jerry M **(SLP)**
Johnston, Gennie S **(SLP)**
Packard, Debra M **(SLP)**
Rea, Dr James R **(SLP)**
Rumbaugh, Mrs Lisa Schubert **(SLP)**
Steimel, Beth Ellen **(SLP)**

Worthington
Blake, Bonnie Marie **(SLP)**
Borus, Dr Judith F **(SLP A)**
Bosse, Mrs Virginia Horne **(SLP)**
Ford, Mrs R Ann **(SLP)**
Harrington, Mrs Jacquelyn Sue **(SLP)**
Johnson, Mrs Christine Richter **(SLP)**
Johnson, Jerry E **(SLP)**
Koenigsknecht, Dr Roy A **(SLP)**
Koudelka, Teri **(A)**
Lewis, Mrs Judy L **(SLP)**
Love, Mrs Joni Emm
Magley, Gail Susan **(SLP)**
Marfurt, Malinda Kay **(SLP)**
Michaelides, Mrs Jackie K
Minard, B Gail **(SLP)**
Mitchell, Mrs Karen K **(A)**
Nipp, Mrs Suzanne S **(SLP)**
Pappas, Cathryn Jean
Rink, Dr Timothy L **(A)**
Roth, Jill Kathleen **(A)**
Schabo, Kathleen K **(SLP)**
Schafer, Susan Mary **(SLP)**
Scott, Pamela Sue B **(SLP)**
Siekmann, Susan N **(SLP)**
Sinden, Nancy L **(SLP)**
Stimpert, Terri Wuthrick **(SLP)**
Tomko, Mrs Sharon Ann **(SLP)**
Weithman, Mrs Jodi Simmonds **(SLP)**
Young, Mrs Amy Bonnell **(SLP)**

Wright Patterson
Prescott, Maj Richard **(A)**

Wyoming
Brooks, Nadine R **(SLP)**
Gerson, Mary **(SLP)**
Wick, Carol Ann **(SLP)**

Yellow Springs
Feely, Rosemary **(SLP)**
Gage, Elizabeth E **(SLP)**

Yorkville
Gaudio, Toni Lynn **(SLP)**

Youngstown
Arnold, Mrs Shirley Ann **(SLP)**
Brady, Dr William A **(SLP)**
Corbett, Mrs Ann Leslie **(SLP)**
Fogarty, Mrs M Maurine **(SLP)**
Garland, Timothy Robert **(SLP)**
Hagberg, Dr Eric N **(A)**
Hallett, Mrs Terry Lynn **(SLP)**
Hardman, Mrs Lorraine M **(SLP)**
Hendricks, Mrs Donna E **(SLP)**
Ingram, Judith L S **(SLP)**
Mentges, Carol J **(SLP)**
Miller, A Elizabeth **(SLP)**
Miller, Erin Louise **(A)**
Miller, Mrs Sandra E **(SLP)**
Monroe, Jeanne Cotters **(SLP)**
Nagy, Mrs MaryJo **(SLP)**
O'Brien, Linda Ann **(SLP)**
Ocarz-Krumpak, Susan L **(SLP)**
Porter, Mrs Christine **(SLP)**
Sebian, Sr Mary Ann **(SLP)**
Sills, Audrey E **(SLP)**
Szari, Janice D **(SLP)**
Thomas, Mrs Carolyn Denise **(SLP)**
Weaver, Mrs Debra Joy **(SLP)**
Weinheimer, Sr LaVerne C **(SLP A)**
Weldele, Dr Frank J **(A)**
Williams, Susan E **(SLP)**

Zanesville
Beam, Mrs Susan Dickey **(A)**
Graham, Mrs Alice D **(SLP)**
Grosshandler, Stacey R **(A)**
Headley, Amy B
Kreider, Thomas N **(A)**
McKee, Bruce L **(SLP)**
Tate, Judith A **(SLP)**
Upton, Mrs Beth M **(SLP)**

OKLAHOMA

Ada
Benham, Mrs Laura L **(SLP)**
Gililland, Mrs Susan V **(SLP)**
Wilson, Mrs Julie A **(SLP)**
Windsor, Shirley M **(SLP)**

Altus
Johnson, Virginia Ann **(SLP)**
Nordman, Donna Lee **(SLP)**
Vincent, Tambra Russom **(SLP)**

Alva
Barton, Johnny L **(SLP)**
Foster, Mrs Kimberly Kay **(SLP)**

Ames
Bisel, Mrs Sheila Dehaas

Anadarko
Bell, Carolyn Baumwart **(SLP)**
Carter, Theresa June
Moran, Patricia Ann Cussen **(SLP)**

Ardmore
Chandler, Burke **(A)**
Johnson, Cindy Smith **(SLP)**
Mashunkashey, Vickie A **(SLP)**

Bartlesville
Barber, Mrs Aagje V Swaay **(SLP)**
Cameron, Mrs Joy Diane **(SLP)**
Dohne, Connie Cox **(A)**
Kennedy, Kim B **(SLP)**
Kisler, Nancy C **(A)**
Kita, Mrs Virginia E **(SLP)**
Loafman, Mrs Debra Gwaltney **(SLP)**
Peters, Mrs Harriet J **(SLP)**
Peters, Robert M **(SLP)**
Sievers, Frankie J **(SLP)**

Bethany
Cain, Mrs Kay Conway **(SLP)**

Bixby
Coody, Mrs Kaylin M **(SLP)**
Curley, Mrs Judy R **(SLP)**
Sundberg, Joan Aline **(SLP)**

Blanchard
Callaway, Noah Mae **(SLP)**

Broken Arrow
Alexander, Mrs Patricia **(SLP)**
Anderson, Jane **(SLP)**
Grindle, Mrs Marsha D **(SLP)**
Lafaver, Joan B **(SLP)**
Romanelli, Mrs Maryann **(SLP)**
Segress, Mrs Carla Jo **(SLP)**
Shaklee, Janet H **(SLP)**
Youngblood, Mrs Janet P **(SLP)**

Carney
Norton, Mrs Sherri Lynnette **(SLP)**

Chandler
Plank, Mrs Karlen Tilus **(SLP)**

Chickasha
Ellis, Colette L **(SLP)**
Hook, Dr Pauline Pepper **(SLP)**

Choctaw
Murray, Mrs Judy Ann **(SLP)**
Wiginton, Mrs Julie Solow **(SLP)**

Claremore
Grimm, Darryl M **(A)**

Cleveland
Blake, Mrs Linda Miller **(SLP)**

Clinton
Andersen, Debra S **(SLP)**
Aneshansley, Mrs Melaine Kim

Coweta
Livingston-Keller, Rachael **(SLP)**

Cushing
Gaudreau, Jeffrey Norman
Hunsucker, Mrs Diann J **(SLP)**

Drumright
Young, Mrs Deborah Dennis **(SLP)**

Duncan
Brunette, Mrs Kim Garrett **(SLP)**
Emerson, Robin C **(SLP)**

Durant
Lee, Lana K **(SLP)**

Edmond
Autry, Mrs Sarah B **(SLP)**
Bodenhamer, Judy H **(A)**
Briody, Rickey Donnetta **(SLP)**
Bull, Marilyn E
Chaumont, Beverly Ann **(SLP)**
Cochran, Dr Corydon E **(SLP)**
Elliott, Linda S **(SLP)**
Fine, Gail P **(A)**
Gales, Charlotte S **(SLP)**
Ganjanathavat, Patty S **(SLP)**
Gardner, Mrs Diane G **(A)**
Gilmore, Mrs Susan E **(SLP)**
Hackworth, Dr Howard Bing **(SLP)**
Ivey, Dr Lillian P **(SLP)**
Leafstedt, Carla Hagemeyer **(SLP)**
McCharen, Martha Sanger
McComb, Kathryn F **(SLP)**
Mills, Jeri Munger **(A)**
Moran, Laurette **(SLP)**
Overton, Rebecca Lynn **(SLP)**
Penland, Mrs Jennifer Eaton **(SLP)**
Ross, Mrs Pamela P **(SLP)**
Sanford, Carol Ann **(SLP)**
Wilkinson, Mrs Cheryl Shipman **(SLP)**

El Reno
Havern, Mrs Amanda **(SLP)**

Elk City
Steele, Judy K **(SLP)**
Walter, Mrs Charlotte **(SLP)**

Enid
Alexander, James H **(A)**
Bodkin, Donna Kay **(SLP)**
Chambers, Katherine E **(SLP)**
Christman, Josephine E **(SLP)**
Donahue, Kathryn K **(SLP)**
Ferguson, Tracey Marie **(A)**
Kelley, Susan Deanne **(SLP)**
King, Mrs Patricia Schovanec **(SLP)**
Lewis, Mrs Louise Y **(SLP)**
Munday, Mrs Becky Sue **(SLP)**
Nimmons, Bonnie W **(SLP)**
Phillips, Merle A **(SLP A)**
Phillips, Mrs Phyllis A **(SLP)**
Ronck, Sharon B **(SLP)**
Thomas, Mrs Claudell F **(SLP)**
Thomas, Mrs Terri Lynn **(SLP)**
Turpin, Mrs Renee E **(SLP)**
Whitton, Leon K **(SLP)**

Eufaula
Pizarro, Shea A **(A)**

Fairfax
Beartrack, Susan K **(SLP)**

Fort Sill
Byrne, 1Lt David C
Cooke, Betty B **(SLP)**

Guthrie
Carey, Ann Grace **(SLP)**
Emmerich, Rhoda Susan **(SLP)**
Wright, Nancy J **(SLP)**

Guymon
Ogan, Donna G **(SLP)**

Hennessey
Kusik, Mrs Lanita J **(SLP)**

Hugo
Mangrum, Mrs Julia Gayle **(SLP)**

Jay
Garrison, Mrs Lola M **(SLP)**

Jenks
Brown, Mrs Rebecca Rhodes **(SLP)**
Buchanan, Lena Faye **(SLP)**
Diehl, Alicia S **(SLP)**
Parrish, Joy Lea **(SLP)**
Schmidt, Ann Eliz **(SLP)**
Spears, Mrs Mary Ann **(SLP)**

Jones
Clemons, Mrs Jeanette W **(SLP)**

Kingfisher
Miller, Mrs Gail **(SLP)**

Kingston
Craig, Mrs Becky Ann **(SLP)**

Lawton
Ahlschlager, Elizabeth Dawn
Ard-Manka, Mrs Sarah Margaret **(A)**
Barron, Mrs Toni Ross **(SLP)**
Blose, Connie **(SLP)**
Bradshaw, Mrs Kelli Diane **(SLP)**
Brehm, Mrs Catharine M
Brown, Mrs Pamela H **(SLP)**
Clark, Elizabeth Moore **(A)**
Gardner, Roni Deann **(SLP)**
Harris, Mrs Nancy B **(SLP)**
Kelly, Debra Parr **(SLP)**
Martin, Deborah J
McGuffin, Mrs Barbara D **(SLP)**
Stafford, Joel Lindsey
Stoneman, Mrs Mary Frances **(SLP)**
Wingfield, Jane Susan

Lindsay
Eubank, Tammi Jo **(SLP)**
Jones, Linda Swindell

Madill
Self, Mrs Deborah L **(SLP)**

Mannford
Earl, Mrs Linda L **(SLP)**
Holsomback, Barbara Jean **(A)**

Marietta
Walker, Clara E **(SLP)**

McAlester
Burrows, Clydeena Gaye **(SLP)**
Ehlen, Patrice J **(A)**
Hassell, M Harden, Jr **(SLP)**
Holloway, Julianne **(SLP)**
Shield, Mrs Lea Anne **(SLP)**
Ward, Robert M **(A)**
Wilkins, Sandra M **(SLP)**

Medford
Good, Mrs Mary J S **(SLP)**

Miami
Taylor, Alicia **(SLP)**

Midwest City
Abrams, Nellie **(SLP)**
Bullard, Joann B **(SLP)**
Demoss, Mrs Wendelyn L **(SLP)**
Elliott, Mrs Sherry Lynn **(SLP)**
Hughes, Diana Fitz **(SLP)**
McLaughlin, Kathy S **(SLP)**
McLaughlin, Dr Scott F **(SLP)**
Redwine, Ruth W **(SLP)**
Reynolds, Mrs Rebecca Birsner **(SLP)**
Rose, Mrs Sheila Kaye **(SLP)**

Moore
Bennett, John M **(SLP)**
Harden, Mrs Jane Eleanor **(SLP)**
Huff, Elaine B **(SLP)**
Over, Mrs Sandra Kay **(A)**

Muskogee
Campbell, Michael Frank **(SLP)**
Cathey, Kimberly Dee **(SLP)**
Dawson, Debby M **(SLP)**
Jefferson, Mary Catherine **(SLP)**
Locke, Sandy R **(SLP)**
Vecchio, Mrs Deborah Strange **(SLP)**
Winston, Kim S **(SLP)**

Norman
Adkins, Mrs Dawna Dutton **(SLP)**
Anderson, Paula Lynette **(SLP)**
Azimi-Bolourian, Carol Lacava **(SLP)**
Burke, Mrs Diane R **(SLP)**
Burns, Lisa Puckett **(SLP)**
Burroughs, Jill A **(SLP)**
Byers, Deborah Kay
Chao, I-Na **(A)**
Cheshier, Mrs Suzanne Smith **(SLP)**
Cummings, Patricia Ann Moore **(SLP)**
Doherty, Patricia M **(SLP)**
Dunn, Mrs Luceen J **(A)**
Earley, Mrs Deborah Ann **(A)**
Eggner, Mrs Ruth S **(SLP)**
Ford, Mrs Linda L **(SLP)**
Gallagher, Mrs Ann M **(SLP)**
Haddad, Synthia S **(SLP)**
Heron, Michael Jon
Hill, Susan K **(SLP)**
Himelick, Thomas Earl **(A)**
Holland, Mrs Diane Marie/Otte **(SLP)**
Hollingsworth, Mrs Cheryl Gay **(SLP)**
Hufstedler, Mrs Laurie C **(SLP)**
Jahnke, Jeanette M **(SLP)**
Jones, Julia Mary **(SLP)**
Lambert, Lorna J **(SLP)**
Lopez, Gilda Irene **(SLP)**
Lynn, Jeannine **(SLP)**
Markum, Mrs Patricia L **(SLP)**
McGuire, Dr Richard A **(SLP)**
Miller, Mrs Rosamond L **(SLP)**
Murray, Nuala Ann **(SLP)**
Newman, M Jeanne **(SLP)**
Nuttall, Dr Edmund C **(SLP)**
Odom, Amy C **(SLP)**
Perry, Terri Lynn **(SLP)**
Reddington, Christine Ann **(SLP)**
Ritchie, Kathryn L **(SLP)**
Schmidt, Mrs Pamela S **(SLP)**
Shaw, Kathie J **(SLP)**
Skov, Mrs Jinda Marie **(SLP)**
Summars, Mrs Lisa Rains **(SLP)**
Telting, Diderika Marie **(SLP)**
Walsh, Katherine **(SLP)**
Weaver, Janet Kathleen **(SLP)**
Winston, Jon A **(A)**
Young, Lisa Gay

Ochelata
Kolts, Mary Hoover **(SLP)**

Okeene
Golliver, Linda M **(SLP)**

Oklahoma City
Abernathy, Mrs Robin C **(SLP)**
Ahaus, Dr William Hoffman **(A)**
Atkinson, Mary Wray **(SLP)**
Barker, Mrs Deborah Anne **(SLP)**
Barry, Dr S Joseph **(A)**
Belling, Erlene D **(A)**
Bergin, Leslie Ann **(SLP)**
Black, Judith W **(SLP)**
Black, Susan G **(SLP)**
Blackburn, Mrs Lennis Rebecca **(SLP)**
Boland, Dr John L, Jr **(SLP)**
Bordeaux, Marcy Annice **(SLP)**
Bottom, Mrs Harriette O **(SLP)**
Bozarth, Gloria A M **(A)**
Bradway, Dr Lauren M **(SLP)**
Brou, Sharon Elizabeth **(SLP)**
Brown, Sarah Z **(SLP)**
Browning, Julia Elizabeth
Brubaker, Judith Jones **(SLP)**
Bryan, Dr George A **(SLP)**
Burnett, Patricia Ann **(A)**
Burroughs, Kathleen Walker **(SLP)**
Butler, Mrs Toni Marie **(SLP)**
Cariker, Mrs Teresa J **(SLP)**
Carter-Forcina, Mrs Greta **(SLP)**
Chess, Tiffany Felts **(SLP)**
Close, Nancy C **(SLP)**
Coe, Thomas E **(SLP)**
Collins, Mrs Georgia B **(SLP)**
Counihan, Dr Donald T **(SLP)**
Counihan, Mrs Marylin A **(SLP)**
Cullinan, Mrs Elnora T **(SLP)**
Cullinan, Dr Walter L **(SLP)**
Cunningham, Jeannette
Dahlgren, Karen B **(SLP)**
Debois, Michelle E **(SLP)**
Dennis, Dr J Michael **(A)**
Dennis, Mrs Judith W **(SLP)**
Dietrich, Susan **(SLP)**
Downing, Carla D **(SLP)**
Edmonds, Mrs Robin Pennell **(SLP)**

Elassal, Mrs Ruth Marie **(SLP)**
Emanuel, Dr Floyd W **(SLP)**
Emerson, Mrs Delores S **(SLP)**
Empie, Kathryn E **(SLP)**
Engelmann, Larry R **(A)**
Evilsizer, Mrs Marjorie J **(SLP)**
Exstrom, Mary I **(SLP)**
Eyer, Dr Julia **(SLP)**
Galbreath, Marilynn Evelyn
Grubbs, Kim Townsdin **(SLP)**
Hall, Rubye Maie **(SLP)**
Harris, William M **(SLP)**
Hawkins, Mrs Michele N **(SLP)**
Higginbothan, Susan Long **(SLP)**
Hoover, Patti Leigh **(SLP)**
Howell, Mrs L J M **(SLP)**
Irwin, Dr Margaret Louise **(SLP)**
Jewell, Mrs Mary Kay **(SLP)**
Johnson, Cherrel **(SLP)**
Kluck, Jana Benge **(SLP)**
Krei, Mrs Barbara Nall **(SLP)**
La Croix, Zane E **(SLP)**
Lacy, Debra D **(SLP)**
Lawton, Kathleen W **(SLP)**
Ledbetter, Dixie Acton **(SLP)**
Ledbetter, Tamra Sue
Lorenz, Lynn U **(SLP)**
Loy, Betty Ann **(A)**
Martin, Elizabeth L **(SLP)**
May, Dr John M **(A)**
McEver, Mrs Janease Graham **(SLP)**
McKaig, Michael Dean **(SLP)**
McKnight, Mrs Roxanne Crum **(SLP)**
Medders, Emily A **(SLP)**
Mencke, Dr Eugene O **(A)**
Messick, Mrs Carolyn M **(SLP)**
Miller, Dr Melvin D **(A)**
Miller, Mrs Susan Lynn **(SLP)**
Monsees, Mrs Harriet Kidwell **(SLP)**
Moore, Jill D **(SLP)**
Murphy, Frieda M **(SLP)**
Nance, Dr Anita L **(SLP)**
Neislar, Susan Kaye **(SLP)**
Nondorf, Sandra B **(SLP)**
Ochsner, Dr Glenda J **(SLP)**
Olson, Marla Lee **(SLP)**
Parke, Mrs Sandra **(A)**
Patrick, Polly S **(A)**
Payne, Neva R **(SLP)**
Peak, Patricia S **(SLP)**
Quillian, Sally L **(A)**
Ray, Mrs Janice K **(SLP)**
Robinson, Mrs Diana Asner **(SLP)**
Rothhammer, Mrs Carma L **(SLP)**
Roueche, James Richard **(SLP)**
Rowan, Mrs Eleanor J **(SLP)**
Rowland, Dr Roy C **(SLP A)**
Royal, Caroline Anne **(SLP)**
Rush, Dathan D **(SLP)**
Ryan, Mrs Mona Boydston **(SLP)**
Scarinzi-Owen, Dr Ann **(SLP)**
Scheer, Becky R **(SLP)**
Schicht, Michele **(SLP)**
Schmaelzle, James G **(A)**
Scott, Paulette
Shadid-Wray, Robin P **(SLP)**
Shapiro, Deborah Ann
Smith, Mrs Joanna T **(SLP)**
Smith, Melanie **(SLP)**
Statham, Sherri Lynn **(A)**
Stout, Connie E **(SLP)**
Strain, Mary K **(SLP)**
Swearingen, Mrs Lisa McDonald **(A)**
Thompson, Rosemary Munday
Trattner, Naoma H **(SLP)**
Underwood, Patricia A **(SLP)**
Varga, Mrs Tamara Elaine
Walford, Janet L
Walker, Julie A **(SLP)**
Walls, Mrs Carol S **(SLP)**
Waychoff, Mrs Tracy Tucker **(A)**
Wayte, Dr Rosemary F **(SLP)**
Wilson, Mrs I Nell **(A)**
Wilson, Dr Linda M **(SLP)**
Wood, Mrs Suzanne Bess **(SLP)**
Zahn, Marsha L **(SLP)**

Okmulgee

Mount, Dr Kay Hand **(SLP)**
O'Shaughnessy, Mrs Nina E **(SLP)**

Pauls Valley

Ice, Sonia G **(SLP)**
Leadford, Mrs Julia Hensley **(SLP)**
McMurtry, Marilyn Holt **(SLP)**
Thornbrue, Sue Ann **(SLP)**

Pocola

Stewart, Linda Pennington **(SLP)**

Ponca City

Bahruth-Poskey, Mary E **(SLP)**
Braden, Mrs Vicki Hillis **(SLP)**
Evans, Mrs Paula S H **(SLP)**
Hamilton, Mrs Gerene Moore **(SLP A)**
Hill, Paul C **(SLP)**
McGuire, Maureen A **(SLP)**
Rogers, Mrs Lucille Volk **(SLP)**
Rogers-Jordan, Mrs Jana Kaye **(A)**
Taylor, Melissa C **(SLP)**
Vanzant, Mrs Nancy P **(SLP)**
White, Cheryl Jouret
White, Marcella Leigh H **(SLP)**
Young, Mrs Mary Sullivan **(SLP)**

Poteau

Pickle, Patricia A **(SLP)**
Slater, Sandra Lanz **(SLP)**

Pryor

Marshall, Ellen Frances **(SLP)**
Smith, Mrs Roblyn Thompson **(SLP)**

Purcell

Lester, Mrs Patricia A **(SLP)**

Ramona

Myers-Brashear, Mrs Melissa **(SLP)**

Sallisaw

Gunter, Shirley Ann **(SLP)**

Sand Springs

Hale, Mrs Karen B **(SLP)**
Harlan, Sharon Elizabeth **(SLP)**
Lambdin, Janis Elaine **(SLP)**
Myers, Leslie Susan **(SLP)**

Sapulpa

Bradley, Clifford R **(SLP)**
Cleveland, Karla P **(SLP)**
Hershberger, Mrs Patty A **(SLP)**

Shattuck

Beeby, Marilyn G **(SLP)**

Shawnee

Baxter, Martha Ann **(SLP)**
Martin, Mrs Beth Miller **(SLP)**
Waddle, Mrs Janis Kay

Snyder

Wesley, Mrs Lynette Ann **(SLP)**

Stillwater

Beeby, Gary James **(SLP A)**
Blake, Mrs Susan C **(SLP)**
Davidson, Anne D **(SLP)**
Hardy, Mrs Deanna C **(SLP)**
Headrick, Mrs Carol Smith **(SLP)**
Koszykowski, Mrs Karen Elizabeth **(SLP)**
Long, Dr Edgarita E **(SLP)**
Marks, Janet A **(SLP)**
Monroe, Dr Nancy J E **(SLP)**
Murray, Mrs Leslie Wright **(SLP)**
Panagos, Dr John M **(SLP)**
Payne, Mrs Nancy R **(SLP)**
Pentz, Dr Arthur L, Jr **(SLP)**
Powell, Mrs Orpha L **(SLP)**
Richardson, Mrs Susan R **(SLP)**
Scott, Dr Cheryl M **(SLP)**
Seitsinger, Mrs Merrisue L **(A)**
Spencer, Marilyn G **(SLP)**
Thompson, Mrs Janet S **(A)**
Turner, Mrs Rebecca Goodwin **(SLP)**
Williams, Mrs Shawn Markey
Wright, Mrs Betty T **(SLP)**

Stillwell

Marshall, David Paul **(A)**
Tibbits, James D **(SLP)**

Stroud

Massey, Mrs E Jeannette **(SLP)**

Sulphur

Bryan, Gerald E **(SLP)**
Johnson, Donald F **(A)**
Powers, Kenneth E **(A)**

Tahlequah

Ainsworth, Dr Stanley H **(SLP A)**
Becker, Sandra K H **(SLP)**
Blenkarn, Mary M **(SLP)**
Burwell, Mrs Linda June **(SLP)**
Frazier, Jamie J
Peake, Mrs Mary L **(SLP)**
Schaefer, Dr Ronald D **(SLP)**

Terlton

Opauski, Marsha Kay **(A)**

Tinker AFB

Prohaska, Ann M **(A)**

Tulsa

Adkins, Gail M **(A)**
Anderson, Debra Sue **(SLP)**
Andrasko, Gay B **(SLP)**
Andrews, Christine Marie **(SLP)**
Ashbaugh, Mrs Judith A **(SLP)**
August, Chandler I **(SLP)**
Auten, Mrs Laura H **(SLP)**
Bales, Mrs Julia Ann **(SLP)**
Barnett, Rebekah Lyn **(A)**
Belvoir, Mary Elizabeth **(SLP)**
Bennett, Becky Bounous **(SLP)**
Bennett, Mrs Carol L M **(SLP)**
Bennett, Mrs Dyann D **(A)**
Berry, Judy O **(SLP)**
Berumen, Sharon **(SLP)**
Bole, Rosalie G **(SLP)**
Bothell, Raymond C **(A)**
Boyd, Janet L **(SLP)**
Boyer, Tracey Dianne **(SLP)**
Boyle, Susan Stark **(A)**
Boyle, Timothy A **(A)**
Brightmire, Mrs Janet Dee **(SLP)**
Brill, Mrs Marilyn **(SLP)**
Bruner, Mrs Thelma J **(SLP)**
Bryant, Mrs Nancy Jackson **(SLP)**
Burns, Joan C **(A)**
Buzzard, Mrs Christine Ann **(SLP)**
Cadogan, Dr Paula M **(SLP)**
Cameron, Yolanda V **(SLP)**
Campbell, Alice L **(SLP)**
Canfield, Elizabeth Cecilia **(SLP)**
Carr, Christopher George **(SLP)**
Christensen, Dr John M **(SLP)**
Cohen, Mrs Janet Kabakoff **(SLP)**
Comer, Carmen Melinda **(SLP)**
Conley, Kathleen **(SLP)**
Crawford, Mrs Barbara P **(SLP)**
Crawford, Joan L **(SLP)**
Crawley, Mrs Kennie J **(SLP)**
Cristiano, Patricia Airyn **(A)**
Curtis, Sandra D **(SLP)**
Davis, Rebecca M **(A)**
Deisenroth, Mrs Patricia L **(SLP)**
Dumond, Donna Lou **(SLP)**
Duncan, Julia Shirk **(A)**
Ellsworth, Mrs Janet B **(SLP)**
Elrod, Mrs Carol Clingan **(SLP)**
Embrey, Dr James E **(A)**
English, Helen Ann **(SLP)**
Fager, Diane Colleen **(SLP)**
Fahle, Jetti Irwin **(SLP)**
Fell, Mary Adrienne **(SLP)**
Finerty, Mrs Mary Ellen **(A)**
Fisher, Vicki Ruff **(A)**
Fonkalsrud, Janice A **(SLP)**
Gates, Mrs Laurie C **(SLP)**
Gawey, Susan Kay
Gerhart, Carrie Sue **(SLP)**
Gimlin, Carol L **(A)**
Glenn, Karin Renee **(SLP)**
Goleski, Leslie Ann **(SLP)**
Goodman, Mrs Nancy Jo **(SLP)**
Gooldy, William H **(SLP)**
Graber, Shannon E **(SLP)**
Hartman, Patricia Joanne **(SLP)**
Hays, Mrs Jenny G **(SLP)**
Hill, Mrs Susan Darling **(SLP)**
Hood, Michele Ruth **(SLP)**
Ingram, Mrs Nancy Murrow **(A)**
Iola, Judith Elaine **(SLP)**
Janssen, Lynda D **(SLP A)**
Johnson, Mrs Lynn A **(SLP)**
Jones-Owens, J Lyndelle **(SLP)**
Kendall, Melody Walsh **(SLP)**
Koehn, Beth **(SLP)**
Lafortune, Mrs Cheryl Collins **(SLP)**
Lambert, Carol A **(A)**
Lang, Dr Stanley R **(A)**
Lewandowski, Mrs Carole C **(SLP)**
Lipe, Barbara C **(SLP)**
Long, Suzanne C **(A)**
Madison, Kathy W **(SLP)**
Marshall, Sue J **(SLP)**
McBee, Gala S **(SLP)**
McElroy, Trecia Lewis **(SLP)**
Merrell, Dr Hal B **(A)**
Mesmer, Lisa H **(A)**
Metzger, Kathleen Marie **(SLP)**
Miller, Candace Johnson
Milton, Mrs Janice Leah
Minson, Mrs Joyce E M **(SLP)**
Momper, Anita F **(SLP)**
Moody, Mrs Mary H **(SLP)**
Munn, Janice C **(SLP)**
Myers, Elizabeth Ann **(SLP)**
Nelson, Mrs Maureen Quealy **(A)**
Oswalt, Mrs Jan L **(SLP)**
Otterstrom, David C **(SLP)**
Otterstrom, Elizabeth **(SLP)**
Overall, Mary Ann **(SLP)**
Parker, Nancy J **(A)**
Paryl, Anita Bell **(SLP)**
Perugino, Melissa C **(SLP)**
Peters, Kristine Louise **(SLP)**
Phillips, Cathy Sue Hawkins **(SLP)**
Plost, Debra L **(SLP)**
Plumb, Kathleen B **(SLP)**
Prescott, Karen Annette **(SLP)**
Price, Jean Albert **(SLP)**
Rains, E Bobbie **(SLP)**
Reed, Lauren C **(SLP)**
Roberson, Kendel E **(SLP)**
Roberts, Linda J **(SLP)**
Robertson, Virginia R **(SLP)**
Russell, Susan **(SLP)**
Seaman, Karen Ricketts **(SLP)**
Sellers, Anita Barbee **(SLP)**
Shalek, Sara E
Simonson, Mrs Donna O **(SLP)**
Sims, Judy K **(SLP)**
Snyder, Kimberly Sue **(SLP)**
Spencer, Jody L **(SLP)**
Standridge, Rebecca E **(SLP)**
Steddum, Mrs Mary Y **(SLP)**
Stice, Linda Sue **(SLP)**
Stone, Mrs Carole R **(SLP)**
Summers, Mrs Debbie Lynn **(SLP)**
Taylor, Diane I P **(SLP)**
Teter, Constance Keenum **(SLP)**
Thomas, Barbara Ann **(SLP)**
Thomas, Susan K **(SLP)**
Thompson, Dr Robert C **(SLP A)**

Vanderlip, Mrs Nancy A **(SLP)**
Veitch, Mrs Genevieve **(SLP)**
Vestal, Kelli Bell **(SLP)**
Walker, Brenda Dodson **(SLP)**
Ward, Mrs Annette Fulton **(SLP)**
Weatherly, Mrs Ann D **(SLP)**
Williams, Becky A **(SLP)**
Wozobski, Bette Schlanger **(SLP)**
Yelton, Donna E **(SLP)**
Youell, Mrs Janice D **(SLP)**

Turpin
Pittman, Mrs Charlotte Leigh

Vinita
Cook, Mrs Katherine D **(SLP)**

Wakita
Miller, Mrs Naida F **(SLP)**

Walters
Hooper, Mrs S Michelle **(A)**
Hooper, Mrs Sandra Delberta **(SLP)**

Weatherford
De Fehr, Mrs Melanie Garner **(SLP)**
Sharp, Mrs Sherrie Lynn **(SLP)**

Webbers Falls
Shackelford, Mary E **(SLP)**

Wetumka
Chastain, Pamela J **(SLP)**

Woodward
Craiger, Dr Pamela A **(A)**
Gill, James M
Moore, Mrs Kerry L **(SLP)**
Sell, Susan Stewart **(SLP)**

Yukon
Arichibald, Cynthia Austin
Beldin, Mrs Nancy J C **(SLP)**
Caraway, Mrs Teresa Heim **(SLP)**
Hallman, Mrs Beverly Jean **(SLP)**
Keel, Franklin D **(A)**
Keel, Mrs Jennifer Lynn W **(SLP)**
Mendenhall, Mrs Janella Annette **(SLP)**
Smith, Mrs Stacy A **(SLP)**
Ward, Suzan Lynette **(SLP)**

OREGON

Albany
Burks, Gregory L **(SLP)**
Dunn, Nancy M **(SLP A)**
Engdall, Carol E **(SLP)**
McCormick, Mrs Wendy Lu **(SLP)**
McNeil, Dr Ellen E **(A)**
McSpaden, Dana Kirsten
Moore, Malinda K **(SLP)**
Onstine-Dill, Joanne **(SLP)**
Peterson, Mrs Susan Evans **(A)**
Rethlefsen, Lola L **(SLP)**
Sea, Louise Marie **(SLP)**

Aloha
Carter, Elisabeth Young **(A)**
Hare, Mrs Valerie Arnold **(SLP)**
Howard, Mrs Julie Marie **(SLP)**
Marks, Susan L N **(SLP)**
McNeal, Mrs Julia Ann Verhey **(SLP)**
Montserrat-Hopple, Mrs Maria **(A)**
Thoma, Nancy Lynn **(SLP)**
Tidwell, Melanie Hall **(SLP)**
Woolley, Linda P **(SLP)**

Ashland
Ackles, Mrs Mary Egan **(SLP)**
Hubka, Beverly J **(SLP)**
Lantello, Debra **(SLP)**
Wasserman, Sandra A F **(SLP)**

Astoria
Dulcich, Mrs Donna Mary **(SLP)**
Ellis, Cynthia E **(SLP)**
Gamache, Gayle Elizabeth **(SLP)**
Laughery, Virginia M **(SLP)**
Sharp, Mrs Dolores S **(SLP)**

Aumsville
Golledge, Mrs Joanna **(SLP)**

Beaverton
Britton, Jean M
Bunker, Vanessa Jow **(SLP)**
Casteel, Dr Robert L **(SLP)**
Collier, Mrs Alice L **(SLP)**
Collins-Lu, Catherine **(SLP)**
Cunningham, Gail Grace **(SLP)**
Davis, Mrs Patricia R **(SLP)**
Engen, Mrs Sharon A **(SLP)**
Feldman, Louise P **(SLP A)**
Gonsalves-Wendt, Diana L **(SLP)**
Greene, Louise H **(SLP)**
Greenholtz-Carrillo, Mrs Debra Lynn **(SLP)**
Hendryx, Teri L **(SLP)**
Henry, James A **(A)**
Henry, Susan Hogue **(A)**
Kienow, Mrs Barbara McGilvray **(SLP)**
Lehman, Karen Jane **(A)**
Marsh, Debra Rose **(SLP)**
Nelsen, Mrs Kristine Kay **(SLP)**
Patterson, Mary Louise **(SLP)**
Reuler, Peggy R **(SLP)**
Rule, Karley Dona **(SLP)**
Schwartz, Katherine L **(SLP)**
Smith, Mrs Lois Reiko
Stewart, Elton L **(SLP)**
Teleck, Verna Margaret **(SLP)**
Warren, Joanne K **(SLP)**
Weybright, Glenn D **(SLP)**
Wood, Julie Ann **(SLP)**

Bend
Daucsavage, Janet Lee **(SLP)**
Jeffers, Mrs Florence K **(SLP)**
Jenks, Dr Randall Julian **(SLP)**
Olson, Mrs Christine C J **(SLP)**
Ricker, Nancy P **(SLP)**
Slaughter, Mrs Mary Lou **(SLP)**
Slothower, Margaret G **(SLP)**
Vranizan, James M, Jr **(SLP)**

Brookings
Anderson, Dr Virgil **(SLP)**
Golding, Mrs Cindy Trotnic **(SLP)**

Brownsville
Nelson, Mrs Kathryn M **(SLP)**

Burns
Howden, Dr Mary E **(SLP)**

Cave Junction
Meengs, Della K **(SLP)**

Clackamas
Liebman, Eve **(SLP)**
Talbert, Linda B **(SLP)**

Coburg
White, Susan Marie

Coos Bay
Banks, Walter G **(SLP)**
Caruso-Davis, Mrs Norma J **(SLP)**
Cummins, Margaret M **(SLP)**
Nunn, Mary P **(SLP)**
Rainey, Chris A **(SLP A)**
Woods, Mrs Donna J **(SLP)**

Coquille
Van Rooyen, Mrs Jennifer Marie **(SLP)**

Cornelius
Dammann, Dr Elly **(SLP)**
Lillywhite, Dr Herold **(SLP)**

Corvallis
Barry, Barbara Emilie **(SLP)**
Camfield, Pamela Jean **(SLP)**
Dennis, Janet B **(SLP)**
Hakanson, Kim M **(SLP)**
Hildebrandt, Dr Emery V **(SLP)**
Johnson, Mrs J Louise
Krivak, Brenda Marie
Latta, Angela Trautman **(SLP)**
Martin, Debra Lynn **(SLP)**
Rudolph, Mrs Judith C **(SLP)**
Sanz, Karen Leslie **(SLP)**
Sharrow, Margaret F **(SLP)**
Vitulli, Deborah
Westbrook, Cathryn J **(SLP)**

Cottage Grove
Abel, Judith S **(SLP)**
Thompson, Sheryl Kesey **(SLP)**

Dallas
Fromherz, Dr Robin Elizabeth

Enterprise
Fechner, Holly Anne **(SLP)**

Eugene
Beggs, Mary Ann **(SLP)**
Bingham, Mrs Virginia W **(SLP)**
Bucher, Nancy Pomeroy **(SLP)**
Christensen, Dr Ned Jay **(SLP A)**
Cripe, Juliann J **(SLP)**
Denney, Janet M **(SLP)**
Ediger, Dr Loyal D **(A)**
Eliason, Mrs M Jane **(SLP)**
Elliott, M Lynn **(A)**
Ford, R Craig **(A)**
George, Linda Louise **(SLP)**
Gerard, Cheryl Burnett **(SLP)**
Giumento, Angela S **(SLP)**
Gjording, Linda L **(SLP)**
Goldish, Susan R **(SLP)**
Hartbauer, Dr Roy Elden **(SLP A)**
Holloway, Mrs Cynthia Lee **(SLP)**
Howard, Mrs Diane M **(SLP)**
Hutton, Mary McCoy **(SLP)**
Johnson, Janice A **(SLP)**
Katz, Nina **(SLP)**
Kerins, Marilyn A **(SLP)**
Leslie, Gail W **(A)**
Lockard, Mrs Cheryl Smith **(SLP)**
Magiera, Beverly D **(SLP)**
Martin, Stephanie Tarrant **(SLP A)**
McDonald, Jane E **(SLP)**
McGhee, Judith L
McGillivray, Mrs Vickie **(SLP)**
McKee, Loralee **(SLP)**
McLean, John M **(SLP)**
McNutt, Eileen Sharon **(SLP)**
Michels, Linda V **(SLP)**
Moller, Mary Scott **(SLP)**
Nelson, Marlene Shapiro **(SLP)**
Nelson, Robert W, Jr **(SLP)**
Nippold, Dr Marilyn A **(SLP)**
Nollkamper, Linda K **(SLP)**
Pauley, Mrs Nancy Maxwell **(A)**
Pearce-Hopper, Mrs Lezlie Kaye **(SLP)**
Pennington, Mrs Carolyn D **(SLP)**
Rawlings-Boyd, Joan **(SLP)**
Reyneke, Mrs Judith Ann Long **(SLP)**
Risbrough, Ned P **(SLP A)**
Roberts, Kathleen Ann **(A)**
Ross, Mrs Dorothy E **(SLP)**
Schaffer, Mrs Carolyn S **(SLP)**
Schwarz, Dr Ilsa Ellen **(SLP)**
Simmons, Mrs Harriet A **(SLP)**
Steele, Merri L **(SLP)**
Thiel, Sharon K **(SLP)**
Turner, Laureen Theresa **(SLP)**
Walkup, Tami K **(SLP)**
Witkin, Bonnie Joyce **(SLP)**
Wittkop, Peggy Ann **(SLP)**
Wood, Dr Kenneth Scott **(SLP A)**

Garibaldi
Hellesto, Pamela J **(SLP)**

Gladstone
Buchanan, Michael S **(SLP)**
Fowler, Mrs Kathy Edmondson **(SLP)**
McMullin, Brent R **(A)**
Moulton, Mrs Christine J **(A)**
Tilden-Browning, Mrs Stacy Ann **(SLP)**
Turner, Nancy N **(SLP)**

Gleneden Beach
Maidlow, Gail Marie **(SLP)**

Glide
Perkett, Vicki Ramee **(SLP)**

Gold Hill
Canode, Melanie E **(SLP)**
Lebrun, Jackie D **(A)**

Grants Pass
Campbell-Evans, Mrs Carolyn L **(SLP)**
Davis, Kelly Jo
Hopper, Nancy C T **(SLP)**
Schmitke, Mrs Linda K **(SLP)**

Gresham
Barbour, Mrs Lloydene J **(SLP)**
Kouba-Monda, Mrs Virginia A **(SLP)**
Nielsen-Ziegler, Mrs Michelle A
Phillips, Mrs Judy **(SLP)**
Sharp, Carrie J **(SLP)**

Halfway
Neal, Ronald Eugene

Helix
Nuzum-Terjeson, Mrs Laurie Patricia

Hermiston
Wood, Mrs Dana Carrillo **(SLP)**

Hillsboro
Buckendorf, Glen R **(SLP)**
Cross, Judith Patricia **(SLP)**
McBurnett, William M, Jr **(SLP)**
McDonald, Ryta E **(SLP)**
Shope, Marie D J **(SLP)**
Swanstrom, Gail J **(A)**

Hood River
Hedin-Peldyak, Kathryn Sue **(SLP)**

Independence
Tebb, Michael Royal **(SLP)**

Ione
Faith-Peterson, Mrs Carol Ann **(SLP)**

Keizer
Carpenter, Stephen J

Klamath Falls
Dubrey, Louis Alpine
Ekman, Mrs Dolores Jean **(SLP)**
Iams, Judith L **(SLP)**
Kaufman, Janis Mae **(SLP)**
Leidwinger, Lewis E **(A)**
Pile, William L **(SLP)**
Welsh, Loren Patricia **(SLP)**
Woods, Dr C Lee **(SLP)**
Woods, Mrs Gay Ann J **(SLP)**

Lake Oswego
Bauer, David A **(SLP)**
Carlson, Dianne Coy **(SLP)**
Cumming, Mrs Kelley Lawson **(SLP)**
Drennan, Pamela Ann **(SLP)**
Favero, Joe C **(SLP)**
Flegel, Cheryl L **(SLP)**
Johnson, Dr Robert M **(A)**
Juergens, Mrs Karen Joy **(SLP)**
Kayser, Mrs Virginia C **(SLP)**
Kirschbaum, Mrs Laurel L **(SLP)**
Kramer, Mrs Judith A **(SLP)**
Kramp, Mrs Lynn M **(SLP)**
Lovelady, Jane **(SLP)**
Martinazzi, Vicci L **(SLP)**
Matejka, Karen A **(A)**
McGuire, Jesse B **(A)**
Mills, Mrs Norma B **(SLP)**
Smithpeter, Mrs Joann V **(SLP)**
Whirt, Mrs Celeste A **(SLP)**
Young, Dr Norton Bruce **(SLP A)**

Lebanon
Huntsinger, Marcy G **(SLP)**
McSpaden, Corlene H **(SLP A)**
McSpaden, Dr Jay B **(A)**

Lincoln City
Hanson, Bernetta O

Madras
Chambers, Nancy C **(SLP)**

McMinnville
Carstensen, Gustav V **(SLP)**
Grinstead, M Jennifer **(SLP)**
Irvin, Mrs Susan Hegel **(SLP)**
Phelps, Richard Allan **(SLP)**

Medford
Amish, Mrs Frances J **(SLP)**
Berger, Phyllis N **(SLP)**
Cool, Marie Hale **(SLP)**
Croly, Richard L **(A)**
Feskens, Cornelius **(SLP)**
Goff, Anne M **(SLP)**
Graham, Susan C M **(SLP)**
Jamieson, Mrs Janet Lorraine **(SLP)**
Marler, Sharon Ellen G **(SLP)**
Olberding, Debra L **(SLP)**
Radich, Diane E **(SLP)**
Strock, William F **(A)**
Wilbur, Mrs Amelia O **(SLP)**

Milwaukie
Arnold-Cockburn, Mrs Shelley **(SLP)**
Chambers, Dorothy R **(SLP)**
Emanuel-Regan, Mrs Valerie **(SLP)**
Hall, Patricia Hennessy **(SLP)**
Hinman, Mrs Marilee Grayce **(SLP)**
Lanier, Janet Crismore **(SLP)**
Otey, Mrs Linda L **(SLP)**
Starr, Kathleen M **(SLP)**
Thompson, Annette L **(SLP)**

Monmouth
Affleck, Christine Anne
Bratten, Julie Ann **(A)**
Dixon, Patricia Eilene **(SLP)**
Emberlin, Lety A
Evans, Dr Evan L **(A)**
Mathews-Ayres, Carol **(SLP)**
McAdam, Daniel L **(A)**
Morrison, Glenda G **(SLP)**
Palmateer, Nadine Smith **(A)**
Silbernagel, Mrs Melinda J
Tracy, Dr John M, III **(SLP)**

Myrtle Creek
Jack-Hannan, Allison R **(SLP)**
Kennedy, Mrs Kathryn Ann/Isaac **(SLP)**
Lawhead, Douglas R **(SLP)**

Newberg
Baumann, Mrs Ann Arends **(SLP)**
Carpenter, Paul E **(SLP)**

Newport
Cornell, Jolynn Ann **(SLP)**
Dewitt, Rich B **(SLP)**
Johnson, Dr Warren Edward **(A)**
Robinson, Sheryl K **(SLP)**
Sawyer, Mrs Marie Y **(SLP)**

North Bend
Desmet, Ann Lahr **(SLP)**
Hammer, Mrs Jean C **(SLP)**

Ontario
Mutterer, Mrs Carol Jean **(SLP)**

Oregon City
Coombes, Susan S **(SLP)**
Mabee, Mrs Ila Pirtle **(SLP)**
Maresh-Ericksen, Bernadette M **(SLP)**
McClellan, Gary E **(A)**

Otis
Nason, Alice T **(SLP)**

Pendleton
Geller, Jean A S **(SLP)**
Hanel, Roxanne Bean **(A)**
Randles, Susan M **(SLP)**
Reese, Carol Doerfler **(SLP)**
Stipe, Marsha M **(SLP)**

Port Orford
Shank, Jean W **(SLP)**

Portland
Abila, Amparo **(SLP)**
Adam, Arlie J **(A)**
Adams, Carol M **(SLP)**
Anderson, Dr Daryl E **(SLP)**
Anderson, Dr Duane I **(SLP A)**
Arwood, Dr Ellyn Lucas **(SLP)**
Arwood, Thomas Wheeler
Asmussen, Anita Ruth **(SLP)**
Baker, Mrs Karin S
Balmforth, Mrs Marlene L **(SLP)**
Barnard, Gail Engels **(SLP)**
Bartels, Mary Jo **(SLP)**
Bates, Karen L **(SLP)**
Blakeley, Dr Robert W **(SLP A)**
Blakely, Thomas L **(SLP)**
Bledsoe, Faith Elizabeth **(SLP)**
Bosler, Sharon A **(SLP)**
Botelho, Jeannie S **(SLP)**
Brockman, Janet L H **(SLP)**
Brown, Antigone Howick
Bryan, Mrs Joanne Salay **(SLP)**
Castner, Marguerite L **(SLP)**
Charuhas, Peter A **(A)**
Charuhas, Sally J T **(SLP)**
Clark, Mrs Charlene E **(SLP)**
Clemens, Denise Leslie **(SLP)**
Cogswell, Mrs Pamela E
Coleman, Dr Ralph O **(SLP A)**
Colvin, Mrs Lyn M **(SLP)**
Conkey, Dr Harlan D **(SLP A)**
Cresswell, Nancy S **(SLP)**
Cridland, Mrs Charlotte Woolley **(SLP)**
Daly, Mary Patricia **(SLP)**
Danzer, Virginia A **(SLP)**
Davidson, Mrs Jacqueline **(SLP)**
Dixon, Mrs Beverly J **(SLP)**
Dolan, Dr Thomas Gordon **(A)**
Dong, Cheryl Diane **(SLP)**
Doucette, Susan Marie **(A)**
Drommond, Ray Earl **(SLP)**
Dudley, Ann F **(SLP)**
Dunn, Julie A **(SLP)**
Erskine, Barbara J **(SLP)**
Fairchild, Michael Henry **(A)**
Fellows, Thelma M **(SLP)**
Fitzpatrick, Barbara N **(A)**
Fong, Carolyn K **(SLP)**
Forman, Monica N **(SLP)**
Fowler, Mrs Lavina P S **(A)**
Fox, Lynn Elizabeth **(SLP)**
Franks, Mrs Anne **(SLP)**
Fried-Oken, Dr Melanie B **(SLP)**
Gayheart, Tamara Lyn **(SLP)**
Gillcrist, Molly M **(SLP)**
Gillespie, Diane Susan **(SLP)**
Gilliland, Vickie A **(SLP)**
Gilman, Leslea A **(A)**
Ginley, Susan Marie **(SLP)**
Goldman, Clifford S **(SLP)**
Goldstein, Dr Karen J **(SLP)**
Golper, Dr Lee Ann C **(SLP)**
Gordon, Mary Ellen **(SLP)**
Grant, Naomi M **(SLP)**
Graville, Mrs Donna Jensen
Gray, Mrs Daria Sovyrda **(SLP)**
Gray, Pamela Sue **(A)**
Gustafson, Margaret Faudree **(A)**
Guyer, Mrs Jo **(SLP)**
Haley-Condon, Mrs Lavon **(SLP)**
Hankerson, Jan C **(A)**
Hannan, Karen Joan **(SLP)**
Hanrahan, Shelley M **(SLP)**
Hansen, Laura Larky **(SLP)**
Haroun, Mrs Deborah Thorsen **(SLP)**
Heath, Dianne G **(A)**
Heisley, Nancy R **(SLP)**
Herrick, Mrs Stephanie A **(SLP)**
Holstein, Janet Laura **(SLP)**
Holterman, Karen Elaine **(SLP)**
Hopkins, Harley J **(SLP)**
Horner, Nancy S **(A)**
Hrdlicka, Jill **(SLP)**
Iverson, Jane Elizabeth **(SLP)**
Jones, Bettie Maxine
Kafton-Minkel, Carol **(SLP)**
Kallen, Deborah **(SLP)**
Keller, Margo I **(SLP)**
Kieburtz, Mrs Nancy Jean **(SLP)**
Kimball, Mrs Carol **(SLP)**
Kollofski, Cindy **(A)**
Kornburg, Mrs Caroline Semler **(SLP)**
Kossover-Wechter, Denise **(A)**
Landsverk, Carolyn J **(SLP A)**
Laskey, Anne Lynn **(SLP)**
Lazere, Mrs Jane P **(SLP)**
Lebow, Catherine **(SLP)**
Lelli, Janet S **(SLP)**
Leonti, Mrs Susan L **(SLP)**
Levinson, Dianne Mihic **(SLP)**
Levinson, Dr Philip J **(SLP)**
Lewis, Kerry E **(SLP)**
Liebowitz, Barbara Joan **(SLP)**
Lilly, Dr David J **(A)**
Looney, Shawn Spangle
Love, Teresa Carnese **(SLP)**
Lyons, Theresa M **(SLP)**
Magers, Mary Alberta
March, Harold H **(SLP)**
Marshall, Dr Robert C **(SLP)**
Mathew, Karen F **(SLP)**
Maurer, Dr James F **(SLP A)**
McCluskey, Mrs Kathryn Marie **(SLP)**
McCoy, Lou Ann **(SLP)**
McDermott, Barbara B **(SLP)**
McDermott, Dr John C **(A)**
McMahon, Joan **(SLP)**
McNee, Mrs Margaret D **(SLP)**
Meek, Merry Mina **(SLP)**
Melum, Arla J **(A)**
Middleton, Mrs Carol L K **(SLP)**
Miller, Jennie L **(SLP)**
Miller, Mrs Sara M **(SLP)**
Mills, Leigh **(A)**
Minear, Kenneth Edward **(SLP)**
Moore, Janie Lee **(SLP)**
Mountain, Catherine Angele **(SLP)**
Mountain, Mary C **(SLP)**
Munson-Davis, Dr Joyce A **(SLP)**
Nauman, Suzanne W **(SLP)**
Nelson, Dr C Donald **(SLP)**
Neuburger, Sandra Ileen P **(SLP)**
Newcombe, Lorna H **(SLP)**
Nicholson, Jane Ann **(SLP)**
Nielsen, Ellen S **(SLP)**
Nonnenkamp, Lucy **(SLP)**
Norris, Dia Vee **(SLP)**
Odell, Lee M **(A)**
O'Hollaren, Mrs Colleen Marie **(SLP)**
Oliver, Sara Ruth Ann
O'Meara, Patricia A **(SLP)**
Osborne, Anne Stewart **(SLP)**
Ouellette, Amelia Wittwer **(SLP)**
Paul, Dr Rhea **(SLP)**
Payne, Rose M **(SLP)**
Peterson, Douglas Scott **(SLP)**
Peterson, Mrs Kay E **(SLP)**
Plapinger, Dr Donald S **(A)**
Polson, Joan C **(SLP)**
Pope, Mrs Lois A **(SLP)**
Prillwitz, David Charles **(SLP)**
Rapp, Gail M **(A)**
Rau, Dr Marie Costa **(SLP)**
Ray, Lorie Renee **(SLP)**
Rentschler, Dr Gary J **(SLP)**
Reuler, Mrs Ellen S **(SLP)**
Riede, Carol Wentworth
Robinson, Sherry A **(SLP)**
Rollins, Dr David T **(A)**
Rosenblum, Judith Fiestal **(SLP)**
Rosenthal, Amy Lynne **(A)**
Rosenthal-Tanzer, Mrs Jo **(SLP)**
Roth, Patrick T **(SLP)**
Rue, Hazel May **(SLP)**
Schechter, Dr Martin A **(A)**
Schienberg, Steven **(SLP)**
Schlesinger, Fern Winkler **(SLP)**
Schnabel, Beverly S **(A)**
Schneider, Diana Rose **(SLP)**
Schroeder, Scott C **(SLP)**
Scollard, Blaise D **(SLP)**
Seligman, Denise M **(SLP)**
Senders, Pamela C **(SLP)**
Shillingburg, Mrs Nancy Freese **(SLP)**
Skalbeck, Dr Gretchen **(A)**
Slater, Mrs Laurie G **(SLP)**
Slingerland, Susan Carol **(SLP)**
Smith, Julie Tackabury **(SLP)**
Smith, Myron Dee **(A)**
Smith, Mrs Sylvia Lee **(SLP)**
Snider, Mrs Mary Ann **(SLP)**
Sokol, Christine Mallard **(SLP)**
Stewart, Farrell **(SLP)**
Stewart, Susan R **(SLP)**
Stocks, Christy Gail
Stout, Patricia E H **(SLP)**
Surbrook, Mrs Janet H **(SLP)**
Talbott, Mrs Carolyn B **(A)**
Tear, Susanne **(SLP)**
Thomas-Kersting, Corinne A **(SLP)**
Thompson, Catherine Anderson **(SLP)**
Thran, Kelly Sue **(SLP)**
Tsugawa, Lance **(SLP)**
Van Horn, Billy J **(SLP)**
Ventura, Dr F Paul **(SLP A)**
Vogelsang, Dr Robert W **(SLP)**
Ware, Kathryn J **(SLP)**
Warlick, Joann **(SLP)**
Wiley, Martha V
Willoughby, Carol D **(SLP A)**
Willoughby, Paul J **(A)**
Winchell, George Corwin **(A)**
Winkler, Mindy R **(SLP)**
Winthrop, Mrs Susan S **(SLP)**
Withers, Mrs Mary T **(SLP)**
Wong, Mrs Marleen N **(SLP)**
Wortham, Mrs Bille Sintek **(A)**
Wuorio, Mrs Judith Kaplan **(SLP)**

Prineville
Smith, Mrs Janlee E **(SLP)**

Rockaway
Diel, Mrs Dorothy L **(SLP)**

Roseburg
Barritt, Virgil C **(SLP)**
Beach, Carol D **(A)**
Holing, John E **(SLP)**

Salem
Adams, Robert J **(SLP)**
Armstrong, Joyce A **(SLP)**
Beck, Allan L **(SLP)**
Brown, Keith O **(SLP)**
Casey, Dr Maureen T **(SLP)**
Derowitsch, Mrs Marlene P **(SLP)**
Fertig, Kurt Robert **(A)**
Fischer, Susan D H **(SLP)**
Fisher, Babette Dean **(SLP)**
Frink, Norman D **(A)**
Gerlinger, Mary Jane **(SLP)**
Gilbert, F Meredith **(SLP)**
Harper, Mrs Sheila Rose **(SLP)**
Harris, Dr Charles Newton **(SLP)**
Herb, Lyman C **(SLP A)**
Hervey, Dr Wesley D **(SLP)**
Kincaid, Kathy K **(SLP)**
Korpela, Mrs Shirley M **(SLP)**

Larson, Glen A **(SLP)**
Little, Mrs Joyce E **(SLP)**
Lockhart, Janet Lee **(SLP)**
Mashaw, Susan L **(SLP)**
Mehr, Dr Allan S **(A)**
Pribnow, Signe Hagen **(A)**
Rice, Donna Marie **(SLP)**
Sanvi, Mrs Jennifer R **(SLP)**
Seavy, Mrs Dorothy J Hoyt **(SLP)**
Severns, Mrs Patty Dorann **(SLP)**
Spicer, Elizabeth Ann
Springer, Mark T **(SLP)**
Stark, Mrs Betsie Dillard **(SLP)**
Steffel, Sue Reedy **(SLP)**
Summers, Steve R **(SLP A)**
Swanson, Mrs Karen L **(SLP)**
Tookey, Mrs Carol **(SLP)**
Triplett, Mrs Marilyn Jean **(SLP)**
Warren, Chuck Nathan **(SLP)**
Warren, Roxanne Williams **(SLP)**
Yetter, Mrs Carol Johnson **(A)**
Zegar, Marcia A **(SLP)**

Seaside
Peets, Mrs Ruth Du Puis **(SLP A)**

Silverton
Rader, Thomas W **(SLP)**

Sisters
Steely, Brian Richard **(SLP)**

Springfield
Allen, Barbara **(SLP)**
Dustrude, Stephen R **(SLP)**
Lorig, Linda R **(SLP)**
Millhollen, Marjory M **(SLP)**
Rock, Deborah M **(SLP)**
Rogers, Mrs Susan G

Stanfield
Clupny, Carol A **(SLP)**
Clupny, Charles Edward **(SLP)**

Sutherlin
Fulton, Richard M **(SLP)**

Tigard
Hoffer, Mrs Dana Lee **(SLP)**
Hoffer, Spencer John **(SLP)**
Horowitz, Alan R **(SLP)**
Owens, Mrs Bonnie L **(SLP)**
Pelson, Dr Rodney O **(A)**
Porter, Jane Boyd **(A)**
Reitter-Turner, Mrs Becky Lee **(SLP)**
Revit, Lawrence Jay
Ross, Carol Frances **(SLP A)**
Vines, Mrs Shannan Hinrichs **(SLP)**

Tillamook
Canfield, Dana W **(SLP)**
Huffman, James Raymond **(SLP)**

Troutdale
Whitten, Carol Ann **(SLP)**
Winning, Mrs Maude I **(SLP)**

Tualatin
Bills, Jennifer Lynn **(SLP)**
Crowell, Mrs Susan Marto **(SLP)**
Eisenbach, Dr Charles R, II **(SLP)**
English, Dr Robert H **(SLP)**
Sullivan, Deborah W **(SLP)**
Winder, Deidre Ann

Warrenton
Tegfeldt, Joyce Ellen **(SLP)**

West Linn
Baker, Mrs Martha E **(SLP)**
Benko, Judy Kadell **(SLP)**
Hickman, Laurel Anne **(SLP)**
Wheeler, Barbara Eleanor **(SLP)**

Westlake
Gunderson, Dr Herbert E **(SLP)**

Weston
Shanks, Carolyn A **(SLP)**

Williams
Morasch, Candace M **(SLP)**

Wilsonville
Piazza, Mrs Candice S **(SLP)**
Wall, Kathryn Ellen **(SLP)**

Winston
Crenshaw, Mrs Nancy L **(SLP)**

Yoncalla
Helmer, Marie C **(SLP)**

PENNSYLVANIA

Abington
Adshead, Mrs Jeanne Weiss **(A)**
Begley, Mrs Michelle M **(SLP)**
Erlich, Eileen V **(SLP A)**
Jubelirer, Mrs Amy R **(SLP)**
Mueller, Alison M
Richardson, D E **(SLP)**

Aliquippa
Bradbury, Rebekah Ann **(SLP)**
Brockmiller, Mrs Faye S **(SLP)**
Durr, Mrs Angela M **(SLP)**
Kush, Christine **(SLP)**
McClure, Mrs Bernadette A Ross **(SLP)**
Peer, Donna L **(SLP)**
Rivetti, Denise Marie **(SLP)**
Ross, Mary Anne **(SLP)**
Saxton, Anne E **(SLP)**
Veness, Deborah Miracle **(A)**
Wauthier, Kelly L **(SLP)**

Allentown
Berson, Mrs Lauren Goldfarb **(SLP)**
Casper, Marie Anne **(SLP)**
Cohen, Alan **(SLP A)**
Conway, Loretta A **(SLP)**
Ehrens, Gail **(SLP)**
Engelson, Mrs Henriette R **(SLP)**
Grabowski, Dr Richard R **(SLP A)**
Holland, Mrs Carolyn Allen **(SLP)**
Howard, Mrs Robin R **(SLP)**
Huryn, Theodore F **(SLP)**
Hutchinson, Lisa Katz **(SLP)**
Irwin, Nedra H **(A)**
Kleckner, Glen T **(A)**
Klingensmith, Judith Kay **(SLP)**
Kramer, Mrs Patricia R **(SLP)**
Kusko, Mrs Cheryl W **(SLP)**
Listwa, Mrs Sharon P **(SLP)**
Louro, Gina P **(A)**
Luchko, Christine D'Altilio **(SLP)**
McKitish, Mrs Dianne M **(SLP)**
Metzger, Jean Frances **(SLP)**
Moran, Alison Jane **(SLP)**
Muhleisen, Mrs Deborah G **(A)**
Ofrichter, Marjorie A **(SLP A)**
Parry, Iola M J **(SLP)**
Roman, Mrs Barbara Johnson **(SLP)**
Sinclair, Mrs Miriam N **(SLP)**
Solomon, Dr Beverly **(SLP)**
Stankoski, Mrs Mary Jean **(SLP)**
Stein, Karin **(SLP)**
Tonini, Ross E **(SLP)**
Walck, Carol Ann **(SLP)**
Widdowson, H Douglas **(A)**

Allison Park
Bistany-Brown, Robin A **(SLP)**
Cosentino, Mary J **(SLP)**
Hepler, Mrs Janet B **(A)**
Murrin, Mary Ruth **(SLP)**
O'Donovan, Mary W **(SLP)**
Schurman, Gary W **(A)**
Spanos, Mrs Katina **(SLP)**
Tiesi, Sharon Reich **(A)**
Weber, Alison Leah **(A)**

Altoona
Bergman, Mrs Lisa Marie
Feather-Grozanick, Pamela **(SLP)**
Gray, Karen Rhea **(A)**
Jubelirer, Mrs Mary-Jo Kann **(SLP)**
Maher, Patricia L **(SLP)**
McDonald, Mrs Gertrude R **(SLP)**
Pennington, Mrs Janet K **(SLP)**
Singer, Dr Jeane Violon **(A)**
Weichel, Kimberly Suzanne **(A)**
Willaman, Kathryn E **(SLP)**

Ambler
Campbell, Mrs Diane Sciullo **(SLP)**
Evans, Joan E **(SLP A)**
Finore, Luanne **(SLP)**
Hamburg, Deborah Susan **(SLP)**
Seidmon, Mrs Nancy Friedman **(SLP)**
Stelzer, Mrs Barbara M **(SLP)**
Wertley, Kathleen M **(SLP)**

Ambridge
Tempalski, Karen **(SLP)**

Andalusia
Clarke, Judith Ann **(A)**
Dougherty Mark, Marie A **(SLP)**

Annville
Pellman, Alton A **(SLP)**
Pulice, Sally A **(SLP)**

Apollo
Callen, Douglas N **(SLP A)**
Dickun, Patricia A **(SLP)**
Fisher, Mrs Terri Lee **(SLP)**
Zabinski, Mrs Denise A **(SLP)**

Ardmore
Barron, Mrs Sara **(A)**
Darby, Kathe Shannon **(SLP)**
Goldman, Mrs Laura G **(SLP)**
Kelly, Edward Joseph **(SLP)**
Robinson, Pauline Katherine **(A)**

Ardsley
Duffin, Marybeth **(SLP)**

Aristes
Baurys, Karl J **(A)**

Arnold
Gawlik, Janice L **(SLP)**

Aston
Burgess, Mrs Valerie Ann **(SLP)**
Madden, Barbara Jane **(A)**

Audubon
Schopman, Nancy Graham **(SLP)**

Avoca
Bartosiewicz, Mrs Sharon Rosa **(A)**

Avondale
Delahanty, Mrs Katherine Dannettel **(SLP)**

Baden
Waters, Mrs Kathleen **(SLP)**

Bala-Cynwyd
Addis, Ann Buckler **(SLP)**
Cohen, Mrs Karen R **(SLP)**
Cohlberg, Nancy K **(SLP)**
Freidman, Helene W **(SLP)**
Genkin, Marian Block **(SLP)**
Gertz, Thea-Gail **(SLP A)**
Hansen, Stanley C **(SLP)**
Robertson, James B **(A)**
Sanders, Deborah Eve **(SLP)**
Shusterman, Karen Lynn **(SLP)**
Wick, Eleanor A **(SLP)**

Bangor
Batson-Magnuson, Mrs Luann **(SLP)**

Barto
Zelinsky, Pamela S **(SLP)**

Bath
Loetzbeier, Mrs Anne H **(SLP)**

Beaver
Mathianas, Mrs Karen Obringer **(SLP)**
Richmond, Thomas E, Jr **(SLP A)**

Beaver Falls
Comin, Mrs Amy Cyphers **(SLP)**
Gilmore, Marian L **(SLP)**
Mooney Majeski, Mrs Sandra L **(SLP)**
Peterson, Dennis A **(A)**
Sokol-Evans, Mrs Sandra A **(SLP)**

Beavertown
Mitchell, Mrs Lisa A **(SLP)**

Bedford
Richardson, Mrs Melissa A **(SLP)**
Whetstone, Clarence E, Jr **(SLP)**

Belle Vernon
Alessio, Charles **(SLP)**
Brightwell, Dr Mary A **(SLP)**
Fecek, Ronald J **(A)**
Fish, Judith A **(SLP)**
Garber, Janice Ritsko **(SLP)**
Hawk, Dorothy M **(A)**
Kruppa, John R **(SLP)**
Woss, Mrs Debra Podvia **(SLP)**

Bellefonte
Johnston, Kathleen A **(SLP)**
Martin, Mrs Marilyn Morse **(SLP)**
Peck, Sandra L **(SLP A)**

Bensalem
Cassidy, Deborah Diane **(SLP)**
De Blander, Mrs Marjorie Ann **(SLP)**
Eisen, Mrs Debra S **(SLP)**
Holly, Susanna Maniace **(SLP)**
Kandel, Mrs Bonnie Daduk **(SLP)**
Kane, Mrs Wendy Louise **(SLP)**
Meltzer-Weller, Cynthia R **(A)**
Miller, Lloyd **(SLP)**
Scott-Casucci, Mrs Robin J
Segall, Linda Susan
Seidman, Jill W **(SLP)**
Snyder, Joan S **(SLP)**
Sperling, Robin Sue **(SLP)**
Weiner-Kaplow, Dawn F **(SLP)**
Witmer, Lila A **(SLP)**

Bentleyville
Blackburn, Mrs Vita Bava **(SLP)**
Karnack, Mrs Romaine S **(SLP)**

Berwyn
Colfelt, Mrs Gail S **(SLP)**
Dougherty, Mrs Barbara B **(SLP)**
Ezickson, Katherine F **(A)**
Hendrickson, Mrs Virginia **(A)**
Maust, Mrs H Madelein **(SLP)**
Owens, Susan C **(SLP)**
Tozer, Cynthia S **(SLP)**
Wilson, Lillian F **(SLP)**

Bethel Park
Babik, Mrs Rebecca A **(SLP)**
Burkhart, John N **(SLP)**
Follett, Michelle Marie **(SLP)**
Graney, Colleen Marie **(SLP)**
Koerth, Rosemarie **(SLP)**
Larner, Mrs Deborah Ann **(SLP)**
Lea, Leeanne Joy **(SLP)**
McCabe, Mrs Melanie S **(SLP)**
Metzler, Robin Sedor **(SLP)**
Pagnanelli, Jacqueline **(SLP)**
Sustich, Linda LaBuda **(SLP)**
Tomko, Mrs Rosemary **(SLP)**
Tulak, John M **(SLP)**

Bethlehem
Arch, Robyn Joan **(SLP)**
Boyko, Nora Ann **(SLP)**
Carrington, Mrs Barbara Brugger **(SLP)**
Conner, Mrs Kelly E **(SLP)**
Delfino, Gregory Daniel **(A)**
Farris, Mrs Kathleen M **(SLP)**
Fullam, Mrs Patricia Williams
Harpster, Mrs Diane N **(SLP)**
Hawkins, Howard S **(A)**

Lee, Mrs Susan D **(SLP)**
Manzek, Mrs Noralee B **(SLP)**
Marsh, Nancy C **(SLP)**
McGinnis, Carolyn S **(A)**
Millett, Mrs Ann Fantauzzi **(SLP)**
Ocampo, Graciela M **(SLP)**
Schimmel, Mrs Judith M **(SLP)**
Sitler, Barbara A **(SLP)**
Topper, Mrs Maureen Gallagher **(SLP)**
Trauger, Mrs Vicki C **(SLP)**
Vail, Mrs Pamela Arnold **(SLP)**

Bethlehem Township
Burke, Mrs Deborah Stirrat **(SLP)**

Birdsboro
Bingaman, Mrs Sharon P **(SLP)**
Jarman, Susan M **(SLP)**
Robinson, Carol Ann **(A)**
Seiger, Mrs Lynann Louise **(SLP)**

Black Lick
Clawson, Bonnie E **(SLP)**

Blairsville
Lenz, Judith A
Richards, Kathleen L

Bloomsburg
Alderfer, Maureen C **(SLP)**
Angelo, Dr Dianne H **(SLP)**
Angelo, Dr Richard **(A)**
Champoux, Dr Ronald Roland **(SLP)**
Collins, Mrs Constance R **(SLP)**
Hauck, Joan **(SLP)**
Lloyd, Mrs Therese H **(SLP)**
Marks, Dr Colleen J **(SLP)**
Miller, Dr Glenn D, Jr **(A)**
Mulligan, Dr Kathleen **(SLP)**
Nettling-Snyder, Mrs Peggy Eileen **(SLP)**
Seip, Mrs Jodi A **(SLP)**
Weitz, Julia M **(SLP)**

Blue Bell
Keidel, Susan M **(SLP)**
McBride, Mrs Janet E **(SLP)**
Smith, Mrs Elaine Genuardi **(SLP)**

Boiling Springs
Giovannitti, Mrs Judith B **(SLP)**

Boothwyn
Chester, Mrs Christine Dallam **(SLP)**
Gensel, Mrs Donna M **(SLP)**

Boyertown
Pender, Mrs Elizabeth A **(SLP)**
Waring, Mrs Margaret L **(SLP)**

Bradford
Costello, Elizabeth M **(SLP)**
Geisler, Mrs Janice L **(SLP)**
Higie, Mrs Pauline G **(SLP)**

Bridgeport
Storrs, Sheila A **(SLP)**

Bridgeville
Banks, Mrs Tabitha Owens **(SLP)**
Capozzoli, Annette T **(SLP)**
Dankovich, Jacqueline **(SLP)**
Kotelnicki-Martin, Deborah Joann **(SLP)**
Kustron, Mrs Janice M **(SLP)**
McChesney, Kathleen Ann
Rothermel, Mrs Carol N **(SLP)**

Bristol
Ballow, Mrs Judith G **(A)**

Brookhaven
Brown-Martin, Mrs Penny I **(SLP)**
Middleton, Rita Danneker
Suppa, Rosanna P **(A)**

Brookville
McPherson, Mrs Wendy B **(SLP)**

Broomall
Cromley, Elisabeth **(SLP)**
Dale, Mrs Beverly H **(SLP)**
Falcone, Sandra H **(SLP)**
Ferri, Cecelia A **(SLP)**
Russo, Mrs Michelle **(SLP)**
Sands, Leslie Leigh **(A)**
Tandarich, Mrs Charon B H **(SLP)**

Brownsville
Bonfanti, Dr Barbara H **(SLP)**

Bryn Mawr
Altschuler, Dr Sherry Levin **(SLP)**
Dabrow, Mrs Lori Michelle **(SLP)**
Goldstein, Mrs Marilyn Karen **(SLP)**
Greenbaum, Mrs Bettsie W **(SLP)**
Heft, Laurel C **(A)**
Keenan, Mrs Patricia M **(SLP A)**
Litwack, Ellen P **(SLP)**
McDonald, Janet M **(SLP)**
Payne, Mrs Ruth T **(SLP)**
Rosen, Mrs Debra L **(A)**
Rosenberg, Sara W **(SLP)**
Wagenheim, Evonne Vaksman **(SLP)**
Wechsler, Mrs Rivi **(SLP)**

Butler
Campbell, Judy Lynn **(SLP)**
Carrig, Edward James **(A)**
Carrig, Mrs Faye **(SLP)**
Dancu, Mrs Rose Defazio **(SLP)**
Evans, Mrs Donna J **(SLP)**
High, Linda Marie
Jarecki, Janis Marie **(SLP)**
Kuehner, Suzanne June **(SLP)**
Mahood, Mrs Gina Marie **(SLP)**
McCormick, Dr Glen P **(SLP A)**
McDougall-Thompson, Mrs Martha **(SLP)**
Robertson, Mrs Valerie H **(SLP)**
Rosenbauer, Diane D **(SLP)**
Stanley, Linda H **(A)**
Todd, Pamela R **(SLP)**
White, Ethel B **(SLP)**
Zitalone, Mrs Kathleen Harder **(SLP)**

California
Dominick, Mrs Diana Marie **(SLP)**
Gismondi, Charles A **(SLP)**
Kaleita, Dr Annette M **(A)**
Nemec, Richard R **(SLP)**
Yates, Albert E **(SLP)**

Cambridge Springs
Gettys, Tina M **(SLP)**
Molrine, Charlotte J **(SLP)**

Camp Hill
Beall, Scott Gregory **(A)**
Brown, Mrs Carol A **(SLP)**
Cherewka, Mrs Michele R **(SLP)**
Church, Mrs Debra L **(SLP)**
Curry, Joseph J **(A)**
Fleegal, Mrs Elaine M
Guild, Jennifer Ann **(SLP)**
Hagenbuch, Roxanne R **(A)**
Lichty, Jill K **(SLP)**
Mroczkowski, Marcia M **(SLP)**
Schreck, Byron L **(SLP)**
Simpson-Steele, Mrs Harriet K **(SLP)**
Tornblom, David H **(SLP A)**

Canadensis
Tischler, Mrs Joan Marie **(SLP)**

Canonsburg
Galbraith, Amy A **(SLP)**
Nalitz, Mrs Noreen A G **(SLP)**

Carlisle
Areeda, Laura A **(SLP)**
Barefoot, Mrs Myrna C **(SLP)**
Campagna, Laurie S **(SLP)**
Dennin, Rebecca Ann **(SLP)**
McIntyre, Christine **(SLP)**
Mira, Mrs Janet C **(SLP)**
Myers, Dorothy E **(SLP)**
Ohl, Jacqueline Z
Powell, Mrs Louise McGinnis **(SLP)**
Ramedia, Mary A **(SLP)**
Robinson, Catherine Ono **(SLP)**
Rowland, Mrs Lillian K **(SLP)**
Schwanger, Joan W **(SLP)**

Carnegie
Gompers, Mrs Cathleen Callahan
Morgan, Terri Ann **(SLP)**
Robson-Brandi, Carol Ann **(SLP)**
Sabo, Diane L **(A)**
Sonntag-Vucich, Mrs Karin Marie **(SLP)**

Carroll Valley
McCarthy, Mary Pat **(SLP)**

Castle Shannon
Belsterling, Ralph John **(SLP A)**

Catasauqua
Hofmann, Mrs Nancy S
Roth, Mrs Hazel F **(SLP)**

Center Valley
Koury-Parker, Dr Danielle I **(SLP)**

Centralia
Jurgill, Carol A **(SLP)**

Centre Hall
Dixon, Henry P **(SLP A)**
Volz, Dr Helen Breon **(SLP)**

Centre Square
Baker, Charlotte Pierce **(SLP)**

Chadds Ford
Deberardinis, Carol S **(SLP)**
Doughten, Mrs Barbara Stern **(SLP)**
Erickson, Mrs Sarah S **(SLP)**
Liebner, Mrs Catherine **(A)**
Williams, Brenda Haas **(SLP)**

Chalfont
Drabyak, Janice Kratz **(SLP)**
Moneta, Deborah K **(SLP)**
Tomlin, Kathryn J **(SLP)**

Chalk Hill
Caldwell, Mary D

Chambersburg
Anderson, Pamala **(SLP)**
Bangs, Mrs Dorothy Z **(SLP)**
De Lullo, Dianne Marie **(SLP)**
Gray, Mrs Marjorie A **(SLP)**
Kaufman, Mrs Nancy W **(SLP)**
McFeely, Susan P **(SLP)**
Metz, Mrs Stephanie S **(SLP)**

Charleroi
Russo, Mrs Barbara Stafura **(SLP)**

Cheltenham
Einhorn, Ellen A **(SLP)**
Finkelstein, Alison Briggs **(SLP)**
Myers, Mindy Fae **(SLP)**
Nordlinger, Vivian M **(SLP)**
Vescovich, Margaret A **(SLP)**

Chester Springs
Goldstein, Mrs Donna Woods **(SLP)**

Cheswick
Bowser, Janice Pivik **(SLP)**
Burgi, Dr Ernest J **(SLP A)**

Childs
McCarthy, Mrs Mary C **(SLP)**

Clairton
Capocciama, John A **(SLP)**
Fabian, Loretta Ann
Francellini, Dr Anthony J **(SLP)**
Medvidovich, Patricia A **(SLP)**
Miller, Rebecca Ward
Pawlesh, Mrs Marina M **(SLP)**
Zehnder, Mrs Barbara Pajak

Clarion
Burge, Heather Lois
Dininny, Dr Donald H **(SLP)**
Kinkead, Rebecca J **(SLP)**
Linnan, Mrs Kathy B **(SLP)**
McAleer, Dr Colleen A **(SLP A)**

Clarks Summit
Basalyga, Mrs Michele Dunne **(SLP)**
Coco, Mrs Bernadette Maria Y **(SLP)**
Dawgert, Mrs Grace F **(SLP)**
Goldenziel, Barbara R **(SLP)**
Kiser, Patricia M **(SLP)**
Klien, Karen Ann **(SLP)**
Russell, Jean Westfall **(SLP)**
Sakovich, Linda Marie **(SLP)**
Sofranko-Noto, Mary A **(SLP)**
Zakar, Linda M **(SLP)**

Clinton
Telega, Mildred C **(SLP)**

Coaldale
Rajnic, Alexine M **(SLP)**

Coatesville
Brubaker, Lynne E **(SLP)**
Conahan, Helen P **(SLP)**
Grubb, Edward N **(SLP)**
Hardy, Mrs Patricia Diemer **(SLP)**
Pellegrino, Patricia Ann
Reach, Lynn **(SLP)**
Tolbert, Alfred J **(SLP)**
Toomey-Brigham, Rosemary **(SLP)**
Whitehair, Mrs Patricia M **(SLP)**

Collegeville
Cooke, Mrs Judith W **(SLP)**
Kirk, Mrs Karen Lee **(SLP)**
Puhak, Mary Louise **(SLP)**

Columbia
Lundy, Mrs Nancy Lynn **(SLP)**

Conneaut Lake
Isenhath, Dr J O **(A)**

Conneautville
Shimek, Mrs Barbara B **(SLP)**

Conshohocken
Ankney, Enid Elaine **(SLP)**
Boardley, Lorraine P **(SLP)**
Donahue-Reese, Mrs Phyllis A **(SLP)**
Fellin, Mrs Paula S **(A)**
Laplaca, Mary Grace **(SLP)**
Molchan, Ann Marie **(SLP)**
Sives, Sheila Mae **(SLP)**

Conyngham
Dobash, Cecelia A **(SLP)**
Kalowsky, Leora B **(SLP)**
Steppling, Mrs Mary Lou G **(SLP)**

Cooksburg
Flaherty, Mrs Sarah M **(SLP)**

Coopersburg
McClatchy, Mrs Callie R **(SLP)**
Mease, Mrs Deborah Kay **(SLP)**
Valent-Matsick, Mrs Nancy Lee **(SLP)**

Coraopolis
Bolea, Mary Kathleen **(SLP)**
Galiyas, Mary Jo **(SLP)**
Johnson, Mrs Nancy S **(SLP)**
McCorry, Mrs Lori Eisenberg **(A)**
Moreau, Vaughn K **(SLP)**
Stein, Dr David W **(SLP)**
Stein, Mrs Karen Goltz **(SLP)**
Suffredini, Doreen Elizabeth **(SLP)**

Corry
Dubois, Barbara Nuss **(SLP)**

Coudersport
Campbell, Robert L **(A)**

Crafton
Bidoli, Diane E **(SLP)**

Cranberry
Hartley, Dr Harold V, Jr **(SLP A)**

Cresco
Lynott, Mrs Cheryl Ann **(SLP)**

Cresson
Bonfanti, Richard T **(SLP A)**

Curwensville
Elensky, Mrs Nancy C **(SLP)**

Dallas
Gurdin, Martha H **(SLP)**

Dallastown
Heft, Mrs Julee H **(SLP)**

Dalton
Di Simoni, Dr Frank G **(SLP)**

Danville
Barna, Mrs Theresa Elizabeth **(A)**
Boscia, Mrs Cathy A **(SLP)**
Chappen, Pamela Lee
Curry, Patricia Zellner **(A)**
Gensemer, Dr Ira B **(SLP)**
Greenwood, Susan Teicher **(SLP)**
Harlor, Mark Y **(SLP)**
Jacobson, Claire Adrienne **(A)**
Jacobson, Dr John T **(A)**
Pierce, Mrs M Lynn **(SLP)**
Pirnot, Dennis V **(A)**
Pope, Kathy Ann **(SLP A)**
Reichard, Mrs Cheryl Lynn **(SLP)**
Smith, Richard M **(SLP)**

Dauphin
Bylotas, Mrs Cynthia L **(SLP)**

Delaware Water Gap
Shuey, Elaine M **(SLP)**

Delmont
Murray, Margaret A **(SLP)**

Delta
Koegel, Mrs Marian T **(SLP)**

Denver
Hall, Mrs Patricia Ann **(SLP)**

Devon
Molloy, Jill Marie **(A)**
Spease, Wendy Kay **(A)**
Townsend, Thomas H **(A)**
Wavrek, Dorothy J **(A)**
Young, Sarah Baldwin
Zweben, Diane Mildred **(SLP)**

Dillsburg
Beard, Kim G **(SLP)**
Bowers, Mrs Louise E **(SLP)**

Dormont
Morrison, Regina Z **(SLP)**

Dover
Lord, Mrs Katharine Berry **(SLP A)**
Trump, Stephanie Ann **(SLP)**

Downingtown
Brewer, Mrs Andrea Polley **(SLP)**
Condon, Mrs Mary Z **(SLP)**
Hess, Barbara Fabo **(SLP)**
Lindsay, Charles Hunter
Lingras, Robyn Levine **(SLP)**
McElwee, Amy Salitsky **(SLP A)**
Pagano, Mrs Janie E **(SLP)**
Revucky, Mrs Mary C **(SLP)**
Stratton, Dr Cleavonne **(SLP)**
Weiss, Cathryn Claudia **(SLP)**

Doylestown
Blaker, Howard Michael
Blaker, Mrs Renee G **(SLP)**
Levithan, Lisa **(SLP)**
Lumadue, Carol E J **(SLP)**
Luskin, Wendy Marie **(SLP)**
Morris-Gonzales, Ellen Kathryn **(SLP)**
Rohovsky, Mrs Karen A **(SLP)**
Timko, Andrew F **(SLP)**
Von Drach, Dr Robert B **(SLP)**
Weatherill, Joy M **(SLP)**
Williams, Mrs Kimberly Ann **(SLP)**
Woods, Martha S **(SLP)**

Dresher
Greis, Sharon M **(SLP)**
Harris, Mrs Cheri Lamont **(SLP)**
Horwitz, Randi B **(SLP)**
Milner, Ruth K **(A)**
Morgan, Mrs Diane B **(SLP)**

Drexel Hill
Anger, Pamela J Mertz **(SLP A)**
Banks, Diane Moody **(SLP)**
Dickter, Ann Ellen **(A)**
Knightly, Carol Ann **(A)**
Turnbull, Kathleen R **(SLP)**
Young, Maxine L **(SLP A)**

Du Bois
Donati, Stephanie **(SLP)**
Foust, Richard W **(A)**
Giordano, John Joseph
Huff, Ronna Lynn
Zbieg, Mrs Mary Elizabeth **(SLP)**

Dunancsville
Martini, Jerry B **(SLP)**

Dunlevy
Byers, Candace Lafferty **(SLP)**

Dunmore
Bonadio, Mary Susan

Dupont
Toczylowski, Corinne A **(SLP)**

East Petersburg
Kornfield, Mrs Roberta T **(SLP)**
Lusaitis, John Robert **(A)**
Young, Lind S **(SLP)**

East Stroudsburg
Ackerman, Dr Robert J **(SLP)**
Caprioli, Corinne Seltzer **(SLP)**
Lilly, Mrs Karen C B **(SLP)**
Nolan, Joan T **(SLP)**
Peterson, Mrs Roberta Kuhns **(SLP)**
Simpson, Mrs Joyce B **(SLP)**
Westheim, Mrs Adrienne **(SLP)**
Williams, Robert L **(A)**

Easton
Bartholomew, Carol I **(SLP)**
Beebe, Mrs Helen Hulick **(SLP)**
DiMatteo, Rhonda Lynn
Dimiceli, Michele A **(SLP)**
Farrar, Karen H **(A)**
Ferguson, Mrs Kate Abbott **(SLP)**
Finnen, Kathleen Ann **(SLP)**
Giel, Mrs Janey Carolyn **(SLP)**
Greenawald, Mrs Lynn A **(SLP)**
Jean, Mrs Jacqueline Willever **(SLP)**
Kaplan, Mrs Helene E **(SLP)**
Pearson, Mrs Helen R **(SLP)**
Westlund, Janet A **(A)**

Ebensburg
Hoffman, Teresa E **(SLP)**
Marcinko, Mrs Michele Brady
Murtha, Susan C
Myers, Mary Jane **(SLP)**
Numer, Linda Jane **(SLP)**
Scanlan, Mrs Carol S **(SLP)**
Wickstrom-Kane, Susan Kay **(SLP)**

Edinboro
Boyd, Marjorie L **(SLP)**
Boylan, John A, Jr **(SLP)**
Dubbs, Patricia J **(SLP)**
Durst, Brenda Adsit **(SLP)**
Forcucci, Dr Richard A **(SLP)**
Hill, Katharine **(SLP)**
Scanlon, Dr Stanley L **(SLP A)**
Simmons, John R **(SLP)**
Tan, Barbara **(SLP)**
Yankovich, Carol Elaine **(SLP)**

Effort
Fisher, Mrs Joanne Marie K **(SLP)**

Elizabethtown
Barney, L Gayle **(SLP)**
Bashista, Mrs Kathleen F **(SLP)**
Reber, Mrs Mary Katharine **(SLP)**

Elkins Park
Brown, Mrs Rose M **(SLP)**
Burkhard, Beth A **(SLP)**
Cohen, Marla S **(A)**
Ellison, Mrs Elaine K **(SLP)**
Kaufman, Diana Kay **(SLP)**
Melnick, Robyn H **(SLP)**
Schaffer, Mrs Kay N **(SLP)**
Schwartz, Mrs Joye R **(A)**
Selbst, Andrea K **(SLP)**
Sobel, Paula R **(SLP)**

Ellwood City
Fornataro, Lisa Marie **(SLP)**
Fox, William L **(SLP)**

Elwyn
Madison Isaac, Sherryl Luane **(A)**

Elysburg
Wasileski, Mrs Anita Arthur **(SLP)**

Emlenton
Miller, Beverly Rycz **(SLP)**

Emmaus
MacOmb, Mrs Carol Krause **(SLP)**
Moll, Denise Zapach **(A)**

Enola
D'Innocenzo, Mrs Maureen M **(SLP)**

Ephrata
Elliehausen, Jennifer Cobb **(SLP)**
Miller, Mrs Sandra Lynne **(SLP)**

Erdenheim
Farber, Mrs Judith S G **(SLP)**
Fetterman, Mrs Sally Ann **(SLP)**

Erie
Adams, Janet Rose **(SLP)**
Adams, Mrs Mary Beth Kane **(SLP)**
Barber, Carol Maynard **(A)**
Briggs, Stephanie C **(SLP)**
Bruce, Peter I **(SLP A)**
Budacki, Robert M **(SLP A)**
Carlin, Mrs Jerri C **(SLP)**
Clinard, Donna Masters **(SLP)**
Cullen, Mrs Barbara Ellen **(SLP)**
Di Luzio, Janice Marie **(SLP)**
Downey, Mrs Jeanne C **(SLP)**
Ehrheart, Natalie Anne **(SLP)**
Ferro, Deborah A **(SLP)**
Gibson, Peter S **(SLP)**
Goldaine, John A **(SLP)**
Grau, Gregory L **(A)**
Hagerty, Mrs Jane Ellen **(SLP)**
Haggerty, Barbara A **(SLP)**
Hamilton, Kathleen E **(SLP)**
Hayes, Mary Fordyce
Holland, Mrs Karen E **(SLP)**
Hrinda, Mrs Mary L **(A)**
Hughes, Mrs Kathleen Homet **(SLP)**
Keenan, Allison Faye **(A)**
Kemp, Martha Jane **(SLP)**
Kibler, Melinda A **(A)**
Kovacic, James **(SLP)**
Laneve, Mrs Cathy Kash **(SLP)**
Lansberry, Carole Miller **(SLP)**
Latzo, Mrs Michele Marie **(SLP)**
Lingenfelter, D C **(SLP A)**
MacIsaac, Mrs Lorri W **(SLP)**
Marin, Mrs Beatriz Gumucio **(SLP)**
Martin, Mrs Kristen Kosisko **(SLP)**
McQuown, Maureen E **(SLP)**
Nagle, Kim Marie **(SLP)**
Peacock, Mrs Deborah T **(SLP)**
Potoker, Dr David R **(SLP)**
Regan, James M **(SLP)**
Rudy, V Susan **(SLP)**
Schaal, Patricia Ann **(SLP)**
Sheppard-Nene, Karen **(SLP)**
Troester, Judith Hill **(A)**
Verdecchia, Julie Marie **(SLP)**
Vogt, Mrs Kathleen Casey **(SLP)**
Warren, Mrs Margaret R **(A)**
Weber, Frank Jacob, III **(SLP)**
Wisinski, Diane J **(SLP)**
Woods, Sr M Lucy **(SLP)**
Wujcik, April Doehrel **(A)**
Yeaney, Mrs Barbara Bayless **(SLP)**

Erwinna
Jurikson-Hankin, Helene Beth

Etters
Duncan, Virginia McNamara **(SLP)**

Evans City
Cornack, Julianna Holme **(SLP)**
Moravek, Mrs Peggy Mulcrone **(SLP)**

Exton
Almy, Judith K **(SLP)**
Suppan, Mrs Josephine **(SLP)**
Suppan, Vincent V **(SLP)**

Fair Oaks
Anderson, Mrs Linda D **(SLP)**

Fairless Hills
Proust, Janice **(SLP)**

Fairview
Bukowski, Mrs Darlene Collins **(SLP)**
Harayda, Debra Sue **(SLP)**

Fairview Village
Piscotty, Michael A **(A)**

Fallentimber
North, Elise Ann **(A)**

Fawn Grove
Dunaway, Kenneth H **(SLP)**

Fayetteville
Doetzer, Kimberly Ann **(SLP)**
Gamby, Mrs Vicki J **(SLP)**

Feasterville
Dewhirst, Susan Watts **(SLP)**
Setzman, Mrs Lynn H **(SLP)**
Tully, Joanne B **(SLP A)**

Felton
Adkins, Laura Westerberg **(SLP)**

Finleyville
Solties, Mrs Barbara Carter

Fleetwood
Heller, Tracy Denise **(SLP)**
Rearden, Eileen Marie **(SLP)**

Flourtown
Adler, Nancy Ford **(SLP A)**
Baum, Mrs Bonnie L **(SLP)**
Murphy, Mrs Laura McNavage **(SLP)**

Forest Hills
Emanuele, Diana Dewey **(SLP)**

Fort Washington
Hickey, Karen **(SLP)**
McClurken, Rita W **(A)**
Olshin, Judith M **(SLP)**
Roper, Julie Marie **(A)**
Russell, Dr Lorraine H **(SLP)**

Forty Fort
Roberts, Janet Lynne **(SLP)**
Rukstalis, Kathleen Grace **(SLP)**
Saporito, Karen Ann **(SLP)**

Foxburg
Smith, Jack H **(SLP)**

Frackville
Swartz, Kristin Kay

Franklin
Eidenmuller, Kirk J **(SLP A)**
Halo, Anna M **(A)**
Kassi, John **(SLP)**
Loeffert, Richard H **(SLP)**

Frazer
Nordsiek, Mrs Sari Biddle **(A)**

Freedom
Cotter, Pricilla M **(SLP)**

Furlong
Hengst, Mrs Judith F **(SLP)**
Stalletti, Mrs Amy Baxter
Victor, Mrs Constance P **(SLP)**

Galilee
Muth, Mrs Lisa A P **(SLP)**

Gettysburg
Coston, Mrs Susan Steinour **(SLP)**
Hollingsworth, Mrs Patricia B **(SLP)**
Keisch, Christine C **(SLP)**
Marschall, Ellen J F **(SLP)**
McQuaide, Marilyn H **(SLP)**
Waybright, Mrs Cheryl J **(SLP)**

Gibsonia
Bond, Linda Chepponis **(SLP)**
Campbell, William J **(A)**
Chalfant, Joyce S **(SLP)**
Johnson, Cynthia P **(SLP)**
Kraynick, Linda I
Perriello, Mrs Miriam A **(SLP)**

Gilbert
Muni-Thompson, Lynnette A **(SLP)**

Gilbertsville
Lovely, Nancy J **(A)**
Moysan, Beth Ann **(A)**
Watson, Bruce W **(SLP)**

Gladwyne
Plastino, Mrs Sue Ellen **(SLP)**

Glen Mills
Melnychuk, Mrs Kathleen **(SLP)**

Glenmoore
Balbierer, Mrs Karen Kingsley **(SLP)**
Brooks, Stanley M **(SLP A)**
Dutton, Mrs Susan R **(SLP)**
Helm, Barbara J **(SLP)**
Mars, Mrs Julie Burkholder **(SLP)**

Glenolden
Bevan, Mrs Joann L **(A)**
Postiglione, Dana M

Glenshaw
Cushman, Mrs Betty B **(SLP)**
Febbraro, Catherine A **(SLP)**
Hofstetter, Mrs Lynn D **(SLP)**
McKibben, Dr Margaret Anne **(SLP)**
Tarantine, Deborah Pauline **(SLP)**
Wood, Margaret **(SLP)**

Glenside
Pacheco, Christophr John **(SLP)**
Rogers, Mrs Ann E **(SLP)**
Ryan, L Margaret **(A)**
Whittinghill, Mrs E Jane **(SLP)**

Gouldsboro
Franklin, Diane **(A)**
Simancek, Gerald E **(SLP)**

Green Lane
Gottwald, Sheryl Ridener **(SLP)**

Greencastle
Wagner, Mrs Susan K **(SLP)**

Greensburg
Dana, Mrs Amy Thompson **(SLP)**
David, Mrs Karen S **(SLP)**
De Angelo, Mrs Maryann P **(SLP)**
Donlon, Mrs Patricia D **(SLP)**
Hewitt, Mrs Loreen Kay **(SLP)**
Krivacek, Paul Louis **(SLP)**
Kubler, Mrs Paula S **(SLP)**
Mains, Sheryl **(SLP)**
Martin, Marlene M **(SLP)**
Plucker, Paul R **(A)**
Repka, Donna L **(SLP)**
Rugh, Caroline Lee **(A)**

Greenville
Nystrom, Mrs Sharon W **(SLP)**
Wilt, Dr Sonya M **(SLP)**

Grindstone
Neil, Mrs Debra Campbell **(SLP)**

Grove City
Black, Mrs Susan K G **(SLP)**
Sigmund, Mrs Claudia J **(SLP)**

Guthriesville
Slater, C Richard **(SLP)**

Gwynedd
Wanger, Cynthia K **(A)**

Gwynedd Valley
Yerger, Josephine C **(SLP)**

Hallstead
Mullins, Paul Leroy **(A)**

Hamburg
Angelo, Robert J **(SLP)**
Kuipers, Kenneth E **(SLP)**
Reinhart, Lori Ann **(SLP)**

Hamlin
Yanick, Dr Paul **(A)**

Hanover
Bridwell, Mrs Carol Pearce **(SLP)**
Crooks, Cynthia M **(SLP)**
Roth, William Russell **(SLP)**
Troxell, Mrs Lucinda B **(SLP)**
Ziegler, Willard D, Jr **(SLP)**

Harborcreek
Leri, Mrs Susan M **(SLP)**

Harleysville
Bonnell-Corcoran, Mrs Catherine **(SLP)**
Heavener, Wren **(SLP)**
McDonnell, Eileen **(SLP A)**
Piccolomini, Marion Marie **(SLP)**

Harmony
Caldwell, Mrs Janine Ann **(SLP)**
Cusick, Joanne **(SLP)**
Hockenberger, Elaine H **(SLP)**

Harrisburg
Arena, Ann Marie **(SLP)**
Bashore, Samuel R **(A)**
Blecker, Rose W **(SLP)**
Brenner, Josephine **(SLP)**
Brenner, Lory L **(A)**
Brittingham, Lisa W **(SLP)**
Cariski, Denise M **(SLP A)**
Cassell, Mrs Mary Anita **(SLP)**
Coleman, Mrs Julia W **(SLP)**
Dell, Elise Louise **(SLP)**
Demko, Sharon R **(SLP)**
Doyle, Mrs Laurie J **(SLP)**
Elliott, Dr John W **(SLP)**
Emanuel, Permelia R **(SLP)**
Engleman, Pearl Ruth **(SLP)**
Errickson, Mrs Christina Ann **(SLP)**
Goepfert, Mrs Gayle Zimmerman **(SLP)**
Haney, Colleen Ann **(SLP)**
Harbeson, Mrs Cynthia J **(SLP)**
Harder, Brenda K **(A)**
Helfman, Mrs Karen Epstein **(SLP)**
Keiser, Mrs Gay K **(SLP)**
Kern, Diane P **(SLP)**
Krieger, Richard C **(A)**
Leiman, Lori I **(A)**
Marinak, Joseph M **(A)**
Mulhall, Alice Marie **(SLP)**
Noone, Mrs Romney M **(SLP)**
Quinn, Wendy M **(SLP)**
Rabin, Mrs Sandra C **(A)**
Ziltz, Mrs Mary Termine **(SLP)**

Hartstown
Laird, James Bryan **(SLP A)**

Hatboro
Ahrens, Sandra F **(SLP)**
Connell, Kathleen Patricia **(SLP)**
Hutt, Donna Marie **(SLP)**
Marinelli, Karen Cook **(SLP)**

Hatfield
Ramspacher, Mrs Kathryn K **(SLP)**

Haverford
Hahn, Shelly E **(SLP)**

Havertown
Afroilan, Mrs Rebecca F **(A)**
Andrews, Mrs Dale Joan **(SLP)**
Benshoof, Patricia G **(SLP)**
Collins, Beth Salvin
Davis, Mrs Phyllis K
Garland, Charlene Mary **(SLP)**
Halpern, Mrs Mindy Orlow **(SLP)**
Isack, Audrey Helen **(SLP)**
Midgette, Laurie L **(A)**
O'Carroll, Mrs Karen Gerber **(SLP)**
Phipps-Kauder, Mrs Tamara **(SLP)**
Rothstein, Mrs Jean Cofsky **(SLP)**
Toll, Mrs Donna Marie **(SLP)**

Hawley
Thomas, Mrs Connie S **(SLP)**

Hazleton
Bognet, Dr Lea Andreuzzi **(SLP)**
Farley, Mrs Linda M **(A)**
Gilgannon, Robert E **(SLP A)**

Hellertown
Moran, Lynn Ryan **(SLP)**
Wolst, Denise Kertsmar **(SLP)**

Hermitage
Biggins, Mrs Nancy Antonino **(SLP)**
Graban, Mrs Elizabeth A R **(SLP)**
Grine, Clifford **(SLP A)**
Shaw, B Dennis **(SLP)**
Ustik, Gary **(SLP)**

Hershey
Boswell, Joanne Elizabeth **(SLP)**
Bucher, Pamela M **(SLP)**
Hess, Mrs Terri Lorene **(SLP)**
Hostetter, Patricia L **(SLP)**
Lankford, Holly M **(A)**
Ott, Penelope A **(SLP)**
Poch, Nancy E **(A)**
Vargo, Dr Steven William **(A)**

Hickory
Scram, Jeanette Ballard **(SLP)**

Hiller
Christopher, Mrs Lynn Rankin **(SLP)**

Holland
Kinnard, Kristi K **(SLP)**
Pate, Louise Ann **(SLP)**
Segal, Lauren Kirsch **(SLP A)**
Staffin, Mrs Andrea Gross **(SLP)**
Whitham, Mrs Nancy Cox **(A)**

Hollidaysburg
Bradley, Mrs Janice Marie **(SLP)**
Decker, Mrs Amy K **(SLP)**
Gerraughty, Mrs Mary E C **(SLP)**
Kanar, Mrs Robin Rochelle **(SLP)**
Mariani, Felix Joseph **(SLP)**
McNamara, Stephen D **(SLP)**

Hollsopple
Vann, Mrs Vicki Jo **(SLP)**

Hollywood
Hartsough, Mrs Diane R **(SLP)**

Homer City
Molestatore, Mrs Patricia Ann **(SLP)**

Homestead
Petro, Geraldine **(SLP)**

Honesdale
Jenkins, Mrs Beverly J **(SLP)**
McDowell, Kathleen Ana **(SLP)**
Milone, Mrs Sheri Sullivan **(SLP A)**
Warren, Sally C **(SLP)**

Hookstown
Joachim, Mrs Amy M **(SLP)**

Horsham
Farnsworth, Mrs Kim Marie **(SLP)**
Feller, Deborah Tint **(SLP)**
McCullough, Maryann Desch **(A)**
Myers, Mrs Nancy McGlynn **(SLP)**
Popp-Dipietro, Debra K **(SLP)**
Shafer, Margaret Payne **(SLP)**
Swarthout, Shelly Jo **(SLP)**

Hummelstown
Knarr, Stacey Collins **(SLP)**
Querry, Mrs Patricia H **(SLP)**
Snyder, Ann Elizabeth **(SLP)**
Wakefield, Mrs Lucille Atkinson **(SLP)**

Hunker
Kintigh, Marcella Louise **(SLP)**

Huntingdon
O'Connor-McManamon, Mrs Erin **(SLP)**
Rousseau, Frank E **(SLP A)**
Van Nest, Devona S **(SLP)**

Huntingdon Valley
Appelbaum, Mrs Beth Rosenau **(SLP)**
Brecher, Adelyn R **(SLP)**
Chud, Mrs Randi L R **(SLP)**
Cooper, Judith Schiller **(SLP)**
Durkin, Teresita Marie **(SLP)**
Epstein, Mrs Sherri Joy **(SLP)**
Fishback, Mrs Inez F **(SLP)**
Fleisher, Ada M **(SLP)**
Glickstein, Mrs Donna Rostow **(SLP)**
Hernes, Mrs Clara G **(SLP)**
Isdaner, Mrs Ellen Kalodner **(SLP)**
Lieberman, Jody **(SLP)**
Messinger, Laura Grabell **(SLP)**
Simon, Bonnie L **(SLP)**
Sitman, Bonnie **(SLP)**
Temin, Donna R **(SLP)**
Temin, Michael B **(SLP)**
Utain, Sharon Beth **(SLP)**

Hustontown
Ferguson, Cindy Louise **(SLP)**

Imperial
Splain, Gay L **(SLP)**

Indiana
Beers, Mrs Kathleen B **(SLP)**
Boone, Mrs Carol A **(SLP)**
Bormann, Nelson H **(SLP)**
Brungard, Dr Maude O **(SLP A)**
Clapper, Mrs Karen Maria **(SLP)**
Empfield, Mrs Dorothy Rae **(SLP)**
Huber, Thomas M **(SLP)**
Kisiday, Cynthia T **(SLP)**
Mease, Richard P **(SLP)**
Mohn, Mrs Nichole Aline **(SLP)**
Nowell, Dr Richard C **(A)**
Nowell, Mrs Susan Polk
Prezant, Fran Pollock **(SLP)**
Reber, Mrs Clarice K **(SLP A)**
Scanga, Connie C **(SLP)**
Shane, Mrs Esther McGeoch **(SLP)**
Turton, Dr Lawrence J **(SLP)**
Vetere, Mrs Mary T **(SLP)**
Wilkerson, Mrs Dorian Lee **(SLP)**
Zorich, Mrs Donna June **(A)**

Irwin
Marting, Debra Abplanalp **(SLP)**

Steele, Mrs Sandra Covell

Jamison
Osgood, Mrs Cheryl Renee **(SLP)**

Jeanette
Seanor, Suzann

Jeffersonville
Centurioni, Dr Kathleen **(A)**
Clancy, Pamela H **(SLP)**
Zawadzki, Louise I **(SLP)**

Jenkintown
Atkins, Mrs Naomi R **(SLP)**
Feskanin, Catherine **(SLP)**
Hauber, Mary D **(SLP)**
Kahn, Betti E **(SLP)**
Madianos, Lorette D **(SLP)**
Pasternack, Lisa G **(SLP)**
Solis-Cohen, Ellen **(SLP)**
Trachtenberg, William **(SLP)**

Jennerstown
Miller, Mrs Judy Lynne **(SLP A)**

Jersey Shore
O'Neill, Mark A **(SLP)**

Jessup
Povanda, Elizabeth Ann **(SLP)**

Johnsonburg
Kanski, Mrs Cynthia R **(SLP)**

Johnstown
Astorino, Marylou **(A)**
Banda, Cynthia Ann **(SLP)**
Bloom, Annette Faye
Dugan, Mrs Elizabeth M **(SLP)**
Elliott, Mrs Kristine M **(SLP)**
Garcia, Carlos E **(SLP)**
Garcia, Emily Medic **(SLP)**
Kane, Dr James K **(A)**
Locher, Tracy Christine
Machella, Mary W **(SLP)**
Matolyak, Joye E **(SLP)**
Pastovic, Cora A **(SLP)**
Patrick, Mrs Velva V **(SLP)**
Petersen, Mrs Cynthia A **(SLP)**
Petersen, David R **(SLP)**
Schrock, Mrs Adeleen S
Skinner, Diane L **(SLP)**
Wertz, Jean B **(SLP)**
Wesner, Mrs Barbara P **(SLP)**
Wojcik-Davidson, Diane J **(A)**

Kane
Anderson, Susan B **(SLP)**
Meckley, Mrs Stacy Lynn **(SLP)**

Kenhorst
Blanski, Mrs Sheree L **(SLP)**

Kennett Square
Hudak, Mrs Diane C **(SLP)**
Krishna, Suzanne **(SLP)**
Nicholson, Mrs Allison W **(SLP)**
Piccora, Mrs Rose Rocco **(SLP)**
Snyder, Diana A **(SLP)**

Kersey
Bruni, Cheryl A **(SLP)**
Lipsey, Mrs Judy M **(SLP)**

King of Prussia
Breslau, Carol **(A)**
Ferguson, Beth W **(SLP)**
Fischer, Roberta J **(SLP)**
Graham-Hartung, Mrs Jacqueline Ann **(SLP)**
Hu, Linda L **(SLP)**
Jaloszynski, Jacqueline M **(SLP A)**
Majdic, Lynn Napkori **(SLP)**
Meitus, Vicki L **(SLP)**
Pollikoff, Francine **(SLP)**

Kingston
Conklin, Gloria Jean **(SLP)**
Hurwitz, Mrs Renee Linda **(SLP)**
Kennedy, Alexanne **(SLP)**
Mutchler, Sharon Louise **(SLP)**
Orlando, Mrs Joann Margaret **(SLP)**
Sieminski, Dr Louis R **(A)**
Wallace, Donald E **(SLP)**

Kittanning
Chemelli, Melanie P
Swast, Mrs Amy L **(SLP)**
Zambotti, Cynthia Lynn **(SLP)**

Knox
Goble, Tamalyn F **(SLP)**

Kutztown
Brasted, Sandra C **(SLP)**
Grim, Virginia S **(A)**
Kondis, Marilyn D **(SLP)**
Patton, Mrs Mary Sabo **(SLP)**
Saras, Loline J **(SLP)**

Lafayette Hill
Cutler, Mrs Rae S **(SLP)**
Duncan, Deborah Suzanne **(SLP)**
Goodman, Mrs Linda B **(SLP)**
Lundy, Mrs Marcia Cohn **(SLP A)**
Nurick, Dr Etta-Lee K **(SLP)**
Paul, Mrs Susan P **(SLP)**
Small, Mrs Audrey Gale **(A)**

Lake Ariel
Averto, Mrs Christine **(SLP)**
Fulton, Mrs Terri Browning **(SLP)**

Lake City
Domowiczo, Faye Hilary **(SLP)**

Lancaster
Beittel, Mrs Marylin P **(SLP)**
Boltik, Mrs Kathleen L **(SLP)**
Chappell, Mrs Linda J **(SLP)**
Christoffel, Mrs Elizabeth Faith **(SLP)**
Crain, Sharon Sapp **(SLP)**
Creamer, Mrs Wendy K **(SLP)**
Day, Margaret C Pecora **(SLP)**
French, Amy Ruhl **(SLP)**
Garfinkel, Mrs Rosalind **(A)**
Hartley, Mrs Carol B **(SLP)**
Kirkpatrick, Mrs Bonita Smith **(A)**
Kozlosky, Michaline **(SLP)**
Lum, Laura S F **(A)**
Mackey, Mrs Virginia R **(SLP)**
McCollom, Herbert F, Jr **(SLP A)**
Millard, Robert T **(SLP)**
Miller, Mrs Lisa C **(SLP)**
Perdeus, Melanie **(SLP)**
Rickard, Lisa R **(A)**
Sabol, Laura R **(SLP)**
Schooling, Mrs Margaret Goldbach **(SLP)**
Siguenza, Philippa M **(SLP)**
Sterner, Marcia Klein **(SLP)**
Williams, Robin Kaye **(SLP)**
Woge, Edward George **(SLP)**
Wright, Mrs Lisa Kay **(SLP)**

Landisville
Rohm, Mrs Cathy S **(SLP)**

Langhorne
Beachler, Jeanne C **(SLP)**
Booher, Deborah E **(SLP)**
Bromer, Mrs Denise Helene **(SLP)**
Brownstein, Shelley L **(SLP)**
Devore, Mrs Estra Joy **(SLP)**
Ference, Linda A Jones **(SLP)**
Gisondi, Nancy Eve **(SLP)**
Harrison, Mrs Susan Smock **(A)**
Kessler, Geraldine **(SLP)**
Kommers, Mary S **(SLP)**
Lassin, Mrs Bonnie Sue **(SLP)**
Lehman, Linda Maurer **(SLP)**
Maks, Wendy W **(SLP)**
Maples, Barbara Milillo **(SLP)**
Mears, Kathleen Lazgin **(SLP)**
Milligan, Terri P **(SLP)**
Sherrin, Mrs Janet R **(SLP)**

Lansdale
Cook, Mrs Suzanne M **(SLP)**
Corradi, Mrs Barbara Jean **(SLP)**
Denneny, Rebecca Jane **(SLP)**
Farrell, Jacqueline **(SLP)**
Geller, Barbara J **(SLP)**
Gordon, Miriam M **(SLP)**
Kane, Michele G **(SLP)**
Kestner, Joanne B **(SLP)**
Kirszbraun, Mrs Arlene F **(SLP)**
Kirts, Mrs Celine F **(SLP)**
Laubach, Mrs Connie L **(SLP)**
Leiss, Dr Robert H **(SLP)**
McGarry, Mrs Amy H **(SLP)**
Mytych, Mrs Mary Beth **(SLP)**
Reiff, Patricia Hartnett **(A)**
Roberts, Kathryn L **(SLP)**
Rogers, Julie F **(SLP)**
Shorr, Mrs Wendy E **(SLP)**
Siegel, Marshall H **(SLP)**
Swartz, Mrs Burnetta Flagg **(SLP)**
Walters, Mrs Florence M **(A)**
Yassi, Rosa Sara **(SLP)**

Lansdowne
Amster, Dr Barbara J **(SLP)**
Barron, Mrs Verna S **(SLP)**
Chapman, Michele D **(SLP A)**
Morris, Mrs Michele Diane **(A)**
Spence, Judith Ann **(SLP A)**

Latrobe
Dillon, Willard H **(SLP)**
Johnson, Mrs Mary J **(SLP)**
Labick, John M **(SLP)**
Leonard, Carol Jane **(SLP)**

Laureldale
Scull, Janet Loeper **(SLP)**

Laverock
Clark, John R, Jr **(SLP)**

Lebanon
Althouse, Susan R **(SLP)**
Brown, Diane L **(A)**
Hughes, Mrs Sharon Kaye **(A)**
Youse, Mrs Lillian A **(SLP)**

Leechburg
George, Mrs Mary J D **(SLP)**

Leesport
Elliot, Elyse M **(SLP A)**

Lehighton
Laky, Mrs Mildred H **(SLP)**

Lemont Furnace
Nickman, Stephanie Ann **(A)**

Lemoyne
Shafer, James L **(A)**

Leola
Bustaque, Mrs Patricia G **(SLP)**
Porreca, Rosemarie A

Levittown
Colflesh, Marie A **(A)**
Goehl, Dr Henry **(SLP)**
Irion, Loretta Snyder **(SLP)**
McMahon, Kathleen Mary **(SLP)**
Morris, Patricia A **(SLP)**

Lewisberry
Kumpf, Donna M **(SLP)**
Martin, Mrs Cheryl Sprout **(A)**

Lewisburg
Himes, Mrs Lori A **(SLP)**
Noyce, Betsy Ann **(SLP)**
Olson, Patricia A **(SLP)**
Pawling, Helen M
Whitman Reynolds, Kathleen Kelly **(SLP)**

Lewistown
Albrecht, Judith L **(SLP A)**
Stomackin, Karen M **(SLP)**
Votral, Karen Ann **(SLP)**

Library
Hines, Marilyn D **(SLP)**
Steimer, Mrs Charlotte Jean **(SLP)**

Lightstreet
Kruse, Dr R J **(SLP)**

Ligonier
Bailey, Mrs Jolan Nagy **(SLP)**
Costello, Thomas J **(SLP)**

Lititz
Fuehrer, Mrs Patricia McElhinny **(SLP)**
Hershey, Wendy Walls **(SLP)**
Kiec-Lehmier, Cheryl **(SLP)**
Kovacs, Colleen Braden **(SLP)**
Rostolsky, Mrs Maureen D **(SLP)**

Lock Haven
Barth, Sherry L **(SLP)**

Lower Burrell
Cirigliano, Paulette **(SLP)**
Gartley, Linda Ann **(SLP)**
Pappafava, Mrs Kathryn B **(SLP)**
Picone, Mrs Janet E **(A)**
Yates, Mrs Judith Ann L **(SLP)**

Lower Merion
Mueller, Evelyn K **(SLP)**

Macungie
Deutsch, Steven M **(SLP)**
Helm, Mrs Alice M **(SLP)**
Lemma, James Dominic **(SLP)**
Ogawa, Patricia Mary **(SLP)**
Soler, Mrs Sandra Gearhart **(SLP)**

Mahanoy City
Dicasimirro, Donna M **(A)**

Malvern
Carr, Mrs Susan A **(A)**
Gallagher-Kubat, Mrs Anne Marie **(SLP)**
Saunders, Elizabeth Lynne **(SLP)**
Valentine, Susan Mairne **(SLP)**

Manchester
Kearns, Mrs Felicia J **(SLP)**

Mansfield
Leiboff, Mrs Jean A **(SLP)**

Maple Glen
Cohen, Linda E **(SLP)**
Jackel, Rebecca B **(SLP)**
Kendrick, Nancy B **(A)**
Rinko, Mrs Ferris D Forman **(SLP)**
Solon, Carol **(SLP)**
Stanford, Marilyn Sachs **(SLP)**
Zieha, Ellen E **(SLP)**

Marietta
Helman, Sally Eberly **(SLP)**

Mars
Adamczyk, Deborah Fischer **(SLP)**
Bortnyik, Mrs Mary M **(SLP)**
Cicholski, Mrs Barbara A **(SLP)**
Gaul, Bridget I
Hourlland, Mrs Sue Ann Elizabeth **(SLP)**
Mattock, Regis A **(SLP)**
Palmer, Mrs Christine **(SLP)**
Reinhart, Kimberly Kay **(A)**
Richards, Bruce L **(SLP)**
Rosato-Ziggas, Mrs Diane M **(SLP)**

Martins Creek
Pribic, Mrs Mary Lou Brinker **(SLP A)**

Marysville
Leonard, Barbara A McCleaf **(SLP)**

Matamoras
O'Donnell, Linda J **(SLP)**

Mc Adoo
McAloose, Jennifer Mary

Mc Kean
Lee, Mrs Susan E **(SLP)**

Mc Kees Rocks
Duggan, Mrs Elaine Tonarelli **(A)**
Schram, Mrs Susan Lex **(SLP)**
Shank, Patricia T **(A)**
Wadsworth, Margaret Marie **(SLP)**

Mc Keesport
Cullen, Mrs Louise W **(SLP)**
Stare, Mrs Tina M **(SLP)**

Mc Murray
Graham, Mrs Brenda Rader **(SLP)**
McGough, Mrs Sandra C **(SLP)**
Morency-Hnat, Mrs Rachelle Anne **(SLP)**
Veraldi, Mrs Janet J **(SLP)**
Webb, Elaine W **(A)**

Meadowbrook
Bookbinder, Mrs Marlene R **(SLP)**

Meadville
Gagliotti, Mrs Michelle Eileen **(A)**
Janes, Mrs Judith E **(SLP)**
Keenan, Robert A

Mechanicsburg
Acker-Bailey, Patricia G **(SLP)**
Almon-Matangos, Mrs Susan Elizabeth **(SLP)**
Atwood, Karen Hoffman **(SLP)**
Beall, Mrs Robbin J **(A)**
Clifford, Mrs Lois J **(SLP)**
Conner, Peggy S **(SLP)**
Ensslen, Mrs Sandra Jadick **(SLP)**
Fry, Mrs Antoinette Deascenti **(SLP)**
Harding, Elizabeth Maurer **(SLP)**
Hunter, Mrs Ann E **(SLP)**
Jones, Mrs Teresa Marie **(SLP)**
Kloske, Mrs Margaret L **(SLP)**
Labuskes, Debra Hettinger **(SLP)**
Lorah, April D **(SLP)**
Miller, Virginia Carol **(SLP)**
Pankuch, Ann L
Polkowski, Mrs Diane Patricia **(SLP)**
Richards, Maribeth J
Shaul, Mrs Cynthia Shock **(SLP)**
Solon, Elizabeth M **(SLP)**
Vandrew, Mrs Karen Singiser **(SLP)**
Wollins, Dr Sally **(A)**

Media
Baker, Margaret L **(SLP)**
Berkowitz, Joyce R **(SLP)**
Bouyer, Penelope **(SLP)**
Cohen, Phyllis **(A)**
Geiger, Leigh Ellen
Harrison, John P **(A)**
Merenda, Irene B **(A)**
Obrien, Mrs Nancy Lou Rhoads **(SLP)**
Oerther, Patricia L **(SLP)**
Solomon-Dworkin, Mrs Marsha **(SLP)**

Melrose Park
Alper, Beth Sheckman **(SLP)**
Feinberg, Mrs Chantal L **(SLP)**
Genter, Ruth Z **(SLP)**
Perlman, Mrs Gail Brenner **(A)**
Weiss, Betty G **(SLP A)**

Mercer
Miller, Mrs Lillie C F **(SLP)**
Shilling, Samuel P **(SLP A)**

Merion
Cohen, Lindy S **(SLP)**
Honigman, Erica J
Kaplan, Mrs Sharon R **(SLP)**
Polishook, Pnina T **(SLP)**
Silverman, Mrs Melanie **(A)**

Merion Station
Creed, Judith S **(SLP)**

Mertztown
Godfriaux, Mrs Lois D **(SLP)**
Kwiatkowski, Mrs Ellen B **(SLP)**
Moon, Dr Susan L **(SLP)**

Middleburg
Sautner, Mrs Elaine Marie **(SLP)**

Middletown
Krzywicki, Joanne K **(SLP)**

Mifflinburg
Coates, Charles J, Jr **(SLP)**
Shively, Louise Ann **(SLP)**

Mifflinville
Lowe, Dr Robert Joel **(SLP)**

Milford
Nagy-Greenberg, Janet **(SLP)**
Nuelle, Kathleen M **(SLP)**

Mill Village
Crawford, Nannette **(SLP)**

Millersville
Peechatka, Barbara Jane **(A)**

Millville
Bankus, Mrs Carol A **(SLP)**
Cosoleto, Catherine Elizabeth **(SLP)**

Milton
Waugh, Janet Elaine **(SLP)**

Mineral Point
Good, Susan Brown **(A)**

Minersville
Rearic, Betsy Jane **(SLP)**

Mohnton
Beil, Janice Krempasky **(SLP)**
Styer, Mrs Jana K **(SLP)**

Mohrsville
Link, Karen E **(SLP)**

Monaca
Homitz, Susan Lynn
Jones, Mrs Charlene A **(A)**
Matuga, Patricia

Monessen
Vesely, Donna M **(SLP)**

Monongahela
Amy, Mrs Sandra L **(SLP)**
Ballein, Kathleen C **(SLP)**
De Stefano, Cheryl Cheroki **(SLP)**

Monroeville
Bloom, Barbara M **(SLP)**
Bodnar, Mrs Kathleen Ann **(SLP)**
Burton, Kathleen Lynn **(SLP)**
Dormer, Natalie Ann **(A)**
Dressler, Mrs Bernice S **(SLP)**
Floyd, Karla Jean **(A)**
Friedland, Sandra M
Gross, Mrs Roxann Diez **(SLP)**
Hartman, Kathleen Ann **(SLP)**
Jones, Dr Betty M E **(SLP)**
Jones, John F **(SLP)**
Kmetz, John W **(SLP)**
Konitzer, Nancy McCue **(SLP)**
Malinowski, Pamela Ann **(SLP)**
Miller, Mrs Gabriella **(SLP)**
Rodgers, Julie Ann **(SLP)**
Truschel, Mrs Mary Joan **(SLP)**
Ulizio, Deborah Lynne **(A)**
Wegrzynek, Lynn Ann **(SLP)**

Mont Clare
Ezell, Robin Ward **(SLP)**

Montoursville
Bower, Loren J **(SLP)**
Hilsher, Mrs Eve A S **(SLP)**
Ranck, Mrs Sheryl Ann **(A)**

Montrose
Ellsworth-Severcool, Mrs Rebecca Anne **(SLP)**

Moosic
Navich, Michelle Ann **(SLP)**

Morgan
Veydt, Nicole **(SLP)**

Morgantown
Petrey, Susan L **(A)**

Morristown
Pomilio, Mrs Carole B **(SLP)**

Morrisville
D'Annibale, Marisa G **(SLP)**
Doran, Catherine Beam **(SLP)**
Ludwig-Macaulay, Anita M **(SLP)**
Roach, April S **(SLP)**
Vernon, Mrs Jean C
Zirlin, Rachel Meisler **(SLP)**

Morton
De Luca, Mrs Paula D **(SLP)**

Moscow
Cortazzo, Mary A **(SLP)**
Rodney, Mrs Patricia Barone **(SLP)**
Stout, Mrs Joann Cooper **(SLP)**

Mount Carmel
Altomare, Diane T
Gownley, Kelly Ann **(SLP)**
Rudock, Michele Gabriele **(A)**

Mount Holly Springs
Leidy, Dr Gerald A **(SLP)**

Mount Lebanon
Barrios, Cynthia Flesher **(SLP)**
Gentile-Lazarchik, Mrs Christine M **(SLP)**
Schiff-Pasekoff, Mrs Deanna **(SLP)**

Mountain Top
Culkin, Mary La Rue **(SLP)**
Gauz, Dr Maurice T **(A)**

Mountville
Blackburn, Mrs Karen D **(SLP)**

Muncy
Kaplan, Holly Sue **(A)**
Muffly, Debra Lowe **(SLP)**

Munhall
Lenkner, Lucretia A **(SLP A)**
Skwarecki, Robert M **(SLP)**

Murrysville
Baumgart, Margaret S **(SLP)**
Dezzutti, Ida L **(SLP)**
Fike, Mrs Barbara C **(A)**
Forys, Mrs Donna R **(SLP)**

Nanticoke
Jacopetti, Mrs Theresa M **(SLP)**

Narberth
Aungst, Dr Lester F, Jr **(SLP)**
Aungst, Mrs Roberta B **(A)**
Brenner-Yborra, Linda S **(SLP)**
Geschke, Kathy M P **(SLP)**
Gold, Wendy M **(SLP)**
Kaplan, Beverly L **(A)**
Tomlinson, Kristine Diegel **(A)**

Natrona Heights
Chase, Susan Leeper **(SLP)**
Daloise, Mrs Shelley L **(SLP)**

Nazareth
Andress, Mrs Marilyn Miller **(SLP)**
Basso, Mrs Barbara May **(A)**
Green, Dr Robert A **(SLP)**
Hellwege, Eileen W **(SLP)**
Rampulla, Mary Louise **(SLP)**

Nesquehoning
Payan, Karen S **(A)**
Sasserath, Richard J **(SLP)**

New Bloomfield
Shawver, Katrina L **(SLP)**

New Britain
Kollinger, Mrs Dorothy P **(SLP)**
McGroarty, Jane L **(SLP)**

New Castle
Bukowski, Mary Davis **(SLP)**
Gibson, Mrs Terry Black **(SLP)**
Haas, Linda Sirianni **(SLP)**
Matheny, Nancy **(SLP)**

New Columbia
Dickson-Dutrow, Mrs Deborah A **(A)**

New Cumberland
Brahm, Jill L **(SLP)**
Chmiola, Mrs Mary Ann **(SLP)**
Dellegrotto, John T **(SLP)**
Dellegrotto, Mrs Mary Anne **(SLP)**
Fox, Mrs Margaret **(SLP)**
McKee, Teresa J **(SLP)**
Paul, Mrs Clara D **(SLP)**
Stillman, Lori Ann **(SLP)**

New Freedom
Libertini, Mrs Kim E **(SLP)**

New Hope
Funke, Mrs Beth Weisberger **(SLP)**
Plonsker, Leslie Schmidt **(SLP)**

New Kensington
Czarnecki, Tama D **(SLP)**
Hammer, David W **(SLP)**
Hanasewych, Mrs Marybeth T **(SLP)**
O'Neill, Mrs Ellen Kester **(SLP)**

New Oxford
Carr, Mrs Georgette **(SLP)**

New Philadelphia
Paukstis, Mrs Patricia F **(SLP)**

New Ringgold
Zehner, Cynthia Louise

Newport
Morrow, Mrs Jeanne Shuster **(SLP)**

Newtown
Balent, Jerilyn W **(A)**
Bevan, Richard C
Jones, Mrs Frances Marie **(SLP)**
November, Mrs Ronni **(SLP)**
Rothschild, Devera R **(SLP)**
Rozzi, Mrs Mary Ruth **(SLP)**
Schulman, Jill Theise **(SLP)**
Weisbein, Mrs Wanda **(SLP)**
Weiss, Mrs Judith Bellin **(SLP)**

Newtown Square
Chafin, Peggy J **(A)**
Dabrowski, Mrs Patricia Anne **(A)**
Keshgegian, Mrs Patrice Anne **(SLP)**
Murphy, Kathleen **(SLP)**
Perfect, Jolene A **(SLP)**
Pittenger, Anne M **(SLP)**
Tonge, Mrs Michele Stolar **(SLP)**

Newville
Black, Mrs Nancy Jane **(SLP)**
Derr, Mrs Martha Pool **(A)**

Norristown
Belkin, Mrs Marlene R **(SLP)**
Block, Mrs Wendy Heller **(SLP)**
Cooper, Karen Jacobs **(A)**
Esposito, Samuel John **(SLP)**
Hughes, Mrs Nancy Marie **(SLP)**
Krais, Janelle Graveline **(SLP)**
Levy, Mrs Susan F **(SLP)**
McFadden, Maureen Ann **(SLP)**
McGinness, Mrs Joanne P **(SLP)**
Morley, Russell D **(SLP)**
Newirth, Jill Ann **(SLP)**
Paolini, Mrs Sheila Incorvati **(SLP)**
Peters, Felicia A **(SLP)**
Phifer, Mrs Cynthia Ann **(SLP)**
Rosato, Lynne A **(SLP)**
Schoch, Candace J **(SLP)**

Wolf, Deborah L **(SLP)**
Young, Dr In Min

North East
Carll, Marcia Marie **(SLP)**
Denne, Mrs Claire M **(SLP)**
Mann, Neal E **(A)**

North Huntingdon
Javor, John M **(SLP)**
Matty, Betty Jean **(SLP)**
Phillips, Mrs Janet Lynn **(SLP)**
Smith, Mrs Rosemary Hanley **(SLP)**
Tragesser, Mrs Dorothy L **(SLP)**
Vitori, Mrs Laurie J **(SLP)**
Wilson, Deborah A **(SLP)**

North Wales
Bowes, Mrs Miriam E D **(SLP)**
Fitzgerald, Debra Adams **(SLP)**
Laquer, Mrs Mary Jane W **(SLP)**
McLaughlin, Jean Marie **(SLP)**
Micucci, Debbie E **(SLP)**
Villwock, Mrs Martha M **(SLP)**

Northampton
Holohan, Jeanette M **(SLP)**

Northumberland
Redington, Mrs Barbara L **(SLP)**

Oakdale
Collins, Linda Marie
Spanier, Cynthia Ann **(SLP)**

Oakmont
Croyle, Mrs Denise A F **(SLP)**
Kaufman, Mary F **(SLP)**
Nelson, Charles T **(A)**
Zalenski, Mrs Jane Reck **(SLP)**

Oil City
Morris, Mrs Julie P **(SLP)**
Wyant, Cathy R **(SLP)**

Old Forge
Giacometti, Mrs Jeanne M B **(SLP)**
Marmo, Deborah Marie F **(SLP)**
Matuszewski, Mrs Domencia **(SLP)**

Orangeville
Woolcock, Mrs Wendy Jane **(SLP)**

Orefield
Fedetz, Mrs Sherri Lee **(A)**

Oreland
Hall, Regina Marie **(SLP)**
Zindel, Elaine M **(SLP)**

Orrtanna
Borger, Harry L **(SLP)**

Orwigsburg
Gaydos, William John **(SLP)**
McClure, Mrs Lisa Marie **(SLP)**

Osceola Mills
Millward, Dorothy D **(SLP)**

Ottsville
Grave, Mrs Jeanette E Page **(A)**
Hammerle, Linda M **(SLP)**

Overbrook Hills
Joblin, Meryl A **(SLP)**

Oxford
Quinlan, Mrs Maureen Patrice **(SLP)**

Palmyra
Spinner, Ann Louise **(SLP)**

Paoli
Goldman, Mrs Marilyn M **(A)**
Kenney, Yvonne C **(SLP)**
Needles, Marita Riener **(SLP)**
Salisbury, Patricia Christoff **(SLP)**
Wenick, Susan Fern **(A)**

Park Hill
Kozel, Monica Marie **(SLP)**

Peckville
Fallon, Katie Helen **(SLP)**
Najaka, Elizabeth Hodovance

Penfield Downs
Herman, Meryl E **(SLP)**

Penllyn
Danforth-Dargie, Mrs Anita Louise **(SLP)**
Dooley, Mrs Constance **(SLP)**

Penn Hills
Weingartner, Susan C **(SLP)**

Penn Valley
Connor, Mrs Margaret M **(A)**
Conston, Marcia E **(SLP)**
Duchin, Dr Sandra W **(SLP)**
Kamin, Alice M R **(SLP)**
Shrut, Mrs Jamisen S **(SLP)**
Zidel, Mrs Marsha Rubin **(SLP)**

Penn Wynne
Wiese, Enid **(SLP)**

Penns Park
Atkinson, Mrs Eleanor R **(SLP)**
Leo, Mrs Ellen Deborah **(SLP)**

Pennsburg
Boone, Mrs Theresa Lynn **(SLP)**

Pennsylvania Furnace
Pringle, Mrs Emily Porter **(SLP)**
Steider, Patricia L **(SLP)**

Pequea
McJunkin, Suzanne R **(SLP)**

Perkasie
Umstead, Mrs Monica Marie **(SLP)**

Perryopolis
Filak, Mrs Patricia C **(SLP)**

Philadelphia
Agins-Bochetto, Paula **(SLP)**
Alson, Leila B **(SLP)**
Altshuler, Dr Morton W **(SLP A)**
Antoniadis, Anastasia **(SLP)**
Ball, Nadine Ann **(SLP)**
Barnes, Ann Marie **(SLP)**
Baron, Mrs Marleen Ann **(SLP)**
Baskin, Barbara Jane **(SLP)**
Becker, Mrs Andrea **(SLP)**
Berenson, Mrs Ann Berlin **(SLP)**
Berg, Jody Lynn **(SLP)**
Berger, Linda S **(SLP)**
Berger-Morra, Rita **(SLP)**
Berman, Sheree Ilene **(SLP)**
Berman, Dr Steven E **(SLP A)**
Berry, Grant A **(A)**
Betley, Nora **(SLP)**
Billups-Morgan, Barbara A **(SLP)**
Blackman, Lisa **(A)**
Blick, Judith M **(SLP)**
Bloom, Anita R **(A)**
Blume, Mrs Annette Harris **(SLP)**
Boettger, Robert Joseph **(SLP)**
Bonanno, Amy **(A)**
Bonderow, Mrs Helene R **(SLP)**
Bordman, Martin **(SLP)**
Bosin, Mrs Debra Isaacman **(SLP)**
Boyd, Judith M **(SLP)**
Brand, Helene Ann **(SLP)**
Brescia, Pamela Annette **(SLP)**
Brind, Myrna K **(SLP)**
Broad, Audrey Fern **(SLP)**
Brodie, Mrs Janet Elizbeth **(SLP)**
Brown, Muriel Ronee **(A)**
Bruton, Peggy B **(SLP)**
Bunnell, Joyce Brown **(A)**
Calbazana, Maya Victoria **(SLP)**
Calio, Victoria Anne **(SLP)**
Camins, Mrs Judith P **(SLP)**
Carner, Mrs Linda D **(SLP)**
Cavitolo, Andrea A **(A)**
Chaplick, Susan C **(SLP)**
Christy, Lloyd Wayne **(A)**
Coaxum, Barbara Ann **(SLP)**
Coffey, M Alexandra **(A)**
Cohen, Lisa Rachelle **(SLP)**
Cohen, Wendy Joy
Comer, Mrs Elaine K **(A)**
Cooper, Katherine **(A)**
Crimi, Mrs Cynthia Squillace
Davidson, Mrs Dora L **(SLP)**
Defrancesco, Miki P **(SLP)**
Deitch, Susan Anne **(A)**
Deolalikar, Padmaja Anil **(A)**
Diamond, Barry S **(SLP)**
Dodge, Paul **(A)**
Domizio-Pilla, Carmella **(SLP)**
Donohoe, Julia M **(SLP)**
Doran, Mari C **(SLP)**
Dorn, Israel Jerome **(SLP)**
Dzuba, Selma S **(SLP)**
Edinburg, Evelyn Jane **(SLP)**
Erby, Sheila A **(SLP)**
Erlbaum, Sheila J **(SLP)**
Fallon, Doris E **(SLP A)**
Faust, Joan C **(SLP)**
Feld, Nancy Sue M A **(SLP)**
Feldherr, Louise B **(SLP A)**
Feldman, Ellen R **(SLP)**
Feldman, Lynn Ann **(SLP)**
Fili, Patricia Iannelli **(SLP)**
Fink, Ruth B **(SLP)**
Frankel, Andrea **(SLP)**
Franklin, Sharon Annette **(SLP)**
Freeman, Melissa Lynn **(SLP)**
Friedman, Lois Ann **(SLP)**
Furman, Mrs Ruth B **(SLP)**
Godshalk, Lori Susan **(SLP)**
Gold, Pennysue
Goldberg, Sandra K **(SLP)**
Gorin, Rae I **(SLP)**
Goss, Mrs Monica Lynn **(SLP)**
Grachen, John J **(SLP)**
Green, Jacquelyn **(SLP)**
Gunning, Dr Mary L E **(SLP)**
Gutierrez-Clellen, Vera Florencia **(SLP)**
Haldeman, Margaret M **(SLP)**
Halfond, Dr Murray M **(SLP)**
Harris, Dr Robert **(SLP A)**
Hauser, Susan S **(SLP)**
Head, Mrs Judy H **(SLP)**
Hensenne, Janet Louise **(SLP)**
Herrick, Dr Helen M **(A)**
Hirshout, Debbie S **(A)**
Hutchinson, Debra A **(SLP)**
Iglesias, Dr Aquiles **(SLP)**
Jacobson, Bonny S **(SLP)**
Jassal, Sat Pal **(A)**
Johnson, Louise C **(SLP)**
Juston, Loretta Adele
Kalix, Joan Smyrl **(SLP)**
Kaplan, David B **(SLP)**
Keels, Edward W **(A)**
Kline, Margaret L **(SLP)**
Komisarof, Miriam S **(SLP)**
Konkle, Dr Dan F **(A)**
Krum, Susan Elizabeth **(A)**
Kujolic, Carolyn Ann
Lacey, Cynthia A **(A)**
Lasensky-Curtin, Judith A **(SLP A)**
Leonard, Cathy Marie **(SLP)**
Leonard, Laurie A **(SLP)**
Lester, Mrs Rochelle Monica **(SLP)**
Letcavage, Noryn Ann **(SLP A)**
Lewis, Brenda S **(SLP)**
Lidell, Stacy C **(SLP)**
Loeper, Sr Donna Jo **(SLP)**
Loigman, Mrs Sonia Spielberg **(SLP)**
Lopez, Alina
Luterman, Dr Barry F **(A)**
Lynch-Kenyon, Mrs Terri **(A)**
MacElrevey, Mary Denise **(SLP A)**
MacIntosh, Rita G **(SLP)**
MacLean, Mrs Carol Pavlick **(SLP)**
Mancinelli, James Mark **(SLP)**
Margolies, Mrs Judy K **(SLP)**
Matsko, Thomas A **(SLP)**
McCarthy, Christine M **(A)**
McGowan, Joy Silverman **(SLP)**
McMenamin, Sr Therese **(SLP)**
McQuaide, Karen Lynn **(A)**
Merson, Dr Richard M **(SLP)**
Mikaelian, Dr Diran O
Miller, Anne H **(SLP)**
Miller, Gerard A **(A)**
Moore, Ellen H **(SLP)**
Morgan, Mrs Tamara Snyder **(A)**
Nathanson, Yale S **(SLP)**
Niemtzow, Patricia **(SLP)**
Oday, Paula A **(SLP)**
Paarmann, Dr Larry Dean
Painter, Lee Mariano **(SLP)**
Palmer, Kimberly Ann **(SLP)**
Palmer, Mrs Maria R **(SLP)**
Petry, Susan M **(SLP)**
Pratt, Robert E, Jr **(A)**
Price, Judith Kalan **(SLP)**
Prinsket, Donnamarie H **(SLP)**
Quinn, Rosemary **(SLP)**
Reses, Nina Arkin
Ripley, Mrs Julie Margaret **(SLP)**
Roberts, Julia L **(SLP)**
Rosenblit-Braunstein, Lori Beth **(SLP)**
Rosenstein, Mrs Tamara P **(SLP)**
Rothstein, Evelyn **(SLP)**
Russo, Kathryn **(SLP)**
Sable, Mrs Randye Hoffman **(SLP)**
Sacks, Gail Karen **(SLP)**
Saenz, Terry I **(SLP)**
Sataloff MD, Joseph
Savitz, Lynne **(SLP)**
Schmidt, Edith W **(SLP)**
Schneider, Mrs Eve **(A)**
Schneier, Mrs Charlene M **(SLP)**
Schwartz, Dr Daniel M **(A)**
Schwartz, Ellen R **(SLP)**
Schwartz, Virginia Anne **(SLP)**
Seidman, Marsha R **(SLP)**
Selber, Stephen M **(SLP)**
Severino, Mrs Elissa W **(SLP)**
Shapiro, Betty Pollack **(SLP)**
Shepard, Dale R **(SLP)**
Silverman, Mrs Shirley **(SLP)**
Slutsky, Dr Sidney S **(SLP)**
Smigo, Therese M Bradley **(SLP)**
Snedden, Susan L
Solot, Cynthia Beth **(SLP)**
Spielberg, Paula G **(SLP)**
Stadler, Jacqueline C **(SLP)**
Staton, Mrs Patricia A
Stepak, Bryna C **(SLP)**
Stephenson-Opsal, Deborah **(SLP)**
Swidler, Arleen G **(SLP)**
Tabbut, Christina Stengel **(SLP)**
Taubman, Miriam **(SLP)**
Thornton, Mrs Kathy Lee **(SLP)**
Topf, A Bridget **(SLP)**
Towne, Dr Carol **(SLP)**
Valentik, Kathleen **(SLP)**
Videlock, Dr Joyce L **(SLP)**
Viggiano, Christine **(SLP)**
Wachs, Diane Kaufman **(SLP)**
Wagner, Marita L **(SLP)**
Walsh, Donna Wright **(SLP)**
Watt, Cydney Harrington **(SLP)**
Weinberg, Susan Oppenheim
Weiss, Mina **(SLP A)**
Welsh, Loretta A **(SLP)**
Wetherbee Taggart, Mrs Maureen A **(SLP)**
Whitman, Mrs Margherita **(SLP)**
Wilson, Mrs Jane C **(SLP)**
Wren, Susan Ann **(SLP)**
Young, Janet L **(SLP)**
Young, Linda L **(SLP)**
Young, William L, Jr **(SLP)**
Zeidner, Mrs Joan D **(SLP)**

Zervas, Mrs Rachel Hyman **(SLP)**
Zulewski, Richard **(SLP)**

Philipsburg

McDonald, Denise Marie **(SLP)**

Phoenixville

Kotula, Ona C **(A)**
Real, Mrs Karen K **(A)**
Reardon, Mrs Catherine **(A)**

Pipersville

Barr-Silk, Mary Jane **(SLP)**

Pittsburgh

Abbott, Nancy Jean **(SLP)**
Angelelli, Dr Roger M **(A)**
Ankney, Teresa M **(SLP)**
Avery, Charlotte B **(A)**
Bakaysza, Mrs Donna **(SLP)**
Barnhart, Susan E **(SLP)**
Bednarik, Patricia Ann **(SLP)**
Beery, Dr Quinter C **(SLP)**
Bell, Mrs Doris C **(SLP)**
Bellissimo, Mary A **(SLP)**
Bendet, Dr Roslyn M **(A)**
Berardino, Mrs Mary Baldi
Biagini, Mrs Elizabeth Duffy **(A)**
Binstock, Eve Renee **(SLP)**
Bird, Linda J **(SLP)**
Black, Carol B **(A)**
Bleil, Mrs Theresa R **(SLP)**
Block, Ina Levine **(SLP)**
Bloom, Mrs Elaine Shapiro **(SLP)**
Bloom, Lawrence A **(SLP)**
Bobrowsky, Dr Gerrian M **(SLP)**
Bonfield, Mrs Marianne Chapas **(SLP)**
Bourgeois, Michelle Suzanne **(SLP)**
Boyd, Miriam R **(SLP)**
Broadus, Sheila C **(SLP)**
Brody, Leslie A **(SLP)**
Brown, Mrs Alice F **(SLP)**
Brunk, Sakina T **(SLP A)**
Brunner, Kathleen Louise **(SLP)**
Brzenk, Donna Blankenshi **(SLP)**
Bucek, Valerie McCann **(SLP)**
Bucholtz, Mrs Joan Goldberg **(SLP)**
Butler, Judith V **(SLP)**
Campbell, Dr Thomas Franklin **(SLP)**
Capezzuto, Vincent A **(SLP)**
Carlins, Mrs Nancy Walsh **(SLP)**
Carlson, Faith **(SLP)**
Carrigan, Victoria Ashoff **(A)**
Caruso, Mary D **(A)**
Castelli, Beth Ann **(SLP)**
Chakurda, Mrs Diane Renee **(SLP)**
Charlton, Ella M
Cherry, Mrs Maureen M **(SLP)**
Chester, Sondra Lee **(SLP)**
Chilia-Hodges, Susan **(A)**
Christy, Mrs Darlene Marie **(SLP)**
Ciccone, Catherine **(SLP)**
Cimino, Mary F **(SLP)**
Cohen, Jerome M **(A)**
Cohn, Dr Ellen Rassas **(SLP)**
Coletta, Mrs Deborah J **(SLP A)**
Conley, Kathleen Scherbick **(A)**
Conley, Mrs Mary Jane Giovengo **(SLP A)**
Connelly, Sr Helen L
Connors, William A **(SLP)**
Conrad, Christie A **(SLP)**
Cook, Donna Walker **(SLP)**
Copeland, Sr Marie Estelle **(A)**
Cotter, Tracy Lynn **(SLP)**
Craig, Sam B
Craig, Dr William N **(A)**
Craven, Candida M **(SLP)**
Cullinan, Maureen Ann **(SLP)**
Cupples, Joseph K **(SLP)**
Dansak, Denise Ann **(SLP)**
De Gregorio, Emmy K **(SLP)**
Dellecker, Cynthia M **(A)**
Dempster, Mrs Del O **(SLP)**
Dess-Schwender, Mrs Amy Lynn **(A)**
Dettore, Marlene G **(SLP)**
Dickinson, Pamela J **(A)**
Dieterle, Joanne M **(SLP)**
Dixon-Ernst, Christine **(A)**
Dobbins, Mrs Patti L **(SLP)**
Doerfler, Dr Leo G **(A)**
Dollaghan, Dr Christine Ann **(SLP)**
Donato, Barbara B **(SLP)**
Doyle, Joyce Gloeckl **(SLP)**
Doyle, Patrick J **(SLP)**
Drummond, Lori Lee **(A)**
Dubner, Mrs Margery M **(SLP)**
Durrant, Dr John D **(A)**
Easterling, Mrs Cathleen Corbin **(SLP)**
Eaton, Helen F **(SLP)**
Ebert, Mrs Pricilla R **(SLP)**
Eckert, Mrs Jill Koch **(SLP)**
Eger, Dr Diane Levy **(SLP A)**
Egolf, Donald B **(SLP)**
Eide, Mrs Sandra Kay **(SLP)**
Eisner, Debra S **(A)**
Elash, Alice I **(SLP)**
Esposito Visgitis, Mrs Nina **(SLP)**
Estomin, Ellen R **(SLP)**
Ezell, Helen K **(SLP)**
Ezzell-Holdcroft, Melissa **(SLP)**
Fabian, Mrs Eulalia W **(SLP)**
Falcone, Mrs Judy Nicholas **(A)**
Fallon, Nancy M **(SLP)**
Feldman, Dr R Michael **(A)**
Ferraro-Saul, Mrs Annette Marie **(SLP)**
Findlay, Dr Robert C **(A)**
Finn, Janis Susan **(SLP)**
Fitzgerald, Sr Rita A **(SLP)**
Francis, Raymond Patrick **(A)**
Frank, Diane Loeb **(A)**
Franks, Thomas **(SLP)**
Frey, Mrs Regina M **(SLP)**
Fromm, Davida S **(SLP)**
Gailliot, Mary L **(SLP)**
Gaulin, Cynthia A **(SLP)**
Georgiana, Beverly Jean **(SLP)**
Giardino, Dorothy Ann
Gilmartin, Kathleen J **(A)**
Glickstein, Dr Joan Katz **(SLP)**
Glover, Mary Jo P **(SLP)**
Goldstein, Howard **(SLP)**
Goldstone, Frances Leigh **(SLP)**
Greenberg, Dr Sylvia **(SLP)**
Greenberger, Mrs Debra Levine **(A)**
Guenther, Mrs Megan Marie **(SLP)**
Guggenheimer, Constance **(SLP)**
Guttman, Mrs Sara R **(SLP)**
Haag, Elizabeth **(SLP)**
Hackworth, Maryann **(SLP)**
Hall, Lisa Blackburn **(SLP)**
Hamorsky, Lynda **(SLP)**
Hanak, Kathleen **(SLP)**
Hanna, Mrs Sylvia K **(SLP)**
Hastings, Eileen **(A)**
Hauser, Julia A **(A)**
Helfrich-Miller, Dr Kathleen R **(SLP)**
Hersh, Susan B **(SLP)**
Hinchliffe, Marie Capozzi **(SLP)**
Hodnik, Mrs Janet Ann **(SLP)**
Hogel, Judith M **(SLP)**
Holland, Dr Audrey L **(SLP)**
Hopkinson, Dr Norma T **(A)**
Horn, Dr Richard M **(SLP)**
Hough, Joanne McAleer **(SLP)**
Hough, Mrs Susan D **(SLP)**
Houth, Karen Kay **(A)**
Hugley-Priori, Martha Ann
Hyre, Rickey J **(A)**
Isacke, Mrs Bonnie W **(SLP)**
Jackson, Susan Theresa
Jardini, Mrs Linda P **(A)**
Johnson, Dr Charlotte E **(SLP)**
Johnson, Mrs Laurie W **(SLP)**
Jozwick-Joseph, Mrs Denise M **(SLP)**
Junker, Mrs Carolyn W **(A)**
Kalla, Mrs Barbara **(SLP)**
Kammersell, Mrs Nancy M **(SLP)**
Kania, Deborah A **(SLP)**
Keefe, Kristen Ann **(SLP)**
Kelly, Kathleen A
Kenyherz, Mrs Janet Z **(SLP)**
Kesterson, Randall K **(A)**
Klein, Susan **(A)**
Klimcheck, Mary Ann
Kohen, Francine P **(SLP)**
Krishnan, Dr Ananthanarayan **(A)**
Kuklewski, Karen Marie **(SLP)**
Kwasniewski, Kenneth James **(SLP)**
Lafferty, Mrs Deborah Ann **(SLP)**
Lambie, Charlene L **(SLP)**
Landesberg, Ann Simpson **(SLP)**
Lang, Mrs Carol E **(SLP)**
Langue, Mrs Jill Silverman **(SLP)**
Levenson, Mrs Sally Kanner
Levine, Mrs Jan W **(SLP)**
Levinson, Renee **(A)**
Limbacher, Maureen **(A)**
Linder, Mrs Barbara C **(SLP)**
Linnelli, Mrs Donna C **(SLP)**
Lippert, Emily Anne **(SLP)**
Los, Mrs Donna Weaver **(A)**
Magnotta, Olive Hughes **(SLP)**
Mahlmann, Dr Jeanne E **(SLP)**
Malloy, Mrs Jacquelynn A **(SLP)**
Marshall, Dr Thomas D **(SLP)**
Martin, Hubert **(SLP)**
Matesich, Charlene **(A)**
Matthews, Hannah **(SLP)**
Matthews, Jack **(SLP)**
McWilliams, Dr Betty J **(SLP)**
Meehan, Mary H **(SLP)**
Mickey, Robin Reid **(SLP)**
Mient, Mrs Mary G **(SLP)**
Mieszkowski, Mrs Gail B **(SLP)**
Miller, Ravenna P **(SLP)**
Mitchell, Karyn S **(SLP)**
Modreck, George A **(A)**
Morelock-Maddamma, Cynthia Elizabeth **(SLP)**
Mormer, Elaine A **(A)**
Morris, Mrs Thelma L **(SLP)**
Musto, Lisa M **(SLP)**
Myers, Mrs Bernita A **(SLP)**
Nakles, Karen Oleyar **(SLP)**
Neustadt, Gail K **(SLP)**
Niren, Mrs Carol Snyder **(SLP)**
Nozza, Robert J **(A)**
Oakley, Mrs Mary Ann **(SLP)**
Orringer, Mrs Maxine Katz **(SLP)**
Ott-Milisits, Lavonne E **(A)**
Owen, Peggy M
Park, Charles R **(SLP)**
Parson, Cynthia Jean
Patterson, Dr M Dean **(SLP A)**
Payne, Dolores Y **(A)**
Pecora, Marian W **(SLP)**
Pennesi, Kathleen **(SLP)**
Pennington, Mrs Ruth M **(SLP)**
Perilman, Ross M **(SLP)**
Perrone, Rosemary Petrovic **(SLP)**
Petruzzelli, Mrs Patricia Graf
Pferdehirt, Evelyn R **(SLP)**
Philbin, Erin Declan **(SLP)**
Phillips, Dana M **(SLP)**
Piehler, Mrs Margaret Forbes **(SLP)**
Pipski, Mary Ann **(SLP)**
Plung, Debbie **(SLP)**
Posch-Baldy, Mrs Vickie L **(SLP)**
Potrocky, Dr Michael G **(SLP)**
Probst, Gretchen E **(A)**
Proto, Josephine **(SLP)**
Queen, Sharon L **(SLP)**
Rankin, Lynn J **(SLP)**
Rector, Kathryn L **(SLP)**
Reihing, Terri Marie **(SLP)**
Rollins, Mrs Rebecca Pinedo **(SLP)**
Rood, Dr Stewart R **(SLP A)**
Rossman, Reva N **(A)**
Roth, Mrs Deborah Darling **(SLP)**
Rothermel, Mrs Barbara Armor **(SLP)**
Rubin, Dr Herbert **(SLP)**
Rucker, Mrs Sandra A **(SLP)**
Rusnak, Elaine M **(SLP)**
Schneider, Beth Ellen **(A)**
Seller, Mrs Carole C **(SLP)**
Seltzer, Dr Herbert N **(SLP)**
Shames, Dr George H **(SLP)**
Shames, Mrs Joan Kramer **(SLP A)**
Shanahan, James H **(A)**
Shepard, Carole Spolar **(SLP)**
Sherman, Eileen R **(SLP)**
Shockey, Kathleen M **(SLP)**
Shultz, Tracy Ann **(SLP)**
Siegfried, Pamela N **(SLP)**
Sinteff, Elizabeth G **(SLP)**
Slaney, Maureen Lee **(SLP)**
Smith, Betty Jo **(SLP)**
Smith, Clyde G **(A)**
Smith, Mrs Elizabeth Kolski **(A)**
Smith, Lisa Jane **(SLP)**
Snyder, Mrs Shelley Henry **(A)**
Soika, Tina M **(SLP)**
Somma, Dolores R **(SLP)**
Stosic, Mrs Patricia Waylonis **(SLP)**
Sung, Dr Jing J **(A)**
Sung, Dr Show Stu **(A)**
Sutherland, Mrs Marcia Evans **(SLP)**
Szekeres, Shirley F **(SLP)**
Szewczyk, Catherine J **(SLP)**
Takacs, Mrs Patricia Ann **(SLP)**
Teig, Mary J **(SLP)**
Territo, Dr Jacqueline M **(SLP)**
Tobin, Mrs Deborrah Johnston **(A)**
Tompkins, Dr Connie A **(SLP)**
Torkos, Gina Pretti **(SLP)**
Vassilaros, Mrs Maria Athena **(SLP)**
Vatz, Claire Santagati **(SLP)**
Vento, Mrs Barbara A **(A)**
Vogl, Beate R **(SLP)**
Volz, Pamela Rosen **(SLP)**
Vukas, Cynthia **(SLP)**
Warshawsky, Mrs Adrienne E **(SLP)**
Weber, Elaine Dorothy **(SLP)**
Weber, Vaughan **(SLP)**
Weiner, Dr Ruth H **(SLP)**
Wey, Mary Jane **(SLP)**
Winkler, Dr Sheila J **(SLP)**
Wunderly, Mrs Joan Lacki **(SLP)**
Young, Mrs Carol M **(SLP)**
Young, Mrs Mary Kathryn **(SLP)**
Zajac, David J **(SLP)**
Zangwill, Estelle R **(SLP)**
Zentz, Cynthia Klobuka **(A)**
Zionts, Mrs Laurie B **(SLP A)**
Zyskowski, Gladys Sophia **(SLP)**

Pittston

Shovlin, Deborah Anne **(SLP)**

Pleasant Hills

Rovito, Mrs Guadalupe M **(SLP)**

Plymouth Meeting

Caplan, Mrs Elyse Spatz **(SLP)**
Hoyes, Angela M **(SLP)**
Stewart, Mrs Donna Smith **(SLP)**

Polk

Kucherawy, David A **(SLP)**

Port Carbon

Schuettler, Mrs Susan Scheaffer **(SLP)**

Portage

Bem, Denise Chippo **(SLP)**

Pottstown

Batten, Mrs Jennifer Swartley **(SLP)**
Brown, Mrs Linda Bell **(A)**
D'Alessandro, Mrs Joan Valevas **(A)**
Granger, Kathleen Theresa **(SLP)**
Hans, Mrs Judith L G **(SLP)**
Harsany, Mrs Leslie Marcus **(SLP)**

Ivory, SarahAnn **(SLP)**
Johnston, Elizabeth **(SLP)**
Roth, Ronal **(SLP)**
Sholly, Ralph G **(SLP)**
Wyler, Mrs Michele R **(SLP)**

Pottsville
Ambrose, David L **(A)**
Hranichny, Kay Lynn **(A)**
Mansell, Mrs Teresa M **(SLP)**

Prosperity
Cooper, Joyce E **(SLP)**
King, Kerry B **(SLP)**

Punxsutawney
Kengersky, Mrs Donna Ann **(SLP)**

Quakertown
Clark, John Richard **(SLP)**
Hollenbach, Ann Yazujian

Quarryville
Kohlbus, Mrs Carin Marie **(SLP)**

Radnor
Alpern, Mrs Ramona L **(SLP)**

Reading
Beck, Mrs Karen S **(SLP)**
Bierly, Mrs Debra Roth **(SLP)**
Boland, Mrs Linda B **(SLP)**
Campbell, Vlacia Z **(SLP)**
Crissup, Larry A **(SLP)**
Crossen, Marcia M **(SLP)**
Exas, Mrs Katherine M **(SLP)**
Ganz, Leslie Lapinski **(SLP)**
Guers, Terry K **(SLP)**
Hook, Marcia Suzanne **(SLP)**
Jacobson, Lucille S **(SLP)**
Johnson, Dr Albert F **(SLP A)**
Kapusta, Mrs Lauri Walting **(A)**
Kaufman, Kathy E **(SLP)**
Kinney, Kimberley Ann **(SLP)**
Klemka, Lisa Michelle **(SLP A)**
Krogulski, Priscilla Mary **(SLP)**
May, Mrs Marilyn P **(SLP)**
Maylath, Mrs Pamela J **(SLP)**
Reese, Robert C, Jr **(SLP)**
Schifalacqua, Christine Victoria **(SLP A)**
Schwartz, Katharine **(SLP)**
Sova, Mrs Carol Frances **(A)**
Swigart, Dr Elca **(A)**
Terway, Joanne **(SLP)**
Ulrich, Mrs Rhonda Bay **(SLP)**
Wendling, Mrs Donna L **(SLP)**
Wolfe, Robert D, Jr **(A)**

Red Hill
Holcombe, Mrs Claire S **(SLP)**

Red Lion
Kaltenborn, J Dean **(SLP)**
Swoboda, Harvey J, Jr **(SLP)**

Reinholds
King, Mrs Peggy A **(SLP)**
Shober, Mrs Gerarda A **(SLP)**

Republic
Kelly, Catherine **(SLP)**

Richboro
Cahill, Mrs Ellen Rauchway **(SLP)**
Gold, Betsy R **(SLP)**
Palmer, Mary A **(SLP)**
Pasker, Ruthann W **(SLP)**

Ridgway
Verbeck, Margaret Mary

Ringtown
Tomtishen, Mrs Louise F **(SLP)**

Robesonia
Starkey, Mary B **(SLP A)**

Rochester
Pezzo, Donna Lee **(SLP)**

Rosemont
Schwartz, Mrs Lorna T **(SLP)**
Weissman, Mrs Cynthia C **(SLP)**

Roslyn
Smith, Dori Jean **(SLP)**
Stolp, Lauren E **(SLP)**

Rothsville
Warner, Joann Marie **(SLP)**

Ruffs Dale
Beck, Janet Ann **(SLP)**

Russell
Lindell, Gloria Jean **(SLP)**

Russellton
Dickson, Mrs Kathleen L **(SLP)**
Dickson, Mark T **(A)**

Rydal
Drubin, Mrs Susan Wikler **(SLP)**
Muller, Mrs Robin W **(SLP)**
Nyman, Marilyn S **(SLP)**
Ripkin, Mindy Perlman **(SLP)**

Sarver
Almquist, Mrs Bonnie Bricker **(SLP)**
Ehrman, Mary Hanz **(SLP)**

Scenery Hill
McAuley, Mrs Nancy C **(SLP)**

Schnecksville
Kowker, Mrs Kathleen Ann **(SLP)**

Schuylkill Haven
Hedges, Mrs MaryAnn

Schwenksville
Caisse, Mrs Karen Lynne **(SLP)**
Szymanski, Deborah A **(SLP)**

Scottdale
Shendge, Mrs Valerie Carroll

Scranton
Belfanti, Mrs Debra J **(SLP)**
Belinski, Theresa M **(SLP)**
Bisset, Dr Janet D **(SLP)**
Costello, Margaret Neary
Flahive, Michael J **(SLP A)**
Graham, Barbara J **(A)**
Harrington, Paul J **(SLP)**
Hinton, Ann Sullivan **(SLP)**
Luciani, Ann Kristen
Mariotti, Mrs Margaret Q **(A)**
Monsky, Ann Lebowitz **(SLP)**
Moreken, Mrs Betty C **(SLP)**
Panebianco, Marcia Lee **(SLP)**
Pendrak, Mrs Rose M **(SLP)**
Prislupski, Mrs Denise T **(A)**
Ruane, Thomas Joseph **(SLP)**
Shrive, Albert **(A)**
Sweda, Mrs Mary T **(SLP)**
Wadas, David A **(A)**
Wintermantel, Patricia **(SLP)**

Secane
Rundbaken, Ann E **(SLP)**

Selinsgrove
James, Anna Maria **(SLP)**
Snyder, Mrs Kristi W **(SLP)**

Sellersville
Fosbenner, Kimberly A **(A)**

Seven Valleys
Neuburger, Marilyn F **(SLP)**
Tucker, Mrs Janice K **(SLP)**

Sewickley
Baker, Mrs Mary G **(SLP)**
Bennett, Mrs Patricia Petrich **(SLP)**
Hermes, Mrs Ellen Valenzi **(SLP)**
Irvin, E C **(SLP)**
Kennedy, Regina M Z **(SLP)**
Miller, Suellen **(SLP)**
Russo, Sharon H **(A)**

Shamokin
Augustine, Joanne **(SLP)**

Sharon
Dzepina, Nada **(A)**

Sharpsville
Balko, John P **(A)**
Sebastian, Linda Lee **(SLP)**

Shavertown
Roman, Mrs Ann C **(SLP)**

Sheffield
Welsh, Mrs Darlene Fay **(SLP)**

Shenandoah
Jacavage, Gene **(A)**

Shermans Dale
Young, Catherine **(A)**

Shillington
Alabovitz, Sanford R **(A)**
Greene, Jill Diamond **(SLP)**
Wool, Sharon Lee **(SLP)**

Shippensburg
McGovern, Mrs Tara Diehl **(SLP)**

Shippenville
Anthony, Mrs Margaret Fuller **(SLP)**
Brown, Dr Jonathan R **(A)**
Simpson, Edwin R **(SLP)**

Shiremanstown
Bailets, Mrs Ann Britt **(SLP)**

Shoemakersville
Wu, Janice K **(A)**

Shrewsbury
Nasim, Abdo G **(SLP)**
Stepanik, Mark J **(SLP)**

Sigel
Brown, Jeffrey L **(SLP)**

Sinking Spring
Brunner, Mrs Karen Hoppman **(SLP)**
Decker, Mrs Hilary McAllister **(SLP)**
Kidron, Charles A **(SLP)**
Nau, Elaine B **(SLP)**
Reilly, Mrs Ida Pedergnana **(SLP)**
Sands, Denise M M **(SLP)**
Toomey, Mrs Carol S **(SLP)**
Williams, Mrs Michelle Kummerer **(SLP)**

Skippack
Gehman, Jane Susan **(SLP)**
Hildebrand, Renee Lynn
Willson, Mrs Jane C **(SLP)**

Slippery Rock
Ellermeyer, Mrs Cynthia Ann **(SLP)**
McGuinness, Gretchen M **(SLP)**
McGuinness, Kevin **(A)**

Somerset
Ogline, Mrs Kathy Harrington **(SLP)**
Rehberg, Barbara Foos **(SLP)**

Souderton
Ashmore, Mrs Susan H **(SLP)**
Novack, Evelyn B **(SLP)**

South Waverly
Angelo, Mrs Valerie T **(SLP)**

South Williamsport
Nordstrom, Mrs Judy A **(SLP)**

Southampton
Bumford, Deborah D **(SLP)**
Goldstein, Julie **(SLP)**
Klebes, Martha S **(SLP)**
Manno, Cecilia J **(SLP)**
Miller, Lindsay N **(SLP)**
Sniscak, Linda J **(SLP)**
Subrahmanyam, Mrs Carol Elizabeth **(SLP)**

Spring City
Klossman, Mrs Patricia N **(SLP)**
Reitnour, Melissa Adsit **(A)**

Spring Grove
Stambaugh, Lora Kay **(SLP)**

Spring House
Garrity, Rosemary Agnes O **(SLP)**

Springboro
Miehl, Frances Margaret

Springfield
Perachio, Jey J **(SLP)**
Pumphrey, Mrs Leslie G **(SLP)**
Silio, Paula M **(SLP)**

St Davids
Bell, Dr Hannah R **(SLP)**
Bertoni, Mrs Martina B **(SLP)**
Griffin, Thomas J **(SLP)**
Meglasson, Katherine **(SLP)**

Star Junction
Peccon, Mrs Sharon Ugolini **(SLP)**

State College
Abbott, Harry D **(SLP)**
Anderson, Carol B **(SLP)**
Bellanti, Carolyn A **(SLP)**
Berlin, Dr Asa J **(SLP)**
Black, Brenda Joyce **(SLP)**
Blood, Dr Gordon W **(SLP)**
Blood, Dr Ingrid M U **(A)**
Bryant, Virginia Anne **(SLP)**
Campbell, Martha I **(SLP)**
Clouser, Richard A **(A)**
Ebbert, Mrs Janet J **(SLP)**
Ferrand, Carole T **(SLP)**
Fluder, Mary B W **(SLP)**
Foreman, Lydia Marie **(SLP)**
Frick, Dr James V **(SLP)**
Gallaher, Dr Alan J **(SLP)**
Gilmer, Karen L **(SLP)**
Klevans, Dr Deborah R **(SLP)**
Lechner, Roberta E **(SLP)**
Lichtig, Christine **(SLP)**
Lucks, Dr Lisa Ellen
McDonald, Eugene T **(SLP)**
Mentzer-Dice, Mrs Joan L **(SLP)**
Michael, Dr Paul L
Mortimer, Mrs Emily Church **(A)**
Nilsen, Barbara S **(SLP)**
O'Keefe, Bernard Michael **(SLP)**
Podol, Mrs Joanne C **(SLP)**
Rekart, Dr Deborah Marie
Sherwood, Patricia **(SLP)**
Siegenthaler, Dr Bruce M **(SLP A)**
Suffolk, Mrs Debra R S **(SLP)**
Turley, William A **(A)**
Weaver, Gayle M **(SLP)**
Webb, Kelly Darleen **(SLP)**
Weiner, Frederick F **(SLP)**
Westlake, Mrs 0ONNA Fridy **(SLP)**
Yevick, Mrs Susan P **(SLP)**

Stoneboro
Graff, Sharon D **(SLP)**
Schleifer, Patricia H **(SLP)**

Strafford
Cohen, Mrs Debra LeShay **(SLP)**
Walker, Cori L S **(A)**

Strattanville
Hays, Mrs Susan E **(SLP)**

Stroudsburg
Chorney, Craig A **(A)**
Dean, Renee **(SLP)**
Field, Mrs Kathleen J **(SLP)**
Gottfried, Nancy E **(SLP)**
Nolan, Brian Christophe **(A)**
Pohutsky, Mrs Joelyne C J **(SLP)**
Smith, Dr Loretta Wagner **(SLP)**

Sugarloaf
Morgan, Mrs Linda M **(SLP)**
Tomkiewicz, Carol C **(SLP)**
Whitebread, Bonnie P **(A)**

Summit Hill
Hosak, Mary Ann **(SLP)**

Swarthmore
Ament, George D, Jr **(SLP)**
High, Mrs Marion L **(SLP)**
Kozubal, Judith A **(A)**
Krieger, Dr Miriam R
Overton, Lynda L **(SLP)**
Putz, Randee I **(A)**
Russell, Joanne Marie **(SLP)**
Tschiderer, Mrs Patricia Archila **(SLP)**
Vaurio, Kathryn P **(SLP)**

Swiftwater
Itsines, Mrs Christina **(SLP)**

Swissvale
Ereditario, Monica A **(A)**

Tamaqua
Yearick, Mrs Ileen H **(SLP)**

Tarentum
Knoch, Mrs Joni K **(SLP)**

Taylor
Gwyn, Robert David **(A)**
Maher, Mrs Sherri Rae **(SLP)**
Mayger-Gwyn, Tara **(SLP)**

Telford
Heckler, Melanie Leigh **(SLP)**
Morriconi, Alfonso **(SLP)**
Price, Mrs Claudia S **(SLP)**

Terre Hill
Zell, Abby B **(SLP)**

Thornton
Borowski, Mrs Marilyn McCormick
Schweitzer, Maureen Cassidy **(SLP)**

Titusville
Nasralla, Mrs Karen K **(SLP)**
Rosenblat, Mrs Bonnie Smith **(A)**

Tobyhanna
Eckles, Dennis Edward **(SLP)**

Towanda
Corbe, Grace Ann

Trafford
Stroebel, Rose Chervenak **(SLP)**

Trappe
Rafuse, Mrs Donna W **(SLP)**

Trevorton
Dunkelberger, Daniel W **(A)**

Trevose
Xanos, Mrs Janet Lynn **(SLP)**

Troy
Kennedy, William W, II **(SLP)**

Turtle Creek
Botti, Mrs Christine Pingree **(SLP)**
Ludwick, Dianne Marie **(A)**

Uniontown
Bowlen, James H **(SLP)**
Goodstein, R Sarah **(SLP)**
Henry, Gretchen B **(A)**
McDaniel, Adalyn R **(SLP)**

University Park
Frank, Dr Thomas Alan **(A)**
Gilbert, Harvey R
Hergenreder, Mrs Patti A **(A)**
Nelson, Dr Jeniece E **(SLP)**
Stouffer, Mrs Jodi L **(SLP)**

Upper Black Eddy
Stalgaitis, Mrs Kathleen **(SLP)**

Upper Darby
Schlosser, Valerie Ashman **(A)**
Sprunger, Margaret Liechty **(SLP)**
Vanston, Marylynn A **(A)**

Upper Gwynedd
Horswill, Mrs Lynn A **(SLP)**

Utica
Foster, Mrs Jacqueline Star **(SLP)**

Valley Forge
Price, Harold A **(SLP)**

Venetia
Mockridge, Candace A **(SLP)**
Rigatti, Carol F **(SLP)**
Snow, Mrs Marsha W **(SLP)**

Verona
Mascaro, Mrs Janet M **(SLP)**

Villanova
Armour, Mrs Betsy Crane **(SLP)**

Wallingford
Benz, Mrs Patricia W **(SLP)**
Byrd, Christina E
Celebre, Mrs Dorothy L **(SLP)**
Kehoe-Murray, Karen L **(A)**
Lewis, Lisa Beth **(A)**
McGoldrick, Catherine **(SLP)**
Peimer, Mrs Fran Lavovitch
Rafter, Kristine Olson **(A)**
Secunda, Lynne G **(SLP)**
Stahle, Mrs Carol Wimmer **(SLP)**
Williams, Thema Johnson **(SLP)**
Wineman, Ellen Frey **(SLP)**

Warminster
Barrett, Mrs Vivian Thompson **(SLP)**
Dranoff, Carol Beth **(SLP)**
Hittner, Roberta A **(SLP)**
Kelly, George J **(SLP)**
Kennedy, Mrs Anne Louise **(A)**
McMenamin, Cathy Elizabeth **(SLP)**
Peck, Mrs Ann Agnes **(SLP)**
Wilkes-Travers, Judith **(SLP)**
Wright, Virginia Thompson **(A)**

Warren
Brennan, Michael E **(SLP)**
Keller, Mrs Kathleen **(SLP)**
Nelson, Mark I **(SLP)**
Topa, Mrs Christine Breen **(SLP)**

Warrington
Batchelor, Mrs Maureen C **(SLP)**
Gauman, Lynn Louise **(SLP)**
Gubernick, Mrs Diane P K **(SLP)**
Murphy, Patrick Maxwell **(A)**

Washington
Backner, Kathleen A **(SLP)**
Garcia, Renee **(SLP)**
Hudock, John F **(A)**
Rutherford, Pamela
Stoy, Mrs Mary Philipps **(SLP)**
Swanik, Mrs Nancy Jane **(SLP)**
Wherry, James Allen, Jr

Washington Crossing
Digeorgio, Mrs Karen M **(SLP)**

Waterford
Bartholme, Susan Elaine **(SLP)**
Loveland, Mrs Christine Kina **(SLP)**

Waymart
Di-Stasio, Mrs Linda C **(SLP)**
King, Mrs Cheryl L **(SLP)**

Wayne
Archer, Mrs Cassandra Apostolou **(SLP)**
Belsky, Mrs Susan K **(SLP)**
Blumberg, Mrs Beverly G **(SLP)**
Demchak, Mary Ann Perry **(SLP)**
Derenzo, Adrianne C **(SLP)**
De Sante, Mrs Mary Ann **(SLP)**
Dryburgh, Susan Zabel **(SLP)**
Farley, Mary J **(SLP)**
Janson, Laura Jean **(SLP)**
Julian, Mrs Cynthia C **(SLP)**
Kornblatt, Mrs Debra Fink **(SLP)**
Satell, Mrs Margaret Cox **(SLP)**
Schanzenbach, Nancy R **(SLP)**
Weintrob, Sharon **(SLP)**
Wisely, Mrs Joanne M M **(SLP)**

Waynesboro
Brown, Mrs Judy Anne **(SLP)**
Nelson, Barbara Gail **(SLP)**

Wellsboro
Albaugh, Julie A **(SLP)**
Strauch, Richard J **(A)**
Westlake, Dr Harold **(SLP)**

Wernersville
Cramp, Carolyn A **(SLP)**
Elliott, Mrs Lori Cross **(SLP A)**
Smith, Robert M **(SLP)**

Wescosville
Ashmar, Sharon Miller **(SLP)**
Dalfonso, Raymond J **(SLP)**
Staiano, Dr Anthony V **(SLP)**

West Alexander
Neugebauer, Freda W **(SLP)**

West Chester
Blanco, Mrs Lorraine R **(A)**
Brandt, Betty C **(SLP)**
Christos, Mrs Sandra Shuman **(SLP)**
Coffey, Jacqueline **(SLP)**
Cottle, Cheri Colleen **(A)**
Domenici, Kathy Jo **(SLP)**
Eberhart, John L **(SLP A)**
Gilbertson, Mrs Anne Marie **(SLP)**
Hanes, Dr Madlyn L **(SLP)**
Harshbarger, Mrs Kim Batson **(SLP)**
Hoberman, Mrs Joyce B **(SLP A)**
Kraut, Mrs Beverly H **(SLP)**
Kryder, Mrs Cynthia Landis **(SLP)**
Kuhn, Ruby M **(SLP)**
Leidy, Dr Gordon Alan **(A)**
Lopez, Susanne R **(SLP)**
Lynn, Doyle L **(SLP)**
Lynn, Mrs Margaret H **(SLP)**
Maxwell, Susan **(SLP)**
McIntosh, Mrs Evelyn Jean **(A)**
McLaughlin, Donna Marie **(SLP)**
McManus, Sharon G **(SLP)**
McNamara, Christine T **(SLP)**
Miller, Marita Murphy **(SLP)**
Monachese, Teresa **(SLP)**
Noll, Heather Alise **(SLP)**
O'Donnell, Mrs Darlene Kay **(SLP)**
Perrin, Dr Kenneth L **(SLP)**
Sapovits, Mrs Cynthia Roddy **(SLP)**
Shurer, Thomas E **(SLP)**
Speaker, Virginia K
Spencer, Amy **(SLP)**
Stigora, Mrs Cynthia Marie **(SLP)**
Stigora, Dr Joseph A **(SLP)**
Stuart, Mrs Elena A **(SLP)**
Trent, Mrs Janice Diane **(A)**
Uschold, Mrs Kathie H **(SLP)**
Walker, Lois Alice **(A)**
Weiss, Dr Michael S
Zabriskie, Mrs Carol J K **(SLP)**

West Grove
Nelson, Mrs Lisa L **(SLP)**
Ritter, Mrs Becky A **(SLP)**

West Homestead
Wyse, Thomas J, Jr **(SLP)**

West Lawn
Green, Mrs Jean Y **(SLP)**
Katz, Mrs Betsy H **(SLP)**

West Mifflin
Mosallem, Lynn C **(SLP)**
Muckle-Davis, Lori K **(SLP)**

West Pittston
Baylor, Charles Morgan **(SLP)**
Fino, Mary A **(A)**

West Reading
Gance, Robert A **(SLP A)**

Westover
Wagner, Kathleen Sparks **(SLP)**

Westtown
Lovrinic, Dr Jean Hahn **(A)**
Lovrinic, Dr William S

Wexford
Baker, Mrs Alyse Otvos **(SLP)**
Davidson, Mrs Jane R **(SLP)**
Moules, Mrs Pamela Susan **(SLP)**
Rabbitt, Barbara Jill **(SLP A)**
Sutton, Sandra W **(SLP)**

White Haven
Flynn, Barbara J **(SLP)**

Whitehall
Bowen, Pamela A **(SLP)**
Honochick, Michele Ann **(SLP)**
Ladmer, Linda A **(SLP)**
Page, Mrs Jane Bickerton **(SLP A)**
Page, Dr John McCue **(A)**
Schappell, Linda **(SLP)**
Snyder, Mrs Beth Alaine
Vancura, Mrs Rebecca Rose **(SLP)**

Wilkes-Barre
Asby, Robert S **(SLP A)**
Barrouk, Marie Martin **(SLP)**
Buczynski, Mary Frances
Ginocchetti, Darlene Erma **(SLP)**
Ginsburgh, Dr Laurel Cooper **(SLP)**
Graham, Melinda A **(SLP)**
Krackenfels, Doreen **(SLP)**
O'Donnell, Brian David
Patchoski, Philip E **(A)**
Preston-Krackenfels, Joan **(SLP)**
Sherbin, Charles S **(SLP)**
Sundbeck, John J **(SLP A)**
Zaborny, Anne M **(SLP)**
Zehel, Dr Zoe **(SLP)**
Zeigler, James Alan **(A)**

Wilkinsburgh
Pashek, Gail V **(SLP)**

Williamsport
Baclawski, Mrs Darlene C **(SLP)**
Bresticker, Mrs Carol Marie **(SLP)**
Duff, Margaret A **(SLP)**
Dzikowski, Kimberly Sue **(A)**
Hoelscher, Susan G **(SLP)**
Pontius, William L **(A)**
Skowronski, George J **(A)**
Weikel, Mrs Stephanie Suzette **(SLP)**

Willow Grove
Berman, Mrs Jennifer Farmer **(SLP)**
Kern, Nelda Jean **(SLP)**

Wind Gap
Williams, Mary Kay **(SLP)**

Windber
Penrod, Alison Dawn **(SLP)**

Wormleysburg
Sullivan, Suzanne **(SLP)**

Wycombe
Connard, Sheryl Johanson **(A)**

Wyncote
Axelrod, Susan Breazzano **(SLP)**
Burns, Arlene G **(SLP)**
Hughes, Margaret E **(A)**
Laucius, Gail **(A)**
Lent, Alexandra **(A)**
Levine, Mrs Nioma K **(SLP)**
Starkweather, Dr C Woodruff **(SLP)**

Wyndmoor
Casciato, Karen Marie **(SLP)**
Gerber, Adele J **(SLP)**
Liddle, Mrs Brenda H **(SLP)**
Park, Patricia **(SLP)**

Wynnewood
Benson, Mrs Bonnie Kramer **(SLP)**
Davis, Mrs Rosemary B **(A)**
Denenberg, Mary E E **(SLP)**
Domers, Hillary S **(SLP)**
Goldberg, Christine Riggott **(SLP)**
Goodman, Kathy Landau **(SLP A)**
Lewison, Mrs Nancy M **(SLP)**
Mancano, Bridget Barnard **(A)**
Quinn, Marion **(SLP)**
Rosen, Mrs Robin L **(A)**
Slott, Shelley H **(SLP)**
Stumacher, Mrs Sharon G **(SLP)**

Wyoming
Pollock, Marianne M **(SLP)**

Wyomissing
Fuoco, Vito Nicholas **(A)**
Greth, Maxine T **(SLP)**
Kaucher, Gail Louise **(A)**
Rossi, Mrs Leisha Moyer **(SLP)**
Rudnick, Marcia E **(SLP)**
Walters, Melissa J **(SLP)**

Yardley
Abrams, Michele R **(A)**
Coyle, Carol Ann **(SLP)**
Cruzan, Mrs Margaret K **(SLP)**
Dolan, Mrs Marie B **(SLP)**
Dordick, Nancy H **(A)**
Ellis, Mrs Rose M Vasta **(SLP)**
Feingold, Mrs Ellen Reisner **(SLP)**
Fletcher, Bonnie Downham **(SLP)**
Kaminski-Thorpe, Carol Ann **(SLP)**
Lehrhaupt, Judith R **(SLP)**
Lilienfeld, Mrs Riselle S **(SLP)**
Linde, Lisa M **(SLP)**
Smith, Mrs Linda Skapura **(SLP)**
Tinker, Mrs Agnes Z **(SLP)**
Waller-Lee, Mrs Rhonda Jean **(SLP)**
Ward, Mrs Susan M **(SLP)**

Yeadon
Aaron, Lee R **(SLP)**
Stewart, Denise Elissa **(A)**

York
Bean, Sandra L **(SLP)**
Bomberger, Victoria E **(SLP)**
Chamberlain, Mrs Karen Shilliday **(SLP)**
Drudy, Michael Edward **(SLP)**
Erdos, Mrs Erda G **(SLP)**
Fullmer, Mrs Sue A D **(SLP)**
Hays, John M **(SLP)**
Hertig, Mrs Carla Ann **(SLP)**
Hollinger, Mrs Dianne S **(SLP)**
Innerst, Mrs Shari Lynn **(SLP)**
Jennerjohn, Mrs Carolyn J **(SLP)**
Koessler, Mrs Susan Grace **(SLP)**
Morton, Mrs Ann N **(SLP)**
O'Fallon, Mrs Celia M K **(SLP)**
Owen-Garber, Diane P **(SLP)**
Riley, Dorlas L **(SLP)**
Rotz, Mrs Marian Babbitt **(SLP)**
Smay, Karen J **(SLP)**
Smolin, Mrs Shirlee J **(SLP)**
Swengel, Kristen E **(SLP)**
Toerper, Mrs Billie Jean **(SLP)**

Youngwood
Crock, Mary Louise **(A)**

Zelienople
Baker, Mrs Dorothy A C **(SLP)**
Blackstone, Barbara **(SLP)**
Hardt, Mrs Marilyn Morgan **(SLP)**
Shenesky, Della Butcher **(SLP)**
Vecchio, Mrs Kathy Ann **(SLP)**

Zion Grove
Snyder, Jean **(SLP)**

PUERTO RICO

Arecibo
De La Rosa, Mrs Elly M **(SLP)**
Salas, Carmen Cecilia **(SLP)**
Santiago, Vilma A **(SLP)**

Bayamon
Beauchamp, Angel Dexter **(A)**
Cruz, Dr Angel R C **(A)**
Negron-Marrero, Sonia Ivette **(SLP)**
Orraca, Neysa Idalia **(A)**
Rodriquez, Mrs Hilda Velez **(A)**
San Miguel, Sonia **(SLP)**

Coamo
Torres, Nelida

Dorado
Padin-Soto, Rafaela **(SLP)**

Fijardo
Haggard, Carolyn S **(SLP)**

Guaynabo
Biamon, Carmen Teresa **(SLP)**
Medina, Mrs Alma Lizette **(SLP)**
Padilla, Teresa Melendez **(SLP)**
Robert, Mrs Betty Swanick **(SLP)**
Strubbe, Esther O **(SLP)**
Torres, Nellie **(SLP)**

Hato Rey
Gonzalez, Carmen L **(SLP)**
Maldonado, Miguel E **(A)**
Vazquez, Rosa I **(SLP)**

Isla Verde
Aleman, Martha M **(SLP)**

Lajas
Acosta, Lorena **(SLP)**

Miramar
Anglero, Olga M

Ponce
Ball, Grace Ann
McDowall, Dr Mark T **(A)**

Rio Grande
Felicier, Mrs Maria De Los A **(SLP)**

Rio Piedras
Anderson, Dr Raquel Teresa **(SLP)**
Bustillo, Maria C **(SLP)**
Colberg, Mrs Carlota M **(SLP)**
Dejesus, Maria M **(SLP)**
Febo-Rodriguez, Tomas **(SLP)**
Gonzalez, Ana M **(SLP)**
Linares-Orama, Dr Nicolas **(SLP)**
Lopez-Valladares, Jose A **(SLP)**
Marcano, Maria Amelia
Oliver-Padilla, Dr German P **(SLP)**
Ossorio-Henriquez, Flor Del R **(SLP)**
Paredes, Mrs Genoveva Cautino
Parodi, Louis M
Pinero, Iris M **(SLP)**
Piza, Maria E **(SLP)**
Quinones-Perez, Aracelis **(SLP)**
Ramos-Pizarro, Carmen Ana **(SLP)**
Roche, Mrs Ada Iris **(SLP)**
Sabo, Ana M **(SLP)**
Santiago, Nydia I **(A)**
Schilling, Mrs Edda Acosta **(SLP A)**
Schnitzer, Dr Marc L **(SLP)**
Shoenut, Dr Blanca M **(SLP A)**

San Juan
Brockmeyer, Mrs Andrea S **(SLP)**
Cancel, Dr Cruz A **(SLP A)**
Gillespie, Dr Robert V **(A)**
Guzman, Luz Rivera **(SLP)**
Kroll, Mrs Mercedes **(SLP)**
Ramos, Luz Martina
Tomassini, Daisy **(SLP)**
Toro, Jaime Irizarry

Santurce
Bonness, Sheryll Lynn **(A)**
Hogan, Dr Donald D **(A)**
Urbistondo, Vincente J

Vega Baja
Velez-Davila, Wanda Damaris

Yauco
Vivaldi, Ann M **(SLP)**

RHODE ISLAND

Adamsville
Jankowski, Mrs Ann Ericsson **(SLP)**
Thomson, Mrs Cynthia M **(SLP)**

Barrington
Cirka, Nancy A **(SLP)**
Curley, Mrs Janet **(SLP)**
Di Matteo, June S **(A)**
Ellis, Mrs Maureen O'Connell **(SLP)**
Faber-Hammond, Gayle **(SLP)**
Farnum, Mrs Marcia Ide **(SLP)**
Fisher, Pamela L **(SLP)**
Hughes, Suzanne W **(SLP)**
McNally, Mrs Michele Gauthier **(SLP)**
Van Deusen, Elaine **(SLP)**
Zwir, Rosalie R **(A)**

Bristol
Bell, Barbara Ann **(SLP)**
Cabral, Mrs Donna M **(SLP)**
Longo, Elizabeth A **(SLP)**

Central Falls
Labrecque, Janet **(SLP)**

Charlestown
Walsh, Mrs Linda H **(SLP)**

Coventry
Dooley-McLaughlin, Patricia Joan **(SLP)**
Fortier, Mrs Claire A **(SLP)**
Squillante, Mrs Susan McHenry **(SLP)**

Cranston
Boriskin, Mrs Ellen Goldman **(SLP)**
Carnevale, Susan C **(SLP)**
Davis, Sheila Lane **(SLP)**
Fitzgerald, Debra Lyn **(SLP)**
Gravell, Alan W **(SLP)**
Harris, Marsha Robin **(A)**
Healey, James Edward **(A)**
Koussa, Mrs Therese **(A)**
MacChio, Elaine A **(SLP)**
McCaleb, Peggy Ann **(SLP)**
Morrissey, Elizabeth **(SLP)**
Murtagh, Mrs Patricia J **(SLP)**
Nonis, Mrs Carol J **(SLP)**
Petrarca, Marilyn A **(SLP)**
Pizzi, Mrs Lisa Marie
Raisner, Susan J **(SLP)**
Reuter, Mrs Ellen R **(SLP)**
Rogers, Annette Piscopo **(SLP)**
Rogers, Robert R **(A)**
Wacks, Mrs Joyce S **(SLP)**

Cumberland
Cunningham, Mrs Marcia Dzaman **(SLP)**
Porter, Donica T **(A)**
Scoffone, Mrs Diane M **(SLP)**

East Greenwich
Keegan, Frances P **(SLP)**
La Chance, Patti A **(SLP)**
Lineberry, Mrs Nancy Caplitcka **(SLP)**
McWeeney, Leeann Di Salvia **(SLP)**
Miller, Bonnie G **(SLP)**
Patterson, Mrs Diane M **(SLP)**
Pierson, Patricia M **(SLP)**

East Providence
Fales, Mrs Cathy Ann **(SLP)**
Glass, Jodi L **(A)**
Maher, Suzanne Rachael **(SLP)**
McCormick, Eileen P **(SLP)**
Prizant, Dr Barry M **(SLP)**
Schuler, Kay A **(SLP)**
Starsoneck, Karen Ann **(SLP)**

Edgewood
Hamilton, Ruth G **(SLP A)**

Exeter
Goodman, David M **(SLP)**

Foster
Geehan, George Ryan **(A)**

Greenville
Gorgone, David John **(SLP)**
Stecher, Catherine **(SLP)**

Harrisville
Siner, Kathleen Read **(SLP)**
Tannock, Joy Ann

Hope
Regan, Dr J Barry **(SLP A)**

Hope Valley
Olean, Elizabeth **(SLP)**

Jamestown
Detour, Christine C **(SLP)**
Ellis, Roberta A **(SLP)**
Gargaro, Janet M **(SLP)**
Geib, Mrs Gladys Gannon **(SLP)**
Morenzi, Mrs Andria R **(SLP)**

Johnston
Lang, Mrs Grace L **(SLP)**

Kenyon
Girard, Kathleen Ann **(SLP)**

Kingston
Beaupre, Dr Walter J **(SLP A)**
Connors, Elizabeth C **(SLP)**
Culatta, Dr Barbara E **(SLP)**
Gates, Jane Krohn **(SLP)**
Hurley, Raymond Michael **(A)**
Naughton, Barbara M **(SLP)**
Oberle, Mrs Barbara S **(SLP)**
Singer, Jay **(A)**
Singer, Roberta N **(A)**
Smith, Mrs Susan Marie **(SLP)**

Lincoln
Hurlburt, Skye
Marcotte, Beth Anne **(SLP)**
McLellan, Elaine A **(SLP)**
Norton, Mrs Margaret S **(SLP)**
Norton, Robert Gerard **(SLP A)**

Manville
Goetz, Mrs Suzanne M **(SLP)**
Poisson, Doris A **(SLP)**

Middletown
Allan, Mrs Maryanne Miller **(SLP)**
Bardorf, Mary Catherine **(SLP)**
Ferguson, Linda S **(A)**
Gorman, Jacqueline **(SLP)**
Woolbright, Wendy Lamont **(SLP)**

Narragansett
Connery, Ellen Gallagher **(SLP)**
Cruise, Mrs Susan Karpe **(SLP)**
Iacono, Mrs Jacqueline **(SLP)**
Johannis, Mrs Joyce Ann **(SLP)**
Montague, Kathryn Marie **(SLP)**
Nash, Maria L
Pratt, Mrs Margaret Spinney **(A)**
Rakovic, Patricia A **(SLP)**
Rubin, Denise J **(SLP)**
Wright, Judith A **(SLP)**

Newport
Craig, Mrs Roberta Preston **(SLP)**
Embleton, Arthur C **(A)**
Sells, Mrs Janet P **(A)**

North Kingstown
Chagnon, Maryann T **(SLP)**
Fournier, Mrs Barbara Elizabeth **(SLP)**
Grubman-Black, Dr Stephen D **(SLP)**
Houle, Karen Rae **(SLP)**
Kalina, Mrs Christine **(SLP)**
Marshall, Mrs Lori J **(SLP)**
Schranz, Mrs Nancy M **(SLP)**
Tobin, Mrs Janet P **(SLP)**
Tobin, William D **(SLP)**

North Providence
Adley, Mrs Luz Marina **(A)**
Bellini, Patricia Iafrate **(SLP)**
Bowen, Mrs Paula Poirier **(SLP)**
Davis, Debra Marie **(SLP)**
Donovan, Mrs Cindy Anne **(SLP)**
Healey, Grace D **(SLP)**
Pensa, Mrs Donna Anne **(SLP)**
Wytrwal, Mrs Sandra Johnson **(SLP)**

North Scituate
Bouchard, Mrs Kathie A **(SLP)**
Burke-Constantineau, Eileen M **(SLP)**
Jakubowski, Barbara **(SLP)**
Normand, Mrs Debra Ann **(SLP)**
Osenkowski, Carolyn Ann **(A)**

North Smithfield
Gramolini, Mrs Christine Ann **(SLP)**
Owre, Mrs Deanne Marquerite **(SLP)**

Pawtucket
Audet, Lisa R **(SLP)**
Basta, Susan Cohick **(SLP)**
Dolan, Leo F **(SLP)**
Fitzpatrick-Joyce, Maureen **(SLP)**
Francisco, Arminda
Haworth, Freda **(SLP)**
Kasden, Stephen Douglas **(SLP A)**
Kayata, Mary Ellen **(SLP)**
Moreau, Leonard J **(SLP)**
Sasnett, Wendy C **(SLP)**

Portsmouth
Corseri, Susan G **(SLP)**
Kielbasa, Mrs Maureen Greichen **(SLP)**
Morley, Elizabeth Hird **(SLP)**
Sargent, Mrs C I **(SLP)**
Short, Mrs Mary Garrity **(SLP)**
Singleton, Karen Mary

Providence
Baird, Diane J **(SLP)**
Belshe, Susan Graham **(SLP)**
Bergin, Eileen Celeste **(A)**
Burgess, Kathleen **(SLP)**
Burke, Grace M **(SLP)**
Chiappinelli, Mrs Margo Ann **(A)**
Corwin-Gotimer, Maria **(SLP)**
Delaney, Patricia Marie **(SLP)**
Di Martino, Marie J G **(SLP)**
Enzer, Susan M **(A)**
Falcone, Cynthia E **(SLP)**
Farber, Laurie B **(A)**
Feyerabend, Lucy **(SLP)**
Finck, Sara V **(SLP)**
Forde, Elizabeth Ann **(SLP)**
Gelch, Joan **(SLP)**
Gozonsky, Mrs Dorothy A **(SLP)**
Grupp, Michael G **(SLP)**
Halvorsen, Jean M **(SLP)**
Kaufman, Elise S **(SLP)**
Kaufman, Sharon F **(SLP)**
Kohring, Mrs Sandra K **(SLP)**
Langhorn, Mary C **(SLP)**
Lataille, Charlene Frances **(SLP)**
Lieberman, Mrs Elaine F **(SLP)**
Luessenhop, Stephanie K **(SLP)**
Lytton, Richard E **(SLP)**
Novack, Dr Harry S **(SLP)**
O'Connor, Mrs Elizabeth **(SLP)**
Palangio, Judy
Peiser, Mrs Libby M **(SLP)**
Prescott, Hope **(SLP)**
Reed, Harriet S **(SLP)**
Rohland, Pamela A **(A)**
Schreffler, Amy E **(SLP)**
Scott, Colleen Gail **(SLP)**
Tancredi, Sandra A **(SLP)**
Tasca, Martha Flynn **(SLP)**
Venezia, Robert **(SLP)**

Riverside
MacPherson, Helen Margaret **(A)**

Rumford
Bartol, Pamela K **(A)**
Gage, Mrs Nancy Arden **(SLP)**
Jenkin, Mrs Cynthia Miranne **(SLP)**
Sachs, Michelle Anne **(SLP)**
Shank, Kathleen Ryan **(SLP)**
Sullivan, Mrs A Constance **(SLP)**

Saunderstown
Goodrich, Mrs Marianne L **(SLP)**
Sherman, Patricia M **(A)**

Slatersville
Miller, Maureen Marie **(A)**

Smithfield
Cavanagh, Elizabeth **(SLP)**

Tiverton
Chew, Elizabeth P **(SLP)**
Fezette, Mrs Susan Lynn **(SLP)**
Mahon, Julia Weiss **(SLP)**

Wakefield
Baldwin, Dr Nona B **(SLP)**
Boyle, Mary Catherine **(SLP)**
Peigelbeck, Will Gary **(A)**
Yrchik-Shoemaker, Mrs Debra A **(SLP)**

Warren
Accardi, Clare Mercier **(SLP)**
Moran, Cynthia Ann **(SLP)**
Pratte, Catherine A **(SLP)**

Warwick
Ahlijanian, Mrs Zarie K **(SLP)**
Brandreth, Shirley Elizabeth **(SLP)**
Carlson, Judith Hammerlind **(SLP)**
Curnett, Jeffrey C **(SLP)**
D'Alfonso, Patricia H **(SLP)**
Doonan, Lesley C S **(SLP)**
Dubois, Cheryl B **(SLP)**
Fitzsimons, Dr Ruth N **(SLP)**
Fordon-Abbott, Irene **(A)**
Furman, Mrs Gayle F **(SLP)**
Furman, Mrs Temma **(SLP)**
Garrahy, Patricia Ellen **(SLP)**
Gerstenblatt, Deborah S **(SLP)**
Gordon, Dora N **(SLP)**
Green, Mrs Hanna **(SLP)**
Lake, Albert E **(A)**
Lake, Kathleen T **(SLP)**
Marquis-Canham, Mrs Celeste **(SLP)**
McEntee, Maureen K **(SLP)**
McMahon, Judith A **(SLP)**
O'Brien, Jane Asprinio **(A)**
Rigney, Kathleen M
Roland, Mrs Barbara Ann **(A)**
Sholes, Gertrude Jozefowicz **(A)**
Siperstein, Mrs Mynde S **(SLP)**
Spencer, Kathleen M
Stoskopf, Colette M **(SLP)**
Venturini, Mrs Susan Parkin **(SLP)**
Zaminer, Marie M **(A)**

West Kingston
Loy, Kent Matthews **(A)**

West Warwick
Lesowski, Kristin Ann **(SLP)**
McGinity, Lori Jean
McMullen, Mrs Maureen

Westerly
Alfiero-Bavasso, Mrs Susan Jane **(SLP)**
Gagnon, Mrs Rachel F **(SLP)**
Mather, Jennifer Leigh **(A)**
Mooney, Darlene Rose **(SLP)**
Newman, Mrs Diane J **(SLP)**
Serra, Marilyn Frances **(SLP)**
Theadore, Mrs Geraldine Liguori **(SLP)**

Wickford
Salisbury, Toni Ann **(SLP)**

Woonsocket
Webster, Cheryl Ann **(SLP)**

SOUTH CAROLINA

Aiken
Costigan, Mrs Carter Rainsford **(SLP)**
Harris, Marcia L **(SLP)**
Lane, Mrs Rhonda Smith **(SLP)**
Looney, Nancy A **(SLP)**
Metts, Marlene **(SLP)**
Seward, Linda H **(A)**
Wright, Cynthia J **(SLP)**
Zapp, Mrs Marlene U **(SLP)**

Anderson
Brandon, Dickey L **(A)**
Burrow, Sandra C **(SLP)**
Farmer, Phyllis Allen **(SLP)**
Gillespie, Mrs Myrtle E **(A)**
Goldman, William H **(SLP A)**
Roscoe, Mrs Lauren **(A)**
Thomason, Mrs Pauline Claire **(SLP)**

Beaufort
Dawsey-Brown, Mrs Deborah **(SLP)**
Fallon, John F **(SLP)**
Johnson, Mrs Ruby Stradford
Settles, Mrs Gloria Harvin **(SLP)**
Widener, Dr Anna H **(A)**
Wright, Karen Jo **(SLP)**

Belton
Babb, Agatha B **(SLP)**

Bennettsville
Nobles, Mrs Penelope M **(SLP)**

Bowman
Summers, Paula Elaine **(SLP)**

Buffalo
Parham, Mrs Lisa L **(SLP)**

Camden
Bishop, Dr Judith Hidding **(SLP)**
Shell, Mrs Claire L F **(SLP)**
Walker, Johnnie C **(SLP)**

Cayce
Metts, Mrs Cheri Cobb **(SLP)**

Chapin
O'Connor, Mrs Pearl May **(SLP)**

Charleston
Ashton, Carol G **(SLP)**
Baran, Lorelei Jeane **(SLP)**
Carle, Timothy D **(SLP)**
Carnell, Dr Claude M, Jr **(SLP)**
Cohen, Stuart L **(A)**
Davidson, Salley Barton **(SLP A)**
Driscoll, Heather **(A)**
Gravino, Mrs Amy W **(SLP)**
Gross, LCdr Allan H **(A)**
Herring, Claudia A **(SLP)**
Hudson, Atwood **(SLP)**
Hufnagle, Katy Kammer **(SLP)**
Kapp, Mrs Helen H **(SLP A)**
Klein, Dr Alan J **(A)**
Landers, Mrs Kristine S **(SLP)**
Larkin, Mrs Mary Ann **(A)**
Leonard, Mrs Cheryl M **(SLP)**
Maddox, Sarah Payne **(SLP)**
Martine, Catherine Jane **(A)**
Matthews, Lois Jean **(A)**
McGuirt, Mrs Janice Spakes **(SLP)**
Mills, John H **(A)**
Morrison, Sandra H **(SLP)**
Newhouse, Susan J **(SLP)**
Poston, Mary Baron **(SLP)**
Rainsford, Evangelyon Holmes **(SLP)**
Reidenbach, Elizabeth **(SLP)**
Richardson, Methlee E **(SLP)**
Schum, Lorianne Katherine **(A)**
Sumter, Mrs Debra Gethers **(SLP)**
Szypulski, Edmund S **(SLP A)**
Szypulski, Mrs Theresha A **(SLP)**
Waldron, Dr Daryle Lee **(A)**
Weathers, Patricia Reed **(A)**

Chester
Owens, Gloria J

Clemson
Fishcer Geldard, Mrs Patricia Von **(SLP)**
Greenstein, Katherine Lodenkamp **(SLP A)**
Pollock, Mrs Carol R **(SLP)**
Powell, Constance **(SLP)**
Silvestro, Mrs Elizabeth Rice **(SLP)**

Clinton
Barber, Russell James
Brondyke, Vicki L **(SLP)**

Cola
Ellis, Mrs Linda A **(SLP)**

Columbia
Agoe, Mrs Lisbeth Ann **(SLP)**
Anderson, Melanie Gayle **(SLP)**
Balfour, Patricia **(A)**
Blackwelder, Mrs Joan B **(SLP)**
Bockhaus, Nancy Jean **(SLP)**
Bogus, Janet Carol **(A)**
Boylston, Eula W **(SLP)**
Burnett, Lynn M **(SLP A)**
Collins, Loralyn Perry **(SLP)**
Cook, Mrs Elizabeth Batson **(SLP)**
Cooper, Dr William A, Jr **(A)**
Coston, Mrs Carol C **(SLP)**
Coston, Dr Gale Norman **(SLP)**
Daniels, Teri Joseph **(SLP)**
Davis, Ellen E **(SLP)**
Edwards, Margaret Susan **(SLP)**
Ewing, Janice Kryski **(SLP)**
Feurstein, Elizabeth **(SLP)**
Frank, Dr Elaine M **(SLP A)**
Gaylord, Mrs Cathy W **(SLP)**
Gore, Mrs Donna W **(SLP)**
Gore, Mrs Leah C **(SLP)**
Gutierrez-Mauzy, Regina Anne **(SLP)**
Hadley, Mrs Carin Bridges **(SLP)**
Halford, Mrs Wilma E **(SLP)**
Halligan, Pamela L W **(A)**
Hawkins, Dr David B **(A)**
Henry, Mrs Geri Spencer **(SLP)**
Hinnant, Elizabeth **(A)**
Honaker, Mrs Jane Griffin **(SLP)**
Huntley, Jill E **(SLP)**
Ickes, Mrs Michelle Ann **(A)**
Jargosch, Debra L **(SLP)**
Johnson, Mrs Michele B **(SLP)**
Jones, Bradley L **(SLP)**
Jones, Mrs E Sharon L **(SLP)**
Kirkwood-Hodge, Alledi J **(SLP)**
Langley, Sharon B **(A)**
Leadbitter, Elizabeth **(A)**
Lee, Carol T **(SLP)**
Lewis, Jennifer **(SLP)**
Lewis, Michael A **(A)**
Long, Karen Madison **(SLP)**
Lyles, Mrs Sarah B J **(SLP)**
McDade, Dr Hiram L **(SLP)**
McDonald, Dr F Douglas **(A)**
McKenzie, Mrs Emma R **(SLP)**
Means, Mrs D Yvonne N **(A)**
Miller, Mrs Louise Gervais **(SLP)**
Minges, Geraldine S **(SLP)**
Monteith, Mrs Martha **(SLP)**
Montgomery, Dr Allen A **(SLP)**
Montgomery, Marcia M **(SLP)**
Moody, Rosemary **(SLP)**

Moore, Dr Sulyn E **(SLP)**
Murphree-Holden, Crystal **(SLP)**
Nagle, Patricia **(SLP)**
Nalty, Lily Neumann **(SLP)**
O'Connor, Alma Elizabeth **(SLP)**
Orange, Mrs Tina Tettenburn **(A)**
Pearlstine, Mrs Edelu G **(SLP)**
Quattlebaum, Patricia D **(SLP)**
Ramsey, Myra G **(SLP)**
Regan, Margaret Elizabeth **(A)**
Reynolds, Linda Estelle **(SLP)**
Robinson, Dorothy Polite **(SLP)**
Roux, Mrs Pam J L
Saleem, Naheed
Simpson, Martha A **(SLP)**
Smith, Karen Gregory **(SLP)**
Sofley, Frances Eckel **(SLP)**
Stahl, Mrs Wendy B **(SLP)**
Streater, James A, Jr **(A)**
Strother, Dorothy K **(SLP)**
Summerson, Deborah N **(SLP)**
Tannenbaum, Sandra **(SLP)**
Tanner, Mrs Carol Jw **(SLP)**
Taylor, Hazel E **(SLP)**
Thomas, Susan Clark **(SLP)**
Thompson, Dr David J **(A)**
Thompson, Judith J **(SLP)**
Thompson, Mrs Lurline Glover
Thompson, Mrs Marie H **(A)**
Toner, Mrs Tommie C **(SLP)**
Varadi, Mrs Carol Anne **(SLP)**
Varnedoe, Danielle Reed **(SLP)**
Wade, Elizabeth Parnell **(A)**
Washington, Hazel Delois
Weiss, Mrs Aileen A **(SLP)**
Weiss, Dr Arthur I **(SLP)**
Wilkes, Mrs Pamela Taylor **(SLP)**

Conway
Booth, Beneature Sander
Gifford, Grace M **(SLP)**
Hasty, Sarah A **(SLP)**
Sloan, Mrs Gayle Y **(SLP)**

Cross Hill
Rogers, Mrs Lisa B **(A)**

Dalzell
Redmond-Tillotson, Barbara **(SLP)**

Darlington
Robandt, Mrs Theresa L **(SLP)**

Easley
Horne, Mrs Laurie Michelle **(SLP)**
Poland, Robert M **(A)**

Edgefield
Sears, Mrs Sara P **(SLP)**

Elgin
Gordon, Mrs Jamie Saltrick **(SLP)**
Tallon, Valerie McDonald **(SLP)**
Tetz, Mrs Shelley Marie/Rand **(SLP)**

Florence
Bennett, Susan G **(SLP)**
Beverly, Brenda Lee **(SLP)**
Cloud, Steven J **(SLP)**
Cocklin, LuAnn J **(SLP)**
Cooper, Sandra Gail **(SLP)**
Gaster, Mrs Lydia Sexton **(SLP)**
Gibbons, Joan Walker **(A)**
Gowin, Jane **(SLP)**
Gwin, Barbara Naser
Harris, Luetta **(SLP A)**
Morales, Diana Carol
Murphy, Mrs Susan Granger **(SLP)**
Nichols, Anne Christine **(SLP)**
Rogers, Janet Alma **(SLP)**
Roth, Mrs Diane Renee **(SLP)**
Schultz, Mrs Kathy Jo **(SLP)**
Silverberg, Barbara Sue **(SLP)**
Stack-McLaughlin, Mrs Eileen Marie **(SLP)**
Thomas, Dr Kenneth P **(A)**
Vincent, Patricia J **(SLP)**
Watson, Linda Ann **(SLP)**
Webb, Ronald J **(SLP)**

Fort Mill
Simpson, Susan K **(SLP)**
Young, Lorie Vaughn

Gaffney
Compton, Roger Lee **(A)**

Georgetown
Kimes, Mrs Patricia Klesel **(SLP)**

Goose Creek
Ciucci, Mrs Rebecca Lee **(A)**
Julian, Mrs Betty R **(SLP)**
Kahrs, Catherine **(SLP)**
Lawler, Terri Ann **(SLP)**
Nattkemper, Mrs Laurie L **(A)**
Singletary, Louise J **(SLP)**

Greenville
Beverung, John William **(SLP)**
Camp, Marcia Winecoff **(A)**
Cantrell, Dr James C **(SLP)**
Coleman, Dr Gerry Watson
Cosgrove, Sarilla B **(SLP)**
Davis, M Sue **(SLP)**
Fischer, Debra K **(SLP)**
Gosselin, Michelle Ann **(SLP)**
Gould, Elaine Dwyer **(SLP)**
Groblewski, Tonjia S **(SLP)**
Grumbine, Mrs Thayer F **(SLP)**
Lucking, Victoria Bradley **(SLP)**
May, Sally L **(SLP)**
Pence, David C **(SLP)**
Quick, Deborah A **(SLP)**
Scarlett, Mrs Deborah S **(SLP)**
Sewell, Natalie B **(SLP)**
Skipper, Sandra Lane **(A)**
Strother, Mrs Jean Downey **(SLP)**
Thompson, Mrs Nancy B **(SLP)**
Trask, Julie G **(SLP)**
Van Patten, Christine K **(SLP)**
Walpool, Thomas W **(SLP)**
Webber, Sharon Green **(SLP)**
Wells, Mrs Judy Haselwood **(SLP)**
Whitesides, Margie Karen **(SLP)**
Whitson, Edward T, Jr **(A)**
Williams, Genice Nix **(A)**
Wise-Siegel, Barbara Lynne **(SLP)**

Greenwood
Bryson, Frances Rebecca **(SLP)**
Dennis, Susan Elizabeth **(A)**
Taylor, Roxie G **(SLP)**

Greer
Edwards, Mrs Mary W **(SLP)**
McPhail, Mrs Barbara E **(SLP)**
Meeks, Mrs Kathryn R **(SLP)**
Morrow, Elise Wilbanks **(SLP)**
Williamson, Mrs Sue Ellen **(SLP)**

Hartsville
Cannarella, Mrs Beverly Tedards **(SLP)**
Crawford, Patricia Lee **(SLP)**
Parish, Deborah Clymer **(SLP)**

Hilton Head
Burdinie, Mrs Heather Turner **(SLP)**
Flory, Susan Williamson **(A)**
Gibbes, Florence W **(SLP)**
Hall, Mrs Diane Hayes **(SLP)**
Lau, Dr Aileen C **(SLP)**
Leboutillier, Mrs Merrianne L **(SLP)**
O'Neal, Linda M **(SLP)**

Hilton Head Island
Markey, Susan Anne **(A)**
Rushing, Robin Ann **(SLP)**
Tracy, Mrs Rebecca T **(SLP)**

Hopkins
Dixon, Sharon B **(SLP)**
Glenn-Watson, Althea **(A)**
Robinette, Connie C **(A)**

Inman
Morgan, Mrs Deborah Jones **(SLP)**

Irmo
Bigiarelli, Michele Ann **(A)**
Bowie, Rosemary Chandler **(SLP)**
Corley, Ellen C **(SLP)**
Jennings, Mrs Carol M **(SLP)**

Isle of Palms
Grieg, Diana H **(SLP)**
Morley, Lisa J **(SLP)**
Stamp, Judith Long **(A)**
Wiseman, Mrs Peggy G **(A)**

Jonesville
Gault, Sharon Tharp **(SLP)**

Ladson
Cripps, Mrs Susan B **(SLP)**
Green, J Michael

Lancaster
Conrad, Mrs Diane F **(SLP)**
Gilmore, Janet Buie **(SLP)**
Stevenson, Rebecca Elliott **(SLP)**
Whitlow, Lucinda A **(SLP)**

Lane
McClorin, Cynthia V **(SLP)**

Laurens
Behrendt, Karen Lynne **(SLP)**
McAlister, Mrs Sarah Long **(SLP)**
Parsons, Deborah Ann **(SLP)**

Leesville
Dickert, Mrs Karen B **(SLP)**

Lexington
Brady, Debbie E **(SLP)**
Clark, Jacqueline Cindy **(SLP)**
Fleming, Mrs Joyce F **(SLP)**
Harris, Mrs Elizabeth T **(SLP)**
McCrarey, Mrs Rebecca Ann **(SLP)**
Whitlock, Mrs Kathleen Staggs **(SLP)**

Lugoff
Bowe, Teresa Gunter **(SLP)**
Quigley, Mrs Anne Sonsmith **(SLP)**

Marion
English, Mrs Wynne Adele **(SLP)**
Mace, Mrs Shirley C **(SLP)**

Mauldin
Harris, Constance B **(SLP)**

Moncks Corner
Gosnell, Mrs Marie Dovre **(SLP)**

Mount Pleasant
Armstrong, Barbara L **(SLP)**
Barnwell, Mrs Elizabeth Ogier **(SLP)**
Cooley, Kathleen Shannon **(SLP)**
Creger, Mrs Alexandra Joan **(SLP)**
Culbertson, Mrs Patti F **(SLP)**
Huff, Mrs Marion Vonkolnitz **(SLP)**
Mills, Janice F **(SLP)**
Parker, Cheryl **(A)**
Schum, Dr Donald Joseph **(A)**
Stuhr, Fonda Carol **(SLP)**
Wilson, Connie S **(SLP)**

Mullins
Mason, Mrs Rachel J **(SLP)**

Myrtle Beach
Benbow, Mrs Pamela Jean **(A)**
Davis-Lary, Andrea S **(SLP A)**
Ginn, Mary E **(SLP)**
Shealy, Candler Leslie **(A)**
Steadman, Dorothy Bates **(A)**

Newberry
Waterfall, Mrs Lorraine M **(SLP)**

Ninety Six
Barnes, Mrs Leigh C **(SLP)**

North
McKinney, Marnette P **(SLP)**

North Augusta
Giess, Suzanne Marie **(A)**
Hopkins, Rebecca B **(A)**
Young, Mrs Jeanette S **(SLP)**

North Charleston
Ficken, Mrs Elizabeth Anne **(SLP)**

Norway
Brown, Mary Beth **(SLP)**
Hannibal, Ruth Renee **(SLP)**

Orangeburg
Ashley, Betty Thomas **(SLP)**
Coleman, Dr Thalia J **(SLP)**
Frishberg, Debra M **(SLP)**
Graves-Rivera, Dr Silvia A **(SLP)**
Griffin, Flavia Ramcharan **(SLP)**
Haynes, Thomas Charles, Jr **(A)**
Huddleston, Delores Jeneal **(SLP)**
Jackson, Janette Rhodes **(SLP)**
Jenkins, Mrs Sharon E F **(A)**
Morrissey, Mrs Emily Rollins **(SLP)**
Myers, Corine C **(SLP)**
Powell, Dr Harold **(SLP)**
Sandifer, Henri D **(SLP)**
Smith, Mrs Tina Thompson **(SLP)**
Tanner, Amgela Maria
Wilson, Gwendolyn D **(A)**

Pauline
Davis, Mrs Catherine C **(A)**

Pawleys Island
Evans, Mrs Coletia Brown **(SLP)**
Maloney, John Stevens
Rogers, Mrs Susan Fulmer **(SLP)**

Piedmont
Freeman, Mrs Cecilia Porter **(SLP)**
Wasilewski, Mrs Nancy A **(SLP)**
Wyatt, Mrs Elizabeth Caroll **(A)**

Port Royal
Main, Kimberly L **(SLP)**

Prosperity
James, Mrs Cynthia Dwyer **(SLP)**

Rock Hill
Alto, Mrs Carolyn L **(A)**
Beard, Dr Anne Evans **(SLP)**
Edwards, Mrs Nancy G **(SLP)**
Fantry, Timothy J **(SLP)**
Hope, Mrs Andrea W **(SLP)**
Kea, Mrs Christa Langston **(SLP)**
Moore, Wendy Ann **(SLP)**
Niedringhaus, Mrs Jacquelyn D **(SLP A)**
Rosso, Dr Louis J **(SLP)**
Sturkey, Clare A P **(SLP)**
Zdenek, Mrs Constance **(SLP)**

Saluda
Wilder, Mrs Martha J **(SLP)**

Santee
Clark, Mrs Patricia H **(SLP)**
Sanders-Jackson, Elaine **(SLP)**

Seneca
Hale, Mrs Terri Kay **(SLP)**
Lusk, Susan Lay **(SLP)**

Simpsonville
Cantrell, Connie Stephens **(SLP)**
Hubbard, Mrs Francine Bruster **(SLP)**
Poole, Mrs Ann Taylor **(SLP)**
Vickerman, Katherine **(SLP)**

Spartanburg
Anderson, Erin Gaye **(SLP)**
Andress, Diane **(SLP)**
Bales, Tammy Lynn **(SLP)**
Breon, Mrs Nanine C **(A)**
Brown, Gwen T **(SLP)**
Browning, Denise Joy **(SLP)**

Casey, Kathleen C **(SLP)**
Chaney, Mrs Gayle Lynn **(A)**
Cleveland, Mrs Lea Niblett **(SLP)**
Dawsey, Ben W **(A)**
Edgemon, Mrs Jenny C **(A)**
Hicks, Mrs Cynthia P **(SLP)**
Hodge, Mrs Laura Fisher **(SLP)**
Holian, Mrs Eva Maria **(SLP)**
Jones, Vivian Booker **(SLP)**
Lankford, Nila Kay **(SLP)**
Ogletree, Nancy Cureton **(SLP)**
Parrish, Mrs Patrice Weimert **(SLP)**
Perkins, Cynthia B **(SLP)**
Prall, Josephine **(A)**
Pruitt, Mrs Joyce D **(SLP)**
Rodriguez, Marcia Weaver **(SLP)**
Stevens, Mrs Donna Shuler **(SLP)**
Taylor, Carolyn F **(SLP)**
Youmans, Patricia L **(SLP)**

St Matthews
Murph, Jennifer Tallulah
Rucker, Mrs Emily Gressette **(SLP)**

Summerville
Burke, Linda Dunneage **(SLP)**
Gatch, Eleanor G **(SLP)**
Haller, Dr Raphael M **(SLP)**
Johnson, Mrs Aleta Marie
Johnson, Mrs Emily C **(A)**
Lusby, Mrs Barbara Peterson **(SLP)**
Martin, Mrs Bonita L **(SLP)**
Miller, Lisa Wigington **(A)**
Monat-Haller, Mrs Rosalyn K **(SLP)**
Morabito, Cindy Palatka **(SLP)**
Potter, Ellen L **(SLP)**
Rich, Wanda M **(SLP)**
Silver, Mrs Valeria Bonnette **(SLP)**

Sumter
Butler, Lucy E
Corley, Virginia M **(A)**
Graham, Gwendolyn Henrietta
Kight, Mrs Carolyn Rizer **(SLP)**
Lyles, Melanie Kay **(SLP)**
McTeer, Vidalia G **(SLP)**
Spann, Melanie H **(SLP)**
Tomchik, Peggy Frances **(SLP)**
White, Mrs Mary H **(SLP)**

Surfside
Ferri, Mrs Deann S **(SLP)**

Taylors
Dickinson, David L **(A)**
Fisher, Karen Lynn T **(SLP)**
Guryan, Mrs Barbara M **(SLP)**
Guryan, Stephen Thomas **(A)**
Hurley, Martin D **(SLP)**
Turley-Shuck, Jeanne C **(SLP)**
Whitley, Mrs Ruth S **(SLP)**

Tega Cay
Hermsen, Mrs Julie B **(SLP)**

Travelers Rest
Arnold, Deborah A **(SLP)**
Fowler, Elbert E **(SLP)**

Trenton
Cassels, Caro M **(SLP)**
Pickett, Mrs Iris H **(SLP)**

Union
Mize, Dr Jean C **(SLP)**
Waddell, Mrs Judith S **(SLP A)**

Walterboro
Johnston, Mrs Tracy R **(SLP)**
Pearcy, Mrs Altha B **(SLP)**

West Columbia
Bailey, Mrs Alice G **(SLP)**
Carney, R John **(SLP)**
Price, Mrs Alyson Duffie
Rickenbaker, Mrs Joyce Brown **(SLP)**
Spires, Karen L **(SLP)**
Sproles, Linda O **(SLP)**

Williston
Stephens, Mrs Harriet Kennedy **(SLP)**

Winnsboro
Fifer, Mrs Gretchen G **(SLP)**

SOUTH DAKOTA

Aberdeen
Cook, Mrs Sheryce Lynn **(SLP)**
Coughlin, Patrick M **(A)**
Froke, Robert A **(A)**
Ronayne, Liza Ann Gingras **(SLP)**
Rux, Mrs Dawn Whites **(SLP)**

Belle Fourche
Madison, Mrs Patricia Trippe **(SLP)**

Beresford
Dolan, Sally Joan **(SLP)**

Box Elder
Bishop, Mrs Mary Greene

Brookings
Charlson, Mrs Teresa Jean **(SLP)**
Kephart, Lucy Rosauer **(SLP)**
Lampson, Joyce M **(SLP)**
Meyer, Dr Edward L **(SLP)**

Canistota
Woltzen, Mrs Carol Ann **(SLP)**

Centerville
Gullickson, Mrs Colleen F **(SLP)**

Custer
Chard, Jan Bryggmanh **(SLP)**
Moore, Jacquelyn **(SLP)**

Deadwood
Apa, Mrs Marty Ann **(A)**

Elk Point
Slattery, Janet Turrou **(SLP)**

Fort Pierre
Wilcox, Mrs Jeri Milner **(SLP)**

Frankfort
Solheim, Tammy Dee

Groton
Fliehs, Joan B **(SLP)**

Hartford
Willer, Mrs Phyllis Lorene **(SLP)**

Hill City
Johnson, Mrs Michele A **(SLP)**

Hot Springs
Berg, Joanne Kaye **(SLP)**
Holloway, Dr Gordon F **(SLP A)**
Jones, W Harold **(SLP)**

Huron
Northrup, Peggy Oevering **(SLP)**

Kadoka
Bonenberger, Pamela L **(SLP)**

Lemmon
Norris, Mrs Linda F **(SLP)**

Madison
Lindsay, Kathleen **(SLP)**

Meckling
Fostvedt, Patricia Ann **(SLP)**

Mitchell
Krall, Mrs Cindy Martin **(SLP)**

Mount Vernon
Hammer, Mrs Verla J **(SLP)**

Parker
Preheim, Michaelene Weidemann **(SLP)**

Pierre
Anderson, Charles A **(SLP)**
Barnett, Deborah S **(SLP)**
Manus, Louis J, Jr **(SLP)**
Monicken-Johnson, Mrs Teresa Marie **(A)**
Roberts, Mrs Kim Meyer **(SLP)**

Porcupine
Miller, Sr Annette Marie **(SLP)**

Presho
Mackey, April F **(SLP)**

Rapid City
Allard, Mrs Elinor T **(SLP)**
Bridgeford, Ethel B **(SLP)**
Brunner, Mrs Patty J **(SLP)**
Colleran, Michael J **(A)**
Dalin, Mrs Tamora Mueller **(SLP)**
Feehan, Mrs Pamela J **(A)**
Feiszli, Marianne **(SLP)**
French, Louise A **(A)**
Gibbens, Theresa Marie **(SLP)**
Gienger, Denny L **(A)**
Hanson, Barbara J **(SLP)**
Larson, Mrs Kendra Sue **(SLP)**
Moore, Lois Ann **(SLP)**
Sachs, Sharon Ann **(A)**
Samuelsen, Ruth A **(SLP)**
Schultz, Lynette Lee **(SLP)**
Shea, Ann Kathleen **(SLP)**
Wilson, Mrs Diane S **(SLP)**

Redfield
Day, Beverly Elaine **(SLP)**
Metzgar, Mrs Kim Marie **(SLP)**
Willis, Mrs Diane Kay **(SLP)**

Salem
Sabers, Mrs Rhonda Kaye

Sioux Falls
Albritton, Dr Evelyn G **(SLP A)**
Allen, Mrs Darla Rae Marie
Bailin, Janet H G **(SLP)**
Bofenkamp, Stewart P **(A)**
Brockevelt, Mrs Susan R **(SLP)**
Clem, Mrs Jane M **(SLP)**
Fields, Tracee Lane **(SLP)**
Finsand, Gail DeeAnn **(SLP)**
Hacecky, Karla R **(SLP)**
Hanavan, Perry C **(A)**
Hedeen, Mrs Maureen Marie **(SLP)**
Heegel, Mrs Melinda A **(A)**
Johnson, Mrs Susan L W **(SLP)**
King, Gregory P **(SLP A)**
Klumpp, Mrs Jean Ann **(SLP)**
Leite, Jane M **(SLP)**
McPherson, James H **(A)**
Nygard, Joni Lea **(SLP)**
Olson, Mrs Patricia Lynn **(SLP)**
Patterson, Dr Mary A **(SLP A)**
Pollard, Mrs Catherine **(SLP)**
Raysby, Cheryl A **(SLP)**
Ruhaak, Linda Ellen **(SLP)**
Scholten, Mrs Connie Lynn
Sigl, Bonnie L **(SLP)**
Slack, Elizabeth Louise **(SLP)**
Spriggs-Blair, Mrs Susan M **(SLP)**
Stanford, Gary D **(A)**
Stuart, Sheela L **(SLP)**
Tjomsland, Lily Clara **(SLP)**
Warren, Geralynn F **(SLP)**
Welk, Mrs Genevieve **(SLP)**
White, Nancy C **(SLP)**
Williams, Mrs Shelley Plath **(SLP)**
Winkleman, Mrs Dorothy E **(SLP)**

Spearfish
Degen, Mrs Elizabeth Crosswait
Lind, Mrs Cheryl G **(SLP)**

Springfield
Weber, Theresa M **(SLP)**

Tyndall
Koan, Margaret A **(SLP)**

Vermillion
Berndt, Alice **(A)**
Clifford, Dr Sylvester **(SLP A)**
Ferris, Karen K **(SLP)**
Flanagin, Mrs Judy Davis **(SLP)**
Hanneman, Launa Kae **(SLP)**
Hoff, Mrs Janet Kay **(SLP)**
Litke, Robert E **(SLP A)**
Lockwood, Dr Dean D **(SLP A)**
Mueller, Mrs Michele Marie **(SLP)**
Newman, Dr Ruth Ann **(SLP)**
Spiegel, Hazel S **(SLP)**
Stuefen, Betty Watkins **(SLP)**
Treon, Dr Martin Avery **(SLP)**
Walters, James E **(SLP)**

Wakonda
Wilcox, Mrs Aneita **(SLP)**

Watertown
Gertsen, Mrs Connie Bard **(SLP)**
Hensler, Eve Lynn **(A)**

Yankton
Highland, Mrs Kristeen H **(SLP)**
Malchow, Mary K **(SLP)**
Pardy, Mrs Crystal Wendt **(SLP)**
Raysby, Julie L
Stanage, Sally Ann **(SLP)**
Strand, Gayle Jean **(SLP)**
Wilcox, Juli **(SLP)**

TENNESSEE

Afton
Moore, Joyce Ann **(SLP)**

Antioch
Ashford, John R **(SLP)**
Drost, Hazel Rose Marie **(SLP)**
Helton, Mrs Elizabeth Sammer **(SLP)**
Hendrix-Crommelin, Kathleen F **(SLP)**
Mosely, Marcella M **(SLP)**
Pleiss, Claire W **(SLP)**
Shields, Mrs Susan Sinnamon **(SLP)**
Trumpy, Carol Jean **(SLP)**
Yeager-Williamson, Mrs Elizabeth Annette **(SLP)**

Athens
Bessom, Mrs Kathy K **(SLP)**

Bartlett
Bonastia, Mrs Lou Rita **(SLP)**
Coltharp, Loretta J **(A)**
Hanhold, Diana Tresa Dyky **(SLP)**
White, Mrs Jennifer W **(SLP)**

Blaine
Sayler, Mrs Mary Ellen **(SLP)**

Bluff City
Carrier, Mrs Elizabeth **(SLP)**

Brentwood
Bergerson, Jane T S **(SLP)**
Browning, Mrs Patricia Ann **(SLP)**
Drennan, Mrs Deborah F **(A)**
Dunkle, Karji L **(SLP)**
Fetters, Mrs Marcia L G **(SLP)**
Hays, Mrs Denise B **(SLP)**
Webb, Dr Wanda G **(SLP)**

Brighton
Wallace, Kathleen P **(SLP)**

Bristol
Fountain-Walls, Mrs Karen Lanore **(SLP)**
Massengill, Dr Raymond, Jr **(SLP)**
Menzel, Otto J **(A)**
Snyder, John C, Jr **(A)**

Brownsville
Moss, Mrs Amy F **(SLP)**
Watson, Cheryl Ann **(A)**

Camden
Waters, Mrs Nancy Suzanne **(SLP)**

Celina
Young, Casey Freeman **(SLP)**

Chattanooga
Abramson, Mrs Myrna G **(SLP)**
Addison, C Lewis **(A)**
Bercaw, Mrs Maggi Delaney **(A)**
Boeninger, Mrs Frances R **(SLP)**
Bourdon, Donna L **(SLP)**
Browning, Mrs Denise Dotts **(SLP)**
Burriss, Mrs Catherine Dandl **(SLP)**
Byrd, Anna Christina **(SLP)**
Cartwright, Cynthia Anne **(SLP)**
Daniel, Lynn **(SLP)**
Dorton, Linda E **(SLP)**
Edmonds, Priscilla E **(SLP)**
Ellis, Mary M **(SLP)**
Fox, Danette L **(SLP)**
Goebel, Mrs Elizabeth **(SLP)**
Hathorne, Dr Howell F **(SLP)**
Hawthorne, Mrs Carole C **(SLP)**
Hess, Mrs Lynn Durham **(SLP)**
Hochrein, Celeste Renee **(SLP)**
Inman-Ebel, Mrs Beverly **(SLP)**
Jenison, Marcia M **(SLP)**
Keith, Mary Russell **(A)**
Kleehammer, Kimberly Smith **(SLP)**
Massey, Claire A **(SLP)**
McEuen, Gayle Appling **(SLP)**
Miller, Diana L **(SLP)**
Miller, Janet E **(SLP)**
Moore, Dana **(SLP)**
Parker, Kenneth C **(A)**
Patton, Susan A **(SLP)**
Polen, William D, Jr **(A)**
Pritchett, Mrs Judy G **(SLP)**
Rhea, Melinda Kaye
Scafe, Mrs Darnell Holler **(A)**
Scott, Mrs Susan M **(SLP)**
Smith, Ruby D **(SLP)**
Stamps, Dennis Earl **(A)**
Stephens, Mrs Jayne **(SLP)**
Stephens, Lynda Jean **(A)**
Stotts, Janet Fay **(SLP)**
Tilford, Michelle Renee **(SLP)**
Wiggins, Mrs Patsy J **(SLP)**
Wilkinson, Mrs Jean M **(SLP A)**

Chuckey
Hoss, Mrs Sarah Vance **(SLP)**

Church Hill
Teague, Mrs Melissa Carol **(SLP)**

Clarksville
Dunham, Mrs Angela Harrah
Fleming, Mrs Marcia D **(SLP)**
Freeman, Dr Barry A **(A)**
Kranich, Jane G **(SLP)**
Moser, Mrs Elizabeth Mills **(SLP)**
Wallace, Mrs Jane Lambert **(SLP)**
Wright, Mrs Mary Catherine **(SLP)**

Cleveland
Brown, Marsha **(SLP)**
Jordan, Mrs Jean Whitlock **(SLP)**
Murphy, Mrs Janice Cox **(SLP)**
Rann, Patti Elfreda **(A)**

Clinton
Grace, Ann Wilson **(SLP)**
Porter, Alicia K **(SLP)**

College Grove
Blews, Mrs Deborah Lyle **(SLP)**

Collierville
Breazeale, Mrs Karen Lynn **(SLP)**

Columbia
McDaniel, Barbara C **(SLP)**
McDaniel, David Michael **(A)**
Pierce, Linda J **(SLP)**
West, Daniel Welch **(A)**

Cookeville
Claeys, Wanda M **(SLP)**
Neal, Mary R **(SLP)**
Nichols, Kim E **(SLP)**
Norwood, Reed **(A)**
Stewart, Dr James Monroe

Cordova
Cox, Benton W, III **(A)**
Francis, Mrs Sherri B **(A)**
Guthrie, Mrs Renee Poteet **(SLP)**
Hanover, Mrs Regina K **(SLP)**
Massey, Elizabeth **(SLP)**
Pike, Connie Moore **(SLP)**
Sanders, Mrs Deanna Dear **(SLP)**
Steinberg, Marilyn A **(A)**
Tackett, Katherine Holland **(A)**

Covington
Goldsmith, Georgie A **(SLP)**

Dayton
Ulrich, Mrs Margaret Littell **(A)**

Dickson
Gray, Joanne M **(SLP)**
Jennings, Mrs Evelyn W **(A)**

Donelson
Faklis, Mrs Holly Lee **(SLP)**

Dover
Jones-Lewis, Beverly L **(A)**

Dyersburg
Armstrong, Mrs Nancy Monack **(A)**
Patterson, Dana Hall

East Ridge
Smith, Karen Denise **(SLP)**
Thomas, Terry A **(SLP)**

Elizabethton
Carrier, Jackie M **(A)**

Elora
Taylor, Lorraine

Fairfield Glade
Gatti, Pamela Jean **(SLP)**

Fall Branch
Smith, Mrs Eileen Ward **(SLP)**

Fayetteville
Conger, Mrs Jane J **(SLP)**

Franklin
Alvey, Mrs Charlene R **(A)**
Bell, Linda C **(SLP)**
Darville, Mrs Lesa Ward **(SLP)**
Fly, Mrs Diane T **(SLP)**
Hansen, Ellen A **(SLP)**
Hessenthaler, Mrs Kerry M **(SLP)**
Johnson, Mrs Grace Kane **(SLP)**
Lammel, Julie K **(SLP)**
Lathrop, Mrs Debra Lantz **(SLP)**
Menefee, John Thomas, II
Summers, Mrs Donna Jo **(A)**
Sweatt, Beverly Leverda **(SLP)**
Taylor, Andrewena **(SLP)**
Trace, Melissa M **(SLP)**
Wolczyk, Vicki R **(SLP)**
Wood, Lynn Rodney **(SLP)**

Gallatin
Buck, Garry Earl **(SLP)**
Diller, Mrs Tomi-Tara K **(SLP)**
Hibbett, Jean P **(SLP)**
Howe, Mrs Pauline Elam
Hutchins, Mrs P Joan **(SLP)**
Roberts, Ruth Ellen **(SLP)**
Rodriguez, Mrs Sandra Lynn
Sanders, Mrs Andrea S **(SLP)**
Sanders, Richard **(A)**

Gatlinburg
Adair, Dr Joe B **(A)**
Adair, Melanie N **(SLP)**

Germantown
Anderson, Robert M **(SLP)**
Bensman, Mrs Harriet L **(SLP)**
Berry, Dr Bill **(SLP)**
Carter, Mrs Margaret Fleming **(SLP)**
Chambelain, Jo Ann K **(SLP)**
Glass, Mrs Nancy E **(SLP)**
Hazen, Mrs Carol A K **(SLP)**
Hodges, Nancy W **(SLP)**
Hunter, Mrs Joyce K **(SLP)**
Inglis, Mrs Marjorie K **(SLP)**
Moore, Jacklyn Minnick **(SLP)**
Riley, Sherri B G **(SLP)**
Spratlin, Mrs Barbara P **(SLP)**
Tatge, Barbara A **(A)**

Goodlettsville
Craig, Mrs Kathryn C **(SLP)**
Lay, Mary Francis **(SLP)**
Ralph, Luwana Diane **(SLP)**

Gray
Burns, Margaret C **(A)**
Lyons, Mrs Shelley Byas **(SLP)**

Greenback
Hester, Joan M **(SLP)**

Greeneville
Dougherty, Betty Sterling
Johnson, Glen W **(A)**

Hampton
Franklin, Leslie Diane **(SLP)**

Harriman
Fraser, Mrs Peggy B **(SLP)**

Hendersonville
Clodius, Anne Patricia **(SLP)**
Cosgrove, Joan N **(SLP)**
Edwards, Mary F **(SLP)**
Garrett, Coy Edwin, Jr **(SLP)**
Good, Mrs Martia B **(A)**
Griffin, Dr Kathleen F **(SLP A)**
Hornbostel, Susan Marie
Irwin, Janet S **(SLP)**
Martin, Mrs Cathryn P **(SLP)**
McClannahan, Sharon K
McConnell, Betty D **(SLP)**
McCord, Christine Jo **(SLP)**
Membrino, Mrs Irene F
Pate, Suzanne M **(SLP)**
Robertson, Lynne Farrar **(SLP)**
Sheffey, Ronald Carl **(SLP)**

Hermitage
Cornetta, Eileen Marie
Ross, Mrs Lajuana Dee **(SLP)**

Hixson
Burroughs, H D Rob, Jr **(SLP)**
Dailey, Mrs Janis A **(A)**
Pecsok, Janet A **(SLP)**
Rice, Barbara D **(SLP)**
Richardson, Mrs Margaret R **(SLP)**
Siler, Mrs Rebecca S **(SLP)**
Wilson, Karen Lee **(SLP)**

Hohenwald
Cook, Mrs Sherri B **(SLP)**

Jackson
Butler, Mrs Linda C **(SLP)**
Gatgens, Mary Lou **(SLP)**
Hale, Diane H **(SLP)**
Hankins, Kathy Dawn
Hightower, Alicia Diane **(SLP)**
Howell, Mrs Nancy Hanks **(A)**
Kerr, Mrs Linda Susan **(SLP)**
Lee, Barbara Dean **(SLP)**
Lowe, Mary Elizabeth **(SLP)**
McClellan, Sherry Jaynes **(SLP)**
Moss, Mrs Arlene S **(A)**
Tabor, Linda Kolwyck **(SLP)**
Teague, Rebecca Lynn **(SLP)**
Wagster, Mrs Cindy M **(SLP)**
Weikel, Mrs Marilyn Lucy **(SLP)**

Jamestown
White, Daniel Raymond **(SLP)**

Joelton
Baker, Carol Putman **(A)**

Johnson City
Babb, Mrs Pamela Bobich **(A)**
Barnes, Mrs Jill Harwood **(A)**
Bowman, Zeph M **(SLP A)**
Copeland, Mrs Pauline B **(SLP A)**
Cox, Mrs Teresa J **(SLP)**
Cradic, Mrs Pamela Sue **(SLP)**
Crews, Lynette Marlowe **(SLP A)**
De Jarnette, Dr Glenda **(SLP)**
Flugrath, Dr James M **(SLP A)**
Freeman, Dr Algeania W **(SLP)**
Garland, Mrs Margaret Ann
Garvin, Mrs Virginia Barbara **(SLP)**
Gold, Dr Saralyn **(A)**
Graunke, Dr W Lloyd **(A)**
Gregory, Mary L **(A)**
Grube, Dr M Marshall **(SLP)**
Hall, Mrs Sharon C
Higgins, Laurie A **(A)**
Johnson, Mrs Doris Emiko
Lucas, Elizabeth Creech **(SLP)**
Lutz, Dennis R **(SLP)**
Overbay, Carolyn H **(SLP)**
Painton, Dr Stephen W **(A)**
Schumaier, Dr Daniel R **(A)**
Sherrod, Mrs Lynn R **(SLP)**
Shirk, Mrs Sandra Potts **(SLP)**
Summers, Mrs Juanita W **(SLP)**
Waddoups, Dr Milo O **(SLP)**
Wood, Dr James Fowle
Wood, Patsy Ruth H **(SLP)**
Worley, Mrs Martha Lundy **(SLP)**
Young, Marilyn J **(A)**

Jonesboro
King, Robert S **(SLP)**
Wilcox, Aneita W D **(SLP)**

Kingsport
Bray, Deirdre **(SLP)**
Brown, Mrs Kathleen Cross **(SLP)**
Burdine, Mrs Martha Jane **(SLP)**
Dodd, Mrs Elizabeth **(SLP)**
Hrivnak, Mrs Brenda Martin **(SLP)**
Maleski, Mrs Diane P **(SLP)**
Pennington, John C **(SLP)**

Kingston
Dutton, Mrs Ada Mullins **(SLP)**
Wilkinson, Sue A C **(SLP)**

Kingston Springs
Bush, Linda Southwick **(SLP)**

Knoxville
Adler, Dr Sol **(SLP)**
Anderson, Mrs Ann Catlett **(SLP)**
Arthur, Deborah W **(A)**
Asp, Dr Carl W **(SLP A)**
Bedwinek, Anne Plummer **(SLP)**
Bennett, Kathy Lee **(SLP)**
Bergin, Dr Kendall R **(SLP)**
Bird, Ann Thomas **(SLP)**
Boden, Laura Canter **(SLP)**
Bower, Marcia Louise **(A)**
Bradley, Denita Hyler **(SLP)**
Browning, Ann L **(SLP)**
Bruce, Mrs Carla Jo **(SLP)**
Buckels, Marcia K **(SLP)**
Burchfield, Samuel B **(A)**
Burman, Mrs Julia Ann **(SLP)**
Butler, Mrs Carol Reedy **(A)**
Carney, Dr Patrick J **(SLP)**
Carroll, James R, Jr **(A)**
Chapman, Iva M **(SLP)**
Chen, Hsiao-Chuan **(A)**
Chohanin, John P **(SLP)**
Coates, Suzanne Lake **(SLP)**
Cole, Mrs Evelyn Brown **(SLP)**

Coleman, Betty D **(SLP)**
Comer, Sherry L **(SLP)**
Commons, Susan D **(SLP)**
Corum, Mrs Susan Smith **(SLP)**
Cox, Mrs Lisa Thurman **(SLP)**
Critcher, Carolyn G **(SLP)**
Crockett, Emily Cary
Crunk, Mrs Anne M **(SLP)**
Cruz, Eduardo **(A)**
Curlee, Mrs Deborah L **(SLP)**
Davis, Cathy Ann **(A)**
Dehart, Mrs Nancy Nunley **(A)**
Dickey, Mrs Margaret Keck **(SLP)**
Diefendorf, Dr Allan O **(A)**
Earl, Dr Dennis Charles **(A)**
Earl, Dr Patricia Wojciak **(A)**
Edwards, Mrs Edith A **(SLP)**
Eskew, Nancy D **(A)**
Ferguson, Mrs Cynthia Perkins **(SLP)**
Ferrell, Charles J **(A)**
Ferrell, Judith Y **(A)**
Fine, Mrs Jan Sliger **(SLP)**
French, Mrs Elsie H **(SLP)**
Fryar, Laura Elizabeth **(SLP)**
Gaul, Vicki Bridges **(SLP)**
Geisen, Helana Sietsma **(A)**
Gibson, Barbara A **(SLP)**
Golik, Maureen Anne
Grater, Mrs Melissa J **(SLP)**
Griffith, Dr Jerry **(SLP A)**
Griffith, Dr Twila E **(SLP)**
Guthrie, Mrs Lynda T **(SLP)**
Hagen-Pilkinton, Karol Lee **(SLP)**
Hake, Mrs Ann S **(SLP)**
Hamby, Dr Ellen I **(SLP)**
Hamilton, Joan M **(SLP)**
Harmon, Lynne F **(SLP)**
Horton, Ann M **(SLP)**
Howard, Ellen Duncan **(SLP)**
Hubbard, Charlotte A **(SLP)**
Hume, Dr Celia Bessel **(SLP)**
Hutchins, Robin P **(SLP)**
Jarvis, Hilary **(A)**
Jennings, Sara Easter **(A)**
Johnson, Carole Elizabeth
Karwowski, Mrs Lucianne Pitard **(SLP)**
Keever, Mrs Aelise H **(SLP)**
King, Deborah A **(SLP)**
Kirby, Wayne H **(A)**
Lawrence, Suzanne M **(SLP)**
Lednicky, Mrs Ann Blaize **(SLP)**
Letowski, Dr Tomasz R
Levy, David H **(A)**
Luper, Dr Harold L **(SLP A)**
Maisel, Clare G **(SLP)**
Marashi, Mrs Melinda O **(SLP)**
Marley-Leedom, Suzanne Marie
McCarver, Melodie Carol **(SLP)**
McDuffie, Mrs Andrea S **(SLP)**
McPherson, Betsy Nan **(SLP)**
Mingledorff, Tracy L
Moreland, Mrs Elizabeth Bondurant **(SLP)**
Nabelek, Dr Anna K
Nelson, Denise Smith **(A)**
Newman, Leslie Suzanne **(SLP)**
Norris, Mary Velvet **(SLP)**
Parsons, Mrs Joanna Dickerman **(SLP)**
Peterson, Dr Harold A **(SLP)**
Phelan-Latimer, Mrs Barbara K **(SLP)**
Pietrick, Julie A **(SLP)**
Pomy, Valerie A **(SLP)**
Pullen, Catherine N **(SLP)**
Ray, Joan P **(SLP)**
Robinson, Karen Lynn
Roettger, Ruby W **(A)**
Rook, Paul D **(A)**
Saffer, Mrs Eva Kinsey **(A)**
Scandlyn, Kay B **(A)**
Scantlin, Dorothy L **(SLP)**
Scariano, Mrs Rebecca Ratliffe **(SLP)**
Schohl, Mrs Betty Jane **(A)**
Sheffield, Leslie Elaine **(SLP)**
Silverstein, Dr Bernard **(SLP)**
Sinclair, Sally W **(SLP)**
Singletary, Mrs Theronne Burlison **(SLP)**
Smith, Mrs Linda T **(SLP)**
Smith, Mrs Maree Nipper **(SLP)**
Spann, E Daniel **(A)**
Stelling, Kelly Ann **(SLP)**
Stone, Sue Sherwood **(A)**
Tolliver, Janey K **(SLP)**
Tronolone, Veronica **(SLP)**
Tucker, Frances M **(SLP)**
Turnbull, Laura Hammond **(A)**
Vantrease, Mrs Carma Morrow **(SLP)**
Wallace, Susan Mervin **(SLP)**
Watkins, Richard B **(A)**
Weaver, Vickie Denise **(SLP)**
Webb, Patricia H **(SLP)**
Whaley, Celeste Patton **(SLP)**
Williams, Danna Duncan **(A)**
Wolfe, Gwendolyn Talley **(SLP)**
Womack, Mrs Bethel Hissom **(SLP)**
Woolley, Margaret L **(SLP)**
Wunschel, Karen L **(SLP)**

Lawrenceburg
Philpot, Mrs Terri Lynn Miller **(SLP)**

Lebanon
Geist, Virginia Sefton **(SLP)**
Lafevor, Mrs Julia S **(SLP)**
Osborn, Mrs Emma Lou **(SLP)**
Phillips, Dr Phyllis **(SLP)**

Lenoir City
Burk, Mrs Anita Manning **(SLP)**
Chandler, Mrs Jill Porter **(SLP)**
Williams, Mrs Harriet Lee

Loudon
Carrouth, Sharon Stamey **(A)**
Lamb, Leigh A **(A)**

Louisville
Millsaps, Mrs Deborah M **(SLP)**
Peterson, Mrs Mary McC **(SLP)**

Madison
Buell, Barbara Sutton **(SLP)**
Hoctor, Maria Noe **(SLP)**
Kaufman, Debra Watson **(SLP)**
Sims, Mrs Gretha Burch

Martin
Cates, Mrs Colleen F **(SLP)**
Damron-Belote, Mrs Dawne A
Murray, Dr Elaine C **(SLP)**

Maryville
Berry, John S
Collins, Mrs Deborah Taylor **(SLP)**
Dawson, Sue A **(A)**
Eby, Mrs Janice Read **(A)**
Lewis, Mary Grady **(SLP)**
Miller, Mrs Vickie Barnes **(A)**
Moffatt, Mrs Karen Baird **(SLP)**
Smuckler, Karen J **(A)**
Waters, Dr Jerry E **(A)**

McMinnville
Hutchins, Lisa Anne **(A)**
Smartt, Joan D **(SLP)**

Medina
Watt, Rhonda J **(SLP)**

Memphis
Acosta, Sharon Trimble **(SLP)**
Alexander, Genevieve C **(A)**
Alexander, Mrs Susan Killen **(SLP)**
Antwine, Brenda M **(SLP)**
Arnovitz, Mrs Laura Mazo **(A)**
Baggs, Terry W **(SLP)**
Barnes, Mrs Kandace Leigh
Batchelor, Mrs Valerie W **(A)**
Beasley, Dr Daniel S **(SLP)**
Boydston, Mrs Anne Elizabeth **(SLP)**
Brookshaw, Neddy R **(SLP)**
Brucks, Jane Ann **(A)**
Burgess, Mrs Bethany J **(A)**
Burroughs, Mrs Beverly W **(SLP)**
Busija, Nancy Barrett **(SLP)**
Caplan, Cheryl Lynn **(A)**
Carmichael, Mrs Virginia **(SLP)**
Chappell, Jennifer Leah
Chesser, Mrs Jody Edwards **(A)**
Connor, Lisa Rae
Cooke, Amy Lou **(SLP)**
Covington, Mrs Jan R **(SLP)**
Cox, Dr Robyn M **(A)**
Crawford, Margie Renee **(A)**
Crislip, Debra Ann **(SLP)**
Crook, Carol M **(SLP)**
Daniel, Margaret Ellen **(SLP)**
De Loach, Betty Ann **(A)**
Dillen, Sue Ann **(SLP)**
Dixon, Carolyn **(SLP)**
Domico, Elizabeth Hutcheson **(A)**
Domico, Dr William D **(A)**
Dubrowski, Richard Michael **(A)**
Dunham, Marilyn J **(SLP)**
Dunlap, Alice **(SLP)**
El-Oqlah, Mrs Sherri Michelle **(A)**
Everingham, Neil Mark **(A)**
Fancher-Cook, Debra **(SLP)**
Fleming, Susan Shaw **(SLP)**
Foster, Suzanne R **(SLP)**
Franks, Renaee **(A)**
Fraser, Malcolm H
Fulmer, Kathy C **(SLP)**
Gavrock, Robbie Angeline **(SLP)**
George, Catherine **(SLP)**
Gilbertson, Margie Lynn **(SLP)**
Gilmore, Christine Anne **(A)**
Gordon, Mrs Elaine K **(SLP)**
Gottlieb, Mrs Dvora Posner **(SLP)**
Gould, Dr Herbert J **(A)**
Green, Mrs Marva J **(A)**
Hackmeyer, Mrs Linda P **(SLP)**
Hall, Vickie L **(A)**
Harris, Deborah G **(SLP)**
Harris, Howard R **(A)**
Heffington, Mrs Mary F **(SLP)**
Henderson, Cathy **(SLP)**
Hentz, Kathryn Elizabeth **(SLP)**
Higginbotham, Peggy Virginia **(SLP)**
Hillard, Sallie Webber **(SLP)**
Hines, Janet Lynn **(SLP)**
Hinkle, Jo-Ann M **(SLP)**
Hinkle, Dr William G **(SLP)**
Hitt, Mrs Toni Leigh **(SLP)**
Holmes, Susan Laurie **(A)**
Hooker, Margaret A **(SLP)**
Hotchkiss, Marcia Wheat **(SLP)**
Howell, Mrs Nellie H **(SLP)**
Howse, Paula R **(SLP)**
Hudson, Karen Sue **(SLP)**
Hughey, Mrs Julianne C **(SLP)**
Hull, Virginia Anne **(A)**
Hustedde, Dr Carol G **(A)**
Isabell, Mrs Terry Lynn **(SLP)**
Isbell, Marie M **(SLP)**
Jeffries, Cheryl Anita **(SLP)**
Kahane, Dr Joel C **(SLP)**
Kamhi, Dr Alan G **(SLP)**
Kish, Edward L **(A)**
Kraft, Stephanie A
Lane, Allison Wilhite **(A)**
Lane, Audrey Lynn **(SLP)**
Larkin, Mrs Ann A **(A)**
Lazarov, Debbie Sue **(SLP)**
Lee, Dr Rene Friemoth **(SLP)**
Lester, Leatrice Burgess **(SLP)**
Lim, Kerk Chan **(A)**
Lopez, Mrs Amye Humphreys **(SLP)**
Madlock, Mrs Rosalind Dewitt **(SLP)**
Manning, Dr Walter Harne **(SLP)**
Manton, Judee Anne
Marsh, Susan A G **(A)**
Mayo, Dr Carolyn M **(SLP)**
Mayo, Robert **(SLP)**
McKinney, Beverly M **(SLP)**
McKown, Mary Frances **(A)**
McNamara, Jean **(SLP)**
McRae, Mrs Martha Polk **(SLP)**
Mendel, Dr Maurice I **(A)**
Miller, Susan L **(SLP)**
Mirro, Janice F **(SLP)**
Montgomery, Barbara S **(SLP)**
Moorhead, Mary Katherine
Nickey, Jeryl M **(SLP)**
Orchik, Dr Daniel J **(A)**
Orlikoff, Dr Robert F **(SLP)**
Page, Olga H **(A)**
Parker, Bobbie H **(SLP)**
Parr, Mrs Patricia Tipton **(SLP)**
Parsons, Sarah S **(SLP)**
Peaster, Mrs Monica Soldevila
Peck, Ronald F **(A)**
Perkins, Denice Jane **(SLP)**
Peterson, Lori Lee **(SLP)**
Phillips, Mrs Elizabeth Marie **(SLP)**
Pollack, Sharon R **(SLP)**
Presley, Emelia Elizabeth **(A)**
Price, Mrs Lee A **(SLP)**
Pusakulich, Kay M **(A)**
Quinter, Valerie Elise **(SLP)**
Rice, Mary W T **(SLP)**
Richardson, Carol M **(SLP)**
Rike, Mrs Ruth **(SLP A)**
Rivera, Izel Marice
Rocconi, Carol Ann **(SLP)**
Ryan, Lori F **(SLP)**
Sanders, Mrs Elizabeth G **(A)**
Sanders, Dr Sara B **(SLP)**
Shapiro, Nancy H **(A)**
Shea, Deborah Longaker **(A)**
Shea, Dr John J
Shelton, Maura Vaughn **(SLP)**
Sherbecoe, Robert L
Short, Cynthia Jo **(A)**
Simmons, Laura Vanita
Simpson, Mrs Mary E **(A)**
Skillion, Kim H **(SLP)**
Sowle, Karolyn Kay **(A)**
Starr, Deborah H **(A)**
Stone-Beasley, Stephanie **(SLP)**
Strange, Sheri Foshee **(SLP)**
Studebaker, Dr Gerald A
Swindell, Carol S **(SLP)**
Taylor, Rebecca Rae **(A)**
Thomas, Jane D **(SLP)**
Thompson, Carol A **(SLP)**
Tribble, Renee **(SLP)**
Tuck, Robin Elizabeth **(A)**
Usdan, Mrs Linda K **(SLP)**
Ward, Louise M **(SLP)**
Wark, Dr David J **(A)**
Wark, Nancy H **(SLP)**
Welch, Mrs Ann H **(SLP)**
White, Mrs Patricia Fincher **(SLP)**
Williams, Mrs Wanda S
Williamson, Mary **(SLP)**
Williamson-Jenkins, Mrs Susan D **(SLP)**
Willis, Yvonne Ingram **(SLP)**
Wine, Mrs Ann Dogan **(SLP)**
Young, Lisa J
Zapala, David A **(A)**

Michie
Fullwood, Mrs Joan Horner **(SLP)**

Milan
Greenhagen, Mrs Pamela **(SLP)**

Morristown
Knight, Mrs Judy W **(A)**
Self, Mrs Lana C C **(SLP)**
Shelton, Dr Doris H **(SLP)**

Mount Juliet
Enstrom, Mrs Janine C **(SLP)**
Harrell, Mrs Lisa Bailey **(SLP)**
Mitchell, Harold R **(SLP)**

Mitchell, Jacqueline **(SLP)**
Robinson, Martha P **(SLP)**

Mountain City
Lefler, Cynthia Ann **(SLP)**

Mountain Home
Turner, Charlcie H **(A)**

Murfreesboro
Arnold, David **(SLP)**
Arnold, Mrs Janice M **(SLP)**
Bratcher, Carole Ann **(SLP)**
Carroll, Charles Randall **(SLP)**
Clark, Dr Bertha Smith **(SLP)**
Daly, Bobbie D **(A)**
Hodge, Mrs Betty A **(SLP)**
Keenan, Dr Joseph S **(SLP)**
La Lance, Linda L **(SLP)**
Mathews, Mrs Bertha B **(SLP)**
Mehta, Annette M **(SLP)**
Seneker, Jeannie Lytton **(A)**
Stewman, W Denette Yarber **(SLP)**
Stockdell, Kenneth G **(A)**
Tuma, Mrs Aleta Dean **(A)**
Westfall, Mary F **(SLP)**

Nashville
Allen, Mrs Suzanne S **(SLP)**
Amberg, Susan Michele **(A)**
Bagli, Dr Zenobia R **(SLP A)**
Baldwin, Martha Lynne **(SLP)**
Barach, Mrs Carol M **(SLP)**
Berry, Bette J **(SLP A)**
Bess, Fred H **(A)**
Biberdorf, Vicki Lynn **(SLP)**
Blake, Patricia E **(A)**
Borchelt, Janet Katherine **(SLP)**
Bratt, Gene W **(A)**
Brewer, Mrs Debra Burnett **(A)**
Brown, Mrs Ginger Hargis **(SLP)**
Brown, Thomas Rodger **(A)**
Bueker, Susan Elizabeth **(SLP)**
Buen, Patricia Marie **(SLP)**
Casey, Patricia F **(SLP)**
Collignon, Margaret Melton **(SLP)**
Coscarelli-Buchanan, Janet E **(SLP A)**
Crandell, Carl C **(A)**
Curtis, Kim Ann **(SLP)**
Davis-Dansky, Mrs Ellen J **(SLP)**
Denton, Elizabeth Muddiman **(SLP)**
Dietrich, Joan M **(SLP)**
Dobey, Phyllis Schmidt **(SLP)**
Duhon, Helen Marie S **(SLP)**
Dunkerley, Mrs Nancy B **(SLP)**
Fainberg, Jolie Carin **(A)**
Farnsworth, Page J **(SLP)**
Fishbein, Mrs Gloria B **(SLP)**
Fitzgerald, Dr Mary T **(SLP A)**
Galloway, Mrs Sallye Martin **(SLP)**
Garrard, Dr Kay Russell **(SLP)**
Gibler, Anne M **(A)**
Gillis, Dr Rita J **(SLP)**
Glackman, Margaret E **(A)**
Gordon, Dr Gaile Andrea **(SLP)**
Griffith, Traci Marie **(SLP)**
Grimm, Mrs Jennifer Herbert **(SLP)**
Hall, Dr James W, III **(SLP A)**
Hausman, Charles H **(SLP)**
Heard, Mrs Sheila Trice
Helmers, Donna Lane **(SLP)**
Henry, Mrs Melissa Carender **(SLP)**
Henry, Melissa Morley **(A)**
Hoffman, Sara G **(SLP)**
Holzen, Mrs Helen K **(A)**
Jackson, Juaquita E **(SLP)**
Jennings, Karen Sue **(SLP)**
Jones, Merrily M **(SLP)**
Josey, Anne F **(A)**
Kennedy, Mrs Patricia P **(SLP)**
Kiefer, Mrs Marlene **(SLP)**
Killyon, Mrs Jeanine L **(SLP)**
Kirshner, Mrs Sheri Weiner **(A)**
Klee, Dr Thomas M
Knight, Jane Sanders **(SLP)**
Koury, Laurie Nash **(SLP)**
Lackey, Mrs Cathy Lynn **(SLP)**
Langston, Mrs Patricia S **(SLP)**
Large, Julie Gwynne **(SLP)**
Lazenby, Mrs Blake B **(A)**
Leftwich, Emily G **(SLP)**
Lewis, Mrs Virginia Morgan **(A)**
Lillie, Sue M **(A)**
Logan, Susan A **(A)**
Love, Dr Russell J **(SLP)**
Lumm, Mrs Crystal Wells **(SLP)**
Lynch, Martha E **(SLP)**
Macon, Cynthia Rutherford **(SLP)**
Mahn, Kathleen E **(SLP)**
Martin, Martha A **(SLP)**
Martin, Michael E **(A)**
Marx, Joann K **(SLP)**
Mattingly, Dr Susan C **(SLP A)**
Mays, Cheryl Ann **(A)**
McConnell, Prof Freeman E **(A)**
McQuain, Johnny D **(SLP)**
Medanich, Melanie **(SLP)**
Moore, Mrs Dawn Marie **(SLP)**
Morgan, Mrs Janet **(SLP)**
Ochs, Dr Marleen G **(A)**
Ohde, Ralph N **(SLP)**
Parham, Dr Janet S **(SLP)**
Parker, J Whitney
Payne, Mrs Virginia Mason **(SLP)**
Peek, Barbara F **(A)**
Powers, Vicki Stafford **(A)**
Prentice, Charlotte Henninger **(A)**
Preston, Donna M **(SLP)**
Rainey, Cheryl Lee
Rhoads, Mrs Marjorie J **(SLP)**
Richardson, Penny Wan **(A)**
Roberts, Valeria A **(A)**
Ruth, Kelley Grace **(SLP)**
Sacks, Mrs Jo-Anne
Sammeth, Dr Carol Anne **(A)**
Sanders, Jay W **(SLP A)**
Schaffer, Mary Ann **(SLP)**
Schwaber, Donna K G **(A)**
Sewell, Dr John C **(SLP)**
Siroky, Denise M
Sitton, Mrs Ann Bradshaw **(A)**
Smith, Mrs Enid Dianne **(A)**
Soucaze, Carole E **(SLP)**
Srinivasan, Mrs Pratibha **(A)**
Stevens, Karen C **(SLP)**
Stillman, Judy L **(SLP)**
Stone, Dr Robert E, Jr **(SLP)**
Sweat, Linda Logan **(SLP)**
Tharpe, Anne M **(A)**
Thompson, Angela M S **(A)**
Tudor, Patricia Lynn **(SLP)**
Warren, Dr Steven Forest
Whitfield, Jennifer B **(SLP)**
Wilson, Deborah Suzanne **(A)**
Woloshen, D **(SLP)**
Yoder, Dr Paul Jorden

New Tazewell
Stanifer, Mrs Jan Weller **(SLP)**

Nolensville
Goodman, Mrs Elizabeth Baskervill **(SLP)**

Norris
Weaver, Amanda S **(SLP)**

Oak Ridge
Blakeman, Anita Dela Garza **(SLP)**
Burkett, Sidney Wright **(SLP)**
Cates, Linda Lee **(SLP)**
Griffin, Elizabeth Barnes **(SLP)**
Hulsey, Carol J **(SLP)**
Keyser, Mrs Nancy S **(SLP)**
Larcher, Elaine W **(SLP)**
Lewis, Mrs Marti C **(SLP)**
Meyer, Beth D **(SLP)**

Old Hickory
Marshall, Mrs Jean M **(SLP)**
Whitefield, Mrs Sylvia H **(SLP)**

Ooltewah
Cates, Ronald T **(A)**
Overmyer, Mrs Claire Lee **(SLP)**
Sajwaj, Mrs Eva M **(SLP)**

Paris
French, Mrs Judy Louise **(SLP)**

Pigeon Forge
Walker, Karen Woodford **(SLP)**

Powell
Hedrick, Mrs Tracy L

Puryear
Veazey, Deborah Paschall **(SLP)**

Ripley
Morris, Mrs Marion G **(SLP)**

Rockford
Byrd, William H, Jr **(A)**
Moore, Robert E **(A)**

Sevierville
Harper, Mrs Elaine D **(SLP)**
Henry, Andrell W **(SLP A)**
Owens, Mrs Alana Howard **(SLP)**

Seymour
Moser, Mrs Claire Blackwell

Shelbyville
Alexander, C Joy **(SLP)**

Signal Mountain
Griffin, Sarah H **(SLP)**
Jonakin, Mrs Karen Benfield **(SLP)**
Peacock, Elizabeth **(SLP)**
Thomas, Mrs Cynthia Stager **(SLP)**
Weishan, Mrs Deborah A **(A)**

Smithville
Williams, Louise Ann **(SLP)**

Somerville
Shelton, Dale Sandusky **(SLP)**

South Pittsburg
Adcock, Ava L **(SLP)**
Matthews, Debbie S **(SLP)**

Sparta
Haston, Judy D
Kay, Mrs Pamela M **(SLP)**
Pearson, Margaret D

Springfield
Gunn, Mrs Melanie W **(SLP)**
White, Vivian Dianne **(SLP)**

Sweetwater
Dycus, Mrs Sarah Archer **(SLP)**

Thompson Station
Miller, Stacy Lee **(SLP)**

Tullahoma
Mitchell, Mrs Louann S **(SLP)**
Waldrop, Teresa Anne **(SLP)**

Whites Creek
Shanks, Mrs Paulette Willie **(SLP)**

TEXAS

Abilene
Ashby, Dr Jon K **(SLP A)**
Atchison, Susan L **(A)**
Austin, Mrs Lynette Blackburn **(SLP)**
Balanay, Mrs Cheryl A **(SLP)**
Bilberry, Tina M **(SLP)**
Boeshart, Linda R **(SLP)**
Breeding, Malesa Smith **(SLP)**
Calderon-Rogers, Mrs Esperanza G **(SLP)**
Craig, Leslie D
Daniels, Mrs Kay Ileene **(SLP)**
Dowdy, Lissa Karen **(A)**
Feemster, Ben David **(SLP)**
Forbis-Stokes, Nancy K **(A)**
Gray, Mrs Louise K **(SLP)**
Grigg, Mrs Ann Marie
Grosvenor, Mrs Terry M **(SLP)**
Haire, Dr Carol D **(SLP)**
Harlow, Mrs Kathie **(SLP)**
Harvey, Patricia Lynn **(A)**
Hatherill, Betsy Weese **(A)**
Hatherill, Dennis L **(A)**
Holland, Jay W **(A)**
Holland, Sue Ann **(A)**
Howard, Dr Karen J **(SLP)**
Jameson, Dean G **(SLP)**
Jones, Mrs Barbara Plunkert **(SLP)**
Killorin, Victoria Stewart **(SLP)**
Kirby, D'Lyla A **(SLP)**
McBride, Martha Louise **(SLP)**
Moore, Anne White **(A)**
Pierson, Sandra Kay **(SLP)**
Price, L Denise D **(A)**
Reece, Teryl Lyn **(SLP)**
Riley, Mrs Karen L **(SLP)**
Schulze, Mrs P Marilyn **(SLP)**
Simek, Marlene Theresa **(A)**
Stephens, Mrs Constance Fiero **(A)**
Stevens, Debralea **(SLP)**
Walker, Mrs Connie K **(SLP)**

Allen
Rice, Vickie Diann **(A)**
Swanson, Mrs Tracy L A **(A)**

Alpine
Hendryx, Mrs Rebecca L **(SLP)**

Alvin
Beardsley, Amy Neel **(SLP)**
Bennett, Barbara E **(SLP)**
Dewitt, Mrs Mary Catherine **(SLP)**
Lachowsky, Mrs Pamela Smith **(SLP)**
Meeks, Peggy N **(SLP)**
Wiesenborn, Mrs Gloria K **(SLP)**

Amarillo
Appleby, Annette **(SLP)**
Barrick, Mrs Marcia Lee **(SLP)**
Besly, Mrs Nancy S **(SLP)**
Boutte, Donna Maria
Brotherton, Gary James
Clark, Jenny Sue **(SLP)**
Clifton, Noel F **(SLP)**
Day, L Karen Carter **(SLP)**
Fleming, Margaret A **(SLP)**
Green, Martha Hazelwood **(SLP)**
Hans, Mrs Patricia G **(A)**
Henry, Mrs Betsy W **(SLP)**
Johnson, Maurita G **(SLP)**
Laccinole, Dr Michael D **(SLP)**
Mason, LaRita **(SLP)**
McMurry, Mrs Claudia **(SLP)**
Moseley, Mrs Donna J **(SLP)**
Ormson, Kerry D **(A)**
Schiebel-Knox, Mrs Cynthia Diane **(SLP)**
Scholl, Mrs Kay L **(SLP)**
Soper, Mrs Heather L **(SLP)**
Thomasson, Jana R'Dean
Tipton, Carol B **(SLP)**
Williams, Jerry O **(SLP)**
Williams, Susan G **(SLP)**

Andrews
Barnett, Mrs Denise Derrick **(SLP)**

Angleton
Ratcliff, Mrs Brenda S **(SLP)**
Seay, Lela Jane **(SLP)**

Argyle
Green, Mrs Joy R **(SLP)**

Arlington
Anderson, Janet E **(SLP)**
Bach, Nancy H **(A)**
Baker, Mrs Beverly H **(SLP)**

Barrera, Deborah E **(SLP)**
Barth, Susan L **(A)**
Bennett, Linda A **(SLP)**
Burkink, Denise Wyman **(SLP)**
Busse, Lu Ann **(A)**
Butler, Mrs Lynne L **(SLP A)**
Colby, Susan L **(SLP)**
Cole, Pamela J **(SLP)**
Combs, Mrs Judith A **(SLP)**
Combs, Raymond B **(A)**
Cortinas, Rochelle M **(SLP)**
Donnelly, Karen L **(A)**
Durand, Elizabeth **(SLP)**
Elston, Mrs Krista Kile **(SLP)**
Eng, Mrs Pearl Q **(SLP)**
Foley, Maureen F **(SLP)**
Fox, Carolyn E **(SLP)**
Gapa, Rhea M Greer **(SLP)**
Garner, Patricia N **(SLP)**
Grabow, Mrs Suzan K **(A)**
Guy, Christine **(SLP)**
Harris, Sheryl L **(SLP)**
Hembree, Mrs Margaret E **(SLP)**
Hildner, Cynthia **(SLP)**
Hopkins, Mrs Diana W **(SLP)**
Humphreys, Paula Louise **(A)**
Hutchings, Mrs Teresa C **(SLP)**
Inman, Nancy L **(SLP)**
Johnson, Mrs Elizabeth Ann **(A)**
Johnson, Richard M **(SLP)**
Keaton, Mrs Larue M **(SLP)**
Kos, Susanne **(A)**
Krueger, Kathy Ann **(SLP)**
Loudamy, Mrs Shelly Renea **(SLP)**
Ludwig, Lynne Marie
Lukach, Sharon D **(A)**
Lynch, Laurel Rebecca **(SLP)**
Lyons, Mrs Denise E **(SLP)**
McCown, Mrs Donna E **(SLP)**
McGovern, Mrs Ella Jo C **(SLP)**
McNairn, Mrs Peggi H **(SLP)**
Nash, Mrs Janice P **(SLP)**
Pitt, Laurel Ann H **(SLP)**
Ragland, Pamela D **(SLP)**
Ratcliff, Mrs Alice **(SLP)**
Reyes, Mrs Belinda Alvarado **(SLP)**
Ritchey, Gilbert G **(A)**
Seher, Donald Matthew **(SLP)**
Shelby, Mrs Tracie Lathram **(SLP)**
Snyder, Mrs Laura Ann **(SLP)**
Spalding, Kathleen J **(SLP A)**
Spurgin, Tracy Gail
Sullivan, Marybeth Bothmann **(SLP)**
Taylor, Dr Kenya S **(SLP A)**
Trevino, Mrs Carmen Hernandez **(SLP)**
Ward, Dianne Gottlieb **(SLP)**
Wiig, Dr Elisabeth H **(SLP A)**
Willingham, Christina Maria **(SLP)**
Woolet, Deborah J **(SLP)**
Wright, Cherry **(SLP)**
Wright, Cynthia L **(SLP)**

Aubrey

Watson, Mrs Margaret Anne **(SLP)**

Austin

Abrahamson, Judy E **(A)**
Abu-Rayyan, Mrs Rebecca G **(SLP)**
Acevedo, Mary Ann **(SLP)**
Allen, Mrs Karen L **(SLP)**
Anderson, Anita J **(A)**
Andregg, Mrs Karen Jan **(A)**
Ashmore, Lear Lee **(SLP)**
Baden, Nancy A **(SLP)**
Bader, Virginia T **(SLP)**
Baker, Nora Mandell **(SLP A)**
Balash, Joan M **(A)**
Barber, Mrs Aleisa Dolloph **(SLP)**
Barnhart, Laura Drewyer **(SLP)**
Beck, Sydney Leighann **(SLP)**
Benners, Ann Ownby **(SLP)**
Berg, Mrs Cecilia A **(SLP)**
Bernhard, Beth A **(SLP)**
Bielitz, Roberta Ann **(SLP)**
Bigham, Caryl L **(A)**
Bingham, Pam **(SLP)**
Bolin, Theresa Richburg **(SLP)**
Brock, Miriam B **(SLP)**
Brooks, Mrs Alta Fann **(SLP)**
Bryant, Marcella Lynn **(SLP)**
Bush, Nancy Marguerite **(SLP)**
Cannito, Dr Michael P **(SLP)**
Carlin, Dr T Walter **(SLP A)**
Carter, Dr C Dwayne **(SLP A)**
Chaligne, Mrs Carol Grimes **(SLP)**
Champlin, Dr Craig A **(A)**
Cherry, Ellen Lee **(SLP)**
Chodorow, Mrs Rowena B **(SLP)**
Cole, Mary H **(SLP)**
Cole, Dr Patricia R **(SLP)**
Cromwell, Mrs McCraw Duncan **(SLP)**
Cutrer, Mrs Cathryn Sue **(SLP)**
Danley, Mrs Judy Harris **(SLP)**
Davis, Barbara L **(SLP)**
Davis, Kimberly M **(SLP)**
Dibrell, Jayne W **(SLP)**
Dickenson, Priscilla **(SLP)**
Dieball, Linda Kaye S **(SLP)**
Dodson, Susan L **(SLP)**
Doering, Rebecca Elaine
Doss, Sharon L **(SLP)**
Drake, Barbara N **(SLP)**
Dunn, Carla **(SLP)**
England, Mrs Carol J **(SLP)**
English, Linda Hammons **(SLP)**
Famiglietti, Lisa **(SLP A)**
Fletcher, Mrs Brenda G **(SLP)**
Flowers, Mrs Marian H **(SLP)**
Foster, Mrs Leah L **(SLP)**
Frost, Darcy K **(SLP)**
Fulton, Mrs Patricia H **(SLP)**
Gardner, Elizabeth Shepherd **(SLP)**
Gershbein, Holly Jane **(SLP)**
Givens, Alan D **(SLP A)**
Granof, Dr Dena H **(SLP)**
Griffith, Mrs Carol Rose **(SLP)**
Groesbeck, Billie J **(SLP A)**
Grote, Barbara Gibbs **(SLP)**
Guerrero, Oralia Ochoa **(SLP)**
Hagood, Linda Wardell **(SLP)**
Halfin, Kimberly Kay
Hamm, Mrs Donna Koho **(SLP)**
Handkins, Jill E **(SLP)**
Hanson, Grace Haen **(SLP A)**
Harren, Mrs Tami Watson **(SLP)**
Harris, Daniel Preston **(SLP A)**
Hatch, Sandra K **(SLP)**
Hawkins, Renae LaJean **(SLP)**
Hays, Dr C Lynne **(SLP)**
Hill, Carol F **(SLP)**
Hiller, Jay Felice **(SLP)**
Hillis, Ann M **(SLP)**
Howell, Jenell L **(SLP)**
Hwang, Dora K **(SLP)**
Jasuta, Stephanie **(SLP)**
Jones, Kathryn S **(A)**
Jorgensen, Carol A B **(SLP)**
Kaufman, Mrs Jennifer R **(A)**
Keesee, Mrs Linda Lee **(SLP)**
Kent, Mrs Ann Kaiser **(SLP)**
Killion, Duree Gail **(SLP)**
Kirk, Joni Rogers **(SLP)**
Knolle, Janie H **(SLP)**
Kopra, Dr Lennart L **(A)**
Krautter, Mary E **(SLP)**
Kuemmel, Robbie E **(SLP)**
Kuta, Joan E **(SLP)**
Lane, Mrs Carol Ann **(SLP)**
Larson, D Jayne **(SLP)**
Lawson, Mrs Donna H **(SLP)**
Leatherwood, Elaine M **(A)**
Leavitt, Ron J **(A)**
Leech, Melissa Frances **(SLP)**
Lenich, Jennifer Komnick **(A)**
Lindamood, Linda Phelps **(SLP)**
Lingo, Mida Evans **(SLP)**
Loera, Barbara G **(SLP)**
Magnera, Dr Georgia Elizabeth **(SLP)**
Markley, Mary F **(SLP)**
Marks, Sheila Gay **(SLP)**
Marquardt, Dr Thomas P **(SLP)**
Martin, Dr Frederick N **(SLP A)**
Martin, Linda D Marquez **(SLP)**
Mata-Pistokache, Mrs Teri **(SLP)**
Mauzy, Mrs Anne **(A)**
Maxwell, Mrs Barbara Hafner **(SLP)**
May, Mona M **(SLP)**
May, Samye Louise **(A)**
McBride, Debra L **(SLP)**
McBroom, Gail B **(SLP)**
McCaffrey, Helen A **(A)**
McFadden, Dr Dennis
McGlothlin, Martha **(SLP)**
McKinney, Susan Aiken **(SLP)**
McNeill, Mrs Donna M D **(SLP)**
Medford, Cydney M **(SLP)**
Menlo, Louise **(SLP)**
Miller, Jean Ellen **(SLP)**
Miller, Mrs Julie L **(SLP)**
Miller, Dr M Lynda **(SLP)**
Milstead, Kim F **(SLP)**
Minton, Denise Casimir **(SLP)**
Minyard, Lisa A **(SLP)**
Miskin, Kathryn Ann **(SLP)**
Mixon, Mrs Carolyn Johnson **(SLP)**
Montgomery, Lillian L **(SLP)**
Moore, Pamela Gale **(SLP)**
Morgan, Nancy Patton **(SLP)**
Neeb, Mrs Amy Warden
Nericcio, Mary Anne **(SLP)**
Nevitt, Amanda L **(A)**
Nevlud, Gail New **(SLP)**
Newton, Dr Lauren **(SLP A)**
Nicols, Joseph C, Jr **(SLP)**
Noble, Bart E **(A)**
Ornelas, Myrna Joy **(SLP)**
Parks, Mrs Janet Elizabeth **(SLP)**
Petit, Marcia Yvette
Pickett, Trenna Jo **(SLP)**
Pittman, Mrs Angela Sadler **(SLP)**
Plasterer, Lisa Rose **(SLP)**
Pokorny, Ellen Brooke **(SLP)**
Powers, Dr Gene R **(SLP)**
Qualls, Tamara Jo **(SLP)**
Radcliffe, Wendy E **(SLP)**
Rasmussen, Rosalie P **(SLP)**
Reinhart, Janet B **(SLP)**
Rhyner-Saulnier, Mary **(SLP)**
Richardson, Dr Alice P **(SLP)**
Robinson, Linda Louise **(SLP)**
Robinson, Mrs Sylvia L **(A)**
Robinson, Thomas W **(SLP)**
Rodriquez, Sara R **(SLP)**
Rogers, Mrs Marilyn B
Rollman, Mrs Cynthia R **(SLP)**
Sanchez, Rachel Lara **(SLP)**
Sargent, Barbara J **(SLP)**
Scherich, Dayl L **(A)**
Schlabach, Sheryl L **(SLP)**
Schumann, Mrs Nancy **(SLP)**
Shaffer, Norma L W **(SLP)**
Sheridan, Anne P **(SLP)**
Sherman, Mrs Saundy C **(SLP)**
Sinast-House, Linda **(SLP)**
Sitzer, Nancy Jane **(SLP)**
Slack, Kay E **(SLP)**
Smith, Mischa Jerine **(SLP)**
Snowden, Patricia H **(SLP A)**
Stahl, Valerie J **(SLP)**
Stinson, Mrs Sylvia Salinas
Stiritz, Lori L **(A)**
Strane, Kim K **(A)**
Stuart, Mrs Loraine G **(SLP A)**
Taipale, Mrs Cynthia Jean **(SLP)**
Tarver, Margaret Miller **(SLP)**
Thibodeau, Mrs Linda Mesloh **(SLP A)**
Thomas, Ann Christine **(SLP)**
Thomas, Mrs Corinne Adele **(SLP)**
Townsend, Mrs Lorrie Blackmon **(SLP)**
Tucker, Mrs Alison Marsh **(SLP)**
Van Kleeck, Dr Anne E **(SLP)**
Villarreal, Jesse J **(SLP)**
Voiers, William D
Walker, Jena W **(SLP)**
Walker, Mrs Pamela Hoover **(SLP)**
Walls, Mrs Brenda K **(SLP)**
Walsh, Cindy Therese **(SLP)**
Waterbury, Olga A **(SLP A)**
Watkins, Christine L **(SLP)**
Watson, Kay E P **(SLP)**
Weber, Mrs Susan Stuckey **(SLP)**
Winkler, Lisa Ellen **(SLP)**
Wood, Dr Mary Lovey **(SLP)**
Woodfin, Shelia T **(SLP)**
Worob, Mrs Phyllis Sacks **(A)**
Wright, Karen A P **(A)**
Wristen, Mrs Martha A **(SLP)**
Zeagler, Mrs Clare Wells **(SLP)**

Azle

Sinclair, Mrs Nancy P **(SLP)**

Barker

Eastham, Mrs Penelope L **(SLP)**

Bay City

Christie, M Michele **(SLP)**
Cumbie, Mrs Janet **(SLP)**
Woods, Carrie Lynn **(SLP)**

Baytown

Butts, Mrs Sandra Dysart **(SLP)**
Carlson, Elizabeth Cranford **(SLP)**
Morton, Natalie L

Beaumont

Achilles, Dr Robert F **(SLP)**
Broussard, Mrs MaryJo L **(SLP)**
Clem, Roger Fair **(A)**
Colgan, Mrs Ellen H **(SLP)**
Cooley, Debra Ann **(A)**
Corrigan, Gayle **(SLP)**
Cowgill, Mrs Susan P **(A)**
Darling, Mrs Christine Petkovsek **(SLP)**
Dawson, Deborah Ann **(SLP)**
Dye, Crisann Louise
Espinosa, Melanie K **(SLP)**
Firestone, Mrs Sharon P **(SLP)**
Gowling, Mrs Jimmye L **(SLP)**
Granitz, Dr David W **(SLP A)**
Gunnarson, Dr Adele Delaine **(A)**
Hillin, Celeste S **(A)**
Hyman, Susan M **(A)**
King, Emily M **(SLP)**
Laurent, Jan Claire **(SLP)**
Lavergne, Mrs Angela Marie **(SLP)**
McGarry, Jane Elizabeth **(SLP)**
Middleton, Mrs Suzanne S **(SLP)**
Moulton, Dr Robert D **(SLP)**
Netterville, Nancy L S **(SLP)**
Olds, Robert E, Jr **(SLP)**
Patterson, Mrs Julie S **(SLP)**
Pederson, Dr Olen T **(SLP A)**
Peiler, Mrs Suzanne Giglio **(A)**
Phelan, Mrs Elizabeth L **(SLP)**
Phelan, James G **(A)**
Phelan, Mark Dufner
Ryall, Judy Lynn
Sarradet, Valerie K **(A)**
Tunteri, Diane Shaffer **(A)**
Wilson, Dr Howard Franklin **(SLP)**

Bedford

Beall, Mrs Shelley Campbell **(SLP)**
Carswell, Mrs Jill B **(SLP)**
Clarkson, Sandra Lynne **(A)**
Dilleshaw, Susan L **(SLP)**
Eastin, Janet S **(SLP)**
Griffin, Mrs Melinda P **(SLP A)**
Haxel, Susan Sjoberg **(SLP)**
Long, Mrs Cathy Brown
Morgan, Jeffrey Lynn **(A)**

Morlier, Mrs Robin Eiserloh **(SLP)**
Noah, Mrs Deborah S **(SLP)**
Parks, Mrs Susan W **(SLP)**
Petric, Roberta Lands **(SLP)**
Sanders, Ann C **(SLP)**
Schneider, Mrs Paula **(SLP)**
Sharp, Mrs Patricia Stone **(SLP)**
Suggs, Laura G **(SLP)**
Underwood, Mrs Debra Drumwright **(SLP)**
Zukoff, Pricilla J **(SLP)**

Beeville
Estrada, Mrs Sylvia A **(SLP)**
Green, Mrs Aleene McKinney **(SLP)**

Bellaire
Jacobus, Mrs Heather J **(SLP)**
Kelty, Mrs Kimberly Renee **(SLP)**
Robert, Mrs Margaret Thompson **(SLP)**
Tuller, Karen Burke **(SLP)**

Bellevue
Zarate, Nora **(SLP)**

Belton
Reed, Mrs Gayle Lynette **(SLP)**
Togami, Joan Allbright **(SLP)**

Benbrook
West, Gayla Beth

Big Foot
Johnson, Georgia S **(SLP)**

Boerne
Lockart-Neilon, Ina Jeane **(A)**
Settle-Strain, Lisa Ann **(SLP)**

Booker
Clark, Lois Diane **(SLP)**

Brenham
Hoffmann, Roland Jules, III **(SLP)**
Kulcak-Studer, Mrs Bridget **(SLP)**
Lather, James E **(SLP)**
Milenki, Kathy Helen **(SLP)**
Nuffer, Mrs Patricia **(SLP)**
Shoup, Nancy L **(SLP)**
Stein, Kristi Lynn **(SLP)**
Stom, Mrs Sylvia Thompson **(A)**
Williams, Mrs Marilyn G **(SLP)**

Brooks AFB
Schleifer, John Gary **(A)**

Brownfield
Zeltmann, Mrs Frances Kay **(SLP)**

Brownsville
Carolan, Mrs Louise W **(SLP)**
Dunne, Mrs Sally A **(SLP)**
Hallock, Keith R **(SLP)**
Polston, Mrs Paula Denise **(SLP)**
Ruiz, Willie **(A)**
Sears-Bode, Deborah **(SLP)**
Van Coppenolle, Mrs Sylvia S **(SLP)**

Brownwood
Butler, Charles Eugene **(A)**
Graves, Martha Taylor **(SLP)**

Bruceville
Rainer, Mrs Deborah F **(SLP)**

Bryan
Bassham, Mrs Geanifer Jo **(SLP)**
Foster, Dr Jean Rizzo **(SLP)**
Goodwin, Patricia B **(SLP)**
Hendrick, Lynn S **(SLP)**
Jones, Mary Elizabeth **(SLP)**
Thrash, Mrs Paula Genice **(SLP)**
Wade, Mrs Cami Lynn **(A)**

Buda
Brown, Gale M **(SLP)**
O'Neal, Joy P **(A)**
Respess, Joyce Ann **(SLP)**
Sowell, Michele McCord **(SLP)**

Bulverde
Cooper, J C, Jr **(A)**
Green, Marilyn S **(SLP)**

Burleson
Boyd, Mrs Jacqueline Compere **(SLP)**
Brashier, Ronda E
White, Mrs Elizabeth Jo **(A)**

Caldwell
Chapman, Ann Yager **(SLP)**

Canadian
Eubank, Andrew B **(SLP)**

Canton
Lambert, Mrs Nancy N **(SLP)**

Canyon Lake
Ellis, Mrs Felinda Trolinder **(SLP)**

Carrollton
Acord, Mrs Tera S **(SLP)**
Anderson, M Lynn **(SLP)**
Bosler, Michelle **(SLP)**
Boyd, Mrs Pamela Dianne W **(SLP)**
Brand, Mrs Bobbye Rennae **(A)**
Brown, Jan Rutledge **(A)**
Bryant, Mrs Patricia A **(SLP)**
Cartrite, Celesta F
Cawyer, Mrs S Annette Schaffner **(SLP)**
Decker, Margaret L **(SLP)**
Freed, Marilyn Shosid **(SLP)**
Kaplan, Karen E **(SLP)**
Lauffenburger, Angela T
Lougeay-Mottinger, Janice W **(SLP)**
Marguglio, Gloriann **(SLP)**
Massey, Mrs Michele Miller **(SLP)**
Matthews, Cheryl L T **(SLP)**
Murph, Jane Vallery **(SLP)**
Ohler, Elizabeth D **(SLP)**
Pennington, Mrs Dixie Freydberg **(SLP)**
Perotti, Diane Marie **(SLP)**
Pullin, Cheryl Ann **(SLP)**
Robenalt, Kathleen S **(SLP)**
Smith, Eloise K **(SLP)**
Welch, Carolyn Louise **(SLP)**
Witt, Mrs Holly Burrell **(SLP)**

Carthage
Kyle, Mildred W **(SLP)**
Martin, Sherry Ann **(SLP)**
Parker, Mrs Jeanette Luce
Vincent, Mrs Carol A **(SLP)**

Castroville
Stinson, Mrs Suzanne B **(SLP)**

Caty
Taylor, Mrs Nancy Jane **(SLP)**

Cedar Creek
Stiles, 524595 C **(SLP)**

Cedar Hill
Vosel, Sherrie Ruth **(A)**

Cedar Park
Burda, Pamela Kay **(A)**
Dolan, Jean Theresa **(SLP)**
Haskins-Kobelan, Mrs Christi Lynn **(SLP)**

Channelview
Keith, Odilia F **(SLP)**
Law, Gail E **(A)**

Chicota
Burk, Mrs Sherri Nell **(SLP)**

Childress
Driver, Althea Allison **(SLP)**
Reeves, Mrs Charlene Baird

Cibolo
Vaughn, Denise Lynn

College Station
Deuermeyer, Mrs Sally P **(SLP)**
Dragga, Linda C **(SLP)**
Fischbuch, Tracy Stanford **(SLP)**
Martinez, Mrs Cynthia Rose **(SLP)**
Riess, Richard L **(A)**
Smith, Mrs Patricia R **(SLP)**
Springer, Anita S **(A)**
Street, Mrs Nancy Anne **(SLP)**
Williams, Mrs Susan M **(SLP)**

Colleyville
Cheek, Linda T **(SLP)**
Harrington, Suzanne M **(SLP)**
Van Natta, Mrs Madeleine Aura Beth **(SLP)**
Vowell, Mrs Mary B **(SLP)**

Colorado City
Nation, Alta G **(SLP)**

Columbus
Johnson, Mrs Virginia C **(SLP)**

Comfort
Crutchfield, Dr Verna Mae **(SLP)**

Commerce
Brister, Dr Frank Lutz, Jr **(A)**
Mills, Mrs Anne E **(SLP)**
Morgan, Mrs Kathleen I **(SLP)**
Sanders, Mrs Kathryn L **(SLP)**

Conroe
Anderson, Mrs Debra P **(SLP)**
Booth, Janette A **(SLP)**
Davis, Mrs Dianne S **(SLP)**
Gereke, Mrs Helene D **(SLP)**
Jennings, Mrs Joan Bormann **(SLP)**
Merritt, Mrs Sharon **(SLP)**
Raica, Anthony N **(A)**
Robison, Connie June **(SLP)**
Schulze, Barbara Gay **(A)**
Tayrien, Mrs Lucille E **(SLP)**

Converse
Davenport, Beverly W **(SLP)**
Kirkpatrick, Tara L **(SLP)**
Stanush, Mrs Priscilla Diane **(SLP)**
Tom, Mrs Rosemarie N **(SLP)**

Copeville
Marder, Linda J

Coppell
Arras, Mrs Patricia Gail **(A)**
Corbeil, Mary Kay **(SLP)**
Pegram, Tamara V **(SLP)**
Rainbolt, Mrs Rebecca M **(SLP)**
Vestri, Jean Barnhart **(SLP)**

Corpus Christi
Corrigan, Mrs Judy A **(A)**
Dietert-Carnes, Denise **(SLP)**
Foster, Isabelle F **(SLP)**
Garza, Mrs Frances F **(SLP)**
Gonzalez, Mrs Odette **(SLP)**
Harris, Barbara E **(SLP)**
Higdon, Lawrence W **(A)**
Hodges, Monette Gregory **(SLP)**
Kent-Udolf, Dr Louise **(SLP)**
Kurz, Olivia Dee **(SLP)**
Magiera, Nancy Snidow **(A)**
O'Hearn, Karen L **(SLP)**
Osterloh, Patricia O'Neal **(SLP)**
Reyna, Gaila Denise **(SLP)**
Rivera, Brenda **(SLP)**
Schroeder, Elaine **(SLP)**
Schumann, Gretchen Rosemond **(SLP)**
Seitz, Jay D **(SLP)**
Sherman, Susan L **(SLP)**
Skarphol, Katherine Rae **(SLP)**
Smith, Mrs Pamela Kennette **(SLP)**
Vara, Mrs Eileen A W **(SLP)**
Voges, Kathryn Biles **(A)**
Waltrip, Susan Grose **(A)**
West, Vicky Nowell **(SLP)**
Woodman, Patricia Anne **(SLP)**
Young, Sandra **(SLP)**

Corsicana
Means, Mrs Pamela Ingram **(SLP)**

Crockett
Kelly, Mrs Deborah R **(SLP)**

Crosby
Joseph, Rosanne Miller **(SLP)**

Crowley
Roupe, Mrs Karla Kay Koch **(SLP)**

Cypress
Gordon, Donna Barclay **(SLP)**

Dallas
Aaron, Mrs Marilyn B **(SLP)**
Abraham, Mrs Sheradine **(SLP)**
Adriance, Carolyn Ruth **(SLP)**
Andrews, Carol L **(SLP)**
Apple, Mrs Jill Elizabeth
Apt, Mrs Norma Abramson **(SLP)**
Arista, Yolanda **(SLP)**
Arnold, Mary Beth Shick **(SLP)**
Askew, Benna L **(SLP)**
Atkinson, Mrs Karen Staicer **(SLP)**
Balay, Catherine Nolan **(SLP)**
Banker, Mrs Melinda Sanders **(SLP)**
Barnum, Rebecca A **(SLP)**
Barrow, Mrs Kathy Glass **(SLP)**
Beaubien, Marilyn R **(A)**
Bernstein, Mrs Phyllis F **(A)**
Bird, Allan K **(SLP)**
Bond, Mrs Suzanne B **(SLP)**
Booth, Frank D **(A)**
Booth, Patricia S **(A)**
Briscoe, Mrs Valerie C **(SLP)**
Brown, Mrs Karen Clinton **(A)**
Brusniak, Mrs Rosario R **(SLP)**
Bryant, Dr Lynda C **(SLP A)**
Burgdorf, Sherrill Arlene **(SLP)**
Burtis, Marguerite **(SLP)**
Burtis, Mary I **(SLP)**
Bush, Martha
Cady, Candace A **(SLP)**
Calvert, Dr Anne S **(A)**
Campbell, Mary G **(SLP)**
Carlberg, Karen S **(A)**
Carlisle, Margaret A **(SLP)**
Carlock, Jenifer Lee **(A)**
Chaney, Victoria Lea **(SLP)**
Chapman, Dr Sandra Bond **(SLP)**
Chase, Kathy K **(A)**
Clark, Mrs Betty Jean **(SLP)**
Clodfelter-Cartier, Mrs Carla **(SLP)**
Coleman, Trudy H **(A)**
Collier, Cynthia Janese
Condon, Karen S **(SLP A)**
Conner, Cathy I **(SLP)**
Copeland, Mrs Katherine Eby **(SLP)**
Cording, Joanne C Algozzino **(SLP)**
Crawford, Sandra G **(SLP)**
Crutcher, Damaris W **(SLP A)**
Culp, Delva Mae **(SLP)**
Dahlgren, Phyllis O **(SLP)**
Davis, Jacqueline Bryant **(SLP)**
Davis, Ruth Norene **(SLP)**
Deahl, Mrs Susan K **(A)**
Dearing, Carol F **(SLP A)**
Deatherage, Violet M **(SLP)**
De Costa, Mrs Linda Anne **(SLP)**
Dodgen, Mrs Lana S **(SLP)**
Doss, Janet M **(SLP)**
Douglas, Joan C G **(SLP)**
Doyle, Mrs Margaret Jill **(SLP)**
Duncan, Mrs Marilyn S **(SLP)**
Dunckel, D Creig **(A)**
Dunlap, Mrs Denise Drace **(SLP)**
Dunn, Julie Ann **(SLP)**
Dyer, Mrs Patricia Lex **(SLP)**
Eastham, Sharon L **(SLP)**
Eidels, Eleanor R **(SLP)**
Ellis, Mrs Deborah T **(SLP)**
Ely, Amy N **(SLP)**
Emory-Pacheco, Christine K **(SLP)**
Everitt, Wanda Huey **(SLP)**
Farrar, Mrs Beverly J Clark **(SLP)**

Ferris, Marilyn M **(SLP)**
Fine, Catherine **(SLP)**
Finitzo, Dr Terese **(A)**
Fink, Janet L **(A)**
Fisher, Mrs Inez Freeney **(A)**
Fleming, Dr Susan G **(SLP)**
Fletcher, Dorothy Isbell **(SLP)**
Flint-Shaw, Mrs Lynn M **(SLP)**
Formby, Ellen S F **(SLP)**
Formichella, Katherine **(SLP)**
Foster, Mrs Suzanne C **(SLP)**
Frank, Cheryl R **(SLP)**
Franklin, Honor **(SLP)**
Freels, Deborah A **(SLP)**
Friel-Patti, Dr Sandy **(SLP)**
Fuller, Diane Michelle **(SLP)**
Gage, Denise Annette **(SLP)**
Gartenberg-Fletcher, Mrs Carol **(SLP)**
Gehm, John R **(A)**
Gehm, Patricia A **(A)**
Gerken, Dr George M
Gholson, Mrs Sibyl G **(SLP A)**
Gibson, Deborah Ann **(SLP)**
Gilbert, Margaret B **(SLP)**
Gill, Mrs Elizabeth Bryant **(A)**
Glover, Lynn K **(SLP)**
Goodman, Mrs Rona B **(SLP)**
Gore, Marcy **(SLP)**
Gorrell, Howard Anthony **(SLP)**
Greenberg, Mrs Lauri R J **(SLP)**
Hancock, Mrs Jimelle Rodgers **(SLP)**
Hardin, Mrs Janice Marie **(SLP)**
Harris, Ann Meador **(SLP)**
Harris, Dr Dean A **(SLP A)**
Harris, Teresa Williamson **(A)**
Harrison, Dr Peggy R **(SLP)**
Harry, Mary Ellen Bret **(SLP)**
Hayes, Deborah Kay **(SLP)**
Haynes, Sara M **(SLP)**
Hein, Dr Sally Lee **(SLP)**
Henry, Donna Therese
Henry, Mrs Patricia M **(SLP)**
Herzer, Mrs Michelle Mizell **(SLP)**
Hill, Carole L **(SLP)**
Hodge, Mrs Marilyn Julia **(SLP)**
Holderby, Gail G **(SLP)**
Horan, Mrs Anne C **(SLP)**
Horn, Mrs Melanie **(A)**
Howard, Lisa Lynn **(SLP)**
Hudson, Jan Elaine **(SLP)**
Hughes, Pamela Jean **(SLP)**
Hurley, Leah Ann **(SLP)**
Hurley, Michele
Isham, Cynthia Rochelle
Jakubik, Dennis M **(SLP)**
Jarvis, Barbara S **(A)**
Jaster, Mary L **(SLP)**
Johns, Dr Donnell F **(SLP)**
Johnson, Clint Daniel **(SLP)**
Kamen, Ruth Saletsky **(SLP)**
Keenan, Kathleen L **(SLP)**
King, Linda Marian **(SLP)**
Kolenovsky, Mrs Gladys W **(SLP)**
Krauss-Lehrman, Patricia L **(SLP)**
Legrow, Lori Novek **(SLP)**
Lipman, Mrs LeAnn Carol **(A)**
Litten, Mrs Janet R **(SLP)**
Little, Jimmie L **(SLP)**
Loch, Lucinda
Lonergan, Mary Ann **(SLP)**
Long, Mrs Laurie Constance **(SLP)**
Lontos, Nancy Bywaters **(SLP)**
MacWilliam, Dalene D **(SLP)**
Martin, Faith Suzanne **(SLP)**
Martin, Maryann Leathem **(SLP)**
Matthews, Cynthia B **(SLP)**
May, Helen M **(SLP)**
McClure, Mrs Mona W **(SLP)**
McDonough, Roberta F **(A)**
McIlwain, Mrs Judith W **(SLP)**
McQuaid, Mrs Patricia W **(SLP)**
Meyer, Mrs Jeanne D **(SLP)**
Millay, Kathleen K **(SLP A)**
Miller, Mrs Louise H **(SLP A)**
Miller, Stephen E **(A)**
Mirmelstein, Mrs Marcy R **(SLP)**
Mitchell, Mrs Ann B **(SLP)**
Mobley, Cynthia L **(SLP)**
Morgan, Mrs Patti A **(SLP)**
Morris, Mrs Kathleen Elizabeth **(SLP)**
Morris, Mrs Shelia D **(SLP)**
Morrison, Mary M **(A)**
Moss, Barbara Ann **(SLP A)**
Musa, Mrs Judith F **(SLP)**
Nevin, Mrs Barbara Anne **(SLP)**
Newman, Mary Katherine
Northrup, Mrs Briseida D **(A)**
Nudleman, Mrs Elisa Mitrani **(SLP)**
Oberlin, Melissa Waller **(A)**
Olson, Sandy L **(SLP)**
Oswalt, Lora S **(SLP)**
Pappas, Mrs Michele Rebecca **(SLP)**
Paul, Alesia Renee **(SLP)**
Paul, Cynthia G **(SLP)**
Payne, Brenda Wildermuth **(SLP)**
Piacenti, Mrs Terri **(SLP)**
Pickrell, Kerry K **(SLP)**
Portley, Rossanna S **(SLP)**
Potyka, Pamela Spencer
Powers, Sally L **(SLP)**
Price, Deborah **(A)**
Puls-Grzybowski, Mrs Beth D **(SLP)**
Purdy, Carol A **(SLP)**
Quarterman, Pamela H **(SLP)**
Ramey, Anna M C **(SLP)**
Ramsey, Mrs Wendy H **(SLP)**
Rauchle, Mrs Judith Lee **(SLP)**
Reese, Janice C **(SLP)**
Reisch, Sandy J **(A)**
Reynolds, R Eric **(A)**
Richardson, Beverly Anne **(SLP)**
Richardson, Lisa G
Rickoff, Mrs Michelle Ann **(SLP)**
Robertson, Jana Renee **(SLP)**
Robinson, Debra L **(SLP)**
Rochon, Carol Joyce **(SLP)**
Roeser, Dr Ross J **(A)**
Rogers, Jodi A **(A)**
Rogers, Mariann **(SLP)**
Ronquillo, Yazmin J **(SLP)**
Rothschild, Mrs Suellen Blum **(SLP)**
Rothstein, Marilyn C **(SLP)**
Saenz, Belinda M **(SLP)**
Santana, Mrs Elizabeth **(SLP)**
Schopfer, Kathryn Humphreys **(SLP)**
Schulze, Mrs Gaynelle Babb **(SLP A)**
Scott, Susan C **(SLP)**
Sears, Carolyn Jean **(A)**
Sekhon, Mrs Laura Jane **(SLP)**
Sharp, Mary Christian **(SLP)**
Shaw, Joan Kain **(SLP)**
Shook, Mrs Jane Ellen **(SLP)**
Shortall, Mrs Ann L **(SLP)**
Shulman, Susan C **(SLP A)**
Silver, Valerie **(SLP)**
Simanonis, Mrs Marcy Koonz
Simonson, Josephine **(SLP)**
Smith, Mrs Kelly Hudspeth **(SLP)**
Sneed, Mrs Donna Doss **(SLP)**
Sowell, Kathy Brakefield **(SLP)**
Spears, Mark Thompson **(A)**
Speed, Mrs Tanya Jo Lennard **(SLP)**
Stanley, Renee L **(SLP)**
Stephens, Phyllis Kay **(A)**
Stephenson, Paul Gregory **(A)**
Stewart, Vicki Eklund **(A)**
Stillman, Dr Robert David
Stone, Carolyn **(A)**
Stroud, Mrs Janice W **(SLP)**
Sullivan, Holly Le Blanc **(SLP)**
Sullivan, Mary Patricia **(SLP)**
Swift, Carol A **(SLP)**
Tackett, Annette Renc
Thomas, Kathy Wright **(SLP)**
Tobe, Mrs Judy Gail **(SLP)**
Tobolowsky, Judith W **(SLP)**
Tolley, Carolyn J **(A)**
Toro, Bridget H **(SLP)**
Tucker, Mrs Connie Montgomery **(SLP)**
Tunney, Pamela Ann **(A)**
Turek, Monica D **(SLP)**
Valentine, Mrs Melinda S **(SLP)**
Varnon, Mrs Suzanne M **(SLP)**
Vitt, Mrs Melissa Engelsmann
Wallace, Beth E **(SLP)**
Walsh, Jeanne M **(SLP)**
Watson, Ben C **(SLP)**
Wells, Mrs Randi S **(SLP)**
Whatley, Mrs Jean Scott **(SLP)**
Wheeler, Mrs Betty K **(SLP)**
Wilson, Nancy M **(SLP)**
Wilson, Phillip L **(A)**
Windhager, Julie Claire **(SLP)**
Winney, Mrs Vernell **(SLP)**
Woods, Mrs Margaret Y **(SLP)**
Wright, Joyce E **(SLP)**
Yates, Rebecca R **(SLP)**
Yellin, M Wende **(A)**
Young, Judy Sue **(SLP)**

Dawn
Stribling, Daulma **(SLP)**

De Soto
Brandenburg, Mrs April Dawn **(SLP)**
Faulk, Emily Anne
Nunn, Will Ann **(SLP)**

Decatur
Stone, Mrs Wanda Jean **(SLP)**

Delrio
Lee, Carol E **(SLP)**

Denison
Brewer, Mrs Claudia Stagner **(SLP)**
Liles, Sara J **(SLP)**
Marburger, Mrs Marianne Rebholz **(SLP)**

Denton
Ballard, Katheryn Lynn **(SLP)**
Batson, Dr Delaina W **(SLP)**
Beamer, Mrs Mary W **(SLP)**
Bulla, Pat O **(SLP)**
Caudle, Chris D **(A)**
Cendroski, Julie Whiting **(A)**
Cohen, Karen E **(SLP)**
Davis, Mrs Rebecca A **(A)**
Gaskill, Benettee Lee **(SLP)**
Gathings, Robert D **(SLP A)**
Gitter, Mary Jane **(SLP)**
Goldmann, Mrs Kathleen M **(SLP)**
Grant, Dr Dorothy E **(SLP A)**
Guess, Lawrence Kevin
Holmes, Dr David **(A)**
Jacquot, Dr Willard S **(SLP A)**
Larson, Dr George W **(SLP)**
Moorer, Mrs Laura Poteet **(SLP)**
Morris, Barbara B **(SLP)**
Mueller, Dr Peter B **(SLP)**
Muncy, Mrs Julie Kehl **(SLP)**
Nelson, Mrs Allison Leigh **(SLP)**
Newman, Gloria Ann **(SLP)**
Oelschlaeger, Dr Mary L **(SLP)**
Riley, Mrs Linda Pitner **(SLP)**
Sallack, Mrs Hilda W **(SLP)**
Scott, Brian Lee
Seabourn, Mrs Beverly Jolene **(SLP)**
Shelton, Dr June Ford **(SLP)**
Smith, Mrs Alice V **(SLP A)**
Smith, Mrs Mary E **(SLP)**
Stream, Dr Kathryn S **(A)**
Stream, Dr Richard W **(A)**
Summers, Patricia Anne **(SLP)**
Taylor, Mrs Lilia Hinojo **(SLP)**
Thomas, Rebecca Nurre **(SLP)**
Willson, Marcia G **(SLP)**

Denver City
Loffler, Mrs Tanya Lambert **(SLP)**

Dickinson
Early, Patricia **(SLP)**

Donna
Gonzales, Maria Diana **(SLP)**

Driftwood
Jakielski, Mrs Kathy Jo **(SLP)**

Duncanville
Anderson, Mrs Emily T **(SLP)**
Bruning, Mrs Annette Cavalli **(SLP)**
Coroneos, Judith Cann **(SLP)**
Herrbold, Mrs Merrie M **(SLP)**
Parsons, Sharon D **(SLP)**
Paul, Mrs Bernice E

Dyess AFB
Galentine, Joy Kimura **(SLP)**

Eagle Pass
Cassie, Dhyan McCollom **(A)**

Eastland
Morren, Mrs Jeanette A
Walley, Mary L **(SLP)**

Edinburg
Leach, Dr Edwin A **(SLP)**
Valles, Luciano, Jr **(SLP)**

El Paso
Allen, Mrs Ana Elena **(SLP)**
Anderson, Juel H **(A)**
Anderson, Susan S **(SLP)**
Bond, Sandra Lynn **(SLP)**
Brand, Madeline **(SLP)**
Burgess, Mrs Laura Frances **(SLP)**
Castillo, Mrs Alma Luisa **(SLP)**
Cenk, Mrs Susan Talavera **(SLP)**
Cleek, Thyra J **(A)**
Cobos, Mrs Anne S **(SLP)**
Daniel, Sarah Weller **(A)**
Daudistel, Mrs Sandra **(SLP)**
Dawson, Ronald E **(SLP)**
Delgado, Mrs Pollie Johnson **(SLP)**
Dennis, Richard A **(A)**
Dictor, Mrs Rona S **(SLP)**
Dodson, Stephanie Karr **(SLP)**
Dovalina, Norma **(SLP)**
Duncan, Mrs Julie Ellen **(SLP)**
Durbin, Christine **(SLP)**
Faulk, Mark Steven
Fisher, Mrs Cathy Lane **(SLP)**
Gore, Carol N **(A)**
Greene, Penny N **(SLP)**
Hazelton, Laura Campbell **(SLP)**
Jaffee, Mrs Susan Ann **(SLP)**
Jones, Mrs Anne G **(SLP)**
Kligman, Mrs Roberta A **(SLP)**
Knott, Mary Carolyn **(SLP)**
Lail, Mrs Lorie Fox **(SLP)**
Lamay, Mrs Linda P **(SLP)**
Lewis, Donna Lee **(SLP)**
Longnecker, Beth Anne **(A)**
Lopez, Arlys N **(SLP)**
Lopez, Mrs Jeanette B **(SLP)**
Mancha, Ellen Padget **(SLP)**
Manigold, Mrs Jo Ann W **(SLP)**
Maynard, Margaret E Ochoa **(SLP)**
McCleskey, Mrs Katrina Sanders
McCowen, Mrs Judith E **(SLP)**
McNiel, Mrs Bernadine Ledwig **(SLP)**
Metz, Mrs Cheryl Lynn **(SLP)**
Middleton, Dr Grace Frederick **(SLP)**
Mooney, Mary L **(SLP)**
Moore, Mrs Edith Young **(SLP)**
Moreno, Mrs Yolanda Flores
Morris, Karen Elaine **(A)**
Munoz, Dr Orlando **(SLP)**
Nehls, Luanne **(SLP)**
Panko, Mrs Alice L **(SLP)**
Patterson, Mrs Ellen Emilia **(SLP)**

Perozzi, Dr Joseph A **(SLP)**
Pirreca, Mrs Marcia S **(SLP)**
Poole, Penny Jean **(SLP)**
Rivas, Mary S **(SLP)**
Rivera, Mary Lou **(A)**
Rodriquez, Rubina Rueda **(SLP)**
Schmidt, Marjorie Thorn **(SLP)**
Shepherd, Mrs Jennifer Felts
Templeman, Janette E **(SLP)**
Van Meter, Mrs Cynthia Louise
Vokes, Jimmie Ann
Voss, Mrs Marsha K **(SLP)**
Waissman, Rachael
Wallace, Diane **(SLP)**
Whittington, Mrs Mitzi J **(SLP)**
Williams, Dr Harold N **(SLP A)**
Wright, Pamela Mabel **(SLP)**

Elgin

Haynie, Jo K **(SLP)**
Meadows, Mrs Jan H **(SLP)**
Wooten, Angela Lathem **(A)**

Ennis

Chancellor, Jana L **(SLP)**
Christian, Jana Lee **(SLP)**
Knize, Mrs Evelyn B **(SLP)**

Euless

Brooks, Mrs Jami Harris
Brown, Beverly Elizabeth **(SLP)**
Combs, Mrs Jami Baker **(SLP)**
Faurot, Judith W **(SLP)**
Hall, Patricia **(SLP)**
Juengerman, Paula J **(SLP)**
MacCammond, Mrs Mickie S, III **(SLP)**
McPherson, Mrs Shirley Smith **(SLP)**
Petersen, Mrs Brenda D **(SLP A)**
Phillips, James W R **(A)**
Symington, Mrs Debbie Lynn **(SLP)**
Watson, Dr Jennifer Barber **(SLP)**

Farmers Branch

Hasfjord, Heidi Annette **(SLP)**
Reed, Paula L **(SLP)**

Farmersville

Bullard, Mrs Billie H **(SLP)**

Farney

Mosher, Mrs Beth **(SLP)**

Flower Mound

Barbee, Jeanette Patterson **(SLP)**
Clark, Jackie Phelps **(A)**
Easler, Rochelle L **(SLP)**
Markello, Mrs Carol G **(SLP)**
Miguel, Dr Shirley A **(SLP)**
Socha-Smith, Karen Marie **(SLP)**

Forney

Fischer, Patricia Lynn **(A)**
Hooper, Mrs Dorothy W **(SLP)**

Fort Hood

Rathke, Maj John J **(A)**
Silber, Kim Marie **(SLP)**
Williams, Capt Barbara Jean **(A)**

Fort Sam Houston

Hight, Nancy G **(A)**
Risher, Timothy B **(A)**

Fort Stockton

Davidson, Ben N **(SLP)**
Walters, Martha Ann **(SLP)**

Fort Worth

Ahrens, Mrs L Ann D **(SLP)**
Allen, Mrs Susan E **(SLP)**
Anderson, Karen C **(SLP)**
Anderson-Smith, Mrs Cheryl Joy
Baca, Ann H **(SLP)**
Baker, Mrs Rita Arlene **(SLP)**
Barry, Nancy W **(SLP)**
Bean, Mrs Patricia A **(SLP)**
Bell, Dr Dorothy M **(SLP A)**
Bernard, Annella K **(SLP)**
Berry, Mrs Patsy A **(SLP)**
Bloxom, Mrs Katie Riddle **(A)**
Carter, Lisa Kay **(A)**
Chesner, Mrs Kathleen Everson **(A)**
Cobb, John C **(A)**
Cook, Gayle W **(SLP)**
Cornelius, Jodie L **(SLP)**
Coulter, Mary Elise **(SLP)**
Davis, Albert L **(A)**
Dickens, Patsy Hill **(SLP)**
Disharoon, Sandra B **(SLP)**
Doyle, Mrs Linda Ann **(SLP)**
Estes, Sandra S **(SLP)**
Farrar, Mrs Lynne Brew **(SLP)**
Gann, Mrs Patsy J **(SLP)**
German, Susan B **(SLP)**
Glaser, Mrs Sherri Lynn **(SLP)**
Gracey, Sally Brown **(SLP)**
Gregory, Susan **(SLP)**
Griffith, Karan Elizabeth **(SLP)**
Guthrie, Terry M **(A)**
Guydon, Dr Audrey Sessom **(SLP)**
Hahn, Mary C **(SLP)**
Haptonstall, Linda C **(SLP)**
Harden, Dr R Joyce **(SLP)**
Harris, Debby J **(SLP)**
Harris, Mrs Nada E **(SLP)**
Helmick, Dr Joseph W **(SLP)**
Hendelman, Mrs Ruth S **(A)**
Hobson, Mrs Susan K **(SLP)**
Holland, Donna J **(SLP)**
Homer, Mrs Susan Olivia **(SLP)**
Houchen, Ronald H **(A)**
Howell, Susan M **(A)**
James, Mrs Rae K **(SLP)**
Johnson, Mrs Carolyn Russell **(SLP)**
Johnson, Gail A **(SLP)**
Johnson, Mrs Rebecca Lynn **(A)**
Johnson, Mrs Sharon J **(SLP)**
Johnston, Valerie Leigh **(SLP)**
Jones, Mrs Irene E **(A)**
Jones, Mrs Kay H **(SLP)**
Kayser, Dr Hortense Garcia **(SLP)**
Kennedy, Mrs Karen Darlene **(SLP)**
Kingsley-Douglas, Susan **(SLP)**
Kohut, Ellen Allen **(SLP)**
Laing, Pamela J **(SLP)**
Lane, Barbara D **(SLP)**
Lanza, Mrs Janet Royer **(SLP)**
Larimore, Mrs Jody Kelly
Lawler, Mrs Marcia Putzel **(SLP)**
Lawrence, Mrs Telete Z **(SLP)**
Leever, Karen N **(SLP)**
Lieberth, Dr Ann K **(SLP A)**
Luft, Cynthia Burt **(SLP)**
Manning, Mrs Marlynn C **(SLP)**
Marshall, Pauline D **(SLP)**
McClean, Marsha D **(A)**
Mershon, Dr Patricia M **(SLP)**
Millikan, Mrs Cynthia Diane **(SLP)**
Minnich, Julie Anne **(SLP)**
Morton, Larry H **(SLP)**
Mower, Mrs Paula T **(SLP)**
Nelson, Sharon S **(SLP)**
Norris, Marylee K **(SLP)**
Odom, Mrs Glenna L **(SLP)**
Omo, Mrs Patricia H **(SLP)**
Orr, Mrs Helen Bohn **(SLP)**
Padilla, Teresa C **(SLP)**
Price, Mrs Dorothy M **(SLP)**
Quick, Victoria Ann **(SLP)**
Rapp, Sharon Beall **(A)**
Rappe, Elizabeth Medlock **(SLP)**
Reece, Paul A **(SLP)**
Roberts, Mrs Gail Forman **(SLP)**
Robinson, Mrs Carolyn C **(SLP)**
Rogers, Janice R **(SLP)**
Ruckriegel, Linda Anne **(A)**
Siler, Mrs Kathy F **(SLP)**
Stocker, Dr Harold S **(SLP)**
Stovall, Wanda W **(SLP)**
Stroup, Mrs Nancy R **(SLP)**
Symon, Mrs Carol H **(SLP)**
Tade, Mrs Wilma Jean **(SLP)**
Tallarico Cutter, Tina **(SLP)**
Terrell, Dr Sandra L **(SLP)**
Tipps, Mrs Deborah L **(SLP)**
Tucker, Mrs E Raylene **(SLP)**
Tucker, Mrs Marsha B **(SLP)**
Ullberg, Mrs Renee Gould **(SLP)**
Van Giesen, Marjorie Fleck **(SLP)**
Waggoner, Mrs Barbara Joyce **(SLP)**
Wallace, Patty Nesom **(SLP)**
Weaver, Marietta B **(SLP)**
Wells, Mrs Cheryl D **(SLP)**
Williams, Rita J **(SLP)**
Wilson, Mrs Carolyn C **(SLP)**
Wright, Mrs China Allen **(A)**
Wright, Mary B **(SLP)**

Fredericksburg

Barsch, Ann E **(A)**
Briery-Leon, Debra J **(A)**
Herzog, Glenn L **(SLP)**

Friendswood

Cress, Sharon T **(SLP)**
Engel, Karen W **(SLP)**
Kling, Mrs Sandra Tiffany **(SLP)**
Noga, Alicia S **(SLP)**
O'Hare, Nancy J **(SLP)**
Taylor, Mrs Kerri Pool **(SLP)**
Williams, Mrs Susan Thomas **(A)**

Frisco

Molidor, Mrs Rebecca A **(SLP)**
Prouty, Mrs Vicki L **(SLP)**

Gainesville

Allen, Mrs Ima Jean **(SLP)**
Cheatham, Mrs Melinda M **(SLP)**
Molloy, Debra A **(SLP)**
Richey, Mrs Vera Crow **(SLP)**
Sharp, Mrs Linda Gayle **(SLP)**

Galveston

Clark-Hill, Mrs Lesley M **(SLP)**
Conde, Rebecca Hart **(SLP)**
Danna, Victoria Lee **(A)**
Dworkin, Dr James Paul **(SLP)**
Fulmer, Mrs Janet Elise **(A)**
Gary, Lucinda Boyd **(A)**
Kampe, Mary Angela **(SLP)**
Lee, Mrs Heidi Marie **(A)**
Lettieri, Teresa Jo **(SLP)**
Levin, C Lynn **(SLP)**
Mundy, Martha R **(A)**
Newland, Mrs Donna L M **(SLP)**
Pruszenski, Malea Anne **(A)**
Reeh, Mrs Hilary L **(A)**
Roberts, Nancy E **(SLP)**
Rusk, Bobbie Leigh **(SLP)**
Stubbs, Stephanie A

Garland

Alt, Mrs Lisa Wojcik
Brown, Mrs Lavonda L **(SLP)**
Brunz, Mrs Susan B
Buckley, Gloria L **(A)**
Conboy, Mrs Joan Carver
Copeland, Dr Alfred Beryl **(A)**
Donaghey, Mrs Trish A **(SLP)**
Evans, Mrs Patricia Ann **(SLP)**
Gardner, Janet Lee **(A)**
Hammer, Susan Annette **(SLP)**
Henson, Mrs Reeda Ruth **(SLP)**
Hibbs, Mrs Pauline Greve **(SLP)**
Hicks, Dr James W, Jr
Hutchinson-Clutter, Margaret L **(A)**
Jonas, Mrs Carol F **(A)**
Kite, LeAnn **(SLP)**
Lambert, Mrs Lynn O **(SLP)**
Lance, Mrs Beverly Ann **(SLP)**
McCormack, Judy J **(SLP)**
McGregor, Joyce E Hansen **(SLP)**
Mosser, Mrs Sharon U **(SLP)**
O'Neill, Kerri R **(SLP)**
Rasor, Mrs Glynn H **(SLP)**
Rivera, Mrs Theresa Ann **(A)**
Ross, Becky L **(SLP)**
Scates, Mrs Penny Barham **(A)**
Sherman, Mrs Lynn W **(SLP)**
Shortino, Mrs Margaret Denise **(SLP)**
Taylor, Kathryn **(SLP)**
Terry, Mrs Diana B **(SLP)**
Valdez, Mrs Elizabeth S
Watkins, Lydia Steiner **(SLP)**
Westbrook, Janice B **(SLP)**
Wilkes, Mrs Deborah Egly **(SLP)**

George West

Moffatt, Mrs Bridgett G **(SLP)**

Georgetown

Bauer, Janetta M **(SLP)**
Eaton, Andrea Sinkking **(SLP)**
McKay, Mrs Janet Lea **(SLP)**
Mickan, Mrs Penny Pierce **(SLP)**
Patterson, Mrs Susan A P **(SLP)**

Gladewater

Ricks, Melissa Ann **(SLP)**

Golden

Gibson, Valori Norris **(SLP)**

Gonzales

McKee, Mrs Lynda C **(SLP)**
Wilson, Robert Lynn **(SLP)**

Graham

Yarbrough, Mrs Donna Lavoy

Granbury

Davis, Helen Handley **(SLP)**
Durant, Mrs Linda Godard **(SLP)**
Smedley, Mrs Elizabeth M **(SLP)**

Grand Prairie

Beaulieu, Jacqueline Johnson **(SLP)**
Erwin, Mrs Judith L **(SLP)**
Geracci, Mrs Jane Marie **(SLP)**
Moser, Ann Allen **(SLP)**
Olvera-vonRabenau, Franz D **(A)**
Scroggin, Mrs Deborah K **(SLP)**
Strueby, Mrs Laurie Culberson

Grapevine

Hailey, Mrs Ann H W **(SLP)**
Phoebus, Brenda Lee **(SLP)**
Sorsby, Mrs Patricia Glass **(SLP)**

Greenville

Ackley, Mrs Dolores Shuler **(SLP)**
Bracken, Maryann P **(SLP)**
Fields, Mrs Sondra Kay **(SLP)**
Fields, Dr Thomas A **(SLP)**
Gill, Dr Cynthia B **(SLP)**
Griffin, Mrs Beverly G **(SLP)**
Kennedy, Mary K W **(SLP)**
Shuler, Mrs Cleta J **(SLP)**
Spivy, Rebecca Ellen S **(SLP)**

Groves

Nicholson, Mrs Deborah Lynne **(A)**
Sullivan, Mrs Jeri Boudreaux **(SLP)**

Harker Heights

Ibbotson, Candace Baumgart **(SLP)**
Privratsky, Mrs Kathy I **(SLP)**

Harlingen

Leal, Sr Lourdes **(SLP)**
McKelvey, Mrs Judy F **(SLP)**
Rath, Roger J **(SLP A)**

Haslet

Carter, Mrs Molly Sue **(SLP)**

Helopes

Shadowens, Dr Melvin R **(A)**

Henderson

Carroll, Mrs Hazel Deason **(SLP)**
Hall, Mrs Beverly Butler **(SLP)**

Hewitt
Maclel, Sabrina Dunham **(SLP)**
Martindale-Whipple, Dr Kathy **(SLP)**
Warren, Mrs Mary Kay **(SLP)**
Wolfe, Mrs Julie Atkins **(SLP)**

High Island
Foerster, Shawn W

Hitchcock
Griffith, Amy Marian **(SLP)**
Sharp, Mrs Janet Sue **(SLP)**

Horizon City
Glover, Mrs Mary Marguerite

Houston
Abbott, Susan Elayne **(A)**
Abrams, Mrs Susan L S **(A)**
Adams, Dr Martin R **(SLP)**
Adams-Ethridge, Donna E **(SLP)**
Adrian, Marjorie R **(SLP)**
Albright, Kathryn Bills **(A)**
Albritton, Mrs Elizabeth Marshall **(SLP)**
Allison, Paula **(A)**
Allred, Elizabeth **(SLP)**
Andersen, Monica K **(A)**
Anderson, Amy Beth **(SLP)**
Anderson, Delmarine **(SLP)**
Anderson, Mary S **(SLP)**
Arceneaux, Judith D **(SLP)**
Arnold, Genevieve **(SLP)**
Aussenberg, Mrs Elizabeth G **(SLP)**
Austin, Mrs Meredith Hall **(SLP)**
Baccaro, Paul Michel **(SLP A)**
Bailey, Lorena **(SLP)**
Baker, Dian Gail **(SLP)**
Bangs, Dr Tina E **(SLP A)**
Barhorst, Annette Marie **(SLP)**
Barnett, Carol Jane **(A)**
Barnhill, Mrs Kathy Harrison **(SLP)**
Barragan, Mrs Connie L **(A)**
Bass, Mrs Emily Anne **(SLP)**
Bass, Pamela M **(SLP)**
Bastidas, Deborah Ann **(SLP)**
Battin, Dr R Ray **(SLP A)**
Bebb, Gretchen E **(SLP)**
Bell, Susan F **(SLP)**
Bender, Martha A M **(SLP)**
Berkowitz, Michael A **(SLP)**
Berryman, Mrs Dolores S **(SLP)**
Besetzny-Holub, Diane Marie **(SLP)**
Bilyeu, Delores Lena **(SLP)**
Blackwelder, Mrs E Diane **(SLP)**
Blaesing, Dr Leslie L **(SLP)**
Blair, Mrs Pamela Sue **(SLP)**
Blankinship, Mrs Becky Tomlinson **(SLP)**
Bollerer, Susan Puryear **(SLP)**
Bonner, Marilou P **(SLP)**
Bonner, Mrs Regina **(SLP)**
Boudreaux, Cynthia Leigh **(SLP)**
Bowman, Julia Beeson **(SLP)**
Brackett, Mrs April Anne **(SLP)**
Brezner, Mrs Diane J L **(SLP)**
Brookshire, Bonnie **(SLP)**
Brown, Dr Denice P **(A)**
Bruce, Melissa C **(SLP)**
Bruchas, Dr Joan K **(SLP)**
Bryant, Jane Elizabeth
Bukauskas, Cynthia Louise **(SLP)**
Burdine, Gayle Janeane **(SLP)**
Burford, Mrs Nancy Grubbs **(SLP)**
Burnham, Mrs Margaret G **(SLP)**
Buse, Mrs Maria Christina **(SLP)**
Buysse, Mrs Miriam Swedberg **(SLP)**
Byrns, Glenda E **(SLP)**
Caell, Teresa A **(SLP)**
Caldwell, Lacey J S **(SLP)**
Califf, Elizabeth Kimberly **(A)**
Callner, Lisa Beth **(SLP)**
Camarata, Mrs Phyllis Ann **(SLP)**
Campbell, Bertha M **(SLP)**
Cardenas-Hagan, Elsa **(SLP)**
Carmichael, Dorothy Harry **(SLP)**
Carnicom, Mrs Ruth C **(SLP)**
Carter, James P **(SLP)**
Carver, Mrs RuthAnn D **(SLP)**
Casassa, Mrs Angela Cassady **(SLP)**
Cascio, Carol F Lowe **(SLP)**
Catlin, Dr Francis Irving **(A)**
Chambliss, Marcia J **(SLP)**
Chapman, Mrs Kristen M **(SLP)**
Chmiel, Rose A **(A)**
Ciolli, Lois Gregory **(SLP)**
Ciro, Linda A B **(SLP)**
Clark, Mrs Judith G **(SLP)**
Clark, Mrs Olivia A **(SLP)**
Cobb, Mrs Jayne Staler
Coe, Sandra L **(A)**
Cohen, Beverly Rose **(SLP)**
Coleman, Jeanne Marie **(SLP)**
Collins, Carol Diane **(SLP)**
Cooper, Mary B **(SLP)**
Corbett, Gioia M
Craig, Cathleen C **(SLP)**
Crosswhite, Mrs Cynthia Lynn R **(SLP)**
Crowley, Mrs Ellen C **(SLP)**
Curl, Mrs Mary Reid **(SLP)**
D'Antoni, Maria L **(SLP)**
Davidson, Mrs Keiko Y **(SLP)**
Davis, Marjorie Renee **(A)**
Davis, Yondle Climer **(SLP)**
Decker, Cathy J S **(SLP)**
De La Cruz, Angel F **(A)**
Delgado-Vilches, Mrs Gloria **(A)**
Delhommer, Mrs Janet A **(SLP)**
Dey-Sigman, Susan **(A)**
Dickerson, Linda H **(SLP)**
Di Donato, Roberta M **(SLP)**
Diekmann, Sharon B **(SLP)**
Dillard, Cindy A **(SLP)**
Dillman, Mary Kathryn
Dinwoodie, Mrs Cheryl Klobnak **(SLP)**
Donaldson, Dr Rita Joyce **(A)**
Dowling, Dr Susann S **(SLP)**
Drewyer, Mrs Martha B **(SLP)**
Duconge, Jean Ann **(A)**
Ducote, Mrs Karen B **(SLP)**
Dunhill-Zannoni, Mrs Moreen Ann **(SLP)**
Durante, Mrs Dace Anita **(SLP)**
Durkee, Mrs Margaret Jill **(SLP)**
Duval, Mrs Sharon Cooper **(SLP)**
Edgley, Mrs Edna B **(SLP)**
Elledge, Mrs Debra L **(SLP)**
Engelman, Mrs Sylvia L **(SLP)**
Falconer, Dr George A **(A)**
Farkas, Audrey **(SLP)**
Farley, Mrs Joyce J **(SLP A)**
Feldman, Mrs Sheryl N **(SLP)**
Fisher, Anna
Fishman, Mrs Hedy F **(A)**
Forbes, Carolyn Elizabeth **(SLP)**
Ford, Renee Jarreau **(SLP)**
Forester, D'Laine **(SLP)**
Fox, Dr Donna R **(SLP)**
Frank, Mrs Carol L **(SLP)**
Frankiewicz, Yvonne G **(SLP)**
Franklin, Barbara S **(SLP)**
Freedman, Sharon Rance **(SLP)**
Furstenberg, Joan F **(A)**
Garrett, Dana Kathryn **(SLP)**
Genuth-Fox, April G **(SLP)**
Gibson, Johanna J **(SLP)**
Gilbert, Catherine **(A)**
Gillespie, Mrs Karen Denise **(SLP)**
Ginyard, Cynthia Melissa **(SLP)**
Goetz, Mrs Celia Drewyer **(SLP)**
Goldstein, Mrs Michele G **(A)**
Goodman, Sarah H **(SLP)**
Gotsdiner, Mrs Nancy Shulak **(SLP)**
Gray, Davon **(SLP)**
Gray, Mrs Eliz Gay **(SLP)**
Gray, Eulalia Rebecca **(SLP)**
Gray, Mrs Margaret H **(SLP)**
Green, Susan K **(SLP A)**
Greenspan, Phyllis **(SLP)**
Griffin-Spears, Mrs Dora M **(SLP)**
Grimes, Karen W **(SLP)**
Grimmett, Mrs Rachel W **(SLP)**
Groginski, Beatrice B **(SLP)**
Grothaus, Mrs Mary Lou McNickle **(SLP)**
Haedicke, Susan Phyllis S **(SLP)**
Hailey, Donna R **(SLP)**
Hale, Suzan L **(SLP)**
Hall, Mrs Diane Carey **(SLP)**
Hall, James Hartmann, Jr **(A)**
Hamburg, Ellen M
Hamner, Constance Elizabeth **(A)**
Handy, Vickie Kay **(SLP)**
Hardy, Edward Robertson, Jr **(SLP)**
Hardy, Maryclare **(SLP)**
Hardy, Mrs Michelle Crudup **(A)**
Harkins, Dr Edwina C **(SLP)**
Harmon, Mrs Brenda Carmickle **(SLP)**
Harris, Mrs Hannah G **(SLP)**
Harris, Katherine Pittenger **(SLP)**
Hartig, Juliana **(A)**
Hartley, Dr Leila L **(SLP)**
Hayward, Floanne J **(SLP)**
Heap, Nancy Jean **(SLP)**
Heffington, Rosalyn E **(SLP)**
Herzog, Dr Jean Talmage **(SLP)**
Hewett, Mrs Jo Murphy **(SLP)**
Higgins, Mrs Kelly Call
Hill, Debra Nell **(SLP)**
Hinze, Mrs Dianna Fake **(SLP)**
Holland, Dr Francine **(SLP)**
Hollier, Adrienne K **(SLP)**
Holmes, Elaine J **(SLP)**
Holmes, Mrs Elizabeth Gossett **(SLP)**
Hong, Li-Jane **(SLP)**
Hubbard, Mrs Frances L **(SLP)**
Hutchinson, Mrs Cheryl Schosek
Hutchison, Kathleen **(A)**
Ipsen, Mrs Peggy Loretta **(SLP)**
Israel, Sherri M **(A)**
Jackson, Audrey A **(SLP)**
Jackson, Janet L
Jackson, Rhonda L **(SLP)**
Jaegli, Mrs Luanne **(SLP)**
Jaffe, Mrs Louise C **(SLP)**
Jeremic, Elisa D **(SLP)**
Jerger, Dr James F **(A)**
Jerger, Dr Susan Wood **(A)**
Jerome, Dr Eldon K **(SLP)**
Johnson, Deloris Marie **(SLP)**
Johnson, Karen Christine **(A)**
Johnson-James, Janet **(SLP)**
Johnson-Sollenne, Jeanene **(SLP)**
Johnson-Thomas, Patricia **(SLP)**
Johnson-Weatherall, Mrs Ruth **(SLP)**
Jones, Mrs Betty Reingold **(SLP)**
Jones, Ruth E M **(SLP)**
Kaufman, Nancy Hope **(SLP)**
Kavanagh, Mrs Heddy Lee **(SLP)**
Kelso, Peggy D **(SLP)**
Kent, Marilyn Louise **(SLP A)**
Kerner, Debra Hanovich **(SLP)**
Kilday, Theresa Claire **(SLP)**
Killion, M'Lizabeth **(SLP)**
Kimpel, M Anne **(SLP)**
Kirk, Mrs Carolyn S **(SLP)**
Klecan-Aker, Joan S **(SLP)**
Kleinworth, Roxie Cummings **(SLP)**
Klinar, Charles A **(A)**
Knowles, Cynthia Dixon **(SLP A)**
Koppelman, Mark Lee **(A)**
Koser, Larry A **(SLP)**
Kraemer, Stacey Fordham **(SLP)**
Kriendler, Mrs Sandra L **(SLP)**
Kupchak, Linda S **(SLP)**
Lafevers, Nancy E **(SLP)**
Larrick, William Raymond **(SLP)**
Larson, Linda J **(SLP)**
LeBlanc-Ward, Mrs Linda Fay **(SLP)**
Levine, Esther S **(SLP)**
Levine, Nancy **(SLP)**
Linklater, Diane K **(SLP)**
Little, Mrs Cheryl D S **(SLP)**
Loiselle, Louise Hathaway **(A)**
Longoria, Margarita L **(SLP)**
Lopez, Beth B **(SLP)**
Loren, Dr Catherine Ann **(SLP)**
Louis, Timothy C **(A)**
Lupo, Judith L **(SLP)**
Lynch, Dr Joan I **(SLP)**
Lynn, Michelle **(SLP)**
Magee, Dorothy Lynn **(SLP)**
Mahle, Mrs Carla Brooks
Malof, Leah Berkowitz
Mancini, Mrs Susan B **(SLP)**
Mann, Mrs Jeri Lynn **(SLP)**
Marotta, Louis Jude **(SLP)**
McAughan, Margaret Ann **(SLP)**
McCants, Diana J **(SLP)**
McCarthy, David Max **(A)**
McClain, Sandra D **(SLP)**
McCoy, Margaret Jane **(A)**
McDonald, Betty Y **(SLP)**
McDonald, Mary O'Farrell **(A)**
McGary, Robin Jo **(A)**
McGlasson, Julie A **(SLP)**
McIngvale, Gayelene K **(SLP)**
McIntyre, Annagail M **(SLP)**
McKee, Sally Bradshaw **(SLP)**
McMillian, Jennifer H **(SLP)**
Meadows, Joseph D **(SLP)**
Meloy, Melette L **(A)**
Milledge, Ruth A **(SLP)**
Miller, Tammi Lynn **(SLP)**
Miller, Teresa Mary **(SLP)**
Miller Wilson, Grace Christine **(SLP)**
Moake, Mary E **(SLP)**
Moheet, Denise M K **(SLP)**
Molinaro, Michelle T **(SLP)**
Moore, Mary Ann **(SLP)**
Morales, Laura Rufina **(SLP)**
Moura, Rosangela **(A)**
Murray, Mrs Herbye Micheale **(SLP)**
Musher, Mrs Karol Katz **(SLP)**
Nager, Mrs Deborah F **(A)**
Narotam, Ruksha
Narun, Mrs Linda R S **(SLP)**
Needle, Lynn **(SLP)**
Neyland, Mrs Ann K **(SLP)**
Ostrow, Rhona E **(A)**
Papangelou-Kakouris, Marina Elvira
Parish, Robbin **(SLP)**
Parker, Mrs Leanne M **(SLP)**
Parrott, Dr Jean O **(SLP)**
Patterson, Mrs Terri Loo **(A)**
Perez, Mrs Denice Gordon **(SLP)**
Person, Beth A **(SLP)**
Pesavento-Braun, Gail Jean **(SLP)**
Peterson, Mrs Jane Carol **(SLP)**
Petrucci-Coley, Teresa M **(SLP)**
Platt, Mrs Mary F **(SLP)**
Pravda, Mrs Linda Friedman **(SLP)**
Preer, Vicki Marie **(SLP)**
Prietto, Anita L **(A)**
Pruitt, Jeanine Blake **(A)**
Ramirez, Mrs Toni G **(SLP)**
Raymond, Marie E **(SLP)**
Rea, Renee Riley **(SLP)**
Reed, Mrs Patricia George **(SLP)**
Rendon, Kristine Lois **(SLP)**
Richards, Amy Briner **(SLP)**
Richards, Mrs Karen Ann **(SLP)**
Ried, Dr Stephanie **(SLP)**
Rivera, Sunshine Lynda **(SLP)**
Robin, Mrs Constance
Robinson, Dana Karol **(SLP)**
Robinson, Sandra Sue **(A)**
Rodriguez, Mrs Maria I G **(SLP)**
Rolph, Teresa K **(SLP)**
Rombakis Crawford, Mrs Georgia **(SLP)**
Ron, Ann Creamer **(SLP)**
Rosenbaum, Alane A **(SLP)**
Rosenfield, David B
Rosenthal, Mary D **(SLP)**

Rosenzweig, Mrs Sue D **(SLP A)**
Rudisill, D Kay **(SLP)**
Rudrauff, Sally Ann **(SLP)**
Ruehle-Kumar, Karen **(SLP)**
Ruiz, Cesar E
Sanders, Johnny Lee **(A)**
Sanders, Mrs Linda B **(SLP)**
Sanford, Mrs Elizabeth Boozer **(A)**
Schilling, Rhonda Ann **(SLP)**
Schuchard, Susan E **(SLP)**
Schuelke, Sandra H **(SLP)**
Schuleman, Mrs Barbara Ann **(SLP)**
Schwartz, Florence **(SLP)**
Scott, Mrs Carol S **(SLP)**
Scott, Saralynn **(SLP)**
Seals, Sharon Skrivanos **(SLP)**
Segal, Mrs Beverly E **(SLP)**
Segal, Sharon **(SLP)**
Seigle, Melanie N **(SLP)**
Seitel, Dr Alan L **(SLP)**
Sekel, Patricia P **(SLP)**
Shirley, Sue A **(SLP)**
Siciliano-Cagle, Anna M **(SLP)**
Siegel, Mrs Christine Earle **(SLP)**
Siff, Mrs Jacqueline **(SLP)**
Sims, Elwin Lawson **(SLP)**
Slade, Christina Louise **(SLP A)**
Sladek, Mrs Brenda K **(SLP)**
Slaten, Mrs Nancy J **(SLP)**
Slipakoff, Mrs Ethel L **(SLP)**
Smarra, Mrs Paula Denise **(SLP)**
Smith, Allison Harmon **(SLP)**
Smith, Mrs Carla Jamison **(SLP)**
Smith, Mrs Sandra B **(SLP)**
Smith-Farach, Sheri **(A)**
South, Laura L **(SLP)**
Sparker, Ann W **(SLP)**
Speerschneider, Jane Marie **(A)**
Spinelli, Francesca M **(SLP)**
Spretnjak, Maureen Lee
Stach, Dr Brad A **(A)**
Stach, Carol Blossom **(SLP)**
Stearns, Agnes T **(SLP)**
Steer, Mrs Elizabeth (Betsy) L **(SLP)**
Stephens, Mrs Janice Clare **(SLP)**
St Jacques, Mrs Patricia Bohac **(SLP)**
Stolzberg, Mrs Hilary M **(SLP)**
Stoner, Wynette Renae **(A)**
Stout, Gayle **(A)**
Strother, Mrs Rebecca Joy **(SLP)**
Stubblefield, Lacinda Kaye **(SLP)**
Sullivan, Gayla K **(A)**
Sutton, Dr Lois **(A)**
Tammone, Karen Lee **(SLP)**
Taylor, Mrs Sherri S **(SLP)**
Tett, Pamela G **(SLP)**
Thaxton, Loree D
Thompson, Dena Fletcher **(SLP)**
Thompson, Mrs Linda Conley **(SLP)**
Till, Kathleen Kiddon **(SLP)**
Timby, Mrs Marsha M **(SLP)**
Todd, Mrs Margaret Florance **(SLP)**
Toman, Mrs Barbara Kessler **(SLP)**
Tompkins, Susan Morgan **(A)**
Toombs, Margaret S **(SLP)**
Unruh, Mrs Jane Barrick **(SLP)**
Upchurch, Mrs Carla Blakley **(SLP)**
Van Haalen, Teresa G **(SLP)**
Vankleeck, Mrs Marilyn M **(A)**
Vavra, Mrs Alicia O R **(SLP)**
Vigilante, Carla **(SLP)**
Viswanath, Nagalapura S **(SLP)**
Walker, Bobbie Lonsford **(SLP)**
Walker, Mrs Roberta A **(SLP)**
Walther, Bonnie J **(SLP)**
Walton, Anne **(SLP)**
Walton, Michael W **(SLP)**
Warren, Kechia Virginia
Waryas, Dr Carol Lynn **(SLP)**
Waryas, Dr Paul Allen **(A)**
Wasson, Miriam I **(SLP)**
Waters, Larry D **(A)**
Waters, Sandra Cristo **(A)**
Waters, Mrs Saundra C **(SLP)**
Watson, Paula Renee **(A)**
Watters, Sandra M **(SLP)**
Webb, Mrs Jeanette C **(SLP)**
Webster, Mrs Lynda F D **(SLP)**
Wells, Barbara **(SLP)**
Wells, Carolyn R **(SLP)**
West, Ronda Shackelford **(SLP)**
Wheeler, Linda Marie
Whitaker, Oreno Faye **(SLP)**
Whitehead, Jean M **(SLP A)**
Wiggins, Mrs Sheri Freeman **(SLP)**
Wilson, Cathy L **(SLP)**
Wilson, Janice A **(SLP)**
Wilson, Mary A
Wilson, Mrs Sabrina Fowler **(SLP)**
Windle, Jill V **(SLP)**
Winn, Barbara B **(SLP)**
Wizig, Mrs Carol Ann **(SLP)**
Woehr, Donna Yancy **(SLP)**
Wofford, Dr Martha J **(A)**
Wong-Chin, Karen **(SLP)**
Wood, Mrs Elizabeth **(SLP)**
Woolfolk, Mrs Elizabeth Carrow **(SLP)**
Wyatt-Engman, Mrs Margaret F **(SLP)**
Wynter, Cecile A **(SLP)**
Yelich, Ann Marie **(A)**
Yonovitz, Dr A
Zafar, Kausar Humayon **(SLP)**
Zirkelbach, Dr Thelma K **(SLP)**
Zylla-Jones, Elizabeth M **(SLP)**

Humble
Fields, Mrs Danell Liberda **(SLP)**
Hasek, Mrs Carol S **(SLP)**
Howlett, Susan J S **(SLP)**
Janak, Judy A **(SLP)**
Marsh, Mary G **(SLP)**
Riley, Janeva S **(SLP)**
Seitz, Mrs Laura L **(A)**
Spalter, Mrs Joanne Belofsky **(SLP)**
White, Gayl A **(SLP)**

Hunt
Storey, Mary F **(SLP)**

Huntsville
Allred, Dr Phillip L **(A)**
Bobruk, Toni S **(SLP)**
Woodward, Lily L **(SLP)**

Hurst
Cochran, Mrs Teresa Walton **(SLP)**
Endebrock, F Andra B **(SLP)**
Pooley, Mrs Mary Ann Shurina **(SLP)**
Ruiz, Judith H **(SLP)**
Staats, Diane M **(SLP)**
Zimmerman, Mrs Sandra J **(SLP)**

Irving
Achilles, Mrs Judith **(SLP)**
Bell, Mrs Lisa Barnes **(SLP)**
Boles, Mrs Susan P **(SLP)**
Bongfeldt, Mary L T **(SLP)**
Brozka, Thomas William **(SLP)**
Butt, Francis V **(SLP)**
Day, Mrs Antoinette Debner **(SLP)**
Dennison, Laura L **(SLP)**
Dunn, Mrs Janice M **(SLP)**
Fehrs, Kelly Lee **(SLP)**
Fellows, Mrs Alice B **(SLP)**
Foy, Kathleen Maureen **(A)**
Gilhooly, Trudi Patricia **(SLP A)**
Gutierrez, Brenda **(SLP)**
Leibensberger, Gail Ruth
Parker, Tammy Stevens **(SLP)**
Porter, Jane W **(A)**
Porter, Todd H **(A)**
Reeves, Gwenlynn Diann **(SLP)**
Roberts, Cindy Abbott **(SLP)**
Sheets, Mrs Pamela M
Staples, Kimberly Anna **(SLP)**
Vance, Cynthia L **(SLP)**
Wehmeyer, Mrs Jan Blair **(SLP)**
Whatoff, Angela Brooke **(SLP)**
Young, Mrs Debbie Marsh **(SLP)**

Katy
Aspelund, Mrs Leanna C **(SLP)**
Brown, Mrs Jane Hughes **(SLP)**
Cregg, Mrs Leesa Suddath **(A)**
Harrison, Mary Sue **(A)**
Holland, Mrs Bonnie B **(SLP)**
Irons, Mrs Patricia Lynn **(SLP)**
Kerr, Mrs Barbara Benson **(SLP)**
Laflure, Mrs Dorothy Drobny **(SLP)**
Lewis, Mrs Jacquelyn B **(SLP)**
Marcin, Mrs Kathy Elaine **(SLP)**
Ritchey, Mrs Lisa Ann **(SLP)**
Stapleton, Jenny **(SLP)**
Wintersteen, Mrs Marylee Darlene **(SLP)**

Keller
Bauer, Mrs Debra B A **(A)**
Sawyer, Mary E **(SLP)**
Warren, Mrs Tracey Lynne

Kenedy
Wiatrek, Susan Long **(SLP)**

Kermit
Hale, Mrs Bernie A **(SLP)**

Kerrville
Gram, Louis E **(SLP)**
Kilcoyne, Claire N **(A)**
Nitishin, Mrs Leah G **(SLP)**

Killeen
De Salle, Jean Marie
Smith, Mrs Deborah M **(SLP)**

Kingsville
Browning, Mrs Cheryl Virginia **(SLP)**
Nixon, Melodee Annette

Kingwood
Barajas, Mrs Dorinda Ann E **(SLP)**
Birleffi, Mrs Judith A **(A)**
Burns, Mrs Karen Billeter **(SLP)**
Butler, Glenda C **(SLP)**
Campbell, Mrs Peggy E **(SLP)**
Chapman, Mrs Robin W **(SLP)**
Grant, Catherine Shirley
Mansfield, Miriam C **(A)**
Murrell, Darlene Y **(SLP A)**
Orf, Mrs Peggy A **(A)**
Sterrett, Mrs Mary Sue **(SLP)**

Kirby
Jaramillo, Aura Elena **(SLP)**

Knoxville
Nicodemus, Barbara **(A)**

La Grange
Kolbe, Joyce B **(SLP)**
Wanke, Mrs Janis Ann **(SLP)**

La Marque
Tinsley, Glen, Jr **(SLP)**

La Vernia
Sutherland, Harrell C, Jr **(A)**

Lackland AFB
Myers, Mrs Karen Elizabeth **(SLP)**
Scott, Kimberly Rae **(SLP)**
Williamson, Capt Angela Starr **(A)**

Lake Dallas
Lovejoy, Donna Akers **(SLP)**

Lake Jackson
Marable, Denise L **(SLP)**
Nunnery, Mrs Karen B **(SLP)**
Putty, Mrs Patricia Isabel **(SLP)**
Salazar-Jaffe, Renee **(SLP)**

Lakehills
Endicott, Dr James E **(A)**

Lancaster
Walters, Mary Ann **(SLP)**

Laredo
Castillo, Elisa Angers **(SLP)**
Gonzales, Norma **(SLP)**
Kimmel, Mrs Theresa Marie **(SLP)**
Potucek, Ann B **(SLP)**
Rush, Mrs Lisa B **(SLP)**
Willett, Mrs Irma Ramos **(SLP)**

Laughlin AFB
Fleenor, Mary D **(SLP)**

League City
Beckler, Mrs Lynn L **(SLP)**
Callis, Lisa A **(SLP)**
Dawson, Gerald J **(A)**
Kapner, Mary **(SLP)**
Laurence, Mrs Elizabeth Wilkey **(SLP)**
Mackey, Mrs Thada W **(SLP)**
Revis, Margret F **(SLP)**
Richards, Dana Williams **(SLP)**
Sadler, Mrs Suzanne M **(SLP)**
Stogner, Mrs Barbara Pate **(SLP)**

Lewisville
Abshier, Victoria Plunkett **(SLP)**
Berquist, Rebecca Bonini **(A)**
Donnell, Adrienne J **(SLP)**
Hawkins-Seely, Jennifer **(A)**
Helfer, Dr Thomas M **(A)**
Lanham, Mrs Tammy Kay **(A)**
Maxfield, Kathrine M **(SLP)**
Stouppe, Mrs Marilyn Ann **(SLP)**

Lindale
Holland, Mrs Susan E **(A)**
Sharron, Anna Carol **(A)**

Livingston
Myers, Lisa Nanette

Llano
Gayler, Barbara C **(SLP)**

Lockhart
Dennis, Mrs Cassandra Chavez
Stromberg, Mrs Sadie G **(SLP)**

Longview
Dickerson, Mrs Nancy Jo **(SLP)**
Gillam, Brenda Gay **(SLP)**
Green, Kelly R **(A)**
Lo, Dawn R **(SLP)**
Magness, Lana Jaton **(SLP A)**
Parada, Mrs Luann Ulmann **(SLP)**
Summers, Mrs Victoria E **(SLP)**
Supercinski, Mrs Becky Reed **(SLP)**

Lorena
Grygar, Janet H **(SLP)**
Muchow, Mary Katherine **(SLP)**

Los Fresnos
Berg, Mrs Ruth R **(SLP)**

Lubbock
Adkins-Smith, Julie S **(SLP)**
Baker, Dorothy E **(SLP)**
Baliga, Mrs Gayathri Bantwal **(SLP)**
Bray, Mrs Katherine J **(SLP)**
Coons, Mrs Pamela Johnson **(SLP)**
Copple, Mrs Karen Sue **(SLP)**
Crabtree, Rebecca Denise **(SLP)**
Cremeens, Penny R **(SLP)**
Daily, Kathryn Ann **(SLP)**
Davidson, Roseanna C
Duval, Mrs Kathryn Mary **(SLP)**
Flynn, Mrs Deborah Ann **(SLP)**
Ford, Janna R **(SLP)**
Frazier, Mary E **(SLP)**
Grunwald, Eleanor Elizabeth **(A)**
Hamill, Dr Teri Anne **(A)**
Hamre, Dr Curtis E **(SLP)**
Harn, Dr William E **(SLP)**
Hart, Patricia **(SLP)**
Ickes, Dr William K **(SLP A)**
Jones, Bobby D **(SLP)**
Keesee, Mrs Denise Renee **(SLP)**

Kennedy, Mrs Jacqueline **(SLP)**
King, Mrs Nelda K **(SLP)**
Kuratko, Charles Patrick **(A)**
Lawton, Suzan Pflug **(SLP)**
Linville, Dr Raymond N **(SLP)**
Mahan, Mrs Carla S
Maki, Ruanna Kuykendall **(SLP)**
Martin, Nancy Stuart **(SLP)**
McGowan, Mrs Neita B **(SLP)**
Mendenhall, Marcia Ann **(SLP)**
Miller-Linville, Beth Ann **(SLP)**
Moore, Mrs Kathanne Kelly **(SLP)**
Morriss, Mrs Debra M
Muma, Diane B **(SLP)**
Muma, John Ronald **(SLP)**
Oliver, Nancy L **(SLP)**
Palmer, Yolanda **(SLP)**
Patton, Gail D **(SLP)**
Patton, Lynda Rolan
Paxton, Mrs Martha Wilder **(A)**
Perl, Diane **(SLP)**
Rudder, Marynell H **(SLP)**
Sancibrian, Cheryl L **(SLP)**
Schwantz, Janet Rector **(SLP)**
Sims, Mrs Frankie B **(SLP)**
Smith, Mrs Evelyn H **(SLP)**
Smolensky, Mrs Terri Allyn **(SLP)**
Soria, Mrs Jeanne Marie **(A)**
Taylor, Anita Kay **(SLP)**
Thompson, Molly Kathleen S **(SLP)**
Turner, Mrs Nancy Aduddell **(SLP)**
Walters, Lynn Perkins **(SLP)**

Lufkin
De Vries, Karen Leigh **(A)**
Krenzke, Lorre **(SLP)**
Long, Susan D **(SLP)**

Luling
Daniels, Kelly Lee **(SLP)**
Zedler, Dr Empress **(SLP)**

Lumberton
Sheffield, Mrs Priscilla Jo **(SLP)**

Magnolia
Gary, Sherry J **(SLP)**

Manchaca
Johnson, Linda Grassel **(SLP)**
Parker, Anna M L **(SLP)**

Manor
Franklin, June Marie **(SLP)**

Mansfield
Minor, Mrs Carla McNeely
Sizer, Mary K **(SLP)**
Walter, Teri A **(SLP)**

Marble Falls
Rogers, Shelley D **(A)**

Marlin
Nolen, Mrs Cynthia Alice **(SLP)**

Marshall
Bober, Sally Bradburn **(SLP)**
Morgan, Alice A **(SLP)**
Thompson, Mrs Margaret R **(SLP)**

Martindale
Haug, Dr C Olaf **(A)**

Mc Allen
Applbaum, Dr Ronald Lee
Denman, Mrs Edna A **(SLP)**
Doyle, Mrs Dorothy G **(SLP)**
Gurwitz, Mrs Bailey A **(SLP)**
Munneke, Mrs Margaret F **(SLP)**
Nelson, Crystal **(SLP)**
Patton, Mrs Melinda Jane **(SLP)**
Raff, Michael J **(A)**
Raff, Nina Zahn **(SLP)**
Singleton, James M **(A)**
Vasseur-Kwech, Virginia Marie **(A)**

Mc Gregor
Anderson, Samantha G **(SLP)**
Schmidt, Mrs Nan Norton **(SLP)**

Mc Kinney
Hilz, Mrs Lani M **(SLP)**
Kellum, Jane M G **(SLP)**
Reynolds, Susan Marie **(A)**
Yetter, Mary Jean **(SLP)**

Mercedes
Stewart, Mrs Susan E B **(SLP)**

Mesquite
Anderson, Lisa Kay
Boling, Mrs Patricia V **(SLP)**
Davis, Christine **(SLP)**
Green, Mrs Lori Yates **(SLP)**
Hale, Tammy Schraeder **(SLP)**
Mitchell, Sarah F **(SLP)**
Phillips, Stacia White **(SLP)**
Wyman, Kristina Kaye **(SLP)**

Mexia
Anders, Linda Dovalina **(SLP)**
Brunette, Gerald Wayne **(A)**
Cashell, Mrs Joyce Mullican **(SLP)**
Dodge, Colleen **(A)**
Lambert, Dr James David **(SLP A)**
Lutz, Mrs Carol M **(SLP)**
Ridge, Denecia Dodson **(SLP)**

Midland
Beall, Mrs Carolyn R **(A)**
Boyd, Mrs Patricia T **(SLP)**
Burton, Cynthia Jane **(SLP)**
Cobb, Mrs Christine **(SLP)**
Cohagan, Amelia A **(SLP)**
Crabtree, Dr Margaret **(SLP)**
Hawkes, Mrs Mary H **(SLP)**
Herndon, Mrs Kirsten S **(SLP)**
Lee, Mrs Loretta B **(SLP)**
Miller, Mrs Sandra Malyn **(SLP)**
Phillips, Kay S **(SLP)**
Purcell, Orland **(A)**
Purcell, Mrs Sheryll R **(SLP)**
Roberson, Mrs Janet Gary **(A)**
Russell, Susan Jeanne **(SLP)**

Midlothian
Moltz, Mrs Candace C **(SLP)**

Mineral Wells
Dickson, Catherine A **(SLP)**
Gibson, Mrs Peggy Carver **(SLP)**

Mission
Ochoa, Bella Linda L **(SLP)**

Missouri City
Bennett, Leann W **(SLP)**
Janik, Mrs Rosa Lee **(SLP)**
Kent, Mrs Sandra Ferguson **(SLP)**
Moseley, Jacqueline **(SLP)**
Mullins, Mrs Marion M **(SLP)**
Polk, Mrs Marian L **(SLP)**
Rodriguez-Bravo, Leticia **(SLP)**
Upchurch, Tamara A **(SLP)**

Monahans
Gay, Mrs Bonnie T **(SLP)**

Montgomery
Kynett, Deanna **(SLP)**

Mount Pleasant
Collins, Martha B **(SLP)**
Koelliker, Deborah Lee **(SLP)**

Nacogdoches
Anson, Holly **(SLP)**
Bankston, Debra W **(SLP)**
Brennan, Tom
Craig, Mrs Karen Louise
Hanke, Gilbert C **(SLP)**
Hartman, Dr Bernard Thomas **(SLP A)**
Herman, Mrs Suzanne Couch **(SLP)**
Legg, Mrs Hettie F **(SLP)**

Morton, Mrs Karen D **(SLP)**
Stanley, Dr Elnita O **(SLP)**

Nash
Sessions, Mrs Jan A **(SLP)**

Navasota
Coleman, Mrs Carole J **(SLP)**

Nederland
Lege, Mrs Niki Smith **(SLP)**
Mistric, Mrs Catherine **(SLP)**
Powell, Mrs Annette S **(SLP)**
Williams, Gerilyn A **(SLP)**

Needville
Kettler, Mrs Sandra D **(SLP)**

New Braunfels
Campbell, Mrs Cynthia G **(SLP)**
Corona, Mrs Diana Marie **(SLP)**
Duran, Margaret **(SLP)**
Gonzalez, Mrs Lisa M **(SLP)**
Hardee, Dr Weldon P **(SLP)**
Laubach, Mrs Victoria H **(SLP)**
Owens, Mrs Karen E I **(SLP)**
Stadt, Vicki L **(SLP)**
Terry, Joanna Lynn **(SLP)**
Wiggins, Mrs Frances A **(SLP)**

Nocona
Holman, Eileen S
Otto, Frances M **(SLP)**

Normangee
Small, Kristi Lynn **(SLP)**

North Richland Hills
Curtis, Mrs Sandra S **(SLP)**
Everett, Mrs Paula L
Harding, Mrs Cynthia B **(SLP)**
Knight, Kathryn Elaine **(SLP)**
Linker, Mrs Elizabeth L
Records, Mrs Bobbye R **(SLP)**

Odem
Stalcup, Rebecca N **(SLP)**

Odessa
Ahnert, Mrs Alice C **(SLP)**
Beard, Mrs Raquel Tomic
Evins, Linda Faye **(SLP)**
Gailey, Clark E **(A)**
Leever, Lynn C **(SLP)**
Munson, Mrs Theresa J **(SLP)**
Owensrson, Mrs Teresa Kay **(A)**
Pro, Mrs Melissa Le Ann **(SLP)**
Rupp, Diana Susan
Russell, Randy P **(SLP A)**
Stanislav, Monica L **(SLP)**
Thorpe, Kellee Ann **(SLP)**
Zamora, Lourdez Dianna

Orange
Shatto, Donna Leta **(A)**
Shearer, Dale C **(SLP)**

Orange Grove
Alsbrooks, Sharon W **(SLP)**
Gonzalez, Zulema Perez **(SLP)**

Overton
Saathoff, Neva M **(SLP)**

Paige
Freeman, Letitia Smith **(SLP)**

Palestine
Burch, Mary Danko **(A)**
Lindsey, Mrs Pamela Sloan **(SLP)**

Palmer
Capps, Mrs Sunshine Williamson **(SLP)**

Pampa
Agee, Mrs Teresa McGowan **(SLP)**
Alexander, Mrs Susan S **(SLP)**
Holt, Barbara A **(SLP)**

Paris
Harlan, Glena R **(SLP)**

Loch, Michael C **(A)**
McCleskey, Mrs Marla G **(SLP)**
Stephenson, Kim Lambert **(SLP A)**
Watson, Mrs Cheryl Ann **(SLP)**

Pasadena
Chessher, Mrs Rita Ann **(SLP)**
Elkins, Mrs Andee Ann **(SLP)**
Koenig, Mrs Marcia L **(SLP)**

Pearland
Cinciripini, Mrs Doreen Dora **(SLP)**
Davis, Shirley J **(SLP)**
Oliver, Terrey A **(A)**
Shatto, Mrs Kathleen C **(SLP)**

Pearsall
Murray, Donna E **(SLP)**

Perryton
Brown, Patricia Benson **(SLP)**

Plainview
Antrobus-Kendall, Sarah A **(SLP)**
Berry, Nina J **(SLP)**
Earls, Mrs Nancy Loree **(SLP)**
Frey, Dr William G **(A)**

Plano
Andrews, Mrs Mary J **(SLP)**
Barbee, Mrs Lynda Jean **(SLP)**
Berg, Mrs Sheryl Swofford **(SLP)**
Bowling, Mary Arrington **(SLP)**
Brennan, Mrs Nancy Ann **(SLP)**
Brink, Lynnette K **(SLP)**
Bushey, Marylou R **(SLP)**
Campbell, Mrs Lauralee F **(SLP)**
Carlsen, Alice F **(A)**
Dawes, Michele Lynn **(SLP)**
Dichmann, Mrs Karla Louise **(SLP)**
Doughty, Mrs Cecile I **(SLP)**
Elmore, Mrs Janice B **(SLP)**
Farr, Lisa Kay
Ford, Jean Marie **(SLP)**
Galley, Mrs Deborah Hager **(A)**
George, Mrs Helen Gillies **(SLP)**
Germeck, Judith J **(SLP)**
Glaze, Mrs Nancy Humphrey **(SLP)**
Gohl, Mrs Glenna G **(SLP)**
Graff, Mrs Beverly L **(SLP)**
Hafemeister, Mrs Linda V **(SLP)**
Hall, Mrs Laurie Dees **(SLP)**
Harrison, Mrs Susan Arnold **(SLP)**
Henriksen, Joellen Jacobs **(SLP)**
Hill, Clara V **(SLP)**
Hudson, Gail C **(SLP)**
Hughes, Mrs Suann **(SLP)**
Jeffries, Mrs Mary Joan P **(SLP)**
Johnsen, Mrs Sue H **(SLP)**
Koelemay, Mrs Fon W **(SLP)**
Krafcheck, Mrs Debbie J **(SLP)**
Krebs, Mrs Leslie B **(SLP)**
Kuusisto, Rita Paal **(SLP)**
Lantz, Mrs Karen G **(SLP)**
Leight, Gilbert **(SLP)**
Lipson-Ticker, Mrs Denise **(A)**
McCormick, Jean Tedford **(SLP)**
McDaniel, Jane R G **(SLP)**
McDonald, Mrs Melanie Dalrymple **(SLP)**
McLeroy, Kathleen **(A)**
McMahan, Mrs Maxine Marilyn **(SLP)**
Mills, Mary Cathleen **(SLP)**
Morgan, Mrs Lori Jean **(SLP)**
Noble, Mrs Leslie Steckbeck **(SLP)**
Nunnery, Betty D **(SLP)**
Oden, Lorin Star **(A)**
Parker, Ruth N **(SLP)**
Price, Mrs Jeanne Virginia
Rentschler, Mrs Pamela Jo **(SLP)**
Russell, Mrs Sharon A **(SLP)**
Ryan, Jodell Newman **(A)**
Shandor, Judith A Sparks **(SLP)**
Shelton, Mrs Susan N **(SLP)**
Silver, Lynn **(SLP)**
Sims, Mrs Elizabeth Asbury **(SLP)**

Socolof, Mrs Gale L **(SLP)**
Starkel, John Philip
Strickland, Mrs Kristie Jensen **(SLP)**
Toal, Carmen S **(SLP)**
Todd, Mrs Deborah S **(SLP)**
Van Loozen, Dorothy Cox **(SLP)**
Walner, Mrs Joan C **(SLP)**
Whelan, Mrs Janice M **(SLP)**
Woods, Mrs Elissa Bennack **(SLP)**
Youngblood, Mrs Brenda K **(SLP)**

Pleasanton

Gebheim, Mrs Janie Fairchilds **(A)**
Williams, Mrs Caroline Miller **(SLP)**

Port Arthur

Beckman, John Thomas
Bolch, Tammie M **(SLP)**
Oldham, Jackson D **(SLP)**
Savell, Paula E **(SLP)**

Port Lavaca

Terasaki, Dr Diana Lynn **(SLP)**

Port Neches

Clark, Mrs Mona Lisa **(SLP)**

Portland

Holt, Mrs Janet Clark
Hopkins, Margot Trushaw **(SLP)**
Langford, Marietta M **(SLP)**
McLeroy, Mrs Carol M **(SLP)**
Rollison, Larry L **(A)**
Stryk, Mrs Rebecca Phillips **(SLP)**

Purdon

Kurland, Mrs Linda Roberts **(SLP)**

Rankin

Kuhlmann, Marcia D **(SLP)**

Redford

Manno, Mrs Carol Eve **(SLP)**

Richardson

Alexander, Mrs Jeran D **(SLP)**
Alfson, Karen K **(SLP)**
Brown, Mrs Lynne M **(SLP)**
Buckner, Mrs Rebecca Ray **(SLP)**
Cobb, Karen L **(SLP)**
Crim, Mrs Sidney A **(SLP)**
Garrett, Margaret Jean **(SLP)**
Gonzalez, Mrs Rebecca C **(SLP)**
Hachtel, Mrs Marsha J **(SLP)**
Hendricks-Godby, Mrs Beverly J **(A)**
Hengstenberg, Kate **(SLP A)**
Hopper, Kay Lynn **(SLP)**
Hummel, Karen S **(SLP)**
Johnstone, Diane B **(SLP)**
Keylon, Mrs Judy G **(SLP)**
King, Carol Leigh **(SLP)**
Kratville, Mrs Carol A D **(SLP)**
Lodwick, Mrs Helen **(SLP)**
MacDonald, Mrs D Hannah **(SLP)**
Marshall, Mrs Phyllis **(SLP)**
Mason, Clarice Jaynes **(SLP)**
McKenna, Teresa E **(SLP)**
McKnight, Mrs Catherine Margaret **(SLP)**
Meek, Kathleen Stauffer **(SLP)**
Musket, Mrs Carolyn H **(A)**
Post, Jimmy D **(A)**
Shaw, Mrs Ann E **(SLP)**
Smith, Shirley Cronin **(SLP)**
Snow, Mrs Billie Reed **(SLP)**
Stamps, Patricia Lynn **(SLP)**
Sudbrink, Pamela Dawn
Taylor, Mrs Cynthia Lee **(SLP)**
Walker, Ann B **(SLP)**
Ward, Mrs Leslie G
Wesley, Carol Lorraine **(SLP)**
White, Mrs Carolyn Martin **(SLP)**
Wolff, Suzanne Gits **(SLP)**

Richmond

Christiana, Diana Grana **(SLP)**
Gurecky, Cynthia S **(SLP)**
Kalinowski, Mrs Linda C **(SLP)**
Pellerin, Robert J **(A)**
Smitheal, Mrs Judith W **(SLP)**
Spittler, Janice **(SLP)**
Stallings, Stephen Scott **(A)**
Wallace, Mrs Dana D **(SLP)**

Richwood

Helling, Celeste Rita
Kriss, Charles Anthony, Jr **(A)**

Richwood Clute

Wilson, Mrs Yvonne H **(SLP)**

Roanoke

Huff, Mrs Brenda Kay **(SLP)**
Johnson, Mrs Deborah K B **(SLP)**
Roach, Sharla B **(A)**

Rockdale

Gebhart, Janice Lou M **(SLP)**

Rockport

Clark, Janice Z **(SLP)**

Rockwall

Abernathy, Mrs Dorothy E **(SLP)**
Henry, Mrs Linda Sue **(SLP)**
Kozlovsky, Eva B **(SLP)**
Spiva, Jane A **(SLP)**
Woodward, Mrs Laura D **(SLP)**
Zerfas, Mrs Terri Bumpas **(SLP)**

Round Rock

Bray, Victor H, Jr **(A)**
Meuse, Dr Sheila A **(SLP)**
Morgan, Mrs Karen Gough **(SLP)**
Wysuph, Mrs Pamela A **(SLP)**

Rowlett

Barnes, Laura Ann **(SLP)**
Newell, Mrs Kathleen Pierson **(SLP)**

Rusk

Harris, Marilyn S **(SLP)**

Salado

Rodriguez, Mrs Debra Jean **(SLP)**

San Angelo

Abbott, Mrs Marcia Staggs **(SLP)**
Bradley, Susan Kay **(A)**
Comstock, Cathryn Lynn **(A)**
Hamilton, Debra Jo **(A)**
Killam, Mrs Doris **(SLP)**
Kulig, Dr Sharon G **(SLP)**
Murphy, Gail E **(SLP)**
Pierce, Dr Sharalee **(SLP)**
Reeves, Mrs Susan D **(SLP)**
Stinnett, Elizabeth A/Simpson **(SLP)**
Welch, Cara Suzette **(A)**
Wilson, Christine M **(SLP)**
Wilson, Mrs Suzan Gayle **(SLP)**
Young, Mrs Nanci Cheryll **(SLP)**

San Antonio

Allen, Tedi **(SLP)**
Barnett, Claudette S **(SLP)**
Barnett, Mary Barbara **(SLP)**
Batezel, Mrs Roxanne Kay **(SLP)**
Bay, Jean E **(SLP)**
Bean, Donald R **(SLP)**
Beard, Maria Cherie
Belsjoe, Frances W **(SLP)**
Bender, Dr Donald R **(A)**
Biggerstaff, Karen Diane **(SLP)**
Billik, Cheryl W **(SLP)**
Bishop, Linda H **(SLP)**
Black-Lawson, Virginia L **(SLP)**
Blase, Mrs Jane Z **(SLP)**
Bloom, Mrs Thea I **(SLP)**
Boone, Kathleen M **(A)**
Borglund, Patricia **(SLP)**
Bragg, Dr Vernon C **(A)**
Brannon, Patricia C **(SLP)**
Breidenbach, Mrs Lynda M **(SLP)**
Brelsford, Jacalyn Lee **(A)**
Bryson, Mrs Marilyn Scott **(SLP)**
Burough, Leallan L **(A)**
Burris, Laura Ann **(A)**
Cantu, Evangeline **(SLP)**
Carssow-Robbins, Cynthia **(SLP)**
Casarez, Sylvia Ann
Ceccatti, Carol Steffler **(SLP)**
Chambers, Mrs Floy Beth **(SLP)**
Chambers, Nancy C **(SLP)**
Charlip, Dr Walter S **(A)**
Cherniss, Mrs Suzan Marie **(SLP)**
Clowe, Gail G **(SLP)**
Constanzo, Cindy A **(SLP)**
Correa, Alma Morales **(SLP)**
Crawford, Cheryle Saunders **(SLP)**
Cutts, Mrs Betty Powell **(A)**
Danford, Roy, Jr **(A)**
Davalos, Lancey H **(SLP)**
Davidson, Jane B **(SLP)**
Davidson, Mrs Leslie Ann **(SLP)**
Delgado-Gaitan, Margaret **(SLP)**
Dellenback, Cynthia H **(SLP)**
Deppensmith, Kathryn McDonald **(A)**
Dielmann, Sharon M **(SLP)**
Dix, Patricia Elizabeth **(SLP)**
Dudich, Tim M **(A)**
Dugger, Mrs Nancy Wray **(SLP)**
Dunham, Ruth J **(SLP)**
Eades, Malinda P
Effenberger, Cynthia Ann **(SLP)**
Elkins, Mrs Suzanne H **(SLP)**
Emge, Marie E **(SLP)**
Enriquez, Mrs Linda Maclas **(SLP)**
Eugenio, Mrs Carolyn S **(SLP)**
Eugenio, Elmo E **(SLP)**
Ferguson, Mrs LaDonna Meeks **(A)**
Fleisig, Mrs Marsha C **(SLP)**
Flores, Mary H **(SLP)**
Flores, Nancy Martinez **(SLP)**
Freeman, Eleanor M **(SLP)**
Gardiner, Paula M R **(SLP)**
Garis, Mrs Marcine **(SLP)**
Garvin, Mrs Susanne B **(SLP)**
Garza, Anna Belinda **(SLP)**
George, Kathryn A **(A)**
Gibson, Virginia S **(SLP)**
Gilchrist, Linda A **(SLP)**
Gioiello-Meyer, Mrs Jacqueline Jean **(SLP)**
Gonzales, Jo Ann **(SLP)**
Gonzalez-Sierra, Maria N **(SLP)**
Goolsby, Mrs Pamela A **(SLP)**
Gooze, Dr Edward C **(SLP)**
Gooze, Mrs Sally Schneir **(SLP)**
Grant, Dr June Myers
Grassman, Mrs Joan C **(SLP)**
Greenwood, Mrs Janet Cain **(SLP)**
Guerrero, Janis Mazurek **(SLP)**
Gureckis, Mrs Kathleen M **(SLP)**
Haag, Terri L S **(SLP)**
Hamlyn, Hugh W **(SLP)**
Harris, Joyce L **(SLP)**
Hayes, Hazel Denise **(SLP)**
Herman, Mrs Louisa M **(SLP)**
Hernandez, Gilbert V **(SLP)**
Hill, Capt Brian J **(A)**
Hogan, Diann Davis **(SLP)**
Holguin, Yolanda Garza **(A)**
Horn, Monica A **(SLP)**
Horney, Kathryn Ruth **(SLP)**
House, Len M **(SLP)**
Hrovat, Susan D **(SLP)**
Irwin, James Ross **(A)**
Johns, Mary Bloomquist **(SLP)**
Johnson, James W **(A)**
Juarez, Irma Estella **(SLP)**
Juarez, Dr Manuela **(SLP)**
Juenke, Dorothy Ebersole **(SLP)**
Keeler, Janice W **(SLP)**
Khan, Linda M L **(SLP)**
Kinion, Renee Louise
Kolb, Karen C **(SLP)**
Kriske, Mrs Lydia Lucio **(SLP)**
Labatt, Mrs Laura M **(SLP)**
L'Armee, Claudette **(SLP)**
Lauder, Edmund **(SLP)**
Lecholop, Carol R **(SLP)**
Lehne, Mrs Kathryn Audette
Lewis, Rosemary M **(SLP)**
Linville, Mrs Debra Devore **(SLP)**
Lovell, Mrs Debra Mase **(SLP)**
Lowery, Dr Scott D **(SLP)**
Luduena, Linda G **(SLP)**
Luthy, Sheila Snell **(SLP)**
Marriott, Mrs Kay Joyce
Martinez, Frieda Bleeck **(SLP)**
Martinez, Mrs Regina Ann **(SLP)**
McClendon, Mrs Carol S **(SLP)**
McDonald, Mrs Ann M **(SLP)**
Mesa, Mrs Linda S **(SLP)**
Miller, Mrs Laurie W **(SLP)**
Moses, Dr Gerald R **(SLP)**
Moses, Mrs Maryann C **(SLP)**
Mullen, Mrs Elisa Celeste **(SLP)**
Napier, Marcia **(SLP)**
Nelson, Loetitia M **(SLP)**
Nelson, Mrs Sally M **(SLP)**
Nemky, Martha T **(SLP)**
O'Connor, Mrs Judy L A **(SLP)**
Offutt, Pamela Gene **(SLP)**
Olberding, Mrs Lucynda R **(SLP)**
Oliver, Mrs Leslie Blackwell **(SLP)**
O'Malley, Mrs Janet B **(SLP)**
Padilla, Belinda Hazel **(SLP)**
Page, Mrs Yvonne **(SLP)**
Patterson, Jean Kraege **(SLP)**
Paynter, Dr Earlene T **(SLP)**
Perkins, Lana L **(SLP)**
Pillow, A Hart **(SLP)**
Pommerening, Mrs Connie E **(SLP)**
Porter, Patricia L **(SLP)**
Powell, Mrs Janna Rhodes **(SLP)**
Prochazka, Katherine Marie **(SLP)**
Pulcifer, Maj Donald E **(SLP A)**
Rane, Dr Robert L **(A)**
Reeves, Deborah A **(A)**
Reilly, Margaret Hoover **(SLP)**
Renfro-Lesley, Rachel Pozniak **(SLP)**
Ribera, John E **(A)**
Riddell, S Frances **(SLP A)**
Ritter, Dr Ronald L **(A)**
Roberson, Mrs Terri Hill **(A)**
Rodriguez, Mary Ruth **(SLP)**
Rosenberg, Arthur L **(SLP)**
Rost, Alan John **(A)**
Ryan, Cathy Elizabeth **(SLP)**
Saenz, Amparo Aida
Salomon, Mrs Judith Zalmanott **(SLP)**
Sanders, Mrs Deborah P **(SLP)**
Sanner, Mrs Joan Ella **(SLP)**
Scharlack, Gaby Ray E **(SLP)**
Schoolcraft, Mary C **(SLP)**
Schrader, Clarence H **(SLP)**
Schultz, Lynette C **(SLP)**
Scruggs, Theresa Babinsky **(SLP)**
Shearn, Nancy Weaver **(SLP A)**
Sheldon, Shelly A **(SLP)**
Sherris, Capt Cari Ann **(SLP A)**
Sierra-Irizarry, Benigno **(A)**
Simpson, Linda Smith **(A)**
Simpson, Mrs Sarah M **(SLP)**
Smith, April Gayle **(SLP)**
Sparkman, Linda L **(SLP)**
Sparks, Mrs Joni F **(SLP)**
Spiser, Holly Kay **(A)**
Spiser, Valarie L **(SLP)**
Starr, Mrs Nancy E **(SLP)**
Stevenson, Michael H **(A)**
Stewart, Barbara Stewart
Sweatt, Mrs M Lynn **(SLP)**
Swiercinsky, Mrs Carol A **(SLP)**
Swinny, Dr Frances R **(SLP)**
Sykes, Barbara T **(SLP)**
Tatum, Pamela E **(SLP)**
Terrell, Joanne M **(SLP)**
Thomas, Mrs Alice F **(SLP)**
Thompson, Heather Lee **(SLP)**

Travers, Capt Denise M **(SLP)**
Trujillo, Denise E **(SLP)**
Tuller, Linda Golden **(SLP)**
Tyler, Melanie **(SLP)**
Tynan, Mary P **(SLP)**
Urbanczyk, Amanda Elizabeth
Uvodic, Kathleen T **(SLP)**
Vogel, Dr Deanie **(SLP)**
Walsh, Karen C **(SLP)**
Warren, Barbara Crownover **(SLP)**
Warren, Mrs Nancy H **(SLP)**
Wasson, Patricia M **(SLP)**
Waterwall, Jeannit Elain **(SLP)**
Webster, Kathy L **(SLP)**
Wessell, Mrs Margery H **(SLP)**
Wester, Linda **(SLP)**
Wheeler, Kathy M **(SLP)**
White, Anne C **(A)**
Wilke, Mrs Debra D **(SLP)**
Winkler, Lois Jeanne **(SLP)**
Wood, Mrs Rebecca Marsh **(SLP)**
Wright, Mrs Anne T **(SLP)**
Young, Mrs Karen L **(SLP)**
Zepeda, Isabel Castillo **(SLP)**
Zuniga, Mrs Deborah Ann

San Marcos
Armstrong, Susan **(SLP)**
Baker, Billie Ruth **(A)**
Boruff, Diane C **(SLP)**
Byrd, Mrs Nancy Sorrentino **(SLP)**
Castilla, Mary Helen
Fletcher, Dr John Lynn
Hethcock, Mrs Laura M **(SLP)**
Hopkins, Mrs Lori Marie **(SLP)**
Howle, Mrs Nell T **(SLP)**
Kosary, Therese Ann **(SLP)**
Mallard, Dr A Dick **(SLP)**
McBryde, Mrs Terri Moore **(SLP)**
McCall, Mrs Carolyn M **(SLP)**
Ward, Dr Doyle G **(SLP)**
Wilson, Sharon A **(SLP)**

Sanger
Murrell, Mrs Karen T **(SLP)**
Stevens, Nancy C **(SLP)**

Schertz
Hollingsworth, Mrs Rita M **(SLP)**

Seabrook
Neff, Mrs Rachel Lynn

Seguin
Henderson, Carol Williams
Selig, Mrs Gertrude Zanar **(SLP)**

Sherman
Chlipala, M Linda **(SLP)**
Collins, Emilie S **(A)**
Deal, Donald Bryan **(A)**
Flowers, Donna Jean **(SLP)**
Fuller, Mrs Charlotte **(SLP)**
Geier, John Glover **(SLP)**
Graham, Paula Patterson **(SLP)**
Quesnel, Leah Kayrin
Sanders, Mrs Cynthia A **(SLP)**
Smith, Sharon Marie

Silsbee
Beck, Mrs Diane Elizabeth **(SLP)**

Sour Lake
Maddox, Mrs Gail G **(SLP)**

Southlake
Samartin, Mrs Lucille P **(SLP)**

Spring
Applegate, Mrs Mary P **(SLP)**
Babington, Vicki L **(SLP)**
Bailey, Mrs Cherie Campagna **(SLP)**
Baker, Kelley D **(SLP)**
Cates, Mrs Laurel B **(SLP)**
Chadwick, Abbie B **(SLP)**
Coleman, Deborah Z
Crowley, Melissa Ann **(SLP)**
Gadler, Judi B T **(SLP)**
Graham, Laura Gates **(SLP)**
Harris, Mrs C Denice **(SLP)**
Kennedy, Jera J **(SLP)**
Krepps, Mrs Cathleen Stowe **(SLP)**
Lutgen, Mrs Kathleen Duerinck **(SLP)**
Steele, Mrs Lisa E **(SLP)**
Stevens, Patricia Hagan **(A)**
Wyatt, Mrs Linda Chatalian **(SLP)**

Spring Branch
Richardson, Mrs Sharon M **(SLP)**

St Hedwig
Friesenhahn, Mrs Denise Simecki **(SLP)**

Stephenville
Dorsett, Susan G **(A)**
Svien, Leonard D **(SLP)**

Sugar Land
Bathey, Janet Rose **(SLP)**
Blakesley, Kathryn Lucier **(SLP)**
Brown, Patricia S **(SLP)**
Crosley, Mrs Pamela Ann
Douthit, Lillian **(SLP)**
English, Sally A D **(SLP)**
Farris, Kathryn B **(SLP)**
Flynn, Vicki H **(A)**
Gilden, Mrs Jan L **(A)**
Glasofer, Mrs Janet T **(SLP)**
Hansen, Luann Tietge **(SLP)**
Harper, Dahlia B S **(SLP)**
Hughes, Deborah Dukes **(SLP)**
Pry, Mrs Erlene B **(SLP)**
Rosenberg, Barbara C **(SLP)**
Rosenzweig, Mrs Margaret C **(SLP)**
Sears, Cynthia Hooker **(A)**
Swanson, Mrs Sharon Kay **(SLP)**
Tardy, Mrs Kathryn K **(SLP)**
Verburg, Mrs Virginia L **(SLP)**
Wall, Mrs Mary Elizabeth **(SLP)**

Sweetwater
Bonner, Mrs Norma T **(SLP)**

Taylor
Morgan, Elizabeth Ash **(SLP)**

Teague
Eppes, Linda F **(SLP)**

Temple
Atwood, Mrs Kathryn P **(SLP)**
Baker, Nancy Mae **(A)**
Beaver, Harold G **(SLP A)**
Dunlop, Dr Jeanette M **(SLP)**
Dunlop, Dr Robert J **(A)**
Elwood, Mrs Joanne F **(SLP)**
Faulkenburg, Kim Rene **(A)**
Jackson, Mrs Laurie Lynn K **(SLP)**
Lorenz, Deborah G **(SLP)**
Lueck, Dr Anne Gillespie **(SLP)**
McClellan, Mrs Lucile E **(SLP)**
Peterson, Dr David D **(SLP)**
Salzman, Virginia H **(SLP)**
Stark, Dr Earl W **(A)**
Venus, Dr Carol A **(SLP)**
Wardell, Ferman N **(A)**

Terrell
Burks, Dr Sheila S **(SLP)**

Texarkana
Burns, Thomas D **(A)**
Campbell, Mrs Mary Alesia **(SLP)**
Carter, Jeannie Snodgrass **(SLP)**
Coleman, Judy F Harmon **(A)**
Houser, Jo M **(SLP A)**
Quebedeaux, Darla Rochelle **(SLP)**
Seals, Mrs Jody Lynn **(A)**
Stanley, Susan Williams **(SLP)**
Wood, Debra Sue **(SLP)**
Young, Mrs Paula Elaine **(SLP)**

Texas City
Fass, Patricia A **(SLP)**

The Colony
Hogg, Mrs Nina Justice **(SLP)**
Kirkpatrick, Mrs Sandra Lee **(SLP)**
Salmon, Mrs Jeannette Wernette **(SLP)**

The Woodlands
Capozzoli, Mrs Kathleen R **(SLP)**
Kuberry, Gjoa **(SLP)**
Lefort, Claudia A **(A)**
Ligas, Michael J **(SLP)**
O'Banion, Mrs Kathryn Lou **(SLP)**
Pacelli, Monica M **(A)**
Samfield, Barbara A **(SLP)**
Vogelhuber, Barbara Wickson **(A)**

Tomball
Wood, Marla K **(SLP)**

Trophy Club
Wheeler, Catherine **(SLP)**

Tyler
Bell, Raylene **(SLP)**
Colley, Mrs Carol A **(SLP)**
Felknor, Gratia Aileen **(SLP)**
Fulcher, Starr Reed **(SLP)**
Garrett, Joan **(SLP)**
Gilliam, Lauren S **(SLP)**
Hicks, Mrs Laurie Leslie **(A)**
Leeper, Nancy S **(SLP)**
Mahaffey, Mrs Joy A **(SLP)**
Mitchell, Judy M **(SLP)**
Moseley, Mrs Faye
Moseley, Dr Mac R **(SLP)**
Murphy, Mrs Donna K **(SLP)**
Pattullo, Anne Cox **(SLP)**
Peterson, Dr Laura N **(SLP)**
Pitts, Mrs Deborah Dailey **(SLP)**
Powell, Mrs Cynthia **(SLP)**
Sanford, Tracey **(SLP)**
Simpson, Rosemary **(A)**
Sloan, Lisa Karen **(SLP)**
Thomas, Susan Ridenhour **(SLP)**
Turner, Charles R
Twomey, David L **(A)**
Ware, Myra Jo **(SLP)**
Weir, Mitzi Hancock **(SLP)**

Universal City
O'Neal, Harriett **(SLP)**
Pass, Barbara B **(SLP)**
Poulsen, Barbara Frantz **(SLP A)**
Scanlon, Mrs Louise **(SLP)**

Uvalde
Nowlin, Dr Joy O **(SLP)**

Vernon
Little, Mrs Patricia S **(SLP)**
Sharp, Margaret Ann **(SLP)**

Victoria
Bischofshausen, Dr Sharon **(SLP)**
Blackshare, Cynthia McDonald
Cire, George E **(A)**
Collins, Lula Mae **(SLP)**
Cox, Mary Steele **(SLP)**
Hopson, Cheryl A **(SLP)**
McAlpine, Mrs Catherine A **(SLP)**
Parrott, Mrs Margaret E **(A)**
Stevenson, Mrs Sandra Jo **(SLP)**
Stryk-Longoria, Mrs Janice **(SLP)**
Worsley, Mrs Martha W **(SLP)**

Vidor
Castilaw, Karen Ballard **(SLP)**

Waco
Balbo, John M **(A)**
Behnke, Sue E **(SLP)**
Bohn, Jane E **(SLP)**
Bradfield, Lisa C **(SLP)**
Carter, Angela N **(SLP)**
Casas, Melody S V **(SLP A)**
Cassel, Debbie **(SLP)**
Cook, Deborah Knowles **(SLP)**
Croyle, Mrs Edana C **(SLP)**
Downing, Karen Dianne **(SLP)**
Elias, Mrs Patricia D **(SLP)**
Gage, Mrs La Vada W Herring **(SLP)**
Gateley, Dr William G **(SLP)**
Grayson, Mrs Danni Leigh **(SLP)**
Johnson, Mrs Ann F **(SLP)**
Johnson, Mrs Cathy J **(SLP)**
Jones, Mrs Priscilla Henderson **(SLP)**
Klaras, Mrs Denise Demaret **(A)**
Lambert, Mrs Alice M **(SLP)**
Martin, Gloria Rodriguez **(SLP)**
Murphy, Mrs Mary Ann **(SLP)**
Powell, Mrs Donna Lynne **(SLP)**
Richards, Dr Allan L **(A)**
Ritter, Michaela J **(SLP)**
Rivers, Dr David L **(SLP)**
Rogers, Crystal F **(SLP)**
Scott, Susan Scoggins **(SLP)**
Simpson, Elizabeth **(SLP)**
Stein, Felisha Glass **(SLP)**
Sterling, Beverly A **(SLP)**
Stewart, Mrs Janice Ann **(SLP)**
Timmons, Mary Catherine **(SLP)**
Velasquez, Mrs Stacy Goodrich **(SLP A)**

Wake Village
Youngblood, Karen W **(SLP)**

Warren
Evans, Patricia Bryan **(SLP)**

Waskom
Grider, Cathy Belcher **(SLP)**

Waxahachie
Hadley, Sarah Catherine **(SLP)**
King, Kayla Rochelle

Weatherford
Bealmear, Dr Mary K **(SLP)**
Stinson, Mrs Myra Livingston **(SLP)**

Webster
Blanchette, Jacqueline Anne **(SLP)**
D'Aniello, Anthony J **(A)**
Frazier, Laura Jane **(SLP)**
Robinson, Mrs Michelle Kimberly
Turner, Linda S **(SLP)**

Wharton
Snelling, Mrs Barbara Oberg **(A)**
Squires, Mrs Regena H **(SLP A)**

White Oak
Phillips, Mrs Trevelyn Mosher **(SLP)**

Whitesboro
Gellinger, Susan L **(SLP)**

Wichita Falls
Bender, Mrs Pamela A Z **(A)**
Bender, Ron G **(SLP)**
Boone, Cyndi Cuba **(SLP)**
Brady, Mrs Ricki I **(SLP)**
Clark, Mrs Beverly L **(SLP)**
Cowart, Gwendolyn **(SLP)**
Hathaway, Mrs Carrie Ristow **(A)**
Henderson, Leesa Simons **(SLP)**
Howald, Mrs Carolyn Frances **(SLP)**
Jackson, Mrs Nina Jim **(SLP)**
Kerr, Rosellen **(SLP)**
Lamb, Mrs Patricia A **(SLP)**
Onstott, Mrs Karla Cummings
Osborn, Mrs Katherine Vahey **(SLP)**
Stewart, Terri S **(SLP)**
Street, Mrs Robin Webb **(SLP)**
Tanaka, Mieko **(A)**
Turner, Paula Marie **(A)**
Varelman, Dian W **(SLP)**
Watkins, Karen J **(A)**
Williams, Martha **(SLP)**

Wimberley
Kelly, Vanessa McIntosh **(SLP)**
Mayne, Mrs Pat L **(SLP)**
Rigby, Susan P **(SLP)**
Rogers, Mercedes **(SLP)**

Winters
Rives, Mrs Mary E B **(SLP)**

Woodlands
Gardner, Mrs Polly J **(SLP)**
Ramirez, Susan Gayle **(SLP)**

Woodville
Cordes, Mrs Dede Gerke **(SLP)**

Wortham
Forrest, Kathleen **(SLP)**

UTAH

American Fork
Blackburn, Mrs Starla Lucido **(SLP)**
Clarke, Shawn Sawyer **(SLP)**
Mecham, Richard W **(SLP)**

Bountiful
Beauregard, Roxann **(SLP)**
Gilbert, Connie Lee **(SLP)**
Gudmundson, Bonnie S **(SLP)**
Johnson, Sandra Stringham **(SLP)**
Mecham, Dr Merlin J **(SLP)**
Nelson, Laurie **(A)**
Paasch, Elaine K **(SLP)**
Pergler, Harold R **(A)**

Brigham City
Chlarson, Leann **(SLP)**

Brighton
Full, Mariette Helene **(SLP)**

Cedar City
McArthur, Madelyn **(SLP)**
Nielsen, Lynn **(SLP)**

Centerville
Holbrook, Sally **(SLP)**
Keller, Karen Leone **(A)**
Leishman, Kim B **(SLP)**
Reitz, Mary Lou D **(A)**
Tea, Mrs Janice S

Cleveland
Player, Mrs Kim Williams **(SLP)**

Derby
Willis, Lisa Jean **(SLP)**

Eden
Agricola, Mrs Susan Merrill **(A)**

Fairview
Smith, Mrs Patricia S **(SLP)**

Farmington
Barton, Mrs Jill H
Ernstrom, Vera J **(SLP)**

Heber
Nielsen, Mrs Elise E **(SLP)**

Helper
Kohlman, Sandra N **(SLP)**

Highland
Russon, Mrs Karen Vincent **(SLP)**
Young, Kathryn Benton **(SLP)**

Hill AFB
Tate, Rebecca C **(SLP)**

Honeyville
Stokes, Orvil J **(SLP)**

Hurricane
Peek, Mrs Michelle S **(SLP)**

Hyrum
Griffith, David L **(SLP)**

Kaysville
Ashmead, Dr Allez M **(SLP)**
Howe, Mrs Marilyn K **(SLP)**
Nielson, Dr Melvin A **(SLP A)**

Kearns
James, Mary Catherine **(SLP)**
Marchant, Calvin R **(SLP A)**

Layton
Barnum, Lawrence Dean **(A)**
Ellibee, Gina Holman **(SLP)**
Magnuson-Jongsma, Mrs Cleo Grace **(SLP)**
Randall, Kurt D **(A)**

Lehi
Vance, Michelle Chamberlai **(SLP)**
Vanwagoner, Richard S **(A)**

Lewiston
Gailey, Terri S **(SLP)**
Littledike, Lila Jaclyn **(SLP)**

Liberty
Smyka, Richard Joseph **(A)**

Logan
Bailey, Mrs Tyyna M
Balcena, Alice M
Berg, Dr Frederick S **(A)**
Blair, Dr James Carson **(A)**
Child, Dee R **(SLP)**
Elsweiler, Mrs Anne Wolters **(SLP)**
Gantz, Mrs Kathryn Snyder **(SLP)**
Giordano-Olson, Mrs Judy A
Jensen, Mrs Janet Kay **(SLP)**
Jensen, Dr Jay R **(SLP)**
Johnson, Dr Thomas Stoddard **(SLP)**
McWhorter, Mrs Sue Jordan **(SLP)**
Pierce, Alesia J **(SLP)**
Rawlins, J'Lene **(SLP)**
Rowland, Cynthia Jane **(SLP)**
Straquadine, Judith E T **(SLP)**
Street, Caroline **(A)**
Strong, Carol D **(SLP)**
Viehweg, Dr Steven H **(A)**
Walton, Patricia A **(SLP)**

Magna
Randolph, Loren J **(A)**

Mendon
Larsen, Mrs Sandra M **(SLP)**

Midvale
Babcock, Susan L **(SLP)**
Logan, Carol Lynn **(A)**
Smith, Laura Lee **(SLP)**
Squire, Shauna K **(SLP)**
Stringham, Roxanne H **(SLP)**

Murray
Anderson, Patricia Lynn
Brown, Laurel O **(SLP)**
Durham, Kathleen E **(SLP)**
Fue, Laurie D **(SLP)**
Hartmann, Barbara V **(SLP)**
Rotman, Mrs Linda Carole **(SLP)**
Sanches, Jean Elizabeth **(SLP)**
Spensko-Arellano, Kelly Sue **(SLP)**

Nephi
Jensen, Darrell L **(SLP)**

North Logan
Seamons-Lindquist, Carla

Ogden
Boman, Tel S **(A)**
Christensen, Gordon V **(SLP)**
Fakhraie, Mrs Kay Davis **(SLP)**
Harward, Stephen B **(A)**
Healey, Mrs Kay Novak **(SLP)**
John, Mrs Valerie L **(SLP)**
Knighton, Robert D **(SLP)**
Lee, Mrs Karen M **(SLP)**
Lundwall, Cherilyn J **(SLP)**
McCaskey, Monica E F **(SLP)**
Neill, Mrs Sara Lee **(SLP)**
Orme, Cheryl L **(SLP)**
Quercia, Mrs Cindy Harvey **(SLP)**
Roberts, Mrs Noreen Hubbard **(SLP)**
Smith, Mrs Frances G **(SLP)**
Vogel, Mrs Lorilyn King **(SLP)**
Weber, Larry Dwayne **(A)**

Orem
Bartholomew, Mrs Karen Case **(A)**
Channell, Mrs Sandy S **(SLP)**
Christensen, Mrs Alyson Aycock **(SLP)**
Dick, Dr William K **(A)**
El Halta, Barbara Ellayne
Gray, Mrs Donna Jean **(SLP)**
Hilton, Dr Laurence M **(SLP)**
Hogan, Mrs Debra D **(SLP)**
Iler, Mrs Becky B **(SLP)**
Sauter, Mrs Gail Louise **(SLP)**
Schaffner, Elaine Merkley **(SLP)**
Schuldt, Marlo E **(SLP)**
Smith, Michele **(SLP)**
Swensen, W Dean **(SLP)**
Thornton, Mrs Cheryl G **(SLP)**
Townsend, Mrs Joan Adams **(SLP)**
Wallace, Thomas Claude **(SLP)**

Park City
Brock, Lala Suzanne **(SLP)**
Jolley, Elaine Braithwait **(A)**

Pleasant Grove
Farnes, Clyde W **(SLP)**
Nielsen, Mrs Cathleen L **(SLP)**

Price
Clark, Sheri E **(SLP A)**
Thomas, Curtis Gerald **(A)**

Providence
McKeehan, Ann Lee **(SLP)**
Miller, Sandra Petersen **(SLP)**
Pond, Mrs Deneen Schneiter **(SLP)**

Provo
Brey, Dr Robert H **(A)**
Channell, Dr Ron W **(SLP)**
Clark, Mrs Lillian N **(SLP)**
Edwards, Karen **(SLP)**
Harris, Dr Richard W **(A)**
Johansen, David Duke **(SLP)**
Jones, Julie **(SLP)**
Kelsch, Carol **(SLP)**
Low, Dr Gordon M **(SLP)**
Lucido, Mrs Bonnie R **(SLP)**
Morley, Dr Alonzo John **(SLP A)**
Newman, Dr Parley W **(SLP)**
Newton, Mrs April Woodward **(SLP)**
Nielson, Mrs Sheila G **(SLP)**
Ravsten, Mrs Mildred T **(SLP)**
Sainio, Seija B **(SLP)**
Sargent, Mrs Shanone Kaye **(SLP)**
Sumner, Ann Swensen **(SLP)**
Ungricht, Susannah
Van Buren, Cynthia A **(SLP)**
Weaver, Dr Ross Maughan **(SLP A)**
Wiscombe, Cheryl Kay **(A)**

Riverton
Coulter, Mrs Lisa Tateoka
Coulter, Lisa Tateoka **(SLP)**

Salt Lake City
Armour, Jill Ann **(SLP A)**
Ashcraft, Paula S **(SLP)**
Barnes, Mrs Kimberly M **(SLP)**
Behnke, Mrs Barbara Johnson **(SLP)**
Bittner, Carol J **(SLP)**
Black, Denise Marie **(SLP)**
Bodily, Sherlene Ann
Boettger, Mrs Jill Hodgett **(SLP A)**
Bohning, Susan A **(A)**
Bowen-Pearson, Patricia **(SLP)**
Bown, Dr Jesse Clinton, Jr **(SLP A)**
Bray, Mrs Jacque Neilson **(SLP)**
Brennan, Anne M **(SLP)**
Bryant, Leslie Bond **(SLP)**
Burruss, Patricia J **(SLP)**
Cannon, Mrs Janet A **(SLP)**
Cantor, Mark Mitchell **(SLP)**
Carlson, Donna M **(SLP)**
Christensen, Mrs Margaret S **(SLP)**
Christensen, Nancy **(SLP)**
Clawson, Coy L **(SLP)**
Clezy, Mrs Gillian M **(SLP)**
Coon, Shonna Stanfill **(SLP)**
Corth, Susan B **(A)**
Cozakos, Nick G **(SLP A)**
Dankowski, Mrs M Korine **(A)**
Darcey, Mrs Molly Mitchell **(SLP)**
Denison, Dr Joyce **(SLP A)**
Denton, Mrs Susan F **(SLP)**
Dieterle, Francis R **(SLP)**
Dove, Heather M **(SLP)**
Driver-Gilchrist, Mrs Mary Elizabeth **(SLP)**
Dwire, Louis Ian **(SLP)**
Eernisse, Claudia C **(SLP)**
Eichwald, John Gary **(A)**
Euston, Kathleen **(SLP)**
Fingerle, Dr Clarence O **(SLP A)**
Fox, C Brent **(A)**
Fox, Mark L
Foye, Mary Dobner **(SLP)**
Goates, Dr Wallace A **(SLP A)**
Goates-Maughan, Dr Joyce S **(SLP)**
Goldstein, Janet K **(SLP)**
Gooch, Gilbert E **(SLP)**
Goudie, Kathryn L **(SLP)**
Gravkin, Karen Jean **(SLP)**
Gurrister, Tom W **(SLP)**
Hanson, Dr Marvin L **(SLP)**
Harward, Richard S **(A)**
Heusner, Donna M S **(SLP)**
Hinerman, Dr Paige **(SLP)**
Howe, Mrs Janet Morse **(SLP)**
Hutchins, Susan S **(A)**
Jacobs, Gary Michael **(A)**
Johnson-Casteel, Linda L **(SLP)**
Kamhoot, Judi Kaye **(A)**
Kazdan, Mrs Phyllis Parks **(SLP)**
Kleinschmidt, Mary Jo **(SLP)**
Koike, Dr Kazunari J **(A)**
Koike, Mary A **(A)**
Kurz, Christine Shaver **(A)**
Lee, Robyn Ladean **(SLP)**
Levitt, Robert Olin **(SLP)**
Lewis, Delinda **(SLP)**
Liston, William J **(SLP A)**
Little, Mrs Deborah Joy **(SLP)**
Lockwood, Mrs Susan Alta **(SLP)**
Lujan, Beverly Ann **(SLP)**
Mahoney, Dr Thomas M **(SLP A)**
Matheny, Mrs Mary Palmer **(SLP)**
McCandless, Phillip Todd
Miller, Pamela Elizabeth **(SLP)**
Morgan, Pamela Lynne **(SLP)**
Newberg, Nanette L **(A)**
Niederhauser, Mrs Diane Lynn **(SLP)**
Nielson, Dr Harriet R **(SLP)**
Noda, Denise D **(SLP)**
Norris, Mrs Patricia Brown
Owens, Cynthia Kay **(SLP)**
Page, Michael Don **(A)**
Paul, Dr L Dixon **(SLP)**
Payne, Mrs Kimberly Ann **(SLP)**
Phillips, Patricia A
Pinborough, Judith A **(SLP)**
Platis, Dr Dean **(SLP A)**
Price-Larson, Marilyn **(SLP)**
Purdy, Julie Kay **(A)**
Radke, Jean M **(A)**
Reed, Georgeanna **(SLP)**
Richardson, Mrs Linda S **(SLP)**
Sachau, Beth Ann **(SLP)**
Schermerhorn, Mark Charles **(SLP)**
Schweitzer, Lisa A **(SLP)**
Scott, C Rex **(A)**
Shenk, Kalomyra C **(SLP)**
Sigvardt, Mrs Dorothy **(SLP)**
Simons-McCandless, Marsha **(A)**
Slusser, Janice Lee K **(A)**
Smith, Dr Dianna M **(A)**
Stanley, Lee Ann **(SLP)**
Strasser, Dr Delbert H **(A)**

Sundstrom, Susan Colleen **(A)**
Tanner, Mrs Donna W **(SLP A)**
Taylor, Mrs Sandra Smith **(SLP)**
Thompson, Christy L **(SLP)**
Van Gend, Patricia Lynn **(SLP)**
Walker, Michael T **(A)**
Watts, Mrs Michelle Therese **(SLP)**
Werts, Jeanne L **(SLP)**
Wester, Derin C **(A)**
Wheeler, Barbara Ann **(SLP)**
Willbrand, Dr Mary L **(SLP)**
Williams, Lynn L **(SLP)**
Wolff, Cissy **(SLP)**
Wollenweber, Robert William **(A)**
Woodruff, Susan A **(SLP)**
Woods, Leslie K **(SLP)**
Wright, Sandra M **(SLP)**
Yanagisawa, Erin Merle **(SLP)**
Zolintakis, Linda **(SLP)**
Zouck, Elizabeth **(SLP)**

Sandy
Almerico, Rebecca Garda **(SLP)**
Almerico, Thomas P **(SLP)**
Alvord, Dr Lynn S **(A)**
Andersen, Allan L **(A)**
Boyd, Evelyn G **(SLP)**
Burns, Judith M **(SLP)**
Condie, Ronda K W **(A)**
Esterreicher, Mrs Carol A **(SLP)**
Fronce, Mrs Marti P **(SLP)**
Handy, Mrs Deborah A **(SLP)**
Hansen, Cassandra **(SLP)**
Harmer, Maj S Dean **(A)**
Jackson, Terri A **(A)**
Massine, Donna White **(SLP A)**
Pater, John R **(A)**
Radley, Mrs Janine G **(SLP)**
Schafer, Deborah Ann **(SLP)**
Stevens, Mrs Janeen Weyland **(SLP)**
Walker, Pamela M **(A)**
Weis, Mary Dvorak
Wright, Mrs Cynthia C **(SLP)**

Santa Clara
Forbes, Kimball B **(A)**

Smithfield
Spriet, Mrs Sheryl Y

South Jordan
Miller, Mrs Randi J **(SLP)**

South Ogden
Simpson, Mrs Marcia A **(SLP)**
Summers, Mrs Geniel Y **(SLP)**

Spanish Fork
Grotegut, Timothy David **(SLP)**
Rust, William L

Springville
Casey, Dawnne Margaret **(SLP)**

St George
Bennion, Martell S **(SLP)**
Lambert, David Armstrong **(SLP)**
Oar, Judy Lee **(SLP)**
Williams, Dr William G **(SLP A)**
Young, Abram O **(SLP)**

Stansbury Park
Loving, Susan H **(SLP)**

Tooele
Wendel, Mrs Karen M S **(SLP)**

Vernal
Kimball, Dr B D **(A)**
Pease, Susan Noble **(SLP)**
Stevens, Helen **(SLP A)**

Wellsville
Fields, Tobey Kempler **(SLP)**

West Jordan
Christensen, Mrs Marlene N **(SLP)**
Dupre, Gerald F **(SLP)**
Leyba, Naomi E **(SLP)**
Reichmann, Shelly Snow **(SLP)**
Sacco, Robert C **(A)**
Sapp, Ann Christine **(SLP)**

West Valley City
Martin, Mrs Cynthia J **(SLP)**
Pappas, Mrs Kristy K **(A)**

VERMONT

Arlington
Nicholson, Mrs June D **(SLP)**

Barnard
Zagar, Linda Louise **(SLP)**

Barre
Stafford, Mary F W **(SLP)**

Bennington
Flewelling, Wayne M **(SLP)**
Gager, David Wayne **(A)**
Hamilton, Helen Voluckas **(SLP)**
Kirkpatrick, Nancy Shay **(SLP)**
MacDonald, Deborah Crabbs **(SLP)**
Wagner, Mrs Amelia A **(SLP)**

Bethel
Orr, Mrs Linda Dean **(SLP)**

Bradford
Wickens, Alice R

Brandon
Fjeld, Carol E **(SLP)**
Pelletier, Mark C **(SLP)**
Pelletier, Mary Anne **(SLP)**

Brattleboro
Bombicino, James T **(A)**
Clark, Katherine Gail **(SLP)**
Kauffman, Catherine **(SLP)**
North, Susan Deary **(SLP)**
Rigano, Paula Jeanne **(A)**
Sweeney, Patrice Moore **(SLP)**

Bristol
Mailloux, Sally S **(SLP)**
Miller, Mrs Linda Boczany

Brookfield
Knight, Mrs Marion H **(SLP)**

Burlington
Amis, Mrs Jane Wiggins **(A)**
Bair, Deborah L **(SLP)**
Baker, Dr Nancy E **(SLP)**
Belin-Frost, Mrs Gayle **(SLP)**
Bono, Joan **(SLP)**
Cohn, Anita Lynne **(SLP)**
Douglas, Priscilla **(A)**
Dzewaltowski, Julie Ann **(SLP)**
Follansbee, Lenore
Golato, June Ellen **(SLP)**
Gomez, Carey C **(SLP)**
Green, Deborah Ellen **(A)**
Guitar, Dr Barry E **(SLP)**
Lubker, Dr James Fredrick
McCauley, Dr Rebecca Joan **(SLP)**
Mulligan, Moira **(SLP)**
Scafa, Gina A **(SLP)**
Smith, Dinah K **(A)**
Stone, F Scott **(SLP)**
Strand, Dr Edythe A **(SLP)**

Calais
Redmond, Mrs Linda D **(SLP)**

Chelsea
Pomerantz, Jilda Colville **(SLP)**

Colchester
Streator, Rondi Elizabeth

Cuttingsville
French, Nancy Mangan **(SLP)**

East Barre
Fritjofson, Mrs Claudia N **(SLP)**

East Burke
Hall, Nancy L **(SLP)**

East Dover
Erway, Dr Ella A **(SLP)**

East Fairfield
Lawyer, Mrs Sharon Harmes **(SLP)**

East Middlebury
Marceau, Mrs Frances Kaldenbach **(SLP)**

East Thetford
Bartoletto, Nancy E **(SLP)**

Enosburg Falls
Libbey, Stephen R **(SLP)**

Essex Junction
Bernardin, Lisa R **(SLP)**
Boles, Larry A **(SLP)**
Going, Joan L **(SLP)**
Houghton, Martha H **(A)**
Smith, Dr Cheryl **(SLP)**

Fair Haven
Gallant, Susanne Marie **(SLP)**
Waitkus, Mrs Nancy A **(SLP)**

Fairfax
Capossela, Mrs Cynthia L **(SLP)**

Glover
Young, Judy D **(SLP)**

Hardwick
Brightenback, Andrea **(SLP)**

Hinesburg
Feidner, Mrs Mary P **(SLP)**
Wargo, Susan Shaw **(SLP)**

Huntington
Hinchey, Carol A **(SLP)**

Jeffersonville
Hopkins-Nash, Mrs Andrea Jackson

Jericho
Boyle, Mrs Lakshmi Joshi **(SLP)**
Nathan, Jane E **(A)**
Peaper, Ruth E **(SLP)**

Johnson
Desell-Lund, Paulette Marie **(SLP)**

Lake Elmore
Agone, Mary Sue **(SLP)**

Ludlow
Remy, Mrs Darlene Robert **(SLP)**

Manchester Village
Ingison, Mrs Dianna Scott **(SLP)**

Middlebury
Fitzpatrick, Mildred S **(SLP)**
Garbose, David Morse **(SLP)**
Jamison, Mrs Robin J R **(SLP)**
Poulin, Doreen **(SLP)**

Milton
La Mora, Christine M **(SLP)**
Mahood, Mrs Lynne Temple **(SLP)**

Montpelier
Elwert, Patricia Rita **(SLP)**
Farnum, H Arthur **(SLP)**
Farnum, Sandra Duncan **(A)**
Keitel, Stephanie **(SLP A)**
Kimmerly, Susan L **(SLP)**
Mayette, Mrs Sue Anne **(SLP)**
Miller-Requarth, Marilyn Ann **(SLP)**
Nelson, Mrs Ann Letitia **(SLP)**
Orrick, Sue S **(SLP)**
Ross, Kate D **(SLP)**

Moretown
Strojny, Mrs Linda A **(A)**

Newfane
Bates, Beverly G **(SLP A)**

Newport
Geraghty, Sheila Ann **(SLP)**

North Bennington
Milchen, Mrs Selma B **(SLP)**
Poppe, Carol **(SLP)**

North Clarendon
Cater, Mrs Kathleen F **(SLP)**

North Ferrisburg
Close, Terry Annn

North Hero
Lantz-Dey, Susan Ann **(SLP)**

Norwich
Aliza, Barbara E **(SLP)**

Pittsford
Calvert-Noble, Mrs Elizabeth Lynn **(SLP)**
Furland, Delores J **(SLP)**

Plainfield
Moran, Mrs Cynthia J **(SLP)**

Pownal
Cook, Juanita W **(SLP)**
Fothergill, Mary E **(SLP)**

Putney
Balakrishnan, Uma **(SLP A)**
Hamm, Marcia G **(SLP)**

Randolph
Bruce, Nancy Van **(SLP)**
Iven, Cari Joanne **(SLP)**
McKeon, Barbara J **(SLP)**
Tucker, Mrs Nancy M **(A)**

Richmond
Emery, Carol Zwycewicz **(SLP)**
Engle, Connie L **(SLP)**
O'Leary, Mrs Stephanie J S **(SLP)**

Rutland
Cohen, Brenda P **(SLP)**
Farenkopf, Doris J **(SLP)**
Hartenstein, Robert W **(A)**
Hull, Karla M **(SLP)**
Jarrosak, Mrs Nancy R **(SLP)**
Kirk, Barbara C **(A)**
Kramer, Dr Mitchell B **(A)**
Probst, Angela Sanders
Reynolds, Beverly A **(SLP)**
Ross, Jean C **(SLP)**
Rotz, Sandra W **(SLP)**
Scott, Mrs Karen Heckman **(SLP)**
Stubbins, Sherry D **(SLP)**
Toner, Susan M **(SLP)**
Williamson, Donna E **(SLP)**

Saxtons River
Campbell, Joan H

Shelburne
Fialkoff, Donna **(SLP)**
Greer, Phyllis S
Hannah, Mrs Kay L **(SLP)**
Hudock, Mrs Victoria Ann **(SLP)**

Shoreham
Bullard, Shirley P **(SLP)**

South Burlington
Devost, Mrs Pamela Conway **(SLP)**
Faulkner, Mrs Marcia J **(SLP)**
Gear, Mrs Nancy H **(SLP)**
Hamrell, Mrs Recille C **(SLP)**
Lehr, Janet S **(SLP)**
Muhr, Diane I **(A)**
Parsley, Alicia **(SLP)**
Sheridan, Patricia E **(SLP)**

South Hero
Bryant, Marilyn Louise **(SLP)**

South Royalton
McCoy, Lois T **(SLP)**

South Strafford
Warner, Klaran Wyn **(SLP)**

Springfield
Svendsen, Mrs Mary Lou **(SLP)**

St Albans
Magnan, Elaine A R **(SLP)**
Simpson, Mrs Claire R **(SLP)**
Slesinski, Carolyn A **(SLP)**

St Johnsbury
Kessler, Mitchell Ray **(SLP)**
Kozlowski, Mrs Colleen Cook **(SLP)**
Perry, Mrs Denise L **(A)**
Wirth, Abigail J **(SLP)**

Sutton
Keizer, Kathleen B **(SLP)**

Thetford
Piotrowski, Patricia **(SLP)**

Underhill
Ellenwood, John **(SLP)**

Underhill Center
Dumoulin, Lyn **(SLP)**
Filak, Mrs Marilyn Kimball **(SLP)**

Waitsfield
Charron-Shea, Maureen H **(SLP)**

Waterbury
Clompus, Edie Merle **(SLP)**

West Newbury
Rosenberg-Arps, Joanne R **(A)**

West Rutland
Geery, Carol J **(SLP)**

Westford
Clark, Diann G **(SLP)**

Westminster
Pirruccello, Kathleen H **(SLP)**

Weston
Andrew, Mrs Margarette White **(SLP)**

Williston
Brooks, Rebecca S **(SLP)**
Burke, Deborah M **(SLP)**
Crane, Mrs Suzanne A **(SLP)**

Windsor
Beecher, Mrs Valerie P **(SLP)**
Loyer, Mrs Barbara C **(SLP)**

Winooski
Fox, Bernard J **(SLP)**
Podhajski, Dr Blanche R **(SLP)**
Toomey, Dr Mary Fran **(SLP)**
Villemaire, Judy A **(SLP)**
Wilson, Dr Mary Sweig **(SLP)**

Woodstock
Kintz, Julia Aileen **(SLP)**
Tobias, Celeste V **(SLP)**

Worcester
Hazouri, Patricia A **(SLP)**

VIRGIN ISLANDS

St Croix
Brandl, Lynne **(SLP)**
Roberts, Karen Ann **(SLP)**

St Thomas
Evans, Sandra L **(SLP)**
Perlich, Catherine Ann **(SLP)**

VIRGINIA

Abingdon
Hunt, Mrs Sharon R **(A)**
Miller-Fritz, Mrs Jayne Ellen **(A)**
Perkins, James Patrick **(SLP)**
Rasnick, Catherine Sue **(SLP)**

Accomac
Weaver, Nancy J **(SLP)**

Alexandria
Baker, Mrs Cynthia S **(SLP)**
Barry, Pamela Jeanne **(SLP)**
Barsoumian, Vergine **(A)**
Beebe, Kary Lynn **(SLP)**
Bell, Constance S **(SLP)**
Blasier, Mrs Martha H **(SLP)**
Bobbitt, Mildred B **(SLP)**
Bradley, Betty **(SLP)**
Bregstone, Mrs Andrea P **(SLP)**
Burns, Wendy Duguid **(SLP)**
Calvert, Mrs Mary Balfour **(SLP)**
Cattaneo, Angela M **(SLP)**
Coggins-Stoltz, Carolyn **(SLP)**
Cole, Mrs Barbara K **(SLP)**
Corazza, Janice A **(SLP)**
Cosgray, Nancy D **(SLP)**
Croak, Tammy Schlim **(SLP)**
Davis, Mrs Delores F **(SLP)**
De Long, Mrs Joan Nelson **(SLP)**
Demello, Mrs Sharon L **(SLP)**
Diehlmann, Tonia Marie **(A)**
Dudley, Jacqueline Hastings **(SLP)**
Dunlap, Alice R **(SLP)**
Ellett, Mrs Lee Withers **(SLP)**
Fielding, Dolores P **(SLP A)**
Giammittorio, Roberta **(SLP)**
Gibbons, Patricia Jenkins **(SLP)**
Gollinger, Dorothy
Gross, Mrs Barbara J
Gulyas, Ann E **(SLP)**
Harre, Mrs Swing S **(SLP)**
Harris, Mrs Beatrice G **(SLP)**
Harrison, Francine K **(SLP)**
Hartsough, Kathleen F **(SLP)**
Henselman, Lynn Wilson **(A)**
Higbe, Mrs Jeanette F **(SLP)**
Holmes, Judy H **(SLP)**
Holtzclaw, Mrs Margaret S **(A)**
Hyre, Mrs Noreen Marie **(SLP)**
Jacobs-Condit, Linda **(A)**
Johns, Dr Elizabeth **(SLP)**
Joyce, Margaret M **(SLP)**
Kennedy, Mrs Lynn G **(SLP)**
Kline, Nancy Lee **(SLP)**
Koenig, Dr Mareile A **(SLP)**
Kurtz-Myers, Mrs Lisa **(SLP)**
Laub, Billie **(SLP)**
Lawson, Kathryn Chaffin **(SLP)**
Lipman, Joan Michelle **(SLP)**
Lipsi, Kathy Ann **(SLP)**
Longstreet, Eric J
Lutz, Margaret Mary **(SLP)**
Mauer, Joanna Marie **(SLP)**
Noel, Helen Patricia **(SLP)**
O'Connell, Maureen Ann **(SLP)**
O'Connor, Sheila Leahy **(SLP)**
Ofcharka, Carol Ann **(SLP)**
Polon, Mrs Marilyn B **(SLP)**
Potts, Paula L **(A)**
Rankell, Gail E **(SLP)**
Rastatter, Dr Mary Doyle **(SLP A)**
Relyea-Conklin, Mrs Rhonda **(SLP)**
Reynolds, Mrs Colette Bartlinski **(SLP)**
Rogers, Mrs Patricia A **(SLP)**
Roland, Mrs Adrienne Chavers **(SLP)**
Ruge, Mrs Mary E **(SLP)**
Schulman-Heffley, Mrs Sharon **(SLP)**
Schwartz, Mrs Alice E **(SLP)**
Shallant, Mrs Robin Blackman **(SLP)**
Shamel-Pertuso, Karen Lee **(SLP)**
Siwek, Marilyn L **(SLP)**
Skelly, Nancy **(SLP)**
Smith, Martha J **(SLP)**
Southard, Mrs Laurie Jones **(SLP)**
Staubach, Lynn Carol **(SLP)**
Steinburg, Susan Palmer **(A)**
Stilwell, Catherine A
Swanson, Lori **(A)**
Thompson, Vivienne F **(SLP)**
Tripp, Karen Anne **(SLP)**
Turkin, Anita Beth **(SLP)**
Tweedie, Dr David **(SLP A)**
Vann, Peter D **(SLP)**
Wade, Barbara J **(SLP)**
Waiss, Sharon L **(SLP)**
Winston, Mrs Susan M **(SLP)**

Amherst
Bolt, Winifred Fitzgerald **(SLP)**
Nicks, Mrs Judith A B **(SLP)**

Annandale
Buchalter-Levitan, Esther **(SLP)**
Campbell, Sylvia L **(SLP)**
Coffee, Mrs Lauren K **(SLP)**
De Longa, Mary P **(SLP)**
Farling, Joyce M **(SLP)**
Fields, Elaine A **(SLP)**
Goebel, Martha D **(SLP)**
Grinage, Diane M **(SLP)**
Hawkins, Jane A **(SLP)**
Irving, Mary Manzione **(SLP)**
Kelley-McCarthy, Leigh Anne **(SLP)**
Langhaus-Herrmann, Terry **(SLP)**
Lebo, Christina Ann F **(A)**
Lillevig, Mrs Diana W **(SLP)**
Lumsden-Boehling, Nancy C **(SLP)**
Massa, Michael V **(A)**
Moore, Katherine Knox **(SLP)**
Nelson, Gloria B **(SLP)**
Pilberg, Rochelle **(SLP)**
Sadler, Mrs Rebecca Eggers **(SLP)**
Tibbetts, Susan H S **(SLP)**
Webster, Beverly Nielsen **(A)**

Arcola
Dower, Nikia Rae **(SLP)**

Ark
Bunch, Carolyn O **(SLP)**

Arlington
Anderson, Joy E
Arnold, Carol Brown
Avezzano, Karen Hillman **(SLP)**
Behrens, Thomas R **(A)**
Brower, Catherine J **(SLP)**
Brown, Alice B **(SLP)**
Brown, Sharon Miller **(A)**
Browne, Tomi Thibodeaux **(A)**
Burford, Sandra I **(SLP)**
Busacco, Dr Debra Ann **(A)**
Campanelli, Dr Peter A **(SLP A)**
Chavoor-Pardes, Mrs Claude Mv **(SLP)**
Cross, Lesley V **(A)**
Demaio, Mrs Diane Dunhoff **(SLP)**
Depasquale, Mrs Jessie Devlin **(SLP)**
Einhorn, Mrs Robin Dubowe **(A)**
Ely, Carolyn R **(SLP)**
Fox, Wendy J **(SLP)**
Frattali, Dr Carol Marie **(SLP)**
Gaines, Donna S **(SLP)**
Garrett, Judith L N **(SLP)**
Garrus, Nancy P **(A)**
Geoffrey, Dr Virginia C **(SLP)**
Hermanoff, Wendy Sue **(SLP)**
Hodapp, Mary E **(SLP)**
Hoofnagle, Robin E **(SLP)**
Hughes, Christine M **(SLP)**
Jacobs, Luann **(SLP)**
Johnson, Diane F **(SLP)**
Johnson, Marilyn Kaye **(SLP)**
Jolly, Sharon T G **(SLP)**
Kester, Mrs Sandra Isaacman **(A)**
Kosh, Mrs Zelda H **(SLP)**
Kubiak, Mrs Margaret Kristen **(A)**
Lore, Dr James I **(SLP A)**
Lowery, Jeffery **(SLP)**
Lukmire, Nan K **(A)**
Lyon, Karen F **(SLP)**
Marsh, Rochelle I **(SLP)**
Mazuzan, Marsinah Anne **(SLP)**
McGrady, Dr Harold J, Jr **(SLP)**
McIntyre, Mrs Patricia A **(SLP)**
Morey, Mrs Kathryn Downs **(SLP)**
Neville, Mrs Katherine McGoldrick **(SLP)**
O'Neil, Denise C **(SLP)**
Porter, Mrs Elaine A **(SLP)**
Samuels, Jessica R **(SLP)**
Saul, Mrs Nancy Q **(SLP)**
Schimmelpfenneg, Nancy Leigh **(SLP)**
Scott, Susanne Manzi **(A)**
Selman, Mrs Elsie M **(SLP)**
Semanchik, Karen **(SLP)**
Shambelan, Michele Ruth **(SLP)**
Singer, Rosalind D **(SLP)**
Syfert, Gretchen Adams **(A)**
Thomas, Beth Fullerton **(SLP)**
Trout, Dr Susan Struve **(SLP)**
Trumbull, Lois King **(SLP)**
Walsh, Kimberly K **(SLP)**
Werner, Mary Kathryn **(SLP)**
Yudson, Mrs Kay C **(SLP)**
Zeese, Mrs Dina Smith **(SLP)**
Zerbst, Ellen S **(SLP)**

Ashland
Luck, Mrs Georgia H **(SLP)**

Bassett
Akers, Susan Gail **(SLP)**
James, Mrs Sheryl G **(SLP)**

Basye
James, Sally Lynn **(SLP)**

Bealeton
Dunham, Mrs Hildy Helene **(SLP)**

Bedford
Deane, Barbara G **(SLP)**

Bena
Kramp, H Ned **(A)**

Bent Mountain
Coffey, Mrs Mary Elisabeth **(SLP)**

Big Stone Gap
Hutson, Kathleen A **(SLP)**

Blacksburg
Piersol, Barbara L **(SLP)**
Scheneman, Mrs Mary A **(SLP)**
Schetz, Mrs Katherine **(SLP)**
Tew, Mrs Lisa E H **(SLP)**
Waldron, Mrs Claire M **(SLP)**
Willis, Mina P **(SLP)**

Blackstone
French, Mrs Connie W **(SLP)**

Bluemont
Suder, Darlene Sue **(SLP)**

Boones Mill
Conway, Mrs Kathleen R **(SLP)**

Boston
Gottlieb, Dr Sidney **(SLP)**

Bracey
Copp, Leslie M **(SLP)**

Bridgewater
Foster, Julie Beard **(SLP)**
Seal, Mrs Brenda C **(SLP)**

Bristol
Barker, Lynette Mae **(SLP)**
Burke, Bonnie F **(SLP)**
Rest, Mrs Deborah C **(SLP)**

Broadway
Bennett, Mrs Linda Angst **(A)**

Burke
Brooks, Mrs Ruth Ann **(SLP)**
Buffardi, Jean R **(SLP)**
Bupp, Mrs Chandler M **(SLP)**

Geiger, Dianne W **(SLP)**
Gordon, Mrs Carol S **(SLP)**
Hargraves, Mrs Tomma S **(SLP)**
Hitz, Mrs Loretta O **(SLP)**
Horner, Mrs Diane S **(SLP)**
Isaacson, Frances **(SLP)**
Kopp, Mrs Christine **(SLP)**
Perry, Mrs Beth Walker **(SLP)**
Pfaff, Kurt T **(A)**
Ryan, Maryann H **(SLP)**
Samuel, Susan Candler **(SLP)**
Shunfenthal, Sherri F **(SLP)**
Stanton, Lydia Dawn **(SLP)**
Stegner, Mrs Sandra N **(SLP)**
Steiner, Mrs Linda M **(SLP)**
Tope, Dolores M
Wiese, Mrs Marie Altmeyer **(SLP)**
Withers, Mrs Lisa D **(SLP)**
Zykorie, Bonnie E **(SLP)**

Capeville
Kundo, Mrs Peggy Diane **(SLP)**

Carrollton
Saunders, Mrs Mary N **(SLP)**

Cartersville
Culbertson, Dr William R, III **(SLP)**

Centreville
Fincher, Cynthia K **(SLP)**
Howell, Mrs Sara W C **(SLP)**
Kieber, Mrs Carol Ann **(SLP)**
Lewis, Valerie Tenney **(SLP)**
Mellott, Mrs Patricia Klimas **(SLP)**
Menking, Mrs Elizabeth Polizos **(SLP)**
Savia, Karen **(SLP)**
Swanson, Nancy F **(A)**

Chantilly
Jones, Mary B **(SLP)**
Morris, Joyce M **(SLP)**
Niccum, Mrs Mary Rose **(SLP)**
Perkins, Sheila R **(SLP)**

Charlottesville
Allaire, Mrs Janet H **(SLP)**
Bonvillian, John D
Bralley, Dr Ralph C **(SLP)**
Brooks, Mrs Barbara A **(A)**
Brown, Mrs Kathleen Wright **(SLP)**
Brown, Lois A **(SLP)**
Bull, Dr Glen L **(SLP)**
Bullock, Mrs Elizabeth Johnson **(SLP)**
Burr, Dr Helen Gunderson **(SLP)**
Caldwell, Margo L **(SLP)**
Chute, Mrs Sharon M **(SLP)**
Cline, Mrs Claire McDaniel **(SLP)**
Cohen, Mrs Elizabeth P
Donaldson, Gail Spaid **(A)**
Easton, Mrs Leslie Ann
Eidson, Sue Ann **(SLP)**
Epstein, Mrs Lillian C **(SLP)**
Ferguson, Julie Kathryn
Flowers, Doris Anita **(SLP)**
Goffen, Robin Layle **(SLP)**
Goodman, Mrs Deborah Brown **(SLP)**
Gordon, Mrs Ellen E **(SLP)**
Hahn, Mrs Milege J **(A)**
Hansborough, Mrs Susan Babecki **(A)**
Heitz, Ann A S **(SLP)**
Higgins, Elizabeth Ruth **(SLP)**
Hildebrand, Debra Lynn **(A)**
Hodges, Annelle Vaden **(A)**
Hogle, Linda S **(SLP)**
Horner, Dr John S **(SLP A)**
Horner, Juliette P **(SLP A)**
Huskey, Marilyn R
Jackson, Mrs Janet Sue **(SLP)**
Jones, Ellen Laetitia **(SLP)**
Koss, Penny Sue **(SLP)**
Lawton, Ellen Lynn **(SLP)**
Ledbetter, Patricia **(SLP)**
Leinbach, Cs Martha A Y **(SLP)**
Lindsay, Mrs Jean Horton **(SLP)**
Lord, Cheryl C **(SLP)**
Marshall, Mrs Linda **(SLP)**
Martin, Mrs Ann O'Neill **(SLP)**
Matt, David W **(SLP)**
Mayer, Nancy E **(SLP)**
McElroy, Margaret D **(SLP A)**
McNally, Geralyn M **(SLP)**
Meyers, Dr Susan C **(SLP)**
Mitch, James L **(SLP)**
Page, Mrs Linda J **(SLP)**
Pearce, Mrs Margaret Muraik **(SLP)**
Richards, Nelda S **(SLP)**
Ringers, Mrs Barbara B **(A)**
Ruth, Dr Roger A **(A)**
Schildwachter, Mrs Allison St C **(SLP)**
Schoeny, Dr Zahrl G **(SLP A)**
Schurrer, Judy S **(SLP)**
Sikorski, Christine **(A)**
Smith, Catherine L **(SLP)**
Stoudt, Dr Ralph J, Jr **(SLP)**
Strawley, Brenda Nelson **(SLP)**
Sturtevant, Janet Evans **(A)**
Sullivan, Mrs Janet Kaminsky **(SLP)**
Swinson, Linda Jean **(A)**
Thomas, Mrs Jean Feddersen **(A)**
Tucker, Denise Anne **(A)**
VanLier, Rebecca Lansing **(SLP)**
Vidrine-Bralley, Jean C **(SLP)**
Woodford, Lee Lucas **(SLP)**

Chesapeake
Belcher, Louise A **(SLP)**
Berrett, Dr M Victor **(A)**
Brothers, Mrs Nancy P S **(SLP)**
Carver, Mrs Joanne Y **(SLP)**
Christensen, Mrs Ann Oddy **(SLP)**
Cobbs, Karen D **(SLP)**
Cox, Mrs Geraline Hinton **(SLP)**
Elder, Sharon Hooper **(A)**
Faircloth, John William **(SLP)**
Grant, Mrs Margie Baucom **(SLP)**
Hammer, Mrs Pamela Smith **(SLP)**
Liedman, James **(SLP)**
Manasco, Mrs Betty Jo P **(SLP)**
Mason, Pamela K **(SLP)**
Matrozzo, Mrs April Joy **(SLP)**
Probst, Dianne Marie **(SLP)**
Reel, Mrs Evelyn E **(SLP)**
Spellman, Mrs Sharon Wilson **(SLP)**
Watts, Vivian G
Wertz, Mrs Mildred B **(SLP)**
Woodruff, Mrs Rebecca Clifton

Chester
Davis, Mrs Karen Moreno **(SLP)**
Fong, Gwenolyn **(SLP)**

Chesterfield
Cluver, Dr Elizabeth **(SLP A)**
Hammack, Mrs Mary Jo **(SLP)**
Potter, Marjorie E **(SLP)**
Prime, Mrs Donna Harris **(A)**
Snider, Elizabeth **(SLP)**
Walker, Susan M **(SLP)**

Chilhowie
Whitely, Mrs Sherri Ranee **(SLP)**

Christiansburg
Calloway, Mary Lee C **(SLP)**
James, Laura S **(SLP)**
Kingma, Lora Leigh **(SLP)**
Ravlin, Mrs Susan A **(SLP)**
Shelor, Mrs Joan White **(SLP)**

Clifton Forge
Crackel, Carol S **(SLP)**
Dotson, Debra R **(SLP)**
Shaw, Nancy L **(SLP)**

Clintwood
Hensley, Mrs Sheila Davis **(SLP)**

Cobbs Creek
Newsome, Peggy W **(SLP)**

Collinsville
Adkins, Lynda Compton **(SLP)**

Colonial Heights
Barber, Linda L **(SLP)**
Brown, Mrs Anna S **(SLP)**

Covington
Byer, Annette Ellen
Fey, Daniel William **(A)**

Crozet
Wagner, Bruce Robert **(A)**

Culpeper
Clore, Susan Christensen **(SLP)**
Jameson, Mrs Michele B **(SLP)**
Meyer, Mrs Courtland Gunn **(SLP)**
Reynolds, Charla L **(SLP)**
Rutkowski, Mrs Leanne H **(SLP)**

Dale City
Black, Mrs Karen Schroeder **(SLP)**
Fetzer, Mrs Barbara J
Schum, Judith A **(SLP)**
Ward, Lisa P **(SLP)**

Danville
Bowman-Nance, Kay L **(SLP)**
Dodson, Gloria Susan **(SLP)**
Getz, Gail C **(SLP)**
Gnewikow, Dr Danny W **(A)**
Marshall, Elizabeth T **(SLP)**
Weiler, Pamela A **(SLP)**
Whitley, Mrs Jennifer W **(SLP)**

Dayton
Morehouse, Katherine **(A)**

Dublin
Dowdy, Brenda Hobbs **(SLP)**

Dumfries
Baltazar, Shirley Amaral **(SLP)**
Rudolph, Mrs Catherine Louise **(SLP)**

Earlysville
Borowitz, Mrs Kathleen C **(SLP)**
Gentry, Mrs Alice Goldsmith **(SLP)**

Elliston
Linkous, Mrs Pamela Thornton **(SLP)**

Evington
Block, Lisa Joan **(SLP)**

Faber
Morris, Dr Suzanne E **(SLP)**

Fairfax
Baron, Rori Faith **(SLP)**
Biggins, Anne R **(SLP)**
Breithaupt, Douglas H **(A)**
Brockbank, Mrs Linda C **(SLP)**
Byrne, Susan C **(SLP)**
Chester, Mrs Mary Louise **(SLP)**
Cofey, Carol J **(SLP)**
Conrad, Mrs Beverly Lazaroff **(SLP)**
Denkinger, Sandra G **(SLP)**
Dias, Molly M **(A)**
Ellis, Mrs Cherrye Hammans **(SLP)**
Estabrook, Marylin H **(SLP)**
Fahey, Mrs Sheryl Eanet **(SLP)**
Fee, Barbara P **(SLP)**
Fellows, Mrs Jane W **(SLP)**
Fernandez, Mrs Jan-Marie S **(SLP)**
Goodrich, Sharon J **(SLP)**
Gray, Judith M **(SLP)**
Hinson, Mrs Troye M **(SLP)**
Howard, Tamaryn Means **(SLP)**
Jones, Dr Julie Kay
Keith, Mrs Melanie P **(SLP)**
Kemmerer, Eileen Ann **(SLP)**
Miller, Mrs Shelby Victoire
Monroe, Alice D **(SLP)**
Morgan, Lynne Clark **(SLP)**
Perry, Mrs Ruthie L **(SLP)**
Rearick, Mrs Sarah Whitsett **(SLP)**
Sklarow, Mrs Mindy E **(SLP)**
Takagi, Dr Yasuaki
Thompson, Beverly B **(A)**
Van Buskirk, Karen Lynn **(SLP)**
Walton, Ruth T **(A)**
Wilder, Carolyn S **(SLP)**

Fairfax Station
Brobst, Mrs Glenda A **(SLP)**
Brown, Mrs Joanne M **(SLP)**
Dendinger, Marcia Lynn **(SLP)**
Eastes, Mrs Dawn Elizabeth **(SLP)**
Eubanks, Mrs Patricia **(SLP)**
Halayko, Mrs Kathleen A **(SLP)**
Hance, Mrs Susan Ellis **(SLP)**
Kaplan, Mrs Lynda **(A)**
Kitchen, Mrs Mary C
Page, Suzanne **(SLP)**
Powell, Mrs Kathy Rein **(SLP)**
Swope, Dr Suzanne **(SLP)**

Falls Church
Andrews, Cheryl H **(SLP)**
Berlin, Nancy L **(A)**
Biles, Patricia Ann
Green, Mrs Twhanna J **(SLP)**
Hurvitz, Judith A **(SLP)**
Jarrett, Marian H **(SLP)**
Jones-McNamara, Mrs Sara **(SLP)**
Martin, Carolyn F **(SLP)**
McCarthy, Dr Geraldine MacAvoy **(SLP)**
Michie, Laura Audia **(SLP)**
Saferstein, Sharon
Santa, Daphne A **(SLP)**
Seidenberg, Karen Hedia **(SLP)**
Slaughter, Marylin M **(A)**
Spielberg, Martin H **(SLP)**
Vitagliano, Mary Louise **(A)**
Wexler, Mrs Hilary P **(SLP)**
White, Joanne Elizabeth **(SLP)**

Farmville
Beck, Dr Robert Nels **(SLP)**
O'Brien, Mrs Martha J **(SLP)**

Fishersville
Farrar-Hersch, Julie A **(A)**
Meyer, Dr Linda Anne **(SLP)**
Mills, Janice Adele **(A)**
Minor, Birdie J **(SLP)**

Floyd
Sholar, Joanne Franck **(SLP)**

Forest
Gallier, Mrs Carole Trent **(SLP)**
Nutter, Mrs Marilyn M **(SLP)**

Fort Belvoir
Dahmer, Susan McVaney **(SLP)**
Fanning, Belinda J **(SLP A)**

Franklin
Bigger, Mrs Ruth Ann W **(A)**
Hunter, Mrs Sue Ann **(SLP)**

Fredericksburg
Altman, Mrs Sharon Demme **(SLP)**
Burgess, Mrs Dawn Thompson **(SLP)**
Conolly, Mrs Elizabeth A Srsic **(SLP)**
Davis, Karen Sue **(SLP)**
Frank, Thomas M **(A)**
Gibert, Ivonne Teresa **(SLP)**
Hinman, Mrs Mary P **(SLP)**
Holt, Mrs Margaret H **(SLP)**
Howerton, Mrs Jan DeMonde **(SLP)**
Jett, Mrs Susanna Tingle **(SLP)**
Johns, Valerie C **(SLP)**
Kuhns, Mrs Linda Lister **(SLP)**
Lanford, Elizabeth Davis **(SLP)**
Lasalle, Lisa Renee
Palgutta, Renea Elaine
Sutherland, Ann Elizabeth **(SLP)**
Thompson, Lisa Mele **(SLP)**
Tiffany, Mrs Sheila Ann **(SLP)**
Winkler, Karen Jean **(SLP)**

Front Royal
Jordan, Lillian H **(SLP)**
Melvin-Hines, Mrs Darshell Devore **(SLP)**
Smith, Mrs Arlene Dawn **(SLP)**

Galax
Sisk, Daina A

Gate City
Parks, Robin S

Glen Allen
Brooks, Mrs Patricia Shaw **(SLP)**
Diver, Kathleen Joan **(SLP)**
Edwards, Kathleen **(SLP)**
Hudgins, Mrs Leslee E **(SLP)**
Humphrey, Mary Lisa **(SLP)**
Welker, Vivian A **(SLP)**

Grafton
Bowen, Mrs Terry T **(A)**

Graves Mill
Menks, Alice H **(SLP)**

Great Falls
Burka, Barbara N **(SLP A)**
Patton, Joseph A **(SLP)**
Rini, Mrs Kathleen S **(SLP)**

Grottoes
Wiley-Shreffler, Yvonne Kay **(SLP)**

Hamilton
Prieston, Mrs Cathy M G **(SLP)**

Hampton
Baumgardner, Ruth E **(SLP)**
Bellefleur, Dr Philip A **(A)**
Clark, Frank E **(SLP)**
Core, Mrs Coleen Shank **(SLP)**
Davis, Mrs Linda Prince **(SLP)**
Destefano, Carla Haymaker **(SLP)**
Gilmore, Mrs Martha R **(A)**
Hebert, Mrs Pamela Pereira **(SLP)**
Holliday, Sarah Ford **(SLP)**
Hurlock, Michael Thomas **(SLP)**
Jarvis, Doris S **(SLP)**
Johnson, Sharon Ann **(SLP)**
Kight, Jana Brown **(A)**
Landon, Connie L **(SLP)**
Murphy, Dr Pollie Saunders **(SLP)**
Schlitt, Robert **(SLP)**
Screen, Dr Robert Martin **(SLP)**
Snaidman, Mrs Patricia J **(SLP)**
Sykes, Susan P **(SLP)**
Walton, Rosemary Rice **(SLP)**
Zambas, Chris S **(A)**

Harrisonburg
Bennett, Dr Clinton **(SLP)**
Booth, Mrs Sara A **(SLP)**
Browning, Mrs Krista B **(SLP)**
Filter, Dr Maynard D **(SLP)**
Harkins, Barbara L **(SLP)**
Harper, Mrs Susan Bowman **(SLP)**
Helton, Mrs Rebecca Elsarelli **(SLP)**
Hinkle, Dr Robert R **(A)**
Lilley, Lois Anne **(SLP)**
Lindberg, Karen W
Matthias, Karen Killian **(SLP)**
Morris, Robert C **(SLP A)**
Nussbaum, Mary Kirby **(SLP)**
Rucker, Leigh-Ann **(A)**
Runyan, Dr Charles M **(SLP)**
Runyan, Sara Elizabeth **(SLP)**
Smith, Mrs Jo Ellyn **(SLP)**
Spangler, Nancy Rebecca **(SLP)**
Stokes, Anne Katherine **(SLP)**
Tanchak, Theresa L **(SLP)**
Williams, Fern Elizabeth **(SLP)**

Hartwood
Stribling, Mrs Catherine **(SLP)**

Hayes
Lenhardt, Dr Martin Louis **(SLP A)**

Herndon
Adams, Leslie Anderson **(SLP)**
Ballato, Mrs Pamela R **(SLP)**
Bonk, Mary Shannon **(SLP)**
Bracken, Annamarie Mariani **(SLP)**
Dera, Dawn C **(SLP)**
DiPlacidi, Mrs Barbara M **(SLP)**
Eisenberg, Mrs Sharon Luber **(SLP)**
English, Susan M **(SLP)**
Hanlon, Joan M **(SLP)**
Keller, Mrs Pamela A **(SLP)**
Mastri, Stephanie Mirchel **(SLP)**
Mullins, Mrs Tina Ruth **(A)**
Quinn, Maureen A **(SLP)**
Schloesser, Mrs Mary Patricia **(SLP)**
Sheese, Mrs Rebecca J **(SLP)**
White, Linda R **(SLP)**
Wolley, Jane K C **(SLP)**

Highland Springs
Cutler, S James **(A)**

Hillsville
Honeycutt, Mrs Carolyn Howlett **(SLP)**
Phillips, Leigh A **(SLP)**
Rudy, Susan Kay **(SLP)**

Hood
Bowman, Ann S **(SLP)**

Hopewell
Chester, Mrs Joyce Rhodes **(SLP)**
Tiller, Mrs Charlene T **(SLP)**

Huddleston
Peters, Barbara C **(SLP)**

Jonesville
Allen, Mary W **(SLP)**

Keswick
Shackelford, Mrs Anne Rushton **(SLP)**

Lake Ridge
Field, Mrs Elizabeth Carol **(A)**
Pizer, Sherry H **(SLP)**

Leesburg
Bardwell, Mrs Marianne K **(SLP)**
Farley, Mrs Dollie O **(SLP)**
Hearst, Mrs Karen Blankenship **(SLP)**
Shelton, Mrs Lesa L Gray **(SLP)**

Lexington
Armor, Robin A **(A)**
Beckley, Mrs Debby P **(SLP)**
Novack, Lesley L **(SLP)**

Linville
Kaiser, Paula Lynn **(SLP)**

Lortonx
Pybus, Edith Connor **(SLP)**

Low Moor
Pillow, Gary L **(A)**

Luray
Tucker, Mrs Sharon Lynn

Lynchburg
Acree, Jo Nell **(A)**
Bolton, Mrs Elizabeth Ann **(SLP)**
Brindle, Barbara R **(SLP)**
Brown, Carol A **(SLP)**
Brown, Mrs Jean Puppe **(SLP)**
Dorsey, Lora D B **(SLP)**
Edwards, Mrs Barbara C **(SLP)**
Edwards, Ernest Calvin **(A)**
Frankenbach, Mrs Glenda Lynn
Garrett, Carol A **(SLP)**
Groover, Mrs Beth Broman **(SLP)**
Hunt, Joanna Ruth
Ickes, Mrs Claire R **(SLP)**
Jordan, Patrick David **(SLP)**
Koch, Carol Anne **(SLP)**
Lane, Kathleen Ann **(SLP)**
Lindamood, Lori Hope **(SLP)**
O'Hara, Virginia R **(SLP)**
Okin, Mrs Deborah Fletcher **(SLP)**
Porter, Mrs Carolyn T **(SLP)**
Rotter, Margaret A **(SLP A)**
Sanders, Elizabeth C **(SLP)**
Staton, Mrs Yvonne Fauber **(SLP)**
Stephens, V Carole **(A)**
Warner, Karen Simpson **(SLP)**
Wassum, Gregory P **(SLP)**
Wassum, Mrs Susan E K **(SLP)**
Wilson, Gregory Scott **(A)**

Madison Heights
Johnson, Raymonde Crennel **(SLP)**

Manakin-Sabot
Evans, Mrs Barbara B **(SLP)**

Manassas
Bombard, Mrs Linda Ann **(SLP)**
Bond, Mrs Nona **(SLP)**
Bugbee, Judith K **(SLP)**
Chichester, Donna J **(SLP)**
Donaldson, Mrs Gillian K **(SLP)**
Figula, Diane A **(SLP)**
Jacobson, Eileen Roberts **(SLP)**
Lunsford, Deborah B **(SLP)**
Muzelak, Mrs Kimberly Ann Booth
Rainville, Mrs Marilyn **(SLP)**
Simmons, Mrs Nanci W **(SLP)**
Talbot, Gwendolyn **(SLP)**

Marion
Huber, Mrs Carol T **(SLP)**

Martinsville
Anderson, Anne F **(SLP)**
Eschenbach, Mrs Cheryl D **(SLP)**
Ezelle, Mrs Nancy C N **(SLP)**
Jones, Mrs Susan C **(SLP)**
McLachlan, Catherine Dunn **(SLP)**

Mathews
Crittenden, Mrs Constance **(SLP)**

Maurertown
Livesay, Alesia Good **(SLP)**

Mc Gaheysville
Klien, Mrs Mary Hewson **(SLP)**
Sistrunk, Mrs Debra Ann **(SLP)**

Mc Lean
Brockett, Mrs Patricia S **(SLP)**
Brown, Janet E **(SLP)**
Glaub, Susan Ann **(SLP)**
Henry, Yvonne M **(SLP)**
Herbers, Suzanne D **(SLP)**
Lambert, Mrs Nancy B **(SLP)**
Leidecker, Catherine Beardsley **(SLP)**
Losey, Sue Ann S **(SLP)**
McCarty, Janet Platt **(SLP)**
McGuinness, Rosemarie Contini **(SLP)**
Overman, Dr Carol Ann **(SLP)**
Palacios, Judith Tuck **(SLP)**
Randall, Joellen M **(SLP)**
Rassiga, Nancy Diane **(SLP)**
Schaefer, Mrs Ellen L **(SLP)**
Shefferman, Ileen S **(SLP)**
Stearns, Martha R **(SLP)**
Visnick, Mrs Joyce Dragash **(SLP)**

Mechanicsville
Alter, Mrs Kathryn Satterfield **(SLP)**
Barnes, Ruth A **(SLP)**
Greenday, Mrs Laura Ann **(SLP)**
Jeremiah, Mrs Kimberly W **(SLP)**
McCallister, Mrs Kimberly Sue **(SLP)**
Munden, Mrs Anne D **(SLP)**

Middletown
Holsinger, Mrs Cynthia M

Midlothian
Barron, Sharon C **(SLP)**
Beach, Woodford A **(SLP)**
Braytenbah, Mrs Marlene **(SLP)**
Brinser, Mrs Chryl C **(SLP)**
Burke, Cabell R **(SLP)**
Condrin, Mrs Susan Loen **(SLP)**
Cook, Ann G **(A)**
Creech, Dr Henry B **(SLP A)**
Dean, Dr Linda May **(A)**
Dewire, Nancy Kirn **(SLP)**
Dimenna, Mrs Deborah G **(SLP)**
Fehling, Roberta Hill **(SLP)**
Goergen, Mrs Joann E **(SLP)**
Hapala, Mrs Susan B **(SLP)**
Harrigan, Mrs Claudia Bakker **(SLP)**
Kleifges, Mrs Elena Munero **(A)**
Loeffler, Kathryn E **(SLP)**
Murphy, Mrs Suzanne McKeever **(SLP)**
Nebera, Rebecca Annette **(SLP)**
Richard, Mrs Holly B **(SLP)**
Smith, Mrs Nancy Brizzie **(SLP)**
Staples, Theresa O **(SLP A)**
Wilson, Mrs Heidi Bergmuelle **(SLP)**

Mineral
Anderson, Vivian Denise **(SLP)**

Monroe
Barnes, Glynda **(SLP)**

Montpelier
Shutt, Mrs Elizabeth Anne **(SLP)**

Mount Crawford
Clark, Mrs Dorothy W **(SLP)**
James, Carol C **(SLP A)**

Mount Holly
Hall, Melanie G **(SLP)**

Narrows
Webb, Mrs Catherine Sparacino **(SLP)**

Nassawadox
Fears, Anita G **(SLP)**

Newport News
Abeyounis, Elizabeth Cardwell **(SLP)**
Adams, Carolyn A **(SLP)**
Bowers, Mrs Linda G **(A)**
Cochrane, Mrs Mary Ellen **(SLP)**
Dennie, Mrs Helen Marcopoulos **(A)**
Familant, Mrs Rosalee P **(SLP)**
Ferrell, Mrs Ann Cooley **(SLP)**
Freeman, Mrs Cheryl H **(SLP)**
Gailey, Dr Platon G **(SLP)**
Graham, Mrs Theoni Savvas **(A)**
Hannon, Mrs Kathleen C
Harris, Nancy Diane
Hecker, Henry C **(A)**
Hertzler, Donna P **(SLP)**
Jones, Cheryl Phillips-W **(SLP)**
Kenney, Rosita L **(SLP)**
Krueger, Michele Sabol
Lasko, Teresa Helen **(SLP)**
Logston, Sharee Lu **(A)**
Mikita, Stephen F **(SLP)**
Norman, Elaine Marie **(SLP)**
Radus, Dr Libby **(SLP)**
Ritchie, Mrs Joyce L **(A)**
Spells-Greene, Mrs Ina Ruth **(SLP)**
Verhoef, Mrs Joan Fernandes **(A)**
Vogt, Mrs Donna Crinklaw **(SLP)**
Walton, Betty Reed **(SLP)**
Zeigler, Laura B **(SLP)**

Norfolk
Abrahamsen, Dr Eileen P **(SLP)**
Adler, Anne Joyce **(A)**
Aurand, Barbara S **(SLP)**
Baker, Mrs Katherine Perez **(SLP)**
Barrett, Ross S **(SLP)**
Bountress, Mrs Martha G **(SLP A)**
Bountress, Dr Nicholas G **(SLP)**
Buck, Mrs Barbara H **(A)**
Coleman, Dr Robert F **(SLP)**
Cooper, Reuben **(SLP)**
Dashiell, Mrs Lynn Purnell **(A)**
De Lucenay, Mrs Cynthia Darlene **(SLP)**
Diamonstein, Beth A **(SLP)**
Elbers, Caroline H G **(SLP)**

Fisher, Deborah Ann **(SLP)**
Flax, Norma J **(SLP)**
Francis, Joseph Helbert **(SLP)**
Francis, Mrs Rosemary Eakes **(SLP)**
French, Richard B **(SLP)**
Gilbert, Janet L **(SLP)**
Greenberg, Mrs Marci Katz **(SLP)**
Gutnick, Dr Howard N **(A)**
Hughes, Mrs Renee M **(SLP)**
Klee, Margaret A **(SLP)**
Laderberg, Mrs Cathy M **(SLP)**
MacDonald, Carol A **(SLP)**
MacKisack-Morin, Eleanor Louise **(SLP)**
McNamara, James Patrick **(SLP)**
Metcalf, Mikealiene Gail **(SLP)**
Moyer, Deborah L **(SLP)**
Murphy, Catherine R **(A)**
Padgett, Ann Midkiff **(SLP)**
Page, John Clifford
Poertner, Mrs Luanne Conrad **(SLP)**
Robinson, Mrs Carol Mauney
Rose, Mrs Susan A **(SLP)**
Saul, Jonathan O **(A)**
Sever, Joseph C, Jr **(A)**
Shields, Dorothy D **(SLP)**
Waters, Kimberly Jane **(SLP)**
Werbowetzki, Cynthia Lynn **(SLP)**
White, Mrs Lynne M
Williams, Debra Elizabeth **(A)**
Wilson, Mrs Joan Powers **(A)**
Zimmer, Barbara J **(SLP)**

Oakton
Gitlow, Caryl **(SLP)**
Lawson, Mrs Dorothy M **(SLP)**
Plummer, Mrs Hazel M **(SLP)**
Smith, Mrs Marsha Burwell **(SLP)**
Williamson, Mrs Darlene S **(SLP)**

Pearisburg
Church, Marie Ahern **(A)**

Petersburg
Allen, Dr Madge B **(SLP)**

Poquoson
Anderson, Mrs Deborah Phillips **(SLP)**

Portsmouth
Cage, Mrs Janiece Lynn **(SLP)**
Coie, John Paul **(A)**
Jones, Rhonda Duman **(SLP)**
Lewis, Steven Edward **(A)**
Rankins, Scott D
Young, Dr Neil M **(A)**

Pulaski
Shomo, Mrs Barbara Patterson **(SLP)**

Purcellville
Hockersmith, Dr Mary J **(SLP A)**
Starliper, Deborah S **(SLP)**

Quantico
McLaurine, Mary A **(SLP)**

Quinton
Harrod, Mrs Patricia **(SLP)**

Radford
Crouse, Beverly T **(SLP)**
Garn-Nunn, Dr Pamela **(SLP)**
Goodman, Mrs Anne Ladd **(SLP)**
Nicely, Dr James E **(SLP)**
Twitchell, Dr Mary C **(SLP)**
Whisonant, Brenda L **(SLP)**

Rawlings
Lafoon, Cynthia Lynn

Remington
Parker, Mrs Sheryl H **(SLP)**

Reston
Amdur, Mrs Judith Ann **(SLP)**
Armentrout, Carolyn Clement **(SLP)**
Boster, Gail Brook **(SLP)**
Doran-Quine, Dr MaryEllen **(SLP)**
Eubanks, Mrs Cynthia E **(SLP)**
Harper, Mary Jan **(SLP)**
Holmberg, Mrs Denise Quinn **(SLP)**
Hopkins, Mrs Anita Freeman **(SLP)**
Jones, Mrs Carol Johnston **(SLP)**
Kendrick, Mrs Marian M **(SLP)**
McNeilly, Mrs Lemmietta Jones **(SLP)**
Morrow, Julia T **(SLP)**
Pathak, Bhama P **(A)**
Ratner, Mrs Barbara M **(SLP)**
Sargent, Mrs Ruth S **(A)**
Schrott, Mrs Ruth G **(SLP)**
Wagner, Susan Adele **(SLP)**
Webb, Mrs Katherine **(SLP)**
Williams, Sheila Carol **(SLP)**
Wilson, Mrs Evelyn L **(SLP)**

Rice
Eiban, Mrs Gloria D **(SLP)**

Rich Creek
Brown, Penny B **(SLP)**

Richmond
Albright, Mrs Paulette A **(SLP A)**
Anderson, Mrs Marcia Alexander **(SLP)**
Andrews, Mrs Jane W **(SLP)**
Ballard, Deborah Denise **(SLP)**
Barnes, Christine Cheryl **(SLP)**
Basinger, Sherry Marie **(SLP)**
Behrendt, Mrs Linda Lane **(SLP)**
Benda, Mary G **(SLP)**
Bernstein, Dr Claire M **(A)**
Blachman, Lynn **(SLP)**
Blanchard, Jane Maxwell **(A)**
Breeding, Brenda Sue **(SLP)**
Brenner, Mrs Joann F **(SLP)**
Browne, Mrs Nancy P **(A)**
Bruce, Mrs Carolyn Walker **(SLP)**
Bruckhart, Mrs Margaret Nissley **(SLP)**
Bryant, Dr Douglas F **(A)**
Bryant, Mrs Kim Christman **(A)**
Burke, Barbara R **(SLP)**
Butts, Dr Frank M **(A)**
Camden, Mrs Rebecca Rankin **(A)**
Card, Mrs Yolonda Baker **(SLP)**
Casey, Kathleen Ferguson **(SLP)**
Casey, Thomas A, Jr **(A)**
Charles, Mrs Patricia D **(SLP)**
Cleary, Mrs Christine Fowler **(SLP)**
Cuff, Martin Daniel
Daniels, Wendy Louise **(SLP)**
Deleo, Monica Rose **(SLP)**
Divizio, Gail Ellen **(SLP)**
Dunton, Virginia Jordan **(SLP)**
Durham, Catherine Therese
Dwyer-Urban, Regina **(SLP)**
Dysert, Mrs Denise H **(SLP)**
Edelstein, Mrs Geraldine Ozark
Eichten, Philip I **(SLP)**
Flinn, Mrs Sally E **(SLP)**
Flowers, Dr Elsie Ann **(SLP)**
Ford, Valerie Sarno **(SLP)**
Fulp, Angela Morgan **(SLP)**
Gareau, Ann M **(SLP)**
Gillespie, Cheryl D **(SLP)**
Goodman, Mrs Julie S **(SLP)**
Gregory, Sharon A **(SLP A)**
Hankammer, Mrs S Bonnie **(SLP)**
Harless, Karen Adams **(SLP)**
Harsh, Betty Anne **(SLP)**
Hurwitz, Mrs Diane Albert
Jenkins, Mrs Sarah **(SLP)**
Johnson, Rebecca C **(SLP)**
Jones, Dr Ronald Count **(A)**
Kaminsky, Mrs Maryann P **(SLP)**
Karam, Marilyn R **(SLP)**
Kelly, Erma F **(SLP)**
King, Dr Michael D **(SLP)**
Klein, Lorraine E **(A)**
Kriegman, Mrs Lois S
Laneve, Natalie Rose **(A)**
Lennox, Barbara E **(SLP)**
Lent, Barbara Claire **(SLP)**
Levine, Mrs Risa F **(SLP)**
Ligon, Judith Carol **(SLP)**
Lingerfelt, Gwendolynn F **(SLP)**
Little, Patricia Wright **(SLP)**
Loughran, Colleen **(A)**
Lowe, M Kathleen **(SLP)**
Macri, Constance Leigh
Marrs, Mrs Elizabeth Gage **(A)**
Marshall, Mrs Robin A H **(A)**
Martino, Nancy L **(SLP)**
Maxwell, Jean A **(SLP)**
May, Diana P **(SLP)**
McGinley, Heather L **(A)**
Metzger, Jayne W **(A)**
Millhiser, Mrs Rochelle D **(SLP)**
Minshew, Susan Ricks **(A)**
Modde, Mrs Karen A
Morris, Susan L **(SLP)**
Murphy, Karla B A **(SLP)**
Nelson, Jane E T **(A)**
Norfleet, Mrs Michele M **(SLP)**
Norvell, Beth Ann Frisk **(SLP)**
Nuckols-Currence, Margaret **(SLP)**
Ogborn, Laurinda L
Oggel, Mrs Linda Lou Shearer **(SLP)**
Oyler-Russell, Mary Elizabeth **(SLP)**
Peek, Emily Francis **(A)**
Proctor, Mrs Lorraine DeStefano **(SLP)**
Ramser, Mrs Angelique Thacker **(SLP)**
Richard, Mrs Sharon Smith **(SLP)**
Rivers, Tracy Irene
Ryals, Dr Brenda Morgan **(A)**
Sale, Mrs Cheryl C **(A)**
Sanford, Mrs Helen J **(SLP)**
Schay, Mrs Nancy Lambdin **(A)**
Schutte, Mrs Melissa W **(SLP)**
Seaton, Mrs Joanne C **(A)**
Semach, Diane L **(SLP)**
Silverman, Robyn D
Sledd, Mrs Lourie S **(A)**
Smit, Mrs Pamela Mills **(SLP)**
Smith, Nancy A **(A)**
Stastny, Mrs Gwynn S **(SLP)**
Steele, William Fredrick **(A)**
Stillerman, Fern **(SLP)**
Taylor, Mrs Patricia Ann **(SLP)**
Trivelpiece, Mrs Ruth Moskowitz **(SLP)**
Ulmer, Mrs Susan Judith **(A)**
Vancey, Mrs Gail Richerson **(SLP)**
Vergales, Phylis Ellen **(A)**
White, Mary Anne **(SLP)**
Williams, Angela Kay
Williams, Nancy Lynne
Wintermeyer, Dana B **(SLP)**
Wooten, Dr Philip Gary
Wright, Susan Meredith **(A)**
Yeamans, Carolyn J **(SLP)**

Roanoke
Barrow, Mrs Mary Hunter **(SLP)**
Beasley, Lillian Elaine **(A)**
Berry-Shawver, Sally Lu **(SLP)**
Brown, Luann **(SLP)**
Buckley, Mrs Katherine Gregory **(SLP)**
Colletti, Laurel Jean **(SLP)**
Cundiff, Phyllis Mae **(SLP)**
Edwards, Ellen C **(SLP)**
Freeman, Margaret H **(SLP)**
Hall, Emily L
Hawkins, Richard R **(A)**
Hopkins, Mrs Mary R **(SLP)**
Ingle, Mrs Bobbie H **(A)**
James, Mrs Mary-Teresa C **(A)**
Kahn, Mary Kay **(SLP)**
Kampf, Pamela D **(SLP A)**
Katz, Mrs Sarabeth B **(SLP)**
King, Linda Johnston **(SLP)**
Lambeth, Robert Scott **(SLP)**
Maranzano, Nanci A **(SLP)**
Mason, Susan Shaw **(SLP)**
Masters, Dr Joseph J **(SLP)**
Maxwell, Martha Lynn **(SLP)**
Miller, Mrs Jennifer Stump **(SLP)**
Moore, George Wayne **(A)**
Olson, Charlene Marie **(SLP)**
Orem, Mrs Ann P **(SLP)**
Peters, Mrs Patricia Myers **(SLP)**
Ridenhour, Michael W **(A)**
Schmitt, Sharon P **(SLP)**
Silverstein, Aditi Eve **(SLP)**
Smithey, Nancy T **(SLP)**
Tinsley, Kerri D **(SLP)**
Trout, Mrs Kimberly L
Wilkinson, Dr Robert J **(SLP)**
Williams, Mrs Deborah A **(SLP)**

Round Hill
Smale, Mrs Ruth **(SLP)**

Rustburg
Wright, Hope Vandegrift **(SLP)**

Salem
Abbanat, Mrs Ginette Rand **(SLP)**
Arm, Janine I **(SLP)**
Cobb, Dr Frederick Edmund **(A)**
Dorsey, Mrs Joan J **(SLP)**
Grove, Mrs Tammy Herring **(SLP)**
Singleton, Susan Kessler **(SLP)**
Whichard, Mrs Susan P **(A)**

Saltville
Carter, Betsy L **(SLP)**

Smithfield
Cypress, Marian Amanda **(SLP)**
Garrett, Mrs Mavis W **(A)**
Saunders, Barbara Gray **(A)**

South Boston
Lacy, Mrs Brigitte Gil **(SLP)**
McBride, Mrs Vivian D **(SLP)**

South Hill
Hicks, Elaine Robin **(SLP)**

Springfield
Baxter, Mrs Theresa G **(SLP)**
Blumberg, Pamela P **(SLP)**
Botuck, Deborah Ann **(SLP)**
Call, Janice Merlo **(SLP)**
Cardenuto, Nancy Jeanne **(SLP)**
Casey, Edith Nmi **(SLP)**
Chadwick, Susan G **(A)**
Chapell, Patti E **(SLP)**
Georger, Diane Duggan **(SLP)**
Grundeman, Mrs Sandra Edson **(SLP)**
MacKie, Mrs Elizabeth Ann **(SLP)**
McKinney, Marcia Ann **(SLP)**
McManus, Natalie Gutow **(SLP)**
Nichols, Diane E **(SLP)**
Paivanas, Susan M K **(SLP)**
Person, Cheryl L **(SLP)**
Priebe, Florence M **(SLP)**
Qualls, Dr Pamela Hammett **(SLP)**
Radke, Mary C Popp **(SLP)**
Rice, Mrs Shannon L **(SLP)**
Rockwood, Mrs Judith D **(SLP)**
Ruelle, Mrs Martha L **(SLP)**
Sarnes, Mrs Diane Bea **(SLP)**
Wall, Mrs Brenda **(SLP)**

Stafford
Johansen, Mrs Sharon H **(SLP)**
Josserand, Mrs Deedra Quay **(SLP)**
Mills, Denise Marie **(A)**
Wanner, Nancy Weakley **(SLP)**

Stanardsville
Layton, Mrs Donna K **(SLP)**
Realy, Janice Scully **(A)**

Staunton
Alexander, Kenmar Campbell **(A)**
Carpenter, Mrs Marilyn S **(SLP)**
Craun-Carey, Mrs Kelly Vivian **(SLP)**
Finnegan, Dr Denis Edward **(SLP)**
Jones-Oleson, Mrs Linda Doreen **(SLP)**
O'Hare, Dr Nancy K **(SLP A)**
Pierce, Linda Kite **(SLP)**

Shifflett, Martha Ellen **(A)**

Stephens City
Powell, Mrs Marsha Stollings **(SLP)**
Rinker, Nancy C **(A)**

Sterling
Casuccio, R Christine **(A)**
Chisholm, Barbara B **(SLP)**
Goode, Mrs Sharon Blackford
Oswald, Mrs Beth A **(SLP)**
Wakefield, Maureen Pohn **(SLP)**
Wilson, Mrs Paula S **(A)**

Sterling Park
Bergman, Mrs Judy Merlin **(SLP)**

Suffolk
Johnson, Mrs Sara Ann **(SLP)**
Smith, Catherine **(SLP)**

Sumerduck
Hampton, Andrea J B **(SLP)**

Sweet Briar
Meadows, Sally B **(SLP)**

Tabb
Blouin, Martha Jo **(SLP)**

Tappahannock
Winslow, Mrs Cynthia C **(SLP)**

Tazewell
Prince, David C

Timberville
Lewis, Mrs Margaret Kyle **(SLP)**

Triangle
Locke, Mrs Miriam G **(SLP)**
Phillips, Frances Carol **(SLP)**

Troutville
Hedrick, Mark Stephen
Welsh, Mrs Pamela S **(SLP)**

Urbanna
Reuse, Alison Foote **(SLP)**

Verona
Ruud, Elizabeth McKee **(SLP)**

Vienna
Atkinson, Dr James Edward
Bell, Mary W **(SLP)**
Bergey, Mrs Patricia S **(SLP)**
Blacklin, Mrs Jerrie Schmalzer **(SLP)**
Bosone, Dr Zilpha T **(SLP)**
Cummings, Janet L **(SLP)**
Eid, Catherine Nasri **(SLP)**
Fairbanks, Kelly Ann **(SLP)**
Fischi, Mrs Barbara M **(SLP)**
Gale, Deborah C **(SLP)**
Herold, Marcia A **(SLP)**
Hine, Patricia Lynne **(SLP)**
Hinman, Mrs Barbara J **(SLP)**
Houston, Mrs Joan H **(SLP)**
Klein, Mrs Camille S **(A)**
Knox, Dr Thomas E
Koches, Mrs Lisa C **(SLP)**
Louick, Mrs Bettye A **(SLP)**
Moore, Mrs Jeneen Graves **(SLP)**
Nelson, Claudia P **(SLP)**
Pendlebury, Mrs Marianne F **(SLP)**
Perrin, Mrs Karen I **(SLP)**
Pryor, Maryann S **(SLP)**
Purcell, Rita Marie **(SLP)**
Rice, Mrs Cheryl E **(A)**
Roman, Mrs Virginia P **(SLP)**
Roselle, Mrs Rebecca S **(SLP)**
Schmauss, Cheryl L **(SLP)**
Shoham, Andrea B **(SLP)**
Stackhouse, Mrs Rhoda J **(SLP)**
Stolarik, Gail A **(SLP)**
Tabor, Mrs Marie A **(SLP)**
Warren, Linda S **(SLP)**
Westbrook, Mrs Mary K **(A)**

Vinton
Beckett, Mrs Rebecca Justus **(SLP)**

Virginia Beach
Apfelbeck, Mrs Jean Glover **(SLP)**
Arney, Mary Shepard **(SLP)**
Barnes, Mrs Mary Jane **(SLP)**
Barrow, Mrs Irene Marie **(SLP)**
Bingham, Mrs Carol Cole **(SLP)**
Bowhers, Mrs Wendy **(SLP)**
Brower, Mrs Joan **(SLP)**
Brupbacher, Mrs Nancy Aldrich **(A)**
Burns, Kathleen Ruth **(SLP)**
Burwell, Cynthia L **(SLP)**
Callender, Mrs Martha M **(SLP)**
Carpenter, Regina M **(SLP)**
Cicotello, Christine
Clark, Mrs Christine M **(SLP)**
Clayton, Mary K **(SLP)**
Coffman, Mrs Robbin K
Cohill, Mary B **(SLP)**
Crawford, Mrs Arleen B **(SLP)**
Cullen, Monica L **(A)**
Davidson, Mrs Anne Massenburg **(SLP)**
Davis, Mrs Margaret B **(SLP)**
Dickman, Mrs Harriet B **(SLP)**
Finkelstein, Mrs Patricia Auerbach **(SLP)**
Gamsey, Helen B **(A)**
Garretson, Dr Carolyn D **(SLP)**
Goldin, Miriam R **(SLP)**
Gray, Marybeth
Hall, Cheryl L **(SLP)**
Harold, Mrs Alma H **(SLP)**
Harrell-Cowell, Mrs Carolyn Denise **(A)**
Harrison, Jan Lanette **(SLP)**
Holt, Connie Smith **(A)**
Holt, Stephanie Virginia **(SLP)**
Jacobs, Mrs Dale H **(SLP)**
Jingst, Judith Ann **(SLP)**
Johnson, Mrs Patricia A **(SLP)**
Jordan, Mrs Jacqueline **(SLP)**
Kane, Christina Marie **(SLP)**
Keally, Mrs Maryann Wilson **(SLP)**
Kilpatrick-Staubus, Jean M **(SLP)**
Leffke, Gary S **(A)**
Lenhart, Mrs Brenda Craig **(SLP)**
Lewis, Yvonne J **(SLP)**
McGinty-Pace, Patricia L **(SLP)**
McKanna, Mrs Susan I **(SLP)**
Michele, Judith Louise **(SLP)**
Mulligan, Marilyn G **(SLP)**
Page, Mrs Ruth M **(SLP)**
Pechan, Paula P **(A)**
Pecorelli, Mrs Judith A **(SLP)**
Pendleton, Anne Zenobia
Pratt, Janet **(SLP)**
Raymer, Mrs Anastasia Moynihan **(SLP)**
Saunders, Mrs Kathleen Duerr **(SLP)**
Schweiger, Mrs Barbara Reese **(SLP)**
Sharp, Jack R **(SLP)**
Sheppard, Angela Dawn **(A)**
Simmons, Mrs A Ferrin **(SLP)**
Sipe, Mrs Linda J **(A)**
Snyders, Cathryn Pearse **(SLP)**
Stallings, Mrs Melody Akers **(SLP)**
Tace, Mrs Heather J
Themides, Michelle Anne **(SLP)**
Vortherms, Mrs Kimberly A **(SLP)**
Weber, Mrs Mary Amelia **(SLP)**
Weingart, Lori **(A)**
White, Mrs Susan G **(SLP)**
Wilkinson, Melissa K
Wynn-Dancy, Margaret L **(SLP)**
Yoshikawa, Courtney Smith **(SLP)**
Zoller, Mrs Valerie Ann

Warrenton
Gauthier, Mrs Mary O **(SLP)**
Morgan, Mrs Ruth Howells **(SLP)**
Payne, Susan Clair **(SLP)**
Phillips, Anne H **(SLP)**
Schwalbach, Mrs Diane Mc Coy **(A)**

Warsaw
Whiteway, Mrs Deborah Hare **(SLP)**

Washington
Dougherty, Mrs Mary Kathryn **(SLP)**

Waynesboro
Preski, Jeanne **(SLP)**
Ratliff, Susan L H **(SLP)**
Sadonis, Cynthia **(A)**
Van Huss, Margaret C **(SLP)**
Yeamans, Elizabeth Louise **(SLP)**

West Point
Barkey-Kasminsky, Mrs Deborah Ann **(SLP)**

Williamsburg
Brumfield, Mrs Katharine **(SLP)**
Grutzner-Martell, Heidi Jo **(SLP)**
Matherne, Roberta T **(SLP)**
Oliver, Lydia Tussey **(SLP A)**
Paul, Dr John E **(SLP)**
Peterson, Alicia Ruth **(A)**
Puffenberger, Mrs Janice K **(SLP)**
Simasek, Mrs Mary Grace **(SLP)**
Turner, Mrs Nancy Wilson **(SLP)**

Winchester
Cardinale, Carol M **(SLP)**
Clay, Teresa H **(SLP)**
Covert, Mrs Kathleen **(SLP)**
Fehr, Eric M **(SLP)**
Fisher, Barbara Cyr **(SLP)**
Franz, Robert J, Jr **(SLP)**
Jennings, Amy Leigh **(A)**
Kwitowski, Mrs Clare N **(SLP)**
Owen, John R **(SLP A)**
Wever, Mrs Jane R **(SLP)**

Wise
Butler, Janice Merrial **(SLP)**
Cole, Mrs Georgeanne **(SLP)**
Helbert, Fredia **(A)**

Woodbridge
Blaemire, Mrs Robin L **(SLP)**
Carini, Mrs Patricia Kane **(SLP)**
Coyle, Jane N **(SLP)**
Ettinger, Donna Proctor **(A)**
Fees, Mrs Margaret Ruffennach **(SLP)**
Gillespie, Mrs Judith B **(SLP)**
Haygood, Mrs Kathy C **(SLP)**
Holmes, Mrs Robyn C **(SLP)**
Jamieson, Mrs Frances Rayman
Keane, Marta M **(SLP)**
Kerr, Mrs Robin R **(SLP)**
Martin, Mrs Joanne Wilbur **(SLP)**
Montalvo, Cathryn F **(SLP)**
Moore, Joseph H **(SLP)**
Narburgh, David H **(SLP)**
O'Neill, Janet J **(SLP)**
Spoth, Mrs Elizabeth Segovia **(SLP)**
Stanaland, Joyce L **(SLP)**
Steinmeyer, Mrs Christine K **(SLP)**
Warnke, Mrs Ann Marie **(SLP)**
Williams, Helen Hargadon **(SLP)**

Woodlawn
Edmonds, Mrs Rebecca L **(A)**
Smith, Douglas M **(SLP)**

Woolwine
Cockram, Mrs Shannon Smith **(SLP)**

Wytheville
Mize, Pamala Dawn **(A)**

Yorktown
Fiskus, Mrs Selwa M **(SLP)**

WASHINGTON

Aberdeen
Akerlund, Paula M **(SLP)**
Kelley, Roberta Ann **(SLP)**
Keltner, Jerry L **(SLP)**

Addy
Drake, Beverly S **(SLP)**

Anacortes
Guderjohn, Lloyd Marvin **(SLP)**
Miller, Mrs Margaret T **(SLP)**

Ardenvoir
Mallon, Christine **(SLP)**

Arlington
Oquist, Mrs Kerstin **(SLP)**
Thordarson, Kathleen Wells **(SLP)**

Auburn
Bradley, Alana K **(SLP)**
Burrows, Heidi Olson **(SLP)**
Ciampi, Mrs Valerie Marie **(SLP)**
Ginn, Sandra Luenn **(A)**
Lix, Jean D **(SLP)**
Primley, Alice A **(SLP)**
Trebay, Dana Victoria **(A)**

Bainbridge Island
Albright, Janet Juracich **(A)**
Blackadar, Sue Helen **(SLP)**
Donahoo, Barbara L **(SLP)**
Goldstein, Mrs Marion B **(SLP)**
Resager, Mrs Barbara W **(SLP)**

Bangor
Rogers, Susan H **(SLP)**

Battle Ground
Saltness, Mrs Lori Jo **(SLP)**
Vander-Ploeg, James **(SLP)**

Belfair
Sleight, Mrs Wendy Corrine S **(SLP)**

Bellevue
Ashcom, Mrs Pamela H **(SLP)**
Azure, Mrs Linda S
Bennett, Mrs Nellie Mae **(SLP)**
Bess-Berg, Mrs Doris F **(SLP)**
Burditt, Gayle J L **(SLP)**
Cook, Anne Mary **(A)**
Dafforn, Rhonda M B **(SLP)**
Delisi, Adele O **(SLP)**
Delplain, Robert C **(SLP A)**
Dohrmann, Mrs Vicki Sue **(SLP)**
Funk, Janis E **(SLP)**
Green, Carol A **(SLP)**
Greenbaum, Annette
Holt, Mrs Jo Anne Nyberg **(SLP)**
Ingerson, Mrs Linda Leigh **(SLP)**
Kadavy, Julie Rice **(SLP)**
Lestz, Mrs Nancy Morris **(SLP)**
List, Catherine Oas **(SLP)**
Lloyd, Janet M **(SLP)**
Luhman, Annalee D **(SLP)**
Malte, Patricia L **(SLP)**
Marques, Corinne L **(SLP)**
Marrs, Mrs Sandra Lorentz **(SLP)**
Matsui, Lisa **(SLP)**
Maule, Bettyjo
McRae, Mrs Carol **(SLP)**
Milstein, Leslie J **(SLP)**
Neu, Mrs Jean H **(SLP)**
Oppfelt, Glenn R **(SLP A)**
Parks, Theresa M C **(SLP)**
Peterson, Nina E **(SLP)**
Prins, Dr David **(SLP)**
Radin, Nona S **(A)**
Redenbaugh, Margaret Ann **(SLP)**
Rettig, Nancy D **(SLP)**
Schild, Mrs Pamela K **(SLP)**
Therriault, Teresa Marie **(SLP)**
Veith, Mary C **(SLP)**
Watson, Louise Gooch **(SLP)**
Wolthausen, Julie Pollock
Wuth, James F **(A)**
Zimmerman, Joseph B **(SLP)**

Bellingham
Ambrose, Mrs Carolyn E **(SLP)**
Anderson, Mrs Lois L **(SLP)**

Banas, Patricia A **(SLP)**
Brown, Mrs Beverly J **(SLP)**
Cahoon-Simon, Mrs Sandra **(SLP)**
Carlile, Mrs Jill Ann **(SLP)**
Chase, Mardi **(A)**
Cunningham, Gary W **(SLP)**
Egan, James P **(A)**
Egan, Dr Katherine S **(SLP A)**
Frederick, Shonie Elizabeth **(A)**
Ganz, Candace K **(SLP)**
Genuit, Christine **(SLP)**
Hess, Gregory R **(A)**
Hunter, Mrs Donna J **(A)**
Hunt-Thompson, Jill **(SLP)**
McRandle, Dr Carol C **(SLP A)**
Montag, Mary M **(SLP)**
Newell, Sharon Lynn
Polen, Dr Samuel B **(SLP)**
Quick, Margaret M **(SLP)**
Ryan, Mrs Rosemary E **(SLP)**
Schinske, Dr Erhart A **(SLP)**
Seilo, Dr Michael T **(SLP A)**
Smith, Janice A **(SLP)**
Solomon, Dr Arthur L **(SLP)**
Webb, Dr Loren L **(A)**
Wells-Weekly, Barbara J **(SLP)**
Zeine, Dr Lina **(SLP)**

Bonney Lake
Knutzen, Mrs Robin H **(SLP)**
Larson, Christine **(SLP)**

Bothell
Bannister, Kay A **(SLP)**
Bentz, Jocelyn Gillen **(SLP)**
Bittner, Mrs Colleen Creason **(SLP)**
Brock, Miriam S **(SLP)**
Demmert, Karen R **(SLP)**
Ellis, Shana **(SLP)**
Jacobson, Mrs Dana B **(SLP)**
Jacobson, Mrs Deborah A **(SLP)**
McCoy, Mary K **(SLP)**
Pietrowski, Mrs Ann Peyser **(SLP)**
Reanier, Mrs Carol Cook **(SLP)**
Schultz, Jean M **(SLP)**
Stenseth, Mrs Natalie W **(SLP)**
Ware, Mrs Virginia A **(SLP)**
Waugh, Patricia F **(SLP)**

Bow
Allen, Debra Betschart **(SLP)**

Bremerton
Black, S K **(SLP)**
Dougherty, Mrs Susan F **(SLP)**
Duke, Mrs Judith Ann **(SLP)**
Flondarina, Mrs Susan B **(SLP)**
Flynn, Mrs Rose Marie **(SLP)**
Foley, Michael Joseph **(A)**
Johnson, Mrs Josephine W **(SLP)**
Keen, Mrs Lynn E **(A)**
Kipps, Helen A **(SLP)**
McMahon, Ann Fleming **(SLP)**
Raszler, Diane W **(A)**
Wax, LCDR James P **(A)**

Buckley
Roberts, Paul E **(SLP)**

Camano Island
Furuheim, Mrs Frances W **(SLP)**

Camas
Downer, Mrs Margaret L **(SLP)**
Lorang-Schmirler, Mrs Karen Marie **(SLP)**

Centralia
Odegard, Thomas B **(A)**

Chehalis
Edwards, Sue J **(SLP)**
Emerick, Mary L **(SLP)**
Gantry, Anita Rae **(SLP)**
Gober, Mrs Karen M **(SLP)**
Harvey, David J **(SLP)**

Chelan
Clare, Laurel Ann **(SLP)**

Cheney
Breitenfeldt, Dr Dorvan H **(SLP)**
Briggs, Robert E **(SLP)**
Craig, Dr J Marvin **(SLP A)**
Hahn, Dr Patricia A **(SLP)**
Haugen, Dr David M **(SLP)**
Mertens, Patricia Lynne **(SLP)**
Russell, Dr Marilyn Margaret **(SLP)**
Sima, Shannon Marie **(SLP)**
Triplett, Mrs Julenne Kay **(SLP)**

Chewelah
Schott-Evans, Mrs Diane M **(SLP)**

Clarkston
Brown, Mrs Melissa Bengtson **(SLP)**

Cle Elum
Toepel, Gail A **(A)**

Clinton
Suhadolnik, Sarah Jane

Colbert
Shafer, Mrs Mary B **(SLP)**

Colfax
Eskelson, Edna Mae **(SLP)**

College Place
Nailor, Audrey
Wood, Clarence A **(SLP)**

Connell
Minor, Mrs Wendy Mary

Deer Harbor
Hutchins, Mrs Kathryn J **(SLP)**

Deer Park
Bowlin-Johnson, Jo Anna **(A)**
Davis, Mrs Susan J **(SLP)**

Duvall
Amend, Mrs Mary J **(SLP)**

East Wenatchee
Kerby, Mary Ellen **(SLP)**

Edmonds
Bohnhoff, Mrs Cathy I **(A)**
Knowles, Mrs Patti Rose **(SLP)**
Knowles-McCall, Mrs Amy S **(A)**
Lindemann, Larisa **(SLP)**
Lubach, Karly S **(SLP)**
Miller, Dr Janice Gritti **(SLP)**
O'Farrell, Deirdre Ann
Rush, Mrs Judith I **(SLP)**

Ellensburg
Franzen, Dr Richard Lyle **(A)**
Geigle, Paula Rae **(SLP)**
Harris, Donald Ray **(SLP)**
Lynch, Linda Lee **(SLP)**
Purcell, Jackie Lianne **(SLP)**

Enumclaw
Northfield, Mrs Jeanne S R **(SLP)**
Warren, Mrs Margaret V **(SLP)**

Ephrata
Dell, Beverly D **(SLP A)**

Everett
Beach, Kimberlee K **(SLP)**
Brade, Mrs Vivian A **(SLP)**
Butler, Mrs Barbara J **(SLP)**
Chagnon, Kathleen J **(SLP)**
Farley, Nancy Petrus
Jevne, Robert B **(SLP)**
Johnson, Joni Lynn **(A)**
Johnson, Kevin Charles **(SLP)**
Knudsen, Nancy Willard **(SLP)**
Mallahan, Michael Stephen **(A)**
Pajak, Nancy Hartman **(A)**
Pearce, Carol Susan **(SLP)**
Quinn, Allison Mary **(A)**
Williams, Mrs Carol Troffer **(SLP A)**

Everson
Lilley, Georgetta Sue **(SLP)**
Sparks, Diane Seydell **(SLP)**

Fairchild AFB
Bennett, Capt Carolyn Sydnee **(A)**

Federal Way
Ayers, Shelley B **(SLP)**
Birmingham, Mrs Elizabeth A **(SLP)**
Chinn, Mrs Gaye Sasaki **(A)**
Cole, Donna Ann **(SLP)**
Geyer, Suzanne T W **(SLP)**
Hartman, Mrs Susan Deck **(SLP)**
Jentges, Helen C **(SLP)**
Johansen, Alice Elizabeth **(SLP)**
Kolbeck, Mrs Cathleen M **(SLP)**
Manning, Dr Charlie C **(SLP A)**
O'Neill, Rosanna Marie **(SLP)**
Schultz, Mrs Cheryl Ann **(SLP)**
Templeman, Mary A **(SLP)**
Torkelsen, Mrs Darla J
Warner, Kimberley Racheal **(SLP)**

Ferndale
Tunnell, John S **(A)**
Williams, Mrs Sharon Louise **(SLP)**

Fort Lewis
Brittain, Mrs Gwen Frutchey **(SLP)**
Magelssen, Liane **(A)**

Fox Island
Dukes, Linda Zehnder **(SLP)**

FPO Seattle
Baumann, Carolyn A
Cowan, Katherine Elizabeth **(SLP)**
Gischia, Mrs Carol Faulkner **(A)**
Kidder, Dr Herman C **(A)**
Levitt, Joyce Barbara **(SLP)**
Markeson, Judith M **(SLP)**
Rovig, Glen W **(A)**
Smith, Mrs Eileen F **(A)**
Smith, Mrs Karen E **(SLP)**
Thomas, Kenneth E **(SLP)**
Wagner, Sylvia Clymer **(SLP)**

Gig Harbor
Berg, Viola G **(SLP)**
Dean, Mrs Diana C **(SLP)**
Drew, Mrs Karin **(SLP)**
Evans, Mrs Candace M **(SLP)**
Mason, Pamela Jean **(SLP)**
Oliver, Mrs Kathy D **(SLP)**
Pearson, Barbara A **(SLP)**
Rosendahl, Pamela DePonty **(SLP)**
Rowe, Colleen M **(SLP)**
Stevens, Jamie H **(SLP)**

Goldendale
Grossman, James S
Monthey, Joanne C

Grandview
Lawrence, Thomas George **(SLP)**

Hoquiam
Scoones, Mark Howard **(A)**

Issaquah
Abate, Mrs Mary A **(SLP)**
Atcheson, Dr Barbara A **(SLP A)**
Baker, Tarrah M **(SLP)**
Brown, Diane D **(SLP)**
Cohn, Susan G **(SLP)**
Flag, Carol L **(SLP)**
Flynn, Lori D **(SLP)**
Kagan, Marcia **(SLP)**
Meyers, Annette L **(SLP)**
Rowe, Katherine Liann **(SLP)**
Saylor, Suzanne P **(SLP)**
Scott, Kathy P **(SLP)**
Seiber, James L **(SLP)**
Weisel, Mrs Christine **(SLP)**
Yalowitz, Jan A **(SLP)**

Kelso
Conaway, Karen B **(SLP)**

Kennewick
Anderson, Mrs Joann Wanda **(SLP)**
Hague, Kevin W **(A)**
Hollenback, Mrs Sylvia D **(SLP)**
Jordan, Mrs Maria Poon **(SLP)**
King, Marilyn O **(SLP)**
Loosveldt, Sylvia L **(SLP)**
Stevenson, Linda L **(SLP)**
Stredwick, Laura Lee **(SLP)**

Kent
Clarke, Mrs Patricia McGinley **(SLP)**
Dooley, Linda Rae **(SLP)**
Harestad, Mrs Carolyn **(SLP)**
Lainoff, Janice S **(SLP)**
Olson, Karin Elizabeth **(SLP)**
Page, Mrs Gwendolyn M **(SLP)**
Prout, Nancy A **(SLP)**
Reister, Gaye McKinnon
Rickert, Nancy E W **(SLP)**
Sponseller, Karen S **(SLP)**
Wagner, Mrs Danette P
Wilkins, Lucinda M **(SLP)**
Williams, Mary H

Kirkland
Barnett-Frazier, Amy Frances **(SLP)**
Brace, Terri L
Callahan, Margaret J **(SLP)**
Cerf, Dr F Ann **(SLP)**
Clark-Hahn, Jannet Eileen **(A)**
Davis, Nancy L **(SLP)**
Downes, Mrs Charlene S **(SLP)**
Gauthier, Sharon V **(SLP)**
Lewis, Judy L **(SLP)**
McCrory, Ana Moran **(SLP)**
Morell, Susan A W **(SLP)**
Norwood, Thomas J **(A)**
Robinson, Kristi Ellice **(SLP)**

La Conner
Erickson, Mrs Susan J **(SLP)**

Lacey
Caldwell, Catherine Lynne
Richeson, Mrs Denice Elaine D **(SLP)**

Lake Stevens
Adams, Mrs Linda G **(SLP)**
Quigley, Mrs Suzanne Marion **(A)**

Langley
Liddell, Richard A **(SLP)**

Leavenworth
Fitz-Armstrong, Dr Linda C **(SLP)**

Liberty Lake
Anderson, Ellen Biddle **(SLP)**
Reed, Kristi Holzheimer **(A)**

Longview
Chapman, Marian Rose **(SLP)**
Healea, Susan Kay **(A)**
Orthel, Susan D **(SLP)**
Ring, Mrs Cosette Laurie
Weed, Suzanne G **(SLP)**

Loon Lake
Johnson, Mrs Doris E **(SLP)**

Lynnwood
Andrews, Claudia B **(SLP)**
Cobb-Cooper, Julie **(SLP)**
Cogley, Wallace H **(SLP)**
Emerling, Lisa Gail
Johnson, Mrs Suzanne **(SLP)**
Patterson, Mrs Elizabeth McCleave **(SLP)**
Rowley, Mrs Cindy Jo **(SLP)**

Manson
Templin, Jessica Leigh

Marysville
Goset, Frederick **(A)**

McHord AFB
Formes-Ackerson, Mrs Carol **(SLP)**

Mead
Norton, Mrs Lynette A **(SLP)**

Medical Lake
Grigar, Mrs Janice G **(SLP)**

Medina
Phillips, Mrs Sylvia Dean **(SLP)**

Mercer Island
Bogle, Janice T **(SLP A)**
Bray, Mrs Mary K **(A)**
Kenfield, Ann E **(SLP)**
Lippke, Mrs Barbara A **(SLP)**
Redd, Mrs Jill **(SLP)**
Spiegelberg, Beverly **(SLP)**
Wright, Anita L **(SLP)**

Metaline Falls
Reed, Mrs Jane Elizabeth **(SLP)**

Mill Creek
Glover, Sherrie M **(SLP)**

Monroe
Swenson, Katharine Freeburg **(SLP)**

Moses Lake
Sisson, Elizabeth Marie **(SLP)**

Mount Vernon
Fish, Mrs Gloria Jane **(SLP)**
Scott, David Michael **(SLP)**
Shulenberger, Kayle A **(SLP)**
Webb, Wendy Stewart **(A)**

Mountlake Terrace
Hall, Ruthann **(SLP)**
Meiser, Amy Maria **(A)**
Mourtada, Mrs Patricia R **(SLP)**

Mukilteo
Campbell, Kelli Sue **(SLP)**
Jones, Mrs Janet Hyde **(SLP)**
Rambo, Mrs Mary H B **(SLP)**
Wendt, Katherine Lynn **(SLP)**

Naches
Glover, Marie E **(SLP)**

Newman Lake
McKinney, Mrs Christine Lee **(SLP)**

Newport
Hall, Suzy D **(SLP)**
Rickey, Mrs Lola Ann **(SLP)**

Nine Mile Falls
Demaris, Mrs Terri M **(SLP)**

North Bend
Rixon, Mrs Shelley Eckels **(SLP)**
Szumlas, Mrs Janet J **(SLP)**

Oak Harbor
Aldridge, Mrs Augusta S **(SLP)**
Porter, Lawrence A **(SLP)**
Reynolds, Julia Winifred **(A)**
Watson, Michael Lyon **(SLP)**

Ocean Shores
Johnson, Reid C **(SLP)**

Okanogan
Bankhead, Lorna Marian **(SLP)**

Olympia
Allsop, Terilee **(SLP)**
Boyce, Mrs Susan H **(SLP)**
Clemens, Karen L **(SLP)**
Foreman, Mrs Karen Lynne **(SLP)**
Foster, Karen K **(SLP)**
Frahm, Caren Bernice **(SLP)**
Gabrielse, Patricia Handley **(SLP)**
Goodwin, Mary Beth
Grubb, Suzanne Shor **(SLP)**
Hancock, Mrs Sally M **(SLP)**
Hansen, Diane Louise **(SLP)**
Harbour, Anita S H **(SLP)**
Kimmel, Barry L **(A)**
Krehbiel, Mary B **(SLP)**
Miranda, Mrs Judith T **(SLP)**
Mose, Mrs Janyce K **(A)**
Ruhl, A Connie (Kuhrt) **(SLP)**
Staiger, Sharon J **(SLP)**
Staton, Robert N **(A)**
Weeks, Patricia Sue **(SLP)**
Woods, Roland E **(SLP)**
Zodrow, Nancy S **(SLP)**

Omak
Werth, Kathryn J **(SLP)**

Othello
Simpson, Mrs Connie V **(SLP)**

Pasco
Grilley, Mrs Beryl H **(SLP)**
Ihrig, Steve **(SLP)**

Port Angeles
Hall, Betty F **(SLP)**
Mather, Mrs Susan O **(A)**
Meier, Gary A **(SLP)**

Port Orchard
Sanders, Mrs Jana S **(SLP)**

Port Townsend
Fitch, Waring J **(A)**
Fraser, Anita Louise **(SLP)**
Pratt, Mrs Kim Loraine **(SLP)**

Poulsbo
Campbell, Mrs Sarabeth Jung **(SLP)**
Fasting, Judith Charlotte **(SLP)**
Haelsig, Mrs Patricia Cahill **(SLP)**
Jensen, Mary P **(SLP)**

Pullman
Bruce, Arden G **(SLP)**
Chermak, Dr Gail D **(A)**
Dengerink, Joan E **(SLP A)**
Finley, Patricia Elaine
Franks, Dr J Richard **(A)**
Howard, Lori Ann **(A)**
Jennings, Mrs Karen Jean Lucas **(SLP)**
Johnson, Dr Jeanne M **(SLP)**
Kam, Elizabeth Y F
Madison, Dr Charles L **(SLP)**
Madison, Nancy K **(A)**
Potter, Dr Robert E **(SLP)**
Seikel, John A **(SLP)**
Wilbourn, Mrs Carmen R **(SLP)**
Wingate, Cicely J **(SLP)**

Puyallup
Bargmeyer, Kurt Erwin
Bene, Mrs Julie Barber **(SLP)**
Brittin, Dr Marie E **(SLP)**
Dixon, Kristen Lynn
Draper, John F **(SLP)**
Hiroo, Vivian F **(SLP)**
Kennedy, Kathleen A **(SLP)**
Loy-Every, Marilyn J **(A)**
Martin, Sandra Kay **(A)**
Reed, Marilyn Nadine **(SLP)**
Scheer, Mrs Judith A **(SLP)**
Yates, Phil P **(SLP)**
Youngman, Patricia Kay **(SLP)**

Randle
Burmeister, Patricia B **(A)**

Redmond
Benner, Mrs Nancy L **(SLP)**
Bolie-Costello, Shila R **(SLP)**
Buettemeier, Cheryl Ann **(SLP)**
Burge, Nancy L **(SLP)**
Canfield, Mrs Marilyn A **(SLP)**
Ellis, Sandra Kase **(A)**
Glenn, Mrs Carol Frances **(SLP)**
Gruen, Karen L **(A)**
Hatheway, Mrs Wendy B **(SLP)**
Killingsworth, Carol A **(A)**
Liljegren, Mrs Susanne F **(SLP)**
Limb, Terence Alford **(A)**
Nevdahl, Martin Ted **(SLP)**
Rasmussen, Mrs Louise Pearl **(SLP)**
Rossi, Carolyn S **(SLP)**
Shrader, Jean **(SLP)**
Solomon, Mrs Jenny A **(SLP)**
Stachowiak, Shirley K **(SLP)**
Welch, Mrs Denise Suzanne **(A)**
Willett, Mrs Donna K **(SLP)**

Renton
Freeman, Ann Marie **(SLP)**
Holm, Marilyn K **(SLP)**
Morgan, Mrs Mary L **(SLP)**
Muto-Coleman, Mrs Dorothy **(A)**
Quaranta, Jolene L
Rash, Mrs Robin Zachow **(SLP)**
Reboli, Jean O
Witkin, Dr Belle Ruth **(SLP)**

Richland
Aiello, Dr Francis A **(A)**
Clark, R Jeanne **(SLP)**
Olson, Romaine A **(SLP)**
Schweiger, Mrs Linda Ann **(SLP)**
Shoop, Mrs Kathryn Kight **(SLP)**
Underwood, Mark A **(SLP)**

Ridgefield
Stohr, Pamela M **(SLP)**

Ritzville
Whitney, Mrs Carolyn J **(SLP)**

Seabeck
Bryant, Judith M **(SLP)**

Seattle
Abdala, Caroline **(A)**
Adams, Leslie J **(SLP)**
Adams, Marsha Lee **(SLP)**
Anderson, Mrs Cynthia R **(SLP)**
Aurich, Carol Diane **(A)**
Baarslag-Benson, Ross Edward **(SLP)**
Bargones, Jill Yvette **(A)**
Barker, Dr Rebecca **(SLP)**
Bergeson, Mrs Rebecca A **(SLP)**
Bergsagel, Mrs Judith Anna **(SLP)**
Bernhardt, Linda Elsie **(SLP)**
Berryman, Mrs Ann Jaleen **(SLP)**
Bjork, Melanie **(SLP)**
Bjorklund, Janet V **(SLP A)**
Blair, Cristine Ann **(SLP)**
Bodding, Heidi L **(SLP)**
Bodily, Noralee **(SLP)**
Boroughs, Kathleen **(SLP)**
Bowes, Ann Jeane **(SLP)**
Bowlus, Rebecca Ann **(A)**
Brazier, Mrs Susan H **(SLP)**
Bridges, Monte L **(SLP)**
Brooks, Carla Ann **(SLP)**
Brown, Jacqueline M **(SLP)**
Burgess, Mrs Mary Ann A **(SLP)**
Burns, Edward M
Caldwell, Gail Olive
Carney, Marilyn Jean **(SLP)**
Carpenter, Dr Robert L **(SLP)**
Carte, Terry Timberlake **(SLP)**
Catlett, Mrs Margaret E
Catterall, Nancy S **(A)**
Chamberlin, Lynn Louise **(SLP)**
Chase, Deborah A **(SLP)**
Clark, Paula Jurnak **(SLP)**
Clumeck, Mary Annetta **(SLP)**
Coggins, Mrs Kathleen Bryan **(SLP)**
Coggins, Dr Truman E **(SLP)**
Coles, Margaret R **(SLP)**
Collins, Janis K **(SLP)**
Collins-Byrne, M **(SLP)**
Cook, Dewanda
Cromwell, Prudence A **(SLP)**
Cropley, Robert W **(A)**
Cullinan, Timothy B **(SLP)**
Culpepper, N Brandt **(A)**
Dacres, Joan L **(SLP)**
Dale, Dr Phillip S
Dalton, Wendy R **(A)**
Dang, Celeste B **(SLP)**
Davis, Carol Williams **(SLP)**
Dawson, Dr Warren R **(SLP A)**
De Castro, Mrs Jennifer Louise **(A)**
Dejmal, Nancy L **(SLP)**
Dewey, Jody A **(SLP)**
Dickenson, Leslie Ann
Dille, Marilyn F **(A)**
Dowden, Patricia A **(SLP)**
Eblen, Linda E **(SLP)**
Edwards, Mrs Dinah Hubbard **(SLP)**
Elrand, Teri Anita **(SLP)**
Eng, Mrs Ruth L **(SLP)**
Engelbrecht, Claire Elizabeth **(SLP)**
Etter, Brenda F **(SLP A)**
Faherty, Amy Susan **(SLP)**
Farrar, Dr Cathy Lucile
Farrier, Lynn Dee **(SLP)**
Feeney, M Patrick **(A)**
Filson, Kay S **(A)**
Fine, Jody E **(A)**
Flowers, Dr Charles Ray **(SLP)**
Flynn, Dale T **(A)**
Folsom, Dr Richard C **(A)**
Fox, Robert James **(A)**
France, Mary Colleen **(SLP)**
Freitas, Richard Joseph **(SLP)**
French, Mrs Sheryl Salzberg **(SLP)**
Fulmer, Charles Virgil, Jr **(A)**
Furuta, Jennifer Satomi **(SLP)**
Gallagher, Elizabeth Bullard **(SLP)**
Gilchrist, Florence S **(SLP)**
Gill, Patricia Ann **(SLP)**
Gorohoff, Mrs Sandra Waters **(SLP)**
Graebner, Mrs Corinne M Anderson **(SLP)**
Grant, G Maura **(SLP)**
Gray, Jennifer L **(A)**
Greenhalgh, Mrs Kathy Bouffard **(SLP)**
Grieser, Dianne Lynne **(SLP)**
Groman, Mrs Fern Rogow **(SLP)**
Guenzel, Cheryl C
Guthrie, Janet **(SLP)**
Hall, Raelene A **(SLP)**
Hall, Randy Margaret **(SLP)**
Hamilton, Susan L **(SLP)**
Harder, Connie B **(SLP)**
Harney, Martha Lynn **(A)**
Harvey, Dr Donald G **(A)**
Hashimoto, Lori A **(SLP)**
Haskell, Dr George B **(A)**
Haslett, Dr Elizabeth J **(A)**
Haukenes, Iva Mae **(SLP)**
Hawk, Andrea J **(SLP)**
Hedges, Joyce Stella **(SLP)**
Heiberger-Hammen, Vicki L **(SLP)**
Helbach, Mary T **(SLP)**
Herren, Mrs Shelley Lynn **(SLP)**
Herrington, Mrs Paula Beckett **(SLP)**
Hetherington, Laurel Jean
Hiraki, Cynthia Kathleen **(SLP)**
Hoerster, Carol **(SLP)**
Holmberg, Tristan L **(A)**
Honsinger, Melissa J Becker **(SLP)**
Hubbard, Carol P **(SLP)**
Ibarra, Claire Kimie **(SLP)**
Jackson, Catherine **(SLP)**
Jaeger, Joan M **(SLP)**
Johnsen, Mrs Marijane **(SLP)**
Johnson, Anita Lee **(A)**
Johnson, Mrs Erin Dawn **(SLP)**
Johnson, Glenn A **(SLP)**
Johnson, Karen L **(SLP)**
Johnson, Kyle C **(A)**
Jones, Debra Leigh **(SLP)**
Jones, Jeri A **(SLP)**
Joyce, Julia Beatrice **(SLP)**
Kays, Linda A **(SLP)**
Kelly, Charleen A **(SLP)**
Kelly, Sheila D **(SLP)**

Kennard, Carol Ann **(SLP)**
Keough, Kristine Marie **(SLP)**
Kovar, Nancy Christine **(SLP)**
Krasny, Lori Ellen **(SLP)**
Kriegsmann, Elinor L **(SLP)**
Kuprenas, Sandra V **(A)**
La Barge-King, Karen Elaine **(SLP)**
Labiak, James M **(A)**
Lambert, Dennis E **(A)**
Lambrecht, Karen J **(SLP)**
Lancaster, Ernest Arthur, Jr **(SLP)**
LaRosa, Janell B **(A)**
Larsen, Dr George Lars **(SLP)**
Larsen, Lori Jean **(SLP)**
Lemay, Laurie Keefe **(SLP)**
Leonard-Fleckman, Star C **(A)**
Leong, Marci Kim **(A)**
Levi, Ellen Carol **(A)**
Lewis, Mrs Johanna L **(SLP)**
Lichtenstadter, Anne Elizabeth **(SLP)**
Liensch, Lynne W **(SLP)**
Livingstone, Deborah Kay **(SLP)**
Loup, C Lorioux **(SLP)**
Luthas, Pamela J **(A)**
MacLean, Sandra C **(A)**
Maher, John J, III **(A)**
Margolis, Wendy M **(A)**
Marshalla, Pamela R **(SLP)**
Matas, Judy A **(SLP)**
Mathers-Schmidt, Barbara A **(SLP)**
Mattheis, Mrs Susan A
McAlerney, Colleen Ann **(SLP)**
McCall, Eleanor T **(SLP)**
McCann, Donna S **(SLP)**
McCombs, Dr Richard P **(A)**
McDaniel, Mary M **(A)**
McDonald, Elizabeth Jean **(SLP)**
McDonald, Judith B **(SLP)**
McGrath, Dr Carl O **(SLP)**
McGrath, Mrs Muiriel Jean **(SLP)**
McHenry, Dr Monica A **(SLP)**
Melvey, Mary K **(SLP)**
Miller, Dr Robert M **(SLP)**
Miner, Dr Adah L **(SLP)**
Minifie, Dr Fred D
Mitsuda, Patricia M **(SLP)**
Moering, Betty C **(SLP)**
Moore, Ann S **(SLP)**
Moore, John Mick **(A)**
Moroney, Patricia Ann **(SLP)**
Morris-Lent, Mrs Valerie Sue **(SLP)**
Moser, Mrs Miriam T **(SLP)**
Neuhart, Julee M **(SLP)**
Oblak, Mrs Susan B **(SLP)**
Oistad, Mrs Georgia M **(SLP)**
Olswang, Dr Lesley B **(SLP)**
Orlando, Mark Stephen **(A)**
Otterholt, Janelle **(SLP)**
Palmer, Dr John M **(SLP A)**
Pankiewicz, Shelley Maria **(A)**
Parker, Mary Catherine **(SLP)**
Partnow, Susan L **(SLP)**
Paul, Wendy **(SLP)**
Peizer, Elaine Rosenstock **(SLP)**
Pendergast, Mrs Kathleen K **(SLP)**
Peters, Mrs Linda D **(SLP)**
Pinder, Gay L **(SLP)**
Platt, Janelle Renee **(SLP)**
Qudsi, Laila
Quint, Janice H **(SLP)**
Rahill, Mrs Valerie Zehnder **(SLP)**
Randall, Carol G **(SLP A)**
Raquer, Linda A **(SLP)**
Rathbone-Meeks, Nancy L **(SLP)**
Rauch-Mahoney, Christine **(A)**
Rees, Dr Thomas S **(A)**
Reich, Dr Alan Richard **(SLP)**
Rickard, Lisa K
Ross, Jennifer Ruth **(SLP)**
Rothwell, Mrs Gail W **(SLP)**
Sacia, Jane A **(SLP)**
Sakai, Connie Sayo **(A)**
Sanborn, Dr E Sue **(A)**
Sansalone, Teresa Nievez **(A)**
Schapire, Irene Sue **(SLP)**
Schwarz, Gail Cahn **(SLP)**
Seline, Gloria Ellen **(SLP)**
Selmar, John W **(SLP)**
Shapley, Dr James **(A)**
Shebly, Sharon K **(SLP)**
Sheehan, Dr Marian **(SLP)**
Shorr, Dr David N
Skalabrin, Theresa Ann **(A)**
Smith, Kathleen M **(SLP)**
Smith, Keoni **(SLP)**
Smith, Mrs Nancy Stecker **(SLP)**
Snow, David Page
Snyder, Dr Jack M **(SLP A)**
Sohlberg, McKay Moore **(SLP)**
Spatola, Glenn J **(A)**
Squires, Mrs Laura Louise **(SLP)**
Stanton, Karen M **(SLP)**
Stenehjem, Bonnie Buchanan **(SLP)**
Stevenson, Marcia B **(SLP)**
Stoel-Gammon, Dr Carol
Stone, Judith R **(SLP)**
Talley, Mrs Mary Ellen **(SLP)**
Teachman, Sandra E
Thomas, Steven Michael **(SLP)**
Thompson, Mrs Diane C **(A)**
Thompson, Dr Gary **(A)**
Thomson, Janet L R **(SLP)**
Tinsley, Shelley **(SLP)**
Tobin, Annette R **(SLP)**
Torgerson, Judith Martha **(A)**
Town, Margaret J **(SLP)**
Van Horne, Mrs Lisa J
Walmsley, Dixie Maas **(SLP)**
Watkins, Alice Lee **(SLP)**
Watts, Donna K **(A)**
Weisleder, Mrs Jenny N
Wichman, Rachel L **(SLP)**
Wiedmer, Beatrix E **(SLP)**
Wilson, Michael J **(A)**
Wilson, Dr Wesley R **(SLP A)**
Wishkoski, Linda Slentz **(SLP)**
Wren, Mrs Thelma I **(SLP)**
Wright, Geri C **(SLP)**
Wyse, Marilyn A **(SLP)**
Yang, Hsu-Chun
Yantis, Mrs Elna M **(SLP)**
Yantis, Dr Phillip A **(A)**
Yonick, Tracey A **(SLP)**
Yorkston, Dr Kathryn M **(SLP)**
Young, Mary B **(SLP)**
Zeches, Jane Teresa **(SLP)**
Zupan, Diane Marie **(SLP)**

Selah
Clark, Kathleen Laurane **(A)**

Sequim
Krantz, Mrs Henrietta C **(SLP A)**
Weiss, Dr Curtis E **(SLP)**

Shelton
Tindall, Reed B **(SLP)**

Snohomish
Brodeur, Mrs Natalie Goodfellow **(SLP)**
Hannley, Elizabeth Ann **(SLP)**
Lee, Mrs Susan K T **(SLP)**
Sasser, Elizabeth K **(SLP)**

Snoqualmie
Wainright, Mrs R LaNell **(SLP)**

South Bend
Spogen, David Roy **(SLP)**

Southworth
Blackburn, Mrs Phyllis G **(SLP)**

Spanaway
Anderson, Karen Lynn **(A)**

Spokane
Ashley, Debra Lynn
Bassett, Sandra S **(SLP)**
Blunk, Sheila L **(SLP)**
Bogarosh, Mrs Lorna Y **(A)**
Boltjes, Mrs Connie Lee **(SLP)**
Bonney, Mrs Carol L **(SLP)**
Brophy, Dr Nancy Hovorka **(SLP)**
Bukaty, Carolyn
Clouse, Mrs Patricia Lynn **(A)**
Coleman, Mrs Cynthia E **(SLP)**
Cunningham, Jane Tubbs **(SLP)**
Driscoll, Karyn Louise **(SLP)**
Endersbe, Mikki Kay **(SLP)**
Evans, Ceanne L **(A)**
Evans, Doreen Ann **(SLP)**
Ferguson, Judith A **(SLP)**
Freese, Mrs Gail Joan **(SLP)**
French, Mrs Leigh Ann **(SLP)**
Gallaher, Mrs Carole B **(SLP)**
Gentry, Mrs Susan M **(SLP)**
Gregg, Rita Ann Cantwell **(SLP)**
Hamilton, Sallie Sederstrom **(SLP)**
Harper, Mrs Linda Dianne **(SLP)**
Hay, Marcella
Heitman, Mrs Robin Marie **(A)**
Hogan, Mrs Kathleen Ann **(SLP)**
Jensen, Mrs Becky J L **(SLP)**
Jones, Vern **(SLP)**
Lacey-Scholze, Brenda A **(SLP)**
Larrigan, Lynn B **(SLP)**
Latta, Mrs Diane C **(SLP)**
Levernier, Mrs Christine Marie **(SLP)**
Lorenz, Mrs Delores Rustad **(SLP)**
Mannix, Mrs Maureen McMahon **(SLP)**
McGrew, Mrs Winifred C **(SLP)**
Melton, Barbara Ann **(A)**
Michels, Mrs Marsha M **(SLP)**
Miller, Warren M **(SLP)**
Mochel, Anne Louise
Morris, Lizbeth T **(SLP)**
Murphy, Mrs Marie B **(SLP)**
O'Connor, Thomas M **(A)**
Omlin, Cynthia Joy H **(SLP)**
Payne, Mrs Patricia Garnsey
Pirttima, Elizabeth Furney **(SLP)**
Power, Leslie D **(SLP)**
Richlie, Mary D **(SLP)**
Seipp, Patsy Leigh **(SLP)**
Shrader-Cory, Mrs Kathleen J **(SLP)**
Shute, Brian James **(SLP)**
Simpson, Joseph Gerard **(A)**
Simpson, Karen Rademaker **(SLP)**
Smith, Kathleen Joan **(SLP)**
Stanton, Dr Fred E **(SLP)**
Stoyko, Mrs Donna Jane **(SLP)**
Strate, Shirlene S **(SLP)**
Trygg, Larry D **(SLP)**
Uppinghouse, Karen Marie **(SLP)**
Warrick, Mrs Debra Mattern **(SLP)**
Weisbrod, Mrs Kathleen Granahan **(SLP)**
Wilder, Mrs Mary K **(A)**
Wolfe, Donald L **(A)**
Young, Mrs Janice J **(SLP)**

Stanwood
Corder, Mrs Betty L **(SLP)**
Lipscomb, Dr David M **(A)**

Steilacoom
Soelling, Mrs Carol Sue **(SLP)**
Taggart-Ross, Mrs Linda **(SLP A)**
Turcotte, Mrs Mary Leclair **(SLP)**

Suquamish
Kroll, Linda J **(SLP)**

Tacoma
Adams, Amanda Wallin **(SLP)**
Aden, Mrs Frances A **(SLP A)**
Anderson, Mrs Janice Ann **(SLP)**
Andrues, James W **(A)**
Baisinger, Dr Wilbur H **(SLP)**
Beckstead, Debra Ann **(SLP)**
Bennett, Audrey **(SLP)**
Blank, Catherine **(SLP)**
Branson, Cynthia W **(SLP)**
Brown, Laurel Jean **(SLP)**
Carpenter, Susan K **(SLP A)**
Castilla-Wilson, Mrs Dora L **(SLP)**
Critchfield-Schultz, Mary L **(SLP)**
Danielson, Maj Richard W **(A)**
Debertin, Mrs Phyllis L **(SLP)**
Getchell, Sandra D **(A)**
Hathaway, Tamara F
Herigstad, Mrs Suzanne Jo **(SLP)**
Hewkin, Steven Kenneth **(A)**
Hoover, Karl M **(A)**
Johnson, Kenneth A **(SLP)**
Jones, Kenneth E **(A)**
Kankelborg, Carol G **(SLP)**
Kelly-Ballweber, Denise **(A)**
Leacy, Mrs Lorelle Barrett **(SLP)**
Legresley, Mrs Kelly G **(SLP)**
Lesniak, Peggy S **(SLP)**
Meadors, Deborah Lynn **(SLP)**
Mindel, Maxine C **(SLP)**
Nelson, Carol L S **(SLP)**
O'Connell-Halloway, Maureen **(SLP)**
Olson, Mrs Mary Crollard **(A)**
Petermann, Mrs Patricia Marie **(A)**
Peterson, Mrs Cathi S **(SLP)**
Phillips, Rita H **(A)**
Post, Mrs Verna Ruth **(SLP)**
Rand, Shann **(A)**
Sprunk-Berlin, Holly Suzanne **(SLP)**
Taylor-Walker, Ophelia **(SLP)**
Thornton, Cathy M **(SLP)**
Tiger, Ruth W **(SLP)**
Veatch, Dr John W **(SLP)**
Volpe, Kathleen A **(SLP)**
Williams, Mrs Lynn Dell
Williams, Mrs Susan S **(SLP)**
Yockey, Kenton L **(SLP)**

Tonasket
Karlberg, Janice M T **(SLP)**
Karlberg, Philip L **(SLP)**

Tukwila
Brislin, Helen Ann **(A)**

Union
Vincent, Vicki Lynn **(SLP)**

Vancouver
Beary-Stolle, Jean **(SLP)**
Beech, Mrs Marjorie M **(SLP)**
Bong, Joanne L **(SLP)**
Book, Sandra Lynn **(A)**
Bowen, Nancy Marie **(A)**
Burres, Pamela Zoe **(SLP)**
Collins, Mary L **(SLP)**
Ehlers, Patricia McShane **(SLP)**
Goggin, Julie Heide **(SLP)**
Greenwell, Mrs Mary Lorene **(SLP)**
Hanson, Rhys E **(SLP A)**
Harding, Mrs Julie Diane **(SLP)**
Harmon, Mrs Mertis M **(SLP)**
Hicks, Al **(A)**
Hollevoet, Catherine **(A)**
Holman, Dr Gary Lynn **(SLP)**
Kimbrough, Mrs Deborah A **(SLP)**
Kirkpatrick, Mrs Mary Jill **(SLP)**
Klinski, Lee N **(SLP)**
Knauf, Mrs Marilyn G **(SLP)**
Matteson, Susan Lori **(SLP)**
May, June E **(SLP)**
Nelly, Mrs Christine Kay **(SLP)**
Peterson, Gwen **(SLP)**
Russell, Mrs Mary M **(SLP)**
Rylander, Robert E **(SLP)**
Sands, Sindy **(SLP)**
Schaefer, James B **(SLP)**
Silver, Sharon Arlene **(SLP)**
Sullivan, Tyece L **(SLP)**
Weeks, Robert Alan **(SLP)**

Vashon
Crudo, Lynn Hilley **(SLP)**

Vaughn
Marra, Mrs Pamela S **(SLP)**

Veradale
Hamilton, Mrs Eilene K **(SLP)**
Hays, Lynette D **(SLP)**
Mattson, Mrs Mary Mueller **(SLP)**
Miller, Mrs Lynn Ann **(SLP)**

Walla Walla
Anderson, Mrs Renata Appel **(A)**
Dunbar, James W **(A)**
Greenwalt, Eileen V **(SLP)**
Hippauf, Mrs Lynette Kay **(SLP)**
Price, Joanne **(A)**
Schneller, Carol Ann **(SLP)**
Smith, Deborah Rowland **(SLP)**
Templeton, Lillian Richeson **(SLP)**
Warren, Mrs Jane Anne **(SLP)**

Wapato
Cable, Della Jane **(SLP)**

Warden
McKamey, Mrs Laura Jo **(SLP)**

Washougal
Cuyler, Juliana S
Kasner, Mrs Lois J **(SLP)**
Warren-Manning, Mrs Debby Anne

Wenatchee
Ciarlo, Debra A **(SLP)**
Moomaw, Douglas Edward **(A)**
Norton-Kavanaugh, Carol **(A)**
Simmons, Patrilla Sue **(SLP)**
Ullrich, Kenneth Albert **(A)**
West, Hazel Hill

West Richland
Bruemmer, Mrs Susan M **(SLP)**
Hollingsworth, Brenda Merritt **(SLP)**

Woodinville
Cooper, Mrs Sherrie J **(SLP)**
Cornwall, Mrs Judith A **(SLP)**
Coulson, Tamara E A **(SLP)**
Meilahn, Kristine **(SLP)**
Mrowca, Mrs Susan Ann **(SLP)**
Munro, Carolyn B **(SLP)**
White, Kristen Mattson **(SLP)**

Woodland
Behrendsen, Mrs Lynn L

Yakima
Beck, Mrs Janet Anderson **(SLP)**
Burkhardt, Linda Mae **(SLP)**
Christensen, Holli J **(A)**
Frank, Mrs Phyllis C **(SLP)**
Hoffman, Mrs Julie Mae **(SLP)**
Jenkins, Debra Lynne **(A)**
John, Martin B **(A)**
Krieger, Mrs Janet Carmichael **(SLP)**
Lowary, Susann M **(SLP)**
Polich, Laure **(SLP)**
Prehm, Mrs Katherine T **(SLP)**
Pryor, Laura Ann **(SLP)**
Rankin Coffin, Robin L **(SLP)**
Sandersen, Marsha Becker **(SLP)**
Sheets, Gregory B **(A)**
Simms, Mrs Barbara O **(SLP)**
Smart, Mrs Nancy Sundahl **(A)**
Strange, Kelley Harmon **(SLP)**
Thompson, James W **(A)**

Zillah
Delp, JoAnn Thomas **(SLP)**
Walker, Mrs Janice L **(SLP)**

WEST VIRGINIA

Alum Creek
Sowards, Mrs Ellen L **(SLP)**

Barboursville
Bickford, Mrs Vernenna Donell **(SLP)**
Chiles, Mrs Michaela B **(SLP)**
George, Mrs Linda M **(SLP)**
McComas, Mrs Karen Leigh **(SLP)**
McComas, Mrs Robin Lynn **(SLP)**

Beckley
Carrico, Mrs Dianna Arlene **(SLP)**
Darby, Mrs Ann M **(SLP)**
Datsko, Mrs Margaret L **(SLP)**
Fink, Mrs Marsha A Smith **(SLP)**
Heffinger, Sharon Lynne **(A)**
Lindsay, Mrs Elissa G **(SLP)**
Long, Lisa Dawn
Walker, Mrs Helen S **(SLP)**
Walker, Randy Wayne **(A)**

Berkeley Springs
Offutt, Suzanne **(SLP)**

Bethany
Weppler, Mrs Cynthia Levelle **(SLP)**

Bluefield
Bourne, Mrs Victoria L **(SLP)**
Constantino, Mrs Kimberli Rumburg **(SLP)**
Hood, Mrs Patricia Ann **(A)**
Hughes, Karen R **(SLP)**
Martin, Paul G **(A)**
Meredith, James E **(SLP A)**
Newman, Valerie Lynne **(A)**
Pullins, Mrs Mary Ann M **(SLP)**
Stewart, Kimberly Jane **(A)**

Boomer
Hill, Mrs Mary Bria **(SLP)**

Brenton
Allen, Rhonda Yvonne **(SLP)**

Bridgeport
Fusco, Mary Lou **(SLP)**
Olness, Mrs June Birkelbach **(SLP)**
Wilbourn, Mrs Carolyn Springer **(SLP)**

Bristol
Richardson, Mrs Debra Heramb **(SLP)**

Buckhannon
Mendicino, Michael

Chapmanville
Conley, Deangela **(SLP)**

Charleston
Barton, Jesse M, Jr **(SLP)**
Campanelli, Mrs Angela L **(SLP)**
Eckhardt, Virginia Lynne **(A)**
Edwards, Janet C **(A)**
Engle, Susan Diane **(A)**
Frail, James H **(A)**
Green, Margaret E **(SLP)**
Harman, Mrs Patricia **(SLP)**
Hoffman, Leah J **(SLP)**
Holland, Mrs Betty R **(SLP)**
Jahnes, Mrs Kim H **(SLP)**
Johnson-Elmore, Fannie Mason
Lustig, Dr Vincent Frank **(SLP A)**
McIlwain, Cheri McDaniel
Miller, Sally L **(SLP)**
Mullett, Carolyn M **(SLP)**
Murray, Cynthia Lee **(A)**
Smith, Dr Rosemary L **(A)**
Stoneking, Brenda Jo
Swisher, Pamela Ann **(SLP)**
Thomas, Carolyn Marie **(A)**
White, Mrs Deborah P **(SLP)**
Woody, Nancy Jean **(A)**

Chester
Pugh, Natalie Jean **(SLP)**

Clarksburg
Baskin, Cynthia Mae **(A)**
Ferrari, Patricia V **(SLP)**
Mancina, Mary Rose **(SLP)**
Squires, Richard L **(A)**

Clay
Shelton, Madelyn L **(SLP)**

Craigsville
Pullins, Mrs Vickie H **(SLP)**

Cross Lanes
Andrews, Frank D **(SLP)**
Peaks, S Darlene **(SLP)**
Poniatowski, Sonja M **(SLP)**

Culloden
Fizer, Mrs Claudia Krebs **(SLP)**

Davisville
Segal, Alan I **(A)**

Dellslow
Dailey, Mary B **(SLP)**

Dunbar
Brenner, Faith Anne **(SLP A)**

Dunmore
Bland, Ruth Anne

Eleanor
Slijepcevic, Jane E **(SLP)**

Elizabeth
Butcher, Dennis James **(SLP)**
Kohner, Pamela K **(SLP)**

Elkins
Trimboli, Barbara H **(SLP)**

Elkview
Bee, Norma M **(SLP)**

Fairmont
Adams, Mrs Patricia S **(A)**
Brooks, Mrs Kathy Marie **(SLP)**
Dewitt, Linda Marie **(A)**
Hadox, Mrs Bonita Bartlett **(SLP)**
Haley, Mrs Deena C **(SLP)**
Joseph, Laura Sue **(SLP)**
Mason, Mrs Nancy Kite **(SLP)**
Murphy, Sharon Rae **(SLP)**
Tekieli, Dr Mary E **(SLP)**
Yanero, Diane Everly **(SLP)**

Fayetteville
Langham, Diane Elizabeth **(SLP)**

Follansbee
Hooper, Franklin E **(SLP)**
Winner, Lori Ann **(SLP)**

Fort Ashby
Kesner, Mrs Catherine I **(SLP)**

Franklin
Kee, Donna Katherine
Sowar, Mrs Deborah Fessenden **(SLP)**

Gallipolis Ferry
Hinds, Ronald Van **(SLP)**

Gassaway
Hart, Mrs Ann L **(SLP)**

Gilbert
Browning, Michael **(SLP)**

Gilboa
Williams, Mrs Amy Patricia **(SLP)**

Glendale
Lewis, Susan R S **(SLP)**

Glenville
Westfall, Patricia D **(SLP)**

Grafton
Cartwright, Lynn Rae **(SLP)**
Everly, Mrs Jaunita A **(SLP)**
Hefferin, Amy Louise **(SLP)**

Harpers Ferry
Gardner, Lela **(SLP)**

Harts
Dingess, Mrs Cheryl Ratliff **(SLP)**

Henderson
Long, Debra Northup

Hillsboro
Wymer, Wanda J **(SLP)**

Huntington
Bockway, Nancy C **(A)**
Campbell, Nausha C **(SLP)**
Carter, Mrs Stephanie Ann **(SLP)**
Chezik, Kathryn H **(SLP)**
Cole, Mrs Catherine D **(SLP)**
Cremeans, Mrs Lura Thern **(SLP)**
Dean, Carolyn A **(A)**
Dollman, Cynthia **(SLP)**
Egnor, Mrs Debra Frances **(SLP)**
Elliott, Rebecca **(SLP)**
Gardner, Dr Pamela R **(SLP)**
Garrett, Dr Ruth E C **(SLP)**
Hogsett, Denise **(SLP)**
Jeter, Mrs Amy Lee **(SLP)**
Jones, Cynthia D **(SLP)**
Knicely, Dena Marie **(SLP)**
Lester, Rhonda A **(A)**
Lovins, Mrs Julia Feola **(SLP)**
Maloy, Mrs Janet Y **(SLP)**
Martin, Mrs Mary Kay C **(SLP)**
McNealy, Karen K **(A)**
Miller, Rebecca Ballard **(SLP)**
Olson, Robert D **(SLP)**
Overholt, Mrs Suzanne Welch **(SLP)**
Ray, Mrs Marsha W **(SLP)**
Reynolds, Mrs Mary E **(SLP)**
Runyon, Mrs Ramona G **(SLP)**
Shumate, Mrs Lena Scurry **(A)**
Shumate, Robert Bradley **(A)**
Smith, David L **(A)**
Sullivan, Betty **(SLP)**
Sullivan, Susan W **(SLP)**
Survance, Mrs Cathi Ann **(SLP)**
Welch, Mrs Sheila Swentzel **(SLP)**

Hurricane
Davis, Mrs Jeanine K **(SLP)**

Institute
Starkey, Mrs Shirley J **(SLP)**

Jane Lew
Lake, Mrs Donna Bland **(SLP)**

Keyser
Mangold, Lorraine S **(SLP)**

Kingwood
Miller, Mrs Mary Kay **(SLP)**
Wallace, Mrs Vicki Rush **(A)**

Lavalette
Johnson, Mrs Lila Kay **(SLP)**

Lewisburg
Fauber, Mrs Lura June **(SLP)**
Ikner, Cynthia Lewis **(A)**
Nelson, Mrs Linda L **(SLP)**
Nelson, William H **(SLP)**
Vandevander, Gary M **(A)**
Youmans, Albert Thomas **(SLP)**

Lindside
Cowder, W Wayne **(SLP)**

Logan
Esposito, Andrea S **(SLP)**
Ferrell, Mrs Catherine Ellen **(SLP)**
Mullins, Vernon N **(A)**
Willis, Mrs Deborah L **(SLP)**

Man
Porter, Kimberly Stickel **(SLP)**

Martinsburg
Carter, Dr John Francis **(SLP)**
Georgiana, Angela Marie **(SLP)**
Gurick, Mrs Cathy **(SLP)**
Kelly, Dorothy Ann **(A)**
Morgan, Debra Lynn **(A)**
Shelton, Mrs Vicki Diane **(SLP)**
Yarnell, Mrs Mary D **(SLP)**
Zagarella, Michael J **(A)**

McMechen
Bosworth, Cathy Lynn **(A)**

Milton
Moul, Laura L **(SLP)**

Mineralwells
Lipsmeyer, Gregory Anderson **(SLP)**

Moorefield
Hammer, Sharon Ciccolella **(SLP)**

Morgantown
Alderson, Tracy Breitbach **(SLP)**
Andes-Viski, Suzanne Evelyn **(SLP)**
Atkins, Dr Carolyn P **(SLP)**
Berryman, Joyce Lanham **(SLP)**
Borsch, Jennifer Kay **(SLP)**
Bowman-Sorine, Marilyn L **(SLP)**
Castellan, Susan B **(SLP)**
Cody, Robert Charles **(A)**
Culberson, Carole Lynne
Haines, Mrs Karen Barr **(SLP)**
Hively, E Antionette **(SLP)**
Hoge, Susan E **(A)**
Hurley, Mrs Holly Ann **(A)**
Ingle, Catherine D **(A)**
Jones, Robin R **(A)**
Kerns, Mrs Cynthia Newton **(A)**
King, Debra Arslain **(SLP)**
Lass, Dr Norman J
Lee-Sheridan, Sharon M **(SLP)**
Lundeen, Dr Conrad **(A)**
Lundeen, Mrs Deedra Jane **(A)**
Marano, Mrs Deborah F **(SLP)**
May, Mrs Gaylene M **(SLP)**
McCabe, Barbara Ann **(A)**
Minor, Mrs Judy Kelley **(SLP)**
Mitchell, Dr Pamela R **(SLP)**
Murabito, Lucia **(SLP)**
Neldon, Mrs Gayle B **(A)**
Olexa-Smith, Mrs Sandra Kaye **(SLP)**
Oramas, Consuelo **(A)**
Patrick, Linda **(SLP)**
Petitte, Mrs Janet J **(A)**
Prichard, Cheryl L **(SLP)**
Ruscello, Dr Dennis M **(SLP)**
Shuster, Dr Linda I **(SLP)**
St Louis, Karen W **(SLP)**
St Louis, Dr Kenneth O **(SLP)**
Stone, Mrs Janet L **(SLP)**
Woodford, Dr Charles M **(SLP A)**

Oak Hill
Klug, Pamela Sue **(A)**

Ona
Ratliff, Patricia Ann **(SLP)**

Parkersburg
Ciesielski, Teresa M **(SLP)**
Corra, Mrs Norabelle Shuman **(SLP)**
Evans, George F **(A)**
Florence, Mary L **(A)**
Hurtz, Mrs Kathryn S **(SLP)**
King-Reeves, Mrs L Carole **(SLP)**
Lemley, Colleen Belle
Mace, Mrs Linda S **(SLP)**
McCauley, Mrs Linda Hall **(SLP)**
Meigs-Haislop, Mrs Amy Jo **(SLP)**
Pacifico, Daneen A **(A)**
Parrish, William C, Jr **(A)**
Swanson, Mrs Barbara Izzett **(SLP)**
Wilson, Mrs Mary Ann D **(SLP)**

Pennsboro
Le Vos, Mrs Sandra Clawson **(SLP)**

Petersburg
Deicas, Wendy Marie **(SLP)**
Harman, Cynthia J **(SLP)**
Shaffer, Chester M **(A)**

Pineville
Justice, Mrs Brenda Sue **(SLP)**

Poca
Dean, Curtis Lawrence **(SLP)**
McClanahan, Mrs Sharon Lynn **(SLP)**
Purvis, Mrs Judie W **(SLP A)**

Point Pleasant
Frye, Devona D **(SLP)**

Princeton
Desmond, Alan Louis **(A)**
Pizzo, Mrs Bonnie Jean **(SLP)**
Shanklin-Shay, Mrs Donna Ruth **(SLP)**
Shrewsberry, Mrs Sonya E **(SLP)**
Spence, Dr Susan Durham **(SLP)**
Vuchetich, Julie Ann **(SLP)**

Ravenswood
Simon, Dee Ann M **(SLP)**

Ripley
Miller, Mrs Nora Kathleen **(SLP)**
Moore, Mrs Pamela Ann **(SLP)**
Nester, Mrs Ann A **(SLP)**
Poling, Mrs Cheryl Rene **(SLP)**
Smith, Deborah L **(SLP)**

Romney
Mathias, Gerald A **(SLP)**

Ronceverte
Moore, Anna Cornell **(SLP)**

Sand Fork
Heater, Mrs Cheryl A **(SLP)**

Shady Spring
McCallister, Robin R **(SLP)**

Shepherdstown
Gordon, Nancy Halstead **(SLP)**
Magee, Janet Clark **(SLP)**
McCort, Tricia Anne **(SLP)**

Sistersville
Ash, Kathryn Lynn

South Charleston
Americo, Peter K **(SLP)**
Basham, Jean Carla **(SLP)**
Harris, Dr Gary D **(A)**
Hartstein, Mrs Janice Cooper **(SLP)**
King, Susan J **(SLP)**
Krinock, Mrs Pamela S **(SLP)**
McDavid, Mary E F **(SLP)**
Potesta, Karen L **(SLP)**
Simmons, Mrs Elizabeth Champe **(SLP)**
Smith, Mrs Keith Ann **(SLP A)**
Trochlil, Margaret A **(A)**
Woods-Groves, Mrs Mary L **(A)**

Spencer
Knight, Linda L **(SLP)**

St Albans
Bonnett, Mrs Marilyn Via
Le Donne, Marianne **(SLP)**
Ulery, Norma Jean **(SLP)**

St Marys
Buck, Robert J **(SLP A)**

Star City
Gallon, Rudolph John **(SLP)**

Summersville
Cox, Dr Geraldine **(SLP)**
Cox, Dr James R **(A)**
Long, Patricia B **(SLP)**

Talcott
Terek-Ball, Linda M **(SLP)**

Thornton
Mead, Mrs Denise M **(SLP)**

Victor
Dever, Deen A **(SLP)**

Vienna
Briggs, Connie D **(SLP)**
Hardman, Teresa Amuso **(SLP)**
Longacre, Mrs Kathleen D **(SLP)**
Shrewsbury, Rosemary G **(SLP)**
Stanley, Ruth J H **(SLP)**

Wardensville
Mathias, Mrs Karen Peterson **(SLP)**

Washington
McManus, Mrs Nancy L **(SLP)**

Weirton
Chiodo, Denise Margaret **(SLP)**
Fowler, Joyce Lynn **(A)**
Mancuso, Robert A **(SLP)**

Wellsburg
Chastel, Penny Jean
Flasko, Deborah Jo **(A)**

West Hamlin
Blankenship, Mrs Jacquelyn Sue **(SLP)**

Weston
Di Thomas, Mary B **(SLP)**
Shaver, Mrs Cinda King

Westover
Lakawicz, Judith Anne **(SLP)**

Wheeling
Basilone, Frank J **(SLP)**
Boyle, Mary Christina **(SLP)**
Breza, Constance M **(SLP)**
Chambers, Lisa Young **(SLP)**
Finsley, Kathy M **(SLP)**
Front, Rosemary M **(SLP)**
Frum, James P **(SLP A)**
Hill, Ellen M **(SLP)**
Hon, Mrs Martha M **(SLP)**
Johnson, Dr Peter Roy **(SLP)**
Kevech, John James **(SLP)**
Kurz, Mary Ann **(SLP)**
Nagel, Ann E **(SLP)**
Rentschler, Fred W **(SLP)**
Riemer, Vernon Dale **(SLP)**
Soltman, Shirley K **(SLP)**
Walker, Glynda Marie **(SLP)**

Williamstown
Armstrong, Mrs Susan J **(SLP)**
Branson, Dr Virginia M **(SLP)**
Burns, Mrs Cinda S C **(SLP)**

Winfield
Adkins, Mrs J Pamela **(SLP A)**

WISCONSIN

Abbotsford
Kramer, Mrs J Beverly **(SLP)**

Agusta
Olson, Joyce A M **(SLP)**

Almond
Reineking, Mrs Mary B **(SLP)**

Altoona
Wetzel, Barbara **(SLP)**

Antigo
Findlay, Cynthia Marie **(SLP)**
Gress, Mrs Susan A
Mc Dougal, Carol Langreck **(SLP)**

Appleton
Andersen, Mrs Julia **(SLP)**
Barina, Jean Louise **(SLP)**
Bogdanow, Janet R **(SLP)**
Borchardt, Mrs Debra Ann **(SLP)**
Borchert, Cynthia Ruth **(A)**
Christiaansen, Mrs Ellen **(SLP)**
Dyer, Mrs Lynn Carew **(SLP)**
Ellisen-Doe, Mrs Katherine M **(SLP)**
Gruner, Pamela J B **(SLP)**
Heffron, Geralyn M **(SLP)**
Horan, Janet M **(SLP)**
Kelnhofer, Cheryl D **(SLP)**
Kopetsky, Marilyn Blick **(SLP)**
Kuba, Janis M **(SLP)**
Larson, Fonda Rae **(SLP)**
Larson, Mary Lynn
Mielke, Mrs Debra Nault **(A)**
Milner, Anna Mae **(SLP)**
Mixdorf, Mrs Carol F T **(SLP)**
Mueller, Cathy Lynn **(SLP)**
Mueller, Lois Goetsch **(SLP)**
Muenster, Ann Powers **(SLP)**
Needham, Ellen C **(SLP)**
Nocito, Mrs Catherine B **(SLP)**
Olson, Mary L **(SLP)**
Otto, Patricia Ann **(SLP)**
Pazak, Kathleen A **(SLP)**
Riederer, Renee A **(SLP)**
Schall-Krokosky, Charlotte **(SLP)**
School, Grace M **(SLP)**
Shudy, Mrs Jane M P **(SLP)**
Stewart, Suzette Marie **(SLP)**
Stoffregen, Tracey Ann **(SLP)**
Thelen, Michael K **(A)**
Tiller, Denise Marie **(SLP)**
Vilker-Krause, Mrs Nancy K
Ward, Mrs Martha Z **(SLP)**
Warden, Rebecca M **(SLP)**
Weiland, Ellen B **(SLP)**

Arpin
Dorshorst, Mrs Margie Ann **(SLP)**

Ashland
Eaton, Karen R **(SLP)**
Hallen, Linda A **(SLP)**
Holzhaeuser, Mrs Mary Jo Dewitte **(SLP)**
Holzhaeuser, William Joseph **(A)**
Traeder, Mrs Maxine D **(SLP)**

Baileys Harbor
Parent, Dawn E **(SLP)**

Balsam Lake
Clark, Cheryl Louise **(SLP)**
Coleman, Joanne P **(SLP)**

Barneveld
Hutson-Nechkosh, Margaret Ruth **(SLP)**

Bayside
Blumenfeld, Mrs Brenda C **(SLP)**
Cohen, Dr Gary S **(SLP)**
Gimbel, Lesley G **(SLP)**
Hawke, Carol J
Loeb, Mrs Marlene L **(SLP)**
Mitz, Mrs Lynda R **(SLP)**

Beaver Dam
Kalinosky, Mrs Sharon Marie **(SLP)**
Koehler, Lisa Claire **(SLP)**
Ruddock, Lisa Jean **(SLP)**
Stupich, Michael C **(A)**

Belleville
Muller, Barbara W **(SLP)**

Beloit
Brossard, Debra Flood **(SLP)**
De Soto, Jane Everhardt **(SLP)**
Eggers, Mrs Leslie Jane **(SLP)**
Jentoft, Richard C **(SLP)**
Walsh, Mary Justina **(SLP)**

Big Bend
Koehler, Mrs Dorothy M **(SLP)**
Mitton, Rosemary P **(SLP)**

Bloomer
Ruff, Jacqueline **(SLP)**

Brookfield
Alberswerth, Linda J M **(SLP)**
Barbour, Mrs Ruth A **(SLP)**
Bastiani, Robert **(SLP)**
Corlew, Dr Marilyn M **(SLP)**
Ertel, Mrs Judith M **(SLP)**
Hahn, Susan Margaret **(SLP)**
Herriges, Catherine Lynn **(A)**
Huntzinger, Mrs Janet H **(SLP)**
Hurley, Connie Lynn

Ilseman, Mrs Carmen B **(SLP)**
Knudten, Lisa A **(SLP)**
Koch, Lynnette J **(SLP)**
McComas, Anne W **(SLP)**
Mulcahy, Mrs Kathryn Salo **(SLP)**
Nelson, James A **(SLP)**
Nitschke, Terilynn
Oliver, Mrs Cynthia Robinson **(SLP)**
Pflieger, Eunice A **(SLP)**
Radtke, Judith W **(SLP)**
Reck, Joelene S **(SLP)**
Riedl, Patricia **(SLP)**
Rose, Mrs Darlene **(SLP)**
Sutton, Marjorie Alice **(SLP)**
Sweeney, Hansine Schumacher **(SLP)**
Theis, Mrs Denice K **(SLP)**
Weber, Mrs Sandra S **(SLP)**
Wright, Dr Laura F **(SLP)**
Young, Karen S **(SLP)**

Brooklyn
Tissot, Mrs Kathleen L **(SLP)**
Wilson, Mrs Carole **(SLP)**

Brown Deer
Hansen, Anne Christine **(SLP)**
Horkan, Ellen S **(SLP)**
Ruhland, Carol A **(SLP)**

Burlington
Bequest, Mrs Julie A **(SLP)**
Brawley, Mary C **(SLP)**
Clark, Mrs Tamara L **(SLP)**
Cramer, Mrs Debra Lynn **(SLP)**
Finley, Anita Trzobiatow **(SLP)**
Gabriel, Mrs Eileen K **(SLP)**
Hansen, James E **(SLP A)**
Hansen, Mrs Marilynn J **(SLP)**
Przybylinski, Donna G **(SLP)**

Caledonia
Canadeo, Lisa **(SLP)**

Cedarburg
Hadler, Joanne W **(SLP)**
Haischer, Mrs Lori G **(A)**
Henke, Mrs Cornella J **(SLP)**
Kacmarynski, Mrs Judith A **(SLP)**
Kamke, Mrs Jo K **(SLP)**
Schulte, William Charles

Chippewa Falls
Clark, Mrs Mary Beth Boos **(SLP)**
Haley, Mrs Judith **(SLP)**
Haut, Mrs Monica Osborne **(SLP)**
Miller, Julia Ann **(SLP)**
Willkom, Bonnie S **(SLP)**

Colfax
Kiesow, James R **(A)**

Colgate
Franzke, Debra T **(SLP)**
Hawker, Mrs Pamela Agnes **(SLP)**
Kossel, Mrs Sylvia K **(SLP)**
Rohs, Mrs Carol M **(SLP)**

Columbus
Chudy-Hesselberg, Mrs Barbara Ann

Crandon
Brockway, Mrs Susan M **(SLP)**

Cuaahy
Liska, Jill M

Cuba City
Parks, Michael F **(SLP)**

Cudahy
Curry, Mrs Dawn Denise **(SLP)**
Kwass, Susan M **(SLP)**
Ludwig, Jeanne Law **(SLP)**
Mysliwy, Julie Thiel **(SLP)**
Stewart, Katherine Priddy **(SLP)**
Wood, Mrs Dorothy H **(SLP)**

Cumberland
Carlson, Mrs Diane J **(SLP)**

Paisley, John M **(SLP)**

Darlington
Peterson, Sue Ellen Cox **(SLP)**

De Forest
Bair, Sharon Mutchler **(SLP)**

De Pere
Heideman-Lenz, Diane **(SLP)**
Waldkirch, Therese M **(SLP)**

Deerfield
Turner, Greg S **(SLP)**
Turner, Mrs Patricia Jo **(SLP)**

Delafield
Akre, Mrs Marie Patricia **(SLP)**
Coakley, Mrs Frieda Truman **(SLP)**
Parrish, Mrs Susan Christine **(SLP)**
Scoufis, Margaret R **(SLP)**

Delavan
Guido, Mrs Mary Krieger **(SLP)**
Kraayeveld, Sandra Jean
Strzelecki, Eve M **(SLP)**

Depere
Hogenson Day, Mrs Wendy J
Laubacher, Marci P **(SLP)**
Wiers, Mrs Kathleen A **(A)**

Dodgeville
Jewell, Mary Carole **(SLP)**
Schraeder, Patricia B **(SLP)**

Dousman
Freer, Cynthia Anne **(SLP)**
Nelson, Mrs Kay E **(SLP)**

Eagle River
Goss, Krista Hill **(SLP)**
Uttech, Shawn Lee **(SLP)**

Eau Claire
Anger, Carol Ann **(SLP)**
Bohn, Patti Claire **(SLP)**
Brandeland, Mrs Marilyn A **(SLP)**
Carpenter, Dr Linda J **(SLP)**
Christian, Mrs Carolyn Brovold **(SLP)**
Christian, Sara Schultz **(SLP)**
Eiten, Leisha R **(A)**
Feakes, Darrel Ray **(A)**
Fields, Mrs Vicki J **(SLP)**
Gregorash, Charysse M **(SLP)**
Hagedorn, Kay E **(SLP)**
Hager, Paul Milton **(SLP)**
Heins, Mrs Patricia P **(SLP)**
Herrell, Judy **(SLP)**
Hintgen, Thomas L **(SLP)**
Johnson, Vicki Lynette **(SLP)**
Jordan, Marjorie J **(A)**
Larson, Dr Vicki Lord **(SLP)**
McAfee, Dena P **(SLP)**
McDougall-Gibbs, Betsy E **(SLP)**
McGuine, Mrs Jane Barden **(SLP)**
McKinley, Nancy L **(SLP)**
McMillen, Dr Margaret H **(SLP)**
McNish, Mrs Lynn M **(SLP)**
Mollerud, Theodore **(A)**
Overson, Joan Sandra W **(SLP)**
Peters, Dr Theodore J **(SLP)**
Peterson, Nancy Marie
Picago, Stanley T **(SLP)**
Retherford-Stickler, Dr Kristine Sue **(SLP)**
Risen, Anne Dachel
Rogers, Caroline I **(SLP)**
Schemm, Donna Kay **(SLP)**
Schimke, Mrs Jean G R **(SLP)**
Schumacher, Mrs Jerelyn Wodill **(A)**
Simpson, Mrs Catherine Norris **(SLP)**
Slota, Mrs Ginger **(SLP)**
Smith, Dr Marshall M **(A)**
Steenson, Juliet B **(SLP)**
Steiner, Dr Sylvia
Suick, Joan M **(SLP)**
Tritz, Lois Catherine **(SLP)**

Tschanz, Mrs Dina Marie **(SLP)**
Tufte, Lori Jean **(SLP)**
Wobosel, Carolyn Mary **(SLP)**
Wolfarth, Dr Donald L

Egg Harbor
Hermann, Mrs Jennifer S **(SLP)**

Eland
Day, Mrs Mary P **(SLP)**

Elk Mound
Holte, Gayle Arnold **(SLP)**
Weix, Mrs Donna Jean **(SLP)**

Elkhorn
Gill-Dorgan, Deborah **(SLP)**
Palmer, Mrs Deborah Ann **(SLP)**

Ellsworth
Fischer, Shelley Jean **(SLP)**
Harris, Michael D **(SLP)**

Elm Grove
Barber, Sr Mary Nora
Burke-Thompson, Maureen **(SLP)**
Denny, Joan Marie **(SLP)**
Faught, Carole A **(SLP)**
Makovec, Julie A **(SLP)**
Mulhaney, Mrs Laurie Elizabeth **(SLP)**
White-Martin, Mrs Bonnie **(SLP)**

Elmwood
Weber, Bonita L **(SLP)**

Emerald
Moore, Mrs Mania F K **(SLP)**

Falls Creek
Zellmer, Mary K **(SLP)**

Fennimore
Johnson, Mrs Mony Coey

Fond Du Lac
Duehring, Bonnie R **(SLP)**
Gifford, Daniel Mark **(SLP)**
Killeen, Alicia M **(SLP)**
Kimpel, Mrs Linda Sue **(SLP)**
Kirschner, Sandra A **(SLP)**
Koerner, Sr Janet E **(SLP)**
Pino-Merriam, Mrs Barbara K **(SLP)**
Regan-Burton, Laurie P **(SLP)**
Sande, Susan Tourdot **(SLP)**
Sheimo, Mrs Diane L **(SLP)**
Tobin, Mrs Denise A **(SLP)**
Vruwink, Debra Lynn **(SLP)**
Wiersema, Gregory N **(A)**

Fontana
Van Diggelen-Cooper, Kathleen **(SLP)**

Fort Atkinson
Casey, Dr Patricia Louise **(SLP)**
Leaver, Mrs Kathleen Ann **(SLP)**
Rasmussen, Randall L **(SLP)**
Rattray, Mrs Kathryn Jean **(SLP)**
Stradinger, Mrs Teresa Carpentier **(SLP)**

Fox Point
Dabrowski, Patricia Duffy **(SLP)**
Gilson, Mrs Norma Lee **(SLP)**
Mann, Mrs Ellen K **(SLP)**
Washer, Mrs Sandra **(SLP)**

Franklin
Carver, Mrs Linda Rose **(SLP)**
Dinger, Mrs Nancy A
Dombeck, Mrs Monica A **(SLP)**
Ellis, Julie Heiman **(SLP)**
Giacalone, Mrs Jeanine Marie **(SLP)**
Heck, Sally Beth **(SLP)**
Kilmer, Mark T **(SLP)**
Lindsay, Ted J **(SLP)**
Liss, Mrs Bonnie S **(SLP)**
Miller, Dr Alfred L **(A)**
Milosch, Lizabeth Lynn **(SLP)**
Sengbusch, Mrs Diane Kittsley **(SLP)**
Tabili-Kilmer, Mrs Julie Anne **(SLP)**

Zeit, Mrs Janice J **(SLP)**

Fredonia
Braun, Mrs Mary Strzelczyk **(SLP)**
Derks, Jane A **(SLP)**
Sadowsky, Mrs Sara L **(SLP)**

Germantown
Richards, Ruth Marie **(SLP)**

Gilman
Peterson, Rosanne B **(SLP)**

Glendale
Clark, Mrs Jo Ann **(SLP)**
Felion, Mrs Elizabeth Ann **(SLP)**
Gruenwald, Susan M **(SLP)**
Hoffman, Mrs Harleene S **(SLP)**
Jakubowski, Allan J **(SLP)**
Kim, Dr Byoung W
Mandel-Herbert, Mrs Jody **(SLP)**
Pearson, Mrs Beth R **(SLP)**
Rothstein, Mrs Sharon H **(SLP)**
Spice, James G **(SLP)**

Grafton
Cekada-Kruesel, Mrs Julie A **(SLP)**
Hickcox, Mrs Barbara J **(SLP)**
Killinger, Pamela J **(SLP)**
Ott, Mrs Diane M **(SLP)**
Perini, Mrs Susan Guddie **(SLP)**

Green Bay
Ackeret, Ruth E **(SLP)**
Arps, Ritalyn K **(SLP A)**
Dictus, Kristine Ann **(SLP)**
Friedrich, Peggy Welsh **(SLP)**
Geiser, Judith Ann **(SLP)**
Hamersky, Daniel Joseph **(SLP)**
Hein, Barbara Phalen **(SLP)**
Hissong, Christine E **(SLP)**
Hunsberger, Deborah N **(SLP)**
Jaekels, Anne L **(SLP)**
Kadulski, Mrs Jane W **(SLP)**
Kenney, Susan P **(A)**
Klatt, Carolyn A **(SLP)**
Kozicki, Michelle M
Krepsky, Dr Judith C **(SLP)**
Krowiorz, Pamela Jeanne **(SLP)**
Kurland, Paul F **(A)**
Ledvina, Mrs Catherine Ann **(SLP)**
Ludwikoski, Steven P **(SLP)**
Monson, Deborah Jean **(SLP)**
Mosnik, Mrs Susan M **(SLP)**
Neilitz, Mrs Frances Glowienka **(SLP)**
O'Brien, Colleen K
Pahl, Mrs Cynthia Rachel **(SLP)**
Pesek, Mrs Elizabeth Ann **(SLP)**
Poels, Kathleen M **(SLP)**
Ricker, Mrs Susan Klingbell **(A)**
Roach, Beth Anne **(SLP)**
Rudeen, Lori L **(SLP)**
Ruef, Carolyn Larson **(SLP)**
Scheer, Debra Ann **(SLP)**
Schleis, Beth Ann
Schlender, Margaret Mary **(SLP)**
Schlitt, Mary M A **(SLP)**
Shalhoub, Amy Jo
Sook, Mrs Cynthia L Ciha **(SLP)**
Soukup, Mrs Lisa Stipe **(SLP)**
Stadelman, Cindy M **(SLP)**
Turner, Mrs Cheryl R **(SLP)**
Vetter-Powell, Mrs Julie **(SLP)**
Wadle, Cherie L **(SLP)**
Weberpal, Molly **(SLP)**

Green Lake
Ogle, Mrs Sharon Kay

Greendale
Birmingham, Barbara Ann **(SLP)**
Cristan, Monica Suzanne **(SLP)**
Dostal, Mrs Susan A H **(SLP)**
Doyle, Mrs Susan Ann **(SLP)**
Erdman, Kathleen B **(SLP)**
Heydon, Susan L **(SLP)**

Marks, Mary Jane **(SLP)**
Towne, Judith Ann **(SLP)**
Westin, Jane C **(SLP)**

Greenfield
Attermeier, Julie A **(SLP)**
Buck, Mrs Susan M **(SLP)**
Fluharty, George M **(SLP)**
Hilber, Mrs Jean S **(SLP)**
Kassees, Kenneth Salim **(SLP)**
Ketterman, Mrs Mary T **(SLP)**
Knuth, Renee Marie **(SLP)**
Napieralski, Linda Moore **(SLP)**
Scherbert, Thomas G **(SLP)**
Schlecht, Mrs Kathleen Marie **(SLP)**
Spankowski, Mrs Geralyn C **(SLP)**
Spitzenberger, Gail M **(SLP)**
Wuenstel, Mrs Peggy Sue **(SLP)**

Hager City
Anderson, Karen L
Baier, Mrs Mary S **(SLP)**
Fridgen, Mary Jean **(SLP)**
Marcks, Erin Alley

Hales Corners
Bjorklund, Tamy F **(SLP)**
Bykowski, Kathleen Adam **(SLP)**
Mahoney, Susan Mary
Markwiese, Beth Mary **(SLP)**
Mehner, Robert O **(SLP)**
Ostergren, Patricia G **(SLP)**
Paruzynski, Thad F **(SLP)**
Wainwright, Patricia Colby **(SLP)**
Zeigler-Waddell, Nancy E **(SLP)**

Hartford
Millikin, Paula A **(SLP)**
Omer, Mrs Elaine Okonek **(A)**

Hawthorne
Noble-Olson, Deborah A **(SLP)**

Hayward
Berger, Vicki J **(SLP)**
Bonicatto, Mrs Corinne H **(SLP)**
Rajala, James S **(SLP)**

Hazel Green
Schuler, Gail Lynn **(SLP)**

Holcombe
Flater, Mrs Paula Paquette **(SLP)**

Hubertus
Whelan, Mrs Debra J **(SLP)**

Hudson
Gardner, Beth Marie Abrahamson **(SLP)**
Griffin-Ziebart, Mrs Susanne Elizabeth
Hansen, John Henry **(SLP)**
Hauser, Carol A
Hole, Mrs Sherri Rae **(SLP)**

Iron River
Williamson, Mrs Rebecca Kinney **(SLP)**

Janesville
Braun, Janet M **(SLP)**
Bruner, Kathryn Ann
English, Betsy A
Gevaart, Mrs Carol C **(SLP)**
Johnson, Mindy O **(SLP)**
Long, Leland L **(SLP A)**
Losching, Mrs Susan Ruth **(SLP)**
MacPherson, Mrs Mary E **(SLP)**
Matulle, Terry V **(A)**
Mowbray, Mary L **(SLP)**
O'Leary, Debra M **(SLP)**
Pike, Susan R
Rasmussen, Mary Janet **(SLP)**
Saltzman, Galen Dean **(SLP)**
Scharenbroch, Mary Schanock **(SLP)**
Weir, Beth
Wood, Elaine Bay **(SLP)**
Wootton, Joan W **(SLP A)**

Jefferson
Gansen, Christi J Pearson **(SLP)**
Johnson, Joyce E **(SLP)**

Johnson Creek
Miller, Mrs Nola Moore **(SLP)**

Kenosha
Aiello, Maribeth Ann
Boris, Carol Jean **(SLP)**
Brown, Carolyn Marie **(SLP)**
Christ, Linda Townsend **(SLP)**
Fetherston, Gerald J **(SLP)**
Fulton, Timothy P **(SLP)**
Herrmann-Brydges, Virginia **(SLP)**
McDevitt, Marcie E **(SLP)**
Perlwitz, Mrs Renee S **(SLP)**
Plous, Mrs Helen C **(SLP)**
Pourchot, Mrs Ann Marie **(SLP)**
Pynckel, Lori Danette **(SLP)**
Randle, Mrs Kathleen Miller **(SLP)**
Rinaldi, Marilyn L
Szynski, Michael John **(A)**
Thibaudeau-Meyers, Camille **(SLP)**
Werve, Kathryn Symons **(SLP)**
Willems, Mrs Sherry G **(SLP)**
Wruck, Dr Kurt **(SLP)**

Kewaskum
Robertson, Mrs Shari Brand **(SLP)**

Kiel
Deibele, Denise Ristow **(SLP)**

La Crosse
Benson, Betty Dilley **(SLP)**
Harms, Helen L **(SLP)**
Hartman, Dr David E **(SLP)**
Joyce, Jeanne M **(SLP)**
Kakuska, Mrs Frances W **(SLP)**
King, Sally **(SLP)**
Monk, Vicki R B **(SLP)**
Monsoor, Mary R **(SLP)**
Palm, Dr David E **(A)**
Peterson, Harry J **(A)**
Retzlaff, Suellen S **(SLP)**
Rone, Mrs Kathleen L **(SLP)**
Sauer, Jacquelyn Ann **(SLP)**
Schmida, Milton Joseph **(A)**
Temple, Vicki L **(SLP)**

Ladysmith
Jacobson, Brenda Rae
Tauchen, Aileen **(SLP)**

Lake Geneva
Donovan, Mrs Cori L **(SLP)**
Host, Leigh **(SLP)**
Lasure, Mrs Laurie Lou **(SLP)**

Lake Mills
Myers, Jeanette Marie **(SLP)**
Ostrander, Elizabeth Larimer **(A)**

Lancaster
Carroll, Nancy L **(SLP)**

Lavalle
Haasch, Kathleen Mary **(A)**

Little Chute
Kons, Jane Marie **(SLP)**
Nelson, Janet R W **(SLP)**
Schumacher, Joyce Ann **(SLP)**

Little Suamico
Poburka, Bruce J **(SLP)**

Luxemburg
Eron, Brenda Kay

Madison
Abbs, James Howard
Allan, Joan **(A)**
Allen, Prudence **(A)**
Bailey, Laura Miller **(SLP)**
Barrett, Kathryn A **(A)**
Becker, Irene M **(SLP)**
Benson, Mrs Janice T **(SLP)**
Best, Sharon Larson **(SLP)**
Biever, Dawn Marie **(SLP)**
Bjorklund, Mrs Joylyn Louise **(SLP)**
Bless, Dr Diane McQueen **(SLP)**
Bonus, Katherine A **(SLP)**
Boser, Sheryl L L **(SLP)**
Bradford-Amrhein, Mrs Denise **(SLP)**
Brasser, Barbara Aylward **(A)**
Brewer, Kathryn A **(A)**
Brown, Kimberly Ann **(A)**
Bruce, Mrs Helen B **(SLP)**
Buchalter, Laurie **(SLP)**
Butler, Marcia T M **(SLP)**
Chapman, Dr Robin S
Chertoff, Keyna Klein **(A)**
Chertoff, Mark E **(A)**
Chial, Dr Michael R
Collins, Dr Michael James **(SLP)**
Connor, Nadine P **(SLP)**
Corbin, Kim M **(SLP)**
Crafton, Marilyn P **(SLP)**
Crews, Mrs Debbie **(SLP)**
Delisle, Dorothy M **(SLP)**
De Nil, Luc F
Denk, Mrs Renee Ritchie **(SLP)**
Depape, Donna J **(SLP)**
Depaul, Roxanne **(SLP)**
Doherty, Mrs Rosalind Tosti **(SLP)**
Donley, Debra J **(SLP)**
Dougall, Ronald N **(SLP)**
Drewry, Mrs Jane V
Dummeyer, Mary Beth **(SLP)**
Dyer, Erin C **(SLP)**
Eckles, Julie Beth **(SLP)**
Eide, Mrs Eunice A **(SLP)**
Ewanowski, Dr Stanley J **(SLP)**
Felckowski, Lynn Marie
Ferrer, Jami **(SLP)**
Filley, Florence S **(SLP A)**
Flynn, Margaret M **(SLP)**
Ford, Dr Charles N
Frazier, Julie A
Frey, Julie Eggleson **(SLP)**
Fruchtman, Amy Beth **(SLP)**
Fry, Debra S **(A)**
Galitski, Maureen E
Gamradt, Julie E **(SLP)**
Garrett, J David **(SLP)**
Gavinski, Janice Lange **(A)**
Gergen, Anne **(A)**
Gibson, Eloise J **(SLP)**
Gill, Dr Gary Dee **(SLP)**
Gillen, Carol A **(SLP)**
Godar, Mrs Cheryl Skovsted **(SLP)**
Godwin, Elizabeth **(SLP)**
Goldstein, Robert **(A)**
Goodenough, Sandra E S **(SLP)**
Gruenewald, Dr Lee John **(SLP)**
Hagen, Jennifer Lynn **(SLP)**
Hamele, Eileen Skelton **(SLP)**
Hansen, Mrs Deborah Lessiter
Hanson, Judith J **(SLP)**
Hartmann, Tamila Ann **(SLP)**
Heide, Veronica **(A)**
Heintzelman, Anne Teresa **(SLP)**
Hellmer, Jill F N **(A)**
Hesketh, Linda J **(SLP)**
Hunker, Dr Chauncey Joseph **(SLP)**
Imhoff-Smith, Georgia Ellen **(SLP)**
James, Dr Sharon L **(SLP)**
Javid, Claudia M **(SLP)**
Johnston, Joann Carol **(SLP)**
Kaemmerle, Ann W **(A)**
Kaplan, Jacqueline L **(SLP)**
Karlovich, Dr Raymond S **(SLP A)**
Kay-Rainingbird, Elizabeth **(SLP)**
Kellman, Mrs Marianne J **(SLP)**
Kellner, Judith Roach **(SLP)**
Kennedy, Catherine **(SLP)**
Kent, Dr Raymond D
Klipsch, Marcia S **(SLP)**
Kloosterboer, Linda Jean **(SLP)**
Kohn, Connie Rae **(SLP)**
Kohn, Lawrence L **(SLP)**
Koschkee, Danna L **(SLP)**
Koth, Margaret A
Kwiatkowski, Joan **(SLP)**
Lafollette, Lisa Marie
Lam, Mrs Barbara B **(SLP)**
Lippert, Mrs Janet C **(SLP)**
Liss, Julie Marie **(SLP)**
Lodholz, Mrs Colleen A **(SLP)**
Lof, Gregory L **(SLP)**
Mackey, Catherine Hadley **(SLP)**
Maron, Linda R **(SLP)**
McCartan, Daniel Edward **(SLP)**
McCaughey, Mrs Vicki Rowe
McCormick, Cecilia M **(SLP)**
McCoy, Christine **(SLP)**
McCrary, Judith Anne
McNeil, Dr Malcolm R **(SLP)**
Michaels, Susan Liz E **(SLP)**
Mikesell, Stephanie L **(SLP)**
Miller, Eric G **(A)**
Miller, Jon F **(SLP)**
Miller, Patricia J **(SLP)**
Morgan, Gary L **(A)**
Morgan, Jane Kirschbaum **(SLP)**
Moses, Mrs Christine Cefalu **(SLP)**
Murphy, Valerie H **(SLP)**
Murray-Branch, Jamie **(SLP)**
Musin, Mrs Charlotte **(SLP)**
Mutchler-Mathias, Karen Sue
Nellis, Robert A **(A)**
Nelson, Dr Lois A **(SLP)**
Notbohm, Heidi L **(SLP)**
Odell, Katharine Hobart **(SLP)**
Otterson, Patricia Ann **(SLP)**
Parry, Laurie J **(SLP)**
Patterson, Jennifer A **(A)**
Peppard, Robert C **(SLP)**
Perkins, Giovanna Frittelli **(SLP)**
Perlman, Abel **(SLP)**
Peterson, John L **(A)**
Podvin, Julie A **(A)**
Pratt, Dr Shelia Rose **(SLP A)**
Punch, Dr Jerry L **(A)**
Reibetanz, Dr Karen R **(SLP)**
Robbins, Dr Joanne **(SLP)**
Robinson, Susan Marie **(SLP)**
Robl, Gwen S **(SLP)**
Roethe, Lynn A **(SLP)**
Rohe, Susan Westervelt **(SLP)**
Roman, Allison Sedey **(SLP A)**
Rosenbek, John C **(SLP)**
Rosin, Margaret Mary **(SLP)**
Rouse, Mrs Ann T **(SLP)**
Ruchti, Lynda Lee **(SLP)**
Salee, Mrs Susan Elizabeth **(SLP)**
Schultz, Michael A
Seeker, Tamara J **(SLP)**
Shriberg, Dr Lawrence D **(SLP)**
Sidler, Mrs Mary E **(SLP)**
Simmons, Kathryn M **(SLP)**
Sinha, Dr Narendra K **(SLP)**
Slansky, Barry L **(SLP)**
Slansky, Pamela M **(SLP)**
Smith, Mary E **(SLP)**
Smithyman, Mrs Jennifer Ann
Steege, Mrs Suzanne E **(SLP)**
Strennen, Mary Lou **(A)**
Swift, Mrs Estelle W **(SLP)**
Topalian, Tracy Ann **(SLP)**
Turco, Tambria Marie **(SLP)**
Tweed, Theodore S **(A)**
Vanderheiden, Dr Gregg C
Veloon, Paulette A **(SLP)**
Verkuilen, Mrs Kathleen Kimmel **(SLP)**
Vernon, Mary Lou **(SLP)**
Vetter, Dolores Kluppel
Wahl, Lisa Hinze **(SLP)**
Wahlton, Raymond E **(SLP A)**
Weatherby, Lynn A **(A)**
Weismer, Susan Ellis **(SLP)**

Weston, Audrey **(SLP)**
Wiley, Terry L **(A)**
Williamson, Linda Lee **(SLP)**
Wilson, Linda A **(SLP)**
Woodward, Sandra H **(A)**
Wyman, Marion Resha **(SLP)**
Young, Carolyn E **(A)**
Zabawski, Charlene J **(SLP)**
Zimmerman, Susan Mary **(SLP)**
Zwaska, Janet Marie **(SLP)**

Manitowoc
Brisbane, Sr Arlene **(SLP)**
Holle, Peggy J **(SLP)**
Johnson, Mrs Paula Tenpas **(SLP)**
Vodicka, Diana Mary **(SLP)**
Wilger, Terese Marie **(SLP)**

Marathon
Fedo-Rosvold, Susan M **(SLP)**
Ruplinger, Kathleen A **(SLP)**

Maribel
Zaffke, Linda O **(A)**

Marinette
Menza, Marie A **(SLP)**
Paczkowski, Mrs Patricia M **(SLP)**

Marion
McLaughlin, Mrs Nancy Cookle **(SLP)**

Marshall
Schwellenbach, Julie Ann **(SLP)**

Marshfield
Bartelt, Rosalyn M **(SLP)**
Berger, Mrs Julie Ann **(A)**
Birmingham, Marie Kay **(SLP)**
Crawford, Mary B **(SLP)**
Hansen, Donald A **(A)**
Holt, Catherine Chun **(A)**
McShane, William Thomas **(SLP)**
Mester, Lori Marie **(SLP)**
Michalski, Mrs Mary J **(SLP)**
Peterson, Jeanette Marie **(SLP)**
Quinn-Padron, Maura **(SLP)**
Strand, Richard L **(A)**
Wiemann, Mrs Janet M **(SLP)**
Workinger, Dr Marilyn Seif **(SLP)**
Wunrow, Jean R **(SLP)**

Mauston
Benson, Mrs Sheri H **(SLP)**

Mayville
Carter, Jane Royer **(SLP A)**
Fanta, Mrs Katherine Ann **(SLP)**
Gumm, Mrs Carolyn K **(SLP)**
Loest, Patricia L **(SLP)**

Mazomanie
Shimon, Debra Ann **(A)**

McFarland
Mooney, Thomas G **(SLP)**
Odell, Brent C **(SLP)**
Odell, Mrs Ruth M **(SLP)**
Toennies, Mrs Joanne Elizabeth **(SLP)**
Tuecke, Susan K **(SLP)**

Medford
Novinska, Mrs Deirdre A **(SLP)**

Menasha
Beck, Judith E **(SLP)**
Boylan, Donna M **(SLP)**
Curtis, Sue Ellen **(SLP)**
Gmeiner-Heinrich, Ann **(SLP)**
Jacobson, Mrs Kathy Jean **(SLP)**
Osborne-Hurley, Mrs Julie E **(SLP)**

Menomonee Falls
Budde, Betty Ion **(SLP)**
Clark-McGowan, Mrs Jill M **(SLP)**
Corsi-Fraundorf, Laura J **(SLP)**
King, Karen Lynn **(SLP)**
Kingsbury, Karen Basting **(SLP)**
Olson, Marilyn R **(A)**
Rauh, Linda A **(SLP)**
Thompson, Julie Kay **(SLP)**

Menomonie
Breitzman, Julie J **(SLP)**
Eitrheim, Amy Jo **(SLP)**
Harvey, Janet L **(SLP)**
Hegna, Wendy S **(SLP)**
King, Dr Thomas W **(SLP)**
Preston, Jodi Weber **(SLP)**
Zengel, Mrs Beverly J **(SLP)**

Mequon
Benedict, Pamela H **(A)**
Bradley, Mrs Roberta Lynn **(SLP)**
Carneol, Susan Oliff **(SLP)**
Chester, Roberta L **(SLP)**
Duncan, Mrs Janice L **(SLP)**
Foley, Mrs Denise Jennings **(A)**
Hare, Mrs Karla P **(SLP)**
Jagla, Mrs Virginia Abraham **(SLP)**
Johnson, Deanna E **(SLP)**
Lukas, Elaine K **(SLP)**
Orcholski, Emil R **(SLP)**
Peck, Mrs Luann English **(SLP)**
Peters, Alma D **(SLP)**
Terrill, Mrs Karen L **(SLP)**
Van Cleave, Mary L **(A)**
Vercoe, Donna M **(SLP)**
Walczak, Necia B **(SLP)**

Merrill
Andreski, Mrs Mary K **(SLP)**
Knapstein, Mary K **(SLP)**
Lewis, James A **(SLP)**

Middleton
Barlow, Virginia L **(SLP)**
Bondi, Mrs Carole Turner **(SLP)**
Glaze, Leslie Ellen **(SLP)**
Hardy, Mary Lynn Z **(SLP)**
Hyland, Jennifer Denise **(SLP)**
Johnson, Beth Ellen **(SLP)**
Lethlean, B Sue **(SLP)**
Metzger, Maria Jusko **(SLP)**
Nathanson, Barbara **(SLP)**
Pauly, Cathie A **(SLP)**
Raupp, Mrs Colleen Campbell **(SLP)**
Schwartz, Scott E **(SLP)**
Weidman, Maja B **(SLP)**

Milton
Brandes, Mrs Polly P **(SLP)**
Massoglia, Ann Tomasin **(SLP)**
Rowe, Mary Grace **(SLP)**
Sierzega, Carol D **(SLP)**
Zummo, Samuel R **(SLP)**

Milwaukee
Ackeret, Mrs Rosalind Marie **(SLP)**
Allen, Patricia Lee **(SLP)**
Anton, Mrs Linda **(SLP)**
Bachtell, Cheryl Lee **(SLP)**
Bakker, Dr Klaas
Baldwin, Kathleen A **(SLP)**
Beecher, Robert Best **(SLP)**
Bell-McGhee, Mary Elizabeth **(SLP)**
Berger, Kathy M
Bhatnagar, Dr Subhash C **(SLP)**
Bischoff, Joanne R **(SLP)**
Block, Ellen Patricia **(A)**
Blom, Mrs Annem G **(SLP)**
Bohlman, Mrs Patricia A **(SLP)**
Bohrman, Sandra A **(SLP)**
Bradburn-Oates, Ann **(SLP)**
Brandriet, Stanley E **(SLP)**
Broeren, Margaret Mary **(SLP)**
Brown, Mrs Julie Anne **(SLP)**
Bruce, Mary Katherine **(SLP)**
Burg, Mrs Linda Sue **(A)**
Busalacchi, Mrs Gail Marie **(SLP)**
Caceres, Milagros Ong **(SLP)**
Carlis, Mrs Kimberly **(SLP)**
Cechal, Patricia Jeanne **(SLP)**
Clark, Mrs Judith A K **(SLP)**
Clay, Mrs Cynthia C **(SLP)**
Colombo, Joanne Marie **(A)**
Conway, Nancy Ann **(SLP)**
Craig, Dr Chie Higuchi **(A)**
Culbertson, Mrs Patricia Marie **(SLP)**
Culver, Mrs Margaret A **(SLP)**
D'Alessio-Caniza, Prudence Dianne **(SLP)**
Daniels, Elizabeth Anne **(SLP)**
Dardis, Mrs Linda L **(SLP)**
Deacy, Denise Bauman **(A)**
Doherty, Mrs Betty **(SLP)**
Dowling, Mrs Frances R **(A)**
Dubin, Mrs Carol Kampner **(SLP)**
Eklund, Adele C **(SLP)**
Eldredge, Christine **(SLP)**
Erickson, Jane F **(SLP)**
Eriksson, Anne-Guri **(SLP)**
Falat, Mrs Barbara Sovey **(SLP)**
Feiss, Mrs Sarah **(SLP)**
Fiedler, Dr Irma Gail **(SLP)**
Fields, Mrs Karen A **(SLP)**
Filipiak, Debra Ann **(SLP)**
Fina, Ruth B **(SLP)**
Fischer, Mrs Cathryn Avallone **(SLP)**
Flood, Mary K **(SLP)**
Franke, Gabrielle Ann **(SLP)**
Fuchs, Mrs Mary D'Amico **(SLP)**
Gardon, Andrea Marie **(A)**
Garvalia, Carrie A
Gaskin, Maura Louise **(SLP)**
Gavin, Dr Kenneth J **(SLP)**
Geiger, Patricia **(SLP)**
Gelin, Mrs Devora D **(SLP)**
George, Audrey C **(SLP)**
Geraghty, Susan Green **(SLP)**
Gies-Zaborowski, Jeanne Ellen **(SLP)**
Gitter, Mrs Kelly Jo **(A)**
Goerner, Mrs Lisa McHugh **(A)**
Goetz, Karen Cox **(A)**
Gorzalski, Mrs Janet A **(SLP)**
Graan, Ellen M **(SLP)**
Gramling, Susan M S **(SLP)**
Grande, Barbara Sue **(SLP)**
Hansen, Joan Bode **(SLP)**
Harris, Laura Lee **(SLP)**
Harris, Paula Dinkins
Hartnett, Laura Lee **(SLP)**
Hartney, Bridget Joan **(SLP)**
Haubner, Colleen C **(SLP)**
Heintz, Janet Lynn **(SLP)**
Henry, Frederick **(SLP)**
Hoehnke, Mrs Valerie Jane **(SLP)**
Ihrig, Karen R **(SLP)**
Jacobson, Mrs Laura L **(SLP)**
Johnson, William B **(SLP)**
Jonas, Mrs Jane M **(SLP)**
Kaucic, Cheryl Ann **(SLP)**
Kirchner-Smudde, Mrs Patricia Lynn **(SLP)**
Kloet, Marilyn Jean **(SLP)**
Koenen, Susan Kathryn
Kolo, Mrs Lori E Solberg **(SLP)**
Kopmeier, Mrs Mary K **(SLP)**
Korabic, Dr Edward W **(A)**
Kowalski, Mrs Susan Swartz **(SLP)**
Kravit, Mrs Deborah S **(SLP)**
Kravitz, Dena S **(SLP)**
Kueht, James D **(SLP)**
Kuhn, Joan C **(SLP)**
Kulpa, Judith I **(SLP)**
Leff, Mrs Ruth B **(SLP)**
Lewis, Sheila Renee **(SLP)**
Linville, Dr Sue Ellen **(SLP)**
Maierle, Victoria M **(SLP)**
Maile-Freese, Jill R **(SLP)**
Maki, Mrs Linda G **(SLP)**
Mann, Mrs Mary Ann **(SLP)**
Maring, Lana J **(SLP)**
Marino, Marcia L **(SLP)**
Marks, Susan M **(SLP)**
Mathewson, David Richard **(SLP)**
Mayo, Robert A **(SLP)**
McCabe, Mrs Barbara Michalak **(SLP)**
McGinn, Nancy **(SLP)**
McIntyre, Mary Elizabeth **(SLP)**
McVann, Owen J **(SLP)**
Mechanic, Janis B **(SLP)**
Minard, Mrs Pamela Dickinson **(A)**
Minix, Paula Vanlaanen **(SLP)**
Moller, Mrs Miriam **(SLP)**
Molter, Mrs Sandra Schneider **(SLP)**
Morris, Oranell D
Mueller, Laura J **(SLP)**
Nadolski, Mark W **(SLP)**
Nathan, Mrs Jeanette **(SLP)**
Newman, Dr Linda Lee **(SLP)**
Niederjohn, Dr Russell J
Olsen, Kathryn Mary **(A)**
Olson, Joan R **(SLP)**
Orlowski, Michalynn **(SLP)**
Orozco, Patricia **(SLP)**
Ostergaard, Sue Ann **(A)**
Payerl, Mrs Christine A **(SLP)**
Payerl, Douglas Gene **(SLP)**
Pecyna Rhyner, Dr Paula M **(SLP)**
Pergande, Mrs Krisann S **(SLP)**
Peterson, Julia Gail **(SLP)**
Piedt, Diane O **(SLP)**
Piette, Joe **(SLP)**
Pike, Sandra M **(SLP)**
Pinter, Mrs Ann R **(SLP)**
Powers-Todt, Mrs Maureen F **(SLP)**
Pozza, Charlyn M **(SLP)**
Pozza, Cynthia Ann **(SLP)**
Puglisi-Creegan, Santina V **(SLP)**
Regan, Mrs Margaret Brady **(SLP)**
Regner, Jennifer C **(SLP)**
Reinick, Mrs Lynn P **(SLP)**
Reitz, Ellen Christine **(SLP)**
Rodgers, Mrs Mary Sue **(SLP)**
Rogers, Martha E **(SLP)**
Ronowski, Laura J **(SLP)**
Rospenda, Mrs Sharon **(SLP)**
Ross-Crabtree, Mrs Vicki L **(SLP)**
Rouleau, Mary L **(SLP)**
Rubenstein, Merilyn B **(SLP)**
Ryan, Stephan B **(A)**
Sapiro, Mrs Vivian A **(SLP)**
Schaning, Helen D **(SLP)**
Schermer, Sheryl Lynn **(SLP)**
Schloss, Cynthia Diane **(SLP)**
Schlosser, Diane K **(SLP)**
Schmidt, Mrs Carol S **(SLP)**
Schmitz, Mrs Nancy J **(SLP)**
Schneider, Kathy Elaine **(SLP)**
Schwebke, Steven Paul **(SLP)**
Scopp-Liegel, Elizabeth Ann **(SLP)**
Shaker, Catherine Shriver **(SLP)**
Shonrock, Cynthia M **(SLP)**
Silverman, Dr Ellen-Marie **(SLP)**
Silverman, Dr Franklin H **(SLP)**
Sokolnicki, Alfred J **(SLP)**
Sommers, Mrs Patricia A **(SLP)**
Soukup, Mrs Nina R **(SLP)**
Starobin, Mrs Caryl W **(SLP)**
Stein, Pamela D **(SLP)**
Steven, Rene Schwalbach **(SLP)**
Streng, Alice H **(A)**
Stringer, Gary K **(SLP)**
Susienka, Cindy Hasenzahl **(SLP)**
Taves-Ruenzel, Mary Elizabeth **(SLP)**
Tikofsky, Mrs Rita **(SLP)**
Tikofsky, Dr Ronald S **(SLP)**
Toyne, Mrs Julie Ann **(SLP)**
Trotter, Paul James **(SLP)**
Turner, Dr Janet E **(SLP)**
Ulrich, Colby Kendro
Vasterling, Margaret M **(SLP)**
Vielgut, Mrs Kathleen Marie
Wallschlaeger, Anne Marie **(SLP)**
Warner, Kathleen Jane **(SLP)**
Warren, Dr Richard M
Wealton, Kate A **(SLP)**
Welsh, Mrs Joan Benner **(SLP)**
Whitson, Sally H **(A)**

Winter, Mrs Susan K **(SLP)**
Wolkober, Martina M **(SLP)**
Woppert, Mrs Diane L **(SLP)**
Worachek-Jarocki, Mary **(SLP)**
Wright, Ferne E **(SLP)**
Yahle, Patricia A **(SLP)**
Yates, Mrs Joan Diane **(SLP)**
Zientara, Mrs Betty K **(SLP)**
Zimmer, Catherine H **(SLP)**
Zimmermann, Mrs Kelly J
Zizzo, Robert **(SLP)**

Minequa
Bassett, Mrs Wendy Bendrick **(SLP)**
Treb, William E **(A)**

Monroe
Knuteson, Mrs Christine Owen **(A)**
MacLeod, Mrs Nancy J **(SLP)**
Ziegler, Mrs Phyliss M **(SLP)**

Monticello
Voegeli, Mrs Beth Carson **(SLP)**

Mosinee
Forsythe, Michelle Rene **(SLP)**

Mukwonago
Carr, Mrs Patricia Etten **(SLP)**

Muscoda
Galdes, Mrs Karen Lee **(SLP)**
Thingvold, Jacqueline Williams **(SLP)**

Muskego
Breitzke, Mrs Juanita L **(SLP)**
Graff, James L **(SLP)**
Shanks, Rosemarie Ann **(SLP)**
Steckel, Mary Clare

Necedah
Kolff, Andrew J

Neenah
Collins, Sherryl Jeannine **(SLP)**
Conradt, Mark **(A)**
Kressner, Kathrine **(SLP)**
Lesselyong, Mrs Lisa Marie **(SLP)**
Lucht, James L **(A)**
Praefke, Mrs Marie H **(SLP)**
Rieck, Cynthia A **(SLP)**
Rouse, Mrs Marie T **(SLP)**
Ward, Mrs Judith H **(SLP)**
Wilder, Mrs Suzanne Marie **(SLP)**

Nekoosa
Hamin, Mrs Amy Lynn **(SLP)**
Kovars, Mrs Louise J **(SLP)**

Nelsonville
Voeks, Dr Susan K **(SLP)**

New Berlin
Batterman, Mrs Laurel Kay **(SLP)**
Breitbach, Idelle J **(SLP)**
Calabresa-Echelard, Mrs Maria Louise **(SLP)**
Heerey, Mary N **(SLP)**
Hotelling, Mrs Renee C **(SLP)**
May, John P **(A)**
Ragonese, Maria Theresa
Rausch, Dr Marie A **(SLP)**
Sessler, Patricia L **(SLP)**
Sylla, Mary Beth **(SLP)**

New Franken
French, Mrs Patricia G **(SLP)**

New Holstein
Cummings, Tara T **(SLP)**

New Lisbon
Raabe, Mrs Ann Hammond **(A)**

New London
Martin, Mrs Deborah S **(SLP)**

New Richmond
Krier, Marcia Ann **(SLP)**

Nonona
Witherell, Mrs Julie Korb **(SLP)**

North Fond Du Lac
Walser, Paula S **(SLP)**

Oak Creek
Gaffney, Lorrie Jeanne **(SLP)**
Hoesl, Lori Sue **(A)**
Klein, Mrs Carolyn G **(SLP)**
Schmidt, Nancy A **(SLP)**
Shallow, Mrs Lisa Kundinger **(SLP)**

Oconomowoc
Frederick, Julie Anne **(SLP)**
Freiberg, Cathlene J
Karenz, Mrs Sandra M **(SLP)**
Kupperman, Dr Gerard L **(A)**
Kupperman, Mrs Suzan L **(SLP)**
Meske, Mrs Pauline L **(SLP)**
Papador, Amalia A **(SLP)**
Radke, Mrs Michelle Lee **(SLP)**
Rohde, Mrs Ruthann **(SLP)**
Schaetz, Doreen **(SLP)**

Oconto Falls
Nypaver, Virginia Ireen **(SLP)**

Onalaska
Anderson, Mrs Judy Annbrenner **(SLP)**
Donlan, Mrs Sharon Askew **(A)**
Heineck, Kristine Marie **(SLP)**
Tushkowski, Mrs Renae **(SLP)**
Uglem, Mrs Linda R H **(SLP)**

Oneida
Frame, Charles Wayne

Oostburg
Wykhuis, Mrs Nicole Nesselroad **(SLP)**

Oregon
Karlsen, Else **(SLP)**
Kirchdoerfer, Diana G **(SLP)**

Oregon City
Schneider, Mrs Kathryn J **(SLP)**

Oshkosh
Ansell, Dr Barbara J **(SLP)**
Ansfield, Mrs Sandra **(SLP)**
Beck, Janice Nutt **(SLP)**
Brown, Sharon Maxine **(SLP)**
Duffy, Mrs Darcy P **(SLP)**
Haushalter, Mrs Phyllis Jayne **(SLP)**
Hayes, Mrs Kathleen Mary
Hermann-O'Keeffe, Katherine **(SLP)**
Holub, Mary M **(SLP)**
Homann, Dr Hal W **(SLP A)**
Kile, Dr Jack E **(A)**
Larson, Doreen A **(SLP)**
Poliak, Mrs Diana R W **(SLP)**
Rossetti, Dr Louis M **(SLP)**
Schade, Mrs Kristine **(SLP)**
Sterkens, Juliette P M **(A)**

Osseo
Boley, Mrs Delesa Fox **(SLP)**
Schwartz, Linda **(SLP)**

Owen
Strand, Joan Marie **(SLP)**

Pardeeville
Ruhland, Mrs Robin Kay **(SLP)**

Park Falls
Kennedy, Timothy J **(SLP)**

Pewaukee
Easterling, Caryn S C **(SLP)**
Heidemann, Kathleen **(SLP)**
Soper-Cotter, Sally J **(SLP)**
Wollner, Barbara A **(SLP)**

Phillips
Olson, Thomas J **(SLP)**

Plainfield
Kuphall, Susan S **(SLP)**

Platteville
Boatright, Mrs Deborah S **(SLP)**
Droessler, Catherine A **(SLP)**
Hoyman, Tami Lyn **(SLP)**
Ollinger, Mary Beth **(SLP)**

Plover
Ronzani, Mrs Judith M **(SLP)**
Weber-Pagel, Vivian **(SLP)**

Plymouth
Obenberger, Nancy Ann **(SLP)**
Rolzin, Mrs Elaine A **(SLP)**

Poynette
Dugolenski, Lynne Giacomino **(SLP)**

Praire Du Chien
Kilbey, Gretchen Carla
Newmann, Mrs Melody L
Schilling, Karen Marie **(SLP)**

Prescott
Howard, Mrs Deborah Ann **(SLP)**

Pulaski
Mannigel, Mrs Pamela A **(SLP)**

Racine
Amundsen, Mrs Judith A **(SLP)**
Barry, Ann Marie **(SLP)**
Beighley, Melody F **(SLP)**
Chu, Diane Elizabeth **(SLP)**
Denning, Jacqueline Ann
Hardiman, Linda Kay **(SLP)**
Hesse, Mrs Kathleen L
Horvath, Mrs Patricia Eileen **(SLP)**
Knox, John Gerard **(A)**
Lee, Dr Bonnie Engel **(SLP)**
Maiers, Mary A **(SLP)**
Mayer, Margaret Jean **(SLP)**
Nelson, Mrs Katherine Van Opens **(SLP)**
Rintelmann, Joan **(SLP)**
Robertson, Christine E **(SLP)**
Rouse, Mrs Jean L B **(SLP)**
Seefeldt, Mariel D **(SLP)**

Rhinelander
Amo, Kathleen Marie **(SLP)**
Hochmuth, Lou A **(SLP)**
Laursen, Mrs Charlene Ann **(SLP)**
O'Brien, Karen S **(SLP)**
Vaughn, Tracey Jane **(SLP)**

Rice Lake
Conroy-Peckham, Kay Marie **(SLP)**
Hanson, Paul E **(SLP)**
Messick, Cheri Fox **(SLP)**
Minell, Jane F **(A)**
Ronning, Mrs Nina M **(SLP)**

Ridgeland
Mattison, Kelly Mack **(SLP)**

Ripon
Berendsen, Mrs Madeline Geary **(SLP)**
Schultz, Susan E **(SLP)**
Worrall, Mrs Christena **(SLP)**

River Falls
Berry, Dr Galen W **(A)**
Bystrom, Susan Kay **(SLP)**
Freeman, Mrs Nancy Lindseth
Giebel, Mrs Linda Ann **(SLP)**
Girtz, Pamela Sue **(SLP)**
Halvorson, Dr Jerome A **(SLP A)**
Harter, Mrs Diana Jones
Hayden, Paul A **(SLP)**
Hirsch, Dr Judith E **(A)**
Justinger, Judith A **(SLP)**
Larsen, William G **(SLP)**
Moelter, Mary Kathryn
Norman, Janell B **(SLP)**
Paulson, Mrs Jill Marie **(SLP)**
Peitso, Mrs Lorraine A **(SLP)**
Peterson, Sally Ann **(SLP)**
Wing, Christine **(SLP)**

Roberts
Meyer, Nancy E M **(SLP)**

Rosholt
Bialzik, Barb J **(SLP)**

Sauk City
Halverson, Teresa K **(SLP)**

Schofield
Edahl, Kristine C **(SLP)**
Johnson, Gayl E **(SLP)**

Seymour
De Bruin, Mrs Mary Noren **(SLP)**

Shawano
Golembiewski, Colleen Marie **(SLP)**
Johnson, Mrs Frances Y **(SLP)**
McDougal, Kathleen A **(SLP)**
Schoenfeld, Julie T **(SLP)**

Sheboygan
Arena, Maria Lynn **(SLP)**
Baalke, Mrs Nancy Wiedmeyer **(SLP)**
Caldwell, Carol S **(SLP)**
Feingold, Mrs Frances H
Hoffmann, Roger E **(SLP)**
James, Mrs Julie Koehn **(SLP)**
McKittrick, Julie Linn **(SLP)**
Neumann, Mrs Suzanne Marie **(A)**
Scharrer, Mrs Ann F **(SLP)**
Tyszka, Dr Frederic A **(A)**
Walker, Fred L **(SLP)**

Sheboygan Falls
Kuhn, Mrs Cheryl Thomas **(SLP)**
Van Himbergen, Lori M **(SLP)**

Shorewood
Battles, James F **(SLP)**
Hodous, Mrs Michele McGuire **(A)**
Miller, Dr George H **(SLP)**
Nording, Lori J **(A)**
Onufrock, Mrs Elizabeth Hamm **(SLP)**
Rindo, Mrs Ellen Sue **(SLP)**
Ritchie, Dr Betty C **(SLP A)**
Weston, Mrs Lucinda C **(SLP)**
Wolfley, Mary Elizabeth **(SLP)**

South Milwaukee
Johnson, Janet Mary

Sparta
Meyer-Boldon, Carol A **(SLP)**
Sherin, Krista **(SLP)**

Spooner
Keown, Therese Marie **(SLP)**
Pearson, Mrs Susan Kay **(SLP)**

Spring Green
Moore, Emily Katharine **(SLP)**

St Croix Falls
Erickson, Charlotte **(SLP)**

St Francis
Michaelis, Lucinda Jane **(SLP)**

Stanley
Seidl, Dennis M **(SLP)**

Star Prairie
White, Margaret R **(SLP)**

Stevens Point
Aylesworth, Dr Donald L **(SLP)**
Balas, Dr Robert F **(A)**
Burkhart, Brian Paul **(SLP)**
Burmesch, Julianna Fisher **(SLP)**
Chappell, Gerald E **(SLP)**
Christensen, Mrs Donna Y **(SLP)**
Dean, Mary Pat **(SLP)**
Fonti, Patti L **(A)**
Fuehrer-Mancl, Joyce Ann
Gallagher, Mrs Constance **(A)**
Glascoe, Dr Gary Jay **(A)**
Johnson, Dr Gerald F **(SLP A)**
Johnson, Mrs Maxine M **(SLP)**

Meyer, Dr William H **(SLP)**
Nash, Dr Dennis B **(SLP)**
Nguyen, Mrs Kathie Rae **(SLP)**
Olson, Dorothy M **(SLP)**
Pratt, Judith E **(SLP)**
Redmond, Jacquelyn Ann
Soat, Lynn A **(SLP)**
Sperberg, Mrs Holly Hofman
Steffen, Mrs Catherine **(SLP)**
Tufts, Dr La Rene C **(SLP A)**
Van Den Heuvel, Denise M **(SLP)**
Wyhuske, Claire M **(SLP)**

Stoughton
Heil, Mrs Judith Meyer **(SLP)**
Johnson, Marie H **(SLP)**
Kleckner, Ann Marie **(SLP)**
Knutson, Mrs Diane K **(SLP)**
Orcutt, Anne Witt **(SLP)**
Smedal, Mrs Heidi Ann **(A)**

Sturgeon Bay
Arbter, Mrs Jody Ann **(SLP)**
Bohn, Eileen Hunziker **(SLP)**
Farrell, Catherine **(SLP)**
Hoffman, Laurie T **(SLP)**

Sturtevant
Armgardt, Mrs Colleen K **(A)**
Klawinski, Donna Marie **(A)**
Pawlowski-Vincer, Mrs Karen **(SLP)**

Sullivan
Melcher, Mrs Keli L

Sun Prairie
Callahan, Angela Marie **(SLP)**
McClain, Thora H **(SLP)**
Rattmann, Janet M **(SLP)**
Taulman, Mrs Cheryl Ann **(SLP)**

Superior
Currie-Heytens, Mrs Desiree Ann **(SLP)**
Kelly, Mrs Linda A **(SLP)**
Nelson, Roberta Lynn **(SLP)**

Suring
Jagodzinski, Mrs Mary Carolyn **(SLP)**

Sussex
Gresch, Anna M K **(SLP)**
Morand, Kate **(SLP)**
Patnode, Margaret Mary **(SLP)**
Voss-Schwartz, Kathleen **(SLP)**

Thiensville
Reuter, Catherine **(SLP)**

Tomah
Baribeau, Larry J **(SLP)**
Jensen, Mrs Debra A R **(SLP)**
Leis-Rossio, Dr Beverly **(SLP A)**
Swallum, Mrs Alice **(SLP)**
Sweeney, Dr Ronald J **(SLP)**

Tomahawk
Hamlin, Mary Lee **(SLP)**
Jarvis, Cynthia Nick **(A)**

Trevor
Gehrke, Shari L **(SLP)**

Union Grove
Nowinski, Mrs Hazel Y **(SLP)**
Roedema, Mrs Laurie Frances **(SLP)**

Unity
Juedes, Mrs Elizabeth **(SLP)**
Runge, Mrs JoAnn Kay **(SLP)**

Verona
Babl, Linda C **(SLP)**
Llorente, Renee Ann **(A)**
Pedersen, Sarah G **(SLP)**
Sauer, Richard C **(A)**

Viroqua
Fortun, Lynn P **(SLP)**
Keeley, Jane Lee **(SLP)**
Leighton, Gregory Scott **(SLP)**

Wales
Stein, Barbara J **(SLP)**

Waterford
Maletzke, Ann M **(SLP)**
Streeter, Amy Beth **(SLP)**

Watertown
Baisden, Terese Horning **(SLP)**
Betts, Jeri-Lynn **(SLP)**
Derleth, Mrs Denyce A
Dopke, Mrs Lynn Constance **(SLP)**
Evans, Virginia F **(SLP)**
Moll, Karla K **(SLP)**
Piper, Mrs Sara Faith **(SLP)**
Ryan, Mrs Marcia Leslie **(SLP)**
Schultz, Pamela A **(SLP)**

Waukesha
Aspan, Mary Ann **(SLP)**
Bache-Wiig, Mrs Barbara J **(SLP)**
Barker, Mary Elizabeth **(SLP)**
Becker, Tim Richard **(A)**
Berman, S Sue **(SLP)**
Blackwell, Suzanne R **(SLP)**
Breneman, Mrs Nancy Palmieri **(SLP)**
Coleman, Mrs Roseann Fasi **(SLP)**
Edwards, Mrs Mary Ann **(SLP)**
Fandel, Susan King **(SLP)**
Fitzgerald, Mary Jo **(SLP)**
Francione, Cindy Marie **(SLP)**
Griffiths, Mary N **(SLP)**
Hanley, Sheila Mary **(A)**
Hansen, Mrs Marie Meagher **(SLP)**
Hase, Meredy **(A)**
Jasinski, Mrs Mary E **(SLP)**
Jones, Margaret E **(SLP)**
Klescewski, Sue **(SLP)**
Kueht, Margaret Lynn **(SLP)**
La Loggia, Mary Messina **(SLP)**
Logan, Patricia Mary **(SLP)**
McGurk, Mary Pat **(SLP)**
Michaels, Kathleen Cichocki **(SLP)**
Morris, Mary W **(SLP)**
Murray, Catherine A **(A)**
Nelson, Karen D'Amico **(A)**
Novotny, Ann Marie **(SLP)**
Perry, June A **(SLP A)**
Raabe, Christine Nitschke **(SLP)**
Reichardt, Mrs Margaret Meyer **(SLP)**
Remmers, Page Peters **(SLP)**
Strong, Gail K **(A)**
Ullrich, Diane Rita **(SLP)**
Waite, Joanne Metzger **(SLP)**
Wheeler, Dale C **(SLP A)**
Willis, Patricia **(SLP)**
Witkowski, Mrs Jane B **(SLP)**

Waunakee
Laffey, Mrs Bonnie Jean **(SLP)**
Tande, Dennis O **(SLP)**

Waupaca
Schwartz, Lori Ann **(SLP)**

Waupun
Redeker, Mrs Janet Wollangk **(SLP)**

Wausau
Bauer, Ann M **(SLP)**
Bowers, Mrs Betty N **(SLP)**
Butzen-Murdock, Mrs Rita A **(SLP)**
Dahlke, Michael G **(A)**
Dietrich, Mrs Cecelia A **(SLP)**
Fisher, Thomas E **(A)**
Freiberg, Christine L **(SLP)**
Huart, Steven A **(A)**
Kittson, Susan A **(SLP)**
Laliberte, Mrs Jeannie S **(SLP)**
Lombardo, James C **(A)**
Mayo, Mrs Patricia Jean **(SLP)**
Miller, Mrs Catherine S **(SLP)**
Miller, Deborah S **(SLP)**
Pankratz, Nancy Stone **(SLP)**
Rademaker, Mrs Barbara K **(SLP)**
Sack, Theresa O **(SLP)**
Salwach, Deborah Lynn **(SLP)**
Trucco, Mrs Corinne R **(SLP)**
Zeihen, Mrs Connie Zaqzebski **(SLP)**

Wautoma
McMahon, Cynthia Marie **(SLP)**

Wauwatosa
Alexander, Dr Rona P **(SLP)**
Berghauer, Jaye R **(SLP)**
Brown, Mrs Beth A **(SLP)**
Cherf, Mrs Laura Ericsen **(SLP)**
Chung, Mrs Jane Ellyn
Conway, Elizabeth Law
Corcoran, Kathleen Ann **(SLP)**
Dineen, Mary Goes **(SLP)**
Farrell, Mrs Susan Torke **(SLP)**
Fehr, Dr Joann D **(SLP A)**
Ford, Susette M **(SLP)**
Fritchen, Susan E
Grimm, Karen Jane **(A)**
Grimm, Mrs Susan S **(SLP)**
Gross, Mrs Nancy T **(SLP)**
Groves, Alix K **(SLP)**
Heckman, Terri Ellyn **(SLP)**
Huebsch-Lessmann, Noreen **(SLP)**
Johnson, Annette Simmon **(SLP)**
Kirchner, Mrs Therese **(A)**
Levenhagen, Tracy Ann **(SLP)**
Lichter, Kathryn M **(SLP)**
Lindner, Ruth Jean
Maegli, Mary **(SLP)**
McMahon-Llaurado, Kathleen D **(SLP)**
Osborn, Debra K **(SLP)**
O'Sullivan, Mary K **(SLP)**
Otten, Mrs Lysbeth M **(SLP)**
Peterson, Susan K **(SLP)**
Pflug-Maslowski, Mrs Susan I **(SLP)**
Podewils, Mrs Jacqueline Ann **(SLP)**
Racinowski, Mrs Darlene H **(SLP)**
Renberg, Gay Scott **(SLP)**
Sarvela, Mrs Junia L **(SLP)**
Scampini, Mrs Deanna L **(SLP)**
Schreiber, Marie Kathryn **(SLP)**
Selck, Mrs Faye A **(SLP)**
Serwe, Mrs Ann Schmitz **(SLP)**
Traut, Mrs Edith M **(SLP)**
Trotter, Dr William D **(SLP)**
Walsh, Mrs Joann M **(SLP)**

Webb Lake
Ralph, Mrs Valerie C **(SLP)**

West Allis
Ash, Pamela Helen **(SLP)**
Grulke, Darlyn K **(SLP)**
Hundt-Loss, Patricia A **(SLP)**
Kulzick, Mary Lynn **(SLP)**
Leahy, Mrs Patricia M **(SLP)**
Sowinski, Mary B **(SLP)**
Wangerin, Kathleen Ann **(SLP)**

West Bend
Dechant, Susan B **(SLP)**
German, Janette S **(SLP)**
Jolitz, Julie Lynne
Kunstman, Mrs Mary J Bahr **(SLP)**
Pulda, Marianne **(SLP)**
Schaub, Michele Mary **(SLP)**
Theys, Mrs Leslie Ann **(SLP)**
Washa, Laura K

West Milwaukee
Belgard, Karen Lyn **(A)**

West Salem
Calvetti, Gwyneth J **(SLP)**
Martin, Sharon Robinson **(A)**
Sarnes, Ann E **(SLP)**
Trochinski, Mrs Barbara A **(SLP)**

Westby
Francis, Mrs Marian Forest **(SLP)**
Lindevig, Kathy Ann

Whitefish Bay
Bluestone, Judith B **(SLP)**
Cirilli, Patti J **(SLP)**
Cole, Mrs Jody L W **(A)**
Degnan, Deborah W **(SLP)**
Dennis, Joanne Mary **(SLP)**
Desmond, Patricia K **(SLP)**
Dibble, Peggy C **(A)**
Doyle, Lynn Horrigan **(SLP)**
Harrington, Mrs Lana L **(SLP)**
Hirsch-Phillips, Lisa **(SLP)**
Hrycyna, Mrs Terry L **(SLP)**
Johnson, Mrs Janet A **(SLP)**
Longstreth, Dana G **(SLP)**
Merklein, Richard A **(A)**
Nelson, Cynthia L **(SLP)**
Nicholas, Patricia Kay **(SLP)**
Osmon, Mrs Jennifer E **(SLP)**
Wildt, Mrs Cathleen Frances **(SLP)**
Wroblewski, Anna Clare **(A)**

Whitehall
Moriarty, Michele Rae **(SLP)**

Whitelaw
Grall, Mrs Mary Bleser **(SLP)**

Whitewater
Chevrette, William **(A)**
Cooper, Mrs Nancy H **(SLP)**
Cordio, Sally Lynn S **(SLP)**
Huer, Dr Mary B **(SLP)**
Pease, Francine **(SLP)**
Wilson, William Arthur

Williams Bay
Mueller, Susan Jane **(A)**

Wilson
Jordahl, Nanette J **(SLP)**
Kielmeyer, Mrs Kristine Marie **(SLP)**

Wind Lake
Dahl, Mrs Sherry Gail
Kohl, Mrs Cynthia Ann **(SLP)**

Winneconne
Lang, Mrs Anne A **(SLP)**

Wisconsin Dells
Marston, Mrs Linda J **(SLP)**
Schulz, Mrs Elizabeth Ruth **(SLP)**

Wisconsin Rapids
Chambers, Mrs Dorothy L **(SLP)**
Lippold, Timothy Alan **(A)**
Parolini, Richard J **(SLP)**
Savela, Kay Dianne **(SLP)**
Spees, Edgar Brian **(SLP)**

Woodruff
Leonard, Dr Ralph **(A)**
Ruebl, Celeste Burnett **(SLP)**
Schussler, Elizabeth **(SLP)**

WYOMING

Aspon
Newcom, Mrs Mary Ann **(SLP)**

Banner
Bourgault, Rachel M **(SLP)**

Buffalo
Larson, Mrs Gladys Jacobson **(SLP A)**
Satter, Mrs Susan Ann **(SLP)**
Wollmuth, Wayne Robert **(SLP)**

Casper
Harrison, Janelle Lee **(SLP)**
Helmick, Mrs Cynthia J **(SLP)**
Hietpas, Mrs Kathleen T **(A)**
Kirkmeyer, Reva D M **(SLP)**
Kostecki, Cami Alayne **(A)**
Loutas, Mrs Shirla S **(SLP)**
Ortiz, J Dennis **(A)**
Sarvey, Mrs Sally H **(SLP)**
Tucker, Mrs Beverly J **(SLP)**

Veltman, Anne Marie **(SLP)**
Wallace-Bates, Mrs Victoria Rose **(SLP)**
Watters, Mrs Mary Jo **(SLP)**

Cheyenne
Arnold, Ruth H **(SLP)**
Atkins, Mrs Pennie L **(SLP)**
Barnes, Mrs Lisa C **(SLP)**
Carpenter, Mrs Susan Carroll **(SLP)**
Carr, Peggy **(SLP)**
Dolence, Mrs Connie A **(SLP)**
Donaldson, Mrs Cathy Fay **(SLP)**
Mellblom, Caron **(SLP)**
Norwood, Mrs Ann M **(SLP)**
Peterson, Kathleen Shanahan **(SLP)**
Rader, Mrs Krista L **(SLP)**
Rulon, Mrs Kristi J
Walter, Arlan E **(A)**

Cody
Brooks, Mrs Jill Elaine **(A)**
Deery, Debra Joines **(SLP)**
Koperski, Ben Joseph **(A)**
Richards, Michael R **(SLP)**
Williams-Beintema, Teresa Marie **(SLP)**

Dayton
Sellar, Barbara Gail **(SLP)**

Dubois
Stephens, Mrs Janet Sanborn **(SLP)**

Elk Mountain
Kennedy, Mrs Robin G R **(SLP)**

Francis E Warren AFB
Walker, Sherry Wilson

Gillette
Harris, Jacqueline **(SLP)**
Lubnau, Kathryn Lee **(SLP)**
Schmidt, Kathryn Jean **(A)**
Short, Susan **(SLP)**

Glendo
Archie, Mrs Lori Longfellow **(SLP)**

Green River
Kessler, Lue Ann **(SLP)**
Stamos-Owen, Mrs Lydia A **(SLP)**

Kemmerer
Bagniefski, Susan Mary **(SLP)**

Lander
Cessna, Mrs Susan Adams **(SLP)**
Kienlen-Trujillo, Mrs Kyle **(SLP)**
McDonnel, Annette **(SLP)**
Murdock, Michael Joseph **(SLP)**

Laramie
Bradley, Jean C **(SLP)**
Burns, Lisa Maria **(SLP)**
Coomes, Mrs Carla Rae **(SLP)**
Donaghy, Dr William C
Gilpin, Mrs Cathy Vanderford **(A)**
Holland, Mrs Judy N
Jacobson, Deborah K **(SLP)**
Jelinek, Dr Janis A **(SLP)**
Jones, Paula L **(A)**
Kohler, Dr R Ramon **(SLP)**
Laws, Dr Douglas W **(A)**
Lindstedt, D Elise **(SLP)**
Logan, Kenneth J **(SLP)**
McDonald, Edward J **(A)**
Primus, Dr Michael A **(A)**
Rimac, Dr Robert T **(SLP)**
Routson, Margueite Elaine **(SLP)**
Sailors, Stephanie Gaye **(SLP)**
Seabeck, Mrs Diana J **(SLP)**
Seville, Mrs Diane Tofini **(SLP)**
Toner, Dr Mary A **(SLP)**
Wood, Carolyn A **(SLP)**

Mountain View
Dolezal, Mrs Laura Kathleen **(SLP)**
Freeman, Mrs Rebecca Peterson **(SLP)**

Newcastle
Doeksen-Gould, Debra **(SLP)**
Ward, Allan R

Powell
Rowley, Thomas William **(SLP)**
Schneider, Kerri Dee **(SLP)**

Ranchester
Noyer, Zama Helene **(A)**

Rawlins
Penney, Mary Louise **(SLP)**

Riverton
Germany, Nena Maria **(SLP)**
Listoe, Kim M **(A)**

Rock Springs
Bakke-Horton, Mary G **(SLP)**
Plant, Susannah **(SLP)**
Proctor, Marlene Koscak **(SLP)**

Sheridan
Andrews, Jo Lynn **(SLP)**
Mischke, Renetta M **(SLP)**
Murphy, Mrs Tempe L C **(SLP)**

Sinclair
Thornton, Mrs Karen Himdmarsh **(SLP)**

Teton Village
Drui, Mrs Patricia **(SLP)**

Thermopolis
Beach, Danna Kay **(SLP)**
Helm, Mrs Vicki B **(SLP)**

Wheatland
Barber, Mrs Sheila J W **(SLP)**
Davis, Alicia M **(SLP)**
Maloney, Ann **(SLP)**

Worland
Munsterteiger, Kay D **(SLP)**

Yellowstone Park
McCaleb, Mrs Mary L **(SLP)**

ANTIGUA

St Johns
Chernin, Florence **(SLP)**

AUSTRALIA

New South Wales

Bayview
Rosen, Dr Jeanette K **(SLP A)**

Bellevue Hill
Bentwood, Mrs Judy J **(SLP)**

Lidcombe
Reed, Dr Vicki A **(SLP)**

Narrabeen
Wray, Elinor C **(SLP)**

Phegans Bay
Francis, Chris **(SLP)**

St Ives
Mitchell, Robin S **(SLP)**

Sydney
Jones-Boon, Gael A **(SLP A)**

Vaucluse Sydney
Bloch, Mrs Joy **(SLP)**

Wallsend
Gresham, Sharon Lea **(SLP)**

Willoughby
Patterson, Margaret K **(SLP)**

Queensland

Brisbane
Moll, Dr Dianne-Lynn L **(SLP)**
Newman, Dr Denis G **(SLP)**

Rockhampton
Vuolo, Mrs Janelle M **(SLP)**

Trinity Beach Cairns
St Martin, Mrs Anne Griggs **(SLP)**

South Australia

Bedford Park
Gilmore, Dr Stuart Irby **(SLP A)**
Rounsefell, Nancy L **(SLP)**

Kingswood
Paterson, Mrs Heather L **(SLP)**

Kybunga
Jenkin, Mrs Laura Snodgrass **(SLP)**

North Adelaide
Kelly, Michael A **(SLP)**

Tasmania

Hobart
Edberg, Judith A **(SLP)**

Sandy Bay
Hostetler, Sheila A **(SLP)**

Victoria

Beaumaris
Hekel, Mrs Marie-Louise Ann **(A)**

Carlton
Erber, Dr Norman Phillip **(A)**
Parsons, Dr Carl L **(SLP)**

Donvale
Dohnt, Debra Williams **(SLP)**

Melbourne
Gorman, Dr Pierre Patrick

West Australia

Claremont
Doull, Linda K **(A)**
Farrant, Prof R H **(A)**

Fremantle
Bain, Donna McDade **(SLP)**
Zubrick, Dr Stephen R **(SLP A)**

Perth
Weeks, Sharon A **(A)**
Wilde, Dr Ronald A **(A)**

Shenton Park
Nathan, Colette **(SLP)**

Wembley
Wilde, Mrs Nancy Jo R **(A)**

AUSTRIA

Salzburg
Eliason, Elizabeth **(SLP)**

BAHAMAS

Nassau
Clarke, Sharon Janette **(SLP)**
Langdon, S Fruzan **(SLP)**

BARBADOS

St James
Pierson, Nancy Bush **(SLP)**

BELGIUM

Brussels
Leonard, Lois M **(SLP)**

BRAZIL

Sao Paulo Sp
Albernaz, Dr Pedro L M

CANADA

Alberta

Airdrie
Nelles, Mrs Teresa M **(SLP)**

Calgary
Brorson, Kent Robert **(SLP)**
Dipalma, Mrs Ann Marie **(SLP)**
Doupe, Mrs Barbara J **(SLP)**
Dunsmore, Caroline E **(SLP)**
Feldman, Naida A **(SLP)**
Gaines, Dr Barbara Hartley **(SLP)**
Giesbrecht, Marilyn P **(SLP)**
Green, Mrs Carol Senoyuit
Hartwig, Mrs Marguerite **(SLP)**
Humphrey, Cynthia T **(SLP)**
Humphreys, Mrs Rita H **(SLP)**
Iceton, Mrs Mary Lou **(SLP)**
Janovcik, Marita Harsanyl **(SLP)**
Jeje, Saeeda S N
Johnson, Lucie M **(A)**
King, Barbara S **(SLP)**
Knowles, Gillian E **(SLP)**
MacKenzie, Dr Elizabeth H **(SLP)**
MacLaren, Suzanne Carol **(A)**
Massarotto, Caroline E **(SLP)**
McCue, Susan Kay **(SLP)**
McDonough, Mrs Alanna May **(SLP)**
McEwen, Beth Ann **(SLP)**
Moore, Thomas **(SLP)**
Nowak, Michele A **(SLP)**
Osinski, Rose Marie **(SLP)**
Pals, Catherine L Vankka **(SLP)**
Patzelt, Rebecca S C
Pearce, Patsy Steig **(SLP)**
Roth, Werner Roland **(A)**
Scott, Janet C **(SLP)**
Tinker, Christine Bolen **(SLP)**
Traboulsi, Mrs Margaret Ann **(A)**
Watters, Mrs Amany **(SLP)**

Camrose
McHan, Kathryn Carson **(SLP)**

Cochrane
Hawkwood, Nielle R **(SLP)**

Drumheller
Ouwens, Nel S **(SLP)**

Edmonton
Blundon, Patricia L H **(SLP)**
Boberg, Dr Einer **(SLP)**
Branch, Mrs Judith L **(SLP)**
Brennan, William P **(A)**
Brown, David Kenneth **(A)**
Burns, Sarah E **(A)**
Catherall, Paul **(SLP)**
Davidson, Mrs Margaret **(SLP)**
Dawson, Wendy R **(SLP)**
Desrochers, Chet M **(A)**
Ennis, Sheila Joan **(SLP)**
Evans, Ruth Ellen **(A)**
Filice, Lori Demeriez **(SLP)**
Gardner, Janet **(SLP)**
Goodman, Susie Lynn **(SLP)**
Gotaas, Christine Elizabeth **(SLP)**
Gough, Dr Kenneth H **(SLP A)**
Greenberg, Dr Frederick R
Haske, Dr Susan Claire **(A)**

Heaton, Mrs Elaine M **(SLP)**
Hodge, Megan M **(SLP)**
Holdgrafer, Dr Gary E **(SLP)**
Hund-Reid, Cecelia M **(SLP)**
Hurtig, Cynthia Ruth **(A)**
Ilott, Dr Helen G **(SLP)**
Johnston, Patricia A **(SLP)**
Kamitomo, Gail A **(SLP)**
Kully-Martens, Deborah A **(SLP)**
Laberge, Mrs Patricia Christine
Lopushinsky, Mrs Anne Martha **(SLP)**
Mansell, Bruce **(A)**
Manz, Mrs Laura
Marxheimer, Mrs Suzette **(SLP)**
McClain, Sara C **(A)**
Meikle-Neelley, Louise D **(SLP)**
Nobleman, Mrs Francie Robins **(SLP)**
O'Sullivan, Avril **(SLP)**
Pendergast, Laurie G **(SLP)**
Rochet, Dr Anne Putnam **(SLP)**
Ryan, Kathryn Riedlinger **(SLP)**
Stewart-Muirhead, Gwyneth Eleanor **(SLP)**
Sutter, Dr Judith Carol **(SLP)**
Thacker, Mrs Susan Jane **(A)**
Throckmorton, Verl John **(A)**
Waine, Zillah Bernidine **(SLP)**
Webster, Dr Michael **(SLP)**
Wilson, Dr Frank B **(SLP A)**

Edson
Wager, Glenda G **(SLP)**

Fairview
Galbreath, Kristen Marie **(SLP)**

Fort McMurray
Leonard-Harper, Gayle S **(SLP)**

Fort Saskatchewan
Commodore, Robert W **(SLP)**
Hagler, Mrs Marian K **(A)**
Hagler, Dr Paul H **(SLP)**

Grande Cache
Simpson, Janet P **(SLP)**

Lethbridge
Lingard, William E **(SLP)**
Simmons, Wendy Margaret **(SLP)**
Witt-Lajeunesse, Alane Kay **(SLP)**

Medicine Hat
Jansson, Mrs Eraine Arndt

Peace River
Heckner, Patricia Ann **(A)**

Red Deer
Cormack, Barbara Jean **(SLP)**
Hitchcock, Mrs Barbara Joan **(SLP)**
Nichols, Anne E **(SLP)**

Spruce Grove
Bakker, Connie Reddick **(SLP)**

St Albert
Dale, Duane A **(SLP)**
Dale, Mrs Margaret Olga R **(SLP)**
Henderson, Isabel C **(SLP)**
Hutchings, Mrs Susan Lorraine **(A)**
Mikus, Mrs Linda D **(SLP)**
Olasker, Kathleen M **(SLP A)**
Olasker, William Bruce **(SLP)**
Packford, Kathy Jean **(A)**

British Columbia

Abbotsford
Casanova, Ruth G **(SLP)**
Delmonico, Rosslyn Jean
Greenwood, Richard Patrick **(A)**

Bella Coola
Stainsby, Leslie Michelle **(SLP)**

Blubber Bay
Suen, Arleen J **(SLP)**

Burnaby
Krowchenko, Laura L **(SLP)**

Clearbrook
Leaney, A Pearl **(SLP)**

Comox
Tremel, Nancy A **(A)**

Coquitlam
Dowswell, Barbara Spindel **(SLP)**
Paranjpe, Meenakshi Anand **(SLP)**

Fort St John
Lam, Vivian Wai Wan **(SLP)**

Garibaldi Hi
Ross, Anne Louise **(SLP)**

Kamloops
Ellis, Donna Marie **(A)**
Nelson, Iris Ripley **(SLP)**
Zordell, John K **(SLP)**

Kelowna
Henderson, Alice H **(SLP)**
Jensen, Kris Kay **(SLP)**
Neyman, Charles E **(SLP A)**
Olson, Patricia **(A)**
Stinnett, Joseph Michael **(A)**

Kitimat
Goutier, Maureen

Langley
Boyd-Whitley, Robert Forrest **(SLP)**
Crawford, Mrs Wendy A W **(SLP)**

MacKenzie
Wachs, Katharine **(SLP)**

Maple Ridge
Rhodes, Don E **(SLP)**

Montrose
Green, Ann S **(SLP)**

Nanaimo
Maltby, Robert L **(SLP)**
Topp, Karen S **(SLP)**

New Westminster
Conlin, Leah T **(A)**
Gelmon, Reesa Lynn

North Delta
Carlaw, Caren Elizabeth **(SLP)**
Hutcheson, Deloris A **(SLP)**
Wormeli, Dale K **(A)**

North Vancouver
Davies, Lorene Catherine **(SLP)**
Sin, Yuen Ming **(SLP)**

Parksville
Ketelsen, Mrs Mary J **(SLP)**

Point Coquitlam
Appleton, Rita Anne **(SLP)**
Martin, Glenn Thomas **(A)**

Port Alberni
Low, Cynthia H **(SLP)**
Rankin, Lorna Janet **(SLP)**

Powell River
Cogswell, Annastacia **(SLP)**

Prince George
Bosnjak, Vesna **(SLP)**
Kulkarni, Shridhar Govind **(A)**
Miller, Karen Teresa **(A)**
O'Neill, Clare Elizabeth **(SLP)**

Revelstoke
Simpson, Carolyn E

Richmond
Berinbaum, Mrs Penelope V **(SLP)**
Burgess, Lucinda Anne **(SLP)**
Katagi, Dr Roland K **(SLP)**
Seeley, Joyce Irene **(SLP)**

Salmon Arm
Cody, Janet Patricia **(A)**
Nussbaum, Jo **(SLP)**
Seaman, Don P
Seaman, Mrs Michelle Gardner

Surrey
Garnett, Catherine Mary **(SLP)**
Jeter-Krasnikoff, Michelle **(SLP)**
Lane, Susan A **(SLP)**
Lowe-Heistad, Mrs Mardi E **(SLP)**

Terrace
Fox, Maureen Theresa

Vancouver
Bennett, Leslie A **(A)**
Blockberger, Susan J **(SLP)**
Borkenhagen, Mrs Anne M **(SLP)**
Braasch, Thomas J **(A)**
Chow, Margaret K **(SLP)**
Clemons, Mrs M Elaine **(SLP)**
Cohen, Garland J **(SLP)**
Davidson, Deborah L **(SLP)**
Delicati, Dawn G **(A)**
Deshpande, Kamal D **(SLP A)**
Droettboom, Mrs M Michelle **(SLP)**
Fisk, Susan B **(SLP)**
Fowler, K Jean **(SLP)**
Gillis, Mrs Heather R **(A)**
Goldenberg, Barry **(SLP)**
Green, Richard B **(SLP)**
Green, Yvonne F **(SLP)**
Heaney, Carol Mary **(SLP)**
Johnston, Dr Judith Rae **(SLP)**
Kahler, Mrs Sally A **(SLP)**
Lamb, Noelle L **(A)**
Lewis, Stephen W **(SLP)**
Lincoln, Laura **(SLP)**
MacMillan, Claudia J **(SLP)**
McDonald, Mrs Maryalyce **(A)**
McDonald, Sharon L **(SLP)**
Mearns-Brown, Mrs Marily Ann **(SLP)**
Muller, George **(A)**
O'Dornan, Sharon Theresa **(SLP)**
Rother, Judy R **(SLP)**
Slind, Mrs Margaret A **(SLP)**
Tatham, Ellen G **(SLP)**
Theimer, Lisa R
Towler, Patience K **(SLP)**
Vaudin, Andrea **(SLP)**
Washington, Dorothy M **(SLP)**
Zipursky, Mrs Myrna A **(SLP)**

Vernon
Coley-Donohue, Mrs Lisa Katherine **(SLP)**
Larsen, Kristine Marie
Laughlin, John Bohan, Jr **(SLP)**
Peltonen, Charles D **(SLP)**
Prem-Stein, Jutta W **(SLP)**

Victoria
Crickmay, Marie C **(SLP)**
Durbach, Miriam H **(SLP)**
Ellis, Dr Leonard **(SLP)**
Frank, Mrs E Stacey **(A)**
Greenberg, Douglas B **(A)**
Harmuth, Phillip C **(SLP)**
Houston, Mrs Melaine Jayne **(SLP)**
Larson, Joy Elspeth **(SLP)**
Lewis, Marlene M **(SLP)**
Lobb, Barbara Routley **(SLP)**
Marshall, Ethel C **(SLP)**
McMullin, Jane A **(SLP)**
Pinch, Diane Kathleen **(SLP)**
Pribilsky, Todd A **(A)**
Richard, Isabel **(SLP)**
Shinto, Marilyn M **(A)**
Unke, Alberta B **(SLP)**
Unke, Paul J **(SLP)**

Westbank
Haynes, Elizabeth Jane **(SLP)**

White Rock
Faraher-Amidon, Christy A **(SLP)**

Manitoba

Brandon
Cayer, Mrs Nicola Jane **(SLP)**
Kille, Judi C **(A)**
Lange, Geraldine A

Dauphin
Ewanchyshyn, Nadine Elizabeth **(SLP)**

East Silkirk
Robertson, Mark Lawrence **(SLP)**

Headingly
Bock, Ruth Elizabeth **(SLP)**

Lorette
McKenzie, Earl V **(A)**

Morden
Cooper, Heather A
Olson, Lori Bastness **(SLP)**

Plap
Prokop, Beverly Jo **(SLP)**

Selkirk
Pitz, Mrs Maria Anna **(SLP)**

St Germaine
Morse, Elizabeth Goss **(SLP)**

Thompson
Frame, Gloria Dianne **(SLP)**

Winnipeg
Alexander, Dr Patrick T **(SLP)**
Baird, Allison J **(SLP)**
Blum, Jacqueline Marci **(SLP)**
Cameron, Darcey A R **(SLP)**
Carefoot, Mrs Nancy J **(SLP)**
Chochinov, Mrs Michelle Ann **(SLP)**
Cowan, Heather E **(A)**
Dashefsky, Mrs Lisa Kowall **(SLP)**
Dunham, Charles R **(SLP)**
Eliuk, Bonnie E **(SLP)**
Evans, Charlotte Johanna **(SLP)**
Furness, Nancy Anne **(SLP)**
Ganes, Cheryl Proceviat **(SLP)**
Gardner, Cheryl L **(SLP)**
Gaudry, Florent P **(A)**
Gerylo, Kathryn S **(SLP)**
Gibb, Susan M **(A)**
Gillespie, Ian Graham **(A)**
Gilmore, Keely J **(SLP)**
Gray, Barbara M **(SLP)**
Gregora, April W **(SLP)**
Gusdal, Sharyn Ann **(SLP)**
Halldorson, Sharon G **(SLP)**
Hawkins, Mrs Kaaren O **(SLP)**
Inglis, Joanne M **(SLP)**
Jackson, Mrs Patricia P **(SLP)**
Jones, Mrs Elizabeth **(SLP)**
Kusamura, Yoshimi **(SLP)**
Lesiuk, Lorraine **(SLP)**
Lockwood, Mette Norma
Lukaszewski, Carolyn A **(SLP)**
Lumsden-Owen, Patricia A **(SLP)**
MacAngus, Shona Jane
MacGill, Debra Anne **(SLP)**
Martin, Mrs Virginia E **(SLP)**
Mills, Marion **(SLP)**
Okrainec, Mrs J Alexa **(SLP)**
Penko, Mrs Maureen **(SLP)**
Schoenhofer, Deborah Heidi **(SLP)**
Shanks, Mrs Karen L **(SLP)**
Smolak, Arlene **(SLP)**
Spack, Cathy M **(SLP)**
Sylwester, John H **(A)**
Thorkelsson, Anne E **(SLP)**
Turner, Janet Lois **(SLP)**
Ward, Betty Jane **(SLP)**

New Brunswick

Fredericton
Lounsbury, Kathrin Ilona **(SLP)**
Stickles, Judith Lee **(SLP)**
Woodworth, Mrs Ruth MacCallum

Moncton
Fuchs, Elizabeth A **(A)**
Gorey, Mary E

St John
Ough, Dwight S **(A)**
Webber, Susan Ann **(SLP)**

Newfoundland

Corner Brook
Werner, James Lee **(A)**

Gander
Duffitt, Deanna V **(SLP)**

Labrador
Atkinson, Mrs Susan Ingram **(SLP)**

Mt Pearl
Taylor, Mrs Kathleen Manuel **(SLP)**

St Johns
Murphy, Jerome E **(A)**

Stephenville
Wong, Helen Fung-Ying

Nova Scotia

Amherst
Stucki, Peter F K **(SLP)**
Yarrow, Joseph **(SLP)**

Bedford
Allard, Elizabeth **(SLP)**

Cape Breton
Hunter, Elizabeth Ann **(SLP)**

Dartmouth
Stager, Dr Sheila V **(SLP)**

Greenwood
Wooley, Margaret E **(SLP)**

Halifax
Armson, Joy M **(SLP)**
Barton, Debbie Elaine **(SLP)**
Campbell, Lynda R **(SLP)**
Cieplinski, Mrs Nancy **(SLP)**
Doyle, Dr Philip C **(SLP)**
Green, Dr Walter B **(SLP A)**
Henrickson, Dr Larry K **(A)**
Jiang, Tao
Mencher, Dr George T **(SLP A)**
Quinton, Janice **(SLP)**
Roda, Vicki A C **(SLP)**
Schmidbauer, Judith A **(SLP)**
Shaw, Elizabeth **(SLP)**
Skarakis-Doyle, Dr Elizabeth **(SLP)**
Stoesz, Barbara **(SLP)**
Wozniak, Linda A **(SLP)**

Hants County
Herx, Dennis A **(A)**

Lr Sackville
Maxwell, Stephen Allen **(A)**

Pictou
Heighton, Mrs Sharon B **(SLP)**

Sydney
Robertson, Jeanne Sheldon **(SLP)**

Tantallon
Merritt, Debra Reynolds **(SLP)**

Windsor Junction
Kienapple, Jean Ann **(A)**

Wolfville
Burton, Mrs Thea Koenig **(SLP)**

Yarmouth
Shediac, Mrs Julie M **(SLP)**

Northwest Territories

Yellowknife
Hanlan, John W **(SLP)**
Moore, Jan Allison **(SLP A)**

Ontario

Agincourt
Kahansky, Karen **(A)**

Ajax
Charles, Malusha Marie **(SLP)**

Almonte
Gareau, Maureen E **(SLP)**

Arva
Mistal, Gregory Joseph **(A)**

Aurora
Bauer, Doris S **(SLP)**

Barrie
Bell, Mrs Alison Louise **(SLP)**
Nixon, Tani M **(A)**
Riggin Springstead, Mary Catherine **(SLP)**
Setchell, Cherryl Mae **(SLP)**

Belleville
Suite, Leslie P

Bimbrook
Zuk, Mrs Cynthia Anne **(SLP)**

Blenheim
Bowden, Dr Ann E **(SLP)**

Bowmanville
Rempel, Susan Anne **(SLP)**

Bramalea
Brassem, Maureen Joy

Brampton
Jordan, Gretchen B **(SLP)**

Brantford
Schmalz, Mary J **(SLP)**
Wyman, Renee Marie **(SLP)**

Burlington
Birch, Mrs Susan J
Lezynski, Jeffrey Mark **(A)**

Camlachie
Greensmith, Mrs Jennifer Margaret

Campbellville
Casali, Janet Louise **(SLP)**

Charing Cross
Hyde, Lawrence Dow **(SLP)**

Chatham
Fotheringham, Lawrence **(SLP)**
Fullowka McCabe, Mrs Debora Lee **(SLP)**
Juba-Jelusic, Karen Louise **(SLP)**
Rounds, Anne E **(SLP)**

Clearwater
Mroczek, Michael R **(SLP)**

Cornwall
Kodama, Sakie

Downsview
Troncho, Mrs Sue A **(SLP)**

Dundas
Bennett, Jerry J **(A)**
Tweedie, Gary L

Eagle River
Hrubecky, Arlene E **(SLP)**

Elliot Lake
Kososki, Carrie Lee **(SLP)**

Etobicoke
Smith, Alison Kelford
Venema, Theodore H **(A)**

Fergus
Farrell, Nancy I **(SLP)**

Fonthill
Coyne, Lesley Bracken **(SLP)**

Fort Erie
Baxter-Fiorella, Alison Elizabeth **(SLP)**

Fort Frances
Asplund, Mrs Janet Pochailo **(SLP)**
Stokes, Ann Marie **(SLP)**

Georgetown
Cole, Tanya Elizabeth **(SLP)**

Gloucester
Tryggvason, Lilyanna Zmijak **(SLP)**
Williams, Cynthia Kathleen

Goulais River
Kruppert-Hayes, Ursula **(SLP)**

Grimsby
Deegan, Mrs Shelley A **(SLP)**
Earle, Mrs Cindy Ann **(SLP)**

Hamilton
Anderson, Deborah Gertrude
Canale-Hess, Jane Ellen **(SLP)**
Head, Mrs Brenda R **(A)**
Heikurinen, Mrs Catherine Tytaneck **(A)**
Hess, Chad Wilson **(SLP)**
Hollingham, Mrs Linda Ferraro **(A)**
Ingrosso, Diana **(SLP)**
Johnson, Nancy Y **(SLP)**
King, Richard N **(SLP)**
Knott, Monica Cathrine **(SLP)**
Lewis, Terry K **(A)**
Loncke, Jane Marie **(SLP)**
Martens, Colleen Finnen **(SLP)**
Merchant, Penelope Watson **(SLP)**
Mileris, Ramona **(SLP)**
Miller-Van Veghel, Mrs Jeri L **(SLP)**
Oehler, Susan Marie **(A)**
Pavey, Carol Elaine **(A)**
Schram, Geraldine Elaine **(SLP)**
Stanley, Gay **(SLP)**
Tutt, Marilyn Louise **(A)**

Holland Lndg
Kasper-Marrello, Marie Yvonne **(SLP)**

Hornby
Lucas, Mary Anne

Islington
Loeffelhardt, Jean **(SLP)**

Kanata
Wawrykow, Margaret Jean **(SLP)**
Wilson, Julie Viola **(SLP)**

Kemptville
Wegner, Mrs Sara R **(SLP)**

Kinburn
Button, Marjorie A **(SLP)**

King City
Stoicheff, Dr Margaret L **(SLP)**

Kingston
Becker, Marianne **(SLP)**
Finch-Williams, Dr Amy **(SLP)**
Gorenko, Alexa Mae **(SLP)**
McGorman, Margot Maureen **(SLP)**

Kirkland Lake
Joseph, Karyn Marie **(SLP)**

Kitchener
Barr, David Joseph **(A)**
Blevis, Lisa S
Cronshaw, Mrs Kayla E D **(A)**
Ladzik, Mrs Kathleen M **(SLP)**
Martin, Mrs Bette J S **(A)**
McFarlane, Jean L **(SLP)**
Morency, Janet M **(A)**

Lansdowne
Cliffe, Mollie D **(SLP)**

Leamington
Dedo-Bailey, Vesna M **(SLP)**

London
Bandur, Donna **(SLP)**
Boyd, Dr John **(SLP)**
Cheesman, Margaret Fern
Cleave, Patricia Lynn **(SLP)**
Clements, Gail Anne **(SLP)**
Corcoran, Donna M **(A)**
Corcoran, Dr Joseph A, Jr **(SLP)**
Donkervoort, Janet B **(SLP)**
Erle, Kerry Denise **(SLP)**
Fey, Dr Marc E **(SLP)**
Fey, Mrs Sandra H **(SLP)**
Fisher, James Ernest **(SLP)**
Fisher, Mrs Randi B **(SLP)**
Foss, Elizabeth Ann **(A)**
Gagne, Dr Jean-Pierre **(A)**
Godden, Anne L **(SLP)**
Gritzan, Mrs Janet Elizabeth
Hawkins, Sarah A
Husband, Susan **(SLP)**
Ikuta, Brenda Laurel
Ivey, Dr Robert G **(A)**
Jadd, Lisa-Gaye Marie **(SLP)**
Johnson, Carla J **(SLP)**
Latham, Mrs Elizabeth **(SLP)**
Lawrence, Jacqueline Deirdre **(SLP)**
Lay, Christine L
Leeper, Dr Herbert Andrew, Jr **(SLP)**
Ling, Dr Daniel
MacKinnon, Elizabeth **(SLP)**
Mencel, Mrs Elizabeth **(SLP)**
Michels, Mrs Suzanne Goenner **(SLP)**
Nicholson, Cynthia Jane **(SLP)**
Norton, Mrs Pamela G **(SLP)**
Pincombe, Mrs Jane Elizabeth
Poluha, Patricia C **(SLP)**
Proudfoot, Mrs Penny Ann **(SLP)**
Raade, Dr Adele Suzanne **(SLP)**
Roy, Louise Michele
Sabourin, Mrs Theresa Mitchell **(SLP)**
Salazer, D Rosine **(SLP)**
Savage, Diane J
Seewald, Dr Richard C **(A)**
Sharpe, Julie Vaughan **(SLP)**
Simner, Mrs Phyllis Starnbach **(SLP)**
Sokol, Janice Lynn
Stouffer, Dr James L **(A)**
Vanderheyden, Denise
Vermeulen, Rosalyn A **(SLP)**
Walker, Danya **(SLP)**
Warr-Leeper, Dr Genese Ann **(SLP)**
Wilkins, Carol Marlene **(SLP)**
Wright-Morrison, Amelia **(SLP)**
Yovetich, Sally Ann **(SLP)**
Yovetich, Dr William S **(SLP)**

Marathon
Dickson, Mrs Christine **(SLP)**

Mississauga
Benziger, Lise M **(A)**
Bergman, Ingrid R **(SLP)**
Galloway, Cheryl Anne **(A)**
Kreuk, Lydia M **(A)**
Semple, Jean Elizabeth **(SLP A)**

Moonbeam
Clinker-Farquhar, Margo S **(SLP)**

Mount Brydges
Sinclair, Rose C

Munster Hamlet
Arab, Margaret Mary

Navan
Sawyer-Woods, Linda M **(SLP)**

Nepean
Levitz, Mrs Ingrid **(SLP)**
Lubinsky-Zubrycky, Mary-Anne **(SLP)**
McVicar, Mrs Denise Yvonne **(SLP)**
Ross, Mrs Lynn E **(SLP)**
Seligman, Dawn L **(SLP)**

New Liskeard
Dawson, Joanne H **(A)**
McKinney, Stephen Kent **(SLP)**

New Market
Kelly, Deborah A **(SLP)**
Victor, Henry P **(A)**

Niagara Falls
Hayden, Heather Lynne **(SLP)**
Kremer, Linda Susan **(SLP)**

North Bay
Bertrand, Mrs Judy Davidson **(A)**
Hewitt, Cecily T **(SLP)**
Laferriere, Darlene Margaret **(SLP)**
Quinones-Nitsch, Mrs Wilma D **(SLP)**

North York
Little, Jane K **(SLP)**
Vosu, Lorraine Wander **(A)**

Oakville
Giroux, Fred A **(SLP)**
Jones-Prus, Mrs Debora **(SLP)**
Morrison, M Elizabeth **(SLP)**
Mullen, Jennifer Olson **(SLP)**
Rosenblum, Melanie R **(SLP)**
Ross, Debbie Faye **(A)**
Trecroce, Mrs Marie Suzanne **(SLP)**
Young, Mrs Michelle **(A)**

Orangeville
Arensberg, Karen Elizabeth **(SLP)**

Orillia
Kudritz, Joann Monica **(A)**
Lauer, Therese P **(A)**

Orleans
Garcia, Linda Jeannette **(SLP)**

Oshawa
Weber, Dr Jack L **(SLP)**
Wunderlich-Croft, Mrs Gabriele **(SLP)**

Ottawa
Caissie, Rachel **(A)**
Fletcher, Mrs Rose **(SLP)**
Gershkovitch, Mrs Beverly J **(SLP)**
Neuss, Deirdre **(SLP A)**
Pierce, Jennifer Lynn **(SLP)**
Pressman, Dr D Elaine **(SLP)**
Roberts, Patricia M **(SLP)**
Schultz, Robert E **(A)**
Simon, Anne E **(SLP)**
Smith, Dr Andree Durieux **(A)**
Sullivan, Patricia Anne **(SLP)**
Wevrick, Mrs Patricia J **(SLP)**
Wood, Lisa Ann **(SLP)**

Owen Sound
Lee, Rebecca Mance **(SLP)**
McInnes, Alison Jean **(SLP)**

Peterborough
Karwandy, Elizabeth R
Rinaldi, Rosa A **(SLP)**
Temple, Linda Anne **(SLP)**
Welland, Richard Joseph

Porcupine
Vanagas-Cote, Susan A **(SLP)**

Richmond Hill
Diamond, Mrs Mona Foster **(SLP)**
Frankel-Freedland, Ellyn **(SLP)**

Rockwood
Honeyman, Susan Jane **(SLP)**

Sarnia
Carmichael, Linda Ann **(SLP)**
Church, Rose May
Crehan, Sheila Mary **(A)**
Friesen, Cheryl V
Manz, Michael J **(A)**

Sault Ste Marie
Lacelle, Dr Barbara D **(SLP)**

Scarborough
Cramb, Debbie A **(A)**
Manji, Shelina T **(SLP)**
Montini, Mrs Maria **(SLP)**
Pike, Marilyn J **(A)**
Thomas-Stonell, Nancy L **(SLP)**
Tse, Dr Sou-Mee **(A)**

South Porcupine
Chaffart, Mrs Lynona Ann

St Catharines
Fernie, Mrs Rosemary Martino
Kroll, Dr Allan **(SLP)**
Lye, Mrs C Kathryn **(SLP)**
Macdonald, Charlene Alexandra Cratt **(SLP)**
Novosel, Lorna M **(SLP)**
Pasnak, Laurie A **(SLP)**
Reynolds, Mrs Danielle Helen **(SLP)**
Smith, Brian E **(SLP)**
Wray, John Anthony **(SLP)**

St Thomas
Dick, Nancy Lee

Stirling
Thompson, Mary-Ellen **(SLP)**

Stratford
Hoste, Christine Marie **(SLP)**

Sudbury
Blythe, Michael E **(A)**

Thornhill
Bedder-Manley, Carrie Elise **(SLP)**
Berger, Shelley Carpman **(SLP)**
Edelstein, Brenda F **(SLP)**
Starr, Noreen

Thorold
Mascitelli, Anna Marie **(SLP)**

Thunder Bay
Ball, Judith K **(SLP)**
Eynon, Diane Perras
Haugen, Rosemary **(SLP)**
Middaugh, Mrs Linda Welch
Ozburn, Mrs Flora C
Shanahan, Mrs Mona Aida **(SLP)**
Shanahan, Patrick E **(SLP)**
Stalker, Janet Sillman **(SLP)**
Woese, Jane Diane

Timmons
Pell, Robert Joseph **(A)**

Toronto
Axelrod, Natalie **(SLP)**
Babbitt, Susan **(SLP)**
Barbiero, Denise Celeste **(A)**
Bartelt, Susan M **(SLP)**
Bauer, Renata **(SLP)**
Bennett, Ida L **(A)**
Blaxley, Lynn R **(SLP)**
Bliss, Bonnie J **(A)**
Bond, Judith Louise **(SLP)**
Boone, Mrs Elaine Marie **(SLP)**
Boyden, Mariln Fay **(A)**
Boyer, Mrs Rosemary Teresa **(SLP)**
Brooks, Cherylan **(A)**
Brown, Mrs Alison Kyro **(SLP)**
Cashman, Marlene Z **(A)**
Chodikoff, Karen Ann
Corbin, Hollis J **(A)**
Davis, Patricia Jane **(A)**
Defrancesco, Marisa **(A)**
Duchowny, Reena Julia **(A)**
Edwards, Carolyn Anne **(A)**
Eidinger, Karen R **(SLP)**
Eisenberg, Robin Ann **(SLP)**
Findlay, Laurie Hamilton **(SLP)**
Fineberg, Miriam Sharon **(A)**
Fraser, D Lynn
Fridman, Anna **(SLP)**
Gannon, Ruth K **(SLP)**
Geller, Mrs Barbara E **(SLP)**
Girolametto, Dr Luigi E **(SLP)**
Gomberg, Marilyn R **(SLP)**
Hayden, Elyse Shumway **(SLP)**
Hayes, Donald Edward **(A)**
Henderson, Sandra M **(SLP)**
Hill, David Allan **(SLP)**
Hollett, Valerie Grace
Horodezky, Mrs Naomi B **(SLP)**
Hotz, Gillian A **(SLP)**
Hufana, Melinda Suyin
Jurecka, Joanne W **(SLP)**
Karasik, Mrs Rozalyn Z **(SLP)**
Kotler, Ava-Lee **(SLP)**
Kukich, Boyana **(SLP)**
Leary, Martha H **(SLP)**
Lewis, Lynda Patricia **(SLP)**
MacKenzie-Stepner, Mary Karen **(SLP)**
Manolson, Ayala A **(SLP)**
Marcon, Doris Louise **(SLP)**
Mastronardi, Mrs Debra Longawa **(SLP)**
Mayerovitch, Julie R **(SLP)**
McClean, Dr Michael D
McDonald, Joan K **(SLP)**
McDonald-Judd, Margaret J **(SLP)**
McEnroe, Catherine **(A)**
Milne, Ruth I **(SLP)**
Moore, Mrs B Jane M **(SLP)**
Patterson, Patricia Ann **(SLP)**
Posluns, Sandy Ellen **(SLP)**
Rapkin, Judy **(SLP)**
Roche, Lorraine M **(SLP)**
Ryan, Kelly Marie
Sadinsky, Priscilla **(SLP)**
Salkovitch, Mrs Barbara L **(SLP)**
Sarfeld, Evelyn A **(SLP)**
Schachter, Alison Donna **(SLP)**
Scott, Laurie Louise **(SLP)**
Shimotakahara, Joanne N **(SLP)**
Shore, Susan Lee **(SLP)**
Silverman, Jan L **(A)**
Sinclair, Mrs Margaret Lunnie **(A)**
Sloan, Nahum **(SLP)**
Sorin, Riva Ann **(SLP)**
Stalker, Catherine Harriette **(SLP)**
Stein, Mrs Marlene C
Storer, Dr Paula Square **(SLP)**
Thelander, Mary J **(SLP)**
Tollos, Sandra Katherine **(A)**
Totten, Holly Lynne **(A)**
Turkstra, Lyn Siobhan
Ushycky, Irene **(SLP)**
Witzel, Dr Mary Anne **(SLP)**
Wolf, Davidah **(A)**
Woodcox, Sharon Christine **(A)**
Wylde, Mrs Barbara J **(SLP)**

Unionsville
Suddick, Mary **(SLP)**

Waterloo
Barnes, Margaret L **(A)**
Stuart, Mrs Lesley A **(SLP)**

Welland
Ruiter, Irma Divera **(SLP)**

West Hill
Ferguson, Mrs Peggy J **(SLP)**
Victor-Beale, Margaret C **(SLP)**

Weston
Sanders-Lofaso, Mrs Jamie Sue **(SLP)**

Whitby
Lloyd, Peggy Allen **(SLP)**
Oye-Shipp, Mrs May Mitsuko **(SLP)**
Wurl, Melinda L **(SLP)**

Willowdale
Boychuk, Mrs Carol A **(A)**
Carlow, Mrs Patricia J **(SLP)**
Demchuk, Mrs Marcia Karen **(SLP)**
Dodgson, Mrs Sandra Elizabeth **(SLP)**
Klasner, Estelle R **(SLP)**
Rubin, Dr Hyla **(SLP)**
Shoom, Mrs Lauren Ann **(SLP)**
Shuster, Cheryl **(SLP)**
Turk, Helen
Vine, Deborah Louise **(SLP)**

Windsor
Baker, Mrs Arlene P
Barden, Randall Glen **(A)**
Barnes, Mrs Cynthia Lillian **(SLP)**
Bebout, Dr Linda Joyce
Carrico, Cheri S **(SLP)**
Fletcher-Levasseur, Susan **(SLP)**
Flynn, Eileen B R **(SLP)**
Kaplan, Dr Netta R **(SLP)**
Kavanaugh, D Jane **(SLP)**
Minton, Sheila Cohen **(SLP)**
Novak, Marie M **(SLP)**
Ribbeck, Karen S **(SLP)**
Saylor, Mrs Diane Patricia **(SLP)**
Simison, Mrs Victoria B **(SLP)**
Sjoli, Karen M
Southern, Toni Jane **(SLP)**
Turton, Mrs Carla Catherine **(SLP)**
Van Den Hoven, Mrs Monica Heffernan **(SLP)**
Vojnovic, Olga
Yadach, Kathleen Young **(SLP)**

Woodbridge
Roberts, Roland James

Woodstock
Almost, Deborah Gilchrist **(SLP)**

Prince Edward Island

Breadalbane
Ferraro, Anne M **(SLP)**

Hunter River
Anderson, Eleanor I **(SLP)**

Quebec

Madar, Mrs Glenda Falovitch **(SLP)**

Cote St Luc
Diamond, Judie Arbess **(SLP)**
Fichman, Mrs Marilyn T **(SLP)**
Rubin, Alanna **(SLP)**
Zavalkoff, Mrs Barbara H **(A)**

Hampstead
Mendelsohn, Mrs Bernice L **(SLP)**

Lachine
Sutton, Ann Colquhoun **(SLP)**

Longueuil
Jazzar, Carol Barbara

Montreal
Anders, Victoria Meighan
Baum, Dr Shari R **(SLP)**
Brunelle, Louise **(A)**
Chan, Mrs Nancy T **(SLP)**
Charan, Dr Kirti Kumar **(A)**
Coderre, Mrs Louise
Cole, Dr Elizabeth B **(A)**
Doehring, Donald G
Gallagher, Dr Tanya M
Gardner, Marsha Lee **(A)**
Huot, Germaine **(SLP)**
Hus, Mrs Yvette **(SLP)**
Ilecki, Dr Henry J **(A)**

Kapusta, Mrs Carol-Lynn
Lucie, Mrs Riel **(A)**
McNutt, Dr James C **(SLP)**
Perigoe, Christina Barris
Schwartz, Dr Sybil J **(SLP)**
Sheetreet, Mrs Pamela B
Shultz, Judith M **(SLP)**
Silverman, Mrs Anita H **(SLP)**
St George, Dr Marilyn F **(A)**
Watkin, Dr Kenneth L
Weiss, Barbara **(A)**

St Lambert
Fortier, Julie L **(SLP)**
Kingston, Mary E **(SLP)**

St Laurent
Sulkes-Segal, Mrs Marcia R **(SLP)**

Ville Lasalle
Cote, Mrs Isabelle

Westmount
Woytowych, William

Saskatchewan

Bredenbury
Bond-Moore, Sharon A **(SLP)**

Estevan
Morissette, Charmaine Lynne **(SLP)**

Humboldt
Cook, Linden S **(SLP)**

Meadow Lake
Downey-Barnhardt, Erin Lynn

Melville
Griffith, Sharon Linda

Moose Jaw
Mitchell, Norma C **(SLP)**

Regina
Chlopan, Lesley Carol **(SLP)**
Elgaard, Mrs Gina Marie **(SLP)**
George, Mrs Pauline J **(SLP)**
Mohr, Ann H O **(SLP)**
Richardson, Lisa Marie **(A)**
Shatford, Jill C **(SLP)**
Tuchscherer, Maria **(SLP)**
Wagner, Valerie A **(SLP)**

Saskatoon
Bockus, Sherry Lee
Dahl, Mrs Beverly Anne **(SLP)**
Ford, Krista K **(SLP)**
Illerbrun, Dr David W **(SLP)**
Kerr, Allison Joan **(SLP)**
Murphy, Mrs Angela M **(SLP)**
Simmie, Mrs Kathy Jo **(SLP)**
Wood, Mrs Gillian Christine

Swift Current
Bateson, Lynn Malene

Yorkton
Malazdrewicz, Edward John
Nolan, Lori A **(SLP)**

CHILE

Santiago
Brown, Mrs Bonnie Kositzky **(SLP)**
Gorski, Cynthia Witt **(SLP)**
Kenaston, Alicia Ann **(SLP)**

COLOMBIA

Bogota
Williamson, Juanita **(SLP)**

DENMARK

Birkerod
Groth, Mrs Jennifer A **(SLP)**

Ebeltoft
Hansen, Roberta H **(A)**

ECUADOR

Quito
Burneo, Dr Cesar A

EGYPT

Cairo
Soliman, Mrs Ann Hisley **(SLP)**
Soliman, Dr Salah M **(A)**

ENGLAND

Brighton
Wilkie, Pamela C **(SLP)**

Bristol
Kirk, Bonnie Jo **(SLP)**

Cambridge
Butterfield, Sally D
Kundrot, Mrs Theresa Marie **(SLP)**
Moore, Dr Brian Cecil

Carlisle Cumbria
Staley, Mrs Patricia C **(SLP)**

Isle of Wight
Acutt, Mrs Margaret S **(SLP)**

London
Hill, Edeen L **(SLP)**
Jans, Mrs Deborah L **(SLP)**
Neves, Mrs Gail M **(SLP)**
Slade, Mrs Marilyn V **(SLP)**
Sohl, Mrs Mary P **(SLP)**
Wade, Helen K **(A)**
Young, Fay Elizabeth **(SLP)**

Shropshire
Crichton, Mrs Linda Jaine **(SLP)**

Surrey
Franklin, Mrs Sandra S **(SLP)**

West Meon
Cafarelli-Dees, Denise L **(A)**

Wiltshire
Montgomery, Karen Lynn **(SLP)**

FRANCE

Paris
Baudoin-Chial, Dr Sonia T **(SLP)**
Comfort, Mrs Carolyn **(SLP)**
Holt, Bonnie Riggs **(SLP)**

GERMANY

Zweibruchen
White, Laurel M D **(SLP)**

GREECE

Athens
Litinas, Nikos
Makrynioti, Athina **(SLP)**
Martin-Hantas, Ann E **(SLP)**

Thessaloniki
Xofillis, Athanasios **(SLP)**

HONG KONG

Cheung Chau Island
Chan, Karen Pui-Lee **(SLP)**

Kowloon
Cheng, Mei-Kuan **(SLP)**

Pokfulam
Whitehill, Tara Loraine **(SLP)**

Tavistock
Baker, Ashley H **(A)**

ICELAND

Reykjavik
Gudmundsdottir, Bryndis Sigfusson **(SLP)**
Ulfsdottir, Thora Saeunn **(SLP)**

Varma
Magnusdottir, Mrs Sigridur **(SLP)**

INDIA

Pune
Mandke, Kalyani Narsinha **(A)**

INDONESIA

Jakarta
Sutadisastra, Rozella J **(SLP)**

IRELAND

Co Dublin
Hynes, Ann P F **(SLP)**

Dublin
Supple, Sr Maria Demontfort **(SLP)**

ISRAEL

Ashdod
Jacoby, Dr David I **(SLP)**

Ashkelon
Shaw, Dr Irwin R **(SLP)**

DN Misgar
Armel, Joyce P **(SLP)**

Emek Hayarden
Kinarti, Ruth

Givatayim
Lewis, Mrs Lesley L **(SLP)**

Haifa
Bar-David, Mrs Dahlia **(SLP A)**
Bentur, Dr Esther Eden **(SLP)**
Fredman, Mrs Marion R **(SLP)**
Yinnon, Mrs Maya **(SLP)**

Jerusalem
Bachi, Dr Ilana **(SLP A)**
Grossbaum, Mrs Dorothy Traub **(SLP)**
Krinkin, Mrs Naomi K **(SLP)**
Lipson, David **(SLP)**
Romm, Marcia K **(A)**
Roskin, Mrs Lessa C **(SLP)**
Sherman, Sura J **(SLP)**
Weiss, Samuel **(A)**
Yunker, Rosalind J **(SLP)**

Netanya
Hoffnung, Dr Steven **(A)**

Petach Tekvah
Toar, Janet W **(SLP)**

Petach-Tikva
Grossman, Joseph **(A)**

Raanana
Brilliant, Mrs Cynthia Gitelman **(SLP)**
Dahm, Barbara Lee **(SLP)**

Ramat Gan
Katz, Mrs Erica J **(SLP)**

Rechovot
Kurz, Mrs Sue E **(SLP)**

Rehovot
Froehlich, Mrs Carole D **(SLP)**

Tel Aviv
Andelman, Mrs Fani **(SLP)**
Bergman, Dr Moe **(A)**

ITALY

Florence
Dalimonte, Mrs Cynthia W **(SLP)**

JAMAICA

Kingston
Sang, Ruth Gooden
Stewart, Cheryl B **(SLP)**

JAPAN

Kanagawa
Nagasawa, Dr Taiko

Kanazawa-Shi
Katsuki-Nakamura, Dr Jun

Saitama-Ken
Kitagawa, Yoko

Sendai
Harley, Mrs Elizabeth Keil **(SLP)**

Takarazuka
Takeda, Dr Keiichi

Tokyo
Denny, Mrs Martha Q **(SLP)**
Draper, Mrs Eileen S **(SLP)**
Haniu, Yohko **(SLP)**
Osawa, Fumiko
Otomo, Kiyoshi
Sasanuma, Dr Sumiko
Watamori, Toshiko S

Tukui City
Kariyasu, Makoto

Yokohama
Itoh, Dr Motonobu
Kamiyama, Dr Goro

KOREA

Dong
Lee, Soon-Hee Park

Seoul
Shin, Moonja

MALAYSIA

Melaka
Kang, Poh-Sim **(SLP)**

Selangor
Abdullah, Shireen B **(SLP)**

MALTA

Fgura
Borg, Carmel Eleno

MEXICO

Coalcalco
Suarez-Marina, Maria Luisa

Edo De
De Erdmann, Mrs Georgina R **(SLP A)**

Jalisco
Puglisi, Dr Elizabeth Antonia

Mexico DF
Neuman, Nilda M **(A)**
Salomon-Friedmann, Regina Ana **(A)**

NETHERLANDS

Amsterdam
Shopwin, Dr Charles D **(SLP)**

Barneveld
Baldwin, Barbara A **(SLP)**

Le Hague
Dempsey, Mrs June M **(SLP)**

NEW ZEALAND

Auckland
Felix, Nancy L **(SLP)**
Glazer, Ellen S **(SLP)**

Dunedin
Smith, Dale K **(A)**

Governors Bay
Spigel, Mrs Susan G **(SLP)**

Wellington 1
Freitag, Leonore **(SLP)**

NORTHERN IRELAND

County Derby
Kerrin, Rosemary G **(SLP)**

NORWAY

Sandviken
Korneliussen, Barbara Ann **(SLP)**

PERU

Callao
Neely, Kathleen R **(SLP)**

PHILIPPINES

Manila
Chin, Mrs Charlotte Y **(SLP)**

PORTUGAL

Funchal
Sandy, Don Glen **(SLP)**

Lisbon
Formaad, Dr William **(SLP A)**
Santos, Maria Emilia

SAUDI ARABIA

Dhahran
Lauten, Kathleen W **(SLP)**

Jeddah
Tenenholtz, Elisabet **(SLP)**

Riyadh
Navia, Marilyn **(A)**
Wilson, Dr Willa Campbell **(SLP)**

Rizadh
Prescod, Dr Stephen V **(A)**

SINGAPORE

Singapore
McCormack, Julie Ellen
Nimelstein, Mrs Ruth L **(SLP)**

SOUTH AFRICA

Cape Province
Reynolds, Louise

Johannesburg
Abrahamsohn, Mrs Freida **(SLP)**
Aron, Prof Myrtle L **(SLP)**
Tuomi, Dr Seppo K **(SLP)**

Pretoria
Goldblum, Mrs Glenn Binder **(SLP)**

Transvall
MacHado, Elisa Celeste

SPAIN

Madrid
Perez, Mrs Carmen A **(A)**

Vitoria-Gasteiz
Larsen, Ulla Tang **(SLP)**

SWEDEN

Lund
Cheney, Mrs Audrey P **(SLP)**
Deaner, Eileen L **(SLP)**

Tullinge
Fritzell, Dr Bjorn

SWITZERLAND

Lutry
Metraux, Ruth W **(SLP)**

Staefa
Buerkli-Halevy, Ora **(A)**

TAIWAN

Taipei
Wu, Jorie T **(SLP)**

THAILAND

Chonburi
Briggs, Linda Jean **(SLP)**

Nakorn Phanom
Gowdy, Mrs Shirley P **(SLP)**

VENEZUELA

Caracas
Behrens, Denise **(SLP)**
Fernandez, Gilda **(A)**
Ferrer, Dr Oscar **(SLP A)**
Hausmann, Linda P **(SLP)**
Terrero, Irene

WEST GERMANY

Bonn
O'Boyle, Mrs Louise M **(SLP)**

Bremen
Smith-Koehler, Robin E **(SLP)**

Darmstadt
Crowley, Alice L **(A)**

Hennef
Schmitz, Marlies **(SLP)**

Malsch
Schlagheck, Mrs Grace Judith **(A)**

Stuttgart
Paine, Sherry Lindsey **(SLP)**

CARLETON
GRAPHICS
A.D.D.S.
South Bend, Indiana